Applied Therapeutics:
THE CLINICAL USE OF DRUGS
Ninth Edition

Editors

Mary Anne Koda-Kimble
Lloyd Yee Young
Brian K. Alldredge
Robin L. Corelli
B. Joseph Guglielmo
Wayne A. Kradjan
Bradley R. Williams

Section Editors

Marcus Ferrone	Solid Organ Transplantation, Nutrition Issues
Patrick R. Finley and Kelly C. Lee	Psychiatric Disorders
Kathleen Hill-Besinque	Women's Health
Pamala Jacobson	Neoplastic Disorders
Myrna Y. Munar	Renal Disorders

Applied Therapeutics:
THE CLINICAL USE OF DRUGS
Ninth Edition

Edited By

Mary Anne Koda-Kimble, PharmD
Professor of Clinical Pharmacy and Dean
TJ Long Chair in Community Pharmacy Practice
School of Pharmacy
University of California, San Francisco
San Francisco, California

Lloyd Yee Young, PharmD
Professor Emeritus
Department of Clinical Pharmacy
School of Pharmacy
University of California, San Francisco
San Francisco, California

Brian K. Alldredge, PharmD
Professor of Clinical Pharmacy
Clinical Professor of Neurology
Departments of Clinical Pharmacy and Neurology
Schools of Pharmacy and Medicine
University of California, San Francisco
San Francisco, California

Robin L. Corelli, PharmD
Professor of Clinical Pharmacy
Department of Clinical Pharmacy
School of Pharmacy
University of California, San Francisco
San Francisco, California

B. Joseph Guglielmo, PharmD
Professor and Chair
TA Oliver Chair in Clinical Pharmacy
Department of Clinical Pharmacy
School of Pharmacy
University of California, San Francisco
San Francisco, California

Wayne A. Kradjan, PharmD, BCPS
Professor and Dean
College of Pharmacy
Oregon State University
Oregon Health & Science University
Corvallis, Oregon

Bradley R. Williams, PharmD, FASCP, CGP
Professor of Clinical Pharmacy and Clinical Gerontology
Titus Family Department of Clinical Pharmacy and Pharmaceutical Economics and Policy
Schools of Pharmacy and Gerontology
University of Southern California
Los Angeles, California

Wolters Kluwer Health | Lippincott Williams & Wilkins
Philadelphia • Baltimore • New York • London
Buenos Aires • Hong Kong • Sydney • Tokyo

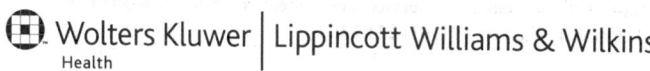

Editor: David B. Troy
Managing Editor: Meredith Brittain, Loftin Paul Montgomery, Jr.
Marketing Manager: Christen Murphy
Production Editor: Julie Montalbano
Designer: Risa Clow
Compositor: Aptara, Inc.

351 West Camden Street
Baltimore, Maryland 21201-2436 USA

530 Walnut Street
Philadelphia, Pennsylvania 19106-3621 USA

Printed in the United States of America.

9 8 7 6 5 4 3 2 1

Library of Congress Cataloging-in-Publication Data

Applied therapeutics : the clinical use of drugs / edited by Mary Anne Koda-Kimble ... [et al.]. – 9th ed.
p. ; cm.
Includes bibliographical references and index.
ISBN 978-0-7817-6555-8
1. Chemotherapy. 2. Pharmacology. I. Koda-Kimble, Mary Anne.
[DNLM: 1. Drug Therapy–methods. WB 330 A651 2009]
RM262.A65 2009
615.5′8–dc22

2008024503

DISCLAIMER

Care has been taken to confirm the accuracy of the information present and to describe generally accepted practices. However, the authors, editors, and publisher are not responsible for errors or omissions or for any consequences from application of the information in this book and make no warranty, expressed or implied, with respect to the currency, completeness, or accuracy of the contents of the publication. Application of this information in a particular situation remains the professional responsibility of the practitioner; the clinical treatments described and recommended may not be considered absolute and universal recommendations.

The authors, editors, and publisher have exerted every effort to ensure that drug selection and dosage set forth in this text are in accordance with the current recommendations and practice at the time of publication. However, in view of ongoing research, changes in government regulations, and the constant flow of information relating to drug therapy and drug reactions, the reader is urged to check the package insert for each drug for any change in indications and dosage and for added warnings and precautions. This is particularly important when the recommended agent is a new or infrequently employed drug.

Some drugs and medical devices presented in this publication have Food and Drug Administration (FDA) clearance for limited use in restricted research settings. It is the responsibility of the health care provider to ascertain the FDA status of each drug or device planned for use in their clinical practice.

To purchase additional copies of this book, call our customer service department at **(800) 638-3030** or fax orders to **(301) 223-2320**. International customers should call **(301) 223-2300**.

Visit Lippincott Williams & Wilkins on the Internet: http://www.lww.com. Lippincott Williams & Wilkins customer service representatives are available from 8:30 am to 6:00 pm, EST.

PREFACE TO THE NINTH EDITION

It has been nearly 35 years since the first edition of *Applied Therapeutics: The Clinical Use of Drugs* was published. The use of case studies served as a founding principle for this innovative text and remains integral to the current edition. Our authors present patient cases that stimulate the reader to integrate and apply therapeutic principles in the context of specific clinical situations. We also strive to provide students and practitioners with a glimpse into the minds of clinicians who are assessing and solving therapeutic problems so that they too can develop and refine their own problem-solving skills. All chapters in this edition have been revised and updated to reflect our changing knowledge of drugs and the application of this knowledge to the therapy of patients.

Today, it is more critical than ever that health care providers make informed decisions regarding the clinical use of drugs. As our population ages, more people carry the burden of multiple chronic diseases. New knowledge about pathophysiology and drug targets has expanded our approaches to drug therapy and, in many cases, polypharmacy has become the standard of care. This, in turn, increases patient exposure to adverse medication events. Meanwhile, we observe a health care system under considerable stress. Shortages of nurses, pharmacists, physicians, and other health care providers interface with remarkable new technologies, increased costs, and decreased access to care. Ironically, the number of disadvantaged and underserved populations continue to increase at a time of remarkable economic growth. This underscores the importance of finding better approaches to managing escalating costs while enhancing the quality of care provided. Systems and approaches to care that guarantee freedom from medical errors (including medication errors) are urgently needed.

The authors have drawn much information from the literature, current standards, and their clinical experiences to share how one might think about making sound and thoughtful therapeutic decisions. *However, it remains the responsibility of every practitioner to evaluate the appropriateness of a particular opinion in the context of the actual clinical situation, keeping in mind any new developments in the field. We strongly urge students and practitioners to consult several appropriate information sources when working with new and unfamiliar drugs.*

Brian K. Alldredge
Robin L. Corelli
B. Joseph Guglielmo
Mary Anne Koda-Kimble
Wayne A. Kradjan
Lloyd Yee Young
Bradley R. Williams

July 2008

PREFACE TO THE FIRST EDITION

In the past decade, new roles for the pharmacist have emerged. More and more frequently the pharmacist is placed in increasingly responsible positions within the health care delivery system. In this capacity (s)he is able to have a significant influence on the quality of health care delivered to the patient. M. Silverman and P. Lee have skillfully assessed the current and future role of the pharmacist in *Pills, Profits and Politics.*[1]

"... It is the pharmacist who can play a vital role in assisting physicians to prescribe rationally, who can help see to it that the right drug is ordered for the right patient at the right time, in the right amounts and with due consideration of costs and that the patient knows how, when and why to use both prescription and non-prescription products.

"It is the pharmacist who has been most highly trained as an expert in drug products, who has the best opportunity to keep up-date on developments in this field and who can serve both physician and patient as a knowledgeable advisor. It is the pharmacist who can take a key part in preventing drug misuse, drug abuse and irrational prescribing."

Many schools of pharmacy have made substantial curriculum changes to prepare their graduates for these responsibilities. Although traditional pharmacy courses have imparted factual information about drugs, they have not enabled the students to apply these facts to the drug therapy of patients. Similarly, traditional pharmacology and medical textbooks do not provide the professional with sufficient information to make a judgment regarding the selection and dosing of a particular product for a specific patient. To arrive at this decision, the clinician must consider a number of patient factors, including age, renal and hepatic function, concurrent disease states and medications and allergies. (S)he must also consider drug product factors, including bioavailability, pharmacokinetics, efficacy, toxicity, risk to benefit ratio, and cost.

We have found that students have most difficulty in *integrating* and *applying* the multiple components of their education to formulate the safest, most rational drug regimen for a given patient. We have also observed that although the student is able to enumerate the adverse effects on a drug, (s)he is unable to recognize or monitor for these effects should they occur in his/her patient.

This text is an outgrowth of the clinical pharmacy courses taught at the University of California and at Washington State University. The major objective of these courses is to enable the student to practice effectively in the clinical setting. Lectures on the pathophysiology and medical management of disease states are supplemented with conferences where students are challenged with drug therapy questions frequently asked by physicians and by case histories, which require drug therapy assessment and the selection of appropriate alternatives. The objective of these conferences and this text is to enable the student to identify relevant factors in drug treatment, such as the probability of whether or not a specific drug is responsible for a patient's symptoms; the clinical significance of a drug interaction; why a specific drug is not achieving therapeutic blood levels; the dose for a patient with multiple disease states.

The success of the conference portion of our courses was a major determinant of the format used for this text; case histories that simulate the actual practice situations and frequently asked therapeutic questions are followed by well-referenced responses.

The authors have drawn much information from their clinical experiences. *It remains the responsibility of every practitioner to evaluate the appropriateness of a particular opinion in the context of the actual clinical situation and with due considerations of any new developments in the field.* Although the authors have been careful to recommend dosages that are in agreement with current standards and responsible literature, we suggest the student or practitioner consult several appropriate information sources when dealing with new and unfamiliar drugs.

[1] Silverman, M. and Lee, PR: *Pills, Profits and Politics*. Berkeley: The University of California Press, 1974. Copyright © 1974, The Regents of the University of California.

ADDITIONAL RESOURCES FOR THE NINTH EDITION

The Ninth Edition of *Applied Therapeutics: The Clinical Use of Drugs* includes additional resources for both instructors and students, available on the book's companion website at http://thePoint.lww.com/KodaKimble9e.

Instructors
Approved adopting instructors will be given access to the following additional resources:

- Image Bank
- PowerPoint Presentations

Students
Resources for students include:

- New Interactive Quiz Bank
- Supplemental Cases
- Answers to Supplemental Cases
- Physiology, Pathophysiology, and Pharmacology Animations

In addition, purchasers of the text can access the searchable Full Text On-line by going to the *Applied Therapeutics: The Clinical Use of Drugs*, Ninth Edition website at http://thePoint.lww.com/KodaKimble9e. See the inside front cover for more details, including the passcode you will need to gain access to the website.

Acknowledgment
Review questions for the Quiz Bank were written by Valerie B. Clinard, Larry N. Swanson, J. Andrew Bowman, Steven M. Davis, Steve Fuller, Dustin Wilson, Sarah McBane, Cynthia J. Johnston, Michelle L. Sharpe, Rebekah R. Arthur Grube, Charles Herring, James Groce, Tracy A. Dewald, Connie Lee Barnes, Nancy Allen-LaPointe, Roy Pleasants, II, Jennifer Schuh, Mary L. Townsend, Matthew T. Harris, Mara Watson, John Murray, Kimberly Lewis, Tina H. Thornhill, Jennifer Smith, Amber Peoples, Kimberly Tamura, Kathey B. Fulton, Melanie W. Pound, D. Byron May, Lydia Mis, Melissa D. Johnson, Andrew J. Muzyk, LeAnne Kennedy, Tara L. Bell, and Laura Bowers.

ACKNOWLEDGMENTS FOR THE NINTH EDITION

We are deeply indebted to the many dedicated people who have given of themselves to complete the ninth edition of this book. As always, we are most grateful to our contributing authors who have been attentive to meeting our stringent time deadlines and unique writing format. We especially thank the following section editors for their truly remarkable support as they edited chapters, assisted authors, and worked with our publishers at Lippincott Williams & Wilkins (LWW): Kathleen Hill-Besinque (Women's Health), Marcus Ferrone (Solid Organ Transplantation, Nutrition Issues), Patrick R. Finley and Kelly C. Lee (Psychiatric Disorders), Pamala Jacobson (Neoplastic Disorders), and Myrna Y. Munar (Renal Disorders).

The work of our editorial assistant and colleague, Loftin (Paul) Montgomery, Jr., is noteworthy. Paul's exceptional patience, attention to detail, and firm guidance helped us all stay on task. This edition would not have come to completion without his partnership. Above all, we are especially grateful for the understanding and support of our spouses (Kimberly, Tom, Deter, Don, Carolyn, Linda, and Marilyn, respectively) during those nights and weekends we spent writing or editing, our children (both young and old), and now our grandchildren.

Finally, we dedicate our work to our students who inspire us and to the many patients we have cared for. Our patients have taught us over and over again how critical it is to tailor our knowledge to their specific circumstances, to listen well, and to welcome them as true partners in their care.

Brian K. Alldredge
Robin L. Corelli
B. Joseph Guglielmo
Mary Anne Koda-Kimble
Wayne A. Kradjan
Lloyd Yee Young
Bradley R. Williams

CONTRIBUTORS

Steven R. Abel, PharmD, FASHP
Assistant Dean for Clinical Programs, Bucke Professor and Head
Department of Pharmacy Practice
Purdue University School of Pharmacy and Pharmacal Sciences
West Lafayette, Indiana

Brian K. Alldredge, PharmD
Professor of Clinical Pharmacy
Associate Dean, Academic Affairs, School of Pharmacy
Clinical Professor of Neurology, School of Medicine
Departments of Clinical Pharmacy and Neurology
University of California, San Francisco
San Francisco, California

Judith Ann Alsop, PharmD
Associate Clinical Professor, Department of Clinical Pharmacy, School of Pharmacy
University of California, San Francisco
Clinical Professor, Department of Pulmonary Medicine, Toxicology, Critical Care
University of California, Davis, Medical Center
San Francisco and Sacramento, California

J. V. Anandan, PharmD, BCPS
Adjunct Associate Professor
Department of Pharmacy Practice, Eugene Applebaum College of Pharmacy and Health Sciences
Wayne State University
Pharmacy Specialist, Department of Pharmacy Practice, Henry Ford Hospital
Detroit, Michigan

Jennifer Ash, PharmD, BCNSP
Assistant Professor of Pharmacy Practice
College of Pharmacy and Health Sciences, Butler University
Nutrition Support Pharmacist, Clinical Pharmacy
Methodist Hospital
Indianapolis, Indiana

Mitra Assemi, PharmD
Associate Professor of Clinical Pharmacy
Department of Clinical Pharmacy
School of Pharmacy
University of California, San Francisco
San Francisco, California

Sara Grimsley Augustin, PharmD, BCPP
Assistant Professor
Clinical and Administrative Sciences
Mercer University Southern School of Pharmacy
Atlanta, Georgia

Francesca T. Aweeka, PharmD
Professor in Residence
Department of Clinical Pharmacy
School of Pharmacy
University of California, San Francisco
San Francisco, California

Andrew D. Barnes, PharmD
Clinical Associate Professor
School of Pharmacy
Clinical Pharmacist, Cardiothoracic Surgery, Departments of Pharmacy and Medicine, University of Washington Medicine
University of Washington
Seattle, Washington

David T. Bearden, PharmD
Clinical Associate Professor
Department of Pharmacy Practice
Oregon State University College of Pharmacy
Portland, Oregon

Sandra Benavides, PharmD
Assistant Professor
Department of Pharmacy Practice, Nova Southeastern University
Clinical Pharmacist, Pediatric Pharmacy Services
Jackson Memorial Hospital
Fort Lauderdale and Miami, Florida

Rosemary Berardi, PharmD, FCCP, FASHP, FAPhA
Professor of Pharmacy
College of Pharmacy, University of Michigan
Clinical Specialist, Gastrointestinal/Liver Diseases, Department of Pharmacy
University of Michigan Medical Center
Ann Arbor, Michigan

Douglas J. Black, PharmD
Associate Professor
School of Pharmacy
University of Washington
Seattle, Washington

KarenBeth H. Bohan, PharmD, BCPS
Assistant Professor, Pharmacy Practice
Wilkes University, Nesbitt College of Pharmacy
Clinical Specialist, Internal Medicine, Department of Pharmacy
Wilkes-Barre General Hospital
Wilkes-Barre, Pennsylvania

Thomas C. Bookwalter, PharmD
Associate Clinical Professor
Department of Clinical Pharmacy, School of Pharmacy and
Clinical Pharmacist, Department of Pharmaceutical Services, UCSF Medical Center
University of California, San Francisco
San Francisco, California

Nicole J. Brandt, PharmD, CGP, BCPP, FASCP
Associate Professor
Department of Pharmacy Practice and Science
School of Pharmacy
University of Maryland at Baltimore
Baltimore, Maryland

Tina Penick Brock, MSPharm, EdD
Lecturer
Department of Practice & Policy, School of Pharmacy, University of London
Adjunct Assistant Professor, Department of Pharmacotherapy & Experimental Therapeutics, School of Pharmacy
University of North Carolina at Chapel Hill
London, United Kingdom and, Chapel Hill, North Carolina, USA

Michael R. Brodeur, PharmD, CGP, FASCP
Associate Professor
Department of Pharmacy Practice, Albany College of Pharmacy
Senior Care Pharmacist, The Eddy-Northeast Health
Albany, New York

Donald F. Brophy, PharmD, MS, FCCP, BCPS
Associate Professor
Department of Pharmacy
School of Pharmacy
Virginia Commonwealth University
Richmond, Virginia

Glen R. Brown, PharmD
Clinical Professor
Department of Pharmaceutical Sciences
University of British Columbia
Critical Care Specialist
Pharmacy Department
St. Paul's Hospital
Vancouver, British Columbia, Canada

Gilbert J. Burckart, PharmD
Associate Director
Office of Clinical Pharmacology
US Food and Drug Administration
Silver Spring, Maryland

Jill S. Burkiewicz, PharmD
Assistant Professor
Director, Primary Care Residency Program Midwestern Univesity
Midwestern University Chicago College of Pharmacy
Clinical Pharmacist, Advocate Health Centers
Downer's Grove, Illinois

Pauline Ann Cawley, PharmD
Clinical Assistant Professor
Department of Clinical Pharmacy, College of Pharmacy, University of Utah
Clinical Pharmacist Specialist, Critical Care
LDS Hospital
Salt Lake City, Utah

James Chan, PharmD, PhD
Assistant Professor
Department of Clinical Pharmacy, School of Pharmacy, University of California, San Francisco
Pharmacy Quality and Outcomes Coordinator, Pharmacy Operations, Kaiser Foundation Hospitals
Kaiser Permanente
San Francisco and Oakland, California

Jennifer C. Y. Chan, PharmD
Clinical Assistant Professor
College of Pharmacy, The University of Texas at Austin
Clinical Associate Professor of Pediatrics and Clinical Assistant Professor of Pharmacology
The University of Texas Health Science Center
San Antonio, Texas

Stanley W. Chapman, MD
Professor of Medicine, Department of Medicine
Director, Division of Infectious Diseases
University of Mississippi Medical Center
University of Mississippi
Jackson, Mississippi

Steven W. Chen, PharmD, FASHP, CDM
Associate Professor
Titus Family Department of Clinical Pharmacy & Pharmaceutical Economics and Policy
School of Pharmacy
University of Southern California
Los Angeles, California

Michael F. Chicella, PharmD
Clinical Coordinator
Department of Pharmacy
Children's Hospital of the King's Daughters
Norfolk, Virginia

Jennifer Chow, PharmD
Pediatric Clinical Specialist
Pharmacy Department
Children's Hospital of the King's Daughters
Norfolk, Virginia

Cary R. Chrisman, PharmD
Clinical Pharmacist, Department of Pharmacy
Methodist Medical Center of Oak Ridge
Assistant Professor, Department of Clinical Pharmacy, College of Pharmacy, University of Tennessee
Oak Ridge and Memphis, Tennessee

Tom E. Christian, BS Pharm, BCPS
Affiliate Faculty
College of Pharmacy, Oregon State University
Clinical Specialist, Pharmacy Infectious Disease Coordinator
Southwest Washington Medical Center
Vancouver, Washington

Tamara E. Claridge, PharmD, BCPS
Pharmacotherapy Specialist
Department of Pharmacy
Tampa General Hospital
Tampa, Florida

John D. Cleary, PharmD
Professor & Vice Chair of Research
Department of Clinical Pharmacy Practice, School of Pharmacy, University of Mississippi
Assistant Professor, Medicine, Department of Infectious Disease
University of Mississippi Medical Center
Jackson, Mississippi

Michelle Condren, PharmD
Associate Professor
Pharmacy: Clinical & Administrative Sciences
College of Pharmacy
University of Oklahoma
Tulsa, Oklahoma

Todd Allen Conner, PharmD
Nephrology Fellow
College of Pharmacy
University of New Mexico
Albuquerque, New Mexico

Amanda H. Corbett, PharmD, BCPS
Clinical Assistant Professor
Division of Pharmacotherapy and Experimental Therapeutics
School of Pharmacy
University of North Carolina
Chapel Hill, North Carolina

Robin L. Corelli, PharmD
Professor of Clinical Pharmacy
Department of Clinical Pharmacy
School of Pharmacy
University of California, San Francisco
San Francisco, California

Timothy W. Cutler, PharmD
Assistant Professor of Clinical Pharmacy
Department of Clinical Pharmacy, School of Pharmacy, University of California, San Francisco
Clinical Pharmacist, Department of Pharmaceutical Services
University of California, Davis Medical Center
San Francisco and Sacramento, California

Kendra M. Damer, PharmD
Assistant Professor of Pharmacy Practice
Department of Pharmacy Practice, Midwestern University, Chicago College of Pharmacy
Clinical Specialist, Infectious Diseases, Pharmacy,
Rush University Medical Center
Chicago, Illinois

Larry H. Danziger, PharmD
Professor
Department of Pharmacy Practice
College of Pharmacy
University of Illinois at Chicago
Chicago, Illinois

Cathi Dennehy, PharmD
Clinical Professor
Department of Clinical Pharmacy
School of Pharmacy
University of California, San Francisco
San Francisco, California

Philip T. Diaz, MD
Associate Professor, Internal Medicine
Medical Director, Pulmonary Rehabilitation
The Ohio State University Medical Center
The Ohio State University
Columbus, Ohio

Betty Jean Dong, PharmD
Professor of Clinical Pharmacy
Department of Clinical Pharmacy, School of Pharmacy
Clinical Pharmacist, Thyroid Clinic, Department of Medicine
University of California, San Francisco
San Francisco, California

Andrew J. Donnelly, PharmD, MBA
Director of Pharmacy Services, Department of Pharmacy
University of Illinois Medical Center at Chicago
Clinical Professor, Department of Pharmacy Practice
College of Pharmacy, University of Illinois Chicago
Chicago, Illinois

Julie Ann Dopheide, PharmD, BCPP
Associate Professor of Clinical Pharmacy
Titus Family Department of Clinical Pharmacy and Pharmaceutical Economics and Policy, Schools of Pharmacy and Medicine, University of Southern California
Los Angeles County and University of Southern California Medical Center
University of Southern California
Los Angeles, California

Richard H. Drew, PharmD, BCPS
Associate Professor
Department of Medicine/Infectious Disease, Duke School of Medicine, Clinical Pharmacist, Medicine/Infectious Disease
Duke Medical Center
Durham, North Carolina

Vicky Dudas, PharmD
Assistant Clinical Professor of Pharmacy, Department of Clinical Pharmacy, School of Pharmacy
Director, Antimicrobial Management Program, Pharmaceutical Services
University of California San Francisco Medical Center
University of California at San Francisco
San Francisco, California

Julie B. Dumond, PharmD
HIV Pharmacology Fellow
School of Pharmacy
University of North Carolina at Chapel Hill
Chapel Hill, North Carolina

Robert E. Dupuis, PharmD, BCPS
Clinical Associate Professor
School of Pharmacy
University of North Carolina at Chapel Hill
Chapel Hill, North Carolina

Sandra B. Earle, PharmD, BCPS
Associate Professor
Department of Pharmaceutical Science
School of Pharmacy
University of Findlay
Findlay, Ohio

Rene A. Endow-Eyer, PharmD, BCPP
Psychiatric Clinical Pharmacy Specialist
Pharmacy Department,
VA San Diego Healthcare System
San Diego, California

Michael E. Ernst, PharmD
Associate Professor (Clinical)
College of Pharmacy
Department of Family Medicine, College of Medicine
The University of Iowa
Iowa City, Iowa

Martha P. Fankhauser, MS Pharm, FASHP, BCPP
Clinical Professor
Department of Pharmacy Practice and Science
University of Arizona College of Pharmacy
College of Pharmacy
The University of Arizona
Tucson, Arizona

Christopher K. Finch, PharmD, BCPS
Critical Care Specialist, Department of Pharmacy
Methodist University Hospital
Associate Professor
Department of Clinical Pharmacy, College of Pharmacy, University of Tennessee
Memphis, Tennessee

Patrick R. Finley, PharmD, BCPP
Professor of Clinical Pharmacy
Department of Clinical Pharmacy
School of Pharmacy
University of California, San Francisco
San Francisco, California

Douglas N. Fish, PharmD, FCCM, FCCP, BCPS
Associate Professor
Department of Clinical Pharmacy, School of Pharmacy, University of Colorado at Denver and Health Sciences Center
Clinical Specialist in Infectious Diseases/Critical Care, Department of Pharmacy, Medical/Surgical Intensive Care Units, Department of Pharmacy
University of Colorado Hospital
Denver, Colorado

Randolph V. Fugit, PharmD, BCPS
Internal Medicine Clinical Specialist, Department of Pharmacy,
Denver Veterans Affairs Medical Center
Adjoint Assistant Professor
Department of Pharmacy Practice, School of Pharmacy, University of Colorado
Denver, Colorado

Victoria Furstenberg, Ferraresi PharmD, FASHP, FCSHP
Director of Pharmacy Services
Pathways Home Health and Hospice
Assistant Professor of Clinical Pharmacy
Department of Clinical Pharmacy, School of Pharmacy
University of California, San Francisco
Sunnyvale and San Francisco, California

Mark W. Garrison, PharmD
Associate Professor
Department of Pharmacotherapy, College of Pharmacy
Washington State University, Spokane
Clinical Pharmacist, Pharmacy Department, Deaconess Medical Center
Spokane, Washington

James J. Gasper, PharmD
Assistant Clinical Professor
Department of Clinical Pharmacy, School of Pharmacy, University of California, San Francisco
Psychiatric Clinical Pharmacist, Department of Pharmacy Services
Community Behavioral Health Services
San Francisco, California

Steven P. Gelone, PharmD
Associate Professor of Community Medicine
Department of Medicine
College of Medicine
Drexel University
Philadelphia, Pennsylvania

Jane Maria Gervasio, PharmD, BCNSP
Associate Professor
Department of Pharmacy Practice, College of Pharmacy and Health Sciences, Butler University
Nutrition Support Pharmacist, Department of Clinical Pharmacy
Methodist Hospital
Indianapolis, Indiana

Jeffery A. Goad, PharmD, MPH
Associate Professor of Clinical Pharmacy
Titus Family Department of Clinical Pharmacy and Pharmaceutical Economics and Policy
School of Pharmacy
University of Southern California
Los Angeles, California

Julie A. Golembiewski, PharmD
Clinical Associate Professor
Department of Pharmacy Practice, College of Pharmacy, University of Illinois at Chicago
Clinical Pharmacist, Anesthesia/Pain, Hospital Pharmacy
University of Illinois Medical Center
Chicago, Illinois

William C. Gong, PharmD, FASHP
Associate Professor of Clinical Pharmacy
Director, Residency and Fellowship Training
Titus Family Department of Clinical Pharmacy and Pharmaceutical Economics & Policy
School of Pharmacy
University of Southern California
Los Angeles, California

Luis S. Gonzales III, PharmD. BCPS
Adjunct Clinical Instructor
Department of Clinical Pharmacy, Mylan School of Pharmacy, Duquesne University
Manager, Clinical Pharmacy Services, Pharmaceutical Care Services
Memorial Medical Centery, Johnstown, Pennsylvania
Pittsburgh, Pennsylvania

Susan Goodin, PharmD, BCPS, BCOP
Associate Professor
Department of Medicine
Robert Wood Johnson Medical School, University of Medicine and Dentistry of New Jersey
Director, Division of Pharmaceutical Sciences
The Cancer Institute of New Jersey
New Brunswick, New Jersey

Mildred D. Gottwald, PharmD
Director, Clinical Science
Sunesis Pharmaceuticals
Volunteer Faculty, Department of Clinical Pharmacy, School of Pharmacy
University of California
San Francisco, California

B. Joseph Guglielmo, PharmD
Professor and Chair
TA Oliver Endowed Chair in Clinical Pharmacy
Department of Clinical Pharmacy
School of Pharmacy
University of California, San Francisco
San Francisco, California

Karen M. Gunning, PharmD, BCPS
Associate Professor (Clinical)
Department of Pharmacotherapy, College of Pharmacy
Department of Family & Preventive Medicine, School of Medicine
University of Utah
Salt Lake City, Utah

Sally Guthrie, PharmD
Associate Professor
Department of Clinical Science, College of Pharmacy, University of Michigan
Clinical Pharmacist
University of Michigan Health System
Ann Arbor, Michigan

Maureen Haas, PharmD, BCPS, BCOP
Clinical Specialist Hematology and Oncology
Winship Cancer Institute
Emory University
Atlanta, Georgia

Mark R. Haase, PharmD, BCPS
Associate Professor of Pharmacy Practice
Department of Pharmacy Practice
School of Pharmacy
Texas Tech University
Amarillo, Texas

Raymond W. Hammond, PharmD, FCCP, BCPS
Associate Dean for Practice Programs
College of Pharmacy
University of Houston
Houston, Texas

Laura B. Hansen, PharmD, FCCP, BCPS
Assistant Professor
Department of Clinical Pharmacy, School of Pharmacy
Clinical Pharmacy Specialist, Department of Family Medicine
University of Colorado at Denver and Health Sciences Center
Denver, Colorado

Jennifer L. Hardman, PharmD
Clinical Assistant Professor
Department of Pharmacy Practice, College of Pharmacy
Department of Obstetrics and Gynecology, University of Illinois Hospital
University of Illinois at Chicago
Chicago, Illinois

R. Donald Harvey, PharmD, BCPS, BCOP
Assistant Professor, Hematology/Oncology
Director, Phase I Unit
Winship Cancer Institute
School of Medicine, Emory University
Atlanta, Georgia

Mary F. Hebert, PharmD, FCCP
Professor
Department of Pharmacy
School of Pharmacy
University of Washington
Seattle, Washington

David W. Henry, MS, BCOP, FASHP
Associate Professor
Department of Pharmacy Practice
School of Pharmacy
University of Kansas Medical Center
Kansas City, Kansas

Richard Neal Herrier, PharmD
Clinical Associate Professor
Department of Pharmacy Practice and Science, College of Pharmacy
University of Arizona
Tucson, Arizona

Karl M. Hess, PharmD
Assistant Professor
Department of Pharmacy Practice
College of Pharmacy
Western University
Pomona, California

Kathleen Hill-Besinque, PharmD
Associate Professor and Director of Experiential Programs
Titus Family Department of Clinical Pharmacy and Pharmaceutical Economics and Policy
University of Southern California School of Pharmacy
Los Angeles, California

Mark T. Holdsworth, PharmD, BCOP
Associate Professor of Pharmacy and Pediatrics
College of Pharmacy
University of New Mexico
Albuquerque, New Mexico

Curtis D. Holt, PharmD
Clinical Professor
Department of Surgery
University of California, Los Angeles
Los Angeles, California

Priscilla P. How, PharmD, BCPS
Clinical Assistant Professor
Department of Pharmacy Practice
College of Pharmacy, University of Illinois at Chicago
Clinical Pharmacist (Nephrology)
Ambulatory Care Pharmacy
University of Illinois Medical Center at Chicago
Chicago, Illinois

Yvonne Huckleberry, PharmD
Clinical Assistant Professor
Department of Pharmacotherapy
College of Pharmacy
Washington State University
Pullman, Washington

Karen Suchanek Hudmon, DrPH, MS, RPh
Associate Professor
Department of Pharmacy Practice
School of Pharmacy & Pharmaceutical Sciences
Purdue University
West Lafayette, Indiana

Matthew Ito, PharmD, FLLP, BCPS
Professor and Chair of Pharmacy Practice
College of Pharmacy
Oregon State University
Oregon Health & Science University
Portland, Oregon

Gail S. Itokazu, PharmD
Clinical Assistant Professor
Department of Pharmacy Practice, College of Pharmacy, University of Illinois at Chicago
Clinical Pharmacist, Department of Medicine
John H. Stroger, Jr. Hospital of Cook County
Chicago, Illinois

Timothy J. Ives, PharmD, MPH, FCCP, BCPS
Associate Professor of Pharmacy,
Division of Pharmacy Practice
School of Pharmacy
University of North Carolina at Chapel Hill
Chapel Hill, North Carolina

Pamala Jacobson, PharmD
Associate Professor, Experimental and Clinical Pharmacology
College of Pharmacy
University of Minnesota
Minneapolis, Minnesota

James S. Kalus, PharmD, BCPS
Assistant Professor
Department of Pharmacy Practice and Science
School of Pharmacy
University of Maryland
Baltimore, Maryland

Angela Kashuba, PharmD
Associate Professor,
School of Pharmacy
University of North Carolina at Chapel Hill
Chapel Hill, North Carolina

Michael B. Kays, PharmD, FCCP
Associate Professor
Department of Pharmacy Practice
School of Pharmacy & Pharmaceutical Sciences
Purdue University
Indianapolis, Indiana

George A. Kenna, PhD, RPh
Assistant Professor of Psychiatry
Center for Alcohol and Addiction Research Brown University
Providence, Rhode Island
Senior Scientific Advisor Tufts Health Care Institute Program on Opiod Risk Management
Boston, Massachusetts
Clinical Pharmacist The Westerly Hospital
Westerly Rhode Island

Jiwon W. Kim, PharmD, BCPS
Assistant Professor of Clinical Pharmacy
Titus Family Department of Clinical Pharmacy and Pharmaceutical Economics and Policy, School of Pharmacy, University of Southern California
Clinical Pharmacist, Department of Pharmacy,
University of Southern California University Hospital
Los Angeles, California

Mark N. Kirstein, PharmD
Assistant Professor
Department of Experimental and Clinical Pharmacology
College of Pharmacy
University of Minnesota
Minneapolis, Minnesota

Kathryn Kiser, PharmD
Clinical Instructor
Pharmach Practice and Experiential Education
School of Pharmacy
Univesity of North Carolina
Chapel Hill, North Carolina

Dusko Klipa, PharmD
Pharmacy Practitioner, Liver Transplant
Instructor in Pharmacy, College of Medicine
Mayo Clinic in Jacksonville
Jacksonville, Florida

Daren L. Knoell, PharmD, FCCP
Associate Professor of Pharmacy and Internal Medicine
Davis Heart and Lung Research Institute
The Ohio State University Medical Center
The Ohio State University
Columbus, Ohio

Mary Anne Koda-Kimble, PharmD
Professor of Clinical Pharmacy and Dean
TJ Long Chair in Community Pharmacy Practice
School of Pharmacy
University of California, San Francisco
San Francisco, California

Wayne A. Kradjan, PharmD
Dean and Professor
College of Pharmacy
Oregon State University
Oregon Health & Science University
Corvallis, Oregon

Donna M. Kraus, PharmD
Pediatric Clinical Pharmacist
Associate Professor of Pharmacy Practice
Departments of Pharmacy Practice and Pediatrics
Colleges of Pharmacy and Medicine
University of Illinois at Chicago
Chicago, Illinois

Lisa A. Kroon, PharmD, CDE
Professor of Clinical Pharmacy
Department of Clinical Pharmacy
School of Pharmacy
University of California, San Francisco
San Francisco, California

Deborah Sako Kubota, PharmD
Formulary Pharmacist
Drug Information Services
Kaiser Permanente Medical Care Program
Downey, California

Samuel Kuperman, MD
Professor
Department of Psychiatry, Carver College of Medicine
Director Division of Child and Adolescent Psychiatry
University of Iowa Hospitals and Clinics
Iowa City, Iowa

Jonathan Lacro, PharmD, BCPS, BCPP
Associate Clinical Professor of Pharmacy
Department of Psychiatry, University of California, San Diego
Clinical Pharmacy Specialist in Psychiatry, Pharmacy Service
University of California San Diego
VA San Diego Healthcare System
San Diego, California

Alan H. Lau, PharmD
Professor
Department of Pharmacy Practice
College of Pharmacy
University of Illinois at Chicago
Chicago, Illinois

Kelly C. Lee, PharmD, BCPP
Assistant Professor of Clinical Pharmacy
Skaggs School of Pharmacy and Pharmaceutical Sciences
University of California San Diego
La Jolla, Californis

Susan H. Lee, PharmD
Associate Professor, School of Pharmacy
University of Washington
Surgery/Trauma Clinical Pharmacist, Department of Pharmacy Services
Harborview Medical Center
Seattle, Washington

Lisa K. Lohr, PharmD, BCPS, BCOP
Clinical Assistant Professor
College of Pharmacy, University of Minnesota
Clinical Leader, Oncology/BMT, Department of Pharmacy Services
University of Minnesota Medical Center, Fairview
Minneapolis, Minnesota

Rex S. Lott, PharmD
Associate Professor of Pharmacy Practice
Department of Pharmacy Practice & Administrative Science, College of Pharmacy, Idaho State University
Mental Health Clinical Pharmacist, Department of Mental Health & Pharmacy
Boise Veterans Affairs Medical Center
Boise, Idaho

Sherry Luedtke, PharmD
Associate Dean, Professional Affairs
Associate Professor, Pharmacy Practice
School of Pharmacy
Texas Tech University Health Science Center
Amarillo, Texas

May C. Mak, PharmD, CGP
Assistant Professor
Titus Family Department of Clinical Pharmacy and Pharmaceutical Economics and Policy, School of Pharmacy, University of Southern California
Manager, Anticoagulation Management Service, Department of Medicine, University of Southern California
Clinical Pharmacist, HIV Adult Service, Los Angeles County Hospital
Los Angeles, California

Joel Marrs, PharmD
Clinical Assistant Professor
Department of Pharmacy Practice, College of Pharmacy, Oregon State University
Clinical Pharmacy Specialist, Pharmacy Department
Oregon Health & Science University Hospital
Portland, Oregon

James W. McAuley, PhD
Associate Professor
Division of Pharmacy Practice and Administration
College of Pharmacy
The Ohio State University
Columbus, Ohio

James P. McCormack, PharmD
Associate Professor
Faculty of Pharmaceutical Sciences
University of British Columbia
Vancouver, British Columbia, Canada

Jeannine S. McCune, PharmD, BCPS, BCOP
Associate Professor, Pharmacy Department
Affiliate Investigator, Clinical Research Division, Fred Hutchinson Cancer Research Center
Clinical Director, Pharmakokinetics Laboratory, Seattle Cancer Care Alliance
University of Washington
Seattle, Washington

Jennifer McNulty, MD
Staff Perinatologist
Long Beach Memorial Medical Center for Women
Associate Clinical Professor, School of Medicine
University of California, Irvine
Long Beach, California

Robert J. Michocki, PharmD, BCPS
Professor
Pharmacy Practice and Science
School of Pharmacy
University of Maryland
Baltimore, Maryland

Robert Keith Middleton, PharmD
Clinical Coordinator
Department of Pharmacy
Saint Clare's Hospital
Weston, Wisconsin

Melissa Mitchell, PharmD
Psychiatry Pharmacy Resident
Pharmacy Department
VA San Diego Healthcare System
San Diego, California

Myrna Y. Munar, PharmD, BCPS
Associate Professor
College of Pharmacy
Oregon State University
Portland, Oregon

Milap C. Nahata, PharmD
Professor and Chair
Pharmacy Practice and Administration, College of Pharmacy
Associate Director, Pharmacy, Ohio State University Medical Center
The Ohio State University
Columbus, Ohio

Jean M. Nappi, PharmD, FCCP, BCPS
Professor of Pharmacy and Clinical Sciences
South Carolina College of Pharmacy
Professor of Medicine, Medical University of South Carolina
Charleston, South Carolina

Paul G. Nolan Jr., PharmD, FCCP, FASHP
Professor
Department of Pharmacy Practice and Science
College of Pharmacy
University of Arizona
Tucson, Arizona

Edith A. Nutescu, PharmD
Clinical Associate Professor
Department of Pharmacy Practice
College of Pharmacy
University of Illinois at Chicago
Chicago, Illinois

Cindy Lea O'Bryant, PharmD, BCOP
Assistant Professor
Department of Clinical Pharmacy, School of Pharmacy, University of Colorado
Clinical Oncology Pharmacist
University of Colorado Health Sciences Center
Denver, Colorado

Judith A. O'Donnell, MD
Associate Professor of Clinical Medicine,
Division of Infectious Diseases, School of Medicine, University of Pennsylvania
Hospital Epidemiologist and Director of Infection Control
Penn Presbyterian Medical Center
University of Pennsylvania Health Care System
Philadelphia, Pennsylvania

Neeta Bahal O'Mara, PharmD
Clinical Pharmacist
Dialysis Clinics, Inc.
North Brunswick, New Jersey

Robert Lee Page II, PharmD, FASCP, BCPS, CGP
Associate Professor
Departments of Clinical Pharmacy and Medicine, UCHSC Schools of Pharmacy and Medicine
Clinical Specialist, Division of Cardiology,
University of Colorado Hospital
Denver, Colorado

Amy Barton Pai, PharmD
Associate Professor (Clinical Pharmacy)
Department of Pharmacy Practice; College of Pharmacy
University of New Mexico
Albuquerque, New Mexico

Louise Parent-Stevens, PharmD, BCPS
Clinical Assistant Professor
Department of Pharmacy Practice
College of Pharmacy
Clinical Pharmacist, Family Medicine Center,
University of Illinois at Chicago
Chicago, Illinois

Patricia L. Parker, PharmD, BCPS
Health Sciences, Assistant Clinical Professor
School of Pharmacy, University of California San Francisco
Clinical Coordinator
Department of Pharmacy, UC Davis Medical Center
San Francisco and Sacramento, California

Margaret M. Pearson, PharmD, MS
Division of Epidemiology, Mississippi State Department of Health
Jackson, Mississippi

Paul P. Perry, PhD
Professor of Pharmacy
Pharmacy Practice Department,
College of Pharmacy, Touro University
Emeritus Professor of Psychiatry
Department of Psychiatry
Carver College of Medicine
University of Iowa
Vallejo, California and, Iowa City, Iowa

Jennifer Tran Pham, PharmD, BCPS
Clinical Assistant Professor
Department of Pharmacy Practice, College of Pharmacy
Neonatal Clinical Pharmacist, Pharmacy Department, University of Illinois Medical Center at Chicago
University of Illinois at Chicago
Chicago, Illinois

David J. Quan, PharmD, BCPS
Health Sciences Associate Clinical Professor
Department of Clinical Pharmacy, School of Pharmacy
Clinical Pharmacist, Pharmaceutical Services, UCSF Medical Center
University of California San Francisco
San Francisco, California

Ralph H. Raasch, PharmD
Associate Professor
Division: Pharmacotherapy and Experimental Therapeutics, School of Pharmacy
Clinical Specialist, Pharmacy Department, University of North Carolina Hospitals
University of North Carolina at Chapel Hill
Chapel Hill, North Carolina

Ellen Rhinard, PharmD, BCPS
Clinical Assistant Professor
Department of Pharmacy
School of Pharmacy, University of Washington
Seattle, Washington

Carol J. Rollins, MS, PharmD
Clinical Associate Professor
Department of Pharmacy Practice and Science, College of Pharmacy
University Medical Center
Clinical Coordinator, Pharmacy Department, University Medical Center
University of Arizona
Tucson, Arizona

Rebecca A. Rottman, PharmD, BCPS, CGP
Clinical Assistant Professor
College of Pharmacy, University of Texas at Austin, University of Texas Health Sciences Center at San Antonio
Geriatrics Clinical Pharmacy Specialist, Department of Pharmacy
South Texas Veterans Health Care System, Audie L. Murphy Division
San Antonio, Texas

Jamila C. Russeau, PharmD, BCPS
Coordinator, Education and Staff Development
Coordinator, PGY-1 Pharmacy Residency
Department of Pharmacy
Mayo Clinic in Jacksonville
Jacksonville, Florida

Tricia M. Russell, PharmD, BCPS, CDE
Assistant Professor
Department of Pharmacy Practice,
Nesbitt School of Pharmacy, Wilkes University
Clinical Specialist, Ambulatory Care, Clinical Pharmacy
Geisinger Medical Group - Lake Scranton
Wilkes-Barre and Scranton, Pennsylvania

Joseph J. Saseen, PharmD, BCPS
Associate Professor
Departments of Clinical Pharmacy and Family Medicine
University of Colorado Health Sciences Center
Schools of Pharmacy and Medicine
University of Colorado at Denver and Health Sciences Center
Aurora, Colorado

Larry D. Sasich, PharmD, MPH, FASHP
Acting Chair
Department of Pharmacy Practice
School of Pharmacy
Lake Erie College of Osteopathic Medicine
Erie, Pennsylvania

Katrina Schwartz, PharmD
Clinical Assistant Professor
Department of Pharmacotherapy
College of Pharmacy
Washington State University
Spokane, Washington

Timothy H. Self, PharmD
Professor of Clinical Pharmacy
Department of Clinical Pharmacy, College of Pharmacy
University of Tennessee
Director, Internal Medicine Specialty Residency, Methodist University Hospital
Memphis, Tennessee

Amy Hatfield Seung, PharmD, BCOP
Clinical Specialist, Hematological Malignancies
Department of Pharmacy
Director, Oncology Specialty Residency
Sidney Kimmel Comprehensive Cancer Center at the Johns Hopkins Hospital
Baltimore, Maryland

Carrie A. Sincak, PharmD, BCPS
Associate Professor
Department of Pharmacy Practice, Chicago College of Pharmacy, Midwestern University
Clinical Pharmacist, Internal Medicine, Pharmacy Department, Loyola University Medical Center
Downers Grove and Maywood, Illinois

Hareleen Singh, PharmD
Clinical Assistant Professor
Department of Pharmacy Practice, College of Pharmacy,
Oregon State University, Oregon Health & Science University
Clinical Pharmacist, Pharmacy Department
VA Medical Center
Portland, Oregon

Jessica Song, M.A., PharmD
Associate Professor, Pharmacy Practice
Thomas J. Long School of Pharmacy and Health Sciences, University of the Pacific
Pharmacy Residency Coordinator, Department of Pharmacy Services
Santa Clara Valley Medical Center
San Jose and Stockton, California

Suellyn J. Sorensen, PharmD, BCPS
Clinical Pharmacy Manager
Clinical Pharmacist, Infectious Diseases
Indiana University Hospital of Clarian Health Partners
Indianapolis, Indiana

Anne P. Spencer, PharmD, BCPS
Associate Professor, Department of Pharmacy and Clinical Sciences
South Carolina College of Pharmacy,
Clinical Specialist, Department of Pharmacy Services,
Medical University of South Carolina
Charleston, South Carolina

Marilyn R. Stebbins, PharmD
Health Sciences Clinical Professor
Department of Clinical Pharmacy, School of Pharmacy, University of California San Francisco
Pharmacy Utilization Director,
Mercy Medical Group, CHW Medical Foundation
San Francisco and Sacramento, California

Irving Steinberg, PharmD
Associate Professor, Clinical Pharmacy & Pediatrics,
Titus Family Department of Clinical Pharmacy and Pharmaceutical Economics & Policy; Director, Division of Pediatric Pharmacotherapy, Department of Pediatrics
Women's and Children's Hospital, Los Angeles County & University of Southern California Medical Center
University of Southern California School of Pharmacy & Keck School of Medicine
Los Angeles, California

Glen L. Stimmel, PharmD
Professor of Clinical Pharmacy and Psychiatry
Titus Family Department of Clinical Pharmacy and Pharmaceutical Economics & Policy
Schools of Pharmacy and Medicine
University of Southern California
Los Angeles, Californa

Sana Sukkari, B Sc Phm, M. Phil
Assistant Professor
Department of Pharmacy Practice
School of Pharmacy
Lake Erie College of Osteopathic Medicine
Erie, Pennsylvania

Kelly M. Summers, PharmD
Assistant Professor of Pharmacotherapy
Department of Pharmacy Practice and Science
School of Pharmacy
University of Maryland at Baltimore
Baltimore, Maryland

David Taber, PharmD
Assistant Professor
Departments of Clinical Pharmacy and Outcomes Science
Clinical Pharmacy Specialist
South Carolina College of Pharmacy, Medical University of South Carolina
Charleston, South Carolina

Yasar Tasnif, PharmD
Assistant Professor
Cooperative Pharmacy Program
The University of Texas—Pan American
University of Texas at Austin, College of Pharmacy
Edinburg, Texas

Daniel J.G. Thirion, M.Sc, PharmD, BCPS
Clinical Assistant Professor
Faculte de Pharmacie, Universite de Montreal
Pharmacist, Internal Medicine Teaching Unit, Pharmacy Department, Hospital Sacre-Coeur de Montreal
Montreal, Quebec, Canada

Toby C. Trujillo, PharmD, BCPS
Associate Professor of Clinical Pharmacy
School of Pharmacy, University of Colorado at Denver Health Sciences Center
Clinical Coordinator
University of Colorado Hospital
Denver, Colorado

Candy Tsourounis, PharmD
Professor of Clinical Pharmacy
Department of Clinical Pharmacy
School of Pharmacy
University of California, San Francisco
San Francisco, California

Kimey Ung, PharmD
Clinical Pharmacist Specialist
Women's Pavillion at Miller Children's Hospital and Long Beach Memorial Hospital
Long Beach, California

Kenneth John Utz, PharmD
Clinical Instructor
Department of Clinical Pharmacy
School of Pharmacy, University of Colorado
Denver, Colorado

John Valgus, PharmD, BCOP
Clinical Assistant Professor
Division of Pharmacotherapy, UNC School of Pharmacy
Clinical Hematology/Oncology Specialist, Department of Pharmacy
University of North Carolina Hospitals and Clinics
Chapel Hill, North Carolina

Geoffrey Wall, PharmD, BCPS, CGP
Associate Professor of Pharmacy Practice
Department of Pharmacy Practice, College of Pharmacy, Drake University
Internal Medicine Clinical Pharamcist, Department of Pharmacy
Iowa Methodist Medical Center
Des Moines, Iowa

Kristin Watson, PharmD, BCPS
Assistant Professor of Pharmacotherapy
Pharmacy Practice and Science Department
School of Pharmacy
University of Maryland
Baltimore, Maryland

Charles Wayne Weart, PharmD, BCPS, FASHP
Professor, Pharmacy and Family Medicine
South Carolina College of Pharmacy
Medical University of South Carolina
Charleston, South Carolina

Timothy Edward Welty, PharmD, FCCP, BCPS
Professor
Department of Pharmacy Practice, McWhorter School of Pharmacy, Samford University
Adjunct Associate Research Professor
Department of Neurology
University of Alabama, Birmingham
Birmingham, Alabama

C. Michael White, PharmD, FCP, PCCP
Associate Professor, Department of Pharmacy Practice
School of Pharmacy, University of Connecticut
Director, Cardiac Pharmacology Service
Hartford Hospital
Hartford, Connecticut

Bradley R. Williams, PharmD, FASCP, CGP
Professor, Clinical Pharmacy & Clinical Gerontology
Titus Family Department of Clinical Pharmacy and Pharmaceutical Economics & Policy
School of Pharmacy, Andrus Gerontology Center
University of Southern California
Los Angeles, California

Dennis M. Williams, PharmD
Associate Professor
Division of Pharmacotherapy & Experimental Therapeutics, School of Pharmacy
Clinical Specialist, Pharmacy Department, UNC Hospitals
University of North Carolina
Chapel Hill, North Carolina

Ann K. Wittkowsky, PharmD, CACP, FASHP, FCCP
Clinical Professor
Department of Pharmacy, School of Pharmacy, University of Washington
Director of Anticoagulation Services, Department of Pharmacy
University of Washington Medical Center
Seattle, Washington

Annie Wong-Beringer, PharmD
Associate Professor, Titus Family Department of Clinical Pharmacy and Pharmaceutical Economics & Policy
School of Pharmacy, University of Southern California
Infectous Diseases Pharmacist
Department of Pharmacy, Huntington Hospital
Los Angeles and Pasadena, California

Lloyd Y. Young, PharmD
Professor Emeritus
Department of Clinical Pharmacy
School of Pharmacy
University of California, San Francisco
San Francisco, California

Wendy Zizzo, PharmD
Adjunct Professor of Behavioral Sciences
Alcohol and Other Drug Studies, San Diego City College
Assistant Clinical Professor of Pharmacy, Department of Clinical Pharmacy, School of Pharmacy
University of California, San Francisco
San Diego and San Francisco, California

Paolo V. Zizzo, D.O.
Assistant Clinical Professor
Department of Medicine, School of Medicine, University of California, San Diego
Clinical Internist, Private Practice
San Diego and Carlsbad, California

TABLE OF CONTENTS

GENERAL PRINCIPLES

CHAPTER 1

Assessment of Therapy and Medication Therapy Management

Marilyn R. Stebbins, Timothy W. Cutler, and Patricia L. Parker

This chapter presents several approaches to assessing drug therapy and provides the framework for medication therapy management services (MTMS) across the continuum of care. The illustrations in this chapter primarily focus on the pharmacist; however, the principles used to assess patient response to drug therapy are of value to all health care providers.

MTMS was first described in the Medicare Modernization Act of 2003 (MMA 2003), which also established the first outpatient prescription drug benefit (also known as Part D) for those eligible for Medicare.[1] MTMS was defined in MMA 2003 as *a program of drug therapy management that may be furnished by a pharmacist and that is designed to assure, with respect to targeted beneficiaries described in clause (ii), that covered Part D drugs under the prescription drug plan are appropriately used to optimize therapeutic outcomes through improved medication use, and to reduce the risk of adverse events, including adverse drug interactions. Such a program may distinguish between services in ambulatory and institutional settings.*

According to MMA 2003, individuals can qualify to receive MTMS if they meet the following three criteria:

1. Take multiple Medicare Part D–covered drugs
2. Have multiple chronic diseases
3. Are likely to incur annual costs of at least $4,000 for all covered Part D drugs

Although MTMS is the term used in MMA 2003 to describe medication management for those eligible under the Medicare Part D benefit, the same approach may be used for any patient. To respond to the need for further clarification of the term MTMS, 11 professional pharmacy associations more formally defined MTMS in a consensus document published in 2004.[2] According to this definition, MTMS could be applied to any patient in a variety of settings. Furthermore, this definition clarifies the type of activities involved in a medication therapy management (MTM) program.

MTMS has a direct relationship to pharmaceutical care. Pharmaceutical care has been described as *the responsible provision of drug therapy to achieve definite outcomes that are intended to improve a patient's quality of life.*[3,4] In fact, MTMS has been described as a service provided in the practice of pharmaceutical care.[5] However, unlike pharmaceutical care, MTMS is recognized by payers, has current procedural technology (CPT) codes specifically for pharmacists, and has several clearly defined interventions. Therefore, MTMS will be the term used to describe the activity of MTM in various patient populations.

Both patient self-care and medication reconciliation are critical aspects of any MTMS encounter regardless of the setting (i.e., inpatient, community, ambulatory, or institutional). Patient self-care is defined by the World Health Organization as those *activities [that] individuals, families, and communities undertake with the intention of enhancing health, preventing disease, limiting illness, and restoring health. These activities are derived from knowledge and skills from the pool of both professional and lay experience. They are undertaken by lay people on their own behalf, either separately or in participative collaboration with professionals.*[6] Patient self-care requires the patient to take responsibility for the illness; however, the help of a professional to structure healthy self-care is important. For example, patients with diabetes who monitor their blood glucose levels regularly and adjust their diet according to the guidelines published from the American Diabetes Association (ADA) would be practicing self-care. Self-care is often the work that the patient performs between visits with the provider. The patient should be involved in his own care to ensure the best outcomes.

Medication reconciliation is the process by which medication prescribing accuracy is ensured from one care setting to another or from one practitioner to another. Although not a new concept to the profession of pharmacy, there has been heightened awareness and intensified effort in this area of practice as a result of the Joint Commission. The Joint Commission is the national accrediting body for hospitals and other health care delivery organizations that has committed to improving patient care through an inspection and evaluation process. Through this process, the Joint Commission holds institutions to national consensus-based standards. In 2005, the Joint Commission announced its National Patient Safety Goal (NPS goal 8A and 8B) to *accurately and completely reconcile medications across the continuum of care*. This NPS goal required institutions to develop and test processes for medication reconciliation and to implement them by January 2006.[7]

The general approach to an MTMS patient encounter in various clinical settings will be discussed in the next sections. Figure 1-1 provides an overview of a patient encounter that includes patient information gathering from various data sources; interviewing the patient while utilizing effective communication skills; assessing the medical illness(es); developing a plan to manage the illness(es); documenting the service (including billing); and monitoring, follow-up, or referral for any additional issues that cannot be resolved during the encounter.

SOURCES OF PATIENT INFORMATION

Successful patient assessment and monitoring requires the gathering and organization of all relevant information.[4,8] The patient (or family member or other representative) is always the primary source of information. The provider asks the patient a series of questions to obtain subjective information that is helpful in making a diagnosis or evaluating ongoing therapy. Likewise, pharmacists, home care nurses, and other providers without direct access to patient data also must obtain subjective data or measure objective physical data to guide recommendations for therapy and to monitor previously prescribed therapy.

Data-Rich Environment

In a "data-rich environment," such as a hospital, long-term care facility, or outpatient medical clinic, a wealth of information is available to practitioners from the medical record, pharmacy profile, and nursing medication administration record (MAR). In these settings, physicians, nurses, and patients are readily available. This facilitates timely, effective communication among those involved in the drug therapy decision-making process. Objective data (e.g., diagnosis, physical examination, laboratory and other test results, vital signs, weight, medications, medication allergies, intravenous flow rates, and fluid balance) are readily available. Likewise, the cases presented throughout this text usually provide considerable data on which to make more thorough assessments and therapeutic decisions. The patient record provides readily available information that is needed to identify and assess medical problems. It is necessary in order to design patient specific care plans and document MTMS. In some settings, patient insurance information is important to help understand the formulary choices and coverage of medications. When billing for MTMS, this insurance information is very important and would be available in a data-rich environment.

Paper Charts

A paper chart may be a source of valuable patient information. Paper charts may exist in a variety of settings, including the hospital, outpatient clinic, or institutional setting. This source of information is considered data rich but does have limitations. Paper charts are organized differently by site and by setting. The information contained in a hospital chart will be different from that contained in an outpatient clinic. Furthermore, it may be difficult to obtain a paper chart, or access may be delayed if another professional is using the chart. Significant data delays may occur in paper charts, as information such as laboratory results, test results, and chart notes may not be placed in the chart for several days after the test or documentation is complete. As a result, it is important to realize the limitations of this data-rich environment and that the information obtained during the patient interview is still extremely important.

Electronic Medical Record

An electronic medical record (EMR) is an electronic version of the paper chart. Once again, these records are available in hospitals, clinics, and institutional settings, but the type of EMR and the organization of information will vary among the different settings and software applications. The EMR provides a wealth of information and is one of the most complete sources of reliable information. Unlike a paper chart, the EMR may be interfaced with the laboratory, pharmacy, and radiology systems so that data is available real time with minimal delays. Unfortunately, clinicians may rely on the EMR too much for the patient information, which could lead to assumptions. For example, a patient who has metformin 500 mg twice daily listed in the EMR may actually be taking the medication once daily. Therefore, the data in the EMR is extremely useful, but it is still important to obtain information directly from the patient.

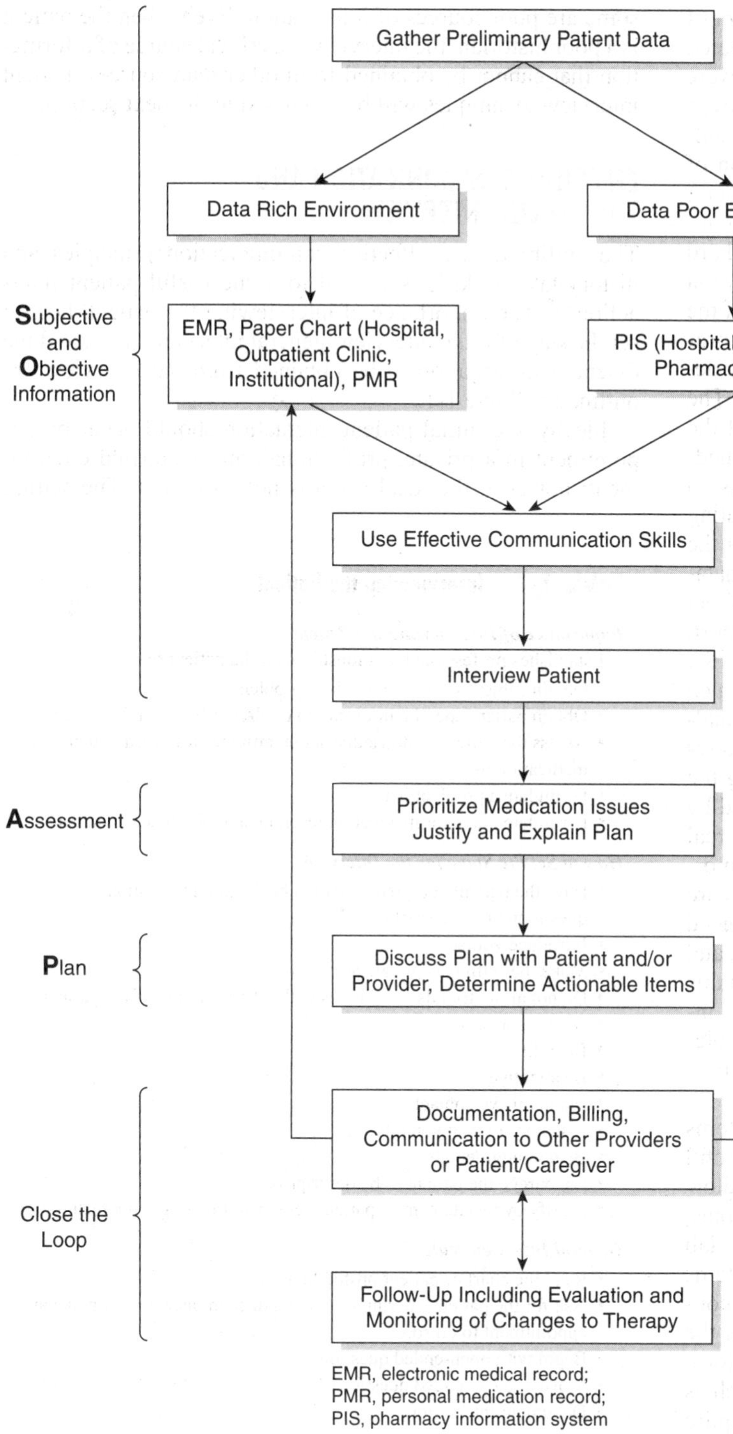

FIGURE 1-1 General approach to a patient encounter.

Data-Poor Environment

In reality, clinicians are often required to make assessments with limited information. Even in a relatively data-poor environment, such as a community pharmacy, valuable sources of information are still available, including (a) the medication profile, (b) patient data, and (c) the patient's insurance coverage information. In addition, it is often possible to consult with the prescriber (or the prescriber's office staff); however, contact may be delayed, and requests for information may be met with resistance due to time constraints or other factors. As illustrated later in this chapter, the successful practitioner can make assessments and intervene on the patient's behalf even in the absence of all the available information.

Pharmacy Information Systems

Pharmacy information systems (PIS) are generally considered data poor. When discussing PIS, it is important to look at both inpatient and outpatient PIS. Pharmacy billing and inventory management were the motivation behind the establishment of the early PIS. These initial systems provided fill lists, generated patient profiles, and produced medication labels, which were valuable to institutional pharmacies as the profession moved toward a unit dose medication distribution system. More modern functionalities allow for some limited documentation of clinical pharmacy activities, but still, this system is data poor. Current work flow for institutions functioning off of PIS consists of medication processing via a physician-generated hard copy medication order, which is provided to the pharmacy via delivery, facsimile, or scanner. After pharmacist review of the medication order for clinical appropriateness, the nurse is provided access to the medication either by direct pharmacy delivery or by means of an automated dispensing system. The nurse ensures that the patient receives the medication at the appropriate time and documents the administration on the medication administration record (MAR). Increased emphasis on patient safety has highlighted the importance of integrating PIS with other computerized systems utilized throughout the inpatient setting. This involves a transition from PIS to a data-rich clinical information system (CIS), which includes direct computerized physician order entry, clinical decision support, EMR, an electronic medication administration record (eMAR), and integration of various ancillary information systems such as pharmacy and laboratory services. Additional functionality incorporates the use of bar code technology, which allows the ability to track and promote quality assurance during the medication administration process. Information generated by the CIS is electronically transmitted to the pharmacy in real time, eliminating lost, illegible, or incomplete medication orders. Improved communication between various health care providers, decreased medication turnaround time, enhanced compliance with medication use policies and formularies, and reductions in medication errors may be benefits seen from this system. Although increasing numbers of institutions are incorporating this technology into their practice settings, implementation of CIS in hospitals has not occurred for numerous reasons, including expense and system complexity.

A variety of outpatient PIS exist. Some of these systems contain only basic data such as the medication profile, refill history, allergies, and insurance information. Other PIS allow the pharmacist to enter information such as progress notes, vital signs (blood pressure [BP], pulse, respirations), and lab results (blood glucose, cholesterol levels), but these systems are rarely linked to an EMR. Therefore, the information contained in the outpatient PIS is dependent on the ability of the pharmacist to obtain the information. As pharmacists perform more advanced services in the community pharmacy (such as immunizations, tobacco cessation, MTMS, etc.) that require documentation of services, the PIS will need to become a more robust source of data.

Especially in a data-poor environment, it is important that the clinician be a proactive interviewer where the interviewer often becomes an investigator. The investigative approach is direct and requires strong problem-solving abilities as well as requires the interviewer to actively listen to the patient. Questions should be formulated to obtain information such as the medication history, actual medication use, patient perception of care, use of over-the-counter (OTC) and natural or herbal products, and health beliefs (cultural or otherwise). This approach with the patient can help to verify and ensure the accuracy of other data sources. Not all patients are reliable historians, and some are poor sources of information. Even when the patient is a poor historian, the interview is a critical source of information that cannot be obtained from other data sources. Patient interview techniques will be discussed in the next section.

EFFECTIVE COMMUNICATION AND THE PATIENT INTERVIEW

The ability to use effective communication principles and history-taking skills is crucial to a successful patient interaction.[4,8] The importance of interviewing the patient, how to set the stage for the interview, general interview rules, and the essential information to be obtained from the interview are outlined in Table 1-1.

Ideally, the initial patient interaction should occur by appointment in a private, professional, and unhurried environment; however, the ideal often is not an option. The setting

Table 1-1 Interviewing the Patient

Importance of Interviewing the Patient

Establishes professional relationship with the patient to:
- Obtain subjective data on medical problems
- Obtain patient-specific information on drug efficacy and toxicity
- Assess the patient's knowledge about, attitudes toward, and pattern of medication use
- Formulate a problem list
- Formulate plans for medication teaching and pharmaceutical care

How to Set the Stage for the Interview
- Have the patient complete a written health and medication questionnaire, if available
- Introduce yourself
- Make the setting as private as possible
- Do not allow friends or relatives without permission of the patient
- Do not appear rushed
- Be polite
- Be attentive
- Maintain eye contact
- Listen more than you talk
- Be nonjudgmental
- Encourage the patient to be descriptive
- Clarify by restatement or patient demonstration (e.g., of a technique)

General Interview Rules
- Read the chart or patient profile first
- Ask for the patient's permission to conduct an interview or make an appointment to do so.
- Begin with open-ended questions
- Move to close-ended questions
- Document interaction

Information to Be Obtained
- History of allergies
- History of adverse drug reactions
- Weight and height
- Drugs: dose, route, frequency, and reason for use
- Perceived efficacy of each drug
- Perceived side effects
- Adherence to prescribed drug regimen
- Nonprescription medication use (including complementary and alternative medications)
- Possibility of pregnancy in women of childbearing age
- Family or other support systems

Adapted from work by Teresa O'Sullivan, PharmD, University of Washington.

may be the pharmacy, a clinic, or the bedside. Regardless of the setting, the process may be expedited by asking or helping the patient to complete a written self-assessment history form (current medical conditions and medications, height, weight, allergies, adverse drug reactions, immunizations, tobacco and alcohol use, pregnancy status, etc.) before obtaining a verbal history. Figure 1-2 presents a sample form.[4]

Communication

Once the self-assessment form is completed and reviewed, the pharmacist can focus on the patient interview. Setting the stage for the interview and getting off to a good start can be accomplished by greeting the patient with a smile, providing formal introductions, and explaining the purpose of the encounter. Asking the patient what expectations she may have will help to ensure that concerns are addressed. At this point, several other key issues may surface. During the interview, language barriers or cultural issues may be identified that need to be addressed. This will also provide an opportunity to look for clues that can help to determine the patient's level of health literacy. These concepts will be discussed later in this section. Specific communication skills that can be used to guide the practitioner through a productive patient interview include the following:

- Effective questioning by using open-ended questions
- Active listening
- Reflective responding
- Careful attention to body language
- Identifying cultural differences and disparities
- Understanding the patient's level of health literacy

Effective questioning techniques include both open- and closed-ended questions. To the extent possible, the practitioner should ask open-ended questions so that the patient is encouraged to explain and elaborate. Skilled use of these questions puts the practitioner in the role of observer, listener, recorder, and prompter and the patient in the role of storyteller. This technique also allows the practitioner to assess quickly the patient's depth of knowledge and understanding of his medications and health situation. For example, at the beginning of the interview, the practitioner may ask, "If there is one thing I can accomplish for you today, what would that be?" Or, perhaps during the interview when discussing adherence to a specific medication, the practitioner may ask, "How many times a day do you take this medication?" or "What time of day do you take this medication?" To conclude the interview, the practitioner may choose to ask, "Just to be sure we haven't missed anything important, what other medication issues have you had since your last visit?" Open-ended questions are asked one at a time with a pause in between each to allow the patient to answer. Closed-ended questions (e.g., those that can be simply answered "yes" or "no") can be used to prompt patients who know little about their health situation and to systematically minimize inadvertent omissions. If closed-ended questioning is used, all "yes or no" responses should be followed with additional questions such as, "Please explain what you experienced."

The patient should be encouraged to do most of the talking, while the practitioner utilizes active listening techniques. In order to be an effective active listener, distractions should be minimized. This may be difficult in certain settings, but finding a private area for the interview, ensuring that mobile phones and pagers are off (or at a minimum set to the silent or vibrate mode), and not allowing interruption from the staff during the visit can all lead to enhanced communication. The active listening technique requires the interviewer to focus on what the patient is saying without interrupting. Providing verbal and nonverbal cues such as "Yes, please go on" or nodding affirmatively lets the patient know that the practitioner is listening.

Reflective responding allows the practitioner to periodically check in with the patient to ensure understanding of what the patient is communicating. This technique demonstrates caring and helps to build a rapport with the patient. An example of reflective responding may be, "From what you have told me, I understand that you are not taking your medications because they are too expensive" or "It seems like you are not having any difficulty taking your new cholesterol medication." By periodically summarizing the information obtained from the patient, the practitioner can clarify and bring closure to one segment of the interview before progressing further.

As the practitioner gains experience and becomes more sophisticated in interviewing patients, subtle clues (e.g., unusual information, observation, and body language) can be used to pursue a line of questioning that could explain an unexpected problem or clarify an existing problem. For example, a patient may become very nervous and fidget when asked to play back what was explained to her, or she may state, "I understood everything you said, and I don't need to waste your time repeating it." This may be a sign that the patient is hearing impaired or has cognitive difficulties that need to be addressed.

Cultural differences and health disparities must also be recognized and addressed for practitioners to achieve successful health outcomes. By definition, cultural competence is a set of congruent behaviors, attitudes, and policies that come together among a group of people, a system, or an agency that enables them to work effectively in cross-cultural situations.[9] There are several core elements to cultural competence:

- Awareness and acceptance of difference
- Awareness of one's cultural values
- Development of knowledge of different cultures
- Understanding the dynamics of difference
- Ability to adapt skills to fit the cultural context of others

Health disparities refer to gaps in the quality of health and health care across racial, ethnic, and socioeconomic groups.[10] These gaps result in worse clinical outcomes, and these differences persist after adjustment for known factors including, but not limited to, social determinants and access to health care. It is generally accepted that disparities can result from three main areas:[11,12]

- From the personal, socioeconomic, and environmental characteristics of different ethnic and racial groups
- From the barriers encountered by certain racial and ethnic groups when trying to enter into the health care delivery system
- From the quality of health care that different ethnic and racial groups receive

In order to provide culturally competent care, practitioners must tailor care to meet the patient's linguistic, cultural, and social needs, recognizing that communication is directly linked to health outcomes. Linguistically, the patient and provider's spoken language, dialects, accents, and speed of the spoken language are important factors that will influence communication.

Name: ______________________________ **Date:** ____________

Mailing Address: ______________________________
street city state zip

Social Security Number: ____________ **Phone: (H)** ____________ **(W)** ____________

DOB: ________ **Height:** ________ **Weight:** ________ **HR:** ________ **BP:** ________

Gender: ________ **Pregnancy Status:** ________

Allergies: ______________________________ **Reactions:** ______________________________

Devises/Alerts: ______________________________

PRESCRIPTION MEDICATION HISTORY

Name/Strength	Directions	Start Date	Stop Date	Physician	Purpose	Effectiveness

OTC USE: Check conditions for which you have used a non-prescription medication.

____ headache
____ eye/ear problems
____ cold/flu
____ allergies
____ sinus
____ cough
____ sleeplessness
____ drowsiness
____ weight loss
____ diarrhea
____ hemorrhoids
____ muscle/joint pain
____ rash/itching/dry skin
____ heartburn/GI upset/gas
____ vitamins
____ herbal products
____ organic products
____ other:

OVER-THE-COUNTER MEDICATION HISTORY

Name/Strength	Directions	Purpose	How Often	Effectiveness

FIGURE 1-2 Patient history form. Reprinted with permission from Rovers JP, Currie JD. *A Practical Guide to Pharmaceutical Care: A Clinical Skills Primer*, Washington, DC: American Pharmacists Association; 2007, p. 61–62.

MEDICAL PROBLEMS: Have you experienced, or do you have: (circle Y or N)

known kidney problems?	Y	N	sores on legs or feet?	Y	N
frequent urinary infections?	Y	N	known blood clot problems?	Y	N
difficulty with urination?	Y	N	leg pain or swelling?	Y	N
frequent urination at night?	Y	N	unusual bleeding or bruising?	Y	N
known liver problems/hepatitis?	Y	N	anemia?	Y	N
trouble eating certain foods?	Y	N	thyroid problems?	Y	N
nausea or vomiting?	Y	N	known hormone problems?	Y	N
constipation or diarrhea?	Y	N	arthritis or joint problems?	Y	N
bloody or black bowel movements?	Y	N	muscle cramps or weakness?	Y	N
abdominal pain or cramps?	Y	N	memory problems?	Y	N
frequent heartburn/indigestion?	Y	N	dizziness?	Y	N
stomach ulcers in the past?	Y	N	hearing or visual problems?	Y	N
shortness of breath?	Y	N	frequent headaches?	Y	N
coughing up phlegm or blood?	Y	N	rash or hives?	Y	N
chest pain or tightness?	Y	N	change in appetite/taste?	Y	N
fainting spells or passing out?	Y	N	walking/balance problems?	Y	N
thumping or racing heart?	Y	N	other problems? ______________	Y	N

MEDICAL HISTORY: Have you or any blood relative had: (mark all that apply)

	self	relative		self	relative
high blood pressure	___	___	heart disease	___	___
asthma	___	___	stroke	___	___
cancer	___	___	kidney disease	___	___
depression	___	___	mental illness	___	___
lung disease	___	___	substance abuse		
diabetes	___	___	other ______________________		

SOCIAL HISTORY: Please indicate your tobacco, alcohol, caffeine and dietary habits.

Nicotine Use

_____ never smoked
_____ packs per day for _____ years
_____ stopped _____ year(s) ago

Alcohol Consumption

_____ never consumed
_____ drinks per day/week
_____ stopped _____ year(s) ago

Caffeine Intake

_____ never consumed
_____ drinks per day
_____ stopped _____ year(s) ago

Diet Restrictions/Patterns

_____ number of meals per day
_____ food restrictions: ______________
____

OTHER INFORMATION/COMMENTS:

____
Pharmacist Signature   Date

FIGURE 1-2 Patient history form *(Continued)*.

Table 1-2 Behaviors Suggestive of Inadequate Health Literacy

- Asking for help
- Bringing someone along who can read
- Inability to keep appointments
- Making excuses like "I forgot to bring my glasses"
- Nonadherence with medications
- Poor adherence to recommended medical interventions
- Postponing making decisions
- Watching others and mimicking behaviors

Whether a personal or impersonal approach to the encounter is culturally acceptable will be important to know. Also, the degree of formality expected, appropriate subjects for conversation, directness, touch, and loudness of conversation may play a role in the success of the encounter. Often overlooked but critically important are health and healing beliefs that the patient and her family or community may have. It is only after these factors are recognized and acknowledged that a practitioner can make recommendations and negotiate a plan with the patient or her caregiver. From a communication standpoint, the practitioner must determine, at a minimum, the preferred mode of communication, the level of literacy, the preferred language, and whether an interpreter or a cultural broker (an individual who shares the cultural identity with the client/patient and can effectively mediate when cross-cultural communication is necessary) is needed.

Health literacy is a component of cultural competence. It was defined in the Institute of Medicine Report in 2004 as the *degree to which individuals have the capacity to obtain, process, and understand basic health information and services needed to make appropriate health decisions.*[13] There are several behaviors or cues that may be suggestive of inadequate health literacy skills that a provider can look for when interacting with patients. These behavioral cues can be found in Table 1-2. There are several communication techniques that may be helpful in determining the level of health literacy and may aid the provider in addressing a patient with inadequate health literacy. These communication techniques are presented in Table 1-3.

In all interactions, the health care provider must treat the patient with respect as well as make every effort to ask questions and receive information in a nonjudgmental way (e.g., "Please tell me how you take your medications" as opposed to "Do you take your medications exactly as prescribed?"). Practitioners who provide MTMS must keep in mind that patients hold them in trust and often share intimate details of their medical and social histories. Thus, practitioners must maintain the confidentiality of that information and share it only with those providers who need this information to provide patient care. Additionally, clinicians must adhere to the regulations set forth by the Health Insurance Portability and Accountability Act (HIPAA) of 1996, which provides standards to protect the security and confidentiality of individually identifiable protected health information (PHI). PHI includes information created during the provision of patient care that can be linked with a specific patient. Examples of PHI include the patient's name, home address, date of birth, medical record number, medical diagnoses, treatment records, prescriptions, and laboratory and test results. Further discussion of the HIPAA regulations is beyond the scope of this chapter; consult the U.S. Department of Health and Human Services website for additional information.

Table 1-3 Communication Tips for Identifying and Addressing Inadequate Health Literacy

- Assess patient's baseline understanding before providing extensive information
- Speak slowly
- Use lay language instead of medical terminology
- Emphasize only 1 to 3 points in any one encounter
- Encourage questions by using the open-ended question approach
- Show or draw pictures to enhance understanding and subsequent recall, if appropriate
- Use the teach-back or show-me method
- Write down important instructions
- Provide useful educational materials
- Be respectful, caring, and sensitive

OBTAINING A PATIENT HISTORY

Those who provide MTMS should develop standardized forms to record patient information obtained from the patient interview. Standardization facilitates quick retrieval of information, minimizes the inadvertent omission of data, and enhances the ability of other practitioners to use shared records.[4,8]

For convenience, the patient interview and record can be divided into sections with subjective and objective data as well as an assessment and plan (including expected outcomes). Components of subjective and objective data are the medical history, drug history, and social history. In some situations, these histories can be supplemented by the generation of flowchart diagrams to monitor changes in specific parameters (e.g., blood glucose concentration, BP, weight) over time. These charts and documentation systems may be incorporated into the EMR, PIS, or a similar electronic platform.

Medical History

The medical history is essential to the provision of MTMS. It can be as extensive as the medical records that are maintained in an institution or physician's office, or it can be a simple patient profile that is maintained in a community pharmacy. The purpose of the medical history is to identify significant past medical conditions or procedures; identify, characterize, and assess current acute and chronic medical conditions and symptoms; and gather all relevant health information that could influence drug selection or dosing (e.g., function of major organs such as the gastrointestinal tract, liver, and kidney, which are involved in the absorption and elimination of drugs; height and weight, including recent changes in either; age and gender; pregnancy and lactation status; and special nutritional needs). Not all interviews require the interviewer to ask for this much general information; however, in a data poor environment, more information is required directly from the patient. A more focused interview may be appropriate in settings where the information required is available electronically or is specific to a single disease state. For example, in an anticoagulation clinic, the information that is elicited from the patient is often specific to the patient's anticoagulation therapy (e.g., bleeding incidents, newly started medications, dietary changes, missed warfarin doses, etc.).

1. P.J., a 45-year-old woman of normal height and weight, states that she has diabetes. What questions might the practitioner ask of P.J. to determine whether type 1 or type 2 disease should be documented in her medical history?

Patients usually can enumerate their medical problems in a general way, but the practitioner often will have to probe more specifically to refine the diagnosis and assess the severity of the condition. Diabetes mellitus is used to illustrate the types of questions that can be used to gather important health information and assess drug therapy. The following questions should generate information that will help to determine whether P.J. has type 1 or type 2 diabetes mellitus.

- **How old were you when you were told you had diabetes?**
- **Do any of your relatives have diabetes mellitus? What do you know of their diabetes?**
- **Do you remember your symptoms? Please describe them to me.**
- **What medications have you used to treat your diabetes?**

When questions such as these are combined with knowledge of the pathophysiology of diabetes, appreciation of the typical presenting signs and symptoms of the disease, and understanding of the drugs generally used to treat both forms of diabetes, meaningful MTM can be provided. Even simple assessments such as the observation of a patient's body size can provide information useful for therapeutic interventions. For example, a person with type 2 diabetes is more likely to be an overweight adult (see Chapter 50).

Medication History

In the community pharmacy setting, patients generally present themselves in one of four ways: (a) with a self-diagnosed condition for which nonprescription drug therapy is sought; (b) with a newly diagnosed condition for which a drug has been prescribed; (c) with a chronic condition that requires refill of a previously prescribed drug or the initiation of a new drug; or (d) on referral from their health plan, provider or self-referral for focused medication therapy review (MTR). In the first and second situations, the practitioner must confirm the diagnosis by using disease-specific questions as illustrated in Question 1. In the third situation, the practitioner uses the same type of questioning as in the first two situations; however, this time the practitioner needs to evaluate whether the desired therapeutic outcomes have been achieved. The practitioner must evaluate the information gleaned during follow-up visits in the context of the history and incorporate it into his or her assessment and medication action plan (MAP). The fourth situation, in which patients require a focused MTR, the medication and medical history information are equally important. Without the medical history, it is not possible to evaluate whether the drug therapy is appropriate, and without an accurate medication history, it is not possible to determine if the patient has reached the desired goals of therapy for her condition. The goal of the medication history is to obtain and assess the following information: the specific prescription and nonprescription drugs that the patient is taking (the latter includes OTC medications, botanicals, dietary supplements, recreational drugs, alcohol, tobacco, and home remedies); the intended purpose or indications for each of these medications; how taken (e.g., route, ingestion in relation to meals), how much, and how often these medications are used; how long these agents have been taken or used (start and stop dates); whether the patient believes that any of these agents are providing therapeutic benefit; whether the patient is experiencing or has experienced any adverse effects that could be caused by each of these agents (idiosyncratic reactions, toxic effects, adverse effects); whether the patient has stopped taking any of the medications for any reason; and allergic reactions and any history of hypersensitivity or other severe reactions to drugs. This information should be as specific as possible, including a description of the reaction, the treatment, and the date of its occurrence.

The approach and process by which the medication history is obtained does not necessarily change based on the setting of the encounter. However, one primary difference in the inpatient setting is the Joint Commission requirement for medication reconciliation. A successful medication reconciliation process consists of a standardized systematic approach, with the initial step in this process involving the collection of the best medication history possible from every patient that enters any point in the health care system. The appropriate health care professional to obtain this information varies widely from one institution to the next, involving an array of individuals. Although pharmacists are uniquely qualified and have demonstrated increased accuracy in acquiring the medication history[14], ultimately, medication reconciliation requires a multidisciplinary effort in which all available resources are integrated into each step of the process where appropriate.[15] Shared accountability by utilizing key members of the health care team such as direct-care nurses, pharmacy technicians, pharmacists, and the prescriber is essential in this process. Once an accurate medication history is obtained, the information is used to ensure that any deviation from prescribing as the patient moves through the health care system is deliberate and based on acute changes in the patient's condition. If a discrepancy is an intended therapeutic decision by the prescribing clinician, appropriate documentation with either the reason for or intention to change, hold, or discontinue the medication should be completed in a manner that is clear to all members of the health care team. Unintentional variances in the lists should be considered as potential medication errors pending clarification from the prescribing clinician.

Since medication errors are most commonly seen at interfaces of care, the essential times to conduct medication reconciliation are when a patient is admitted to, transferred within (setting, service, practitioner, or level of care change), or discharged from a health care facility.[16,17] A crucial final step in the reconciliation process and a vital piece of MTMS occurs at discharge to avoid therapeutic duplication, drug interactions, and omissions of medications that may have been discontinued or placed on hold during hospitalization. On departure from the health care facility, a complete list of the patient's medications must be communicated to the patient and the next provider of service regardless of whether it is within or outside the organization. It is important to realize that efforts to implement a medication reconciliation process should not focus simply on fulfilling a Joint Commission standard but that this process allows for informed prescribing decisions and creates a safer environment for patients by improving the accuracy of medication administration throughout the continuum of care.

Perhaps the most important aspect of the medication history is to ensure that no assumptions related to medication use go unverified with the patient. The provider should ask questions related to how the current medication therapy is actually taken by the patient. The interviewer should then compare the use of medications as defined by the patient to the prescription information on the bottle or in the PIS/EMR. This information may identify discrepancies or misunderstandings between the prescriber and patient. As discussed previously, the patient may not have adequate health literacy, and the interpretation of the medication instructions printed on the bottle or described by a health professional may not be understandable to a patient. The review of the medication history is an opportune time to identify and clarify such misunderstandings.

2. P.J. has indicated that she is injecting insulin to treat her diabetes. What questions might be asked to evaluate P.J.'s use of and response to insulin?

The following types of questions, when asked of P.J., should provide the practitioner with information on P.J.'s understanding about the use of and response to insulin.

Drug Identification and Use

- **What type of insulin do you use?**
- **How many units of insulin do you use?**
- **When do you inject your insulin in relationship to meals?**
- **Where do you inject your insulin? (Rather than the more judgmental question, "Do you rotate your injection sites?")**
- **Please show me how you usually prepare your insulin for injection. (This request of the patient requires the patient to demonstrate a skill.)**
- **What, if anything, keeps you from taking your insulin as prescribed?**

Assessment of Therapeutic Response

- **How do you know if your insulin is working?**
- **What blood glucose levels are you aiming for?**
- **How often and when during the day do you test your blood glucose concentration?**
- **Do you have any blood glucose records that you could share with me?**
- **Would you show me how you test your blood glucose concentration?**
- **What is your understanding of the hemoglobin A_{1c} blood test?**
- **When was the last time you had this test done?**
- **What were the results of the last hemoglobin A_{1c} test?**

Assessment of Adverse Effects

- **Do you ever experience reactions from low blood glucose?**
- **What symptoms warn you of such a reaction?**
- **When do these typically occur during the day?**
- **How often do they occur?**
- **What circumstances seem to make them occur more frequently?**
- **What do you do when you have a low blood glucose?**

The patient's responses to these questions on drug use, therapeutic response, and adverse effects will allow a quick assessment of the patient's knowledge of insulin and whether she is using it in a way that is likely to result in blood glucose concentrations that are neither too high nor too low. The responses to these questions also should provide the practitioner with insight about the extent to which the patient has been involved in establishing and monitoring therapeutic outcomes. Based on this information, the practitioner can begin to formulate the patient's therapeutic plan.

Social History

The social history is used to determine the patient's occupation and lifestyle; important family relationships or other support systems; any particular circumstances (e.g., a disability) or stresses in her life that could influence the MAP; and attitudes, values, and feelings about health, illness, and treatments.

3. A patient's occupation, lifestyle, insurance status, ability to pay, and attitudes often can determine the success or failure of drug therapy. Therefore, P.J.'s prescription drug coverage, nutritional history, her level of activity or exercise in a typical day or week, the family dynamics, and any particular stresses that may affect glucose control need to be documented and assessed. What questions might be asked of P.J. to gain this information?

Work

- **Describe a typical work day and a typical weekend day.**

Insurance/Cost

- **What type of prescription drug coverage do you have? What are the copays for your insulin and diabetic supplies? How often do you go without your insulin or supplies due to cost?**

Exercise

- **Describe your exercise habits. How often, how long, and when during the day do you exercise? Describe how you change your meals or insulin when you exercise.**

Diet

- **How many times per day do you usually eat? Describe your usual meal times.**
- **What do you usually eat for each of your main meals and snacks?**
- **Are you able to eat at the same time each day?**
- **What do you do if a meal is delayed or missed?**
- **Who cooks the meals at home? Does this person understand your dietary needs?**
- **How often do you eat meals in a restaurant?**
- **How do you order meals in a restaurant to maintain a proper diet for your diabetes? (*Note:* This is asked of patients who frequently dine in restaurants.)**

Support Systems

- **Who else lives with you? What do they know about diabetes? How do they respond to the fact that you have diabetes? How do they help you with your diabetes management? Does it ever strain your relationship? What are the issues that seem to be most troublesome? (*Note:* These questions apply equally to the workplace or school setting. Often, the biggest barrier to multiple daily injections is refusal of the patient to inject insulin while at work or school.)**

Table 1-4 Elements of the Problem Oriented Medical Record[a]

Problem name: Each "problem" is listed separately and given an identifying number. Problems may be a patient complaint (e.g., headache), a laboratory abnormality (e.g., hypokalemia), or a specific disease name if prior diagnosis is known. When monitoring previously described drug therapy, more than one drug-related problem may be considered (e.g., nonadherence, a suspected adverse drug reaction or drug interaction, or an inappropriate dose).Under each problem name, the following information is identified:

Subjective	Information that explains or delineates the reason for the encounter. Information that the patient reports concerning symptoms, previous treatments, medications used, and adverse effects encountered.These are considered nonreproducible data because the information is based on the patient's interpretation and recall of past events.
Objective	Information from physical examination, laboratory results, diagnostic tests, pill counts, and pharmacy patient profile information.Objective data are measurable and reproducible.
Assessment	A brief but complete description of the problem, including a conclusion or diagnosis that is supported logically by the above subjective and objective data. The assessment should not include a problem/diagnosis that is not defined above.
Plan	A detailed description of recommended or intended further workup (laboratory radiology, consultation), treatment (e.g., continued observation: physiotherapy, diet, medications, surgery), patient education (self-care, goals of therapy, medication use and monitoring), monitoring, and follow-up relative to the above assessment.

[a] Sometimes referred to as the *SOAP* (subjective; objective, assessment, plan) note.

Attitude

- **How do you feel about having diabetes?**
- **What worries or bothers you most about having diabetes? (*Note:* Participate in the patient's care. This approach is likely to enhance the patient–provider relationship, which should translate into improved care.)**

APPROACH TO AND ASSESSMENT OF PATIENT THERAPY

The provider–patient encounter will vary based on the location and type of services provided and access to necessary information. However, the general approach to the patient encounter should follow the problem-oriented medical record (POMR). Organizing information according to medical problems (e.g., diseases) helps to break down a complex situation (e.g., a patient with multiple medical problems requiring multiple drugs) into its individual parts.[3,4] The medical community has long used a *POMR* or *SOAP note* to record information in the medical record or chart by using a standardized format (Table 1-4). Each medical problem is identified, listed sequentially, and assigned a number. *Subjective* data and *objective* data in support of each problem are delineated, an *assessment* is made, and a *plan* of action identified. The first letter of the four key words (subjective, objective, assessment, and plan) serve as the basis for the SOAP acronym.

The POMR is a general approach and helps to focus the encounter, which provides a structure for the documentation of the services provided. The following section will describe the POMR and SOAP note in more detail.

Problem List

Problems are listed in order of importance and are supported by the subjective and objective evidence gathered during the patient encounter. Each problem in the list can then be given an identifying number. All subsequent references to a specific problem can be identified or referenced by that number (e.g., "problem 1" or simply "1"). These generally are thought of in terms of a diagnosed disease, but they also may be a symptom complex that is being evaluated, a preventive measure (e.g., immunization, contraception), or a cognitive problem (e.g., nonadherence). Problems should be identified based on the practitioner's level of understanding. For example, the symptoms of "difficulty breathing at night" or "two-pillow orthopnea" are consistent with the symptom complex of heart failure (HF); however, these symptoms could be assessed as individual problems if the student or practitioner is unaware of the association of these symptoms with HF. Any condition that requires a unique management plan should be identified as a problem to serve as a reminder to the practitioner that treatment is needed for that problem. Different settings and activities or clinical services will determine the priority of the problems identified.

Medical problems can be *drug related*, including prescribing errors, dosing errors, adverse drug effects, adherence issues, and the need for medication counseling. Drug-related problems may be definite (i.e., there is no question that the problem exists) or possible (i.e., further investigation is required to establish whether the problem really exists). The most commonly encountered types of drug-related problems are listed in Table 1-5.[4,8]

The distinction between medical problems and drug-related problems sometimes is unclear, and considerable overlap exists. For example, a medical problem (i.e., a disease, syndrome, symptom, or health condition) can be prevented, cured, alleviated, or exacerbated by medications. When assessing drug therapy, several situations could exist: treatment is appropriate and therapeutic outcomes have been achieved; drugs that have been selected are ineffective or therapeutic outcomes are partially achieved; dosages are subtherapeutic or medication is taken improperly; an inappropriate drug for the medical condition being treated has been prescribed or is being used; or the condition is not being treated.

Likewise, a drug-related problem can cause or aggravate a medical problem. Such drug-related problems could include hypersensitivity reactions; idiosyncratic reactions; toxic reactions secondary to excessive doses; adverse reactions (e.g., insulin-induced hypoglycemia or weight gain); drug-drug, drug-disease, drug-laboratory test, and drug-lifestyle interactions; or polypharmacy (using multiple medications), which may increase the risk of adverse drug events.[18]

Subjective and Objective Data

Subjective and objective data in support of a problem are important because assessment of patients and therapies requires the gathering of specific information to verify that a

Table 1-5 Drug-Related Problems

Drug Needed (also referred to as no drug)
Drug indicated but not prescribed; a medical problem has been diagnosed, but there is no indication that treatment has been initiated (maybe it is not needed)
Correct drug prescribed but not taken (nonadherence)
Wrong/Inappropriate Drug
No apparent medical problem justifying the use of the drug
Drug not indicated for the medical problem for which it has been prescribed
Medical problem no longer exists
Duplication of other therapy
Less expensive alternative available
Drug not covered by formulary
Failure to account for pregnancy status, age of patient, or other contraindications
Incorrect nonprescription medication self-prescribed by the patient
Recreational drug use
Wrong Dose
Prescribed dose too high (includes adjustments for renal and hepatic function, age, body size)
Correct prescribed dose but overuse by patient (overadherence)
Prescribed dose too low (includes adjustments for age, body size)
Correct prescribed dose but underuse by patient (underadherence)
Incorrect, inconvenient, or less-than-optimal dosing interval (consider use of sustained-release dosage forms)
Adverse Drug Reaction
Hypersensitivity reaction
Idiosyncratic reaction
Drug-induced disease
Drug-induced laboratory change
Drug Interaction
Drug-drug interaction
Drug-food interaction
Drug-laboratory test interaction
Drug-disease interaction

problem continues to exist or that therapeutic objectives are being achieved. Subjective data refer to information provided by the patient or another person that cannot be confirmed independently. This is the data most commonly obtained during a patient interview. Objective data refer to information observed or measured by the practitioner (e.g., laboratory tests, BP measurements). The objective data is most commonly obtained from the EMR or paper chart (data-rich-environment). However, some objective data can be obtained in data-poor-environments. In the absence of a medical record, weight, height, pulse, BP, blood glucose readings, and other objective information can be gathered during the provider–patient encounter.

4. P.N., a 28-year-old man, has a BP of 140/100 mmHg. What is the primary problem? What subjective and objective data support the problem, and what additional subjective and objective data are not provided but usually are needed to define this particular problem?

The primary problem is hypertension. No subjective data are given. The objective data are the patient's age, gender, and BP of 140/100 mmHg. Each of these is important in designing a patient-specific therapy plan. Because hypertension often is an asymptomatic disease (see Chapter 13), subjective complaints such as headache, tiredness or anxiety, shortness of breath (SOB), chest pain, and visual changes usually are absent. If long-term complications such as rupturing of blood vessels in the eye, glomerular damage, or encephalopathy were present, subjective complaints might be blurring or loss of vision, fatigue, or confusion. Objective data would include a report by the physician on the findings of the chest examination (abnormal heart or lung sounds if secondary HF has developed), an ocular examination (e.g., presence of retinal hemorrhages), and laboratory data on renal function (blood urea nitrogen, creatinine, or creatinine clearance). To place these complications in better perspective, the rate of change should be stated. For example, the serum creatinine has increased from a level of 1 mg/dL 6 months ago to a value of 3 mg/dL today. Vague descriptions such as "eye changes" or "kidney damage" are of little value, because progressive damage to these end organs results from uncontrolled high BP, and disease progression needs to be monitored more precisely.

5. D.L., a 36-year-old construction worker, tripped on a board at the construction site 2 days ago, sustaining an abrasion of his left shin. He presents to the emergency department with pain, redness, and swelling in the area of the injury. He is diagnosed as having cellulitis. What is the primary problem? What subjective and objective data support the problem? What additional subjective and objective data are not provided but usually are needed to define this particular problem?

The primary problem is cellulitis of the left leg. Useful pieces of subjective information are D.L.'s description of how he injured his shin at a construction site and his current complaints of pain, redness, and swelling. The fact that he was at a construction site is indirect evidence of a possible dirty wound. Further information must be obtained about how he cleaned the wound after the injury and whether he has received a booster dose of tetanus toxoid within the past 10 years. Objectively, the wound is on the left shin. No other objective data are given. Additional data to obtain would be to document the intensity of the redness on a one-to-four-plus scale, the size of the inflamed area as described by an area of demarcation, the circumference of his left shin compared with his right shin, the presence or absence of pus and any lymphatic involvement, his temperature, and a white blood cell count with differential.

6. C.S., a 58-year-old woman, has had complaints of fatigue, ankle swelling, and SOB, especially when lying down, for the past week. Physical examination shows distended neck veins, bilateral rales, an S_3 gallop rhythm, and lower extremity edema. A chest radiograph shows an enlarged heart. She is diagnosed as having HF and is being treated with furosemide and digoxin. What is/are the primary problem(s)? What subjective and objective data support the problem(s)? What additional subjective and objective data are not provided but usually are needed to define this (these) particular problem(s)?

The primary problem is systolic HF. Subjectively, C.S. claims to be experiencing fatigue, ankle swelling, and SOB, especially when lying down. She claims to have been taking furosemide and digoxin. An expanded description of these symptoms and her medication use would be helpful. The findings on physical examination and the enlarged heart on chest radiograph are objective data in support of the primary problem of HF. In addition, other objective findings that would help in her assessment would be the pulse rate, BP, serum creatinine, serum potassium concentration, and digoxin blood level and a more thorough description of the rales on lung examination, extent of neck vein distension, and degree of leg edema. Pharmacy records could be screened to determine current dosages and refill patterns of the medications.

In this case, a second primary problem may be present. Current recommendations for the management of HF include use of an angiotensin-converting enzyme (ACE) inhibitor before or concurrent with digoxin therapy. Thus, a possible drug-related problem is the inappropriate choice of drug therapy ("wrong drug"). The patient and/or prescriber should be consulted to ascertain whether an ACE inhibitor has been used previously, if any contraindications exist, or if possible adverse effects were encountered.

Assessment

After the subjective and objective data have been gathered in support of specific listed problems, the practitioner should assess the acuity, severity, and importance of these problems. She should then identify all factors that could be causing or contributing to the problem. The assessment of the severity and acuity is important because the patient expects relief from the symptoms that are of particular concern at this time. During the initial encounter with a patient, it might be discovered that the medical problem is only a symptom complex and that a diagnosis is needed to more accurately identify the problem and further define its severity.

The assessment is usually performed during or immediately following the data gathering while the provider keeps in mind evidence-based practices. For example, if diabetes is assessed and pertinent subjective data (medication history, social history, diet and exercise, etc.) and objective data exist (labs like glycosylated hemoglobin [A_{1c}], low-density lipoprotein cholesterol [LDL-C], BP, etc.), then the assessment of diabetes may be to determine if the patient is meeting the goals for the disease as defined by the ADA. If the patient is not at goal, then the explanation of the reasons why would be described in the assessment, and the plan would then be centered on helping that patient get to goal. Sometimes, the distinction between subjective information provided by the patient and assessments made by the practitioner are confused in the POMR. What the patient reveals belongs in the subjective data, and how the provider interprets it belongs in the assessment. For example, a patient stating that she is having difficulty affording her medications belongs in the subjective information. However, a patient appearing to have difficulty affording her medications belongs in the assessment, as it is the provider's interpretation of what the patient has stated.

Drug Therapy Assessment

A responsibility of the practitioner is to monitor the response of patients to prescribed therapeutic regimens. The purpose of drug therapy monitoring is to identify and solve drug-related problems and to ensure that all therapeutic objectives are being achieved. Unless proven otherwise, the medical diagnosis should be assumed to be correct. On occasion, the diagnosis may not be readily apparent, or a drug-induced problem may have been diagnosed incorrectly as being a disease entity.

Nurses, pharmacists, physicians, physician assistants, and other health care practitioners share the responsibility to assess and monitor patient drug therapy. For the pharmacist, the drug therapy assessment may occur in many practice settings, including the community pharmacy while dispensing or refilling prescriptions or counseling patients, during MTMS encounters, assessing therapy for the hospitalized patient, through medication reconciliation, or as part of routine monthly evaluations of patients residing in long-term care facilities. Many states have enacted legislation allowing pharmacists to develop collaborative drug therapy agreements with physicians for disease state management of common disorders such as asthma, diabetes, dyslipidemia, and hypertension. Additional services commonly provided by pharmacists through collaborative drug therapy agreements include anticoagulation monitoring, emergency contraception, and immunizations.[5] These services often involve more detailed drug therapy assessment and may occur within or outside the traditional pharmacy setting. Regardless, the patient's need (this should be the primary consideration), time constraints, working environment (a determinant of the amount of patient information that is available), and practitioner's skill level governs the extent of monitoring. Similarly, the exact steps used to monitor therapy and the order in which they are executed need to be adapted to a practitioner's personal style. Thus, the examples given in this chapter should be used by the reader as a guide rather than as a recipe in a cookbook.

Plan

After the problem list is generated, subjective and objective data are reviewed, and the severity and acuity of the problems are assessed and prioritized, the next step in the problem-oriented (i.e., SOAP) approach is to create a plan, which at the minimum should consist of a diagnostic plan and a MAP that includes patient education. The plan is the action that was justified in the assessment. The plan is clear and direct and does not require explanation (this should be explained in the assessment). For example, if a patient is experiencing constipation while taking an opioid pain reliever, the plan would be to recommend a stool softener and stimulant laxative such as docusate sodium and bisacodyl. The plan should also include any follow-up that would be necessary related to the action taken.

Patient Education

Educating patients to better understand their medical problem(s) and treatment is an implied goal of all treatment plans. This process is categorized as the development of a patient education plan. The level of teaching has to be tailored to the patient's needs, health literacy, willingness to learn, and general state of health and mind. The patient should be taught the knowledge and skills needed to achieve and evaluate his therapeutic outcome. An important component of the patient education plan emphasizes the need for patients to follow prescribed treatment regimens.

The POMR will allow the provider to focus the interview and encounter independent of the site or service offered. The POMR facilitates documentation of the provision of MTMS across multiple sites and services (across the continuum of care).

The next few sections will discuss how to approach MTMS in various clinical settings.

MEDICATION THERAPY MANAGEMENT SERVICES IN THE COMMUNITY PHARMACY/AMBULATORY SETTING

The core elements of MTMS have been described by the American Pharmacists Association (APhA) and the National Association of Chain Drug Stores.[19] According to these organizations, the core elements of MTMS should include the following components:

1. Medication Therapy Review (MTR)
2. Personal Medication Record (PMR)
3. Medication Action Plan (MAP)
4. Intervention and referral
5. Documentation of services/Billing for services

Medication Therapy Review (MTR)

The MTR may be a comprehensive review in which the provider reviews all of the medications the patient is currently taking, or it may be a focused review of one medication-related issue such as an adverse event. Examples of services provided during the MTR are described in Table 1-6. MTR is dependent on the information that is available from the patient or other data sources. Community pharmacies may be a data-poor environment, and access to necessary information may be limited. In some ambulatory clinics, the provider may have access to the EMR (data-rich environment). Regardless of the setting, a necessary tool to help with the gathering of the medication information is the PMR. This medication record should be updated after any change in medication therapy and should be shared with other health care providers. The patient is responsible for the upkeep of the PMR, but the PMR requires periodic review by the pharmacist or other provider. The goal of this record is to promote self-care and ownership of the medication regimen.[19] The PMR should be used at all levels of care, thereby facilitating the medication reconciliation process required across the continuum of care. An example of a PMR is shown in Figure 1-3.

Table 1-6 Examples of Services Provided During a Medication Therapy Review

- Assess the patient's health status
- Assess cultural issues, health literacy, language barriers, financial status, and insurance coverage or other patient characteristics that may affect the patient's ability to take medications appropriately
- Interview the patient or caregiver to assess, identify, and resolve actual or potential adverse medication events, therapeutic duplications, untreated conditions or diseases, medication adherence issues, and medication cost considerations
- Monitor medication therapy, including response to therapy, safety, and effectiveness
- Monitor, interpret, and assess patient laboratory values, especially as they relate to medication use/misuse
- Provide education and training on the appropriate use of medications
- Communicate appropriate information to other health professionals, including the use and selection of medication therapy

Adapted from reference 19.

Once the patient interview has occurred and the PMR has been updated, the provider may still require information to make an assessment. In such cases, the provider must do his best with the available information, or may obtain missing information such as the medical history or objective data from other providers. Lack of objective information is common in the community pharmacy setting, and the ability to address all problems effectively may be limited in this data-poor environment. In some encounters, obtaining the necessary information may take the entire visit, necessitating a follow-up encounter.

Medication Action Plan (MAP)

If adequate information is available to assess the current problem, a MAP should be developed. Because the MAP is patient centered and is prioritized based on the urgency of need, the provider and the patient should develop it together. An example of a MAP can be seen in Figure 1-4.

The MAP often describes the intervention performed in an MTM encounter and may serve as documentation that can be

Patient: M.C. ALLERGIES: None Type of reaction: N/A		Primary Physician: Dr. Sara Smith (555-3971)				Pharmacist: Mary Doe (555-5551)	Date Prepared: 4/2/08		Date Updated: 5/2/08
Start Date	**Medication (generic)**	**Dosage**	**Route**	**Times per Day**	**Scheduled Times**	**Purpose for Use**	**Remarks**	**Prescriber (Phone)**	**Stop Date**
1/2/08	(lisinopril)	40 mg	By mouth	Once	9 a.m.	High blood pressure		Sara Smith, MD (555-3971)	
1/2/08	(metoprolol)	50 mg	By mouth	Twice	9 a.m. and 9 p.m.	High blood pressure		Sara Smith, MD (555-3971)	
1/2/08	(glipizide)	5 mg	By mouth	Once	9 a.m.	Diabetes	Take 30 minutes prior to breakfast	Sara Smith, MD (555-3971)	
1/2/08	(propoxyphene/ acetaminophen)	100 mg/650 mg	By mouth	Up to four times a day if needed	9 a.m., 2 p.m., 9 p.m., 2 a.m.	Back pain	Take with food. Do not take this medicine with other acetaminophen products (Tylenol®). Do not take this medication unless you have pain.	Sara Smith, MD (555-3971)	
4/2/08	Crestor® (rosuvastatin)	40 mg	By mouth	Once	9 a.m.	Cholesterol		Ted Hart, MD (555-1234)	
Bring this Personal Medication Record with you to all visits with health care providers and if you are admitted to a hospital. Contact your pharmacist regarding questions or updates.									

FIGURE 1-3 Example of a Personal Medication Record (PMR).

My Medication – Related Action Plan	
Patient:	M.C.
Provider (Phone):	Dr. Sara Smith (555-3971)
Pharmacy/Pharmacist (Phone):	RiteMart/Mary Doe, PharmD (555-5551)
Date Prepared:	May 2, 2008

The list below has important Action Steps to help you get the most from your medications. Follow the checklist to help you work with your pharmacist and providers to manage your medications AND make notes of your actions next to each item on your list

Action Steps ⟶ What I need to do...	**Notes ⟶ What I did when I did it...**
☐ **For your muscle weakness and soreness** Stop Crestor® (rosuvastatin) 40 mg. We asked Dr. Hart to change to a lower dose or different agent such as simvastatin. Obtain blood test from Dr. Hart's office. Follow-up with Dr. Hart in 2 days.	
☐ **Medicine Cost** We have asked Dr. Hart to stop Crestor® (rosuvastatin) as it is too expensive. A generic medicine such as simvastatin will costs you less and was recommended to Dr. Hart as an alternative. Continue to ask your pharmacist and doctor if the medications you are taking are covered by your Medicare Part D plan and if there are any alternatives that might be less expensive for you.	
☐ **For Pain** Talk to Dr. Sara Smith about other pain medicines because the Darvocet® (propoxyphene and acetaminophen) may not work as well as other choices. Some choices might include other medicines such as Vicodin® (hydrocodone and acetaminophen), over the counter acetaminophen, or medicines like naproxen or ibuprofen.	

My next appointment with my pharmacist is on: __________ (date) at ______ ☐AM ☐PM

This form is based on forms developed by the American Pharmacist Association and the National Association of Chain Drug Store Foundation. Reproduced with permission from APhA and NACDS Foundation.

FIGURE 1-4 Example of a Medication Action Plan (MAP).

shared with the patient and other health care providers (like the PMR). The primary purpose of the MAP is to make the action plan patient centered and to provide the patient with documentation of what they need to do next in the action plan. It also provides space for the patient to document what they did related to this action and when they did it. In some instances, the MAP may involve referral to another provider (a physician or pharmacist with additional qualifications) if the issue is beyond the scope of the intervening pharmacist. Some reasons for referral may include diabetes education by a certified diabetes educator, diagnosis of a new or suspected medical condition, or laboratory testing that may be beyond the scope of the pharmacist.

Coordination of care is a key element of MTMS and MTR.[2] This may include improving the communication between the patient and other health care providers, enhancing the patient's understanding of his health issues or concerns, maximizing health insurance coverage, advocating on behalf of the patient to get needed medications utilizing available resources and programs, and various other functions that will improve the patient's understanding of their health care environment and promote self-care. Coordination of care may be the primary action taken on behalf of the patient and may be included in the MAP.

Documentation of Services

The development of a documentation process is a necessary component of MTMS.[19] Documentation should be standardized and based on the POMR format. All appropriate records, including the PMR and MAP, should be shared with other providers to promote communication and continuity of care. If the encounter requires follow-up, the documentation should reflect the timing of the follow-up care, and any expectations of the patient and providers should be included. Thorough documentation of the encounter allows all providers to quickly assess the progress of the patient and determine that the desired outcome has been achieved.

Billing for Medication Therapy Management Services

Although billing for MTMS is not universally accepted by all payers, the introduction of the national provider identifier (NPI) and pharmacist-specific current procedural terminology (CPT) codes may soon make this a reality.[5,20] The implementation of Medicare Part D in 2006 allowed pharmacists in pharmacies contracted with prescription drug plans to provide MTMS to plan-identified Medicare recipients. Pharmacists bill these plans through the contracted pharmacy by using their individual NPI and one of three CPT codes. The NPI number designates the provider to be paid, and the CPT determines the amount of payment based on the services rendered. The CPT codes specific to pharmacists providing MTMS include the following:

CPT 99605: Initial face-to-face assessment or intervention by a pharmacist with the patient for 1 to 15 minutes
CPT 99606: Subsequent face-to-face assessment or intervention by a pharmacist with the patient for 1 to 15 minutes
CPT 99607: Each additional 15 minutes spent face-to-face by a pharmacist with the patient; used in addition to 99605 or 99606

Although the NPI number and CPT codes allow pharmacists to bill for MTMS, the reimbursement varies by plan and negotiated contract and is beyond the scope of this text. Pharmacists have also developed patient self-pay reimbursement strategies as well as contracts with self-insured employers and state-run Medicaid programs to provide services.[21,22]

7. M.C. is a 76-year-old female who comes to an appointment at the community pharmacy with her daughter for a focused MTR. She has a Medicare Part D prescription drug plan and is asking for help with her medication costs. She indicates that she has type 2 diabetes, hypertension, back pain, and hyperlipidemia. Her medications include lisinopril 40 mg once daily, metoprolol 50 mg twice daily, glipizide 5 mg once daily, propoxyphene/acetaminophen 100 mg/650 mg one tablet every 6 hours as needed for pain, and rosuvastatin 40 mg once daily. M.C. tells you that she has trouble paying for her rosuvastatin (tier 3, $60 copayment) and would rather have something generic that costs less (tier 1, $5 copayment). Further, she complains of muscle soreness and weakness over the last 3 weeks. What objective information can be obtained in a community pharmacy setting? What is the primary problem? What additional information is necessary to determine the cause of her problem? How would a clinician assess and document her problem(s) in a SOAP format?

Although generally not considered a data-rich environment, increasing amounts of objective information can be gathered during the patient encounter at a community pharmacy. Specifically, information such as weight, BP, temperature, and fingerstick glucose and cholesterol levels can be measured if indicated for this patient. This information may be useful to the community pharmacist when performing the MTR in order to determine if the medications are achieving the desired therapeutic outcomes. Although the patient presented for MTR, the primary complaint is the patient's self-reported muscle weakness and soreness over the last 3 weeks. It is impossible to determine if this problem is a medication-related adverse event, because she did not provide a medication history or PMR. Assuming that M.C. is a patient of this pharmacy, the practitioner could gather the necessary medication history from the PIS. Because the patient is present, this is a good opportunity to develop a PMR with M.C. While developing the PMR with the patient, the practitioner should gather additional information from M.C. about her medication use. For example, the name of one of M.C.'s medicines could be read with the practitioner continuing to ask open-ended questions such as, "How do you take this medication?" "What is your routine for taking your medication?" and "What types of problems, if any, have you had while using this medication?" This process will help to quickly identify any medication discrepancies between the pharmacy computer system and the patient's understanding of medication administration. If discrepancies are noted, the practitioner can clarify them with M.C. right away as part of the intervention. The PMR should also include a section to list medication allergies. The type of reaction should also be included on the PMR so that other providers will know the severity of the medication allergy (i.e., intolerance vs. anaphylactic reaction).

Based on data gathered from the pharmacy computer and M.C., a PMR (depicted in Fig. 1-3) could be developed. Once the PMR has been developed, the provider will have more information to determine if the current problem is medication related. Unfortunately, reviewing the medications alone often does not provide enough information to determine if M.C. is experiencing a medication-related event. Further questioning may be necessary. M.C. should be asked questions such as "How often do you experience muscle weakness and soreness?" "Which muscles are hurting?" "Show me where the problem is," "What do you think is causing the problem?" or "Describe the problem you are experiencing in more detail." Asking questions related to the onset of her symptoms of muscle soreness and weakness will help to determine whether this is a medication-related problem.

Based on this questioning and the PMR, the practitioner can develop an assessment of the current problem that she is experiencing. As indicated on the PMR, M.C. started rosuvastatin most recently. The initiation of this medication corresponds to the onset of her recent soreness and weakness. HMG-coA reductase inhibitors like rosuvastatin are known to cause myositis, or muscle breakdown, which may lead to weakness and muscle soreness. Furthermore, the prescribed dose is high for a female of M.C.'s age. Based on this information, an assessment of the problem can be pursued. If rosuvastatin is the suspected agent, the plan would include actions necessary to solve the problem or to determine if rosuvastatin is the cause of her muscle soreness and weakness. Unfortunately, all of the necessary information is not available (e.g., her baseline cholesterol, serum creatinine, liver function tests, or creatine kinase levels) to develop a formal plan of action to resolve the adverse medication event. However, part of the plan may be to obtain the labs necessary to identify or act on the adverse medication event. An example of the documentation of the SOAP note follows.

PRIMARY PROBLEM:
Muscle soreness and weakness (possible adverse medication event)

SUBJECTIVE:
M.C. reports weakness and soreness, predominantly in her legs over the past 3 weeks. She has difficulty rising from her chair after sitting for long periods and describes the

pain as aching. The patient reports taking her medications as prescribed and rarely misses a dose.

OBJECTIVE:

Total Cholesterol: 137 mg/dL; LDL-C: 56 mg/dL; HDL: 54 mg/dL; Triglycerides: 136 mg/dL

Temperature: 98.5°F

ASSESSMENT:

M.C. has muscle weakness and soreness in her large muscle groups. She is currently at the recommended LDL-C goal level for a person with diabetes and hypertension per NCEP ATP III guidelines (very-high-risk LDL-C goal is <70 mg/dL).[23] Her current lipid therapy is rosuvastatin 40 mg once daily, which was started by her cardiologist 4 weeks ago. The initiation of rosuvastatin 40 mg correlates to the timing of her muscle soreness and weakness. HMG-coA reductase inhibitors (i.e., rosuvastatin) are known to cause myositis/myalgias, and this patient is at particular risk given her age, gender, and starting dose. It is possible that the rosuvastatin could be causing her muscle soreness and weakness. Other lipid-lowering agents could be tried or the dose of rosuvastatin could be reduced, which might eliminate or reduce this adverse event. A creatine kinase level should be obtained to determine the severity of the myositis. A serum creatinine should also be measured, as myositis can lead to renal damage and rhabdomyolisis in severe cases; however, this is usually accompanied by fever and other symptoms that the patient is not currently experiencing.

PLAN:

- Discussed the possibility of an adverse medication event, which included the signs and symptoms of myalgias and myositis.
- Contacted Dr. Hart (M.C.'s cardiologist) to discuss the current problem with rosuvastatin.
- Per discussion with Dr. Hart, will obtain a creatine kinase level and serum creatinine.
- Discontinue rosuvastatin per the pharmacist recommendation. Dr. Hart agreed that M.C. should temporarily stop her rosuvastatin until her laboratory values are reviewed.
- Alternative dosing of rosuvastatin 5 mg or another equivalent agent (atorvastatin 10 mg or simvastatin 20 mg) was discussed with Dr. Hart.
- M.C. is to see Dr. Hart in the cardiology clinic in 2 days to discuss the laboratory values and alternative therapies.
- Discussed the entire plan with M.C., and she verbalized understanding of steps that she is to take with respect to her current medication-induced problem.

8. Based on M.C.'s medication profile, what other problems can be identified with her medication therapy? What can be done to address these issues?

There are three remaining issues that may need to be addressed. The first issue relates to the pain medicine (propoxyphene/acetaminophen) that M.C. is taking. It is well documented that propoxyphene is not an effective opioid pain reliever, and it may lead to increased adverse events in the elderly.[24] Other prescription medications such as hydrocodone/acetaminophen or nonprescription medication such as acetaminophen alone or nonsteroidal anti-inflammatory drugs could be used to help treat M.C.'s pain (see Chapters 8 and 99). Second, it is not clear from the current information if the various providers are communicating. It is the responsibility of the pharmacist to help coordinate care between multiple prescribers as described by the APhA MTMS consensus document.[2] Therefore, it is important to be sure that both providers (Drs. Smith and Hart) receive a copy of the documentation of the issues addressed during the visit (SOAP note).

Table 1-7 Cost Containment Strategies

Patient with Prescription Drug Coverage

- Maximize generic drugs
- Maximize formulary coverage
  - Switch to agents covered on the least expensive formulary tier
- If patient has Medicare Part D, determine eligibility for low-income subsidy through the Social Security Administration
- Consider mail-order prescription programs

Uninsured Patient

- Use low-cost generic programs (e.g., Rx Outreach, Wal-Mart, Target generic programs)
- Switch to therapeutically equivalent lower-cost brand name drugs when generics are unavailable
- Consider tablet splitting, if appropriate
- Consider pharmaceutical industry–sponsored patient assistance programs
- Determine if the patient is eligible for Medicaid, Medicare, Medicare Part D, or other assistance programs

Finally, M.C. came into the pharmacy asking for help with her medication costs. In order to assess this problem, it is important to ask if there are specific cost issues with a particular drug or if it is her overall medication regimen that causes her concern. Another important question to ask is if she has stopped taking any medications or changed the way that she takes her medications due to cost. Many patients will discuss cost and adherence issues with their pharmacist, because the point of sale for medications occurs at the pharmacy. However, they may not discuss this problem with the prescriber. Cost and nonadherence due to cost may be medication-related problems that the pharmacist must communicate to the prescriber on behalf of the patient. In assessing drug cost, there are several steps that can be taken. First, determine the patient's ability to pay for medications; implement low-cost, medically appropriate interventions targeted to patient needs; facilitate enrollment into relevant benefit programs; and confirm medication changes with the patient and prescribers (Table 1-7).

For M.C., the rosuvastatin is her biggest concern, as it costs $60 per month and her Medicare Part D plan lists it as a nonpreferred (tier 3) agent on the formulary. With the possible discontinuation of her rosuvastatin, it is important for the pharmacist to anticipate her need for an alternative lipid-lowering agent and to determine if there are cost-effective formulary alternatives that may be appropriate. This information can then be relayed to the prescriber. Furthermore, the alternative lipid-lowering formulary choice can be integrated into the plan developed for the primary issue of muscle soreness and weakness (see Question 7 above). The integration of multiple problems is a complicated but important aspect of the MAP.

9. What additional information can be provided to M.C. at this time?

As discussed previously, an important part of MTMS involves the MAP. The MAP is a document that may empower the patient and promote self-care. The information on the MAP is important for both the patient and provider and facilitates communication among multiple providers. When a patient presents the PMR and MAP to all providers, complex medication information can be shared across the continuum of care. An example of M.C.'s MAP is included in Figure 1-4.

Because extensive information was communicated to the patient and other providers, follow-up (phone or face-to-face) would be appropriate and necessary to determine the resolution to the medication-related issues identified. Follow-up should occur in a timely manner, likely after M.C. has obtained the necessary labs and has been evaluated by her cardiologist as outlined in the plan. The follow-up should include questions related to the changes that were (or were not) made based on the practitioner recommendations and any new issues that have surfaced. Follow-up should be considered after any encounter in which an action plan is developed in order to determine if the medication-related problem has been resolved. Additionally, problems may be identified and prioritized during the initial visit but, due to time constraints, may not be addressed. A follow-up visit allows for assessment of these problems.

10. Assuming that the pharmacy provider had an NPI number and a contract with M.C.'s Medicare Part D prescription drug plan, how could the 30 minutes spent with M.C. be billed to her insurance?

Provided that M.C. was identified by her Medicare prescription drug plan as eligible for MTMS, the practitioner could bill for the 30-minute encounter. Using the practitioner's NPI number and the appropriate CPT codes, the practitioner could bill for one CPT 99605 (for the first 15 minutes of initial face-to-face MTM encounter) and one CPT 99607 (for an additional 15 minutes spent with the patient in a face-to-face MTM encounter). M.C.'s Medicare Part D plan may require the practitioner to bill the prescription drug plan initially, and then the plan would pay the community pharmacy directly instead of reimbursing the individual pharmacist. Documentation of the visit would need to be stored at the site of the encounter in case any information was requested from M.C.'s prescription drug plan.

MEDICATION THERAPY MANAGEMENT IN THE ACUTE CARE SETTING

11. M.C. has just been hospitalized in a large medical center for renal failure and urosepsis. The pharmacist has access to the medical chart, nursing record, MAR, and a computer that directly links to the clinical laboratory. The pharmacists at this facility assess the patient's drug therapy and routinely provide clinical pharmacokinetic monitoring. How would the pharmacist approach M.C. differently in this inpatient setting compared with the pharmacist in Question 7 who worked in a community pharmacy?

Similar to the outpatient setting, the SOAP format is often used when documenting the encounter of the hospitalized patient; however, obtaining the information needed poses unique challenges. In this setting, subjective information may be more difficult to obtain at the time of assessment in those patients presenting with cognitive impairment resulting from their acute condition, such as the seriously ill or injured. Objective data, on the other hand, is more readily available and retrievable with access to pharmacy, laboratory, and other medical record information. On admission to the health care facility, the medication reconciliation process should be initiated to identify any variances in the admission orders when compared with the patient's home medication list. With acute medical problems superimposed on chronic conditions, it is not unusual to have new medications added and home medications held, changed, or discontinued.

Assessing the appropriateness of drug therapy requires a basic understanding of both pharmacokinetic (e.g., absorption, distribution, metabolism, and elimination of the drug) and pharmacodynamic (e.g., the relief of pain with an analgesic or reduction of BP with an antihypertensive agent) principles. This detailed assessment and monitoring is dependent on the availability of robust patient and laboratory data. The inpatient setting is a relatively data-rich environment where access to needed information is generally readily available. Knowledge of the patient's height, body weight, and hepatic and renal functions are essential for proper dosage considerations. The type of hospitalized patient will vary from the short-stay, otherwise healthy elective surgery patient to the critically ill, hemodynamically compromised patient. The pharmacist must be intimately aware of how pharmacokinetics and pharmacodynamics can be markedly altered throughout the hospitalization or disease-state process in each patient evaluated. This heightened awareness will allow for timely interventions and minimize medication errors resulting from improper or delayed dosage adjustments as the clinical status of the patient changes. Drug level monitoring may be suitable for certain medications and are of great clinical value; nevertheless, it is important to take into consideration clinical response to drug therapy along with the assessment of a specific laboratory value. Accurate interpretation of any drug level requires review of the nursing MAR (or eMAR), evaluating time of drug administration to that of serum sample acquisition. When serum drug levels are obtained, they must be reviewed for validity before alterations in medication regimens are made. If a serum drug concentration seems unusually high or low, the clinician must consider all of the various factors that might influence the serum concentration of the drug in that particular patient. When the reason for an unexpected abnormal serum drug concentration is not apparent, the test should be repeated before considering a dose change that may cause supra- or subtherapeutic concentrations resulting from erroneous data.

When M.C. was seen in the community pharmacy, the pharmacist assessed her chronic conditions (diabetes, hypertension, and hyperlipidemia and her cost issues), and her drug therapy. Monitoring in the community pharmacy–based MTM program will occur at regular time intervals and is less sensitive to the day-to-day changes of the patient. However, in the inpatient setting, M.C. has acute conditions (renal failure and urosepsis) superimposed on her chronic conditions. Monitoring of medication therapy will occur frequently, resulting in a dynamic treatment plan for her acute and chronic conditions.

Although the inpatient setting is relatively data rich, the information gathered and the assessment and plan formulated in the facility must be communicated to other providers once the patient is discharged. At a minimum, communication of the patient's new medication therapy regimen (or PMR) should be communicated to the patient's primary care physician and pharmacist. This step in the process (medication reconciliation) is important to ensure appropriate medication use across the continuum of care.

CONCLUSION

Interventions in any setting require interdisciplinary communication, assessment of patient-specific needs, and documentation of the visit. The health care system is complicated, and it is often difficult for the patient to effectively navigate. Consistency and follow through are important to both patients and other providers regardless of MTMS setting. As illustrated in Figure 1-1, communication to the patient, documentation by using the SOAP note and the MAP, and follow-up are all closely correlated. To develop a successful action plan, information must be gathered in an organized and concise fashion. This information, if properly documented and shared with other providers, will help in the provision of care to the patients served within the health care system.

ACKNOWLEDGMENT

The authors acknowledge Mary Anne Koda-Kimble, Wayne Kradjan, Robin Corelli, Lloyd Young, B. Joseph Guglielmo. and Brian Alldredge for their contributions to previous editions of this chapter.

REFERENCES

1. Medicare Prescription Drug, Improvement, and Modernization Act of 2003 (MMA). Cost and Utilization Management; Quality Assurance; Medication Therapy Management Program. Public Law 108–173. Section 101, Subpart 2, Sec. 1860-D49(c). Enacted December 8, 2003.
2. Bluml BM. Definition of medication therapy management: development of profession wide consensus. *J Am Pharm Assoc* 2005;45:566.
3. Hepler CD, Strand LM.Opportunities and responsibilities in pharmaceutical care. *Am J Hosp Pharm* 1990;47:533.
4. Rovers JP, Currie JD eds. *A Practical Guide to Pharmaceutical Care: A Clinical Skills Primer*, Washington, DC: American Pharmacists Association; 2007.
5. Isetts BJ, Buffington DE. CPT code-change proposal: national data on pharmacists medication therapy management services. *J Am Pharm Assoc* 2007;47:491.
6. World Health Organization. Health Education in Self-care: Possibilities and Limitations. Geneva, Switzerland; 1983.
7. Hospitals National Patient Safety Goals. Joint Commission on Accreditation of Healthcare Organizations. Available at: http://www.jointcommission.org. Accessed June 1, 2008.
8. Cipolle RJ et al., eds. *Pharmaceutical Care Practice: The Clinician's Guide*. New York: McGraw-Hill; 2004.
9. U.S. Department of Health and Human Services (HHS), Office of Minority Health. National Standards for Culturally and Linguistically Appropriate Services in Health Care. Final Report. Washington, DC; March 2001. Available at: http://www.omhrc.gov/clas/. Accessed June 1, 2008.
10. U.S. Department of Health and Human Services (HHS), Healthy People 2010. *National Health Promotion and Disease Prevention Objectives. Conference Ed. in Two Vols*. Washington, DC; January 2000.
11. Henry J. Kaiser Family Foundation (KFF). A synthesis of the literature: racial and ethnic differences in access to medical care; October 1999.
12. Goldberg J et al. Understanding Health Disparities. Health Policy Institute of Ohio; November 2004:6.
13. Nielson-Bohlman L, Panzer A, Kindig DA, eds, *Health Literacy: A Prescription to End Confusion*. Washington, DC: National Academy Press; 2004.
14. Nester TM, Hale LS. Effectiveness of a pharmacist-acquired medication history in promoting patient safety. *Am J Health Syst Pharm* 2002;59:2221.
15. Varkey P et al. Multidisciplinary approach to inpatient medication reconciliation in an academic setting. *Am J Health Syst Pharm* 2007;64:850.
16. Forster AJ et al. The incidence and severity of adverse events affecting patients after discharge from the hospital. *Ann Intern Med* 2003;138:1617.
17. Beers MH et al. The accuracy of medication histories in the hospital medical records of elderly persons. *J Am Geriatr Soc* 1990;38:1183.
18. Hanlon JT et al. Adverse drug events in high risk older outpatients. *J Am Geriatr Soc* 1997;45:945.
19. American Pharmacists Association and National Association of Chain Drug Stores Foundation. Medication therapy management in pharmacy practice: core elements of an MTM service model. Version 2.0. *J Am Pharm Assoc* 2008;48:341.
20. HIPAA Administrative Simplification: Standard Unique Identifier for Health Care Providers; Final Rule. Federal Register. Department of Health and Human Services. 45 CFR Part 162; July 23, 2004.
21. Cranor CW et al. The Asheville Project: long-term clinical and economic outcomes of community pharmacy diabetes care program. *J Am Pharm Assoc* 2003;43:173.
22. Chrischilles EA et al. Evaluation of the Iowa Medicaid pharmaceutical case management program. *J Am Pharm Assoc* 2004;44:337.
23. Grundy SM et al. Implications of recent trials for the National Cholesterol Education Program Adult Treatment Panel III guidelines. *Circulation* 2004;110:227.
24. Fick DM et al. Updating the Beers criteria for potentially inappropriate medication use in older adults. *Arch Intern Med* 2003;163:2716.

CHAPTER 2

Interpretation of Clinical Laboratory Tests

Catrina R. Schwartz and Mark W. Garrison

This chapter provides the reader with an overview of laboratory tests commonly used in clinical medicine. Specialized laboratory tests, which are used to monitor specific disease states or specific drug therapies, are integrated into the case histories, questions, and answers in the disease-specific chapters of this book. Over-the-counter, or patient-directed laboratory tests, are briefly presented at the end of this chapter because these are being used to a greater extent. The most recent edition of a comprehensive laboratory textbook should be reviewed when comprehensive understanding of clinical laboratory tests is required.[1]

GENERAL PRINCIPLES

Generally, laboratory tests should be ordered only if the results of the test will affect decisions about the care of the patient. The serum, urine, and other bodily fluids can be analyzed routinely; however, the economic cost of obtaining these data must always be balanced by benefits to patient outcomes.

Normal Values

Clinical laboratory test results that appear within a predetermined range of values are referred to as "normal," and those outside this range are typically referred to as "abnormal." Laboratory findings, both normal and abnormal, can be helpful in assessing clinical disorders, establishing a diagnosis, assessing drug therapy, or evaluating disease progression. In addition, baseline laboratory tests are often necessary to evaluate disease progression and response to therapy or to monitor the development of toxicities associated with therapy.

Clinical laboratories can analyze sample specimens by different laboratory methods; therefore, each laboratory has its own set of normal values. Consequently, clinicians should rely on normal values listed by their own clinical laboratory facility when interpreting laboratory tests.

Laboratory Error

A variety of factors can interfere with the accuracy of laboratory tests. Patient-related factors (e.g., age, gender, weight, height, time since last meal) can affect the range of normal values for a given test. Laboratory-based issues can also influence the accuracy of laboratory values. For example, a specimen can be spoiled because of improper handling or processing (e.g., hyperkalemia due to hydrolysis of a blood specimen); because it was taken at a wrong time (e.g., fasting blood glucose level taken shortly after a meal); because collection was incomplete (e.g., 24-hour urine collection that does not span a full 24-hour period); Errors also can arise due to faulty or poor quality reagents (e.g., improperly prepared, outdated); due to technical errors (e.g., human error in reading result, computer-keying error); due to interference from medical procedures (e.g., cardioconversion increases creatine kinase [CK] serum concentrations); due to dietary effects (e.g., rare meat ingestion can cause a false-positive guaiac test); and because medications can interfere either with the testing procedure or by their pharmacologic effects (e.g., thiazides can increase the serum uric acid concentration, β-agonists can reduce serum potassium concentrations). Clinicians might not be aware of when laboratory-related issues arise. As a result, laboratory findings must always be interpreted carefully, and the validity of a test result questioned when it does not seem to correlate with a patient's clinical status.

Units of Measure

The International System of Units (SI) reports clinical laboratory values using the metric system. For example, the basic unit of mass for the SI system, the *mole* is not influenced by the added weight of salt or ester formulations. The mole, therefore, is technically and pharmacologically more meaningful than the gram because each physiological reaction occurs on a molecular level. Nevertheless, efforts to implement the SI system internationally for laboratory test reports have been resisted in the United States. Despite adopting SI transition policies in the late 1980s,[2,3] major American medical journals have since reverted back to the traditional units for laboratory test reporting. The "normal" values for common blood chemistry tests are presented in both conventional units and SI units, along with "conversion factors" to interchange traditional and SI units in Tables 2-1 (blood chemistry reference values) and 2-2 (hematologic laboratory tests). Formulas for converting conventional units to SI units are also available in the primary literature.[4,5]

ELECTROLYTES AND BLOOD CHEMISTRIES

Sodium

Normal: 135–145 mEq/L or mmol/L

Sodium is the predominant cation of extracellular fluid (ECF). Only a small amount of sodium (~5 mEq/L) is in intracellular fluid (ICF). Along with chloride, potassium, and water, sodium is important in establishing serum osmolarity and osmotic pressure relationships between ICF and ECF. Dietary intake of sodium is balanced by renal excretion of sodium, which is regulated by aldosterone (enhances sodium reabsorption), natriuretic hormone (increases excretion of sodium), and antidiuretic hormone (enhances reabsorption of free water). An increase in the serum sodium concentration could suggest either impaired sodium excretion or volume contraction. Conversely, a decrease in the serum sodium concentration to less-than-normal values could reflect hypervolemia, abnormal sodium losses, or sodium starvation. Although healthy individuals are able to maintain sodium homeostasis without difficulty, patients with kidney failure, heart failure, or pulmonary disease often encounter sodium and water imbalance. In adults, changes in serum sodium concentrations most often represent water imbalances rather than sodium imbalances. Hence, serum sodium concentrations are more reflective of a patient's fluid status rather than sodium balance.

Hyponatremia

Hyponatremia can result from dilution of the sodium concentration in serum or from a total body depletion of sodium. The finding of hyponatremia implies that sodium has been diluted throughout all body fluids because water moves freely across cell membranes in response to oncotic pressures. Dilutional hyponatremia occurs when the ECF compartment expands without an equivalent increase in sodium. Some clinical conditions (e.g., cirrhosis, congestive heart failure, renal impairment), as well as the administration of osmotically active solutes (e.g., albumin, mannitol), are commonly associated with dilutional hyponatremia. Hyponatremia that results from sodium depletion presents as a low serum sodium concentration in the absence of edema. Sodium-depletion hyponatremia can be caused by mineralocorticoid deficiencies, sodium-wasting renal disease, or replacement of sodium-containing fluid losses with nonsaline solutions.

Hypernatremia

Hypernatremia represents a state of relative water deficiency and, therefore, excessive concentrations of sodium in all body fluids (hypertonicity). Hypernatremia can be caused by the loss of free water, loss of hypotonic fluid, or excessive sodium intake. Free water loss is uncommon, except in the presence of diabetes insipidus. Gastroenteritis is the most common cause of hypotonic fluid loss in infants and the elderly. Increased retention of sodium in patients with hyperaldosteronism can also increase serum sodium concentrations. Excessive salt intoxication is usually accidental or iatrogenic and most commonly results from inappropriate intravenous administration of hypertonic salt solutions. Some β-lactam antibiotics (e.g., ticarcillin) contain a modest sodium load and can cause fluid overload when high dosages are administered.

The primary defense against hypertonicity is thirst and subsequent fluid intake. Hypernatremic syndromes, therefore, usually occur in patients who are unable to drink sufficient fluids. For example, infants who cannot demand fluid are at greatest risk for the development of hypernatremia. Similarly, patients, who are vomiting, comatose, or not allowed oral fluids are at risk for hypernatremia.

1. M.C., a 61-year-old woman with no known drug allergies (NKDA) is hospitalized with a chief complaint of increasing shortness of breath (SOB) and orthopnea over the past week. She has been treated previously for heart failure and has not taken any

Table 2-1 Blood Chemistry Reference Values

Laboratory Test	Normal Reference Values: Conventional Units	SI Units	Conversion Factor	Comments
Electrolytes				
Sodium	135–145 mEq/L	135–145 mmol/L	1	Low sodium is usually due to excess water (e.g., ↑ serum antidiuretic hormone) and is treated with water restriction. ↑ in severe dehydration, diabetes insipidus, significant renal and GI losses.
Potassium	3.5–5 mEq/L	3.5–5 mmol/L	1	↑ with renal dysfunction, acidosis, K-sparing diuretics, hemolysis, burns, crush injuries. ↓ by diuretics, alkalosis, severe vomiting and diarrhea, heavy NG suctioning.
CO_2 content	22–28 mEq/L	22–28 mmol/L	1	Sum of HCO_3 and dissolved CO_2. Reflects acid–base balance and compensatory pulmonary (CO_2) and renal (HCO_3) mechanisms. Primarily reflects HCO_3.
Chloride	95–105 mEq/L	95–105 mmol/L	1	Important for acid–base balance. ↓ by GI loss of chloride-rich fluid (vomiting, diarrhea, GI suction, intestinal fistulas, overdiuresis).
BUN	8–18 mg/dL	2.8–6.4 mmol/L	0.357	End product of protein metabolism, produced by liver, transported in blood, excreted renally. ↑ in renal dysfunction, high protein intake, upper GI bleeding, volume contraction.
Creatinine	0.6–1.2 mg/dL	50–110 μmol/L	88.4	Major constituent of muscle; rate of formation constant; affected by muscle mass (lower with aging); excreted renally. ↑ in renal dysfunction. Used as a primary marker for renal function (GFR).
CrCl	75–125 mL/min	1.25–2.08 mL/sec	0.01667	Reflects GFR; ↓ in renal dysfunction. Used to adjust dosage of renally eliminated drugs.
Glucose (fasting)	70–110 mg/dL	3.9–6.1 mmol/L	0.05551	↑ in diabetes or by adrenal corticosteroids. Important to obtain fasting glucose level.
Glycosylated hemoglobin	<5%	<5%	1	Used to assess average blood glucose over 1–3 months. Helpful for monitoring chronic blood glucose control in patients with diabetes. Values >8% seen in patients with poor glucose control.
Calcium–total	8.8–10.2 mg/dL	2.20–2.55 mmol/L	0.250	Regulated by body skeleton redistribution, parathyroid hormone, vitamin D, calcitonin. Affected by changes in albumin concentration. ↓ by hypothyroidism, loop diuretics, vitamin D deficiency; ↑ in malignancy and hyperthyroidism.
Calcium–unbound	4.5–5.6 mg/dL	1.13–1.4 mmol/L	0.250	Physiologically active form. Unbound "free" calcium remains unchanged as albumin fluctuates. Total calcium ↓ when albumin ↓.
Magnesium	1.6–2.4 mEq/L	0.8–1.20 mmol/L	0.5 1	↓ in malabsorption, severe diarrhea, alcoholism, pancreatitis, diuretics, hyperaldosteronism (symptoms of weakness, depression, agitation, seizures, hypokalemia, arrhythmias). ↑ in renal failure, hypothyroidism, magnesium-containing antacids.
Phosphate[a]	2.5–5 mg/dL	0.8–1.60 mmol/L	0.323	↑ with renal dysfunction, hypervitaminosis D, hypocalcemia, hypoparathyroidism. ↓ with excess aluminum antacids, malabsorption, renal losses, hypercalcemia, refeeding syndrome.
Uric acid	2–7 mg/dL	0.12–0.42 mmol/L	0.06	↑ in gout, neoplastic, or myeloproliferative disorders, and drugs (diuretics, niacin, low-dose salicylate, cyclosporine).
Proteins				
Prealbumin	15–36 mg/dL	150–360 mg/L	10	Indicates acute changes in nutritional status, useful for monitoring TPN.
Albumin	4–6 g/dL	40–60 g/L	10	Produced in liver; important for intravascular osmotic pressure. ↓ in liver disease, malnutrition, ascites, hemorrhage, protein-wasting nephropathy. May influence highly protein-bound drugs.
Globulin	2.3–3.5 g/dL	23–35 g/L	10	Active role in immunologic mechanisms. Immunoglobulins ↑ in chronic infection, rheumatoid arthritis, multiple myeloma.
Enzymes				
CK	0–150 units/L	0–2.5 μkat/L	0.01667	In tissues that use high energy (skeletal muscle, myocardium, brain). ↑ by IM injections, MI, acute psychotic episodes. Isoenzyme CK-MM in skeletal muscle; CK-MB in myocardium; CK-BB in brain. MB fraction >5%–6% suggests acute MI.
CK-MB	0–12 units/L	0–0.2 μkat/L	0.01667	
cTnI	<0.03 ng/mL	<0.03 μg/L	1	More specific than CK-MB for myocardial damage, elevated sooner and remains elevated longer than CK-MB. cTnI >2.0 suggests acute myocardial injury.

(continued)

Table 2-1 Blood Chemistry Reference Values *(Continued)*

Laboratory Test	*Normal Reference Values* Conventional Units	*Normal Reference Values* SI Units	*Conversion Factor*	*Comments*
Enzymes (*continued*)				
Myoglobin	<90 μg/L	<90 mcg/L	1	Early elevation (within 3 hr), but less specific for myocardial compared to CK-MB.
Homocysteine	4–15 μmol/L	4–15 μmol/L	1	Damages vessel endothelial, which may increase the risk for cardiac disease. Associated with deficiencies in folate, vitamin B_6, and vitamin B_{12}.
LDH	100–190 units/L	1.67–3.17 μkat/L	0.01667	High in heart, kidney, liver, and skeletal muscle. Five isoenzymes: LD1 and LD2 mostly in heart, LD5 mostly in liver and skeletal muscle, LD3 and LD4 are non-specific. ↑ in malignancy, extensive burns, PE, renal disease.
BNP	<100 pg/mL	<100 ng/L	1	BNP >500 ng/L indicates left ventricular dysfunction. Released from heart with ↑ workload placed on heart (e.g., CHF).
CRP	0–1 mg/dL	0–10 mg/L	10	Nonspecific indicator of acute inflammation. Similar to ESR, but more rapid onset and greater elevation. CRP >3 mg/dL increases risk of cardiovascular disease.
Liver Function				
AST	0–35 units/L	0–0.58 μkat/L	0.01667	Large amounts in heart and liver; moderate amounts in muscle, kidney, and pancreas. ↑ with MI and liver injury. Less liver specific than ALT.
ALT	0–35 units/L	0–0.58 μkat/L	0.01667	From heart, liver, muscle, kidney, pancreas. ↑ negligible unless parenchymal liver disease. More liver specific than AST.
ALP	30–120 units/L	0.5–2.0 μkat/L	0.01667	Large amounts in bile ducts, placenta, bone. ↑ in bile duct obstruction, obstructive liver disease, rapid bone growth (e.g., Paget disease), pregnancy.
GGT	0–70 units/L	0–1.17 μkat/L	0.01667	Sensitive test reflecting hepatocellular injury; not helpful in differentiating liver disorders. Usually high in chronic alcoholics.
Bilirubin–total	0.1–1 mg/dL	1.7–17.1 μmol/L	17.1	Breakdown product of hemoglobin, bound to albumin, conjugated in liver. Total bilirubin includes direct (conjugated) and indirect bilirubin. ↑ with hemolysis, cholestasis, liver injury.
Bilirubin–direct	0–0.2 mg/dL	0–3.4 μmol/L	17.1	
Miscellaneous				
Amylase	35–120 units/L	0.58–2.0 μkat/L	0.01667	Pancreatic enzyme; ↑ in pancreatitis or duct obstruction.
Lipase	0–160 units/L	0–2.67 μkat/L	0.01667	Pancreatic enzyme, ↑ acute pancreatitis, elevated for longer period than amylase.
PSA	0–4 ng/mL	0–4 mcg/L	1	↑ in benign prostatic hypertrophy (BPH) and also in prostate cancer. PSA levels of 4–10 ng/mL should be worked up. Risk of prostate cancer increased if free PSA/total PSA <0.25.
TSH	2–10 μunits/mL	2–10 m units/L	1	↑ TSH in primary hypothyroidism requires exogenous thyroid supplementation.
Cholesterol				
Total	<200 mg/dL	<5.2 mmol/L	0.02586	Desirable = Total <200; LDL 70–160 (depends on risk factors); HDL >45 mg/dL; ↑ LDL or ↓ HDL are risk factors for cardiovascular disease. Consult NCEP and ATP guidelines for most current target goals and description of patient risk factors.
LDL	70–160 mg/dL	<3.36 mmol/L	0.02586	
HDL	>45 mg/dL	>1.16 mmol/L	0.02586	
Triglycerides (fasting)	<160 mg/dL	<1.80 mmol/L	0.0113	↑ by alcohol, saturated fats, drugs (propranolol, diuretics, oral contraceptives). Obtain fasting level.

[a] Phosphate as inorganic phosphorus.

ALP, alkaline phosphatase; ALT, alanine aminotransferase; AST, aspartate aminotransferase; ATP, Adult Treatment Panel; BNP, brain natriuretic peptide; BPH, benign prostatic hypertrophy; BUN, blood urea nitrogen; CHF; congestive heart failure; CK, creatine kinase (formerly known as creatine phosphokinase); CrCl, creatinine clearance; CRP, C-reactive protein; cTnI, cardiac troponin I; ESR, erythrocyte sedimentation rate; GFR, glomerular filtration rate; GGT, gamma-glutamyl transferase; GI, gastrointestinal; HDL, high-density lipoprotein; IM, intramuscularly; LDH, lactate dehydrogenase; LDL, low-density lipoprotein; MI, myocardial infarction; NCEP, National Cholesterol Education Program; NG, nasogastric; PE, pulmonary embolism; PSA, prostate-specific antigen; SI, International System of Units; TPN, total parenteral nutrition; TSH, thyroid-stimulating hormone.

Table 2-2 Hematologic Laboratory Values

Laboratory Test	Normal Reference Values: Conventional Units	Normal Reference Values: SI Units	Comments
RBC count			
• Male	4.3–5.9 × 10^6/mm^3	4.3–5.9 × 10^{12}/L	
• Female	3.5–5.0 × 10^6/mm^3	3.5–5.0 × 10^{12}/L	
Hct			↓ with anemias, bleeding, hemolysis. ↑ with polycythemia, chronic hypoxia.
• Male	39%–49%	0.39–0.49 1[a]	
• Female	33%–43%	0.33–0.43 1[a]	
Hgb			Similar to Hct.
• Male	14–18 g/dL	140–180 g/L	
• Female	12–16 g/dL	120–160 g/L	
MCV	76–100 μm^3	76–100 fL[b]	Describes average RBC size; ↑ MCV = macrocytic, ↓ MCV = microcytic.
MCH	27–33 pg	27–33 pg	Measures average weight of Hgb in RBC.
MCHC	33–37 g/dL	330–370 g/L	More reliable index of RBC hemoglobin than MCH. Measures average concentration of Hgb in RBC. Concentration will not change with weight or size of RBC.
Reticulocyte count (adults)	0.1%–2.4%	0.001–0.024 1[a]	Indicator of RBC production; ↑ suggests ↑ number of immature erythrocytes released in response to stimulus (e.g., iron in iron-deficiency anemia).
ESR			Nonspecific; ↑ with inflammation, infection, neoplasms, connective tissue disorders, pregnancy, nephritis. Useful monitor of temporal arteritis and polymyalgia rheumatica.
• Male	0–20 mm/hr	0–20 mm/hr	
• Female	0–30 mm/hr	0–30 mm/hr	
WBC count	3.2–9.8 × 10^3/mm^3	3.2–9.8 × 10^9/L	Consists of neutrophils, lymphocytes, monocytes, eosinophils, and basophils; ↑ in infection and stress.
ANC	>2,000 mm^3		ANC = WBC × (% neutrophils +% bands)/100; if <500 ↑ risk infection, if >1,000 ↓ risk infection.
Neutrophils	54%–62%	0.54–0.62 1[a]	↑ in neutrophils suggests bacterial or fungal infection. ↑ in bands suggests bacterial infection.
Bands	3%–5%	0.03–0.05 1[a]	
Lymphocytes	25%–33%	0.25–0.33 1[a]	
Monocytes	3%–7%	0.03–0.07 1[a]	
Eosinophils	1%–3%	0.01–0.03 1[a]	Eosinophils ↑ with allergies and parasitic infections.
Basophils	<1%	<0.01 1[a]	
Platelets	130–400 × 10^3/mm^3	130–140 × 10^9/L	<100 × 10^3/mm^3 = thrombocytopenia; <20 × 10^3/mm^3 = ↑ risk for severe bleeding.
Iron			
• Male	80–180 mcg/dL	14–32 μmol/L	Body stores two-thirds in Hgb; one-third in bone marrow, spleen, liver; only small amount present in plasma. Blood loss major cause of deficiency.
• Female	60–160 mcg/dL	11–29 μmol/L	↑ needs in pregnancy and lactation.
• TIBC	250–460 mcg/dL	45–82 μmol/L	↑ capacity to bind iron with iron deficiency.

[a] With the SI, the concept of number fraction replaces percentage. Thus, for mass fraction, volume fraction, and relative quantities, the unit "1" is used to replace former units.
[b] fL, femtoliter; femto, 10^{-15}; pico, 10^{-12}; nano, 10^{-9}; micro, 10^{-6}; milli, 10^{-3}.
ANC, absolute neutrophil count; ESR, erythrocyte sedimentation rate; Hct, hematocrit; Hgb, hemoglobin; MCH, mean corpuscular hemoglobin; MCHC, mean cell hemoglobin concentration; MCV, mean cell volume; RBC, red blood cell; SI, International System of Units; TIBC, total iron-binding capacity; WBC, white blood cell.

medication over the past 2 weeks. M.C. has severe (4+) pedal edema and is in respiratory distress. Laboratory tests were ordered and reported back as follows: sodium (Na), 123 mEq/L (normal, 135–145); potassium (K), 4.1 mEq/L (normal, 3.5–5.0); chloride (Cl), 90 mEq/L (normal, 95–105); carbon dioxide (CO_2), 28 mEq/L (normal, 22 to 28); blood urea nitrogen (BUN), 30 mg/dL (normal, 8–18); serum creatinine (SCr), 1.3 mg/dL (normal, 0.6–1.2); and fasting glucose, 100 mg/dL (normal, 70–110). Why should M.C. not be given sodium chloride to return her serum sodium concentration to a normal value?

[SI units: Na, 123 mmol/L; K, 4.1 mmol/L; Cl, 90 mmol/L; CO_2, 28 mmol/L; BUN, 10.7 mmol/L; SCr, 115 μmol/L; glucose, 5.5 mmol/L]

All body fluids are in osmotic equilibrium, and changes in serum sodium concentration are associated with shifts of water into and out of cells. M.C. has 4+ pedal edema and heart failure; her serum concentration of sodium is probably low because her plasma volume is increased relative to sodium. The serum sodium concentration in this case does not reflect total body sodium content. The usual treatment for this type of hyponatremia is salt and water restriction combined with diuresis in an attempt to remove the excess fluid associated with M.C.'s heart failure (see Chapters 11 and 18).

Potassium

Normal: 3.5–5.0 mEq/L or mmol/L

Sodium is the major cation in the ECF, and potassium is the major intracellular cation in the body. The potassium ion in the ECF is filtered freely at the glomerulus of the kidney, reabsorbed in the proximal tubule, and secreted into the distal segments of the nephron. Because the majority of potassium is sequestered within cells, a serum potassium concentration is not a good measure of total body potassium. Intracellular potassium, however, cannot be measured easily. Fortunately, the clinical manifestations of potassium deficiency (e.g., fatigue, drowsiness, dizziness, confusion, electrocardiographic changes, muscle weakness, muscle pain) correlate well with serum concentrations. The serum potassium concentration is buffered and can be within normal limits despite abnormalities in total body potassium. During potassium depletion, potassium moves from the ICF into the ECF to maintain the serum concentration. When the serum concentration decreases by a mere 0.3 mEq/L, the total body potassium deficit is approximately 100 mEq. Serum potassium concentrations, therefore, can be misleading when interpreted in isolation from other considerations, and assumptions should not be made as to the status of total body potassium concentration based solely on a serum concentration measurement.

Hypokalemia

The kidneys are responsible for about 90% of daily potassium loss (~40–90 mEq/day), and the remaining 10% of potassium excretion each day is managed by the gastrointestinal (GI) system and the dermatologic system (i.e., sweating). The kidneys, however, only have a limited ability to conserve potassium. Even when potassium intake has ceased, the urine will contain at least 5 to 20 mEq of potassium per 24 hours. Therefore, prolonged intravenous therapy with potassium-free solutions in a patient unable to obtain potassium in foods (e.g., nothing by mouth [NPO] patient) can result in hypokalemia. Hypokalemia can also be induced by osmotic diuresis (e.g., mannitol, glucosuria), thiazide or loop diuretics, excessive mineralocorticoid activity, or protracted vomiting. Although the fluid secreted along most of the upper GI tract contains only modest amount of potassium (i.e., 5–20 mEq/L), vomiting can induce hypokalemia because of the combined effect from decreased food intake, loss of acid, alkalosis, and loss of sodium. The loss of large amounts of colonic fluid through severe diarrhea can cause potassium depletion because fluid in the colon is high in potassium content (i.e., 30–40 mEq/L). Insulin and stimulation of β_2-adrenergic receptors can also induce hypokalemia because both increase the movement of potassium into cells from the extracellular fluid.

Hyperkalemia

Hyperkalemia most commonly results from decreased renal excretion of potassium, excessive exogenous potassium administration (especially when combined with a potassium-sparing diuretic), or excessive cellular breakdown (e.g., hemolysis, burns, crush injuries, surgery, infections). Metabolic acidosis also can induce hyperkalemia as hydrogen ions move into cells in exchange for potassium and sodium. Abnormal potassium concentrations in the serum primarily affect excitability of nerve and muscle tissue (e.g., myocardial tissue). As a result, arrhythmias can be induced by hyperkalemia or hypokalemia. Potassium also affects some enzyme systems, acid–base balance, as well as carbohydrate and protein metabolism.

2. J.S., a 17-year-old female (NKDA) with type 1 diabetes mellitus, is hospitalized for ketoacidosis. Her fasting blood glucose was 802 mg/dL normal, 70–110), her urine output was 140 mL/hour (normal, 50), and her urine was positive (4+) for glucose and ketones. J.S.'s blood pH was 7.1 (normal, 7.4), and her serum potassium concentration was 4.1 mEq/L (normal, 3.5–5.0). Although J.S.'s serum potassium concentration is normal, why is her serum potassium of concern?

[SI units: glucose, 44.5 mmol/L (normal, 3.9–6.1); K, 4.1 mmol/L]

Treatment of J.S.'s diabetic ketoacidosis without supplemental potassium could result in significant hypokalemia. When the pH of the blood is acidic, potassium shifts out of cells in response to increased concentrations of intracellular hydrogen ion. J.S.'s total-body potassium concentration is decreased as a result of both glycosuria and polyuria. Her serum potassium concentration, however, appears "normal" because acidosis has shifted potassium from intracellular storage sites into the circulating plasma volume. When her acidosis and hyperglycemia are treated, potassium ions will return intracellularly. If supplemental potassium is not provided, the serum potassium concentration will decrease dramatically. As a very general guideline, for every 0.1 decrease in pH from 7.4, the serum potassium concentration will be falsely elevated by about 0.6 mEq/L. Understanding J.S.'s pH is 7.1, her serum potassium concentration (4.1 mEq/L) will actually be closer to 2.3 mEq/L (i.e., 0.6 mEq/L × three 0.1 units = 1.8 mEq/L) when the acidosis is corrected.

Carbon Dioxide Content

Normal: 22–28 mEq/L or mmol/L

The CO_2 content in the serum represents the sum of the bicarbonate concentration (HCO_3) and the concentration of dissolved CO_2 in the serum. The dissolved CO_2 represents a relatively small component of total CO_2 content, making CO_2 essentially a measure of the bicarbonate concentration in serum. Chloride and bicarbonate are the primary negatively charged anions that offset the positively charged cations (i.e., sodium, potassium).

Although several buffer systems (e.g., hemoglobin [Hgb], phosphate, protein) participate in regulating pH within physiological limits, the carbonic acid-bicarbonate system is the most important. From a clinical standpoint, most disturbances of acid–base balance result from imbalances of the carbonic acid-bicarbonate system. The importance of bicarbonate in maintaining physiological pH is presented in Chapter 10.

Chloride

Normal: 95–105 mEq/L or mmol/L

Chloride is the principal inorganic anion of the ECF; changes in chloride concentration are usually related to sodium concentration in an effort to maintain a neutral charge. The serum chloride concentration per se has no real diagnostic significance. In fact, the only real reason for measuring the serum chloride is to validate the serum sodium concentration. The relationship between serum concentrations of sodium, bicarbonate, and chloride is described by Equation 2-1, where *R* represents the anion gap:

$$Cl^- + HCO_3^- + R = Na^+ \qquad \textbf{2-1}$$

As with bicarbonate, chloride contributes to maintaining acid–base balance. A decreased serum chloride concentration often accompanies metabolic alkalosis, whereas an increased serum chloride concentration may be indicative of a hyperchloremic metabolic acidosis. The serum chloride concentration, however, can also be slightly decreased in acidosis if organic acids or other acids are the primary cause of the acidosis. *Hyperchloremia*, in the absence of metabolic acidosis, is seldom encountered because chloride retention is usually accompanied by sodium and water retention. *Hypochloremia* can result from excessive GI loss of chloride-rich fluid (e.g., vomiting, diarrhea, gastric suctioning, intestinal fistulas). Because chloride ions are renally excreted with cations, hypochloremia may also result from significant diuresis.

Anion Gap

The *R* factor, or anion gap (AG), represents the contribution of unmeasured acids, such as lactate, phosphates, sulfates, and proteins. As displayed in Equation 2-1, a patient's anion gap is determined by subtracting the primary anions (Cl and HCO_3) from the primary cation (Na). Some clinicians include potassium in this determination and subtract the anions from both major cations (Na and K). A normal anion gap is typically <12 mEq/mL if potassium is not incorporated in the calculation or <16 mEq/mL if potassium is considered.

An elevated anion gap may be indicative of a metabolic acidosis caused by an increase in lactic acids, ketoacids, salicylic acids, methanol, or ethylene glycol. A low anion gap may be the result of reduced concentrations of unmeasured anions (e.g., hypoalbuminemia) or from systematic underestimation of serum sodium (e.g., hyperviscosity of myeloma). Again, see Chapter 10 for a more detailed discussion of the clinical use of the anion gap.

Blood Urea Nitrogen

Normal: 8–18 mg/dL or 2.8–6.4 mmol/L

Urea nitrogen is an end product of protein metabolism. It is produced solely by the liver, is transported in the blood, and is excreted by the kidneys. The serum concentration of urea nitrogen (i.e., BUN) is reflective of renal function because the urea nitrogen in blood is filtered completely at the glomerulus of the kidney, and then reabsorbed and tubularly secreted within nephrons. Acute or chronic renal failure is the most common cause of an elevated BUN. Although the BUN is an excellent screening test for renal dysfunction, it does not sufficiently quantify the extent of renal disease. In addition, several nonrenal factors such as unusually high protein intake and conditions that increase protein catabolism (or upper GI bleeding) can increase the BUN concentration. A patient's hydration status will also influence BUN; a water deficit tends to concentrate the urea nitrogen, and a water excess dilutes the urea nitrogen. The ratio of BUN to SCr can also be of clinical use. A normal ratio is roughly 15:1. Ratios >20:1 are observed in patients with decreased blood flow to the kidney (e.g., prerenal disease such as dehydration or conditions involving reduced cardiac output) or conditions involving increased protein in the blood (e.g., dietary intake or an upper GI bleed). Situations where the BUN:SCr ratio is <15:1 are seen in patients with renal failure, significant malnourishment (decreased intake of protein), or severe liver disease where the liver is no longer able to form urea.

3. Why is the BUN abnormal for M.C. (from question 1)?

The BUN serum concentration in M.C. is somewhat increased, perhaps because of inadequate renal perfusion secondary to her heart failure. Her renal function could also be more severely compromised than one would anticipate from her slightly increased BUN value because of dilution by increased ECF volume. Therefore, M.C.'s renal status should be further evaluated.

Creatinine

Normal: 0.6–1.2 mg/dL or 50–110 μmol/L

Creatinine is derived from creatine and phosphocreatine, major constituents of muscle. Its rate of formation for a given individual is remarkably constant and is determined primarily by an individual's muscle mass or lean body weight. Therefore, the SCr concentration is slightly higher in muscular subjects, but unlike the BUN, it is less directly affected by exogenous factors or liver impairment. Once creatinine is released from muscle into plasma, it is excreted renally almost exclusively by glomerular filtration. A decrease in the glomerular filtration rate (GFR) results in an increase in the SCr concentration. Thus, careful interpretation of the SCr concentration is used widely in the clinical evaluation of patients with suspected renal disease.

A doubling of the SCr level roughly corresponds to a 50% reduction in the GFR. This general rule of thumb only holds true for steady-state creatinine levels.[5]

4. M.C. was given digoxin 0.125 mg/day, and a SCr was ordered to further assess her renal function. The clinical laboratory determined her SCr was 1.2 mg/dL. Although this laboratory test result is within normal limits, why does it not clearly indicate normal renal function for M.C.?

[SI unit: SCr, 106 μmol/L]

A SCr of 1.2 mg/dL in M.C. does not necessarily reflect normal renal function. As patients become older, muscle mass represents a smaller proportion of total weight, and creatinine production is decreased. Furthermore, the SCr concentration in female patients is generally 0.2 to 0.4 mg/dL (85%–90%) less than for males because females have relatively smaller kidneys. Because M.C. is a 61-year-old woman, a creatinine clearance (CrCl) determination would more accurately reflect her renal function status.

Creatinine Clearance

Normal: 75–125 mL/minute or 1.25–2.08 mL/second

Because creatinine is cleared almost exclusively through the glomerulus in the kidney, CrCl can be used as a clinically useful measure of a patient's GFR. CrCl serves as a valuable clinical parameter because many renally eliminated drugs are dose adjusted based on the patient's renal function. To determine actual CrCl, the patient's urine is collected over a 24-hour period, and the concentration of urine creatinine (mg/dL), total volume of urine collected over the 24-hour period (mL/minute), and SCr (mg/dL) are determined. The patient-specific, measured CrCl is determined using Equation 2-2:

$$\text{Measured 24 hr CrCl}_{(\text{mL/min})} = \frac{[\text{Urine conc}_{(\text{mg/dL})}] \times [\text{Total urine volume}_{(\text{mL/min})}]}{\text{SCr}_{(\text{mg/dL})}} \qquad \textbf{2-2}$$

Unfortunately, urine collections are time consuming and expensive, and incomplete collections can substantially underestimate renal function. In lieu of measuring actual CrCl, simplistic equations are commonly used to estimate a patient's CrCl. The following Cockcroft-Gault[7] formula incorporates age, body weight, and SCr. Typically, clinicians use ideal body weight (IBW) in the calculation of estimated CrCl; however, actual body weight (ABW) may be used when ABW is less than IBW. Equation 2-3 has the highest correlation and the greatest accuracy in patients with SCr concentrations <1.5 mg/dL[8]:

$$\text{Estimated CrCl for males (mL/min)} = \frac{(140 - \text{Age})\ (\text{Body weight in kg})}{(72)\ (\text{SCr}_{(\text{mg/dL})})} \qquad \textbf{2-3}$$

The Cockcroft-Gault formula must be multiplied by 85% to calculate CrCl for females. Another commonly used approach to estimating CrCl is the Jelliffe method,[9] shown in Equation 2-4:

$$\text{Estimated CrCl for Males (mL/min/1.73 m}^2) = \frac{98 - [(0.8)\ (\text{Age} - 20)]}{\text{SCr}_{(\text{mg/dL})}} \qquad \textbf{2-4}$$

This Jelliffe formula must be multiplied by 90% to calculate CrCl for females. The use of this method substantially underestimates CrCl for patients with SCr values <1.5 mg/dL,[10] whereas Cockcroft-Gault appears to have the highest correlation and greatest accuracy in patients with SCr values <1.5 mg/dL.[8] For patients with liver dysfunction, all methods of calculating CrCl from a SCr value are associated with significant overpredictions of CrCl.[10] Thus, methods for predicting CrCl should be used cautiously when attempting to adjust drug dosages in patients with liver disease.

5. A 24-hour CrCl determination was ordered for E.S., a 63-year-old, 60-kg man. The following data were returned from the clinical laboratory: total collection time was 24 hours; total urine volume, 1,000 mL; urine creatinine concentration, 42 mg/dL; and SCr, 1.7 mg/dL. Determine both the measured and the estimated CrCl for E.S. based on the given data, and compare and contrast these results.

[SI units: SCr, 150 μmol/L]

Using Equation 2-2, E.S. has a 24-hour measured CrCl of approximately 17 mL/minute. His estimated CrCl is 38 mL/minute using the Cockcroft-Gault method (Equation 2-3). Based on both methods, E.S.'s ability to clear renally eliminated drugs is impaired. An incomplete collection of urine over the 24-hour period or possible mishandling of the specimen can be possible explanations for the lower value seen with the measured CrCl. Because E.S. had an elevated SCr of 1.7 mg/dL, the accuracy of the Cockcroft-Gault estimation might also be compromised.

Glucose

Normal: 70–110 mg/dL or 3.9–6.1 mmol/L

The fasting glucose concentration in the ECF is regulated closely by homeostatic mechanisms to provide body tissues with a ready source of energy. Insulin and glucagon play a critical role in this complex process. Because plasma glucose concentrations fluctuate in response to ingestion of meals, most glucose concentrations are measured in either the fasting state or the postprandial state, depending on the type of information desired. Generally, normal glucose values refer to the plasma glucose concentration in the fasting state. The specific laboratory assay of blood sugar determinations must also be considered because different assay methods vary in their specificity and sensitivity to glucose. Glucose testing using whole blood from capillary finger sticks is used in conjunction with blood glucose metering devices for patients with diabetes. Whole blood measurements using these devices are typically 15% lower than corresponding plasma glucose levels.

Glycosylated Hemoglobin

Hgb is the oxygen-carrying component of the red blood cell (RBC). Over the functional life span of RBCs (~4 months), glucose molecules irreversibly bind to Hgb which results in glycosylated Hgb (A1c). The concentration of Hgb A1c, therefore, reflects a patient's average blood glucose concentration over the life span of circulating RBCs. In contrast, fasting glucose serum concentrations can fluctuate acutely based on either meals or insulin use. As a result, measurement of Hgb A1c concentrations provides a much better tool for evaluating chronic diabetes therapy. In a patient without diabetes, about 5% of Hgb is glycosylated; however, poorly controlled patients with diabetes can have A1c values greatly exceeding 8%. In one study of patients with elevated A1c values, every 1% reduction in the elevated A1c reduced the risk of microvascular complications by 37% and reduced the risk of acute myocardial infection by 14%.[11] The interpretation of serum concentrations of plasma glucose, Hgb A1c, and other related laboratory tests is presented in Chapter 50.

Hyperglycemia and Hypoglycemia

Hyperglycemia and hypoglycemia are nonspecific signs of abnormal glucose metabolism. Diabetes mellitus is the most common cause of hyperglycemia. Insufficient carbohydrate intake because of a missed meal is the most common cause of hypoglycemia in a patient receiving insulin or another hypoglycemic medication.

6. T.C., a 68-year-old male, visits his endocrinologist to assess control of his type 2 diabetes. His average blood sugar over the past 90 days recorded via his blood glucose monitor is 217 mg/dL. However, T.C.'s Hgb A1c was 9%, which correlates with an average glucose concentration of roughly 240 mg/dL. T.C. is confused that these values are different because he routinely ensures his blood glucose machine is calibrated and coded properly. Why is the laboratory average different?

[SI units: glucose, 13.5 mmol/L]

T.C. should not be alarmed with the difference in these values. His blood glucose monitor is probably working properly and adequately measuring fluctuations in his plasma glucose concentrations. However, the monitor may be reflecting a lower average glucose concentration due to the timing of his daily testing for glucose. For example, measuring blood glucose in a fasting state more frequently than after mealtime could contribute to lower average concentrations because fasting values are typically lower than postprandial concentrations. The A1c is more indicative of his average blood sugar control over the past 90 days than the 90-day average recorded by his blood glucose monitor. A higher concentration of glucose in the blood positively correlates to a higher glycosylated Hgb. This value is typically reported as a percentage, with approximately 5% (100 mg/dL) considered as normal in a person without diabetes. As the A1c percentage increases, each point raises the corresponding blood glucose value by about 35 mg/dL (e.g., 8% = 205 mg/dL, 9% = 240 mg/dL).

Osmolality

Normal: 280–300 mOsm/kg or mmol/kg

The osmolality of a solution is a measure of the number of osmotically active ions (i.e., particles present) per unit of solution. It is the total number of particles in the solution, not the weight of the particle or the nature of the particle that determines osmolality. Because one mole of a substance contains 6×10^{23} molecules, equimolar concentrations of all substances in the undissociated state exert the same osmotic pressure. A mole of an ionized compound such as NaCl contributes twice as many particles in solution as one mole of an undissociated compound such as glucose. In most situations, the primary determinants of serum osmolality in the ECF are sodium (and its accompanying anions), glucose, and BUN. If one corrects for the concentrations of glucose and BUN, the serum concentration of sodium closely mirrors the serum osmolality.

A simplified formula (Equation 2-5) useful for rule-of-thumb calculations is as follows:

$$\text{Osmolarity}^* = 2[\text{Na}^+] + \frac{[\text{Glucose}]}{20} + \frac{[\text{BUN}]}{3} \qquad \textbf{2-5}$$

*Osmolarity is measured in mOsm/kg H_2O

Serum osmolarity is useful when evaluating fluid and electrolyte disorders, particularly sodium imbalances. An increase in the measured serum osmolarity, relative to the calculated osmolarity, can be attributed to an increase in the number of solutes, a reduction in the amount of free water (e.g., patients with significant dehydration), or perhaps laboratory error. The difference between the measured serum osmolality and the calculated serum osmolality is commonly referred to as the "osmol gap" (see Chapter 11).

MULTICHEMISTRY PANELS

SMA-7, SMA-12, Chem Profile-20

7. What are the advantages and disadvantages of biochemical profiles such as the SMA-7, SMA-12, and Chem Profile-20 ordered for M.C. (from question 1)?

The SMA-7, SMA-12, and Chem Profile-20 are compilations of 7, 12, or 20 biochemical tests that analyze blood chemistries on large-volume, automated instruments. The abbreviation SMA refers to "sequential multiple analyzer." Such tests are routinely obtained because they quickly provide basic information concerning organ function at relatively low cost. If abnormal values are noted, additional tests can be ordered to further investigate specific organ function. Nevertheless, routine use of biochemical profiles is controversial. When biochemical profiles are ordered without regard for the clinical evidence in an individual patient (i.e., routine testing is done on all patients on admission to a hospital), there is no evidence that these tests have improved patient care, lessened hospital costs, or shortened lengths of stay.

The SMA-7 panel typically analyzes a patient's sodium, potassium, chloride, CO_2, BUN, SCr, and glucose concentrations. This particular blood chemistry panel provides rapid insight to a patient's serum electrolytes, acid–base status, renal function, and metabolic state. An abbreviated method to report the SMA-7 used commonly by clinicians is shown in the following figure.

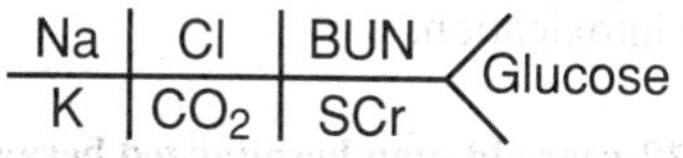

If an SMA-12 is ordered instead of the SMA-7 panel, the additional tests usually include serum concentrations of albumin, total protein, bilirubin, alkaline phosphatase, and calcium. A Chem Profile-20 provides eight more tests, such as phosphorus, cholesterol, triglycerides, uric acid, iron, lactic dehydrogenase (LDH), aspartate aminotransferase (AST), and alanine aminotransferase (ALT). These eight tests provide additional information for a general evaluation of metabolism, cardiovascular risk factors, and liver function, not provided by the SMA-7 or SMA-12 profiles. The cost of a Chem Profile-20 is seldom much greater than that of an SMA-7 or SMA-12 because of the automated nature of these tests. The particular grouping of tests included in various chemistry panels may vary with different clinical laboratories.

Calcium

Normal: 8.8 to 10.2 mg/dL or 2.20 to 2.55 mmol/L

The total calcium content resides primarily in the bone, with only about 1% freely exchangeable with that in the ECF. This reservoir of calcium in bones maintains the concentration of calcium in the plasma constant despite pronounced changes in the external balance of calcium. If the homeostatic factors (i.e., parathyroid hormone, vitamin D, calcitonin) that regulate the calcium content of body fluid are intact, a patient can lose 25% to 30% of total body calcium without a change in the concentration of calcium ion in the plasma.

About 40% of the calcium in the ECF is bound to plasma proteins (especially albumin); 5% to 15% is complexed with phosphate and citrate; and about 45% to 55% is in the unbound, ionized form. Most laboratories measure the total calcium concentration, although it is the free, ionized calcium concentration that is important physiologically, and the form that is closely regulated physiologically. Most laboratories are also able to measure the ionized form of calcium (4.5–5.6 mg/dL or 1.13–1.4 mmol/L).

A reduced calcium concentration usually implies a deficiency in either the production or the response to parathyroid hormone or vitamin D. The abnormality in the parathyroid hormone system might result from hypomagnesemia, hypoparathyroidism, or pseudohypoparathyroidism. The abnormality in the vitamin D system can be caused by decreased nutritional intake; decreased absorption of vitamin D secondary to gastrectomy, chronic pancreatitis, or small bowel disease; decreased production of 25-hydroxycholecalciferol due to liver disease; increased metabolism of 25-hydroxycholecalciferol because of enzyme-stimulating drugs (e.g., phenobarbital, phenytoin, rifampin); or decreased production of 1,25-dihydroxycholecalciferol due to chronic renal disease. Patients with low concentrations of magnesium also typically have low serum concentrations of calcium, and hypomagnesemia must be corrected before the calcium concentration can be adequately addressed.

Elevated calcium concentrations are commonly associated with malignancy or metastatic diseases. Other causes of hypercalcemia include hyperparathyroidism, Paget disease, milk-alkali syndrome, granulomatous disorders, thiazide diuretics, and vitamin D intoxication.

8. V.C. is a 38-year-old man hospitalized because of obtundation, somnolence, and severe alcohol intoxication. He has NKDA, and his laboratory tests revealed the following: albumin, 2.0 g/dL (normal, 4–6); Ca, 6.8 mg/dL (normal, 8.8–10.2); total bilirubin, 10.8 mg/dL (normal, 0.1–1.0); serum AST, 280 units/L (normal, 0–35); and alkaline phosphatase, 240 units/L (normal, 30–120). Why is calcium treatment inappropriate despite V.C.'s apparent low serum concentration of calcium?

[SI units: albumin, 20 g/L; Ca, 1.7 mmol/L; total bilirubin, 184.6 μmol/L; AST, 4.67 μkat/L; alkaline phosphatase, 4 μkat/L]

This case presentation provides insufficient patient data to make a conclusion concerning treatment. However, it does illustrate the importance of treating the patient as a whole, not as a specific laboratory value. Because calcium in the serum is partially bound to plasma proteins (mostly albumin), the serum calcium concentration is affected by the concentration of these plasma proteins. If the albumin concentration is low, the reported serum calcium will generally be less than the lower limit of normal. A useful method to estimate a corrected value for serum calcium in the presence of a low serum albumin is to use the following guideline: the total serum calcium will decrease by 0.8 mg/dL for each decrease of 1.0 g/dL in serum albumin concentration. V.C.'s serum albumin concentration is about 3.0 mg/dL less than "normal" (i.e., 5.0 mg/dL – 2.0 mg/dL = 3.0 mg/dL). Therefore, his correct serum calcium would be approximately 9.2 mg/dL (i.e., [3.0 mg/dL of albumin × 0.8] added to his reported serum calcium of 6.8 mg/dL). The "corrected" serum calcium concentration falls within the normal range, and V.C. should not be treated with calcium based on the available data. Direct measurement of ionized calcium is independent of albumin concentration, making it unnecessary to correct calcium concentrations in the presence of hypoalbuminemia. Unfortunately, some clinical laboratories do not have the capability of measuring ionized calcium.

Magnesium

Normal: 1.6–2.4 mEq/L or 0.8–1.2 mmol/L

Magnesium is primarily an intracellular electrolyte that, together with potassium and calcium, helps maintain a neutral charge within the cell. Magnesium also serves an important metabolic role in the phosphorylation of adenosine triphosphate (ATP).

A primary cause of *hypomagnesemia* is malnourishment. Toxemia in pregnancy is associated with hypomagnesemia. Hypomagnesemia needs to be corrected before attempting to correct hypokalemia or hypocalcemia. Attempts to replace potassium or calcium in patients with hypomagnesemia will be ineffective until the low magnesium concentrations are adequately addressed. Excessive ingestion of magnesium-containing antacids can lead to *hypermagnesemia*. Increased concentrations of magnesium are also observed in patients with reduced renal function. Hypermagnesemia can slow conduction in the heart, prolong PT intervals, and widen the QRS complex.

Phosphate

Normal: 2.5 to 5.0 mg/dL or 0.80 to 1.60 mmol/L

The extracellular concentration of phosphate as inorganic phosphorus is the prime determinant of the intracellular concentration, which in turn is the source of phosphate for ATP and phospholipid synthesis. Intracellular phosphate is also important in the regulation of nucleotide degradation.

The ECF concentration of phosphate is influenced by parathyroid hormone, intestinal phosphate absorption, renal function, bone metabolism, and nutrition. Moderate *hypophosphatemia* is encountered by malnourished patients (especially when anabolism is induced), patients who excessively use antacids (aluminum-containing antacids bind phosphorus in the GI tract), chronic alcoholics, and septic patients. Clinical consequences of severe hypophosphatemia involve nervous system dysfunction, muscle weakness, rhabdomyolysis, cardiac irregularities, and dysfunction of leukocytes and erythrocytes. *Hyperphosphatemia* is most commonly caused by renal insufficiency, although increased vitamin D, hypoparathyroidism, and advanced malignancies are also significant causes.

Uric Acid

Normal: 2.0 to 7.0 mg/dL or 0.12 to 0.42 mmol/L

Uric acid is an end product of purine metabolism. It serves no biological function, is not metabolized, and must be excreted renally. Gout is usually associated with increased serum concentrations of uric acid and deposits of monosodium urate.

Increased serum uric acid concentrations can result from either a decrease in urate excretion (e.g., renal dysfunction) or excessive urate production (e.g., increased purine metabolism resulting from cytotoxic therapy of neoplastic or myeloproliferative disorders). Low serum uric acid concentrations are inconsequential and are usually reflective of drugs that have hypouricemic activity (e.g., high dosages of salicylates). The determinants of the serum concentration of uric acid, the clinical implications of hyperuricemia, and the therapeutic management of uric acid disorders are presented in Chapter 42.

PROTEINS

Prealbumin

Normal: 15 to 36 mg/dL or 150 to 360 mg/L

Prealbumin is one of the primary proteins in circulation, but it accounts for a relatively small percentage of the circulating proteins. It is also referred to as "thyroxine-binding prealbumin (TBPA)" due to its role as a transport mechanism for triiodothyronine (T_3) and thyroxine (T_4). However, prealbumin is most frequently used to monitor patients at risk for poor nutrition (e.g., patients with eating disorders, HIV, or patients receiving total parenteral nutrition). Compared to the relatively long half-life of albumin (about 3 weeks), the half-life of prealbumin is only 1 to 2 days. This shorter half-life provides a more accurate reflection of acute changes in protein synthesis and catabolism. Prealbumin, therefore, is an effective and useful marker of immediate nutritional status. Hepatic disease and malnutrition are associated with decreases in both albumin and prealbumin. Hodgkin disease, pregnancy, chronic renal disease, and corticosteroid use can increase prealbumin serum concentrations.

Albumin

Normal: 4 to 6 g/dL or 40 to 60 g/L

Albumin, produced by the liver, contributes approximately 80% of serum colloid osmotic pressure. As a result, hypoalbuminemic states are commonly associated with edema and transudation of ECF. A lack of essential amino acids from malnutrition or malabsorption, or impaired albumin synthesis by the liver, can result in decreased serum albumin concentrations. Most forms of hepatic insufficiency are associated with decreased synthesis of albumin. Albumin can be lost directly from the blood because of hemorrhage, burns, or exudates, or it may be lost directly into the urine because of nephrosis. Serum albumin concentrations seldom increase, but increases may be noted in volume depletion or shock, or immediately after the administration of large amounts of intravenous albumin. In addition to its diagnostic value, the serum albumin concentration is an important consideration in the therapeutic monitoring of drugs and electrolytes that are highly protein bound (e.g., phenytoin, digoxin, calcium). In cases of severe hypoalbuminemia, determination of the "free" or unbound concentration of these entities might be necessary for an accurate assessment of drug therapy.

Globulin

Normal: 2.3 to 3.5 g/dL or 23 to 35 g/L

In addition to albumin, globulin is another primary plasma protein. Whereas albumin principally functions to maintain serum oncotic pressure, globulins play an active role in immunologic processes. The globulins can be separated into several subgroups such as α, β, and γ. The γ-globulins can be separated further into various immunoglobulins (e.g., IgA, IgM, IgG). Chronic infection or rheumatoid arthritis can increase immunoglobulin levels, and fractionation of immunoglobulins can provide useful information in the evaluation of immune disorders. When immunoglobulins are separated by electrophoresis, elevations of one or several in a specific pattern can suggest a diagnosis of multiple myeloma, a plasma cell malignancy. Because globulin is not manufactured solely by the liver, the ratio of albumin to globulin (the A/G ratio) is changed in patients with liver disease. Changes in this ratio result from decreased albumin concentration and a compensatory increase in globulin concentration.

ENZYMES

Enzyme activity is typically expressed in terms of international units (IU), where one IU is the enzyme amount needed to catalyze the conversion of 1 μmol of substrate per minute. The analogous expression in SI terms involves the term katal (kat). One katal is the amount of enzyme to catalyze 1 mol of substrate per second, making 1.0 μkat the amount for 1.0 μmol/second. Based on this information, the conversion between μkat and IU is 1 μkat = 60 IU.

Creatine Kinase

Normal: 0 to 150 units/L or 0 to 2.5 μkat/L

The CK enzyme, formerly known as creatine phosphokinase, catalyzes the transfer of high-energy phosphate groups in tissues that consume large amounts of energy (e.g., skeletal muscle, myocardium, brain). The serum concentration of CK can be increased by strenuous exercise, intramuscular injections of drugs that are irritating to tissue (e.g., diazepam, phenytoin), acute psychotic episodes, crush injuries, or myocardial damage.

CK is composed of M and B subunits, which are further divided into three isoenzymes: MM, BB, and MB. The CK-MM isoenzyme is found predominantly in skeletal muscle, the CK-BB in the brain, and the CK-MB in the myocardium. Myocardial CK activity consists of 80% to 85% CK-MM and 15% to 20% CK-MB. Noncardiac tissues that contain large amounts of CK have either CK-MM or CK-BB. The MB fraction is rare in tissues other than the myocardium.

CK-MB typically begins to increase 3 to 6 hours after an acute myocardial infarction (MI), peaks at 12 to 24 hours, and accounts for about 5% or more of the total CK.[12] Myocardial damage appears to correlate with the amount of CK-MB released into the serum (i.e., the higher the amount of CK-MB, the more extensive the myocardial injury). Although CK-MB levels >25 units/L are usually associated with an MI,[13] the absolute amount can vary, depending on the assay method. Generally, if the amount of CK-MB exceeds 6% of the total, myocardial injury has presumably occurred. Analysis of CK-MB provides a rapid, sensitive, specific, cost-effective, and definitive means of detecting MI.[14]

9. S.G., a 44-year-old woman, appears at the emergency department of a local hospital, with complaints of sudden-onset chest pain, diaphoresis, and nausea that began about 1 hour ago. S.G describes her pain as severe and not relieved by position change, antacids, or nitroglycerin. An electrocardiogram (ECG) reveals changes consistent with an acute MI. The total CK serum concentration is 118 units/L (normal, <150) and the CK-MB is 5 units/L (normal, <12). S.G. was admitted to the coronary care unit to rule out an acute MI. Why are the total CK and CK-MB serum concentrations within the normal range in S.G., despite clear evidence supporting an acute MI?

[SI units: CK, 1.97 μkat/L; CK-MB, 0.08 μkat/L]

The total CK and CK-MB are both within the normal range for S.G.; however, an MI cannot be excluded. CK serum concentrations usually do not rise above normal values until 4 to 8 hours after myocardial injury and usually peak in about 12 to 24 hours. About 10% of patients with suspected MIs fail to demonstrate an increase in the total CK, although serial CK-MB fractions will be increased. When CK-MB is >6% of total CK, an MI has probably occurred even if the total CK is not elevated.[12]

Troponin

Normal: 0 to 0.03 ng/mL or 0 to 0.03 mcg/L

10. How can myocardial enzymes be detected earlier than 4 to 8 hours after myocardial injury?

Troponins are proteins that mediate the calcium-mediated interaction of actin and myosin within muscles. There are two cardiac-specific troponins, cardiac troponin I (cTnI) and cardiac troponin T (cTnT). Whereas cTnT is present in cardiac and skeletal muscle cells, cTnI is present only in cardiac muscle.[15,16] Compared with the detection of CK-MB, the presence of troponin I is a more specific and sensitive indicator of myocardial damage.[17] Furthermore, the concentration of cTnI increases within 2 to 4 hours of an acute MI, enabling clinicians to quickly initiate appropriate therapy. Troponin also remains elevated for about 10 days compared to the 2- to 3-day elevation typically observed with CK-MB. cTnI levels >2.0 ng/mL are suggestive of acute myocardial tissue injury. The use of troponin as a primary diagnostic test for acute MI is becoming widely accepted as a standard.[17] (See Chapter 17.)

Myoglobin

Normal: 0 to 90 mcg/L

Myoglobin, a protein in heart and skeletal muscle cells, provides oxygen to working muscles. When muscle is damaged, myoglobin is released into the bloodstream. As a cardiac biomarker, myoglobin concentrations in serum rise within 3 hours after insult to the myocardial tissue, peak in about 8 to 12 hours, and return to normal in about a day. Because myoglobin serum concentrations rise more quickly than CK-MB after myocardial injury, it can be of value in helping rule out MI in the emergency department. Myoglobin serum concentrations, however, tend to be less specific for myocardial tissue compared to CK-MB. Trauma or ischemic injury to noncardiac tissue can increase serum myoglobin. Because troponin serum concentrations in serum also increase rapidly after myocardial damage, troponin is often preferred over myoglobin as a biomarker of cardiac damage.

Homocysteine

Normal: 4 to 15 μmol/L

Patients with deficiencies in folate, vitamin B_6, or vitamin B_{12} tend to have elevated serum levels of homocysteine. Homocysteine is believed to have a destructive affect on vascular epithelium. Over time, patients with elevated homocysteine levels (>12 μmol/L) are believed to be at increased risk for cardiac disease.[18] Screening individuals with a positive family history for elevated homocysteine or those with atherosclerosis without typical risk factors or increased lipids has been advocated. Understanding the association between increased homocysteine levels and specific vitamin deficiencies, supplementation of folate, B_6 and B_{12} has been used clinically. However, data are too limited to suggest this approach reduces the incidence of acute MI or stroke.

Lactate Dehydrogenase

Normal: 100 to 190 units/L or 1.67 to 3.17 μkat/L

The enzyme, lactate dehydrogenase (LDH), is present in the heart, kidney, liver, and skeletal muscle. It is also abundantly present in erythrocytes and lung tissue. Because increased serum concentrations of LDH can be associated with diseases in many different organs and tissues, the diagnostic usefulness of an LDH determination is somewhat limited. There are, however, five isoenzymes of LDH. Although most tissues contain all five isoenzymes, some tissues have a predominance of one of the isoenzymes. LDH_1 and, to a lesser extent, LDH_2 predominate in the heart. Skeletal muscle and the liver have a predominance of LDH_5. LDH_3 and LDH_4 are found in a variety of tissues, including the lungs, RBCs, kidneys, brain, and pancreas. Consequently, identifying specific isoenzymes can increase the diagnostic usefulness of serum LDH determinations. For example, the elevated serum LDH associated with MI consists mostly of LDH_1 and LDH_2, whereas with acute liver disease there is a greater proportion of LDH_4 and LDH_5. Unfortunately, these isoenzyme patterns are not necessarily typical of all myocardial or liver diseases. With the availability of other myocardial enzymes, LDH as a diagnostic tool is used less frequently.

Brain Natriuretic Peptide

Normal: 0 to 100 pg/mL or 0 to 100 ng/L

Brain natriuretic peptide (BNP) is released from the heart when increased demands are placed on the myocardial tissue. Elevations in BNP are indicative of patients with congestive heart failure (CHF). In an effort to reduce workload on the heart, BNP counteracts the renin-angiotensin-aldosterone system and causes vasodilatory effects, along with natriuresis (increased excretion of sodium), all geared at reducing blood volume. Patients with some degree of CHF typically have BNP levels >100 ng/L. BNP levels >500 ng/L represent definite left ventricular dysfunction, and further evaluation is warranted to more fully characterize the extent of impaired cardiac function.[19] The beneficial aspects of endogenous BNP have prompted marketing the recombinant BPN product, nesiritide (Natrecor). Nesiritide is approved for the treatment of acute decompensated heart failure in patients with dyspnea at rest.[20]

C-Reactive Protein

Normal: 0 to 1.0 mg/dL or 0 to 10 mg/L

C-reactive protein (CRP) is a nonspecific, acute-phase reactant that is helpful in the diagnosis and monitoring of inflammatory processes (e.g., rheumatoid arthritis) and infections. CRP is produced by the liver in response to an inflammatory process. Although an elevation in CRP indicates the presence of an acute inflammatory event, the nonspecific nature of the test does little to identify the cause or location of the inflammation. CRP is similar to an older test, erythrocyte sedimentation rate (ESR), but it tends to be more sensitive then ESR and is also associated with a more rapid and greater response to acute inflammation. A potential use of CRP is in the diagnosis of acute MI and as a risk factor for cardiovascular disease. Patients with CRP levels <1.0 mg/dL are considered to be at low risk, whereas patients with CRP levels >3.0 mg/dL are at increased risk for cardiovascular disease.[21] Because viral infections do not typically increase in CRP serum concentrations, the use of CRP as a diagnostic tool to differentiate viral versus bacterial meningitis might be clinically helpful. For example, a CRP value within the normal range could help exclude a diagnosis of bacterial meningitis.

LIVER FUNCTION TESTS

Aspartate Aminotransferase

Normal: 0 to 35 units/L or 0 to 0.58 μkat/L

The AST enzyme, formerly called "serum glutamic oxaloacetic transaminase," is abundant in heart and liver tissue and moderately present in skeletal muscle, the kidney, and the pancreas. In cases of acute cellular injury to the heart or liver, the enzyme is released into the blood from the damaged cells. In clinical practice, AST determinations have been used to evaluate myocardial injury and to diagnose and assess the prognosis of liver disease resulting from hepatocellular injury. The serum AST level is increased in more than 95% of patients after an MI. However, the increase in AST does not occur until 4 to 6 hours after the onset of myocardial injury. Peak AST concentrations are seen in the serum after 24 to 36 hours, returning to the normal range in about 4 to 5 days. The magnitude of the peak AST levels approximate the extent of myocardial damage (see Chapter 17).

Serum AST values are elevated significantly in patients with acute hepatic necrosis, whether caused by viral hepatitis or a hepatotoxin (e.g., carbon tetrachloride). In these situations, the serum concentrations of both AST and ALT will be increased, even before the appearance of clinical symptoms (e.g., jaundice). The AST and ALT serum concentrations can be increased by as much as 100 times greater than the usual upper limits of normal in the presence of parenchymal liver disease. Patients with intrahepatic cholestasis, posthepatic jaundice, or cirrhosis usually experience more moderate elevations of AST, depending on the extent of cell necrosis. The AST serum concentration is usually higher than that of ALT in patients with cirrhosis, and the AST increase is usually about four to five times greater than the upper limit of normal.

Alanine Aminotransferase

Normal: 0 to 35 units/L or 0 to 0.58 μkat/L

The ALT enzyme, formerly called "serum glutamic pyruvic transaminase," is found in essentially the same tissues that have high concentrations of AST. However, elevations in serum ALT are more specific for liver-related injuries or diseases. Although ALT is relatively more abundant in hepatic tissue versus cardiac tissue than AST, the liver still contains 3.5 times more AST than ALT. Serum concentrations of both AST and ALT increase when disease processes affect liver cell structure, but ALT concentrations are not significantly increased as a result of an acute MI. Evaluating the ratio of ALT to AST can be potentially useful, particularly in the diagnosis of viral hepatitis. The ALT/AST ratio frequently exceeds 1.0 with alcoholic cirrhosis, chronic liver disease, or hepatic cancer. However, ratios <1.0 tend to be observed with viral hepatitis or acute hepatitis, which can be useful when diagnosing liver disease.

Alkaline Phosphatase

Normal: 30 to 120 units/L or 0.5 to 2.0 μkat/L

The alkaline phosphatases (ALPs) constitute a large group of isoenzymes that play important roles in the transport of sugar and phosphate. These isoenzymes of ALP have different physiochemical properties and originate from different tissues (e.g., liver, bone, placenta, intestine). In normal adults, ALP is derived primarily from liver and bone. Although only small amounts of ALP are present in the liver, this enzyme is secreted into the bile, and substantially elevated ALP serum concentrations can be seen with mild intrahepatic or extrahepatic biliary obstruction. Thus, the presence of early bile duct abnormalities can result in elevated ALP before increases in the serum bilirubin are observed. Drug-induced cholestatic jaundice (e.g., chlorpromazine or sulfonamides) can increase serum ALP concentrations. In mild cases of acute liver cell damage, ALP levels are seldom elevated. Even in cirrhosis, ALP concentrations are variable and depend on the degree of hepatic decompensation and obstruction. Serum ALP concentrations are an excellent indicator of space-occupying lesions in the liver, primarily due to disruption of biliary canaliculi within the liver.[22]

The osteoblasts in bone produce large amounts of ALP, and marked serum elevations can be seen in Paget disease, hyperparathyroidism, osteogenic sarcoma, osteoblastic cancer metastatic to bone, and other conditions of pronounced osteoblastic activity. The serum ALP is increased during periods of rapid bone growth (e.g., infancy, early childhood, healing bone fractures) and during pregnancy because of the contributions of the placenta and fetal bones.

11. L.M., a 59-year-old female currently taking atorvastatin 40 mg daily for hypercholesterolemia, complains of fatigue and myalgia over the past week since her last prescription refill. On assessment, her primary care provider determines she has been taking an incorrect dose. Instead of cutting an 80-mg tablet in half, she has been taking the entire tablet, thereby effectively doubling her dose. The physician orders liver function tests (LFTs), CK, and SCr to evaluate her myalgia. Laboratory results indicate the following: AST, 51 units/L (normal, <35); ALT, 72 units/L (normal, <35); ALP, 82 units/L (normal, 30–120); CK, 216 units/L (normal, <150); and SCr, 1.4 mg/dL (normal, 0.6–1.2). Why are these laboratory results of sufficient concern to warrant discontinuation of atorvastatin?

[SI units: AST, 0.85 μkat/L; ALT, 1.2 μkat/L; ALP 1.37 μkat/L; CK, 3.6 μkat/L; SCr 123.8 μmol/L]

L.M.'s LFTs are elevated and are of concern, particularly in light of her other signs and symptoms. Statins have been implicated in causing elevations in LFTs on initiation of therapy and with dose increases. LFTs can be increased by up to three times the upper limit of normal. In the absence of jaundice or other clinical signs and symptoms, reduction of her atorvastatin dose will generally be sufficient in returning LFTS to normal values without adverse sequelae. L.M.'s values will likely return to baseline when her atorvastatin dose is reduced to 40 mg or discontinued. Additional monitoring after intervention would be indicated to confirm whether her LFTs stabilize or whether a trend of elevations is noted on multiple occasions. CK serum concentrations can also be increased in response to muscle injury or myalgia. When CK increases ten times the upper limit of normal, myopathy should be suspected. L.M.'s CK is mildly increased at this time, but not at an alarming value.

Gamma-Glutamyl Transferase

Normal: 0 to 70 units/L or 0 to 1.17 μkat/L

Although the enzyme gamma-glutamyl transferase (GGT) is found in the kidney, liver, and pancreas, its major clinical value is in the evaluation of hepatobiliary disease. An increase in the serum concentration of GGT parallels the increase of ALP in obstructive jaundice and infiltrative disease of the liver. However, increased ALP in the presence of a normal GGT is more suggestive of muscular or bone-related issues. GGT is one of the more sensitive liver enzymes for identifying biliary obstruction and cholecystitis. Because GGT is a hepatic

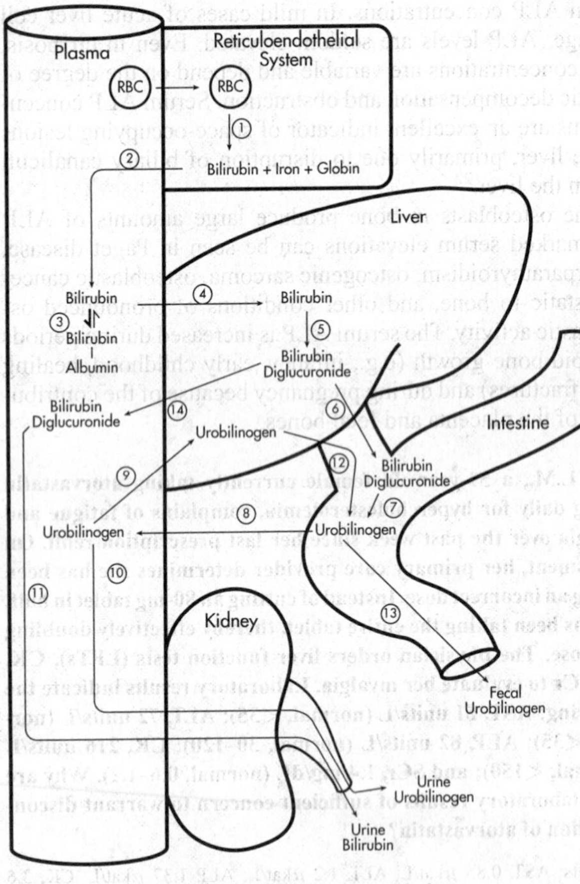

FIGURE 2-1 Bilirubin metabolism.

microsomal enzyme, tissue concentrations increase in response to microsomal enzyme induction by alcohol and other drugs (e.g., carbamazepine, phenobarbital, phenytoin). As a result, GGT is a sensitive indicator of recent or chronic alcohol exposure.

Bilirubin

Total Bilirubin—Normal: 0.1 to 1.0 mg/dL or 1.7 to 17.1 μmol/L
Direct (Conjugated) Bilirubin—Normal: 0 to 0.2 mg/dL or 0 to 3.4 μmol/L

Bilirubin is primarily a breakdown product of Hgb and is formed in the reticuloendothelial system (Fig. 2-1, step 1). It is then transferred into the blood (step 2), where it is almost completely bound to serum albumin (step 3). When bilirubin arrives at the sinusoidal surface of the liver cells, the free fraction is rapidly taken up into the cell (step 4) and converted primarily to bilirubin diglucuronide (step 5). A monoglucuronide is also formed that is metabolized predominantly to the diglucuronide. The conjugated bilirubin diglucuronide is then excreted into the bile (step 6) and appears in the intestine, where bacteria convert most of it to urobilinogen (step 7). The majority of urobilinogen is destroyed or excreted in the feces (step 13), but a small portion is reabsorbed into the blood (step 8) and either reabsorbed into the liver (step 9) and subsequently excreted into the bile (step 12) or excreted into the urine (step 10). Urobilinogen is responsible for the straw color of the urine and the yellowish-brown color of the feces. The mechanism by which conjugated bilirubin in the liver cell is transferred to the blood (step 14) is not well understood. However, in many types of liver disease, conjugated (direct) bilirubin is present in increased concentrations in the blood. When this concentration exceeds 0.2 to 0.4 mg/dL, bilirubin will begin to appear in the urine (step 11). Unconjugated (indirect) bilirubin is water insoluble and is highly bound to serum albumin; both factors account for its lack of excretion in the urine.[23]

Hyperbilirubinemia

12. A.R., a 42-year-old man with a 2-year history of hypertension controlled with hydrochlorothiazide and a 1-year history of Parkinson disease controlled by carbidopa/levodopa, is hospitalized after an episode of orthostatic hypotension. Admitting laboratory results show a hematocrit (Hct) of 27% (normal, 39–49). Because A.R. had a long history of alcoholism, additional laboratory tests were obtained. His results were as follows: total bilirubin, 3.5 mg/dL (normal, 0.1–1.0); direct bilirubin, 0.5 mg/dL (normal, <0.2); ALP, 40 units/L (normal, 30–120); AST, 32 units/L (normal, <35); and ALT, 27 units/L (normal, <35). Based on this information and Figure 2-1, what are three major causes of increased bilirubin in adults, and what might be the most logical cause of increased bilirubin in A.R.?

[SI units: Hct, 0.27; total bilirubin, 59.8 μmol/L; direct bilirubin, 8.6 μmol/L; ALP, 0.67 μkat/L; AST, 0.53 μkat/L; ALT, 0.45 μkat/L]

Increases in serum bilirubin can be categorized into three primary causes. First, hepatocellular injury interferes with the ability of the liver to conjugate bilirubin, leading to a disproportional increase of total bilirubin relative to the direct bilirubin (i.e., the indirect bilirubin will be increased). The normal AST and ALT values observed with A.R. indicate that hepatocellular damage is not likely the cause of the increased bilirubin. Therefore, a diagnosis of hepatocellular damage cannot be confirmed by the serum bilirubin concentrations alone. Second, hyperbilirubinemia can involve cholestatic or obstructive (posthepatic) causes. Blockage of the bile duct secondary to cholelithiasis (gallstone) or tumor will tend to increase conjugated (direct) bilirubin. In obstructive causes of hyperbilirubinemia, mild elevations in AST and ALT, as well as marked increase in ALP and GGT, are usually observed. Furthermore, increased excretion of excess conjugated bilirubin in the urine commonly results in dark brown–colored urine. Again, the clinical scenario illustrated with A.R. does not appear to support a cholestatic component as the cause of his increased bilirubin (ALP is within the normal range, and his direct bilirubin is only slightly elevated). The third primary cause of increased serum bilirubin involves hemolysis (prehepatic). In cases where erythrocytes are rapidly hemolyzed (e.g., sickle cell disease, drug-induced hemolysis), serum concentrations of indirect bilirubin increase. If the liver is conjugating and eliminating bilirubin normally, total bilirubin will increase out of proportion to the direct bilirubin, and the other LFTs will appear normal. This appears evident in A.R.'s case, making hemolysis the likely cause of his hyperbilirubinemia.

MISCELLANEOUS TESTS

Amylase and Lipase

Amylase (35–120 units/L or 0.58–2.0 μkat/L) and lipase (0–160 units/L or 0–2.67 μkat/L) are enzymes produced in the pancreas and secreted into the duodenum to assist in the digestive process. Amylase is responsible for breaking down complex carbohydrates into simple sugars and is also found in the saliva. Significant elevations in serum amylase are observed in patients with acute pancreatitis or pancreatic duct obstruction. Amylase levels tend to rise 6 to 48 hours after onset of the disease and usually return to normal 3 days after the acute event. In chronic pancreatitis or obstruction, amylase levels may remain elevated for longer periods. Other nonpancreatic conditions (e.g., bowel perforation, biliary disease, perforated peptic ulcer, ectopic pregnancy, mumps) can be associated with elevated serum amylase levels.

Lipase is responsible for breaking down triglycerides into fatty acids. Elevated serum lipase levels are also suggestive of pancreatic disease and tend to be more specific for pancreatic disease than amylase. The onset of lipase elevation is similar to amylase; however, lipase typically remains elevated for 5 to 7 days and can be useful in diagnosing patients in later stages of pancreatic disease. Narcotics (e.g., morphine) can constrict the sphincter of Oddi and increase serum concentrations of amylase and lipase.

Prostate-Specific Antigen

Normal: 0 to 4 ng/mL or 0 to 4 mcg/L

Prostate-specific antigen (PSA) is a protease glycoprotein produced almost exclusively by prostate epithelial cells. Serum concentrations of PSA are increased when the normal prostate glandular structure is disrupted by benign or malignant tumor or inflammation. More than half of the men with benign prostatic hyperplasia have elevated serum PSA concentrations. PSA is also a valuable parameter for staging and monitoring the progression and response to therapy of prostate cancer.[24]

PSA serum concentrations increase after prostatic manipulation such as digital rectal examination (DRE), transrectal ultrasound, cystoscopy, or biopsy of the prostate. In addition, serum PSA will increase 24 to 48 hours following ejaculation. Although elevated serum concentrations of PSA can occur in men with benign prostatic hyperplasia, concentrations tend to be higher and encountered more often in men with cancer. As a result, the American Cancer Society[25] and the American Urological Association[26] currently recommend that health care providers offer a PSA blood test and DRE yearly to men older than 50 years. For men considered to be at high risk (family history or African American men), testing at age 45 years is suggested. Combination of both PSA and DRE were more effective in detecting prostate cancer than either test alone.

The serum half-life of PSA is 2 to 3 days, but serum PSA concentrations can remain high for several weeks after manipulation of the prostate. Men with PSA levels between 4 and 10 ng/mL should be evaluated further for potential prostate cancer. Circulating serum PSA is bound to plasma proteins, and the capability exists to measure both total and free (unbound) PSA concentrations. Increased risk of prostate cancer has been observed in men with a free PSA-to-total PSA ratio of <0.25.[27] An aggressive approach to localize prostate cancer for men with life expectancies more than 10 years is now favored.[24,28] The diagnosis and treatment of prostate cancer is presented in Chapter 91.

Thyroid-Stimulating Hormone

Normal: 2 to 10 μ units/L or m units/L

Thyroid-stimulating hormone (TSH) is commonly used to monitor exogenous thyroid replacement therapy in individuals diagnosed with primary hypothyroidism. In addition, TSH may also be measured in conjunction with T_4 levels to diagnose this condition or secondary hypothyroidism. Causes of secondary hypothyroidism typically arise from damage, such as trauma or tumors, to the hypothalamus or pituitary gland. Secretion of thyroid-releasing hormone (TRH) and TSH are substantially impaired or absent due to this damage. Conversely, primary hypothyroidism occurs in response to low levels of T_3 and T_4. Reduced levels stimulate TRH and TSH release in absence of the negative feedback typically exerted by normal levels of T_3 and T_4; as a result, increased TSH is noted.

Exogenous thyroid replacement therapy balances TSH secretion to achieve a euthyroid state. Individuals taking inappropriate replacement doses will exhibit alterations in TSH levels. In the absence of other clinical influences or interactions, a high TSH level indicates the need to supplement with additional thyroid medication, whereas a low TSH supports the reduction in exogenous supplementation. Causes of primary hypothyroidism include congenital defects, idiopathic hypothyroidism, thyroiditis (inflammation of the thyroid gland), or antithyroid medications. Chapter 49 provides a more detailed discussion of the clinical implications of altered thyroid laboratory findings.

Cholesterol and Triglycerides

A detailed discussion of hypercholesterolemia and lipid disorders is provided in Chapter 12. For convenience, the current range of desired values for total cholesterol (TC), low-density lipoproteins (LDLs), high-density lipoproteins (HDLs), and fasting triglycerides (TGs) has been incorporated in Table 2-1. The reader is referred to Chapter 12 or to National Cholesterol Education Program and Adult Treatment Panel guidelines for a detailed description on the topic.[29]

HEMATOLOGY

There are several different hematologic cell types that originate from the hematopoietic stem cell. Each cell line has a defined role and unique contribution to the overall homeostatic process, and may be found in the bone marrow, lymph system, or blood. Typically, routine clinical laboratory testing involves measuring concentrations of mature myeloid cells found in the blood. Figure 2-2 illustrates the various lineages derived from the hematopoietic stem cell.[30] The cells derived via the myeloid linage are the focus of the following discussion. Readers are encouraged to refer to Sections 18 (Chapters 86 and 87) and 19 (Chapters 88 to 92) to gain further understanding of the clinical relevance of lymphoid and myeloid cells (Fig. 2-2).

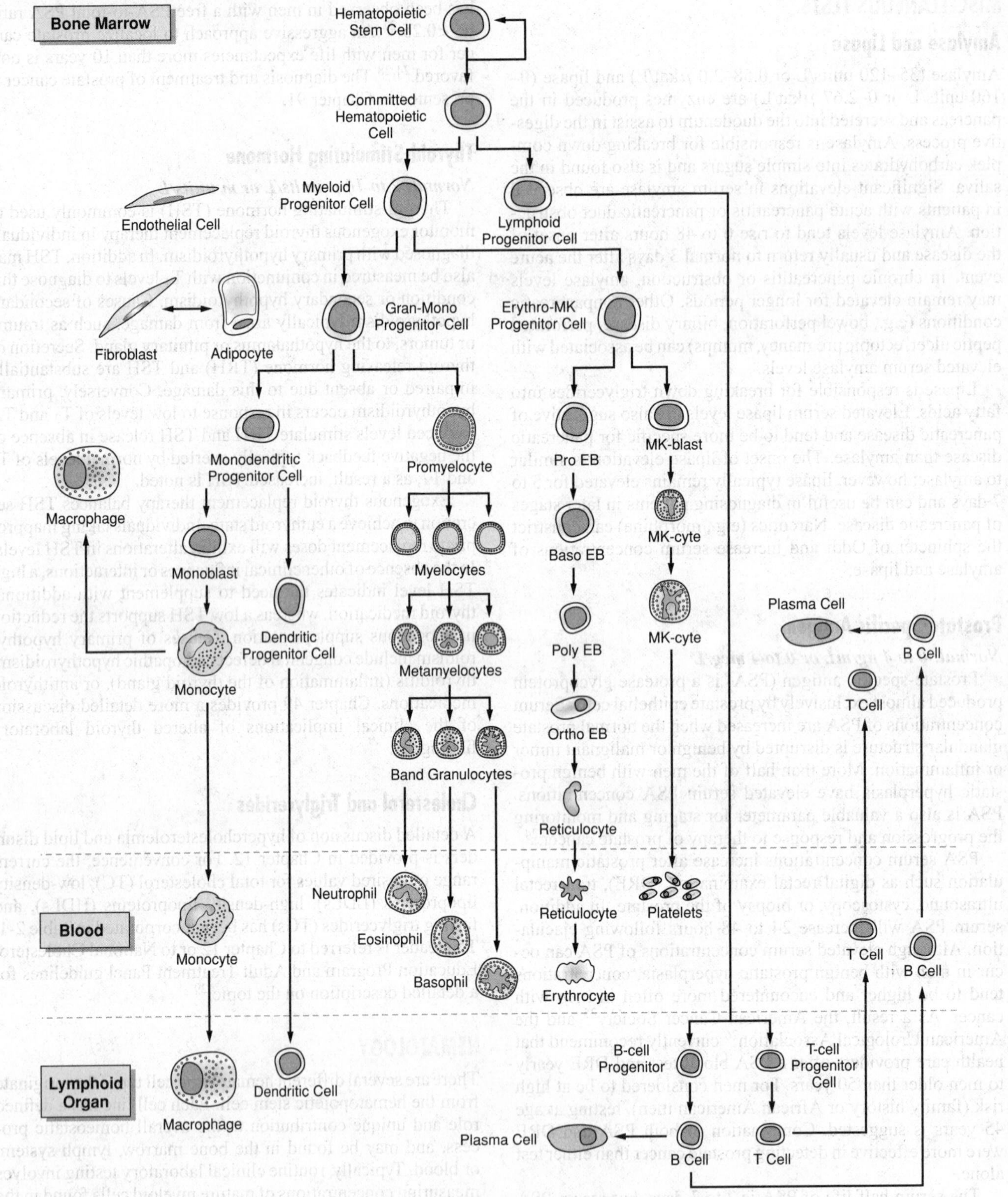

Bone Marrow
Hematopoietic Stem Cell
Committed Hematopoietic Cell
Myeloid Progenitor Cell
Lymphoid Progenitor Cell
Endothelial Cell
Gran-Mono Progenitor Cell
Erythro-MK Progenitor Cell
Fibroblast
Adipocyte
Monodendritic Progenitor Cell
Promyelocyte
Pro EB
MK-blast
Macrophage
Monoblast
Myelocytes
Baso EB
MK-cyte
Plasma Cell
Dendritic Progenitor Cell
Poly EB
MK-cyte
B Cell
Metamyelocytes
Monocyte
T Cell
Ortho EB
Band Granulocytes
Reticulocyte
Neutrophil
Reticulocyte
Platelets
Blood
Eosinophil
T Cell
B Cell
Monocyte
Basophil
Erythrocyte
B-cell Progenitor
T-cell Progenitor Cell
Lymphoid Organ
Dendritic Cell
Macrophage
Plasma Cell
B Cell
T Cell

FIGURE 2-2 Hematopoietic stem cell lineage.

Complete Blood Count

The complete blood count (CBC) is one of the most commonly ordered clinical laboratory tests. A CBC measures the RBCs, Hgb, Hct, mean cell volume (MCV), mean cell Hgb concentration (MCHC), and total white blood cells (WBCs). Depending on the laboratory, an order for a CBC may also include platelets, reticulocytes, or leukocyte differential. An abbreviated method of noting hematologic parameters in clinical practice is noted in the following figure. In addition, a list of hematologic laboratory values is presented in Table 2-2.

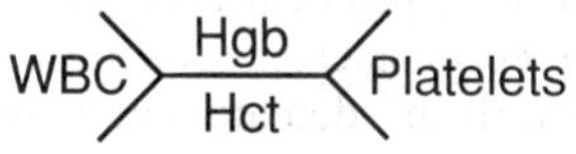

Red Blood Cells (Erythrocytes)

Males—Normal: 4.3 to 5.9 × 10^6/mm^3 or 4.3 to 5.9 × 10^{12}/L
Females—Normal: 3.5 to 5.0 × 10^6/mm^3 or 3.5 to 5.0 × 10^{12}/L

Erythrocytes or RBCs are produced in the bone marrow, released into the peripheral blood, circulated for approximately 120 days, and cleared by the reticuloendothelial system. The primary function of RBCs is to transport oxygen to tissues. The concentration of RBCs in the blood can be measured to detect anemia, calculate RBC indices, or calculate the Hct. Hct and Hgb concentrations are generally used to monitor quantitative changes in RBCs.

Hematocrit

Males—Normal: 39% to 49% or 0.39 to 0.49 I
Females—Normal: 33 to 43% or 0.33 to 0.43 I

Hct (packed cell volume) is determined by centrifuging a capillary tube of whole blood and comparing the height of the settled RBCs to the height of the column of whole blood. The percentage of RBCs to the blood volume is the Hct. A decrease in Hct may result from bleeding, the bone marrow suppressant effects of drugs, chronic diseases, genetic alterations in RBC morphology, or hemolysis. An increase in Hct may result from hemoconcentration, polycythemia vera, or polycythemia secondary to chronic hypoxia.

Hemoglobin

Males—Normal: 14 to 18 g/dL or 140 to 180 g/L
Females—Normal: 12 to 16 g/dL or 120 to 160 g/L

Hgb is the oxygen-carrying compound contained in RBCs. Therefore, total Hgb concentration primarily depends on the number of RBCs in the blood sample. As mentioned with Hct, medical conditions that impact the number of RBCs will also affect Hgb concentration. As discussed previously, glycosylated Hgb (A1c) is a related test used to monitor diabetes mellitus.

Red Blood Cell Indices

RBC indices (also known as Wintrobe indices) are useful in the classification of anemias. These indices include the MCV, the mean cell hemoglobin (MCH), and the MCHC. These indices are calculated in Equations 2-6 to 2-8:

$$\text{MCV} = \frac{\text{Hct} \times 1{,}000}{\text{RBC (in millions}/\mu\text{L)}} = 76 - 100 \text{ (in } \mu\text{m}^3 \text{ or fL)} \qquad \textbf{2-6}$$

$$\text{MCH} = \frac{\text{Hgb (in g/dL} \times 10)}{\text{RBC (in millions}/\mu\text{L)}} = 27 - 33 \text{ (in pg)} \qquad \textbf{2-7}$$

$$\text{MCHC} = \frac{\text{Hgb (in g/dL)}}{\text{Hct}} = 33 - 37 \text{ (in g/dL)} \qquad \textbf{2-8}$$

Mean Cell Volume

The MCV detects changes in cell size. A decreased MCV indicates a microcytic cell, which can result from iron-deficiency anemia. A large MCV indicates a macrocytic cell, which can be caused by a vitamin B_{12} or folic acid deficiency. Underlying disease states (e.g., habitual alcohol ingestion, chronic liver disease, anorexia nervosa, hypothyroidism, reticulocytosis, hematologic disorders) may also present with an elevated MCV secondary to deficiencies in these vitamins.[31] The MCV can be normal in a patient with a "mixed" (microcytic and macrocytic) anemia. Note that a direct assessment of a blood smear via microscopic examination is the gold standard for confirming RBC size.

Mean Cell Hemoglobin

The MCHC is a more reliable index of RBC Hgb than MCH. The former measures the concentration of Hgb, whereas the latter measures the weight of Hgb in the average RBC. In normochromic anemias, changes in the size of RBCs (MCV) are associated with corresponding changes in the weight of Hgb (MCH), but the concentration of Hgb (MCHC) remains normal. Changes in the Hgb content of RBCs alter the color of these cells. Thus, hypochromic refers to a decrease in RBC Hgb, reflected by reduced MCHC, and may indicate iron-deficiency anemia. Conversely, hyperchromic RBCs have an elevated MCHC due to the presence of greater amounts of Hgb. Hyperchromic cells are not commonly encountered.[32]

13. C.U., a 58-year-old chronic alcoholic, was hospitalized after a barroom brawl. A CBC was ordered, and the following RBC indices were noted: MCV, 108 μm^3; MCH, 38 pg; and MCHC, 34 g/dL. How should these indices be interpreted in C.U.?

[SI units: MCV, 108 fL; MCH, 38 pg; MCHC, 340 g/L]

Usually, the MCH and MCV are both increased and the MCHC is normal in macrocytic anemias associated with vitamin B_{12} or folic acid deficiency. The MCH is increased because the RBCs have increased in size; however, the concentration of Hgb (MCHC) has not changed. This characteristic picture is illustrated in the alcoholic patient, C.U., who is likely to have a dietary folic acid deficiency. If C.U.'s indices were normal (normocytic, normochromic) and if anemia was present (decreased Hgb or Hct), acute blood loss from injuries he sustained in the brawl should be considered. If the anemia seems to be more chronic in nature, alcohol-induced bone marrow suppression should be considered (see Chapters 28 and 84).

Reticulocytes

Adults—Normal: 0.1% to 2.4% of RBCs or 0.001 to 0.024 I

Reticulocytes are young, immature erythrocytes (RBCs). The reticulocyte count measures the percentage of these new cells in the circulating blood. An increase in the number of reticulocytes implies an increased number of erythrocytes are being released into the blood in response to a stimulus. Because erythrocytes regenerate rapidly, reticulocytosis can be noted within 3 to 5 days after hemolysis or after a hemorrhagic episode. Appropriate treatment of anemias caused by iron, vitamin B_{12}, or folic acid deficiencies should result in an increased reticulocyte count. Caution must be exercised in the interpretation of reticulocyte counts. Changes in the number of RBCs will result in proportional changes in the reticulocyte count because the latter is reported as a percentage of the number of RBCs.

Erythrocyte Sedimentation Rate

Males—Normal: 0 to 20 mm/hour
Females—Normal: 0 to 30 mm/hour

The ESR is the rate at which erythrocytes settle to the bottom of a test tube through the forces of gravity and in response to fibrinogen levels in the blood. The ESR is a nonspecific value and may be increased abnormally in acute and chronic inflammatory processes, acute and chronic infections, neoplasms, infarction, tissue necrosis, rheumatoid-collagen disease, dysproteinemias, nephritis, and pregnancy. Laboratory technique can affect the sedimentation rate substantially.[22] Because many factors can enhance the settling rate of RBCs, moderate to marked elevation of the ESR merely indicates an inflammatory component to a disease state. An increased ESR in the setting of a normal physical examination is usually transitory and is rarely the harbinger of serious occult disease.[33]

White Blood Cells

Normal: 3.2 to 9.8 × 10^3/mm^3 or 3.2 to 9.8 × 10^9/L

Leukocytes or WBCs are comprised of five different types of cells. Neutrophils are the most abundant of the circulating WBCs, followed in order of frequency by lymphocytes, monocytes, eosinophils, and basophils. The neutrophils, eosinophils, basophils, and monocytes are formed from stem cells in the bone marrow. Lymphocytes are formed primarily in the lymph nodes, thymus, spleen, and, to a lesser extent, bone marrow (Fig. 2-2). Each WBCs has unique functions, and it is best to consider them independently rather than collectively as "leukocytes."[34] Ultimately, all WBCs contribute to host defense mechanisms. A convenient mnemonic for remembering the various types of WBCs is "Never Let Monkeys Eat Bananas" (N = neutrophils; L = lymphocytes; M = monocytes; E = eosinophils; and B = basophils).

Neutrophils

Normal: 54% to 62% of WBC

The terms "polys," "segs," "polymorphonuclear neutrophils," and "granulocytes" are synonymous with the term "neutrophil" in clinical practice. The number of neutrophils is commonly increased during bacterial or fungal infections because these cells are essential in killing invading microorganisms. While the bone marrow increases production of new leukocytes, there is also an increase in the number of circulating immature neutrophils (e.g., bands); this phenomenon is commonly referred to as a "left shift," which suggests bacterial infection.[32]

However, neutrophils are also important in the pathogenesis of tissue damage in some noninfectious diseases, such as rheumatoid arthritis, inflammatory bowel disease, asthma, MI, or gout.[35] Increased neutrophils or neutrophilia can also be encountered during metabolic toxic states (e.g., diabetic ketoacidosis, uremia, eclampsia) and during physiological response to stress (e.g., physical exercise, childbirth). Drugs (e.g., epinephrine, corticosteroids) can also cause significant neutrophilia, primarily by demargination from blood vessel walls.

Agranulocytosis and Absolute Neutrophil Count

The condition involving decreased neutrophils, or neutropenia, is defined as a neutrophil count of <2,000 cells/mm^3; agranulocytosis refers to severe neutropenia. The degree of neutropenia is often expressed by the absolute neutrophil count (ANC). The ANC is defined as the total number of granulocytes (polymorphonuclear leukocytes and band forms) present in the circulating pool of WBCs and can be calculated as WBC × (% neutrophils + % bands)/100. Generally, the risk of infection is low when the ANC exceeds 1,000/mm^3; however, the risk of infection increases significantly when the ANC is <500/mm^3. The risk of developing bacteremia is increased further as the ANC decreases to <100/mm^3, a condition commonly referred to as "profound neutropenia" (see Chapter 68). The most common causes of neutropenia are metastatic carcinoma, lymphoma, and chemotherapeutic agents.

Lymphocytes

Normal: 25% to 33% of WBC

Lymphocytes constitute the second most common WBC in circulating blood. These leukocytes respond to foreign antigens by initiating the immune defense system. The vast majority of lymphocytes is located in the spleen, lymph nodes, and other organized lymphatic tissue. The lymphocytes circulating in blood represent <5% of the total amount in the body.

There are two major types of lymphocytes. T lymphocytes (thymic dependent) participate in cell-mediated immune responses, and B lymphocytes (bone marrow derived) are responsible for humoral antibody responses. Therefore, diseases affecting lymphocytes primarily manifest themselves as immune deficiency disorders that render the patient unable to defend against normal pathogens (see Chapter 69) or as autoimmune diseases in which immune responses are directed against the body's own cells.[34]

Increased numbers of lymphocytes on a white count differential sometimes accompany lymphoma (see Chapter 90) and viral infections such as infectious mononucleosis, mumps, and rubella. A relative lymphocytosis is sometimes encountered when the total lymphocytes have remained constant despite a decline in the total neutrophils.

Monocytes

Normal: 3% to 7% of WBC

Monocytes are formed in the bone marrow and are the precursors to macrophages and antigen-presenting cells (dendritic cells), which are found in the body's tissues.[36] Macrophages and dendritic cells are phagocytic cells that engulf foreign antigens or dead or dying cells. Dendritic cells also present fragments of antigens to T and B lymphocytes. Monocytosis may be observed in mononucleosis, subacute bacterial endocarditis, malaria, and tuberculosis, as well as during the recovery phase of some infections.

Eosinophils

Normal: 1% to 3% of WBC

Because eosinophils have surface receptors that bind IgG and IgE, they can modify reactions associated with IgG- and IgE-mediated degranulation of mast cells. Primary lysosomal granules, small dense granules, and specific or secondary granules are the three types of granules found within eosinophils. The latter granules account for most of the biological activity of eosinophils and are toxic to parasites, tumor cells, and some epithelial cells.[37]

Eosinophils have phagocytic activity, catalyze the oxidation of many substances, facilitate killing of micro-organisms, initiate mast cell secretion, protect against various parasites, and play some role in host defense. Eosinophilia is probably most commonly associated with allergic reactions to drugs, allergic disorders (e.g., hay fever, asthma, eczema), invasive parasitic infections (e.g., hookworm, schistosomiasis, trichinosis), collagen vascular diseases (e.g., rheumatoid arthritis, eosinophilic fasciitis, eosinophilic-myalgia syndrome), and malignancies (e.g., Hodgkin disease).[38–40]

Basophils

Normal: <1% of WBC

During infection or inflammation, basophils leave the blood and mobilize as mast cells to the affected site and release granules. These granules contain histamine, serotonin, prostaglandins, and leukotrienes. Degranulation results in an increased blood flow to the site and may compound inflammatory processes. An increase in basophils commonly accompanies allergic and anaphylactic responses, chronic myeloid leukemia, myelofibrosis, and polycythemia vera. A decrease in the number of basophils is generally not readily apparent because of the small number of these cells in the blood.[34]

14. R.L., a 45-year-old man, is hospitalized with a sustained high fever of 39.4°C, SOB, and pleurisy. His cough is productive of rusty sputum, and he appears to be in acute distress. The results of the CBC and leukocyte differential are as follows: total WBC count, 18,000/mm^3; neutrophils, 76%; bands, 13%; lymphocytes, 10%; monocytes, 0; eosinophils, 1%; and basophils, 0. On the basis of this laboratory report and other findings, a diagnosis of pneumococcal pneumonia is suspected. How is R.L.'s laboratory report consistent with bacterial infection?

[SI units: WBC, 1.8 × 10^9/L; neutrophils, 0.76; bands, 0.13; lymphocytes, 0.10; eosinophils, 0.01]

WBCs are the host's chief defense system, and the neutrophil is the main component of that system. During bacterial infections, the leukocyte count and the neutrophils are generally increased, and a left shift (increase in bands) may be noticeable. The percentage of other types of WBCs is decreased proportionately because the number of neutrophils is increased.

As the infection progresses, the percentage of band cells may decrease as a result of an increase in the number of neutrophils that have a longer half-life. This decrease in bands does not necessarily indicate improvement. A decrease in the percentage of neutrophils with a decrease in the total WBC count is characteristic of effective antibiotic therapy.

15. S.Q., a 35-year-old woman, was treated for 7 days with dicloxacillin for cellulitis of the left leg. On the eighth day, an allergic urticarial rash developed. The CBC showed a total leukocyte count of 10,000/mm^3 with 6% eosinophils. What is the significance of this eosinophil count?

[SI units: WBC, 1.0 × 10^9/L; eosinophils, 0.06]

In the clinical setting, absolute leukocyte counts may be used in conjunction with normal reference values. Absolute counts are calculated by multiplying the percentage of each individual cell by the total leukocyte count. Eosinophils are usually increased in allergic reactions; therefore, a drug-induced hypersensitivity reaction is a strong probability in S.Q., with an absolute count of 600 eosinophils/mm^3 (i.e., 6% of 10,000 leukocytes). The clinician should be suspicious of an allergic drug reaction when absolute eosinophil counts exceed 300 cells/mm^3. Eosinophils may increase before, after, or concurrent with other evidence of allergy (e.g., rash). Eosinophilia without evidence of allergy is not sufficient cause to discontinue a suspected medication unless the eosinophilia is significant (i.e., >2,000 cells/mm^3). In addition, the absence of eosinophilia certainly does not rule out an allergic diagnosis in a patient exhibiting clear clinical manifestations of an apparent allergic reaction.

Thrombocytes

Normal: 130 to 400 × 10^3/mm^3 or 130 to 400 × 10^9/L

Appropriate platelet (i.e., thrombocyte) function is essential to blood clotting. Decreased platelet counts or thrombocytopenia may lead to petechiae, ecchymosis, and spontaneous hemorrhage. Causes include decreased platelet production, accelerated destruction, loss from excessive bleeding/trauma, dilution of blood samples secondary to blood transfusion, sequestration secondary to hypersplenism, disseminated intravascular coagulation, infection, or systemic lupus erythematosus. Malignancy, rheumatoid arthritis, iron-deficiency anemia, polycythemia vera, and postsplenectomy syndromes are the most common causes of elevated platelet counts or thrombocytosis.

Coagulation Studies

The control of bleeding depends on the formation of a platelet plug and the formation of a stable fibrin clot. The formation of this clot, the complex interactions of plasma proteins and clotting factors, and the clinical application of laboratory tests of coagulation are described in Chapter 15. The prothrombin time (PT), international normalized ratio (INR), and activated partial thromboplastin time (aPTT) are used to diagnose coagulation abnormalities or to monitor the effectiveness of patients receiving anticoagulation therapy. When used to assess drug therapy, achieving a value outside the "normal" range is in fact a therapeutically desirable outcome. These tests are described briefly in this chapter, with the understanding that the reader will refer to Chapter 15 to gain the appropriate perspective on the clinical applicability of these tests.

Activated Partial Thromboplastin Time

aPTT measures the intrinsic clotting system, which depends on factors VIII, IX, XI, and XII and the factors involved in the final common pathway of the clotting cascade (factors II, X, and V). The typical control ranges from 35 to 45 seconds. aPTT is commonly used to monitor unfractionated heparin therapy.

Prothrombin Time

Prothrombin is synthesized in the liver and is converted to thrombin during the blood clotting process. Thrombin formation is the critical event in the hemostatic process because thrombin creates fibrin monomers that ultimately assemble into a clot and stimulates platelet activation. The PT test directly measures the activity of clotting factors VII, X, prothrombin (factor II), and fibrinogen. Automated laboratory instruments measure PT by recording the time required for the blood to clot after tissue thromboplastin has been added to the patient's blood sample. The reference range depends on the specific laboratory, but is usually between 10 and 12 seconds when rabbit brain thromboplastin is used.

International Normalized Ratio

Although INR is the recommended method to accurately monitor anticoagulant therapy, several potential problems have been identified with the INR system. Because of the variable sensitivity of thromboplastin reagents to decreases in specific clotting factors, there may be a lack of reliability of the INR system when it is used at the onset of warfarin therapy and for screening for a coagulopathy. Despite these potential problems with the INR system, the American College of Chest Physicians unanimously recommends using the INR system of reporting during initiation and maintenance of anticoagulant therapy.[41] However, attempts to standardize laboratory reporting have not completely eliminated the variability observed between different laboratories, so clinicians must be cautious when interpreting coagulation parameters obtained for more than one institution.

The INR is calculated using Equation 2-9, where the prothrombin ratio (PTR) is the ratio between the patient's PT and the laboratory's control PT, and the ISI is the international sensitivity index. Commercial manufacturers quantify the ISI for the specific thromboplastin reagent used in each lot and report this information in the product package insert. For a thorough review on the monitoring of anticoagulant therapy, see Chapter 15.

$$\text{INR} = \left\{\frac{\text{PT(patient)}}{\text{PT(control)}}\right\}^{\text{ISI}} = \text{PTR}^{\text{ISI}} \qquad \textbf{2-9}$$

URINALYSIS

A standard urinalysis begins with simple observation of the color and the gross general appearance of the urine specimen. The urine pH and specific gravity are then recorded. Formed elements in the urine are examined microscopically, and the urine is searched routinely for pathologically significant substances that are normally not present (e.g., glucose, blood, ketones, bile pigments).

Gross Appearance of the Specimen

The concentrated, first-morning urine specimen is usually analyzed to eliminate effects of undue dilution as a result of water intake. The color should be slightly yellow, depending on the degree of dilution, and the appearance should be clear. The appearance of the urine may reveal clouds of crystals, bilirubin, blood, porphyrins, proteins, food or drug colorings, or melanin. Discolored urine is abnormal. A red coloration of the urine may be imparted by blood, porphyria, or ingestion of phenolphthalein. A brown urine color may be caused by the acid hematin of blood or from melanin pigments. Excessive excretion of urobilinogen or the effects of drugs such as rifampin or phenazopyridine may cause a dark orange urine color. A blue to blue-green color of the urine may result from the systemic administration of methylene blue.

Specimen pH

When freshly produced, urine is normally mostly acidic (pH 4.6–8). Alkaline urine may indicate an aged specimen, systemic alkalosis, failure of renal acidifying mechanisms, or infection in the urinary tract.

Specific Gravity

A normal morning urine specimen should have a specific gravity of 1.020 to 1.025. The upper end of this range is close to the maximal concentrating ability of the kidney. Glomerular filtrate has a specific gravity of 1.010, and a urine of such a low specific gravity, under conditions of restricted water intake, would suggest failure of renal concentrating mechanisms. When water intake is not restricted, specific gravity readings are difficult to interpret.

Protein

Proteinuria is a classic sign of renal injury and a matter of concern. If proteinuria is found during the evaluation of a patient with a nonrenal illness, it suggests that the disease may also involve the kidneys (i.e., hypertension, diabetes).[42] A healthy adult generally excretes 30 to 130 mg/day of protein into the urine.

Protein in a urine sample is generally tested qualitatively on a random urine sample by a dipstick method and is usually reported on a scale of 0 (<30 mg/dL), 1+ (30–100 mg/dL), 2+ (100–300 mg/dL), 3+ (300–1,000 mg/dL), and 4+ (>1,000 mg/dL). A positive qualitative test for urine protein should be repeated after a few days because transient proteinuria can accompany various physiological and pathological states, even when kidney function is normal. Therefore, patients with CHF, seizures, or febrile illnesses and normal renal function need not undergo invasive renal function tests if the proteinuria is modest and likely to be transient. Another qualitative evaluation of proteinuria can be performed in about 2 weeks to confirm the diagnosis of transient proteinuria.[43] If subsequent qualitative test results are positive, a 24-hour urine sample should be collected to quantitatively test for protein and creatinine (see Creatinine Clearance section). In patients with a normal 24-hour urinary protein concentration, previous positive qualitative test results probably represent either false-positive results or a transient phenomenon.[42]

Microscopic Examination

The urine sediment is examined for RBCs, WBCs, casts, yeast, crystals, and epithelial cells.

RBCs should be absent in normal urine, although one or two RBCs per high-power field (HPF) would still be considered in the normal range. Bleeding or clotting disorders, some collagen diseases, and various bladder, urethral, and prostatic conditions may cause microscopic hematuria. In females, vaginal blood occasionally contaminates the urine specimen, but the presence of numerous squamous epithelial cells should be sufficient to alert clinicians to this artifact.

WBCs should be virtually absent in normal urine, although up to five WBCs/HPF would still be in the normal range. The presence of WBCs in the urine usually suggests an acute infection in the urinary tract (see Chapter 64). Some noninfectious inflammatory diseases of the kidney, ureter, or bladder may also contribute WBCs to the urine sediment.

Casts are composed of proteinaceous or fatty material that outlines the shape of the renal tubules where they were deposited. The presence of casts in the urine must be interpreted in light of other factors related to the kidney and its function; however, fatty casts, RBC casts, and WBC casts are always significant. RBC casts usually suggest glomerular injury, and WBC casts suggest tubular or interstitial injury. Lipid casts with proteinuria are characteristic findings in patients with the nephrotic syndrome.[44] The finding of hyaline casts alone in the presence of proteinuria suggests a renal origin for the protein. Hyaline or granular casts alone, however, only suggest some defect in factors that affect cast formation, and are therefore difficult to interpret.

Crystals may originally appear as a cloud in the urine. Their formation is pH dependent, and they often appear only as the urine cools to room temperature or in concentrated urine. In acid urine, crystals may be uric acid or calcium oxalate; in alkaline urine, they may be phosphates. Crystals per se are not highly significant, although they may reflect a tendency toward the formation of renal calculi (see Chapter 30).

16. R.C. is a 23-year-old man who was diagnosed with type 1 diabetes mellitus about 10 years ago; until now, his diabetes has been well controlled with an aggressive insulin regimen. His sister brings him to the emergency department with a 3-day history of fever, chills, dysuria, malaise, and some confusion. He also complains of nausea and vomiting and a poor appetite. Because he has not been able to keep any food down for about 48 hours, he has not taken his insulin. A finger stick blood glucose is 545 mg/dL, and a stat midstream urinalysis and Gram stain indicate the following: pH 5.2; appearance cloudy; specific gravity 1.033; urine protein 3+; urine glucose 4+; urine ketones positive; urine bacteria 4+; urine WBC, too numerous to count (TNTC); squamous epithelial, few per HPF; urine nitrite positive; and Gram stain, numerous gram-negative rods. What objective data from the urinalysis indicate that R.C. is critically ill?

[SI unit: glucose, 30.3 mmol/L]

The cloudy appearance of R.C.'s urine indicates the presence of bacteria, protein, and WBCs, which is substantiated by the data (4+ bacteria, 3+ protein, and TNTC WBCs). The lack of a significant amount of squamous epithelial cells, the presence of a significant amount of nitrite-producing bacteria, and the Gram stain indicate a clean-catch urine specimen

Table 2-3 FDA and Non–FDA-Approved Products Available for Patient-Directed Monitoring or Testing

Blood Chemistry	Fertility—Female
Blood glucose monitors	Ovulation tests (LH)
Glycosylated hemoglobin (A1c)	Pregnancy tests (hCG)
Lipids (TC, HDL, LDL, TG)	Menopause tests (FSH)
Prothrombin (PT, INR)	Maternity testing (DNA)
	Hormone tests (estrogen, progesterone, testosterone)
Screening for Disease or Infection	**Drugs of Abuse**
Middle ear monitor (otitis media)	Alcohol
Urinary tract infection	Nicotine
Urine dipsticks	THC (marijuana)
Glucose, ketones, specific gravity, blood, pH, protein, nitrite, leukocytes	Cocaine
Anemia (Hgb)	Opiates
Hepatitis C	Amphetamines
HIV	Methamphetamines
Kidney disease (microalbuminuria)	PCP-phencyclidine
Thyroid (TSH)	Barbiturates
Fecal occult blood test	Benzodiazepines
Fertility—Male	MDMA (ecstasy)
Fertility tests (sperm counts)	
Paternity testing (DNA)	
Hormone tests (testosterone, DHEA)	

A1c, glycosylated hemoglobin; DHEA, dehydroepiandrosterone; FDA, U.S. Food and Drug Administration; FSH, follicle-stimulating hormone; hCG, human chorionic gonadotropin; HDL, high-density lipoprotein; Hgb, hemoglobin; INR, international normalized ratio; LDL, low-density lipoprotein; LH, luteinizing hormone; MDMA, 3′4-methylelenedioxy-methamphetamine; PCP, phencyclidine; PT, prothrombin time; TC, total cholesterol; TG, triglyceride; THC, tetrahydrocannabinol; TSH, thyroid-stimulating hormone.

and a urinary tract infection (UTI) involving gram-negative organisms. Because the renal threshold of glucose is typically 180 mg/dL, the presence of 4+ glucose in the urine indicates that the blood glucose concentration significantly exceeds this figure (substantiated by blood glucose of 545 mg/dL). Acidification of the urine and ketonuria occur after the release of ketone bodies into the bloodstream after the breakdown of fatty acids for energy utilization. It is likely that R.C. has a severe UTI and, most likely, diabetic ketoacidosis. (See Chapters 50 and 64 for thorough discussions of diabetes, diabetic ketoacidosis, and UTIs.)

PATIENT-DIRECTED MONITORING AND TESTING

Often patient-directed self-monitoring is an essential component to successful management of certain disease states such as blood pressure monitoring for hypertension and blood glucose monitoring for diabetes mellitus. When used appropriately, data obtained from these monitoring devices can be used by health care providers and consumers to initiate or modify therapies accordingly.

Additional laboratory, self-monitoring tests or devices are also available for consumers to purchase for independent testing or screening purposes at home (Table 2-3). Some products provide an immediate result, whereas others require submitting a completed kit to a laboratory for analysis. Samples may be obtained from various sources, including urine, blood, saliva, stool, or hair samples. In 1992, sales of over-the-counter diagnostic tests in the United States were $750 million. By 2002, sales jumped to $2.8 billion annually.[45] The incidence of consumers using these products has significantly increased and likely will continue to climb due to increased access via the Internet as well as additional tests becoming available.

In the United States, some, but not all, patient-directed tests have been approved by the U.S. Food and Drug Administration (FDA). A current listing of approved products is available though the FDA's Office of In Vitro Diagnostic Device Evaluation and Safety (OIVD) and can be accessed online at http://www.fda.gov/cdrh/oivd/.[46] Consumers should be cautioned about the accuracy of tests that have not been approved and the validity of all test results, especially for diagnostic purposes, because many factors can impact or interfere with the sensitivity (probability of obtaining a positive result when sample is truly positive) and specificity (probability of obtaining a negative result when the sample is truly negative). Follow-up assessment with a health care provider should be encouraged to confirm or refute patient-directed test results. provides examples of tests available. Readers are encouraged to refer to the *Handbook of Nonprescription Drugs* for a detailed description of commonly used patient-directed tests.[47]

REFERENCES

1. McPherson RA, Pincus MR. Henry's Clinical Diagnosis and Management by Laboratory Methods. 21st ed. Philadelphia: WB Saunders Company; 2006.
2. Evans PC, Cleary JD. SI units—are we leaders or followers? [editorial]. *Ann Pharmacother* 1993;27:97.
3. Vaughan LM. SI units: is it pass the mass but hold the mole? [editorial]. *Ann Pharmacother* 1993;29:99.
4. Laposata M. *SI Unit Conversion Guide.* Boston: NEJM Books; 1992.
5. Kratz A, Lewandrowski KB. Case records of Massachusetts General Hospital normal reference laboratory values. *N Engl J Med* 1998;339:1063.
6. Winter ME et al. *Basic Clinical Pharmacokinetics.* 4th ed. Baltimore: Lippincot Williams & Wilkins; 2004.
7. Cockcroft DW, Gault MH. Prediction of creatinine clearance from serum creatinine. *Nephron* 1976; 16:31.
8. Rhodes PJ et al. Evaluation of eight methods for estimating creatinine clearance in men. *Clin Pharm* 1987;6:399.
9. Jelliffe RW. Creatinine clearance: bedside estimate. *Ann Intern Med* 1973;79:604.
10. Hull JH et al. Influence of range of renal function and liver disease on predictability of creatinine clearance. *Clin Pharmacol Ther* 1981;29:516.
11. Stratton IM et al. Association of glycaemia with macrovascular and microvascular complications of type 2 diabetes (UKPDS 35): prospective observational study. *BMJ* 2000;321:405.
12. Lee TH, Goldman L. Serum enzyme assays on the diagnosis of acute myocardial infarction. *Ann Intern Med* 1986;105:221.
13. White RD et al. Diagnostic and prognostic significance of minimally elevated creatine kinase-MB in suspected acute myocardial infarction. *Am J Cardiol* 1985;55:1478.
14. Roberts R. Where, oh where has the MB gone? *N Engl J Med* 1985;313:1081.
15. Hamm CW. New serum markers for acute myocardial infarction. *N Engl J Med* 1994;331:607.
16. Chapelle JP. Cardiac troponin I and troponin T: recent players in the field of myocardial markers. *Clin Chem Lab Med* 1999;37:11.
17. Malasky BR, Alpert JS. Diagnosis of myocardial injury by biochemical markers: problems and promises. *Cardiol Rev* 2002;10:306.
18. Rasouli ML et al. Plasma homocysteine predicts progression of atherosclerosis. *Atherosclerosis* 2005;181:159.
19. Cardarelli R, Lumicao TG Jr. B-type natriuretic peptide: a review of its diagnostic, prognostic, and therapeutic monitoring value in heart failure for primary care physicians. *J Am Board Fam Pract* 2003;16:327.
20. Natrecor (nesiritide). *Prescriber information.* Mountain View, CA: Scioc Inc.; January 2007.
21. Ridker PM et al. Novel risk factors for systemic atherosclerosis: a comparison of C-reactive protein, fibrinogen, homocysteine, lipoprotein(a), and standard cholesterol screening as predictors of peripheral arterial disease. *JAMA* 2001;285:2481.
22. Ravel R. *Clinical Laboratory Medicine: Clinical Application of Laboratory Data.* 6th ed. St. Louis, MO: Mosby; 1995.
23. Schmid R. Bilirubin metabolism in man. *N Engl J Med* 1972;285:703.
24. Barry MJ. Prostate-specific-antigen testing for early diagnosis of prostate cancer. *N Engl J Med* 2001; 344:1373.
25. Smith RA et al. American Cancer Society guidelines for the early detection of cancer: update of the early detection guidelines for prostate, colorectal, and endometrial cancers. *CA Cancer J Clin* 2001;51:38.
26. American Urological Association. Prostate-specific-antigen (PSA) best practice policy. *Oncology (Huntingt)* 2000;14:267.
27. Catalona W et al. Use of the percentage of free prostate-specific antigen to enhance differentiation of prostate cancer from benign prostatic disease: a prospective multicenter clinical trial. *JAMA* 1998;279:1542.
28. Lange PH. New information about prostate-specific antigen and the paradoxes of prostate cancer. *JAMA* 1995;273:336.
29. Stone NJ et al. Recent National Cholesterol Education Program Adult Treatment Panel III update: adjustments and options. *Am J Cardiol* 2005;96(4A):53E.
30. Greer J et al. *Wintrobe's Clinical Hematology.* 11th ed. Philadelphia: Lippincott Williams & Wilkins; 2004.
31. Keenan WF. Macrocytosis as an indicator of human disease. *J Am Board Fam Pract* 1989;2:252.
32. Henry JB, ed. *Clinical Diagnosis and Management by Laboratory Methods.* 20th ed. Philadelphia: WB Saunders; 2001.
33. Sox HC, Liang MH. The erythrocyte sedimentation rate. *Ann Intern Med* 1986;104:515.
34. Winkelstein A et al. *White Cell Manual.* 5th ed. Philadelphia: FA Davis; 1998.
35. Malech HL, Gallin JI. Neutrophils in human diseases. *N Engl J Med* 1987;317:687.
36. Cline MG et al. Monocytes and macrophages: functions and diseases. *Ann Intern Med* 1978;88:78.
37. Beeson PB. Cancer and eosinophilia. *N Engl J Med* 1983;309:792.
38. Butterworth AE, David JR. Eosinophil function. *N Engl J Med* 1981;304:154.
39. Clauw DJ et al. Tryptophan-associated eosinophilic connective-tissue disease. *JAMA* 1990;263:1502.
40. Dombrowicz D, Capron M. Eosinophils, allergy and parasites. *Curr Opin Immunol* 2001;13:716.
41. Seventh ACCP consensus conference on antithrombotic and thrombolytic therapy: evidence based guidelines. *Chest* 2004;126(Suppl):204S.
42. Abuelo JG. Proteinuria: diagnostic principles and procedures. *Ann Intern Med* 1983;98:186.
43. Reuben DB et al. Transient proteinuria in emergency medical admissions. *N Engl J Med* 1982;306:1031.
44. Morrin PAF. Urinary sediment in the interpretation of proteinuria. *Ann Intern Med* 1983;98:254.
45. Demetrakakes P. Health kit packaging helps consumers feel at home with self-care: packaging for home health monitoring devices combines healthcare concerns with appeal to both consumers and retailers—medical packaging. Food & Drug Packaging 2003; February.
46. U.S. Food and Drug Administration (FDA), Office of In Vitro Diagnostic Device Evaluation and Safety (OIVD) Web site. Available at: www.fda.gov/cdrh/oivd/. Accessed April 10, 2008.
47. Rosenthal WM, Briggs GC. Home testing and monitoring devices. In: Berardi RR et al., eds. *Handbook of Nonprescription Drugs.* 14th ed. Washington, DC: American Pharmaceutical Association; 2004:1179.

CHAPTER 3

Herbs and Nutritional Supplements

Cathi Dennehy and Candy Tsourounis

INTRODUCTION

During the 1990s, the terms "alternative," "complementary," "unconventional," and "integrative" described health care practices that were not commonly taught or practiced by health care providers in the United States.[1] Today, these practices are more widely accepted within the mainstream of care, so the terms "complementary" or "integrative" are most commonly used to describe them. These terms more accurately reflect the combined use of complementary therapies and conventional medicine. Some complementary therapies used today include homeopathy, massage therapy, aromatherapy, acupuncture, acupressure, herbs and supplements, reflexology, and chiropractic care. This chapter focuses on dietary supplements, one of the most common forms of complementary care.[1,2]

In the United States, the popularity and use of herbs and dietary supplements has increased significantly since 1994. This has led to an estimated $17.8 billion market for these products. The U.S. Food and Drug Administration (FDA) estimates that there are more than 29,000 different dietary supplements available to consumers, with an estimated 1,000 new products introduced to the market annually. Given the vast demand for these products, consumers need accurate information on their safety and effectiveness so they can make informed choices.

According to one national survey, consumers often do not discuss the use of dietary supplements with their health care providers because they believe their providers know little or nothing about these products and are biased against them.[3] This practice can be hazardous if the consumer is self-treating a serious disorder with a dietary supplement for which more effective therapies exist, or if the supplement interacts with a particular medication or exacerbates a disease state. Indeed, nearly 16% of prescription drug users also report having taken a dietary supplement at the same time.[4] Many consumers believe so strongly in the potential health benefits of certain dietary supplements that they would continue taking them even if they were proven to be ineffective.[3] This emphasizes the importance of open communication with patients regarding their health care needs and beliefs and, in particular, their use of these products. One study found that consumers who use alternative health care practices were not necessarily dissatisfied with their medical care.[5] Instead, alternative health care was more consistent with their way of life and attitudes toward health and living.

This chapter is designed to provide an evidence-based approach and critical analysis of the scientific literature on herbal and other supplements. The quality of the scientific literature in this area varies significantly, in that many studies suffer from flaws in study design, statistical analysis, small sample size, bias, and blinding. When possible, the recommendations made are designed to be in the best interest of the patient. Providing consumers with quality information will help them make educated decisions related to their care.

Although many products are available on the market, this chapter addresses some of the more common herbal and nutritional supplements. A summary of the products reviewed in this chapter appears in Table 3-1.

German Commission E

The prevalence of dietary supplement use in Europe far exceeds that of the United States. Therefore, it is not surprising that one of the first groups to examine the safety and efficacy of herbal products was established in Germany. In 1978, the German Commission E, an expert panel composed of physicians, toxicologists, pharmacists, pharmacologists, biostatisticians, and others, was assembled by the German Federal Health Agency.[6] Its purpose was to review the available clinical information on herbs and to determine which ones achieved "reasonable certainty of efficacy and absolute safety."[7] More than 300 herbs and herbal combinations were reviewed by the German Commission E, and its findings were published in the German *Bundesanzeiger*, which is similar to the *Federal Register*.[7] This information was translated and published in English by the American Botanical Council. Today, the German Commission E monographs are used to a limited degree because much more evidence exists in the form of controlled trials for many of the popular dietary supplements.

Dietary Supplement Health and Education Act

In 1994, the U.S. Congress passed a bill that revolutionized the market for nonprescription drugs. The Dietary Supplement Health and Education Act (DSHEA) of 1994 (PL 103-417) was created to regulate dietary supplements: botanicals, vitamins, minerals, tissue extracts, and amino acids.[8] The DSHEA has special provisions that regulate dietary supplements as foods, removing them from regulation as pharmaceuticals. Manufacturers of dietary supplements can make labeling claims without submitting evidence to the FDA, but they are responsible for the truthfulness of those claims. The FDA cannot remove a product from the market unless the product is proven to pose a serious or unreasonable risk to consumers. In contrast, pharmaceuticals must demonstrate a significant degree of safety and efficacy before they are approved for marketing. These differences have led to the rapid growth of the dietary supplement industry.

The terms used in this chapter to refer to dietary supplements differ from the FDA definition. Herbal remedy (botanical) is used to refer to any product derived from a plant source. Nutritional supplement is used to refer to vitamins, minerals, cofactors, enzymes, amino acids, and others. Despite the legal classifications and variations in nomenclature, dietary supplements are indeed drugs in that they do alter the structure and function of the body for the treatment or prevention of disease.

Product Labeling

Product labeling refers to both the label of the actual product and any accompanying written information. The labeling on a product must conform to the provisions in the Code of Federal Regulations for foods,[8] which states that the principal display panel (PDP) must contain the name of the product and the contents in net weight. Other information about the product is located on the information panel, usually found to the right of the PDP. Currently, not all supplements on the market conform to these regulations, especially if they are imported from other countries. As of March 23, 1999, specific labeling requirements were required for all products sold as dietary supplements. The rules require manufacturers to include the terms "dietary supplement" as part of the name of the product. For example, vitamin C is sold as "Vitamin C Dietary Supplement." Ingredient requirements also changed. Products are

Table 3-1 Summary of Herbal Products and Nutritional Supplements Reviewed

Herbal/Nutritional Supplement	Proposed Indication(s)	Authors' Interpretation of Level of Evidence for Use in a Clinical Setting[a]	Dosing
Garlic	Hyperlipidemia	Promising	Standardized to contain 1.3% alliin or 0.6% allicin (600–900 mg powdered garlic/day in two to three divided doses) Equivalent to 1.8–2.7 g fresh garlic daily (one clove is approximately 3 g)
Allium sativum	Hypertension	Doubtful	
	Antiplatelet	Promising	
	Antiatherosclerotic	Promising	
	Cancer prevention	Investigational	
	Antitumor/antiproliferative	Unknown	
	Antimicrobial	Investigational	
	Diabetes/hypoglycemia	Doubtful	
Ginkgo	Dementia	Promising	Ginkgo biloba extract standardized to contain 22%–24% flavone glycosides and 5%–7% terpene lactones (120–240 mg/day in two or three divided doses)
Ginkgo biloba	Peripheral vascular disease	Promising	
	Stress/anxiety	Unknown	
	Short-term memory	Doubtful	
	Tinnitus/hearing loss	Promising	
	Sexual dysfunction	Investigational	
St. John's wort	Mild to moderate depression	Promising	Alcoholic extract standardized to contain at least 0.3% hypericin or 5% hyperforin (900 mg/day in three divided doses)
Hypericum perforatum	Antiviral	Investigational	
	Wound healing (topical)	Unknown	
Echinacea	Cold treatment	Promising	6–9 mL of *E. purpurea* fresh-pressed juice or 900 mg/day of *E. pallida* root (1:5 tincture, 50% ethanol); administer in divided doses (e.g., 15–30 drops of *E. purpurea* juice equivalent to 0.75–1.5 mL, two to five times daily)
Echinacea purpurea	Cold prophylaxis	Doubtful	
Echinacea pallida	Urinary tract infection (supportive treatment)	Unknown	
	Wound healing	Unknown	
Saw palmetto	Benign prostatic hyperplasia	Promising	Lipophilic extract standardized to contain 85%–95% fatty acids and sterols; 160 mg BID
Serenoa repens			
Panax ginseng	Adaptogen	Unknown	*P. ginseng* extract standardized to contain at least 7% ginsenosides; 1–2 g of the crude root or its equivalent (1 g of crude root is equivalent to 200 mg of the extract)
	Ergogenic	Unknown	
	Immune modulation	Promising	
	Anticancer/antitumor	Promising	
	Diabetes/hypoglycemia	Promising	
	Hyperlipidemia	Unknown	
	Hypertension/cardiovascular	Unknown	
	Erectile dysfunction/infertility	Investigational	
Glucosamine	Osteoarthritis	Promising	500–1,000 mg TID; 1,500 mg once daily
	Wound healing	Doubtful	
	Antioxidant	Investigational	
Shark cartilage	Anticancer	Doubtful	1 g/kg/day or 80–100 g/day given in three divided doses
	Antimicrobial	Doubtful	*ZGG:* 13.3 mg Q 2 hr while awake
Zinc	Common cold	Promising	*ZG:* 23 mg Q 2 hr while awake
	Allergic rhinitis	Investigational	*ZA:* 10 mg Q 2 hr while awake
Melatonin	Jet lag	Doubtful	*Jet lag:* 5–8 mg IR the evening of departure and for 3–5 days after
	Insomnia	Promising	
	Reproduction	Investigational	*Insomnia:* 0.3–5 mg once nightly for sleep onset
	Antioxidant	Investigational	Higher dosages may be required for sleep maintenance
	Immune modulation	Investigational	
	Anticancer	Investigational	
	Aging	Doubtful	
	Depression	Doubtful	
Coenzyme Q10	Hypertension	Promising	100–120 mg daily; given in two to three divided doses
	Heart failure	Promising	50–150 mg daily in two to three divided doses

HIV, Human immunodeficiency virus; IR, immediate release; ZA, zinc acetate; ZG, zinc gluconate; ZGG, zinc gluconate-glycine.

[a]Promising: A sufficient number of double-blind, placebo-controlled studies have been conducted that indicate an effect may exist.

Investigational: Studies have indicated promising results in animal models or in epidemiologic studies. Small trials in humans may currently be underway.

Unknown: There is an equivalent amount of scientific evidence, which shows both positive and negative results of studies that have been conducted and indicates positive findings but was generally of poor study design, or there is a relative lack of trials that have been performed for this indication.

Doubtful: Studies that have been conducted have generally shown no effect.

required to include a "Supplement Facts" panel similar to the "Nutrition Facts" panels used for many processed foods. The labels contain information on as many as 14 ingredients when present in "significant amounts." Examples include sodium, calcium, iron, ascorbic acid, and other vitamins and minerals. If the product was derived from a plant, the product identifies the part of the plant used and the Latin binomial. Similarly, for nonherbal dietary supplements, the source of the substance is listed: animal, human, and synthetic. When the ingredients exceed 100% of the dietary reference intake (DRI) for that vitamin or mineral, the product is referred to as high potency. DRI is a general term for nutrient requirements in a population. The DRI differs from the recommended dietary allowance (RDA) in that the RDA is based on individual nutrient requirements rather than population requirements.

The most significant labeling change requires that for each essential nutrient listed on a dietary supplement label, the "% Daily Value" must be provided. The "% Daily Value" is based on the RDA; for example, a supplement containing 60 mg vitamin C is considered to provide 100% of the daily value for adults. However, the problem is that the RDAs are based on 1968 nutrition recommendations. For example, the recommended calcium intake based on the RDA is too low for most adults, including postmenopausal women. For postmenopausal women, the National Institutes of Health recommends 1,200 mg of calcium daily, whereas the RDA for adults is 800 mg. In this example, an 800-mg dose represents 100% of the daily value for calcium. However, based on the new calcium requirements, the value is closer to 67%. The National Academy of Sciences is updating the human nutrient requirements for vitamins, minerals, and antioxidant dietary supplements. Substances such as choline, betaine, glutamic acid, inositol, and botanicals are considered nonessential nutrients for health. These products are added to supplements and are easily identified on a product label that states that the "% Daily Value" has not been established.

Structure-Function Claims

Manufacturers of dietary supplements can make only "structure-function" claims, which describe the role of a supplement intended to affect the structure or function in humans. These claims characterize the documented mechanism by which a supplement acts to maintain such structure or function, provided that such statements are not disease claims. For example, if a supplement claims to increase the release of macrophages, the structure affected is the "macrophage" and the function is "an increase in release." In this way, the manufacturer is not claiming that the supplement is treating an upper respiratory tract infection. Under the DSHEA, manufacturers who make structure-function claims on product labels must also include the following disclaimer, "This statement has not been evaluated by the FDA. This product is not intended to diagnose, treat, cure or prevent any disease." Consequently, a product can claim that it "enhances memory," but it cannot claim that it "treats dementia." Manufacturers who want to use a structure-function claim must inform the FDA no later than 30 days after the product is marketed. The manufacturer must be able to substantiate the claim, but is not required to submit supporting evidence to the FDA or make the evidence publicly available.

Fraudulent claims are common in the dietary supplement field. Phrases such as "miracle cure" suggest that the product is a cure for a disease, whereas terms such as "detoxify" and "purify" are vague and misleading. The most troubling labeling claims suggest that these products are free of side effects. If a dietary supplement is potent enough to cause a beneficial effect, it is also able to cause a side effect.

Supplement Labeling

Consumers may receive informational leaflets on a particular supplement at the time of purchase. The informational leaflets might consist of an article, a newsletter, a summary, or other written document. The quality of the information provided is not reviewed by the FDA, an expert panel, or other authority. The DSHEA specifies that dietary supplement labeling excludes accompanying written information from regulation when the information (a) is not false or misleading, (b) does not promote a particular manufacturer or brand, (c) is physically separate from the dietary supplement, and (d) does not have other information appended to it.[8] It is difficult to enforce these provisions. Consequently, the information distributed to consumers may be false, biased, inaccurate, or misleading.

Product Formulations

Herbal remedies come in a variety of formulations, some of which include teas, extracts, oil macerations, and fresh expressed juice or tinctures.

Teas: Infusions, Decoctions, and Cold Maceration

Teas are prepared by drying the herb, which is then marketed in its coarse cut form or in tea bags. In general, tea formulations have not been studied in a randomized, controlled fashion because they are difficult to mask.[7]

Thus, empirical data have been used to establish indications for use.[7] Teas can be prepared by infusion, decoction, or cold maceration. The most common preparation, infusion, involves steeping the herb in boiling hot water for up to 10 minutes and then straining. To prepare a decoction, the herb is placed in cold water and the combination is heated to a boil, steeped for up to 10 minutes, and then strained. Macerations are prepared by letting the herb stand in water at room temperature for many hours before straining.

Extracts

The term "extraction" is used when a portion of the herb or the entire herb is processed for the purpose of concentration. Extractions are formulated as fluids, powders, solids, and volatile oils. Extraction of the dried herb with ethanol, water, or both is used to make fluid extracts.[7] Fluid extracts, which use alcohol as a solvent, are further classified as tinctures. Evaporation of the solvent is used to prepare solid and powder extracts.[7] Either distillation or lipophilic extraction can be used to prepare volatile oils.[7]

Oil Maceration and Fresh-Pressed Juice or Tincture

Oil macerates can be prepared with fresh or dried herbs. In either case, similar to tea macerations, the herb is allowed to stand in oil (e.g., vegetable oil) to macerate at room temperature for many hours before straining. Fresh-pressed juice is prepared by macerating the herb in water and then squeezing the juice from it.[7] Fresh herbal tinctures can also be prepared by using an alcohol-based solvent.

Good Manufacturing Practices

In the United States, pharmaceutical manufacturers are required by law to conform to strict standards. Good manufacturing practices (GMPs) were designed to protect consumers from contamination and improper conditions during manufacturing. Dietary supplements are not required by law to conform to the same level of GMPs as pharmaceutical manufactures. Under the DSHEA, dietary supplements are subject to current GMP in production, packing, or holding human food.[8] These guidelines include maintenance of buildings and facilities, food handler requirements, and safety standards. Products imported from other countries are more difficult to regulate. Consequently, problems related to product purity, potency, and contamination have been documented in the scientific literature.[9] Often, neither the distributor nor the consumer have any assurance that product content matches the labeling claims. Adulteration, whether intentional or accidental, is dangerous and puts the public health in jeopardy. In an attempt to begin addressing this issue, the U.S. Pharmacopeia (USP) established a program called the Dietary Supplement Verification Program (DSVP). This program helps establish ingredient quality and other standards unique to herbs and dietary supplements. Participation in the program is voluntary. Manufacturers who meet the DSVP criteria will be allowed to carry the USP-certified seal on their labels. This will help consumers distinguish a particular manufacturer's product as having the highest quality standards for content. Other organizations have established similar programs including Consumer Lab and the National Sanitation Foundation. Importantly, none of these programs address issues of pharmacologic safety or efficacy.

In 2007, more than 10 years after the DSHEA was enacted, the FDA issued a final rule on proposed changes to dietary supplement GMPs. The proposed changes in GMPs standards came after significant pressure from stakeholders and consumers. Among the various changes, dietary supplements must now be manufactured in a quality manner, without contaminants or impurities, and need to be labeled accurately. These changes in GMPs will indeed help better regulate manufacturing. To allow manufacturers time to comply, a long phase-in period has been developed. Larger supplement manufacturers are required to comply by June 2008 and smaller manufacturers by 2009 or later. In response, manufacturers have expressed concern regarding the cost of these changes, which may mean that these added costs are likely be passed on to the consumer.

One of the most important changes to the supplement industry involves the Dietary Supplement and Non-Prescription Drug Consumer Protection Act (PL 109-462), which was signed into law on December 22, 2006. This law requires manufacturers, packers, or distributors of dietary supplements to submit serious adverse event reports to the FDA based on specific information that they receive from the public. Under this law, serious adverse events may include death, a life-threatening situation, an inpatient hospitalization, a persistent or significant disability or incapacity, or a congenital anomaly or birth defect, or one that requires medical or surgical intervention to prevent such serious outcomes (based on reasonable medical judgment). This law will help better characterize the frequency at which serious adverse events associated with herbs and supplements are reported. More important, it may help alert the FDA to serious adverse event trends so appropriate corrective action may be taken.

Given the popularity of dietary supplements, unscrupulous companies have attempted to cut costs through product adulteration. This is especially true of herbs that are expensive to acquire or that take years to cultivate. As a consequence of adulteration, the product could fail to have the desired effect, could cause serious side effects, or could interact with other drugs. Although some of the hazards may be mitigated by the new GMP requirements, some hazards may endure, including those related to the appropriate cultivation and accurate identification of botanicals.

Herbal Hazards

Consumers sometimes believe that "natural" products available without a prescription must also be safe.[10] Often, this is not the case because hazards can be introduced during the collection and manufacturing process or, unknowingly, by the patient. Other hazards can result from toxic components within the herb.

Manufacturing Hazards (Adulteration)

In some cases, substances that do not appear on the package labeling may be introduced into a product, either deliberately or by accident. For example, plant misidentification resulted in renal failure in up to 100 women who ingested a Chinese herbal diet aid. In this case, *Stephania tetrandra* was replaced with a nephrotoxic herb, *Aristolochia fangchi.*[11] Similar cases of misidentification have resulted in digitalis poisoning.[12]

High levels of heavy metals (e.g., lead, mercury, arsenic) have been observed in some traditional Chinese and Ayurvedic (Indian) herbal remedies.[13,14] A recent survey of 260 Asian products distributed in the United States revealed that high levels of heavy metals or adulterants were present in 83 products (32%).[9] In these cases, the amounts exceeded the recommended maximum amounts set by the USP. Heavy metal toxicity has resulted in cases of anemia, hepatitis, and death.[13,14]

There are many reports of toxicity caused by adulterated products. In the United States, an outbreak of eosinophilic myalgia syndrome occurred in patients using the nutritional supplement L-tryptophan.[15] An aniline-derived contaminant was later found to be the cause. Cases of digitalis poisoning prompted the chemical analysis of an herbal product advocated for bowel cleansing. *Digitalis lanata* was isolated from the plantain (plantago) portion of the product.[11] Adulteration of herbal remedies with prescription drugs such as diazepam, nonsteroidal anti-inflammatory drugs (NSAIDs), hydrochlorothiazide, and steroids has been observed as well.[16]

Direct Hazards: Products to Avoid or Use Cautiously

Products associated with severe adverse reactions are listed in Table 3-2.[17–26] Herbs containing pyrrolizidine alkaloids generally should be avoided because they are metabolized to pyrroles, which are hepatotoxic. Ephedrine and ephedrine-containing products can increase the risk of stroke, myocardial

Table 3-2 Hazards Associated With Some Nutritional Supplements

Supplement/Latin Binomial	References	Associated Clinical Use[a]	Toxicity	Recommendation
Comfrey rhizome, roots, leaves *Symphytum* spp.	6, 10, 17, 18	Internal digestive aid External wound healing	Pyrrolizidine alkaloids—hepatotoxicity	Avoid ingestion. External application only. Limit use to 4–6 wk. Do not use on unbroken skin.
Coltsfoot flower, leaves *Tussilago farfara*	6, 10, 17	Upper respiratory tract infections	Pyrrolizidine alkaloids—hepatotoxicity	Avoid herb, root, or flower products. Leaf can be used as an external anti-inflammatory agent. Limit use to 4–6 wk.
Germander leaves, tops *Teucrium chamaedrys*	10, 17, 19	Diet aid	Hepatotoxicity	Avoid
Borage leaves, tops *Borago officinalis*	6, 10, 17	Anti-inflammatory, diuresis	Pyrrolizidine alkaloids—hepatotoxicity	Avoid
Chaparral leaves, twigs *Larrea tridentata*	10, 17, 20	Anti-infective, antioxidant, anticancer	Hepatotoxicity	Avoid
Sassafras root bark *Sassafras albidum*	17	Tonic, blood thinner	Safrole oil—hepatocarcinogen in animal studies	Avoid
Aconite (found in some Chinese herbal remedies) *Aconitum* spp.	21	Analgesic	Alkaloids—cardiac and central nervous system toxicity	Avoid
Kava *Piper methysticum*	22	Anxiety	Hepatotoxicity	Avoid
Pennyroyal extract from *Mentha pulegium* or *Hedeoma pulegoides*	10, 23	Digestive aid, induction of menstrual flow, abortifacient	Pulegone and its metabolite—hepatic and renal failure	Avoid
Life root, whole plant *Senecio aureus*	17	Induction of menstrual flow	Pyrrolizidine alkaloids—hepatotoxicity	Avoid
Poke root, root of plant *Phytolacca americana*	17	Antirheumatic	Hemorrhagic gastritis	Avoid
Jin Bu Huan (a Chinese herbal remedy)	24	Analgesic, sedative	Hepatotoxicity—mechanism unknown, but levotetrahydropalmatine is structurally similar to pyrrolizidine alkaloids	Avoid
Aristolochic acid *Aristolochia* spp.	24	Weight loss	End-stage renal failure	Avoid
Ephedra ma huang, *Ephedra* spp.	27	Weight loss, stimulant, bronchodilation	Extension of pharmacologic effects	Avoid use in patients in whom stimulant effects could be harmful (e.g., hypertension, diabetes, heart disease, anxiety, hyperthyroidism)
Royal jelly from the honeybee *(Apis mellifera)*	25	Tonic	IgE-mediated bronchospasm, and anaphylaxis in patients with atopy or asthma	Avoid use in patients with history of asthma, atopy, or allergies
Guar gum *Cyamopsis psorabides* or *tetragonolobus*	10, 26	Weight loss, diabetes, hypercholesterolemia	Esophageal, small bowel obstruction	Avoid

[a] Associated clinical use is based on patient report at time of event or reported use in listed references.

infarction (MI), and seizures. Many cases of adverse events, including fatalities in otherwise healthy adults, have prompted several countries and individual states to ban the sale of ephedra-containing products. Currently, ephedra-containing products carry a warning indicating the risks in people with certain health conditions.[27]

Hazards Introduced by the Consumer

Consumers should not exceed the doses recommended on the package label because overuse may lead to toxicity. Indirect toxicity can occur if consumers attempt to self-treat serious disorders. In general, dietary supplements should not be used to treat cancer or serious infection if more effective therapies exist. However, if the patient is terminally ill and the supplement provides relief, use may be justified. Use during pregnancy, during lactation, or in children should also be avoided because the products have not been adequately studied for safety in these vulnerable patient populations.

Patient Recommendations

General recommendations regarding the use of herbal products are outlined in Table 3-3. These may be used when counseling patients on product selection and appropriate use. Many of

Table 3-3 Guidelines for Selecting or Recommending on Herbal Remedy or Dietary Supplement Product

- Read all labels carefully.
- Never share these products with others.
- Avoid using in children.
- Avoid if you are pregnant, nursing, or trying to become pregnant.
- Never take more than the recommended amount listed on the label.
- Do not select a product that does not have dosing recommendations on the label.
- Avoid products that do not carry a lot number or expiration date.
- Discard products 1 year from the date of purchase when no other expiration date present.
- Select products that list the manufacturer's name, address, and telephone number.
- Speak to your health care professional if you are trying to treat a life-threatening condition, such as cancer or HIV.
- If you are taking a prescription medicine, do not take an herbal remedy or dietary supplement for the same condition.
- Avoid taking multiple-ingredient preparations; select single-ingredient products that list the strength per dose.
- Do not store these products in a medicine cabinet or glove compartment; store them in a dry environment out of direct sunlight and humidity.
- The term "natural" does not mean safe; be diligent and report any unusual experiences to your doctor or pharmacist.
- Store products away from young children and pets.
- Always inform your health care provider of the products you are taking; keep a list if necessary or bring them with you to your appointment.
- Do not take these products with alcohol until you know it is safe to do so or are familiar with the effects.
- Check with your health care provider if you are taking "blood thinning" drugs; some products may interact.
- Never use these products in place of proper rest and nutrition; eat a balanced diet.
- Do not expect a cure or unrealistic results; these agents are not "cure-alls."
- If it sounds too good to be true, it probably is; use discretion when evaluating claims.

the recommendations are conservative because data on quality, safety, and efficacy of these products, specifically in special patient populations, are unavailable. These recommendations are not intended to promote use, but rather to educate patients and practitioners. Each decision should be made on an individual basis with the best interest of the patient in mind.

GARLIC (*ALLIUM SATIVUM*)

Garlic Formulations

1. M.J., a 65-year-old obese man, is concerned about his cholesterol and wants to start taking garlic. What types of commercial preparations are available, and how is garlic standardized? Which formulations are preferred?

Preparations of Garlic and Active Constituents

A variety of organosulfur compounds in garlic have been reported to have therapeutic effects. Fresh bulbs contain all of these compounds, but their potency varies depending on how the plant was grown, harvested, and stored. The type and amount of organosulfur compounds in commercial preparations also varies based on the manufacturing process.[28]

Di-allyl-disulfide-oxide, or allicin, is responsible for the characteristic odor of garlic, and some garlic products (e.g., dried garlic powders) may be standardized to this ingredient or its precursor, alliin. Specifically, when bulb garlic is crushed, chewed, or chopped, the odorless precursor, S-allyl-L-cysteine sulfoxide, or alliin, is exposed to the enzyme allinase, and allicin and other thiosulfinates are formed.[29] Allinase is a very unstable enzyme that can be destroyed by heat and stomach acid.[28] Allicin is oil soluble and highly volatile, and is easily converted into the other odorous oil-soluble compounds: diallylsulfides (DASs), vinyl dithiins, and ajoenes.[28]

There are four main types of commercial garlic products, and their content is based on how they are prepared. Dried garlic powders contain both water and oil-soluble organosulfur compounds, and will likely be standardized to alliin content or state an allicin-generating capacity on the packaging.[7,28] Enteric coating of powdered formulations may prevent allinase degradation in the stomach and improve allicin release into the small intestine, minimizing the odor.[29] Powdered formulations have been widely studied in clinical trials. The most common was standardized to 1.3% alliin or 0.6% allicin (based on allicin-releasing ability).[6] Oil-based preparations that have been steam distilled contain oil-soluble DASs, but no water-soluble compounds.[28] Macerated oil preparations, which are made without heating, contain oil-soluble DASs, vinyl dithiins, and ajoenes.[28] Both steam-distilled oil preparations and macerated oil preparations have been poorly studied in clinical trials. Fermented or aged garlic extracts, which are odor free, predominantly contain water-soluble compounds such as S-allylcysteine (SAC) and may carry standardization for this compound.[7,28] Aged garlic extracts have also been studied in clinical trials.

Consumers wanting to use garlic can begin by adding it to their diet. Those who want to use a supplement are best advised to choose a product that has been studied in clinical trials and demonstrated benefits in one or more therapeutic areas. These would include standardized powdered garlic or standardized aged garlic extract.

Antihyperlipidemic Effects

2. M.J. weighs 105 kg and is 6 ft tall. He rarely exercises and eats a diet high in fat; his medication profile indicates that he has been taking benazepril (Lotensin) 10 mg PO daily for 2 years. M.J.'s doctor has recommended a diet and exercise program. On questioning, he recalls his cholesterol values from last month: total cholesterol, 290 mg/dL; high-density lipoprotein cholesterol (HDL-C), 30 mg/dL; low-density lipoprotein cholesterol (LDL-C), 230 mg/dL; and triglycerides (TG), 150 mg/dL. Can garlic significantly improve M.J.'s lipid profile?

Many studies have examined the lipid-lowering effects of garlic, but only a few have included sample sizes of more than 100 subjects.[30,31] For this reason, the antihyperlipidemic properties of garlic are largely based on published meta-analyses.[32,33]

A meta-analysis and systematic review suggests a small but favorable effect of garlic on hyperlipidemia, lowering total cholesterol by 4% to 6%. In the presence of dietary controls, however, this effect became insignificant.[32] Trials varied in the type of garlic product used and in the duration of treatment. The most common formulation was a dried powdered preparation known as Kwai. Studies that lasted up to 12 weeks showed significant reductions in total cholesterol; however, these benefits became insignificant at 20 to 24 weeks.[32,33] It was initially hypothesized that variations in efficacy seen in more recent trials may be related to the poor allicin-releasing ability of some powdered formulations marketed after 1993.[29] This notion, however, was dispelled with the results of a recent clinical trial.[30] This trial randomized 192 adults with a baseline LDL-C of 130 to 190 mg/dL to receive either 4 g of raw garlic, 1,400 mg of standardized powdered garlic with proven allicin-releasing ability (Garlicin), 1.8 g of aged garlic extract (Kyolic), or placebo for 6 months. None of the garlic groups had significant benefits on LDL-C as compared to placebo at the study end point.

Mechanism of Action

In vitro inhibition of hepatic 3-hydroxy-3methylglutaryl coenzyme A (HMG-CoA) reductase has been observed and is considered the primary mechanism for garlic's antihyperlipidemic action.[34] Inhibition of later steps in cholesterol synthesis has also been observed, but this effect requires garlic concentrations exceeding those achieved with normal or long-term human consumption.[34] Garlic also has multiple organosulfur compounds that act as antioxidants and could be beneficial in preventing oxidation of LDL-C.[35] Whether these mechanisms apply in humans remains uncertain.

3. Is M.J. a candidate for garlic?

M.J. should be advised that dietary modification and exercise are the best ways to reduce cholesterol without pharmacotherapy. His high total cholesterol and LDL-C and low HDL-C are not likely to be significantly lowered by the limited effect, if any, of garlic. As already noted, the benefits of garlic remain questionable because only small numbers of patients have been evaluated. Furthermore, its benefit in people who are already modifying their diets may be insignificant.

Hypotensive Activity

4. M.J. decides to purchase garlic and tells you that he will also begin the diet and exercise plan his doctor recommended. M.J. is taking benazepril (Lotensin) for hypertension. Do you have any additional questions or concerns?

Although there have been no drug–drug interactions reported for garlic and benazepril, M.J. should be aware that a few trials have reported a lowering of blood pressure (BP) following garlic use. Overall, however, it is unlikely that the effects of garlic on BP are clinically meaningful, so M.J. should not have to monitor his BP more often than usual after initiating a garlic supplement.

A review of 30 randomized controlled trials measuring BP outcomes concluded that although several trials reported significant reductions in BP using within group comparisons with at least 4 weeks of use, statistical significance was only achieved in three trials when compared to placebo. Among these three trials, the systolic blood pressure (SBP) was reduced by approximately 3% and the diastolic blood pressure (DBP) by 2% to 7%.[33] Stimulation of nitric oxide (NO) synthesis (a potent vasodilator), inhibition of angiotensin-converting enzyme, and reductions in intracellular calcium have all been observed in vitro and may be responsible for this effect.[36–38]

Antiatherosclerotic Effects

5. T.L. is a 70-year-old man with a history of coronary artery disease (CAD) and peripheral vascular disease. He began taking warfarin (Coumadin) after a stroke 2 months ago. His other medications include metoprolol (Lopressor) 50 mg PO daily, simvastatin (Zocor) 20 mg PO daily, and isosorbide dinitrate (Isordil) 20 mg PO TID. T.L.'s friend told him that garlic might help his heart condition. Is there any evidence that garlic is beneficial in treating CAD?

The antiatherosclerotic effects of garlic are largely based on its potential to reduce coronary risk factors of hyperlipidemia, hypertension, platelet aggregation, LDL-oxidation, and fibrin formation (see question 6). Reductions in atherosclerotic lesions, atherosclerotic cell proliferation, aortic collagen accumulation, and vascular damage caused by oxidized LDL have been observed in garlic-treated animals fed a cholesterol-rich diet.[38]

Only a few clinical trials have evaluated the effect of garlic in patients with CAD.[39–41] A double-blind, placebo-controlled trial randomized patients with advanced atherosclerotic plaques and at least one risk factor for CAD to receive 900 mg/day of powdered garlic or placebo. At 2 years, plaque volume in the carotid and femoral arteries was significantly reduced by 5% to 18% in the treatment group.[39] A small pilot trial also demonstrated a reduction in the progression of coronary calcification (a marker of atherosclerosis progression) in patients who received aged garlic extract and statin therapy as compared to placebo and statin therapy over the course of 1 year.[40]

Antiplatelet and Thrombolytic Effects

6. You inform T.L. that garlic may reduce coronary risk factors for CAD, but that its effectiveness in treating CAD has not been adequately studied in humans. Nevertheless, T.L. wants to take garlic. Do you have any concerns about T.L.'s use of garlic given his current medication profile?

Studies evaluating the effects of garlic on platelets have generally observed a decrease in platelet aggregation.[33,38,41] Significant increases in fibrinolytic activity have also been observed in some trials with chronic ingestion of garlic for ≥14 days.[33,38] Serum fibrinogen levels, however, do not appear to be significantly altered.[33] Small sample size, use of variable garlic preparations, and variable study duration have made drawing definitive conclusions from these studies difficult.

Mechanism of Action

Allicin and adenosine have antiplatelet effects in vitro.[42,43] However, because both of these compounds are metabolized in vivo, antiplatelet effects have been attributed to DASs, particularly diallyltrisulfide (DATS) and ajoene,[42,43] although ajoene is unlikely to play a role when fresh or powdered preparations are used.[42] These metabolites may inhibit thromboxane formation and platelet aggregation in response to various activating factors, such as collagen, adenosine diphosphate, and epinephrine.[41,43] Stimulation of NO synthesis may also play a role because NO is a potent inhibitor of platelet aggregation and adhesion.[36]

In summary, T.L. should be told that garlic might increase his risk for bleeding. He should be advised not to initiate garlic supplements because he is currently taking warfarin. A few cases of increased international normalized ratios (INRs) have been reported in patients stabilized on warfarin who initiated garlic supplements. If T.L. still wants to try garlic, he should watch for signs and symptoms of bleeding, and have his INR tested within a few weeks of initiating the product.

Other Effects of Garlic

Anticarcinogenic/Antitumor Effects

Several epidemiologic case control studies have reported a reduced incidence of stomach, esophageal, and colorectal cancers in patients who consumed high amounts of raw, cooked, or both raw and cooked garlic as a food.[44] A meta-analysis also supported the effect of consuming garlic and a reduced incidence of both stomach and colorectal cancers with a relative risk estimate of 0.54 and 0.67, respectively.[45] Interestingly, one of the largest studies to examine the use of garlic supplements as opposed to garlic foods did not find a protective cancer benefit. Specifically, 120,852 Netherlanders, ages 55 to 69 years, were followed for 3.3 years for the development of cancer. Overall, there was no association between garlic supplement use and a lower risk of lung, breast, or colorectal cancer.[45]

In vivo animal studies looking at the anticarcinogenic properties of garlic have focused on the water-soluble constituent, SAC, and the lipid-soluble diallylsulfide (DAS) constituents, particularly DAS, diallyldisulfides (DADS), and DATSs.[44,46] In vivo animal studies show inhibition of procarcinogens for multiple cancer types (e.g., colon, skin, breast, esophagus, lung, liver, renal) using DAS or DADS.[44] Mechanisms of cancer prevention observed for garlic constituents include enhanced activity of phase II detoxification enzymes such as glutathione-S-transferases, which aid in the detoxification of carcinogens, and decreased activity of phase I drug-metabolizing enzymes such as cytochrome P450, involved in carcinogen activation.[44,46] Inhibition of DNA adduct formation, antioxidant effects, and induction of apoptosis are other mechanisms that have been observed.[44] In vitro garlic also inhibited the growth of *Helicobacter pylori,* a known risk factor in the development of stomach cancer.[46]

Tumor growth inhibition has been observed in vitro and in animal models with garlic constituents.[46,47] A review of studies involving the antiproliferative effects of garlic in animals speculated that usefulness in humans would be limited based on the difficulty in controlling the growth of established tumors and the small numbers of cells that could be inhibited.[47] Whether the concentrations of garlic constituents used to inhibit tumor growth could be achieved or tolerated in humans is also of concern.

Anti-Infective Effects

Garlic has antibacterial, antifungal, antiprotozoal, and antiviral properties in vitro.[48,49] Allicin has been identified as the primary anti-infective component.[48] Today, the availability of potent antimicrobials limits the use of garlic as an anti-infective in industrialized countries.

Antidiabetic/Hypoglycemic Effects

Some studies have reported that garlic has a hypoglycemic effect.[33] However, others, including two trials in patients with type 2 diabetes mellitus, failed to find an effect.[33] Until further research confirms a consistent effect on blood glucose, garlic should not be used to treat diabetes. Furthermore, patients with diabetes who take garlic need not monitor their blood sugar more frequently than normal.

Adverse Drug Reactions/Drug Interactions

An observational study of 2,010 patients taking 900 mg/day of garlic for 16 weeks found the following incidence of side effects: 6% nausea, 1.3% hypotension, and 1.1% allergy.[7] A dose-ranging study of the odiferous effects of enteric-coated garlic found that 14 days of garlic, 1,200 mg, resulted in a 50% incidence of perceived odor. Doses of 300 to 900 mg were associated with a 36% to 45% incidence of perceived odor, respectively.[7]

Contact dermatitis has been reported most often in people who frequently handle raw garlic (e.g., cooks, farmers).[50] The reaction is preceded by an eczematous rash, followed by the potential for desquamation and hyperkeratosis of the palms.[50] Rarely, allergic conjunctivitis, allergic rhinitis, and bronchospasm have been reported.[7]

The antiplatelet effects of garlic have been cited as a risk factor for postoperative bleeding.[51,52] A case report of a spinal epidural hematoma in a previously healthy patient suggested that the patient's use of four cloves per day of raw garlic may have been the cause.[52] Patients should be advised to avoid garlic 7 to 10 days before and after surgery.

There have been few reported drug–drug interactions between garlic and other medications. As already noted, patients taking anticoagulants and BP medications should be monitored closely. A 50% reduction in the bioavailability of saquinavir also has been reported.[53] Ritonavir, however, was not similarly affected.[54]

Pharmacokinetics and Dosing

In healthy adults who consumed 500 mg of aged garlic extract (Kyolic), peak plasma SAC levels were detected 1 hour after administration. The half-life and excretion times for SAC were 10 and 30 hours, respectively.[55] In a separate study, N-acetyl-S-allyl-L-cysteine was detected in the urine of healthy adults who consumed 200 mg of powdered garlic extract (Kwai).[56]

Patients wanting to reduce the possibility of garlic odor should purchase an enteric-coated formulation. A daily dosage of 600 to 900 mg of powdered garlic in two to three divided doses is recommended.[7] A dose of 900 mg of powdered garlic is equivalent to 2.7 g or 1 clove of fresh garlic per day. Products should be standardized for alliin or allicin content if they are powdered. The recommended standard is an alliin concentration of 1.3% or an allicin content of 0.6%. Aged garlic extracts may indicate that they are standardized by SAC content on the package label, but no accepted percentage standard has been established.

GINKGO (*GINKGO BILOBA*)

Neuroprotection

7. E.B., a 22-year-old woman, comes to the pharmacy to purchase *G. biloba* for her 80-year-old grandmother. E.B.'s grandmother has difficulty recalling past events and often becomes disoriented and anxious. Her grandmother was recently diagnosed as having cerebral insufficiency (CI) secondary to early Alzheimer disease (AD), but the neurologist suggested waiting before initiating donepezil (Aricept) because she has a history of low BP and dizziness when standing. E.B. heard that *G. biloba* may be helpful for patients with AD. Her grandmother's medications include aspirin 325 mg PO daily and buspirone (BuSpar) 2.5 mg PO TID. Do any clinical data demonstrate *G. biloba's* efficacy in the treatment of AD?

CI includes a variety of clinical symptoms, some of which can include confusion, poor concentration and memory, forgetfulness, fatigue, depression, anxiety, vertigo, tinnitus, and hearing loss.[57] Many of these symptoms are said to be relieved by *G. biloba* extract (GBE). Studies using GBE for CI conducted before 1991 assessed efficacy based on improvements in clinical symptoms and tests designed to assess cognitive improvement.[7] In 1991, the German Commission E developed new criteria for evaluation of nootropic (i.e., cognition-enhancing) therapies. It recommended that clinical improvement be based on three distinct levels of observation involving (a) patients' and families' impression of effect on daily living, (b) objective testing of cognitive performance, and (c) clinicians' impressions of symptomatic improvement.[7] Newer clinical trials have met this recommendation by using the following standardized outcome measures, respectively: the Geriatric Evaluation by Relatives Rating Instrument, the standardized Alzheimer's Disease Assessment Scale for cognition (ADAS-cog), and the Clinical Global Impression of Change (CGIC) scale.[7]

The most recent systematic review and meta-analysis of ginkgo for patients with dementia or cognitive decline was published in 2002.[57] Only randomized, double-blind controlled trials that compared ginkgo to placebo and involved patients with acquired cognitive impairment or any severity of dementia were included. Thirty-three trials were included and ranged in length from 3 to 52 weeks. All but one study used a standardized ginkgo extract (i.e., 24% flavone glycosides and 6% terpene lactones), and most used a daily dose of 200 mg or less (range 80–600 mg/day). Small but significant improvements in the ADAS-cog were observed for doses <200 mg at 12 and 52 weeks and for any dose at 12 and 24 weeks. Small but significant improvements were also noted for activities of daily living (ADL) for doses <200 mg at 12, 24, and 52 weeks. The CGIC scale was associated with significant benefits at doses <200 mg at 12 weeks and doses >200 mg at 24 weeks.

A large-scale trial comparing the efficacy of ginkgo to an acetylcholinesterase inhibitor for Alzheimer dementia has yet to be conducted. A small three-arm trial did compare 160 mg GBE, 5 mg donepezil, or placebo, and showed significant and equivalent benefits for both treatment arms compared to placebo.[58] However, a Cochrane Collaboration meta-analysis that looked at efficacy based on cognitive function changes, found that ginkgo was less effective than prescription donepezil, rivastigmine, and galantamine.[59]

Current research is aimed at determining the preventative potential of ginkgo in dementia. Two large-scale prevention trials are underway with results expected in 2010: the Ginkgo Evaluation of Memory study and the GuidAge study.[60,61] These studies will attempt to address whether use of a standardized ginkgo extract can delay the mean time to onset of Alzheimer dementia and delay the advancement of cognitive decline in persons age 70 years or older who have either mild cognitive impairment or have consulted a physician for a memory complaint. Both trials will include approximately 3,000 people and last 5 or more years.

8. Is E.B.'s grandmother a candidate for GBE? If so, how long should therapy be continued?

E.B.'s grandmother has been diagnosed with AD of mild severity. Clinical studies suggest that GBE may have some benefit for dementia of mild to moderate severity, but further research should be conducted to firmly establish efficacy. GBE is an option for E.B.'s grandmother, but her primary care provider should be informed if she initiates therapy. The optimal dosage and duration of therapy is unknown, but no significant adverse events have been noted in studies that have treated subjects with GBE for up to 1 year.[57]

Mechanism of Action

9. What are the proposed mechanisms of action for the neuroprotective effects of *G. biloba*?

Cerebral ischemia, oxidative stress, and neuronal degeneration are believed to be involved in the pathogenesis of dementia and dementia of the Alzheimer's type. A prominent feature of AD is the development of neuritic plaques and neurofibrillary tangles in the areas of the brain that control cognition and emotion. Neurochemical imbalances also develop as cholinergic, adrenergic, and gamma-aminobutyric acid (GABA)-aminergic neurons are lost.[62]

The mechanism of *G. biloba*'s action as a neuroprotective agent has been examined in many in vitro and some in vivo studies. Potential mechanisms include improved blood flow, antioxidant effects, antagonism of platelet-activating factor (PAF), alterations in neurotransmitter concentrations and binding sites, and inhibition of amyloid-beta (Abeta) fibrils.[63–68] If GBE can decrease inflammation and improve blood flow through PAF antagonism, decrease oxidation through its antioxidant and radical scavenging properties, affect neurotransmission in humans as it does in animals, and inhibit the aggregation and toxicity of Abeta fibrils, it may be clinically meaningful for patients like E.B.'s grandmother who have AD.

Preparations and Active Constituents

10. E.B.'s grandmother loves tea. Will a tea formulation of *G. biloba* be beneficial?

G. biloba is prepared from the leaves of the Ginkgo tree.[6] The active constituents include a flavonoid fraction (kaempferol, quercetin, and isorhamnetin) and a terpene fraction (ginkgolides A, B, C, J, and M, and bilobalide).[63] These compounds require concentration for optimal potency. The German Commission E recommends an herb:extract ratio of 50:1, which means that 50 parts of ginkgo leaf are used to generate 1 part of extract.[7] Extracts should be standardized to contain 22% to 27% flavone glycosides and 5% to 7% terpene lactones.[7] Although crude leaf teas are available, they are unlikely to be beneficial because of their low potency. Standardization for flavones and terpenes should be indicated on the package labeling.

Stress and Anxiety

11. E.B.'s grandmother is taking buspirone (BuSpar). Can GBE be used as a substitute for buspirone to treat her anxiety?

GBE has exhibited physiological stress-relieving properties in rodent models that differ from those of classic anxiolytics and antidepressants.[67] In rats, an 8-day treatment of GBE reduced corticosterone synthesis by reducing adrenal peripheral-type benzodiazepine receptor expression. This receptor has been linked to the stress response through enhanced steroid production.[67] In humans, exposure to physiological or psychological stress can result in steroid production. GBE may control the stress response by minimizing this elevation in steroids and promoting a more "normal" circulating corticosteroid level. GBE may improve cognitive deficiency, and anxiety is considered one of many symptoms associated with cognitive deficiency.

A recent randomized, double-blind, placebo-controlled study of GBE in generalized anxiety disorder (GAD) and adjustment disorder with anxious mood (ADWAM), also suggests significant benefits for both disorders.[69] In this study, 170 patients with GAD or ADWAM received placebo, GBE 480 mg, or GBE 240 mg for 1 month. Intention-to-treat analysis on the Hamilton Rating Scale for Anxiety (HAMA) showed significantly lower HAMA scores for both treatment groups compared to placebo and a significant dose–response effect.

Despite promising results of this former study, few trials have evaluated GBE as a monotherapy for GAD, and no trials have compared it to a benzodiazepine or buspirone. Therefore, GBE should not be used as a substitute for buspirone in E.B.'s grandmother. The potency and effectiveness of GBE as an antianxiety or antistress agent need to be studied further before it can be recommended for this indication.

Intermittent Claudication

12. E.B.'s grandmother has always had a problem with "poor circulation" in her legs, which limits her ability to walk. Will *G. biloba* help this problem?

Although GBE may improve vascular insufficiency through enhanced blood flow, there is less literature to support its use for complications of peripheral arterial occlusive disease (PAOD) than there is for dementia.[7] Two recent meta-analyses involving eight and nine randomized, double-blind, placebo-controlled trials evaluated GBE for intermittent claudication, a painful symptom of PAOD. Both concluded that GBE was more effective than placebo at improving pain-free walking distance.[70,71] The weighted mean improvement in walking distance for GBE versus placebo was approximately 34 m. Effective dosing ranged from 120 to 160 mg/day for 24 weeks.

The clinical effect of GBE has been compared with the prescription drug, pentoxifylline (Trental). One meta-analysis suggested the improvement in pain-free walking distance was comparable, with an increase of 45% for GBE and 57% for pentoxyfylline.[72] However, this analysis is disputed by another one in which GBE improved pain-free walking distance by 32 m versus 138 m for pentoxyfylline.[73] In summary, GBE may enhance E.B.'s grandmother's ability to walk longer distances.

Pharmacokinetics, Dosing, and Onset

13. What are the pharmacokinetic characteristics of GBE? What dose should be recommended for E.B.'s grandmother? When can beneficial effects be expected?

Pharmacokinetic parameters have been reported for the flavonoid fraction of ginkgo, ginkgolides A and B, and bilobalide.[74] Kinetics for the ginkgolides and bilobalide were determined following a single 80-mg oral dose of GBE. Single-dose kinetics for the flavonoid fraction were determined following the oral administration of equivalent doses of GBE (dose not stated) in capsules, drops, or tablets.[74] All GBE constituents studied were well absorbed (>60%) and reached peak concentrations within 1 to 3 hours. Half-life ranged from 2 to 6 hours for all constituents. Studies in animals identified many routes of clearance: 38% appeared in expired air, 22% in urine, and 29% in feces.

The recommended dosage of GBE is 120 to 240 mg/day taken orally in two to three divided doses.[7] GBE is available as 40-, 60-, and 120-mg capsules or tablets. Studies in patients with CI suggest that clinical benefits may not be observed for 4 to 6 weeks.

Adverse Drug Reactions/Drug Interactions

14. Should E.B. be warned of any adverse effects or drug interactions with GBE?

Adverse effects associated with GBE are minimal. An evaluation of >10,000 individuals who took GBE for at least 3 months found that only 183 patients (1.69%) reported adverse events.[7] All reported side effects occurred with a frequency of >0.5%. Ranked in order from the most to the least common, they included nausea, headache, stomach upset, diarrhea, allergy, anxiety, and insomnia.[7]

Case reports suggest an association between GBE use and the development of hemorrhage, especially when used in combination with aspirin or warfarin (Coumadin).[75,76] Patients should be monitored for bleeding when taking antiplatelet or anticoagulant medications based on these case reports and discontinue ginkgo at least 7 to 10 days before or after surgery. E.B.'s grandmother should not use ginkgo in combination with aspirin. Ginkgo should also be avoided in patients with a history of epilepsy or seizures. Case reports of seizures associated with ginkgo are likely due to product contamination with ginkgo seeds, which are known to contain an epileptogenic neurotoxin.[77] Coma has occurred following the use of ginkgo in combination with trazodone (Desyrel).[78]

Short-Term Memory

15. C.S. is a college student and has a big test in 4 days. Can GBE improve her memory?

A number of randomized, double-blind, placebo-controlled studies in healthy young (age 20–30 years) and older (age older than 50 years) adults have looked at the effect of GBE on memory.[79–82] In general, improvements were undetectable, inconsistent, and limited to a small fraction of cognitive tests.[79–81] Some argue that beneficial effects, even though limited, seem more likely to occur following acute administration of very high doses of GBE (e.g., one 360–600-mg dose) in young adults or chronic administration of lower doses (<200 mg/day) in older adults. A recent systematic review involving seven single-dose and eight chronic-dose randomized clinical trials in healthy adults (without cognitive impairment) concluded that ginkgo was not effective for memory enhancement.[82]

C.S. should be informed that GBE is unlikely to improve her memory for her upcoming examination. Its benefits on memory are limited to persons with mild cognitive impairment or Alzheimer dementia.

Other Indications

16. What other conditions might be improved by the use of GBE?

GBE has been used for several other conditions, but in most cases only a few studies have been conducted, or results have been conflicting. The use of GBE for tinnitus has been studied with conflicting results.[83] A review of five randomized trials (including four placebo-controlled trials) for this indication generally reported significant improvement in audiometry or the severity score.[83] A separate Cochrane review of GBE for tinnitus found that GBE is likely to be ineffective for primary tinnitus, which usually stems from a cochlear problem. However, it may be beneficial for tinnitus associated with cognitive insufficiency, which is caused by vascular insufficiency or a neural metabolic disorder.[84]

GBE has been less well studied for use in macular degeneration, erectile dysfunction, antidepressant-induced sexual dysfunction, and acute mountain sickness.[85–88] GBE cannot be recommended for these indications until more definitive clinical studies are completed. The most recently published, well-designed trials cast doubt on the efficacy of GBE for acute mountain sickness or erectile dysfunction of any etiology.[86–88]

ST. JOHN'S WORT (*HYPERICUM PERFORATUM*)

Depression

17. G.C., a 47-year-old man, heard that St. John's wort can be used to treat depression. He is tired of the side effects associated with prescription antidepressants and wants to try this herb. G.C. was diagnosed with major depression of moderate severity 2 years ago and was treated with fluoxetine (Prozac) 40 mg PO daily, which he discontinued after 2 months because it caused sexual dysfunction. G.C. never returned to the physician because he believed that his symptoms had improved. However, for the past few months, he has noted recurrent symptoms of lethargy, insomnia, poor appetite, a feeling of hopelessness, and a general disinterest in pleasurable activities. Assuming that G.C.'s depression is moderate in severity, is there any evidence that hypericum is a safe and effective alternative to prescription antidepressants for this indication?

Systematic reviews and meta-analyses evaluating the efficacy of hypericum or St. John's wort in the treatment of depression have been published.[89–92] The Hamilton Depression Scale (HAMD) was the primary tool used to assess response in a majority of these studies.[89–92] The HAMD score is based on a 17- to 21-item survey of the patient's somatic symptoms in which a score of 18 to 24 is indicative of modest depression.[90] Treatment response in these studies was typically defined as a HAMD score of <10 or a 50% drop in the HAMD score by the study end point.[90]

The most recent systematic review and meta-analysis included 37 randomized, double-blind, controlled trials published from 1979 to 2002.[90] Most patients were defined as having mild to moderate depression and were treated with 900 mg/day of hypericum (range, 240–1,800 mg/day) for 4 to 12 weeks. Twenty-six trials compared hypericum to a placebo, while 14 compared it to a reference treatment (tricyclic antidepressant in 7 trials or serotonin reuptake inhibitor [SSRI] in 7 trials). Overall, hypericum was more effective than placebo. In the placebo-controlled trials, benefits tended to be greatest in studies that were smaller in sample size and not restricted to major depression (response rate, 6.13). In larger, more precise placebo-controlled trials that were restricted to major depression, benefits were smaller (response rate, 1.15). A subanalysis comparing hypericum to reference treatments demonstrated equivalence (response rate, 1.01), even when it was limited to comparisons to SSRIs (relative response, 0.98). All but one of these latter trials included patients with major depressive disorder. Adverse effects and study drop-outs were consistently more likely to occur with prescription antidepressants than with hypericum.

There have been three three-arm trials assessing the efficacy of hypericum in comparison to a placebo and an SSRI in patients with moderate to severe depression (baseline HAMD of at least 20).[93–95] The largest trial compared 900 mg of hypericum to 20 mg of citalopram or placebo in 388 patients over 6 weeks. Equivalent, significant reductions in the HAMD score were observed for both treatment groups compared to placebo.[93] Surprisingly, in the other two trials, neither the hypericum arm nor the SSRI arm were superior to placebo in reducing HAMD scores at 4 to 8 weeks.[94,95] CGIC scores, however, were significantly improved in one of these two trials for the SSRI arm,[94] while remission rates were significantly improved for both the hypericum and the SSRI arms in the other trial.[95]

Additional two-arm trials comparing the efficacy of hypericum to either a placebo[96,97] or an SSRI[98,99] in moderate to severe depression have been published since the most recent systematic review and meta-analysis. Hypericum was significantly more effective than placebo and equally effective to its

SSRI comparison in these trials. Both SSRI comparator trials had a duration of 6 months, representing the longest treatment period to date.

In summary, hypericum is effective in mild to moderate depression and has a more tolerable side effect profile than prescription antidepressants. It may be an alternative for patients, such as G.C., who are unwilling or unable to tolerate the side effects of prescription antidepressants. The efficacy of hypericum in severely depressed patients is still uncertain and should be further studied before it is recommended. In addition, hypericum should not be recommended for patients who have experienced suicidal ideation, therapy resistance, or complicated depressive courses.

Mechanism of Action

18. What is the mechanism of action for St. John's wort in depression?

In vitro and animal studies have been conducted to evaluate the antidepressant mechanism for St. John's wort.[100,101] Originally, the hypericin constituent was reported to have monoamine oxidase inhibitor qualities based on in vitro data, but this has not been affirmed.[100] Recent attention has focused on hyperforin and its structural analog, adhyperforin, as the primary antidepressant constituents in the extract.[100,101] In vitro hyperforin equally inhibits the reuptake of serotonin, dopamine, norepinephrine, GABA, and L-glutamate.[100] Unlike other antidepressants, hyperforin does not act as a competitive antagonist at transmitter binding sites to decrease reuptake; instead, it attenuates the sodium gradient to alter neurotransmitter transport. This could also explain why its effects on neurotransmitters are less specific than with other antidepressants. Hypericum can also affect the density of neurotransmitter binding sites. In rats, chronic administration of hypericum results in a significant downregulation of cortical beta-receptors and an upregulation of serotonin $5HT_2$ receptors.[100] Many prescription antidepressants also downregulate cortical beta-receptors, and electroconvulsive treatment, a highly effective antidepressant treatment, upregulates $5HT_2$ receptors.[100]

19. How should G.C. be advised regarding his request for St. John's wort?

G.C. should be advised against self-treatment of his depressive symptoms without first consulting his physician. Although G.C. did not tolerate fluoxetine, he did report temporary relief of symptoms, indicating that a reduction in dosage may be an option. In addition, there are a variety of other atypical antidepressants (e.g., bupropion [Wellbutrin], duloxetine [Cymbalta], venlafaxine [Effexor]) that G.C. may be able to tolerate. It is unclear what level of depression G.C. is currently experiencing. Although he was diagnosed as being moderately depressed 2 years ago, his relapse of symptoms is concerning, warranting re-evaluation of his depressive state. The long-term benefits of treatment with hypericum remain unknown because study durations typically lasted 8 to 12 weeks.[89–92]

Adverse Drug Reactions/Drug Interactions

20. One month later, G.C.'s physician indicates that he has improved on a lower dosage of fluoxetine 20 mg PO daily. However, G.C. still has complaints consistent with depression and wants to try St. John's wort. Is it safe to use St. John's wort in combination with a prescription antidepressant? Are there any adverse effects that G.C. should watch for?

There have been no clinical studies evaluating the combined use of prescription antidepressants and hypericum. Because the mechanism of action for hypericum is still unclear, it would be wise to avoid its combined use with agents that could enhance adrenergic or serotonergic neurotransmission (e.g., amphetamines, phenylephrine or phenylpropanolamine, antidepressants, triptans). There have been case reports of possible "serotonergic syndrome" in patients who began taking hypericum 600 to 900 mg/day in combination with prescription antidepressants, a prescription triptan, and buspirone (BuSpar).[102–104] Almost all of these patients reported symptoms such as nausea, vomiting, dizziness, headache, restlessness/anxiety, and confusion within 2 to 4 days of initiating hypericum. All symptoms resolved with discontinuation of hypericum, and in two cases, cyproheptadine, a serotonin antagonist, was administered. In another case report, a patient developed sedative hypnotic symptoms when hypericum was used in combination with paroxetine (Paxil).[104] The latter is an unexpected reaction given the proposed mechanism for these agents.

Mania, hypomania, anxiety, autonomic arousal, and psychotic relapse have been reported in patients taking hypericum.[105] In most cases, patients had a history of psychiatric illness (e.g., panic disorder, posttraumatic stress disorder, mania, schizophrenia, severe depression) but were not taking psychiatric medications. One woman had initiated hypericum within 1 week of discontinuing sertraline, so an additive effect may have occurred.

Hypericum induces multiple cytochrome P450 isoenzymes (e.g., 3A4, 2D6, 2C8, 2C9, 2C19)[106] as well as the activity of the P-glycoprotein drug transporter, which is responsible for drug excretion from cells. The extent of enzyme induction may be related to the hyperforin constituent.[106] There are multiple case reports of patients who experienced a reduction in efficacy or serum drug concentration of digoxin, theophylline, cyclosporine, warfarin, indinavir, nevirapine, amitriptyline, midazolam, simvastatin, tacrolimus, oral contraceptives, and other medications after beginning hypericum therapy.[106] Patients using these medications or medications that are essential to their health should avoid hypericum or initiate therapy under the direction of a physician.

Few side effects have been reported in people taking standard doses of hypericum in postmarketing surveillance studies. It is estimated that hypericum is ten times less likely to elicit side effects as compared to standard antidepressants.[107] The most common side effects are gastrointestinal (GI) disturbances, sensitivity to light and other skin symptoms, and agitation.[107]

Other adverse effects that have been observed in at least one case report and may have been caused by hypericum include hypertension and hypertensive crisis, sexual dysfunction, elevated thyrotropin levels, withdrawal symptoms after 1 month of use, cardiovascular collapse during anesthesia, delayed emergence from anesthesia, and seizures associated with an overdose attempt.[104,108–110] Photosensitization is a rare side effect caused by the hypericin constituent in St. John's wort.[107] The effect has been observed more commonly in animals that ingest large amounts of the plant and can include symptoms such as blisters, burns, restlessness, seizures, and death.[107] In humans, phototoxic reactions are rare at recommended doses up to 1,800 mg/day; they occur more often in patients with HIV who are receiving parenteral hypericin or taking the extract while undergoing laser treatment.[111–113] Hypericin enhances the oxidation of lens proteins in the eye, which could lead to the formation of cataracts.[114] Sunglass protection is therefore advisable. If high doses of hypericum are ingested acutely (e.g., in a suicide attempt), sun exposure should be avoided for 1 week because of hypericin's long half-life.[7]

Case reports of possible "serotonin syndrome" when St. John's wort was used in combination with other prescription antidepressants should be brought to the physician's attention. If he still wants to proceed with St. John's wort therapy, G.C. should monitor himself for symptoms of GI upset, anxiety/restlessness, and skin reactions. He should also wear sunscreen, sunglasses, and protective clothing, and avoid prolonged sun exposure. Warning patients to avoid tyramine-containing foods when taking hypericum is unnecessary based on in vitro data showing low levels of MAO inhibition.

Preparations and Active Constituents

21. What factors should G.C. consider when selecting a product? What type of product would you recommend?

St. John's wort is prepared from the dried above-ground parts of the plant.[6] A variety of constituents have been isolated, including flavonoids, bioflavonoids, tannins and proanthocyanidins, xanthones, phloroglucinols (e.g., hyperforin, pseudohyperforin), phenolic acid, volatile oils, napthodianthrones (e.g., hypericin, pseudohypericin), sterols, vitamins, and choline.[6] Products are typically standardized by the hypericin content, even though it is unlikely to be the sole active constituent.[100] Hyperforin, which represents 2% to 4% of the crude herbal drug, could be the primary antidepressant constituent,[100] although a combination of chemicals is likely involved.

A dried alcoholic extract can be prepared by extraction with ethanol or methanol and is the formulation most commonly used in the treatment of depression.[7] Dried alcoholic extracts should contain no <0.3% hypericin or 1% to 6% hyperforin.[7,100]

G.C. should be told that alcoholic extracts have been used most often in clinical studies reporting antidepressant efficacy.[7] In addition, although the active constituents are unknown, total hypericin and hyperforin content are still considered markers of pharmaceutical quality and should be indicated on the package labeling.[7]

Pharmacokinetics and Dosing

22. What is known about the pharmacokinetics of hypericin and hyperforin? What dosage should be recommended, and when can G.C. expect to see a reduction in his symptoms for depression?

Pharmacokinetic parameters have been determined for the hypericin, pseudohypericin, and hyperforin constituents of hypericum.[115–117] Results after single- and multiple-dose oral kinetics indicate an apparent linear relationship for hypericin and pseudohypericin with doses up to 3.6 g of hypericum.[115] Both hypericin and pseudohypericin are poorly bioavailable (14% and 21%, respectively).[116] There is a 2-hour lag time in the onset of action for hypericin compared with 30 minutes for psuedohypericin.[116] Time to peak levels are also delayed for hypericin compared with pseudohypericin (6.0–7.1 hours vs. 3.2–3.5 hours).[115] At steady state, the half-life of hypericin is increased substantially from its single-dose value of 27.5 to 29.1 hours to 41.7 hours.[115] The half-life of pseudohypericin is less affected and increased from 16.1 to 19.4 hours to 22.8 hours.[115] Hypericin and pseudohypericin appear to be completely cleared by the liver because neither the primary compounds nor their glucuronide or sulfate metabolites have been detected in urine.[116]

Hyperforin demonstrates linear pharmacokinetics after single doses of up to 600 mg of hypericum.[117] Larger doses of up to 1,200 mg resulted in serum concentrations that were less than what would have been expected with linear extrapolation. Pharmacokinetic parameters for hyperforin after a single dose of 300, 600, and 1,200 mg of hypericum (enriched to 5% hyperforin) revealed a lag time in the onset of action of 1 hour, a 9-hour half-life, and a time to peak of 3 hours. Half-life increased to 16 hours with multiple dosing of 900 mg of the extract for 8 days, but no accumulation occurred.

Hypericum extract 900 mg/day was the dosage most commonly used in clinical studies of mild to moderate depression.[89–92] Each tablet is formulated to contain 300 mg of hypericum with 0.3% hypericin or 1% to 6% hyperforin and is administered three times daily.[89–92] Although hyperforin is now considered a primary antidepressant constituent, most commercial preparations do not always bear this standardized marker. Patients should be told that 2 to 4 weeks is required for onset of effect.[89–92]

Other Indications

23. What other conditions have been treated with hypericum?

In the past, hypericum was used as a topical agent for wound healing, an effect that was believed to be mediated by the astringent properties of the tannin constituents.[7] The hyperforin constituent also inhibits the growth of various gram-positive bacteria in vitro.[118] Despite these properties, the use of hypericum oil for wound healing is now considered obsolete.[7]

In vitro hypericin and pseudohypericin have demonstrated antiviral properties against enveloped viruses such as HIV-1, cytomegalovirus, and herpes simplex virus.[116] The antiviral effect of St. John's wort is dose dependent and enhanced by exposure to light.[116] The mechanism may involve the generation of singlet oxygen radicals and damage to the viral envelope.[116] Antiviral efficacy has been assessed in patients with AIDS, but the dosages required for antiretroviral activity were generally high.[111] An intravenous (IV) formulation of the isolated hypericin constituent was used and caused phototoxicity in most patients.[111] Until more research is conducted, hypericin and hypericum extract cannot be recommended for the treatment of AIDS.

In vitro studies indicate that hypericin inhibits the growth of a variety of cancer cell types.[119] Photoactivation is required to enhance its antiproliferative effects.[119] Phase I trials in humans are currently underway. Hypericum extract has also been studied in the treatment of seasonal affective disorder, depression with somatic symptoms, reactive depression, premenstrual syndrome, and neuropathy. Additional research is required before hypericum can be recommended for these indications.[6,7,120]

ECHINACEA (*ECHINACEA PURPUREA*)

Preparations and Active Constituents

Many different factors have contributed to the variability in marketed echinacea products, including product content (e.g., parts used, addition of other non-*Echinacea* plant species), method of extraction, and the formulation most likely to trigger biological activity.[121] Three species of *Echinacea* have been evaluated in clinical studies for their immune-stimulating effects: *Echinacea purpurea, Echinacea angustifolia,* and *Echinacea pallida.* Chemical studies conducted before 1990 often confused the botanical identity of these different species, especially *E. pallida* and *E. angustifolia,* making interpretation of therapeutic properties among individual species more difficult.[7] Furthermore, *E. angustifolia* and *E. pallida* have been the predominant species evaluated in chemical analysis, whereas *E. purpurea* was most often used for testing in clinical trials.[121]

In 1992, the German Commission E approved the root of *E. pallida* and the above-ground parts of *E. purpurea* for clinical use.[6] The commission recommends that the root of *E. pallida* be manufactured as a water-alcohol extract (1:5 tincture, 50% ethanol), whereas the above-ground parts of *E. purpurea* must be manufactured as a fresh-pressed juice in 22% ethanol by volume as a preservative (e.g., Echinacin, Echinaguard).[6] Echinacea may stimulate the lymph tissue in the mouth.[7] Although this mechanism of action remains to be proven, such an assumption would indicate preference for a liquid buccal tablet formation versus other formulations.[7]

Although chemically distinct, *E. purpurea, E. pallida,* and *E. angustifolia* share some common fractions; however, these common fractions can still vary in concentration and individual chemical components based on the plant parts used, the species being studied, and the type of formulation. All three species contain a lipophilic fraction (e.g., alkamides, polyacetylenes), water-soluble polysaccharides, caffeol conjugates (e.g., echinacoside, chicoric acid, caffeic acid), and flavonoids.[6,122] The alkamides, chicoric acid, and polysaccharides have been recognized most often for possible immune-modulating effects.[122,123] Alkamides are largely absent in the root of *E. pallida* while polyacetylenes are present.[122] Among the caffeol conjugates, echinacoside is mainly found in the roots of *E. angustifolia* and *E. pallida,* while cichoric acid is found in the above-ground parts of *E. purpurea.*[122] Various constituents have also been studied for possible anti-infective, antioxidant, and anti-inflammatory properties.[121,122,124]

Cold Treatment

24. A.T. is an otherwise healthy 32-year-old man who wants to purchase echinacea. Over the past 2 days, A.T. has had symptoms consistent with a new onset cold: a sore throat, stuffy nose, and general body aches. He is not taking any other over-the-counter or prescription medications and asks you if echinacea will shorten the duration of his cold symptoms.

Clinical trials evaluating the efficacy of echinacea in the relief of respiratory infections have been complicated by product heterogeneity (use of echinacea in combination with other herbs or vitamins and minerals, use of different *Echinacea* species, different methods of formulation, and whether cold symptoms were acquired naturally or following rhinovirus inoculation).[125,126] Placebo control is also complicated by the distinctive flavor of liquid formulations of echinacea.

Fortunately, there have been recent reviews and meta-analysis to help differentiate which echinacea formulations are preferable. In one review, 14 randomized, placebo-controlled trials were evaluated.[125] All trials used either an echinacea monopreparation (10 studies) or a combination product (4 studies) that included echinacea for the prevention or treatment of the common cold. Five studies involved the use of Echinaguard or Echinacin (Madaus AG, Cologne, Germany), which are standardized ethanolic extracts of the above-ground parts of *E. purpurea*. Both persons who acquired the cold naturally (11 studies) or through inoculation (3 studies) were also included. Meta-analysis showed a 58% decrease in the incidence of cold and a reduction in cold duration of 1.25 days. Although there was heterogeneity among the trials, no significant publication bias was detected. The benefits of echinacea remained significant for cold incidence with a trend toward reduced duration, when only monopreparations were evaluated. Limiting the analysis to preparations involving Echinaguard or Echinacin also showed a significant 56% reduction in cold incidence.

The Cochrane Collaboration performed a separate review of echinacea in the treatment and prevention of the common cold (i.e., studies involving inoculation with rhinovirus were excluded).[126] Sixteen randomized trials with 22 comparisons of echinacea to placebo (19 trials), no treatment (2 trials), or another herbal preparation (1 trial) were included. No significant benefits were observed when echinacea was used prophylactically as a preventative agent. When echinacea was used as a treatment at the onset of cold symptoms, significant improvements were more frequently observed for echinacea compared to placebo. The authors concluded that there was evidence to support a beneficial effect of echinacea for cold treatment, specific to monopreparations involving the above-ground parts of *E. purpurea.*

A.T. should be informed that the use of echinacea in the treatment of cold symptoms is still under investigation. However, the evidence to date is positive when the above-ground parts of the *E. purpurea* plant are used. Cold symptoms and duration may be reduced when echinacea is taken early in the course of illness. Echinacea is not a cure for the common cold. Adequate hydration, proper nutrition, and rest are also important during this period.

Mechanism of Action

25. What is echinacea's purported mechanism of action in the abatement of cold symptoms?

Both in vitro and in vivo studies suggest that echinacea has an immune-modulating effect. In vitro studies have been conducted using murine and human macrophages. Using a purified polysaccharide fraction of *E. purpurea,* significant increases in polymorphonuclear (PMN) cell activation; macrophage activation; macrophage cytotoxicity against tumor and bacterial target cells; and macrophage secretion of interleukin (IL)-1, IL-6, tumor necrosis factor-alpha (TNF-α), and reactive oxygen intermediates were observed.[121,127] In vivo the polysaccharide fraction enhanced immune activation in mice against fungal and bacterial pathogens.[121] In healthy volunteers, IV administration of the polysaccharide fraction enhanced PMN activity, macrophage activity, and migration of cells from bone marrow to peripheral blood.[127] Although the mechanisms described for the parenterally administered polysaccharide fraction of *E. purpurea* may not be applicable to the oral formulation used commercially, the water-soluble (polysaccharide-containing) fraction still seems to exert a superior immunostimulant response as compared to the fraction extracted with organic solvents.[123]

Few studies have evaluated the mechanism of action of echinacea in its commercially available form. One in vitro study showed a significant increase in the production of IL-1, IL-6, IL-10, and TNF-α by human phagocytes in the presence of *E. purpurea* juice.[128] In vitro natural killer (NK) cell and antibody-dependent cell cytotoxicities were also enhanced by *E. purpurea* extract in both healthy and immunocompromised patients.[129] However, in vivo, only enhancement of phagocytic activity, total circulating white blood cells, monocytes, neutrophils, and NK cells has been noted with the use of *E. purpurea* formulations.[121,130] Another study failed to find an effect of an orally administered *E. purpurea* juice on either cytokine expression or phagocytosis in 40 healthy volunteers over 14 days as compared to placebo.[131]

Echinacea's mechanism of action remains uncertain. Immune modulation or stimulation may play a role, but to date, only enhancement of phagocytic activity has been observed in humans. Future studies using the orally administered commercial formulations are required to determine if cytokine activity is enhanced in vivo as it is in vitro for humans.

Pharmacokinetics and Dosing

26. What is known about the pharmacokinetics of echinacea? What dose should be recommended for A.T.?

The pharmacokinetic parameters of echinacea indicate that the alkamide fraction is detectable in human plasma after oral administration of a combined *E. angustifolia* and *E. purpurea* combination root extract (liquid or tablet), while caffeic acid conjugates were not detectable in plasma and are likely not bioavailable.[132] Pharmacokinetic parameters of some individual alkamides also have been documented.[122]

Echinacea dosing for the supportive treatment of colds or upper respiratory infections is 6 to 9 mL/day of fresh-pressed juice preserved in ethanol prepared from the above-ground parts of *E. purpurea* (e.g., Echinaguard) or 900 mg/day of *E. pallida* root (1:5 tincture, 50% ethanol).[7] Both preparations are administered in divided doses (e.g., 15–30 drops of *E. purpurea* juice, equivalent to 0.75–1.5 mL, two to five times daily). Appropriate dosing should be indicated on the package labeling. The German Commission E recommends that neither preparation be used for longer than 8 weeks because the mechanism for reported immune modulation is unclear.[6] However, studies as long as 12 weeks have been conducted without serious adverse effects.[121] External preparations should contain no <15% *E. purpurea* fresh-pressed juice.[6]

Adverse Drug Reactions/Drug Interactions

27. Should A.T. be warned of any adverse effects caused by echinacea?

Toxic effects were not observed in animals given supratherapeutic parenteral and oral formulations of *E. purpurea* juice.[133] In vitro mutagenicity and carcinogenicity studies were also negative.[133] In humans, flu-like symptoms (e.g., fever, shivering, headache, vomiting) have been reported infrequently after parenteral administration.[134] This reaction may be caused by stimulation of phagocytes, cytokine production, or a transient decrease in lymphocyte counts immediately after parenteral administration.[135] Few adverse effects have been associated with oral dosing. Unpleasant taste and upset stomach have been reported infrequently.[134] Hypersensitivity reactions (anaphylactoid, bronchospasm, rash) have been reported more commonly in patients with pre-existing allergic rhinitis, atopy, or asthma, as well as in patients with no pre-existing allergic history.[134] One large-scale trial also found a significantly higher incidence of rash (~5%) in pediatric patients taking oral echinacea.[126]

There are no reported drug–drug interactions for *E. purpurea* or *E. pallida.*[6] Theoretically, however, echinacea should be avoided in patients taking immunosuppressive medications (e.g., cyclosporin, steroids). Because of the high alcohol content of certain preparations, patients taking drugs known to cause an Antabuse-like reaction (e.g., metronidazole [Flagyl], griseofulvin [Fulvicin], chlorpropamide [Diabinese]) should be warned of this effect.

Cold Prophylaxis

28. A.T. purchases a product called Echinaguard, a fresh-pressed juice formulation preserved in alcohol made from the above-ground parts of *E. purpurea.* Two days later, he indicates that his partner, who has had HIV for 6 years, wants to use echinacea to protect himself from A.T.'s cold. His partner's most recent CD4+ lymphocyte count was 300 cells/mm^3, and his viral load is undetectable. How would you advise A.T.?

Randomized, double-blind, placebo-controlled trials have generally failed to observe a prophylactic benefit of echinacea in reducing the frequency of the common cold.[125,126] A.T.'s partner should be informed that the prophylactic benefit of echinacea has not been established. Instead, he should be advised to wash his hands frequently and avoid close contact with A.T. while he is symptomatic.

States of Immune Deficiency

29. Could echinacea have other beneficial or harmful effects on A.T.'s partner who is HIV positive? What are the contraindications to its use?

Because the immune-modulating effects of echinacea are still being evaluated, it is unclear how this herb will affect the immune status of patients with HIV infection. On the one hand, echinacea may enhance immune function, and this could be viewed as beneficial. In vitro analysis using cells from patients with AIDS showed enhancement of NK cell activity by *E. purpurea* extract.[129] NK cells, in turn, can have a cidal effect on HIV-infected cells.[129] On the other hand, replication of HIV may also be stimulated by other effects of echinacea: enhancement of TNF-α levels and T-lymphocyte activation.[121] Therefore, until the effects of echinacea are clearly defined, it should not be used by patients who have HIV for any prolonged length of time. Short-term use of echinacea for 7 to 10 days at the onset of cold symptoms, however, is unlikely to be harmful.

Additional disorders have been cited by the German Commission E as contraindications to echinacea use. Many of these disorders could be activated by immunostimulation, such as multiple sclerosis, tuberculosis, leukosis, collagen disorders (i.e., rheumatoid arthritis), and other autoimmune disorders.[6] As further clinical research is conducted, these contraindications may be removed.

Other Indications

30. What other conditions have been treated with echinacea?

Echinacea has been used to enhance hematologic recovery after chemotherapy, but this use is investigational. Two studies used intramuscular *E. purpurea* juice in combination with thymostimulin (an immune-enhancing thymic hormone) after low-dose cyclophosphamide (Cytoxan) therapy.[136,137] In both studies, patients had advanced stage hepatocellular or colorectal cancer, and sample sizes were small. Although certain immune parameters were significantly increased, it was unclear whether thymostimulin or echinacea was predominantly responsible. A pilot study investigated the effect of *E. purpurea* polysaccharides on leukocyte counts before and during chemotherapy. Patients had advanced gastric cancers, and no benefits were observed from the intervention.[138]

The German Commission E recommends *E. purpurea* but not *E. pallida* for the "supportive treatment of lower *urinary tract infections*."[6] This indication is largely based on (a) studies performed in the 1950s using parenteral echinacea preparations and (b) unpublished studies performed by the manufacturer (Madaus) using echinacea lozenges in patients with respiratory and urinary tract infections (UTIs).[135] Despite support by the German Commission E, the use of echinacea for UTIs requires further clinical study. To date, most clinical trials have used injectable formulations of echinacea, which are not commercially available, and have lacked high-quality study design.[135]

Echinacea has also been evaluated for the treatment of recurrent vaginal candidiasis and recurrent genital herpes. In a nonrandomized, open-label study involving 203 women with recurrent vaginal candidiasis, patients received 6 days of topical econazole (Spectazole) with or without a 10-week course of subcutaneous, IV, intramuscular, or oral fresh-pressed juice of *E. purpurea*.[121,135] Recurrence rates in patients receiving echinacea versus econazole alone were significantly lower, 5% to 16.7% versus 60%, respectively. The other trial was randomized and double-blinded and evaluated 50 patients with recurrent genital herpes. Patients received 6 months of an *E. purpurea* extract (Echinaforce) or placebo, but no benefits were observed at the end of the study.[139]

Historically, echinacea has been used for wound healing by Native Americans.[7] The German Commission E has approved *E. purpurea* for the topical treatment of "poorly healing wounds and ulcerations."[6] In vitro echinacea has many effects that are compatible with a variety of possible anti-inflammatory effects. These include inhibition of enzymes involved in the inflammatory process (e.g., cyclo-oxygenase, 5-lipo-oxygenase, hyaluronidase) and a reduction in free radical formation.[121] In animals, echinacea reduces skin inflammation in response to chemical irritants.[121] Although topical anti-inflammatory effects have been demonstrated, there are no well-designed published trials in humans supporting this indication.[121] Thus, the use of echinacea for wound healing requires further research.

SAW PALMETTO (*SERENOA REPENS*)

Background

Prostate growth is largely dependent on the enzymatic conversion of testosterone to dihydrotestosterone (DHT) by 5α-reductase. Elevated DHT levels have been observed in patients with benign prostatic hyperplasia (BPH).[140] Prostatic growth factors, focal inflammation, and upregulation of androgen receptors may also be involved in the hyperplasia of prostatic stroma.[140] Prostatic enlargement can lead to physical obstruction of the urethra and symptoms of urinary hesitancy, dribbling, incomplete bladder emptying, straining, and decreased urinary flow.[141] In addition, α-mediated adrenergic innervation of the prostate smooth muscle and bladder neck can lead to vasoconstriction and further compression of the urethra.[141] This dynamic component of BPH can account for up to 40% of the prostatic tone exerted on the urethra and can contribute to urinary symptoms.[141] Disease progression may lead to UTIs, urinary retention, hematuria, renal insufficiency, and bladder dysfunction from poor detrusor contractility or instability.[140,141]

The American Urological Association (AUA) Symptom Index is the standard scale for prostate symptom assessment.[142] Using this validated symptom scale, seven questions are scored from 0 to 5, and the total sum is used to classify disease progression as mild (0–7), moderate (8–18), or severe (19–35).[142] The International Prostate Symptom Score (I-PSS) is the European equivalent of the AUA Symptom Index and is also used to assess BPH.[143] Prostatic enlargement may often be detected by digital rectal examination; a prostate size $>$20 g is considered abnormal.[141] Urinary flow rate is the most frequent objective test used to assess bladder outlet obstruction.[142] Although peak flow rate can vary with age or voided volume, a guideline for classification of prostatism is mild (15–20 mL/second), moderate (10–14 mL/second), and severe ($<$10 mL/second).[142] Prostate-specific antigen (PSA) values, produced by both benign and malignant prostate cells, can be used to detect prostate abnormalities.[141] Normal PSA values range between 0 and 4 ng/mL. However, PSA values may also be within normal limits in patients with BPH or prostate cancer; therefore, they are not a truly specific marker for either disease.[141] The reader is referred to Chapter 101 for more information.

31. B.F. is a 70-year-old man who presents to the ambulatory care clinic for a follow-up visit with his primary care provider. B.F. was recently referred to the urology clinic for symptoms of frequent urination, urgency, dysuria, and decreased urinary flow. Additional objective tests performed by the urologist included a urinalysis and a peak urinary flow rate. Prostate cancer was ruled out on rectal examination. Results of B.F.'s examination included: AUA score, 12 out of 35; PSA, 3.2 ng/mL; estimated prostate weight, 32 g; peak urinary flow, 12 mL/second; normal urinalysis; BP, 110/60 mm Hg; heart rate (HR), 70 beats/minute; and normal renal function. B.F. has no other medical problems and is not taking any other prescription medications. How would you rate the severity of B.F.'s BPH? What objective parameters contribute to this rating?

Based on B.F.'s AUA score, his disease is of moderate severity. Objective parameters include his increased prostate size of 32 g and a restricted urinary flow of 12 mL/second. Subjective symptoms of dysuria, urgency, and frequent urination should not be used as tools to assess disease severity because both obstructive and irritative symptoms of BPH often wax and wane.[141]

Treatment Options for Benign Prostatic Hyperplasia

32. B.F. is extremely bothered by his symptoms and wants to know the treatment options available besides the minimally invasive procedures and surgical procedures described by his urologist. What are these options?

Because B.F. has moderate disease, a number of treatment options are available. Generally, patients with mild to moderate disease are afforded the "watchful waiting" option, which means that the patient's symptoms are monitored for disease progression.[141] This option is recommended because over a 5-year period, 45% of patients will have no deterioration, 40% will improve, and 15% will deteriorate.[142] The dynamic nature of BPH also has been noted in placebo studies of 2 to 24 weeks' duration in which 42% of patients improved, 46% had no change, and 12% had worsening of symptoms.[142] Patients such as B.F. who are significantly bothered by their symptoms and are requesting nonsurgical treatments are candidates for prescription medications such as alpha-adrenergic antagonists (e.g., terazosin [Hytrin], doxazosin [Cardura], tamsulosin [Flomax], alfuzosin [Uroxatral]) and 5α-reductase inhibitors (e.g., finasteride [Proscar], dutasteride [Avodart]).[142] Dutasteride inhibits isoenzyme types 1 and 2 of 5-alpha-reductase and has been shown to reduce serum DHT levels more effectively (93% vs. 70%) than finasteride, which only inhibits isoenzyme type 2 of 5α-reductase.[144] Saw palmetto, a phytotherapeutic agent, has also been advocated for the treatment of BPH by many physicians in Europe.[140]

Finasteride is most effective in patients with prostate volumes >40 mL and may be no more effective than placebo in patients with prostate volumes <30 mL, which is why the drug class of 5α-reductase inhibitors is often reserved for persons with moderate to severe BPH.[144] B.F.'s prostate volume of 32 mL makes him a poor candidate for finasteride. His BP of 110/60 mmHg is also a concern if α-blockers are prescribed, because they reduce BP in both hypertensive and nonhypertensive patients.[142] Terazosin and doxazosin carry a slightly greater risk of orthostasis as a side effect than the other α-blockers.[144] If alpha-blockers were initiated, B.F.'s BP would have to be monitored closely. Tamsulosin is more specific for the α-1a- and α-1d-receptor subtypes and is less likely to result in orthostasis. The α-1a-receptor subtype is very specific to the prostate (~70% of the adrenergic receptor mRNA).[145] If B.F. is initiated on α-blockers, he should be counseled about first-dose syncope and monitoring his BP when beginning therapy. B.F. should arise slowly from the sitting or lying position, especially when getting out of bed in the morning.

Preparations and Active Constituents

33. Because terazosin was covered under B.F.'s health plan, his doctor started him on this as a first-line agent. B.F. returns to the clinic 1 week later complaining of intolerable dizziness. The primary care physician is considering switching B.F.'s prescription to tamsulosin. This prescription would cost more, so B.F. is considering saw palmetto due to his financial constraints. What are the active ingredients and mechanism of action of saw palmetto?

Saw palmetto berry is composed of many constituents; the active ingredients, however, are as yet unknown.[143] Permixon, the brand most commonly used in Europe, contains 90% free and 7% esterified fatty acids.[143] Phytosterols (i.e., β-sitosterol, campesterol, stigmasterol, cycloartenol, lupeol, lupenone, methylcycloartenol), aliphatic alcohols, polyprenoic compounds, and flavonoids also are present.[143,146] Reported pharmacologic activity may reside in the lipophilic fraction.[140] Saw palmetto is commercially formulated as a concentrated fat-soluble extract that is standardized to contain 85% to 95% fatty acids and sterols.

Mechanism of Action

Early in vitro studies suggested that saw palmetto had antiandrogenic properties. In human foreskin, fibroblasts, and rat prostate cell lines, saw palmetto competitively inhibited DHT binding to cytosolic and nuclear receptors.[140,146] Unlike finasteride, which inhibits 5-α-reductase type 2, saw palmetto inhibited type 1, and, in some cases, both isoforms of the enzyme in vitro.[140,146] Additional mechanisms that have been observed in vitro include inhibition of prostatic growth factors and inflammatory mediators produced by the 5-lipo-oxygenase pathway (e.g., leukotrienes) and α-1-adrenoreceptor antagonism.[140,146]

In vivo, saw palmetto reduced estrogen- and androgen-stimulated prostate growth in rats.[147] However, in healthy males, 1 week of treatment failed to influence 5-α-reductase activity, DHT levels, and testosterone levels when compared with finasteride.[140] Eight days of treatment also had no effect on α_1-adrenoreceptor antagonism in healthy men.[148] In men with BPH, saw palmetto failed to influence plasma levels of testosterone, follicle-stimulating hormone (FSH), and luteinizing hormone after 1 month of treatment.[140] PSA levels were also unaffected by saw palmetto after 6 months of treatment, suggesting a lack of 5-α-reductase activity.[143] Contrary to these reports, some studies in men with BPH report significant reductions in epidermal growth factor, DHT production, and antiestrogenic activity with 3 months of treatment.[149] These reductions were comparable to that observed with 3 months of finasteride therapy. In summary, the mechanism of action of saw palmetto on the prostate remains unclear, but it is likely to involve a number of different processes. More clinical research is required to confirm previously published reports.

34. B.F.'s primary care physician is still unsure whether to initiate tamsulosin or saw palmetto. Are there any clinical trials that have evaluated the efficacy of saw palmetto in the treatment of BPH? How does the effect of saw palmetto compare with the other prescription drugs for BPH? Would it benefit B.F.? If so, what dosage should be used?

A meta-analysis looked at 21 randomized controlled trials conducted between 1966 and 2002 involving saw palmetto for BPH.[150] There were more than 3,000 participants: 1,408 in trials of saw palmetto versus placebo and 1,701 in trials of saw palmetto versus another treatment medication. Urinary symptom scale scores were reported in 13 studies and revealed an absolute improvement of 28% for saw palmetto versus placebo. The weighted risk ratio for patient- and physician-rated symptomatic improvement was 1.76 and 1.72, respectively. The weighted mean difference for nocturia and peak urine flow between saw palmetto and placebo were 0.76 times/evening and 1.86 mL/second. Saw palmetto and finasteride produced similar absolute improvements in urinary peak flow and I-PSS scores. Saw palmetto was typically administered at a dose of 320 mg/day for a mean of 13 weeks.

In contrast, a newer double-blind clinical trial randomized 225 men with moderate to severe symptoms of BPH to 320 mg of saw palmetto daily or placebo. After 1 year, there were no significant differences between groups on either the AUA Symptom Index or any secondary outcomes such as prostate size, urinary flow, quality of life, or residual urinary volume.[151]

Small comparative trials of saw palmetto versus prazosin and alfuzosin have been conducted in patients with mild to moderate BPH.[152,153] The prazosin study was not analyzed statistically, but in both treatment groups symptoms improved at 3 months. Improvements were slightly greater for prazosin 2 mg orally twice a day versus saw palmetto 320 mg/day in the 41 patients studied.[152] A shorter 3-week trial compared saw palmetto 320 mg/day with alfuzosin 2.5 mg PO TID in 63 patients.[153] A standardized scale, the Boyarsky rating scale, was used for symptomatic assessment. Improvements in symptom score (38.8% vs. 26.9%), obstructive score (37.8% vs. 23.1%), and peak urinary flow (71.8% vs. 48.4%) all favored alfuzosin over saw palmetto.

A large double-blind, randomized comparative trial of saw palmetto and tamsulosin also exists.[154] This 1-year trial compared 320 mg/day of saw palmetto to 0.4 mg/day of tamsulosin among 811 men with moderate BPH. The primary end points were the I-PSS score and maximal urinary flow. All outcomes were significantly improved in both groups to a similar degree. Approximately 80% of those treated had improved I-PSS scores. A smaller 6-month open-label comparative trial also showed tamsulosin 0.4 mg, saw palmetto 320 mg, and tamsulosin plus saw palmetto to be of comparable efficacy in improving I-PSS scores in patients with moderate to severe BPH.[155]

A large comparative trial of saw palmetto 320 mg/day and finasteride 5 mg/day was conducted in 1,098 patients.[143] The 6-month trial used the I-PSS rating scale to evaluate BPH symptoms in patients with mild to moderate disease. Objective parameters included peak urinary flow, prostate volume, and PSA levels. Quality of life and sexual dysfunction were also assessed. Both treatment groups had significant improvements in I-PSS score, quality of life, and peak urinary flow on study completion. PSA was reduced by 41% by finasteride but was unaffected by saw palmetto. Finasteride significantly reduced prostate volume (18%) compared with saw palmetto (6%). Sexual dysfunction was significantly more frequent with finasteride (+9%) than with saw palmetto (–6%).

Although impressive in size, the latter trial had methodologic shortcomings. There was no placebo control, and the study lasted only 6 months. Because clinical improvement with finasteride continues for 6 to 12 months into treatment, a longer follow-up period of 1 year may have revealed a significant difference between treatment groups.[156] In addition, enrollment in this comparative study required a prostate volume >25 mL. As previously noted, finasteride is generally reserved for patients with a prostate volume >40 mL and may be no more effective than placebo in patients with a prostate volume <30 mL.[144] Therefore, without a placebo arm, the clinical response observed in both treatment groups may be no greater than placebo. Saw palmetto had a lower incidence of sexual dysfunction, which was significant but not of substantial magnitude. Absolute percentages for side effects of erectile dysfunction and decreased libido, respectively, were 2.8% and 3.0% for finasteride and 1.5% and 2.2% for saw palmetto.

In summary, saw palmetto may improve overall urinary tract symptoms by approximately 28% compared with placebo.[150] In comparative trials, saw palmetto demonstrated similar efficacy to finasteride at 6 months, tamsulosin at 1 year, and a slightly reduced efficacy versus other α-blockers at 1 and 3 months.[143,152–154,156] The benefits of saw palmetto extending beyond 1 year remain uncertain because of short study durations. B.F. may benefit from saw palmetto because it has a quick onset of action (4 weeks) that is similar to α-blockers (4–6 weeks) but shorter than finasteride (6 months).[142,146] B.F.'s low BP and financial constraints also make saw palmetto a reasonable choice. The dose of saw palmetto used most often in trials of patients with BPH was 320 mg/day, taken as 160 mg orally twice a day. The German Commission E recommends 1 to 2 g of saw palmetto berry or 320 mg of lipophilic extract.[6] The lipophilic extract is available as 80- and 160-mg tablets and capsules.

If B.F. does not achieve any symptomatic relief by 6 weeks, another therapy should be instituted. Saw palmetto is not indicated for severe BPH or prostate cancer. B.F. should continue to schedule regular follow-up visits with his primary care physician to continuously assess the need for saw palmetto.

Adverse Drug Reactions/Drug Interactions

35. B.F. begins saw palmetto therapy. Two days later, he complains of stomach upset after ingesting the herb. What adverse effects and drug interactions are associated with saw palmetto?

Is stomach upset a common reaction, and is there anything that can be done to minimize it?

To date, no drug–drug interactions have been reported for saw palmetto, but a small number of side effects have been observed in clinical trials. In the comparative study involving 1,098 patients, saw palmetto–associated side effects occurring with an incidence of 1% to 3% included hypertension, decreased libido, abdominal pain, erectile dysfunction, back pain, urinary retention, and headache.[143] Additional complaints that occurred with an incidence of <1% were diarrhea, flulike symptoms, nausea, constipation, and dysuria.[143]

B.F. should be assured that this type of reaction has occurred before in patients taking saw palmetto. To minimize stomach upset, B.F. can try taking the herb with food. If his stomach upset does not resolve, he should inform his primary care physician so another treatment can be considered.

Pharmacokinetics

36. What is known about the pharmacokinetics of saw palmetto? Will administration with food affect the absorption or the overall efficacy of the herb?

Few pharmacokinetic trials have been performed with saw palmetto. Single-dose kinetics were evaluated in 12 fasting men who ingested 320 mg of the herb. Peak plasma levels were reached in 1.5 hours, and the elimination half-life was 1.9 hours.[140] No trials have been conducted evaluating the effect of food on bioavailability or efficacy. Tissue distribution of saw palmetto has been studied in rats.[140] Saw palmetto supplemented with oleic acid, lauric acid, or β-sitosterol revealed tissue concentrations that were greater in the prostate than other genital organs or the liver.

GINSENG (*PANAX* SPP.)

Preparations and Active Constituents

37. A.J., an overweight 55-year-old man with type 2 diabetes mellitus, hypercholesterolemia, and hypertension, has come to the pharmacy to purchase a dietary supplement to boost his energy. His current medications include simvastatin (Zocor) 10 mg PO daily, metformin (Glucophage) 750 mg PO BID, and benazepril (Lotensin) 10 mg PO daily. His current laboratory values are total cholesterol, 225 mg/dL; LDL-C, 185 mg/dL; HDL-C, 30 mg/dL; TG, 110 mg/dL; and BP 150/80 mmHg. There have been no changes to A.J.'s medication regimen in the past year. A.J. has no family history of coronary heart disease. He states that he has been under a lot of stress lately and has not been feeling as energetic as he normally does. He selects two herbal products, both of which claim to enhance energy. The first is a combination herbal product containing bitter orange as the primary ingredient; the other is labeled "Siberian ginseng." There are so many ginseng products that A.J. asks you if there is any difference between his current selection and the other bottles labeled "Panax."

There are a variety of species of ginseng, many of which are distinguished by their country of origin. Some of these include *Panax ginseng* C.A. Meyer (Chinese or Korean variety), *Panax quinquefolius* (American variety), *Panax japonicus* C.A. Meyer (Japanese variety), and *Panax notoginseng* (Sanchi variety).[157] Thirty different triterpenoid saponin glycosides known as "ginsenosides" have been isolated from ginseng.[157] Additional constituents include polysaccharides, flavonoids, daucosterin, mucilaginous substances, amino acids, bitter substances, vitamins, choline, pectin, fatty oil, and ethereal oil.[158] Composition may vary between different species or within the same species when cultivated at different locations. The ginsenosides are believed to be responsible for many of the reported effects and can be subdivided into three main categories based on their chemical structure: oleanolic acid, panaxadiol, and panaxatriol types.[157] Individual saponins have been further classified and are chemically designated by the letter "R" followed by a subscript letter, number, or both.[7] It is generally the root of the plant that is used for commercial manufacturing; the length of time required for maturation of ginseng root and optimal ginsenoside levels is 5 to 6 years.[158] For this reason, and due to overharvesting, commercial supply can be scarce, leading to higher prices and a greater risk of plant substitution or suboptimal ginsenoside content.[159] Rg_1 and Rb_1 are considered standardized markers of ginsenoside content in both American and Chinese or Korean *P. ginseng* roots; however, the ratio of Rg_1:Rb_1 is higher in Asian ginseng than in American ginseng, which leads to different pharmacologic properties between these two species.[160] Both *P. ginseng* extract and crude herb formulations are recommended by the German Commission E.[6] Ginseng extract should be standardized to contain at least 4% ginsenosides.[6] Crude herb products are available as fresh ginseng (younger than 4 years of age), peeled and dried white ginseng (4–6 years of age), or steamed and dried red ginseng (older than 6 years of age).[158] The latter products may be further processed into powder, extract, or tea formulations.

Other plants that have been reported to have similar clinical effects to ginseng but are not of the *Panax* species include *Eleutherococcus senticosus* (Siberian ginseng) and *Pfaffia paniculata* (Brazilian ginseng).[161] Both species lack the characteristic ginsenosides of the *Panax* species but contain eleutherosides and pfaffosides, respectively.[161] Siberian ginseng was developed as a substitute for the *Panax* species by the former Soviet Union. Many of the clinical studies for Siberian ginseng have been published in the Russian language, making them less available to the scientific community.[6] Both the *Panax* species and *Eleutherococcus* are approved by the German Commission E as "a tonic to counteract weakness and fatigue, as a restorative for declining stamina and impaired concentration, and as an aid to convalescence."[6]

Therefore, A.J. should be informed that Siberian ginseng is not part of the *Panax* species and contains no ginsenosides. However, both preparations are approved for the treatment of similar conditions in Europe. In general, *P. ginseng* C.A. Meyer may be a superior choice because it has been studied more thoroughly by the scientific community and carries a marker of standardization based on its ginsenoside content.

38. Given A.J.'s clinical presentation, what concerns would you have before recommending a ginseng product?

A.J.'s fatigue may be a symptom of poor glucose control. Thus, his recent blood glucose measurements should be reviewed, and his glycosylated hemoglobin (A1c) level should be checked. In addition, A.J. should be asked about other symptoms that can cause a loss of energy such as depression (e.g.,

Table 3-4 Adaptogenic Mechanisms Reported for Ginseng and Its Constituents Based on In Vitro and Animal Studies

References	Mechanism	Adaptogenic Quality
162	↓ Adrenal catecholamine release	Antistress
163	↑ Adrenocorticotropin hormone and corticosterone release, agonist at glucocorticoid receptor	Antistress
162	Centrally mediated enhancement of $GABA_A$, inhibition of substance P	↓ Psychological and pain-mediated stress
157, 162	↑ Central levels of acetylcholine, increase serotonin, norepinephrine, and dopamine in the cerebral cortex	Nootropic
158, 162	Reversal of tolerance and dependence to morphine by decreasing dopamine receptor supersensitivity	↓ Narcotic tolerance and dependence
157	Anti-inflammatory, possibly mediated through anticomplement activity	↓ Acute and chronic inflammation
157	Antioxidant	↓ Cellular damage in states of hypoxia
157	Promotes neurite growth, increase proliferation of neuronal progenitor cells, protects against agents causing neuronal cell death, inhibits N-methyl-D-aspartate (NMDA) and non-NMDA glutamate receptors	Neuronal protection
157	↑ Endothelial nitric oxide and inhibits prostacyclin production	Vasoregulatory effect
157, 158	↓ Platelet aggregation, ↓ (TXA_2), and platelet-activating factor (PAF); ↑ effect of aggregation inhibitors; cGMP, cAMP	Antiplatelet activity
157	↑ Insulin release, number of insulin receptors, and insulin sensitivity	Improved glucose homeostasis
157	Induced mRNA expression for IL-2, IL-1α IFN-γ, and GM-CSF; activated B and T cells, NK cells, and macrophages	Immunomodulation
157	↓ Tumor angiogenesis, ↑ tumor cell apoptosis (death)	↓ Tumor metastasis

GM-CSF, granulocyte-macrophage colony-stimulating factor; IL, interleukin; NK, natural killer.

appetite, quality of sleep), a cold (e.g., congestion, runny nose, sore throat), or hypothyroidism (e.g., constipation, cold intolerance, weight gain).

Mechanism of Action

39. A.J. states that his most recent A1C was 8% (normal, 4%–6%). He performs fingerstick blood glucose measurements twice daily and values range between 130 and 160 mg/dL. He has no other symptoms suggestive of hyperglycemia or other conditions associated with fatigue. A.J. asks for your assistance in choosing between the supplements he has selected. What claims are made for each of these supplements, and how does the proposed mechanism of action for each of these agents affect your recommendation?

A.J. has selected a combination product that contains bitter orange (*Citrus aurantium*) as its primary ingredient. Bitter orange contains synephrine, a sympathomimetic that is similar to ephedrine and has the potential to increase HR and BP. Sympathomimetics act as central nervous system (CNS) stimulants to boost energy; they also constrict blood vessels and raise glucose levels. Because these effects could worsen A.J.'s hypertension and diabetes, he should avoid the use of this combination supplement.

Ginseng has been labeled as an "adaptogen," which refers to the body's ability to normalize itself when exposed to stressful or noxious stimuli. Adaptogenic properties that have been reported for ginseng include stress relief, improved mood and cognitive function, enhanced physical performance, immune modulation, improved cardiovascular function, antidiabetic activity, anticancer effects, and protection against liver damage.[6] The postulated mechanism of action in humans is based on the results of in vitro and animal studies. This extrapolation may be premature because many studies used formulations (e.g., individual ginsenosides or polysaccharides) and routes of administration (e.g., parenteral) that differ from commercially available formulations. Some of the mechanisms reported for ginseng are listed in Table 3-4.[157,158,162,163] Based on these mechanisms, A.J. has no contraindications to ginseng and may or may not benefit from its reported homeostatic effects on glucose control and BP. Of the two supplemental products A.J. has selected, *P. ginseng* would be the preferred agent.

Ergogenic and Nootropic Effects

40. A.J. agrees to avoid the ephedra-containing supplement but wants to know what types of benefits he can expect once he initiates ginseng.

The effects of ginseng on physical (ergogenic) and mental (mood, nootropic) performance have been inconsistent. In 83 healthy patients, 200 to 400 mg/day of *P. ginseng* extract (Ginsana, G115) or placebo for 8 weeks failed to show a significant benefit on positive affect, negative affect, or total mood disturbance.[164] A larger 9-week, double-blind study in 127 healthy patients using 400 mg/day of standardized *P. ginseng* extract (Gerimax) failed to show consistent enhancement of cognitive function.[165] A series of tests were used to assess psychomotor function, attention and concentration, learning and memory, and abstraction. Significant improvements occurred for the abstraction test and the auditive reaction test (one of three tests designed to assess psychomotor function). Studies evaluating an acute dosing effect of ginseng (Ginsana, G115) have also produced inconsistent findings. In a double-blind, placebo-controlled, crossover study, the cognitive benefits of ginseng in doses of 200, 400, or 600 mg were evaluated in 20 healthy young adults. Only the 400-mg ginseng arm showed significant improvements at 1, 2.5, 4, and 6 hours after dosing.[166]

Many human studies evaluating the ergogenic effects (i.e., parameters of muscular oxygen utilization and workload) of ginseng have been criticized for their poor methodology.[167] Well-designed trials involving small numbers of healthy patients (8–38) have been performed. *P. ginseng* extract (Ginsana, G115) at dosages of 200 to 400 mg/day or 8 to 16 mg/day of *P. quinquefolius* extract for 1 to 8 weeks failed to improve parameters of oxygen consumption, blood lactic acid concentration, or respiration under conditions of submaximal or maximal exercise.[168–170] Many studies reporting positive ergogenic effects were not placebo controlled.[167] Those that were blinded and reported benefit were of small sample size (12–30 patients) and conducted in athletes; significant improvements in oxygen uptake, recovery heart rate, and endurance were noted.[167]

Combination products of *P. ginseng* extract (G115) complexed with vitamins, minerals, and trace elements also have been used to assess adaptogenic properties.[171–174] The dosage of ginseng extract used in these studies ranged from 40 to 80 mg/day for up to 12 weeks. Unfortunately, only one study used a control group, which accounted for the effects of vitamins, minerals, and trace elements.[174] Without such a control, the effects of ginseng cannot be distinguished from the other nutritional elements in the product. Ergogenic benefits were observed in one of these studies.[172] In two other studies, quality of life was assessed.[171,174] In 390 patients, 80 mg/day of extract significantly improved one of three scales used to assess quality of life.[171] A subgroup analysis revealed that patients with the lowest quality of life scores had the greatest benefit. In contrast, 80 mg/day of extract in 49 sick and geriatric patients failed to influence cognitive function or somatic symptoms.[173] The only study that used an appropriate control group was conducted in 625 patients, 501 of whom completed the trial. Ginseng extract (40 mg/day) significantly improved quality of life based on an 11-item questionnaire.[174]

A.J. should be told that the reported ergogenic, cognitive, and quality of life benefits of ginseng have not occurred with any consistency. Some studies reported significant effects, whereas others demonstrated no effect. Dosages of *P. ginseng* extract ranged from 40 to 600 mg/day.

Glucose Homeostasis

41. To what degree will A.J.'s diabetes, hypertension, and hyperlipidemia be affected by ginseng?

Both *P. quinquefolius L*, American ginseng, and *P. ginseng*, Korean or Chinese variety, have been studied in small randomized clinical trials for their effects on glucose in diabetic or nondiabetic patients.[175,176] In 19 patients with type 2 diabetes mellitus, use of red *P. ginseng* 6 g/day (divided doses three times daily 40 minutes before meals) resulted in significant reductions ($p < 0.05$) in two of three fasting indices and five of seven indices following a 75-g oral glucose tolerance test compared to placebo. The primary outcome, A1C was not significantly altered versus placebo and averaged 6.5% in both groups over the 12-week study.[176] A separate trial evaluated American ginseng for its effect on postprandial blood sugar levels.[175] Both nondiabetic subjects and subjects with type 2 diabetes mellitus had significant drops in postprandial blood sugar values when 3 g of ginseng was taken 40 minutes before a meal, compared with placebo. A significant drop also was observed in patients with diabetes, but not in healthy subjects, when ginseng was taken at the time of the meal. A recent systematic review also suggests that both American ginseng and *P. ginseng* can reduce blood glucose. Fifteen studies (13 randomized and 2 nonrandomized were included), sample sizes were small (36 or less patients in 14 trials), and overall 9 of the 15 trials showed significant reductions in blood glucose using either American or *P. ginseng* monopreparations.[177] A.J. should continue to check his blood glucose regularly and report any changes to his doctor.

Cardiac and Lipid Homeostasis

Some studies suggest that ginseng may have a beneficial effect on blood pressure (BP) and lipid profiles, but results are inconclusive.[177] Although vasodilatory effects of *P. ginseng* have been observed in animal models, effects in humans have been less consistent. A systematic review of 12 studies (7 randomized, 5 nonrandomized) primarily involving *P. ginseng* ($N = 11$) and its effects on BP showed largely insignificant reductions. Dosing among all trials varied from 40 mg to 4.5 g/day of ginseng. When benefits were observed, they were limited to small changes in systolic or diastolic blood pressure (SBP or DBP) of less than 4% among the randomized trials, which is also unlikely to be clinically meaningful in persons with hypertension.

In contrast, a rise in BP was reported after chronic ingestion (>1 month) of ginseng and Siberian ginseng products.[178] Patients developing hypertension typically consumed an average of 3 g of ginseng root per day,[178] but many of these patients also consumed caffeinated beverages, which may have contributed to the hypertension. Furthermore, no chemical analysis was performed for product content.

The effects of ginseng on serum lipid levels have also been the subject of a recent review.[177] Nine studies (four randomized, five nonrandomized) were included. A majority involved monopreparations of *P. ginseng* ($N = 6$) and variable dosing (80 mg to 9 g/day), and were of small sample size (24 patients or less in six trials). A majority of trials ($N = 5$) showed a significant improvement in one or more lipid parameters, but given the heterogeneity among the trials, it is unclear if these effects are reproducible or clinically meaningful.

A.J. should be informed that hypotensive and antihyperlipidemic effects of ginseng have not been clearly demonstrated. A.J.'s current BP and lipid values are elevated despite prescription therapy, and he has several other cardiovascular risk factors, including his age, diabetes, hypertension, and low HDL-C. A.J.'s dosages of simvastatin and benazepril should be increased, and he should monitor his BP more frequently after initiating ginseng. Any episodes of hypotension or hypertension should be discussed with his physician.

Immune Modulation

42. A.J. has received his flu shot already. Will taking ginseng further decrease his risk of catching the flu this season?

Ginseng is under investigation as an immune modulator. In vitro ginseng appeared to have a greater effect on stimulating lymphocyte proliferation in elderly versus young patients.[179] A lack of effect on leukocyte and lymphocyte counts was also observed in vivo when 300 mg/day of *P. ginseng* extract was studied for 8 weeks in young and healthy adults.[180] However, other research has shown significant enhancement of immune function in healthy patients.[181] Eight weeks of aqueous or standardized *P. ginseng* extract significantly increased PMN cell chemotaxis, phagocytosis fraction and index, intracellular killing, total lymphocytes (T3), T-helper (T4) subset, suppressor cells (T8), and NK cell activity.[181] Both time to effect and degree of immune stimulation were superior in the standardized versus the aqueous extract group.[181] The largest study to date using a *P. ginseng* product as a cold preventative was performed in 227 patients. Influenza vaccine was administered with and without 100 mg/day of *P. ginseng* extract (Ginsana). Forty-two cases of influenza were reported in the vaccination-only group versus 15 in the vaccination and ginseng group at 12 weeks. Antibody titers and NK cell activity were also significantly enhanced at 8 and 12 weeks in the ginseng group.[182]

Two recent randomized, double-blind trials have shown a similar and significant preventative effect on cold frequency and duration among seniors taking American ginseng 400 mg for 4 months (1 month prior and 3 months after receiving the flu shot).[183,184] Benefits may not just be limited to taking the herb while receiving the flu shot, however, as a separate randomized, double-blind study ($N = 279$ persons) of American ginseng 400 mg over 4 months also found significant benefits. The total number of colds was reduced overall and significantly so in persons with at least two colds over the 4-month study period.[185] A significant reduction in cold duration (34.5% less) and symptom severity (31% less) was also observed among all ginseng users who contracted a cold. Thus, ginseng may indeed decrease A.J.'s risk for catching the flu this season.

43. J.L. is a 32-year-old woman with a history of multiple sclerosis who last had an exacerbation 6 months ago. She would like to initiate ginseng to improve her athletic performance in an upcoming race. How would you advise J.L.?

Multiple sclerosis is an autoimmune disorder, and ginseng may enhance cytokine expression and stimulate the immune system. Although the German Commission E does not contraindicate the use of ginseng in patients with autoimmune disorders, it is reasonable to avoid ginseng in patients with multiple sclerosis and other immune system disorders (AIDS, collagen vascular disease, etc.), given the possibility of immune activation.

Anticarcinogenic/Antitumor Effects

44. R.B. is a 32-year-old woman who has a strong family history of stomach cancer. She has heard that ginseng can prevent cancer. Is there any evidence of this effect?

Animal studies have demonstrated anticarcinogenic properties for ginseng. In long-term experiments, ranging in duration from 28 to 56 weeks, ginseng significantly reduced procarcinogen-induced lung adenoma and hepatoma in mice.[186] The incidence and proliferation of tumors was also reduced.[186]

In humans, two large-scale epidemiologic trials observed reductions in the incidence of cancer in patients consuming ginseng.[186] Evaluation of 921 cancer patients and 605 controls on an oncology service in Korea found a direct correlation between ginseng intake and the risk for cancer development.[187] The odds ratio with no ginseng intake was 1.0. This was reduced to 0.6 in patients who consumed ginseng one to three times per year, and to 0.36 if consumption was increased to once per month or more. Duration of ginseng use also correlated to cancer development. At 1, 3, and 5 years of use, the odds ratio for cancer development was 0.64, 0.36, and 0.31, respectively. Fresh ginseng juice or slices and white ginseng tea had no influence on cancer risk, but fresh and white ginseng extract, white ginseng powder, and red ginseng did. Types of cancers that were reduced included oral, pharyngeal, esophageal, gastric, colorectal, hepatic, pancreatic, laryngeal, pulmonary, and ovarian. There were no reductions in breast, cervical, bladder, or thyroid cancer.

A larger prospective study of 4,634 patients compared the quantity of ginseng ingested to future cancer development.[187] The relative risk of cancer development was significantly lower in individuals who consumed ginseng more often. The relative risk for consumption once per month or more was 0.34. Stomach and lung cancers were significantly reduced. In both epidemiologic studies, other patient-specific variables could have influenced cancer development. Although smoking was taken into account, diet, environmental carcinogen exposure, and sexual behavior were not.

In summary, R.B. can be told that ginseng extract or powder may reduce her risk of developing stomach cancer. However, it should not be considered a cure for cancer. The greatest benefit is associated with frequent consumption (once or more per month) and long duration of use. If a fresh formulation is used, it should be manufactured as an extract because other formulations showed no benefit.

Erectile Dysfunction, Fertility, and Sex Hormones in Men

45. B.J. is a 45-year-old man with a history of mild alcohol-induced liver dysfunction, bipolar disorder, and recent intermittent episodes of erectile dysfunction. B.J. has been alcohol free for 2 years, and clinically his bipolar disorder has been stabilized with lithium (Lithobid) for 10 years. He has never been evaluated for sexual dysfunction. His current laboratory values include lithium, 1.0 mEq/L; AST, 80 U/L (normal, 5–40 U/L); ALT, 60 U/L (normal, 7–35 U/L); alkaline phosphatase, 100 U/L (normal, 30–120 U/L); albumin, 3.0 g/dL (normal, 4–6 g/dL); and an INR of 1.3. B.J. read that ginseng can alleviate symptoms of sexual dysfunction; he wants to purchase a bottle. How would you instruct this patient?

Ginseng may enhance fertility and erectile dysfunction in men. In one study, 46 patients with oligoasthenospermia and 20 controls were treated with 4 g/day of *P. ginseng* extract.[188] Sperm number and motility were significantly enhanced, and testosterone, dihydrotestosterone, FSH, and luteinizing hormone levels were increased compared with controls after 3 months of use. In another placebo-controlled, double-blind, crossover study of 45 men, 2,700 mg of red *P. ginseng* extract significantly enhanced parameters of erectile dysfunction compared with placebo (60% vs. 20%, respectively) after 8 weeks of treatment.[189] Nitrogen oxide release has been suggested as a possible mechanism of action.[157]

Although preliminary studies suggest that ginseng might improve fertility and erectile dysfunction, more research is needed. Because B.J.'s erectile dysfunction is of recent onset, he should be evaluated by his physician before initiating any treatment. If ginseng is initiated for sexual dysfunction, patients should be informed that efficacy cannot be assured.

Adverse Drug Reactions/Drug Interactions

46. B.J.'s physician was unable to find any physical abnormalities to explain his temporary erectile dysfunction. Therefore, he would like to try ginseng to alleviate his symptoms. What are the side effects and drug–drug interactions that have been associated with ginseng? Are any of these of concern in B.J.?

CNS stimulation, insomnia, hypertension, and nervousness have been reported in patients using ginseng and Siberian ginseng products.[178] Additional case reports of irritability, sleeplessness, and manic behavior have been observed in patients with a history of psychiatric illness taking ginseng in combination with other psychiatric medications (i.e., lithium, neuroleptics, phenelzine [Nardil]).[190] In these cases, product analysis was not performed, and adulteration could have occurred. However, in animal studies ginseng has altered corticosterone release, neurotransmitter function, and pain modulation (Table 3-4). Because B.J. has a history of bipolar disorder, he and his physician should be informed of these reports. If B.J. initiates ginseng, he should be alert for changes in mood and discuss these with his physician if they occur.

Additional drug–drug interactions that have been reported include a case report of diuretic resistance in a patient using a germanium-containing ginseng product.[190] Germanium, which has been associated with renal dysfunction, was considered to be the cause.[190] Elevated digoxin levels were observed in a patient consuming Siberian ginseng.[191] This may have been the result of contamination of Siberian ginseng products with *Periploca sepium* (silk vine), which contains cardiac glycosides.[192] In another case report, ginseng was associated with a probable reduction in warfarin efficacy,[190] and in animals, antiplatelet properties have been observed (Table 3-4). Antiplatelet properties could increase bleeding risk in patients taking other antiplatelet or anticoagulant medications, so this combination should be avoided. Preoperative and postoperative patients should also be advised to discontinue ginseng 7 to 10 days before and after surgery. Case reports of Stevens-Johnson syndrome and cerebral arteritis have occurred after standard and supratherapeutic (25 g fresh root) ginseng doses, respectively.[190] Finally, because ginseng has been shown to possibly enhance the immune system response, persons with autoimmune disorders should not use ginseng chronically.[181]

The German Commission E lists no drug–drug interactions, contraindications, or adverse events associated with the use of *P. ginseng*.[6] However, high BP has been listed as a contraindication to the use of Siberian but not *P. ginseng*.[6] Adulteration cannot be ruled out in most adverse events and drug interactions that have been reported. Product analyses were not performed.

Sex Hormones in Women

47. Does ginseng have any "hormonal effects" in women?

In women, ginseng has been reported to have weak estrogenic activity.[190] In vivo case reports of vaginal bleeding and mastalgia have occurred after the acute or chronic use of ginseng products.[190] In one of these cases, rechallenge with the ginseng product resulted in a return of the bleeding and a reduced plasma FSH level.[190] Neonatal androgenization was reported after a mother's use of Siberian ginseng.[193] This was later discredited when product analysis revealed the presence of *P. sepium* (silk vine) as a contaminant.[194]

Pharmacokinetics and Dosing

48. What is known about the pharmacokinetics of ginseng? What doses are generally recommended?

After oral dosing of red, white, and *P. ginseng* extract, urinary excretion of 20(S)-protopanaxadiol and 20(S)-protopanaxatriol ginsengosides was >2%.[195] Elimination half-life ranged between 13.5 and 17.0 hours based on urinary excretion data.[195] After single-dose administration, a linear relationship was observed between the amount of ginseng ingested and the rate of ginsenoside excretion. Steady-state excretion of ginsenosides after multiple daily doses was achieved in 5 days.[195] These data provide some information regarding the absorption and excretion of ginsenosides in humans, but the primary route of metabolism and excretion of ginsenosides requires further investigation.

The dose of *P. ginseng* recommended by the German Commission E is 1 to 2 g of the crude root or its equivalent; 1 g of crude root is equivalent to 200 mg of the extract.[169] Ginsana is a standardized extract of *P. ginseng* that has been used in some clinical trials and can be found in the United States. Dosing for Siberian ginseng is 2 to 3 g of crude root or its equivalent. The commission recommends limiting the continuous use of these agents to 3 months.[6]

GLUCOSAMINE/CHONDROITIN

Background

Glucosamine has been promoted for use alone and in combination with chondroitin to treat and prevent osteoarthritis (OA). Both glucosamine and chondroitin were used in veterinary medicine for years prior to their use in humans. Glucosamine is said to strengthen cartilage, and chondroitin is commonly advocated as a product that decreases cartilage breakdown. Both products have been studied clinically as a way to prevent cartilage breakdown, specifically in knee osteoarthritis.

Human Cartilage

Human cartilage is a connective tissue composed of cartilage cells (chondrocytes) and the extracellular matrix. The extracellular matrix accounts for nearly 90% of articular cartilage[196] and is predominantly avascular. Chondrocyte nutrients and waste products are transported by diffusion through the blood supply of trabecular bone, blood, synovial fluid, and the perichondrium.[197] Chondrocyte nutrients help build the extracellular matrix.

The extracellular matrix of cartilage serves as the anchor for chondrocytes and imparts structural stability. Fibronectin, produced by fibroblasts, is also found within the extracellular matrix and is responsible for many cell repair processes.

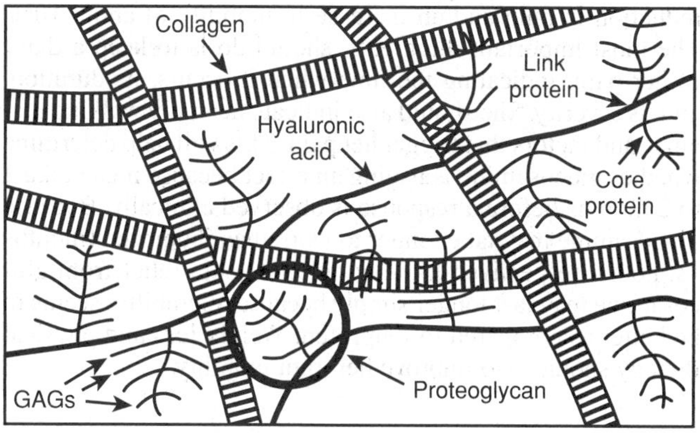

FIGURE 3-1 GAG and PG structures in human cartilage.

The extracellular matrix is a mesh of connective tissue that is composed of collagen, hyaluronic acid, and proteoglycans (PGs).

PGs are macromolecules composed of a protein core covalently linked to sulfated glucosaminoglycan (GAG) side chains. The PG structure resembles a "bottle brush" appearance. In articular cartilage, two types of GAGs are linked to the protein core: chondroitin sulfate and keratan sulfate. Hyaluronate serves as a link protein, which is bound to the PG subunit ionically (Fig. 3-1). The strength of articular cartilage largely depends on collagen, hyaluronate, and the GAGs of the PG aggregates (mostly chondroitin). Chondroitin imparts tensile strength, whereas PGs impart compressive strength. During cartilage synthesis, cations and water are bound to PG. This forms a viscous layer, which cushions and lubricates the joint.

Pharmacology

Glucosamine is an amino monosaccharide and is a product of glucose metabolism via the hexosamine pathway. Glucosamine is found in many human tissues and is a substrate for PG synthesis. Glucosamine is the rate-limiting step in GAG synthesis (Fig. 3-2). Glucosamine increases sulfate uptake, increases production of PG synthesis, and blocks matrix metalloprotease enzymes, which are catabolic enzymes.[198] Exogenous glucosamine sulfate is taken into cells and enters the extracellular matrix through diffusion, where it is incorporated into cartilage.[197] The sulfate salt component, as well as glucosamine, is necessary for the production of PG. Although the exact mechanism of glucosamine uptake has not been determined, PG channels have been suggested as a pathway of entry into the synovial fluid and chondrocytes.[197]

Osteoarthritis (OA)

OA is characterized by a loss of PGs and GAGs and an increase in cartilage degradation, leading to joint stiffness and decreased elasticity.[199] In early OA, GAG synthesis increases.[200] PG aggregates, consisting of noncovalently linked PGs to a single monomer of hyaluronic acid, tend to be smaller and contain a lower proportion of PGs than that found in patients without OA.[201]

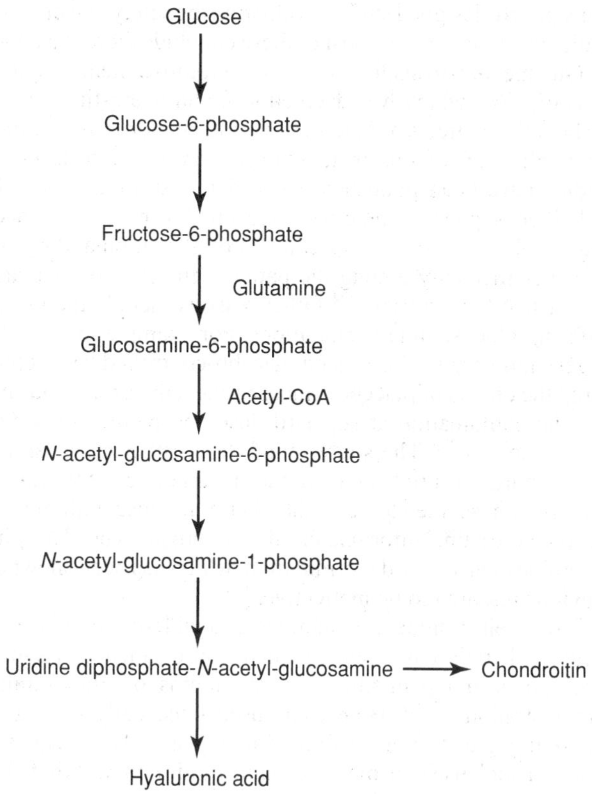

FIGURE 3-2 Biosynthesis of glucosamine, chondroitin, and hyaluronic acid.

Pharmacokinetics

Approximately 26% of oral glucosamine is absorbed after first-pass metabolism.[202] Glucosamine displays linear pharmacokinetics at oral doses of 750 mg, 1,500 mg, and 3,000 mg daily.[198] It is distributed into tissues (kidneys, liver, articular cartilage) and incorporated into plasma proteins and other structures. The volume of distribution approaches 2.5 L, and the elimination half-life following oral glucosamine administration averages 15 hours.[198,202] Unmetabolized and unbound glucosamine is predominantly eliminated in the urine. Unabsorbed glucosamine is largely eliminated by the fecal route. Although the exact amount has not been quantified, glucosamine is also metabolized to carbon dioxide and excreted through the lungs as expired air.[202]

49. K.E. is a 66-year-old obese woman with type 2 diabetes (managed with diet) who has had OA of the left knee for 10 years. She is 5 ft 4 in. and weighs 95 kg (ideal body weight, 55 kg). Five years ago, her knee pain responded to maximum doses of acetaminophen (Tylenol), but it has progressively worsened over the past 2 years. Radiographic examination of the left knee reveals osteophyte formation and articular space narrowing. K.E. is currently taking ibuprofen 400 mg TID, which provides only moderate relief of her pain. She would like to try glucosamine because a friend told her that it would help alleviate knee pain and increase her mobility. What is the clinical evidence for using glucosamine in osteoarthritis?

Glucosamine is widely used by many adults with OA, including older adults. The scientific literature is replete with many poorly designed studies evaluating the safety and efficacy of glucosamine for OA; most of these conclude there is a benefit. One meta-analysis found an overall improvement in symptoms of 30%, which was deemed to be an overestimation of the beneficial effects of glucosamine and chondroitin.[203] Since the publication of this meta-analysis, several well-designed studies have been published, some demonstrating a benefit, and others suggesting no effect. Reasons for these differences may involve inadequate concealment of allocation and significant heterogeneity among the patients enrolled, particularly in industry-funded trials.[204] Other reasons include the use of differing glucosamine formulations. For example, one of the largest and very well-designed placebo-controlled trials compared the effects of placebo, glucosamine, chondroitin sulfate, and the combination at standard doses on painful knee OA over 6 months.[205] The study found that neither glucosamine nor chondroitin sulfate alone reduced pain effectively, and the combination seemed to be slightly better in those with moderate to severe pain. Unfortunately, the investigators used the glucosamine hydrochloride formulation, which has been shown in previous research to be ineffective.[206]

Two well-designed, randomized, double-blind, placebo-controlled trials have demonstrated improvements in symptom scores and pain after 2 to 3 months of glucosamine administration.[207,208] Both trials used once daily dosing of 1,500 mg glucosamine sulfate for 3 years. The Lequesne index, a tool used to measure pain, minimum walking distance, and movement limitation in ADL, was used to measure efficacy. The Western Ontario and McMaster Universities knee osteoarthritis index (WOMAC) was used to assess severity of joint pain, stiffness, and physical function. Patients enrolled had similar baseline OA disease of mild to moderate severity, as measured by radiograph and the Lequesne and WOMAC rating scales. Statistically significant improvements in symptoms and joint space narrowing were observed in patients receiving glucosamine sulfate. Improvements in joint space narrowing were observed at 1 year and continued to improve at 3 years. The patients receiving placebo experienced progression of joint space narrowing and worsening symptom scores. In both studies, the use of rescue medications (e.g., acetaminophen, NSAIDs) was variable and inconsistent between the glucosamine and placebo groups. Interestingly, there was little correlation between structural joint improvements (as seen on radiograph) and symptom improvement. This finding is commonly accepted in the treatment of OA; symptom relief can occur independently of structural changes.

One study compared the effects of glucosamine 500 mg TID to ibuprofen 400 mg TID.[209] Hospitalized patients were treated for active OA of the knee for 4 weeks. Pain scores were significantly lower in those patients receiving ibuprofen at week 1; by week 2, pain score improvements were similar for both groups. Ibuprofen resulted in fast-onset pain relief, but glucosamine had a slower onset of action. Because the study was only 4 weeks long, it is unclear how long efficacy would be maintained in both groups. Nearly 35% of patients taking ibuprofen experienced GI side effects compared to 6% taking glucosamine.

K.E. should be advised that oral glucosamine may help prevent the breakdown of cartilage and may alleviate some of her pain long term, but it will not cure OA. It is unlikely that she will experience a 30% improvement in her symptoms; however, it is possible. A more realistic goal would be to see a reduction in pain and an increase in mobility of about 10%. The most important thing K.E. should do is to keep a diary of her pain, indicating the time when it occurs, its duration, and its severity. She should also indicate her daily walking distance and factors that trigger her pain. This will help determine whether glucosamine is having an effect because it can take 1 to 2 months before a response is observed clinically. Because glucosamine may take longer to work than ibuprofen (months vs. hours, respectively), the duration of pain relief from glucosamine may last longer simply because tolerability seems to be better as compared to ibuprofen. Weight loss and physical therapy should also improve her joint mobility.

Nonsteroidal Anti-Inflammatory Drug Combination Therapy

50. Can glucosamine be used in conjunction with NSAIDs to treat OA pain?

Combined glucosamine and NSAID therapy has not been studied, but because there are significant side effects associated with NSAID use in elderly patients like K.E., the decision to use them should be weighed against her risks for GI bleeding or ulceration, renal dysfunction, and pain severity. Because the analgesic effects of glucosamine are not seen immediately,[207] combined use with ibuprofen may help alleviate acute pain. She should be instructed to use the lowest effective dose of ibuprofen and to take it with food or milk. After 7 to 21 days, K.E. may consider discontinuing NSAID therapy while continuing glucosamine monotherapy. In any case, she should review her treatment decision with her primary care provider.

Product Selection

51. K.E. is concerned that some glucosamine sulfate formulations pose a risk to people with shellfish allergies. Is this true?

Glucosamine is predominantly derived from chitin, which is found in yeast, fungi, and marine invertebrates. In the United States, the primary source is from shellfish such as shrimp, scallops, and lobster. Because quality control issues have been a real concern in the purity of supplements in the Untied States, people with shellfish allergies have been told to avoid products derived from chitin. Interestingly, no reports of allergic reactions have been reported in shrimp-allergic individuals taking glucosamine sulfate. Many people believe that the allergens are found in the meat of crustaceans rather than in the exoskeleton and that this may account for the lack of allergic reactions. Other explanations may involve the method of glucosamine purification and formulation, suggesting that proper manufacturing would ultimately destroy allergenic constituents. One study compared the potential for allergic reactions in shrimp-allergic adults who ingested 1,500 mg of shrimp-derived or synthetic-derived glucosamine.[210] The study concluded that no subjects experienced immediate or delayed allergic reactions (24 hours) following the ingestion of either product. This suggests that allergenicity from properly formulated glucosamine products should not pose a risk in susceptible adults.

52. K.E. is determined to try glucosamine but is confused about which product to select because the ingredients vary. Which glucosamine product should K.E. use?

In the United States, glucosamine is widely available in grocery stores, health food stores, and pharmacies as an over-the-counter dietary supplement. Many salts of glucosamine are available, including glucosamine sulfate, glucosamine hydrochloride, and glucosamine hydroiodide. Glucosamine sulfate is the preferred product because the sulfate salt is required for GAG synthesis and is the most widely studied.[211] The formulations of glucosamine sulfate that have been used in clinical trials are Dona, Viartril-S, or Xicil, all of which are manufactured by Rottapharm in Italy. Dona can be purchased directly from the manufacturer's website. Several other formulations have proven to be of high quality and purity; look for products with the USP seal of approval on the package labeling. Glucosamine hydroiodide may be problematic in patients with undiagnosed thyroid disease or in those taking thioamides and therefore should be avoided. Glucosamine hydrochloride has been studied for OA knee pain for 3 months and was found to be ineffective in improving mobility and joint function as compared with placebo.[206] The only statistically significant improvements noted were in subjective pain relief and objective knee improvements on radiographic examination. Therefore, the value of glucosamine hydrochloride remains unknown. Many oral preparations also contain *N*-acetylglucosamine (NAG), which is a GAG intermediate. However, exogenous NAG is poorly used by cells and is believed to be a poor substrate for kinase phosphorylation, which is needed for GAG synthesis.[212] The role of NAG in preventing OA has not been determined.

Other ingredients added to glucosamine products include herbs, amino acids, sodium, selenium and potassium salts, zinc, copper, manganese, and vitamins. Some of these ingredients are added to make the product more attractive to consumers. Others are added because they are essential cofactors for GAG synthesis. For example, manganese is added because nutritional deficiencies have been associated with bone and joint malformations. Ascorbic acid is added because it is an essential cofactor for collagen synthesis; the objective is to ensure that collagen synthesis occurs at an effective rate.[213] There is no evidence, however, that these added ingredients are necessary in patients who eat a balanced diet. Sodium and potassium are added to increase glucosamine stability.

Chondroitin Sulfate

Dietary supplement manufacturers often combine chondroitin sulfate with glucosamine because it is believed to inhibit cartilage-destroying enzymes called "matrix metalloproteases." Chondroitin sulfate is the most abundant GAG in articular cartilage and consists of repeating units of glucosamine and aminosugars. Whether chondroitin is absorbed intact from the GI tract remains controversial. Chondroitin is likely broken down into individual glucosamine monomers and absorbed via the GI tract. Clinical evidence supports this mechanism.[214–216] In one study, chondroitin (400 mg orally TID) appeared to be as effective as diclofenac sodium (Voltaren), 50 mg orally TID, in relieving the pain associated with OA.[214] Patients experienced a recurrence of pain when either therapy was discontinued. Patients receiving chondroitin appeared to have better long-term control of pain, but they were allowed to continue therapy for 3 months versus 1 month for diclofenac (Voltaren) therapy. A recent meta-analysis supports chondroitin efficacy. However, the authors concluded that chondroitin effectiveness was overestimated in clinical studies.

In summary, the benefits of these combination products have not been adequately studied in clinical trials. One of the largest multicenter studies mentioned previously set out to assess the value of adding chondroitin sulfate to glucosamine.[205] Specifically, this study compared the effects of placebo to glucosamine, chondroitin sulfate, glucosamine with chondroitin sulfate, and celecoxib. Unfortunately, the investigators used glucosamine hydrochloride instead of glucosamine sulfate, making the study outcome less than ideal. The group of patients using chondroitin sulfate alone did experience a small but insignificant improvement in knee OA pain. The group receiving both glucosamine hydrochloride and chondroitin sulfate experienced a similar insignificant outcome. In a subgroup analysis, the authors concluded that the combination may be effective in patients with moderate-to-severe knee pain rather than those with milder disease. This finding is contrary to what many experts have advocated: beginning therapy in early disease to help preserve cartilage form and function as compared to beginning therapy in the later stages when little to no functional cartilage remains. Whether to begin glucosamine/chondroitin in early disease or late disease is still unclear. Until more information is known, K.E. should select a product containing glucosamine sulfate, chondroitin sulfate, or both. Any of these products may help her symptoms. Keep in mind that the addition of other ingredients might increase the potential for adverse effects and may add to the cost of the product.

Dosing

53. What is the most effective dose for glucosamine/chondroitin?

Dose–response studies have not been conducted. The most commonly studied oral daily glucosamine dose is 1,500 mg/day. The most commonly studied dose for chondroitin sulfate is 1,200 mg/day. In clinical trials, glucosamine has been administered as either 500 mg TID or 1,500 mg given once daily with or without meals. Chondroitin sulfate has also been administered as 400 mg TID or 1.200 mg/day. Given that adherence is better with once daily administration as compared to three times daily, K.E. should consider taking either supplement or both once daily.

Adverse Drug Effects

54. K.E. has been experiencing stomach upset while taking ibuprofen. Will glucosamine cause stomach upset or other serious side effects?

Although adverse effects of glucosamine have not been systematically studied, information can be gleaned from patient reports in four clinical trials[207,208,217,218] and one uncontrolled study.[219] Overall, glucosamine appears to be well tolerated and better tolerated than NSAIDs. The most commonly reported adverse symptoms involve the GI tract and include constipation, epigastric pain, tenderness, heartburn, diarrhea, and nausea.[207,208,217,218,220] Therefore, K.E. should be told that glucosamine is well tolerated compared with NSAIDs, but it may also produce symptoms of GI irritation. Taking glucosamine with food may prevent GI irritation. Because K.E. already is complaining of stomach upset while taking ibuprofen and is at high risk for GI bleeding secondary to NSAID use, she should be referred to her primary care provider for further evaluation before she adds glucosamine to her regimen.

Animal studies suggest glucosamine increases blood glucose and insulin resistance. This finding raised serious concerns for adults with diabetes using glucosamine for OA. Many studies have been carried out using both oral and IV formulations. Oral glucosamine administration is unlikely to affect blood sugar, particularly in patients who do not have diabetes.[221] Glucosamine acts intracellularly and not extracellularly, which may explain why blood glucose levels are unaffected. In those patients with undiagnosed disease or impaired glucose tolerance, it is possible that glucosamine may contribute to abnormal blood glucose values.[222] Until more information is available, patients like K.E. with diabetes mellitus or glucose intolerance who use glucosamine should monitor their blood sugar regularly.

55. Are there any known drug interactions with glucosamine?

Although drug–drug interactions have not been formally evaluated, no significant drug interactions have been reported to date. One case report exists that suggests an interaction between warfarin and glucosamine/chondroitin.[223] In this case, a 69-year-old patient with atrial fibrillation was stable on 47.5 mg of warfarin weekly with an INR between 2 and 3. After 4 weeks of self-initiated 3,000 mg of glucosamine and 2,400 mg of chondroitin daily (six capsules of Cosamin DS), the patient's INR increased from 2.58 to 4.52. The dose of Cosamin DS is twice what is recommended in the literature and what is typically used in clinical trials. Because glucosamine is a component of heparin and chondroitin is a small component of danaparoid (a low-molecular-weight heparinoid), it is possible that there may be an additive pharmacodynamic effect. However, this does not explain the increase in INR, which is not affected by heparin-like activity. Whether these higher-than-normal doses enhanced warfarin action is not known. More research is needed to assess the effect of this high dose on warfarin pharmacology. Finally, the purity of the Cosamin DS product was not assessed to rule out contaminants as the cause. At this point, the use of glucosamine/chondroitin with warfarin is not contraindicated, but the INR should be monitored at the start of therapy and during any dose adjustments.

SHARK CARTILAGE

Background

Shark cartilage has been advocated for many disorders, including cancer, psoriasis, diabetic retinopathy, neurovascular glaucoma, inflammation, Kaposi sarcoma, and arthritic pain. It has also been said to have antimicrobial properties[224] and antioxidant effects,[225] neither of which is well studied. Shark cartilage is derived from the elastic cartilage found in the endoskeleton of sharks. The spiny dogfish shark (*Aqualus acanthias*) is the primary source of commercial shark cartilage products in the United States. Native shark cartilage contains three components: chondrocytes (cartilage cells), water, and an extracellular matrix. Shark cartilage dietary supplements contain various proteins, including collagen, proteoglycans (PGs), phospholipids, sterols, and a variety of minerals (calcium, phosphorus, sodium, magnesium, potassium, zinc, iron). Chondroitin-6-sulfate appears to be one of the primary PGs found in shark cartilage, although it is not known whether this is the active ingredient. Various angiogenesis inhibitors have been identified and extracted from native shark cartilage. It is unknown if these are present or active in commercially available shark cartilage supplements.

Two popular brands of shark cartilage advocated for their antineoplastic effects include BeneFin and Neovastat, the latter being the most studied. The proposed antineoplastic activity of shark cartilage or its glycoprotein extracts is based on its ability to block two main pathways that contribute to angiogenesis: matrix metalloproteases and the vascular endothelial growth factor signaling pathway. Results have been inconsistent, however.[226–235] Angiogenesis, or the development of new blood vessels, is an important process in wound healing, building of the corpus luteum, embryonic development, and solid tumor growth and metastases. Unfortunately, whether commercially available dietary supplements actually contain active angiogenesis inhibitors is not known.

Most disturbing is that in June 1997, the FDA sent a warning letter to Lane Labs, the manufacturer of BeneFin, to stop promoting BeneFin for the treatment of cancer. Despite the warnings, the company persisted, and in 1999, FDA was granted the authority to impose a permanent injunction against Lane Labs to stop selling the supplement for the treatment of cancer. Lane Labs had to refund consumers for the cost of the supplement. Shark cartilage, however, is available today and is marketed for its proteoglycan (glucosamine and chondroitin) and calcium content.

56. S.N., a 51-year-old woman, was recently diagnosed with stage III colon cancer. She has had two previous adenomatous polyps removed, and her recent colonoscopy revealed adenocarcinoma of the colon. S.N. recently watched a television news program that claimed shark cartilage is a cure for cancer. She is currently awaiting surgery and will be receiving adjuvant chemotherapy, fluorouracil (Adrucil), and levamisole (Ergamisol). She would like to start taking shark cartilage. Is shark cartilage effective as an anticancer agent?

There is limited information on the effectiveness of shark cartilage or its extracts in the prevention or cure of cancer. Shark cartilage is available in liquid, powder, tablets, and a variety of unique capsule formulations. Each formulation of shark cartilage requires unique processing. Two common methods of processing shark cartilage involve creating an aqueous extract or a dry powder formulation. Among the commercially available shark cartilage dietary supplements, little information is provided to consumers about the type of extract or the extent of the processing. This is important because dosing recommendations vary among the various formulations, and limited data exist regarding an effective dose. One aqueous extract derived from shark cartilage (Neovastat AE-941) has been studied in a phase II renal cell carcinoma study.[236] In this study, Neovastat was given to 22 patients as a twice daily oral preparation. The study began using 60 mL/day; subsequently, some patients received a higher dose, 240 mL/day, based on tolerability. The only responders included two patients receiving 240 mL/day who survived 14 months compared with 7 months for those taking 60 mL/day. Although this study suggests that Neovastat had a favorable effect, the degree of improvement was minimal. Furthermore, the open label design makes these findings difficult to interpret. In one preliminary 16-week study in Cuba, only 3 of 29 patients with cancer responded to an unknown formulation of shark cartilage. Although the findings were not published, the National Cancer Institute reviewed the data and concluded that the results were "incomplete and unimpressive."[237] One unpublished clinical trial evaluated the effect of 80 to 100 g of shark cartilage powder self-administered orally or rectally daily in 70 subjects with cancer (type of cancer and other concomitant therapy unspecified). After 8 weeks, 10 of 20 patients who had been evaluated reported an improvement in quality of life, pain, and appetite; 4 showed partial or complete responses to therapy.[237]

Another study described the use of shark cartilage in 60 adult patients with advanced cancers (16 breast, 16 colon, 14 lung, 8 prostate, 3 lymphoma, 1 brain, 2 unknown) that were resistant to conventional therapies and had objective measurable disease.[238] Life expectancy was $\geq$12 weeks, and none of the patients had received recent or concomitant cancer chemotherapy. All patients received shark cartilage 1 g/kg/day given in three divided doses. After 12 weeks, 47 patients were evaluated for efficacy and toxicity. Five patients dropped out due to GI side effects. Quality-of-life scores did not improve after 12 weeks of therapy, and no complete or partial responses were noted. Based on these findings, shark cartilage did not alter disease progression.

The current scientific literature does not support the use of commercially available shark cartilage dietary supplements for the treatment of any type of cancer, including colon cancer. More importantly, many of the commercially available shark cartilage dietary supplements contain only binding agents or fillers. Therefore, without reliable dose–response data and bioavailability studies, it is difficult to determine whether these products have true antiangiogenic activity. If S.N. decides to use shark cartilage in combination with her chemotherapy, she should be told that it is not a cancer cure. Furthermore, the effect of shark cartilage on the activity of any other drugs she may be taking or the course of her disease is unknown.

Product Selection, Dosage, and Administration

57. If S.N. chooses to use shark cartilage, what type of product should she use and how should she be advised to take it?

There is no evidence that one formulation or source of shark cartilage is superior to another. However, the product selected should not have been exposed to excessive heat during the manufacturing process because this may denature any active proteins.[239,240] This information can be obtained only by contacting the manufacturer directly because dietary supplement labels often do not disclose the specific formulation type.

Clinically, shark cartilage has been administered orally and rectally. The most commonly recommended oral dose is 1 g/kg/day.[238,239] The GI absorption of shark cartilage has not been studied, and skeptics suggest that substantial oral absorption of its macromolecular constituents (40% proteins; 5%–20% GAGs) is unlikely because they will be destroyed by GI enzymes. However, others argue that the active ingredient is unknown, and one GAG, chondroitin, has been shown to undergo significant intestinal absorption.[241] For these reasons, some advocate using products that have been pulverized to the finest particle size.[239] To avert enzymatic degradation, maximize absorption, and minimize GI irritation, shark cartilage has also been administered as a retention enema for 25 minutes. The recommended mixture is 20 g of bulk shark cartilage powder diluted in 20 mL of tepid water. In the lay press, "colonic cleansing" has been recommended before the retention enema to clear the bowel of fecal material and to enhance absorption. This practice is dangerous, can cause dehydration, and should not be used.

Adverse Effects

58. Are there any adverse effects associated with this product? Does S.N. have any contraindications to its use?

S.N. should be warned to watch for GI upset, the most common dose-limiting side effect of shark cartilage.[239] Diarrhea, constipation, indigestion, and taste disturbances have also been observed. Most striking, however, is the unpleasant "fishy" odor of the supplement. Shark cartilage may also contain calcium; therefore, patients taking calcium supplements along with shark cartilage may need to adjust their calcium supplementation. Two cases of hepatitis have also been reported.[242] In one case, the patient was also taking oral comfrey, which is known to be hepatotoxic. Use of other hepatotoxic agents, including alcohol, acetaminophen, and prescription medications, was not described. While taking shark cartilage, S.N. should report any changes in stool or urine color, flulike symptoms, and fatigue. Because the cause of these effects is unknown, S.N. should discontinue use and discard any product that has changed in color, odor, or consistency.

S.N. does not have any contraindications to the use of this product. These include situations in which neovascularization is crucial for tissue growth and repair, such as fetal development (pregnancy), wound healing, and normal growth (infants and children). Drug interactions with shark cartilage have not been identified or reported.

59. Does shark cartilage interact with other medicines?

No formal drug interaction studies have been conducted with shark cartilage, and no interactions have been reported to date. Shark cartilage should be used cautiously in patients receiving anticoagulants because certain proteins isolated from shark cartilage resemble the structure of heparin and other endogenous human proteins that enhance the effects of tissue plasminogen activator.[242] Similar to glucosamine/chondroitin, the potential for a pharmacodynamic interaction with warfarin exists, although no studies are currently available. At this point, there is no contraindication to using shark cartilage along with warfarin because close INR monitoring is implemented at the start of therapy and during any dose adjustments.

ZINC

Background

Zinc is a trace element that serves as an enzymatic cofactor and protects cell membranes from lysis through complement activation and toxin release.[243] Many salt forms of zinc are available, including acetate (2A), gluconate (2G), gluconate-glycine (2GG), ascorbate, aspartate, orotate, sulfate, and chloride.

Each formulation varies in solubility, palatability, and zinc ion (Zn^{2+}) release characteristics. Zn^{2+} in zinc acetate (ZA), zinc gluconate (ZG), and zinc gluconate-glycine (ZGG) has been studied clinically for its role in treating the common cold.

Mechanism of Action

The mechanism of action of Zn^{2+} ions is controversial but may involve a combination of several actions. In vitro studies have shown that Zn^{2+} ions interfere with the formation of rhinoviral capsid proteins, preventing viral replication.[244–246] Zn^{2+} ions also block binding of human rhinovirus to intracellular adhesion molecule-1 (ICAM-I), which subsequently interferes with the inflammatory process.[247] ICAM-1, an immunoglobulin present on the surface of endothelial and epithelial cells, serves as a receptor for the human rhinovirus. However, Zn^{2+} ions do not seem to affect mature rhinoviruses.[245] Other research suggests that Zn^{2+} induces interferon-γ production in human white blood cell cultures.[248] At physiological serum concentrations, zinc has been shown to inhibit histamine release from mast cells and basophils.[249] An astringent or drying effect on mucus-producing goblet cells may contribute to the efficacy of Zn^{2+} in treating the common cold.[250] Finally, Zn^{2+} ions have been shown to inhibit depolarization and impulse transmission in the trigeminal and facial nerves, leading to cold symptom relief in 1 to 3 minutes.[251]

The role for zinc lozenges in the symptomatic relief of the common cold is based on Zn^{2+} release characteristics. Once released into the oral and nasal passages, Zn^{2+} ions are at supraphysiological concentrations, causing an osmotic gradient.[247] This gradient is believed to cause the transfer of Zn^{2+} ions from the mouth to the nasal and mucosal passages, sometimes referred to as a biological closed electric circuit (BCEC), where they prevent rhinoviral binding and activation.[247,252] The Zn^{2+} cation appears to be the most effective form of zinc for the common cold because it may interact with the electronegative cell surfaces in the oropharyngeal cavity. The administration of zinc products that release neutral or negatively charged Zn has been associated with a worsening of symptoms.[253,254] Neutral zinc may decrease transport through the BCEC, and negatively charged zinc may be repelled by mucosal cell surfaces.

Common Cold

The discovery that zinc may help treat the common cold occurred in 1979. A 3-year-old girl with acute lymphocytic leukemia suffering from a cold was taking ZG tablets to help stimulate lymphocyte responses after chemotherapy. Instead of swallowing the tablet whole, she let it dissolve in her mouth. The next day, her cold symptoms were gone.[255] This finding led researchers to begin studying ZG for the treatment and prevention of the common cold.[256,257]

Many studies have been conducted on the effects of zinc and the common cold.[258] These studies have generated controversy and received a great deal of scrutiny. In addition to study design flaws, much of the criticism involves limitations in the nature of common cold. Study design flaws include poor placebo matching (blinding), lack of randomization information and power analysis, small sample size, variations in dosage, frequency of administration, time of first dose, varying patient populations, lack of patient follow-up, and disparity in excipients or flavoring agents used. Other drawbacks that limit the applicability of the results involve a lack in documentation of rhinovirus infection, variations in the time of year studied, variations in location of study, differences in inoculum, and concomitant medication use.

Systematic Review

One comprehensive systematic review analyzed 14 placebo-controlled studies on the use of zinc for the treatment of the common cold.[258] The review focused on explicit criteria necessary to ensure valid experimental study design. The criteria included validated case definition (cold symptoms), quantifiable hypotheses, sample size, randomized allocation, double-blinding, proof of blinding, adherence, drop-out rates, intent-to-treat analyses, methods of statistical analysis, and measurements of probability. These criteria are critical because many of the zinc studies had been criticized for not following appropriate study design methods. The authors identified that seven studies found a positive effect for zinc, and seven studies reported no effect. Among the studies concluding zinc had a positive effect on the common cold, only one study met all 11 criteria listed previously. This is concerning because it implies that the benefits observed with zinc may have been due to chance or possibly due to flawed study design. The most common study design flaw was not using an intent-to-treat analysis. Among the zinc lozenge and nasal spray studies, two fulfilled all study criteria; however, one found a positive effect, and one found no effect of zinc. Other research suggests that the inclusion of citric acid, tartaric acid, mannitol, and sorbitol may prevent Zn^{2+} release. In all, drawing any conclusions from these studies is very difficult given study heterogeneity, lack of consistent study design, and variations in zinc delivery and zinc formulation. Explaining these variables to consumers may be overwhelming; therefore, consumers should know that more studies are needed. The formulation of zinc and the delivery method may all play a role in effectiveness.

60. C.D. is a 32-year-old woman suffering from a "cold." She complains of a sore throat, runny nose, and nasal stuffiness that began yesterday and has worsened since. Today, she developed watery eyes and sneezing. She is taking pseudoephedrine tablets (30 mg Q 8 hr PRN) for her nasal stuffiness. She is not immunocompromised and states that she does not have any other medical problems. She denies headaches, nausea, vomiting, cough, or myalgias and fever. An oral temperature taken at home is 98°F (37°C). She would like to try zinc lozenges for her cold symptoms. Are zinc lozenges appropriate for this patient?

Although many viruses are associated with the common cold, rhinovirus is involved in 30% to 50% of community-acquired colds.[259,260] C.D.'s symptoms began yesterday and have worsened today. The rapid onset is consistent with rhinovirus infections because the majority of viral replication is complete 1 day before symptom onset.[261] Peak symptoms usually appear 2 to 3 days after infection. C.D. is not complaining of headache, sinus pain, fever, fatigue, or myalgias, symptoms that are typically associated with influenza or respiratory syncytial virus. These symptoms usually develop more slowly over the course of ≥5 days. C.D. should see an improvement in her symptoms within 1 to 2 weeks because the common cold is self-limiting. C.D.'s symptoms began yesterday, so she is still a candidate for zinc therapy. In studies that have documented efficacy, improvements in cold symptoms have been seen when zinc therapy is started within 1 to 2 days of symptom onset.[252,256,262] C.D. states that she wants rapid relief of her cold symptoms. Zinc may help relieve these symptoms, but the onset of relief varies. In clinical trials, zinc therapy appeared to shorten the subjective duration of respiratory symptoms by 1 to 2 days. Remind C.D. that zinc lozenges are not a cure for the common cold. They also do not replace rest, proper nutrition, and hydration.

Product Selection and Dosing

61. C.D. wants to know which product to select. Many formulations of zinc are available. What should C.D. know about zinc dosing and administration for the common cold?

Various zinc formulations have been used to deliver Zn^{2+}, including zinc lozenges; nasal gels delivered as nasal sprays; and zinc nasal swabs, gum, and oral chews.

Clinical trials have used oral ZA, ZG, and ZGG, but adequate study blinding has been a problem because zinc lozenges have a characteristic taste that is difficult to mask. Various excipients and fillers have been used to overcome the flavor: citrate, tartaric acid, and mannitol-sorbitol mixtures. These products resulted in a tightly bound zinc complex, as measured by high stability constants, preventing the release of Zn^{2+}.[247] Based on its theoretical Zn^{2+} release characteristics, ZGG was studied. Some research suggests ZGG releases approximately 90% to 93% of the available Zn^{2+} in the mouth,[263] whereas other investigators have found that ZGG does not release any Zn^{2+} in the mouth at physiological pH as measured by zinc ion availability (ZIA).[264] The ZIA method was developed to measure the amount of Zn^{2+} released under physiological conditions in the mouth and oropharyngeal areas.[264] Based on this principle, the ZIA values were estimated for each formulation used in clinical trials and varied based on rate of lozenge dissolution, dosage, and excipients used. ZIA values do not correspond to statistically significant treatment outcomes or to statistically significant changes in the duration of common colds. The clinical relevance of this method is controversial and is currently being evaluated.

Four randomized, double-blind, placebo-controlled trials have examined the effects of zinc gluconate nasal gel on the duration and severity of common cold symptoms.[265–268] Three studies have used the same formulation called Zicam. One study inoculated healthy volunteers with the rhinovirus,[267] and the other two studies evaluated efficacy in naturally acquired colds. All patients were instructed to begin using the spray within 24 to 48 hours of the onset of cold symptoms. They were further instructed to spray one dose into each nostril every 4 hours for as long as they experienced cold symptoms. In all but one study, zinc nasal gel significantly reduced the duration of cold symptoms. The average symptom duration was 2 to 4 days in the zinc group versus 6 to 9 days in the placebo. Side effects were reported equally in the zinc and placebo groups and included a slight tingling or burning sensation. Other side effects included nasal tenderness, dry nose, dry mouth, dysgeusia, and epistaxis.

Another similar trial used a nasal spray containing 0.12% zinc (as zinc sulfate heptahydrate).[268] Patients were instructed to administer two inhalations into each nostril four times daily until the symptoms resolved, up to a maximum of 14 days. After the treatment period, there were no differences in the time to symptom resolution or cold duration; however, the zinc group did have a lower symptom score compared to placebo. The efficacy of zinc nasal spray appears similar to oral zinc lozenges, although zinc lozenges have been studied to a greater extent than zinc nasal spray. More research is needed to determine the best zinc formulation and method of administration in the common cold. Currently, both oral lozenges and nasal sprays appear to be equally effective.

In summary, C.D. should select a zinc formulation that has been shown to release Zn^{2+} readily in the mouth and oropharyngeal areas, but it is currently unclear which of the zinc products can best accomplish this. Oral ZGG, ZG, and ZA as well as nasal sprays seem to be somewhat effective; however, concerns regarding nasal sprays and permanent anosmia make the nasal sprays undesirable. C.D. should select an oral product that she finds the most palatable, convenient, and affordable.

Dosage

The commercially available zinc nasal spray (Zicam) has been administered as one spray in each nostril four times daily while awake. All zinc lozenges studied have been administered every 2 hours while awake. Although the most effective ZGG oral dose has not been established, 13.3-mg lozenges were used in clinical trials. C.D. may benefit from taking one 13.3-mg ZGG lozenge every 2 hours while awake. A higher ZGG dosage may be used, but may be associated with poor palatability. If C.D. chooses to take a ZA formulation, she should select a product with at least 10 mg of ZA per lozenge. If she prefers to take a ZG formulation, each lozenge should contain at least 23 mg of elemental zinc. For any zinc lozenge product selected, C.D. should let the lozenges dissolve completely in her mouth without chewing or swallowing them. C.D. should continue taking the lozenges every 2 hours while awake for the duration of her cold symptoms. Most clinical studies have continued Zicam for up to 10 days and zinc lozenge therapy from 5 to 10 days, or until symptoms have completely resolved. C.D. should be reminded that neither zinc nasal spray nor zinc lozenges are a cure for the common cold. If she does not see an improvement in her symptoms after 10 days or if she develops a fever, purulent sputum, vomiting, or diarrhea, she should stop taking the zinc product and seek medical care.

Adverse Effects

62. What are the side effects of zinc lozenges? What should C.D. expect?

The most common side effects associated with zinc lozenges are related to poor palatability, often resulting in poor adherence and sometimes discontinuation. Other common side effects include nausea, taste disturbances, and mouth irritation. Vomiting, diarrhea, mouth sores, and stomach distress have also been reported. These symptoms are more likely to occur with higher doses of zinc (23 mg every 2 hours).[253,254,256] One acute overdose of ZG resulted in nausea and vomiting and an elevated serum zinc level.[269] Despite a total ingestion of 4.2 g, no caustic effects were observed. If C.D. develops nausea, she should try taking the lozenges after a meal.

63. Are the zinc nasal sprays, gels, and swabs tolerated better than zinc lozenges?

Zinc nasal sprays have been associated with permanent anosmia (loss of smell), which has also led to taste disturbances. The reaction has been described as follows: the solution is applied to the nares and sniffed, a burning sensation lasting minutes to hours occurs. Nearly 48 hours later, anosmia has developed.[270] In October 2004, the FDA received more than 100 complaints about zinc nasal sprays and anosmia. The manufacturers of zinc nasal sprays argue that there is no evidence their products cause anosmia and that anosmia may be caused by many other factors. Given the severity of this side effect, zinc nasal sprays, gels, and swabs that are applied directly to the nasal passages cannot be recommended at this time. If C.D. is interested in trying zinc nasal gel, she should be discouraged and directed to any of the other oral formulations.

Long-Term Safety

64. C.D. returns to the pharmacy 1 month later. She wants to take zinc lozenges again to treat another cold. Is it safe for C.D. to reinitiate zinc lozenges? What are the long-term concerns associated with zinc?

In clinical trials, the average duration of therapy for zinc lozenges has varied between 5 and 10 days or until symptom resolution. Zinc lozenges should be used only for colds of short duration. Currently, there is no information documenting the degree of systemic absorption, resistance to treatment, or cumulative effects of zinc lozenges. Because the amount of elemental zinc absorbed from zinc lozenges has not been measured, the consequences of long-term use are unclear. Studies of elemental zinc supplementation at oral dosages of 150 mg twice daily for 6 weeks did not have adverse consequences.[271] However, with chronic use, oral zinc has resulted in copper and other nutrient imbalances because zinc is an effective copper chelator.[272] C.D. may begin another course of zinc therapy if she follows the same treatment recommendations mentioned previously and does not exceed the dosing recommendations.

Pregnancy and Lactation

65. The following year, C.D. wants to know if she can safely take zinc lozenges for her cold if she is pregnant. What should C.D. know about the safety of zinc lozenges during pregnancy or lactation?

Women who are pregnant or nursing should avoid zinc lozenges because subjects who were pregnant or lactating were excluded from study enrollment. C.D. should attempt to manage her cold symptoms without medications if possible. A humidifier may help her congestion, and adequate hydration is especially important.

Efficacy in Children

66. L.P. is a 5-year-old girl who has caught a cold from her brother. L.P.'s mother wants to give her child zinc lozenges. Has the efficacy of zinc lozenges been evaluated in children?

Only two prospective studies to date have assessed the value of zinc lozenges in children.[256,273] Dosing in these trials was estimated based on the empiric adult dose. For children weighing <27 kg, a dose of 11.5 mg (as ZG) was given every 2 hours while awake.[256] ZGG doses were estimated based on average body surface area and corresponding year in school (at the expected age). Children in school grades 1 to 6 received 10 mg ZGG five times per day. Children in school grades 7 to 12 received 10 mg six times per day.[273] Unfortunately, variations in both the formulation and the dose produced conflicting results. The 11.5-mg ZG lozenge, although higher in dose, resulted in a higher incidence of withdrawals because of taste disturbances and poor mucosal tolerability. The ZGG lozenges were better tolerated, but did not shorten the duration of cold symptoms in children. In children, lozenge flavor is especially important in ensuring medication adherence. Macknin et al. attempted to characterize the amount of time missed from school because of colds.[273] Although children taking zinc lozenges returned to school sooner than those taking placebo, this difference was not statistically significant. Because a dose–response relationship in children has not been established, dosing of zinc lozenges in children is empiric; adverse effects are similar for both children and adults.

Various formulations of zinc specifically marketed to children are now available. These formulations include zinc gluconate bubble gum, zinc lollipops, and sugarfree zinc lozenges. None of these formulations have been specifically studied in children for the relief of the common cold and should not be recommended. L.P.'s mother should be advised to ensure that L.P. gets adequate hydration and nutrition, and to monitor her temperature.

Zinc Deficiency

67. Can zinc lozenges be used to supplement the normal dietary intake of zinc?

Zinc is an essential component in hundreds of cellular and enzymatic processes. The recommended dietary allowance for adult males is 15 mg.[274] Some researchers suspect that zinc lozenges correct an underlying zinc deficiency and therefore strengthen the immune response. In developing countries, zinc deficiencies have been documented in both children and adults.[275] In the United States, zinc deficiencies have been described in the elderly and in premenopausal women.[276,277] Many of the clinical manifestations of zinc deficiency (growth retardation, poor appetite, mental lethargy, delayed wound healing, susceptibility to infection) are reversible after supplementation. Therapeutic zinc supplementation at dosages of 150 mg/day for 1 to 3 months reverses these effects. The amount of elemental zinc delivered in a 7-day course of zinc lozenges given at the maximum recommended dose is about 1.9 g, but because it is unknown how much of the dose is absorbed systemically, these lozenges should not be used to correct nutritional deficiencies. The average U.S. diet provides 10 to 15 mg of zinc.[278] Patients should eat a balanced diet containing foods rich in zinc: red meats, eggs, whole grains, legumes, oysters, and other shellfish.[279] Otherwise, a multiple vitamin with minerals should be adequate to prevent zinc deficiency.

Allergic Rhinitis

68. S.L. is a 38-year-old man who read on the Internet that zinc lozenges alleviate the symptoms of allergic rhinitis. S.L. knows that zinc has been studied for the common cold to relieve nasal congestion and rhinitis. Currently, he is taking loratadine (Claritin) 10 mg PO daily. Should S.L. take zinc lozenges for his allergic rhinitis symptoms?

Some patients enrolled in the clinical trials for the common cold experienced "antiallergic effects" after zinc lozenge administration,[251,252] but there are no studies that have evaluated this effect in people with allergic rhinitis. Some literature suggests that Zn^{2+} interferes with the inflammatory process by inhibiting leukocyte migration. The expression of ICAM-1, an adhesion molecule, is increased during an allergic response, and its expression has been correlated with an increased migration of neutrophils and eosinophils.[251] Because Zn^{2+}can prevent ICAM-1 expression, it may therefore inhibit the inflammatory process; Zn^{2+} also may have antihistaminic effects.[249] If S.L. decides to take zinc lozenges for his allergic rhinitis, he should be told that Zn^{2+} has antihistaminic properties. Although the degree of systemic antihistaminic effects has not been measured clinically, S.L. should be made aware of possible additive effects with his antihistamine.[251] Symptoms to look for include excessive dryness and irritation of the oral and nasal passages and headache. Because there is no clinical information on the use of zinc lozenges for allergic rhinitis, it cannot be recommended.

MELATONIN

Background

Melatonin is an endogenous hormone that is secreted by the pineal gland, located at the base of the brain. Melatonin secretion is primarily controlled by daylight and darkness and corresponds to typical sleep–wake hours. Darkness stimulates melatonin release. Secretion increases progressively after the onset of darkness, usually between 9 PM and 4 AM; peak melatonin levels occur between 2 AM and 4 AM.

Melatonin has received orphan drug status to regulate the sleep cycle in blind patients who have no light perception.[280] In the United States, it is sold as a dietary supplement as 0.1-, 0.3-, 1-, 5-, and 10-mg oral tablets or capsules in immediate-release (IR) and various sustained-release (SR) formulations. Synthetic formulations of melatonin are available and should be used exclusively. Animal-derived or human-derived products carry a risk for viral transmission, contamination, and variable potency. Melatonin has been used for jet lag, insomnia, aging, depression, reproduction, HIV, and a variety of cancers. Other uses include cluster headache prophylaxis and use in nightshift workers and children. Possible antianxiety and analgesic-like effects have led to an increased use of melatonin before and after medical and surgical procedures, including abdominal hysterectomy. Melatonin is being investigated aggressively for use in children undergoing magnetic resonance imaging (MRI) and computed tomography (CT) scans and in children with neurodevelopmental disabilities. Many studies evaluating the effects of melatonin for sleep are limited by small sample size, incomplete information, and inadequate laboratory monitoring. In addition, short treatment duration and variable dosing schedules make treatment recommendations difficult. Many treatment recommendations are based on pharmacologic principles, rather than clinical evidence.

Pharmacokinetics

The effects of several medications on melatonin levels have been studied, as have the pharmacokinetics of endogenous and exogenous melatonin (Tables 3-5 and 3-6). After administration of an 80-mg oral dose, melatonin levels peaked between 60 and 150 minutes and returned to normal in 8 to 19 hours. Melatonin disposition is characterized by a rapid distribution phase followed by an elimination phase. The initial half-life is

Table 3-5 Effect of Various Drugs on Endogenous Melatonin Secretion

Drug Name	Reference	Direction of Change
NSAIDs	Murphy et al.[a]	↓
Fluvoxamine	Skene et al.[b]	↑
Desipramine	Farney et al.,[c] Skene et al.[c]	↑
Fluoxetine	Childs et al.[d]	↓
Tryptophan	Namboodiri et al.[e]	↑
Corticotropin-releasing hormone	Kellner[f]	↓
Sodium valproate	Childs et al.[d]	↓
Clonidine	Kennedy et al.[g]	
Yohimbine	Kennedy et al.[g]	
Atenolol	Cowen et al.[h]	↓
Propranolol	Rommel and Demisch,[i] Vaughan et al.[j]	↓
Scopolamine	Vaughan et al.[j]	↓
Isoproterenol	Vaughan et al.[j]	↓
Zolpidem	Copinschi et al.[k]	
Pyridoxine	Luboshitzky et al.[l]	

[a] Murphy PJ et al. Nonsteroidal anti-inflammatory drugs alter body temperature and suppress melatonin in humans. *Physiol Behav* 1996;59:133.
[b] Skene DJ et al. Comparison of the effects of acute fluvoxamine and desipramine administration on melatonin and cortisol production in humans. *Br J Clin Pharmacol* 1994;37:181.
[c] Farney C et al. Acute treatment with desipramine stimulates melatonin and 6-suphatoxy melatonin production in man. *Br J Clin Pharmacol* 1986;22:73.
[d] Childs PA et al. Effect of fluoxetine on melatonin in patients with seasonal affective disorder and matched controls. *Br J Psychiatry* 1995;166:196.
[e] Namboodiri MA et al. 5-Hydroxyptophan elevates serum melatonin. *Science* 1983;221:659.
[f] Kellner M et al. Corticotropin-releasing hormone inhibits melatonin secretion in healthy volunteers: a potential link to low-melatonin syndrome in depression? *Neuroendocrinology* 1997;65:284.
[g] Kennedy SH et al. Melatonin responses to clonidine and yohimbine challenges. *J Psychiatry Neurosci* 1995;20:297.
[h] Cowen PJ et al. Atenolol reduces plasma melatonin concentration in man. *Br J Clin Pharmacol* 1983;15:579.
[i] Rommel T, Demisch L. Influence on chronic beta-adrenoreceptor blocker treatment on melatonin secretion and sleep quality in patients with essential hypertension. *J Neural Transm Gen Sect* 1994;95:39.
[j] Vaughan GM et al. Nocturnal elevation of plasma melatonin and urinary 5-hydroxyindoleacetic acid in young men: attempts at modification by brief changes in environment lighting and sleep and by autonomic drugs. *J Clin Endocrinol Metab* 1976;42:752.
[k] Copinschi G et al. Effects of bedtime administration of zolpidem on circadian and sleep-related hormonal profiles in normal women. *Sleep* 1995;18:417.
[l] Luboshitzky R et al. The effect of pyridoxine administration on melatonin secretion in normal men. *Neuroendocrinol Lett* 2002;23:213.

Table 3-6 Mean Nocturnal Levels of Circulating Melatonin

Age	*Mean Melatonin Levels*
First 6 mo of life	27.3 pg/mL (0.12 nmol/L)
1–3 yr	329.5 pg/mL (1.43 nmol/L)
15–20 yr	62.5 pg/mL (0.27 nmol/L)
70–90 yr	29.2 pg/mL (0.13 nmol/L)

estimated to be 2 minutes, and the elimination half-life is 20 to 50 minutes.[281] Other research has shown that doses of 0.05, 0.5, and 5 mg have mean elimination half-lives of 65, 43, and 70 minutes, respectively.[282,283]

Endogenous melatonin is metabolized in the liver to 6-hydroxy-melatonin and excreted as sulfate and glucuronide conjugates.[281] In 22 patients with liver cirrhosis, endogenous melatonin serum levels were significantly elevated compared with age-matched controls.[284] A positive correlation between total bilirubin and daytime melatonin level was also seen.[284] As expected, the elimination half-life of exogenous melatonin increased from 44 to 97 minutes, on average, in people with liver cirrhosis.[285] Competition with bilirubin for elimination, decreased liver blood flow, or decreased activity of the enzyme, 6-β-hydroxylase, may also contribute to these observations.[284] Other research has suggested that the endogenous production rate of melatonin appears to be reduced in patients with liver cirrhosis.[285]

The oral bioavailability of melatonin ranges between 40% and 70% for dosages that vary from 2.5 to 100 mg. Food may enhance the absorption somewhat, resulting in higher mean plasma levels compared with those achieved when taken in the fasting state.[285]

Jet Lag (Rapid Time Zone Change)

Transmeridian air travel results in dysregulation of the sleep–wake cycle until the circadian secretion of melatonin adjusts to the new time zone (2–14 days). Adaptation is generally more difficult or slower for older patients when traveling eastward and when multiple time zones are crossed. The most common symptoms of jet lag include GI disturbances and insomnia, particularly daytime sleepiness and frequent awakenings during the night. Maximizing exposure to daylight can enhance symptom recovery.[286]

69. S.T., a 33-year-old female flight attendant, complains of sleep disturbances, loss of mental alertness, and daytime drowsiness. Every 2 weeks, she travels from Los Angeles, California, to London, England, and on to Auckland, New Zealand. A friend recommended melatonin. How should S.T. manage her symptoms? Can melatonin help?

S.T. is experiencing the classic symptoms of rapid and multiple time zone changes, which have caused an abrupt shift in her sleep–wake cycle. Usually, time to adjust to the new time zone and proper sleep hygiene is the only treatment necessary. However, because S.T. is a flight attendant and has to repeat this schedule on a regular basis, her body has little time to adapt, and she is likely to suffer from jet lag symptoms on a more long-term basis.

Clinical trials have evaluated 5 to 8 mg of IR melatonin for jet lag.[287–291] Although these studies included a small number of participants, patients reported subjective improvements in symptoms, including decreased daytime fatigue, normal sleep patterns, energy, alertness, and mood. Subjects who took 5 mg of IR melatonin up to 3 days before departure seemed to have a worse recovery of jet lag symptoms (decreased energy and alertness) than those who began taking the medication on arrival in the new time zone. This difference was not statistically significant. The largest study assessed the effects of melatonin in 257 patients traveling across six time zones.[292] Subjects were randomized to receive placebo or one of three melatonin regimens. Melatonin was administered as 0.5 mg at bedtime, 5 mg at bedtime, or 0.5 mg on a "shifting schedule." The shifting schedule was designed to mimic the circadian release of melatonin throughout the sleep–wake cycle; one dose was taken on the evening of departure and then at 1 hour earlier each night for 6 days. By day 6, the melatonin dose corresponded to the natural melatonin peak time. No differences were observed at all time points among patients receiving any melatonin dosage or placebo. No statistical differences were observed in total sleep time, napping, sleep onset, or other symptoms. Melatonin possesses some hypnotic effects, which may help S.T. However, improvement in jet lag symptoms seems to be more closely related to resynchronization by regular light–dark stimuli. Therefore, S.T. should also maximize her exposure to daylight and implement proper sleep hygiene techniques, which include going to bed at the same time each night and avoiding caffeine and daytime naps.

The optimal dose and timing of melatonin administration have not been determined, but S.T. may benefit from 5 mg of the IR formulation beginning on the evening of departure and then for the next 1 to 3 days after arrival at the destination.

Although melatonin is relatively well tolerated, she should be advised to watch for daytime drowsiness, tachycardia, dysthymia, and headache.[287–290,293] One case of acute psychosis, one case of retrograde amnesia, and two cases of melatonin-induced erythematous plaques have been reported.[294–296] Because melatonin can cause drowsiness, S.T. should use caution when performing tasks that require full alertness 30 minutes to 2 hours after a dose, and she should avoid alcohol or other CNS depressants. The long-term effects of melatonin administration have not been studied.

70. S.T. is trying to become pregnant. Is it safe for her to continue taking melatonin now or when she becomes pregnant? Should S.T. take melatonin while breast-feeding?

Melatonin has been shown to inhibit ovulation when administered in combination with a progestin. Therefore, S.T. should avoid taking melatonin while trying to conceive because high dosages (75–300 mg/day) may inhibit ovulation.[297] Although it is unknown whether lower dosages (0.5–5 mg daily) can alter conception or pose a threat to the fetus, she should avoid taking any drugs while trying to become pregnant and during her pregnancy. Instead, she should try to control her jet lag symptoms through sleep hygiene.

S.T. also should avoid taking melatonin while breast-feeding because it may suppress prolactin secretion and diminish the production of breast milk.[298]

Insomnia

71. T.X. is a 75-year-old woman who complains of insomnia and daytime fatigue. On further questioning, it becomes clear that T.X. falls asleep early (around 9 PM) and wakes up at about the same time each morning (6 AM). However, she wakes up two to three times each night and has difficulty getting back to sleep. Will melatonin help?

Insomnia is a subjective awareness of inappropriate sleep. Patients may complain of difficulty falling asleep (sleep onset), staying asleep, sleep maintenance (as in T.X.'s case), or arising too early (early morning awakening). Melatonin has been studied in the treatment of various sleep disorders, including delayed sleep-phase syndrome (DSPS) and insomnia. Many studies have documented the hypnotic effect of melatonin in improving sleep onset, duration, and quality when administered to healthy volunteers.[299–303] Increases in rapid eye movement sleep have also been documented.[299] One study demonstrated that peak hypnotic effects vary based on the time of day melatonin is ingested, suggesting that light is an important factor for efficacy. Melatonin 5 mg orally caused peak hypnotic effects within 3 hours when taken at noontime compared to 1 hour when taken at 9 PM.[299]

However, these studies are limited by small sample size, inadequate monitoring, and poor study design. Dosing, patient age, timing of drug administration, randomization, study duration, and type of monitoring have varied greatly. Many of the clinical studies failed to establish a relationship between low endogenous melatonin levels and insomnia at study onset. In addition, the cause of the sleep disorder is often not defined or stated, or is confounded by other disease states. Some patients with DSPS, for example, also had a diagnosis of depression, and sleep disturbances often subside in this population once antidepressant therapy is initiated. Larger studies are needed to determine the effect of patient age, dosage, duration of therapy, and sleep disorder etiology on melatonin efficacy. According to one meta-analysis that combined these studies, pooled data from melatonin trials were found to be significantly heterogenous. Despite this, statistically significant improvements in sleep quality have been observed.[303] Improvements in sleep-onset latency (time to fall asleep), sleep efficiency, and sleep duration have all been reported in patients taking melatonin.

Insomnia in the Elderly

As illustrated by T.X., sleep maintenance is the most prevalent sleep-related disorder in patients older than 65 years of age, occurring in approximately 30% of the elderly population.[283] Sleep-onset insomnia is less common (19%), followed by early morning awakening (18.8%).[283] Because melatonin serum levels can be low in elderly patients who suffer from insomnia, some have theorized that use of a SR formulation will correct the low levels and prevent sleep maintenance insomnia. Although elderly patients taking 0.5 mg of SR or IR products experienced significant improvements in sleep onset, the SR formulation did not improve total sleep time. In fact, the effectiveness of melatonin administration on improving total sleep time (sleep maintenance) has been inconsistent. In older ambulatory adults between 55 and 80 years of age, consistent improvements have been seen in sleep quality, sleep latency, and morning alertness with the 2-mg SR formulation.[304,305] Interestingly, there is no evidence of rebound insomnia or withdrawal effect on discontinuation of melatonin.[305] It is unknown which formulation of melatonin is superior for sleep maintenance insomnia; however, subjective improvements have been consistent across all studies. Because melatonin may improve morning alertness and quality of sleep, and given that there are few risks associated with its use, T.X. can try the lowest dose of melatonin (either IR or SR) at bedtime to see if it will maintain her sleep. The dosage can be gradually escalated to 5 mg.

72. R.R. is a 28-year-old male medical student who has been having trouble falling asleep for the past week. He attributes his insomnia to stress because he has to take his medical licensing examination in 2 weeks. He wants to know if melatonin will help him get to sleep without feeling "hung-over" the next day. Will melatonin help?

Melatonin has not been systematically studied in people with insomnia caused by stress, even though it is a common etiology. R.R. wants to achieve adequate rest but also wants to avoid the "hang-over" effects associated with antihistamines contained in over-the-counter sleep medications or prescription sedative-hypnotics. R.R. will likely benefit from melatonin because it has been shown to improve sleep onset. Because he does not experience early morning awakenings, an IR formulation of melatonin should be sufficient. IR melatonin has a short half-life and has not been associated with significant daytime drowsiness or a "hang-over" effect. R.R. should start with the lowest effective dose, 0.3 mg, if possible. If he has no response in 30 to 60 minutes, he may take a repeat dose as needed. Although melatonin is considered relatively safe with few dose-related side effects, using the minimal effective dose is best. Melatonin should only be used 30 minutes before the desired bedtime. There is some evidence that up to 6 months of continuous melatonin use may decrease semen quality in otherwise healthy males. Thus, if R.R. is planning to start a family, he may want to avoid using melatonin. Instead, he should try to follow proper sleep hygiene techniques. For example, he should avoid staying up all night studying, and he should try to maximize his exposure to daylight while awake.

Anticancer Effects

73. J.T. is a 47-year-old woman who currently is taking tamoxifen for breast cancer. She recently read that melatonin may have antitumor effects. What evidence exists for this claim? Would melatonin be effective in her case?

The antitumor effects of melatonin have been studied in vitro and in small clinical trials involving patients with metastatic breast cancer, malignant melanoma, and glioblastoma.[306] In all these cancers, some beneficial effect has been observed, which may be related to melatonin's immune-modulating or antioxidant effects. With regard to breast cancer, in vitro studies have shown that melatonin decreases estrogen-binding capacity and the expression of estrogen receptors in the MCF-7 breast cancer cell line; it also inhibits the growth of epithelial breast cancer cells.[306] In a clinical trial, patients with metastatic breast cancer refractory to tamoxifen displayed a slower progression of disease when given melatonin than patients receiving tamoxifen alone, regardless of estrogen-receptor status.[307] Melatonin also may lessen the cytotoxicity associated with chemotherapy or radiation therapy.[306] These effects are linked to neurohormonal changes at the level of the cell (e.g., modulating membrane excitability, increasing cellular repair, conserving ATP, blocking nitric oxide synthesis). Nonetheless, more study is needed to better define the effects of melatonin based on the severity and type of cancer as well as on duration of disease. Melatonin may have some beneficial effects in J.T.'s case, but she should add this therapy only in consultation with her oncologist, who is in the best position to evaluate its effects on her disease progression. Dosages of 20 to 40 mg/day have been used.

COENZYME Q10

Background

Coenzyme Q10 is a cofactor found in cell membranes, serum, and lipoproteins. It is also known as ubiquinone or, in its reduced form, ubiquinol. As its name implies, it is ubiquitous, being found in small amounts in soybeans, walnuts, almonds, oils, fruits, and spinach. It is also found in various organ meats (heart, liver, kidney, spleen, pancreas) and skeletal muscle. Biochemically, coenzyme Q10 protects mitochondrial proteins and DNA from free-radical damage and serves as an electron carrier of the electron transport chain in the inner mitochondrial membrane. This is an important process in that it is the last step in aerobic respiration that results in ATP generation. For this reason, coenzyme Q10 has been studied for its role in many different conditions, including cardiovascular disorders, Alzheimer's disease (AD), breast cancer, gum disease, and Parkinson disease, among others.

Pharmacokinetics

Coenzyme Q10 is absorbed slowly from the GI tract because it has a high molecular weight and low water solubility.[308] For this reason, many coenzyme Q10 formulations have been designed to maximize absorption often by including a lipophilic vehicle such as vitamin E. Following a single dose, there is a two-peak pattern at 6 and 24 hours. The first peak corresponds to the parent compound, and the second peak corresponds to the metabolite, ubiquinol. Typical adult serum concentrations vary from 0.7 to 1 mcg/mL; the clinical significance of these levels is unknown.[309] Coenzyme Q10 is best absorbed when taken with food, and higher levels have been observed when it is chewed with a high-fat food such as peanut butter.[310] Within cells, most of the coenzyme Q10 (40%–50%) is found in mitochondria within the inner mitochondrial membrane. Whether coenzyme Q10 is metabolized is unknown; however, it is distributed to the liver and incorporated into very low density lipoprotein. Coenzyme Q10 is predominantly excreted via the biliary tract and, therefore, more than 60% of an oral dose is recovered in the feces.[308]

Prevention of Statin-Induced Myopathy

74. J.S. is a 55-year-old male in otherwise good health diagnosed with "high cholesterol" 3 years ago. He states that his LDL cholesterol was 149 mg/dL at the time of diagnosis, but now, after starting simvastatin (a statin drug), his LDL cholesterol is 95 mg/dL. His LDL is under control, but he wants to know if he should begin taking coenzyme Q10 to help prevent statin-related myopathy.

Statins reduce cholesterol production by inhibiting the enzyme HMG-CoA reductase, which is also involved in the synthesis of coenzyme Q10. Initiating statin therapy has been associated with a decrease in coenzyme Q10 serum concentrations, which may block the critical steps in muscle cell energy generation, possibly leading to statin-related myopathy.[311] A reduction in serum concentrations does not always correlate with a reduction in intramuscular concentrations, which may play a greater role in statin-related myopathy. It is unknown whether the reduction in intramuscular coenzyme Q10 leads to statin myopathy or if the myopathy itself causes cellular damage that reduces intramuscular coenzyme Q10. In addition, the type of statin used and the dose of the statin may also play a role. In one small double-blind study, the effect of coenzyme Q10 supplementation was evaluated in patients taking various statins who also had developed myopathy symptoms.[312] Patients received either coenzyme Q10 100 mg/day or vitamin E 400 IU/day for 30 days. After 30 days, the patients taking coenzyme Q10 had statistically significant reductions in muscle pain intensity, whereas the vitamin E group had no change in muscle pain intensity. Although this study suggests a benefit, larger studies are needed to determine when to initiate coenzyme Q10 (e.g., preventative treatment compared to active treatment once myopathy has developed). Given that coenzyme Q10 is relatively safe, however, there is no clinical harm in J.S. using it while taking simvastatin, although the cost may be significant. It is important to let J.S. know that myopathy may still occur rarely with a statin, even while taking coenzyme Q10. He should be instructed that the risk for myopathy from statin therapy is very low compared to the beneficial reduction of morbidity and mortality that has been demonstrated in large, well-designed studies. He should be instructed to report any unusual or unexplained muscle pain to his provider.

Hypertension

75. F.T. is a 75-year-old male with stage 1 hypertension. F.T. measures his blood pressure at home, and since beginning enalapril 20 mg and hydrochlorothiazide 25 mg, his BP readings have improved from 150/95 to 130/85 mmHg. His provider has encouraged him to implement lifestyle modifications to further improve his BP, in particular to increase his physical activity and to minimize his daily consumption of alcohol. F.T. drinks a six-pack of beer after dinner at least nightly while watching television. A friend of his heard that taking coenzyme Q10 can help lower BP, and F.T. wants to try it.

Adults with hypertension have been found to have lower levels of endogenous coenzyme Q10. This has led to speculation that a deficiency in endogenous coenzyme Q10 levels may lead to the development of hypertension. There are many causes of hypertension; however, low endogenous coenzyme Q10 levels have not been studied well enough to make this link. In early clinical trials, small but significant reductions in SBP and DBP (7–10 mmHg) were observed after 8 to 10 weeks of coenzyme Q10 supplementation.[313] This led researchers to believe that coenzyme Q10 possessed antihypertensive properties because of its antioxidant and vasodilatory effects.[313] One large meta-analysis of 12 clinical trials included 362 hypertensive patients and found a BP-lowering benefit of coenzyme Q10. Although this meta-analysis included both well-designed and poorly designed trials (open-labeled, uncontrolled, with and without concomitant antihypertensive therapy), the reductions in blood pressure were consistent across all studies. In three well-designed randomized, controlled trials, coenzyme Q10 supplementation significantly lowered SBP (17 mmHg) and DBP (8 mmHg) compared to no change in the placebo groups.

F.T. should be informed that coenzyme Q10 has the potential to further lower his BP; however, whether this reduction will help him reach his goal (<120/80 mmHg) is still unknown. More research is needed to assess the true value of using coenzyme Q10 either alone or in combination with other antihypertensive medications. More importantly, F.T. should be encouraged to decrease his daily alcohol consumption and increase his physical activity. These lifestyle modifications will not only improve his hypertension but may also contribute to a healthier lifestyle. Finally, because F.T. is not at his goal BP, he should continue his regular doctor appointments because small-dose adjustments to his medications may be necessary. He should continue to self-monitor his BP at home and maintain a log of his BP readings.

Heart Failure

76. S.A. is a 54-year-old male with nonischemic cardiomyopathy diagnosed in 2005. He has never had an MI but does have a history of dyslipidemia and is a current smoker (1 pack per day for 20 years) and heavy drinker (beer and spirits on most days of the week). S.A. was diagnosed to have New York Heart Association (NYHA) Class I disease (left ventricular ejection fraction [LVEF] = 25%) and is currently asymptomatic. He is taking ramipril 5 mg PO twice daily. S.A. read about the benefits of coenzyme Q10 in heart failure (HF) and would like to initiate therapy. What are the benefits of coenzyme Q10 in HF?

Studies have suggested that patients with HF have decreased levels of coenzyme Q10, so a deficiency may contribute to its progression. Early studies have demonstrated improvements in hemodynamic parameters (increases in ejection fraction and end diastolic volume) following coenzyme Q10 therapy.[314] Other studies demonstrated improvements in subjective signs and symptoms of heart failure, including edema, liver enlargement, resting dyspnea, and heart palpitations.[315] Unfortunately, many of these studies are outdated in that enrolled patients were not taking ACE inhibitors or β-blockers, which have been shown to improve morbidity and mortality in patients with HF. In addition, many studies used nonstandard or noninvasive methods to assess disease progression. Coenzyme Q10 may offer a small benefit to patients with mild to moderate heart disease (NYHA Class II–III) without ischemia. Initiating coenzyme Q10 later at more severe stages of disease appears to have little to no effect.[315] Because S.A. does not have ischemia and is still asymptomatic, it is unknown just how much subjective or objective benefit he may experience. When data from studies are combined, a statistically significant improvement in ejection fraction of 4% has been suggested.[315] Because his disease is in the early stages, it is possible that coenzyme Q10 may offer him some benefit because he still has adequate functional heart muscle.

Dosing

There is no established dosing for coenzyme Q10; however, clinical trials have used varied doses, depending on the indication. For most indications, the typical daily dose averages 100 mg/day. For the treatment of hypertension, daily doses ranged from 100 to 120 mg daily.[313] In patients with HF, 50 to 150 mg daily in two or three divided doses have been used.[314] Dosing recommendations may vary among manufacturers; this depends on the formulation and the lipid vehicle used to deliver the coenzyme Q10. For most products, however, multiple daily doses are required to ensure adequate replacement. If S.A. wants to use coenzyme Q10 for his HF, a dose of 100 mg daily in divided doses is appropriate. More importantly, S.A. should limit his alcohol intake and if motivated to quit smoking, he should enroll in a smoking cessation program. S.A. should continue taking ACE inhibitors because they are recommended for patients who are asymptomatic and have an LVEF <40%.

Side Effects

Coenzyme Q10 is very well tolerated with very few side effects reported. In clinical trials, the most common side effects were GI discomfort, including diarrhea, nausea, heartburn, and appetite suppression, occurring with an incidence of <1%.[316] These side effects abated when the dose was reduced or coenzyme Q10 was discontinued. Other side effects included irritability, agitation, headache, and dizziness.[316] Thrombocytopenia, skin rash, and pruritus have also been reported in <0.5% of patients. Ascribing many of these infrequent side effects to coenzyme Q10 is very difficult because many of the studies were conducted when the purity of these products was unknown. Other rare case reports of flu-like symptoms, photophobia, and thrombocytopenia have not been definitely linked to the supplement.

Drug Interactions

Coenzyme Q10 may interact with warfarin leading to a subtherapeutic INR. Coenzyme Q10 is structurally related to menaquinone, also known as vitamin K2. As a result, coenzyme Q10 is believed to have procoagulant effects. Several case reports describe a subtherapeutic INR in patients taking stable doses of warfarin after beginning coenzyme Q10 therapy.[317] Because the potential interaction may have undesirable effects on coagulation, patients should be advised to avoid coenzyme Q10 while taking warfarin. In some patients, the combination may be safely used, provided the patient agrees to more frequent monitoring of INR values, especially during the first month of therapy. In addition, adherence to both warfarin and coenzyme Q10 should be encouraged and maintained throughout the course of therapy.

Because coenzyme Q10 has purported antihypertensive effects, it is reasonable to consider additive antihypertensive effects when combined with prescription antihypertensives.

The most significant effects would be encountered during therapy initiation or following antihypertensive dose increases.

77. D.P. is a 66-year-old woman with a history of atrial fibrillation and no history of bleeding. She has been taking warfarin 7 mg once daily for 2 months, and her INR values have been therapeutic, ranging from 2 to 2.5 (target 2–3). She arrives in clinic today asking whether she should begin coenzyme Q10 for its antioxidant effects to help with her atrial fibrillation.

In D.P.'s case, the desire to initiate coenzyme Q10 is based on its antioxidant effects. Engaging D.P. in a discussion about the need for antioxidant effects would be helpful. If D.P. is committed to using coenzyme Q10 while continuing warfarin, she should be informed that her INR may become subtherapeutic, placing her at risk for a thromboembolic event unless adjustments are made to her warfarin. More frequent monitoring and a change in warfarin dose may be required. D.P. should also know that the antioxidant contributions from coenzyme Q10 have not been studied in patients with atrial fibrillation.

REFERENCES

1. Eisenberg DM et al. Trends in alternative medicine use in the United States, 1990–1997. *JAMA* 1998; 280:569.
2. Balluz LS et al. Vitamin and mineral supplement use in the United States: results from the third national health and nutrition examination survey. *Arch Fam Med* 2000;9:258.
3. Blendon RJ et al. American's views on the use and regulation of dietary supplements. *Arch Intern Med* 2001;161:805.
4. Kaufman DW et al. Recent patterns of medication use in the ambulatory adult population of the United States: the Sloan survey. *JAMA* 2002;287:337.
5. Astin JA. Why patients use alternative medicine: results of a national study. *JAMA* 1998;279:1548.
6. Blumenthal et al., eds. Herbal Medicine: Expanded German Commission E Monographs. *Integrative Medicine Communications*; 2000.
7. Schulz V et al. Rational Phytotherapy: A Physician's Guide to Herbal Medicine. Berlin, NY: Springer-Verlag; 2004.
8. Dietary Supplement Health and Education Act (DSHEA) of 1994 (PL 103–417), 103rd Congress, 2nd session report 103–410, January 25, 1994.
9. Marcus DM, Grollman AP. Botanical medicines—the need for new regulations. *N Engl J Med* 2002; 347:2073.
10. Ernst E. Harmless herbs? A review of the recent literature. *Am J Med* 1998;104:170.
11. De Smet PAGM. Herbal remedies. *N Engl J Med* 2002;347:2046.
12. Brustbauer R, Wenisch C. Bradycardic atrial fibrillation after consuming herbal tea. *Dtsch Med Wochenschr* 1997;122:930.
13. Ernst E, Coon JT. Heavy metals in traditional Chinese medicines: a systematic review. *Clin Pharmacol Ther* 2001;70:497.
14. Ernst E. Heavy metals in traditional Indian remedies. *Eur J Clin Pharmacol* 2002;57:891.
15. Blackburn WD Jr. Eosinophilia myalgia syndrome. *Semin Arthritis Rheum* 1997;26:781.
16. Ernst E. Adulteration of Chinese herbal medicines with synthetic drugs: a systematic review. *J Int Med* 2002;252:107.
17. Tyler VE. What pharmacists should know about herbal remedies. *J Am Pharm Assoc* 1996;NS36: 29.
18. Rode D. Comfrey toxicity revisited. *Trends Pharmacol Sci* 2002;23:497.
19. Polymeros D et al. Acute cholestatic hepatitis caused by *Teucrium polium* (golden germander) with transient appearance of antimitochondrial antibody. *J Clin Gastroenterol* 2002;34:100.
20. Shad JA et al. Acute hepatitis after ingestion of herbs. *South Med J* 1999;92:1095.
21. Chan TY. Incidence of herb-induced aconite poisoning in Hong Kong: impact of publicity measures to promote awareness among the herbalists and the public. *Drug Saf* 2002;25:823.
22. Russmann S et al. Kava hepatotoxicity. *Ann Intern Med* 2001;135:68.
23. Anderson IB et al. Pennyroyal toxicity: measurement of toxic metabolite levels in two cases and review of the literature. *Ann Intern Med* 1996;1234:726.
24. McRae CA et al. Hepatitis associated with Chinese herbs. *Eur J Gastroenterol Hepatol* 2002;14:559.
25. Leung R et al. Royal Jelly consumption and hypersensitivity in the community. *Clin Exp Allergy* 1997;27:333.
26. Lewis J Esophageal and small bowel obstruction from guar gum-containing "diet pills": analysis of 26 case reports reported to the Food and Drug Administration. *Am J Gastroenterol* 1992;87:1424.
27. Bent S et al. The relative safety of ephedra compared with other herbal products. *Ann Intern Med* 2003;138:468.
28. Amagase H. Significance of garlic and its constituents in cancer and cardiovascular disease. *J Nutr* 2006;136:716S.
29. Lawson LD, Gardner CD. Composition, stability and bioavailability of garlic products used in a clinical trial. *J Agric Food Chem* 2005;53:6254.
30. Gardner CD et al. Effect of raw garlic vs. commercial garlic supplements on plasma lipid concentrations in adults with moderate hypercholesterolemia: a randomized, clinical trial. *Arch Intern Med* 2007;167:346.
31. Breithaupt-Grogler K et al. Protective effect of chronic garlic intake on elastic properties of aorta in the elderly. *Circulation* 1997;96:2649.
32. Stevinson C et al. Garlic for treating hypercholesterolemia: a meta-analysis of randomized clinical trials. *Ann Intern Med* 2000;133:420.
33. Ackermann RT et al. Garlic shows promise for improving some cardiovascular risk factors. *Ann Intern Med* 2001;161:813.
34. Liu L, Yeh YY. S-alk(en)yl cysteines of garlic inhibit cholesterol synthesis by deactivating HMG-CoA reductase in cultured rat hepatocytes. *J Nutr* 2002;132:1129.
35. Chung LY. The antioxidant properties of garlic compounds: allyl cysteine, alliin, allicin, and allyl disulfide. *J Med Food* 2006;9:205.
36. Al-Qattan KK et al. Nitric oxide medicates blood pressure lowering effect of garlic in the two-kidney, one-clip model of hypertension. *J Nutr* 2006;136(3 Suppl):774S.
37. Sharifi AM et al. Investigation of antihypertensive mechanism of garlic in 2K1C hypertensive rat. *J Ethnopharmacol* 2003;86:219.
38. Banerjee SK, Maulik SK. Effect of garlic on cardiovascular disorders: a review. *Nutr J* 2002;1:1.
39. Koscielny J et al. The antiatherosclerotic effect of *Allium sativum*. *Atherosclerosis* 1999;144:237.
40. Budoff MJ et al. Inhibiting progression of coronary calcification using aged garlic extract in patients receiving statin therapy: a preliminary study. *Prev Med* 2004;985.
41. Bordia A et al. Effect of garlic (*Allium sativum*) on blood lipids, blood sugar, fibrinogen, and fibrinolytic activity in patients with coronary artery disease. *Prostaglandins Leukot Essent Fatty Acids* 1998;58:257.
42. Agarwal KC. Therapeutic actions of garlic constituents. *Med Res Rev* 1996;16:111.
43. Makheja AN, Bailey JM. Antiplatelet constituents of garlic and onion. *Agents Actions* 1990;29: 360.
44. Shukla Y, Kalra N. Cancer chemoprevention with garlic and its constituents. *Cancer Lett* 2007;247: 167.
45. Fleischauer AT et al. Garlic consumption and cancer prevention: meta-analysis of colorectal and stomach cancers. *Am J Clin Nutr* 2000;72:1047.
46. Thomson M, Ali M. Garlic (*Allium sativum*): a review of its potential use as an anti-cancer agent. *Curr Cancer Drug Targets* 2003;3:67.
47. Lau BHS et al. *Allium sativum* (garlic) and cancer prevention. *Nutr Res* 1990;10:937.
48. Ankri S, Mirelman D. Antimicrobial properties of allicin from garlic. *Microbes Infect* 1999;2:125.
49. Harris JC et al. Antimicrobial properties of *Allium sativum* (garlic). *Appl Microbiol Biotechnol* 2001;57:282.
50. Jappe U et al. Garlic-related dermatoses: case report and review of the literature. *Am J Contact Dermatol* 1999;10:37.
51. Petry JJ. Garlic and postoperative bleeding. *Plast Reconstr Surg* 1995;96:483.
52. Rose KD et al. Spontaneous spinal epidural hematoma with associated platelet dysfunction from excessive garlic ingestion: a case report. *Neurosurgery* 1990;26:880.
53. Piscitelli SC et al. The effect of garlic supplements on the pharmacokinetics of saquinavir. *Clin Infect Dis* 2002;34:234.
54. Gallicano K et al. Effect of short-term administration of garlic supplements on single-dose ritonavir pharmacokinetics in healthy volunteers. *Br J Clin Pharmacol* 2003;55:199.
55. Kodera Y et al. Physical, chemical and biological properties of S-allylcysteine, an amino acid derived from garlic. *J Agric Food Chem* 2002;50:622.
56. De Rooij BM et al. Urinary excretion of N-acetyl-S-allyl-L-cysteine upon garlic consumption by human volunteers. *Arch Toxicol* 1996;70:635.
57. Birks J et al. *Ginkgo biloba* for cognitive impairment and dementia (Cochrane review). In: *The Cochrane Library*, Issue 4, 2002. Oxford: Update Software
58. Mazza M et al. *Ginkgo biloba* and donepezil: a comparison in the treatment of Alzheimer's dementia in a randomized, placebo-controlled double-blind study. *Eur J Neurol* 2006;13:981.
59. Kurz A, Van Baelen B. *Ginkgo biloba* compared with cholinesterase inhibitors in the treatment of dementia: a review based on meta-analysis by the Cochrane Collaboration. *Dement Geriatr Cogn Disord* 2004;18:217.
60. DeKosky ST et al. The Ginkgo Evaluation of Memory (GEM) study: design and baseline data of a randomized trial of *Ginkgo biloba* extract in prevention of dementia. *Contemp Clin Trials* 2006;27:238.
61. Vellas B et al. The GuidAge Study: methodological issues. A 5-year, double-blind, randomized trial of the efficacy of EGb 761 for prevention of Alzheimer's disease in patients over 70 with a memory complaint. *Neurology* 2006;67(Suppl 3):S6.

62. Rathman KL, Conner CS. Alzheimer's disease: clinical features, pathogenesis and treatment. *Ann Pharmacother* 2007;41:1499.
63. Maclennan KM et al. The CNS effects of *Ginkgo biloba* extracts and ginkgolide B. *Progr Neurol* 2002;67:235.
64. Mehlsen J et al. Effects of a *Ginkgo biloba* extract on forearm haemodynamics in healthy volunteers. *Clin Physiol Funct Imaging* 2002;22:375.
65. Diamond BJ et al. *Ginkgo biloba* extract: mechanisms and clinical indications. *Arch Phys Med Rehabil* 2000;81:668.
66. Pietri S et al. *Ginkgo biloba* extract (EGb 761) pretreatment limits free radical-induced oxidative stress in patients undergoing bypass surgery. *Cardiovasc Drugs Ther* 1997;11:121.
67. Amri H et al. Transcriptional suppression of the adrenal cortical peripheral-type benzodiazepine receptor gene and inhibition of steroid synthesis by ginkgolide B. *Biochem Pharmacol* 2003;65:717.
68. Bastianetto S, Quirion R. Egb 761 is a neuroprotective agent against B-amyloid toxicity. *Cell Mol Biol* 2002;48:693.
69. Woelk H et al. *Ginkgo biloba* special extract EGb 761 in generalized anxiety disorder and adjustment disorder with anxious mood: a randomized, double-blind, placebo-controlled trial. *J Psychiatr Res* 2007;41:472.
70. Pittler MH, Ernst E. *Ginkgo biloba* extract for the treatment of intermittent claudication: a meta-analysis of randomized trials. *Am J Med* 2000;108:276.
71. Horsch S, Walther C. *Ginkgo biloba* special extract EGb 761 in the treatment of peripheral arterial occlusive disease (PAOD)—a review based on randomized, controlled studies. *Int J Clin Pharmacol Therapeut* 2004;42:63.
72. Letzel H, Schoop E. *Gingko biloba* extract EGb 761 and pentoxifylline in intermittent claudication. *Vasa* 1992;21:403.
73. Moher D et al. Pharmacological management of intermittent claudication: a meta-analysis of randomized trials. *Drugs* 2000;59:1057.
74. Wojcicki J et al. Comparative pharmacokinetics and bioavailability of flavonoid glycosides of *Ginkgo biloba* after a single oral administration of three formulations to healthy volunteers. *Meter Med Pol* 1995;27:141.
75. Hauser D et al. Bleeding complications precipitated by unrecognized *Ginkgo biloba* use after liver transplantation. *Transpl Int* 2002;15:377.
76. Vaes LP, Chyka PA. Interactions of warfarin with garlic, ginger, gingko, or ginseng: nature of the evidence. *Ann Pharmacother* 2000;34:1478.
77. Hasegawa S et al. Ginkgo nut intoxication in a 2-year-old male. *Pediatr Neurol* 2006;35:275.
78. Galluzzi S et al. Coma in a patient with Alzheimer's disease taking low dose trazodone and *Ginkgo biloba*. *J Neurol Neurosurg Psych* 2000;68:679.
79. Burns NR et al. *Ginkgo biloba*: no robust effect on cognitive abilities or mood in healthy young or older adults. *Hum Psychopharmacol Clin Exp* 2006;21:27.
80. Mix JA, Crews WD Jr. A double-blind, placebo-controlled, randomized trial of *Ginkgo biloba* extract Egb 761 in a sample of cognitively intact older adults: neuropsychological findings. *Hum Psychopharmacol* 2002;17:267.
81. Kennedy DO et al. Modulation of cognition and mood following administration of single doses of *Ginkgo biloba*, ginseng or ginkgo/ginseng combination in healthy young adults. *Physiol Behav* 2002;75:739.
82. Canter PH, Ernst E. *Ginkgo biloba* is not a smart drug: an updated systematic review of randomized clinical trials testing the nootropic effects of *G. biloba* in healthy people. *Hum Psychopharmacol* 2007;22:265.
83. Ernst E, Stevinson C. *Ginkgo biloba* for tinnitus: a review. *Clin Otolaryngol* 1999;24:164.
84. Hilton M, Stuart E. *Ginkgo biloba* for tinnitus (Cochrane review). In: *The Cochrane Library*, Issue 2, 2004. Oxford: Update Software.
85. Evans JR. Ginkgo extract for age-related macular degeneration (Cochrane review). In: *The Cochrane Library*, Issue 3, 2000. Oxford: Update Software.
86. Gertsch JH et al. Randomized, double-blind, placebo-controlled comparison of *Ginkgo biloba* and acetazolamide for prevention of acute mountain sickness among Himalayan trekkers: the prevention of high altitude illness trial (PHAIT). *BMJ* 2004;328:797.
87. Chow T et al. *Ginkgo biloba* and acetazolamide prophylaxis for acute mountain sickness: a randomized, placebo-controlled trial. *Arch Intern Med* 2005;165:296.
88. Wheatley D. Triple-blind, placebo-controlled trial of *Ginkgo biloba* in sexual dysfunction due to antidepressant drugs. *Hum Psychopharmacol Clin Exp* 2004;19:545.
89. Whiskey E et al. A systematic review and meta-analysis of *Hypericum perforatum* in depression: a comprehensive clinical review. *Int Clin Psychopharmacol* 2001;16:239.
90. Linde K et al. St John's wort for depression: meta-analysis of randomised controlled trials. *Br J Psychiatry* 2005;186:99.
91. Williams JW et al. A systematic review of newer pharmacotherapies for depression in adults: evidence report summary. *Ann Intern Med* 2000; 132:743.
92. Werneke U et al. How effective is St John's wort? The evidence revisited. *J Clin Psychiatry* 2004;65:611.
93. Gastpar M et al. Comparative efficacy and safety of a once-daily dosage of hypericum extract STW3-VI and citalopram in patients with moderate depression: a double-blind, randomised, multicenter, placebo-controlled study. *Pharmacopsychiatry* 2006;39:66.
94. Hypericum Depression Trial Study Group. Effect of *Hypericum perforatum* (St John's wort) in major depressive disorder: a randomized controlled trial. *JAMA* 2002;287:1807.
95. Bjerkenstedt L et al. Hypericum extract LI 160 and fluoxetine in mild to moderate depression: a randomized, placebo-controlled, multi-center study in outpatients. *Eur Arch Psychiatry Clin Neurosci* 2005;255:40.
96. Uebelhack R et al. Efficacy and tolerability of hypericum extract STW3-VI in patients with moderate depression: a double-blind, randomized, placebo-controlled clinical trial. *Adv Ther* 2004;21:265.
97. Kasper S et al. Superior efficacy of St John's wort extract WS 5570 compared to placebo in patients with major depression: a randomized, double-blind, placebo-controlled, multi-center trial. *BMC Med* 2006;4:14.
98. Gastpar M et al. Efficacy and tolerability of hypericum extract STW3 in long-term treatment with a once daily dosage in comparison with sertraline. *Pharmacopsychiatry* 2005;38:78.
99. Anghelescu IG et al. Comparison of hypericum extract WS 5570 and paroxetine in ongoing treatment after recovery from an episode of moderate to severe depression: results from a randomized multicenter study. *Pharmacopsychiatry* 2006;39:213.
100. Muller WE. Current St John's wort research from mode of action to clinical efficacy. *Pharmacol Res* 2003;47:101.
101. Butterweck V, Schmidt M. St John's wort: role of active compounds for its mechanism of action and efficacy. *Wien Med Wochenschr* 2007;157:356.
102. Dannawi M. Possible serotonin syndrome after combination of buspirone and St John's wort. *J Psychopharmacol* 2002;16:401.
103. Bonetto N et al. Serotonin syndrome and rhabdomyolysis induced by concomitant use of triptans, fluoxetine and hypericum. *Cephalalgia* 2007;Sept 15 (e-pub ahead of print).
104. Izzo AA, Ernst E. Interactions between herbal medicines and prescribed drugs: a systematic review. *Drugs* 2001;61:2163.
105. Stevinson C, Ernst E. Can St John's wort trigger psychoses? *Int J Clin Pharmacol Ther* 2004;42:473.
106. Xie HG, Kim RB. St John's wort-associated drug interactions: short-term inhibition and long term induction? *Clin Pharmacol Ther* 2005;78:19.
107. Schulz V. Safety of St John's wort extract compared to standard antidepressants. *Phytomedicine* 2006;13:199.
108. Bhopal JS. St John's wort induced sexual dysfunction. *Can J Psych* 2001;46:456.
109. Dean AJ et al. Suspected withdrawal syndrome after cessation of St John's wort. *Ann Pharmacother* 2003;37:150.
110. Karalapillai DC, Bellomo R. Convulsions associated with an overdose of St John's wort. *MJA* 2007;186:213.
111. Gulick RM et al. Phase I studies of hypericin, the active compound in St. John's wort, as an antiretroviral agent in HIV-infected adults. *Ann Intern Med* 1999;130:510.
112. Schempp CM et al. Effect of oral administration of *Hypericum perforatum* extract (St John's wort) on skin erythema and pigmentation induced by UVB, UVA, visible light and solar simulated radiation. *Phytother Res* 2003;17:141.
113. Cotterill JA. Severe phototoxic reaction to laser treatment in a patient taking St John's wort. *J Cosmet Laser Ther* 2001;3:159.
114. Schey KL et al. Photooxidation of lens—crystallin by hypericin (active ingredient in St John's wort). *Photochem Photobiol* 2000;72:200.
115. Brockmoller J et al. Hypericin and pseudohypericin: pharmacokinetics and effects on photosensitivity in humans. *Pharmacopsychiatry* 1997; 30(Suppl 2):94.
116. Kerb R et al. Single-dose and steady-state pharmacokinetics of hypericin and pseudohypericin. *Antimicrob Agents Chemother* 1996;40:2087.
117. Biber A et al. Oral bioavailability of hyperforin from hypericum extracts in rats and human volunteers. *Pharmacopsychiatry* 1998;31:36.
118. Reichling J et al. A current review of the antimicrobial activity of *Hypericum perforatum* L. *Pharmacopsychiatry* 2004;34(Suppl 1):S116.
119. Agostinis P et al. Hypericin in cancer treatment: more light on the way. *Int J Biochem Cell Biol* 2002;34:221.
120. Stevinson C, Ernst E. A pilot study of *Hypericum perforatum* for the treatment of premenstrual syndrome. *Br J Obstet Gynecol* 2000;107:870.
121. Barrett B. Medicinal properties of echinacea: a critical review. *Phytomedicine* 2003;10:66.
122. Barnes J et al. *Echinacea* species (*Echinacea angustifolia* (DC.) Hell., *Echinacea pallida* (Nutt.) Nutt., *Echinacea purpurea* (L.) Moench): a review of their chemistry, pharmacology and clinical properties. *Pharm Pharmacol* 2005;57:929.
123. Pillai S et al. Use of quantitative flow cytometry to measure ex vivo immunostimulant activity of echinacea: the case for polysaccharides. *J Alt Complement Med* 2007;13:625.
124. Sloley BD et al. Comparison of chemical components and anti-oxidant capacity of different *Echinacea* species. *J Pharm Pharmacol* 2001;53:849.
125. Shah SA et al. Evaluation of echinacea for the prevention and treatment of the common cold: a meta-analysis. *Lancet* 2007;7:473.
126. Linde K et al. Echinacea for preventing and treating the common cold (Cochrane review). In: *The Cochrane Library*, Issue 2, 2007. Oxford: Update Software.
127. Roesler J et al. Application of purified polysaccharides from cell cultures of the plant *Echinacea purpurea* to test subjects mediates activation of the phagocyte system. *Int J Immunopharmacol* 1991;13:931.
128. Burger R et al. Echinacea induced cytokine production by human macrophages. *Int J Immunopharmacol* 1997;19:371.
129. See DM et al. In vitro effects of echinacea and ginseng on natural killer and antibody-dependent cell cytotoxicity in healthy subjects and chronic fatigue

syndrome or acquired immunodeficiency syndrome patients. *Immunopharmacology* 1997;35:229.
130. Goel V et al. A proprietary extract from the echinacea plant (*Echinacea purpurea*) enhances systemic immune response during a common cold. *Phytother Res* 2005;19:689.
131. Schwarz E et al. Effect of oral administration of freshly pressed juice of *Echinacea purpurea* on the number of various subpopulations of B- and T-lymphocytes in healthy volunteers: results of a double-blind, placebo-controlled cross-over study. *Phytomedicine* 2005;12:625.
132. Matthias A et al. Comparison of echinacea alkylamide pharmacokinetics between liquid and tablet preparations. *Phytomedicine* 2007;Feb 6 (e-pub ahead of print).
133. Mengs U et al. Toxicity of *Echinacea purpurea*: acute, subacute and genotoxicity studies. *Arzneimittelforschung* 1991;41:1076.
134. Huntley AL et al. The safety of herbal medicinal products derived from *Echinacea* species: a systematic review. *Drug Saf* 2005;28:387.
135. Parnam MJ. Benefit–risk assessment of the squeezed sap of the purple coneflower (*Echinacea purpurea*) for long term oral immunostimulation. *Phytomedicine* 1996;3:95.
136. Lersch C et al. Stimulation of the immune response in outpatients with hepatocellular carcinomas by low doses of cyclophosphamide (LDCY), *Echinacea pupurea* extracts (Echinacin) and thymostimulin. *Arch fur Geschwulstforschung* 1990;60:379.
137. Lersch C et al. Nonspecific immunostimulation with low doses of cyclophosphamide (LDCY), thymostimulin, and *Echinacea purpurea* extracts (Echinacin) in patients with far advanced colorectal cancers: preliminary results. *Cancer Invest* 1992;10:343.
138. Melchart D et al. Polysaccharides isolated from *Echinacea purpurea* herbal cell cultures to counteract undesired effects of chemotherapy: a pilot study. *Phytother Res* 2002;16:138.
139. Vonau B et al. Does the extract of the plant *Echinacea purpurea* influence the clinical course of recurrent genital herpes? *Int J STD AIDS* 2001;12:154.
140. Koch E. Effects from fruits of saw palmetto (*Sabal serrulata*) and roots of stinging nettle (*Urtica dioica*): viable alternatives in the medical treatment of benign prostatic hyperplasia and associated lower urinary tract symptoms. *Planta Med* 2001;67:489.
141. Thorpe A, Neal D. Benign prostatic hypertrophy. *Lancet* 2003;361:1359.
142. Oesterling JE. Benign prostatic hyperplasia. *Drug Ther* 1995;332:99.
143. Carraro JC et al. Comparison of phytotherapy (Permixon) with finasteride in the treatment of benign prostate hyperplasia: a randomized international study of 1,098 patients. *Prostate* 1996;29:231.
144. Beckman TJ, Mynderse LA. Evaluation and medical management of benign prostatic hyperplasia. *Mayo Clin Proc* 2005;80:1356.
145. Lowe F. Role of the newer alpha-1 adrenergic receptor antagonists in the treatment of benign prostatic hyperplasia-related lower urinary tract symptoms. *Clin Ther* 2004;26:1701.
146. Buck AC. Is there a scientific basis for the therapeutic effects of *Serenoa repens* in benign prostatic hyperplasia? Mechanisms of action. *J Urol* 2004;172:1792.
147. Paubert-Braquet M et al. Effect of the lipidosterolic extract of *Serenoa repens* (Permixon) and its major components on basic fibroblast growth factor induced proliferation of cultures of human prostate biopsies. *Eur Urol* 1998;33:340.
148. Goepel M et al. Do saw palmetto extracts block human alpha-1 adrenoceptor subtypes in vivo? *Prostate* 2001;46:226.
149. Di Silverio et al. Response of tissue androgen and epidermal growth factor concentration to the administration of finasteride, flutamide and *Serenoa repens* in patients with benign prostatic hyperplasia (BPH). *Eur Urol* 1996;30(Suppl 2):96.
150. Wilt T et al. *Serenoa repens* for benign prostatic hyperplasia (Cochrane review). In: *The Cochrane Library*, Issue 4, 2002. Oxford: Update Software.
151. Bent S et al. Saw palmetto for benign prostatic hyperplasia. *N Engl J Med* 2006;354:557.
152. Semino AM et al. Symptomatic treatment of benign hypertrophy of the prostate: comparative study of prazosin and *Serenoa repens*. *Arch Exp Urol* 1992;45:211.
153. Grasso M et al. Comparative effects of alfuzosin versus Serenoa repens in the treatment of symptomatic benign prostatic hyperplasia. *Arch Exp Urol* 1995;48:97.
154. Debruyne F et al. Comparison of a phytotherapeutic agent (Permixon) with an alpha-blocker (tamsulosin) in the treatment of benign prostatic hyperplasia: a one year randomized international study. *Eur Urol* 2002;41:497.
155. Hizli F, Uygur MC. A prospective study of the efficacy of *Serenoa repens*, tamsulosin, and *Serenoa repens* plus tamsulosin treatment for patients with benign prostate hyperplasia. *Int Urol Nephrol* 2007;39:879.
156. Denis LJ. Editorial review of "Comparison of phytotherapy (Permixon) with finasteride in the treatment of benign prostatic hyperplasia: a randomized international study of 1,098 patients." *Prostate* 1996;29:241.
157. Radad K et al. Use of ginseng in medicine with emphasis on neurodegenerative disorders. *J Pharmacol Sci* 2006;100:175.
158. Zhou W et al. Molecular mechanisms and clinical applications of ginseng root for cardiovascular disease. *Med Sci Monit* 2004;10:187.
159. Cui J et al. What do commercial ginseng products contain? *Lancet* 1994;344:134.
160. Schlag EM, McIntosh MS. Ginsenoside content and variation among and within American ginseng (*Panax quinquefolius* L.) populations. *Phytochemistry* 2006;67:1510.
161. Vignano C, Ceppi E. What is in ginseng? *Lancet* 1994;344:619.
162. Attele AS et al. Ginseng pharmacology: multiple constituents and multiple actions. *Biochem Pharmacol* 1999;58:1685.
163. Nocerino E et al. The aphrodisiac and adaptogenic properties of ginseng. *Fitoterapia* 2000;71:S1.
164. Cardinal BJ, Engels HJ. Ginseng does not enhance psychological well being in healthy, young adults: results of a double-blind, placebo-controlled, randomized clinical trial. *J Am Dietetic Assoc* 2001;101:655.
165. Sorenson H, Sonne J. A double-masked study of the effects of ginseng on cognitive functions. *Curr Ther Res* 1996;57:959.
166. Kennedy DO, Scholey AB. Ginseng: potential for the enhancement of cognitive performance and mood. *Pharmacol Biochem Behav* 2003;75:687.
167. Bahrke MS, Morgan WR. Evaluation of the ergogenic properties of ginseng: an update. *Sports Med* 2000;29:113.
168. Allen JD et al. Ginseng supplementation does not enhance healthy young adults' peak aerobic exercise performance. *J Am Coll Nutr* 1998;17:462.
169. Vogler BK et al. The efficacy of ginseng: a systematic review of randomized clinical trials. *Eur J Clin Pharmacol* 1999;55:567.
170. Engels HJ. Effects of ginseng on secretory IgA performance and recovery from interval exercise. *Med Sci Sports Exerc* 2003;35:690.
171. Wiklund I et al. A double-blind comparison of the effect on quality of life of a combination of vital substances including standardized ginseng G115 and placebo. *Curr Ther Res* 1994;55:32.
172. Pieralisi G et al. Effects of a standardized ginseng extract combined with dimethylaminoethanol bitartrate, vitamins, minerals, and trace elements on physical performance during exercise. *Clin Ther* 1991;13:373.
173. Thommessen B, Laake K. No identifiable effect of ginseng (Gericomplex) as an adjuvant in the treatment of geriatric patients. *Aging Clin Exp Res* 1996;8:417.
174. Caso Marasco A et al. Double-blind study of a multivitamin complex supplemented with ginseng extract. *Drugs Exp Clin Res* 1996;22:323.
175. Vuksan V et al. Herbal remedies in the management of diabetes: lessons learned from the study of ginseng. *Nutr Metab Cardiovasc Dis* 2005;15:149.
176. Vuksan V et al. Korean red ginseng (*Panax ginseng*) improves glucose and insulin regulation in well-controlled, type 2 diabetes: results of a randomized, double-blind, placebo-controlled study of efficacy and safety. *Nutr Metab Cardiovasc Dis* 2006;July 21 (e-pub ahead of print).
177. Buettner C et al. Systematic review of the effects of ginseng on cardiovascular risk factors. *Ann Pharmacother* 2005;39:83.
178. Siegel RK. Ginseng abuse syndrome. *JAMA* 1979;241:1614.
179. Liu J et al. Stimulatory effect of saponin from *Panax ginseng* on immune function of lymphocytes in the elderly. *Mech Ageing Dev* 1995;83:43.
180. Srisurapanon S et al. The effect of standardized ginseng extract on peripheral blood leukocytes and lymphocyte subsets: preliminary study in young healthy adults. *J Med Assoc Thai* 1997;80(Suppl 1):S81.
181. Scaglione F et al. Immunomodulatory effects of two extracts of *Panax ginseng* C.A. Meyer. *Drugs Exp Clin Res* 1990;16:537.
182. Scaglione F et al. Efficacy and safety of a standardized ginseng extract G115 for potentiating vaccination against the influenza syndrome and protection against the common cold. *Drugs Exp Clin Res* 1996;22:65.
183. McElhaney JE et al. Efficacy of COLD-fX in the prevention of respiratory symptoms in community-dwelling adults: a randomized, double-blinded, placebo-controlled trial. *J Alt Complement Med* 2006;12:153.
184. McElhaney JE et al. A placebo-controlled trial of a proprietary extract of North American ginseng (CVT-E002) to prevent acute respiratory illness in institutionalized older adults. *J Am Geriatr Soc* 2004;52:13.
185. Predy GN et al. Efficacy of an extract of North American ginseng containing poly-furanosyl-pyranosyl-saccharides for preventing upper respiratory tract infections: a randomized controlled trial. *CMAJ* 2005;173:1043.
186. Yun TK. Experimental and epidemiological evidence on non-organ specific cancer preventative effect of Korean ginseng and identification of active compounds. *Mutat Res* 2003;63:523.
187. Yun TK. Panax ginseng: a non-organ specific cancer preventative. *Lancet Oncol* 2001;2:49.
188. Salvatti G et al. Effects of *Panax ginseng* C.A. Meyer on male fertility. *Panminerva Medica* 1996;38:249.
189. Hong B et al. A double-blind, crossover study evaluating the efficacy of Korean red ginseng in patients with erectile dysfunction: a preliminary report. *J Urol* 2002;168:2070.
190. Coon J, Ernst E. *Panax ginseng*: a systematic review of adverse effects and drug interactions. *Drug Saf* 2002;25:323.
191. McRae S. Elevated digoxin levels in a patient taking digoxin and Siberian ginseng. *Can Med Assoc J* 1996;155:293.
192. Awang DVC. Siberian ginseng toxicity may be case of mistaken identity [letter]. *Can Med Assoc J* 1996;155:1237.
193. Koren G et al. Maternal ginseng use associated with neonatal androgenization [letter]. *JAMA* 1990;264:1828.
194. Awang DVC. Maternal use of ginseng and neonatal androgenization [letter]. *Can Med Assoc J* 1991;266:363.
195. Cui JF et al. Gas chromatographic-mass spectrometric determination of 20(S)-protopanaxadiol and 20(S)-protopanaxatriol for study on human urinary excretion of ginsenosides after ingestion of ginseng preparations. *J Chromatogr B Biomed Sci Appl* 1997;689:349.

196. Howell DS et al. Biochemical changes in cartilage relevant to the cause and management of osteoarthritis. *Rheumatology* 1982;7:29.
197. Cumming GJ et al. Permeability of composite chondrocyte-culture millipore membranes to solutes of varying size and shape. *Biochem J* 1979;181:257.
198. Persiani S. Glucosamine oral bioavailability and plasma pharmacokinetics after increasing doses of crystalline glucosamine sulfate in man. *Osteoarthritis Cartilage* 2005;13:1041.
199. Kempson GE et al. Patterns of cartilage stiffness on normal and degenerate human femoral heads. *J Biomech* 1971;4:597.
200. Mankin HJ et al. Biochemical and metabolic abnormalities in articular cartilage from osteoarthritic human hips. II. Correlation of morphology with biochemical and metabolic data. *J Bone Joint Surg* 1971;53A:523.
201. Tenenbaum J et al. Biochemical and biomechanical properties of osteoarthritic dog cartilage. *Arthritis Rheum* 1979;22:666.
202. Setnikar I et al. Pharmacokinetics of glucosamine in man. *Arzneimittelforschung* 1993;43:1109.
203. McAlindon TE et al. Glucosamine and chondroitin for treatment of osteoarthritis: a systematic quality assessment and meta-analysis. *JAMA* 2000;283:1469.
204. Vlad SC et al. Glucosamine for pain in osteoarthritis. *Arthritis Rheum* 2007;56:2267.
205. Clegg DO et al. Glucosamine, chondroitin sulfate, and the two in combination for painful knee osteoarthritis. *N Engl J Med* 2006;354:795.
206. Houpt JB et al. Effect of glucosamine hydrochloride in the treatment of pain of osteoarthritis of the knee. *J Rheumatol* 1999;26:2423.
207. Reginster JY et al. Long-term effects of glucosamine sulphate on osteoarthritis progression: a randomized, placebo-controlled trial. *Lancet* 2001;357:251.
208. Pavelka K et al. Glucosamine sulfate use and delay of progression of knee osteoarthritis. *Arch Intern Med* 2002;162:2113.
209. Müller-Fassbender H et al. Glucosamine sulfate compared to ibuprofen in osteoarthritis of the knee. *Osteoarthritis Cartilage* 1994;2:61.
210. Villacis J et al. Do shrimp-allergic individuals tolerate shrimp-derived glucosamine? *Clin Exp Allergy* 2006;36:1457.
211. Bassleer C et al. In-vitro evaluation of drugs proposed as chondroprotective agents. *Int J Tissue React* 1992;14:231.
212. Karzel K, Domenjoz R. Effects of hexosamine derivatives and uronic acid derivative on glycosaminoglycan metabolism of fibroblast cultures. *Pharmacology* 1971;5:337.
213. Leach RM. Role of manganese in mucopolysaccharide metabolism. *Fed Proc* 1971;30:991.
214. Morreale P et al. Comparison of the antiinflammatory efficacy of chondroitin sulfate and diclofenac sodium in patients with knee osteoarthritis. *J Rheumatol* 1996;23:1385.
215. Palmieri L et al. Metabolic fate of exogenous chondroitin sulphate in the experimental animal. *Arzneimittelforschung* 1990;40:319.
216. Conte A et al. Biochemical and pharmacokinetic aspects of oral treatment with chondroitin sulfate. *Arzneimittelforschung* 1995;45:925.
217. Vajranetra P. Clinical trial of glucosamine compounds for osteoarthritis of knee joints. *J Med Assoc Thai* 1984;67:409.
218. Vaz AL. Double-blind clinical evaluation of the relative efficacy of ibuprofen and glucosamine sulphate in the management of osteoarthrosis of the knee in out-patients. *Curr Med Res Opin* 1982; 8:145.
219. Pujalte JM et al. Double blind clinical evaluation of oral glucosamine sulphate in the basic treatment of osteoarthritis. *Curr Med Res Opin* 1980;7:110.
220. Tapadinhas MJ et al. Oral glucosamine sulphate in the management of arthrosis: report on a multicentre open investigation in Portugal. *Pharmatherapeutica* 1982;3:157.
221. Stumpf JL et al. Effect of glucosamine on glucose control. *Ann Pharmacother* 2006;40:694.
222. Biggee BA et al. Effects of oral glucosamine sulphate on serum glucose and insulin during an oral glucose tolerance test of subjects with osteoarthritis. *Ann Rheum Dis* 2007;66:260.
223. Rozenfeld V et al. Possible augmentation of warfarin effect by glucosamine-chondroitin. *Am J Health Syst Pharm* 2004;61:306.
224. Moore KS et al. Squalamine: an aminosterol antibiotic from the shark. *Proc Natl Acad Sci USA* 1993;90:1354.
225. Gomes EM et al. Shark-cartilage containing preparation protects cells against hydrogen peroxide induced damage and mutagenesis. *Mutat Res* 1996;367:203.
226. Lee A, Langer R. Shark cartilage contains inhibitors of tumor angiogenesis. *Science* 1983;221:1185.
227. Pettit GR, Ode RH. Antineoplastic agents L: isolation and characterization of sphyrnastatins 1 and 2 from the hammerhead shark *Sphyrna lewini*. *J Pharm Sci* 1977;66:757.
228. McGuire TR et al. Antiproliferative activity of shark cartilage with and without tumor necrosis factor-alpha in human umbilical vein endothelium. *Pharmacotherapy* 1996;16:237.
229. Eisenstein R et al. The resistance of certain tissue to invasion. III. Cartilage extracts inhibit the growth of fibroblasts and endothelial cells in culture. *Am J Pathol* 1975;81:337.
230. Pauli BU et al. Regulator of tumor invasion by cartilage-derived anti-invasion factor in vitro. *J Natl Cancer Inst* 1981;67:65.
231. Moses MA et al. Isolation and characterization of an inhibitor of neovascularization from scapular chondrocytes. *J Cell Biol* 1992;119:475.
232. Moses MA et al. Identification of an inhibitor of neovascularization from cartilage. *Science* 1990;248:1408.
233. Cataldi JM, Osbourne DL. Effects of shark cartilage on mammary neovascularization in-vivo and cell proliferation in-vitro. *FASEB J* 1995;9:A135.
234. Langer R et al. Control of tumor growth in animals by infusion of an angiogenesis inhibitor. *Proc Natl Acad Sci USA* 1980;77:4331.
235. Sipos EP et al. Inhibition of tumor angiogenesis. *Ann NY Acad Sci* 1994;732:263.
236. Batist G et al. Neovastat (AE 941) in refractory renal cell carcinoma patients: report of a phase II trial with two dose levels. *Ann Oncol* 2002;13:1259.
237. Mathews J. Media feeds frenzy over shark cartilage as cancer treatment. *J Natl Cancer Inst* 1993;85:1190.
238. Miller DR et al. Phase I/II trial of the safety and efficacy of shark cartilage in the treatment of advanced cancers. *J Clin Oncol* 1998;16:3649.
239. Lane IW, Comac L. Sharks Don't Get Cancer: How Shark Cartilage Can Save Your Life. Garden City, NY: Avery; 1992.
240. Markman M. Shark cartilage: the Laetrile of the 1990s. *Cleve Clin J Med* 1996;63:179.
241. Volpi N. Physico-chemical properties and the structure of dermatan sulfate fractions purified from plasma after oral administration in healthy human volunteers. *Thromb Haemost* 1996;75:491.
242. Ashar B, Vargo E. Shark cartilage induced hepatitis. *Ann Intern Med* 1996;125:780.
243. Pasternak A. A novel form of host defense: a membrane protection by Ca++ and Zn++. *Biosci Rep* 1987;7:81.
244. Geist FC et al. In vitro activity of zinc salts against human rhinoviruses. *Antimicrob Agents Chemother* 1987;31:622.
245. Korant BD et al. Zinc ions inhibit replication of rhinoviruses. *Nature* 1974;248:588.
246. Korant BD, ButterWorth BE. Inhibition by zinc of rhinovirus protein cleavage: interaction of zinc with capsid proteins. *J Virol* 1976;18:298.
247. Novick SG et al. How does zinc modify the common cold? Clinical observations and implications regarding mechanisms or action. *Med Hypotheses* 1996;46:295.
248. Salas M, Kirchner H. Induction of interferon-gamma in human leukocyte cultures stimulated by Zn++. *Clin Immunol Immunopathol* 1987;45: 139.
249. Marone G et al. Physiological concentrations of zinc inhibit the release of histamine from human basophils and lung mast cells. *Agents Actions* 1986;18:103.
250. Eby GA. Handbook for Curing the Common Cold: The Zinc Lozenge Story. Austin, TX: George Eby Research; 1994.
251. Novick SG et al. Zinc-induced suppression of inflammation in the respiratory tract, caused by infection with human rhinovirus and other irritants. *Med Hypotheses* 1997;49:347.
252. Godfrey JC et al. Zinc gluconate and the common cold: a controlled clinical study. *J Int Med Res* 1992;20:234.
253. Farr BM et al. Two randomized controlled trials of zinc gluconate lozenge therapy of experimentally induced rhinovirus colds. *Antimicrob Agents Chemother* 1987;31:1183.
254. Douglas RM et al. Failure of effervescent zinc acetate lozenges to alter the course of upper respiratory tract infection in Australian adults. *Antimicrob Agents Chemother* 1987;31:1263.
255. Eby GA. Zinc lozenges as cure for common colds. *Ann Pharmacother* 1996;30:1336.
256. Eby GA et al. Reduction in duration of common colds by zinc gluconate lozenges in a double-blind study. *Antimicrob Agents Chemother* 1984;25:20.
257. Al-Nakib W et al. Prophylaxis and treatment of rhinovirus colds with zinc gluconate lozenges. *J Antimicrob Chemother* 1987;20:893.
258. Caruso TJ et al. Treatment of naturally acquired common colds with zinc: a structured review. *Clin Infect Dis* 2007;45:569.
259. Jennings LC, Dick EC. Transmission and control of rhinovirus colds. *Eur J Epidemiol* 1987;3:327.
260. Makela MJ et al. Viruses and bacteria in the etiology of the common cold. *J Clin Microbiol* 1998;36: 539.
261. Gwaltney JM. Rhinovirus In: Mandell GL et al., eds. *Principles and Practice of Infectious Diseases.* New York: Churchill Livingstone; 1995:1656.
262. Mossad SB et al. Zinc gluconate lozenges for treating the common cold: a randomized, double-blind, placebo-controlled study. *Ann Intern Med* 1996;125:81.
263. Hirt M et al. Zinc nasal gel for the treatment of common cold symptoms: a double-blind, placebo controlled trial. *Ear Nose Throat J* 2000;79:778.
264. Mossad SB. Effect of zincum gluconicum nasal gel on the duration and symptom severity of the common cold in otherwise healthy adults. *Q J Med* 2003;96:35.
265. Turner RB. Ineffectiveness of intranasal zinc gluconate for prevention of experimental rhinovirus colds. *Clin Infect Dis* 2001;33:1865.
266. Belongia EA et al. A randomized trial of zinc nasal spray for the treatment of upper respiratory illness in adults. *Am J Med* 2001;111:103.
267. Zarembo JE et al. Zinc (II) in saliva: determination of concentrations produced by different formulations of zinc gluconate lozenges containing common excipients. *J Pharm Sci* 1992;81:128.
268. Eby GA. Zinc ion availability: the determinant of efficacy in zinc lozenge treatment of common colds. *J Antimicrob Chemother* 1997;40:483.
269. Lewis MR, Kokan L. Zinc gluconate: acute ingestion. *J Toxicol Clin Toxicol* 1998;36:99.
270. Alexander TH et al. Intranasal zinc and anosmia: the zinc-induced anosmia syndrome. *Laryngoscope* 2006;116:217.
271. Chandra RK. Excessive intake of zinc impairs immune responses. *JAMA* 1984;252:1443.
272. Pfeiffer CC et al. Effect of chronic zinc intoxication on copper levels, blood formation and polyamines. *Orthomol Psychiatry* 1980;9:79.
273. Macknin ML et al. Zinc gluconate lozenges for treating the common cold in children: a randomized controlled trial. *JAMA* 1998;279:1962.
274. Committee on Dietary Allowances, Food and Nutrition Board. *Recommended Dietary Allowances.*

Washington, DC: National Academy of Sciences; 1980.
275. Prasad AS. Zinc: the biology and therapeutics of an ion. *Ann Intern Med* 1996;125:142.
276. Prasad AS. Zinc: an overview. *Nutrition* 1995; 11:93.
277. Yokoi K et al. Iron and zinc nutriture of premenopausal women: associations of diet with serum ferritin and plasma zinc disappearance and of serum ferritin with plasma zinc and plasma zinc disappearance. *J Lab Clin Med* 1994;124:852.
278. Sandstead HH. Zinc nutrition in the United States. *Am J Clin Nutr* 1973;26:1251.
279. Mineral elements. In: Howe PS, ed. *Basic Nutrition in Health and Disease: Including Selection and Care of Good.* 7th ed. Philadelphia: Saunders; 1981: 107.
280. Kastrup H, ed. *Facts and Comparisons.* St. Louis, MO: Facts and Comparisons.
281. Waldhauser F et al. Bioavailability of oral melatonin in humans. *Neuroendocrinology* 1984;39: 307.
282. Deacon S, Arendt J. Melatonin-induced temperature suppression and its acute phase-shifting effects correlate in dose-dependent manner in humans. *Brain Res* 1995;688:77.
283. Hughes RJ et al. The role of melatonin and circadian phase in age-related sleep-maintenance insomnia: assessment in a clinical trial of melatonin replacement. *Sleep* 1998;21:52.
284. Iguchi H et al. Melatonin serum levels and metabolic clearance rate in patients with liver cirrhosis. *J Clin Endocrinol Metab* 1982;54:1025.
285. Lane EA, Moss HB. Pharmacokinetics of melatonin in man: first pass hepatic metabolism. *J Clin Endocrinol Metab* 1985;61:1214.
286. Daan S, Lewy AJ. Scheduled exposure to daylight: a potential strategy to reduce "jet lag" following transmeridian flight. *Psychopharmacol Bull* 1984;20:566.
287. Petrie K et al. Effect of melatonin on jet lag long haul flights. *Br Med J* 1989;298:705.
288. Claustrat B et al. Melatonin and jet lag: confirmatory result using a simplified protocol. *Biol Psychiatry* 1992;32:705.
289. Arendt J et al. Alleviation of jet lag by melatonin: preliminary results of a controlled double blind study. *Br Med J* 1986;292:1170.
290. Petrie K et al. A double-blind trial of melatonin as a treatment for jet lag in international cabin crew. *Biol Psychiatry* 1993;33:526.
291. Edwards BJ et al. Use of melatonin in recovery from jet-lag following an eastward flight across 10 time-zones. *Ergonomics* 2000;43:1501.
292. Spitzer RL et al. Jet lag: clinical features, validation of a new syndrome-specific scale, and lack of response to melatonin in a randomized, double-blind trial. *Am J Psychiatry* 1999;156:1392.
293. Arendt J et al. Some effects of jet lag and their alleviation by melatonin. *Ergonomics* 1987;30:1379.
294. Force RW et al. Psychotic episode after melatonin. *Ann Pharmacother* 1997;31:1408.
295. Bardazzi F et al. Fixed drug eruption due to melatonin. *Acta Derm Venereol* 1997;78:69.
296. Badia P et al. Effects of exogenous melatonin on memory, sleepiness and performance after a 4-hour nap. *J Sleep Res* 1996;5:11.
297. Voordouw BCG et al. Melatonin and melatonin-progestin combinations alter pituitary-ovarian function in women and can inhibit ovulation. *J Clin Endocrinol Metab* 1992;74:108.
298. Arendt J et al. Chronic, timed, low-dose melatonin (MT) treatment in man: effects on sleep, fatigue, mood and hormone rhythms. *EPSG Newslet* 1984;(Suppl)5:51.
299. Tzischinsky O, Lavie P. Melatonin possesses time-dependent hypnotic effects. *Sleep* 1994;17:638.
300. Wurtman RJ, Zhdanova I. Improvement of sleep quality by melatonin. *Lancet* 1995;346:1491.
301. Dollins AB et al. Effect of inducing nocturnal serum melatonin concentrations in daytime on sleep, body temperature and performance. *Proc Natl Acad Sci USA* 1994;91:1824.
302. James SP et al. The effect of melatonin on normal sleep. *Neuropsychopharmacology* 1987;1:41.
303. Brzezinski A et al. Effects of exogenous melatonin on sleep: a meta-analysis. *Sleep Med Rev* 2005;9:41.
304. Wade AG et al. Efficacy of prolonged release melatonin in insomnia patients aged 55–80 years: quality of sleep and next-day alertness outcomes. *Curr Med Res Opin* 2007;23:2597.
305. Lemoine P et al. Prolonged-release melatonin improves sleep quality and morning alertness in insomnia patients aged 55 years and older and has no withdrawal effects. *J Sleep Res* 2007;16:372.
306. Hoang BX et al. Neurobiological effects of melatonin as related to cancer. *Eur J Cancer Prev* 2007;16:511.
307. Lissoni P et al. Modulation of cancer endocrine therapy by melatonin: a phase II study of tamoxifen alone. *Br J Cancer* 1995;71:854.
308. Greenberg S, Frishman WH: Co-enzyme Q10: a new drug for cardiovascular disease. *J Clin Pharmacol* 1990;30:596.
309. Lockwood K et al. Partial and complete regression of breast cancer in patients in relation to dosage of coenzyme Q10. *Biochem Biophys Res Commun* 1994;199:1504.
310. Langsjoen PH et al. Treatment of hypertrophic cardiomyopathy with coenzyme Q10. *Mol Aspects Med* 1997;18(Suppl):S145.
311. Marcoff L et al. The role of coenzyme Q10 in statin-associated myopathy: a systematic review. *J Am Coll Cardiol* 2007;49:2231.
312. Caso G et al. Effect of coenzyme Q10 on myopathic symptoms in patients treated with statins. *Am J Cardiol* 2007;99:1409.
313. Rosenfeldt FL et al. Coenzyme Q10 in the treatment of hypertension: a meta-analysis of the clinical trials. *J Hum Hypertens* 2007;21:297.
314. Singh U et al. Coenzyme Q10 supplementation and heart failure. *Nutr Rev* 2007;65:286.
315. Sanden S et al. The impact of coenzyme Q10 on systolic function in patients with chronic heart failure. *J Card Fail* 2006;12:464.
316. Baggio E et al. Italian multicenter study on the safety and efficacy of coenzyme Q10 as adjunctive therapy in heart failure (interim analysis). *Clin Invest* 1993;71:145.
317. Heck AM et al. Potential interactions between alternative therapies and warfarin. *Am J Health-Syst Pharm* 2000;57:1221.

CHAPTER 4

Anaphylaxis and Drug Allergies

Robert K. Middleton and Paul M. Beringer

Adverse drug reactions occur in approximately 30% of hospitalized patients, and 3% of all hospitalizations are a result of adverse drug reactions. Allergic drug reactions account for 5% to 20% of all observed adverse drug reactions.[1–4] In one study of >36,000 hospitalized patients, 731 adverse events were identified, with 1% being severe, life-threatening, allergic reactions.[5] The potential morbidity and mortality associated with allergic drug reactions is great, although they occur infrequently.

Definition

The appropriate diagnosis and treatment of a patient experiencing an allergic reaction necessitates differentiation between *allergic reactions* from other *adverse drug reactions*. One approach divides adverse reactions into those that are "predictable, usually dose dependent, and related to the pharmacologic actions of the drug" and those that are "unpredictable, often dose independent, and are related to the individual's immunologic response or to genetic differences in susceptible patients."[1] Under this classification, drug allergy or drug hypersensitivity is an unpredictable adverse drug reaction that is immunologically mediated.[1,2,6]

Predisposing Factors

Factors known to affect the incidence of allergic reactions can be categorized as being drug or patient related.[7]

Age and Gender

Children are less likely to become sensitized than adults, presumably because younger age is likely to be associated with less cumulative drug exposure.[6–9] More female than male patients experience allergic reactions (up to 2.3:1), although this may vary by type of reaction, drug, patient age, and setting.[10,11]

Genetic Factors

Patients with histories of allergic rhinitis, asthma, or atopic dermatitis who develop a systemic drug reaction tend to react more severely than others.[7,8,12] Familial occurrences of allergic reactions, although rare, have been reported. For example, erythema multiforme was described in three of five siblings treated with thiabendazole.[13] Ethnic predisposition to drug allergy is increasingly recognized. Whites are more likely to develop hypersensitivity reactions to abacavir than nonwhites, and blacks are more susceptible to angioedema from angiotensin-converting enzyme (ACE) inhibitors than are other ethnic groups.[14,15] A patient's ability to metabolize a drug is influenced by his or her genetic makeup and may affect the incidence of allergic reactions. *Pharmacogenetics* (i.e., the study of genetically determined variability to drug response) often centers on drug-metabolizing enzymes because many drugs are metabolized by enzymes that are encoded by variations in DNA sequences or genetic polymorphisms.[16]

Acetylator phenotype (e.g., fast acetylator or slow acetylator) is genetically determined, and several variations in the gene encoding for *N*-acetyltransferase (NAT) are recognized.[16] The slow acetylator phenotype is an autosomal recessive trait. Slow acetylators are at risk for sulfonamide hypersensitivity and also are more likely to develop antinuclear antibodies (ANA) and symptoms of systemic lupus erythematosus (SLE) when treated with procainamide or hydralazine.[17] Drug-induced lupus can be considered an allergic reaction because of its association with an immune response, as evidenced by an increase in ANA.

Anticonvulsant hypersensitivity syndrome, characterized by fever, generalized rash, lymphadenopathy, and internal organ involvement, is most associated with aromatic anticonvulsants (e.g., phenytoin, phenobarbital, and carbamazepine) and is more common in patients with a heritable deficiency in epoxide hydrolase.[18] This syndrome also is known as *drug hypersensitivity syndrome* and as *DRESS syndrome* (**d**rug **r**ash with **e**osinophilia and **s**ystemic **s**ymptoms). A genetic defect also might be responsible for a serum sicknesslike reaction to cefaclor.[18]

Numerous polymorphisms are known for the CYP isoenzyme family that catalyzes the oxidative metabolism of hundreds of drugs. The best studied of these are variations in genes that encode for CYP2D6, CYP2C9, CYP2C19, and CYP3A4. Examples of the phenotypic expression of these variations include poor metabolizers (who possess nonfunctional alleles and have reduced metabolic activity) and ultrarapid metabolizers (who have multiple copies of functional genes and have enhanced metabolic activity).[16] Genetic differences in CYP-metabolizing enzymes might explain the predisposition to drug allergy and hypersensitivity of some individuals, as well as other forms of drug toxicity and drug response.

Whereas genetic polymorphism in drug metabolizing enzymes is responsible for some allergic reactions, gene variations in the major histocompatibility complex (MHC) perhaps are more significant.[14] For example, dermatologic reactions and thrombocytopenia to gold and toxicity to penicillamine are linked to the presence of the HLA-DR3 allele in the MHC; severe cutaneous reactions to allopurinol are linked to presence of the HLA-B*5801 allele in the Han Chinese population, and the potentially life-threatening hypersensitivity syndrome seen with abacavir is strongly associated with the HLA-B*5701, HLA-DR7, and HLA-DQ3 haplotype.[14,17–21] In the latter case, presence of this haplotype in patients predicted abacavir hypersensitivity 100% of the time, whereas its absence had a 97% negative predictive value.[19] This haplotype appears more commonly in whites than in other ethnic groups and explains the predisposition of whites to this severe reaction. Genetic screening of patients for this haplotype before initiating abacavir therapy has significantly reduced the occurrence of hypersensitivity reactions.[22] In the future, it is hoped genes that are involved in life-threatening hypersensitivity reactions (e.g., anaphylaxis, hepatotoxicity, blood dyscrasias, Stevens-Johnson syndrome, toxic epidermal necrolysis) will be identified.

Associated Illness

Although genes clearly play a role in hypersensitivity reactions, environmental factors (e.g., concomitant illness) also are implicated. For example, the incidence of maculopapular rash with ampicillin therapy is significantly higher in patients with Epstein-Barr virus infections (e.g., infectious mononucleosis), lymphocytic leukemia, or gout.[2,7] Infection with herpes virus or Epstein-Barr virus also has been linked to DRESS syndrome;[23,24] and the occurrence of reactions to trimethoprim-sulfamethoxazole in patients who are HIV positive is about 10-fold higher than in the HIV-negative population.[14]

Previous Drug Administration

A previous history of an allergic reaction to a drug being considered for treatment, or one that is immunochemically similar, is the most reliable risk factor for development of a subsequent allergic reaction.[6,7] A commonly encountered example is the patient with a history of penicillin allergy, in whom all structurally related penicillin compounds should be avoided, and in whom the possibility of a hypersensitivity reaction should be considered when using other β-lactam antibiotics.[7]

Drug-Related Factors

The dose, frequency of exposure, and route of administration can influence the incidence of drug allergy. For example, penicillin-induced hemolytic anemia (see Question 6 in Chapter 87: Drug-Induced Blood Disorders) requires high and sustained drug concentrations.[9] In β-lactam antibiotic IgE sensitivity, frequent intermittent courses, rather than continuous therapy, are more likely to result in drug sensitization.[16] The route of administration is important in terms of the risk of both sensitization and allergic reaction in a previously sensitized person. Topical administration carries the greatest risk of sensitization, whereas the oral route is the least sensitizing. Intramuscular administration is more sensitizing than the intravenous (IV) route. In a patient who is already sensitized to a specific medication, the risk of an allergic reaction to that medication is greatest when it is given IV and least when given orally. This is thought to be a function of the rate of drug delivery.[7]

Pathogenesis

Allergic drug reactions cannot be attributed to a single immunopathologic mechanism. Traditionally, an allergic drug reaction was thought occur in two phases: initial sensitization and subsequent elicitation.[25] Most drugs are small molecules (<1000 Da) and are unable to stimulate an immune response. Sensitization occurs as a result of covalent binding of a drug or a metabolite to a carrier protein in a process referred to as *haptenization*.[2,3,6,12,25] This drug–protein (or drug metabolite–protein) complex is sufficiently large to induce the production of drug-specific T or B lymphocytes and IgM, IgG, and IgE. On re-exposure to the drug, the patient is likely to present with allergic symptoms.[16] Allergic reactions to β-lactam antibiotics occur by this mechanism. This theory, however, cannot explain several allergic phenomena. For instance, some chemically inert drugs (i.e., drugs that cannot form stable covalent bonds and do not have reactive metabolites) can still elicit an allergic response. Lidocaine and mepivacaine are examples. Furthermore, some patients have a strong allergic reaction to a drug on initial exposure, and some allergic reactions rapidly occur following drug exposure, a time period shorter than expected for the development of new antibodies. To account for some of these observations, other models for explaining allergic reactions have been proposed. The direct *pharmacological interaction* or P-I concept offers one explanation for these observations. This model suggests that some drugs are able to bind directly to T-cell receptors in a reversible, noncovalent manner. The drug–T-cell receptor complex interacts with MHC molecules, leading to activation and expansion of T cells that are directed against the drug.[26] On the other hand, the *danger hypothesis* proposes idiosyncratic drug reactions are the result of damaged or stressed cells that release "danger signals." Danger signals may be cytokines (e.g., interleukins, tumor necrosis factors) that act as co-stimulants to trigger an immune response once released. Similar to the P-I concept, neither covalent binding of drug to a carrier protein nor prior drug exposure is a prerequisite for an allergic response with the danger hypothesis. Rather, the drug itself, or a reactive metabolite, directly induces cell injury or stress, causing the release of danger signals. Once the drug is discontinued, generation of danger signals cease, and the clinical manifestations of the allergic reaction resolve.[27] Undoubtedly, the processes involved in allergic reactions are complex and might include some combination of each theory. Interested readers are referred to more in-depth reviews.[28,29]

Drugs as Allergens and Immunologic Classification

Allergic drug reactions can be classified into one of four types (Table 4-1).[6,7]

TYPE I: ANAPHYLACTIC REACTIONS

Anaphylactic reactions are acute, generalized reactions that occur when a previously sensitized person is re-exposed to a particular antigen. Reactions range in severity from pruritus and urticaria to bronchospasm, respiratory distress, laryngeal edema, circulatory collapse, and death. Anaphylactic reactions to antibiotics and radiographic contrast media reportedly occur in 1 in every 5,000 exposures, 10% of which are fatal.[30] Initial exposure to an antigen results in production of specific IgE antibodies. On re-exposure, antigen interacts with antibodies bound to the surface of mast cells or basophils, causing the release of histamine and other mediators.[25] A period of several weeks is required after initial exposure and sensitization before an anaphylactic reaction can be elicited; once sensitized, however, an anaphylactic response can be elicited within minutes as a result of existing antibodies. In addition, an anaphylactic response can occur on re-exposure to small amounts of drug administered by any route.[25,30–32] Reactions that clinically resemble anaphylaxis, but do not involve immunologic mediators (antibodies), are termed *anaphylactoid reactions.*

TYPE II: CYTOTOXIC REACTIONS

Cytotoxic reactions involve the interaction of IgG or IgM and can occur by three different mechanisms (Table 4-1). Common clinical manifestations of cytotoxic reactions include hemolytic anemia, thrombocytopenia, and granulocytopenia. Penicillin-induced hemolytic anemia is the best-known example of a cytotoxic drug reaction (see Question 6 in Chapter 87: Drug-Induced Blood Disorders). This reaction typically appears after 7 days of high-dose therapy.[9,33,34]

TYPE III: IMMUNE COMPLEX–MEDIATED REACTIONS

Immune complex-mediated reactions result from the formation of drug–antibody complexes in serum, which often deposit in blood vessel walls, resulting in activation of complement and endothelial cell injury.[30] Also referred to as *serum sickness,* these reactions typically manifest as fever, urticaria, arthralgia, and lymphadenopathy 7 to 21 days after exposure.[9,35]

TYPE IV: CELL-MEDIATED (DELAYED) REACTIONS

In cell-mediated (delayed) reactions, antigen binds with sensitized T cells. Contact dermatitis is the most common manifestation of cell-mediated reactions, although systemic reactions can occur. The variety of clinical manifestations of delayed hypersensitivity has been attributed to distinct patterns of cytokine release and effector-cell recruitment, based on the type of T cells stimulated. For example, hypersensitivity reactions involving T-helper 1 cells are induced by interferon-γ and interleukin-2, whereas reactions involving T-helper 2 cells employ interleukins 4 and 5. Each pattern of cytokine release recruits specific effector cells, such as macrophages, neutrophils, or other T cells, and is responsible for the unique clinical manifestations of the reaction. Based on this new understanding, type IV reactions have been reclassified as type IVa, type IVb, type IVc, and type IVd, corresponding to four unique patterns of T-cell and effector-cell involvement.[36]

An understanding of the immunologic mechanism can be helpful in the diagnosis and treatment of an allergic reaction; however, the exact immunologic mechanism is unknown for many allergic reactions to drugs. In addition, patients often

Table 4-1 Immunopathologic Classification of Allergic Drug Reactions

Immunologic Class	*Antibody*	*Mechanism*	*Common Clinical Manifestations*
Type I (anaphylactic)	IgE	Drug-hapten reacts with IgE antibody on the surface of mast cells and basophils, resulting in the release of mediators	Anaphylaxis
Type II (cytotoxic)	IgG	*Hapten–cell reaction:* Drug interacts with cell surfaces, resulting in the formation of an immunogenic complex and the production of antibodies	Hemolytic anemia
–	IgM	*Immune complex reaction:* Drug reacts with antibody in circulation, forming a complex that with complement binds to the cell, resulting in injury (hematologic reactions only)	Granulocytopenia
–	–	*Autoimmune reaction:* Drug induces autoantibody production against red blood cells	Thrombocytopenia
Type III (immune complex)	IgG	Same as type II immune complex reactions (nonhematologic reactions)	Serum sickness
Type IVa-d (cell mediated)	–	Interaction of sensitized T lymphocytes with drug antigen	Contact dermatitis

Adapted from reference 6, with permission.

Table 4-2 Clinical Features of Allergic Drug Reactions

- Have no correlation with known pharmacologic properties of the drug
- Require an induction period on primary exposure but not on readministration
- Can occur with doses far below therapeutic range
- Often include a rash, angioedema, serum sickness syndrome, anaphylaxis, and asthma
- Occur in a small proportion of the population
- Disappear on cessation of therapy and reappear after readministration of a small dose of the suspected drug(s) of similar chemical structure
- Desensitization may be possible

Reprinted from reference 2, with permission.

present with several symptoms characteristic of more than one of the reactions described above. The use of many drugs concurrently also makes it difficult to identify the drug responsible for the reaction. Therefore, a careful drug history and diagnostic tests (e.g., wheal and flare, *in vitro* detection of drug-specific IgE antibodies) often are necessary for an appropriate diagnosis and treatment of a patient.

Diagnosis

Distinctive Features of Allergic Reactions

The first step in the diagnosis of an allergic drug reaction is to recognize and differentiate it from other adverse drug reactions. This can be accomplished by having a good understanding of the distinctive features of allergic drug reactions (Table 4-2).[2,6]

1. J.A., a 73-year-old woman, is admitted from a nursing home with an infected decubitus ulcer. Cultures reveal *Staphylococcus aureus,* which is sensitive to oxacillin, cefazolin, and vancomycin. On questioning, J.A. reports having experienced a rash to penicillin in the past. Her current medications include oral docusate 100 mg twice daily (BID), oral enalapril 5 mg every morning, oral prednisone 20 mg daily, and oral ibuprofen 800 mg three times daily (TID). What information should be obtained to determine whether J.A.'s rash represents an allergic drug reaction?

The single most informative diagnostic procedure for allergic drug reactions is a detailed drug history (Table 4-3), which is helpful in obtaining the information necessary to determine whether a reaction represents a drug allergy and in identifying the culprit drug. In inquiring about prior allergic and medication encounters, it is important to document the drugs to which the patient has or has not previously reacted. This can sometimes alert the clinician about certain types of compounds to which the patient is likely to react. In addition, the acquired information allows the clinician to characterize the drug reaction and to appreciate how such a reaction might be manifested in the patient on exposure to the same, or an immunologically similar, compound in the future.

Table 4-3 Detailed Drug History

- Prior allergic and medication encounters
- Nature and severity of reaction
- Temporal relationships between drugs and reaction (dose, date initiated, duration)
- Prior exposure to the same or structurally related medications subsequent to the reaction
- Effect of drug discontinuation
- Response to treatment
- Prior diagnostic testing or rechallenge
- Route of administration
- Other medical problems (if any)

From references 3 and 32, with permission.

The temporal relationship between drugs and reactions often is the strongest piece of evidence implicating an allergic reaction to a particular agent. Drugs that the patient has received for long continuous periods before the onset of a reaction are less likely to be implicated than drugs that have been recently initiated or restarted.[37] Equally important is to determine when an adverse reaction has occurred. Many compounds have been reformulated over the years, resulting in removal of sensitizing impurities (e.g., penicillin, vancomycin). Therefore, it is possible that re-exposure to the agent will not result in an adverse event. Inquiring about whether the patient has received the drug since the first episode by asking the patient about other brands or names of other drugs in the same class (e.g., amoxicillin, ampicillin) will assist in determining whether the patient is likely to react to the drug on re-exposure. It usually is helpful to chart all the drugs the patient is currently taking, their dose, and start and stop dates of use. This can be compared with the onset and disappearance of the reaction.

2. On further questioning, J.A. reports having experienced an urticarial rash in the past when given ampicillin for a kidney infection approximately 2 years ago. The rash developed over her entire body less than a day after starting the antibiotic and disappeared 2 days after discontinuation. Her treatment course was completed with ciprofloxacin. She denies having had a viral infection at the time of the rash to ampicillin. She does not recall having experienced any adverse effects when she received penicillin before this reaction. No other recent changes in her treatment regimen were made before the occurrence of the rash. Why is it likely that J.A. is allergic to penicillin?

Several useful pieces of information gleaned from the drug history obtained from J.A. can be used to determine the likelihood of an allergic reaction to penicillin. J.A.'s rash appeared less than a day after initiation of ampicillin and other drugs had not been added; therefore, the rash probably was caused by ampicillin.

Another important method of identifying a potential drug-induced allergic reaction is to examine the patient's medication list to determine whether the patient is receiving an agent that commonly is implicated in causing the exhibited allergic manifestation. For example, amoxicillin and ampicillin are two of the top three drugs implicated in drug-induced rash.[10]

J.A. received penicillin previously without experiencing any adverse effects until an urticarial rash (a relatively common allergic manifestation) developed on subsequent exposure. This sequence of events follows the typical pattern of an allergic reaction. Allergic reactions require an induction period to sensitize the person to the antigen; however, once sensitized, allergic symptoms typically occur immediately on re-exposure.[37]

Therefore, a prior exposure to the same or structurally related compounds needs to be documented.

Finally, it is important to evaluate other medical problems that can elicit or mimic a reaction resembling drug allergy (see above section "Associated Illness"). Rashes to ampicillin commonly occur in patients with concurrent Epstein-Barr virus infection.[19] J.A. denies having a viral infection at the time of her rash, thereby, strengthening the case that the rash was likely a manifestation of an allergic reaction.

Skin Testing

3. Why might skin testing for penicillin allergy be appropriate (or inappropriate) for J.A.?

Although J.A.'s elicited medication history strongly suggests that she is allergic to penicillin, a skin test and a drug rechallenge would more firmly establish her drug allergy. For many years, skin-testing antigen for penicillin was commercially available as penicilloyl polylysine (Pre-Pen). Although the manufacturer (Hollister-Stier, Spokane, Washington) of penicilloyl polylysine voluntarily withdrew it from the market in 2004, AllerQuest (West Hartford, CT) obtained the legal rights and has been working to market it in the United States and Canada.[38] Penicillin skin testing using Pre-Pen (also known as PPL [penicilloyl polylysine]) is a safe and effective procedure (Table 4-4), with <1% of positive responders developing systemic reactions.[34] In those in whom a false–negative response occurred, reactions were mild and, in most cases, did not require drug discontinuation.[33,34] Skin testing with PPL identifies 80% of patients allergic to penicillin. When the penicilloyl derivative is supplemented with skin tests for the minor determinants of penicillin,[33] 99.5% of penicillin-allergic patients can be identified. When 34 purportedly "penicillin-allergic patients," who subsequently tested negative to penicillin skin-tests, needed β-lactam antibiotics during hospitalization, no allergic drug reactions occurred.[39]

Penicilloyl, the primary metabolite of penicillin, is referred to as the major determinant. The other derivatives, including the parent compound (penicillin), are referred to as minor determinants. The terms *major determinant* and *minor determinant* refer to the frequency of antibody formation to these antigenic penicillin metabolite–protein complexes. These terms do *not* describe the severity of the allergic reaction. Indeed, the major determinant is thought to be responsible for accelerated reactions, but not anaphylaxis. The minor determinants are responsible for anaphylaxis and immediate systemic reactions.

Penicillin and its metabolites become antigenic when combined with proteins and can precipitate a hypersensitivity reaction in a patient on re-exposure. In patients with a history of penicillin hypersensitivity, skin test reactivity is affected by the length of time since the allergic reaction and by the nature of the past reaction. Skin test positivity is greatest 6 to 12 months after a reaction and decreases with time. Skin test positivity in one study was found to be only 40% of patients with a history of anaphylaxis, 17% with urticaria, and 7% for maculopapular rashes.[33] Skin testing should not be performed in patients receiving antihistamines because they block the response to the antigen and can result in misinterpretation. In patients receiving antihistamines (i.e., H_1- or H_2-receptor antagonists) or when skin testing is not possible because of severe skin disease, *in vitro* assays to detect drug-specific IgE antibodies have been developed for the major and minor determinants of penicillin.

Table 4-4 Penicillin Skin Testing Procedure

Agent	*Procedure*	*Interpretation*
Penicilloyl polylysine (Pre-Pen)	Scratch test one drop of full-strength solution (6 to 10^{-5} mol/L)[a]	*No wheal or erythema after 10 minutes:* proceed with intradermal test.
Major determinant		*Wheal or erythema within 10 minutes:* choose alternative agent, desensitization if no other alternatives exist
Penicilloyl polylisine (Pre-Pen)	Intradermal test: 0.01 to 0.02 mL PPL (Pre-Pen).[a] Saline: negative control Histamine: positive control (optional; useful if it is suspected that patient may be anergic)	Negative response: induration size similar or less than saline control Positive response: induration 14 mm or more greater than saline control with or without erythema: choose alternative agent, desensitization if no other alternatives exist
Penicillin G potassium (>1 week old) most important of the minor determinants	Scratch test one drop of 10,000 U/mL solution	Same as scratch test with PPL (see above)
Penicillin G potassium	Intradermal test:0.002 mL 10,000 U/mL solution	Same as intradermal test with PPL (see above)
–	Serial testing with 10, 100, or 1,000 U/mL solutions can be performed in those with strong history or serious reactions	

[a]The penicilloyl derivative of penicillin conjugated to polylysine (PPL) is administered initially as a scratch test. If no wheal or erythema develops, then intradermal testing is performed.

From Schwarz Pharma Kremers Urban Company, Milwaukee, WI, with permission.

Note: as of 2004, Pre-Pen is no longer commercially marketed in the United States. It is anticipated that Pre-Pen will be re-introduced in 2008. From reference 38.

To determine whether skin testing is appropriate for J.A., the risks and benefits must be weighed. Because the time of the last reaction was approximately 2 years ago, J.A. may still retain some skin test positivity if the previous reaction was truly an allergic reaction to ampicillin. Testing with PPL (major determinant) and penicillin (minor determinant) could be useful in determining whether J.A. is likely to develop an urticarial or anaphylactic reaction to penicillin or its derivatives. That J.A. is currently receiving prednisone should not alter the interpretation of the skin test results because the corticosteroids minimally affect the IgE-mediated immediate hypersensitivity reactions. The risks of developing serious systemic reactions to penicillin skin testing are minimal.

The benefit of penicillin skin testing for J.A., however, is questionable because she could be treated with an antibiotic other than a penicillin. The most practical approach to penicillin-allergic patients is simply to avoid the drug. Therefore, the patient's drug history should always be evaluated carefully. In the unlikely situation in which treatment with a penicillin is essential, penicillin skin testing would be useful.

Cross-Reactivity

4. J.A. received a scratch test with PPL, which was negative; however, an intradermal test was positive. What treatment options are available to J.A. for her infection?

All penicillin derivatives should be avoided because J.A. had a positive skin-test reaction. Skin tests are not commercially available for cephalosporins and other β-lactam antibiotics. Although cephalosporin-skin testing (i.e., prick followed by intradermal instillation) using 0.01 mL of a concentration of 2 mg/mL of the cephalosporins in normal saline has been proposed by some, no prospective studies have evaluated this approach.[40] Therefore, clinicians must rely on cross-reactivity data to determine whether a nonpenicillin β-lactam antibiotic (e.g., a cephalosporin) can be used in a penicillin-allergic patient.

In one study, about 50% of patients with a history of penicillin allergy exhibited hypersensitivity reactions to the β-lactam antibiotic, imipenem (Primaxin).[33] Cross-reactivity (i.e., cross-antigenicity) occurs between penicillin and cephalosporins in 5% to 15% of patients;[33,34] however, the true incidence of cross-reactivity is considerably less because these percentages were derived based on the recollection of patients of an allergic history rather than by objective skin tests.

The cross-reactivity between penicillins and cephalosporins formerly was attributed primarily to their common β-lactam chemical-ring structure; however, side-chain–specific reactions are now recognized to be responsible for a significant portion of allergic reactions within and between the penicillin and cephalosporins families.[40–42] In a study of 30 patients with immediate allergic reactions to cephalosporins, <20% reacted to penicillin determinants (i.e., skin test positivity, radioallergosorbent testing [RAST] positivity, or both).[41] (RAST is a radioimmune test to detect IgE antibodies responsible for hypersensitivity.) This cross-reactivity between penicillin and cephalosporins is significantly less than earlier reports (up to 50%); however, the results of this study could be attributable to the greater use of third-generation, rather than the first-generation cephalosporins, which share more chemical structure similarities with the penicillins. Additional support for the importance of side-chain–specific reactions of β-lactams comes from observational data noting that 30% of patients with immediate reactions to penicillins were selective for amoxicillin.[43] These data suggest relatively low cross-reactivity between penicillins and third-generation cephalosporins. The risk of a serious allergic reaction with the use of an advanced-generation cephalosporin in a penicillin-allergic patient might be no greater than the risk of any alternative antibiotic.[42] Some patients also have multiple drug allergies and could manifest an allergic reaction to these drugs (and others that are not β-lactams) in a manner similar to their penicillin reaction.[33]

Although desensitization with an appropriate cephalosporin is a potential option for J.A., her infection is not life-threatening, and the organism is probably sensitive to other antimicrobial agents. In this case, it would be more prudent to treat J.A. with a non–β-lactam antibiotic. If J.A.'s skin tests to cephalosporin were undertaken, and had been negative, she could receive a cephalosporin despite her positive history beginning with a cautiously administered small (i.e., "test") initial dose.[33]

GENERALIZED REACTIONS

Drug allergies can be grouped into three categories: generalized reactions, organ-specific reactions, and pseudoallergic reactions. Generalized reactions involve multiple organ systems and variable clinical manifestations. Anaphylactic reactions, serum sickness reactions, drug-induced fever, drug-induced vasculitis, and autoimmune drug reactions are the generalized drug reactions presented in this chapter.

Anaphylaxis

5. L.P., a 43-year-old man, is brought to the emergency department (ED) with a chief complaint of a hand wound received while defending himself during an attempted robbery. Physical examination reveals a man in moderate distress with a 3.5-inch laceration on the palm of his right hand, requiring sutures. L.P.'s history is notable for migraine headaches, which are managed with atenolol 25 mg once daily; adult-onset diabetes, controlled with diet; and multiple scars from wounds obtained during a barroom brawl 2 years before admission. He has no known allergies. The wound is cleansed and 1% lidocaine is infiltrated around the laceration in preparation for suturing. Four minutes after the lidocaine injections, L.P. notes tingling and pruritus of both his hands and feet, and appears flushed. Three minutes later he complains of light-headedness, difficulty breathing, and a lump in his throat. His vital signs at this time are blood pressure (BP) 80/40 mmHg (nl, 130/85); heart rate 75 beats/minute (normal, 60); and respiratory rate 27 breaths/minute (normal, 12). Chest auscultation reveals restricted airflow and stridor. Anaphylaxis is the diagnosis and emergency treatment is started. What subjective and objective evidence support the diagnosis of anaphylaxis in L.P.?

Anaphylaxis is an acute, clinical syndrome that results from the rapid release of immunologic mediators from tissue mast cells and peripheral blood basophils. The symptoms of anaphylaxis vary widely, depending on the route of exposure, rate of exposure, and dose of allergen.[30,32,44,45] Symptoms usually begin within minutes of exposure, as in L.P., and most reactions occur within 1 hour. On rare occasions, anaphylaxis can appear several hours after exposure and late phase or biphasic attacks have occurred 8 to 12 hours after the initial attack. In general, the severity of the anaphylaxis is directly proportional to the speed of onset. L.P. displays symptoms in many of the organs commonly involved in anaphylaxis. Although almost any organ system can be affected, the cutaneous, gastrointestinal (GI), respiratory, and cardiovascular systems are involved most frequently, either singly or in combination.[30,32,44,45] These "shock organs" contain the largest number of mast cells and are the most highly affected.

L.P. exhibits erythema (flushed appearance) and complains of pruritus of his hands and feet, both common initial symptoms of anaphylaxis; the groin also is commonly affected. These symptoms can progress to urticaria and angioedema, especially of the palms, soles, periorbital tissue, and mucous membranes. L.P. describes the early manifestations of angioedema (laryngeal edema) with complaints of a lump in his throat (this also may be described as throat tightness or constriction by some patients).

The upper and lower respiratory tracts also can be involved during an anaphylactic event. L.P. exhibits stridor, indicating upper airway involvement. Hoarseness is another sign of upper respiratory tract involvement. In addition, L.P. is tachypneic with poor airflow, suggesting his lower airway also is affected. L.P. does not display wheezing or acute emphysema, which are further clues of lower airway involvement. Respiratory symptoms can lead to suffocation and death.[44] In one autopsy series, laryngeal edema accounted for 25% of the fatalities and acute emphysema for another 25% of the deaths.[46] Cardiovascular symptoms also are ominous. Cardiovascular collapse and hypotensive shock (anaphylactic shock) are caused by peripheral vasodilation, enhanced vascular permeability, leakage of plasma, low cardiac output, and intravascular volume depletion. Thus, hypotension, as seen with L.P., is a common cardiac manifestation. Tachycardia also commonly occurs in patients with cardiac complications of anaphylaxis. L.P. does not show a significant increase in heart rate, however, he is taking the β-blocker atenolol. Other cardiac manifestations of anaphylaxis include a direct cardiodepressant effect and various electrocardiographic changes, including arrhythmias and ischemia.

Athough not demonstrated by L.P., common GI manifestations such as abdominal cramping, diarrhea (which can be bloody), nausea, and vomiting also are manifested during an anaphylactic reaction.[30,32,44] In summary, L.P.'s rapid onset and progression of symptoms involving multiple organ systems (i.e., cutaneous, respiratory, and cardiovascular systems) are consistent with an anaphylactic reaction. L.P.'s anaphylaxis is a severe reaction given its speed of onset, the number of organ systems involved, and the degree of involvement. In particular, his respiratory and cardiovascular symptoms indicate a potentially life-threatening reaction.

6. What is the likely cause of L.P.'s anaphylactic event?

Anaphylaxis occurs through one of three mechanisms.[30] In the first type of reaction, exposure to a foreign protein, either in its native state or as a hapten conjugated to a carrier protein, causes IgE-antibody formation. The IgE antibodies then bind to receptors on mast cells and basophils. On reexposure, the antigen stimulates cellular degranulation through both antigen-IgE antibody formation and cross-linking, which result in massive release of preformed immunologic mediators from the mast cells and basophils. Histamine is the major mediator of anaphylaxis and the primary preformed cellular constituent. Histamine has multiple effects and is likely responsible for vasodilation, urticaria, angioedema, hypotension, vomiting, abdominal cramping, and changes in coronary flow.[32] Leukotrienes (e.g., leukotrienes C_4 and D, also known as slow-reacting substance of anaphylaxis [SRS-A]), platelet activating factor, and prostaglandins are generated rapidly as a result of cellular degranulation, and other mediators of anaphylaxis (e.g., tryptase, chymase, heparin, and chondroitin sulfate) are released as well.[30,44] Anaphylactic reactions to *Hymenoptera* venom (e.g., bee stings), insulin, streptokinase, penicillins, cephalosporins, local anesthetics, and sulfonamides occur through this IgE-mediated mechanism.

Anaphylaxis also can occur via a second mechanism. This involves the formation of immune complexes that activate the complement system and the subsequent formation of anaphylatoxins C3a, C4a, and C5a. Such anaphylatoxins can directly stimulate mast cell and basophil degranulation and mediator release.

The third mechanism by which substances, such as radiocontrast media and other hyperosmolar agents, can cause anaphylaxis is by the direct stimulation of mediator release (primarily histamine). The pathway by which this occurs is as yet unknown, but it is independent of IgE and complement.

Lastly, when no distinct mechanism can be associated with an anaphylactic event, the term *idiopathic recurrent anaphylaxis* is applied.[30,45]

L.P.'s anaphylactic episode, most likely, is related to the first mechanism (i.e., IgE-antibody formation). Specifically, L.P. probably received lidocaine when the wounds he sustained 2 years ago were sutured. Exposure to lidocaine at that time probably stimulated IgE-antibody formation. Following reexposure to lidocaine during this admission, antibody–antigen complexes were formed, resulting in cellular degranulation and anaphylaxis. The temporal relationship of L.P.'s anaphylactic reaction to the administration of lidocaine also strongly implicates lidocaine as the precipitating agent. Furthermore, L.P. was not exposed to agents known to cause anaphylaxis by one of the other known mechanisms.

7. Given L.P.'s signs and symptoms and the presumed cause of his anaphylactic reaction, how should he be treated?

Effective management of anaphylaxis requires quick recognition and aggressive therapeutic intervention because of the immediate life-threatening nature of the reaction, as illustrated by L.P. The severity of the anaphylactic reaction must be assessed quickly, the probable causative agent determined, the administration of the offending substance discontinued, and the absorption of the offending agent minimized. All of these interventions must be undertaken promptly and the clinical status of the patient closely monitored. Vital signs, cardiac and pulmonary function, oxygenation, cardiac output, and tissue perfusion in particular must be immediately and continuously assessed.[30,44] In an attempt to minimize further systemic absorption of the anaphylaxis-inducing drug, L.P.'s wound should be thoroughly flushed with normal saline because the lidocaine that was infiltrated around his wound is the probable cause of his anaphylactic reaction.

L.P. is showing signs of anaphylactic shock and peripheral vasodilation, which must be managed immediately. Epinephrine is the drug of choice for the pharmacologic management of anaphylaxis and for all major or severe allergic reactions. It also can be used for the symptomatic relief of minor adverse allergic reactions. The α-adrenergic effects of epinephrine increase systemic vascular resistance and increase blood pressure. These actions counter the vasodilating and hypotensive effects of histamine and the other mediators of anaphylaxis. In addition, the β-adrenergic effects of epinephrine promote bronchodilation and increase cardiac rate and contractility. Epinephrine also inhibits the release of mediators from basophils and mast cells.

The route of epinephrine administration is important. If anaphylaxis is not severe or life threatening, or if vascular access cannot be readily obtained, epinephrine can be administered intramuscularly (IM) or subcutaneously (SC). Although IM epinephrine injections into the thigh achieve higher epinephrine concentrations more rapidly than do SC or IM injections into the arm,[47] the rate and extent of absorption from IM and SC routes of epinephrine administration have not been studied in patients undergoing an anaphylactic reaction.[48] Epinephrine should be administered IV in cases of anaphylaxis that progress to shock because low cardiac output and intravascular volume depletion from shock decrease tissue perfusion and possibly the absorption of SC or IM injections. In animal studies, the benefits of intermittent IV boluses of epinephrine are short lived and a continuous infusion of epinephrine provides optimal results.[49] In L.P.'s case, an IV line should be placed immediately and an epinephrine infusion prepared by mixing 1 mg (1 mL) of a 1:1000 dilution of epinephrine in 250 mL of normal saline to make a concentration of 4 mcg/mL. The infusion should start at 1 to 4 mcg/min and be titrated to clinical response, with a maximal rate of 10 mcg/min.[48]

At the same time, another IV line should be established and normal saline infused at a rate sufficient to maintain perfusion to vital organs. Normal saline is the preferred crystalloid because it stays in the intravascular space longer than does dextrose and does not contain lactate (e.g., Lactated Ringer's solution), which could worsen metabolic acidosis. Circulating blood volume can decrease by as much as 50% in the first 10 minutes of anaphylactic shock because of vasodilation and fluid shifting from the intravascular to the extravascular space.[48] Therefore, vigorous fluid resuscitation might be necessary (e.g., 1 to 2 L of normal saline at a rate of 5 to 10 mL/kg in the first 5 minutes). Cerebral perfusion, as evidenced by adequate mentation, must always take precedence over BP readings when managing shock. Some evidence suggests poor outcomes in patients who are in an upright position during anaphylactic shock. Pumphrey[50] studied 38 deaths from anaphylactic shock and, in 10 cases where postural information was documented, patients died after being moved to an upright position. Four deaths occurred immediately after changing position. Movement of the patient from a supine to an upright position during shock possibly worsened already poor venous return, causing a sudden decrease in cardiac filling and subsequent circulatory collapse.[50] Thus, placing a patient in the Trendelenburg position (patient supine, inclined approximately 45 degrees with head at the lower end and legs at the upper end) might improve survival by enhancing perfusion to vital organs.

The effect of L.P.'s atenolol also must be considered. Patients taking a β-blocker, whether cardioselective or not cardioselective, could experience more severe episodes and more refractory episodes of anaphylaxis than patients not taking a β-blocker. This effect might be caused by a blunted response to epinephrine when given to treat anaphylaxis, resulting in refractory hypotension, bradycardia, and bronchospasm.[48] If L.P.'s BP and heart rate do not substantially improve shortly after initiating epinephrine, IV glucagon, which can stimulate heart rate and cardiac contractility independent of β-adrenergic blockade, should be given (Table 4-5). Inhaled β-agonists, H_1- and H_2-receptor antagonists, corticosteroids, and aminophylline commonly also are used to supplement the actions of epinephrine. In light of L.P.'s severe pulmonary reaction, he should receive oxygen as well as a nebulized β-agonist (e.g., albuterol). If L.P.'s respiratory status fails to improve after pharmacologic intervention, intubation must be considered. Atenolol would not be expected to diminish the effect of albuterol because atenolol is a $\beta 1$ cardioselective β-blocker and the dose is low. Because histamine is the primary mediator of anaphylaxis, IV administration of an antihistamine such as diphenhydramine, 50 mg every 6 hours until the reaction resolves, is warranted. Similarly, giving an H_2-receptor antagonist is reasonable. Because L.P. is not receiving any drugs known to interact with cimetidine and because he has no diseases that require dose adjustment, cimetidine may be given as outlined in Table 4-5.

Lastly, given the severity of his reaction and his pulmonary involvement, L.P. is a candidate for IV corticosteroids. Methylprednisolone, 125 mg every 6 hours for four doses, might be beneficial and is associated with minimal risk. Although commonly used, the indications and doses for corticosteroid administration in the treatment of anaphylaxis are not well defined. The effect of methylprednisolone on L.P.'s diabetes is not a factor because his clinical status is life-threatening. Once stabilized, L.P. should be transferred to a critical care setting and monitored for a minimum of 24 hours because relapses of the anaphylactic reaction can occur.[30,32,44,45]

Serum Sickness

Serum sickness is a type III hypersensitivity reaction that results from the production of antibodies directed against heterologous protein or drug haptens with subsequent tissue deposition. The typical presentation of serum sickness (Table 4-6) includes fever, cutaneous eruptions (95%), lymphadenopathy, and joint symptoms (10%–50%).[51–54] Symptoms usually occur 1 to 2 weeks after exposure, but accelerated reactions can occur within 2 to 4 days in previously sensitized persons. Laboratory data are relatively nonspecific and are of little diagnostic value. For example, the erythrocyte sedimentation rate (ESR) and the serum concentration of circulating immune complexes usually are increased. Complements C3 and C4 are often low, while activation products C3a and C3a desarginine are elevated. Urinalysis might reveal proteinuria, hematuria, or an occasional cast.[51–54]

In most cases, serum sickness reactions are mild and self-limiting and resolve within a few days to weeks after

Table 4-5 Drug Therapy of Anaphylaxis

Drug	Indication	Adult Dosage	Complications
Initial Therapy			
Epinephrine	Hypotension, bronchospasm, laryngeal edema, urticaria, angioedema	0.3 to 0.5 mL of 1:1,000 IM or SC Q 5 min PRN 3–5 mL of 1:10,000 IV over 5 min Q 10–20 min PRN. 1 mL of 1:1,000 in 250 mL of normal saline IV at a rate of 1–10 mcg/min (preferred over intermittent injections) 3 to 5 mL of 1:10,000 intratracheally Q 10–20 min PRN	Arrhythmias, hypertension, nervousness, tremor
Oxygen	Hypoxemia	40%–100%	None
Metaproterenol	Bronchospasm	0.3 mL of 5% solution in 2.5 mL of saline via nebulizer (i.e., 15 mg)	Arrhythmias, hypertension, nervousness, tremor
Or Albuterol	–	0.5 mL of 0.5% solution in 2.5 mL of saline via nebulizer (i.e., 2.5 mg)	–
Or Isoetharine	–	0.5 mL of 1% solution in 2 mL of saline via nebulizer (i.e., 5 mg)	–
IV fluids	Hypotension	1 L of normal saline Q 20–30 min PRN (rates as high as 1–2 mL/kg/min may be necessary)	Pulmonary edema, CHF
Secondary Therapy[a]			
Antihistamines	Hypotension, urticaria		–
H_1-receptor antagonists	–	Diphenhydramine 25–50 mg IV, IM, PO Q 6–8 h PRN Hydroxyzine 25–50 mg IM or PO Q 6–8 h PRN	Drowsiness, dry mouth, urinary retention; may obscure symptoms of continuing reaction
H_2-receptor antagonists		Cimetidine 300 mg IV over 3–5 min or PO Q 6–8 h PRN Ranitidine 50 mg IV over 3–5 min Q 8 h PRN or 150 mg PO BID PRN	– –
Corticosteroids	Bronchospasm; patients undergoing prolonged resuscitation or severe reaction	Hydrocortisone sodium succinate 100 mg IM or IV Q 3–6 h for two to four doses or Methylprednisolone sodium succinate 40–125 mg IV Q 6 hrs for two to four doses	Hyperglycemia, fluid retention
Aminophylline	Bronchospasm	6 mg/kg loading dose (if necessary) IV over 30 min followed by 0.3–0.9 mg/kg/hr as a maintenance dose[b]	Arrhythmias, nausea, vomiting, nervousness, seizures
Norepinephrine	Hypotension	4 mg in 1 L dextrose 5% IV at a rate of 2–12 mcg/min	Arrhythmias, hypertension, nervousness, tremor
Glucagon[c]	Refractory hypotension	1 mg IV over 5 minutes, followed by 5–15 mcg/min in fusion	Nausea, vomiting

[a] Although not effective during acute anaphylaxis, these agents may reduce or prevent recurrent or prolonged reactions.
[b] Doses are for aminophylline; to convert to theophylline, multiply by 0.8. Lower rates may be required in elderly patients, those taking medications that reduce aminophylline metabolism, those with hepatic dysfunction, and those with HF. Higher doses may be required in younger patients or cigarette smokers.
[c] Glucagon may be particularly useful in patients taking β-adrenergic blockers, because it can increase both cardiac rate and contractility regardless of β-adrenergic blockade.
Choice of agent and starting doses should be patient-specific, weighing safety and efficacy.
HF, heart failure; IM, intramuscularly; IV, intravenously; Q, every; PO, orally; PRN, as needed; SC, subcutaneously.
Adapted from references 30, 44, and 45, with permission.

withdrawal of the inciting agent. Antihistamines and aspirin can be used to relieve pruritus and arthralgias. In severe cases, corticosteroids might be used and can be tapered over 10 to 14 days.[51,52–54] Serum sickness reactions are rare because of the infrequent use of foreign serum today;[52] however, reactions to specific agents continue to be reported (Table 4-7).

Drug Fever

8. M.M., a 47-year-old ill-appearing woman, is hospitalized with a 3-day history of difficulty breathing, left-sided chest pain on inspiration, fever, chills, and a productive cough. Her medical history is significant only for hypertension, well controlled on

Table 4-6 Hypersensitivity Reactions to Drugs: Serum Sickness

Clinical Manifestations	Fever, cutaneous eruptions (95% of cases), lymphadenopathy, and joint systems (10%–50%). Onset 1–2 weeks after exposure, 2–4 days in sensitized individuals. Laboratory data relatively nonspecific: elevated ESR and circulating immune complexes. Complements C3 and C4 are often low, whereas activation products C3a and C3a desarginine are elevated. RF sometimes present. UA may reveal proteinuria, hematuria, or an occasional cast.
Prognosis	Usually mild and self-limiting. Most resolve within a few days to weeks after withdrawal of inciting agent.
Treatment	Aspirin and antihistamines can relieve arthralgias and pruritus. Corticosteroids may be required for severe cases and tapered over 10–14 days.

ESR, erythrocyte sedimentation rate; RF, rheumatoid factor; UA, urinalysis.
From references 51–54, with permission.

Table 4-7 Allergic Reactions to Drugs

Serum Sickness[52,145,159–177]

6-Mercaptopurine	Furazolidone	Itraconazole
Antithymocyte globulin	Hemophilus B vaccine	Minocycline
Carbamazepine	Indomethacin	Pentoxifylline
Cefaclor	Intravenous immune globulin	Phenytoin
Ciprofloxacin		Rabies vaccine
Fluoxetine	Iron dextran	–

Drug Fever[55–66]

Allopurinol	Epinephrine	Para-aminosalicylate
Aminoglycosides	Folate	Penicillins
Amphetamine	Griseofulvin	Phenytoin
Amphotericin B	Heparin	Procainamide
Anesthetics, inhaled	Hydralazine	Propylthiouracil
Antacids	Hydroxyurea	Quinidine
Anticholinergics	Ibuprofen	Quinine
Antihistamines	Imipenem	Ranitidine
Antilymphocyte globulin	Insulin	Rifampin
Antineoplastics	Interferon	Salicylates
Azathioprine	Iodides	Streptokinase
Barbiturates	Isoniazid	Streptomycin
Bleomycin	Iron dextran	Sulfonamides
Carbamazepine	Macrolide antibiotics	Sulindac
Cephalosporins	Mebendazole	Tacrolimus
Chloramphenicol	Metoclopramide	Tetracyclines
Cimetidine	Methyldopa	Tolmetin
Clofibrate	Monamine oxidase inhibitors	Triamterene
Cocaine		Trimethoprim
Corticosteroids	Muromonab-CD3	Sulindac
Cyclosporine	Neuroleptics	Vancomycin
Chloramphenicol	Nifedipine	Vitamins
Diazoxide	Nitrofurantoin	–
Digoxin	Oral contraceptives	

Drug-Induced Vasculitis[67,73,178–209]

Allopurinol	Mefloquine	Ritodrine
Azathioprine	Methotrexate	Sotalol
Carbamazepine	Naproxen	Sulfadiazine
Cephalosporins	Nizatidine	Terbutaline
Cimetidine	Ofloxacin	Torsemide
Ciprofloxacin	Penicillin	Trimethadione
Clarithromycin	Phenytoin	Valproate
Furosemide	Phenylbutazone	Vitamins
Hydralazine	Pneumococcal vaccine	Warfarin
Hydrochlorothiazide	Procainamide	Zidovudine
L-Tryptophan	Propylthiouracil	–

Autoimmune Drug Reactions[74–77,80,87–89,210–247]

Anticonvulsants	Interferon	Procainamide
β-Blockers	Isoniazid	Quinidine
Chlorpromazine	Methyldopa	Sulfasalazine
Estrogen	Minocycline	Terbinafine
Hydralazine	Penicillamine	Zafirlukast

hydrochlorothiazide; she has no known drug allergies. M.M.'s physical findings on admission are temperature 38°C; respirations 20 breaths/minute; left-sided crackles heard on auscultation; oxygen saturation 85% on room air; and heart rate 85 beats/minute. A chest radiograph reveals an infiltrate in her left lower lobe. Her white blood cell (WBC) count is 17,500 cells/mm^3 (normal, 5,000–10,000) with the following differential: polymorphonuclear neutrophil leukocytes (PMN), 83% (normal, 45%–79%); bands, 12% (normal, 0%–5%); lymphocytes, 10% (normal, 16%–47%); basophils, 0% (normal, 0%–1%); and eosinophils, 1% (normal, 1%–2%). Community-acquired pneumonia is the diagnosis, and M.M. is empirically started on ceftriaxone 1 g IV daily, azithromycin 500 mg IV every 24 hours, and oxygen at 2 L/minute. Other medications include oral acetaminophen 325 mg every 4–6 hours as needed for temperature >38°C, oral famotidine 20 mg twice daily, and oral hydrochlorothiazide 12.5 mg daily. Seventy-two hours later, M.M. is breathing without pain at a respiratory rate of 12 breaths/minute, her lungs are clear to auscultation, and her oxygen saturation is 98% on room air. She appears much better and offers no new complaints. Her temperature over the previous 48 hours has ranged from 38.6°C–40°C, her pulse has ranged from 90–100 beats/minute, and her WBC count is 22,000 with the following differential: PMN, 89%; bands, 5%; lymphocytes, 12%; basophils, 0%; and eosinophils, 7%. Drug-induced fever is considered. What evidence supports this diagnosis? What is the mechanism for drug fever?

Drug fever is described as a febrile reaction to a drug without cutaneous symptoms and is estimated to occur in 3% to 5% of inpatients.[55] Drug fever can be challenging to identify and can be misinterpreted as a new infectious process or failure of an existing infection to respond to treatment. Such failure to recognize a drug fever can lead to prolonged hospitalization and unnecessary tests or medications. Table 4-8 lists the characteristics of hypersensitivity drug-induced fever. The most important finding in the case of M.M. is her clinical improvement with respect to her pulmonary status despite a high-grade fever and persistent leukocytosis; she also appears healthier than expected if she had an untreated infection. Whereas a drop in her WBC count would be anticipated given her improving respiratory function, her WBC count remains elevated, consistent with hypersensitivity drug fever. Notably, her eosinophil count is increased, a frequent sign of hypersensitivity reactions. Despite her high-grade fever, she has a relative bradycardia; that is, her heart rate is not as elevated as expected

Table 4-8 Hypersensitivity Reactions to Drugs: Drug-Induced Fever[56–58,60–62,65,66]

Frequency	True frequency is unknown because fever is a common manifestation and almost any drug can cause fever. estimate is that 3%–5% of hospitalized patients experiencing adverse drug reaction suffer from drug fever alone or as part of multiple symptoms.
Clinical Manifestations	Temperatures may be 38°C or higher and do not follow a consistent pattern. Although patients may have high fevers with shaking chills, patients generally have few symptoms or serious systemic illness. Skin rash (18%), eosinophilia (22%), chills (53%), headache (16%), myalgias (25%), and bradycardia (11%) can occur in patients with drug fever. Onset of fever after exposure to the offending agent is highly variable, ranging from an average of 6 days for antineoplastics to 45 days for cardiovascular agents. Occurrence of fever is independent of the dose of the offending agent.
Treatment	Although drug fever can be treated symptomatically (e.g., with antipyretics, cooling blankets), stopping the offending agent is the only therapy that will eliminate fevers. Patients generally defervesce within 48–72 hours of stopping the suspect drug.
Prognosis	Drug fever is usually benign, although one review (57) found a mean increased length of hospitalization of 9 days per episode of drug fever. Rechallenge with the offending drug usually results in rapid return of the fever. Although re-exposure to the suspect drug was previously thought to be potentially hazardous, there is little risk of serious sequelae.

if an infectious process were ongoing. Further, the timing of the symptoms favors a drug-induced fever (i.e., within days of starting a new medication). A definitive diagnosis can be made only by stopping the suspected offending agent, however, because fever generally resolves within 48 to 72 hours if a rash is not present. When a rash is present, however, the fever may persist for several days after stopping the implicated drug.

Drug fever can be caused by various mechanisms, although it is ascribed most commonly to a hypersensitivity reaction. Other mechanisms include the pharmacologic action of the drug (e.g., cell destruction from antineoplastic agents releases endogenous pyrogens); altered thermoregulatory function (e.g., increased metabolic rate from thyroid hormone); decreased sweating from drugs with anticholinergic properties (e.g., atropine, tricyclic antidepressants, phenothiazines); drug-administration-related fever (e.g., amphotericin B, bleomycin); and idiosyncratic reactions (e.g., neuroleptic malignant syndrome from haloperidol, malignant hyperthermia from inhaled anesthetics).[55,56]

9. What agent is the most likely cause of drug fever in M.M.?

Most of the information available on drug fever is based on case reports or small case series, and the only critical appraisal of the literature[57] is not consistent with information found in other reports. Furthermore, the literature is inconsistent with regard to the frequency of drug fever (e.g., very common, common, uncommon) and such descriptions are not supported by good clinical data. Nevertheless, some drugs are more commonly associated with drug fever than others. These include anti-infectives as a class (especially β-lactam antibiotics), antiepileptics (especially barbiturates and phenytoin), and antineoplastics. Other causes of drug fever include amphotericin B; antihistamines (except diphenhydramine); anticholinergics and drugs with anticholinergic properties (e.g., tricyclic antidepressants, phenothiazines); asparaginase; bleomycin; hydralazine; interferon; methyldopa; muromonab CD-3; para-aminosalicylic acid; procainamide; quinidine; quinine; and drugs containing a sulfonamide moiety (including antibiotics, stool softeners, and diuretics).[55–66] A more complete listing of drugs associated with fever is presented in Table 4-7.

In M.M.'s case, ceftriaxone or the macrolide, is the most likely cause of her ongoing fever, given the timing of the reaction relative to beginning the antibiotics and the frequency of febrile reactions attributed to them, especially to β-lactam antibiotics. Febrile reactions have not been associated with acetaminophen, and famotidine is rarely a cause of fever without other symptoms of an allergic reaction. Although diuretics such as hydrochlorothiazide can cause fever, M.M. was taking this medication before admission without any ill effects, making this drug an unlikely culprit.

10. How should M.M.'s drug fever be treated? Can M.M. receive cephalosporins in the future?

Because M.M. has responded clinically, her antibiotics should be discontinued and her fever curve, WBC count, heart rate, and respiratory status followed. An oral antibiotic from another drug class (e.g., a fluoroquinolone) should be started to complete a 7- to 10-day antibiotic course of therapy. Acetaminophen and other antipyretics should be avoided unless M.M. becomes uncomfortable from the fever because they can mask the response to the discontinuation of her antibiotics.

As with any hypersensitivity reaction, rechallenge with the offending drug can cause a similar, or sometimes greater, response. In M.M.'s case, re-exposure to ceftriaxone (or another β-lactam antibiotic) or a macrolide might cause a febrile reaction. It is unclear, however, how large the risk of re-exposure truly is. Although drug fever sometimes precedes more serious hypersensitivity reactions, evidence suggests there may be little risk to re-exposure. Should M.M. require ceftriaxone (or another β-lactam or macrolide antibiotic) in the future, it would be prudent to administer the drug in a setting where M.M. can be monitored, at least initially, to ensure prompt treatment if an immediate hypersensitivity reaction develops.

Hypersensitivity Vasculitis

11. M.G., a 26-year-old woman with cystic fibrosis, is admitted for treatment of pneumonia. Sputum cultures obtained before admission reveal *Alcaligenes xylosoxidans* sensitive only to minocycline and chloramphenicol. M.G. is initiated on appropriate doses of these two antibiotics for a 2-week course. On day 8 of therapy, M.G. begins to complain of a rash on her legs. Physical examination reveals palpable purpura and a maculopapular rash on both lower extremities. Laboratory data reveal an elevated ESR and leukocytosis. What is the likely cause of M.G.'s rash and laboratory abnormalities?

M.G.'s presentation is suggestive of a diagnosis of hypersensitivity vasculitis. Hypersensitivity vasculitis, also called *cutaenous leukocytoclastic angiitis* (CLA), is characterized by

Table 4-9 1990 Criteria for the Classification of Hypersensitivity Vasculitis

Criteria[a]	*Definition*
Age at disease onset >16 yrs	Development of symptoms after age 16
Medication at disease onset	Medication was taken at the onset of symptoms that may have been a precipitating factor
Palpable purpura	Slightly elevated purpuric rash over one or more areas of the skin; does not blanch with pressure and not related to thrombocytopenia
Maculopapular rash	Flat and raised lesions of various sizes over one or more areas of the skin
Biopsy including arteriole and venule	Histologic changes showing granulocytes in a perivascular or extravascular location

[a]The diagnosis of hypersensitivity vasculitis can be made if a patient exhibits at least three of these criteria.
Adapted from reference 248, with permission.

inflammation of the small blood vessel walls. These reactions occur when immune complex deposition within the small veins and arterioles activates complement, causing the release of chemotactic factors. These factors attract polymorphonuclear cells that cause vessel damage.[67–69]

Drug-Induced Vasculitis

Approximately 20% of cases of cutaneous vasculitis are believed to be drug-related.[70] Table 4-7 lists the more commonly implicated drugs; interested readers are referred to more in-depth reviews.[71,72] The diagnosis of hypersensitivity vasculitis is based on five clinical criteria (Table 4-9), three of which must be present.[73] M.G. meets three of the five criteria, including age >16 years, palpable purpura, and a maculopapular rash. In addition, minocycline, a medication that she was taking at the onset of the rash, has been associated with serum sickness and vasculitic-type reactions. Onset of symptoms typically occurs 7 to 10 days after initiation of drug therapy, but can occur sooner on re-exposure. Purpuric papules and macular eruptions, the most commonly observed findings, are usually symmetric and occur on the extremities (Table 4-10).[68] Hypersensitivity vasculitis can involve multiple organ systems. Renal damage, ranging from microscopic hematuria to nephrotic syndrome and acute renal failure, is common in patients with disseminated disease.[68] An enlarged liver with elevated enzymes is indicative of hepatocellular involvement. Although the lungs and ears can be involved as well, clinical manifestations are usually mild.[68] Arthralgia also is commonly observed. Laboratory examinations usually show nonspecific abnormalities of inflammation such as an elevated ESR and leukocytosis. In patients with cystic fibrosis experiencing acute pneumonia, these laboratory abnormalities already could be present and, therefore, will not be helpful in establishing the diagnosis of hypersensitivity vasculitis in M.G.

Table 4-10 Hypersensitivity Reactions to Drugs: Clinical Manifestations of Drug-Induced Vasculitis

- Palpable purpura and maculopapular rash occurring symmetrically on the extremities
- Multiple organ systems may be involved:
  Renal: microscopic hematuria to nephrotic syndrome and acute renal failure
  Liver: enlarged liver, elevated enzymes, and arthralgias
- Laboratory data usually show nonspecific abnormalities of inflammation: elevated erythrocyte sedimentation rate and leukocytosis. Peripheral eosinophilia may be present and serum complement concentrations can be low. Histologic findings on biopsy reveal granulocytes in venule or arteriole walls
- Onset typically 7–10 days after initiation of therapy

From references 51, 177, 241, 237, with permission.

12. What additional workup could be performed to confirm the diagnosis of drug-induced vasculitis in M.G.?

In addition to the previous workup, other laboratory and diagnostic procedures might demonstrate peripheral eosinophilia and low serum complement concentrations. A biopsy, which typically reveals granulocytes in the wall of a venule or arteriole and eosinophils at any location, would provide more definitive information.[73]

13. How should M.G.'s hypersensitivity vasculitis be treated?

The first step is to discontinue the minocycline therapy. Drug-induced vasculitic reactions typically resolve on their own without additional interventions. If the reaction is severe, corticosteroids can be used.

Autoimmune Drug Reactions

14. R.F., a 24-year-old white male medical student, has been treated for 5 months with isoniazid because of a positive skin test for tuberculosis. He now is in clinic with complaints of new-onset myalgias and arthralgias. Laboratory values obtained the morning of the visit are within normal limits except for a positive ANA titer and an elevated ESR. What is the likely cause of R.F.'s symptoms and laboratory abnormalities?

Some drugs can induce an autoimmune process characterized by the presence of autoantibodies and, in some instances, clinical features of an autoimmune disorder. A drug-induced syndrome resembling SLE usually is characterized by myalgias, arthralgias, positive ANA titers, and an elevated ESR (Table 4-11). All of these characteristics are manifested by R.F.

Drug-induced SLE was first recognized over 50 years ago in a group of patients taking hydralazine for antihypertensive therapy.[74] Subsequently, isoniazid, chlorpromazine, anticonvulsants, β-adrenergic blockers, quinidine, methyldopa, penicillamine, and sulfasalazine also have been implicated (Table 4-7); however, hydralazine and procainamide have been the drugs most frequently associated with this syndrome.[75–78] An exact incidence of drug-induced lupus is difficult to ascertain because of changing patterns of drug use.

15. How can the diagnosis of drug-induced lupus be differentiated from SLE in R.F.?

In contrast to idiopathic SLE, drug-induced lupus is less likely to affect females and blacks.[76] Individuals with a slow

Table 4-11 Hypersensitivity Reactions to Drugs: Autoimmune Drug-Induced Lupus

Frequency	Less likely to affect females and blacks than idiopathic SLE. Drug-induced lupus is more common in individuals with slow acetylator phenotype.
Clinical Manifestations	Milder disease than idiopathic SLE. Arthralgias, myalgias, fever, malaise, pleurisy, and slight weight loss. Mild splenomegaly and lymphadenopathy. *Onset:* usually abrupt, occurring several months to years after continuous therapy with the offending drug. *Appearance*: Classic butterfly malar rash, discoid lesions, oral mucosal ulcers, Raynaud's phenomenon, and alopecia are unusual features with drug-induced lupus as opposed to idiopathic SLE. *Laboratory studies*: positive ANA (predominantly single-stranded DNA and antihistone antibodies), anemia, and elevated erythrocyte sedimentation rate. Many patients demonstrate ANA without development of lupus disease. It is, therefore, not necessary to discontinue therapy in asymptomatic patients with positive ANA.
Treatment	Clinical features subside and disappear days to weeks after discontinuation of the offending drug. Serologic tests resolve more slowly. ANA may persist for a year or longer.
Prognosis	Drug-induced lupus does not predispose to development of idiopathic SLE. Lupus-inducing drugs do not appear to increase the risk of exacerbation of idiopathic SLE. Long-term treatment with interferon-λ may, however, worsen pre-existing SLE.

ANA, antinuclear antibody; SLE, systemic lupus erythematosus.
From references 74–88, 249, with permission.

acetylator phenotype have a greater tendency to develop drug-induced lupus; ANA following exposure to lupus-inducing drugs also appear more rapidly.[79,80] In general, drug-induced lupus is a milder disease than idiopathic SLE. Many patients with drug-induced lupus, however, could fulfill the diagnostic criteria for SLE according to the American Rheumatism Association.[81] Arthralgias or myalgias accompanied by a positive ANA test can be the only clinical features for some patients with drug-induced lupus. Symptoms usually appear abruptly after several months to years of continuous therapy with the offending drug. Common complaints include fever, malaise, arthralgias, myalgias, pleurisy, and slight weight loss. Mild splenomegaly and lymphadenopathy have been reported occasionally. The classic butterfly malar rash, discoid lesions, oral mucosal ulcers, Raynaud's phenomenon, and alopecia are unusual features in drug-induced lupus in contrast to idiopathic SLE. In addition, the central nervous system and kidneys rarely are affected.[76] Laboratory abnormalities commonly include anemia and an elevated ESR. The evidence supporting a diagnosis of drug-induced lupus in R.F. includes white male predominance, abrupt onset and relatively mild symptomatology, and lack of the classic butterfly malar rash. More definitive tests include determining whether antibodies to single-stranded (indicative of drug-induced lupus) or double-stranded DNA (indicative of SLE) are present.

16. Should ANA have been monitored in an effort to detect drug-induced lupus at an earlier stage in this patient?

No. Although all patients with symptomatic drug-induced lupus test positive for ANA (which consist predominantly of single-stranded DNA and antihistone antibodies),[76] many patients taking lupus-inducing drugs become ANA positive without going on to develop lupus. In patients treated with procainamide, about 50% to 75% are positive for ANA after 12 months and 90% after 2 years or more of continuous therapy; only 10% to 20% of those patients actually develop lupus symptoms.[82–84] Similarly, up to 44% of patients are ANA positive after 3 years of hydralazine therapy, but drug-induced lupus occurs in only 6.7% of patients after 3 years of treatment.[85] It is not necessary to discontinue therapy in asymptomatic patients with positive ANA because most of them will never develop clinical symptoms.[76]

17. How should R.F.'s drug-induced lupus be treated?

Musculoskeletal complaints can be treated with aspirin or nonsteroidal anti-inflammatory drugs (NSAID). More severe symptoms from pleuropulmonary or pericardial involvement may require the use of corticosteroids.[77] Clinical features of drug-induced lupus usually subside and disappear in days to weeks with discontinuation of the offending drug. Occasionally, these symptoms linger or recur over a course of several months before eventually disappearing. Serologic tests tend to resolve more slowly: ANA may persist for a year or longer.[76,86] Drug-induced lupus does not predispose patients to the subsequent development of idiopathic SLE.[87] In most instances, lupus-inducing drugs do not increase the risk of exacerbation of idiopathic SLE[88]; however, long-term treatment with isoniazid may worsen pre-existing SLE.[89] R.F. has not yet completed his 6- to 9-month course of isoniazid therapy. An alternative agent should be prescribed for R.F. for at least an additional month and preferentially for up to 4 more months (see Chapter 61: Tuberculosis).

ORGAN-SPECIFIC REACTIONS

The drug allergies in this chapter have been grouped into categories of generalized reactions, organ-specific reactions, and pseudoallergic reactions. The generalized reactions have been described above, the organ-specific hypersensitivity drug reactions affecting the blood, liver, lung, kidney, and skin are described next, and pseudoallergic reactions follow.

Blood: Immune Cytopenias

Drug-induced immune cytopenias (e.g., granulocytopenia, thrombocytopenia, hemolytic anemia) result from type II-mediated allergic reactions (Table 4-1). A drug or drug metabolite binds to the surface of blood elements such as granulocytes, platelets, and red blood cells. IgG or IgM antibodies are formed and are directed against the drug or drug metabolite bound to the cell (i.e., hapten-cell reaction).[9] The immune complex and autoimmune mechanisms for hemolytic anemia are presented in Chapter 87, Drug-Induced Blood Disorders. Typical symptoms associated with immune thrombocytopenia include chills, fever, petechiae, and mucous membrane bleeding. Granulocytopenia generally manifests with chills, fever, arthralgias, and a precipitous drop in the leukocyte count. Symptoms of hemolytic anemia can be subacute or acute and can be sufficiently severe to cause renal failure. Coombs' test is useful in identifying antibodies bound to red cells or circulating immune complexes directed against red cells. Antibiotics are the most commonly implicated class of drugs causing either neutropenia or hemolytic anemia. (See Chapter 87 for a more complete description of the immune cytopenias.)

Liver

Hypersensitivity reactions involving the liver can be classified as cholestatic or cytotoxic. Jaundice is usually the first sign of a cholestatic reaction, in addition to pruritus, pale stools, and dark urine. Cholestatic reactions usually are reversible on discontinuation of the offending agent.

Cytotoxic reactions can involve hepatocellular necrosis or steatosis and can result in irreversible damage if not recognized early. (See Chapter 29: Adverse Effects of Drugs on the Liver, for a discussion of hypersensitivity reactions involving the liver.)

Lung

Pulmonary manifestations of drug hypersensitivity include asthma and infiltrative reactions. Asthma typically occurs as part of a generalized systemic reaction. Most reactions to drugs that involve asthma alone represent a pharmacologic side effect rather than a true allergic reaction.

Infiltrative reactions typically develop 2 to 10 days after exposure and manifest with cough, dyspnea, fever, chills, and malaise.[6] Infiltrative reactions vary in presentation from eosinophilic pneumonitis to acute pulmonary edema. (See Chapter 25: Drug-Induced Pulmonary Disorders, for a discussion of hypersensitivity reactions to specific drugs.)

Kidney

The most common hypersensitivity reaction involving the kidney is interstitial nephritis. Typical findings include fever, rash, and eosinophilia. Methicillin is the drug most commonly associated with interstitial nephritis, however, penicillins, sulfonamides, and cimetidine also have been implicated in renal hypersensitivity reactions.[6,9] (See Chapter 30: Acute Renal Failure, for an analysis of hypersensitivity reactions to specific drugs that adversely affect the kidney.)

Skin

Adverse reactions involving the skin are the most common clinical manifestation of drug allergy. Although several different types of cutaneous reactions are possible, most drug-induced skin eruptions can be classified as erythematous, morbilliform, or maculopapular in appearance.[9] In a surveillance study of drug-induced skin reactions, amoxicillin was the most common cause, followed by trimethoprim-sulfamethoxazole and ampicillin. Overall, allergic skin reactions were identified in 2% of hospitalized patients.[10]

Treatment of skin reactions includes discontinuation of the offending drug and general supportive care. (See Chapter 38: Dermatotherapy and Drug-Induced skin disorders.)

PSEUDOALLERGIC REACTIONS

18. C.C., a 37-year-old man with no known allergies, is hospitalized for treatment of methicillin-resistant *S. aureus* (MRSA) bacteremia associated with an infected central line. His medical history is significant for short-bowel syndrome requiring parenteral nutrition and one previous episode of MRSA line infection successfully treated with vancomycin. Similar to his last admission, vancomycin 750 mg IV over 60 minutes every 12 hours is begun. A trough level taken after the fifth dose, however, is 5 mg/L and the vancomycin dose is doubled to 1,500 mg IV every 12 hours, to be administered at the same rate. Fifteen minutes after the new dose of vancomycin is begun, C.C. experienced hypotension (100/70 mmHg), tachycardia (85 beats/minute), generalized pruritus, and facial flushing. C.C. is diagnosed as having a pseudoallergic reaction to vancomycin. What subjective and objective data in C.C. are important in differentiating vancomycin pseudoallergic reaction from a true allergic reaction?

Pseudoallergic reactions are drug reactions that exhibit clinical signs and symptoms of an allergic response, but are not immunologically mediated.[90] They can manifest as relatively benign symptoms or as severe, life-threatening events indistinguishable from anaphylaxis (Table 4-12).[90] The latter response is described as an anaphylactoid reaction because it resembles true anaphylaxis, but does not involve IgE-antibody formation.[9,90] The risk of such potentially severe reactions needs to be considered when prescribing agents known to be associated with anaphylactoid reactions. For example, the prophylactic use of antibiotics such as ciprofloxacin to prevent meningococcal infections during an outbreak was associated with a relatively high rate (1:1,000) of serious anaphylactoid reactions.[91] This would be of potentially greater importance in the setting of a mass prophylaxis program to combat exposure to anthrax. Unlike true allergic reactions, which require an induction period during which a patient becomes sensitized to an antigen, pseudoallergic reactions can occur on the first exposure to a drug. The development of pseudoallergic reactions can be dose related, manifesting when large doses of the drug are administered, when the dose is increased, or when the rate of IV administration is increased.[6]

C.C. has experienced a common pseudoallergic reaction to vancomycin, usually referred to as the "red man syndrome" or "red neck syndrome," which primarily occurs when large doses of vancomycin are administered rapidly. Differentiating between a true allergic response and a pseudoallergic response can be difficult because the signs and symptoms can be indistinguishable. For example, each of the symptoms experienced by C.C. (flushing, tachycardia, pruritus, and hypotension) is caused by histamine release and can occur during an anaphylactic episode. To conclusively determine the cause of the reaction would require immunologic testing for antibodies to the suspect drug or agent, which is not always possible or practical. In this case, C.C. had uneventfully received vancomycin

Table 4-12 Hypersensitivity Reactions to Drugs: Pseudoallergic Reactions

Frequency	Highly variable, depending on the agent involved. For example, up to 30% of patients taking aspirin develop a cutaneous pseudoallergic response. On the other hand, pseudoallergic reactions to other agents, such as phytonadione and thiamine, are rare.
Clinical Manifestations	Range from benign reactions (e.g., pruritus and flushing) to a life-threatening clinical syndrome indistinguishable from anaphylaxis
Treatment	Pseudoallergic reactions are treated the same as true allergic reactions (i.e., according to the clinical presentations of the patient). Thus, some reactions simply may require removal of the suspect agent, whereas some anaphylactoid reactions may require aggressive therapy (e.g., epinephrine, antihistamines, corticosteroids).
Prognosis	As with true allergic reactions, patients who have experienced a pseudoallergic drug reaction may have a similar reaction on re-exposure. The severity of response may lessen, however, with repeated administration. Furthermore, for some drugs, the frequency and severity of the reaction also may be influenced by the dose or rate of intravenous (IV) administration. Pretreatment regimens to reduce the frequency and the severity of responses have been developed for some drugs well known to cause pseudoallergic reactions (e.g., radiocontrast media).

From references 5, 9, 90, 91, 93, 94, 100, 111, 250–257, with permission.

previously and has tolerated five doses during this hospitalization; therefore, it is unlikely that the reaction is immunologically mediated (i.e., a true allergic reaction). Furthermore, the reaction occurred after an increase in his vancomycin dose, which further supports the diagnosis of a pseudoallergic reaction.

19. Why did vancomycin cause a pseudoallergic reaction in C.C.?

Two general mechanisms have been proposed for pseudoallergic reactions: complement activation and direct histamine release.[30]

Complement activation is secondary to immune complex formation, leading to the production of C3a, C4a, and C5a. These anaphylatoxins directly stimulate tissue mast cell and basophil degranulation and the subsequent release of neurochemical mediators. Radiocontrast media, whole blood and blood products, and protamine cause pseudoallergic reactions via this mechanism of complement activation.[90]

Pseudoallergic reactions from *direct drug-induced histamine release* occur through an as yet unknown pathway. Direct drug-induced release of histamine does not involve complement activation or IgE-antibody formation. Several drugs (e.g., vancomycin, protamine, radiocontrast media, opiates, pentamidine, phytonadione, deferoxamine) are known to directly stimulate histamine release.[6,90]

Some drugs (e.g., radiocontrast media and protamine) cause pseudoallergic reactions via both complement activation and direct-histamine release mechanisms. Furthermore, some drugs (e.g., vancomycin, quaternary ammonium muscle relaxants, and ciprofloxacin) can cause both true allergic reactions and pseudoallergic reactions.[3]

20. How should C.C.'s pseudoallergic reaction be treated? Does treatment of pseudoallergic reactions differ from that of true allergic reactions?

The first step in treating C.C.'s reaction is to eliminate the underlying cause. Thus, his vancomycin infusion should be held until the reaction resolves. Because the reaction is histamine mediated, administration of an antihistamine such as diphenhydramine 50 mg IV is warranted. Observation of his BP and heart rate is mandatory. IV fluids should be administered if his BP continues to fall or fails to stabilize. Patients with allergic reactions should be treated based on their clinical signs and symptoms, regardless of the mechanism behind the reaction. Thus, for all intents and purposes, pseudoallergic reactions are treated in the same manner as true allergic reactions.

21. Can C.C. continue to receive vancomycin? How can future reactions be prevented?

It is not necessary to discontinue vancomycin therapy in C.C. This reaction can be prevented by administering smaller doses of the drug more frequently (e.g., 1,000 mg every 8 hours rather than 1,500 mg every 12 hours) or infusing the dose over a longer interval, typically 2 hours. Alternatively, pretreatment with an antihistamine 1 hour before vancomycin administration is effective. In addition, tachyphylaxis to vancomycin-induced red man syndrome is independent of pretreatment with antihistamine and is another characteristic that differentiates a pseudoallergic reaction from a true allergic reaction. Pretreatment regimens to prevent pseudoallergic reactions to various other drugs (e.g., radiocontrast media) also are well described and can be effective.

22. What other drugs are commonly associated with pseudoallergic reactions?

Many other agents have been associated with pseudoallergic reactions, as shown in Table 4-13. Some of the agents more commonly associated with pseudoallergic reactions are described next.

Aspirin/Nonsteroidal Anti-inflammatory Drugs (NSAIDs)

After penicillins, aspirin is the drug most commonly reported as causing "allergic" reactions. Reactions to aspirin can be divided into three broad categories: respiratory reactions, cutaneous manifestations, and anaphylaxis. None of these reactions has been consistently associated with IgE.[92]

Respiratory. The prevalence of bronchospasm with rhinoconjunctivitis is 0% to 28% in children with aspirin sensitivity. In adult asthmatics, the prevalence of aspirin sensitivity ranges from 5% to 20%. The prevalence of aspirin sensitivity during aspirin challenge in adult asthmatics with a history of aspirin-induced respiratory reaction ranges from

Table 4-13 Pseudoallergic Reactions

Acetylcysteine[254]	Immune globulin[90]	Phytonadione[90]
ACE inhibitors[100]	Iron dextran[260]	Polyoxyethylated castor oil (Cremophor EL, a solubilizing agent used in parenteral drugs such as cyclosporine, paclitaxel)[258,259]
Angiotensin II–receptor blocking agents[101–109]	Iron sucrose[261]	Protamine[9]
Aspirin[93,94]	Methotrexate[262]	Quaternary ammonium muscle relaxants[5,90]
β-Adrenergic blockers[90]	Minocycline[263]	Radiocontrast media[111]
Ciprofloxacin[5,252,255,256]	Narcotic analgesics[90]	Reserpine[90]
Cisplatin[264]	NSAID[92,93]	Sodium ferric gluconate[265]
Corticosteroids[266,267]	Ondansetron[253,257]	Thiamine[92]
COX-2 inhibitors[95]	Paclitaxel[268]	Vancomycin[9,251]
Deferoxamine[90]	Pentamidine[90]	

66% to 97%.[93,94] Symptoms usually occur within 30 minutes to 3 hours of ingestion. The triad seen in many sensitive patients is aspirin sensitivity, nasal polyps, and asthma. All potent inhibitors of cyclooxygenase can cause respiratory symptoms in aspirin-sensitive patients. Thus, patients who react to aspirin should be considered sensitive to NSAIDs, and vice versa. Weak cyclooxygenase inhibitors, such as acetaminophen, choline magnesium salicylate, propoxyphene, salicylamide, salsalate, and sodium salicylate, are generally well tolerated in patients with aspirin sensitivity.[92]

Cutaneous. The prevalence of cutaneous reactions to aspirin depends on the type of reaction and the population studied. For example, urticaria-angioedema occurs in 0.5% of children, 3.8% of the general adult population, and in 21% to 30% of patients with a history of chronic urticaria. Disease activity at the time of aspirin challenge plays an important role in those with a history of chronic urticaria. In one study, 70% of patients whose urticaria was active at the time of challenge reacted to aspirin, compared with only 6.6% of patients whose urticaria was not active at the time of challenge. Furthermore, aspirin or NSAID may aggravate preexisting urticaria.[92–94] Other dermatologic reactions to aspirin occur with less frequency: for example, eczema, purpura, and erythema multiforme occur in 2.4%, 1.5%, and 1% of the population, respectively.

Anaphylaxis. The true prevalence of aspirin or NSAID-induced anaphylaxis is unknown, but may range from 0.07% of the general population to 10% of patients with anaphylactic symptoms. Although IgE is not consistently associated with aspirin or NSAID-related reactions (including anaphylaxis), aspirin- or NSAID-induced anaphylaxis shares three characteristics with immune-mediated anaphylaxis that point to IgE as a cause. First, the reaction occurs after two or more exposures to the offending agent, suggesting that preformed IgE antibodies are responsible. Second, patients do not have underlying nasal polyposis, asthma, or urticaria. Third, the patient who reacts to aspirin or a single NSAID can tolerate a chemically unrelated NSAID, suggesting that a drug-specific IgE antibody has been formed.[92,95]

The NSAIDs that selectively inhibit cyclooxygenase-2 (COX-2) while sparing cyclooxygenase-1 (COX-1) include celecoxib, rofecoxib, and valdecoxib, among others. Celecoxib is the only COX-2 inhibitor or "coxib" currently marketed in the United States. Selective inhibition of COX-2 provides anti-inflammatory effects while minimizing the renal effects, GI toxicity, and antiplatelet effects seen with inhibition of COX-1. Aspirin and older NSAIDs are nonselective inhibitors of cyclooxygenase, inhibiting both COX-1 and COX-2. Anaphylactoid or hypersensitivity reactions have been reported with celecoxib and it appears that the rate of hypersensitivity is comparable to that of traditional NSAIDs.[95] Notably, celecoxib prescribing information states that, as with any NSAID, use is contraindicated in patients who have experienced asthma, urticaria, or allergic-type reactions after taking aspirin or other NSAIDs. Several reports, however, describe successful administration of celecoxib and other COX-2 selective agents to patients with aspirin-sensitive asthma or a history of hypersensitivity reactions to traditional NSAIDs, and evidence suggests that inhibition of COX-1 rather than COX-2 is key to initiating these events.[96–99] Nevertheless, COX-2 selective agents can still elicit allergic responses by other means (e.g., IgE-mediated hypersensitivity). Thus, appropriate precautions and monitoring should be followed when initiating therapy in any patient with a history of allergic reactions to aspirin or other NSAIDs.

Angiotensin-Converting Enzyme Inhibitors and Angiotensin II–Receptor Blockers

23. K.J., a 48-year-old woman, seeks care at an urgent care center. She presents with impaired speech, but is able to swallow; she has red and swollen lips and tongue, and puffy eyes. Her medical history includes hypertension, atrial fibrillation, and a new diagnosis of hypercholesterolemia (plasma cholesterol 290 mg/dL). Although her BP had been well controlled on hydrochlorothiazide, her diuretic was discontinued about 3 weeks ago because of its effect on cholesterol, and enalapril 5 mg daily was started. K.J. also takes a multivitamin (one tablet each day) and warfarin (5 mg daily). Her physical examination shows BP 130/87 mmHg; heart rate 70 beats/minute; lungs clear to auscultation and percussion; respirations 12 breaths/minute; and skin without rash or urticaria. Her condition is attributed to angioedema induced by enalapril. What is angioedema, and what evidence supports this diagnosis? What is the mechanism behind angioedema?

Angioneurotic edema (angioedema) manifests as local erythematous edema, which frequently involves the tongue, lips, eyelids, and mucous membranes of the mouth, nose, and throat. Drugs can cause this anaphylactoid reaction. For example, ACE inhibitors have been associated with this adverse effect in about 0.1% to 0.2% of individuals treated with this drug. It is not dose related and occurs with all ACE inhibitors. K.J. presents with classic symptoms of angioedema and does not have symptoms of a true anaphylactic reaction, further strengthening the diagnosis of drug-induced angioedema. Symptoms of angioedema usually occur within the first week of starting therapy, although they can occur at any time. Thus, although angioedema developed 3 weeks after K.J. began enalapril, the temporal relationship is reasonable.

The precise mechanism of angioedema remains unclear. Studies suggest, however, that increased concentrations of bradykinin, elevated levels of complement 1-esterase inactivator (an enzyme that inhibits complement activation), histamine-mediated reactions, and deficiencies in carboxypeptidase N, α_1-antitrypsin, and complement C4 may be involved.[92,100,101] (See Chapter 18: Heart Failure.)

24. How should K.J. be treated? Would an angiotensin receptor blocker (ARB) be an appropriate substitute for her ACE inhibitor?

Although angioedema can be life-threatening, symptoms are usually mild and resolve within hours to days of stopping the offending drug. More severe reactions can progress to laryngospasm, laryngeal swelling, and airway obstruction and must be treated emergently with appropriate measures to maintain airway patency. Antihistamines and corticosteroids are commonly prescribed, but the validity of this treatment needs substantiation. K.J. does not need to be hospitalized because her respirations are not compromised and she is not experiencing swallowing difficulty; however, she should be kept under observation at the urgent care center to ensure that her angioedema does not worsen. After this is established, she can be sent home with a prescription for diphenhydramine 25 mg orally every 6 hours for 24 hours, with instructions to seek emergent help if her breathing or swallowing becomes difficult. She should be instructed to discontinue her enalapril, follow up with her primary physician as soon as possible, and to request her community pharmacist to record this adverse reaction to enalapril into her drug profile at the pharmacy. Because angioedema occurs with all ACE inhibitors, K.J. must avoid all drugs in this class.

Angioedema with ARB also has been reported,[102–109] although with less frequency than with ACE inhibitors. Many of the cases of ARB-induced angioedema involved patients with a history of ACE inhibitor-induced angioedema, but this is not consistently the case. Similar to the ACE inhibitors, angioedema to ARB can occur at any time during treatment. In K.J.'s case, it would be best to avoid ARB and ACE inhibitors. Instead, other antihypertensive agents that have little effect on cholesterol (e.g., calcium channel blockers) should be used.

25. Are there other pseudoallergic reactions that occur with ACE inhibitors and ARB?

Besides angioedema, cough is a pseudoallergic reaction caused by ACE inhibitors. It may occur in up to 39% of patients after 1 week to 6 months of therapy. Interestingly, it is more common in nonsmokers than in smokers; the incidence does not increase in patients with chronic airway disease or asthma. Cough is more common in women than men, is not dose related, and, as with angioedema, occurs with all ACE inhibitors.[92,100,101,110] Several mechanisms appear to be responsible, including inhibition of the breakdown of bradykinin in the lung and increases in local mediators of inflammation such as prostaglandins and substance P. Although many approaches to the management of ACE-induced cough have been proposed,[101] angiotensin II-receptor blocking agents are the most promising alternative. Cough can occur with ARB, but the frequency appears to be no more than that of placebo. Furthermore, most direct comparative trials between ARB and ACE inhibitors demonstrate that the frequency of cough with ARB is much lower than with ACE inhibitors.[101]

Radiocontrast Media

Radiocontrast media are widely used diagnostic agents, exceeding 10 million administrations annually.[92] Adverse reactions to radiocontrast media include nausea, flushing, BP changes, bronchospasm, urticaria, angioedema, cardiac arrhythmias, convulsions, angina, and symptoms indistinguishable from true anaphylaxis. The cause of radiocontrast media reactions remains unknown, although histamine release, complement activation, and direct toxic effects on end organs might all play a role. These adverse effects are classified as pseudoallergic reactions because evidence does not support IgE mediation of these reactions. The overall incidence of reaction to radiocontrast media is 0.7%–13%, depending on the type of agent selected and whether the patient was pretreated before administration.[111] Conventional, ionic, high-osmolality contrast media produce reactions in 4%–13% of recipients, whereas nonionic, low-osmolality agents produce fewer reactions (0.7%–3.1%). Estimates of the mortality rate associated with the administration of contrast media varies widely from 1:15,000–1:117,000.[92,111]

Patients with a history of a pseudoallergic reaction to contrast media are at increased risk for future reactions with repeat exposure. Several pretreatment regimens have been developed to minimize such occurrences. For example, 32 mg of oral methylprednisolone given 12 and 2 hours before a procedure involving a high-osmolality contrast medium can reduce the reaction rate by up to 45% in some patients.[111] Another pretreatment regimen uses oral prednisone 50 mg taken 13 hours, 7 hours, and 1 hour before the procedure, plus diphenhydramine 50 mg orally or intramuscularly 1 hour before the examination.[112] This latter regimen lowers the occurrence of pseudoallergic reactions to high-osmolality contrast media, even in high-risk patients (i.e., those with a history of severe anaphylactoid reactions).

Narcotic Analgesics

Some opiates stimulate histamine release and, thereby, cause hypotension, tachycardia, facial flushing, increased sweating, or pruritus. Severe reactions are uncommon, however. In many cases, the opiate can be continued with administration of an antihistamine to treat the symptoms. If the reaction is significant, a non-narcotic alternate analgesic may be considered, or an opiate that does not cause histamine release can be substituted. Morphine and meperidine cause the greatest histamine release in both *in vitro* and *in vivo* studies. Codeine, hydromorphone, oxycodone, and butorphanol stimulate histamine release less commonly; and levorphanol, fentanyl, sufentanil, methadone, and oxymorphone have little to no effect on histamine levels. One of the more frequent reactions to epidurally or intrathecally administered opiates is pruritus, which does not appear to be mediated by histamine because narcotics that do not release histamine (e.g., fentanyl, sufentanil) still cause pruritus after spinal administration. Furthermore, the pruritus tends to develop several hours after the opiate has been administered, when serum levels of histamine are insignificant. The cause of pruritus from spinal opiates remains unclear. The reaction can be managed with antihistamines and low-dose naloxone or nalbuphine, while continuing with the spinal narcotic.[90]

Protamine

Protamine sulfate, a low-molecular weight protein that is a component of some insulin preparations, is used extensively to neutralize heparin during cardiac procedures. In one study, 11% of patients receiving protamine during cardiac surgery experienced an adverse reaction (e.g., angioedema, wheezing, erythema, urticaria). Severe hypotension and shock leading to death have also been reported. The mechanism of these severe reactions is unknown, but might be pseudoallergic and IgE mediated.[9,92]

Iron-Dextran Injection

Iron-dextran injection is a solution of ferric hydroxide (InFeD) or ferric oxyhydroxide (Dexferrum) complexed with low-molecular weight dextran. Iron dextran is used in the treatment of iron deficiency when oral iron preparations cannot be used or are ineffective. This is most commonly seen in patients with anemia of chronic renal failure, particularly those treated with epoetin alfa or darbepoetin and undergoing hemodialysis (Chapter 31: Chronic Kidney Disease). Iron-dextran injection is associated with a wide spectrum of adverse events (e.g., chest pain, hypotension, hypertension, abdominal pain, nausea, vomiting, weakness, syncope, backache, arthralgias, myalgias, hypersensitivity reactions). Hypersensitivity reactions can be manifested as urticaria, sweating, dyspnea, rash, fever, and as anaphylactoid reactions, which can be fatal. Consistent with a nonimmunologic mechanism, hypersensitivity reactions to iron dextran are not dose related and can occur with the first drug exposure.[113] Serious life-threatening anaphylactoid reactions occur in 0.6% to 0.7% of patients treated with iron dextran; serious reactions that prevent further administration occur in 2.47% of recipients.[114] Although the cause of the hypersensitivity reactions from iron dextran is unclear, it is attributed to the dextran component. Anaphylaxis from dextran, when used as a volume expander, has been reported.[114] A test dose of iron dextran should be administered to assess tolerance, before administration of the full dose. Nevertheless, hypersensitivity reactions have been reported despite successful tolerance to a test dose, rendering this practice unreliable.

Two nondextran parenteral iron products are available in the United States: sodium ferric gluconate (Ferrlecit) and iron sucrose, also known as iron saccharate (Venofer). Both agents have a better safety profile than iron dextran. Baile et al.[115] reviewed abstracted reports of adverse reactions made to the U.S. Food and Drug Administration (FDA) between 1997 and 2002 to compare adverse event reporting rates between all parenteral iron products. These researchers categorized reactions according to the standard adverse event dictionary used by FDA. Because of differences between dosing of the products, results were reported per 100-mg dose equivalents (DE). The researchers found the reporting rate for all adverse reactions was 29.2, 10.5, and 4.2 reports per million 100 mg DE for iron dextran, sodium ferric gluconate, and iron sucrose, respectively. The reporting rate for anaphylactoid reactions was 0.87, 0.46, and 0.0 per million 100 mg DE, respectively. There were 0.6 reports of anaphylaxis per million 100 mg DE of iron dextran; no reports exist of anaphylaxis for sodium ferric gluconate or iron sucrose.[115] Another study used data reported to the FDA MedWatch program between 2001 and 2003 to determine the odds of adverse events between all four parenteral iron products. Relative to the InFeD brand of iron dextran, patients receiving sodium ferric gluconate or iron sucrose were half as likely to experience an allergic reaction or any adverse drug event (ADE). An equal risk existed of experiencing an allergic reaction, or any ADE, between sodium ferric gluconate and iron sucrose. Odds ratios between the Dexferrum brand of iron dextran and sodium ferric gluconate or iron sucrose were not reported. Although sodium ferric gluconate and iron sucrose were safer than iron dextran, at least one death and five life-threatening ADE were reported with each of the four agents studied, underscoring that risks are associated with any parenteral iron product.[116]

Both sodium ferric gluconate and iron sucrose cause fewer hypersensitivity reactions, including anaphylactoid reactions, and appear to be safer than iron dextran. The decision to give patients who are to receive parenteral iron preparation a test dose will depend on the product used. All patients receiving iron dextran should receive a test dose to assess tolerance. Neither sodium ferric gluconate nor iron sucrose requires a test dose per their prescribing information. It appears iron dextran-tolerant patients have little risk of experiencing a serious hypersensitivity or anaphylactoid reaction to sodium ferric gluconate or iron sucrose injection and can safely be given one of these products without a prior test dose. Similarly, patients who have never received any parenteral iron product can be administered sodium ferric gluconate or iron sucrose for injection without a prior test dose. Although studies support the safety of both sodium ferric gluconate and iron sucrose for injection in iron dextran-sensitive patients, such patients may be at increased risk for an anaphylactoid reaction or other serious hypersensitivity response, and test dosing in this population may be reasonable. Regardless of whether a test dose is administered for any of the parenteral iron products, close monitoring of the patient following drug administration is necessary and the availability of resuscitative medication and personnel trained to evaluate and address anaphylaxis is prudent.

LATEX ALLERGY

Natural latex is a milky fluid consisting of extremely small particles of rubber obtained from the rubber tree. Natural rubber includes all products made from, or containing, natural latex.[117] Many products commonly used in health care (e.g., gloves, BP cuffs, catheters, injection ports, rubber stoppers of medication vials) are made wholly or in part of latex. Over the past several years, the significance of latex allergy has become clear as cases of allergic reactions, some life-threatening, have been reported.[117] Health professionals must recognize the types of reactions latex can cause and must know how to minimize patient exposure to latex. Also, preparing parenteral drugs for latex-allergic patients can be difficult because of the number of materials involved that may contain latex.

Health professionals are at significant risk for developing latex allergy because of their frequent exposure to latex products. Other groups at risk for developing latex allergy are workers in businesses that manufacture latex products, patients with spina bifida; and people with allergies to avocado, potato, banana, tomato, chestnuts, kiwi fruit, and papaya.[117]

Three types of reactions to latex have been described: irritant contact dermatitis, allergic contact dermatitis (chemical sensitivity dermatitis), and immediate hypersensitivity.[117,118]

Irritant contact dermatitis is the most common reaction to latex and manifests as dry, itchy, irritated areas of the skin. This is not a true allergic reaction to latex.[117]

Allergic contact dermatitis is a delayed hypersensitivity reaction caused by exposure to chemicals added during the processing and manufacturing of latex. A rash, similar to that seen with poison ivy, usually begins 24 to 48 hours after exposure and may progress to oozing blisters.[117]

Immediate hypersensitivity to proteins in the latex is an IgE-mediated allergic response. The reaction can begin within minutes of exposure to latex or occur hours later. Symptoms vary from mild skin redness, hives, and itching to respiratory involvement (runny nose, sneezing, itchy eyes, trouble breathing, asthma). Rare cases of anaphylactic shock have been described.[117] Reports of the prevalence of latex allergy vary from 1% to 6% of the general population and 8% to 12% of health care workers. Latex allergy is diagnosed by obtaining an accurate description of the reaction and establishing a temporal relationship to latex exposure. Diagnostic kits are available to detect latex antibodies as well as to aid in the diagnosis of allergic contact dermatitis.[117,118]

Health care practitioners, particularly those in settings in which IV or intramuscular medications are administered, may be faced with preparing parenteral products for a latex-allergic patient. This often poses a challenge because latex is in many of the materials used to prepare parenteral products (e.g., rubber stoppers on medication vials, injection ports on IV bags, rubber plungers for syringes, IV transfer sets).[117,118] Many manufacturers are now preparing products in a latex-free form, which simplifies drug preparation. Furthermore, manufacturers of medical devices are now required to identify on their labels which products have natural latex and which have dry natural rubber.[119] Many institutions have instituted policies on the preparation of parenteral products for the "latex-sensitive" person. Readers are referred to these references for the details of these procedures.[118,120–123]

PREVENTION AND MANAGEMENT OF ALLERGIC REACTIONS

26. A.M., a 40-year-old woman, is hospitalized with a diagnosis of community-acquired pneumonia. Her medical history is noncontributory except for an uneventful course of ampicillin 6 months before admission for an ear infection. A.M. is empirically treated with cefuroxime 0.75 g IV every 8 hours. On day 2 of therapy, she develops a raised pruritic maculopapular rash on her back, abdomen, and upper extremities. Antacid, docusate sodium, albuterol by metered-dose inhaler, and multivitamins were initiated on the same day as the cefuroxime. How should A.M.'s allergic reaction be managed? How might her allergic reaction have been prevented?

When examining methods to prevent allergic reactions, three possibilities exist: (a) the patient has unknowingly been sensitized to a drug and experiences an allergic reaction on receiving the same or a similar drug again; (b) the patient has a history of an allergic reaction to a medication and mistakenly receives the same or a similar medication a second time and again develops an allergic reaction; and (c) the patient has a history of an allergic reaction to a medication and intentionally receives the same or similar medication again. As in the first situation, A.M.'s allergic reaction was unpredictable and, therefore, could not be prevented. To prevent future allergic reactions (i.e., the second situation), however, A.M.'s reaction should be well documented in the medical chart and pharmacy records. In addition, all patients should undergo a thorough drug history on hospitalization. Careful attention should be paid to differentiating drug intolerance (e.g., stomach upset) from true allergic reactions, and any allergic reactions elicited during an interview should be documented appropriately. Adequate communication of allergic reactions is the single most important method of preventing their occurrence.

As described earlier, the first step in managing an allergic reaction is to determine its cause. Given A.M.'s history of exposure to ampicillin, the timing of the reaction, and the low frequency of allergic reactions to her other medications, cefuroxime are the most likely candidates. Second, a decision regarding whether to stop the suspect drug should be made. This decision must be based on the severity of the reaction, the condition being treated, and the availability of suitable alternatives. When possible, an equally effective alternative drug should be substituted for the suspect agent, preferably one that is immunologically distinct to avoid cross-sensitivity (see Question 4 for a discussion of cross-reactivity).[124] If a suitable alternative exists, the offending agent should be stopped and the reaction treated symptomatically if necessary. In the case of A.M., another antimicrobial (e.g., azithromycin, clarithromycin, trimethoprim-sulfamethoxazole) could be substituted for cefuroxime (Chapter 60: Respiratory Tract Infections) and her symptoms treated with an oral or parenteral antihistamine, as well as a low-potency topical corticosteroid if necessary.

Some cases are described by the third situation: a patient develops an allergic reaction (or has a well-documented history of drug allergy), and it is inappropriate or not possible to change to an alternative drug. If the sensitivity reaction is severe or life-threatening, desensitization should be considered (Questions 27 to 30); premedication to prevent or minimize anaphylaxis is not effective.[3] If the reaction is minor (e.g., pruritus, rash, or GI symptoms), premedication or management of the reaction with antiallergy medications (e.g., antihistamines) might be sufficient to allow completion of therapy. It is rare in such cases for the reaction to progress to more serious allergic symptoms such as anaphylaxis;[124] however, suppression of allergic symptoms should be undertaken cautiously because many immunologic reactions are not IgE mediated and may progress to serious reactions, despite treatment. In general, allergy suppression should be reserved for prevention of mild reactions that are known or strongly suspected to be IgE mediated.[3,124]

Desensitization

β-Lactams

27. K.A. is a 24-year-old primigravida in her eighth week of pregnancy with a history of angioedema secondary to penicillin. Her initial pregnancy screening revealed a positive Venereal Disease Research Laboratory (VDRL) reaction and a fluorescent treponemal antibody absorption (FTA-Abs) titer of 1:64. K.A. denies a history of genital lesions, currently does not exhibit clinical signs or symptoms of syphilis, and denies previous treatment for syphilis. Based on the serologic evidence and her history, a diagnosis of early latent syphilis is made. Current treatment guidelines indicate that penicillin is the drug of choice for K.A. How can a possible reaction to penicillin be prevented in K.A.? Is premedication an alternative to preventing a reaction?

Acute desensitization (or hyposensitization) is the process of administering gradually increasing doses of a drug over hours or days in an effort to develop clinical tolerance.[1,3,6,34,124] This process has been used successfully to reintroduce drugs to patients with known allergic reactions in situations in which no alternatives exist. It is most commonly used in patients with IgE-mediated hypersensitivity and is well described for penicillin-allergic patients. Desensitization, however, is not useful in preventing late penicillin reactions and should not be attempted in patients who have experienced severe dermatologic reactions such as exfoliative dermatitis.[34] Because K.A.'s reaction to penicillin may be potentially severe, premedication is not an option and desensitization to penicillin should be started. (See Chapter 65: Sexually Transmitted Diseases, for alternative therapy.)

28. How should K.A. be desensitized? Why should she be skin tested before desensitization?

If possible before desensitization is begun, K.A. should be skin tested (see Questions 3 and 4) to confirm her penicillin allergy.[3,34,124] Patients who have a positive history of penicillin allergy, but whose skin tests are negative, can receive full therapeutic doses without desensitization with little risk of developing an allergic reaction. One author, for example, reported only one case of acute anaphylaxis in a skin test-negative patient given full therapeutic doses of penicillin in >1,500 skin tests; similar results have been reported by other investigators.[34,124] If skin testing cannot be performed or if K.A.'s skin test is positive, desensitization should be initiated. Acute oral desensitization to penicillin and other β-lactam antibiotics is well established; one such protocol is outlined in Table 4-14, although others have been used successfully.[125–128]

Table 4-14 β-Lactam Oral Desensitization Protocol

Stock Drug Concentration (mg/mL)[a]	Dose No.	Amount (mL)	Drug Dose (mg)	Cumulative Drug (mg)
0.5	1[b]	0.05	0.025	0.025
0.5	2	0.10	0.05	0.075
0.5	3	0.20	0.10	0.175
0.5	4	0.40	0.20	0.375
0.5	5	0.80	0.40	0.775
5.0	6	0.15	0.75	1.525
5.0	7	0.30	1.50	3.025
5.0	8	0.60	3.00	6.025
5.0	9	1.20	6.00	12.025
5.0	10	2.40	12.00	24.025
50	11	0.50	25.00	49.025
50	12	1.20	60.00	109.025
50	13	2.50	125.00	234.025
50	14	5.00	250.00	484.025

[a]Dilutions using 250 mg/5 mL of pediatric suspension.
[b]Oral dose doubled approximately every 15 to 30 min..
Adapted from references 125 and 127, with permission.
Dosing for the oral protocol is arbitrary and should be adjusted for individual patients based on the clinical sensitivity and the desired drug dose end point.

The oral route for β-lactam desensitization is preferred to the parenteral route because (a) exposure by the oral route is less likely to cause a systemic allergic reaction than parenteral exposure; (b) fatal anaphylaxis from oral β-lactam drug therapy is rare; (c) preformed polymers and conjugates of penicillin major and minor determinants to penicillium proteins are not well absorbed after oral administration; (d) blood levels rise gradually, favoring univalent haptenation (appearance of multivalent hapten–carrier conjugates, on the other hand, is gradual); and (e) fatal or life-endangering reactions have not occurred using current methods. In addition, oral desensitization can be accomplished over several hours.[3] If oral desensitization is not possible (e.g., if oral absorption is questionable), parenteral desensitization can be instituted. Although the subcutaneous and intramuscular routes have been used, the IV route is quicker and allows better control over the rate and concentration of drug administered, and any untoward reaction can be detected promptly and treated rapidly.[3,6,9] Table 4-15 outlines an IV β-lactam desensitization protocol. Oral and parenteral desensitization methods have not been compared formally, however. Patients should not be premedicated before desensitization, because this may prevent detection of minor allergic responses that may precede more serious reactions. In addition, desensitization should be performed in a setting where emergency resuscitative equipment and personnel are readily available.[124] Thus, K.A. should undergo oral desensitization as outlined in Table 4-14 if her skin test is positive or if skin testing cannot be performed.

29. Is K.A. at risk for an allergic reaction during desensitization? If desensitization is successful, is she at risk for a reaction during full-dose penicillin therapy?

Acute β-lactam desensitization, regardless of the route or protocol chosen, is not without risk. Approximately 5% of patients experience mild cutaneous reactions during desensitization, although one study reported reactions in 20% of patients during oral desensitization.[3,128] If a reaction occurs during the desensitization procedure itself, the reaction may be treated and desensitization continued using lower doses, increased intervals between doses, or both, after the reaction has abated. Severe, fatal reactions during desensitization are rare.[3]

Uneventful β-lactam desensitization, however, does not guarantee patients will be without reaction during full-dose therapy. Approximately 25% to 30% of patients experience a mild reaction during therapy, whereas 5% experience

Table 4-15 β-Lactam Intravenous Desensitization Protocol

Stock Drug Concentration (mg/mL)[a]	Dose No.[b]	Amount per 50 mL (mg/mL)[c]	Cumulative Drug (mg)
0.005	1	0.0001	0.005
0.025	2	0.0005	0.030
0.125	3	0.0025	0.155
0.625	4	0.0125	0.780
3.125	5	0.0625	3.905
15.625	6	0.3125	19.530
31.25	7	0.625	50.780
62.50	8	1.25	113.280
125.00	9	2.5	238.280
250.00	10[d]	5.0	488.280

[a]Stock drug solutions are prepared using serial dilutions of the desired goal (e.g., 500 mg of β-lactam). Doses one through five represent fivefold dilutions; doses six through ten represent twofold dilutions.

[b]Interval between doses is 1 to 30 minutes. If desensitization is interrupted for >2 half-lives of the β-lactam, desensitization should be repeated.

[c]Mix 1 mL of stock drug solution in 50 mL 5% dextrose/0.225 normal saline or other compatible solution. Infuse each dose over 20–45 minutes. Dilution volume may vary with patient age and weight.

[d]If all 10 doses are administered and tolerated, the remainder of a full therapeutic dose of the β-lactam should be administered.

Adapted from reference 269, with permission.

Dosing for the IV protocol is arbitrary and should be adjusted for individual patients based on the clinical sensitivity and the desired drug dose end point.

Table 4-16 Oral Trimethoprim-Sulfamethoxazole Desensitization Protocol

Hour	Trimethoprim Component (Concentration or Tablet)	Volume	Dose of TMP-SMZ
0	0.0008 mg/mL	5 mL	0.004/0.02 mg
1	0.008 mg/mL	5 mL	0.04/0.2 mg
2	0.08 mg/mL	5 mL	0.4/2 mg
3	0.8 mg/mL	5 mL	4/20 mg
4	8 mg/mL	5 mL	40/200 mg
5	160 mg	1 tablet	160/800 mg

Stock solution of trimethoprim-sulfamethoxazole (TMP-SMZ) may be prepared by appropriate dilutions of the commercially available suspension (8 mg trimethoprim/40 mg sulfamethoxazole per mL) with simple syrup or distilled water.

Adapted reference 151, with permission.

This protocol should serve as a guide only. Obtaining informed consent from the patient before initiating desensitization is advisable.

more severe reactions, including drug-induced serum sickness, hemolytic anemia, or nephritis.[3] Reaction rates are no different in severely ill or pregnant patients compared with stable or nonpregnant patients, although those with cystic fibrosis may be more difficult to desensitize because of their high frequency of allergic reactions.[3,128,129] Despite the occurrence of reactions, full-dose therapy is possible for most desensitizations, but suppression of the reaction (e.g., by diphenhydramine) may be required.[3]

30. If K.A. requires penicillin at a later date, will she need to undergo desensitization again? What is chronic desensitization?

The desensitized state, once achieved, will persist for approximately 48 hours after the last full dose of antibiotic; after this time, drug sensitivity will return.[3] Thus, if K.A. requires future courses of penicillin, she will need to undergo desensitization once again. In some cases, those requiring long-term antibiotic therapy (e.g., for endocarditis), those who may require β-lactams at a future date (e.g., those with cystic fibrosis), or those who have occupational exposure to β-lactams, maintenance of the desensitized state can be considered. Chronic twice-daily dosing of oral penicillin has safely resulted in "chronic desensitization." Similar to acute desensitization, once therapy is interrupted, the allergic state returns.[3,9]

Other Drugs

31. Have patients allergic to drugs besides β-lactams been desensitized successfully?

Although most experience with desensitization is with penicillin and other β-lactams, desensitization also has been accomplished with various other drugs, including rifampin,[130] isoniazid,[130] acyclovir,[131] sulfasalazine,[132–135] aminoglycosides,[129] vancomycin,[136,137] and several others.[138–150] Interestingly, not all of these cases represent IgE-mediated hypersensitivity reactions. Acute desensitization, which has until recently been used to manage only IgE-mediated reactions, appears to be effective in other forms of immunopathology.[3] For example, reactions to trimethoprim-sulfamethoxazole commonly occur in patients infected with HIV and may not be IgE mediated. Yet, successful desensitization to trimethoprim-sulfamethoxazole is increasingly common, given its role in treating and preventing *Pneumocystis jiroveci* pneumonia.[3]

One procedure for trimethoprim-sulfamethoxazole desensitization[151] is outlined in Table 4-16, although several other protocols have been used successfully.[9,152–157] Although mild to moderate reactions can occur (e.g., fever, mild skin rash), patients may complete desensitization successfully by suppressing the reaction with antihistamines, reducing the dose to the highest level previously taken without a reaction until the reaction subsides, or both.[152,154,155] As with the β-lactams, before desensitization for any medication is undertaken, alternative therapies should be sought and used if possible. Furthermore, desensitization is contraindicated if the reaction is a serious dermatologic response, such as toxic epidermal necrolysis or Stevens-Johnson syndrome. Last, desensitization should be undertaken only in an appropriate setting by experienced personnel, because severe reactions can develop.[158]

REFERENCES

1. DeSwarte RD. Drug allergy: problems and strategies. *J Allergy Clin Immunol* 1984;74(Pt 1):209.
2. Assem E-SK. Drug allergy and tests for its detection. In: Davies DM, ed. *Textbook of Adverse Drug Reactions.* 4th ed. New York: Oxford University Press; 1991:689.
3. Sullivan TJ. Drug allergy. In: Middleton E Jr et al., eds. *Allergy. Principles and Practices.* 4th ed. St. Louis: Mosby; 1993:1726.
4. Jick H. Adverse drug reactions: the magnitude of the problem. *J Allergy Clin Immunol* 1984;74:555.
5. Classen DC et al. Computerized surveillance of adverse drug events in hospital patients. *JAMA* 1991;266:2847.
6. Van Arsdel PP Jr. Drug hypersensitivity. In: Bierman CW et al. eds. *Allergic Diseases from Infancy to Adulthood.* 2nd ed. Philadelphia: WB Saunders; 1988:684.

7. Van Arsdel PP Jr. Classification and risk factors for drug allergy. *Immunol Allergy Clin North Am* 1991;11:475.
8. Adkinson NF Jr. Risk factors for drug allergy. *J Allergy Clin Immunol* 1984;74:567.
9. Anderson JA. Allergic reactions to drugs and biological agents. *JAMA* 1992;268:2845.
10. Bigby M et al. Drug-induced cutaneous reactions. *JAMA* 1986;256:3358.
11. Gomes ER et al. Epidemiology of hypersensitivity drug reactions. *Curr Opin Allergy Clin Immunol* 2005;3:309.
12. Parker CW. Drug allergy. *N Engl J Med* 1975; 292(Pt 1-3):511.
13. Johnson-Reagan L et al. Severe drug rashes in 3 siblings simultaneously. *Allergy* 2003;58:445.
14. Pirmohamed M. Genetic factors in the predisposition to drug-induced hypersensitivity reactions. *AAPS J* 2006;8:E20.
15. Morimoto T et al. An evaluation of risk factors for adverse drug events associated with angiotensin-converting enzyme inhibitors. *J Eval Clin Pract* 2004;10:499.
16. Ma MK et al. Genetic basis of drug metabolism. *Am J Health Syst Pharm* 2002;59:2061.
17. Breathnach SM. Mechanisms of drug eruptions: Part I. *Australas J Dermatol* 1995;36:121.
18. Svensson CK et al. Cutaneous drug reactions. *Pharmacol Rev* 2000;53:357.
19. Mallal S et al. Association between presence of HLA-B*5701, HLA-DR7, and HLA-DQ3 and hypersensitivity to HIV-1 reverse-transcriptase inhibitor abacavir. *Lancet* 2002;359:722.
20. Evans WE et al. Pharmacogenomics: drug disposition, drug targets, and side effects. *N Engl J Med* 2003;348:538.
21. Hung SI et al. HLA-B*5801 allele as a genetic marker for severe cutaneous adverse reactions caused by allopurinol. *Proc Natl Acad Sci U S A* 2005;102:4134.
22. Lucas A et al. HLA-B*5701 screening for susceptibility to abacavir hypersensitivity. *J Antimicrob Chemother* 2007;59:591.
23. Tas S et al. Herpesviruses in patients with drug hypersensitivity syndrome: culprits, cofactors, or innocent bystanders? *Dermatology* 2006;213: 273.
24. Tas S et al. Management of drug rash with eosinophila and systemic symptoms (DRESS syndrome); an update. *Dermatology* 2003;206:353.
25. de Weck AL. Pharmacological and immunochemical mechanisms of drug hypersensitivity. *Immunol Allergy Clin North Am* 1991;11:461.
26. Gerber BO et al. Cellular mechanisms of T cell mediated drug hypersensitivity. *Curr Opin Immunol* 2004;16:732.
27. Seguin B et al. The danger hypothesis applied to idiosyncratic drug reactions. *Curr Opin Allergy Clin Immunol* 2003;3:235.
28. Pichler WJ et al. Pharmacological interaction of drugs with immune receptors: the p-i concept. *Allergology International* 2006;55:17.
29. Matzinger P. The danger model: a renewed sense of self. *Science* 2002;296:301.
30. Bochner BS et al. Anaphylaxis. *N Engl J Med* 1991; 324:1785.
31. Yunginger JW. Anaphylaxis. *Ann Allergy* 1992;69: 87.
32. Marquardt DL et al. Anaphylaxis. In: Middleton E Jr et al., eds. *Allergy. Principles and Practices.* 4th ed. St. Louis: Mosby; 1993:1365.
33. Shepherd GM. Allergy to β-lactam antibiotics. *Immunol Allergy Clin North Am* 1991;11:611.
34. Lin RY. A perspective on penicillin allergy. *Arch Intern Med* 1992;152:930.
35. Gruchalla RS et al. In vivo and in vitro diagnosis of drug allergy. *Immunol Allergy Clin North Am* 1991;11:595.
36. Meth MJ et al. Phenotypic diversity in delayed hypersensitivity: an immunologic explanation. *Mt Sinai J Med* 2006;73:769.
37. Weiss ME. Drug allergy. *Med Clin North Am* 1992;76:857.
38. Pre-Pen Update. Available at http://www.allerquest.com/availability.html. Accessed March 20, 2008.
39. Perencevich EN et al. Benefits of negative penicillin test results persist during subsequent hospital admissions. *Clin Infect Dis* 2001;32:317.
40. Romano A et al. Immediate hypersensitivity to cephalosporins. *Allergy* 2002;57(Suppl 72):52.
41. Romano A et al. Immediate allergic reactions to cephalosporins: cross-reactivity and selective responses. *J Allergy Clin Immunol* 2000;106: 1177.
42. Robinson JL et al. Practical aspects of choosing an antibiotic for patients with a reported allergy to an antibiotic. *Clin Infect Dis* 2002;35:261.
43. Blanca M et al. Side-chain-specific reactions to beta-lactams: 14 years later. *Clin Exp Allergy* 2002;32:192.
44. Fath JJ et al. The therapy of anaphylactic shock. *Drug Intell Clin Pharm* 1984;18:14.
45. Atkinson TP et al. Anaphylaxis. *Med Clin North Am* 1992;76:841.
46. Delage C et al. Anaphylactic deaths: a clinicopathologic study of 43 cases. *J Forensic Sci* 1972;17: 525.
47. Lieberman P. Use of epinephrine in the treatment of anaphylaxis. *Curr Opin Allergy Clin Immunol* 2003;3:313.
48. Joint Task Force on Practice Parameters. The diagnosis and management of anaphylaxis: an updated practice parameter. *J Allergy Clin Immunol* 2005;115(3 Supple 2):S483.
49. Brown SGA. Cardiovascular aspects of anaphylaxis: implications for treatment and diagnosis. *Curr Opin Allergy Clin Immunol* 2005;5:359.
50. Pumphrey RS. Fatal posture in anaphylactic shock. *J Allergy Clin Immunol* 2003;112:451.
51. Buhner D et al. Serum sickness. *Dermatol Clin* 1985;3:107.
52. Lawley TJ et al. A study of human serum sickness. *J Invest Dermatol* 1985;85(Suppl):129S.
53. Erffmeyer JE. Serum sickness. *Ann Allergy* 1986;56:105.
54. Lin RY. Serum sickness syndrome. *Am Fam Physician* 1986;33:157.
55. Johnson DH et al. Drug fever. *Infect Dis Clin North Am* 1996;10:85.
56. Tabor PA. Drug-induced fever. *Drug Intell Clin Pharm* 1986;20:413.
57. Mackowiak PA et al. Drug fever: a critical appraisal of conventional concepts. *Ann Intern Med* 1987;106:728.
58. Young EJ et al. Drug-induced fever: cases seen in the evaluation of unexplained fever in a general hospital population. *Rev Infect Dis* 1982;4:69.
59. Lossos IS et al. Hydroxyurea-induced fever: case report and review of the literature. *Ann Pharmacother* 1995;29:132.
60. Cunha BA. Drug fever. *Postgrad Med* 1986;80:123.
61. Hofland SL. Drug fever: is your patient's fever drug-related? *Crit Care Nurse* 1985;5:29.
62. Hiraide A et al. IgE-mediated drug fever due to histamine H_2-receptor blockers. *Drug Safe* 1990;5:455.
63. Cunha BA et al. Fever in the intensive care unit. *Infect Dis Clin North Am* 1996;10:185.
64. Fischer SA et al. Fever in the solid organ transplant patient. *Infect Dis Clin North Am* 1996;10:167.
65. Lipsky BA et al. Drug fever. *JAMA* 1981;245:851.
66. Kumar KL et al. Drug fever. *West J Med* 1986;144: 753.
67. Singhal PC et al. Hypersensitivity angiitis associated with naproxen. *Ann Allergy* 1989;63:107.
68. Calabrese LH. Differential diagnosis of hypersensitivity vasculitis. *Cleve Clin J Med* 1990;57:506.
69. Semble EL et al. Vasculitis: a practical approach to management. *Postgrad Med* 1991;90:161.
70. Carlson JA et al. Cutaneous vasculitis update: small vessel neutrophilic vasculitis syndromes. *Am J Dermatopathol* 2006;28:486.
71. Carlson JA et al. Cutaneous vasculitis update: diagnostic criteria, classification, epidemiology, etiology, pathogenesis, evaluation, and prognosis. *Am J Dermatopathol* 2005;27:504.
72. ten Holder SM et al. Cutaneous and systemic manifestations of drug-induced vasculitis. *Ann Pharmacother* 2002;36:130.
73. Drory VE et al. Hypersensitivity vasculitis and systemic lupus erythematosus induced by anticonvulsants. *Clin Neuropharmacol* 1993;16:19.
74. Gilliland BC. Drug-induced autoimmune and hematologic disorders. *Drug Allergy* 1991;11: 525.
75. Wandl UB et al. Lupus-like autoimmune disease induced by interferon therapy for myeloproliferative disorders. *Clin Immunol Immunopathol* 1992;65:70.
76. Skaer TL. Medication-induced systemic lupus erythematosus. *Clin Ther* 1992;14:496.
77. Vyse T et al. Sulphasalazine-induced autoimmune syndrome. *Br J Rheumatol* 1992;31:115.
78. Perry HJ et al. Relationship of acetyltransferase activity to antinuclear antibodies and toxic symptoms in hypertensive patients treated with hydralazine. *J Lab Clin Med* 1970;76:114.
79. Tan EM et al. The 1982 revised criteria for the classification of systemic lupus erythematosus. *Arthritis Rheum* 1982;25:1271.
80. Woosley RL et al. Effect of acetylator phenotype on the rate at which procainamide induces antinuclear antibodies and the lupus syndrome. *N Engl J Med* 1978;298:1157.
81. Blomgren SE et al. Antinuclear antibody induced by procainamide. *N Engl J Med* 1969;281:64.
82. Henningsen NC et al. Effects of long-term treatment with procainamide. *Acta Med Scand* 1975; 198:475.
83. Kowsowsky BC et al. Long-term use of procainamide following acute myocardial infarction. *Circulation* 1973;47:1204.
84. Cameron HA et al. The lupus syndrome induced by hydralazine: a common complication with low-dose treatment. *BMJ* 1984;189:410.
85. Anderson JA et al. Allergic reactions to drugs and biologic agents. *JAMA* 1987;258:2891.
86. Blomgren SE et al. Procainamide-induced lupus erythematosus: clinical and laboratory observations. *Am J Med* 1972;52:338.
87. Solinger AM. Drug-related lupus. Clinical and etiologic considerations. *Rheum Dis Clin North Am* 1988;14:187.
88. Machold KP et al. Interferon-gamma induced exacerbation of systemic lupus erythematosus. *J Rheumatol* 1990;17:831.
89. Alarcon-Segovia D et al. Clinical and experimental studies on the hydralazine syndrome and its relation to SLE. *Medicine* 1967;46:1.
90. Van Arsdel PP Jr. Pseudoallergic drug reactions. Introduction and general review. *Immunol Allergy Clin North Am* 1991;11:635.
91. Burke P et al. Allergy associated with ciprofloxacin. *BMJ* 2000;320:679.
92. deShazo RD et al. Allergic reactions to drugs. *JAMA* 1997;278:1895.
93. Manning ME et al. Pseudoallergic drug reactions. Aspirin, nonsteroidal anti-inflammatory drugs, dyes, additives, and preservatives. *Immunol Allergy Clin North Am* 1991;11:659.
94. Stevenson DD et al. Sensitivity to aspirin and nonsteroidal anti-inflammatory drugs. In: Middleton E Jr et al., eds. *Allergy. Principles and Practices.* 4th ed. St. Louis: Mosby; 1993:1747.
95. Berkes EA. Anaphylactic and anaphylactoid reactions to aspirin and other NSAIDs. *Clin Rev Allergy Immunol* 2003;24:137.
96. Woessner KM et al. The safety of celecoxib in patients with aspirin-sensitive asthma. *Arthritis Rheum* 2002;46:2201.
97. Szczeklik A et al. Safety of a specific COX-2 inhibitor in aspirin-induced asthma. *Clin Exp Allergy* 2001;31:219.
98. Pacor ML et al. Safety of rofecoxib in subjects with a history of adverse cutaneous reactions to aspirin and/or non-steroidal anti-inflammatory drugs. *Clin Exp Allergy* 2002;32:397.
99. Quiralte J et al. Safety of selective cyclooxygenase-2 inhibitor rofecoxib in patients with NSAID-

induced cutaneous reactions. *Ann Allergy Asthma Immunol* 2002;89:63.
100. Israili ZH et al. Cough and angioneurotic edema associated with angiotensin-converting enzyme inhibitor therapy. A review of the literature and pathophysiology. *Ann Intern Med* 1992;117:234.
101. Pylypchuk GB. ACE-inhibitor-versus angiotensin II blocker-induced cough and angioedema. *Ann Pharmacother* 1998;32:1060.
102. Cha YJ et al. Angioedema due to losartan. *Ann Pharmacother* 1999;33:936.
103. Rivera JO. Losartan-induced angioedema. *Ann Pharmacother* 1999;33:933.
104. Rupprecht R et al. Angioedema due to losartan. *Allergy* 1999;4:81.
105. van Rijnsoever EW et al. Angioneurotic edema attributed to the use of losartan. *Arch Intern Med* 1998;158:2063.
106. Frye CB et al. Angioedema and photosensitive rash induced by valsartan. *Pharmacotherapy* 1998;18:866.
107. Sharma PK et al. Angioedema associated with angiotensin II receptor antagonist losartan. *South Med J* 1997;90:552.
108. Boxer M. Accupril- and Cozaar-induced angioedema in the same patient. *J Allergy Clin Immunol* 1996;98:471.
109. Acker CG et al. Angioedema induced by the angiotensin II blocker losartan. *N Engl J Med* 1995;333:1572.
110. Alderman CP. Adverse effects of the angiotensin-converting enzyme inhibitors. *Ann Pharmacother* 1996;30:55.
111. Lasser EC. Pseudoallergic drug reactions. Radiographic contrast media. *Immunol Allergy Clin North Am* 1991;11:645.
112. Greenberger PA et al. Two pretreatment regimens for high-risk patients receiving radiographic contrast media. *J Allergy Clin Immunol* 1984;74:540.
113. Fishbane S et al. The safety of intravenous iron dextran in hemodialysis patients. *Am J Kidney Dis* 1996;25:529.
114. Michael B et al. Sodium ferric gluconate complex in hemodialysis patients: adverse reactions compared to placebo and iron dextran. *Kidney Int* 2002;61:1830.
115. Baile GR et al. Hypersensitivity reactions and deaths associated with intravenous iron preparations. *Nephrol Dial Transplant* 2006;20:1443.
116. Chertow GM et al. Update on adverse drug events associated with parenteral iron. *Nephrol Dial Transplant* 2006;21:378.
117. DHHS (NIOSH) Publication No. 97-135: Preventing allergic reactions to natural rubber latex in the workplace. June 1997.
118. Senst BL et al. Latex allergy. *Am J Health Syst Pharm* 1997;54:1071.
119. Thompson CA. Medical devices with latex to become easier to identify. *Am J Health Syst Pharm* 1998;55:2059.
120. Kim KT et al. Implementation recommendations for making health care facilities latex safe. *AORN J* 1998;67:615.
121. Rice SP et al. Preparation of latex-safe sterile products. *Am J Health Syst Pharm* 1998;55:1466.
122. Au AL et al. Important points to note when preparing nutritional admixtures for latex-sensitive patients. *Am J Health Syst Pharm* 1997;54:2128.
123. McDermott JS et al. Procedures for preparing injectable medications for latex-sensitive patients. *Am J Health Syst Pharm* 1997;54:2516.
124. Wedner HJ. Drug allergy prevention and treatment. *Immunol Allergy Clin North Am* 1991;11:679.
125. Sullivan TJ et al. Desensitization of patients allergic to penicillin using orally administered β-lactam antibiotics. *J Allergy Clin Immunol* 1982;69:275.
126. Sullivan TJ. Antigen-specific desensitization of patients allergic to penicillin. *J Allergy Clin Immunol* 1982;69:500.
127. Wendel GD Jr et al. Penicillin allergy and desensitization in serious infections during pregnancy. *N Engl J Med* 1985;312:1229.
128. Stark BJ et al. Acute and chronic desensitization of penicillin-allergic patients using oral penicillin. *J Allergy Clin Immunol* 1987;79:523.
129. Earl HS, Sullivan TJ. Acute desensitization of a patient with cystic fibrosis allergic to both beta-lactam and aminoglycoside antibiotics. *J Allergy Clin Immunol* 1987;79:477.
130. Holland CL et al. Rapid oral desensitization to isoniazid and rifampin. *Chest* 1990;98:1518.
131. Henry RE et al. Successful oral acyclovir desensitization. *Ann Allergy* 1993;70:386.
132. Bax DE et al. Sulphasalazine in rheumatoid arthritis: desensitizing the patient with a skin rash. *Ann Rheum Dis* 1986;45:139.
133. Purdy BH et al. Desensitization for sulfasalazine skin rash. *Ann Intern Med* 1984;100:512.
134. Toila V. Sulfasalazine desensitization in children and adolescents with chronic inflammatory bowel disease. *Am J Gastroenterol* 1992;87:1029.
135. Taffet SL et al. Desensitization of patients with inflammatory bowel disease to sulfasalazine. *Am J Med* 1982;73:520.
136. Lerner A et al. Desensitization to vancomycin [Letter]. *Ann Intern Med* 1984;100:157.
137. Lin RY. Desensitization in the management of vancomycin hypersensitivity. *Arch Intern Med* 1990;150:2197.
138. Tenant-Flowers M et al. Sulphadiazine desensitization in patients with AIDS and cerebral toxoplasmosis. *AIDS* 1991;5:311.
139. de la Hoz Caballer B et al. Management of sulfadiazine allergy in patients with acquired immunodeficiency syndrome. *J Allergy Clin Immunol* 1991;88:137.
140. Greenberger PA et al. Management of drug allergy in patients with acquired immunodeficiency syndrome. *J Allergy Clin Immunol* 1987;79:484.
141. Walz-LeBlanc BAE et al. Allopurinol sensitivity in a patient with chronic tophaceous gout: success of intravenous desensitization after failure of oral desensitization. *Arthritis Rheum* 1991;34:1329.
142. Fasm AG et al. Desensitization to allopurinol in patients with gout and cutaneous reactions. *Am J Med* 1992;93:299.
143. Knight A. Desensitization to aspirin in aspirin-sensitive patients with rhino-sinusitis and asthma: a review. *J Otolaryngol* 1989;18:165.
144. Lumry WR et al. Aspirin-sensitive asthma and rhinosinusitis: current concepts and recent advances. *Ear Nose Throat J* 1984;63:102.
145. Vincent A et al. Serum sickness induced by fluoxetine. *Am J Psychiatry* 1991;148:1602.
146. Smith H et al. Adverse reactions to carbamazepine managed by desensitization [Letter]. *Lancet* 1985;1:753.
147. Carr A et al. Allergy and desensitization to zidovudine in patients with acquired immunodeficiency syndrome. *J Allergy Clin Immunol* 1993;91:683.
148. Kurohara ML et al. Metronidazole hypersensitivity and oral desensitization. *J Allergy Clin Immunol* 1991;88:279.
149. Rassiga AL et al. Cytarabine-induced anaphylaxis. Demonstration of antibody and successful desensitization. *Arch Intern Med* 1980;140:425.
150. Thompson DM et al. Prolonged desensitization required for treatment of generalized allergy to human insulin [Letter]. *Diabetes Care* 1993;16:957.
151. Gluckstein D et al. Rapid oral desensitization to trimethoprim-sulfamethoxazole (TMP-SMZ) use in prophylaxis for *Pneumocystis carinii* pneumonia in patients with AIDS who were previously intolerant to TMP-SMZ. *Clin Infect Dis* 1995;20:849.
152. Smith RM et al. Trimethoprim-sulfamethoxazole desensitization in the acquired immunodeficiency syndrome [Letter]. *Ann Intern Med* 1987;106:335.
153. Hughes TE et al. Co-trimoxazole desensitization in bone marrow transplant [Letter]. *Ann Intern Med* 1986;105:148.
154. Torgovnick J et al. Desensitization to sulfonamides in patients with HIV infection [Letter]. *Am J Med* 1990;88:548.
155. Kletzel M et al. Trimethoprim-sulfamethoxazole oral desensitization in hemophiliacs infected with human immunodeficiency virus with a history of hypersensitivity reactions. *Am J Dis Child* 1991;145:1428.
156. Finegold I. Oral desensitization to trimethoprim-sulfamethoxazole in a patient with acquired immunodeficiency syndrome. *J Allergy Clin Immunol* 1986;78:905.
157. White MV et al. Desensitization to trimethoprim sulfamethoxazole in patients with acquired immune deficiency syndrome and *Pneumocystis carinii* pneumonia. *Ann Allergy* 1989;62:177.
158. Sher MR et al. Anaphylactic shock induced by oral desensitization to trimethoprim/sulfamethoxazole (TMP-SMZ) [Abstract]. *J Allergy Clin Immunol* 1986;77:133.
159. Andersen JM et al. Serum sickness associated with 6-mercaptopurine in a patient with Crohn's disease. *Pharmacotherapy* 1997;17:173.
160. Wolfe MS et al. Serum sickness with furazolidone. *Am J Trop Med Hyg* 1978;27:762.
161. Dukes MNG, ed. *Meylers Side Effects of Drugs*. 12th ed. Amsterdam: Elsevier Science Publishers; 1992.
162. Cunningham E et al. Acute serum sickness with glomerulonephritis induced by antithymocyte globulin. *Transplantation* 1987;43:309.
163. Bielory L et al. Human serum sickness: a prospective analysis of 35 patients treated with equine antithymocyte globulin for bone marrow failure. *Medicine* 1988;67:40.
164. Bielory L et al. Cutaneous manifestations of serum sickness in patients receiving antithymocyte globulin. *J Am Acad Dermatol* 1985;13:411.
165. Panwalker AP et al. Serum sickness associated with cefoxitin and pentoxifylline therapy. *Drug Intell Clin Pharm* 1986;20:953.
166. Igarashi M et al. An immunodominant haptenic epitope of carbamazepine detected in serum from patients given long-term treatment with carbamazepine without allergic reaction. *J Clin Immunol* 1992;12:335.
167. Ferraccioli G et al. Indomethacin-related serum sickness-like illness with IgM lambda cryoparaprotein. *Acta Haematol* 1985;73:45.
168. Haruda F. Phenytoin hypersensitivity: 38 cases. *Neurology* 1979;29:1480.
169. Josephs SH et al. Phenytoin hypersensitivity. *J Allergy Clin Immunol* 1980;66:166.
170. Tomsick RS. The phenytoin syndrome. *Cutis* 1983;32:535.
171. Reynolds RD. Cefaclor and serum sickness-like reaction. *JAMA* 1996;276:950.
172. Comenzo RL et al. Immune hemolysis, disseminated intravascular coagulation, and serum sickness after large doses of immune globulin given intravenously for Kawasaki disease. *J Pediatr* 1992;120:926.
173. Tomas S et al. Ciprofloxacin and immunocomplex-mediated disease. *J Intern Med* 1991;230:550.
174. Slama TG. Serum sickness-like illness associated with ciprofloxacin. *Antimicrob Agents Chemother* 1990;34:904.
175. Bielory L. Serum sickness from iron-dextran administration. *Acta Haematol* 1990;83:166.
176. Miller LG et al. A case of fluoxetine-induced serum sickness. *Am J Psychiatry* 1989;146:1616.
177. Park H et al. Serum sickness-like reaction to itraconazole. *Pharmacotherapy* 1998;32:1249.
178. Rustmann WC et al. Leukocytoclastic vasculitis associated with sotalol therapy. *J Am Acad Dermatol* 1998;38:111.
179. Bear RA et al. Vasculitis and vitamin abuse. *Arch Pathol Lab Med* 1982;106:48.
180. Martinez-Taboada VM et al. Clinical features and outcome of 95 patients with hypersensitivity vasculitis. *Am J Med* 1997;102:186.
181. Suh JG et al. Leukocytoclastic vasculitis associated with nizatidine therapy. *Am J Med* 1997;102: 216.
182. Grunwald MH et al. Allergic vasculitis induced by hydrochlorothiazide: confirmation by mast cell degranulation test. *Isr J Med Sci* 1989;25:572.
183. Mitchell GG et al. Cimetidine-induced cutaneous vasculitis. *Am J Med* 1983;75:875.

184. Huminer D et al. Hypersensitivity vasculitis due to ofloxacin. *BMJ* 1989;299:303.
185. Jungst G, Mohr R. Side effects of ofloxacin in clinical trials and in postmarketing surveillance. *Drugs* 1987;34(Suppl 1):144.
186. Palop-Larea V et al. Vasculitis with acute kidney failure and torsemide. *Lancet* 1998;352:1909.
187. Kanuga J et al. Ciprofloxacin-induced leukocytoclastic vasculitis with cryoglobulinemia [Abstract]. *Ann Allergy* 1991;66:76.
188. Choe U et al. Ciprofloxacin-induced vasculitis. *N Engl J Med* 1989;320:257.
189. Stubbings J et al. Cutaneous vasculitis due to ciprofloxacin. *BMJ* 1992;305:29.
190. Hannedouche T et al. Penicillin-induced hypersensitivity vasculitides. *J Antimicrob Chemother* 1987;20:3.
191. Gavura SR et al. Leukocytoclastic vasculitis associated with clarithromycin. *Ann Pharmacother* 1998;32:543.
192. Kamper AM et al. Cutaneous vasculitis induced by sodium valproate. *Lancet* 1991;337:497.
193. Lin RY. Unusual autoimmune manifestations in furosemide-associated hypersensitivity angiitis. *NY State J Med* 1988;88:439.
194. Leung AC et al. Phenylbutazone-induced systemic vasculitis with crescentic glomerulonephritis. *Arch Intern Med* 1985;145:685.
195. Reynolds NJ et al. Hydralazine predisposes to acute cutaneous vasculitis following urography with iopamidol. *Br J Dermatol* 1993;129:82.
196. Fox BC et al. Leukocytoclastic vasculitis after pneumococcal vaccination. *Am J Infect Control* 1998;26:365.
197. Tanay A et al. Dermal vasculitis due to Coumadin hypersensitivity. *Dermatologica* 1982;165:178.
198. Knox JP et al. Procainamide-induced urticarial vasculitis. *Cutis* 1988;42:469.
199. Torres RA et al. Zidovudine-induced leukocytoclastic vasculitis. *Arch Intern Med* 1992;152:850.
200. Travis WD et al. Hypersensitivity pneumonitis and pulmonary vasculitis with eosinophilia in a patient taking an L-tryptophan preparation. *Ann Intern Med* 1990;112:301.
201. Stankus SJ et al. Propylthiouracil-induced hypersensitivity vasculitis presenting as respiratory failure. *Chest* 1992;102:1595.
202. Wolf D et al. Nodular vasculitis associated with propylthiouracil. *Cutis* 1992;49:253.
203. Carrasco MD et al. Cutaneous vasculitis associated with propylthiouracil therapy. *Arch Intern Med* 1987;147:1677.
204. Arellano F et al. Allopurinol hypersensitivity syndrome. *Ann Pharmacother* 1993;27:337.
205. Enat R et al. Hypersensitivity vasculitis induced by terbutaline sulfate. *Ann Allergy* 1988;61:275.
206. Bergman SM et al. Azathioprine and hypersensitivity vasculitis. *Ann Intern Med* 1988;109:83.
207. Simonart T et al. Cutaneous necrotizing vasculitis after low-dose methotrexate therapy for rheumatoid arthritis: a possible manifestation of methotrexate hypersensitivity. *Clin Rheumatol* 1997;16:623.
208. Steinmetz JC et al. Hypersensitivity vasculitis associated with 2-deoxycoformycin and allopurinol therapy. *Am J Med* 1989;86:499.
209. Scerri L et al. Mefloquine-associated cutaneous vasculitis. *Int J Dermatol* 1993;32:517.
210. Alarcon-Segovia D et al. Antinuclear antibodies in patients on anticonvulsant therapy. *Clin Exp Immunol* 1972;12:39.
211. Jacobs JC. Systemic lupus erythematosus in childhood. Report of 35 cases, with discussion of 7 apparently induced by anticonvulsant medication, and of prognosis and treatment. *Pediatrics* 1963;32:257.
212. Bleck TP et al. Possible induction of systemic lupus erythematosus syndrome by valproate. *Epilepsia* 1990;31:343.
213. Ahuja GK et al. Drug-induced SLE: primidone as a possible cause. *JAMA* 1966;198:201.
214. Drory VE et al. Carbamazepine-induced systemic lupus erythematosus. *Clin Neuropharmacol* 1989;12:115.
215. Livingston S et al. Carbamazepine in epilepsy. Nine-year follow-up with special emphasis on untoward reactions. *Dis Nerv Syst* 1974;35:103.
216. Livingston S et al. Systemic lupus erythematosus. Occurrence in association with ethosuximide therapy. *JAMA* 1968;204:185.
217. Ronnblom LE et al. Possible induction of systemic lupus erythematosus by interferon-alpha treatment in a patient with a malignant carcinoid tumour. *J Intern Med* 1990;227:207.
218. Schilling PJ et al. Development of systemic lupus erythematosus after interferon therapy for chronic myelogenous leukemia. *Cancer* 1991;68:1536.
219. Greenberg JH et al. Drug-induced systemic lupus erythematosus. *JAMA* 1972;222:191.
220. Lee SL et al. Drug-induced systemic lupus erythematosus. A critical review. *Semin Arthritis Rheum* 1975;6:83.
221. Perry HM. Late toxicity to hydralazine resembling systemic lupus erythematosus or rheumatoid arthritis. *Am J Med* 1973;54:58.
222. Kendall MJ et al. Quinidine-induced systemic lupus erythematosus. *Postgrad Med J* 1970;46:729.
223. Cohen MG et al. Two distinct quinidine-induced rheumatic syndromes. *Ann Intern Med* 1988; 108:369.
224. West SG et al. Quinidine-induced lupus erythematosus. *Ann Intern Med* 1984;100:840.
225. Burlingame RW et al. Anti-histone antibody induction by drugs implicates autoimmunization with nucleohistone [Abstract]. *Arthritis Rheum* 1980;32(Suppl 4):S22.
226. Dubois EL et al. Chlorpromazine-induced systemic lupus erythematosus. *JAMA* 1972;221:595.
227. Fabius AJM et al. Systemic lupus erythematosus induced by psychotropic drugs. *Acta Rheumatol Scand* 1971;17:137.
228. Goldman LS et al. Lupus-like illness associated with chlorpromazine. *Am J Psychiatry* 1980;137:1613.
229. Quismorio FP et al. Antinuclear antibodies in chronic psychotic patients treated with chlorpromazine. *Am J Psychiatry* 1975;132:1204.
230. Harrington TM et al. Systemic lupus-like syndrome induced by methyldopa therapy. *Chest* 1981;79:696.
231. Dupont A et al. Lupus-like syndrome induced by methyldopa. *BMJ* 1982;285:693.
232. Perry HM Jr et al. Immunologic findings in patients receiving methyldopa: a prospective study. *J Lab Clin Med* 1971;78:905.
233. Nordstrom DM et al. Methyldopa-induced systemic lupus erythematosus. *Arthritis Rheum* 1989;32:205.
234. Griffiths ID, Kane SP. Sulphasalazine-induced lupus syndrome in ulcerative colitis. *BMJ* 1977;2:1188.
235. Crisp AJ et al. Sulphasalazine-induced systemic lupus erythematosus in a patient with Sjögren's syndrome. *J R Soc Med* 1980;73:60.
236. Carr-Locke D. Sulfasalazine-induced lupus syndrome in a patient with Crohn's disease. *Am J Gastroenterol* 1982;77:614.
237. Clementz GL et al. Sulfasalazine-induced lupus erythematosus. *Am J Med* 1988;84:535.
238. Rafferty P et al. Sulphasalazine-induced cerebral lupus erythematosus. *Postgrad Med J* 1982;58:98.
239. Meier CR et al. Postmenopausal estrogen replacement therapy and risk of developing systemic lupus erythematosus or discoid lupus. *J Rheumatol* 1998;25:1515.
240. Elkayam O et al. Minocycline-induced autoimmune syndromes: an overview. *Semin Arthritis Rheum* 1999;28:392.
241. Holmes S et al. Exacerbation of systemic lupus erythematosus induced by terbinafine. *Br J Dermatol* 1998;139:1133.
242. Chalmer A et al. Systemic lupus erythematosus during penicillamine therapy for rheumatoid arthritis. *Ann Intern Med* 1982;97:659.
243. Finekl TH et al. Drug-induced lupus in a child after treatment with zafirlukast (Accolate). *J Allergy Clin Immunol* 1999;103:533.
244. Lahita R et al. Antibodies to nuclear antigens in patients treated with procainamide or acetylprocainamide. *N Engl J Med* 1979;301:1382.
245. Roden DM et al. Antiarrhythmic efficacy, pharmacokinetics and safety of N-acetylprocainamide in human subjects: comparison with procainamide. *Am J Cardiol* 1980;46:463.
246. Stec GP et al. Remission of procainamide-induced lupus erythematosus with N-acetylprocainamide therapy. *Ann Intern Med* 1979;90:799.
247. Booth RJ et al. Beta-adrenergic-receptor blockers and antinuclear antibodies in hypertension. *Clin Pharmacol Ther* 1982;31:555.
248. Calabrese LH et al. The American College of Rheumatology 1990 criteria for the classification of hypersensitivity vasculitis. *Arthritis Rheum* 1990;33:1108.
249. Morrow JD et al. Studies on the control of hypertension by hyphex. II. Toxic reactions and side effects. *Circulation* 1953;8:829.
250. Culver CA et al. Probable anaphylactoid reaction to a pyrethrin pediculicide shampoo. *Clin Pharm* 1988;7:846.
251. Polk RE. Anaphylactoid reactions to glycopeptide antibiotics. *J Antimicrob Chemother* 1991; 27(Suppl B):17.
252. Davis H et al. Anaphylactoid reactions reported after treatment with ciprofloxacin. *Ann Intern Med* 1989;111:1041.
253. Chen M et al. Anaphylactoid-anaphylactic reactions associated with ondansetron [Letter]. *Ann Intern Med* 1993;119:862.
254. Bonfiglio MF et al. Anaphylactoid reaction to intravenous acetylcysteine associated with electrocardiographic abnormalities. *Ann Pharmacother* 1992;26:22.
255. Deamer RL et al. Hypersensitivity and anaphylactoid reactions to ciprofloxacin. *Ann Pharmacother* 1992;26:1081.
256. Soetikno RM et al. Ciprofloxacin-induced anaphylactoid reaction in a patient with AIDS [Letter]. *Ann Pharmacother* 1993;27:1404.
257. Kossey JL et al. Anaphylactoid reactions associated with ondansetron. *Ann Pharmacother* 1994;28:1029.
258. Liau-Chu M et al. Mechanism of anaphylactoid reactions: improper preparation of high-dose cyclosporine leads to a bolus infusion of Cremophor EL and cyclosporine. *Ann Pharmacother* 1997;31:1287.
259. Volcheck GW et al. Anaphylaxis to intravenous cyclosporine and tolerance to oral cyclosporine: case report and review. *Ann Allergy Asthma Immunol* 1998;80:159.
260. Faich G et al. Sodium ferric gluconate complex in sucrose: safer intravenous iron therapy than iron dextrans. *Am J Kidney Dis* 1999;33:464.
261. Ferrlecit (sodium ferric gluconate complex in sucrose injection) prescribing information. Watson Pharma, Inc. November 2001.
262. Alkins SA et al. Anaphylactoid reactions to methotrexate. *Cancer* 1996;77:2123.
263. Okano M et al. Anaphylactoid symptoms due to oral minocycline. *Acta Derm Venerol* 1996;76:164.
264. Hebert ME et al. Anaphylactoid reactions with intraperitoneal cisplatin. *Ann Pharmacother* 1995;29:260.
265. Coyne DW et al. Sodium ferric gluconate complex in hemodialysis patents. II. Adverse reactions in iron dextran-sensitive and dextran-tolerant patients. *Kidney Int* 2003;63:217.
266. Valdivieso R et al. Pseudo-allergic reactions to corticosteroids: diagnosis and alternatives. *J Invest Clin Immunol* 1995;5:171.
267. Kamm GL et al. Allergic-type reactions to corticosteroids. *Ann Pharmacother* 1999;33:451.
268. Essayan DM et al. Successful parenteral desensitization to paclitaxel. *J Allergy Clin Immunol* 1996;97(1 Pt 1):42.
269. Borish L et al. Intravenous desensitization to beta-lactam antibiotics. *J Allergy Clin Immunol* 1987;80:314.

CHAPTER 5

Managing Acute Drug Toxicity

Judith A. Alsop

This chapter reviews common strategies for the evaluation and management of drug overdoses and poisonings. Information for the management of specific drug overdoses is best obtained from a poison control center (reached by dialing 1-800-222-1222 anywhere in the United States).

Epidemiologic Data

American Association of Poison Control Centers and Drug Abuse Warning Network

Toxicity secondary to drug and chemical exposure commonly occurs in children; however, the incidence of exposure to specific agents and the severity of outcomes varies based on the population studied (Table 5-1).[1–3] The number of reported toxic exposures in the United States in 2005 was approximately 2.42 million, according to the American Association of Poison Control Centers (AAPCC).[3] In most cases, little or no toxicity was associated with the exposure. About 22% received treatment at a health care facility, only 5.6% reported moderate or severe symptoms, and 1,261 resulted in fatalities. According to the Drug Abuse Warning Network (DAWN), 1.4 million U.S. emergency room visits involved drug misuse or abuse in the year 2005. Of those cases, 56% involved illicit drug use.[4]

These disparate statistics from two national sources underscore the difficulty in determining the true incidence of poisoning and overdoses.[5] Nevertheless, epidemiologic data are useful in identifying trends and in instigating public health interventions. For example, from 2001 to 2002, the number of inhalant abuse cases reported by DAWN increased 187%, identifying the need for additional education about inhalant abuse toxicity.[6] From 2004 to 2005, after inhalation education programs, inhalant abuse decreased by 54%.[4]

Age-Specific Data

Stratifying patients by age can be useful in assessing the likelihood of severe toxicity from an exposure. For example, most unintentional ingestions by children 1 to 6 years of age occur because children are curious, becoming more mobile and beginning to explore their surroundings, and often putting objects or substances into their mouths. According to AAPCC data, 50.9% of all reported poisonings occur in children younger than 6 years of age.[3] Fortunately, exposures usually involve the ingestion of relatively small amounts of a single substance. In one report, only 10.5% of pediatric poisoning cases were treated in a health care facility; the remaining cases were managed at home.[3] In actuality, severe toxicities in young children from ingestions are relatively uncommon.

AAPCC epidemiologic data also report medication errors, which in the pediatric population, commonly result from confusing units of measurement (e.g., teaspoons vs. milliliters or tablespoons vs. teaspoons), incorrect formulation or concentration administered, dispensing cup errors, and incorrect formulation or concentration dispensed from the pharmacy.[3]

In children younger than 6 years of age, the reasons for toxic exposure to medications are less clear.[7] Adolescent children generally have poor knowledge of the toxicity of medications and can overdose themselves unintentionally.[8] The potential for suicide attempts or intentional substance abuse, however, should not be ignored in older children or adults. These intentional overdoses commonly involve mixed exposures to illicit drugs, prescribed medications, or ethanol, and are associated with more severe toxicity and death than unintentional toxic exposures.

In geriatric patients, overdoses tend to have a greater potential for severe adverse effects, compared with overdoses in other age groups, because the elderly are more likely to have underlying illnesses, and more often have access to a variety of potentially dangerous medications.[10] More than 40% of patients age 65 or older take five medications per week and 12% use ten or more medications weekly.[11] In 2005, 16% of fatalities from toxic ingestions involved patients older than 60 years.[3]

Information Resources

Computerized Databases

A vast number of substances can be involved in a poisoning or overdose, and reliable data about the contents of products,

Table 5-1 Substances Most Frequently Involved in Poisoning Exposures[a]

All Ages	Children Younger Than 6 Years	Adults Older Than 19 Years	Fatalities
Analgesics	Cosmetics and personal care products	Analgesics	Analgesics
Cosmetics and personal care products	Cleaning substances	Sedative/hypnotics/antipsychotics	Sedative/hypnotics/antipsychotics
Cleaning substances	Analgesics	Cleaning substances	Antidepressants
Sedative/hypnotics/antipsychotics	Foreign bodies	Antidepressants	Stimulants and street drugs
Foreign bodies	Topical products	Bites, envenomations	Cardiovascular drugs
Cold and cough preparations	Cough and cold preparations	Cardiovascular drugs	Alcohols
Topical preparations	Plants	Alcohols	Anticonvulsants
Pesticides	Pesticides	Pesticides	Antihistamines
Antidepressants	Vitamins	Cosmetics and personal care products	Fumes/gases/vapors
Bites, envenomations	Antihistamines	Food products/food poisoning	Muscle relaxants
Cardiovascular drugs	Antimicrobials	Hydrocarbons	Hormones and hormone antagonists
Antihistamines	GI preparations	Chemicals	Chemicals
Alcohols	Arts, crafts, office supplies	Fumes/gases/vapors	Unknown drug
Plants	Hormones and hormone antagonists	Anticonvulsants	Cleaning substances
Antimicrobials	Electrolytes and minerals	Antihistamines	GI preparations

[a]Despite a high frequency of involvement, these substances are not necessarily the most toxic, but may reflect ready access.
Adapted from reference 3. These poisoning exposures are listed in order of frequency encountered.

toxicities of substances, and treatment approaches need to be readily accessible. POISINDEX, a computerized database,[12] provides information on thousands of drugs by brand name, generic name, and street name, as well as foreign drugs, chemicals, pesticides, household products, personal care items, cleaning products, poisonous insects, poisonous snakes, and poisonous plants. Annual subscriptions to POISINDEX, updated quarterly, are expensive and are generally available only in large medical centers.[13]

Printed Publications

Textbooks and manuals also provide useful clinical information about the presentation, assessment, and treatment of toxicities. *Goldfrank's Toxicologic Emergencies*[14] and the pocket-size *Poisoning & Drug Overdose*[15] are valuable, inexpensive alternatives to computerized database programs. Books, however, are less useful than computerized databases because information must be condensed and cannot be updated as frequently. Some drug package inserts also refer to treatment of acute toxicities; however, the information can be inadequate or inappropriate.[16]

Poison Control Centers

Poison control centers provide the most cost-effective and accurate information to health care providers and to the general public.[17,18] Poison centers are usually staffed by trained poison information specialists who have a pharmacy, nursing, or medical background. Physician backup is provided 24 hours a day by board-certified medical toxicologists. The nonphysician clinical toxicologists, pharmacists, and nurses who staff poison control centers are certified as specialists in poison information by the AAPCC or as clinical toxicologists by the American Board of Applied Toxicology.[19]

The poison information specialist must accurately and efficiently assess event-specific toxicity by telephone, without the benefit of direct observation of the patient; and communicate this assessment along with treatment information quickly, accurately, and professionally in a reassuring manner. Subsequent to the telephone consultation, the poison control center staff should initiate follow-up calls to determine the effectiveness of the recommended treatment, the need for additional evaluation or treatment, and the outcome.[20,21]

Effective Communication

Effective communication is essential to the assessment of potential poisonings. In most situations, the person seeking guidance on the management of a potentially toxic exposure is the parent of a small child who may have ingested a substance. The caller is usually anxious about the child and may feel guilty about the exposure. To calm the caller, the health care provider should quickly reassure the parent that telephoning for assistance was appropriate and that the best assistance possible will be provided.[20] If English is not the first language of the caller, or if there are other communication barriers, solutions must be found to enhance outcomes. Most poison centers subscribe to translation services or have bilingual staff to communicate with non–English-speaking callers. Poison centers also have TTY equipment to serve the hearing and speech impaired populations.

Once calm, effective communication is established, the health care provider should first determine whether the patient is conscious and breathing and has a pulse. If life-threatening symptoms have occurred, the caller should call for emergency services. If the health care provider does not have the knowledge or resources to provide poison information, he or she should refer the caller to the closest poison control center. Information on the location and phone number of the nearest poison control center can be found on the Internet at www.aapcc.org or by calling 1-800-222-1222. The call is automatically transferred to the poison center that serves the caller's area in the United States.

GENERAL MANAGEMENT

Supportive Care and "ABCs"

Management of poisoned or overdosed patients is primarily based on symptomatic and supportive care. Specific antidotes exist only for a small percentage of the thousands of potential drugs and chemicals that could cause a poisoning. The first aspect of patient management should always be basic support of airway, breathing, and circulation (the "ABCs"). The assessment and treatment of the potentially poisoned patient can be separated into seven primary functions: (a) gathering history of exposure, (b) evaluating clinical presentation (i.e., toxidromes), (c) evaluating clinical laboratory patient data, (d) removing the toxic source (e.g., gastrointestinal [GI] decontamination), (e) considering antidotes and specific treatment, (f) enhancing systemic clearance, and (g) monitoring outcome.[22–24]

Gathering History of Exposure

Comprehensive historical information about the toxic exposure should be gathered from as many different sources as possible (e.g., patient, family, friends, prehospital health care providers). This information should be compared for consistency and evaluated relative to clinical findings and laboratory results. The patient's history of the exposure is often inaccurate and should be confirmed with objective findings.[22,23,25] For example, a patient who presents at the emergency department (ED) with a supposed hydrocodone and carisoprodol overdose is expected to be lethargic or comatose. If the patient arrives wide awake with tachycardia and agitation, the caregiver should suspect exposure to other substances. This would be the case whenever the patient's symptoms are not consistent with the history presented.

Specific information should be sought concerning the patient's state of consciousness, symptoms, probable intoxicant(s), maximum amount and dosage form(s) of substance ingested, as well as when the exposure occurred. Medications, allergies, and prior medical problems also should be ascertained to facilitate development of treatment plans (e.g., a history of renal failure may indicate the need for hemodialysis to compensate for decreased renal drug clearance).[22,23]

Evaluating Clinical Presentation and Toxidromes

A thorough physical examination is needed to characterize the signs and symptoms of overdose, and should be conducted serially to determine the evolution or resolution of the patient's intoxication. An evaluation of the presenting signs and symptoms can provide clues on the drug class causing the toxicity, confirm the historical data surrounding the toxic exposure, and suggest initial treatment.[26,27] The patient may be asymptomatic on presentation, even though a potentially severe exposure has occurred, if absorption of the drug or toxic substance is incomplete or if the substance has not yet metabolized to a toxic substance.[28]

Characteristic toxidromes (i.e., a constellation of signs and symptoms consistent with a syndrome) can be associated with some specific classes of drugs.[23,26,27] The most common toxidromes are those associated with anticholinergic activity, increased sympathetic activity, and central nervous system (CNS) stimulation or depression. The *anticholinergic* drugs can increase heart rate, increase body temperature, decrease GI motility, dilate pupils, and produce drowsiness or delirium. *Sympathomimetic* drugs can increase CNS activity, heart rate, body temperature, and blood pressure (BP). *Opioids, sedatives, hypnotics*, and *antidepressants* can depress the CNS, but the specific class of CNS depressant often cannot be easily identified by a specific constellation of symptoms. Classic findings may not be present for all drugs within a therapeutic class. For example, opioids generally induce miosis, but meperidine can produce mydriasis. Furthermore, the association of symptoms with a particular class of toxic substances is difficult when more than one substance has been ingested. Practitioners should not focus only on the specific clinical findings associated with a toxidrome; rather, they should consider all subjective and objective data gathered from the history of exposure, the patient's medical history, physical examination, and laboratory findings.

Interpretation of Laboratory Data

DRUG SCREENS

A urine drug screen can be useful in identifying the presence of drugs and their metabolites in selected patients. Although a urine drug screen is not indicated in all cases of drug overdose, it can be useful in a patient with coma of unknown etiology, when the presented history is inconsistent with clinical findings, or when more than one drug might have been ingested.[24,29,30]

PHARMACOKINETIC CONSIDERATIONS

The absorption, distribution, metabolism, and elimination of drugs in the overdosed patient can be quite different than when the drug is taken in usual therapeutic doses.[31] The pharmacodynamic and pharmacokinetic behavior of drugs can be substantially altered by large drug overdoses, especially with drugs that exhibit dose-dependent pharmacokinetics. The rate of drug absorption is generally slowed by large overdoses, and the time to reach peak serum drug concentrations can be delayed.[32] For example, peak serum concentrations of phenytoin can be delayed for 2 to 7 days after an orally ingested overdose.[33,34] The volume of distribution of an overdosed drug can be increased, and when usual metabolic pathways become saturated, secondary clearance pathways can be important. For example, large overdoses of acetaminophen saturate glutathione mechanisms of metabolism, resulting in hepatotoxicity.[35]

When the pharmacokinetic parameters of an overdosed drug are altered, serial plasma concentration measurements can better define the absorption, distribution, and clearance phases of the ingested substance. Pharmacokinetic parameters that have been derived from therapeutic doses should not be used to predict whether absorption is complete or to predict the expected duration of intoxication caused by large overdoses.[31,36–38]

Decontamination

After the airway and the cardiopulmonary system are supported, efforts should be directed toward removing the toxic substance from the patient (i.e., decontamination).[22,39] Decontamination presumes that both the dose and the duration of toxin exposure are important in determining the extent of toxicity and that prevention of continued exposure will decrease toxicity.[28] This intuitive concept is clearly relevant to ocular, dermal, and respiratory exposures, when local tissue damage is the primary problem. Respiratory decontamination involves removing the patient from the toxic environment and providing fresh air or oxygen to the patient. Decontamination of skin and eyes involves flushing the affected area with large volumes of water or saline to physically remove the toxic substance from the surface.[22,23]

GASTROINTESTINAL DECONTAMINATION

Because most poisonings and overdoses result from oral ingestions, measures to decrease or prevent continued GI absorption have commonly been used to limit the extent of exposure.[22,23,28,40] GI decontamination should be considered if the ingestion is large enough to produce potentially significant toxicity, or if the potential severity of the ingestion is unknown and the time since ingestion is <1 hour. The following methods have been used: (a) evacuate gastric contents by emesis or gastric lavage, (b) administer activated charcoal as an adsorbent to bind the toxic substance remaining in the GI tract, (c) use cathartics or whole bowel irrigation (WBI) to increase the rectal elimination of unabsorbed drug, or (d) combine any of these methods.

The efficacy of GI decontamination varies, depending on when the process is initiated relative to the time of ingestion, dose ingested, and other factors. Furthermore, ipecac-induced emesis, gastric lavage, cathartics, and activated charcoal are not directly associated with improved patient outcomes.[41–46]

The most appropriate method for GI tract decontamination remains unclear because sound comparative data for different methods of GI decontamination are unavailable. Clinical research in healthy subjects, by necessity, must use nontoxic doses of drugs. Studies using nontoxic doses are not applicable to the overdose situation because alterations in GI absorption can occur with large doses. In addition, low-dose studies generally rely on pharmacokinetic end-points such as peak plasma concentrations, area under the plasma concentration-time curve, or quantity of drug recovered from the urine.[41,42,44–46] In contrast, clinical studies of GI decontamination methods in patients who have ingested toxic doses of a substance use clinical outcomes or a directional change in serum drug concentrations.[41,42,45,46] These latter trials are not standardized with respect to the dose ingested or to the time interval between drug ingestion and GI decontamination.

Ipecac-Induced Emesis and Gastric Lavage

Ipecac-induced emesis and gastric lavage primarily remove substances from the stomach; and their efficacy is affected significantly by the time the ingested substance remains in the stomach. Gastric lavage or ipecac-induced emesis is most effective when implemented within 1 hour of the ingestion (i.e., before the substance moves past the stomach into the intestine).[41,42]

The commonly used adult gastric lavage tube (36F) has an internal diameter too small to allow recovery of large tablet or capsule fragments and an even smaller diameter lavage tube is used for children.[42] Gastric lavage may be useful only if large amounts of a liquid substance were ingested and the patient arrived within 1 hour of the ingestion.[42] Unfortunately, most patients arrive in the ED more than an hour after ingestion, when absorption of the toxic substance from the stomach has most likely already occurred. As a result, the efficacy of these procedures in overdose situations is minimal. Studies have not confirmed that use of gastric lavage or ipecac-induced emesis improves the outcome of the patient.[40–42]

Established Guidelines

The American College of Emergency Physicians has published guidelines for the initial evaluation, diagnosis, stabilization, and management of patients who present with acute toxic ingestions,[22] and the American Academy of Clinical Toxicology (AACT), along with the European Association of Poisons Centres and Clinical Toxicologists (EAPCCT) and other organizations, have published position papers on GI decontamination.[41–46]

The AACT and EAPCCT clinical guidelines state that ipecac syrup and gastric lavage should not be routinely used.[41,42] In addition, the American Academy of Pediatrics no longer supports the use of ipecac syrup routinely as a home treatment of poisoning and advocates that ipecac syrup already in the home should be discarded safely.[47] As a result, the use of ipecac to induce vomiting in both the home and the health care setting has been curtailed significantly.

Activated Charcoal

In 1963, a review article concluded that activated charcoal was the most valuable agent available for the treatment of poisoning.[48] This conclusion was based only on studies in fasting patients who had nontoxic exposures. Nevertheless, data from those studies were extrapolated to poisoned patients. Since then, activated charcoal has become the preferred method of GI decontamination for the treatment of toxic ingestions.[22,27,40,43,49–51] If administered within 1 hour of the ingestion, the adsorption of substances to charcoal prevents absorption. It is assumed that adsorption of the toxin prevents toxicity and improves patient outcome, especially if the risk to the patient is low.[43]

Vomiting with aspiration of activated charcoal occurs in about 5% of patients who receive activated charcoal.[43,51–53] The resulting pulmonary problems can be due to aspiration of acidic stomach contents and/or the charcoal. Decreased oxygenation can occur immediately, or pulmonary effects can occur later.[54–56] Adult respiratory distress syndrome has resulted after the unintentional instillation of charcoal into the lung.[51] Aspiration of charcoal can result in chronic lung disease or fatalities, whereas the toxic exposure, for which the charcoal was administered, is often not lethal or even serious.[53,57]

Cathartics

Sorbitol (a cathartic) was often administered with the activated charcoal to enhance passage of the charcoal-substance complex through the GI tract. However, decreased transit time through the bowel has not been proven to decrease absorption, probably because drug absorption does not take place in the large bowel.[44] Sorbitol is also associated with an increased incidence of vomiting and aspiration.[19] Hypernatremia can also develop subsequent to the administration of repeat doses of activated charcoal with sorbitol.[58,59] Currently, most EDs use aqueous activated charcoal mixtures rather than charcoal-sorbitol combinations. Cathartics are not effective as GI decontaminants, and their use is no longer advised.[22,43,44]

Whole Bowel Irrigation

Whole Bowel Irrigation (WBI) with a polyethylene glycol–balanced electrolyte solution (e.g., Colyte, GoLYTELY) can successfully remove substances from the entire GI tract over several hours. WBI is effective with ingestions of sustained-release dosage forms, as well as substances that form bezoars (concretions of tablets or capsules), such as ferrous sulfate or phenytoin.[23,45,60] WBI is also indicated when the toxic agent is not adsorbed by activated charcoal (e.g., body-packer packets, lithium, iron, potassium).[22,23,45,60] This method of GI decontamination takes much longer to complete and is associated with poor patient adherence because large volumes of fluid (2 L/hour for adults until the effluent is clear) need to be ingested for this to be effective.[60] A nasogastric (NG) tube, however, can be inserted, and the WBI fluid mixture can be administered via this NG tube.[45]

Antidotes and Specific Treatments

An antidote, a drug that neutralizes the toxicity of another substance, is useful if it does not produce even greater hazards for the patient. Some antidotes can displace a drug from receptor sites (e.g., naloxone for opioids, flumazenil for benzodiazepines),[61,62] and some can inhibit the formation of toxic metabolites (e.g., *N*-acetylcysteine [NAC] for acetaminophen, fomepizole for methanol). Some treatments are highly effective for the management of individual drug overdoses, but they do not meet the definition of an antidote. For example, sodium bicarbonate is used to treat the cardiotoxicity arising from tricyclic antidepressant (TCA) overdoses, and benzodiazepines are used to treat CNS toxicity associated with cocaine and amphetamine overdoses.[23,63–65]

Enhancing Systemic Clearance

Hemodialysis and manipulation of urine pH can enhance the clearance of substances. Hemodialysis can successfully treat some specific intoxications (e.g., methanol, ethylene glycol, aspirin, lithium). Hemodialysis can also be used in patients with severe acid–base or renal dysfunction.[40] Alkaline diuresis can enhance the elimination of drugs such as aspirin and phenobarbital.[66]

Monitoring Outcome

Selecting the appropriate parameters and length of time to monitor a patient who has been exposed to a toxic agent requires knowledge of toxic effects and the time course of the intoxication.[28] Most patients who are at risk for moderate or severe toxicity should be monitored in an intensive care unit (ICU) with careful assessments of cardiac, pulmonary, and CNS function.[67]

ASSESSMENT OF SALICYLATE INGESTION

Gathering a History

1. M.O., the mother of a 4-year-old child, states that her daughter, D.O., has ingested some aspirin tablets. What additional information should be obtained from or given to M.O. at this time?

Obtaining an initial assessment of the patient's status is essential. The caller's telephone number should be obtained in the event that the call is disconnected, initial recommendations need to be modified, or subsequent follow-up is needed. The health care provider should ask for patient-specific information with questions that are nonthreatening and nonjudgmental. The caller should be reassured that calling for help was the right thing to do.

Evaluating Clinical Presentation

2. On further questioning, M.O. states that D.O. is crying and complaining of a stomachache. Otherwise, the child appears to be normal. The daughter was found sitting on the bathroom floor with an aspirin bottle in her hand and some partially chewed tablets on the floor next to her. The child had the same look on her face that she does when she eats things that she does not like. M.O. reports that she can see white tablet material gummed on the child's teeth. The mother was gone no more than 5 minutes and had asked her 5- and 6-year-old sons to watch their sister. What additional information is needed to correctly assess the potential for toxicity?

To determine the potential toxicity for an unintentional ingestion, it is important to assess the presence of symptoms and to identify the substance ingested. Inquiries should begin with open-ended questions to determine the facts that the caller is certain of versus what may have been assumed. The answers usually point to more specific information that is needed to accurately assess the exposure.[20]

D.O.'s symptoms presently are not life threatening. Her behavior is consistent with being scared in response to the mother's anxiety. Once it has been established that the child does not need immediate life-saving treatment, the caller is generally more willing and able to answer additional questions.

M.O. already has provided information about the child's symptoms; however, more information is needed to determine the identity of the ingested substance, the time of ingestion, the brand of aspirin (to ensure that the product is not an aspirin-combination or even an aspirin-free formulation), the dosage form, the number of dosage units in a full container, and the number of remaining dosage units in the container. The parent should be careful to look for tablets under beds, rugs, or other locations out of sight (e.g., wastepaper baskets, toilets, pet food dishes, pockets). The dosage forms in the container should be identical in appearance, and the contents should be what are stated on the label. Information concerning the child's weight and health status, as well as whether the child is taking other medications, is also important. The child's weight is useful in determining the maximum mg/kg dose of aspirin that was ingested.

When more than one child is present during an ingestion incident, the caller should be questioned as to whether other children also could have participated in the ingestion. In this situation, the children could have shared equally in the missing dosage units of drug, all of the drug could have been fed to one child, or all of the drug could have been ingested by the oldest or most aggressive child. When it is unclear how many missing dosage units of a substance might have been ingested among a group of children, each child should be evaluated and managed as if he or she may have ingested the total missing quantity.

Triage of Call

3. The caller, M.O., has now determined that a total of five tablets each containing 325 mg/tablet of aspirin are missing from the bottle. Because M.O. recalls having taken two aspirin tablets from this bottle, it is not likely that her daughter took more than three tablets. M.O. states that D.O. weighs 36 lb. What treatment is needed for this child?

The maximum dose of aspirin ingested by this child is likely to be much less than the minimum dose required to produce significant symptoms based on an assumption that this 4-year-old girl is of average weight for her age (i.e., 36 lb or ~16 kg). A dose of 150 mg/kg of aspirin is the smallest dose at which treatment or assessment at a health care facility is necessary.[68,69] D.O. is likely to have ingested a maximum of 975 mg of aspirin (i.e., three 325-mg tablets), which is about 60 mg/kg (975 mg divided by 16 kg). If this child is healthy, takes no medications, and is not allergic to aspirin, the child does not need any treatment. With this history of ingestion, the only adverse effect that might occur is some mild nausea. Providing information to the mother that her child had not ingested a toxic amount will be reassuring.

For many years, aspirin was the most common cause of unintentional poisoning and poisoning deaths among children.[69–71] However, safety closure packaging and reduction of the total aspirin content in a full bottle of children's aspirin to approximately 3 g has steadily reduced the frequency of pediatric aspirin poisoning and deaths.[70–72] Although acute aspirin poisoning remains a problem, the largest percentage of life-threatening intoxications now results from therapeutic overdose.[68] Therapeutic overdoses occur when a dose is given too frequently, when both parents unknowingly dose the child with the drug, or when too large a dose is given. Therapeutic overdoses are especially a problem if the situation continues for a period of time and the drug is able to accumulate.[68]

Outcome for M.O.

Follow-up telephone consultations on toxic ingestions is important to identify children who unexpectedly develop symptoms that might need to be treated. A telephone call to M.O. 6 to 24 hours after her initial call would be appropriate to follow up on the child. On a call back to M.O., the parent stated that she gave D.O. lunch at the appropriate time. D.O. then watched cartoons, took her usual nap, and remained asymptomatic.

Acute and Chronic Salicylism

Signs and Symptoms

4. V.K., a 65-year-old, 55-kg woman with a history of chronic headaches has taken 10 to 12 aspirin tablets a day for several months. On the evening of admission, she became lethargic,

disoriented, and combative. Additional history revealed that she ingested up to 100 aspirin tablets on the morning of admission (about 10 hours earlier) in a suicide attempt. She complained of ringing in her ears, nausea, and three episodes of vomiting. Vital signs were BP 140/90 mmHg, pulse 110 beats/minute, respirations 36 breaths/minute, and temperature 102.5°F. V.K.'s laboratory data obtained on admission were as follows: serum sodium (Na), 148 mEq/L (normal, 135–153); potassium (K), 2.8 mEq/L (normal, 3.5–5.5); chloride (Cl), 105 mEq/L (normal, 95–105); bicarbonate, 10 mEq/L (normal, 24–31); glucose, 60 mg/dL (normal, 70–110); blood urea nitrogen (BUN), 35 mg/dL (normal, 5–25); and creatinine, 2.2 mg/dL (normal, 0.5–1.4). Arterial blood gas (ABG) values (room air) were as follows: pH, 7.25; P_{CO_2}, 20 mmHg; and P_{O_2}, 95 mmHg. A serum salicylate concentration measured approximately 12 hours after the acute ingestion was 88 mg/dL. Her hemoglobin was 9.6 g/dL (normal, 12–16 g/dL for females) with a hematocrit of 28.9% (normal, 37%–47% for females) and a prothrombin time (PT) of 16.4 seconds (normal, 10–13 seconds). Is her ingestion high risk?

The symptoms and severity of salicylate intoxication depend on the dose consumed; the patient's age; and whether the ingestion was acute, chronic, or a combination of the two.[71,73,74] This case illustrates an acute ingestion in someone who has also chronically ingested aspirin. Acute ingestion of 150 to 300 mg/kg of aspirin is likely to produce mild to moderate intoxication, >300 mg/kg indicates severe poisoning, and >500 mg/kg is potentially lethal.[68,69] V.K., who ingested approximately 600 mg/kg, has taken a potentially lethal dose. Chronic salicylate intoxication is usually associated with ingestion of >100 mg/kg/day for more than 2 days.[68,69] V.K. has been taking 70 mg/kg/day for her headaches in addition to her acute ingestion. V.K. demonstrates many of the findings typical of severe acute salicylism (see next two questions and answers). Her outcome does not look good because she is elderly and has taken a potentially lethal amount of aspirin.

Pathophysiology of Salicylate Intoxication

5. Describe the pathophysiology and clinical features of acute and chronic salicylism.

Toxicity from salicylate exposure results in direct irritation of the GI tract, direct stimulation of the CNS respiratory center, stimulation of the metabolic rate, lipid and carbohydrate metabolism disturbances, and interference with hemostasis.[68,69,71,73,74] Toxic doses of salicylate directly stimulate the medullary respiratory center leading to nausea, vomiting, tinnitus, delirium, tachypnea, seizures, and coma, and influence several key metabolic pathways.[68,71–75] Direct stimulation of the respiratory drive increases the rate and depth of ventilation, which can result in primary respiratory alkalosis. The respiratory alkalosis causes increased renal excretion of bicarbonate, resulting in decreased buffering capacity. The patient usually presents with a partially compensated respiratory alkalosis.[68,72,73,75] Hypokalemia can result from increased GI and renal losses of potassium, as well as from systemic alkalosis.[68,73,74]

Although marked metabolic and neurologic abnormalities are most commonly observed in young children with advanced salicylate intoxication, adolescents or adults acutely poisoned with a large dose can develop these symptoms as well.[68,72,73] Acute salicylism in a young child often takes a more severe course than that typically seen in adults. After acute ingestion, children quickly pass through the phase of pure respiratory alkalosis. Renal bicarbonate loss secondary to respiratory alkalosis reduces the buffering capacity more profoundly in a child and facilitates the development of metabolic acidosis.[68,71,73,75]

Salicylates have toxic effects on several biochemical pathways that contribute to metabolic acidosis and other symptoms.[68,73–75] Mitochondrial oxidative phosphorylation is uncoupled and results in an impaired ability to generate high-energy phosphates, increased oxygen use and carbon dioxide production, increased heat production and hyperpyrexia, increased tissue glycolysis, and increased peripheral demand for glucose. Salicylates also inhibit key dehydrogenase enzymes within the Krebs cycle, resulting in increased levels of pyruvate and lactate. The increased demand for peripheral glucose causes increased glycogenolysis, gluconeogenesis, lipolysis, and free fatty acid metabolism. The latter results in enhanced formation of ketoacids and ketoacidosis.[71,75]

The patient may become severely volume depleted through several mechanisms.[68,73–75] Hyperthermia and hyperventilation produce increased insensible water loss, vomiting may promote GI fluid losses, and the solute load caused by altered glucose metabolism results in an osmotic diuresis. Depending on the patient's acid–base balance and net fluid and electrolyte intake and output, serum sodium and potassium concentrations may be normal, elevated, or decreased. Hypernatremia and hypokalemia are most common.[71,73]

Blood glucose concentration is usually normal or slightly elevated, although hypoglycemia may accompany chronic salicylism (e.g., as illustrated by V.K.) or occur late in acute intoxication. CNS glucose levels can be markedly reduced in the presence of normal blood glucose concentrations because increased CNS glucose utilization to generate high-energy phosphate exceeds the rate at which glucose can be supplied.[68,71,73,75]

Other manifestations of severe acute salicylism include a variety of neurologic signs and symptoms: disorientation, irritability, hallucinations, lethargy, stupor, coma, and seizures.[67,71] Hyperthermia may be marked and can result in the inappropriate administration of aspirin as an antipyretic. Coagulopathy can occur because of impaired platelet function, hypoprothrombinemia, reduced factor VII production, and increased capillary fragility, especially when taken chronically.[73–75] Pulmonary edema and acute renal failure also can occur, but the former occurs more commonly after chronic intoxication.[73,75,76]

Chronic salicylism symptoms are similar to acute intoxications. However, patients with chronic exposures may have less GI symptoms but generally appear more ill and have more CNS symptoms.[69,77] In both adults and children, the principal signs of chronic salicylism are a partially compensated metabolic acidosis, increased anion gap, ketosis, dehydration, electrolyte loss, hyperventilation, tremors, agitation, confusion, stupor, memory deficits, renal failure, and seizures.[71,73,74,78] The severity of CNS manifestations is related to the cerebrospinal fluid (CSF) salicylate concentration.[72,73] This may increase in the presence of systemic acidosis because a greater fraction of salicylate is unionized and can cross the blood–brain barrier. Therefore, metabolic acidosis is especially dangerous in a salicylate-intoxicated patient.[71,73]

Unless the history of salicylate intake is specifically sought, the problem may not be immediately apparent, especially in the elderly in whom such findings are likely to be attributed to other causes (e.g., encephalitis, meningitis, diabetic ketoacidosis, myocardial infarction).[24,73,77] Delay in diagnosis has been associated with increased mortality.[24,68,73,77] Unfortunately, plasma salicylate concentrations do not correlate well with the degree of poisoning in chronically intoxicated patients, and it is more important to treat the patient's clinical status than his or her salicylate concentration.[68] Death in patients with salicylism, whether acute or chronic, results from CNS and/or cardiac dysfunction, or pulmonary edema.[71,73,77]

Assessment of Toxicity

6. What signs, symptoms, and laboratory values in V.K. are consistent with salicylate intoxication?

V.K. demonstrates many of the findings typical of severe acute salicylism. Hyperventilation has resulted from the direct respiratory stimulant effects of salicylate and as compensation for her metabolic acidosis (P_{CO_2}, 20 mmHg; pH, 7.25; serum bicarbonate, 10 mEq/L; respiratory rate, 36 breaths/minute). Hypokalemia (2.8 mEq/L) in the presence of metabolic acidosis represents severe potassium depletion because of increased renal and possibly GI losses. Hyperpyrexia caused by salicylate is present in V.K., although an infectious cause also must be considered. Her neurologic symptoms of lethargy, disorientation, and combativeness, as well as tinnitus, nausea, and vomiting, are commonly seen in severe salicylate intoxication. In addition, being elderly and taking a lethal amount of aspirin bodes ill for this patient's outcome.

Laboratory Evaluation

7. What objective evaluations should be assessed in a patient with presumed salicylate intoxication?

V.K.'s workup illustrates a thorough initial patient evaluation. Laboratory evaluation should include ABG values, serum electrolytes, BUN, serum creatinine, blood glucose, and a complete blood count (CBC).[71,73,74] Urine should be tested for specific gravity and pH.[71] In symptomatic patients, a prothrombin (PT), international normalized ratio (INR), and partial thromboplastin times (PTT) are useful to assess the presence of salicylate-induced coagulopathy. Vitals signs should be monitored for an increased respiratory rate and hyperpyrexia.[72,73] Physical examination should include an evaluation of chest x-ray, cardiopulmonary and neurologic function, and measurement of urine output.[73]

A salicylate blood concentration should be obtained 6 hours after an acute ingestion at a known time, immediately and 6 hours after an acute ingestion of an unknown time, and immediately and every 2 to 6 hours in symptomatic patients.[24,65,71,73,79] Repeat a serum salicylate measurement every 4 to 6 hours to verify that the original concentration represented a peak level and that the salicylate level is decreasing rather than increasing.[24,68,71,74,79] Obtaining the units of measurement on salicylate serum concentrations is essential because different laboratories report concentrations in different units (e.g., mg/dL, mcg/mL, mmol/L). An incorrect interpretation of the salicylate unit of measurement can result in overestimates or underestimates of the severity.[24]

Historically, the Done-nomogram was used to determine the degree of toxicity from a known single acute salicylate ingestion by plotting the serum salicylate concentration by time since the ingestion.[80] However, clinical symptoms and laboratory findings are more useful in identifying the degree of acute intoxication, assessing patient prognosis, and guiding therapy.[79] In case of chronic ingestions, the nomogram is not useful, and other parameters such as acid–base and electrolyte balance should be used to determine severity of the case.[68,71]

The Done-nomogram is also not useful in certain situations such as ingestion of enteric-coated or sustained-release salicylate products, when the time of ingestion is unknown, or when the patient is acidemic or has renal failure.[71,73,74,79–81] The nomogram is probably not useful when salicylate serum concentrations are measured more than 12 hours after ingestion. Serum concentrations obtained less than 6 hours after ingestion in acute ingestion situations are also difficult to interpret because the drug level has not yet peaked and can result in an underestimation of the eventual degree of intoxication.[68,71,78,81] Salicylate concentrations can continue to rise over approximately 24 hours if a large amount has been taken or if enteric-coated tablets have been ingested. Enteric-coated tablets can clump together forming a bezoar that slowly releases drug into the gut.[73,79] The Done-nomogram is no longer used because of these difficulties in interpreting salicylate concentrations.[24]

Management

8. What would be a reasonable management plan for V.K.?

Management of salicylate intoxication depends on the degree of acid–base and electrolyte disturbances.[68,71,73] Activated charcoal is not indicated for V.K because the ingestion occurred about 10 hours ago and she has a somewhat altered mental status.[43] The risk of aspiration is greater than the value of possibly adsorbing any remaining aspirin from the GI tract. In addition, V.K. already has symptoms of salicylate poisoning, indicating that the aspirin has already been absorbed. V.K.'s hypokalemia, acidosis, and hypoglycemia must be corrected, and is probably best accomplished through the administration of intravenous (IV) hypotonic saline-dextrose solutions combined with potassium supplementation. This solution is administered at a rate that replaces the patient's deficits and keeps pace with continued losses.[68,71,73–75] Care should be taken to avoid overzealous fluid therapy, which can predispose the patient to cerebral or pulmonary edema.[73,75] Administration of an IV dextrose bolus is also indicated because V.K. is also hypoglycemic (60 mg/dL).[71,73,75]

SODIUM BICARBONATE

It is important to correct V.K.'s acidosis because acidosis will increase CSF salicylate concentrations.[72,73] Correction of acidosis can be accomplished by adding sodium bicarbonate to her IV fluids.[68,71–74] V.K.'s serum sodium and potassium concentrations should be monitored closely.[80] It is essential to provide adequate ventilation to prevent respiratory alkalosis. With a respiratory rate of 36 breaths/minute, placing the patient on a ventilator to assist with breathing might be considered. However, forced mechanical ventilation can interfere with the patient's need to compensate to maintain the serum pH. Patients on ventilators can become severely acidotic, which can result in death because of an inability to compensate adequately.[71,82]

SEIZURES

Seizures are not evident in V.K. but can be encountered in cases of severe salicylate poisoning. Seizures generally carry a poor prognosis and are indicative of severe salicylate intoxication that requires hemodialysis.[71] Other treatable causes of seizures (e.g., marked alkalosis, hypoglycemia, hyponatremia) can be present in individuals such as V.K. and should be ruled out. If seizures occur, benzodiazepines are the drugs of choice for treatment.[71]

COAGULOPATHY AND HYPERTHERMIA

Coagulopathy generally responds to vitamin K_1, which should be given if the PT or INR is prolonged.[71] GI bleeding or other hemorrhage can occur, but not commonly.[71,73,74] Mild hyperthermia usually does not require therapy, but cooling fans and mist may be required for extremely elevated temperatures.[71,75]

PULMONARY EDEMA

Noncardiogenic pulmonary edema commonly occurs in salicylate intoxications, especially when the overdose is attributable to chronic ingestions.[71,73,76] Pulmonary edema is associated with a high incidence of neurologic symptoms in patients and can occur even without fluid overload.[73,76] Increased alveolar capillary membrane permeability, prostaglandin effects, and a metabolic interaction with platelets releasing membrane permeability substances are the primary mechanisms for the cause of pulmonary edema associated with salicylate overdose.[76] Treatment is aimed at reducing salicylate levels via alkalinization or hemodialysis.[76]

ALKALINE DIURESIS

9. What measures will enhance salicylate elimination? Which of these may be indicated in V.K.?

Forced alkaline diuresis and hemodialysis can enhance the excretion of salicylate in overdose situations.[68] Hemodialysis is preferred because it can also correct fluid and electrolyte imbalances.[73,76,78] Sodium bicarbonate is recommended for alkaline diuresis to reduce the arterial pH with the goal of minimizing salicylate transport into the CNS.[72,73,75]

Although large doses of sodium bicarbonate together with forced fluids can enhance the renal elimination of the weak acid and shorten its half-life, this treatment does not favorably influence the morbidity or mortality of patients with salicylism. Alkaline diuresis can also place the patient at risk for sodium and fluid retention, as well as pulmonary edema, if too much fluid is given too quickly.[71,73,74,76] Furthermore, whether the urine can be adequately alkalinized (pH >7) in severely intoxicated pediatric patients has been questioned because of the large acid load that is excreted.[68,71,72] Nevertheless, urine alkalinization with sodium bicarbonate should be attempted in severely salicylate-intoxicated adult patients such as V.K.

Potassium replacement in patients receiving alkaline diuresis is essential.[71,73,75] These patients may require large amounts of potassium supplementation due to renal wasting of potassium. The risk for pulmonary edema can be minimized if this is done without forcing fluids.[71,73,74,75]

Hemodialysis should be considered in patients who show progression of severe salicylate intoxication and seizure activity, renal failure, or plasma salicylate concentrations in the potentially fatal range.[68,73,74,76,78] Patients with a chronic exposure, with acidosis, or CNS symptoms, and who are elderly or ill, are high-risk patients and should be considered for early dialysis.[73,78] Because V.K. has many of the risk factors, she is a candidate for emergent hemodialysis.

Clinical Outcome of Patient V.K.

A repeat salicylate level 6 hours later (18 hours after ingestion) had increased to 93 mg/dL. Her chemistry panel revealed serum sodium (Na), 144 mEq/L (normal, 135–153); potassium (K), 2.1 mEq/L (normal, 3.5–5.5); chloride (Cl), 100 mEq/L (normal, 95–105); bicarbonate, 9 mEq/L (normal, 24–31); glucose, 78 mg/dL (normal, 70–110); creatinine, 4.8 mg/dL (normal, 0.5–1.4); and BUN, 42 mg/dL (normal, 5–25). Her hemoglobin was now 8.5 g/dL (normal, 12–16 for females) with a hematocrit of 23% (normal, 37%–47% for females) and a PT of 16.6 seconds (normal, 10–13 seconds). V.K.'s pH on blood gases remained in the 7.2 to 7.3 range. Urinary alkalinization was attempted with a high-dose IV sodium bicarbonate infusion in an attempt to reach a urine pH of 7.5. However, her urine pH never increased above pH 5.6. V.K. became fluid overloaded and developed dyspnea. She was placed on a ventilator with worsening of her symptoms. A chest radiograph showed pulmonary edema. V.K. became confused and agitated, pulling at her IV lines and trying to get out of bed. Nephrology was consulted to provide emergent hemodialysis to correct the acidosis, electrolyte abnormalities, and fluid overload. As the catheter was being placed, the patient had a tonic-clonic seizure. Diazepam 10 mg IV was administered, and the seizure stopped. At this time, the patient was unresponsive. The NG tube revealed the presence of copious amounts of bright red blood. She was rushed to surgery for an emergency laparotomy. On the way to the operating room, she had another seizure, went into respiratory arrest, coded, and could not be resuscitated.

ASSESSMENT OF IRON INGESTION

Gathering History and Communications

10. The grandmother of R.F., a 20-month-old boy, calls the ED of a nearby hospital because her grandson is vomiting and appears to have been playing with some green tablets. The child was left alone in his room for about 15 minutes to take a nap. Why might the consultation with this grandmother be expected to be more difficult than the consultation in question 1?

Phone calls to a health care provider, a health care facility, or a poison control center from individuals other than the parent are usually more difficult to manage. The caller may not be able to provide all patient-specific information needed (e.g., patient weight, chronic medications) to accurately assess the drug ingestion. Supplemental information is often needed from a parent. Furthermore, nonparent callers tend to be more upset over an unintentional ingestion and may have more difficulty than a parent in taking decisive action.

Triage of Call

11. Despite additional questioning, the grandmother cannot identify the tablets and cannot find any labeling or empty medicine containers that could help in the tablet identification. R.F. is still

vomiting, and some of the vomitus is green-colored like the tablets. There are three children in the household and two adults who take medications for various chronic illnesses. According to the grandmother, R.F. is healthy, and no one else in the household currently has the "flu" or other GI illness. The child's mother gave birth 3 weeks ago and is now at her obstetrician's office for a postnatal visit. What recommendations could be provided to this grandmother at this time?

With this history, the practitioner should consider whether the information presented by R.F.'s grandmother is consistent with a drug ingestion and whether this incident is likely to be associated with a significant adverse outcome. Most 2-year-old children experience limited toxicity with unintentional drug ingestions because only a relatively small amount of substance is usually ingested. Nevertheless, some substances (e.g., methanol, ethylene glycol, nicotine, caustic substances, camphor, chloroquine, clonidine, diphenoxylate-atropine, theophylline, oral hypoglycemic agents, calcium channel blockers, tricyclic antidepressants [TCAs]) can produce significant toxicity when only small amounts are ingested.[83,84]

Although the history of drug ingestion in R.F. is somewhat vague, the description of a green tablet, the vomiting of green material, and the recent pregnancy of his mother suggests possible ingestion of prenatal iron tablets. Because this exposure would be categorized as an unknown toxicity with a realistic potential for severe toxicity if iron tablets were ingested, R.F. should bring the child to the ED for evaluation. Depending on the distance to the hospital and the anxiety level of the grandmother, the practitioner might want to instruct the grandmother to call for emergency medical services transportation rather than relying on other means of transportation. She should be instructed to take the green tablets to the ED along with the child so the tablets can be identified. Other medications that are in the house should also be taken to the ED, and the mother should be contacted at the obstetrician's office.

Substance Identification

12. R.F.'s mother has been contacted and has confirmed that the only green tablets in the house are her prenatal iron supplements. She is in close proximity to the hospital and will await the arrival of her son. R.F. arrived 20 minutes later along with one green tablet and an empty prescription container that was found by his older brother. R.F. is still vomiting but is awake and alert with a heart rate of 125 beats/minute, a respiratory rate of 28 breaths/minute, a temperature of 99.1°F, and pulse oximetry of 99%. How can the maximum potential severity of this ingestion be estimated at this time?

R.F.'s vital signs, when corrected for age, are normal. Attention should now focus on identifying the ingested substance and the maximum potential severity of the ingestion. Although this case involves an unknown ingestion, with a possibility of being a severe iron intoxication, the identity of the tablets still has not been verified. Therefore, R.F. must be carefully assessed, and the ingestion history reaffirmed.

All solid dosage prescription drugs are required by the U.S. Food and Drug Administration (FDA) to have identification markings. Reference books (e.g., *Facts and Comparisons, Physicians Desk Reference*),[85] computerized databases (e.g., IDENTIDEX),[86] and the product manufacturers can assist in identifying solid dosage forms. The imprint code markings on the green tablet brought to the ED with R.F., the empty medication container, and the mother's assistance should be sufficient to correctly identify the tablet. The identification of this green tablet will most likely establish the toxicity potential because most childhood ingestions usually involve only one substance. Once the tablet has been identified, the maximum number of tablets ingested should be estimated. The label on the empty medication container should provide information on the identity and number of tablets dispensed. If the medication container is unlabeled, the date the prescription was obtained, the number of estimated doses taken, and the number currently remaining in the medication container can be used to approximate the maximum number of tablets that were ingested.

R.F.'s vital signs and symptoms should be monitored at frequent intervals to evaluate whether his clinical status is consistent with expectations based on the suspected ingestion. Nausea, vomiting, diarrhea, and abdominal pain are commonly encountered early in the course of iron intoxication.[87–92] The absence of symptoms, however, should not be interpreted as an indication that a poisoning has not occurred, especially if the patient is being evaluated within a short time after the presumed ingestion.[87,89–92]

Evaluating Severity of Toxicity

13. R.F. weighs 22 lb, appears to be in no apparent distress, and has stopped vomiting. About 30 mL of dark-colored vomitus was recovered, but no tablets are seen, and testing demonstrates that no blood is present in the vomitus. A maximum of 11 tablets were ingested based on the bottle label and the mother's recall. What degree of toxicity should be expected in R.F.?

The potential severity of ingestion can be estimated for commonly ingested drugs such as acetaminophen,[93] salicylates,[69] iron,[87] and TCAs[94] because of well-established dose–toxicity relationships. Acute elemental iron ingestions of <20 mg/kg are usually nontoxic, 20 to 60 mg/kg doses result in mild to moderate toxicity, and >60 mg/kg doses are severe and potentially fatal.[88,90,92]

The label on the prescription medication container, as well as independent verification of the tablet by R.F.'s mother and the tablet imprint, indicate that each tablet contained 300 mg of ferrous sulfate in an enteric-coated formulation. Because the dose–toxicity relationship of iron is based on the amount of elemental iron ingested, knowledge of the specific iron salt is important in calculating the ingested dose. Ferrous sulfate contains 20% elemental iron, ferrous gluconate contains 12%, and ferrous fumarate contains 33%.[87,88,90,91] Therefore, each 300-mg ferrous sulfate tablet contains 60 mg of elemental iron. R.F. ingested a maximum of 11 enteric-coated ferrous sulfate 300-mg tablets and he weighs 22 lb (10 kg); therefore, his ingestion of ~66 mg/kg of iron places him at risk of severe toxicity. Although R.F.'s only symptom is vomiting at this time, absorption could be delayed because he ingested an enteric-coated formulation.

Abdominal Radiographs

14. R.F. is expected to experience potentially severe toxicity from his ingestion of iron. Why would an abdominal radiograph

(x-ray) be useful to verify the number of iron tablets that were actually ingested?

Radiodense substances (e.g., iron, enteric-coated tablets, chloral hydrate, phenothiazines, heavy metals), theoretically, can be visualized in the GI tract by an abdominal radiograph.[94] The ability of a radiograph (x-ray) to demonstrate the presence of a radiodense substance, however, depends on the dosage form, concentration, and the molecular weight of the substance. The intact dosage form can often be detected if the tablet has not already disintegrated or dissolved.[95] Less than one-third of pediatric abdominal radiographs show positive evidence of tablets or granules after iron poisoning.[96]

Keep in mind that children are more likely than adults to chew tablets rather than swallow them whole, and false-negative results can occur even when whole tablets have not already started to disintegrate. If the tablets were chewed, an abdominal radiograph to verify the number of ingested iron tablets is not likely to be useful. However, an abdominal radiograph after the completion of GI decontamination can help assess whether additional decontamination is needed.[95]

Gastrointestinal Decontamination

15. Why would gastric lavage and/or activated charcoal not be indicated for the management of R.F.'s iron ingestion?

When selecting a GI decontamination method, one should consider the substance ingested, maximum potential toxicity expected from the drug dosage form, potential time course of toxicity, time elapsed between ingestion and the initiation of treatment, symptoms, and physical examination findings. Decontamination with activated charcoal is not indicated because R.F. has ingested iron tablets, which do not adsorb to activated charcoal.[50,87,97] Gastric lavage would also not be effective because the removal of large undissolved iron tablets from the stomach is limited by the small internal diameter of the gastric lavage tube, especially in pediatric patients.[97,98]

Whole Bowel Irrigation

16. What other method of GI decontamination should be considered for R.F.?

WBI with a polyethylene glycol electrolyte solution can be considered in this case. WBI fluid can be administered orally, or infused by NG tube at a rate of 1.5 to 2 L/hour for adults and at a rate of 500 mL/hour for children.[99,100] Although the large volume of fluid to be ingested over a short period of time (several hours) and the frequent association of the nausea and vomiting often result in poor patient compliance, R.F. is hospitalized and the fluid can be infused by NG tube if needed. WBI should be continued until the rectal effluent is clear, which may take many hours.[99,100]

Monitoring Effectiveness of Treatment

17. How should the effectiveness of GI decontamination be assessed in the ED?

The simplest method of assessing GI decontamination is to visually inspect the return fluid from the WBI. Increasing serum iron concentrations, deteriorating clinical status, or evidence of radiodense tablets in the GI tract on abdominal radiograph would warrant more aggressive treatment.[88–90,96]

Serum Iron Concentrations

18. At this time, R.F. has no evidence of CNS or cardiovascular symptoms that can occur with toxic iron ingestions. He did have one large dark-colored diarrheal stool that tested negative for blood. A serum iron concentration, obtained about 3 hours after the ingestion, was 470 mcg/dL (normal, 60–160 mcg/dL). What conclusions as to severity or likely clinical outcome can be derived from this serum concentration?

The serum iron concentration provides an indication as to whether more aggressive therapy is needed.[92,96,101] The higher than normal serum iron concentration confirms the suspicion that R.F. has ingested iron tablets despite both his current lack of serious symptoms and the absence of tablet evidence in the rectal effluent or abdominal radiograph.

The time course of absorption is probably the most difficult pharmacokinetic parameter to evaluate with toxic ingestions. For example, drug concentrations can continue to rise after an overdose despite GI decontamination.[89,91,92,101] This prolongation of absorption time is even further complicated when sustained-release or enteric-coated dosage formulations have been ingested because the onset of symptoms is unpredictable.[90]

R.F.'s serum iron concentration of 470 mcg/dL at this time suggests a serious ingestion because peak serum iron concentrations >500 mcg/dL are usually predictive of significant toxicity.[89–92,96,101] This single serum iron concentration, however, does not provide information as to whether the serum concentration is rising or declining nor when the serum iron concentration will peak as a result of his iron ingestion.[102] Iron tablets may also clump together and form a concretion or bezoar. Bezoar formation can result in prolonged absorption and delay the onset of toxicity.[89,92] Samples for peak serum iron concentration should be obtained 4 to 6 hours after ingestion.[90–92] Although R.F.'s serum iron concentration was measured approximately 3 hours after ingestion, another serum iron measurement in 2 to 4 hours is needed because he ingested an enteric-coated formulation.

Blood Glucose, White Blood Cell Count, and Total Iron Binding Capacity

19. R.F. had WBI administered through the NG tube for 4 hours until the rectal effluent was clear. At this time, R.F. began to vomit numerous times and became drowsy and fussy. A second serum iron concentration was ordered (i.e., 6 hours after ingestion). What other laboratory tests could be helpful in assessing the potential toxicity of iron in R.F.?

Blood glucose concentrations and white blood cell (WBC) counts usually are increased when serum iron concentrations are >300 mcg/dL. A WBC count >15,000/mm^3 and a blood glucose concentration >150 mg/dL within 6 hours of an ingestion generally suggest a greater likelihood of severe iron intoxication.[88] These tests provide supplemental confirmation of iron intoxication and can be useful in medical facilities in which serum iron concentrations cannot be obtained. Sensitivity of these tests are low (about 50%), and treatment should not be based on a WBC and glucose concentration alone.[89–91,96] These laboratory tests are not routinely monitored in iron poisoning because of the poor sensitivity.[90]

It was once believed that if the serum iron concentration exceeded the total iron binding capacity (TIBC) concentration, it would be a substantiate iron toxicity. The correlation between the TIBC concentration and iron toxicity, however, has not held up, and the TIBC test is no longer used to monitor iron toxicity.[92]

Stages of Iron Toxicity

20. It is now 6 hours since R.F. ingested the iron tablets. His second serum iron concentration is not yet available. He continues to be fussy and drowsy but has missed his usual afternoon nap. He has several more episodes of vomiting. Why is R.F.'s relatively mild course at this time not particularly reassuring?

The time between the ingestion of an overdose of drugs and the development of severe toxicity is often delayed. It is unclear in some cases why there is an asymptomatic period, but it may be secondary to delayed absorption of the ingested drug, the time required for the drug distribution, or the time needed to form a toxic metabolite. Consequently, R.F. may still develop further symptoms of severe toxicity. Four distinct stages of symptoms can be encountered with iron toxicity.[87–92]

Stage I

Stage I symptoms usually occur within 6 hours of ingestion. During this time, nausea, vomiting, diarrhea, and abdominal pain are encountered and are probably secondary to the erosive effects of iron on the GI mucosa. The caustic effects of free iron can cause bleeding as evidenced by blood in the vomitus and stool. In more severe intoxications, CNS and cardiovascular toxicity can be present during Stage I.[89–92]

Stage II

The second stage of iron toxicity is characterized as a period of decreasing symptoms and an apparent improvement in the clinical condition. This stage can last for up to 12 to 24 hours after the ingestion and could be misinterpreted as resolving toxicity. This stage might represent the time needed for the absorbed iron to distribute throughout the body before systemic symptoms develop.[87] Alternatively, this stage might merely reflect patients who did not receive treatment early in the course of intoxication and appeared to be well before systemic effects developed.[86] It is unknown why this stage of apparent improvement occurs with iron toxicity. In most severe cases, Stage II is not encountered and the patient's condition continues to progressively deteriorate.[89,92]

Stage III

Stage III generally occurs 12 to 48 hours after iron ingestion and is characterized by CNS toxicity (e.g., lethargy, coma, seizures) and cardiovascular toxicity (e.g., hypotension, shock, pulmonary edema). Metabolic acidosis, hypoglycemia, hepatic necrosis, renal damage, and coagulopathy can be experienced at this stage.[89–92]

Stage IV

The final stage is apparent 4 to 6 weeks after acute iron ingestion and consists of late-appearing GI tract sequelae that are secondary to the initial local toxicity. In this stage, prior tissue damage can progress to gastric scarring and strictures at the pylorus, resulting in permanent abnormalities of GI function.[89–92]

Patients can present to the health care facility in any stage of iron toxicity and can have a fatal outcome in any stage. Assigning a stage of toxicity should not be based on time since ingestion, but instead should be based on clinical symptoms.[91]

Deferoxamine Chelation

21. The clinical laboratory has reported that the second serum iron concentration that was obtained 6 hours after ingestion from R.F. has increased from 470 to 553 mcg/dL. He has continued to vomit. R.F.'s mother states that the child looks "pale" to her. What criteria are most important in determining whether the antidote deferoxamine should be administered to R.F.?

[SI units: 84.18 and 99.04 μmol/L, respectively]

Deferoxamine (Desferal) chelates iron by binding ferric ions in plasma to form the iron complex ferrioxamine.[90] Deferoxamine prevents iron toxicity at a cellular level by removing iron from mitochondria.[88] Unfortunately, a relatively small amount of iron is bound (approximately 9 mg of iron to 100 mg of deferoxamine).[102,103] The iron-deferoxamine complex primarily is excreted renally as ferrioxamine.[88,90,91] Renal elimination of the ferrioxamine usually results in a pinkish-orange urine, often described as "vin rose."[88,90,91] Deferoxamine therapy should be initiated when serum iron concentrations exceed 500 mcg/dL and when symptoms of iron toxicity (e.g., GI symptoms, hemorrhage, coma, shock, seizures) are present.[88–91] R.F. is experiencing symptoms, he presumably ingested up to 66 mg/kg of elemental iron, and iron absorption appears to be ongoing based on the increase in his serum iron concentration. Therefore, R.F. should be treated with deferoxamine.

Deferoxamine Dose

22. What dose of deferoxamine should be prescribed for R.F., and how should it be administered?

Deferoxamine is more effective when administered intravenously as a constant infusion due to the short half-life of the deferoxamine (76 ± 10 minutes).[89,91,102] Clinically, a slow IV infusion is preferred over intramuscular (IM) administration because the dose administered can be better controlled, is less painful, and is better absorbed than an intramuscularly administered dose.[91,92] Deferoxamine 15 mg/kg/hour is usually administered in a continuous IV infusion; however, doses up to 45 mg/kg/hour have been used in patients with severe iron poisoning.[89–92,102] Hypotension can result from administering IV boluses of deferoxamine too rapidly.[89,90,92,102,103] According to the manufacturer, the total deferoxamine dose should not exceed 6 g every 24 hours when administered to adults or children, but adverse effects have not been seen in patients who received more than 6 g every 24 hours.[91,103]

If IV access is not readily available or if the patient is transported to another medical facility for treatment, deferoxamine should be administered intramuscularly.[88,103] The usual IM dose of deferoxamine for the treatment of acute iron intoxication is 90 mg/kg, not to exceed a maximum of 1 g per dose.[103]

The dose can be repeated every 4 to 12 hours, depending on the clinical status of the patient.[103] Pain at the injection site, as well as induration, is common after IM administration.[91,103]

Deferoxamine should be initially administered to R.F. at a rate of about 8 mg/kg/hour, and his clinical status should be monitored closely. If the dose is tolerated, the rate can be increased every 5 minutes until the desired dose of 15 mg/kg/hour is achieved.[89]

Monitoring and Discontinuation

23. R.F. is admitted to the pediatric ICU 1 hour after the initiation of a deferoxamine infusion at 8 mg/kg/hour. How should deferoxamine therapy be monitored, and when should it be discontinued?

The rate of deferoxamine infusion should be increased if symptoms of severe iron toxicity develop, and the dosage should be decreased if adverse effects develop.[89,90,92,103] The infusion of deferoxamine should be continued until the serum iron concentration is $<$100 mcg/dL and symptoms of iron toxicity are no longer present.[103] Patients will require chelation therapy for about 1 to 2 days, depending on the severity of symptoms.[89–91] Chelation therapy that continues longer than necessary should be avoided because deferoxamine infusion for more than 24 hours has been associated with the development of acute respiratory distress syndrome.[89–91]

The urine color change to "vin rose" indicates ferrioxamine in the urine.[88,82] The disappearance of the "vin rose" color should not be used as a reliable marker of adequacy of deferoxamine therapy because not all patients experience vin rose urine.[88,92] There is no correlation between amount of iron ingested, serum iron concentration, and the urine color change.[88]

Deferoxamine can interfere with some laboratory methods used to measure serum iron concentrations and cause falsely low values.[88,89,101,104] To monitor serum iron concentrations when deferoxamine has been started, using atomic absorptive spectroscopy is recommended.[103] When deferoxamine is initiated, the clinical laboratory should be contacted to clarify whether deferoxamine will interfere with their serum iron analysis.

Outcome of Patient R.F.

R.F. was admitted to pediatric ICU overnight and treated with a constant infusion of deferoxamine at 15 mg/kg/hour for 13 hours. His GI symptoms were no longer apparent, he became more alert, and his vitals signs were stable. An analysis of a free iron blood sample the next morning revealed a serum iron level of 67 mcg/dL. He was discharged home that afternoon.

[SI units: 11.99 μmol/L]

ASSESSMENT OF CENTRAL NERVOUS SYSTEM DEPRESSANT VERSUS ANTIDEPRESSANT INGESTION

Validation of Ingestion

24. T.C., a 34-year-old unconscious woman, was found lying on the couch with a suicide note. The note stated that she had ingested 25 of her pills. On discovering T.C. unresponsive, T.C.'s 15-year-old daughter called paramedics. When the paramedics arrived, T.C.'s heart rate was 145 beats/minute, BP was 105/65 mmHg, and respirations were 12 breaths/minute and shallow. T.C. was found in a pool of vomitus. T.C. responded only to painful stimuli. The paramedics immediately started an IV line after completing their assessment of her ABCs. Why should the drug overdose information from this suicidal patient be validated?

Assessing the accuracy of historical information in adult drug exposures is difficult, and many health care professionals question the validity of information, especially from suicidal patients.[22–26] The ingestion history could be inaccurate because the patient's altered mental status might prevent accurate recollection of what occurred. She may also try to intentionally mislead health care providers to minimize appropriate care. The supposition that the drug overdose history from a patient is unreliable is based on studies demonstrating poor correlation between stated drug ingestions and urine drug test results.[23–26,29,30,105]

Urine drug screens generally detect all recent drug and substance use, rather than just an overdosed drug. Urine drug screen results, therefore, are not reliable indicators of acute exposures. Every effort should be made to validate the history with information from other sources. In suicidal patients, one should consider all drugs that may have been available to the patient, as well as the patient's presenting symptoms, laboratory tests, and information obtained from family members, police, paramedics, and other individuals who know the patient.[22–26]

Interventions by Protocol

25. In addition to managing the ABCs, what pharmacologic interventions should be authorized for the paramedics to administer to T.C. in addition to the initiation of an IV solution?

Glucose and Thiamine

Emergency medical service personnel often have protocols directing them to treat patients who are unconscious from an unknown cause. These protocols generally include administration of glucose, thiamine, and naloxone.[23,26,61,106] If paramedics cannot measure a blood glucose concentration immediately, T.C. should be given 50 mL of 50% dextrose to treat possible hypoglycemia. The risks of hyperglycemia from this dose of glucose are negligible relative to the significant benefits if the patient is hypoglycemic. Thiamine should be administered concurrently with glucose because glucose can precipitate the Wernicke-Korsakoff complex in thiamine-deficient patients[107] (see Chapter 84). Wernicke's encephalopathy is a reversible neurologic disturbance consisting of generalized confusion, ataxia, and ophthalmoplegia. Korsakoff's psychosis is believed to be irreversible and is associated with a more prolonged deficiency of thiamine.[107,108]

This unconscious patient should also be evaluated for blood loss, hypoxia, and evidence of head trauma.[22]

Naloxone

The pure opiate antagonist, naloxone, is indicated for the treatment of respiratory depression induced by opioids,[106,109] but many emergency medical service protocols authorize paramedics to routinely administer naloxone to all patients with decreased mental status.[109] Naloxone reportedly has reversed coma and acute respiratory depression in intoxicated patients who have no evidence of opiate use.[60,108] The response of these patients to naloxone might have been secondary to opioids that were not detected by the urine toxicology screens (e.g., oxycodone, fentanyl). Drug-induced CNS depression usually waxes and wanes, and reports of naloxone success in patients who have not used opioids could also have been the result of responses to needle sticks, movement, or other stimuli rather than to naloxone.

Administering naloxone to an opioid-addicted patient can result in withdrawal symptoms (e.g., agitation, combativeness, vomiting, diarrhea, lacrimation, rhinorrhea) that can further complicate the intoxication picture.[61] Small doses of naloxone should be administered initially to determine the patient's response to this medication. Violent and aggressive behavior can be precipitated when sudden increased consciousness is induced by naloxone.[24] This can complicate emergency care in an emergency transport vehicle and put caregivers and patients at risk for trauma.[61]

Initial Treatment

26. The paramedics arrive at the ED with T.C. 30 minutes after her daughter called them. T.C.'s heart rate in the ED is 148 beats/minute, BP is 90/55 mmHg, and respirations have decreased from 12 breaths/minute, spontaneous and shallow, to 7 breaths/minute, with assisted ventilation from a bag-valve mask. T.C. remains unresponsive. The paramedics were unable to find any prescriptions or other medications in the house. Her daughter believed that her mother was taking medication for depression, but she could not be more specific. The police will notify T.C.'s husband and try to obtain additional information about the ingested substance. What initial treatment should be provided for T.C. in the ED?

T.C. should be intubated and mechanically ventilated with 100% oxygen because of her shallow, slow respirations and the likelihood that vomitus could have been aspirated into her lungs. The blood pressure taken by the paramedics was 105/65 mmHg and now is 90/55 mmHg. A bolus of IV fluid should be administered to T.C. to determine whether an increase in her intravascular fluid volume will increase her blood pressure and improve her mental status.[22,39]

Antidotes

27. T.C.'s husband reports that T.C. is under the care of a psychiatrist for depression and two previous suicide attempts. He does not know the identity of her medication, but attempts are underway to contact T.C.'s psychiatrist. What antidotes can be administered in the ED for diagnostic purposes? Should flumazenil (Romazicon) be administered?

Theoretically, antidotes such as naloxone, flumazenil, deferoxamine, and antidigoxin FAB fragments could be administered in a hospitalized setting to identify an unknown toxin.[24,59,110] However, the costs, time required for administration, and increased risks from these antidotes preclude their use for diagnostic purposes without some plausible suspicion of a specific drug ingestion. Although naloxone and flumazenil can reverse CNS depression caused by opioids and benzodiazepines, respectively, their use is not appropriate without historical, clinical, or toxicologic laboratory findings, which suggest that one of these drugs is a cause of T.C.'s intoxication.

Organ System Evaluations

28. How can the initial physical assessment, using an organ systems approach, help in identifying the drugs ingested by T.C.?

The patient's ABCs and CNS and cardiopulmonary functions should be assessed with special attention to clinical manifestations that suggest ingestion of a specific class of drugs.[26,39] For example, T.C.'s history of depression suggests that antidepressants, antipsychotics, lithium, and/or benzodiazepines are candidates for ingestion in her case. An organ system evaluation will help determine whether these (or other) drugs might have been ingested. Nonprescription medications such as aspirin, acetaminophen, decongestants, and antihistamines, which are commonly available in most households, should also be considered because adult drug ingestions usually involve more than one drug.

Central Nervous System Function

Changes in CNS function are probably the single most common finding associated with drug intoxication.[26] CNS depression or stimulation, seizures, delirium, hallucinations, coma, or any combination of these can be manifested in intoxicated patients. CNS changes can be the direct result of an ingested drug or may be additive to other underlying CNS processes or medical conditions. Many drug overdoses can produce different clinical manifestations at various times during the intoxication and different doses can produce different effects as well.[26,65]

Drugs with anticholinergic properties can produce disorientation, confusion, delirium, and visual hallucinations early in the course of the intoxication; coma can become apparent as toxicity progresses. Generally, overdoses with anticholinergic drugs do not produce true hallucinations, but rather pseudohallucinations. When a patient with an intact baseline mental status presents with psychosis, paranoia, or visual hallucinations, CNS stimulants such as cocaine or amphetamines should be considered.[26,63] Drug intoxication–induced alterations in CNS function are initially difficult to distinguish from those caused by underlying psychiatric disorders, trauma, hypoxia, or metabolic disorders, such as hepatic encephalopathy or hypoglycemia. However, with the passage of time, decreased CNS function secondary to drug toxicity is more likely to wax and wane in severity in contrast to the more constant CNS depression that occurs with significant trauma or metabolic disorders. Drug toxicity also rarely produces focal neurologic findings. Changes in pupil size, reflexes, and vital signs can provide insights into the pharmacologic class of drug involved in the intoxication.[24,26,27]

CNS depression, seizures, disorientation, and other CNS changes that are commonly associated with drugs likely to be prescribed by psychiatrists should be evaluated carefully in T.C. For example, T.C.'s pupil size would most likely be dilated if she had ingested a TCA because of the anticholinergic effects of these drugs. TCA intoxications can also cause myoclonic spasms.[26] These spasms are often difficult to differentiate from seizure activity caused by TCA overdoses, although the spasms are often asymmetric and more persistent.[111]

Cardiovascular Function

Assessment of heart rate, rhythm, conduction, and measurements of hemodynamic function can also be used to help identify the type of drug ingested. For example, overdoses of sympathomimetic drugs usually increase heart rate. Overdoses of cardiac glycosides or beta-blockers can slow the heart rate. Although drugs can increase or decrease heart rate directly, indirect cardiac effects (e.g., reflex tachycardia in response to hypotension) also need to be considered. Abnormal heart rates produced by drug overdoses are usually not treated unless hypotension or severe dysrhythmias are precipitated.[26,39]

Pulmonary Function

Evaluating the rate and depth of respiration and the effectiveness of gas exchange in an intoxicated patient can also help identify drugs that might have been ingested. For example, a decrease in respiratory rate is commonly associated with the ingestion of CNS depressants. An increased respiratory rate and depth is generally associated with CNS stimulant toxicity. An increase in respiratory rate can also be secondary to respiratory compensation for a drug-induced metabolic acidosis.[26] Aspiration of gastric contents after vomiting is a common event in drug ingestions. Aspiration pneumonitis is the most common pulmonary abnormality associated with significant intoxications.[43] Noncardiogenic acute pulmonary edema has been associated with drug overdoses of salicylates[75–78] (especially with chronic intoxications) and the use of drugs of abuse (e.g., cocaine and heroin).[112–119]

Temperature Regulation

Body temperature is an important and sometimes overlooked parameter when assessing potential intoxications.[24,39] Decreased mental status is often associated with a loss of thermoregulation, and this results in a body temperature that falls or increases toward the ambient temperature. Increased body temperature (hyperthermia) caused by overdoses of CNS stimulants (e.g., cocaine, amphetamines, ecstasy), salicylates, hallucinogens (e.g., phencyclidine), or anticholinergic drugs or plants (e.g., jimsonweed) can have serious consequences.[24,26,39] Body temperature should be measured rectally to obtain an accurate representation of core body temperature.[120]

Hyperthermia caused by drug overdoses is commonly encountered in hot, humid environments or when the intoxication is associated with physical exertion, increased muscle tone, or seizures. In these patients, it is important to obtain renal function tests (e.g., BUN, serum creatinine) and a serum creatine kinase (CK) measurement to determine whether rhabdomyolysis has occurred secondary to breakdown of muscle tissue.[24,39,120]

Gastrointestinal Function

The GI tract should be assessed for decreased motility because drug absorption can be delayed or prolonged.[26,121] When this is the case, decontamination may be beneficial after an oral ingestion even if a long period of time has elapsed since the ingestion. The presence of blood in either emesis or stool may signal ingestion of a GI irritant or caustic substance.[122]

Skin and Extremities

The physical examination should include a thorough evaluation of the body surfaces. Look for causes of trauma that may also explain the patient's condition. Examination of the skin and extremities can provide evidence of drug intoxication, especially with IV or subcutaneous drug injection needle marks.[24] Drugs can be hidden in the rectum or vagina.[24] Look for drug patches (e.g., fentanyl) on hidden areas of the body such as the back of the neck or scrotum. Fluid-filled bullae at gravity-dependent sites that have been in contact with hard surfaces for a long time suggest prolonged coma.[26] Muscle tone also should be assessed.[26] Increased tone or myoclonic spasms can be caused by some drug overdoses (e.g., TCAs) and can produce rhabdomyolysis or hyperthermia.[26,120] Dry, hot, red skin may also be an indication of anticholinergic toxicity.[26,39]

In summary, an organ system assessment of T.C. can provide useful insights into the identity of drugs that might have been ingested, the viability of organ function that might have been adversely affected, and the treatment that should be instituted.

Laboratory Tests

29. What laboratory tests should be ordered for T.C.?

The laboratory assessment of an intoxicated patient should be guided by the history of the events surrounding the ingestion, clinical presentation, and past medical history.[22,123] The status of oxygenation, acid–base balance, and blood glucose concentration must be determined, especially in patients with altered mental status such as T.C.[39] Oxygenation can be assessed initially by pulse oximetry, and acid–base status by ABGs and serum electrolyte concentrations.[23,123,124] T.C. was given oxygen and a bolus of IV fluid on her arrival at the ED. Paramedics administered glucose during her transportation to the ED.

A medical history of organ dysfunction or medical disorders (e.g., diabetes, hypertension) that can damage organs of elimination (e.g., kidney, liver) will also guide the need for laboratory tests. A serum creatinine concentration and liver function tests (e.g., aspartate aminotransferase [AST], alanine aminotransferase [ALT]) should be ordered. Other more specific tests reflective of her past medical history can be ordered subsequent to dialogue with her psychiatrist. A CBC, complete chemistry panel, serum osmolality, and other baseline laboratory tests should be obtained.[26] Pregnancy tests should be considered in female patients of childbearing age because unwanted pregnancies are common causes of overdose.[124]

A baseline electrocardiogram (ECG) should be obtained when exposure to a cardiotoxic drug is suspected or whenever the cardiovascular or hemodynamic status is altered.[23,39,124] A 12-lead ECG should be ordered because T.C. is likely to have ingested a psychotropic agent. Continuous cardiac monitoring should be instituted because of the significant cardiotoxicity associated with overdoses of these agents. Patients with severe TCA overdoses frequently present with symptoms of coma, tachycardia with a prolonged QRS segment, seizures, hypotension, and respiratory depression.[125–128]

A chest radiograph is useful when the potential exists for either direct pulmonary toxicity or aspiration.[23] A chest radiograph is indicated because T.C. had vomitus in her mouth and

TCAs are associated with the development of acute respiratory distress syndrome and pulmonary edema.[125,129,130]

Qualitative Screening

30. Why should (or should not) T.C.'s urine and blood be screened to assist in identifying the ingested substance?

Toxicology laboratory testing can be used to identify the substances involved in a toxic exposure, to exclude substances, or to measure the concentration of substances in serum or other biological fluids.[24,123,124] The identification and quantification of compounds should be considered as two distinct types of toxicologic testing.[24,131] *Qualitative* screening, intended to identify unknown substances, must be able to identify which substance or class of substances, is involved in the toxic exposure. *Quantitative* testing is similar to therapeutic drug monitoring in that the presence of the substance usually is known, and the question being answered is how much is present.[24]

Screening various biological fluids suspected of having high concentrations of a parent drug and its metabolites can identify unknown substances. Urine is screened much more commonly than blood, whereas gastric fluid is rarely evaluated. A urine drug screen is preferred to a blood drug screen because urine generally contains a higher concentration of a drug and its metabolites than other body fluids.[132]

When reviewing the results of urine screening panels for drugs and other substances, one must remember that the presence of a substance in urine is not necessarily related to a concurrent toxicity. A positive result on a urine screening panel merely indicates that the patient has ingested or has been exposed to the substance, but it does not differentiate between toxic and nontoxic doses. If a drug and its metabolites are eliminated slowly into the urine over a prolonged period of time, and if the testing methodology detects small concentrations of the substance, urine drug screening could identify the presence of a substance days, weeks, or even months after the exposure (e.g., marijuana).[24,124]

It is important to know which drugs/substances are tested at a given laboratory. Many laboratories restrict the number of drugs for which they test because 15 drugs account for more than 90% of all drug overdoses.[29] Some urine toxicology screens only detect common drugs of abuse (e.g., amphetamines, barbiturates, benzodiazepines, cocaine, marijuana, opioids).[124] Some drugs of abuse are not detected on routine drug screening (e.g., gamma hydroxybutyrate, ketamine, flunitrazepam).[24] Some analyses detect only antibodies to drug metabolites. For example, a benzodiazepine screen detects oxazepam, a common benzodiazepine metabolite. However, alprazolam and lorazepam are not metabolized to oxazepam and will not be detected in a urine screen. Likewise, an opioid screen may not detect the synthetic opioids such as fentanyl and methadone.[124]

Results of qualitative toxicology screening tests are difficult to interpret. False negatives, false positives, cross-reactivity with related drugs, chronicity of exposure, and length of time since last exposure all complicate results.[124] Urine toxicology screen results rarely change clinical management of the patient. Monitoring mental status, cardiovascular and respiratory status, and other laboratory parameters provide better clues than the results of a urine toxicology screen.[23,24,123,124,131]

Toxicology screening can be appropriate when the history of a suspected toxic exposure is unavailable, inaccurate, or inconsistent with the clinical findings.[24] However, it is important to know which drugs are detected on a given toxicology screen.[124] A comprehensive qualitative urine drug screen can be considered for T.C. because information about the substance(s) she ingested is not yet known.

Quantitative Testing

31. Why should a quantitative toxicology laboratory test be ordered (or not ordered) for T.C. as well?

Following a qualitative urine analysis for drugs, a quantitative analysis of drug concentration in blood can help determine the severity of toxicity and the need for aggressive interventions (e.g., hemodialysis).[24,30,124,131] Quantitative tests are especially useful when assessing the potential toxicity of drugs with delayed clinical toxicity or when the toxicity primarily is caused by metabolites (e.g., ethylene glycol, methanol). Furthermore, the concentration of a drug in serum is sometimes much more predictive of end-organ damage than clinical findings (e.g., acetaminophen effect on the liver).

Quantifying the amount of drug in serum is useful when (a) the concentration of the substance correlates with toxic effects, (b) the turnaround time for results is rapid, and (c) treatment can be guided by the serum concentration.[29,123,131] To aid in the care of poisoned patients, stat quantitative serum concentrations of acetaminophen, carbamazepine, carboxyhemoglobin, digoxin, ethanol, ethylene glycol, iron, lithium, methanol, methemoglobin, phenobarbital, and theophylline should be available at laboratories of large health care facilities.[23,24,30,123,131]

When blood samples are collected to quantitate potentially intoxicating substances, as much information as possible should be obtained about the time course of events to determine whether absorption and distribution of the substance is complete. Serial samples may be needed to determine whether significant absorption is still occurring.[28] In contrast to the interpretation of therapeutic serum concentrations of chronically administered drugs, the serum concentration of a substance ingested in an overdose will not be at steady state.

Quantitative toxicologic testing will not benefit T.C. at this point in time because the identity of the ingested substance is unknown. Nevertheless, a serum ethanol concentration could be useful in this case because alcohol is often ingested concurrently in overdose situations.[123] Most poison centers also recommend obtaining a quantitative acetaminophen level on all intentional ingestions because serious hepatotoxicity can occur if acetaminophen ingestion is missed.[24,123,124]

Assessment

32. T.C.'s clinical status has not changed over the past 10 minutes. A urine toxicology screen, blood acetaminophen, blood alcohol, and ABGs have been ordered. The 12-lead ECG shows a prolonged QRS interval of 0.14 seconds (normal, <0.1 seconds). No antidotes have been administered. T.C.'s physical examination did not detect any evidence of trauma to her head. Her pupils were dilated and slowly responsive to light, and her bowel sounds were

hypoactive. What conclusions can be made at this time with regard to the likely substance ingested by T.C.?

Although the ingested substance still has not been specifically identified, the available data provide some clues as to the likely pharmacologic class of drug that was ingested. The presence of CNS depression (T.C. is unresponsive), slowed ventricular conduction (prolonged QRS on ECG), tachycardia (heart rate, 148 beats/minute), hypotension (BP, 90/55 mmHg), decreased GI motility (hypoactive bowel sounds), and the history of a possible depressive illness (history from husband and daughter) are all consistent with a TCA drug overdose. The antidepressant could have been ingested alone or with other agents.

Antidepressant Toxicities

33. How would the different toxicities of the various available antidepressants affect the treatment of T.C.?

The major pharmacologic effects and toxicities of the antidepressants are similar for all drugs within the same class. When a specific drug within a therapeutic class has not yet been identified, the overdose should be managed as if the ingested drug can produce the most severe toxicity of any drug in the class. In this light, T.C.'s presumed antidepressant drug overdose should be evaluated and managed initially as TCA (e.g., amitriptyline) ingestion.[127,133] Antidepressants with different structures and actions (e.g., trazodone [Desyrel], fluoxetine [Prozac], sertraline [Zoloft]) generally do not produce toxicity as severe as that of the TCAs.[127,133,134]

Gastrointestinal Decontamination

34. If a TCA ingestion is presumed, why might GI decontamination be appropriate at this time?

The longer GI decontamination is delayed relative to the time of ingestion, the less effective it is likely to be because drug absorption will already have occurred. Because the time of ingestion is unknown and T.C. is unresponsive, she probably already has absorbed significant amounts of the drug, making her more vulnerable to aspiration. Furthermore, T.C. might already have aspirated because she was found in a pool of vomitus. TCA overdoses can also induce seizures, which would be a relative contraindication to GI decontamination. In consideration of these concerns, some would not support GI decontamination for T.C.[41,42,43,44,52–55]

Others might support GI decontamination because TCAs have strong central and peripheral anticholinergic properties that slow GI emptying, which could result in erratic absorption and delayed toxicity. Furthermore, TCAs have a large volume of distribution (10–50 L/kg), and both the parent drug and its metabolite undergo enterohepatic recirculation. The half-life of TCAs in overdose situations is 37 to 60 hours.[94] For those reasons, activated charcoal could be reasonably administered in an effort to adsorb any drug that may not yet be absorbed from the GI tract.[50]

Repeated doses of activated charcoal have been used to increase the elimination of TCAs because of the long half-life of TCAs and the enterohepatic recirculation. In clinical studies, multiple-dose activated charcoal has increased the elimination of amitriptyline, but the data are insufficient to support or exclude the use of this therapy.[46]

Monitoring Efficacy

35. How should the effectiveness of GI decontamination be monitored in T.C.?

If activated charcoal is administered, T.C. must first be intubated to protect her airway, and the charcoal must be administered via NG tube because she is unconscious. The insertion of the NG tube could stimulate the gag reflex; thereby, causing emesis and possible aspiration. T.C.'s lung sounds should be monitored closely to determine if aspiration pneumonitis is developing, particularly because T.C. was found unconscious and had already vomited.

Activated charcoal, especially in multiple doses, can produce ileus, GI obstruction, or intestinal perforation, especially when administered to patients who have ingested drugs that slow GI motility.[46,50,97] Bowel sounds must be monitored frequently to determine that an ileus is not developing. Once the patient passes a charcoal-laden stool, the activated charcoal can be considered to have successfully passed through the GI tract.

Sodium Bicarbonate and Hyperventilation

36. According to T.C.'s psychiatrist, he prescribed amitriptyline 100 mg at bedtime for her severe depression. How does this new information alter T.C.'s treatment plan?

This information confirms the assumptions that a TCA was ingested, and it also specifically identifies the probable ingested drug. In TCA ingestions, severe toxicity has been associated with doses of 15 to 25 mg/kg.[94] T.C. ingested a total of 2,500 mg based on her suicide note that said she took 25 tablets. If she weighs about 60 kg and was truthful about the amount taken, she ingested a significantly toxic dose (about 42 mg/kg).

On the ECG, TCA toxicity will exhibit as tachycardia with prolongation of the PR, QTc and QRS intervals, ST and T wave changes, and abnormalities of the terminal 40-millisecond vector.[94,111,125,128,135–138] TCAs have anticholinergic, adrenergic, and quinidinelike membrane effects on the heart.[111,125,127,133,136] It is believed that the anticholinergic effect causes the tachycardia and the quinidinelike effect causes the ECG changes.

In addition, TCAs are sodium channel blockers.[139] Sodium channel blockade slows the maximum uptake stroke of phase 0 of the action potential and decreases automaticity. Blockade decreases conduction velocity in the Purkinje fibers, which increases the QRS interval.[136] Myocardial depression, ventricular tachycardia, and ventricular fibrillation are the most common causes of death from TCAs.[128] Therefore, admission to the ICU with continuous cardiac monitoring is essential for T.C.[135]

The primary therapy for reversing ventricular arrhythmias and conduction delays is alkalinization of the serum and sodium loading by administrating IV hypertonic sodium bicarbonate.[111,125,127,128,136,137,140] Indications for sodium bicarbonate include hypotension, prolonged QRS segment (longer than 100 milliseconds), right bundle branch block, and wide complex tachycardia.[127,137] Alkalinization increases serum protein binding of the TCAs and thereby reduces the amount of free active drug (probably a minor consideration).[111,125,128,137] Correction of the serum pH is beneficial because underlying acidosis increases TCA cardiotoxic effects.[137] Furthermore, sodium bicarbonate has been found useful even in patients with a normal pH because sodium bicarbonate purportedly overcomes the sodium channel blockade and decreases cardiotoxicity.[137,139]

Based on T.C.'s tachycardia and a widened QRS segment on ECG, she should be treated with IV sodium bicarbonate with the goal of achieving an arterial pH of 7.5 to 7.55.[128,137] Sodium bicarbonate could have been administered earlier because the suspicion of an antidepressant overdose was strong initially, her ECG demonstrated QRS prolongation and worsening myocardial conduction, and her BP continued to decline from the time she was first seen by the paramedics. The use of IV sodium bicarbonate could introduce the risk of sodium overload and subsequent pulmonary edema, if not monitored closely.[94,138] An alternate is to hyperventilate the patient to a pH of 7.5 by adjusting her ventilator setting, and in this manner, decrease the cardiotoxicity of the TCA.[125,128,138]

The combination of IV bicarbonate and mechanical ventilation is more likely to produce severe alkalemia. Careful and frequent monitoring of the serum pH of patients on dual therapy is essential.[125,139]

Monitoring Efficacy

37. How should the sodium bicarbonate therapy in T.C. be monitored?

Many patients intoxicated with TCAs present with severe acidosis. Large doses of sodium bicarbonate may be required to normalize the arterial pH. The efficacy of sodium bicarbonate administration can be evaluated by monitoring acid–base status using ABGs, especially if the patient is also being ventilated mechanically.[125,139,140]

A bolus of sodium bicarbonate (1 mEq/mL) should be administered IV as a bolus of 1 to 2 mEq/kg over a 1- to 2-minute period. Continuous ECG monitoring is needed to monitor results of the bolus on cardiac abnormalities. Repeat bolus doses are administered as needed until the QRS interval narrows and tachycardia slows. Blood pH should be tested after several boluses to determine if a target pH of 7.5 to 7.55 has been obtained.[137] At a minimum, ABGs should be determined within an hour of starting sodium bicarbonate therapy to determine pH response to the bicarbonate.[140] Bolus bicarbonate can be followed by a constant sodium bicarbonate infusion of 150 mEq sodium bicarbonate per liter to maintain an alkaline pH.[137] ABGs must be monitored frequently to ensure a response.[125,139,140] Serial ECGs to measure the QRS interval can evaluate the efficacy of sodium bicarbonate. A prolonged QRS interval will generally narrow to normal after the systemic pH has been increased to about 7.5.[140]

Seizures

38. T.C. gradually developed more severely altered mental status and became comatose, not responding even to painful stimuli. She suddenly experienced a tonic-clonic seizure, which lasted about 2 minutes and terminated spontaneously. Should anticonvulsant therapy be initiated for T.C. at this time?

CNS toxicity is common in TCA overdoses. Symptoms include agitation, hallucinations, coma, myoclonus, and seizures.[111,125–128] Seizures can cause significant increases in acidosis and increase cardiotoxicity. Indeed, seizures are often seen immediately prior to cardiopulmonary arrest. Due to the severe consequences of prolonged seizures, aggressive drug treatment with rapid onset of action is indicated, and benzodiazepines are the drugs of choice to treat these seizures.[125,128]

Drug overdose–induced grand mal seizures are most commonly single seizures that terminate before drug therapy can be administered.[127] Seizure activity is not expected to persist; therefore, instituting long-term anticonvulsant therapy is not indicated. However, if her seizure did not stop within 1 to 2 minutes, a benzodiazepine would have been indicated.[111,125,127] The onset of action of phenobarbital is too delayed for managing acute seizures, and phenytoin is usually ineffective in treating drug toxicity–related seizures.[111] After a seizure, the patient may become more acidotic and hypotensive.[128] Blood gases and ECG changes should be monitored immediately after a seizure.

Interpretation of Urine Screens

39. T.C.'s BP fell to 88/42 mmHg and dopamine was started. Her pH on repeat ABGs was 7.26. T.C.'s ECG normalized after the administration of 150 mL of sodium bicarbonate by IV bolus. After dopamine, her BP increased to 102/68 mmHg, and seizure activity ceased. The urine drug screen results were positive for amitriptyline and nortriptyline. Acetaminophen and alcohol were not detected in her blood. Does the presence of nortriptyline indicate that T.C. has ingested other drugs in addition to her combination of amitriptyline?

Nortriptyline is a metabolite of amitriptyline and, therefore, was identified on the urine drug screen. Metabolites, as well as the parent compound, are often identified on comprehensive urine drug screens.[124]

Duration of Hospitalization

40. How long should T.C. be monitored?

T.C. should be admitted to the ICU and monitored until all evidence of CNS and cardiovascular toxicity has been reversed.[111] There is some controversy over how long symptomatic patients should be observed. Some believe symptomatic patients need cardiac monitoring for 24 hours post ingestion.[127] Some believe TCA overdose patients need to be monitored until they are symptom free for 24 hours because of a few reports of late development of symptoms.[128] However, 98% of signs of cardiotoxicity and arrhythmias are seen within the first 24 hours post TCA ingestion.[111,126] Because the incidence of late-occurring symptoms is rare, most patients are discharged after they are fully awake.[125] After the toxicity has completely resolved, T.C. should be evaluated by a psychiatrist to determine whether she should be admitted for inpatient treatment of her suicidal tendencies.[125–127]

Outcome of Patient T.C.

T.C. had no further seizure activity. She remained on a dopamine infusion for 8 hours and required several more boluses of IV sodium bicarbonate. The next afternoon, she started to awaken with her family at the bedside. She was tearful and expressed regret that her suicide attempt was not successful. She repeatedly told her family that they would be better off without her. Her psychiatrist saw her, and arrangements were made to transfer her to an in-patient psychiatric hospital once she was medically cleared.

ASSESSMENT OF ACETAMINOPHEN INGESTION

Mechanism of Hepatotoxicity

41. L.P., a 23-year-old woman who is about 32 weeks pregnant, presents to the ED 5 hours after ingesting 50 acetaminophen 500-mg tablets. She is depressed and hoped to end her pregnancy by ingesting acetaminophen. Her pregnancy was unplanned, and she has received no prenatal care. L.P. has vomited spontaneously four times since the ingestion and is complaining of abdominal pain; her heart rate is 100 beats/minute, BP is 100/70 mmHg, and temperature is 97.5°F. L.P. does not have any chronic diseases, and the remainder of her medical history is unremarkable. How does an overdose of acetaminophen cause toxicity?

Acetaminophen is metabolized in the liver by glucuronidation and sulfation. The mixed-function oxidase system cytochrome P450(CYP)2E1 metabolizes a portion of the acetaminophen to the highly reactive metabolite N-acetyl-p-benzoquinoneimine (NAPQI). In therapeutic doses, this metabolite is detoxified in the liver by glutathione. At toxic serum acetaminophen concentrations, the glucuronidation and sulfation metabolic pathways become saturated. Usually, NAPQI is detoxified by conjugation with glutathione, but increased amounts of the toxic metabolite deplete hepatic glutathione stores. When glutathione stores are decreased to about 30% of normal, the toxic metabolite binds to liver cells, resulting in the characteristic centrilobular hepatic necrosis seen in acetaminophen overdoses.[141–144]

Complication of Pregnancy

42. How does L.P.'s pregnancy change the management of her acetaminophen ingestion?

Pregnancy does not alter the initial approach to the assessment or treatment of potentially toxic ingestions, and assessment should focus initially on the mother.[144,145] Overdoses during pregnancy are often associated with attempted abortions, depression, prior loss of a child/children, potential loss of a lover, and/or economic reasons.[146,147] Intentional ingestions of analgesics, prenatal vitamins, iron, psychotropics, and antibiotics account for 74% of the overdoses during pregnancy.

The fetus is at risk when the mother overdoses on acetaminophen because acetaminophen crosses the placenta. The fetal liver can oxidize acetaminophen to its hepatotoxic metabolite by 14 weeks of gestation.[141] However, the ability of the fetal liver has only about 10% of the capability of the adult liver to metabolize acetaminophen. The fetal liver can conjugate acetaminophen with both glutathione and sulfate, but detoxification by glutathione conjugation appears to be decreased.[148,149]

In studies of maternal acetaminophen toxicity, most of the pregnant women survived without damage to themselves or their babies. However, there were also maternal and fetal deaths as a result of the overdoses.[148,150] Acetaminophen overdoses during pregnancy did not appear to increase the risk for birth defects or adverse pregnancy outcome unless the mother suffered severe toxicity, emphasizing the need to treat the mother promptly.[141,148]

Gastrointestinal Decontamination

43. What GI decontamination should be initiated for L.P.?

L.P.'s acetaminophen ingestion occurred 5 hours ago; therefore, the drug is likely to be totally absorbed, and no GI decontamination should be initiated.

Estimating Potential Toxicity

44. How should the potential toxicity of the acetaminophen ingestion be assessed in L.P.?

Serum acetaminophen concentrations better predict acetaminophen-induced hepatotoxicity than the dose of acetaminophen acutely ingested.[151,152] The Matthew-Rumack nomogram (Fig. 5-1) is used in the United States to assess the potential for hepatotoxicity from acute overdoses of acetaminophen.[152] The treatment line is defined by a serum acetaminophen concentration of 200 mcg/mL at 4 hours after acetaminophen ingestion and 30 mcg/mL at 15 hours post ingestion on a semilogarithmic graph.[144] The serum acetaminophen concentration is plotted on a graph against the time of ingestion.[152] The nomogram predicts the probability that the AST or ALT will be >1,000 IU/L and can be used to guide therapy by indicating whether a specific acetaminophen

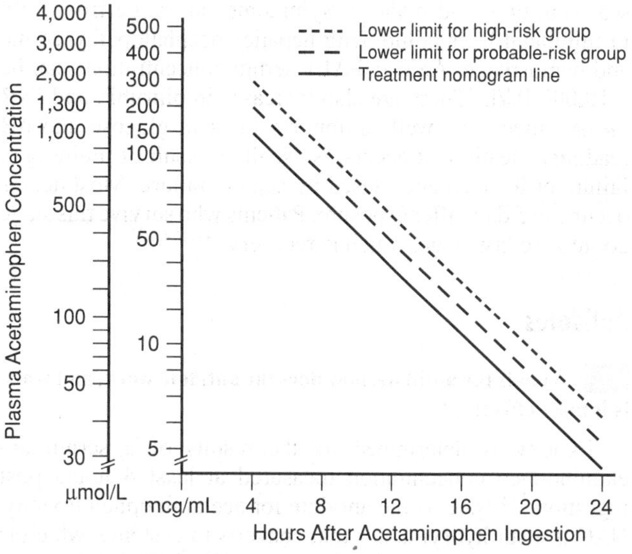

FIGURE 5-1 Nomogram for interpretation of severity of acetaminophen poisoning. (Copyright © 2001 Massachusetts Medical Society. All rights reserved.)

concentration is in the toxic range.[153] The nomogram is useful only for acute ingestions because it underestimates the potential for toxicity in chronic acetaminophen ingestions. It should be noted that although the nomogram is used to plot acetaminophen concentrations for all patients, it has been validated only in healthy nonalcoholic adult patients.[144]

Acetaminophen Treatment Nomogram

45. When is the preferred time to measure a serum acetaminophen concentration?

Acetaminophen absorption generally is complete within 1.5 to 2.5 hours after ingestion of solid or liquid dosage forms.[152] The Matthews-Rumack nomogram is not applicable before 4 hours post ingestion because it is based on complete drug absorption.[153] Most clinical laboratories can complete their assays and report acetaminophen serum concentration results within 2 hours.

Stages of Acetaminophen Toxicity

46. What are the clinical signs and symptoms of acetaminophen toxicity?

Early detection of an acetaminophen overdose is difficult because there are no characteristic early diagnostic findings. Toxicity appears in stages that may overlap and are not clear cut. About 30 minutes to 24 hours post ingestion, the patient may exhibit anorexia, nausea, vomiting, malaise, and diaphoresis that can easily be attributed to other causes. The second stage of acetaminophen toxicity occurs about 24 to 48 hours post ingestion and is the stage in which hepatotoxicity develops. Hepatotoxicity is universal by 36 hours post ingestion. An AST measurement is the most sensitive measure of hepatotoxicity. AST abnormalities always precede evidence of actual liver impairment.[144,154,155]

In the third stage, 72 to 96 hours post ingestion, maximum liver dysfunction is evident with the return of anorexia, nausea, vomiting, and malaise. Symptoms can range from mild to fulminant liver failure with hepatic encephalopathy, coma, and hemorrhage. AST and ALT serum concentrations can be >10,000 IU/L. There are also increases in bilirubin and INR measurements, as well as abnormalities in glucose and pH readings. Death, if it occurs, is usually a result of multiorgan failure or hemorrhage caused by hepatic failure. Most deaths occur 3 to 5 days after exposure. Patients who survive this stage go into the last stage, which is recovery.[144,154,155]

Antidotes

47. What is the antidote, how does the antidote work, and when is it most effective?

Toxicity is determined by the results of a serum acetaminophen concentration measured at least 4 hours post ingestion.[152] NAC is the antidote for acetaminophen toxicity. NAC is a sulfhydryl donor that converts to cysteine, which is subsequently converted to glutathione.[141,155,156] NAC acts as a glutathione substitute and directly combines with the toxic acetaminophen metabolite, NAPQI, reducing it to a nontoxic cysteine conjugate.[154] NAC can also substitute for sulfation, which increases the nontoxic metabolism through that route as well. NAC increases intrahepatic microcirculation and is believed to possess hepatoprotective properties showing some value even after liver damage has already occurred.[141,155]

Instituting therapy early with NAC is essential. When NAC is started within 8 to 10 hours of the ingestion, hepatotoxicity resulted in only 1.6% of cases. If NAC treatment is delayed, especially longer than 16 hours post ingestion, the efficacy of NAC treatment declines dramatically.[141,144,148,155–157] In patients who were started on NAC more than 10 hours after ingestion, 53% developed liver damage.[144,156,157]

Safety of *N*-Acetylcysteine in Pregnancy

48. Is NAC safe to use during pregnancy?

Acetaminophen overdose in pregnant women should be managed in the same manner as in nonpregnant patients.[141,144,148] If the life of the mother is not saved, the fetus will not survive (unless the child is near term and is emergently delivered); therefore, attention to the mother must be foremost. NAC therapy is not contraindicated in pregnant patients and might be helpful because it crosses the placenta and can protect the fetus from hepatotoxicity.[141,148]

NAC therapy appears to be protective for both mother and fetus.[141,144,155,157] When used as an antidote for acetaminophen overdose in pregnancy, NAC did not appear to result in toxic effects to the fetus.[141,144,158] The probability of fetal death was increased with the delay in NAC treatment after overdose and with acetaminophen overdose early in gestation.[144,148,155]

Route of Administration of *N*-Acetylcysteine

49. The 6-hour acetaminophen concentration in L.P. was 245 mcg/mL. By what route should NAC be administered?

This concentration of acetaminophen at 6 hours is above the treatment line on Figure 5-1. Because there is some delay from the time of ingestion to presentation at the emergency department and L.P. has already had vomiting, it will be more difficult for L.P. to tolerate oral NAC. For this reason, IV NAC is recommended.

A FDA-approved sterile, pyrogenfree formulation of NAC is available in the United States as Acetadote.[156,159] The use of IV NAC is not completely risk free because of a possible anaphylactoid reaction during the first dose of the IV NAC. The incidence of adverse reactions ranges from 14.3% to 23%. Asthmatic patients and patients with ectopy should receive the drug slowly and carefully, watching for symptoms of a reaction.[159]

A majority of the adverse reactions included nausea, vomiting, urticaria, flushing, and pruritus. Bronchospasm, angioedema, hypotension, and death have occurred, although rarely so, and must be carefully monitored for when the IV route is being used.[156,160,161] Most reactions occur during or just after the first 15 minutes of the antidote infusion and appear to be dose related.[161] The first dose of IV NAC is usually administered over 60 minutes instead of 15 minutes, even though a study comparing adverse reactions in the two infusion rates did not show clinically significant differences.[159,162]

Intravenous *N*-Acetylcysteine

50. How is NAC given intravenously?

The FDA-approved IV NAC protocol is the same 20-hour dosing regimen used in Europe, known as the Prescott protocol.[156,157,159] A 150 mg/kg loading dose of NAC in 5% dextrose is infused intravenously slowly over 60 minutes while watching for symptoms of a possible anaphylactoid reaction. This is followed by a maintenance dose of 50 mg/kg infused over 4 hours, and then followed with a 100 mg/kg dose infused over 16 hours. This regimen provides a total of 300 mg/kg NAC over the 20 hours after the loading dose.[159] As soon as the patient is able to tolerate oral administration, the patient can be switched to oral NAC therapy. Oral therapy is as effective as IV therapy as long as it is started early in the course. In addition, oral therapy is much less expensive.[163]

Oral *N*-Acetylcysteine

51. What should be the dosing regimen for oral NAC?

The standard oral NAC protocol is based on the original clinical studies.[153] The loading dose of NAC is 140 mg/kg orally using either the 10% or 20% mucolytic solutions that were formulated for inhalation therapy. Seventeen additional maintenance doses of 70 mg/kg of NAC are administered at 4-hour intervals after the initial dose for a total of 72 hours of therapy. This provides a total of 1,330 mg/kg NAC over 72 hours.[156,164] Because oral NAC contains a sulfhydryl group, the substance has a very disagreeable taste and smell (like rotten eggs) that commonly results in nausea and vomiting for the patient. To mask the unpleasant taste and odor, NAC is diluted to a concentration of 5% using a carbonated beverage or fruit juice.[153] Because the entire dose of oral NAC passes through the liver, high concentrations are produced, which is seen as an advantage of oral therapy.[156]

Shorter oral NAC regimens are currently being used based on the efficacy of IV therapy.[165,166] Short course oral NAC follows the same 20-hour time course as IV NAC. Patients receive the usual 140 mg/kg oral loading dose of NAC, followed by 70 mg/kg every 4 hours for 5 additional doses (20 hours of therapy). Serum acetaminophen, liver function tests, and INR are repeated at 20 hours after the loading dose, which is after the fifth maintenance dose. If 20-hour liver function tests and coagulation studies are normal and the acetaminophen level is below the lower limits of detection, NAC can be stopped. A repeat set of liver function tests is recommended at 36 hours after ingestion. In other versions of the 20-hour NAC therapy, the dosage regimen is the same, but the laboratory studies are measured initially, at 16, 36, and 48 hours post ingestion.[166]

Efficacy of *N*-Acetylcysteine

52. Which route of NAC administration is more effective?

There has been no proven evidence that one route of NAC administration is superior.[155,156,167] Patient outcome after an acetaminophen overdose depends more on the time after the ingestion that treatment begins rather than on the route of administration of NAC. Patients who are started on NAC within 8 to 10 hours post ingestion, regardless of the route, rarely develop hepatotoxicity. Patients who present late or have a delay in the time of NAC treatment have higher rates of hepatoxicity.[141,155,156,163,164,168]

In one comparative study of IV NAC to oral NAC therapy, both were effective in reducing hepatotoxicity when therapy was initiated within 10 hours after ingestion. Vomiting delayed oral administration of the drug, but IV administration resulted in significantly longer delays in instituting therapy.[168] IV NAC avoids the problems of the vomiting patient, but oral NAC is safer. Oral NAC is associated with nausea and vomiting, whereas IV NAC is associated with bronchospasm, urticaria, and angioedema during administration.[141,155]

Starting oral NAC may take less time to prepare than IV NAC therapy and is less expensive. If the patient presents early after an acetaminophen ingestion and does not have nausea and vomiting, oral therapy would be indicated. If the patient presents late (more than 10 hours post ingestion) with signs and symptoms of hepatotoxicity along with intractable nausea and vomiting, IV NAC should be instituted at once.[156,164]

Monitoring Efficacy of *N*-Acetylcysteine

53. How should the efficacy of NAC therapy be monitored in L.P.?

The effectiveness of NAC intervention in L.P. should be monitored by daily assessment of her acetaminophen concentration (as long as it is still measurable), AST, ALT, total bilirubin, glucose, and INR. The AST and ALT serum concentrations typically increase within 36 hours (range: 24–72 hours) after ingestion.[155,168] As the hepatic damage continues, the liver enzymes may peak at several thousand units, even with NAC therapy. In most patients, AST and ALT begin to decline after 3 days and then return to baseline values.[155]

In a small number of patients, usually those who presented late after the ingestion, fulminant hepatic failure may develop. In general, symptoms of severe or persistent acidosis, coagulopathy, a significantly increased serum creatinine, and grade III to IV encephalopathy are consistent with fatal outcomes in patients with fulminant hepatic failure. Liver transplantation might be a consideration for these patients.[144,169–172]

Duration of *N*-Acetylcysteine Therapy

54. How long should NAC administration be continued?

The original NAC dosing protocol was based on an assumption that the half-life of acetaminophen was 4 hours. After five half-lives (20 hours), the acetaminophen should be metabolized and NAC could be discontinued. A NAC dose of 6 mg/kg/hour was determined to be necessary based on the rate of glutathione turnover relative to NAPQI production. To ensure that patients received an adequate NAC dose, the FDA recommended that this dose be changed to 18 mg/kg/hour for 72 hours.[173] This recommendation serves as the basis for the traditional 72-hour oral course of NAC therapy.

When using the traditional 72-hour oral course of NAC, therapy can be discontinued if the liver function tests are trending toward normal, other laboratory tests (i.e., coagulation studies, glucose, pH, bilirubin) are within normal ranges, and acetaminophen is no longer present in the serum. As long as acetaminophen is present, it can be metabolized to NAPQI and cause further toxicity.[155,165,173] Continued NAC will not be harmful to the patient and can be beneficial.

When using the shorter 20-hour course of oral NAC, if liver function tests and coagulation studies are normal and the 20-hour acetaminophen concentration can no longer be measured in the serum, NAC therapy can be stopped.[166] However, if 20-hour liver function tests or coagulation studies are abnormal, or if the 20-hour acetaminophen concentration measurement reveals acetaminophen still present in the serum, NAC therapy should be continued for at least another 24 hours. These laboratory tests should be repeated every 24 hours, and the patient's progress must be monitored closely. If the patient is not improving, NAC should be continued until the patient recovers, receives a liver transplant, or dies.[144]

At this time, there is no consensus as to the best route of NAC administration, optimal dosage regimen, or optimal length of therapy.[155,156,173] There is consensus, however, that NAC therapy must be instituted within 10 hours post ingestion.[141,155,156,163,164,168] For patients who do not exhibit any signs of hepatotoxicity, shorter-course NAC therapy reduces the amount of NAC administered to the patient, decreases the quantity of laboratory tests, shortens hospital stay, and is less costly.[156,165,173]

N-Acetylcysteine Toxicity

55. How should the toxicity of NAC therapy be monitored in L.P.?

With the exception of vomiting, oral NAC is remarkably safe and has not been associated with toxicity.[141,155,156] Oral NAC must be retained for a minimum of 1 hour post ingestion to be successfully absorbed. If L.P. vomits within an hour after her oral NAC dose, the dose should be repeated. If she experiences protracted vomiting, administration of antiemetic drugs (e.g., ondansetron, metoclopramide) or placement of a duodenal feeding tube can improve GI tolerance.[156,174,175] If the patient cannot tolerate oral liquids, NAC therapy should continue via IV administration.

IV NAC therapy has been associated with anaphylactoid reactions in up to 14% of the patients. Although most reactions are not severe, bronchospasm, angioedema, and respiratory arrest have been reported.[141,155,156,173] Patients should be monitored for allergic and anaphylactoid reactions when NAC is administered intravenously. Most reactions can be avoided by infusing the NAC loading dose slowly over 1 hour.[141,155,156]

Outcome of Patient L.P.

L.P. continued to have nausea and vomiting and had difficulty tolerating liquids. IV NAC was continued. An obstetrics consultation was requested to evaluate L.P.'s pregnancy. Fetal monitoring was instituted during her hospital admission. A sonogram was taken of the baby. Once L.P. saw her baby's image from the sonogram, her depressed mood seemed to lift. Approximately 36 hours post ingestion, her acetaminophen level was no longer detectable, and her liver function tests showed a mild elevation of her AST at 274 U/L and an ALT of 188 U/L (normal AST and AST values, 8–45 U/L). Her INR and total bilirubin values were normal at 0.7 seconds (normal INR time, 8–1.2) and 0.8 mg/dL (normal total bilirubin in adults, 0.3–1.0 mg/dL), respectively.

L.P. was seen by a psychiatrist. She was scheduled for counseling and prenatal classes. L.P. seemed eager to attend the classes, and she talked enthusiastically about the baby when family members came to visit. Because of L.P.'s pregnancy, the decision was made to continue NAC for a full 72-hour course with the goal of protecting the fetal liver as much as possible. Six weeks later, she had a normal delivery of a healthy 6-lb, 1-oz baby girl.

SUMMARY

Unfortunately, there is no "cookbook" method to treat all poisoned patients. Each exposure is unique: the patients, substances, symptoms, time of exposure, and circumstances differ in each case. Treatment of the poisoned patient often involves controversy because solid, evidence-based science to support a given decision is frequently lacking. When challenged with a poisoning exposure, consult with a poison control center. By calling 1-800-222-1222, the call will be connected to the poison center nearest your location. Consultation is available 24 hours a day nationwide.

REFERENCES

1. Woolf AD, Lovejoy FR. Epidemiology of drug overdose in children. *Drug Saf* 1993;9:291.
2. Madden MA. Pediatric poisoning: recognition, assessment, and management. *Crit Care Nurs Clin North Am* 2005;17:395.
3. Lai MW et al. 2005 Annual report of the American Association of Poison Control Centers National Poisoning and Exposure Database. *Clin Toxicol* 2006;44:803.
4. Substance Abuse and Mental Health Services Administration, Office of Applied Studies. Drug Abuse Warning Network 2005: National Estimates of Drug-Related Emergency Department Visits. DAWN Series: D-29, DHHS Publication No. (SMA) 07-4256, Rockville, MD; 2007.
5. Blanc PD et al. Surveillance of poisoning and overdose through hospital discharge coding, poison control center reporting, and the drug abuse warning network. *Am J Emerg Med* 1993;11:14.
6. Substance Abuse and Mental Health Services Administration, Office of Applied Studies. Emergency Department Trends from the Drug Abuse Warning Network, Final Estimates 1995–2002. Department of Health and Human Services, DAWN Series: D-24, DHHS Publication No. (SMA) 03-3780, Rockville, MD; 2003.
7. Dean B, Krenzelok EP. Adolescent poisoning: a comparison of accidental and intentional exposures. *Vet Hum Toxicol* 1998;30:579.
8. Huott MA, Storrow AB. A survey of adolescents' knowledge regarding toxicity of over-the-counter medications. *Acad Emerg Med* 1997;4:214.
9. Meyers S. Bracing for boomers, hospital gets ready for next geriatric generation. Available at: http://www.hospitalconnect.com/hospitalconnect_app/search/article.jsp?dcrpath=AHANEWS/AHANewsArticle/data/AHA_News_070528_Bracing_boomers&domain=AHNews. Accessed July 5, 2008.
10. National Institute of Mental Health. Older adults: depression and suicide facts. Available at: www.nimh.nih.gov/publicat/elderlydepsuicide.cfm. Accessed June 6, 2007.
11. Forjuoh SN et al. Physician response to written feedback on a medication discrepancy found with their elderly ambulatory patients. *J Am Geriatr Soc* 2005;53:2173.
12. Klasco RK, ed. *POISINDEX System.* Greenwood Village, CO: Vol. 132, expires 6/2007.
13. Caravati EM, McElwee NE. Use of clinical toxicology resources by emergency physicians and its impact on poison control centers. *Ann Emerg Med* 1991;20:147.
14. Goldfrank LF et al. *Goldfrank's Toxicologic Emergencies.* 8th ed. New York: McGraw-Hill; 2006.
15. Olson KR. *Poisoning and Drug Overdose.* 5th ed. New York: McGraw-Hill; 2007.
16. Mullen WH et al. Incorrect overdose management advice in the Physicians Desk Reference. *Ann Emerg Med* 1997;29:255.
17. Harrison DL et al. Cost-effectiveness of regional poison control centers. *Arch Intern Med* 1996;156:2661.
18. Miller TR, Lestina DC. Costs of poisonings in

the United States and savings from poison control centers: a benefit-cost analysis. *Ann Emerg Med* 1997;29:239.
19. Committee on Poison Prevention and Control Board on Health Promotion and Disease Prevention, Institute of Medicine of the National Academies. Poison control center activities, personnel, and quality assurance. *Forging a poison prevention and control system*, Chapter 5. Washington, DC: The National Academies Press; 2004.
20. Ford PS. A telephone history taking and poisoning care process. *Vet Hum Toxicol* 1981;23:428.
21. Veltri JC. Regional poison control services. *Hosp Forum* 1982;17:1469.
22. American College of Emergency Physicians. Clinical policy for the initial approach to patients presenting with acute toxic ingestion or dermal or inhalation exposure. *Ann Emerg Med* 1995;25:570.
23. Kulig K. Current concepts—initial management of ingestions of toxic substances. *N Engl J Med* 1992;326:1677.
24. Eldridge DL, Holstege CP. Utilizing the laboratory in the poisoned patient. *Clin Lab Med* 2006;26:13.
25. Wright N. An assessment of the unreliability of the history given by self-poisoned patients. *Clin Toxicol* 1980;16:381.
26. Olson KR et al. Physical assessment and differential diagnosis of the poisoned patient. *Med Toxicol* 1987;2:52.
27. Nice A et al. Toxidrome recognition to improve efficiency of emergency urine drug screens. *Ann Emerg Med* 1988;17:676.
28. Spyker DA, Minocha A. Toxicodynamic approach to management of the poisoned patient. *J Emerg Med* 1988;6:117.
29. Mahoney JD et al. Quantitative serum toxic screening in the management of suspected drug overdose. *Am J Emerg Med* 1990;8:16.
30. Hepler BR et al. Role of the toxicology laboratory in the treatment of acute poisoning. *Med Toxicol* 1986;1:61.
31. Sue YJ, Shannon M. Pharmacokinetics of drugs in overdose. *Clin Pharmacokinet* 1992;23:93.
32. Buckley NA et al. Controlled release drugs in overdose: clinical consideration. *Drug Saf* 1995;12:73.
33. Mellick LB et al. Presentations of acute phenytoin overdose. *Am J Emerg Med* 1989;7:61.
34. Chaikin P, Adir J. Unusual absorption profile of phenytoin in a massive overdose case. *J Clin Pharmacol* 1987;27:70.
35. Mitchell JR et al. Acetaminophen-induced hepatic injury: protective role of glutathione in man and rationale for therapy. *Clin Pharm Ther* 1974;16:676.
36. Rosenberg J et al. Pharmacokinetics of drug overdose. *Clin Pharmacokinet* 1981;6:161.
37. Baud FJ. Pharmacokinetic-pharmacodynamic relationships: how are they useful in human toxicology? *Toxicol Lett* 1998;102-103:643.
38. Weisman RS. Toxicokinetics in the ED. *Emerg Med* 1984; May 15.
39. Greene SL et al. Acute poisoning: understanding 90% of cases in a nutshell. *Postgrad Med J* 2005;81:204.
40. Vale JA. Reviews in medicine–clinical toxicology. *Postgrad Med J* 1993;69:19.
41. Krenzelok EP, Vale JA. Position statement: ipecac syrup. *Clin Toxicol* 2004;42:133.
42. Vale JA. Position statement: gastric lavage. *Clin Toxicol* 2004;42:933.
43. American Academy of Clinical Toxicology and European Association of Poisons Centres and Clinical Toxicologists. Position paper: single-dose activated charcoal. *Clin Toxicol* 2005;43:61.
44. Barceloux GD et al. Position statement: cathartics. *Clin Toxicol* 2004;42:243.
45. Tenebein M. Position statement: whole bowel irrigation. *Clin Toxicol* 2004;42:843.
46. Vale JA et al. Position statement and practical guidelines on the use of multi-dose activated charcoal in the treatment of acute poisoning. *Clin Toxicol* 1999;37:731.
47. Committee on Injury, Violence and Poison Prevention. American Academy of Pediatrics policy statement: poison treatment in the home. *Pediatrics* 2003;112:1182.
48. Holz LE, Holz PH. The black bottle. *Pediatrics* 1963;63:306.
49. Derlet RW, Albertson TE. Activated charcoal's past, present and future. *West J Med* 1986;145:493.
50. Neuvonen PJ, Olkkola KT. Oral activated charcoal in the treatment of intoxications, role of single and repeated doses. *Med Toxicol* 1988;3:33.
51. Bond GR. The role of activated charcoal and gastric emptying in gastrointestinal decontamination: a state-of-the-art review. *Ann Emerg Med* 2002;39:273.
52. Harris CR, Filandrinos D. Accidental administration of activated charcoal into the lung: aspiration by proxy. *Ann Emerg Med* 1993;22:1470.
53. Graff GR et al. Chronic lung disease after activated charcoal aspiration. *Pediatrics* 2002;109:959.
54. Elliot CG et al. Charcoal lung aspiration of activated charcoal. *Chest* 1989;96:672.
55. Givens T et al. Pulmonary aspiration of activated charcoal: a complication of its misuse in overdose management. *Pediatr Emerg Care* 1992;8:137.
56. Golej J et al. Severe respiratory failure following charcoal application in a toddler. *Resuscitation* 2001;49:315.
57. Tomaszewski C. Activated charcoal treatment or toxin? *Clin Toxicol* 1999;37:17.
58. Gazda-Smith E, Synhavsky A. Hypernatremia following treatment of theophylline toxicity with activated charcoal and sorbitol. *Arch Intern Med* 1990;150:689.
59. Allerton JP, Strom JA. Hypernatremia due to repeated doses of charcoal-sorbitol. *Am J Kidney Dis* 1991;17:581.
60. Tenebein M. Whole bowel irrigation as a gastrointestinal decontamination procedure after acute poisoning. *Med Toxicol* 1988;3:77.
61. Hoffman RS, Goldfrank LR. The poisoned patients with altered consciousness-controversies in the use of the "coma cocktail." *JAMA* 1995;274:562.
62. Trujillo MH et al. Pharmacologic antidotes in critical care medicine: a practical guide for drug administration. *Crit Care Med* 1988;26:377.
63. Goldfrank LR, Hoffman RS. The cardiovascular effects of cocaine. *Ann Emerg Med* 1991;20:165.
64. Wrenn K et al. Profound alkalemia during treatment of tricyclic antidepressant overdose. *Am J Emerg Med* 1992;10:553.
65. Olson KR et al. Seizures associated with poisoning and drug overdose. *Am J Emerg Med* 1993;11:565.
66. Garrettson LK, Geller RJ. Acid and alkaline diuresis: when are they of value in the treatment of poisoning? *Drug Saf* 1990;5:220.
67. Kulling P, Persson H. Role of the intensive care unit in the management of the poisoned patient. *Med Toxicol* 1986;1:375.
68. Temple AR. Acute and chronic effects of aspirin toxicity and their treatment. *Arch Intern Med* 1981;141:364.
69. Chyka PB et al. Salicylate poisoning: an evidence based consensus guideline for out of hospital management. *Clin Toxicol* 2007;45:95.
70. Clarke A, Walton WW. Effect of safety packaging on aspirin ingestion by children. *Pediatrics* 1979;63:687.
71. Done AK, Temple AR. Treatment of salicylate poisoning. *Mod Treat* 1971;8:528.
72. Done AK. Aspirin overdosage: incidence, diagnosis, and management. *Pediatrics* 1978;62:890.
73. Yip L et al. Concepts and controversies in salicylate toxicity. *Emerg Med Clin North Am* 1994;12:351.
74. Notarianni L. A reassessment of the treatment of salicylate poisoning. *Drug Saf* 1992;7:292.
75. Temple AR. Pathophysiology of aspirin overdosage toxicity, with implications for management. *Pediatrics* 1978;62:873.
76. Heffner JE, Sahn SA. Salicylate-induced pulmonary edema: clinical features and prognosis. *Ann Intern Med* 1976;85:745.
77. Anderson RJ et al. Unrecognized adult salicylate intoxication. *Ann Intern Med* 1976;85:745.
78. Bailey RB, Jones SR. Chronic salicylate intoxication: a common cause of morbidity in the elderly. *J Am Geriatr Soc* 1989;37:556.
79. Dargan PI et al. An evidence based flowchart to guide the management of acute salicylate (aspirin) overdose. *Emerg Med J* 2002;19:206.
80. Done AK. Salicylate intoxication: significance of measurements of salicylate in blood in cases of acute ingestion. *Pediatrics* 1960;26:800.
81. Dugandzic RM et al. Evaluation of the validity of the Done nomogram in the management of acute salicylate intoxication. *Ann Emerg Med* 1989;18:1186.
82. Greenberg MI. Deleterious effects of endotracheal intubation in salicylate poisoning. *Ann Emerg Med* 2003;41:583.
83. Koren G. Medications which can kill a toddler with one tablet or teaspoonful. *Clin Toxicol* 1993;31:407.
84. Litovitz T, Manoguerra A. Comparison of pediatric poisoning hazards: an analysis of 3.8 million exposure incidents: a report from the American Association of Poison Control Centers. *Pediatrics* 1992;89:999.
85. Cada DJ, ed. *Drug Facts and Comparisons 2007.* St. Louis: Wolters Kluwer; 2007.
86. Klasco RK, ed. *INDENTIDEX System.* Greenwood Village, CO: Thomson Micromedex; Vol. 132, expires 6/2007.
87. Manoguerra AS et al. Iron ingestion: an evidence-based consensus guideline for out-of-hospital management. *Clin Toxicol* 2005;43:553.
88. Klein-Schwartz W et al. Assessment of management guidelines: acute iron ingestion. *Clin Pediatr* 1990;29:316.
89. Fine JS. Iron poisoning. *Curr Probl Pediatr* 2000; 30:71.
90. McGuigan MA. Acute iron poisoning. *Pediatr Ann* 1996;25:33.
91. Mills KC, Curry SC. Acute iron poisoning. *Emerg Med Clin North Am* 1994;12:397.
92. Banner W, Tong TG. Iron poisoning. *Pediatr Clin North Am* 1986;33:393.
93. Clark RF et al. Safety of childhood acetaminophen overdose. *Ann Emerg Med* 2001;37:115.
94. Woolf AD et al. Tricyclic antidepressant poisoning: an evidence based consensus guideline for out-of-hospital management. *Clin Toxicol* 2007;44: 203.
95. Jaeger RW et al. Radiopacity of drugs and plants in vivo-limited usefulness. *Vet Hum Toxicol* 1981;23(Suppl 1):2.
96. James JA. Acute iron poisoning: assessment of severity and prognosis. *J Pediatr* 1970;77:117.
97. Perrone J et al. Special considerations in gastrointestinal decontamination. *Emerg Med Clin North Am* 1994;12:285.
98. Kulig K et al. Management of acutely poisoned patients without gastric emptying. *Ann Emerg Med* 1985;14:562.
99. Tenebein M. Whole bowel irrigation as a gastrointestinal decontamination procedure after acute poisoning. *Med Toxicol* 1988;3:77.
100. Tenebein M. Whole bowel irrigation in iron poisoning. *J Pediatr* 1987;111:142.
101. Chyka PA et al. Serum iron concentrations and symptoms of acute iron poisoning in children. *Pharmacotherapy* 1996;16:1053.
102. Lovejoy FH. Chelation therapy in iron poisoning. *J Toxicol Clin Toxicol* 1982–1983;19:871.
103. Engle JP et al. Acute iron intoxication: treatment controversies. *Drug Intell Clin Pharm* 1987;21:153.
104. Helfer RE, Rodgerson DO. The effect of deferoxamine on the determination of serum iron and iron-binding capacity. *J Pediatr* 1966;68:804.
105. Ingelfinger JA et al. Reliability of the toxic screen in drug overdose. *Clin Pharmacol Ther* 1981;29:570.
106. Yealy DM et al. The safety of prehospital naloxone administration by paramedics. *Ann Emerg Med* 1990;19:902.
107. Watson AJS et al. Acute Wernicke's encephalopathy precipitated by glucose loading. *Ir J Med Sci* 1981;150:301.
108. Zubaran C et al. Wernicke-Korsakoff syndrome. *Postgrad Med J* 1997;73:27.

109. Handal KA et al. Naloxone. *Ann Emerg Med* 1983;12:438.
110. Weinbroum A et al. Use of flumazenil in the treatment of drug overdose: a double-blind and open clinical study in 110 patients. *Crit Care Med* 1996; 24:199.
111. Callaham M. Tricyclic antidepressant overdose. *J Am Coll Emerg Phys* 1979;8:413.
112. Ettinger NA, Albin RJ. A review of the respiratory effects of smoking cocaine. *Am J Med* 1989;87:664.
113. Finkle BS, McCloskey KL. The forensic toxicology of cocaine (1971 to 1976). *J Forens Sci* 1978; 23:173.
114. Lora-Tamayo C et al. Cocaine-related deaths. *J Chromatogr* 1994;674:217.
115. Kline JN, Hirasuna JD. Pulmonary edema after freebase cocaine smoking-not due to an adulterant. *Chest* 1990;97:1009.
116. Cucco RA et al. Nonfatal pulmonary edema after "freebase" cocaine smoking. *Am Rev Respir Dis* 1987;136:179.
117. Duberstein JL, Kaufman DM. A clinical study of an epidemic of heroin intoxication and heroin-induced pulmonary edema. *Am J Med* 1971;51:704.
118. Warner-Smith M et al. Morbidity associated with non-fatal heroin overdose. *Addiction* 2002;97:963.
119. Sporer KA, Dorn E. Heroin-related noncardiogenic pulmonary edema. *Chest* 2001;120:1628.
120. Chan TC et al. Drug-induced hyperthermia. *Crit Care Clin* 1997;13:785.
121. Albertson TE et al. A prolonged severe intoxication after ingestion of phenytoin and phenobarbital. *West J Med* 1981;135:418.
122. Knopp R. Caustic ingestions. *J Am Coll Emerg Phys* 1979;8:329.
123. Dawson AH, Whyte IM. Therapeutic drug monitoring in drug overdose. *Br J Clin Pharmacol* 1999;48:278.
124. Hoffman RJ, Nelson L. Rational use of toxicology testing in children. *Curr Opin Pediatr* 2001;13: 183.
125. Crome P. Poisoning due to tricyclic antidepressant overdosage, clinical presentation and treatment. *Med Toxicol* 1986;1:261.
126. Callaham M, Kassel D. Epidemiology of fatal tricyclic antidepressant ingestion: implications of management. *Ann Emerg Med* 1985;14:1.
127. Dziukas L, Cameron P. Management of antidepressants in overdose. *CNS Drugs* 1994;2:367.
128. Frommer DA et al. Tricyclic antidepressant overdose. *JAMA* 1987;257:521.
129. Guharoy SR. Adult respiratory distress syndrome associated with amitriptyline overdose. *Vet Hum Toxicol* 1994;36:316.
130. Shannon M, Lovejoy FS. Pulmonary consequences of severe tricyclic antidepressant ingestion. *Clin Toxicol* 1987;25:443.
131. Sohn D, Byers J. Cost effective drug screening in the laboratory. *Clin Toxicol* 1981;18:459.
132. Garriott JC. Interpretive toxicology. *Clin Lab Med* 1983;3:367.
133. Henry JA. Epidemiology and relative toxicity of antidepressant drugs in overdose. *Drug Saf* 1997;16:374.
134. Phillips S et al. Fluoxetine versus tricyclic antidepressants: a prospective multicenter study of antidepressant drug overdoses. *J Emerg Med* 1997;15:439.
135. Singh N et al. Serial electrocardiographic changes as a predictor of cardiovascular toxicity in acute tricyclic antidepressant overdose. *Am J Ther* 2002;9:75.
136. Pentel P, Benowitz N. Efficacy and mechanism of action of sodium bicarbonate in the treatment of desipramine toxicity in rats. *J Pharmacol Exp Ther* 1984;230:12.
137. Shannon M, Liebelt EL. Toxicology reviews: targeted management strategies for cardiovascular toxicity from tricyclic antidepressant overdose: the pivotal role for alkalinization and sodium loading. *Pediatr Emerg Care* 1998;14:293.
138. Kingston ME. Hyperventilation in tricyclic antidepressant poisoning. *Crit Care Med* 1979; 7:550.
139. Wrenn K et al. Profound alkalemia during treatment of tricyclic antidepressant overdose: a potential hazard of combined hyperventilation and intravenous bicarbonate. *Am J Emerg Med* 1992;10:553.
140. Seger DL et al. Variability of recommendations for serum alkalinization in tricyclic antidepressant overdose: a survey of U.S. poison center medical directors. *Clin Toxicol* 2003;41:331.
141. Kozer E, Koren G. Management of paracetamol overdose: current controversies. *Drug Saf* 2001;24:503.
142. Davis M et al. Paracetamol overdose in man: relationship between pattern of urinary metabolites and severity of liver damage. *Q J Med* 1976;45:181.
143. Corcoran GB et al. Evidence that acetaminophen and N-hydroxyacetaminophen form a common arylating intermediate, N-acetyl-benzoquinoneimine. *Mol Pharmacol* 1980;18:536.
144. Zed P, Krenzelok E. Treatment of acetaminophen overdose. *Am J Health Syst Pharm* 1999;56:1081.
145. Rayburn W et al. Drug overdose during pregnancy: an overview from a metropolitan poison control center. *Obstet Gynecol* 1984;64:611.
146. Czeizel A, Lendvay A. Attempted suicide and pregnancy [letter]. *Am J Obstet Gynecol* 1989;161:497.
147. Lester D, Beck AT. Attempted suicide and pregnancy. *Am J Obstet Gynecol* 1988;158:1084.
148. Riggs BS et al. Acute acetaminophen overdose during pregnancy. *Obstet Gynecol* 1989;74:247.
149. Rollins DE et al. Acetaminophen: potentially toxic metabolite formed by human fetal and adult liver microsomes and isolated fetal liver cells. *Science* 1979;205:1414.
150. McElhatton PR et al. Paracetamol poisoning in pregnancy: an analysis of the outcomes of cases referred to the teratology information service of the national poisons information service. *Hum Exp Toxicol* 1990;9:147.
151. Prescott LF et al. Plasma-paracetamol half-life and hepatic necrosis in patients with paracetamol overdosage. *Lancet* 1971;1:519.
152. Rumack BH, Matthew H. Acetaminophen poisoning and toxicity. *Pediatrics* 1975;55:871.
153. Rumack NH et al. Acetaminophen overdose: 662 cases with evaluation of oral acetylcysteine treatment. *Arch Intern Med* 1981;141:380.
154. Linden CH, Rumack BH. Acetaminophen overdose. *Emerg Med Clinic North Am* 1984;2:103.
155. Anker AL, Smilkstein MJ. Acetaminophen: concepts and controversies. *Emerg Med Clinic North Am* 1994;12:335.
156. Prescott L. Oral or intravenous N-acetylcysteine for acetaminophen poisoning? *Ann Emerg Med* 2005;45:409.
157. Prescott LF. Treatment of severe acetaminophen poisoning with intravenous acetylcysteine. *Arch Intern Med* 1981;141:386.
158. Bronstein AC, Rumack BH. Acute acetaminophen overdose during pregnancy: review of fifty-nine cases. *Vet Hum Toxicol* 1984;26:401.
159. Product information: Acetadote (acetylcysteine) injection labeling. Nashville, TN: Cumberland Pharmaceuticals, Inc.; 2006.
160. Smilkstein MJ at al. Acetaminophen overdose: a 48-hour intravenous N-acetylcysteine treatment protocol. *Ann Emerg Med* 1991;20:1058.
161. Bailey B, McGuigan MA. Management of anaphylactoid reactions to intravenous N-acetylcysteine. *Ann Emerg Med* 1998;31:710.
162. Kerr F et al. The Australasian clinical toxicology investigators collaboration randomized trial of different loading infusion rates of N-acetylcysteine. *Ann Emerg Med* 2005;45:402.
163. Smilkstein MJ et al. Efficacy of oral N-acetylcysteine in the treatment of acetaminophen overdose: analysis of national multicenter study (1976–1985). *N Engl J Med* 1988;319:1557.
164. Buckley NA et al. Oral or intravenous N-acetylcysteine: which is the treatment of choice for acetaminophen (paracetamol) poisoning? *Clin Toxicol* 1999;37:759.
165. Woo OF et al. Shorter duration of oral N-acetylcysteine therapy for acute acetaminophen overdose. *Ann Emerg Med* 2000;35:363.
166. Yip L, Dart RC. A 20-hour treatment for acute acetaminophen overdose. *N Engl J Med* 2003; 348:2471.
167. Clarke S. Oral or intravenous antidote for paracetamol overdose. *Emerg Med J* 2002;19:247.
168. Perry HE, Shannon MW. Efficacy of oral versus intravenous N-acetylcysteine in acetaminophen overdose: results of an open-label clinical trial. *J Pedatr* 1998;132:149.
169. Bernal W et al. Use and outcome of liver transplantation in acetaminophen-induced acute liver failure. *Hepatology* 1998;27:1050.
170. Mitchell I et al. Earlier identification of patients at risk from acetaminophen-induced acute liver failure. *Crit Care Med* 1998;26:279.
171. Gow PJ et al. Paracetamol overdose in a liver transplantation centre: an 8-year experience. *J Gastroenterol Hepatol* 1999;14:817.
172. Harrison PM et al. Serial prothrombin time as prognostic indicator in paracetamol induced fulminant hepatic failure. *Br Med J* 1990;301:964.
173. Kociancic T, Reed MD. Acetaminophen intoxication and length of treatment: how long is long enough. *Pharmacotherapy* 2003;23:1052.
174. Wright RO et al. Effect of metoclopramide dose on preventing emesis after oral administration of N-acetylcysteine for acetaminophen overdose. *Clin Toxicol* 1999;37:35.
175. Reed MD, Marx CM. Ondansetron for treating nausea and vomiting in the poisoned patient. *Ann Pharmacother* 1994;28:331.

CHAPTER 6

End-of-Life Care

Victoria F. Ferraresi and Thomas C. Bookwalter

HOSPICE AND PALLIATIVE CARE

Terminology

Hospice care and *palliative care* are similar, but distinct, terms sharing the common belief that, "the relief of suffering is a long standing, central, and fully legitimate aim of medicine." *End-of-life care* refers to both hospice care and palliative care. The basic principle of end-of-life care is to optimize the quality of life for the patient and family in the last weeks and months of life, as well as to provide support beyond the end of life into bereavement.

Palliative care, which includes hospice care, is ideally introduced early in the disease progression to provide support to patients with a serious chronic or life-threatening illness. The word "palliation," derived from the Latin word "pallium" (a cloak), has been defined as "treatment to reduce the violence of a disease."[1] The World Health Organization defines palliative care as an approach that improves the quality of life of patients and their families who are facing a life-threatening illness, by preventing and relieving suffering through early identification and impeccable assessment and treatment of pain and other physical, psychosocial, and spiritual problems.[2] Palliative care

- Affirms life and regards dying as a normal process
- Provides relief from pain and other distressing symptoms
- Intends neither to hasten nor postpone death
- Integrates the psychological and spiritual aspects of patient care
- Offers a support system to help patients live as actively as possible until death
- Uses a team approach to address the needs of the patient and his or her family during the patient's illness and to provide bereavement counseling when indicated[3]

The provision of palliative care by interdependent health team members composed of physicians, nurses, pharmacists, social workers, and others has been successful in meeting the unique needs of patients with difficult or terminal illnesses.[4–10]

Hospice, originally a place or way station for people making a pilgrimage, is considered both a philosophy of care and a place to deliver care. *Hospice care* can be delivered in a building designated as a hospice, in the patient's home, or in a facility where the patient resides. As a programmatic model for delivering palliative care, hospice care provides a team approach to the individualized symptom management (e.g., pain), as well as psychosocial, emotional, and spiritual support for the patient and his or her family and caregivers during the last months of life.[11]

Medicare Hospice Benefit

According to estimates of the National Hospice and Palliative Care Organization, there were approximately 4,100 hospice programs in the United States in 2005. In that year, more than 1.2 million patients received hospice services, with approximately 800,000 deaths, or one-third of all deaths, in the United States occurring under hospice care. Hospices provided care for patients with various terminal illnesses (e.g., cancer [46% of all admissions], heart disease [12%], dementia [9.8%], debility [9.2%], lung disease [7.5%]). Pediatric patients accounted for <1% of the hospice population, although the number of pediatric programs is growing. About 80% of hospice patients were 65 years of age or older, and one-third were 85 years or older. Under the Medicare Hospice Benefit, 82.4% of hospice patients received coverage in 2005.[11]

The Medicare Hospice Benefit, implemented in 1983, is funded from Part A (the hospital portion) of Medicare.[12] Patients are eligible for this benefit if, in the opinion of two physicians (i.e., patient's primary care physician and hospice medical director), the natural course of their disease will result in death within 6 months. Other insurance payers generally follow this criterion. In electing this benefit, patients must agree to relinquish their regular Medicare benefits, as they relate to the terminal illness, and agree not to seek curative treatment. This benefit links all care related to the terminal illness to the selected hospice program, which coordinates and provides the care. Hospice programs, therefore, have some latitude to establish policy on what they will and will not pay for within the context of the Medicare Hospice Conditions of Participation.[13] Hospice care is provided at four levels as follows, all of which

Table 6-1 Example of Hospice Daily Payment Rates for Routine Level of Care, 2008 Fiscal Year (October 1, 2007–September 30, 2008)

	A Unadjusted Payment Rate (B + C)	B Nonlabor Portion	C Labor Portion	D Wage Index	E Adjusted Labor Portion (C × D)	F Total Daily Payment (B + E)
San Francisco, CA	$135.11	$42.28	$92.83	1.6166	$150.07	**$192.35**
Jefferson City, MO	$135.11	$42.28	$92.83	0.8882	$82.45	**$124.73**

From references 15 and 16.

can be modified based on a patient's condition or caregiving needs:

- Routine level of care (day-to-day care in the home)
- Continuous level of care used when more skilled care in the home is required
- General inpatient care (reimbursement for a hospital stay related to symptoms that cannot be managed in the home)
- Respite care (up to 5 days in a skilled nursing facility) to give the caregiver a break or respite

Patients may freely visit their primary care provider (i.e., physician or nurse practitioner) for any reason, including reasons unrelated to their terminal illness. The primary care provider will be paid directly by Medicare. Patients may choose to use their Medicare benefits for other unrelated illnesses or to revoke their election to the Medicare Hospice Benefit at any time (e.g., to pursue curative treatment or seek treatment outside the hospice plan of care). Patients may at a later date, choose to return to hospice care or change to a different hospice program, without restrictions or loss of benefits.[14]

Hospice programs receive a fixed daily payment to provide all care related to the terminal diagnosis (e.g., medications, supplies, durable medical equipment, procedures, home health aides, provider visits, spiritual care, bereavement services). The reimbursement rates for the four levels of hospice care under the Medicare Hospice Benefit are established each summer for the following fiscal year, effective October 1.[15] A baseline reimbursement rate is set, along with an adjustment for wage differentials based on the local cost of living.[16] As an example, Table 6-1 shows the different reimbursement rates for the provision of routine level of care in San Francisco, California, and Jefferson City, Missouri.

Historically, hospice reimbursement rates have been low and have not kept pace with rising costs. Programs generally have high costs at the start of care because of personnel costs involved in the admission, assessment, and development of the initial plan of care, and obtaining medications, medical equipment, and medical supplies. High costs are also encountered nearer to the end of life, when new problems can appear and symptoms often intensify. In addition, it is becoming more common for patients to be referred to hospice when death is imminent. Median lengths of stay have declined, from 71.8 days during the Medicare demonstration project (1980–1982) to 26 days in 2005 (i.e., half of all patients in 2005 were on service <26 days, half were on longer).[11,17–19] Furthermore, drug costs have outpaced increases in hospice reimbursement by at least a factor of two based on the average wholesale price (AWP) and wholesale acquisition cost (WAC). These variables (i.e., referrals to hospice later in the course of terminal illness, higher costs at the start of care, shortened lengths of stay, higher drug costs) have placed intense pressure on hospice programs to manage expenses.

Management of Drug Costs

Because it is difficult to influence the time when patients are referred to hospice, the duration of time in hospice care, or the inherently higher costs when patients are first enrolled into hospice, the management of drug costs has taken a high priority in providing cost-effective hospice care. Table 6-2 illustrates historical reimbursement rates and how drug costs have proportionately consumed a larger portion of the Medicare reimbursement received by hospice programs since the inception of the Medicare Hospice Benefit.

Most hospices pay for prescriptions obtained from retail pharmacies based on the AWP of a drug. The AWP is determined by pharmaceutical manufacturers and is published as RED BOOK products[27] or by First Databank.[28] Although widely used, the AWP is often criticized as an inflated, artificial index, with drug markups as high as 1,000% over true acquisition costs.[29] In 2001, drug costs consumed 13.4% of hospice reimbursement, and, presumably, this percentage has increased since that year given the disparity in the rise of drug costs compared to hospice reimbursements.[30] Controlling drug costs, therefore, is a critical component of fiscal management for hospice programs.

Well-trained clinical pharmacists can affect the fiscal margins of hospice programs by discouraging inappropriate use of medications, establishing evidence-based formularies, promulgating prior authorization policies for specific targeted drugs, establishing policies for adhering to the use of generic drugs, and managing the quantities of medications to be dispensed. In addition to managing drug expenditures, pharmacists provide drug information both to patients and providers, and work integrally with other members of the hospice health care team to improve the safe and effective use of medications.

Referral to Hospice

Eligibility

1. M.P. is an 89-year-old woman referred to hospice for end-stage Alzheimer's dementia (AD). She lives in a residential care home for the elderly with a hired caregiver. Her husband has been unable to care for her at home for some time because she requires full assistance with all activities of daily living. She was recently hospitalized with aspiration pneumonia and a urinary tract infection, and completed a course of intravenous vancomycin and Zosyn. Her past medical history includes osteoporosis, coronary artery disease, chronic obstructive pulmonary disease (COPD),

Table 6-2 Drug Costs in Relation to Hospice Reimbursement (Routine Level of Care)

Year	Unadjusted Daily Reimbursement[15,20–26]	% Annual Rate Increase	Average Annual Price Increase for Most Widely Used Brand Name Drugs[31–33]		Hospice Per Diem Drug Costs[30]	Drug Costs as % of Reimbursement[30]
			WAC	AWP		
1983	$46.25	NA			$1.06	2.3%
1999	$97.11	110%*			$2.48	2.5%
2000	$101.84	4.9%	4.1%	6.0	NA	NA
2001	$101.84	0%	4.7%	6.0	$15.72	13.4%
2002	$110.42	8.4%	6.1%	6.0		
2003	$114.20	3.4%	7.0%	6.0, 6.5		
2004	$118.08	3.4%	7.1%	6.0		
2005	$121.98	3.3%	6.0%	(21.6%, 2001–2004)		
2006	$126.49	3.7%	6.2%			
2007	$130.79	3.4%				
2008	$135.11	3.3%				

WAC, wholesale acquisition cost (manufacturer's list price to wholesalers); AWP, average wholesale price (determined by manufacturer).
*For a 16-year period.

hypercholesterolemia, and hypothyroidism. She is not oriented to person, place, or date. Her speech is unintelligible or nonsensical. She cannot feed herself, but will eat the thick pureed food that is fed to her. She is bed-bound and incontinent of urine and stool. She is agitated at times, especially at night. Her Palliative Performance Scale (PPS) is 30%. Weight is 112 lb, decreased from 135 lb a year ago, and a recent serum albumin is 2.2 g/dL. What criteria does M.P. meet for eligibility for hospice services under the Medicare Hospice Benefit?

Patients with chronic diseases (e.g., Alzheimer disease, Parkinson disease, stroke, heart failure, lung disease) can be sufficiently ill and debilitated to need custodial care, but might not be sufficiently ill to meet the definition of a terminal illness. This differentiation between terminally ill versus chronically ill requiring custodial care is important because in order to qualify for hospice services under the Medicare Hospice Benefit, patients must be at a stage where death is expected within the next 6 months. For cancer diagnoses, the presence of widespread metastatic disease may make this prognosis more easily evident. However, for other chronic diseases, this is not as clear.

The Medicare fiscal intermediaries have issued criteria to assist in the determination of eligibility for hospice care, as well as criteria to meet a 6-month terminal prognosis for a number of diseases. These criteria, or local coverage determinations (LCDs), provide guidelines for meeting an overall decline in clinical status, for meeting non-disease-specific data to establish a baseline, for establishing the effect of comorbidities (e.g., renal failure, liver disease), and for the submission of documentation for having met criteria. Criteria have been established for patients with cancer and noncancer diagnoses, and these criteria are used in the determination of eligibility for service and reimbursement.[14,34] Criteria for the noncancer diagnoses have been developed for amyotrophic lateral sclerosis, dementia due to Alzheimer's disease and related disorders, heart disease, HIV disease, liver disease, pulmonary disease, stroke, coma of any etiology, and acute and chronic renal disease.

The determination of whether M.P. meets eligibility requirements for Medicare Hospice Benefits must be based on the established LCDs for dementia due to Alzheimer's disease. These criteria are as follows:

- Stage 7 or beyond, according to the Functional Assessment Staging Scale
  - Stage 7A: Can speak six or fewer intelligible words in a day or during an interview
  - Stage 7B: Speech ability limited to the use of a single intelligible word in a day or during an interview
  - Stage 7C: Cannot ambulate without assistance
  - Stage 7D: Cannot sit up without assistance
  - Stage 7E: Loss of ability to smile
  - Stage 7F: Loss of ability to hold head up independently
- Unable to ambulate without assistance
- Unable to dress without assistance
- Unable to bathe without assistance
- Urinary and fecal incontinence, intermittent or constant
- No consistently meaningful verbal communication; stereotypical phrases only or the ability to speak is limited to six or fewer intelligible words
- One of the following within the past 12 months: aspiration pneumonia; pyelonephritis or upper urinary tract infection, septicemia, decubitus ulcers (multiple, stages 3 and 4), fever (recurrent after antibiotic treatment)
- Inability to maintain sufficient fluid and caloric intake with 10% weight loss during the previous 6 months or serum albumin <2.5 g/dL

The PPS score (Table 6-3) gradates the extent of disability and can be used to assist in the determination of hospice eligibility.[35] M.P. meets the previous criteria and is eligible for hospice because of her Alzheimer disease. She clearly is debilitated. She is unable to speak intelligently, cannot feed herself, is not oriented to time or place, incontinent of urine and stool, has lost about 20% of her weight during the past year, has a serum albumin of 2.2 g/dL, and has a PPS rating of 30% (i.e., totally bed-bound, unable to do any activity, confused). In addition, she has a number of comorbidities, experienced a recent episode of aspiration pneumonia, and finished a course of antibiotic therapy.

Table 6-3 Palliative Performance Score (PPSv2) version 2

PPS Level	*Ambulation*	*Activity and Evidence of Disease*	*Self-Care*	*Intake*	*Conscious Level*
100%	Full	Normal activity and work No evidence of disease	Full	Normal	Full
90%	Full	Normal activity and work Some evidence of disease	Full	Normal	Full
80%	Full	Normal activity with effort Some evidence of disease	Full	Normal or reduced	Full
70%	Reduced	Unable to do normal job/work Significant disease	Full	Normal or reduced	Full
60%	Reduced	Unable to do hobby/house work Significant disease	Occasional assistance necessary	Normal or reduced	Full or Confusion
50%	Mainly sit/lie	Unable to do any work Extensive disease	Considerable assistance required	Normal or reduced	Full or confusion
40%	Mainly in bed	Unable to do most activity Extensive disease	Mainly assistance	Normal or reduced	Full or drowsy ± confusion
30%	Totally bed-bound	Unable to do any activity Extensive disease	Total care	Normal or reduced	Full or drowsy ± confusion
20%	Totally bed-bound	Unable to do any activity Extensive disease	Total care	Minimal to sips	Full or drowsy ± confusion
10%	Totally bed-bound	Unable to do any activity Extensive disease	Total care	Mouth care only	Drowsy or coma ± confusion
0%	Death				

From reference 35; adapted with permission of the Victoria Hospice Society.

Medication Management

2. M.P. has no known allergies. Her current medications are memantine (Namenda) 10 mg BID, aspirin 81 mg once daily, alendronate (Fosamax) 10 mg daily, esomeprazole (Nexium) 20 mg daily, lovastatin (Mevacor) 20 mg with dinner, megestrol 40 mg/mL (Megace) 5 mL (200 mg) BID, levothyroxine (Synthroid) 0.1 mg daily, multivitamin daily, beclomethasone (Vanceril) metered-dose inhaler (MDI) one puff daily, albuterol 2.5 mg/ipratropium 0.5 mg (DuoNeb) via nebulizer Q 4 hr PRN for wheezing or shortness of breath, acetaminophen 325 to 650 mg Q 6 hr PRN for mild pain or fever, olanzapine (Zyprexa) 5 mg HS PRN for agitation, milk of magnesia 30 mL PO daily for constipation, and a bisacodyl (Dulcolax) suppository 10 mg Q 3 days PRN if no bowel movement. What is your assessment of M.P.'s medication regimen? Which medications are the hospice required to provide, and which might be discontinued?

Hospices are required to provide (pay for) medications related to the terminal diagnosis for the palliation of symptoms within the hospice plan of care (POC). The POC is the individualized plan of treatment developed for each patient formulated at the start of care and updated regularly by the interdisciplinary group (IDG). The Conditions of Participation mandate that the IDG be composed of a physician, registered nurse, social worker, and a pastoral or other counselor.[13] A registered nurse coordinates the implementation of the POC. Some hospice program IDGs have incorporated a pharmacist into the group to review medication issues.

The large array of medications being taken by M.P. is similar to the lists of medications of many hospice patients. These patients are often elderly, have a long history of several chronic medical conditions, and have been taking multiple medications for past and present medical conditions. In most cases, the medication lists of patients who are admitted into a hospice program have seldom been reviewed, updated, or modified in light of the present medical situation. Admission to a hospice program represents a change in the level of care and is a most appropriate time for a review of all medications to ascertain the necessity of each, with the goal of optimizing efficacy and minimizing the potential for adverse effects, medication errors, and inappropriate costs.

Because M.P. is to be enrolled into a hospice program, her care should not be focused on curative treatments, but rather on the management of discomforting symptoms and on improving her quality of life in the time remaining. M.P.'s medications should be analyzed with the goal of simplification. Unnecessary medications should be discontinued and alternatives added to manage two or more symptoms concurrently. The following changes should be considered:

Acetaminophen. This analgesic is often helpful in relieving mild pain, particularly in immobile elderly patients. A trial of around-the-clock acetaminophen could be helpful.

Albuterol/ipratropium combination. The hospice program is not required to pay for medications related to M.P.'s COPD because it is not related to her LCD for Alzheimer's disease. Nevertheless, this combination inhalation formulation should be continued if she is able to participate in her nebulizer treatments and they improve her breathing.

Alendronate. This bisphosphonate drug can be discontinued because the treatment of osteoporosis is not an important consideration at this terminal stage of her life nor is it in the hospice plan of care. Thus, hospice would not cover it. Furthermore, M.P. is bed-bound; alendronate should be ingested in the upright position, and patients should remain upright after taking the medication to decrease the risk of alendronate-induced esophageal irritation. Pain that she may experience from osteoporosis can be treated with analgesics.

Aspirin. The low-dose aspirin is intended to decrease the risk of cardiovascular clotting. The aspirin will not increase M.P.'s comfort or quality of life. Although the aspirin would not be covered by her Medicare benefit, it can be continued unless her primary care provider prefers its discontinuation.

Beclomethasone MDI. This patient is not functioning well cognitively (i.e., not oriented to time, person, or place) and would be unable to effectively time the inhalation of a breath to the actuation of her MDI. A systemic corticosteroid (e.g., prednisone) might improve her COPD symptoms and also improve her appetite and sense of well-being. The potential for adverse effects is modest with short-term corticosteroid use.

Bisacodyl, Milk of Magnesia. Constipation in hospice patients is common because of decreased gastrointestinal motility with advanced age, decreased physical activity, lack of adequate fiber and fluid intake, and use of constipating medications (e.g., opioids, anticholinergics, psychotropic agents).[36] The milk of magnesium, with an occasional bisacodyl suppository, is a good laxative regimen for this patient. If an opioid is later prescribed for M.P., a mild stimulant laxative (e.g., senna) with a stool softener (e.g., Colace) would be indicated. If stool softeners, stimulants, and saline laxatives are ineffective in resolving opioid-induced constipation, oral sorbitol or lactulose (10 g/15 mL) in 30-mL dosages can be prescribed up to four doses a day if needed. (Sorbitol would be preferred because it is more cost effective.) Mineral oil 30 mL daily is an option if the stool is hard; however, mineral oil would not be optimal for M.P. because of her recent history of aspiration pneumonia. In cases of refractory constipation, the oral ingestion of naloxone, an injectable opioid antagonist, can reverse opioid-induced constipation by antagonizing opioid effects within the gastrointestinal tract without affecting systemic analgesic because naloxone is poorly absorbed orally. The usual starting dose of naloxone for the management of opioid-induced constipation is 0.4 to 0.6 mg PO Q 6 hr. Naloxone doses of 2.4 mg PO Q 6 hr have been used, but have been associated with opioid withdrawal symptoms.[37]

Esomeprazole. This proton-pump inhibitor (PPI) would probably be unnecessary because alendronate-induce esophageal-gastrointestinal irritation would not be an issue subsequent to its discontinuation. If a PPI, however, is needed, nonprescription generic omeprazole is preferred because it is <20% of the cost of Nexium.[38]

Levothyroxine. This thyroid medication should be continued until M.P. is no longer able to swallow. This medication, however, would not be covered under her hospice Medicare benefit, which is based on her Alzheimer's disease, rather than other thyroid end-of-life disease (e.g., cancer).

Lovastatin. Cholesterol-lowering agents are not necessary during the last 6 months of life and should be discontinued. Lovastatin would not improve the quality of life of M.P. at this stage of her terminal illness and would not be covered by her hospice benefit.

Megestrol. The progesterone derivative, megestrol, in doses of 400 to 800 mg daily, can substantially stimulate appetite.[39] If undernourished hospice patients have a desire to eat more, many hospice patients will provide megestrol, regardless of whether it will be covered by the Medicare hospice benefit. It is unclear, however, whether stimulation of appetite in a cognitively impaired patient will result in weight gain or improved nutritional status. Because the benefits in this situation are unclear, the potential of adverse effects (e.g., venous thrombosis) of megestrol needs to be considered, especially in M.P., who is not ambulatory and had been taking low-dose aspirin for prevention of cardiovascular clotting.

Memantine. Because the NMDA (N-methyl-D-aspartate) antagonist, memantine, has been modestly effective in improving performance in patients with moderate-to-severe Alzheimer's disease,[40,41] it is probably of limited utility for M.P. It would be reasonable to discontinue M.P.'s memantine subsequent to discussion with appropriate hospice team members and M.P.'s family.

Multivitamins. and other nutritional supplements are unlikely to improve M.P.'s comfort or quality of life. The discontinuation of these drugs would simplify medication administration, decrease the potential for medication errors, and decrease costs.

Olanzapine. An antipsychotic (e.g., olanzapine, haloperidol, chlorpromazine) is often prescribed to manage the agitation and confusion encountered by patients with dementia. At the time of admission to hospice, patients may be receiving atypical agents (e.g., olanzapine). Small doses of the more typical antipsychotics, such as haloperidol (Haldol) and chlorpromazine (Thorazine), can also be very useful in treating opioid-induced nausea and vomiting[42] and would be covered by M.P.'s Medicare Hospice Benefit. Chlorpromazine would be preferable when more sedation is desired.

SYMPTOM MANAGEMENT

The American College of Physicians has developed clinical guidelines, based on a systematic review of evidence and on a report by the Agency for Healthcare Research and Quality, to improve palliative care at the end of life. These guidelines provide strong recommendations for the regular assessment of patients at the end of life for symptoms of pain, dyspnea, and depression, and for therapies of proven effectiveness for these symptoms. For patients with cancer, these include the use of opioids, nonsteroidal anti-inflammatory drugs, and bisphosphonates for pain; tricyclic antidepressants, selective serotonin reuptake inhibitors, and psychosocial interventions for depression; and opioids for unrelieved dyspnea and oxygen for short-term relief of hypoxemia. The guidelines do not address other variables of palliative care at the end-of-life or the management of other matters (e.g., nutritional support) because the quality of evidence is limited rather than because other issues or symptoms are unimportant.[43]

3. As soon as the hospice admission and assessment is completed, the nurse develops a plan for symptom management and orders a comfort kit for M.P. Why are the components in this kit useful?

Some hospices use a general comfort kit that contains specific medications to manage symptoms commonly encountered by most hospice patients, or they order medications to treat anticipated symptoms for a specific patient. These medications are placed in the home or facility in which the patient resides. This facilitates the availability of medications to patients who encounter anticipated symptoms and are convenient when caregivers are instructed by the patient's primary

Table 6-4 Symptom Prevalence in Advanced Cancer

	% of Patients with Stated Symptom				
Symptom	Vainio and Auvinen[46] (%)	Curtis et al.[48] (%)	Donnelly and Walsh[47] (%)	Conill et al.[45] (First Evaluation) (%)	Conill et al.[45] (Second Evaluation) (%)
Pain	51	NR	64	52.3	30.1
Nausea/vomiting	21	32/25	36/23	26.1/18.8	23/10.2
Dyspnea	19	41	51	39.8	46.6
Constipation	23	40	51	49.4	55.1
Insomnia	9	NR	NR	34.7	28.4
Delirium	NR	NR	NR	NR	NR
Anorexia	30	55	74	68.2	80.1
Fatigue	NR	NR	NR	NR	NR
Weight loss	39	NR	NR	NR	NR
Weakness	51	NR	NR	76.7	81.8
Confusion	8	NR	NR	30.1	68.2
Dry mouth	NR	NR	NR	61.4	69.9
Dysphagia	NR	NR	NR	27.8	46.0
Anxiety	NR	20	23	50.6	45.5
Depression	NR	31	40	52.8	38.6
Diarrhea	NR	NR	NR	8.0	6.8

NR, not reported.

care provider to provide the medication to the patient. Patients living with a life-threatening illness or nearing the end-of-life can encounter as many as 53 symptoms.[44] In one study, patients ($n = 176$) experienced an average of 6.6 to 6.8 distressing symptoms during the last week of life.[45] In general, the prevalence of each symptom is difficult to measure and demonstrates a high degree of variability. The prevalence of pain (43%–80%) in cancer patients, for example, varies with the primary site of advanced cancer.[45] Patients with terminal illnesses also experience nausea and vomiting (4%–44%), dyspnea (15%–79%), constipation (4%–65%), insomnia (7%–28%), delirium (4%–85%), anorexia (6%–74%), weight loss (58%–77%), and fatigue (13%–91%).[45–47] The disparity in symptom prevalence (Table 6-4) may be attributed to a host of variables (e.g., study design, patient population, underlying disease, inconsistent definitions). The occurrence of symptoms, however, can vary significantly, even within the last week of life, and the need for frequent assessments of patients cannot be overemphasized. Morphine, lorazepam, haloperidol, prochlorperazine suppositories, and an anticholinergic agent are commonly ordered for hospice patients.

Morphine. Every hospice cancer patient should have a short-acting opioid available for the palliation of unrelieved dyspnea and pain. Although morphine can cause respiratory depression, small doses are very effective in controlling dyspnea by multiple mechanisms: vasodilation, reduced peripheral vascular resistance, inhibition of baroreceptor responses, reduction of brainstem responsiveness to carbon dioxide (the primary mechanism of opioid-induced respiratory depression), and lessened reflex vasoconstriction caused by increased blood P_{CO_2} levels. Opioids can also reduce the anxiety associated with dyspnea and might also act directly on opioid receptors present in the airways[49–51] (Table 6-5).

Hospice patients generally do not have an easily accessible port (i.e., an IV line) into which medications can be easily administered. As a result, medications are primarily administered orally and, occasionally, by sublingual, buccal, transdermal, rectal, or subcutaneous (if an infusion is warranted) routes of administration. When patients lose the ability to swallow near the end of life (or have a condition that precludes swallowing), the sublingual or buccal routes of administration are the most useful, especially if drugs are lipophilic. Morphine is

Table 6-5 Treatment of Dyspnea at End-of-Life

Nonpharmacologic methods	Pursed lip breathing Upright position Relaxation Meditation Use of a fan or open window to circulate air over the face
Pharmacologic therapy	**Systemic opioids (short acting)** in small doses given orally, sublingually, or via injection can be given Q 1–2 hr PRN. **Long-acting agents** can be added to supplement routine use short-acting opioids. **Inhaled opioids** deliver medication via nebulization directly into the airway, avoiding first-pass metabolism, allowing use of smaller doses, and minimizing side effects such as drowsiness. May cause local histamine release, leading to bronchospasm. Use nonpreserved sterile injectable products. More cumbersome and expensive due to use of nebulizer and nonpreserved parenteral products. Agents: morphine 2.5–10 mg in 2 mL 0.9% NaCl hydromorphone 0.25–1 mg in 2 mL 0.9% NaCl fentanyl 25 mcg in 2 mL 0.9% NaCl Generally given Q 2–4 hr PRN for breathlessness. **Benzodiazepines** are useful for the anxiety associated with breathlessness.

From references 49–51.

hydrophilic, and although some of it might be absorbed across the mucous membranes, the primary clinical effect probably results from gastrointestinal absorption after the drug has trickled down the back of the throat.

Oral morphine sulfate (OMS), in a concentration of 20 mg/mL, is commonly packaged in a 30-mL bottle at the beginning of hospice care. This bottle of morphine can provide sixty 10-mg doses, and at this concentration, only 0.5 mL of morphine needs to be administered. Oxycodone or hydromorphone, in comparable adjusted doses, can be substituted for morphine when needed.

Lorazepam. A short-acting benzodiazepine (e.g., lorazepam 0.5 mg Q 4 hr PRN) is useful for the treatment of anxiety. Patients, especially those with respiratory symptoms, can experience episodes of extreme anxiety near the end-of-life. Caution should be used in not overusing these drugs in the elderly because they can increase the risk of falling or cause paradoxical reactions and worsen delirium or restlessness.

Haloperidol. Small doses of haloperidol (e.g., 0.5–1 mg) are useful for the treatment of restlessness, delirium, or nausea and vomiting.

Prochlorperazine. When patients cannot take oral medications to manage nausea and vomiting, rectal suppositories of prochlorperazine are often effective. Although drug therapy needs to consider the etiology of the nausea and vomiting, prochlorperazine is generally a good initial agent.

Anticholinergic. As death approaches, patients can have difficulty in clearing pharyngeal secretions, and as a result, generate a sound commonly known as a death rattle.[52] Although patients are often unconscious at this point, this sound can be very distressing to those nearby. An anticholinergic (e.g., glycopyrrolate, hyoscyamine, scopolamine, atropine) can be administered in an attempt to dry these pharyngeal secretions. This treatment modality is usually initiated after the patient has become obtunded; if begun too early, patients might develop problems with thickened bronchial or pulmonary secretions, tachycardia, delirium, dry mouth, or other adverse anticholinergic effects. Glycopyrrolate, available in a tablet or injectable formulation, is a good choice for an anticholinergic because it minimally crosses the blood–brain barrier. The 1-mg tablets could be crushed and placed under the tongue Q 8 hr. Hyoscyamine is available as oral tablets, capsules, oral sustained-release tablets, sublingual tablets, oral liquid, oral solution, and injection. Either the sublingual tablets or oral solution of hyoscyamine can be given in a 0.125- to 0.25-mg dose sublingually Q 4 hr PRN. Scopolamine-transdermal patches have a slow onset of action (blood levels are detected 4 hours after application)[53] and are of limited utility in this situation. The oral administration of atropine ophthalmic solution 1% is convenient to administer and is cost effective. Assuming that 20 drops is approximately equivalent to 1 mL, patients can be given 0.5 to 1 mg (1–2 drops) of the atropine ophthalmic solution PO Q 4 hr PRN. Families and caregivers must be instructed not to use this in the eye.

4. The patient's nurse has difficulty finding OMS available from a pharmacy and difficulty in finding a pharmacy willing to accept a faxed prescription. Why is morphine so difficult to obtain?

Providing relief for pain or other symptoms with opioids is often difficult due to numerous barriers. Patients and caregivers are often fearful of opioids, or mistakenly believe these medications will cause addiction or hasten death.[54] Pharmacists can create barriers by not having opioids in the pharmacy, sometimes due to fear of robbery, fear of investigation by drug regulatory agencies, or insufficient appreciation of the usefulness of opioids in pain management and palliative care.[55] Pharmacists, who are inexperienced in providing service to hospice patients, might not be knowledgeable of federal regulations governing the provision of controlled substances to hospice patients. Federal statutes, as well as most state statutes, permit prescriptions for Schedule II controlled substances for hospice patients to be faxed. According to the Code of Federal Regulations (21CFR1306.11) paragraph (g): "A prescription prepared in accordance with Sec. 1306.05 written for a Schedule II narcotic substance for a patient enrolled in a hospice care program certified and/or paid for by Medicare under Title XVIII or a hospice program which is licensed by the state may be transmitted by the practitioner or the practitioner's agent to the dispensing pharmacy by facsimile. The practitioner, or the practitioner's agent, will note on the prescription that the patient is a hospice patient. The facsimile serves as the original written prescription for purposes of this paragraph (g) and it shall be maintained in accordance with Sec. 1304.04(h)."[56]

The process of ordering controlled substances for use by hospice patients at home can take many hours, and sometimes as much as an entire day. Hospice providers should anticipate possible difficulties when placing orders for Schedule II controlled-substance medications.

PAIN MANAGEMENT

5. G.G., a 40-year-old woman, is admitted to hospice with stage IV ovarian cancer, metastatic to pelvis, liver, and lungs. She was diagnosed after many months of nonspecific complaints of gastric distress and bloating. On laparotomy, she was staged as stage III and underwent a total abdominal hysterectomy and bilateral salpingo-oophorectomy and tumor debulking at that time. She has undergone subsequent chemotherapy and repeated tumor debulkings. In the past 6 months, her weight has decreased from 175 lb to 153 lb (she is 52 in. tall). Her primary complaints are constant nausea, constipation, and gripping abdominal pain, which she characterizes as burning and twisting. She quantifies the pain as 8/10 (on a 0- to 10-point scale) and describes the pain as one that moves into her groin and leg. Her family is unhappy about the drowsiness she experiences from her medications; they believe she is overmedicated. She has no known allergies. Current medications are Duragesic transdermal system 75 mcg/hour Q 72 hr, Kadian 50 mg PO once daily (sustained-release morphine intended for once daily administration), DSS 250 mg daily, Prevacid 30 mg PO daily, and lorazepam 0.5 mg Q 4 hr PRN nausea and anxiety. What is your assessment of her pain management regimen?

G.G. is currently using two long-acting opioids (i.e., Duragesic, Kadian), but is still unable to achieve relief of her pain, which is probably neuropathic pain (burning and twisting). The use of two long-acting agents is duplicative and should be replaced with one opioid. Methadone would be a better a long-acting agent because it has activity against neuropathic pain (see Chapter 8). When converting the fentanyl (i.e., Duragesic transdermal) and Kadian to methadone, the following should be considered: (a) patient compliance and ability to follow prescription directions, (b) use of an appropriate conversion formula, (c) converting a transdermal formulation of fentanyl to an oral opioid formulation, and (d) a supplemental opioid for breakthrough pain.

Due to its long and variable elimination half-life, the dose of methadone should generally be adjusted only once every 4 to 6 days, and patients must be able and willing to precisely follow directions for its use. Although formulas and tables are available to assist practitioners in the conversion of a short-acting morphine formulation to long-acting methadone, these have caused problems.[57,58] A better, safer conversion plan is to use the methadone prescribing information[59] and to follow a general rule of thumb not to exceed 30 mg of morphine as an initial oral dose.[60]

Total Daily Baseline Oral Morphine Dose (i.e., Dose of Morphine Equivalents)	*Estimated Daily Oral Methadone Requirement (as % of Total Daily Morphine Dose)*
<100 mg	20%–30%
100–300 mg	10%–20%
300–600 mg	8%–12%
600–1,000 mg	5%–10%
>1,000 mg	<5%

Once the conversion is made, the calculated dose is adjusted and the dosing interval is set at every 12, 8, or 6 hours, based on patient age, previous use of opioids, and current clinical status. Clinical judgment is vital in individualizing a regimen for each patient based on his or her needs.

Before calculating the conversion to methadone for G.G., an important consideration in patients using transdermal fentanyl is an assessment of its absorption.[61] The fentanyl from the transdermal system is absorbed through several layers of the skin and deposited in the subcutaneous fat, from which it is absorbed into the systemic circulation. It is generally observed that transdermal fentanyl is not effective in very thin, cachectic patients. In those cases, the conversion would be made without including the fentanyl. The patch would be removed at initiation of the first methadone dose and supplemented with medication for breakthrough pain if needed. In patients using multiple patches, one patch can be removed every 3 days. Despite weight loss, G.G. (52 in. and 153 lb) is not cachectic, and the fentanyl should be included when calculating the conversion of her current opioid dose to a comparable methadone dose. In this patient, her sustained morphine formulation (i.e., Kadian 50 mg PO TID) is equivalent to 150 mg/day of oral morphine. Her fentanyl transdermal system 75 mcg/hour is equivalent to about 150 mg of oral morphine equivalent/day. Her total morphine equivalents (MEs) per day = 150 mg + 150 mg = 300 mg. Using a 1:5 ratio for conversion of MEs to methadone, the calculated dose of oral methadone for this patient should be about 60 mg/day.

Although G.G. is relatively young, has been using opioids for some time, and has severe pain (quantified at 8/10), a methadone dose of 20 mg Q 8 hr (i.e., 60 mg/day) might be excessive. She should be treated with 15 mg of methadone PO Q 8 hr (45 mg/day), and the dose increased, if needed, based on her clinical response. This smaller initial dose would accommodate for some incomplete cross-tolerance from the morphine and fentanyl, and for any fentanyl that remains in her system over the next several days. Patients who have been on much higher doses of opioids, alternatively, can be converted over a period of several days (e.g., converting one-third of the previous daily dose of opioid every 3 days). This is an especially useful method for converting opioid doses for thin, cachectic patients who have been on multiple transdermal patches. A clinician should be in touch with G.G. frequently during the first several days after her conversion to methadone. A telephone call should be made 2 to 4 hours after the first dose to assess for efficacy and toxicity (primarily somnolence, confusion, or nausea). If pain relief does not last for the entire dosing interval, it can be adjusted, or G.G. can be instructed to take an extra dose of methadone.

An added benefit in changing to methadone for G.G. is a financial one for the hospice. Outpatient prices for long-acting opioids based on AWP are very steep and significantly add to hospice costs. The prudent use of methadone can improve overall pain management and keep costs in check. When methadone is not appropriate, generic extended-release morphine is a good second choice. Transdermal fentanyl should be reserved for patients who cannot take oral medication or for when there are significant compliance issues. OxyContin should be used only when patients cannot tolerate morphine or have other contraindications to its use. By converting to methadone, G.G.'s daily cost for the opioid alone will decrease from $33.41/day (i.e., $16.86 for Kadian and $16.55 for Duragesic) to $0.48 or less based on the AWP prices listed in the table.

Average Wholesale Price (AWP) of Long-Acting Opioids[38] for 1-Day Supply (Equivalent to Oral Morphine 150 mg/day)

OxyContin 120 mg (40-mg tablets × 3)	$17.61
Kadian 150 mg (50-mg capsules × 3)	$16.86
Duragesic 75 mcg ($49.65/patch ÷ 3 = 1 day's dose)	$16.55
Avinza 150 mg (60 mg + 90 mg, one capsule of each)	$15.63
Fentanyl transdermal 75 mcg ($40.23 ÷ 3)	$13.41
MS Contin 75 mg BID (15 mg + 60 mg, two of each)	$10.94
Morphine-ER 75 mg BID (15 mg + 60 mg, two of each)	$8.40
Methadone 30 mg (10 mg × 3)	$0.48

From RED BOOK for Windows, Thompson Micromedex, Vol. 44, April 2007.

G.G. will also need something for breakthrough pain. Some practitioners use small doses of methadone, 2.5 mg or 5 mg, as often as Q 3 hr. This is a good choice in a well-supervised (i.e., inpatient) setting with nurses familiar with the use of methadone. However, if caregivers treat methadone as if it were morphine, which is much more commonly used for breakthrough pain, the risk of overmedicating the patient is very real. This can have disastrous consequences, especially in frail, elderly patients. Because G.G. tolerated morphine well in the past, 30 mg or 1.5 mL of OMS 20 mg/mL can be prescribed Q 2–4 hr PRN for breakthrough pain because she is not in an inpatient setting.

Aggressive Symptom Management and Palliative Sedation

6. D.V., a 35-year-old man with gastric cancer metastasized to the esophagus with periaortic involvement is hospitalized. He

was diagnosed 10 months ago, and his disease has progressed despite multiple courses of chemotherapy (most recently, irinotecan and Erbitux). A double-lumen peripherally inserted central catheter line has been inserted. He has lost 65 lb since diagnosis, weighs 150 lbs at 6 ft tall, and presents with abdominal pain, severe nausea, vomiting, obstipation (intractable constipation), and general malaise. D.V. describes his pain as a 7/10 in intensity and as "burning like a knife through my stomach." He uses 50 to 75 patient-controlled analgesia (PCA) bolus doses Q 24 hr. He has no other medical problems. D.V. is referred to hospice care because he and his wife have agreed to stop chemotherapy and do not want to go back to the hospital. He states a history of allergic reactions to morphine, ondansetron, and diphenhydramine, although these reactions are not noted. He is presently receiving hydromorphone 2 mg/hour in an IV infusion with 1 mg PCA bolus dose Q 5 min, hydromorphone 4 mg PO Q 4 hr PRN pain, fentanyl transdermal 275 mcg/hour Q 3 day, ketamine 20 mg PO Q 3 hr, senna two tablets PO BID, docusate sodium 250 mg PO BID, MiraLax 17 g PO daily, lactulose 15 mL PO PRN constipation, lorazepam 2 mg PO Q 4 hr PRN nausea or vomiting, metoclopramide 10 mg Q 6 hr PRN nausea or vomiting, promethazine 25 mg IV Q 4 hr PRN nausea or vomiting, baclofen 10 mg Q 8 hr as needed for hiccups, and Protonix 40 mg once daily. What is your assessment of his medication regimen?

D.V.'s drug regimen is unnecessarily complicated for a patient at home. It may be possible to simplify it by looking at each problem anew. His pain is poorly managed as evidenced by his complaint of pain intensity at 7/10 (on a scale of 0–10), the use of multiple opioids, and the use of excessive PCA boluses. Once an infusion with PCA dosing is started, there is no need to continue other long-acting opioids (i.e., transdermal fentanyl), or oral agents for breakthrough pain. The PCA doses are serving as the rescue doses for breakthrough pain, and pain relief should be titrated using this method alone. Once pain is well controlled, an oral long-acting agent can be considered if the patient is able to swallow. To do otherwise creates a chaotic approach. Patients reporting allergic reactions to opioids should be carefully asked to describe the precise nature of the purported allergic reaction. True allergies to opioids are rare; patients often refer to an adverse reaction as an allergy or have experienced an effect from the histamine release that is associated with opioids. Hydromorphone, especially injectable hydromorphone, is much more expensive than morphine and is best reserved for use in patients who have a genuine allergy to morphine.

Although D.V. had been prescribed ketamine Q 3 hr in the hospital, it is unrealistic to expect that this can be continued in the home setting. D.V. and his wife would probably be glad to discontinue it and replace it with an alternative due to his need to be dosed Q 3 hr.

D.V.'s constipation is currently treated with multiple medications within the same therapeutic class. It would be more prudent to maximize the use of a single agent within a category, rather than using two at less than the maximally recommended dose. D.V. can use a higher dose of senna (up to four tablets BID), and then, if necessary, add sorbitol (which is more cost effective than lactulose).

D.V. also takes multiple medications for his nausea and vomiting. The injectable promethazine can be converted to suppositories for use at home. He had also been directed to take lorazepam for his nausea and vomiting; however, benzodiazepines are not effective antiemetics. They are given to manage the anxiety associated with nausea and vomiting, and are particularly useful in managing the anticipatory nausea and vomiting that is commonly encountered during chemotherapy administration. Metoclopramide can be useful for D.V.'s nausea and vomiting if his physical examination reveals hypoactive bowel sounds. It is also useful for treating hiccups, and the need for baclofen can be reassessed.

7. **A few days after arriving home, D.V. asks his hospice nurse, "Can't you just give me something to end it all?" He has not been sleeping well, is tired of taking so many medications, and wants to alleviate the burden he feels he is imposing on his wife.**

In patients who are terminally ill, suffering may continue despite maximal palliative efforts. As a result, practitioners continually encounter patients' requests for the ending of their lives because of overwhelming suffering. Although controversial, most clinicians are significantly averse to this practice both ethically and legally.[62–67] State and national professional organizations have not been helpful in providing guidance for managing this ultimate end-of-life decision. Each clinician, therefore, must rely on his or her own ethics to decide whether to participate in facilitating a patient's death. Although substantial numbers of clinicians can imagine situations in which assisted suicide would be acceptable, few are willing to actively participate in the ending of a patient's life.[68,69]

In a small number of patients, it may be desirable to reduce suffering by the thoughtful use of medications to induce sedation. It is not appropriate to increase opioid doses to achieve the desired sedated state. Medications used successfully to induce sedation for these patients include benzodiazepines, barbiturates, and phenothiazines. No drug or drug class is superior to any other for this use.[70]

A trial of palliative sedation with lorazepam could be initiated at a rate of 2 mg/hour and gradually increased if needed to as much as 6 mg/hour. Although palliative sedation has a small potential to shorten life, the need to relieve terminal agitation could justify this risk. Palliative sedation should only be initiated as a last resort in severe cases not responsive to other palliative measures, and only after thorough discussion of the important clinical and ethical issues with the patient, family, and other clinical team members.

8. **Repeated increases in the hydromorphone infusion basal rate (he is now at 25 mg/hour) had little effect on managing D.V.'s pain, and his consistent use of up to 120 PCA attempts over 24 hours reflects his continued pain. He describes the intensity of his pain as 8/10 (on a 0–10 scale). Before considering palliative sedation, what other therapeutic interventions can be implemented for D.V.?**

Before considering palliative sedation, patients should be thoroughly assessed for insomnia and depression. Underlying reasons for insomnia should be explored and treated. Poor pain management is often to blame. In this patient, lidocaine 0.5 to 1 mg/kg/hour administered intravenously or subcutaneously might be useful to assist in the management of his severe neuropathic pain.[71–75] Lidocaine purportedly interrupts pain transmission by blocking sodium channels (see Chapter 8).

Clinical Result. D.V. was started on lidocaine 1 mg/kg/hour intravenously. A bolus dose was not given due to the short half-life of lidocaine. Overnight, his use of hydromorphone boluses dropped to one. He now reported his pain as 1/10 and slept through the night for the first time in months. Over the next 2 days, the hydromorphone basal rate was tapered to 5 mg/hour. He did not develop any toxicity, such as perioral numbness, metallic taste, or somnolence. D.V. continued on lidocaine, using no hydromorphone boluses for the next 2 weeks until he died at home, surrounded by his family.

RESOURCES FOR HOSPICE AND PALLIATIVE CARE

The following websites are resources for practitioners who want more information on hospice and palliative care:

- American Academy of Hospice and Palliative Medicine (AAHPM): www.aahpm.org/
- Center to Advance Palliative Care (CAPC): www.capc.org/
- Centers for Medicare & Medicaid Services (CMS): www.cms.hhs.gov/center/hospice.asp
- End-of-Life/Palliative Education Resource Center (EPERC): www.eperc.mcw.edu/staff.htm
- Hospice Foundation of America (HFA): www.hospicefoundation.org/
- Innovations in End-of-Life Care (an international journal of leaders in end-of-life care): www2.edc.org/lastacts/
- International Association for Hospice & Palliative Care (IAHPC): www.hospicecare.com/
- MedlinePlus Hospice Care: www.nlm.nih.gov/medlineplus/hospicecare.html
- National Hospice and Palliative Care Organization (NHPCO): www.nhpco.org/
- Pallimed, A Hospice and Palliative Medicine Blog: www.pallimed.org
- The Population-based Palliative Care Research Network (PoPCRN): www.uchsc.edu/popcrn/
- U.S. Department of Veterans Affairs, Office of Geriatrics and Extended Care, Hospice and Palliative Care: www1.va.gov/geriatricsshg/page.cfm?pg=65

REFERENCES

1. Lamers W. Defining hospice and palliative care: some further thoughts. *J Pain Palliat Care Pharmacother* 2002;16:65.
2. Doyle D et al. Introduction. In: Doyle D, et al., ed. *The Oxford Textbook of Palliative Medicine.* Oxford: Oxford University Press; 1993:3.
3. Sepulveda C et al. Palliative care: the World Health Organization's global perspective. *J Pain Sympt Man* 2002;24:91.
4. Lipman AG. Drug therapy in terminally ill patients. *Am J Hosp Pharm* 1975;32:270.
5. Berry JI et al. Pharmaceutical services in hospices. *Am J Hosp Pharm* 1981;38:1010.
6. Arter SG et al. Hospice care and the pharmacist. *Am Pharm* 1987;NS27:32.
7. Bonomi AE et al. Cancer pain management: barriers, trends, and the role of pharmacists. *Am J Pharm Assoc* (Wash) 1999;39:558.
8. Lucas C et al. Contribution of a liaison clinical pharmacist to an inpatient palliative care unit. *Palliat Med* 1997;11:209.
9. Hanif N. Role of the epalliative care unit pharmacist. *J Palliat Care* 1991;7:35.
10. Wagner J, Goldstein E. Pharmacist's role in loss and grief. *Am J Hosp Pharm* 1977;34:490.
11. National Hospice and Palliative Care Organization (NHPCO). NHPCO facts and figures 2005 findings. Available at: www.nhpco.org/i4a/pages/Index.cfm?pageid=3274. Accessed July 9, 2007.
12. National Hospice and Palliative Care Organization (NHPCO). History of hospice care. Available at: www.nhpco.org/i4a/pages/index.cfm?pageid=3285. Accessed April 10, 2008.
13. Electronic Code of Federal Regulations. Title 42—Public Health, Chapter IV—Centers for Medicare & Medicaid Services, Department of Health and Human Services, Part 418—Hospice Care. Available at: www.access.gpo.gov/nara/cfr/waisidx_04/42cfr418_04.html. Accessed April 10, 2008.
14. Fine P, Mac Low C. Hospice Referral and Care: Practical Guidance for Clinicians. Medscape CME/CE. Available at: www.medscape.com/viewprogram/3345_pnt (membership required). Accessed April 10, 2008.
15. Centers for Medicaid & Medicare Services, Department of Health and Human Services. CMS Manual System: Pub 100-04 Medicare Claims Processing: Transmittal 1280. Change Request 5685. June 29, 2007. Available at: www.cms.hhs.gov/transmittals/downloads/R1280CP.pdf. Accessed April 10, 2008.
16. Centers for Medicaid & Medicare Services, Department of Health and Human Services. 42 CFR Part 418. Medicare Program; Hospice Wage Index for Fiscal Year 2008. Available at: www.cms.hhs.gov/MLNProducts/downloads/cms-1539-p.pdf. Accessed April 10, 2008.
17. Brinbaum HG, Kidder D. What does hospice cost? *Am J Pub Health* 1984;74:689. Available at www.pubmedcentral.nih.gov/picrender.fcgi?artid=165167&blobtype=pdf. Accessed July 25, 2007.
18. NHPCO Facts and Figures on Hpspice Care in America, January 2001. Available at: www.kued.org/productions/journey/how/factsheet0101.pdf. Accessed July 24, 2007.
19. GAO Report to Congressional Requesters. More beneficiaries use hospice but for fewer days of care. Available at: www.gao.gov/archive/2000/he00182.pdf. Accessed July 26, 2007.
20. National Hospice and Palliative Care Organization. Archived Rates & Indices. Available at: www.nhpco.org/i4a/pages/index.cfm?pageid=4727. Accessed April 15, 2008.
21. Department of Health and Human Services, Health Care Financing Administration. Program Memorandum Intermediaries. Transmittal A-00-38. Change Request 1235. June 2000. Change in Hospice Payment Rates, Update to the Hospice Cap, Revised Hospice Wage Index and Hospice Pricer. Available at: www.cms.hhs.gov/transmittals/downloads/A003860.PDF. Accessed April 15, 2008.
22. Fiscal Year 2003 Hospice Payment Rates, Cap and Wage Index. Available at: www.cms.hhs.gov/transmittals/downloads/A02059.pdf. Accessed July 23, 2007.
23. Department of Health and Human Services, Health Care Financing Administration. Program Memorandum Intermediaries. Transmittal A-03-57. Change Request 2797. July 3, 2003. Medicare Program—Update to the Hospice Payment Rates, Hospice Cap, Hospice Wage Index and the Hospice Pricer for FY 2004. Available at: www.cms.hhs.gov/Transmittals/Downloads/a03057.pdf. Accessed April 15, 2008.
24. Department of Health and Human Services, Centers for Medicaid & Medicare Services. CMS Manual System. Publication 100-04: Medicare Claims Processing. Transmittal 606. Change Request 3386. July 15, 2005. Medicare Program—Update to the Hospice Payment Rates, Hospice Cap, Hospice Wage Index and the Hospice Pricer for FY 2005. Available at: www.cms.hhs.gov/Transmittals/downloads/R606CP.pdf. Accessed April 15, 2008.
25. Department of Health and Human Services, Centers for Medicaid & Medicare Services. CMS Manual System. Publication 100-04: Medicare Claims Processing. Transmittal 663. Change Request 3977. August 26, 2005. Update to the Hospice Payment Rates, Hospice Cap, Hospice Wage Index and the Hospice Pricer for FY 2006. Available at: www.cms.hhs.gov/transmittals/downloads/R663CP.pdf. Accessed April 15, 2008.
26. Department of Health and Human Services, Centers for Medicaid & Medicare Services. CMS Manual System. Publication 100-04: Medicare Claims Processing. Transmittal 1094. Change Request 5254. October 27, 2006. Update to the Hospice Payment Rates, Hospice Cap, Hospice Wage Index and the Hospice Pricer for FY 2007. Available at: www.cms.hhs.gov/transmittals/downloads/R1094CP.pdf. Accessed April 15, 2008.
27. RED BOOK Drug References. Available at: www.micromedex.com/products/redbook/. Accessed April 10, 2008.
28. First Databank Drug Pricing Products. Available at: www.firstdatabank.com/products/. Accessed April 10, 2008.
29. U.S. District Court, District of Massachusetts. In re Pharmaceutical Industry Average Wholesale Price Litigation, M.D.L. No. 1456, Civil Action No. 01-12257-PBS. June 21, 2007. Available at: www.prescriptionaccess.org/docs/AWP-6-21-07-Order.pdf. Accessed April 10, 2008.
30. Cheung L et al. The Costs of Hospice Care: An Actuarial Evaluation of the Medicare Hospice Benefit. August 1, 2001. New York: Milliman USA, Inc. Available at: www.nhpco.org/files/members/TheCostsofHospiceCare-Millman.pdf. Accessed April 10, 2008.
31. AARP Public Policy Institute. Data Digest: Trends in Manufacturer Prices of Brand-Name Prescription Drugs Used by Older Americans—2006 Year-End Update. March 2007. Washington, DC: AARP. Available at: http://assets.aarp.org/rgcenter/health/dd154_drugprices.pdf. Accessed April 15, 2008.
32. Families USA. Sticker Shock: Rising Prescription Drug Prices for Seniors. June 2004. Available at: www.familiesusa.org/assets/pdfs/Sticker_Shock5942.pdf. Accessed April 15, 2008.
33. U.S. Government Accountability Office. Report to Congressional Requesters. Prescription Drugs:

Price Trends for Frequently Used Brand and Generic Drugs from 2000 through 2004. GAO 05-779. August 2005. Available at: www.gao.gov/new.items/d05779.pdf. Accessed April 15, 2008.
34. Local Coverage Determination (LCDs): Indications and Limitations of Coverage and/or Medical Necessity. Available at: www.ugsmedicare.com/providers/LMRP/HospiceREVISED10-01-06.asp. Accessed July 9, 2007.
35. Victoria Hospice Society. Palliative Performance Scale (PPSv2), version 2. Victoria, British Columbia, Canada: Victoria Hospice Society; 2001. Available at: http://www.npcrc.org/usr_doc/adhoc/functionalstatus/Palliative%20Performance%20Scale%20(PPSv2).pdf. Accessed April 10, 2008.
36. Beckwith MC. Constipation in palliative care patients. In: Lipman AG et al., eds. *Evidence Based Symptom Control in Palliative Care.* New York: Haworth Press; 2000:47.
37. Meissner W et al. Oral naloxone reverses opioid-associated constipation. *Pain* 2000;84:105.
38. RED BOOK for Windows, Thompson Micromedex, Vol. 44, April 2007.
39. Lipman AG, Tyler LS. Anorexia and cachexia in palliative care patients. In: Lipman AG et al., eds. *Evidence Based Symptom Control in Palliative Care.* New York: Haworth Press; 2000:11.
40. American Academy of Hospice and Palliative Medicine. Peer-Reviewed Educational Materials. Morrison LJ, Liao S. Fast Fact and Concept #174. Dementia Medications in Palliative Care. Available at: www.aahpm.org/cgi-bin/wkcgi/view?status=A%20&search=334&id=695&offset=0&limit=25. Accessed April 15, 2008.
41. Anon. Memantine. *Med Lett Drugs Ther* 2003; 45:73.
42. Jackson KC, Lipman AG. Delirium in palliative care patients. In: Lipman AG et al., eds. *Evidence Based Symptom Control in Palliative Care.* New York: Haworth Press; 2000:59.
43. Qaseem A et al. Evidence-based interventions to improve the palliative care of pain, dyspnea, and depression at the end of life: a Clinical Practice Guideline from the American College of Physicians. *Ann Intern Med.* 2008;148:141.
44. Doyle D et al. Oxford Textbook of Palliative Medicine. 2nd ed. Oxford: Oxford University Press; 1998:1283.
45. Conill C et al. Symptom prevalence in the last week of life. *J Pain Sympt Man* 1997;14:328.
46. Vainio A, Auvinen A. Prevalence of symptoms among patients with advanced cancer: an international collaborative study. Symptom Prevalence Group. *J Pain Sympt Man* 1996;12:3.
47. Donnelly S, Walsh D. The symptoms of advanced cancer. *Semin Oncol* 1995;22:67.
48. Curtis EB et al. Common symptoms in patients with advanced cancer. *J Palliat Care* 1991;7:25.
49. Ferraresi VF. Inhaled opioids for the treatment of dyspnea. *Am J Health Syst Pharm* 2005;62:319.
50. Gutstein HB, Akil H. Opioid analgesics. In: Hardman JG et al., eds. *Goodman & Gilman's: The Pharmacological Basis of Therapeutics.* 10th ed. New York: McGraw-Hill; 2001:569.
51. Zebraski SE et al. Lung opioid receptors: pharmacology and possible target for nebulized morphine in dyspnea. *Life Sci* 2000;66:2221.
52. American Academy of Hospice and Palliative Medicine. Peer-Reviewed Educational Materials. Bickel K, Arnold R. Fast Fact and Concept #109: Death rattle and oral secretions. Available at: www.aahpm.org/cgibin/wkcgi/view?status=A%20&search=165&id=522&offset=0&limit=25. Accessed April 15, 2008.
53. Transderm Scop Prescribing Information. Available at: www.transdermscop.com/infomed_prescribing.htm#clinical. Accessed April 15, 2008.
54. Portenoy RK et al. Opioid use and Survival at the end of life: a survey of a hospice population. *J Pain Sympt Man* 2006;32:532.
55. Joranson DE, Gilson AM. Pharmacists' knowledge of and attitudes toward opioid pain medications in relation to federal and state policies. *J Am Pharm Assoc* 2001;41:213.
56. Code of Federal Regulations. 21CFR1306.11(g). Available at: http://www.gpoaccess.gov/cfr/retrieve.html. Accessed April 15, 2008.
57. Lacy CF et al., eds. Lexi-Comp's Drug Information Handbook. 11th ed. Hudson, OH: Lexi-Comp, Inc.; 2003.
58. Drug Facts and Comparisons. 60th ed. St. Louis, MO: Facts and Comparisons; 2006.
59. Dolophine Hydrochloride CII Prescribing Information. Columbus, OH: Roxane Laboratories, Inc. Available at: www.fda.gov/cder/foi/label/2006/006134s028lbl.pdf. Accessed April 15, 2008.
60. Bruera E, Sweeney C. Methadone use in cancer patients with pain: a review. *J Palliat Med* 2002;5:127.
61. Duragesic Prescribing Information. Available at: www.fda.gov/cder/foi/label/2005/19813s039lbl.pdf. Accessed July 28, 2007.
62. Cato MA et al. Perspective on ASHP's assisted-suicide policy. *Am J Health Syst Pharm* 1999; 56:1672.
63. ASHP statement on pharmacist decision-making on assisted suicide. *Am J Health Syst Pharm* 1999; 56:1661.
64. Dixon KM, Kier KL. Longing for mercy, requesting death: pharmaceutical care and pharmaceutically assisted death. *Am J Health Syst Pharm* 1998;55:578.
65. Hamerly JP. Views on assisted suicide. Perspectives of the AMA and the NHO. *Am J Health Syst Pharm* 1998;55:543.
66. Brock D Death and dying. In: Vaeatch R ed. *Medical Ethics.* Boston: Jones and Bartlett, 1989: 329.
67. Veatch RM. The pharmacist and assisted suicide. *Am J Health Syst Pharm* 1999;56:260.
68. Vivian J et al. Michigan pharmacists' attitudes about medically assisted suicide. *J Mich Pharm* 1993;31:490.
69. Rupp MT, Isenhower HL. Pharmacists' attitudes toward physician-assisted suicide. *Am J Hosp Pharm* 1994;51:69.
70. Cowan JD, Walsh D. Terminal sedation in palliative medicine: definition and review of the literature. *Support Care Cancer* 2001;9:403.
71. McCleane G. Intravenous Lidocaine: An Outdated or Underutlized Treatment for Pain? *J Pall Med* 2007;10:798.
72. Ferrante FM, Paggioli J, Cherukuri S, Arthur GR. The analgesic response to intravenous lidocaine in the treatment of neuropathic pain. *Anesth Analg* 1996;82:91.
73. Bruera E, Ripamonti C, Brenneis C, Macmillan K, Hanson J. A randomized double-blind crossover trial of intravenous lidocaine in the treatment of neuropathic cancer pain. *J Pain Symptom Manage* 1992;7:138.
74. Ferrini R, Paice JA. How to Initiate and Monitor Infusional Lidocaine for Severe and/or Neuropathic Pain. *J Support Oncol* 2004;2:90. Available at: www.supportiveoncology.net/journal/articles/0201090.pdf. Accessed January 13, 2008.
75. Thomas J. Parenteral Lidocaine for Neuropathic Pain. *Fast Fact and Concept.* Available at: www.eperc.mcw.edu/fastFact/ff_180.htm. Accessed January 13, 2008.

CHAPTER 7

Nausea and Vomiting

Lisa Lohr

Nausea and vomiting are unpleasant symptoms caused by self-limiting disorders or serious conditions such as cancer. These symptoms can range from mild, short-lived nausea to continuing severe emesis and retching. In addition to the suffering involved, uncontrolled vomiting can lead to dehydration, electrolyte imbalances, malnutrition, aspiration pneumonia, and esophageal tears. Nausea and vomiting often reduce food intake and can impair a person's ability to care for themselves. Significant reductions in quality-of-life scores have been demonstrated in cancer patients with chemotherapy-induced nausea and vomiting compared with patients who did not have those symptoms. Clinicians can improve the care of patients by recommending appropriate preventive medications in situations where nausea and vomiting can be predicted (e.g., postoperative, chemotherapy-induced and radiation-induced symptoms). In addition, by assuring appropriate use of rescue antiemetics, clinicians can help reduce existing symptoms.

PATHOPHYSIOLOGY AND NEUROTRANSMITTERS

The neurophysiology of the emetic response is complex, with multiple organs and neurotransmitters involved. The emetic response can be described in three phases: nausea, vomiting, and retching. *Nausea* is the subjective feeling of the need to vomit. It includes an unpleasant sensation in the mouth and stomach and can be associated with salivation, sweating, dizziness, and tachycardia. *Vomiting* is the forceful expulsion of the stomach contents through the mouth, but is preceded by the relaxation of the esophageal sphincter, contraction of the abdominal muscles, and temporary suspension of breathing. *Retching* is the rhythmic contraction of the abdominal muscles without actual emesis. It can accompany nausea, or occur before or after emesis.

Nausea and vomiting are caused by many disorders. Central nervous system (CNS) causes include increased intracranial pressure, migraine, brain metastases, vestibular dysfunction, alcohol intoxication, and anxiety. Infectious disease causes include viral gastroenteritis, food poisoning, peritonitis, meningitis, and urinary tract infections. Metabolic causes include hypercalcemia, uremia, hyperglycemia, and hyponatremia. Gastrointestinal disorders, such as gastroparesis, bowel obstruction, distention, and mechanical irritation, can cause nausea and vomiting. Among the many medications that can cause nausea and vomiting are cancer chemotherapy, antibiotics, antifungals, and opiate analgesics.

The CNS, the peripheral nervous system, and the gastrointestinal (GI) tract are all involved in initiating and coordinating the emetic response. In the CNS, the vomiting center (VC) receives incoming signals from other parts of the brain and the GI tract and then coordinates the emetic response by sending signals to the effector organs. The VC is located in the medulla oblongata of the brain, near the nucleus tractus solitarius (NTS). The VC is stimulated by neurotransmitters released from the chemoreceptor trigger zone (CTZ), the GI tract, the cerebral cortex, the limbic system, and the vestibular system (Fig. 7-1). The major neurotransmitter receptors associated with the emetic response include serotonin (the 5-hydroxytryptamine type 3) receptors, neurokinin-1 receptors, and dopamine receptors. Other receptors involved include corticosteroid, acetylcholine, histamine, cannabinoid, gabaminergic, and opiate receptors. Many of these receptors are targets for antiemetic therapy.

In the CNS, the CTZ is located in the area postrema on the floor of the fourth ventricle in the brainstem; it lies outside the blood–brain barrier. When the CTZ senses toxins and noxious substances in the blood and cerebrospinal fluid, it triggers the emetic response by releasing neurotransmitters that travel to the VC and the NTS. The major neurotransmitter receptors involved in this pathway include serotonin, dopamine, and neurokinin-1.

The GI system also plays a large part in the initiation of the emetic response. The GI tract contains enterochromaffin cells in the GI mucosa. When these cells are damaged by chemotherapy, radiation, or mechanical irritation, serotonin is released, which can stimulate the vagal afferents as well as directly stimulate the VC and NTS. The vomiting center then propagates the emetic response.

The cerebral cortex and limbic system can stimulate the emetic center in response to emotional states such as anxiety, pain, and conditioned responses (anticipatory nausea and vomiting). The neurotransmitters involved in this pathway are less well understood. Disorders of the vestibular system, such as vertigo and motion sickness, stimulate the VC through acetylcholine and histamine release.

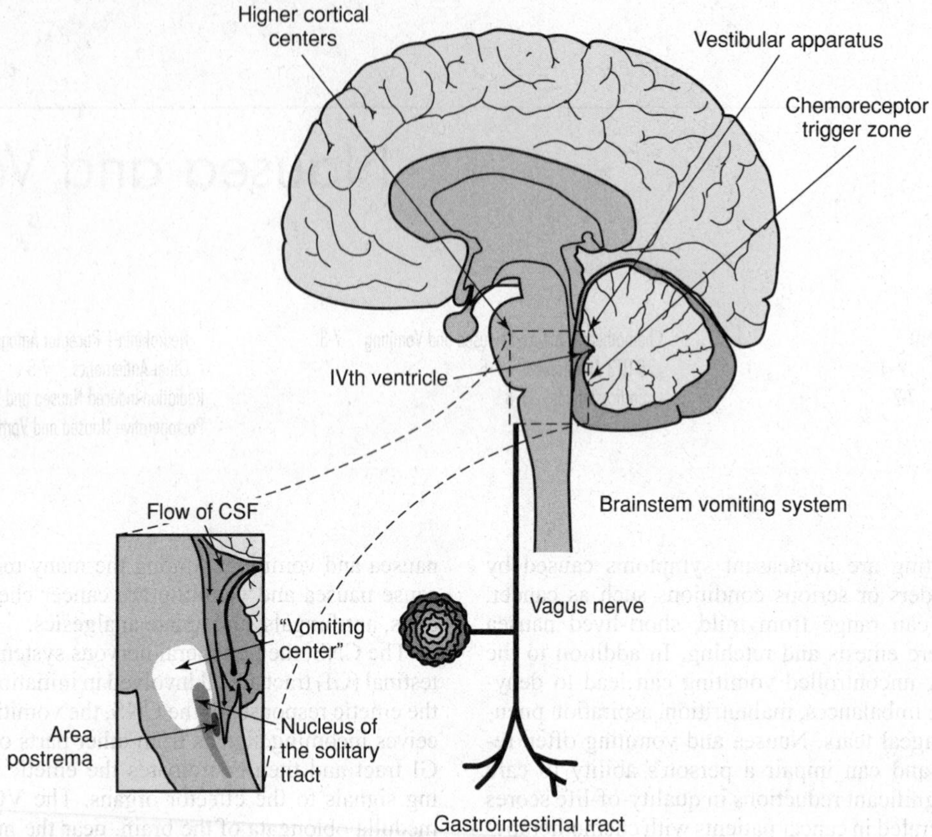

FIGURE 7-1 Vomiting center.

Pharmacotherapy of Emesis

The initial evaluation of the patient with nausea and vomiting should include the onset of symptoms; the severity and duration of symptoms; hydration status; precipitating factors; current medical conditions and medications; and food and infectious contacts. The etiology of the nausea and vomiting should be determined, if possible, so that underlying conditions can be treated specifically. Supportive treatment should be initiated, if needed, including fluid and electrolyte replacement. If the nausea and vomiting is mild and self-limited, antiemetic therapy may not be required. For others, however, the appropriate antiemetic therapy will depend on the patient and the etiology of the nausea and vomiting.

Motion Sickness

1. P.C. is a 27-year-old woman who has no significant medical history, with the exception of moderate dysmenorrhea and motion sickness associated with travel by air. Previously, she has taken dimenhydrinate before airplane trips with moderate success. She is engaged to be married, and she and her fiancé have decided on a week-long Caribbean cruise for their honeymoon. P.C. is concerned that she may also develop sea sickness and that dimenhydrinate may not control her symptoms, particularly in the event of rough weather at sea. Will P.C. be at higher risk for motion sickness?

The symptoms of motion sickness occur in response to an unusual perception of real or apparent motion. In these situations, there is sensory conflict about body position or motion through the visual, vestibular, or body proprioceptors. Acetylcholine is thought to be the primary neurotransmitter involved in signaling the VC, as is histamine, to a lesser extent. Adrenergic stimulation can block this transmission. Symptoms begin with stomach discomfort and progress to salivation changes, sweating, dizziness, lethargy, retching, and emesis. The risk of motion sickness is low in children <2 years of age. The risk is highest in children and adolescents, and higher in females than males. In some individuals, sensitivity to motion sickness diminishes over time. Travel by boat is most likely to cause symptoms; air, car, and train travel is less likely.[1,2] Because of P.C.'s history and her travel plans, she is at high risk for recurrence of her motion sickness symptoms.

Nonpharmacologic measures or natural remedies may be useful for reducing motion sickness. These include riding in the middle of the boat or plane where the motion is less dramatic; lying in a semirecumbent position; fixing the vision on the horizon; avoiding reading; and closing the eyes if below deck or in the cabin. Many people recommend keeping active on a ship to "get their sea-legs" faster through habituation. The effectiveness of acupressure at the P6 point of the wrist (about three fingerbreadths above the wrist) is unclear. A controlled-stimulus trial compared two brands of wristbands with placebo; neither band was more effective than placebo in preventing symptoms of motion sickness.[3] Studies of ginger preparations also are equivocal. The action of ginger may be of promotion of gastric emptying and not on the vestibular system.[4,5]

2. For P.C., what medications are available to prevent and treat motion sickness symptoms?

Anticholinergic agents and antihistamines that cross the blood–brain barrier effectively prevent and treat motion sickness.[1,2] In general, these medications are more effective in preventing than treating established symptoms. 5-hydoxytryptamine 3 (5-HT3) receptor antagonists and neurokinin-1 (NK-1) receptor antagonists have not been shown to be effective in preventing motion sickness[6,7] and are very costly. Nonsedating antihistamines are not as effective as other antihistamines because they do not sufficiently cross the blood–brain barrier.[1] Scopolamine has been well studied for the prevention of motion sickness and is highly effective.[8] In a controlled trial, scopolamine was more effective than promethazine and both were more effective than placebo, meclizine, or lorazepam.[9] Scopolamine is available as a topical patch, which bypasses the problem of GI symptoms associated with motion sickness. Scopolamine is less likely than dimenhydrinate to effect psychomotor performance.[10] Table 7-1 describes medications effective for motion sickness, including the recommended use and the adult doses. The severity of the stimulus is highly dependent on the individual and also varies with the weather and with position in the plane or boat.

Because P.C. is a susceptible individual in a moderate-severe stimulus situation, prevention with a scopolamine patch applied behind the ear every 3 days, starting 6 to 8 hours before departure should be recommended. If she experiences breakthrough symptoms, dimenhydrinate or promethazine can be recommended as well. She should be advised about the potential adverse effects of these agents, which include drowsiness, confusion, and dry mouth.

Chemotherapy-Induced Nausea and Vomiting

3. M.C., a 54-year-old woman with breast cancer, is in the clinic today to receive her first cycle of "AC" (doxorubicin and cyclophosphamide) chemotherapy. She will receive paclitaxel and trastuzumab after the completion of the AC. Her chemotherapy doses will be intravenous (IV) doxorubicin 60 mg/m^2 plus cyclophosphamide 600 mg/m^2 IV for one dose on day 1 of each cycle. This will be repeated every 21 days for four cycles. M.C. does not drink alcohol or smoke. Her only other medical condition is adult onset diabetes, which is controlled with metformin and diet. She has had four children, now all grown, and had substantial morning sickness with each of her pregnancies. M.C.'s neighbor has told her that all chemotherapy causes severe nausea and vomiting. How likely is M.C. to experience nausea and vomiting?

Chemotherapy-induced nausea and vomiting (CINV) occurs in many patients receiving chemotherapy for cancer. The mechanisms of the emetic response described at the beginning of this chapter apply to CINV as well. The major neurotransmitter receptors involved in these pathways include serotonin, NK-1 and dopamine receptors. CINV can occur in different patterns. Acute phase CINV symptoms occur within a few hours after the administration of the chemotherapy. These symptoms often peak several hours after administration and can last for

Table 7-1 Medications for Prevention or Treatment of Motion Sickness in Adults

Medication (Trade name)	*Dosage*	*Recommended Use*	*Adverse Effects*
Scopolamine (Transderm-Scop)	1.5 mg TOP behind the ear Q 3 days. Apply at least 3 hrs (preferably 6–8 hrs) before exposure	Long term exposure (>6 hrs) of moderate-intense stimulus. Alternative treatment for shorter or milder stimulus.	Dry mouth, drowsiness, blurred vision, confusion, fatigue, ataxia
Dimenhydrinate (Dramamine)	50–100 mg PO Q 4–6 h (max 400 mg/day). May be taken PRN or on scheduled basis if required.	Short- or long-term exposure to mild to moderate stimulus. Alternative for other situations.	Drowsiness, dry mouth, thickening of secretions, dizziness
Promethazine (Phenergan)	25 mg PO Q 4–6 h. May be taken PRN or on scheduled basis if required. 25–50 mg IM Q 4–6 h for established severe symptoms. May be taken PRN or on scheduled basis if required.	In combination with dextroamphetamine for short exposure of intense stimulus. Alternative for other situations.	Drowsiness, orthostatic hypotension, dry mouth
Meclizine (Antivert, Bonine)	12.5–50 mg PO Q 6–24 h. May be taken PRN or on scheduled basis if required.	Alternative for mild stimulus or in combination for moderate to severe stimulus	Drowsiness, dry mouth, thickening of secretions, dizziness
Dextroamphetamine (Dexedrine)	5–10 mg PO Q 4–6 h. May be taken PRN or on scheduled basis if required.	In combination with promethazine for short exposure of intense stimulus.	Restlessness, abuse potential, insomnia, overstimulation, tachycardia, palpitations, hypertension
Cyclizine (Marezine)	50 mg PO Q 4–6 h (max 200 mg/day). May be taken PRN or on scheduled basis if required.	Alternative for mild stimulus situations.	Drowsiness, dry mouth,

IM, intramusculare; PO, oral; PRN, as needed; Q, every; TOP, topically.
Adapted from reference 2, with permission.

the first 24 hours. Some antineoplastic agents can also cause nausea and vomiting symptoms for a longer period of time after chemotherapy administration. Delayed CINV symptoms peak in about 2 to 3 days and can last 6 to 7 days. Some patients who have received previous chemotherapy treatments may experience a conditioned response in which they have symptoms even before the chemotherapy starts. This is called *anticipatory nausea and vomiting* and it is difficult to treat because it is primarily triggered by poor nausea and vomiting control in previous cycles. Breakthrough nausea and vomiting occur if the primary prophylactic antiemetics fail to work completely. Of course, regardless of the time course and cause, these are very distressing, unpleasant, and disruptive symptoms for the patient.

The likelihood of CINV depends on several factors.[11] Patient-related factors that increase the risk of acute-phase CINV include age <50 years, female gender, poor control of symptoms in prior cycles, history of motion sickness or nausea with pregnancy, anxiety, or depression. A significant history of alcoholism actually protects against CINV. Delayed symptoms are more common in women and in those who have had poor emetic control in the acute phase.

Recently, a new predictive model has been developed to identify patients at highest risk for serious CINV symptoms.[12] The predictive factors most associated with acute CINV symptoms included age, disease site and stage, comorbid conditions, chemotherapy agent (Table 7-2), absence of alcohol abuse, increasing number of chemotherapy cycles, and nonprescription

Table 7-2 Emetogenicity of Selected Antineoplastic Agents

High Emetogenicity (> 90% of patients developing nausea or vomiting [N/V])	*Antineoplastic*
	Altretamine (PO)
	Cisplatin (IV) ($\geq$50 mg/m^2)
	Cyclophosphamide (IV) ($\geq$1,500 mg/m^2)
	Dacarbazine (IV)
	Dactinomycin (IV)
	Mechorethamine (IV)
	Procarbazine (PO)
	Combination of doxorubicin/cyclophosphamide or epirubicin/cyclophosphamide (IV)
Moderate Emetogenicity (30% to 90% of patients developing N/V)	
	Aldesleukin (IV) (>12–15 million units)
	Amifostine (IV)
	Arsenic Trioxide (IV)
	Carboplatin (IV)
	Cisplatin (IV) (<50 mg/m^2)
	Cyclophosphamide (PO)
	Cyclophosphamide (IV) (<1,500 mg/m^2)
	Cytarabine (IV) (>1g/m^2)
	Daunorubicin (IV)
	Doxorubicin (IV)
	Epirubicin (IV)
	Etoposide (PO)
	Idarubicin (IV)
	Ifosfamide (IV)
	Imantinib (PO)
	Irinotecan (IV)
	Methotrexate (IV) (250 mg to >1 g/m^2)
	Oxaliplatin (IV)
	Temozolamide (PO)
Low Emetogenicity (10% to 30% of patients developing N/V)	*Antineoplastic*
	Bortezomib (IV)
	Capecitabine (PO)
	Cetuximab (IV)
	Cytarabine (IV) (100–200 mg/m^2)
	Docetaxel (IV)
	Etoposide (IV)
	Fluorouracil (IV)
	Gemcitabine (IV)
	Lapatinib (PO)
	Mitoxantrone (IV)
	Methotrexate (IV) (<1g/m^2)
	Paclitaxel (IV)
	Panitumumab (IV)
	Pemetrexed (IV)
	Topotecan (IV)
	Trastuzumab (IV)
	Vorinostat (IV)
Minimal Emetogenicity (< 10% of patients developing N/V)	
	Bevacizumab (IV)
	Bleomycin (IV)
	Chlorambucil (PO)
	Dasatinib (PO)
	Decitabine (IV)
	Erlotinib (PO)
	Fludarabine (IV)
	Gefitinib (PO)
	Gemtuzumab ozogamicin (IV)
	Hydroxyurea (PO)
	Lenalidomide (PO)
	Methotrexate (PO)
	Nelarabine (IV)
	Rituximab (IV)
	Sorafenib (PO)
	Sunitinib (PO)
	Thalidomide (PO)
	Thioguanine (PO)
	Vinblastine (IV)
	Vincristine (IV)
	Vinorelbine (IV)

Adapted from references 11, 13, 14, with permission.

drug use. The factors associated with increased delayed CINV included age, type of antiemetics used, prior nausea and vomiting, including that with pregnancy, increasing number of chemotherapy cycles, previous acute CINV, and nonprescription drug use.

Chemotherapy-related factors also predict the likelihood of symptoms. Factors, such as shorter infusion time, higher dose, and more chemotherapy cycles, increase the risk of CINV. With multiday chemotherapy regimens, the symptoms usually peak on about the third to fourth day of chemotherapy, when the acute symptoms caused by the later days' doses are overlapping with the delayed symptoms from the first days' doses. The most predictive factor, however, is the chemotherapy agent's inherent ability to cause CINV, or its emetogenicity.[11–14] Antineoplastics that are most likely (>90% of patients) to cause symptoms are classified as highly emetogenic chemotherapy. Agents that cause nausea and vomiting in 30% to 90% of patients are classified as moderate-risk agents. Low emetogenicity agents cause symptoms in 10% to 30% of patients. Other chemotherapy agents have a minimal risk, causing CINV in <10% of patients. Table 7-2 lists selected chemotherapy agents in the various emetogenicity classes. References differ in the estimation of emetic risk for some antineoplastic agents. Note, for some agents, that the emetogenicity depends on the dosage used.

Certain antineoplastic agents are more likely to cause delayed CINV symptoms. These include cisplatin, carboplatin, cyclophosphamide, doxorubicin, epirubicin, and ifosfamide. Patients receiving more than one of these agents are at high risk for delayed symptoms.

Most chemotherapy agents are given in combinations, rather than as single agents. Estimating the emetogeniticity of chemotherapy combinations has always been difficult. One method[15] using a mathematical formula for estimating the total effect, is based on a five-level classification of emetogenicity. No method has been prospectively evaluated or unanimously accepted, however. Chemotherapy regimens that contain cyclophosphamide and an anthracycline, such as doxorubicin, are highly emetogenic (symptoms in >90% of patients.) The primary literature should be examined for the incidence of nausea and vomiting for established chemotherapy combination regimens. In the absence of specific information regarding the risk of CINV in certain combinations, the antiemetic regimen should be geared toward the chemotherapy agent with the highest emetogenicity level given on that day.[11,14,16] For example, for a chemotherapy combination with one agent with a high risk and one with a moderate risk, the antiemetic regimen should be appropriate for the high-risk chemotherapy agent.

Antiemetic efficacy, or complete emetic response, is usually defined as no emesis and no nausea or only mild nausea in the first 24 hours after chemotherapy administration. With currently recommended antiemetic regimens, most but not all patients will be protected from emesis in the acute phase (first 24 hours). Nausea, however, is more difficult to control. In addition, delayed CINV symptoms are more difficult to prevent.

4. Our patient, M.C., is at high risk for acute CINV. Her personal risk factors include female gender, history of morning sickness with pregnancy, and being a nondrinker. The chemotherapy regimen she will receive (cyclophosphamide and doxorubicin) is highly emetogenic in the acute phase and also has a high risk of delayed symptoms. What antiemetics are available for M.C.?

Appropriate antiemetic therapy is based on the emetogenicity of the chemotherapy regimen and patient risk factors. Because the pathophysiologic response of nausea and vomiting involves many neurotransmitters, combinations of antiemetics from different therapeutic classes will be more effective in most situations than a single agent. The predominant classes of antiemetics used for CINV include serotonin (5HT3) antagonists, the neurokinin-1 antagonist and corticosteroids.

5-HT3 Antagonists

The 5-HT3 antagonists inhibit the action of serotonin in the GI tract and the CNS and thereby block the transmission of emetic signals to the VC. Serotonin antagonists are both highly effective and have minimal side effects. Several agents in this class are now available: ondansetron, granisetron, dolasetron, and palonosetron. Dosages of these agents are shown in Table 7-3. These agents have been widely studied and some commonalities have emerged. All of these agents have a threshold effect and so a sufficiently large dose must be given to block the relevant receptors. The dose-response curve is relatively flat, such that escalating doses do not enhance efficacy. When given in appropriate doses, all of these agents have similar efficacy for acute CINV, with response rates ranging from about 60% to 80%, depending on study design.[11,14,17–19] The effectiveness of each of these agents is enhanced by the addition of dexamethasone. The response rate increases by about 15% to 20% in regimens that include dexamethasone and a 5-HT3 antagonist.[20,21] Oral and IV 5-HT3 administration are equally effective assuming the patient can take oral medications. The side effects of the 5-HT3 antagonists are similar and fairly mild and include headache, constipation, diarrhea, and transient elevations of liver function tests. These agents are one component of optimal antiemetic prophylaxis for acute CINV, but are not more effective than agents from other classes (notably dexamethasone, aprepitant, or prochlorperazine) for delayed CINV.[22–25] Serotonin antagonists, therefore, are not recommended for delayed CINV.

Palonosetron, the newest member of the serotonin antagonist family, is distinguished by its longer elimination half-life than others in its class. Palonosetron was compared with single doses of ondansetron or dolasetron in two trials of moderately emetogenic chemotherapy and in one trial of highly emetogenic chemotherapy.[26–28] In each of these trials, palonosetron resulted in the same or higher complete response rate (no emesis and no use of rescue medication in the acute or delayed phase) than that of the comparator agents, but methodologic concerns limit the conclusions. In two of these trials, corticosteroid administration was allowed, but not required, although dexamethasone is recommended for prophylaxis for moderately and highly emetogenic chemotherapy. Prophylaxis with dexamethasone for delayed symptoms was not included. These trials essentially compared palonosetron with placebo for the delayed phase, because the comparator was not continued for the 3 days. Palonosetron has not been compared with other serotonin antagonists where dexamethasone dosing was included for both the acute and delayed phase.[14] In addition, it has

Table 7-3 Antiemetic Agents for Chemotherapy-Induced Nausea and Vomiting (CINV)

Medication (Trade name)	*Class*	*Indication/Phase*	*Dose in Adults (doses should be given 30–60 minutes before chemotherapy)*	*Dose in Pediatrics*
Aprepitant (Emend)	NK-1 antagonist	Acute/Delayed	125 mg PO on day 1, 80 mg PO on days 2,3	
Dexamethasone (Decadron)	Corticosteroid	Acute (high emetogenicity)	12 mg (if with aprepitant) or 20 mg IV or PO	
		Acute (moderate emetogenicity)	8 mg IV or PO	
		Acute (low emetogenicity)	4–8 mg IV or PO	
		Delayed	8 mg PO daily days 2–4 (when with aprepitant)	
Dolasetron	Serotonin antagonist	Acute	IV: 100 mg or 1.8 mg/kg PO: 100–200 mg	1.8 mg/kg IV or PO
Dronabinol (Marinol)	Cannabinoid	Breakthrough	2.5–10 mg PO TID to QID	
Droperidol (Inapsine)	Butyrophenone	Breakthrough	0.625–1.25 mg IV Q 4–6 h PRN	50–60 mcg/kg/dose
Granisetron (Kytril)	Serotonin antagonist	Acute	IV:1 mg or 0.01 mg/kg PO: 2 mg	0.01 mg/kg/dose
Haloperidol (Haldol)	Butyrophenone	Breakthrough	0.5–1 mg PO, IV, or IM Q 6 h PRN	
Metoclopramide (Reglan)	Dopamine antagonist	Breakthrough	10–20 mg PO or IV Q 6 h PRN	0.1 mg/kg/dose
Lorazepam (Ativan)	Benzodiazepine	Breakthrough	0.5–2 mg PO, IV, IM, or SL Q 6 h PRN	0.05 mg/kg/dose
Nabilone (Cesamet)	Cannabinoid	Refractory CINV	1–2 mg PO BID (max 2 mg PO TID)	
Olanzapine (Zyprexa)	Serotonin/dopamine antagonist	Acute/delayed/breakthrough	2.5–10 mg PO QHS	
Ondansetron (Zofran)	Serotonin antagonist	Acute (moderate or high emetogenicity)	IV: 8–12 mg or 0.15 mg/kg PO: 16–24 mg PO	0.15 mg/kg Q 4 h ×3 doses or 0.45 mg/kg single dose
Palonosetron (Aloxi)	Serotonin antagonist	Acute/delayed	IV: 0.25 mg	
Prochlorperazine (Compazine)	Dopamine antagonist	Breakthrough	5–10 mg (up to 20 mg) PO, IV, IM Q 4–6 h PRN	>2 yo: 0.1–0.15 mg/kg/dose
Promethazine	Dopamine antagonist	Breakthrough	12.5–25 mg PO, IV, IM, PR Q 4–6 h PRN	>2 yo: 0.25–1 mg/kg/dose

BID, twice daily; IM, intramuscular; IV, intravenous; PO, oral; PR, rectal; PRN, as needed; QHS, every night; QID, four times daily; TID, three times daily.
Adapted from references 11, 14, 16, with permission.

not been compared with regimens containing other 5-HT3 antagonists (in the delayed setting), dexamethasone, and aprepitant. One group of researchers described a three-drug combination of palonosetron, dexamethasone, and aprepitant in a noncomparative, phase II study, and found that the three-drug combination was safe and effective.[29] Whether palonosetron is equivalent or superior to other 5-HT3 antagonists will be determined by trials that compare palonosetron with a 5-HT3 antagonist, with both treatment arms consisting of dexamethasone and aprepitant in the acute and delayed phases.

Palonosetron is normally administered as a single 0.25 mg IV dose before chemotherapy. Repeated dosing within 1 week is not approved by the U.S. Food and Drug Administration (FDA). With its long elimination half-life, palonosetron should be effective for at least a few days, but little data are published regarding repeated doses. Palonosetron has been studied in a three-dose regimen (administration on days 1, 3, 5) for multiday chemotherapy in a noncontrolled trial published only in abstract form.[30] This regimen appeared to be safe and effective, but was not compared with any other regimen.

Other serotonin antagonists, including tropisetron, ramosetron, lerisetron, and others,[31,32] are under development and study.

It is difficult to identify the serotonin antagonist with the highest overall cost-effectiveness because drug acquisition costs vary between the inpatient and outpatient clinics and from institution to institution. Costs of the different agents should be compared at each practice site to determine the preferred agent.

Corticosteroids

The mechanism of action of corticosteroids as antiemetics has not been fully determined. Some suggest that corticosteroids may decrease serotonin release, antagonize serotonin receptors, or activate corticosteroid receptors in the NTS of the medulla in the CNS.[20] Many studies validate the effectiveness of corticosteroids in the prophylaxis of CINV symptoms. Efficacy with both dexamethasone and methylprednisolone has been described, but dexamethasone is much more widely studied and utilized. Dexamethasone improves the antiemetic control of serotonin antagonists by about 15% to 20%.[20,21] In addition, dexamethasone is one of the cornerstone agents used to prevent delayed CINV. It is inexpensive and available in both IV and oral formulations.

The optimal dose of dexamethasone with different emetic stimuli has been studied in two controlled trials. For moderately emetogenic chemotherapy in the acute phase, a single 8-mg dose was as effective as larger doses or prolonged administration.[33] In the setting of highly emetogenic cisplatin-based chemotherapy, higher doses of 12 or 20 mg were superior to doses of 4 and 8 mg.[34] If used with aprepitant, the lower 12-mg prechemotherapy dose is recommended because of inhibition of steroid metabolism by aprepitant (see the neurokinin-1 receptor antagonist section).[14] For prevention of delayed CINV symptoms, the most commonly used dose of dexamethasone is 8 mg twice daily on days 2 and 3 after chemotherapy without aprepitant. The dose should be reduced to 8 mg daily when used with aprepitant.

Corticosteroids are sometimes underutilized because of the potential risk of side effects. The adverse effects of corticosteroids include insomnia, jitteriness, increased appetite, GI distress, and perineal irritation if the IV dose is infused too quickly.[20] For most patients, however, dexamethasone is well tolerated, especially because the therapy is typically short term at lower doses. Hyperglycemia can occur, especially in patients with pre-existing diabetes. These patients should be advised to monitor their glucose levels more frequently and contact their practitioner if the levels remain elevated. In the nondiabetic patient, hyperglycemia is rare. Tapering the corticosteroid dose after the end of treatment for CINV is usually unnecessary because the duration of therapy is short. Rare patients who have withdrawal-like symptoms may, however, benefit from a short taper.

Corticosteroids also have antitumor properties and are a part of the antineoplastic regimen for some malignancies, such as lymphoma, lymphoid leukemia, and myeloma. In these cases, no need is seen to administer additional dexamethasone for the antiemetic protection; however, the corticosteroid should be administered before the rest of the chemotherapy to provide antiemetic activity. If aprepitant is part of an antiemetic regimen in a situation where the corticosteroid is given for antitumor reasons, the dose of the corticosteroid should not be reduced.[14]

Neurokinin-1 Receptor Antagonists

The potential use of NK-1 receptor antagonists as antiemetics became apparent when the role of substance P in the peripheral and CNS was recognized in the emetic stimulus pathway. Aprepitant, the first NK-1 receptor antagonist available, has been studied for the prevention of CINV caused by moderately and highly emetogenic chemotherapy. Aprepitant is usually given as a 3-day oral regimen 125 mg on day 1 and 80 mg on days 2 and 3. Early trials determined that aprepitant could not replace a serotonin antagonist, but that it would be used best in conjunction with corticosteroids and a serotonin antagonist.

Aprepitant was studied in two phase III trials for the prevention of CINV with highly emetogenic cisplatin-based chemotherapy.[35,36] In both of these trials, aprepitant (or placebo) was added to a standard antiemetic regimen of ondansetron on day 1 and dexamethasone on days 1 through 4. The patients treated with aprepitant showed improved complete response rates (no emesis, and no use of rescue medications) by about 20%, in both the acute and delayed phases. In a recent reanalysis,[37] investigators found that the aprepitant-containing regimens were more effective in women than in men, which is fortunate because women have more acute and delayed symptoms than men.

Aprepitant was also studied in the prevention of CINV caused by moderately emetogenic chemotherapy.[38] Patients in the treatment arm were given aprepitant, ondansetron, and dexamethasone on day 1 plus aprepitant on days 2 and 3. The patients in the control arm were given ondansetron and dexamethasone on day 1, plus ondansetron on days 2 and 3. The rate of complete response (no emesis and no use of rescue medications) was higher in the aprepitant arm in both the acute and delayed phases. Dexamethasone, however, is one of the most effective agents for delayed CINV symptoms and it was not used in either arm for the delayed phase. In essence, aprepitant was not compared with the standard of care for the delayed phase. The results may not have been significant if a proper comparator had been used.

The effects of aprepitant seem to be maintained over four cycles of chemotherapy in patients receiving moderately emetogenic chemotherapy.[39] The addition of aprepitant to the antiemetic regimen on cycle 2 (even when it was omitted from cycle 1) also seems to improve control of CINV symptoms.[40,41] For patients who have had inadequate response to an antiemetic regimen that did not include aprepitant, it may be useful to add it in later cycles.

The efficacy of aprepitant for the control of delayed CINV symptoms was confirmed in a trial that included 489 patients comparing a standard aprepitant regimen (aprepitant, ondansetron, and dexamethasone on day 1, followed by aprepitant and dexamethasone on days 2 and 3, and dexamethasone on day 4) to a nonaprepitant regimen (ondansetron and dexamethasone on days 1 through 4) in patients receiving highly emetogenic chemotherapy.[42] The aprepitant-containing regimen offered superior control of CINV in the acute, delayed, and overall time periods. The study confirmed that aprepitant is a better choice than a serotonin antagonist during the delayed phase of CINV.

Aprepitant is generally well tolerated with mild side effects, including fatigue, hiccups, headache, and diarrhea.[35,36,38,42] The overall adverse effects in standard aprepitant-containing regimens are not appreciably different from regimens without aprepitant.[35–38,42] A potential disadvantage of aprepitant is the unavailability of an IV formulation.

Aprepitant is metabolized by the CYP3A4 enzyme system. It is a moderate inhibitor and inducer of CYP3A4, and an inducer of CYP2C9.[11,43,44,45] Consequently, several drugs potentially interact with aprepitant. The most commonly encountered interaction is with the corticosteroids. Aprepitant increases the area under the curve of dexamethasone such that the dexamethasone dose (when used as an antiemetic) should be reduced by about one-half of the usual dose when these drugs are used together.[46] The effect is greatest when the corticosteroid is administered orally.[11,43–47] When the corticosteroid is also given as part of the antitumor regimen, however, the dose should not be reduced because of concern that the antineoplastic activity might be compromised.[14] Aprepitant may also enhance warfarin metabolism by inducing CYP2C9. International normalized ratio (INR) values in patients treated with warfarin and the standard aprepitant regimen are significantly reduced, especially on day 8 of the chemotherapy cycle.[48] The patient's coagulation status after aprepitant administration should be monitored, especially during the 7- to 10-day time period. The dosage of warfarin should be adjusted if the INR is high or low. Several chemotherapy agents (paclitaxel, etoposide, paclitaxel, ifosfamide, irinotecan, imatinib, vinca alkaloids, and others) are metabolized by the CYP3A4 enzyme system and the metabolism of these agents may be altered by aprepitant. Aprepitant was used in clinical trials with some of these agents. Caution is warranted, however, because the clinical relevance of this effect is not known.[18] Other drugs that may interact with aprepitant include oral contraceptives, itraconazole, terfenadine, and phenytoin.[43,44,47]

A new investigational NK-1 receptor antagonist, casopitant, has been studied for the prevention of CINV symptoms in patients receiving moderately and highly emetogenic chemotherapy in preliminary phase II/III trials using doses of 50 to 150 mg daily.[49,50] The initial results suggest that further trials with this agent are warranted.

Other Antiemetics

Medications from other drug classes have also been used as antiemetics for CINV. These include dopamine antagonists (prochlorperazine, promethazine), benzodiazepines (lorazepam), butyrophenones (droperidol, haloperidol), benzamides (metoclopramide), and cannabinoids. Many of these agents were used widely until more effective antiemetic agents became available. These agents remain useful for breakthrough symptoms or for patients who are refractory to standard therapy. The appropriate dosages and indications for these agents are shown in Table 7-3. Many of these agents have more side effects than standard agents, especially sedation and extrapyramidal side effects, such as dystonia and akathesia. Lorazepam is commonly used as a rescue antiemetic. Its mechanism of action as an antiemetic is not completely understood, but it may involve disruption of the cortical impulses to the VC, as well as anxiolytic activity. Because each patient has an individualized response to medicines, additional options for rescue antiemetics are needed.

Olanzapine is an atypical antipsychotic agent that antagonizes several serotonin and dopamine receptors as well as other neurotransmitter receptors. Its antiemetic action was first described in patients with refractory nausea or vomiting and advanced cancer.[51–53] Preliminary studies have shown that olanzapine prevents acute and delayed CINV associated with moderately and highly emetogenic chemotherapy.[54–57] In these trials, the complete response rate to antiemetic regimens containing olanzapine with dexamethasone plus either granisetron or palonosetron was 100% in the acute phase and 75% to 80% in the delayed phase. The usual dose of olanzapine ranges from 2.5 to 10 mg daily for control of refractory symptoms. The dose used in the CINV studies was 5 to 10 mg daily starting up to 2 days before the chemotherapy cycle. The common side effects of olanzapine include sleepiness, dry mouth, and dizziness, although these were not significant in the preliminary reports. Olanzapine is a good choice for control of refractory CINV symptoms, but further study is warranted before it should be routinely recommended for prophylaxis of CINV.

Cannabinoids have long been used for refractory nausea and vomiting. This is based on the effect of the CNS cannabinoid receptors on the CTZ, the NTS, and the VC.[58] Small trials have shown conflicting effectiveness in the prevention of CINV.[59,60] A new oral cannabinoid, nabilone, has recently been approved for the treatment of CINV in patients who do not respond adequately to other antiemetics.[58] Cannabinoids are associated with side effects, such as drowsiness, dry mouth, dysphoria, vertigo, and euphoria. Although some patients have a clear preference for, and good response to, cannabinoids, side effects and a lack of pronounced efficacy limit their use in the general population of chemotherapy patients. These agents are usually reserved for patients who do not have adequate relief from other rescue medications, such as phenothiazines, benzodiazepines, or olanzapine.

Another agent being investigated for the control of CINV is gabapentin in doses of 300 to 900 mg daily for 5 days or more, combined with standard antiemetic regimens.[61,62] In preliminary studies, gabapentin improved control of CINV symptoms and was well tolerated. Further studies are needed to define the role of gabapentin in CINV.

5. M.C. is at high risk for acute nausea and vomiting and for delayed symptoms as well. What would be the most appropriate antiemetic regimen for M.C.?

The optimal prophylactic antiemetic regimens depend on the emetic risk of the chemotherapy regimen. Treatment guidelines have been developed by several groups, including the American Society of Clinical Oncology (ASCO), the National Comprehensive Cancer Network (NCCN), and the Multinational Association of Supportive Care in Cancer (MASCC). These evidence- and consensus-based guidelines, which are largely in agreement with their recommendations, are summarized in Table 7-4.

For multiday chemotherapy regimens, prophylaxis with a serotonin antagonist and dexamethasone should be offered for each day that moderately or highly emetogenic chemotherapy is administered.[11,14,16] Aprepitant might be useful in these situations, although it has not been studied in this context. Preliminary studies indicated that aprepitant was safe to administer for a total of 5 days. If multiday chemotherapy regimens have a high risk of delayed symptoms, then therapy for the delayed symptoms should be continued for at least 2 to 3 days after the last chemotherapy administration.

For M.C., the best regimen would include a single dose of a serotonin antagonist plus dexamethasone 12 mg oral or IV plus oral aprepitant 125 mg on day 1, then oral dexamethasone 8 mg on days 2 through 4 and oral aprepitant 80 mg on days 2 and 3. She should be offered medications for breakthrough CINV symptoms, such as prochlorperazine and lorazepam. She should be warned of the potential adverse effects of dexamethasone, especially hyperglycemia, and counseled to check her blood sugars more frequently and contact her physician if they remain elevated. M.C. should be advised to maintain a record of her symptoms and contact her physician if the breakthrough medications are not working or if she cannot keep fluids down.

Modern antiemetic regimens can achieve complete emetic control in about 70% to 90% of patients, but the response rate is lower for delayed CINV symptoms. If CINV symptoms are not adequately controlled, alterations in the antiemetic regimen should be made for the next cycle. Suggestions include

Table 7-4 Recommended Antiemetic Regimens by Emetogenicity of Chemotherapy Regimen

Emetogenicity Potential	Acute Phase (doses should be given 30–60 min before chemotherapy)	Delayed Phase	Breakthrough
High (>90% of patients)	Day 1: single dose 5-HT3 antagonist + dexamethasone + aprepitant	Dexamethasone days 2–4 + aprepitant days 2–3	One to two agents for PRN use
Moderate (30%–90% of patients) with high risk of delayed CINV (i.e., cyclophosphamide plus doxorubicin)	Day 1: single dose 5-HT3 antagonist + dexamethasone + aprepitant	Dexamethasone days 2–4 + aprepitant days 2–3	One to two agents for PRN use
Other moderate regimens (30%–90% of patients)	Day 1: single dose 5-HT3 antagonist + dexamethasone	None	One agent for PRN use
Low (10%–30% of patients)	Single dose dexamethasone or metoclopramide or prochlorperazine	None	Either none or one agent for PRN use
Minimal (<10%)	None	None	Usually none

5-HT3, 5 hydroxytryptamine type 3; CINV, chemotherapy-induced nausea and vomiting; PRN, as needed.
Adapted from references 11, 14, 16, with permission.

upgrading to the next higher emetogenicity level recommendation, adding aprepitant if not already given, and scheduling agents from other pharmacologic classes.

Many patients may benefit from nondrug therapy for CINV symptoms, especially for anticipatory nausea and vomiting and anxiety. Techniques include guided imagery, hypnosis, relaxation techniques, systematic desensitization, and music therapy.[63] Acupuncture and acupressure techniques have been investigated for use in CINV and some patients benefit from their use. The use of acupressure devices that stimulate the P6 point on the wrist have been proposed; however, in a controlled trial in patients with breast cancer, it was not found to be helpful.[64] If patients are troubled by CINV symptoms, it is recommended that they refrain from heavy meals for 8 to 12 hours before the chemotherapy. They should also avoid heavy, greasy foods and food with strong aromas. Chewing gum can mask the metallic taste, which some patients perceive. Dry, salty foods can also help settle the stomach.

Radiation-Induced Nausea and Vomiting

6. E.G. is a 54-year-old man with newly diagnosed head and neck cancer who will receive radiation therapy concurrently with chemotherapy containing cisplatin and fluorouracil. His daily (Monday through Friday) radiation treatments will last for 6 weeks. He has a heavy smoking history (35 pack-years) and "quit" last week, although it is not going well. After E.G.'s nausea and vomiting from the chemotherapy subsides, is he at risk for developing radiation-induced nausea and vomiting?

Radiation therapy can cause nausea and vomiting through the same basic pathways that chemotherapy does. Radiation induced nausea and vomiting (RINV) affects 40% to 80% of patients receiving radiation therapy. The risk of RINV depends on several factors, namely the size and area to be irradiated. Patients whose radiation areas >400 cm^2 are more likely to have significant RINV symptoms. Total body irradiation (associated with hematopoietic stem cell transplantation) causes RINV in >90% of patients. Patients receiving radiation to the upper abdominal area experience nausea and vomiting about 50% to 80% of the time. Radiation to other areas of the body is less likely to cause nausea and vomiting. E.G is not at high risk for developing RINV, because his radiation site will be in the head and neck region.

Just as with CINV, symptoms caused by radiation can be prevented with serotonin antagonists, corticosteroids, or both. Evidence- and consensus-based recommendations have been published by several multidisciplinary groups and are shown in Table 7-5. High-risk RINV is best treated with a combination of a serotonin antagonist and a corticosteroid.[65,66,67] Patients receiving radiotherapy in the moderate risk group can receive either prophylaxis or rescue therapy with a serotonin antagonist. Because E.G. is unlikely to develop radiation-induced symptoms, he does not need prophylaxis with a serotonin antagonist. If he develops symptoms later, rescue therapy with a dopamine antagonist or a serotonin antagonist should be offered.

Postoperative Nausea and Vomiting

7. E.W. is a 48-year-old woman who is scheduled for a laparoscopic cholecystectomy. The scheduled duration of her surgery is less than an hour. Her medical history includes hypertension. She does not have a history of motion sickness and she is a nonsmoker. E.W. has never had surgery before. Her sister-in-law had severe

Table 7-5 Prophylaxis for Radiation-Induced Nausea and Vomiting

Emetic Risk	Radiation Area	Recommendation
High (>90%)	Total body irradiation	Prophylaxis with a serotonin antagonist + dexamethasone
Moderate (60%–90%)	Upper abdomen	Prophylaxis with a serotonin antagonist
Low (30%–60%)	Lower thorax, pelvis, cranium (radiosurgery), craniospinal region	Prophylaxis or rescue with a serotonin antagonist
Minimal (<30%)	Head or neck, extremities, cranium, breast	Rescue with a dopamine antagonist or a serotonin antagonist

Adapted from references 11, 14, 16, 65, with permission.

nausea and vomiting after an outpatient surgical procedure last year and E.W. is worried that it might happen to her. What is E.W.'s risk of having postoperative nausea and vomiting? What can be done to reduce her risk and how can symptoms be treated if they occur?

Postoperative nausea and vomiting (PONV) is a common complication of surgery, affecting 25% to 30% of all patients, but up to 80% of patients in high risk groups. In surgical patients, PONV can lead to hospitalizations, stress on the surgical closure, hematomas, and aspiration pneumonitis. Patient-related, surgical and anesthetic factors can increase the risk of PONV.[68,69] Some of the patient risk factors include female gender, history of motion sickness, nonsmoking status, obesity, and a history of PONV. Some surgical risk factors for PONV include long duration of surgery and type of surgical procedure (e.g., laparoscopy, ear-nose-throat procedures, gynecologic surgeries, and strabismus repair). Anesthetic risk factors include the use of volatile anesthetics or nitrous oxide (as opposed to IV propofol) and the use of intraoperative or postoperative opioids. Children are twice as likely to develop PONV as adults.[68,70] The risk increases with the child's age but declines after puberty.[68,70]

Certain anesthesia practices may reduce the risk of PONV. These include use of regional anesthesia (instead of general anesthesia), use of intraoperative oxygen, hydration and avoidance of nitrous oxide, and volatile anesthesia therapy.[68–70,72]

Several risk factor models have been studied to correlate these factors into recommendations for prevention and therapy. One model is both simple and practical.[69,71] This model uses the following risk factors: female gender, history of PONV or motion sickness, nonsmoking status, surgery >60 minutes in duration, and the use of intraoperative opioids. If the patient has none or one risk factor, the risk of PONV is about 10% to 20%; no prophylaxis is necessary unless there is a medical risk for emesis. If the patient has two or more risk factors, the incidence increases to 40% to 80%; prophylaxis with one or two medications is warranted. E.W. has at least two risk factors (female, nonsmoker) and may have more if her surgery lasts longer than expected or if she receives intraoperative or postoperative opioids. She has a moderate to high risk of PONV.

An optimal prophylactic regimen for PONV matches medication choice with the patient's risk level.[68–70,72] Appropriate choices for monotherapy include droperidol, a serotonin antagonist, or dexamethasone. Patients at the highest risk for PONV should be given prophylaxis with a combination of two to three antiemetics. Dual therapy choices include a serotonin antagonist plus either droperidol or dexamethasone. Triple therapy would combine a serotonin antagonist plus dexamethasone plus droperidol. Because E.W. has a moderate to high risk for PONV, a combination of a serotonin antagonist and dexamethasone would be a good choice for prophylactic therapy.

The most effective and commonly used medications for the prevention of PONV include serotonin antagonists, dexamethasone, droperidol, and combinations of these agents. No appreciable difference is found in efficacy or adverse effects between the serotonin antagonists; therefore, the costs of the different agents should be taken into consideration when selecting therapy. Droperidol has long been used for PONV, but concerns have been raised about the rare occurrence of QT prolongation and *torsades de pointes*.[72,73] Most clinicians believe droperidol to be a safe, especially when doses are not excessive (up to 1.25 to 2.5 mg/dose for adults and up to 75 mcg/kg/dose for children).[68,73,74] The mechanism by which dexamethasone protects against PONV is unclear, but its efficacy has been shown in many trials.[68,70,72] Combinations of medications with different mechanisms of action are more effective than monotherapy. Aprepitant, has been studied in the prevention of PONV. Two studies recently compared oral aprepitant

Table 7-6 Medications for Prevention and Treatment of Postoperative Nausea and Vomiting (PONV)

Medication	*Prophylactic Dose*	*Treatment or Rescue Dose*
Aprepitant	Adults: 40 mg PO within 3 hrs before induction of anesthesia	
Dexamethasone	Adults: 4–10 mg at the start of induction of anesthesia Pediatrics: 0.15 mg/kg/dose	Adults: 2–4 mg IV
Dolasetron	Adults: 12.5 mg IV at end of surgery Pediatrics: 0.35 mg/kg/dose	Adults: 12.5 mg IV
Droperidol	Adults: 0.625–1.25 mg IV at end of surgery Pediatrics: 50–75 mcg/kg/dose	Adults: 0.625–1.25 mg IV or IM Q 4–6 h Pediatrics: 10–30 mcg/kg/dose (max 100 mcg/kg/dose)
Metoclopramide	Adults: 10 mg IV at end of surgery	Adults: 10–20 mg IV or IM Q 6 h
Granisetron	Adults: 0.35–1 mg IV at end of surgery	Adults: 0.1 mg
Ondansetron	Adults: 4–8 mg IV at end of surgery Pediatrics: 0.05–0.1 mg/kg/dose	Adults: 1 mg IV Q 8 h Pediatrics: 0.05–0.1 mg/kg/dose
Prochlorperazine	Adults: 5–10 mg IV at end of surgery	Adults: 5–10 mg IV or IM Q 4–6 h Pediatrics: 0.13 mg/kg/dose
Promethazine	Adults: 12.5–25 mg IV at end of surgery	Adults: 12.5–25 mg IV or IM Q 4–6 h Pediatrics (>2 yrs): 0.25–0.5 mg/kg/dose
Scopolamine	Adults: 1.5 mg TOP evening before or at least 4 hrs before end of surgery	

IM, intramuscular; IV intravenous; PO, oral; Q, every; TOP, topical.
Adapted from references 68–70, 72, with permission.

40 mg or 125 mg with IV ondansetron 4 mg.[45,74] These trials showed equivalency between the two doses of aprepitant and slight superiority over ondansetron in the proportion of patients without nausea, vomiting, or the use of rescue medications. Aprepitant, however, is significantly more expensive than generic ondansetron or dexamethasone, which is a consideration. Aprepitant's role in PONV has yet to be determined. Dexamethasone and serotonin antagonist combinations have been well studied and are highly effective.[68,70,72,74] Dosages for the prophylaxis and treatment of PONV are shown in Table 7-6. 5-HT3 antagonists and droperidol seem to be more effective when given at the end of surgery. Corticosteroids are best given before the induction of anesthesia.[68,72]

Several methods for nonpharmacologic techniques for the prevention of PONV have been studied and have been shown to be effective, at least in some patient populations. These include acupuncture, transcutaneous nerve stimulation, acupressure at the P6 wrist point, hypnosis, and aroma therapy with isopropyl alcohol. Ginger remedies were not found to be more effective than placebo for PONV.[68]

Even with appropriate prophylaxis for PONV, some patients will experience breakthrough symptoms and require rescue therapy. Patients who have not received prophylaxis with a serotonin antagonist can be offered a low dose of a serotonin antagonist for rescue. For rescue, only about one-quarter of the prophylaxis dose is needed.[68] Serotonin antagonists have a fairly flat dose response and larger doses (ondansetron 4 to 8 mg) have not been found to be more effective for treatment of PONV than lower doses (ondansetron 1 mg).[68,74] For all patients who have breakthrough symptoms, it is important to choose an antiemetic from a different pharmacologic class than the agents used for prophylaxis.[69,72] Droperidol, promethazine, metoclopramide, and prochlorperazine are commonly used as rescue medications. If E.W. had breakthrough nausea, droperidol would be a good choice for rescue therapy.

REFERENCES

1. Shupak A et al. Motion sickness: advances in pathogenesis, prediction, prevention, and treatment. *Aviat Space Environ Med* 2006;77:1213.
2. Committee to Advise on Tropical Medicine and Travel (CATMAT). Statement on Motion Sickness. *Can Commun Dis Rep* 2003;29:1.
3. Miller KE et al. Efficacy of acupressure and acustimulation bands for the prevention of motion sickness. *Aviat Space Environ Med* 2004;75:227.
4. Golding JF et al. Motion sickness. *Curr Opin Neurol* 2005;18:29.
5. Lien HC et al. Effects of ginger on motion sickness and gastric slow-wave dysrhythmias induced by circular vection. *Am J Physiol Gastrointest Liver Physiol* 2003;284:G481.
6. Levine ME et al. The effects of serotonin (5-HT3) receptor antagonists on gastric tachyarrhythmia and the symptoms of motion sickness. *Aviat Space Environ Med* 2000;71:1111.
7. Reid K et al. Comparison of the neurokinin-1 antagonist GR205171, alone and in combination with the 5HT3 antagonist ondansetron, hyoscine and placebo in the prevention of motion-induced nausea in man. *Br J Clin Pharmacol* 2000;50:61.
8. Spinks AB et al. Scopolamine for preventing and treating motion sickness. *Cochrane Database Syst Rev* 2004;CD002851.
9. Dornhoffer J et al. Stimulation of the semicircular canals via the rotary chair as a means to test pharmacologic countermeasures for space motion sickness. *Otol Neurotol* 2004;25:740.
10. Gordon CR et al. The effects of dimenhydrimate, cinnarizine and transdermal scopolamine on performance. *J Psychopharmacol* 2001;15:167.
11. Ettinger DS et al. Antiemesis: clinical practice guidelines in oncology. *Journal of the National Comprehensive Cancer Network* 2007;5:12.
12. Petrella T et al. Identifying patients at high risk for moderate to severe nausea and vomiting following chemotherapy: the development and validation of a prediction tool for the practicing oncologist [Abstract]. *Support Care Cancer* 2006;14:598.
13. Grunberg SM et al. Evaluation of new antiemetic agents and definition of antineoplastic agent emetogenicity—an update. *Support Care Cancer* 2005;13:80.
14. Kris MG et al. American Society of Clinical Oncology guideline for antiemetics in oncology: update 2006. *J Clin Oncol* 2006;24:2932.
15. Hesketh PJ et al. Proposal for classifying the acute emetogenicity of cancer chemotherapy. *J Clin Oncol* 1997;15:103.
16. The Antiemetic Subcommittee of the Multinational Association of Supportive Care in Cancer (MASCC). Prevention of chemotherapy- and radiotherapy-induced emesis: results of the 2004 Perugia International Antiemetic Consensus Conference. *Ann Oncol* 2006;17:20.
17. Hamadani M et al. Relative efficacy of various 5-hydroxytyptamine receptor antagonists in the prevention and control of acute nausea and vomiting associated with platinum-based chemotherapy [Abstract]. *J Clin Oncol* 2006;24:8623.
18. Jordan K et al. Comparative activity of antiemetic drugs. *Crit Rev Oncol Hematol* 2007;61:162.
19. Jordan K et al. A meta-analysis comparing the efficacy of four 5-HT3-receptor antagonists for acute chemotherapy-induced emesis. *Support Care Cancer* 2007;15:1023.
20. Grunberg SM. Antiemetic activity of corticosteroids in patients receiving cancer chemotherapy: dosing, efficacy, and tolerability analysis. *Ann Oncol* 2007; 18:233.
21. Ioannidis JP et al. Contribution of dexamethasone to control of chemotherapy-induced nausea and vomiting: a meta-analysis of randomized evidence. *J Clin Oncol* 2000;18:3409.
22. Lindley C et al. Prevention of delayed chemotherapy-induced nausea and vomiting after moderately high to highly emetogenic chemotherapy. *Am J Clin Oncol* 2005;28:270.
23. Hickok JT et al. 5-hydroxytryptamine receptor antagonists versus prochlorperazine for control for delayed nausea caused by doxorubicin: a URCC CCOP randomized controlled trial. *Lancet Oncol* 2005;6:765.
24. Gelling O et al. Should 5-hydroxytryptamine-3 antagonists be administered beyond 24 hours after chemotherapy to prevent delayed emesis? Systemic re-evaluation of clinical evidence and drug cost implications. *J Clin Oncol* 2005;23:1289.
25. Lachaine J et al. Cost-efficacy analysis of ondansetron regimens for control of emesis induced by non-cisplatin, moderately emetogenic chemotherapy. *Am J Health Syst Pharm* 2002;59:1837.
26. Gralla R et al. Palonosetron improves prevention of chemotherapy-induced nausea and vomiting following moderately emetogenic chemotherapy: results of a double-blind randomized phase III trial comparing single doses of palonosetron with ondansetron. *Ann Oncol* 2003;14:1570.
27. Eisenberg P et al. Improved prevention of moderately emetogenic chemotherapy-induced nausea and vomiting with palonosetron, a pharmacologically novel 5HT3 antagonist. *Cancer* 2003;98:2473.
28. Aapro MS et al. A phase II, double-blind, randomized trial of palonosetron compared with ondansetron in preventing chemotherapy-induced nausea and vomiting following highly emetogenic chemotherapy. *Ann Oncol* 2006;17:1441.
29. Grote R et al. Combination therapy for chemotherapy-induced nausea and vomiting in patients receiving moderately emetogenic chemotherapy: palonosetron, dexamethasone, and aprepitant. *Journal of Supportive Oncology* 2006;4:403.
30. Brames MJ et al. Efficacy and safety of multiple-day palonosetron with dexamethasone for prevention of cinv in patients receiving 5-day cisplatin-regimens for germ cell cancer [Abstract]. *Support Care Cancer* 2006;14:601.
31. Shi Y et al. Ramosetron versus ondansetron in the prevention of chemotherapy-induced gastrointestinal side effects: a prospective randomized controlled study. *Chemotherapy* 2007;53:44.
32. Navari RM et al. Emerging drugs for chemotherapy-induced emesis. *Expert Opinion on Emerging Drugs* 2006;11:137.
33. The Italian Group for Antiemetic Research. Randomized, double-blind, dose-finding study of dexamethasone in preventing acute emesis induced by anthracyclines, carboplatin, or cyclophosphamide. *J Clin Oncol* 2004;22:725.
34. The Italian Group for Antiemetic Research. Double-blind, dose-finding study of four intravenous doses of dexamethasone in the prevention of cisplatin-induced acute emesis. *J Clin Oncol* 1998;16:2937.
35. Hesketh PJ et al. The oral neurokinin-1 antagonist aprepitant for the prevention of chemotherapy-induced nausea and vomiting: a multinational, randomized, double-blind, placebo-controlled trial in patients receiving high-dose cisplatin-the aprepitant 052 study group. *J Clin Oncol* 2003;21:4112.
36. Poli-Bigelli S et al. Addition of the neurokinin-1 antagonist aprepitant to standard antiemetic therapy improves control on chemotherapy-induced nausea and vomiting. *Cancer* 2003;97:3090.
37. Hesketh PJ et al. Combined data from two phase III trials of NK-1 antagonist aprepitant plus a 5HT3 antagonist and a corticosteroid for prevention of chemotherapy-induced nausea and vomiting: effect of gender on treatment response. *Support Care Cancer* 2006;14:354.
38. Warr DG et al. Efficacy and tolerability of aprepitant for the prevention of chemotherapy-induced nausea and vomiting in patients with breast cancer after moderately emetogenic chemotherapy. *J Clin Oncol* 2005;23:2822.
39. Herrstedt J et al. Efficacy and tolerability of aprepitant for the prevention of chemotherapy-induced

nausea and emesis over multiple cycles of moderately emetogenic chemotherapy. *Cancer* 2005;104:1548.

40. Hesketh PJ et al. Aprepitant as salvage antiemetic therapy in breast cancer patients receiving doxorubicin and cyclophosphamide (AC) [Abstract]. *J Clin Oncol* 2006;24:8618.
41. Oechsle K et al. Aprepitant as salvage therapy in patients with chemotherapy-induced nausea and emesis refractory to prophylaxis with 5-HT3 antagonists and dexamethasone. *Onkologie* 2006;29:557.
42. Schmoll HJ et al. Comparison of an aprepitant regimen with a multiple-day ondansetron regimen, both with dexamethasone, for antiemetic efficacy in high-dose cisplatin treatment. *Ann Oncol* 2006;17:1000.
43. Massaro AM et al. Aprepitant: a novel antiemetic for chemotherapy-induced nausea and vomiting. *Ann Pharmacother* 2005;39:77.
44. Shadle, CR et al. Evaluation of potential inductive effects of aprepitant on cytochrome P4503A4 and 2C9 activity. *J Clin Pharmacol* 2004;44:215.
45. Diemunsch PA et al. NK1 antagonist aprepitant vs. ondansetron for prevention of PONV: combined data from 2 large trials [Abstract]. *Anesthesiology* 2006;105:A125.
46. McCrea JB et al. Effects of the neurokinin-1 receptor antagonist aprepitant on the pharmacokinetics of dexamethasone and methylprednisolone. *Clin Pharmacol Ther* 2003;74:17.
47. Dando TM et al. Aprepitant: a review of its use in the prevention of chemotherapy-induced nausea and vomiting. *Drugs* 2004;64:777.
48. Depre M et al. Effect of aprepitant on the pharmacokinetics and pharmacodynamics of warfarin. *Eur J Pharmacol* 2005;61:341.
49. Arpornwirat W et al. Multi-center, randomized, double-blind, ondansetron-controlled, dose-ranging, parallel group trial of the neurokinin-1 receptor antagonist casopitant mesylate for chemotherapy-induced nausea/vomiting in patients receiving moderately emetogenic chemotherapy [Abstract]. *J Clin Oncol* 2006;24:8512.
50. Rolski J et al. Randomized phase II trial of the neurokinin-1 receptor antagonist casopitant mesylate with ondansetron/dexamethasone for chemotherapy-induced nausea/vomiting in patients receiving highly emetogenic chemotherapy [Abstract]. *J Clin Oncol* 2006;24:8513.
51. Srivastava M et al. Olanzapine as an antiemetic in refractory nausea and vomiting in advanced cancer. *J Pain Symptom Manage* 2003;25:578.
52. Jackson WC et al. Olanzapine for intractable nausea in palliative care patients. *J Palliative Med* 2003;6:251.
53. Passik SD et al. A pilot exploration of the antiemetic activity of olanzapine for the relief of nausea in patients with advanced cancer and pain. *J Pain Symptom Manage* 2002;23:526.
54. Navari RM et al. A phase II trial of olanzapine for the prevention of chemotherapy-induced nausea and vomiting: a Hoosier Oncology Group study. *Support Care Cancer* 2005;13:529.
55. Passik SD et al. A retrospective chart review of the use of olanzapine for the prevention of delayed emesis in cancer patients. *J Pain Symptom Manage* 2003;25:485.
56. Navari RM, et al. A phase II trial of olanzapine for the prevention of chemotherapy induced nausea and vomiting (CINV). *J Clin Oncol* 2006;24:8608.
57. Passik SD et al. A phase I trial of olanzapine (Zyprexa) for the prevention of delayed emesis in cancer patients: a Hoosier Oncology Group study. *Cancer Invest* 2004;22:383.
58. Slatkin NE. Cannabinoids in the treatment of chemotherapy-induced nausea and vomiting: beyond prevention of acute emesis *J Support Case* 2007;5(53):1.
59. Meiri E et al. Dronabinol treatment of delayed chemotherapy-induced nausea and vomiting. *J Clin Oncol* 2005;23:8018.
60. Meiri E et al. Efficacy of dronabinol alone and in combination with ondansetron versus ondansetron alone for delayed chemotherapy-induced nausea and vomiting. *Curr Med Res Opin* 2007;23:533.
61. Guttuso Jr T et al. Effect of gabapentin on nausea induced by chemotherapy in patients with breast cancer. *Lancet* 2003;361:1703.
62. Menendez-Leal A, et al. Is gabapentin effective for preventing delayed nausea and vomiting after moderately and highly emetogenic chemotherapy [Abstract]. *J Clin Oncol* 2006;24:18575.
63. Figueroa-Moseley C, et al. Behavioral interventions in treating anticipatory nausea and vomiting. *Journal of the National Comprehensive Cancer Network* 2007;5:44.
64. Roscoe JA et al. Acustimulation wrist bands are not effective for the control of chemotherapy-induced nausea in women with breast cancer. *J Pain Symptom Manage* 2005;29:376.
65. National Cancer Institute of Canada Clinical Trials Group (SC19). 5-hydroxytryptamine-3 receptor antagonist with or without short-course dexamethasone in the prophylaxis of radiation induced emesis: a placebo-controlled randomized trial of the National Cancer Institute of Canada Clinical Trials Groups (SC19). *J Clin Oncol* 2006;24:3458.
66. Abdelsayed GG. Management of radiation-induced nausea and vomiting. *Exp Hematol* 2007;35:34.
67. Urba S. Radiation-induced nausea and vomiting. *Journal of the National Comprehensive Cancer Network* 2007;5:60.
68. Gan TJ et al. Consensus guidelines for managing postoperative nausea and vomiting. *Anesth Analg* 2003;97:62.
69. Golembiewski J et al. Prevention and treatment of postoperative nausea and vomiting. *Am J Health Syst Pharm* 2005;62:1247.
70. Kovac AL. Prevention and treatment of postoperative nausea and vomiting. *Drugs* 2000;59:213.
71. Apfel CC et al. A simplified risk score for predicting postoperative nausea and vomiting. *Anesthesiology* 1999;91:693.
72. Wilhelm SM et al. Prevention of postoperative nausea and vomiting. *Ann Pharmacol* 2006;40:68.
73. McKeage K et al. Intravenous droperidol: a review of its use in the management of postoperative nausea and vomiting. *Drugs* 2006;66:2123.
74. Leslie JB, Gan TJ. Meta-analysis of the safety of 5-HT3 antagonists with dexamethasone or droperidol for prevention of PONV. *Ann Pharmacother* 2006;40:856.
75. Gan TJ et al. A randomized, double-blind comparison of the NK1 antagonist, aprepitant, versus ondansetron for the prevention of postoperative nausea and vomiting. *Anesth Analg* 2007;104:1082.
76. Kazemi-Kjellberg F et al. Treatment of established postoperative nausea and vomiting: a quantitative systematic review. *BMC Anesthesiology* 2001;1:2.

CHAPTER 8

Pain and Its Management

Dusko Klipa and Jamila C. Russeau

Pain is an unpleasant sensation that can negatively affect all areas of a person's life, including comfort, thought, sleep, emotion, and normal daily activity. Chronic, untreated pain can disturb quality of life and social functioning and disrupt employment. The pain sensation results from complex phenomena that involve physical perception as well as the emotional reaction to the perception. Physiologic variables (e.g., tissue injury) and psychological variables (e.g., anxiety) influence a person's reaction to pain. Ascending neural pathways transfer electrochemical pain signals from the periphery to the central cortex where perception occurs, whereas descending pathways may attenuate or modulate signaling back to the site where the pain is felt. The pain sensation is therefore the net effect of complicated interactions of ascending and descending neural pathways with biochemical and electrochemical processes.

Pain is categorized according to its cause, location, duration, and clinical features. The most simplistic categorization involves differentiating brief-duration (acute) pain from long-lasting (chronic) pain syndromes. Acute pain serves a useful purpose of alerting an individual to an injury and initiating a reflex withdrawal from a noxious or offensive stimulus. In contrast, persistent (chronic) pain serves no biologic protective purpose and can cause undue stress and suffering. Pain was formerly believed to be merely a symptom and not a diagnosis. Recent advances in molecular biology and the understanding of neural mechanisms have demonstrated, however, that chronic pain can lead to long-lasting changes in the nervous system, a phenomenon known as *neural plasticity*. This concept is particularly important to the understanding of chronic pain because it helps explain difficulties observed in treating various painful conditions. Although initially considered static, pain processes are now realized to be plastic. Such changes therefore define a disease or process that induces physiologic change in the body. Regardless of its origin, however, pain requires a thorough evaluation to determine the underlying cause. By definition, pain is a subjective experience. Therefore, the patient is the only person who can best describe the intensity and character of pain. Pain is whatever the experiencing person says it is, existing wherever he or she says it does.

Because pain is a variable and personal experience, it is difficult to describe completely and measure objectively. The clinician, therefore, must guard against personal biases, which can interfere with treatment. It is important also to rely on tools, such as pain scales, to communicate with patients and understand the extent of their pain. Such tools allow clinicians to objectively measure the clinical results of their interventions. Most often with chronic painful conditions, total pain elimination is not a realistic goal, owing to the nervous system changes described above. Instead, a more attainable objective is reducing pain to a tolerable predetermined level as agreed on by consensus of the patient and clinician. A person with chronic pain should expect to achieve pain reduction with the ultimate objective of increasing daily function (e.g., activities of daily living) and minimizing suffering.

Mechanisms of Pain

Transduction, Transmission, Modulation, and Perception

Pain sensation involves a series of complex interactions between peripheral nerves and the central nervous system (CNS). This process is modulated by excitatory and inhibitory neurotransmitters released in response to stimuli. Such stimuli can be physical, psychological, or both. An example of a physical stimulus is a burn or cut to the skin. In a short time, local reactions occur in the damaged area that initiate the release of chemical mediators involved in inflammation. This is followed by sensitization of the nerve endings, which ultimately send signals to the sensory cortex of the brain. Nociception, or the sensation of pain, is composed of four basic processes: transduction, transmission, modulation, and perception (Fig. 8-1).[1]

Transduction is the process by which noxious stimuli are translated into electrical signals at peripheral receptor sites. This begins when nociceptors (free nerve endings located throughout the skin, muscle, and viscera) are exposed to a sufficient quantity of mechanical, chemical, or thermal noxious stimuli.[2,3] In addition, a variety of chemical compounds (e.g., histamine, bradykinin, serotonin, prostaglandins and, substance P) are released serially from damaged tissues and can activate or sensitize nociceptors.[2,3] Serotonin has the additional action of modulating the peripheral release of primary afferent neuropeptides that are responsible for neurogenic inflammation. These neuropeptides include substance P, calcitonin gene-related peptide, and neurokinin A.[2,3]

Transmission involves the propagation of an electrical signal along neural membranes. Stimuli, such as prostaglandins and inflammatory mediators, change the permeability of the membrane, producing an influx of sodium and an efflux of potassium, thereby depolarizing neuronal membranes. Electrical impulses are transmitted to the spinal cord via two primary afferent nerve types: myelinated A-fibers and unmyelinated C-fibers. The A-delta fiber is responsible for rapidly conducting electrical impulses associated with thermal and mechanical stimuli to the dorsal horn of the spinal cord. A-delta fibers release excitatory amino acids, such as glutamate, which activate α-amino-3-hydroxy-5-methylisoxazole-4-propionic acid (AMPA) receptors located on dorsal horn neurons.[2,4] Transmission of signals along these fibers results in sharp or stabbing sensations that alert the subject to an injury or insult to tissue. CNS input rapidly produces reflex signals, such as musculoskeletal withdrawal, to prevent further injury.[5]

The smaller, unmyelinated C-fibers respond to mechanical, thermal, and chemical stimuli and conduct electrical impulses to the spinal cord at a much slower rate compared with myelinated A-delta fibers. C-fibers, which also terminate in the dorsal horn, release the excitatory amino acids, glutamate and aspartate. Unlike A-fibers, C-fibers also release peptides, such as substance P, neurokinin A, somatostatin, galanin, and calcitonin gene-related peptide (CGRP).[5] The role of these peptides is not completely understood. Substance P is known to activate neurokinin-1 receptors, which may play a role in increasing excitability of spinal cord neurons.[5,6] Transmission of electrical impulses via C-fibers results in pain that is dull, aching, burning, and poorly localized or diffuse. This type of pain is known as *second* pain because it is perceived after the first pain sensation.

Once dorsal horn receptors are activated, electrical signals are further propagated to the thalamus, primarily via the spinothalamic tract. From the thalamus, signals are sent to the cortex and other regions of the brain for processing and interpretation.

Modulation of nociceptive information occurs quickly between descending inhibitory pathways from the thalamus and brainstem and interneurons in the dorsal horn. Neurons from the thalamus and brainstem release inhibitory neurotransmitters, such as norepinephrine, serotonin, γ-aminobutyric acid (GABA), glycine, endorphins, and enkephalins, which block substance P and other excitatory neurotransmitter activity on primary afferent fibers.[7]

The conscious awareness, or *perception*, of pain is the end result of this complex cascade of actions. The perception of pain involves not only nociceptive processes, but also physiologic and emotional responses, which contribute significantly to the sensation that is ultimately experienced by the person.[7] The perception of pain may be influenced by abnormal generation or processing of electrical pain signals and by the

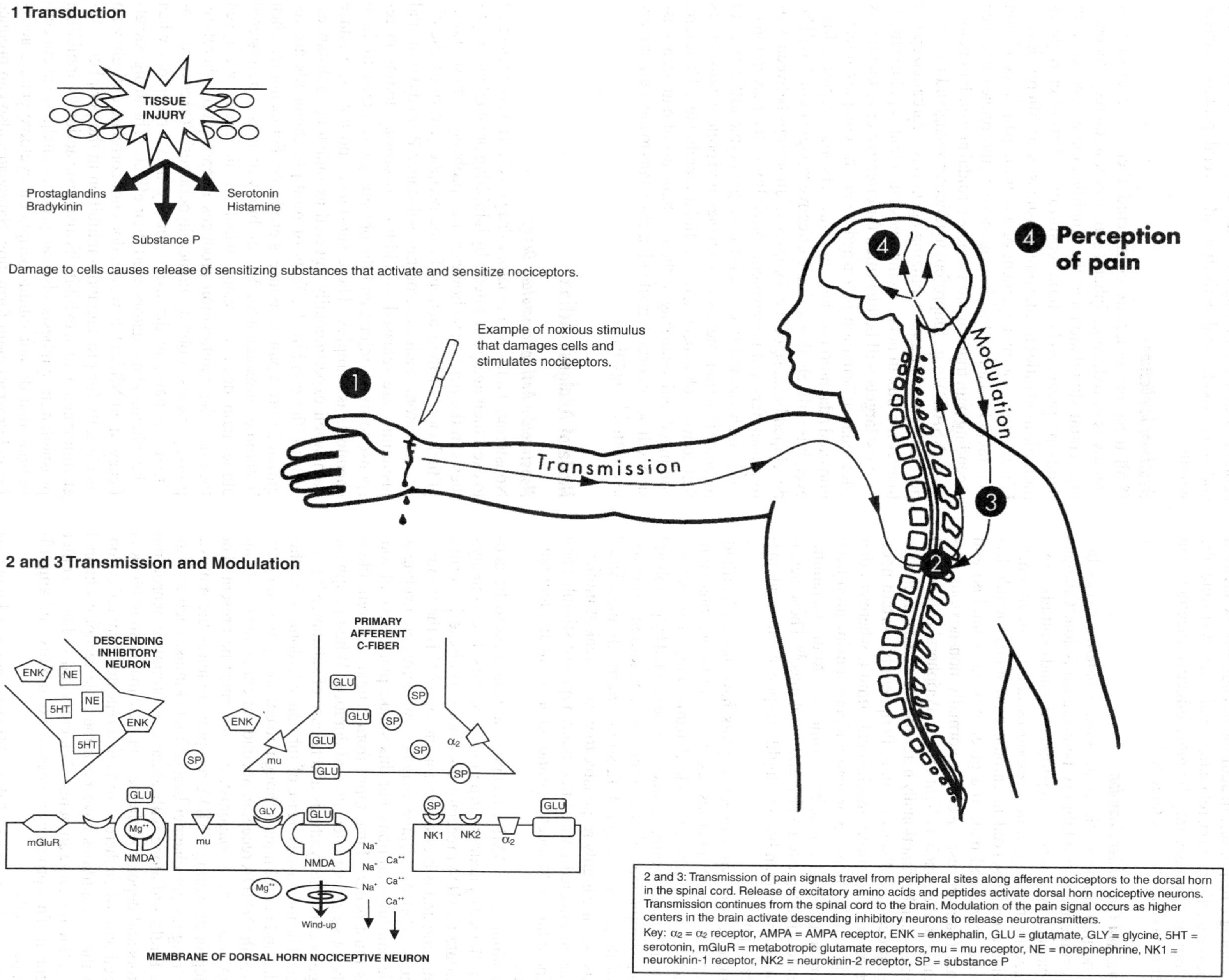
1 Transduction
TISSUE INJURY
Prostaglandins
Bradykinin
Serotonin
Histamine
Substance P
Damage to cells causes release of sensitizing substances that activate and sensitize nociceptors.
Example of noxious stimulus that damages cells and stimulates nociceptors.
1
Transmission
Modulation
4 Perception of pain
4
3
2
2 and 3 Transmission and Modulation
DESCENDING INHIBITORY NEURON
ENK
NE
5HT
PRIMARY AFFERENT C-FIBER
GLU
SP
mu
α2
GLY
mGluR
Mg++
NMDA
NK1
NK2
Na+
Ca++
Wind-up
MEMBRANE OF DORSAL HORN NOCICEPTIVE NEURON
2 and 3: Transmission of pain signals travel from peripheral sites along afferent nociceptors to the dorsal horn in the spinal cord. Release of excitatory amino acids and peptides activate dorsal horn nociceptive neurons. Transmission continues from the spinal cord to the brain. Modulation of the pain signal occurs as higher centers in the brain activate descending inhibitory neurons to release neurotransmitters.
Key: α2 = α2 receptor, AMPA = AMPA receptor, ENK = enkephalin, GLU = glutamate, GLY = glycine, 5HT = serotonin, mGluR = metabotropic glutamate receptors, mu = mu receptor, NE = norepinephrine, NK1 = neurokinin-1 receptor, NK2 = neurokinin-2 receptor, SP = substance P

FIGURE 8-1 Transduction, transmission, modulation, and perception of pain following a noxious stimulus. (Adapted from McCaffery M, Pasero C. *Pain: Clinical Manual.* St. Louis: Mosby; 1999, with permission.)

psychological framework created by the patient's temporal affective state or from previous painful experiences. Therefore, treatment that includes drug therapy to alter the nociceptive and physiologic responses, in addition to cognitive-behavioral strategies (e.g., distraction, relaxation, and imagery) to alter the psychological response, may be more effective together than if either intervention is used alone.[8]

Peripheral and Central Sensitization

Under normal homeostatic conditions, a balance exists between excitatory and inhibitory neurotransmission. Changes in this balance may occur both peripherally and centrally, however, leading to exaggerated responses and sensitization.[8,9] Examples often observed in chronic pain states include hyperalgesia (enhanced pain to a given noxious stimulus) and allodynia (pain in response to a normally non-noxious mechanical stimulus, such as light touch). Peripheral and central nociceptors can be functionally heterogeneous and can change through processes of sensitization. Peripherally, certain nociceptors respond to strong mechanical stimuli, whereas other normally "silent" nociceptors can undergo sensitization from exposure to prostaglandins, bradykinin, serotonin, histamine, adenosine triphosphate (ATP), and cytokines.[10] These sensitized nociceptors then become highly responsive to weak mechanical stimuli.[11]

Centrally, two types of nociceptors have been identified. Nociceptive-specific neurons respond only to noxious stimuli, such as heat, whereas wide dynamic range neurons respond to noxious stimuli, but also may be excited by peripheral mechanostimulation.[11,12] In chronic pain conditions, populations of these neurons can shift, so that normally inactivated neurons become highly responsive to various weak stimuli.[2,11] The person affected notices that many types of stimuli elicit pain, including light touch or minor changes in ambient temperature.

On stimulation, AMPA receptors are the first to be activated, followed by neurokinin peptide receptors. The *N*-methyl-D-aspartate (NMDA) receptor does not participate in normal transmission and is blocked by magnesium.[5,13] If the stimulus continues, NMDA receptors may become activated, leading to chronic painful conditions. For this to take place, several conditions must occur.[5] First, input from primary afferent fibers must be of sufficient intensity and duration. When peripheral damage occurs, the synthesis and release of substance P is increased. The increased release of substance P, along with other peptides and neurokinins is thought to enhance glutamate activation of the NMDA receptor. Second, for glutamate to activate NMDA receptors, a coagonist, glycine, must be present. The last step in activating NMDA receptors requires the removal of the magnesium channel block. Tachykinins, such as substance P released along with glutamate, stimulate neurokinin receptors and depolarize the neuron. The magnesium block is removed only when there is sufficient repeated depolarization. When these conditions have been met, the receptor channel opens, allowing large amounts of calcium and sodium to enter the neuron. This produces excessive excitability and amplification of signals.

This initial activation of the NMDA receptor is known as *wind-up*. Wind-up progressively increases the number and response of nociceptive neurons in the dorsal horn without any change of input to the spinal cord.[5,13] In fact, this process can continue after peripheral input has stopped. With continued nociceptive input, spread occurs activating nearby receptors, known collectively as *metabotropic glutamate receptors*.[4,7] Central sensitization occurs when NMDA and neurokinin receptors are activated, along with increases of cyclic nucleotides and nitric oxide, and activation of several protein kinases within.[11]

Treatment Implications

If all these processes are considered, then the goal of pain therapy is to reduce peripheral sensitization, thereby decreasing central stimulation and the amplification associated with wind-up, spread, and central sensitization. This often requires multiple modalities to interrupt transmission at different levels. For example, the management of a chronic painful condition may include treatment with an opiate (e.g., morphine) to reduce ascending pain transmission, a nonsteroidal anti-inflammatory drug (NSAID) (e.g., ibuprofen) to reduce prostaglandin formation, and a membrane-stabilizing agent (e.g., carbamazepine) to alter ion flux in nerve membranes and blunt depolarization.

New targets will be identified for effective drug therapy as additional information is learned about the complex interactions and adaptations of neurotransmitters and receptors. However, it is unlikely that a single effective "magic bullet" will be developed because of the complex relationships between neurotransmitters and interpatient variability in the perception of pain. Such variability can arise from genotypic differences in receptor function, metabolic enzymes, and protein transporters that convey substances across cellular membranes. Therefore, continued understanding of the mechanisms of pain transmission will be important in allowing clinicians to most effectively use available agents.

Mode of Analgesic Action

Nonsteroidal Anti-Inflammatory Drugs

Nonsteroidal anti-inflammatory drugs (NSAID) are presumed to exert their analgesic effects by inhibiting prostaglandin synthesis in the periphery; however, this probably is an oversimplified view of their action. In the periphery, various chemical mediators, such as serotonin, substance P, bradykinin, and histamine, are released in addition to prostaglandins in response to tissue injury, and the physiologic response to these chemicals is complex. These substances do not all produce pain when experimentally injected as individual substances. Instead, the combined effects of multiple chemicals are required before a pain response is produced. For example, when histamine, prostaglandin E_2, or bradykinin is administered alone, pain does not result; when all the agents are given together, the combination produces intense pain. Therefore, prostaglandins probably induce hyperalgesia (excessive sensitivity to pain) in the local sensory nerve receptors when other chemical mediators exert their effects. The analgesic efficacy of an NSAID, however, does not correlate entirely with its capacity for prostaglandin inhibition in the periphery. Acetaminophen, which exhibits its analgesic action by inhibiting prostaglandin synthesis, also can produce analgesia at concentrations that do not inhibit peripheral cyclooxygenase activity and prostaglandin formation. Salicylates also can produce analgesia at concentrations that do not inhibit peripheral cyclooxygenase activity and prostaglandin formation. Therefore, the exact mechanism of NSAID analgesia has yet to be elucidated; however, the analgesic effect of NSAID is likely central in origin and involves substance-P receptors of the neurokinin-1 type and glutamate receptors of the NMDA type in addition to central prostaglandin inhibition. Because spinal administration of NSAIDs reduces the hyperalgesia evoked by spinal substance P and NMDA, the action of the NSAID appears to be independent of peripheral inflammation. NSAID actions through GABAergic pathways, arachidonic acid byproducts, and AMPA receptors also are being studied. Aspirin, the prototypical NSAID, has demonstrated synergistic activity with endogenous opioids at opioid receptors as well as enhancing serotonin's effects in the central nervous system.[14,15]

Opiates

Opiates can attach to one or more of five opioid receptors: the μ-, δ-, ε-, κ-, and σ-receptors. These receptors can be differentiated further into subtypes (e.g., μ_1, μ_2, δ_1, δ_2, κ_1, κ_2, and κ_3). Animal models suggest that as many as seven subtypes of μ-receptors may exist, but it is not known how many of these can be found in humans. Stimulation of μ_1-receptors may be responsible for the desired effects of supraspinal analgesia, and stimulation of μ_2-receptors may lead to unwanted consequences such as respiratory depression, euphoria, constipation, and physical dependence. Some κ-receptors, as well as δ- and ε-receptors, also mediate analgesic response, although the role of ε-receptors is not fully understood. Autonomic stimulation, dysphoria, and hallucinations may be caused by σ-receptors. These are not considered true opioid receptors, but may interact with some opioid-like agents.

The effect of opiates on these receptor subtypes is gradually being discovered. Morphine can stimulate μ_1-, μ_2-, and κ-receptors, and perhaps this ability to stimulate multiple receptors accounts for morphine's mixed analgesic and side effect profile. Pure opiate antagonists (e.g., naloxone) occupy opiate receptors without eliciting a direct response and block the access of opiate agonists, such as morphine, to these receptors. As a result, pure narcotic antagonists block both the desired and undesired opiate effects. Pentazocine and butorphanol (both mixed agonist–antagonists) produce analgesia through stimulation of κ-receptors, but cause unwanted dysphoria and hallucinations through their effect on σ-receptors. Pentazocine and butorphanol also block access of morphine to μ-receptors, leading to withdrawal symptoms in individuals who are physically dependent on morphine or its analogs.

In the spinal cord, the highest concentration of opioid receptors is located around the C-fiber terminal zones in the lamina 1 of the dorsal horn and the substantia gelatinosa. The μ-opioid receptors constitute approximately 70% of the total receptor population; δ- and κ-receptors account for 24% and 6% of the population, respectively. μ-Receptors also are located in the afferent terminals. Because morphine has a 50 times higher affinity for the μ-receptor than for the δ- or κ-receptors, it is a very effective analgesic. The pharmacologic action of opioids depends on the availability of opioid receptors, and the cutting of peripheral nerves leads to degeneration and loss of opioid receptors in the nerve itself. As a result, postamputation pain often is not relieved by morphine or other opioids.

Opioids produce analgesia by three main mechanisms[16]:

- Presynaptically, opioids reduce the release of inflammatory transmitters (e.g., tachykinin, excitatory amino acids, and peptides) from the terminals of afferent C-fiber neurons after activation of opioid receptors.
- Opioids also can reduce the activity of output neurons, interneurons, and dendrites in the neuronal pathways by means of postsynaptic hyperpolarization.
- Opioids also inhibit neuronal activity via GABA and enkephalin neurons in the substantia gelatinosa.

Analgesic Adjunctive Agents

Analgesic medications often are prescribed concurrently with other drugs to enhance analgesia or to treat pain exacerbations. These adjunctive medications are most often used in the management of chronic pain, particularly when the dose of the primary analgesic has been optimized or when the underlying condition has progressed and is no longer adequately controlled by the primary analgesic agent. Other adjuvant agents may be added to analgesic therapy to reduce side effects, such as excessive sedation, nausea and vomiting, or constipation. The most common drug classes used as adjunctive analgesic agents are corticosteroids, anticonvulsants, heterocyclic antidepressants, α_2-adrenergic agonists, NMDA receptor antagonists, local and oral anesthetics or antiarrhythmics, antihistamines and neuroleptics. Adjunct analgesic agents may be used as the primary analgesic agent in the treatment of neuropathic pain syndromes, where the usefulness of opioids is under debate. Neuropathic pain syndromes do not respond to NSAIDs.

Corticosteroids, such as dexamethasone, are useful in reducing pain associated with cerebral and spinal cord edema and in treating refractory neuropathic pain and bone pain, particularly metastatic bone pain. Corticosteroids may also provide other beneficial effects, such as mood elevation, antiemetic activity, and appetite stimulation.[17]

Antidepressants are commonly used to treat neuropathic pain (e.g., diabetic neuropathy, postherpetic neuralgia) and pain associated with insomnia or depression.[18] They are used to treat fibromyalgia, a syndrome characterized by diffuse muscle and joint pain, which is thought to result from central dysregulation. Their analgesic effect is independent of their antidepressant effect. Postulated mechanisms of action involve blockade of norepinephrine reuptake, antagonism of histamine and muscarinic cholinergic receptors, α-adrenergic blockade, or suppression of C-fiber evoked activity in the spinal cord.[19]

Anticonvulsants; antiarrhythmics; α_2-adrenergic antagonists; and the NMDA receptor antagonists, ketamine and dextromethorphan, also have been used to manage neuropathic pain with varying degrees of success. Antihistamines, such as hydroxyzine and promethazine, are often prescribed postoperatively to augment the analgesic effects of opioid agents. Hydroxyzine may provide minimal analgesia, whereas little evidence exists to confirm analgesic action for promethazine.[20] The addition of phenothiazines and antihistamines may be useful in alleviating opioid-induced nausea and vomiting; however, these agents may potentiate orthostatic hypotension, respiratory depression, sedation, and extrapyramidal side effects.[21] Use of these agents should not be a substitute for appropriate doses of opioid analgesics.

Classification of Pain

Acute Pain

Pain immediately following an injury to the body is considered to be *acute pain*, whereas pain lasting beyond the expected healing time, or persistent pain that does not respond to usual pain control methods, is defined as *chronic pain*. Acute pain serves a useful purpose in minimizing the extent of injury by causing an organism to recoil from a noxious or harmful stimulus. In most cases, the objective physical findings associated with acute pain can be localized directly to the site of injury. Injury to nerves on visceral organ systems can present as diffuse, poorly differentiated, referred pain.

Acute pain is usually self-limiting and typically subsides when the injury heals. Untreated or inadequately treated pain can evoke physiologic hormonal responses that alter circulation and tissue metabolism; these can also produce tachypnea, tachycardia, widening of the pulse pressure, and increased sympathetic nervous system activity. Inadequately treated pain can produce significant psychological stress responses and compromise the body's immune system by provoking release of endogenous corticosteroids. Decreased range of motion, diminished pulmonary vital capacity, and a compromise in the overall well-being of a person secondary to poorly treated pain can delay recovery after surgery or trauma. Acute pain is often exacerbated by anxiety and secondary reflex musculoskeletal spasms.

Acute pain should always be aggressively managed, even before a definitive cause is known. In patients with traumatic head injury, medications should be withheld until a full neurologic workup can be performed because they can interfere with cognitive function. Patients with acute abdominal pain also may have pain medications withheld until a diagnosis is made; however, several studies support early pain management.[22,23] When pain is relieved, the patient is more comfortable and better able to cooperate with the history, physical examination, and diagnostic procedures. Postoperative and other acute pain syndromes often are ignored or inadequately treated, however. Part of the tendency to undertreat pain is the reluctance of caregivers to prescribe opiates for fear of causing addiction. Addiction to opioids is essentially nonexistent when these drugs are prescribed for acute pain, and withholding appropriate pain treatment causes needless patient suffering.

Chronic Pain

The origins of chronic pain may be neurogenic, nociceptive, psychiatric, or idiopathic. As will be presented later, it is important to further differentiate chronic pain syndromes into those that are associated with malignancy from those that are not. All forms of chronic pain share some common characteristics, however. Unlike acute pain, which prompts the afflicted individual to avoid further injury or seek help, chronic pain usually serves no benefit to the individual. Chronic pain can be episodic or continuous, or a combination of both. A patient may feel constant pain and also experience exacerbations of more intense pain at various times. Chronic pain can cause a person to feel "trapped" inside of his or her body, distinguished only by more painful and less painful days. Chronic pain often is destructive to the host by deteriorating quality of life, functional ability, spiritual and psychological well-being, interpersonal relationships, and financial status.[17] Chronic pain also can cause changes in appetite, psychomotor retardation, irritability, social withdrawal, sleep disturbances, and depression. The patient often cannot remember an existence free of pain and is convinced that the pain will be present until death. In short, chronic pain can become an all-consuming focus of the patient's life.

The key to successful chronic pain management rests on prevention and elimination of unnecessary suffering and despair. Chronic pain management should consider the applicability of cognitive interventions (relaxation technique, self-hypnosis, psychiatric therapy) as well as physical manipulations (local application of heat, cold, massage, electrical nerve stimulation, acupuncture, and physical therapy). Pharmacologic agents (antidepressants, antiarrhythmics, anticonvulsants, major tranquilizers, and longer-acting opioids), regional anesthesia (local anesthetic blocks with or without corticosteroids or chemical neurolysis), surgical interventions (spinal decompression, release of nerve entrapment), and spinal analgesia (intraspinal opioids or local anesthetic agents) are also warranted.[24,25]

PAIN ASSOCIATED WITH MALIGNANCY (CHRONIC MALIGNANT PAIN)

Chronic malignant pain can have a combination of acute, intermittent, or constant components. Although the pain is chronic, it can have elements of acute pain when tissue damage continues from tumor infiltration. Nerve destruction, chemotherapy, radiation therapy, and surgery also contribute to malignant pain. Occasionally, chronic malignant pain has only minimal or no associated objective clinical physical findings, and may be erroneously dismissed by inexperienced clinicians.

Anticipation by the patient that malignant pain will be continuous leads to anxiety, depression, and insomnia.[26] These destructive feelings can accentuate the patient's perception of pain. Inadequately treated chronic malignant pain can become progressively more severe and cause relentless suffering. Persistent pain can accelerate the deterioration of the patient's physical and psychological condition more than the malignancy itself.

The most important aspect of chronic malignant pain management is a logical and systematic approach with the goal of pain alleviation (or minimization) and prevention. A primary element of this approach is patient access to health care and pain management information. It is the duty of all health care providers to effectively assess their patients' pain management needs and to make appropriate referrals or therapeutic changes.

CHRONIC NONMALIGNANT PAIN

Pain not associated with a malignant disease and lasting >6 months or beyond the healing period is considered to be chronic nonmalignant pain. This pain also has been called *chronic benign pain,* an obvious misrepresentation, because pain is never benign when it causes patient suffering. Chronic nonmalignant pain is recognized as a serious health problem that affects millions of people worldwide and carries far-reaching social implications.[27] The development of treatment guidelines is difficult because of the heterogeneity of causes. For most types of chronic pain, initial therapy is often conservative. Failure of conservative therapy may necessitate the use of more potent analgesics. The use of opiates in this patient population is controversial; however, increasing data support opiate use in psychologically healthy patients.[28,29] Because chronic pain affects many aspects of a patient's life, a multidisciplinary approach that addresses effective drug therapy and comprehensive rehabilitation often provides greater relief to the patient than drug therapy alone.

Much of the difficulty encountered in pain management arises when clinicians are not sufficiently educated or trained in dealing with the complex pharmacologic and psychosocial

Table 8-1 Common Causes of Analgesic Treatment Failure

Problem	Potential Impact on Pain Management	Example
1. Inappropriate or unknown diagnosis	Improper medication selection	Using a nonsteroidal anti-inflammatory drug (NSAID) for abdominal pain that may be related to a gastrointestinal bleed
2. Misunderstanding of pharmacology or pharmacokinetics	Overestimating potency or half-life	Dosing an opioid less frequently than necessary to provide adequate relief
3. Inadequate management of adverse effects	Patient may discontinue therapy or misuse over-the-counter remedies	Patient suffers constipation from antidepressants and uses daily bisacodyl
4. Fear of addiction	Physician or patient or caregiver may withhold medications	Evidence of tolerance after chronic use of opioids may be mistaken for addiction
5. Unrealistic goals for therapy	Patient will not be satisfied with pain management regimen and may seek other care	Patient states a desire to be "pain free" following significant nerve injury
6. Irrational polypharmacy	Over- or under-use of appropriate therapies	Patient with neuropathic pain using three different opioids without any adjuncts in the regimen
7. Patient barriers	Patient cannot understand appropriate medication use or other pain management modalities	• Language or comprehension deficits • Cognitive deficits: patient cannot remember regimen • Physical impediments to using medicines appropriately • Cultural barriers (e.g., stoicism)
8. Lack of understanding of pathophysiology of pain	Limitations of health care providers' ability to adequately relieve pain	Drugs that show benefit in animal models are not useful for human pain conditions

problems associated with chronic pain. Often the clinician fails to listen to the patient or fails to recognize clues to the subtle nature of the patient's pain complaints. Drug selection often is irrational and doses are frequently inadequate. An unfortunate tragedy occurs when clinicians occasionally withhold adequate analgesia because of a misunderstood fear of addiction, or when a patient refuses medications because of a similar fear of addiction.[30,31]

General Treatment Principles

Pain is one of the most common reasons for which patients seek medical attention, yet it remains significantly undertreated despite the availability of effective medications and other therapies.[32,33]

Table 8-1 lists eight common causes of treatment failure when using analgesics.[34] In general, the reasons include a lack of understanding of pain management principles or the pharmacologic properties of the drugs; an overestimation of the risk of addiction by both patients and caregivers; or poor communication between the patient and medical personnel. A number of steps to overcome these barriers are described in the succeeding section.

Effective analgesic therapy begins with an accurate assessment of the patient. The Pain Intensity and Pain Distress Scales (Figures 8-2 and 8-3, respectively) can help clinicians assess pain. When obtaining a pain history, it is important to gather details about the pattern, duration, location, and character of the pain. Pain intensity should be measured using an appropriate pain scale (Figs. 8-2 and 8-3) according to the patient's ability to communicate.[17,24] Factors that exacerbate or relieve pain should be assessed. The names and amounts of all analgesics that the patient is taking should be documented as well as their effectiveness. In addition, other medical problems and medications should be documented, including over-the-counter and nonprescription remedies. A patient fearful of being accused of analgesic abuse might be reluctant to give an accurate drug use history unless a trusting relationship can be established.

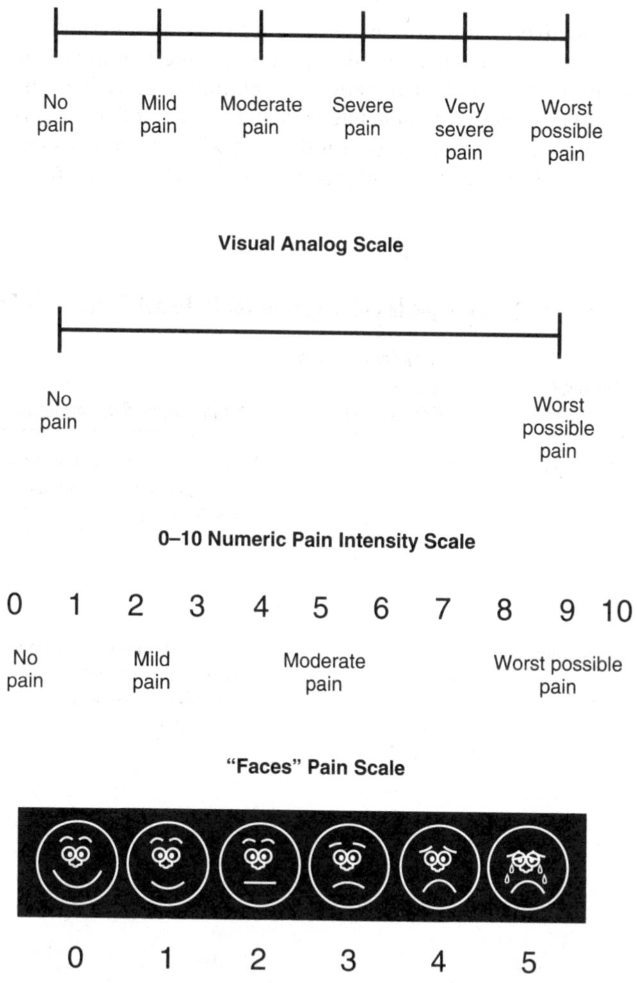

FIGURE 8-2 Pain intensity scales. (Adapted from Patt RB. *Cancer Pain*. Philadelphia: JB Lippincott; 1993; and Wong DL. *Whaley and Wong's Essentials of Pediatric Nursing*. St. Louis: Mosby; 1997, with permission.)

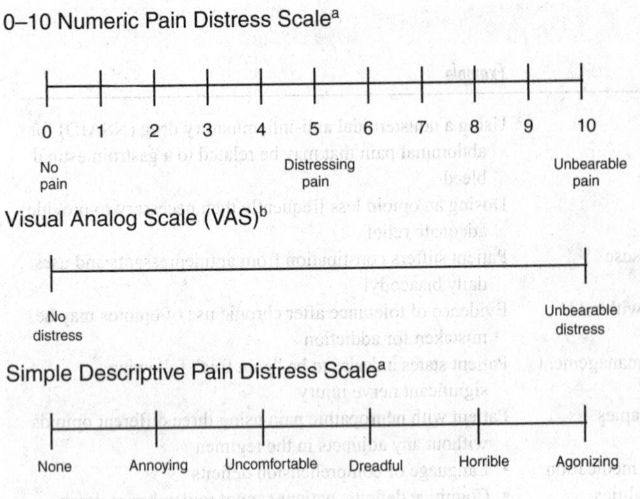

[a]If used as a graphic rating scale, a 10-cm baseline is recommended.
[b]A 10-cm baseline is recommended for VAS scales.

FIGURE 8-3 Pain distress scales.

Effective treatment considers the cause, duration, and intensity of pain and matches the appropriate intervention to the situation. The goal of therapy is to eliminate or reduce the pain to the lowest tolerable intensity and prevent it from recurring, rather than waiting to treat the pain when it becomes unbearable. The patient should predetermine this lowest tolerable level with the health care provider based on a pain scale that is mutually understood. Guidelines from the World Health Organization, summarized in Table 8-2, can be useful when choosing initial therapy.[35] It is also important to consider the clinical situation when determining analgesic selection or whether the painful condition requires analgesic therapy. For example, it would be irrational to use morphine to treat the severe abdominal cramping pain associated with constipation, because morphine can worsen the constipation. If pain is the result of a fracture, then stabilization and immobilization, in addition to appropriate analgesics, will reduce pain in the affected bone. Once a pain regimen is initiated, frequent reassessment will determine whether the goals of therapy are being met and whether they address any emerging side effects. Drug selection, doses, routes of administration, and dosing frequency should be adjusted as needed until the goals of therapy are met. In treating acute, severe postoperative pain, it may be necessary to begin with a potent opiate analgesic and then gradually reduce the dose based on the patient's clinical response.

When treating chronic pain, elimination and prevention of pain is best accomplished by using analgesics at fixed time intervals ("time-contingent") rather than on an as-needed basis. The traditional as-needed analgesic dosing schedule is inadequate much of the time, leading to greater 24-hour drug intake and a pattern of stepwise increases in dosage. Therefore, most pain management specialists now administer, or at least offer, analgesics to their patients on a schedule, at least for the first few days until pain requirements can be adequately assessed. In patients with severe acute or malignant pain, however, scheduled analgesics alone may not be adequate without additional

Table 8-2 Example Initial Regimens for Different Pain Levels Based on Guidelines From the World Health Organization (WHO)

Pain Level Description	*Typical Corresponding Numerical Rating (0 to 10 Scale)*	*WHO Therapeutic Recommendations*	*Example Medicines for Initial Therapy*	*Comments*
"Mild" pain	1–3	Nonopioid analgesic: taken on a regular schedule, not as needed (prn)	• Acetaminophen 650 mg every 4 hr • Acetaminophen 1,000 mg every 6 hr • Ibuprofen 600 mg every 6 hr	• Consider adding adjunct analgesic or using an alternate regimen if pain not reduced in 12 days • Consider step up if pain not relieved by two different regimens
"Moderate" pain	4–6	Add opioid for moderate pain (e.g., moderate potency analgesic). Use on a schedule, not prn	• Acetaminophen 325 mg/codeine 60 mg every 4 hr • Acetaminophen 325 mg/Oxycodone 5 mg every 4 hr • Tramadol 50 mg every 6 hr	• Consider adding adjunct analgesic or using an alternate regimen if pain not reduced in 12 days • Consider step up if pain not relieved by two different regimens
"Severe" pain	7–10	Switch to a high potency (strong) opioid; administer on a regular schedule	• Morphine 15 mg every 4 hr • Hydromorphone 4 mg every 4 hr • Morphine controlled release 60 mg every 8 hr	• Consider alternate regimen (e.g., different strong opioid) if pain not reduced in 12 days • Consider increased dose of strong opioid, or addition of nonopioid agents, if pain not adequately relieved by two regimens

Adapted from the World Health Organization, http://www.who.int/cancer/palliative/painladder/en/.

analgesics for breakthrough episodes. Until the dosage is stabilized, all patients who are receiving analgesics should be monitored closely for efficacy of analgesia as well as untoward side effects. Successful pain management can also include the use of nonpharmacologic measures, such as ensuring that the patient receives adequate rest and emotional support. Physical and occupational therapy may be useful to help improve strength or mobility and to ensure that no barriers at home or work exist that can interfere with the patient's activities of daily living.[28]

Anxiety and guilt often complicate the management of pain. Patients sometimes become anxious, fearing that their pain will become uncontrollable or that they will become addicted to opiates. Also, patients sometimes feel guilty about taking opioids for their pain because of the negative social connotations associated with these drugs. They may feel that they have failed their clinicians' expectations. Therefore, patient education about the rational use of analgesics is imperative. Pain can be managed best when trust and communication exist between the caregiver and the patient, known as a *therapeutic alliance*. Patients must feel comfortable telling caregivers whenever their pain needs arise, and caregivers must respond appropriately and in a timely fashion. Good communication between caregivers and patients can alleviate anxiety and guilt regarding patients' pain needs.

Patient-specific characteristics (e.g., age, gender, race, organ dysfunction, and comorbidities) play an important role in the response to pharmacotherapy, ranging from subtherapeutic effect to toxicities. A genetic polymorphism of the cytochrome P450 system significantly contributes to inconsistency of patient response to drug therapy.[36] Based on CYP 450 enzymatic activity, patients may be classified as poor metabolizers, intermediate metabolizers, extensive metabolizers, and ultrarapid metabolizers. Such variations in drug metabolism have been correlated to a range of effective doses and occurrence of toxicities. This has been observed with different drug classes, including opioids.[36]

Codeine is a prodrug that is metabolized to morphine, a more potent analgesic, by CYP2D6. This particular enzyme is known to have variable presence among individuals, leading to insufficient analgesia in poor metabolizers.[37]

Tramadol, a synthetic opioid, exerts its full analgesic effect when the parent compound is converted to O-desmethyltramadol via CYP2D6. Consequently, it has been demonstrated that, in the postoperative setting, poor metabolizers do not exhibit equal analgesia when compared with extensive metabolizers.[37]

Polymorphism of CYP 450 is not the only target of pharmacogenomic research. Genetic variations that contribute to opioid, cannabinoid, NMDA, dopamine, and serotonin receptor expression, as well as drug transporters, are also subjects of further research. Their effect on response to pharmacotherapy has not yet been elucidated.[37]

In the near future, when genetic testing becomes economically feasible for widespread use, clinicians will utilize this information in their decision process to prevent toxicities and optimize pharmacotherapy.[37]

Analgesic Selection

The selection of an analgesic must be individualized for each patient, depending on the cause and chronicity of the pain as well as the patient's age and concomitant medical conditions that may alter drug response. Furthermore, the clinical response of the patient dictates future dose adjustment, route, and desired dosing interval. The selection of an opioid for the management of severe acute and chronic malignant pain must always include consideration of morphine or one of the other potent opioids; however, the role of NSAID should not be overlooked. Adjunctive analgesic medications, such as antidepressants or anticonvulsants, are often added because chronic nonmalignant pain can be associated with sympathetic dysfunction and neuropathies. An NSAID is the analgesic of choice in the management of mild to moderate pain involving musculoskeletal tissues and also are extremely effective in the management of pain from bony neoplastic metastasis. Neurogenic pain often responds better to tricyclic antidepressants (TCA) than to opioids. Neuropathic pain may not be relieved by opioids until the dose is high enough to also cause significant side effects.

If the maintenance dose of an opioid analgesic is too high, the patient can become oversedated and less functional. In extreme cases, patients may become bedridden from excessive opiate use. When given the choice of eliminating the last trace of discomfort at the cost of some sensorial clouding, patients invariably select full alertness and the continued presence of some pain.[38,39] Patients who are receiving opioids also need to be monitored for deterioration in vital signs (pulse and respiratory rate), constipation, and urinary retention. Stool softeners and other prophylactic measures, such as stimulant laxatives, may be required. Similarly, a patient who is receiving NSAID or adjunctive analgesics should be monitored for possible untoward side effects associated with such medications.

Orally or transdermally administered analgesics allow a patient a greater degree of independence and control over daily activities than parenteral administration by maximizing mobility. Similar advantages can be obtained with an intravenous (IV) infusion device, particularly a portable programmable infusion pump. Regular parenteral administration by other routes can be difficult and painful in cachectic patients.

Low to Moderate Potency (Mild) Analgesics

The nonsteroidal anti-inflammatory analgesics have a relatively flat dose-response effect when contrasted with opioids, reaching maximal analgesia at low to moderate doses. In contrast to opiate analgesics, higher doses of NSAIDs do not produce greater analgesia. These drugs are frequently prescribed at doses in excess of the effective maximal analgesic dose, however, because the duration of analgesia can increase with higher doses. For example, ibuprofen given 600 mg every 6 hours produces a similar analgesic effect as 400 mg given every 4 hours. The total daily dose is the same, but side effects are experienced more often with larger doses. Although NSAIDs have both analgesic and anti-inflammatory properties, it is often difficult to differentiate between these effects in published studies or during clinical use in patients, as the time courses of each effect overlap.

All of the NSAIDs, including ibuprofen (Motrin), naproxen (Naprosyn), naproxen sodium (Anaprox), diflunisal (Dolobid), diclofenac (Voltaren), diclofenac potassium (Cataflam), nabumetone (Relafen), ketoprofen (Orudis), flurbiprofen (Ansaid), ketorolac (Toradol), and others, provide analgesia equivalent or superior to that of aspirin[40,41] or acetaminophen codeine 60 mg combined with a variety of mild to moderate painful conditions.[42,43] As with the opioid analgesics, the duration of action of an NSAID does not correlate well with the serum half-life of the drug. Likely, this is because the analgesic effect arises from central mechanisms, and is related to the exposure of the CNS to adequate drug levels. Patient response should guide the clinician in selecting dosing intervals of these agents, especially when they are combined with opioids.

Opioid Analgesics

In general, opioids are more effective for treating severe pain than nonopioid analgesics such as NSAIDs, although the range of potencies is wide with this class of medicines. They are generally recommended for moderate to severe pain intensity and are used in chronic pain syndromes that are refractory to other classes of agents.

An intramuscular (IM) dose of 10 mg/70 kg of morphine sulfate provides significant analgesia in approximately 70% of patients with severe pain. The remaining 30% of patients require higher doses,[44] which not only increase the intensity and duration of analgesia, but also the incidence of side effects. Morphine dosage requirements also vary with the severity of pain, individual perceptions of pain, age, opioid tolerance or previous exposure, and the presence of concomitant diseases. Thus, single parenteral analgesic doses of morphine ranging from 4 to >20 mg are used to treat acute pain and parenteral doses as high as 200 mg/hour have been required to treat end-stage malignant pain in patients who have developed tolerance.

A 10-mg parenteral dose of morphine is the historical reference standard by which all other opioid analgesics are compared. Therefore, morphine equivalents are often used when calculating analgesic doses for other opioids. The duration of analgesia of an opioid correlates partially with its serum half-life, but also with the dose, route of administration, and the distribution characteristics of the drug.[45] For example, methadone has a very long serum half-life of 24 hours, but its duration of analgesia is only about 6 hours. On the other hand, single daily doses of methadone are retained on opiate receptors in the brain long enough to prevent abstinence symptoms for 24 hours in opiate abusers. When used for pain management, the long half-life of methadone may contribute to cumulative effects and drug toxicity such as QTc prolongation. When methadone is administered epidurally, its duration of analgesia is short because of its high lipophilicity that promotes rapid redistribution from the epidural space into systemic circulation, and consequently, metabolic clearance. Conversely, morphine has a relatively short duration of analgesia when administered parenterally, but when it is administered epidurally, it has a long duration of analgesia because of its low lipophilicity, which inhibits its redistribution from the epidural space.

The administration of opioid analgesics is frequently complicated by the need to convert between different routes of administration or different opioid formulations. The approximate equianalgesic doses of parenteral and oral opioid analgesics are listed in Table 8-3. The specific oral-to-parenteral ratios of these drugs also are listed in Table 8-3; however, the precision of these ratios is controversial, in part because of the methodologies used to infer these "equivalencies." For example, most investigators maintain that the oral-to-parenteral ratio for morphine is 6:1, but some hospice clinicians maintain that morphine's oral-to-parenteral ratio is closer to 2:1. Such confusion may result from differences in the design of single-dose versus multiple-dose clinical trials. First-pass hepatic metabolism may be greater in single-dose clinical studies than in multiple-dose studies because first-pass metabolic pathways can become saturated with repeated doses. Furthermore, the accumulation of the active metabolite morphine-6-glucuronide after chronic dosing may contribute to the clinically observed differences. When all factors are taken into account, the bioavailability of oral morphine varies from 17% to 70% of a dose; therefore, it is reasonable to expect individual patient response to be highly variable.[46,47] No matter which ratio the clinician uses, the dosing must be guided by the patient's clinical response and frequent clinical reassessment.

If an opioid analgesic is to be substituted with another opioid, the equivalent doses as listed in Table 8-3 can be used as an approximate guide to dosage conversions unless the patient has developed tolerance. Cross-tolerance between opioid analgesics exists, but is often not complete. Therefore, calculated doses may be reduced by as much as 50% when interchanging different opioids. This is especially true when switching to methadone from other opioids.[48] Patient comfort is the goal, and the response of the patient should always be the basis for dosage adjustments. Whenever a new opioid analgesic is initiated, the patient's response should be assessed within the first few hours because the initial dose of the new analgesic is only correctly estimated about half the time. Frequent reassessment of clinical responses should facilitate dosage adjustments and control the patient's pain more quickly.

The analgesic efficacy of propoxyphene and combinations of acetaminophen with propoxyphene 65 mg remains controversial. Most double-blind studies demonstrate no advantage of propoxyphene alone over aspirin, acetaminophen, or codeine in relieving various types of pain.[49,50] This lack of benefit conflicts with the observation that propoxyphene in combination with acetaminophen remains a commonly prescribed regimen in the United States. This may be partially explained by an additive or synergistic effect when opioids are combined with nonopioid analgesics. Another possible explanation is the tendency of many patients to take more than the prescribed doses. Because propoxyphene has a 13-hour half-life, repeated doses taken every 4 to 6 hours for several days can result in significant drug accumulation. Furthermore, analgesic assessments of propoxyphene efficacy have been based primarily on single-dose studies,[51] while most patients take as many as 10 to 12 tablets daily. Propoxyphene has significant CNS effects. At lower dosages, propoxyphene can produce mild CNS depressant effects. At higher dosages, however, it can have an amphetaminelike stimulant effect and, in overdoses, propoxyphene can produce seizures. As with other opioid analgesics, propoxyphene can produce physical dependence.

As with all opioid analgesics, patients taking propoxyphene need to be warned about the risks of concurrent alcohol use, the operation of equipment or machinery requiring mental acuity, and the potential for agitation and sleeplessness when the medication is discontinued abruptly after prolonged use. In addition to effects on the CNS, propoxyphene has been associated with hypoglycemia in patients with renal dysfunction.[52]

Table 8-3 Properties of Opioid Analgesics

	Parenteral Dose (mg)	Oral Equivalent	Routes	Onset (min)	Duration (hr)	$t_{1/2}$ (hr)	Notes
Opioid Agonists for Moderate to Severe Pain (mu Receptor Agonists)							
Phenanthrenes							
Morphine (various)	10	30	PO, parenteral, PR	IV: 5 PO: 60	3–6	2–3	Sustained release PO preparations available
Hydromorphone (Dilaudid)	1.5	7.5	PO, parenteral, PR	See morphine	3–6	2–4	
Levorphanol (Levo-Dromoran)	2	4	PO, SC, IM	30–90	4–6	4–16	Accumulates with chronic dosing
Oxymorphone (Numorphan)	1.5	N/A	Parenteral, PR	10–90	3–6	3–4	
Phenylpiperidines							
Fentanyl (Sublimaze)	0.1	N/A	IV, spinal, buccal, patch	10	1–2	3–4	Nonlinear kinetics with repeat dosing
Sufentanil (Sufenta)	10 mcg	N/A	Parenteral, spinal	10	2–4		Duration may be dose-related
Diphenylheptanes:							
Methadone (Dolophine)	10	5	PO, SC, IM	60	6–8	21–25	Accumulates with chronic dosing
Opiods for Mild to Moderate Pain (mu Agonists)							
Phenanthrenes							
Codeine (various)	120	200	PO, parenteral, PR	See morphine	3–6		
Hydrocodone (various)	N/A	30	PO		30–60	3–4	
Oxycodone (various)	N/A	20	PO		30–60	4–6	
Dihydrodeine (various)	N/A	30	PO		30–60	4–6	
Phenylpiperidines							
Meperidine (Demerol)	100	400	PO, parenteral	15–60	1–3	3–4	Normeperidine is a CNS irritant
Partial Agonists/Antagonists (mu and/or Kappa Agonists With or Without mu Antagonism)							
Buprenorphine (Buprenex)	0.3	N/A	SC, IV, IM	1–5	4–6	2–3	Not naloxone reversible
Butorphanol (Stadol)	2	N/A	SC, IV, IM, intranasal	15–45	3–4		Dysphoric
Nalbuphine (Nubain)	10	N/A	SC, IV, IM	1–5	4–6	2–3	Respiratory ceiling
Opioid Antagonists							
Naloxone (Narcan)	0.40.8	N/A	IV	10	2–3	1–1.5	
Naltrexone (Trexan)	N/A	50	PO	30–60	24–72	9–17	Duration dose-dependent

NOTE: Most analgesic equivalents were derived from single dose studies.
CNS, central nervous system; IM, intramuscular; IV, intravenous; N/A, not applicable; PO, orally; PR, by rectum; SC, subcutaneously.
Adapted from *Principles of Analgesic Use in the Treatment of Acute Pain and Cancer Pain.* 5th ed. Glenview, IL: American Pain Society; 2003:1417, with permission.

Differentiating Between Clinical Opioid Use and Drug Abuse

When using opiates to treat severe pain lasting more than a few days, several phenomena can occur. The terms used to describe these phenomena are *tolerance, physical dependence,* and *pseudoaddiction.* Clinicians must understand the differences and the context in which these phenomena occur to differentiate between expected developments and drug abuse. Much of the fear and reluctance to use opioid analgesics result from misunderstandings of these natural events by clinicians, patients, and caregivers.

Tolerance to the analgesic effects of opiates is a common physiologic finding that results from neuroadaptation by the body during chronic use.[53] It may be seen after several days of therapy and can be first recognized by a decrease in the duration of analgesia. Patients who develop tolerance require an increase in the opiate dose to achieve the same level of analgesia. Tolerance to opiates occurs fairly slowly, but should be anticipated in all patients requiring continuous opiate therapy, such as critical care patients or patients with chronic painful conditions. These types of patients should be informed that the need for increasing doses is an expected occurrence and does not indicate addiction.

Physical dependence is a natural physiologic process that occurs with chronic opioid administration.[53] Signs and symptoms of physical dependence are summarized in Table 8-4 and are seen only when opiates are stopped abruptly or the

Table 8-4 Signs and Symptoms of Opiate Physical Dependence

1. Rhinorrhea (runny nose)
2. Lacrimation (tearing)
3. Hyperthermia, chills
4. Muscle aches (myalgia)
5. Emesis, diarrhea, gastrointestinal cramping
6. Anxiety, agitation, hostility
7. Sleeplessness

Symptoms begin within 6 hours for short-acting opioids (e.g., morphine) and generally peak in approximately 36–48 hours. Symptoms of abstinence usually subside within 3 to 7 days (average, 5 days). With methadone, however, abstinence syndrome develops more slowly, and is less severe, but protracted. Opioid antagonists or mixed agonist–antagonist drugs can precipitate abstinence in some patients after chronic or subchronic opioid exposure.

dose is markedly decreased. Physical dependence does not indicate addiction, and the difference should be made clear to patients and their caregivers. The symptoms of physical dependence may be observed in critical care patients who have their doses of opioid analgesics tapered too rapidly or in patients requiring chronic opioid therapy who are unable to obtain an adequate supply of medication or who are undertreated. Unintentional physical withdrawal can also occur if metabolic enzyme inducers, such as phenytoin, are added to a chronic pain regimen. Early symptoms of abstinence can include irritability and restlessness, and onset occurs within 6 to 24 hours of the time the last opioid dose was administered. Later, a person develops chills, sweating, joint and muscle pains, and gastrointestinal (GI) distress, including emesis and diarrhea with abdominal cramping. The time of onset is correlated to the drug's half-life, to the average doses required by an individual, and to the pattern and history of opioid dosing. For example, abstinence induced by tolerance to hydrocodone (a drug with a short half-life) can be anticipated to develop in 4 to 6 hours after the last dose, whereas with methadone it may not occur for 24 to 48 hours after the last dose. Similarly, the abstinence syndrome can last longer when associated with long-acting agents. For short-acting agents (e.g., hydrocodone or oxycodone), abstinence may resolve within 48 to 72 hours, whereas for drugs such as methadone, it may last as long as several days. Mood swings, myalgia, and arthralgia can persist for as long as several weeks after the last dose of an opioid.

Addiction to opioid analgesics is characterized by a dysfunctional pattern of use for purposes other than alleviation of pain. It may involve adverse consequences of opioid use, loss of control over their use, and preoccupation with obtaining opioids despite the presence of adequate analgesia. It is important to realize that tolerance and physical dependence may or may not be present in addiction and that the presence of tolerance and physical dependency does not imply addiction. *Pseudoaddiction* is an important type of behavior that clinicians must understand and recognize because it can easily be misinterpreted as addiction.[53] Pseudoaddictive behaviors may be seen in patients with severe, unrelieved pain. These behaviors can mimic those seen with addiction. Patients become preoccupied with obtaining opioids; however, their underlying focus is on finding relief for their pain. Their fear of not having an adequate amount of medication available to control their pain may result in medication hoarding. When patients with pseudoaddiction are provided adequate analgesia, the behaviors that mimic addiction resolve, the medications are used as prescribed, and the patient's daily functioning increases.[53]

If opioid misuse is suspected, pharmacists can help both patients and prescribers develop appropriate care plans by being vigilant for warning signs that the patient is not adhering to a care plan. These include prescriptions from multiple physicians or phone calls from unknown prescribers; rapid or unsanctioned escalation of dosing requirements, particularly for nonmalignant pain syndromes; frequent excuses for running out of medication early or requests for "vacation" supplies; lack of requests for adjunct analgesic refills (e.g., antidepressants, anticonvulsants); extreme polypharmacy with multiple CNS depressants or multiple habituating substances; and injecting oral medicines or chewing matrix formulations. Persons demonstrating these traits may require referral to an appropriate substance abuse program.[54]

ACUTE PAIN

Analgesic Goals

1. E.T. is a 36-year-old woman recovering from the surgical repair of a left tibia fracture following a motor vehicle accident. She is otherwise healthy, with no other medical conditions. Her medication history reveals no drug allergies or history of recreational drug use, and occasional use of oral ibuprofen 400 mg every 6 hours as needed for menstrual cramps. Postoperatively, E.T. received acetaminophen 325 mg with codeine 30 mg, two tablets orally every 3 hours for pain; however, this analgesic regimen was inadequate for controlling her pain. After extensive complaints, E.T.'s analgesic medication was replaced with two tablets of hydrocodone 5 mg with acetaminophen 500 mg every 4 hours. Despite these changes, E.T. continues to complain of pain. Vital signs indicate the following: respiratory rate, 24 breaths/minute; heart rate, 110 beats/minute; blood pressure (BP), 140/85 mmHg. She rates the intensity of her pain as 8 on a 10-point scale. What is your assessment of E.T.'s pain and what are reasonable analgesia goals for E.T.?

The current analgesic regimen has not provided E.T. with adequate pain relief based on her pain evaluation rating of 8 on a 10-point scale. Physiologic responses to pain include autonomic findings, such as increased respirations, heart rate, and BP. The apparent analgesic failure in E.T. can be attributed to several factors. First, the choice of medication may not be effective for her level of pain, or she may simply require more analgesics than anticipated. Standard analgesic dosage recommendations are only conservative estimates of average initial doses. Ultimately, analgesic dosing must be tailored to the specific needs of the patient. Patients with compromised metabolic function may need smaller doses, whereas patients with extensive injuries may require larger doses. Acute pain always should be aggressively treated.

After an initial analgesic has been administered, the patient should be assessed frequently, and doses should be adjusted quickly in response to inadequate pain control or excessive sedation. The dose of an analgesic should be modified before a patient feels the need to express significant discomfort from pain. E.T.'s complaints of significant pain intensity may also be influenced by anxiety that commonly accompanies inadequate pain relief. E.T.'s possible anxiety over the current surgical outcome could intensify her pain because pain and anxiety are reinforcing phenomena. For most patients, pain is synonymous with injury. When an injury has been repaired and the patient continues to experience pain, the patient's anxiety and fear can intensify pain sensations. The use of pain distress scales, as shown in Figure 8-3, may be more useful for evaluating pain in patients with significant anxiety.[24] The use of distraction or relaxation techniques can also help make E.T. more comfortable.

The goal for managing acute pain is to keep the patient as comfortable as possible while minimizing possible untoward adverse effects from the analgesic. It is important for the clinician to discuss the pain management plan with the patient, establish goals of therapy, address patient concerns, and evaluate patient understanding. Use of pain rating scales, as shown in Figure 8-2, should be reviewed with the patient, and a pain rating goal that is acceptable to the patient should be determined. The importance of factual reporting should be emphasized to the patient. This helps eliminate behaviors of stoicism or exaggeration.[24] Appropriate goals for E.T. would be a pain rating of <4 of 10-point scale, a return of vital signs toward her baseline values, and reduced anxiety. Only appropriate analgesic selection, careful follow-up evaluations, and rational analgesic dosage adjustments can accomplish these goals.

Combination Analgesics

2. Is the choice of acetaminophen with hydrocodone appropriate for E.T.?

Acetaminophen and opioid analgesics provide pain relief by different mechanisms of action and it is reasonable to use both for their additive or synergistic effects when managing pain. Acetaminophen with hydrocodone is a fixed-dose combination, however, and these combination drug formulations decrease dosing flexibility and frequently lead to unintended toxic side effects. The combination of acetaminophen 500 mg and hydrocodone 5 mg given two tablets every 4 hours can result in the patient receiving 6 g of acetaminophen in a 24-hour period. Chronic administration of acetaminophen in doses exceeding 5 g/day has been associated with hepatic enzyme changes. Short-term use of 6 g of acetaminophen daily for a few days in patients without risk factors (e.g., alcoholism, malnutrition, concurrent administration of hepatic-enzyme inducers) is usually safe.[55] If patients need to use acetaminophen-containing combination analgesics frequently throughout the day, then it is important to consider products that contain lower amounts of acetaminophen. Several NSAIDs also have been associated with hepatotoxicity.[56] Acetaminophen and NSAIDs should be avoided in patients who have severe liver disease, as evidenced by elevated liver transaminases, a low serum albumin, or a prolonged prothrombin time. If acetaminophen is to be used at all in patients with impaired hepatic function, doses must be limited to <2 to 3 g/24 hours.

E.T. should have been initiated on a more potent analgesic to control her pain. Analgesic combinations of acetaminophen with either codeine 30 mg or hydrocodone 5 mg are effective for mild to moderate pain (e.g., 5 on a 10-point scale), but these combinations are less than adequate for moderately severe to severe pain, unless the opioid dose is increased. Because E.T.'s pain has not been successfully controlled with either acetaminophen with codeine or acetaminophen with hydrocodone, it would be reasonable to start her on oral morphine 30 mg every 4 hours. If she is unable to tolerate oral medications following surgery, then morphine 4 mg IV every 2 to 3 hours can be used instead. Although the use of IM administration is often prescribed, many clinicians discourage the use of this route because of erratic or unpredictable absorption with some opiates and additional pain caused from the injection itself.

After initiation of morphine, E.T. should be evaluated in a few hours for pain relief and adverse effects. The dose or dosing interval should be adjusted if either is found to be inadequate. Sometimes, changing to an alternative opiate may be indicated if analgesia is still inadequate or unwanted side effects are experienced. Until an individual's response to a particular opioid is known, it is wise for the clinician to formulate a back-up plan with an alternative opiate regimen.

An NSAID such as ibuprofen or naproxen also may be used adjunctively for E.T.'s pain. Although an NSAID alone usually is inadequate for controlling moderate to severe pain, they have additive analgesic effects when combined with opiates. In E.T., the prescriber should also consider the risk of bleeding after surgical intervention owing to the antiplatelet effect of NSAIDs. The cyclooxygenase-2 (COX-2) NSAIDs appear to have minimal antiplatelet effects, and may be considered if surgery or trauma presents a high risk of bleeding.

Equianalgesic Dosing of Opioid Analgesics

3. How should E.T.'s hydrocodone dose be converted to oral morphine?

Hydrocodone 20 mg orally is approximately equal to morphine 30 mg (Table 8-3). Therefore, 10 mg of hydrocodone as originally ordered for E.T. is equal to an oral morphine dose of approximately 15 mg, or 5 mg of morphine by injection. This dose of morphine would likely be inadequate for E.T. because her pain is not controlled by this equivalent dose. Thus, E.T. should be started on oral morphine 30 mg every 4 hours around-the-clock for the first 24 hours, then changed to as-needed dosing afterward. Inflammation caused by trauma often peaks around 48 to 72 hours following the inciting event, so pain is expected to decrease dramatically after this period.

Managing Side Effects of Opioid Analgesics

4. E.T. complains of itching after three doses of morphine, but shows no sign of rash. What can be done to alleviate the problem?

Opioid analgesics infrequently cause pruritic rashes due to true allergic-type reactions. In contrast, when administered parentally they commonly stimulate local histamine release from mast cells and cause a local wheal, burning, itching, and erythema at the site of injection. Similarly, systemic release of histamine after both oral and parenteral administration of opioids can produce either localized or generalized flushing and itching. Although histamine related reactions occur frequently and may be confused with an allergic reaction, true opioid allergies are infrequent. When they do occur, they are IgE-dependent.[57] Coadministration of diphenhydramine (Benadryl) or hydroxyzine (Vistaril) prevents histamine-induced itching and also provides antianxiety effects that may add to morphine's analgesic benefit.

Chemically, there are three distinct structural categories of opioids: the *phenanthrenes* (morphine, codeine, hydrocodone, hydromorphone, dihydrocodeine, oxycodone, oxymorphone, levorphanol, nalbuphine, butorphanol, dezocine, and dihydrocodeine), the *phenylpiperidines* (meperidine, fentanyl, alfentanil, sufentanil, and remifentanil), and the *phenylheptanones* or *diphenylheptanes* (methadone, levomethadyl, and the weak analgesic, propoxyphene). Allergic reactions may cross-manifest within the same chemical structural class, but are less likely between classes. Thus, in patients with true allergic reactions, treatment can be instituted with a product from one of the other chemical groups. For example, if E.T. was allergic to morphine, she could be switched to fentanyl.

5. What other adverse effects from morphine should be monitored for in E.T.? What preventive measures should be considered?

The most common side effects reported with the use of opioid analgesics are nausea, vomiting, itching, and constipation.

These are expected untoward opioid effects and, with some care, they can be managed or minimized. These first three symptoms of nausea, vomiting, and itching can all be minimized by antihistamines, such as diphenhydramine or hydroxyzine 25 to 50 mg orally every 6 hours as needed. If drowsiness from the antihistamine is excessive when used in combination with the opioid, a nonsedating antihistamine such as fexofenadine can be substituted. Persistent and more problematic symptoms may require switching to an alternative opioid analgesic.

The best method for treating opioid-induced constipation is prevention. Postsurgical patients are especially susceptible to this effect because their GI motility is already slowed from decreased physical activity and from anesthetic agents received during surgery. Morphine and other opioids suppress the propulsive peristaltic action of the colon, increase colonic and anal sphincter tone, and reduce the reflex relaxation response to rectal distention. These actions, combined with decreased normal sensory stimuli for defecation because of their CNS-depressant actions, contribute to opioid-induced constipation. Stool softeners are effective in keeping the bowel contents moist, but do not stimulate bowel peristaltic propulsion. Only the stimulant laxatives and prokinetic agents can increase bowel propulsive activity. When opioid analgesics are initiated, a stimulant laxative plus stool softener should also be given. E.T. will be receiving morphine orally around the clock and would probably benefit from two tablets of senna 8.6 mg daily in combination with docusate sodium 200 mg twice daily. If constipation persists, osmotic laxatives, such as lactulose or sodium phosphate enema, may be added to draw water into the lumen of the bowel, which would cause distention and peristalsis.

Postoperative ileus frequently is exacerbated by opioid analgesics, but opioids rarely produce ileus or bowel obstruction alone without other underlying physiologic causes. Oral naloxone 0.4 to 1.2 mg every 6 hours has been used with some success in preventing opioid-induced constipation. Unlike parenteral naloxone, oral naloxone is poorly absorbed systemically (25%) and, therefore, will not interfere with analgesic effect unless doses are high.[58,59] An oral naloxone formulation is not yet commercially available, but the parenteral preparation can be administered orally if needed. The oral naloxone requirement rarely exceeds 2.4 mg every 6 hours. At higher dosages, systemic antagonist effects can occur, resulting in decreased analgesia in addition to the local intestinal effects. Other opioid antagonists, such as methylnaltrexone, are currently being investigated and may provide an alternative to oral naloxone.[60]

6. On the third day of her morphine treatment, E.T. appears agitated. Could her agitation be attributed to her morphine?

Although opioids are CNS depressants, they can cause CNS excitation, especially if the patient receives large doses for a prolonged period. Anxiety, agitation, irritability, motor restlessness, tremors, involuntary twitching, and myoclonic seizures have been associated with meperidine, morphine, and hydromorphone, but not methadone, although methadone may rarely cause myoclonus. For meperidine and morphine, the CNS toxicity correlates to accumulation of their active metabolites, normeperidine and morphine-6-glucuronide, respectively. Because both of these metabolites are cleared renally, patients with renal insufficiency are at greatest risk, but toxicity can also occur when high doses are administered frequently in patients with normal renal function.[59,61] With meperidine, the problem is compounded by the 17-hour half-life of normeperidine. In patients with normal renal function, avoiding doses in excess of 60 mg/hour of meperidine, 100 mg/hour of morphine, or 40 mg/hour of hydromorphone minimizes CNS toxicity.

The treatment of opioid-induced CNS irritability should include discontinuation of the opioid analgesic and treatment with a benzodiazepine. Myoclonic seizures resulting from meperidine administration are sometimes preceded by involuntary twitching in the extremities and can be averted by discontinuing the meperidine. Seizures induced by meperidine are resistant to naloxone, but respond to anticonvulsants such as phenytoin or diazepam. Because E.T. has normal renal function and her morphine dose is not excessive, it is unlikely that she is suffering from morphine-induced CNS effects. It is more likely that she is starting to recover from her surgery and is anxious from her environment. Nevertheless, it may be time to start reducing her morphine dose if her pain is well controlled.

Ketorolac

7. Could parenteral ketorolac (Toradol) be given to E.T. instead of the morphine?

For patients such as E.T. with acute severe pain, an opioid such as oral or parenteral morphine or hydromorphone should be the first-line agent for pain management. As E.T.'s pain severity decreases, however, an NSAID may be considered for treating mild to moderate pain.

Because it is the only available injectable NSAID in the United States, ketorolac is sometimes used as an alternative to opioids. Although ketorolac is indicated for the short-term management of moderate to severe pain, it should not be substituted for appropriate opioid analgesics for the management of acute postoperative pain.[62,63] Ketorolac is most beneficial in postoperative pain if it is used in combination with the opioids instead of as monotherapy. Parenteral formulations of NSAIDs are no more effective than oral formulations given in equivalent doses (e.g., ibuprofen 600 mg orally every 6 hours is equally as effective as 15 to 30 mg parenteral ketorolac).[64] Ketorolac also has been associated with several cases of serious postsurgical bleeding. Although ketorolac could be effective in relieving E.T.'s pain, it is no more effective than morphine. Patients receiving ketorolac should be monitored for typical NSAID side effects, especially postsurgical bleeding.

The NSAIDs cause sodium retention and can also block prostaglandin-induced vasodilation in patients with compromised renal blood flow. Thus, NSAIDs should be used with caution in patients with heart failure, hypovolemia, dehydration or any other conditions that compromise renal blood flow and increase the risk of developing renal toxicity.

Nonsteroidal Anti-Inflammatory Drug Selection

8. Two days later, E.T. is ready to be discharged from the hospital. Although her pain is much improved, she still has mild to moderate intermittent pain. The pain management team is planning to send her home with an NSAID to treat her pain. Is any one NSAID analgesic superior to the others?

In all probability, all NSAIDs, not just those with an approved indication for the treatment of mild to moderate pain, have analgesic properties. The superiority of any particular NSAID for a particular patient cannot be predicted, and no one NSAID has been demonstrated to have superior analgesia over any other. Nevertheless, patients who fail to benefit from one NSAID can respond to a different NSAID. Therefore, an NSAID should be selected based on the patient's previous history of response, efficacy, safety, and cost. Ibuprofen and other proprionic acids have a long history of safety and are available as less costly generic products. (See Chapter 43, Rheumatic Disorders, for a more detailed discussion of the clinical use of NSAIDs.)

When selecting one of these agents, the clinician must be aware of the considerable risk of systemic side effects. Although GI side effects are the most common, NSAIDs have caused undesirable nervous system, otic, ocular, hematologic, renal, hepatic, and cardiovascular adverse effects.

Several large randomized, controlled trials prompted the U.S. Food and Drug Administration (FDA) in 2004 to withdraw rofecoxib, a selective COX-2 inhibitor, from the market because of increased cardiovascular risk associated with a prolonged period of use. At the same time, questions were also raised about the safety of nonselective NSAIDs. When compared with the selective COX-2 inhibitor, celecoxib, naproxen was linked to increased risk for cardiovascular events after approximately 3 years of therapy. This emerging knowledge, on a previously unrecognized problem, prompted the FDA to emphasize a warning for all NSAIDs regarding an increased risk for cardiovascular events. Until further data are available, these drugs should be initiated at the lowest effective dose for the shortest period of time.[65]

9. If E.T. had a history of asthma, would an NSAID be safe to use?

Aspirin and essentially all other NSAIDs can induce bronchospasm and other allergic manifestations in patients with a history of asthma, allergic rhinitis, and nasal polyps. An asthma history alone is not a reason to withhold an NSAID. If, however, a patient describes an asthma-like response (shortness or breath, wheezing, cough, laryngospasm) following aspirin or other NSAID ingestion, no drugs from this class should be used in the future.

The risk of using aspirin or other NSAID in patients with chronic bronchitis, emphysema, or in asthmatics without nasal polyps or history of drug-induced bronchospasm is less clear. If E.T. had a history of asthma, then an NSAID should be used cautiously.[64,66] Acetaminophen does not induce bronchospasm and is safe to give to patients with obstructive airways disease, including a history of NSAID induced asthma.

Analgesic Nephrotoxicity

10. What are the risks of analgesic nephropathy from NSAID use in E.T.?

Analgesic overuse is a common cause of chronic interstitial nephritis (CIN) and may account for approximately 5% of the cases of chronic renal failure in the United States. Historically, aspirin and phenacetin in combination were thought to be the causative agent for most cases of CIN; however, acetaminophen, aspirin,[67] and other NSAIDs[68,69] also have been implicated. Acetaminophen-induced renal toxicity is almost always accompanied by concomitant serum hepatic transaminase changes and generally is associated with acute acetaminophen intoxication.[70] Most cases of interstitial nephritis seem to be related to both dose and duration of NSAID therapy.[71,72] (Also see Chapter 30, Acute Renal Failure.)

The NSAID's effect on renal function may be twofold. NSAIDs can directly damage renal tubules and can also reduce renal blood flow by inhibiting prostacyclin. Prostacyclin modifies renal function in response to the effects of endogenous vasoconstrictors (e.g., norepinephrine and angiotensin II), especially if the patient is volume depleted, has been taking diuretics, or is elderly. Renal insufficiency may occur in 20% of patients with one or more of these identifiable risks who also take NSAIDs.[73,74] Patients with cirrhosis and ascites[75] and patients with significantly altered hemodynamic status can experience as much as a 50% decrease in creatinine clearance (ClCr) when treated with indomethacin (Indocin)[76,77] or ibuprofen (Motrin). Some subjects with normal renal function experience profound changes in glomerular filtration rate when taking indomethacin concurrent with triamterene (Dyrenium).[78]

For E.T., who is fairly young and healthy without risk factors, the potential for NSAID-induced renal toxicity is quite low. Her renal function still should be monitored, however, if she is to be placed on an NSAID for more than a few days because she has recently undergone surgery and may have relative volume depletion.

NSAID Use in Renal Disease

11. If E.T. was currently exhibiting renal dysfunction, what NSAID could be used?

Sulindac (Clinoril) and nabumetone (Relafen) have been reported to cause less renal insufficiency because of the absence of active urinary nephrotoxic metabolites. These two NSAIDs can still decrease renal blood flow in patients at risk and can cause renal dysfunction via hypersensitivity reactions unrelated to their effects on renal blood flow. Although sulindac and nabumetone appear to be preferred over other NSAIDs in patients with renal dysfunction, clinical experience is not as great with these two drugs relative to other NSAIDs.

Possible drug-induced nephrotic syndrome has been reported with indomethacin (Indocin), ibuprofen (Motrin), naproxen (Naprosyn), phenylbutazone (Butazolidin), fenoprofen (Nalfon), sulindac (Clinoril), and tolmetin (Tolectin). In particular, fenoprofen was implicated in 71% of 31 cases.[79] The prognosis for recovery of renal function is excellent, although some patients require treatment with corticosteroids.[80] It is unclear whether patients with pre-existing renal dysfunction are at any greater risk of developing further drug-induced abnormalities, but most clinicians consider it a relative contraindication.

Opioids

Patient-Controlled Analgesia

12. T.J., a 52-year-old woman, has had posterior spinal fusion with instrumentation because of severe scoliosis that compromised her respiratory function and quality of life. She has just been transferred to the ward from the postanesthetic recovery critical care unit. She is now crying and complaining of

severe pain not relieved by intramuscular meperidine 75 mg every 3 hours. T.J. has no known drug allergies. She has a history of taking acetaminophen 500 mg with hydrocodone 7.5 mg two tablets every 3 hours before admission. Why would a patient-controlled analgesia (PCA) device be useful for T.J.?

The current dose of meperidine is high and carries the risk of CNS side effects. PCA is a technique whereby patients self-administer narcotics by using a preprogrammed mechanical infusion device attached to tubing that delivers the drug to the patient through an IV or subcutaneous needle or catheter. Basically, the patient depresses a button to activate the PCA controller to deliver a preset dose of opiate medication. This prevents the need to call a nurse or other caregiver when pain arises and also obviates the problem of drug doses that are not ordered sufficiently frequently. The controller is preprogrammed to establish "lock-out" periods that prevent the pump from delivering a dose if the patient presses the button too often. Safeguards against accidental overdose are instituted by adjusting the concentration of drug in the controller or the duration of the lock-out period. Either of these variables can be adjusted to fit the patient's analgesic needs. Caution must be taken to instruct parents of children or adolescents appropriately on the use of the PCA device, lest they inadvertently administer an excess amount of medication. In general, family members should not act as "surrogates" in helping patients control their pain with a PCA device.

Numerous programmable PCA devices are available, most of which provide intermittent self-boluses of drug, with or without continuous infusion. Some systems use syringe pump technology and others an IV pump system. Compact devices are convenient for ambulatory use. T.J.'s pain can be managed with a PCA device for as long as she is able to comprehend the operation of the device. Most postoperative patients require a basal continuous IV infusion of opioid in addition to intermittent boluses during the first 24-hour period. The need for continuous basal infusion usually diminishes after 24 to 48 hours. PCA is most useful in the first 3 to 5 postoperative days when the patient has the most severe pain. After this initial critical period, the pain can readily be managed with oral analgesic doses. The PCA allows T.J. to have control over her pain. She will determine how often and when the opioid analgesic is delivered, and she can titrate the dose to a level of comfort or side effects that is acceptable to her.

OPIOID SELECTION FOR USE IN PCA

13. What opioid analgesics could be used in T.J.'s PCA device?

Most of the commonly prescribed parenteral opioids can be used in a PCA, but fentanyl, hydromorphone, and morphine are used most frequently. Meperidine is used less frequently because of the problems with the normeperidine metabolite discussed earlier. (See Table 8-5 for dosing guidelines.) Morphine usually is recommended first, followed by hydromorphone, fentanyl, and meperidine. If the patient has a history of morphine intolerance (e.g., itching or nausea), alternative agents, such as hydromorphone, should be initiated. Most of the opioids used for PCA have a broad range of acceptable doses with the exception of meperidine, which has a narrow dosing range because the active normeperidine metabolite can

Table 8-5 Recommended Doses of Opioid Analgesics

Initial Doses	*Adult Oral Dose (mg)*	*Child Oral Dose (mg/kg)*
Opioid Agonists for Moderate to Severe Pain (mu Receptor Agonists)		
Morphine(various)	15–30	0.30
Hydromorphone (Dilaudid)	4–8	0.06
Levorphanol (Levo-Dromoran)	2–4	0.04
Methadone (Dolophine)	5–10	0.20
Opioids for Mild to Moderate Pain (mu Agonists)		
Codeine (various)	30–60	0.51
Hydrocodone (various)	5–10	N/A
Oxycodone (various)	5	0.1
Tramadol (Ultram)	50–100	NR
Meperidine (Demerol)	Not recommended (NR)	

Patient Controlled Analgesia (PCA) (Parenteral)	*Usual Initial Dose (mg)*	*Dose Range (mg)*	*Interval Range (min)*
Morphine	1.0	0.5–2.0	6 (5–10)
Hydromorphone	0.2	0.04–0.4	6 (5–10)
Fentanyl	0.01 (10 g)	0.01–0.05	6 (5–10)

Example: A morphine PCA with a 1.0-mg initial dose that allows a patient to self-administer an additional 1 mg every 6 minutes provides a dosing range of 1–11 mg/hr available medication.

N/A, not applicable.

Adapted from *Principles of Analgesic Use in the Treatment of Acute Pain and Cancer Pain*. 5th ed. Glenview, IL: American Pain Society; 2003:1417 and 1420, with permission.

accumulate, even at normal therapeutic doses. Meperidine also has only a 3-hour half-life and perhaps an even shorter duration of action as an analgesic.[81] Therefore, meperidine is unsuitable for treatment of acute severe pain when the analgesic requirement is exceedingly high or when patients have impaired renal function. Fentanyl can be a safer alternative to meperidine.

Patient controlled analgesia is used most commonly for administering opioids IV and, on rare occasions, subcutaneously. Subcutaneous opioid administration is limited by the fluid volume needed to deliver the drug. A subcutaneous infusion of 1 mL/hour is universally accepted; however, slightly larger volumes is acceptable in some patients. Highly concentrated morphine solutions (e.g., 60 mg/mL) must be compounded to permit maximal doses for these patients. Alternatively, hydromorphone (Dilaudid HP) at concentrations of 10 mg/mL can be used. When necessary, hydromorphone powder can be purchased and higher concentrations can be prepared (maximal concentration of 40 mg/mL can be achieved), but it is unknown whether concentrations that exceed those of commercial products increase local tissue irritation or other untoward effects.[82,83] Because no contraindications exist, T.J. should be started on IV morphine in her PCA pump.

14. What dosing regimen should be recommended for use for T.J.'s PCA pump?

An appropriate order for PCA must include the name of the drug, solution concentration, dose for self-bolus, lock-out period, continuous basal dose, hourly maximal dose limit, and dose and frequency for breakthrough pain. An example of a PCA order for T.J. would include the following:

Morphine sulfate	1 mg/mL
Self-dose	1 mg (1 mL) IV
Lock-out time	6 minutes
Basal dose	1 mg/hour (1 mL/hour) IV
Dose for breakthrough	1 mg IV every 20 minutes as needed for pain
1-hour limit total	12 mg IV

15. How often should monitoring occur for T.J.'s PCA therapy?

Although T.J. has a history of opiate use, it is imperative that appropriate monitoring tools be in place to assess her response to therapy. Even at therapeutic doses, opiate analgesics can depress respiration, alter heart rate, and lower blood pressure. Therapeutic monitoring should be more frequent within the first 24 hours, when opioid effects are less predictable. Typical assessments include blood pressure, pulse, respiratory rate, oxygen saturation, and visual analog and sedation scale scores. An appropriate monitoring pattern for T.J. may include the following:

Holding parameters for PCA:
Respiratory rate <10 breaths/minute, OR
Systolic blood pressure <90 mmHg

T.J. should be assessed at the initiation of the PCA dose and then at regular intervals (every 30 minutes, twice; every hour, twice; then every 4 hours) unless she becomes unstable or pain increases.

DOSE CONVERSION BETWEEN OPIOID ANALGESICS

16. T.J. has requested another analgesic agent because of excessive sedation. She currently needs 10 mg of morphine per hour from her PCA. How should T.J. be converted to another PCA opioid analgesic?

The IV equivalent of morphine 10 mg/hour is approximately equal to hydromorphone 2 mg/hour, meperidine 100 mg/hour, or fentanyl 100 mcg/hour (Table 8-3). Meperidine is not a viable alternative for T.J. because the equivalent meperidine dose of 100 mg/hour exceeds the maximal recommended dose of 60 mg/hour. The remaining options are either hydromorphone or fentanyl PCA. Examples of options for PCA orders include either of the following:

Fentanyl	10 mcg/mL
Self-dose	10 mcg (1 mL) IV
Lock-out dose	6 minutes
Basal dose	10 mcg/hour (1 mL/hour) IV
Breakthrough pain	10 mcg intravenously every 20 minutes as needed for pain
1-hour limit total	120 mcg IV

Hold parameters for PCA: Respiratory rate <10 breaths/minute or, systolic blood pressure <90 mmHg

OR

Hydromorphone	0.2 mg/mL
Self-dose	0.2 mg (1 mL) IV
Lock-out dose	6 minute
Basal dose	0.2 mg/hour (1 mL/hour) IV
Breakthrough pain	0.2 mg IV every 20 minutes as needed for pain
1-hour limit total	2.4 mg IV

Hold parameters for PCA: Respiratory rate <10 breaths/minute or systolic blood pressure <90 mmHg

As always, T.J. should be re-evaluated in 2 hours after changing the PCA, and doses should be adjusted at that time.

CONVERSION FROM PCA TO ORAL OPIOIDS

17. Forty-eight hours later, T.J.'s requirement for hydromorphone has decreased significantly. Her requirement has averaged 0.5 mg hydromorphone/hour in the last 12 hours. How should T.J. be converted to oral opioid analgesics?

Patient controlled analgesia is rarely used beyond 72 hours postoperatively,[84] and continuous basal infusions frequently are discontinued after the first 24 hours. Transition to oral opioid analgesics from PCA should occur as soon as the patient is able to tolerate oral intake of solids. Oral opioid analgesia usually is given every 3 to 4 hours for convenience, as well as allowing time for drug absorption. Conversion to oral from parenteral opioids is best achieved based on the total opioid requirement during the previous 24-hour period. For T.J., the total 24-hour IV hydromorphone (0.5 mg/hour) required was 12 mg, which is roughly equivalent to IV morphine 60 mg, methadone 18 mg, or levorphanol 12 mg. Alternatively, the 24-hour oral equivalent doses are as follows: morphine 180 mg, methadone 18 mg, levorphanol 24 mg, or hydromorphone 48 mg. Levorphanol, with its long duration of action and a lower incidence of GI side effects, would be a good oral agent to use for T.J. The levorphanol dose for T.J. would be 4 mg every 4 hours. A period of 4 to 6 hours of PCA overlapping dosing of oral opioids is recommended to allow equilibration of the oral medicines, but the PCA's continuous basal infusion should be stopped as soon as the oral dose is given.

Tapering of Opioid Analgesics

18. How should T.J.'s opioid analgesics be tapered?

Most patients gradually decrease their activation of a PCA pump as soon as their acute pain begins to subside. In instances in which patients have not decreased their PCA pump use, the dose may safely be reduced by 15% to 20% each day without precipitating symptoms of abstinence. For T.J., the oral levorphanol regimen should be changed to an as-needed schedule once the pain has stabilized. For most patients, a scheduled opioid taper is not essential unless the total daily requirement is in excess of 160 mg of oral morphine (or its equivalent) or if opioid use is prolonged. T.J. should be able to be converted to acetaminophen 325 mg with codeine 30 mg (or an equivalent opioid preparation) once her oral levorphanol has been completely discontinued.

Pain Management in the Opioid-Dependent Patient

19. If T.J. had a history of heroin and cocaine abuse, how would her pain treatment be modified?

Pain management in an IV drug abuser is not difficult as long as the clinician does not judge the patient's behavior or interject personal values into the decision-making process. As with any patient, the goal is to provide as much comfort as possible. Concerns over opiate abuse or addiction are not relevant when treating acute pain, although the clinician must recognize the potential for physical tolerance of opioids and adjust medication doses accordingly.

The first step in the treatment of a patient with a history of substance abuse is to try to determine the amount of illicit drugs the patient has been using, being alert to the possible abuse of multiple drugs in varying quantities.[85] Patients who have a history of opiate (heroin) and stimulant (cocaine) use are likely to demonstrate a much greater tolerance to opiates than a patient who has been using opiates alone. Some evidence indicates that cross-tolerance can occur between cocaine and some opiates, but not to methadone.[86]

The primary goal is to control the patient's pain. A combination of methadone titrated to prevent withdrawal and to provide background analgesia plus a short-acting opioid analgesic dosed adequately to prevent breakthrough pain can be used. If T.J. had a history of substance abuse, she could start with methadone 20 to 40 mg/day in four equally divided doses depending on how much heroin had been used (see Chapter 83, Drug Abuse). The methadone would prevent heroin withdrawal and possibly provide additional analgesia. Because her actual pain requirements are unknown, she also would be placed on a PCA with an agent such as morphine or hydromorphone. It is always important to reassess the patient 1 to 2 hours after starting the analgesic regimen for signs of withdrawal, clinical response, and toxicity, and then titrate the doses of both the methadone and hydromorphone accordingly, although it is best to adjust one medication at a time.[87] The final amount required may be higher than doses typically used in opioid-naïve patients. Conversely, some patients may exaggerate their history of prior drug use and will be quite sensitive to the prescribed therapy. Long-term management should include offering the patient appropriate referrals to drug treatment centers, but the final responsibility should rest with the patient.

Use of Opioids in Recovering Addicts

20. Should opioid analgesics be prescribed to recovering opiate addicts?

Acute opioid use in the hospitalized setting is unlikely to cause opioid addiction; the rate of addiction from clinical opioid use is much less than 1%. Unless it is the patient's choice not to use opioids, no rational reason to avoid them exists. Often the patient's fear of addiction can be alleviated by thorough education. The clinician should have a therapeutic contract with the patient that includes pain management as well as opioid tapering on the resolution of the acute pain (see Chapter 83, Drug Abuse).

Use of Opioids in Renal Disease

21. What adjustments in analgesic dosing would be required if T.J. had an estimated creatinine clearance of 30 mL/minute?

Uremia can produce CNS changes, which can cause patients with renal disease to be more sensitive to the CNS depressant effects of opioids. As discussed in Question 6, some opioids have active metabolites that are renally excreted, and uremia or significant renal disease can lead to their accumulation. For example, the active metabolites of meperidine and morphine (normeperidine and morphine-6-glucuronide, respectively) are renally excreted. Both of these active metabolites can cause CNS excitation; in particular, normeperidine can precipitate tonic-clonic seizures. Therefore, meperidine should be avoided in uremic patients, but other opioids can be used as long as the clinician is aware of the potential toxicities, the patient is closely monitored, and the dosage is properly titrated. For T.J., hydromorphone PCA could still be a reasonable choice for the management of her acute pain; however, a continuous basal infusion would be unnecessary in a patient with significant renal dysfunction. As with all patients receiving opioid analgesics, close monitoring and follow-up care are essential.

Obstetric Pain: Special Considerations for Opioid Analgesia

EPIDURALS

22. M.T., a 28-year-old woman who has been in labor for 10 hours, is experiencing strong, erratic contractions at 5- to 15-minute intervals. Her cervix is minimally dilated, suggesting that delivery is still several hours away. Her pain is severe and, if it continues, may compromise her ability to assist in the labor and delivery process. A single, 50 mcg epidural dose of fentanyl is ordered for M.T. by anesthesia. What guidelines are necessary for the safe use of epidural opioids?

Fentanyl and morphine are frequently administered epidurally during labor and during lower extremity surgical procedures (e.g., cesarean delivery, total joint replacements) because they have limited systemic effects and long durations of analgesic action.[88] Epidural analgesia has also been used in thoracic surgery.[89] A single dose of morphine 2 to 10 mg given epidurally may provide analgesia for >12 hours.[90] Respiratory depression can occur 1 to 3 hours after the administration of epidural morphine and can be readily reversed by naloxone. Facial or generalized pruritus also can occur hours after the administration of epidural morphine. If pruritus does occur, it can be controlled with low doses of IM or IV naloxone 0.02 to 0.08 mg without reversing the analgesic effect of the epidural morphine. Frequent monitoring of vital signs is essential after the administration of epidural opioids. Always be vigilant for delayed signs of toxicity, because their onset occurs up to several hours after the administration of the opioid.

Besides morphine, fentanyl (Sublimaze), sufentanil (Sufenta), and buprenorphine (Buprenex) also have been used epidurally. The duration of analgesia of epidurally administered opioids depends less on the serum half-life of the opioid than on the lipid solubility of the drug. The more lipophilic the opioid, the shorter its duration because these agents rapidly diffuse out of the epidural space. In contrast, the more hydrophilic opioids remain in the epidural space longer. For example, methadone, which is highly lipophilic, has a very short duration of activity when administered epidurally despite a long serum half-life of 24 hours.[91,92] For M.T., fentanyl is a good choice because it has a fairly long duration of analgesia but will not produce significant systemic effects that would compromise the fetus through transplacental migration. Also, the duration of fentanyl is sufficiently short that it will not unnecessarily delay maternal postpartum recovery. A single 50 mcg dose of epidural fentanyl was given to M.T. through an epidural catheter and complete analgesia was achieved.

Spinal Analgesia in Opioid-Dependent Patients

23. Why would spinal opioid analgesia still be appropriate if M.T. is opioid dependent?

Previous opioid use has minimal influence on epidural doses. Opioid-dependent patients can achieve adequate analgesia from epidural opioids, but their physical opioid dependency will not be satisfied. In fact, despite adequate analgesia, an opioid-dependent patient may exhibit symptoms of opiate withdrawal. These include restlessness, insomnia, nervousness, irritability, sweating, and GI hypermotility (nausea, emesis, and diarrhea). If withdrawal symptoms occur, they can be treated effectively by systemic administration of morphine or other opioids. Without treatment, such symptoms may persist for a few days. The dose of the systemic opioids varies with the patient's previous level of opioid dependence, and doses need to be adjusted accordingly. It would be appropriate to start M.T. on a short-acting opioid, such as meperidine 10 mg IV every 15 to 20 minutes, until the symptoms of withdrawal subside. This may be somewhat hazardous because the incidence of respiratory depression in the first 24 hours may be increased when opioids are administered by simultaneous epidural and systemic routes.[93] Therefore, longer-acting opioids, such as methadone or levorphanol, should be avoided. The respiratory depression can be treated with the opioid antagonist naloxone, but the dose must be limited to 0.1 mg increments given IV to avoid precipitation of an acute withdrawal syndrome and reversal of analgesia. The naloxone dose can be repeated and the dose titrated to the desired clinical response.

Clonidine for Opioid Withdrawal Symptoms

24. If M.T. was opioid dependent, what are the alternatives for management of the symptoms of physical withdrawal while she is treated with epidural opioids?

Clonidine (Catapres) 0.2 to 1.2 mg/day can effectively suppress the signs and symptoms of opioid withdrawal without eliciting other opioid effects.[94,95] The specific dose must be individualized for each patient to avoid hypotension, dry mouth, or drowsiness.[96,97] Clonidine also can be given sublingually or transdermally in equivalent doses. Clonidine transdermal patches of 3.5, 7.0, and 10.5 cm^2 deliver 0.1, 0.2, and 0.3 mg of clonidine, respectively, over a 24-hour period. Approximately 24 hours must elapse before steady-state plasma concentrations of clonidine are attained from the patches.[98,99] Therefore, supplemental oral or sublingual[96] clonidine 0.1 mg every 6 to 12 hours must be administered during the first 24 hours of the application of the transdermal patches. Clonidine transdermal patches should be used to treat the signs of physical opioid withdrawal only when these symptoms are expected to be severe or prolonged. In addition, clonidine is available for epidural administration and has been used in combination with opioids alone or with opioids and local anesthetics for epidural analgesia. For M.T., who is in labor, clonidine should be avoided owing to the risk of hypotension and possible adverse effects on the fetus. A shorter-acting opioid should be used as in Question 23.

SYSTEMIC OPIOIDS DURING LABOR

25. Should M.T. be given a systemic analgesic rather than epidural analgesia?

If possible, CNS depressants should be avoided during labor because they can compromise fetal vital functions.[100,101] Nevertheless, if an analgesic is deemed necessary, then an agent that meets the following criteria should be chosen: (a) provides adequate pain relief; (b) has little effect on the course or duration of labor; and (c) affects fetal vital signs minimally during labor, delivery, and postpartum phases. Meperidine and fentanyl meet most of these criteria and, therefore, are frequently preferred over other opioids in obstetrics when given in small, frequent parenteral injections or through a PCA.[102,103] As with all opioid analgesic use, close monitoring of the patient for analgesia and untoward effects is essential.

Although meperidine and fentanyl seem to have only minimal residual effects on the neonate at analgesic doses, adverse effects, such as respiratory depression, can still occur.[104,105] According to an early neonatal neurobehavioral scale, meperidine broadly depressed most measured neonatal activities on the first and second days of life.[106] Nevertheless, if the contractions are very strong, erratic, and prolonged early in the course of labor (as with M.T.), a short-acting analgesic (e.g., meperidine) could be useful to blunt the labor pain and calm the mother, so that she can regain control over her contractions and conserve her energy for the actual delivery.

Butorphanol (Stadol) also has minimal effects on fetal and neonatal function and is a reasonable alternative to meperidine or fentanyl in this situation.[107] All potent analgesics should be administered IM or subcutaneously because IV administration is associated with more neonatal and fetal depression because of the high peak serum concentration achieved by this route.[108,109] Pentazocine has similar effects as butorphanol, but is seldom used because of local tissue reactions at the site of IM or subcutaneous injections. Pentazocine and butorphanol are mixed opiate-agonists/antagonists and can precipitate acute withdrawal reactions in some opiate-dependent individuals. As a result, these drugs need to be used cautiously, if at all, in the opiate-addicted population (see Question 27).

If neonatal respiratory difficulties are manifested as a result of opioid analgesics administered during labor, they can be reversed with naloxone (Narcan). For M.T., meperidine 50 mg IM was given with good clinical response. As with all opioid analgesics, the dose has to be adjusted after an evaluation of the patient's history and clinical findings. Analgesic doses always should be individualized for the specific patient.

Variability in Intramuscular Meperidine Absorption

26. M.T. achieved excellent analgesia from the first dose of meperidine 50 mg IM, but she started to complain that subsequent doses produced variable pain relief, and she accused the nurse of giving her placebos. What are some of the explanations for this problem?

The most common cause of variable clinical response after an IM meperidine injection is erratic bioavailability after repetitive injections at the same site. The absorption of meperidine from an injection can vary by as much as 30% to 50% after repeated IM administrations. Other considerations include tachyphylaxis, progression of an underlying disease (e.g., in patients with cancer), and the possibility of opioid diversion by the patient or someone else through dilution or removal of active drug from its container.

Special Consideration for Using Partial Agonist and Antagonist Opioid Analgesics

27. What are precautions for using partial agonist and antagonist opioids for analgesia in M.T.?

Pentazocine, butorphanol, dezocine, and nalbuphine are partial agonist/antagonist opioid analgesics. Besides exhibiting agonist analgesic effects, they all possess opiate antagonist properties as well. Generally, they act as agonists at κ-opiate receptors and as antagonists at μ-opiate receptors, which explains their ability to simultaneously produce analgesia and precipitate withdrawal symptoms. Pentazocine has an opioid antagonist effect equal to 1/50 of nalorphine; 80 mg has been known to precipitate abstinence in patients who have been given opioids for chronic pain. If a partial opiate agonist is instituted in a patient previously taking a pure agonist, the dose should be increased gradually, and the patient should be observed closely for symptoms of abstinence. If possible, the pure agonist opioid should be withdrawn gradually. If the agonist dose is fairly low and the patient has not been on the drug for >10 days, then the patient can be changed over to pentazocine. In this situation, the patient may experience mild diaphoresis, but should not have significant withdrawal symptoms. A drug-free period of 2 days before the institution of pentazocine also has been suggested, but this is impractical for a patient in pain.

When partial agonist/antagonist opioid analgesics are being considered, the risk of unpleasant psychotomimetic side effects must be weighed against the benefits. For example, butorphanol-induced dysphoric responses are well documented.[110,111] A 2-mg dose of butorphanol was associated with an 18% incidence of psychic disturbance, and a 4-mg dose with a 33% incidence. Pentazocine (Talwin) also is associated with a higher incidence of psychotomimetic reactions than traditional opiate agonist analgesics. Hallucinations occurred in 24 of 65 patients (37%) who received 40 to 50 mg of IM pentazocine. In another trial, psychic changes occurred in 1.7% of patients receiving morphine versus 11.4% of patients treated with pentazocine. In comparison, nalbuphine (Nubain) and other analgesics induce much less psychotomimetic effect than butorphanol or pentazocine.[112,113] Therefore, a partial agonist/antagonist opioid analgesic should be used in M.T. only if she cannot tolerate the available shorter-acting opioid agonist analgesics.

Tramadol

28. What is the purported advantage of tramadol (Ultram) over other opioid analgesics and NSAID?

Tramadol, a centrally acting analgesic with weak opioid agonist properties, activates monoaminergic spinal inhibition of pain. The *O*-demethylated metabolite of tramadol has a higher affinity for opioid receptors than the parent drug; however, after a single oral dose, the binding of tramadol to the μ-opioid receptor is overshadowed by its nonopioid analgesic effects.[114] The tolerance and dependence potential of tramadol during treatment for up to 6 months appear to be low; however, the possibility of dependence with long-term use cannot be excluded entirely.[115] Tramadol is indicated for the treatment of moderate to severe pain, but analgesia is not superior to other opiate analgesics.[116,117] It, however, has a lower incidence of respiratory depression or significant GI dysmotility than most traditional opioids.

Tramadol is well tolerated in short-term use. Doses range from 50 to 100 mg orally every 4 to 6 hours and should not exceed 400 mg/day.[118] As with other opiate agonists, the principal adverse effects are sedation, dizziness, nausea, vomiting, dry mouth, constipation, and sweating; however, the potential for respiratory depression is low. Seizures have occurred during therapy with recommended doses. Seizure risk increases with doses >500 mg/day and in patients taking concurrent selective serotonin-reuptake inhibitors (SSRI), tricyclic antidepressants (TCA), and other opiate agonists.[119,120] Tramadol should be used cautiously in patients taking drugs known to lower the seizure threshold, such as monoamine-oxidase inhibitors or antipsychotic agents. In addition, patients with epilepsy, head trauma, metabolic disorders, alcohol or drug withdrawal, or CNS infections may be at increased risk for seizures with tramadol therapy.[118] Tramadol also has SSRI-like properties that can initially overshadow the opiate effect in some patients. Therefore, instead of sedation, patients may experience excitation. For more on drug interactions with tramadol, see Question 69.

CHRONIC MALIGNANT PAIN

Goal of Malignant Pain Management

29. A.J., a 68-year-old man, was diagnosed with metastatic prostate cancer 6 months ago. Now he is admitted for excessive sedation and respiratory rate of eight breaths per minute. A.J.'s admitting diagnosis is possible opioid overdose. A.J. was started on a fentanyl patch 100 mcg/hour 24 hours ago by his physician because of spinal pain not adequately relieved by oral acetaminophen 325 mg and oxycodone 5 mg every 3 hours. The fentanyl patch was removed 86 hours ago, and A.J. is again complaining of his spinal pain radiating to his buttocks and left leg. A.J. is currently awake and alert and relates that his pain level is at 9 of 10 on the pain scale. What is the goal in managing A.J.'s pain?

The goal in treating pain of terminal illness is comfort and an acceptable (to the patient) level of consciousness. Opioids should not be withheld for fear of addiction or that the dose may be too high. Instead, the dose should be titrated based on the patient's clinical response. Ideally, the patient should be comfortable and voice no complaints when questioned about his or her level of activity and alertness. Under these conditions, any dosage reductions or changes in therapy serve no purpose, even if the patient is receiving doses several times those typically used to treat acute pain. To emphasize, clinicians should focus attention on their patients' clinical response rather than on an arbitrary list of doses or ideal number of medications. The immediate goal for A.J. is to break the cycle of pain and to rapidly achieve the greatest degree of comfort possible.

Indications for Use of Fentanyl Patches

30. What special considerations are necessary for use of fentanyl transdermal patches in patients such as A.J.?

Transdermal fentanyl can be used to effectively manage chronic cancer pain. Because of the nature of the transdermal delivery system, the onset of analgesia may be delayed by 6 to 12 hours after placement of the patch.[121,122] On removal of the patch, the fentanyl deposited in the subcutaneous tissue continues to release active drug for approximately another 8 to 12 hours. These delays in onset on application and in offset after removal of the transdermal patch discourage use of the patch except for patients who require a steady maintenance analgesic dose. The transdermal patches do not provide sufficient flexibility in dosing to manage rapidly changing analgesic needs. Even after stabilized on a given drug regimen, patients with cancer pain always should be given an immediate-onset opioid analgesic (e.g., morphine elixir or solution) to take as needed for management of breakthrough pain.[123] If the need for breakthrough drugs becomes frequent, the underlying dosage regimen should be reassessed and the doses increased as appropriate. Fentanyl absorption from the patches can be affected by body temperature, and unintentional overdoses can occur with hyperthermia.[124]

A patient given fentanyl patches must be instructed to dispose of used patches appropriately to prevent inadvertent access by children or household animals. Fentanyl patches were thought to be safe from diversion and abuse, but the drug enclosure membrane can be removed and active drug accessed.[125]

31. What other delivery system options are available for A.J. to manage his breakthrough pain?

Oral transmucosal delivery of fentanyl offers the advantage of controlling pain relatively quickly without being invasive. Oral transmucosal delivery systems deliver drug with a relatively rapid onset and increased bioavailabillity compared with GI absorption. Because this route delivers medication into the bloodstream so quickly, it is imperative that the relative potency of this agent is understood.[126,127]

Morphine

Use of Oral Morphine

32. What oral dose of morphine should be selected for A.J.?

The usual initial dose for morphine is 30 mg orally every 3 hours (Table 8-5), but A.J. has been receiving acetaminophen with oxycodone for an unknown length of time and likely has some degree of opioid tolerance. His response to morphine should be monitored carefully 1 to 2 hours after his initial dose and the dose adjusted appropriately. If A.J. experiences clinical signs of overdose (excessive sedation and somnolence, low respiratory rate), the dose should be decreased; however, if he is still uncomfortable after the 2 hours, an additional 30 mg should be given at once and subsequent doses increased by 10 mg to a total of 40 mg every 3 hours. A.J.'s response should be the primary criterion for determining the dose, and the pharmacokinetics of the drug should determine the dosing interval. Frequent reassessment of A.J.'s pain status and level of consciousness is essential.

When the pain has been relieved, the dose of morphine often can be decreased. Ideally, only one clinician should assume responsibility for coordinating frequent monitoring of the patient's level of awareness and pain control. Once the pain has been controlled, single-day dosage adjustment should be sufficient. If the dose is changed, then it should be reassessed within the first 2 hours to prevent unnecessary exposure to pain or adverse effects. Most oral opioids reach maximal analgesic effect within the first 2 hours after administration, but for longer-acting opioid analgesics such as methadone, the patient should be monitored for several days because of potential drug accumulation.

Tolerance, Dependence, and Addiction

33. Should tolerance, dependence, and addiction to morphine be an issue in A.J.?

Tolerance and physical dependence should be anticipated and discussed openly with patients who are receiving chronic opioid analgesia. Tolerance occurs when a given dose no longer produces the same effect over time. For patients with a malignant disease, it is difficult to differentiate between tolerance and increased pain from disease progression. A.J. should be instructed to inform his clinicians when his pain regimen becomes ineffective. Escalating doses of opioid analgesics should be expected and should not deter the clinician from continuing with analgesic therapy. The need for increasing doses, however, should serve as a warning that alternative analgesic or adjunct agents need to be considered.

Physical dependence should also be anticipated. It should be explained to A.J. that this is a natural adaptation process of the body that occurs with opiates. The signs and symptoms of dependence are seen when abrupt withdrawal or a marked decrease in opioid administration occurs. Therefore, it is important that A.J. receive an adequate supply of medication to prevent exacerbating withdrawal symptoms caused by difficulties in obtaining medication or missed doses. The potential for dependency to opioid analgesics should never prevent the clinical use of opioid analgesics in malignant disease.

Addiction is a compulsive behavior relating to drug procurement and use. Addiction from clinical opioid use for the treatment of pain is rare. Misunderstanding by clinicians and caregivers regarding the difference between tolerance, dependence, and addiction is common and often results in undertreatment of painful conditions.[128,129] Addiction is not an issue in patients requiring opiates for the treatment of chronic malignant pain. Tolerance and dependence should be expected and should in no way be misconstrued as evidence of addiction.

Use of Sustained-Release Morphine

34. A.J.'s pain was controlled on 40 mg of morphine solution orally every 3 hours, but he is now complaining of the frequency of the morphine dose. He wishes to have the therapy changed to allow fewer daily doses so that he may have longer periods of rest. What can be done about A.J.'s request?

Several controlled release opioid formulations are available for this patient. Morphine is available in four different formulations: MS Contin, Oramorph SR, Kadian, and Avinza. Oxycodone is also available as extended release tablet (OxyContin). Pharmacokinetic profiles differ among formulations of which clinicians need to be aware. Avinza and Kadian provide 24-hour sustained release of morphine, which leads to less fluctuation in drug levels, and therefore less frequent dosing. Avinza is always dosed once daily, whereas Kadian can be given once or twice a day. MS Contin, Oramorph SR, and OxyContin are usually dosed twice daily, whereas some patient may require doses three times a day. Whenever converting patients from one sustained-release (SR) product to a short-acting opioid, it is important to remember that SR formulations (e.g., Kadian and Avinza) will deliver morphine up to 36 hours from the last dose. This warrants intensive monitoring, especially in patients who received high doses for long periods of time.

These opioid formulations have been a target of misuse and abuse. When altering its delivery system, daily drug supply can be released immediately, potentially causing overdose and death. It is important to remember that sustained release formulations should not be crushed and chewed. Kadian and Avinza capsules can be opened and sprinkled over applesauce; however, the integrity of the beads must not be altered.

A.J.'s daily morphine requirement of 320 mg can be provided by use of an SR dosage form given every 8 to 12 hours. However, direct conversion of doses from oral morphine solutions or other immediate-release dosage forms to SR tablets often leads to oversedation initially, particularly during the first hours of the dosing period. Therefore, the SR dose should be reduced by 25% to 240 mg/day (320 mg × 75%) for A.J. This can be given as 90 mg every 8 hours or as 120 mg every 12 hours. SR morphine is available as 15-, 30-, 60-, 100-, and 200-mg tablets and 20-, 50-, and 100-mg capsules. When starting a patient on oral SR preparations, it often is desirable to try an every-8-hour regimen to prevent the initial sedation that often is associated with the larger individual doses of the 12-hour regimen. Likewise, when larger doses are needed, 8-hour dosing intervals usually cause less sedation than 12-hour intervals (i.e., during the first 2 hours of the dosing period). Some patients also may have more breakthrough pain at the end of the 12-hour dosing interval. Careful assessment of the patient's response and toxicity by the clinician is the most essential ingredient between success and failure with either product in managing the patient's pain.

Rectal Use of Morphine Suppositories and Sustained-Release Tablets

35. Several weeks later, A.J. is no longer able to swallow his medication because of worsening of an existing esophageal stricture. What are alternatives for giving A.J. his required daily analgesic?

In addition to the parenteral routes already presented, morphine can be administered as an oral solution or via a rectal suppository. The absorption of the rectal suppository is at least comparable to, or better than that of, the morphine solution.[130,131] If A.J. was stabilized on 240 mg/day of SR morphine, the initial morphine suppository dose also should be 240 mg/day. The duration of action of morphine suppositories is similar to that of morphine solution and therefore must be administered every 3 to 4 hours. For A.J., the starting dose is 30 mg rectally every 3 hours. Other agents, such as hydromorphone (Dilaudid) and codeine, are also available as suppositories. The equianalgesic doses of these agents for A.J. (Table 8-3) would be 6 and 10 mg, respectively. SR oral morphine tablets also can be used for rectal administration. The rectal absorption of SR tablets is comparable to the oral route of administration.[132,133] There is no maximal dose for opioid analgesics for the management of pain of a terminal disease, but there is a limit to how many suppositories or tablets the patient can hold rectally.

Oral Infusion

36. Because A.J. was unable to swallow, he agreed to have a gastrostomy feeding tube placed by a general surgeon. He is now being fed through the tube at a rate of 50 mL/hour. Morphine sulfate solution is added to each feeding bag to deliver 10 mg/hour. He also is receiving amitriptyline (Elavil) 150 mg at bedtime, naproxen suspension 250 mg four times a day (QID), and lorazepam (Ativan) 4 mg three times a day (TID) via the feeding tube. A.J. is reasonably alert and is only slightly uncomfortable. Are there any problems associated with placing A.J.'s morphine in the feeding formula?

No reason exists why morphine cannot be given in this manner. The obvious questions about drug stability, solubility, and binding to proteins in the feeding formula do not appear to present a problem because A.J. has been receiving morphine in this manner for the past several days. The dose of morphine (240 mg/day) is apparently not causing undesirable effects, and A.J. is quite comfortable. Administering morphine as a continuous oral infusion at night while he is sleeping is perhaps the best method to ensure restful, pain-free sleep.

Tricyclic Antidepressants

37. What are the indications for amitriptyline in A.J.'s treatment regimen?

Tricyclic antidepressants have been used experimentally at low to moderate doses as an adjunct to analgesic pain control. These agents may alter psychological responses to pain, have intrinsic analgesic activity, and may potentiate opioid analgesics.[134] European investigations noted an 82% overall response rate to these agents.[135] Imipramine (Tofranil) relieved cancer and surgical pain in approximately 75% to 80% of patients, and doxepin (Sinequan) relieved pain completely in approximately half of 16 depressed, patients with chronic pain.[136] Tension headaches also were improved with 25 to 100 mg of doxepin.[129] Imipramine 50 to 200 mg/day or amitriptyline 10 to 40 mg/day alone or in combination with fluphenazine (Prolixin) have also been investigated for neuropathic pain.[137] Neuroleptic agents have fallen out of general use, however, for chronic pain syndromes because of their potential for extrapyramidal syndromes (EPS) and other long-term effects. TCA and methadone combination also have been used successfully for the long-term management of chronic phantom limb pain (see Questions 49 and 51).[138] For A.J., the choice of TCA is limited, because of his inability to swallow. A few TCA, however, are available as oral suspensions (doxepin and nortriptyline). Therefore, it would be reasonable to continue A.J.'s present TCA therapy.

Methadone

Guidelines

38. The decision has been made to use oral methadone to treat A.J.'s pain. What are guidelines for the safe use of methadone in treating cancer pain?

Clinical experience with the use of methadone for cancer pain is favorable.[139] The patient's physical and mental condition should be monitored closely, and clinicians should be aware of the long elimination half-life of methadone. Repeated dosing with methadone requires decreasing the dose when comfort is achieved to prevent drug accumulation and overdose. Methadone is 85% bound to serum proteins, and its average plasma half-life is approximately 23 hours, with a range of 13 to 47 hours. Therefore, the drug is tightly bound and only slowly released from its binding sites. Plasma levels of methadone can continue to rise for up to 10 days after an increase in dose.

The duration of analgesia, however, does not correlate to the serum half-life, and multiple doses must be given each day. The absolute amount of methadone in plasma, although it undoubtedly affects sedation and respiratory depression, is not a factor in the magnitude of analgesic response. Nevertheless, analgesic effects are obtained only while methadone plasma levels are above a certain individualized concentration. Most patients can be maintained on doses of methadone every 6 or 8 hours after pain control is achieved, but the drug often must be given every 4 hours or administered with another short-acting opioid analgesic during the first day or two of therapy to control pain.[140] Alternatively, methadone loading with larger doses for the first few doses can accomplish rapid analgesia at the onset of methadone administration. However, this carries a higher risk of rapid drug accumulation and excessive drowsiness. Thus, loading doses must be reduced after the first one to two doses.

The necessity for shorter dosing intervals during the initiation of methadone can cause clinicians who are unfamiliar with the long half-life of methadone to adjust doses too frequently or to maintain a patient at an inappropriately high dose after initial pain control is achieved. This can threaten the patient with dangerous drug accumulation. A scenario that often is repeated is one in which analgesia and patient comfort are achieved after 2 or 3 days of gradually increasing doses. On days 4 and 5, the patient becomes increasingly sedated and on day 6 alarmingly so. The drug is then discontinued, or the opioid antagonist naloxone (Narcan) is administered. Suddenly, the patient is no longer sedated, but the pain has reappeared. This sudden reversal of sedation may be short lived. Because the half-life of methadone is much longer than that of naloxone, the patient can still slip back into sedation once the naloxone is cleared from the plasma in 1 to 2 hours.[141] Elderly and severely debilitated patients may require smaller doses of methadone for pain control; therefore, caution must be exercised when methadone is used in these patients.[142]

Dosing

39. What dose of methadone should be prescribed to treat A.J.'s pain?

To convert A.J.'s dose of morphine to an equivalent dose of methadone, use Table 8-3 as a standard reference for comparison. A.J.'s 10-mg every hour oral morphine sulfate solution dose is estimated to be approximately equivalent to 10 mg every 3 hours of morphine IM. On a single-dose basis, IM doses of methadone and morphine are equally potent; however, with repeated doses on a chronic basis, the duration of methadone activity is approximately four times longer than that of morphine. Therefore, the total daily parenteral methadone dose will be only one-fourth that of parenteral morphine. In this case, A.J. would require 20 mg/day of IM methadone. Because oral methadone is only 75% as effective as methadone IM,[143] A.J. should receive approximately 7.5 mg of methadone orally every 6 hours. Approximately 5 to 10 days will elapse before the full methadone effect is realized, unless loading doses equal to twice that of the maintenance analgesic dose are used for the first two doses. These two larger doses accelerate the process of reaching the steady-state concentration. Breakthrough pain should be anticipated despite around-the-clock dosing of methadone, especially immediately after the conversion from other opioids. Because of long half-life and risk of accumulation, additional methadone doses should not be used as a breakthrough drug. Instead, morphine or oxycodone would be reasonable choices to treat A.J.'s breakthrough pain before methadone reaches its steady-state and maintenance dose can be safely increased.

Continuous Intravenous Morphine Infusion

40. Three months later, A.J. is again hospitalized because of a compression fracture of his spine. He is cachectic and weighs only 87 pounds. He has been receiving 20 mg of morphine IM every 3 hours since his admission. His pain is bothersome and his loss of muscle mass is not conducive to IM injections. What would be a reasonable IV analgesic program for A.J.?

Continuous IV infusions of morphine are superior to IM injections in maintaining a pain-free condition in cancer and surgical patients.[144,145] In one study, six of eight children with cancer experienced complete pain control with 0.025 to 2.6 mg/kg/hour of morphine for 1 to 16 days.

A.J. has been receiving 160 mg of morphine daily, which is approximately 7 mg/hour. His initial IV infusion dose of morphine should be increased to 8 mg/hour because his pain is still bothersome. When 500 mg of morphine sulfate is added to 500 mL of 5% dextrose in water, the resulting 1-mg/mL solution can be infused IV at 8 mL/hour to deliver the 8-mg/hour dose. In addition, an order should be written for a 4-mg IV bolus of morphine every hour as needed for signs of pain or discomfort.

The supplemental bolus doses of IV morphine will facilitate subsequent adjustments of the continuous infusion rate. At the end of a predetermined period of time, the number of milligrams of drug that were administered by constant infusion is added to 1.5 times the number of milligrams of drug used in supplemental bolus doses. This amount of drug is then divided by the elapsed interval of time, thereby calculating the new infusion rate. For example, if at the end of 6 hours A.J. has received five supplemental doses of 4 mg each, then (6 hours at 8 mg/hour) plus (1.5×5 doses of 4 mg) = 78 mg per

6 hours. The new infusion rate should then be 13 mg/hour, and the new supplemental doses should be 6 mg (approximately equal to the amount of drug normally infused in 30 minutes) every hour as needed. Continual assessment of the patient and hourly adjustments of dose are probably superior to the method outlined previously, but the aforementioned method may be more practical for the busy clinician.

Pentazocine

41. Why should pentazocine (Talwin) not be used in treating cancer pain?

The use of agonist/antagonists also should be avoided because of poor oral efficacy and because of the particularly disturbing nature of the psychotomimetic side effects in patients who are already fearful and anxious. Furthermore, pentazocine is a "ceiling" drug; that is, doses cannot be greatly increased to treat increasing pain without greatly increasing the incidence or severity of side effects.

Hydroxyzine or Phenothiazine

42. Would coadministration of either hydroxyzine or phenothiazine be beneficial for A.J.'s pain?

The addition of hydroxyzine (Vistaril, Atarax) to an analgesic regimen is thought to potentiate the analgesia of the opioid analgesic.[20,146,147] Whether this is a true analgesic effect or a consequence of its sedating properties is unclear. An additional benefit related to the antihistamine properties of hydroxyzine is prevention of opiate-induced nausea and itching.

Phenothiazines, as with antihistamines, often are administered concomitantly with opioids to "enhance" analgesia. Claims of enhanced analgesia are not supported by well-designed studies, however. Many of these studies lack double-blinding, cross-over of patients, placebo control, or appropriate instruments capable of evaluating pain. Another problem in the design of studies evaluating the combination of a phenothiazine or antihistamine with an opioid is the failure to differentiate between analgesia and sedation. Two excellent reviews summarize the studies that demonstrate analgesia with antihistamines and discuss the proposed mechanisms of action.[148,149]

All phenothiazines, except for methotrimeprazine, initially demonstrated antianalgesic effects in experimental pain studies. Clinicians now realize that experimental pain is not a completely valid model to assess the response of a patient in pain. These studies could not assess the anxiolytic properties of the phenothiazines and the effect a reduction in anxiety has on pain perception. Furthermore, cancer and chronic pain cause anxiety, and anxiety worsens pain perception and, consequently, pain severity. This reinforcement cannot be overestimated and helps explain the apparent benefit many patients obtain from the combination of hydroxyzine with an opioid.

Adrenal Corticosteroids

43. Why might corticosteroids be useful for A.J.'s spinal pain?

Patients who have spinal metastatic disease often obtain pain relief with corticosteroids. This is thought to be because of a combination of direct anti-inflammatory effects and a reduction of pressure from edema around affected nerves. A short course of dexamethasone at a dose of 4 mg orally or IV four times daily with rapid tapering should be considered for A.J.[150]

Corticosteroid response may decrease with repeated use, but a single short-course therapy often can produce a significantly prolonged effect. Dexamethasone is most often used because of its long duration of action and lack of mineralocorticoid effects. Other corticosteroids may be substituted for the dexamethasone, however, using a conversion table to calculate equivalent doses.

Nonsteroidal Anti-Inflammatory Drugs

44. Why should the use of an NSAID be considered for A.J.'s spinal pain?

Pain from tumor metastasis to bone is particularly distressing and difficult to treat. Although the most effective therapy for the relief of bone pain is radiation to the site of the pain,[151] prostaglandin inhibitors may be another reasonable alternative to increased doses of opioids. Osseous metastases induce the production of prostaglandins that can cause osteolysis, sensitize free nerve endings, and augment pain perception. NSAIDs effectively decrease prostaglandin and endoperoxide production and may be useful in treating metastatic bone pain if administered on a scheduled basis. Usual analgesic doses of NSAIDs often are effective, but maximal therapeutic doses may be necessary. Some specialists in treating cancer pain advocate doses considerably larger than the manufacturers' recommendations. Sometimes IV ketorolac is used for this purpose.[152] In extremely painful cases, IV ketorolac has been used as a continuous infusion for managing metastatic bone pain.[152] Beside an NSAID, strontium, and radiopharmaceuticals (e.g., phosphorus 32, strontium 89, samarium 153, rhenium 186, and tin 117m) have been used to treat metastatic bone pain, but occasionally with limited benefit. Nevertheless, they can be considered for severe bony metastatic pain unresponsive to corticosteroids or an NSAID.

CHRONIC NONMALIGNANT PAIN

Goal of Therapy

45. W.C., a 38-year-old man, has been disabled for the past 2 years because of an injury to his cervical spine sustained while operating a forklift at a warehouse. He is currently taking oral oxycodone 5 mg with acetaminophen 325 mg (Percocet) two tablets QID as needed for severe pain, codeine 30 mg with acetaminophen 325 mg (Tylenol #3) or hydrocodone 5 mg with acetaminophen 325 mg (Lorcet-5) two tablets QID as needed for less severe pain, and diazepam 10 mg TID for neck spasms. W.C. describes the pain as sharp and stabbing, and the spasms in his neck are his most troublesome problem. The spasms become severe if he stops taking the diazepam, and the pain starts to build 2 hours after taking the opioids. W.C. currently is seeing an internist and an orthopedic surgeon who prescribed his analgesics. W.C. also has

undergone several cervical discectomies and vertebral fusion with minimal pain relief. What are the treatment goals in W.C.?

Opioid use for chronic nonmalignant pain remains the most controversial issue facing clinical pain management. Not only is opioid efficacy subject to debate, but, in addition, the potential for opioid dependency creates considerable hesitation on the part of many prescribers.[153,154] Although neuropathic pain may respond to opioids, high dosages are often needed.[155] Opioid analgesics should be considered only after the patient has received and failed adequate trials of an NSAID or other analgesic agents. In addition, patients should be evaluated for physical interventions, such as muscle strengthening or conditioning exercises that may improve their clinical situation, before becoming over-reliant on opioids for pain management. As with any chronic pain management, time-contingent dosing (fixed dose and interval) is superior to as-needed dosing. If an opioid is used to manage chronic pain, a longer-acting agent (e.g., SR morphine, methadone, levorphanol) should be used to minimize fluctuations in serum concentrations. Patients should be monitored closely for both efficacy and toxicity.

Shorter-acting opioid analgesics often can complicate chronic nonmalignant pain management by exacerbating the pain perception because of fluctuating serum concentrations and the production of opioid withdrawal hyperalgesia when serum concentrations are low. Analogous withdrawal effects can occur with sedative-hypnotics and antispasmodics as well, particularly those with relatively short half-lives.

Before any therapeutic modality is initiated, the primary caregiver and the patient must have a written agreement that includes provisions for a single prescriber; monitoring of serum drug concentrations; urine or blood substance abuse screening; as well as an agreement to inform all current and future health care providers regarding pain management, and termination of service. There should be only one prescriber for all of W.C.'s medications, and all of his health care providers must be informed of the therapeutic plans. The immediate goal of pain management for W.C. is to consolidate his analgesic regimen to a time-contingent, longer-acting opioid. Longer-term goals should include withdrawal of diazepam, consideration of opioid withdrawal, and institution of alternative analgesic adjuncts (antidepressants or membrane stabilizers). Psychological evaluation and support should supplement pharmacologic therapy. The overall therapeutic goal for W.C. is pain control and pain reduction, but not total pain elimination. He should be able to conduct activities of daily life with minimal discomfort, and ideally be able to return to gainful employment in some capacity, even if his work duties are modified.

Analgesic Consolidation

46. W.C. relates that he has been taking up to 18 tablets of various opioid analgesics daily. How should his pain be managed?

Chronic opiate use can lead to dependence as well as tolerance. The immediate need is to stabilize W.C.'s pain, but a longer-term goal should include analgesic tapering if tolerated. Evidence from pain studies in animal models, and in longitudinal studies of humans, indicate that chronic opioid use can lead to changes in the CNS that result in hyperalgesia. It is not known if this effect is drug- and time-dependent.[156,157]

Tapering is not likely to be achieved quickly, however. W.C. should be started on an opiate tapering regimen after his pain is stabilized, and this process should occur within 24 hours after the analgesic dose has stabilized. The first step in opiate analgesic tapering is opiate consolidation. As in this case, the patient often is receiving several analgesics unnecessarily. A longer-acting opioid analgesic should be used for W.C. to minimize the pain and analgesia fluctuations. One method is to sum his total opioid use per day during the past several weeks and then convert to an equivalent dose of either methadone or SR morphine. Alternatively, an arbitrary dose, such as oral methadone 5 mg every 6 hours, could be started, and all of his current analgesics could be discontinued. If this dose is insufficient, a temporary dosage increase may be necessary. The long half-life of methadone will be beneficial when instituting opioid tapering.

Alternative analgesic adjuncts, such as antidepressants or anticonvulsants, should also be considered and introduced at this time. Opiate consolidation in W.C. would also serve to reduce his exposure to acetaminophen. He is currently taking three different acetaminophen-containing products. Although concern for opioid dosing emphasizes a balance between benefits and risks from the opioids, the risk of either short-term overdose or cumulative effects from acetaminophen (e.g., liver or renal toxicity) should not be overlooked. W.C. should be instructed not to exceed 4 to 5 g/day of acetaminophen from all sources, including analgesic and cold/sinus medications products he may be purchasing over the counter.

Opioid Tapering and Withdrawal

47. How rapidly can opiate analgesics be discontinued in a patient such as W.C. without precipitating withdrawal symptoms?

W.C. would benefit from long-term multidisciplinary pain management that includes behavioral therapy as well as medication adjustments. An acute pain opiate analgesic dose can be decreased in hospitalized patients by 20% daily without precipitating opiate withdrawal symptoms; but in a patient such as W.C., who has been taking opiate analgesics for an extended period of time, the decrease in analgesic dose will have to be much more gradual. In chronic opiate dependence, the opioid dose can be decreased by approximately 10% every 3 to 5 days without inducing withdrawal symptoms. The addition of clonidine can also improve the overall opioid tapering process, because it may impart analgesic effects while assisting in controlling abstinence symptoms.

Managing Opioid Overdose

48. W.C. accidentally received an excessive dose of methadone leading to a respiratory rate of 8 breaths/minute and excessive sedation. How should he be treated?

Methadone can accumulate when converting from short-acting opioids to this longer-acting opioid unless careful attention is paid to the differences in pharmacokinetic properties. Because methadone has a long half-life, steady-state plasma levels may not be achieved for 5 to 10 days. In W.C., the challenge is to treat the respiratory depression induced by methadone without interfering with the desired analgesic effects and without precipitating narcotic withdrawal. Opioid toxicity is not life threatening if it is managed immediately. Naloxone reverses opioid-induced CNS sedation and respiratory depression after overdose of all opiates except buprenorphine. W.C. should be given naloxone 0.1 mg parenterally at 2- to 3-minute intervals until the desired effect (improved respiration rate and increased alertness) is achieved. Because methadone has a long half-life, the naloxone dose may need to be repeated every 15 to 20 minutes, sometimes for several hours, until the methadone toxicity dissipates. Overly aggressive dosing of naloxone can cause agitation and exaggerated responses to pain. The methadone dose will have to be adjusted accordingly if too much naloxone has been administered.

In the event of a massive overdose of opioid analgesics, naloxone can be given as a continuous infusion of 0.2 mg/hour to 0.4 mg/hour. In light of the low incidence of side effects from naloxone, it might be reasonable to start with a loading dose of 0.8 mg and a higher infusion dose such as 0.4 mg/hour, followed by subsequent dosage adjustments, depending on clinical response. The same approach may be utilized for the treatment of overdose with extended release formulations of opioids. As intermittent naloxone may reverse the immediate effect of opioids on receptors, extended release formulation would continue to deliver more drug and, therefore, further the effects of overdose. The required duration of naloxone infusion will vary, depending on the specific opioid and the amount involved.[158,159]

A longer-acting opiate antagonist, nalmefene (Revex), may provide an alternative to naloxone. Approved for the use of conscious sedation reversal and management of opioid overdose, nalmefene may be most beneficial in overdoses of methadone or propoxyphene where repeated administration of antagonists is necessary because of their long elimination half-lives.[160] Nalmefene has a long half-life (8–11 hours) compared with naloxone (1–1.5 hours). Although fewer doses of nalmefene may be needed to reverse opioid intoxication, studies have not shown any difference in efficacy between nalmefene and naloxone.[160,161]

NEUROPATHIC PAIN

49. R.L., a 40-year-old, generally healthy woman, suffered a superficial laceration of her left arm at work from a broken glass window. The initial laceration has since healed without complications, but now she is referred for evaluation of pain management because of persistent intolerable pain in her left arm and hand. Physical examination reveals allodynia (pain resulting from a non-noxious stimulus to normal skin) in her left hand and arm. What caused R.L.'s condition, and how would you manage her pain pharmacologically?

Hyperalgesia after a minor injury is well described, but the pathogenic basis of such pain is not understood. In these afflicted patients, the pain threshold is decreased and stimuli response in the affected region is increased. This persistent pain also can be associated with changes in regional cutaneous blood flow, osteoporosis, swelling, changes in regional temperature, and atrophic musculocutaneous changes in the affected region without demonstrable nerve injury. In the affected areas, pain is elicited by even the slightest mechanical or thermal stimuli. This painful hyperalgesic condition, known as, *reflex sympathetic dystrophy,* or *chronic regional pain syndrome* (CRPS) has been attributed to sympathetic excess and has been called *sympathetically maintained pain* (SMP) by some. It also can be the result of other central or peripheral mechanisms that are independent of the sympathetic nervous system. SMP may partially respond to pharmacologic agents that interfere with the α-adrenergic function; therefore, it would be expected to respond to clonidine, prazosin, phenoxybenzamine, or guanethidine. Some symptoms of these syndromes may respond to other classes of pharmacologic agents, such as steroids and NSAIDs, TCAs, anticonvulsants, antiarrhythmics, or local anesthetics.

α_2-Agonists

50. R.L.'s CRPS will be managed by a sympathoplegic agent. What doses of clonidine or prazosin will be required for pain management in R.L.?

The α_2-agonists (e.g., clonidine) are useful in the management of SMP. They act by reversing the excessive sympathetic adrenergic response at central and peripheral receptors and by reversing local vasoconstriction with improvement in blood flow. Clonidine has analgesic effects when administered either systemically or locally at the spinal level. The α_1-antagonist, prazosin, also has been used in the management of SMP. The dosages for clonidine and prazosin are 0.2 to 0.6 mg/day and 1 to 6 mg/day, respectively, in two to three equally divided doses. The major disadvantage of these agents is their side effects, especially hypotension and exacerbation of depression.[162] In addition, rapid development of tachyphylaxis has been noted. Clonidine 0.1 mg orally four times daily would be a good starting dose for R.L., but the final dose must be titrated based on the patient's clinical response or side effects.

Tricyclic Antidepressants

51. What types of pain are most responsive to antidepressants? Is there any advantage of using one antidepressant over another for pain management in patients such as R.L.?

The analgesic properties of TCAs are independent of their antidepressant properties. Depression, however, often accompanies chronic pain, which in turn, often exacerbates a patient's response to pain and inability to cope with pain-induced lifestyle changes.[163,164] Thus, the antidepressant may interrupt this cycle of events. TCAs produce analgesia directly through modulation of the descending inhibitory nerve pathway by either altering serotonin or norepinephrine neurotransmission. They are also believed to reduce pain through local anesthetic (sodium-channel blocking) effects. Another secondary benefit of some TCAs is their sedative effect, which can help the patient sleep and reduce feelings of anxiety.

Antidepressants have been most widely studied in patients with diabetic neuropathy and postherpetic neuralgia.[165,166] They also have some value in deafferentation pain (central pain resulting from loss of spinal afferent nerve pathway), phantom limb pain, human immunodeficiency virus (HIV) neuropathy,[167] postsurgical pain,[168,169] fibromyalgia, and chronic pain associated with depression. They also have limited usefulness in the management of lower back pain, radiation neuropathy, and direct malignant nerve infiltration.

Clinical data for the management of pain is most extensive for amitriptyline, but other TCAs also have been used for this purpose.[160,170] Data on the use of SSRIs, such as fluoxetine, paroxetine, and sertraline, are limited.[171] The major disadvantage associated with the use of TCAs is their side-effect profile, which includes sedation, anticholinergic effects, and cardiotoxicity (quinidinelike widening of QRS on electrocardiogram [ECG]). Sedation and anticholinergic effects are less severe with secondary amine TCAs (desipramine, nortriptyline) than with tertiary amine TCAs, such as amitriptyline and doxepin. Weight gain can be a limiting factor as well.[172,173] In patients such as R.L., who have no histories of cardiac problems, a TCA can be helpful in pain management. Whether TCAs should be used to treat pain in the elderly population remains controversial because these agents also can produce cognitive impairment and hypotension.[174]

52. L.K., a 46-year-old woman with diabetes mellitus, is admitted to the hospital with pain that involves both hands and feet and which is associated with symptoms of pain, burning sensation, numbness, and tingling. Physical examination reveals only that pinprick sensation in the hands and feet is lessened.

Another class of antidepressants, the serotonin-norepinephrine reuptake inhibitors, duloxetine hydrochloride and venlafaxine provide an alternative for patients whose use of a TCA may be limited because of side effects. These drugs act by providing dual reuptake inhibition of both serotonin and norepinerhrine transporters with weak affinity for the dopamine transporter. The most frequently observed side effects with duloxetine are nausea, vomiting, constipation, somnolence, dry mouth, increased sweating, loss of appetite, and weakness. The immediate-release version of venlafaxine is associated with more CNS and somatic side effects, but the extended-release version of this medication is more tolerable with the main side effect being gastrointestinal disturbances. The optimal dose of duloxetine is 60 mg/day with 150 to 225 mg/day being an effective dose for venlafaxine.[175,176]

Anticonvulsants and Antiarrhythmics

53. What other alternatives are there for the management of L.K.'s neuropathic pain?

Anticonvulsants have been used frequently in the management of neuropathic pain with varying success. In randomized-controlled studies, gabapentin and pregabalin have improved symptoms of diabetic neuropathy and postherpetic neuralgia.[177,178] Doses of gabapentin up to 3,600 mg/day or greater may be required in some patients, whereas the range for pregabalin is from 150 to 600 mg/day. Additionally, higher doses of gabapentin are generally well tolerated compared with pregabalin. Gabapentin requires more individualization in patients because doses are slowly titrated to pain control. Pregabalin can be titrated more rapidly and has a short onset of action (<1 week), which may require less combination therapy in some patients. The most common side effects of gabapentin and pregabalin include dizziness, somnolence, peripheral edema, and dry mouth.[176,179]

HEAD INJURY AND OPIOID ANALGESIA

54. M.C., a 24-year-old male hemophiliac, is admitted to the emergency department (ED) with several minor lacerations, contusions, and painful hemarthrosis secondary to a bicycle accident. Meperidine 50 mg IV was ordered and he was transferred to the medical ward for further evaluation. There, M.C. was given antihemophilic factor. He also was given meperidine 50 to 75 mg IV every 3 hours, as needed, for pain. What was the danger in administering an opioid to M.C. in the ED or shortly after he was admitted?

Opioid analgesics generally are avoided in patients with head injury for the following reasons: (a) opioid-induced pupillary changes, nausea, and general CNS clouding can mask or confuse the neurologic evaluation; (b) head injury potentiates the respiratory depressant effects of opioids; (c) opioids induce carbon dioxide retention, which in turn causes vasodilation of cerebral arteries and an increase in cerebrospinal fluid pressure that might already be elevated because of head injury[180,181]; (d) opioids in excessive doses can mask internal organ injury; and (e) morphine and meperidine can produce further hypotension in patients who have blood loss caused by trauma. These potential complications, however, should not preclude the use of a short-acting opioid, such as fentanyl, for pain control in emergency situations, especially when the patient's clinical condition and analgesic responses are monitored closely. If fentanyl is to be used, small but frequent IV doses are preferred over single, large boluses (see Table 8-5 for starting doses). The final dose is based on the patient's analgesic and toxic responses. It would be reasonable to start M.C. on fentanyl 25 to 50 mcg IV every 30 to 60 minutes followed by analgesic titration.

MYOCARDIAL PAIN

55. C.P., a 65-year-old man with a history of angina pectoris, is brought to the ED with a suspected acute myocardial infarction (MI). Meperidine 25 mg IV is prescribed for pain control. Would another analgesic be preferred over pentazocine in C.P.?

This dose of meperidine might be effective for analgesia; however, meperidine has variable hemodynamic effects in patients with hemodynamic instability, whereas fentanyl and morphine's effects are more predictable. Butorphanol (Stadol) and pentazocine can increase pulmonary vascular resistance and pulmonary artery pressure.[182,183] Furthermore, pentazocine can produce idiosyncratic hypotensive episodes, which could be disastrous in these patients. Therefore, these agents should be avoided after MI.

Morphine does not increase myocardial wall tension or oxygen consumption and does not affect cardiac dimensions. Morphine also can decrease heart rate and induces only minimal orthostatic changes in blood pressures. In postsurgical patients who are volume depleted, the orthostatic effect of morphine can be quite dramatic, however. Sedative and emetic effects of morphine are comparable to methadone, but may be greater than those of meperidine or hydromorphone. Methadone, hydromorphone, buprenorphine, and nalbuphine affect the cardiovascular system in a manner similar to that of morphine.[183]

In summary, although all the aforementioned agents are effective analgesics, pentazocine and butorphanol cause greater cardiovascular effects and can exacerbate an acute MI by increasing the cardiac workload and oxygen consumption. Therefore, morphine remains the preferred agent. (See Chapter 17, Myocardial Infarction, for further discussion.)

COLIC PAIN

Biliary Colic

56. B.C., a 42-year-old man, is admitted for severe, intermittent right upper quadrant pain accompanied by nausea, vomiting, and clay-colored stools. The differential diagnosis is biliary colic versus acute pancreatitis. Two doses of meperidine 100 mg IM 3 hours apart fail to ease the pain. What other potent analgesics are preferred in this situation?

Opioid analgesics can induce smooth-muscle spasms in the sphincter of Oddi and thereby increase intrabiliary pressure.[184,185] The resulting intraductal back pressure can aggravate pain symptoms and increase the serum concentrations of amylase 5 to 10 times above the control value.[186] Although it often is claimed that meperidine is less likely than morphine to cause spasm of the sphincter of Oddi, no clear evidence indicates the superiority of one agent over the other.[187] Significant increases in intrabiliary pressures of patients receiving fentanyl (Sublimaze), morphine, meperidine, pentazocine (Talwin), butorphanol (Stadol), and oxycodone are documented.[188,189]

In one study,[190] buprenorphine (Buprenex) did not increase biliary pressure, but further controlled investigations are needed to substantiate this finding. Generally, biliary pressure increases and spasm begins within 5 minutes of parenteral opioid administration. These effects peak within 20 to 60 minutes, and values gradually return to normal over 1 to 2 hours.[191,192] Because the reported severity, intensity, and duration of biliary hypertension vary greatly, it is unlikely that any agent presently available has a clear advantage over another.[187]

Opioid-induced biliary hypertension and sphincter of Oddi spasm can be reversed by parenteral glucagon or naloxone.[191,193] It is still unclear whether orally administered naloxone will have similar effects, although orally administered naloxone prevented opioid-induced constipation in one study.[194] It is unclear whether B.C. is having more pain because of an adverse drug effect or primary failure of meperidine. Because no consistent way exists to measure intraductal pressure clinically, it is recommended that he be given a longer-acting opioid, such as methadone 5 mg IV every 8 hours for pain.

Renal Colic

57. M.J., a 36-year-old woman with a history of urolithiasis, comes to the ED because of severe flank pain along with microscopic hematuria. She is diagnosed with renal colic by the ED physician who wishes to treat her pain with meperidine 100 mg IM, but M.J. does not want to take opioids. What can M.J. be given for her severe pain from her renal colic?

Renal colic is extremely painful, and patients often require parenteral opioid analgesics. No significant clinical difference is seen between any of the opioids for this type of acute analgesic indication. Because M.J. does not want to receive opioids, the choice of analgesics is limited. The parenteral nonsteroidal analgesic ketorolac is likely to be the best alternative.[195] It would be appropriate to start M.J. on ketorolac 15 mg IV every 6 hours as an alternative to the opioids for acute analgesia.

LIVER DISEASE AND ANALGESIA

58. A.A., a 54-year-old man with alcoholic cirrhosis, severe ascites, and mild jaundice, has been hospitalized with severe right upper quadrant abdominal pain. His stools are guaiac positive, and he occasionally has bright red blood present at the rectum secondary to hemorrhoids. He was placed on oral lactulose 30 g QID when the protein content of his diet was increased. Although he has a history of hepatic encephalopathy, he is currently alert and receiving only spironolactone 200 mg/day and prophylactic lactulose. What problems can arise when administering opioid analgesics to patients such as A.A.?

Morphine can induce electroencephalogram (EEG) changes similar to those associated with impending hepatic encephalopathy when administered to patients with hepatic cirrhosis.[196] These morphine-induced EEG changes cannot be correlated with alkalosis, hypokalemia, or increased blood ammonia levels, and the mechanism is unknown.

Because most opioid analgesics are significantly metabolized in the liver, their serum levels can accumulate if dosing intervals are not adjusted in patients with decreased hepatic function.[197,198] The oral bioavailability of some of the opioids also can be increased because of a decreased hepatic first-pass effect.[199] The opioids with the greatest first-pass effect or a high extraction ratio have the greatest variability in bioavailability. For example, oral morphine and meperidine have a higher extraction ratio than methadone and, therefore, are more likely to be absorbed unpredictably in patients with severe liver disease. In these patients, methadone is most likely to be absorbed consistently when administered orally.

It would be reasonable to treat A.A.'s pain with a single, modest dose of parenteral morphine, but subsequent doses should await the reappearance of signs of pain to prevent the possible precipitation of hepatic encephalopathy. Careful monitoring of A.A. is essential to minimize risk while maximizing analgesia. The clinician should remember that any CNS depressant can trigger significant problems in a patient such as A.A. If an oral opioid is to be used, then methadone will be a good choice because of its more consistent bioavailability. Although methadone has a long half-life, it is still safer to use orally than morphine. All opioid analgesics should be given in small, frequent, on-demand doses in patients such as A.A. Time-contingent dosing of opioids should be avoided in patients with liver disease because of the risk of drug accumulation. A.A. can be given methadone 2.5 mg no more often than every 6 hours, as needed, accompanied by close monitoring.

RESPIRATORY DISEASE AND ANALGESIA

59. C.T., a 65-year-old man admitted to the hospital with a hip fracture, has a history of chronic obstructive pulmonary disease (COPD). On admission, C.T. has a nonpurulent productive cough and wheezing. His medical history includes several episodes of pneumonia. Morphine sulfate 6 to 10 mg IM every 3 hours is ordered for his severe hip pain. What risks are associated with

using morphine in C.T.? Are there better alternative potent analgesics?

Systemic opioids remain the first-line agents in managing pain in patients with COPD. Careful monitoring orders also should be written along with the opioid orders. Morphine and all other opioid analgesics can depress respiration when given in therapeutic doses and should be used cautiously in patients with advanced respiratory disease and decreased respiratory function. Respiratory rate, tidal volume, and sensitivity to hypercapnia or hypoxemia are all decreased by opioid analgesics.[200] Although all opioids and agonists produce respiratory depression at therapeutic doses, there appears to be a ceiling effect to the respiratory depression caused by butorphanol (Stadol), nalbuphine (Nubain), and buprenorphine (Buprenex) at higher doses.[201,202] Increased doses of these compounds do not further depress respiration and still provide increased analgesia. The antagonist naloxone reverses the respiratory difficulty (and analgesia) produced by nalbuphine and butorphanol. Although respiratory depression caused by buprenorphine is uncommon, naloxone does not reverse buprenorphine's effects predictably.[203] Ventilatory support is the only treatment.

Because C.T. is in severe pain, a lower dosage of morphine should be used initially. Opioids do not always depress respiration when dosed correctly and, in some instances, they actually can improve respiratory function in patients who have recently had a thoracotomy. These patients often are afraid to breathe deeply because of the pain elicited by such activity. The analgesic phenothiazine, methotrimeprazine, nerve block, or epidural anesthetics also can be used with fewer respiratory effects than systemic morphine.[204,205] Alternatively, morphine PCA should be considered for C.T., because PCA will allow him to self-administer small, frequent doses, thereby reducing the possibility of opioid-induced respiratory depression.

60. **During his admission, C.T. mentions that he was recently diagnosed with sleep apnea. Would your approach to C.T.'s pain management change?**

Patients with sleep apnea must be carefully monitored when receiving pain medications and sedation, especially via the parenteral route.

Sleep apnea generally can be described as prolonged apneic episodes during sleep that can be attributed to relative hypotonia of upper pharyngeal muscles. These muscles play an important role in patency of the airway.

During an apneic episode, arterial oxygen saturation falls and carbon dioxide concentration rises, which stimulates arousal by the autonomic nervous system alerting the patient to breathe. This can occur multiple times during sleep and often is unnoticed by a patient with sleep apnea. In severe disease, patients may experience cardiac dysrhythmias owing to repeated falls in oxygen saturation. Chronic and untreated sleep apnea can lead to pulmonary and systemic hypertension, cor pulmonale, and cardiopulmonary arrest.[206] Clinicians must exercise caution when providing pain management to patients with sleep apnea. Opioid administration causes relaxation of upper respiratory tract muscles as well as a decrease in the sensitivity to rising CO_2. The ability to maintain an open airway is already compromised in a patient with sleep apnea. As a result, patients with sleep apnea may experience respiratory failure, cardiac arrhythmias, and even death.[206]

Currently, there are no published guidelines on pain management of patients with sleep apnea. It is prudent that C.T. receive continuous cardiac and oxygen saturation monitoring while being treated with opioids. Continuous positive airway pressure (CPAP) may be used to prevent hypoxic episodes caused by opioids.[207] Short acting opioids would be preferred if C.T.'s pain can be adequately controlled with these agents.

Use of buprenorphine, a partial opioid agonist, for severe pain in patients with sleep apnea has been postulated, but published clinical trials are lacking. Concomitant use of an NSAID and acetaminophen is recommended to reduce opioid requirements.[206]

OPIATES IN SPECIAL AGE GROUPS

Advanced Age

61. **B.V., a 75-year-old woman, is seen in the office for a routine physical examination. She has a history of osteoarthritis in both knees, osteoporotic vertebral disease, and peptic ulcer disease. In addition to estrogen and calcium supplementation, B.V. takes acetaminophen 650 mg every 4 hours during the day for general discomfort and ibuprofen 400 mg every night to "help [her] sleep." What further information should be assessed before modifying B.V.'s drug therapy?**

Chronic pain can have a significant impact on daily functioning and quality of life and should be recognized as a significant problem requiring prompt attention. Chronic pain is common in older adults and may easily go unrecognized and untreated. Painful conditions affecting bones and joints often develop as people age. These conditions provide a chronic source of pain and are often incurable. Approximately one of five older adults takes analgesic medications regularly and more than half of these patients have taken prescription analgesics for >6 months. Prevalence rates for chronic pain among community-dwelling older people have been estimated to be between 25% and 50%.[208] Studies of nursing home residents have documented similar rates for chronic nonmalignant pain and also have shown a consistent trend toward undertreatment with analgesics.[209,210]

Clinical practice guidelines have been developed for the management of chronic pain in older persons.[208] All older patients should be assessed for evidence of chronic pain as well as for acute pain that may indicate a new illness or exacerbation of a chronic condition. Older patients may be reluctant to report pain because they may fear the consequences of a diagnostic workup. Older adults may also perceive pain to be synonymous with serious disease or death.[208] When providing a history, they may not use the word "pain" to describe how they feel. Instead, they may describe their discomfort as "aching, soreness, burning, or tightness." Finally, patients with dementia or language deficits may not be able to communicate the presence of pain. In these individuals and others, grimacing or other unusual behavior may provide clues to the presence of pain.

B.V. should receive a comprehensive assessment that includes a complete medical history and physical examination to determine any new underlying causes of pain, sensory deficits, or neurologic abnormalities. Physical function and pain associated with activities of daily living should be assessed as well as her psychosocial function to evaluate her for depression and to understand her social network and support system. A thorough evaluation of current pain should be performed to characterize her pain and to determine the patterns of her analgesic use and their effectiveness. The medication history should be reviewed for potential drug side effects and interactions. B.V.'s use of ibuprofen should be further evaluated, because older patients who use NSAID chronically have a higher frequency of GI bleeding, especially if they have a previous history of this condition.[208]

62. When asked, B.V. states that her current pain level is a 7 on a 10-point scale, and that it can vary from 4 to 8 during the day. It is usually better after rest and worsens later in the day, especially after physical exertion. Although she takes acetaminophen and ibuprofen regularly, they do not effectively reduce her pain. B.V. realizes that her current medical condition will probably not allow her to be completely pain free and states that a pain level of 3 would be acceptable. Would opiate analgesics be appropriate to control B.V.'s pain?

The use of opioid analgesic for chronic nonmalignant pain is controversial. The usefulness of this class of drugs should not be overlooked, however, and may provide fewer risks than long-term or high-dose NSAID therapy. The doses needed are often much smaller than those needed to treat chronic malignant pain. Older patients often experience greater pain relief from opioid analgesics than do younger patients, probably because both the extent and duration of analgesia are enhanced in this group.[211,212] Older patients achieve higher-than-expected plasma opioid levels (compared with younger patients) after IM or IV administration. Physiologic changes associated with aging, such as decreases in lean body mass, renal function, plasma proteins, hepatic blood flow, and hepatic metabolism,[213,214] may be responsible for the enhanced activity of opioids in older patients.[215]

When initiating opioid or adjunct analgesics in older patients, it is important to remember the phrase "start low and go slow." Because B.V. has underlying conditions that cause continuous pain, time-contingent dosing will be more beneficial. An appropriate initial regimen for B.V. using oxycodone HCl 2.5 mg and acetaminophen 325 mg would be one tablet orally every 6 hours, with one tablet every 4 hours as needed. This would provide continuous analgesic therapy throughout the day and allow B.V. flexibility to take an additional dose before activities that may exacerbate her pain. B.V. should be instructed to discontinue taking ibuprofen and to avoid other products containing acetaminophen. B.V. may also respond to tramadol 25 to 50 mg (i.e., 1/2–1 tablet) every 8 hours for her pain, because it has shown efficacy equivalent to NSAIDs in osteoarthritis pain. This agent can be considered as an alternative to a high-potency analgesic, but still presents a risk of dizziness and drowsiness.

B.V. should be monitored closely for sedation that could affect her concentration and ability to perform her activities of daily living. Because older patients are more sensitive to the constipating side effects of opioids, a bowel regimen consisting of a stimulant laxative and stool softener should be started at the beginning of therapy. Patients also should be encouraged to maintain good fluid intake and to include fruits and vegetables that are high in fiber in their diet. B.V.'s therapy should be adjusted based on careful monitoring for efficacy and side effects.

Neonates and Children

63. M.M., a 2-day-old, 3-kg girl, has just had bowel surgery for congenital bowel atresia. How should pain management be approached for M.M.?

Many misconceptions exist about the management of pain in the pediatric population. Historically, infants and children have been undertreated for pain and painful procedures. This is partly because of difficulty in communicating with, and evaluating pain, in children, particularly those who are nonverbal. It was also believed that children did not experience pain in the same way as adults do. Significant advances have been made in the understanding of children's pain perception, and assessment tools designed for different stages of development and communication abilities are available.[216,217] Nevertheless, misconceptions still exist, ranging from the amount of pain a child should experience after a painful procedure to the fear of addiction. Inadequately treated pain can interfere with the healing process, increase heart and respiratory rates, reduce oxygen saturation, and induce hyperglycemia and metabolic acidosis. Increased morbidity and mortality associated with unrelieved pain has been documented in neonates undergoing cardiac surgery.[218] The reality is that infants and children experience pain just as adults do and should receive appropriate medication and doses to treat their pain.

64. What would be a rational pain management plan for M.M.?

Because M.M. has had significant GI surgery, severe pain should be anticipated and prevented. Therefore, use of opiates, such as morphine or fentanyl, would be appropriate in this situation. Children appear to mature very early with respect to morphine metabolism. Infants as young as 5 months of age show very similar pharmacokinetic parameters as adults; however, morphine concentrations in patients younger than 2.4 months are five times higher than in older patients because of slower metabolic clearance and a lower central compartment volume of distribution.[219] The dosing of morphine in children is similar to adults on a milligram-per-kilogram basis, but children <5 months of age may require less-frequent dosing. The use of opiates in infants and children does not lead to addiction. Critically ill children who are receiving opiates for long periods of time develop tolerance and physical dependence and exhibit signs and symptoms of withdrawal if opiates are weaned too quickly, which however, should not preclude pediatric patients from receiving opiates.

An appropriate initial dosing regimen for M.M. would be fentanyl 1 mcg/kg IV every 4 hours with 1 mcg/kg every 2 hours as needed for breakthrough pain. When using parenteral morphine preparations in infants, close attention should be given to the preparation used and the age of the infant. Parenteral morphine preparations are available with and without preservatives. Infants <3 months of age are more susceptible to respiratory depression caused by an allergic reaction to the sulfites or to CNS irritation induced by benzyl alcohol. Thus, neonates and infants <3 months of age should receive only preservative-free morphine. When choosing a route of administration, attention should be given to the patient's clinical condition. Although oral routes are preferred, they may not be appropriate immediately following surgery. Opiates are frequently administered IM; however, IM administration offers no advantage over IV and causes much more pain and distress. Children receiving repeated IM injections often deny the presence of pain to avoid the injection.[217] Therefore, IV administration is the preferred parenteral route in pediatric patients.

Assessment of pain and relief in M.M. is more challenging because she is unable to verbalize specific information. Careful attention to behavioral responses, such as crying characteristics, crying duration, facial expressions, visual tracking, response to stimuli, and body movement, will be most useful in assessing pain and relief in M.M.[216,217] Heart rate, respiratory rate, blood pressure, and presence of diaphoresis can provide useful clues to M.M.'s level of pain or comfort and can alert the clinician to potential side effects. Careful monitoring, together with adjustments to the dose and frequency of administration, provides optimal therapy.

MORPHINE-INDUCED NAUSEA AND VOMITING

65. J.J., a 48-year-old woman, has advanced inoperable cervical cancer. The physician has ordered 30 mg of oral morphine solution every 4 hours for pain, but she has vomited after each dose despite apparently adequate doses of prochlorperazine. What can be done to relieve pain in J.J. who vomits after oral morphine?

Morphine and its derivatives induce nausea and vomiting by stimulating the chemoreceptor trigger zone (CTZ). Although the CTZ is stimulated initially, subsequent doses of morphine generally suppress the vomiting center. Because the incidence of nausea (40%) and vomiting (15%) increases in ambulatory patients, a vestibular component also is likely to be involved. If the vomiting is vestibular in origin, instructing J.J. to lie quietly, with as little head motion as possible for an hour or two, often will help. The nausea usually persists for 48 to 72 hours.[220]

Levorphanol (Levo-Dromoran) may cause less nausea and vomiting than other potent opioid analgesics at equianalgesic doses and might be an alternative to morphine if the aforementioned recommendations are ineffective in modifying J.J.'s nausea and vomiting. An equipotent dose of levorphanol for J.J., according to Table 8-3, would be 4 mg. The reported duration of action of levorphanol is 6 hours, longer than that of morphine.[221]

Adjunctive drugs such as droperidol, prochlorperazine, hydroxyzine, scopolamine, and diphenhydramine have been used successfully to control opioid-induced nausea and vomiting. Patients who are extremely sensitive to this opioid-induced effect have to be placed on concurrent or scheduled antiemetics; transdermal scopolamine can be used for this purpose. Although much more costly, agents such as ondansetron may also be useful in patients who have contraindications to the use of phenothiazines or butyrophenones.

USE OF CENTRAL NERVOUS SYSTEM STIMULANTS

66. D.H., a 34-year-old man, is diagnosed with acquired immunodeficiency syndrome (AIDS) and Kaposi's sarcoma. He was discharged from the hospital with a prescription for oral morphine solution, 30 mg every 3 hours. He has been relatively pain free for about a month, but now returns to the clinic complaining of excessive morning sedation. He cannot reduce his morphine dose because the pain makes him too uncomfortable. What therapeutic intervention can be used to alleviate D.H.'s problem of excessive morning sedation?

Limited clinical data suggest that a morning dose of methylphenidate (Ritalin) or dextroamphetamine (Dexedrine) could both relieve opioid-induced drowsiness and potentiate analgesia.[222] Less sleepiness has been associated with these combinations than with opioid analgesics alone, and a 10-mg dose of amphetamine combined with the opioid analgesic improved pain tolerance more than the analgesic alone.[223,224] Although these studies involved only single doses, these agents should cause sufficient CNS stimulation to obviate morning drowsiness. D.H. should try a morning dextroamphetamine dose of 5 to 20 mg. A somewhat smaller dose may be added around noon if he desires increased alertness in the late afternoon and early evening hours. Another alternative would be to switch D.H. to an opioid analgesic that is less sedating. Drugs such as hydromorphone, levorphanol, methadone, and fentanyl often produce the desired clinical response in a patient such as D.H.[225]

IMPORTANT DRUG INTERACTIONS

Phenytoin and Methadone

67. B.D., a 32-year-old man, has an 18-year history of chronic pain in the right hip as a result of a motor vehicle accident. He has a long problem list that includes grand mal seizures and gastric ulcer disease. In the past, he has been treated with a variety of opioid analgesics on an as needed schedule, which resulted in escalating drug requirements and a complex regimen of multiple-ingredient drugs (e.g., Percocet, Tylenol #3, Vicodin). B.D.'s attending physician prescribed methadone 10 mg every 6 hours several weeks ago. This switch was initially very successful, but B.D. now presents with symptoms suggestive of opioid withdrawal and poor pain control despite good compliance to his methadone regimen. A note in his chart indicates that B.D. saw a neurologist recently who started him on phenytoin therapy. What important drug–drug interactions might explain this rather complex case?

Phenytoin (Dilantin) induces cytochrome P450 (CYP) 3A4 isoenzymes that are responsible for the clearance of methadone, and can thereby decrease serum concentrations of methadone and precipitate symptoms of withdrawal.[226,227] The methadone dose should be increased to 20 mg every 6 hours, and a note should be made in the chart that the doses will need to be reduced if the phenytoin is discontinued for any reason. After his dose has been increased, B.D. should be watched closely for the next several days for drug-induced drowsiness because the long half-life of methadone can produce accumulation.

Cimetidine and Methadone

68. One week later, B.D.'s wife calls and says that he is very drowsy and that his speech has started to slur. On further questioning, his wife notes that B.D. restarted oral cimetidine 400 mg TID for symptoms of gastritis. She confirms that B.D. has been taking oral methadone 20 mg every 6 hours. What may explain B.D.'s symptoms of apparent opioid toxicity?

Cimetidine (Tagamet) inhibits CYP3A4 isoenzymes, thereby decreasing the metabolism of methadone and potentially subjecting patients to toxic levels. B.D. also could be reaching serum methadone steady-state levels at this time. He should be instructed to withhold the methadone until his mental status returns to baseline; then, the dose of methadone needs to be decreased to 10 mg every 6 hours. When adding cimetidine to existing methadone therapy, methadone doses need to be decreased; the doses should be increased again if cimetidine is subsequently withdrawn.[228]

Similar precautions need to be instituted for other CYP3A4 inhibitors, such as antiretroviral agents, ketoconazole or fluconazole, erythromycin, and other agents.

Codeine Interactions With CYP2D6 Inhibitors

Tramadol and SSRI

69. T.R. is a 42-year-old man who suffered a right tibial fracture requiring pinning and external fixation. He is now able to ambulate with crutches. Before discharge from the hospital, four acetaminophen 500 mg with hydrocodone 5-mg tablets throughout the day provided good pain control. At the time of discharge, T.R.'s pain regimen was changed to acetaminophen 325 mg with codeine 60 mg, two tablets orally every 3 to 4 hours, owing to his pharmacy benefit limitations. T.R. calls your office because the acetaminophen with codeine is not controlling his pain even when he takes two tablets every 3 hours. T.R. also is taking oral paroxetine 20 mg every morning for his chronic depression. His physician is considering switching his medication to tramadol or acetaminophen with oxycodone. What changes in T.R.'s therapy can be recommended to provide better pain control?

Codeine is metabolized to morphine in the liver by CYP2D6 isoenzymes. Concurrent administration of codeine with agents that inhibit the CYP2D6 system, such as paroxetine, fluoxetine, amiodarone, and ritonavir, may reduce the conversion of codeine to morphine and influence drug response.[229] In addition, this isoenzyme shows genetic polymorphism and individuals may demonstrate ultrarapid, extensive, or poor metabolism. Recognition of these potential drug interactions is important because concurrent administration of CYP2D6 inhibitors may make some patients appear to be poor metabolizers and less responsive to codeine, which, in fact, may not be true.

Oxycodone, hydrocodone, and tramadol are also substrates for the CYP2D6 isoenzyme. Although a potential interaction exists between oxycodone and paroxetine, little evidence at this time indicates that oxycodone requires conversion to an active metabolite via the 2D6 pathway to be an effective analgesic. However, tramadol is partially metabolized by CYP2D6 and has an active metabolite. Concurrent administration with a CYP2D6 inhibitor could potentially reduce analgesic activity.[229]

Coadministration of tramadol and paroxetine could potentially cause more serious problems in this patient. Tramadol has SSRI-like activity because it decreases the synaptic reuptake of norepinephrine and serotonin. Coadministration with SSRI agents, such as paroxetine, fluoxetine, fluvoxamine, and citalopram, can put the patient at risk for serotonin syndrome.[230] Signs and symptoms associated with serotonin syndrome include diaphoresis, chest pain, tachycardia, hypertension, confusion, psychosis, agitation, and tremor. Neurotoxicity can be severe and may progress to seizures or coma. Therefore, tramadol is not a good choice for this patient.

Similarly, tramadol can interact with the antimigraine agents known as "triptans," because their mode of action includes enhancing serotonin activity centrally. Therefore, combinations of tramadol, SSRI, or triptans are relatively contraindicated and require close and judicious monitoring.

It would be reasonable to consider either acetaminophen with oxycodone or hydrocodone for pain control in this patient, especially because he has experienced good pain control with the hydrocodone preparation in the past.

PRIMARY DYSMENORRHEA

70. P.O., a 27-year-old woman, is seen in the primary care clinic because of severe abdominal pain secondary to her menstrual periods. She reports having pain-free menstrual periods only once or twice yearly. She has been diagnosed as having primary dysmenorrhea with no other gynecologic pathology being found. How should P.O.'s menstrual pain be treated?

Primary dysmenorrhea is a common gynecologic disorder affecting 60% to 80% of women at some time in their life.[231] Pain usually occurs 2 to 12 hours before the commencement of menstrual flow, but it can occur simultaneously with, or a few hours after, the beginning of menstruation. It reaches maximal intensity at 2 to 24 hours, then decreases over the next few days.[232] Primary dysmenorrhea is associated with increases in endometrial and circulatory prostaglandins. Thus, NSAIDs, which alter the production of the prostaglandins, are frequently used to manage primary dysmenorrhea. The dosages required for the treatment of primary dysmenorrhea usually are higher than those used for analgesia, but frequently a single dose is sufficient to terminate the dysmenorrhea pain. On some occasions, frequent, high doses may be required.

The best time to initiate an NSAID remains controversial. Some clinicians recommend beginning drug therapy a few days before the start of menses; others argue that the prostaglandins are not stored and, therefore, prefer to initiate drug therapy only after the start of menses. Pretreatment with an NSAID carries the risk of fetal drug exposure during early pregnancy. Studies comparing pretreatment with dosing at the onset of menses show no difference in the analgesia between either of the regimens.[233,234] (Also see Chapter 47, Treatment of Menstrual and Menstrual-Related Disorders.) P.O. should be instructed to take 600 to 800 mg of ibuprofen at the onset of menses or when discomfort begins. Repeat dosages of 400 to 600 mg may be taken every 4 to 6 hours as needed. If this regimen is ineffective, she can take the first dose 1 to 2 days before the first day of menses is expected.

HEADACHES

71. M.K., a 32-year-old man, is complaining of severe headaches that occur at least once every 2 weeks. He takes two Excedrin extra-strength tablets (acetaminophen 250 mg, aspirin 250 mg, and caffeine 65 mg) every 2 hours until the headache starts to ease and sometimes requires a cumulative dose of up to 16 tablets. Migraine and vascular headaches have been ruled out in M.K.

Would one of the nonsalicylate NSAIDs be more efficacious for M.K.? Are there any other considerations in managing M.K.'s headache? Is caffeine an effective analgesic for headaches?

Headaches are common, afflicting nearly everyone at some time during their life. The incidence of headache is higher in females and increases with age; 10% of headaches develop into chronic disabling conditions. For M.K., who self-medicates chronically with large doses of acetaminophen, the concern is toxicity from the analgesics. Chronic use of both NSAID analgesics and caffeine (either as single agents or in combination) can possibly precipitate withdrawal ("rebound") headaches on discontinuation. Although NSAIDs are not considered habituating, accumulating evidence indicates that chronic intake of peripheral-acting analgesics can perpetuate the underlying pain syndrome. In the case of M.K., it is important to consider the possibility of caffeine withdrawal headache as well, because he is taking a caffeine-containing combination product. Other dietary sources of caffeine ingestion from coffee, tea, and other foods should be determined as well.

Caffeine is used in analgesic combination products because it has both a CNS stimulant and a vasoconstrictive effect, which may reverse some of the headache symptoms. The value of caffeine, especially in the small quantities found in most pain relievers, has been controversial. A meta-analysis and subsequent study conclude, however, that caffeine does add to the analgesic effect of aspirin and acetaminophen.[235,236]

Acute headache can be managed with parenteral ketorolac, but it is not a viable alternative for chronic headache management.[237] M.K.'s headaches may resolve on gradual withdrawal of NSAID analgesics and caffeine, but this process is slow and requires the clinician's as well as the patient's determination to stay with the treatment plan. (Also see Chapter 53, Headache.)

PROCEDURAL PAIN

72. C.T., a 26-year-old woman, injured her left knee during a fall while skiing. After immobilizing her left knee and using ice therapy, most of her swelling has subsided. She is now seen in the outpatient surgical center for an arthroscopic evaluation of her knee. She is very concerned that the lidocaine that is to be used to anesthetize her knee is going to produce pain, because she has had a bad experience with regional lidocaine injections. What can be recommended to reduce the pain associated with lidocaine infiltration?

Lidocaine injection is quite acidic and can produce local irritation and pain during the infiltration procedure before the anesthetic effect takes place. Because this is a common complaint, C.T.'s concerns should be taken seriously. A simple solution is to neutralize the lidocaine injection solution by adding 1 mL of 1 mEq/mL sodium bicarbonate to 9 mL of 1% to 2% lidocaine before injecting C.T.[238,239] Because lidocaine is stable over a wide range of pH values, the bicarbonate will not reduce its efficacy of local anesthetic blockade. This technique should not be used with other local anesthetics, however, because they may be subject to rapid degradation by basic agents.

TOPICAL ANESTHETICS AND ANALGESICS

73. J.G., a 6-year-old boy, is being treated for osteomyelitis of his foot as a result of a skate boarding accident. Because of the need for long-term antibiotic therapy, he requires occasional IV access replacement. He is very fearful of the procedure because of the associated pain. What can be offered to J.G. to reduce his discomfort?

Insertion of a venous catheter often produces significant discomfort and pain, but there is no reason C.T. has to endure it. Topical lidocaine–prilocaine cream (EMLA) can provide good pain relief during catheter insertion for minor surgical procedures such as circumcision and skin grafts.[240,241] The cream must be applied 30 to 60 minutes before the procedure with an occlusive dressing; the anesthetic effect lasts approximately 60 to 120 minutes.[242] A smaller-gauge catheter also may reduce the amount of pain associated with the venipuncture.[243]

REFERENCES

1. Fields HL. *Pain.* New York: McGraw-Hill; 1987:364.
2. Heller PH et al. Peripheral neural contributions to inflammation. In: Fields HL et al., eds. *Pharmacological Approach to the Treatment of Chronic Pain. Progress in Pain Research and Management.* Seattle: IASP Press; 1994:31.
3. Dickenson AH. The roles of transmitters and their receptors in systems related to pain and analgesia. In: Max M, ed. *Pain 1999: an updated review.* Seattle: IASP Press; 1999:381.
4. Wilcox GL. Pharmacology of pain and analgesia. In: Max M, ed. *Pain 1999: an updated review.* Seattle: IASP Press; 1999:573.
5. Dickenson AH et al. Mechanisms of chronic pain and the developing nervous system. In: McGrath PJ et al., eds. *Chronic and Recurrent Pain in Children and Adolescents. Progress in Pain Research and Management.* Seattle: IASP Press; 1999:5.
6. Besson JM. The neurobiology of pain. *Lancet.* 1999;353:1610.
7. Golianu B et al. Pediatric acute pain management. *Pediatr Clin N Am* 2000;47:559.
8. McCaffery M et al. *Pain: Clinical Manual.* St. Louis: Mosby; 1999:15.
9. Woolf CJ et al. Neuropathic pain: aetiology, symptoms, mechanisms, and management. *Lancet* 1999;353:1959.
10. McMahon SB et al. Silent afferents and visceral pain. In: Fields H et al., eds. *Pharmacological Approach to the Treatment of Chronic Pain. Progress in Pain Research and Management.* Seattle: IASP Press; 1994:11.
11. Willis WD Jr. Introduction to the basic science of pain and headache for the clinician: physiological concepts. In: Max M, ed. *Pain 1999: an updated review.* Seattle: IASP Press; 1999:561.
12. Price DP et al. Central neural mechanisms of normal and abnormal pain state. In: Fields HL et al., eds. *Pharmacological Approach to the Treatment of Chronic Pain. Progress in Pain Research and Management.* Seattle: IASP Press; 1994:61.
13. Dickenson AH. NMDA receptor antagonists as analgesics. In: Fields HL et al., eds. *Pharmacological Approach to the Treatment of Chronic Pain. Progress in Pain Research and Management.* Seattle: IASP Press; 1994:173.
14. Pini LA et al. Serotonin and opiate involvement in the antinociceptive effect of acetylsalicylic acid. *Pharmacology* 1997;54:84.
15. Sandrini M et al. Central antinociceptive activity of acetylsalicylic acid is modulated by brain serotonin receptor subtypes. *Pharmacology* 2002;65: 1937.
16. Dickenson AH. Where and how do opioids act? Proceedings of the 7th World Congress on Pain. *Progress in Pain Research and Management* 1994;2:525.
17. Clinical Practice Guideline, Cancer Pain Management. U.S. Department of Health and Human Services, Agency for Health Care Policy and Research. AHCPR Pub. Rockville, MD; 1994.
18. Porternoy RK. Opioids and adjuvant analgesics. In: Max M, ed. *Pain 1999: an updated review.* Seattle: IASP Press; 1999:3.
19. Max MB et al. Effects of desipramine, amitriptyline, and fluoxetine on pain in diabetic neuropathy. *N Engl J Med* 1992;326:1250.
20. Beaver WT et al. Comparison of the analgesic effects of morphine, hydroxyzine, and their combination in patients with postoperative pain. In: Bonica JJ et al., eds. *Advances in Pain Research and Therapy.* New York: Raven Press; 1976:553.
21. American Pain Society. Principles of analgesic use in the treatment of acute and chronic cancer pain. 2nd ed. *Clin Pharm* 1990;9:601.

22. LoVecchio F et al. The use of analgesics in patients with acute abdominal pain. *J Emerg Med* 1997;15:775.
23. Pace S et al. Intravenous morphine for early pain relief in patients with acute abdominal pain. *Acad Emerg Med* 1996;3:1086.
24. Clinical Practice Guideline, Acute Pain Management. U.S. Department of Health and Human Services, Agency for Health Care Policy and Research. AHCPR Pub. No. 92-0032. Rockville, MD; 1992.
25. Krames ES. Intrathecal infusional therapies for intractable pain: patient management guidelines. *J Pain Symptom Manage* 1993;8:36.
26. Skevington SM. The relationship between pain and depression: a longitudinal study of early synovitis. Proceedings of the 7th World Congress on Pain. *Progress in Pain Research and Management* 1994;2:201.
27. Gureje O et al. Persistent pain and well-being: a World Health Organization study in primary care. *JAMA* 1998;280:147.
28. Ashburn MA et al. Management of chronic pain. *Lancet* 1999;353:1865.
29. Rowbotham MC et al. Oral opioid therapy for chronic peripheral and central neuropathic pain. *N Engl J Med.* 2003 Mar 27;348:1223.
30. Weissman DE. Doctors, opioids, and the law: the effect of controlled substances regulations on cancer pain management. *Semin Oncol* 1993;20(2 Suppl 1):53.
31. Hill CS Jr. The barriers to adequate pain management with opioid analgesics. *Semin Oncol* 1993;20(2 Suppl 1):1.
32. Weinstein SM et al. Physicians' attitudes toward pain and the use of opioid analgesics: results of a survey from the Texas Cancer Pain Initiative. *South Med J* 2000;93:479.
33. Sloan PA et al. Cancer pain assessment and management by housestaff. *Pain* 1996;67:475.
34. Foley KM. The treatment of cancer pain. *N Engl J Med* 1985;313:84.
34a. World Health Organization. Cancer pain relief and palliative care. Report of a WHO expert committee [World Health Organization Technical Report Series, 804]. Geneva, Switzerland: World Health Organization; 1990.
35. World Health Organization guidelines at http://www.who.int/cancer/palliative/painladder/en/.
36. Fishbain et al. Genetic testing for enzymes of drug metabolism: does it have clinical utility for pain medicine at the present time? A structured review. *Pain Med* 2004;5:81.
37. Stamer UM et al. Genetics and variability in opioid response. *Eur J Pain* 2005;101.
38. Claiborne R. A patient looks at pain and analgesia. *Hosp Pract* 1982;17:21.
39. Donovan BD. Patient attitudes to postoperative pain relief. *Anesthesia and Intensive Care* 1983;11:125.
40. Cooper SA et al. Comparative analgesic potency of aspirin and ibuprofen. *J Oral Surg* 1977;35:898.
41. Winter L Jr et al. Analgesic activity of ibuprofen (Motrin) in postoperative oral surgical pain. *Oral Surg Oral Med Oral Pathol* 1978;45:159.
42. Heidrich G et al. Efficacy and quality of ibuprofen and acetaminophen plus codeine analgesia. *Pain* 1985;22:385.
43. Indelicato PA et al. Comparison of diflunisal and acetaminophen with codeine in the treatment of mild to moderate pain due to strains and sprains. *Clin Ther* 1986;8:269.
44. Lasagna L. Analgesic methodology: a brief history and commentary. *J Clin Pharmacol* 1980;20(Pt. 2):373.
45. Levine J et al. Relationship of duration of analgesia to opioid pharmacokinetic variables. *Brain Res* 1983;289:391.
46. Hammack JE et al. Use of orally administered opioids for cancer-related pain. *Mayo Clin Proc* 1994;69:384.
47. Davis T et al. Comparative morphine pharmacokinetics following sublingual, intramuscular, and oral administration in patients with cancer. *Hospice* 1993;9:85.
48. Crews JC et al. Clinical efficacy of methadone in patients refractory to other mu-opioid receptor agonist analgesics for management of terminal cancer pain. Case presentations and discussion of incomplete cross-tolerance among opioid agonist analgesics. *Cancer* 1993;72:2266.
49. Miller RR. Propoxyphene: a review. *Am J Hosp Pharm* 1977;34:413.
50. Li Wan Po A et al. Systematic overview of coproxamol to assess analgesic effects in addition of dextropropoxyphene to paracetamol. *BMJ* 1997; 315:1565.
51. Beaver WT. Analgesic efficacy of dextropropoxyphene and dextropropoxyphene-containing combinations: a review. *Human Toxicology* 1984; 3(Suppl):191S.
52. Almirall J et al. Propoxyphene-induced hypoglycemia in a patient with chronic renal failure. *Nephron* 1989;53:273.
53. Savage SR. Chronic pain and the disease of addiction: the interfacing roles of pain medicine and addiction medicine. In: Max M, ed. *Pain 1999: an updated review.* Seattle: IASP Press; 1999:115.
54. Portenoy RK. Opioid therapy for chronic nonmalignant pain: a review of critical issues. *J Pain Symptom Manage* 1996;11:203.
55. Lewis JH. Hepatic toxicity of nonsteroidal antiinflammatory drugs. *Clin Pharm* 1984;3:128.
56. Seeff LB et al. Acetaminophen hepatotoxicity in alcoholics. A therapeutic misadventure. *Ann Intern Med* 1986;104:399.
57. Baldo BA et al. Chemistry of drug allergenicity. *Curr Opin Allergy Clin Immunol* 2001;1:327.
58. Longo WE et al. Prokinetic agents for lower gastrointestinal motility disorders. *Dis Colon Rectum* 1993;36:696.
59. Laizure SC. Considerations in morphine therapy. *Am J Hosp Pharm* 1994;51:2042.
60. Chun-Su Y et al. Methylnaltrexone for reversal of constipation due to chronic methadone use: a randomized controlled trial. *JAMA* 2000;283:367.
61. Clark RF. Meperidine: therapeutic use and toxicity. *J Emerg Med* 1995;13:797.
62. Catapano MS. The analgesic efficacy of ketorolac for acute pain. *J Emerg Med* 1996;14:67.
63. Neighbor ML et al. Intramuscular ketorolac vs oral ibuprofen in emergency department patients with acute pain. *Acad Emerg Med* 1998;5:118.
64. Tramer MR et al. Comparing analgesic efficacy of non-steroidal antiinflammatory drugs given by different routes in acute and chronic pain: a qualitative systematic review. *Acta Anaesthesiol Scand* 1998;42:71.
65. Chaiamnuay S et al. Risks versus benefits of cyclooxygenase-2-selective nonsteroidal antiinflammatory drugs. *Am J Health Syst Pharm* 2006;63:1837.
66. Hallen H et al. The nasal reactivity in patients with nasal polyps. *ORL J Otorhinolaryngol Relat Spec* 1994;56:276.
67. Muther RS et al. Aspirin-induced depression of glomerular filtration rate in normal humans: role of sodium balance. *Ann Intern Med* 1981;94:317.
68. Schoch PH et al. Acute renal failure in an elderly woman following intramuscular ketorolac administration. *Ann Pharmacother* 1992;26:1233.
69. Pearce CJ et al. Renal failure and hyperkalemia associated with ketorolac tromethamine. *Arch Intern Med* 1993;153:1000.
70. Epstein M. Renal prostaglandins and the control of renal function in liver disease. *Am J Med* 1986;80(Suppl 1A):46.
71. Zipser RD et al. Implication of nonsteroidal antiinflammatory drug therapy. *Am J Med* 1986;80 (Suppl 1A):78.
72. Brater DC. Drug–drug and drug-disease interactions with nonsteroidal anti-inflammatory drugs. *Am J Med* 1986;80(Suppl 1A):62.
73. Dunn MJ et al. Renal effects of drugs that inhibit prostaglandin synthesis. *Kidney Int* 1980;18:609.
74. Blackshear JL et al. NSAID-induced nephrotoxicity, avoidance, detection and treatment. *Drug Ther Hosp* 1983;(Nov.):47.
75. Zipser RD et al. Prostaglandins: modulators of renal function and pressor resistance in chronic liver disease. *J Clin Endocrinol Metab* 1979;48: 895.
76. Donker AJ et al. The effect of indomethacin on kidney function and plasma renin activity in man. *Nephron* 1976;17:288.
77. Walsche JJ et al. Acute oliguric renal failure induced by indomethacin. Possible mechanism. *Ann Intern Med* 1979;91:47.
78. Favre L et al. Reversible renal failure from combined triamterene and indomethacin. *Ann Intern Med* 1982;96:317.
79. Stillman MT et al. Adverse effects of nonsteroidal anti-inflammatory drugs on the kidney. *Med Clin North Am* 1982;68:371.
80. Finkelstein A et al. Fenoprofen nephropathy: lipoid nephrosis and interstitial nephritis. A possible T-lymphocyte disorder. *Am J Med* 1982;72:81.
81. Fung DL et al. A comparison of alphaprodine and meperidine pharmacokinetics. *J Clin Pharmacol* 1980;20:37.
82. Poniatowski BC. Continuous subcutaneous infusions for pain control. *Journal of Intravenous Nursing* 1991;14:30.
83. Lang AH et al. Treatment of severe cancer pain by continuous infusion of subcutaneous opioids. *Recent Results Cancer Res* 1991;121:51.
84. Sawaki Y et al. Patient and nurse evaluation of patient-controlled analgesia delivery systems for postoperative pain management. *J Pain Symptom Manage* 1992;7:443.
85. Shaffer HJ et al. Patterns of substance use among methadone maintenance patients. Indicators of outcome. *J Subst Abuse Treat* 1992;9:143.
86. Gossop M et al. Severity of dependence and route of administration of heroin, cocaine and amphetamines. *Br J Addict* 1992;87:1527.
87. Hoffman M et al. Pain management in the opioid-addicted patient with cancer. *Cancer* 1991;68:1121.
88. Rickford WJ et al. Epidural analgesia in labour and maternal posture. *Anaesthesia* 1983;38:1169.
89. Conacher ID et al. Epidural analgesia following thoracic surgery. A review of two years' experience. *Anaesthesia* 1983;38:546.
90. Adu-Gymafi Y et al. High dose epidural morphine for surgical analgesia. *Middle East J Anaesthesiol* 1985;8:165.
91. Haynes SR et al. Comparison of epidural methadone with epidural diamorphine for analgesia following caesarean section. *Acta Anaesthesiol Scand* 1993;37:375.
92. Jacobson L et al. Intrathecal methadone: a dose-response study and comparison with intrathecal morphine 0.5 mg. *Pain* 1990;43:141.
93. Krames ES. Intrathecal infusional therapies for intractable pain: patient management guidelines. *J Pain Symptom Manage* 1993;8:36.
94. Uhde TW et al. Clonidine suppresses the opioid abstinence syndrome without clonidine-withdrawal symptoms: a blind inpatient study. *Psychiatry Res* 1980;2:37.
95. Bond WS. Psychiatric indications for clonidine: the neuropharmacologic and clinical basis. *J Clin Psychopharmacol* 1986;6:81.
96. Gold MS et al. Opiate withdrawal using clonidine. A safe, effective and rapid non-opiate treatment. *JAMA* 1980;243:343.
97. MacGregor TR et al. Pharmacokinetics of transdermally delivered clonidine. *Clin Pharmacol Ther* 1985;38:278.
98. Arndts D et al. Pharmacokinetics and pharmacodynamics of transdermally administered clonidine. *Eur J Clin Pharmacol* 1984;26:78.
99. Clark HW et al. Clonidine transdermal patches: a recovery oriented treatment of opiate withdrawal. *California Society for the Treatment of Alcohol Other Drug Dependency News* 1986;13:1.
100. Kanto J et al. Obstetric analgesia: pharmacokinetics and its relation to neonatal behavioral and adaptive functions. *Biological Research in Pregnancy and Perinatology* 1984;5:23.
101. Mirkin BL. Perinatal pharmacology: placental

transfer, fetal localization, and neonatal disposition of drugs. *Anesthesiology* 1975;43:156.
102. Nation RL. Drug kinetics in childbirth. *Clin Pharmacokinet* 1980;5:340.
103. Jepson HA et al. The Apgar score: evolution, limitations, and scoring guidelines. *Birth* 1991;18:83.
104. Bardy AH et al. Objectively measured perinatal exposure to meperidine and benzodiazepines in Finland. *Clin Pharmacol Ther* 1994;55:471.
105. Nimmo WS et al. Narcotic analgesics and delayed gastric emptying during labour. *Lancet* 1975; 1: 890.
106. Refstad SO et al. Ventilatory depressions of the newborn of women receiving pethidine or pentazocine. *Br J Anaesth* 1980;52:265.
107. Atkinson BD et al. Double-blind comparison of intravenous butorphanol (Stadol) and fentanyl (Sublimaze) for analgesia during labor. *Am J Obstet Gynecol* 1994;171:993.
108. Isenor L et al. Intravenous meperidine infusion for obstetric analgesia. *J Obstet Gynecol Neonatal Nurs* 1993;22:349.
109. Rosaeg OP et al. Maternal and fetal effects of intravenous patient-controlled fentanyl analgesia during labour in a thrombocytopenic patient. *Can J Anaesth* 1992;39:277.
110. Galloway FM et al. Comparison of analgesia by intravenous butorphanol and meperidine in patients with post-operative pain. *Can Anaesth Soc J* 1977;24:90.
111. Ameer B et al. Drug therapy reviews: evaluation of butorphanol tartrate. *Am J Hosp Pharm* 1979;36:1683.
112. Sprigge JS et al. Nalbuphine versus meperidine for post-operative analgesia: a double-blind comparison using the patient controlled analgesic technique. *Canadian Anaesthesiology Society Journal* 1983;30:517.
113. Young RE. Double-blind placebo controlled oral analgesic comparison of butorphanol and pentazocine in patients with moderate to severe post-operative pain. *J Int Med Res* 1977;5:422.
114. Dayer P et al. The pharmacology of tramadol. *Drugs* 1994;47(Suppl 1):3.
115. Lee CR et al. Tramadol: a preliminary review of its pharmacodynamic and pharmacokinetic properties, and therapeutic potential in acute and chronic pain states. *Drugs* 1993;46:313.
116. Stubhaug A et al. Lack of analgesic effect of 50 and 100 mg oral tramadol after orthopaedic surgery: a randomized, double-blind, placebo and standard active drug comparison. *Pain* 1995;62:111.
117. Moore PA et al. Tramadol hydrochloride: analgesic efficacy compared with codeine, aspirin with codeine, and placebo after dental extraction. *J Clin Pharmacol* 1998;38:554.
118. Ortho-McNeil Pharmaceuticals, Inc. Ultram package insert. Raritan, NJ: April, 1998.
119. Spiller HA et al. Prospective multicenter evaluation of tramadol exposure. *J Toxicol* 1997; 35:361.
120. Tobias JD. Seizures after tramadol overdose. *South Med J* 1997;90:826.
121. Portenoy RK et al. Transdermal fentanyl for cancer pain. Repeated dose pharmacokinetics. *Anesthesiology* 1993;78:36.
122. Payne R. Transdermal fentanyl: suggested recommendations for clinical use. *J Pain Symptom Manage* 1992;7(3 Suppl):S40.
123. Calis KA et al. Transdermally administered fentanyl for pain management. *Clin Pharm* 1992;11: 22.
124. Rose PG et al. Fentanyl transdermal system overdose secondary to cutaneous hyperthermia. *Anesth Analg* 1993;77:390.
125. DeSio JM et al. Intravenous abuse of transdermal fentanyl therapy in a chronic pain patient. *Anesthesiology* 1993;79:1139.
126. Lichtor JL et al. The relative potency of oral transmucosal fentanyl citrate compared with intravenous morphine in the treatment of moderate to severe postoperative pain. *Anesth Analg* 1999;89:732.
127. Cephalon Incorporated. Fentora package insert. Salt Lake City, UT: Jun, 2006.
128. Cohen FL. Postsurgical pain relief: patients' status and nurses' medication choices. *Pain* 1980;9:265.
129. Morland TJ et al. Doxepin in the prophylactic treatment of mixed 'vascular' and tension headache. *Headache* 1979;19:382.
130. Westerling D et al. Absorption and bioavailability of rectally administered morphine in women. *Eur J Clin Pharmacol* 1982;23:59.
131. Westerling D. Rectally administered morphine: plasma concentration in children premedicated with morphine in hydrogel and in solution. *Acta Anaesthesiol Scand* 1985;29:653.
132. Babul N et al. Pharmacokinetics of two novel rectal controlled-release morphine formulations. *J Pain Symptom Manage* 1992;7:400.
133. Wilkinson TJ et al. Pharmacokinetics and efficacy of rectal versus oral sustained-release morphine in cancer patients. *Cancer Chemother Pharmacol* 1992;31:251.
134. Feinmann C. Pain relief by antidepressants: possible modes of action. *Pain* 1985;23:1.
135. Kocher R. The use of psychotropic drugs in the treatment of chronic, severe pain. *Eur Neurol* 1976; 14:458.
136. Ward NG et al. The effectiveness of tricyclic antidepressants in the treatment of coexisting pain and depression. *Pain* 1979;7:331.
137. Adler RH. Psychotropic agents in the management of chronic pain. *Journal of Human Stress* 1978;4:15.
138. Urban BJ et al. Long-term use of narcotic/antidepressant medication in the management of phantom limb pain. *Pain* 1986;24:191.
139. Fainsinger R et al. Methadone in the management of cancer pain: a review. *Pain* 1993;52:137.
140. Fainsinger R et al. Methadone in the management of cancer pain: a review. *Pain* 1993;52:137.
141. Berkowitz BA. The relationship of pharmacokinetics to pharmacological activity: morphine, methadone and naloxone. *Clin Pharmacokinet* 1976;1:219.
142. Symonds P. Methadone and the elderly. *BMJ* 1977;1:512.
143. Gourlay GK et al. A comparative study of the efficacy and pharmacokinetics of oral methadone and morphine in the treatment of severe pain in patients with cancer. *Pain* 1986;25:297.
144. Miser AW et al. Continuous intravenous infusion of morphine sulfate for control of severe pain in children with terminal malignancy. *J Pediatr* 1980;96:930.
145. Church JJ. Continuous narcotic infusions for relief of postoperative pain. *BMJ* 1979;1:977.
146. Hupert C et al. Effect of hydroxyzine on morphine analgesia for the treatment of postoperative pain. *Anesth Analg* 1980;59:690.
147. Stambaugh JE Jr et al. Analgesic efficacy and pharmacokinetic evaluation of meperidine and hydroxyzine, alone and in combination. *Cancer Invest* 1983;1:111.
148. Rumore MM et al. Clinical efficacy of antihistaminics as analgesics. *Pain* 1986;25:7.
149. Rumore MM et al. Analgesic effects of antihistaminics. *Life Sci* 1985;36:403.
150. Vecht CJ. Clinical Management of brain metastasis. *J Neurol* 1998;245:127.
151. Campa JA 3rd et al. The management of intractable bone pain: a clinician's perspective. *Semin Nucl Med* 1992;22:3.
152. Miller LJ et al. Pain management with intravenous ketorolac. *Ann Pharmacother* 1993;27:307.
153. Terman GW et al. A case of opiate-insensitive pain: malignant treatment of benign pain. *Clin J Pain* 1992;8:255.
154. Goldman B. Use and abuse of opioid analgesics in chronic pain. *Can Fam Physician* 1993;39:571.
155. Bowsher D. Pain syndromes and their treatment. *Curr Opin Neurol Neurosurg* 1993;6:257.
156. Mercadante S et al. Hyperalgesia: an emerging iatrogenic syndrome. *J Pain Symptom Manage* 2003;26:769.
157. Sjögren P et al. Hyperalgesia and myoclonus in terminal cancer patients treated with continuous intravenous morphine. *Pain* 1993;55:93.
158. Romac DR. Safety of prolonged, high-dose infusion of naloxone hydrochloride for severe methadone overdose. *Clin Pharm* 1986;5:251.
159. Lewis JM et al. Continuous naloxone infusion in pediatric narcotic overdose. *Am J Dis Child* 1984;138:944.
160. Wang DS et al. Nalmefene: a long-acting opioid antagonist. Clinical implications in emergency medicine. *J Emerg Med* 1998;16:471.
161. Kaplan JL et al. Double-blind, randomized study of nalmefene and naloxone in emergency department patients with suspected narcotic overdose. *Ann Emerg Med* 1999;34:42.
162. Quan DB et al. Clonidine in pain management. *Ann Pharmacother* 1993;27:313.
163. Sullivan MJ et al. The treatment of depression in chronic low back pain: review and recommendations. *Pain* 1992;50:5.
164. Herr KA et al. Depression and the experience of chronic back pain: a study of related variables and age differences. *Clin J Pain* 1993;9:104.
165. Gonzales GR. Postherpes simplex type 1 neuralgia simulating postherpetic neuralgia. *J Pain Symptom Manage* 1992;7:320.
166. Max MB et al. Effects of desipramine, amitriptyline, and fluoxetine on pain in diabetic neuropathy. *N Engl J Med* 1992;326:1250.
167. Penfold J et al. Pain syndromes in HIV infection. *Can J Anaesth* 1992;39:724.
168. Kerrick JM et al. Low-dose amitriptyline as an adjunct to opioids for postoperative orthopedic pain: a placebo-controlled trial. *Pain* 1993;52:325.
169. Dillin W et al. Analysis of medications used in the treatment of cervical disk degeneration. *Orthop Clin North Am* 1992;23:421.
170. Onghena P et al. Antidepressant-induced analgesia in chronic non-malignant pain: a meta-analysis of 39 placebo-controlled studies. *Pain* 1992;49:205.
171. Max MB et al. Effects of desipramine, amitriptyline, and fluoxetine on pain in diabetic neuropathy. *N Engl J Med* 1992;326:1250.
172. Acton J et al. Amitriptyline produces analgesia in the formalin pain test. *Exp Neurol* 1992;117:94.
173. Panerai AE et al. Antidepressants in cancer pain. *J Palliat Care* 1991;7:42.
174. Conn DK et al. Pattern of use of antidepressants in long-term care facilities for the elderly. *J Geriatr Psychiatry Neurol* 1992;5:228.
175. Goldstein DJ et al. Duloxetine vs. placebo in patients with painful diabetic neuropathy. *Pain* 2005;116:109.
176. Attal N. et al. EFNS guidelines on pharmacological treatment of neuropathic pain. *Eur Neurol* 2006;13:1153.
177. Backonja M et al. Gabapentin for the symptomatic treatment of painful neuropathy in patients with diabetes mellitus. *JAMA* 1998;280:1831.
178. Rowbotham M et al. Gabapentin for the treatment of postherpetic neuralgia: a randomized controlled trial. *JAMA* 1998;280:1837.
179. Dubinsky RM et al. Practice parameter: treatment of postherpetic neuralgia: an evidence-based report of the Quality Standards Subcommittee of the American Academy of Neurology. *Neurology* 2004;63:959.
180. Smith AL et al. Cerebral blood flow and metabolism: effects of anesthetic drugs and techniques. *Anesthesiology* 1972;36:378.
181. Albanese J et al. Sufentanil increases intracranial pressure in patients with head trauma. *Anesthesiology* 1993;79:493.
182. Vandam LD. Drug therapy: butorphanol. *N Engl J Med* 1980;302:381.
183. Scott DH et al. Haemodynamic changes following buprenorphine and morphine. *Anaesthesia* 1980;35:957.
184. Gaensler EA et al. A comparative study of the action of Demerol and opium alkaloids in relation to biliary spasm. *Surgery* 1948;23:211.
185. Chisholm RJ et al. Narcotics and spasm of the sphincter of Oddi. A retrospective study of operative cholangiograms. *Anaesthesia* 1983;38: 689.

186. Radnay PA et al. Common bile duct pressure changes after fentanyl, morphine, meperidine, butorphanol, and naloxone. *Anesth Analg* 1984; 63:441.
187. Radnay PA et al. The effect of equi-analgesic doses of fentanyl, morphine, meperidine and pentazocine on common bile duct pressure. *Anaesthesist* 1980;29:26.
188. Staritz M et al. Effect of modern analgesic drugs (tramadol, pentazocine, and buprenorphine) on the bile duct sphincter in man. *Gut* 1986;27:567.
189. Economou G et al. A cross-over comparison of the effect of morphine, pethidine, pentazocine, and phenazocine on biliary pressure. *Gut* 1971; 12:216.
190. Hopton DS et al. Action of various new analgesic drugs on the human common bile duct. *Gut* 1967;8:296.
191. McCammon RL et al. Reversal of fentanyl induced spasm of the sphincter of Oddi. *Surg Gynecol Obstet* 1983;156:329.
192. McCammon RL et al. Naloxone reversal of choledochoduodenal sphincter spasm associated with narcotic administration. *Anesthesiology* 1978; 48:437.
193. McLean ER Jr et al. Cholangiographic demonstration of relief of narcotic-induced spasm of the sphincter of Oddi. *Am Surg* 1982;48:134.
194. Sykes NP. Oral naloxone in opioid-associated constipation [Letter]. *Lancet* 1991;337:1475.
195. Larsen LS et al. The use of intravenous ketorolac for the treatment of renal colic in the emergency department. *Am J Emerg Med* 1993;11:197.
196. Hoyampa AM Jr et al. The disposition and effects of sedatives and analgesics in liver disease. *Ann Rev Med* 1978;29:205.
197. Klotz U et al. The effect of cirrhosis on the disposition and elimination of meperidine in man. *Clin Pharmacol Ther* 1974;16:667.
198. Roberts RK et al. Drug prescribing in hepatobiliary disease. *Drugs* 1979;17:198.
199. Pond SM et al. Enhanced bioavailability of pethidine and pentazocine in patients with cirrhosis of the liver. *Aust NZ J Med* 1980;10:515.
200. Lehmann KA et al. CO_2-response curves as a measure of opiate-induced respiratory depression. Studies with fentanyl. *Anaesthesist* 1983;32:242.
201. Gal TJ et al. Analgesic and respiratory depressant activity of nalbuphine: a comparison with morphine. *Anesthesiology* 1982;57:367.
202. Nagashima H et al. Respiratory and circulatory effects of intravenous butorphanol and morphine. *Clin Pharmacol Ther* 1976;19:738.
203. Heel RC et al. Buprenorphine: a review of its pharmacological properties and therapeutic efficacy. *Drugs* 1979;17:81.
204. Bailey CJ et al. Epidural morphine infusion. Continuous pain relief. *AORN J* 1984;39:997.
205. Jones SF, White A. Analgesia following femoral neck surgery. Lateral cutaneous nerve block as an alternative to narcotics in the elderly. *Anaesthesia* 1985;40:682.
206. Ostermeier et al. Three sudden postoperative respiratory arrests associated with epidural opioids in patients with sleep apnea. *Anesth* Analg1997;2: 452.
207. Jain SS et al. Perioperative treatment of patients with obstructive sleep apnea. *Curr Opin Pulm Med* 2004;10:482.
208. American Geriatrics Society Panel on Chronic Pain in Older Persons. Clinical practice guidelines: the management of chronic pain in older persons. *J Am Geriatr Soc* 1998;46:635.
209. Won A et al. Correlates and management of nonmalignant pain in the nursing home. *J Am Geriatr Soc* 1999;47:936.
210. Fox PL et al. Prevalence and treatment of pain in older adults in nursing homes and other long-term care institutions: a systematic review. *Can Med Assoc J* 1999;160:329.
211. Faherty BS et al. Analgesic medication for elderly people post-surgery. *Nurs Res* 1984;33:369.
212. McCaffery M. Narcotic analgesia for the elderly. *Am J Nurs* 1985;85:296.
213. Cohen JL. Pharmacokinetic changes in aging. *Am J Med* 1986;80:31.
214. Ouslander JG. Drug therapy in the elderly. *Ann Intern Med* 1981;95:711.
215. Harkins SW et al. Pain and the elderly. *Adv Pain Res Ther* 1984;7:103.
216. Beyer JE et al. The assessment of pain in children. *Pediatr Clin N Am* 1989;36:837.
217. LaFleur CJ et al. School-age child and adolescent perception of the pain intensity associated with three word descriptors. *Pediatric Nursing* 1999;25:45.
218. Anand KJS et al. Halothane-morphine compared with high-dose sufentanil for anesthesia and postoperative analgesia in neonatal cardiac surgery. *N Engl J Med* 1992;326:1.
219. Olkkola KT et al. Kinetics and dynamics of postoperative intravenous morphine in children. *Clin Pharmacol Ther* 1988;44:128.
220. Gutner LB et al. The effects of potent analgesics upon vestibular function. *J Clin Invest* 1952; 31:259.
221. Dixon R et al. Levorphanol: pharmacokinetics and steady-state plasma concentrations in patients with pain. *Res Commun Chem Pathol Pharmacol* 1983;41:3.
222. Forrest WH et al. Dextroamphetamine with morphine for the treatment of postoperative pain. *N Engl J Med* 1977;296:712.
223. Twycross RG et al. Long-term use of morphine in advanced cancer. *Adv Pain Res Ther* 1976;1:653.
224. Webb SS et al. Toward the development of a potent, nonsedating, oral analgesic. *Psychopharmacol* 1978;60:25.
225. Yee JD et al. Dextroamphetamine or methylphenidate as adjuvants to opioid analgesia for adolescents with cancer. *J Pain Symptom Manage* 1994;9:122.
226. Tong TG et al. Phenytoin-induced methadone withdrawal. *Ann Intern Med* 1981;94:349.
227. Bernard SA et al. Drug interactions in palliative care. *J Clin Oncol* 2000;18:1780.
228. Sorkin EM et al. Cimetidine potentiation of narcotic action. *Drug Intelligence and Clinical Pharmacy* 1983;17:60.
229. Poulsen L et al. The hypoalgesic effect of tramadol in relation to CYP2D6. *Clin Pharmacol Ther* 1996;60:636.
230. Egberts AC, et al. Serotonin syndrome attributed to tramadol addition to paroxetine therapy. *Int Clin Psychopharmacol* 1997;12:181.
231. Caufriez A. Menstrual disorders in adolescence: pathophysiology and treatment. *Horm Res* 1991;36:156.
232. Mackinnon GL et al. Current concepts in the management of primary dysmenorrhea. *Can Pharm J* 1982;1150:3.
233. Mehlisch DR. Double-blind crossover comparison of ketoprofen, naproxen, and placebo in patients with primary dysmenorrhea. *Clin Ther* 1990;12:398.
234. Shapiro SS et al. The effect of ibuprofen in the treatment of dysmenorrhea. *Curr Ther Res Clin Exp* 1981;30:327.
235. Laska E et al. Caffeine as an analgesic adjuvant. *JAMA* 1984;251:1711.
236. Migliardi J et al. Caffeine as an analgesic adjuvant in tension headache. *Clin Pharm Ther* 1994;56: 576.
237. Harden RN et al. Ketorolac in acute headache management. *Headache* 1991;31:463.
238. Roberts JE et al. Improved peribulbar anaesthesia with alkalinization and hyaluronidase. *Can J Anaesth* 1993;40:835.
239. Smith SL et al. The importance of bicarbonate in large volume anesthetic preparations. Revisiting the tumescent formula. *J Dermatol Surg Oncol* 1992;18:973.
240. Benini F et al. Topical anesthesia during circumcision in newborn infants. *JAMA* 1993;270:850.
241. Young SS et al. EMLA cream as a topical anesthetic before office phlebotomy in children. *South Med J* 1996;89:1184.
242. Farrington E. Lidocaine 2.5%/prilocaine 2.5% EMLA cream. *Pediatric Nursing* 1993;19:484.
243. Gershon RY et al. Intradermal anesthesia and comparison of intravenous catheter gauge. *Anesth Analg* 1991;73:469.

CHAPTER 9

Perioperative Care

Andrew J. Donnelly and Julie A. Golembiewski

The operating room (OR) is one of the most medication-intensive settings in a hospital. During the perioperative period (broadly defined as the preoperative, intraoperative, and post-operative periods), a patient may receive many medications. Most of these medications are used primarily in the OR setting and have limited application elsewhere in the institution. For other medications, their use in the OR may differ from that seen in other patient care areas. The OR is unique in that a significant number of the medications are administered as single doses by the anesthesia care provider (e.g., physician, nurse anesthetist). To ensure continuity of care of the surgical patient, health care providers from all settings (e.g., acute care, home health care, extended care) should have a basic understanding of perioperative drug therapy.

This chapter reviews seven major classes of medications used during the perioperative period: preoperative medications, intravenous (IV) anesthetic agents, volatile inhalation agents, neuromuscular blocking agents, local anesthetics, antiemetic agents, and analgesic agents. The clinical use of cardioplegia solution is also presented. The chapter concludes with a presentation of economic considerations associated with the use of anesthesia-related medications.

PREOPERATIVE MEDICATIONS

Administration of preoperative medications (premedicants) to patients can be thought of as the start of their operative course. Many different medications are used preoperatively and can be grouped into the following classes: benzodiazepines, opioids, anticholinergics, dissociative anesthetics, gastric motility stimulants, H_2-receptor antagonists, antacids, and α-2 agonists.

A key point concerning preoperative medication is that not all patients will require premedicants. A preoperative evaluation by the anesthesia provider ensures that the patient is medically prepared for surgery (e.g., pre-existing medical conditions such as diabetes, hypertension, or asthma are controlled or stabilized), allows the provider to discuss the most appropriate anesthetic and postoperative pain management options with the patient, and helps reassure and educate the patient. Preoperative assessment by an anesthesia provider is an important component of the patient's preparation for surgery. Patients should be assessed individually regarding their need for pharmacologic premedication. If required, premedicants should be selected based on patient-specific needs. Administration of a standard preoperative regimen to all patients should be avoided. Furthermore, the anesthesia provider and the surgeon must determine whether the patient should take his or her regularly scheduled medications the morning of surgery. These medications are often necessary to maintain the patient's physiological condition. The decision to continue or withhold chronic medications before surgery depends on the surgical procedure (e.g., major vs. minor), the patient's current medical condition, the pharmacological effect of the medication, and the potential for drug interactions with anesthetics. Medications that cause bleeding, excessive hemodynamic effects, or withdrawal symptoms are the most problematic. Antihypertensives, bronchodilators, tricyclic antidepressants, selective serotonin reuptake inhibitors, corticosteroids, thyroid preparations, anxiolytics, and anticonvulsants are generally continued up to, and including, the morning of surgery. Alternatively, medications that increase the risk for bleeding (e.g., aspirin, nonsteroidal anti-inflammatory drugs [NSAIDs], warfarin, clopidogrel) may need to be discontinued up to 7 days or more before surgery. Finally, patients with suppression of the pituitary-adrenal axis (e.g., patients currently or recently taking corticosteroids) may not be able to respond to surgical stress. Hydrocortisone can be administered intravenously before surgery, with subsequent doses dependent on the estimated amount of surgical stress and the need for supraphysiological steroid replacement in the postoperative period.

Goals of Premedication

A major goal of premedication is to decrease the patient's fear and anxiety about his or her upcoming surgery. In addition to reducing anxiety, premedication is used for a variety of other reasons. Medications can be used before surgery to produce sedation, provide analgesia, produce amnesia, facilitate a smooth anesthetic induction, reduce anesthetic requirements, prevent autonomic responses resulting in intraoperative hemodynamic stability, decrease salivation and secretions, reduce gastric fluid volume, and/or increase gastric pH. Table 9-1 lists medications commonly used preoperatively and their major indications, routes of administration, and dosages.[1–5] Midazolam is by far the most commonly used premedicant.

Selection Criteria

Factors to consider when selecting a preoperative drug for a patient include his or her American Society of Anesthesiologists (ASA) physical status class, medical conditions, degree of anxiety, age, surgical procedure to be performed, length of procedure, postoperative admission status (e.g., inpatient vs. outpatient), drug allergies, previous experience with medications, and concurrent drug therapy. The ASA physical status classification system classifies patients as I through V. ASA-I patients are healthy with little medical risk, whereas ASA-V patients have little chance of survival. Severe systemic disorders (e.g., uncontrolled diabetes mellitus, coronary artery disease) are present in ASA-III through ASA-V patients. Selection of preoperative medications in this group of patients will be more difficult. These patients generally have limited physiological reserve; thus, administration of a cardiovascular depressant agent, for example, can be harmful. Furthermore, these patients will be taking a significant number of medications; hence, chances for drug interactions are increased. The patient's other medical conditions are important to consider to prevent the administration of contraindicated medications. For example, the benzodiazepines are contraindicated in pregnancy.[3] A patient's age will play a role in the response seen with premedicant administration. The elderly are often more sensitive to preoperative opioids and benzodiazepines, as well as to the central nervous system (CNS) effects of anticholinergic agents.[6]

Familiarity with the surgery to be performed will aid in selecting appropriate premedicants. In surgical cases in which painful procedures (e.g., vascular cannulation, peripheral nerve block) will be performed on the patient, an analgesic premedicant may be warranted. The length and type of the procedure is important to consider when selecting premedicants. For example, a patient undergoing emergency surgery who has not fasted is often administered a nonparticulate antacid because he or she is at risk for aspiration of gastric contents.[1] Likewise, in short duration, outpatient surgery, agents with a long duration of action should be avoided because residual effects can prolong discharge time. Some drugs should not be administered to patients because of drug allergies; however, genuine allergies must be differentiated from adverse effects. For example, patients often state allergies to opioids after having experienced nausea and vomiting, which are common adverse effects of these drugs. A patient's previous experience with premedicants can assist in agent selection. If a medication has caused trouble in the past, it should be avoided. Finally, it is important to review the patient's current drug therapy before selecting an agent to prevent potentially harmful drug interactions.

Table 9-1 Indications, Routes of Administration, and Doses of Preoperative Agents[a]

Agent	Indications	Routes of Administration	Doses[b]
Benzodiazepines			
Diazepam (Valium)	Anxiolysis, amnesia, sedation	PO	*Adults:* 5–10 mg
Lorazepam (Ativan)	Anxiolysis, amnesia, sedation	PO	0.025–0.05 mg/kg (range, 1–4 mg for adults)
		IV	*Adults:* 0.025–0.04 mg/kg; *pediatrics:* 0.01–0.03 mg/kg (titrate dose; max: 2 mg)
Midazolam (Versed)	Anxiolysis, amnesia, sedation	PO	*Adults:* 20 mg; *pediatrics:* 0.5–0.75 mg/kg (max: 20 mg)
		IM	*Adults:* 0.07–0.08 mg/kg (max: 10 mg); *pediatrics:* 0.1–0.15 mg/kg (max: 10 mg)
		IV	*Adults:* 1–2.5 mg (titrate dose); *pediatrics:* 0.025–0.05 mg/kg (titrate dose)
		IN	*Pediatrics:* 0.2 mg/kg (max: 15 mg)
Opioids			
Morphine	Analgesia, sedation	IM	*Adults:* 2–4 mg; *pediatrics:* 0.02–0.05 mg/kg
		IV	Titrate dose
Fentanyl (Sublimaze)	Analgesia, sedation	IV	Adults: 25–100 mcg (titrate dose); *pediatrics:* 0.05–2 mcg/kg
Anticholinergics			
Atropine (A)	Antisialagogue (S > G > A), sedation (S > A > G)	IM/IV	*Adults:* 0.4–0.6 mg; *pediatrics:* 0.02 mg/kg IM, 0.01 mg/kg IV (max: 0.4 mg)
Scopolamine (S)	Sedation, amnesia, antisialagogue	IM/IV	*Adults:* 0.2–0.4 mg; *pediatrics:* 0.02 mg/kg IM, 0.01 mg/kg IV (max: 0.4 mg)
Glycopyrrolate (G) (Robinul)	Antisialagogue	IM/IV	*Adults:* 0.2–0.3 mg; *pediatrics:* 0.005–0.01 mg/kg (max: 0.3 mg)
Dissociative Anesthetics			
Ketamine (Ketalar)[c]	Sedation, amnesia, analgesia	PO	*Pediatrics:* 3–6 mg/kg
		IM	*Adults:* 3–4 mg/kg; *pediatrics:* 2–4 mg/kg
		IV	*Adults:* 0.5–1 mg/kg
Gastric Motility Stimulants			
Metoclopramide (Reglan)	Reduce gastric volume, antiemetic	PO	*Adults:* 10 mg; *pediatrics:* 0.15 mg/kg
		IV	*Adults:* 0.1–0.2 mg/kg (10–20 mg); *pediatrics:* 0.1–0.15 mg/kg
H_2-Receptor Antagonists			
Cimetidine (Tagamet)	↑ Gastric pH	PO	*Adults:* 300 mg; *pediatrics:* 7.5 mg/kg
		IV	*Adults:* 300 mg; *pediatrics:* 7.5 mg/kg
Ranitidine (Zantac)	↑ Gastric pH	PO	*Adults:* 150 mg; *pediatrics:* 2 mg/kg
		IV	*Adults:* 50 mg; *pediatrics:* 0.5–1 mg/kg
Famotidine (Pepcid)	↑ Gastric pH	PO	*Adults:* 40 mg; *pediatrics:* 0.5 mg/kg
		IV	*Adults:* 20 mg; *pediatrics:* 0.25 mg/kg
Nizatidine (Axid)	↑ Gastric pH	PO	*Adults:* 150 mg
Nonparticulate Antacids			
Sodium citrate/citric acid (Bicitra)	↑ Gastric pH	PO	*Adults:* 30 mL
α-2 Agonists			
Clonidine (Catapres)	Anxiolysis, potentiate action of anesthetic agents, sedation, analgesia	PO	*Adults:* 0.2 mg; *pediatrics:* 0.002–0.004 mg/kg (max: 0.2 mg)

[a] General dosage guidelines; doses must be individualized based on patient-specific parameters.
[b] Doses listed are for agents when used as sole premedicant; doses may need to be reduced if premedicants are administered in combination (e.g., opioids, benzodiazepines).
[c] The duration and depth of sedation from ketamine is determined by the dose and route of administration. Low dosages (0.025–0.075 mg/kg IV or 2–3 mg/kg IM) should produce light sedation for a short period. Higher dosages will produce deep sedation to the point of general anesthesia. In addition, airway reflexes are depressed, increasing the patient's risk for aspiration. An anesthesia care provider should be present, and resuscitative/suction equipment should be readily available.
IM, intramuscular; IN, intranasal; IV, intravenous; PO, oral.
Adapted from references 1–5.

Timing and Routes of Administration

The timing and route of administration is almost as important as the choice of the agent. For optimal results, the agent's peak effects should occur before the patient arrives in the OR suite. This will require the agent to be administered at varying times before surgery, depending on the route of administration. Preoperative agents are administered by several routes: IV, intramuscular (IM), oral (PO), and intranasal (IN). As a general rule, agents administered by the IV route produce the fastest onset of action and are often given after the patient arrives in the OR, whereas medications administered via the IM route are usually administered 30 to 60 minutes before the patient arrives in the OR. If possible, the IM route should be avoided because it is painful and undesirable for the patient. Onset of peak effect is the slowest with PO administration of agents, which should be administered 60 to 90 minutes before the patient's scheduled arrival in the OR.[1]

Drug Interactions

Preoperative medications can interact with one another, as well as with drugs the patient is receiving currently or will receive in the OR. These drug interactions can be advantageous and intentionally produced, or they can be problematic. For example, patients must be closely monitored when they concurrently receive a benzodiazepine and an opioid for premedication due to synergistic respiratory and cardiovascular adverse effects.[1] The α-2 agonists, however, can reduce the requirements for inhalational anesthetics and opioids.[4]

Administration of a Premedicant

1. K.J., a 21-year-old man, is scheduled to undergo a laparoscopic hernia repair on an outpatient basis under general anesthesia. This is the first time K.J. has undergone surgery, and he is highly anxious in the preoperative area. Should K.J. receive premedication, and, if so, what medication(s) should be administered?

The administration of a preoperative sedative to a patient undergoing outpatient surgery was formerly controversial; however, with midazolam, the delayed recovery and discharge that had been associated with agents used in the past (e.g., lorazepam, triazolam, temazepam) is less of a concern. Midazolam should be titrated to the desired effect (in increments of 0.5–1 mg IV), with the average adult generally requiring 2 mg IV. Elderly patients who receive as little as 0.5 mg midazolam intravenously can experience decreased oxygen saturation in the preoperative period and longer recovery time in the postanesthesia care unit (PACU) following short duration surgery.[7] Midazolam premedication produces sedation and provides anterograde amnesia and anxiolysis,[7,8] which can be problematic if these effects continue into the postoperative period when outpatients are provided with discharge instructions. In children, premedication with oral midazolam can reduce both the child's and the parents' anxiety during the preoperative period,[8] the likelihood of a child's distress at induction of anesthesia,[9] and the manifestation of negative behavioral changes in the child during the first 7 postoperative days.[10] The use of oral midazolam premedication in children who are undergoing outpatient surgery, however, can delay discharge.[9] Therefore, nonpharmacologic approaches to reduce anxiety must be optimized. If explanation of upcoming events and reassurance by the anesthesia provider has not sufficiently allayed K.J.'s anxiety, small titrated doses of IV midazolam can be administered.

Aspiration Pneumonitis Prophylaxis

Definition

Aspiration pneumonitis, although uncommon, is a potentially fatal condition that occurs as a result of regurgitation and aspiration of gastric contents. Aspiration of undigested or semidigested gastric contents into the respiratory tract can cause obstruction and an inflammatory response. Acute chemical pneumonitis and subsequent acute lung injury (aspiration pneumonitis) can result from aspiration of acidic gastric secretions.[11] Aspiration of gastric contents is also an important risk factor for the development of adult respiratory distress syndrome (ARDS).[12] Historically, a gastric pH of <2.5 and a gastric volume >25 mL (0.4 mL/kg) have been accepted as the cutoff values that place the patient at greater risk for severe pneumonitis should aspiration occur. However, in clinical practice, the values commonly used are a gastric pH <3.5 and gastric volume >50 mL, with pH appearing to be a greater determinant of morbidity than volume.[13]

Risk Factors

Patients at greatest risk for regurgitation and aspiration include those with increased gastric acid, elevated intragastric pressure, gastric or intestinal hypomotility, digestive structural disorders, neuromuscular incoordination, and depressed sensorium. These can include pregnant patients, obese patients, and trauma patients, as well as patients with a hiatal hernia, gastroesophageal reflux, esophageal motility disorders, or peptic ulcer disease.[14] Diabetic patients with reflux symptoms or poor glucose control may also benefit from pharmacologic prophylaxis.[15] In addition to having delayed gastric emptying, obese patients will often present with increased abdominal pressure and an abnormal airway; both factors predispose these individuals to aspiration. Hormonal changes in pregnant patients account for delayed gastric emptying and relaxation of the lower esophageal sphincter. An increase in intra-abdominal pressure is also seen in pregnant patients. Labor can increase gastrin levels, increasing gastric volume and acidity as well as delaying gastric emptying. Patients undergoing emergency surgery frequently have full stomachs because they have not had time to fast appropriately.

Rapid sequence induction, effective application of cricoid pressure, maintaining a patent upper airway, avoiding inflation of the stomach with anesthetic gases, inserting a large-bore gastric tube once the airway has been secured, as well as the use of regional anesthesia when possible, are probably the most important measures the anesthesia provider can take to reduce the patient's risk of aspiration.[16,17] Administration of pharmacologic aspiration prophylaxis is not cost effective and does not reduce morbidity or mortality in healthy patients undergoing elective surgery. Administration of pharmacologic aspiration prophylaxis should, however, be considered to prevent morbidity (e.g., ARDS) in patients at risk for aspiration.

Medications

Many medications (e.g., antacids, gastric motility stimulants, H_2-receptor antagonists) can reduce the risk of pneumonitis if aspiration occurs. These drugs, with the possible exception of metoclopramide, are relatively free of adverse effects and have a favorable risk–benefit profile.

ANTACIDS

Antacids, effective in raising gastric pH to >3.5,[1] should be given as a single dose (30 mL) approximately 15 to 30 minutes before induction of anesthesia. Nonparticulate antacids (e.g., sodium citrate/citric acid [Bicitra]) are the agents of choice because the suspension particles in particulate antacids can act as foci for an inflammatory reaction if aspirated and increase the risk of pulmonary damage.[18] Antacids have two major advantages when used for aspiration pneumonitis prophylaxis; there is no "lag time" for onset of activity, and antacids are effective on the fluid already in the stomach. Their major disadvantages are (a) a short-acting buffering effect that is not likely to last as long as the surgical procedure (sodium citrate must be administered no more than 1 hour before induction of anesthesia, with its duration possibly dependent on gastric emptying); (b) the potential for emesis (due to their lack of palatability); (c) the possibility of incomplete mixing in the stomach; and (d) their administration adds fluid volume to the stomach.[19,20]

GASTRIC MOTILITY STIMULANTS

The gastric motility stimulant, metoclopramide (Reglan), has no effect on gastric pH or acid secretion. This agent reduces gastric volume in predisposed patients (e.g., parturients, obese patients) by promoting gastric emptying. Preoperative metoclopramide increases lower esophageal sphincter pressure and reduces gastric volume.[3,21] Metoclopramide should be administered 60 minutes before induction of anesthesia when given orally. When given by the IV route, metoclopramide should be administered 15 to 30 minutes before induction of anesthesia. The effects of metoclopramide on gastric emptying have been variable, especially when used with other agents. For example, the concomitant administration of anticholinergics (e.g., glycopyrrolate, atropine), or prior administration of opioids, can reduce lower esophageal sphincter pressure, which can offset the effects of metoclopramide on the upper gastrointestinal (GI) tract.[22]

H_2-RECEPTOR ANTAGONISTS

H_2-receptor antagonists reduce gastric acidity and volume by decreasing gastric acid secretion. Unlike antacids, the H_2-receptor antagonists do not produce immediate effects. Onset time for these agents when administered orally is 1 to 3 hours; good effects will be seen in 30 to 60 minutes when administered intravenously.[3] Oral doses of the H_2-receptor antagonists should not be crushed and given via a nasogastric tube at the time of surgery. As already mentioned, onset of action is not immediate. Furthermore, administration of tablets introduces particulate matter into the stomach, which can be detrimental if aspirated. Duration of action of H_2-receptor antagonists is also important because the risk of aspiration pneumonitis extends through emergence from anesthesia. After IV administration, the cimetidine (Tagamet) dose should be repeated in 6 hours if necessary, whereas therapeutic concentrations of ranitidine (Zantac) and famotidine (Pepcid) persist for 8 and 12 hours, respectively.[3] Although cimetidine is associated with more adverse reactions than famotidine or ranitidine, this is probably not clinically significant because only one or two doses of the agent are given.[1]

PROTON-PUMP INHIBITORS

Proton-pump inhibitors (PPIs) (omeprazole, rabeprazole, lansoprazole, esomeprazole, and pantoprazole) act at the final site of gastric acid secretion, making these agents very effective in suppressing acid secretion. When the effects of preoperative IV pantoprazole on gastric pH and volume were compared with IV ranitidine and placebo, both pantoprazole and ranitidine significantly reduced the volume and increased the pH of gastric contents when compared to placebo (saline). There was no difference, however, between the pantoprazole and ranitidine groups.[23] Therefore, there appears to be no need to use the more expensive PPIs in patients at risk for pulmonary aspiration.

Choice of Agent

2. D.W., a 5′4″, 95-kg, 38-year-old woman, ASA-II, is scheduled to undergo a laparoscopic cholecystectomy under general anesthesia. D.W. has type 2 diabetes. Physical examination is normal except for an abnormal airway, which is anticipated to complicate intubation. Her medications include glipizide and an antacid for dyspepsia. The procedure is scheduled as a same-day surgery. What factors predispose D.W. to aspiration, and what premedication, if any, should D.W. receive for aspiration prophylaxis?

D.W. has several factors that place her at risk for aspiration. She is obese with an abnormal airway. She also has diabetes and reports symptoms of dyspepsia that are relieved by antacids. These conditions will predispose D.W. to increased abdominal pressure, delayed gastric emptying, and increased risk of regurgitation. Her abnormal airway may delay intubation, increasing the amount of time D.W. is susceptible to aspiration. Therefore, aspiration prophylaxis with medications that buffer gastric acid and reduce gastric volume is prudent for D.W. Because D.W.'s surgery is scheduled as a same-day surgery, D.W. will arrive at the hospital or surgical center approximately 90 minutes before the start of surgery. Although oral agents, in general, are less expensive than their parenteral counterparts, cimetidine 300 mg (Tagamet), famotidine 40 mg (Pepcid), or ranitidine 150 mg (Zantac) should be administered approximately 1 to 2 hours before induction of anesthesia to effectively decrease gastric acidity. Hence, due to time constraints, cimetidine 300 mg, famotidine 20 mg, or ranitidine 50 mg should be administered intravenously 30 to 60 minutes before induction of anesthesia in D.W. A nonparticulate antacid such as sodium citrate/citric acid solution (Bicitra) 30 mL PO can be administered to D.W. immediately before entering the OR rather than, or in addition to, an H_2-receptor antagonist.

3. C.T., a 28-year-old woman, ASA-I, is admitted for an emergency cesarean section under general anesthesia. She is otherwise healthy and currently taking no medications. Why is C.T. susceptible to aspiration pneumonitis, and what preoperative medications would be appropriate to help prevent this adverse event from occurring in her?

C.T. is at an increased risk for aspiration and the possible development of pneumonitis because she is pregnant and about to undergo emergency surgery. In the obstetric patient, preoperative administration of the nonparticulate antacid, sodium citrate, or a H_2-receptor antagonist can effectively reduce gastric acidity. Furthermore, the administration of a nonparticulate antacid before C-section can reduce maternal complications. Metoclopramide, however, can reduce peripartum nausea and vomiting. Therefore, an appropriate regimen for C.T. would include both sodium citrate/citric acid solution (Bicitra) 30 mL PO and metoclopramide 10 mg IV. Famotidine (or another H_2-receptor antagonist) can be given instead of, or in addition to, the sodium citrate/citric acid solution. There is not sufficient time to administer famotidine and metoclopramide orally because of their slower onsets of action when administered by this route. Sodium citrate/citric acid solution provides immediate protection by raising gastric pH, metoclopramide will help reduce the increased gastric volume commonly seen in pregnant patients, and famotidine will provide sustained coverage throughout the surgery. These agents have not been shown to have detrimental effects on the fetus.[24]

INTRAVENOUS ANESTHETIC AGENTS

General Anesthesia

General anesthesia is a state of drug-induced unconsciousness. Other components of general anesthesia include amnesia, analgesia, immobility, and attenuation of autonomic responses to noxious stimuli.[25] Drugs used to induce general anesthesia should produce unconsciousness rapidly and smoothly while minimizing any cardiovascular changes. Table 9-2 lists additional desirable, as well as undesirable, characteristics of an IV induction agent. Although currently available IV induction agents possess many of the desirable characteristics, no agent is free of the undesirable effects. An IV induction agent is commonly administered for initiation of general anesthesia. Drugs commonly used for IV induction include ultrashort-acting barbiturates (thiopental, methohexital), etomidate, and propofol. The synthetic opioids (fentanyl, sufentanil, alfentanil, and remifentanil), benzodiazepines (primarily midazolam), and ketamine are less frequently used. Propofol can also be used to maintain general anesthesia, as drugs that do not accumulate during repeat or continuous dosing are ideal choices for maintenance therapy. When used at dosages lower than those necessary for unconsciousness, some of the IV anesthetic agents can be used to produce sedation for monitored anesthesia care or regional anesthesia, as well as in the medical procedure units and intensive care units (ICUs). Table 9-3 lists common clinical uses for IV anesthetic agents.

Table 9-2 Characteristics of an Intravenous Induction Agent

Desirable Characteristics	*Undesirable Characteristics*
Water soluble	Histamine release
Stable in solution	Hypersensitivity reaction
Small volume required for dose	Local toxicity at injection site
Rapid, smooth onset of action	Pain on injection
Predictable effect	Adverse central nervous system effects
High therapeutic index	
Analgesic	Adverse cardiovascular effects
Amnestic	
Short duration to awakening	Active metabolites
Rapid full recovery	
Availability of reversal agent	

Table 9-3 Common Clinical Uses of IV Anesthetic Agents

Etomidate (Amidate)	**Midazolam (Versed)**
IV induction	Anxiolysis
Ketamine (Ketalar)[a]	Amnesia
Analgesia	Sedation
Sedation	**Propofol (Diprivan)**[a]
IV induction	Sedation
IM induction	IV induction
Methohexital (Brevital)[a]	Maintenance of general anesthesia
IV induction	**Thiopental**
Sedation	IV induction

[a] Dose-dependent effects; sedation at lower doses, anesthesia at higher doses.
IV, intravenous; IM, intramuscular.

Mechanisms of Action

Most IV anesthetic agents produce CNS depression by action on the γ-aminobutyric acid (GABA) benzodiazepine chloride ion channel receptor. GABA is the principal inhibitory neurotransmitter in the CNS. The barbiturates bind to a receptor site on the GABA-receptor complex, reducing the rate of dissociation of GABA from its receptor. This results in increased chloride conductance through the ion channel, nerve cell hyperpolarization, and inhibition of nerve impulse transmission. Barbiturates can directly activate the chloride channels by mimicking the action of GABA. Benzodiazepines also bind to this GABA-receptor complex and their subsequent potentiation of the inhibitory action of GABA is well described. At large doses, most of the benzodiazepine receptors will be occupied, and hypnosis (unconsciousness) will occur. The site of action of etomidate (Amidate) and propofol (Diprivan) is also at the GABA receptor, with etomidate augmenting GABA-gated chloride currents and propofol enhancing the activity of the GABA-activated chloride channel. Ketamine (Ketalar) acts at a different site than other induction agents. It produces dissociation between the cortex and the thalamus within the limbic system, resulting in a dissociative state; that is, the patient appears to be detached from his or her surroundings. Unlike anesthesia produced by other agents (e.g., propofol for induction followed by sevoflurane/nitrous oxide/oxygen for maintenance) where the patient's eyes are closed resembling normal sleep, a ketamine-anesthetized patient's eyes are often open and move from side to side. Ketamine also produces analgesia and amnesia in patients.[26]

Pharmacokinetics

The onset and duration of effect are the most important pharmacokinetic properties of IV anesthetic agents when used for induction of anesthesia. In general, the commonly used IV induction agents have a rapid onset of action and short clinical duration, with the short clinical duration resulting from redistribution of the drug from the brain to other tissue sites (e.g., muscle, fat). Using the barbiturates as an example, thiopental

Table 9-4 Pharmacokinetic Comparison of Common Intravenous Anesthetic Agents

Drug	Half-Life (hours)	Onset (seconds)	Clinical Duration (minutes)[a]	Hangover Effect[b]
Etomidate (Amidate)	2–5	≤30	3–12	+
Ketamine (Ketalar)	1–3	30–60	10–20	++ – +++[c]
Methohexital (Brevital)	4	≤30	5–10	+
Midazolam (Versed)	1–4	30–90	10–20	+++[d]
Propofol (Diprivan)	0.5–7	≤45	5–10	0 – +
Thiopental (Pentothal)	11	≤30	5–10	++

[a] Time from injection of agent to return to conscious state.
[b] Residual psychomotor impairment after awakening.
[c] When ketamine is administered as the induction agent (e.g., 5–10 mg/kg IM).
[d] When midazolam is administered as the induction agent (e.g., 0.15 mg/kg IV).
Adapted from references 26–28.

and methohexital undergo maximal brain uptake within 30 seconds of injection as a result of their high lipophilicity and high rate of blood flow to the brain. This is followed by a decline over the next 5 minutes to half of the initial peak brain concentration, predominately through drug redistribution. As a result, patients awaken in <10 minutes after a single induction dose of thiopental, despite a half-life of approximately 11 hours. Because cumulative effects can be seen after repeat or continuous dosing of barbiturates due to fat deposition and storage, these drugs make poor choices for maintenance of general anesthesia. The degree to which metabolism plays a role in the clinical duration of IV induction agents is variable; rapid metabolism can be a significant factor in the relatively shorter duration to full recovery of propofol.[26] Table 9-4 compares the pharmacokinetic properties of IV anesthetic agents.[26–28]

Adverse and Beneficial Effects

IV anesthetic agents can produce a variety of adverse and beneficial effects other than loss of consciousness (e.g., cardiovascular depression or stimulation, pain on injection, nausea and vomiting, respiratory depression or stimulation, CNS cerebroprotection or excitation, adrenocorticoid suppression). Table 9-5 compares the relative significance of these effects among available agents.[26–28] The most troublesome are usually cardiovascular effects or CNS excitation reactions. Contribution to postoperative nausea and vomiting (PONV) and "hangover" can be significant and may delay full recovery and patient discharge from the PACU. This is of particular concern in the ambulatory surgery setting because the patient will be discharged home. CNS effects can include hiccups, myoclonus, seizure activity, euphoria, hallucinations, and emergence delirium. The cerebroprotective effect produced by barbiturates, etomidate, and propofol results from a reduction in cerebral blood flow secondary to cerebral vasoconstriction. As a result, cerebral metabolic rate, cerebral blood flow, and intracranial pressure are reduced.[26–28] This effect is useful if these drugs are available in therapeutic concentrations at a time of potential cerebral ischemia. Thiopental, for example, has been given during deep hypothermic circulatory arrest to minimize the possibility of ischemic events.

Agent Selection

The selection of an IV anesthetic agent should be determined based on patient characteristics, circumstances associated with surgery, and cost. Patient characteristics may include history of PONV, allergy profile, psychiatric history, or cardiovascular status. Circumstances associated with surgery that could influence the choice of IV anesthetic include the postoperative admission status (inpatient vs. outpatient), placement of an IV line, duration of surgery, and extubation status at the end of

Table 9-5 Adverse Effects and Costs of Intravenous Induction Agents

Adverse Effect	Etomidate (Amidate)	Ketamine (Ketalar)	Methohexital (Brevital)	Midazolam (Versed)	Propofol (Diprivan)	Thiopental (Pentothal)
Adrenocorticoid suppression	+[a]	–	–	–	–	–
Cerebral protection	+	–	+	+	+	+
Cardiovascular depression	–	–	++	+	++	++
Emergence delirium or euphoria	–	++	–	–	+	–
Myoclonus	+++	+	++	–	+	+
Nausea/vomiting	+++	++	++	+	–	++
Pain on injection	++	–	+	–	++	+
Respiratory depression	++	–	++	+/++	++	++
Relative cost	++	++	+++	+	+	+++

[a] Not shown to be clinically significant in single dose.
+ to ++++, likelihood of adverse effect relative to other agents (or increasing cost for cost comparison); –, no effect.
Adapted from references 26–28.

the procedure. The cost of induction agents varies, with older agents (e.g., thiopental, methohexital) priced higher per single induction dose than newer agents (e.g., etomidate, propofol).

Propofol Use in Ambulatory Surgery: Antiemetic Effect and Full Recovery Characteristics

4. K.T., a 19-year-old girl, ASA-I, is admitted to the ambulatory surgery center for strabismus surgery to correct misalignment of her extraocular muscles. She is otherwise healthy, and all laboratory values obtained before surgery are within normal limits. The duration of K.T.'s surgery is anticipated to be approximately 90 minutes. Which IV induction agent should be used?

Propofol (Diprivan) is a good choice here for several reasons. Strabismus surgery is considered highly emetogenic because operative manipulation of extraocular muscles triggers the release of dopamine, serotonin, and acetylcholine (Ach) in the chemoreceptor trigger zone (CTZ) through the oculoemetic reflex.[29] Therefore, precautions should be taken to reduce the possibility of nausea and vomiting postoperatively. Propofol produces the lowest incidence of PONV when compared with other IV induction agents and the volatile inhalation agents; it has even been associated with a direct antiemetic effect.[30] This effect does not preclude the need for prophylactic antiemetic therapy, but may contribute to the avoidance of emesis in K.T. Furthermore, ambulatory surgery demands rapid, full recovery from general anesthesia. Propofol, etomidate, and methohexital produce less of a hangover than other IV induction agents. Propofol, in particular, is associated with a more rapid recovery of psychomotor function and a patient-perceived superior quality of recovery.[28] Propofol also offers advantages for maintenance of anesthesia in this case, and it does not accumulate when administered as a continuous infusion.

Etomidate Use in Cardiovascular Disease

5. L.M., a 73-year-old man, ASA-IV, is in need of repair of an abdominal aortic aneurysm. During a preoperative evaluation a few days before surgery, his blood pressure (BP) was 160/102 mmHg, and his medical records revealed hypertension that was poorly controlled by hydrochlorothiazide 25 mg daily and metoprolol XL (Toprol) 100 mg daily. He also has angina that occasionally requires treatment with SL nitroglycerin. An exercise stress test showed electrocardiogram changes at a moderate exercise load. Two days before the elective aneurysm repair was scheduled, L.M. presented to the emergency department (ED) with a 4-hour history of severe back pain. His surgeon believes that there is a high likelihood that the aneurysm is leaking or expanding and schedules surgery immediately. What is the best plan for L.M.'s anesthetic induction and maintenance?

L.M. has significant cardiovascular disease, and care should be taken to minimize any cardiovascular depression, tachycardia, or hypertension during induction and maintenance of anesthesia. Of the currently available induction agents, etomidate has the most stable cardiovascular profile[28] and is associated with minimal cardiovascular depression. Opioids generally produce minimal cardiovascular effects and could potentially be used for induction. Thiopental, propofol, and ketamine can cause hemodynamic changes and are best avoided in L.M. Etomidate would be an excellent choice for induction, followed by isoflurane (with low-dose opioids) to maintain anesthesia. Although opioid-based anesthetics provide cardiovascular stability, the doses required to maintain anesthesia can prolong the duration of respiratory depression, which might necessitate postoperative mechanical ventilation.

Methohexital for Electroconvulsive Therapy

6. T.B., a 33-year-old woman, ASA-I, will undergo an electroconvulsive therapy (ECT) procedure for treatment of her severe, medication-resistant depression. T.B. is scheduled to go home within 1 to 2 hours after the procedure, which will be performed under general anesthesia. What IV induction agent should be used?

ECT procedures are an important method of treatment of severe and medication-resistant depression, mania, and other serious psychiatric conditions. During the ECT procedure, an electrical current is applied to the brain, resulting in an electroencephalographic (EEG) spike and wave activity, a generalized motor seizure, and acute cardiovascular response. For an optimal therapeutic (antidepressant) response, T.B.'s seizure activity should last from 25 to 50 seconds. General anesthesia is administered to ensure amnesia, prevent bodily injury from the seizure, and control the hemodynamic changes. When selecting an IV induction agent, its effect on EEG seizure activity, its ability to blunt the hemodynamic response to ECT, and its recovery profile (e.g., short time to discharge, nonemetogenic) are important considerations. Because most IV induction agents have anticonvulsant properties, small doses must be used to allow adequate seizure duration. Methohexital is considered the gold standard. Propofol, in smaller doses, can also be used. Combining a short-acting opioid such as remifentanil with propofol will allow a small dose of propofol to be used and the seizure duration to be prolonged. Although etomidate does not adversely affect the seizure duration, the hemodynamic response to ECT is accentuated because etomidate is cardiovascularly stable and cannot blunt the cardiovascular response to ECT. In addition, it can cause nausea and vomiting, resulting in delayed recovery. Midazolam reduces seizure activity, and ketamine increases the risk of delayed recovery by producing nausea and ataxia.[31,32] Therefore, methohexital, in a dose of 0.75 to 1 mg/kg IV, can be administered because it will not affect the seizure duration or prolong T.B.'s recovery time. Alternatively, a small dose of propofol (0.75 mg/kg) and remifentanil (up to 1 mcg/kg) are also appropriate.

Ketamine Use in Pediatrics

7. R.L., a 4-year-old boy, ASA-II, is scheduled for a painful debridement and dressing change that is anticipated to take approximately 15 minutes. He is brought to the procedure room near the OR along with his parents and is in distress over parting from them. He currently has no IV line in place. How could sedation and analgesia be provided to R.L.?

Ideally, analgesia should be provided without the need to start an IV and, for children with a high level of separation anxiety, in the presence of a parent. Although ketamine can be given intramuscularly, administration by this route is painful and not optimal. However, it might be preferable to starting an IV in R.L. for a short, painful procedure. At relatively low doses (3 or 4 mg/kg IM), ketamine produces analgesia and a compliant patient who is not heavily sedated. Intubation is unnecessary because ketamine causes little or no respiratory depression. Ketamine, however, can produce a dissociative stare and nystagmus, random movements of the head and extremities, and tonic/clonic movements. R.L.'s parents should be informed about these potential effects. An anticholinergic drug (e.g., glycopyrrolate) can be given along with ketamine to counteract its sialagogue effect. Ketamine use has expanded to EDs because of the quality of sedation and analgesia and the short duration of action (<30 minutes) associated with this drug. Appropriate guidelines for use of ketamine in this setting should be followed.[33]

Delirium and hallucinations are unusual adverse effects of ketamine that occur in 10% to 30% of patients on awakening from anesthesia. Emergence reactions (e.g., dreaming, illusions, sense of floating out of body) vary in severity; occur within hours of awakening from anesthesia; and occur more often in adults, females, frequent dreamers, patients with personality disorders, and patients receiving high doses of ketamine (>2 mg/kg) by rapid IV administration. These reactions can be attenuated by prophylactic administration of benzodiazepines.[28,33] R.L. is at very low risk for an emergence reaction based on age, gender, dose, and route of ketamine administration; therefore, benzodiazepines are not needed in R.L.

VOLATILE INHALATION AGENTS

Currently, four volatile inhalation agents are available for use in the United States: desflurane, sevoflurane, isoflurane, and enflurane, with the latter being less commonly used in clinical practice than the other three. The volatile inhalation agents are unique in that they can produce all components of the anesthetic state, to varying degrees (e.g., minimal, if any, analgesia). Immobility to surgical stimuli and amnesia is postulated to be the predominant effect produced by these agents. Unlike IV anesthetic agents, these drugs are administered into the lungs via an anesthesia machine, and as a result, it is easy to increase or decrease drug levels in the body. The anesthetist can estimate, with the use of technology, the anesthetic partial pressure at the site of action (brain); this helps the anesthetist maintain an optimal depth of anesthesia.[34]

Although the volatile inhalation agents could, theoretically, be used to produce general anesthesia by themselves, it is much more common to use a combination of drugs intended to take advantage of smaller doses of each drug while avoiding the disadvantages of high doses of individual agents. This practice is referred to as *balanced anesthesia*. For example, midazolam is used routinely to produce sedation, anxiolysis, and amnesia, whereas the administration of a barbiturate (e.g., thiopental) or other IV anesthetic agent (e.g., propofol), followed by administration of a neuromuscular blocking agent (e.g., succinylcholine), can induce rapid loss of consciousness and muscle relaxation to facilitate endotracheal intubation. Volatile inhalation agents provide maintenance of general anesthesia, along with reflex suppression (e.g., lowering BP and heart rate) and some muscle relaxation. Opioids (e.g., fentanyl) also can induce reflex suppression, thereby lowering total anesthetic requirements. Subsequent doses of a nondepolarizing neuromuscular blocking drug might be necessary to provide adequate relaxation for surgery.

Uses

The volatile inhalation agents are primarily used in clinical practice to maintain general anesthesia. Sevoflurane also can be used to induce general anesthesia via a face mask because of its low pungency. Desflurane and sevoflurane, because of their low blood solubility, are ideally suited for maintenance of general anesthesia in ambulatory surgery patients and for inpatients when rapid wake-up is desired (e.g., neurosurgery procedures).

Site/Mechanism of Action

The goal of inhalation anesthesia is to develop and maintain a satisfactory (anesthetizing) partial pressure of anesthetic in the brain, which is the site of anesthetic action.[34] Although the mechanism of action of the volatile inhalation agents is not fully understood, these agents are believed to disrupt neuronal transmission in discrete areas throughout the CNS by either blocking excitatory, or enhancing inhibitory, transmission through synapses. Ion channels (especially GABA receptors) are likely targets of volatile inhalation anesthetic agent action.[25]

Anesthesia Machine and Circuit

A basic understanding of the anesthesia machine and circuit is helpful to understanding many of the concepts associated with the administration of volatile inhalation agents. Three parts of the anesthesia machine are critically important for the administration of volatile inhalation anesthetics. The *flow meters* regulate the amount of nitrous oxide (an anesthetic gas), air, and oxygen delivered to the patient. The *vaporizers* regulate the concentration of volatile inhalation agent administered to the patient, whereas the *carbon dioxide absorber*, which contains either soda lime or Baralyme, removes carbon dioxide from exhaled air. The first step in the administration of a volatile inhalation agent to a patient is to begin the flow of background gases. Flow is measured in liters per minute. A mixture of nitrous oxide and oxygen is commonly used. This gas mixture flows to one of the vaporizers, where a portion of it enters the vaporizer and "picks up" the anesthetic vapor of the volatile inhalation agent. The concentration of volatile inhalation agent delivered by the vaporizer is proportional to the amount of gas mixture passing through it, which is regulated by adjusting the vaporizer's concentration dial. The gas and anesthetic vapor mixture exits the vaporizer and continues through the anesthetic circuit, where it is ultimately delivered to the patient via an endotracheal tube or face mask. The exhaled air from the patient, which contains the volatile inhalation agent and carbon dioxide, is returned to the circuit. If a semiclosed circle breathing system is being used, rebreathing of the exhaled volatile agent can occur if the fresh gas flow rate is low enough (e.g., ≤2 L/minute).[35]

Table 9-6 Pharmacologic and Pharmacokinetic Properties of the Volatile Inhalation Agents

Property/Effect	*Desflurane*	*Sevoflurane*	*Isoflurane*	*Enflurane*
MAC in O_2 (adults)	6.0	1.71	1.15	1.7
Blood/gas partition coefficient[a]	0.42	0.69	1.46	1.91
Brain/blood partition coefficient[b]	1.29	1.7	1.6	1.4
Muscle/blood partition coefficient[c]	2.02	3.13	2.9	1.7
Fat/blood partition coefficient[d]	27.2	47.5	45	36
Metabolism	0.02%	3%	0.2%	2%
Molecular weight (g)	168	201	184.5	184.5
Liquid density[e]	1.45	1.505	1.496	1.517

[a] The greater the blood/gas partition coefficient, the greater the blood solubility.
[b] The greater the brain/blood partition coefficient, the greater the brain solubility.
[c] The greater the muscle/blood partition coefficient, the greater the muscle solubility.
[d] The greater the fat/blood partition coefficient, the greater the fat solubility.
[e] Density determined at 25°C for desflurane, isoflurane, and enflurane and at 20°C for sevoflurane.
MAC, minimum alveolar concentration to prevent movement in 50% of subjects.
Adapted from reference 34.

Potency

Potency of the volatile inhalation agents is compared in terms of minimum alveolar concentration (MAC). MAC is the alveolar concentration of anesthetic at one atmosphere that prevents movement in 50% of subjects in response to a painful stimulus (e.g., surgical skin incision).[34] The lower an agent's MAC, the greater is the anesthetic potency. A value of 1.3 MAC is required to produce immobility in 95% of patients, whereas 1.5 MAC is required to block the adrenergic response to noxious stimuli.[34] Furthermore, the inhalation agents are additive in their effects on MAC; the addition of a second agent reduces the required concentration of the first agent. For example, when desflurane, isoflurane, and sevoflurane are administered with 60% to 70% nitrous oxide, their MAC values decrease from 6%, 1.15%, and 1.71% to 2.38%, 0.56%, and 0.66%, respectively.[34] Of the volatile inhalation agents routinely used, isoflurane has the lowest MAC and desflurane the highest (Table 9-6).[34]

Chemical Stability

Desflurane and isoflurane are very stable compounds and are not broken down by the moist soda lime or Baralyme contained in the carbon dioxide absorber of the anesthesia machine. Sevoflurane degrades in the presence of carbon dioxide absorbent to multiple by-products, with compound A being most important. In rats, compound A has caused nephrotoxicity,[36] but no clinically significant changes in serum creatinine and blood urea nitrogen (BUN) have been demonstrated in human studies.[37–39] The administration of sevoflurane at low flow rates is one of the major factors that increases compound A concentration. The U.S. Food and Drug Administration (FDA) requires that the sevoflurane package insert contain a warning that sevoflurane exposure should not exceed 2 MAC hours at flow rates of 1 to <2 L/minute, and flow rates <1 L/minute are not recommended. Nevertheless, even when low fresh gas flows are used for long periods of time and exposure to compound A was high, the levels of compound A are much less than what is believed to be a toxic level.[40]

Unlike sevoflurane, desflurane, isoflurane, and enflurane can react with dry carbon dioxide absorbent to produce carbon monoxide.[41] The water content of the absorbent is the major factor leading to the production of carbon monoxide.[42] When these agents pass through dry absorbent, carbon monoxide is produced. This situation is most commonly encountered on a Monday morning in an anesthesia machine that has been idle during the weekend and has had a continuous flow of fresh gas through the absorbent. Carbon monoxide production can be prevented by ensuring that only fully hydrated absorbent is used.

The newer alkali hydroxide-free carbon dioxide absorbents containing calcium hydroxide (vs. sodium or potassium hydroxide) make the chemical stability of volatile inhalation agents in the absorbent not a clinical concern. In an in vitro study of one of these absorbents (Amsorb), compound A levels were no higher than those found in sevoflurane itself when it was passed through this absorbent at a low flow rate (1 L/minute). Likewise, carbon monoxide production was negligible when desflurane, isoflurane, or enflurane passed through an anhydrous form of this absorbent.[43]

Pharmacokinetics

A series of anesthetic partial pressure gradients beginning at the anesthesia machine serve to drive the volatile inhalation agent across barriers to the brain. These gradients are as follows: anesthesia machine > delivered > inspired > alveolar > arterial > brain. The alveolar partial pressure provides an indirect measurement of the anesthetic partial pressure in the brain because the alveolar, arterial, and brain partial pressures rapidly equilibrate.[34]

Factors that influence the uptake and distribution of a volatile inhalation agent include the inspired concentration of the agent, alveolar ventilation, solubility of the agent in the blood (blood/gas partition coefficient), blood flow through the lungs, distribution of blood to individual organs (levels rise most rapidly in highly perfused organs—brain, kidney, heart, liver), solubility of the agent in tissue (tissue/blood partition coefficient), and mass of tissue.[34] If all other factors are equal, agents with low solubilities will equilibrate quickly and, as a result, have a faster wash-in (onset). Solubility is also a factor in the elimination of volatile inhalation agents, in addition to metabolism and extent of tissue equilibration. Low-solubility agents are more rapidly washed out (eliminated) because more of the agent is removed from the blood in one passage through the lungs.[34] As can be seen in Table 9-6, desflurane has the lowest solubility of any of the volatile inhalation agents, with sevoflurane's solubility being lower than isoflurane's for blood and muscle. As a result of their low solubility, quicker responses to intraoperative concentration changes are seen with desflurane and sevoflurane as well as a faster emergence and awakening from anesthesia and a more rapid return to normal motor function and judgment when compared with isoflurane.[44–46]

As seen in Table 9-6, the metabolism of the volatile inhalation agents varies (e.g., desflurane is metabolized least). An important point is that metabolism does not alter the rate of induction or maintenance of anesthesia because the amount of anesthetic administered to the patient greatly exceeds its uptake.[34] Metabolism of sevoflurane has resulted in peak inorganic fluoride levels $>100\ \mu$mol/L.[38] Historically, a fluoride level of 50 μmol/L has been used as a cut-off for potential nephrotoxicity based on reports of methoxyflurane-associated nephrotoxicity at levels $>50\ \mu$mol/L.[47] Despite this, sevoflurane has not been demonstrated to produce nephrotoxicity. Potential reasons for this include the fact that sevoflurane's low blood gas solubility may limit the degree of its metabolism once the anesthetic is discontinued and that sevoflurane, unlike methoxyflurane, undergoes minimal renal defluorination.[48] In clinical studies examining the preanesthetic and postanesthetic serum creatinine and BUN values in patients receiving sevoflurane anesthesia, clinically significant renal damage in patients with normal renal function has not been reported, nor has renal function worsened in patients with stable renal insufficiency or in those undergoing hemodialysis.[49–51]

Pharmacologic Properties

All volatile inhalation agents depress ventilation (with an elevation of $Pa{CO_2}$) and dilate constricted bronchial musculature in a dose-dependent manner. As mentioned previously, sevoflurane can be used for mask induction of general anesthesia because it is not as pungent as desflurane, isoflurane, or enflurane. Administration of a pungent agent by mask for induction can cause coughing, breath-holding, laryngospasm, and salivation in the patient. All volatile inhalation agents depress myocardial contractility and decrease arterial BP in a dose-dependent manner. Isoflurane can increase heart rate, so cardiac output is usually maintained. Sevoflurane produces little increase in heart rate, so cardiac output may not be as well maintained as with isoflurane. Although enflurane can increase heart rate, cardiac output is usually decreased. Desflurane can produce sympathetic nervous system activation, resulting in a transient increase in BP and heart rate, when concentrations are rapidly increased.[52] The sympathetic nervous system activation may be due to stimulation of medullary centers via receptors in the upper airway and lungs.[53] Enflurane can sensitize the myocardium to the arrhythmogenic effects of epinephrine. The volatile inhalation agents decrease cerebral metabolic rate and produce cerebral vasodilation, resulting in increased cerebral blood flow and volume. Enflurane can cause epileptiform activity that can result in clinical tonic-clonic seizures. All volatile inhalation agents produce muscle relaxation and potentiate the actions of the neuromuscular blocking agents. The volatile inhalation agents relax uterine smooth muscle, which can contribute to perinatal blood loss. All volatile inhalation agents have been implicated as triggers of malignant hyperthermia (MH) and are contraindicated in MH-susceptible patients. Finally, all volatile inhalation agents are associated with postoperative nausea, vomiting, and shivering.[34,47]

Drug Interactions

Opioids, benzodiazepines, α-2 agonists, and neuromuscular blocking agents potentiate the effects of the volatile inhalation agents. Thus, their administration permits use of lower dosages of the volatile inhalents, thereby reducing their potential for adverse effects.

Economic Considerations

The following items must be considered when examining the costs associated with the administration of volatile inhalation agents from an institutional perspective: cost of the volatile inhalation agent (including waste), cost of the equipment necessary to administer the volatile inhalation agent, cost of adjuvants used to treat adverse effects of the volatile agent, and time spent in the OR and PACU.

The cost of a volatile agent depends on (a) the cost per milliliter of the liquid anesthetic, (b) the amount of vapor generated per milliliter, (c) the amount of volatile agent that must be delivered from the anesthesia machine to sustain the desired alveolar concentration, and (d) the flow rate of the background gases.[54] Items a and b are, for the most part, constant, with price increases or decreases occurring periodically. Because desflurane and sevoflurane are less soluble in blood and tissue than isoflurane, lower amounts of these agents will need to be delivered to the alveoli to attain the desired anesthetic depth.[54] The flow rate of background gases is a major determinant of the cost; as flow rate increases, the amount of anesthetic consumed per time increases.[55] The following formula is frequently used to calculate the cost of volatile inhalation agent used:

$$\text{Cost used} = (\text{PFTMC})/(2412d)$$

where P is vaporizer concentration (%), F is fresh gas flow (L/minute), T is time (minute), M is molecular weight of the agent, C is the cost of the agent ($/mL), and d is the density of the agent.[56] The use of low flow rates can result in substantial reductions in the volatile anesthetic drug cost per case. An important point to keep in mind when comparing only the cost of the volatile inhalation agents themselves (e.g., excluding any benefits in terms of cost reduction that may be realized by a quicker discharge from the recovery room) is that the low-solubility volatile agents have to be administered at low flow rates to prevent their cost from being substantially higher than that of the more traditional agents (e.g., isoflurane) when administered at rates of 2 to 3 L/minute.

The cost of purchasing new vaporizers and upgrading or replacing agent analyzers that are used to administer and monitor volatile inhalation agents, respectively, can be significant. These costs become a concern when a new product is introduced onto the market.

Medications used to treat adverse effects associated with the volatile inhalation agents include β-blockers, opioids, benzodiazepines, vasopressors, and antiemetic agents. Antiemetic agents are routinely used to prevent and/or treat the PONV seen with the volatile inhalation agents. Intraoperative use of volatile inhalation agents is a leading cause of early (within the first 2 hours following surgery) postoperative vomiting.[57] Although the administration of an antiemetic agent adds costs,[58] it is significantly less than the cost of an unanticipated admission to the hospital secondary to PONV.

The use of low-solubility volatile inhalation agents can significantly reduce the overall net cost of the surgical procedure by reducing the time patients spend in the OR and PACU. This concept is discussed at the end of this chapter.

Desflurane Use for Maintenance of General Anesthesia

Sympathetic Nervous System Activation

8. C.K., a 26-year-old man, ASA-I, is scheduled to undergo a laparoscopic hernia repair on an outpatient basis. During his preoperative evaluation on the morning of surgery, his BP was 115/75 mmHg, and his heart rate was 70 beats/minute. The surgery is expected to last <2 hours, so a propofol induction is planned followed by maintenance of general anesthesia with desflurane without nitrous oxide. After induction of anesthesia, the desflurane concentration on the vaporizer was rapidly increased to 8%. Within 1 minute of the concentration increase, C.K.'s BP increased to 148/110 mmHg, and his heart rate increased to 112 beats/minute. What could be causing C.K.'s increased BP and heart rate, and how could it have been prevented?

Desflurane can produce sympathetic nervous system activation with a resultant increase in BP and heart rate under certain circumstances. One of these is the rapid increase of desflurane concentration to 1.1 MAC as seen with C.K.[59] This hemodynamic response can be attenuated by the IV administration of fentanyl approximately 5 minutes before the increase in desflurane concentration.[60] Fentanyl is a good choice because it effectively blunts the increase in heart rate and BP, while having minimal cardiovascular depressant and postoperative sedative effects. Alternatively, nitrous oxide can be administered with desflurane, thereby allowing the desflurane concentration to be maintained at <1 MAC (6%).

Emergence Agitation in Children

9. P.F., a 3-year-old child, ASA-I, is undergoing a tonsillectomy. General anesthesia will be induced and maintained with sevoflurane and nitrous oxide. His surgery was uneventful, with a duration of 30 minutes. He was awakened from anesthesia and transferred to the postanesthesia care unit to recover. Shortly after he arrived, P.F. became extremely restless and began crying. The nurse and his mom were unable to console him. Could this reaction be attributed to sevoflurane, and, if so, can it be prevented?

Emergence agitation following the administration of the short-acting inhaled anesthetics, desflurane and sevoflurane, is fairly common, with a reported incidence as high as 80%.[61] Emergence agitation is more common in young children, and its cause is not clear. Children become restless, cry, and exhibit involuntary physical activity that can result in self-injury. Caring for a child experiencing emergence agitation is difficult and very upsetting to the caregiver and the parents of the child. Premedication with oral midazolam[62] and administering analgesics to minimize postoperative pain[63] may reduce the incidence. A small dose of dexmedetomidine (0.3 mcg/kg IV), an α-2 agonist with sedative and analgesic properties, after induction of anesthesia reduces the incidence of emergence agitation, without prolonging recovery in children undergoing sevoflurane anesthesia.[64] Although desflurane cannot be used to induce general anesthesia, switching to desflurane for maintenance of anesthesia following sevoflurane induction effectively reduces the severity of emergence agitation when it occurs.[65]

NEUROMUSCULAR BLOCKING AGENTS

Uses

Neuromuscular blocking agents are one of the most commonly used classes of drugs in the OR. They are used primarily as an adjunct to general anesthesia to facilitate endotracheal intubation and to relax skeletal muscle during surgery under general anesthesia.[66] Skeletal muscle relaxation optimizes the surgical field for the surgeon and prevents patient movement as a reflex response to surgical stimulation. Neuromuscular blocking agents are also used in the ICU to paralyze mechanically ventilated patients.[67] An important point to remember is that neuromuscular blocking agents have no known effect on consciousness or pain threshold. Consequently, adequate sedation and analgesia must be ensured when neuromuscular blocking agents are administered to ICU patients.

Mechanism of Action

When two molecules of Ach bind to the Ach subunits of the nicotinic cholinergic receptors located on the motor nerve end plate, the Ach receptor undergoes a conformational change that allows the influx of sodium and potassium into the muscle cell, the membrane depolarizes, and the muscle contracts. Neuromuscular blocking agents bind to these subunits and effectively block normal neuromuscular transmission. Two classes of neuromuscular blocking agents exist based on their mechanism of action: depolarizing and nondepolarizing. Succinylcholine, the only depolarizing neuromuscular blocking agent in clinical use today, acts like Ach to depolarize the membrane. Because succinylcholine is not metabolized as quickly as Ach at the neuromuscular junction, its action at the nicotinic receptor persists longer than Ach. Succinylcholine causes a persistent depolarization of the motor end plate because the sodium channels cannot reopen until the motor end plate repolarizes. As a result, sustained skeletal muscle paralysis occurs. The paralysis produced by depolarizing agents is preceded initially by fasciculations (transient twitching of skeletal muscle). The nondepolarizing neuromuscular blocking agents act as competitive antagonists to Ach at the Ach subunits of the nicotinic cholinergic receptors, thereby preventing Ach from binding and causing depolarization of the muscle membrane and muscle contraction.[66,68]

Table 9-7 Classification of Neuromuscular Blocking Agents

Agent	Type of Block	Clinical Duration of Action[a]	Structure
Atracurium (Tracrium)	–	Intermediate	Benzylisoquinolinium
Cisatracurium (Nimbex)	–	Intermediate	Benzylisoquinolinium
Pancuronium (Pavulon)	–	Long	Steroidal
Rocuronium (Zemuron)	–	Intermediate	Steroidal
Succinylcholine (Anectine, Quelicin)	+	Ultrashort	Acetylcholine-like
Vecuronium (Norcuron)	–	Intermediate	Steroidal

[a]Time from injection of agent to return to twitch height to 25% of control (time at which another dose of agent will need to be administered to maintain paralysis); in general, clinical duration of a standard intubating dose of ultrashort agents ranges from 3 to 5 minutes, intermediate agents from 30 to 40 minutes, and long agents from 60 to 120 minutes.
+, depolarizing; –, nondepolarizing.
Adapted from reference 69.

Monitoring Neuromuscular Blockade

In addition to clinical assessment (e.g., lack of movement) by the anesthesia provider and the surgeon, the degree of neuromuscular blockade produced by neuromuscular blocking agents is monitored by nerve stimulation with a peripheral nerve stimulator. Most commonly, the ulnar nerve is electrically stimulated, and the response of the innervated muscle, the adductor pollicis in the thumb, is visually assessed. Adequate neuromuscular blockade is present when the train-of-four (four electrical stimulations of 2 Hz delivered every 0.5 seconds) count is 1/4 or 2/4 (one or two visible muscle twitches out of a possible four twitches).[67]

Classification

Neuromuscular blocking agents are commonly classified by the type of blockade produced (depolarizing vs. nondepolarizing), chemical structure (steroidal compound, Ach-like, benzylisoquinolinium compound), or duration of action (ultrashort, intermediate, long), as listed in Table 9-7.[69]

Adverse Effects

The underlying mechanisms for the cardiovascular adverse effects of neuromuscular blocking agents are listed in Table 9-8 and include blockade of autonomic ganglia (hypotension), blockade of muscarinic receptors (tachycardia), and/or release of histamine from circulating mast cells (hypotension).[68–70] In general, the steroidal compounds exhibit varying degrees of vagolytic effect, whereas the benzylisoquinolinium compounds are associated with varying degrees of histamine release. Although not reported as a problem when used short term in the OR, the use of neuromuscular blocking agents in ICU patients for extended periods can result in prolonged neuromuscular blockade or acute quadriplegic myopathy syndrome, albeit infrequently.[68] Of the currently available neuromuscular blocking agents, cisatracurium (Nimbex) and vecuronium (Norcuron) are devoid of clinically significant cardiovascular effects and are the agents of choice for patients with unstable cardiovascular profiles.[66,68,69] Succinylcholine (Anectine, Quelicin) is associated with a significant number of adverse effects, including hyperkalemia; arrhythmias; fasciculations; muscle pain; myoglobinuria; trismus; phase II block; and increased intraocular, intragastric, and intracranial pressures.[69,70] Succinylcholine, like inhalational anesthetics, can trigger MH.[68] Of these adverse effects, bradycardia, hyperkalemia (which can trigger arrhythmias and cardiac arrest in patients at risk), and MH crisis are severe and potentially life-threatening reactions. Nevertheless, succinylcholine is still used today because of its rapid onset and ultrashort duration of action as well as its ability to be administered intramuscularly in children in an emergent situation when IV access has not been established.

Drug Interactions

Several drugs interact with neuromuscular blocking agents. The volatile inhalation agents potentiate the neuromuscular

Table 9-8 Causes of Cardiovascular Adverse Effects of Neuromuscular Blocking Agents

Agent	Histamine Release[a]	Autonomic Ganglia	Vagolytic Activity	Sympathetic Stimulation
Atracurium[a] (Tracrium)	++	–	–	–
Cisatracurium (Nimbex)	–	–	–	–
Pancuronium (Pavulon)	–	Weak block	++	++
Rocuronium[b] (Zemuron)	–	–	+	–
Succinylcholine (Anectine, Quelicin)	+	Stimulates	–	–
Vecuronium (Norcuron)	–	–	–	–

[a]Histamine release is dose and rate related; cardiovascular changes can be lessened by minimizing dose and injecting agent slowly.
[b]Produces an increase in heart rate of approximately 18% with intubating dose of 0.6 mg/kg; effect usually transient and resolves spontaneously.
+ – ++, likelihood of developing the cardiovascular adverse effect relative to the other agents; –, no effect.
Adapted from references 68–70.

blockade produced by nondepolarizing agents, thereby allowing a lower dose of the latter to be used when administered concomitantly. Other agents reported to potentiate the effects of neuromuscular blocking agents include the aminoglycosides, clindamycin, magnesium sulfate, quinidine, furosemide, lidocaine, amphotericin B, and dantrolene. Carbamazepine, phenytoin, corticosteroids (chronic administration), and theophylline antagonize the effects of neuromuscular blocking agents.[68,69] By appropriately monitoring the patient and dosing the neuromuscular blocking agent to effect, significant problems from drug interactions can be minimized.

Reversal of Neuromuscular Blockade

The action of neuromuscular blocking agents ceases spontaneously as plasma concentrations decline or when anticholinesterases (e.g., neostigmine, edrophonium, pyridostigmine) are administered. Anticholinesterases inhibit the enzyme acetylcholinesterase, which degrades Ach, and are used to reverse paralysis produced by nondepolarizing agents. Anticholinergic agents are coadministered (in same syringe) with the anticholinesterases to minimize other cholinergic effects (e.g., bradycardia, bronchoconstriction, salivation, increased peristalsis, nausea, vomiting) caused by the increase in Ach concentration. Atropine is routinely administered with edrophonium, and glycopyrrolate with neostigmine or pyridostigmine, to take advantage of similar onset times and durations of action.[66,67,69] Reversal of neuromuscular blockade, as a general rule, is not attempted until spontaneous recovery is well established. Before extubation, adequacy of reversal is assessed with the use of a peripheral nerve stimulator and by clinical assessment of the patient (e.g., ability to sustain head lift for 5 seconds).[69,70]

A new reversal agent, sugammadex, is currently under development that may eliminate some of the issues currently seen with the anticholinesterases. Sugammadex, a modified cyclodextrin, encapsulates steroidal (e.g., rocuronium) neuromuscular blocking agents, thereby preventing them from acting at the neuromuscular junction. It produces a rapid recovery from neuromuscular blockade, even when administered during profound blockade, and does not appear to have any serious adverse effects.[71]

Pharmacokinetics and Pharmacodynamics

Rapid Sequence Induction

10. R.D., a 36-year-old man, ASA-I, is admitted through the ED for an emergency appendectomy. R.D. is otherwise healthy, has no drug allergies, and is currently taking no medications. All laboratory values are normal. Admission notes reveal that R.D. ate dinner approximately 2 hours earlier. Because of this, the anesthesia provider plans to perform a rapid sequence induction using the Sellick maneuver. Which neuromuscular blocking agent would be most appropriate for R.D.?

Rapid sequence induction is indicated for patients at risk for aspiration of gastric contents should regurgitation occur. Patients who have recently eaten (with a full stomach), morbidly obese patients, or patients with a history of gastroesophageal reflux are at risk for aspiration, as is the case for R.D. The goal of rapid sequence induction is to minimize the time during which the airway is unprotected by intubating the patient as fast as possible (e.g., within 60 seconds). In this technique, the patient is preoxygenated, after which an IV induction agent is administered, followed immediately by a neuromuscular blocking agent. Manual ventilation of the patient is not attempted after administration of these agents. Apnea occurs as the neuromuscular blocking agent takes effect; therefore, a neuromuscular blocking agent with as rapid an onset as possible is required to produce adequate intubating conditions as quickly as possible. The Sellick maneuver is often used during rapid sequence induction. It is performed by placing downward pressure on the cricoid cartilage, which compresses and occludes the esophagus and helps prevent passive regurgitation of gastric contents into the trachea. Intubation is then performed within 60 seconds.

Table 9-9 lists the onset times of normal intubating doses and other information pertaining to the use of neuromuscular blocking agents.[67–70] Succinylcholine has the fastest onset time, which makes it an appropriate agent to use in rapid sequence induction.[72]

Table 9-9 Pharmacokinetic and Pharmacodynamic Parameters of Action of Neuromuscular Blocking Agents

Agent	*Cl (mL/kg/min)*	*Vd_{ss} (L/kg)*	*Half-Life (minutes)*	*ED95 (mg/kg)*	*Intubating Dose[a,b] (mg/kg)*	*Onset[c] (minutes)*	*Clinical Duration of Action of Initial Dose (minutes)*
Atracurium[d] (Tracrium)	5–7	0.2	20	0.2–0.25	0.4–0.5	2–3	25–30
Cisatracurium (Nimbex)	4.6	0.15	22	0.05	0.15–0.2	2–2.5	50–60
Pancuronium (Pavulon)	1–2	0.3	80–120	0.07	0.04–0.1	3–5	80–100
Rocuronium[d] (Zemuron)	4.0	0.3	60–70	0.3	0.6–1.2	1–1.5	30–60
Succinylcholine[d] (Anectine, Quelicin)	37	0.04	0.65	0.25	1.5	1	5–10
Vecuronium[d] (Norcuron)	4.5	0.4	50–70	0.05–0.06	0.1	2–3	25–30

[a] Dose when nitrous oxide-opioid technique is used.
[b] Intermittent maintenance doses to maintain paralysis, as a general rule, will be approximately 20% to 25% of the initial dose.
[c] Time to intubation.
[d] Also can be administered as a continuous infusion to maintain paralysis. Suggested infusion ranges under balanced anesthesia are atracurium, 4–12 mcg/kg/min; cisatracurium, 1–2 mcg/kg/min; rocuronium, 6–14 mcg/kg/min; succinylcholine, 50–100 mcg/kg/min; vecuronium, 0.8–2 mcg/kg/min.
Cl, clearance; ED95, effective dose causing 95% muscle paralysis; Vd_{ss}, steady-state volume of distribution.
Adapted from references 67–70.

Because R.D. is an otherwise healthy man with no contraindications to the use of succinylcholine, this agent should be used.

Depolarizing Agent Contraindications

11. What would be your choice of a neuromuscular blocking agent if R.D. presents with a history of susceptibility to MH, and why?

Succinylcholine is contraindicated in patients with skeletal muscle myopathies; after the acute phase of injury (i.e., 5–70 days after injury) following major burns, multiple trauma, extensive denervation of skeletal muscle, or upper motor neuron injury; in children and adolescents (except when used for emergency tracheal intubation or when the immediate securing of the airway is necessary); and in patients with a hypersensitivity to the drug.[66,69] Succinylcholine can also trigger MH and is absolutely contraindicated in MH-susceptible patients.[73]

The nondepolarizing neuromuscular blocking agents are safe to use in MH-susceptible patients.[74] Rocuronium (Zemuron) has the fastest onset time of the nondepolarizing agents, although it is slightly slower than succinylcholine.[70] The onsets of the remaining intermediate and long duration agents can be shortened by increasing the dose, which not only results in a faster onset of action but also prolongs the duration of action. Rocuronium's time to maximum blockade, for example, can be reduced to 60 seconds with an initial dose of 1.2 mg/kg (vs. a normal initial dose of 0.6 mg/kg). Increasing the dose from 0.6 mg/kg to 1.2 mg/kg, however, will prolong the clinical duration from approximately 30 minutes to at least 60 minutes.[75] Rocuronium, with its rapid onset of action, would be a suitable alternative to succinylcholine in R.D.'s case. Its longer clinical duration of action could be a concern if the airway cannot be secured immediately or if the procedure is shorter than the duration of an intubating dose of rocuronium. Because this procedure will last longer than the duration of muscle relaxation provided by the intubating dose of rocuronium, this is not a concern.

Routes of Elimination

12. M.M., a 70-year-old woman, ASA-IV, is scheduled to undergo a 2-hour GI procedure. Pertinent laboratory findings are aspartate aminotransferase (AST), 272 U/L (normal, 5–45 U/L); alanine aminotransferase (ALT), 150 U/L (normal, 5–37 U/L); BUN, 40 mg/dL (normal, 8–21 mg/dL); serum creatinine (SrCr), 1.8 mg/dL (normal, 0.5–1.1 mg/dL); albumin, 2.6 g/dL (normal, 3.5–5.0 g/dL); and bilirubin, 0.74 mg/dL (normal, 2–18 mg/dL). Which neuromuscular blocking agent would you recommend for M.M.?

[SI units: AST, 4.5 μkat/L; ALT, 2.5 μkat/L; BUN, 14.28 mmol/L; SrCr, 159 μmol/L; albumin, 26 g/L; bilirubin, 12.7 mol/L]

When selecting a neuromuscular blocking agent, one of the factors that must be considered is the patient's renal and hepatic function. Neuromuscular blocking agents often depend on the kidneys and liver for varying amounts of their metabolism and excretion (Table 9-10).[66,67,70] Some agents, however, are primarily metabolized by plasma cholinesterase (pseudocholinesterase), Hofmann elimination (a nonbiological process that does not require renal, hepatic, or enzymatic function), and/or nonspecific esterases.

Hofmann elimination is a pH- and temperature-dependent process unique to atracurium (Tracrium) and cisatracurium (Nimbex). One of the products produced by Hofmann elimination is laudanosine, a CNS stimulant in high concentrations. Laudanosine undergoes renal and hepatic elimination. Due to the short-term use of atracurium and cisatracurium in the OR, accumulation of laudanosine with resultant seizure activity is not a concern, even in patients with end-stage renal failure.[76] Because plasma cholinesterase levels may be decreased in patients with renal or hepatic dysfunction, the duration of action of succinylcholine could be prolonged. The increased duration of action of succinylcholine in patients with low levels of normal plasma cholinesterase is not clinically significant. Atypical plasma cholinesterase can increase the duration of action of succinylcholine significantly.[77]

Unchanged neuromuscular blocking agents and their metabolites are excreted by the renal or biliary routes. The duration of action of the renally eliminated agent, pancuronium, will be increased in patients with renal failure. Vecuronium's duration of action can be increased in patients with liver disease, particularly when larger doses (0.2 mg/kg) are administered, reflecting impaired metabolism or excretion rather than termination of effect by redistribution.[78] Although the main route of elimination of rocuronium is hepatobiliary, the duration of action of rocuronium can be significantly prolonged in chronic renal failure.[79]

Because M.M. has evidence of both significant renal and hepatic impairment, cisatracurium or atracurium would be appropriate choices for a neuromuscular blocking agent because their properties are not altered significantly by renal and hepatic failure. Furthermore, because these agents have an

Table 9-10 Elimination of Neuromuscular Blocking Agents

Agent	*Renal*	*Hepatic*	*Biliary*	*Plasma*
Atracurium (Tracrium)	10%		NS	Hofmann elimination, ester hydrolysis
Cisatracurium (Nimbex)	NS		NS	Hofmann elimination
Pancuronium (Pavulon)	80%	10%	5%–10%	
Rocuronium (Zemuron)	10%–25%	10%–20%	50%–70%	
Succinylcholine (Anectine, Quelicin)				Plasma cholinesterase
Vecuronium (Norcuron)	15%–25%	20%–30%	40%–75%	

NS, not significant.
Adapted from references 66, 67, and 70.

intermediate duration of action, they can easily be used in a 2-hour procedure. The availability of generic atracurium makes this agent a more economic choice; however, the greater propensity of atracurium to cause histamine release with resultant hypotension makes cisatracurium the most appropriate choice in this 70-year-old, ASA-IV patient.

LOCAL ANESTHETICS

Local and Regional Anesthesia

Some surgical procedures can be performed under regional anesthesia (anesthesia selective for part of the body, such as the area near the surgical site) rather than general anesthesia (total body anesthesia with the patient rendered unconscious). Epidural, spinal (intrathecal), IV regional, peripheral nerve block, topical, or local infiltration anesthesia can be chosen, depending on the location of the surgical site, extent of the surgery, patient health and physical characteristics, coagulation status, duration of surgery, and the desires and cooperativeness of the patient. For epidural anesthesia, the local anesthetic is administered into the epidural space, which is located between the dura and the ligament covering the spinal vertebral bodies and disks. To provide spinal anesthesia, the local anesthetic is injected into the cerebrospinal fluid within the subarachnoid (intrathecal) space. By injecting a local anesthetic in the tissue near a specific nerve or nerve plexus, anesthesia can be provided for a carotid endarterectomy (cervical plexus), upper extremity surgery (brachial plexus), or hand surgery (ulnar, median and/or radial nerve). Regional anesthesia can be selected to reduce or avoid the likelihood of complications such as postoperative pain, nausea, vomiting, and laryngeal irritation, or dental complications, all of which are associated with general anesthesia. Peripheral nerve block may be selected over general, spinal, or epidural anesthesia because it is not associated with bowel obstruction or urinary retention, and it provides postoperative analgesia (particularly when long-acting local anesthetics are used).[80] Potential advantages of spinal or epidural anesthesia include reduction of the stress response to surgery, improvement in cardiac function in patients with ischemic heart disease, fewer postoperative pulmonary complications, potentially favorable effects on coagulation (lower risk of venous thrombosis), and the ability to continue epidural analgesia into the postoperative period.[81] Disadvantages of spinal, epidural, or peripheral nerve block include the additional time and manipulations required to perform it, possible complications or pain from invasive catheter placements or injections, slow onset of effect, possible failure of technique, and toxicity from absorption of the drugs administered. Local infiltration anesthesia can be used to provide localized anesthesia to allow a minor procedure (e.g., a deep laceration repair) to be performed.

Uses of Local Anesthetic Agents

Local anesthetics are a mainstay of analgesia because they prevent the initiation or propagation of the electrical impulses required for peripheral and spinal nerve conduction. These agents can be administered by all routes previously discussed, depending on the drug chosen. Table 9-11 lists the common uses of currently available local anesthetics.[82,83] Local anesthetics are often given in combination with other agents, such as sodium bicarbonate (to increase the speed of onset and reduce pain on local infiltration), epinephrine (to prolong the duration of action and to delay vascular absorption of the local anesthetic, thereby minimizing plasma concentration and systemic toxicity), or opioids (to provide analgesia by a different mechanism of action).

Mechanism of Action

The two structural classes of local anesthetics are characterized by the linkage between the molecule's lipophilic aromatic group and hydrophilic amine group: amides and esters. Both amide and ester classes provide anesthesia and analgesia by reversibly binding to and blocking the sodium channels in nerve membranes, thereby decreasing the rate of rise of the action potential such that threshold potential is not reached. As a result, propagation of the electrical impulses required for nerve conduction is prevented. The axonal membrane blockade that results is selective depending on the drug, the concentration and volume administered, and the depth of nerve penetration.

Table 9-11 Clinical Uses of Local Anesthetic Agents

Agent	*Primary Clinical Use*
Esters	
Chloroprocaine (Nesacaine)	Epidural
Cocaine	Topical
Procaine (Novocain)	Local infiltration, spinal
Tetracaine (Pontocaine)	Topical, spinal
Amides	
Bupivacaine (Marcaine, Sensorcaine)	Local infiltration, nerve block, epidural, spinal
Etidocaine (Duranest)	Local infiltration, nerve block, epidural
Levobupivacaine (Chirocaine)	Local infiltration, nerve block, epidural
Lidocaine (Xylocaine)	Local infiltration, nerve block, spinal, epidural, topical, intravenous regional
Mepivacaine (Carbocaine, Polocaine)	Local infiltration, nerve block, epidural
Ropivacaine (Naropin)	Local infiltration, nerve block, epidural

Adapted from references 82 and 83.

C fibers (pain transmission and autonomic activity) appear to be the most easily blocked, followed by fibers responsible for touch and pressure sensation (A-α, A-β, and A-Δ), and finally, those responsible for motor function (A-α and A-β). At the most commonly used doses and concentrations, some non–pain-transmitting nerve fibers are also blocked. The blockade of sensory, motor, or autonomic (sympathetic, parasympathetic) fibers may result in adverse effects such as paresthesia, numbness and inability to move extremities, hypotension, and urinary retention. Systemic effects (e.g., seizures or cardiac arrhythmias) are related to the inherent cardiac and CNS safety margins of these drugs.[82,83]

Ropivacaine, like bupivacaine, has a long duration of action. Higher plasma concentrations of ropivacaine are required to produce mild CNS toxicity (lightheadedness, tinnitus, numbness of the tongue) in volunteers, when compared with bupivacaine. In animal studies, ropivacaine was found to be less cardiotoxic than bupivacaine. In addition, ropivacaine may produce less motor blockade than bupivacaine.[84] As a result, some anesthesia providers believe ropivacaine is safer than bupivacaine. However, inadvertent intravascular administration of ropivacaine can produce significant CNS toxicity (seizures), emphasizing the importance of ensuring appropriate placement of the local anesthetic solution by the anesthesia provider.

Allergic Reaction

Most adverse effects to local anesthetics are manifestations of excessive plasma concentration (systemic toxicity) of the local anesthetic. Localized hypersensitivity reactions (e.g., local erythema, edema, dermatitis) to local anesthetics are rare. Ester-type local anesthetic agents (benzocaine, procaine, tetracaine) produce most of the allergic reactions, which is probably caused by their metabolite, para-aminobenzoic acid (PABA). True (systemic) allergy to amide-type local anesthetics is extremely rare and may be due to the preservative (methylparaben or other substances that are structurally similar to PABA) or to accidental intravascular injection of an epinephrine-containing local anesthetic. Because amide-type local anesthetics do not undergo metabolism to a PABA metabolite, a patient with a known allergy to an ester-type local anesthetic can safely receive an amide-type agent.[82,83,85] It is best to administer a preservative-free, epinephrine-free preparation to a patient with a known allergy to a local anesthetic.

Toxicity

Factors that influence the toxicity of local anesthetics include the total amount of drug administered, presence or absence of epinephrine, vascularity of the injection site, type of local anesthetic used, rate of destruction of the drug, age and physical status of the patient, and interactions with other drugs. Systemic absorption of the local anesthetic is positively correlated with the vascularity of the injection site (IV > epidural > brachial plexus > subcutaneous). End-stage pregnancy, older age (e.g., the elderly), significant hepatic/renal dysfunction, and advanced heart failure can result in either higher peak levels or accumulation of local anesthetic with continued or repeat dosing. In general, local anesthetic doses should be reduced in patients with these conditions.[86]

Toxic levels of local anesthetics are most often achieved by unintentional intravascular injection, which result in excessive plasma concentrations. Systemic toxicity of local anesthetics involves the CNS and cardiovascular system. Patients may initially complain of tinnitus, lightheadedness, metallic taste in their mouth, tingling, numbness, and dizziness. Hypotension may occur. These symptoms can quickly be followed by tremors, seizures, arrhythmias, unconsciousness, and cardiac/respiratory arrest as plasma levels rise.[82,87]

Physicochemical Properties Affecting Action

The potency of a local anesthetic is primarily determined by the degree of lipid solubility. Local anesthetics such as bupivacaine are highly lipid soluble and can be given in concentrations of 0.25% to 0.5%. Less lipid-soluble agents, such as lidocaine, require concentrations of 1% to 2% for many anesthetic techniques.

Amide-type local anesthetics are metabolized primarily by microsomal enzymes in the liver. The cytochrome P450 enzyme system is involved in the metabolism of lidocaine (CYP3A4), levobupivacaine (CYP3A4, CYP1A2), and ropivacaine (CYP3A2, CYP3A4, and CYP1A2). Agents that induce or inhibit these enzymes could affect the metabolism, and therefore the plasma concentration, of these drugs. Ester-type local anesthetics are hydrolyzed by plasma cholinesterase and, to a lesser extent, cholinesterase in the liver.[82,83]

Differences in the clinical activity of local anesthetics are explained by other physicochemical properties such as protein binding and pK_a (the pH at which 50% of the drug is present in the unionized form and 50% in the ionized form). Agents that are highly protein bound typically have a longer duration of action. Agents with a lower pK_a typically have a faster onset of action.[83]

Choice of local anesthetic is based on the duration of the surgical procedure (e.g., the duration of analgesia required). Usually, a local anesthetic that will, at least minimally, outlast the duration of surgery with a single injection is chosen; a continuous infusion can also be administered for titration of effect with shorter-acting agents. Important physicochemical and pharmacokinetic properties of local anesthetics are shown in Table 9-12.[82,83]

Regional Anesthesia in High-Risk Patients

13. M.S., a 52-year-old, 5′9″, 105-kg black man, is undergoing an emergent minor hand repair procedure after a fall-related injury. His medical history is positive for type 1 diabetes mellitus for 41 years, angina, and hypertension. On OR admission, laboratory values of note are plasma glucose, 240 mg/dL, and BP, 145/92 mmHg. His sister tells the anesthesia provider that he has been having increasing difficulty walking up stairs and, of late, is often short of breath. The anesthesia provider chooses to provide regional anesthesia via an axillary block; the anticipated duration of surgery is 2 hours. M.S. agrees with this plan. Why is this a good plan for M.S., and which local anesthetic should be chosen?

[SI unit: glucose, 13.3 mmol/L]

With his medical conditions of diabetes, angina, and hypertension, M.S. is at risk for complications from general

Table 9-12 Physicochemical and Pharmacokinetic Properties of Local Anesthetic Agents

Agent	pK_a	Potency	Toxicity	Onset	Duration[a]	Maximum Recommended Dose[b] Plain (mg)	With Epinephrine (mg)
Esters							
Cocaine[c]	–	–	–	–	–	1.5 mg/kg	–
Chloroprocaine (Nesacaine)	9.1	Low	Very low	Very fast	Short	800	1,000
Procaine (Novocain)	8.9	Low	Low	Fast	Short	400	600
Tetracaine (Pontocaine)	8.4	High	Moderate	Slow	Very long	100 (topical)	200
Amides							
Bupivacaine (Marcaine, Sensorcaine)	8.1	High	High	Slow	Long	175	225
Etidocaine (Duranest)	7.9	High	Moderate	Fast	Very long	300	400
Levobupivacaine (Chirocaine)	8.1	High	Moderate	Slow	Long	150	
Lidocaine (Xylocaine)	7.8	Moderate	Moderate	Fast	Moderate	300	500
Mepivacaine (Carbocaine, Polocaine)	7.7	Moderate	Moderate	Moderate	Moderate	300	500
Ropivacaine (Naropin)	8.1	High	Moderate	Slow	Long	300	–

[a]Depends on factors such as injection site, dose, and addition of epinephrine. In general, a short duration is <1 hour, a moderate duration is 1–3 hours, and a long/very long duration of action is 3–12 hours when the local anesthetic is administered without epinephrine.
[b]Maximum recommended single dose for infiltration or peripheral nerve block in 70-kg adults.
[c]Topical use only; concentrations >4% are not recommended due to increased risk for systemic adverse effects.
Adapted from references 82 and 83.

anesthesia. General anesthesia is not absolutely necessary in this localized surgery. Regional anesthesia would be beneficial in M.S. because it does not disrupt autonomic function. In addition, his diabetes and obesity, and possibly full stomach (emergency surgery, diabetic gastroparesis), place him at significant risk for aspiration during induction or emergence from general anesthesia. An axillary block with a local anesthetic could provide M.S. with adequate anesthesia and analgesia during and after his procedure.

The local anesthetic of choice is one with a duration at least that of the anticipated surgery and with a good safety profile should systemic absorption inadvertently occur. A local anesthetic containing epinephrine would increase the agent's duration of action and reduce the systemic absorption; however, such an agent is not indicated in M.S. because of his diabetes (peripheral vascular effects) and hypertension (added effect from catecholamine administration). Lidocaine as a single injection without epinephrine has a duration of action that may be too short for M.S.'s procedure. Mepivacaine, an intermediate-acting local anesthetic, or bupivacaine, a long-acting agent, would be appropriate choices to use in M.S.

Alkalinization of Local Anesthetics

15. T.F., a 22-year-old man, is scheduled for a hernia repair. He has never undergone surgery and is very anxious. In the preoperative area, the nurse chooses to locally infiltrate 1% lidocaine to reduce the pain and discomfort from IV catheter placement. She injects a small amount of lidocaine under the skin. T.F. flinches and complains of pain from the injection. Can anything be done to speed the onset and reduce the pain from injection of lidocaine?

The onset of action of local anesthetics depends on their pK_a. Drugs with pK_as closest to body pH (7.4) will have the fastest onset because a high percentage of the local anesthetic molecules will be unionized and therefore able to cross the nerve membranes to their intracellular site of action. Local anesthetics are formulated in solutions with acidic pHs to optimize their shelf-lives. When sodium bicarbonate is added to local anesthetic solutions, the pH is increased, the percentage of unionized drug is increased, and the onset of local anesthetic action can be shortened considerably. The amount of bicarbonate added to the solution depends on the pH of the local anesthetic agent. Because too much sodium bicarbonate will precipitate the local anesthetic, a dose of 0.1 mEq (0.1 mL of a 1 mEq/mL concentration) of sodium bicarbonate is added to 10 mL of bupivacaine, whereas 1 mEq (1 mL of a 1 mEq/mL concentration) is added to 10 mL of lidocaine. Furthermore, alkalinized lidocaine can be significantly less painful for subcutaneous injection before IV catheter placement when compared with lidocaine at pH 5 (its pH in the commercially available vial).[88]

CARDIOPLEGIA SOLUTION

Use in Cardiac Surgery

Hypothermic, hyperkalemic cardioplegia solution was first used in open heart surgery in the 1970s and enjoys widespread clinical use today. Cardioplegia solution is infused into the coronary vasculature to produce an elective diastolic cardiac arrest. Inducing cardiac arrest, or cardioplegia, helps protect the myocardium while providing the surgeon with a still, bloodless operative field and a flaccid heart on which to work. Cardioplegia solution is administered via the cardiopulmonary bypass pump (a heart-lung machine) through specialized circuits.

During open heart surgery, the heart is excluded from normal circulation by diverting venous blood away from the right atrium via gravity drainage and by clamping the aorta. Systemic circulation of blood is maintained through the use of the cardiopulmonary bypass pump; a cannula is placed in the aorta distal to the clamp and carries oxygenated blood from the pump to the patient. The blood circulates through the body and is returned to the cardiopulmonary bypass pump through cannulas inserted into the superior and inferior venae cava.

Delivery Methods

Cardioplegia solution is delivered to the coronary circulation by three approaches: antegrade, retrograde, or combination antegrade/retrograde. With antegrade administration, the solution is administered via a cannula placed in the aortic root, whereas with retrograde administration, the cannula is placed in the coronary sinus.[89] The commonly used combination approach eliminates problems such as the nonhomogeneous distribution of cardioplegia solution, which can occur with the antegrade approach, while still ensuring a rapid arrest (arrest produced by retrograde administration is not as fast as antegrade).[90,91] This approach has significantly reduced patient morbidity when compared with antegrade administration, especially in high-risk patients requiring reoperation.[90]

Phases of Cardioplegia

Cardioplegia can be divided into three phases: induction of arrest, maintenance of arrest, and reperfusion (immediately before aortic unclamping). Cardioplegia solution is used routinely during the induction and maintenance phases, and reperfusion solution is used at the end of surgery before aortic unclamping. The solutions used in each phase may differ in composition and characteristics.

Goal of Treatment

Cardioplegia solution is used to prevent myocardial ischemic damage that can occur during the induction and maintenance of arrest, whereas reperfusion solution is used to help prevent and minimize the destructive phenomena that can occur during reperfusion. Myocardial ischemia can result in a number of detrimental changes to the heart, including rapid cellular conversion from aerobic to anaerobic metabolism, high-energy phosphate (e.g., adenosine triphosphate [ATP]) depletion, intracellular acidosis, calcium influx, and myocardial cell membrane disruption. Destructive changes that can occur during reperfusion include intracellular calcium accumulation, explosive cell swelling, and inability to use delivered oxygen.[92] Chemical components are added to cardioplegia solution to counteract the specific cellular effects of ischemia and the cellular events that can occur during reperfusion.

Cardioplegia Solution Vehicles

The chemical composition of a cardioplegia solution depends on the vehicle used: blood or crystalloid. Each has advantages and disadvantages, as can be seen in Table 9-13.[89,90,93] Blood, because of its many advantages, is the vehicle most commonly used. Blood cardioplegia provides oxygen while the heart is arrested, proteins in blood maintain osmotic pressures closer to normal and are capable of serving as buffers, and endogenous oxygen-free radical scavengers are beneficial during reperfusion.[93] The disadvantages listed for blood have not been shown to occur during clinical use of blood-based cardioplegia solution. The patient's own hemodiluted blood from the extracorporeal circuit is used. Blood-based cardioplegia solution delivery systems include commercially available microprocessor-controlled pumps that are capable of directly injecting an additive into the blood as well as more conventional systems that deliver a fixed ratio of blood with a premixed crystalloid cardioplegia solution. Ratios of blood to crystalloid composition range from 1:1 to 16:1. The concentration of additives in the crystalloid solution must be tailored to the specific delivery ratio used to prevent accidental overdosage or underdosage. A commonly used ratio in clinical practice today is 4:1; in other words, the blood-based cardioplegia solution being delivered to the patient contains four parts blood to one part crystalloid solution. Therefore, the concentration

Table 9-13 Advantages and Disadvantages of Cardioplegia Solution Vehicles

Vehicle	*Advantages*	*Disadvantages*
Blood	Oxygen-carrying capacity	Possible sludging at low temperatures
	Active resuscitation	Possible unfavorable shift in oxyhemoglobin association curve
	Reduction in systemic hemodilution	Potential for poor distribution of solution beyond coronary stenoses
	Minimize reperfusion damage	Possible red blood cell crenation
	Provision of inherent buffering, oncotic, and rheologic effects	Impaired visualization
	Provision of physiological calcium concentration	
	Presence of endogenous oxygen-free radical scavengers	
Crystalloid	History of effectiveness	Minimal oxygen-carrying capacity
	Ease of solution preparation	Possible damage of coronary endothelium
	Low cost	Reduced efficacy (compared with blood) in preserving left ventricular function postoperatively
	Minimal potential for capillary obstruction	Systemic hemodilution
		Possible role in production of late myocardial fibrosis

Adapted from references 89, 90, and 93.

of additives contained in the crystalloid solution is five times greater than that actually delivered to the patient due to the dilution of this solution with blood before it reaches the patient. Furthermore, with blood-based cardioplegia solution, there is a reduced need to place additives in the crystalloid component of the solution. For example, calcium and magnesium need not be added to the crystalloid component because sufficient quantities are contained in blood.

Common Characteristics

Most cardioplegia solutions have certain basic characteristics in common. Crystalloid cardioplegia solutions are made hyperosmolar to help minimize myocardial edema associated with cardiac arrest and are usually made slightly basic to compensate for the metabolic acidosis that accompanies myocardial ischemia. Cardioplegia solutions are traditionally chilled to a temperature of 4°C to 8°C before being infused into the coronary circulation. Hypothermia decelerates the metabolic activity of the heart, reduces myocardial oxygen demand and the detrimental effects seen with myocardial ischemia, and helps maintain cardiac arrest.[94,95] However, hypothermia can also produce deleterious effects on the heart, including impaired mitochondrial energy generation and substrate utilization, membrane destabilization, and the need for a longer period of reperfusion to rewarm the heart, which can increase the chances of reperfusion injury. In an effort to minimize the adverse consequences of hypothermia, the use of normothermic cardioplegia solution for induction of arrest (with cardioplegia maintained with a hypothermic solution) and the administration of a normothermic reperfusion solution before aortic cross-clamp removal was demonstrated to improve myocardial metabolic and functional recovery in energy-depleted hearts.[93] The benefits seen with this technique prompted investigators to study the use of intermittent, normothermic (37°C) cardioplegia. Positive results were reported with this technique and included a decreased incidence of perioperative myocardial infarction (MI) and need for intra-aortic balloon pump (IABP) support, as well as a lower incidence of postoperative low cardiac output syndrome.[96,97] However, studies examining the use of normothermic cardioplegia solution have not consistently demonstrated a decrease in mortality or perioperative MI when compared with hypothermic cardioplegia solution. With normothermic cardioplegia, a major concern is that not as much protection from ischemia is provided during the time that cardioplegia solution is not being infused as that provided with the use of hypothermic solution. Furthermore, when compared with hypothermic cardioplegia solution, warm cardioplegia is associated with a greater use of crystalloid and α-agonists to maintain perfusion pressure, higher total volumes of cardioplegia, increased use of high-potassium cardioplegia to stop periodic episodes of electrical activity, a higher incidence of systemic hyperkalemia, and lower systemic vascular resistance.[98] In an attempt to reduce problems seen with normothermic cardioplegia, the use of tepid (29°C) cardioplegia solution has been advocated. When compared with hypothermic techniques, tepid cardioplegia resulted in greater left and right ventricular stroke work indices (slightly less than normothermic cardioplegia) and a much faster recovery of myocardial function.[99,100] Currently, a combination normothermic/hypothermic technique is still used more frequently in practice. Additional work is needed in this area.

Additives

Table 9-14 presents additives commonly used in cardioplegia and/or reperfusion solutions, the reason for their addition, and frequently used concentrations.[89,90] In addition to these additives, several other classes of agents continue to be examined for their usefulness in cardioplegia and/or reperfusion solutions.

Oxygen-free Radical Scavengers

Oxygen-free radicals (e.g., superoxide anion, hydrogen peroxide, free hydroxyl radical) are released during the sudden reintroduction of oxygen to ischemic tissue during reperfusion. They have been implicated in myocyte death, reperfusion-induced arrhythmias, and prolonged left ventricular dysfunction after reperfusion.[92] The addition to reperfusion solution of drugs that inhibit oxygen-free radical production or degrade free radicals (e.g., mannitol, deferoxamine, allopurinol) has been demonstrated to reduce post-reperfusion myocardial injury and other free radical-induced surgical complications.[101–103] An advantage of using blood-based cardioplegia solution is that blood contains endogenous oxygen-free radical scavengers (e.g., catalase, superoxide dismutase, glutathione).[104]

Adenosine

Adenosine is an endogenous nucleoside that is released from the ischemic myocardium during the catabolism of ATP. It protects the heart from ischemic and reperfusion injury and may have a role in ischemic preconditioning. Adenosine produces the majority of its effects through interaction at the adenosine A1, A2, and A3 receptors. Stimulation of A1 receptors causes activation of the ATP-sensitive potassium channel (K-ATP), ultimately resulting in positive chronotropic and dromotropic effects, antiadrenergic effects, stimulation of glycogenolysis, and stimulation of neutrophil adherence. Stimulation of A2 receptors results in vasodilation, renin release, inhibition of neutrophil adherence to endothelium, and inhibition of superoxide generation. The physiological effects of stimulation of A3 receptors include inhibition of neutrophil adherence to endothelium.[105] The cardioprotective effects during preconditioning are believed to be the result of K-ATP channel activation. Preliminary results of a phase II trial found that adenosine may improve postoperative hemodynamic function and possibly reduce morbidity and mortality when patients receive IV adenosine immediately before and after aortic cross-clamping in addition to cold blood cardioplegia containing 2 mM adenosine.[106] However, further multicenter studies are needed to identify patients who will benefit the most from adenosine and whether adenosine will definitively reduce the incidence of MI or death following open heart surgery.

L-Arginine

Ischemia results in decreased formation of nitric oxide; nitric oxide helps prevent neutrophils from adhering to the vascular endothelial cells. Neutrophil adhesion to the coronary endothelium is a prerequisite for neutrophil activation and accumulation in the myocardium. Activated neutrophils may be a

Table 9-14 Commonly Used Cardioplegia Solution Additives

Additive	*Frequently Used Concentration*[a]	*Function*
Amino acid substrates (glutamate/aspartate[b])	11–12 mL/L[c]	Improves myocardial metabolism; improves metabolic and functional recovery in energy-depleted hearts
Calcium	At least trace amounts (0.1 mEq/L)	Maintains integrity of myocardial cell membrane; prevents "calcium paradox"[d]
Chloride	90–110 mEq/L	Establishes a solution similar in composition to extracellular fluid
CPD solution	12 mL/L[e] 45 mL/L[c]	Chelates calcium in blood-based cardioplegia solution to produce safe levels of hypocalcemia for rapid diastolic arrest; limits postischemic calcium accumulation and improves postischemic performance
Glucose	5–10 g/L safely used	Helps achieve desired osmolarity of solution; serves as a metabolic substrate for the heart
Magnesium	32 mEq/L	Reduces magnesium loss during ischemia; reduces calcium influx and potassium efflux during ischemia; has a weak arresting action on heart
Potassium	15–30 mEq/L[f]	Induces rapid diastolic arrest
Sodium	120–140 mEq/L	Necessary for protective action of potassium; establishes a solution similar in composition to extracellular fluid
Sodium bicarbonate or THAM	Variable; added until desired pH is obtained	Provides buffering capacity; helps maintain physiologically normal pH range; counters acidosis produced by ischemia

[a] Concentration delivered to patient; concentration dependent on other cardioplegia solution additives (concentration of any one additive may be changed by inclusion of other additives).
[b] Not commercially available in parenteral formulation; each milliliter of solution contains 178.4 mg monosodium L-glutamate and 163.4 mg monosodium L-aspartate (for preparation directions, see reference 89).
[c] Warm, blood-based induction and reperfusion solutions.
[d] Calcium paradox is a condition that results in rapid consumption of high-energy phosphates, extensive ultrastructural damage of myocardial cells, and myocardial contracture; it results from an influx of calcium into the myocardial cells, resulting from the introduction of a calcium-containing perfusate (i.e., blood) into the system during reperfusion after the use of a cardioplegia solution completely lacking in calcium.
[e] Cold, blood-based induction and maintenance solutions.
[f] Lower concentrations (5–10 mEq/L) used during maintenance phase.
CPD, citrate-phosphate-dextrose; THAM, trishydroxymethylaminomethane.
Adapted from references 89 and 90.

major source of oxygen-free radical production. They enhance degranulation and the release of proteases, which cause cellular damage, and they adhere to microvascular endothelium or embolize in the microcirculation. Nitric oxide–dependent vasodilation and inhibition of neutrophil activity are believed to play important roles in preventing reperfusion damage after ischemia.

L-arginine is a nitric oxide donor and may have a role as a supplement to cardioplegia and/or reperfusion solutions. Animal studies have demonstrated benefits (reduction in oxygen-free radical formation, restoration of endothelial function) from the addition of L-arginine to cardioplegia solutions.[107–109] Limited trials in patients undergoing coronary artery bypass grafting have demonstrated that the addition of L-arginine (7.5 g/500 mL) to blood cardioplegia reduced the release of cardiac troponin T, a marker of myocardial ischemia.[110]

Potassium

16. W.D., a 64-year-old man, ASA-III, is scheduled to undergo a coronary artery bypass graft. W.D.'s serum potassium concentration is 4 mEq/L. A blood-based cardioplegia solution is ordered for the patient with the concentration of potassium in the crystalloid component to be 76 mEq/1,000 mL. Cold induction (e.g., chilled cardioplegia solution) using a delivery system of four parts blood to one part cardioplegia solution will be used. On administration of the solution to W.D., cardiac arrest was not achieved. A STAT chemical analysis of the crystalloid solution revealed that it contained no potassium. Why is this consistent with the findings in W.D.?

Failure to see immediate arrest within 1 to 2 minutes after the administration of cardioplegia solution can be due to several factors, including incomplete aortic clamping, aortic insufficiency, and failure to have a potassium concentration sufficient to produce arrest. Because W.D.'s cardioplegia solution contained no potassium, a direct cause-and-effect relationship can be made to the inability to achieve an arrest.

The major role of potassium in cardioplegia solution is to induce a rapid diastolic arrest by blocking the inward sodium current and initial phases of cellular depolarization. This results in cessation of electromechanical activity and helps preserve ATP and creatine phosphate stores for postischemic work. A delivered potassium concentration in the range of 15 to 20 mEq/L is used most commonly. This concentration has consistently produced asystole while minimizing adverse effects (e.g., tissue damage, systemic hyperkalemia). Potassium concentrations >40 mEq/L alter myocardial cell membranes, allow extracellular calcium to enter the cell, and raise energy demands.[111] In laboratory studies, high concentrations of potassium (>100 mEq/L) increase myocardial contracture and wall tension, a condition referred to as *stone heart syndrome.*[112] Varying concentrations of potassium are used in the cardioplegia solution, depending on the phase of cardioplegia. As previously discussed, a high concentration of potassium is required to induce arrest, whereas lower concentrations (e.g., 5–10 mEq/L) are sufficient to maintain arrest.[113] On first glance, the concentration of potassium ordered in W.D.'s blood-based cardioplegia solution appears excessive. However, the concentration delivered to the coronary circulation is slightly <20 mEq/L if one considers that the potassium contribution from the blood component of this blood-based cardioplegia solution is approximately 4 mEq/L and that from the crystalloid component is approximately 15 mEq/L (76 mEq/L ÷ 5). This highlights the importance of knowing the delivery ratio being used for the administration of blood-based cardioplegia solution.

Amino Acids: Normothermic, Blood-Based Cardioplegia Solution

17. T.E., a 55-year-old man, ASA-IV, is admitted to the hospital with an MI. He is currently in the coronary care unit and is scheduled for myocardial revascularization surgery. He has poor left ventricular function (cardiac output, 2.2 L/minute [normal, 4–6 L/minute]; pulmonary capillary wedge pressure, 25 mmHg [normal, 5–12 mmHg]; left ventricular ejection fraction, 25% [normal, >60%]), and is on an IABP for circulatory support. In addition to being on the IABP, he is receiving dopamine and milrinone. A diagnosis of cardiogenic shock is made. What type of cardioplegia solution should T.E. receive during his revascularization surgery?

Normothermic (37°C), blood-based cardioplegia and reperfusion solutions containing the amino acids glutamate and aspartate have been advocated for the induction and reperfusion phases of cardioplegia in patients with ischemic hearts (e.g., extending MI, cardiogenic shock, hemodynamic instability) or those with advanced left or right ventricular hypertrophy or dysfunction.[114–116] Glutamate and aspartate, Krebs' cycle precursors, are added to cardioplegia solution to counteract the depletion of Krebs' cycle intermediates during myocardial ischemia and to enhance energy production during reperfusion.[114,116,117] These agents enhance oxidative metabolism optimally at normothermia (37°C).[117]

With this technique, cardioplegia induction is accomplished with an infusion of the normothermic, blood-based cardioplegia solution over 5 minutes. Normothermia optimizes the rate of cellular repair, whereas glutamate and aspartate improve oxygen utilization capacity.[103] The normothermic solution is immediately followed by a 5-minute infusion of hypothermic, blood-based cardioplegia solution. Cardioplegia is maintained with hypothermic, blood-based solution. Normothermic reperfusion solution is administered for 3 to 5 minutes immediately before aortic unclamping (reperfusion). The administration of normothermic solution at the conclusion of surgery is referred to by some as a *hot shot.* It is believed to result in early resumption of temperature-dependent mitochondrial enzymatic function and to allow energy supplies to be channeled into cellular recovery rather than electromechanical work. This results in improved hemodynamic and myocardial metabolic recovery.[117,118]

T.E., with his poor myocardial function, is a suitable candidate to receive amino acid–enriched, normothermic, blood-based cardioplegia solution and reperfusion solution during the induction and reperfusion phases of cardioplegia, respectively.

ANTIEMETIC AGENTS AND POSTOPERATIVE NAUSEA AND VOMITING

Impact of Postoperative Nausea and Vomiting

PONV is a relatively common (overall incidence, 25%–30%) yet highly undesirable anesthetic and surgical outcome. Patients who develop PONV are greatly dissatisfied with their surgical experience and require additional resources such as nursing time and medical/surgical supplies. PONV typically lasts <24 hours; however, symptom distress can continue at home, thereby preventing the patient from resuming normal activities or returning to work.[119] It is important to remember that nausea is a separate subjective sensation and is not always followed by vomiting. Nausea can be as or more distressing to patients as vomiting.

Mechanisms of and Factors Affecting Postoperative Nausea and Vomiting

The vomiting center is reflex activated through the chemoreceptor trigger zone (CTZ). Input from other sources can also stimulate the vomiting center. Afferent impulses from the periphery (e.g., manipulation of the oropharynx or GI tract), the cerebral cortex (e.g., unpleasant tastes, sights, smells, emotions, hypotension, pain), and the endocrine environment (e.g., female gender) can also stimulate the vomiting center. In addition, disturbances in vestibular function (e.g., movement after surgery, middle ear surgery) can stimulate the vomiting center via direct central pathways and the CTZ. Neurotransmitter receptors that play an important role in impulse transmission to the vomiting center include dopamine type 2 (D_2), serotonin ($5HT_3$), muscarinic cholinergic (M_1), histamine type 1 (H_1), and neurokinin type 1 (NK_1) (Fig. 9-1).[119–125] The vestibular apparatus is rich in M_1 and H_1 receptors. Opioid analgesics can activate the CTZ, as well as the vestibular apparatus, to produce nausea and vomiting.[119–122]

PONV is probably not caused by a single event, entity, or mechanism; instead, the cause is likely to be multifactorial. Factors that place a patient at risk for developing PONV in adults include female gender, history of PONV and/or motion sickness, nonsmoking status, use of opioids, type of surgery, duration of surgery, and general anesthesia with inhalation anesthetic agents and/or nitrous oxide.[126] For children, risk factors for postoperative vomiting include duration of surgery ≥30 minutes, age ≥3 years, strabismus surgery, and a history of postoperative vomiting in the child or PONV in the mother, father, or siblings.[125] Unlike adults, nausea is not easily measured in children and hence not routinely assessed.

18. J.E., a 34-year-old, 55-kg woman, is scheduled to undergo a gynecologic laparoscopy under general anesthesia on an outpatient basis. She has had one previous surgery, has no known medication allergies, and is a nonsmoker. On questioning, she reports that she developed PONV following her first surgery. Her physical examination is unremarkable. Is J.E. a candidate for prophylactic antiemetic therapy?

J.E. has several risk factors that make her susceptible to developing PONV. Adult women are two to three times more likely than adult men to develop PONV. Previous PONV also

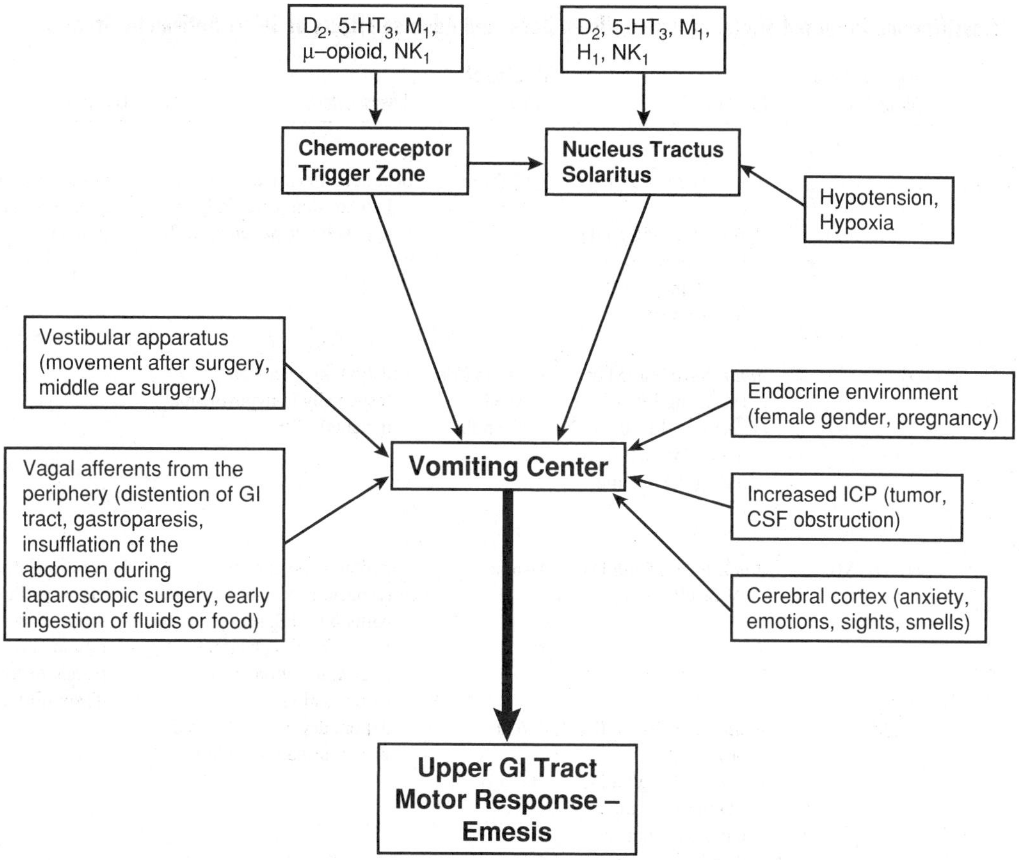

FIGURE 9-1 Mechanisms and neurotransmitters of postoperative nausea and vomiting. The chemoreceptor trigger zone (CTZ) is located in the area postrema of the midbrain. The vomiting center is also located in the midbrain, close to the nucleus tractus solaritus (NTS) and the area postrema. The CTZ, NTS, and area postrema are rich in 5-HT_3, H_1, M_1, D_2, and μ-opioid receptors. Antiemetic agents used to manage postoperative nausea and vomiting block one or more of these receptors. D_2, dopamine type 2 receptor; 5-HT_3, serotonin type 3 receptor; M_1, muscarinic cholinergic type 1 receptor; NK_1, neurokinin type 1 receptor; H_1, histamine type 1 receptor; GI, gastrointestinal; ICP, intracranial pressure; CSF, cerebral spinal fluid. *Source:* Adapted from references 119–125.

increases the likelihood of developing PONV threefold. In addition, a nonsmoking status increases the risk of developing PONV. The type of procedure J.E. is undergoing (gynecologic laparoscopy) places her at a higher risk for developing PONV. Finally, J.E. is scheduled for general anesthesia, which is also associated with a greater risk of PONV when compared with regional anesthesia. Because of the presence of many risk factors, J.E. is at high risk and should be administered at least two prophylactic antiemetic agents. Patients undergoing surgery view PONV as a highly undesirable consequence, thereby reducing their overall level of satisfaction.

Prevention of Postoperative Nausea and Vomiting: Choice of Agent

19. Which antiemetic drugs would be most appropriate for J.E., and when should they be administered?

Antiemetic drugs can be classified as antimuscarinics (scopolamine, promethazine, diphenhydramine), serotonin antagonists (ondansetron, dolasetron, granisetron), benzamides (metoclopramide), butyrophenones (droperidol), phenothiazines (prochlorperazine), and the NK_1 antagonist, aprepitant. These drugs exert their antiemetic effects primarily by blocking one central neurotransmitter receptor. Dopamine antagonists include the benzamides, butyrophenones, and phenothiazines. Ondansetron, granisetron, and dolasetron block $5HT_3$ receptors of vagal afferent nerves in the GI tract and in the CTZ. Antimuscarinics likely exert their antiemetic effect by blocking Ach in the vestibular apparatus, vomiting center, and CTZ. The proposed site of action, usual adult dose, and select adverse effects of the commonly used antiemetic drugs for prevention and treatment of PONV are summarized in Table 9-15.[3,119,121,125–127]

Butyrophenones

Droperidol possesses significant antiemetic activity, with IV doses of 0.625 to 1.25 mg effectively preventing PONV. Droperidol is more effective for nausea than vomiting, even at a dose as low as 0.3 mg. Droperidol has an onset of action of 3 to 10 minutes, with peak effects seen at 30 minutes. Doses of 0.625 or 1.25 mg often prevent PONV for up to 24 hours.

Table 9-15 Classification, Proposed Site(s) of Action, Usual Dose, and Adverse Effects of Select Antiemetic Drugs

Antiemetic Drug	*Proposed Receptor Site of Action*	*Usual Dose*[a]	*Duration of Action*	*Adverse Effects*	*Comments*
Butyrophenones					
Droperidol (Inapsine)	D_2	*Adult:* 0.625–1.25 mg IV *Pediatric:* 20–50 μg/kg IV for prevention; 10–20 mcg/kg IV for treatment	≤12–24 hr	Sedation, dizziness, anxiety, hypotension (especially in hypovolemic patients), EPS	Monitor ECG for QT prolongation/torsades de pointes
Phenothiazines					
Prochlorperazine (Compazine)	D_2	*Adult:* 5–10 mg IM or IV; 25 mg PR *Pediatric*[b]: 0.1–0.15 mg/kg IM, 0.1–0.13 mg/kg PO, 2.5 mg PR	4–6 hr (12 hr when given PR)	Sedation, hypotension (especially in hypovolemic patients), EPS	
Antimuscarinics					
Promethazine (Phenergan)	D_2, H_1, M_1	*Adult:* 6.25–25 mg IM, IV, or PR[c]	4–6 hr	Sedation, hypotension (especially in hypovolemic patients), EPS, serious tissue injury from inadvertent arterial injection or IV extravasation	Limit concentration to 25 mg/mL; dilute in 10–20 mL saline, inject through a running line, and advise patient to report IV site discomfort
Diphenhydramine (Benadryl)	H_1, M_1	*Adult:* 12.5–50 mg IM or IV *Pediatric:* 1 mg/kg IV, PO (max: 25 mg for children younger than 12 years)	4–6 hr	Sedation, dry mouth, blurred vision, urinary retention	
Scopolamine (Transderm Scop)	M_1	*Adult:* 1.5 mg transdermal patch	72 hr[d]	Sedation, dry mouth, visual disturbances, dysphoria, confusion, disorientation, hallucinations	Apply at least 4 hr before end of surgery; wash hands after handling patch; not appropriate for children, elderly, or patients with renal/hepatic impairment
Benzamides					
Metoclopramide (Reglan)	D_2	*Adult:* 10–20 mg IV *Pediatric:* 0.25 mg/kg IV	≤6 hr	Sedation, hypotension, EPS	Consider for rescue if N/V is believed to be due to gastric stasis; reduce dose to 5 mg in renal impairment; give slow IV push
Serotonin Antagonists					
Ondansetron (Zofran)	5-HT_3	*Adult:* 4 mg IV *Pediatric:* 0.05–0.1 mg/kg IV	Up to 24 hr	Headache, lightheadedness, QT prolongation	
Dolasetron (Anzemet)	5-HT_3	*Adult:* 12.5 mg IV *Pediatric:* 0.35 mg/kg IV	Up to 24 hr	Headache, lightheadedness, QT prolongation	
Granisetron (Kytril)	5-HT_3	*Adult:* 0.35 mg–1 mg IV *Pediatric:* Not known	Up to 24 hr	Headache, lightheadedness, QT prolongation	
Palonosetron (Aloxi)		*Adult:* 0.075 mg IV	Up to 24 hr	Bradychardia, headache, QT prolongation	
NK_1 Antagonists					
Aprepitant (Emend)	NK_1	*Adult:* 40 mg PO up to 3 hr before surgery	Up to 24 hr	Headache	

Table 9-15 Classification, Proposed Site(s) of Action, Usual Dose, and Adverse Effects of Select Antiemetic Drugs (Continued)

Antiemetic Drug	Proposed Receptor Site of Action	Usual Dose[a]	Duration of Action	Adverse Effects	Comments
Other					
Dexamethasone (Decadron)	None	*Adult:* 4–8 mg IV *Pediatric:* 0.15 mg/kg IV	Up to 24 hr	Genital itching, flushing, hyperglycemia	

[a]Unless otherwise indicated, pediatric doses should not exceed adult doses.
[b]Children >10 kg or older than 2 years only. Change from IM to PO as soon as possible. When administering PR, the dosing interval varies from 8 to 24 hours, depending on the child's weight.
[c]Maximum of 12.5 mg in children younger than 12 years.
[d]Remove after 24 hours. Instruct patient to thoroughly wash the patch site and their hands.
5-HT_3, serotonin type 3 receptor; D_2, dopamine type 2 receptor; ECG, electrocardiogram; EPS, extrapyramidal symptoms (e.g., motor restlessness or acute dystonia); H_1, histamine type 1 receptor; IV, intravenous; IM, intramuscular; M_1, muscarinic cholinergic type 1; N/A, not applicable; N/V, nausea and/or vomiting; PO, orally (by mouth); PR, per rectum.
Adapted from references 3, 119, 121, and 125–127.

The duration of action of a 0.3-mg dose, however, is short lived, with repeated doses often necessary. Droperidol is most effective when administered near the end of surgery. Adverse effects include sedation (especially at doses ≥2.5 mg), anxiety, hypotension, and, rarely, restlessness or other extrapyramidal (EP) reactions.[128] Because of its effectiveness and cost, droperidol has historically been used extensively as a first-line agent. However, in December 2001, the FDA strengthened warnings regarding adverse cardiac events following droperidol administration. With the new warning to perform continuous 12-lead electrocardiographic monitoring before and for 2 to 3 hours following administration of droperidol, it became an issue, from both expense and logistical viewpoints, to administer droperidol to an outpatient, patient in the PACU (recovery room), or patient in an unmonitored bed. Because low-dose droperidol has been used for >30 years to prevent PONV, many anesthesia providers challenged the decision of the FDA to issue this "black box" warning.[129] Nuttall et al.[130] retrospectively examined whether low-dose droperidol administration increased the incidence of torsades de pointes (TdP) in patients undergoing general surgery. Of the 16,791 patients exposed to droperidol, no patient experienced TdP. The authors concluded that the FDA's black box warning for low-dose droperidol is excessive and unnecessary.

Benzamides

Metoclopramide, in doses of 10 to 20 mg, has been used in the prevention and treatment of PONV. However, variable results have been seen with this agent.[131] For maximum benefit, metoclopramide must be administered near the end of surgery (secondary to its rapid redistribution after IV administration); 10 mg IV administered at the beginning of surgery is not effective. Adverse effects of metoclopramide include drowsiness and EP reactions, such as anxiety and restlessness. Metoclopramide should be administered by slow intravenous injection over at least 2 minutes to minimize the risk of EP reactions and cardiovascular effects such as hypotension, bradycardia, and supraventricular tachycardia.

Serotonin Antagonists

Ondansetron (4 mg IV) was the first $5HT_3$ antagonist to receive an indication for PONV. Dolasetron (12.5 mg IV) and granisetron (1 mg IV) are also approved for preventing and treating PONV. Palonosetron (0.075 mg IV) is approved for the prevention of PONV for up to 24 hours following surgery. As a general rule, serotonin antagonists are consistently more effective in reducing vomiting rather than nausea.[132] Ondansetron and dolasetron are equally efficacious in preventing PONV.[133] A single dose of ondansetron, dolasetron, or granisetron provides acute relief and can protect against nausea and vomiting for up to 24 hours after administration. For optimal efficacy, serotonin antagonists should be administered near the end of surgery. Adverse effects are minimal and include headache, constipation, and elevated liver enzymes. Because of their good efficacy and adverse effect profile, serotonin antagonists are recommended as first-line therapy.[125]

Dexamethasone

Dexamethasone is frequently used as an antiemetic in patients undergoing highly emetogenic chemotherapy. Its mechanism of action as an antiemetic is not well understood, particularly in the surgical setting. When compared to placebo, a prophylactic dose of dexamethasone is antiemetic in high-risk patients. It is most effective in preventing late PONV (up to 24 hours). Adverse effects in otherwise healthy patients are minimal and include headache, dizziness, drowsiness, constipation, and muscle pain.[134] Because of its good efficacy and adverse effect profile (from a single dose), dexamethasone is also recommended as first-line therapy.[125] Unlike droperidol and the serotonin antagonists, dexamethasone is most effective when administered at the beginning of surgery (immediately before induction).[135]

Phenothiazines

Prochlorperazine has been used successfully to prevent PONV. Prochlorperazine (10 mg IM) was found to have superior efficacy (less nausea and vomiting, as well as less need for rescue antiemetics) when compared with ondansetron for preventing PONV.[136] Prochlorperazine may cause sedation, EP reactions, and cardiovascular effects. Because it has a short duration of action, multiple doses may be necessary.

Antimuscarinics

Scopolamine blocks afferent impulses at the vomiting center and blocks Ach in the vestibular apparatus and CTZ.

Transdermal scopolamine is useful for prevention of nausea, vomiting, and motion sickness. Compared with placebo, transdermal scopolamine effectively reduces the incidence of emetic symptoms.[137] Common side effects include dry mouth and visual disturbances. Patients can also have trouble correctly applying the patch. It is important to apply the patch before surgery because its onset of effect is 4 hours. Patients should also be instructed to wash their hands after applying the patch and to dispose of the patch properly.

Neurokinin-1 Antagonists

Aprepitant is the first NK_1 antagonist to be approved for prevention of PONV. Aprepitant has a long half-life and is administered orally prior to surgery. For prevention of PONV in patients undergoing abdominal surgery, aprepitant was similar in efficacy (defined as no vomiting and no use of rescue antiemetics in the first 24 hours following surgery) to ondansetron. Aprepitant, however, was significantly more effective than ondansetron in preventing vomiting at 24 and 48 hours after surgery. Aprepitant was well tolerated, with adverse effects similar to ondansetron.[138]

Combination of Agents

As discussed, droperidol, serotonin antagonists, dexamethasone, and transdermal scopolamine effectively prevent PONV. However, these agents fail to prevent PONV in approximately 20% to 30% of patients. Most of the agents effectively block one receptor believed to be involved in the activation of the vomiting center. However, because the cause of PONV is likely multifactorial, a combination of antiemetic agents (from different classes) is more efficacious for preventing PONV in a high-risk patient. In a factorial trial of six interventions for prevention of PONV in more than 5,000 high-risk patients undergoing surgery, patients were randomly assigned to 1 of 64 possible combinations of six different prophylactic interventions: 4 mg IV ondansetron or no ondansetron; 4 mg IV dexamethasone or no dexamethasone; 1.25 mg IV droperidol or no droperidol; propofol or a volatile inhalation anesthetic agent; nitrous oxide or nitrogen (i.e., no nitrous oxide); and remifentanil (an ultrashort-acting opioid) or fentanyl (a short-acting opioid).[139] Each antiemetic agent intervention (ondansetron, dexamethasone, droperidol) had similar efficacy and reduced the risk of PONV by about 26%. The risk was further reduced when a combination of any two antiemetics was administered, with no difference between the various combinations of agents. The risk was the lowest when all three antiemetic agents were administered.

For prophylaxis of PONV, J.E. should receive at least two antiemetic agents because she is at high risk for developing PONV. Dexamethasone 4 mg IV can be administered at the beginning of surgery (just after induction of anesthesia) and 4 mg IV ondansetron should be administered approximately 30 minutes before the end of surgery. If an alternative agent (to ondansetron and dexamethasone) or third agent is warranted, a transdermal scopolamine patch can be placed within 2 hours before the induction of general anesthesia. The addition of transdermal scopolamine to ondansetron for prevention of PONV significantly reduces PONV, as well as supplemental antiemetic requirements.[140]

Treatment of Postoperative Nausea and Vomiting

20. J.E. is taken to surgery. Anesthesia is induced with propofol and maintained with sevoflurane. Fentanyl is administered intraoperatively for analgesia. A prophylactic dose of dexamethasone is administered at the beginning of surgery, and ondansetron is administered near the end of surgery. Neuromuscular blockade produced by vecuronium is reversed with neostigmine and glycopyrrolate. In the recovery room, J.D. becomes nauseated and has several emetic episodes. What do you recommend?

Although dexamethasone and ondansetron are effective for both prevention and treatment of PONV, a rescue antiemetic is more efficacious if it works by a different mechanism of action.[141] Prophylactic dexamethasone and/or ondansetron can be effective for up to 24 hours. If nausea and emetic episodes occur in the recovery room, the prophylactic antiemetic agents were ineffective. Phenothiazines (prochlorperazine) and benzamides (metoclopramide) block dopaminergic stimulation of the CTZ, making these agents appropriate for J.E. Prochlorperazine may be preferred because metoclopramide's primary effect is in the GI tract rather than the CTZ. Diphenhydramine or promethazine, which blocks Ach receptors in the vestibular apparatus, as well as histamine receptors that activate the CTZ, would also be appropriate choices for rescue for J.E. Because excessive sedation could delay J.E.'s discharge from the ambulatory surgery center, doses should not exceed 25 mg IV for promethazine and 50 mg IV for diphenhydramine. In addition, it is important to assess J.E. for postoperative factors that could increase the likelihood of PONV. If postural hypotension is present, IV fluids and ephedrine would be appropriate therapy. Postoperative pain must also be assessed because PONV is directly related to the degree of postoperative pain; a threefold higher frequency of PONV has been reported in ambulatory surgery patients with postoperative pain.[142]

Anesthetic Agents With a Low Incidence of Postoperative Nausea and Vomiting

21. How could J.E.'s anesthetic regimen have been modified to reduce the likelihood of PONV?

Several changes could be made in the anesthetic regimen to reduce the likelihood of PONV. When propofol is used for both induction and maintenance of anesthesia, it reduces the risk of PONV similar to the administration of a single antiemetic.[139] Because perioperative administration of opioids is associated with PONV, the use of NSAIDs (oral agents preoperatively and postoperatively, parenteral ketorolac intraoperatively and postoperatively), when appropriate, can reduce the need for postoperative opioids. In addition, surgical wound infiltration with a long-acting local anesthetic, such as bupivacaine, should also be used, as needed, to reduce postoperative incisional pain.

ANALGESIC AGENTS AND POSTOPERATIVE PAIN MANAGEMENT

Acute Pain

Surgery causes injury to the body, resulting in acute pain. Specifically, the tissue trauma from surgery directly stimulates nociceptors (receptors in the periphery that detect damaging or unpleasant stimuli, inflammation, pressure, and/or temperature). In addition, tissue injury causes the release of inflammatory mediators (e.g., prostaglandins, substance P) that sensitize and activate nociceptors. Sensitized nociceptors amplify the pain impulse by generating nerve impulses more readily and more often; this is called "peripheral sensitization." The pain impulse then travels from the periphery to the dorsal horn of the spinal cord. From here, the pain impulse ascends to higher centers in the brain, which results in the patient "feeling" the pain. Because both cortical and limbic systems are involved and social and environmental influences are present, the same surgery can result in significant individual differences in pain perception. Persistent bombardment of the dorsal horn with pain impulses from the periphery results in central sensitization ("wind-up"), where there is increased firing of dorsal horn neurons. Clinically, when these two processes occur, the patient will experience a lower pain threshold, both at the site of injury and in the surrounding tissue. When this occurs, pain may be prolonged beyond the usual expected duration following surgery. If central sensitization is prolonged, permanent changes in the CNS can occur. Clinically, this can result in postoperative pain that is hard to manage.[143,144]

The degree of pain usually depends on the magnitude of the surgery[145] and the patient's level of fear and anxiety. Patients vary in their response to pain (and interventions) and in their personal preferences toward pain management. Acute pain usually resolves when the injury heals (hours to days). Unrelieved acute postoperative pain has detrimental physiological and psychological effects, including impaired pulmonary function (leading to pulmonary complications); thromboembolism; tachycardia; hypertension and increased cardiac work; impairment of the immune system; nausea, vomiting, and ileus; chronic pain; and anxiety, fatigue, and fear.[146]

Adequate pain assessment and management are essential components of perioperative care. Education of patients and families about their roles, as well as the limitations and side effects of pain treatments, is critical to managing postoperative pain. Pain management must be planned for and integrated into the perioperative care of patients. Proactive planning includes obtaining a pain history based on the patient's own experiences with pain; determining the patient's pain goal; and anticipating preoperative, intraoperative, and postoperative pain therapies. The intensity and quality of pain, as well as the patient's response to treatment and the degree to which pain interferes with normal activities, should be monitored. Ideally, pain should be prevented by treating it adequately because once established, severe pain can be difficult to control.

Management Options

Effective postoperative pain management should provide subjective pain relief while minimizing analgesic-related adverse effects, allow early return to normal daily activities, and minimize the detrimental effects from unrelieved pain. The following techniques can be used to manage postoperative pain: (a) systemic administration of opioids, NSAIDs, and acetaminophen; (b) on-demand administration of IV opioids, also known as *patient-controlled analgesia* (PCA); (c) epidural analgesia (continuous and on-demand, usually with an opioid/local anesthetic mixture); (d) local nerve blockade such as local infiltration or peripheral nerve block; and (e) application of heat or cold, guided imagery, music, relaxation, or other nonpharmacologic intervention. Local anesthetics, opioids, acetaminophen, and NSAIDs can be used alone or in combination to create the optimal analgesic regimen for each patient based on factors such as efficacy of the agent to reduce pain to an acceptable level, type of surgery, underlying disease, adverse effects, and cost of therapy. For patients experiencing mild to moderate postoperative pain, local anesthetic wound infiltration or peripheral nerve blockade, or administration of a nonopioid analgesic such as an NSAID or acetaminophen are appropriate approaches to analgesia. For moderate postoperative pain, a less potent oral opioid, such as hydrocodone or codeine, is added. For moderate to severe pain following more invasive surgery, an IV opioid (e.g., morphine, hydromorphone), an epidural containing a local anesthetic and opioid, or a peripheral nerve block with local anesthetic is necessary. (For more information about general pain management, see Chapter 8.) Analgesia for acute pain in the perioperative setting is best achieved by using a multimodal (balanced) approach with a combination of two or more analgesic agents that have different mechanisms of action or that are administered by different techniques.[146]

Patient-Controlled Analgesia

ADVANTAGES

22. J.A., a 50-year-old, 5′4″, 50-kg woman, is immediately postoperative from a total abdominal hysterectomy for a neoplasm. Her laboratory values are remarkable for a SrCr of 1.3 mg/dL (normal, 0.6–1.0 mg/dL). She is allergic to penicillin. She will be admitted to the postsurgical floor for a planned stay of 2 to 3 days. What mode of pain management should be chosen for J.A.?

PCA is a popular method of administering analgesics and offers several advantages over traditional IM or IV opioid dosing. Patients treated with intermittent IM or IV dosing of opioids "as needed" can experience severe pain because the serum opioid concentration is allowed to fall to less than the minimum effective analgesic concentration (the concentration that provides approximately 90% pain relief). In addition, high peak plasma opioid concentrations can be seen with this administration method, often resulting in excessive nausea, vomiting, or sedation, as well as respiratory depression. Small, frequent opioid doses, as seen in PCA, minimize the peaks and valleys in serum concentrations seen with relatively larger intermittent IM or IV doses. This is helpful in avoiding adverse effects associated with high peak serum concentrations and inadequate pain relief caused by subtherapeutic serum concentrations. Small, frequent, patient-controlled dosing of opioids is efficacious because opioids have a steep sigmoidal dose–response curve for analgesia, resulting in the ability of a small opioid dose to move the plasma concentration from being subtherapeutic to above the minimum effective plasma concentration that will provide effective pain relief.[147,148] In terms of safety, analgesia occurs at lower opioid dosages than sedation, and sedation generally precedes respiratory depression.[149] Therefore, if a patient becomes sedated, self-administration of additional patient-controlled bolus doses will stop, allowing the serum opioid concentration to fall to a safe level.

Therapy can be individualized by using small doses of opioids at preset intervals (e.g., 1 mg morphine every 8 minutes), with the patient in control of his or her analgesic administration. An infusion pump, with a programmed on-demand dose (the dose the patient can self-administer) and number of minutes between allowable doses (lock-out interval), is equipped with a button that the patient presses to receive a dose. IV bolus is the most common PCA route, with opioids being the drugs of choice to provide postoperative analgesia. The epidural route can also be used in select patients.

If the patient is educated to use PCA properly, it can be used to alleviate anticipated pain before movement or physical therapy in a pre-emptive fashion. J.A. has undergone a procedure for which moderate-to-severe pain is expected in the immediate postoperative period. J.A.'s pain requirement in the immediate postoperative period could be met with PCA opioid administration after first administering a bolus dose of opioid, which is titrated to achieve the appropriate level of analgesia. When her opioid requirements decline or when she can tolerate oral intake, she can then be switched to oral analgesics.

PATIENT SELECTION

23. J.A.'s surgeon decides to prescribe PCA for postoperative pain management. How should J.A. be evaluated for her ability to appropriately participate in her analgesic administration?

Patients receiving PCA therapy must be able to understand the concept behind PCA and to operate the drug administration button. J.A. must be alert and oriented before being put in control of her own pain management. She must be able to comprehend verbal and/or written instructions regarding the function and safety features of the infusion pump and how to titrate drug as needed for satisfactory analgesia. PCA has been used successfully in children, generally after ages 8 or 9 (adjusting doses appropriately) and in elderly patients. PCA is not indicated in patients who are expected to require parenteral opioids for analgesia for <24 hours because these patients will generally be able to tolerate oral analgesics shortly after surgery.

PATIENT INSTRUCTIONS

24. J.A. is nervous about giving herself an overdose while using PCA. What instructions should be provided to her?

Patients often worry about the safety of PCA, which can lead to reluctance to provide themselves with adequate pain relief. J.A. should be informed that if she administers too large of an amount of the prescribed opioid analgesic, she should fall asleep. Because she is asleep, she will not press the button. When this adverse effect of the opioid has worn off, she will wake up (plasma opioid level has fallen back into or below the therapeutic range). This is an important safety feature of PCA and is the reason family members must not push the button for the patient. However, J.A. should also know that she may have to press the button several times (after the lock-out interval has passed) before her pain is relieved. She must also be informed that she may require a larger PCA dose, so it is important for J.A. to assess her pain relief from the "usual" dose most patients are initially started on following surgery. Accurate pain assessment following her prescribed dose is critical for ensuring that her dose is sufficient to provide the desired level of analgesia. She should also understand the possible adverse effects of her PCA medication and what can be done to prevent and treat these effects, as well as the advantages of providing herself with adequate analgesia (e.g., early ambulation). Finally, she should be told of the negligible risk of "narcotic" addiction from short-term PCA use and be given ample opportunity to ask questions.

CHOICE OF AGENT

25. Meperidine is ordered for J.A.'s PCA. Is this a reasonable drug choice for her?

Ideally, opioids for PCA administration have a rapid onset and intermediate duration of action (30–60 minutes), with no accumulation, ceiling effect, or adverse effects. The physicians, nurses, and pharmacists involved with the care of the patient should be familiar with the drug selected for PCA. Morphine is by far the most common choice for PCA, although other opioids such as fentanyl and hydromorphone can be used. Drug choice is based on past patient experiences, allergies, adverse effects, and special considerations, such as renal function. Meperidine has a metabolite, normeperidine, which is renally excreted; has a long half-life; and can cause cerebral irritation and excitation. Symptoms of CNS toxicity from normeperidine include agitation, shaky feelings, delirium, twitching, tremors, and myoclonus/tonic-clonic seizures. These symptoms can be seen when meperidine is administered in higher doses and/or for a prolonged period.[150,151] The presence of renal insufficiency increases the risk of accumulation of normeperidine.[150] Meperidine also inhibits serotonin reuptake and has a fairly high serotonergic potential. The risk of a patient developing the serotonin syndrome is greater when meperidine is coadministered with another drug that has moderate or high serotonergic potential (e.g., fluoxetine, fluvoxamine, paroxetine, venlafaxine).[152] For these reasons, meperidine is a poor choice for analgesia, particularly for J.A. who has diminished renal function. Morphine is conjugated with glucuronide in hepatic and extrahepatic sites (particularly the kidney) to its two major metabolites, morphine-3-glucuronide and morphine-6-glucuronide; both metabolites are excreted primarily in the urine. Morphine-6-glucuronide is an active metabolite that can accumulate in patients with renal failure, resulting in prolonged analgesia, sedation, and respiratory depression.[153] Because of J.A.'s diminished renal function, morphine should probably be avoided because other options exist. Hydromorphone is not metabolized to an active 6-glucuronide metabolite, and fentanyl is metabolized to inactive metabolites. Either hydromorphone or fentanyl is an appropriate analgesic choice for J.A. Hydromorphone is chosen. Table 9-16 lists common doses and lock-out intervals for drugs administered by PCA.[154–156]

DOSING

26. J.A. was not receiving an opioid prior to surgery (e.g., she is opioid naive). What dose of hydromorphone and what lock-out interval should be used for her initial PCA pump settings?

If J.A. is experiencing pain before PCA has been initiated, she should receive a loading dose of IV hydromorphone titrated to achieve baseline pain relief (usually up to 1 mg). Once adequate analgesia is achieved, demand doses of 0.2 mg with a lock-out interval of 8 minutes would be a good choice to

Table 9-16 Adult Analgesic Dosing Recommendations for Intravenous Patient-Controlled Analgesia[a]

		Demand Dose (mg)		
Drug	Usual Concentration	Usual	Range	Lock-Out Interval (min)
Fentanyl (as citrate) (Sublimaze)	10 μg/mL	0.01–0.02	0.01–0.05	4–8
Hydromorphone hydrochloride (Dilaudid)	0.2 mg/mL	0.2–0.3	0.1–0.5	5–10
Morphine sulfate	1 mg/mL	1–2	0.5–3	5–10

[a] Analgesic doses are based on those required by a healthy 55- to 70-kg, opioid-naive adult. Analgesic requirements vary widely between patients. Doses may need to be adjusted because of age, condition of the patient, and prior opioid use.
Adapted from references 154–156.

maintain analgesia for this opioid-naive patient. If J.A.'s pain is not relieved after two to three demand doses within 1 hour, the demand dose can be increased to 0.3 mg.

USE OF A BASAL INFUSION

27. After the first postoperative evening, J.A. tells you that she had a terrible time sleeping. She describes waking up in pain frequently, despite pressing her PCA button many times. She rates her pain as moderate to severe in intensity and fairly constant. A review of the history on her PCA device reveals successful delivery of 9 mg of hydromorphone (30 demand doses, 0.3 mg each) over the past 12 hours. J.A. is not sedated and reports no adverse effects from hydromorphone. How can J.A.'s pain management be improved?

Many PCA infusion pumps offer a continuous infusion setting for a basal infusion during intermittent dosing. Use of a basal (continuous) infusion has not been shown to improve analgesia and likely increases the risk of adverse effects (due to the potential of an opioid overdose in some patients). Therefore, routine basal (continuous) infusion of opioids cannot be recommended for acute pain management. In an opioid-naïve patient such as J.A., however, continuing to increase the demand dose increases the risk of excessive sedation and respiratory depression (due to high peak levels). Also, J.A. describes her pain as moderate to severe in intensity and fairly constant in nature when she does not regularly push the demand button. For J.A., a continuous infusion would be beneficial. As a rule of thumb, an opioid-naïve patient experiencing acute pain (that can change quickly) should only receive about one-third of her average hourly usage as a continuous infusion or 1 mg/hour of morphine (or its equivalent, which would be 0.2 mg/hour for hydromorphone). For J.A., begin a continuous infusion of 0.2 mg/hour hydromorphone in addition to her demand dose of 0.3 mg every 8 minutes. Because the onset of action of hydromorphone is about 5 minutes, shortening the lock-out interval is not a good idea because J.A. could access the next dose of hydromorphone before the effects of the initial dose can be appreciated. That could lead to significant adverse effects, such as excessive sedation and respiratory depression.

ADVERSE EFFECTS

28. The next day, J.A. requested only a few demand doses and reports adequate pain relief with her PCA, but now complains of feeling slightly groggy and nauseated. Bowel sounds are noted on physical examination, and J.A. plans to try to take clear liquids later that morning. What are the adverse effects of PCA opioids, and how can J.A.'s complaints be addressed?

Opioids given by PCA can produce adverse effects similar to those given by other parenteral routes. Sedation, confusion, euphoria, nausea and vomiting, constipation, urinary retention, and pruritus can be experienced, and these can be managed by dose adjustments or pharmacologic intervention. Respiratory depression is very rare with PCA opioid administration.[155] However, elderly patients, patients with severe underlying systemic disease or pre-existing respiratory compromise, and those who are receiving other sedative-hypnotics concomitantly are predisposed to respiratory depression.[148] Technical problems must also be ruled out. The PCA pump should be checked to ensure that it is delivering the correct drug and dose, programming should be checked for accuracy (e.g., drug concentration, dosing interval), and the opioid reversal agent naloxone must be readily available. Monitoring for efficacy and adverse effects of PCA therapy should include pain intensity and quality, response to treatment, number of on-demand requests, analgesic consumption, BP, heart rate, respiratory rate, and level of sedation, as well as the presence of other adverse effects of opioids such as nausea and itching.

J.A.'s PCA hydromorphone dose could be reduced to manage her sedation and nausea. However, her pain control must be carefully reassessed to ensure efficacy of the newly lowered dose. An order for an antiemetic could also be provided. NSAIDs (ketorolac IM/IV or other NSAID orally) are not sedating; thus, they could be added to the analgesic regimen to provide analgesia and allow a reduction in her opioid dose. However, because of J.A.'s compromised renal function, NSAIDs should be administered with caution and in lower doses (e.g., 15 mg IM/IV ketorolac). Before administering ketorolac, J.A.'s hydration status should be evaluated to ensure that she is not hypovolemic.[157] If J.A. is able to take fluids orally, PCA should be discontinued and oral analgesics administered as needed. As healing occurs, her pain intensity should lessen, and oral opioid/acetaminophen products should manage her pain adequately.

Epidural Analgesia

29. T.M., a 69-year-old man, enters the surgical ICU after surgery for colorectal cancer (lower anterior resection, urethral stents, ileorectal pull-through). His pain is managed through a lumbar epidural catheter. What are the benefits and risks of epidural analgesia, and why was this approach to postoperative analgesia chosen for T.M.?

ADVANTAGES AND DISADVANTAGES

Epidural analgesia can offer superior pain relief over traditional parenteral (IM and IV PCA) analgesia.[158] Continuous epidural infusions offer an advantage over intermittent epidural injections because peak and trough concentrations of drugs are avoided. Epidural catheter placement is an invasive procedure that can result in unintentional dural puncture, causing postdural puncture headache, insertion site inflammation or infection, and, rarely, catheter migration during therapy and epidural hematoma.[155]

PATIENT SELECTION

Epidural analgesia should be chosen based on the need for good postoperative pain relief and reduced perioperative physiological responses. Postoperative pain should be localized at an appropriate level for catheter placement in the lumbar or thoracic location of the epidural space. Patients undergoing abdominal, gynecologic, obstetric, colorectal, urologic, lower limb (e.g., major vascular), or thoracic surgery are excellent candidates for epidural pain management. Absolute contraindications to epidural analgesia include severe systemic infection or infection in the area of catheter insertion, known coagulopathy, significant thrombocytopenia, recent or anticipated thrombolytic therapy, full (therapeutic) anticoagulation, uncorrected hypovolemia, patient refusal, and anatomical abnormalities that make epidural catheter placement difficult or impossible.[159] T.M. is a good candidate for epidural analgesia based on the severity of pain associated with his surgery and the surgical procedure.

CHOICE OF AGENT AND MECHANISMS OF ACTION

30. What drug or drug combination can be used for T.M.'s epidural infusion? What are the mechanisms of action of the analgesics commonly administered in the epidural space?

Opioids and local anesthetics are administered alone or in combination in epidural infusions. Opioids in the epidural space are transported by passive diffusion and the vasculature to the spinal cord, where they act at opioid receptors in the dorsal horn. After epidural administration, opioids can reach brainstem sites by cephalad movement in the cerebrospinal fluid. In addition, lipophilic opioids (fentanyl, sufentanil) have substantial systemic absorption from the epidural space.[153,160] Opioids selectively block pain transmission and have no effect on nerve transmission responsible for motor, sensory, or autonomic function.[161] Local anesthetics, however, act on axonal nerve membranes crossing through the epidural space to produce analgesia by blocking nerve transmission. Depending on the drug, concentration, and depth of nerve penetration, local anesthetics also produce sensory, motor, or autonomic blockade (see Local Anesthetics section). Table 9-17 describes the spinal actions, efficacy, and adverse effects of opioids and local anesthetics administered by the epidural route.[154,159,160,162]

Most often, opioids and local anesthetics are combined in the same solution because these two classes of drugs act synergistically at two different sites to produce analgesia, allowing the administration of lower doses of each drug to reduce the risk of adverse effects while providing effective analgesia. Table 9-18 lists the drugs, concentrations, and typical infusion rates for epidural administration.[155,156,160,161,163] Bupivacaine is commonly chosen as the local anesthetic agent because it can preferentially block sensory fibers (producing analgesia) without significantly blocking motor fibers.[155] The choice of opioid is based on pharmacokinetic differences among the available agents. Onset, duration, spread of agent in the spinal fluid (dermatomal spread), and systemic absorption are affected by the lipophilicity of the drug.[162] Highly lipophilic opioids such as fentanyl and sufentanil have a faster onset of action, a shorter duration of action (from a single dose), less dermatomal spread, and much greater systemic absorption. Morphine, which is relatively hydrophilic, has a slower onset of action, longer duration of action, greater dermatomal spread and migration to the brain, and less systemic absorption.[160,162] However, after several hours of epidural infusion, the dermatomal (regional) effect of fentanyl is lost, and analgesia is achieved because of a therapeutic plasma concentration. Morphine, however, retains its spinal mechanism of action.[160] The lipophilicity of hydromorphone is intermediate between fentanyl and morphine. Clinically, hydromorphone has a faster onset and shorter duration than morphine. Its site of action is likely spinal.[164] A

Table 9-17 A Comparison of the Spinal Actions, Efficacy, and Adverse Effects of Opioids and Local Anesthetics[a]

	Opioids	Local Anesthetics
Actions		
Site of action	Substantia gelatinosa of dorsal horn of spinal cord[b]	Spinal nerve roots
Modalities blocked	"Selective" block of pain conduction	Blockade of sympathetic pain fibers; can cause loss of sensation and motor function
Efficacy		
Surgical pain	Partial relief	Complete relief possible
Labor pain	Partial relief	Complete relief
Postoperative pain	Fair/good relief	Complete relief
Adverse effects	Nausea, vomiting, sedation, confusion, pruritus, constipation/ileus, urinary retention, respiratory depression	Hypotension, urinary retention, loss of sensation, loss of motor function resulting in inability to ambulate

[a] Epidurally administered morphine and local anesthetics exert their effects mainly by a spinal mechanism of action; lipophilic opioids such as fentanyl and sufentanil achieve therapeutic plasma concentrations when administered epidurally.
[b] And/or other sites where opioid receptor-binding sites are present.
Adapted from references 154, 159, 160, and 162.

Table 9-18 Adult Analgesic Dosing Recommendations for Epidural Infusion

Drug Combinations or Drug[a]	Infusion Concentration[b]	Usual Infusion Rate[b]
Morphine + bupivacaine	25–100 μg/mL (M) 0.5–1.25 mg/mL (B)	4–10 mL/hr
Hydromorphone + bupivacaine	3–20 μg/mL (H) 0.5–1.25 mg/mL (B)	4–10 mL/hr
Fentanyl + bupivacaine	2–10 μg/mL (F) 0.5–1.25 mg/mL (B)	4–10 mL/hr
Sufentanil + bupivacaine	1 μg/mL (S) 0.5–1.25 mg/mL (B)	4–10 mL/hr
Morphine	100 μg/mL	5–8 mL/hr

[a]Use only preservative-free products and preservative-free 0.9% sodium chloride as the admixture solution.
[b]Exact concentrations and rates are institution specific. Initial concentration and/or rate often depend on the age and general condition of the patient.
M, morphine; B, bupivacaine; H, hydromorphone; F, fentanyl; S, sufentanil.
Adapted from references 155, 156, 160, 161, and 163.

comparison of the pharmacokinetic properties important to epidural opioids is found in Table 9-19.[155,158,162,163] T.M. should receive a combination of opioid and local anesthetic, such as fentanyl and bupivacaine, as an epidural infusion for postoperative pain management.

31. Fentanyl/bupivacaine is chosen for T.M. How should this be prepared, and what infusion rate should be chosen?

Fentanyl and bupivacaine are commonly admixed in 0.9% sodium chloride (usual concentration ranges are found in Table 9-18). Concentrations are often institution specific and depend on the rate of administration. Preservative-free preparations of each drug should be used because neurologic effects are possible with inadvertent subdural administration of large amounts of benzyl alcohol or other preservatives. Strict aseptic technique should be used when admixing and administering an epidural solution.

The rate of administration is chosen empirically based on the anticipated analgesic response, the concentration of opioid in the admixture, and the potential for adverse effects. Usually, a rate of 4 to 10 mL/hour is adequate; the epidural space can safely handle up to approximately 20 mL/hour of fluid. An initial infusion rate of 5 to 8 mL/hour would be reasonable for T.M., with titration based on efficacy and adverse effects.

ADVERSE EFFECTS

32. Two hours after initiation of his fentanyl/bupivacaine epidural infusion, T.M. experiences discomfort in the form of an itchy feeling on his nose, torso, and limbs. Is this related to his epidural infusion?

Pruritus has been associated with almost all opioids, with a significantly greater frequency when the opioid is administered as an epidural infusion rather than by IV administration.[165] This effect is usually seen within 2 hours and is probably dose related. It generally subsides as the opioid effect wears off and can be more of a problem with continuous epidural administration of opioids or when opioids are administered via PCA. Although pruritus from opioids is probably μ-receptor mediated and not histamine mediated,[166] antihistamines (e.g., diphenhydramine) can provide symptomatic relief. Alternatively, very small doses of opioid antagonists (e.g., naloxone 0.04 mg) can be used to effectively reverse opioid adverse effects, such as pruritus, but not analgesia. Due to naloxone's short duration of action, repeat doses or a continuous infusion may be necessary.

Other adverse effects possible with epidural opioids include nausea, vomiting, sedation, confusion, constipation, ileus, urinary retention, and respiratory depression. Although rare, respiratory depression from epidural opioids is the most dangerous adverse effect. Respiratory depression can occur as long as 12 to 24 hours after a single bolus of morphine[160,162] or within hours to 6 days after beginning a continuous infusion of fentanyl/bupivacaine.[167] Typically, regular assessments of sedation level and rate and depth of respirations safely detect respiratory depression from opioids.[148,160] As with parenteral opioid administration, risk factors for opioid-related respiratory depression include severe underlying systemic

Table 9-19 Pharmacokinetic Comparison of Common Epidural Opioid Analgesics

Agent	Partition Coefficient[a]	Onset of Action of Bolus (minutes)	Duration of Action of Bolus (hours)	Dermatomal Spread
Fentanyl (Sublimaze)	955	5	3–6	Narrow
Hydromorphone (Dilaudid)	525	15	6–17	Intermediate
Morphine Sulfate (Duramorph)	1	30	12–24	Wide
Sufentanil (Sufenta)	1,737	5	4–7	Narrow

[a]Octanol/water partition coefficient; used to assess lipophilicity; higher numbers indicate greater lipophilicity.
Adapted from references 155, 158, 162, and 163.

disease or pre-existing respiratory compromise, concomitant use of other sedative-hypnotics (e.g., benzodiazepines, opioids administered by another route), and older age. As a result, reduced doses should be used in patients with these risk factors. Adverse effects of epidural local anesthetics include hypotension, urinary retention, lower limb paresthesias or numbness, and lower limb motor block. Depending on the degree of numbness and motor block, the patient may have difficulty ambulating. Monitoring for efficacy and adverse effects of epidural analgesia should include pain intensity and quality, response to treatment, number of on-demand requests (if PCA is being used), analgesic consumption, BP, heart rate, respiratory depth and rate, level of sedation, urinary output, presence of numbness/tingling, inability to raise legs or flex knees/ankles (lumbar epidural placement), and temperature.

ADJUNCTIVE KETOROLAC USE

33. On the second postoperative day, T.M. is able to rest comfortably when undisturbed, while receiving treatment with a lumbar epidural infusion of fentanyl 3 μg/mL and bupivacaine 1.25 mg/mL at a rate of 8 mL/hour. However, when he is moved at the change of each nursing shift, he complains of significant pain. Increasing the rate of his epidural infusion was tried, but caused unacceptable pruritus and sedation. How can T.M.'s intermittent pain needs be addressed?

The use of additional analgesics for breakthrough pain may be necessary in patients receiving continuous epidural infusion. T.M.'s intermittent pain could be managed by patient-controlled epidural analgesia. Like IV PCA, patient-activated epidural boluses can be administered to control pain during movement. Alternatively, ketorolac, an injectable NSAID, may be considered for T.M.; it does not contribute to respiratory depression, sedation, or pruritus and effectively treats moderate-to-severe pain. The analgesic effects of NSAIDs are additive with the opioids and can lower postoperative pain scores. Patient selection for ketorolac therapy should consider renal function, plasma volume and electrolyte status, GI disease, risk of bleeding, and concomitant drugs and therapies such as epidural analgesia.

ADJUNCTIVE ANTICOAGULANT ADMINISTRATION

34. The surgeon has determined that T.M. is at risk for developing postoperative venous thromboembolism. Enoxaparin 40 mg SC QD has been ordered postoperatively. What are the risks of enoxaparin in this situation? What are reasonable precautions?

Prolonged therapeutic anticoagulation appears to increase the risk of epidural and spinal hematoma formation, which can lead to long-term or permanent paralysis. Administration of antiplatelet or anticoagulant drugs in combination with low-molecular-weight heparin (LMWH) results in an even greater risk of perioperative hemorrhagic complications, including spinal hematoma. These findings have led to concern for the safety of spinal and epidural anesthesia and analgesia in patients receiving LMWH. Important considerations for managing a patient being administered LMWH and receiving continuous epidural analgesia are (a) the time of catheter placement and removal relative to the timing (and peak effect) of LMWH administration, (b) total daily dose of LMWH, and (c) the dosing schedule of LMWH.[168] For T.M., the epidural catheter is already in place and the LMWH is started postoperatively as a single daily dose. It is safe to leave the epidural catheter in place as long as the first dose of LMWH is administered 6 to 8 hours postoperatively. The second dose should be administered no sooner than 24 hours after the first dose. The timing of the catheter removal is of the utmost importance; it should be delayed for at least 10 to 12 hr after the last dose of LMWH, with subsequent dosing occurring a minimum of 2 hours after the catheter has been removed. There may be a greater risk of spinal hematoma when LMWH is administered twice a day. For that reason, if Q 12 hr enoxaparin is required, the catheter should be removed, and the first dose of LMWH administered at least 2 hours after catheter removal.[168] Because T.M. is receiving prophylactic daily enoxaparin, his catheter should be removed no earlier than 10 hours after his last dose of enoxaparin, with his next dose administered no earlier than 2 hours after catheter removal.

MULTIMODAL PAIN MANAGEMENT

35. W.W., a 36-year-old male, arrives at the ambulatory surgery center for an inguinal hernia repair. This procedure will be performed under local anesthesia, with sedation as needed, and is expected to be completed within 30 minutes. His medical and surgical histories are unremarkable. He is not currently taking any medication and reports no drug allergies. Following discharge from the ambulatory surgery center, how should W.W.'s postoperative pain be managed?

In general, one would expect that the greater the magnitude of the surgical trauma, the greater the patient's postoperative pain.[145] For minor surgical procedures (e.g., inguinal hernia repair, breast biopsy), there is minimal surgical trauma, and the patient goes home shortly after surgery. For intermediate surgical procedures (e.g., total abdominal hysterectomy, laparoscopic cholecystectomy), short-term hospitalization is often necessary to observe the patient's recovery and manage his or her pain. Patients undergoing major surgery (e.g., bowel resection, thoracotomy) experience a significant surgical stress response that can significantly increase postoperative morbidity. Effective pain management is essential.

If pain is mild in intensity, a nonopioid analgesic such as acetaminophen or an NSAID is appropriate. If pain is moderate in intensity or not controlled with acetaminophen or an NSAID, a low-potency opioid combination (e.g., acetaminophen with hydrocodone or codeine) is used. When pain is moderate to severe in intensity, a more potent opioid (e.g., morphine, oxycodone) is necessary. If a fixed combination of opioid and nonopioid is used, the total daily dose administered to the patient is limited by the maximum allowable daily dose of the nonopioid (e.g., acetaminophen, ibuprofen).

Multimodal or "balanced" analgesia is often used to provide postoperative analgesia. It is difficult to optimize postoperative pain relief, to the point of achieving normal function, by using one drug or route of administration. By using two or more drugs that work at different points in the pain pathway, additive or synergistic analgesia can be achieved and adverse effects reduced because doses are lower and side effect profiles are different. Opioids are a mainstay of analgesic therapy for moderate-to-severe pain. However, opioids are often associated with intolerable adverse effects (e.g., nausea, vomiting,

Table 9-20 Commonly Used Analgesic Drugs and Nonpharmacologic Techniques for Postoperative Pain Management

Type of Agent	*Examples*	*Potential Adverse Effects*
Local anesthetics	Peripheral nerve block, tissue infiltration, wound instillation	Tingling, numbness, residual motor weakness, hypotension, CNS and cardiac effects from systemic absorption
NSAIDs	Ketorolac (IV, IM, oral), ibuprofen (oral), naproxen (oral), celecoxib (oral)	GI upset, edema, hypertension, dizziness, drowsiness, GI bleeding, operative site bleeding (not celecoxib)
Other nonopioids	Acetaminophen (oral, rectal)	GI upset, hepatotoxicity
Nonpharmacologic	Transcutaneous electrical nerve stimulation, acupuncture	Skin irritation, discomfort
	Ice or cold therapy	Excessive vasoconstriction, skin irritation
	Distraction, music, deep breathing for relaxation	
Less potent opioids	Hydrocodone + acetaminophen, codeine or oxycodone + acetaminophen	Nausea, vomiting, constipation, rash, sedation, mental confusion, hallucinations, respiratory depression
More potent opioids	Morphine (IV, epidural), hydromorphone (IV, epidural), fentanyl (IV, epidural), oxycodone (oral)	Nausea, vomiting, pruritus, constipation, rash, sedation, mental confusion, hallucinations, respiratory depression

CNS, central nervous system; NSAIDs, nonsteroidal anti-inflammatory drugs; IV, intravenous; IM, intramuscular; GI, gastrointestinal.
Adapted from references 145, 146, and 169–172.

constipation, itching, sedation). Maximizing the use of nonopioid analgesics generally results in less need for opioids and improved analgesia (Table 9-20).[145,146,169–172] When compared to morphine alone, the addition of an NSAID following major surgery reduces pain intensity and 24-hour morphine consumption. As a result, the incidence of morphine-related adverse effects of nausea, vomiting, and sedation is also reduced. Although the risk of surgical bleeding from nonselective NSAIDs is low, the risk can be increased in certain settings (e.g., after tonsillectomy).[169]

For W.W., the anticipated surgical trauma is minor, and he will recover at home. The surgeon will inject a long-acting local anesthetic (e.g., bupivacaine) into the tissues surrounding the surgical field. This will provide intraoperative anesthesia at the surgical site and postoperative analgesia until the effects of bupivacaine wear off. Then, W.W. will likely require a less potent opioid (e.g., hydrocodone, codeine) combined with acetaminophen for pain control. If his pain is not controlled or his pain is mild in intensity, W.W. may take an NSAID (e.g., ibuprofen 200 or 400 mg Q 4–6 hr PRN or naproxen 220 mg Q 12 hr PRN).

ECONOMIC ISSUES

It is still common to find several anesthesia-related medications (e.g., sevoflurane, rocuronium) on an institution's top 25 expenditure list. Because of this, these medications are often targeted for cost-containment activities (e.g., appropriate flow rate for sevoflurane, use of vecuronium in place of rocuronium when appropriate).[173–177] Although many anesthetic agents do not appear to be excessively expensive when looking at individual patient use, large dollar savings can be realized because of the thousands of patients that are anesthetized per year in a hospital.

Value-Based Anesthesia Care

When trying to reduce costs in the perioperative setting, one should not focus solely on using the least expensive technology, piece of equipment, or drug. This strategy can lead to unacceptable patient outcomes and higher total costs. The importance of looking at the "big picture" has been recognized by the anesthesiology profession since the early 1990s when they put forth the concept of value-based anesthesia care, which seeks the best patient outcomes at the most reasonable costs. The advantages and disadvantages of the technique or drug are balanced against all costs associated with the surgical experience.[178]

Total Costs of Surgical Stay

In one study, anesthesia costs, including medication use, accounted for 6% of the total costs for inpatient surgery, with approximately 50% being variable. Hence, modifying medication selection can impact, at most, 3% of the total costs associated with surgery. However, OR costs, including the costs of the PACU, accounted for 37% of the total costs of surgery, with approximately 44% being variable. Therefore, modifying practices that influence these costs can impact total cost by up to 16%.[179] In another study, labor costs were estimated to be two orders of magnitude greater than anesthesia maintenance costs for a 60-minute outpatient procedure; therefore, a major component of cost-containment efforts should be directed at the reduction of labor costs by streamlining OR time and shortening PACU discharge time.[180] Methods to reduce a patient's PACU stay may allow personnel reductions and/or reassignment of staff during slow periods. These studies highlight the opportunity for cost reduction in the perioperative setting by focusing on nonmedication costs and support the concept of fast-track anesthesia.

Fast-Track Anesthesia

Throughput is a major issue in most hospitals today. The perioperative setting is often targeted as needing improvement. Fast-track anesthesia, if successfully implemented, can help with throughput issues. The goal of fast tracking is to accelerate the movement of the patient through the perioperative experience (OR, PACU, and/or ICU). It has been promoted to improve patient satisfaction, to improve OR and PACU efficiency, and to lower the costs of the surgical experience. Several developments have facilitated the fast-track process and include the wide-scale use of less invasive surgical procedures (e.g., laparoscopy), the incorporation of new monitoring techniques to allow better titration of anesthesia (e.g., "consciousness" monitors),[181] and the use of short-acting, fast-emergence anesthetic agents to reduce wake-up times and drug hangovers. Although medication costs may be higher with fast-track anesthesia, fast tracking can improve clinical and financial outcomes in both inpatient and outpatient settings. Fast tracking cardiac surgery patients has resulted in quicker extubation, reduced length of stay, reduced ICU readmission rate, and a 25% cost reduction.[182,183] Furthermore, fast-track cardiac surgery patients have a decreased health care resource usage for at least 1 year following discharge.[184] In a landmark outpatient study, fast tracking was implemented in five surgical centers and resulted in annual net savings from $50,000 to $160,000, with no significant differences in patient outcomes.[185,186] In this study, outpatients meeting a well-defined set of criteria were allowed to skip phase I recovery and proceed directly to phase II from the OR. Phase I recovery can be considered an ICU-type environment. Patients are taken here from the OR to recover hemodynamically and fully regain consciousness; this requires intensive nursing care (usually one nurse to two patients). Once patients are awake, hemodynamically stable, and able to sit upright, they are moved to phase II recovery to finish the recovery process. In this setting, the nurse–patient ratio is 1:3, or greater if nurse assistants are employed. The low-solubility, volatile inhalation agents (desflurane, sevoflurane) are ideally suited for fast tracking in the outpatient setting.[181,187]

Thus, the goal for the cost-effective use of medications in the perioperative setting is a net reduction in the cost of surgical procedures (either the result of a lower overall medication cost or process modifications such as fast tracking) by taking advantage of the medications' properties and keeping in mind that patients' outcomes should not be negatively impacted and, ideally, should be improved.

REFERENCES

1. Hata TM, Moyers JR. Preoperative medication. In: Barash PG et al., eds. *Clinical Anesthesia*. Philadelphia: Lippincott Williams & Wilkins; 2006: 475.
2. Cravero J, Kain ZN. Pediatric anesthesia. In: Barash PG et al., eds. *Clinical Anesthesia*. Philadelphia: Lippincott Williams & Wilkins; 2006:1205.
3. Donnelly AJ et al. *Anesthesiology & Critical Care Drug Handbook*. Hudson, OH: Lexi-Comp, Inc.; 2006.
4. Scholz J, Tonner PH. α-2-Adrenoreceptor agonists in anaesthesia: a new paradigm. *Curr Opin Anaesthesiol* 2000;13:437.
5. Friedberg BL. Propofol ketamine anesthesia for cosmetic surgery in the office suite. *Int Anesthiol Clin* 2003;41:39.
6. Muravchick S. Anesthesia for the geriatric patient. In: Barash PG et al., eds. *Clinical Anesthesia*. Philadelphia: Lippincott Williams & Wilkins; 2006:1219.
7. Fredman B et al. The effect of midazolam premedication on mental and psychomotor recovery in geriatric patients undergoing brief surgical procedures. *Anesth Analg* 1999;89:1161.
8. Kain ZN et al. Parental presence during induction of anesthesia versus sedative premedication: which intervention is more effective? *Anesthesiology* 1998;89:1147.
9. Holm-Knudsen RJ et al. Distress at induction of anaesthesia in children: a survey of incidence, associated factors and recovery characteristics. *Paediatr Anaesth* 1998;8:383.
10. Kain ZM et al. Postoperative behavioral outcomes in children: effects of sedative premedication. *Anesthesiology* 1999;90:758.
11. Marik PE. Aspiration pneumonitis and aspiration pneumonia. *N Engl J Med* 2001;344:665.
12. Fowler AA et al. Adult respiratory distress syndrome: risk with common predispositions. *Ann Intern Med* 1983;98:593.
13. Rocke DA et al. At risk for aspiration: new critical values of volume and pH? *Anesth Analg* 1993;76:666.
14. Pisegna JR, Martindale RG. Acid suppression in the perioperative period. *J Clin Gastroenterol* 2005;39:10.
15. Jellish WS et al. Effect of metoclopramide on gastric fluid volumes in diabetic patients who have fasted before elective surgery. *Anesthesiology* 2005;102:904.
16. Rosenblatt WH. Airway management. In: Barash PG et al., eds. *Clinical Anesthesia*. Philadelphia: Lippincott Williams & Wilkins; 2006:595.
17. Minami H, McCallum RW. The physiology and pathophysiology of gastric emptying in humans. *Gastroenterology* 1984;86:1592.
18. Schneck H, Scheller M. Acid aspiration prophylaxis and caesarian section. *Curr Opin Anaesthesiol* 2000;13:261.
19. Lim SK, Elegbe EO. The use of single dose of sodium citrate as a prophylaxis against acid aspiration syndrome in obstetric patients undergoing caesarean section. *Med J Malaysia* 1991;46:349.
20. Schmidt JF et al. The effect of sodium citrate on the pH and the amount of gastric contents before general anesthesia. *Acta Anaesthesiol Scand* 1984;28:263.
21. American Society of Anesthesiologists. Practice guidelines for preoperative fasting and the use of pharmacologic agents to reduce the risk of pulmonary aspiration. *Anesthesiology* 1999;90:896.
22. Ng A, Smith G. Gastroesophageal reflux and aspiration of gastric contents in anesthetic practice. *Anesth Analg* 2001;93:494.
23. Memis D et al. The effect of intravenous pantoprazole and ranitidine for improving preoperative gastric fluid properties in adults undergoing elective surgery. *Anesth Analg* 2003;97:1360.
24. American Society of Anesthesiologists Task Force on Obstetric Anesthesia. Practice Guidelines for Obstetric Anesthesia. *Anesthesiology* 2007; 106:843.
25. Evers AS, Crowder CM. Cellular and molecular mechanisms of anesthesia. In: Barash PG et al., eds. *Clinical Anesthesia*. Philadelphia: Lippincott Williams & Wilkins; 2006:111.
26. White PF, Romero G. Nonopioid intravenous anesthesia. In: Barash PG et al., eds. *Clinical Anesthesia*. Philadelphia: Lippincott Williams & Wilkins; 2006:334.
27. Stoelting RK, Hillier SC. Nonbarbiturate intravenous anesthetic drugs. *Pharmacology and Physiology in Anesthetic Practice*. Philadelphia: Lippincott Williams & Wilkins; 2006:155.
28. Reves JG et al. Intravenous nonopioid anesthetics. In: Miller RD, ed. *Anesthesia*. Philadelphia: Elsevier; 2005;317.
29. Greenwald MJ et al. Extraocular muscle surgery. In: Krupin T, Holker AE, eds. *Complications of Ocular Surgery*. St. Louis, MO: Mosby; 1993.
30. Borgeat A et al. Subhypnotic doses of propofol possess direct antiemetic effects. *Anesth Analg* 1992;74:539.
31. Souter KJ. Anesthesia provided at alternate sites. In: Barash PG, et al. eds. *Clinical Anesthesia*. Philadelphia: Lippincott Williams & Wilkins; 2006:1331.
32. Ding Z, White PF. Anesthesia for electroconvulsive therapy. *Anesth Analg* 2002;94:1351.
33. Green SM, Kraus B. Clinical practice guidelines for emergency department ketamine dissociative sedation in children. *Ann Emerg Med* 2004;44; 460.
34. Ebert TJ, Schmid PG III. Inhalation anesthesia. In: Barash PG et al., eds. *Clinical Anesthesia*. Philadelphia: Lippincott Williams & Wilkins; 2006; 384.
35. Brockwell RC, Andrews JJ. Inhaled anesthetic delivery systems. In: Miller RD, ed. *Anesthesia*. Philadelphia: Elsevier; 2005;273.
36. Gonsowski CT et al. Toxicity of compound A in rats. *Anesthesiology* 1994;80:556.
37. Mazze RI et al. The effects of sevoflurane on serum creatinine and blood urea nitrogen concentrations: a retrospective, twenty-two-center, comparative evaluation of renal function in adult surgical patients. *Anesth Analg* 2000;90:683.
38. Eger EI II et al. Dose-related biochemical markers of renal injury after sevoflurane versus desflurane anesthesia in volunteers. *Anesth Analg* 1997;85:1154.
39. Karasch ED et al. Assessment of low-flow sevoflurane and isoflurane effects on renal function using sensitive markers of tubular toxicity. *Anesthesiology* 1997;86:1238.
40. Bito H et al. Effects of low-flow sevoflurane on renal function: comparison with high-flow sevoflurane anesthesia and low-flow isoflurane anesthesia. *Anesthesiology* 1997;86:1231.
41. Frink EJ et al. Production of carbon monoxide using dry Baralyme with desflurane, enflurane, isoflurane, halothane, or sevoflurane anesthesia in pigs. *Anesthesiology* 1996;85:A1018.
42. Fang ZX et al. Carbon monoxide production from degradation of desflurane, enflurane, isoflurane, halothane, and sevoflurane by soda lime and Baralyme. *Anesth Analg* 1995;80:1187.
43. Murray MM et al. Amsorb: a new carbon dioxide absorbent for use in anesthetic breathing systems. *Anesthesiology* 1999;91:1342.
44. Philip BK et al. A multicenter comparison of maintenance and recovery with sevoflurane or isoflurane for adult ambulatory anesthesia. *Anesth Analg* 1996;83:314.
45. Beaussier M et al. Comparative effects of desflurane and isoflurane on recovery after long lasting anesthesia. *Can J Anaesth* 1998;45:429.
46. Ebert TJ et al. Recovery from sevoflurane anesthesia: a comparison to isoflurane and propofol anesthesia. *Anesthesiology* 1998;89:1524.
47. Stoelting RK. *Pharmacology and Physiology in Anesthetic Practice*. Philadelphia: Lippincott-Raven; 1999:36.

48. Karasch ED et al. Human kidney methoxyflurane and sevoflurane metabolism: intrarenal fluoride production as a possible mechanism of methoxyflurane nephrotoxicity. *Anesthesiology* 1995;82:689.
49. Conzen PF et al. Low-flow sevoflurane compared with low-flow isoflurane anesthesia in patients with stable renal insufficiency. *Anesthesiology* 2002;97:578.
50. Higuchi H et al. Renal function in patients with high serum fluoride concentrations after prolonged sevoflurane anesthesia. *Anesthesiology* 1995;83:449.
51. Nishiyama T et al. Inorganic fluoride kinetics and renal tubular function after sevoflurane anesthesia in chronic renal failure patients receiving hemodialysis. *Anesth Analg* 1996;83:574.
52. Morgan Jr GE et al. *Inhalational anesthetics. Clinical Anesthesiology*. New York: Lange Medical Books/McGraw-Hill; 2002:127.
53. Muzi M et al. Site(s) mediating sympathetic activation with desflurane. *Anesthesiology* 1996;85:737.
54. Weiskopf RB, Eger EI. Comparing the costs of inhaled anesthetics. *Anesthesiology* 1993;79:1413.
55. Smith I. Cost considerations in the use of anesthetic drugs. *Pharmacoeconomics* 2001;19:469.
56. Rosenberg MK et al. Cost comparison: a desflurane-versus propofol-based general anesthetic technique. *Anesth Analg* 1994;79:852.
57. Apfel CC et al. Volatile anesthetics may be the main cause of early, but not delayed postoperative vomiting: a randomized, controlled trial of factorial design. *Br J Anaesth* 2002;88:659.
58. Tang J et al. Antiemetic prophylaxis with sevoflurane anesthesia: a comparison with propofol in the office setting. *Anesth Analg* 2000;90:519.
59. Ebert TJ, Muzi M. Sympathetic hyperactivity during desflurane anesthesia in healthy volunteers. *Anesthesiology* 1993;79:444.
60. Weiskopf RB et al. Fentanyl, esmolol, and clonidine blunt the transient cardiovascular stimulation induced by desflurane in humans. *Anesthesiology* 1994;81:1350.
61. Kulka PJ et al. Clonidine prevents sevoflurane-induced agitation in children. *Anesth Analg* 2001; 93:335.
62. Lapen SL et al. Effects of sevoflurane anesthesia on recovery in children: a comparison with halothane. *Paediatr Anaesth* 1999;9:299.
63. Galinkin JL et al. Use of intranasal fentanyl in children undergoing myringotomy and tube placement during halothane and sevoflurane anesthesia. *Anesthesiology* 2000;93:378.
64. Ibacache ME et al. Single-dose dexmedetomidine reduces agitation after sevoflurane anesthesia in children. *Anesth Analg* 2004;98:60.
65. Mayer J et al. Desflurane anesthesia after sevoflurane inhaled induction reduces severity of emergence agitation in children undergoing minor ear-nose-throat surgery compared with sevoflurane induction and maintenance. *Anesth Analg* 2006; 102:400.
66. Bevan DR. Neuromuscular blocking agents. In: Barash PG, et al., eds. *Clinical Anesthesia*. Philadelphia: Lippincott Williams & Wilkins; 2006:421.
67. McManus MC. Neuromuscular blockers in surgery and intensive care: part 2. *Am J Health-Syst Pharm* 2001;58:2381.
68. McManus MC. Neuromuscular blockers in surgery and intensive care: part 1. *Am J Health-Syst Pharm* 2001;58:2287.
69. Naguib M, Lien CA. Pharmacology of muscle relaxants and their antagonists. In: Miller RD, ed. *Anesthesia*. Philadelphia: Elsevier; 2005:481.
70. Sethee JS, Dunn PF. Neuromuscular blockade. In: Dunn PF, ed. *Clinical Anesthesia Procedures of the Massachusetts General Hospital*. Philadelphia: Lippincott Williams & Wilkins; 2007:190.
71. Fields AM, Vadivelu N. Sugammadex: a novel neuromuscular blocker inhibiting agent. *Curr Opin Anaesthesiol* 2007;20:307.
72. Sparr HJ. Choice of muscle relaxant for rapid-sequence induction. *Eur J Anaesth* 2001;23 (Suppl):71.
73. Strazis KP, Fox AW. Malignant hyperthermia: a review of published cases. *Anesth Analg* 1993;77: 297.
74. Malignant Hyperthermia Association of the United States. Anesthetic agent choice for the MH-susceptible patient. Available at: http://medical.mhaus.org/index.cfm/fuseaction/Content.Display/PagePK/AnestheticList.cfm. Accessed April 17, 2008.
75. Zemuron product information, Organon USA, Inc., July 2005.
76. Grigore AM et al. Laudanosine and atracurium concentrations in a patient receiving long-term atracurium infusion. *Crit Care Med* 1998;26:180.
77. Viby-Mogenson J. Succinylcholine neuromuscular blockade in subjects homozygous for atypical plasma cholinesterase. *Anesthesiology* 1981;55: 429.
78. Hunter JM et al. The use of different doses of vecuronium in patients with liver dysfunction. *Br J Anaesth* 1985;57:758.
79. Lewis KS et al. Prolonged neuromuscular blockade associated with rocuronium. *Am J Health-Syst Pharm* 1999;56:1114.
80. Hartmannsgrube MWB, Atanassoff PG. Regional anesthesia versus general anesthesia: does it make a difference? *Semin Anesth* 1998;17:58.
81. Bode RH Jr, Lewis KP. Con: regional anesthesia is not better than general anesthesia for lower extremity revascularization. *J Cardiothorac Vasc Anesth* 1994;8:118.
82. Liu SS, Joseph Jr RS. Local anesthetics. In: Barash PG et al., eds. *Clinical Anesthesia*. Philadelphia: Lippincott Williams & Wilkins; 2006:453.
83. Jin P, Min JC. Local anesthetics. In: Dunn PF, et al., eds. *Clinical Anesthesia Procedures of the Massachusetts General Hospital*. Philadelphia: Lippincott Williams & Wilkins; 2007:238.
84. Markham A, Faulds D. Ropivacaine: a review of its pharmacology and therapeutic use in regional anesthesia. *Drugs* 1996;52:429.
85. Heauner JE. Local anesthetics. *Curr Opin Anaesthesiol* 2007;20:336.
86. Rosenberg PH et al. Maximum recommended doses of local anesthetics: a multifactorial concept. *Reg Anesth Pain Med* 2004;29:564.
87. Singh P, Lee JS. Cardiovascular and central nervous system toxicity of local anesthetics. *Semin Anesth* 1998;17:18.
88. Nuttall GA et al. Establishing intravenous access: a study of local anesthetic efficacy. *Anesth Analg* 1993;950.
89. Donnelly AJ, Djuric M. Cardioplegia solutions. *Am J Hosp Pharm* 1991;48:2444.
90. Golembiewski J, Bourtsos N. Cardioplegia solution. *J Pharm Pract* 1993;6:182.
91. Chitwood W et al. Complex valve operations: antegrade versus retrograde cardioplegia? *Ann Thorac Surg* 1995;60:815.
92. Loop FD et al. Myocardial protection during cardiac operations: decreased morbidity and lower cost with blood cardioplegia and coronary sinus perfusion. *J Thorac Cardiovasc Surg* 1992;104:608.
93. Buckberg GD. Myocardial protection: an overview. *Semin Thorac Cardiovasc Surg* 1993;5:98.
94. Griepp RB et al. The superiority of aortic cross-clamping with profound local hypothermia for myocardial protection during aorta-coronary bypass grafting. *J Thorac Cardiovasc Surg* 1975;70:995.
95. Barden C, Hansen M. Cold versus warm cardioplegia: recognizing hemodynamic variations. *Dimens Crit Care Nurs* 1995;14:114.
96. Lichtenstein SV et al. Warm heart surgery. *J Thorac Cardiovasc Surg* 1991;101:269.
97. Naylor CD et al. Randomized trial of normothermic versus hypothermic coronary bypass surgery. *Lancet* 1994;343:559.
98. Christakis GT et al. A randomized study of the systemic effects of warm heart surgery. *Ann Thorac Surg* 1992;54:449.
99. Hayashida N et al. The optimal cardioplegic temperature. *Ann Thorac Surg* 1994;58:961.
100. Hayashida N et al. Tepid antegrade and retrograde cardioplegia. *Ann Thorac Surg* 1995;59:723.
101. Drossos G et al. Deferoxamine cardioplegia reduces superoxide radical production in human myocardium. *Ann Thorac Surg* 1995;59:169.
102. Ferreira R et al. Reduction of reperfusion injury with mannitol cardioplegia. *Ann Thorac Surg* 1989;48:77.
103. Bical O et al. Comparison of different types of cardioplegia and reperfusion on myocardial metabolism and free radical activity. *Circulation* 1991;84(5 Suppl):375.
104. Lapenna D et al. Blood cardioplegia reduces oxidant burden in the ischemic and reperfused human myocardium. *Ann Thorac Surg* 1994;57:1522.
105. Vinten-Johansen J et al. Broad-spectrum cardioprotection with adenosine. *Ann Thorac Surg* 1999;68:1942.
106. Mentzer R et al. Adenosine myocardial protection: preliminary results of a phase II clinical trial. *Ann Surg* 1999;229:643.
107. Engelman DT et al. Critical timing of nitric oxide supplementation in cardioplegic arrest and reperfusion. *Circulation* 1996;94(Suppl II):407.
108. Mizuno A et al. Endothelial stunning and myocyte recovery after reperfusion of jeopardized muscle: a role of L-arginine blood cardioplegia. *J Thorac Cardiovasc Surg* 1997;113:379.
109. Izhar U et al. Cardioprotective effect of L-arginine in myocardial ischemia and reperfusion in an isolated working rat heart model. *J Cardiovasc Surg* 1998;39:321.
110. Carrier M et al. Cardioplegic arrest with L-arginine improves myocardial protection: results of a prospective randomized clinical trial. *Ann Thorac Surg* 2002;73:837.
111. Tyers GFO. Cardioplegic additives: a critical review. In: Engleman RM, Levitsky S, eds. *A Textbook of Clinical Cardioplegia*. Mount Kisco, NY: Futura; 1982:139.
112. Rich TL, Brady AJ. Potassium contracture and utilization of high-energy phosphates in rabbit heart. *Am J Physiol* 1974;226:105.
113. O'Riordain DS et al. Low potassium cardioplegia: its effect on the incidence of complete heart block following cardiac surgery. *Ir J Med Sci* 1989;158:257.
114. Rosenkranz ER et al. Warm induction of cardioplegia with glutamate-enriched blood in coronary patients with cardiogenic shock who are dependent on inotropic drugs and intra-aortic balloon support. *J Thorac Cardiovasc Surg* 1983;86:507.
115. Pisarenki OI et al. Glutamate-blood cardioplegia improves ATP preservation in human myocardium. *Biomed Biochem Acta* 1987;46:499.
116. Teoh KH et al. The effect of lactate infusion on myocardial metabolism and ventricular function following ischemia and cardioplegia. *Can J Cardiol* 1990;6:38.
117. Buckberg GD. Strategies and logic of cardioplegic delivery to prevent, avoid, and reverse ischemic and reperfusion damage. *J Thorac Cardiovasc Surg* 1987;93:127.
118. Teoh KH et al. Accelerated myocardial metabolic recovery with terminal warm blood cardioplegia. *J Thorac Cardiovasc Surg* 1986;91:888.
119. Golembiewski J et al. Prevention and treatment of postoperative nausea and vomiting. *Am J Health-Syst Pharm* 2005;62:1247.
120. ASHP therapeutic guidelines on the management of nausea and vomiting in adult and pediatric patients receiving chemotherapy or radiation therapy or undergoing surgery. *Am J Health-Syst Pharm* 1999;56:729.
121. Kovac AL. Prevention and treatment of postoperative nausea and vomiting. *Drugs* 2000;59:213.
122. Watcha MF, White PF. Postoperative nausea and vomiting. *Anesthesiology* 1992;77:162.
123. Haynes GR, Bailey MK. Postoperative nausea and vomiting: review and clinical approaches. *South Med J* 1996;89:940.
124. Fukuda K. Intravenous opioid anesthetics. In: Miller RD, ed. *Anesthesia*. Philadelphia: Elsevier; 2005:379.
125. Gan TJ et al. Consensus guidelines for managing

postoperative nausea and vomiting. *Anesth Analg* 2003;97:62.
126. Eberthart LHJ et al. The development and validation of a risk score to predict the probability of postoperative vomiting in pediatric patients. *Anesth Analg* 2004;99:1630.
127. Taketomo CK et al. *Pediatric Dosage Handbook*. Hudson, OH: Lexi-Comp, Inc.; 2006.
128. Henzi I et al. Efficacy, dose-response, and adverse effects of droperidol for prevention of postoperative nausea and vomiting. *Can J Anaesth* 2000;47:537.
129. Gan TJ et al. FDA "black-box" warning regarding use of droperidol for postoperative nausea and vomiting: is it justified? *Anesthesiology* 2002;97:287.
130. Nuttall GA et al. Does low-dose droperidol administration increase the risk of drug-induced QT prolongation and torsades de pointes in the general surgical population. *Anesthesiology* 2007;107:531.
131. Domino KD et al. Comparative efficacy and safety of ondansetron, droperidol, and metoclopramide for preventing postoperative nausea and vomiting: a meta-analysis. *Anesth Analg* 1999;88:1370.
132. Tramer MR et al. Efficacy, dose–response, and safety of ondansetron in prevention of postoperative nausea and vomiting. *Anesthesiology* 1997;87:1277.
133. Zarate E et al. A comparison of the costs and efficacy of ondansetron versus dolasetron for antiemetic prophylaxis. *Anesth Analg* 2000;90:1352.
134. Henzi I et al. Dexamethasone for the prevention of postoperative nausea and vomiting: a quantitative systematic review. *Anesth Analg* 2000;90:186.
135. Wand JJ et al. The effect of timing of dexamethasone administration on its efficacy as a prophylactic antiemetic for postoperative nausea and vomiting. *Anesth Analg* 2000;91:136.
136. Chen JJ et al. Efficacy of ondansetron and prochlorperazine for the prevention of postoperative nausea and vomiting after total hip replacement or total knee replacement procedures. *Arch Intern Med* 1998;158:2124.
137. Kranke P et al. The efficacy and safety of transdermal scopolamine for the prevention of postoperative nausea and vomiting: a quantitative systematic review. *Anesth Analg* 2002;95:133.
138. Diemunsch P et al. Single-dose aprepitant versus ondansetron for the prevention of postoperative nausea and vomiting: a randomized, double-blind phase III trial in patients undergoing open abdominal surgery. *Br J Anaesth* 2007;99:202.
139. Apfel CFC et al. A factorial trial of six interventions for prevention of postoperative nausea and vomiting. *N Engl J Med* 2004;350:2441.
140. Jones S et al. The effect of transdermal scopolamine on the incidence and severity of postoperative nausea and vomiting in a group of high-risk patients given prophylactic intravenous ondansetron. *AANA J* 2006;74:127.
141. Kovac AL et al. Efficacy of repeat intravenous dosing of ondansetron in controlling postoperative nausea and vomiting: a randomized, double-blind, placebo-controlled multicenter trial. *J Clin Anesth* 1999;11:453.
142. Sinclair DR et al. Can postoperative nausea and vomiting be predicted? *Anesthesiology* 1999;91:109.
143. Reuben SS, Buvanendran A. Preventing the development of chronic pain after orthopaedic surgery with preventive multimodal analgesic techniques. *J Bone Joint Surg* 2007;89:1343.
144. Rowlingson JC. Acute pain management revisited. *IARS Rev Course Lectures* 2002:92.
145. Carpenter RL. Optimizing postoperative pain management. *Am Fam Physician* 1997;56:835.
146. Kehlet H, Wilmore D. Multimodal strategies to improve surgical outcome. *Am J Surg* 2002;183:630.
147. Grass JA. Patient-controlled analgesia. *Anesth Analg* 2005;101:S44.
148. Etches RC. Patient-controlled analgesia. *Surg Clin North Am* 1999;79:297.
149. Pasero C, McCaffery M. Monitoring sedation: it's the key to preventing opioid-induced respiratory depression. *Am J Nurs* 2002;102:67.
150. Mernes ER, Hare BD. Meperidine neurotoxicity: three case reports and a review of the literature. *J Pharm Care Pain Sympt Control* 1993;1:5.
151. Kaiko RF et al. Central nervous system excitatory effects of meperidine in cancer patients. *Ann Neurol* 1983;13:180.
152. Mason PJ et al. Serotonin syndrome: presentation of 2 cases and a review of the literature. *Medicine* 2000;79:201.
153. Austrup ML, Korean G. Analgesic agents for the postoperative period. *Surg Clin North Am* 1999;79:253.
154. Lubenow TK et al. Management of acute postoperative pain. In: Barash PG et al., eds. *Clinical Anesthesia*. Philadelphia: Lippincott Williams & Wilkins; 2006:1405.
155. Wu CL. Acute postoperative pain. In: Miller RD, ed. *Anesthesia*. Philadelphia: Elsevier; 2005:2729.
156. Ginsberg B, Latta KS. Acute pain management. In: Lipman AG, ed. *Pain Management for Primary Care Clinicians*. Bethesda, MD: American Society of Health-System Pharmacists; 2004:123.
157. Ketorolac tromethamine injection U.S.P. Bedford, OH: Bedford Laboratories; 2006.
158. Dolin SJ et al. Effectiveness of acute postoperative pain management: I. evidence from published data. *Br J Anaesth* 2002;89:409.
159. Bernards CM. Epidural and spinal anesthesia. In: Barash PG et al., eds. *Clinical Anesthesia*. Philadelphia: Lippincott Williams & Wilkins; 2006:691.
160. Cerda SE, Eisenach JC. Intrathecal and epidural opioids. *Semin Anesth* 1997;16:92.
161. Rawal N. Epidural and spinal opioids for postoperative analgesia. *Surg Clin North Am* 1999;79:313.
162. Cousins MJ, Mather LE. Intrathecal and epidural administration of opioids. *Anesthesiology* 1984;61:276.
163. DeLeon-Casasola OA, Lema MJ. Postoperative epidural opioid analgesia: what are the choices? *Anesth Analg* 1996;83:867.
164. Lui S et al. Intravenous versus epidural administration of hydromorphone: effects on analgesia and recovery after radical retropubic prostatectomy. *Anesthesiology* 1995;82:682.
165. Bromage PR et al. Nonrespiratory side effects of epidural morphine. *Anesth Analg* 1982;61:490.
166. Ko MC, Naughton NN. An experimental itch model in monkeys: characterization of intrathecal morphine-induced scratching and antinociception. *Anesthesiology* 2000;92:795.
167. Scott DA et al. Postoperative analgesia using epidural infusions of fentanyl with bupivacaine. *Anesthesiology* 1995;83:727.
168. American Society of Regional Anesthesia and Pain Medicine (ASRA). Consensus statements. Second consensus conference on neuraxial anesthesia and anticoagulation. Regional anesthesia in the anticoagulated patient: defining the risks. April 25–28, 2002. Available at: www.asra.com/consensus-statements/2.html. Accessed April 22, 2008.
169. Elia N et al. Does multimodal analgesia with acetaminophen, nonsteroidal anti-inflammatory drugs, or selective cyclooxygenase-2 inhibitors and patient-controlled analgesia morphine offer advantages over morphine alone? *Anesthesiology* 2005;103:1296.
170. McCaffery M, Pasero C. *Pain Clinical Manual*. St. Louis, MO: Mosby; 1999.
171. White PF. The role of non-opioid analgesic techniques in the management of pain after ambulatory surgery. *Anesth Analg* 2002;94:577.
172. Crews JC. Multimodal pain management strategies for office-based and ambulatory procedures. *JAMA* 2002;288:629.
173. Lubarsky DA et al. The successful implementation of pharmaceutical practice guidelines. *Anesthesiology* 1997;86:1145.
174. Szocik JF, Learned DW. Impact of a cost containment program on the use of volatile anesthetics and neuromuscular blocking drugs. *J Clin Anesth* 1994;6:378.
175. Gillerman RB, Browning RA. Drug use inefficiency: a hidden source of wasted health care dollars. *Anesth Analg* 2000;91:921.
176. Bastron RD, Vallamaria FJ. Use of practice parameters to control drug costs. *Anesthesiology* 1995;83:A1059.
177. Freund PR et al. Cost-effective reduction of neuromuscular blocking drug expenditures: a two year follow-up. *Anesth Analg* 1997;84:537.
178. Orkin FK. Moving toward value-based anesthesia care. *J Clin Anesth* 1993;5:91.
179. Macario A et al. Where are the costs in perioperative care? Analysis of hospital costs and charges for inpatient surgical care. *Anesthesiology* 1995;83:1138.
180. Lubarsky DA et al. A comparison of maintenance drug costs of isoflurane, desflurane, sevoflurane, and propofol with OR and PACU labor costs during a 60 minute outpatient procedure. *Anesthesiology* 1995;83:A1035.
181. Song D et al. Titration of volatile anesthetics using bispectral index facilitates recovery after ambulatory anesthesia. *Anesthesiology* 1997;87:842.
182. Cheng DCH et al. Early tracheal extubation after coronary artery bypass graft surgery reduces costs and improves resource use. *Anesthesiology* 1996;85:1300.
183. Cheng DCH et al. Morbidity outcome in early versus conventional tracheal extubation after coronary artery bypass graft surgery: a prospective randomized controlled trial. *J Thorac Cardiovasc Surg* 1996;112:755.
184. Cheng DCH et al. Randomized assessment of resource use in fast-track cardiac surgery 1 year after hospital discharge. *Anesthesiology* 2003;98:651.
185. Apfelbaum JL et al. Bypassing the PACU: a new paradigm in ambulatory surgery. *Anesthesiology* 1997;87:A32.
186. Apfelbaum JL et al. Eliminating intensive postoperative care in same-day surgery patients using short-acting anesthetics. *Anesthesiology* 2002;97:66.
187. Song D et al. Fast-track eligibility after ambulatory anesthesia: a comparison of desflurane, sevoflurane, and propofol. *Anesth Analg* 1998;86:267.

CHAPTER 10

Acid-Base Disorders

Luis S. Gonzalez and Raymond W. Hammond

Understanding the etiology of a clinically important acid-base disturbance is important because therapy generally should be directed at the underlying cause of the disturbance rather than merely the change in pH. Severe acid-base disorders can affect multiple organ systems: cardiovascular (e.g., impaired contractility, arrhythmias), pulmonary (e.g., impaired oxygen delivery, respiratory muscle fatigue, dyspnea), renal (e.g., hypokalemia, nephrolithiasis), or neurologic (e.g., decreased cerebral blood flow, seizures, coma).

ACID-BASE PHYSIOLOGY

To protect body proteins, acid-base balance must be tightly controlled in an attempt to maintain a normal extracellular pH of 7.35 to 7.45 and an intracellular pH of approximately 7.0 to 7.3.[1] This narrow range is maintained by complex buffer systems, ventilation to expel CO_2, and renal elimination of acids and reabsorption of HCO_3^{-2}. At rest, about 200 mL of CO_2, and even more during exercise, is transported from the tissues and excreted in the lungs.[3] Whereas HCO_3^- is only responsible for about 36% of intracellular buffering, it provides about 86% of the buffering activity in extracellular fluid (ECF).[1] Extracellular fluid contains approximately 350 mEq HCO_3^-, which buffers generated H^+.

$$HCO_3^- + H^+ \Leftrightarrow H_2CO_3 \qquad \textbf{(10-1)}$$

Hydrogen ion (H^+) combines with HCO_3^- and shifts the equilibrium of Equation 10-1 to the right. In the proximal renal tubule lumen, carbonic anhydrase catalyzes the dehydration of H_2CO_3 to CO_2 and H_2O, which are absorbed into the tubule cell, as illustrated in Equation 10-2 and Figure 10-1. Within the tubule cell, H_2O dissociates into H^+ and OH^-. The H^+ is then secreted into the lumen by a Na^+-H^+ exchanger. Carbonic anhydrase then catalyzes the combination of OH^- and CO_2 to HCO_3^-, which is carried into the circulation by a $Na^+HCO_3^-$ cotransporter.[4]

$$HCO_3^- + H^+ \Leftrightarrow H_2CO_3 \overset{CA}{\Leftrightarrow} CO_2\ (\text{dissolved}) + H_2O \qquad \textbf{(10-2)}$$

To maintain acid-base balance, the kidney must reclaim and regenerate all the filtered HCO_3^-. The daily amount that must be reabsorbed can be calculated by the product of the glomerular filtration rate (GFR) and the HCO_3^- concentration in ECF (180 L/d GFR × 24 mEq/L HCO_3^- = 4,320 mEq/day).[1] The proximal tubule reabsorbs about 85% of the filtered HCO_3^-. The loop of Henle and the distal tubule reabsorb about 10%.[5] Acid salts, such as HPO_4^- (pK_a of 6.8), which have a pK_a greater than the pH of the urine (titratable acids) can accept a proton and be excreted as the acid, thus regenerating an HCO_3^- anion.[5] Sulfuric acid and other acids with a pK_a <4.5 are not titratable. Protons from these acids must be combined with another buffer to be secreted. Glutamine deamination in proximal tubular cells forms NH_3 that accepts these protons. In the collecting tubule, the NH_4^+ produced is lipid insoluble, trapping it in the lumen and causing its excretion, eliminating the proton, and allowing for regeneration of HCO_3^-.[4–6] Figure 10-2 is a simplified illustration of the buffering of these acids.

The daily metabolism of carbohydrates and fats generates about 15,000 mmol of CO_2. Although CO_2 is not an acid, it reversibly combines with H_2O to form carbonic acid (i.e., H_2CO_3). Respiration prevents the accumulation of volatile acid

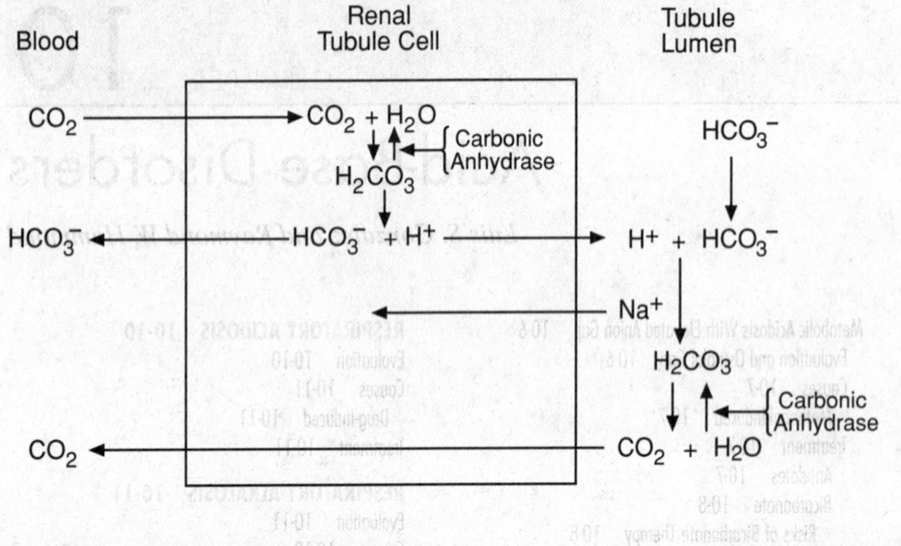

FIGURE 10-1 **Renal tubular bicarbonate reabsorption.**

through the exhalation of CO_2. Metabolism of proteins and fats results in several fixed acids and bases. Amino acids such as lysine and arginine have a net positive charge and serve as acids. Compounds, such as glutamate, aspartate, and citrate, have a negative charge. In general, animal proteins contain more sulfur and phosphates, producing an acidic diet. Vegetarian diets consist of more organic anions, resulting in a more alkaline diet.[7] Normally, fatty acids are metabolized to HCO_3^-; however, during starvation or diabetic ketoacidosis, they may be incompletely oxidized to acetoacetate and β-hydroxybutyric acid.[6] The typical diet generates a net nonvolatile acid load of about 70 to 100 mEq of H^+ (1.0–1.5 mEq/Kg) per day.[1,8] Renal excretion of 70 mEq in 2 L of urine each day would require a pH of 1.5. Because the kidney cannot produce a pH less than 4.5, most of this fixed acid load must be buffered. The primary buffers for renal net acid excretion are NH_3-NH_4^+ and titratable buffers, such as HPO_4^--$H_2PO_4^{2-}$, as mentioned above.[7] The correct assessment of acid-base disorders begins with an evaluation of appropriate laboratory data and an understanding of the physiologic mechanisms responsible for maintaining a normal pH.

Laboratory Assessment

Laboratory data used to evaluate acid-base status are arterial pH, arterial carbon dioxide tension ($PaCO_2$), and serum bicarbonate (HCO_3^-).[9–11] These values are obtained routinely with an arterial blood gas (ABG) determination. Acid-base abnormalities occur when the concentration of $PaCO_2$ (an acid) or HCO_3^- (a base) is altered. ABG measurements also include the arterial oxygen tension (PaO_2); however, this value does not directly influence decisions regarding acid-base abnormalities. Normal ABG values are listed in Table 10-1. When arterial pH is <7.35, the patient is considered acidemic, and the process that caused acid-base imbalance is called *acidosis*. Conversely, when the arterial pH is >7.45, the patient is considered alkalemic, and the causative process is *alkalosis*. The process is further defined as respiratory in cases of an inappropriate elevation or depression of $PaCO_2$ or metabolic with an inappropriate rise or fall in serum HCO_3^-.

Acid-base balance is normally maintained by the primary extracellular buffer system of HCO_3^--CO_2. Components of this buffer system are measured routinely to assess acid-base

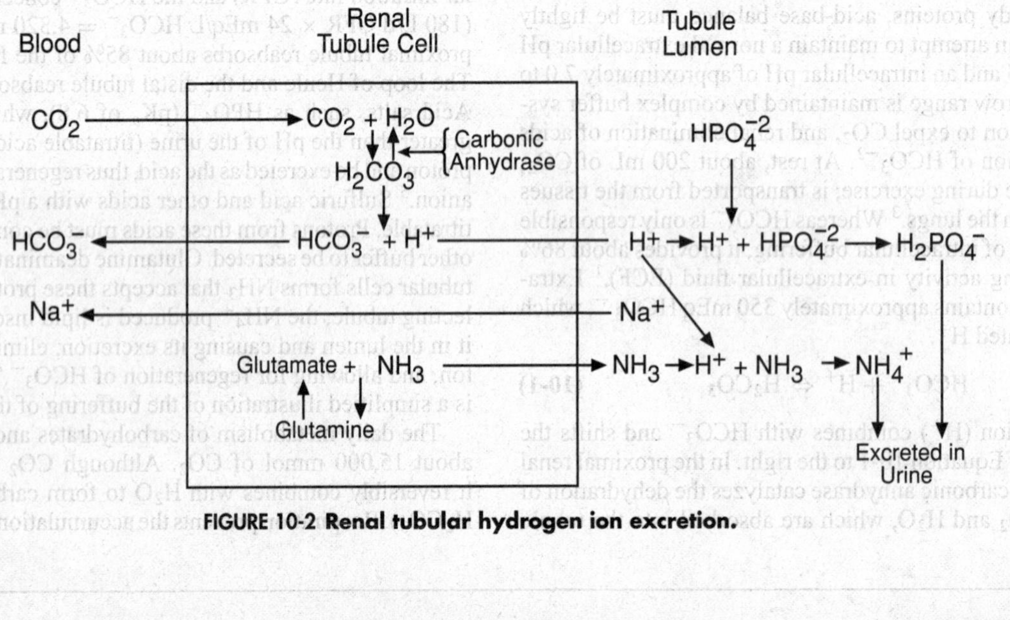

FIGURE 10-2 **Renal tubular hydrogen ion excretion.**

Table 10-1 Normal Arterial Blood Gas (ABG) Values

ABGs	Normal Range
pH	7.36–7.44
Pao_2	90–100 mmHg
$Paco_2$	35–45 mmHg
HCO_3^-	22–26 mEq/L

status. Other extracellular buffers (e.g., serum proteins, inorganic phosphates) and intracellular buffers (e.g., hemoglobin, proteins, phosphates), however, also contribute significant buffering activity.[1,7–10] Serum electrolytes are obtained to calculate the anion gap, an estimate of the unmeasured cations and anions in serum. The anion gap helps determine the probable cause of a metabolic acidosis.[6,10,12–29] Urine pH, electrolytes, and osmolality help to further differentiate among the possible causes of metabolic acidosis.[10,30–34]

Acid-Base Balance, Carbon Dioxide Tension, and Respiratory Regulation

In aqueous solution, carbonic acid (i.e., H_2CO_3 formed through the reaction described in Equation 10-1) reversibly dehydrates to form carbon dioxide (CO_2) and water (H_2O) as shown in Equation 10-2.

The enzyme carbonic anhydrase (CA), present in red blood cells, renal tubular cells, and other tissues, catalyzes the interconversion of carbonic acid and carbon dioxide. Some of the carbon dioxide produced by dehydration of carbonic acid remains dissolved in plasma, but most exists as a volatile gas:

$$HCO_3^- + H^+ \Leftrightarrow H_2CO_3 \overset{CA}{\Leftrightarrow} CO_2\text{ (dissolved)} + H_2O$$
$$\uparrow\downarrow \qquad (10\text{-}3)$$
$$k \times CO_2\text{ (gas)}$$

In Equation 10-3, k is a solubility constant that has a value of approximately 0.03 in plasma at body temperature.[2,34] Virtually all the carbonic acid in body fluids is in the form of carbon dioxide. Therefore, the $Paco_2$, a measure of carbon dioxide gas, is directly proportional to the amount of carbonic acid in the HCO_3^-/H_2CO_3 buffer system. The normal range for $Paco_2$ is 35 to 45 mmHg.

The lungs can rapidly exhale large quantities of carbon dioxide and thereby contribute significantly to the maintenance of a normal pH. Carbon dioxide formed through the reaction described in Equation 10-3 diffuses easily from tissues to capillary blood and from pulmonary capillary blood into the alveoli where it is exhaled from the body.[3] Pulmonary ventilation is regulated by peripheral chemoreceptors (located in the carotid arteries and the aorta) and central chemoreceptors (located in the medulla). The peripheral chemoreceptors are activated by arterial acidosis, hypercarbia (elevated $Paco_2$), and hypoxemia (decreased Pao_2). Central chemoreceptors are activated by cerebrospinal fluid (CSF) acidosis and by elevated carbon dioxide tension in the CSF.[3] Activation of these chemoreceptors stimulates the respiratory control center in the medulla to increase the rate and depth of ventilation, which results in increased exhalation of carbon dioxide.

Bicarbonate and Renal Control

As described in the acid-base physiology section above, the kidneys are responsible for regulating the serum bicarbonate concentration. This is accomplished through two important and interrelated functions. First, they must reabsorb the bicarbonate that undergoes glomerular filtration and is present in the renal tubular fluid. Second, the kidneys must excrete hydrogen ions released from nonvolatile acids. Both functions are important in preventing systemic acidosis.

One mechanism of bicarbonate reabsorption in the proximal renal tubule is illustrated in Figure 10-1. Carbonic anhydrase catalyzes intracellular formation of carbonic acid (H_2CO_3) from carbon dioxide (CO_2) and water in the renal tubular cell. The carbonic acid then dissociates to form H^+ and HCO_3^-. The H^+ ion is secreted into the lumen of the tubule in exchange for a sodium ion (Na^+), and the bicarbonate from the renal tubule cell is reabsorbed into the capillary blood. Inside the lumen, carbonic acid is reformed from secreted H^+ and filtered HCO_3^-. Carbonic anhydrase present inside the lumen (on the brush border membrane of the cell) catalyzes conversion of carbonic acid to carbon dioxide that can readily diffuse back into the blood. Thus, the net result is reabsorption of sodium and bicarbonate. Although a hydrogen ion is secreted into the lumen in this process, no net excretion of acid occurs because of the reabsorption of carbon dioxide.[4–6] Figure 10-2 illustrates H^+ excretion by the kidney. This process was discussed in the physiology section above.

In clinical practice, the serum bicarbonate concentration usually is estimated from the total carbon dioxide content when the serum concentration of electrolytes are ordered on an electrolyte panel or calculated from the pH and $Paco_2$ on an ABG determination. These estimations of the serum bicarbonate concentration are more convenient than directly measuring serum bicarbonate. The total carbon dioxide content that is reported on serum electrolyte panels is determined by acidifying serum to convert all the bicarbonate to carbon dioxide and measuring the partial pressure of CO_2 gas. Approximately 95% of the total carbon dioxide content is bicarbonate. The serum bicarbonate concentration reported on ABG results is calculated from the patient's pH and $Paco_2$ using the Henderson-Hasselbalch equation (Equation 10-4). This calculated bicarbonate concentration should be within 2 mEq/L of the measured total carbon dioxide. The normal range of serum bicarbonate using these methods is 22 to 26 mEq/L.[10]

Bicarbonate:Carbonic Acid Ratio

The relationship between the pH and the concentrations of the acid-base pairs in buffer systems is described by the Henderson-Hasselbalch equation:

$$pH = pK + \log \frac{[base]}{[acid]} \qquad (10\text{-}4)$$

The pK_a is the negative logarithm of the equilibrium constant for the buffer reaction. The pK for the carbonic acid–bicarbonate buffer system is 6.1. Because most of the carbonic acid in plasma is in the form of carbon dioxide gas, the concentration of acid [acid], can be estimated as $Paco_2$ multiplied by 0.03 (the solubility constant, k, in Equation 10-3). The concentration of base [base] is equal to the serum bicarbonate concentration. Using these values, Equation 10-4 can be rewritten as follows:

$$pH = 6.1 + \log \frac{(HCO_3^-)}{(0.03)(Paco_2)} \quad \textbf{(10-5)}$$

As shown by Equation 10-5, the arterial pH will be 7.40 when the ratio of HCO_3^-:H_2CO_3 is approximately 20:1. Note that it is the *ratio* of bicarbonate to the carbon dioxide tension and not the absolute concentration of these factors that determines the arterial pH. Therefore, if the serum bicarbonate concentration and the carbon dioxide tension are increased or decreased proportionately, the ratio remains fixed and the pH is not affected.[33–36]

EVALUATION OF ACID-BASE DISORDERS

Acid-base disorders should be evaluated using a stepwise approach.[32,33]

1. Obtain a detailed patient history and clinical assessment.
2. Check the arterial blood gas, sodium, chloride, and HCO_3^-. Identify all abnormalities in pH, $Paco_2$, and HCO_3^-.
3. Determine which abnormalities are primary and which are compensatory based on pH.
   a. If the pH is <7.40, then a respiratory or metabolic acidosis is primary.
   b. If the pH is >7.40, then a respiratory or metabolic alkalosis is primary.
   c. If the pH is normal (7.40) and there are abnormalities in $Paco_2$ and HCO_3^-, a mixed disorder is probably present because metabolic and respiratory compensations rarely return the pH to normal.
4. Always calculate the anion gap. If ≥20, a clinically important metabolic acidosis is usually present even if the pH is within a normal range.[37]
5. If the anion gap is increased, calculate the excess anion gap (anion gap −10). Add this value to the HCO_3^- to obtain corrected value.[38]
   a. If corrected value >26, a metabolic alkalosis is also present.
   b. If corrected value is <22, a nonanion gap metabolic acidosis is also present.
6. Consider other laboratory tests to further differentiate the cause of the disorder.
   a. If the anion gap is normal, consider calculating the urine anion gap.
   b. If the anion gap is high and a toxic ingestion is expected, calculate an osmolal gap.
   c. If the anion gap is high, measure serum ketones and lactate.
7. Compare the identified disorders to the patient history and begin patient-specific therapy.

METABOLIC ACIDOSIS

Metabolic acidosis is characterized by loss of bicarbonate from the body, decreased acid excretion by the kidney, or increased endogenous acid production. Two categories of simple metabolic acidosis (i.e., normal anion gap and increased anion gap) are listed in Table 10-2. The anion gap (AG) represents the concentration of unmeasured negatively charged substances (anions) in excess of the concentration of unmeasured positively charged substances (cations) in the extracellular fluid. The concentrations of total anions and cations in the body are equal because the body must remain electrically neutral. Most clinical laboratories, however, measure only a portion of these ions (i.e., sodium, chloride [Cl^-], and bicarbonate). The concentrations of other negatively and positively charged substances, such as potassium (K^+), magnesium (Mg^{2+}), calcium (Ca^{2+}), phosphates, and albumin, are measured less often. The concentration of unmeasured anions normally exceeds the concentration of unmeasured cations by 6 to 12 mEq/L and the anion gap can be calculated as follows:

$$\text{Anion gap} = Na^+ - (Cl^- + HCO_3^-) \quad \textbf{(10-6)}$$

Table 10-2 Common Causes of Metabolic Acidosis

Normal AG	Elevated AG
Hypokalemic	*Renal Failure*
Diarrhea	*Lactic Acidosis*
Fistulous disease	(see Table 10-5)
Ureteral diversions	*Ketoacidosis*
Type 1 RTA	Starvation
Type 2 RTA	Ethanol
Carbonic anhydrase inhibitors	Diabetes mellitus
Hyperkalemic	*Drug Intoxications*
Hypoaldosteronism	Ethylene glycol
Hydrochloric acid or precursor	Methanol
Type 4 RTA	Salicylates
Potassium-sparing diuretics	
Amiloride	
Spironolactone	
Triamterene	

AG, anion gap; RTA, renal tubular acidosis.

Of the unmeasured anions, albumin is perhaps the most important. In critically ill patients with hypoalbuminemia, the calculated AG should be adjusted using the following formula: adjusted AG = AG + 2.5 × (normal albumin – measured albumin in g/dL), where a normal albumin concentration is assumed to be 4.4 g/dL.[19–22] For example, a hypoalbuminemic patient (serum albumin, 2.4 g/dL) with early sepsis and lactic acidosis might have a calculated AG of 11 mEq/L; however, after the calculation is corrected for the effect of the abnormal serum albumin concentration, the presence of elevated AG acidosis is more prominent (the calculated AG is adjusted: $AG_{(adjusted)}$ = 11 mEq/L + 2.5 × [normal albumin – measured albumin] = 16 mEq/L).

Metabolic acidosis with a normal AG (e.g., hyperchloremic metabolic acidosis) usually is caused by loss of bicarbonate and can be further characterized as hypokalemic or hyperkalemic.[5,31,34,39–50] Diarrhea can result in severe bicarbonate loss and a hyperchloremic metabolic acidosis. Elevated AG metabolic acidosis usually is associated with overproduction of organic acids or with decreased renal elimination of nonvolatile acids.[34,51–53] Increased production of organic acids (e.g., formic, lactic acids) is buffered by extracellular bicarbonate with resultant consumption of bicarbonate and appearance of an unmeasured anion (e.g., formate, lactate).[32,51,52] The decrement in serum bicarbonate approximates the increment in the AG, the latter being a good estimate of the circulating anion level. Prolonged hypoxia results in lactic acidosis.

Uncontrolled diabetes mellitus or excessive alcohol intake with starvation can cause ketoacidosis. In the case of renal failure, the capacity for H^+ secretion diminishes, resulting in metabolic acidosis.[39] The accompanying increased AG results from decreased excretion of unmeasured anions such as sulfate and phosphate.[26]

Normal Anion Gap (Hyperchloremic) Metabolic Acidosis

Evaluation

1. A.B., a 27-year-old, 60-kg woman, is hospitalized for evaluation of weakness. She has a history of bipolar affective disorder and reports recent ingestion of paint from the walls of her house. A.B.'s only current medication is lithium carbonate 300 mg TID. On admission, she appears weak and apathetic and complains of anorexia. Laboratory tests reveal the following: serum Na, 143 mEq/L (normal, 135–145 mEq/L); K, 3.0 mEq/L (normal, 3.5–5.0 mEq/L); Cl, 121 mEq/L (normal, 95–105 mEq/L); albumin, 4.4 g/dL (normal, 3.6–5.0 g/dL); pH, 7.28 (normal, 7.35–7.45); $Paco_2$, 26 mmHg (normal, 35–45 mmHg); HCO_3^-, 12 mEq/L (normal, 22–26 mEq/L); and urine pH, 5.5. A.B.'s urine pH following an ammonium chloride (NH_4Cl) 0.1 g/kg IV load is <5.1. A bicarbonate load of 1 mEq/kg infused IV over 1 hour induces bicarbonaturia (urinary pH, 7.0) and lowers the serum potassium to 2.0 mEq/L. Her blood pH only increased to 7.31. Assess A.B.'s acid-base status.

[SI units: Na, 143 mmol/L (normal, 135–145); K, 3.0 and 2.0 mmol/L, respectively (normal, 3.5–5.0); Cl, 121 mmol/L (normal, 95–105); albumin, 44 g/L (normal, 36–50); $Paco_2$, 3.5 kPa (normal, 4.7–6.0); HCO_3^-, 12 mmol/L (normal, 22–26)]

Using a stepwise approach, we see that A.B.'s history gives a clue to the cause for her acidosis. The low pH is consistent with a metabolic acidosis because her CO_2 and HCO_3^- are both reduced (Table 10-2). Alterations in pH resulting from a primary change in serum bicarbonate are metabolic acid-base disorders. Specifically, metabolic acidosis is associated with a decrease in serum HCO_3^- and decreased pH, whereas metabolic alkalosis is associated with an increase in serum HCO_3^- and increased pH. In respiratory disorders, the primary change occurs in the $Paco_2$. If A.B. had a decrease in pH and increase in $Paco_2$, a respiratory acidosis would be present. Because A.B. has a low $Paco_2$ and decreased serum HCO_3^-, she has a metabolic acidosis. In most cases of metabolic acidosis or alkalosis, the lungs compensate for the primary change in serum HCO_3^- concentration by increasing or decreasing ventilation. Most stepwise approaches would next suggest the evaluation of whether the decrease in $Paco_2$ of 14 mmHg for A.B. is consistent with respiratory compensation (Table 10-3). A primary decrease in the serum bicarbonate to 12 mEq/L should result in a compensatory decrease in the $Paco_2$ by 12 to 17 mmHg (Table 10-3). A.B.'s $Paco_2$ has fallen by 14 mmHg (normal, 40 mmHg; current, 26 mmHg), confirming that normal respiratory compensation has occurred. When values for $Paco_2$ or serum HCO_3^- fall outside of normal compensatory ranges, either a mixed acid-base disorder, inadequate extent of compensation, or inadequate time for compensation should be suspected.

Nomograms, especially ones that are different for acute and chronic disorders, are inherently difficult to memorize, however, and are often not available to the clinician at the point of care. Following the stepwise approach advocated above will enable clinicians to identify most clinically important disorders without needing to depend on tables or formulas.

Table 10-3 Normal Compensation in Simple Acid-Base Disorders

Disorder	*Compensation*[a]
Metabolic acidosis	$\downarrow Paco_2$ (mmHg) = 1.0 – 1.2 × HCO_3^- (mEq/L)
Metabolic alkalosis	$\uparrow Paco_2$ (mmHg) = 0.5 – 0.7 × $\uparrow HCO_3^-$ (mEq/L)
Respiratory acidosis	
Acute	$\uparrow HCO_3^-$ (mEq/L) = 0.1 × $\uparrow Paco_2$ (mmHg)
Chronic	$\uparrow HCO_3^-$ (mEq/L) = 0.4 × $\uparrow Paco_2$ (mmHg)
Respiratory alkalosis	
Acute	$\downarrow HCO_3^-$ (mEq/L) = 0.2 × $\downarrow Paco_2$ (mmHg)
Chronic	$\downarrow HCO_3^-$ (mEq/L) = 0.4–0.5 × $\downarrow Paco_2$ (mmHg)

[a] Based on change from normal HCO_3^- = 24 mEq/L and $Paco_2$ = 40 mmHg.

Causes

2. What are potential causes of metabolic acidosis in A.B.?

Steps 4 to 7 of the stepwise approach in the evaluation of acid base disorders (see above) are used to further determine the cause of the acid-base disorder. In patients with metabolic acidosis, calculation of the AG serves as a first step in classifying the metabolic acidosis and provides additional information about conditions that might be responsible for the acid-base disorder. A.B.'s calculated AG is 10 mEq/L (Equation 10-6). Thus, A.B. has hyperchloremic metabolic acidosis with a normal AG.

The common causes of metabolic acidosis are presented in Table 10-2.[5,10,51] Normal AG metabolic acidosis usually is caused by gastrointestinal loss of bicarbonate (diarrhea, fistulous disease, ureteral diversions); exogenous sources of chloride (normal saline infusions); or altered excretion of hydrogen ions (renal tubular acidosis). A.B. reports a history of both paint ingestion (perhaps lead-based paint) and chronic use of lithium. Both lead and lithium have been associated with the development of renal tubular acidosis.[31,54]

RENAL TUBULAR ACIDOSIS

3. How do the results of NH_4Cl and sodium bicarbonate ($NaHCO_3$) loading help identify the type of renal tubular acidosis in A.B.?

Renal tubular acidosis (RTA) is characterized by defective secretion of hydrogen ion in the renal tubule with essentially normal GFR. Many medical conditions and chemical substances have been associated with RTA (Table 10-4).[31,34] The recognized forms are type 1 (distal), type 2 (proximal), and type 4 (distal, hypoaldosterone). Type 1 RTA is caused by a defect in the distal tubule's ability to acidify the urine; type 2 by altered urinary bicarbonate reabsorption in the proximal tubule; and type 4 by hypoaldosteronism and impaired ammoniagenesis.[31,48]

Evaluation of bicarbonate reabsorption during bicarbonate loading and of response to acid loading by infusion of ammonium chloride is useful in distinguishing between the various

Table 10-4 Common Causes of Lactic Acidosis

Type A	Type B
Anemia	Diabetes mellitus
Carbon monoxide poisoning	Liver failure
Congestive heart failure	Renal failure
Shock	Seizure disorder
Sepsis	Leukemia
	Drugs
	Didanosine
	Ethanol
	Isoniazid
	Metformin
	Methanol
	Salicylates
	Zidovudine

types of RTA. In healthy subjects, approximately 10% to 15% of the filtered bicarbonate escapes reabsorption in the proximal tubule but is reabsorbed in more distal segments of the nephron. Therefore, urine bicarbonate excretion is negligibly small, and urine pH is maintained between 5.5 and 6.5.

Type 2 (proximal) RTA is associated with a decrease in proximal tubular bicarbonate reabsorption. The distal tubular cells partially compensate for this defect by increasing bicarbonate reabsorption, but urinary bicarbonate excretion still is increased. As occurred with A.B., serum HCO_3^- concentration in patients with type 2 RTA may acutely fall below a threshold of 15 but then stabilize around 15 mEq/L.[10,31] At this point, distal bicarbonate delivery no longer is excessive, allowing the distal nephron to acidify the urine appropriately and excrete acid in the form of titratable ammonia and phosphate.

In type 1 (distal) RTA, a defect in net hydrogen ion secretion, results from a back-diffusion of H^+ from the tubule lumen to the tubule cell. Patients with type 1 RTA cannot reduce their urine pH below 5.5 even when systemic acidosis is severe.[48]

A.B.'s response to the acid (NH_4Cl) load demonstrates an ability to acidify the urine (i.e., pH <5.1), which helps rule out type 1 RTA. During bicarbonate loading in patients with type 2 RTA, serum bicarbonate concentration is increased and abnormally large amounts of bicarbonate are again delivered to the distal tubule. Its hydrogen secretory processes are overwhelmed, resulting in bicarbonaturia. Administration of bicarbonate to A.B. produced bicarbonaturia and an elevation in urine pH (7.0), with low blood pH (7.31). These findings indicate that the reabsorption of bicarbonate in the proximal tubule is impaired, which is characteristic of type 2 RTA. Type 4 (hypoaldosterone) RTA is unlikely given her initial serum potassium of 3.0 mEq/L.

LEAD-INDUCED

4. What is the cause of A.B.'s proximal RTA?

The most likely cause of A.B.'s proximal RTA is her exposure to presumably lead-based paint (Table 10-4). The pathogenesis of lead-induced type 2 RTA is unclear. Some studies suggest that carbonic anhydrase deficiency in the proximal tubule is the major factor, but these data are inconclusive.

5. Why is A.B. hypokalemic?

Bicarbonate wasting in proximal RTA is associated with sodium loss, extracellular fluid reduction, and activation of the renin-angiotensin-aldosterone axis. Aldosterone increases distal tubular sodium reabsorption and greatly augments potassium and hydrogen ion secretion. This results in potassium wasting, which explains A.B.'s hypokalemia.[55] When plasma bicarbonate achieves steady-state, less bicarbonate reaches the distal tubule, and the stimulus for aldosterone release is removed. Therefore, A.B. experiences only a mild depletion of potassium body stores. When A.B. is exposed to bicarbonate loading, the renin-angiotensin-aldosterone axis is reactivated, and hypokalemia worsens. In addition, raising the concentration of bicarbonate in the blood drives potassium intercellularly, and contributes to her hypokalemia.

Treatment

6. What treatment is indicated for A.B.?

Although it is rare for patients with type 2 RTA to develop severe acidosis and potassium depletion chronically, it is not uncommon in an acute situation such as this. A.B. has a bicarbonate deficit; thus, she should be treated with alkali replacement, and the offending agent, if confirmed to be lead, should be removed concurrently. Her serum potassium is also dangerously low and bicarbonate correction could further decrease it. A.B. needs potassium supplementation. The clinician should obtain hourly blood samples for electrolytes until her potassium is >3.5 mEq/L. In adults such as A.B., chronic treatment often is not needed because acidosis is self-limited. A.B., however, should be treated with sodium bicarbonate until proximal RTA resolves. Very large doses of bicarbonate (6–10 mEq/kg/day) would be required to increase serum bicarbonate to the normal range.[10] In adults with proximal RTA, however, the goal is to increase serum bicarbonate to no more than 18 mEq/L.[31] Bicarbonate can be provided as sodium bicarbonate tablets (8 mEq/600-mg tablet) or Shohl's solution. Shohl's solution, USP, contains 334 mg citric acid and 500 mg sodium citrate per 5 mL. Sodium citrate is metabolized to sodium bicarbonate in the liver. Shohl's solution provides 1 mEq of sodium and 1 mEq of bicarbonate per milliliter of solution. Therapy for A.B. should be initiated with 1 mEq/kg/day. The clinician should monitor A.B.'s lithium levels while she is receiving alkali therapy. Sodium ingestion might increase renal lithium excretion and exacerbate her bipolar disorder. Because of severe hypokalemia resulting from alkali administration, supplemental potassium as chloride, bicarbonate, acetate, or citrate salts also should be administered.

Metabolic Acidosis With Elevated Anion Gap

Evaluation and Osmolal Gap

7. G.D., a 34-year-old, 60-kg man, is brought to the emergency department (ED) by the police in a semicomatose state. He was found lying on the floor of his hotel room 30 minutes ago. G.D. has a long history of alcohol abuse. In the ED, supine blood pressure (BP) is 120/60 mmHg, pulse is 100 beats/minute, and respiratory rate is 40 breaths/minute. G.D.'s pupils are reactive, and mild papilledema is noted. Laboratory tests reveal the following: serum Na, 140 mEq/L (normal, 135–145 mEq/L); K, 5.8 mEq/L (normal,

3.5–5.0 mEq/L); Cl, 103 mEq/L (normal, 95–105 mEq/L); blood urea nitrogen (BUN), 25 mg/dL (normal, 10–26 mg/dL); creatinine, 1.4 mg/dL (normal, 0.7–1.4 mg/dL); and fasting glucose, 150 mg/dL (normal, 70–105 mg/dL). ABG include pH, 7.16 (normal, 7.35–7.45); Pa_{CO_2}, 23 mmHg (normal, 35–45); HCO_3^-, 8 mEq/L (normal, 22–26). His toxicology screen is negative for alcohol and his serum osmolality is 332 mOsm/kg (normal, 280–295).

What acid-base disturbance is present in G.D., and what are possible causes of the disorder?

[SI units: Na, 140 mmol/L; K, 5.8 mmol/L; Cl, 103 mmol/L; BUN, 8.9 mmol/L (normal, 3.57–9.28); creatinine, 124 mmol/L (normal, 62–124); fasting glucose, 8.3 mmol/L (normal, 2.8–5.8); Pa_{CO_2}, 3.1 kPa; HCO_3^-, 8 mmol/L; osmolality, 332 mmol/kg (normal, 280–295)]

G.D. has an acidosis (pH, 7.16; HCO_3^-, 8 mEq/L) with a large AG (29 mEq/L). Subtracting 10 from the anion gap of 29 and adding this value to his serum bicarbonate concentration (see Step 5 in above section on evaluation of acid base disorders) yields a value of 27, suggesting no other metabolic abnormality is present.

An elevated AG metabolic acidosis often indicates lactic acidosis resulting from intoxications (e.g., salicylates, acetaminophen, methanol, ethylene glycol, paraldehyde, metformin) or ketoacidosis induced by diabetes mellitus, starvation, or alcohol.[14,29,33,39,52,56–61] The sixth step in the stepwise approach leads to the consideration of additional laboratory tests that may be helpful in the differential diagnosis of an elevated AG. These include serum ketones, glucose, lactate, BUN, creatinine, and plasma osmolal gap.[33] Osmolal gap is defined as the difference between measured serum osmolality (SO) and calculated SO using Equation 10-7.

$$\text{Calculated SO (mOsm/Kg)} = 2 \times Na^+(\text{mEq/L}) + \frac{Glucose(mg/dL)}{18} + \frac{BUN(mg/dL)}{2.8} \quad \textbf{(10-7)}$$

When the difference between measured and calculated SO is >10 mOsm/kg, the presence of an unmeasured osmotically active substance, such as ethanol, methanol, or ethylene glycol, should be considered.[33,61,62] G.D.'s calculated SO is 297 mOsm/kg, compared with the measured value of 332; therefore, his osmolal gap is 35 mOsm/kg. An increase in the anion gap and osmolal gap, without diabetic ketoacidosis or chronic renal failure, suggests the possibility of metabolic acidosis resulting from a toxic ingestion.[33] On the basis of G.D.'s presentation (papilledema, history of alcohol abuse, increased osmolal gap, increased AG metabolic acidosis), methanol intoxication should be considered.

Causes

METHANOL-INDUCED

8. How would G.D.'s methanol intake induce metabolic acidosis with an elevated anion AG?

Methanol intoxication results in the formation of two organic acids, formic and lactic acid, which consume bicarbonate with production of an AG metabolic acidosis. Alcohol dehydrogenase in the liver metabolizes methanol to formaldehyde and then to formic acid. The formic acid contributes to the metabolic acidosis and also is responsible for the retinal edema and blindness associated with methanol intoxication.[33,34,61]

Table 10-5 Classification of Metabolic Alkalosis

Saline-Responsive	*Saline-Resistant*
Diuretic therapy	Normotensive
Extracellular volume contraction	Potassium depletion
Gastric acid loss	Hypercalcemia
Vomiting	Hypertensive
Nasogastric suction	Mineralocorticoids
Exogenous alkali administration	Hyperaldosteronism
Blood transfusions	Hyperreninism
	Licorice

Serum lactic acid concentrations also are increased in patients with methanol intoxication.[33] Lactic acidosis classically has been divided into type A, which is associated with inadequate delivery of oxygen to the tissue, and type B, which is associated with defective oxygen utilization at the mitochondrial level (Table 10-5). Although these distinctions often are not clear, the lactic acidosis caused by methanol intoxication is most consistent with the type B variety.[63]

Treatment

9. How should G.D.'s methanol intoxication be managed acutely?

ANTIDOTES

In addition to expert management of G.D.'s airway, breathing, and circulation, therapy should be directed toward treatment of the underlying cause and may include additional supportive management. Ethanol and fomepizole (Antizol) compete with methanol for alcohol dehydrogenase binding sites.[34,61–65] Because ethanol and fomepizole have much greater affinity for alcohol dehydrogenase than methanol, these agents may reduce the conversion of methanol to its toxic metabolite, formic acid. The unmetabolized methanol then is excreted by the lungs and kidneys. Fomepizole can be given intravenously (IV) as a 15 mg/kg loading dose over 30 minutes, followed by bolus doses of 10 mg/kg Q 12 hr. Because of induction of metabolism of fomepizole, doses should be increased to 15 mg/kg every 12 hours if therapy is required beyond 2 days.[61] Fomepizole is usually continued until the serum methanol concentration is <20 mg/dL (6.2 mmol/L). Adverse effects of fomepizole are relatively mild, consisting of headache, nausea, dizziness, agitation, metallic taste, abnormal smell, and rash. Because of its high cost and infrequent use, some hospitals might not have fomepizole readily available. In such cases, ethanol is an alternative. Administration of IV ethanol as an antidote can be technically difficult and may produce central nervous system (CNS) depression.[61,64] For patients with methanol toxicity, an IV loading dose of 0.6 gm/kg ethanol solution can be administered over 30 minutes, followed by a continuous infusion of about 150 mg/kg/hour for drinkers and 70 mg/kg/hour for nondrinkers. Serum ethanol concentration should be maintained >100 mg/dL.[34,63] Charcoal may be considered to bind other agents that may be co-ingested.[34,66]

When other low-molecular-weight toxins, such as ethanol or ethylene glycol, are not present, the serum methanol level can be estimated by multiplying the patient's osmolal gap by a standardized conversion factor of 2.6. G.D.'s osmolal gap of

35 mOsm/L, therefore, may reflect a methanol level of ~91 mg/dL (35 mOsm/L ×2.6). When methanol blood levels are higher than 50 mg/dL, hemodialysis is indicated to rapidly reduce concentrations of methanol and its toxic metabolite. The dosage of fomepizole or ethanol should be increased in patients receiving hemodialysis to account for the increased elimination of these antidotes.[34,63] Ethylene glycol poisoning can also be treated by using fomepizole or ethanol.

BICARBONATE

Severe acidosis causes reduced myocardial contractility, impaired response to catecholamines, and impaired oxygen delivery to tissues as a result of 2,3-diphosphoglycerate depletion. For this reason, some clinicians have judiciously administered IV sodium bicarbonate to patients with metabolic acidosis in an attempt to raise the arterial pH to about 7.20.[67–69] If IV sodium bicarbonate is given, the amount required to correct serum HCO_3^- and arterial pH can be estimated using Equation 10-8 as follows:

$$\text{Bicarbonate dose (mEq)} = 0.5\ (\text{L/kg}) \times \text{Body Weight (kg)} \times \text{Desired increase in serum } HCO_3^-\ (\text{mEq/L}) \quad \textbf{(10-8)}$$

Bicarbonate distributes to approximately 50% of total body weight (thus, the factor of 0.5 L/kg in Equation 10-8). To prevent overtreating, bicarbonate doses should only attempt to increase the bicarbonate concentration by 4 to 8 mEq/L (see Question 10).[68] For G.D., the dose required to raise serum bicarbonate from 8 to 12 mEq/L amounts to 120 mEq of bicarbonate (0.5 L/kg × 60 kg × 4 mEq/L; Equation 10-8). Clinical assessment of the effect of bicarbonate can be determined about 30 minutes after administration.[68] Arterial pH and serum bicarbonate concentrations should be obtained before any additional therapy.

Risks of Bicarbonate Therapy

10. What are the risks of G.D.'s bicarbonate therapy?

Concerns about the risks of bicarbonate administration and the failure of studies to demonstrate significant short-term benefits have raised questions about the appropriateness of bicarbonate therapy in metabolic acidosis, particularly in ketoacidosis and lactic acidosis caused by cardiac arrest or other hypoxic events.[69–76] Bicarbonate administration can result in overalkalinization and a paradoxical transient intracellular acidosis. Whereas arterial pH can increase rapidly following bicarbonate administration, intracellular pH increases more slowly because of slow penetration of the negatively charged bicarbonate ion across cell membranes. The bicarbonate in plasma, however, is converted rapidly to carbonic acid, and the carbon dioxide tension increases as a result (Equation 10-2). Because CO_2 diffuses into cells more rapidly than HCO_3^-, the intracellular $HCO_3^-:CO_2$ ratio decreases, resulting in a decrease in intracellular pH. This intracellular acidosis will persist as long as bicarbonate administration exceeds the CO_2 excretion; therefore, adequate tissue perfusion and ventilation must be provided in patients with diminished CO_2 excretion (e.g., cardiac or pulmonary failure).[71]

Overalkalinization also will cause a shift to the left in the oxygen-hemoglobin dissociation curve. This shift increases hemoglobin affinity for oxygen, decreases oxygen delivery to tissues, and potentially increases lactic acid production and accumulation.[34] Sodium bicarbonate administration also can cause hypernatremia, hyperosmolality, and volume overload; however, the excessive sodium and water retention usually can be avoided by the administration of loop diuretics.[34,62] Hypokalemia is another potential adverse effect of bicarbonate therapy. Acidosis stimulates movement of potassium from intracellular to extracellular fluid in exchange for hydrogen ions. When acidosis is corrected, potassium ions move intracellularly, and hypokalemia can occur. This translocation of potassium tends to reduce serum potassium levels by ~0.4 to 0.6 mEq/L for each 0.1 unit increase in pH, although wide interpatient variability in this relationship exists.[5,8] In G.D. and other patients with organic acid intoxications, raising extracellular pH helps to provide a gradient to shift the toxin from the CNS and "trap" it into the blood and urine, enhancing elimination. To prevent the risks of bicarbonate therapy, G.D.'s mental status, serum sodium and potassium levels, and ABG should be monitored.

ALTERNATIVE ALKALINIZING THERAPY

Although sodium bicarbonate is the most commonly used agent to raise arterial pH, alternative therapies are available. Sodium lactate and acetate have been used in select patients; however, these agents, which require metabolic conversion to bicarbonate, are associated with many of the same risks as sodium bicarbonate (i.e., sodium and fluid overload, overalkalinization, carbon dioxide production).[39]

Tromethamine acetate (THAM), a sodium-free organic amine with a pH of 8.6, is available commercially as a 0.3 M (36 mg/mL) solution for IV administration. THAM can combine with hydrogen ions from carbonic acid and lactic, pyruvic, or other metabolic acids; however, its role in the management of metabolic acidosis needs clarification. THAM may produce hyperkalemia in patients with renal impairment and is contraindicated in anuric or uremic patients. Administration of THAM also has been associated with other serious side effects, including respiratory depression, increased coagulation times, and hypoglycemia.[77–80] Carbicarb and dichloroacetate have been used investigationally in the treatment of metabolic acidosis.[39,63,81] Carbicarb and THAM are better than bicarbonate at improving extracellular pH and bicarbonate and intracellular pH, while not increasing CO_2; however, neither has yet resulted in better patient outcomes.[5,24,71] Hemofiltration and "continuous renal replacement" therapies have been advocated for patients with lactic acidosis, especially in Europe; however, their roles need further study.

METABOLIC ALKALOSIS

Metabolic alkalosis is associated with an increase in serum bicarbonate concentration and a compensatory increase in $PaCO_2$ (caused by hypoventilation). The two general classifications of metabolic alkalosis, saline-responsive and saline-resistant (Table 10-6), are usually distinguishable based on an assessment of the patient's volume status, BP, and urinary chloride concentration.

Saline-responsive metabolic alkalosis is associated with disorders that result in the loss of chloride-rich, bicarbonate-poor fluid from the body (e.g., vomiting, nasogastric suction, diuretic therapy, cystic fibrosis). Physical examination

Table 10-6 Common Causes of Respiratory Acidosis

Airway Obstruction	***Cardiopulmonary***
Foreign body aspiration	Cardiac arrest
Asthma	Pulmonary edema or infiltration
COPD	Pulmonary embolism
Adrenergic blockers	Pulmonary fibrosis
CNS Disturbances	***Neuromuscular***
Cerebral vascular accident	Amyotrophic lateral sclerosis
Sleep apnea	Guillain-Barré syndrome
Tumor	Myasthenia gravis
CNS depressant drugs	Hypokalemia
Barbiturates	Hypophosphatemia
Benzodiazepines	Drugs
Opioids	Aminoglycosides
	Antiarrhythmics
	Lithium
	Phenytoin

CNS, central nervous system; COPD, chronic obstructive pulmonary disease.

may reveal volume depletion (e.g., orthostatic hypotension, tachycardia, poor skin turgor), and the urinary chloride concentration often will be <10 to 20 mEq/L (although urine chloride levels may be >20 mEq/L in patients with recent diuretic use).[10,35,82]

Severe hypokalemia or excessive mineralocorticoid activity can result in a saline-resistant metabolic alkalosis, but this disorder is rare in comparison with saline-responsive metabolic alkalosis. Saline-resistant metabolic alkalosis should be suspected in alkalemic patients with evidence of increased ECF volume, hypertension, or high urinary chloride values (>20 mEq/L) without recent diuretic use.[10,82]

Evaluation

11. K.E., a 60-year-old, 50-kg woman, was admitted to the hospital 4 days ago with peripheral edema and pulmonary congestion consistent with a congestive heart failure exacerbation. Since admission, she has been treated aggressively with furosemide 80 to 120 mg IV daily, which has generated approximately 3 L of urine output each day. Her chest radiograph findings and peripheral edema now show considerable improvement with diuresis; however, she now complains of dizziness when she gets out of bed to go to the bathroom. Physical examination reveals a tachycardic (heart rate [HR], 100 beats/minute), a thin elderly woman with poor skin turgor and slight muscle weakness. K.E.'s electrocardiogram shows flattened T waves and U waves. Laboratory tests reveal the following: serum Na, 138 mEq/L; K, 2.5 mEq/L; Cl, 92 mEq/L; creatinine, 0.9 mg/dL; BUN, 28 mg/dL; pH, 7.49; $Paco_2$, 46 mmHg; and HCO_3^-, 34 mEq/L. Urine Cl concentration is 60 mEq/L.

What acid-base disorder is present in K.E.?

[SI units: Na, 138 mmol/L; K, 2.5 mmol/L; Cl, 92 mmol/L; creatinine, 79.6 mmol/L; BUN, 10 mmol/L; $Paco_2$, 6.1 kPa; HCO_3^-, 34 mmol/L; urine Cl, 60 mmol/L]

Using the stepwise approach to the evaluation of acid-base disorders as previously described, K.E.'s elevated pH is consistent with alkalosis. Furosemide-induced diuresis may be a clue to her acid-base disorder. The increased serum HCO_3^- and increased $Paco_2$ suggest primary metabolic alkalosis with respiratory compensation. K.E.'s anion gap is 12, suggesting no additional metabolic acid-base abnormalities are present. A $Paco_2$ of 46 mmHg suggests normal respiratory compensation for metabolic alkalosis. Appropriate treatment of the metabolic alkalosis should return her $Paco_2$ to normal if there is no underlying pulmonary disease.

Causes

Diuretic-Induced

12. What is the most likely cause of K.E.'s acid-base imbalance?

Common causes of metabolic alkalosis are listed in Table 10-6. The hypokalemic, hypochloremic, metabolic alkalosis in K.E. most likely is the result of diuretic-induced volume contraction. The incidence of this adverse effect is influenced by the type, dose, and dosing frequency of the diuretic.

Diuretics cause metabolic alkalosis (sometimes referred to as a "contraction alkalosis") by the following mechanisms. First, they enhance excretion of sodium chloride and water, resulting in extracellular volume contraction. Volume contraction alone will cause only a modest increase in plasma bicarbonate; however, volume contraction also stimulates aldosterone release. Aldosterone increases distal tubular sodium reabsorption and induces hydrogen ion and potassium secretion, resulting in alkalosis and hypokalemia. In addition, hypokalemia induced by diuretics will stimulate intracellular movement of hydrogen ions to replace cellular potassium, producing extracellular alkalosis. Hypochloremia also is important in sustaining metabolic alkalosis. In a hypochloremic state, sodium will be reabsorbed, accompanied by bicarbonate generated by secreted hydrogen (Fig. 10-1).[82–84]

Treatment

13. How should K.E.'s acid-base imbalance be corrected and monitored?

Treatment of metabolic alkalosis depends on removal of the cause. K.E.'s diuretic therapy should be temporarily discontinued until her volume status and electrolytes can be restored. The initial goal is to correct fluid deficits and replace chloride and potassium by infusing sodium and potassium chloride. As long as hypochloremia exists, renal bicarbonate excretion will not occur and the alkalosis will not be corrected.[83] The severity of alkalosis dictates how rapidly fluid and electrolytes should be administered. In patients with hepatic or renal failure or congestive heart failure, infusion of large volumes of sodium and potassium salts can produce fluid overload or hyperkalemia. Thus, fluid and electrolyte replacement should proceed cautiously and these patients should be monitored closely for these complications.

Potassium chloride should be administered to correct K.E.'s hypokalemia. The amount of potassium required to replace total body stores is difficult to determine accurately because 98% of the potassium in the body is intracellular. Although wide variation exists, for each 1 mEq/L decrease in K^+ from an ECF concentration of 4 mEq/L, the total body K^+ deficit is about 4 to 5 mEq/kg.[10] K.E.'s serum potassium is 2.5 mEq/L, which correlates with a decrease of about 350 mEq in total body potassium stores. K.E. should be treated with the chloride salt to ensure potassium retention and correction of alkalosis. Potassium replacement can be achieved over several days with supplements of 100 to 150 mEq/day given either orally in divided doses or as a constant IV infusion. K.E.'s laboratory tests for BUN, creatinine, chloride, sodium, and potassium should be monitored during sodium and potassium chloride therapy. As noted above, hypercapnia should disappear after correction of the alkalemia, which can be confirmed with an ABG, if clinically indicated.

14. What other agents are available to treat K.E.'s alkalosis if fluid and electrolyte replacement does not correct the arterial pH?

Patients unresponsive to sodium and potassium chloride therapy or those at risk for complications with these agents can be treated with acetazolamide, hydrochloric acid (HCl), or a hydrochloric acid precursor. The most commonly used agent is acetazolamide, a carbonic anhydrase inhibitor that blocks hydrogen ion secretion in the renal tubule, resulting in increased excretion of sodium and bicarbonate. Although the serum bicarbonate concentration often improves with acetazolamide, metabolic alkalosis may not completely resolve. Other concerns with the use of acetazolamide include its ability to promote kaliuresis and its relative lack of effect in patients with renal dysfunction.[82,85,86]

A solution of 0.1 N HCl may be administered to patients who require rapid correction of alkalemia. The dose of HCl is based on the bicarbonate excess using Equation 10-9, where the factor 0.5 × body weight (kg), represents the estimated bicarbonate space.[10,82,83,85]

$$\text{Dose of HCl (mEq)} = 0.5 \times \text{Body Weight (kg)} \times (\text{plasma bicarbonate} - 24) \quad \textbf{(10-9)}$$

Parenteral hydrochloric acid is prepared extemporaneously by adding the appropriate amount of 1 N HCl through a 0.22-micron filter into a glass bottle containing 5% dextrose or normal saline. The dilute solution should be administered via central venous catheter in the superior vena cava to reduce the risk of extravasation and tissue damage. The infusion rate should not exceed 0.2 mEq/kg/hour.[85] ABG should be monitored at least every 4 hours during the infusion. HCl should not be added to total nutrient solutions.[86]

Precursors of hydrochloric acid, such as ammonium and arginine hydrochloride, are not recommended.[82] The adverse effect profile of these agents has significantly limited their role.[85] Ammonium hydrochloride is metabolized to HCl and NH_3 in the liver. Severe ammonia intoxication with CNS depression can occur during rapid infusion of ammonium hydrochloride or in patients with liver disease.[82] Arginine can cause rapid shifts in potassium from the intracellular to extracellular space, resulting in dangerous hyperkalemia.[82]

RESPIRATORY ACIDOSIS

Respiratory acidosis occurs as a result of inadequate ventilation by the lungs. When the lungs do not excrete CO_2 effectively, the $Paco_2$ rises. This elevation in $Paco_2$ (a functional acid) causes a fall in pH (Equations 10-3 and 10-5). Common causes of respiratory acidosis are listed in Table 10-7. They generally can be categorized into conditions of airway obstruction, reduced stimulus for respiration from the CNS, failure of the heart or lungs, and disorders of the peripheral nerves or skeletal muscles required for ventilation.[87]

Table 10-7 Common Causes of Respiratory Alkalosis

CNS Disturbances	***Pulmonary***
Bacterial septicemia	Pneumonia
Cerebrovascular accident	Pulmonary edema
Fever	Pulmonary embolus
Hepatic cirrhosis	***Tissue Hypoxia***
Hyperventilation	High altitude
Anxiety-induced	Hypotension
Voluntary	CHF
Meningitis	***Other***
Pregnancy	Excessive mechanical ventilation
Trauma	Rapid correction of metabolic acidosis
Drugs	
Progesterone derivatives	
Respiratory stimulants	
Salicylate overdose	

CHF, congestive heart failure; CNS, central nervous system.

Evaluation

15. B.B., a 56-year-old man, is admitted to the hospital for treatment of an exacerbation of chronic obstructive pulmonary disease (COPD). He complains of worsening shortness of breath and increased production of sputum for the past 3 days. He has also noted a mild headache, a flushed feeling, and drowsiness within the past 24 hours. He has a history of COPD, hypertension, coronary artery disease, and low back pain. Current medications are ipratropium (Atrovent) inhaler two puffs QID, salmeterol (Serevent) dry powder inhaler one inhalation BID, hydrochlorothiazide 25 mg daily, diltiazem (Cardizem LA) 240 mg daily, and diazepam (Valium) 5 mg TID PRN for back pain.

Vital signs include respiratory rate of 16 breaths/minute and HR of 90 beats/minute. Diffuse wheezes and rhonchi are heard on chest auscultation. Laboratory tests reveal the following: Na, 140 mEq/L; K, 4.0 mEq/L; Cl, 100 mEq/L; pH, 7.32; $Paco_2$, 58 mmHg; Pao_2, 58 mmHg; and HCO_3^-, 29 mEq/L. B.B's baseline ABG at the physician's office last month was pH, 7.35; $Paco_2$, 51 mmHg; Pao_2, 62 mmHg; and HCO_3^-, 28 mEq/L.

Which of B.B.'s signs and symptoms are consistent with the diagnosis of respiratory acidosis?

[SI units: Na, 138 mmol/L; K, 2.5 mmol/L; Cl, 92 mmol/L; $Paco_2$, 7.7 and 6.8 kPa; Pao_2, 7.7 and 8.3 kPa; HCO_3^-, 29 and 28 mmol/L]

A stepwise evaluation reveals a respiratory acidosis. A history of COPD and physical findings of dyspnea, headache, drowsiness, and flushing support the ABG evaluation. Respiratory acidosis also can cause more severe symptoms, including CNS effects, such as disorientation, confusion, delirium, hallucinations, and coma. These CNS abnormalities probably are partly caused by the direct effects of carbon dioxide. Hypoxemia (decreased Pao_2), which commonly accompanies respiratory acidosis, also contributes to these symptoms. Elevated $Paco_2$ causes cerebral vascular dilation, resulting in headache caused by increased blood flow and increased intracranial pressure. Cardiovascular effects typically include tachycardia, arrhythmias, and peripheral vasodilation.[88]

16. Is the respiratory acidosis present in B.B. consistent with an acute or a chronic disorder?

Following the stepwise approach, it is determined that B.B. has a respiratory acidosis. He has a normal AG. Comparing his current to previous values (e.g., pH, $Paco_2$, HCO_3^-), it appears B.B. has an acute on chronic respiratory acidosis since his baseline $Paco_2$ was 51 mmHg with an acute worsening to 58 mmHg. In respiratory acidosis, increased renal reabsorption of bicarbonate compensates for the increase in $Paco_2$; however, at least 48 to 72 hours are needed for this compensatory mechanism to become fully established.[10] Patients with COPD commonly present with an "acute-on-chronic" respiratory acidosis similar to B.B.

Causes

17. What potential causes of respiratory acidosis are present in B.B.?

Respiratory acidosis often is caused by airway obstruction, as shown in Table 10-7.[87,88] Chronic obstructive airway disease is a common cause of both acute and chronic respiratory acidosis. Upper respiratory tract infections, such as acute bronchitis, can worsen airway obstruction and produce acute respiratory acidosis.

Drug-Induced

B.B.'s drug therapy also may be contributing to respiratory insufficiency. Many drugs (Table 10-7) decrease ventilation, but usually these drugs only significantly affect patients who are predisposed to respiratory problems because of underlying diseases. Because B.B. has COPD, he may be more sensitive to drugs affecting respiration. The benzodiazepines, barbiturates, and opioids minimally decrease respiration in normal subjects and in most patients with COPD when given usual therapeutic doses. These drugs, however, can cause significant respiratory insufficiency when administered either in large doses or in combination with other respiratory depressant drugs.[88] B.B.'s diazepam may be contributing to hypoventilation and respiratory acidosis and should be withdrawn from his regimen. Nonselective adrenergic blocking drugs should not be used in patients with COPD.

Treatment

18. How should B.B.'s respiratory acidosis be treated?

As with most cases of respiratory acidosis, treatment primarily involves correction of the underlying cause of respiratory insufficiency. In this case, treatment of acute bronchospasm with ipratropium or an α-adrenergic agent, such as inhaled albuterol, is warranted. Corticosteroids, such as methylprednisolone (60–125 mg Q 6–12 hr initially) are commonly used in hospitalized patients with acute exacerbations of COPD.[89] Antibiotic therapy with a β-lactam or β-lactamase inhibitor should be considered in hospitalized patients producing purulent, large-volume secretions.[90] B.B's respiratory status should be monitored closely during his hospitalization. If the acidosis, hypercarbia, or associated hypoxemia worsen, noninvasive positive pressure ventilation or intubation with mechanical ventilation may be required.[68]

Treatment with IV sodium bicarbonate is not recommended in most cases of acute respiratory acidosis because of the risks associated with bicarbonate therapy (see Question 10) and because an absolute deficiency of bicarbonate is not present. When the excess CO_2 is excreted, arterial pH should return to normal. Hypercapnia should not be overcorrected, because hypocapnia results in decreased lung compliance, increases dysfunctional surfactant production, and shifts the oxyhemoglobin dissociation curve to the left, restricting the release of oxygen to tissues.[75,76,91]

RESPIRATORY ALKALOSIS

Respiratory alkalosis usually is not a severe disorder. Excessive rate or depth of respiration results in increased excretion of carbon dioxide, a fall in $Paco_2$, and a rise in arterial pH. Common causes of respiratory alkalosis are presented in Table 10-8. Many conditions can cause respiratory alkalosis by stimulating respiratory drive in the CNS. In addition, pulmonary diseases can stimulate receptors in the lung to increase ventilation, and conditions that decrease oxygen delivery to tissues also can stimulate ventilation, causing respiratory alkalosis.[92,93]

Evaluation

19. S.P., a 35-year-old, 60-kg woman, is admitted for treatment of presumed bacterial pneumonia. She was in good health until 24 hours before presentation when she noted a fever; onset of a productive cough with thick, yellowish sputum; and chest pain on deep inspiration. She has taken aspirin 650 mg Q 4 hr since the onset of fever, with mild relief. Since arriving in the ED, she has become anxious and lightheaded and has developed tingling in her hands, feet, and lips. Vital signs include the following: temperature, 38°C; respiratory rate, 24 breaths/minute; HR, 110 beats/minute; and BP, 135/70 mmHg. Physical examination reveals dullness to percussion, rales, and decreased breath sounds over the left lower lung field.

Laboratory findings include the following: serum Na, 135 mEq/L; Cl, 105 mEq/L; pH, 7.49; $Paco_2$, 30 mmHg; Pao_2,

Table 10-8 Laboratory Values in Simple Acid-Base Disorders

Disorder	*Arterial pH*	*Primary Change*	*Compensatory Change*
Metabolic acidosis	↓	$\downarrow HCO_3^-$	$\downarrow Paco_2$
Respiratory acidosis	↓	$\uparrow Paco_2^-$	$\uparrow HCO_3^-$
Metabolic alkalosis	↑	$\uparrow HCO_3^-$	$\uparrow Paco_2$
Respiratory alkalosis	↑	$\downarrow Paco_2^-$	$\downarrow HCO_3^-$

90 mmHg; and HCO_3^-, 22 mEq/L. Gram stain of sputum reveals 25 white blood cells (WBC) per high-power field and many gram-positive diplococci. WBC count is 15,400 cells/mm^3 (normal, 3,500–10,500 cells/mm^3) with a left shift. A left lower lobe infiltrate is seen on chest radiograph.

What acid-base disorder is present in S.P.?

[SI units: $Paco_2$, 4.0 kPa; Pao_2, 12.0 kPa; HCO_3^-. 22 mmol/L; other SI units are: Na, 135 mmol/L; Cl, 105 mmol/L]

Steps 1 to 3 in the evaluation of the ABG values, as described previously, indicate a respiratory alkalosis (increased pH, decreased $Paco_2$). The history and physical findings of deep, rapid breathing and tingling sensations are clues to the etiology. This disorder is most likely acute because her HCO_3^- concentration is normal. She does not have an AG. If a large AG was present, it would suggest she has a coexisiting metabolic acidosis, possibly caused by salicylate intoxication (see below).

20. Which of S.P.'s signs and symptoms are consistent with the diagnosis of acute respiratory alkalosis?

Respiratory alkalosis typically produces paresthesias of the extremities and perioral region, lightheadedness, confusion, decreased mental acuity, and tachycardia.[5,6,10] Increased rate and depth of respiration may be evident. Simple respiratory alkalosis rarely produces life-threatening abnormalities.

Causes

21. What is the cause of the acid-base disorder in S.P.?

Common causes of respiratory alkalosis are listed in Table 10-8.[5,6,10,92–94] Based on physical examination, laboratory findings, and chest radiograph, S.P. appears to have an acute bacterial pneumonia. Pneumonia and other pulmonary diseases can result in stimulation of ventilation and respiratory alkalosis, even with a normal Pao_2, as in this case. The anxiety S.P. is experiencing also may be contributing to respiratory alkalosis by producing the familiar anxiety-hyperventilation syndrome. Although salicylate intoxication is a potential cause of respiratory alkalosis because of the direct respiratory stimulant effect of salicylate,[94] S.P. displays few other symptoms of salicylate intoxication (e.g., nausea, vomiting, tinnitus, altered mental status, elevated AG metabolic acidosis). The total aspirin dose reportedly ingested (65 mg/kg over 24 hours) is not large enough to be associated with significant risk for toxicity.

Treatment

22. What is the appropriate treatment for S.P.'s respiratory alkalosis?

Similar to respiratory acidosis, treatment of respiratory alkalosis usually involves correcting the underlying disorder. Initiation of appropriate antibiotic therapy is indicated in this case. Simple respiratory alkalosis is unlikely to cause life-threatening symptoms, although mortality rates for critically ill patients with this disorder can be high.[88] The well-known remedy of rebreathing expired air from a paper bag for treatment of hyperventilation associated with anxiety appears to be effective for this cause of respiratory alkalosis and may be helpful for S.P.

MIXED ACID-BASE DISORDERS

Evaluation

23. B.L., a 58-year-old man, transferred from a nursing home 2 days previously, is disorientated and lethargic. He was doing well until 1 week before admission, when the staff noted that he was somnolent. He progressively became more lethargic and could no longer remember the names of other persons. B.L. has a history of alcoholic cirrhosis, non–insulin-dependent diabetes mellitus, and hypertension. Medications before admission were nadolol 80 mg QD, isosorbide mononitrate 20 mg BID, glyburide 10 mg QD, and spironolactone 50 mg BID. On admission, B.L. was disoriented to person, place, and time and was difficult to arouse. Vital signs include the following: temperature, 37°C; respirations, 16 breaths/minute; HR, 70 beats/minute; and BP, 154/92 mmHg. Physical examination revealed asterixis and mild ascites. Laboratory studies included the following: Na, 133 mEq/L; K, 4.3 mEq/L; Cl, 106 mEq/L; BUN, 5 mg/dL; creatinine, 0.7 mg/dL; fasting glucose, 150 mg/dL; albumin, 3.2 g/dL (normal, 3.6–5.0 g/dL); and ammonia, 120 μmol/L (normal, 19–43 μmol/L); ABG: pH, 7.43; $Paco_2$, 30 mmHg; Pao_2, 90 mmHg; and HCO_3^-, 19 mEq/L.

On admission, spironolactone was increased to 75 mg BID and lactulose 60 mL PO QID was started for treatment of hepatic encephalopathy. Within the first 24 hours of lactulose therapy, B.L. produced four loose, watery stools; however, his mental status worsened to the point of being unresponsive, his BP dropped to 100/60 mmHg, and his breathing became labored and eventually required mechanical ventilation. At the time of intubation, his laboratory values were Na, 136 mEq/L; K, 4.5 mEq/L; Cl, 105 mEq/L; BUN, 10 mg/dL; creatinine, 1.2 mg/dL; arterial pH, 7.06; $Paco_2$, 48 mmHg; Pao_2, 58 mmHg; and HCO_3^-, 13 mEq/L. Gram stain of peritoneal fluid revealed many WBC and gram-negative rods; the diagnosis of spontaneous bacterial peritonitis with possible septicemia is made.

Describe B.L.'s acid-base status on admission and at the current time.

[SI units: Na, 133 and 136 mmol/L; K, 4.3 and 4.5 mmol/L; Cl, 106 and 105 mmol/L; BUN, 1.8 and 3.6 mmol/L; creatinine, 62 and 106 mmol/L; fasting glucose, 8.3 mmol/L; albumin, 32 g/L; $Paco_2$, 4.0 and 6.4 kPa; Pao_2, 12.0 and 7.7 kPa; HCO_3^-, 19 and 13 mmol/L]

An evaluation of B.L.'s ABG using steps 1 and 2 (in the section on evaluation of acid-base disorders) reveals abnormal $Paco_2$ and serum bicarbonate values, suggesting the existence of an underlying acid-base abnormality. The direction of change in his $Paco_2$ and serum HCO_3^- along with a pH of 7.43 suggests a respiratory alkalosis is a primary disorder. His calculated AG of 8 is not increased. Examination of the ranges of expected compensation in Table 10-3 reveals that these values are indeed consistent with chronic respiratory alkalosis (serum HCO_3^- decreased by 0.5 mEq/L for each 1-mmHg drop in $Paco_2$). B.L.'s history of alcohol-induced liver disease is consistent with the diagnosis of chronic respiratory alkalosis (Table 10-8).[8,10]

The second set of ABG reveals severe acidosis. B.L.'s serum bicarbonate has fallen from 19 to 13 mEq/L, and his $Paco_2$

has increased acutely from 30 to 48 mmHg. Because these values have changed in opposite directions, a mixed acid-base abnormality should be suspected.

The diagnosis of a mixed, metabolic and respiratory acidosis can be confirmed by applying the stepwise approach outlined previously. If the acidosis was purely metabolic in nature, a serum HCO_3^- of 13 mEq/L should result in hyperventilation and a low $Paco_2$. B.L's $Paco_2$ of 48 mmHg is high, which would be consistent with coexistent respiratory acidosis. The anion gap is 18, indicating an AG metabolic acidosis is present. The excess AG (AG − 10 = 8) added to B.L's gap of 18 yields a corrected HCO_3^- of 26 which is normal. This suggests no additional metabolic disturbances are present.

Causes

24. What are possible causes for the mixed acidosis in B.L.?

The AG should be calculated in all patients with a metabolic acidosis. B.L.'s calculated AG has increased from 8 to 18 mEq/L (11 and 21 mEq/L, respectively, after adjusting for hypoalbuminemia), suggesting that an elevated AG acidosis is now present. Septicemia from bacterial peritonitis can produce profound hypotension, which leads to tissue hypoperfusion, generation of lactic acid, and a subsequent elevation in the AG. Other causes of elevated AG metabolic acidosis can be excluded with additional laboratory data (e.g., serum ketones, glucose, osmolal gap).

Although diarrhea and spironolactone should be considered in the differential diagnosis, these are usually associated with hyperchloremic, normal AG metabolic acidosis (Table 10-2).[95] The coexisting respiratory acidosis is most likely the result of B.L.'s altered mental status and his diminished respiratory drive.

25. Over the next 6 hours, B.L.'s hepatic encephalopathy, peritonitis, and acid-base disorders are aggressively treated with lactulose, antibiotics, fluids, and mechanical ventilation. His most recent ABG reveals the following: pH, 7.45; $Paco_2$, 24 mmHg; Pao_2, 90 mmHg; and HCO_3^-, 16 mEq/L. Ventilator settings are assist-control mode at 16 breaths/minute, tidal volume 700 mL, and inspired oxygen concentration 40%. B.L. is noted to be more awake, anxious, and initiating 25 to 30 breaths/minute. Describe the current acid-base status and probable cause.

[SI units: $Paco_2$, 3.2 kPa; Pao_2, 12.0 kPa; HCO_3^-, 16 mmol/L]

Evaluation of the ABG reveals a pH at the upper limit of normal with significant decreases in both $Paco_2$ and serum HCO_3^- concentration. This clinical scenario is most consistent with a mixed, acute respiratory alkalosis and ongoing metabolic acidosis. The time frame in which B.L.'s $Paco_2$ decreased from 48 to 24 mmHg is consistent with acute respiratory alkalosis. B.L.'s low serum HCO_3^- suggests ongoing metabolic acidosis as a result of his septicemia. The metabolic acidosis should improve with time, given adequate antibiotic therapy and supportive measures that maintain BP and increase oxygen delivery to the tissues.

The acute respiratory alkalosis in this case is most likely caused by the mechanical ventilator, B.L.'s anxiety, or sepsis. In the assist-control mode, any inspiratory effort by B.L. results in delivery of a full assisted breath by the ventilator.[96] B.L.'s anxiety and resultant tachypnea are stimulating the ventilator to hyperventilate him, producing excessive CO_2 excretion and respiratory alkalosis. Appropriate changes in therapy may include use of an anxiolytic, analgesic if needed to treat pain, changing the ventilator mode, or probably a combination of these strategies.

REFERENCES

1. Androgue HE et al. Acid-base physiology. *Respir Care* 2001;46:328.
2. Rose BD et al. Acid-base physiology. In: Rose BD et al., eds. *Clinical Physiology of Acid-Base Disorders.* 5th ed. New York: McGraw-Hill; 2001:299.
3. Ganong WF. *Review of Medical Physiology.* 22nd ed. New York: McGraw-Hill; 2005.
4. Rose BD et al. Regulation of acid-base balance. In: Rose BD et al., eds. *Clinical Physiology of Acid-Base Disorders.* 5th ed. New York: McGraw-Hill; 2001:325.
5. Bongard FS et al. Fluids, electrolytes, & acid-base. In: Bongard FS, ed. *Current Critical Care Diagnosis & Treatment.* 3rd ed. New York: McGraw Hill; 2007:14.
6. Gluck SL. Acid-base. *Lancet* 1998;352:474.
7. Alpern RJ et al. Renal acid-base transport. In: Schrier RW, ed. *Diseases of the Kidney and Urinary Tract.* 8th ed. Philadelphia: Lippincott Williams & Wilkins; 2006:203.
8. Rose BD et al. Introduction to simple and mixed acid-base disorders. In: Rose BD et al., eds. *Clinical Physiology of Acid-Base Disorders.* 5th ed. New York: McGraw-Hill; 2001:535.
9. Ravel R. *Clinical Laboratory Medicine: Clinical Application of Laboratory Data.* 6th ed. St. Louis: Mosby; 1995:393.
10. Fukagawa M et al. Fluid & electrolyte disorders. In: Tierney LM Jr, ed. *Current Medical Diagnosis & Treatment.* 46th ed. New York: McGraw-Hill; 2007: 839.
11. Kelly AM et al. Venous pH can safely replace arterial pH in the initial evaluation of patients in the emergency department. *Emerg Med J* 2001;18: 340.
12. Paulson WD et al. Wide variation in serum anion gap measurements by chemistry analyzers. *Am J Clin Pathol* 1998;110:735.
13. Story DA et al. Estimating unmeasured anions in critically ill patients: anion-gap, base-deficit, and strong-ion-gap. *Anesthesia* 2002;47:1102.
14. Balasubramanyan N et al. Unmeasured anions identified by the Fencl-Stewart method predict mortality better than base excess, anion gap, and lactate in patients in the pediatric intensive care unit. *Crit Care Med* 1999;27:1577.
15. Fencl V et al. Stewart's quantitative acid-base chemistry: applications in biology and medicine. *Respir Physiol* 1993;91:1.
16. Stewart PA. Modern quantitative acid-base chemistry. *Can J Physiol Pharmacol* 1983;61:1444.
17. Cusack RJ et al. The strong ion gap does not have prognostic value in critically ill patients in a mixed medical/surgical adult ICU. *Intensive Care Med* 2002;28:864.
18. Wooten EW. Strong ion difference theory: more lessons from physical chemistry [Letter]. *Kidney Int* 1998;54:1769.
19. Salem MM et al. Gaps in the anion gap. *Arch Intern Med* 1992;152:1625.
20. Fencl V. Reliability of the anion gap [Letter]. *Crit Care Med* 2000;28:1693.
21. Jurado RL et al. Low anion gap. *South Med J* 1998;91:624.
22. Carvounis CP et al. A simple estimate of the effect of the serum albumin level on the anion gap. *Am J Nephrol* 2000;20:369.
23. Yaron T. Calculating the anion gap for patients with acidosis and hyperglycemia [Letter]. *Ann Intern Med* 1998;129:753.
24. Borawski J et al. Hemoglobin level is an important determinant of acid-base status in hemodialysis patients. *Nephron* 2002;90:111.
25. Lorenz JM et al. Serum anion gap in the differential diagnosis of metabolic acidosis in critically ill newborns. *J Pediatr* 1999;135:751.
26. Oster JR et al. Metabolic acidosis with extreme elevation of anion gap: case report and literature review. *Am J Med Sci* 1999;317:38.
27. Matsumoto LC et al. Anion gap determination in preeclampsia. *Obstet Gynecol* 1998;91:379.
28. Kirschbaum B et al. The anion gap associated with pregnancy-induced hypertension. *Clin Nephrol* 2000;53:264.
29. Chang CT et al. High anion gap metabolic acidosis in suicide: don't forget metformin intoxication-two patients' experiences. *Renal Fail* 2002;24:671.
30. Annerose H et al. Acid-base and endocrine effects of aldosterone and angiotensin II inhibition in metabolic acidosis in human patients. *J Lab Clin Med* 2000;136:379.
31. Smulders YM et al. Renal tubular acidosis: pathophysiology and diagnosis. *Arch Intern Med* 1996; 156:1629.
32. Fall PJ. A stepwise approach to acid-base disorders: practical patient evaluation for metabolic

acidosis and other conditions. *Postgrad Med* 2000; 107:249.
33. Kraut JA et al. Approach to patients with acid-base disorders. *Respir Care* 2001;46:392.
34. Rose BD et al. Metabolic acidosis. In: Rose BD, et al., eds. *Clinical Physiology of Acid-Base Disorders.* 5th ed. New York: McGraw-Hill; 2001:578.
35. Breen PH. Arterial blood gas and pH analysis: clinical approach and interpretation. *Anesthesiol Clin North Am* 2001;19:835.
36. Sirker AA et al. Acid-base physiology: the traditional and the modern approaches. *Anesthesia* 2002; 57:348.
37. Gabow PA et al. Diagnostic importance of an increased serum anion gap. *N Engl J Med* 1980;303: 854–858.
38. Goodkin DA et al. The role of the anion gap in detecting and managing mixed metabolic acid-base disorders. *Clin Endocrinol Metab* 1984;13:333–349.
39. Swenson ER. Metabolic acidosis. *Respir Care* 2001;46:342.
40. DuBose TD. Hyperkalemic metabolic acidosis. *Am J Kidney Dis* 1999;33:xlv.
41. Doberer D et al. Dilutional acidosis: an endless story of confusion [Letter]. *Crit Care Med* 2003;31: 337.
42. Kellum JA. Dilutional acidosis: an endless story of confusion: the author replies [Author Reply]. *Crit Care Med* 2003;31:338.
43. Stephens RCM et al. Saline-based fluids can cause a significant acidosis that may be clinically relevant [Letter]. *Crit Care Med* 2000;28:3375.
44. Waters J. Saline-based fluids can cause a significant acidosis that may be clinically relevant [Letter]. *Crit Care Med* 2000;28:3376.
45. Waters JH et al. Cause of metabolic acidosis in prolonged surgery. *Crit Care Med* 1999;27:2142.
46. Izzedine H et al. Drug-induced Fanconi's syndrome. *Am J Kidney Dis* 2003;41:292.
47. Schoolwerth AC et al. Renal metabolism. In: Schrier RW, ed. *Diseases of the Kidney and Urinary Tract.* 7th ed. Philadelphia: Lippincott Williams & Wilkins; 2001:228.
48. Daphnis E et al. Isolated renal tubular disorders: molecular mechanisms and clinical expression of disease. In: Schrier RW, ed. *Diseases of the Kidney and Urinary Tract.* 7th ed. Philadelphia: Lippincott Williams & Wilkins; 2001:620.
49. Verheist D et al. Fanconi syndrome and renal failure induced by tenofovir: a first case report. *Am J Kidney Dis* 2002;40:1331.
50. Kamel KS et al. A new classification for renal defects in net acid excretion. *Am J Kidney Dis* 1997;29; 136.
51. Prough DS. Physiologic acid-base and electrolyte changes in acute and chronic renal failure patients. *Anesthesiol Clin North Am* 2000;18:809.
52. Luft FC. Lactic acidosis update for critical care clinicians. *J Am Soc Nephrol* 2001;12:S15.
53. Kellum JA. Metabolic acidosis in the critically ill: lessons from physical chemistry. *Kidney Int* 1998;43(Suppl 66):S81.
54. Boton R et al. Prevalence, pathogens, and treatment of a renal dysfunction associated with chronic lithium therapy. *Am J Kidney Dis* 1987;10:329.
55. Gill JR et al. Correction of renal sodium loss and secondary aldosteronism in renal tubular acidosis with bicarbonate loading. *Clin Res* 1961;9:201.
56. Bell AJ et al. Acute methyl salicylate toxicity complicating herbal skin treatment for psoriasis. *Emerg Med* 2002;14:188.
57. Koulouris Z et al. Metabolic acidosis and coma following a severe acetaminophen overdose. *Ann Pharmacother* 1999;33:1191.
58. Moyle GJ et al. Hyperlactatemia and lactic acidosis during antiretroviral therapy: relevance, reproducibility and possible risk factors. *AIDS* 2002;16: 1341.
59. Reynolds HN et al. Hyperlactatemia, increased osmolar gap, and renal dysfunction during continuous lorazepam infusion. *Crit Care Med* 2000;28:1631.
60. Caravaca F et al. Metabolic acidosis in advanced renal failure: differences between diabetic and nondiabetic patients. *Am J Kidney Dis* 1999;33:892.
61. Brent J et al. Fomepizole for the treatment of methanol poisoning. *N Engl J Med* 2001;344:424.
62. Hanston P et al. Ethylene glycol poisoning treated by intravenous 4-methylpyrazole. *Intensive Care Med* 1998;24:736.
63. Halperin ML et al. *Fluid, Electrolyte, and Acid-Base Physiology.* 3rd ed. Philadelphia: WB Saunders; 1999:73.
64. Brent J et al. Fomepizole for the treatment of ethylene glycol poisoning. *N Engl J Med* 1999;340:832.
65. Poldelski V et al. Ethylene glycol-mediated tubular injury: identification of critical metabolites and injury pathways. *Am J Kidney Dis* 2001;38:339.
66. Rao RB et al. Acid-base disorders [Letter]. *N Engl J Med* 1998;338:1626.
67. Hood V et al. Mechanisms of disease: protection of acid-base balance by regulation of acid production. *N Engl J Med* 1998;339:819.
68. Androgue HJ et al. Management of life-threatening acid-base disorders: first of two parts. *N Engl J Med* 1998;338:26.
69. Androgue HJ et al. Acid-base disorders [Letter]. *N Engl J Med* 1998;338:1626.
70. Marik P et al. Acid-base disorders [Letter]. *N Engl J Med* 1998;338:1626.
71. Kraut JA et al. Use of bas in the treatment of severe acidemic states. *Am J Kidney Dis* 2001;38:703.
72. Laffey JG. Acid-base disorders in the critically ill. *Anesthesia* 2002;57:183.
73. Levy MM. Evidence-based critical care medicine. *Crit Care Clin* 1998;14:458.
74. Vukmir RB et al. Sodium bicarbonate in cardiac arrest: a reappraisal. *Am J Emerg Med* 1996;14: 192.
75. Laffey JG et al. Carbon dioxide and the critically ill: too little of a good thing? *Lancet* 1999;354:1283.
76. Laffey JG et al. Buffering hypercapnic acidosis worsens acute lung injury. *Am J Respir Crit Care Med* 2000;161:141.
77. Nahas GG et al. Guidelines for the treatment of acidemia with THAM. *Drugs* 1998;55:191.
78. Kallet RH et al. The treatment of acidosis in acute lung injury with tris-hydroxymethyl aminomethane (THAM). *Am J Respir Crit Care Med* 2000;161: 1149.
79. Nahas GG et al. More on acid-base disorders [Letter]. *N Engl J Med* 1998;339:1005.
80. Androgue HJ et al. More on acid-base disorders [Letter]. *N Engl J Med* 1998;339:1005.
81. Leung JM et al. Safety and efficacy of intravenous Carbicarb in patients undergoing surgery: comparison with sodium bicarbonate in the treatment of mild metabolic acidosis. *Crit Care Med* 1994;22:1540.
82. Rose BD et al. Metabolic alkalosis. In: Rose BD et al., eds. *Clinical Physiology of Acid-Base Disorders.* 5th ed. New York: McGraw-Hill;, 2001:551.
83. Galla JH. Metabolic alkalosis. *J Am Soc Nephrol* 2000;11:369.
84. Khanna A et al. Metabolic alkalosis. *Respir Care* 2001;46:354.
85. Adrogue H et al. Management of life-threatening acid-base disorders. *N Engl J Med* 1998;338:107.
86. Bistrian BR et al. Acid-base disorders [Letter]. *N Engl J Med* 1998;338:1626.
87. Rose BD et al. Respiratory acidosis. In: Rose BD, et al., eds. *Clinical Physiology of Acid-Base Disorders.* 5th ed. New York: McGraw-Hill; 2001:647.
88. Epstein SK et al. Respiratory acidosis. *Respir Care* 2001;46:366.
89. Niewoehner DE et al. Effect of systemic glucocorticoids in exacerbations of chronic obstructive pulmonary disease. *N Engl J Med* 1999;340(25): 1941–1947.
90. Global Initiative for Chronic Obstructive Pulmonary Disease. Global strategy for the diagnosis, management, and prevention, of chronic obstructive pulmonary disease. Executive Summary, 2005. www.goldcopd.com. Accessed March 17, 2007.
91. Laffey JG et al. Medical progress: hypocapnia. *N Engl J Med* 2002;347:43.
92. Foster GT et al. Respiratory alkalosis. *Respir Care* 2001;46:384.
93. Brandon JOW et al. Hormone replacement therapy causes a respiratory alkalosis in normal postmenopausal women. *J Clin Endocrinol Metab* 1999;84:1997.
94. Rose BD et al. Respiratory alkalosis. In: Rose BD, et al., eds. *Clinical Physiology of Acid-Base Disorders.* 5th ed. New York: McGraw-Hill; 2001: 673.
95. Milionis HJ et al. Acid-base abnormalities in a patient with hepatic cirrhosis. *Nephrol Dial Transplant* 1999;14:1599.
96. Tobin MJ. Current concepts: mechanical ventilation. *N Engl J Med* 1994;330:1056.

CHAPTER 11

Fluid and Electrolyte Disorders

Alan H. Lau and Priscilla P. How

BASIC PRINCIPLES

Body Water Compartments and Electrolyte Composition

In newborns, approximately 75% to 85% of the body weight is water. After puberty, the percentage of water per kilogram of weight decreases as the amount of adipose tissue increases with age.[1,2] Body water constitutes 50% to 60% of the lean body weight (LBW) in adult men but only 45% to 55% in women because of their greater proportion of adipose tissue. The water content per kilogram of body weight further decreases with advanced age.

Two-thirds of the total body water resides in the cells (intracellular water). The extracellular water can be divided into different compartments: the interstitial fluid (12% LBW) and the plasma (5% LBW) are the two major compartments. Other compartments of the extracellular fluid include the connective tissues and bone water, the transcellular fluids (e.g., glandular secretions), and other fluids in sequestered spaces, such as the cerebrospinal fluid.[1]

The electrolyte composition differs between the intracellular and extracellular compartments. Potassium (K), magnesium (Mg), and phosphate (PO_4) are the major ions in the intracellular compartment, whereas sodium (Na), chloride (Cl), and bicarbonate (HCO_3) are predominant in the extracellular space.[2] Water travels freely across the cell membranes of most parts of the body. The cell membrane, however, is only selectively permeable to solutes. The impermeable solutes are osmotically active and can exert an osmotic pressure that dictates the distribution of water between fluid compartments. Water moves across the cell membrane from a region of low osmolality to one of high osmolality. Net water movement ceases when osmotic equilibrium occurs. Each fluid compartment contains a major osmotically active solute: potassium in the intracellular space and sodium in the extracellular fluid. The volumes of the two compartments reflect the asymmetrically larger number of solute particles or osmoles inside the cells.[2,3]

The capillary wall separates the interstitial fluid from plasma. Because sodium moves freely across the capillary wall, its concentration is identical across both sides of the wall. Therefore, no osmotic gradient is generated, and water distribution between these two spaces is not affected. Plasma proteins, which are confined in the vascular space, are the primary osmoles that affect water distribution between the interstitium and the plasma.[2] In contrast, urea, which traverses both the capillary walls and most cell membranes, is osmotically inactive.[2,3]

Plasma Osmolality

Osmolality is defined as the number of particles per kilogram of water (mOsm/kg). It is determined by the number of particles in solution and not by particle size or valence. Nondissociable solutes, such as glucose and albumin, generate 1 mOsm/mmol of particles; and dissociable salts, such as sodium chloride liberate two ions in solution to produce 2 mOsm/mmol of salt. The osmolality of body fluid is maintained between 280 and 295 mOsm/kg. Because all body fluid compartments are isoosmotic, plasma osmolality reflects the osmolality of total body water. Plasma osmolality can be measured by the freezing point depression method, or estimated by the following equation, which takes into account the osmotic effect of sodium, glucose, and urea[2,3]:

$$P_{OSM} = 2(\text{Na})(\text{mmol/L}) + \frac{\text{Glucose (mg/dL)}}{18} + \frac{\text{BUN (mg/dL)}}{2.8} \quad \textbf{11-1}$$

This equation predicts the measured plasma osmolality within 5 to 10 mOsm/kg. Although urea contributes to the measured osmolality, it is an ineffective osmole because it readily traverses cell membranes and, therefore, does not cause significant fluid shift within the body. Hence, the effective plasma osmolality (synonymous with tonicity, the portion of total osmolality that has the potential to induce transmembrane water movement) can be estimated by the following equation:

$$P_{OSM} = 2(\text{Na})(\text{mmol/L}) + \frac{\text{Glucose (mg/dL)}}{18} \quad \textbf{11-2}$$

An osmolal gap exists when the measured and calculated values differ by >10 mOsm/kg[4]; it signifies the presence of unidentified particles. When the individual solute has been identified, its contribution to the measured osmolality can be estimated by dividing its concentration (mg/dL) by one-tenth of its molecular weight. Calculating the osmolal gap is used to detect the presence of substances, such as ethanol, methanol, and ethylene glycol, which have high osmolality. Occasionally, the osmolal gap can also result from an artificial decrease in the serum sodium secondary to severe hyperlipidemia or hyperproteinemia.

1. J.F., a 31-year-old man, is admitted to the inpatient medicine service for methanol (molecular weight, 32) intoxication. Routine laboratory analysis reveals the following: Na, 145 mEq/L (normal, 134–146); K, 3.4 mEq/L (normal, 3.5–5.1); Cl, 105 mEq/L (normal, 92–109); carbon dioxide (CO_2), 20 mEq/L (normal, 22–32); blood urea nitrogen (BUN), 10 mg/dL (normal, 8–25); creatinine, 1.1 mg/dL (normal, 0.5–1.5); and glucose, 90 mg/dL (normal, 60–110). The blood methanol concentration was 108 mg/dL, and the measured plasma osmolality was 333 mOsm/kg. What is J.F.'s calculated osmolality? Are other unidentified osmoles present?

[SI units: Na, 135 mmol/L; K, 3.4 mmol/L; Cl, 105 mmol/L; CO_2, 20 mmol/L; BUN, 3.57 mmol/L; creatinine, 97.4 μmol/L; glucose, 5.0 mmol/L; methanol, 33.7 mmol/L]

Using Equation 11-1, J.F.'s total calculated osmolality is as follows:

$$P_{OSM} = 2(145\ \text{mEq/L}) + \frac{90\ \text{mg/dL}}{18} + \frac{10\ \text{mg/dL}}{2.8} \quad \textbf{11-A}$$
$$= 290 + 5 + 3.6$$
$$= 299\ \text{mOsm/kg}$$

$$\text{Osmolal gap} = 333\ \text{mOsm/kg} - 299\ \text{mOsm/kg} \quad \textbf{11-B}$$
$$= 34\ \text{mOsm/kg}$$

In J.F., the entire osmolal gap can be accounted for by the presence of the methanol (because 108 mg/dL of methanol will provide 108/3.2 = 33.7 mOsm/kg). It is unlikely, therefore, that other unmeasured osmoles are present (e.g., ethylene glycol, isopropanol, and ethanol). The laboratory determination of osmolality measures the total number of osmotically active particles but not their permeability across the cell membrane. Methanol increases plasma osmolality but not tonicity because the cell membrane is permeable to methanol. Therefore, no net water shift occurs between the intracellular and extracellular compartments. Conversely, mannitol, which is confined to the extracellular space, contributes to both plasma osmolality and tonicity.

Tubular Function of Nephron

The kidney plays an important role in maintaining a constant extracellular environment by regulating the excretion of water and various electrolytes. The volume and composition of fluid filtered across the glomerulus are modified as the fluid passes through the tubules of the nephron.

The renal tubule is composed of a series of segments with heterogeneous structures and functions: the proximal tubule, the medullary and cortical thick ascending limb of Henle's loop, the distal convoluted tubule, and the cortical and medullary collecting duct[2] (Fig. 11-1). The mechanism for sodium reabsorption is different for each nephron segment, but is generally mediated by carrier proteins or channels located on the luminal membrane of the tubule cell.[2] Na^+-K^+-ATPase (adenosine triphosphatase) actively pumps sodium out of the renal tubule cell in exchange for potassium in a 3:2 ratio. Hence, the intracellular sodium concentration is kept at a low level. The potassium that is pumped into the cell leaks back out through potassium channels in the membrane, rendering the cell interior electronegative. The low intracellular sodium concentration and a negative intracellular potential produce a favorable gradient for passive sodium entry into the cell.[3] The Na^+-K^+-ATPase also indirectly provides the energy for active sodium transport and the reabsorption and secretion of other solutes across the luminal membrane of the renal tubule.

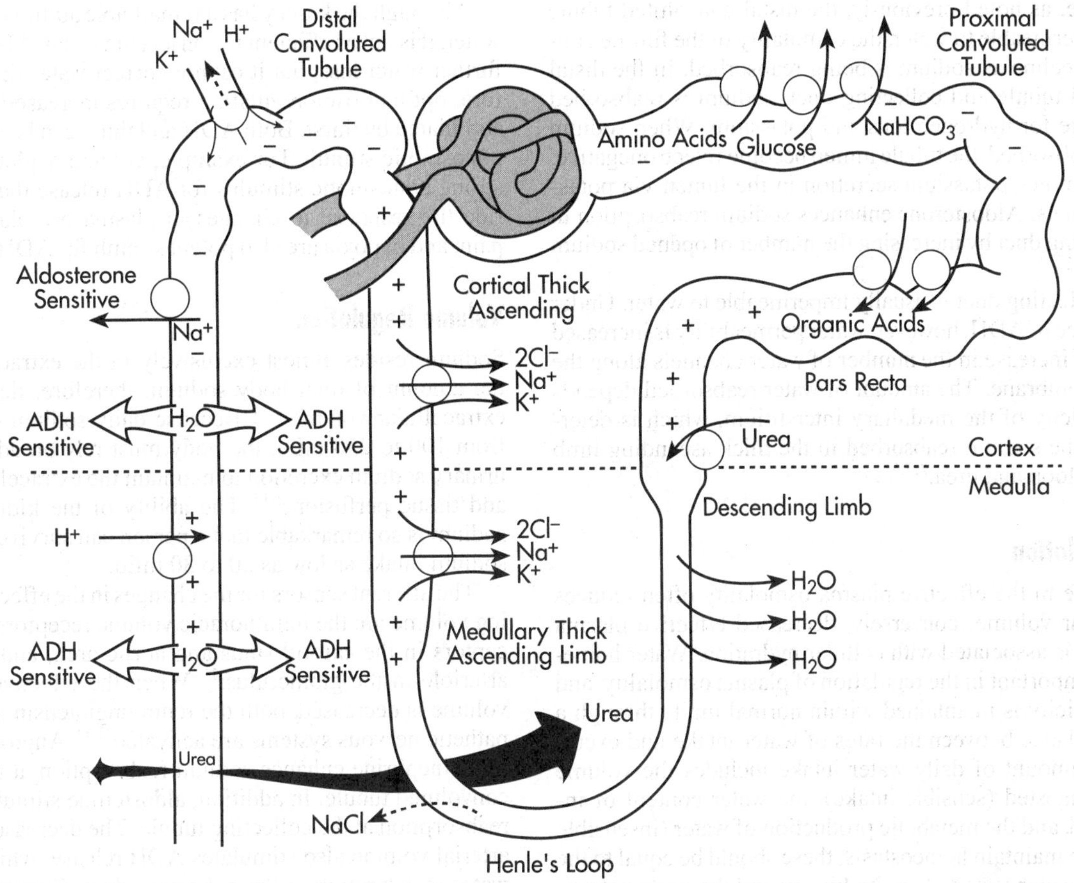

FIGURE 11-1 Sites of tubule salt and water absorption. Sodium is reabsorbed with inorganic anions, amino acids, and glucose in the proximal tubule against an electrical gradient that is lumen negative. In the late part of the proximal tubule (pars recta), sodium and water are reabsorbed to a lesser extent and organic acids (hippurate, urate) and urea are secreted into the urine. The electrical potential is lumen positive in the pars recta. Water, but not salt, is removed from tubule fluid in the thin descending limb of Henle's loop, but in the ascending portion salt is reabsorbed without water, rendering the tubule fluid hyposmotic with respect to the interstitium. Sodium, chloride, and potassium are reabsorbed by the medullary and cortical portions of the ascending limb; the lumen potential is positive. Sodium is reabsorbed and potassium and hydrogen ions are secreted in the distal tubule and collecting ducts. Water absorption in these segments is regulated by antidiuretic hormone (ADH). The electrical potential is lumen negative in the cortical sections and positive in the medullary segments. Urea is concentrated in the interstitium of the medulla and assists in the generation of maximally concentrated urine. (From reference 23, with permission.)

The distal segments are mainly involved in the reabsorption of sodium and chloride ions and the secretion of hydrogen and potassium ions.[2]

Iso-osmotic reabsorption of the glomerular filtrate occurs in the proximal tubule such that two-thirds of the filtered sodium and water and 90% of the filtered bicarbonate are reabsorbed. The Na^+-H^+ antiporter (exchanger) in the luminal membrane is instrumental in the reabsorption of sodium chloride, sodium bicarbonate, and water. The reabsorption of most nonelectrolyte solutes, such as glucose, amino acids, and phosphates, are coupled to sodium transport.[2,5]

Both the thick ascending limb of Henle's loop and the distal convoluted tubule serve as the diluting segments of the nephron because they are impermeable to water. Sodium chloride is extracted from the filtrate without water. Sodium transport in both of these segments is flow dependent and varies with the amount of sodium ions delivered from the proximal segments of the nephron. Decreased sodium ions in the tubular fluid will limit sodium transport in the thick ascending limb of Henle's loop and the distal convoluted tubule.[2,6]

Reabsorption of sodium in the thick ascending limb of Henle's loop accounts for approximately 25% of the total sodium reabsorption. Sodium, chloride, and potassium are reabsorbed by the medullary and cortical portions of the ascending limb, but the leakage of reabsorbed potassium ions back into the tubular lumen, via potassium channels, makes the tubular lumen electropositive. This electrical gradient promotes the passive reabsorption of cations, such as sodium, calcium, and magnesium, in the distal convoluted tubules. Because the thick ascending limb of Henle's loop is impermeable to water, it contributes to the interstitial osmolality in the medulla. This high osmolality is key to the reabsorption of water by the medullary portion of the collecting duct under the influence of antidiuretic hormone (ADH, vasopressin). Therefore, the thick ascending limb of Henle's loop is important for both urinary concentration and dilution.[6]

Because, as noted previously, the distal convoluted tubule also is impermeable to water, the osmolality of the filtrate continues to decline as sodium is being reabsorbed. In the distal convoluted tubule and collecting duct, sodium is reabsorbed in exchange for hydrogen ions and potassium. When sodium ions are reabsorbed, the tubule lumen becomes electronegative, which promotes potassium secretion in the lumen via potassium channels. Aldosterone enhances sodium reabsorption in the collecting duct by increasing the number of opened sodium channels.[2,7]

The collecting duct is usually impermeable to water. Under the influence of ADH, however, water permeability is increased through an increase in the number of water channels along the luminal membrane. The amount of water reabsorbed depends on the tonicity of the medullary interstitium, which is determined by the sodium reabsorbed in the thick ascending limb of Henle's loop and urea.[2,7,8]

Osmoregulation

An increase in the effective plasma osmolality often reduces intracellular volume; conversely, decreased effective plasma osmolality is associated with cellular hydration. Water homeostasis is important in the regulation of plasma osmolality, and plasma tonicity is maintained within normal limits through a delicate balance between the rates of water intake and excretion. The amount of daily water intake includes the volume of water ingested (sensible intake), the water content of ingested food, and the metabolic production of water (insensible intake).[2] To maintain homeostasis, these should be equal to the amount of water excreted by the kidney and the gastrointestinal (GI) tract (sensible loss) plus water lost from the skin and respiratory tract (insensible loss).[2,3]

Changes in plasma tonicity are detected by osmoreceptors in the hypothalamus, which also houses the thirst center and is the site for ADH synthesis.[9,10] When the plasma tonicity falls below 280 mOsm/kg as a result of water ingestion, ADH release is inhibited,[2] water is no longer reabsorbed in the collecting duct, and a large volume of dilute urine is excreted. Conversely, when the osmoreceptors in the hypothalamus sense an increased plasma osmolality, ADH is released to increase water reabsorption. A small volume of concentrated urine is then excreted. The threshold for ADH release is 280 mOsm/kg, and maximal ADH secretion occurs when the plasma osmolality is 295 mOsm/kg.[9] Thus, urine osmolality varies from 50 mOsm/kg in the absence of ADH to 1,200 mOsm/kg during maximal ADH release. The volume of urine produced depends on the solute load to be excreted, as well as the urine osmolality[2,3,9,10]:

$$\text{Urine volume (L)} = \left(\frac{\text{Solute load (mOsm)}}{\text{Urine osmolality (mOsm/kg)}}\right) \qquad \textbf{11-3}$$

$$\left(\frac{1}{\text{Density of water (kg/L)}}\right)$$

Therefore, for a typical daily solute load of 600 mOsm:

$$= \left(\frac{600\text{ mOsm}}{50\text{ mOsm/kg}}\right)\left(\frac{1}{1\text{ kg/L}}\right) = 12\text{ L} \qquad \textbf{11-C}$$

$$= \left(\frac{600\text{ mOsm}}{1{,}200\text{ mOsm/kg}}\right)\left(\frac{1}{1\text{ kg/L}}\right) = 0.5\text{ L} \qquad \textbf{11-D}$$

Although the kidney has a remarkable ability to excrete free water, it is not as efficient in conserving water. ADH minimizes further water loss, but it cannot correct water deficits. Therefore, optimal osmoregulation requires increased water intake stimulated by thirst. Both ADH and thirst can be stimulated by nonosmotic stimuli. For example, volume depletion is such a strong nonosmotic stimulus for ADH release that it can override the response to changes in plasma osmolality. Nausea, pain, and hypoxia are also potent stimuli for ADH secretion.[11]

Volume Regulation

Sodium resides almost exclusively in the extracellular fluid; the amount of total body sodium, therefore, determines the extracellular volume.[2,11] Because daily sodium intake varies from 100 to 250 mEq, the body must rely on adjustments in urinary sodium excretion to maintain the extracellular volume and tissue perfusion.[2,11] The ability of the kidney to retain sodium is so remarkable that a person can survive with a daily sodium intake as low as 20 to 30 mEq.

The afferent sensors for the changes in the effective circulating volume are the intrathoracic volume receptors, the baroreceptors in the carotid sinus and aortic arch, and the afferent arteriole in the glomerulus.[11] When the effective circulating volume is decreased, both the renin-angiotensin and the sympathetic nervous systems are activated.[2,11] Angiotensin II and norepinephrine enhance sodium reabsorption at the proximal convoluted tubule. In addition, aldosterone stimulates sodium reabsorption at the collecting tubule. The decrease in effective arterial volume also stimulates ADH release, which enhances water reabsorption at the collecting duct. Conversely, after a salt load, the increases in atrial pressure and renal perfusion pressure suppress the production of renin and, subsequently, angiotensin II and aldosterone. The release of atrial natriuretic peptide secondary to increased atrial filling pressure and intrarenal production of urodilation increase urinary excretion of the excess sodium.[12,13]

Although the kidney can excrete a 20-mL/kg water load in 4 hours, only 50% of the excess sodium is excreted in the first day.[3] Sodium excretion continues to increase until a new steady state is reached after 3 to 4 days, when intake equals output.[3,12] It is important to recognize that osmoregulation and volume regulation occur independently of each other.[2,3] The two homeostatic systems regulate different parameters and possess different sensors and effectors. Both systems can be activated simultaneously, however.

DISORDERS IN VOLUME REGULATION

Sodium Depletion

2. A.B., a 17-year-old girl, presented to the emergency department (ED) with complaints of anorexia, nausea, vomiting, and generalized weakness for the past 3 days. She denied other medical problems and had not used any medications. On examination, her supine blood pressure (BP) was 105/70 mm Hg, with a pulse of 80 beats/min. Her standing BP was 85/60 mm Hg with a pulse of 100 beats/min, and she complained of feeling dizzy when she stood up. Her mucous membranes were dry but her skin turgor was normal. The jugular vein was flat, and peripheral or sacral edema was not present. Laboratory blood tests showed serum Na,

134 mEq/L (normal, 134–146); K, 3.5 mEq/L (normal, 3.5–5.1); Cl, 95 mEq/L (normal, 92–109); total CO_2 content, 35 mEq/L (normal, 22–32); BUN, 18 mg/dL (normal, 8–25); creatinine, 0.8 mg/dL (normal, 0.5–1.5); and glucose, 70 mg/dL (normal, 60–110). Random urinary Na was 40 mEq/L, K was 40 mEq/L, and Cl was <15 mEq/L. The hemoglobin (Hgb) was 14 g/dL (normal, 12–16), and white cell and platelet counts were normal. Why were the clinical and laboratory data in A.B. consistent with an assessment of volume depletion?

[SI units: serum Na, 134 mmol/L; K, 3.5 mmol/L; Cl, 95 mmol/L; CO_2, 35 mmol/L; BUN, 5.7 mmol/L; creatinine, 70.72 μmol/L; glucose, 3.9 mmol/L; urine Na, 40 mmol/L; K, 40 mmol/L; Cl, <15 mmol/L; Hgb, 140 g/L]

The signs and symptoms in A.B. were consistent with volume depletion. The loss of gastric fluid owing to vomiting and decreased oral intake secondary to anorexia had led to moderate to severe volume depletion. There were orthostatic changes in both her BP (a drop in systolic BP of 20 mm Hg) and pulse (an increase of 20 beats/minute). The dry mucous membranes, the flat jugular vein, and the absence of edema support volume depletion as well, and dizziness on standing indicates extracellular volume depletion.[14] Her hypochloremic metabolic alkalosis was probably initiated by loss of acidic gastric contents through vomiting. Her volume depletion increased renal bicarbonate reabsorption, which perpetuated the metabolic alkalosis. The decreased renal perfusion brought about by volume depletion enhanced proximal tubular reabsorption of urea, resulting in an increased BUN:creatinine ratio (prerenal azotemia). When renal perfusion is decreased and the renin-angiotensin-aldosterone system is activated, the proximal reabsorption of sodium and chloride is increased. A.B.'s urinary sodium is therefore <10 mEq/L.[15] Excretion of the poorly permeable bicarbonate ions, however, results in obligatory urinary sodium loss to maintain luminal electroneutrality. A.B.'s urinary sodium was therefore elevated (40 mEq/L). In this situation, the urinary chloride remained low, and this is a better index of volume status.[15] Both urinary sodium and chloride are elevated, however, in patients using diuretics, in those undergoing osmotic diuresis, and in those with underlying renal disease or hypoaldosteronism, even in the face of volume depletion. Physical examination should therefore be conducted as part of the volume status assessment. A.B.'s volume depletion increased the concentration of red blood cells, which could explain her slightly elevated Hgb concentration of 14 g/dL.

3. How should A.B.'s volume depletion be managed?

The etiology of A.B.'s vomiting should be sought and the cause removed. Because the patient is neither hypernatremic nor hyponatremic, normal saline should be administered intravenously to replenish the extracellular volume and improve tissue perfusion.[2,14] If the patient is hypernatremic (having a greater deficit of water than solute), half-isotonic saline (1/2NS) or dextrose solution, which contains more free water, should be administered. In contrast, hyponatremic hypovolemic patients have a greater deficit of solute than water; isotonic or hypertonic saline should then be given. The amount of volume deficit is often difficult to ascertain. Because A.B. was severely orthostatic, 1 or 2 L of fluid can be given over 2 to 4 hours. The subsequent rate of infusion will depend on A.B.'s response and the prevailing symptoms. The clinician should monitor her body weight, skin turgor, supine and upright BP, jugular venous pressure, urine output, and urine chloride concentration to assess the adequacy of volume repletion. Because the treatment goal is to achieve a positive fluid balance, the infusion rate should be 50 or 100 mL/hour in excess of the sum of urine output, insensible losses, and other losses, such as emesis and diarrhea.[2]

Sodium Excess

4. L.J., a 45-year-old man, presented to the clinic with complaints of swollen legs and puffy eyelids. He also noticed that his urine had been foamy recently. On examination, his BP was 180/100 mm Hg and his pulse was 80 beats/minute. Bilateral periorbital edema and 2+ bilateral pitting edema up to the thigh were noted. On auscultation, his heart was normal and his lungs had bilateral crackles. His jugular venous pressure was elevated at 10 cm H_2O. Laboratory tests revealed serum Na, 132 mEq/L (normal, 134–146); K, 3.8 mEq/L (normal, 3.5–5.1); Cl, 100 mEq/L (normal, 92–109); bicarbonate, 26 mEq/L (normal, 22–32); BUN, 40 mg/dL (normal, 8–25); creatinine, 2.5 mg/dL (normal, 0.5–1.5); glucose, 120 mg/dL (normal, 60–110); and albumin, 2 g/dL (normal, 3.4–5.4). The serum transaminases, alkaline phosphatase, and bilirubin were within normal limits. The serum cholesterol level was 280 mg/dL (normal, <200), and the triglyceride level was 300 mg/dL (normal, 30–200). Urinalysis showed specific gravity of 1.015 (normal, 1.002–1.030), pH 7.0 (normal, 4.6–7.9), protein >300 mg/dL, oval fat bodies, and fatty casts. The 24-hour urinary protein excretion was 6 g and the measured creatinine clearance (Cl_{Cr}) was 40 mL/minute L.J. was taking no medications and he denied illicit drug use. Hepatitis B serology and human immunodeficiency virus (HIV) antibody were negative. The impression was anasarca (total body edema) secondary to nephrotic syndrome. What is nephrotic syndrome? What could be the cause of L.J.'s sodium excess state?

[SI units: Na, 132 mmol/L; K, 3.8 mmol/L; Cl, 100 mmol/L; bicarbonate, 26 mmol/L; BUN, 14.3 mmol/L; serum creatine (SrCr), 221 μmol/L; glucose, 6.7 mmol/L; albumin, 20 g/L; cholesterol, 7.24 mmol/L; triglyceride, 3.4 mmol/L; protein, 3 g/L; Cl_{Cr}, 0.67 mL/second]

Nephrotic syndrome is characterized by hypoalbuminemia, urine protein excretion >3.5 g/day, hyperlipidemia, lipiduria, and edema.[16,17] The heavy proteinuria is a result of damage to the selective barrier of the glomerulus. The causes of nephrotic syndrome are multiple and diverse.[16] The cause of nephrotic syndrome can be idiopathic (primary glomerular disease) or secondary to chronic systemic diseases (e.g., diabetes mellitus, amyloidosis, sickle cell anemia,[18] lupus), cancer (e.g., multiple myeloma, Hodgkin's disease), infections (e.g., HIV,[19] hepatitis B, syphilis, malaria), intravenous (IV) drug abuse, and medications (e.g., gold, penicillamine, captopril, nonsteroidal anti-inflammatory drugs [NSAID][20]).

A heavy urinary protein loss results in various extrarenal complications.[16,17] Hypoalbuminemia reduces plasma oncotic pressure and contributes to the increased hepatic synthesis of both albumin and lipoproteins. This, coupled with the decreased catabolism of lipoproteins, resulted in L.J.'s hyperlipidemia.[16,21] Loss of inhibitors of coagulation in the urine predispose these patients to thromboembolism.[16] Specific therapy of nephrotic syndrome ranges from simple removal of the offending medication and treatment of the underlying infection, to the use of immunosuppressive agents in specific glomerular diseases.

The edematous state (L.J.'s anasarca) results from changes in both capillary hemodynamics and renal sodium and water retention.[22] The hypoalbuminemia (2 g/dL) and proteinuria (>300 mg/dL) produced an imbalance in the Starling forces across the capillary wall, namely the hydrostatic and oncotic pressures in the capillary and interstitial compartments. The reduced capillary oncotic pressure favors movement of fluid from the vascular space into the interstitium.[23] This leads to contraction of the effective arterial blood volume, which in turn activates humoral, neural, and hemodynamic mechanisms that signal the kidney to retain sodium and water.[24,25] This *underfill hypothesis* has been challenged by data suggesting that hypoalbuminemia plays a minor role in nephrotic edema[26,27] and the observation that patients with nephrotic syndrome can have increased, normal, or decreased plasma volumes.[23]

A defect in the intrarenal sodium handling mechanism that causes inappropriate sodium retention also contributes to nephrotic edema.[23,26] According to this *overflow hypothesis,* proteinuric renal disease leads to increased sodium reabsorption in the distal nephron. The mechanism is not well defined but may be related to cellular resistance to atrial natriuretic peptide.[23] Thus, a sodium excess state occurs and edema results. It is likely that the interaction between the "underfill" and "overflow" mechanisms results in the production of nephrotic edema.[28] Patients with severe hypoalbuminemia (i.e., serum albumin level <1.5 g/dL) who have a severe reduction in plasma oncotic pressure are most likely to exhibit evidence of the underfill phenomenon.[22]

5. How should L.J.'s sodium excess state be managed?

The etiology of L.J.'s nephrotic syndrome should be identified for specific treatment. Although L.J.'s serum sodium concentration of 132 mEq/L is low, it reflects dilution secondary to fluid excess. Salt restriction is therefore important to control L.J.'s generalized edema.[23] For most nephrotic patients, modest dietary sodium restriction to approximately 50 mEq/day may be sufficient to maintain neutral sodium balance.[22,23] For nephrotic patients who are very sodium avid (urine sodium concentration <10 mEq/L), sufficient restriction is difficult to achieve. Thus, slowing the rate of edema formation rather than hastening its resolution should be the goal of therapy for these patients.[23] Bedrest reduces orthostatic stimulation of the renin-angiotensin-aldosterone and sympathetic systems, thereby favoring the movement of interstitial fluid into the vascular space.[23] The central blood volume is thus increased and natriuresis and diuresis are facilitated. Prolonged bedrest might, however, predispose these hypercoagulable patients to thromboembolism.[16] Similarly, use of support stockings may reduce the stimulation for sodium retention by redistributing blood volume to the central circulation.[23,29]

Diuretics

Usually, loop diuretics are the mainstay of therapy in the management of nephrotic edema.[2,23] In most of these patients, the edema can be removed safely with rapid diuresis without compromising the systemic circulation, probably because of the rapid refilling of the plasma volume by interstitial fluid.[23] Nevertheless, as the edema resolves, the rate of fluid removal and weight loss should be decreased to avoid compromising the effective circulating volume. The patient should be monitored for the development of orthostatic hypotension.

Infusions of albumin can expand the plasma volume; however, it is expensive, the relief is temporary, and it should therefore be used only for resistant edema.[30] In patients who are resistant to the aforementioned measures, extracorporeal fluid removal, namely ultrafiltration, may be necessary.[23,31]

L.J. was initially treated with IV furosemide 60 mg twice daily and placed on a low-sodium (50 mEq), low-fat, high–complex-carbohydrate diet that consisted of 0.8 g/kg protein of high biologic value with additional protein to match gram-per-gram of urinary protein loss. Fluid was restricted to 1,000 mL/day.[32] He had 5 L of diuresis in 2 days, with resolution of respiratory symptoms and a reduction in the anasarca. Parenteral furosemide was discontinued on the fifth day of hospitalization and oral furosemide 120 mg twice daily was started. After a total weight loss of 12 kg, he was then discharged with instructions to maintain the diet and oral furosemide.

DISORDERS IN OSMOREGULATION

Hyponatremia

Serum sodium concentration reflects the ratio of total body sodium to total body water and is not an accurate indicator of total body sodium. Both hyponatremia and hypernatremia can occur in the presence of a low, normal, or high total body sodium.[33,34] Because the kidney can excrete >12 to 16 L of free water daily, hyponatremia does not occur unless the water intake overwhelms the kidney's ability to excrete free water (e.g., psychogenic polydipsia),[35,36] or free water excretion is impaired.[2,37]

Free water formation requires a normal glomerular filtration rate (GFR), the reabsorption of sodium chloride without water in the thick ascending limb of Henle's loop and the distal convoluting tubule, and the excretion of a dilute urine in the absence of ADH[37] (Fig. 11-1). Therefore, hyponatremia can occur when the kidney's diluting ability is exceeded or impaired owing to volume depletion and nonosmotic stimulation of ADH release or inappropriate stimulation of ADH production.[2,37]

Although plasma sodium is the primary determinant of plasma tonicity, hyponatremia does not always represent hypotonicity.[2,37] In patients with severe hyperlipidemia or hyperproteinemia (e.g., multiple myeloma), pseudohyponatremia can occur because the increased amounts of lipids and proteins displace plasma water, which sodium ions dissolve in, resulting in a lower concentration of sodium per unit volume of plasma.[34,37,38] Normally, water accounts for 93% of the plasma volume, and lipids and proteins make up the rest.[37] The increase in plasma lipid and protein contents expands plasma volume, displaces water, and increases the percentage of solids in plasma.[34,37] Because sodium is distributed only in the aqueous phase, the sodium content per liter of the newly recomposed plasma is thus decreased and the plasma sodium concentration is reduced.[34,37,38] The sodium concentration in plasma water remains the same, however. Because osmolality depends on the solute concentration in plasma water, serum osmolality remains unchanged.[34] Indeed, the measured osmolality is normal. Another example of isotonic hyponatremia can be found when a large volume of isotonic mannitol irrigant is used during prostate surgery.[34,37] Absorption of the irrigation solution can result in severe hyponatremia but normal osmolality. In contrast, use of large amounts of isotonic sorbitol and isotonic, or slightly hypotonic, glycine solutions during urologic surgery can cause the hypotonicity as a late complication.[34,37] Similar to mannitol, sorbitol and isotonic glycine initially distribute only in the extracellular space, resulting in hyponatremia without a change in osmolality.[37] Unlike mannitol, both sorbitol and glycine are later metabolized, leaving water behind to result in hypotonicity. The severe hypotonic hyponatremia, in conjunction with the neurotoxic effects of glycine and its metabolites, puts the patient at significant risk for severe neurologic symptoms (Table 11-1).[37,39]

Table 11-1 Clinical Presentation and Treatment of Hyponatremia

Na^+ and H_2O Status	*Clinical Presentation/Cause*	*Treatment*
Edematous, Fluid Overload (Hypervolemic, Hypotonic)		
↑ Total Body Na^+ –↑↑ Total Body H_2O	*Cirrhosis/CHF/nephrotic syndrome:* A ↓ in renal blood flow activates renin angiotensin system. ↑ aldosterone leads to ↑ Na^+, and ↑ ADH leads to free H_2O retention. Urine Na^+ is low (0–20 mEq/L) and urine osmolality ↓. Diuretics can induce paradoxical effects on urine Na^+ and osmolality. This form also can occur in patients with renal failure who drink excessive amounts of water. Patients have symptoms of fluid overload (ascites, distended neck veins, edema).	Fluid and Na+ restriction. Correct underlying disorder (e.g., paracentesis for ascites). Diurese cautiously; avoid ↓ ECF and accompanying ↓ tissue perfusion. ↑ BUN may indicate overly rapid diuresis.
Nonedematous Hypovolemic (Hypotonic with ECF Depletion)		
↓↓ Total Body Na^+ ↓ Total Body H_2O	Occurs in: *GI fluid loss (e.g., diarrhea) with hypotonic electrolyte-poor fluid replacement, overdiuresis, "third spacing," Addison's disease, renal tubular acidosis, osmotic diuresis.* Replacement of fluid losses with solute-free fluid predisposes these patients to hyponatremia. Kidneys concentrate urine to conserve fluid (urine Na^+ <10 mEq/L). Symptoms: nonedematous; ECF depletion (collapsed neck veins, dehydration, orthostasis). Neurologic symptoms: (See Hyponatremia: Symptoms in text).	Discontinue diuretics. Replace fluid and electrolyte (especially K^+) losses. 0.9% saline preferred unless Na^+ deficit severe, then use 3%–5% saline. See footnote *a* for method of estimating Na^+ deficit.
Nonedematous, Normovolemic (Normovolemic, Hypotonic)		
↓ Total Body Sodium ↑ Total Body H_2O	*SIADH[a]*: Hyponatremia, hypo-osmolality, renal Na^+ wasting (>40 mEq/L), absence of fluid depletion, $U_{osm} > P_{osm}$, normal renal and adrenal function. Free H_2O retained while Na^+ lost. *Causes:* (a) ADH production (infectious disease, vascular disease, cerebral neoplasm, cancer of lung, pancreas, duodenum); (b) exogenous ADH administration; (c) drugs; (d) psychogenic polydipsia.	*Conivaptan:* Loading dose of 20 mg IV over 30 minutes, followed by 20 mg IV as continuous infusion over 24 hours for an additional 1 to 3 days; may titrate up to maximal dose of 40 mg/day; maximal duration is 4 days after the loading dose. Dedicated IV line recommended and site of peripheral IV lines should be changed every 24 hours. *Chronic treatment:* Restrict fluids to less than urine loss. *Demeclocycline* (300–600 mg BID) induces reversible diabetes insipidus. *Emergency treatment* for unresponsive patients includes *furosemide* diuresis to achieve negative H_2O balance with careful replacement of Na^+ and K^+ using hypertonic saline solutions.[b] See footnote *b* for method of calculating TBW excess and type of solutions to use.

[a]Estimate Na deficit: (mEq) = (0.5 L/kg × wt in kg) (Na desired - Na observed), where 0.5 L/kg is volume of distribution (Vd) of Na in the body. Rate of Na and fluid repletion used depends on severity. Mild: replace with NS. First one-third over 6 to 12 hours at a rate of <0.5 mEq/L/hr, remaining two=thirds over 24 to 48 hours. Severe (e.g., seizures): Use 3% to 5% saline, rate gauged by patient's ability to tolerate Na and volume load. Monitor CNS function, skin turgor, BP, urine Na, signs of Na/H_2O overload, especially in patients with cardiovascular, renal, and pulmonary disease.

[b]Total body water (TBW) = 0.5 L/kg × wt in kg. TBW excess = TBW − TBW (observed serum NA)/(desired serum NA)

ADH, antidiuretic hormone; BID, twice daily; BUN, blood urea nitrogen; CHF, congestive heart failure; ECF, extracellular fluid; GI, gastrointestinal; IV, intravenous; NS, normal saline (0.9% Na); SIADH, syndrome of inappropriate ADH.

Remove estimated excess free water with IV furosemide (1 mg/kg). Repeat as necessary. Because furosemide generates a urine that resembles 0.5% NaCl, urine losses of Na and K must be carefully measured and replaced hourly with hypertonic salt solutions. *Correction rate:* 1 to 2 mEq Na/hr in symptomatic patients; 0.5 mEq/hr in asymptomatic patients.

6. T.T., a 23-year-old man with end-stage renal disease caused by diabetic nephropathy, is receiving chronic ambulatory peritoneal dialysis. Because of dietary and fluid noncompliance, T.T. complained of shortness of breath (SOB) and his dialysis prescription was adjusted to include six cycles of 2.5% peritoneal dialysis solutions. Today, his laboratory values are Na, 128 mEq/L (normal, 134–146); K, 4 mEq/L (normal, 3.5–5.1); Cl, 98 mEq/L (normal, 92–109); total CO_2, 24 mmol/L (normal, 22–32); BUN, 50 mg/dL (normal, 8–25); creatinine, 6 mg/dL (normal, 0.5–1.5); and glucose, 600 mg/dL (normal, 60–110). Evaluate T.T.'s plasma osmolality. What is the etiology of T.T.'s hyponatremia?

[SI units: Na, 128 mmol/L; K, 4 mmol/L; Cl, 98 mmol/L; CO_2, 24 mmol/L; BUN, 17.85 mmol/L; creatinine, 530.4 μmol/L; glucose, 33.3 mmol/L]

T.T.'s effective plasma osmolality is calculated to be 289 mOsm/L, of which 33 mOsm/L is contributed by the hyperglycemia. The slow utilization of glucose, because of the lack of insulin, causes water to move from the intracellular compartment into the plasma space because of the increased tonicity, thereby lowering the plasma sodium concentration.[34,37] Despite the lowered plasma sodium concentration, the plasma osmolality is normal because of hyperglycemia. Hence, no symptoms attributable to hypo-osmolality are observed. Indeed, when serum glucose is normalized with insulin and hydration, the serum sodium level will increase to approximately 136 mEq/L. For each 100-mg/dL increment in serum glucose, serum sodium decreases by 1.3 to 1.6 mEq/L.[34,37] Use of hypertonic mannitol or glycine solutions in patients with cerebral edema also results in a hyperosmolar hyponatremia.[34]

Hypotonic Hyponatremia With Decreased Extracellular Fluid

7. Q.B., a 30-year-old male athlete who has had multiple bouts of diarrhea over the last several days, has been drinking Gatorade to keep himself from getting dehydrated. His vital signs are supine BP, 145/80 mm Hg, and pulse, 70 beats/minute; standing BP, 128/68 mm Hg, and pulse, 90 beats/minute. Respiratory rate (RR) was 12 breaths/minute, and he was afebrile. His skin turgor was mildly decreased and laboratory data were Na, 128 mEq/L (normal, 134–146); K, 3.0 mEq/L (normal, 3.5–5.1); Cl, 100 mEq/L (normal, 92–109); bicarbonate, 17 mEq/L (normal, 24–31); BUN, 27 mg/dL (normal, 8–25); and creatinine, 1.2 mg/dL (normal, 0.5–1.5). Urinary Na and Cl were both <10 mEq/L. Assess Q.B.'s electrolyte and fluid status. What is the etiology of Q.B.'s hyponatremia?

[SI units: plasma Na, 128 mmol/L; K, 3 mmol/L; Cl, 100 mmol/L; bicarbonate, 17 mmol/L; BUN, 7.14 mmol/L; creatinine, 106.1 μmol/L; urinary Na, <10 mmol/L; Cl, <10 mmol/L]

Q.B. has true hypotonic hyponatremia with extracellular fluid depletion, suggesting that his total body sodium deficit is greater than that of total body water.[34] His poor skin turgor, orthostasis, prerenal azotemia, and low urinary sodium are consistent with volume depletion. The urinary sodium concentration helps distinguish between renal and nonrenal losses that result in the sodium and water deficits.[15,34,40] When the plasma volume is depleted, the urinary sodium concentration is <10 mEq/L, suggesting appropriate renal sodium conservation.[15] This is usually seen in patients such as Q.B. with GI fluid loss as in vomiting, diarrhea, or profuse sweating.[34,37,40] Other causes of hypotonic hyponatremia are less likely in Q.B. They include surreptitious cathartic abuse and "third spacing," or accumulation of extracellular fluid in the abdominal cavity during acute pancreatitis, ileus, or pseudomembranous colitis.[37,40] If the urinary sodium is >20 mEq/L in the face of volume depletion, renal salt wastage should be considered.[15,37,40] The potential causes of this latter problem include diuretic use,[41–44] adrenal insufficiency,[44] and salt-wasting nephropathy[35] (e.g., chronic interstitial nephritis, medullary cystic disease, polycystic kidney disease, obstructive uropathy, and cisplatin toxicity[44,45]). In patients with renal insufficiency, neither the urinary sodium nor chloride concentration is a reliable index of volume status.[15]

Volume depletion leads to increased reabsorption of sodium and water in the proximal tubule and, thus, decreased sodium delivery to the diluting segments for free water formation.[34,37,40] Decreased effective arterial volume is also a potent nonosmotic stimulus for ADH release.[9,10] These factors combine to dampen the ability of the kidney to form dilute urine and result in high urine osmolality despite a low serum sodium concentration.[34,37,40] Although the fluid lost in diarrhea is hypotonic, it is the replacement of fluid loss with an even more hypotonic fluid such as Gatorade or tap water that causes hyponatremia in patients such as Q.B.[37,40]

Q.B.'s diarrhea probably caused loss of potassium and bicarbonate through the GI tract, resulting in hypokalemia and hyperchloremic metabolic acidosis. The potassium depletion can sensitize ADH secretion in response to hypovolemic stimuli, and the hypokalemia also can lead to hyponatremia.[37] The cellular efflux of potassium causes cellular uptake of sodium, further reducing the serum sodium concentration.

8. How should Q.B.'s hyponatremia be treated?

The treatment of hypovolemic hyponatremia involves sodium replacement to correct the deficit. The sodium deficit can be estimated by the following formula:

$$\text{Na Deficit} = \text{Vd of Na} \times \text{Patient Weight (Desired} - \text{Current Na concentration)} \quad \text{11-4}$$

$$= (0.5\ \text{L/kg})(70\ \text{kg})(140 - 125\ \text{mEq/L}) \quad \text{11-E}$$
$$= 525\ \text{mEq}$$

Approximately one-third of the deficit can be replaced over the first 12 hours at a rate of <0.5 mEq/L/hour. The remaining amounts can be administered over the next several days.

The use of isotonic sodium chloride solution is ideal for the treatment of volume-depleted hyponatremia. As renal perfusion is restored, free water will be excreted with appropriate retention of sodium.[40] Because Q.B. has only mild volume depletion, oral replacement fluids can be given. Oral solutions containing both electrolyte and glucose[46] or rice-based solutions[47] are ideal for the management of persistent fluid loss. Glucose not only provides calories but also promotes the intestinal absorption of ingested sodium.[48] Because the rice-based solution provides more glucose and amino acids, both of which can promote intestinal sodium absorption, it is more effective than glucose alone.[2,48]

In patients with renal salt wasting, the ongoing daily sodium loss also should be taken into consideration when estimating the amount of replacement. Potassium should be given to correct hypokalemia, thereby reducing the hyponatremia as well. The serum sodium concentration may rise faster than expected because as tissue perfusion is restored, sodium delivery to the distal tubules will increase and ADH secretion will be suppressed appropriately.[34,37,40] In the absence of ADH, increased free water excretion will improve the serum sodium concentration faster than initially estimated.

Hypervolemic Hypotonic Hyponatremia

9. T.W., a 55-year-old man with a longstanding history of alcoholic liver cirrhosis, is admitted to the hospital for worsening SOB. His medical history includes portal hypertension, esophageal varices, and noncompliance with dietary restriction and medications. His BP is 120/60 mm Hg; pulse, 100 beats/minute; RR, 20 breaths/minute. He is afebrile. Physical examination reveals a jaundiced man in respiratory distress. His jugular vein is flat and lung examination reveals bilateral basal rales. Abdominal examination shows tense ascites with hepatomegaly and spider angiomas (telangiectasias resembling a spider). He has 1+ pedal edema bilaterally. Laboratory data on admission are Na, 127 mEq/L (normal, 134–146); K, 3.4 mEq/L (normal, 3.5–5.1); Cl, 95 mEq/L (normal, 92–109); total CO_2 content, 24 mEq/L (normal, 22–32); BUN, 10 mg/dL (normal, 8–25); SrCr, 1.2 mg/dL (normal, 0.5–1.5); and albumin, 2.5 g/dL (normal, 3.5–5.4). Urine Na was <10 mEq/L, and osmolality was 380 mOsm/L (normal, 250–1,000). Identify the possible causes of hyponatremia in T.W. and discuss its pathophysiology. How should he be treated?

[SI units: serum Na, 127 mmol/L; K, 3.4 mmol/L; Cl, 95 mmol/L; CO_2, 24 mmol/L; BUN, 3.57 mmol/L; SrCr, 106.1 μmol/L; albumin, 25 g/L; urine, Na <10 mmol/L]

T.W. had no history of vomiting or diarrhea and had stopped using diuretics before admission. The physical findings of ascites and bilateral edema are not consistent with volume depletion but indicate a sodium-excess state. Both sodium and water retention take place, but the disproportionate accumulation of ingested water relative to sodium leads to hyponatremia.[34,37,40]

Cirrhotic patients who are susceptible to develop hyponatremia have a decreased effective arterial blood volume.[24,37,46,47] The low urinary sodium concentration suggests that the effective arterial blood volume was decreased.[15] The high urinary osmolality in the face of hypotonic hyponatremia suggests, however, that the release of ADH has been stimulated, impairing free water excretion. Peripheral vasodilation causes decreases in systemic arterial BP despite a normal to high cardiac output. This, along with splanchnic venous pooling and decreased oncotic pressure secondary to hypoalbuminemia, decreases renal perfusion in patients such as T.W. with cirrhosis.[22,28,46] Decreased renal perfusion activates the renin-angiotensin-aldosterone system, the sympathetic nervous system, and the release of ADH. Reabsorption of sodium and water in the proximal tubules is enhanced, diminishing sodium and water delivery to the distal segments of the nephron. The diluting capacity of the kidney is thus impaired. Increased secretion of antidiuretic hormone also promotes free water reabsorption at the collecting tubule and contributes to the hyperosmolality of urine and hyponatremia. The hypervolemic hyponatremia also is seen in patients with congestive heart failure (CHF) and nephrotic syndrome[24–28] and in patients with chronic renal disease who drink excessive amounts of water.[37,40] (See Chapter 18, Heart Failure.) As the GFR decreases, distal delivery of sodium is reduced and the ability to generate free water is impaired. In addition, the capacity to conserve sodium is impaired in these patients.[15]

Most patients who are edematous and hyponatremic are asymptomatic, but the degree of hyponatremia probably reflects the severity of the underlying disease.[46,47,49] Unless an acute decrease in serum sodium occurs, rapid therapeutic correction is not warranted.[37,40,46,47,50] Water restriction, the mainstay of therapy, is determined by the degree of hyponatremia and the severity of symptoms. Sodium restriction and judicious use of diuretics may help reduce the edematous state, but the patient must be monitored closely to avoid prerenal azotemia, which suggests overaggressive diuresis. Furthermore, diuretics can induce or worsen hyponatremia and volume depletion by impairing the diluting capacity of the kidney.[43–47]

T.W. had abdominal paracentesis to relieve respiratory discomfort with no sequelae. He was then prescribed a 1,000-mg sodium diet, and water was restricted to 500 mL/day. Diuretic therapy was resumed.

Normovolemic Hypotonic Hyponatremia

10. C.C., a 50-year-old man who was diagnosed recently with small-cell lung carcinoma, was brought to the ED by his family because he had become progressively lethargic and stuporous over the past week. Laboratory data revealed the following: serum Na, 110 mEq/L (normal, 134–146); K, 3.6 mEq/L (normal, 3.5–5.1); Cl, 78 mEq/L (normal, 92–109); bicarbonate, 22 mEq/L (normal, 24–31); BUN, 10 mg/dL (normal, 8–25); SrCr, 0.9 mg/dL (normal, 0.5–1.5); glucose, 90 mg/dL (normal, 60–110); serum osmolality, 230 mOsm/kg (normal, 274–296); urine osmolality, 616 mOsm/kg (normal, 250–1,000); and urine Na, 60 mEq/L. Arterial blood gas (ABG) examination at room air showed pH, 7.38 (normal, 7.35–7.42); P_{CO_2}, 38 mm Hg (normal, 35–45); and P_{O_2}, 80 mm Hg (normal, 80–100). On physical examination, C.C. was normotensive, appeared to be euvolemic, and had no edema detected. Review of his medical records showed normal adrenal and thyroid function. C.C. was currently not using any medications. On admission to the ward, C.C. weighed 60 kg and was given 1 L of normal saline, after which his serum sodium concentration was 108 mEq/L. Identify the cause of hyponatremia in C.C. and describe its pathophysiology.

[SI units: serum Na, 110 mmol/L; K, 3.6 mmol/L; Cl, 78 mmol/L; bicarbonate, 22 mmol/L; BUN, 3.57 mmol/L; SrCr, 79.6 μmol/L; glucose, 5.0 mmol/L; serum osmolality, 230 mmol/kg; urine osmolality, 616 mmol/kg; urine Na, 60 mmol/L; P_{CO_2}, 5.1 kPa; P_{O_2}, 853.1 mmol/L; serum Na, 108 mmol/L]

In a patient with hypo-osmolar hyponatremia with a volume status that is apparently normal, the differential diagnosis[40] includes hypothyroidism,[51] cortisol deficiency,[52] a reset osmostat,[53] psychogenic polydipsia,[36,38] and the syndrome of inappropriate antidiuretic hormone secretion (SIADH),[54–56] which is a diagnosis of exclusion. C.C.'s normal thyroid and adrenal function tests exclude hypothyroidism and cortisol insufficiency as causes of his hyponatremia. The inappropriately elevated urine osmolality (>100 mOsm/kg) is inconsistent with psychogenic polydipsia or a reset osmostat, because free water excretion is usually not impaired in these disorders. These findings, in addition to a urine sodium concentration >40 mEq/L and a normal acid–base and potassium balance, are consistent with SIADH.[37,55,56]

In SIADH, the ADH secretion is considered inappropriate because of its persistence in the absence of appropriate osmotic and hemodynamic stimuli. Water ingestion is essential to the development of hyponatremia in SIADH because persistent ADH activity impairs water excretion, resulting in expansion of body fluids and hypo-osmolar hyponatremia. Edema rarely is apparent because only one-third of the retained water resides in the extracellular space and the sodium homeostatic mechanisms are intact.[34,40] The extracellular fluid expansion activates volume receptors and results in natriuresis. At steady state, urinary sodium excretion reflects sodium intake and is usually >40 mEq/L, as in C.C.'s case. Nonetheless, if sodium intake is reduced severely, the urinary sodium concentration may become <40 mEq/L.[37]

The causes of SIADH are diverse and are shown in Table 11-1. Four different patterns of inappropriate ADH release have been identified.[37] No correlation has been found between these patterns and the underlying causes of SIADH, however. Mechanisms for drug-induced SIADH include ADH-like action on the collecting tubule, central stimulation of ADH release, and potentiation of the ADH effect.[37,57] Small-cell lung carcinoma is the most likely cause of C.C.'s SIADH.

11. Why was C.C.'s serum sodium concentration lower after the saline infusion?

Isotonic sodium chloride solution (154 mEq/L each of Na and Cl ions, or 308 mOsm/L) initially will increase the plasma sodium concentration because its osmolality is higher than C.C.'s.[58] C.C., however, has a relatively fixed urine osmolality of 616 mOsm/kg owing to persistent ADH activity; thus, he must excrete an osmolar load of 616 mOsm in a volume of 1,000 mL of urine at steady state. Because a total of 1 L of fluid containing 308 mOsm was administered, all the solutes were excreted in 500 mL of urine output, and 500 mL of free water was retained to cause a further dilution of sodium and a reduction in serum sodium concentration.[37,58]

Neurologic Manifestations

12. Why are C.C.'s neurologic manifestations characteristic of hyponatremia?

As the plasma osmolality declines, the osmotic gradient created across the blood–brain barrier favors the movement of water into the brain and other cells.[37,40] Water movement from the cerebrospinal fluid into the cerebral interstitium results in cerebral edema. Brain swelling is limited by the meninges and cranium, however, giving rise to increased intracranial pressure and neurologic symptoms. The degree of cerebral overhydration and the rapidity of its development appear to correlate with the severity of symptoms.[37,40]

When hyponatremia develops in <2 to 3 days or the rate of decline in serum sodium >0.5 mEq/L/hour, the situation is regarded as acute.[37,59,60] The patient often becomes symptomatic when serum sodium concentration falls to 125 mEq/L; early complaints include nausea, vomiting, and malaise.[37,61] Severe symptoms occur more commonly when the serum sodium falls to <120 mEq/L and the rate of decline >0.5 mEq/L/hour. The patient may present with headache, tremors, incoordination, delirium, lethargy, and obtundation. As the serum sodium drops below 110 to 115 mEq/L, seizure and coma may result.[37,61] On occasion, severe brain edema leads to transtentorial herniation and eventually death. Women, especially those who are premenopausal, apparently are more susceptible to the development of severe neurologic symptoms and irreversible neurologic damage than are men.[62,63]

In contrast to acute hyponatremia, patients who are chronically hyponatremic are usually asymptomatic.[37,59] If present, symptoms are usually vague and nonspecific and tend to occur at lower serum sodium concentrations than those associated with symptomatic acute hyponatremia.[37,59,61] The patient may experience anorexia, nausea, vomiting, muscle weakness, and cramps. Irritability, hostility, confusion, and personality changes also may be seen. At extremely low sodium levels, stupor and, rarely, seizures have been reported.

Brain Adaptation to Hyponatremia

The difference in symptoms between acute and chronic hyponatremia is related to cerebral adaptation to hypotonicity. Two adaptive mechanisms are important in minimizing cerebral edema.[37,40,64,65] First, *cerebral overhydration* increases the hydrostatic pressure in the cerebral interstitium, which results in the movement of fluid from the cerebral interstitial space to the cerebrospinal fluid. Second, the *extrusion of intracellular solutes* reduces cellular osmolality, which in turn enhances water movement out of the cells. Sodium and potassium ions are the initial solutes extruded, followed over a period of hours to days by osmolytes such as inositol, glutamine, glutamate, and taurine.[64] Therefore, when the serum sodium concentration falls faster than the onset of brain osmotic adaptation processes, serious and permanent neurologic damage can occur.[37,40,64,65] On the other hand, when hyponatremia develops over 2 to 3 days, symptoms are not usually seen unless the serum sodium concentration is reduced markedly.

It is often difficult to determine the acuity and chronicity of hyponatremia. Unless an obvious cause for acute hyponatremia is found, assume that the condition is chronic.[37,59,60,65] A rapid decline in serum sodium concentration usually suggests that hypotonic fluid was administered to a patient with a condition that overwhelms or impairs renal water excretion. These conditions include psychogenic polydipsia[35,36]; postoperative hyponatremia[62,63,66,67]; postprostatectomy syndrome[39]; and administration of thiazide diuretics,[41,42] parenteral cyclophosphamide,[68] oxytocin,[69] and arginine vasopressin or its analogs.[57] C.C.'s symptoms appear to have developed over 7 days and are consistent with chronic hyponatremia.

Rate of Correction of Hyponatremia

13. How should C.C.'s hyponatremia be managed?

C.C.'s water excess should be calculated to estimate the amount of water that should be removed to achieve the desired sodium concentration.

$$\text{Water excess} = \text{TBW} - \text{TBW}\left(\frac{\text{Observed serum Na}}{\text{Desired serum Na}}\right) \quad \textbf{11-5}$$

$$= 30\text{ L} - 30\text{ L}\left(\frac{110\text{ mEq/L}}{120\text{ mEq/L}}\right) \quad \textbf{11-F}$$

$$= 2.4\text{ L}$$

$$\text{where TBW} = (0.5\text{ L/kg})(60\text{ kg}) = 30\text{ L} \quad \textbf{11-G}$$

The treatment of hyponatremia has been controversial. Severe hyponatremia is associated with high rates of morbidity and mortality, but its treatment can also result in morbidity. The rate of correction has been implicated as the main cause of complications.[59–61,65,70–72]

It takes time for the brain to lose osmolytes to reduce cerebral swelling during hyponatremia; conversely, the rate of reaccumulation of these osmolytes must keep pace with the rise in serum sodium concentration to avoid brain dehydration and damage. Indeed, rapid correction of hyponatremia can cause a constellation of neurologic findings known as *osmotic demyelination syndrome* (ODS).[71,72] Clinical manifestations usually are delayed and occur 1 to several days after the treatment has been started. Neurologic findings include transient behavioral changes, seizures, akinetic mutism in mild cases, and features of a pontine disorder in severe cases (pseudobulbar palsy, quadriparesis, and coma). In some patients, the damage is irreversible, and central pontine myelinolysis can be documented in fatal cases. Patients at greatest risk for osmotic demyelination are those with severe hyponatremia lasting >2 days and those in whom the rate of correction of hyponatremia is >12 mEq/L in any 24-hour period.[65,71,72] Hypokalemia, which was found in about 90% of patients with ODS associated with rapid hyponatremia correction, has been suspected as a predisposing factor in the development of ODS.[72] Because the etiology of this complication is unclear, it may be beneficial to correct the hypokalemia before correcting the severe hyponatremia.[72]

Retrospective reviews suggest that acute hyponatremia can be treated safely at a rate of 1 mEq/L/hour initially, until the serum sodium concentration reaches 120 mEq/L. Thereafter, the rate of correction should be reduced to ≤0.5 mEq/L/hour, such that an increment in sodium concentration does not exceed 12 mEq/L in the first 24 hours.[59,73] Slow correction is indicated for severe chronic hyponatremia. No neurologic complications were seen in patients with severe hyponatremia when the average rate of correction to serum sodium was <0.55 mEq/L/hour or when the increase in serum sodium was <12 mEq/L in 24 hours or <18 mEq/L in 48 hours.[73]

In C.C., the serum sodium concentration should be raised to approximately 120 mEq/L at a correction rate of approximately 0.5 mEq/L/hour, using hypertonic saline and furosemide. Serum sodium concentrations should be monitored closely because the equation for calculating water excess does not take into account insensible loss, which can increase the rate of sodium correction.

The use of normal saline is not useful in C.C. because he excretes salt normally (urine Na, 60 mEq/L). C.C.'s sodium deficit is as follows:

$$(0.5\text{ L/kg})(60\text{ kg})(120 - 110\text{ mEq/L}) = 300\text{ mEq} \quad \textbf{11-H}$$

Because 1 L of 3% sodium chloride solution contains 513 mEq of sodium, approximately 600 mL of 3% saline solution, which contains 308 mEq of sodium, will be required to correct the sodium deficit. The recommended serum sodium concentration correction rate is 0.5 mEq/L/hour; therefore, a minimum of 20 hours will be needed to raise the serum sodium concentration by 10 mEq/L (from 110–120 mEq/L). The amount of sodium replacement to safely increase the serum sodium concentration can be determined by the product of the rate of replacement (0.5 mEq/L/hour) and total body weight (TBW) (30 L, Equation 11-G)—that is, 15 mEq/hour. The maximal rate of infusion of 3% saline, which contains 0.513 mEq/mL of sodium, is therefore 29.2 mL/hour [15 mEq/hour]/[0.513 mEq/mL]). A rate of 25 mL/hour, therefore, is appropriate to safely replace C.C.'s sodium deficit.

Because calculations for water excess and sodium deficits are only approximations, the patient's serum osmolality, serum sodium, and clinical response must be monitored closely. Urinary losses can be replaced with 3% sodium chloride solution and appropriate amounts of potassium.

Chronic Management of the Syndrome of Inappropriate Antidiuretic Hormone Secretion

The SIADH is usually transient if the underlying cause can be removed. Chronic SIADH can occur, however, as illustrated by C.C. Water restriction sufficient to create a negative water balance is the primary therapy and should be attempted first.[37,40] In general, all fluids, not just water, should be included in the restriction. Salt intake, however, should not be reduced or solute depletion can occur. The extent of fluid restriction depends on urine output, the amount of insensible water loss, and urine osmolality. For a given amount of solute excretion, patients with a high urine osmolality require a smaller volume of urine (i.e., more water retained) than those with a lower urine osmolality (i.e., less water retained). Hence, more stringent water restriction is required in patients with a high urine osmolality. Commonly, several days of restriction are needed before a significant increase in plasma osmolality is observed.

When fluid restriction fails to reverse the hypo-osmolar state or when the patient is unwilling or unable to comply with the severe fluid restriction, drugs that antagonize the effect of ADH can be used.[37,40] These include loop diuretics,[74,75] demeclocycline,[76] and lithium.[77] Furosemide, 20 to 40 mg/day, reduces urine osmolality by blocking the concentrating ability of the kidney.[74] Demeclocycline and lithium directly impair the response to ADH at the collecting tubule, inducing nephrogenic diabetes insipidus.[76,77] Demeclocycline (300–600 mg twice daily) is usually better tolerated than lithium. Its effect on water excretion is delayed for a few days and it dissipates over a similar period of time after the drug is stopped. Nephrotoxicity has been reported with its use in patients with cirrhosis.[78] Limited data suggest that phenytoin may inhibit ADH secretion, but its effectiveness is questionable.[82] Urea can correct hypo-osmolality by increasing solute-free water excretion and reducing urinary sodium excretion.[83] It has been used effectively, at 30 to 60 g/day, both short and long term, to reduce the need for fluid restriction.[84] An IV formulation of urea is available commercially; however, for oral administration, 30 g of urea crystals can be dissolved in 10 mL of aluminum-magnesium antacid (Maalox) and 100 mL of water. Alternatively, orange juice or other strongly flavored liquids can be used to improve palatability.

Vasopressin Receptor Antagonists

Vasopressin receptor antagonists (VRA), also known as the "vaptans" or "aquaretic agents," comprise a new class of agents used for the treatment of hyponatremia. Arginine vasopressin (AVP), a neuropeptide hormone, plays an important role in maintaining serum osmolality, as well as circulatory and sodium homeostasis.[85] AVP exerts its physiologic effects by acting on V_{1A}, V_2, and V_{1B} receptors, causing effects such as vasoconstriction,[86,87] water excretion,[88] and corticotropin release, [89] respectively. V_2 receptors are located in the renal collecting tubules and they mediate the antidiuretic effects of AVP. Antagonism of the V_2 receptors results in aquaresis, a unique solute-free and electrolyte-sparing (sodium and potassium) water excretion by the kidneys. Because circulating levels of AVP is elevated in SIADH, cirrhosis, and heart failure, VRA would be beneficial in the management of hyponatremia associated with these conditions.

Currently, conivaptan, a mixed V_{1A} and V_2 receptor antagonist, is the only VRA approved by the FDA for the treatment of euvolemic and hypervolemic hyponatremia in hospitalized patients.[85] Randomized, double-blind, placebo-controlled trials have demonstrated its efficacy in increasing serum sodium concentrations in patients with euvolemic and hypervolemic hyponatremia associated with SIADH and heart failure, respectively.[90,91] Its use is restricted to a short-term (4 days) inpatient use only and it is administered as an IV infusion. Close monitoring of serum sodium concentration is necessary to prevent overly rapid correction of hyponatremia and central pontine myelinolysis that may ensue. Because conivaptan is a potent inhibitor of the CYP3A4 enzyme, drug interaction with medications that undergo CYP3A4-mediated metabolism is possible.[85] In addition, infusion-site reactions with conivaptan are common caused by the organic solvent, polypropylene glycol.

Tolvaptan, lixivaptan, and satavaptan are three other VRA that are selective for the V_2 receptor. Being orally active, they are useful in patients who require chronic therapy or when oral therapy is preferred. Because of their selectivity for the V_2 receptor, these agents should have less effect on lowering blood pressure and may be more suitable for use in patients with low to normal blood pressure, such as those with heart failure or cirrhosis. Tolvaptan has been shown to increase serum sodium concentration significantly and correct hyponatremia in patients with SIADH, chronic heart failure, or cirrhosis.[92] It has also been studied most extensively in chronic heart failure where reduction of edema and weight, as well as normalization of serum sodium concentrations, were shown.[93,94] To date, the use of tolvaptan in heart failure does not, however, appear to result in any overall mortality benefit.[95] Lixivaptan has been studied in patients with hyponatremia from heart failure and cirrhosis where the results showed significant increase in aquaresis and serum sodium concentrations.[96–98] When satavaptan was administered to patients with hyponatremia caused by SIADH, normalization of serum sodium concentrations or an increase by $\geq$5 mEq/L was observed.[99] Adverse effects of these agents include thirst, dry mouth, polyuria, and blood pressure reduction. Additionally, all three agents are inhibitors of the CYP3A4 enzyme.

The VRA should be used in hyponatremic patients with mild to moderately severe neurologic symptoms. Not only have they been shown to maintain normal serum sodium concentrations both short- and long-term, their aquaretic effect could also reduce or eliminate the need for fluid restriction normally required of the patients.[100,101] The effectiveness of VRA to correct euvolemic and hypervolemic hyponatremia has now been shown. Their long-term safety with chronic use and their potential benefits on morbidity and mortality, however, need to be assessed.

Hypernatremia

Hypernatremia can occur under the following conditions: (a) normal total body sodium with pure water loss, (b) low total body sodium with hypotonic fluid loss, and (c) high total body sodium as a result of pure salt gain.[102] Therefore, as in hyponatremia, it is important to assess the volume status of the extracellular fluid when evaluating hypernatremia.

Pure water loss can result from the inability of the kidney to conserve water (diabetes insipidus) or from extrarenal water loss through the respiratory tract or the skin.[103] Usually, pure water loss does not cause hypernatremia unless the thirst center is damaged or access to free water is limited.[102]

Hypotonic fluid loss can occur renally as a result of osmotic diuresis, use of loop diuretics, postobstruction diuresis, or intrinsic renal disease. Extrarenally, hypotonic fluid loss can result from diarrhea, vomiting, burns, and excessive sweating.

Pure salt gain can result from the use of hypertonic saline during abortion, sodium bicarbonate administration during cardiopulmonary resuscitation, hypertonic feedings in infants, and, rarely, mineralocorticoid excess.

The management of hypernatremia includes correcting the underlying cause of the hypertonic state, replacing the water deficits, and administering adequate water to match ongoing losses.[102] The pure water deficit can be estimated as follows:

$$\text{Water deficit} = \text{Normal TBW} - \text{Present TBW} \qquad \textbf{11-6}$$

$$= 0.6\,(\text{LBW}) - \left(\frac{\text{Normal Na concentration}}{\text{Present Na concentration}}\right) 0.6\,(\text{LBW}) \qquad \textbf{11-I}$$

$$= 0.6\,(\text{LBW}) \left[1 - \left(\frac{\text{Normal Na concentration}}{\text{Present Na concentration}}\right)\right]$$

The rate at which hypernatremia should be corrected depends on the severity of symptoms and degree of hypertonicity. Too rapid correction can precipitate cerebral edema, seizures, and irreversible neurologic damage, and it can be fatal. For asymptomatic patients, the rate of correction probably should not exceed changes of 0.5 mEq/L/hour in plasma sodium. A rule of thumb is to replace half the calculated deficit with hypotonic solutions over 12 to 24 hours. Any ongoing water loss, including insensible loss, also should be replenished while carefully monitoring the patient's neurologic status. The remaining deficit can then be replaced over the ensuing 24 to 48 hours. Concomitant solute deficits and ongoing solute losses should also be replaced as appropriate. If hypernatremia is caused only by pure water loss, free water can be administered as 5% dextrose in water. Half-normal or quarter-normal saline is used if a sodium deficit is also present. In patients with hypotension or shock, the effective arterial blood volume should be restored with normal saline or colloids before the plasma tonicity is corrected.

CLINICAL USE OF DIURETICS

Diuretics reduce sodium chloride reabsorption in the kidney tubules, thereby increasing urine volume. Enhanced solute and fluid excretion can be initiated through osmotic diuresis or inhibition of transport in the kidney tubules. Diuretics are categorized according to the sites within the kidney tubules where they inhibit sodium reabsorption. (See Chapter 13, Essential Hypertension, and Chapter 31, Chronic Renal Failure.)

Loop Diuretics

The loop diuretics, furosemide, bumetanide, torsemide, and ethacrynic acid, are the most potent diuretics available. They are also known as *high-ceiling diuretics* because they can inhibit the reabsorption of up to 20% to 25% of the filtered sodium load. The loop diuretics act in the medullary and cortical portion of the thick ascending limb of Henle's loop. Sodium and chloride transport through the Na^+-K^+-$2Cl^-$ carrier in the luminal membrane is inhibited. Reabsorption of calcium and magnesium is reduced secondary to the reduction in sodium chloride transport. The loop diuretics also possess a vasodilatory effect that can contribute to their diuretic activity.

Thiazide Diuretics

The thiazide diuretics are a group of structurally similar compounds that share a common mechanism of action. Several other sulfonamide diuretics that differ chemically, such as chlorthalidone, indapamide, and metolazone, also have diuretic effects similar to the thiazides. The primary site of action of these diuretics is at the proximal portion of the distal tubule. Sodium reabsorption via the Na^+-Cl^- cotransporter is blocked through competition with the Cl^- site of the transporter. Some of these agents, such as chlorothiazide, may also reduce sodium transport in the proximal tubule. The contribution of this effect toward net diuresis is negligible, however, because the sodium ions that are not reabsorbed in the proximal tubule will subsequently be reabsorbed in Henle's loop. Thiazide diuretics can enhance the reabsorption of calcium ion through a direct action on the early distal tubule. Therefore, these agents are useful to reduce calciuria in patients with kidney stones. In contrast, magnesium excretion is increased by the thiazides, which may result in hypomagnesemia.

Potassium-Sparing Diuretics

Spironolactone, Triamterene, and Amiloride

Spironolactone, triamterene, and amiloride are potassium-sparing diuretics that inhibit sodium reabsorption in the cortical collecting tubules through different mechanisms. Spironolactone (Aldactone) is a competitive receptor-site antagonist of aldosterone in the distal segment of the renal tubule and is indicated especially for patients with hyperaldosteronism secondary to decreased renal perfusion. Patients with hyperaldosteronism can be identified by urinary electrolyte screening, which shows high urine potassium excretion with concomitant diminished or absent urine sodium excretion. By serving as an aldosterone antagonist, spironolactone inhibits sodium reabsorption and decreases the excretion of potassium and hydrogen ions. Dosages as high as 200 to 400 mg/day may be needed to induce natriuresis in patients with hyperaldosteronism.

In contrast to spironolactone, triamterene and amiloride reduce the passage of sodium ions through the luminal membrane, independent of aldosterone activity, by directly acting on sodium and potassium transport processes in the distal renal tubular cells. Triamterene and amiloride offer the advantage of a more rapid onset of action than spironolactone.

The initial effects of spironolactone are usually delayed for 2 or 3 days, and several additional days are needed to attain maximal diuretic effect. This delay is caused partly by the formation of an active metabolite, canrenone, which accounts for approximately 70% of the antimineralocorticoid activity of spironolactone. The elimination half-life of canrenone is 13.5 to 24 hours in normal subjects and is prolonged in patients with chronic liver disease (59 hours [range, 32–105 hours]) or CHF (37 hours [range, 19–48 hours]).[104] Although the elimination half-life of canrenone is prolonged in these patients, plasma canrenone concentrations do not differ significantly from those in normal subjects because assay methods for canrenone are nonspecific and include measurement of both active and inactive metabolites.[105,106]

Triamterene (Dyrenium) is absorbed incompletely from the GI tract. The drug has a short half-life of 1.5 to 2.5 hours. The total body clearance is high because of rapid and extensive metabolism by the liver. Both the parent compound and the metabolite undergo biliary and renal excretion. As with spironolactone, the hepatic metabolism of triamterene can be altered in patients with cirrhosis.[107] The diuretic effect of triamterene begins within 2 to 3 hours of administration, with a maximal duration of 12 to 16 hours.

Amiloride (Midamor) does not undergo hepatic metabolism; approximately 50% of amiloride is excreted in the urine unchanged and the remainder is recovered in the stool as unabsorbed drug or through biliary excretion. Serum amiloride concentrations peak 3 hours after oral ingestion, and the half-life is 6 hours. Although commonly administered doses are in the range of 2.5 to 10 mg, diuresis increases over a much greater range. The onset of action is 2 hours, with maximal effects at 4 to 6 hours. Duration of action is dose dependent and ranges from 10 to 24 hours. Amiloride does not undergo hepatic metabolism, and the drug can accumulate in patients with renal insufficiency.

The maximal amount of filtered sodium that can be excreted through the action of potassium-sparing diuretics is approximately 1% to 2%. Their natriuretic activity, therefore, is relatively limited compared with the thiazide and loop diuretics. These agents are often used concurrently with thiazide and loop diuretics to reduce potassium loss. Spironolactone is especially useful in patients with liver cirrhosis and ascites, who are likely to have high levels of aldosterone.

Acetazolamide

Acetazolamide inhibits carbonic anhydrase, an enzyme that mediates the excretion of sodium, bicarbonate, and chloride ions in the proximal tubule. Use of the drug will increase urine pH owing to the increased excretion of bicarbonate ion. The net diuretic and natriuretic effects are limited, similar to those of the potassium-sparing diuretics. Because of the drug's proximal site of action, the sodium ions that are not reabsorbed will subsequently be reclaimed in Henle's loop and the distal tubule. In addition, metabolic acidosis associated with the use of acetazolamide diminishes its diuretic effect.

Osmotic Diuretics

Osmotic diuretics are nonreabsorbable solutes in the kidney tubule. They act primarily in the proximal tubule, where the osmotic pressure they generate impedes the reabsorption of water and solutes. Unlike other diuretics, the amount of water loss exceeds the concurrent loss of sodium and potassium. Mannitol has been used in the early treatment of oliguric postischemic acute renal failure to increase urine output. Urea, another osmotic diuretic, and mannitol are used to reduce intracranial pressure through cellular dehydration.

Complications of Diuretic Therapy

Disturbances in fluid, electrolyte, and acid–base balance are common side effects associated with diuretic therapy. These side effects, including hypokalemia, are discussed in detail in Chapter 13, Essential Hypertension; Chapter 18, Heart Failure; and Chapter 42, Gout and Hyperuricemia. Two complications, hyponatremia and metabolic alkalosis and acidosis, are, however, discussed in the following section because of their specific relevance to fluid balance.

Hyponatremia

Thiazides induce diuresis by inhibiting sodium and water reabsorption in the kidney tubule. Because both sodium and water are lost, overdiuresis *per se* is not expected to cause hyponatremia. Instead, hyponatremia represents a dilution of plasma sodium by excess free water caused by volume depletion-induced ADH activity. The enhanced ADH secretion increases free water reabsorption, resulting in hyponatremia. Large doses of diuretic, excessive water drinking, and severe sodium intake restriction all will accentuate the hyponatremia. Elderly patients are susceptible to this diuretic-induced complication.

Metabolic Alkalosis and Acidosis

Metabolic alkalosis often occurs in conjunction with potassium depletion secondary to diuretic use. The diuretic-induced contraction of extracellular fluid volume stimulates the secretion of aldosterone, which promotes the absorption of sodium and the retention of hydrogen ions in the kidney tubule. The net urinary loss of hydrogen ions into the urine results in metabolic alkalosis. Generally, reducing the dose of the diuretic will restore the acid–base balance.

Acetazolamide causes metabolic acidosis by inhibiting carbonic anhydrase, which results in urinary excretion of sodium bicarbonate. Spironolactone, amiloride, and triamterene can cause hyperchloremic metabolic acidosis because of their ability to decrease potassium and hydrogen ion tubular secretion. Patients with renal dysfunction or those taking potassium supplements or angiotensin-converting enzyme inhibitors, which reduce aldosterone secretion, are at increased risk for developing hyperkalemia and metabolic acidosis.

POTASSIUM

Homeostasis

The total amount of potassium stored in the body is approximately 45 to 55 mEq/kg and varies with age, gender, and muscle mass. Lower total body potassium is found in older adults, females, and individuals with a low lean body mass-to-fat ratio. Potassium is distributed unevenly between the intracellular and extracellular compartments: 98% of the total body potassium resides in the intracellular compartment, predominantly the muscle, and only 2% is found in the extracellular space.[34,99,109] The disproportionate intracellular distribution of potassium is maintained by the Na^+-K^+-ATPase pump, which transports sodium out of the cell in exchange for potassium.[108–111] The cell membrane resting potential is determined by the ratio of intracellular-to-extracellular potassium concentrations. As this ratio increases, hyperpolarization of the cell membrane occurs. Conversely, cellular depolarization results when the ratio decreases. In both situations, generation of the action potential is impaired.

The plasma potassium concentration is maintained within a narrow range: 3.5 to 5.0 mEq/L. Although the plasma potassium concentration can be affected by the total body potassium store, total body potassium excess or deficit cannot be estimated accurately based solely on the plasma concentration. In fact, a normal plasma potassium concentration does not imply normal total body potassium because multiple factors affect the plasma potassium concentration independent of total body potassium.[108]

Potassium homeostasis is maintained by both renal and extrarenal processes. The renal process regulates total body potassium by matching potassium excretion to dietary intake (external balance),[112] whereas the extrarenal process regulates potassium distribution across cell membrane (internal potassium balance).[108,110]

The normal daily intake of potassium ranges between 50 and 100 mEq. Approximately 90% of the ingested potassium is eliminated by the kidneys and approximately 10% is eliminated via the GI tract.[112] Potassium is filtered freely through the glomerulus and then reabsorbed. By the time the filtrate reaches the distal convoluted tubule, >90% of filtered potassium has already been reabsorbed. The amount of potassium excreted is determined by distal tubular potassium secretion in the principal cells of the cortical collecting duct, which is under the influence of aldosterone. Hyperkalemia, increased potassium load, and angiotensin II can all stimulate aldosterone secretion.[108]

Factors that affect renal potassium excretion include tubular flow, sodium delivery to the distal segments of the nephron, the presence of poorly absorbable anions that increase luminal electronegativity, acid–base status, and aldosterone activity.[96] Potassium excretion increases during hyperkalemia and decreases during potassium depletion. Excretion of an acute potassium load is a slow process, with only half the potassium load excreted in the first 4 to 6 hours. Lethal hyperkalemia would ensue were it not for the extrarenal process that regulates intracellular–extracellular potassium distribution.[108]

The Na^+-K^+-ATPase pump, which extrudes sodium from the cell in exchange for potassium, is pivotal in maintaining internal potassium balance.[111] Different hormonal factors regulate the activity of the Na^+-K^+-ATPase pump, namely insulin, catecholamines, and aldosterone. Insulin, the most important regulator, enhances potassium uptake by muscle, liver, and adipose tissue by stimulating Na^+-K^+-ATPase[114] Indeed, basal insulin secretion is essential for potassium homeostasis.[108] Whereas β_2-adrenergic agonists activate the Na^+-K^+-ATPase pump via cyclic adenosine monophosphate (cAMP) and cause hypokalemia, α-adrenergic stimulation promotes hepatic potassium release and causes hyperkalemia.[115] Epinephrine, an α- and β-agonist, causes a transient increase in plasma potassium (α-agonism) followed by a more sustained decrease in plasma potassium (β-agonism).[115,116] Besides its kaliuretic effect and enhanced potassium secretion in the colon, aldosterone also stimulates Na^+-K^+-ATPase.

Other factors that affect the transcellular distribution of potassium include systemic pH, plasma tonicity, and exercise.[108,111] The effect of *acid–base balance* on potassium distribution is not readily predictable and depends on both the nature and the direction of the underlying disorder. The concomitant effect of the acid–base disorder on renal potassium excretion further complicates the relationship between plasma potassium concentration and pH.[108,117] In acute inorganic acidosis, plasma potassium concentration increases by 0.2 to 1.7 mEq/L per 0.1-U decrease in pH. Chronic inorganic metabolic acidosis usually is associated, however, with hypokalemia because of urinary potassium loss associated with both proximal (type II) and distal (type I) renal tubular acidosis.[108,117] In contrast, organic acidosis commonly has no effect on potassium distribution.[118] Other associated factors in the organic acidosis may, however, affect cellular potassium distribution.[117] For example, hyperglycemia in diabetic ketoacidosis may increase the serum potassium concentration because of the hypertonic effect of glucose.[119] Hypertonicity causes cell shrinkage and increases the intracellular to extracellular fluid potassium gradient, favoring potassium egress. Acute metabolic alkalosis only modestly decreases the plasma potassium concentration: 0.3 mEq/L for each 0.1-U pH increment.[108,117] As with chronic metabolic acidosis, chronic metabolic alkalosis causes profound renal potassium wasting and is associated with hypokalemia. Respiratory acid–base disorders usually are associated with less significant changes in plasma potassium concentration than are metabolic acid–base disorders.[117] Exercise often causes an increase in the serum potassium concentration to a degree that varies with the intensity of the exercise.[120]

Hypokalemia

Etiology

14. J.P., a 60-year-old woman, presents to the ED with complaints of malaise, generalized weakness, nausea, and vomiting for 3 days. Her medical history includes hypertension for 20 years. J.P.'s current medications include hydrochlorothiazide 25 mg/day and nifedipine XL 30 mg/day. She has not been able to take her medications in the past few days, however, because of vomiting. J.P. denies recent diarrhea or use of laxatives. Her BP is 130/70 mm Hg with a pulse of 80 beats/minute while sitting, and 120/70 mm Hg with a pulse of 95 beats/minute on standing. Physical examination reveals a thin, older woman with poor skin turgor, dry mucous membranes, and a flat jugular vein. T-wave flattening is noted on the electrocardiogram (ECG). Laboratory tests show serum Na, 138 mEq/L (normal, 134–146); K, 2.1 mEq/L (normal, 3.5–5.1); Cl, 100 mEq/L (normal, 92–109); bicarbonate, 32 mEq/L (normal, 24–31); BUN, 30 mg/dL (normal, 18–25); creatinine, 1.2 mg/dL (normal, 0.5–1.5); and glucose, 100 mg/dL (normal, 60–110). ABG shows pH 7.50 (normal, 7.35–7.45); P_{CO_2}, 45 mm Hg (normal, 35–45); and P_{O_2}, 70 mm Hg (normal, 80–100) at room air. Urine electrolytes are Na, 30 mEq/L; K, 60 mEq/L; and Cl, <15 mEq/L. The patient's presentation is consistent with gastroenteritis. What are the causes of J.P.'s hypokalemia?

[SI units: serum Na, 138 mmol/L; K, 2.1 mmol/L; Cl, 100 mmol/L; bicarbonate, 32 mmol/L; BUN, 10.7 mmol/L; creatinine, 106.1 μmol/L; glucose, 5.55 mmol/L; P_{CO_2}, 6.0 kPa; P_{O_2}, 9.33 kPa; urine Na, 30 mmol/L; K, 60 mmol/L; Cl, <15 mmol/L]

When evaluating hypokalemia, the clinician should determine whether the hypokalemia is a result of low intake, increased cellular uptake of potassium, or excessive loss of potassium via the kidneys, GI tract, or skin.[34,121] History and physical evidence of potassium depletion; medication history (including use of over-the-counter medicines); and assessment of the patient's BP, extracellular volume, and concurrent acid–base status can provide clues to the causes of hypokalemia.[34,121]

Because J.P. has been unable to eat for the past few days, decreased oral intake may have contributed to her hypokalemia. Because most foods are rich in potassium, however, inadequate intake rarely is the sole cause of potassium depletion unless inappropriate and continued renal or extrarenal losses occur, or potassium intake is severely restricted to <10 to 15 mEq/day.[121] Alkalosis,[117] insulin administration,[108] hypertonic solution administration, periodic paralysis,[122] β_2-agonists,[123] barium poisoning,[124] and treatment of megaloblastic anemia with vitamin B_{12}[125] all have been associated with increased cellular potassium uptake (Table 11-2). Although the relationship between the degree of hypokalemia and increase in blood pH varies widely,[117] J.P.'s metabolic alkalosis probably enhances the cellular uptake of potassium. The transcellular shift of potassium should not result in total body potassium depletion, however.

The GI tract is an important site of potassium loss, particularly through vomiting and diarrhea. Because the potassium content of gastric secretion (5–10 mEq/L) is much less than that of the intestinal secretion (up to 90 mEq/L),[121] loss of a large volume of gastric secretion is needed to produce substantial potassium depletion. Potassium deficit induced by vomiting, however, is commonly secondary to renal potassium loss, especially within the initial 24 to 48 hours.[126] The loss of hydrogen ion in gastric juice results in an elevated plasma bicarbonate concentration. The increased amount of bicarbonate ion, as a nonreabsorbable anion, increases water delivery to the distal nephron and enhances sodium reabsorption and potassium secretion, resulting in hypokalemia. The potassium wasting is often transient, because increased proximal reabsorption of sodium and bicarbonate will result in diminished bicarbonate delivery to the distal site. Reduced potassium excretion will ensue, commonly within 48 to 72 hours. Subsequent potassium

Table 11-2 Drugs That Most Commonly Induce Hypokalemia

Drug	Mechanism	Predisposing Factors
Acetazolamide	Marked ↑ in renal K^+ loss	Most profound with short-term therapy
Amphotericin	Renal K^+ loss (renal tubular acidosis)	Concurrent piperacillin, ticarcillin
β_2-agonists	Intracellular shift of K^+	
Cisplatin	Renal K^+ loss secondary to renal tubular damage	May be dose related but can occur after a single 50-mg/m^2 dose
Corticosteroids	Renal K^+ loss. Enhanced Na^+ reabsorption at distal tubule and collecting ducts in exchange for K^+ and H^+	Supraphysiologic doses of agents with moderate to strong mineralocorticoid activity (e.g., prednisone, hydrocortisone)
Insulin with glucose	Intracellular shift of K^+	Predictable effect when insulin administered to patients with diabetic ketoacidosis' combination used to treat hyperkalemia
Penicillins (piperacillin, ticarcillin)	High Na^+ load and nonreabsorbable anions can ↑ K^+ loss	Was more common with carbenicillin when it was available; newer penicillins are used in lower doses; less likely to produce hypokalemia
Thiazide and loop diuretics	Renal K^+ loss. ↑ Na^+ delivery to the late distal tubule, resulting in Na^+ resorption in exchange for K^+	Patients with hyperaldosteronism (e.g., cirrhosis, CHF) predisposed; may be dose related

CHF, Congestive heart failure.

loss will then be primarily consequent to gastric secretion removal.

The absence of diarrhea in J.P. excludes the GI tract as the source of potassium loss. Potassium loss through the skin also is unlikely in J.P. because the potassium concentration of sweat is <10 mEq/L. Therefore, profuse sweating, such as that induced by vigorous exercise in a hot, humid environment, or severe burns are needed to cause substantial loss.

J.P.'s inappropriately high urinary potassium concentration indicates that the kidney is the source of the potassium loss.[34,121] The urinary potassium concentration is a good marker for differentiating various hypokalemic syndromes. A urinary potassium excretion of <20 mEq/day suggests extrarenal potassium loss. Renal potassium wastage cannot be excluded, however, unless the low urinary potassium excretion is accompanied by a sodium intake of at least 100 mEq/day, because a low-sodium diet can reduce renal potassium excretion.[34] In J.P., the metabolic alkalosis and hypovolemia promote renal potassium wastage.[34,121] The distal delivery of a large sodium bicarbonate load and increased aldosterone activity (from hypovolemia) enhance potassium secretion and severely impair the kidney's ability to conserve potassium. The hydrochlorothiazide, which J.P. had been taking until 3 days before admission, could also have induced hypokalemia through volume depletion, hypochloremic metabolic alkalosis, and renal potassium wastage. The diuretic is unlikely, however, to be the cause for J.P.'s hypokalemia because she has stopped taking the medication, and this is reflected by the low urinary chloride concentration.[15] Bartter's syndrome, which presents as normotension, hypokalemia, hypochloremic metabolic alkalosis, and renal potassium wastage, is characterized by impaired renal sodium and chloride reabsorption. The low urinary chloride concentration in J.P. can rule out Bartter's syndrome. Other causes of hypokalemia are listed in Table 11-2.

In an asymptomatic hypokalemic patient with no apparent causes for potassium depletion or transcellular redistribution, pseudohypokalemia should be excluded before pursuing an intensive evaluation.[104] Spurious hypokalemia can occur in leukemic patients whose leukocyte count ranges from 100,000 to 250,000 cells/μL.[127] The potassium in serum is taken up by the large number of leukemic cells when the blood specimen is allowed to stand at room temperature.

Clinical Manifestations

15. What clinical manifestations of hypokalemia are evident in J.P.?

The clinical presentation of hypokalemia, which depends on the severity of potassium depletion, is a result of changes in cell membrane polarization.[121] Patients are usually asymptomatic when the plasma potassium level is 3.0 to 3.5 mEq/L, but they may complain of malaise, weakness, fatigue, and myalgia. J.P.'s muscle weakness and ECG changes reflect the muscular and cardiac manifestations of hypokalemia, respectively.[128,129]

Potassium depletion can lead to hyperpolarization of myocardial cells and a prolonged refractory period. When serum potassium concentrations fall below 3 mEq/L, T-wave flattening, straight tubule segment depression, and prominent U waves are seen on the ECG.[129] Mild hypokalemia (potassium concentration of 3.0–3.5 mEq/L) is potentially arrhythmogenic in patients with underlying coronary artery disease. The incidence of ventricular arrhythmia increases with the degree of hypokalemia. Patients without underlying heart disease may be susceptible to these myocardial effects during exercise, especially if the patient's pre-exercise potassium concentration is <3.5 mEq/L, because the potassium concentration may drop below 3.0 mEq/L as a result of β_2-adrenergic receptor-mediated cellular potassium uptake.[121] Potassium depletion may also increase the BP,[122] which can be lowered with potassium supplementation.[130]

When the serum potassium concentration is <2.5 to 3.0 mEq/L, muscle weakness, cramps, general malaise, fatigue, restless leg syndrome, and paresthesia can occur, probably because potassium is necessary for vasodilation in skeletal muscle. In addition, severe potassium depletion (<2.5 mEq/L) can result in elevation of serum creatine phosphokinase, aldolase, and aspartate aminotransferase levels. Rhabdomyolysis can ensue when the serum potassium concentration falls below 2.0 mEq/L.[121,128]

Chronic potassium depletion can alter renal function and structure, which can manifest as decreased GFR and renal blood flow, disturbance in tubular sodium handling, impaired urinary concentrating ability with polydipsia, and ADH-resistant nephrogenic diabetes insipidus.[104,114] Reversible pathologic changes include renal hypertrophy and epithelial vacuolization of the proximal convoluted tubule. Interstitial scarring and tubular atrophy have been reported with prolonged potassium depletion.[121]

Other effects of hypokalemia and potassium depletion include decreased insulin secretion resulting in carbohydrate intolerance,[131] metabolic alkalosis, and increased renal ammoniagenesis, which may play a role in the development of hepatic encephalopathy.[132]

Treatment

16. How should J.P.'s hypokalemia be treated?

J.P.'s protracted vomiting should be corrected, and fluids and electrolytes (sodium, potassium, and chloride) should be replaced to correct the volume deficit, hypokalemia, and hypochloremic metabolic alkalosis. Hydrochlorothiazide should continue to be withheld.

The amount of potassium deficit and the rate of continued potassium loss should be determined to guide replacement therapy. It has been estimated that a 1-mEq/L fall in serum potassium from 4 to 3 mEq/L represents a total body deficit of approximately 200 mEq. When the serum potassium falls below 3 mEq/L, the total body deficit increases by 200 to 400 mEq for each 1-mEq/L reduction in serum concentration. Other data suggest that even greater degrees of potassium loss can occur: a deficit of 100 mEq per 0.27-mEq/L fall in the serum potassium concentration.[109] Transcellular redistribution of potassium may, however, significantly alter the relationship between serum concentration and total body deficit.[121] Therefore, potassium repletion should be guided by close monitoring of serum concentrations and analysis of J.P.'s urine for potassium content to help assess the need for additional replacement.

The route of potassium administration depends on the acuity and severity of hypokalemia,[133] but oral supplementation is usually preferred. The parenteral route is indicated for patients who cannot tolerate high dosages of oral potassium supplements and for those with severe or symptomatic hypokalemia. J.P.'s potassium deficit is estimated to be 300 to 500 mEq, but because she is only moderately symptomatic, aggressive therapy is not indicated. Potassium chloride can be added to her IV fluid in a concentration of 40 mEq/L and infused at a rate that does not exceed 10 mEq/hour. For patients with life-threatening, hypokalemia-induced arrhythmias or those with a serum potassium level <2.0 mEq/L, a more concentrated potassium solution (60 mEq/L) can be infused at a rate not exceeding 40 mEq/hour. A solution that is too concentrated or a rate of infusion that is too rapid would likely cause phlebitis in the peripheral veins and could cause arrhythmias, especially when administered through a central line. The potassium concentration should be monitored every 4 hours, more frequently in patients with severe potassium depletion or when a rapid infusion is given.[134] ECG monitoring is mandatory to identify life-threatening hyperkalemia.

Parenteral potassium can be given as chloride, acetate, or phosphate. The chloride salt is preferred in J.P., who has concurrent hypochloremic metabolic alkalosis. The acetate preparation is useful in cases of concomitant metabolic acidosis. Potassium phosphate is in order if hypophosphatemia coexists. In the latter condition, the serum calcium concentration should also be monitored because hypocalcemia may ensue. Glucose solution should be avoided as the vehicle because glucose-induced insulin secretion will promote intracellular potassium uptake.[136]

Once J.P.'s potassium levels are replenished and she can take medicine by mouth, oral potassium chloride can be started (see Chapters 13, Essential Hypertension, and 18, Heart Failure).

Hyperkalemia

Etiology

17. A.B., a 25-year-old woman with type 1 diabetes and hypertension, returns to the clinic for follow-up. Her BP is 170/90 mm Hg with a pulse of 80 beats/minute, and her physical examination is remarkable for 2+ pedal edema. Laboratory tests show plasma Na, 135 mEq/L (normal, 134–146); K, 5.8 mEq/L (normal, 3.5–5.1); Cl, 108 mEq/L (normal, 92–109); total CO_2, 20 mEq/L (normal, 22–32); BUN, 28 mg/dL (normal, 8–25); creatinine, 2 mg/dL (normal, 0.5–1.5); and glucose, 200 mg/dL (normal, 60–110). Current medications include oral captopril 25 mg three times daily (TID), Dyazide one capsule daily, human isophane (NPH) insulin 30 units subcutaneously (SC) every morning, and ibuprofen 200 mg as needed (PRN) for menstrual cramps. She uses a salt substitute occasionally. What is the etiology of her hyperkalemia?

[SI units: Na, 135 mmol/L; K, 5.8 mmol/L; Cl, 108 mmol/L; total CO_2, 20 mmol/L; BUN, 10 mmol/L; creatinine, 176.8 μmol/L; glucose, 11.1 mmol/L]

Before conducting any extensive evaluation to identify the etiology of hyperkalemia, the serum potassium concentration ought to be repeated to confirm the presence of hyperkalemia. Also to be ruled out are the different causes of spurious hyperkalemia, which can result from severe leukocytosis ($>500{,}000/mm^3$),[136] thrombocytosis ($>750{,}000/mm^3$),[137] or hemolysis within the blood collection tube.[138] *Pseudohyperkalemia* is a test-tube phenomenon that occurs when potassium is released from leukocytes, platelets, or erythrocytes during blood coagulation. These disorders can be confirmed easily by comparing serum (clotted) and plasma (unclotted) potassium concentrations from the same blood sample. The two values should agree within 0.2 to 0.3 mEq/L. Improper tourniquet technique, causing strangulation of the patient's arm before blood sampling, may also result in spurious hyperkalemia.[139]

Identifying the etiology of hyperkalemia can be approached systematically by considering possible disturbances in internal and external potassium balance. The former involves transcellular flux of potassium from the intracellular to the extracellular space, whereas the latter involves either increased intake, including increased endogenous potassium load (e.g., rhabdomyolysis,[140] tumor lysis syndrome[141]), or decreased elimination. A thorough medication history is important to identify drugs associated with hyperkalemia.[142–144] (Also see Chapter 31, Chronic Renal Failure, for additional information on hyperkalemia.)

A dietary history should ascertain whether A.B.'s consumption of potassium-rich foods, salt substitutes, or potassium supplements has increased. Dietary intake alone will *not* induce hyperkalemia unless renal excretion is impaired. Usually, the GFR must be <10 to 15 mL/minute, unless there is concurrent hypoaldosteronism or distal tubular potassium secretory defects.[1] A.B.'s renal insufficiency is mild, with an estimated Cl_{Cr} of 40 mL/minute.

Conditions associated with low renin and aldosterone, which usually present as hyperkalemia and hyperchloremic metabolic acidosis, decrease potassium excretion by the kidneys. These include diabetes (present in A.B.),[145] obstructive uropathy, sickle cell disease, lupus nephritis, and various tubulointerstitial diseases (e.g., gouty nephropathy, analgesic nephropathy). Adrenal insufficiency presents commonly with hyperkalemia because of mineralocorticoid deficiency.[146] A.B.'s poorly controlled hyperglycemia may cause movement of potassium-rich fluid from the intracellular space to the extracellular space because of the increased tonicity. Elevating the plasma tonicity by 15 to 20 mOsm/kg will increase the plasma potassium concentration by 0.8 mEq/L.[147] Patients with diabetes, mineralocorticoid deficiency, or end-stage renal failure, which commonly results in hyporeninemic hypoaldosteronism, are particularly susceptible.

A.B. is also taking several medications that may impair her ability to excrete potassium. Captopril indirectly decreases aldosterone secretion by decreasing the formation of angiotensin II.[148] Ibuprofen inhibits prostaglandin production as well as renin and aldosterone secretion.[149] Other drugs that cause hyperkalemia by impairing renin and aldosterone production include angiotensin II receptor antagonists,[150] β-adrenergic blockers,[151] lithium,[152] heparin,[153–155] and pentamidine.[140] Triamterene, the diuretic in Dyazide, inhibits tubular potassium secretion, as do amiloride, spironolactone, high-dose trimethoprim,[156,157] cyclosporine,[158] tacrolimus,[159] and digitalis preparations.[160] By inhibiting Na^+-K^+-ATPase, digitalis decreases tubular potassium secretion and reduces cellular potassium uptake. Arginine,[161] succinylcholine,[162] β-adrenergic blockers, α-adrenergic agonists, and hypertonic solutions also cause hyperkalemia by impairing transcellular potassium distribution into the intracellular space.

Clinical Manifestations

18. V.C., a 44-year-old woman with chronic renal failure, returns to the outpatient unit for routine hemodialysis with complaints of severe muscle weakness. Her vital signs are BP, 120/80 mm Hg; pulse, 90 beats/minute; RR, 20 breaths/minute; and temperature, 98°F. Laboratory data are serum K, 8.9 mEq/L (normal, 3.5–5.1); total CO_2, 15 mmol/L (normal, 22–32); BUN, 60 mg/dL (normal, 8–25); creatinine, 9 mg/dL (normal, 0.5–1.5); and glucose, 100 mg/dL (normal, 60–110). The ECG reveals an increased PR interval and a widened QRS complex. What clinical manifestations of hyperkalemia are evident in V.C.?

[SI units: K, 8.9 mmol/L; total CO_2, 15 mmol/L; BUN, 21.42 mmol/L; creatinine, 795.6 μmol/L; glucose, 5.55 mmol/L]

Hyperkalemia decreases the intracellular-to-extracellular potassium ratio. Hence, the resting membrane potential becomes less negative and moves closer to the threshold excitation potential. Muscle weakness and flaccid paralysis result when the resting membrane potential approaches the threshold potential, rendering the excitable cells unable to sustain an action potential.

The cardiac toxicity of hyperkalemia is a major cause of morbidity and mortality, with ECG findings paralleling the degree of hyperkalemia. When plasma potassium >5.5 to 6.0 mEq/L, narrow, peaked T waves and a shortened QT interval are seen. As the plasma potassium concentration increases further, the QRS complex widens and the P-wave amplitude decreases. As the level reaches 8 mEq/L, the P-wave disappears and the QRS complex continues to widen and merge with the T wave to form a sine wave pattern. If these ECG changes are not recognized and no treatment is initiated, ventricular fibrillation and asystole will ensue. Hyponatremia, hypocalcemia, and hypomagnesemia all reduce the threshold potential, thereby increasing the patient's susceptibility to the cardiac effects of hyperkalemia.[140] V.C.'s muscle weakness, ECG, chronic renal failure, and serum potassium concentration all are consistent with severe hyperkalemia.

Treatment

19. How should V.C.'s hyperkalemia be treated?

Hyperkalemia with ECG changes requires urgent treatment. Three therapeutic modalities are available: (a) agents that antagonize the cardiac effects of hyperkalemia, (b) agents that shift potassium from the extracellular into the intracellular space, and (c) agents that enhance potassium elimination. Considering V.C.'s severe ECG changes, calcium should be administered at a dose of 10 to 20 mL of 10% calcium gluconate IV over 1 to 3 minutes. Calcium counteracts the depolarizing effect of hyperkalemia by increasing the threshold potential, thus making it less negative and moving it away from the resting potential. The onset of action occurs in a few minutes, but the effect is short-lived, lasting approximately 15 to 60 minutes. The dose can be repeated in 5 minutes if ECG changes do not resolve and as needed afterward for recurrence. With no response after the second dose, additional attempts, however, are not beneficial. When the hyperkalemia presents with a digitalis overdose, calcium should be used cautiously because it can worsen the cardiotoxic effects of digoxin.[140,163]

Because the serum potassium concentration is not affected by calcium administration, maneuvers should be employed to shift potassium from plasma into the cells. Three modalities are available: insulin and glucose, β_2-agonists, and sodium bicarbonate.

Insulin rapidly shifts potassium into the cell in a dose-dependent fashion. The maximal effect occurs at insulin concentrations >20 to 40 times the basal levels. Therefore, endogenous insulin secreted in response to dextrose administration is insufficient, and exogenous insulin must be administered.[108] Although high concentrations of dextrose may worsen hyperkalemia, particularly in diabetic patients because intracellular potassium may be shifted to the extracellular space owing to the elevated plasma tonicity,[164] it is always administered with insulin to prevent hypoglycemia. Regular insulin (5–10 units) can be given with 50 mL of 50% dextrose as IV boluses, followed by a continuous infusion of 10% dextrose at 50 mL/hour to prevent late hypoglycemia.[109] In dialysis patients susceptible to developing fasting hyperkalemia, 20 units of insulin can be added to 1 L of 10% dextrose and administered at a rate of 50 mL/hour to prevent the hyperkalemia.[165] The insulin–dextrose combination lowers serum potassium by direct stimulation of cellular potassium uptake and potentiates the potassium-lowering effect of β-adrenergic stimuation.[165] The reduction in potassium is apparent 15 to 30 minutes after the start of the therapy and persists for 4 to 6 hours.[140] In a diabetic patient who is both hyperkalemic and hyperglycemic, insulin alone may be insufficient. If the patient has end-stage renal disease, the insulin–glucose combination is more predictable in lowering plasma potassium concentrations than sodium bicarbonate.[109,163,165]

β_2-Agonists, by binding with the β_2-adrenoreceptor to activate adenylyl cyclase, have an additive effect with the insulin–dextrose combination in decreasing serum potassium. When albuterol nebulization is used alone, the hypokalemic effect may be inconsistent.[166] Although side effects of albuterol nebulization are minimal, these agents can cause tachycardia and should be used cautiously in patients with underlying coronary artery disease.[167] Although not commercially available, IV albuterol has a faster onset of action (30 vs. 90 minutes).[168] In contrast, nebulization is easier to set up and is less likely to be associated with tachycardia, but multiple doses are often necessary to attain an adequate response. In conjunction with the insulin–dextrose combination, albuterol (20 mg dissolved in 4 mL of saline) can be administered by nebulization and inhaled over 10 minutes to further decrease serum potassium if necessary.[169]

Although sodium bicarbonate has long been recommended for the acute treatment of hyperkalemia, its efficacy in this setting has been questioned.[109,163] The usual dose, 44 to 50 mEq, is infused slowly over 5 minutes and repeated in 30 minutes when necessary. Alternatively, it can be added to dextrose and saline solution to form an isotonic sodium bicarbonate infusion.[170] The hypokalemic effect is variable and may be delayed up to 4 hours, and it is reportedly ineffective in patients on maintenance hemodialysis. Although bicarbonate therapy is not a reliable option in the acute management of hyperkalemia, it may be beneficial in patients with severe metabolic acidosis (pH <7.20).[109] Potential complications of sodium bicarbonate therapy are volume overload and metabolic alkalosis.

The definitive treatment of hyperkalemia is removal of potassium from the body. Sodium polystyrene sulfonate (SPS) with sorbitol is an ion-exchange resin that binds potassium in the bowel and enhances its excretion in the stools.[171] Each gram of SPS exchanges 0.5 to 1.0 mmol of potassium for an equal amount of sodium. SPS can be administered orally or rectally; the latter route is preferred in the symptomatic hyperkalemic patient because intestinal potassium exchange occurs mainly in the ileum and colon. A dose of 50 g of SPS in sorbitol can be given as an enema, retained for at least 30 to 60 minutes, at 4- to 6-hour intervals. For nonemergent removal of body potassium, 15 to 60 g of SPS with sorbitol suspension can be given orally, which can be repeated as needed. The onset of action is approximately 1 to 2 hours after administration. The major side effects are GI intolerance, including diarrhea and sodium overload, and, rarely, intestinal necrosis.[172]

Hemodialysis is the most efficient way to remove potassium; potassium clearance by peritoneal dialysis is lower than for hemodialysis.[173] The hypokalemic effect is immediate and lasts for the duration of dialysis[163]; however, the amount of potassium removed is variable.[174] Dialysis with a glucose-free dialysate will remove 30% more potassium than one containing 200 mg/dL of glucose.[175]

Table 11-3 summarizes the treatment alternatives for hyperkalemia.

Although V.C. is receiving chronic maintenance hemodialysis, the severe cardiac effects of hyperkalemia she experienced warrant immediate institution of the aforementioned measures while awaiting preparation for dialysis. Loop diuretics, which enhance kaliuresis, are rarely useful in managing severe hyperkalemia, especially in patients with renal dysfunction.

Table 11-3 Treatment of Hyperkalemia

Drug	*Mechanism*	*Dose*	*Comment*
Ca gluconate	Reverse cardiotoxicity caused by K^+	10 to 20 mL 10% Ca gluconate IV over 1 to 3 min; may repeat once.	*Onset:* 1 to 3 min *Duration:* 30 to 60 min. [K^+] remains unchanged
Insulin and glucose	Redistribution of K^+ intracellularly	5 to 10 units regular insulin with 50 mL 50% dextrose, then $D_{10}W$ infused at 50 mL/hr[a]	*Onset:* 15 to 30 min *Duration:* several hours Watch for hypoglycemia and hypokalemia. Does not ↓ total body K^+
β_2-agonists (e.g., albuterol)	Redistribution of K^+ intracellularly	Oral: 2 or 4 mg TID-QID Inhalation: 20 mg in 4 mL saline via nebulizer	*Onset:* 30 to 60 min *Duration:* 2 hrs
Sodium polystyrene sulfonate (SPS)	Cationic binding resin. 1 g of resin binds 0.5 to 1 mEq K^+ in exchange for Na^+	*Oral:* 15 to 20 g with 20 to 100 mL 70% sorbitol Q 4 to 6 hr; PRN preferred *Retention enema:* 50 g in 50 mL (70% sorbitol and 150 mL H_2O) Retain 30 min and follow with nonsaline irrigation	*Onset:* Slow; 50 g will lower [K^+] by 0.5 to 1 mEq/L over 4 to 6 hrs; watch for Na^+ overload (100 mg Na^+/1 g SPS)
$NaHCO_3$	Redistribution of K^+ intracellularly	50 mEq IV over 5 min Repeat PRN	*Onset:* variable, ≈30 min May work best in acidosis Watch for Na^+ overload and hyperosmolar state No change in total body K^+
Dialysis	Removal of K^+		Use as last resort

[a]Glucose unnecessary in patients with high glucose concentrations.
BID, twice daily; IV intravenous; PRN, as needed; QID, four times daily.

After V.C.'s condition stabilized, she admitted to eating a lot of fruits in the past few days. Because noncompliance with dietary potassium restriction is the most common cause for acute and chronic hyperkalemia in a dialysis patient, V.C. should be counseled to consume potassium-rich foods in moderation. Medications that impair V.C.'s extrarenal potassium handling should be avoided. If V.C. remains chronically hyperkalemic, SPS will then be needed, probably three or four times weekly. If hyperkalemia is associated with metabolic acidosis, however, an alkalinizing agent should be added to maintain a serum bicarbonate concentration of about 24 mEq/L.

CALCIUM

Homeostasis

Healthy adults have approximately 1,400 g of calcium in the body, of which >99% is stored in bone. Nonetheless, the 0.1% of the total body calcium that is in the plasma and extravascular fluid plays a critical role in many physiologic and metabolic processes. Calcium is important in maintaining nerve tissue excitability and muscle contractility. It regulates the secretory activities of exocrine and endocrine glands and serves as a cofactor for enzyme systems and the coagulation cascade. It also is an essential component of bone metabolism.

Plasma calcium concentration is normally maintained within a relatively narrow range: 8.5 to 10.5 mg/dL. This is accomplished through a complex interaction between parathyroid hormone (PTH), vitamin D, and calcitonin, as well as the effect of these hormones on calcium metabolism in bone, the GI tract, and the kidneys.

Normally, about 40% of the plasma calcium is protein bound, primarily to albumin, and is nondiffusible.[125] Of the 60% that is diffusible, about 13% is complexed to various small ligands: phosphate, citrate, and sulfate. The remaining 47% is ionized, free, and physiologically active. Changes in serum protein concentration will alter the concentrations of both protein-bound and total calcium. Therefore, the serum albumin concentration needs to be monitored to adequately interpret the total serum calcium concentration. Each 1-g/dL increase in serum albumin concentration is expected to increase the protein-bound calcium by 0.8 mg/dL, thus increasing the total serum calcium concentration by the same amount. The total serum calcium therefore can be corrected by the following equation:

$$\text{Correct Ca} = \text{Observed Ca} + 0.8\,(\text{Normal albumin} - \text{Observed albumin}) \qquad \text{11-7}$$

Calcium is also bound to plasma globulins: 0.16 mg of calcium for each gram of globulin. When the total globulin concentration exceeds 6 g/dL (normal, 2.3–3.5 g/dL), moderate hypercalcemia may be seen. Changes in pH have an effect on calcium protein binding: acidosis decreases calcium binding, resulting in an increase in free calcium fraction, whereas an increase in pH reduces the amount of ionized calcium. Changes in serum phosphate and sulfate concentrations are expected to alter the fraction of ionized calcium because of the formation of calcium complexes with these anions. The presence of abnormal plasma proteins with a high affinity for calcium binding, as in patients with multiple myeloma, also affects the preceding equation for serum calcium concentration correction.[176]

Serum calcium concentration is regulated by the combined effect of GI absorption and secretion, renal reabsorption, and turnover of the skeletal calcium pool. Several hormones, such as PTH, 1,25-dihydroxyvitamin D_3, and calcitonin, have significant effects on these processes. Balanced diets generally contain 600 to 1,000 mg of calcium, although the minimum daily requirement is 400 to 500 mg. Calcium is primarily absorbed in the duodenum and jejunum via saturable and nonsaturable processes.[177] The nonsaturable process is diffusive in nature and varies with luminal calcium concentration. The saturable carrier-mediated component is stimulated by 1,25-dihydroxyvitamin D_3. Absorption of calcium is enhanced when the calcium intake is low and also when the demand is increased, such as in pregnancy and when total body calcium is depleted. Conversely, protein deficiency can reduce intestinal calcium absorption, presumably because of the reduced amount of specific calcium-binding protein.[178] Calcium also is secreted into the bowel lumen, which may account for the presence of a negative calcium balance when there is no oral calcium intake.[179]

The portion of plasma calcium that is not bound to protein is filtered by the glomerulus. Approximately 97% to 99.5% of the filtered calcium is reabsorbed: 60% in the proximal tubule, 20% in the ascending limb, 10% in the distal tubule, and 3% to 10% in the collecting duct. Approximately 20% of the calcium in the kidney tubule is ionized, whereas the remainder is bound to cations such as citrate, sulfate, phosphate, and gluconate. The extent of calcium resorption depends on the presence of specific cations and also on the urine pH, which affects the fraction of calcium bound to cations. Passive reabsorption at the proximal convoluted tubule is linked closely to sodium transport and is increased by extracellular fluid contraction and decreased by volume expansion. At the proximal straight tubule, the transport process is active and dissociable from sodium and water transport. PTH increases the calcium reabsorption at the distal tubule and also at the collecting duct independent of sodium reabsorption. Acidosis can also increase renal calcium excretion by inhibiting tubule reabsorption and by increasing the ultrafiltrable calcium through reduced binding of calcium to plasma proteins. Conversely, alkalosis promotes calcium protein binding, thus reducing the amount of ultrafiltrable calcium. It also induces hypocalciuria independent of PTH. Phosphorus administration reduces renal calcium excretion, whereas phosphorus depletion increases urinary calcium elimination. Normally, approximately 50 to 300 mg of calcium is excreted by the kidneys daily, but this can be increased to 600 mg/day.[180]

The other important factor regulating plasma calcium concentration is bone metabolism. The rate of bone turnover and calcium resorption is influenced by PTH, 1,25-dihydroxyvitamin D_3, and calcitonin.

Hypercalcemia

Etiology

20. A.C., a 62-year-old woman, is brought to the hospital by family members because she has become more lethargic and unresponsive over the past several days. Approximately 4 years ago, she underwent a radical mastectomy and node dissection followed by radiation and chemotherapy for breast carcinoma. Despite several courses of chemotherapy, she developed metastasis to the bone.

About 1 week before this admission, A.C. complained of fatigue, muscle weakness, and anorexia. Since then, she has spent most of her time in bed and has had very limited oral intake. Medications taken before admission included hydrochlorothiazide, oral morphine sulfate, and tamoxifen. Physical examination reveals a dehydrated, cachectic woman responsive only to painful stimuli. Vital signs include BP, 100/60 mm Hg, and RR, 16 breaths/minute. Pertinent laboratory values are Na, 138 mEq/L (normal, 134–146); K, 4.5 mEq/L (normal, 3.5–5.1); Cl, 99 mEq/L (normal, 92–109); CO_2, 33 mEq/L (normal, 22–32); BUN, 40 mg/dL (normal, 8–25); creatinine, 1.2 mg/dL (normal, 0.5–1.5); Ca, 19 mg/dL (normal, 8.0–10.4); P, 4.5 mg/dL (normal, 2.6–4.6); and albumin, 3.0 g/dL (normal, 3.5–5.4). The ECG revealed a shortened QT interval. What are the common causes of hypercalcemia? Which of these might be responsible for the hypercalcemia seen in A.C.?

[SI units: Na, 138 mmol/L; K, 4.5 mmol/L; Cl, 99 mmol/L; CO_2, 33 mmol/L; BUN, 14.3 mmol/L; creatinine, 106.1 μmol/L; Ca, 4.75 mmol/L; P, 1.45 mmol/L; albumin, 30 g/L]

MALIGNANCY

Malignancy and primary hyperparathyroidism are the most common causes for hypercalcemia. Hematologic malignancies, such as multiple myeloma, tend to be responsible for more hypercalcemia than solid tumors. Cancer of the breast, lung, head, and neck and renal cell carcinoma, are solid tumors commonly associated with hypercalcemia. Malignancy can cause paraneoplastic hypercalcemia secondary to bone metastasis, which results in increased bone resorption. Alternatively, patients may develop hypercalcemia in the absence of bone metastasis owing to the production of osteolytic humoral factors by the tumor. The mediators secreted may be PTH, PTH-like substances, prostaglandins, cytokines, transforming growth factor-α, and tumor necrosis factor.[181]

HYPERPARATHYROIDISM

Hyperparathyroidism is the other common cause of hypercalcemia. Although the etiology of primary hyperparathyroidism is unclear, women tend to develop the condition more frequently, especially in the fourth to sixth decades of life. Approximately 75% of patients have a single adenoma, whereas much smaller percentages of patients have multiglandular disease, hyperplasia, or carcinoma.[180] Other conditions that can result in hypercalcemia include postkidney transplantation, immobilization, vitamin A intoxication, hyperthyroidism, Addison's disease, and pheochromocytoma. Hypercalcemia can also occur secondary to increased intestinal calcium absorption because of vitamin D intoxication, sarcoidosis, and other granulomatous diseases. Use of thiazide diuretics, lithium, estrogens, and tamoxifen, as well as excessive calcium ingestion together with alkali (milk-alkali syndrome), may result in hypercalcemia.

A.C.'s breast cancer bone metastasis, volume contraction, and use of hydrochlorothiazide and tamoxifen may all contribute to her hypercalcemia.

Clinical Manifestations

21. How is hypercalcemia manifested in A.C.?

The clinical presentations of hypercalcemia vary substantially among patients, but the severity of the symptoms correlates well with free calcium concentrations.[182] The specific presentation depends on the rate of serum calcium concentration elevation, the presence of malignancy, the PTH concentration, and the patient's age. Concurrent electrolyte and metabolic abnormalities and underlying diseases also will have an effect. Because calcium is an important regulator of many cellular functions, hypercalcemia can produce abnormalities in the neurologic, cardiovascular, pulmonary, renal, GI, and musculoskeletal systems. As seen in A.C., the signs and symptoms can be nonspecific: fatigue, muscle weakness, anorexia, thirst, polyuria, dehydration, and a shortened QT interval on the ECG.

The effect of hypercalcemia on the central nervous system includes lethargy, somnolence, confusion, headache, seizures, cerebellar ataxia, altered personality, acute psychosis, depression, and memory impairment. The neuromuscular manifestations include weakness, myalgia, hyporeflexia or areflexia, and arthralgia.

Symptoms of impaired renal function include polyuria, nocturia, and polydipsia. These may reflect a defective concentrating ability, possibly because of resistance to the effects of ADH.[183] The GFR may be decreased because of afferent arteriolar vasoconstriction, and if hypercalcemia is prolonged, nephrolithiasis, nephrocalcinosis, chronic interstitial nephritis, and renal tubular acidosis may be present. Hypermagnesuria and metabolic alkalosis may also be observed.[180]

Calcium has a positive inotropic effect and reduces heart rate, similar to cardiac glycosides. ECG changes indicative of slow conduction, with prolonged PR and QRS intervals and shortened QT intervals, are commonly seen. In severe hypercalcemia, increased QT intervals, widened T waves, and arrhythmia may be present.[180,184]

The GI symptoms of hypercalcemia are related primarily to the depressive action of calcium on smooth muscle and nerve conduction. Constipation, anorexia, nausea, and vomiting result from reduced GI motility and delayed gastric emptying. Duodenal ulcer can occur because of increased acid and gastrin secretion. Pancreatitis can occur during acute hypercalcemia owing to the blockade of the pancreatic ducts caused by intraductal calcium deposits.[180] Proteolytic enzymes may also be activated by calcium to cause tissue damage. Both ulcer disease and pancreatitis are more common in hypercalcemia associated with primary hyperparathyroidism; they are less likely to be seen in patients with malignancy-induced hypercalcemia.[184]

Treatment

22. After vigorous fluid resuscitation with IV saline, combined saline and furosemide diuresis was instituted in A.C. Her serum calcium concentration declined very slowly, prompting the use of calcitonin. Despite initial success, the serum calcium concentration rose to pretreatment values within 24 hours. Higher dosages of calcitonin could have been attempted at this point; however, plicamycin was used instead. Her serum calcium concentration finally stabilized at 8 mg/dL (normal, 8.0–10.4) after several days of therapy. What was the rationale for each of these regimens? What other agents are available for hypercalcemia treatment?

Several therapeutic approaches are used to lower serum calcium concentration: increasing urinary calcium excretion, inhibiting release of calcium from bone, reducing intestinal calcium absorption, and enhancing calcium complex formation with chelating agents. The underlying disease that causes the hypercalcemia should also be treated if possible. The specific

Table 11-4 Treatment of Hypercalcemia

Intervention	Dose	Comment
Saline and furosemide	1 to 2 L NS; then furosemide 80 to 100 mg Q 2 to 4 hr Establish and maintain normovolemia Other electrolytes as needed.	Saline diuresis and volume expansion depresses Ca^{++} reabsorption in tubules. Lowers $[Ca^{++}]$ within 24 hrs. Treatment of choice in patients without CHF or renal failure.
Calcitonin	4 IU/kg SC or IM Q 12 hr ↑ Dose or use another therapy if unresponsive after 24 hrs (*Max:* 8 IU/kg Q 6 hr)	Inhibits osteoclast resorption and renal reabsorption of calcium. Preferred second-line agent because it has a rapid onset (6 hrs) and is nontoxic. It can be used safely in CHF and renal failure. Nausea is the major adverse effect. Tolerance occurs in 24 to 72 hrs. Concomitant plicamycin can lead to hypocalcemia. Only the salmon-derived product is available.
Plicamycin	25 mg/kg/day IV over 4 to 6 hrs; repeat PRN in 48 hrs *Renal failure:* 12.5 mg/kg	Inhibits osteoclast bone resorption. Onset 24 to 48 hrs; duration 3 to 14 days. Common side effects: N/V, minimized by slow IV. Because the dose is 10% of an antineoplastic dose, cytotoxic effects less severe. Obtain baseline renal and hepatic function, platelet counts.
Gallium nitrate	100 to 200 mg/m^2/day infused IV over 24 hrs for 5 days (depending on severity of hypercalcemia) If calcium levels return to normal before 5 days, therapy may be discontinued	Inhibits bone resorption. Patients should be well hydrated during therapy. A urine output of ~2 L/day should be maintained owing to risk for nephrotoxicity (10%).
Biphosphonates (etidronate, pamidronate)	Etidronate: 7.5 mg/kg IV QD × 3 days over at least 2 hrs Maintenance: 20 mg/kg/day PO Pamidronate: 60 to 90 mg IV over 4 hrs × 1 Repeat in 7 days PRN	Inhibits osteoclast reabsorption in malignancy state. Efficacy 75% to 100%. Onset 48 hrs. Duration, days. Concomitant hydration is imperative. Do not use in renal failure. Adverse effects: ↑ P, ↑ SrCr, N/V (oral).
Zoledronic acid	Doses: 4 mg IV administration over 15 min	Potent effect on bone resorption. Preferred biphosphonate for hypercalcemia of malignancy. May have promising effects on skeletal complications secondary to bone metastasis.
Phosphate	IV $PO^{=}_4$ not recommended PO $PO^{=}_4$ gradually titrate to 30 to 60 mmol/day (1–3 g/day in divided doses)	Inhibits bone resorption; soft tissue calcification. IV onset 24 hrs, but not drug of choice. Oral agents used for chronic therapy. Contraindicated in renal failure.
Corticosteroids	Prednisone 60 to 80 mg/day Hydrocortisone 5 mg/kg/day IV × 2–3 days	Impair GI absorption and bone resorption. Onset several days. Best in patients with multiple myeloma, vitamin D intoxication, granulomatous conditions. Can be used in CHF, renal failure.
Indomethacin	75 to 150 mg/day	Reports of efficacy are mixed.

CHF, congestive heart failure; GI, gastrointestinal; IM, intramuscular; IV, intravenous; NS, normal saline; N/V, nausea and vomiting; PO, oral; PRN, as needed; QD, every day; SC, subcutaneously; SrCr, serum creatinine.

treatment used depends on the serum ionized calcium concentration, the presenting signs and symptoms, and the severity and duration of hypercalcemia. Immediate therapy was needed for A.C., who had symptoms consistent with severe hypercalcemia.

Specific interventions are described in the following paragraphs, but as an overview, hydration and diuresis with furosemide generally are the first steps in the acute treatment of hypercalcemia. If these measures fail to reduce the serum calcium concentration adequately, several other agents can be added. Calcitonin provides a rapid onset of hypocalcemic effect, but its duration of action is relatively short. Thus, one of the bisphosphonates could be used to elicit a longer hypocalcemic response. Gallium nitrate is an alternative to plicamycin without such toxic effects. Other agents, such as inorganic phosphates, glucocorticoids, and prostaglandin inhibitors, also have been used to treat hypercalcemia with varying success (Table 11-4).

HYDRATION AND DIURESIS

As noted, the first-line emergency treatment for hypercalcemia is hydration and volume expansion. Most patients with hypercalcemia are volume depleted because of the accompanying polyuria, nausea, and vomiting. Normal saline 1 to 2 L is commonly given to correct the fluid deficit and to expand extracellular volume, which will increase urinary calcium excretion by increasing the GFR and inhibiting calcium reabsorption in the proximal tubule. Because both sodium and calcium are reabsorbed at the same site in the proximal tubule, saline hydration will reduce the reabsorption of both cations simultaneously. A.C. was hypotensive and appeared dehydrated; therefore, saline hydration was used initially to treat the hypercalcemia. In patients who have renal failure or CHF, saline hydration and forced diuresis should be avoided.

After adequate volume repletion has been established, IV furosemide can be administered to augment calciuresis. Furosemide blocks the reabsorption of sodium, chloride, and calcium at the thick ascending limb of Henle's loop. Doses of 80 to 100 mg every 2 to 4 hours can be used until a sufficient decline of the serum calcium concentration is attained.[185] Smaller doses (20–40 mg) commonly are given to avoid the significant loss of fluid and electrolytes caused by the more aggressive regimen. Adequate amounts of sodium, potassium, magnesium, and fluid should be used to replace any therapy-induced electrolyte abnormalities. Fluid balance as well as serum and urine concentrations of these electrolytes must be monitored closely. Urine flow must be maintained and the renal loss of sodium chloride must be replaced to preserve the calciuric effect of furosemide.[186] In A.C., the decline of serum calcium concentration was slow, possibly because of inadequate restoration of plasma volume, replacement of renal sodium loss, or both. More aggressive hydration with adequate sodium replacement will ensure that the efficacy of furosemide is not compromised.

CALCITONIN

Calcitonin can be used when saline hydration and furosemide diuresis fail to lower serum calcium concentration adequately or when their use is contraindicated. Calcitonin reduces serum calcium concentration by inhibiting osteoclastic bone resorption. It may also increase the renal excretion of calcium and phosphorus. Only the salmon-derived calcitonin product is available in the United States.

The serum calcium concentration is often reduced several hours after calcitonin is administered, and the response may last approximately 6 to 8 hours. If used with plicamycin, the effect is additive and can lead to hypocalcemia. The drug is relatively nontoxic compared with agents such as plicamycin and organic phosphates and may be used in patients with dehydration, CHF, or renal failure.[186] Nausea, vomiting, diarrhea, and facial flushing are the more common side effects; soreness and inflammation at the injection site may also be seen.[181] Because of the potential for developing a hypersensitivity reaction to salmon calcitonin, the manufacturer recommends skin testing with 1 IU of the salmon calcitonin before the first dose. As seen in A.C., tolerance to the hypocalcemic effect of calcitonin can develop after 24 to 72 hours of therapy. This "escape phenomenon" may be secondary to the altered responsiveness of the hormone receptors and might be prevented by concurrent use of corticosteroids.[187] After long-term therapy, antibodies may develop as well.[173]

The dosage of salmon calcitonin is 4 IU/kg given SC or intramuscularly (IM) every 12 hours; the maximal dosage is 8 IU/kg every 6 hours. The hypocalcemic response is often limited, and serum calcium concentration seldom drops to the normal range.[188]

PLICAMYCIN

Plicamycin (Mithramycin) is an antibiotic resembling actinomycin D, which was used to treat refractory testicular cancer. With the advent of cisplatin-based regimens, plicamycin is now used primarily to treat hypercalcemia. It inhibits RNA synthesis, which suppresses osteoclast-mediated calcium resorption from bone. The drug is effective for hypercalcemia associated with breast cancer, myelomas, lung, renal cell, or parathyroid carcinoma, and hypervitaminosis D.

The recommended dosage of plicamycin is 25 mcg/kg infused over 4 to 6 hours. Generally, a response is seen within 24 to 48 hours, and most patients attain normocalcemia after a single dose.[174] The response lasts 3 to 14 days or longer in some patients. If an adequate response is not obtained, the dose can be repeated 48 hours later.

Many serious adverse effects are associated with plicamycin therapy. The drug is usually well tolerated at the lower doses used for hypercalcemia treatment, which is only one-tenth the antineoplastic dose.[188] Nausea and vomiting are common side effects that can be minimized by infusing the drug slowly and by using an antiemetic such as prochlorperazine. The drug is a vesicant and should be administered as a dilute solution to minimize the injury associated with extravasation. Other toxicities include impaired platelet function, proteinuria, azotemia, bone marrow suppression, and elevated hepatic transaminases.[189] Plicamycin can also cause hepatic toxicity, nephrotoxicity, and dose-related acute hemorrhagic syndrome. Because the drug is excreted primarily through the kidneys, impaired renal function may increase the risk for adverse effects.[180] Renal and hepatic function and platelet count should be assessed before and during therapy.

Plicamycin's side effect profile may potentiate the toxic effects of chemotherapeutic agents used to treat patients with malignancy-induced hypercalcemia. Thus, its use is limited to patients unresponsive to other antiresorptive agents. It also is used intermittently to take advantage of its relatively long duration of action. In addition, the drug should not be used in patients with severe hepatic or renal dysfunction, thrombocytopenia, or coagulopathies or those who are dehydrated or receiving myelosuppressive chemotherapy.[186]

BISPHOSPHONATES

Bisphosphonates are synthetic analogs of pyrophosphate that form stable bonds that are resistant to phosphatase degradation during osteoclast-mediated bone mineralization and resorption. The compounds adsorb to the hydroxyapatite crystals of the bone, inhibiting their growth and dissolution. In addition, the compounds may have a direct effect on the osteoclasts.

The two distinct pharmacologic classes of bisphosphonates that exist have different mechanisms of action. Etidronate, which does not contain any nitrogen atom, is metabolized to cytotoxic, nonhydrolyzable adenosine triphosphate (ATP) analogs. In contrast, nitrogen-containing bisphosphonates, such as pamidronate and zoledronic acid, inhibit the prenylation of proteins and have potent inhibitory effects on osteoclast-mediated bone resorption.[190] In addition, they induce apoptosis of osteoclasts as well as certain tumor cells. Further antitumor activities may be mediated through their inhibitory effect on angiogenesis, stimulation of the γ-T-cell fraction in blood, and reduction of cancer cells' adherence to bone matrix. At present, etidronate, pamidronate, and zoledronic acid are approved in the United States for the treatment of hypercalcemia secondary to malignancy.

Etidronate

Etidronate is administered in doses of 7.5 mg/kg for 3 consecutive days by IV infusion over 2 to 4 hours. Response may be seen after 1 to 2 days, and normocalcemia is expected to be attained in most patients, with response sustained for >10 days.[191] Because of the inconvenient dosing schedule as well as variability in its duration of action, other bisphosphonates are now preferred for the treatment of hypercalcemia of malignancy. In addition, etidronate may inhibit bone mineralization, a property not shared by other bisphosphonates.

Pamidronate

Pamidronate is more potent than etidronate as an inhibitor of bone resorption, but it has negligible effect on bone mineralization. For moderate hypercalcemia (albumin-corrected serum calcium concentration of 12.0–13.5 mg/dL), a single dose of 60 to 90 mg of pamidronate is commonly infused over 3 to 4 hours. For severe hypercalcemia (albumin-corrected serum calcium concentration >13.5 mg/dL), the dose is 90 mg. The advantages of pamidronate are that it requires only a single dose and produces a superior response compared with three doses of etidronate.[192]

If the hypercalcemia recurs, the etidronate or the pamidronate regimen may be repeated after an interval of ≥7 days. Etidronate (20 mg/kg/day by mouth) may be given to prolong the normocalcemic duration, but nausea and vomiting are common with the oral therapy. Long-term treatment may result in osteomalacia; however, the limited life expectancy of most patients may diminish the significance of this adverse effect.

Etidronate use has resulted in renal failure,[193] which probably is caused by the formation of biphosphonate–calcium complexes in the serum.[194] Because pamidronate requires a lower molar concentration to produce a comparable hypocalcemic effect, it is less likely to impair renal function. In fact, pamidronate has been given to a limited number of patients with end-stage renal disease without adverse consequence.[194]

Zoledronic Acid

Among the bisphosphonates approved for the treatment of hypercalcemia of malignancy, zoledronic acid has the most potent effect on bone resorption. It is superior to pamidronate with respect to the number of complete responses, time needed to attain calcium normalization, and duration of effect.[196] Because 8-mg doses were not superior to 4-mg, 4-mg doses are administered IV over 15 minutes.[197] The drug is well tolerated at 4-mg doses. Zolendroic acid's superior efficacy and convenience of administration make it the preferred biphosphonate for hypercalcemia of malignancy. Emerging studies show that zoledronic acid also may have promising effects in reducing skeletal complications secondary to bone metastasis associated with breast cancer, prostate cancer, non–small-cell lung cancer, and multiple myeloma.[197]

GALLIUM NITRATE

Gallium is a naturally occurring group IIIa heavy metal. In addition to its antitumor activity and potential for use as a chemotherapeutic agent, it has been shown to be effective in the treatment of moderate to severe hypercalcemia of malignancy. Hypocalcemia is induced primarily via the inhibition of bone resorption and reduction in urinary calcium excretion.[198] Several clinical studies have shown the effectiveness of gallium nitrate in the treatment of cancer-related hypercalcemia when compared with agents such as calcitonin and bisphosphonates.[198–202] The recommended dose is 100 to 200 mg/m^2/day as a continuous infusion for 5 days. Vigorous hydration is necessary to prevent nephrotoxicity. In general, its clinical use is limited by the inconvenient method of administration, significant risk of nephrotoxicity, and cost.

PHOSPHATE

Inorganic phosphates lower the serum calcium concentration by inhibiting bone resorption. They also promote the deposition of calcium salts ($CaHPO_4$) in the bone and soft tissue. If given orally, phosphate reduces intestinal calcium absorption by forming a poorly soluble complex in the bowel lumen and also by decreasing the formation of active vitamin D through enzyme inhibition.[203]

When given IV, phosphate is very effective, but renal failure and extensive extraskeletal calcifications are a concern. For these reasons, IV phosphate is not the agent of choice for acute treatment of hypercalcemia.

Oral phosphate (1–3 g/day in divided doses) may be used for long-term maintenance therapy, with the optimal dose determined by serum calcium concentrations. Nausea, vomiting, and diarrhea are common problems, especially when the daily dose exceeds 2 g. Soft tissue calcification is also a concern, and hyperphosphatemia and hypocalcemia can occur if the dose is not titrated appropriately. Phosphate therapy should not be given to patients with hyperphosphatemia or renal failure because it can cause further deterioration of renal function. Accumulation of the potassium and sodium salts in phosphate preparations may also present a therapeutic problem in certain patients.

CORTICOSTEROIDS

Several possible mechanisms exist that may explain the hypocalcemic effect of corticosteroids. Vitamin D_3-mediated intestinal calcium absorption may be impaired[204] and the action of osteoclast-activating factor, which mediates bone resorption in malignancy, may be inhibited. Corticosteroids also may have a direct cytolytic effect on tumor cells and inhibit the synthesis of prostaglandins (see Prostaglandin Inhibitors). Prednisone (60–80 mg/day) is given initially, with subsequent dosage reduction based on the calcemic response. Alternatively, hydrocortisone (5 mg/kg/day for 2–3 days) may be given. The hypocalcemic effect will not be apparent for at least 1 to 2 days. Patients with hematologic malignancies and lymphomas tend to have a better response than those with solid tumors. Corticosteroids are also effective in treating hypercalcemia associated with vitamin D intoxication,[205] sarcoidosis,[206] and other granulomatous conditions. They are not generally used for long-term therapy because of their potential for serious adverse reactions.

PROSTAGLANDIN INHIBITORS

Because prostaglandins of the E series, especially PGE_2, may be responsible for hypercalcemia associated with some malignancies, NSAID may be useful for a select group of patients with hypercalcemia. For example, indomethacin is effective in lowering the serum calcium concentration in patients with renal cell carcinoma, but not in patients with other types of malignancy.[192] Indomethacin, 75 to 150 mg/day, can be tried in patients unresponsive to other therapy, especially when it is used as part of palliative treatment for cancer pain.

PHOSPHORUS

Homeostasis

Phosphorus is found primarily in bone (85%) and soft tissue (14%); <1% of the total body store resides in the extracellular fluid. Virtually all of the "free" or active phosphorus exists as phosphates in the plasma. Most clinical laboratories, however, measure and express the concentrations of elemental phosphorus contained in the phosphate molecules. One millimole of phosphate contains 1 mmol of phosphorus, but 1 mmol of phosphate is three times the weight of 1 mmol of phosphorus. Therefore, it is incorrect to equate a certain milligram weight of phosphorus as the same milligram weight of phosphate. Of the total plasma phosphorus, 70% exists as the organic form and 30% as the inorganic form. Organic phosphorus, primarily phospholipids and small amounts of esters, is bound to proteins. About 85% of inorganic phosphorus, or orthophosphate, is unbound or "free." The relative amounts of the two orthophosphate components, $H_2PO_4^-$ and HPO_4^{2-}, vary with the pH. At pH 7.40, the ratio of the two species is 1:4, giving rise to a composite valence of 1.8 for the orthophosphate. Serum phosphate concentrations reported by clinical laboratories reflect only the inorganic portion of the total plasma phosphate. To avoid confusion related to the pH effect on valence, phosphate concentrations are reported as mg/dL or mmol/dL rather than mEq/volume.

The normal range of serum phosphate concentration in healthy adults is 2.7 to 4.7 mg/dL. The value is higher in children, possibly because of the increased amount of growth hormone and the reduced amount of gonadal hormones.[208] In postmenopausal women, the range is slightly higher; however, it is lower in older men. The serum phosphate concentration is also affected by dietary intake. Phosphate-rich foods can transiently increase the serum phosphate concentration. In contrast, glucose decreases the serum phosphate concentration because of the flux of sugar and phosphate into cells and because of the phosphorylation of glucose. Similarly, administration of insulin and epinephrine decreases the serum phosphate concentration because of their effects on glucose. The serum concentration of phosphate is reduced in alkalosis and increased in acidosis.[209]

A balanced diet contains 800 to 1,500 mg/day of phosphorus. Both the organic and inorganic forms of phosphorus are present in food substances. Most of the phosphorus in milk is the organic form, whereas the phosphorus in meat, vegetable, and other nondairy sources represents organic forms bound to proteins, lipids, and sugars, which usually are hydrolyzed before absorption.[210] In general, 60% to 65% of the phosphorus ingested is absorbed, mostly in the duodenum and jejunum through an energy-dependent, saturable, active process.[211] Phosphorus absorption is linearly related to the dietary intake when the intake is 4 to 30 mg/kg/day.[156] The amount of phosphorus ingested probably is the most important factor in determining net absorption. Phosphorus absorption is also stimulated during periods of increased demand, such as active growth and pregnancy.[212] Increased intake of calcium and magnesium and concurrent use of aluminum hydroxide antacids may reduce phosphorus absorption owing to formation of a nonabsorbable complex.[213] In addition, absorption is also affected by vitamin D, PTH, and calcitonin.[208]

Renal phosphorus excretion depends on the dietary phosphorus intake. Normally, >85% of the filtered phosphate load is reabsorbed; however, the fractional urinary excretion can vary from 0.2% to 20%.[159] Renal phosphate excretion is also affected by acid–base balance, extracellular fluid volume, and calcium and glucose concentrations.[208] In addition, PTH, thyroid hormone, thyrocalcitonin, vitamin D, insulin, glucocorticoid, and glucagon can also alter renal phosphate excretion.[208]

Hypophosphatemia

Etiology

23. M.R., a 72-year-old woman, was admitted to the hospital with a 1-week history of increasing malaise, confusion, and decreased activity. M.R. has a history of CHF, hypertension, type 2 diabetes, and peptic ulcer disease. She was receiving hydrochlorothiazide, Maalox, sucralfate, and insulin. She is febrile and in significant respiratory distress. ABG results at admission were pH 7.5 (normal, 7.36–7.44); Po_2, 42 mm Hg (normal, 80–90); and Pco_2, 20 mm Hg (normal, 34–46). Respiratory function continued to deteriorate, requiring intubation and mechanical ventilation. Serum electrolytes are Na, 128 mEq/L (normal, 134–146); K, 3.6 mEq/L (normal, 3.5–5.1); Cl, 96 mEq/L (normal, 92–109); CO_2, 23 mEq/L (normal, 22–32); glucose, 320 mg/dL (normal, 60–110); and phosphorus (P), 0.9 mg/dL (normal, 2.4–4.6). What may have contributed to the low serum phosphorus concentration in M.R.?

[SI units: Na, 128 mmol/L; K, 3.6 mmol/L; Cl, 96 mmol/L; CO_2, 23 mmol/L; glucose, 17.8 mmol/L; P, 0.29 mmol/L]

Hypophosphatemia can develop as the result of a phosphorus deficiency or secondary to a net flux of phosphorus out of the plasma compartment without a total body deficit. Moderate hypophosphatemia is defined as a serum phosphorus concentration of 1.0 to 2.5 mg/dL. A concentration of <1.0 mg/dL, as in M.R., is considered severe.[214] The extent of hypophosphatemia may not be assessed accurately by a single plasma phosphorus concentration determination because of diurnal variation.[215] Patients receiving large doses of mannitol may have pseudohypophosphatemia owing to the binding of mannitol with molybdate, which is used in the calorimetric assay for phosphorus.[216]

Hypophosphatemia is commonly caused by conditions that impair intestinal absorption, increase renal elimination, or shift phosphorus from the extracellular to the intracellular compartments. Hypophosphatemia secondary to low dietary phosphorus is exceedingly rare because phosphorus is ubiquitous.[208] In addition, renal phosphorus excretion is reduced and intestinal phosphorus absorption is increased to prevent a deficiency state.[159,217] Starvation in itself does not result in severe hypophosphatemia because the phosphorus content in plasma and muscles is often normal. Hypophosphatemia, however, can develop during refeeding with a high-calorie diet low in phosphorus. Therefore, hyperalimentation without phosphorus supplementation is likely to cause severe hypophosphatemia.[218]

Impaired phosphorus absorption secondary to malabsorptive conditions, prolonged nasogastric suction, and protracted vomiting can also result in hypophosphatemia. In M.R., the use of aluminum- and magnesium-containing antacids may further reduce phosphorus absorption. The antacids bind with endogenous and exogenous phosphorus in the GI tract and cause severe hypophosphatemia in patients with or without renal failure.[219] In addition, M.R. was taking sucralfate, which can bind phosphorus in the GI tract.[220] Similarly, iron preparations can bind phosphorus.[221]

Hyperglycemia-induced osmotic diuresis and diuretic use may have increased the renal loss of phosphorus in M.R. Other conditions associated with renal phosphorus wasting include renal tubular acidosis, hyperparathyroidism, hypokalemia, hypomagnesemia, and extracellular volume expansion.[208] None of these situations, however, was evident in M.R. Shifting of phosphorus into the intracellular compartment by glucose or insulin and profound respiratory alkalosis, especially during alcoholic withdrawal, may also have contributed to M.R.'s hypophosphatemic state.[222,223]

24. What other conditions are commonly associated with hypophosphatemia?

Diabetic ketoacidosis, chronic alcoholism, chronic obstructive airway disease, and extensive thermal burns are other conditions commonly associated with hypophosphatemia.[224,225] They are characterized by a combination of factors that result in phosphate loss and intracellular phosphate use. In patients with diabetic ketoacidosis, metabolic acidosis enhances the movement of phosphate from the intracellular compartment to plasma, whereas the concurrent osmotic diuresis secondary to hyperglycemia increases the renal elimination of extracellular phosphate.[226] The net result is a depletion of total body stores. Correction of the acidosis and administration of insulin then promotes the rapid uptake of phosphorus by tissues, and volume repletion dilutes the extracellular concentration. This sequence of events can ultimately lead to severe hypophosphatemia. The hypophosphatemia associated with chronic alcoholism and acute alcohol intoxication is also thought to be related to several factors, including reduced intestinal phosphorus absorption caused by vomiting, diarrhea, and antacid use; repeated acidosis that results in increased urinary phosphate excretion; and a shift of phosphorus into cells because of respiratory alkalosis. Renal phosphorus wasting can also result from hypomagnesemia or as a direct effect of alcohol.[227]

Clinical Manifestations

25. What are the signs and symptoms associated with hypophosphatemia?

The clinical effects associated with chronic phosphorus depletion are often insidious and gradual in onset. In contrast, a rapid decline in plasma phosphorus concentrations results in sudden and serious organ dysfunction. Most of the effects can be attributed to impaired cellular energy stores and tissue hypoxia secondary to depletion of ATP or erythrocyte 2,3-diphosphoglycerate (2,3-DPG).[228] Severe hypophosphatemia can result in generalized muscle weakness, confusion, paresthesias, seizures, and coma. In addition, reduced cardiac contractility, hypotension, respiratory failure, and rhabdomyolysis have been observed with acute severe hypophosphatemia.[208] Chronic phosphorus depletion has been associated with decreased mentation; muscle weakness; osteomalacia; rickets; anorexia; dysphagia; cardiomyopathy; tachypnea; reduced sensitivity to insulin; and dysfunction of red blood cells, white blood cells, and platelets. Renal function is altered, as manifested by hypophosphaturia, hypercalciuria, hypermagnesuria, bicarbonaturia, and glycosuria. M.R.'s decreased mentation, weakness, and respiratory failure are consistent with severe hypophosphatemia.

Treatment

26. How can phosphate depletion be assessed? Outline a treatment regimen that would effectively and safely correct the phosphorus deficit in M.R. How should her therapy be monitored?

Phosphorus resides primarily in the intracellular space; the amount in the extracellular fluid is only a small percentage of the total body store. Because the patient's pH, blood glucose concentration, and insulin availability may affect phosphorus distribution, it is difficult to determine the magnitude of the phosphorus deficit based on the serum concentration alone. As discussed, a patient may have hypophosphatemia secondary to a rapid shift of phosphorus into the intracellular space without a total body deficit. The duration of the hypophosphatemia is often limited because it may be corrected by renal phosphorus conservation and oral intake of phosphorus-containing foods. Aside from serum phosphorus concentrations, urinary phosphorus excretion may be used to further assess the phosphorus deficit. Typically, renal phosphorus excretion is severely limited in patients with significant deficits. A phosphorus excretion of <100 mg/day (fractional phosphorus excretion <10%) confirms appropriate renal phosphorus conservation when the serum phosphorus is <2 mg/dL. It also suggests a nonrenal etiology (e.g., impaired GI absorption) or some type of internal redistribution (e.g., respiratory alkalosis).[229]

Prophylactic supplementation should be used in situations that predictably increase the risk for developing hypophosphatemia. These include patients who are receiving total parenteral nutrition or large doses of antacids for an extended period, alcoholic patients, and those with diabetic ketoacidosis.

The specific treatment of hypophosphatemia depends on the presence of signs and symptoms, as well as the anticipated duration and severity of hypophosphatemia. In an asymptomatic patient with mild hypophosphatemia (1.5–2.5 mg/dL) who has no evidence of phosphorus depletion, phosphorus supplementation is generally not necessary because the condition is usually self-limited.[208] In other patients with mild and moderate hypophosphatemia who have evidence of phosphorus deficit, oral supplementation is the safest and preferred mode of replacement. Skim or low-fat milk is a convenient source of phosphorus and calcium. Whole milk, because of its high fat content, can cause diarrhea if a large amount is consumed. Several oral phosphorus preparations can be used in patients who cannot tolerate milk products.

When hypophosphatemia is severe, as in M.R., or when the patient is vomiting or unable to take oral medication, parenteral phosphorus replacement is needed. Several empiric regimens have been evaluated. IV administration of 0.08 to 0.5 mmol/kg body weight of phosphorus over 4 to 12 hours is safe and effective in restoring the serum phosphorus concentration.[230,231] More aggressive regimens, such as infusion over 30 minutes to 2 hours, have also been suggested for critically ill and surgical patients.[232,233] Parenteral phosphorus replacement should be stopped once the serum phosphorus concentration reaches 2.0 mg/dL and also when oral supplementation is started. In general, no more than 32 mmol (1 g) of phosphorus should be administered IV in a 24-hour period. Regardless of the regimen used, serum phosphorus, calcium, and magnesium concentrations should be monitored closely because IV phosphorus administration can induce hyperphosphatemia quite rapidly, as well as hypocalcemia and hypomagnesemia. Monitoring of urine phosphorus concentration also helps determine the adequacy of therapy. Metastatic soft tissue calcification, hypotension, and, depending on the preparation used, potassium, sodium, or volume overload may occur. This could be significant in patients such as M.R. who have a history of CHF and hypertension. Therefore, renal function and volume status should be monitored during therapy. Diarrhea, a common dose-related side effect of oral phosphorus replacement, can be minimized by diluting the supplement and slowly titrating the dose. Large doses can also result in metabolic acidosis.[230]

Phosphorus can be administered orally in doses of 30 to 60 mmol/day, usually given in two to four divided doses to minimize GI adverse events, using any commercially available oral supplement (e.g., Fleet or Neutra-Phos). Fleet Phospho-Soda (5 mL twice daily) delivers 40 mmol/day of phosphorus. Skim milk, the preferred agent for diluting the supplement, contains approximately 7 mmol of phosphorus/cup and provides calcium and potassium as well.

In M.R., oral supplementation was not feasible because she had intermittent diarrhea and vomiting. Potassium phosphate 15 mmol (providing 22 mEq of potassium) was therefore infused IV in 250 mL of 0.45% saline over 12 hours. The regimen was repeated once until the serum phosphorus concentration reached 2 mg/dL. Oral supplementation with Fleet Phospho-Soda then was begun by adding one teaspoonful twice daily to her enteral tube feeding.

Hyperphosphatemia

Refer to the section on "Secondary hyperparathyroidism and renal osteodystrophy" in Chapter 31 "Chronic Renal Failure."

MAGNESIUM

Homeostasis

Magnesium is an intracellular cation found primarily in bone (65%) and muscle (20%). Only 2% of the total body store of 21 to 28 g (1,750–2,400 mEq) is located in the extracellular compartment. Serum magnesium concentrations, therefore, do not reflect the total magnesium body store accurately. In healthy adults, the serum magnesium concentration is 1.80 to 2.40 mEq/L, with approximately 20% of the serum magnesium bound to proteins.

Magnesium plays an important role in different metabolic processes, particularly in energy transfer, storage, and utilization. Cation deficiency can impair many ATP-mediated energy-dependent cellular processes as well as the action of phosphatases.[234] Magnesium is necessary for many enzymes involved in the metabolism of carbohydrate, fat, and protein, as well as RNA aggregation, DNA transcription, and degradation. The normal operation of many sodium, proton, and calcium pumps and the regulation of potassium and calcium channels are all dependent on the availability of intracellular magnesium.[235,236] In addition, adequate magnesium stores are needed to maintain normal neuronal control, neuromuscular transmission, and cardiovascular tone.

The average diet in North America contains about 20 to 30 mEq of magnesium.[237] The daily requirement is approximately 18 to 33 mEq for young persons and 15 to 28 mEq for women.[238] Normally, 30% to 40% of the elemental magnesium is absorbed, primarily in the jejunum and ileum. However, absorption may be increased to 80% in deficiency states and reduced to 25% during high magnesium intake. In patients with uremia, GI absorption of magnesium is decreased; however, absorption in the jejunum can be normalized by physiologic doses of 1α,25-dihydroxyvitamin D_3.[239] In addition, PTH also modulates magnesium absorption.[240]

Magnesium is eliminated primarily by the kidneys; only 1% to 2% of the endogenous magnesium is eliminated by the fecal route.[179] The magnitude of renal removal is determined by GFR and tubular reabsorption. Approximately 20% to 30% of the tubular reabsorption takes place in the proximal tubule, whereas Henle's loop, primarily the thick ascending limb, is responsible for up to 65% of the total reabsorption.[241] Only about 5% to 6% of the filtered magnesium is generally eliminated in the urine. The extent of magnesium reabsorption changes in parallel with sodium reabsorption, which is affected by the extracellular fluid volume. The renal threshold for urinary magnesium excretion is 1.3 to 1.7 mEq/L, which is similar to the normal plasma magnesium concentration. Slight changes in plasma magnesium concentration, therefore, may substantially alter the amount of magnesium excreted in the urine.[242]

Urinary magnesium reabsorption is affected by many factors, including sodium balance; extracellular fluid volume; serum concentrations of magnesium, calcium, and phosphate; and metabolic acidosis and alkalosis.[243] Concurrent use of loop and osmotic diuretics will also modulate the reabsorption.[144,245] Hormones, such as PTH, and possibly calcitonin, glucagon, and mineralocorticoids may affect the routine maintenance of magnesium balance as well.[246–248]

Hypomagnesemia

Etiology

27. R.J., a 61-year-old man, is admitted to the hospital because of trauma to his forehead after falling at home. He has a long history of conditions related to his alcohol abuse: liver disease, ascites, seizures, pancreatitis, and malabsorption. R.J. complained of abdominal pain, nausea, vomiting, and diarrhea for the past several days. At admission, R.J. was confused, apprehensive, and combative, and he had marked tremors. He also had delirium, as evidenced by hallucinations, screaming, and delusions, and he was having multiple tonic-clonic seizures. The medical record revealed that R.J. had been taking furosemide for the last 2 months. Pertinent laboratory test results obtained at admission were K, 2.5 mEq/L (normal, 3.5–5.1); Mg, 0.8 mEq/L (normal, 1.6–2.8); and creatinine, 0.8 mg/dL (normal, 0.5–1.5). Phenytoin was administered for seizure control and R.J. was placed on nasogastric suction. Fluid restriction was instituted and furosemide therapy was continued to control his ascites. What are the circumstances that have contributed to R.J.'s hypomagnesemia?

[SI units: K, 2.5 mmol/L; Mg, 0.4 mmol/L; creatinine, 70.72 μmol/L]

Magnesium body stores are difficult to assess because magnesium is primarily an intracellular ion, and serum magnesium concentrations do not provide an accurate indication of the total body load. In fact, cellular magnesium depletion may be present with low, normal, or even high serum magnesium concentrations.[249,250] Conversely, hypomagnesemia may be seen without a net loss of body magnesium. Refeeding after starvation will result in increased trapping of magnesium by newly formed tissue, resulting in hypomagnesemia. Similarly, acute pancreatitis and parathyroidectomy can cause hypomagnesemia without a net loss of the cation.[251,252]

The prevalence of hypomagnesemia in ambulatory and hospitalized patients was found to be approximately 6% to 12%.[253] The incidence increased to 42% in patients who were hypokalemic[254] and to 60% to 65% in those under intensive care.[255] Multiple risk factors and clinical conditions can contribute to the high rate of hypomagnesemia in critically ill patients.

Magnesium depletion and hypomagnesemia can develop owing to GI, renal, and endocrinologic causes. Depletion can occur in patients whose dietary magnesium intake is severely restricted[256] and in those who have protein calorie malnutrition.[257] Also at risk are patients who receive prolonged parenteral nutrition[258] and those who undergo prolonged nasogastric suction.[259] Hypomagnesemia may be present in patients who have increased magnesium requirements, such as pregnant women and infants.[260] Conditions associated with steatorrhea, such as nontropical sprue and short-bowel syndrome, can result in reduced GI magnesium absorption. Insoluble magnesium soaps may be formed in the GI tract because of the presence of unabsorbed fat.[261] Hypomagnesemia can also occur in patients with a bowel resection[262] and severe diarrhea.[263] A rare genetic disorder has also been reported in patients with defective GI magnesium absorption.[264] An impaired carrier-mediated magnesium transport system is believed to be responsible for the symptomatic deficiency, which requires high oral magnesium intake to overcome the defect.

Renal magnesium wasting can be caused by a primary defect or be secondary to systemic factors. A rare form of renal magnesium wasting is congenital.[265] Various drugs can induce hypomagnesemia through increased renal loss: cisplatin,[266] aminoglycosides,[267] cyclosporine,[268] and amphotericin B.[269] Use of loop and thiazide diuretics can also result in hypomagnesemia, which can be reversed with the concurrent use of amiloride or triamterene. Magnesium depletion can be associated with phosphate depletion,[270] calcium infusion,[271] and ketoacidosis.[272] Acute and chronic ingestion of alcohol will result in increased renal magnesium loss.[204,273] Various endocrinologic disorders, such as SIADH,[274] hyperthyroidism,[275] hyperaldosteronism,[248] and postparathyroidectomy,[276] are also associated with hypomagnesemia.

R.J. could be hypomagnesemic for many reasons. His long history of alcohol use, malnutrition, and malabsorption may all have contributed to his magnesium deficit. The vomiting and diarrhea that he experienced could have reduced GI magnesium absorption. Use of furosemide and nasogastric suction while in the hospital could also have exacerbated his magnesium depletion through renal and GI losses, respectively.

Clinical Manifestations

28. What are the clinical manifestations of hypomagnesemia in R.J.?

Magnesium depletion can result in abnormal function of the neurologic, neuromuscular, and cardiovascular systems. Hypomagnesemia lowers the threshold for nerve stimulation, resulting in increased irritability. Typical findings include Chvostek's and Trousseau's signs, muscle fasciculation, tremors, muscle spasticity, generalized convulsions, and possibly tetany. The patient may experience weakness, anorexia, nausea, and vomiting, as seen in R.J. Hypokalemia, hypocalcemia, and alkalosis may be present as well. In patients who are moderately depleted, changes in the ECG include widening of the QRS complex and a peaking T wave.[277] In severe depletion, a prolonged PR interval and a diminished T-wave may be seen. Ventricular arrhythmias also have been reported in some patients.[278]

Treatment

29. Outline a regimen to replenish the body stores of magnesium for R.J., and develop a monitoring plan to assess efficacy and potential adverse effects.

The specific regimen for magnesium replenishment depends on the clinical presentation of the patient. Symptomatic patients require more aggressive parenteral therapy, whereas oral replacement may suffice for asymptomatic hypomagnesemia. Patients with life-threatening symptoms, such as seizures and arrhythmias, need immediate magnesium infusion. Because serum magnesium concentrations do not reflect total body stores, symptoms are more important determinants of the urgency and aggressiveness of therapy.

The body stores of magnesium must be replenished slowly. Serum magnesium concentrations may return to the normal range within the first 24 hours, but total replenishment of body stores may take several days. Furthermore, approximately 50% of the administered IV dose of magnesium will be excreted in the urine.[279] Because the threshold for urinary magnesium excretion is low, the abrupt increase in serum magnesium after an IV dose will result in increased urinary magnesium excretion despite a total body magnesium deficit. Conversely, in patients with renal insufficiency, decreased excretion of magnesium will place the patient at risk for hypermagnesemia. A reduced rate of magnesium administration and frequent monitoring of serum magnesium concentrations are therefore necessary in patients with renal dysfunction.

Oral replacement of magnesium is indicated for asymptomatic patients with mild depletion. Magnesium-containing antacids, Milk of Magnesia, and magnesium oxide are effective choices for replacement. Sustained-release preparations, such as Slow Mag (containing magnesium chloride) and Mag-Tab SR (containing magnesium lactate), are preferred, however. With 5 to 7 mEq (2.5–3.5 mmol or 60–84 mg) of magnesium per tablet, six to eight tablets should be given daily in divided doses for severe magnesium depletion. For mild and asymptomatic disease, two to four tablets per day may be sufficient.[280] A diet high in magnesium (cereals, nuts, meat, fruits, fish, legumes, and vegetables) also will help replenish body stores and prevent depletion.[281]

For patients with symptomatic hypomagnesemia, such as R.J., parenteral magnesium replacement is indicated. The magnesium deficit in patients with chronic alcoholism is estimated to be 1 to 2 mEq/kg.[282] Because up to half of the IV magnesium dose will be excreted in the urine during replacement, approximately 2 to 4 mEq/kg will be needed to replenish R.J.'s body store.[279] One milliequivalent per kilogram of magnesium, as magnesium sulfate 10% solution, should be administered IV in the first 24 hours. Half of this amount is given in the first 3 hours, and the remaining half is infused over the rest of the day. This dose may be repeated to keep the serum magnesium concentration >1.0 mg/dL.[280] Later on, 0.5 mEq/kg of magnesium may be replenished daily for up to 4 additional days.[279,283] Magnesium can be given IM as 50% solution, but the injections are painful and potentially sclerosing, and multiple administrations are needed. Therefore, the IV route is the preferred mode of parenteral administration. For patients with symptomatic hypomagnesemia who are unstable, such as those experiencing seizures or life-threatening arrhythmias, 16 mEq of magnesium sulfate may be administered as a short IV infusion over 2 minutes, followed by 16 mEq over 20 minutes, then 16 to 24 mEq over 2 to 4 hours.[279,284]

After IV magnesium administration, the patient should remain in a supine position to avoid hypotension. He should be monitored carefully for marked suppression of deep tendon reflexes (Mg, 4–7 mEq/L); ECG, BP, and respiration changes; and high serum magnesium levels. Facial flushing, a sensation of warmth, and sweatiness may result from vasodilation secondary to a rapid magnesium infusion.[279] Particular caution is warranted in patients with renal impairment, in whom the rate of magnesium should be reduced. These patients should be monitored frequently to avoid toxicities related to hypermagnesemia. IV magnesium should also be administered cautiously in patients with severe atrioventricular heart block or bifascicular blocks because magnesium possesses pharmacologic properties similar to calcium channel blockers.[279,284]

In patients who develop hypomagnesemia secondary to a thiazide or loop diuretic, amiloride may be added to reduce renal magnesium loss by increasing reabsorption in the cortical collecting tubule.[280]

30. Over the initial 2 days of hospitalization, R.J. received 3 mEq/kg of IV magnesium sulfate. However, his serum magnesium concentration remained <1.5 mEq/L (normal, 1.5–2.6). What might have contributed to the lack of favorable response to the magnesium therapy?

The total amount of magnesium administered to R.J. over the past 2 days was higher than the usual recommended rate (4–5 days) of magnesium replenishment, leading to renal excretion of a large portion of the dose.[286] Furthermore, the use of nasogastric suction and furosemide have increased the magnesium loss during the replacement period, and hypokalemia may have reduced the effectiveness of magnesium replacement. In a patient whose serum magnesium concentration does not increase after appropriate magnesium therapy, a 24-hour urine collection to assess magnesium renal excretion can be helpful. A low urinary magnesium concentration is consistent with magnesium depletion, whereas high urinary magnesium excretion in the presence of hypomagnesemia suggests renal magnesium wasting.

Hypermagnesemia

Etiology

31. J.O., a 63-year-old man with renal insufficiency, was admitted to the hospital because of increasing weakness over the past several days. J.O. began taking a magnesium–aluminum hydroxide antacid several times daily 2 weeks ago when he developed stomach upset. Physical examination reveals hypotension and depressed deep tendon reflexes. The ECG reveals prolonged PR and QRS intervals. The serum magnesium concentration is 6.5 mEq/dL (normal, 1.6–2.8). What is the most likely cause of hypermagnesemia in J.O.?

[SI unit: Mg, 3.25 mmol/L]

Because the kidney is the primary route of magnesium elimination, renal impairment is a virtual requisite for hypermagnesemia (see Chapter 31, Chronic Renal Failure). A common cause of hypermagnesemia is the use of magnesium-containing medications, such as antacids and laxatives, by patients with impaired renal function, including older adults. When a patient with renal failure, such as J.O., takes magnesium-containing medications, the serum magnesium concentration can increase substantially, resulting in toxicities. Hypermagnesemia may be seen when the creatinine clearance drops below 30 mL/minute; an inverse relationship is observed between the serum magnesium concentrations and the creatinine clearances.[287] Hypermagnesemia is also seen in patients with acute renal failure during the oliguric phase, but not the diuretic phase.[288] Other potential causes of hypermagnesemia include adrenal insufficiency,[234] hypothyroidism,[289] lithium,[289] magnesium citrate used as a cathartic for drug overdose,[290] and parenteral magnesium given for pre-eclampsia.[291]

Clinical Manifestations

32. Describe the usual clinical presentation of a patient with hypermagnesemia.

An elevated magnesium serum concentration alters the normal function of the neurologic, neuromuscular, and cardiovascular systems. When the serum magnesium concentration is >4 mEq/L, deep tendon reflexes are depressed; they are usually lost at >6 mEq/L. Flaccid quadriplegia can develop when the concentration is >8 to 10 mEq/L. Respiratory paralysis, hypotension, and difficulty in talking and swallowing may also be present.[293] Changes in the ECG may include a prolonged PR interval and widening of the QRS complex. Complete heart block may be seen at concentrations of approximately 15 mEq/L. In mild hypomagnesemia, the patient may experience nausea and vomiting.

Drowsiness, lethargy, diaphoresis, and altered consciousness may be present at higher serum magnesium concentrations. J.O.'s increasing weakness, hypotension, depressed deep tendon reflexes, andECG findings are consistent with hypermagnesemia.

Treatment

33. How should J.O.'s hypermagnesemia be treated?

If magnesium-containing medications are discontinued in patients with hypermagnesemia, the serum magnesium concentration will usually return to the normal range through renal elimination. When potentially life-threatening complications are present, as in J.O., 5 to 10 mEq of IV calcium should be administered to antagonize the respiratory and cardiac manifestations of magnesium.[291,292] The dose of the calcium can be repeated as necessary because its effect is short lived. In patients with good renal function without life-threatening complications, IV furosemide, plus 0.45% sodium chloride to replace lost urine volume, will enhance urinary magnesium excretion while preventing volume depletion. Hemodialysis or peritoneal dialysis is indicated for patients with significant renal function impairment and possibly for those with severe hypermagnesemia.

REFERENCES

1. Fanestil DD. Compartmentation of body water. In: Narins RG, ed. *Maxwell & Kleeman's Clinical Disorders of Fluid and Electrolyte Metabolism*. 5th ed. New York: McGraw-Hill; 1994:3.
2. Rose BD. Renal function and disorders of water and sodium balance. In: Rubenstein E et al., eds. *Scientific American Medicine*. New York: Scientific American Inc., 1994;Section 10:1.
3. Rose BD. Introduction to disorders of osmolality. In: Rose BD et al., eds. *Clinical Physiology of Acid-Base and Electrolyte Disorders*. 5th ed. New York: McGraw-Hill; 2001.
4. Oster JR et al. Hyponatremia, hypo-osmolality, and hypotonicity: tables and fables. *Arch Intern Med* 1999;159:333.
5. Rose BD. Proximal tubule. In: Rose BD et al., eds. *Clinical Physiology of Acid-Base and Electrolyte Disorders*. 5th ed. New York: McGraw-Hill; 2001.
6. Rose BD. Loop of Henle and the countercurrent mechanism. In: Rose BD et al., eds. *Clinical Physiology of Acid-Base and Electrolyte Disorders*. 5th ed. New York: McGraw-Hill; 2001.
7. Rose BD. Functions of the distal nephron. In: Rose BD et al., eds. *Clinical Physiology of Acid-Base and Electrolyte Disorders*. 5th ed. New York: McGraw-Hill; 2001.
8. Sands JM et al. Vasopressin effects on urea and water transport in inner medullary collecting duct subsegments. *Am J Physiol* 1987;253:F823.
9. Gines P et al. Vasopressin in pathophysiological states. *Semin Nephrol* 1994;14:384.
10. Zerbe RL et al. Osmotic and nonosmotic regulation of thirst and vasopressin secretion. In: Narins RG, ed. *Maxwell & Kleeman's Clinical Disorders of Fluid and Electrolyte Metabolism*. New York: McGraw-Hill; 1994.
11. Rose BD. Regulation of the effective circulating volume. In: Rose BD et al., eds. *Clinical Physiology of Acid-Base and Electrolyte Disorders*. 5th ed. New York: McGraw-Hill; 2001.
12. Goetz KL. Renal natriuretic peptide (urodilatin?) and atriopeptin: evolving concepts. *Am J Physiol* 1991;261:F921.
13. Goetz K et al. Evidence that urodilatin, rather than ANP, regulates renal sodium excretion. *J Am Soc Nephrol* 1990;1:867.
14. Rose BD. Hypovolemic states. In: Rose BD et al., eds. *Clinical Physiology of Acid-Base and Electrolyte Disorders*. 5th ed. New York: McGraw-Hill; 2001.
15. Rose BD. Meaning and application of urine chemistries. In: Rose BD et al., eds. *Clinical Physiology of Acid-Base and Electrolyte Disorders*. 5th ed. New York: McGraw-Hill; 2001.
16. Kaysen GA. Proteinuria and the nephrotic syndrome. In: Schrier RW, ed. *Renal and Electrolyte Disorders*. 6th ed. Philadelphia: Lippincott Williams & Wilkins; 2003.
17. Harris RE et al. Extrarenal complications of the nephrotic syndrome. *Am J Kidney Dis* 1994;23:477.
18. Saborio P et al. Sickle cell nephropathy. *J Am Soc Nephrol* 1999;10:187.
19. Klotman PE. HIV-associated nephropathy. *Kidney Int* 1999;56:1161.
20. Feinfeld DA et al. Nephrotic syndrome associated with the use of the nonsteroidal anti-inflammatory drugs: case report and review of the literature. *Nephron* 1984;37:174.
21. Kaysen GA et al. New insights into lipid metabolism in the nephrotic syndrome. *Kidney Int* 1999;56(Suppl 71):S18.
22. Chonko AM et al. Treatment of edema states. In: Narins RG, ed. *Maxwell & Kleeman's Clinical Disorders of Fluid and Electrolyte Metabolism*. 5th ed. New York: McGraw-Hill; 1994:545.
23. Glassock RJ. Management of intractable edema in nephrotic syndrome. *Kidney Int* 1997;51(Suppl 58):S75.
24. Schrier RW. Body fluid volume regulation in health and disease: a unifying hypothesis. *Ann Intern Med* 1990;113:155.
25. Schrier RW. An odyssey into the milieu Interieur: pondering the enigmas. *J Am Soc Nephrol* 1992;2:1549.
26. Brown EA et al. Sodium retention in nephrotic syndrome is due to an intrarenal defect: evidence from steroid-induced remission. *Nephron* 1985;39:290.
27. Koomans HA et al. Renal function during recovery from minimal lesion nephrotic syndrome. *Nephron* 1987;47:173.
28. Schrier RW et al. A critique of the overfill hypothesis of sodium and water retention in the nephrotic syndrome. *Kidney Int* 1998;53:1111.
29. Bank N. External compression for the treatment of resistant edema. *N Engl J Med* 1980;302:969.
30. Davidson AM et al. Salt-poor human albumin in the management of nephrotic syndrome. *BMJ* 1974;1:481.
31. Fancheld P et al. An evaluation of ultrafiltration as treatment of diuretic-resistant edema in nephrotic syndrome. *Acta Med Scand* 1985;17:127.
32. Yeun JY et al. The nephrotic syndrome: nutritional consequences and dietary management. In: Mitch WE et al., eds. *Handbook of Nutrition and the Kidney*. 4th ed. Philadelphia: Lippincott Williams & Wilkins; 2002.
33. Soupart A et al. Therapeutic recommendations for management of severe hyponatremia: current concepts on pathogenesis and prevention of neurologic complications. *Clin Nephrol* 1996;46:149.
34. Narins RG et al. Diagnostic strategies in disorders of fluid, electrolyte and acid-base homeostasis. *Am J Med* 1982;72:496.
35. Goldman MB et al. Mechanisms of altered water metabolism in psychotic patients with polydipsia and hyponatremia. *N Engl J Med* 1988;318:397.
36. Illowsky B et al. Polydipsia and hyponatremia in psychiatric patients. *Am J Psychiatry* 1988;145:6.
37. Sterns RH et al. Hyponatremia: pathophysiology, diagnosis, and therapy. In: Narins RG, ed. *Maxwell & Kleeman's Clinical Disorders of Fluid and Electrolyte Metabolism*. New York: McGraw-Hill; 1994.
38. Weisberg LS. Pseudohyponatremia: a reappraisal. *Am J Med* 1989;86:315.
39. Rothenberg DM et al. Isotonic hyponatremia following transurethral prostate resection. *J Clin Anesth* 1990;2:48.
40. Faber MD et al. Common fluid-electrolyte and acid-base problems in the intensive care unit: selected issues. *Semin Nephrol* 1994;14:8.
41. Ashraf N et al. Thiazide-induced hyponatremia associated with death or neurologic damage in outpatients. *Am J Med* 1981;70:1163.
42. Ashouri SD. Severe diuretic induced hyponatremias in the elderly. *Arch Intern Med* 1986;146:1355.
43. Shah PJ, Greenburg WM. Water intoxication precipitated by thiazide diuretics in polydipsic psychiatric patients. *Am J Psychiatry* 1991;48:1424.
44. Vassal G et al. Hyponatremia and renal sodium wasting in patients receiving cisplatinum. *Pediatr Hematol Oncol* 1987;4:337.
45. Hutchison FN et al. Renal sodium wasting in patients treated with cisplatin. *Ann Intern Med* 1988;108:21.
46. Vaamonde CA. Renal water handling in liver disease. In: Epstein M, ed. *The Kidney in Liver Disease*. Baltimore: Williams & Wilkins; 1988.
47. Papadakis MA et al. Hyponatremia in patients with cirrhosis. *Q J Med* 1990;76:675.
48. Carpenter CCJ et al. Oral rehydration therapy: the role of polymeric substrates. *N Engl J Med* 1988;319:1346.
49. Leier CV et al. Clinical relevance and management of the major electrolyte abnormalities in congestive heart failure: hyponatremia, hypokalemia, and hypomagnesemia. *Am Heart J* 1994;128:564.
50. Gore SM et al. Impact of rice-based oral rehydration solution on stool output and duration of diarrhea: meta-analysis of 13 clinical trials. *BMJ* 1992;304:287.
51. Allon M et al. Renal sodium and water handling in hypothyroid patients: the role of renal insufficiency. *J Am Soc Nephrol* 1990;1:205.
52. Linas SL et al. Role of vasopressin in the impaired water excretion of glucocorticoid deficiency. *Kidney Int* 1980;18:58.
53. DeFronzo RA et al. Normal diluting capacity in hyponatremic patients: reset osmostat or variant of SIADH. *Ann Intern Med* 1975;82:811.
54. Schwartz WB et al. Syndrome of renal sodium loss and hyponatremia probably resulting from inappropriate secretion of antidiuretic hormone. *Am J Med* 1957;23:529.
55. Bartter FC et al. The syndrome of inappropriate secretion of antidiuretic hormone. *Am J Med* 1967;42:790.
56. Cooke RC et al. The syndrome of inappropriate antidiuretic hormone secretion (SIADH): pathophysiologic mechanisms in solute and volume regulation. *Medicine* 1979;58:240.
57. Marchioli CC et al. Paraneoplastic syndromes associated with small cell lung cancer. *Chest Surg Clin N Am* 1997;7:65.
58. Rose BD. New approaches to disturbances in the plasma sodium concentration. *Am J Med* 1986;81:1033.
59. Cluitmans FHM et al. Management of severe hyponatremia: rapid or slow correction? *Am J Med* 1990;88:161.
60. Sterns RH. The treatment of hyponatremia: first, do no harm. *Am J Med* 1990;88:557.
61. Gross P. Treatment of severe hyponatremia. *Kidney Int* 2001;60:2417.
62. Arieff AI. Hyponatremia, convulsions, respiratory arrest, and permanent brain damage after elective surgery in healthy women. *N Engl J Med* 1986;314:1529.
63. Ayus JC et al. Postoperative hyponatremic encephalopathy in menstruant women. *Ann Intern Med* 1992;117:891.
64. Lien Y et al. Study of brain electrolytes and organic osmolytes during correction of chronic hyponatremia: implications for the pathogenesis of central pontine myelinolysis. *J Clin Invest* 1991;88:303.
65. Berl T. Treating hyponatremia: damned if we do and damned if we don't. *Kidney Int* 1990;37:1006.
66. Chung HM et al. Post-operative hyponatremia. *Arch Intern Med* 1986;314:1529.
67. Cochrane JPS et al. Arginine vasopressin release following surgical operations. *Br J Surg* 1981;68:209.
68. DeFronzo RA et al. Water intoxication in man after cyclophosphamide therapy. Time course and relation to drug activation. *Ann Intern Med* 1973;78:861.
69. Morgan DB et al. Water intoxication and oxytocin infusion. *Br J Obstet Gynaecol* 1977;84:6.
70. Cheng JC et al. Long-term neurologic outcome in psychogenic water drinkers with severe symptomatic hyponatremia: the effect of rapid correction. *Am J Med* 1990;88:561.
71. Laureno R et al. Pontine and extrapontine myelinolysis following rapid correction of hyponatremia. *Lancet* 1988;1:1439.
72. Lohr JW. Osmotic demyelination syndrome following correction of hyponatremia: association with hypokalemia. *Am J Med* 1994;96:408.
73. Sterns RH et al. Neurologic sequelae after treatment of severe hyponatremia: a multicenter perspective. *J Am Soc Nephrol* 1994;4:1522.
74. Decaux G. Treatment of the syndrome of inappropriate secretion of antidiuretic hormone by long-loop diuretics. *Nephron* 1983;35:82.
75. Decaux G et al. Treatment of the syndrome of inappropriate secretion of antidiuretic hormone with furosemide. *N Engl J Med* 1981;304:329.
76. Cherill DA et al. Demeclocycline treatment in the syndrome of antidiuretic hormone secretion. *Ann Intern Med* 1975;83:654.
77. White MG et al. Treatment of the syndrome of inappropriate secretion of antidiuretic hormone with lithium carbonate. *N Engl J Med* 1975;292:390.

78. Miller PD et al. Plasma demeclocycline levels and nephrotoxicity: correlation in hyponatremic cirrhotic patients. *JAMA* 1980;243:2513.
79. Palm C et al. V2-vasopressin receptor antagonists-mechanism of effect and clinical implication in hyponatraemia. *Nephrol Dial Transplant* 1999;14:2559.
80. Guyader D et al. Pharmacodynamic effects of a nonpeptide antidiuretic hormone V2 antagonist in cirrhotic patients with ascites. *Hepatology* 2002;36:1197.
81. Wong F et al. A vasopressin receptor antagonist (VPA-985) improves serum sodium concentration in patients with hyponatremia: a multicenter, randomized, placebo-controlled trial. *Hepatology* 2003;37:182.
82. Decaux G et al. Lack of efficacy of phenytoin in the syndrome of inappropriate antidiuretic hormone secretion of neurological origin. *Postgrad Med J* 1989;65:456.
83. Decaux G et al. 5-year treatment of the chronic syndrome of inappropriate secretion of ADH with oral urea. *Nephron* 1993;63:468.
84. Decaux G et al. Hyponatremia in the syndrome of inappropriate secretion of antidiuretic hormone. Rapid correction with urea, sodium chloride, and water restriction. *JAMA* 1982;247:471.
85. Ali F et al. Therapeutic potential of vasopressin receptor antagonists. *Drugs* 2007;67:847.
86. Verbalis JG. Vasopressin V2 receptor antagonists. *J Mol Endocrinol* 2002;29:1.
87. Thibonnier M et al. The basic and clinical pharmacology of nonpeptide vasopressin receptor antagonists. *Annu Rev Pharmacol Toxicol* 2001;41:175.
88. Knepper MA. Molecular physiology of urinary concentrating mechanism: regulation of aquaporin water channels by vasopressin. *Am J Physiol* 1997;272:F3.
89. Burrell LM et al. Vasopressin receptor antagonism—a therapeutic option in heart failure and hypertension. *Exp Physiol* 2000;85:259S.
90. Verbalis JG et al. Novel vasopressin V-1A and V2 antagonist (conivaptan) increases serum sodium concentration and effective water clearance in patients with hyponatremia. *Circulation* 2004;110:723.
91. Ghali J. Efficacy and safety of oral conivaptan: a V1A/V2 vasopressin receptor antagonist, assessed in a randomized, placebo-controlled trial in patients with euvolemic or hypervolemic hyponatremia. *J Clin Endocrinol Metab* 2006;91:21.
92. Schrier RW et al. Tolvaptan, a selective oral vasopressin V2-receptor antagonist, for hyponatremia. *N Engl J Med* 2006;355:2099.
93. Gheorghiade M et al. Vasopressin V2-receptor blockade with tolvaptan in patients with chronic heart failure: results from a double-blind, randomized trial. *Circulation* 2003;107:2690.
94. Gheorghiade M et al. Effects of tolvaptan, a vasopressin antagonist, in patients hospitalized with worsening heart failure: a randomized controlled trial. *JAMA* 2004;291:1963.
95. Gheorghiade M et al. Short term clinical effects of tolvaptan, an oral vasopressin antagonist, in patients hospitalized for heart failure: The EVEREST Clinical Status Trials. *JAMA* 2007;297:1332.
96. Abraham WT et al. Aquaretic effect of lixivaptan, an oral, non-peptide, selective V2 receptor vasopressin antagonist, in New York Heart Association functional class II and III chronic heart failure patients. *J Am Coll Cardiol* 2006;47:1615.
97. Wong F et al. A vasopressin receptor antagonist (VPA-985) improves serum sodium concentration in patients with hyponatremia: a multicenter, randomized, placebo-controlled trial. *Hepatology* 2003;37:182.
98. Gerbes AL et al. Therapy of hyponatremia in cirrhosis with a vasopressin receptor antagonist: a randomized double-blind multicenter trial. *Gastroenterology* 2003;124:933.
99. Soupart A et al. Successful long-term treatment of hyponatremia in syndrome of inappropriate antidiuretic hormone secretion with SR 121 463B, an orally active, nonpeptide, vasopressin V-2 receptor antagonist. *J Am Soc Nephrol* 2004;15:563A.
100. Schrier RW et al. Tolvaptan, a selective oral vasopressin V2-receptor antagonist, for hyponatremia. *N Engl J Med* 2006;355:2099.
101. Verbalis JG et al. Conivaptan, a novel arginine vasopressin antagonist, produced aquaresis and increased serum sodium concentration in patients with heart failure and euvolemic or hypervolemic hyponatremia. *Crit Care Med* 2006;33(Suppl):A170.
102. Morrison G et al. Hyperosmolal states. In: Narins RG, ed. *Maxwell & Kleeman's Clinical Disorders of Fluid and Electrolyte Metabolism*. 5th ed. New York: McGraw-Hill; 1994.
103. Snyder NA et al. Hypernatremia in elderly patients: a heterogeneous, morbid, and iatrogenic entity. *Ann Intern Med* 1987;107:309.
104. Beerman B et al. Clinical pharmacokinetics of diuretics. *Clin Pharmacokinet* 1980;5:221.
105. Merkus F. Is canrenone the major metabolite of spironolactone? *Clin Pharm* 1983;2:209.
106. Sklath H et al. Spironolactone: a re-examination. *DICP. Ann Pharmacother* 1990;24:52.
107. Pruitt AW et al. Variations in the fate of triamterene. *Clin Pharmacol Ther* 1977;21:610.
108. Sterns RH et al. Internal potassium balance and the control of the plasma potassium concentration. *Medicine* 1981;60:339.
109. Allon M. Treatment and prevention of hyperkalemia in end-stage renal disease. *Kidney Int* 1993;43:1197.
110. Perrone RD et al. Regulation of extrarenal potassium metabolism. In: Narins RG, ed. *Maxwell & Kleeman's Clinical Disorders of Fluid and Electrolyte Metabolism*. 5th ed. New York: McGraw-Hill; 1994.
111. Salem MM et al. Extrarenal potassium tolerance in chronic renal failure: implications for the treatment of acute hyperkalemia. *Am J Kidney Dis* 1991;18:421.
112. Field MJ et al. Regulation of renal potassium metabolism. In: Narins RG, ed. *Maxwell & Kleeman's Clinical Disorders of Fluid and Electrolyte Metabolism*. 5th ed. New York: McGraw-Hill; 1994:147.
113. Wright FS. Renal potassium handling. *Semin Nephrol* 1987;7:174.
114. Sterns RH et al. The disposition of intravenous potassium in normal man: the role of insulin. *Clin Sci* 1987;73:557.
115. Williams ME et al. Impairment of extrarenal potassium disposal by alpha-adrenergic stimulation. *N Engl J Med* 1984;311:345.
116. Rosa RM et al. Adrenergic modulation of extrarenal potassium disposal. *N Engl J Med* 1980;302:431.
117. Androgue HJ et al. Changes in plasma potassium concentration during acute acid-base disturbances. *Am J Med* 1981;71:456.
118. Oster JR et al. Plasma potassium response to acute metabolic acidosis induced by mineral and nonmineral acids. *Miner Electrolyte Metab* 1980;4:28.
119. Androgue HJ et al. Determinants of plasma potassium levels in diabetic ketoacidosis. *Medicine* 1986;65:163.
120. Hazeyama Y et al. A model of potassium efflux during exercise of skeletal muscle. *Am J Physiol* 1979;236:R83.
121. Krishna GG et al. Hypokalemic states. In: Narins RG, ed. *Maxwell & Kleeman's Clinical Disorders of Fluid and Electrolyte Metabolism*. 5th ed. New York: McGraw-Hill; 1994.
122. Johnsen T. Familial periodic paralysis with hypokalemia. *Dan Med Bull* 1981;28:1.
123. Moravec MD et al. Hypokalemia associated with terbutaline administration in obstetrical patients. *Anesth Analg* 1980;59:917.
124. Kethersid TL et al. Dialysate potassium. *Semin Dial* 1991;4:46.
125. Moore EW. Ionized calcium in normal serum, ultrafiltrates and whole blood determined by ion-exchange electrode. *J Clin Invest* 1970;49:318.
126. Kassirer JP et al. The response of normal man to selective depletion of hydrochloric acid: factors in the genesis of persistent gastric alkalosis. *Am J Med* 1966;40:10.
127. Adams PC et al. Exaggerated hypokalemia in acute myeloid leukemia. *BMJ* 1981;282:1034.
128. Knochel JP. Neuromuscular manifestations of electrolyte disorders. *Am J Med* 1982;75:521.
129. Surawicz B. Relationship between electrocardiogram and electrolytes. *Am Heart J* 1967;73:814.
130. Smith SR et al. Potassium chloride lowers blood pressure and causes natriuresis in older patients with hypertension. *J Am Soc Nephrol* 1992;2:1032.
131. Helderman JH et al. Prevention of the glucose intolerance of thiazide diuretics by maintenance of the body potassium. *Diabetes* 1983;32:106.
132. Tizianello A et al. Renal ammoniagenesis in humans with chronic potassium depletion. *Kidney Int* 1991;40:772.
133. Stanaszek WF et al. Current approaches to management of potassium deficiency. *Drug Intell Clin Pharm* 1985;19:176.
134. Kruse JA et al. Rapid correction of hypokalemia using concentrated intravenous potassium chloride infusions. *Arch Intern Med* 1990;150:613.
135. Kunin AS et al. Decrease in serum potassium concentration and appearance of cardiac arrhythmias during infusion of potassium with glucose in potassium-depleted patients. *N Engl J Med* 1962;266:228.
136. Bronson WR et al. Pseudohyperkalemia due to release of potassium from white blood cells during clotting. *N Engl J Med* 1966;274:369.
137. Ingram RH Jr et al. Pseudohyperkalemia with thrombocytosis. *N Engl J Med* 1962;267:895.
138. Mather A et al. Effects of hemolysis on serum electrolyte values. *Clin Chem* 1960;6:223.
139. Romano AT et al. Mild forearm exercise during venipuncture and its effect on potassium determinations. *Clin Chem* 1977;2:303.
140. DeFronzo RA et al. Clinical disorders of hyperkalemia. In: Narins RG, ed. *Maxwell & Kleeman's Clinical Disorders of Fluid and Electrolyte Metabolism*. 5th ed. New York: McGraw-Hill; 1994:697.
141. Cohen LF et al. Acute tumor lysis syndrome. *Am J Med* 1980;68:486.
142. Perazella MA. Drug-induced hyperkalemia: old culprits and new offenders. *Am J Med* 2000;109:307.
143. Reston RA et al. University of Miami Division of Clinical Pharmacology therapeutic rounds: drug-induced hyperkalemia. *Am J Ther* 1998;5:125.
144. Rimmer et al. Hyperkalemia as a complication of drug therapy. *Arch Intern Med* 1987;147:867.
145. DeFronzo RA. Hyperkalemia and hyporeninemic hypoaldosteronism. *Kidney Int* 1980;17:118.
146. Fraser R. Disorders of the adrenal cortex: their effects on electrolyte metabolism. *Clin Endocrinol Metab* 1984;13:413.
147. Kurtzman NA et al. A patient with hyperkalemia and metabolic acidosis. *Am J Kidney Dis* 1990;15:333.
148. Reardon LC et al. Hyperkalemia in outpatients using angiotensin-converting enzyme inhibitors. How much should we worry? *Arch Intern Med* 1998;158:26.
149. Schlondorff D. Renal complications of nonsteroidal anti-inflammatory drugs. *Kidney Int* 1993;44:643.
150. Bakris GL et al. ACE inhibition or angiotensin receptor blockade: impact on potassium in renal failure. VAL-K Study Group. *Kidney Int* 2000;58:2084.
151. Lundborg P. The effect of adrenergic blockade on potassium concentrations in different conditions. *Acta Med Scand* 1983;672(Suppl):121.
152. Goggans FC. Acute hyperkalemia during lithium treatment of manic illness. *Am J Psychiatry* 1980;137:860.
153. Abdel-Raheem MM et al. Effect of low-molecular-weight heparin on potassium homeostasis. *Pathophysiol Haemost Thromb* 2002;32:107.
154. Oster JR et al. Heparin-induced aldosterone suppression and hyperkalemia. *Am J Med* 1995;98:575.
155. Briceland LL et al. Pentamidine-associated nephro-

toxicity and hyperkalemia in patients with AIDS. *DICP* 1991;25:1171.
156. Velazquez H et al. Renal mechanisms of trimethoprim-induced hyperkalemia. *Ann Intern Med* 1993;119:296.
157. Alappan R et al. Trimethoprim-sulfamethoxazole therapy in outpatients: is hyperkalemia a significant problem? *Am J Nephrol* 1999;19:389.
158. Caliskan Y et al. Cyclosporine-associated hyperkalemia: report of four allogeneic blood stem-cell transplant cases. *Transplantation* 2003;75:1069.
159. Woo M et al. Toxicities of tacrolimus and cyclosporin A after allogeneic blood stem cell transplantation. *Bone Marrow Transplant* 1997;20;1095.
160. Bismuth C et al. Hyperkalemia in acute digitalis poisoning: prognostic significance and therapeutic implications. *Clin Toxicol* 1973;6:153.
161. Bushinsky DA et al. Life-threatening hyperkalemia induced by arginine. *Ann Intern Med* 1978;89:632.
162. Cooperman LH. Succinylcholine-induced hyperkalemia in neuromuscular disease. *JAMA* 1970; 213:1867.
163. Blumberg A et al. Effect of various therapeutic approaches on plasma potassium and major regulating factors in terminal renal failure. *Am J Med* 1988;85:507.
164. Nicolis GL et al. Glucose-induced hyperkalemia in diabetic subjects. *Arch Intern Med* 1981;141:49.
165. Allon M et al. Effect of insulin-plus-glucose with or without epinephrine on fasting hyperkalemia. *Kidney Int* 1993;43:212.
166. Wong SL et al. Albuterol for the treatment of hyperkalemia. *Ann Pharmacother* 1999;33:103.
167. Allon M. Hyperkalemia in end stage renal disease: mechanism and management. *J Am Soc Nephrol* 1995;6:1134.
168. Liou HH et al. Hypokalemic effects of intravenous infusion or nebulization of salbutamol in patients with chronic renal failure: comparative study. *Am J Kidney Dis* 1994;23:266.
169. Allon M et al. Albuterol and insulin for treatment of hyperkalemia in hemodialysis patients. *Kidney Int* 1990;38:869.
170. Gutierrez R et al. Effect of hypertonic versus isotonic sodium bicarbonate on plasma potassium concentrations in patients with end-stage renal disease. *Miner Electrolyte Metab* 1991;17:291.
171. Scherr L et al. Management of hyperkalemia with a cation-exchange resin. *N Engl J Med* 1961;264:115.
172. Gestman BB et al. Intestinal necrosis associated with postoperative orally administered sodium polystyrene sulfonate in sorbitol. *Am J Kidney Dis* 1992;20:159.
173. Brown ST et al. Potassium removal with peritoneal dialysis. *Kidney Int* 1973;4:67.
174. Sherman RA et al. Variability in potassium removal by hemodialysis. *Am J Nephrol* 1986;6:284.
175. Ward RA et al. Hemodialysate composition and intradialytic metabolic acid-base and potassium changes. *Kidney Int* 1987;32:129.
176. Lindgarde F et al. Hypercalcemia and normal ionized serum calcium in a case of myelomatosis. *Ann Intern Med* 1973;78:396.
177. Favus MJ. Transport of calcium by intestinal mucosa. *Semin Nephrol* 1981;1:306.
178. LeRoith D et al. Bone metabolism and composition in the protein-deprived rat. *Clin Sci* 1973;44:305.
179. Bourdeau JE et al. In: Narins RG, ed. *Maxwell & Kleeman's Clinical Disorders of Fluid and Electrolyte Metabolism*. 5th ed. New York: McGraw-Hill; 1994:243.
180. Benabe JE et al. Disorders of calcium metabolism. In: Narins RG, ed. *Maxwell & Kleeman's Clinical Disorders of Fluid and Electrolyte Metabolism*. 5th ed. New York: McGraw-Hill; 1994:1009.
181. Mundy GR. Pathophysiology of cancer-associated hypercalcemia. *Semin Oncol* 1990;17(Suppl 5):10.
182. Ladenson JH et al. Relationship of free and total calcium in hypercalcemic conditions. *J Clin Endocrinol Metab* 1979;48:393.
183. Beck N et al. Pathogenetic role of cyclic AMP in the impairment of urinary concentrating ability in acute hypercalcemia. *J Clin Invest* 1974;54:1049.
184. Bajorunas DR. Clinical manifestations of cancer-related hypercalcemia. *Semin Oncol* 1990;17(Suppl 5):16.
185. Suki WN et al. Acute treatment of hypercalcemia with furosemide. *N Engl J Med* 1970;283:836.
186. Davidson TG. Conventional treatment of hypercalcemia of malignancy. *Am J Health Syst Pharm* 2001;58(Suppl 3):S8.
187. Minstock ML et al. Effect of calcitonin and glucocorticoids in combination on the hypercalcemia of malignancy. *Ann Intern Med* 1980;93:269.
188. Ritch PS. Treatment of cancer-related hypercalcemia. *Semin Oncol* 1990;17(Suppl 5):26.
189. Green L et al. Hepatic toxicity of low doses of mithramycin in hypercalcemia. *Cancer Treatment Reports* 1984;68:1379.
190. Major P. The use of zoledronic acid, a novel, highly potent bisphosphonate, for the treatment of hypercalcemia of malignancy. *Oncologist* 2002;7:481.
191. Ryzen E et al. Intravenous etidronate in the management of malignant hypercalcemia. *Arch Intern Med* 1985;145:449.
192. Gucalp R et al. Comparative study of pamidronate disodium and etidronate disodium in the treatment of cancer-related hypercalcemia. *J Clin Oncol* 1992;10:134.
193. Bounameaux HM et al. Renal failure associated with intravenous diphosphonates. *Lancet* 1983;1: 471.
194. Francis MD et al. Acute intravenous infusions of disodium dihydrogen (1-hydroxy-ethylidene) diphosphonate: mechanisms of cytotoxicity. *J Pharm Sci* 1983;73:1097.
195. Morton AR. Bisphosphonates for the hypercalcemia of malignancy in end-stage renal disease. *Semin Dialysis* 1994;7:76.
196. Major P et al. Zoledronic acid is superior to pamidronate in the treatment of hypercalcemia of malignancy: a pooled analysis of two randomized, controlled clinical trials. *J Clin Oncol* 2001;19:558.
197. Brenson JR. Advances in the biology and treatment of myeloma bone disease. *Am J Health-Syst Pharm* 2001;58(Suppl 3):S16.
198. Warrell RP Jr et al. Metabolic effects of gallium nitrate administered by prolonged infusion. *Cancer Treatment Reports* 1985;69:653.
199. Warrell RP Jr et al. Gallium nitrate inhibits calcium resorption from bone and is effective treatment for cancer-related hypercalcemia. *J Clin Invest* 1984;73:1487.
200. Warrell RP Jr et al. Gallium nitrate for treatment of refractory hypercalcemia from parathyroid carcinoma. *Ann Intern Med* 1987;107:683.
201. Warrell RP Jr et al. Gallium nitrate for acute treatment of cancer-related hypercalcemia. A randomized, double-blind comparison to calcitonin. *Ann Intern Med* 1988;108:669.
202. Warrell RP Jr et al. A randomized double-blind study of gallium nitrate compared with etidronate for acute control of cancer-related hypercalcemia. *J Clin Oncol* 1991;9:1467.
203. Haussler MR et al. Basic and clinical concepts related to vitamin D metabolism and action. *N Engl J Med* 1977;297:974.
204. Kalbfleisch JM et al. Effects of ethanol administration on urinary excretion of magnesium and other electrolytes in alcoholic and normal subjects. *J Clin Invest* 1963;42:1471.
205. Streck WF et al. Glucocorticoid effects in vitamin D intoxication. *Arch Intern Med* 1979;139:974.
206. Baughman RP et al. Sarcoidosis. *Lancet* 2003;361: 1111.
207. Smith BJ et al. Prostaglandins and cancer. *Ann Clin Lab Sci* 1983;13:359.
208. Dennis VW. Phosphate disorders. In: Kokko JP et al., eds. *Fluids and Electrolytes*. 3rd ed. Philadelphia: WB Saunders; 1996:359.
209. Harrison HE et al. The effect of acidosis upon renal tubular reabsorption of phosphate. *Am J Physiol* 1941;134:781.
210. Moog F et al. Phosphate absorption and alkaline phosphatase activity in the small intestine of the adult mouse and of the chick embryo and hatched chick. *Comp Biochem Physiol* 1972;42A: 321.
211. Fox J et al. Stimulation of duodenal and head absorption of phosphate in the chick by low-calcium and low-phosphate diets. *Calcif Tissue Int* 1978;26:243.
212. Brommage R et al. Vitamin D-independent intestinal calcium and phosphorus absorption during reproduction. *Am J Physiol* 1990;259:G631.
213. Sheikh MS et al. Reduction of dietary phosphorus absorption by phosphorus binders. *J Clin Invest* 1989;83:66.
214. Levine BS et al. Hypophosphatemia and hyperphosphatemia: clinical and pathologic aspects. In: Narins RG, ed. *Maxwell & Kleeman's Clinical Disorders of Fluid and Electrolyte Metabolism*. 5th ed. New York: McGraw-Hill; 1994:1045.
215. Portale AA et al. Dietary intake of phosphorus modulates the circadian rhythm in serum concentration of phosphorus: implications for the renal production of 1,25-dihyroxyvitamin D. *J Clin Invest* 1987;80:1147.
216. Eisenbrey AB et al. Mannitol interference in an automated serum phosphate assay. *Clin Chem* 1987; 33:2308.
217. Lee DBN et al. Effect of phosphorus depletion on intestinal calcium and phosphorus absorption. *Am J Physiol* 1979;236:E451.
218. Crook MA et al. The importance of the refeeding syndrome. *Nutrition* 2001;17:632.
219. Lotz M et al. Evidence for phosphorus depletion syndrome in man. *N Engl J Med* 1968;278: 409.
220. Roxe DM et al. Phosphate-binding effects of sucralfate in patients with chronic renal failure. *Am J Kidney Dis* 1989;13:194.
221. Cox GJ et al. The effects of high doses of aluminum and iron on phosphorus metabolism. *J Biol Chem* 1931;92:11.
222. Marwich TH et al. Severe hypophosphatemia induced by glucose-insulin-potassium therapy: a case report and proposal for altered protocol. *Int J Cardiol* 1988;18:327.
223. Stein JH et al. Hypophosphatemia in acute alcoholism. *Am J Med* 1996;252:78.
224. Fiaccadori E et al. Hypophosphatemia in course of chronic obstructive pulmonary disease: prevalence, mechanisms, and relationships with skeletal muscle phosphorus content. *Chest* 1990;97:857.
225. Lennquist S et al. Hypophosphatemia in severe burns. *A prospective study. Acta Chirurgica Scandiavica* 1979;145:1.
226. Kebler R et al. Dynamic changes in serum phosphorus levels in diabetic ketoacidosis. *Am J Med* 1985;79:571.
227. Massry SG. The clinical syndrome of phosphate depletion. *Adv Exp Med Biol* 1978;103:301.
228. Lichtman MA et al. Reduced red cell glycolysis, 1,2-diphosphoglycerate and adenosine triphosphate concentration and increased hemoglobin-oxygen affinity caused by hypophosphatemia. *Ann Intern Med* 1971;74:562.
229. Narins RG et al. Diagnostic strategies in disorders of fluid, electrolyte and acid-base homeostasis. *Am J Med* 1982;72:496.
230. Subramanian R et al. Severe hypophosphatemia. Pathophysiologic implications, clinical presentations, and treatment. *Medicine* 2000;79:1.
231. Rubin MF et al. Hypophosphatemia: pathophysiological and practical aspects of its therapy. *Semin Nephrol* 1990;10:536.
232. Rosen GH et al. Intravenous phosphate repletion regimen for critically ill patients with moderate hypophatemia. *Crit Care Med* 1995;23:1204.
233. Charron T et al. Intravenous phosphate in the intensive care unit: More aggressive repletion regimens for moderate and severe hypophosphatemia. *Intensive Care Med* 2003;29:1273.
234. Wacker WEC et al. Magnesium metabolism. *N Engl J Med* 1968;278:658.
235. Kurachi Y et al. Role of intracellular Mg^{2+} in the activation of muscarinic K^+ channel in cardiac atrial cell membrane. *Pflugers Arch* 1986;407:572.

236. White RE et al. Magnesium ions in cardiac function. Regulator of ion channels and second messengers. *Biochem Pharmacol* 1989;38:859.
237. Seelig MS. The magnesium requirement by the normal adult: summary and analysis of published data. *Am J Clin Nutr* 1964;14:212.
238. Jones JE et al. Magnesium requirements in adults. *Am J Clin Nutr* 1967;20:632.
239. Schmulen AC et al. Effect of 1,25-$(OH)_2D_3$ on jejunal absorption of magnesium in patients with chronic renal disease. *Am J Physiol* 1980;238:G349.
240. Heaton FW. The parathyroid glands and magnesium metabolism in the rat. *Clin Sci* 1965;28:543.
241. Quamme GA. Renal magnesium handling: new insights in understanding old problems. *Kidney Int* 1997:52.
242. Massry SG et al. Renal handling of magnesium in the dog. *Am J Physiol* 1969;216:1460.
243. Lennon EJ et al. A comparison of the effects of glucose ingestion and NH_4Cl acidosis on urinary calcium and magnesium excretion in man. *J Clin Invest* 1970;49:1458.
244. Quamme GA. Effect of furosemide on calcium and magnesium transport in the rat nephron. *Am J Physiol* 1981;241:F340.
245. Wong NLM et al. Effects of mannitol on water and electrolyte transport in the dog kidney. *J Lab Clin Med* 1979;94:683.
246. Morel F. Sites of hormone action in the mammalian nephron. *Am J Physiol* 1981;240:F159.
247. Massry SG et al. The hormonal and non-hormonal control of renal excretion of calcium and magnesium. *Nephron* 1973;10:66.
248. Horton R et al. Effect of aldosterone on the metabolism of magnesium. *Clin Endocrinol Metab* 1962;22:1187.
249. Lim P et al. Tissue magnesium levels in chronic diarrhea. *J Lab Clin Med* 1977;80:313.
250. Alfrey AC et al. Evaluation of body magnesium stores. *J Lab Clin Med* 1974;84:153.
251. Thoren L. Magnesium metabolism. *Proc Surg* 1971;9:131.
252. Potts JT et al. Clinical significance of magnesium deficiency and its relationship to parathyroid disease. *Am J Med Sci* 1958;235:205.
253. Jackson CE et al. Routine serum magnesium analysis: correlation with clinical state in 5100 patients. *Ann Intern Med* 1968;69:743.
254. Rasmussen HS et al. Intravenous magnesium in acute myocardial infarction. *Lancet* 1986;1:234.
255. Chernow B et al. Hypomagnesemia in patients in post-operative intensive care. *Chest* 1989;95:391.
256. Shils ME. Experimental human magnesium depletion. *Medicine* 1969;118:61.
257. Caddell JL et al. Studies in protein-calorie malnutrition. 1: Chemical evidence for magnesium deficiency. *N Engl J Med* 1967;276:533.
258. Flink EB et al. Magnesium deficiency after prolonged parenteral fluid administration and after chronic alcoholism, complicated by delirium tremens. *J Lab Clin Med* 1954;43:169.
259. Baron DN. Magnesium deficiency after gastrointestinal surgery and loss of excretions. *Br J Surg* 1960;48:344.
260. Coons CM et al. The retention of nitrogen, calcium, phosphorus and magnesium by pregnant women. *J Biol Chem* 1930;86:1.
261. Booth CC et al. Incidence of hypomagnesaemia in intestinal malabsorption. *BMJ* 1963;2:141.
262. Hallberg DAG. Magnesium problems in gastroenterology. *Acta Med Scand* 1981;661:62.
263. Thoren L. Magnesium deficiency in gastrointestinal fluid loss. *Acta Chirurgica Scandiavica* 1963;306(Suppl.):1.
264. Milla PJ et al. Studies in primary hypomagnesemia: evidence for defective carrier-mediated small intestinal transport of magnesium. *Gut* 1979;20:1028.
265. Evans RA et al. The congenital magnesium-losing kidney: report of two patients. *Q J Med* 1981;197:39.
266. Lam M et al. Hypomagnesemia and renal magnesium wasting in patients treated with cisplatin. *Am J Kidney Dis* 1986;8:164.
267. Keating MJ et al. Hypocalcemia with hypoparathyroidism and renal tubular dysfunction associated with aminoglycoside therapy. *Cancer* 1977;39:1410.
268. Wong NLM et al. Cyclosporin-induced hypomagnesaemia and renal magnesium wasting in rats. *Clin Sci* 1988;75:505.
269. Barton CH et al. Renal magnesium wasting associated with amphotericin B therapy. *Am J Med* 1984;77:471.
270. Coburn JW et al. Changes in serum and urinary calcium during phosphate depletion. Studies on mechanisms. *J Clin Invest* 1970;49:1073.
271. Quamme GA et al. Magnesium transport in the nephron. *Am J Physiol* 1980;8:393.
272. Butler AM et al. Metabolic studies in diabetic coma. *Trans Assoc Am Phys* 1947;60:102.
273. Flink EB et al. Magnesium deficiency after prolonged parenteral fluid administration and after chronic alcoholism, complicated by delirium tremens. *J Lab Clin Med* 1954;43:169.
274. Hellman ES et al. Abnormal water and electrolyte metabolism in acute intermittent porphyria: transient inappropriate secretion of antidiuretic hormone. *Am J Med* 1962;32:734.
275. Tapley DF. Magnesium balance in myxedematous patients treated with triiodothyronine. *Johns Hopkins Medical Journal* 1955;96:274.
276. Heaton FW et al. Magnesium metabolism in patients with parathyroid disorders. *Clin Sci Mol Med* 1963;25:475.
277. Seelig MS. Magnesium deficiency and cardiac dysrhythmia. In: Seelig MS, ed. *Magnesium Deficiency in Pathogenesis of Disease*. New York: Plenum; 1980:219.
278. Iseri LT. Magnesium and cardiac arrhythmias. *Magnesium* 1986;5:111.
279. Oster JR et al. Management of magnesium depletion. *Am J Nephrol* 1988;8:349.
280. Agus Z. Hypomagnesemia. *J Am Soc Nephrol* 1999;10:1616.
281. Alfrey AC. Normal and abnormal magnesium metabolism. In: Schrier RW, ed. *Renal and Electrolyte Disorders*. 6th ed. Philadelphia: Lippincott Williams & Wilkins; 2003.
282. Flink EB. Magnesium deficiency in alcoholism. Alcoholism: clinical and experimental research. *Alcohol Clin Exp Res* 1986;10:590.
283. Flink EB. Therapy of magnesium deficiency. *Ann NY Acad Sci* 1969;162:901.
284. Sachter JJ. Magnesium in the 1990s: implications for acute care. *Topics in Emergency Medicine* 1992; 14:23.
285. Iseri LT et al. Magnesium: nature's physiologic calcium blocker. *Am Heart J* 1984;108:188.
286. Rude RK et al. Renal tubular maximum for magnesium in normal, hyperparathyroid, and hypoparathyroid man. *J Clin Endocrinol Metab* 1980; 51:1425.
287. Coburn JW et al. The physicochemical state and renal handling of divalent ions in chronic renal failure. *Arch Intern Med* 1967;124:302.
288. Massry SG et al. Divalent ion metabolism in patients with acute renal failure: studies on the mechanisms of hypocalcemia. *Kidney Int* 1974;5:437.
289. Mordes JP et al. Excess magnesium. *Pharmacol Rev* 1978;29:273.
290. Jones J et al. Cathartic-induced magnesium toxicity during overdose management. *Ann Emerg Med* 1986;15:1214.
291. Pritchard JA. The use of magnesium ion in the management of eclamptogenic toxemias. *Surg Gynecol Obstet* 1955;100:131.
292. Alfrey AC et al. Hypermagnesemia after renal homotransplantation. *Ann Intern Med* 1970;73:367.

CARDIAC AND VASCULAR DISORDERS

Wayne A. Kradjan
SECTION EDITOR

CHAPTER 12

Dyslipidemias, Atherosclerosis, and Coronary Heart Disease

Matthew K. Ito

Dyslipidemias (one or more abnormalities of blood lipids) produce atherosclerosis, which in turn produces coronary heart disease (CHD) and coronary artery disease (CAD). Successful management of dyslipidemias alters the natural course of atherosclerosis and prevents CHD as well as other forms of atherosclerosis. This is the simple but profound notion behind the modern approach to reducing the incidence of the nation's number-one killer. The challenge for the clinician is to know how to assess the patient's CHD risk, to understand lipid-modulating therapies, to match the intensity of treatment with the patient's risk, and to implement treatments that meet and maintain treatment goals. The principal focus of this chapter is on providing the information required to meet this challenge.

Lipid Metabolism and Drug Effects

The journey begins with acquiring an understanding of how lipids are formed, transported, and utilized; how these processes can go awry; and how our therapies alter these aberrant processes. At the center of these processes are cholesterol, triglycerides (TG), and phospholipids. Of these three, cholesterol plays the central role in the pathogenesis of atherosclerosis. Cholesterol is a naturally occurring sterol that is essential for life. It is the precursor molecule for the formation of bile acids (which are required for absorption of nutrients), the synthesis of steroid hormones (which provide important modulating effects in the body), and the formation of cell membranes. TG are an important source of stored energy in adipose tissue. TG are synthesized from three molecules of fatty acids esterified to glycerol. Phospholipids are a class of lipids formed from fatty acids, a negatively charged phosphate group, nitrogen containing alcohol, and a glycerol backbone. Phospholipids are essential for cellular function and the transport of lipids in the circulation by forming a membrane bilayer of lipoproteins (discussed below).

In Vivo Cholesterol Synthesis

Cells derive cholesterol in two ways: by intracellular synthesis or by uptake from the systemic circulation. Within each cell, cholesterol is synthesized through a series of biochemical steps, many of which are catalyzed by enzymes (Fig. 12-1). One important and early step in its synthesis is the conversion of hydroxymethylglutaryl-coenzyme A (HMG-CoA) to mevalonic acid. The enzyme HMG-CoA reductase catalyzes this step. One of the most effective therapies developed to date for managing dyslipidemias (i.e., HMG-CoA reductase inhibitors or statins) interferes with this enzyme and thereby reduces the cellular synthesis of cholesterol. Other catalytic enzymes involved in the biosynthesis of cholesterol, including HMG-CoA synthase and squalene synthase, have been targets in the search for therapies to reduce cholesterol synthesis. Drugs modifying these enzymes, however, caused more, not less, atherosclerotic disease. For example, a drug released for cholesterol lowering in the 1950s, MER 29, interfered with a late step in cholesterol biosynthesis and effectively reduced cellular cholesterol production, but caused a toxic accumulation of desmosterol and other cholesterol precursors that resulted in the development of cataracts and myocardial ischemia.

Intracellular cholesterol is stored in an esterified form. Free cholesterol is converted to this ester form through the action of the enzyme acetyl CoA acetyl transferase (ACAT). Two forms of ACAT have been identified. ACAT1 is present in many tissues, including inflammatory cells, whereas ACAT2 is present in intestinal mucosa cells and hepatocytes. ACAT2 is required for the esterification and absorption of dietary cholesterol from the gut. In theory, inhibition of this enzyme should reduce the absorption of dietary cholesterol, the secretion of cholesterol by the liver, and even the uptake and storage of circulating cholesterol in inflammatory cells in the arterial wall. Several inhibitors of ACAT have been developed. These inhibitors do not appear to reduce atherosclerosis, however.[1]

Lipoproteins

The second way cells obtain cholesterol is by extracting it from the systemic circulation. The source of this cholesterol is the liver, where it is synthesized and secreted into the systemic circulation. Because cholesterol and other fatty substances are insoluble in water, they are formed into complexes (particles) in the hepatocyte and gut before being secreted into the aqueous medium of the blood. These particles contain an oily inner lipid core made up of cholesterol esters and TG and an outer hydrophilic coat made up of phospholipids and unesterified cholesterol (Fig. 12-2). The outer coat also contains at least one protein, which provides the ligand for interaction with receptors on cell surfaces. The presence of a central lipid core and an outer protein gives rise to the name of these particles, *lipoproteins*.

The three major lipoproteins found in the blood of fasting (10–12 hours) patients are very-low-density lipoprotein (VLDL), low-density lipoprotein (LDL), and high-density lipoprotein (HDL).[2] These particles vary in size, composition, and accompanying proteins (Table 12-1).

VERY-LOW-DENSITY LIPOPROTEINS

Very-low density lipoprotein particles are formed in the liver (Fig. 12-2). They normally contain 15% to 20% of the total blood cholesterol concentration and most of the total blood TG concentration. The concentration of cholesterol in these particles is approximately one fifth of the total TG concentration; thus, if the total TG concentration is known, the VLDL-cholesterol (VLDL-C) level can be estimated by dividing total TG by 5. VLDL particles are large and appear to play only a small role in the pathogenesis of atherosclerosis.

VLDL REMNANTS

As VLDL particles flow through capillaries, some of their TG content is removed through the action of the enzyme lipoprotein lipase. Drugs that enhance the activity of lipoprotein lipase (i.e., fibrates) increase the delipidization process and lower blood TG levels. The removed TG is converted to fatty acids and stored as an energy source in adipose tissue. As TG are removed, the VLDL particle becomes progressively smaller and relatively more cholesterol rich. The particles formed through this process include small VLDL particles (called remnant VLDL), intermediate-density lipoproteins (IDL), and LDL (Fig. 12-2). Approximately 50% of the remnant VLDL and IDL particles are removed from the systemic circulation by receptors on the surface of the liver (receptors called LDL or B-E receptors); the other 50% are converted into LDL particles.

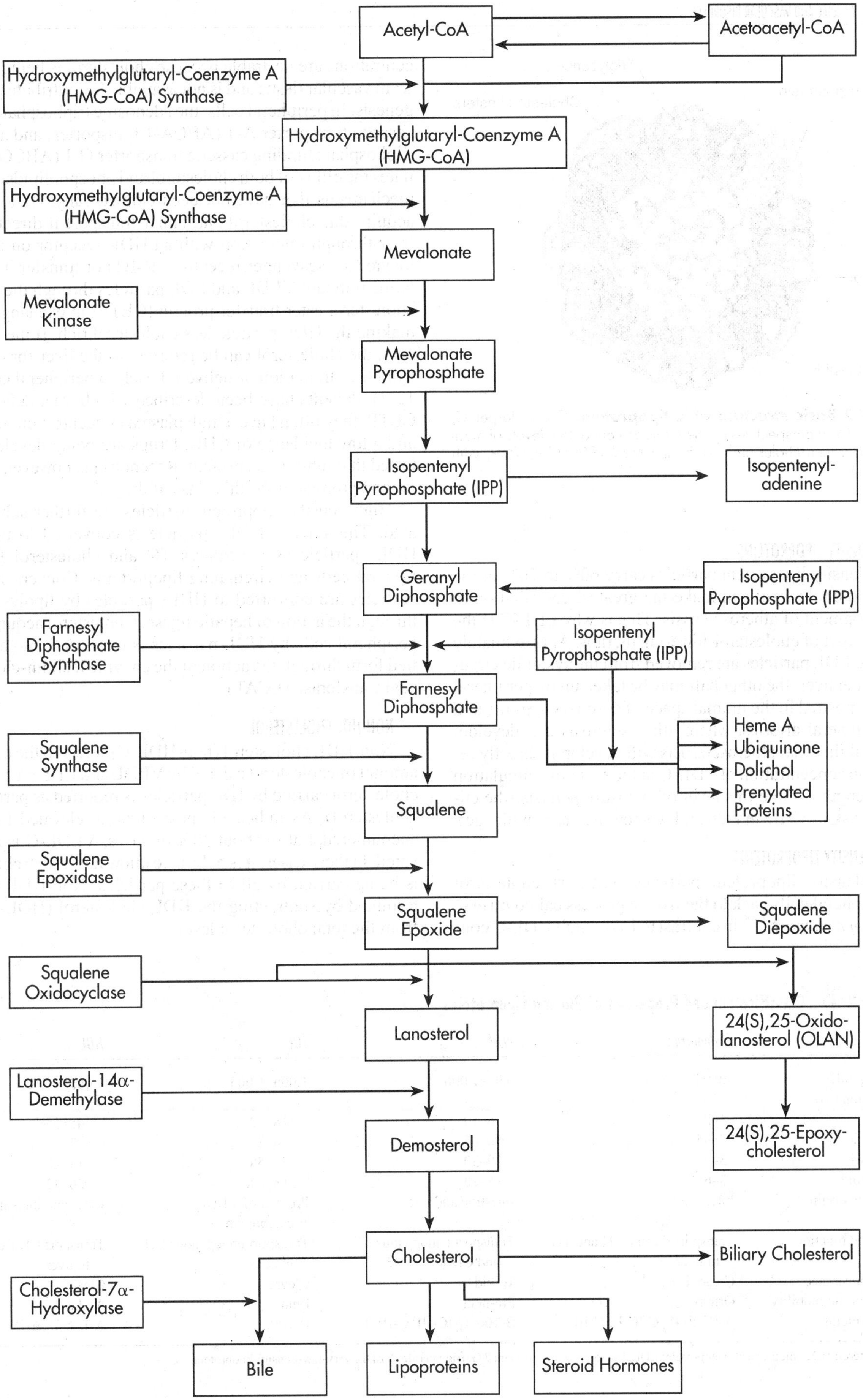

FIGURE 12-1 Biosynthetic pathway of cholesterol.

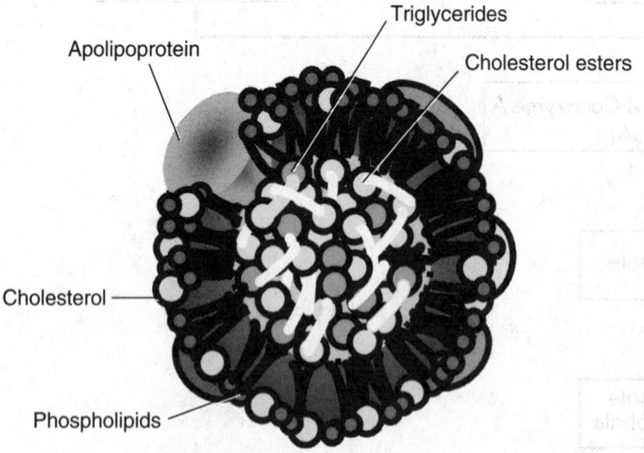

FIGURE 12-2 Basic structure of a lipoprotein. (From Harper C, Jacobsen T. New perspectives on the management of low levels of high-density lipoprotein cholesterol. *Arch Inter Med* 1999;159;1049, with permission.)

LOW-DENSITY LIPOPROTEINS

Low-density lipoprotein particles carry 60% to 70% of the total blood cholesterol and make the greatest contribution to the development of atherosclerosis. This is why LDL-C is the primary target of cholesterol-lowering therapy. Approximately half of the LDL particles are removed from the systemic circulation by the liver; the other half may be taken up by peripheral cells or deposited in the intimal space of coronary, carotid, and other peripheral arteries, where atherosclerosis can develop. The probability that atherosclerosis will develop is directly related to the concentration of LDL-C in the systemic circulation and the length of time this level of exposure persists (the cumulative risk of CHD in men and women increases with age).

HIGH-DENSITY LIPOPROTEINS

High-density lipoprotein particles transport cholesterol from peripheral cells back to the liver, a process called *reverse cholesterol transport*.[3–5] In contrast to LDL, high HDL-C concentrations are desirable because cholesterol is being removed from vascular tissue and is not available to contribute to atherogenesis. In peripheral cells, the adenosine triphosphate binding cassette transporter A-1 (ABCA-1 transporter) and adenosine triphosphate binding cassette transporter G-1 (ABCG-1) facilitates the efflux of both cholesterol and phospholipids. Through mechanisms that have not been defined fully, HDL particles acquire this cholesterol and either transport it directly to the liver through interaction with an HDL receptor on the hepatocyte (the scavenger receptor, SR-B1) or transfer it to circulating remnant VLDL and LDL particles through the action of cholesterol ester transfer protein (CETP) in exchange for TG making the HDL particle less cholesterol rich. If the latter occurs, the cholesterol can be returned to the liver for clearance from the circulation or delivered back to peripheral cells (Fig. 12-3). Patients have been described who have a deficiency of CETP; they often have a high plasma concentration of HDL-C and a low incidence of CHD. Drugs are being developed and tested that inhibit this protein. Recent trials, however, have not looked promising for this class of drugs.[6]

High-density lipoprotein particles are further subfractionated. The smaller HDL_3 particle is converted to the larger HDL_2 particle as it acquires TG and cholesterol from peripheral cells and circulating lipoproteins. Conversely, HDL_2 particles are converted to HDL_3 particles by lipolysis of TG through the action of hepatic lipase. Cholesterol acquired from peripheral cells by HDL particles is converted into an esterified form through the action of the enzyme lecithin-cholesterol acyl transferase (LCAT).

NON-HDL CHOLESTEROL

Non-HDL cholesterol (non-HDL-C) refers to the combined amount of cholesterol carried by VLDL and LDL particles (the cholesterol carried by IDL particles is reported as part of LDL cholesterol). As indicated, most often an elevated LDL-C is encountered, but in about 30% of cases, VLDL-C is also elevated. In these cases, it is helpful to know how much cholesterol is being carried by all of these particles. Non-HDL-C is determined by subtracting the HDL-cholesterol (HDL-C) level from the total cholesterol level.

Table 12-1 Classification and Properties of Plasma Lipoproteins

	Chylomicron	*VLDL*	*LDL*	*HDL*
Density (g/mL)	<0.94	0.94–1.006	1.006–1.063	1.063–1.210
Composition (%)				
Protein	1–2	6–10	18–22	45–55
Triglyceride	85–95	50–65	4–8	2–7
Cholesterol	3–7	20–30	51–58	18–25
Phospholipid	3–6	15–20	18–24	26–32
Physiologic origin	Intestine	Intestine and liver	Product of VLDL catabolism	Liver and intestine
Physiologic function	Transport dietary CH and TG to liver	Transport endogenous TG and CH	Transport endogenous CH to cells	Transport CH from cells to liver
Plasma appearance	Cream layer	Turbid	Clear	Clear
Electrophoretic mobility	Origin	Pre-beta	Beta	Alpha
Apolipoproteins	A-IV, B-48, C-IC-II, C-III	B-100, C-IC-III, C-III, E	B-100, (a)	A-I, A-II, A-IV

CH, cholesterol; HDL, high-density lipoprotein; LDL, low-density lipoprotein; TG, triglyceride; VLDL, very-low-density lipoprotein.

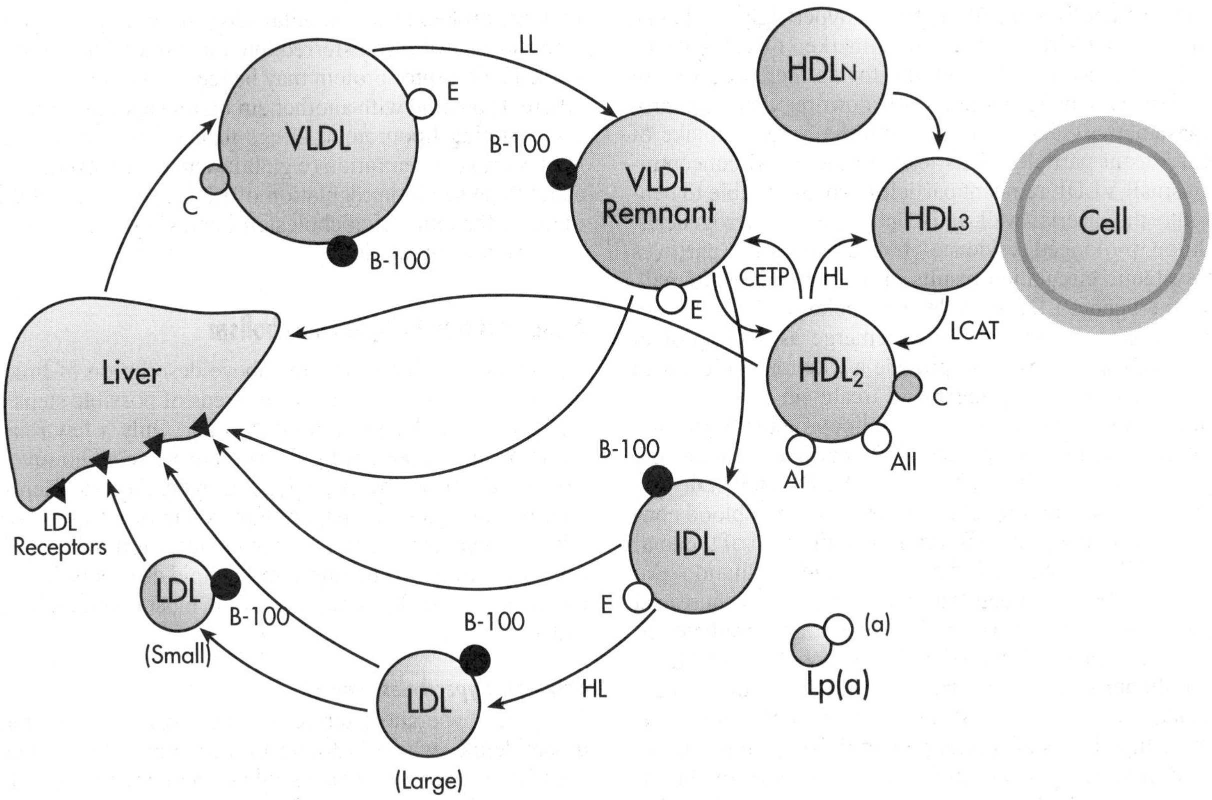

FIGURE 12-3 The lipoproteins, apolipoproteins, and enzymes involved in the transport of cholesterol and triglycerides. HDL, high-density lipoprotein; IDL, intermediate-density lipoprotein; LDL, low-density lipoprotein; VLDL, very-low-density lipoprotein.

CHYLOMICRONS

Unlike the lipoproteins that transport cholesterol from the liver to peripheral cells and back (endogenous system), chylomicrons transport fatty acids and cholesterol derived from the diet or synthesized in the intestines from the gut to the liver (exogenous system) (Fig. 12-3 and Table 12-1). Chylomicrons are large, TG-rich lipoproteins. As they pass through capillary beds on the way to the liver, some of the TG content is removed through the action of lipoprotein lipase in a manner similar to that described for TG removal from VLDL particles. In the rare individual who has a lipoprotein lipase deficiency, this removal process is faulty and TG levels in the blood become very high (e.g., 1,000 to 5,000 mg/dL).

Following a fatty meal, the number of chylomicron particles (and therefore the concentration of TG) is high. If the patient fasts for 10 to 12 hours, however, chylomicrons will have time to be removed from the blood. TG concentrations obtained during fasting reflect TG that is produced by the liver and carried in VLDL and other remnant particles (unless the patient has a rare chylomicron clearance disorder). This is why patients are asked to fast before a lipoprotein profile is obtained. A blood sample that is rich in chylomicrons (and to a lesser extent VLDL particles) appears turbid; the higher the TG level, the more turbid the sample. If the sample from a patient with hyperchylomicronemia is refrigerated, chylomicrons will float to the top and form a frothy white layer, whereas smaller VLDL stay suspended below.

Apolipoproteins

Each lipoprotein particle contains proteins on its outer surface called *apolipoproteins* (Fig. 12-3 and Table 12-1). These proteins have three functions: (*a*) provide structure to the lipoprotein, (*b*) activate enzyme systems, and (*c*) bind with cell receptors.[2] Abnormal metabolism of apolipoproteins, even in the face of seemingly normal blood cholesterol levels, can result in faulty enzyme activity or cholesterol transport and an increased risk of atherosclerosis. Because of this, lipid specialists often assess blood levels of apolipoproteins to evaluate dyslipidemic patients fully, especially those who have a family history of premature CHD. The five most clinically relevant apolipoproteins are A-I, A-II, B-100, C, and E.

Very-high-density lipoprotein particles contain apolipoproteins B-100, E, and C (Fig. 12-3). The B and E proteins are ligands for LDL receptors (also called *B-E receptors*) on the surface of hepatocytes and peripheral cells. Linkage allows the transfer of cholesterol from the circulating lipoprotein into the cell through absorptive endocytosis and cellular uptake of the particle. Defects in these proteins reduce their ability to bind with receptor proteins. This results in defective clearance of lipoproteins from the systemic circulation and increased levels of circulating cholesterol.

Apolipoprotein C-II (Apo C-II) is a cofactor for lipoprotein lipase (LPL). By activating LDL, Apo C-II stimulates the hydrolysis of TG from lipoprotein particles in the capillary beds. Deficiencies of C-II apolipoproteins result in faulty TG metabolism and ultimately in hypertriglyceridemia. Apolipoprotein C-III has become a marker of atherogenic dyslipidemia (described below) and for an increased risk of atherosclerosis. Apolipoprotein C-III downregulates lipoprotein lipase activity and interferes with the hepatic uptake of VLDL remnant particles. This leads to increased concentrations of small VLDL remnant particles, which are able to penetrate into the arterial wall and contribute to atherogenesis. In addition, prolonged residence of VLDL and LDL particles in the systemic circulation results in the formation of small, highly atherogenic LDL particles (see below).[7] With further research, apolipoprotein C-III may emerge as an important marker of atherosclerosis and provide a way for clinicians to identify patients requiring aggressive treatment.

Remnant VLDL particles retain apolipoproteins B-100 and E during the delipidization process; LDL particles contain only apolipoprotein B-100 (Fig. 12-3). Each VLDL and LDL particle contains one apolipoprotein B-100. Thus, the blood concentration of apolipoprotein B-100 is an indication of the total *number* of VLDL and LDL particles in the circulation. An increased number of lipoprotein particles (i.e., an increased apolipoprotein B-100 concentration) is a strong predictor of CHD risk. The ratio of non–HDL-C (total cholesterol–HDL-C) to apolipoprotein B-100 gives an estimate of the cholesterol contained in each VLDL and LDL particle. Some patients have high levels of apolipoprotein B-100 (suggesting an increased number of VLDL and LDL particles in the circulation), even though their cholesterol level is in the desirable range. These patients have an increased risk of atherosclerosis. A apolipoprotein B-100:LDL-C ratio greater than 1 is also an indicator of the presence of small, dense LDL—particles that convey a higher CHD risk than larger LDL particles.

High-density lipoprotein particles contain apolipoproteins A-I, A-II, and C. A-I protein activates LCAT, which catalyzes the esterification of free cholesterol in HDL particles. Levels of apolipoprotein A-I have a stronger inverse correlation with CHD risk than apolipoprotein A-II levels. HDL particles that contain only A-I apolipoproteins (LpA-I) are associated with a lower CHD risk than are HDL particles containing both A-I and A-II (LpA-I, A-II).[8]

LDL Receptor

The uptake of cholesterol into peripheral and hepatic cells is accomplished by the binding of apolipoproteins B-100 and E on circulating lipoproteins to cell-surface LDL receptors. The synthesis of LDL receptors is stimulated by a low intracellular cholesterol concentration.[8] Within the cell, the receptor protein travels from the mitochondria (where it is synthesized) to the cell surface (where it migrates to an area called the *coated pits*). Once in this position, it is capable of binding with lipoproteins that contain apolipoprotein E or B-100, including VLDL, remnant VLDL, IDL, and LDL. Because remnant VLDL and IDL particles contain both B-100 and E proteins, they may have a higher affinity for LDL receptors than do LDL particles, which contain only the B protein. Furthermore, drugs that increase the synthesis of LDL receptors (e.g., statins) can increase the clearance of both VLDL remnant particles and LDL particles from the circulation. This would account for their ability to reduce serum TG levels as well as cholesterol levels. After these proteins are bound, the lipoproteins undergo endocytosis and are taken up by lysosomes, where they are broken into elemental substances for use by the cell. The cholesterol is transferred into the intracellular cholesterol pool. The receptor protein may be returned to the cell surface, where it can bind with another circulating apolipoprotein E- or B-containing lipoprotein. Drugs that reduce the intracellular cholesterol concentration (e.g., bile acid resins, ezetimibe, and statins) cause the upregulation of LDL receptors and thereby increase the removal of cholesterol-carrying lipoproteins from the systemic circulation.

Abnormalities in Lipid Metabolism

As can be imagined from the above description of lipid synthesis and transport, literally hundreds of possible steps could malfunction and cause a lipid disorder. Only a few relatively common and important lipid disorders are seen, however. The first two described below, polygenic hypercholesterolemia and atherogenic dyslipidemia, are largely the result of an interaction between genes and lifestyle choices; following these are several prominent, but rarer familial lipid disorders. Table 12-2 summarizes the characteristics of the most common lipid disorders.

Polygenic Hypercholesterolemia

Polygenic hypercholesterolemia, the most prevalent form of dyslipidemia, which is found in more than 25% of the U.S. population, is caused by a combination of environmental (e.g., poor nutrition, sedentary lifestyle) and genetic factors (thus, the term "polygenic"). Saturated fatty acids in the diet of these patients can reduce LDL receptor activity, thus reducing the clearance of LDL particles from the systemic circulation. As a result, patients with polygenic hypercholesterolemia have mild to moderate LDL-C elevations (usually in the range of 130 to 250 mg/dL), but no unique physical findings are seen. Family history of premature CHD is present in approximately 20% of cases. These patients are effectively managed with dietary restriction in saturated fats and cholesterol and by drugs that lower LDL-C levels (i.e., statins, bile acid sequestrants, niacin, and ezetimibe).

Atherogenic Dyslipidemia

Atherogenic dyslipidemia is found in about 25% of patients who have a lipid disorder. It is characterized by a moderate TG elevation (150 to 500 mg/dL; indicative of the increased presence of VLDL remnant particles), a low HDL-C level (<40 mg/dL); and a moderately high LDL-C level (including increased concentrations of small-dense LDL particles). Most commonly, these patients are either overweight or obese with increased waist circumference, hypertensive, and insulin resistant with or without diabetes and are said to have the *metabolic syndrome*.

Patients who are obese or have diabetes have an increased mobilization of fatty acids from adipose cells to the systemic circulation, which leads to increased TG synthesis and secretion of VLDL particles by the liver. Often these particles contain apolipoprotein C-III, which interferes with the action of lipoprotein lipase, thus retarding lipolysis of TG from VLDL particles. This results in the formation of TG-rich VLDL remnant particles. TG from these particles is exchanged with cholesterol esters from HDL under the influence of CETP, which means the VLDL remnant particles become enriched

Table 12-2 Characteristics of Common Lipid Disorders

Disorder	Metabolic Defect	Lipid Effect	Main Lipid Parameter	Diagnostic Features
Polygenic hypercholesterolemia	↓LDL clearance	↑LDL-C	LDL-C: 130–250 mg/dL TG: 150–500 mg/dL	None distinctive
Atherogenic dyslipidemia	↑VLDL secretion, ↑C-III synthesis ↓LPL activity ↓VLDL removal	↑TG ↑Remnant VLDL ↓HDL ↑Small, dense LDL	HDL-C: <40 mg/dL	Frequently accompanied by central obesity or diabetes
Familial hypercholesterolemia (heterozygous)	Dysfunctional or absent LDL receptors	↑LDL-C	LDL-C: 250–450 mg/dL	Family history of CHD, tendon xanthomas
Familial defective apoB-100	Defective ApoB on LDL and VLDL	↑LDL-C	LDL-C: 250–450 mg/dL	Family history of CHD, tendon xanthomas
Dysbetalipoproteinemia (type III hyperlipidemia)	ApoE2:E2 phenotype, ↓VLDL remnant clearance	↑Remnant VLDL, ↑IDL	LDL-C: 300–600 mg/dL TGs: 400–800 mg/dL	Palmar xanthomas, tuberoeruptive xanthomas
Familial combined hyperlipidemia	↑ApoB and VLDL production	↑CH, TG, or both	LDL-C: 250–350 mg/dL TGs: 200–800 mg/dL	Family history, CHD Family history, Hyperlipidemia
Familial hyperapobetalipoproteinemia	↑ApoB production	↑ApoB	ApoB: >125 mg/dL	None distinctive
Hypoalphalipoproteinemia	↑HDL catabolism	↓HDL-C	HDL-C: <40 mg/dL	None distinctive

ApoB, apolipoprotein B; ApoE, apolipoprotein E; CH, cholesterol; CHD, coronary heart disease; IDL, intermediate-density lipoprotein; LDL, low-density lipoprotein; LDL-C, low-density lipoprotein cholesterol; TGs, triglycerides; VLDL, very-low-density lipoprotein.

with cholesterol whereas HDL particles lose cholesterol (and gain TG) (Fig. 12-3). TG is also exchanged from VLDL remnant particles with cholesterol esters from LDL particles. Thus, VLDL remnants become even more cholesterol enriched and LDL becomes TG enriched. The cholesterol-enriched, small VLDL remnant particle is atherogenic. TG-rich LDL and HDL particles undergo lipolysis catalyzed by hepatic lipase to remove TG, leaving small, cholesterol ester-deficient LDL particles (called *small dense LDL*) that are highly atherogenic and a reduction in HDL-C from the loss of apolipoprotein A-I by the kidneys.[9]

Patients with atherogenic dyslipidemia can often be effectively managed with weight reduction and increased physical activity. If needed, drugs that enhance the removal of remnant VLDL and small dense LDL particles (i.e., statins) and that lower TG levels (i.e., niacin or fibrates) are effective in the management of these cases.

Familial Hypercholesterolemia

Familial hypercholesterolemia (FH) is the classic lipid disorder of defective clearance. This autosomal dominant disorder is strongly associated with premature CHD.[10,11] Heterozygotes (1 of 500 people in the United States) of this disorder inherit one defective LDL receptor gene. Consequently, these persons possess approximately half the number of functioning LDL receptors and double the LDL-C level of unaffected patients (i.e., LDL-C of 250 to 450 mg/dL).[12,13] Clinically, heterozygous FH patients may deposit cholesterol in the iris, leading to arcus senilis. Cholesterol also deposits in tendons, particularly the Achilles' tendon and extensor tendons of the hands, leading to tendon xanthomas. The clinical diagnosis of FH is established by documenting a very high LDL-C level, a strong family history of premature CHD events, and the presence of tendon xanthomas. Untreated heterozygous FH patients have approximately a 5% chance of a myocardial infarction (MI) by age 30, a 50% chance by age 50, and an 85% chance by age 60. The mean age of death in untreated male heterozygotes is in the mid 50s; for untreated female heterozygotes, it is in the mid 60s.[14]

Homozygotes (1 of 1,000,000 people in the United States) for this disorder inherit a defective LDL receptor gene from both parents and generally have LDL-C levels >500 mg/dL. This rare disorder results in CHD by age 10 to 20 years. Because these individuals have lost the ability to clear cholesterol-carrying lipoproteins from the circulation, apheresis (analogous to dialysis for the kidney patient) is required to help remove these atherogenic particles.

Familial defective apolipoprotein B-100 (FDB) is a genetic disorder clinically indistinguishable from heterozygous FH. These patients have normally functioning LDL receptors, but a defective apolipoprotein B-100, which results in reduced binding to LDL receptors and reduced clearance of LDL particles from the systemic circulation.[15,16] As with FH, LDL-C levels are 250 to 450 mg/dL.[15,17,18] Presumably, the apolipoprotein E and half of the apolipoprotein B in heterozygous FDB patients function normally, providing mechanisms for removal of these lipoproteins from the systemic circulation. Clinical diagnosis of FDB, as FH, is based on a very high LDL-C level, a family history of premature CHD, and tendon xanthomas. The definitive diagnosis requires molecular screening techniques.

Familial Dysbetalipoproteinemia

Familial dysbetalipoproteinemia (also called *type III hyperlipidemia* and *remnant disease*) is caused by poor clearance of VLDL and chylomicron particles from the systemic circulation.[19] Apolipoprotein E is necessary for the normal clearance of these particles. It is inherited as an E2, E3, or E4 isoform from each parent. The E2 isoform has a low binding affinity for the LDL receptor. Thus, individuals with an apolipoprotein E2:E2 phenotype have delayed clearance of

VLDL remnant (and possibly chylomicron) particles from the circulation and a reduced conversion of IDL to LDL particles. A lipid disorder, however, usually does not result unless triggered by other metabolic problems (e.g., diabetes, hypothyroidism, or obesity). Clinically, these patients have high cholesterol (owing to an enrichment of cholesterol esters in VLDL remnant particles), high TG (usually in the range of 400 to 800 mg/dL), and a VLDL-C:TG ratio >0.3.[20] Some patients have palmar xanthomas (yellow-orange discoloration in the creases of the palms and fingers) and tuberoeruptive xanthomas (small, raised lesions in areas of pressure, particularly the elbows and knees). A personal and family history of premature atherosclerotic vascular disease often is present. As noted above, these patients often have diabetes mellitus, hypertension, obesity, and hyperuricemia.

Familial Combined Hyperlipidemia

Familial combined hyperlipidemia (FCHL) is the classic example of a dyslipidemia caused by increased production of lipoproteins. For reasons that are not clear, patients with FCHL overproduce apolipoprotein B-containing particles, VLDL, and LDL.[21–23] Many patients have an elevated apolipoprotein B-100 level.[24] As the name implies, patients with this disorder may have hypercholesterolemia (usually in the range of 250 to 350 mg/dL), or hypertriglyceridemia (usually between 200 and 800 mg/dL) or a combination of both (usually with a low HDL-C level). First-degree relatives of these individuals frequently have a lipid disorder. A family history of premature CHD is often present as well. Patients with FCHL commonly are overweight and hypertensive and also may have diabetes or hyperuricemia. A diagnosis of FCHL is presumed in patients who have increased cholesterol or TG levels, a strong family history of premature CHD, and a family history of dyslipidemia.

Familial Hyperapobetalipoproteinemia

Familial hyperapobetalipoproteinemia is a variant of FCHL. This disorder is characterized by increased hepatic production of apolipoprotein B in the absence of other lipid abnormalities.[25] These patients have acceptable LDL-C and TG levels and a family history of CHD. Their apolipoprotein B-100 concentration is usually >125 mg/dL, indicating an increase in the *number* of cholesterol-carrying lipoprotein particles. It is likely that FCHL and hyperapobetalipoproteinemia are related disorders, both resulting from excessive secretion of apolipoprotein B-100 containing lipoproteins.[26]

Hypoalphalipoproteinemia

Low HDL-C (<40 mg/dL; hypoalphalipoproteinemia) without an increase in TG level is fairly uncommon, but is associated with increased CHD risk.[27,28] Little, however, is known about the precise molecular defect causing this problem, although genetic influences undoubtedly are involved.[29] Recently, Tangier disease, which is characterized by low HDL-C, orange tonsils, and hepatosplenomegaly, has been linked to a defect in the ABCA-1 transporter responsible for the efflux of cholesterol from peripheral cells. The inherited tendency to have low HDL-C is accentuated by lifestyle factors such as obesity, smoking, and lack of exercise. Despite strong epidemiologic evidence showing an inverse relationship between HDL-C and CHD, clinical trials demonstrating a benefit of raising isolated low HDL-C with drugs are lacking. What has been shown is that lowering LDL-C in patients with low HDL-C reduces CHD risk.[30] It is anticipated that therapies to raise HDL-C will become available and can be tested to see if they reduce CHD risk also.

Rationale for Treating Dyslipidemia

Scientific data from animal studies, genetic studies, epidemiologic studies, and clinical trials support the link between cholesterol, atherosclerosis, and CHD. This collective body of knowledge resoundingly supports a critical role for cholesterol in the pathogenesis of atherosclerosis. Even more important, in clinical trials the lowering of blood cholesterol levels has been consistently associated with reduced CHD, whether the blood cholesterol was reduced by drug, diet, or surgical means. Even the most vigorous cholesterol-lowering approach does not result in the complete amelioration of CHD, however, suggesting that other causes are in play. Some of the significant literature on the pathogenesis of atherosclerosis and clinical trials establishing the link between blood cholesterol and CHD is summarized below.

Pathogenesis of Atherosclerosis

Circulating cholesterol has a central role in the pathogenesis of atherosclerosis. Even the name *atherosclerosis* depicts this (from the Latin *athero* ["porridge-like"] and *sclerosis* ["fibrous-like"]. Atherosclerotic lesions begin with the accumulation of cholesterol from LDL and VLDL remnant particles in the intimal space (Fig. 12-4). The reason this occurs is unknown, but in some way it appears directly related to the level of circulating cholesterol and the provocation by risk factors such as hypertension, smoking, diabetes, stress, and genetic predisposition. An important finding is that native LDL *per se* does not contribute to the development of atherosclerosis;

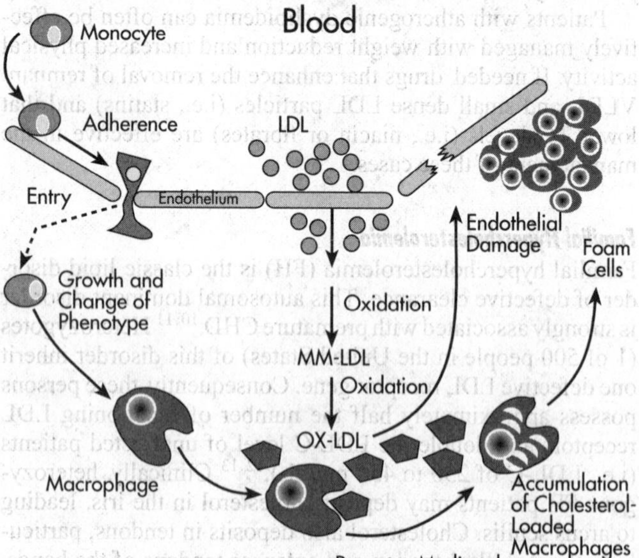

FIGURE 12-4 Some of the steps involved in the development of the fatty streak. LDL, low-density lipoprotein.

instead, LDL must be modified (e.g., oxidized) before it becomes a factor in causing atherosclerosis.

Soon after taking up residence in the subendothelial space, LDL is modified primarily by oxidation. Simultaneously, monocyte adhesion molecules are released from endothelial cells on the surface of the lumen.[31,32] They cause circulating monocytes to attach to the intact endothelial surface, and then chemoattractants cause these monocytes to squeeze between endothelial cells into the intima (Fig. 12-4).[33]

Once recruited, the monocytes are converted to activated macrophage cells, which begin to ingest modified LDL and remnant VLDL particles. These modified particles are taken up by special scavenger or acetyl-LDL receptors on the surface of macrophage cells.[34] Modified LDL serves as another chemoattractant for circulating monocytes, thus causing more monocytes from the systemic circulation to take up residence in the intima. It also inhibits the mobility of resident macrophage cells (blocking the egress of these cells from the intima); macrophage cells become a cytotoxic agent (causing damage to the endothelium).[31] As the uptake of modified LDL into macrophage cells continues, the cells become laden with lipid, grow in size, and eventually become *foam cells* (Fig. 12-4 and Fig. 12-5).

Early in the process, the monocellular layer surrounding the lumen (the endothelium) becomes dysfunctional. Notably, the release of nitric oxide from these cells is impaired, which results in vasoconstriction and ischemic symptoms. Regulation of blood cholesterol levels and management of other risk factors restore endothelial function, nitrous oxide release, and the vasodilatory response.

The accumulation of foam cells in the intimal space below the endothelium eventually results in a raised lesion, the *fatty streak,* which is widely recognized as the precursor to atherosclerosis. Fatty streaks transform the once smooth endothelial surface of the artery into a lumpy, uneven surface. As this process continues, an atherosclerotic plaque is formed. In the initial stages, this plaque is characterized by a large lipid core made up of macrophage (foam) cells filled with cholesterol along the surface and at the shoulders of the lesion (Fig. 12-5).

During plaque growth, a number of cells (including macrophages, endothelial cells, platelets, and smooth muscle cells) secrete chemoattractant and growth factors, which cause smooth muscle cells from the media to migrate upward and proliferate near the luminal surface.[35] Collagen synthesis is increased. This leads to conversion of atherosclerotic lesions that initially are weak and unstable (because they contain a large lipid core surrounded by a thin fibrous cap) to become strong and hard (because they contain a small inner lipid core and much collagen, and matrix). At any given time, atherosclerosis at various stages of development can be found all along the arterial tree in susceptible patients (Fig. 12-4).

As atherosclerotic lesions grow, the coronary artery remodels. Lesions initially grow away from the lumen toward the media, thus preserving the luminal opening and ensuring normal blood flow. Late in the growth of the lesion, however, the

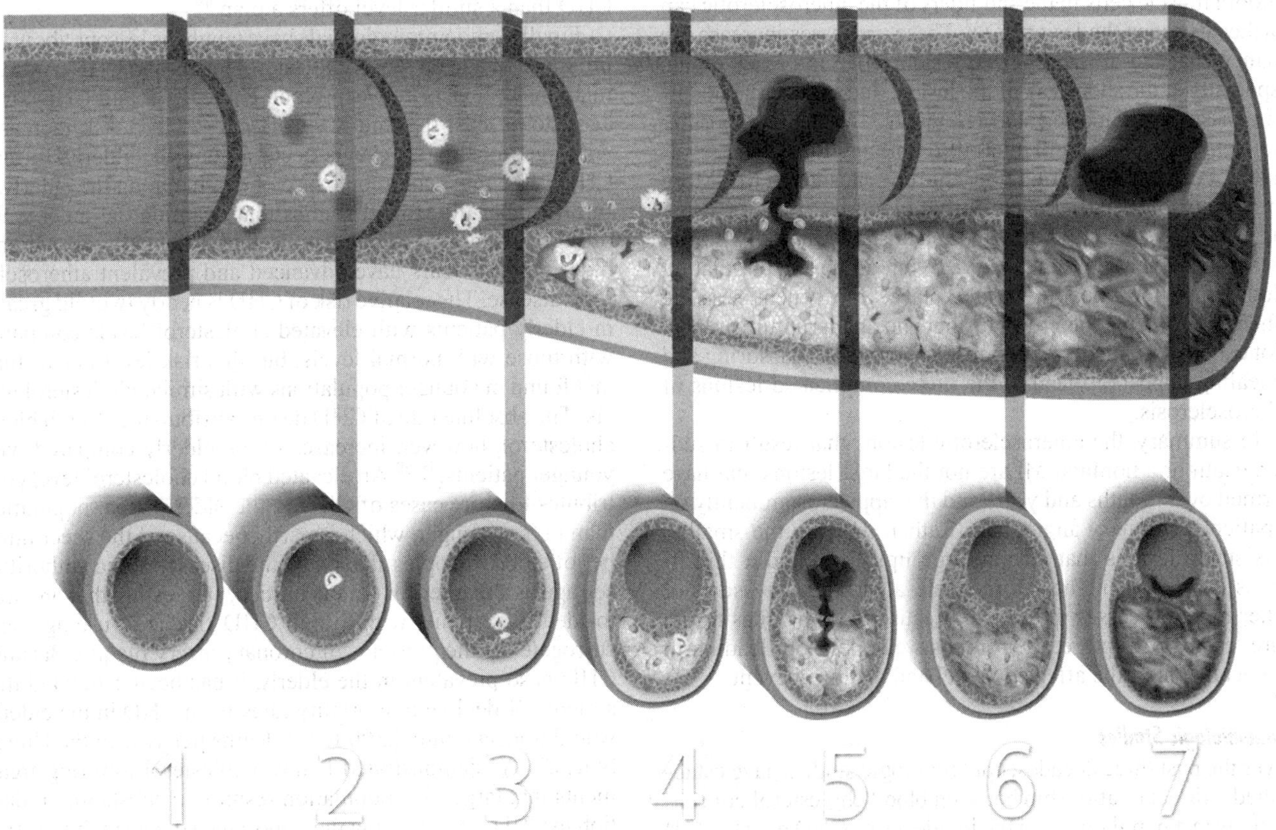

FIGURE 12-5 Initiation, progression, and complication of human coronary atherosclerotic plaque.

luminal space is invaded and becomes progressively narrowed as the atherosclerotic lesion grows.

Similar to the stages of development, atherosclerotic lesions exist along a continuum from vulnerable lesions that can rupture and cause a thrombosis to older, rigid lesions that will not rupture. The younger lesions occupy only the intimal space, whereas the older lesions may protrude into the luminal space. In examining the coronary angiogram of a patient, evidence of stenosis (narrowing of the lumen) indicates the presence of older, more advanced lesions. When these lesions are seen, other lesions distal to the narrowing are likely to be present. They are younger and more susceptible to erosion or rupture, which can cause a thrombosis. In fact, the culprit lesion that results in an MI is usually not at the site of the greatest stenosis, but distal to it.[36]

A number of processes cause younger lesions to become unstable; most of these are a part of an active inflammatory process. The uptake of cholesterol by activated macrophage cells is one of these processes. Chemoattractants, such as monocyte chemoattractant protein-1 (MCP-1), adhesion molecules, and a family of T-cell substances, participate in the migration of monocytes into the intima. Macrophage colony-stimulating factor (M-CSF) contributes to the differentiation of blood monocytes into macrophage cells. T cells elaborate inflammatory cytokines that stimulate macrophages, endothelial cells, and smooth muscle cells. Activated macrophage cells produce proteolytic enzymes that degrade collagen and weaken the fibrous cap.[37] The release of metalloproteinase enzymes causes the destruction of connective tissue and renders the atherosclerotic lesion vulnerable to rupture. Apoptosis (cell death) of smooth muscle cells in the shoulders of the atherosclerotic cap further weakens the lesion.[38–43] These processes increase the chance that the atherosclerotic lesion will rupture or erode, especially at the shoulders of the lesion, and expose the underlying tissue to circulating blood elements.[44] With this exposure, platelets may adhere and microthrombi may form. The resultant clot can occlude blood flow entirely, causing an MI. More commonly, only partial occlusion of blood flow occurs, causing transient ischemic symptoms and unstable angina. The clot creates a barrier between the underlying tissue and circulating blood and allows healing to take place. Subsequently, as the atherosclerotic plaque grows further and again ruptures, a new clot can form to mend the lesion. This process of fissuring and rehealing appears to lead to the more complicated lesions of atherosclerosis.

In summary, the atherosclerotic lesions that result in sudden death or a nonfatal MI are not the large lesions that have formed over months and years and that appear prominently on a patient's coronary angiogram. Rather, they are the smaller, less stable lesions that have a large lipid core and a thin fibrous cap.[45] When shear forces, elevated blood pressure, or other toxic processes in the artery cause these plaques to fissure, erode, or rupture, a thrombosis can develop, leading to the occlusion of the affected vessel and a clinical event.

Epidemiologic Studies

Over the past three decades, epidemiologic studies have established a direct relationship between blood cholesterol concentrations in a population and the incidence of CHD events.[46–48] For every 1% increase in blood cholesterol levels, a 1% to 2% increase exists in the incidence of CHD. HDL-C has an inverse relationship with CHD. For every 1% *decrease* in HDL-C levels, a 1% to 2% *increase* in the risk of CHD events occurs.[49]

Other epidemiologic trials have demonstrated the influence of environmental versus genetic factors on cholesterol levels and CHD incidence. One of the most revealing studies comes from the Honolulu Heart Study, which reported that Japanese individuals who had very low cholesterol levels and a low CHD death rate experienced a rise in cholesterol levels as well as the incidence of CHD when they migrated to Hawaii and subsequently to the west coast of the United States.[50] Similarly, Mexicans who live close to the U.S. border have cholesterol levels and a CHD incidence that is similar to those of U.S. residents, whereas those living in the southern part of Mexico have a lower cholesterol level and a lower incidence of CHD.

Gender differences have been the focus of other epidemiologic studies. Before menopause, the incidence of CHD in women is low,[51,52] but after menopause the rate of CHD in women parallels that of men. In fact, the prevalence of CHD in women is ultimately similar to that in men; it is just displaced by about 10 years.[48,53] Whereas men begin to experience CHD events in their 50s and 60s, women experience it in their 60s and 70s. Eventually, CHD causes nearly as many deaths in women as it does in men.[54] In fact, CHD is the cause of more deaths in women than all forms of cancer combined, including cancer of the breast, ovary, and cervix. Furthermore, the presence of diabetes in a woman with dyslipidemia negates whatever protection she may have had before menopause and is associated with a very high incidence of CHD events.[55,56] Conversely, a high HDL-C level may offer women more protection from CHD than a similar level offers a man.[49]

Finally, epidemiologic trials have taught us lessons about the influence of age on blood cholesterol levels and CHD. A direct relationship exists between blood cholesterol and CHD at all ages, to at least the mid 80s.[57] Because CHD risk increases with age, most CHD events occur among the elderly. In fact, CHD is the most common cause of death among the elderly.[58] Intravascular ultrasound studies that examine the inner walls of coronary arteries demonstrate that practically all patients older than 70 years have advanced and prevalent atherosclerotic disease. The relative risk of CHD is nearly twofold greater in elderly patients with elevated cholesterol levels compared with those with normal levels, but this risk level is less than that found in younger populations with similar cholesterol levels. The absolute rate of CHD deaths attributable to high blood cholesterol, however, increases in the elderly compared with younger patients.[58,59] An elevated blood cholesterol level contributes to more cases of CHD in the older patient population than in the younger, which is partly because of the sheer number of elderly people affected by the disease. Some authorities see age as a marker for plaque burden, suggesting that one way to identify patients with a high CHD risk is to use age as a surrogate for the presence of coronary artery plaque. Because CHD is so prevalent in the elderly, it has been estimated that a mere 1% decline in mortality rates from CHD in the elderly would translate into 4,300 fewer deaths per year in the United States.[60] As demonstrated below, cholesterol-lowering treatments that target this population result in a substantial reduction in CHD, underscoring the importance of age in forecasting a high risk of future CHD events.

Clinical Trials

ANGIOGRAPHIC REGRESSION TRIALS

Based on animal, epidemiologic, and genetic studies, the direct relationship between blood cholesterol levels and CHD events was established. The critical hypothesis that remained to be proven before cholesterol-lowering therapies could be widely recommended was that lowering blood cholesterol levels would reduce CHD risk. The proof for this hypothesis was ultimately demonstrated in clinical trials. The initial test of this hypothesis involved angiographic trials that sought to demonstrate that by lowering blood cholesterol levels, coronary stenosis visualized on coronary angiography would regress.[61–78] Much to the surprise of investigators, this did not occur. In fact, more commonly, cholesterol lowering seemed only to slow lesion progression.

Despite these disappointing results, angiographic trials taught many important lessons. They demonstrated that aggressive lipid lowering caused lesions to progress at a slower rate regardless of the vascular bed under study, including coronary,[62–70,73,74,76–78] carotid,[71,72,75] and femoral arteries.[67,75] They established that this effect was achieved regardless of the lipid-lowering therapy deployed: diet and other lifestyle modification,[64] lipid-lowering drugs,[7,30,38–43,62,63,66,69–77] or ileal bypass surgery.[61] They also suggested that the more aggressive the lipid lowering, especially if it resulted in >60% reduction in LDL-C, the greater the chance of plaque regression.[79,80]

The reason early angiographic studies failed to demonstrate lesion regression was not because this process did not occur, but because the methodology could not detect it. Angiograms outline the lesion from the outside of the coronary artery. Because atherosclerotic lesions initially remodel outward away from the lumen, as explained above, the lumen would appear normal until the late stage of atherosclerosis plaque development. Thus, lesions that were visible on a coronary angiogram were the older, more rigid lesions that were less likely to change with lipid-lowering therapy. Younger lesions, which were not visualized in a coronary angiogram, may well have regressed, however. Recent investigations of the contour of the inner lining of the lumen using intravascular ultrasound report that lipid lowering does cause widespread plaque regression without any change in lumen size.[81]

Angiographic studies were the first to suggest that lipid-modifying therapy could alter the composition of plaque. As summarized earlier, plaques are initially characterized by a large lipid core and a thin fibrous cap; these lesions are more susceptible to rupture.[32,44] Additionally, these lesions are small, usually <50% the size of the lumen diameter. Angiographic studies revealed that the lesions that caused MI were not the large ones that caused substantial stenosis, but the smaller lesions. Subsequently, pathology studies performed during autopsies on patients who had died following MI showed that these smaller lesions were lipid laden and had thin fibrous caps.

Although angiographic trials were primarily designed to study coronary angiograms, they reported fewer CHD events in treated patients. Most of these observations did not reach statistical significance because of the small numbers of patients in the study and the relatively short (1 to 3 years) duration of observation. When these studies were combined, the message was clear, however: cholesterol lowering was associated with fewer CHD events.[45] These results set the stage for the larger clinical trials.

CHOLESTEROL-LOWERING CLINICAL TRIALS

Proof of whether LDL-C lowering reduces CHD events has been demonstrated by well-designed, large, placebo-controlled clinical trials. Since the early 1990s, the results of a dozen or more major clinical trials have conclusively demonstrated the value of lipid-modifying therapy to prevent CHD events (Table 12-3).

The first of these, the Lipid Research Clinics Coronary Primary Prevention Trial,[82] showed that a relatively modest 10% reduction in cholesterol levels with the bile acid sequestrant cholestyramine compared with placebo over a 5-year period reduced CHD deaths and nonfatal MI by an impressive 19%. The results of this study launched the modern era of cholesterol management to reduce CHD risk.

Secondary Prevention

Beginning in the mid 1990s, the results of clinical trials with the more potent cholesterol-lowering statins were reported. Five of these (4S,[83] CARE,[84] LIPID,[90] TNT,[85] and IDEAL[86]) were secondary prevention trials (i.e., they were conducted in patients with known CHD). In 4S, CARE, and LIPID, CHD death and nonfatal MI occurred in 13% to 22% of placebo-treated patients over 5 years, compared with event rates of 10% to 14% with statin therapy. Total mortality was reduced significantly in two of these trials. Fewer revascularization procedures were required in patients receiving statin therapy; also 31% fewer strokes occurred.[87] This important and unexpected finding suggests that the same mechanisms by which statins affect coronary atherosclerosis may be operable in extracranial carotid atherosclerosis. It also demonstrates that patients who have atherosclerosis in one vascular bed (e.g., the coronary vessels) are likely to have atherosclerosis in other vascular beds, and that cholesterol-lowering treatment can have beneficial effects throughout the vascular tree. Finally, these studies demonstrate that LDL-C–lowering therapy not only improves the quality of life (by preventing MI, strokes, and revascularization procedures), but can also prolong life (by delaying deaths from any cause). Most recently, the TNT and IDEAL trials demonstrated additional cardiovascular benefit for lowering LDL-C substantially <100 mg/dL in patients with stable CHD. These two trials randomized patients to either high-dose (atorvastatin 80 mg) statin therapy or moderate-dose (atorvastatin 10 mg or simvastatin 20 mg) statin therapy with an approximate follow-up period of 5 years. In both trials, more intensive lowering of LDL-C significantly <100 mg/dL was associated with a reduction in CHD. The results of these two trials allowed the Writing Group for the cholesterol guidelines (see below) to lower the target goal of LDL-C in patients with CHD to <70 mg/dL.[88,89]

Likewise, the Heart Protection Study (HPS)[91] extended the results of the earlier statin trials (4S,[83] CARE,[84] LIPID[90]). The HPS included 20,536 patients with a history of CHD or cerebrovascular disease (stroke or transient ischemic attacks), peripheral vascular disease, or diabetes not considered by their general practitioner to have a clear indication for statin therapy because of relatively low baseline cholesterol levels (mean

Table 12-3 Randomized Endpoint Trials With Cholesterol-Lowering Therapies

Trial	*Intervention*	*LDL-C: Initial (On Rx)*	*LDL-C Changes %)*	*Placebo CHD Rate (%)[a]*	*CHD Event Reduction (%)*
CHD and CHD Risk Equivalent Patients					
4S[83]	Simvastatin 20–40 mg	188 (117)	↓35	21.8	↓34
LIPID[90]	Pravastatin 40 mg	150 (112)	↓25	15.9	↓24
CARE[84]	Pravastatin 40 mg	139 (98)	↓32	13.2	↓24
Post-CABG[250]	Lovastatin/Resin	136 (98)	↓39	13.5	↓24
HPS[91]	Simvastatin 40 mg	131 (89)	↓32	11.8	↓24
PROSPER[249]	Pravastatin 40 mg	147 (97)	↓34	12.7	↓19
TNT[85]	Atorvastatin 80 mg	152 (77)	↓49	—	↓22
	Atorvastatin 10 mg	152 (98)	↓35	—	
IDEAL[86]	Atorvastatin 80 mg	121 (77)	↓33	—	↓20
	Simvastatin 20 mg	121 (104)	↓14	—	
ALLHAT[99]	Pravastatin 40 mg	146 (105)	↓28	—	↓9
	Usual care	146 (130)	↓11	—	
Acute Coronary Syndrome Patients					
MIRACL[93,94]	Atorvastatin 80 mg	124 (72)	↓42	—	↓26[b]
AVERT[95]	Atorvastatin 80 mg	145 (77)	↓42	—	↓36[b]
PROVE IT[96]	Atorvastatin 80 mg	106 (62)	↓51	—	↓16
	Pravastatin 40 mg	106 (95)	↓22	—	
Patients Without Evidence of CHD					
LRC-CPPT[82]	Resin	205 (175)	↓15	9.8	↓19
WOSCOPS[97]	Pravastatin 40 mg	192 (142)	↓26	14.9	↓31
Tex/AFCAPS[100]	Lovastatin	150 (115)	↓25	3.0	↓40
ASCOT[98]	Atorvastatin 10 mg	132 (85)	↓31	4.7	↓50[c]
CARDS[105]	Atorvastatin 10 mg	117 (77)	↓34	5.5	↓37[d]

CHD, coronary heart disease; LDL-C, low density lipoprotein cholesterol; Rx, drug therapy.
[a]Placebo CHD rate: nonfatal myocardial infarction and CHD death.
[b]Ischemic events.
[c]Estimated 5-year CHD risk reduction.
[d]Acute coronary events.

LDL-C was 131 mg/dL). Of note, with the exception of the patients with a history of CHD, this grouping of patients is designated by the National Cholesterol Education Program's Adult Treatment Panel III (NCEP ATP-III) as being a "CHD equivalent population" because their risk of a CHD event is >20% in a 10-year period.[92] Treatment with simvastatin therapy for 5 years reduced LDL-C to 89 mg/dL and lowered the future risk of a CHD event in each of these populations by about 24% compared with placebo. By coincidence, the results of the HPS support the NCEP ATP-III recommendation for aggressive management of cholesterol in patients at high-risk for CHD events without established CHD. The CHD event reduction was achieved equally in men and women; in all age groups, including those ages 75 to 85 years; and regardless of the baseline LDL-C, including those with initial levels <100 mg/dL.

Trials carried out in patients with acute coronary syndromes have also demonstrated CHD risk reduction (Table 12-3). The MIRACL study randomized patients presenting to the hospital with unstable angina or non–Q-wave MI to statin therapy or placebo for 4 months. This resulted in a 24% reduction in symptomatic ischemia requiring emergency hospitalization and a 60% reduction in nonfatal strokes in those receiving the statin.[93,94] The AVERT study evaluated statin-based medical management versus revascularization and usual medical care in patients who had stable CAD and were candidates for a revascularization procedure. After 18 months of therapy, the statin-treated group had 36% fewer cases of ischemia requiring hospitalization compared with placebo-treated patients.[95] These studies show that intervention with a statin in patients with acute coronary syndromes can have important effects on ischemic symptoms in a relatively brief time after beginning therapy. The CHD risk reductions reported in the 5-year clinical trial were evident within the first 1 to 2 years of statin therapy and were significantly different from placebo after 5 years of treatment. More recently, PROVE-IT[96] was designed to determine if intensive LDL-C lowering with atorvastatin (80 mg) would reduce major coronary events to a greater extent compared with less-intensive LDL-C lowering with pravastatin (40 mg) in patients who had been hospitalized for an acute coronary syndrome. Following 2 years of treatment, mean LDL-C in patients randomized to atorvastatin (80 mg) and pravastatin (40 mg) were 62 mg/dL and 95 mg/dL, respectively. The composite cardiovascular endpoint (death from any cause, MI, documented unstable angina requiring rehospitalization, revascularization, and stroke) was significantly reduced by 16% with atorvastatin compared with pravastatin. Both treatments were well tolerated; however, elevations in alanine aminotransferase were threefold higher in patients treated with atorvastatin compared with pravastatin.

Primary Prevention

Five trials with statin therapy have been reported in patients without evident CHD (i.e., primary prevention) but with multiple CHD risk factors. WOSCOPS, which included men who had two or more CHD risk factors, found that CHD events and revascularization procedures were reduced by 31% and 37%, respectively, in those receiving statin therapy for 5 years; total mortality was reduced 22% ($P < 0.051$).[97] The ASCOT trial, which included men and women with hypertension and an average of 3.7 other CHD risk factors, reported that CHD events were reduced by 36% and strokes by 27% after only 3.3 years of statin treatment.[98] Similarly, the ALLHAT trial enrolled 10,355 hypertensive patients with moderately elevated hypercholesterolemia with at least one additional CHD risk factor and randomized them to nonblinded treatment with pravastatin or usual care for 4.8 years.[99] The results, however, were in contrast to those found in the ASCOT trial, likely because of the high use of nonstudy statin in the usual-care group (30%) and only a 77% adherence to pravastatin in the treatment group. This likely resulted in the total cholesterol difference between the two groups of only 9.6% and a nonsignifiant reduction in CHD deaths and nonfatal MI of 9%. The TexCAPS/AFCAPS trial was important because it included the lowest risk population, with an estimated 10-year CHD risk of only 6%. Despite this relatively low CHD risk, the composite endpoint (i.e., fatal and nonfatal MI, sudden cardiac death, and unstable angina) was reduced by 37%, fatal and nonfatal MI were reduced by 40%, and unstable angina was reduced by 32%, with 5 years of statin treatment.[100] Significant reductions in CHD events were seen in women, older patients, and diabetic patients, emphasizing the value of treatment in these populations.

Lowering LDL-C by other means also reduces CHD events.[61] For example, LDL-C lowering with ileal bypass surgery in the POSCH study resulted in a 40% reduction of CHD events compared with the groups not having this surgery.[61] These studies suggest that effective LDL-C lowering by any means can reduce CHD risk.

Taken together, the results of these trials demonstrate that LDL-C lowering reduces the risk of a CHD event in patients at practically any level of risk. In the aggregate, common CHD events, including sudden CHD deaths and nonfatal MI, were reduced by 25% to 40%. Revascularization procedures were reduced by 25% to 50%. Strokes were reduced by an average of 15% in primary prevention patients and 32% in secondary prevention patients.[87] In fact, essentially all known adverse consequence of atherosclerosis has been reduced with lipid-lowering therapy. In some of these studies, especially those in patients at very high risk for CHD, total mortality was significantly reduced. These trials show that aggressive lipid lowering improves the quality as well as the length of life. In addition, in patients with stable CHD and those having had an acute coronary event, aggressive lowering of LDL-C to <70 mg/dL provides further protection from CHD events. The protective effects are illustrated by a plot of the relative risk of CHD and LDL-C levels, which shows a log-linear relationship (Fig. 12-6)[89] which suggest the optimal level of LDL-C is far below 70 mg/dL (the relative risk is set at 1.0 for LDL-C = 40 mg/dL). This log-linear relationship is consistent with epidemiologic data, clinical trials, and population data.[101] Evidence from hunter-gatherer populations who still follow their indigenous lifestyles show no evidence for atherosclerosis into the seventh and eighth decades of life and their estimated LDL-C are approximately 50 to 75 mg/dL. The above cumulative evidence has led the NCEP ATP III to define the "optimal" LDL-C level as <100 mg/dL and a reasonable goal of <70 mg/dL for all patients with CHD.[88,89]

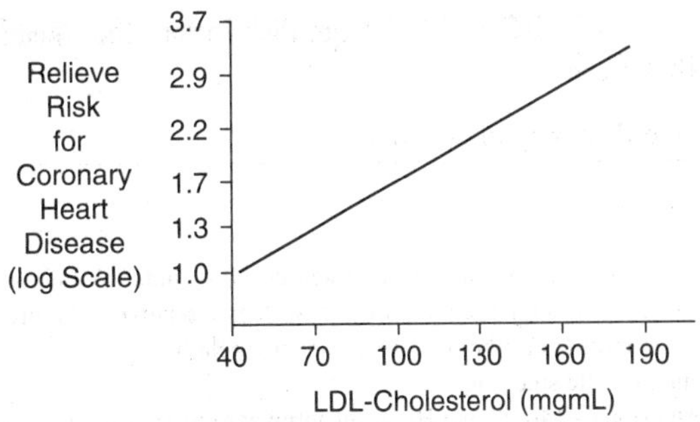

FIGURE 12-6 Log-linear relationship between LDL-C levels and relative risk for CHD. (Adapted from Grundy SM, et al. Coordinating Committee of the National Cholesterol Education Program. Implications of recent clinical trials for the National Cholesterol Education Program Adult Treatment Panel III guidelines. *Arterioscler Thromb Vasc Biol* 2004;24:e149–61, with permission.)

Patients with Diabetes

Diabetic patients have a very high risk of macrovascular disease (i.e., CHD) as well as microvascular disease (e.g., retinopathy). Investigations have shown that diabetic patients with no history of CHD have the same risk of a future CHD event as do nondiabetic patients who have experienced an MI (approximately 20% risk in 7 years).[102] Close management of blood glucose levels appears to reduce microvascular disease, but not CHD.[103,104] Because of this, NCEP ATP III and the American Diabetic Association (ADA) considered patients with diabetes to be a CHD risk equivalent (>20% 10-year CHD risk) and recommended that these patients be treated with aggressive lipid-modifying therapy to an LDL-C goal of <100 mg/dL.[92] Findings from the above clinical trials demonstrate that a reduction in CHD events with lipid-modifying therapy is of a similar or greater magnitude in diabetic patients compared with nondiabetic patients.[90,105] This supports the NCEP ATP III recommendation for aggressive management of diabetic patients.[92]

Global CHD Risk Identification

The large number of clinical trials available illustrates the continuum of risk in patients with CHD (secondary prevention) and those without (primary prevention). In fact, the CHD risk in these two populations overlaps considerably. In secondary prevention patients, atherosclerosis is known to be present and the risk of a subsequent event is great. In primary prevention patients with multiple risk factors, atherosclerosis is likely present and that this increases the risk of a future CHD event. In fact, some primary prevention patients have so many risk factors that they reach the level of a "CHD risk equivalent" as defined by the NCEP ATP III guidelines, denoting a >20% CHD risk in 10 years.[92] Others have only a few or no accompanying CHD risk factors and have a low to moderate future risk of a CHD event. Thus, the decision of how aggressively to treat patients begins with an assessment of their global CHD risk.

Table 12-4 NCEP ATP III Major Risk Factors That Modify LDL-C Goals

Positive Risk Factors (↑Risk)
Age: Male ≥45 yr
Female: ≥55 yr
Family history of a premature CHD (definite MI or sudden death before 55 yr in father or other male first-degree relative or before 65 yr in mother or other female first-degree relative)
Current cigarette smoking
Hypertension (≥140/90 mm Hg or on antihypertensive drugs)
Low HDL-C (<40 mg/dL)
Negative Risk Factor (↓Risk, protective)
High HDL-C (≥60 mg/dL)

Expert Panel on Detection, Evaluation, and Treatment of High Blood Cholesterol in Adults, 2001.[92]

Note: Presence of diabetes mellitus is considered a CHD risk equivalent (see Table 12-7). It is not included in counting the number of risk factors because its presence automatically qualifies the patient for aggressive treatment whether or not true CHD is manifest.

CHD, coronary heart disease; HDL-C, high-density lipoprotein cholesterol; MI, myocardial infarction.

The first step is to identify patients who have two or more risk factors and no CHD and CHD risk equivalent history (Table 12-4). The next step is to assess their global CHD risk with an instrument such as that illustrated in Figure 12-7 from the Framingham Heart Study.[92] (It is not necessary to conduct a global risk assessment of CHD patients, as their risk is known to be >20% in 10 years.) Patients with a very high risk of a future CHD event (e.g., diabetic patients and those with a global risk of >20% in 10 years) can be considered a CHD equivalent and given aggressive LDL-C–lowering treatment with the same LDL-C goal as applied to patients who have experienced a CHD event (i.e., an LDL-C treatment goal of <100 mg/dL).[106] Those with <20% risk of a CHD event in 10 years can be given lifestyle modification and drug therapy, if needed, to reach an intermediate LDL-C goal (<130 mg/dL).

This approach of assessing a patient's CHD risk and matching the intensity of treatment is illustrated in the cases that follow.

TG-LOWERING CLINICAL TRIALS

Five clinical trials have tested TG-lowering therapies (fibrates and niacin) in randomized endpoint trials involving patients who generally had baseline TG levels of 150 to 500 mg/dL and HDL-C <40 mg/dL (Table 12-5). The Helsinki Heart Study studied 4,081 men without CHD and found a 34% reduction in CHD death and nonfatal MI after 5 years of gemfibrozil therapy compared with placebo.[107] *Post hoc* analysis of this study showed that the group of patients with TG >200 mg/dL and an LDL:HDL ratio >5.0 (generally with LDL-C >194 mg/dL and HDL-C <40 mg/dL) accounted for 71% of the CHD reduction achieved in the entire study, although the group represented only 10% of the total study population[108] (Table 12-5). The VA-HIT (HDL Intervention Trial) studied 2,531 men with a history of CHD and low HDL-C levels (mean HDL-C level, 32 mg/dL) and reported a 22% reduction in CHD events with gemfibrozil therapy. The authors reported that approximately 25% of this risk reduction resulted from the 6% increase in HDL-C.[109] The Bezafibrate Infarction Prevention (BIP) trial studied CHD patients with a lipid profile similar to the patients in the Tex/AFCAPS trial (high LDL-C, low HDL-C, normal TG) and reported an insignificant 9% reduction in CHD events associated with an 18% increase in HDL-C and a 21% reduction in TG.[110] A post hoc analysis of this trial found that patients who had TG levels of >175 and 200 mg/dL had significant CHD event reductions of 22% and 40%, respectively. The FIELD study investigated the effects of fenofibrate versus placebo with an average follow-up of 5 years on CHD events in patients with type 2 diabetes with a mean baseline LDL-C, HDL-C, and triglyceride level of 119 mg/dL, 42 mg/dL, and 153 mg/dL, respectively.[111] Similar to the BIP trial, this trial failed to demonstrate a significant reduction in major coronary events (11% reduction in risk; $P = 0.16$) in patients randomized to fenofibrate. Because this trial allowed changes in therapy at the discretion of the patient's primary care physician, significantly more patients receiving placebo

Table 12-5 Randomized Endpoint Trials With Triglyceride-Lowering Therapies

Trial	*Intervention*	*Lipids: Initial (On Rx)*	*Lipid Changes (%)*	*Placebo CHD Rate (%)*	*CHD Event Reduction (%)*
HHS[107]	Gemfibrozil	LDL-C: 189 (170 TG: 178 (116) HDL-C: 47 (52)	↓10 ↓35 ↑11	4	↓34
VA-HIT[226]	Gemfibrozil	LDL-C: 111 (113) TG: 161 (115) HDL-C: 32 (34)	0 ↓31 ↑6	22	↓22
BIP[110]	Bezafibrate	LDL-C: 148 (138) TG: 145 (115) HDL-C: 35 (41)	↓7 ↓21 ↑18	15	↓9.4
FIELD[111]	Fenofibrate	LDL-C: 119 (94) TG: 154 (130) HDL-C: 42 (44)	↓6 ↓22 ↑1	6	↓11
CDP[112]	Niacin	TC: 250 (235) TG: 480 (354)	↓10 ↓26	30	↓13

CHD, coronary heart disease; HDL, high-density lipoprotein cholesterol; LDL-C, low-density lipoprotein cholesterol; Rx, drug therapy; TG, triglyceride.

(17%) compared with fenofibrate (8%) were taking nonstudy lipid-lowering agents. This may have partially accounted for the study results.

The current outcome evidence for fenofibrate and gemfibrozil (bezafibrate is not available in the United States) reasonably supports their use as second-line agents in type 2 diabetes and secondary prevention with low HDL-C, respectively. In addition, post hoc analyses suggest that patients with atherogenic dyslipidemia obtain CHD risk reduction with fibrate therapy. The risk reduction may be similar to that achieved with statins, although no head-to-head trials exist to refute or affirm this. This presents a dilemma for the clinician: When presented with a patient who has atherogenic dyslipidemia, which is the drug of choice, a statin or fibrate? Some guidance to this question will be provided during the case discussions that follow.

Only one placebo-controlled endpoint study is available for niacin (Table 12-5). The study was completed in men who had had a prior MI and mixed hyperlipidemia. After 5 years of niacin therapy, the CHD event rate was reduced by 13%.[112] Fifteen years after the start of the study, and 9 years after the study was terminated, the investigators reported that total mortality was 11% lower in the men in the niacin arm, suggesting that any period of lipid-modifying treatment may translate into a long-term benefit.[112] Combination therapy with niacin plus a statin has been studied in patients with CHD with low HDL-C and normal LDL-C.[113] Compared with a mean 3.9% progression in coronary stenosis with placebo, niacin–simvastatin therapy was associated with a mean regression of 0.4% ($P < 0.001$). The authors posited that event reduction with this combination should be equivalent to the sum of the LDL-C reduction and the HDL-C increase. In the study, LDL-C was reduced by 42% and HDL-C was increased by 26%, and the composite endpoint of death from coronary causes, MI, stroke, or revascularization for worsening ischemia was reduced 60% with the niacin–statin combination ($P = 0.02$).

Niacin has long been an intriguing drug to lipid specialists. It is one of the few drugs that positively affects each component of the lipid profile (LDL-C, TG, and HDL-C). It is the best therapy available to raise HDL-C and one of the best at lowering TG. It is logical to expect that these effects would translate into substantial CHD risk reduction. It is especially interesting to speculate on how these effects may combine to offer better risk reduction, especially when combined with one of the statins. This hypothesis is being evaluated in the ongoing AIM HIGH study.

Mechanisms of CHD Risk Reduction

Given the consistent relationship between lowering blood cholesterol and reducing CHD events, the question arises, "what is the mechanism of this protection?" Scientists are offering many new and exciting answers to this question. At present, it appears that the reduction in CHD with lipid-altering therapy is mediated through, or at least tracked by, a reduction in cholesterol levels. In addition to lowering blood cholesterol levels, statins and other lipid-altering therapies produce other, so-called pleiotropic, effects that may partly explain their CHD-reducing capability.[114]

One way in which cholesterol lowering may reduce CHD is by changing atherosclerotic plaque from "high risk" lesions with a large lipid core, thin fibrous cap, and many cholesterol-filled macrophage cells along the shoulders of the lesion to "lower risk" lesions with a small lipid core and much connective tissue and smooth muscle matrix throughout. The lesion does not appear to change much in size, or at least not in ways that can be visualized on an arteriogram. The harder lesion created with lipid lowering is much less likely to rupture or erode, however, thus reducing the risk of forming an occluding clot and producing CHD events.

Lipid lowering may also affect endothelial function. Evidence indicates that high LDL-C levels cause "endothelial dysfunction," as evidenced by a lowered ability of coronary arteries to dilate. Cholesterol lowering by practically any means restores endothelial function. Many studies have demonstrated improvement in brachial artery reactivity and coronary artery dilation when cholesterol levels are reduced.[115–120] Positron emission tomography (PET) scans demonstrate improved blood flow and reduced areas of ischemia throughout the myocardium in patients receiving lipid-altering therapy.[117,118] These effects may have important clinical benefits. In patients with CAD, cholesterol lowering reduces the number of ST-segment depressions recorded during a 48-hour electrocardiogram (ECG) Holter monitor study.[121,122] Therapy with a statin can also reduce ischemic events requiring acute management, a potential effect of restored endothelial function.[95]

Cholesterol lowering might also combat the inflammation that accompanies atherogenesis. Early in the development of plaques, monocyte-derived macrophages are recruited to engulf modified LDL particles, and in every stage of the disease, specific subtypes of T lymphocytes are present.[36,42] At various stages, cytokines, chemokines, and growth factors are released. Inflammatory processes may be especially active just before or after the plaque ruptures. Several investigators have attempted to identify markers of inflammation that may signal an increased risk of a CHD event. One promising marker is high-sensitivity C-reactive protein (hs-CRP). An elevated hs-CRP level predicts a high risk of future CHD events and appears to add to the risk predicted by LDL-C alone.[123] A subanalysis of the CARE trial reported that high levels of hs-CRP forecast CHD risk in patients on placebo, but this was attenuated and nonsignificant in patients assigned to pravastatin, suggesting that statin treatment has an anti-inflammatory effect.[124] The American Heart Association (AHA) has recently recommended that measurement of the hs-CRP level be considered in a patient with two or more risk factors as a way to further characterize the patient's future CHD risk.[125]

Cost-Effectiveness

Several cost-effectiveness analyses of lipid-lowering therapies have been conducted.[126–129] One variable used in these analyses is the cost per years of life saved (YOLS). Analyses of other prophylactic measures to reduce CHD risk, such as the use of aspirin in patients after MI and the treatment of mild hypertension with antihypertensive drugs, indicate that it costs up to $50,000 per YOLS to treat these patients. Our society has accepted this level of expenditure as cost-effective. Analyses of cholesterol-lowering treatment in clinical trials have found that drug treatment of high-risk patients for secondary prevention costs approximately $12,000 per YOLS, whereas treatment of high-risk patients for primary prevention costs approximately $25,000 per YOLS. In the 4S study, the cost saved in reduced hospital days by treatment was so great that simvastatin was estimated to cost only $0.28 per day (an 88% savings).[130] In another analysis of the cost of treating patients to their NCEP goal in an office setting, atorvastatin was found to cost the least, approximately $1,064 per year, in combined expenses for drugs, office visits, and laboratory monitoring.[131] These analyses support aggressive (i.e., drug and lifestyle) treatment of CHD and high-risk patients with lipid-lowering therapy.

HYPERCHOLESTEROLEMIA

Evaluation of the Lipoprotein Profile

1. T.A., a 43-year-old premenopausal woman, is screened with a lipid profile during an annual medical evaluation. She has never taken cholesterol-lowering medication and currently takes only a multivitamin daily. She has had no symptoms of coronary, carotid, or peripheral vascular disease. She has a 20-pack/year history of smoking and exercises four times a week, without physical limitations. T.A. states that she follows a low-fat, low-cholesterol diet. Her father is alive and well at age 71, with a normal cholesterol level. Her mother had an MI at age 47 and died at age 57 from a second event. Her grandfather died of an MI at age 52; a sister has hypercholesterolemia and is taking simvastatin. Pertinent physical findings are weight, 125 lb; height, 63 in; blood pressure (BP), 120/82 mm Hg; pulse, 66 beats/min and regular; carotid pulses symmetric bilaterally without bruits; no neck masses; no abdominal bruit; and no evidence of tendon xanthomas. Pertinent laboratory findings, obtained after a 12-hour fast, show total cholesterol, 290 mg/dL; TG, 55 mg/dL; HDL-C, 55 mg/dL; LDL-C, 224 mg/dL; non-HDL-C, 235; plasma glucose, 96 mg/dL (normal, 60 to 115); thyroid-stimulating hormone (TSH), 0.92 IU/mL (normal, 0.4 to 6.2); alanine aminotransferase (ALT), 11 U/L (normal, 6 to 34); aspartate aminotransferase (AST), 8 U/L (normal, 9 to 34); blood urea nitrogen (BUN), 12 mg/dL (normal, 4 to 24); creatinine, 1.0 mg/dL (normal, 0.4 to 1.1); and a negative urinalysis. What is your assessment T.A.'s lipid panel results?

[SI units: total cholesterol, 7.5 mmol/L; TG, 0.62 mmol/L; HDL-C, 1.42 mmol/L; LDL-C, 5.79 mmol/L; glucose, 5.33 mmol/L; TSH, <100 units; ALT, 0.18 μkat/L; AST, 0.13 μkat/L; BUN, 4.28 mmol/L urea; creatinine, 88.4 μmol/L]

T.A.'s LDL-C is considered "very high" (>190 mg/dl); NCEP defines the optimal LDL-C as <100 mg/dL.[92] Her HDL-C is right at the average HDL-C for a woman and her TG is normal (<150 mg/dL) (Table 12-6). In most cases, it is wise to repeat the lipid profile to be sure the first results are not atypical. However, T.A.'s LDL-C is so high a repeat test is not likely to change the assessment. Thus, in this case, a second test is optional.

While it is possible to measure LDL-C directly, it is common for many laboratories to calculate LDL-C. Total cholesterol, HDL-C, and TG are measured directly and then the following formula (Friedwald equation) is applied to calculate LDL-C:

$$\text{LDL-C} = \text{Total Cholesterol} - (\text{HDL-C} + \text{VLDL-C})$$

Because the ratio of cholesterol to TG in LDL is 1:5, VLDL-C is estimated by dividing the total TG level by 5. Thus, the formula is rewritten as:

$$\text{LDL-C} = \text{Total Cholesterol} - (\text{HDL-C} + \text{TG}/5)$$

Table 12-6 NCEP ATP III Classifications of Blood Lipids[92]

LDL-Cholesterol	
<100 mg/dL	Optimal
100–129 mg/dL	Near optimal or above optimal
130–159 mg/dL	Borderline high
160–189 mg/dL	High
≥190 mg/dL	Very high
Total Cholesterol	
<200 mg/dL	Desirable
200–239 mg/dL	Borderline high
≥240 mg/dL	High
HDL-Cholesterol	
<40 mg/dL	Low
≥60 mg/dL	High
Triglycerides	
<150 mg/dL	Normal
150–199 mg/dL	Borderline high
200–499 mg/dL	High
>500 mg/dL	Very high

HDL, high-density lipoprotein; LDL, low-density lipoprotein.

Applying the formula to T.A.'s lipid profile, the calculated LDL-C is 224 mg/dL.

$$\begin{aligned}\text{LDL-C} &= \text{Total Cholesterol} - (\text{HDL-C} + \text{TG}/5)\\ &= 290 - (55 + 55/5)\\ &= 224 \text{ mg/dL}\end{aligned}$$

If the TG level is >400 mg/dL, the formula for estimating VLDL-C is not accurate and, therefore, LDL-C cannot be calculated. An accurate LDL-C measurement also requires that the patient fast for 10 to 12 hours. This provides sufficient time for exogenous TG, carried by chylomicrons, to be cleared from the systemic circulation (provided the patient does not have hyperchylomicronemia). Most laboratories can measure LDL-C directly and should be asked to do so when the TG is >400 mg/dL or the patient has not fasted.

Non–HDL-C is calculated by the following formula:

$$\text{Non-HDL-C} = \text{Total Cholesterol} - \text{HDL-C}$$

For T.A.:

$$\begin{aligned}\text{Non-HDC-C} &= 290 \text{ mg/dL} - 55 \text{ mg/dL}\\ &= 235 \text{ mg/dL}\end{aligned}$$

Secondary Causes of High Blood Cholesterol

2. Is there any evidence that T.A.'s elevated LDL-C is secondary to other conditions or concurrent drug therapy?

As a routine, every new patient with hypercholesterolemia should be evaluated for four things in the following order: (1) secondary causes of the high cholesterol level, (2) familial disorders, (3) presence of CHD and CHD equivalents, and (4) CHD risk factors.

Conditions that can produce lipid abnormalities (i.e., secondary causes) include diabetes mellitus, hypothyroidism, nephrotic syndrome, and obstructive liver disease. Selected drugs can also produce lipid abnormalities (Table 12-7). When

Table 12-7 Drug-Induced Hyperlipidemia

	Effect on Plasma Lipids			
	Cholesterol (%)	Triglycerides (%)	HDL-C (%)	Comments
Diuretics				
Thiazides	↑5–7% initially ↑0–3% later	↑30–50	↑1	Effects transient; monitor for long-term effects
Loop	No change	No change	↓ to 15	
Indapamide	No change	No change	No change	
Metolazone	No change	No change	No change	
Potassium-sparing	No change	No change	No change	
β-blockers				
Nonselective	No change	↑20–50	↓10–15	Selective β-blockers have greater effects than nonselective; β-blockers with ISA or α-blocking effects are lipid neutral
Selective	No change	↑15–30	↓5–10	
α-Blocking	No change or ↓	No change	No change	
α-Agonists and antagonists (e.g., prazosin and clonidine)	↓0–10%	↓ 0–20	↑0–15	In general, drugs that affect α-receptors ↓cholesterol and ↑HDL-C
ACE inhibitors	No change	No change	No change	
Calcium channel blockers	No change	No change	No change	
Oral contraceptives				
α-Monophasics	↑5–20	↑10–45	↑15 to ↓15	Effects caused by reduced lipolytic activity and/or ↑VLDL synthesis; mainly caused by progestin component; estrogen alone protective
α-Triphasics	↑10–15	↑10–15	↑5–10	
Glucocorticoids	↑5–10	↑15–20		
Ethanol	No change	↑up to 50	↑	Marked elevations can occur in patients who are hypertriglyceridemic
Isotretinoin	↑5–20	↑50–60	↓10–15	Changes may reverse 8 wk after stopping drug
Cyclosporine	↑15–20	No change	No change	

ACE, angiotensin-converting enzyme; HDL-C, high-density lipoprotein cholesterol; ISA, intrinsic sympathomimetic activity.

one of these secondary causes is identified, it should be managed first, as this may resolve the lipid abnormality.

In T.A.'s case, no secondary causes are evident. Her blood glucose level does not indicate the presence of diabetes; her TSH level does not indicate hypothyroidism; her ALT and AST levels are within acceptable levels, suggesting normal liver function; and her BUN, creatinine, and urinalysis are acceptable, signifying normal renal function. She is not taking any drugs that could have contributed to her cholesterol elevation.

Familial Forms of Hypercholesterolemia

3. Could T.A. have an inherited form of hyperlipidemia?

T.A.'s history is consistent with polygenic hypercholesterolemia, the form of hypercholesterolemia that affects 98% of patients with hypercholesterolemia. As described previously, polygenic hypercholesterolemia is suspected when the patient's LDL-C is 130 to 250 mg/dL and no evidence seen of tendon xanthomas (Table 12-2). A family history of CHD is present in approximately 18% of these patients and is a strong finding in T.A.'s case. Polygenic hypercholesterolemia is caused by a combination of nutritional and genetic factors that reduce the clearance of LDL particles from the plasma. It is impossible to determine which of these factors are causing hypercholesterolemia in a given patient by simply examining the lipoprotein profile. If the patient's blood lipids normalize with a low-fat diet, however, one can assume that the diet is a major etiologic factor for that person. Conversely, if little or no change is seen in blood cholesterol levels after dietary modification, genetics likely significantly influences the patient's elevated cholesterol. In most cases, a relatively equal contribution is made by genetic factors and environment on cholesterol elevations.

CHD and CHD Risk Equivalents

4. Does T.A. have evidence of CHD or a CHD risk equivalent?

A search for CHD starts with a good medical history of symptomatic coronary artery disease, but is quickly followed with a broader search for atherosclerotic disease in other artery beds, including the arteries of the limbs and carotid arteries[92] (Table 12-8). If detected in one site, atherosclerosis is likely to be present in all or most vessels, and it is associated with a five- to sevenfold higher risk of a major coronary event.[132–134]

The patient should be asked about a history of myocardial ischemia (exercise-induced angina), prior MI (i.e., severe angina with elevated cardiac creatine phosphokinase [CPK] or characteristic ECG changes), history of revascularizations (i.e., coronary artery bypass surgery, angioplasty with percutaneous transluminal coronary angioplasty or stent placement), or history of hospitalization due to unstable angina

Table 12-8 NCEP APT III Definitions of CHD and CHD Risk Equivalents[92]

Clinical CHD
Myocardial ischemia (angina)
Myocardial infarction
Coronary angioplasty and/or stent placement
Coronary bypass graft
Prior unstable angina
Carotid artery disease
Stroke history
Transient ischemic attack history
Carotid stenosis >50%
Peripheral arterial disease
Claudication
ABI >0.9
Abdominal aortic aneurysm
Diabetes mellitus

Estimated global CHD risk >20% in 10 years for any of the factors above.
ABI, ankle:brachial blood pressure index; CHD, coronary heart disease.

(see Table 12-8). The presence of any of these findings is associated with a very high (>20%) risk of a CHD death or nonfatal MI in the next 10 years; the risk approaches 40% if unstable angina and stroke are also considered. None of these signs are present in T.A.

The evaluation can stop here, but some would advocate continuing the search with noninvasive procedures, even if the patient has not experienced symptoms (Table 12-9). The case for pursuing these evaluations is more convincing in patients who have a high probability of atherosclerosis because of the presence of multiple risk factors or a strong family history of premature CHD events. One noninvasive evaluation is exercise testing with either ECG monitoring for signs of ischemia or pharmacologic perfusion imaging (e.g., exercise thallium). Because these tests are expensive and not widely available, they are reserved for selected use. Even if the results are found to be normal, atherosclerosis is not ruled out because both tests are designed to detect flow-limiting disease, and atherosclerosis can be present without causing obstructions in luminal blood flow.[92]

Table 12-9 Emerging CHD Risk Factors[92]

Noninvasive Evaluations for Subclinical Atherosclerosis	*Blood Tests*
Exercise ECG	Lipoprotein(a)
Myocardial perfusion imaging	Small, dense LDL
Stress echocardiography	Apolipoprotein B (particle concentration)
Carotid intimal-medial thickness (IMT)	High-sensitivity CRP (and other inflammatory markers)
Electron beam computed tomography (EBCT)	Homocysteine
	HDL subspecies
	Apolipoprotein A-1
	Apolipoprotein B:C-III
	Thrombogenic factors (e.g. fibrinogen, PAI-1, t-PA)

CRP, C-reactive protein; ECG, electrocardiogram; HDL, high-density lipoprotein cholesterol; LDL-C, low-density lipoprotein cholesterol; t-PA, tissue plasminogen activator.

In recent years, electron beam computed tomography and spiral computed tomography have been used to detect calcium in coronary vessels. The presence of coronary calcium suggests the presence of old atherosclerotic plaque. If old disease is present, then it is likely that younger, more vulnerable plaques are also present. This test is simple, quick, and noninvasive, but it is relatively expensive and not widely available. High coronary calcium volume scores can add to the prediction of future coronary events based on traditional risk factor assessment.[92] Use of these tests is particularly helpful in modifying the assessment of risk in patients with multiple risk factors. In T.A.'s case, her strong family history could support obtaining an electron beam computed tomography evaluation. If she has a significantly positive calcium volume score, more aggressive medical therapy could be considered.

A good history should also probe for evidence of atherosclerotic vascular disease in peripheral vessels. Patients with flow-limiting atherosclerosis in peripheral vessels often describe claudication (pain and weakness in the limb muscles) after walking a distance (Chapter 14, Peripheral Vascular Disorders). NCEP recommends that patients >50 years of age be evaluated with an ankle:brachial index (ABI). This index is determined by measuring the systolic blood pressure of the brachial, posterior tibia, and dorsalis pedis arteries using a handheld Doppler device and dividing the higher of the two ankle systolic blood pressures by the higher of two systolic brachial pressures.[92] An ABI of <0.9 constitutes the diagnosis of peripheral vascular disease (PVD; also called peripheral arterial disease or PAD). Finding atherosclerosis in peripheral vessels probably means it is present in coronary arteries as well. In fact, most patients with PVD die of a CHD event. Further, most patients with PVD have a very high (>20%) risk of a CHD event in the next 10 years, and so are said to have a CHD risk equivalent.

The clinician should also evaluate the patient for atherosclerosis in the carotid vessels by asking about signs and symptoms of transient ischemic attacks (TIA) and strokes (see Chapter 15, Peripheral Vascular Disorders). On the physical examination, the carotid vessels should be evaluated for the presence of a bruit (indicative of a space-occupying lesion in the carotid vessel). If a bruit is present, further evaluation with carotid duplex imaging is indicated to detect stenotic lesions. Some authorities recommend performing carotid sonography to measure the intimal-medial thickness. This test is safe and simple but relatively expensive and not widely available. Intimal-medial thickness results correlate with the severity of coronary atherosclerosis. Patients who have experienced a stroke or TIA have a >20% 10-year risk of experiencing a CHD event and so are also considered a CHD risk equivalent. Patients found to have a stenosis of >50% in their carotid vessel, even if asymptomatic, have a >20% 10-year CHD risk and again can be considered a CHD risk equivalent. Patients found to have an increased intimal-medial thickness, suggesting the presence of subclinical atherosclerosis, may also have a high

CHD risk and, therefore, are candidates for more aggressive medical therapy.[92]

Other conditions that confer a >20% risk of a CHD event in the next 10 years, and thus are considered by NCEP to be CHD risk equivalents, include abdominal aortic aneurysm and the diagnosis of diabetes. More will be said about diabetes below. T.A. does not have evidence of CHD or a CHD risk equivalent.

CHD Risk Factors

5. Does T.A. have CHD risk factors, and what is her global CHD risk?

Patients who are found to have CHD or CHD risk equivalent do not need a risk factor assessment to establish their LDL-C treatment goal; the presence of CHD or a CHD risk equivalent satisfies that. These patients, however, should have an appraisal of risk factors so that risk factor modification can be incorporated in the overall treatment plan. For patients who do not have CHD or a CHD risk equivalent, risk factor counting and global risk assessment is important to establish treatment goals and approaches.

Begin this process by counting the number of risk factors present (Table 12-4). Patients with either zero or one risk factor most likely have a low risk of a CHD event in the next 10 years and are assigned an LDL-C goal of <160 mg/dL. Patients with two or more risk factors have a moderate to high risk, depending on the number and type of risk factors present. NCEP recommends that patients who have two or more risk factors be further evaluated using the Framingham-based global risk assessment tool (Fig. 12-7) to define the 10-year risk. Patients with two or more risk factors have an LDL-C goal of <130 mg/dL. The clinician, however, has the option to treat these patients to reach <100 mg/dL depending on clinical judgment of the patient's absolute risk and potential benefit if that patient's Framingham calculated 10-year CHD risk is between 10% and 20%. The presence of modifiable risk factors should become the target of any risk-reduction treatment program.

T.A. has two CHD risk factors: current cigarette smoking and a family history of premature CHD. She thus has an LDL-C treatment goal of <130 mg/dL (Table 12-10). T.A. is found to have a 5% 10-year CHD risk, which is several times greater than the average risk for women her age but below the threshold where aggressive drug treatment is indicated (i.e., >10% CHD risk in 10 years). If she were not a smoker, her 10-year CHD risk estimate would be 1%, illustrating the prominent influence that smoking has on her future risk of a CHD event.

Based on this assessment and assuming that the noninvasive assessments performed on her, if any, were negative, T.A. should be counseled on diet and exercise and strongly advised to stop smoking. Because of its strong effect on her risk, smoking cessation should be a primary focus of her risk-reduction program. If these measures fail to bring her LDL-C to her treatment goal of <130 mg/dL and her LDL-C remains ≥160 mg/dL, drug therapy should be considered (Table 12-10). If she stopped smoking, however, she would have only one risk factor (family history), and her new LDL-C goal would be <160 mg/dL. In this case, drug therapy would be considered only if the LDL-C remains ≥190 mg/dL.

Therapy for Lowering Cholesterol Levels

Diet Therapy

6. What dietary changes should be recommended to T.A.?

The centerpiece of treatment for high blood cholesterol is a diet low in saturated fat and cholesterol. The therapeutic lifestyle change (TLC) diet recommended by NCEP restricts total fat intake to 25% to 35% of calories, saturated fats to <7% of calories, and dietary cholesterol to 200 mg/day (Table 12-11).[92] The TLC diet is aggressive and requires instruction by a dietitian, nurse, or other health professional well versed in nutrition counseling. The TLC diet is also flexible and allows for modification of carbohydrate and monounsaturated fat intake according to the individual patient's needs. The goals presented by the TLC diet are minimal goals, and some patients will want to exceed them, even to the point of following a "vegetarian" diet. This is permissible, as long as the diet is nutritionally balanced.

When saturated fat is removed from the diet, it is important to understand what should be given in replacement. In the overweight or obese patient, it may be appropriate to do nothing, because a reduction in saturated fat is a good way to lower calories and encourage weight loss.

In individuals who are close to their ideal weight, such as T.A., replacing saturated fats with carbohydrates may not be the best choice. Increased intake of sugar and highly refined starches, as found in the many low-fat, high-calorie snack foods, may actually increase weight and reduce HDL-C as well as LDL-C.[135] More importantly, a low-fat, high-carbohydrate diet has not been shown to reduce the risk of CHD. Consumption of complex carbohydrates is recommended, however, and could be a replacement for saturated fat calories in a TLC diet.

Replacing saturated fat with unsaturated fats, especially monounsaturated fats (e.g., canola, olive oil products) and omega-3 polyunsaturated fats (e.g., fish oil sources), is highly desirable.[136] This is the diet of the Mediterranean people, who have a low incidence of CHD, and has the advantage of lowering LDL-C without affecting HDL-C. In fact, in a major randomized clinical trial in which it was compared with a "prudent Western-type diet," the Mediterranean diet was associated with a >70% reduction in cardiovascular endpoints and total mortality, a result that exceeds that achieved by our best lipid-lowering drug trials.[137] This study alone illustrates how important it is to initiate a good diet in hyperlipidemic patients, even with the availability of very potent, highly efficacious, and safe drugs to lower serum cholesterol levels.

In western society, diets high in protein and saturated fats and low in carbohydrates (e.g., Atkins Diet) promise quick weight loss and other health effects. Although these diets can reduce lipid levels and cause weight loss, they are not nutritionally sound and may even be unhealthy. Patients should be advised to avoid them.

T.A. is likely to need help in translating the dietary recommendations of a TLC diet into practical terms and concepts that she can easily implement in her everyday life. Two approaches can be used to achieve this: (*a*) teach her to count calories or (*b*) provide general guidance in the selection of low-fat foods.

The more sophisticated patient may want to count calories or grams of total and saturated fat per day. The first step in

Estimate of 10-Year Risk for Men

(Framingham Point Scores)

Age	Points
20-34	−9
35-39	−4
40-44	0
45-49	3
50-54	6
55-59	8
60-64	10
65-69	11
70-74	12
75-79	13

Total Cholesterol	Points				
	Age 20-39	Age 40-49	Age 50-59	Age 60-69	Age 70-79
<160	0	0	0	0	0
160-199	4	3	2	1	0
200-239	7	5	3	1	0
240-279	9	6	4	2	1
≥280	11	8	5	3	1

	Points				
	Age 20-39	Age 40-49	Age 50-59	Age 60-69	Age 70-79
Nonsmoker	0	0	0	0	0
Smoker	8	5	3	1	1

HDL (mg/dL)	Points
≥60	−1
50-59	0
40-49	1
<40	2

Systolic BP (mmHg)	If Untreated	If Treated
<120	0	0
120-129	0	1
130-139	1	2
140-159	1	2
≥160	2	3

Point Total	10-Year Risk %
<0	<1
0	1
1	1
2	1
3	1
4	1
5	2
6	2
7	3
8	4
9	5
10	6
11	8
12	10
13	12
14	16
15	20
16	25
≥17	≥30

10-Year risk ____ %

A

Estimate of 10-Year Risk for Women

(Framingham Point Scores)

Age	Points
20-34	−7
35-39	−3
40-44	0
45-49	3
50-54	6
55-59	8
60-64	10
65-69	12
70-74	14
75-79	16

Total Cholesterol	Points				
	Age 20-39	Age 40-49	Age 50-59	Age 60-69	Age 70-79
<160	0	0	0	0	0
160-199	4	3	2	1	1
200-239	8	6	4	2	1
240-279	11	8	5	3	2
≥280	13	10	7	4	2

	Points				
	Age 20-39	Age 40-49	Age 50-59	Age 60-69	Age 70-79
Nonsmoker	0	0	0	0	0
Smoker	9	7	4	2	1

HDL (mg/dL)	Points
≥60	−1
50-59	0
40-49	1
<40	2

Systolic BP (mmHg)	If Untreated	If Treated
<120	0	0
120-129	1	3
130-139	2	4
140-159	3	5
≥160	4	6

Point Total	10-Year Risk %
<9	<1
9	1
10	1
11	1
12	1
13	2
14	2
15	3
16	4
17	5
18	6
19	8
20	11
21	14
22	17
23	22
24	27
≥25	≥30

10-Year risk ____ %

B

FIGURE 12-7 A: Estimate of 10-year risk for men. B: Estimate of 10-year risk for women.

Table 12-10 NCEP ATP III and AHA/ACC LDL-C Goals and Cutpoints for Therapeutic Lifestyle Changes (TLC) and Drug Therapy[88,89,92]

Risk Category	*LDL-C Goal*	*LDL-C at which to Initiate TLC*	*LDL-C at which to Consider Drug Therapy*[a]
CHD or CHD risk equivalents (10-year risk >20%)	<100 mg/dL (Reasonable goal <70 mg/dL)[c]	>100 mg/dL	>100 mg/dL (<100 mg/dL, consider drug options)[b]
2+ risk factors (10-year risk 10% to 20%)	<130 mg/dL (Optional goal <100 mg/dL)	>130 mg/dL	>130 mg/dL (100–129 mg/dL; consider drug options)[d]
2+ risk factors (10-year risk <10%	<130 mg/dL	>130 mg/dL	>160 mg/dL
<2 risk factors[e]	<160 mg/dL	>160 mg/dL	190 mg/dL (160–189 mg/dL, LDL-C lowering drug therapy is optional)

[a] For all patients without CHD: LDL-C lowering medications should be initiated at a dose that is consistent with at least a 30% to 40% reduction in LDL-C levels. The use of lower doses just to barely attain the LDL-C goal would not be a prudent use of medications.
[b] The clinician may select niacin or fibrate therapy if patient has high triglycerides and or low HDL-C. The decision to lower LDL-C with drug therapy is optional based on available clinical trial evidence.
[c] All patients with CHD: When LDL-C <70 mg/dL is not achievable because high baseline LDL-C levels, it generally is possible to achieve reductions of >50% by either statins or LDL-C lowering drug combinations.
[d] The decision to lower LDL-C with drug therapy to achieve an LDL-C <100 mg/dL is optional based on available clinical trial evidence.
[e] Patients with <two risk factors usually have a 10-year risk of <10%, and therefore do not need a 10-year risk assessment.
CHD, coronary heart disease; LDL-C, low-density lipoprotein cholesterol.

teaching a patient to do this is to determine his or her daily caloric requirements, adjusted for his or her level of activity. The average caloric requirement for women is 1,800 calories/day; for men it is 2,500 calories/day. Based on this, T.A. should be instructed to keep her total fat intake to 450 to 630 calories/day (25% to 35% of calories) and saturated fat to <126 calories/day (<7% of total calories). Converting fat calories to grams (i.e., dividing calories by 9 calories/g), T.A. should be instructed to restrict her total fat intake to <50 to 70 g/day and saturated fat to <14 g/day.

Once these calculations have been made, the next step is to teach T.A. how to determine the grams of saturated and unsaturated fat contained in the foods she eats by reading food labels and referring to reference charts or books that list the nutritional content of foods. A good source for this nutrition information is the National Institutes of Health website on Therapeutic Lifestyle Change (http://www.nhlbi.nih.gov) under the Health Information icon). This site contains information on the TLC diet, a 10-year risk calculator, recipes, a virtual grocery store, a cyberkitchen, a fitness room, and a resource library. The AHA sites (www.americanheart.org and www.deliciousdecisions.org) provide equally good information on risk assessment, a cholesterol tracker, low-fat recipes, and guidance for eating in restaurants, cooking, and fitness.

Table 12-11 NCEP ATP III Therapeutic Lifestyle Change Diet[92]

Nutrient	*Recommended Intake*
Total fat	25–35% of total calories
Saturated fat	<7% of total calories
Polyunsaturated fat	Up to 10% of total calories
Monounsaturated fat	Up to 20% of total calories
Carbohydrate	50–60% of total calories
Fiber	20–30 g/day
Cholesterol	<200 mg/d
Protein	Approx. 15% of total calories

For patients who are not able or willing to count calories or grams, general instruction on how to select low-fat foods and control portion sizes of higher-fat foods would provide an alternative approach. Principles to teach include the following:

- Eat less high-fat food (especially food high in saturated fats).
- Replace saturated fats with monounsaturated fats and fish oils whenever possible.
- Eat less high-cholesterol food.
- Choose foods high in complex carbohydrates (starch and fiber).
- Attain and maintain an acceptable weight.

T.A. should be counseled to recognize and minimize the three main sources of saturated fats in her diet: meat products, dairy products, and oils used in processed foods and cooking.

All meat products, including beef, pork, and poultry, contain fat. Much of the fat is visible and should be trimmed off before consumption. The remaining fat is contained within the meat and can be limited by (*a*) selecting the leanest meat (e.g., lean beef, skinless chicken, fish), (*b*) limiting portion size to about the size of a deck of playing cards (no more than 6 oz/day), and (*c*) cooking the meat in a manner that allows the fat to drip away from the meat (i.e., broiling, grilling).

High-fat dairy products are made with whole milk (~4% fat); low-fat alternatives are made with skim or 1% milk (which contain all of the nutrient value of whole milk products). T.A. should be taught to substitute low-fat alternatives for high-fat products—for example, by choosing soft margarine (or no fatty spread at all) instead of stick butter (note that unsaturated fats exist normally in liquid form and saturated fats in solid form); nonfat creams rather than whole milk creams; low-fat or nonfat soft cheese (e.g., cottage cheese) rather than natural or processed hard cheese (including cream cheese); skim milk rather than whole milk; light or nonfat sour cream rather than regular sour cream; and nonfat frozen yogurt rather than ice cream. She also should avoid or limit cream sauces on meats and vegetables and creamy soups.

Products prepared with coconut, palm, or palm kernel oils, as well as lard and bacon fat contain a high concentration of saturated fats, and intake should be restricted. In their place, products made with monounsaturated fats (e.g., olive oil, canola oils) or polyunsaturated fats (especially oils that contain omega-3 fatty acids) may be substituted. Monounsaturated fats have little or no effect on blood lipids, and polyunsaturated fats actually may help reduce total cholesterol. Although unsaturated fats do not elevate cholesterol levels, they are sources of dense calories and, therefore, may contribute to the development of obesity and hypertriglyceridemia. Also, when the "good" (unsaturated) oils are partially hydrogenated (i.e., saturated to make them solid, as in some margarine products), they take on the character of saturated oils and may raise cholesterol levels. These are called *trans fatty acids*. Major sources of saturated and trans fatty acids include cakes, pies, cookies, chips, and crackers. T.A. should be advised to avoid or limit not only saturated fats, but also trans fatty acids by reading food labels.

It is best not to give the patient a list of foods to avoid; this aversive approach is likely to fail. Rather, good instruction about a low-fat diet should teach the patient how to make good selections. Any food, even a high-fat food, is not prohibited as long as portion size and frequency of use are controlled.

Another dietary approach to lowering blood cholesterol is to use dietary adjuncts. For example, adding 5 to 10 g of viscous fiber (e.g., guar, pectin, oat gum, psyllium) or other dietary sources of fiber (e.g., vegetables, legumes, whole grains, fruits) to the diet daily will aid in lowering blood cholesterol levels about 5% on average. Also, plant stanol and sterol esters have been made available in margarine and salad dressing products (Benecol and Total Control) and can lower LDL-C 5% to 15% when the equivalent of one tablespoonful is ingested one to three times a day. They act by reducing the absorption of cholesterol in the intestine. The estimated cumulative percent reduction in LDL-C achievable through therapeutic lifestyle changes is between 20% and 30%.

T.A. will need to follow a low-fat diet indefinitely to sustain its benefit. For this reason, it might be necessary to have T.A. work with a registered dietitian or other professional who understands low-fat, low-cholesterol diets and who can give her personalized instruction. Particularly important is instruction on how to shop for and prepare low-fat foods and how to select low-fat foods in restaurants.

EFFECT ON LDL-C

7. What changes in T.A.'s LDL-C can be expected if she follows a TLC diet?

Serum cholesterol is reported to be reduced by an average of 3% to 14% in males who restrict saturated fat to <10% of calories; a slightly smaller response is attained in women, perhaps because their intake of saturated fats is generally lower than that of men.[138–140] Patients who can restrict saturated fat intake to <7% of daily calories should experience an additional 3% to 7% average reduction. Most patients can attain at least a 5% reduction in cholesterol levels with a TLC diet, some patients much more. If dietary adjuncts are added, LDL-C may be lowered by an additional 5% to 15%.

Patients' response to a low-fat diet is variable. In some patients, blood cholesterol levels fall substantially, whereas in others practically no change occurs. Response to a low-fat diet depends on many factors, including the patient's dietary habits before implementing the low-fat diet, the patient's adherence with the diet, the degree to which the patient restricts fats and cholesterol, and the influence of genetic factors. The patient should not be discouraged if LDL-C levels do not change much or at all despite close adherence to the diet. The Mediterranean diet, for example, which is high in monounsaturated fats and fiber, has no appreciable effect on blood lipids, but can still reduce cardiovascular disease and mortality by 70%.[137] Patients who adhere to a low-fat diet might also respond to lower doses of lipid-lowering drugs.

Because T.A. is a woman and was following a low-fat diet before her diagnosis, a TLC diet is not likely to have a substantial effect on her blood cholesterol levels. It would be prudent to have her maintain a 3-day diary of everything she eats to allow a more objective view of her eating habits. If there are ways for her to improve her diet, this approach will reveal them.

Other Lifestyle Changes

8. What other modifications in behavior are prescribed in the TLC program?

Weight reduction in the overweight patient can reduce LDL-C and is a key component to the TLC plan. A 5- to 10-lb weight loss, for example, can up to double the LDL-C reduction achieved with a low saturated fat diet alone.[138] The predominant effect of weight loss is a reduction in serum TG and a small increase in HDL-C, however.[141] In addition, weight reduction may offset the risk of developing hypertension and diabetes. The initial goal of a weight loss program is to reduce body weight by approximately 10% within about 6 months.[142] This is best achieved by restricting total daily energy consumption through a reduction in saturated and trans fatty acid intake and by increasing physical exercise. A normal weight is defined as a body mass index (BMI) between 18.5 and 24.9, and a desirable waist circumference is <40 inches for male patients and <35 inches for female patients.[142] Because T.A. has an acceptable weight, these considerations do not apply.

Smoking cessation substantially reduces the risk of CHD, pulmonary disease, and cancer and is a central component of a TLC program. This is an important consideration in T.A. The CHD risk she has from smoking is greater than the risk she has from her LDL-C elevation. By stopping smoking, T.A. will not only reduce her blood cholesterol levels slightly, but will also substantially alter her risk profile. Because most patients gain weight when they stop smoking and because weight gain may worsen lipid levels, plans need to be made to alter her diet and increase physical activity to counter these effects.

Increasing physical activity should be a component of the treatment of any patient with high blood cholesterol. Regular physical exercise may reduce TG and VLDL-C levels, raise HDL-C levels slightly, promote weight loss or maintenance of desired weight, lower BP, and cause favorable changes in coronary blood flow.[143] Regular aerobic exercise (e.g., brisk walking, jogging, swimming, bicycling, and tennis) should be prescribed in terms of amount (e.g., walking 4 miles), intensity (e.g., walking 4 mph), and frequency (walking each day if possible, but at least three times a week). T.A. states that she is already physically active. The level of her activity should be documented and enhancements recommended if needed.

Goal of Therapy

9. **A lipid profile obtained 12 weeks after T.A. initiated a TLC diet and exercise program and had stopped smoking revealed an LDL-C level of 195 mg/dL; HDL-C and TG did not differ from baseline values. What is your assessment of the need for additional lipid-modifying treatment?**

[SI units: LDL-C, 5.40, 5.43, and 5.17 mmol/L, respectively]

Based on her initial assessment, T.A.'s LDL-C goal is <130 mg/dL; drug therapy can be considered if her LDL-C is >160 mg/dL (Table 12-10). She has stopped smoking, however, and now has a global CHD risk of 1% in the next 10 years. Thus, her LDL-C goal today is <160 mg/dL. While she is not currently smoking, it may take a year or more for the associated risk to fully dissipate. NCEP recommends that drugs be considered in patients with fewer than two risk factors if their LDL-C remains ≥160 mg/dL after implementing a TLC plan. Realistically, this is a therapeutic gray area where clinical judgment must be exercised. T.A. has a relatively low risk of CHD despite her current LDL-C level, supporting a decision to maximize TLC and withhold lipid-lowering drug therapy until her CHD risk rises to a high level. Her strong family history suggests, however, there is more to the story than LDL-C alone.

Emerging Risk Factors

10. **To help determine whether to initiate lipid-lowering drug therapy in T.A., is there value in ordering additional laboratory tests to identify possible emerging risk factors?**

As mentioned in question 4, noninvasive tests, such as ABI, carotid intimal-medial thickness, and electron beam computed tomography, can uncover evidence of subclinical atherosclerotic disease and help the clinician decide whether to pursue more aggressive therapy with lipid-lowering drugs. In addition, the clinician can measure several specialized laboratory tests of emerging risk factors to help with these decisions (Table 12-9). In T.A.'s case, a global risk assessment indicating about a 1% risk of a CHD event in 10 years and her strong family history for premature CHD events present conflicting information. Measuring one or more of the emerging risk factors may help focus the treatment decision in one direction or another.

Lp(a) (pronounced "el, pea, little a") appears to be an independent risk factor for CHD, although this is not a universal finding.[144] This very small cholesterol-containing lipoprotein particle contains the apolipoprotein(a). Its structure suggests that it could be an important source of cholesterol for the formation of atherosclerosis as well as a stimulus for thrombogenic mechanisms. High Lp(a) levels suggest a high CHD risk and support a more aggressive approach to lowering LDL-C. Evidence has shown that lowering LDL-C aggressively can overcome the increased CHD risk predicted by an elevated Lp(a) level. The only drug that can lower Lp(a) is niacin, but no studies have shown that giving niacin to these patients reduces CHD risk.

Apolipoprotein B is a marker for the number of atherogenic lipoproteins (VLDL and LDL) in the circulation. It is a strong predictor of CHD risk, at least as strong as LDL-C. It is a surrogate for LDL-C, but provides different information.[145] Some specialists prefer to use apolipoprotein B levels rather than, or in addition to, LDL-C in treating patients. Apolipoprotein B levels are usually disproportionately high in patients with high TG, although they may also parallel LDL-C levels. There is a genetic dyslipidemia that is characterized by increased apolipoprotein B levels (increased particle number) and normal LDL-C levels. Based on this information, it appears reasonable to measure apolipoprotein B to gain additional information.

Severe elevations in homocysteine are positively correlated with CHD risk, especially in patients with inherited forms of hyperhomocysteinemia.[146] Several clinical trials are underway to determine whether treating moderate hyperhomocysteinemia will lower CHD events. High levels of homocysteine are easily treated with folic acid; the recent fortification of foods with folic acid is predicted to substantially reduce homocysteine levels. NCEP ATP III does not recommend homocysteine measurements in risk assessment to modify LDL-C goals because panel members were uncertain of the relationship between homocysteine levels and CHD risk.[92] It may be useful in patients such as T.A. when searching for causes of a strong family history of CHD.

Increasingly, it is recognized that atherosclerosis is a chronic inflammatory disease. Thus, markers of inflammation have been sought to measure arterial inflammation. The marker that has emerged from this search is hs-CRP. Many observational studies have found that hs-CRP predicts a two- to fourfold increase in CHD risk over what is predicted by LDL-C alone.[123] Recently, the AHA has recommended that hs-CRP levels between 3 and 10 be considered suggestive evidence of a chronic inflammatory disease.[125] Levels >10 suggest the presence of an acute inflammation caused by infection, trauma, connective tissue disease, or other causes; in this case, the hs-CRP measurement should be repeated after 6 weeks.

T.A. was found to have a slightly elevated apolipoprotein B level (135 mg/dL) (which is consistent with her elevated LDL-C level), normal Lp(a) and homocysteine levels, and an hs-CRP of 4.7 mg/dL. An hs-CRP >3.0 is consistent with the presence of a chronic inflammatory disease, possibly atherosclerosis. Some clinicians believe that these findings would support more aggressive LDL-C lowering therapy in T.A.

Drug Therapy

11. **L.W. is a 53-year-old man with a LDL-C of 200 mg/dL. He states that he follows a low saturated fat diet and jogs 2 miles three times a week. He does not smoke and has no family history of premature CHD. His high BP is under marginal control with enalapril 10 mg/day (BP, 134/88 mm Hg). His glucose level is 80 mg/dL (normal). He does not have hypothyroidism. His total cholesterol is 261 mg/dL, HDL-C is 45 mg/dL (normal average for a man), LDL-C is 200 mg/dL, and TG level is 80 mg/dL. No secondary or familial causes of his hypercholesterolemia are evident, and his physical examination findings are normal. Is L.W. a candidate for cholesterol-lowering drug therapy?**

[SI unit: LDL-C, 5.17 mmol/L]

According to NCEP guidelines, L.W. has two CHD risk factors: male >45 years and a diagnosis of hypertension; this makes his LDL-C goal <130 mg/dL (Tables 12-4 and 12-6). Because he has two risk factors, his global risk was assessed (Fig. 12-7). L.W was found to have a 12% risk of a CHD event in the next 10 years and has an optional LDL-C treatment goal of <100 mg/dL. With two risk factors and an estimated

Table 12-12 Drugs of Choice for Dyslipidemia

Lipid Disorder	Drug of Choice	Alternative Agents	Combination Therapy
Polygenic hypercholesterolemia	Statin	Resin, ezetimibe, niacin Combination	Statin-ezetimibe, statin-resin, resin-niacin, statin-niacin
Familial hypercholesterolemia or severe polygenic hypercholesterolemia	Statin (high-dose)	–	Statin-ezetimibe, statin-resin, resin-niacin, statin-niacin, statin-ezetimibe-niacin, statin-resin-niacin
Atherogenic dyslipidemia	Statin, niacin, fibrate[a]	Statin, niacin, fibrate[a]	Statin-niacin, niacin-resin, niacin-fibrate
Isolated low HDL	Statin	Niacin	Statin-niacin

[a] Use cautiously because there is an increased risk of myopathy.
HDL, high-density lipoprotein.

10-year risk assessment between 10% and 20%, he is a candidate for cholesterol-lowering drug therapy in addition to therapeutic lifestyle change (Table 12-10).

BILE ACID RESINS AND CHOLESTEROL ABSORPTION INHIBITORS

12. The NCEP recognizes four drug categories for lowering LDL-C: bile acid resins, cholesterol absorption inhibitors, niacin, and the statins.[92] Which of these is preferred to treat L.W. (Table 12-12)?

Bile acid resins have appeal in the management of hypercholesterolemia because they have a strong safety record established from years of use, effectively lower LDL-C, and demonstrated the ability to reduce CHD events in the Coronary Primary Prevention Trial.[82,147] Resins are not absorbed from the gastrointestinal (GI) tract and thus lack systemic toxicity. They are available in powder and tablet forms. They reduce total and LDL cholesterol in a dose-dependent manner (Table 12-13). LDL-C is reduced approximately 15% with 5 g (1 packet) daily of colestipol (Colestid) powder (equivalent to 4 g of cholestyramine [Questran]), 23% with 10 g/day, and 27% with 15 g/day.[147] Therapy should be initiated with one packet, scoop, or tablet of resin daily (Table 12-14). The reduction achieved is inversely proportional to the baseline, untreated LDL-C level.[148] Thus, patients with a moderate cholesterol elevation (such as L.W.) will have a greater relative reduction than if the LDL-C were higher.

The older resins are not well tolerated, however, because of numerous GI side effects and the unpleasant granular texture of the powder. A new bile acid resin, colesevelam (WelChol), is available in 0.625-g tablets; the daily dose is six tablets (3.8 g) administered in one or two divided doses daily. Although the tablets are large and difficult for some patients to swallow, the product is much easier to administer and, owing in part to a smaller total daily dose, less susceptible to cause GI side effects than the older products. The standard daily dose reduces LDL-C by 15% to 18%.

Mechanism of Action

The resins are anion exchange agents that bind bile acids in the intestinal lumen and cause them to be eliminated in the stool.[149] By disrupting the normal enterohepatic recirculation of bile acids from the intestinal lumen to the liver, the liver is stimulated to convert hepatocellular cholesterol into bile acids. This in turn causes a reduction in the concentration of cholesterol in the hepatocyte, prompting the upregulation of LDL receptor synthesis. Finally, circulating LDL-C levels are lowered by binding to the newly formed LDL receptors on the liver surface. This mechanism has appeal not only because it effectively lowers LDL-C but also because it is additive with

Table 12-13 Dose-Related LDL-C Lowering of Major Drugs

Drug[a]	Daily Dosage	LDL-C Lowering (%)
Bile acid resins (colestipol)	5 g	−15
	10 g	−23
	15 g	−27
Bile acid resin (Cosevelam)	3.8 g	−15
	4.5 g	−18
Ezetimibe[151]	10 mg	−18 to −22
Ezetimibe/Simvastatin	10 mg/10 mg	−45
	10 mg/20 mg	−52
	10 mg/40 mg	−55
	10 mg/80 mg	−60
Niacin (crystalline)[155]	1,000 mg	−6
	1,500 mg	−13
	2,000 mg	−16
	3,000 mg	−22
Niaspan	1,000 mg	−9
	1,500 mg	−14
	2,000 mg	−17
Atorvastatin[167]	10 mg	−39
	20 mg	−43
	40 mg	−50
	80 mg	−60
Fluvastatin[167]	20 mg	−22
	40 mg	−24
	80 mg	−34
Lovastatin[167]	20 mg	−24
	40 mg	−34
	80 mg	−40
Pravastatin[167]	10 mg	−22
	20 mg	−32
	40 mg	−34
	80 mg	−37
Rosuvastatin	10 mg	−46
	20 mg	−52
	40 mg	−55
Simvastatin[167]	5 mg	−26
	10 mg	−30
	20 mg	−38
	40 mg	−41
	80 mg	−47

[a] Numbers following drugs are references.

Table 12-14 Dosages of Selected Lipid-Modulating Drugs

Drug	Initial Dosage	Usual Dosage	Maximal Dosage	Comment
Cholestyramine	4 g before main meal	4 g BID before heaviest meals	8 g BID before heaviest meals	May prescribe 24 g/day, but few patients can tolerate.
Colestipol	5 g powder or 2 g tabs QD before main meal	5 g of powder or 4 g of tabs BID before heaviest meals	10 g powder or 8 g of tabs BID before heaviest meals	May prescribe 30 g of powder per day, but few patients can tolerate.
Colesevelam	6 –0.63-g tablets per day	Same	7 × 0.63-g tablets/day	Less bulk is associated with less gastrointestinal intolerance.
Niacin	100–125 BID with food	750–1,000 mg BID	1,500 mg BID	Dosages up to 6 g/day have been used, but few can tolerate. Dosages may be increased 200–250 mg/day every 3–7 days until desired dosage has been obtained.
Niaspan	500 mg q HS	1,000–2,000 mg q HS	2,000 mg q HS	Increase dose by 500 mg daily Q 4 wks.
Atorvastatin	10–40 mg QD	10–40 mg QD	80 mg QD	Administer any time of day.
Fluvastatin	20–40 mg QHS	20–40 mg QHS	40 mg BID 80 mg XL QD	Modified-release form (XL) has similar efficacy but has less bioavailability (and less risk of adverse effects).
Lovastatin	20 mg with dinner	20–40 mg with dinner	40 mg BID	Administration with food increases bioavailability. BID dosing provides greater LDL-C lowering efficacy than QD.
Pravastatin	10–40 mg QD	10–40 mg QD	80 mg QD	Administer with food to reduce dyspepsia.
Rosuvastatin	10–20 mg QD	10–20 mg QD	40 mg QD	Administer any time of the day.
Simvastatin	20–40 mg Q pm	20–40 mg Q pm	80 mg Q pm	Administer with food to reduce dyspepsia.
Gemfibrozil	600 mg BID	Same	Same	
Fenofibrate[a]	67–201 mg QD	Same	201 mg QD	

[a]Multiple formulations are available and doses do vary.

other therapies to lower cholesterol. For example, combining a drug that reduces hepatocellular cholesterol biosynthesis (e.g., statins) with a resin that interferes with bile acid recycling can cause a substantial upregulation of LDL receptors and enhance removal of cholesterol from the blood.[10]

Adverse Effects

The disadvantage of the older resins (i.e., colestipol or cholestyramine) is their side effects. These resins often cause GI symptoms, including constipation, bloating, epigastric fullness, nausea, and flatulence[147] (Table 12-15). Colesevelam is associated with less GI intolerance. If one of the older resins is prescribed, the patient should be instructed to mix the resin powder in noncarbonated, apple juice or pulpy juices such as orange juice[150]; to swallow it without engulfing air (administering it through a straw may help avoid air entrapment); and to maintain an adequate intake of fluids and fiber in the diet.

The older resins also can *raise* TG levels by 3% to 10% or more, especially in patients with high TG levels; this appears to be less of a problem with colesevelam. Reduction in the absorption of fat-soluble vitamins and folic acid has been reported with high dosages of resins, but this is rarely a problem in otherwise healthy patients consuming a nutritionally balanced diet. The older resins also can reduce the absorption of digitoxin (but not digoxin), warfarin, thyroxine, thiazide diuretics, beta-blockers, and presumably other anionic drugs. This interaction can be minimized by administering other drugs 1 hour before or 4 hours after the resin dose. Colesevelam appears to have a high specificity for binding with bile acids and not with other anionic drugs, including warfarin; thus, it may be safely administered with other drugs.

Based on this summary, no contraindications exist to the use of resin therapy in L.W. Colesevelam, which can safely be taken along with his BP medication and is less likely to cause intolerable symptoms, would be the preferred choice. Colesevelam therapy, however, is unlikely to achieve the desired 30% to 40% reduction in LDL-C levels needed by L.W. As shown in Table 12-11, it lowers LDL-C only about 20% on average, which is not sufficient to reduce L.W.'s LDL-C from 200 mg/dL to <130 mg/dL (or <100 mg/dL as an optional goal).

EZETIMIBE

Ezetimibe represents a class of lipid-altering drugs called cholesterol absorption inhibitors. One advantage of this compound is its ability to reduce LDL-C by an action in the gut, with minimal systemic exposure. This suggests that the drug may be very safe, much like the resins. It is administered once a day as a 10-mg tablet.

Ezetimibe reduces LDL-C by 18% to 22%, but has little effect on TG or HDL-C.[151] In combination with a statin, it demonstrates an additive effect, enhancing LDL-C lowering by an additional 10% to 20%. In fact, when added to a low dose of a statin, the net LDL-C reduction can be similar to the lowering achieved with the maximal dose of the statin.[152] When added to the maximal dose of a statin, it causes further LDL-C reduction, an effect important in patients with very high LDL-C levels requiring substantial reduction to achieve treatment goals.

Table 12-15 Monitoring Parameters, Adverse Effects, and Drug Interactions with Major Cholesterol-Lowering Drugs

Drug	Adverse Effects	Drug Interactions	Monitoring Parameters
Resin	Indigestion, bloating, nausea, constipation, abdominal pain, flatulence	GI binding and reduced absorption of anionic drugs (warfarin, β-blockers, digitoxin, thyroxine, thiazide diuretics); administer drugs 12 hr before or 4 hr after resin	Lipid profile Q 4–8 wk until stable dose; then Q 6–12 mo long term. Check TG level after stable dose achieved, then as needed.
Niacin	Flushing, itching, tingling, headache, nausea, gas, heart-burn, fatigue, rash, worsening of peptic ulcer, elevation in serum glucose and uric acid, hepatitis, and elevation in hepatic transaminase levels	Hypotension with BP-lowering drugs such as α-blockers possible; diabetics taking insulin or oral agents may require dosage adjustment because of increase in serum glucose levels	Lipid profile after 1,000–1,500 mg/day and then after stable dosage achieved; then Q 6–12 mo long term. LFT at baseline and Q 6–8 wk during dose titration; then as needed for symptoms. Uric acid and glucose at baseline and again after stable dose reached (or symptoms produced), more frequently in diabetic patients.
Statins	Headache, dyspepsia, myositis (myalgia, CPK >10 times normal), elevation in hepatic transaminase levels	Increased myositis risk with concurrent use of drugs that inhibit or compete for P450 3A4 system (e.g., cyclosporine, erythromycin, calcium blockers, fibrates, nefazodone, niacin, ketoconazole); risk greater with lovastatin and simvastatin; caution with concurrent fibrate or niacin use; lovastatin increases the pro-time with concurrent warfarin	Lipid profile 4–8 wk after dose change, then Q 6–12 mo long term. LFT at baseline, in 3 months, and periodically thereafter. CPK at baseline and if the patient has symptoms of myalgia.

BP, blood pressure; CPK, creatinine phosphokinase; GI, gastrointestinal; LFT, liver function tests; TC, total cholesterol; TG, triglyceride.

Mechanism of Action

Cholesterol that is ingested in the diet and circulated through the bile from the liver is actively reabsorbed in the intestines. Once transported across the intestinal lumen into the enterocyte, it is combined with TG and apolipoprotein B48 to form chylomicron particles that transport the lipids through the lymphatic system to the hepatocyte. The TG and cholesterol can then be packaged into VLDL particles and secreted into the systemic circulation.

Ezetimibe interferes with the active absorption of cholesterol from the intestinal lumen into the enterocyte by binding to the Niemann-Pick C1 Like 1 (NPC1L1) transporter, which is a cholesterol transporter responsible for the uptake of dietary and biliary cholesterol into the small intestine. By interfering with the absorption of cholesterol, about 50% less cholesterol is transported from the intestines to the liver by the chylomicrons. This causes an upregulation in hepatic cholesterol synthesis, which is diverted to the intestines via the bile to replenish the cholesterol available for absorption processes. It also causes an upregulation of hepatic LDL receptors and increased clearance of circulating VLDL and LDL particles. The net effect of the inhibition of cholesterol absorption in the gut is approximately a 70% increase in GI sterol excretion, a 50% reduction in hepatic cholesterol concentration, a 90% increase in hepatic cholesterol synthesis, and approximately a 20% increase in LDL-C taken up from the systemic circulation via upregulated LDL receptors.[153]

Ezetimibe also inhibits the absorption of sitosterol, a plant sterol, from the gut, resulting in about a 40% reduction in blood sitosterol levels. The occurrence of sitosterolemia is rare, but patients who have it have a high CHD risk. Ezetimibe provides one of the first effective treatments for this rare disorder.

Adverse Effects

Ezetimibe's side effects include diarrhea, arthralgias, cough, and fatigue. These occur no more frequently with ezetimibe than they do with placebo. Whether used alone or together with a statin, no increases in liver function abnormalities have been reported nor any cases of myopathy or rhabdomyolysis. As with resin therapy, ezetimibe can safely reduce the LDL-C by about 20%, which is not likely to be sufficient to reduce L.W.'s LDL-C to his goal of <130 mg/dL (or <100 mg/dL as an optional goal).

NIACIN

Clinical Use

Niacin (or nicotinic acid) is a water-soluble B vitamin that can improve the levels of all serum lipids. Favorable attributes are low cost, a long history of use, and clinical trial evidence that it can reduce CHD events.[112,113,154] Crystalline (immediate-release) niacin lowers LDL-C levels by 15% to 25% and TG 30% to 60% and raises HDL-C levels 20% to 35%[154–156] (Tables 12-13 and 12-16). Reduction in LDL-C follows a linear relationship to dose: Doses need to be increased to 2 to 3 g/day to reduce LDL-C levels by 20% to 25%. Conversely, the increase in HDL-C and reduction in TG follows a curvilinear relationship with dose: Low to moderate doses (i.e., 1 to 2 g/day) can increase HDL-C by 25% and lower TG by 30% to 40%[155] (Table 12-13, Fig. 12-8). Crystalline niacin should be started at a low level (e.g., 250 mg in two or three divided doses daily) and slowly titrated as tolerated (e.g., daily doses increased by 250 mg every 3 to 7 days) to a maximum of 3,000 mg/day (Table 12-14). Higher doses have been used but are associated with unpleasant side effects. Niacin is also the only drug that lowers Lp(a), with reductions being as great as 30%.[157] Its metabolite, nicotinamide, has no effect on

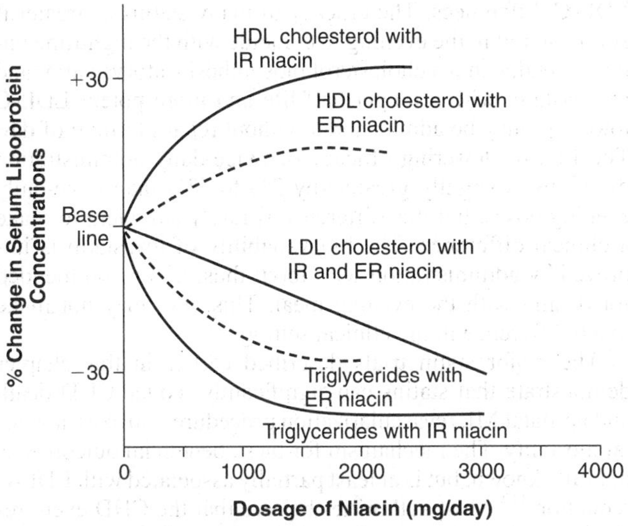

FIGURE 12-8 Dose-related effects of niacin on lipoproteins. (From Knopp RH. Drug treatment of lipid disorders. *N Engl J Med* 1999;341:498, with permission.)

cholesterol and should not be used as a substitute to lower side effects.

Sustained-release (timed-release) dosage forms of niacin were developed to reduce the flushing side effects associated with crystalline niacin. These products are sold as a dietary supplement ostensibly for treating niacin deficiency, but are mistakenly purchased by patients to treat high blood cholesterol. These products may have slightly greater LDL-C–lowering efficacy at each dose level and slightly less HDL-C and TG effects compared with crystalline niacin, but they cannot be recommended because of a substantially increased risk of liver toxicity at higher dosages (see Adverse Effects).

An extended-release dosage form of niacin, Niaspan, is available by prescription to treat elevated cholesterol and TG levels and appears to be better tolerated than either the crystalline or sustained-release forms. Niaspan releases niacin over an 8- to 12-hour period, a feature that turns out to be important in improving its side effect profile, and it has the efficacy pattern of crystalline niacin. It lowers LDL-C by 10% to 15% and TG by 20% to 30%, and it raises HDL-C by 15% to 25% with daily doses between 1,000 and 2,000 mg. Daily doses of Niaspan should not exceed 2,000 mg/day to reduce the risk of liver side effects.

Mechanism of Action

Niacin inhibits the mobilization of free fatty acids from peripheral adipose tissue to the liver, which, either alone or together with other hepatic effects, results in reduced synthesis and secretion of VLDL particles by the liver.[158] This explains its effectiveness in lowering TG levels. Because LDL is a VLDL degradation product, reducing the secretion of VLDL particles secondarily lowers the LDL-C level. Niacin reduces the amount of apolipoprotein A-I extracted and catabolized from HDL during the hepatic uptake of cholesterol, thus preserving the structural and functional integrity of HDL particles.[159] As a result, cholesterol-deficient apolipoprotein A-I–containing

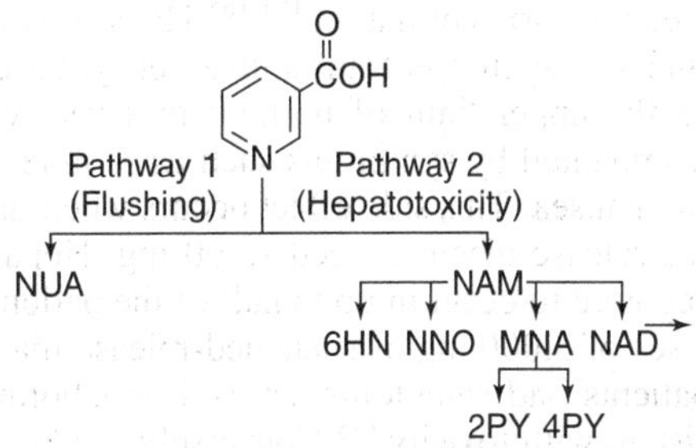

FIGURE 12-9 Niacin metabolism. NAM, nicotinamide; NUA, nicotin-uric acid. (From Piepho RW. The pharmacokinetics and pharmacodynamics of agents proven to raise high-density lipoprotein cholesterol. *Am J Cardiol* 2000;86(Suppl):35L, with permission.)

HDL particles are recirculated from the liver to the peripheral cells, maintaining HDL levels and enhancing reverse cholesterol transport.[160]

Adverse Effects

The differences in release characteristics among various niacin products are important because they determine how the drug is metabolized, in turn influencing the side effect profile of the product. Niacin is metabolized through two separate metabolic pathways (Fig. 12-9).[161] The nicotinamide (NAM) pathway is a high-affinity, low-capacity pathway. Crystalline niacin quickly saturates this pathway and is predominately metabolized through the high-capacity conjugation pathway. The flushing effect with crystalline niacin results from prostaglandin-mediated vasodilation associated with the formation of nicotinuric acid (NUA) by the conjugation pathway. In contrast, sustained-release niacin is slowly absorbed and preferentially metabolized via the NAM pathway. Because of this, sustained-release niacin rarely causes flushing, but it can cause serious, dose-related hepatotoxicity because of the formation of toxic metabolites of the NAM pathway. Niaspan, with its intermediate absorption rate, has a more balanced metabolism between the two pathways. The result is less flushing and less risk of hepatotoxicity, at least with daily doses of >2 g.

The main drawbacks to crystalline niacin therapy are frequent, bothersome vasodilation-related side effects: flushing, itching, and headache[155,156,162] (Table 12-15). Practically every patient will experience these side effects, at least transiently.[163] These symptoms can be reduced by having patients take doses with food and by taking 325 mg of aspirin 30 minutes before the morning dose of niacin (to inhibit prostaglandin synthesis, which is thought to mediate these side effects).[164] Use of Niaspan can further reduce these symptoms, and administering it once daily at bedtime can diminish the patient's awareness of flushing symptoms. Niacin also can cause fatigue and a variety of GI symptoms, including nausea, dyspepsia, and activation of peptic ulcer. As with flushing, GI side effects are minimized by taking the drug with food. Other less common, though potentially troublesome, side effects of niacin are hyperuricemia, gout, and transient worsening of glucose tolerance in some diabetic patients (Table 12-15).

The most worrisome side effect associated with niacin is hepatotoxicity, which is associated almost exclusively with the sustained-release forms of niacin.[155,165] Hepatotoxicity is detected by an increase in liver transaminase enzymes exceeding three times the upper limit of normal; in severe cases, this can be accompanied by symptoms such as fatigue, anorexia, malaise, and nausea. This side effect occurs when daily doses of sustained-release niacin exceed 1,500 mg. Hepatotoxicity has been reported to occur in up to half of the patients titrated to daily doses of 3,000 mg of sustained-release niacin; many of these patients had symptoms, as well as laboratory findings, consistent with toxicity.[155] Conversely, <1% of patients titrated up to 2,000 mg/day of Niaspan have elevated liver function tests. Rare cases of fulminant hepatitis have been reported with sustained-release niacin. Niacin-induced hepatotoxicity appears to be completely reversible when the drug is discontinued.

Because of the hepatotoxic effects of sustained-release niacin and the flushing side effects of crystalline niacin, Niaspan is the preferred form of niacin for general use. It can be safely used in a daily dose up to 2,000 mg. An estimated 30% of patients experience flushing symptoms that will cause them to discontinue therapy.

No apparent contraindications are seen to the use of niacin in L.W. Niacin, however, would not be expected to lower his LDL-C by the 35% to 50% required to reach his treatment goal of <130 mg/dL or <100 mg/dL (optional goal), respectively.

STATINS

Clinical Use

The group of drugs with the most potent cholesterol-lowering potential is composed of the statins. They lower LDL-C by approximately 20% to 40% with initial doses and 35% to 60% with maximal doses[166,167] (Table 12-13). Statins also reduce TG levels by 15% to 45% and increase HDL-C modestly (5% to 8%) (Table 12-16). The LDL-C lowering achieved is dose dependent and log linear. Low dosages produce substantial LDL-C–lowering effects, and with each doubling of the daily dose, LDL-C is lowered an additional 6% to 7% on average (Table 12-13).

The currently available statins are atorvastatin (Lipitor), fluvastatin (Lescol), lovastatin (Mevacor), pravastatin (Pravachol), rosuvastatin (Crestor), and simvastatin (Zocor). Rosuvastatin provides the most substantial LDL-C lowering, followed by atorvastatin, simvastatin, lovastatin, pravastatin, and fluvastatin in descending order. With clinical trial evidence that lower LDL-C levels are associated with less CHD, higher initial doses of these statins are being advocated, thus blurring these LDL-C differences. The efficacy of many statins is greater if administered in the evening to coincide with the nighttime upturn in endogenous cholesterol biosynthesis; atorvastatin, and rosuvastatin with a longer half-life and more potent LDL-C lowering, may be administered without regard to time of day. The LDL-C–lowering efficacy of twice-daily administration of statins is slightly greater (by 2% to 4%) than once-daily evening doses, but this difference is rarely sufficient to make a clinical difference. The bioavailability of lovastatin is improved by administration with food; thus, it is recommended for dosing with the evening meal. This, too, may not make much difference in the clinical setting.

The major statin trials described earlier in this chapter demonstrate that statins can significantly reduce CHD death and nonfatal MI, revascularization procedures, strokes, and total mortality. The mechanism for these beneficial outcomes is not fully known, but is at least partially associated with LDL-C reduction.[114] Most authorities believe that the CHD event reduction with statins is a class effect and can be accomplished with any of the available statins. This, coupled with their favorable safety profile and their potency in lowering LDL-C, supports the NCEP ATP III recommendation that statins are the drugs of first choice to lower cholesterol and reduce CHD risk.[92,168]

Table 12-16 Average Effects of Selected Drugs on Lipoprotein Cholesterol and Triglycerides

Drug	*LDL (%)*	*HDL (%)*	*TG (%)*
Resin	−15–30	±3	+3–10
Ezetimibe	−18–22	+0–2	−0–5
Niacin	−15–30	+20–35	−30–60
Statin	−25–60	+5–15	−10–45
Fibrates	±10–25	+10–30	−30–60

HDL, high-density lipoprotein; LDL, low-density lipoprotein; TG, triglycerides.

Mechanism of Action

Statins competitively inhibit the enzyme responsible for converting HMG-CoA to mevalonate in an early, rate-limiting step in the biosynthetic pathway of cholesterol (Fig. 12-1).[10] Reduction in hepatocellular cholesterol prompts an upregulation of LDL receptor proteins and thus increases the clearance of circulating LDL particles from the blood. The TG-lowering effects appear to be produced in two ways: by an increase in the clearance of VLDL and VLDL remnant particles from the systemic circulation (by the upregulation of LDL receptors) and by a reduced secretion of VLDL particles from the liver.[169–171] All statins have the ability to lower TG levels. Their TG-lowering efficacy is related, however, to their LDL-C–lowering effectiveness (thus, statins with greater LDL-C–lowering efficacy will have greater TG-lowering efficacy) and to the patient's baseline TG level (the higher the TG level, the greater the percentage of reduction produced by the statin).

Adverse Effects of Statins

13. L.W.'s physician decides to start therapy with 20 mg/day of simvastatin. Several days after starting the drug, he played tennis for the first time in several years. The next morning he experiences new leg and arm pain. He had been warned that statins can cause muscle damage. He does not complain of any other side effects since starting the drug. Could this be a side effect of simvastatin? Should he discontinue the therapy?

Statins are well tolerated by most patients. Headache; myalgias (without CPK changes); and GI symptoms, including dyspepsia, flatus, constipation, and abdominal pain, occasionally are experienced[166,172,173] (Table 12-15). These symptoms are usually mild and disappear with continued therapy. The statin side effects receiving the most attention include increases in liver function tests and myopathy. These two problems are described in detail below.

Statins can cause an elevation in transaminase enzyme levels of more than three times the upper limit of normal in 1% to 1.5% of patients in a dose-dependent manner. The transaminase level can return to normal spontaneously even with continued statin therapy. Similarly, elevations in transaminase will return to normal if the statin is discontinued. Rechallenge with the same or a different statin after enzymes have returned to normal limits is acceptable. If the drug is tolerated on rechallenge, it can be continued; recurrence of transaminase elevation warrants further evaluation of other potential causes. No cases of hepatic failure or liver transplant associated with statin therapy have been reported, leading many to conclude that transaminase elevations are relatively unimportant and not associated with worrisome adverse consequences.

The potential for muscle toxicity is a different matter. Myositis, defined as the presence of muscle symptoms, including aches, soreness, or weakness (i.e., myalgia), *and* an increase in serum CPK >10 times the upper limit of normal, occurs in approximately 0.1% to 1% of patients in a dose-dependent manner. Routine monitoring of CPK levels is unnecessary; rather, unexplained symptoms of muscle aches, weakness, or soreness should prompt a CPK evaluation. If myositis is present, a careful history is necessary to rule out usual causes (i.e., trauma, increased physical activity). If no explanation is present for the findings and the CPK is elevated, the statin should be withdrawn until CPK levels return to normal. Occasionally, symptoms of myalgia are bothersome to the patient, even with a normal CPK, resulting in discontinuation of the statin. Once symptoms subside, statin therapy can be restarted, preferably with a different statin. Myositis is more likely to occur with high systemic concentrations of the statin and when there is a provocation for the event (e.g., hypothyroidism, trauma, or flulike syndromes). Myositis has also been reported more often when a statin is combined with gemfibrozil or when a drug is given concurrently that can increase blood levels of the statin, such as a macrolide antibiotic (e.g., erythromycin). Cases of rhabdomyolysis, myoglobinuria, and acute tubular necrosis have been reported in patients receiving statin therapy. Most of these cases have occurred with high doses, in patients with impaired renal or hepatic function, in older individuals, or when statins are used in combination with interacting drugs.

Drug interactions with statins that result in higher blood levels of the statin or an active metabolite can increase the risk of myositis. Statins that depend on the P450 3A4 enzyme system to be metabolized are most vulnerable to this interaction (i.e., lovastatin, simvastatin, and to a lesser extent atorvastatin). Fluvastatin is metabolized by the P450 2C9 system and, therefore, is more vulnerable to interactions with drugs that directly inhibit 2C9 or act as competitive inhibitors (substrates) for this alternate system. Rosuvastatin is metabolized minimally (i.e., about 10%) by 2C9 to less active metabolites. Pravastatin undergoes isomerization in the gut to a relatively inactive metabolite. Variability of gastric metabolism has been shown to be associated with the LDL-C–lowering effects of pravastatin.[174] Some of the more commonly encountered drugs that inhibit the 3A4 enzyme system are azole antifungals (itraconazole, ketoconazole, and miconazole), certain calcium channel blockers (diltiazem and verapamil), macrolide antibiotics (clarithromycin and erythromycin), protease inhibitors (ritonavir), and antidepressants (nefazodone). Drugs that are substrates for the 3A4 system include certain benzodiazepines (alprazolam, midazolam, triazolam), calcium channel blockers (especially diltiazem), carbamazepine, cisapride, cyclosporine, estradiol, felodipine, loratadine, quinidine, and terfenadine. When these substrate drugs are used together with simvastatin or lovastatin (and to a lesser extent atorvastatin), systemic blood levels of the statin may be increased because of competitive inhibition of the 3A4 enzymes, and this may increase the risk for myositis. Inhibitors of 2C9 isoenzymes include alprenolol, diclofenac, hexobarbital, tolbutamide, and warfarin.

It is preferable to avoid the combined use of interacting drugs with statins. If the patient requires a short course of therapy with a potentially interacting drug (e.g., erythromycin), the statin should be discontinued during this period and restarted when the course has been completed. If an interacting drug must be used long term (e.g., cyclosporine) with a statin, the lowest effective dose of the statin should be selected, with careful monitoring of muscle symptoms. If myositis occurs, it is quickly reversible when the statin is discontinued.

Caution should also be exercised when adding gemfibrozil with a statin to treat patients with high blood cholesterol and TG. Gemfibrozil interferes with the glucuronidation of statins, thereby interfering with their renal clearance. This interaction results in two- to fourfold increases in systemic statin levels and has been demonstrated with all statins except fluvastatin. Because the interaction has not been reported to occur with fenofibrate, it is the preferred fibrate to add to a statin when treating patients with a mixed lipid disorder.

Hospitalizations and deaths caused by rhabdomyolysis led to the withdrawal of one statin, cerivastatin, from the market, punctuating the importance of this potential side effect. Cerivastatin at its top dosage of 0.8 mg daily caused a significantly higher incidence of myotoxicity than other currently marketed statins. Additionally, when interacting drugs or gemfibrozil were added to this dose of cerivastatin, many cases of severe muscle toxicity and rhabdomyolysis occurred. The U.S. Food and Drug Administration (FDA) subsequently observed that factors that appeared to raise the risk of severe muscle toxicity and rhabdomyolysis with cerivastatin included older individuals (especially women), small body frame, reduced renal function, multiple organ diseases, and use of multiple concurrent medications, particularly those known to interact with statins. Whenever these factors are present in a patient receiving a statin, it is advisable to use the lowest effective statin dose, to avoid or use with caution interacting drugs, and to monitor the patient carefully. It is also advisable not to unduly frighten the patient with dire warnings about the potential for this side effect; it occurs only rarely, especially when these drugs are used responsibly in the manner described.

Lovastatin and rosuvastatin may prolong the prothrombin time in patients receiving coumarin anticoagulants concurrently; this effect is not caused by pravastatin. Statins should not be used in patients with active liver disease or those who are (or hope to become) pregnant because of potential hazards to the fetus.

Based on this information, it is unlikely that simvastatin is causing any serious side effects. His muscle pain is most likely the result of heavy exercise that is not part of his usual pattern of exercise. If the muscle soreness persists for more than the expected 2 to 3 days or worsens, he should report it to his doctor to determine if measuring a CPK level is necessary.

14. Was simvastatin a good choice for L.W? Was the dose appropriate?

A statin is the preferred drug for L.W. He is not receiving a potentially interacting drug and has no apparent contraindication to its use. Further, it is more likely than a resin, ezetimibe, or niacin to help him reach his LDL-C goal. In selecting the specific statin for the patient, it is assumed, for reasons previously stated, that all statins are equally safe and have a similar potential to reduce CHD events. The characteristic that differentiates the statins is their ability to lower LDL-C (Tables 12-13 and 12-16). Given the minimum of a 35% reduction required to achieve L.W.'s LDL-C goal, it would be preferable to select the statin with the greatest LDL-C–lowering potency, such as simvastatin, atorvastatin, or rosuvastatin. At 20 mg/day of simvastatin, 10 mg/day of atorvastatin, or 10 mg/day of rosuvastatin, LDL-C is reduced by an average of 39%, indicating that 50% of patients will experience at least this level of LDL-C reduction. Starting therapy with even higher doses (i.e., rosuvastatin 20 mg, simvastatin 40 mg or atorvastatin 20 mg) will increase the chance of reaching L.W.'s minimal treatment goal of <130 mg/dL. For now the 20 mg starting dose of simvastatin given to L.W. is reasonable. He should be assessed for success in achieving his lipid goal in about 6 weeks.

Fiber

15. What role can supplemental fiber play in the treatment of L.W.?

Increasing fiber intake in the diet or adding supplemental fiber in the form of psyllium (Metamucil), oat bran, gums, or other products might temporarily aid in LDL-C reduction. When given to a patient who is following a low-fat diet, the LDL-C reduction is modest (usually about 5%). A dietary supplement of fiber would make little overall contribution to L.W.'s treatment, although appropriate fiber intake in the form of fresh fruits, beans, and vegetables is highly advisable. Overuse of fiber is associated with bothersome GI symptoms, including flatulence and bloating.

Fish Oils

16. Is there a role for fish oil supplements in L.W.'s treatment?

Fish oils predominantly contain polyunsaturated (omega-3) fatty acids, which lower TG levels significantly (30% to 60%) but have variable effects on cholesterol levels. They serve little value in achieving LDL-C reduction, as is needed by L.W. As noted, however, under the discussion of diet, consumption of foods rich in omega-3 fatty acids (e.g., fish) several times a week has been associated with a reduced risk of heart disease, and they are recommended as part of a low-fat diet. Supplements of fish oils demonstrated a reduction in CHD events in several large clinical trials.[175] Commercial sources of fish oils vary in their content. The fish oil supplements used in the GISSI study, which demonstrated a CHD risk reduction, contained 850 mg of eicosapentaenoic acid (EPA) and docosahexanoic acid (DHA). Fish oils are most useful in the treatment of patients who have hypertriglyceridemia and who cannot achieve adequate control with conventional TG-lowering drugs (niacin and a fibrate) alone. The CHD risk reduction with fish oils appears to be caused by an antiarrhythmic effect and not a change in atherosclerosis, because sudden CHD deaths are the outcome primarily affected by fish oil therapy.

Postmenopausal Drug Therapy

17. C.M. is a 57-year-old woman whose last menses occurred 2 years ago. She follows a TLC diet and participates in an aerobic exercise program three times a week. She has a strong family history of CHD (her father died suddenly at age 59 and her 43-year-old brother has had a heart attack). Her mother is alive at age 78, but lives in a nursing home because of a hip fracture last year. C.M. does not have diabetes or hypertension; she smokes half a pack of cigarettes per day. Her mean BP for the last two visits is 142/88. She does not have hypothyroidism. Her lipid profile is total cholesterol, 260 mg/dL; LDL-C, 186 mg/dL; HDL-C, 58 mg/dL; and TG, 78 mg/dL. C.M. has no evidence of secondary or familial dyslipidemia or atherosclerotic vascular disease on her physical examination. She has not had a hysterectomy. She complains of frequent daily hot flashes and night sweats. Does C.M. need cholesterol-lowering drug therapy, and if so, with which drug? Is she a candidate for estrogen replacement therapy?

[SI units: LDL-C, 5.17 mmol/L; HDL-C, 1.5 mmol/L; and TG, 0.88 mmol/L]

Being postmenopausal, whether natural, surgical, or premature, is associated with an increased CHD risk. C.M. has three risk factors: postmenopausal status, smoking, and family history of premature CHD (Table 12-4). Because she has two or more risk factors, her LDL-C goal is <130 mg/dL. An assessment of her global risk (Fig. 12-6B) indicates that she has an 11% risk of a CHD event in the next 10 years. Because her global risk is between 10% and 20%, the option is to treat her LDL-C to <100 mg/dL. Because her mean LDL-C after diet is still 186 mg/dL, she will require a 46% reduction to achieve her goal. Until recently, C.M. would have been a candidate for estrogen therapy before (or instead of) other cholesterol-lowering drugs. Estrogen is known to improve lipid and lipoprotein profiles and was thought to provide cardioprotective effects as well as minimizing osteoporosis and menopausal symptoms. Today, with new data in hand, this approach has changed.

Estrogen Replacement Therapy

CONSIDERATIONS FOR USE IN HYPERCHOLESTEROLEMIA

18. What are the considerations for using estrogen therapy in C.M. to reduce her CHD risk?

Epidemiologic studies report up to 50% lower CHD rates in women who use estrogens compared with those who do not.[176–179] A meta-analysis of 31 case-control, cross-sectional, and cohort studies found an overall relative risk of 0.56 (i.e., a 44% lower rate of CHD in estrogen users compared with nonusers).[180] The difference in CHD rates between estrogen users and nonusers is even greater in women who have developed CHD.[178,181] Despite calls for caution,[182] the epidemiologic evidence of lower CHD risk was so impressive and consistent that many authorities supported the use of estrogen therapy as a first-line treatment to reduce CHD risk in dyslipidemic, postmenopausal women, especially if they were experiencing menopausal symptoms or were at risk from osteoporosis.

Following the reports of the Heart and Estrogen/Progestin Replacement Study (HERS) and the Women's Health Initiative (WHI), this position has changed. HERS evaluated 2,763 women with known CHD.[183] The active treatment group received conjugated equine estrogen (0.625) and medroxyprogesterone (2.5) mg/day (Prempro) for 5 years. Compared with placebo, the hormone replacement therapy (HRT) regimen lowered LDL-C by 11% and increased HDL-C by 10%. At the conclusion of the study, no difference was seen between the groups with regard to CHD death and nonfatal MI (the primary study outcome measure) or total mortality. Of greatest concern was a 52% *increase* in CHD events during the first year of the study. By the fourth and fifth years of the study, HRT-treated women had 33% *fewer* CHD events, but this difference was not sufficiently great to counter the first-year results. Venous thromboembolic events occurred in 0.6% of treated women compared with 0.2% in placebo-treated women; the incidence of gallbladder disease was 38% greater in HRT-treated than in placebo-treated patients. No significant differences were found between the groups with respect to breast cancer, endometrial cancer, or fracture. Study investigators searched for explanations of these surprising results, but ultimately concluded that in this well-controlled study of estrogen therapy in CHD women, estrogen provided no benefit and may have caused harm.

Subsequently, the WHI reported the results of a 5.2-year, randomized, placebo-controlled study of the same estrogen/progestin product in 16,608 postmenopausal women who had no prior evidence of CHD.[184] The study was stopped before its planned 8.5-year duration because the rate of invasive breast cancer exceeded the stopping boundary. Investigators reported the following negative outcomes: a 29% increase in CHD events (nonfatal MI or CHD death), a 26% increase in breast cancer, a 41% increase in stroke, and a twofold increase in pulmonary embolism. Positive outcomes included a 37% reduction in colorectal cancer, a 17% reduction in endometrial cancer, a 34% reduction in hip fracture, and an 8% reduction in death from non-CHD causes. These relative changes in risk camouflage a low overall absolute risk of harmful study events. That said, however, the absolute excess risk of adverse events during the study was 19 per 10,000 person-years, supporting an overall conclusion that the risks of estrogen/progestin (Prempro) therapy exceeded the benefits among healthy postmenopausal women. Because the whole purpose of healthy women taking a therapy is to preserve health and prevent disease, this study provides further strong evidence that women should not receive combination estrogen/progestin therapy for long-term use to prevent CHD. It should be noted that the WHI study arm with postmenopausal women taking estrogen alone was not stopped prematurely, suggesting that the adversities reported above were caused by the progestin component of the combination and not to the estrogen. Nonetheless, until further data are available, long-term use of estrogen for lipid management is not recommended. Short-term (1 to 2 years) use for relief of C.M.'s menopausal symptoms is acceptable.

Alternative Lipid Therapy for Postmenopausal Women

19. If C.M. should not be started on estrogen/progestin therapy, what should she be given?

C.M.'s risk of dying of CHD is as great as it is for a male patient. Further, her risk rises after menopause in a log-linear manner parallel to men (although behind men by about 10 years). The Heart Protection Study and a meta-analysis of most of the major statin trials has shown strong evidence that postmenopausal women benefit from lipid-lowering treatment just as much as men[91,185] (Table 12-3). For all of these reasons, C.M. is a candidate for lipid-modifying therapy. Because she requires a 46% reduction to achieve her LDL-C goal of <100 mg/dL, a statin with sufficient LDL-C–lowering potency to achieve this target (i.e., simvastatin, atorvastatin, or rosuvastatin) would be the drug of choice or a statin combined with another drug (see below). Even if the decision is made by her and her gynecologist to initiate short-term HRT to reduce vasomotor symptoms, a statin will still be needed to reduce her LDL-C to the goal level and to reduce her CHD risk.

Familial Hypercholesterolemia

20. D.E. is a 45-year-old man with no evidence of CHD. His father and grandfather both died suddenly from apparent heart attacks in their early 50s, but D.E. has no other CHD risk factors. He has no evidence of secondary causes of dyslipidemia. On physical examination, he is noted to have bilateral corneal arcus and bilateral Achilles' tendon xanthomas; the rest of his examination findings are normal. Likewise, his laboratory test results are within normal limits, except for the following lipid profile: total cholesterol, 440 mg/dL; TG, 55 mg/dL; HDL-C, 55 mg/dL; and LDL-C, 374 mg/dL. What form of hypercholesterolemia does D.E. most likely have? Is he a candidate for drug therapy at this time?

[SI units: total cholesterol, 11.38 mmol/L; TGs, 0.62 mmol/L; HDL-C, 1.42 mmol/L; LDL-C, 9.67 mmol/L]

The combination of a very high LDL-C, tendon xanthomas, corneal arcus, and a strong family history of premature CHD is consistent with a diagnosis of familial hypercholesterolemia (FH) (Table 12-2). The risk of a CHD event in the next 10 years associated with FH is very high, well in excess of 20%. Thus, it is not necessary to conduct a global risk assessment, because the diagnosis of the genetic disorder defines his risk. Although D.E. has bilateral tendon xanthomas, this finding would not necessarily be detected in all 45-year-old patients because it takes time for xanthomas to develop. With a strong family history and a very high LDL-C level independent of the presence or absence of xanthomas, however, it is still presumed that the person has either FH or severe polygenic hypercholesterolemia. Thus, he deserves aggressive lipid management to reduce his high CHD risk. D.E. should be given therapy to lower his LDL-C to 130 mg/dL, lower if possible. To achieve this goal, D.E. will require a 65% LDL-C reduction, which almost assuredly will require combination drug therapy in addition to a low-fat diet. Because this is a genetically induced lipid abnormality, a low-fat diet alone will not correct the problem; in fact, diet may have little effect on his LDL-C.

Combination Drug Therapy

21. What cholesterol-lowering drugs should be combined to manage D.E.'s lipid disorder?

As stated previously, four drugs effectively reduce LDL-C: a statin, a resin, ezetimibe, and niacin (Table 12-12). When two or more of these are combined, an additive LDL-C–lowering effect is achieved. Combinations of niacin and resin result in LDL-C reductions of 32% to 43%;[62] a statin and a resin lower LDL-C by 45% to 55%,[63] and ezetimibe plus a statin reduces LDL-C by 46% to 70%.[152,186] LDL-C reductions of 50% to 60% are possible when the three-drug regimen of a statin plus resin plus niacin is used.[187,188]

The major limiting factor in combining drugs is side effects. Niacin and the older resins both cause bothersome side effects to the extent that 25% to 50% of patients cannot tolerate them. The use of Niaspan rather than crystalline niacin may reduce the vasodilatory side effects, however, and the use of colesevelam rather than one of the older resins should reduce GI intolerance.[189] The combination of a statin and niacin is said to be associated with an increased risk of myositis, although this risk appears to be very low.[190] The combination of a statin and ezetimibe is the one best tolerated and offers the most convenient once-a-day dosing of the possible combinations. This is the combination that was selected for D.E.

INITIATING THERAPY

22. How should combined therapy with a statin and ezetimibe be initiated in D.E.?

Given the amount of LDL-C lowering needed to reach D.E.'s LDL-C goal, it is reasonable to select one of the more potent LDL-C–lowering statins (e.g., simvastatin, atorvastatin, or rosuvastatin) and to start with a high daily dose (40 mg/day). Before therapy is initiated, baseline liver function tests and CPK levels should be obtained (Table 12-15). Renal function should be assessed because impaired renal clearance of the statin or its active metabolite could result in increased systemic levels, which might increase the risk of myotoxicity. LDL-C levels should be evaluated in about 6 weeks, when the maximal effect of the statin is anticipated. If the LDL-C is within 6% of D.E.'s goal, the dosage of the statin may be advanced to 80 mg as this should be sufficient to achieve the goal. If the LDL-C is >6% below goal, however, ezetimibe (10 mg) daily should be added to the regimen. This should add an additional 10% to 20% LDL-C–lowering effect.[186] D.E. should be seen in another 6 weeks for further LDL-C evaluation. Alternatively, the patient can be started on a fixed combination product of simvastatin and ezetimibe (Table 12-14).

If D.E. does not achieve his goal with this two-drug combination, the addition of a third drug should be considered. Choices are to add a bile acid resin, such as colesevelam, or niacin. Presently, no study has described the efficacy of an ezetimibe, resin, and statin combination. Theoretically, the combination should be effective, but a limit may exit to how much hepatic LDL receptors can be upregulated. Niacin has been successfully added as a third drug in a regimen and provides a 10% to 15% additional LDL-C–lowering effect when titrated to about 2,000 mg/day.

ADDING A THIRD LIPID-LOWERING DRUG TO THE REGIMEN

23. How should niacin be initiated in D.E., and what monitoring is required?

Before niacin therapy is started (and after its maximal dosage is reached), liver function tests should be evaluated (Table 12-15). Patients with an active peptic ulcer or liver disease should not receive niacin. Niacin can increase glucose levels by 10% to 20% in some diabetic patients or patients with impaired fasting glucose levels, necessitating careful monitoring of glucose control. None of these issues is a factor in D.E.

The addition of niacin to D.E.'s statin and ezetimibe regimen should be initiated with low doses that are slowly titrated upward to allow tolerance to develop at each dosage level (Table 12-14). D.E. should be given as much control over niacin administration as possible. Crystalline niacin can be started at 250 to 300 mg/day, administered in two or three divided doses. Thereafter, daily dosages can be increased every 3 to 7 days in the following sequence: 500, 1,000, 1,500, 2,000, and 3,000 mg. Niaspan is initiated at 500 mg at bedtime and increased every 7 days to 1,000 mg, 1,500 mg, and 2,000 mg daily as tolerated by the patient. The over-the-counter sustained-release niacin dosage form is not recommended because of its increased risk of causing hepatotoxicity.

D.E. should be warned about the vasodilatory symptoms associated with niacin use (facial flushing, itching, rash) and reassured that these symptoms are not dangerous and that tolerance should develop after several weeks of therapy. He should be advised to take 325 mg of aspirin or another prostaglandin-inhibiting drug 30 minutes before the morning dose of crystalline niacin or the bedtime dose of Niaspan to decrease these symptoms. Taking each dose with food will help to reduce flushing and GI symptoms. Instruction can also be provided to reduce doses if necessary to manage bothersome symptoms. He should be encouraged to call his clinician whenever troublesome symptoms occur.

Several weeks after the 1,500-mg/day dosage is reached (Table 12-14), the patient should be evaluated for achievement of the LDL-C goal and side effects. If the LDL-C goal is not achieved with 1,500 mg/day, further increments can be made up to the maximal tolerated dose or a ceiling dose of 3,000 mg of crystalline niacin or 2,000 mg of Niaspan. In addition to a fasting lipid profile, laboratory tests of liver function, glucose, and uric acid may be indicated.

MIXED HYPERLIPIDEMIA

Assessing the Patient With Mixed Hyperlipidemia

24. B.C., a 56-year-old man, experienced acute chest pain 3 months ago and was admitted to the local hospital with a diagnosis of unstable angina. His only known medical problem was hypertension treated with enalapril 10 mg QD. His lipid profile on admission was total cholesterol, 235 mg/dL; HDL-C, 30 mg/dL; LDL-C, 165 mg/dL; and TG, 300 mg/dL. He underwent a cardiac catheterization, which revealed a 90% stenotic lesion in his left anterior ascending artery. A drug-coated stent was placed without difficulty. He was subsequently discharged on simvastatin 40 mg QHS, ezetimibe 10 mg QD, ASA 325 mg QD, propranolol 40 mg BID, and enalapril 10 mg QD.

Today, he weighs 220 lb, is 6 feet tall (ideal body weight [IBW], 140 to 185 lb), and has a waist circumference of 42 inches. He has lost 10 lb since his MI by following a low-fat diet and an exercise program. He swims 1 mile three times a week without symptoms of cardiac ischemia, and he drinks two glasses of wine each evening with dinner. His father died at age 58 of an MI (lipids unknown). He has never smoked. Pertinent physical findings include BP 148/90 mm Hg; heart rate 60 regular; arcus senilis; carotid pulses equal without bruits; and chest clear to auscultation without cardiomegaly. Laboratory tests disclose normal thyroid-stimulating hormone levels, normal renal and liver function, and a fasting glucose level of 120 mg/dL. His urinalysis was normal. The lipid profile while taking the above regimen is total cholesterol, 143 mg/dL; TG, 210 mg/dL; HDL-C, 33 mg/dL; and LDL-C, 68 mg/dL.

What is your assessment of B.C.'s lipids and lipoprotein cholesterol concentrations?

[SI units: glucose, 6.66 mmol/L; total cholesterol, 3.7 mmol/L; TG, 2.37 mmol/L; HDL-C, 0.85 mmol/L; LDL-C, 1.76 mmol/L]

According to NCEP guidelines, B.C. has reached the "reasonable" LDL-C treatment goal (<70 mg/dL) for a patient with a history of CHD.[88,89] (Table 12-10). The LDL-C should be confirmed with a second lipid profile (because of biologic and analytical variability). According to NCEP guidelines, his TG level remains high (200 to 500 mg/dL) and his HDL-C is low (<40 mg/dL) (Table 12-6). The lipid profile obtained during his hospitalization can be interpreted in a normal manner, because it was drawn within 24 hours of his acute coronary event. Profiles drawn after 24 hours are generally lower, however, than pre-event levels and remain so for several weeks.

Based on his recent CHD event, B.C. has a >20% chance of a recurrent CHD event in the next 10 years. He is therefore considered to be a high-risk, CHD risk equivalent patient. Additionally, B.C. has several risk factors for CHD that add to his risk: family history, male >45 years, high BP, and low HDL-C. His fasting blood sugar is defined as impaired fasting glucose (i.e., a fasting value 110 to 126 mg/dL). Some clinicians would consider him to be diabetic, given how close he is to the definition of diabetes (fasting blood sugar >126 mg/dL). Evaluation of HgA1c and a glucose tolerance test are indicated to further define B.C.'s diabetes state.

B.C. was appropriately treated with a statin (as well as antiplatelet, angiotensin-converting enzyme [ACE] inhibitor, and beta-blocker therapy) and a TLC diet and exercise program to achieve an LDL-C <70 mg/dL. In such a high-risk patient, therapeutic interventions should not be delayed. Not only will the initiation of drug treatment in the hospital setting provide risk-reducing benefit, but the patient is more likely to relate this therapy to his acute event and adhere to it.[189]

Although B.C. has reached his LDL-C goal, the job of reducing his CHD risk is not complete. The next step is to evaluate the CHD risk associated with the high TG level and, if indicated, develop a plan to address it (Table 12-17).

Relation of Triglycerides to Coronary Heart Disease

25. Does the increased TG level in B.C. indicate an increased CHD risk?

The exact role that TG play in the pathogenesis of CHD is under intense investigation. Most epidemiologic studies have found that a high TG level is an independent risk factor for CHD when evaluated with univariate analysis. When other lipid abnormalities, such as increased LDL-C or low HDL-C, are included in a multivariate analysis, TG often lose their independent predictive power.[191] Part of the reason for this is the close interrelationship between lipids. Patients with high TG levels almost always have a low HDL-C, which also predicts CHD risk.[192,193] In addition, elevated TG levels are associated with increased levels of TG-rich lipoproteins (i.e., remnant VLDL particles) and small, dense LDL particles.[9,194] These particles are atherogenic and mediate a higher CHD risk than associated with an elevated LDL-C alone.[195–198] When epidemiologic studies were combined, a meta-analysis found that TG independently predicted CHD risk, even after adjustment for other lipid risk factors.[199] High TG levels are also found in certain familial disorders, including dysbetalipoproteinemia and familial combined hyperlipidemia, which carry increased CHD risk.[19,200] Additionally, hypertriglyceridemia is associated with a procoagulant state, which promotes coronary thrombosis.[194]

Paradoxically, very high TG levels (>500 mg/dL) are not commonly associated with an increased CHD risk, but do cause an increased risk of pancreatitis, especially when levels exceed 1,000 mg/dL. Often, a genetic defect in lipoprotein lipase is present in these cases that impairs the removal of TG from TG-rich particles (VLDL and chylomicrons). These particles do not become enriched with cholesterol and, therefore, are not often atherogenic.[200,201] If the blood sample is stored in the refrigerator overnight, a thick creamy layer often appears on the surface, indicating the presence of chylomicrons. Although most patients with very high TG remain free of CHD throughout their lives, some develop it.[191]

On the other hand, patients such as B.C., with TG in the borderline to high range (150 to 500 mg/dL), have an increased CHD risk because they likely have atherogenic TG-rich lipoproteins (Table 12-6). Characteristically, B.C. has a high TG level and a low HDL-C and is likely to also have elevated remnant VLDL-C and small dense LDL levels. This is the profile of atherogenic dyslipidemia described earlier in this chapter and is linked to a high CHD risk. This is exemplified by the placebo groups in the HIT and BIP trials, two studies that included patients with mixed hyperlipidemia. Untreated subjects had CHD event rates of 15% to 22% in 5 to 6 years, respectively.[110,111]

Atherogenic Dyslipidemia

26. Why does atherogenic dyslipidemia occur? How should the clinician assess and treat atherogenic dyslipidemia?

Patients such as B.C. with borderline high or high TG levels (Table 12-6) secrete large numbers of TG-enriched VLDL particles from the liver. One reason for this is increased levels of nonesterified fatty acids in the systemic circulation that come from adipose cells (especially in patients with central obesity). The liver clears these fatty acids and is stimulated to increase the synthesis of triglycerides.[202]

A second reason for the increased secretion of VLDL particles is an upregulation of the gene expression for microsomal

Table 12-17 Treatment Targets for Patients Who Have Achieved Their LDL-C Goal and Have a Triglyceride Level >200 mg/dL and Meet Criteria for the Metabolic Syndrome

Patient Category	*LDL-C Treatment Target*	*Non-HDL-C Treatment Target*	*Apolipoprotein B Treatment Target*
CHD or CHD risk equivalent	<100 mg/dL	<130 mg/dL	<90 mg/dL
(Reasonable target for patients with CHD)	<70 mg/dL	<100 mg/dL	<70 mg/dL
No CHD, >2 risk factors	<130 mg/dL	<160 mg/dL	<110 mg/dL
No CHD, <2 risk factors	<160 mg/dL	<190 mg/dL	<130 mg/dL

CHD, coronary heart disease; HDL, high-density lipoprotein cholesterol; LDL-C, low-density lipoprotein cholesterol.

triglyceride transfer protein (MTP) that is caused by the elevated insulin levels in these patients.[203] MTP is responsible for assembling VLDL particles in the hepatocyte. It brings together TG, cholesterol, and apolipoproteins to form the VLDL particle. This mechanism suggests a molecular basis for the link between insulin resistance and increased VLDL secretion. One way of telling that there are increased numbers of lipoprotein particles in the systemic circulation is to measure apolipoprotein B. One apolipoprotein B is attached to each VLDL and LDL particle. An increased apolipoprotein B level indicates an increased number of particles. Patients with a high apolipoprotein B level have a high risk of CHD.

With the increase in VLDL particles, plasma levels of apolipoprotein C-III also increase. Apolipoprotein C-III has two detrimental effects. It interferes with the normal removal of TG from VLDL by reducing the action of lipoprotein lipase. This reduces lipolysis and increases the concentration of TG in the VLDL particle. The second negative effect of apolipoprotein C-III is an interference with the normal removal of VLDL particles from the circulation via LDL receptors on the hepatocytes.[202]

TG-rich VLDL particles interact with other circulating lipoproteins through the action of cholesterol ester transfer protein. Through this protein, a molecule of cholesterol ester is exchanged from circulating HDL and LDL particles for a molecule of TG from VLDL particles. With time, the HDL particles give up >50% of their cholesterol content and become enriched with TG. This results in low HDL-C levels. VLDL becomes more enriched with cholesterol and simultaneously smaller in size, close to the size of LDL, and thus more atherogenic (both because of its smaller size and its higher cholesterol content). LDL particles take on more TG than normal. Subsequently, under the influence of hepatic lipase, TG is removed from LDL particles, leaving a very small particle that is deficient in cholesterol and TG, but is present in great numbers. Because of their small size and concentration, small, dense LDL particles are very atherogenic.

The net result of the above mechanisms is a high VLDL-C, low HDL-C, and increased small, dense LDL, a lipid triad termed *atherogenic dyslipidemia*. How does the clinician measure this in the clinical setting? VLDL-C and VLDL-TG levels are not available from most clinical laboratories, however. Several companies provide measurements of particle size, but these are not widely available and do not yet relate to a reference standard; particle size measurements are best reserved for research purposes at present. The clinician can measure apolipoprotein B as an indicator of the number of atherogenic particles; these levels are available from most clinical laboratories. A much easier, more accessible measure is non–HDL-C. Non–HDL-C is the product of VLDL-C and LDL-C and is determined by subtracting HDL-C from total cholesterol. NCEP recommends that non–HDL-C be determined in patients who have a TG >200 mg/dL after attaining their LDL-C goal.[92] Once the patient is at his or her LDL-C goal, any elevation in non–HDL-C will result from an increase in VLDL-C. Because VLDL-C levels are normally <30 mg/dL, non–HDL-C treatment goals are set 30 mg/dL above LDL-C treatment goals (Table 12-17). Included in the same table are alternative apolipoprotein B treatment goals that have been recommended by authorities.[204] Note that non–HDL-C levels can be determined from a nonfasting sample measuring only total cholesterol and HDL-C, thus making it very convenient for the clinician to make these measurements any time of the day without regard to food intake.

Secondary Causes of Hypertriglyceridemia

27. In addition to an assessment of B.C.'s lipid profile, what other evaluations should be made?

One of the questions that should be answered routinely when evaluating patients with lipid disorders: Is there a secondary cause of the patient's lipid disorder? Secondary causes of hypertriglyceridemia include chronic renal failure; diabetes mellitus; alcohol use and abuse; a sedentary lifestyle; obesity; and the use of TG-raising drugs, including β-blockers, estrogens, and glucocorticoids (Table 12-7). B.C. has a normal TSH level, normal liver and renal function test results, and a normal urinalysis. His blood glucose is elevated into the impaired fasting glucose range, which can be associated with impaired TG metabolism, as described earlier. In addition, he is overweight, with much of the weight distributed around his waist (i.e., a waist circumference >40 inches). Patients who have truncal obesity often overproduce TG and oversecrete VLDL particles, thereby raising their TG level. The HDL-C is inversely reduced. This would appear to be an important factor affecting TG levels in B.C. A reduction in weight through an exercise program and a low-calorie, low saturated fat, and low-carbohydrate diet would be one of the most effective ways to improve B.C.'s glucose level, raise his HDL-C, and lower his TG level.

Light to moderate alcohol intake, defined as up to two drinks per day (1 drink = 5 oz wine, 12 oz beer, or 1.5 oz 80-proof liquor), as is practiced by B.C., has been associated with lower CHD rates. The observed reduction in CHD among light to moderate alcohol drinkers is consistently on the order of 40% to 60% in epidemiologic trials.[205,206] Available epidemiologic evidence supports arguments of causality.[207,208] It is problematic, however, to recommend alcohol consumption for CHD prevention. From a public health point of view, the adverse consequences of alcohol consumption are great and may outweigh the benefits gained. One known adverse consequence of alcohol consumption is hypertriglyceridemia, especially when alcohol is abused, but it may be seen with only moderate intake as well. Even though B.C.'s alcohol intake appears moderate, it may be contributing to his hypertriglyceridemia, so a period of abstinence is warranted to determine whether this is the case.

Use of a β-blocker could also raise TG levels (Table 12-7) and might be a contributing factor in B.C.'s lipid profile. He already had a high TG level on admission to the hospital before starting propranolol therapy, however. In this case, the beta-blocker is providing an important health benefit that probably outweighs the small risk posed by its effect of TG levels. More probably, B.C.'s weight and impaired glucose are the key factors contributing to his increased TG level and are the logical places to start when attempting to correct secondary causes of elevated TG levels.

Metabolic Syndrome

28. B.C. has a combination of obesity, impaired fasting glucose, and hypertension in addition to atherogenic dyslipidemia. What is the significance of this constellation of findings?

Not only does B.C. have CHD and a combination of lipid abnormalities that substantially raise his risk of CHD, but he also has a number of nonlipid risk factors that raise it as well.[209] These factors include obesity, impaired fasting glucose, and hypertension. Most of B.C.'s excess weight is concentrated around his waist. This central distribution of fat may reflect an excess of intra-abdominal fat, which in turn may influence the development of atherogenic dyslipidemia, as already described.[210] An increased outflow of fatty acids from intra-abdominal TG stores may provide the substrate for increased hepatic TG synthesis and VLDL secretion. This could explain B.C.'s elevated TG level.

Abdominal obesity also is strongly associated with insulin resistance.[202,211] Insulin resistance leads to mild hyperglycemia, and the pancreas responds by increasing insulin secretion; hyperinsulinemia results.[212,213] Some genetically predisposed patients are not able to secrete sufficient insulin to overcome this resistance and they develop impaired glucose metabolism or diabetes. The presence of a fasting blood sugar between 110 and 126 mg/dL in B.C. suggests impaired glucose metabolism and probably insulin resistance (with hyperinsulinemia).[214]

B.C. has hypertension. The beta-blocker and ACE inhibitor he is receiving to reduce his CHD risk also help lower his blood pressure. According to the most recent guidelines, B.C. still has stage I hypertension (systolic BP 140 to 159 mm Hg); his untreated BP may be higher.[215] Before concluding inadequate BP control, however, BP readings should be obtained on at least two other occasions and adherence to therapy documented. Abdominal obesity and insulin resistance also are commonly associated with high BP and could be a factor in B.C.[216,217] The exact mechanisms for this remain speculative.

What emerges from the preceding discussion is the strong possibility that B.C.'s risk factors are not independent, but rather represent a constellation of medical problems that have a common pathway. This pathway may be related to insulin resistance.[216,218] NCEP called this constellation the *metabolic syndrome*.[92] Other names given the same problem in the literature are *syndrome X, the deadly quadrangle, insulin resistance syndrome,* and *Reavan's syndrome.*[197,198,207,213,216,218] Metabolic syndrome is diagnosed when any three of the factors listed in Table 12-18 are present. The syndrome is associated with a substantial increase in CHD risk; the exact level of risk should be determined by using the risk-scoring charts in Figure 12-7. B.C. has the metabolic syndrome by having met all five criteria in Table 12-18. Weight loss, especially loss of visceral abdominal adiposity, will be the centerpiece of his nondrug treatment program. The goal is for weight reduction to correct, or at least substantially improve, his blood glucose, TG, and HDL-C levels and BP.

Table 12-18 Clinical Identification of the Metabolic Syndrome

Presence of any three of the following:	
• Waist Circumference	
• Men	≥40 inches (>35 inches for Asian-Americans)
• Women	≥35 inches (>31 inches for Asian-Americans)
• Triglycerides	≥150 mg/dL (or on drug treatment for elevated triglycerides)
• High-density lipoprotein cholesterol (HDL-C)	
• Men	<40 mg/dL (or on drug treatment for reduced HDL-C)
• Women	<50 mg/dL (or on drug treatment for reduced HDL-C)
• Blood pressure (systolic/diastolic)	≥130/≥85 (or on drug treatment for hypertension)
• Fasting glucose	>110 mg/dL (or on drug treatment for elevated glucose)

Hypertension Management With Atherogenic Dyslipidemia

29. If B.C.'s BP elevation persists after lifestyle changes are made, how should he be treated?

Consideration of antihypertensive therapy in a patient with dyslipidemia should take into account how BP-modifying drugs affect blood lipids. As noted above, the propranolol B.C. is receiving can elevate TG levels, but the benefit in post-MI prophylaxis warrants its continued use.[215] Substitution of a β-blocker with intrinsic sympathomimetic activity (e.g., pindolol) or a mixed alpha-beta-blocker (e.g., labetalol) may have less adverse effect on lipids (Table 12-7), but their benefits for post-MI prophylaxis are unproved.

The ACE inhibitor B.C. currently is receiving for his hypertension has a neutral effect on serum lipids. His BP is not under good control, however, so an adjustment to his antihypertensive regimen is in order. One of the best drugs to reduce BP in patients receiving an ACE inhibitor is a thiazide diuretic.[215] Although thiazides can increase blood cholesterol levels (Table 12-7), these effects usually are small, especially with long-term use. The thiazide dose should be kept low (i.e., 12.5 mg/day) to minimize the effect on his blood lipids. Calcium channel blockers (e.g., ACE inhibitors) are lipid neutral and are possible alternatives to a thiazide.

Treatment of the Metabolic Syndrome

CHOLESTEROL-LOWERING AND WEIGHT-LOSS DIET

30. What nondrug therapies should be implemented to help B.C. achieve his treatment goals?

B.C. needs to lose weight in addition to lowering his LDL-C and non–HDL-C levels. Effective weight loss and subsequent weight maintenance could substantially or fully correct his atherogenic dyslipidemia, lower his BP, reduce his waist circumference, and correct his blood glucose. He has already shown progress, having lost 10 pounds since his MI 3 months ago. He appears to be following a low-fat diet, which undoubtedly has helped him lose weight. He needs to lose more weight and needs to modify his lipids further, however. A more rigorous restriction of saturated fats might help him accomplish these goals. This will also substantially reduce total daily calories, because fats contain 9 calories/g. Restriction of saturated fat calories will encourage weight loss and will reduce TG levels; however, it may also reduce HDL-C levels. If saturated fat calories are replaced with polyunsaturated fats, HDL-C usually does not change and may increase. An increase in carbohydrate intake will increase TG and may cause weight gain. Therefore, in a weight-loss diet for the metabolic syndrome, saturated fats and carbohydrates should generally both be restricted. This level of complexity supports the involvement of a registered dietitian who can provide expert advice and practical meal planning.

DRUG THERAPY FOR THE METABOLIC SYNDROME

31. If weight loss and an exercise program are insufficient to fully correct B.C.'s lipid disorder, it is appropriate to consider drug therapy. What lipid-modulating drugs should be considered?

In patients with the metabolic syndrome and not at their non–HDL-C goal, four drugs are used: statins, statins combined with ezetimibe, niacin, or a fibrate. The statin combined with ezetimibe given to B.C. has achieved his primary treatment goal, an LDL-C <70 mg/dL. It has also reduced his TG level about 30% and raised his HDL-C level modestly, both typical effects of statins. His non–HDL-C is 110 mg/dL (goal <100 mg/dL). The reduction in non–HDL-C with each dose doubling of a statin is about 6%. Thus, an increase in the daily dose of simvastatin from 40 mg to 80 mg per day would be expected to reduce B.C.'s non–HDL-C level from 110 mg/dL to approximately 103 ng/dL, not likely sufficient to achieve his non–HDL-C goal of <100 mg/dL (Table 12-17). A more potent statin, such as atorvastatin or rosuvastatin, lowers LDL-C, non–HDL-C, and TG more than simvastatin and may achieve B.C.'s treatment goal with daily doses of 40 to 80 mg or 10 to 20 mg, respectively.

An alternative is to add a third drug (niacin, bile acid resin, or fibrate) to his simvastatin and ezetimibe to achieve the non–HDL-C treatment goal. Adding another drug, however, can increase side effects while adding complexity to, and increasing cost of, the regimen.

The bile acid resins will add 10% to 20% additional LDL-C lowering when added to a statin; non–HDL-C will be lowered nearly as much. Much of the reduction in non–HDL-C will be from a reduction in LDL-C, however. VLDL-C and TG levels may not change or may even increase with a bile acid resin. This effect of resins is most pronounced in patients such as B.C. with hypertriglyceridemia.

Niacin generally enhances VLDL-C and TG lowering (up to double the amount) and substantially increases HDL-C levels when added to a statin.[219] The effects on VLDL-C, TG, and HDL-C with niacin follow a curvilinear pattern such that substantial changes in these parameters can be achieved with modest daily doses of niacin (1 to 1.5 g/day) (Fig. 12-8). Thus, when niacin is added to a statin, it need not be titrated to maximal doses, which might in turn increase patient tolerance of niacin. In one study, the addition of 750 mg/day of niacin to simvastatin extended the reduction in TG from 26% to 31% and in VLDL-C from 28% to 44%, while increasing HDL-C from 13% to 31%.[220] The principal concern with niacin in patients with the metabolic syndrome is its potential to worsen glucose metabolism. Several recent studies in subjects with and without diabetes have shown that niacin causes transient increases in fasting glucose and glycosylated hemoglobin levels in about a third of patients. These increases return to baseline levels in about 6 weeks, presumably because of adjustments made to the subject's diabetic therapy.[204,221] Investigators with the Coronary Drug Project reported that fasting and 1-hour postprandial blood glucose levels were increased in patients assigned to niacin, but this metabolic change did not adversely effect CHD risk reduction. In fact, nonfatal MI after 6 years of therapy and all-cause death after 15 years of therapy was reduced by 11% and 9%, respectively, among study patients with a 1-hour postprandial glucose of <140 mg/dL compared with reductions of 21% and 14% among patients with a 1-hour postprandial glucose of >220 mg/dL.[222] Nonetheless, it is important to use appropriate doses of insulin or oral hypoglycemics in patient with inadequately controlled diabetes.

FIBRIC ACID DERIVATIVES

32. What are the characteristics of gemfibrozil and fenofibrate that would qualify either drug for use in B.C.?

Clinical Use

Gemfibrozil (Lopid) and fenofibrate (TriCor) (and the other fibric acid derivative available in the United States, clofibrate [Atromid S]) lower TG levels by 20% to 50% and in patients with hypertriglyceridemia, raise HDL-C by 10% to 15%[223–227] (Table 12-16). Gemfibrozil generally lowers LDL-C by 10% to 15%, but in patients with both hypercholesterolemia and hypertriglyceridemia it may have no effect on (or may actually increase) LDL-C levels. Fenofibrate lowers LDL-C by 15% to 25%.[228] This effect is blunted in patients with combined hypercholesterolemia and hypertriglyceridemia, but an LDL-C reduction of 10% to 15% is still expected.[223,224,228,229]

Gemfibrozil and fenofibrate are both indicated for the reduction of TG levels in patients with hypertriglyceridemia.[219] In patients who have TG levels >1,000 mg/dL and are at risk for developing pancreatitis, fibrates, along with niacin, are the drugs of choice. Similarly, in patients with familial dysbetalipoproteinemia, fibric acid derivatives are highly effective and are considered the drugs of choice. Fibrates also have a place in the management of combined or mixed hyperlipidemia. Support for this comes primarily from the results of the Helsinki Heart Study and the HIT trials, in which gemfibrozil combined with diet therapy was associated with a reduction in CHD deaths and nonfatal MI.[107,109] These positive outcomes are attributed to significant reductions in serum TG (and, therefore, a reduction in TG-rich VLDL remnants and in small, dense LDL) and an increase in HDL-C. Persons most likely to benefit are those with diabetes or the lipid triad found in patients with the metabolic syndrome.[230,231]

Mechanism of Action

Fibrates activate peroxisome proliferator-activated receptors alpha (PPARα), which explains most of their effects on blood lipids.[232] PPARα receptors are located in the nucleus of cells and are ligand-dependent transcription factors that regulate target gene expression. Stimulation of PPARα suppresses the gene responsible for synthesis of apolipoprotein C-III and stimulates the gene responsible for LDL receptor synthesis.[232,233] As a result, lipolysis of TG from VLDL particles and the removal of these particles via hepatic LDL receptors is enhanced. Stimulation of PPARα also increases fatty acid oxidation, which reduces the synthesis of TG in the liver, and this in turn reduces the TG content of secreted VLDL particles.[233] Stimulation of PPARα may increase the synthesis of apolipoprotein A-1, the critical building block of nascent HDL, thereby enhancing reverse cholesterol transport. Research also suggests that fibrates stimulate the expression of ABC_1 transporters in macrophage cells, which are responsible for bringing cholesterol from within the cell to the cell surface, where it can be taken up by nascent HDL particles and removed from these cells.[232]

Adverse Effects

33. Gemfibrozil and fenofibrate appear to have a similar mechanism of action. What factors might lead to choice of one agent over the other?

Gemfibrozil and fenofibrate are usually well tolerated. Gemfibrozil causes mild GI symptoms (nausea, dyspepsia, abdominal pain) in about one third of patients. Fenofibrate causes a rash in 2% to 4% of patients. Fibrate therapy can also cause muscle side effects, including myositis and rhabdomyolysis.[234] Most cases of muscle toxicity have been reported with gemfibrozil, especially when it is used in combination with a statin. Recent studies reveal that the area under the blood-concentration curve of most statins is increased two- to fourfold when given concurrently with gemfibrozil. These effects are not seen with fenofibrate. The mechanism causing this interaction appears to be related to an interference by gemfibrozil with the glucuronidation of statins and thereby a reduction in statin renal clearance from the systemic circulation.[235,236] This supports the preferential use of fenofibrate over gemfibrozil when a combination with a statin is indicated in managing cases such as B.C. with a mixed hyperlipidemia. Patients who receive gemfibrozil or fenofibrate therapy alone or in combination with a statin should be monitored for symptoms of muscle soreness and pain. If these symptoms emerge, a CPK level should be obtained. A CPK level >10 times the upper limit of normal, along with muscle symptoms, supports a diagnosis of myositis. The presence of myositis is an indication to withdraw fibrate therapy, provided other possible causes are not apparent, such as increased physical exercise or a recent trauma or fall.

Gemfibrozil increases biliary secretion of cholesterol, which increases the lithogenicity of bile and results in the development of cholesterol gallstones. Presumably, the same effect occurs with all fibrates.

The results of three major primary prevention trials have raised questions about the safety of fibrates. In the World Health Organization trial, clofibrate reduced nonfatal MI by 25%, but caused an increase in total mortality.[237,238] As a result, its use has declined markedly in the United States. Some of these deaths may have been related to gallstone disease.[237] In the Helsinki Heart Study, gemfibrozil reduced fatal and nonfatal MI by 37%, but was associated with a slight increase in non-CHD mortality such that there was no net reduction in total mortality.[108] In a 3.5-year follow-up to this study, total mortality in patients given gemfibrozil was increased because of an increase in non-CHD mortality. Follow-up evaluations of nongemfibrozil therapies were associated with continued event reduction.[112] In the HIT trial, death from CHD was significantly reduced by 22% with gemfibrozil, but total mortality was not.[109] In the FIELD study, fenofibrate did not significantly reduce CHD deaths and nonfatal MI compared with placebo. In addition, more patients receiving fenofibrate had pancreatitis or a pulmonary embolism compared with those given placebo.[111] Fenofibrate was also evaluated against placebo in 418 patients with diabetes and at least one visible lesion on angiographic evaluation in the DAIS trial.[239] The trial was not powered to examine clinical endpoints, but fewer events, including deaths, occurred in the fenofibrate group. Taken together, the clinical trial evidence for the fibric acid derivatives is not as robust as with the statins. The data supporting the use of gemfibrozil in the primary and secondary prevention setting has been established. In contrast, clear improvements in CHD-related outcomes is still lacking for fenofibrate. Thus, these data support the use of fibric acid derivatives as second-line agents, with the exception in patients with hypertriglyceridemia.

DRUG SELECTION FOR MANAGING ATHEROGENIC DYSLIPIDEMIA

34. Given these considerations, what drugs are indicated for B.C.?

One approach would be to replace simvastatin with atorvastatin or rosuvastatin, as mentioned previously. This should attain both the LDL-C and non–HDL-C goals. Alternatively, consideration could be given to adding a TG-lowering (i.e., non–HDL-C lowering) drug such as niacin or fenofibrate. Gemfibrozil should be avoided, given its documented pharmacodynamic drug interaction with statins and the increased risk of muscle toxicity. Both niacin and fenofibrate effectively lower TG by 30% to 50%; more importantly, they reduce VLDL-C and small dense LDL and raise HDL-C (Table 12-16). Both alter the mechanisms responsible for atherogenic dyslipidemia, although the effect of PPARα agonism has a broader and more fundamental effect on these mechanisms. Fibrate therapy is not likely to worsen B.C.'s impaired fasting glucose, whereas niacin might do so. Fenofibrate is certainly more tolerable than niacin: About 30% of niacin-treated patients cannot tolerate its vasodilatory side effects. Niacin is less expensive and has demonstrated CHD risk reduction alone or together with a statin in major clinical trials. Given these considerations, it is obvious that there is no one correct choice; the choice will be based on individual preferences.

INITIATING COMBINATION DRUG THERAPY FOR ATHEROGENIC DYSLIPIDEMIA

35. How should combined therapy with a statin and fenofibrate be initiated in B.C.? What monitoring is required?

Fenofibrate can be added as a 200-mg/day capsule and the lipid profile rechecked in 6 to 8 weeks. A lower daily dose of 67 mg should be selected for patients with impaired renal function and in patients >65 years, because creatine clearance declines with older age. As with all lipid-altering therapies, patients should be instructed on the purpose of the medication and its expected effects on blood lipids and on CHD risk reduction. They should be encouraged to remain adherent with the regimen to sustain its effects on serum lipids and, thereby, attain its CHD risk-reducing benefit. Withdrawal, even after a long period of consistent cholesterol control, will likely result in a return of blood lipids to pretreatment levels. Patients should be counseled to call a health professional if they experience any untoward symptoms, especially muscle soreness or discomfort or a rash. A CPK level should be obtained whenever a patient experiences symptoms of myositis (muscle soreness and aches).

LOW HDL-C

36. J.M. is a 59-year-old man who has no history of CHD or a CHD risk equivalent. He has no known medical problems. He does not smoke. His mother had an ischemic episode at age 70 and subsequently had coronary artery bypass surgery. There is no other family history of CHD. J.M. eats a diet low in saturated fat and is sedentary. His physical examination is unremarkable: BP, 122/82 mm Hg, heart rate, 66 regular. He weighs 206 lb and is 6 feet tall (BMI 28). His laboratory values are fasting blood glucose, 80 mg/dL; total cholesterol, 137 mg/dL; LDL-C, 84 mg/dL; TG, 120 mg/dL; HDL-C, 29 mg/dL. Should J.M. be treated for his low HDL-C?

J.M. has two CHD risk factors (age and low HDL) and a LDL-C goal of <130 mg/dL. His NCEP CHD risk is 6% in 10 years, mostly because of his age. His LDL-C is well within his treatment goal. His TG are in the normal range. Epidemiologic studies clearly link low HDL-C with increased CHD events, especially in those over age 50. These studies show that a 1% decrease in HDL-C is associated with a 1% to 2% increase in CHD risk. Most commonly, low HDL-C is secondary to a number of lifestyle and medical conditions (Table 12-19). Of these conditions, overweight, physical inactivity, and a diet very low in fat may play a part in J.M.'s low HDL-C. Patients who substantially restrict saturated fats have lower HDL-C levels as well as LDL-C. A careful dietary history would be important to determine whether this is occurring with J.M. Vegetarians who have a low LDL-C and low BP have a low CHD risk despite having a low HDL-C. Increasing intake of monounsaturated fats and lowering carbohydrate intake is one maneuver to raise HDL-C. An obvious approach to improving J.M.'s HDL-C is to encourage him to increase his physical activity.

In addition to secondary causes, there are rare primary (genetic) causes of low HDL-C. Some are associated with increased CHD risk, whereas others are not. Tangier disease is associated with a reduction in the ABC_1 transporter that moves cholesterol out of peripheral cells. Patients with Tangier disease have characteristic orange tonsils as well as splenomegaly and neuropathy. Fish-eye disease is characterized by corneal opacification and an HDL deficiency. About a third of patients with fish-eye develop CHD. Patients with apolipoprotein A-1_{Milano} have very low HDL-C levels, but live well into their ninetieth decade, apparently because their reverse cholesterol transport is very efficient. J.M. does not appear to have any of these disorders. Importantly, he also does not have a family history of premature CHD. This suggests that his low HDL-C is not caused by a genetic abnormality associated with an increased CHD risk.

Table 12-19 Factors Causing Low HDL-C

Secondary Causes
- Hypertriglyceridemia
- Obesity (visceral fat)
- Physical inactivity
- Type 2 diabetes
- Smoking
- Very-low-fat diet
- Drugs
  - β-blockers
  - Androgenic steroids
  - Androgenic progestins

Primary (Genetic) Causes
- Apo A-1
  - Apo A-1 mutations (e.g., ApoA-1_{Milano})
- LCAT
  - Complete LCAT deficiency
  - Partial LCAT deficiency (fish-eye disease)
- ABC A-1
  - Tangier disease
  - Familial hypoalphalipoproteinemia (some families)
- Unknown genetic etiology
  - Familial hypoalphalipoproteiniemia (most families)
  - Familial combined hyperlipidemia with low HDL-C
  - Metabolic syndrome

ABC A-1, adenosine triphosphate binding cassette A-1; Apo A, apolipoproteins; HDL-C, High-density lipoprotein cholesterol; LCAT, lecithin-cholesterol acyl transferase.

What makes cases of patients such as J.M. difficult to manage is that little clinical trial evidence indicates that raising low levels of HDL-C with diet or drugs will reduce CHD risk. Part of the problem is that no effective drugs substantially and specifically increase HDL-C. Niacin has the most substantial raising effect (mean increases of 25% to 35%). Fibrates also raise HDL-C by 10% to 20%, but they may also raise LDL-C in patients with hypertriglyceridemia. The available evidence indicates that aggressive LDL-C lowering is the most powerful way to reduce CHD risk in patients with low HDL-C. In fact, the lower the HDL-C level, the greater the CHD risk reduction with statin therapy.[240] Based on this evidence, NCEP recommended aggressive LDL-C lowering with a statin in patients with a low HDL-C.[92] In cases of isolated low HDL-C (without hypertriglyceridemia), NCEP recommended lifestyle modification with weight reduction and increased physical activity and the empiric use of HDL-C– raising drugs (niacin or a fibrate), if indicated, to reduce CHD risk.[92]

It would be prudent to encourage J.M. to lose weight and especially to adopt a more physically active lifestyle. This will help his overall well-being. Because he lacks a family history

Table 12-20 Randomized Clinical Trials of Vitamin E Supplementation and CHD Events

Investigator/Reference	*Number of Subjects*	*Vitamin E Dose (U)*	*Population*	*Follow-Up (yrs)*	*Relative Risk*
Rapola[247]	29,133	50	Males, no CHD	4.7	0.9 (NS)
Stephens[248]	2,002	400 and 800	Males and females, with CHD	1.4	0.53
Vitamo	27,271	50	Males, no CHD	6.1	0.98 (NS)
GISSI[175]	2,830	300	Males and females, with CHD	3.5	0.95 (NS)
HOPE[249]	9,541	400	Males and females, high risk	4.5	1.05 (NS)
HPS[91]	20,536	600 (+ vitamin C and β-carotene)	Males and females, with CHD	5.0	1.02 (NS)

CHD, coronary heart disease; NS, not significant.

of premature CHD or associated CHD risk factors, his CHD risk would appear to be low and not supportive of an aggressive effort to raise his low HDL-C. If he did have a family history of premature CHD, a more aggressive approach, particularly with increased physical activity and possibly niacin therapy, would be advisable.

ANTIOXIDANT THERAPY

37. Should antioxidants, such as vitamin E or beta-carotene, be considered in the management of hyperlipidemic patients, especially patients who have developed CHD?

Only oxidized (or otherwise modified) LDL is taken up by macrophage cells in the initial phase of atherogenesis. This observation has led to the supposition that drugs that have antioxidant properties might reduce or block the development of atherosclerosis. Vitamins E, C, and beta-carotene (the precursor of vitamin A) have antioxidant properties and have been variably recommended to prevent CHD.[241]

Studies in hypercholesterolemic animals have demonstrated that antioxidants, such as probucol, can reduce the development of atherosclerosis.[241,242] In humans, oxidized LDL-C has been detected in atheromatous lesions, and circulating antibodies to oxidized LDL have also been detected.[243,244] In epidemiologic studies, people who frequently used beta-carotene and vitamin E had 35% to 50% fewer CHD events.[245,246] When the hypothesis that antioxidant therapy will prevent CHD events was tested in well-controlled, randomized clinical trials, however, no benefit was observed. For example, vitamin E, whether administered in low, moderate, and high daily doses, either as monotherapy or combined with other antioxidants, failed to demonstrate a CHD risk-reducing effect during clinical trials involving close to 100,000 patients (Table 12-20).[91,175,247–249] The latest, and one of the largest of these trials, the Heart Protection Study, prescribed vitamin E (600 U) plus beta-carotene or placebo daily for 5 years to 20,536 high-risk individuals. No demonstrable benefit was shown, whether measured as CHD death, nonfatal MI, stroke, or revascularization procedures and whether or not the study population had a history of CHD, stroke, peripheral vascular disease, or diabetes. Further, no change was seen in the incidence of cancer, another claim of potential benefit for antioxidant therapy. These results effectively close the door on the use of antioxidant therapy for the prevention of CHD events. Future randomized clinical trials will have to demonstrate a benefit before these products can be recommended.

HYPERCHYLOMICRONEMIA

38. M.B., an asymptomatic woman, is screened with a lipoprotein profile during an annual physical evaluation by her primary care provider. She has non–insulin-dependent diabetes, which is treated with 60 U/day of NPH insulin. M.B. is approximately 20% overweight. Her fasting lipoprotein profile is total cholesterol, 234 mg/dL; TG, 2,300 mg/dL; HDL-C, 24 mg/dL; and LDL-C (direct measured), 160 mg/dL. Fasting blood glucose is 290 mg/dL.

What is the assessment of M.B.'s CHD risk, and what treatment, if any, should she be given?

[SI units: total cholesterol, 6.05 mmol/L; TG, 25.97 mmol/L; and HDL-C, 0.62 mmol/L]

Patients with fasting TG >500 mg/dL have an increase in TG-rich chylomicron and VLDL particles. TG elevations of this magnitude typically increase the risk of pancreatitis, but usually not atherosclerosis and CHD. On the other hand, patients with type II diabetes have a high CHD risk. Thus, it is possible that M.B. has two lipid disorders, one causing hyperchylomicronemia and a second causing the typical pattern of atherogenic dyslipidemia. There is no way of knowing whether M.B. has atherogenic dyslipidemia until her TG levels are lowered. Because of the life-threatening nature of TG levels of this magnitude, the priority in treating this patient is to first lower her TG to as close to normal as possible, then assess her LDL.

Most likely, she has an inherited deficiency of lipoprotein lipase, which is the most common cause of very high TG levels. TG levels this high can also be triggered by uncontrolled diabetes mellitus, alcohol abuse, obesity, or drugs, including estrogens, beta-blockers, and steroids. Treatment of these patients should be aggressive. One of the first steps is to improve her diabetes control, because this alone may normalize lipid levels. A TG-lowering diet (severe carbohydrate restriction), fish oil supplementation, and drug therapy (gemfibrozil or fenofibrate or niacin) should be initiated. If the patient has symptoms of pancreatitis, she should be treated in the hospital. In the absence of symptoms, outpatient management is possible, but frequent follow-up and aggressive therapy are indicated. Once the TG level is reduced to <400 mg/dL, a calculated LDL-C can be determined; if it is >100 mg/dL, therapy with a statin or other suitable lipid-modifying agent should be initiated to achieve a LDL-C level <100 mg/dL.

REFERENCES

1. Nissen SE et al. ACAT Intravascular Atherosclerosis Treatment Evaluation (ACTIVATE) Investigators. Effect of ACAT inhibition on the progression of coronary atherosclerosis. *Engl J Med* 2006;354:1253.
2. Eisenberg S. Metabolism of apolipoproteins and lipoproteins. *Curr Opin Lipidol* 1990;1:205.
3. Kwiterovich PO. The metabolic pathways of high-density lipoprotein, low-density lipoprotein, and triglycerides: a current review. *Am J Cardiol* 2000;86(Suppl):5L.
4. Barter P. High-density lipoproteins and reverse cholesterol transport. *Curr Opin Lipidol* 1993; 4:210.
5. Brewer HB, Santamarina-Fofo S. New insights into the role of the adenosine triphosphate-binding cassette transporters in high-density lipoprotein metabolism and reverse cholesterol transport. *Am J Cardiol* 2003;91(Suppl):3E.
6. Nissen SE et al. ILLUSTRATE Investigators. Effect of torcetrapib on the progression of coronary atherosclerosis. *N Engl J Med.* 2007;356:1304.
7. Hodis HN et al. Triglyceride-rich lipoproteins and the progression of coronary artery disease. *Curr Opin Lipidol* 1995;6:209.
8. Schmitz G, Williamson E. High-density lipoprotein metabolism, reverse cholesterol transport and membrane protection. *Curr Opin Lipidol* 1991;2: 177.
9. Austin MA et al. Low-density lipoprotein subclass patterns and risk of myocardial infarction. *JAMA* 1988;260:1917.
10. Brown MS, Goldstein JL. A receptor-mediated pathway for cholesterol homeostasis. *Science* 1986;232:34.
11. Goldstein JL, Brown MS. Familial hypercholesterolemia. In: Scriver CR et al, eds. *The Metabolic Basis of Inherited Disease.* New York: McGraw-Hill; 1989:1215.
12. Hobbs HH et al. Molecular genetics of the LDL receptor gene in familial hypercholesterolemia. *Hum Mutat* 1992;1:445.
13. Hobbs HH et al. Deletion of the gene for the low-density-lipoprotein receptor in a majority of French Canadians with familial hypercholesterolemia. *N Engl J Med* 1987;317:734.
14. Mabuchi H et al. Development of coronary heart disease in familial hypercholesterolemia. *Circulation* 1989;79:225.
15. Soria LF et al. Association between a specific apolipoprotein B mutation and familial defective apolipoprotein B-100. *Proc Natl Acad Sci USA* 1989;86:587.
16. Vega GL, Grundy SM. In vivo evidence for reduced binding of low-density lipoproteins to receptors as a cause of primary moderate hypercholesterolemia. *J Clin Invest* 1986;78:1410.
17. Innerarity TL et al. Familial defective apolipoprotein B-100: a mutation of apolipoprotein B that causes hypercholesterolemia. *J Lipid Res* 1990;31:1337.
18. Innerarity TL et al. Familial defective apolipoprotein B-100: low-density lipoproteins with abnormal receptor binding. *Proc Natl Acad Sci USA* 1987;84:6919.
19. Mahley RW, Rall SC Jr. Type III hyperlipoproteinemia (dysbetalipoproteinemia): the role of apolipoprotein E in normal and abnormal lipoprotein metabolism. In: Scriver CR et al., eds. *The Metabolic Basis of Inherited Disease.* 6th ed. New York: McGraw-Hill; 1991:1195.
20. Brewer HB Jr et al. Type III hyperlipoproteinemia: diagnosis, molecular defects, pathology, and treatment. *Ann Intern Med* 1983;98:623.
21. Kissebah AH et al. Integrated regulation of very low density lipoprotein triglyceride and apolipoprotein-B kinetics in man: normolipemic subjects, familial hypertriglyceridemia, and familial combined hyperlipidemia. *Metabolism* 1981;30:856.
22. Haffner SM et al. Metabolism of apolipoprotein B in members of a family with accelerated atherosclerosis: influence of apolipoprotein E-3/E-2 pattern. *Metabolism* 1992;41(3):241.
23. Cortner JA et al. Familial combined hyperlipidemia: use of stable isotopes to demonstrate overproduction of very low-density lipoprotein apolipoprotein B by the liver. *J Inherit Metab Dis* 1991;14(6):915.
24. Austin MA et al. Bimodality of plasma apolipoprotein B levels in familial combined hyperlipidemia. *Atherosclerosis* 1992;92:67.
25. Sniderman A, Cianftone K. Substrate delivery as a determinant of hepatic ApoB secretion. *Arterioscler Thromb* 1993;13:629.
26. Sniderman A et al. From familial combined hyperlipidemia to hyperapoB: unraveling the overproduction of hepatic apolipoprotein B. *Curr Opin Lipidol* 1992;3:137.
27. Rifkind BM. High-density lipoprotein cholesterol and coronary artery disease: survey of the evidence. *Am J Cardiol* 1990;66:3A.
28. Miller M, Kwiterovich PO Jr. Isolated low HDL-cholesterol as an important risk factor for coronary heart disease. *Eur Heart J* 1990;11(Suppl H):9.
29. Genest JJ Jr et al. Prevalence of familial lipoprotein disorders in patients with premature coronary artery disease. *Circulation* 1992;85:2025.
30. Campeau L et al. Aggressive cholesterol lowering delays saphenous vein graft atherosclerosis in women, the elderly, and patients with associated risk factors. NHLBI Post Coronary Artery Bypass Graft Clinical Trial. *Circulation* 1999;99:3241.
31. Steinberg D et al. Beyond cholesterol: modification of low-density lipoprotein that increases its atherogenicity. *N Engl J Med* 1989;320:915.
32. Davies MJ et al. Atherosclerosis: inhibition or regression as therapeutic possibilities. *Br Heart J* 1991;65:302.
33. Faggiotto A et al. Studies of hypercholesterolemia in the nonhuman primate. I. Changes that lead to fatty streak formation. *Arterioscler Thromb* 1984;4: 323.
34. Witztum JL, Steinberg D. Role of oxidized low-density lipoprotein in atherogenesis. *J Clin Invest* 1991;88:1785.
35. Ross R, Agius L. The process of atherogenesis: cellular and molecular interaction: from experimental animal models to humans. *Diabetologia* 1992;35(Suppl 2):34.
36. Libby P. Current concepts of the pathogenesis of the acute coronary syndromes. *Circulation* 2001;104:365.
37. Libby P et al. Inflammation and atherosclerosis. *Circulation* 2002;105:1135.
38. Henderson EL et al. Death of smooth muscle cells and expression of mediators of apoptosis by T-lymphocytes in human abdominal aortic aneurysms. *Circulation* 1999;99:96.
39. Galina K et al. Evidence for increased collagenolysis by interstitial collagenases-1 and -3 in vulnerable human atheromatous plaques. *Circulation* 1999;99:2503.
40. Libby P. Molecular basis of the acute coronary syndromes. *Circulation* 1995;91:2844.
41. Ridker PM. Inflammation, infection, and cardiovascular risk. How good is the clinical evidence? *Circulation* 1998;97:1671.
42. Ross R. Atherosclerosis: an inflammatory disease. *N Engl J Med* 1999;340:115.
43. Libby P et al. Novel inflammatory markers of coronary risk. Theory versus practice. *Circulation* 1999;100:1148.
44. Fuster V et al. The pathogenesis of coronary artery disease and acute coronary syndromes. *N Engl J Med* 1992;326:242.
45. Brown BG et al. Lipid lowering and plaque regression. New insights into prevention or plaque disruption and clinical events in coronary disease. *Circulation* 1993;87:1781.
46. Neaton JD et al. Serum cholesterol level and mortality findings for men screened in the Multiple Risk Factor Intervention Trial. *Arch Intern Med* 1992;152:1490.
47. Jacobs D et al. Report of the conference on low blood cholesterol: mortality associations. *Circulation* 1992;86:1046.
48. Castelli WP. Epidemiology of coronary heart disease: the Framingham Study. *Am J Med* 1984; 76:4.
49. Gordon DJ et al. High-density lipoprotein cholesterol and cardiovascular disease: four prospective American studies. *Circulation* 1989;79:8.
50. Kagan A et al. Epidemiologic studies of coronary heart disease and stroke in Japanese men living in Japan, Hawaii and California: demographic, physical, dietary and biochemical characteristics. *J Chronic Dis* 1974;27:345.
51. Rosenberg L et al. Myocardial infarction in women under 50 years of age. *JAMA* 1983;250:2801.
52. Rosenberg L et al. Myocardial infarction and cigarette smoking in women younger than 50 years of age. *JAMA* 1985;253:2965.
53. Castelli WP et al. Cardiovascular risk factors in the elderly. *Am J Cardiol* 1989;63:12H.
54. Thom TJ. Cardiovascular disease mortality among United States women. In: Eaker ED et al., eds. *Coronary Heart Disease in Women.* New York: Haymarket Doyma; 1987.
55. Garg A, Grundy SM. Management of dyslipidemia in NIDDM. *Diabetes Care* 1990;13:153.
56. Kannel WB. Lipids, diabetes, and coronary heart disease: insights from the Framingham Study. *Am Heart J* 1985;110:1100.
57. Kannel WB, Gordon T. Evaluation of cardiovascular risk in the elderly. The Framingham Study. *Bull NY Acad Med* 1978;54:573.
58. Manolio TA et al. Cholesterol and heart disease in older persons and women. Review of an NHLBI workshop. *Ann Epidemiol* 1992;2:161.
59. Malenka DJ, Baron JA. Cholesterol and coronary heart disease: the importance of patient-specific attributable risk. *Arch Intern Med* 1988;148:2247.
60. LaRosa JC et al. The cholesterol facts: a summary of the evidence relating dietary fats, serum cholesterol, and coronary heart disease. *Circulation* 1990;81:1721.
61. Buchwald H et al. Effect of partial ileal bypass surgery on mortality and morbidity from coronary heart disease in patients with hypercholesterolemia: report of the Program on the Surgical Control of Hyperlipidemias (POSCH). *N Engl J Med* 1990;323:946.
62. Blankenhorn DH et al. Beneficial effects of combined colestipol-niacin therapy on coronary atherosclerosis and coronary venous bypass grafts. *JAMA* 1987;257:3233.
63. Brown G et al. Regression of coronary artery disease as a result of intensive lipid-lowering therapy in men with high levels of apolipoprotein B. *N Engl J Med* 1990;323:1289.
64. Ornish D et al. Can lifestyle changes reverse coronary heart disease: the Lifestyle Heart Trial. *Lancet* 1990;336:129.
65. Watts GF et al. Effects on coronary artery disease of lipid-lowering diet, or diet plus cholestyramine, in the St. Thomas' Atherosclerosis Regression Study (STARS). *Lancet* 1992;339:563.
66. Kane JP et al. Regression of coronary atherosclerosis during treatment of familial hypercholesterolemia with combined drug regimens. *JAMA* 1990;264:3007.
67. Duffield RGM, et al. Treatment of hyperlipidemia retards progression of symptomatic femoral atherosclerosis. A randomized controlled trial. *Lancet* 1983;ii:639.
68. MAAS Investigators. Effect of simvastatin on coronary atheroma: the Multicentre Anti-Atheroma Study (MAAS). *Lancet* 1994;344:633.
69. Waters D et al. Effects of monotherapy with an HMG-CoA reductase inhibitor on the progression of coronary atherosclerosis as assessed by serial quantitative arteriography. The Canadian Coronary Atherosclerosis Intervention Trial. *Circulation* 1994;89:959.

70. Haskell WL et al. Effects of intensive multiple risk factor reduction on coronary atherosclerosis and clinical cardiac events in men and women with coronary heart disease. The Stanford Coronary Risk Intervention Project (SCRIP). *Circulation* 1994;89:975.
71. Furberg CD et al. Pravastatin, lipids, and major coronary events. *Am J Cardiol* 1994;73:1133.
72. Furberg CD et al. Effect of lovastatin on early carotid atherosclerosis and cardiovascular events. *Circulation* 1994;90:1679.
73. Blankenhorn DH et al. Coronary angiographic changes with lovastatin therapy. The Monitored Atherosclerosis Regression Study (MARS). *Ann Intern Med* 1993;119:969.
74. Pitt B et al. Pravastatin limitation of atherosclerosis in the coronary arteries (PLACI): reduction in atherosclerosis progression and clinical events. *J Am Coll Cardiol* 1995;26:1133.
75. Salonen R et al. Kuopio atherosclerosis prevention study (KAPS). A population-based primary prevention trial of the effect of LDL lowering on atherosclerotic progression in carotid and femoral arteries. *Circulation* 1995;92:1758.
76. Jukema JW et al. Effects of lipid lowering by pravastatin on progression and regression of coronary artery disease in symptomatic men with normal to moderately elevated serum cholesterol levels. The Regression Growth Evaluation Statin Study (REGRESS). *Circulation* 1995;91:2528.
77. Herd JA et al. Effects of fluvastatin on coronary atherosclerosis in patients with mild to moderate cholesterol elevations (Lipoprotein and Coronary Atherosclerosis Study [LCAS]). *Am J Cardiol* 1997;80:278.
78. The Post Coronary Artery Bypass Graft Trial Investigators. The effect of aggressive lowering of low-density lipoprotein cholesterol levels and low-dose anticoagulation on obstructive changes in saphenous-vein coronary-artery bypass grafts. *N Engl J Med* 1997;336:153.
79. Thompson GR. What targets should lipid-modulating therapy achieve to optimise the prevention of coronary heart disease? *Atherosclerosis* 1997; 131:1.
80. Nissen SE et al. ASTEROID Investigators. Effect of very high-intensity statin therapy on regression of coronary atherosclerosis: the ASTEROID trial. *JAMA* 2006;295:1556.
81. Takagi T et al. Intravascular ultrasound analysis of reduction in progression of coronary narrowing by treatment with pravastatin. *Am J Cardiol* 1997;79:1673.
82. Lipid Research Clinics Program. The Lipid Research Clinics Coronary Primary Prevention Trial results. I: Reduction in incidence of coronary heart disease. *JAMA* 1984;251:351.
83. Scandinavian Simvastatin Survival Study (4S) Group. Randomised trial of cholesterol lowering in 4444 patients with coronary heart disease. *Lancet* 1994;344:1383.
84. Sacks FM et al. The effect of pravastatin on coronary events after myocardial infarction in patients with average cholesterol levels. *N Engl J Med* 1996;335:1001.
85. LaRosa JC et al. Treating to New Targets (TNT) Investigators. Intensive lipid lowering with atorvastatin in patients with stable coronary disease. *N Engl J Med* 2005;352:1425.
86. Pedersen TR et al. Incremental Decrease in End Points Through Aggressive Lipid Lowering (IDEAL) Study Group. High-dose atorvastatin vs. usual-dose simvastatin for secondary prevention after myocardial infarction: the IDEAL study: a randomized controlled trial. *JAMA* 2005;294: 2437.
87. Crouse JR III, et al. Reductase inhibitor monotherapy and stroke prevention. *Arch Intern Med* 1997;157:1305.
88. Smith SC Jr et al. AHA/ACC; National Heart, Lung, and Blood Institute. AHA/ACC guidelines for secondary prevention for patients with coronary and other atherosclerotic vascular disease: 2006 update: endorsed by the National Heart, Lung, and Blood Institute. *Circulation* 2006;113:2363.
89. Grundy SM et al. Coordinating Committee of the National Cholesterol Education Program. Implications of recent clinical trials for the National Cholesterol Education Program Adult Treatment Panel III guidelines. *Arterioscler Thromb Vasc Biol* 2004;24:e149-61.
90. The Long-Term Intervention with Pravastatin in Ischaemic Disease (LIPID) Study Group. Prevention of cardiovascular events and death with pravastatin in patients with coronary heart disease and a broad range of initial cholesterol levels. *N Engl J Med* 1998;339:1349.
91. Heart Protection Study Collaborative Group. MRC/BHF Heart Protection Study of cholesterol lowering with simvastatin in 20,536 high-risk individuals: a randomized placebo-controlled trial. *Lancet* 2002;360:7.
92. Expert Panel on Detection, Evaluation, and Treatment of High Blood Cholesterol in Adults. Third Report of the National Cholesterol Education Program (NCEP) Expert Panel on detection, evaluation, and treatment of high blood cholesterol in adults (Adult Treatment Panel III). Final Report. *Circulation* 2002;106:3143. Executive Summary in *JAMA* 2001:2486.
93. Schwartz GG et al. Effects of atorvastatin on early recurrent ischemic events in acute coronary syndromes. The MIRACL study: a randomized controlled trial. *JAMA* 2001;285:1711.
94. Waters DD et al. Effects of atorvastatin on stroke in patients with unstable angina or non-Q-wave myocardial infarction. A Myocardial Ischemia Reduction with Aggressive Cholesterol Lowering (MIRACL) substudy. *Circulation* 2002;106:1690.
95. Pitt B et al. Aggressive lipid-lowering therapy compared with angioplasty in stable coronary artery disease. *N Engl J Med* 1999;341:70.
96. Cannon CP et al. Pravastatin or Atorvastatin Evaluation and Infection Therapy-Thrombolysis in Myocardial Infarction 22 Investigators. Intensive versus moderate lipid lowering with statins after acute coronary syndromes. *N Engl J Med* 2004;350:1495-504.
97. West of Scotland Coronary Prevention Study Group. Influence of pravastatin and plasma lipids on clinical events in the West of Scotland Coronary Prevention Study (WOSCOPS). *Circulation* 1998;97:1440.
98. Sever PS et al. Prevention of coronary and stroke events with atorvastatin in hypertensive patients who have average or lower-than-average cholesterol concentrations, in the Anglo-Scandinavian Cardiac Outcome Trial-Lipid Lowering Arm (ASCOT-LLA): A multicentre randomized controlled trial. *Lancet* 2003;361:1149.
99. ALLHAT Officers and Coordinators for the ALLHAT Collaborative Research Group. The Antihypertensive and Lipid-Lowering Treatment to Prevent Heart Attack Trial. Major outcomes in moderately hypercholesterolemic, hypertensive patients randomized to pravastatin vs usual care: The Antihypertensive and Lipid-Lowering Treatment to Prevent Heart Attack Trial (ALLHAT-LLT). *JAMA* 2002;288:2998.
100. Downs JR et al. Primary prevention of acute coronary events with lovastatin in men and women with average cholesterol levels. Results of AFCAPS/TexCAPS. *JAMA* 1998;279:1615.
101. O'Keefe JH Jr et al. Optimal low-density lipoprotein is 50 to 70 mg/dl: lower is better and physiologically normal. *J Am Coll Cardiol* 2004;43:2142–2146.
102. Haffner SM et al. Mortality from coronary heart disease in subjects with type 2 diabetes and in nondiabetic subjects with and without prior myocardial infarction. *N Engl J Med* 1998;339:229.
103. The Diabetes Control and Complications Trial Research Group. The effect of intensive treatment of diabetes on the development and progression of long-term complications in insulin-dependent diabetes mellitus. *N Engl J Med* 1993;329:977.
104. UK Prospective Diabetes Study (UKPDS) Group. Intensive blood-glucose control with sulphonylureas or insulin compared with conventional treatment and risk of complications in patients with type 2 diabetes (UKPDS 33). *Lancet* 1998;352:837.
105. Colhoun HM et al. CARDS investigators. Primary prevention of cardiovascular disease with atorvastatin in type 2 diabetes in the Collaborative Atorvastatin Diabetes Study (CARDS): multicentre randomised placebo-controlled trial. *Lancet* 2004;364:685.
106. Grundy SM. Primary prevention of coronary heart disease. Integrating risk assessment with intervention. *Circulation* 1999;100:988.
107. Frick MH et al. Helsinki Heart Study: primary-prevention trial with gemfibrozil in middle-aged men with dyslipidemia. Safety of treatment, changes in risk factors, and incidence of coronary heart disease. *N Engl J Med* 1987;317:1237.
108. Manninen V et al. Joint effects of serum triglyceride and LDL cholesterol and HDL cholesterol concentrations on coronary heart disease risk in the Helsinki Heart Study: implications for treatment. *Circulation* 1992;85:37.
109. Rubins HB et al. Gemfibrozil for the secondary prevention of coronary heart disease in men with low levels of high-density lipoprotein cholesterol. *N Engl J Med* 1999;341:410.
110. The BIP Study Group. Secondary prevention by raising HDL cholesterol and reducing triglycerides in patients with coronary heart disease. The Bezafibrate Infarction Prevention Study. *Circulation* 2000;102:21.
111. Keech A et al. FIELD study investigators. Effects of long-term fenofibrate therapy on cardiovascular events in 9795 people with type 2 diabetes mellitus (the FIELD study): randomised controlled trial. *Lancet* 2005;366:1849.
112. Canner PL et al. for the Coronary Drug Project Research Group. Fifteen-year mortality in coronary drug project patients: long-term benefit with niacin. *J Am Coll Cardiol* 1986;8:1245.
113. Brown BG et al. Simvastatin and niacin, antioxidant vitamins, or the combination for the prevention of coronary disease. *N Engl J Med* 2001;345:1583.
114. Ito MK et al. Statin-associated pleiotropy: possible beneficial effects beyond cholesterol reduction. *Pharmacotherapy.* 2006;26:85S.
115. Vogel RA et al. Effect of a single high-fat meal on endothelial function in healthy subjects. *Am J Cardiol* 1997;79:350.
116. O'Driscoll G et al. Simvastatin, an HMG-coenzyme reductase inhibitor, improves endothelial function within 1 month. *Circulation* 1997;95:1126.
117. Gould KL et al. Short-term cholesterol lowering decreases size and severity of perfusion abnormalities by positron emission tomography after dipyridamole in patients with coronary artery disease. *Circulation* 1994;89:1530.
118. Baller D et al. Improvement in coronary flow reserve determined by positron emission tomography after 6 months of cholesterol-lowering therapy in patients with early stages of coronary atherosclerosis. *Circulation* 1999;99:2871.
119. Treasure CB et al. Beneficial effects of cholesterol-lowering therapy on coronary endothelium in patients with coronary artery disease. *N Engl J Med* 1995;332:481.
120. Anderson TJ et al. The effect of cholesterol-lowering and antioxidant therapy on endothelium-dependent coronary vasomotion. *N Engl J Med* 1995;332:488.
121. Andrews TC et al. Effect of cholesterol reduction on myocardial ischemia in patients with coronary disease. *Circulation* 1997;95:324.
122. Van Boven AJ et al. Reduction of transient myocardial ischemia with pravastatin in addition to the conventional treatment in patients with angina pectoris. *Circulation* 1996;94:1503.
123. Ridker PM. Clinical application of C-reactive protein for cardiovascular disease detection and prevention. *Circulation* 2003;107:363.
124. Ridker PM et al. Inflammation, pravastatin, and the

risk of coronary events after myocardial infarction in patients with average cholesterol levels. *Circulation* 1998;98:839.
125. Pearson TA et al. Markers of inflammation and cardiovascular disease. Application to clinical and public health practice. A statement for healthcare professionals from the Centers for Disease Control and Prevention and the American Heart Association. 2003;107:499.
126. Schulman KA et al. Reducing high blood cholesterol level with drugs: cost-effectiveness of pharmacologic management. *JAMA* 1990;264:3025.
127. Goldman L et al. Cost-effectiveness of HMG-CoA reductase inhibition for primary and secondary prevention of coronary heart disease. *JAMA* 1991;265:1145.
128. Weinstein MC et al. Forecasting coronary heart disease, mortality, and cost: the coronary heart disease policy model. *Am J Public Health* 1987;77:1417.
129. Weissfeld JL et al. A mathematical representation of the expert panel's guidelines for high blood cholesterol case-finding and treatment. *Med Decis Making* 1990;10:135.
130. Pederson TR et al. Cholesterol lowering and the use of healthcare resources. Results of the Scandinavian Simvastatin Survival Study. *Circulation* 1996;93:1796.
131. Koren MJ et al. The cost of reaching National Cholesterol Education Program (NCEP) goals in hypercholesterolaemic patients. A comparison of atorvastatin, simvastatin, lovastatin, and fluvastatin. *Pharmacoeconomics* 1998;1:59.
132. Pekkanen J et al. Ten-year mortality from cardiovascular disease in relation to cholesterol level among men with and without preexisting cardiovascular disease. *N Engl J Med* 1990;322:1700.
133. Criqui MH et al. Mortality over a period of 10 years in patients with peripheral arterial disease. *N Engl J Med* 1992;326:381.
134. Salonen JT, Salonen R. Ultrasonographically assessed carotid morphology and the risk of coronary heart disease. *Arterioscler Thromb* 1991;11:1245.
135. Katan MB et al. Beyond low-fat diets. *N Engl J Med* 1997;337:563.
136. Leaf A. Dietary prevention of coronary heart disease. The Lyon Diet Heart Study. *Circulation* 1999;99:733.
137. de Lorgeril M et al. Mediterranean diet, traditional risk factors, and the rate of cardiovascular complications after myocardial infarction. Final Report of the Lyon Diet Heart Study. *Circulation* 1999;99:779.
138. Caggiula AW et al. The Multiple Risk Factor Intervention Trial (MRFIT). IV: Intervention on blood lipids. *Prev Med* 1981;10:443.
139. Ramsay LE et al. Dietary reduction of serum cholesterol concentration: time to think again. *BMJ* 1991;303:953.
140. Boyd NF et al. Quantitative changes in dietary fat intake and serum cholesterol in women: results from a randomized, controlled trial. *Am J Clin Nutr* 1990;52:470.
141. Wood PD et al. Changes in plasma lipids and lipoproteins in overweight men during weight loss through dieting as compared with exercise. *N Engl J Med* 1988;319:1173.
142. The Expert Panel. Executive summary of the clinical guidelines on the identification, evaluation, and treatment of overweight and obesity in adults. *Arch Intern Med* 1998;158:1855.
143. Wood PD et al. The effects of plasma lipoproteins of a prudent weight-reducing diet, with or without exercise, in overweight men and women. *N Engl J Med* 1991;325:461.
144. Danesh J et al. Lipoprotein (a) and coronary heart disease: meta-analysis of prospective studies. *Circulation* 2000;102:1082.
145. Bloch S et al. Apolipoprotein B and LDL cholesterol: which parameter(s) should be included in the assessment of cardiovascular risk? *Ann Biol Clin (Paris)* 1998;56(5):539.
146. Malinow MR et al. Homocysteine, diet, and cardiovascular diseases: a statement for healthcare professionals for the Nutrition Committee, American Heart Association. *Circulation* 1999;99:178.
147. Lipid Research Clinics Program. The Lipid Research Clinics Coronary Primary Prevention Trial results. II: The relationship of reduction in incidence of coronary heart disease to cholesterol lowering. *JAMA* 1984;251:365.
148. Superko HR et al. Effectiveness of low-dose colestipol therapy in patients with moderate hypercholesterolemia. *Am J Cardiol* 1992;70:135.
149. Einarsson K et al. Bile acid sequestrants: mechanisms of action on bile acid and cholesterol metabolism. *Eur J Clin Pharm* 1991;40(Suppl 1):S53.
150. Ito MK et al. Acceptability of cholestyramine and colestipol formulations in three common vehicles *Clin Pharm* 1991;10:138.
151. Bays HE et al. Ezetimibe Study Group. Effectiveness and tolerability of ezetimibe in patients with primary hypercholesterolemia: pooled analysis of two phase II studies. *Clin Ther* 2001;23:1209.
152. Davidson MH et al. Ezetimibe co-administered with simvastatin in patients with primary hypercholesterolemia. *J Am Coll Cardiol.* 2002;40:2125.
153. Sudhop T et al. Inhibition of intestinal cholesterol absorption by ezetimibe in humans. *Circulation* 2002;106:1943.
154. Coronary Drug Project Research Group. Clofibrate and niacin in coronary heart disease. *JAMA* 1975;231:360.
155. McKenney JM et al. A comparison of the efficacy and toxic effects of sustained- vs. immediate-release niacin in hypercholesterolemic patients. *JAMA* 1994;271:672.
156. Drood JM et al. Nicotinic acid for the treatment of hyperlipoproteinemia. *J Clin Pharmacol* 1991;31:641.
157. Carlson LA et al. Pronounced lowering of serum levels of lipoprotein Lp(a) in hyperlipidemic subjects treated with nicotinic acid. *J Intern Med* 1989;226:271.
158. Grundy SM et al. Influence of nicotinic acid on metabolism of cholesterol and triglycerides in man. *J Lipid Res* 1981;22:24.
159. Sakai T et al. Niacin, but not gemfibrozil, selectively increases LP-A1, a cardioprotective subfraction of HDL, in patients with low HDL cholesterol. *Arterioscler Thromb Vasc Biol* 2001;21:1783.
160. Jin FY et al. Niacin decreases removal of high-density lipoprotein apolipoprotein A-I but not cholesterol ester by Hep G2 cells: implication for reverse cholesterol transport. *Arterioscler Thromb Vasc Biol* 1997;17:2020.
161. Piepho RW. The pharmacokinetics and pharmacodynamics of agents proven to raise high-density lipoprotein cholesterol. *Am J Cardiol* 2000;86(Suppl):35L.
162. Henkin Y et al. Niacin revisited: clinical observations on an important but underutilized drug. *Am J Med* 1991;91:239.
163. Knopp RH et al. Contrasting effects of unmodified and time-release forms of niacin on lipoproteins in hyperlipidemic subjects: clues to mechanism of action of niacin. *Metabolism* 1985;34:642.
164. Wilkin J et al. Aspirin blocks nicotinic acid-induced flushing. *Clin Pharmacol Ther* 1982; 31:478.
165. Rader JI et al. Hepatic toxicity of unmodified and time-release preparations of niacin. *Am J Med* 1992;92:77.
166. Hunninghake DB et al. Efficacy and safety of pravastatin in patients with primary hypercholesterolemia. II: Once-daily versus twice-daily dosing. *Atherosclerosis* 1990;85:219.
167. Jones P et al. Comparative dose efficacy study of atorvastatin versus simvastatin, pravastatin, lovastatin, and fluvastatin in patients with hypercholesterolemia (The Curves Study). *Am J Cardiol* 1998;81:582.
168. Grundy SM et al. Guide to primary prevention of cardiovascular diseases. A statement for health care professionals for the task force on risk reduction. *Circulation* 1997;95:2329.
169. Grundy SM et al. Influence of combined therapy with mevinolin and interruption of bile-acid reabsorption on low-density lipoproteins in heterozygous familial hypercholesterolemia. *Ann Intern Med* 1985;103:339.
170. Ginsberg HN et al. Suppression of apolipoprotein B production during treatment of cholesteryl ester storage disease with lovastatin: implications for regulation of apolipoprotein B synthesis. *J Clin Invest* 1987;80:1692.
171. Arad Y et al. Effects of lovastatin therapy on very low-density lipoprotein triglyceride metabolism in subjects with combined hyperlipidemia: evidence for reduced assembly and secretion of triglyceride-rich lipoproteins. *Metabolism* 1992;41:487.
172. Hunninghake DB et al. Efficacy and safety of pravastatin in patients with primary hypercholesterolemia. I: A dose-response study. *Atherosclerosis* 1990;85:81.
173. Dujovne CA et al. Expanded Clinical Evaluation of Lovastatin (EXCEL) study results. IV: Additional perspectives on the tolerability of lovastatin. *Am J Med* 1991;91(Suppl 1B):25S.
174. Ito MK. Effects of extensive and poor gastrointestinal metabolism on the pharmacodynamics of pravastatin. *J Clin Pharmacol* 1998;38:331-6.
175. GISSI Prevenzione Investigators. Dietary supplementation with omega-3 polyunsaturated fatty acids and vitamin E after myocardial infarction: results of the GISSI-Prevenzione trial. *Lancet* 1999;354:447.
176. Stampfer MJ et al. Post-menopausal estrogen therapy and cardiovascular disease: ten-year follow-up from the Nurses Health Study. *N Engl J Med* 1991;325:756.
177. Barrett-Connor E, Bush TL. Estrogen and coronary heart disease in women. *JAMA* 1991;265:1861.
178. Grady D et al. Hormone therapy to prevent disease and prolong life in postmenopausal women. *Ann Intern Med* 1992;117:1016.
179. Grodstein F et al. Postmenopausal hormone therapy and mortality. *N Engl J Med* 1997;336:1769.
180. Stampfer MJ, Colditz GA. Estrogen replacement therapy and coronary heart disease: a quantitative assessment of the epidemiologic evidence. *Prev Med* 1991;20:47.
181. Gruchow HW et al. Postmenopausal use of estrogen and occlusion of arteries. *Am Heart J* 1988;115(5):954–63.
182. The Writing Group for the PEPI trial. Effects of estrogen or estrogen/progestin regimens on heart disease risk factors in postmenopausal women. The Postmenopausal Estrogen/Progestin Interventions (PEPI) trial. *JAMA* 1995;273:199.
183. Hulley S et al. Randomized trial of estrogen plus progestin for secondary prevention of coronary heart disease in postmenopausal women. *JAMA* 1998;280:605.
184. Writing Group for the Women's Health Initiative Investigators. Risks and benefits of estrogen plus progestin in healthy postmenopausal women. Principal results from the Women's Health Initiative randomized controlled trial. *JAMA* 2002;288:321.
185. LaRosa JC et al. Effects of statins on risk of coronary disease. A meta-analysis of randomized controlled trials. *JAMA* 1999;282:2340.
186. Ballantyne CM et al. Effect of ezetimibe coadministered with atorvastatin in 628 patients with primary hypercholesterolemia: a prospective, randomized, double-blind trial. *Circulation* 2003;107:2409.
187. Brown BG et al. Moderate dose, three-drug therapy with niacin, lovastatin, and colestipol to reduce low-density lipoprotein cholesterol <100 mg/dL in patients with hyperlipidemia and coronary artery disease. *Am J Cardiol* 1997;80:111.
188. Brown BG et al. Very intensive lipid therapy with lovastatin, niacin, and colestipol for prevention of death and myocardial infarction: a 10-year Familial Atherosclerosis Treatment Study (FATS) follow-up [abstract]. *Circulation* 1998;98:I-635.
189. Grundy SM et al. When to start cholesterol-lowering therapy in patients with coronary heart disease. A statement for healthcare professionals from the American Heart Association Task

Force on Risk Reduction. *Circulation* 1997;95:1683.

190. Tobert JA et al. Clinical experience with lovastatin. *Am J Cardiol* 1990;65:23F.
191. NIH Consensus Development Panel on Triglyceride, High-Density Lipoprotein, and Coronary Heart Disease. Triglyceride, high-density lipoprotein, and coronary heart disease. *JAMA* 1993;269:505.
192. Gordon DJ, Rifkind BM. High-density lipoprotein—the clinical implications of recent studies. *N Engl J Med* 1989;321:1311.
193. Grundy SM et al. The place of HDL in cholesterol management. A perspective from the National Cholesterol Education Program. *Arch Intern Med* 1989;149:505.
194. Grundy SM, Vega GL. Two different views of the relationship of hypertriglyceridemia to coronary heart disease. Implications for treatment. *Arch Intern Med* 1992;152:28.
195. Reardon MF et al. Lipoprotein predictors of the severity of coronary artery disease in men and women. *Circulation* 1985;71:881.
196. Steiner G et al. The association of increased levels of intermediate-density lipoproteins with smoking and with coronary heart disease. *Circulation* 1987;75:124.
197. Grundy SM. Small LDL, atherogenic dyslipidemia, and the metabolic syndrome. *Circulation* 1997;95:1.
198. Grundy SM. Hypertriglyceridemia, atherogenic dyslipidemia, and the metabolic syndrome. *Am J Cardiol* 1998;81(4A):18B.
199. Austin MA et al. Hypertriglyceridemia as a cardiovascular risk factor. *Am J Cardiol* 1998;81(4A):7B.
200. Brunzell JD et al. Plasma lipoproteins in familial combined hyperlipidemia and monogenic familial hypertriglyceridemia. *J Lipid Res* 1983;24:147.
201. Lamarche B et al. Small, dense low-density lipoprotein particles as a predictor of the risk of ischemic heart disease in men. Prospective results from the Quebec Cardiovascular Study. *Circulation* 1997;95:69.
202. Ginsberg HN. Insulin resistance and cardiovascular disease. *J Clin Invest* 2000;106:453.
203. Sato R et al. Sterol regulatory element-binding protein negatively regulates microsomal triglyceride transfer protein gene transcription. *J Biol Chem* 1999;274:24714.
204. Grundy SM. Approach to lipoprotein management in 2001 National Cholesterol Guidelines. *Am J Cardiol* 2002;90 (8A):11i.
205. Marmot M, Brunner E. Alcohol and cardiovascular disease: the status of the U-shaped curve. *BMJ* 1991;303:565.
206. Jackson R, Beaglehole R. The relationship between alcohol and coronary heart disease: is there a protective effect? *Curr Opin Lipidol* 1993;4:21.
207. Steinberg D et al. Davis conference, alcohol and atherosclerosis. *Ann Intern Med* 1991;114:967.
208. Klatsky AL et al. Alcohol and mortality: a ten-year Kaiser-Permanente experience. *Ann Intern Med* 1981;95:139.
209. Assmann G, Schulte H. Triglycerides and atherosclerosis: results from the Prospective Cardiovascular Munster Study. In: Gotto AM Jr, Paoletti R, eds. *Atherosclerosis Reviews*. Vol. 22. New York: Raven; 1991:51.
210. Fujioka S et al. Contribution of intra-abdominal fat accumulation to the impairment of glucose and lipid metabolism in human obesity. *Metabolism* 1987;36:54.
211. Barakat HA et al. Influence of obesity, impaired glucose tolerance, and NIDDM on LDL structure and composition. Possible link between hyperinsulinemia and atherosclerosis. *Diabetes* 1990;39:1527.
212. Bierman EL. Atherogenesis in diabetes. *Arterioscler Thromb* 1992;12:647.
213. DeFronzo RA, Ferrannini E. Insulin resistance. A multifaceted syndrome responsible for NIDDM, obesity, hypertension, dyslipidemia, and atherosclerotic cardiovascular disease. *Diabetes Care* 1991;14:173.
214. American Diabetes Association. Screening for type 2 diabetes. *Diabetes Care* 1998;21:S20.
215. Chobanian AV et al. The seventh report of the Joint National Committee on prevention, detection, evaluation, and treatment of high blood pressure. The JNC 7 Report. *JAMA* 2003;289:2560.
216. Reaven GM. Insulin resistance and compensatory hyperinsulinemia: role in hypertension, dyslipidemia, and coronary heart disease. *Am Heart J* 1991;121:1283.
217. Gwynne J. Clinical features and pathophysiology of familial dyslipidemic hypertension syndrome. *Curr Opin Lipidol* 1992;3:215.
218. Reaven GM. Role of insulin resistance in human disease. *Diabetes* 1988;37:1595.
219. Gingsburg HN. Hypertriglyceridemia: new insights and new approaches to pharmacologic therapy. *Am J Cardiol* 2001;87:1174.
220. Stein EA et al. Efficacy and tolerability of low-dose simvastatin and niacin, alone and in combination, in patients with combined hyperlipidemia: a prospective trial. *J Cardiovasc Pharmacol Ther* 1996;1:107.
221. Elam MB et al. Effect of niacin on lipid and lipoprotein levels and glycemic control in patients with diabetes and peripheral arterial disease. The ADMIT study: a randomized trial. *JAMA* 2000;284:1263.
222. Canner PL et al. Benefits of niacin by glycemic status in patients with healed myocardial infarction (from the Coronary Drug Project). *Am J Cardiol* 2005;95(2):254-257.
223. Hunninghake DB, Peters JR. Effect of fibric acid derivatives on blood lipid and lipoprotein levels. *Am J Med* 1987;83:44.
224. Manttari M et al. Effect of gemfibrozil on the concentration and composition of serum lipoproteins: a controlled study with special reference to initial triglyceride levels. *Atherosclerosis* 1990;81:11.
225. Rubins HB, Robins SJ. Effect of reduction of plasma triglycerides with gemfibrozil on high-density-lipoprotein-cholesterol concentrations. *J Intern Med* 1992;231:421.
226. Vega GL, Grundy SM. Comparison of lovastatin and gemfibrozil in normolipidemic patients with hypoalphalipoproteinemia. *JAMA* 1989;262:3148.
227. Miller M et al. Effect of gemfibrozil in men with primary isolated low high-density lipoprotein cholesterol: a randomized, double-blind, placebo-controlled, crossover study. *Am J Med* 1993;94:7.
228. Brown WV et al. Effects of fenofibrate on plasma lipids. Double-blind, multicenter study in patients with type IIA or IIB hyperlipidemia. *Arteriosclerosis* 1986;6:670.
229. Manninen V et al. Relation between baseline lipid and lipoprotein values and the incidence of coronary heart disease in the Helsinki Heart Study. *Am J Cardiol* 1989;63:42H.
230. American Diabetic Association. Management of dyslipidemia in adults with diabetes. *Diabetes Care* 1998;21(Suppl 1):S36.
231. Grundy SM et al. Diabetes and cardiovascular disease. A statement for healthcare professionals from the American Heart Association. *Circulation* 1999;100:1134.
232. Berger J, Moller DE. The mechanisms of action of PPARa. *Annu Rev Med* 2002;53:409.
233. Grundy SM, Vega GL. Fibric acids: effects on lipids and lipoprotein metabolism. *Am J Med* 1987;83:9.
234. Pierce LR et al. Myopathy and rhabdomyolysis associated with lovastatin-gemfibrozil combination therapy. *JAMA* 1990;264:71.
235. Prueksaritanont T et al. Effects of fibrates on metabolism of statins in human hepatocytes. *Drug Metab Dispos* 2002;30:1280.
236. Prueksaritanont T et al. Mechanistic studies on metabolic interactions between gemfibrozil and statins. *J Pharmacol Exp Ther* 2002;301:1042.
237. Committee of Principal Investigators. World Health Organization. WHO cooperative trial on primary prevention of ischaemic heart disease using clofibrate to lower serum cholesterol: mortality follow-up. *Lancet* 1980;2:379.
238. Committee of Principal Investigators. A co-operative trial in the primary prevention of ischaemic heart disease using clofibrate. *Br Heart J* 1978;40:1069.
239. Diabetes Atherosclerosis Intervention Study Investigators. Effect of fenofibrate on progression on coronary-artery disease in type 2 diabetes: the Diabetes Atherosclerosis Intervention Study, a randomised study. *Lancet* 2001;357:905.
240. Gotto AM et al. Relationship between baseline and on-treatment lipid parameters and first major coronary events in the Air Force/Texas Coronary Atherosclerosis Prevention Study (TexCAPS/AFCAPS). *Circulation* 2000;101:477.
241. Parthasarathy S et al. Probucol inhibits oxidative modification of low-density lipoprotein. *J Clin Invest* 1986;77:641.
242. Kita T et al. Probucol prevents the progression of atherosclerosis in Watanabe heritable hyperlipidemic rabbits, and animal models for familial hypercholesterolemia. *Proc Natl Acad Sci USA* 1987;84:5928.
243. Parums D et al. Serum antibodies to oxidized low-density lipoprotein and ceroid in chronic periaortitis. *Arch Pathol Lab Med* 1990;114:383.
244. Salonen JT et al. Autoantibody against oxidized LDL and progression of carotid atherosclerosis. *Lancet* 1992;339:883.
245. Gaziano JM et al. Beta-carotene therapy for chronic stable angina [abstract]. *Circulation* 1990;82:III-201.
246. Stampfer MJ et al. A prospective study of vitamin E supplementation and risk of coronary disease in women [abstract]. *Circulation* 1991;86:I-463.
247. Rapola JM et al. Effect of vitamin E and beta-carotene on the incidence of angina pectoris: a randomized, double-blind, controlled trial. *JAMA* 1996;275:693.
248. Stephens NG et al. Randomised controlled trial of vitamin E in patients with coronary disease: Cambridge Heart Antioxidant Study. *Lancet* 1996;347:781.
249. The Heart Outcomes Prevention Evaluation (HOPE) Study Investigators. Vitamin E supplementation and cardiovascular events in high-risk patients. *N Engl J Med* 2000;342:154.
250. Shepherd J et al. PROSPER study group. PROspective Study of Pravastatin in the Elderly at Risk. Pravastatin in elderly individuals at risk of vascular disease (PROSPER): A randomised controlled trial. *Lancet* 2002;360:1623.

CHAPTER 13

Essential Hypertension

Joseph J. Saseen

INTRODUCTION

Approximately 72 million Americans have hypertension, also called high blood pressure (BP).[1] It is estimated that approximately 30% of adult Americans have hypertension, making it the most frequently encountered chronic medical condition.[2,3] It is also one of the most significant risk factors for cardiovascular (CV) morbidity and mortality resulting from target-organ damage to blood vessels in the heart, brain, kidney, and eyes. These complications can manifest as either atherosclerotic vascular disease or other forms of CV disease. The exact etiology of essential hypertension is unknown; however, lifelong management with lifestyle modifications and pharmacotherapy are needed.

Awareness, treatment, and control of hypertension are not optimal. Based on the most recent data from the National Health and Nutrition Examination Survey (NHANES), 2003–2004, approximately 76% of patients who truly have hypertension are diagnosed with this medical condition, leaving many patients undiagnosed. Similarly, only 65% of people with hypertension are receiving some form of treatment. Ultimately, the most disappointing statistic is that only 37% of patients with hypertension, including those who have undiagnosed hypertension, have controlled BP (liberally defined as both systolic BP <140 mmHg and diastolic BP <90 mmHg).[2] When just patients with the diagnosis of hypertension are considered, 63% have controlled BP.[4] Similarly, when only those patients who are treated for hypertension are considered, 57% have controlled BP.[2] These BP control estimates actually underestimate the magnitude of this problem, because many patients require more aggressive BP control than <140/90 mmHg. Improvements in diagnosing, treating, and overall management of hypertension are desperately needed.

Blood Pressure (BP)

During systole, the left ventricle contracts, ejecting blood systemically into the arteries, causing a sharp rise in arterial BP. This is the systolic BP (SBP). The left ventricle then relaxes during diastole, and arterial BP decreases to a trough value as blood returns to the right atria and ventricle of the heart from the venous system. This is the diastolic BP (DBP). When recording BP (e.g., 120/76 mmHg), the numerator refers to SBP and the denominator refers to DBP. BP has a predictable diurnal rhythm, with fluctuations throughout the day. Values are lowest during the nighttime, sharply rise starting in the early morning, and peak in the late morning to early afternoon. These fluctuations are less pronounced in the black population and may be absent in patients with secondary hypertension.

Mean arterial pressure (MAP) is sometimes used to represent BP. MAP collectively reflects both SBP and DBP, with one-third of the pressure from SBP and two-thirds from DBP. It is calculated using the following equation (Eq. 13-1):

$$\text{MAP} = ([\text{SBP}] \cdot [1/3]) + ([\text{DBP}] \cdot [2/3]) \qquad \textbf{(13-1)}$$

The Seventh Report of the Joint National Committee on Detection, Evaluation, and Treatment of High Blood Pressure (JNC7), published in 2003, classifies BP based on systolic and diastolic values (Table 13-1).[5] Hypertension is defined as an elevated SBP, DBP, or both. A clinical diagnosis of hypertension is based on the mean of two or more properly measured seated BP measurements taken on two or more occasions. This mean BP is also used initially to classify and stage hypertension. The JNC7 classification includes normal BP, prehypertension, stage 1 hypertension, and stage 2 hypertension. Qualitative terms (e.g., mild, moderate, high-normal, severe) are not recommended, and should not be used.

Table 13-1 Classification and Management of Blood Pressure (BP) in Adults[5,a]

Classification	*SBP[a] (mmHg)*	*DBP[a] (mmHg)*
Normal	<120	and <80
Prehypertension	120–139	or 80–89
Stage 1 hypertension	140–159	or 90–99
Stage 2 hypertension	≥160	or ≥100

[a] Classification is determined based on highest BP category.
DBP diastolic blood pressure; SBP, systolic blood pressure.

Pathophysiology of BP Regulation

Various neural and humoral factors are known to influence and regulate BP.[6] These include the adrenergic nervous system (controls α- and β-receptors), the renin-angiotensin-aldosterone system (RAAS) (regulates systemic and renal blood flow), renal function and renal blood flow (influences fluid and electrolyte balance), several hormonal factors (adrenal cortical hormones, vasopressin, thyroid hormone, insulin), and the vascular endothelium (regulates release of nitric oxide, bradykinin, prostacyclin, endothelin). Knowledge of these mechanisms is important in understanding antihypertensive drug therapy. BP is normally regulated by compensatory mechanisms that respond to changes in cardiac demand. An increase in cardiac output (CO) normally results in a compensatory decrease in total peripheral resistance (TPR); likewise, an increase in TPR results in a decrease in CO. These events regulate MAP, as is represented in the following equation (Eq. 13-2):

$$\text{MAP} = \text{CO} \cdot \text{TPR} \qquad \textbf{(13-2)}$$

Adverse changes in BP can occur when these compensatory mechanisms are not functioning properly. It has been suggested that in hypertension an initial increase in fluid volume increases CO and arterial pressure. Eventually, with long-standing hypertension, it is believed that TPR increases so that CO returns to normal.

The kidney plays an important role in the regulation of arterial pressure, especially through the RAAS. Decreases in BP and renal blood flow, volume depletion or decreased sodium concentration, and an activation of the sympathetic nervous system can all trigger an increased secretion of the enzyme renin from the cells of the juxtaglomerular apparatus in the kidney. Renin acts on angiotensinogen to catalyze the formation of angiotensin-1. Angiotensin-converting enzyme (ACE) converts angiotensin-1 to angiotensin-2 (see Figs. 18-1 and 18-6 in Chapter 18, Heart Failure). Angiotensin-2 is a potent vasoconstrictor that acts directly on arteriolar smooth muscle and also stimulates the production of aldosterone by the adrenal glands. Aldosterone causes sodium and water retention and the excretion of potassium. Several factors influence renin release, especially those that alter renal perfusion. Lastly, the resultant increase in BP results in suppression of renin release through negative feedback.

Approximately 20% of patients with essential hypertension have lower-than-normal plasma renin activity (PRA), whereas approximately 15% have PRA concentrations that are higher than normal. Those with normal to high PRA should theoretically be more responsive to drug therapies that target the RAAS (e.g., ACE inhibitors or β-adrenergic blockers). Patients with low PRA may be more responsive to diuretic therapy. Measuring PRA is not readily available in most clinical settings, however, and is not advocated as a practical means for selection of drug therapy.

Arterial BP also is regulated by the adrenergic nervous system, which causes contraction and relaxation of vascular smooth muscle. Stimulation of α-adrenergic receptors in the central nervous system (CNS) results in a reflex decrease in sympathetic outflow causing a decrease in BP. Stimulation of postsynaptic α_1-receptors in the periphery causes vasoconstriction. α-Receptors are regulated by a negative feedback system; as norepinephrine is released into the synaptic cleft and stimulates presynaptic α_2-receptors, further norepinephrine release is inhibited. This negative feedback results in a balance between vasoconstriction and vasodilatation. Stimulation of postsynaptic β_1-receptors located in the myocardium causes an increase in heart rate and contractility, whereas stimulation of postsynaptic β_2-receptors in the arterioles and venules results in vasodilation.

A direct association exists between sodium and BP. Patients with a high dietary sodium intake have a greater prevalence of hypertension than those with a low sodium intake. The mechanism by which hypertension is caused by an increase in sodium intake is hypothesized to involve natriuretic hormone (not to be confused with A- and B-type natriuretic peptides associated with heart failure). Natriuretic hormone is potentially increased to facilitate sodium and water excretion in response to an increase in renal sodium retention and extracellular fluid volume. Natriuretic hormone might also cause an increase in intracellular sodium and calcium, resulting in increased vascular tone and hypertension. This hypothesis has not been definitively proved, however.

Epidemiologic evidence and clinical trials have demonstrated an inverse relationship between calcium and BP. One proposed mechanism for this relationship involves an alteration in the balance between intracellular and extracellular calcium. Increased intracellular calcium concentrations can increase peripheral vascular resistance, resulting in increased BP.

A decrease in potassium has been associated with an increase in peripheral vascular resistance. In theory, diuretic-induced hypokalemia could counteract some of the hypotensive effects of diuretic therapy, but this has not been well studied. It is important, however, that potassium concentrations be maintained within the normal range because hypokalemia increases the risk of CV events, such as sudden death, and increases the risk of metabolic side effects (hyperglycemia) associated with diuretics.

Insulin resistance and hyperinsulinemia also have been associated with hypertension. Kaplan[6] suggests that insulin resistance is responsible for the frequent coexistence of diabetes, dyslipidemia, hypertension, and abdominal obesity. This is also referred to as the *metabolic syndrome*.[7] Although the exact role of insulin resistance in the development of hypertension is still evolving, it is clear that these factors are intertwined and increase CV risk.

The vascular epithelium is a dynamic system in which vascular tone is regulated by numerous substances. As noted previously, angiotensin-2 promotes vasoconstriction of the vascular epithelium. Several other substances regulate vascular tone, however. Nitric oxide (NO) is produced in the endothelium and is a potent vasodilatory chemical that relaxes the vascular epithelium. The NO system has been firmly established as an important regulator of arterial BP. Hypothetically, some patients with hypertension have an intrinsic deficiency in NO release and inadequate vasodilation, which could contribute to hypertension and its vascular complications.

Factors that regulate BP are well understood and continue to evolve, but the cause of essential hypertension is still unknown. It is currently impossible to target therapy to specific abnormalities. Antihypertensive therapy should be determined on outcome-based clinical data that demonstrate reductions in hypertension-associated complications, as is discussed later in this chapter.

Cardiovascular (CV) Risk and BP

Direct correlations between BP values and risk of CV disease have been established based primarily on epidemiologic data. Beginning at a benchmark BP of 115/75 mmHg, the risk of CV disease doubles with every increment of 20/10 mmHg.[5] There is a significant increase in risk of CV events in patients with prehypertension BP values versus normal BP values.[8] Clinically, it is important to note that incremental elevations in SBP are more predictive of CV disease than elevations in DBP for patients older than 50 years of age. Within this population, elevated SBP is often the primary BP abnormality. Therefore, SBP is the target of evaluation and intervention for most patients with hypertension.[5,9] In younger patients with hypertension, elevated DBP may be the only BP abnormality present.

Measuring BP

AUSCULTATORY METHOD

Blood pressure measurement should be standardized to minimize variability in readings. The American Heart Association (AHA) technique for auscultatory BP measurement (Table 13-2) should be used in most patients.[10] Correct BP measurements require that the clinician listen through a stethoscope that is placed over the brachial artery for the appearance of the five phases of the Korotkoff sounds. Each sound has distinct features, which are depicted in Figure 13-1.[10]

BP MONITORING OUTSIDE THE OFFICE

Blood pressure values measured outside the office should be considered in the overall treatment of patients with hypertension, but definitive routine use cannot be universally recommended. The major clinical trials that have established that appropriate treatment of hypertension reduces morbidity and mortality rates used office-based BP measurements. Therefore, office-based BP measurements are still considered the gold standard values that guide antihypertensive drug therapy.

Ambulatory blood pressure monitoring (ABPM) typically measures BP every 15 to 30 minutes throughout the day using a monitoring device. This form of specialized monitoring is indicated for patients with suspected white-coat hypertension, and also may be helpful in patients with apparent

Table 13-2 Auscultatory Method for Measuring BP in Adults as Recommended by the AHA[10]

1. **PATIENT:** Patient should be seated for 5 minutes with arm bared, unrestricted by clothing, and supported at heart level. Smoking or food ingestion should not have occurred within 30 minutes before the measurement.
2. **CUFF:** An appropriately sized cuff should be chosen. The internal inflatable bladder width should be at least 40% and the bladder length at least 80% of the upper arm circumference. The cuff should be wrapped snugly around the arm with the center of the bladder over the brachial artery.
3. **MONITOR:** Measurements should be taken with a correctly calibrated mercury sphygmomanometer, an aneroid manometer, or a validated electronic device.
4. **PALPATORY METHOD:** The palpatory method should be used to estimate SBP. The cuff is inflated while simultaneously palpating the radial pulse on the cuffed arm and observing the manometer. The point at which the radial pulse is no longer palpable is the estimated SBP. The cuff is then deflated rapidly.
5. **KOROTKOFF SOUNDS:** The head of the stethoscope, ideally using the bell, should be positioned over the brachial artery, and each earpiece placed in the clinician's ear. The cuff should then be rapidly inflated to 20 to 30 mmHg above the estimated SBP from the palpatory method. The cuff is slowly deflated at a rate of 2 mmHg per second while simultaneously listening for phase 1 (the first appearance of sounds) and phase 5 (the disappearance of sounds) Korotkoff sounds while the clinician is observing the manometer. When the pressure is 10 to 20 mmHg below phase 5, the cuff can be rapidly deflated.
6. **DOCUMENTATION:** BP values should always be recorded. The BP values (SBP/DBP) should be recorded using even numbers (rounded up from an odd number) along with the patient's position (seated, standing or supine), arm used, and cuff size.
7. **REPEAT:** A second measurement should be taken after at least 1 minute in the same arm. If the readings differ by >5 mmHg, additional measurements should be obtained. The mean of these values should be used to make clinical decisions. BP should be taken in both arms at the initial visit with the BP taken in the arm with the higher reading at subsequent visits.

AHA, American Heart Association; BP, blood pressure; DBP, diastolic blood pressure; SBP, systolic blood pressure

drug resistance, hypotensive symptoms while receiving antihypertensive therapy, episodic hypertension, and autonomic dysfunction.[10] ABPM values are typically lower than office-based measurements. Patients with hypertension have average values of >135/85 mmHg while awake and >120/75 mmHg while asleep. Therefore, the threshold for acceptable values is lower than that obtained during office-based measurements. Evidence indicates that ABPM recordings can predict clinical outcomes, as does traditional office-based and home-based BP measurements. The utility of using ABPM to evaluate antihypertensive treatment is limited, however.[10]

Home BP measurements can provide information on response to therapy and may help improve adherence to therapy and goal BP achievement in some patients.[5,11] Home measurement devices (e.g., electronic monitors, auscultatory monitors) need to be routinely checked for accuracy. As is the case with ambulatory monitoring, patients with average home BP values >135/85 mmHg are considered hypertensive. Wrist or finger devices that measure BP are not accurate and should not be used.

Types of Hypertension

Essential Hypertension

Most patients with hypertension have essential hypertension (also known as primary hypertension), with no identifiable cause for their disorder.

Secondary Hypertension

Patients with secondary hypertension have a specific identified cause for elevated BP (Table 13-3). Although only 5% to 10% of those among the hypertensive population have secondary hypertension, further diagnostic evaluation should occur if physical or laboratory findings are consistent with a secondary cause (Table 13-4). Secondary causes are potentially correctable. Further diagnostic workup also should be considered in patients who do not respond to increasing doses of antihypertensive medication or who have a sudden increase in BP or accelerated or malignant hypertension.[5,6] A thorough review of prescription medications, nonprescription medications, and supplements should be conducted to rule out potential causes of BP elevations.

Pseudohypertension

The possibility of pseudohypertension should be considered when measuring BP in elderly patients. In pseudohypertension, blood vessels become stiff and thick because of calcification and resist compression from the bladder of the inflatable BP cuff. Greater pressure is then needed to occlude the artery, and this results in an inaccurate overestimation of SBP. Osler's maneuver is used to detect pseudohypertension. A BP cuff is inflated above the SBP while palpating the brachial or radial arteries to determine whether the pulseless artery is still palpable. If the artery is still palpable, the patient might have pseudohypertension. Pseudohypertension is thought to be relatively rare.

White-Coat Hypertension

White-coat hypertension describes patients who have consistently elevated BP values measured in a clinical environment in the presence of a health care professional (e.g., physician's office), yet when measured elsewhere or with 24-hour ambulatory monitoring, BP is not elevated.[10] Home BP monitoring or 24-hour ABPM is warranted in patients suspected of having white-coat hypertension to differentiate this from true hypertension. The commonly used definition is a persistently elevated average office blood pressure of >140/90 mmHg and an average awake ambulatory reading of <135/85 mmHg. The label *white-coat hypertension* applies only to patients without target-organ disease who are not on antihypertensive therapy. It is estimated to be present in 15% to 20% of people with stage 1 hypertension.[10]

Significant controversies surround white-coat hypertension. Although this does not represent a clinical diagnosis, patients with white-coat hypertension are at risk for developing clinically relevant hypertension. Moreover, data suggest that patients with white-coat hypertension are at a higher risk for CV disease than normotensive patients.[12] The decision to treat or not treat white-coat hypertension, however, is controversial. Indeed, many patients enrolled in the landmark clinical trials that demonstrated reductions in CV morbidity and mortality with antihypertensive therapy had white-coat hypertension.

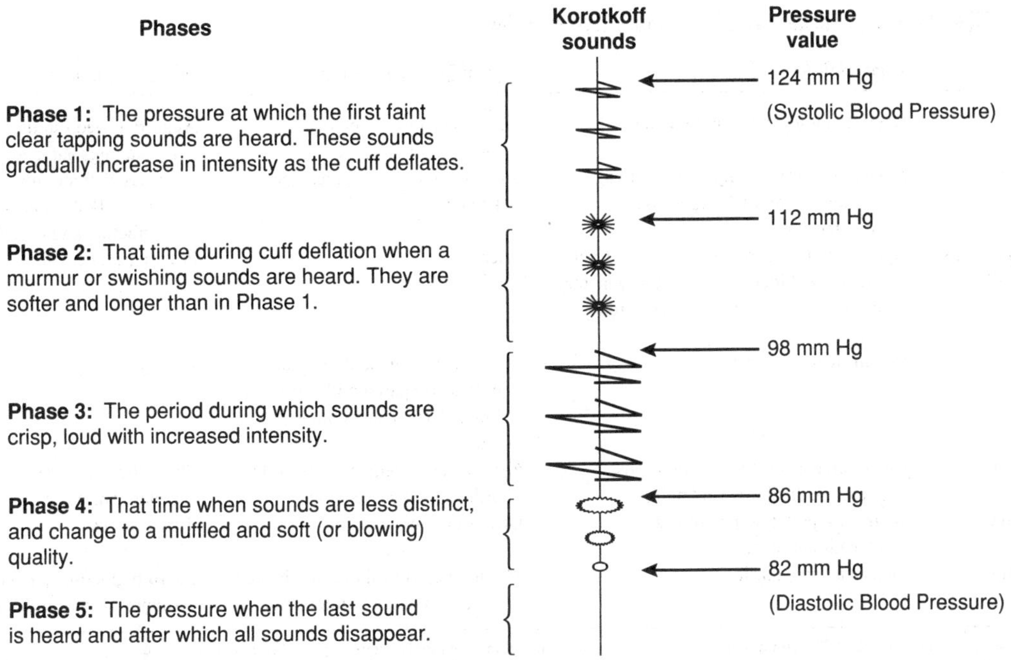
Phases
Korotkoff sounds
Pressure value
Phase 1: The pressure at which the first faint clear tapping sounds are heard. These sounds gradually increase in intensity as the cuff deflates.
124 mm Hg
(Systolic Blood Pressure)
112 mm Hg
Phase 2: That time during cuff deflation when a murmur or swishing sounds are heard. They are softer and longer than in Phase 1.
98 mm Hg
Phase 3: The period during which sounds are crisp, loud with increased intensity.
Phase 4: That time when sounds are less distinct, and change to a muffled and soft (or blowing) quality.
86 mm Hg
82 mm Hg
(Diastolic Blood Pressure)
Phase 5: The pressure when the last sound is heard and after which all sounds disappear.

FIGURE 13-1 Phases of the Korotkoff sounds heard when indirectly measuring blood pressure.

At minimum, patients with white-coat hypertension should be treated with lifestyle modifications, and need to be closely monitored with a device that can measure BP outside the clinic environment if they are not treated with antihypertensive drug therapy.

Hypertensive Crises

Hypertensive crises are situations when measured BP values are markedly elevated, typically in the upper range of stage 2 hypertension (>180/110 mmHg). They are classified as either a hypertensive emergency (with acute or progressive target-organ damage) or urgency (without acute or progressive target-organ damage).[6] Hypertensive emergencies require hospitalization for immediate BP lowering using intravenous (IV) medications and intraarterial BP monitoring. Examples of acute target-organ damage include encephalopathy, myocardial infarction (MI), unstable angina, pulmonary edema, eclampsia, stroke, head trauma, life-threatening arterial bleeding, aortic dissection, severe retinopathy, or acute kidney failure. Hypertensive urgencies do not require immediate BP lowering; instead, BP should be slowly reduced within 24 hours (but not generally to goal BP so quickly) following drug therapy recommendations for stage 2 hypertension (see Chapter 20, Hypertensive Emergencies). The optimal rate of BP lowering in hypertensive emergencies and urgencies is less clear, however.

Table 13-3 Secondary Causes of Hypertension[5]

Chronic Kidney Disease
Chronic Steroid Therapy and Cushing's Syndrome
Coarctation of the Aorta
Drug-Induced or Drug-Related
• Adrenal steroids
• Alcohol in excess
• Amphetamines and anorexiants (e.g., phentermine, sibutramine)
• Cocaine and other illicit drugs
• Cyclosporine and tacrolimus
• Erythropoietin
• Licorice (including some chewing tobacco)
• Nonsteroidal anti-inflammatory drugs and COX-2 inhibitors
• Oral contraceptives
• Oral decongestants (e.g., pseudoephedrine)
• Some over-the-counter supplements (e.g., ephedra, ma huang, bitter orange)
Pheochromocytoma
Primary Aldosteronism
Renovascular Disease
Sleep Apnea
Thyroid or Parathyroid Disease

Hypertension Management

Hypertension is treated with both lifestyle modifications and pharmacotherapy. The JNC7 has been considered the "gold standard" consensus guidelines for the management of hypertension in the United States. The 2007 American Heart Association (AHA) scientific statement regarding the treatment of hypertension is now considered the most up-to-date and evidence-based guideline.[9] The AHA 2007 guidelines provide more aggressive BP goals and pharmacotherapy recommendations based on more recent evidence. Of note, the 2007 European Society of Hypertension/European Society of Cardiology also recommend more aggressive BP goals and recommendations, analogous to the AHA 2007 recommendations.[13] The overall principles common to these guidelines are to implement lifestyle modifications in addition to pharmacotherapy to control BP in patients with hypertension. The presence of specific complications of hypertension or comorbidities (sometime referred to as "compelling indications") in any given patient should be considered when selecting specific

Table 13-4 Clinical Findings Suggestive of Secondary Hypertension

Causes	*Historical Findings*	*Physical Examination Finding*	*Laboratory Finding*
Sleep apnea	Daytime fatigue and somnolence	Large neck circumference; overweight or obese	Abnormal sleep studies with frequent awakenings and anoxic episodes
Renovascular disease	Moderate or severe high BP before age 30 or after 55; rapidly progressive hypertension	Abdominal bruits; funduscopic hemorrhages	Suppressed or stimulated plasma renin activity; IVP (rapid sequence); digital subtraction angiography
Renoparenchymal disease	Dysuria, polyuria, nocturia; urinary tract infections; kidney stones; family history of polycystic or other types of kidney disease	Edema	Proteinuria; hematuria; bacteriuria
Coarctation of the aorta	Intermittent claudication	Diminished or absent femoral pulses compared with carotids; lower SBP in leg compared with arm	–
Pheochromocytoma	Paroxysmal headaches, palpitations, sweating, dizziness, and pallor	Nervousness, tremor, tachycardia, orthostatic hypotension	Clonidine suppression tests[a]; high urine metanephrine or vanillylmandelic acid
Primary aldosteronism	Weakness, polyuria, polydipsia, intermittent paralysis	Orthostatic hypotension	Hypokalemia
Cushing's syndrome	Menstrual irregularity	Moon face; truncal obesity; buffalo hump; hirsutism; violet striae	↑ serum glucose; ↑ plasma cortisol after suppression with dexamethasone

[a]Failure of plasma catecholamines to ↓ by 50% within 3 hr of administration of 0.3 mg clonidine highly suggests pheochromocytoma.
BP, blood pressure; IVP, intravenous pyelogram; SBP, systolic blood pressure.

pharmacotherapy to treat hypertension. These issues are discussed later in this chapter.

Goals

The overarching goal of treating hypertension is to reduce associated morbidity and mortality. These manifest as hypertension-associated complications (Table 13-5), which includes atherosclerotic vascular disease and other forms of CV disease. Clinical presentation of such complications can be as an acute CV event (e.g., MI), or development of a chronic medical condition (e.g., chronic kidney disease [CKD]). Hypertension-associated complications are the primary causes of death in patients with hypertension. Several risk factors for complications have been identified. These are considered major CV risk factors that increase the likelihood of developing hypertension-associated complications, not hypertension.

FRAMINGHAM RISK SCORING

Estimating individual risk for CV disease is essential for all patients with hypertension. In the United States, Framingham risk scoring is considered an appropriate way to predict individual 10-year risk for coronary artery disease (CAD), also referred to as coronary heart disease (CHD) (see Fig. 12.7, Chapter 12, Dyslipipidemias, Atherosclerosis, and Coronary Heart Disease). All patients with hypertension who do not have a history of hypertension-associated complications (Table 13-5) or diabetes, (considered a CAD risk equivalent condition) should have Framingham risk scoring because their 10-year risk can be low or moderate risk (<10%), moderately high risk (10%–20%), or high risk (>20%).[14] Identifying patients with Framingham risk scores ≥10% is clinically relevant because more aggressive antihypertensive treatment is

Table 13-5 Hypertension-Associated Complications and Major Cardiovascular Risk Factors for Complications

Hypertension-Associated Complications

- Atherosclerotic Vascular Disease:
  - Coronary artery disease (sometimes called coronary heart disease)
    - Myocardial infarction [MI]
    - Acute coronary syndromes
    - Chronic stable angina
  - Carotid artery disease:
    - Ischemic stroke
    - Transient ischemic attack
  - Peripheral arterial disease
  - Abdominal aortic aneurysm
- Other forms of CV disease
  - Left ventricular dysfunction (heart failure)
  - Chronic kidney disease
  - Retinopathy

Major CV Risk Factors

- Advanced age (>55 yr for men, >65 yr for women)
- Cigarette smoking
- Diabetes mellitus
- Dyslipidemia
- Family history of premature atherosclerotic vascular disease (men <55 yr or women <65 yr)
- Hypertension
- Kidney disease (microalbuminuria or estimated GFR <60 mL/min)
- Obesity (BMI ≥30 kg/m^2)
- Physical inactivity

BMI, body mass index; CV, cardiovascular; GFR, glomerular infiltration rate.

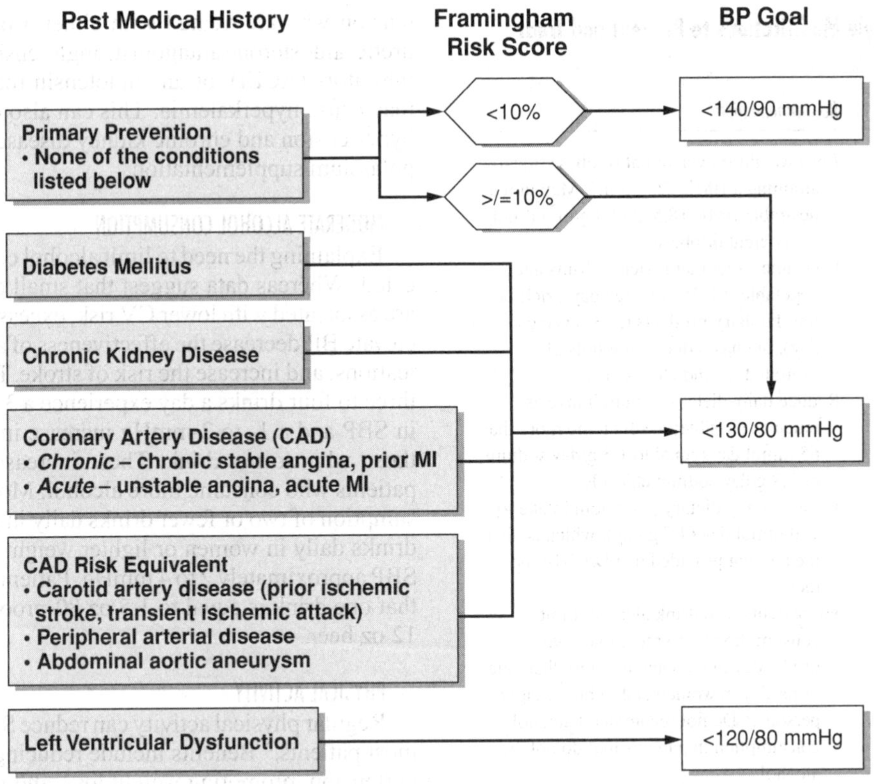

FIGURE 13-2 Goal BP determination based on patient specific history and cardiovascular risk assessment. BP, blood pressure.

needed in this population according to 2007 AHA guidelines.[9] For patients with hypertension-associated complications or diabetes, Framingham risk scoring is not needed because 10-year risk of CAD is assumed to be >20%.

GOAL BP VALUES

The surrogate goal of treating hypertension is to achieve goal BP values. Patients with hypertension have a BP goal of either <140/90, <130/80, or <120/80 mmHg (Fig. 13-2). Patients with estimated 10-year risk of CAD of <10%, based on Framingham scoring, have a goal BP of <140/90 mmHg. In general, all other patients, have a goal BP of <130/80 mmHg. More aggressive BP goals are recommended in these patients because they are at higher risk for hypertension-associated complications, and lowering BP to this level has been shown to maximize risk reduction, particularly in patients with diabetes or CKD.[15,16] If patients have a history of left ventricular dysfunction (also known as systolic heart failure), a BP goal of <120/80 mmHg is recommended.[9] Although elevated SBP is more predictive of CV disease than DBP for most patients,[5] goal achievement requires reduction of both SBP and DBP to goal values. Control of SBP is imperative and this usually results in control of DBP. Clinicians should follow these recommendations and be appropriately aggressive with therapy despite the tendency to accept BP values that are close to, but not at, the goal.

Lifestyle Modifications

Lifestyle modifications are the cornerstone of management for preventing and treating hypertension. In 2006, the AHA published new guidelines for lifestyle modifications that include both diet and exercise.[17,18] These are summarized in Table 13-6. Engaging in these modifications is encouraged for all persons to prevent the development of hypertension; however, they are recommended as a component of first-line therapy in all patients with prehypertension, and in all patients with a diagnosis of hypertension regardless of whether their BP values are at goal or not (Table 13-1).[5,9] Independent of BP lowering, CV risk may also be reduced.

WEIGHT REDUCTION

Weight loss as small as 5% to 10% of body weight in overweight individuals may significantly lower CV risk. For most patients, an average weight loss of 10 kg can reduce SBP by 5 to 20 mmHg.[5]

DASH EATING PLAN

The DASH (Dietary Approaches to Stop Hypertension) diet is rich in fruits, vegetables, and low-fat dairy foods, coupled with reduced saturated and total fat.[19] This diet can substantially reduce BP (8–14 mmHg in SBP for most patients) and yield similar results to single drug therapy. The low-fat component of this diet is important because weight loss is more readily achieved by a reduced calorie diet (fats contribute more calories per gram than do either carbohydrates or protein) and lowered fat intake also reduces the risk of CV disease by lowering cholesterol.

DIETARY SODIUM RESTRICTION

The average American intake of sodium is >6 g/day. Restricting sodium is reasonable for patients with prehypertension or hypertension, and current recommendations

Table 13-6 Lifestyle Modifications to Prevent and Treat Hypertension[7,17,18]

Modification	*Recommendation*
Weight management	Lose weight if overweight or obese, ideally attaining a BMI <25 kg/m^2. Maintain a desirable BMI (18.5–24.9 kg/m^2) if not overweight or obese.
Adopt DASH-type dietary patterns	Consume a diet that is rich in fruits and vegetables (8–10 servings/day), rich in low-fat dairy products (2–3 servings/day), but has reduced amounts of saturated fat and cholesterol
Reduced sodium intake	Reduce daily dietary sodium intake as much as possible; ideally to no more than 65 mmol/day (equal to 1.5 g/day sodium, or 3.8 g/day sodium chloride)
Increased dietary potassium intake	Increase daily dietary potassium intake to 120 mmol/day (4.7 g/day), which is also the amount provided in a DASH-type diet.
Moderation of alcohol consumption	For patients who drink alcohol, limit consumption to no more than two drinks/day in men and no more than one drink/day in women and lighter-weight persons.[a] Do not recommend alcohol consumption in patients that do not drink alcohol.
Regular physical activity	Regular moderate-intensity aerobic physical activity; at least 30 min of continuous or intermittent 5 days/wk, but preferably daily.

[a]Note: one drink is defined as 12 oz of regular beer, 5 oz of wine (12% alcohol), and 1.5 oz of 80-proof distilled spirits.
BMI, body mass index; DASH, Dietary Approaches to Stop Hypertension.

to restrict daily sodium intake to no more than 1.5 g is lower than what has traditionally been recommended. Some clinicians may argue that the efficacy of implementing sodium restriction in patients with hypertension may vary. Evidence from clinical trials has shown, however, that sodium restriction provides mean reductions in BP of 5/2.7 mmHg in patients with hypertension.[18] Some populations (diabetics, blacks, and elderly persons) respond better to sodium restriction than the general population, but all patients with hypertension should be instructed to reduce their sodium intake. They should be counseled not to add salt to foods, and to avoid or minimize ingestion of processed or packaged foods, foods with high sodium content, and nonprescription drugs containing sodium (see Chapter 18, Heart Failure).

INCREASED POTASSIUM INTAKE

A new recommendation from the AHA is to increase dietary potassium intake.[18] Adhering to a DASH eating plan will usually assure an intake of the recommended 4.7 g daily. Dietary supplementation should be the primary strategy to increase potassium. Implementing potassium supplementation outside of dietary sources for the sole purpose of lowering BP should be avoided because of potential harm from hyperkalemia. Moreover, potassium supplementation in patients with hypertension who are treated with either a potassium-sparring diuretic, aldosterone antagonist, angiotensin-converting-enzyme inhibitors (ACEI), or an angiotensin receptor blocker (ARB) may cause hyperkalemia. This can also occur in patients with hypertension and chronic kidney disease who are treated with potassium supplementation.

MODERATE ALCOHOL CONSUMPTION

Explaining the need to limit alcohol consumption is complicated. Whereas data suggest that small daily doses of ethanol are associated with lower CV risk, excessive alcohol intake can elevate BP, decrease the effectiveness of antihypertensive medications, and increase the risk of stroke. Patients who consume three to four drinks a day experience a 3- to 4-mmHg increase in SBP and a 1- to 2-mmHg increase in DBP compared with those who do not drink. These increases are even higher in patients who consume more alcohol. Moderating alcohol consumption of two or fewer drinks daily in men and one or fewer drinks daily in women or lighter weight persons can decrease SBP approximately 2 to 4 mmHg. Patients should be instructed that one drink is equal to 1.5 oz 80-proof whiskey, 5 oz wine, 12 oz beer.

PHYSICAL ACTIVITY

Regular physical activity can reduce SBP by 4 to 9 mmHg in most patients.[5] Benefits include reducing the incidence of hypertension, promoting weight loss, and improving overall CV fitness. Most patients with hypertension can safely increase their aerobic activity. Those with more severe forms of target-organ damage (e.g., angina, previous MI) may, however, need a medical evaluation before increasing their activity level. Physical activity should occur for at least 30 minutes, at least 5 days of the week, but preferably daily. Aerobic exercise such as walking, running, cycling, swimming, and cross-country skiing, are examples of recommended physical activity.

Pharmacotherapy

Numerous clinical trials have demonstrated that antihypertensive pharmacotherapy generally reduces the risk of hypertension-associated complications (e.g., CV morbidity and mortality).[5,9] This evidence is the foundation for the 2003 JNC7 and 2007 AHA consensus guidelines, which recommend specific evidence-based pharmacotherapy recommendations based on patient-specific medical history and CV risk (Fig. 13-3).

As is recommended in the 2007 AHA guidelines, evidence supports the use of an ACEI, ARB, calcium channel blocker (CCB), thiazide diuretic, or a two-drug combination for first-line therapy for primary prevention patients.[9,20] This is in contrast to the 2003 JNC7 guidelines that placed preference on using a thiazide diuretic over other agents for most patients, and also included a β-blocker as a potential first-line option.[5] Evidence obtained since the 2003 JNC7 guidelines demonstrates, however, that, for first-line treatment in primary prevention patients, β-blocker therapy is not as effective in reducing CV events compared with ACEI, ARB, CCB, or thiazide diuretic therapy.[21] Moreover, newer evidence also suggests that the reductions in CV events with ACEI, ARB, CCB, or thiazide diuretic are comparable so that one agent is not automatically preferred over another.[20]

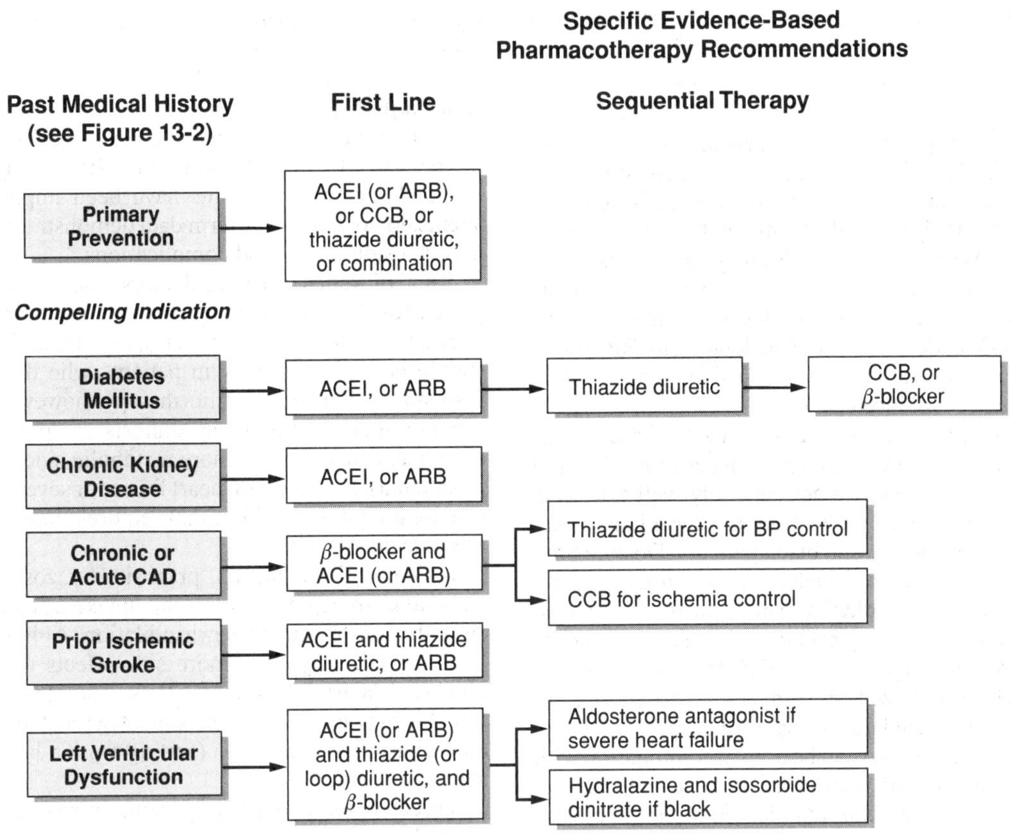

FIGURE 13-3 Recommended pharmacotherapy based on clinical trials evidence demonstrating long term reductions in morbidity and/or mortality in patients with hypertension and specific comorbid conditions and cardiovascular risk. Combination therapy with two antihypertensive drugs is an option for patients with stage 1 hypertension (see Table 13-1) and is strongly recommended in patients with stage 2 hypertension. ACEI, angiotensin converting enzyme inhibitor; ARB, angiotensin receptor blocker; CAD, coronary artery disease; CCB, calcium channel blocker.

Pharmacotherapy has been evaluated in patients with one of several comorbid conditions considered compelling indications for specific pharmacotherapy. The selection of pharmacotherapy in such patients is much more prescriptive than in primary prevention patients, and is outlined in Figure 13-3. These recommendations are based on evidence demonstrating reduced risk of CV events in patients with both hypertension and the compelling indication.

FIRST-LINE AGENTS

Angiotensin Converting Enzyme Inhibitors (ACEIs)

The ACEIs directly inhibit angiotensin-converting enzyme and, therefore, block the conversion of angiotensin-1 to angiotensin-2. This action reduces angiotensin-2–mediated vasoconstriction and aldosterone secretion, and ultimately lowers BP. Because additional pathways exist for the formation of angiotensin-2, ACEIs do not completely block the production of angiotensin-2. These agents generally do not cause metabolic effects. Hyperkalemia is possible, however, and potassium concentrations should be monitored. Patients with chronic kidney disease or volume depletion may be more susceptible to hyperkalemia or to further kidney dysfunction. Bradykinin accumulates in some patients because inhibiting ACE prevents the breakdown and inactivation of bradykinin. Although this may lead to additive vasodilation by releasing nitrous oxide, bradykinin can also cause a dry cough in some patients. Cough is the most frequent, yet harmless side effect of ACEI therapy.

Angiotensin Receptor Blockers (ARBs)

The newest antihypertensive agents are ARBs. They modulate the RAAS by directly blocking the angiotensin-2 type 1 receptor site. Therefore, they block angiotensin-2–mediated vasoconstriction and aldosterone release. Overall, ARBs are very well tolerated. They do not affect bradykinin and, therefore, do not cause a dry cough as do the ACEI. Because aldosterone is blocked, monitoring of potassium is important to avoid hyperkalemia.

Calcium Channel Blockers (CCBs)

The CCBs are pharmacologically complex. They reduce calcium entry into smooth muscles, cause coronary and peripheral vasodilation, and lower BP. All decrease cardiac contractility (except amlodipine and felodipine). Dihydropyridine CCBs are primarily vasodilators that can cause a reflex tachycardia. Non-dihydropyridine CCBs (verapamil and diltiazem) directly block the AV node, decrease heart rate, decrease cardiac contraction, and have some vasodilatory effects. Side effects depend on the individual CCB used, but can include flushing, peripheral edema, tachycardia, bradycardia or heart block, and constipation.

Thiazide Diuretics

Diuretics, particularly thiazide diuretics, such as hydrochlorothiazide (HCTZ), have been extensively studied in large clinical trials for hypertension. They have historically been the most commonly prescribed antihypertensive agents in the United States. When initially started, they induce a natriuresis that causes diuresis and decreases plasma volume. Diuresis usually decreases after chronic use with some of these agents, especially with thiazide diuretics. The long-term BP lowering effects are maintained because of a sustained decrease in peripheral vascular resistance (PVR).

Overwhelming evidence from large outcome-based clinical trials indicates that diuretic therapy reduces morbidity and mortality rates.[5,9,20,22] Diuretics are generally well tolerated, and most can be given once daily. They are especially effective in lowering BP in elderly and black patients. Dose-related metabolic alterations (e.g., hypokalemia, hyperuricemia, hyperglycemia, hypercholesterolemia) can occur with diuretics. These effects were particularly problematic when high doses were used many years ago (e.g., HCTZ 100–200 mg/day), but are drastically minimized by using lower doses that are now considered the standard of care (e.g., HCTZ 12.5–25 mg).[22,23] Thiazide diuretics can be used in combination with a potassium-sparing diuretic, such as triamterene or amiloride, to minimize any potential potassium depletion, not necessarily to provide a greater reduction in BP. Other biochemical changes in glucose and cholesterol are minimal and mostly transient with low-dose therapy.

SECOND-LINE AGENTS

β-Blockers

β-Blockers have several direct effects on the CV system. They can decrease cardiac contractility and output, lower heart rate, blunt sympathetic reflex with exercise, reduce central release of adrenergic substances, inhibit norepinephrine release peripherally, and decrease renin release from the kidney. All these contribute to their antihypertensive effects. Adverse metabolic effects include altered lipids and increased glucose concentrations. Similar to diuretics, these changes are generally temporary, however, and have minimal to no clinical significance. These agents were considered first-line for the treatment of most patients with hypertension in older JNC guidelines.[24] They are now only considered first-line for patients with CAD or left ventricular dysfunction.[9] In primary prevention patients, they should be used as add-on therapy in combination with the other first-line agents (ACEI, ARB, CCB, or thiazide diuretic).

Aldosterone Antagonists

Spironolactone and eplerenone are aldosterone antagonists, also classified as potassium-sparing diuretics. Potent blockade of the aldosterone receptor inhibits sodium and water retention, and inhibits vasoconstriction. Hyperkalemia, a known dose-dependent effect with these agents, is more prominent in patients with chronic kidney disease or in patients taking a concurrent ACEI or ARB. The incidence of hyperkalemia may be greater with eplerenone compared with spironolactone because eplerenone is a more specific aldosterone blocker. Gynecomastia is a side effect of spironolactone that does not occur with eplerenone.

OTHER AGENTS

Many older antihypertensive drug classes should primarily be used to provide additional BP lowering after first-line and second-line agents have been implemented. These agents do not have long-term data demonstrating reductions in hypertension-associated complications.

Loop diuretics (furosemide, torsemide) can be used for hypertension. When dosed appropriately, they can provide BP reductions similar to what is seen with a thiazide diuretic. They should be used primarily in patients who do not adequately respond to thiazide diuretic therapy, however, because they are more potent at inducing diuresis compared with thiazide diuretics, and can cause more metabolic side effects (e.g., hypokalemia). Patients with heart failure or severe chronic kidney disease are patients who might require a loop diuretic instead of a thiazide diuretic.

α-Blockers (doxazosin, prazosin, terazosin) attach to peripheral α_1-receptors, inhibit the uptake of catecholamines in smooth muscle, and cause vasodilation. Although effective in lowering BP, they have more side effects than diuretics, β-blockers, ACEIs, ARBs, or CCBs. The most prominent side effect is hypotension, which is most evident after the first dose and with postural changes (arising from a lying position to a standing position).

Direct vasodilators (hydralazine, minoxidil) work on the arterial vasculature. They are considered last-line therapy, reserved for patients with specific indications or those with very difficult-to-control BP. Fluid retention and reflex tachycardia are frequent side effects. Concomitant therapy with both a diuretic and an agent that lowers heart rate (a β-blocker, diltiazem, or verapamil) is usually needed.

Central α_2-agonists (e.g., clonidine, methyldopa) work in the vasomotor centers of the brain where they stimulate inhibitory neurons, and decrease sympathetic outflow from the CNS. The resultant decrease in PVR and cardiac output lowers BP. These agents commonly cause anticholinergic side effects (e.g., sedation, dizziness, dry mouth, fatigue) and possibly sexual dysfunction. Although α_2-agonists lower BP, they often cause fluid retention and, ideally, they should be used in combination with a diuretic.

Adrenergic antagonists (reserpine, guanadrel, guanethidine) are not frequently used to treat hypertension. Reserpine depletes catecholamines from storage granules to then decrease BP. Potential advantages include low cost and once daily dosing. High doses are associated with more side effects, but low-dose reserpine (0.05–0.1 mg/day), when used as third-line therapy has been shown to be well tolerated. Because of the potential for fluid retention, reserpine requires concurrent diuretic therapy. Guanadrel and guanethidine have numerous significant adverse effects and should be avoided.

NEW ANTIHYPERTENSIVE AGENTS

Aliskiren, approved in 2007, is the first direct renin inhibitor. Other agents within this drug class should become available in the future. Similar to an ACEI or ARB, this agent blocks the RAAS. It is approved for treatment of hypertension, and has been studied in combination with an ACEI or ARB. Because it is a new antihypertensive drug class, however, its exact role in the treatment of hypertension will continue to evolve as clinical experience is obtained.

CLINICAL EVALUATION

Patient Presentation

1. D.C. is a 44-year-old black man who presents to his primary care provider with a chief complaint that his BP was measured at an employee health screening last month and he was told he has "stage 1 hypertension" at that time. His provider has never told him that he has hypertension. He has been advised, however, to lose weight and exercise more. His medical history is significant for allergic rhinitis. His BP was 144/84 and 146/86 mmHg when measured last year at work during an employee health screening. D.C.'s father had hypertension and died of an MI at age 54. His mother had diabetes and hypertension and died of a stroke at age 68. D.C. smokes one pack per day of cigarettes and thinks that his BP might be high because of job-related stress. He does not believe that he really has hypertension. D.C. does not engage in any regular form of exercise and does not restrict his diet in any way, although he knows he should lose weight.

Physical examination shows he is 175 cm tall, weighs 108 kg (body mass index [BMI], 35.2 kg/m^2), BP is 148/88 mmHg (left arm) and 146/86 mmHg (right arm) while sitting, heart rate is 80 beats/minute and regular. Six months ago, his BP values were 152/88 mmHg and 150/84 mmHg when he was seen by his primary care provider for allergic rhinitis. Funduscopic examination reveals mild arterial narrowing, arteriovenous nicking, with no exudates or hemorrhages. The other physical examination findings are essentially normal.

Laboratory examination reveals the following values: blood urea nitrogen (BUN), 24 mg/dL (normal, 7–20 mg/dL); serum creatinine (SrCr), 1.0 mg/dL (normal, 0.5–1.2 mg/dL); fasting glucose, 105 mg/dL (normal, 60–99 mg/dL); potassium (K), 4.4 mEq/L (normal, 3.5–5.2 mEq/L); uric acid, 6.5 mg/dL (normal, 2.0–7.0 mg/dL); total cholesterol 196 mg/dL (normal, <200 mg/dL), low-density lipoprotein cholesterol (LDL-C), 131 mg/dL (normal, <130 mg/dL, optimal <100 mg/dL); high-density lipoprotein cholesterol (HDL-C), 32 mg/dL (normal, >40 mg/dL for men), and triglycerides 170 mg/dL (normal, <150 mg/dL). An electrocardiogram (ECG) and chest radiograph reveal mild left ventricular hypertrophy (LVH). What is the proper assessment of D.C.'s BP based on this information?

D.C. has uncontrolled stage 1 hypertension. He has had elevated BP values, measured in clinical environments, and meets the diagnostic criteria for hypertension because two or more of his BP measurements are elevated on separate days. SBP values are consistently stage 1, whereas DBP values are all in the prehypertension range. The higher of the two classifications is used to classify hypertension.[5]

2. Why does D.C. have hypertension?

D.C.'s has essential hypertension; therefore the exact cause is not known. He has several characteristics (e.g., family history of hypertension, obesity) that may have increased his chance of developing hypertension. Race and sex also influence the prevalence of hypertension. Across all age groups, blacks have a higher prevalence of hypertension than do whites and Mexican Americans.[25] Similar to other forms of CV disease, hypertension is more severe, more likely to include hypertension-associated complications, and occurs at an earlier age in black patients.

Patient Evaluation and Risk Assessment

Evaluation of patients with hypertension has multiple purposes. First, the presence and absence of hypertension-associated complications and major CV risk factors (Table 13-5) must be assessed. Second, secondary causes of hypertension (Table 13-3), if present, should be identified and managed accordingly. Third, concomitant medical conditions (e.g., diabetes), and lifestyle habits should be evaluated so that they can be used to guide therapy.

Hypertension-Associated Complications

3. Does D.C. have hypertension-associated complications?

A complete physical examination to evaluate hypertension-associated complications includes examination of the optic fundi; auscultation for carotid, abdominal, and femoral bruits; palpation of the thyroid gland; heart and lung examination; abdominal examination for enlarged kidney, masses, and abnormal aortic pulsation; lower extremity palpation for edema and pulses; and neurologic assessment. Routine laboratory assessment after diagnosis should include the following: ECG; urinalysis; fasting glucose; hematocrit; serum potassium, creatinine, and calcium; and a fasting lipid panel. Optional testing may include measurement of urinary albumin excretion or albumin-to-creatinine ratio, or additional tests specific for secondary causes if suspected.

D.C. does not yet have hypertension-associated complications. He is exhibiting early signs, however, based on his physical examination that, if left untreated, will likely develop into such complications. These early signs have likely evolved from his longstanding, poorly controlled hypertension. D.C.'s ECG revealed LVH indicating early cardiac damage. Although the gold standard for confirming LVH is with echocardiography, this confirmatory procedure is not necessary unless symptoms are present indicating that LVH has progressed to left ventricular dysfunction (e.g., peripheral edema, shortness of breath). His funduscopic examination reveals mild arterial narrowing and AV nicking, early signs of retinopathy and atherosclerosis. D.C.'s serum creatinine is normal, ruling out overt chronic kidney disease. Additional testing for microalbuminuria is needed, however, to confirm that he does not have early stage kidney disease.

4. Which forms of hypertension-associated complications might D.C. develop?

Hypertension adversely affects many organ systems, including the heart, brain, kidneys, peripheral circulation, and eyes. These are summarized in Table 13-5. Damage to these systems resulting from hypertension is termed *hypertension-associated complications*, *target-organ damage*, or *CV disease*. There are often misconceptions about the terms CV disease and CAD. CV disease encompasses the broad scope of all forms of *hypertension-associated complications*. CAD is simply a subset of CV disease and refers specifically to disease related to the coronary vasculature, including ischemic heart disease and MI. Hypertension-associated complications and major risk factors for developing such complications should be assessed by a thorough patient history, a complete physical examination, and laboratory evaluation.

Hypertension can affect the heart either indirectly, by promoting atherosclerotic changes, or directly, via pressure-related effects. Hypertension can promote CV disease and increase the risk for *ischemic events,* such as angina and MI. Antihypertensive therapy has been shown to reduce the risk of these coronary events. Hypertension also promotes the development of LVH, which is a myocardial (cellular) change, not an arterial change. These two conditions often coexist, however. It is commonly believed that LVH is a compensatory mechanism of the heart in response to the increased resistance caused by elevated BP. LVH is a strong and independent risk factor for CAD, left ventricular dysfunction, and arrhythmias. A finding of LVH does not necessarily indicate the presence of left ventricular dysfunction, but is a risk for progression to left ventricular dysfunction (see Chapter 18, Heart Failure), which is a major cardiac outcome of hypertension. This may be caused by repeated ischemia, excessive ventricular hypertrophy, or pressure overload. Ultimately, left ventricular dysfunction results in a decreased ability to contract (systolic dysfunction) or an inability of the heart to fill (diastolic dysfunction).

Hypertension is one of the most frequent causes of cerebrovascular disease.[25] Cerebrovascular signs can manifest as transient ischemic attacks, ischemic strokes, multiple cerebral infarcts, and hemorrhages. Residual functional deficits caused by stroke are among the most devastating forms of hypertension-associated complications. Clinical trials have demonstrated that antihypertensive therapy can significantly reduce the risk of both initial and recurrent stroke.[5] A sudden, prolonged increase in BP also can cause hypertensive encephalopathy, which is classified as a hypertensive emergency.

The glomerular filtration rate (GFR) is used to estimate kidney function, which declines with aging. This rate of decline is greatly accelerated by hypertension. Hypertension is associated with nephrosclerosis, which is caused by increased intraglomerular pressure. It is unknown whether a primary kidney lesion with ischemia causes systemic hypertension or whether systemic hypertension directly causes glomerular capillary damage by increasing intraglomerular pressure. Regardless, chronic kidney disease, whether mild or severe, can progresses to kidney failure (stage 5 chronic kidney disease) and the need for dialysis. Although studies have demonstrated that aggressive BP control is the most important strategy to slow the rate of kidney function decline,[26] it may not be entirely effective in slowing the progression of renal impairment in all patients.

Chronic kidney disease is staged based on estimated GFR values.[26] Moderate (stage 3) kidney disease is defined as a GFR 30 to 59 mL/minute/1.73 m^2, severe (stage 4) is 15 to 29 mL/minute/1.73 m^2, and kidney failure is <15 mL/minute/ 1.73 m^2 or the requirement of dialysis. In hypertension, moderate kidney disease or worse (estimated GFR <60 mL/minute) is considered a hypertension-associated complication. An estimated GFR <60 mL/minute corresponds approximately to a serum creatinine concentration of >1.5 mg/dL in an average man and >1.3 mg/dL in an average woman. This level of kidney compromise lowers an individual's BP goal to <130/ 80 mmHg. The presence of albuminuria (>300 mg albumin in a 24-hour urine collection or 200 mg albumin/g creatinine on a spot urine measurement) also indicates significant chronic kidney disease. Achieving the more aggressive goal is a strategy to minimize the rate of progression to kidney failure. (Note: These definitions of the stages of kidney disease and albuminuria will be used throughout the remaining cases in this chapter.)

Kidney function can be approximated by calculating a patient's creatinine clearance using the Cockcraft-Gault equation, or by estimating GFR using the Modification of Diet in Renal Disease (MDRD) equation. The Cockcroft-Gault equation is a universally accepted way to estimate kidney function and requires knowledge of the patient's serum creatinine clearance, ideal body weight, and gender (see Fig. 30-1, Chapter 30 Acute Renal Failure). Estimating GFR using the MDRD equation is more reflective of true kidney function, however, and is needed to stage chronic kidney disease (see Fig. 30-2, Chapter 30 Acute Renal Failure).[26] Serum creatinine concentration, age, race, and sex are needed with the MDRD equation.[26,27]

Peripheral arterial disease is another form of atherosclerotic vascular disease that is considered target-organ damage. It is equivalent in CV risk to CAD.[5] Risk factor modifications, BP control, and antiplatelet agent(s) are needed to decrease progression. Complications of peripheral arterial disease can include infection and necrosis, which in some cases require revascularization procedures or extremity amputation.

Hypertension causes retinopathies that can progress to blindness. Retinopathy is evaluated according to the Keith, Wagener, and Barker funduscopic classification system. Grade 1 is characterized by narrowing of the arterial diameter, indicating vasoconstriction. Arteriovenous (AV) nicking is the hallmark of grade 2, indicating atherosclerosis. Longstanding, untreated hypertension or accelerated hypertension also can cause cotton wool exudates and flame hemorrhages (grade 3). In severe cases, papilledema occurs, and this is classified as grade 4.

Major Risk Factors

5. Which major CV risk factors are present in D.C.?

Hypertension is one of nine major CV risk factors identified by the JNC7. These are not necessarily risk factors for developing essential hypertension; rather, they increase the risk of hypertension-associated complications such as CHD or CAD (Table 13-5). D.C. has multiple CV risk factors: smoking, dyslipidemia, family history of premature atherosclerotic vascular disease, hypertension, obesity, and physical inactivity.

6. What is D.C.'s Framingham risk score and how is this valuable to his overall treatment?

D.C. is considered a primary prevention patient because he does not yet have any hypertension-associated complications or compelling indications. He has multiple major CV risk factors, however, and Framingham risk scoring is needed to determine his BP goal value (Fig. 13-2) and to guide choice of pharmacotherapy (Fig. 13-3) and to provide an overall prognosis for his hypertension. Using the Framingham risk calculator (see Fig. 13.7, Chapter 13, Dyslipidemias, Atherosclerosis, and Coronary Heart Disease), D.C. has an 8% risk of developing CHD (or CAD) over the next 10 years.[28] This is considered moderate risk, and because it is < 10%, his BP goal is <140/90 mmHg.[9,14] This risk will increase as he ages, and especially if he does not modify his risk factors. This estimation helps justify aggressive approaches to reduce CV risk, which includes lifestyle modifications and pharmacotherapy.

Many of D.C.'s risk factors are modifiable. He has a history of cigarette smoking. This significantly increases his CV risk and may reduce the efficacy of antihypertensive therapy. Smoking cessation may not independently lower D.C.'s BP, but it will decrease his overall risk of CV disease. D.C. is obese based on his BMI. His sedentary lifestyle (lack of physical activity) and dietary patterns have likely contributed to his obesity. A more focused patient interview on diet and exercise would be helpful to reinforce the assumption that he has a sedentary lifestyle. D.C.'s abnormal cholesterol values (especially his elevated LDL-C) increase his CV risk and lipid-lowering therapy should be considered because intervention trials have repeatedly shown that lowering LDL-C can decrease the risk of CHD and other forms of hypertension-associated complications (see Chapter 12, Dyslipidemias, Atherosclerosis, and Coronary Heart Disease).[14,28] Based on Framingham estimates, risk increases with higher SBP values.[28] Patients with untreated hypertension have an increased CHD risk related to the degree of BP elevation. Even if D.C.'s BP were controlled with antihypertensive therapy, he would have a lower, but still elevated risk.

Advanced age, depending on sex, is considered a major CV risk factor. Although CV disease in the elderly age is not considered premature, increasing age increases the risk of hypertension-associated complications. Premenopausal women are at low risk for CV disease. CV risk in women increases significantly after menopause, however, similar to the increased risk in men. Therefore, cutoff values for age as a risk factor in men and women are separated by 10 years (>55 years for men, >65 years for women). At age 50, D.C. does not yet have this risk factor. Premature CV disease in first-degree relatives (i.e., parents and siblings) should be identified because it is a major CV risk factor. D.C. has a significant family history of premature CHD as evidenced by his father's death of an MI before the age of 55.

PRINCIPLES OF TREATMENT

Goals of Therapy

7. What are the goals of treating D.C.?

The ultimate overarching goal of therapy is to lower hypertension-associated morbidity and mortality. Control of BP is currently the most feasible clinical endpoint used to guide therapy, which can be thought of as a surrogate goal that is a means to attain the overarching goal. D.C.'s goal BP is <140/90 mmHg because he is a primary prevention patient with a Framingham risk score of 8%, meaning that of 100 patients similar to D.C., 8 will have CAD within the next 10 years. Pharmacotherapy principles to achieve these goals include selecting a treatment regimen with antihypertensive agent(s) that have been proved to reduce morbidity and mortality, complemented by appropriate lifestyle modifications.

Health Beliefs and Patient Education

8. What patient education should be provided to D.C. regarding his disease?

Provision of thorough patient education is needed to ensure that D.C. understands his disease and its complications (Table 13-7). This should comprehensively include information on disease, treatment, adherence, and complications. Several approaches can be effective, but all methods should include direct communication between a clinician and the patient. Multidisciplinary approaches to disease state management in hypertension can effectively utilize a team of different clinicians. Clinicians can be physicians, nurse practitioners, physician assistants, pharmacists, dietitians, or exercise physiologists. Providing education in a face-to-face manner is most common, but the key components in patient education may be delivered via indirect interactions (e.g., on the telephone).

Recommendations should be tailored to the patient's specific needs. For example, some patients are able to comprehend the importance of achieving controlled BP by reading written materials, whereas others understand this only after implementing self-BP monitoring. The patient education process must be continuous throughout the duration of therapy. Not all aspects need to be discussed during each clinical interaction. Careful selection of both written and verbal information is needed so that patients are not overwhelmed or frightened by too much information. It is important that clinicians review all materials provided to patients to identify the source of information, assess ease of reading, and identify omitted information and sources of confusion or anxiety (e.g., drug side effects). Patients' needs can also change over time as their disease or circumstances change, and different strategies might be necessary to enhance education and adherence.

Table 13-7 Patient–Provider Interactions for Hypertension

Patient Education

- Assess patient's understanding and acceptance of the diagnosis of hypertension
- Discuss patient's concerns and clarify misunderstandings
- When measuring BP, inform the patient of the reading both verbally and in writing
- Assure patient understands their goal BP value
- Ask patient to rate (1–10) his or her chance of staying on treatment
- Inform patient about recommended treatment, including lifestyle modification. Provide specific written information using standard brochures when available
- Elicit concerns and questions and provide opportunities for patient to state specific behaviors to carry out treatment recommendations
- Emphasize:
  - the need to continue treatment
  - that control does not mean cure
  - elevated BP is usually not accompanied by symptoms

Individualize Treatment Regimens

- Include the patient in decision-making
- Simplify the regimen to once-daily dosing, whenever possible
- Incorporate treatment into patient's daily lifestyle
- Set realistic short-term objectives for specific components of the medication and lifestyle modification plan
- Encourage discussion of diet and physical activity, adverse drug effects and concerns
- Encourage self-monitoring with validated BP devices
- Minimize the cost of therapy, when possible
- Discuss adherence at each clinical encounter
- Encourage gradual sustained weight loss

BP, blood pressure.

Patients such as D.C. often incorrectly explain BP elevation as stress related. A certain percentage of patients may have an increase in BP because of anxiety, as seen in those with white-coat hypertension. Most patients with essential hypertension, however, will have an elevated BP regardless of their stress level. D.C. should be informed about the cause of his disease and the lack of correlation between stress or symptoms and high BP. Most importantly, D.C. needs to realize that elevated BP is almost always asymptomatic, but can cause serious long-term complications. It is essential that he understand the chronic nature of hypertension and the need for long-term therapy. Otherwise, he may adhere to the prescribed treatment only when he "feels his BP is high" or during stressful events.

Some patients believe they can control their BP by stress management rather than with prescribed therapy (lifestyle modifications and antihypertensive agents). Controlled trials have not consistently proven that stress management is beneficial in hypertension.[29] It is important to determine the patient's health beliefs and attitudes and to educate him or her about the etiology and management of hypertension to promote BP control.

Another common myth patients believe is that treating hypertension commonly leads to fatigue, lethargy, and sexual dysfunction. This misconception can be a limiting factor in appropriate management. Clinical trials have repeatedly reported that quality of life is better with active medication than with placebo.[30,31] Data have indicated that as many as 27% of men with hypertension have erectile dysfunction.[32] Although many believe this to be a side effect of their medication, and incidence rates may vary between certain antihypertensive agents and classes, erectile dysfunction is likely caused by penile arterial changes (probably atherosclerosis), which is related to uncontrolled or untreated hypertension.[32]

Benefits of Treatment

9. Does antihypertensive therapy reduce the incidence of hypertension-associated complications?

Without a doubt, antihypertensive therapy reduces the risk of CV disease and CV events in patients with hypertension. Numerous landmark placebo-controlled studies have clearly demonstrated these benefits. The first large-scale trial, published in 1967, was the Veterans Administration (VA) study in men with DBP between 115 and 129 mmHg.[33] This study was prematurely stopped because benefits of treatment were so dramatic. Antihypertensive therapy significantly reduced cerebral hemorrhage, MI, left ventricular dysfunction, retinopathy, and kidney disease. Other landmark placebo-controlled studies, mostly from the 1980s and 1990s, have evaluated antihypertensive therapy in patients with less severe hypertension (DBP, 90–109 mmHg) and have shown a reduced risk of stroke, ischemic heart disease, left ventricular dysfunction, progression to more severe hypertension, and death.[22,24] Long-term, placebo-control studies evaluating morbidity and mortality in hypertension are not only unnecessary, but are considered unethical because treatment is definitively beneficial.

10. Will D.C.'s early signs of hypertension-associated complications improve or reverse with appropriate BP control?

Most antihypertensive drugs reduce LVH through varying mechanisms. It is logical that regression of LVH is desirable, but this remains unproved. Theoretically, myocardial function might be compromised when hypertrophied muscle regresses in size because of the increased ratio of collagen to muscle. Nonetheless, until proved otherwise, regression of LVH in D.C. is desirable.

Reductions in BP can reverse many of the changes associated with D.C.'s retinopathy. In particular, studies have demonstrated that the risk of retinopathy in diabetic patients increases significantly when the DBP is >70 mmHg and that control of BP can slow this progression. D.C. has an elevated fasting glucose indicating prediabetes, but he does not have diabetes. Regardless, lowering BP is desirable for anticipated beneficial effects on his retinopathy.

HYPERTENSION MANAGEMENT

Lifestyle Modifications

11. Should D.C. start antihypertensive drug therapy, or should lifestyle modifications be his primary treatment?

It is reasonable to assume that lifestyle modifications can partially help D.C. achieve his BP goal. Previous JNC guidelines recommended lifestyle modifications for 6 to 12 months before starting drug therapy in patients with few to no risk factors and no hypertension-associated complications, and no compelling indications (i.e., primary prevention patients with Framingham risk scores of <10%).[24] The 2007 European guidelines recommend lifestyle modifications alone to treat hypertension for only "several weeks" before starting drug therapy in patients with stage 1 hypertension who have "moderate" CV risk (i.e., one to two risk factors), and for "several months" in patients with stage 1 hypertension who are at "low" CV risk (i.e., no additional risk factors).[13] D.C. has several major risk factors for developing hypertension-associated complications, and has early evidence of hypertension-associated complications. Lifestyle modifications are germane to the appropriate treatment of hypertension, but they have not been shown to prevent CV disease in patients with hypertension.[9] As recommended in the AHA and the European Society of Hypertension/European Society of Cardiology guidelines from 2007, initiation of drug therapy should not be delayed unnecessarily, especially for patients with CV risk factors.[9,13] Because D.C. has stage 1 hypertension with multiple risk factors, both lifestyle modifications (Table 13-6) and drug therapy should be implemented simultaneously.

Modalities that Lower BP

12. Which lifestyle modifications should be recommended for D.C. to lower his BP?

Weight reduction with dietary modifications and physical activity, sodium restriction, and smoking cessation are the most apparent lifestyle modifications for D.C. A thorough patient interview includes a diet history to quantify his intake of total calories, sodium, fat, and cholesterol. A social history should also be obtained to determine alcohol consumption and to confirm cigarette use. Based on these interviews, customized recommendations can be made.

The DASH diet should be strongly encouraged in D.C. Publications such as Facts About the DASH Eating Plan, are readily available on the National Heart, Lung and Blood Institute (NHLBI) website (http://www.nhlbi.nih.gov/guidelines/hypertension/index.htm) and are written in language easily understood by most patients. D.C.'s BMI of $\geq$30 kg/m^2 classifies him as obese. He needs >16-kg weight loss to lower his weight classification to overweight. As little as a 5% to 10% loss in weight (5–11 kg) will provide global health benefits. Strategies that increase his aerobic activity, in addition to diet, can augment weight loss.

The role of supplementation with calcium, and magnesium in hypertension is unclear. Therefore, these should not be routinely recommended in patients with hypertension for the purpose of lowering BP. Caffeine ingestion has been associated with an acute elevation in BP; however, these elevations appear to be transient. Limitations on caffeine intake are not recommended unless caffeine ingestion is detrimental for other medical reasons (e.g., cardiac arrhythmias, panic attacks).

Other CV Risk Reduction Strategies

13. Aside from treating hypertension, which other CV risk reduction strategies should be recommended in D.C.?

SMOKING CESSATION

Smoking is an important and significant modifiable major CV risk factor. Cigarette smoking independently has been shown to increase CV and overall mortality, and cessation can decrease the incidence of CV disease.[34] Although smoking may not chronically alter BP, it can blunt the response to certain antihypertensive medications. Hypertensive smokers should be continually educated about the risks associated with cigarette smoking and directed to behavior modification programs that can assist smoking cessation efforts (see Chapter 85, Tobacco Use and Dependence).

LOW-DOSE ASPIRIN

Low-dose aspirin therapy (81 mg daily) provides antiplatelet effects that reduce the risk of MI. This is available over the counter, and is recommended by consensus guidelines for primary prevention patients with a Framingham risk score of $\geq$10% to reduce the risk of a CV event.[35] It is also recommended in all secondary prevention patients who have a history of atherosclerotic vascular disease to reduce the risk of recurrent CV events or CV disease.[36] Patients with an absolute contraindication to aspirin therapy (e.g., aspirin allergy, gastrointestinal bleed, aspirin-induced bronchoconstriction) should not receive aspirin therapy. Aspirin can cause an increased risk of bleeding, is subject to many potential drug interactions, and can possibly cause gastrointestinal side effects. Using enteric coated aspirin products, and using low dose can minimize the risk of these potential complications. Based on D.C.'s current Framingham risk score, he is not yet a candidate for low-dose aspirin.

CONTROLLING OTHER COMORBID DISEASES

In addition to treating hypertension and lowering BP to goal, controlling other comorbidities is recommended to further reduce the risk of CV events. When present, dyslipidemia, diabetes mellitus, obesity, and any other forms of CV disease should be diligently treated and controlled. D.C. does have dyslipidemia (he has elevated LDL-C, low HDL-C, and elevated triglycerides), and his CV risk would be reduced with better control of this condition (see Chapter 12, Dyslipidemias, Atherosclerosis, and Coronary Heart Disease).

Pharmacotherapy for Primary Prevention Patients

Evidence-Based Recommendations

14. Which treatment principles need to be considered when choosing an initial antihypertensive agent for D.C.?

Selecting an antihypertensive drug is difficult considering the numerous choices. All antihypertensive agents can effectively lower BP. Depending on the dose used, pressure reductions are similar.[37] BP reduction, however, is only a surrogate endpoint of therapy that does not necessarily reflect overall efficacy. Reducing hypertension-associated complications is the ultimate goal of treatment. Evidence-based medicine is the conscientious, explicit, and judicious use of current best evidence in making decisions about the care of individual patients.[38] Practicing evidence-based medicine in hypertension requires a balance between weighing the findings from outcome-based studies showing reduced hypertension-associated complications and considering specific drug therapies for each patient's individual situation.

15. Which antihypertensive agent is appropriate as first-line treatment in D.C.?

The JNC7 report from 2003, supplemented by more recent evidence in the AHA 2007 guidelines, outlines pharmacotherapy recommendations that follow an evidence-based approach.[5,9] These recommendations are based on the interpretation of clinical trials. Although the JNC7 recommended a thiazide diuretic, either alone or in combination with another antihypertensive (depending on hypertension stage), as the initial drug choice for most patients, recent evidence demonstrates that either an ACEI, ARB, CCB, thiazide diuretic, or certain combinations of these agents is a reasonable first-line drug therapy option for primary prevention patients (Fig. 13-3).[5,9] This recommendation is based on the propensity of data showing reduced morbidity and mortality with these drug classes.[20–22] For patients with a *compelling indication* (Fig. 13-3), the choice of pharmacotherapy is more specific, and is discussed later in this chapter. D.C. does not have a compelling indication for specific pharmacotherapy, and is considered a primary prevention patient. Thus, treatment with either an ACEI, ARB, CCB or thiazide diuretic is considered acceptable according to the most recent evidence-based guidelines.[9]

Traditional landmark placebo-controlled hypertension studies conducted in the 1980s (the Systolic Hypertension in the Elderly Program [SHEP],[39] Swedish Trial of Old Patients with Hypertension [STOP-hypertension],[40] and Medical Research Council [MRC][41]) established that treating hypertension produces significant reductions in CV events (e.g., stroke, MI) and mortality. These traditional landmark trials utilized thiazide diuretic-based therapy and, thus, thiazide diuretics have been the quintessential antihypertensive agent for most patients. Subsequently, several clinical trials evaluating newer agents (ACEI, ARB, and CCB) have provided additional evidence on

CV event reduction.[42–63] Most of these trials do not include a placebo group (because it is unethical to use placebo in long-term studies); rather, they use an active antihypertensive agent as the comparator (usually a thiazide diuretic or β-blocker). In those studies in which newer antihypertensive agents were compared with thiazide diuretics, very similar effects were seen.

16. Should D.C. be placed on a monotherapy or two drug therapy as his initial regimen?

A monotherapy approach is reasonable for D.C., because his BP is classified as stage 1 (Fig. 13-3). Monotherapy with an agent from one of these classes will likely reduce his BP to <140/90 mmHg because his SBP is within 10 mmHg of his goal value. This is not the common scenario; many patients present with stage 2 hypertension and, thus, require two antihypertensive agents from the start. Two-drug therapy using low doses typically lowers BP more effectively than high-dose monotherapy, and may reduce the risk of drug-related side effects compared with high-dose monotherapy.[64] Initial treatment with two drugs are not needed because D.C. does not have stage 2 hypertension and, in contrast to most patients with hypertension, can feasibly attain goal with one agent.[5,9]

Special Populations

BLACK PATIENTS

17. D.C. is black. Should his race influence the selection of an antihypertensive regimen?

Black patients have a higher incidence of hypertension, hypertension-associated complications, and an increased need for combination therapy to achieve and maintain BP goals.[25,65] As monotherapy, it is well documented that a thiazide diuretic or a CCB is highly effective in lowering BP in black patients. Conversely, ACEI, ARB, or β-blocker monotherapy is less effective in lowering BP in black patients compared with white patients. When these agents are used in combination, especially with a thiazide diuretic, BP lowering is greatly improved. This information may aid in selecting one drug option over another in a primary prevention patient, but does not apply to black patients with compelling indications, where choice of therapy follows an evidence-based approach to selection.

The Hypertension in African American Working Group (HAAWG) of the International Society on Hypertension in Blacks has treatment guidelines that are similar to the JNC7 and 2007 AHA hypertension guidelines with respect to lifestyle modifications and pharmacotherapy.[5,9,65] These guidelines, however, highlight that attaining BP goal values is more challenging in blacks, and usually requires more aggressive initiation of pharmacotherapy. They also identify that black patients are at higher risk of side effects with ACEI (both angioedema and cough) compared with whites.[45]

D.C. does not have any compelling indications for specific antihypertensive drug therapy. His first-line treatment options are an ACEI, ARB, CCB, or thiazide diuretic. Monotherapy with either a thiazide diuretic or a CCB would be very effective in BP lowering; either of these two drugs is an acceptable treatment option for him.

VERY ELDERLY PATIENTS

18. How is treatment of hypertension in an elderly patient different than in a younger patient? Are there any special precautions for lowering BP too much?

Older patients with hypertension (>65 years of age) have the lowest rates of BP control, and this rate decreases in even older populations.[25] Very elderly patients (>75 years of age), similar to black patients, respond best to thiazides and CCBs and less to ACEIs, ARBs, and β-blockers. However, it is unclear whether these small differences in BP lowering are clinically significant, so they should be viewed as medical myths rather than definitive realities.

Isolated Systolic Hypertension

Isolated systolic hypertension (ISH) is defined as an elevated SBP (>140 mmHg) with a "normal" DBP (<90 mmHg).[5] This pattern of hypertension is most common in patients >65 years of age and incurs a significant risk for CV disease. It was once thought that patients with ISH required high SBP to ensure normal perfusion of the heart and brain and that treating ISH would further lower DBP and worsen organ perfusion. Evidence clearly demonstrates, however, that treating ISH reduces the risk of CV events.[39,42,49]

The care of patients with ISH, including the very elderly, should follow the same general hypertension care principles that apply to all patients, with two exceptions. The first exception is that lower doses should be used when first starting therapy. The second is that initial drug therapy, even with stage 2 hypertension, should only be started with monotherapy. Drug doses can be gradually increased as tolerated and combination therapy subsequently used to achieve recommended BP goals.[5,9] In earlier JNC recommendations, thiazide diuretics and long-acting dihydropyridine CCB were preferred based on the evidence of reduced hypertension-associated complications.[39,40,42] The JNC7 recommends that selection of pharmacotherapy in elderly patients be according to the same general treatment philosophies as for other patients with hypertension. Although lower starting doses may be needed to minimize the risk of side effects, elderly patients eventually need standard treatment doses and often require combination therapy to reach and maintain their BP goals.

Few data exist evaluating antihypertensive therapy in the very elderly (i.e., patients >75 years). These patients are underrepresented in most clinical trials. A meta-analysis evaluating landmark clinical trials in hypertension indicates that antihypertensive therapy in patients who were age 80 and older reduced the risk of stroke, but not necessarily all cause mortality.[66] The Hypertension in the Very Elderly Trial (HYVET) is a placebo-controlled, randomized trial evaluating the effect of antihypertensive pharmacotherapy in patients with hypertension age 80 years and older.[67] This trial was halted prematurely, after only 1.8 median years, owing to significant reductions in both stroke and overall mortality in the treatment arm.[68] The HYVET provides the most compelling evidence that treatment of hypertension in the very elderly provides significant benefits.

Absence of a J-Curve

Data from observational studies generated concern that there is a "J-curve" phenomenon where lowering BP too far may

Table 13-8 Additional Considerations in Antihypertensive Drug Choice[a]

Antihypertensive Agent	Situations with Potentially Favorable Effects	Situations with Potential Unfavorable Effects[b]	Avoid Use
ACEI	Low-normal potassium, prediabetes, microalbuminuria in patients without diabetes	High-normal potassium or hyperkalemia	Pregnancy, bilateral renal artery stenosis, history of angioedema
ARB	Low-normal potassium, prediabetes, microalbuminuria in patients without diabetes	High-normal potassium or hyperkalemia	Pregnancy, bilateral renal artery stenosis
CCB: dihydropyridine	Raynaud's syndrome, elderly patients with isolated systolic hypertension, cyclosporine induced hypertension	Peripheral edema, left ventricular dysfunction (all except amlodipine and felodipine), high-normal heart rate or tachycardia	
CCB: nondihydropyridine	Raynaud's syndrome, migraine headache, arrhythmias, high-normal heart rate or tachycardia	Peripheral edema, low-normal heart rate	Second or third degree heart block, left ventricular dysfunction
Thiazide diuretic	Osteoporosis or at increased risk for osteoporosis, high-normal potassium	Gout, hyponatremia, prediabetes (as monotherapy), low-normal potassium	

[a]Never to replace recommendations because of a compelling indication.
[b]May use but requires diligent monitoring.
High-normal refers to patients in the high end of the normal range, but not above the range.
Low-normal refers to patients in the low end of the normal range, but not below the range.
ACEI, angiotensin converting enzyme inhibitor; ARB, angiotensin-2 receptor blocker; CCB, calcium channel blocker.

be harmful.[69,70] These data found that CAD events were decreased as expected when DBP was reduced to approximately 85 mmHg. Below this level, however, the risk of events actually increased.

The J-curve phenomenon is a medical myth. The data used to establish this phenomenon are observations from retrospective evaluations and, therefore, cannot establish cause and effect. The J-curve has been associated only with CAD events, not stroke or kidney impairment. For stroke prevention and kidney impairment, data consistently suggest that the lower the BP the better, unless BP reductions are too abrupt or are excessive. If the J-curve has any validity, it would occur when BP is reduced much lower than the therapeutic range. Furthermore, patients with very low BP may have other illnesses that predispose them to coronary events (e.g., autonomic dysfunction, volume depletion).

Controlled evidence disputes the J-curve. The Hypertension Optimal Treatment (HOT) trial was a prospective clinical trial designed to evaluate lower BP goals and CV events (challenging the J-curve).[16] More than 18,700 patients were randomized to goal DBP values of <90 mmHg, <85 mmHg, or <80 mmHg. The risks for major CV disease events were the lowest when treatment BP was <139/83 mmHg. The risk for cerebrovascular events was lowest at a treatment BP of <142/80 mmHg. Only in patients with ischemic heart disease and diabetes did the lowest risk occur at a DBP <80 mmHg. A significant increase in events was not seen in patients with lower BP values. Therefore, the HOT trial does not support the concept of a J-curve.

Additional Considerations

19. Multiple pharmacotherapy options are equally recommended in a primary prevention patient. What additional considerations help to select an agent for a specific patient?

It cannot be emphasized enough that selecting pharmacotherapy should follow an evidence-based philosophy. In patients with compelling indications, certain antihypertensive drug classes are recommended in place of other options. In patients without compelling indications, additional factors (e.g., other diseases, cost, serum electrolytes, prior intolerances or allergies) are considered when selecting a drug class (Table 13-8). These are particularly helpful when selecting initial therapy for a primary prevention patient who has more than one acceptable drug class as a therapeutic option. It can also be helpful when selecting add-on therapy to further lower BP. These are discussed later in this chapter.

The costs of treating hypertension and related complications are substantial to patients and health systems.[71] Costs attributed to drug acquisition are small in comparison to expenses for laboratory evaluations, office visits, and medical care for hypertension-associated complications. Whenever possible, affordable regimens that do not compromise efficacy should be designed. Generic antihypertensive products are less expensive than brand-name products, and all first- and second-line antihypertensive classes, except ARB, have generic alternatives. The frequency of administration must also be considered because it can influence patients' adherence to regimens. Once-daily administration maximizes compliance and is most desirable. All major antihypertensive drug classes offer a once-daily product, so optimizing regimen administration is very feasible.

Pharmacotherapy for Patients with Compelling Indications

Throughout the remainder of this chapter the term *compelling indications* will be used frequently. Compelling indications are defined as comorbid diseases for which specific antihypertensive classes are indicated based on evidence from clinical trials. Although these clinical trials may not have evaluated hypertension-related complications alone, they show significant benefits in reducing CV morbidity or mortality that warrants their use in a hypertensive patient with a given compelling indication (Fig. 13-3). A BP goal of <130/80 mmHg is recommended in patients with a compelling indication, with an even lower goal of <120/80 mmHg recommended if the compelling indication is left ventricular dysfunction.

Diabetes

Kidney disease and CV disease are both considered long-term complication of diabetes and hypertension-associated complications. Patients with diabetes are at high risk for these complications. Evidence shows that treatment with antihypertensive agents (ACEI, ARB, CCB, thiazide diuretics, and even β-blockers) in patients with diabetes reduces risk of CV events, and progression of kidney disease.[72] When compared head-to-head, ACEI are superior to dihydropyridine CCB at reducing CV events.[53,54] Subanalyses of larger clinical trials further support CV event reduction with ACEI and ARB[73,74] (see Chapter 50, Diabetes Mellitus). Therefore, initial antihypertensive therapy for a patient with diabetes should ideally consist of an ACEI or ARB first-line. A thiazide diuretic as add-on agent, followed by either a CCB or β-blocker as the next add-on therapy, should be used to provide additional BP lowering when needed. Aggressive BP control is indicated in diabetes (e.g., <130/80 mmHg) to minimize the risk of hypertension-associated complications.[5,16,72] To get to this BP goal, however, two or more antihypertensive drugs are almost always needed.[72,75]

Chronic Kidney Disease

Chronic kidney disease initially presents with microalbuminuria (30–299 mg albumin in a 24-hour urine collection) that can progress over several years to overt kidney failure.[26] Progression is accelerated in the presence of both hypertension and diabetes. ACEI or ARB therapy should be used first-line in these patients because both have been shown to reduce the progression of chronic kidney disease in type 1 diabetes,[76] in type 2 diabetes,[50,56–58] and in those without diabetes.[60,75,77] For purposes of hypertension management, patients have chronic kidney disease sufficiently significant to be considered a compelling indication with a goal BP of <130/80 mmHg if they have one of the following three criteria: (a) an estimated GFR <60 mL/minute/1.73 m^2 based on MDRD calculation (calculator available at: http://www.kidney.org/professionals/KDOQI/gfr_calculator.cfm); (b) a serum creatinine >1.3 mg/dL in women or >1.5 in men because this roughly correlates to a GFR estimation of <60 mL/minute/1.73 m^2; or (c) albuminuria (>300 mg/day on a 24-hour urine collection or total protein-to-creatinine ratio >200 mg/g on a spot urinalysis).[5] These patients typically require three or more antihypertensive agents, within which an ACEI or ARB should be the foundation of the drug therapy regimen.[60,75]

Chronic and Acute CAD

The two most common forms of chronic CAD, post-MI and chronic stable angina, are considered compelling indications.[5,9] The American College of Cardiology (ACC)/AHA have guidelines for these conditions that recommend treatment with a β-blocker, followed shortly thereafter by the addition of an ACEI.[36,78] β-Blockers (those without intrinsic sympathomimetic activity [ISA]) decrease the risk of a subsequent MI or sudden cardiac death by decreasing the adrenergic burden on the heart,[79,80] and progression of atherosclerosis.[81] ACEI therapy promotes cardiac remodeling, improves cardiac function, and reduces the risk of CV events.[82,83] An ARB should be used as an alternative in patients who do not tolerate an ACEI, because fewer data exist that assess the long-term impact of an ARB on CV events compared with an ACEI in this setting.[9,78] If additional BP reduction is needed, a thiazide diuretic can be added to the core regimen of a β-blocker with an ACEI (or ARB). If an additional agent is needed to treat ischemic symptoms for patients with chronic stable angina, a dihydropyridine CCB can be added to this core regimen. If a β-blocker cannot be used because of intolerance or contraindication, a nondihydropyridine CCB (verapamil or diltiazem) can be used as an alternative.

Acute CAD, also called *acute coronary syndrome*, includes unstable angina, non–ST-segment elevation MI, and ST-segment elevation MI.[9] The ACC/AHA guidelines for these conditions indicate a β-blocker as first-line pharmacotherapy.[84,85] Patients must be hemodynamically stable, however, before starting a β-blocker. The addition of an ACEI (or ARB as an alternative) is recommended if an anterior MI is present, if left ventricular dysfunction is present, if the patient has diabetes, or if additional BP lowering is needed.[9] Most patients with an acute coronary syndrome will have one of these considerations for an ACEI (or ARB). Similar to chronic CAD, a thiazide diuretic can be added for further BP lowering. A dihydropyridine CCB can be added if ischemic symptoms are present. If a β-blocker cannot be used because of intolerance or contraindication, a nondihydropyridine CCB (verapamil or diltiazem) can be used as an alternative.

Prior Stroke

A history of a prior ischemic stroke (the predominant etiology of most cases of stroke) is considered a form of noncoronary atherosclerotic vascular disease and a compelling indication for specific antihypertensive drug therapy to lower the risk of a recurrent stroke. In fact, ischemic stroke is the only form of noncoronary atherosclerotic vascular disease for which specific antihypertensive drug therapy has been shown to reduce recurrent CV events. Lowering BP to goal in patients with a history of stroke is beneficial once patients have stabilized after their acute event. Specifically, the combination of an ACEI with a thiazide diuretic is documented to reduce the incidence of recurrent stroke.[46] Similarly, an ARB-based regimen has been shown to reduce the incidence of recurrent stroke more effectively than a dihydropyridine CCB-based treatment regimen.[63] Therefore, based on these data, either an ACEI with a thiazide diuretic, or ARB-based therapy is considered an appropriate first-line pharmacotherapy option for patients with a history of a prior ischemic stroke. Because dihydropyridine CCB-based therapy has also been shown to reduce the risk of ischemic stroke in patients with hypertension (albeit less than with an ARB),[42] a dihydropyridine CCB is a good add-on option for combination therapy.

Left Ventricular Dysfunction

Left ventricular dysfunction (sometimes called *systolic heart failure* or *chronic heart failure*) is a common complication of hypertension in which cardiac contractility is compromised. This compelling indication has the lowest BP goal of <120/80 mmHg. If patients are optimally treated with the combination of pharmacotherapy options recommended by both the 2007 AHA hypertension guidelines and ACC/AHA heart failure guidelines, they will likely attain this strict BP goal and experience reduced CV morbidity and mortality.[9,86]

Standard first-line therapy for left ventricular dysfunction should included a three-drug combination of an ACEI, a diuretic (either a thiazide or loop, depending on kidney function and need for diuresis), and a β-blocker. ACEI have numerous landmark clinical trials showing reduced morbidity and mortality rates and diuretics provide primarily symptomatic relieve of edema.[86] As left ventricular dysfunction progresses, loop diuretics are almost always needed instead of a thiazide diuretic because they produce more pronounced diuresis. β-Blocker therapy is a component of standard first-line therapy for left ventricular dysfunction because numerous clinical trials have demonstrated reduced morbidity and mortality when added to ACEI with diuretic therapy.[79,87,88] According to evidence-based medicine principles, only metoprolol, carvedilol, and bisoprolol are indicated for left ventricular dysfunction. Other β-blockers (e.g., atenolol) should not be used in patients with left ventricular dysfunction because they do not have supporting data demonstrating they reduce CV event rates in these patients. Before adding a β-blocker in a patient recently started on an ACEI and diuretic, the patient should be hemodynamically stable. As discussed in detail in Chapter 18 (Heart Failure), it is important to start with very low doses of a β-blocker, then slowly titrating upward over several weeks to the recommended dosing range for left ventricular dysfunction.

Based on evidence demonstrating reduced risk of CV events, additional antihypertensive agents reduce CV risk in this patient population. An aldosterone antagonist (spironolactone, eplerenone) can be added to a standard first-line regimen in patients with severe left ventricular dysfunction.[9,89,90] Similarly, the combination of hydralazine with isosorbide dinitrate can be added in black patients.[91] An ARB should be used as an alternative for patients intolerant to an ACEI,[92,93] or in addition to standard first-line treatment for left ventricular dysfunction.[94] Speculation was that an ARB would be even better than an ACEI in left ventricular dysfunction,[95] but when compared head-to-head, ACEIs were found to provide better outcomes.[96]

Implementing Pharmacotherapy

Monotherapy

Starting with one drug to treat hypertension is optimal when initial BP is close to goal values. When using a standard dose of a first-line antihypertensive agents (an ACEI, ARB, CCB, or thiazide diuretic), and even with β-blockers, the average reduction in SBP/DBP is only10/5 mmHg.[64] This has been termed by some as the "10 over 5" rule.

Two general approaches to monotherapy exist. The stepped-care approach to monotherapy is where a single agent is selected with the dose increased until BP is controlled, the maximal dose is reached, or dose-limiting toxicity occurs. If the goal BP is not achieved, a second drug from a different class is added. Theoretically, this process can be continued, if necessary, until three or even four drugs are used in combination. The Veterans Affairs (VA) Cooperative Studies Group on Antihypertensive Agents evaluated the ability of a monotherapy in attaining a BP of <140/90 mmHg using one of several antihypertensive agents in patients with stage 1 or 2 hypertension.[30] Less than 60% of patients reached a DBP <90 mmHg with this approach when doses were titrated up to the maximal dosage. After 1 year, approximately 50% actually maintained a DBP of <90 mmHg. Therefore, monotherapy is limited in its ability to attain goal BP values for many patients, especially those with higher baseline BP values.

With the sequential therapy approach, monotherapy is initiated and titrated to the maximal dose as needed. If goal BP is not achieved, an alternative agent is selected to replace the first. Combination drug therapy is reserved for patients who do not achieve goal BP values after the second agent. Sequential therapy seems most appropriate when the first drug is either poorly tolerated or results in minimal reduction in BP. The VA Cooperative Studies Group on Antihypertensive Agents also evaluated sequential therapy. Only an additional 49% of the nonresponders to the first agent achieved a DBP <90 mmHg when switched to a second drug.

Combination Therapy

Starting therapy with two drugs is strongly encouraged for patients far from their BP goal, such as patients who have stage 2 hypertension.[5,9] This approach is also an option for patients closer to their BP goal, who have compelling indications for two drugs, or have BP goals of <130/80 mmHg or <120/80 mmHg. It is justified by the observation that most patients with hypertension have not attained goal BP values, and most patients require two or more agents.[5] In contrast to high-dose monotherapy, low-dose, two-drug combination therapy provides greater BP lowering with a lower risk of side effects.[64]

IDEAL COMBINATIONS

When selecting a second agent as add-on therapy for BP reduction, a thiazide diuretic should usually be considered if it was not the first drug added. This does not always apply if the second drug is being added to treat a compelling indication, although most patients will respond to a two-drug regimen if it includes a diuretic.[5] Thiazide diuretics are very effective in lowering BP when used in combination with most other antihypertensive agents. Similarly, the combination of an ACEI or ARB with a CCB is also very effective in lowering BP. By appropriately selecting combination regimens, many patients can achieve a BP goal of <140/90 mmHg with two drugs. It is not uncommon, however, to require three or more drugs to attain a goal BP of <130/80 mmHg or lower.

ORTHOSTATIC HYPOTENSION

Orthostatic hypotension occurs when standing upright results in a SBP decrease >10 mmHg and is accompanied by dizziness or fainting.[5] This is a risk of rapid BP lowering. Orthostatic hypotension is more frequent in very elderly patients (especially those with ISH), diabetes, autonomic dysfunction, and in patients taking certain drugs (diuretics, nitrates, α-blockers, phosphodiesterase inhibitors use in erectile dysfunction, or psychotropic agents). Combination therapy can still be used in these patients, but close evaluation is needed. Dose titration should be gradual with caution applied to minimize the risk of hypotension and to avoid volume depletion. Moreover, initial therapy with two drugs should be avoided in this population owing to the increased risk of orthostatic hypotension.

Monitoring Therapy

Four aspects of treatment must always be considered: (a) BP response to attain goal, (b) adherence with lifestyle modifications and pharmacotherapy, (c) progression to hypertension-associated complications, and (d) drug-related toxicity.

Blood pressure control should be evaluated 1 to 4 weeks after starting or modifying therapy for most patients. BP usually begins to fall within 1 to 2 weeks of starting an agent, but steady-state antihypertensive effects typically take up to 4 weeks. If patients have experienced a hypertensive crisis, evaluation should occur sooner. For example, hypertensive emergencies are triaged for hospitalized care, and BP response is evaluated with continuous monitoring. For patients with hypertensive urgency (BP values in the upper range of stage 2 hypertension without signs of acute target-organ damage), BP response to treatment should be assessed ideally within 3 days.

Two BP values should be measured each time to evaluate response, with the average of the two used to make a proper assessment. If dehydration or orthostatic hypotension is suspected, BP measurements should be made in both the seated and standing positions to detect orthostatic changes. For routine monitoring, measuring BP in the seated position is sufficient. Home BP monitoring values should be considered when they are available. They, however, normally are slightly lower (5 mmHg) than clinic values even in patients without white-coat hypertension. For example, patients with a goal BP value of <140/90 mmHg should have home measurements that are <135/85 mmHg.[5]

All patients should be questioned in a nonthreatening manner regarding adherence to lifestyle modifications and drug therapy. This is especially important for complex regimens, when drug intolerance is likely, or when financial constraints hinder acquisition of medications. Medical evaluation to assess hypertension-associated complications and drug side effects is essential. The presence of new hypertension-associated complications may necessitate modification of therapy. Drug therapy may require changes based on the need to treat a compelling indication or attain a new BP goal. The presence of drug-related side effects might similarly result in the need to modify therapy.

CLINICAL SCENARIOS

Diuretics

20. B.A. is a 62-year-old woman who is postmenopausal, does not smoke, and never drinks alcohol. Since being diagnosed with hypertension, she has modified her diet, begun routine aerobic exercise, and has lost 10 kg over the past 18 months. She now weighs 72 kg and is 165 cm tall. Her present BP is 142/94 mmHg (144/92 when repeated) and has consistently remained near this value over the past year. Her BP when first diagnosed was 150/98 mmHg. No evidence is found of LVH or retinopathy. Urinalysis is negative for protein. Other laboratory tests are normal, except for dyslipidemia. B.A. has no health insurance and is concerned about the cost of therapy, and pays full price for all of her medications. Her Framingham risk score is 22%. She takes over-the-counter calcium with vitamin D (she has osteoporosis) and is to start hydrochlorothiazide (HCTZ) for hypertension. Is this an appropriate first-line treatment for her?

This patient has hypertension that is considered uncontrolled. Because of her elevated Framingham risk score, a BP goal of <130/80 mmHg is recommended.[9] She is a primary prevention patient without compelling indications. An ACEI, ARB, CCB, or thiazide diuretic is acceptable first-line treatment options. A thiazide diuretic is optimal for her. It is the most inexpensive treatment option, and may also benefit her osteoporosis (Table 13-8). Several types of diuretics are used to manage hypertension (Table 13-9). All lower BP, with the primary differences being duration of action, potency of diuresis, and potential for electrolyte abnormalities.

Table 13-9 Diuretics in Hypertension

Category	*Selected Products*	*Usual Dosage Range (mg/day)*	*Dosing Frequency*
Thiazide	Chlorthalidone (Hygroton)	12.5–25	Daily
	Hydrochlorothiazide (Esidrix, Hydrodiuril, Microzide)	12.5–25	Daily
	Indapamide (Lozol)	1.25–5	Daily
	Metolazone (Zaroxolyn)	2.5–10	Daily
	Metolazone (Mykrox)	0.5–1.0	Daily
Loop	Bumetanide (Bumex)	0.5–4	BID
	Furosemide (Lasix)	20–80	BID
	Torsemide (Demadex)	2.5–10	Daily
Potassium-sparing	Amiloride (Midamor)	5–10	Daily to BID
	Triamterene (Dyrenium)	50–100	Daily to BID
Combination	Triamterene/Hydrochlorothiazide (Maxide, Dyazide)	37.5/25–75/50	Daily
	Spironolactone/Hydrochlorothiazide (Aldactazide)	25/25–50/50	Daily
	Amiloride/Hydrochlorothiazide (Moduretic)	5–10/50–100	Daily
Aldosterone antagonist	Eplerenone (Inspra)	50–100	Daily to BID
	Spironolactone (Aldactone)	25–50	Daily to BID

BID, twice daily.

Thiazides

Thiazide diuretics are the drugs of choice for hypertension based on landmark data using these types of diuretics. Similar to loop diuretics, an initial diuresis is experienced. After approximately 4 to 6 weeks of thiazide diuretic therapy, diuresis dissipates, however, and is supplanted by a decrease in PVR, which is responsible for sustaining antihypertensive effects. HCTZ and chlorthalidone have been used in several major outcome trials, including the ALLHAT.[5,22,45,47] HCTZ, which is most frequently used in the United States, is very inexpensive and is dosed once daily. Chlorthalidone may be slightly more potent on a milligram per milligram basis, but this difference has questionable clinical relevance. The usual starting dose of HCTZ or chlorthalidone is a low-dose of 12.5 mg once daily. A maintenance dose of 25 mg once daily can effectively lower BP and has a low incidence of side effects.[22,30,37] The propensity of evidence showing benefit with thiazide diuretics is with low-dose therapy, considered to be the equivalent of HCTZ or chlorthalidone 12.5 to 25 mg daily.[22]

Loop Diuretics

Loop diuretics produce a more potent diuresis, a smaller decrease in PVR, and less vasodilation than thiazide diuretics. Therefore, a thiazide is more effective at lowering BP than loop diuretics in most patients. Loop diuretics are usually the diuretics of choice for patients with severe chronic kidney disease (an estimated GFR <30 mL/minute/1.73 m^2), left ventricular dysfunction, or severe edema because potent diuresis is often needed in these patients. Furosemide has a short duration of effect and should be given twice daily when used in hypertension, whereas torsemide can be given once daily.

Potassium-Sparing Diuretics

Potassium-sparing diuretics should be reserved primarily for patients who develop hypokalemia while on a thiazide diuretic. With low-dose thiazide diuretics, <25% of patients develop hypokalemia and most cases are not severe. Potassium-sparing diuretics do not provide significant BP-lowering effects when used alone or in combination with a thiazide. Several fixed-dose products are available that include HCTZ with a potassium-sparing agent. Empirically starting all patients with hypertension treated with a diuretic on one of these fixed-dose combination products to avoid hypokalemia is not rational unless baseline serum potassium is in the low-normal range.

21. How should a thiazide diuretic be started in B.A.?

B.A. has stage 1 hypertension and monotherapy with a thiazide diuretic is rational. Evidence supports the use of thiazide diuretics in primary prevention patients, and she has no contraindications to this therapy (Table 13-10). B.A. does have dyslipidemia, but thiazide diuretics are unlikely to have a clinically significant effect on cholesterol when used in low doses.[23,97] An appropriate starting dose of HCTZ for B.A. is 12.5 or 25 mg daily. She has no additional risks for orthostatic hypotension, so starting at the higher 25 mg daily is safe, and will have a better chance of lowering her BP to <130/80 mmHg than the lower 12.5-mg dose. Most antihypertensive agents provide a 10 mmHg reduction in SBP and 5 mmHg reduction in DBP with a standard starting dose, with less than this amount as additional BP lowering with each dose-doubling thereafter.[64]

Patient Education

22. B.A. is prescribed HCTZ 25 mg daily. How should she be counseled regarding this therapy?

Several counseling points regarding hypertension are summarized in Table 13-7. Some patients disregard lifestyle modifications when they start antihypertensive therapy, so she should be encouraged to continue lifestyle modification to maximize her response to drug therapy. Drug-specific counseling for diuretics includes informing B.A. that diuretics effectively lower BP and risk of CV events. Taking her daily dose at about the same time each morning is best to minimize nocturia and provide consistent effects. Patients experience increased urination when starting this medicine, but this diminishes with time. Missed doses should be taken as soon as possible within the same day, but doubling doses the next day is not recommended. B.A. should be informed of the potential for hypokalemia which is easily identified and managed, and the need for routine monitoring of serum potassium. She should be counseled on the signs and symptoms of electrolyte abnormalities (e.g., leg cramps, muscle weakness) and encouraged to report these to her health care provider if they occur. Increasing dietary intake of potassium-rich foods (i.e., bananas, orange juice) to minimize electrolyte depletion is an option to minimize potassium loss. This should be encouraged only with thiazide and loop diuretics, because a potassium-enhanced diet could contribute to hyperkalemia with potassium-sparing agents.

23. After 4 weeks of HCTZ 25 mg daily, B.A. returns for evaluation without complaints. She has not missed a dose, is still exercising, and is following the DASH diet. Her BP values are 132/82 and 130/84 mmHg. Her serum potassium is 3.8 mEq/L (normal, 3.5–5.2 mEq/L), uric acid is 7.3 mg/dL (normal, 2.0–7.5 mg/dL), fasting glucose is 99 mg/dL (normal, 60–99 mg/dL), and the other laboratory values are unchanged. One month ago, her potassium was 4.0 mEq/L, uric acid was 6.8 mg/dL, and fasting glucose was 95 mg/dL. What is your assessment from the data given regarding efficacy and toxicity?

[SI units: K, 3.8 mmol/L (normal, 3.5–5.2 mmol/L); uric acid, 432 mmol/L (normal, 119–476 mmol/L); and glucose, 5.6 mmol/L (normal, 3.3–6.1 mmol/L)]

Despite significant improvements with lifestyle modifications before starting HCTZ and apparent adherence with taking her HCTZ dose as directed, B.A.'s goal BP of <130/80 mmHg has not been met based on today's BP average of 131/83 mmHg. No new signs of hypertension-associated complications are seen. She should be encouraged to continue with her current efforts, but other interventions are now indicated.

Potassium Loss

Adverse reactions with low-dose thiazide diuretics (e.g., HCTZ 12.5–25 mg daily) are minimal compared with high-dose therapy (HCTZ ≥50 mg daily). Moreover, most side effects with low-dose thiazide diuretic therapy has been shown to be similar to placebo,[37] and have similar tolerability compared with other first-line drug therapy options.[30] Increased urination usually subsides after the first few weeks of therapy with thiazide diuretics, but this is sometimes a cause for nonadherence,

Table 13-10 Side Effects and Contraindications of Antihypertensive Agents

	Side Effects			
	Innocuous but Sometimes Annoying	*Potentially Harmful*	*Usually Requires Cessation of Therapy, at Least Temporarily*	*Contraindications*
Thiazide diuretics	Increased urination (at onset of therapy), muscle cramps, hyperuricemia (without gout), GI disturbances	Hypokalemia,[a] hyperglycemia, hypovolemia, pancreatitis, photosensitivity, hypercholesterolemia, hypertriglyceridemia, hyperuricemia with gout, orthostatic hypotension (more frequent in elderly)	Hypercalcemia, azotemia, skin rash (cross-reacts with only certain sulfonamide allergies), purpura, bone marrow depression, lithium toxicity in patients on lithium therapy	Persistent anuria or oliguria, advanced kidney failure
Loop diuretics	Increased urination, muscle cramps, hyperuricemia (less than with thiazides), GI disturbances	Hypokalemia,[a] hyperglycemia, hypovolemia, pancreatitis, hypercholesterolemia, hypertriglyceridemia, hearing loss with large IV doses orthostatic hypotension (more frequent in elderly)	Hyponatremia, hypocalcemia, azotemia, skin rash (cross-reacts with only certain sulfonamide allergies), photosensitivity, lithium toxicity in patients on lithium therapy	
ACEI	Dizziness, dry cough	Orthostatic hypotension (more frequent in elderly treated with a diuretic), increased serum creatinine, increased potassium	Angioedema, severe hyperkalemia, increase in serum creatinine >35%	Bilateral renal artery stenosis, volume depletion, hyponatremia, pregnancy, history of angioedema
ARB	Dizziness	Orthostatic hypotension (more frequent in elderly treated with a diuretic), increased serum creatinine, increased potassium	Severe hyperkalemia, increase in serum creatinine >35%	Bilateral renal artery stenosis, volume depletion, hyponatremia, pregnancy
CCB: dihydropyridines	Dizziness, headache, flushing	Peripheral edema, tachycardia.	Significant peripheral edema	Left ventricular dysfunction (not with amlodipine or felodipine)
CCB: nondihydropyridines	Dizziness, headache, constipation	Bradycardia	Heart block, left ventricular dysfunction, interactions with certain drugs	Left ventricular dysfunction, second- or third-degree heart block, sick sinus syndrome
β-Blocker	Bradycardia, weakness, exercise intolerance	Masking the symptoms of hypoglycemia in diabetes, hyperglycemia, aggravation of peripheral arterial disease, erectile dysfunction, increased triglycerides, decreased HDL-C	Left ventricular dysfunction (not with carvedilol, metoprolol, bisoprolol), bronchospasm in patients with asthma	Severe asthma, second- or third-degree heart block, acute left ventricular dysfunction exacerbation, coronary artery disease for agents with intrinsic sympathomimetic activity
Aldosterone antagonist	Menstrual irregularities (spironolactone only) or gynecomastia (spironolactone only)	Increased potassium	Hyperkalemia, hyponatremia	Kidney failure. kidney impairment (for eplerenone: CrCl <50 mL/min, or type 2 diabetes with proteinuria, and elevated or creatinine >1.8 in women, >2.0 in men), hyperkalemia, hyponatremia

[a]Routine use of potassium supplements and/or concurrent potassium sparing diuretics should be discouraged unless hypokalemia is documented, the patient is taking digoxin, or potassium is in the low-normal range in a patient at risk for prediabetes or diabetes.

ACEI, angiotensin converting enzyme inhibitor; ARB, angiotensin-2 receptor blocker; CCB, calcium channel blocker; CrCl, creatinine clearance; GI, gastrointestinal; HDL-C, high-density lipoprotein cholesterol; IV, intravenous.

especially in elderly patients who fear incontinence. Signs and symptoms of metabolic changes, such as hypokalemia, hyperglycemia, or hyperuricemia, should be evaluated. B.A.'s serum potassium has dropped and uric acid has risen. These are small changes that are consistent with thiazide-induced abnormalities. B.A. should be questioned about muscle cramps or weakness, which can be associated with decreases in potassium.

24. Is B.A.'s decrease in potassium concerning? If so, how should this be managed?

Most total body potassium is intracellular (~98%). Thiazide can reduce serum potassium concentrations. This can result in potassium serum concentrations in the low end of the normal range, but overt hypokalemia is not common. Most often, thiazide diuretic-induced hypokalemia is mild, with serum potassium concentrations reaching a nadir within the first month of therapy and generally remaining stable thereafter.[30,97] HCTZ in doses of 12.5, 25, and 50 mg daily can decrease serum potassium by an average of 0.21, 0.34, and 0.5 mEq/L, respectively.[23,97]

SUBCLINICAL POTASSIUM DECREASES

The clinical significance of small potassium decreases when serum potassium concentrations are still in the normal range is controversial. B.A.'s potassium has dropped slightly and her current serum concentration is in the low end of the normal range. Patients treated with a thiazide diuretic who experience the greatest decreases in potassium also experience the greatest increases in glucose values.[98] It is optimal to maintain serum potassium (in milliequivalent per liter [mEq/L]) in the middle to high end of the normal range (e.g., between 4.0 and 5.0 mEq/L in patients treated with thiazide diuretics.[99] This may minimize the risk, albeit small, of increasing fasting glucose concentrations, and possibly development of type 2 diabetes, which has been demonstrated in patients treated with thiazide diuretics.[100] Keeping serum potassium concentrations in this 4.0 to 5.0 mEq/L range can be accomplished by administering the thiazide diuretic in combination with a potassium-sparing diuretic or an ACEI, ARB, or aldosterone antagonist if additional BP lowering is needed.[98,99]

B.A.'s BP is still not at goal. Adding either an ACEI or ARB is the most reasonable option to both control her BP and minimize the decrease in potassium. She should be encouraged to continue a low-salt diet. Her potassium and BP should be re-evaluated in 4 weeks.

HYPOKALEMIA

25. When is potassium supplementation needed to manage diuretic-induced hypokalemia?

B.A.'s potassium is still within the normal range. Potassium replacement is not indicated. Diuretic-associated hypokalemia, however, should be treated when serum concentrations are below normal regardless of whether symptoms (weakness and muscle cramps) are present. Serum potassium should be measured at baseline and within 4 weeks of initiating therapy or after increasing diuretic doses. Other conditions, such as chronic diarrhea, high-dose corticosteroid use, and hyperaldosteronism, can contribute to hypokalemia.

Potassium-rich foods (e.g., dried fruit, bananas, potatoes, avocados) may help prevent subclinical decreases in potassium, but they cannot be used as sole therapy to correct hypokalemia. For instance, one medium-size banana has 11.5 mEq of potassium. The usual replacement dose of prescribed potassium chloride is 20 to 40 mEq/day but can range from 10 to more than 100 mEq/day. Potassium chloride, bicarbonate, gluconate, acetate, and citrate salts are available as single ingredients and as components of combination products. Potassium chloride (KCl) preparations are generally preferred, however. Oral potassium supplements are available in liquid, enteric-coated, and slow-release preparations. Slow-release formulations are preferred because they cause fewer gastrointestinal adverse effects than other preparations.

OTHER METABOLIC ABNORMALITIES

26. B.A.'s glucose and uric acid both increased after starting HCTZ. Are these changes clinically significant?

An increase in fasting glucose is a recognized complication of diuretic therapy, but the magnitude of increase is both variable and dose dependent. Patients with diabetes and prediabetes exhibit the greatest glucose increases, and patients without diabetes exhibit the smallest increases. When increases in serum glucose concentration occur in patients without diabetes, they are typically on average 3.6 to 6.7 mg/dL after multiple years of thiazide diuretic therapy.[30,45,97] It appears that these changes are not clinically relevant because CV events are reduced despite these changes.

Diabetes is not a contraindication to the use of diuretics; rather, it is actually a compelling indication for a diuretic (Fig. 13-3). Risk of CV events is reduced in patients treated with a thiazide who have diabetes.[5,39,45,75] Altering diet or the dose of diabetes medications can manage hyperglycemia if it occurs in these patients.

B.A. does not have a strong family history of diabetes, and her fasting glucose concentration is still considered normal. Her fasting glucose values should be documented and monitored at least once a year to detect any increases.

Thiazide and loop diuretics can increase serum uric acid concentrations in a dose-dependent fashion. This is more problematic with thiazide diuretics than with loop diuretics. Increased proximal tubular renal reabsorption, decreased tubular secretion, or increased postsecretory reabsorption of uric acid contribute to diuretic-induced hyperuricemia. Thiazide-induced hyperuricemia is usually small ($\leq$0.5 mg/dL) and is not clinically significant in most patients.[23,97] For patients without a history of gout, increases in uric acid serum concentrations are not clinically relevant. For patients with a history of gout, especially those not on preventive antihyperuricemic therapy (allopurinol, probenecid), any increase in serum uric acid usually requires a decrease in dose or possibly discontinuation of the diuretic. If acute gouty arthritis is precipitated, then treatment of gout, discontinuation of the diuretic, or both should be considered. Very few patients have to discontinue a thiazide diuretic secondary to exacerbation of gout.[101] A history of gout is not a contraindication to diuretic therapy but is a potentially unfavorable effect. B.A.'s serum uric acid concentration is elevated, but switching to a different agent or

Table 13-11 Reasons for not Attaining Goal Blood Pressure Despite Antihypertensive Pharmacotherapy

Drug Related	*Health Condition or Lifestyle Related*	*Other*
Nonadherence	Volume overload	Improper blood pressure measurement
Inadequate antihypertensive dose	Excess sodium intake	Resistant hypertension
Inappropriate antihypertensive combination therapy	Volume retention from chronic kidney disease	
Inadequate diuretic therapy	Secondary disease causes (Table 13-3)	
Secondary drug-induced causes (Table 13-3)	Obesity	
	Excessive alcohol intake	

lowering the dose of HCTZ is unnecessary because she is not symptomatic.

27. How much will HCTZ alter B.A.'s cholesterol values?

Dyslipidemia is a potential side effect of diuretic therapy. Alterations are characterized by small increases in LDL-C and small increases in triglycerides. Dietary fat restrictions help minimize, but do not necessarily prevent, these effects. Contrary to other biochemical disturbances, diuretic-induced changes in the lipid profile are not dose related, but overall changes are small. Many clinical trials lasting more than 1 year have shown that hypercholesterolemia and hypertriglyceridemia with diuretic therapy is not sustained with prolonged use.[23,97] Even if these changes are persistent, they are not clinically significant with the doses of thiazide diuretics used for hypertension because the absolute changes are very small. Diuretic therapy should never be avoided in patients with dyslipidemia. B.A. should continue to use her HCTZ.

28. What other metabolic abnormalities should be considered because of B.A.'s thiazide diuretic therapy?

Hyponatremia is a serious, yet infrequent adverse effect of diuretics. Changes in sodium concentrations are usually small, and patients are usually asymptomatic. Decreased renal excretion of free water, inappropriate antidiuretic hormone secretion, urinary sodium loss, and depletion of magnesium and potassium may all contribute to diuretic-induced hyponatremia. Hyponatremia, especially severe hyponatremia (<120 mEq/L), which rarely occurs with diuretic therapy, definitely requires discontinuation of the diuretic when present.

Hypomagnesemia is an often-overlooked metabolic complication of diuretic therapy. Both thiazide and loop diuretics increase urinary excretion of magnesium in a dose-dependent manner. Symptoms of significant hypomangnesemia include muscle weakness, muscle tremor or twitching, mental status changes, and cardiac arrhythmias (including torsades de pointes). Presence of these symptoms would necessitate magnesium supplementation. Hypomagnesemia frequently coexists with hypokalemia. Unless hypomagnesemia is corrected, potassium replacement therapy for hypokalemia can be ineffective, even when high doses of potassium are given.

Thiazide diuretics decrease urinary calcium excretion and have been used to prevent stone formation in patients with calcium-related kidney stones. The resulting systemic retention of calcium does not result in elevated serum calcium concentrations and does not place patients at risk for hypercalcemia. This effect, however, may be beneficial in women at risk for osteoporosis (e.g., postmenopausal) such as B.A. or in patients with osteoporosis. Unlike thiazide diuretics, loop diuretics increase renal clearance of calcium and are used for acute management of severe hypercalcemia.

Reasons for Inadequate BP Control

29. What are common reasons for inadequate patient response to antihypertensive pharmacotherapy?

The classification of B.A.'s current BP is prehypertension, but this is misleading and not helpful in her treatment at this point. She has uncontrolled hypertension because her BP values are above her goal of <130/80 mmHg. The full antihypertensive effect of HCTZ has been achieved since she has been on her current dose for 4 weeks. She has had a response, but it still is inadequate. Potential reasons for an inadequate response, or lack of attaining BP goal values, with an antihypertensive should be considered before choosing to modify her drug therapy regimen (Table 13-11). Evaluation requires a comprehensive medication history and medical evaluation to rule out identifiable causes, in particular nonadherance to the prescribed dosing regimen. Based on the given information, her BP measurements appear accurate, and the BP reduction she has experienced is typical and predictable. Her kidney function is good and no evidence exists of edema, so volume overload is unlikely. There are no apparent secondary causes of elevated BP. It is reasonable to conclude that B.A. needs additional therapy to achieve her goal BP. It is very common that most patients require two or three antihypertensive agents to attain BP goal values, especially when goal values are <130/80 mmHg.

Modifying Therapy

B.A.'s present dose of HCTZ is appropriate and should not be increased to the maximal recommended dose of 50 mg daily (considered high-dose therapy). An increased risk exists of side effects and minimal to no additional BP lowering occurs when increasing from 25 to 50 mg of HCTZ.[22,102] B.A.'s potassium dropped to 3.8 mEq/L with HCTZ, and further dosage increases may produce significant hypokalemia (<3.5 mEq/L) requiring supplementation. Her hyperuricemia may also be worsened. Discontinuing HCTZ and starting a different agent is an option, but is not ideal for several reasons. HCTZ lowered her BP; it is known to reduce CV events is inexpensive, and may benefit her osteoporosis. Hypokalemia might lead some clinicians to switch to another agent, possibly because of a higher propensity to increase glucose, but her potassium is still within the normal range, and the addition of an ACEI or ARB will favorably affect her potassium.

Two-Drug Regimens

The role of two-drug regimens in the treatment of hypertension is very clear. Most patients require multiple agents for BP control, especially in populations with BP goals of <130/80 mmHg or lower. Both the JNC7 and AHA guidelines strongly recommend two-drug regimens as initial therapy for patients in stage 2 hypertension, and also cite a two-drug regimen as an option for initial therapy in stage 1 hypertension.[5,9,65,75]

Adding a second agent to B.A.'s regimen is needed to reduce BP to her goal of <130/80 mmHg. Because she is a primary prevention patient, three potential add-on antihypertensive agents that are considered first-line include an ACEI, ARB, or CCB. Ideally, a combination of two drugs with different mechanisms of action should be selected to produce a complementary effect to lower BP.

COMBINATIONS THAT INCLUDE A THIAZIDE

Thiazide diuretics, when combined with several agents (especially an ACEI, ARB, and even a β-blocker), result in additive antihypertensive effects that are independent of reversing fluid retention. Diuretics reduce BP initially by decreasing fluid volume, but maintain their antihypertensive effects by lowering PVR. BP lowering, however, can stimulate renin release from the kidney and activate the RAAS. This compensatory mechanism is an in vivo attempt to neutralize BP changes and regulate fluid loss. An ACEI or an ARB blocks the RAAS, explaining why combinations of these agents with diuretics are additive. One mechanism by which β-blockers reduce BP is by suppressing renin release and activity, resulting in additive BP lowering in combination with a thiazide diuretic. Certain nondiuretic antihypertensive agents (i.e., aliskiren, reserpine, arterial vasodilators, and centrally acting agents) can eventually cause significant sodium retention and increased fluid volume. These agents should ideally be given in combination with a diuretic to maximize BP lowering.

LESS EFFICACIOUS COMBINATIONS

The combination of an ACEI or ARB with a β-blocker provides less additional BP lowering compared with other combination regimens. The primary mechanism of action of an ACEI or ARB is to decrease the effects of angiotensin-2. Less angiotensin-2 is produced when PRA is suppressed by β-blockers. Therefore, if the angiotensin-2–mediated BP effects are suppressed by a β-blocker, adding a β-blocker to an ACEI or ARB might not result in a highly additive effect. Although this combination may not be highly additive, it is often used when multiple conditions or compelling indications require treatment with each of these agents (e.g., hypertension with CAD, left ventricular dysfunction).[5]

Other combinations are only minimally effective at producing significant BP lowering compared with monotherapy. An ACE in combination with an ARB may be used in left ventricular dysfunction or in patients with certain forms of very advanced chronic kidney disease. Absent these conditions, however, this combination is minimally effective at producing significant BP lowering. Similarly, the use of a dihydropyridine CCB in combination with a nondihydropyridine CCB may lower BP, but the overlapping mechanism of action results in less than ideal reductions in BP. These combinations should be used as last-line alternative combinations when BP reduction is the only purpose for using combination therapy.

FIXED-DOSE COMBINATION PRODUCTS

Several fixed-dose combination products are available (Table 13-12). Although individual dose titration is not easy with fixed-dose combination products, their use can reduce the number of tablets or capsules taken by patients. This can benefit patients by promoting adherence, which may increase the likelihood of achieving or maintaining goal BP values.

Table 13-12 Common Combination Antihypertensive Agents

Combination Type	*Fixed-Dose Combination*	*Unit Strengths (mg/mg)*
ACEI with thiazide diuretic	Benazepril/HCTZ (Lotensin HCT)	5/6.25, 10/12.5, 20/12.5, 20/25
	Captopril/HCTZ (Capozide)	25/15, 25/25, 50/15, 50/25
	Enalapril/HCTZ (Vaseretic)	5/12.5, 10/25
	Lisinopril/HCTZ (Prinzide, Zestoretic)	10/12.5, 20/12.5, 20/25
	Moexipril/HCTZ (Uniretic)	7.5/12.5, 15/25
	Quinapril/HCTZ (Accuretic)	10/12.5, 20/12.5, 20/25
ARB with thiazide diuretic	Candesartan cilexetil/HCTZ (Atacand HCT)	16/12.5, 32/12.5
	Eprosartan mesylate/HCTZ (Teveten HCT)	600/12.5, 600/25
	Irbesartan/HCTZ (Avalide)	150/12.5, 300/12.5, 300/25
	Losartan potassium/HCTZ (Hyzaar)	50/12.5, 100/12.5, 100/25
	Olmesartan medoxomil/HCTZ (Benicar HCT)	20/12.5, 40/12.5, 40/25
	Telmisartan/HCTZ (Micardis HCT)	40/12.5, 80/12.5, 80/25
	Valsartan/HCTZ (Diovan HCT)	80/12.5, 160/12.5, 160/25, 300/12.5, 300/25
ACEI with CCB	Amlodipine besylate/Benazepril hydrochloride (Lotrel)	2.5/10, 5/10, 5/20, 10/20, 5/40, 10/40
	Enalapril/Felodipine (Lexxel)	5/5
	Trandolapril/Verapamil (Tarka)	2/180, 1/240, 2/240, 4/240
CCB with ARB	Amlodipine/Valsartan (Exforge)	5/160, 5/320, 10/160, 10/320
	Amlodipine/Olmesartan medoxomil (AZOR)	5/20, 5/40, 10/20, 10/40

ACEI, angiotensin converting enzyme inhibitor; ARB, angiotensin-2 receptor blocker; CCB, calcium channel blocker; HCTZ, hydrochlorothiazide.

Most fixed-dose combinations include a thiazide diuretic and many are available generically. Other fixed-dose combination products combine a CCB with either an ACEI or ARB. These combinations, similar to a thiazide with an ACE or ARB, are highly effective in lowering BP. Use of fixed-dose combination products should continue to increase because the 2007 AHA guidelines recommend lower BP goals for many populations, more combination products are available, and the bottom line is that many patients need multiple agents to attain their BP goal. Clinicians should be comfortable with choosing a fixed-dose combination product in an attempt to simplify regimens and expedite goal achievement. An economic advantage may even exist to using a fixed-dose combination if it allows the patient to receive two drugs for one medication copayment.

B.A. is a candidate for a thiazide-containing fixed-dose combination product. Many options exist because nearly all of these combinations utilize a 12.5 and 25 mg hydrochlorothiazide dose. Cost should be considered because this is a concern for B.A. She has no compelling indications that require selection of a specific second antihypertensive drug class. The most attractive second agent for her is either an ACEI or an ARB. B.A. has no reason to avoid a CCB, and this would be a reasonable second agent. An ACEI or ARB is more reasonable, however, because these agents may blunt some of the potassium loss that she has experienced, and may also delay progression to type 2 diabetes.[99,100,103] After this second agent is added to her regimen, her BP, serum potassium, and serum creatinine should be reassessed in 2 to 4 weeks.

Step-Down Therapy

30. T.J., a 58-year-old man has a 10-year history of hypertension. He has been treated with lisinopril/hydrochlorothiazide 20/25 mg daily and amlodipine 10 mg daily for more than 2 years and his BP has been well controlled during this time. He has no compelling indications for specific antihypertensive agents and has no hypertension-associated complications. His Framingham risk score is 18% and his BP is 118/74 and 116/72 mmHg. He denies any problems, dizziness, or difficulties with his medications. Should his antihypertensive therapy be changed to reduce his medication doses and/or possibly discontinue some of his medications?

Few patients with hypertension can later have their BP medications slowly withdrawn, resulting in normal BP values for weeks or months following discontinuation of their medications. This is called *step-down therapy*. It is not a feasible option for most patients with hypertension. Primary prevention patients with a goal BP $<140/90$ mmHg who have very well-controlled BP for at least 1 year might be eligible for a trial of step-down therapy. This option should not be considered for patients who have a Framingham risk score $\geq 10\%$, compelling indications, or hypertension-associated complications.

Step-down therapy consists of attempting to gradually decrease the dosage, number of antihypertensive drugs, or both without compromising BP control. Abrupt or large dosage reductions should be avoided because of the risk of rapid return of uncontrolled blood pressure and even rebound surges in blood pressure. In particular, rapid withdrawal of a β-blocker or an α_2-agonist (e.g., clonidine) can be problematic owing to increased receptor sensitivity following long-term receptor up-regulation (see Question 60).

Step-down therapy is most often plausible for patients who have lost significant amounts of weight or have drastically changed their lifestyle. Any attempt at step-down therapy must be accompanied by scheduled follow-up evaluations because BP values can rise over months to years after drug discontinuation, especially if lifestyle modifications are not maintained.

Step-down therapy in T.J. is not an option. Although he does not have compelling indications or hypertension-associated complications, he is considered a high CV risk primary prevention patient based on his Framinghan risk score. Although his BP might be viewed as "low," he does not have symptomatic hypotension, and his BP is considered normal.

ACEI

31. A.R. is a 49-year-old black woman with type 2 diabetes mellitus. She started lisinopril 10 mg daily 4 weeks ago when her BP values were consistently in the high end of the stage 1 hypertension range (156/98 mmHg). Since then, she has had weekly BP measurements and her values have averaged 142/85 mmHg despite strict adherence to her lifestyle modifications. Her BP today is 144/84 mmHg (140/88 when repeated), and her heart rate is 78 beats/minure. She is not a smoker, and her BMI is 29 kg/m^2 (considered overweight). Her latest hemoglobin A1C was 8.5% (goal for diabetes is $<$7%). All her laboratory test results, including kidney function, are within normal limits, except that her spot urine albumin-to-creatinine ratio is 80 mg/g (4 weeks ago it was 90 mg/g). How long should A.R. take lisinopril before her BP response is evaluated?

The ACEI lower BP primarily by causing peripheral arterial vasodilation without significant changes in cardiac output, heart rate, or GFR. The principal activity of an ACEI is through inhibition of the RAAS. ACEIs are believed to provide unique CV benefits by improving endothelial function, promoting LVH regression and collateral vessel development, and improving insulin sensitivity.[104,105] The effects on renal blood flow and glomerular filtration are complex, depending on sodium balance and if renal artery stenosis is present.

Pharmacotherapy Considerations

Several ACEIs are currently marketed for the management of hypertension (Table 13-13). Some agents are primarily renally eliminated (benazepril, enalapril, lisinopril, quinapril, ramipril); others have mixed hepatic and renal elimination (captopril, fosinopril, perindopril, trandolapril), and moexipril is almost completely hepatically eliminated. These characteristics may be important when selecting a product in patients with unstable organ function. Other differences, such as a slower rate of elimination, a longer duration of action, prolonged onset of action with prodrugs, and a slower dissociation from binding sites, have been described. These differences, however, have not been shown to have major clinical importance.

The time to reach steady-state BP conditions is similar to what is seen with other antihypertensive agents. Following the initiation of therapy, it may take several weeks before the full antihypertensive effects of these drugs are observed. Therefore, evaluating BP response 2 to 4 weeks after starting or

Table 13-13 ACEI in Hypertension

Drug	Usual Starting Dose[a] (mg/day)	Usual Dosage Range (mg/day)	Dosing Frequency
Benazepril (Lotensin)	10	20–40	Daily to BID
Captopril (Capoten)	25	50–100	BID to TID
Enalapril (Vasotec)	5	10–40	Daily to BID
Fosinopril (Monopril)	10	20–40	Daily
Lisinopril (Prinivil, Zestril)	10	20–40	Daily
Moexipril (Univasc)	7.5	7.5–30	Daily to BID
Perindopril (Aceon)	4	4–16	Daily
Quinapril (Accupril)	10	20–80	Daily to BID
Ramipril (Altace)	2.5	2.5–20	Daily to BID
Trandolapril (Mavik)	1	2–4	Daily

[a] Starting dose may be decreased 50% if patient is volume depleted, in acute heart failure exacerbation, or are very elderly (≥75 yrs).
ACEI, angiotensin converting enzyme inhibitor; BID, twice daily; TID, three times daily.

changing the dose of an ACEI is appropriate. A.R. has been taking lisinopril for 4 weeks, and her present BP should be used to determine whether she has attained goal. Both her BP range over the past few weeks and today's average BP are above her goal of <130/80 mmHg (because she has diabetes).

Most ACEI are dosed once daily in hypertension (Table 13-13). Captopril is the only one for which at least twice daily dosing is needed. In general, most ACEI, if used in equivalent doses, are considered interchangeable.

32. Why should A.R. have serum potassium and serum creatinine monitored while on lisinopril therapy?

The ACEI can increase serum potassium as a result of aldosterone reduction. Potassium increases with ACEI monotherapy are very small and typically do not result in hyperkalemia. This risk is increased, however, when used in patients with significant chronic kidney disease (estimated GFR <60 mL/minute/1.73 m^2), or when used in combination with other drugs that can also raise potassium (i.e., an ARB, potassium-sparing diuretics, aldosterone antagonists). ACEI therapy can also cause a small increase in serum creatinine, owing to decreased vasoconstriction of the efferent arteriole in the kidney. This results in a small decrease in GFR that may be realized as a small increase in serum creatinine. One common mistake is to discontinue an ACEI when there is a modest rise in serum creatinine. Increases in serum creatinine of up to 35% from the baseline creatinine value are safe and anticipated. In these patients, the ACEI should be continued because they are more likely to benefit from the renal protective effects.[75] An ACEI can, however, also cause acute renal compromise (primarily in a small subset of patients with bilateral renal artery stenosis). In these patients, the increase in serum creatinine will be much greater than 35% and would necessitate discontinuing ACEI therapy.

Serum potassium and serum creatinine need to be monitored because of A.R.'s ACEI therapy. This should be done 2 to 4 weeks after starting ACEI therapy or increasing the dose. This is the same time frame at which BP should also be measured.

33. A.R.'s lisinopril dose is increased to 20 mg daily. Although A.R. did not experience hypotension when she first started lisinopril, will this doubling of her dose place her at risk for significant hypotension?

Patients who are either very elderly, volume depleted, or have a heart failure exacerbation may experience a significant first-dose response to an ACEI. This can manifest as orthostatic hypotension, dizziness, or possibly syncope. The increased pretreatment activity of the RAAS, coupled with acute blockade of this system by an ACEI, explains this effect. These patients should initiate ACEI therapy at half the normal dose (Table 13-13), and be slowly titrated up to standard doses.

Concurrent diuretic therapy may predispose some patients to first-dose hypotension. When ACEIs were first approved, dosing guidelines recommended starting at half the standard dose of the ACEI, decreasing the dose of the diuretic, or stopping the diuretic before initiating the ACEI. This was owing to fear that BP would sharply and acutely drop. These recommendations are not necessary unless the patient is hemodynamically unstable (volume depleted, hyponatremic, or poorly compensated heart failure), or very elderly. A.R. does not have any of these characteristics; thus, she did not experience first-dose hypotension. Currently, she does not have these characteristics and can safely increase her dose of lisinopril without fear of significant hypotension.

34. Will an ACEI work in A.R. because she is black?

ACEI monotherapy is more effective at lowering BP in young white patients than in black or elderly patients.[30] Elderly and black patients are more likely to have low renin hypertension, which may partially explain some of the differences in response. Nevertheless, many of these patients still respond to ACEI as monotherapy. Combination therapy, especially with a diuretic, can often overcome the race- or age-related differences in BP response to an ACEI. In patients whose conditions do not adequately respond to an ACEI, the addition of a low-dose diuretic (e.g., HCTZ 12.5 mg) can significantly enhance the antihypertensive effect.[24] Thiazide diuretic use results in compensatory increases in renin. An ACEI in combination with a thiazide is considered a very additive antihypertensive combination through complementary mechanisms.

When an antihypertensive agent is being selected as initial monotherapy in a primary prevention black patient, an ACEI should generally not be chosen. A thiazide diuretic or CCB is preferred. If a compelling indication, such as left ventricular dysfunction, diabetes, or chronic kidney disease is present, an ACEI is a drug of choice. When selecting initial combination therapy in a primary prevention black patient, a combination of an ACEI with either a thiazide or a CCB can be selected. Of note, black patients have a two- to four-fold increased risk of angioedema and cough compared with whites.[45] Although this does not preclude ACEI use in black patients, it requires patient education regarding these potential side effects.

A.R. should not be treated as a primary prevention patient. She has type 2 diabetes mellitus, which is a compelling indication for an ACEI. She also has microalbuminuria, which further justifies ACEI use as a first-line therapy. A.R. is also above her goal BP of <130/80 mmHg. Although an ACEI is ideal treatment, a monotherapy approach is not expected to get her to goal. She has had some BP reduction from lisinopril, and the dose could be increased to the maximum, but she will likely require the addition of a second agent, preferably a thiazide diuretic (Fig. 13-3).

Compelling Indications

Angiotensin-converting enzyme inhibitor therapy is recommended for all compelling indications, either as first-line therapy or as a component of sequential add-on therapy. Evidence has clearly demonstrated reduction in hypertension-associated complications in patients with these medical conditions. ACEIs are also useful as a first-line treatment option for primary prevention patients, including those who may not adequately respond to other therapies, or those who cannot take other first-line agents owing to contraindications or adverse reactions (e.g., patients with asthma, gout).

DIABETES

Angiotensin-converting enzyme inhibitor therapy is strongly recommended first-line to manage hypertension in diabetes based on evidence showing reduced hypertension-associated complications, including CV events and kidney disease.[5,72] In particular, a substudy of the Heart Outcomes Prevention Evaluation (HOPE) study showed that in 3,577 patients with diabetes, ramipril significantly reduced CV events and overt nephropathy.[50] Additional clinical trials' data have demonstrated that the combination of an ACEI with a thiazide diuretic significantly reduces the risk of major CV events and death in patients with type 2 diabetes and hypertension.[106] These data further reinforce the role of ACEI in patients with diabetes and hypertension, and also the benefits of combination therapy in this population.

An added benefit of ACEI in diabetes is that they do not have metabolic adverse effects on glucose as may other agents. Moreover, the favorable effects on insulin resistance result in a lower risk of progressing to type 2 diabetes in patients with hypertension who do not have diabetes, when compared with thiazide diuretics, a CCB or β-blockers.[103]

CHRONIC KIDNEY DISEASE

The ACEI protect the kidney from the unrelenting deterioration that occurs with chronic kidney disease, hypertension, and diabetes.[5,72,75] Therefore, these agents are first-line options in chronic kidney disease. Chronic kidney disease is characterized by increased intraglomerular pressure and mesangial cell proliferation, which leads to proteinuria and a progressive decline in kidney function. Reductions in renal blood flow cause the kidneys to increase renin release, thus activating the RAAs. This action constricts the efferent renal arteriole to preserve glomerular pressure, but may aggravate further renal impairment.

The ACEI preferentially dilate the efferent arteriole, which relieves intraglomerular pressure. Data suggest that ACEI may have unique renal preservation properties, making chronic kidney disease a compelling indication for ACEI therapy. Some of the risk reduction is also related to systemic BP lowering.[26]

Patients with diabetes are at risk for nephropathy. This is especially true in type 1 diabetes. Evidence indicates that ACEI therapy reduces progression to severe chronic kidney disease and kidney failure in patients with type 1 diabetes and proteinuria.[76] ACEI therapy also reduces worsening of proteinuria in patients with type 2 diabetes and proteinuria,[75] but evidence showing progression to severe chronic kidney disease or failure is not available. Nonetheless, ACEI therapy is considered highly effective and is strongly recommended as a compelling indication in both type 1 and type 2 diabetes.

CHRONIC AND ACUTE CAD

Angiotensin-converting enzyme inhibitor therapy is recommended first-line treatment in all patients with chronic CAD (post-MI, chronic stable angina) and acute CAD (non–ST-segment elevation MI, ST-segment elevation MI).[36,78,84,85] This is in addition to β-blocker therapy. The benefits of ACEI therapy in patients with CAD is a reduced risk of CV events that is independent of both LV function and BP. ACEI therapy will not provide anti-ischemic effects. Therefore, the role of ACEI therapy in CAD is as an add-on to a β-blocker to reduce CV risk, but not to treat underlying ischemic symptoms.

PRIOR STROKE

The perindopril protection against recurrent stroke study (PROGRESS) was a double-blind, placebo-controlled evaluation of an ACEI in combination with a thiazide diuretic for 4 years in 6,105 patients with a history of stroke or transient ischemic attack.[46] Hypertensive and nonhypertensive patients were included. The incidence of stroke and total major vascular events were significantly reduced with the combination regimen, and reductions were seen regardless of baseline BP or reduction in BP. These data justify the compelling indication to use an ACEI (in combination with a thiazide diuretic) to reduce recurrence of stroke in patients who have had a stroke.

LEFT VENTRICULAR DYSFUNCTION

Angiotensin-converting enzyme inhibitors reduce morbidity and mortality in patients with left ventricular dysfunction.[86] Standard therapy for left ventricular dysfunction consists of a diuretic with an ACEI followed by the addition of a β-blocker. Although either an ARB or an aldosterone antagonist can reduce morbidity and mortality in patients with left ventricular dysfunction, either one of these agents may ideally be used in addition to standard therapy. Therefore, ACEI with diuretic therapy is the first-line intervention in patients with hypertension with left ventricular dysfunction. In general, the CV benefit of ACEI therapy in left ventricular dysfunction is considered a class effect, and ACEI are used interchangeably at equivalent dosages in these patients.[9]

Other Considerations

Although an ACEI may not lower BP as well in elderly patients as in young patients, this is also true for black patients when compared with white patients. BP lowering, however, is only a surrogate marker of overall effectiveness of antihypertensive agents. The ability of an ACEI to reduce CV events appears to be equal across all of these patient populations.[48] Therefore, the overall tendency to avoid ACEI therapy because it might not be as effective in lowering BP should not be a consideration in selecting therapy when an ACEI is compellingly indicated in an elderly patient or in a black patient. This should be a consideration when selecting initial monotherapy to treat hypertension in a primary prevention patient who is either elderly or black; a thiazide diuretic or CCB would be a better initial agent as monotherapy than an ACEI (or ARB) with respect to BP lowering. When an ACEI (or ARB) is used in combination with a thiazide diuretic or CCB, however, the differences in BP lowering are less apparent because the additive antihypertensive effect of using these combinations neutralizes any differences in response that are based on age or race.[64]

35. **A.R. has microalbuminuria based on her spot urine. ACEI therapy may help preserve her kidney function, but is there a risk that ACEI can also cause acute renal dysfunction?**

The ACEIs are effective in patients with hypertension-associated renal disease. They are contraindicated, however, in bilateral renal artery stenosis, pregnancy, and volume depletion (Table 13-10). They should be used cautiously in patients who have suspected bilateral renal artery stenosis, or in those who have stenosis in a solitary kidney after nephrectomy. In these patients, high angiotensin concentrations maintain renal blood flow. Acute renal dysfunction can occur when an ACEI is started. Because it is often not known if a patient has bilateral renal artery stenosis, problems with ACEI can be minimized by starting with recommended doses and careful monitoring of serum creatinine within 4 weeks of starting therapy. Modest elevations in serum creatinine that are <35% (for baseline creatinine values <3.0 mg/dL) do not warrant changes.[75] These changes might even be expected in some patients. If greater increases occur, ACEI therapy should be stopped. Patients with elevated serum creatinine at baseline (up to 3.0 mg/dL) may particularly benefit from the vasodilatory effects of ACEI in the kidney, but definitely require close monitoring. A.R.'s renal function tests were normal after 4 weeks of lisinopril therapy. She is not experiencing any kidney-related adverse effects from lisinopril.

36. **What are the risks of using ACEIs in women of childbearing age?**

Because ACEI are teratogenic in the second and third trimester,[107] their use in pregnancy is contraindicated. Moreover, their use in women of child-bearing potential is discouraged. If used in this population, patient education should be explicitly clear regarding risks to the fetus, which include potentially fatal hypotension, anuria, renal failure, and developmental deformities. A highly effective form of contraception should be strongly recommended.

ARB

37. **Four weeks after increasing lisinopril to 20 mg daily, A.R.'s BP is 126/78 mmHg (128/76 mmHg when repeated). Her serum potassium and creatinine are unchanged from previous values. Her husband states, however, that she has had a persistent dry cough for the past few months that sometimes keeps them both awake at night. She has no additional signs suggesting upper respiratory infection or left ventricular dysfunction. Should A.R.'s lisinopril be replaced with an ARB?**

A well-known side effect of ACEI is a nonproductive, dry cough, which can occur in up to 15% of patients.[108] Patients may describe this as a tickling sensation in the back of the throat that commonly occurs late in the evening. This is distinctly different from the cough associated with left ventricular dysfunction, which is associated with crackles and rales (on auscultation) that may be wet and productive. ACEI-related cough subsides with discontinuation. Many agents have been used to treat an ACEI cough with poor results. The best treatment option for a patient with an intolerable ACEI cough is to switch agents. For A.R., switching to an ARB would likely eliminate the dry cough and still be considered an acceptable first-line treatment option for her hypertension considering her history of diabetes.[9,72] ARB therapy would also have similar benefits to an ACEI considering her microalbuminuria.

ARBs are considered first-line options for primary prevention patients and have data demonstrating reductions in CV events.[9,20,22] Seven of these agents are commercially available as brand-name only products (Table 13-14). Fixed-dose combination products with HCTZ are also available (Table 13-12).

Table 13-14 ARB in Hypertension

Drug	Starting Dose[a] (mg/day)	Usual Dosage Range (mg/day)	Dosing Frequency
Candesartan cilexetil (Atacand)	16	8–32	Daily to BID
Eprosartan mesylate (Teveten)	600	600–800	Daily to BID
Irbesartan (Avapro)	150	75–300	Daily
Losartan potassium (Cozaar)	50	25–100	Daily to BID
Olmesartan medoxomil (Benicar)	20	20–40	Daily
Telmisartan (Micardis)	40	20–80	Daily
Valsartan (Diovan)	80–160	80–320	Daily

[a] Starting dose may be decreased 50% if patient is volume depleted, very elderly, or taking a diuretic.

ARB, angiotensin-2 receptor blocker; BID, twice daily; TID, three times daily.

38. **How exactly do ACEIs and ARBs differ in regard to their mechanism of action?**

Pharmacologic Differences between an ACEI and an ARB

Unlike ACEIs, ARBs specifically bind to angiotensin-2 receptors in vascular smooth muscle, adrenal glands, and other tissues. As a result, access of angiotensin-2 to its receptors is blocked and angiotensin-2–mediated vasoconstriction and aldosterone release is prevented, resulting in BP reduction. Reduction in intraglomerular blood flow and pressure is mediated by angiotensin-2 actions in the efferent arteriole of the kidney. ARBs do not affect bradykinin, therefore dry cough does not occur.

Considerable investigation has focused on describing the pharmacologic differences between the angiotensin-2 type 1 and type 2 receptors. Stimulation of the type 1 receptor causes vasoconstriction, salt and water retention, and vascular remodeling. Other deleterious effects from type 1 receptor stimulation include myocyte and smooth muscle hypertrophy, fibroblast hyperplasia, cytotoxic effects in the myocardium, altered gene expression, and possible increased concentrations of plasminogen activator inhibitor. Stimulation of the type 2 receptor results in antiproliferative actions, cell differentiation, and tissue repair when stimulated.

Theoretically, an ideal antihypertensive agent would block only type 1 and not type 2 receptors as is the case with currently marketed ARBs. Therefore, it is possible that an ARB would be superior to an ACEI in reducing hypertension-associated complications because ACEIs ultimately decrease stimulation of both type 1 and type 2 receptors by decreasing production of angiotensin-2. This argument is purely speculative and is not supported by clinical trial data. The Ongoing Telmisartan Alone and in Combination with Ramipril Global Endpoint Trial (ONTARGET) was a prospective, double-blind, randomized controlled trial that directly compared ARB and ACEI therapy.[109] After a median of 56 months, the incidence of CV events was similar with both treatments. Therefore, as a class, ARBs are as effective as other antihypertensive agents for BP lowering. Similar to ACEI, combinations with a thiazide diuretic are highly efficacious in lowering BP.

Compelling Indications

39. Under what circumstances would an ARB be a better initial antihypertensive agent than an ACEI?

DIABETES

Patients with diabetes should be treated with either an ACEI or ARB. ARB-based treatment regimens have been shown in clinical trials to reduce the progression of diabetic nephropathy.[72] These benefits are similar to what is seen with ACEI, but only among patients with type 2 diabetes who have microalbuminuria. ARB-based therapy contains the only antihypertensive agents for which evidence shows reduced kidney failure in patients with type 2 diabetes who have diabetic nephropathy with albuminuria (not microalbuminuria) and elevated serum creatinine.[56] Therefore, for patients with type 2 diabetes and advanced nephropathy, evidence supports ARB therapy as the primary antihypertensive agent, ahead of ACEI therapy.

CHRONIC KIDNEY DISEASE

An ARB, similar to an ACEI, minimizes damage that occurs with chronic kidney disease. Both ACEIs and ARBs preferentially dilate the efferent arteriole, which relieves intraglomerular pressure. Thus, chronic kidney disease is a compelling indication for ARB therapy. For nondiabetic kidney disease, less evidence supports ARB use, and these agents should be reserved as alternatives to an ACEI.

CHRONIC AND ACUTE CAD

Angiotensin receptor blocker therapy is a reasonable alternative to ACEI therapy in patients with CAD. Data are very limited, however. For patients post-MI, ARB therapy has been evaluated, and is an option for patients with intolerable side effects from an ACEI. For patients with chronic stable angina or acute coronary syndromes, long-term data evaluating effects on CV events are not available.

PRIOR STROKE

Angiotensin receptor blocker therapy is an evidence-based alternative to the combination of an ACEI with a thiazide diuretic in patients with a history of ischemic stroke or transient ischemic attack. In the Morbidity and Mortality after Stroke Eprosartan Compared with Nitreadipine for Secondary Prevention (MOSES) study, ARB-based therapy reduced the incidence of recurrent stroke more than dihydropyridine CCB-based therapy in a large number of patients with cerebrovascular disease.[63] Based on these data, prior stroke (ischemic stroke) is a compelling indication for ARB therapy.

LEFT VENTRICULAR DYSFUNCTION

Pharmacologic blockade of the renin-angiotensin-aldosterone system in left ventricular dysfunction is of paramount importance. An ARB is a reasonable alternative in patients with hypertension and left ventricular dysfunction who cannot tolerate an ACEI (e.g., those who experience cough).[93] They should, however, never be empirically used in place of an ACEI, because ACEI therapy is considered superior to ARB therapy in patients with left ventricular dysfunction.[86] As sequential add-on therapy for patients with left ventricular dysfunction who are already treated with the standard regimen of a diuretic with an ACEI and β-blocker, ARB therapy has been proved to reduce risk of CV events.[94] Clinicians should be aware that if an ARB is used in combination with an ACEI, a significant increase in risk of side effects exists, particularly hyperkalemia.[109,110]

Other Considerations

ARB VERSUS ACEI

Monitoring requirements, contraindications, and side effects (other than cough) are the same for ARBs and ACEIs. Because of the potential hyperkalemia and acute renal dysfunction, serum creatinine and potassium should be monitored. Both drug classes are contraindicated in pregnancy and in patients with bilateral renal artery stenosis or volume depletion. Acute hypotension is possible when starting ARB therapy in patients with hyponatremia, volume depletion, or left ventricular dysfunction exacerbation.

40. If A.R. experienced angioedema from lisinopril, would treatment with an ARB be contraindicated?

A history of ACEI angioedema is not a contraindication to ARB therapy. The cross-reactivity between angioedema with an ACEI and ARB is not exactly known. The best available data come from the Candesartan in Heart Failure: Assessment of Reduction in Mortality and Morbidity (CHARM)-alternative study where 39 patients with left ventricular dysfunction and a history of ACEI angioedema were treated long term with ARB therapy.[93] Only one of these patients experienced repeat angioedema that required discontinuation of the ARB. This small cross-reactivity rate has been demonstrated in other evaluations.[111] Therefore, cross-reactivity appears possible, but unlikely.

When the benefits of an agent that blocks the RAAS is needed (e.g., left ventricular dysfunction, diabetes, chronic kidney disease), an ARB is a reasonable alternative for patients with ACEI angioedema. The ACC/AHA guidelines recommend an ARB in patients who have experienced angioedema from an ACEI.[86] Nonetheless, patients with a history of ACEI angioedema should be counseled regarding the small potential for recurrent angioedema if treated with an ARB.

CCB

41. How do dihydropyridine CCB differ from the nondihydropyridine CCB, verapamil and diltiazem?

Table 13-15 Pharmacologic Actions of CCB

	Nondihydropyridines		
	Verapamil	Diltiazem	Dihydropyridines
Peripheral vasodilation	+	+	++
Heart rate	−−	−	+
Cardiac contractility	−−	−	0/−[a]
Atrioventricular nodal conduction	−	−	0
Coronary blood flow	+	+	++

[a]No significant decreases are seen with amlodipine or felodipine.
+, increase; ++, marked increase; −, decrease; −−, marked decrease; 0, no change.
CCB, calcium channel blocker.

Calcium channel blockers are very effective in lowering BP. Elderly and black patients have greater BP reduction with a CCB than with other agents (β-blockers, ACEIs, ARBs). The addition of a diuretic to a CCB provides additive antihypertensive effects. CCBs do not alter serum lipids, glucose, uric acid, or electrolytes and they do not aggravate asthma or peripheral vascular disease.

A heterogeneous drug class, all CCBs inhibit the movement of extracellular calcium, but there are two primary subtypes: dihydropyridines and nondihydropyridines (i.e., diltiazem and verapamil). Each has distinctly different pharmacologic effects that are summarized in Table 13-15.

Dihydropyridines

Dihydropyridines are potent vasodilators of peripheral and coronary arteries. They do not block artrioventricular (AV) nodal conduction and do not effectively treat arrhythmias. Moreover, the potent vasodilation associated with most dihydropyridines can induce a reflex tachycardia. With the exception of amlodipine and felodipine, dihydropyridines can decrease cardiac contractility and should be avoided in patients with left ventricular dysfunction. Side effects of dihydropyridines are related to their potent vasodilatory effects, such as reflex tachycardia, headache, flushing, and peripheral edema.

Nondihydropyridines

The nondihydropyridines, diltiazem and verapamil, are similar. Relative to dihydropyridines, they are only moderately potent vasodilators, but they directly decrease AV nodal conduction and have negative inotropic actions. The blockade of AV nodal conduction can slow heart rate and is the basis for their use in treating supraventricular arrhythmias (e.g., atrial fibrillation). Most patients only have a modest decrease in heart rate. However, heart block (first-, second-, or third-degree) is a potential adverse effect, especially with large doses.

Verapamil and diltiazem are considered safe and effective antihypertensives. Both should be avoided in patients with second- or third-degree heart block. Under these circumstances, a dihydropyridine can be used if a CCB is needed. Verapamil and diltiazem should also be avoided in patients with left ventricular dysfunction because they can significantly reduce cardiac contractility. Diltiazem has a lower incidence of constipation than verapamil.

Formulations

Several CCB are available for the treatment of hypertension. They are listed in Table 13-16.

IMMEDIATE-RELEASE NIFEDIPINE

42. A 68-year-old man has a new prescription for immediate-release nifedipine 10 mg three times daily for newly diagnosed hypertension. He has no contraindications to CCB therapy. Why should immediate-release nifedipine not be used to treat his hypertension?

Most dihydropyridines, except amlodipine, are formulated as sustained-release products to provide 24-hour effects.

Table 13-16 CCB in Hypertension[a]

Drug	Usual Dosage Range (mg/day)	Dosing Frequency
Nondihydropyridines[b]		
Diltiazem, sustained-release (Cardizem CD, Cartia XT, Dilacor XR, Dilt-CD, Diltia XT, Taztia XT, Tiazac)	120–480	Daily
Diltiazem, extended-release (Cardizem LA)[c]	120–540	Daily
Verapamil, sustained-release (Calan SR, Isoptin SR, Verelan)	180–480	Daily to BID
Verapamil, controlled-onset extended-release (Covera HS)[c]	180–480	QHS
Verapamil, chronotherapeutic oral drug absorption system (Verelan HS)[c]	100–400	QHS
Dihydropyridines		
Amlodipine, immediate-release tablet (Norvasc)	2.5–10	Daily
Felodipine, extended-release tablet (Plendil)	2.5–10	Daily
Isradipine, controlled-release tablet (DynaCirc CR)	5–20	Daily
Nicardipine, sustained-release capsule (Cardene SR)	60–120	BID
Nifedipine, sustained-release[d] tablet (Procardia XL, Adalat CC)	30–90	Daily
Nisoldipine, extended-release tablet (Sular)	17–34	Daily

[a]Immediate release (IR) diltiazem, nifedipine, and verapamil should be avoided in hypertension.
[b]Many long acting products exist, but vary in release characteristics. Thus, they are not directly interchangeable using a mg/mg conversion.
[c]"Chronotherapeutic" agents; because they use different delivery systems, they are not interchangeable products.
[d]Only sustained-release nifedipine is approved for hypertension. Immediate release should be avoided.
BID, twice daily; QHS, every night; CCB, calcium channel blocker.

Nifedipine has a very short half-life, and is available as an immediate-release capsule. It was once used to quickly reduce BP in hypertensive urgencies, but it should never be used for this indication. Immediate-release nifedipine, given sublingually or orally, has been associated with several adverse effects such as severe hypotension, cerebral ischemia, acute MI, fetal distress, conduction abnormalities, and even death. The rapid and potent hypotensive effect can "steal" blood flow from coronary arteries, induce reflex tachycardia, and acutely decrease cardiac contractility. Immediate-release nifedipine is not approved for the treatment of hypertension, and the Cardiorenal Advisory Panel of the U.S. Food and Drug Administration (FDA) concluded that the use of immediate-release nifedipine is neither safe nor efficacious.[112] Immediate-release dihydropyridines that are short acting, especially nifedipine, should be avoided. Even with verapamil and diltiazem, once-daily, sustained-release formulations are preferred for hypertension.

SUSTAINED-RELEASE FORMULATIONS

43. C.F. is a 60-year-old man with a history of hypertension, asthma, and type 2 diabetes. His hypertension has been treated with HCTZ 25 mg daily, controlled-onset, extended-release verapamil 240 mg daily (Covera HS), and ramipril 10 mg daily for the past 5 years. Today his BP is 124/74 mmHg (128/72 mmHg when repeated), and his heart rate is 64 beats/minute C.F. is interested in a generic alternative for his controlled-onset, extended-release verapamil, such as sustained-release verapamil. What are the differences between these two verapamil products, and are they interchangeable?

All CCBs have short half-lives, except amlodipine. Immediate-release forms require multiple daily doses to provide 24-hour effects. Sustained-released formulations are preferred when a CCB is used to treat hypertension. Various sustained-release delivery devices are available. Serum drug concentrations differ between sustained-release CCBs, but the overall BP-lowering effects are usually similar. Nonetheless, most of these products that include the same drug are not AB rated by the Food and Drug Administration (FDA) as equivalent and identical. Insurance formularies often require therapeutic substitution between these agents. Therapeutic interchange with sustained-release diltiazem products or with chronotherapeutic verapamil, however, are not equivalent using a milligram-per-milligram conversion. Therapeutic substitution between these products may result in variable BP-lowering effects if not adjusted appropriately. BP and heart rate monitoring should occur within 2 weeks of interchanging sustained-release CCBs.

CHRONOTHERAPEUTIC CCB

Blood pressure has a predictable circadian rhythm characterized by a sharp rise in pressure starting in the early morning, peaking in the mid to late morning, followed by a gradual decrease to lowest values during early to mid-nighttime. Importantly, MI incidence also has a circadian rhythm in which events are most frequent during the time of the early morning BP surge. Chronopharmacology is the concept of recognizing circadian rhythms of disease and targeting drug delivery to blunt such rhythms. The prevailing assumption is that targeting BP reduction according to the circadian rhythm can maximally reduce the risk of CV events.

Two sustained-release verapamil products (Covera HS and Verelan PM) and one verapamil product (Cardizem LA) are chronotherapeutically designed to target the circadian BP rhythm. These formulations are dosed primarily at bedtime, have a delayed drug release for a period of hours, followed by slow delivery of drug that starts just before the morning BP surge, with no delivery during the early evening. The two verapamil products use different delivery devices and are not interchangeable with each other or other long-acting verapamil products, using a milligram-to-milligram conversion. Cardizem LA is similarly not interchangeable with other long-acting diltiazem products. Therapeutic substitution between products must involve close monitoring.

The scientific rationale supporting chronotherapy in hypertension is only hypothetical. Evidence from the Controlled Onset Verapamil Investigation of Cardiovascular Endpoints (CONVINCE) trial shows that chronotherapeutic verapamil is similar, but not better than, a thiazide diuretic- or β-blocker–based regimen in reducing hypertension-associated complications.[43] C.F. has achieved his goal BP of <130/80 mmHg with his present verapamil product. It is ideal to continue using this product. If a switch occurs, however, his present verapamil 240 mg daily should be changed to sustained-release generic verapamil 240 mg daily. This conversion requires BP and heart rate monitoring in 2 weeks to detect whether BP remains controlled after the switch, because these two products are not identical and are not AB rated as interchangeable.

Compelling Indications

DIABETES

44. Why is diabetes a compelling indication for a CCB?

Calcium channel blockers are recommended as options to treat hypertension in patients with diabetes because they have been shown to reduce risk of CV events.[5,72] They do not affect glucose. Evidence showing reduced CV events with CCB in patients with diabetes is not, however, as convincing as that seen with an ACEI, ARB, or thiazide diuretics. The results of the Fosinopril versus Amlodipine Cardiovascular Events Randomized Trial (FACET) and Appropriate Blood pressure Control in Diabetes (ABCD) trial suggest that ACEI have more CV protection than CCB.[53,54]

Nondihydropyridine CCB (particularly diltiazem) may slow the progression of chronic kidney disease, although evidence is not as extensive or definitive as it is with an ACEI or ARB. The proposed mechanism is dilation of the afferent and efferent arterioles, which would decrease intraglomerular pressure. Dihydropyridines have unclear effects on progression of kidney disease. The prevailing opinion is that the renal protective effects of an ACEI and ARB are superior to a CCB.

The primary role of a CCB in the management of hypertension in diabetes is ideally as a component of sequential add-on therapy, after an ACEI or ARB and a thiazide diuretic. Because the BP goal in diabetes is <130/80 mmHg, most patients with diabetes need three or more antihypertensives to achieve this goal. A CCB is frequently needed in this population.

CHRONIC CAD

45. A.P. is a 71-year-old man with a BP of 168/90 mmHg (170/90 mmHg when repeated) and a heart rate of 88 beats/minute. He has a history of chronic stable angina that is controlled with sublingual nitroglycerin as needed. He also has severe asthma that is worsened with β-blocker therapy. He currently has no chest pain, and his ECG shows no acute ischemia. Other laboratory results are within normal range, except his serum creatinine is 1.3 mg/dL (normal, 0.5–1.2 mg/dL). Is a CCB appropriate for A.P.? If yes, which type is preferred?

Calcium channel blockers are compellingly indicated in chronic CAD (i.e., chronic stable angina) as an alternative to a β-blocker, or as sequential add-on therapy to a β-blocker for patients who require additional anti-ischemic effects.[78] Alternatives to β-blockers are needed when contraindications or intolerances to β-blockers are present. Sustained-release CCB formulations or long-acting products (i.e., amlodipine) are always preferred for outpatient management of these patients. A nondihydropyridine is preferred in chronic CAD when used as an alternative to a β-blocker, whereas a dihydropyridine is preferred when CCB therapy is used in addition to a β-blocker.

First developed to treat ischemic heart disease, CCBs were later proved to be effective in hypertension. Nondihydropyridine CCBs decrease myocardial oxygen demand, improve myocardial blood flow, and have negative inotropic and chronotropic effects. All these may benefit patients with CAD. Dihydropyridine CCBs are similar, but do not lower heart rate, and have less negative inotropic effects. They can be used in patients with chronic CAD and possibly acute CAD, but verapamil and diltiazem are preferred when a CCB is used in place of a β-blocker. Moreover, dihydropyridine CCBs are not particularly helpful in patients with acute CAD.

Therapy with a CCB is preferred in A.P., because β-blockers worsened his severe asthma. Verapamil will lower his elevated heart rate and BP as well as treat his angina. Constipation, which may be more prominent in an elderly patient, is the most frequent side effect. Of all the CCBs, constipation is most commonly associated with verapamil, but can be countered with dietary changes or bulk-forming laxatives. Similar to other antihypertensive agents, a low dose (120–180 mg daily) should be used initially and slowly titrated at 2- to 4-week intervals.

Additional Populations

ISOLATED SYSTOLIC HYPERTENSION

46. T.C. is a 76-year-old woman with hypertension and dyslipidemia. Her Framingham risk score is 25%. She has been treated with HCTZ 25 mg daily for several years, and she is very compliant with this regimen. Her BP values are 164/76 mmHg (168/78 mmHg when repeated). She has no other evidence of hypertension-associated complications, and no compelling indications. Her laboratory values and ECG are all normal. Amlodipine 5 mg daily is added to her regimen. What are the benefits of using a CCB to treat T.C.'s hypertension?

T.C. has isolated systolic hypertension. This should be managed according to the general patient care principles for hypertension. Thiazide diuretics have traditionally been considered first-line for this population based on historical data demonstrating CV event lowering in elderly patients with isolated systolic hypertension. The SHEP trial proved that treating ISH in the elderly is beneficial and established thiazide diuretic-based regimens as first-line agents.[39] Long-acting dihydropyridine CCBs have been shown to reduce CV events in patients with isolated systolic hypertension also. The Systolic hypertension in Europe (Syst-Eur) study was similar to the SHEP trial, but used a nitrendipine-based (a long-acting dihydropyridine CCB similar to long-acting nifedipine) regimen instead of a thiazide diuretic-based regimen.[42] A dihydropyridine CCB is an appropriate add-on therapy for T.C. to control her BP and reduce her risk of CV events.

EDEMA FROM DIHYDROPYRIDINE CCB

47. One month later, T.C.'s BP is down to 148/70 mmHg (150/70 when repeated). She is tolerating her amlodipine, except she has noticed her ankles are both swollen. She has never had this problem before. A compete cardiovascular examination is conducted and no signs found of left ventricular dysfunction or other hypertension-associated complications that would explain this new peripheral edema. Her amlodipine therapy is identified as the cause of this edema. How should her edema be managed? Should her HCTZ be replaced with a loop diuretic, should her amlodipine be stopped, or is there another approach to manage this side effect?

Peripheral edema with CCB therapy, especially a dihydropyridine CCB, is a dose-dependent side effect. It is a direct result of the potent peripheral arterial vasodilation. When there is not equal vasodilation on the venous vasculature, a risk exists for leaking though the capillaries in the legs and, thus, an increased risk of peripheral edema. The best way to manage this side effect is to reduce the dose of the dihydropyridine, or to add an agent that blocks the RAAS to decrease the effects of angiotensin-2, which will result in venous vasodilation. Adding either an ACEI or ARB can be used to accomplish this with the added benefit of further lowering BP. Clinicians should note that using diuretics for the primary purpose of treating peripheral edema that is secondary to CCB use is not recommended, and is not effective.

T.C.'s BP is not at her goal of <130/80 mmHg. Therefore, additional drug therapy is needed. Her best option is to add an ACEI or ARB. This will provide a more balanced pressure gradient across her peripheral vasculature by providing vasodilation of both the arteries and veins. She has otherwise tolerated amlodipine, so no urgent need exists to discontinue this agent. Moreover, lowering the dose of amlodipine to 2.5 mg is an option, but she would still require the addition of a third agent.

ADDITIONAL POPULATIONS

Calcium channel blockers may also have potential benefits for other conditions. Diltiazem and verapamil can be used in atrial fibrillation, atrial flutter, and supraventricular arrhythmias owing to their ability to block the AV node and lower heart rate. Verapamil is effective in migraine prophylaxis. Patients with Raynaud's syndrome can obtain symptomatic relief from the peripheral vasodilation associated with a dihydropyridine CCB. Lastly, CCBs are effective in treating cyclosporine-induced hypertension, but should be used cautiously because verapamil and diltiazem increase cyclosporine concentration.

Table 13-17 Common β-Blockers in Hypertension

Drug	Usual Dosage Range (mg/day)	Dosing Frequency	Half-life (hr)	β_1 Selectivity	Lipid Solubility
Atenolol (Tenormin)	25–100	Daily to BID	6–7	++	Low
Carvedilol (Coreg)	12.5–50	BID	6–10	0	High
Carvedilol (Coreg CR)	10–80	daily	6–10	0	High
Labetalol (Trandate, Normodyne)	200–800	BID	6–8	0	Moderate
Metoprolol tartrate (Lopressor)	100–400	BID	3–7	+	Moderate to high
Metoprolol succinate (Toprol XL)	25–400	Daily	3–7	+	Moderate to high
Nebivolol (Bystolic)	5–10	Daily	12–19	++	High
Propranolol (Inderal, Inderal LA, InnoPran XL)	40–180	Daily (LA and XL) or BID	3–5	0	High

BID, twice daily.

Other Considerations

LEFT VENTRICULAR DYSFUNCTION

48. Why are nondihydropyridine CCB contraindicated in patients left ventricular dysfunction (systolic heart failure)?

Calcium channel blockers, especially nondihydropyridines, decrease cardiac contractility owing to negative inotropic effects. This is most pronounced with verapamil, but is also present with diltiazem and with some dihydropyridines (Table 13-15). In left ventricular dysfunction, the primary physiologic problem is decreased cardiac contractility. Using a CCB in this population can exacerbate left ventricular dysfunction owing to the direct negative inotropic effects, or reveal left ventricular dysfunction that has not yet been diagnosed.

When patients with left ventricular dysfunction require a CCB to treat another condition (i.e., angina or uncontrolled hypertension), amlodipine or felodipine may be used. Amlodipine and felodipine are the only CCB that have been convincingly shown to be safe in left ventricular dysfunction and may be used if needed for either angina or hypertension. Unlike many other antihypertensive agents, they do not, however, protect against left ventricular dysfunction-related mortality.[113]

β-Blockers

49. E.K. is a 78-year-old black man with a history of hypertension, who was hospitalized for an acute MI 2 months ago. He has been treated with metoprolol succinate 50 mg daily and lisinopril 20 mg daily since then. Today his BP readings are 148/92 and 146/90 mmHg, and his heart rate is 80 beats/minute. He denies side effects from his medications. Because E.K. is black and elderly, will β-blocker therapy be effective in lowering his BP?

β-Blockers reduce morbidity and mortality in patients with certain compelling indications.[5,9] These include left ventricular dysfunction, CAD, and diabetes. β-Blocker therapy should not be the primary antihypertensive agent for primary prevention patients, but is an effective alternative add-on agent for primary prevention patients to lower BP. Elderly and black patients may have less BP reduction than young or white patients. E.K. is elderly and might have more BP reduction with another agent (i.e., thiazide diuretic or CCB), but these points are moot in E.K. Age and race should never deter use of a β-blocker when a compelling indication is present. E.K. has history of a recent MI, which is a compelling indication for a β-blocker as first-line therapy.[5,9,36,84,85]

Pharmacologic Differences

Many different β-blockers are available (Table 13-17). Clinically important differences relate primarily to cardioselectivity, intrinsic sympathomimetic activity (ISA), relative lipid solubility, and benefit-to-risk in left ventricular dysfunction. These differences might be useful when selecting an individual agent.

CARDIOSELECTIVITY

50. What are the advantages of using a cardioselective β-blocker to treat E.K.'s hypertension?

β_1-Adrenergic receptors are primarily located in the heart, and β_2-adrenergic receptors are in the lungs, kidneys, and peripheral arteriolar endothelium. Low-affinity β_1-receptors are also present in the lung, and low-affinity β_2-receptors are present in the heart. Some β-blockers demonstrate relative cardioselectivity with greater antagonism of cardiac β_1-receptors and less activity on β_2-receptors in the lung or bronchial tissue. Selectivity is not absolute, however, because it is dose-dependent. For instance, asthma has been precipitated even with cardioselective agents when they are used in higher doses, but not with low to moderate doses.

Nonselective β-blockers potentially have the disadvantage of blunting the symptoms of hypoglycemia in patients with diabetes. β_2-Blockade from nonselective β-blockers can lead to unopposed β_1-induced peripheral vasoconstriction. This may worsen Raynaud's phenomenon, peripheral arterial disease, or hypertension caused by catecholamine-producing tumors (pheochromocytoma). Despite these shortcomings, nonselective β-blockers are preferred in patients with non-CV indications for β-blocker therapy, such as migraine prophylaxis or essential tremor. Absent these indications, cardioselective β-blockers are preferred. E.K. is taking metoprolol for CV indications (hypertension and post-MI). Metoprolol, being a cardioselective agent, is appropriate therapy for E.K.

INTRINSIC SYMPATHOMIMETIC ACTIVITY

51. Why should acebutolol, carteolol, penbutolol, and pindolol not be used in E.K.?

Pure β-blockers occupy the β-receptor, inhibiting stimulatory catecholamine access while exerting no effect on their own. β-Blockers with ISA, such as acebutolol, carteolol, penbutolol, and pindolol, partially stimulate β-receptors while attached to this receptor, but much less than a pure agonist. When given to a patient with a slow resting heart rate, ISA β-blockers can increase the heart rate. Conversely, these agents can slow heart rate in patients with resting or exercise-induced tachycardia, because β-blocking properties predominate.

β-Blockers with ISA are theoretically less likely to cause bradycardia, bronchospasm, reduced cardiac output, peripheral vasoconstriction, and increased plasma lipids than nonselective β-blockers. Nonetheless, these agents still might worsen asthma and should never be used in patients with left ventricular dysfunction or CAD because they can worsen these conditions as a result of their agonist properties. No role exists for ISA β-blockers in the treatment of hypertension. Because E.K. has a history of MI, a β-blocker with ISA (e.g., acebutolol) is contraindicated.

LIPID SOLUBILITY

Lipophilic β-blockers (e.g., propranolol) have a larger volume of distribution and undergo more extensive first-pass hepatic metabolism than hydrophilic β-blockers. Highly hydrophilic β-blockers (e.g., atenolol) are primarily excreted by the kidneys and may require lower doses in patients with severe chronic kidney disease. Highly lipophilic agents theoretically penetrate the CNS more extensively and readily than hydrophilic agents. It is possible that lipophilic agents are associated with increased CNS side effects. Comparative studies, however, have not demonstrated significant differences between low to moderate doses of lipophilic and hydrophilic β-blockers. High lipid-soluble drugs are hepatically cleared. A high lipid-soluble β-blocker is desirable for migraine prophylaxis because of better CNS penetration.

Compelling Indications

DIABETES

52. Diabetes is a compelling indication for β-blocker therapy. What role do β-blockers play in treatment and why is caution sometimes recommended when using these drugs in patients with diabetes?

β-Blockers reduce coronary events, progression of kidney disease, and stroke in patients with diabetes.[72] Their role in treating hypertension in diabetes is as sequential add-on therapy, after an ACEI or ARB and thiazide diuretic. Their role in therapy is similar to that of CCB. These drugs can, however, inhibit insulin secretion and infrequently cause hyperglycemia. In patients with prediabetes, a theoretical higher risk exists of progressing to diabetes than with CCB, ACEI, or ARB therapy based on these changes in insulin sensitivity.[103] Therefore, in patients with diabetes, unless another compelling indication is present for a β-blocker (e.g., left ventricular dysfunction or CAD), a CCB should be used ahead of a β-blocker.

All β-blockers can mask symptoms of impending hypoglycemia associated with epinephrine release (e.g., palpitations, tremor, hunger), but do not prevent hypoglycemia-related sweating. Although they do not cause hypoglycemia, nonselective β-blockers can worsen a hypoglycemic episode and may prolong recovery from hypoglycemia. The risk of masking and potentiating hypoglycemia is not a contraindication. Although β-blockers are best avoided in insulin dependent type 1 diabetes, they can be used if other agents fail or if concurrent diseases are present that justify the use of a β-blocker. Because hypoglycemia is less common in patients with type 2 diabetes who do not require insulin, β-blockers are less likely to create adverse effects in this population.

All patients with diabetes who use β-blockers should be monitored carefully with regular glucose measurements and targeted patient education about how the signs and symptoms of hypoglycemia can change. Nonselective β-blockers should be avoided in patients with tightly controlled diabetes, especially those receiving insulin therapy. If a β-blocker is needed to control BP, or treat a compelling indication in diabetes, a cardioselective agent is preferred.

53. Why are β-blockers so strongly recommended in patients with a history of CAD?

CHRONIC AND ACUTE CAD

Overwhelming evidence supports β-blocker therapy in all forms of CAD.[5,9,36,78,84,85] β-Blockers prolong survival and reduce the risk of recurrent CV events. These agents are considered first-line agents, but are often underutilized in this population because of perceived contraindications. Patients with relative contraindications to β-blocker therapy (e.g., chronic pulmonary disease), however, do indeed benefit from β-blocker therapy if they have CAD. All patients, even if they have controlled BP, should receive a β-blocker post-MI unless they have demonstrated intolerance or have an absolute contraindication. In addition to lowering BP, β-blockers reduce heart rate, contractility, and myocardial oxygen demand. Therefore, they also relieve ischemic symptoms and β-blocker therapy is essential therapy in many patients with CAD.

LEFT VENTRICULAR DYSFUNCTION

54. β-blockers decrease cardiac contractility. Why then do they benefit patients with left ventricular dysfunction?

β-Blockers decrease cardiac contractility, and reduce cardiac output when first initiated. In patients with left ventricular dysfunction, the primary physiologic abnormality is decreased contractility. Therefore, using a β-blocker seems pharmacologically flawed. Extensive research has shown, however, that slow introduction of certain β-blockers using doses much lower than what is used for BP lowering (i.e., carvedilol 3.125 mg twice daily and metoprolol 12.5 mg daily), followed by very slow and careful titration up to high dose, actually improves cardiac function. Cardiac β-receptor upregulation occurs, and the detrimental compensatory tachycardia and excessive catecholamine release is halted. The end result is decreased morbidity and mortality.[86] β-Blocker therapy is compellingly indicated in left ventricular dysfunction. β-blockers are the third of three agents that comprise standard therapy for patients with left ventricular dysfunction.

55. Which β-blockers should be used in patients with left ventricular dysfunction?

Metoprolol and carvedilol are FDA approved for left ventricular dysfunction based on evidence showing reduced CV events and mortality.[86] When β-blockers are used in patients with both hypertension and left ventricular dysfunction, one of these two agents should be selected following dose recommendations as approved for left ventricular dysfunction (start with a low dose followed by gradual titration upward). Bisoprolol also has been evaluated in left ventricular dysfunction, and demonstrates similar benefits, but is less frequently used.

Additional Considerations

56. Atenolol is the most frequently prescribed β-blocker in hypertension. Why is it not beneficial in left ventricular dysfunction?

When the entire body of evidence evaluating β-blockers and their ability to lower CV events, especially in CAD is examined, a paucity of data are found that independently evaluated atenolol in left ventricular dysfunction.[114] Moreover, some data suggests that atenolol is inferior to other β-blockers (e.g., metoprolol) in ability to reduce CV risk.[21] Perhaps the problem with atenolol is dosing. It is nearly always dosed once daily in hypertension. Its half-life, however, is similar to immediate-release formulations of metoprolol or carvedilol, which are both dosed twice daily (Table 13-17). It is possible that the lack of long-term beneficial data with atenolol might be influenced by improper dosing. Because of this uncertainty, clinicians should select β-blockers, such as metoprolol or carvedilol, instead of atenolol when initiating β-blocker therapy in patients with hypertension. Alternatively, twice daily dosing of atenolol might be a more ideal utilization of this particular agent.

57. How severe are the metabolic side effects associated with β-blocker use?

β-Blockers are associated with adverse metabolic alterations and bothersome side effects that limit their universal use. The incidence of other adverse reactions (e.g., sexual dysfunction) is lower, however, than popular medical myth suggests. Adverse reactions are dose-dependent and are minimized with low to moderate doses.

Nonselective β-blockers have been associated with increased serum triglycerides and reductions in HDL-C. Agents with ISA have little or no effects on lipids, whereas cardioselective β-blockers have intermediate effects. Similar to diuretics, these changes are often not sustained with chronic therapy. β-Blockers have definitively been shown to lower morbidity and mortality, so their effects on cholesterol have little clinical significance. If a β-blocker is indicated in a patient with dyslipidemia, HDL-C and fasting triglyceride values should be monitored.

58. What other noncardiovascular conditions are responsive to β-blockers in patients with concurrent hypertension?

β-Blockers have potential benefits in other conditions. They slow the rate of cardiac conduction, a benefit in patients with paroxysmal supraventricular tachycardia or atrial fibrillation. They are also used in patients with tachycardia and anxiety from mitral valve prolapse, or preoperative hypertension. Finally, β-blockers are effective in treating other noncardiac conditions, such as thyrotoxicosis, essential tremor, and migraine prophylaxis.

59. How should monitoring of heart rate be used to optimize β-blocker therapy?

β-Blockers decrease conduction through both the SA and AV node. Lowering of the resting heart rate can be used as a marker of response. While receiving β-blocker therapy, heart rate should ideally be controlled to a resting pulse rate of no less than 60 beats/minute to avoid heart block. First-degree heart block may be present when the heart rate is <60 beats/minute, but normal conduction is maintained. β-Blocker therapy should, under most circumstances, be reduced if this occurs. Second- and third-degree heart block result in heart rates typically <55 and <40 beats/minute, respectively, with abnormal cardiac conduction. β-Blocker therapy should be decreased or stopped if either of these two situations occur. Failure to achieve a lowered resting pulse could indicate inadequate dosage (i.e., need for a higher dose) or poor patient adherence to the prescribed regimen. If the BP goal has been obtained, however, this is more important than lowered pulse response.

60. What is the harm associated with abruptly discontinuing β-blocker therapy? How should clinicians treat patients who must have β-blocker therapy discontinued?

Chronic β-blocker therapy upregulates the expression of β-receptors. This does not, however, result in a rise of BP while the β-blocker continues to occupy the receptors. If β-blocker therapy is abruptly stopped, however, rebound hypertension can occur because more β-receptors are available to be activated, causing cardiac stimulation and vasoconstriction. Symptoms of rebound hypertension can include headache, tachycardia, and possibly anxiety. Patients with ischemic heart disease can have significant increases in angina frequency if β-blockers are abruptly stopped. If a β-blocker requires discontinuation, rebound hypertension or ischemia can be avoided by gradually tapering the dose by 50% for 3 days and then another 50% for 3 days. Replacing one β-blocker with another at an equivalent dose should not cause rebound hypertension.

Alternative Antihypertensive Agents

61. R.R. is a 62 year-old man with a long-standing history of hypertension. He has not yet experienced any hypertension-associated complications or target organ damage. He does not have a history of diabetes, does not smoke, and his Framingham risk score is 13%. He has been treated with HCTZ 25 mg daily, amlodipine/valsartan 10/320 mg daily, and carvedilol 12.5 mg twice daily for one year. He is very adherent with these medications, measures his BP at home every day, and follows recommended lifestyle modifications as diligently as possible. He has tried other medications that resulted in intolerances (quinapril caused angioedema, doxazosin caused dizziness, clonidine caused a dry mouth). His BP has never been <130/80 mmHg, which is his goal. All secondary causes of hypertension have been ruled out. His BP today is 150/90 mmHg (152/92 when repeated), heart rate is 60 beats/minute, serum potassium is 4.2 mEq/L, and serum creatinine is 1.1 mg/dL. He is 183 cm tall, and weighs 85 kg. What other options are available for R.R.? Does he have resistant hypertension?

Several alternative agents (Table 13-18) are available to treat difficult-to-control hypertension or resistant hypertension. Resistant hypertension is defined as that in which patients fail to attain their BP goal while treated with a three-drug regimen that utilizes full antihypertensive doses, one of which is a diuretic.[5] In reality, this represents a hypertensive population that is likely to use four or five drugs to treat hypertension.

Table 13-18 Alternative Antihypertensive Agents

Drugs/Mechanism of Action	Usual Dosage Range (mg/day)	Dosing Frequency
Aldosterone Antagonists (see Table 13-9)		
α_1-Blockers		
Doxazosin (Cardura)	1–8	Daily
Prazosin (Minipress)	2–20	BID to TID
Terazosin (Hytrin)	1–20	Daily to BID
Direct Renin Inhibitor		
Aliskiren (Tekturna)	150–300	Daily
α_2-Agonists (Central)		
Clonidine (Catapres)	0.1–0.8	BID
Clonidine Transdermal (Catapres TTS)	0.1–0.3	Once weekly
Methyldopa (Aldomet)	250–1,000	BID
Arterial Vasodilators		
Hydralazine (Apresoline)	25–100	BID
Minoxidil (Loniten)	2.5–80	Daily to BID
Adrenergic Neuron Blockers		
Reserpine (Serpasil)	0.05–0.25	Daily

BID, twice daily; TID, three times daily.

R.R. meets the definition of resistant hypertension. He has already failed to respond to, or tolerate, several drug classes that typically are associated with reductions in hypertension-associated complications. His HCTZ, amlodipine, and valsartan are all at the maximal doses. Carvedilol could be increased to 25 mg twice daily, but this should not be done because his heart rate is 60 beats/minute and increasing this dose would place him at risk for bradycardia. To attain his BP goal of <130/80 mmHg (appropriate because of his elevated Framingham score), an alternate agent, other than clonidine, should be selected because he did not tolerate it in the past.

Alternative agents should not be used as monotherapy in the treatment of nearly all patients' hypertension because they have not been shown to reduce hypertension-associated complications. They should primarily be used as last-line agents in combination with the aforementioned antihypertensive agents that reduce morbidity and mortality.

Aldosterone Antagonists

Spironolactone and eplerenone are aldosterone antagonists. Technically, these are potassium-sparing diuretics and can increase potassium and cause hyperkalemia. When used in hypertension, increases in potassium are small in most patients. This risk increases, however, in patients with chronic kidney disease or when used in combination with an ACEI or ARB.

62. Would it be safe to add spironolactone 25 mg daily to R.R.'s regimen?

Spironolactone is especially useful as an add-on therapy in patients with resistant hypertension. Spironolactone 25 mg daily is a reasonable addition to R.R.'s regimen. His potassium is in the normal range, but could increase after adding spironolactone. Therefore, it should be monitored 2 to 4 weeks after it is started to assure R.R. does not develop hyperkalemia. Eplerenone is more specific than spironolactone in aldosterone blockade. Compared with spironolactone, gynecomastia is not a frequent side effect. The incidence of hyperkalemia is greater with eplerenone, however. When used for hypertension, eplerenone is contraindicated in populations at high risk for hyperkalemia: type 2 diabetes with microalbuminuria, an estimated creatinine clearance <50 mL/minute, or elevated serum creatinine (>1.8 mg/dL in women and >2.0 mg/dL in men).

These agents are indicated for hypertension, but their greatest use is in left ventricular dysfunction. This is considered a compelling indication because of evidence showing reduced morbidity and mortality.[89,90] In studies to date, eplerenone reduced mortality in patients with left ventricular dysfunction soon after MI, whereas spironolactone was beneficial in patients with more severe left ventricular dysfunction.[89,90] Although it is logical to add an aldosterone inhibitor to R.R.'s regimen based on the presence of heart failure, the antihypertensive effect may still not be sufficient for him to reach his BP goal.

α-Blockers

63. J.L. is a 64-year-old man with hypertension and peripheral arterial disease. His BP is 138/84 mmHg (136/86 mmHg when repeated). His current antihypertensive regimen is HCTZ 25 mg daily and nifedipine extended release (ER) 60 mg daily. J.L. is not completely adherent with lifestyle modifications, but insists he is doing the best he can. He has been experiencing frequent nocturia, difficulty in starting urination, and a decrease in his urinary flow for the past several months and is diagnosed with benign prostatic hyperplasia (BPH). J.L.'s physician is considering changing one of his antihypertensive agents to an α-blocker. How do α-blockers compare with other agents in reducing CV events?

α-Blockers are not first-line agents in the management of hypertension. The ALLHAT trial, as discussed previously, originally included an α-blocker (doxazosin) treatment arm. Interim results after a mean follow-up of 3.3 years revealed that doxazosin had a statistically higher risk of combined CV disease and heart failure when compared with chlorthalidone.[115] Therefore, the ALLHAT data show that thiazide diuretic therapy is more protective against hypertension-associated complications than is α-blocker therapy. This study did not include a placebo group; therefore, to conclude that doxazosin is harmful is inaccurate. For J.L., discontinuing HCTZ or nifedipine to start an α-blocker is not prudent. It may be appropriate, however, to add an α-blocker to his regimen because he is above his goal BP of <130/80 mmHg (appropriate because he has peripheral arterial disease) and is already treated with two first-line agents (thiazide diuretic and CCB). Adding an ACEI or ARB, or even a β-blocker, would be reasonable considerations, but an α-blocker will also provide symptomatic benefit to his BPH.

64. How would adding an α-blocker to J.L.'s treatment regimen affect his BPH?

An α-blocker can potentially improve the symptoms of BPH by reducing urethral tone and alleviating bladder outlet obstruction. Terazosin and doxazosin are both approved for the treatment of symptoms caused by BPH. Prazosin can be used, but requires more frequent dosing. Decreased symptoms of BPH with α-blockers are dose-related, and titration to high doses is often needed. This increases the risk of side effects, such as orthostatic hypotension. In J.L., an α-blocker will lower his BP and might also relieve his urinary symptoms.

65. J.L. prefers to try doxazosin rather than undergo surgery to relieve his symptoms of BPH. How should this agent be started?

For J.L., it would be best to add a low dose of doxazosin to his present two-drug regimen. Based on his tolerance of the new drug and BP response, it can be titrated up. One of his other antihypertensive agents can be decreased if he becomes hypotensive. The initial dose of doxazosin should not exceed 1 mg daily and it should be given at bedtime. This can minimize orthostatic hypotension (i.e., profound hypotension, dizziness, and possible fainting), which is the most frequent side effect of α-blockers. This complication is most pronounced with the first dose, but can persist in some patients. The dose can be increased to symptom control based on BP and tolerability.

66. What patient education should be provided to J.L. about the potential adverse effects of doxazosin?

α-Blockers are relatively well tolerated if dosed appropriately. J.L. could experience side effects, such as drowsiness, headache, weakness, palpitations from reflex tachycardia, and nausea, but these do not occur in all patients. Patients starting an α-blocker should be instructed to take the initial dose at bedtime and to anticipate a first-dose effect, in which they may experience orthostatic hypotension. Specifically, patients should be counseled to rise more slowly from a seated or supine position.

Mixed α/β-Blockers

67. R.P. is a 68-year-old man with hypertension and a history of ischemic stroke (1 year ago). Two months ago, his BP values were 164/94 mmHg and 162/98 mmHg, with a heart rate of 62 beats/min while on atenolol 50 mg daily. He was started on benazepril/HCTZ 10/12.5 mg daily 2 months ago. His BP today is 142/82 mmHg (144/82 mmHg when repeated). All his laboratory values are normal except his serum creatinine, which is 1.9 mg/dL (normal, 0.5–1.2 mg/dL). J.L. has implemented lifestyle modification to the best of his ability. Because R.P.'s BP is still not at goal (<130/80 mmHg because of his history of ischemic stroke), could his atenolol be replaced with an agent such as labetalol and carvedilol?

Labetalol and carvedilol are nonselective β-blockers that also have α_1-receptor blocking activity. Their antihypertensive effects are only somewhat similar to a combination of a nonselective β-blocker (e.g., propranolol) with an α_1-antagonist (e.g., terazosin). Dosing recommendations are listed in Table 13-17.

These agents produce vasodilation and can cause more adverse reactions than β-blocker or α-blocker monotherapy. The same precautions and typical contraindications relevant to β-blockers apply to these agents because they basically are nonselective β-blockers (Table 13-10). Unlike pure β-blockers, however, both carvedilol and labetalol may be safer to use in patients with peripheral arterial disease because unopposed peripheral α-constriction does not occur.

Carvedilol is approved for both hypertension and left ventricular dysfunction. Carvedilol has been shown to reduce morbidity and mortality in a wide range of patients with left ventricular dysfunction.[79,88] Labetalol and carvedilol have no clear advantage over other β-blockers in most patients with hypertension, and patients might experience α-blocker–related side effects (e.g., orthostatic hypotension). If R.P. had the compelling indication of left ventricular dysfunction, switching to carvedilol would be reasonable. His heart rate is between 60 and 70 beats/minute, so this indicates he is adherent with atenolol. Increasing the atenolol dose to 100 mg daily is not wise because it may induce heart block. Atenolol is renally eliminated, so his present dose is probably causing more BP lowering than usual doses based on his chronic kidney disease. Increasing his ACEI will help to control both his BP and preserve his kidney function. This can be done without increasing his HCTZ by switching his fixed-dose combination product to benazepril/HCTZ 20/12.5 mg daily or simply increasing both the ACE and HCTZ by doubling his current dose.

Direct Renin Inhibitors

68. How is aliskiren different than an ACEI or ARB?

Aliskiren is the first oral direct renin inhibitor.[116] Agents within this new antihypertensive drug class inhibit the RAAS at the first step of this system, which results in reduced plasma renin activity and BP lowering. This is different than both the inhibition of angiotensin-2 production from ACEI therapy and the inhibition of angiotensin-2 seen with ARB therapy. Aliskiren has a 24-hour half-life that allows for once-daily dosing. Its primary route of elimination is through biliary excretion as unchanged drug.

Some similarities and some differences exist among the side effects associated with aliskiren when compared with ACEIs and ARBs. Similarly, aliskiren should not be used in pregnancy because of the known teratogenic effects from blocking the RAAS system. Increases in serum creatinine and serum potassium have been associated with aliskiren similar to ACEI and ARB therapy, mediated by the inhibition of angiotensin-2 vasoconstrictive effects on the efferent arterioles of the kidney, and blocking of aldosterone. Monitoring of serum creatinine and serum potassium should be done in patients treated with aliskiren, particularly in those treated with the combination of aliskiren and an ACEI, ARB, potassium-sparing diuretic, or aldosterone antagonist. Angioedema has been reported in patients treated with aliskiren, but the exact prevalence is unknown.

69. What is the role of aliskiren in treating hypertension? Can patients treated with either an ACEI or ARB have aliskiren added to their drug regimen?

The exact role of aliskiren treatment of hypertension is unclear. It is approved as monotherapy or in combination therapy. The BP reductions with aliskiren as monotherapy are similar to those seen with an ACEI, ARB, or CCB (specifically amlodipine). Aliskiren provides additive BP lowering when used in combination with HCTZ, ACEI, ARB, and CCB. Its efficacy in combination with maximal doses of ACEI is unknown, however. Studies evaluating long-term effects on CV events and progression of diabetic nephropathy are currently underway. Therefore, aliskiren is considered an alternative antihypertensive agent at this time because of unknown long-term effects on hypertension-associated complications.

Central α_2-Agonists

CLONIDINE

70. T.M. is a 37-year-old man. He is a truck driver with a 5-year history of hypertension. His Framingham risk score is <10% and

he does not have hypertension-associated complications or any compelling indications. Secondary causes have been ruled out. His regimen is losartan/HCTZ 100/25 mg daily and sustained-release diltiazem 240 mg daily. Other antihypertensive drugs have failed because of various side effects (captopril and lisinopril caused a dry cough, atenolol and carvedilol caused fatigue, nifedipine and amlodipine caused edema, and terazosin caused orthostasis). T.M. has been adherent to his present medications and lifestyle modification, but has been unable to quit smoking. His clinic and home BP values have been similar and averaged 150/95 mmHg for the past 3 months. Clonidine 0.1 mg twice daily is added to his regimen. How can both an α_2-agonist and α_1-antagonists be effective antihypertensive agents?

The antihypertensive effects of α_2-agonists (Table 13-18) are attributed to their central α_2-agonist activity. Stimulation of α_2-receptors in the CNS inhibits sympathetic outflow (via negative feedback) to the heart, kidneys, and peripheral vasculature, resulting in peripheral vasodilation. Although the α_2-agonists are effective as monotherapy, they are not first-line therapy for the treatment of hypertension because of their potential side effects and a lack of evidence showing reductions in morbidity and mortality.

α_2-Agonists are most effective when used with a diuretic because they all can cause fluid retention. Ideally, they should be used in combination with agents that have different mechanisms of action and with agents that do not affect other central adrenergic receptors. Clonidine can cause rebound hypertension when abruptly stopped. T.M.'s occupation may place him at risk for this complication if he misses doses because of unusual work hours or prolonged travel.

71. How should T.M.'s clonidine dose be titrated?

Clonidine should be started at a low dosage and gradually increased to achieve optimal BP lowering with minimal side effects. It is started as 0.1 mg twice daily, with 0.1 or 0.2 mg/day increases every 2 to 4 weeks until BP goal is achieved or side effects appear. Clonidine also is available as a transdermal patch, which releases the medication at a controlled rate over 7 days, and may have fewer side effects than the oral dosage form. The onset of initial BP effect may be delayed for 2 to 3 days after application; thus, rebound hypertension might occur when oral clonidine is switched to transdermal. To prevent this, an oral dose should be taken on the first day that the transdermal patch is used. Anticholinergic side effects, such as sedation and dry mouth, are the most frequent and bothersome side effects of clonidine. These are especially problematic in elderly patients.

72. After several weeks, T.M.'s BP is 138/84 mmHg with clonidine 0.2 mg twice daily. However, he is now experiencing daytime somnolence and dry mouth. What other α_2-agonists are available?

METHYLDOPA

Methyldopa has been extensively evaluated and is considered safe in pregnancy. Therefore, it is recommended as a first-line agent when hypertension is first diagnosed during pregnancy.[117] Beyond that, little role exists for methyldopa in the management of hypertension. The usual initial dose is 250 mg administered twice daily up to 2,000 mg/day. Methyldopa causes side effects similar to those associated with clonidine, including sedation, lethargy, postural hypotension, dizziness, dry mouth, headache, and rebound hypertension. These may decrease with continued use. Other significant side effects include hemolytic anemia and hepatitis. Although these are both rare, they necessitate discontinuing the medication.

OTHERS

Guanfacine and guanabenz have a high incidence of side effects. These agents can cause dry mouth, sedation, dizziness, orthostatic hypotension, insomnia, constipation, and impotence. Guanfacine has a long half-life and may have less rebound hypertension than other α_2-agonists. The adverse effects of other α_2-agonists (methyldopa, guanfacine, and guanabenz) are nearly identical to that of clonidine. In general, patients who do not tolerate one α_2-agonist will not tolerate the others. An antihypertensive agent from a different class (aldosterone antagonist, aliskiren, reserpine or an arterial vasodilator) should be chosen for T.M.

Reserpine

73. What is the role of reserpine in the contemporary management of hypertension?

Reserpine is one of the oldest antihypertensive agents currently available. It is extremely effective in lowering BP when added to a thiazide diuretic. Reserpine is inexpensive, and is dosed once daily. Several of the landmark trials that demonstrated reduced morbidity and mortality with BP lowering in hypertension used reserpine. The SHEP trial used reserpine as a second-step agent added to chlorthalidone in patients who could not take atenolol.[39]

Low-dose reserpine (0.05–0.1 mg once daily) is effective at lowering BP and has significantly fewer side effects compared with high doses. Reserpine can cause nasal stuffiness in many patients. Gastrointestinal ulcerations have been reported, but they are associated with either parenteral administration or very large doses. T.M. is a candidate for low-dose reserpine. He is already taking a thiazide diuretic, which should always be used with reserpine, and his therapeutic options are limited. Of all the agents remaining for T.M., other than aliskiren, reserpine has the most favorable side effect profile.

Many clinicians avoid reserpine because of the myth that it can cause depression. This fear was generated from case reports in the 1950s when very high doses (0.5–1.0 mg/day) were used. Furthermore, many of the patients described in these cases would not meet modern criteria for depression; rather, they would be described as oversedated. When reserpine is limited to a maximum of 0.25 mg daily, depression is no more frequent than with other antihypertensive agents.

Arterial Vasodilators

HYDRALAZINE

74. C.M. is a 56-year-old woman with a history of hypertension and severe chronic kidney disease (estimated GFR of 14 mL/minute/1.73 m^2). Her antihypertensive regimen consists of torsemide 40 mg daily, amlodipine/olmesartan 10/40 mg daily, metoprolol succinate 200 mg daily, and lisinopril 40 mg daily. She started hydralazine 50 mg twice daily 4 weeks ago when her BP was 148/92 and 146/90 mmHg. She has been very compliant, and her BP is now 136/88 mmHg with a heart rate of 82 beats/minute. Her lung fields are clear, with 1+ bilateral pitting edema. Serum electrolytes are within normal limits. Why was hydralazine used in this patient?

Hydralazine causes direct relaxation of arteriolar smooth muscle with little effect on the venous circulation. Arterial vasodilators are infrequently used, except for patients with severe chronic kidney disease. In this population, hypertension is difficult to control and often requires four or five agents. Severe chronic kidney disease results in increased renin release and increased fluid retention. Potent vasodilation, in combination with diuresis, is often effective in lowering BP under these conditions. Potent vasodilation, however, stimulates the sympathetic nervous system and results in a reflex tachycardia, increased PRA, and fluid retention. Thus, the hypotensive effectiveness of direct arterial vasodilators can quickly diminish with time when used as monotherapy. To prevent this effect, arterial vasodilators should always be used in combination with both a β-blocker to counteract reflex tachycardia and a diuretic, often a loop diuretic if used in severe chronic kidney disease, to minimize fluid retention.

75. After 18 months, C.M.'s hydralazine dose is 150 mg twice daily, and her BP is at goal. She now complains of joint pain in both her right and left hands, which extends to the wrists, and generalized weakness with frequent fevers. What is a possible explanation for C.M.'s subjective complaints?

C.M.'s symptoms are consistent with drug-induced lupus (DIL). Hydralazine is one of the most common agents reported to cause DIL. Musculoskeletal pains are the most frequent symptoms, but systemic symptoms (e.g., pericardial effusion and chest pain) and rash may also occur. Hydralazine doses as low as 100 mg/day can cause DIL, and the risk significantly increases when >200 mg/day is used.

76. What objective data can be obtained to confirm the suspicion of DIL?

Laboratory tests are used to establish a diagnosis of DIL. A positive antinuclear antibody (ANA) is a common finding in 70% to 100% of those with long-term hydralazine exposure. Only a small percentage of these patients, however, will experience symptoms of DIL. A positive ANA test without symptoms of DIL does not warrant stopping hydralazine, so routine ANA testing is not necessary. The typical ANA pattern in DIL is diffuse and directed against single-stranded DNA (ss-DNA), not against double-stranded DNA (ds-DNA), as is the case with systemic lupus erythematosus (SLE). Other common laboratory findings include an elevated erythrocyte sedimentation rate (ESR), lupus erythematosus (LE) cells, and a false–positive serologic test finding for syphilis.

Patients with DIL from hydralazine rarely develop serious complications, which include blood dyscrasias such as leukopenia, and thrombocytopenia. Renal complications are not frequently associated with DIL. Of all causative agents associated with DIL, hydralazine, however, has the highest incidence of kidney dysfunction. A serum creatinine should be obtained to identify any elevations, and a urinalysis should be conducted to monitor for signs of proteinuria and hematuria. In C.M., these tests may not be helpful because she has severe chronic kidney disease.

77. Laboratory findings for C.M. showed a positive ANA (diffuse), a white blood cell count of 3,500/mm^3, and an ESR of 45 mm/hour. DIL is diagnosed. How should this drug-induced toxicity be managed?

Hydralazine should be discontinued. Symptoms should begin to subside within days or weeks and complete resolution of symptoms can be expected; however, a positive ANA may persist for several months.

MINOXIDIL

78. How should C.M.'s BP be managed?

C.M.'s BP responded to hydralazine, so she would likely benefit from another arterial vasodilator. Minoxidil, a potent arterial vasodilator, is similar to hydralazine with regard to causing reflex tachycardia, increased cardiac output, increased PRA, and fluid retention. Therefore, concomitant β-blocker and diuretic therapy is required. Minoxidil should be reserved for patients such as C.M. who have severe chronic kidney disease or have resistant hypertension.

79. How should C.M. be counseled regarding the use of minoxidil for her hypertension?

Hypertrichosis is a common adverse effect of oral minoxidil, occurring in 80% to 100% of patients. The hair growth is not associated with an endocrine abnormality and begins within the first few weeks. It commonly occurs on the temples, between the eyebrows, on the cheeks, and on the pinna of the ear. Hair growth can extend to the back of the legs, arms, and scalp with continued use. Some patients, especially women, find the hypertrichosis so intolerable that they stop treatment. Topical minoxidil is an approved therapy for male pattern baldness, but topical administration does not provide BP-lowering effects.

Fluid retention with minoxidil is common, presenting as edema and weight gain. If adequate diuresis is not maintained during minoxidil therapy, left ventricular dysfunction may be precipitated or worsened. This also occurs with hydralazine. The compensatory reflex tachycardia with minoxidil also may precipitate angina in patients who have, or are at risk for, coronary artery disease.

REFERENCES

1. Rosamond W et al. Heart disease and stroke statistics—2007 update: a report from the American Heart Association Statistics Committee and Stroke Statistics Subcommittee. *Circulation* 2007;115(5):e69.
2. Ong KL et al. Prevalence, awareness, treatment, and control of hypertension among United States adults 1999–2004. *Hypertension* 2007:49:69.
3. Prevalence of actions to control high blood pressure—20 states, 2005. *MMWR Morb Mortal Wkly Rep* 2007;56:420.
4. Wang YR et al. Outpatient hypertension treatment, treatment intensification, and control in Western Europe and the United States. *Arch Intern Med* 2007;167:141.
5. Chobanian AV et al. The seventh report of the Joint National Committee on Prevention, Detection, Evaluation, and Treatment of High Blood Pressure. *Hypertension* 2003;42:1206.
6. Kaplan NM. *Kaplan's Clinical Hypertension.* 9th ed. Philadelphia: Lippincott Williams & Wilkins; 2006.
7. Grundy SM et al. Diagnosis and Management of the Metabolic Syndrome. An American Heart Association/National Heart, Lung, and Blood Institute Scientific Statement. Executive Summary. *Circulation* 2005;112:2735.
8. Vasan RS et al. Impact of high-normal blood pressure on the risk of cardiovascular disease. *N Engl J Med* 2001;345:1291.
9. Rosendorff C et al. Treatment of hypertension in the prevention and management of ischemic heart disease: a scientific statement from the American

Heart Association Council for High Blood Pressure Research and the Councils on Clinical Cardiology and Epidemiology and Prevention. *Circulation* 2007;115:2761.
10. Pickering TG et al. Recommendations for blood pressure measurement in humans and experimental animals. Part 1: blood pressure measurement in humans: a statement for professionals from the Subcommittee of Professional and Public Education of the American Heart Association Council on High Blood Pressure Research. *Circulation* 2005;111:697.
11. Mehos BM et al. Effect of pharmacist intervention and initiation of home blood pressure monitoring in patients with uncontrolled hypertension. *Pharmacotherapy* 2000;20:1384.
12. Glen SK et al. White-coat hypertension as a cause of cardiovascular dysfunction. *Lancet* 1996; 348:654.
13. Mancia G et al. 2007 Guidelines for the Management of Arterial Hypertension: The Task Force for the Management of Arterial Hypertension of the European Society of Hypertension (ESH) and of the European Society of Cardiology (ESC). *J Hypertens* 2007;25:1105.
14. Grundy SM et al. Implications of recent clinical trials for the National Cholesterol Education Program Adult Treatment Panel III guidelines. *Circulation* 2004;110:227.
15. Lazarus JM et al. Achievement and safety of a low blood pressure goal in chronic renal disease. The Modification of Diet in Renal Disease Study Group. *Hypertension* 1997;29:641.
16. Hansson L et al. Effects of intensive blood-pressure lowering and low-dose aspirin in patients with hypertension: principal results of the Hypertension Optimal Treatment (HOT) randomised trial. HOT Study Group. *Lancet* 1998;351:1755.
17. Lichtenstein AH et al. Diet and lifestyle recommendations revision 2006: a scientific statement from the American Heart Association Nutrition Committee. *Circulation* 2006;114:82.
18. Appel LJ et al. Dietary approaches to prevent and treat hypertension: a scientific statement from the American Heart Association. *Hypertension* 2006; 47:296.
19. Appel LJ et al. A clinical trial of the effects of dietary patterns on blood pressure. DASH Collaborative Research Group. *N Engl J Med* 1997;336:1117.
20. Turnbull F. Effects of different blood-pressure lowering regimens on major cardiovascular events: results of prospectively-designed overviews of randomized trials. *Lancet* 2003;362:1527.
21. Wiysonge C et al. Beta-blockers for hypertension. *Cochrane Database Syst Rev* 2007:CD002003.
22. Psaty BM et al. Health outcomes associated with various antihypertensive therapies used as first-line agents: a network meta-analysis. *JAMA* 2003;289: 2534.
23. Lakshman MR et al. Diuretics and beta-blockers do not have adverse effects at 1 year on plasma lipid and lipoprotein profiles in men with hypertension. Department of Veterans Affairs Cooperative Study Group on Antihypertensive Agents. *Arch Intern Med* 1999;159:551.
24. The sixth report of the Joint National Committee on Prevention, Detection, Evaluation, and Treatment of High Blood Pressure. *Arch Intern Med* 1997;157:2413.
25. American Heart Association. Heart disease and stroke statistics—2007 update: a report from the American Heart Association statistics committee and stroke statistics subcommittee. *Circulation* 2007;115:e69.
26. K/DOQI clinical practice guidelines for chronic kidney disease: evaluation, classification, and stratification. Kidney Disease Outcome Quality Initiative. *Am J Kidney Dis* 2002;39:S1.
27. National Kidney Foundation. MDRD GFR Calculator (with SI units). Available at: http://www.kidney.org/professionals/KDOQI/gfr_calculator.cfm. Accessed July 29, 2007.
28. Executive Summary of The Third Report of The National Cholesterol Education Program (NCEP) Expert Panel on Detection, Evaluation, And Treatment of High Blood Cholesterol In Adults (Adult Treatment Panel III). *JAMA* 2001;285:2486.
29. Anonymous. The effects of nonpharmacologic interventions on blood pressure of persons with high normal levels. Results of the Trials of Hypertension Prevention, Phase I. *JAMA* 1992;267:1213.
30. Materson BJ et al. Single-drug therapy for hypertension in men: a comparison of six antihypertensive agents with placebo. The Department of Veterans Affairs Cooperative Study Group on Antihypertensive Agents. *N Engl J Med* 1993;328:914.
31. Grimm RH Jr et al. Relationships of quality-of-life measures to long-term lifestyle and drug treatment in the Treatment of Mild Hypertension Study. *Arch Intern Med* 1997;157:638.
32. Jensen J et al. The prevalence and etiology of impotence in 101 male hypertensive outpatients. *Am J Hypertens* 1999;12:271.
33. Veterans Administration Cooperative Study Group on Antihypertensive Agents. Effects of treatment on morbidity in hypertension: results in patients with diastolic blood pressures averaging 115 through 129 mmHg. *JAMA* 1967;202:1028.
34. The Tobacco Use and Dependence Clinical Practice Guideline Panel, Staff, and Consortium Representatives. A clinical practice guideline for treating tobacco use and dependence: a U.S. Public Health Service report. *JAMA* 2000;283:3244.
35. Saseen JJ. ASHP therapeutic position statement on the daily use of aspirin for preventing cardiovascular events. *Am J Health Syst Pharm* 2005;62: 1398.
36. Smith SC et al. AHA/ACC guidelines for secondary prevention for patients with coronary and other atherosclerotic vascular disease: 2006 update endorsed by the National Heart, Lung, and Blood Institute. *J Am Coll Cardiol* 2006;47:2130.
37. Neaton JD et al. Treatment of Mild Hypertension Study. Final results. Treatment of Mild Hypertension Study Research Group. *JAMA* 1993;270:713.
38. Sackett DL et al. Evidence based medicine: what it is and what it isn't. *BMJ* 1996;312:71.
39. SHEP Cooperative Research Group. Prevention of stroke by antihypertensive drug treatment in older persons with isolated systolic hypertension. Final results of the Systolic Hypertension in the Elderly Program (SHEP). *JAMA* 1991;265:3255.
40. Dahlof B et al. Morbidity and mortality in the Swedish Trial in Old Patients with Hypertension (STOP-Hypertension). *Lancet* 1991;338:1281.
41. MRC Working Party. Medical Research Council trial of treatment of hypertension in older adults: principal results. *BMJ* 1992;304:405.
42. Staessen JA et al. Randomised double-blind comparison of placebo and active treatment for older patients with isolated systolic hypertension: the Systolic Hypertension in Europe (Syst-Eur) Trial Investigators. *Lancet* 1997;350:757.
43. Black HR et al. Principal results of the Controlled Onset Verapamil Investigation of Cardiovascular End Points (CONVINCE) trial. *JAMA* 2003;289:2073.
44. Dahlof B et al. Cardiovascular morbidity and mortality in the Losartan Intervention For Endpoint reduction in hypertension study (LIFE): a randomised trial against atenolol. *Lancet* 2002;359:995.
45. ALLHAT Officers and Coordinators for the ALLHAT Collaborative Research Group. Major outcomes in high-risk hypertensive patients randomized to angiotensin-converting enzyme inhibitor or calcium channel blocker vs. diuretic: the Antihypertensive and Lipid-Lowering Treatment to Prevent Heart Attack Trial (ALLHAT). *JAMA* 2002;288:2981.
46. PROGRESS Collaborative Group. Randomised trial of a perindopril-based blood-pressure-lowering regimen among 6,105 individuals with previous stroke or transient ischaemic attack. *Lancet* 2001;358:1033.
47. Wing LM et al. A comparison of outcomes with angiotensin-converting-enzyme inhibitors and diuretics for hypertension in the elderly. *N Engl J Med* 2003;348:583.
48. Hansson L et al. Randomised trial of old and new antihypertensive drugs in elderly patients: cardiovascular mortality and morbidity the Swedish Trial in Old Patients with Hypertension-2 study. *Lancet* 1999;354:1751.
49. Wang JG et al. Chinese trial on isolated systolic hypertension in the elderly. Systolic Hypertension in China (Syst-China) Collaborative Group. *Arch Intern Med* 2000;160:211.
50. Heart Outcomes Prevention Evaluation Study Investigators. Effects of ramipril on cardiovascular and microvascular outcomes in people with diabetes mellitus: results of the HOPE study and MICRO-HOPE substudy. *Lancet* 2000;355:253.
51. Hansson L et al. Randomised trial of effects of calcium antagonists compared with diuretics and beta-blockers on cardiovascular morbidity and mortality in hypertension: the Nordic Diltiazem (NORDIL) study. *Lancet* 2000;356:359.
52. Hansson L et al. Effect of angiotensin-converting-enzyme inhibition compared with conventional therapy on cardiovascular morbidity and mortality in hypertension: the Captopril Prevention Project (CAPPP) randomised trial. *Lancet* 1999;353:611.
53. Estacio RO et al. The effect of nisoldipine as compared with enalapril on cardiovascular outcomes in patients with non-insulin-dependent diabetes and hypertension. *N Engl J Med* 1998;338:645.
54. Tatti P et al. Outcome results of the Fosinopril versus Amlodipine Cardiovascular Events Randomized Trial (FACET) in patients with hypertension and NIDDM. *Diabetes Care* 1998;21:597.
55. Efficacy of atenolol and captopril in reducing risk of macrovascular and microvascular complications in type 2 diabetes: UKPDS 39. UK Prospective Diabetes Study Group. *BMJ* 1998;317:713.
56. Brenner BM et al. Effects of losartan on renal and cardiovascular outcomes in patients with type 2 diabetes and nephropathy. *N Engl J Med* 2001;345:861.
57. Lewis EJ et al. Renoprotective effect of the angiotensin-receptor antagonist irbesartan in patients with nephropathy due to type 2 diabetes. *N Engl J Med* 2001;345:851.
58. Parving HH et al. The effect of irbesartan on the development of diabetic nephropathy in patients with type 2 diabetes. *N Engl J Med* 2001;345:870.
59. Dickstein K et al. Effects of losartan and captopril on mortality and morbidity in high-risk patients after acute myocardial infarction: the OPTIMAAL randomised trial. Optimal Trial in Myocardial Infarction with Angiotensin II Antagonist Losartan. *Lancet* 2002;360:752.
60. Wright JT Jr. et al. Effect of blood pressure lowering and antihypertensive drug class on progression of hypertensive kidney disease: results from the AASK trial. *JAMA* 2002;288:2421.
61. Dahlof B et al. Prevention of cardiovascular events with an antihypertensive regimen of amlodipine adding perindopril as required versus atenolol adding bendroflumethiazide as required, in the Anglo-Scandinavian Cardiac Outcomes Trial-Blood Pressure Lowering Arm (ASCOT-BPLA): a multicentre randomised controlled trial. *Lancet* 2005;366:895.
62. Julius S et al. Outcomes in hypertensive patients at high cardiovascular risk treated with regimens based on valsartan or amlodipine: the VALUE randomised trial. *Lancet* 2004;363:2022.
63. Schrader J et al. Morbidity and Mortality After Stroke, Eprosartan Compared with Nitrendipine for Secondary Prevention: principal results of a prospective randomized controlled study (MOSES). *Stroke* 2005;36:1218.
64. Law MR et al. Value of low dose combination treatment with blood pressure lowering drugs: analysis of 354 randomised trials. *BMJ* 2003;326:1427.
65. Douglas JG et al. Management of high blood pressure in African Americans: consensus statement of the Hypertension in African Americans Working Group of the International Society on Hypertension in Blacks. *Arch Intern Med* 2003;163:525.

66. Gueyffier F et al. Antihypertensive drugs in very old people: a subgroup meta-analysis of randomised controlled trials. INDANA Group. *Lancet* 1999;353:793.
67. Bulpitt C et al. Hypertension in the Very Elderly Trial (HYVET): protocol for the main trial. *Drugs Aging* 2001;18:151.
68. Beckett NS et al. Treatment of hypertension in patients 80 years of age or older. *N Engl J Med* 2008; 358:1887.
69. Farnett L et al. The J-curve phenomenon and the treatment of hypertension: is there a point beyond which pressure reduction is dangerous? *JAMA* 1991;265:489.
70. Voko Z et al. J-shaped relation between blood pressure and stroke in treated hypertensives. *Hypertension* 1999;34:1181.
71. Cutler DM et al. The value of antihypertensive drugs: a perspective on medical innovation. *Health Aff* 2007;26:97.
72. Standards of medical care in diabetes—2007. *Diabetes Care* 2007;30(Suppl 1):S4.
73. Lindholm LH et al. Cardiovascular morbidity and mortality in patients with diabetes in the Losartan Intervention for Endpoint reduction in hypertension study (LIFE): a randomised trial against atenolol. *Lancet* 2002;359:1004.
74. Niskanen L et al. Reduced cardiovascular morbidity and mortality in hypertensive diabetic patients on first-line therapy with an ACE inhibitor compared with a diuretic/beta-blocker-based treatment regimen: a subanalysis of the Captopril Prevention Project. *Diabetes Care* 2001;24:2091.
75. Bakris GL et al. Preserving renal function in adults with hypertension and diabetes: a consensus approach. National Kidney Foundation Hypertension and Diabetes Executive Committees Working Group. *Am J Kidney Dis* 2000;36:646.
76. Lewis EJ et al. The effect of angiotensin-converting-enzyme inhibition on diabetic nephropathy. The Collaborative Study Group. *N Engl J Med* 1993;329:1456.
77. The GISEN Group (Gruppo Italiano di Studi Epidemiologici in Nefrologia). Randomised placebo-controlled trial of effect of ramipril on decline in glomerular filtration rate and risk of terminal renal failure in proteinuric, non-diabetic nephropathy. *Lancet* 1997;349:1857.
78. Gibbons RJ et al. ACC/AHA 2002 guideline update for the management of patients with chronic stable angina—summary article: a report of the American College of Cardiology/American Heart Association Task Force on Practice Guidelines (Committee on the Management of Patients With Chronic Stable Angina). *Circulation* 2003;107:149.
79. Dargie HJ. Effect of carvedilol on outcome after myocardial infarction in patients with left-ventricular dysfunction: the CAPRICORN randomised trial. *Lancet* 2001;357:1385.
80. Anonymous. A randomized trial of propranolol in patients with acute myocardial infarction. I. Mortality results. *JAMA* 1982;247:1707.
81. Sipahi I et al. Beta-blockers and progression of coronary atherosclerosis: pooled analysis of 4 intravascular ultrasonography trials. *Ann Intern Med* 2007;147:10.
82. Yusuf S et al. Effects of an angiotensin- converting-enzyme inhibitor, ramipril, on cardiovascular events in high-risk patients. The Heart Outcomes Prevention Evaluation Study Investigators. *N Engl J Med* 2000;342:145.
83. Pfeffer MA et al. Effect of captopril on mortality and morbidity in patients with left ventricular dysfunction after myocardial infarction. Results of the survival and ventricular enlargement trial. The SAVE Investigators. *N Engl J Med* 1992;327: 669.
84. Anderson JL et al. ACC/AHA 2007 guidelines for the management of patients with unstable angina/non ST-elevation myocardial infarction: a report of the American College of Cardiology/American Heart Association Task Force on Practice Guidelines (Writing Committee to Revise the 2002 Guidelines for the Management of Patients With Unstable Angina/Non ST-Elevation Myocardial Infarction): developed in collaboration with the American College of Emergency Physicians, the Society for Cardiovascular Angiography and Interventions, and the Society of Thoracic Surgeons: endorsed by the American Association of Cardiovascular and Pulmonary Rehabilitation and the Society for Academic Emergency Medicine. *Circulation* 2007;116:e148.
85. Antman EM et al. ACC/AHA guidelines for the management of patients with ST-elevation myocardial infarction—executive summary: a report of the American College of Cardiology/American Heart Association Task Force on Practice Guidelines (Writing Committee to Revise the 1999 Guidelines for the Management of Patients With Acute Myocardial Infarction). *Circulation* 2004;110:588.
86. Hunt SA. ACC/AHA 2005 guideline update for the diagnosis and management of chronic heart failure in the adult: a report of the American College of Cardiology/American Heart Association Task Force on Practice Guidelines (Writing Committee to Update the 2001 Guidelines for the Evaluation and Management of Heart Failure). *J Am Coll Cardiol* 2005;46:e1.
87. Effect of metoprolol CR/XL in chronic heart failure: Metoprolol CR/XL Randomised Intervention Trial in Congestive Heart Failure (MERIT-HF). *Lancet* 1999;353:2001.
88. Packer M et al. Effect of carvedilol on survival in severe chronic heart failure. *N Engl J Med* 2001; 344:1651.
89. Pitt B et al. Eplerenone, a selective aldosterone blocker, in patients with left ventricular dysfunction after myocardial infarction. *N Engl J Med* 2003; 348:1309.
90. Pitt B et al. The effect of spironolactone on morbidity and mortality in patients with severe heart failure. Randomized Aldactone Evaluation Study Investigators. *N Engl J Med* 1999;341:709.
91. Taylor AL et al. Combination of isosorbide dinitrate and hydralazine in blacks with heart failure. *N Engl J Med* 2004;351:2049.
92. Cohn JN et al. A randomized trial of the angiotensin-receptor blocker valsartan in chronic heart failure. *N Engl J Med* 2001;345:1667.
93. Granger CB et al. Effects of candesartan in patients with chronic heart failure and reduced left-ventricular systolic function intolerant to angiotensin-converting-enzyme inhibitors: the CHARM-Alternative trial. *Lancet* 2003;362:772.
94. McMurray JJ et al. Effects of candesartan in patients with chronic heart failure and reduced left-ventricular systolic function taking angiotensin-converting-enzyme inhibitors: the CHARM-Added trial. *Lancet* 2003;362:767.
95. Pitt B et al. Randomised trial of losartan versus captopril in patients over 65 with heart failure (Evaluation of Losartan in the Elderly Study, ELITE). *Lancet* 1997;349:747.
96. Pitt B et al. Effect of losartan compared with captopril on mortality in patients with symptomatic heart failure: randomised trial—the Losartan Heart Failure Survival Study ELITE II. *Lancet* 2000;355:1582.
97. Savage PJ et al. Influence of long-term, low-dose, diuretic-based, antihypertensive therapy on glucose, lipid, uric acid, and potassium levels in older men and women with isolated systolic hypertension: the Systolic Hypertension in the Elderly Program. SHEP Cooperative Research Group. *Arch Intern Med* 1998;158:741.
98. Zillich AJ et al. Thiazide diuretics, potassium, and the development of diabetes: a quantitative review. *Hypertension* 2006;48:219.
99. Carter BL et al. Development of diabetes with thiazide diuretics: the potassium issue. *J Clin Hypertens* 2005;7:638.
100. Barzilay JI et al. Fasting glucose levels and incident diabetes mellitus in older nondiabetic adults randomized to receive 3 different classes of antihypertensive treatment: a report from the Antihypertensive and Lipid-Lowering Treatment to Prevent Heart Attack Trial (ALLHAT). *Arch Intern Med* 2006;166:2191.
101. Langford HG et al. Is thiazide-produced uric acid elevation harmful? Analysis of data from the Hypertension Detection and Follow-up Program. *Arch Intern Med* 1987;147:645.
102. Freis ED. The efficacy and safety of diuretics in treating hypertension. *Ann Intern Med* 1995; 122:223.
103. Elliott WJ et al. Incident diabetes in clinical trials of antihypertensive drugs: a network meta-analysis. *Lancet* 2007;369:201.
104. O'Keefe JH et al. Should an angiotensin-converting enzyme inhibitor be standard therapy for patients with atherosclerotic disease? *J Am Coll Cardiol* 2001;37:1.
105. Frohlich ED et al. The heart in hypertension. *N Engl J Med* 1992;327:998.
106. Patel A et al. Effects of a fixed combination of perindopril and indapamide on macrovascular and microvascular outcomes in patients with type 2 diabetes mellitus (the ADVANCE trial): a randomised controlled trial. *Lancet* 2007;370:829.
107. Cooper WO et al. Major congenital malformations after first-trimester exposure to ACE inhibitors. *N Engl J Med* 2006;354:2443.
108. Luque CA et al. Treatment of ACE inhibitor-induced cough. *Pharmacotherapy* 1999;19:804.
109. Yusuf S et al. Telmisartan, Ramipril, or both in patients at high risk for vascular events. *N Engl J Med* 2008;358:1547.
110. Phillips CO et al. Adverse effects of combination angiotensin II receptor blockers plus angiotensin-converting enzyme inhibitors for left ventricular dysfunction: a quantitative review of data from randomized clinical trials. *Arch Intern Med* 2007; 167:1930.
111. Cicardi M et al. Angioedema associated with angiotensin-converting enzyme inhibitor use: outcome after switching to a different treatment. *Arch Intern Med* 2004;164:910.
112. Grossman E et al. Should a moratorium be placed on sublingual nifedipine capsules given for hypertensive emergencies and pseudoemergencies? *JAMA* 1996;276:1328.
113. Packer M et al. Effect of amlodipine on morbidity and mortality in severe chronic heart failure. Prospective Randomized Amlodipine Survival Evaluation Study Group. *N Engl J Med* 1996;335:1107.
114. Freemantle N et al. Beta Blockade after myocardial infarction: systematic review and meta regression analysis. *BMJ* 1999;318:1730.
115. ALLHAT Collaborative Research Group. Major cardiovascular events in hypertensive patients randomized to doxazosin vs. chlorthalidone: the antihypertensive and lipid-lowering treatment to prevent heart attack trial (ALLHAT). *JAMA* 2000;283:1967.
116. Staessen JA et al. Oral renin inhibitors. *Lancet* 2006;368(9545):1449.
117. National High Blood Pressure Education Program Working Group Report on High Blood Pressure in Pregnancy. *Am J Obstet Gynecol* 1990;163:1691.

CHAPTER 14

Peripheral Vascular Disorders

Anne P. Spencer and C. Wayne Weart

Peripheral Arterial Disease

Peripheral arterial disease (PAD) is a common and sometimes painful complications from stenosis or occlusion in the peripheral arteries of the legs, usually caused by atherosclerosis. Some clinicians and patients have characterized claudication pain as "angina" of the legs. When considering the risk factors and pathology of intermittent claudication (IC), the association with coronary disease becomes clear.

Intermittent claudication is described as aching, cramping, tightness, or weakness of the legs, which usually occurs during exertion. Claudication pain is relieved when the physical activity is discontinued. Numbness or continuous pain in the toes or foot may be present, indicating tissue ischemia, which can lead to ulceration. IC is a painful condition that can severely limit the patient's mobility and lead to tissue necrosis or amputation of the affected limb. Many patients with PAD, however, are asymptomatic or have atypical lower limb symptoms, such as leg fatigue, difficulty walking, or similar nonspecific complaints. Because symptoms of IC develop gradually, patients may not seek medical attention until the condition is advanced.

Epidemiology

Peripheral arterial disease is a relatively common condition that affects men and women equally, with a prevalence of 12%,[1] although men have a twofold increased prevalence of symptomatic IC.[2] The annual incidence of IC increases dramatically with age (Table 14-1). Most patients with PAD are largely asymptomatic, although their risk of developing symptoms of IC in the future is greatly increased. In a population with only a 2% prevalence of IC symptoms, 11.7% of patients had detectable large vessel atherosclerosis of the lower extremities.[3] This disparity between IC symptoms and the presence of PAD contributes to the observation that 50% to 90% of patients with IC do not mention the symptoms to their physician. Patients attribute the symptoms of IC to normal walking difficulties associated with aging, not a medical condition requiring treatment.[4]

Risk factors for developing occlusive PAD are similar to those for coronary artery disease. Longstanding diabetes is the most significant risk factor, with 30% of patients with diabetes affected by PAD.[5] PAD is five times more common in patients with diabetes than in patients without diabetes; in diabetics, it develops at a younger age and progresses more rapidly. Each 1% increase in glycosylated hemoglobin is associated with a 28% risk of incident PAD.[6] Other risk factors include cigarette smoking, hypertension, dyslipidemia, hyperhomocysteinemia, and C-reactive protein.[7] Hypertriglyceridemia is a more significant risk factor for PAD than for coronary artery disease, and this may partially explain the increased prevalence of PAD in patients with diabetes.[8]

Cigarette smoking has a higher correlation with the development of IC pain than any other risk factor, and the risk increases dramatically with the number of cigarettes smoked per day and the duration of smoking history.[9] In patients with other cardiovascular risk factors, including hypertension or diabetes, smoking further increases the rate of claudication development. Smoking confers a sevenfold increase in risk for PAD compared with nonsmokers. In contrast, the risk of coronary artery disease is only increased twofold in smokers. Thus, the mechanism by which cigarette smoking causes damage may be different for these two vascular diseases.[10]

Epidemiologic studies show that IC is nonprogressive in 75% of patients over a period of 4 to 9 years. The other 25% of patients with IC have worsening painful ischemic episodes over this period. Although rare, more serious complications can occur. Ischemic tissue changes, ulceration, and gangrene can accompany advanced peripheral atherosclerosis. Amputation of the affected limb may be necessary in up to 5% of

Table 14-1 Annual Incidence of Intermittent Claudication by Age[3]

Age Group (yr)	*Annual Incidence (%)*
40	2.0
50	4.2
60	6.8
70	9.2

patients with claudication.[11] The presence of two independent risk factors, such as diabetes and cigarette smoking, has an additive effect on the risk for the development of progressive IC and serious limb complications (Table 14-2).

During a relatively short 2-year follow-up of a population with IC, 3.6% of patients died, whereas 22% experienced a nonfatal cardiovascular event (defined as any cardiac, cerebral, or peripheral vascular event). Furthermore, 26% experienced a decline in their walking capability during the same time frame.[12,13] Although a relatively small fraction of patients died during the 2-year observation period, it is paramount to recognize that severe, short-term morbidity is highly likely in this patient population. IC clearly reflects generalized atherosclerosis and is associated with considerable morbidity.

Pathophysiology

Intermittent claudication, and its associated pain and impaired mobility, is the predominant complication of occlusive PAD. The major cause of occlusive PAD is arteriosclerosis obliterans, defined as the development of atherosclerotic plaques in the peripheral vasculature. These plaques develop as a result of endothelial activation associated with conditions such as dyslipidemia, diabetes mellitus, hypertension, and tobacco use. Plaques result in the proliferation of vascular smooth muscle, with subsequent damage to the vascular structure. The damaged endothelium of the vasculature has impaired vasodilatory capabilities because secretion of nitric oxide, also known as endothelium-derived relaxing factor, is decreased and secretion of vasoconstrictive substances, such as endothelin, are increased. Both defects impede blood flow to the extremities. In addition, growth of atherosclerotic lesions can physically limit blood flow. Exercise may induce IC symptoms in patients who have lesions with >50% stenosis, whereas patients with lesions of >80% stenosis can have pain at rest. The lesions themselves can be unstable and rupture, or adjacent smaller vessels experiencing high hemodynamic pressure caused by nearby plaques may rupture. Either situation can lead to acute vascular occlusion, analogous to unstable angina or acute myocardial infarction (MI) in coronary arteries.[14]

Table 14-2 Long-Term Incidence of Outcomes in Patients With Intermittent Claudication[11,12]

Patient Population	*Abrupt Limb Ischemia (%)*	*Amputation (%)*
All patients	23	7
Diabetics	31	11
Smokers	35	21

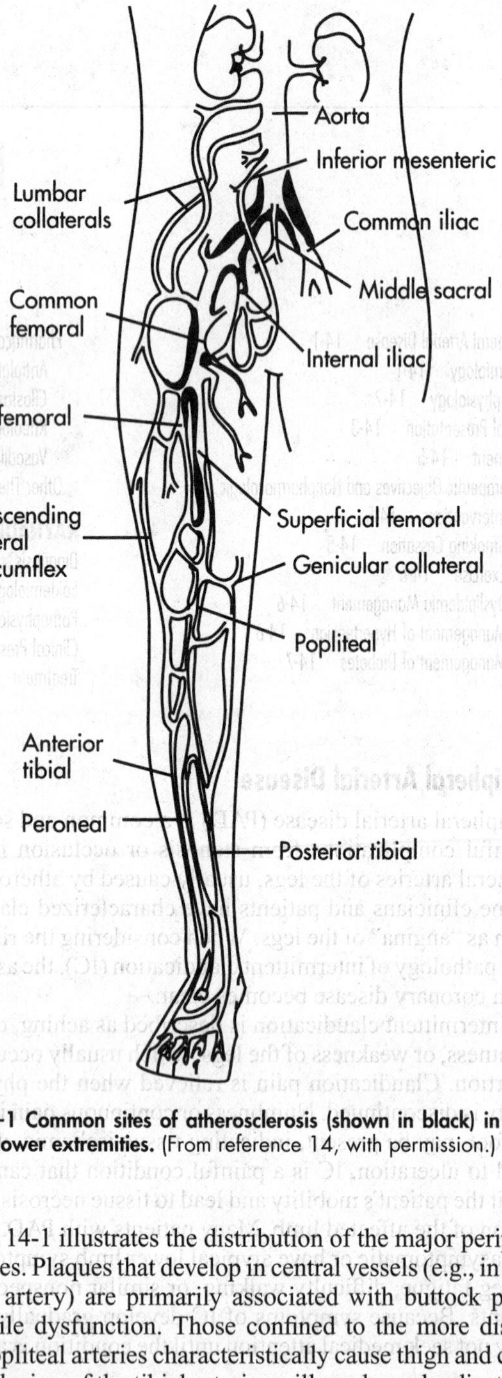

FIGURE 14-1 Common sites of atherosclerosis (shown in black) in the aorta and lower extremities. (From reference 14, with permission.)

Figure 14-1 illustrates the distribution of the major peripheral arteries. Plaques that develop in central vessels (e.g., in the ilioaortic artery) are primarily associated with buttock pain and erectile dysfunction. Those confined to the more distal femoropopliteal arteries characteristically cause thigh and calf pain. Occlusion of the tibial arteries will produce claudication pain in the foot. When more than one artery bed is affected by severe atherosclerosis, symptoms of IC will be diffuse. Symptoms of IC indicate an inadequate supply of arterial blood to peripheral muscles. Exercise, including walking, increases the metabolic demands of the muscles and can lead to claudication pain. Reduced blood supply to the muscles results from changes in perfusion pressures and vascular tone caused by atherosclerosis.

Atherosclerosis can impair the microcirculation of the peripheral muscles by altering the pressure gradient needed for perfusion of the capillaries (Fig. 14-2). When obstruction develops, perfusion of tissue distal to the stenotic lesion relies on collateral blood flow. Collateral circulation consists of new

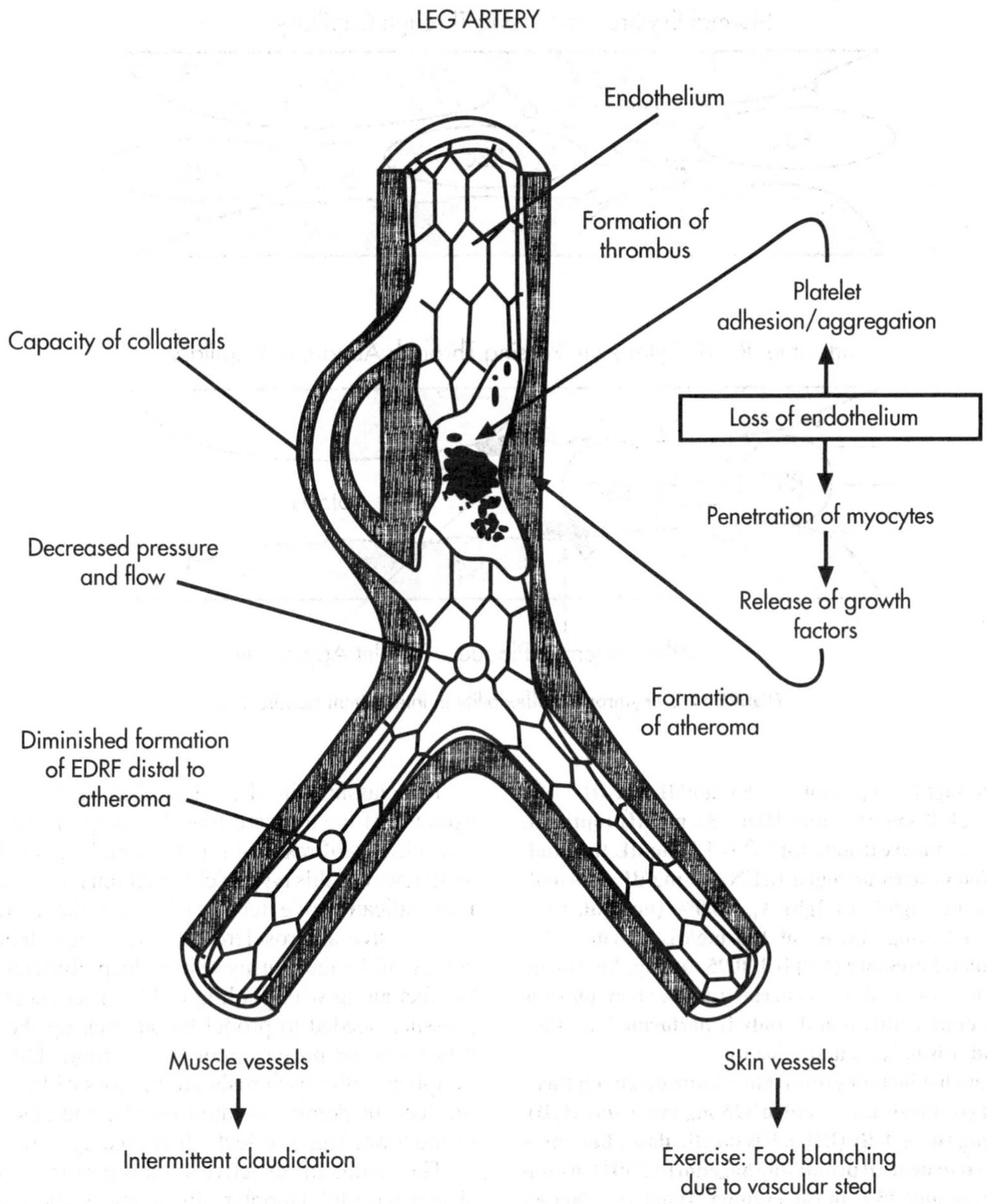

FIGURE 14-2 Consequences of occlusive atherosclerotic disease in the lower limbs. EDRF, endothelium-derived relaxing factor. (From reference 169, with permission.)

blood vessels that develop to carry blood around the occluded area.

Erythrocyte deformability is an important factor for in vitro capillary perfusion.[15,16] In areas free of compromised blood flow, normal red blood cells (RBCs) have the ability to deform when passing through a small capillary. By aligning themselves in a planar manner, the RBCs also reduce the viscosity of the blood suspension, enabling them to pass smoothly through the capillary. In many patients with IC, RBCs have a marked decrease in this intrinsic ability to deform, which results in increased blood viscosity. This defect is promoted by chronic tissue ischemia and hypoxia caused by increased intracapillary leukocyte adherence, platelet aggregation, and activation of complement and clotting factors.[14] The vascular responses to hypoxia are detrimental because this sequence of events further inhibits blood flow and oxygen delivery to the tissues (Fig. 14-3).

Clinical Presentation

1. J.S. is a 54-year-old, 100-kg man with a history of type 2, insulin-treated diabetes mellitus, angina, dyslipidemia, and tobacco use. His chief complaint today is right upper thigh pain while walking around the block. The pain has gradually increased over the past 12 months, but only recently has become intolerable. The pain is relieved within minutes after he stops walking. J.S. smokes 1.5 packs of cigarettes a day.

His most recent laboratory results are significant for total cholesterol, 290 mg/dL (optimal, <200 mg/dL); fasting

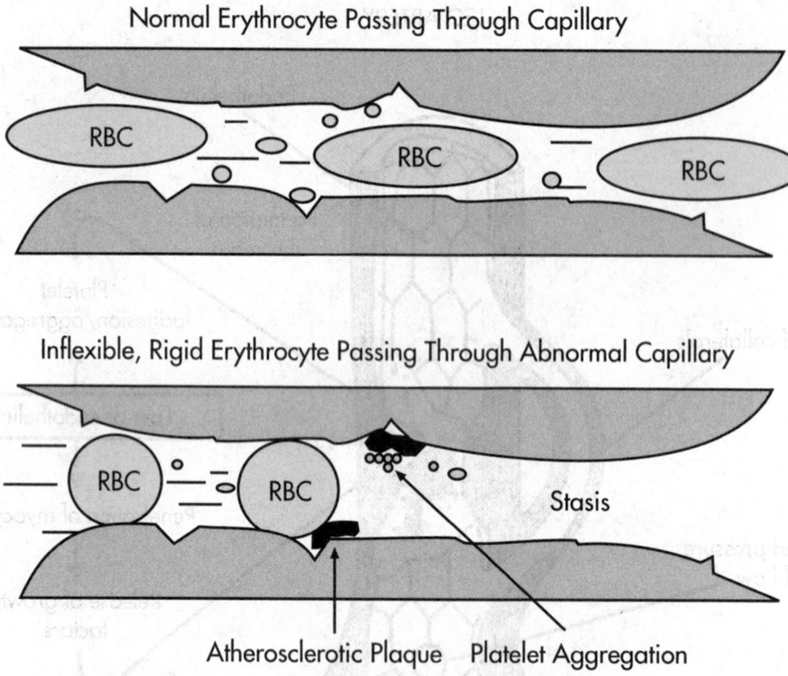

FIGURE 14-3 Erythrocyte inflexibility in intermittent claudication.

triglycerides, 350 mg/dL (optimal, <150 mg/dL); LDL, 188 mg/dL (optimal, <100 mg/dL); and HDL, 32 mg/dL (optimal, >40 mg/dL). His serum creatinine (SrCr) is 1.0 mg/dL (normal, 0.7–1.5 mg/dL), blood urea nitrogen (BUN) 15 mg/dL (normal, 8–20 mg/dL), and hemoglobin (Hgb) A_{1c} 10.0% (normal, 5%–6%), and he has a fasting glucose of 150 mg/dL (normal, 70–115 mg/dL). His blood pressure (BP) is 170/95 mmHg, heart rate (HR) is 89 beats/minute, and his posterior tibial artery pulse is not palpable. A Doppler ultrasound study is performed, and his ankle:brachial index is 0.7 (normal, >0.90).

J.S.'s medication list includes isosorbide dinitrate 20 mg three times daily (TID) (while awake), aspirin 325 mg every day (QD), and enalapril 10 mg twice daily (BID). His insulin doses have progressively increased to neutral protamine hagedorn (NPH) insulin 40 U in the morning and 35 U in the evening. What risk factors and elements of J.S.'s presentation are compatible with a diagnosis of IC?

[SI units: total cholesterol, 7.49 mmol/L (optimal, <3.88 mmol/L); triglycerides, 3.95 mmol/L (optimal, <2.26 mmol/L); LDL, 4.86 mmol/L (normal, <2.58 mmol/L); HDL, 0.83 mmol/L (normal, >1.04 mmol/L); SrCr, 60 mmol/L; BUN, 5.3 mmol/L; HgbA1c, 0.1, glucose 8.3 mmol/L]

J.S.'s medical history illustrates classic risk factors for vascular occlusion and IC, including dyslipidemia (specifically hypertriglyceridemia), diabetes, hypertension, and tobacco use. In particular, his diabetes is not adequately controlled based on elevated HgbA1c and fasting glucose levels, and he is obese. This constellation of disorders is known as the *metabolic syndrome*. These factors, along with smoking, commonly are seen together and have been linked with hyperinsulinemia and accelerated atherosclerosis (Fig. 14-4).[17,18] The presence of angina indicates coronary artery disease, so it is not surprising that he has peripheral vascular occlusion as well.

The classic pain of IC described by J.S. is associated with exercise of the affected muscle group(s) and subsides with a few minutes of rest and reperfusion. IC pain also can occur at rest; however, this type of claudication pain is less common and is an indication of extensive disease. Other common symptoms of extensive atherosclerosis include cold feet and persistent aching of the feet during rest or sleep. Restricted blood flow to the feet along with pooling of blood secondary to inadequate pressure needed to propel blood back up the leg can lead to rubor (red or purple color of the foot). Other indicators of peripheral atherosclerosis are the loss of hair from the top of the feet, thickening of the toenails, and absence of sweating of the lower legs and feet, all caused by poor circulation.[14]

The results of objective studies performed on J.S. are consistent with IC. Doppler ultrasound of the spine is helpful in

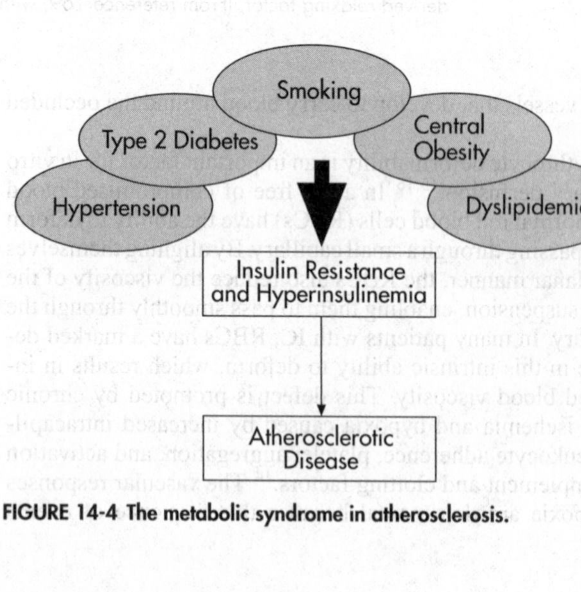

FIGURE 14-4 The metabolic syndrome in atherosclerosis.

Table 14-3 Severity of Arterial Obstruction As Assessed by Ankle:Brachial Index[27]

Severity	*Ankle:Brachial Index*[a]
Normal	>0.90
Mild	0.70–0.89
Moderate	0.50–0.69
Severe	>0.50

[a]Ankle:brachial index is the systolic blood pressure in the ankle divided by the systolic blood pressure in the arm.

excluding pseudoclaudication caused by spinal stenosis and other neurogenic or musculoskeletal causes of leg pain. Ultrasound also is useful to measure BP of the lower extremities. An ankle:brachial index (ABI) of 0.7 means that the ankle systolic BP reading is only 70% of the systolic pressure in the brachial artery supplying blood to the arm. In patients with IC, this is caused by atherosclerotic obstruction of blood flow in the lower limbs and subsequent decreased perfusion pressures in the ankle compared with the arm (Table 14-3). The lower the ABI, the more blood flow to the extremities is compromised and the greater the severity of symptoms. An ABI <0.9 is diagnostic for peripheral arterial disease. Also, loss of the posterior tibial pulse, as seen in J.S., is common in those with peripheral vascular occlusion.

Treatment

Therapeutic Objectives and Nonpharmacologic Interventions

2. What is the therapeutic objective in treating J.S.? What interventions should be initiated to prevent claudication pain and arrest progression of the disease?

The specific treatment goals for J.S. are prevention of further claudication pain, lessening the current pain he experiences, arresting the progression of underlying disease, and decreasing his risk of any cardiovascular event. Achieving these goals will provide J.S. with the best chance of avoiding further mobility impairment, amputation, and cardiovascular events such as stroke or MI. An important concept that should be stressed when explaining these treatment goals to J.S. is that all his diseases are closely interrelated, and that a beneficial intervention for one disease is beneficial for all. Interventions that can be initiated include diet modification and weight loss, control of his diabetes, hypertension therapy optimization, and dyslipidemia therapy. The American College of Cardiology and American Heart Association have published guidelines that thoroughly evaluate the interventions and medications that have been used to treat IC and PAD.[7] Table 14-4 summarizes these recommendations. The two most important things that J.S. can do for his IC are summed up in five words: "Stop smoking and keep walking."[19]

SMOKING CESSATION

The importance of smoking cessation cannot be overemphasized to patients with IC. It is the most important modifiable factor in preventing the development of rest pain, prolonged limb ischemia, and the need for amputation. Several studies document improved survival and decreased amputation rates in patients with IC who stopped smoking compared with patients who continue to smoke.[20,21] Other benefits, such as improved treadmill walking distance, decreased progression to symptoms, and decreased complications following vascular reconstructive surgery, have been shown in patients who are able to quit smoking compared with patients who continue to smoke.[7,20,22–24] It is also the intervention that will decrease J.S.'s claudication pain most rapidly. If J.S. is able to stop smoking, his risk of developing rest pain or requiring limb amputation will be very low. He also will decrease his risk of MI and mortality by three- and fivefold, respectively. Table 14-5 summarizes the risk of cigarette smoking and the value of smoking cessation on cardiovascular complications.

Table 14-4 Medical Treatment of Peripheral Arterial Disease and Expected Outcomes[7,168]

Intervention	*Improve Leg Symptoms?*	*Prevent Systemic Complications?*
Smoking cessation	Yes	Yes
Exercise	Yes	No
Cilostazol	Yes	No
Statin drugs	Yes	Yes
Angiotensin-converting enzyme inhibitors	Yes	Yes
Blood pressure control	No	Yes
Antiplatelet therapy[a]	No	Yes

[a]Aspirin or clopidogrel.

Many pharmacologic products and strategies are available to aid patients such as J.S. to stop smoking (see Chapter 84, Treatment of Tobacco Use and Dependence). Many are nicotine replacement products, which can be administered as a nasal spray, chewed as a gum, consumed as a lozenge, or absorbed through a transdermal patch. If these are needed to help him stop smoking, their use is warranted. Nicotine itself has harmful effects on the vasculature via catecholamine release and vasoconstriction, however, and it may play a role in endothelial damage and atherosclerosis progression.[25] Medications that do not contain nicotine, such as bupropion (Zyban) and varenicline (Chantix), and smoking cessation counseling or support groups should be used as necessary to help the patient stop smoking.

Table 14-5 Patient Outcomes Based on Smoking Status After Intermittent Claudication Diagnosis[11,20]

Outcome	*Length of Follow-up (yr)*	*Patient Population*	
		Current Smokers (%)	*Past Smokers (%)*[a]
Rest pain	7	16	0
Myocardial infarction	10	53	11
Amputation	5	11	0
Mortality	10	54	18

[a]Quit after intermittent claudication diagnosis.

EXERCISE

An individualized and supervised exercise program has been endorsed for patients with PAD and will benefit J.S.'s other risk factors as well.[7] The pain associated with IC results in decreased mobility, and because of deconditioning from lack of exercise, patients with IC may slowly become dependent on others for activities of daily living. An exercise program is the most effective way to both preserve and increase mobility. It is more effective than the best pharmacologic therapy currently available.[26] The ideal exercise program consists of walking for a minimum of 30 to 45 minutes at least three times a week.[7] J.S. should walk as fast and far as he can until the pain becomes severe; he should then wait until the pain subsides, and then resume walking.[27] At first, J.S. may experience several painful episodes during each exercise session, but these should gradually decrease as the beneficial effects of exercise therapy begin to emerge. Studies have documented that this type of exercise program can more than double the pain-free distance a patient with IC is able to walk.[28] Several surgical options are available for patients, including surgical bypass of the affected arteries, in addition to angioplasty and stenting. An appropriate exercise program results in superior outcomes compared with angioplasty and stenting, and equal in terms of walking distance compared with surgery. Significant complications and mortality are associated with surgery, however, and when all outcomes are considered, an exercise program is far more advantageous than surgery.[28] For all patients able to walk, an exercise program should be supervised and individually designed, and the patient should understand the importance of exercise to his or her continued mobility.[26]

Rheologic abnormalities of increased blood viscosity, impaired RBC filterability, hyperaggregation, and polycythemia (elevated hematocrit) have been shown to return to normal in many patients with IC who participate in a regular exercise program.[29] Exercise may offset the need for pharmacologic intervention. The potential mechanisms by which exercise benefits patients with IC are listed in Table 14-6.

DYSLIPIDEMIA MANAGEMENT

3. Is lipid-lowering therapy indicated for J.S.?

Because IC is a consequence of atherosclerosis, arresting the progression of J.S.'s atherosclerotic disease is important (see Chapter 12, Dyslipidemias, Atherosclerosis, and Coronary Heart Disease). The initiation of the nutritional and exercise recommendations outlined in the Therapeutic Lifestyle Changes (TLC) guidelines,[30] as well as cholesterol-lowering agents, are the cornerstones for attaining this goal. Considerable data suggest that aggressive dietary and pharmacologic management of dyslipidemia, particularly lowering low-density lipoprotein cholesterol (LDL-C), leads to regression of atherosclerotic lesions in the coronary and carotid vasculature.[31–33] In contrast, relatively few prospective data exist about the effect of successful lipid-lowering therapy on the regression or stabilization of peripheral lesions, or on clinical events in patients with PAD. A *post hoc* analysis of a large lipid-lowering study in subjects with known coronary artery disease treated with simvastatin, however, demonstrated a significant decrease in new or worsening IC, suggesting that benefit is seen in the prevention of clinically symptomatic PAD in high-risk patients.[34] Another study randomized patients with known arterial disease of various types to simvastatin 40 mg daily or placebo. After 5 years, a 15% decrease was found in noncardiac revascularizations, including amputations, among the patients receiving simvastatin.[35] Short-term outcomes (e.g., 6 months to 1 year), such as improved walking distance and walking time, have also been documented with simvastatin 40 mg/day.[36,37]

A meta-analysis of 698 subjects from several small, randomized trials using a variety of lipid-lowering therapies in patients with PAD demonstrated reduced severity of claudication and decreased disease progression as measured by angiography. A decrease in mortality was also seen, but this did not reach statistical significance.[38] Limited data suggest high Lp(a) lipoprotein concentrations may be particularly important in the development of PAD.[39]

All patients with evidence of atherosclerotic disease and a LDL cholesterol >100 mg/dL (SI: 2.6 mmol/L) are candidates for a lipid-lowering regimen according to the National Cholesterol Education Program (NCEP).[30] J.S. has angina and lower extremity atherosclerosis, both of which indicate a need for aggressive lipid lowering. His LDL-C is 180 mg/dL, so a reduction of almost 50% is desired. Lowering triglycerides and raising HDL-C are secondary goals in J.S. and can be reassessed after his LDL goal has been reached and the effect of therapy on these parameters is measured. In addition to an aggressive dietary management program, an hydroxymethylglutaryl-coenzyme A (HMG-CoA) reductase inhibitor agent should be prescribed as initial therapy for J.S. HMG-CoA reductase inhibitors, exercise, and the American Heart Association diet will all improve his LDL-C level. They also have beneficial effects on triglycerides and HDL-C, and the need for additional therapy can be assessed after the impact of these measures is determined. Because of a lack of outcome data with many of the available agents for dyslipidemia, a fibric acid derivative is the best alternative or additional agent if lipid goals are not met with statin therapy.[7]

Table 14-6 Primary Mechanisms of Symptom Improvement With Exercise Therapy in Intermittent Claudication[26]

Decrease of blood viscosity
Metabolic changes in the muscle
Improved muscle metabolism
Improved oxygen extraction
Improved endothelial function and microcirculation
Decreased occurrence of ischemia and inflammation
Atherosclerosis risk factors improved via:
Weight loss
Glycemic control
Blood pressure control
Increased high-density lipoprotein (HDL)
Decreased triglycerides
Decreased thrombotic tendency

MANAGEMENT OF HYPERTENSION

4. J.S.'s BP is elevated to 170/95 mmHg despite enalapril therapy. Because he has angina, and his HR is 89, a β-adrenergic blocker is considered. Are there alternative antihypertensive therapies that might be preferable for J.S.?

J.S.'s hypertension has likely contributed to the development of his atherosclerosis and PAD. Hypertension has been associated with deficiencies in the synthesis of vasodilating substances, such as prostacyclin, bradykinin, and nitric oxide, by the endothelial cells lining the vasculature. Hypertension also increases concentrations of vasoconstricting substances, such as angiotensin II. An increase in vascular tone can alter local hemodynamics, especially in the presence of a stenotic lesion. Although it has not been determined whether normalization of BP has a positive effect on IC, it is well established that uncontrolled BP, as in J.S., results in vascular complications such as MI and stroke. In light of J.S.'s numerous risk factors for these complications, improved management of his hypertension is warranted.

β-blockers are frequently cited as contraindicated in patients with IC owing to the potential for unopposed α-adrenergic–mediated vasoconstriction during peripheral β-blockade. Evidence to document worsening IC by β-blockade is lacking, however. Overall, controlled studies have been inconclusive, although, a meta-analysis of placebo-controlled trials and studies with control groups concludes that β-blockers do not worsen claudication.[40]

Angiotensin-converting enzyme (ACE) inhibitors are first-line agents in patients with PAD.[7] Compared with other antihypertensive agents, more data document their beneficial effects in these patient populations. Compared with placebo, walking distance is increased with both perindopril and ramipril in patients with PAD.[41,42] The Heart Outcomes Prevention Evaluation (HOPE) study of the ACE inhibitor ramipril versus placebo included >4,000 patients with PAD, and this subgroup derived benefit in terms of decreased mortality, MI, and stroke.[43]

Because J.S. has both hypertension and diabetes, his BP goal is <130/80.[44] He is already taking an ACE inhibitor, which is an excellent initial antihypertensive choice in a patient with diabetes and PAD. The dose of enalapril could be increased, or a low-dose diuretic, such as hydrochlorothiazide or chlorthalidone, could be added. This combination is synergistic and should be very effective in reducing J.S.'s BP.[45,46] Other options include a calcium channel blocker or a β-blocker, both of which are useful in patients such as J.S. with angina. If J.S. develops angina symptoms with exercise as a result of sympathetic stimulation, a β-blocker may be required to permit participation in an exercise program that could greatly benefit his IC.

MANAGEMENT OF DIABETES

5. Will improving J.S.'s diabetes control slow the progression of his PAD? What changes in his diabetes management do you recommend?

Patients with type 2 diabetes mellitus are able to minimize macrovascular and microvascular complications of their disease with aggressive pharmacologic glucose control.[6,47,48] Insulin, sulfonylurea, or metformin therapy have a beneficial effect on slowing the development of the microvascular complications of diabetes, such as retinopathy and nephropathy. Metformin has specifically been shown to further reduce the occurrence of macrovascular complications such as stroke or myocardial infarction compared with therapy with insulin or sulfonylureas in obese patients with type 2 diabetes.[47]

Table 14-7 Effect of Diabetes Mellitus on Intermittent Claudication Outcomes After 5 Years[10]

	Patients With Diabetes (%)	Patients Without Diabetes (%)
Mortality	49	23
Major amputation	21	3
Deterioration	35	19

J.S.'s diabetes is a significant risk factor for progression to further ischemic events (Table 14-7). He has a twofold greater risk of death and a sevenfold greater risk of amputation compared with a patient without diabetes. Although a specific benefit on IC has not been demonstrated, it seems prudent to initiate or continue aggressive diabetes management in patients with type 2 diabetes mellitus and IC. The addition of metformin to J.S.'s therapy could improve his blood glucose control and decrease his risk of vascular complications. This agent will favorably affect hepatic glucose production and insulin sensitivity and could result in weight loss. The addition of a short-acting insulin before meals is another possible intervention. It is hoped that J.S. can reach his hemoglobin A1c goal of <7% and a fasting blood glucose of 90 to 130 mg/dL with diet, exercise, and metformin therapy, in addition to his standing dose of insulin.[49] It would also be helpful to have J.S. check his blood glucose before meals, 1 to 2 hours after meals, and at bedtime and to keep a log of the results. This may help improve understanding of his medication and nutrition therapies and help guide future therapy changes.

J.S. also must take proper care of his feet to prevent ulcerative complications of IC. He should be encouraged to keep his feet warm, dry, and moisturized and to wear properly fitted shoes and perform daily foot inspections.[7] He should seek medical attention immediately for minor trauma to his feet or legs.[4] These measures can reduce the incidence of amputation in patients with diabetes.

Pharmacologic Therapies

ANTIPLATELET THERAPIES

6. Is the aspirin that J.S. is taking beneficial for preventing further complications of IC? Would a newer agent such as clopidogrel offer any advantage over aspirin?

Aspirin is one of several antiplatelet agents that may be considered for indefinite use in patients such as J.S. with IC. A paucity of studies has directly addressed the effects of aspirin on IC symptoms. Rather, most available data address the impact of aspirin on overall cardiovascular morbidity and mortality. Aspirin exerts its antiplatelet effect by irreversibly inhibiting cyclooxygenase. This enzyme is essential for the production of thromboxane A_2, a stimulus for platelet aggregation. Although aspirin has no direct effect on plaque regression, it does prevent and retard the role platelets play in the thrombogenic events that occur in the vicinity of atherosclerotic plaques.[50] Aspirin is an effective antithrombotic agent at dosages ranging from 50 to 1,500 mg daily. The minimal dosages proved to decrease cardiovascular events are 75 to 150 mg daily, with the higher dosage showing benefit in active processes, such as acute ischemic stroke[51] and acute MI.[52] A dosage of 75 mg daily has demonstrated benefit in patients with hypertension[53] and stable angina.[54] No evidence indicates that these "low doses" are any more or any less effective than dosages of 900 to 1,500 mg daily.[55]

Aspirin is mandatory in patients with vascular disease of any origin (this includes stroke, MI, PAD, and angina). At dosages of 75 to 150 mg/day, it decreases vascular death by approximately 15% and all serious vascular events (MI, stroke, or vascular death) by approximately 20% in high-risk patients, including those with PAD.[55] In patients with PAD, aspirin can delay the progression of established lesions as assessed by angiography. When used for primary prevention of cardiovascular disease in men, aspirin decreased the need for arterial reconstructive surgery needed because of PAD.[56] Whether aspirin has any beneficial effects on walking distance or claudication pain in patients with IC has not been studied, however.

Because all dosages of aspirin are similarly efficacious in decreasing vascular events in this patient population, side effects determine the dose chosen. Although few studies have directly compared varying doses, side effects appear to be dose related. Aspirin 30 mg daily results in less minor bleeding compared with approximately 300 mg daily,[57] and 300 mg daily results in fewer GI side effects compared with 1,200 mg daily.[58] Therefore, J.S. should take the lowest effective dose of aspirin; for convenience, 81 mg daily. Of note, J.S.'s hypertension should be controlled before initiating aspirin therapy to decrease the small increased incidence of cerebral hemorrhage associated with its use.[59]

Ticlopidine is a thienopyridine derivative that blocks adenosine 5′-diphosphate (ADP) receptors on platelets, and decreases platelet-fibrinogen binding.[60] Several studies document its efficacy in patients with PAD on endpoints such as walking distance, cardiovascular death, and the need for revascularization surgery.[61,62] Diarrhea is a common side effect, however, and hematologic toxicities (neutropenia and rarely, thrombotic thrombocytopenic purpura) further limit its use.[63,64] Clopidogrel, an antiplatelet agent with the same mechanism of action as ticlopidine but with an improved safety profile, has largely replaced ticlopidine when thienopyridine therapy is desired. The effects of clopidogrel on specific PAD outcomes are not known, but it has been compared with aspirin in patients with known atherosclerotic disease. Dosages of 75 mg daily significantly reduced cardiovascular endpoints by approximately 25% compared with aspirin in this patient population.[65] In fact, the treatment effect was most pronounced in the subgroup that had PAD, leading to the suggestion that clopidogrel may be preferable in the patient population with PAD. No measure was taken of clopidogrel's effect on walking distance or claudication pain, however, nor have these results been replicated. The combination of aspirin and clopidogrel was compared with aspirin alone in >15,000 patients at high risk of vascular events, of whom >20% had a history of PAD, and approximately 10% had IC.[66,67] In this large study that assessed cardiovascular endpoints, no benefit was found to dual antiplatelet therapy with aspirin and clopidogrel.[67] Thus, clopidogrel is an appropriate alternative to aspirin in patients unable to take aspirin therapy, perhaps owing to a serious allergy.[7] It should not be used in addition to aspirin, however, because the risk of bleeding and increased cost are not outweighed by any measurable vascular benefit.[67]

CILOSTAZOL

7. Are there any medications that can be used to increase the walking abilities of patients with IC?

Cilostazol is one of the few agents approved by the U.S. Food and Drug Administration (FDA) specifically for the treatment of IC. Several studies have confirmed that at a fixed dose of 100 mg twice daily of cilostazol increases walking distance by approximately 50%,[68–70] and that discontinuation of cilostazol resulted in a decline in function.[71] This drug possesses antiplatelet and vasodilitory effects mediated by the inhibition of phosphodiesterase III.[72] Some in vitro observations suggest that these pharmacologic effects of cilostazol are particularly pronounced at the blood–vessel interface,[72] which may explain its particular efficacy in the patient population with PAD. Studies that included quality-of-life measurements have found that cilostazol improved overall quality of life in these patients.[68,73] Additionally, a small improvement was seen in ABI with chronic cilostazol therapy.[74] Despite these positive findings with cilostazol, several drawbacks exist to its use. It is contraindicated in patients with heart failure, because other phosphodiesterase inhibitors cause excess mortality in patients with heart failure, presumably owing to increased arrhythmias.[75] Other common side effects include headache, occurring in up to one-third of patients, and loose stools or diarrhea.[69,76] Cilostazol is a cytochrome P450 3A4 substrate; therefore, any inhibitor of this enzyme system may substantially increase cilostazol levels.

Cilostazol is an importance advance in the treatment of IC. It is the first pharmacologic agent to demonstrate a consistent effect on a significant source of IC disability: walking and mobility measures. Although no data address its impact on other important endpoints, such as amputation and revascularization procedures or cardiovascular events, it should be added to J.S.'s existing medication regimen at a dosage of 100 mg twice daily to attenuate his symptoms of IC. It is hoped that its addition to smoking cessation, exercise, and optimal blood pressure and glycosylated hemoglobin attainment will result in good long-term symptomatic and vascular event outcomes.

RHEOLOGIC AGENTS

8. Has pentoxifylline been shown to be efficacious in patients such as J.S.? How does this drug benefit patients with IC?

Pentoxifylline, a methylxanthine derivative, is one of the few agents approved by the FDA for the treatment of IC. The exact mechanism of action is unclear; however, it appears to decrease blood viscosity by decreasing fibrinogen, improving the deformability of both red and white blood cells, and eliciting antiplatelet effects.[77] Although the theoretic and in vitro data on pentoxifylline are unique and positive, the data demonstrating clinical usefulness of this agent are controversial. In general, the improvements in walking distances from study to study are unpredictable, and the clinical importance of the sometimes minimal increases in walking distances is not clear (e.g., pain-free walking of approximately 30 m greater than with placebo).[78] Some experts assert that these potential benefits of questionable clinical significance are not worth the expense of drug therapy or the GI side effects.[40,79] Because the therapy is of questionable benefit, the expense and potential for side effects are rarely justified.

Pentoxifylline's role in IC therapy is limited. It may have a role in patients who are unable to engage in exercise therapy or in patients with markedly reduced walking distances, in whom any small increase in walking distance would greatly improve the patient's level of activity.[80] It also may be tried in patients who have not gained the desired benefit from smoking cessation and exercise therapy. A 2-month trial of pentoxifylline is adequate to determine if the patient will benefit from the therapy.[27] J.S. is not severely debilitated, and the benefits of smoking cessation, exercise therapy, and cilostazol have not been fully realized. Therefore, pentoxifylline therapy should be withheld until his response to these well-proven therapies has been determined and the need for further improvement in walking distance is established.

VASODILATORS

9. J.S. is already taking isosorbide dinitrate for his angina. Because IC is made worse by vasoconstriction, should another vasodilating agent be added to treat both his hypertension and IC?

The use of vasodilators for J.S. would at first appear to be a logical pharmacologic intervention to prevent claudication pain. Vasodilators, including isosorbide dinitrate, directly or indirectly relax blood vessel walls and increase both skin and muscle blood flow as long as cardiac output is maintained. With obstructive arterial disease, however, vessels are sclerotic and unable to dilate any further. As a result, relatively healthy collateral vessels dilate to a greater extent than diseased vessels and blood flow is redistributed (shunted) away from areas that have the greatest need. Blood pressure and perfusion paradoxically drop even further in the affected tissues. This process is known as the *steal phenomenon*.

Numerous vasodilators (i.e., prostaglandin-E1, prostacyclin, isoxsuprine, papaverine, ethaverine, cyclandelate, niacin derivatives, reserpine, guanethidine, methyldopa, tolazoline, nifedipine, L-carnitine) have been used to treat IC. None, however has convincingly or consistently improved exercise performance, despite earlier beliefs that they were effective.[81,82] ACE inhibitors are the exception to this rule, as discussed above, and their beneficial effects are likely independent of their vasodilator properties. One small, controlled study demonstrated improvement in walking distance with verapamil, a calcium channel blocker, compared with placebo in patients with IC.[83] Thus, although vasodilators have generally been eliminated from the treatment of IC and related obstructive vascular disorders,[14] verapamil may be an agent with vasodilating properties that is useful in patients with IC.

Smoking cessation, an exercise program, and cilostazol are the interventions that should reduce J.S.'s symptoms of IC to the greatest degree. After these three measures have been implemented and the impact of the modified BP regimen, which should definitely continue to include an ACE inhibitor, has been assessed, the addition of verapamil could be considered. Verapamil is a cytochrome P450 3A4 inhibitor, and would be expected to increase concentrations of cilostazol. The magnitude of this interaction has not been characterized, nor has its impact on efficacy and bleeding events been assessed. Based on the necessity of cilostazol therapy in J.S., the poorly characterized benefits of verapamil in IC, and the plethora of other antihypertensive and antianginal agents, avoidance of verapamil is prudent in this patient. If additional BP or antianginal effects are needed, β-blockade or amlodipine can be initiated, or the nitroglycerin dose can be increased (see Chapter 16, Ischemic Heart Disease: Anginal Syndromes).

Other Therapeutic Alternatives

10. The sales clerk at a health food store told J.S. that several nutritional supplements and herbal products would improve his circulation so that he could walk better. He is considering buying ginkgo biloba. Does ginkgo or any other herbals or vitamins really work?

Several herbs and vitamins have been used to treat IC, but most have not been rigorously studied. To complicate matters, many studies are published in foreign journals, making access and interpretation of the data challenging.

Ginkgo biloba is one of the few herbal therapies with double-blind, placebo-controlled trials to support its use. A meta-analysis of eight trials representing data from 385 patients reported a mean increase in pain-free walking of 34 m (a 47% increase) with a median dosage of 160 mg daily for 6 months.[84] It has been proposed that ginkgo's therapeutic value is related to its antiplatelet properties.[85] Gingko is generally well tolerated with no major side effects, except for an increased risk of bleeding as would be expected with any platelet inhibitor.[86] Occasionally, mild GI upset or headache have been reported.[87] Although the treatment benefit is modest, a consistent trend in benefit is seen and the side effects are minor.

Vitamin E has been advocated for the treatment of intermittent claudication for many years.[88] Only a few very small, poorly controlled studies, however, support its ability to improve blood flow and walking distance.[89,90] Vitamin E has not prevented cardiovascular events in patients with both established coronary artery disease and risk factors for cardiovascular disease.[90–92] Although it is generally not harmful at dosages of 400 to 800 IU/day, vitamin E is unlikely to offer any symptomatic relief or long-term protection from cardiovascular events to J.S.

Patients with IC have decreased intramuscular carnitine levels, and this impairs oxidative metabolism in skeletal muscle.[93,94] Exogenous propionyl-L-carnitine, 1 to 2 g/day, improves energy production in ischemic muscles. Small studies have demonstrated beneficial effects on walking distances[95,96] and quality of life[97] in patients with IC. Although it is not approved by the FDA, similar agents, such as levocarnitine, are available in the United States. Limited data suggest its effects are less than those seen with propionyl-L-carnitine.[96]

With the abundance of proved, therapeutic measures to be initiated in J.S., the use of relatively poorly studied and unsubstantiated alternative products is not warranted. If debilitating symptoms are still present after adequate trials of the proved therapies, then ginkgo biloba may be considered. J.S. should inform his doctors and pharmacist if he uses any of these agents so they can anticipate the inevitable drug interactions (e.g., ginkgo biloba plus antiplatelet drugs) and to allow for appropriate assessment and monitoring.

11. Three years have passed, and J.S. stopped smoking 6 months ago. His symptoms of IC have remained fairly stable, until the recent development of a nonhealing ulcer on his toe. What options

are there for J.S. if nonpharmacologic and pharmacologic interventions are not sufficient?

Surgical intervention eventually may be necessary for persistent and complicated disease. Because success rates for preventing amputation and postsurgical complications vary from institution to institution, surgery should be considered only for severely ischemic limbs and should be performed in a hospital with a good history of success.[98] Arterial bypass grafting and percutaneous transluminal angioplasty of the femoral or iliac arteries, similar to cardiac revascularization, are two procedures that can be performed. Angioplasty is beneficial in patients with localized disease, especially in the iliac or superficial femoral arteries, and should be considered in patients who truly are incapacitated by their activity limitations.[99] Angioplasty $\pm$ stent deployment, atherectomy, and the use of drug-eluting stents in the peripheral arteries are all options.[7] The results obtained are based on several factors, including the vascular bed affected, the technique used, and the degree of occlusive disease. Interestingly, angioplasty has not decreased the number of amputations, yet costs for revascularization procedures have doubled.[100] The more invasive reconstructive arterial (bypass) surgery can be used if diffuse lesions preclude the use of localized angioplasty. The true benefits and pitfalls of these skilled interventions remain unclear.

Emergency surgical intervention may be required if acute, persistent ischemia develops. This is frequently owing to a thrombosis associated with advanced atherosclerosis, although other causes, such as cardiac emboli, cannot be excluded.[80] Both surgical thrombectomy and localized thrombolytic administration[101] with tissue-plasminogen activator (t-PA) or urokinase have equal success in alleviating acute limb-threatening ischemia.[102,103]

RAYNAUD'S PHENOMENON

Raynaud's disease, first described by Maurice Raynaud in 1862,[104] remains largely a medical enigma today. This disorder is essentially an exaggerated vasospastic response to cold or emotion. The digits initially turn white, indicating ischemia; then blue, signaling deoxygenation; and finally, digits appear red when reperfusion occurs.[105] It is usually limited to the skin of the hands and fingers, but can also occur in the feet. Between attacks, the digits may appear cool and moist or normal. This abrupt and discomforting phenomenon can be brought on by exposure to cold or emotional stress, both likely mediated through an exaggerated sympathetic response to the precipitating stimuli. Although both IC and Raynaud's phenomenon are disorders of the peripheral arterial circulation, they differ significantly in that IC results primarily from atherosclerotic obstruction, whereas Raynaud's disease is caused by vasospasm.

Diagnosis

This disorder can be separated into primary Raynaud's phenomenon, indicating an idiopathic origin, and secondary Raynaud's. Secondary Raynaud's consists of signs and symptoms of Raynaud's phenomenon in the presence of an associated disease or condition, most commonly a connective tissue disorder, such as scleroderma, rheumatoid arthritis, or systemic lupus erythematosus. Primary Raynaud's disease is diagnosed only when secondary causes have been excluded.[106] Common criteria for the diagnosis of primary Raynaud's phenomenon are listed in Table 14-8. The diagnosis is generally a subjective one, consisting of clinical signs and symptoms, and simply reflects cold hands, feet, or both without normal recovery following a cold stimulus or emotional stress.[107] In unaffected individuals, a cold provocation should result in some mottling and cyanotic changes in the hands, with recovery once the stimuli are removed. In patients with Raynaud's phenomenon, however, the same cold provocation causes closure of the digital arteries, which produces a sharply demarcated pallor and cyanosis of the digits that persists despite removal of the stimulus.[107] The most reliable objective method to measure artery closure during an attack is the finger systolic BP[108]; however, subjective diagnostic criteria are most commonly and easily employed to diagnose Raynaud's phenomenon.

Table 14-8 Diagnosis of Primary Raynaud's Phenomenon[113]

Vasospastic attacks caused by cold or emotional stress
Symmetric attacks involving both hands
No evidence of digital ulcerations, pitting, or gangrene
Normal nailfold capillaries
No suggestion of a secondary cause
A negative antinuclear test
A normal sedimentation rate

Epidemiology

In general, the prevalence of Raynaud's phenomenon is about 3% to 4% across several ethnic groups[106]; however, it may be as high as 20% in some geographically defined populations.[109] It is more common in women than men, tends to affect young patients, and has a higher prevalence in patients with family members who also experience Raynaud's phenomenon. An onset in the teenage years suggests primary Raynaud's phenomenon, whereas an onset after 30 years of age suggests a secondary cause.[110] Secondary Raynaud's phenomenon is usually associated with a connective tissue disorder, but several other conditions may predispose individuals to its development. These include occupational-related exposures to vibratory machinery (e.g., drills, grinders, chain saws) that cause neural damage,[111] vinyl chloride, or hand trauma.[112,113] The diagnosis of primary Raynaud's phenomenon is accurate approximately 85% of the time. The remaining 15% will manifest a connective tissue disorder during the next decade, and will most likely occur in individuals with serum antinuclear antibodies and thickened fingers.[114] Raynaud's phenomenon can also be associated with medications, including β-adrenergic blocking agents, ergots, cytotoxic drugs, and interferon, all of which can induce vasoconstriction.[115,116] Although avoidance of β-adrenergic blocking agents in patients with Raynaud's phenomenon appears prudent, no discernible effect, as measured by skin temperature and blood flow, was found with the administration of both selective and nonselective β-blockers to patients with Raynaud's phenomenon.[116] Raynaud's phenomenon not associated with a connective tissue disorder is often transient, and does not interfere with daily activities.[117] The effect of smoking on Raynaud's phenomenon has yielded conflicting results. Overall, there appears to be a negligible effect of smoking on the prevalence of Raynaud's phenomenon, the incidence of attacks, and digital blood flow.[118,119]

Pathophysiology

The blood vessels of the digital skin, which have a prime role in the regulation of body temperature, are supplied with vast amounts of sympathetic vasoconstricting nerves.[106] Cold-induced vasospastic attacks in patients with primary Raynaud's phenomenon involve a heightened vasoconstriction of these digital arteries that is mediated by α_2-adrenergic receptor.[120] The cause of this exaggerated response to cold stimuli is unknown; however, several plausible mechanisms involving peripheral α_2-adrenoreceptors could result in an intense vasoconstriction. These include an increased (a) number of α_2-adrenoreceptors, (b) temperature sensitivity of the α_2-adrenoreceptors, and (c) activity of the α_2-adrenergic intracellular signal-transduction pathway.[110] The mechanism of secondary Raynaud's phenomenon is also not known, but it is thought to be similar to primary Raynaud's phenomenon. The α_2-adrenoreceptor aberrancy may be the result of arterial damage induced by an associated disease state, such as a connective tissue disorder.[110] It is also possible that serotonin receptors (S_2) play a role in Raynaud's phenomenon. Serotonin agonists have caused decreased finger blood flow and, conversely, antagonists have increased digital blood flow.[121] Clinically, a patient with Raynaud's disease will present with a waxy pallor of one or more of the fingers after the sudden decrease of arterial blood flow. Hemoglobin desaturation occurs with static venous blood flow and causes the digit or digits to have a cyanotic appearance. The attack subsides over time, and the affected arteries vasodilate. As the skin temperature increases, classic rubor, or reddening of the afflicted area, will be seen. Many patients will be observed to have pallor only during the initial attack, in which the digits take on a white or yellow, sometimes patchy, appearance. In most cases, the ischemia produced by the phenomenon does not have important consequences; however, in severe cases, atrophy of the skin, irregular nail growth, and wasting of the tissue pads can occur.[106]

Clinical Presentation

12. F.K., a 39-year-old man, presents today with a 4-day history of left hand pain. He notes that the third digit of his left hand is "cold and somewhat blue," especially in the distal area. The other areas of his hand have recovered, but the distal portion of the digit remains cyanotic and numb. He has used acetaminophen and warm-water soaks without success. He is a construction worker who uses his hands "quite a bit" in his work. He has a history of gastroesophageal reflux and has no allergies. His social history is significant for smoking 1.5 packs of cigarettes a day for 19 years. On physical examination, his extremities reveal appropriate sensation of the forearm and hand. Some blue areas are noted on the distal portion on the third phalanx, with no other signs and symptoms. When F.K.'s opposite hand was placed in cold water, several white splotches appeared and he experienced tingling in this hand as a result of the cold-water exposure. He is diagnosed as having Raynaud's phenomenon. Does F.K. present with primary or secondary Raynaud's phenomenon?

F.K. presents with what is most likely secondary Raynaud's phenomenon owing to one of several potential underlying causes. His clinical presentation is classic for Raynaud's phenomenon, with vasospasm, pallor, and a cyanotic overtone. The diagnosis is confirmed by the cold-water test, which indicates that the vasospastic attack is precipitated by cold exposure. He has a work history that may easily include hand trauma and the use of vibrating machinery, and his age also suggests secondary Raynaud's phenomenon. Because of its association with connective tissue disorders, other laboratory tests such as an antinuclear antibody (ANA) and sedimentation rate should be checked.

Treatment

Nonpharmacologic Management

13. What conservative measures can be taken with F.K. to prevent or decrease the painful vasospasm of Raynaud's disease?

Most patients with both primary and secondary Raynaud's phenomenon will respond to conservative management. Avoiding cold stimuli is the primary treatment. F.K. should be instructed to protect his hands and fingers from exposure by using mittens and insulated wrappers when handling cold drinks. Although protecting his hands is important, he must also protect other parts of the body from cold exposure to prevent a sympathetic response, which may trigger symptomatic vasoconstriction in his hands. This includes layering his clothing when working outside in cold weather. He should avoid medications that can induce vasoconstriction, particularly sympathomimetics, clonidine, serotonin receptor agonists, and ergot preparations.[113] He should be encouraged to stop smoking, which will avoid smoking-induced vasoconstriction and provide an overall positive health benefit. The impact of smoking cessation on Raynaud's phenomenon, however, actually appears to be negligible.[118,119]

F.K. has new-onset and relatively mild Raynaud's phenomenon. For others who have more severe symptoms and manifestations, especially patients with underlying connective tissue disorders, it is important to immediately and aggressively manage any ulcers that develop on the digits and to be extremely vigilant in detecting infected digits. Antibiotic therapy should be initiated if necessary.[122]

Calcium Channel Blockers

14. Nifedipine extended-release 30 mg QD is ordered for F.K. What is the rationale for using a calcium channel blocker in this case?

Drugs can be used to treat primary and secondary Raynaud's phenomenon if it interferes with the patient's ability to work or perform daily activities or if digital lesions develop. Most proposed treatments for Raynaud's are, however, variably effective; they introduce the risk for significant side effects and may be expensive. Drug therapy should always be in addition to nonpharmacologic measures.

Calcium channel blockers decrease calcium ion influx and prevent smooth muscle contraction, especially vascular responses evoked by cold exposure. Nifedipine, a potent peripheral vasodilating calcium channel blocker, has become the drug of choice in patients with Raynaud's disease not controlled by conservative measures. In primary Raynaud's phenomenon, ten or more episodes per week are common. Nifedipine therapy results in an approximate 50% decrease in the number of attacks, in addition to a decrease in severity by one-third.[123] Patient's with secondary Raynaud's phenomenon experience a similar decrease in attack severity, and also obtain a decrease in number of attacks with nifedipine therapy. Because their baseline number of attacks per week often exceeds 20, the relative benefit is not as great as with primary Raynaud's phenomenon, averaging approximately a 25% decrease in weekly episodes.[124] Doses of 10 to 30 mg three times daily of immediate-release nifedipine are beneficial,[125,126] although higher doses, if tolerated, may be required for maximal benefit.[127] Most clinicians administer nifedipine as an extended-release formulation to increase convenience and decrease side effects such as dizziness, headache, facial flushing, and peripheral edema, which can occur in up to 50% of patients,[128] and this practice is supported by several clinical studies.[129–131] Even the extended-release preparation of nifedipine can cause bothersome edema owing to dilation of the precapillary bed.

Although less thoroughly studied than nifedipine, other vasoselective calcium channel blockers (CCBs), such as amlodipine, felodipine, isradipine, and nisoldipine decrease the frequency and severity of ischemic attacks.[132–135] Patients who do not benefit from nifedipine likely will not benefit by switching to another CCB. Patients who cannot tolerate the side effects of nifedipine (e.g., ankle edema) might benefit by switching to another CCB.

F.K. should be warned of the potential side effects with nifedipine therapy, especially dizziness associated with hypotension, and should return in 2 weeks for assessment. A 30-mg daily dose of extended-release nifedipine is a reasonable starting dose. He should be instructed to keep a diary documenting the number of attacks he experiences and details surrounding each attack, such as time course and precipitating factors. In addition to the usual side effects mentioned above, F.K. should be aware that his symptoms of gastroesophageal reflux could worsen with nifedipine therapy, which can cause a decreased lower esophageal sphincter pressure. This side effect should be specifically assessed at his follow-up appointment.

Other Therapeutic Agents

15. What other drugs may be tried if F.K. cannot tolerate the calcium channel blocker?

Other than CCBs, no proven therapy for Raynaud's phenomenon exists. Many agents, however, have been used based on minimal data and anecdotal reports. The α_1-adrenergic antagonists are one such class of drugs. Prazosin, 1 mg three times a day, yielded moderate benefit in two-thirds of patients in two small studies.[136,137] Side effects of prazosin are significant at maximal doses and include dizziness, edema, fatigue, and orthostasis. The longer-acting α_1-adrenergic antagonist terazosin was evaluated in one small study and it improved symptomatology as well as objective measures of blood flow.[138] No sufficient data with this class of drugs exist to routinely recommend their use in patients with Raynaud's phenomenon.

Several therapeutic approaches are being vigorously investigated, and show promise as future therapies for Raynaud's phenomenon. These include the intravenous prostanoids, iloprost and alprostadil, which enhance nitric oxide-mediated vasodilation[139]; endothelin antagonists, such as bosentan[140]; and oral phosphodiesterase inhibitors, such as sildenafil[141] and vardenafil,[142] which also promote vasodilation. Because of side effects, extreme cost, and administration difficulties, these agents are only being studied in the most severe secondary Raynaud's phenomenon cases with digital ulcers or other systemic complications associated with connective tissue diseases. If benefit is proved, however, it will shed light onto the pathogenesis of the disorder, and perhaps lead to therapies appropriate for the larger population with Raynaud's phenomenon.

The ACE inhibitors act as vasodilators and have been investigated in several small studies. ACE inhibitors and angiotensin receptor blockers, however, do not appear to have any beneficial effects in patients with Raynaud's phenomenon.[143] Fluoxetine, a selective serotonin reuptake inhibitor, was shown in one study to reduce the symptoms of Raynaud's phenomenon.[144] It is hypothesized to exert its effect by depleting platelet serotonin, rendering the platelet unable to release a significant amount of the vasoconstrictive serotonin during activation and aggregation.

The application of nitroglycerin (NTG) ointment to the hands of patients with Raynaud's disease has been tried since the mid-1940s. High doses of NTG ointment (3.5 inches) three times a day applied to the hands for 6 weeks resulted in fewer and less severe attacks.[145] Transdermal NTG patches also provide some benefit, although headaches may be a limiting factor.[146] The potential for tolerance developing to the nitrates for this indication has not been studied. Because the data supporting nitrate use in the management of Raynaud's phenomenon are sparse, these agents should be discontinued after 2 to 3 weeks if no benefit is observed.[122] Alternative therapies, such as ginkgo biloba and L-arginine, have also been studied in small trials with positive results; however, larger trials are needed to confirm the findings before these therapies can be recommended.[147,148]

All patients with Raynaud's phenomenon should be counseled regarding cold avoidance and other protective measures. A CCB, nifedipine if tolerated, should be initiated if conservative measures are ineffective and titrated to the highest tolerated dose and symptom resolution. Combination therapies have not been investigated, but another agent, such as an α_1-adrenergic antagonist, may be considered in addition to the CCB if symptom resolution is not satisfactory and side effects permit.

NOCTURNAL LEG MUSCLE CRAMPS

Nocturnal leg muscle cramps are idiopathic, involuntary contractions occurring at rest that cause a visible and palpable knot in the affected muscle. This type of muscle cramp usually afflicts middle-aged to elderly persons and is a distressing and painful condition. Its cause is unknown. The two primary hypotheses that attempt to explain the pathophysiology propose neurologic impairments. One involves a central nervous system impairment of γ-aminobutyric acid (GABA)[149] and the other, an impaired peripheral response to muscle lengthening.[150] Although the incidence of nocturnal cramps is unknown, some data indicate it is very common. In a survey of veterans (95% men averaging 60 years of age), 56% complained of leg cramps, with 12% having cramping nearly every night[151]; 36% of these veterans were also attempting some type of drug treatment for their symptoms. A survey of a general population revealed that the prevalence of nocturnal leg cramps was 37% in people >50 years of age, and increased to 54% in people

>80 years of age. The prevalence in men and women is equal.[152] Nocturnal leg cramps are associated with lower extremity atherosclerosis, coronary artery disease, and peripheral neurologic deficits.[152,153]

Clinical Presentation

16. E.A., a 62-year-old woman, complains of cramps in her left calf that began last night around 10 PM. The cramping occurred several times throughout the night and has resolved slowly since she arose this morning. These nighttime cramping episodes occur frequently, are very painful, and cause her calf muscle to become "knotted." She denies any trauma, fever, or chills, has no other medical problems, and takes no medications. The pain is not associated with walking. The physical examination is unremarkable and her vital signs are stable. An extended chemistry panel and thyroid function tests are within normal limits. E.A. works at an elementary school and walks up and down stairs throughout the day. Her physician associates the pain with nocturnal leg cramps. What characteristics differentiate E.A.'s nocturnal leg cramps from other pain syndromes?

Benign nocturnal leg cramps usually occur in the early hours of sleeping; they are asymmetric and are not exclusive to, but primarily affect, the calf muscle and small muscles of the foot. These cramps are not associated with exercise, specific electrolyte or laboratory abnormalities, or medication use. Nocturnal cramps occurs with the further contraction of a muscle already in its most shortened position. For example, sleeping in the supine position may place the calf and ventral foot muscles in their most shortened and vulnerable position, predisposing these muscles to contract.[154]

For diagnosis and treatment, true muscle cramps first should be distinguished from other causes of muscle cramping, including drug-induced cramps (Table 14-9). The onset of cramps at rest is characteristic of ordinary leg cramps and is the primary symptom used for diagnosis. Clinical signs of sodium depletion, hyper- and hypothyroidism, tetany, and lower motor neuron disease should be evaluated. Laboratory measurements such as standard electrolytes and thyroid function tests can help rule out some of these other conditions.

Table 14-9 Other Causes of Muscle Cramps[154,155,161]

Drug-Induced Cramps	*Biochemical Causes*	*Other*
Alcohol	Dehydration	Contractures
Antipsychotics (dystonia)	Hemodialysis	Diabetes
β-agonists (e.g., albuterol, terbutaline, salbutamol)	Hypocalcemia	Lower motor neuron disease
	Hypokaelmia	
Cimetidine	Hypomagnesemia	Peripheral vascular disease
Clofibrate	Hyponatremia	
Diuretics	Uremia	Tetany
Lithium		Thyroid disease
Narcotic analgesics		
Nicotinic acid		
Nifedipine		
Penicillamine		
Statins		
Steroids		

Treatment

Therapeutic Objectives and Nonpharmacologic Interventions

17. What are the therapeutic objectives in treating E.A.? What nonpharmacologic recommendations can be made?

The primary treatment goal is to prevent this uncomfortable condition. Sufferers of leg cramps are commonly advised to stretch out the afflicted muscle or perform dorsiflexion of the feet throughout the day and before bedtime, but this therapeutic modality has sparse, uncontrolled data in the literature and cannot be relied on to be helpful.[155] Patients are also warned to avoid plantar flexion while sleeping by hanging the feet over the edge of the bed when sleeping on the stomach. Once a cramp occurs, the goal is to relieve the cramp as quickly as possible. Acute therapy consists of dorsiflexion (grasping the toes and pulling them upward in the opposite direction of the cramp). This can be accomplished with the hands, by walking, or by leaning toward a wall while standing 2 feet away from it, maintaining the feet flat on the floor.[154]

Quinine

18. E.A. is amenable to the recommended stretching practices, and will avoid plantar flexion during sleep. She returns in 3 months, and reports a minor decrease in the attack frequency, but not severity. Her sleep is being affected 2 to 3 nights/week, and she feels it is affecting her performance as a teacher. She remembers her aunt taking a "pill" for her leg cramps. Is there any medication that may help relieve her symptoms?

Quinine is the most frequently prescribed medication for nocturnal leg cramps and was once a nonprescription product. In 1995, the FDA stated that quinine was not considered safe and effective for nocturnal leg cramps[156] and discontinued its over-the-counter status. Physicians can still prescribe quinine for the treatment of nocturnal leg cramps because it is commercially available and indicated for the treatment of malaria. The FDA, however, has clearly stated quinine should not be used for nocturnal leg cramps because of an unfavorable risk:benefit ratio.

Quinine has been used to treat nocturnal leg cramps since the 1940s, when four patients suffering from leg cramps experienced marked improvement in symptoms after being treated with quinine.[157] When given placebo, their symptoms apparently worsened. Quinine may exert a beneficial effect by increasing the refractory period of skeletal muscle and by decreasing the excitability of the motor endplate. Despite its frequent use, significant controversy exists over its benefit. Only a few small controlled trials have been conducted, with mixed conclusions. A meta-analysis was published in 1998 that included both published and unpublished data addressing the efficacy of quinine in the treatment of leg cramps.[158] Pooled data from 659 patients indicated that quinine, at 200 to 325 mg/day, reduced the severity and average number of cramps experienced in a 4-week period from 17.1 to 13.5. Thus, the efficacy of quinine is proved; however, the magnitude of benefit is rather small, and the risks associated with quinine therapy for a benign condition must also be considered. Of note, a recent study that randomized patients to quinine cessation reported no effect on nocturnal leg cramp frequency (e.g., no worsening of symptoms).[159]

Before initiating quinine, prophylactic stretching and alteration of sleeping position should be tried and evaluated. Additionally, modifiable causes of cramps should be explored and addressed. If these measures do not result in adequate relief, therapy with quinine can be considered if the patient is fully aware of the risks, appreciates the small benefit she can expect, and has no medications or conditions that place her at increased risk of adverse effects.

Precautions With Quinine

19. What side effect information should both the physician and E.A. know about before initiation of quinine therapy? How long should therapy be continued?

If quinine therapy is successful, E.A. should see a decrease in the severity and frequency of her cramping attacks. Quinine is available in the United States only as the 324 mg sulfate salt, as the brand name Qualaquin. One tablet should be taken in the evening. Cinchonism, a syndrome that includes nausea, vomiting, blurred vision, tinnitus, and deafness, is a dose-related side effect of quinine.[154] Tinnitus alone occurs in up to 3% of patients.[158] With overdose, central nervous system manifestations, such as headache, confusion, and delirium, can occur. Self-limiting rashes that resolve with drug discontinuation have been described.[154] The unpredictable and life-threatening side effect of thrombocytopenia was the impetus for the FDA to ban the over-the-counter status of this preparation. Thrombocytopenia has been estimated to occur in up to 1 of 1,000 patients taking quinine.[156] Care should also be taken with the use of quinine because its clearance is decreased in the elderly,[160] and several drugs decrease its clearance, such as cimetidine, verapamil, amiodarone, and alkalinizing agents.[161] Each of these could increase the risk of quinine dose-related side effects, specifically the central nervous system manifestations. Quinine can also produce toxic levels of digoxin, phenobarbital, and carbamazepine[161] and is contraindicated in patients with G6PD deficiency.

E.A. should be instructed to take the dose of quinine with food to minimize GI irritation. If a response is not seen within 2 weeks, it should be discontinued in light of the potentially serious side effects.[154] E.A. should be instructed to keep a diary documenting the frequency of the cramping episodes so that its efficacy can be objectively assessed.

Other Therapies

20. Are there other treatment options for E.A.?

Electrolyte replacement (e.g., sodium, potassium, calcium, magnesium) may be indicated if specific deficiencies are noted or if the onset of cramping is associated with a recent initiation or dosage increase of diuretic therapy. Prophylactic use of other pharmacologic agents has been attempted, but their use is mostly anecdotal. Diphenhydramine, riboflavin, carbamazepine, methocarbamol, and phenytoin have been used empirically,[154] but no data support their use in nocturnal leg cramps. Vitamin E has been recommended, but one controlled study with 800 IU/day of vitamin E showed no benefit.[162] Verapamil has been shown in an open-label trial of eight elderly patients to relieve quinine-resistant cramps. A dose of 120 mg of verapamil at bedtime was used, and relief was seen after 6 days of treatment.[163] Similar results were reported from a similar small study using diltiazem.[164] A small study found benefit associated with vitamin B complex administration for nocturnal leg cramps, but no quantification of a decrease in the number of cramps was provided.[165] Two small crossover studies suggested that chronic magnesium administration is not effective for the treatment of nocturnal leg cramps.[166,167]

Although nocturnal leg cramps are relatively benign, they do cause considerable discomfort. Nonpharmacologic measures should be maximized before drug therapy is contemplated. If drug therapy is warranted, quinine is the only agent with proved benefit, but the potential for side effects, especially in the elderly population, is very real. Careful patient selection, patient education, and vigilant monitoring for side effects should all be used to minimize the occurrence and progression of adverse effects from quinine.

REFERENCES

1. Criqui M et al. The prevalence of peripheral arterial disease in a defined population. *Circulation* 1985;71:210.
2. Kannel WB et al. Update on some epidemiologic feature of intermittent claudication. *J Am Geriatr Soc* 1985;33:13.
3. Caspary L. Epidemiology of vascular disease. *Dis Manage Health Outcomes* 1997;2:9.
4. Boccalon H. Intermittent claudication in older patients. *Drugs Aging* 1999;14:247.
5. Kannel WB et al. Diabetes and cardiovascular disease: the Framingham study. *JAMA* 1979;241:2035.
6. UK Prospective Diabetes Study (UKPDS) group. Intensive blood-glucose control with sulfonylureas or insulin compared with conventional treatment and risk of complications in patients with type 2 diabetes (UKPDS 33). *Lancet* 1998;352:837.
7. Hirsch AT et al. ACC/AHA guidelines for the management of patients with peripheral arterial disease (lower extremity, renal, mesenteric and abdominal aorta): executive summary: a report of the American College of Cardiology/American Heart Association Task Force on Practice Guidelines *J Am Coll Cardiol* 2006;47:1239.
8. MacGregor AS et al. Role of systolic blood pressure and plasma triglycerides in diabetic peripheral arterial disease. *Diabetes Care* 1999;22:453.
9. Willigendael EM et al. Influence of smoking on incidence and prevalence of peripheral arterial disease. *J Vasc Surg* 2004;40:1158.
10. Price JF et al. Relationship between smoking and cardiovascular risk factors in the development of peripheral arterial disease and coronary artery disease. *Eur Heart J* 1999;20:344.
11. McDaniel CD et al. Basic data related to the natural history of intermittent claudication. *Ann Vasc Surg* 1989;3:273.
12. Hertzer N. The natural history of peripheral vascular disease. *Circulation* 1991;83:112.
13. Brevetti G et al. Intermittent claudication and risk of cardiovascular events. *J Vasc Dis* 1998;49:843.
14. Rockson SG et al. Peripheral arterial insufficiency: mechanisms, natural history, and therapeutic options. *Adv Intern Med* 1998;43:253.
15. Weed RI. The importance of erythrocyte deformability. *Am J Med* 1970;49:147.
16. Braasch D. Red cell deformability and capillary blood flow. *Physiol Rev* 1971;51:679.
17. Kaplan NM. The deadly quartet. Upper body obesity, glucose intolerance, hypertriglyceridemia, and hypertension. *Arch Intern Med* 1989;149:1514.
18. Sowers JR. Insulin resistance, hyperinsulinemia, dyslipidemia, hypertension, and accelerated atherosclerosis. *Clin Pharmacol* 1992;32:529.
19. Housley E. Treating claudication with five words. *BMJ* 1988;296:1483.
20. Jonason T et al. Cessation of smoking in patients with intermittent claudication: effects on the risk of peripheral vascular complications, myocardial infarction, and mortality. *Acta Med Scand* 1987;221:253.
21. Faulkner KW et al. The effect of cessation of smoking on the accumulative survival rates of patients with symptomatic peripheral vascular disease. *Med J Aust* 1983;1:217.
22. Wiseman S et al. Influence of smoking and plasma factors on patency of femoralpopliteal vein grafts. *BMJ* 1989;299:643.
23. Quick CRG et al. Measured effect of stopping smoking on intermittent claudication. *Br J Surg* 1982;69:524.

24. Hughson WG et al. Intermittent claudication: factors determining outcome. *BMJ* 1978;1:1377.
25. Powell JT. Vascular damage from smoking: disease mechanism at the arterial wall. *Vasc Med* 1998;3:21.
26. Stewart K et al. Exercise training for claudication. *N Engl J Med* 2002;347:1941.
27. Gray BH et al. Vascular claudication: how to individualize treatment. *Cleve Clin J Med* 1997;64:492.
28. Leng GC et al. Exercise for intermittent claudication. *Cochrane Database of Syst Rev* 2000;2: CD000990.
29. Ernst E et al. Intermittent claudication, exercise, and blood rheology. *Circulation* 1987;76:1110.
30. Summary of the third report of the National Cholesterol Education Program (NCEP) Expert Panel on Detection, Evaluation, and Treatment of High Blood Cholesterol in Adults (Adult Treatment Panel III). *JAMA* 2001;285:2486.
31. Brown G et al. Regression of coronary artery disease as a result of intensive lipid lowering therapy in men with high levels of lipoprotein b. *N Engl J Med* 1990;323:1289.
32. Blankenhorn DH et al. Beneficial effects of combined colestipol-niacin therapy on coronary atherosclerosis and coronary venous bypass grafts. *JAMA* 1987;257:3233 [published erratum appears in *JAMA* 1988 May13;259:2698].
33. Blankenhorn DH et al. Coronary angiographic changes with lovastatin therapy. The Monitored Atherosclerosis Regression Study (MARS). The MARS Research Group. *Ann Intern Med* 1993;119:969.
34. Pedersen TJ et al. Effect of simvastatin on ischemic signs and symptoms in the Scandinavian Simvastatin Survival Study (4S). *Am J Cardiol* 1998;81:333.
35. MRC/BHF heart protection study of cholesterol lowering in 20,536 individuals: a randomised placebo-controlled trial. *Lancet* 2002;360:7.
36. Mondillo S et al. Effects of simvastatin on walking performance and symptoms of intermittent claudication in hypercholesterolemic patients with peripheral vascular disease. *Am J Med* 2003;114: 359.
37. Aronow WS et al. Effect of simvastatin versus placebo on treadmill exercise time until the onset of intermittent claudication in older patients with peripheral arterial disease at six months and at one year after treatment. *Am J Cardiol* 2003;2:711.
38. Leng G et al. Lipid-lowering for lower limb atherosclerosis. *Cochrane Database Syst Rev* 2000;2:CD000123.
39. Hiatt W. Medical treatment of peripheral arterial disease and claudication. *N Engl J Med* 2001; 334:1608.
40. Radack K et al. Beta-adrenergic blocker therapy does not worsen intermittent claudication in subjects with peripheral arterial disease. A meta-analysis of randomized controlled trials. *Arch Intern Med* 1991;151:1769.
41. Lip GYH et al. Treatment of hypertension in peripheral arterial disease. *Cochrane Database Syst Rev* 2003;2:CD003075.
42. Ahimastos AA et al. Ramipril markedly improves walking ability in patients with peripheral arterial disease. *Ann Intern Med* 2006;144:660.
43. The Heart Outcomes Prevention Evaluation Study Investigators. Effects of an angiotensin converting enzyme inhibitor, ramipril, on cardiovascular events in high-risk patients. *N Engl J Med* 2000;342:145.
44. Chobanian A et al. The Seventh Report of the Joint National Committee on Prevention, Detection, Evaluation, and Treatment of High Blood Pressure. *JAMA* 2003;289:2560.
45. Ismail N et al. Renal disease and hypertension in non-insulin-dependent diabetes mellitus. *Kidney Int* 1999;55:1.
46. Rodgers P. Combination drug therapy in hypertension: a rational approach for the pharmacist. *J Am Pharm Assoc* 1998;38:469.
47. UK Prospective Diabetes Study (UKPDS) Group. Effect of intensive blood-glucose control with metformin on complications in overweight patients with type 2 diabetes (UKPDS 34). *Lancet* 1998;352:854.
48. Goede P et al. Multifactorial intervention and cardiovascular disease in patients with type 2 diabetes. *N Engl J Med* 2003;348:383.
49. American Diabetes Association. Standards of medical care for patients with diabetes mellitus. *Diabetes Care* 2003;26 (Suppl 1):S33.
50. Patrono C et al. Platelet active drugs: the relationship among dose, effectiveness and side effects. *Chest* 1998;114:470S.
51. Chen ZM, et al. CAST: randomised placebo-controlled trial of early aspirin use in 20,000 patients with acute ischemic stroke. *Lancet* 1997;349: 1641.
52. Second International Study of Infant Survival Collaborative Group. Randomised trial of intravenous streptokinase, oral aspirin, both, or neither among 17,187 cases of suspected acute myocardial infarction: ISIS-2. *Lancet* 1988;2:349.
53. Hansson L et al. Effects of intensive blood-pressure lowering and low-dose aspirin in patients with hypertension: principle results of the Hypertension Optimal Treatment (HOT) randomised trial. *Lancet* 1998;351:1755.
54. Juul-Moller S et al. Double-blind trial of aspirin in primary prevention of myocardial infarction in patients with stable chronic angina pectoris. The Swedish Angina Pectoris Aspirin Trial (SAPAT) Group. *Lancet* 1992;340:1421.
55. Antithrombotic Trialists' Collaboration. Collaborative meta-analysis of randomised trials of antiplatelet therapy for prevention of death, myocardial infarction, and stroke in high risk patients. *BMJ* 2002;324:71.
56. Goldhaber S et al. Low-dose aspirin and subsequent peripheral arterial surgery in the physician's health study. *Lancet* 1992;340:143.
57. The Dutch TIA trial study group. A comparison of two doses of aspirin (30 mg vs. 283 mg a day) in patients after a transient ischemic attack or minor ischemic stroke. *N Engl J Med* 1992;325:1261.
58. Farrell B et al. The United Kingdom transient ischemic attack (UK-TIA) aspirin trial: final results. *J Neurol Neurosurg Psychiatry* 1991;54:1044.
59. Meade T et al. Determination of who may derive most benefit from aspirin in primary prevention: subgroup results from a randomised controlled trial. *BMJ* 2000;321:13.
60. Sharis P et al. The antiplatelet effects of ticlopidine and clopidogrel. *Ann Intern Med* 1998;129:394.
61. Arcan J et al. Ticlopidine in the treatment of peripheral occlusive arterial disease. *Sem Thromb Hemost* 1989;15:167.
62. Balsano F et al. Ticlopidine in the treatment of intermittent claudication: a 21 month double-blind trial. *J Lab Clin Med* 1989;114:84.
63. Love B et al. Adverse haematological effects of ticlopidine. *Drug Saf* 1998;19:89.
64. Chen D et al. Thrombotic thrombocytopenic purpura associated with ticlopidine use: a report of 3 cases and review of the literature. *Arch Intern Med* 1999;159:311.
65. CAPRIE Steering Committee. A randomised, blinded, trial of clopidogrel versus aspirin in patients at risk of ischaemic events (CAPRIE). *Lancet* 1996;348:1329.
66. Bhatt DL et al. A global view of atherothrombosis: baseline characteristics in the clopidogrel for high atherothrombotic risk and ischemic stabilization, management and avoidance (CHARISMA) trial. *Am Heart J* 2005;150:401.
67. Bhatt DL et al. Clopidogrel and aspirin versus aspirin alone for the prevention of atherothrombotic events. *N Engl J Med* 2006;354:1706.
68. Beebe H et al. A new pharmacologic treatment for intermittent claudication: results of a randomized multicenter trial. *Arch Intern Med* 1999;159:2041.
69. Money S et al. Effect of cilostazol on walking distances in patients with intermittent claudication caused by peripheral vascular disease. *J Vasc Surg* 1998;27:267.
70. Dawson D et al. Cilostazol has beneficial effects in treatment of intermittent claudication. *Circulation* 1998;98:678.
71. Dawson D et al. The effect of withdrawal of drugs treating intermittent claudication. *Am J Surg* 1999;178:141.
72. Jacoby D et al. Drug treatment of intermittent claudication, Drugs 2004;64:1657.
73. Regensteiner JG et al. Effect of cilostazol on treadmill walking, community-based walking ability, and health-related quality of life in patients with intermittent claudication due to peripheral arterial disease: meta-analysis of six randomized controlled trials. *J Am Geriatr Soc* 2002;50:1939.
74. Mohler ER et al. Effects of cilostazol on resting ankle pressures and exercise-induced ischemia in patients with intermittent claudication. *Vasc Med* 2001;6:151.
75. Cruickshank J. Phosphodiesterase III inhibitors: long-term risks and short-term benefits. *Cardiovasc Drugs Ther* 1993;7:655.
76. Thompson PD et al. Meta-analysis of results from eight randomized, placebo-controlled trials on the effect of cilostazol on patients with intermittent claudication. *Am J Cardiol* 2002;90:1314.
77. Samlaska C et al. Pentoxifylline. *J Am Acad Dermatol* 1994;30:603.
78. Frampton JE et al. Pentoxifylline. A review of its therapeutic efficacy in the management of peripheral vascular and cerebrovascular disorders. *Drugs Aging* 1995;7:480.
79. Ward A et al. Pentoxifylline: a review of its pharmacokinetic and pharmacodynamic properties, and its therapeutic efficacy. *Drugs* 1987;34:50.
80. Jackson MR et al. Antithrombotic therapy in peripheral arterial occlusive disease. *Chest* 1998;114: 666S.
81. Cameron HA et al. Drug treatment of intermittent claudication: a critical analysis of the methods and findings of published clinical trials, 1965–1985. *Br J Clin Pharmacol* 1988;26:569.
82. Reiter M et al. Prostanoids for intermittent claudication. *The Cochrane Database of Syst Rev* 2003;4:CD000986.
83. Bagger JP et al. Effect of verapamil in intermittent claudication. A randomized, double-blind, placebo controlled, cross-over study after individual dose-response assessment. *Circulation* 1997;95:411.
84. Pittler M et al. Ginkgo biloba extract for the treatment of intermittent claudication: a meta-analysis of randomized trials. *Am J Med* 2000;108:276.
85. Campbell W et al. Lipid-derived autocoids. In: Hardman J et al., eds. *Goodman and Gillman's The Pharmacological Basis of Therapeutics*. New York: McGraw-Hill; 1996:601.
86. Kincheloe L. Gynecological and obstetric concerns regarding herbal medicinal use. In: Miller L et al., eds. *Herbal Medicines: A Clinician's Guide*. New York: Pharmaceutical Product Press; 1998:279.
87. Newall C et al. Herbal Medicine: A Guide for Health Care Professionals. London: The Pharmaceutical Press; 1996:138.
88. Haeger K. Long-time treatment of intermittent claudication with vitamin E. *Am J Clin Nutr* 1974;27: 1179.
89. Williams H et al. Alpha tocopherol in the treatment of intermittent claudication. *Surg Gynecol Obstet* 1971;132:662.
90. Stephens N et al. Randomised controlled trial of vitamin E in patients with coronary artery disease: Cambridge Heart Antioxidant Study (CHAOS). *Lancet* 1996;347:781.
91. GISSI-Prevenzione Investigators. Dietary supplementation with n-3 polyunsaturated fatty acids and vitamin E after myocardial infarction: results of the GISSI Preventione Trial. *Lancet* 1999;354:447.
92. The Heart Outcomes Prevention Evaluation Study Investigators. Vitamin E supplementation and cardiovascular events in high-risk patients. *N Engl J Med* 2000;342:154.
93. Brevetti G et al. Muscle carnitine deficiency in patients with severe peripheral vascular disease. *Circulation* 1991;84:1490.

94. Hiatt W et al. Skeletal muscle carnitine metabolism in patients with unilateral peripheral arterial disease. *J Appl Physiol* 1992;73:346.
95. Brevetti G et al. European multicenter study on propionyl-L-carnitine in intermittent claudication. *J Am Coll Cardiol* 1999;34:1618.
96. Brevetti G et al. Superiority of L-propionyl-carnitine vs. L-carnitine in improving walking capacity in patients with peripheral vascular disease: an acute, intravenous, double-blind, cross-over study. *Eur Heart J* 1992;13:251.
97. Brevetti G et al. Effect of propionyl-L-carnitine on quality of life in intermittent claudication. *Am J Cardiol* 1997;79:777.
98. Coffman J. Intermittent claudication: be conservative. *N Engl J Med* 1991;325:577.
99. Pentecost M et al. Guidelines for peripheral percutaneous transluminal angioplasty of the abdominal aorta and lower extremity vessels: a statement for health professionals from a special writing group of the Councils on Cardiovascular Radiology, Arteriosclerosis, Cardiothoracic and Vascular Surgery, Clinical Cardiology, and Epidemiology and Prevention, the American Heart Association. *Circulation* 1994;89:511.
100. Tunis S et al. The use of angioplasty, bypass surgery and amputation in the management of peripheral vascular disease. *N Engl J Med* 1991;325: 556.
101. Working Party on Thrombolysis in the Management of Limb Ischemia. Thrombolysis in the management of lower limb peripheral arterial occlusion—a consensus document. *Am J Cardiol* 1998;81: 207.
102. Nilsson L et al. Surgical treatment versus thrombolysis in acute arterial occlusion: a randomised controlled study. *Eur J Vasc Surg* 1992;6:189.
103. Ouriel K et al. A comparison of thrombolytic therapy with operative revascularization in the initial treatment of acute peripheral arterial ischemia. *J Vasc Surg* 1994;19:1021.
104. Raynaud M. On local asphyxia and symmetrical gangrene of the extremities. In: Barlow T, ed. *Selected Monographs, 121.* London: The Syndenham Society; 1888:1.
105. Herrick AL. Pathogenesis of Raynaud's phenomenon. *Rheumatology* 2005;44:587.
106. Shepard F et al. Primary Raynaud's disease. In: *Vascular Diseases of the Limbs: Mechanisms and Principles of Treatment.* St. Louis: Mosby Yearbook; 1993:153.
107. Gasser P et al. Evaluation of reflex cold provocation by laser Doppler flowmetry in clinically healthy subjects with a history of cold hands. *Angiology* 1992;43:389.
108. Nielson S. Raynaud's phenomena and finger systolic blood pressure during cooling. *Scand J Clin Lab Invest* 1978;38:765.
109. Maricq H et al. Geographic variation in the prevalence of Raynaud's phenomenon: a five region comparison. *J Rheumatol* 1997;24:879.
110. Wigley F et al. Raynaud's phenomenon. *Rheum Dis Clin North Am* 1996;22:765.
111. Stoyneva Z et al. Current pathophysiological views on vibration-induced Raynaud's phenomenon. *Cardiovasc Res* 2003;57:615.
112. Belch J. Raynaud's phenomenon. *Cardiovasc Res* 1997;33:25.
113. Wigley F. Raynaud's phenomenon. *N Engl J Med* 2002;347:1001.
114. Ziegler S et al. Long-term outcome of primary Raynaud's phenomenon and its conversion to connective tissue disease: a 12-year retrospective patient analysis. *Scand J Rheumatol* 2003;32:346.
115. Schapira D et al. Interferon-induced Raynaud's syndrome. *Semin Arthritis Rheum* 2002;32:157.
116. Franssen C et al. The influence of different beta-blocking drugs on the peripheral circulation in Raynaud's phenomenon and in hypertension. *J Clin Pharmacol* 1992;32:652.
117. Suter LG et al. The incidence and natural history of Raynaud's phenomenon in the community. *Arthritis Rheum* 2005;52:1259.
118. Goodfield M et al. The acute effects of cigarette smoking on cutaneous blood flow in smoking and nonsmoking subjects with and without Raynaud's phenomenon. *Br J Rheumatol* 1990;29:89.
119. Palesch Y et al. Association between cigarette and alcohol consumption and Raynaud's phenomenon. *J Clin Epidemiol* 1999;52:321.
120. Freedman R et al. Blockade of vasospastic attacks by alpha 2-adrenergic but not alpha1-adrenergic antagonists in idiopathic Raynaud's disease. *Circulation* 1995;92:1448.
121. Coffman J et al. Serotonergic vasoconstriction in human fingers during reflex sympathetic response to cooling. *Am J Physiol* 1988;254:H889.
122. Belch J et al. Pharmacotherapy of Raynaud's phenomenon. *Drugs* 1996;52:682.
123. Thompson AE et al. Calcium channel blockers for primary Raynaud's phenomenon: a meta-analysis. *Rheumatology* 2005;44:145–50.
124. Thompson AE et al. Calcium-channel blockers for Raynaud's phenomenon in systemic sclerosis. *Arthritis Rheum* 2001;44:1841.
125. Smith C et al. Controlled trial of nifedipine in the treatment of Raynaud's phenomenon. *Lancet* 1982;2:1299.
126. Rodeheffer R et al. Controlled double-blind trial of nifedipine in the treatment of Raynaud's phenomenon. *N Engl J Med* 1983;308:880.
127. Boin F et al. Understanding, assessing and treating Raynaud's phenomenon. *Curr Opin Rheumatol* 2005;17:752.
128. Landry G et al. Current management of Raynaud's syndrome. *Adv Surg* 1996;30:333.
129. Finch M et al. A double-blind cross-over study of nifedipine retard in patients with Raynaud's phenomenon. *Clin Rheumatol* 1988;7:359.
130. Waller D et al. Clinical and rheological effects of nifedipine in Raynaud's phenomenon. *Br J Clin Rheumatol* 1986;22:449.
131. Raynaud's Treatment Study Investigators. Comparison of sustained-release nifedipine and temperature biofeedback for treatment of primary Raynaud's phenomenon. Results from a randomised clinical trial with 1-year follow-up. *Arch Intern Med* 2000;160:1101.
132. Leppert J et al. The effect of isradipine, a new calcium-channel antagonist, in patients with primary Raynaud's phenomenon: a single-blind dose- response study. *Cardiovasc Drugs Ther* 1989;3:397.
133. La Civita L et al. Amlodipine in the treatment of Raynaud's phenomenon. *Br J Rheumatol* 1993; 32:524.
134. Schmidt J et al. The clinical effect of felodipine and nifedipine in Raynaud's phenomenon. *Eur J Clin Pharmacol* 1989;37:191.
135. Kallenberg C et al. Once-daily felodipine in patients with primary Raynaud's phenomenon. *Eur J Clin Rheumatol* 1991;40:313.
136. Wollersheim H et al. Double-blind, placebo controlled study of prazosin in Raynaud's phenomenon. *Clin Pharmacol Ther* 1986;40:219.
137. Wollersheim H et al. Dose-response study of prazosin in Raynaud's phenomenon: clinical effectiveness versus side effects. *J Clin Pharmacol* 1988;28:1089.
138. Paterna S et al. Raynaud's phenomenon: effects of terazosin. *Minerva Cardioangiol* 1997;45:215.
139. Marasini B et al. Comparison between iloprost and alprostadil in the treatment of Raynaud's phenomenon. *Scand J Rheumatol* 2004;33:253.
140. Humbert M et al. Successful treatment of systemic sclerosis digital ulcers and pulmonary arterial hypertension with endothelin receptor antagonist bosentan. *Rheumatology* 2003;42:191.
141. Fries RF et al. Sildenafil in the treatment of Raynaud's phenomenon resistant to vasodilator therapy. *Circulation* 2005;112:2980.
142. Caglayan E et al. Phosphodiesterase type 5 inhibition is a novel therapeutic option in Raynaud disease. *Arch Int Med* 2006;166:231.
143. Challenor V. Angiotensin converting enzyme inhibitors in Raynaud's phenomenon. *Drugs* 1994;48:864.
144. Coleiro B et al. Treatment of Raynaud's phenomenon with the selective serotonin reuptake inhibitor fluoxetine. *Rheumatology* 2001;40:1038.
145. Franks A. Topical glyceryl trinitrate as adjunctive treatment in Raynaud's disease. *Lancet* 1982;1:76.
146. Teh L et al. Sustained-release transdermal glyceryl trinitrate patches as a treatment for primary and secondary Raynaud's phenomenon. *Br J Rheumatol* 1995;34:636.
147. Rembold CM et al. Oral L-arginine can reverse digital necrosis in Raynaud's phenomenon. *Mol Cell Biochem* 2003;244:139.
148. Muir AH et al. The use of ginkgo biloba in Raynaud's disease: a double-blind placebo-controlled trial. *Vasc Med* 2002;7:265.
149. Obi T et al. Muscle cramps as the result of impaired GABA function-an electrophysiological and pharmacological observation. *Muscle Nerve* 1993;16:1228.
150. Bertolasi L et al. The influence of muscle lengthening on cramps. *Ann Neurol* 1993;33:176.
151. Oboler S et al. Leg symptoms in outpatient veterans. *West J Med* 1991;155:256.
152. Naylor J et al. A general population survey of rest cramps. *Age Ageing* 1994;23:418.
153. Haskell S et al. Clinical epidemiology of nocturnal leg cramps in male veterans. *Am J Med Sci* 1997;313:210.
154. Leclerc K et al. Benign nocturnal leg cramps. Current controversies over use of quinine. *Postgrad Med* 1996;99:177.
155. Butler JV et al. Nocturnal leg cramps in older people. *Postgrad Med J* 2002;78:596.
156. Drug products for the treatment and/or prevention of nocturnal leg cramps for over-the-counter human use. *Fed Reg* 1994;59:432.
157. Moss H et al. Use of quinine for relief of "night cramps" in the extremities. *JAMA* 1940;115:1358.
158. Man-So-Hing M et al. Quinine for nocturnal leg cramps: a meta-analysis including unpublished data. *J Gen Intern Med* 1998;13:600.
159. Coppin RJ et al. Managing nocturnal leg cramps: calf-stretching exercises and cessation of quinine treatment. *Br J Gen Prac* 2005;55:186.
160. Krishna S et al. Pharmacokinetics of quinine, chloroquine, and amodiaquine: clinical implications. *Clin Pharmacokinet* 1996;30:263.
161. Brasic J. Should people with nocturnal leg cramps drink tonic water and bitter lemon? *Psychol Report* 1999;84:355.
162. Connolly P et al. Treatment of nocturnal leg cramps: a crossover trial of quinine vs vitamin E. *Arch Intern Med* 1992;152:1877.
163. Baltodano N et al. Verapamil vs. quinine in recumbent nocturnal leg cramps in the elderly. *Arch Intern Med* 1988;148:1969.
164. Voon W et al. Diltiazem for nocturnal leg cramps. *Age Ageing* 2001;30:91.
165. Chan P et al. Randomized, double-blind, placebo-controlled study of the safety and efficacy of vitamin B complex in the treatment of nocturnal leg cramps in elderly patients with hypertension. *J Clin Pharmacol* 1998;38:1151.
166. Frusso R et al. Magnesium for the treatment of nocturnal leg cramps: a crossover randomized trial. *J Fam Pract* 1999;48:868.
167. Roffe C et al. Randomised, cross-over, placebo controlled trial of magnesium citrate in the treatment of chronic persistent leg cramps. *Med Sci Monitor* 2002;8:CR326.
168. Hankey GJ et al. Medical treatment of peripheral arterial disease. *JAMA* 2006;295:547.
169. Krajewski LP et al. Atherosclerosis of the aorta and lower-extremity arteries. In: Young JS et al., eds. *Peripheral Vascular Diseases.* St. Louis: Mosby; 1996:208.

CHAPTER 15

Thrombosis

Ann K. Wittkowsky and Edith A. Nutescu

GENERAL PRINCIPLES

Thrombosis is the process involved in the formation of a fibrin blood clot. Both platelets and a series of coagulant proteins (clotting factors) contribute to clot formation. An *embolus* is a small part of a clot that breaks off and travels to another part of the vascular system. Damage is caused when the embolus becomes trapped in a small vessel, causing occlusion and leading to ischemia or infarction of the surrounding tissue. Normal clot formation maintains the integrity of the vasculature in response to injury, but pathological clotting can occur in many clinical settings. Abnormal thrombotic events include deep venous thrombosis (DVT) and its primary complication, pulmonary embolism (PE), as well as stroke and other systemic manifestations of embolization of clots that form within the heart. Anticoagulant drug therapy is aimed at preventing pathological clot formation in patients at risk and at preventing clot extension and/or embolization in patients who have developed thrombosis. This chapter emphasizes arterial and venous thromboembolic disease and the use of heparin and warfarin as anticoagulants. Chapters 17, 18, and 55 provide more in-depth discussions of thrombolytic agents and antiplatelet therapy.

Etiology of Thromboembolism

Three primary factors influence the formation of pathological clots and are described in a model referred to as Virchow's triad (Fig. 15-1).[1] First, abnormalities of blood flow that cause venous stasis can result in DVT, which can progress to PE if embolization occurs. Intracardiac stasis of blood can also result in clot formation within the heart chambers, and embolization of intracardiac thrombi may lead to stroke or other systemic manifestations. Abnormalities of blood vessel walls, such as those that occur in injury or trauma to the vasculature, are a second source of thrombus formation. The presence of foreign material within the vasculature, including artificial heart valves and central venous catheters, is also thrombogenic and, like vascular injury, represents the presence of an abnormal surface in contact with blood. Finally, hypercoagulability resulting from alterations in the availability or the integrity of blood-clotting components or naturally occurring anticoagulants also represents a significant risk factor for thromboembolic disease.[2]

Clot Formation

The intact endothelial lining of blood vessels normally repels platelets and inhibits clot formation through secretion of numerous inhibitory substances. Damage to the endothelium leads to exposure of circulating blood to subendothelial substances, and this results in a complex series of events, including platelet adhesion, activation, and aggregation, followed by activation of the clotting cascade. These events result in formation of a fibrin clot.[3]

Platelet Adhesion, Activation, and Aggregation

Endothelial damage leads to exposure of blood to subendothelial collagen and phospholipids, resulting in platelet adhesion to the surface. von Willebrand factor serves as the binding ligand and for platelet adhesion, via the glycoprotein I (GPI) receptor on the platelet surface. Adhered platelets become activated and release numerous compounds, including adenosine diphosphate and thromboxane A_2, which stimulate platelet aggregation. Fibrinogen serves as the binding ligand for platelet aggregation, via the GPIIb/IIIa receptor on the platelet surface.[4]

Clotting Cascade

Transformation of the relatively unstable platelet plug (i.e., the aggregated platelets) to a stable fibrin clot occurs as a result of an imbalance between other procoagulant and anticoagulant factors. In addition to stimulating the platelet response, endothelial damage results in activation of the clotting cascade (Fig. 15-2). The extrinsic pathway of the clotting cascade is activated by the release of thromboplastin (tissue factor) from endothelial cells. Tissue factor converts factor VII to factor VII_a, which mediates the activation of factor X. The intrinsic pathway of the clotting cascade is activated by exposure of factor XII to subendothelial components exposed during vessel injury. The intrinsic pathway mediates factor X activation via a chain of events initiated by factor XI. The distinction between these pathways is primarily an in vitro phenomenon; in vivo, the two pathways are activated simultaneously.

Once stimulated, both the extrinsic and intrinsic pathways activate the common pathway of the clotting cascade via factor X. Activated forms of factors V and VIII serve independently to accelerate this process. The final steps include conversion of factor II (prothrombin) to factor II_a (thrombin), with eventual formation of a stable fibrin clot.

Naturally occurring inhibitors of clotting factors play a role in localizing fibrin formation to the sites of injury and in maintaining the fluidity of circulating blood. Table 15-1 outlines these clotting inhibitors and their primary actions. In

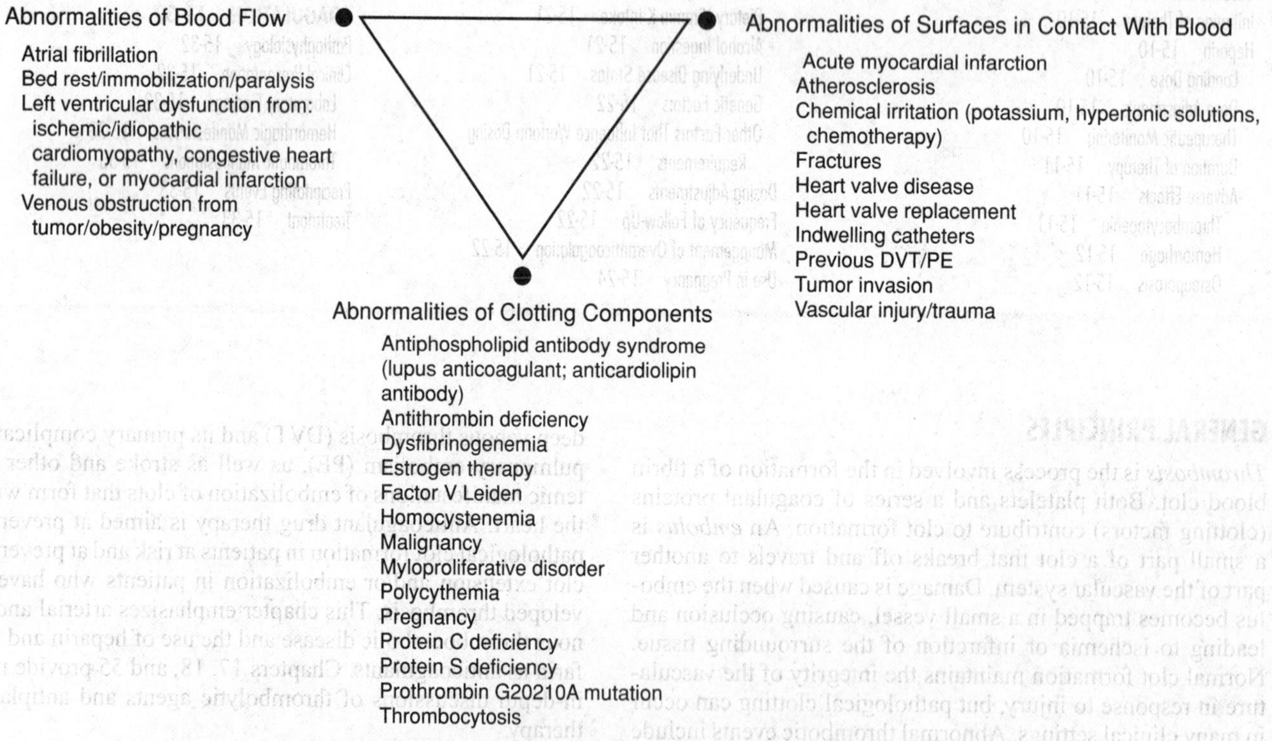

FIGURE 15-1 Risk factors for thromboembolism. DVT, deep venous thrombosis; PE, pulmonary embolism.

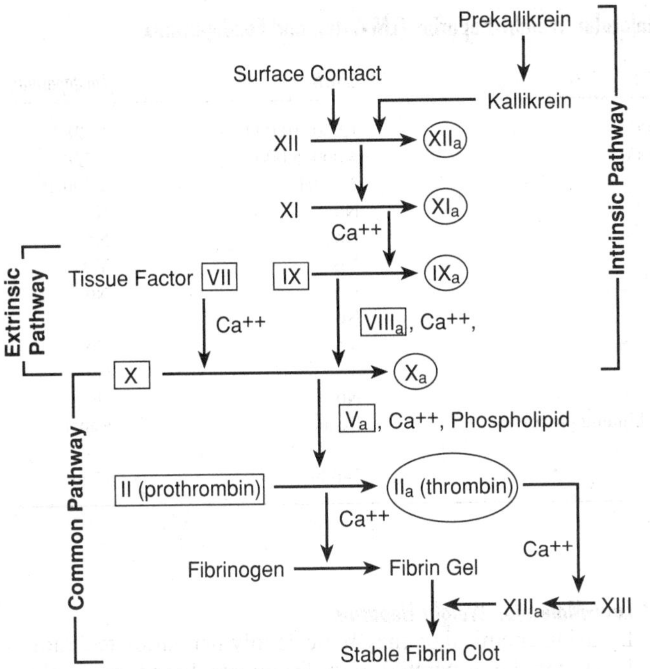

FIGURE 15-2 Simplified clotting cascade. Components in ovals are influenced by heparin; components in boxes are influenced by warfarin.

addition, the fibrinolytic system is involved in degradation of fibrin clots. The actions of both clotting inhibitors and the fibrinolytic system prevent excessive coagulation. Thus, the process of clot formation is dynamic and involves various factors that can stimulate, inhibit, and dissolve a fibrin clot.

Pathological Thrombi

Pathological thrombi are sometimes classified according to location and composition. Arterial thrombi are composed primarily of platelets, although they also contain fibrin and occasional leukocytes. Arterial thrombi generally occur in areas of rapid blood flow (i.e., arteries) and are typically initiated by spontaneous or mechanical rupture of atherosclerotic plaques (see Chapter 18). Venous thrombi are found primarily in the venous circulation and are composed almost entirely of fibrin and erythrocytes. Venous thrombi have a small platelet head and generally form in response to either venous stasis or vascular injury after surgery or trauma. The areas of stasis prevent dilution of activated coagulation factors by normal blood flow.

The selection of an antithrombotic agent may be influenced by the type of thrombus to be treated. The anticoagulants heparin, low-molecular-weight heparins, factor X_a inhibitors, and warfarin are used in the treatment and prevention of both arterial and venous thrombi. Drugs that alter platelet function (e.g., aspirin), alone and in combination with anticoagulants, are used in the prevention of arterial thrombi. Fibrinolytic agents are used for rapid dissolution of thromboemboli, most notably during myocardial infarction (MI).

Table 15-1 Inhibitors of Clotting Mechanisms

Inhibitor	*Target*
Antithrombin	Inhibits factors IIa, IXa, and Xa
Protein S	Cofactor for activation of protein C
Protein C	Inactivates factors Va and VIIIa
Tissue factor pathway inhibitor	Inhibits activity of factor VIIa
Plasminogen	Converted to plasmin via tissue plasminogen activator
Plasmin	Lyses fibrin into fibrin degradation products

Pharmacology of Antithrombotic Agents

Heparin

Heparin is a rapid-acting anticoagulant that is administered parenterally. Standard heparin (unfractionated heparin [UFH]) is a heterogeneous mixture of glycosaminoglycans of varying molecular weights obtained from bovine lung or porcine intestinal mucosa (Table 15-2). The action of heparin is facilitated by its binding to the naturally circulating anticoagulant antithrombin (AT), a serine protease also referred to as heparin cofactor. Binding of heparin to AT accelerates the anticoagulant effect of AT. The heparin–AT complex attaches to and irreversibly inactivates factor II_a (thrombin) and factor X_a, as well as activated factors IX, XI, and XII (Fig. 15-3).[5] Approximately one-third of the molecules present in UFH bind to AT and provide the anticoagulant properties of heparin. The remaining two-thirds of the heparin molecules bind to plasma proteins and to endothelial cells, saturable processes that contribute to the dose-dependent pharmacokinetic profile of the drug and limit its bioavailability. In addition to its anticoagulant effects, heparin inhibits platelet function and increases vascular permeability; these properties contribute to the hemorrhagic effects of heparin.

In cases of acute DVT or PE, the clotting cascade has been activated, generating abnormal quantities of thrombin and fibrin. In these situations, thrombin must be inactivated directly, a process that may require relatively large doses of heparin. However, when the clotting cascade is in a normal balance, it is possible to indirectly inactivate thrombin with smaller heparin doses by complexing factor X_a. Because of the amplification effect of the clotting cascade, inactivation of relatively small amounts of factor X_a indirectly prevents the production of large quantities of thrombin. This phenomenon is the basis for low-dose heparin prophylaxis after surgery or in cases of prolonged bed rest or immobilization.

Heparin may be administered intravenously (IV) by continuous infusion, or subcutaneously (SC), although its bioavailability is significantly reduced by SC administration. Intramuscular administration should be avoided because of the potential for hematoma formation.

After IV administration, the anticoagulant effect of heparin is noted immediately. During active thromboembolism, the high concentration of clotting factors necessitates a higher concentration of heparin to neutralize them. This increased dosing requirement may also be related to continuing thrombin formation on the surface of the thrombus. Once endothelialization (localization and incorporation of the clot into the vascular endothelium) of the clot begins and the concentration of clotting factors decreases, dosing requirements typically decrease. Considerable variability in dosing requirements among patients necessitates routine therapeutic monitoring to maintain an appropriate intensity of anticoagulation with heparin. The primary laboratory test for monitoring therapeutic heparinization is the activated partial thromboplastin time

Table 15-2 Comparison of Unfractionated Heparin (UFH), Low-Molecular-Weight Heparins (LMWHs), and Fondaparinux

Property	*UFH*	*LMWH*	*Fondaparinux*
Molecular weight range[a]	3,000–30,000	1,000–10,000	1,728
Average molecular weight[a]	12,000–15,000	4,000–5,000	1,728
Anti-X_a:anti-II_a activity	1:1	2:1–4:1	>100:1
aPTT monitoring required	Yes	No	No
Inactivation by platelet factor 4	Yes	No	No
Capable of inactivation of platelet-bound factor X_a	No	Yes	Yes
Inhibition of platelet function	++++	++	No
Increases vascular permeability	Yes	No	No
Protein binding	++++	+	No
Endothelial cell binding	+++	+	No
Dose-dependent clearance	Yes	No	No
Primary route of elimination	1. Saturable binding processes 2. Renal	Renal	Renal
Elimination half-life	30–150 min	2–6 hr	17 hr

[a]Measured in daltons.
Adapted from references 6 and 7.

(aPTT) (see Tests Used to Monitor Antithrombotic Therapy section).

The plasma half-life of heparin varies from 30 to 150 minutes, but the half-life increases with increasing doses. Heparin is cleared by extensive binding to plasma proteins and endothelial cells, saturable processes that explain both its nonlinear kinetics and the variability in dosing requirements among patients. Additional clearance occurs by transfer to the reticuloendothelial system, with ultimate elimination controlled by the kidneys.

Low-Molecular-Weight Heparins

By using chemical or enzymatic depolymerization techniques, UFH can be separated into fragments based on molecular weight.[6] Several low-molecular-weight heparin (LMWH) molecules have been isolated and commercially marketed as anticoagulants. The LMWH products available in the United States are dalteparin (Fragmin), enoxaparin (Lovenox), and tinzaparin (Innohep). These products have replaced the use of UFH in many clinical situations. These compounds differ substantially from UFH with respect to molecular weight,

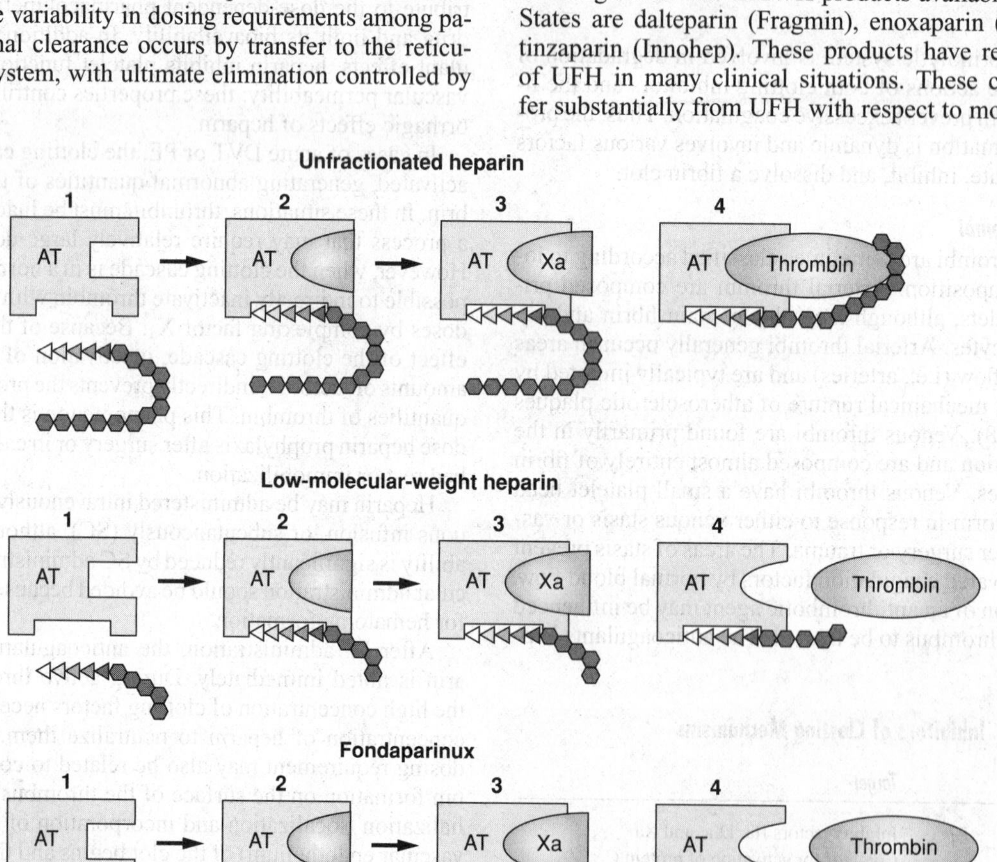

FIGURE 15-3 Mechanism of action of heparin, low-molecular-weight heparins, and fondaparinux (see text for details). Reprinted from reference 5, with permission.

antithrombotic and pharmacokinetic properties, adverse effect profiles, and monitoring requirements (Table 15-2).

To inactivate factor X_a, only the AT component of the heparin–AT complex is required to bind to factor X_a (Fig. 15-3). Both the longer, high-molecular-weight fragments of UFH and the shorter, low-molecular-weight fragments of LMWHs are capable of inactivating factor X_a. However, to inactivate factor II_a (thrombin), both the heparin component and the AT component of the heparin–AT complex are required to bind to factor II_a. This binding requires heparin molecules of at least 18 saccharide units in length, which are less prevalent in LMWHs. Therefore, the anti-X_a properties of LMWHs are more significant than their anti-II_a properties. The resultant antithrombotic effect does not prolong the aPTT, meaning that these compounds do not require laboratory monitoring to ensure a therapeutic effect.

Additional advantages of LMWHs over UFH are explained by their reduced binding affinity for plasma proteins and endothelial cells. These compounds display improved bioavailability after SC injection, a predictable dose response, and a longer pharmacodynamic effect compared with UFH. In general, these compounds are administered subcutaneously every 12 to 24 hours at fixed doses. Many LMWH products have been studied in the prevention and treatment of thromboembolic disease (Table 15-3). They differ significantly in their molecular weight distributions, methods of preparation, and the ratio of anti-X_a:anti-II_a activities, as well as in their pharmacokinetic and pharmacodynamic characteristics.

Fondaparinux

Fondaparinux (Arixtra) is a selective indirect factor X_a inhibitor that is indicated for the prevention of venous thrombosis associated with orthopedic surgery and abdominal surgery, and for the treatment of deep vein thrombosis and pulmonary embolism.[6,7] It is a synthetic derivative of the five-residue saccharide sequence found in both UFH and LMWH that binds to AT to inactivate factor X_a with no direct impact on factor IIa. This agent has a long elimination half-life, allowing for once-daily SC administration at a fixed dose without the need for routine coagulation monitoring.

Direct Thrombin Inhibitors

Argatroban, lepirudin (Refludan), and bivalirudin (Angiomax) are direct thrombin inhibitors that are used as alternative anticoagulants in patients with heparin-induced thrombocytopenia.[8] (Table 15-4). These agents are administered by continuous infusion and require aPTT monitoring for appropriate dosing adjustments. Bivalirudin is also used in patients undergoing percutaneous coronary intervention. This

Table 15-3 Low-Molecular-Weight Heparin Products Available in the United States

Generic Name	Brand Name	Average Molecular Weight (range)[a]	Anti-X_a:Anti-II_a Activity
Dalteparin	Fragmin	5,000 (2,000–9,000)	2.0:1
Enoxaparin	Lovenox	4,500 (3,000–8,000)	2.7:1
Tinzaparin	Innohep	4,500 (3,000–6,000)	1.9:1

[a] Measured in daltons.

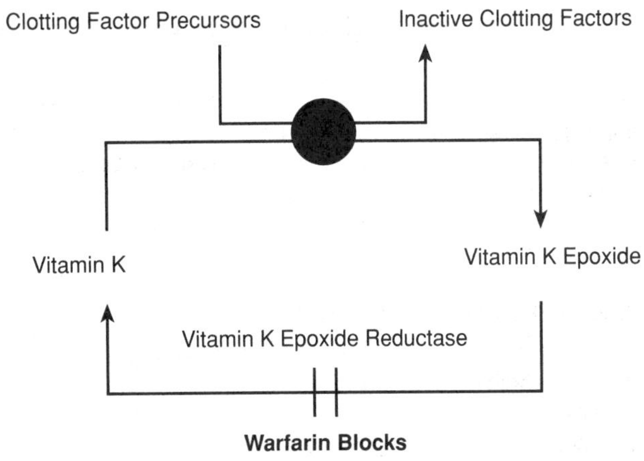

FIGURE 15-4 Mechanism of action of warfarin.

agent appears to be associated with a lower rate of hemorrhagic complications than UFH and may reduce the need for concurrent therapy with glycoprotein IIb/IIIa receptor antagonists[9].

Warfarin

Warfarin is an oral anticoagulant with a delayed onset of effect that acts as a vitamin K antagonist. Vitamin K is essential for the conversion (carboxylation) of precursors to clotting factors II, VII, IX, and X into inactive clotting factors and for the synthesis of protein C and protein S. During factor conversion, vitamin K is oxidized to inactive vitamin K epoxide (Fig. 15-4). In the nonanticoagulated patient, vitamin K epoxide is in reversible equilibrium with vitamin K, but this equilibrium is disrupted in patients taking oral anticoagulants. Warfarin (Coumadin) interferes with the hepatic recycling of vitamin K by inhibiting vitamin K epoxide reductase (VKOR), the enzyme that converts vitamin K epoxide to vitamin K.[10] The accumulation of vitamin K epoxide reduces the effective concentration of vitamin K and reduces the synthesis of coagulation factors. Concentrations of clotting factors II, VII, IX, and X are diminished gradually at rates commensurate with their elimination half-lives (Table 15-5). Thus, the onset of the anticoagulant effect of warfarin is delayed. It takes approximately 5 to 7 days to reach a steady state of anticoagulation after warfarin therapy is initiated or after dosing changes. Protein C and its cofactor protein S are also vitamin K dependent, and these proteins are depleted by warfarin at rates dependent on their elimination half-lives.

Warfarin is rapidly and completely absorbed in the upper gastrointestinal (GI) tract by passive diffusion, with nearly 100% bioavailability. Peak absorption of warfarin occurs in 60 to 120 minutes. It is approximately 99% bound to serum albumin. The volume of distribution (Vd) for warfarin is 12.5% of body weight. This small volume of distribution is consistent with the extensive binding of warfarin to albumin. The primary laboratory test for monitoring warfarin therapy is the prothrombin time (PT). No correlation appears to exist between PT and the dose of warfarin, the total warfarin concentration, or the free warfarin concentration among individuals, although in individual patients, an increasing dose of warfarin will increase the serum concentration (free and total) and the PT.

Warfarin is administered orally as a racemic mixture containing equal parts of the enantiomers R(+)-warfarin and S(−)-warfarin. The S(−)-isomer is 2.7 to 3.8 times more potent

Table 15-4 Pharmacologic and Clinical Properties of Direct Thrombin Inhibitors

	Lepirudin	*Bivalirudin*	*Argatroban*
Route of administration	IV or SC (BID)	IV	IV
FDA-Approved Indication	Treatment of thrombosis in patients with HIT	Patients with UA undergoing PTCA; PCI with provisional use of GPI; Patients with or at risk of HIT/HITTS undergoing PCI.	Treatment of thrombosis in patients with HIT; Patients at risk for HIT undergoing PCI
Binding to Thrombin	Irreversible at catalytic site and exosite-1	Partially reversible at catalytic site and exosite-1	Reversible at catalytic site
Half-Life in healthy subjects	1.3–2 hrs	25 min	40–50 min
Monitoring	aPTT (IV) SCr/CrCL	aPTT/ACT SCr/CrCL	aPTT/ACT Liver Function
Clearance	Renal	Enzymatic (80%) Renal (20%)	Hepatic
Antibody Development	Antihirudin antibodies in up to 40%–60% of patients	May cross-react with antihirudin antibodies	No
Effect on INR	Slight increase	Slight increase	Increase
Initial dose for HIT	HITTS: Bolus[a]: 0.4 mg/kg, up to a maximum of 110 kg, given over 15 to 20 seconds Infusion: 0.15 mg/kg/hr HIT: no bolus; 0.1 - mg/kg/hr infusion	No bolus Infusion: 0.15mg/kg/hr	No bolus Infusion: 2mcg/kg/min[b] *In critically ill patients: consider lower infusion rat of 0.5–1 mcg/kg/min*
Initial dose for PCI	NA	Bolus: 0.75mg/kg Infusion: 1.75mg/kg/hr	NA
Dosing if renal impairment	Bolus[a]: 0.2 mg/kg (bolus dose is best avoided in patients with renal impairment) Infusion: CrCL 45–60: 0.075 mg/kg/hr CrCL 30–44: 0.045 mg/kg/hr CrCL 15–29: 0.0225 mg/kg/hr CrCL< 15: no bolus; avoid or stop infusion HD: stop infusion & additional IV bolus doses of 0.1 mg/kg every other day should be considered if the aPTT ratio falls below 1.5	PCI: Bolus: no dose adjustment Infusion: CrCL < 30: 1 mg/kg/hr HD:0.25mg/kg/hr HIT: No bolus Infusion: CrCL < 30: 0.08mg/kg/hr HD:0.02mg/kg/hr	CrCL < 30: mean doses of 0.8 mcg/kg/min have been reported; Note: Dose adjustment not required per product information but recent literature support dose adjustment as above.
Dosing if hepatic impairment	Dose adjustment not required	Dose adjustment not required	Initiate at 0.5 mcg/kgmin then titrate to aPTT 1.5–3.0 x baseline

[a] Initial IV bolus ONLY recommended when life-threatening thrombosis is present.
[b] Recent reports indicate that lower initial infusion rates of ~ 1.5mcg/kg/min may be more appropriate
IV, intravenous; SC, subcutaneous; PO, oral; bid, twice daily; qd, daily; HIT, heparin induced thrombocytopenia; HITTS, heparin induced thrombocytopenia and thrombosis syndrome; DVT, deep vein thrombosis; THA, total hip arthroplasty; UA, unstable angina; PTCA, percutaneous transluminal coronary angioplasty; PCI, percutaneous coronary intervention;; GPI, glycoprotein IlbIlla inhibitor; VTE, venous thromboembolism; AF, atrial fibrillation; aPTT, activated partial thromboplastin time; SCr, serum creatinine; CrCL, creatinine clearance; ACT, activated clotting time; HD, hemodialysis

as an anticoagulant than the R(+)-isomer, has a longer elimination half-life, and is primarily metabolized by cytochrome P450 (CYP)-2C9. Comparatively, R(+)-warfarin is metabolized by primarily by CYP1A2 and CYP3A4. Many drugs interact with warfarin by stereoselectively inhibiting the metabolism of either the R(+)-isomer or the S(−)-isomer (see Drug Interactions section). Genetic expression of CYP2C9 influences the rate of metabolism of warfarin and thus impacts dosing requirements to meet a particular therapeutic end point.[11] Variability in genetic expression of VKORC1 (the C1 subunit on the gene that codes for VKOR) also influences dosing requirements in patients taking warfarin.[12] Testing for CYP2C9 and VCORC1 genotype are being evaluated as a method to determine warfarin dosing requirement, but will not ready for clinical use until randomized controlled trials confirm that this method of dosing improves patient outcomes and is cost effective.

Tests Used to Monitor Antithrombotic Therapy

Before the initiation of antithrombotic therapy, an assessment of coagulation status is necessary. The clinician should obtain a baseline platelet count and hematocrit (Hct), as well as evaluate the baseline integrity of the extrinsic and intrinsic coagulation pathways with PT and aPTT, the tests used to monitor warfarin and heparin, respectively.

Prothrombin Time/International Normalized Ratio

The PT is prolonged by deficiencies of clotting factors II, V, VII, and X, as well as by low levels of fibrinogen and very high

Table 15-5 Elimination Half-Lives of Vitamin K–Dependent Clotting Factors

Clotting Factors	*Half-Life (hours)*
II	42–72
VII	4–6
IX	21–30
X	27–48
Protein C	9
Protein S	60

levels of heparin. It reflects alterations in the extrinsic and common pathways of the clotting cascade, but not in the intrinsic system.[13] The PT is measured by adding calcium and tissue thromboplastin to a sample of plasma from which platelets have been removed by centrifugation. The time to clot formation is detected by automated instruments using light-scattering techniques that measure optical density. The mean normal PT, obtained by averaging a number of PT results from nonanticoagulated subjects, is approximately 12 seconds for most reagents.

The thromboplastins used in PT monitoring are extracted from various tissue sources by a number of techniques and prepared for commercial use as reagents. Unfortunately, thromboplastins are not standardized among manufacturers or among batches of reagent produced by the same manufacturer, leading to significant variability in PT results for anticoagulated patients.[14] To standardize PT results, the World Health Organization developed a system by which all commercially available thromboplastins are compared with an international reference thromboplastin and then assigned an International Sensitivity Index (ISI). This value is used to mathematically convert PT to the international normalized ratio (INR) by exponentially multiplying the PT ratio to the power of the ISI of the thromboplastin being used in the laboratory to measure the test ($INR = [PT\ patient/PT\ mean\ normal]^{ISI}$). The ISI of the international reference thromboplastin is 1.0.

INR is the internationally recognized standard for monitoring warfarin therapy. Current recommendations for intensity of oral anticoagulation therapy for accepted clinical indications are summarized in Table 15-6. Regular-intensity therapy is defined as dosing warfarin to reach a goal INR of 2.5 (range, 2.0–3.0) and is appropriate for most settings that require the prevention and/or treatment of thromboembolic disease. High-intensity therapy is used in mechanical valve replacement and certain situations of thromboembolic recurrence, despite adequate anticoagulation, and is defined as dosing warfarin to reach a goal INR of 3.0 (range, 2.5–3.5).

Activated Partial Thromboplastin Time

The aPTT reflects alterations in the intrinsic pathway of the clotting cascade and is used to monitor heparin therapy.[15] The test is performed by adding a surface-activating agent (kaolin or micronized silica), a partial thromboplastin reagent (phospholipid; platelet substitute), and calcium to the plasma sample. Mean normal values vary among reagents, but typically fall between 24 and 36 seconds.

Like PT, the aPTT is a highly variable test based on differences among commercially available partial thromboplastin reagents. However, a system equivalent to the INR has not been developed for standardization of aPTT results. Heparinization to prolong the aPTT to 1.5 to 2.5 times the mean normal value historically was considered adequate to prevent propagation or extension of thrombus, but is no longer recommended because it is not appropriate for all reagents and testing systems. Instead, the aPTT should be calibrated for each reagent lot and coagulometer, and a reagent-specific therapeutic range in seconds determined that corresponds to therapeutic heparin levels of 0.3 to 0.7 U/mL by factor X_a inhibition (anti-X_a activity).[6,16]

Anti-X_a Activity

Although LMWHs do not require coagulation monitoring to ensure an appropriate antithrombotic effect or to adjust dosing, certain clinical situations may require evaluation of the anti-X_a activity of LMWHs.[17] Because these agents are eliminated renally, patients with severe renal failure may accumulate LMWHs, leading to an increased risk of hemorrhagic complications and necessitating evaluation of anti-X_a activity. LMWHs are dosed according to total body weight, but clinical trials have included only limited numbers of obese patients. Therefore, it may be appropriate to monitor anti-X_a activity in these patients. Anti-X_a activity should also be evaluated in patients who experience unexpected bleeding complications secondary to anticoagulation with LMWHs, and in pregnant patients in whom LMWHs are used for treatment or prevention of thrombosis.

Anti-X_a activity is measured using a chromogenic assay that is expensive and of limited availability. Peak activity levels should be obtained approximately 4 hours after a SC dose of LMWH, with empiric dosing adjustments to maintain a level of roughly 0.5 to 1.0 U/mL for therapeutic anticoagulation.[6,18] Like other measures of hemostasis, results vary considerably, requiring both instrument- and method-specific determination of therapeutic ranges.

DEEP VENOUS THROMBOSIS

Clinical Presentation

Signs and Symptoms

1. L.N., a 76-year-old, obese (92 kg, 6 ft tall) man, was admitted to the hospital 3 days ago for management of recurrent angina. He was started on a nitroglycerin drip and confined to bed rest with gradual increases in his oral antianginal medications. On the third day of hospitalization, he noted progressive swelling and soreness of the right calf. He denied shortness of breath (SOB), cough, or chest pain. His medical history includes coronary artery disease, MI at ages 55 and 67, and hypercholesterolemia. His medications are diltiazem CD (Cardizem CD) 360 mg/day PO, isosorbide mononitrate (Imdur) 120 mg/day PO, atenolol (Tenormin) 50 mg/day PO, aspirin 325 mg/day PO, and simvastatin (Zocor) 5 mg PO Q pm. Initial laboratory values include Hct, 36.5% (normal, 42%–52%); PT, 10.8 seconds (INR, 1.0); aPTT, 23.6 seconds (normal, 24–36); and platelet count, 255,000/mm^3 (normal, 150,000–300,000). What signs and symptoms demonstrated by L.N. are consistent with DVT?

[SI units: Hct, 0.365 (normal, 0.42–0.52); platelet count, 255 × 10^9/L (normal, 150–300)]

One of the most reliable, although nonspecific, physical findings of DVT is unilateral leg swelling that often is

Table 15-6 Optimal Therapeutic Range and Duration of Anticoagulation

Indication	*Target INR (Range)*	*Duration*	*Comment*
Atrial Fibrillation (AF)/Atrial Flutter			
Age older than 65 years with no risk factors	None	Chronic	Use aspirin 325 mg QD alone
Age 65–75 years with no risk factors	2.5 (2.0–3.0)	Chronic	Or aspirin 325 mg QD
Age older than 75 years OR any risk factor [hx TIA/stroke/TE; HTN; poor LV fxn; mitral valve dz; valve replacement]		Chronic	
Precardioversion (AF or flutter >48 hours)	2.5 (2.0–3.0)	3 weeks	
Postcardioversion (in NSR)	2.5 (2.0–3.0)	4 weeks	
Cardioembolic Stroke			
With risk factors for stroke [AF, CHF, LV dysfxn; mural thrombus, hx TIA/stroke/TE]	2.5 (2.0–3.0)	Chronic	
Following embolic event despite anticoagulation	2.5 (2.0–3.0)	Chronic	Add antiplatelet therapy
Left Ventricular Dysfunction			
Ejection fraction <30%	2.5 (2.0–3.0)	Chronic	
Transient, following myocardial infarction <30%	2.5 (2.0–3.0)	3 months	With aspirin 81 mg QD
Following embolic event despite anticoagulation <30%	2.5 (2.0–3.0)	Chronic	Add antiplatelet therapy
Myocardial Infarction (MI)			
Following anterior MI	2.5 (2.0–3.0)	3 months	With aspirin 81 mg QD
Following inferior MI with transient risk(s) [AF; CHF, LV dysfxn, mural thrombus, hx TE]	2.5 (2.0–3.0)	3 months	With aspirin 81 mg QD
Following initial tx with persistent risks	2.5 (2.0–3.0)	Chronic	With aspirin 81 mg QD
Thromboembolism (DVT, PE)			
Treatment/prevention of recurrence (including calf vein and upper extremity DVT)			
• Transient risk factors	2.5 (2.0–3.0)	3 months	
• Idiopathic/first episode	2.5 (2.0–3.0)	6–12 months	Consider chronic therapy
• Recurrent VTE	2.5 (2.0–3.0)	Chronic	
• With malignancy	2.5 (2.0–3.0)	Chronic	Preceded by LMWH × 3–6 months
• Hypercoagulable state	2.5 (2.0–3.0)	6–12 months	Consider chronic therapy
• Two or more thrombophilic conditions	2.5 (2.0–3.0)	12 months	Consider chronic therapy
• Antiphospholipid antibody syndrome	2.5 (2.0–3.0)	12 months	Consider chronic therapy
• With recurrent VTE or other risk factors	2.5 (2.0–3.0)	12 months	Consider chronic therapy
Chronic thromboembolic pulmonary hypertension	2.5 (2.0–3.0)	Chronic	
Cerebral venous sinus thrombosis	2.5 (2.0–3.0)	3–6 months	
Valvular Disease			
Aortic valve disease	2.5 (2.0–3.0)	Chronic	
• With mobile atheroma or aortic plaque >4 mm			
Mitral valve prolapse, regurgitation, or annular calcification			
• With AF or hx systemic embolization	2.5 (2.0–3.0)	Chronic	
• With recurrent TIA despite ASA therapy	2.5 (2.0–3.0)	Chronic	
Rheumatic mitral valve disease			
• With AF, hx systemic embolization, or LA >5.5 cm	2.5 (2.0–3.0)	Chronic	
• S/p embolic event despite anticoagulation	2.5 (2.0–3.0)	Chronic	With aspirin 81 mg QD
Valve Replacement—Bioprosthetic			
Aortic	2.5 (2.0–3.0)	3 months	Followed by aspirin (or aspirin alone)
Mitral	2.5 (2.0–3.0)	3 months	Followed by aspirin 81 mg QD
Aortic or mitral			
• With LA thrombus	2.5 (2.0–3.0)	3 months	Followed by aspirin 81 mg QD
• With prior history systemic embolism	2.5 (2.0–3.0)	3–12 months	Followed by aspirin 81 mg QD
• With atrial fibrillation	2.5 (2.0–3.0)	Chronic	
Following systemic embolism	2.5 (2.0–3.0)	Chronic	With aspirin 81 mg QD

Continued

accompanied by warmth and local tenderness or pain.[19] A tender, cordlike entity caused by venous obstruction can sometimes be palpated in the affected area. L.N. presented with the sudden onset of swelling along with soreness, but without evidence of a cord. Discoloration of the affected limb, including pallor from arterial spasm, cyanosis from venous obstruction, or a reddish color from perivascular inflammation, may also occur. The presence or absence of a positive Homans' sign (pain behind the knee or calf on dorsiflexion of the foot) is rarely helpful in making the diagnosis because it is present in only about 30% of patients with DVT. Many patients (>50%) can present with asymptomatic disease, but even asymptomatic

Table 15-6 Optimal therapeutic range and duration of anticoagulation (continued)

Valve Replacement—Mechanical			
Aortic			
• Bileaflet St Jude	2.5 (2.0–3.0)	Chronic	
• Bileaflet Carbomedics/tilting disk Medtronic Hall			
~ In NSR, with nl EF, and nl LA size	2.5 (2.0–3.0)	Chronic	
~ all others	3.0 (2.5–3.5)	Chronic	
• Tilting disk (all other brands)	3.0 (2.5–3.5)	Chronic	
• Ball and cage/caged disk	3.0 (2.5–3.5)	Chronic	With aspirin 81 mg qd
Mitral			
• Bileaflet or tilting disk	3.0 (2.5–3.5)	Chronic	
• Ball and cage/caged disk	3.0 (2.5–3.5)	Chronic	With aspirin 81 mg qd
With additional risk factors or following TE event	3.0 (2.5–3.5)	Chronic	Add aspirin 81 mg qd

INR, international normalized ratio; QD, once daily; hx, history; TIA, transient ischemic attack; TE, thromboembolism; HTN, hypertension; LV, left ventricular; fxn, function; DZ, disease; NSR, normal sinus rhythm; CHF, congestive heart failure; dysfxn, dysfunction; tx, therapy; DVT, deep vein thrombosis; PE, pulmonary embolism; VTE, venous thromboembolism; LMWH, low molecular weight heparin; ASA, aspirin; LA, left artium; s/p, status post; nl, normal.

patients can have long-term complications such as recurrent DVT or postthrombotic syndrome. Because symptoms of DVT are nonspecific, the diagnosis must be confirmed by objective testing.[20]

Risk Factors

2. What risk factors does L.N. exhibit that are associated with DVT?

The diagnosis of DVT depends not only on the presenting signs and symptoms, but also on the presence of risk factors. A summary of risk factors for thromboembolism is presented in Figure 15–1. L.N. has presented with obesity and immobilization (i.e., prolonged bed rest), two important risk factors for thromboembolism. It is common for more than one risk factor to be present in patients who develop DVT, and these factors are cumulative in their effect.[21]

Diagnosis

3. How should the final diagnosis of DVT be made in L.N.?

After evaluation of the signs and symptoms of DVT and consideration of risk factors for the development of thrombus, a definitive diagnosis should be made. Diagnostic strategies should include an assessment of pretest clinical probability (clinical suspicion), D-dimer assay (an evaluation of the presence of fibrin degradation products, indicative of clot formation), and noninvasive imaging tests.[22]

Despite its limitations as a single diagnostic tool, clinical assessment can improve the diagnostic accuracy of noninvasive testing. A clinical prediction rule, such as the Wells criteria, takes into account signs, symptoms, and risk factors to categorize patients as being at low, intermediate, or high probability of having a DVT (Table 15-7).[23,24] The D-dimer test can be used in conjunction with clinical evaluation or a clinical prediction rule to help "rule out" DVT in patients with a low clinical suspicion, and thus decrease the need for imaging tests in these patients.[25] A D-dimer should not be tested if the clinical suspicion is high because diagnostic imaging is indicated in these patients.

The most common noninvasive test is duplex scanning, which combines B-mode imaging or color flow imaging with Doppler ultrasonography to visualize veins and thrombi while investigating flow patterns.[19] Other noninvasive testing options include ^{125}I-fibrinogen leg scanning (injection of radiolabeled fibrinogen followed by scanning to detect areas of accumulation corresponding to thrombosis), impedance plethysmography (use of pneumatic cuffs to detect leg blood volume changes associated with thrombosis), and Doppler ultrasonography alone (use of a transducer to audibly detect venous flow changes indicative of thrombosis). Each option differs with respect to sensitivity, specificity, and cost. Venography (radiographic visualization of the involved vessels with injection of radiocontrast material), an invasive diagnostic test, is the most sensitive and specific method for diagnosis of DVT, but exposes patients to the risks associated with contrast material.[23]

Treatment

Baseline Information

4. What additional baseline data should be obtained before administering anticoagulants to L.N.?

Table 15-7 Clinical Model for Evaluating the Pretest Probability of Deep Vein Thrombosis[a]

Clinical Characteristic	*Score*
Active cancer (cancer treatment within previous 6 months, or currently on palliative treatment)	1
Paralysis, paresis, or recent plaster immobilization of the lower extremities	1
Recently bedridden for ≥3 days, or major surgery within the previous 12 weeks requiring general or regional anesthesia	1
Localized tenderness along the distribution of the deep venous system	1
Entire leg swollen	1
Calf swelling at least 3 cm larger than that on the asymptomatic side (measured 10 cm below tibial tuberosity)	1
Pitting edema confined to the symptomatic leg	1
Collateral superficial veins (nonvaricose)	1
Previously documented deep vein thrombosis	1
Alternative diagnosis at least as likely as deep vein thrombosis	−2

[a]Clinical probability of DVT: low <0; moderate 1–2; high >3. In patients with symptoms in both legs, the more symptomatic leg is used.
Adapted from references 22 and 24.

In addition to assessing the integrity of the clotting process with platelet count, Hct, PT, and aPTT, the patient's baseline renal function should also be evaluated and documented because some anticoagulants are renally eliminated. Generally, it is unnecessary to type and cross-match blood, but if this information is available, it should be recorded. Baseline values are used for comparison with the parameters that will be used in monitoring both therapeutic and adverse effects of anticoagulant therapy.

Initiation of Therapy

5. Duplex scanning reveals clot formation in L.N.'s right calf extending to the right thigh. He does not exhibit signs of PE. What is the appropriate therapy for L.N., and how should it be initiated?

Prompt and optimal anticoagulant therapy is indicated to minimize thrombus extension and its vascular complications, as well as to prevent PE. Treatment options include IV UFH therapy initiated with a loading dose followed by a continuous infusion, adjusted-dose SC UFH, or LMWH or fondaparinux administered by SC injection.[26] Because L.N. currently is hospitalized, IV UFH is selected for initial treatment of his DVT.

Heparin

LOADING DOSE

6. L.N.'s medical resident ordered a heparin bolus dose of 5,000 units (U) IV, to be followed by a continuous infusion of 1,000 U/hour. Is this heparin dosing regimen appropriate?

A loading dose of heparin is required for several reasons. Based on pharmacokinetic principles, a therapeutic serum level will be achieved more quickly; thus, pharmacodynamic and therapeutic responses to help prevent progression of clot will occur rapidly. Second, a relative resistance to anticoagulation exists during the active clotting process. Therefore, a larger initial dose generally is necessary to achieve a therapeutic effect.

Although many clinicians historically used standardized doses of heparin for initiation of therapy (e.g., 5,000-U loading dose; 1,000-U/hour maintenance dose), this approach can result in significant delays in reaching a therapeutic intensity of anticoagulation. Body weight represents the most reliable predictor of heparin dosing requirement. For nonobese patients, the use of the actual body weight is recommended to calculate the initial UFH dose. In obese patients, the use of the actual body weight is controversial, and the use of an adjusted-dosing weight is recommended by some experts.[27] Compared with standardized dosing, weight-based dosing (80-U/kg loading dose; 18-U/kg/hour initial infusion rate) increases the frequency of therapeutic aPTT at 6 hours and at 24 hours, and decreases the risk of recurrent venous thromboembolism (VTE).[28–30]

Initial heparin loading doses of 70 to 100 U/kg followed by an infusion rate of 15 to 25 U/kg/hour are commonly recommended. Selection of the lower or upper dosage range is guided by the severity of the patient's symptoms and his or her potential sensitivity to adverse effects. For this 92-kg patient, a midrange loading dose of 7,400 U (92 kg × 80 U/kg), followed by a continuous infusion of 1,700 U/hour (92 kg × 18 U/kg per hour), is recommended. Loading doses are typically rounded to the nearest 500 U and maintenance infusion rates to the nearest 100 U for convenience of administration.

DOSE ADJUSTMENTS

7. The orders for L.N. were rewritten by his attending physician. Based on the data that follow, explain the variability in laboratory results. (At this institution, aPTT values of 60–100 seconds correspond with heparin plasma concentrations of 0.3–0.7 U/mL determined by antifactor X_a assay.)

Time	*APTT (seconds)*	*Heparin Dosage Order*
0800	31 (baseline)	7,400-U bolus followed by 1,700-U/hour infusion
0900	130	Hold infusion for 30 minutes, then to 1,500 U/hour
1500	40	Rebolus with 2,400 U, then to 1,700 U/hour
2100	85	Continue at 1,700 U/hour; recheck aPTT Q AM

Although the aPTT drawn 1 hour after the initiation of the maintenance infusion (9 AM) demonstrates excessive prolongation of the aPTT (130 seconds), this value is most likely explained by inappropriate timing of the test. When aPTT values are drawn too soon after a heparin bolus dose (i.e., before the maintenance infusion has achieved a steady-state concentration in serum), they are predictably very high, but are not associated with a bleeding risk and do not accurately reflect the anticipated level of anticoagulation in the patient. To ensure accuracy, the clinician should obtain aPTT values no sooner than 6 hours after a bolus dose or any change in the infusion rate. Even results obtained at 6 hours may be excessively prolonged in some patients because of the dose-dependent pharmacokinetic characteristics of heparin.

L.N.'s heparin dose was decreased at 0900 based on this prolonged, yet inappropriately timed, value. A repeat aPTT at 3 PM was only 40 seconds. The decrease in the dosage to 1,500 U/hour and the repeat aPTT of 40 seconds reflect near steady-state conditions because 6 hours have elapsed since the dosage change. Because the aPTT was subtherapeutic at 3 PM (40 seconds), administration of a smaller repeat bolus dose (2,400 U) and an increase in the maintenance infusion to 1,700 U/hour was the correct course of action. Subsequent aPTT values reflected therapeutic anticoagulation.

Dosing nomograms or protocols have been recommended for adjustment of heparin dosing based on aPTT results.[6,31] Nomogram-based dosing reduces the time to reach therapeutic range compared with empiric dosing.[31] After initiation based on patient weight, dosing adjustments may also be weight based or may simply be made in units per hour. A heparin dosing nomogram specific for a reagent with a therapeutic aPTT range of 60 to 100 seconds (and used in the adjustment of heparin doses for L.N.) is illustrated in Table 15-8.

Responses to changes in infusion rates of heparin are not always linear, and to some extent, heparin doses are adjusted by trial and error. As the patient's condition improves after several days and endothelialization of the clot occurs, heparin dosing requirements may decrease.

THERAPEUTIC MONITORING

8. How should L.N.'s heparin therapy be monitored?

Once baseline clotting parameters have been established and a loading dose of heparin has been administered, the aPTT should be measured routinely to guide subsequent dosing adjustments. The aPTT should be evaluated no sooner than

Table 15-8 Heparin Dosing Nomogram[a]

1. Suggested loading dose
   - Treatment of DVT/PE: 80 U/kg(rounded to nearest 500 U)
   - Prevention, including cardiovascular indications:70 U/kg (rounded to nearest 500 U)
2. Suggested initial infusion
   - Treatment of DVT/PE: 18 U/kg/hr (rounded to nearest 100 U)
   - Prevention, including cardiovascular indications: 15 U/kg/hr (rounded to nearest 100 U)
3. First aPTT check: 6 hours after initiating therapy
4. Dosing adjustments: per chart below (rounded to nearest 100 U)

aPTT[b] (seconds)	Heparin Bolus	Infusion Hold Time	Infusion Rate Adjustment	Next aPTT
<40	4,000 U	0	Increase by 200 U/hr	In 6 hr
40–59	2,000 U	0	Increase by 100 U/hr	In 6 hr
60–100	0	0	None	Q am
101–110	0	0	Decrease by 100 U/hr	In 6 hr
111–120	0	0	Decrease by 200 U/hr	In 6 hr
>120	0	30 minutes	Decrease by 200 U/hr	In 6 hr

[a]University of Washington Medical Center.
[b]Based on aPTT reagent-specific therapeutic range of 60–100 sec corresponding to a plasma heparin concentration of 0.3–0.7 U/mL determined by antifactor X_a activity.

6 hours after the loading dose or after any changes in infusion rate, as noted previously. If dosing is stable, the aPTT should be evaluated once daily (Table 15-8).

Additional monitoring parameters for heparin therapy include evaluation for potential adverse reactions and possible therapeutic failure. Hct and platelet count should be checked every 1 to 2 days. L.N. should be examined for signs of bleeding, as well as for signs and symptoms associated with thrombus extension and PE. Finally, if unusual or unexpected aPTT results are reported, the clinician should consider the possible influence of solution preparation errors, infusion pump failure, infusion interruption, and administration or charting errors in the assessment of L.N.'s heparin therapy.[32]

DURATION OF THERAPY

9. How long should heparin therapy be continued in L.N.?

Adherence of a thrombus to the vessel wall and subsequent endothelialization usually takes 7 to 10 days. However, anticoagulation therapy must generally continue for 3 to 6 months to prevent recurrent thrombosis.[26] Warfarin is preferred for this long-term anticoagulation because it can be administered orally, and it is generally initiated on the same day as heparin. The long elimination half-life of warfarin and the long elimination half-lives of clotting factors II and X necessitate a prolonged period of overlap between warfarin and heparin. Heparin is, therefore, continued for ≥5 days and until the INR is >2 and stable. Heparin therapy should not be discontinued before at least 5 days even if the INR is therapeutic before then because of the time required for adequate elimination of factors II and X by warfarin and the time required to reach its full antithrombotic potential. Shortening the duration of heparin therapy is associated with an increased risk of recurrent thrombosis.

ADVERSE EFFECTS

10. On day 2 of heparin therapy, L.N.'s complete blood count reveals a platelet count of 180,000/mm^3, decreased from 255,000/mm^3 at baseline. What is a reasonable explanation for this thrombocytopenia, and how should it be managed?

Thrombocytopenia

Thrombocytopenia induced by heparin has two distinct presentations.[8] Heparin-associated thrombocytopenia (HAT) occurs as a direct effect of heparin on platelet function, causing transient platelet sequestration and clumping with reductions in platelet count, but usually remaining >100,000/mm^3. This reversible form of thrombocytopenia occurs within the first several days of heparin therapy. Patients remain asymptomatic, and platelet counts return to normal even when heparin therapy is continued. L.N.'s reduction in platelet count is somewhat modest and likely represents HAT. His platelet count should be monitored daily, and heparin therapy should be continued.

Reductions in platelet count of >50% from baseline suggest the development of heparin-induced thrombocytopenia (HIT), a more severe immune-mediated reaction with a typical delay in onset of 5 to 14 days after the initiation of heparin therapy. In contrast, "immediate-onset" HIT can occur rapidly (within 24 hours of UFH initiation) in patients previously exposed to heparin. In addition, delayed-onset HIT has also been reported, where the development of thrombocytopenia begins several days after heparin has been stopped in patients naive to UFH.[33]

In the immune-mediated reaction, heparin binds to an IgG antibody to form a heparin–antibody complex that then binds to platelets, leading to significant platelet aggregation. The observed thrombocytopenia is the result of drug-induced platelet aggregation as opposed to platelet destruction or bone marrow suppression. The diagnosis of immune-mediated HIT is made based on clinical findings supplemented by laboratory tests confirming the presence of antibodies to heparin or platelet activation induced by heparin.[8]

The overall incidence of HIT is <3% after 5 days of UFH use, but the cumulative incidence can be as high as 6% after 14 days of continuous heparin use. HIT occurs more frequently with bovine lung heparin than with heparin derived from porcine gut mucosa, and also with prolonged IV UFH use versus SC UFH.[8,33] Despite its low incidence, HIT is a life-threatening condition with high morbidity and mortality. Platelet aggregation secondary to HIT can lead to significant venous and arterial thrombosis, as well as thromboembolic stroke, acute MI, skin necrosis, and thrombosis of other major arteries. Amputation is necessary in up to 25% of patients, and mortality approaches 25% to 30% (see Chapter 87).

In patients who develop HIT, heparin therapy should be stopped immediately, and treatment with an alternative anticoagulant should be initiated.[8,33] Although associated with a lower risk of HIT (<1%) than UFH, LMWH products are contraindicated in patients with HIT because of a high incidence of immunologic cross-reactivity with heparin.[8] The future use of heparin in patients with HIT, especially in the first 3 to 6 months following the diagnosis, should be avoided. Treatment options include the direct thrombin inhibitors argatroban, lepirudin and bivalirudin, although only the first two are U.S. Food and Drug Administration (FDA) approved for this indication. The dose of lepirudin and argatroban should be titrated based on aPTT testing, and both are administered by IV infusion. Although some clinicians prefer argatroban because it has a shorter half-life and lower cost when compared to lepirudin, both agents are considered equally suitable for the initial treatment of HIT. Bivalirudin also appears to be a promising emerging alternative for the treatment of HIT due to its short-half life, low immunogenicity, minimal effect on INR, and enzymatic metabolism. Various patient-related factors—such as the presence of renal or hepatic dysfunction; prior exposure to lepirudin; and drug availability, cost, and institutional preference—should be used to select the most appropriate and agent[8,34] (Table 15-4).

11. On day 3 of heparin therapy, L.N.'s Hct has dropped from a baseline of 36.5% to 29%, and blood is noted in his urine. Describe an approach to evaluate and interpret this event.

Hemorrhage

Bleeding is the most common adverse effect associated with heparin. A summary of eight inception cohort studies reporting heparin-associated bleeding found the absolute frequency of fatal, major, and all (major or minor) bleeding to be 0.4%, 6%, and 16%, respectively.[35] The corresponding average daily frequencies were 0.05% for fatal bleeding, 0.8% for major bleeding, and 2% for major or minor bleeding; cumulative risk increased with the duration of therapy. The most common sites for heparin-associated bleeding are soft tissues, the GI and urinary tracts, the nose, and the oral pharynx.

In addition to length of therapy, many factors influence the risk of bleeding during heparinization, including advanced age, serious comorbid illnesses (heart disease, renal insufficiency, hepatic dysfunction, cerebrovascular disease, malignancy, and severe anemia), and concomitant antithrombotic therapy.[36] The incidence of UFH-associated bleeding complications is minimal with SC prophylactic doses, but higher (2%–4%) with therapeutic doses given via IV infusion. Soft tissue bleeding commonly occurs at sites of recent surgery or trauma. Previously undiagnosed abnormalities, including malignancy and infection may be identified in some patients with GI or urinary tract bleeding associated with heparin therapy.

The influence of the intensity of heparinization on bleeding risk is controversial. Although an elevated aPTT has historically been considered a risk factor for bleeding complications, several investigators have been unable to substantiate a relationship between supratherapeutic aPTT values and hemorrhagic effects.[36] In addition, bleeding episodes can occur when coagulation test results are within the therapeutic range. These conflicting results may be explained in part by the influence of additional risk factors for bleeding and by the effect of heparin on platelet function and vascular permeability.

L.N. has developed hematuria despite an acceptable intensity of anticoagulation. He should be questioned and examined for the presence of nose bleeding (epistaxis), increased tendency to bruise (ecchymosis), bright red blood in the stool (hematochezia), black or tarry stool (melena), or coughing up of blood (hemoptysis). Blood pressure and pulse, both sitting and standing, should be obtained to determine whether orthostasis representing blood loss is present. A thorough evaluation of the urinary tract may reveal a previously unknown abnormality that will explain the bleeding episode.

12. What other side effects of heparin should be considered in L.N.?

Osteoporosis

The development of osteoporosis has been associated with administration of >20,000 U/day of heparin for 6 months or longer.[37] Various mechanisms have been suggested, but the underlying pathophysiology of this rare adverse effect remains unclear. Affected patients may present with bone pain and/or radiographic findings suggestive of fractures. The possibility of osteoporosis should be considered in patients receiving long-term, high-dose heparin therapy such as pregnant patients or elderly patients.

Hyperkalemia

Although rare, hyperkalemia has been attributed to heparin-induced inhibition of aldosterone synthesis. Hypoaldosteronism leading to hyperkalemia has been described with both high-dose and low-dose heparin therapy, may occur as quickly as within 7 days after initiation of heparin therapy, and appears to be reversible after discontinuation of heparin.[6] Patients with diabetes or renal failure may be at greatest risk.

Hypersensitivity Reactions

Other rarely occurring adverse effects associated with heparin include generalized hypersensitivity reactions, such as urticaria, chills, fever, rash, rhinitis, conjunctivitis, asthma, and angioedema, as well as priapism and a reversible temporal alopecia.[6]

ADJUSTED-DOSE SUBCUTANEOUS ADMINISTRATION

13. By day 4 of heparinization, IV access for L.N. has become difficult. What alternatives can be considered?

The most common strategy for treatment of venous thrombosis in hospitalized patients without IV access is the use of SC LMWH (see question 15). Another alternative is SC administration of unfractionated heparin with adjustment of dosing to maintain a therapeutic aPTT.[26,38] Typically, SC heparin is administered at 12-hour intervals, and aPTT is monitored at the mid-dosing interval (i.e., 6 hours after a dose). Due to lower bioavailability if the SC route of administration is used, the initial SC UFH dose should be approximately 10% to 20% higher than the corresponding IV dose required to maintain therapeutic effect.

Table 15-9 Heparin Protocol for Adjusted-Dose Subcutaneous Administration[a]

Initial Dosage

1. Initial therapy with adjusted-dose SC heparin
   a. Give SC heparin 240 U/kg STAT.
   b. Check first aPTT 6 hours after first dose.
   c. Adjust dosing per chart below.
2. Conversion from continuous infusion heparin to adjusted-dose SC heparin
   a. Calculate total 24-hour heparin requirement necessary to maintain therapeutic aPTT.
   b. Divide 24-hour heparin requirement by 2 and increase this dose by an additional 10%–20% to determine initial Q 12 hours SC dosing requirement.
   c. Discontinue IV heparin and administer initial Q 12 hr SC dose within 1 hr.
   d. Check first aPTT 6 hr after first dose.
   e. Adjust dosing per chart below.
3. Conversion from warfarin to adjusted-dose SC heparin
   a. Discontinue warfarin.
   b. Give 240 U/kg SC heparin within 24 hr.
   c. Check first aPTT 6 hr after first dose.
   d. Adjust dosing per chart below.

Dosing Adjustments

aPTT[b] *(seconds)*	*Dosing Adjustment*[c]	*Next aPTT*
<40	Increase by 48 U/kg Q 12 hr	6 hr after dose
40–59	Increase by 24 U/kg Q 12 hr	6 hr after dose
60–100	No change	Q am
101–120	Decrease by 12 U/kg Q 12 hr	6 hr after dose
121–140	Decrease by 24 U/kg Q 12 hr	6 hr after dose
>140	Decrease by 36 U/kg Q 12 hr	6 hr after dose

[a]University of Washington Medical Center.
[b]Based on aPTT reagent-specific therapeutic range of 60–100 sec corresponding to a heparin concentration of 0.3–0.7 U/mL determined by antifactor X_a activity.
[c]Rounded to nearest 500 U.
SC, subcutaneous; aPTT, activated partial thromboplastin time; Q, every; IV, intravenous.

For L.N., whose current heparin dosage is 1,700 U/hour, the initial SC heparin dose would be 22,500 U (1,700 U/hour × 12 hours plus a 10% increase and rounded to the nearest 500 U). L.N.'s aPTT should be checked 6 hours after the first dose, with adjustment of dosing as necessary. A weight-based dosing nomogram, specific for a reagent with a therapeutic aPTT range of 60 to 100 seconds, is described in Table 15-9.

More recent data support the efficacy of weight based SC UFH (initial dose of 333 U/kg followed by 250 U/kg every 12 hours) *without routine aPTT monitoring* for the treatment of acute VTE. Although not yet ready for wide implementation because data are only based on one trial, the use of weight-based, unmonitored SC UFH has the potential to simplify the way acute VTE is treated.[39]

REVERSAL OF EFFECT

14. P.B. is a 64-year-old woman with DVT. On day 4 of heparin therapy, she received 25,000 U of heparin during a 1-hour period as a result of an infusion pump malfunction. The infusion was stopped and within 30 minutes, she became diaphoretic and hypotensive. Bright red blood was evident on rectal examination, and a large retroperitoneal mass was noted. How should the excessive heparin effect be reversed?

P.B. has definite signs of hemorrhage from the GI tract, a site of bleeding associated with considerable mortality. Heparin should be discontinued immediately, and treatment should include maintenance of fluid volume and replacement of clotting factors with whole blood, fresh frozen plasma, or clotting factor concentrates. If hemorrhage had not been present and the only manifestation of overdose had been a prolonged aPTT, administration of heparin simply could have been discontinued, permitting the effects to clear within a few hours.

Protamine can be used to neutralize heparin by forming an inactive protamine–heparin complex.[40] Protamine has a rapid onset of action, with effects lasting about 2 hours. Protamine sulfate is infused slowly over 3 to 5 minutes, as a 1% solution at a dose of 1 mg for each 100 U of heparin administered, but only if it is given within 30 minutes of discontinuation of heparin administration. The maximum single recommended dose of protamine is 50 mg, but doses may be repeated if bleeding persists. If protamine therapy is delayed, dosing should be based on the estimated amount of heparin remaining, taking into consideration the elimination half-life of heparin. Response to protamine therapy can be assessed by a return of the aPTT to baseline. Adverse effects associated with protamine include systemic hypotension secondary to rapid administration; anaphylaxis characterized by edema, bronchospasm, and cardiovascular collapse; and catastrophic pulmonary vasoconstriction[41] (see Chapter 4).

LOW-MOLECULAR-WEIGHT HEPARIN

15. H.K. is a 32-year-old woman who presents to the emergency department (ED) complaining of right calf pain of 1 day's duration. She denies trauma to the calf but reveals that she has just

Table 15-10 Dosing of Low-Molecular-Weight Heparin and Fondaparinux for the Treatment of Venous Thromboembolism

Dalteparin	*Enoxaparin*	*Tinzaparin*	*Fondaparinux*
100 U/kg SC Q 12 hr OR 200 U/kg SC Q 24 hr	1 mg/kg SC Q 12 hr OR 1.5 mg/kg SC Q 24 hr	175 U/kg SC Q 24 hr	5 mg SC Q 24 hr if weight <50 kg 7.5 mg SC Q 24 hr if weight 50–100 kg 10 mg SC Q 24 hr if weight >100 kg

returned to the United States from Australia on a lengthy flight. She has no significant medical history, has no family history of clotting disorders, and takes no medications. A duplex ultrasound is positive for DVT, and immediate anticoagulation is indicated. What therapeutic alternative to hospitalization for UFH is available for this patient?

Historically, UFH was the initial treatment of choice for acute DVT. However, LMWHs have now emerged as more convenient and practical treatment alternatives to UFH.[26] In addition, meta-analysis data suggest that LMWH results in fewer deaths, major hemorrhages, and recurrent VTE when compared to UFH.[42] Weight-based, once- or twice-daily SC dosing of LMWHs provides a consistent anticoagulant effect that does not require aPTT monitoring.[43] Based on these advantages, outpatient use of LMWH has become the most common approach to treatment of uncomplicated DVT. Home treatment is safe and effective and improves the overall physical and social functioning of patients being treated for DVT.[44] The drug costs associated with LMWH treatment are much higher than the costs of UFH, but overall costs to health care systems are significantly reduced when patients can be treated at home rather than in the hospital.[45] The synthetic pentasaccharide, fondaparinux, can be considered as an alternative treatment option to the LMWHs as it has been shown to be as effective and safe as LMWH in the treatment of DVT.[46] Fondaparinux has the benefit that, to date, HIT has not been associated with its use.[47]

For H.K. to be treated at home with LMWH, she or a family member must be willing and able to administer SC injections, and she must be able to return for frequent follow-up visits, particularly during the first week while warfarin therapy is initiated. In addition, her health care insurance should cover the cost of the drug, or she must be able to pay out of pocket. Contraindications to home treatment of DVT include a pre-existing condition that requires hospitalization, clinical symptoms of PE and/or hemodynamic instability, recent or active bleeding, and end-stage renal disease.

H.K. meets the eligibility requirements for home treatment and is interested in self-injection of LMWH at home, with support from her partner, for initial treatment of DVT. Possible treatment options and doses for H.K. are listed in Table 15-10. However, most institutional formularies carry only a single LMWH product, with formulary decisions based on FDA-approved indications and clinical data supporting use for treatment and prevention of thromboembolism in various settings. In this case, enoxaparin is the LMWH available for use. The usual dosing of enoxaparin for treatment of DVT is 1 mg/kg total body weight SC Q 12 hours, rounded to the nearest 10-mg increment. Once-daily dosing, at 1.5 mg/kg SC Q 24 hours is also an option, but this strategy is inferior to twice-daily dosing in patients with malignancy or obesity.[48] In addition, results from a meta-analysis suggest that hemorrhage and recurrent VTE are less likely to occur with twice-daily dosing of LMWH as compared to once-daily dosing, thus raising further controversy around the routine use of once-daily dosing.[43]

Because LMWHs are eliminated renally, patients with significant renal impairment require dose reductions.[49] The degree of drug accumulation can vary between the various LMWH preparations, thus specific guidelines for dose adjustments will be agent specific[50–52] (Table 15-11). Some experts suggest monitoring of antifactor X_a activity to rule out accumulation of LMWHs in patients with renal impairment.[53,54] Fondaparinux is also renally excreted and is contraindicated in patients with creatinine clearance <30 mL/minute. Data with the use of LMWH and fondaparinux for the prevention and treatment of VTE in patients on hemodialysis is lacking; thus, UFH is the recommended treatment option in these patients.

16. What systems must be in place for H.K.'s home treatment to be successful? What is the role of the pharmacist or other caregiver in her therapy?

H.K. should be weighed to determine her dose of enoxaparin. Because she is not obese and does not have a malignancy, a 1.5-mg/kg dose once daily can be considered for convenience

Table 15-11 Dosing of Low-Molecular-Weight Heparins (LMWHs) in Patients With Renal Impairment (CrCL <30 mL/min[a])

LMWH	*Dalteparin*	*Enoxaparin*	*Tinzaparin*
Product information recommendations	Use with caution	Prophylaxis—30 mg SC daily Treatment—1 mg/kg SC daily	Use with caution
Dosing suggestions based on agent-specific pharmacokinetic observations	CrCL <30[a] mL/min: no dose adjustment needed up to 1 week For use longer than 1 week, consider monitoring of anti-X_a activity and adjust dose if accumulation is noted CrCL 30–50 mL/min: no dose adjustment needed	CrCL <30[a] mL/min: Consider a 40%–50% dose decrease and subsequent monitoring of anti-X_a activity CrCL 30–50 mL/min: Consider a 15%–20% dose decrease with prolonged use (longer than 10–14 days) and subsequent monitoring of anti-X_a activity	CrCL <30[a] mL/min: consider a dose decrease of 20% and subsequent monitoring of anti-X_a activity CrCL 30–50 mL/min: no dose adjustment needed

[a]In patients with a CrCL <20 mL/min, data are very limited and use of unfractionated heparin is suggested.

of administration. Dosing is typically rounded to the nearest 10 mg based on the availability of prefilled syringes. At 64 kg, H.K. will receive 100 mg SC Q 24 hours. Warfarin therapy is initiated concurrently to expedite the conversion to oral treatment.

H.K. must be taught to self-administer enoxaparin by SC injection. Patient education resources, including videotaped instructions and written materials, should supplement hands-on instruction. H.K. will administer the first dose of enoxaparin in the ED with the assistance of a pharmacist. She should also be given prescriptions for enoxaparin and warfarin that must be filled immediately at the pharmacy of her choice.

H.K. should be instructed regarding the potential adverse effects of LMWH therapy (bleeding, thrombocytopenia, pain and bruising at the injection site), required laboratory monitoring, and the expected duration of anticoagulation. At baseline, Hct, INR, renal function, and platelet count should be determined. Platelets will continue to be monitored at least every 2 to 3 days while the patient is receiving LMWH therapy. Platelet counts will be monitored up to 10 to 14 days or for as long as the patient is receiving LMWH therapy, whichever is sooner. H.K. can expect to continue enoxaparin therapy for a minimum of 5 days. If by day 5 her INR is therapeutic and stable, enoxaparin can be discontinued. Oral anticoagulation with warfarin will continue for 3 to 6 months.[26]

To ensure the safety and efficacy of home treatment, H.K. should be provided with the names and telephone numbers of the health care providers who will assume responsibility for her care, including her primary physician and her anticoagulation management team. No patient should be sent home with LMWH without an adequate follow-up plan.

Prevention

17. D.F., a 63-year-old obese woman, is to undergo elective abdominal surgery for treatment of diverticulitis. She has a medical history significant for mild hypertension, currently controlled by enalapril 10 mg QD (blood pressure, 135/85 mmHg), and peripheral vascular disease. What therapeutic interventions might decrease the risk of DVT or PE in D.F.?

Surgical procedures represent a significant risk factor for DVT formation. All hospitalized patients, including both surgical and nonsurgical patients, should be stratified for risk of DVT based on the presence of various factors.[21,55,56] Risk stratification is used to select the most appropriate therapeutic interventions to prevent DVT, and thereby reduce the risk of fatal PE. These interventions include both mechanical and pharmacologic strategies.

Nonpharmacologic Measures

Mechanical interventions aimed at preventing venous stasis and increasing venous return include the use of elastic compression stockings, as well as leg elevation, leg exercises, and early postoperative ambulation. Intermittent pneumatic compression (IPC) of the leg muscles, using inflatable cuffs applied to the calf and thigh, represents another alternative for the prevention of DVT.[21]

Pharmacologic Measures

Fixed, low-dose unfractionated heparin (LDUFH), administered as 5,000 U SC Q 8 to 12 hr depending on the indication, is an inexpensive and effective pharmacologic approach to DVT prevention in the setting of venous stasis, in medical patients, or after certain surgical procedures. Because low-dose heparin inactivates factor X_a without a direct effect on factor II_a, the aPTT is not prolonged, and therefore, aPTT monitoring is unnecessary. Bleeding complications are minimized using this dosing regimen.

Fixed-dose SC LMWH and fondaparinux are alternative approaches for preventing DVT. Enoxaparin 30 mg SC Q 12 hr or 40 mg SC once daily, dalteparin 2,500 to 5,000 IU SC once daily, and fondaparinux 2.5 mg SC once daily are effective strategies, although enoxaparin has been studied for a larger number of indications. Current recommendations for prevention of VTE based on risk stratification are presented in Table 15-12.[21]

D.F. is at high risk for DVT and PE, not only because of general surgery, but also because of her age (older than 40 years) and the presence of other risk factors for VTE (obesity, peripheral vascular disease, and probable postoperative immobilization). Options for DVT prevention include SC heparin at 5,000 U Q 8 hr or a LMWH (enoxaparin 40 mg SC QD, or dalteparin 2,500 IU initial dose followed by 5,000 IU SC QD). The first dose should be administered several hours preoperatively, and dosing should continue postoperatively until she is fully ambulatory. If bleeding risk is of concern, IPC could be used as an alternative.

PULMONARY EMBOLISM

Clinical Presentation

18. D.J. is a 38-year-old, 90-kg man. Several days ago, he developed a swollen left calf, which was painful and warm. This swelling gradually increased, affecting the entire left leg to the groin and prompting him to seek medical attention. In the ED, he also notes the recent onset of right-sided pleuritic chest pain without SOB or hemoptysis. His medical history includes a gastric ulcer 4 years ago, treated medically without recurrence. Physical examination reveals a pleasant, obese man with an enlarged left leg and mild to moderate tenderness in the entire leg. Chest examination reveals a loud, pulmonary heart sound (P_2). Vital signs include blood pressure, 150/85 mmHg; heart rate, 100 beats/minute; and respiratory rate, 28 breaths/minute and regular. Laboratory data include Hct, 26.7% (normal, 45%–52%); SCr 1.1 mg/dL (normal, 0.8–1.2); and arterial blood gases (on room air) Po_2, 72 mmHg (normal, 75–100); Pco_2, 30 mmHg (normal, 35–45); and pH 7.48 (normal, 7.35–7.45). The chest radiograph and lung scan (ventilation-perfusion [V/Q] scan) are highly suggestive of PE. An angiogram was not performed. The electrocardiogram (ECG) shows sinus tachycardia. The venogram is positive for defects in the ileofemoral vein. Coagulation test results include PT, 11.2 seconds (INR, 1.0); aPTT, 28 seconds; and platelet count, 248,000/mm^3 (normal, 150,000–350,000). What subjective and objective evidence in D.J. is compatible with PE?

[SI units: Hct, 0.267 (normal, 0.45–0.52); platelets, 248 × 10^9/L (normal, 150–300)]

Signs and Symptoms

The clinical diagnosis of PE is often difficult to make because of the nonspecificity of symptoms.[57] The most commonly observed subjective symptoms are dyspnea, pleuritic

Table 15-12 Prevention of Venous Thromboembolism (VTE)[21]

General surgery	
Low risk	Early ambulation
Moderate risk	LDUH Q 12 hr, LMWH QD, IPC, or GCS
High risk	LDUH Q 8 hr, LMWH QD, or IPC
Highest risk	LMWH QD, Fondaparinux QD, Warfarin (INR 2–3), or IPC/GCS + LDUH/LMWH
Gynecologic surgery	
Brief procedures (<30 min)	Early ambulation
Laparoscopic surgery with additional VTE risk factors	LDUH Q 12–Q 8 hr, or LMWH QD, or IPC/GCS
Major surgery for benign disease and no other risk factors	LDUH Q 12 hr, LMWH QD, or IPC
Major surgery for malignancy, or additional VTE risk factors	LDUH Q 8 hr; or LMWH QD; or IPC; or LDUH/LMWH + IPC/GCS.
Urologic surgery	
Low-risk procedures	Early ambulation
Major open procedures	LDUH Q 12–Q 8 hr, LMWH QD, IPC/GCS
Highest-risk patients	LDUH Q 12–Q 8 hr or LMWH QD + IPC/GCS
Orthopedic surgery	
Hip replacement	Fondaparinux, or LMWH QD or BID, or warfarin (INR 2–3)
Knee replacement	Fondaparinux, or LWMH BID, or warfarin (INR 2–3)
Hip fracture surgery	Fondaparinux, or LMWH BID, or warfarin (INR 2–3); IPC/GCS if anticoagulation therapy is contraindicated.
Trauma	LMWH BID; IPC/GCS if anticoagulation is delayed or contraindicated.
Acute spinal cord injury	LMWH BID, or LMWH/LDUH + IPC/GCS
Neurosurgery	IPC/GCS ± LDUH Q 12 hr, or LMWH QD
Acutely medically ill	LDUH Q 8–12 hr or LMWH QD

LDUH, low-dose unfractionated heparin (5,000 U SC Q 8–12 hr); LMWH, low-molecular-weight heparin (enoxaparin 40 mg SC QD or 30 mg SC Q 12 hr; dalteparin 2,500–5,000 IU SC QD); Fondaparinux (2.5 mg SC QD); GCS, graduated compression stockings; IPC, intermittent pneumatic compression.
Low risk: minor surgery, age younger than 40 years, and no additional risk factors for VTE. Moderate risk: minor surgery and additional risk factors for VTE; surgery, age 40–60 years, and no other risk factors for VTE. High risk: surgery with age older than 60 years, or age 40–60 years with additional risk factors for VTE. Highest risk: surgery in patients with multiple risk factors for VTE (age older than 40 years, cancer, prior VTE); orthopedic surgery, trauma.

chest pain, apprehension (anxiety or a feeling of impending doom), and cough. Hemoptysis occurs occasionally. The objective signs most commonly observed are tachypnea at a rate of ≥20 breaths/minute, tachycardia of ≥100 beats/minute, accentuated pulmonary component of the second heart sound (P_2), and rales. DVT precedes PE in 80% or more of patients. A combination of these signs and symptoms provides further evidence for acute PE. D.J. has presented with pleuritic chest pain, tachycardia, tachypnea, loud P_2, and a decrease in Po_2; therefore, he may have developed PE.

Diagnosis

Because the clinical signs and symptoms of PE are difficult to distinguish from many other medical conditions, further evaluation is necessary.[57,58] Chest radiograph, ECG, and arterial blood gas (alveolar-arterial oxygen gradient [A-a gradient]) abnormalities are often present in patients with PE, but like clinical signs and symptoms, they are somewhat nonspecific. Although pulmonary angiography has been considered the gold standard for diagnosis of PE, it is an invasive procedure that is expensive and technically difficult to perform. In addition, the contrast material used can be toxic or irritating, and some patients are unable to tolerate the procedure. Noninvasive tests such as V/Q lung scans and computed tomography (CT) scans are useful and the most frequently used diagnostic procedures to document the presence of PE. Lung scans that incorporate an assessment of perfusion, or regional distribution of pulmonary blood flow, and ventilation are referred to as V/Q scans; they involve both the injection and the inhalation of radiolabeled compounds. Test results are expressed as a high, intermediate, or low probability of PE. When ventilation (air movement) is normal over an area that shows abnormal perfusion (blood flow), a V/Q mismatch exists, and PE is highly probable. If a matched defect is noted (abnormal ventilation over an area of abnormal perfusion), another disease state, such as chronic obstructive airway disease, is more likely.

As in the case of DVT, clinical assessment can improve the diagnostic accuracy of noninvasive tests such as CT or VQ scanning.[23,58] Validated assessment tools can be used to stratify patients into high, moderate, and low probability of a PE[59] (Table 15-13). In patients with a low clinical probability of PE, measuring a high-sensitivity D-dimer can be considered, and if negative, PE can be ruled out eliminating the need of further imaging studies.[23,60] In patients with a moderate to high clinical probability of PE, diagnostic imaging studies should be performed.[23]

A positive lung scan (D.J. had one highly suggestive of PE) or a positive pulmonary angiogram would confirm the presence of a PE. If the results of the clinical assessment and the noninvasive scan are discordant, angiography should be performed to aid in making the definitive diagnosis. Nonetheless, when the diagnosis of PE is suspected, anticoagulation should be initiated immediately while awaiting results of more definitive

Table 15-13 Clinical Model for Evaluating the Pretest Probability of Pulmonary Embolism (PE)[a]

Clinical Characteristic	*Score*
Cancer	+1
Hemoptysis	+1
Previous PE or deep vein thrombosis (DVT)	+1.5
Heart rate >100 beats/min	+1.5
Recent surgery or immobilization	+1.5
Clinical signs of DVT	+3
Alternative diagnosis less likely than PE	+3

[a] Clinical probability of PE: low, 0–1; moderate, 2–6; high, ≥7.
From reference 58.

diagnostic procedures. Mortality associated with PE has been documented to be as high as 17.5% over 3 months.[61]

Treatment

19. What anticoagulant strategy should be initiated for D.J.?

Treatment options for PE include IV UFH therapy initiated with a loading dose followed by a continuous infusion, or a LMWH or fondaparinux administered by SC injection.[26,62] UFH therapy could be started in D.J. with a loading dose of 7,200 U (80 U/kg × 90 kg), followed by continuous infusion of 1,600 U/hour (18 U/kg/hour × 90 kg). Monitoring of the aPTT would be used to adjust dosing to maintain treatment within the therapeutic range (Table 15-8).

The alternative to UFH for treatment of PE is the use of a SC LMWH[63,64] or SC fondaparinux[65] (Table 15-10). D.J. could receive fixed-dose enoxaparin 90 mg SC Q 12 hr (1 mg/kg Q 12 hr–90 kg). Generally, PE should not be treated on an outpatient basis.[63] In this case, LMWH or fondaparinux would be used during the complete hospital course, or only for partial outpatient therapy in selected lower-risk and stable patients who may be discharged early.

The use of thrombolytic therapy should be reserved for patients with acute massive embolism, who are hemodynamically unstable (SBP <90 mmHg) and at low risk for bleeding.[26]

Warfarin

TRANSITION FROM HEPARIN/LMWH THERAPY

20. When should warfarin be administered, and how should the transition be accomplished?

Either heparin or LMWH/fondaparinux therapy should be continued for at least 5 days in the setting of PE, and until warfarin therapy is therapeutic and stable. Warfarin should be started on the first day of hospitalization and continued for a minimum of 3 to 6 months or longer, if indicated. However, a delay in the initiation of warfarin may be acceptable in the setting of an anticipated extended hospitalization, recent or anticipated surgery or other invasive procedures, or a medical condition with the potential for uncontrolled bleeding.[26,63]

There are several reasons to overlap heparin and warfarin therapy. The onset of warfarin activity depends not only on its inherent pharmacokinetic characteristics (half-life >36 hours), but also on the rate of elimination of circulating clotting factors. Although warfarin inhibits production of the vitamin K–dependent clotting factors, previously synthesized clotting factors must be eliminated at rates that correspond with their elimination half-lives (Table 15-5). Approximately four half-lives are required for these factors to reach a new steady state after their production is inhibited, so the effect of warfarin can be delayed for several days. Initial increases in the INR reflect only reductions in factor VII activity, but full anticoagulation with warfarin requires adequate suppression of factors II and X, which have significantly longer elimination half-lives. By overlapping a quick onset anticoagulant such as heparin or LMWH with warfarin therapy, adequate anticoagulation can be continued with heparin/LMWH until warfarin therapy reaches a therapeutic intensity.[10,66]

In addition to suppressing the synthesis of the vitamin K–dependent clotting factors, warfarin also inhibits the formation of the naturally occurring anticoagulant protein C and its cofactor, protein S. In patients with congenital protein C or protein S deficiency, initial warfarin therapy can suppress these proteins to concentrations that may result in hypercoagulability with possible thrombus extension, unless concurrent heparin therapy provides adequate anticoagulation.[67] To prevent these complications, heparin and warfarin therapy should overlap.

Heparin therapy has been observed to prolong the INR,[68] and warfarin can prolong the aPTT by several seconds.[69] Thus, interference with laboratory tests should be considered in the evaluation of the intensity of anticoagulation during the overlap of heparin and warfarin therapy.

INITIATION OF THERAPY

21. In an effort to discharge D.J. from the hospital as soon as possible, an initial dose of warfarin 10 mg PO Q pm for 3 days has been ordered. Is such a "loading dose" reasonable? What would be a more appropriate approach to initiating therapy?

Initiation of warfarin dosing is complex because dosing requirements vary significantly among individuals. Daily doses as low as 0.5 mg and as high as 20 mg or more may be required in individual patients to reach a therapeutic INR.[70] Two methods for initiation of warfarin therapy have been developed.[71] The average daily dosing method relies on an understanding that although dosing requirements for warfarin vary significantly among patients, an average dosing requirement of 4 to 5 mg/day of warfarin is necessary to maintain an INR of 2.0 to 3.0. When the average daily dosing method is used for initiation of warfarin therapy, patients are typically started at 4 to 5 mg daily, with dosing adjustments as necessary until the therapeutic goal is reached. However, patients who may be more sensitive to the effects of warfarin (Table 15-14) are expected to require lower dosages of warfarin. In these patients, therapy should be initiated at 1 to 3 mg daily, with subsequent dosing adjustments as necessary. Several dosing algorithms, using a 4- to 5-mg initiation dose, have been developed to aid with dosing decisions after the first few doses of warfarin have been administered.[72–74] Another popular dosing algorithm used a 10-mg initiation dose for the first 2 days, with the INR on day 3 used to guide dosing on days 3 and 4, and the INR on day 5 used to guide the next three doses[75] (Fig. 15-5). Although

Table 15-14 Factors That Increase Sensitivity to Warfarin

Age older than 75 years
Clinical congestive heart failure
Clinical hyperthyroidism
Decreased oral intake
Diarrhea
Drug–drug interactions
Elevated baseline INR
End-stage renal disease
Fever
Hepatic disease
Hypoalbuminemia
Known CYP2C9 variant
Malignancy
Malnutrition
Postoperative status

INR, international normalized ratio.

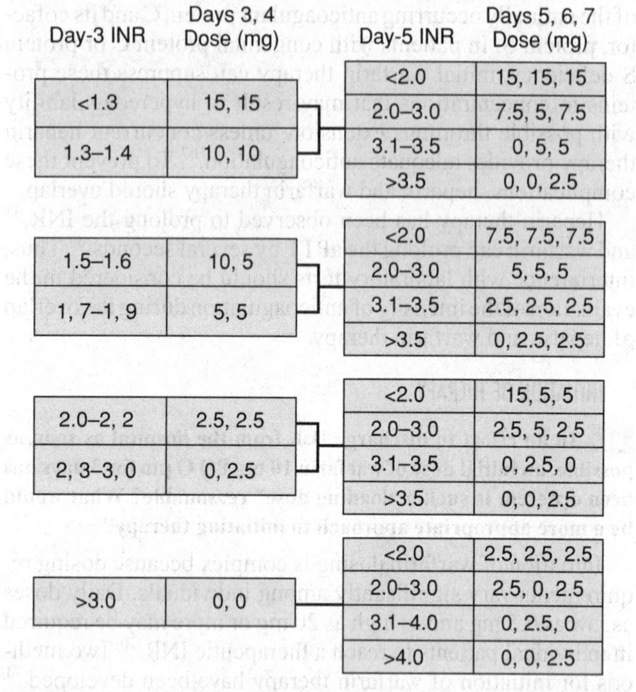
Day-3 INR
Days 3, 4 Dose (mg)
Day-5 INR
Days 5, 6, 7 Dose (mg)
<1.3 | 15, 15
1.3–1.4 | 10, 10
<2.0 | 15, 15, 15
2.0–3.0 | 7.5, 5, 7.5
3.1–3.5 | 0, 5, 5
>3.5 | 0, 0, 2.5
1.5–1.6 | 10, 5
1, 7–1, 9 | 5, 5
<2.0 | 7.5, 7.5, 7.5
2.0–3.0 | 5, 5, 5
3.1–3.5 | 2.5, 2.5, 2.5
>3.5 | 0, 2.5, 2.5
2.0–2, 2 | 2.5, 2.5
2, 3–3, 0 | 0, 2.5
<2.0 | 15, 5, 5
2.0–3.0 | 2.5, 5, 2.5
3.1–3.5 | 0, 2.5, 0
>3.5 | 0, 0, 2.5
>3.0 | 0, 0
<2.0 | 2.5, 2.5, 2.5
2.0–3.0 | 2.5, 0, 2.5
3.1–4.0 | 0, 2.5, 0
>4.0 | 0, 0, 2.5

FIGURE 15-5 Warfarin initiation dosing algorithm based on starting with 10-mg doses on days 1 and 2. Reprinted from reference 75, with permission.

using this dosing algorithm helps achieve a therapeutic INR more quickly than using a 5-mg initial dose, these findings may not the generalizable to all patient populations because the patients evaluated were relatively healthy, young outpatients.[76] The 10-mg initiation dose may lead to overanticoagulation and heightened bleeding risk in elderly and ill patients with multiple medical problems.[77] Average daily dosing is often used to initiate therapy in ambulatory patients; in this case, the first INR should be evaluated within 3 to 5 days of initiation of warfarin therapy. In hospitalized patients, it is more common to evaluate the INR daily during initiation of therapy.

Flexible initiation of warfarin is an alternative approach for starting therapy that is based on evaluating the rate of increase in the INR and making daily dosing adjustments based on daily INR evaluation, with a goal of determining the eventual maintenance dosing requirement. A popular flexible initiation nomogram is presented in Table 15-15.[78,79] Using this nomogram, warfarin can be initiated with either a 10-mg or a 5-mg starting dose, with daily dosing adjustments based on the rate of increase in the INR. Flexible initiation does not necessarily shorten the time to reach the goal INR, and initiating therapy with a 10-mg dose as described in some protocols may be associated with an increased risk of early overanticoagulation in certain patients. Nonetheless, these methods offer a more individualized approach to initiation of therapy.

The baseline INR for D.J. was 1.0. Using the flexible initiation protocol presented in Table 15-15, the first dose of warfarin should be 10 mg administered in the evening on the first day of hospitalization. Subsequent INR values obtained daily will guide dosing requirements until a therapeutic INR is reached. The order for warfarin 10 mg orally every evening for three doses should be discontinued and replaced with daily orders for warfarin and INR monitoring.

Table 15-15 Flexible Initiation Dosing Protocol for Warfarin Dosing, Including 10- and 5-mg Starting Dose Options

Day	*INR*	*10-mg Initiation Dose*	*5-mg Initiation Dose*
1		10 mg	5 mg
2	<1.5	7.5–10 mg	5 mg
	1.5–1.9	2.5 mg	2.5 mg
	2.0–2.5	1.0–2.5 mg	1–2.5 mg
	>2.5	0	0
3	<1.5	5–10 mg	5–10 mg
	1.5–1.9	2.5–5 mg	2.5–5 mg
	2.0–2.5	0–2.5 mg	0–2.5 mg
	2.5–3.0	0–2.5 mg	0–2.5 mg
	>3.0	0	0
4	<1.5	10 mg	10 mg
	1.5–1.9	5–7.5 mg	5–7.5 mg
	2.0–3.0	0–5 mg	0–5 mg
	>3.0	0	0
5	<1.5	10 mg	10 mg
	1.5–1.9	7.5–10 mg	7.5–10 mg
	2.0–3.0	0–5 mg	0–5 mg
	>3.0	0	0
6	<1.5	7.5–12.5 mg	7.5–12.5 mg
	1.5–1.9	5–10 mg	5–10 mg
	2.0–30	0–7.5 mg	0–7.5 mg
–	>3.0	0	0

INR, international normalized ratio.
Reprinted from reference 78, with permission.

INTENSITY OF THERAPY

22. What is the goal INR for D.J., and how long should anticoagulation be administered?

In patients with DVT or PE, warfarin doses that prolong the PT to an INR of 2.0 to 3.0 is defined as "low-intensity therapy." This therapeutic range is recommended to maximize the antithrombotic effect of warfarin while minimizing potential bleeding complications associated with excessive anticoagulation.[10]

DURATION OF THERAPY

Once formed, clots adhere to the vessel wall. Thus, the first step in resolution of a thrombus involves covering the clot with a layer of endothelial cells to prevent additional platelet aggregation at the site of vessel injury. This endothelialization process generally takes 7 to 10 days to be completed. Initial anticoagulant treatment is used to prevent clot extension while allowing adequate endothelialization to occur. Continued anticoagulation prevents further clotting.

The appropriate duration of warfarin therapy is based on the likelihood of a recurrent venous thromboembolic event and also the risk of bleeding in each patient. The presence of concurrent risk factors for VTE and the specific circumstances that triggered the initial thrombotic event all have to be taken into account. Patients with unprovoked (idiopathic) DVT or PE, like in the case of D.J., should be treated for at least 6 to 12 months, but considered for indefinite therapy as their likelihood of having a recurrent event can be as high as 30% over 5 years.[26,63] Patients with DVT or PE associated with transient

Table 15-16 Duration of Anticoagulation Therapy in Patients With Venous Thrombosis (Deep Vein Thrombosis and/or Pulmonary Embolism)

Patient Characteristic	Duration of Therapy	Comments
First episode of venous thromboembolism (VTE) secondary to a transient (reversible) risk factor	At least 3 months	Recommendation applies to both proximal and calf vein thrombosis
First episode of VTE and cancer	6 months (indefinite therapy or until cancer is resolved should be considered)	Low-molecular-weight heparin is recommended over warfarin
First episode of idiopathic VTE with or without a documented hypercoagulable abnormality	At least 6–12 months (indefinite therapy may be considered)	Continue warfarin therapy after 12 months if patient is low risk for bleeding
First episode of VTE with documented antiphospholipid antibodies or two or more thrombophilic abnormalities	12 months to indefinite	The risk–benefit of indefinite therapy should be reassessed at periodic intervals
First episode of VTE with documented deficiency of antithrombin, protein C, protein S, factor V Leiden or prothrombin 20210 gene mutation, homocystinemia, elevated factor VIII	6–12 months; indefinite for idiopathic thrombosis	The risk–benefit of indefinite therapy should be reassessed at periodic intervals
Second episode or recurrent VTE	Indefinite	

Adapted from reference 26.

or reversible risk factors are usually treated for 3 to 6 months, as the risk of recurrence is lower (approximately 10% over 5 years). In patients with recurrent DVT/PE and patients with persistent risk factors, including AT deficiency, protein C or protein S deficiency, factor V Leiden, prothrombin gene mutation, antiphospholipid antibody syndrome, or other hypercoagulable states, including malignancy, warfarin treatment should be continued indefinitely[26,63] (Table 15-16).

ADVERSE EFFECTS

23. What possible adverse effects from warfarin therapy should be considered in D.J., and how should they be monitored?

Hemorrhage

Bleeding is the most common adverse effect associated with warfarin. A summary of experimental and observational inception cohort studies determined that the average annual frequency of fatal, major, and all (major or minor) bleeding in patients treated with warfarin was 0.6%, 3%, and 9.6%, respectively.[35] However, wide variation in bleeding frequencies has been reported, probably because of differences in patient characteristics, treatment protocols, and the definition and assessment of bleeding among trials.

Warfarin-associated bleeding most commonly occurs in the nose, oral pharynx, and soft tissues, followed by the GI and urinary tracts. Hemarthrosis (bleeding into joint spaces) and retroperitoneal and intraocular bleeding represent less common hemorrhagic complications of warfarin therapy.[35,36] As with heparin, GI and urinary tract bleeding associated with warfarin is often caused by previously undiagnosed lesions. Menstrual blood flow may be increased and prolonged in patients taking anticoagulants. This problem may be clinically significant if there is an underlying pathological condition (ovarian cysts, uterine fibroids. or polyps) resulting in abnormal vaginal bleeding.

Although it is uncommon, intracranial bleeding resulting in hemorrhagic stroke represents the most common cause of fatal bleeding associated with warfarin therapy. Rates of intracranial hemorrhage associated with anticoagulants have been estimated to range from 0.3% to 2%, and up to 60% are fatal.[80]

Many factors influence the risk of hemorrhagic complications associated with warfarin. The frequency of bleeding is higher in the first 3 months of therapy than during subsequent months.[81] Unlike heparin, the intensity of anticoagulation with warfarin directly influences the risk of bleeding, including intracranial hemorrhage.[82] Other patient-specific variables that influence the risk of warfarin-associated bleeding include a history of GI bleeding, serious comorbid disease (including malignancy), and concomitant therapy with aspirin or nonsteroidal anti-inflammatory drugs (NSAIDs).[35,36]

The influence of age on bleeding risk is controversial. Older patients are known to require lower dosages of warfarin than younger patients to reach a therapeutic intensity of anticoagulation.[83] Inherent vitamin K deficiency or age-related differences in stereoisomeric disposition of warfarin may explain why older patients are more sensitive to the effects of warfarin and, therefore, require lower dosages than younger patients. This increased sensitivity to the effect of warfarin is not the result of differences in pharmacokinetic characteristics of warfarin between older and young patients, including protein binding and metabolism. It is also not related to gender, weight, underlying medical conditions, or the presence of interacting drugs. Nonetheless, increased sensitivity to warfarin does not imply an increased bleeding risk if older patients are managed appropriately.

Some studies have reported that age is an independent risk factor for bleeding, whereas others have suggested that age alone does not increase bleeding risk.[84] However, in two studies in which comprehensive anticoagulation monitoring and follow-up were provided through anticoagulation management services, elderly patients did not experience an increased incidence of major bleeding.[85,86] However, other reports suggest that advanced age is linked to an increased risk of warfarin-related intracranial hemorrhage, even when patients are managed in an anticoagulation clinic setting.[82]

Hemorrhagic risk assessment can be used to predict bleeding risk during anticoagulant therapy. A popular bleeding index scoring system assigns level of risk based on the presence of age older than 65 years, history of GI bleeding, history of stroke, and one or more of four comorbid conditions: recent MI, anemia (Hct <30), renal insufficiency (Scr >1.5), and diabetes.[87]

The cumulative risk of major bleeding at 48 months in low-, intermediate-, and high-risk patients was 3%, 12%, and 53%, respectively. The bleeding index can be useful in making decisions about management of drug interactions, overanticoagulation, bridge therapy for invasive procedures, and other issues that may present during anticoagulant therapy.

Bleeding complications in D.J. can be minimized by careful attention to the signs and symptoms of bleeding by the patient and his caregivers, maintenance of the INR within the therapeutic range, avoidance of therapy with concomitant drugs known to increase the risk of bleeding or to increase the INR, and routine outpatient follow-up for INR monitoring and clinical assessment.

Skin Necrosis

Warfarin-induced skin necrosis is a rare, but serious adverse effect of oral anticoagulation, occurring in approximately 0.01% to 0.1% of patients treated with warfarin.[88,89] Patients present within 3 to 6 days of the initiation of warfarin therapy with painful discoloration of the breast, buttocks, thigh, or penis. The lesions progress to frank necrosis with blackening and eschar. Skin necrosis appears to be the result of extensive microvascular thrombosis within subcutaneous fat and has been associated with hypercoagulable conditions, including protein C or protein S deficiency. In these patients, rapid depletion of protein C before depletion of vitamin K–dependent clotting factors during early warfarin therapy can result in an imbalance between procoagulant and anticoagulant activity, leading to initial hypercoagulability and thrombosis. Adequate heparinization during initiation of warfarin can prevent the development of early hypercoagulability.

Warfarin therapy should be discontinued in patients who develop skin necrosis. However, subsequent warfarin therapy is not necessarily contraindicated if it is required for treatment or prevention of thromboembolic disease.[88] In patients with protein C or protein S deficiency and a history of skin necrosis, warfarin therapy can be restarted at low dosages as long as therapeutic heparinization has been achieved. Therapy is maintained until the INR has been within the therapeutic range for 72 hours. Supplementation of protein C through administration of fresh frozen plasma also may be indicated.

Purple Toe Syndrome

Purple toe syndrome is a rarely reported adverse effect that typically occurs 3 to 8 weeks after the initiation of warfarin therapy and is unrelated to intensity of anticoagulation.[89] Patients initially present with painful discoloration of the toes that blanches with pressure and fades with elevation. The pathophysiology of this syndrome has been related to cholesterol microembolization from atherosclerotic plaques, leading to arterial obstruction. Because cholesterol microembolization has been associated with renal failure and death, warfarin therapy should be discontinued in patients who develop purple toe syndrome.

PATIENT EDUCATION

24. B.H. is a 30-year-old woman newly diagnosed with idiopathic DVT. Before anticoagulation is initiated, appropriate laboratory tests are drawn to evaluate the possibility of a hypercoagulable state. She will be treated as an outpatient with enoxaparin 1.5 mg/kg SC QD and started on warfarin 4 mg PO QD using the average daily dosing method. Her primary care physician would like her to receive follow-up care in the medical center's pharmacist-managed anticoagulation clinic. What information should B.H. receive regarding the benefits of formal anticoagulation management services?

One of the keys to successful oral anticoagulant therapy is appropriate outpatient management. In comparison with routine medical care, management of warfarin therapy by anticoagulation clinics is associated with significant reductions in bleeding and thromboembolic complications, with reductions in the rates of warfarin-related hospital admissions and ED visits, and with outcome-based cost savings for health care organizations.[90,91] Pharmacist-managed anticoagulation clinics offer many benefits for the management of anticoagulation therapy, including improved dosing regulation, continuous patient education, early identification of risk factors for adverse events, and timely intervention to avoid or minimize complications. B.H.'s referral to a pharmacist-managed anticoagulation clinic is likely to improve her overall satisfaction with care and to improve her clinical outcomes.

25. At her initial visit to the anticoagulation clinic, B.H. will receive extensive education about her warfarin therapy. What information should be conveyed to her by her anticoagulation provider to ensure the safety and efficacy of warfarin therapy?

Successful warfarin therapy depends on the active participation of knowledgeable patients.[10] The anticoagulant effect of warfarin is influenced by various factors, and fluctuations in the intensity of the anticoagulant effect of warfarin can increase the risk of both hemorrhagic complications and recurrent thromboembolism.[92] Pharmacists and other providers can improve adherence to the medication schedule, as well as ensure the safety and efficacy of warfarin therapy, by providing appropriate education to patients treated with this agent.

Key elements that form the basis of a thorough patient education program for warfarin therapy are listed in Table 15-17.

Table 15-17 Key Elements of Patient Education Regarding Warfarin

Identification of generic and brand names
Purpose of therapy
Expected duration of therapy
Dosing and administration
Visual recognition of drug and tablet strength
What to do if a dose is missed
Importance of prothrombin time/INR monitoring
Recognition of signs and symptoms of bleeding
Recognition of signs and symptoms of thromboembolism
What to do if bleeding or thromboembolism occurs
Recognition of signs and symptoms of disease states that influence warfarin dosing requirements
Potential for interactions with prescription and over-the-counter medications and natural/herbal products
Dietary considerations and use of alcohol
Avoidance of pregnancy
Significance of informing other health care providers that warfarin has been prescribed
When, where, and with whom follow-up will be provided

INR, international normalized ratio.

This information may be conveyed through written teaching materials, videotaped instruction, individual or group discussion, or a combination of these approaches. Many useful educational tools are available from the manufacturers of warfarin.

B.H. should receive extensive education about warfarin therapy in an individual teaching session or an organized education program. A wallet card, medical bracelet, or alternative method of identifying her as a patient treated with warfarin should be provided. The health care provider who assumes responsibility for her outpatient warfarin therapy will need to provide continuing reinforcement of the essential elements of medication information at each follow-up visit.

FACTORS INFLUENCING DOSING

26. After receiving 6 days of enoxaparin therapy and six doses of warfarin 4 mg/day PO, B.H.'s INR is 2.4. Enoxaparin is discontinued, and B.H. is instructed to continue her current dosage of warfarin. She is scheduled to return to the anticoagulation clinic in 1 week for re-evaluation. At that time, her INR is 1.7. What factors might account for this change in the intensity of anticoagulation?

Patients should always be questioned about their understanding of the prescribed dose and their adherence to the prescribed regimen. Questions might include, "what dose of the medication have you been taking?", or "what time of the day do you take your medication?", or "how many times in the last week did you miss a dose of your medication?" If there is no evidence of misunderstanding of the correct dose or of noncompliance, numerous other factors should be considered that are known to influence warfarin dosing requirements in individual patients during both initiation and maintenance phases of therapy. Changes in dietary vitamin K intake, alcohol use, underlying disease states, genetic factors, and concurrent medications can significantly change the intensity of therapy, resulting in the need for dosing adjustments to maintain the INR within the therapeutic range.

Dietary Vitamin K Intake

The two primary sources of vitamin K in humans are the biosynthesis of vitamin K_2 (menaquinone) by intestinal bacteria and dietary intake of vitamin K_1 (phytonadione). The U.S. recommended daily allowance for vitamin K is 70 to 140 mcg/day, and the typical Western diet provides approximately 300 to 500 mcg/day.[93] Vitamin K is found in high concentrations in certain foods, including green leafy vegetables (asparagus, broccoli, Brussels sprouts, cabbage, cauliflower, chick peas, collard greens, endive, kale, lettuce, parsley, spinach, and turnip greens), soy milk, certain oils, certain nutritional supplements, and multiple vitamin products. Green tea and chewing tobacco are other significant sources of vitamin K.

Variations in vitamin K intake have been linked to INR fluctuations in patients taking warfarin.[94,95] In addition, diets high in vitamin K content have been associated with acquired warfarin resistance, defined as excessive warfarin dosing requirements to reach a therapeutic INR range.[96] Numerous cases have also been reported in which patients previously stabilized with warfarin experienced elevations in INR with or without hemorrhagic complications when dietary sources of vitamin K were eliminated. Conversely, reductions in INR with or without thromboembolic complications have been reported in patients in whom dietary sources of vitamin K have been added.

These data illustrate the potential clinical significance of dietary changes in patients taking warfarin. To minimize these potential effects, B.H. should be counseled to maintain a *consistent* intake of dietary vitamin K.[97] Her final warfarin maintenance dose will be partially influenced by her typical diet. However, restriction of dietary vitamin K intake is unnecessary, except in cases of significant resistance to the anticoagulant effect of warfarin. B.H. should be aware of the types of foods and supplements that contain large quantities of vitamin K, and should be counseled to maintain a consistent diet, to avoid bingeing with foods high in vitamin K content, and to report significant dietary changes to her health care provider. Appropriate assessment and follow-up are essential to prevent hemorrhagic or thromboembolic complications that may arise from changes in INR resulting from dietary alterations.

Alcohol Ingestion

Chronic alcohol ingestion has been associated with induction of the hepatic enzyme systems that metabolize warfarin. Therefore, warfarin dosing requirements are sometimes higher in alcoholic patients. Conversely, acute ingestion of large amounts of alcohol can slow warfarin metabolism through competitive inhibition of metabolizing enzymes, leading to elevations in INR and an increased risk of bleeding complications.[98,99] Despite some reports linking low amounts of alcohol to an elevated INR,[100] in general it is believed that moderate intake of alcoholic beverages is not associated with alterations in the metabolism or the therapeutic effect of warfarin as measured by INR. Patients taking warfarin should be educated to limit their alcohol consumption to less than one to two alcoholic beverages per day. Chronic drinkers should be counseled to limit their drinking and maintain a regular pattern to avoid fluctuations in INR.[97] B.H. does not need to abstain from drinking alcoholic beverages in moderation, but she should be counseled to avoid the sporadic ingestion of large amounts of alcohol.

Underlying Disease States

The presence or exacerbation of various medical conditions can also influence anticoagulation status.[101] Diarrhea-associated alterations in intestinal flora can reduce vitamin K absorption, resulting in elevations in INR. Fever enhances the catabolism of clotting factors and can increase INR. Heart failure, hepatic congestion, and liver disease can also cause significant elevations in INR because of a reduction in warfarin metabolism. End-stage renal disease is associated with decreased CYP2C9 activity, resulting in lower warfarin dose requirements.

Thyroid function can influence warfarin therapy significantly. Hypothyroidism decreases the catabolism of certain clotting factors, increasing their availability and producing a relative refractoriness to warfarin therapy. This results in the need for increased dosages to reach a therapeutic INR. The addition of thyroid supplementation in these patients reverses the influence of hypothyroidism and can lead to significant elevations in INR unless the warfarin dose is reduced. Conversely, hyperthyroidism increases the catabolism of clotting factors, leading to an increased sensitivity to warfarin. Frequent monitoring of and adjustments in warfarin therapy are necessary in patients with changing thyroid function.

Genetic Factors

Cytochrome-P450 2C9 genotype[102,103] and VKOR[12,104] haplotype have been shown to correlate with the dose of warfarin required for effective anticoagulation. Patients with variant expression of CYP2C9 have a lower warfarin dose requirement and their risk of overanticoagulation is higher during therapy. Dosing algorithms that incorporate CYP2C9 genotype and VKOR1 haplotype along with other patient characteristics to predict warfarin maintenance doses are being tested.[105] It still remains to be determined whether pharmacogenomic-based dosing will improve clinical outcomes.

Other Factors That Influence Warfarin Dosing Requirements

Acute physical or psychological stress has been reported to increase INR.[106] Increased physical activity has also been reported to increase the warfarin dosing requirement.[107] Smoking can induce CYP1A2, which may increase warfarin metabolism in certain patients, resulting in increased dose requirements.[108] Due to its high vitamin K content, chewing smokeless tobacco can suppress the INR response.[109]

27. How should B.H. be assessed and evaluated at this clinic appointment?

At each clinic visit, regardless of the INR result, all factors that may influence B.H.'s anticoagulation status should be evaluated carefully, including adherence with the warfarin dose schedule. A patient assessment nomogram (Fig. 15-6) is a helpful tool to assist with patient evaluation.

The accuracy and reliability of the INR test should be also considered. B.H. should be assessed thoroughly for signs and symptoms of thromboembolism and hemorrhage. Detailed questions should be asked to determine whether any changes in diet, alcohol intake, underlying disease states, concurrent medications, or other factors have occurred.

DOSING ADJUSTMENTS

28. After a thorough assessment, it is determined that B.H. has adhered to her prescribed warfarin dosage schedule and that there is no apparent explanation to account for her reduction in INR. How should her warfarin dosage be adjusted?

When overanticoagulation or underanticoagulation is verified, an adjustment in warfarin dosing may be necessary. Figures 15-7 and 15-8 describe approaches to warfarin dosing adjustments for both regular-intensity and high-intensity maintenance therapy. Typically, dosing adjustments of 5% to 20% of the total daily dose (or the total weekly dose) are appropriate to reach the therapeutic range.[110] Because warfarin does not follow linear kinetics, small adjustments in dose can lead to large INR changes, thus large dose adjustments (i.e., greater than or less then 20% of the total weekly dose) are not recommended. These maintenance dosing guidelines should only be applied to patients who have reached a steady-state dose and not in the initiation phase of therapy.

Because B.H. is currently taking 4 mg daily, an adjustment of 10% would increase her dosage to approximately 4.5 mg/day. This dosing adjustment can be made by having her take one 4-mg tablet and half of a 1-mg tablet each day (same daily dosing) or by having her take 6 mg 2 days per week and 4 mg all other days of the week (alternate-day dosing). Patient preference and the likelihood of confusion about different tablet sizes versus different doses on different days of the week should be the primary considerations when selecting a dosing method.[111]

FREQUENCY OF FOLLOW-UP

29. B.H. agrees to increase her warfarin dosage to 4.5 mg/day. A new prescription for 1-mg tablets is written for her, and she is instructed about the use of these tablets. When should her INR be reassessed and her anticoagulation status, including physical assessment, be re-evaluated?

It will take several days for her warfarin level to reach a new steady state because of the long elimination half-lives of both warfarin and the vitamin K–dependent clotting factors. Her INR should be rechecked approximately 1 week after a dosing adjustment has been made. Once a stable dose has been reached, patient assessment and INR monitoring should occur every 4 to 6 weeks. However, if B.H. displays any signs of medical instability or nonadherence, a follow-up schedule of every 1 to 2 weeks is indicated (Table 15-18).

MANAGEMENT OF OVERANTICOAGULATION

30. E.M., who has been taking warfarin for 6 months with good laboratory control, noted a slight pink color to his urine. In the ED, an INR of 5.6 was reported. His Hct and hemoglobin (Hgb) were both within normal limits, as were his vital signs. A stool Hemoccult test was negative, but urinalysis revealed >50 red blood cells per high-power field. How should this adverse effect of warfarin be treated in E.M.?

Management of overanticoagulation depends on the clinical presentation of the patient. In the case of an elevated INR without bleeding complications, interruption of warfarin therapy by holding one or two doses until the INR returns to the therapeutic range is usually sufficient.[112] Minor bleeding complications accompanied by an elevated INR can be also managed by withholding warfarin therapy for a short period until bleeding resolves. In either case, the patient should be questioned to determine a possible cause for overanticoagulation, including intake of extra doses of warfarin, changes in diet or alcohol intake, changes in underlying medical conditions, or the use of other medications. In some cases, no apparent explanation is identified. Depending on the cause, a reduction in the maintenance dosing of warfarin may be necessary.

The time required for INR to return to the therapeutic range after warfarin is withheld depends on several patient characteristics. Advanced age, lower warfarin maintenance dose requirements, and higher INR are associated with increased time for INR correction.[113] Other factors that can prolong the time for INR to return to the therapeutic range include decompensated heart failure, active malignancy, and recent use of medications known to potentiate warfarin.

To shorten the time to correction of overanticoagulation, an alternative approach is to withhold warfarin and administer a small dose of vitamin K (phytonadione)[10] (Table 15-19). An oral dose of 1 to 2.5 mg can correct overanticoagulation in 24 to 48 hours without causing prolonged resistance to warfarin therapy, a problem commonly seen with larger (10-mg) doses of vitamin K.[114] Intramuscular administration is contraindicated due to the risk of hematoma formation, and SC administration of vitamin K is not recommended because of variable absorption.[115]

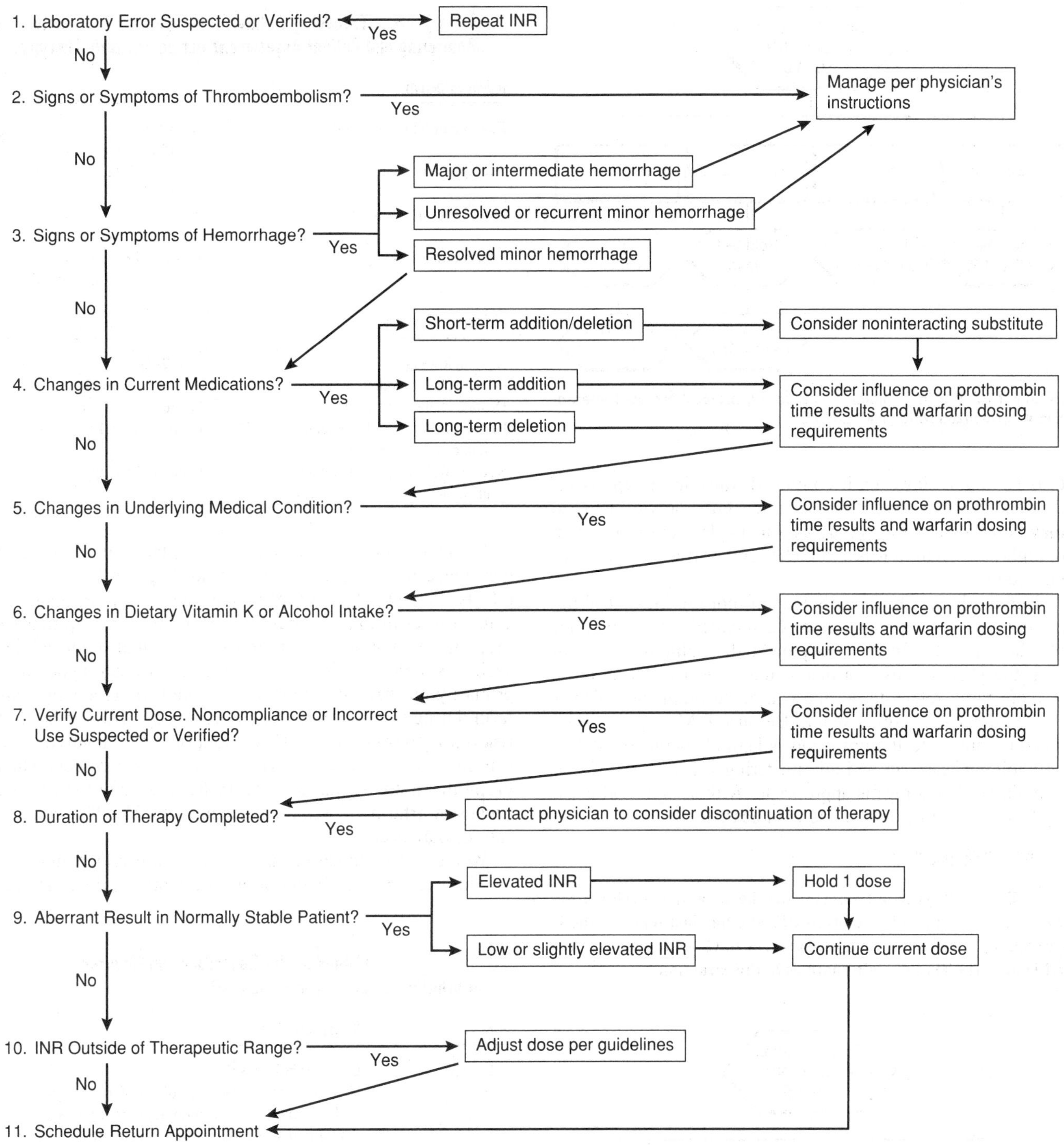

FIGURE 15-6 Assessment nomogram for patients taking warfarin.

IV doses of 0.5 to 1 mg of vitamin K can correct overanticoagulation within 24 hours.[116] This approach is also useful for reversal of therapeutic anticoagulation prior to invasive procedures and can be used to correct overanticoagulation in high-risk cases. IV vitamin K should be diluted and administered by slow infusion over 30 to 60 minutes to prevent flushing, hypotension, and cardiovascular collapse.[117] Although these symptoms resemble anaphylaxis, the mechanism of this adverse response is unclear: it is not known if it is caused by phytonadione or by the vehicle in which phytonadione is formulated. If this adverse reaction occurs, administration of epinephrine may be indicated, as well as other standard measures to support blood pressure and maintain the airway.

Rapid reversal of warfarin therapy is indicated in the setting of major, life-threatening bleeding. Fresh frozen plasma or factor concentrates to replace clotting factors will decrease the INR for 4 to 6 hours and should be administered as needed with careful monitoring of volume status. Supplementation with high-dose IV vitamin K (10 mg) may also be indicated. IV administration will reverse the effects of warfarin within

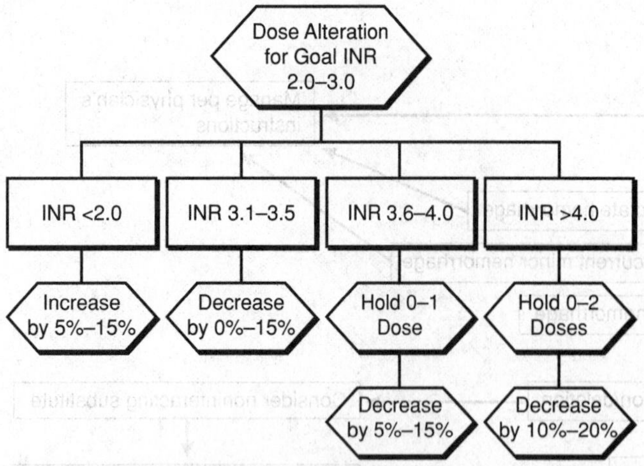

FIGURE 15-7 Warfarin maintenance dosing protocol for goal international normalized ratio (INR) 2.0–3.0.

6 to 12 hours. However, if continued warfarin therapy is indicated when bleeding resolves, anticoagulation with heparin may be necessary for as long as 7 to 14 days until the effect of high-dose vitamin K is diminished and warfarin responsiveness returns.

Hematuria may be an early sign of more serious bleeding, but in many cases this condition is associated with only minor bleeding episodes. In a reliable patient, discontinuing warfarin until the INR returns to a therapeutic level usually suffices. A more rapid return to normal can be accomplished if low-dose vitamin K is administered. Because E.M. appears to be bleeding only into the urine and is hemodynamically stable, withholding warfarin and administering a low dose of oral vitamin K (1–2.5 mg) is appropriate. A thorough workup to evaluate the source of bleeding is indicated.

USE IN PREGNANCY

31. E.S., a 30-year-old woman, has been taking warfarin for continuing therapy of a resolved PE. She has just learned she is pregnant. What effects might warfarin have on the fetus? Are UFH or LMWHs safer alternatives in this situation?

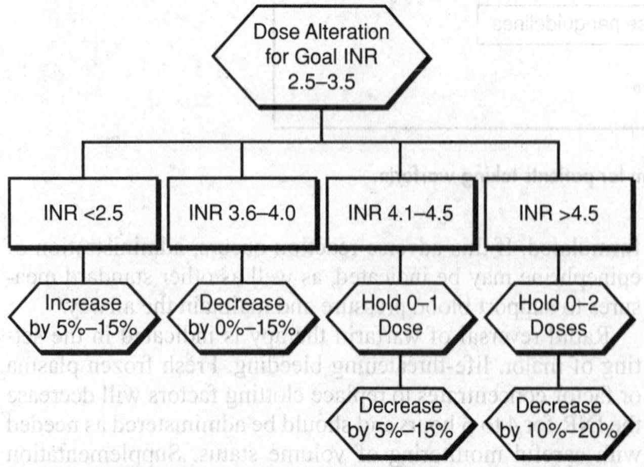

FIGURE 15-8 Warfarin maintenance dosing protocol for goal international normalized ratio (INR) 2.5–3.5.

Table 15-18 Frequency of International Normalized Ratio Monitoring and Patient Assessment During Warfarin Therapy

Initiation Therapy	
Flexible initiation method	Daily through day 4, then within 3–5 days
Average daily dosing method	Within 3–5 days, then within 1 week
After hospital discharge	If stable, within 3–5 days; if unstable, within 1–3 days
First month of therapy	Every 1–4 days until therapeutic, then weekly
Maintenance Therapy	
Dose held today	In 1–2 days
Dosage change today	Within 1–2 weeks
Dosage change <2 weeks ago	Within 2–4 weeks
Routine follow-up of medically stable and reliable patients	Every 4–6 weeks
Routine follow-up of medically unstable or unreliable patients	Every 1–2 weeks

Coumarin anticoagulants cross the placental barrier and may place the fetus at risk for hemorrhage and teratogenic effects.[118] Up to 30% of pregnancies that involve exposure to coumarin result in abnormal liveborn infants, and up to 30% in spontaneous abortion or stillbirth. Congenital abnormalities such as stippled calcifications and nasal cartilage hypoplasia primarily occurred in infants born to mothers receiving warfarin during the first trimester of pregnancy, with the highest risk during weeks 6 to 12. Other abnormalities, involving the central nervous system and eyes, are more likely to occur when the mother is taking warfarin later in the pregnancy. In addition, because warfarin crosses the placenta, fatal bleeding complications may occur.

Women of childbearing age who require anticoagulation should be counseled about options for contraception. Patients

Table 15-19 Guidelines for Reversal of an Elevated International Normalized Ratio (INR)

INR	*Recommendation*
<5	Lower or hold dose.
5–8.9	Hold one or two doses, or hold dose and give vitamin K (<5 mg orally). If more rapid reversal is required, use 2–4 mg. Repeat vitamin K (1–2 mg orally) if INR is still elevated at 24 hr.
≥9	Hold warfarin and give vitamin K (5–10 mg orally). Use additional vitamin K, if necessary.
Serious bleeding with high INR	Hold warfarin and give vitamin K (10 mg slow IV infusion) supplemented with fresh frozen plasma, prothrombin complex concentrate, or recombinant factor VIIa. May repeat vitamin K every 12 hr, if necessary.
Life-threatening bleeding	Hold warfarin and give prothrombin complex concentrates or recombinant factor VIIa supplemented with vitamin K (10 mg slow IV infusion). Repeat as necessary.

From reference 10.

Table 15-20 Recommendations for Anticoagulation During Pregnancy

Clinical Situation	*Peripartum Options*	*Postpartum*
1. Prophylaxis		
Known hypercoagulable state with no prior history of VTE	• Surveillance • Minidose UFH • Prophylactic LMWH	Warfarin to INR 2–3 for 4–6 weeks with UFH/LMWH overlap until INR >2.0
Single prior episode of VTE associated with transient risk factors, not receiving long-term anticoagulants	• Surveillance	Warfarin to INR 2–3 for 4–6 weeks with UFH/LMWH overlap until INR >2.0
Single prior episode of idiopathic or thrombophilia-related VTE, not receiving long-term anticoagulants	• Surveillance • Minidose UFH • Moderate-dose UFH • Prophylactic LMWH	Warfarin to INR 2–3 for 4–6 weeks with UFH/LMWH overlap until INR >2.0
Multiple prior episodes of VTE and/or receiving long-term oral anticoagulants for VTE	• Adjusted-dose UFH • Prophylactic LMWH • Full-dose LMWH	Long-term warfarin to INR 2–3 with UFH/LMWH overlap until INR >2.0
Long-term oral anticoagulants for mechanical valve replacement	• Adjusted-dose UFH • Full-dose LMWH	Long-term warfarin to prior INR goal with UFH/LMWH overlap until INR above lower limit of therapeutic range
2. Treatment of VTE that occurs during pregnancy	• IV UFH for ≥5 days, followed by adjusted-dose UFH • Full-dose LMWH	Warfarin to INR 2–3 for a minimum of 6 weeks with UFH/LMWH overlap until INR >2.0

VTE, venous thromboembolic disease; UFH, unfractionated heparin; LMWH, low-molecular-weight heparin; INR, international normalized ratio.
Minidose UFH: 5,000 U SQ Q 12 hr. Moderate-dose UFH: adjusted to 0.1–0.3 U/mL anti-X_a activity. Adjusted-dose UFH: adjusted to maintain therapeutic aPTT at mid-dosing interval. Prophylactic LMWH: enoxaparin 40 mg SQ QD or dalteparin 5,000 U SQ QD. Full-dose LMWH: enoxaparin 1 mg/kg SQ Q 12 hr or dalteparin 200 IU/kg and adjusted throughout pregnancy to maintain 4-hour postinjection anti-X_a activity level of 0.5–1.2 U/mL (VTE) or approximately 1.0 U/mL (mechanical valves).

who become pregnant while receiving warfarin should be informed of the risks of continued anticoagulation to the fetus, as well as the risk to themselves of discontinuing anticoagulation.

Other options for pregnant women who require anticoagulation include UFH and LMWHs.[118] Because these agents do not cross the placenta, they are preferred over warfarin for use in pregnancy. UFH is typically recommended because it has been used extensively during pregnancy. However, many clinical trials have validated the safety and efficacy of LMWHs in the prevention and treatment of DVT and PE during pregnancy.[119] These agents represent an alternative to UFH, with advantages as previously described. When used at full doses for the treatment of VTE during pregnancy, dosing must be adjusted throughout the pregnancy to account for the expected increase in the body weight of the mother and the reported increase in clearance of LMWH during pregnancy.[120]

In pregnant patients with mechanical heart valves, there is controversy regarding the use of LMHWs.[121] Several cases of valvular thrombosis and of maternal and fetal death have been reported. These cases may be the result of underdosing of LMWH and UFH.[118] Table 15-20 describes recommendations for anticoagulation during and after pregnancy for various conditions.

After being informed of the risks associated with warfarin, E.S. decided to continue her pregnancy and to begin anticoagulation with UFH. Warfarin therapy should be discontinued immediately and UFH initiated using SC treatment doses as previously described, or by continuous IV infusion. Dosing adjustments may be required throughout pregnancy as determined by aPTT monitoring. Potential adverse effects of UFH use, including hemorrhage, thrombocytopenia, and osteoporosis, should be monitored appropriately.

SC heparin should be discontinued 24 hours before elective induction of labor and resumed as soon as bleeding from delivery has been controlled. IV heparin should be discontinued 6 hours before delivery. Warfarin therapy can then be safely reinitiated. If spontaneous labor occurs, protamine can be used to reverse the effect of UFH. Warfarin is not secreted in breast milk; therefore, E.S. can safely breast-feed.

PREVENTION OF CARDIOGENIC THROMBOEMBOLISM

Atrial Fibrillation

Anticoagulation Before Cardioversion

32. C.D., a 68-year-old woman with hypertension, presents to the cardiology clinic complaining of several days of fatigue and a "racing heart." On physical examination, her pulse is irregularly irregular, and her heart rate is approximately 120 beats/minute. Using ECG, a diagnosis of atrial fibrillation is made and cardioversion planned. Should C.D. be anticoagulated before cardioversion?

In atrial fibrillation, compromised atrial activity and atrial enlargement causes stasis of blood within the atria and the left atrial appendage, often resulting in atrial thrombus formation. Atrial thrombus formation increases the risk of systemic embolization; clinical manifestations include arterial embolization of the extremities or embolization of the splenic, renal, or abdominal arteries. However, the most prevalent site of embolization is the cerebral arterial system, resulting in transient ischemic attack or stroke with potentially devastating neurologic and functional impairment.[122]

Both direct current cardioversion and pharmacologic cardioversion using antiarrhythmic drugs expose patients with atrial fibrillation to an initial short-term increase in stroke risk from embolization secondary to resumption of normal atrial mechanical activity (see Chapter 20). Data from a prospective cohort study of 437 patients noted a stroke incidence of 5.3% in patients with atrial fibrillation who were cardioverted without prior anticoagulation, but a significant reduction in stroke incidence to 0.8% was noted if patients who had received cardioversion were anticoagulated.[123] In addition to preventing the development of new atrial thrombi, anticoagulation allows any thrombus that may be present to endothelialize and adhere to the atrial wall so that the thromboembolic risk is minimized. Based on the assumed time course of thrombus development, as well as the presumed time course of clot endothelialization, patients who have been in atrial fibrillation for 48 hours should receive 3 weeks of therapeutic anticoagulation with warfarin to a target INR of 2.5 (range, 2.0–3.0) before cardioversion is attempted.[122] Despite a lower risk of stroke than that associated with atrial fibrillation, patients with atrial flutter should be treated similarly.

Whether C.D. has been in atrial fibrillation for 48 hours is not known; therefore, she requires a 3-week course of therapeutic anticoagulation with a goal INR range of 2.0 to 3.0 before cardioversion is attempted. If C.D. cannot tolerate her heart symptoms despite control of the ventricular response rate, her medical team might consider immediate cardioversion without anticoagulation if transesophageal echocardiography (TEE) is used to rule out left atrial thrombi. TEE is much mores sensitive than transthoracic echocardiography to visualize the left atrium and the left atrial appendage.

In a clinical trial, 1,222 patients with atrial fibrillation of more than 2 day's duration were randomly assigned to either treatment guided by TEE findings or to conventional precardioversion anticoagulation.[124] Patients assigned to conventional treatment and patients in the TEE group in whom thrombus was detected received a 3-week course of warfarin prior to cardioversion. Patients without detectable thrombus by TEE were cardioverted without precardioversion anticoagulation. All patients received 4 weeks of postcardioversion anticoagulation. Thromboembolic rates were identical between patients who received conventional treatment and those whose treatment was guided by TEE (0.5% vs. 0.8%, $p = 0.5$).

Anticoagulation After Cardioversion

33. After 3 weeks of regular-intensity warfarin therapy, C.D. is successfully cardioverted. Should warfarin be discontinued?

Despite normalization of atrial electrical activity, restoration of effective atrial mechanical activity after cardioversion of atrial fibrillation can be delayed for up to 3 weeks. In addition, a significant number of patients with atrial fibrillation who initially are successfully cardioverted revert to atrial fibrillation during the first month. Both of these factors contribute to the recognized delay in stroke presentation after cardioversion in patients with atrial fibrillation. For these reasons, anticoagulation with warfarin should be continued after cardioversion for a minimum 4 weeks.

Anticoagulation for Paroxysmal, Permanent, or Persistent Atrial Fibrillation

34. Two weeks after successful cardioversion, C.D. presents to the ED with chest palpitations and light-headedness. An ECG is evaluated, and atrial fibrillation is diagnosed again. What decisions regarding anticoagulation need to be made?

ANTICOAGULATION IN VALVULAR ATRIAL FIBRILLATION

Atrial fibrillation secondary to valvular heart disease has historically been recognized as a significant risk factor for stroke. Patients with atrial fibrillation who have a history of rheumatic mitral valve disease have a 17-fold higher incidence of stroke than in matched controls. Patients with valvular atrial fibrillation require long-term, regular-intensity anticoagulation to a target INR of 2.5 (range, 2.0–3.0) to prevent thromboembolism and stroke.[122,125]

ANTICOAGULATION IN NONVALVULAR ATRIAL FIBRILLATION

Nonvalvular heart disease is the most common cause of atrial fibrillation and, like valvular heart disease, represents a significant risk for stroke in patients with atrial fibrillation. Five clinical trials have substantiated the role of warfarin in the primary prevention of systemic embolization and stroke in chronic, nonvalvular atrial fibrillation.[126] All five trials compared warfarin with a placebo and were terminated before completion because of the substantial benefit of warfarin. In comparison with a placebo, warfarin significantly reduced the risk of stroke from approximately 5% per year to approximately 2% per year, with an average relative risk reduction of 67%. Based on the results of these trials, long-term anticoagulation with warfarin to a goal INR of 2.5 (range, 2.0–3.0) is recommended in patients like C.D., who have atrial fibrillation secondary to nonvalvular heart disease.[122,125]

Several clinical trials have attempted to define the comparative efficacy of warfarin versus aspirin in the prevention of stroke associated with atrial fibrillation.[127] Compared with a placebo or control, aspirin decreases the risk of stroke in patients with atrial fibrillation. However, that reduction is not as substantial as the reduction seen with warfarin. In clinical trials comparing warfarin and aspirin, the risk reduction associated with warfarin is significantly larger than that of aspirin. However, aspirin may be appropriate in certain patients at low risk for stroke associated with atrial fibrillation (Table 15-6).

The decision to continue long-term anticoagulation with warfarin in C.D. should be based on an evaluation of the likelihood that her atrial fibrillation will become chronic with a paroxysmal, persistent, or permanent presentation, as well as an assessment of her risk of stroke compared with her risk of warfarin-associated bleeding complications. Because of her age and history of hypertension, the appropriate strategy should be long-term warfarin therapy with a goal INR of 2.5 (range, 2.0–3.0).

Cardiac Valve Replacement

Mechanical Prosthetic Valves

35. D.L., a 56-year-old woman with a history of rheumatic mitral valve disease, has undergone mitral valve replacement. A St. Jude (bileaflet mechanical) valve has been implanted, and heparin

therapy is initiated postoperatively. Does D.L. require continued anticoagulation with warfarin?

Mechanical prosthetic valves confer a significant thromboembolic risk by providing a foreign surface in contact with blood components on which platelet aggregation and thrombus formation can occur. Valvular thrombosis can impair the integrity of valve function and can lead to embolization with systemic manifestations, including stroke.[128] The incidence of thromboembolic complications depends on the type of artificial valve (caged ball [Starr-Edwards] > tilting disk [Medtronic-Hall; Bjork-Shiley] > bileaflet [St. Jude]), as well as the anatomical position of the replacement (dual valve replacement > mitral > aortic).[129]

Long-term anticoagulation is required in patients with mechanical valve replacement because it significantly reduces the risk of stroke and other manifestations of systemic embolization. Trials comparing different intensities of oral anticoagulation with warfarin in mechanical valve replacement helped identify the intensity of anticoagulation that protects against thromboembolic risk, while reducing the incidence of hemorrhagic complications.[129,130] Patients with a St. Jude bileaflet valve in the aortic position should receive long-term anticoagulant therapy with warfarin to a target INR of 2.5 (range, 2.0–3.0).[128,131] For all other mechanical valve types in the aortic position, and for any mechanical mitral valve replacement, chronic warfarin therapy with a target INR of 3.0 (range, 2.5–3.5) is recommended.[128,131] The concurrent use of low-dose aspirin (81 mg daily) is recommended for patients with additional risk factors for systemic embolization (atrial fibrillation, left ventricular dysfunction, a history of prior systemic embolism, or a hypercoagulable condition), unless the patient has a significant risk for bleeding or a history of aspirin intolerance.

Bioprosthetic Valves

36. **E.K., an 86-year-old woman with a history of symptomatic aortic stenosis, has received a bioprosthetic (mammalian) aortic valve replacement. Is anticoagulant therapy required in E.K.?**

Prosthetic heart valves extracted from mammalian sources (porcine or bovine xenografts; homografts) are significantly less thrombogenic than mechanical prosthetic valves. The period of greatest thromboembolic risk appears to be during the first 3 months after implantation. Therefore, short-term, regular-intensity, preventive anticoagulation to an INR of 2.5 (range, 2.0–3.0) is recommended.[128,131] After this period, long-term aspirin therapy (minimum dose, 162 mg/day) is indicated. However, oral anticoagulation should be continued long term in patients with concurrent atrial fibrillation, a history of systemic embolism, or evidence of atrial thrombus at surgery.

BRIDGE THERAPY

Management of Anticoagulation Around Invasive Procedures

37. **C.G. is a 43-year-old woman with a history of valvular heart disease associated with Marfan syndrome. She has a St. Jude mitral valve replacement and is anticoagulated with warfarin 7.5 mg once daily to a goal INR range of 2.5 to 3.5. Recently, she has complained of episodic rectal bleeding despite adequate anticoagulation. She is scheduled for colonoscopy in several weeks. Her gastroenterologist calls you at the anticoagulation clinic to determine the most appropriate plan for reversal of her warfarin prior to the procedure. What are the options?**

When an invasive procedure is planned, it is often necessary to reverse the effects of warfarin to minimize the risk of bleeding complications associated with the procedure, which can be worsened by the presence of an anticoagulant. It can take several days for the anticoagulant effect of warfarin to be reversed after discontinuation of the drug, but in that period of time, a patient may be at risk for thromboembolic complications associated with underanticoagulation. *Bridge therapy* is the term that refers to the use of a relatively short-acting injectable anticoagulant (UFH, LMWH) as a substitute for warfarin prior to and immediately following an invasive procedure.[132] Because UFH and LMWH have shorter elimination half-lives than warfarin, they can be stopped just prior to the invasive procedure without increasing the risk of bleeding associated with the procedure. In addition, because of their shorter onset of effect, they can be used when warfarin is restarted and until the INR reaches the therapeutic range.

Although bridge therapy has not been studied in randomized clinical trials, there are multiple options, many of which have been evaluated in case series, observational studies, and nonrandomized trials involving patients with various indications for anticoagulation, including valve replacement.[133–135] The choice of a bridge therapy strategy depends on the risk of bleeding associated with continued anticoagulation for the surgery or procedure to be performed and on the risk of thromboembolism associated with underanticoagulation in the patient in question. Individualized risk assessment and bridge therapy planning are necessary for each patient who may require temporary discontinuation of warfarin.

Because the use of IV UFH for bridge therapy requires hospitalization, there has been considerable interest in using LMWH on an outpatient basis for this purpose. Clinical outcomes in patients bridged with LMWH or UFH are similar, and overall costs are lower for LMWH because of the avoidance of hospital admission, despite higher drug costs.[136] UFH, however, may be appropriate in patients with significant renal impairment, or in patients without third-party prescription coverage who cannot afford the drug cost of LMWH. A guideline for bridge therapy based on the risk of thromboembolism and on renal function is presented in Table 15-21.

Because C.G. has a mechanical mitral valve replacement, her risk of thromboembolism associated with underanticoagulation is considered high. Therefore, warfarin should not simply be withheld; instead, she should receive bridge therapy with an injectable anticoagulant. Her renal function is normal, and her health care insurance covers injectable drugs. Therefore, her plan will include early discontinuation of warfarin 3 to 5 days prior to the procedure, and substitution with enoxaparin 1 mg/kg Q 12 hr when the INR falls below the lower limit of the therapeutic range. The last dose of enoxaparin should be given no later than 24 hours prior to the procedure to minimize the risk of bleeding at the time of the procedure. After the procedure, warfarin should be restarted at her usual dose, and enoxaparin should be continued until the INR is >2.5.

Table 15-21 Bridge Therapy Guidelines for Invasive Procedures

Thrombolic Risk	*Renal Function*	*Bridge Therapy*
HIGH • Afib with moderate/high stroke risk per CHAD2 score, or with concurrent valve replacement or mitral stenosis • Hx stroke/TIA • Any hypercoagulate state • Mechanical valve • hx DVT/PE <3 months ago	CLcr >30	• Hold warfarin for 3–5 days preprocedure (decision predicated on age, dosing requirement, and other comorbid conditions associated with prolonged time for reversal) OR hold warfarin 2–3 days preprocedure and administer vitamin K 2.5 mg PO 2 days preprocedure (may repeat on day 1) • Initiate UFH SQ/IV or LMWH when INR falls below lower limit of therapeutic range • Stop IV UFH 6 hr preprocedure or stop SQ UFH/LMWH 24 hr preprocedure • Resume UFH/LMWH 12–24 hr postprocedure (decision predicated on postop assessment of bleeding risk) and continue until INR above lower limit of therapeutic range • Resume warfarin 12–24 hr postprocedure at usual maintenance dose (decision predicated on postprocedure assessment of bleeding risk)
	CLcr <30	• Last dose of warfarin on day 3 preprocedure • Vitamin K 2.5 mg PO on day 2 preprocedure • Admit on day 1 preprocedure and begin IV UFH (70 U/kg bolus, 15 U/kg/hr infusion and adjust per inpatient protocol) • If INR above 1.5 on day 1, give vitamin K 1 mg IV • Stop IV UFH 6 hr preprocedure • Resume UFH 12–24 hr postprocedure (decision predicated on postprocedure assessment of bleeding risk) and continue until INR above lower limit of therapeutic range • Resume warfarin 12–48 hr postprocedure at usual maintenance dose (decision predicated on postop assessment of bleeding risk)
LOW • Afib with low/moderate stroke risk per CHADS2 score • Dilated cardiomyopathy with no hx thrombosis • hx DVT/PE >3 months ago	All patients	• Hold warfarin for 3–5 days preprocedure OR hold warfarin for 2–3 days preprocedure and administer vitamin K 2.5 mg PO 2 days preprocedure (may repeat on day 1) • Resume warfarin 12–48 hr postprocedure at usual maintenance dose (decision predicated on postop assessment of bleeding risk)

Management of Anticoagulation Around Dental Procedures

38. J.Y. is a 76-year-old man with a history of hypertension, hypercholesterolemia, adult-onset diabetes, and atrial fibrillation. He receives warfarin 2.5 mg on Monday, Wednesday, and Friday and 5 mg on all other days for stroke prevention. He is scheduled to have a tooth removed, and his dentist has recommended that warfarin be withheld for 5 days prior to the procedure. He calls his anticoagulation provider for advice. What is your response?

Based on his medical history, A.V. is considered at moderate to high risk for stroke. If his warfarin were to be discontinued for 5 days prior to this dental procedure, he would require bridge therapy with inpatient UFH or outpatient LMWH prior to the procedure, and afterward until his INR reached 2.0. However, for many dental procedures, it is often not necessary to withhold warfarin.[137] Oral bleeding can be prevented or controlled using a combination of local measures, including cold water rinse, local pressure (biting on gauze or tea bags [which release tannins, causing local vasoconstriction]), additional suturing, or electrocautery. Other options include packing the site with gelatin sponges (Gelfoam) or absorbable oxycellulose (Surgicel), or applying microcrystalline collagen (Avitene), topical thrombin, or a fibrin adhesive.

A mouth rinse of 5% tranexamic acid or 5% aminocaproic acid can also be used to control oral bleeding.[138] Patients are instructed to hold 10 mL of the rinse in their mouths for 2 minutes, 30 minutes prior to the procedure, and then to repeat every 2 hours as needed afterward until bleeding is resolved. Table 15-22 describes guidelines for the management of warfarin around dental procedures based on the bleeding risk of the procedure.

The simple extraction planned for A.V. does not require discontinuation of his warfarin therapy. The anticoagulation clinic provider should call the dentist to offer suggestions regarding local prevention and control of oral bleeding. A.V. should be cautioned to avoid hot liquid, vigorous mouthwashes, hard foods, and NSAIDs and other antiplatelet agents during the first 24 to 48 hours after his tooth extraction.

DRUG INTERACTIONS

Interactions With Legend Drugs

39. D.G., a 72-year-old man, received a Bjork-Shiley tilting disk mitral valve prosthesis 5 years ago. He has been anticoagulated with warfarin 6 mg/day with good control. He is allergic to ampicillin and has gastric intolerance to tetracycline. Yesterday, he was seen in an acute-care clinic with symptoms of an acute prostatic infection and prescribed one double-strength tablet of trimethoprim-sulfamethoxazole (TMP-SMX) BID for 10 days. How will the combination of warfarin and TMP-SMX (Bactrim, Septra) affect D.G.'s anticoagulation control? Should his warfarin dosage be adjusted or another drug substituted for TMP-SMX?

Drug interactions with warfarin occur by a number of different mechanisms and can have a significant impact

Table 15-22 Suggestions for Anticoagulation Management Before and After Dental Procedures[a]

	Low Bleeding Risk	*Moderate Bleeding Risk*	*High Bleeding Risk*
Procedure	• Supragingival scaling • Simple restorations • Local anesthetic injections	• Subgingival scaling • Restorations with subgingival preparations • Standard root canal therapy • Simple extractions • Regional injection of local anesthetics	• Extensive surgery • Apicoectomy (root removal) • Alveolar surgery (bone removal) • Multiple extractions
Suggestions	• Do not interrupt warfarin treatment • Use local measures to prevent/control bleeding	• Interruption of warfarin treatment is not necessary • Use local measures to prevent or control bleeding *Consult with dentist to determine comfort with use of local measures to prevent bleeding when anticoagulation is not interrupted*	• May need to reduce international normalized ratio or return to normal hemostasis • Follow bridge therapy guidelines for invasive procedures based on risk of thromboembolism

[a]University of Washington Medical Center Anticoagulation Clinics.

on the anticoagulant effect of warfarin.[139–141] Elevations or reductions in INR have been observed when interacting drugs are added to or discontinued from the medication regimens of patients taking warfarin or when used intermittently. Clinically significant hemorrhagic or thromboembolic complications can result. Careful selection of both prescription and nonprescription medications, appropriate INR monitoring, and detailed patient education regarding drug interactions are important interventions for pharmacists caring for patients taking warfarin. A summary of drugs that interact with warfarin, including mechanisms of interaction and effect on INR, is provided in Table 15-23.

Although warfarin is highly bound to protein, primarily to albumin, and can be displaced from protein-binding sites by a number of weakly acidic drugs, these interactions typically do not result in clinically significant elevations in PT/INR.[142] Warfarin displaced from protein-binding sites is readily available for elimination by hepatic metabolism, resulting in increased clearance without a significant change in the free drug concentration.

Other types of interactions with warfarin are much more significant. Pharmacodynamic interactions are those that alter the physiology of hemostasis, particularly interactions that influence the synthesis or degradation of clotting factors or that increase the risk of bleeding through inhibition of platelet aggregation. Pharmacokinetic interactions influence the absorption and metabolism of warfarin, and many clinically significant interactions with warfarin occur when warfarin metabolism is induced or inhibited. Interactions involving agents known to influence the hepatic microsomal enzyme systems responsible for the metabolism of the more potent S(−)-warfarin (CYP2C9) are potentially more significant than those that influence the enzymes that metabolize R(+)-warfarin (CYP1A2, CYP3A4).[141]

Sulfamethoxazole can increase the effect of warfarin significantly by stereoselectively inhibiting the metabolism of the more potent S(−)-enantiomer of warfarin.[139] Potentiation of warfarin activity after inhibition of metabolism usually takes several days, and the effect may be slow to resolve once the offending agent is discontinued. In addition, fever associated with the infection for which TMP-SMX has been prescribed may enhance the catabolism of vitamin K–dependent clotting factors, resulting in an accentuated hypoprothrombinemic response. This effect will dissipate as the fever abates with antibiotic therapy.

For D.G., the best choice would be to discontinue TMP-SMX. Because ampicillin and tetracycline are contraindicated, either a first-generation cephalosporin or TMP alone may be used. Oral quinolones should be avoided because they also carry the risk of potentiating the anticoagulant effect of warfarin. Careful monitoring of the INR should continue because the introduction of any changes in treatment, as well as the acute illness, may alter the patient's response to warfarin therapy.

If noninteracting alternatives are not clinically appropriate, the concomitant use of interacting agents is not an absolute contraindication in patients taking warfarin. TMP-SMX can be prescribed if D.G. is monitored frequently and carefully, with adjustment of warfarin dosages as necessary to maintain his INR within the therapeutic INR range of 2.5 to 3.5 and with attention to potential hemorrhagic complications. No initial change in the dosage of warfarin should be made because it may take several days for the interaction to become apparent. The INR should be repeated within 3 days, with warfarin dosing adjustments and subsequent monitoring guided by initial INR results.

40. D.R. is a 39-year-old woman recovering from unexplained ventricular fibrillation several weeks ago with significant, but improving, neurologic deficits. A defibrillator system has been implanted, with amiodarone 400 mg/day added for suppressive antiarrhythmic therapy. As a result of being immobile during her hospitalization, she developed a DVT and has been receiving heparin for 5 days. A full 3-month course of anticoagulation is indicated. How will amiodarone influence D.R.'s anticoagulation?

Amiodarone appears to inhibit the hepatic metabolism of warfarin, resulting in significant increases in the INR in patients previously stabilized on warfarin therapy and in whom amiodarone is added.[143] Elevations in INR typically occur within 1 week and stabilize after approximately 1 month of combination therapy. These patients require frequent monitoring with downward adjustments in warfarin dose by as much as 50% or more.

In the case of D.R., warfarin is to be added to pre-existing amiodarone therapy. The use of a drug known to interact with warfarin is not an absolute contraindication to the addition of warfarin. Warfarin therapy should begin using a flexible initiation protocol or average daily dosing method, but with the expectation that D.R.'s INR will likely increase at a rate

Table 15-23 Drug Interactions

Mechanism	Effect on International Normalized Ratio	Drugs/Drug Classes	
Increased synthesis of clotting factors	Decreased	Vitamin K	
Reduced catabolism of clotting factors	Decreased	Methimazole	Propylthiouracil
Induction of warfarin metabolism	Decreased	Alcohol(chronic use)	Fosphenytoin[a]
		Aminoglutethimide	Glutethimide
		Barbiturates	Griseofulvin
		Bosentan	Nafcillin
		Carbamazepine	Phenytoin[a]
		Dicloxacillin	Primidone
		Ethchlorvynol	Rifampin
Reduced absorption of warfarin	Decreased	Cholestyramine	Sucralfate
		Colestipol	
Unexplained mechanisms	Decreased	Ascorbic acid	Corticosteroids
		Azathioprine	Cyclosporin Mercapto purine
Increased catabolism of clotting factors	Increased	Thyroid hormones	
Protein binding displacement	Increased	Chloral hydrate	
Decreased synthesis of clotting factors	Increased	Cefamandole	Cefoperazone
		Cefotetan	Moxalactam
		Cefmetazole	Vitamin E
Impaired vitamin K production by GI flora	Increased	Broad-spectrum antibiotics	
Inhibition of warfarin metabolism	Increased	Acetaminophen	Isoniazid
		Alcohol (acute use)	Macrolide antibiotics
		Allopurinol	Metronidazole
		Amiodarone	Omeprazole
		Azole antifungals	Phenytoin[a]
		Capecitabine	Propafenone
		Celecoxib	Quinidine
		Chloramphenicol	Rofecoxib
		Cimetidine	SSRIs
		Disulfiram	Statins
		Fluoroquinolone antibiotics	Sulfa antibiotics
		Fluorouracil	Zafirlukast
		Fosphenytoin[a]	
Additive anticoagulant response	Increased	Direct thrombin inhibitors	Low molecular weight heparins
		Heparin	Thrombolytic agents
Unexplained mechanism	Increased	Androgens	Gemcitabine
		Clofibrate	Gemfibrozil
		Cyclophosphamide	Influenza virus vaccine
		Fenofibrate	Mesalamine
Increased bleeding risk	No effect	Aspirin/acetylated salicylates	Cyclo-oxygenase 2 inhibitors
		Clopidogrel/ticlopidine	Glycoprotein IIb/IIIa antagonists
			NSAIDS

[a] Reported to both increase and decrease PT/INR.

faster than if she were not taking amiodarone and that her maintenance dosing likely will be significantly lower than if she were not taking amiodarone concurrently. Frequent monitoring will be required for D.R. to establish a maintenance dose because she may not yet have a steady-state amiodarone level.

If amiodarone therapy is discontinued while D.R. is anticoagulated, frequent monitoring will also be necessary. However, the effect of amiodarone on warfarin metabolism can continue for several months after amiodarone is discontinued because of amiodarone's long elimination half-life and large volume of distribution. Gradual increases in warfarin dosing requirements over weeks to months have been observed after discontinuation of amiodarone.

41. M.G., a 67-year-old woman, was recently diagnosed with bursitis of the right shoulder. A course of anti-inflammatory medication is recommended by her doctor. M.G. is taking warfarin

12.5 mg/day for a history of chronic atrial fibrillation. What could be prescribed for M.G.'s shoulder pain that would not significantly interact with the warfarin she is taking?

This question illustrates one of the most difficult therapeutic dilemmas for a patient taking warfarin. All NSAIDs have the potential to cause gastric irritation by inhibiting cytoprotective prostaglandins, thereby providing a focus for GI bleeding. In addition, most NSAIDs inhibit platelet aggregation, which compromises effective clotting and can lead to bleeding complications.[144] Some NSAIDs (phenylbutazone, sulfinpyrazone, mefenamic acid) may also have specific pharmacokinetic interactions with warfarin that can increase the hypoprothrombinemic effect of warfarin.

These effects can increase the risk of hemorrhagic complications significantly in patients taking warfarin who are prescribed concurrent NSAID therapy. In a retrospective cohort study of patients age 65 years or older, the risk of hospitalization for bleeding peptic ulcer disease was approximately three times higher for patients taking concurrent warfarin and an NSAID versus patients taking either drug alone, and almost 13 times higher than in patients taking neither warfarin nor an NSAID.[145] Warfarin therapy is considered a relative contraindication to NSAID use.

In patients like M.G. who require combination therapy, clinical experience suggests that ibuprofen (Motrin), naproxen (Naprosyn), or nabumetone (Relafen) are somewhat better tolerated than other NSAIDs with respect to additive hemorrhagic complications, particularly for short-term use. Alternative agents include the nonacetylated salicylates such as salsalate or choline salicylate. These agents have minimal effect on platelet aggregation compared with other salicylates. However, all patients requiring combined warfarin and NSAID therapy should be followed closely and observed routinely for signs and symptoms of bleeding, with frequent stool testing for GI bleeding. Patients should be counseled to avoid additional NSAID use, including use of aspirin, and to seek assistance from a pharmacist to prevent inadvertent NSAID use when selecting over-the-counter medications.

The analgesic and antipyretic of choice in patients taking warfarin is acetaminophen, which has not been consistently shown to increase the risk of bleeding. However, in a controversial case-control study of patients taking warfarin, acetaminophen use of >2,275 mg/week was an independent risk factor for developing an INR >6.0.[146] Controls were matched for age, gender, and race, but patients had a higher frequency of febrile illness and reduced oral intake, factors that may influence the INR independently as well as account for acetaminophen use. Acetaminophen may increase the INR by inhibition of CYP1A2 metabolism of R(+)-warfarin, but this effect has not been reported consistently.[147] Appropriate monitoring and assessment of patients taking concurrent warfarin and acetaminophen, either routinely or as needed, is sufficient to detect any potential interaction.

Interactions With Natural Products/Dietary Supplements

42. K.P. is a 32-year-old woman who developed a left lower extremity DVT after sustaining a skiing injury 1 month ago. She has been taking warfarin 5 mg on Monday, Wednesday, and Friday and 7.5 mg on all other days of the week. She has maintained stable INRs between 2.0 and 3.0 for the last 2 weeks. She has no known medical problems and takes no other medications. However, she has felt increasingly lethargic since her accident and feels that she cannot participate fully in physical therapy because of fatigue. She is interested in taking an herbal supplement to increase her level of energy. How should she be counseled?

Dietary supplements, including herbal medicinals, amino acids, and other nonprescription products, are not tested before marketing for interactions with other medications, including warfarin.[97] Little is known about their interactive properties, other than published case reports of varying quality. In addition, dietary supplements are not required to meet *United States Pharmacopeia* standards for tablet content uniformity. Therefore, the actual ingredients and quantity of ingredients of a given product may change from batch to batch, and different products produced by different manufacturers may also differ substantially. These limitations influence the availability and reliability of information regarding potential interactions between warfarin and dietary supplements.

Table 15-24 lists dietary supplements reported to influence INR or suspected to interact with warfarin based on known or implied properties.[141] Because of limited information regarding the full extent of possible interactions with dietary supplements, including herbal medicinals, it is appropriate to counsel patients taking warfarin to avoid use of these products. However, a large percentage of patients may not report their use of dietary supplements to health care providers. Ongoing, detailed evaluation of all current medications including dietary supplements is necessary to prevent potential adverse effects

Table 15-24 Drug Interactions with Dietary Supplements

Mechanism	*Effect*	*Supplement*
Inhibition of warfarin metabolism	Increased INR	Chinese wolf berry Cranberry juice Grapefruit juice
Contain coumarin derivatives	Increased INR	Dan shen Dong quai Fenugreek
Unknown	Increased INR	Curbicin Devil's claw Glucosamine-chondroitin Melatonin Papaya extract Quilinggao
Inhibition of platelet aggregation	Increased bleeding	Garlic Ginger Ginkgo
Contain vitamin K/derivatives	Decreased INR	Coenzyme q10 Green tea Some multivitamins
Induction of CYP3A4	Decreased INR	St. John's wort
Unknown	Decreased INR	Ginseng Melatonin

associated with interactions between warfarin and dietary supplements.

DISSEMINATED INTRAVASCULAR COAGULATION

Pathophysiology

43. W.K., a 63-year-old woman, was admitted to the intensive care unit with respiratory failure secondary to acute PE. She required ventilatory support until 48 hours ago, when she was extubated. At that time, aspiration was suspected, but no antibiotic coverage was prescribed. Within the last 24 hours, W.K. developed tachycardia (heart rate, 120 beats/minute), tachypnea (respiratory rate, 30 breaths/minute), and a fever to 39°C. Sepsis was suspected, broad-spectrum antibiotic coverage was started, and W.K. was reintubated. Because of the sudden appearance of bright red blood per rectum and through her nasogastric tube, a coagulation screen was ordered. Until this time, all coagulation parameters had been within normal limits. Now the results show platelets, 43,000/mm^3 (normal, 150,000–350,000); PT, 24 seconds (mean normal, 12); aPTT, 76 seconds (mean normal, 34); thrombin time, 48 seconds (normal, 16–27); fibrinogen, 60 mg/dL (normal, 150–400); and fibrin degradation products, 580 ng/mL (normal, <250). The diagnosis of disseminated intravascular coagulation (DIC) is made. How does the pathophysiology of DIC explain these hematologic abnormalities?

[SI units: platelets, 43 × 10^9/L (normal, 150–300), and fibrinogen, 0.6 g/L (normal, 1.5–4)]

Thrombosis in response to endothelial damage or the presence of an altered surface in contact with blood components is a localized phenomenon. Thrombus formation occurs at the site of injury or abnormality, where procoagulant and anticoagulant mechanisms, as well as fibrinolytic and antifibrinolytic mechanisms, are regulated. The term *localized extravascular coagulation* describes the site-specific nature of venous and arterial thrombosis.

In contrast, DIC is a diffuse response to systemic activation of the coagulation system (Fig. 15-9).[148] Circulating thrombin converts fibrinogen to fibrin, resulting in fibrin deposition within the microcirculation. Clinical manifestations of microvascular thrombosis are the result of tissue ischemia resulting from thrombotic occlusion of small and midsize vessels.

The presence of systemic circulating thrombin causes simultaneous systemic activation of the fibrinolytic system, resulting in circulating plasmin within the systemic circulation. Plasmin causes systemic lysis of fibrin to fibrin degradation products and results in hemorrhagic complications.

Bleeding manifestations of DIC occur not only as a result of systemic fibrinolysis, but also secondary to thrombocytopenia, clotting factor deficiency, and platelet dysfunction. Circulating thrombin promotes platelet aggregation, resulting in thrombocytopenia as platelet aggregates deposit in the microcirculation. Circulating plasmin degrades clotting factors as well as fibrin, and the presence of fibrinogen degradation products from fibrinolysis inhibits platelet function. Normal mechanisms of platelet and clotting factor synthesis are unable to compensate for this consumption. In essence, the patient shows paradoxical bleeding secondary to overactivation and eventual consumption of available clotting factors and platelets.

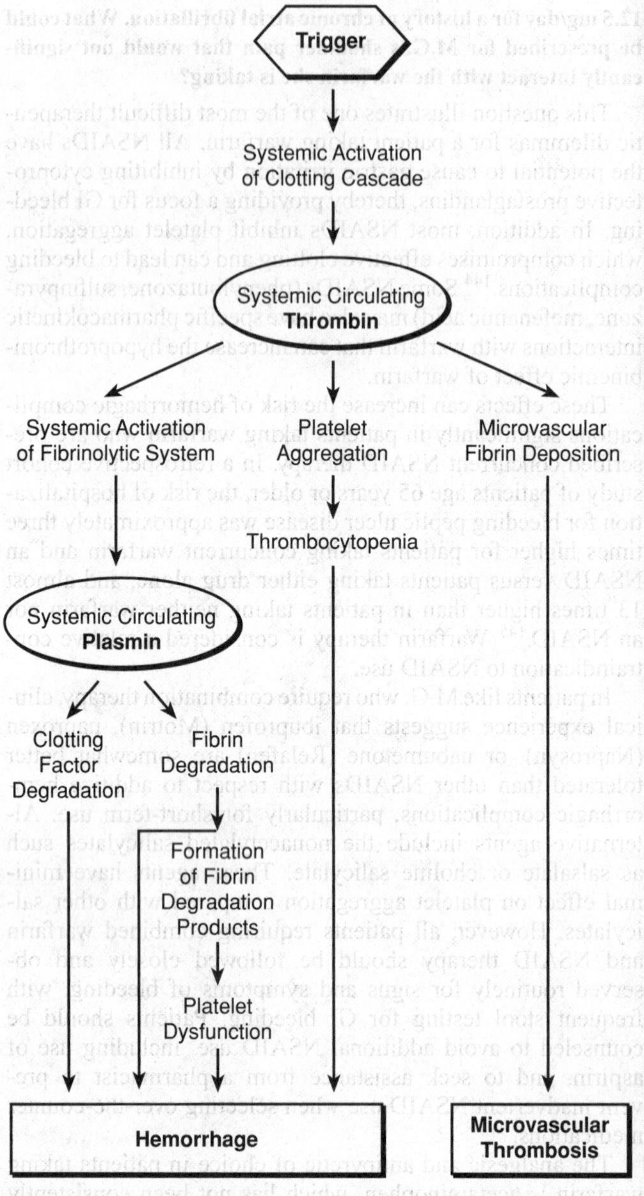

FIGURE 15-9 Pathophysiology of disseminated intravascular coagulation.

Clinical Presentation

44. What subjective and objective evidence in W.K. is consistent with the diagnosis of acute DIC?

Laboratory Findings

Many coagulation laboratory abnormalities occur in DIC.[149] The PT/INR, aPTT, and thrombin time are increased because clotting factors, as well as antithrombin and proteins C and S, are consumed more quickly than they can be replenished by hepatic synthesis. Platelet count is diminished secondary to thrombin-mediated platelet aggregation. Fibrinogen is reduced as a result of plasmin-mediated fibrinolysis, with an elevation in fibrinogen degradation products including D-dimer, indicative of a fibrinolytic state. A peripheral smear will often show thrombocytopenia and red blood cells fragmented by exposure to microcirculatory fibrin (schistocytes).

Table 15-25 International Society on Thrombosis and Haemostasis Disseminated Intravascular Coagulation (DIC) Scoring System

Does the patient have an underlying disorder known to be associated with DIC? (if YES, continue with scoring)

Laboratory Test	*Result*	*Point Score*
Platelet count	>100,000	0
	<100,000	1
	<50,000	2
Fibrin-related markers	No increase	0
	Moderate increase	2
	Strong increase	3
PT (vs. baseline)	<3 seconds	0
	3–6 seconds	1
	>6 seconds	2
Fibrinogen	>1 g/L	0
	<1 g/L	1
TOTAL SCORE	≥5	Compatible with over DIC (repeat daily)
	<5	Suggestive but nonaffirmative for nonovert DIC (repeat in 1–2 days)

PT, prothrombin time.
From reference 150.

Table 15-26 Clinical Conditions Associated With Disseminated Intravascular Coagulation

Infectious Diseases	**Obstetric States**
Aspergillosis	Amnionic fluid embolism
Bacterial infections	Eclampsia
Candidiasis	Retained dead fetus
Cytomegalovirus	Septic or saline abortion
Fungal infections	**Tissue Injury**
Gram-negative sepsis	Burns
Gram-positive sepsis	Crush injuries
Hepatitis	Extensive surgery
Histoplasmosis	Multiple trauma
Miscellaneous infections	**Vascular Disorders**
Mycobacteria malaria	Aortic aneurysm
Mycoplasma	Giant hemangioma
Psittacosis	**Miscellaneous**
Rocky Mountain spotted fever	Acidosis
Varicella	Anaphylaxis
Viral infections	Acute respiratory distress syndrome
Intravascular Hemolysis	Cardiopulmonary bypass
Hemolytic transfusion reactions	Hematologic disorders
Massive transfusions	Heat stroke
Minor hemolysis	Hepatic disease
Malignancy	Hypoperfusion
Myeloproliferative diseases	Hypovolemia
Solid tumor	Severe allergic reaction
	Snake bites
	Transplant rejection

The International Society of Thrombosis and Haemostasis Overt DIC Scoring System, based on laboratory values observed in patients suspected of having DIC, is used in the diagnosis of DIC (Table 15-25).[150] There is a strong correlation between increasing DIC score and 28-day mortality.[151]

Hemorrhagic Manifestations

As illustrated by W.K., hemorrhagic manifestations are the predominant clinical finding in DIC.[148] Bleeding can occur at sites of injury, including surgical incisions, venipuncture sites, nasogastric tubes, or gastric ulcers. However, spontaneous bleeding also occurs from intact sites or organ systems. Spontaneous ecchymosis, petechiae, epistaxis, hemoptysis, hematuria, and GI bleeding are commonly encountered. Intracranial, intraperitoneal, and pericardial bleeding may also occur.

Thrombotic Manifestations

Thrombotic manifestations of DIC result in the obstruction of blood flow to multiple organ systems. The resultant ischemic damage to end organs, including the skin, kidneys, brain, lungs, liver, eyes, and GI tract, can result in multisystem failure. Despite the severity of hemorrhagic complications, microvascular thrombosis represents a significant cause of morbidity and mortality in patients with acute DIC.

Precipitating Events

45. What events may have precipitated the development of DIC in W.K.?

DIC is a pathological syndrome triggered by disease states or conditions that activate coagulation systemically rather than locally.[149] The presence of thrombin within the systemic circulation can be triggered by systemic endothelial damage (e.g., bacterial endotoxin), by systemic contact activation of the clotting cascade (e.g., cardiopulmonary bypass), or by the release of procoagulants into the systemic circulation (e.g., malignancy). Table 15-26 presents an abbreviated list of disorders associated with the development of DIC. Although the most likely stimulus for DIC in W.K. is sepsis, both hypoxia and acidosis associated with respiratory compromise may also have contributed.

Treatment

46. Over the course of several hours, W.K. has developed more severe GI bleeding. Her Hct has fallen from 43% to 35%. What treatment course should be pursued? Should heparin therapy be given?

The most important element of treatment in patients with DIC is alleviation of the underlying cause to eliminate the stimulus for continued thrombosis and hemorrhage.[152] For W.K., this involves appropriate antibiotic therapy, as well as supportive measures to correct or prevent the hemodynamic, respiratory, and metabolic manifestations of shock. Fluid replacement, maintenance of blood pressure and cardiac output, and adequate oxygenation are essential components of the treatment of patients with DIC.

The selection of other therapies aimed at correcting the hemorrhagic or thrombotic manifestations of DIC are controversial and to some extent depend on whether hemorrhagic manifestations or thrombotic complications predominate in the clinical presentation. Initial treatment in patients with hemorrhage involves replacement of clotting components that have been consumed in DIC, guided by coagulation laboratory data.[153]

Transfusion of platelets, fresh frozen plasma (containing all clotting factors), and/or cryoprecipitate (containing factor VIII and fibrinogen) may be necessary, with close monitoring of platelet count and fibrinogen level.

Several approaches to restoring the inherent anticoagulant pathways that are disrupted in DIC have been attempted. Transfusion of AT concentrates may improve survival in DIC associated with sepsis.[154] Recombinant thrombomodulin was associated with a higher degree of resolution of DIC compared to heparin in a randomized clinical trial, but it is not yet commercially available.[155] Recombinant activated protein C (drotrecogin), which lowered mortality in patients with sepsis in the Prowess Trial, had its most significant impact on mortality in the subgroup of sepsis patients who had DIC.[156,157]

Anticoagulation with heparin in patients with DIC is controversial. In theory, because the initial pathological event in DIC is activation of the clotting system with formation of intravascular thrombin, the antithrombin activity of heparin should prevent further fibrin deposition and subsequent activation of fibrinolysis. However, randomized trials have not been conducted to confirm this potential benefit, and the role of heparin remains controversial. Emerging anticoagulants that are targeted more specifically at the underlying pathophysiology of thrombosis in DIC, recombinant tissue factor pathway inhibitor, and recombinant nematode anticoagulant protein c2 are being studied in phase II and phase III clinical trials, but are not yet part of routine care of patients with DIC.[152]

Finally, the use of the antifibrinolytic agents tranexamic acid and aminocaproic acid to control bleeding is relatively contraindicated. These agents may worsen the thrombotic complications of DIC, particularly if heparin is not used concurrently. However, antifibrinolytic therapy or recombinant activated factor VII (NovoSeven) may be used in patients with life-threatening bleeding who fail to respond to replacement of clotting components or to heparinization.

REFERENCES

1. Haines ST, Bussey HI. Thrombosis and the pharmacology of antithrombotic agents. *Ann Pharmacother.* 1997;29:892.
2. Simioni P et al. Inherited thrombophilia and venous thromboembolism. *Semin Thromb Hemost* 2006;32:700.
3. Colman RW et al. Overview of hemostasis. In: Colman RW et al., eds. Hemostasis and Thrombosis: Basic Principles and Clinical Practice. 5th ed. Philadelphia: Lippincott Williams & Wilkins; 2006.
4. George JN et al. Overview of platelet structure and function. In: Colman RW et al., eds. Hemostasis and Thrombosis: Basic Principles and Clinical Practice. 5th ed. Philadelphia: Lippincott Williams & Wilkins; 2006.
5. Nutescu E, Racine E. Traditional versus modern anticoagulant strategies: summary of the literature. *Am J Health-System Pharm* 2002;59(Suppl 6):s7.
6. Hirsh J, Raschke R. Heparin and low molecular weight heparin: the 7th ACCP conference on antithrombotic and thrombolytic therapy. *Chest* 2004;126(Suppl 3):188.
7. Petitou M et al. The synthetic pentasaccharide fondaparinux: first in a class of antithrombotic agents that selectively inhibit coagulation factor Xa. *Semin Thromb Hemost* 2002;28:393.
8. Warkentin TE, Greinacher A. Heparin-induced thrombocytopenia: recognition, treatment, and prevention: the seventh ACCP conference on antithrombotic and thrombolytic therapy. *Chest* 2004;126(3 Suppl):311S.
9. Lincoff AM et al. Bivalirudin and provisional glycoprotein IIb/IIIa blockade compared with heparin and planned glycoprotein IIb/IIIa blockade during percutaneous coronary intervention. *JAMA* 2003;289:853.
10. Ansell J. The pharmacology and management of the vitamin K antiagonists: the 7th ACCP conference on antithrombotic and thrombolytic therapy. *Chest* 2004;126(Suppl 3):204.
11. Wittkowsky AK. Pharmacogenomics and the management of oral anticoagulation. *Curr Hematol Rep* 2004;3:363.
12. Rieder MJ et al. Effect of VKORC1 haplotypes on transcriptional regulation and warfarin dose. *N Engl J Med* 2005;352:2285.
13. Kitchen S, Preston FE. Standardization of prothrombin time for laboratory control of oral anticoagulant therapy. *Semin Thromb Hemost* 1999; 25:17.
14. Bussey HI et al. Reliance on prothrombin time ratios causes significant errors in anticoagulation therapy. *Arch Intern Med* 1992;152:278.
15. Nelson DE. Current considerations in the use of the aPTT in monitoring unfractionated heparin. *Clin Lab Sci* 1999;12:359.
16. Olson JD et al. College of American Pathologists Conference XXXI on laboratory monitoring of anticoagulant therapy: laboratory monitoring of unfractionated heparin therapy. *Arch Pathol Lab Med* 1998;122:782.
17. Samama MM, Poller L. Contemporary laboratory monitoring of low-molecular-weight heparins. *Clin Lab Med* 1995;15:119.
18. Laposata M et al. College of American Pathologists Conference XXXI on laboratory monitoring of anticoagulant therapy: the clinical use and laboratory monitoring of low-molecular-weight heparin, danaparoid, hirudin and related compounds, and argatroban. *Arch Pathol Lab Med* 1998;122:799.
19. Haines ST, Bussey HI. Diagnosis of deep vein thrombosis. *Am J Health Syst Pharm* 1997;54:66.
20. Kahn SR. The clinical diagnosis of deep venous thrombosis: integrating incidence, risk factors, and symptoms and signs. *Arch Intern Med* 1998;158: 2315.
21. Geerts WH et al. Prevention of venous thromboembolism: the seventh ACCP conference on antithrombotic and thrombolytic therapy. *Chest* 2004;126(3 Suppl):338S.
22. Scarvelis D, Wells PS. Diagnosis and treatment of deep-vein thrombosis. *CMAJ* 2006;175:1087.
23. Qaseem A et al. Joint American Academy of Family Physicians/American College of Physicians Panel on Deep Venous Thrombosis/Pulmonary Embolism. Current diagnosis of venous thromboembolism in primary care: a clinical practice guideline from the American Academy of Family Physicians and the American College of Physicians. *Ann Fam Med* 2007;5:57.
24. Wells PS et al. Value of assessment of pretest probability of deep-vein thrombosis in clinical management. *Lancet* 1997;350:1795.
25. Wells PS et al. Evaluation of D-dimer in the diagnosis of suspected deep-vein thrombosis. *N Engl J Med* 2003;349:1227.
26. Buller HR et al. Antithrombotic therapy for venous thromboembolic disease: the seventh ACCP conference on antithrombotic and thrombolytic therapy. *Chest* 2004;126(3 Suppl):401S.
27. Schwiesow SJ et al. Use of a modified dosing weight for heparin therapy in a morbidly obese patient. *Ann Pharmacother* 2005;39:753.
28. Raschke RA. A weight-based heparin dosing nomogram compared with a "standard-care" nomogram: a randomized controlled trial. *Ann Intern Med* 1993;119:874.
29. Hull RD et al. The importance of initial heparin treatment on long-term clinical outcomes of antithrombotic therapy: the emerging theme of delayed recurrence. *Arch Intern Med* 1997;157: 2317.
30. Anand SS et al. Recurrent venous thrombosis and heparin therapy: an evaluation of the importance of early activated partial thromboplastin times. *Arch Intern Med* 1999;159:2029.
31. Gunnarson PS et al. Appropriate use of heparin: empiric vs. nomogram-based dosing. *Arch Intern Med* 1995;155:526.
32. Hylek E et al. Challenges in the effective use of unfractionated heparin in the hospitalized management of acute thrombosis. *Arch Intern Med* 2003;163:621.
33. Arepally GM, Ortel TL. Clinical practice: heparin-induced thrombocytopenia. *N Engl J Med* 2006;355:809.
34. Nutescu EA et al. New anticoagulant agents: direct thrombin inhibitors. *Clin Geriatr Med* 2006; 22:33.
35. Landefeld CS, Beyth RJ. Anticoagulation-related bleeding: clinical epidemiology, prediction and prevention. *Am J Med* 1993;85:315.
36. Levine MN et al. Hemorrhagic complications of anticoagulant treatment: the seventh ACCP conference on antithrombotic and thrombolytic therapy. *Chest* 2004;126(3 Suppl):287S.
37. Barbour LA et al. A prospective study of heparin-induced osteoporosis in pregnancy using bone densitometry. *Am J Obstet Gynecol* 1994;170:862.
38. Hommes DW et al. Subcutaneous heparin compared with continuous intravenous heparin administration in the initial treatment of deep vein thrombosis: a meta-analysis. *Ann Intern Med* 1992;116:279.
39. Kearon C et al. Comparison of fixed-dose weight-adjusted unfractionated heparin and low-molecular-weight heparin for acute treatment of venous thromboembolism. *JAMA* 2006;296:935.
40. Schulman S, Bijsterveld NR. Anticoagulants and their reversal. *Transfus Med Rev* 2007;21:37.
41. Haverkamp D et al. The use of specific antidotes as a response to bleeding complications during anticoagulant therapy for venous thromboembolism. J Thromb Haemost 2003;1:69.
42. Van Dongen CJ et al. Fixed dose subcutaneous low molecular weight heparins versus adjusted

dose unfractionated heparin for venous thromboembolism [review]. *Cochrane Database Syst Rev* 2004;4:CD001100.
43. Van Dongen CJ et al. Once versus twice daily LMWH for the initial treatment of venous thromboembolism [review]. *Cochrane Database Syst Rev* 2003;1:CD003074.
44. Segal JB et al. Outpatient therapy with low molecular weight heparin for the treatment of venous thromboembolism: a review of efficacy, safety, and costs. *Am J Med* 2003;115:298.
45. Rodger MA et al. The outpatient treatment of deep vein thrombosis delivers cost savings to patients and their families compared to inpatient therapy. *Thromb Res* 2003;112:13.
46. Matisse Investigators. Fondaparinux or enoxaparin for the initial treatment of symptomatic deep vein thrombosis: a randomized trial. *Ann Intern Med* 2004;140:867.
47. Dager WE et al. Special considerations with fondaparinux therapy: heparin-induced thrombocytopenia and wound healing. *Pharmacotherapy* 2004;24(7 Pt 2):88s.
48. Merli G et al. Subcutaneous enoxaparin once or twice daily compared with intravenous unfractionated heparin for treatment of venous thromboembolic disease. *Ann Intern Med* 2001;134:191.
49. Lim W et al. Meta-analysis: low-molecular-weight heparin and bleeding in patients with severe renal insufficiency. *Ann Intern Med* 2006;144:673.
50. Shprecher AR et al. Peak antifactor X_a activity produced by dalteparin treatment in patients with renal impairment compared with controls. *Pharmacotherapy* 2005;25:817.
51. Siguret V et al. Elderly patients treated with tinzaparin (Innohep) administered once daily (175 anti-X_a IU/kg): anti-X_a and anti-IIa activities over 10 days. *Thromb Haemost* 2000;84:800.
52. Sanderink GJ et al. Pharmacokinetics and pharmacodynamics of the prophylactic dose of enoxaparin once daily over 4 days in patients with renal impairment. *Thromb Res* 2002;105:225.
53. Wittkowsky AK, Nutescu EA. Thrombosis: treatment and prevention in patients with chronic illness. In: Schumock G et al., eds. Pharmacotherapy Self-Assessment Program. 5th ed. Kansas City: American College of Clinical Pharmacy. 2005;VIII(Chronic Illnesses):169 .
54. Harenberg J. Is laboratory monitoring of low molecular weight heparin therapy necessary? Yes. *J Thromb Haemost* 2004;2:547.
55. Caprini JA et al. Effective risk stratification of surgical and nonsurgical patients for venous thromboembolic disease. *Semin Hematol* 2001;38(2 Suppl 5):12.
56. Heit JA. Related articles, links venous thromboembolism: disease burden, outcomes and risk factors. *J Thromb Haemost.* 2005;3:1611.
57. Dalen JE. Pulmonary embolism: what have we learned since Virchow? Natural history, pathophysiology, and diagnosis. *Chest* 2002;122:1440.
58. Wells PS. Advances in the diagnosis of venous thromboembolism. *J Thromb Thrombolysis* 2006; 21:31.
59. Chagnon I et al. Comparison of two clinical prediction rules and implicit assessment among patients with suspected pulmonary embolism. *Am J Med* 2002;113:269.
60. Kearon C et al. An evaluation of D-dimer in the diagnosis of pulmonary embolism: a randomized trial. *Ann Intern Med* 2006;144:812.
61. Goldhaber SZ et al. International Cooperative Pulmonary Embolism Registry detects high mortality rate. *Circulation* 1997;96(Suppl 1):1.
62. Weitz JI. Emerging anticoagulants for the treatment of venous thromboembolism. *Thromb Haemost* 2006;96:274.
63. Snow V et al. Management of venous thromboembolism: a clinical practice guideline from the American College of Physicians and the American Academy of Family Physicians. *Ann Intern Med* 2007;146:204.
64. Quinlan DJ et al. Low-molecular-weight heparin compared with intravenous unfractionated heparin for treatment of pulmonary embolism: a meta-analysis of randomized, controlled trials. *Ann Intern Med* 2004;140:175.
65. Buller HR et al. Subcutaneous fondaparinux versus intravenous unfractionated heparin in the initial treatment of pulmonary embolism. *N Engl J Med* 2003;349:1695.
66. Hirsh J et al. American Heart Association/ American College of Cardiology Foundation guide to warfarin therapy. *J Am Coll Cardiol* 2003; 41:1633.
67. D'Angelo A et al. Relationship between international normalized ratio values, vitamin K–dependent clotting factor levels and in vivo prothrombin activation during the early and steady phases of oral anticoagulant treatment. *Hematologica* 2002;87:1074.
68. Leech BF, Carter CJ. Falsely elevated INR results due to the sensitivity of the thromboplastin reagent to heparin. *Am J Clin Pathol* 1998;109:764.
69. Kearon C et al. Effect of warfarin on activated partial thromboplastin time in patients receiving heparin. *Arch Intern Med* 1998;158:1140.
70. James AH et al. Factors affecting the maintenance dose of warfarin. *J Clin Pathol* 1992;45:704.
71. Wittkowsky AK. *Warfarin*. In: Murphy J (ed). Clinical Pharmacokinetics (4th Edition). American Society of Health System Pharmacists; Bethesda, 2007.
72. Pengo V et al. A simple scheme to initiate oral anticoagulant treatment in outpatients with nonrheumatic atrial fibrillation. *Am J Cardiol* 2001; 88:1214.
73. Siguret V et al. Initiation of warfarin therapy in elderly medical inpatients: a safe and accurate regimen. *Am J Med* 2005;118:225.
74. Tait RC, Sefcick A. A warfarin induction regimen for out-patient anticoagulation in patients with atrial fibrillation. *Br J Haematol* 1998;101:450.
75. Kovacs MJ et al. Prospective assessment of a nomogram for the initiation of oral anticoagulant therapy for outpatient treatment of venous thromboembolism. *Pathophysiol Haemost Thromb* 2002;32:131.
76. Kovacs MJ et al. Comparison of 10 mg and 5 mg warfarin initiation nomograms together with low molecular weight heparin for outpatient treatment of acute venous thromboembolism. *Ann Intern Med* 2003;138:714.
77. Eckhoff CD et al. Initiating warfarin therapy: 5 mg versus 10 mg. *Ann Pharmacother* 2004;38:2115.
78. Crowther MA et al. Warfarin: less may be better. *Ann Intern Med* 1997;127:332.
79. Crowther MA et al. A randomized trial comparing 5-mg and 10-mg warfarin loading doses. *Arch Intern Med* 1999;159:46.
80. Hart RG et al. Oral anticoagulants and intracranial hemorrhage: facts and hypotheses. *Stroke* 1995;26:1471.
81. Palareti G et al. Bleeding complications of oral anticoagulant treatment: an inception-cohort, prospective collaborative study (ISCOAT). *Lancet* 1996;348:423.
82. Fang MC et al. Advanced age, anticoagulation intensity, and risk for intracranial hemorrhage among patients taking warfarin for atrial fibrillation. *Ann Intern Med* 2004;141(10):745.
83. Garcia D et al. Warfarin maintenance dosing patterns in clinical practice: implications for safer anticoagulation in the elderly population. *Chest* 2005;127:2049.
84. Beyth RJ, Landefeld CS. Anticoagulants in older patients: a safety perspective. *Drugs Aging* 1995;6:45.
85. Beyth RJ et al. A multicomponent intervention to prevent major bleeding complications in older patients receiving warfarin. *Ann Intern Med* 2000;133:687.
86. Copland M et al. Oral anticoagulation and hemorrhagic complications in an elderly population with atrial fibrillation. *Arch Intern Med* 2001;161: 2125.
87. Fihn SD et al. The risk for and severity of bleeding complications in elderly patients treated with warfarin. The National Consortium of Anticoagulation Clinics. *Ann Intern Med* 1996;124:970.
88. Chan YC et al. Warfarin-induced skin necrosis. *Br J Surg* 2000;87:266.
89. Sallah S. Warfarin and heparin-induced skin necrosis and the purple toe syndrome: infrequent complications of anticoagulant treatment. *Thromb Haemost* 1997;78:785.
90. Chiquette E et al. Comparison of an anticoagulation clinic with usual medical care. *Arch Intern Med* 1998;185:1641.
91. Witt DM et al. Effect of a centralized clinical pharmacy anticoagulation service on the outcomes of anticoagulation therapy. *Chest* 2005;127:1515.
92. Fihn SD et al. Risk factors for complications of chronic warfarin therapy: a multicenter study. *Ann Intern Med* 1993;118:511.
93. Booth SL et al. Food sources and dietary intakes of vitamin K-1 (phylloquinone) in the American diet: data from the FDA Total Diet Study. *J Am Diet Assoc* 1996;96:149.
94. Franco V et al. Role of dietary vitamin K intake in chronic oral anticoagulation: prospective evidence from observational and randomized protocols. *Am J Med* 2004;116:651.
95. Sconce E et al. Patients with unstable control have a poorer dietary intake of vitamin K compared to patients with stable control of anticoagulation. *Thromb Haemost* 2005;93:872.
96. Booth SL et al. Vitamin K: a practical guide to the dietary management of patients on warfarin. *Nutr Rev* 1999;57(9 Pt 1):288.
97. Nutescu EA et al. Warfarin and its interactions with foods, herbs and other dietary supplements. *Expert Opin Drug Saf* 2006;5:433.
98. Weathermon R, Crabb DW. Alcohol and medication interactions. *Alcohol Res Health* 1999;23:40.
99. Ha CE et al. Investigation of the effects of ethanol on warfarin binding to human serum albumin. *J Biomed Sci* 2000;7:114.
100. Havrda DE et al. Enhanced antithrombotic effect of warfarin associated with low-dose alcohol consumption. *Pharmacotherapy* 2005;25:303.
101. Demirkan K et al. Response to warfarin and other oral anticoagulants: effects of disease states. *South Med J* 2000;93:448.
102. Higashi M et al. Influence of CYP2C9 genetic variants on the risk of overanticoagulation and of bleeding events during warfarin therapy. *JAMA* 2002;287:1690–1698.
103. Aithal GP et al. Warfarin dose requirement and CYP2C9 polymorphisms. *Lancet* 1999;353:1972.
104. DAndrea G et al. A polymorphism in the VCORC1 gene is associated with interindividual variability in the dose-anticoagulant effect of warfarin. *Blood* 2005;105:645.
105. Sconce EA et al. The impact of CYP2C9 and VCORC1 genetic polymorphism and patient characteristics upon warfarin dose requirements: proposal for a new dosing regimen. *Blood* 2005;1-6:2329.
106. Hawk TL, Havrda DE. Effect of stress on International Normalized Ratio during warfarin therapy. *Ann Pharmacother* 2002;36:617.
107. Shibata Y et al. Influence of physical activity on warfarin therapy. *Thromb Haemost* 1998;80:203.
108. Zevin S, Benowitz NL. Drug interactions with tobacco smoking: an update. *Clin Pharmacokinet* 1999;36:425.
109. Kuykendall JR et al. Possible warfarin failure due to interaction with smokeless tobacco. *Ann Pharmacother* 2004;38:595.
110. Gage BF et al. Management and dosing of warfarin therapy. *Am J Med* 2000;109:481.
111. Wong W et al. Influence of warfarin regimen type on clinical and monitoring outcomes in stable patients in an anticoagulation management service. *Pharmacotherapy* 1999;19:1385.
112. DeZee KJ et al. Treatment of excessive anticoagulation with phytonadione (vitamin K). *Arch Intern Med* 2006;166:391.

113. Hylek EM et al. Clinical predictors of prolonged delay in return of the International Normalized Ratio to within the therapeutic range after excessive anticoagulation with warfarin. *Ann Intern Med* 2001;135:393.
114. Weibert RT et al. Correction of excessive anticoagulation with low-dose oral vitamin K_1. *Ann Intern Med* 1997;125:959.
115. Crowther MA et al. Oral vitamin K lowers the international normalized ratio more rapidly than subcutaneous vitamin K in the treatment of warfarin-associated coagulopathy: a randomized, controlled trial. *Ann Intern Med* 2002;137;251.
116. Hung A et al. A prospective randomized study to determine the optimal dose of intravenous vitamin K in reversal of over-warfarinization. *Br J Haematol* 2001;113:839.
117. Shields RC et al. Efficacy and safety of intravenous phytonadione (vitamin K1) in patients on long-term oral anticoagulant therapy. *Mayo Clin Proc* 2001;76:260.
118. Bates SM et al. Use of antithrombotic agents during pregnancy. *Chest* 2004;126(Suppl 3):627.
119. Laurent P et al. Low-molecular-weight heparins: a guide to their optimum use in pregnancy. *Drugs* 2002;62:463.
120. Greer IA. Anticoagulants in pregnancy. *J Thromb Thrombolysis* 2006;21:57.
121. James AH et al. Low-molecular-weight heparin for thromboprophylaxis in pregnant women with mechanical heart valves. *J Matern Fetal Neonatal Med* 2006;19:543.
122. Singer DE et al. Antithrombotic therapy in atrial fibrillation. The 7th ACCP conference on antithrombotic and thrombolytic therapy. *Chest* 2004;126(Suppl 3):429.
123. Bjerkelund CJ et al. The efficacy of anticoagulant therapy in preventing embolism related to DC electrical conversion of atrial fibrillation. *Am J Cardiol* 1969;23:208.
124. Klein AL et al. Use of transesophageal echocardiography to guide cardioversion in patients with atrial fibrillation. *N Engl J Med* 2001;344:1411.
125. Fuster V et al. ACC/AHA/ESC 2006 guidelines for the management of patients with atrial fibrillation. *Circulation* 2006;114:e257.
126. Atrial Fibrillation Investigators. Risk factors for stroke and efficacy of antithrombotic therapy in atrial fibrillation: analysis of pooled data from five randomized controlled trials. *Arch Intern Med* 1994;154:1449.
127. Atrial Fibrillation Investigators. The efficacy of aspirin in patients with atrial fibrillation: analysis of pooled data from three randomized trials. *Arch Intern Med* 1997;157:1237.
128. Salem DN et al. Antithrombotic therapy in valvular heart disease-native and prosthetic. *Chest* 2004;126(Suppl 3):457.
129. Cannegeiter SC et al. Optimal oral anticoagulant therapy in patients with mechanical heart valves. *N Engl J Med* 1995;333:11.
130. Saour JN et al. Trial of different intensities of anticoagulation in patients with prosthetic heart valves. *N Engl J Med* 1990;322:428.
131. Bonow RO et al. ACC/AHA 2006 guidelines for the management of patients with valvular heart disease. *Circulation* 2006;114:84.
132. Dunn A. Perioperative management of oral anticoagulation: when and how to bridge. *J Thromb Thrombolysis* 2006;21:85.
133. Douketis JD et al. Low molecular weight heparin as bridging anticoagulation during interruption of warfarin: assessment of a standardized periprocedural anticoagulation regimen. *Arch Intern Med* 2004;164:1319.
134. Kovacs MJ et al. Single-arm study of bridging therapy with low molecular weight heparin for patients at risk of arterial embolism who require temporary interruption of warfarin. *Circulation* 2004;110:1658.
135. Sypropouos AC et al. Clinical outcomes of unfractionated heparin or low molecular weight heparin as bridging therapy in patients on long-term oral anticoagulants: the REGIMEN registry. *J Thromb Haemost* 2006;4:1246.
136. Spyropoulus AC et al. Costs and clinical outcomes associated with low molecular weight heparin versus unfractionated heparin for perioperative bridging receiving long term oral anticoagulant therapy. *Chest* 2004;125:1642.
137. Scully C, Wolff A. Oral surgery in patients on anticoagulant therapy. *Oral Surg Oral Med Oral Pathol Oral Radiol Endod* 2002;94:57.
138. Patatanian E, Fugate SE. Hemostatic mouthwashes in anticoagulated patients undergoing dental extraction. *Ann Pharmacother* 2006;40:2205.
139. Hansten PD, Wittkowsky AK. Warfarin drug interactions. In: Ansell J et al., eds. Managing Oral Anticoagulant Therapy: Clinical and Operational Guidelines. 2nd ed. Gaithersburg, MD: Aspen; 2002.
140. Holbrook AM et al. Systematic overview of warfarin and its drug and food interactions. *Arch Intern Med* 2005;165:1095.
141. Wittkowsky AK. Drug interactions with oral anticoagulants. In: Colman RW et al., eds. Hemostasis and Thrombosis: Basic Principles and Clinical Practice. 5th ed. Philadelphia: Lippincott Williams & Wilkins; 2006.
142. Sands CD et al. Revisiting the significance of warfarin protein-binding displacement interactions. *Ann Pharmacother* 2002;36:1642.
143. Kerin NZ et al. The incidence, magnitude and time course of the amiodarone-warfarin interaction. *Arch Intern Med* 1988;148:1779.
144. Chan TYK. Adverse interactions between warfarin and nonsteroidal antiinflammatory drugs: mechanisms, clinical significance, and avoidance. *Ann Pharmacother* 1995;29:1274.
145. Shorr RI et al. Concurrent use of nonsteroidal antiinflammatory drugs and oral anticoagulants places elderly persons at high risk for hemorrhagic peptic ulcer disease. *Arch Intern Med* 1993;153:1665.
146. Hylek EM et al. Acetaminophen and other risk factors for excessive warfarin anticoagulation. *JAMA* 1998;279:657.
147. Kwan D et al. The effects of acetaminophen on pharmacokinetics and pharmacodynamics of warfarin. *J Clin Pharmacol* 1999;39:68.
148. Levi M. Current understanding of disseminated intravascular coagulation. *Br J Haematol* 2004;124:567.
149. Levi M et al. The diagnosis of disseminated intravascular coagulation. *Blood Rev* 2002;16:217.
150. Taylor FBJ et al. Towards definition, clinical and laboratory criteria, and a scoring system for disseminated intravascular coagulation. *Thromb Haemost* 2001;86:1327.
151. Bakhtiari K et al. Prospective validation of the International Society of Thrombosis and Haemostasis scoring system for disseminated intravascular coagulation. *Crit Care Med* 2004;32:2416.
152. Levi M, deJonge E, van der Poll T. New treatment strategies for disseminated intravascular coagulation based on current understanding of the pathophysiology. *Ann Med* 2004;36:41.
153. deJone E et al. Anticoagulation factor concentrates in disseminated intravascular coagulation: rationale for use and clinical experience. *Semin Thromb Hemost* 2001;27:667.
154. Wiedermann CJ, Kaneider NC. A systematic review of antithrombin concentrate use in patients with disseminated intravascular coagulation of severe sepsis. *Blood Coag Fibrinolysis* 2006;17:521.
155. Saito H et al. Efficacy and safety of recombinant human soluble thrombomodulin (ART-123) in disseminated intravascular coagulation: results of a phase III, randomized, double-blind clinical trial. *J Thromb Haemost* 2007;5:31.
156. Bernard GR et al. Efficacy and safety of recombinant human activated protein C for severe sepsis. N Engl J Med 2001;344;699.
157. Dhainaut JF et al. Treatment effects of drotrecogin alfa (activated) in patients with severe sepsis with or without overt disseminated intravascular coagulation. *J Thromb Haemost* 2004;2:1924.
158. Beyth RJ et al. Prospective evaluation of an index for predicting risk of major bleeding in outpatient treated with warfarin. *Am J Med* 1998;105:91.

CHAPTER 16

Ischemic Heart Disease: Anginal Syndromes

Toby C. Trujillo and Paul E. Nolan

Angina pectoris, whether stable or unstable, is one common manifestation of coronary heart disease (CHD). Other manifestations can include myocardial infarction (MI), heart failure (HF), arrhythmias, as well as sudden cardiac death. By far the most common cause of CHD is narrowing of the coronary arteries through the presence of atherosclerotic plaques, or coronary artery disease (CAD). Because angina is a marker for underlying heart disease, its management is of great importance.

Definitions

Angina pectoris is a "clinical syndrome characterized by discomfort in the chest, jaw, shoulder, back, or arm."[1,2] Although angina is typically brought on by exertion and relieved by nitroglycerin (NTG), its presentation is variable. At one extreme, angina occurs predictably with strenuous exercise; at the other, angina can develop unexpectedly with little or no exertion.

Patients who have a reproducible pattern of angina that is associated with a certain level of physical activity have *chronic stable angina* or exertional angina. In contrast, patients with unstable angina experience new-onset angina or a change in their angina intensity, frequency, or duration.[3] Both chronic stable angina and unstable angina often reflect underlying atherosclerotic narrowing of coronary arteries. Classic Prinzmetal's variant angina, or vasospastic angina, occurs in patients without CHD; it is caused by a spasm of the coronary artery that decreases myocardial blood flow.[3,4] When coronary vasospasm occurs at the site of a fixed atherosclerotic plaque, mixed angina can result.[3]

Silent (asymptomatic) myocardial ischemia, which can result in transient changes in myocardial perfusion, function, or electrical activity, is detected on an electrocardiogram (ECG) in most patients with angina.[3,5] The patient, however, does not experience chest pain or other signs of angina (e.g., jaw pain, shortness of breath [SOB]) during these episodes. Silent myocardial ischemia also can occur in patients with no angina history (see Chapter 18, Myocardial Infarction).

Epidemiology

Cardiovascular disease (CVD) is the leading cause of death in the United States (U.S.), and death caused by CHD is responsible for approximately half of all deaths from CVD. *Chronic stable angina* is the first clinical sign of CHD in approximately 50% of patients.[3,6] CVD remains the leading cause of death in the U.S. despite a decline in the death rate from CVD in the late 20th century. The incidence of angina is difficult to assess because it often is unrecognized by patients and physicians. Current estimates are that of the 16,000,000 patients with CHD, approximately 9,100,000 have chronic stable angina.[6]

Although CHD accounts for one of every five deaths in the United States, individual mortality varies according to the patient's age, gender, cardiovascular risk profile, myocardial contractility, coronary anatomy, and specific anginal syndrome. The annual mortality rate increases as the number of coronary vessels with high-grade atherosclerotic lesions increases. Patients with left main coronary artery disease have an increased mortality rate compared with patients without left main CAD. Similarly, patients with diminished left ventricular (LV) function (ejection fraction [EF] <50%) have higher mortality rates compared with patients without impaired LV function.

In addition to the high morbidity and mortality associated with CHD, the economic cost to the U.S. health care system is substantial. Total direct and indirect costs associated with CHD are estimated to be $156.4 billion.[6]

Coronary Anatomy

Figure 16-1 illustrates the normal distribution of the major coronary arteries, although variation is common from individual to individual. The anterior and lateral portions of the left ventricle receive blood flow from the left coronary artery, usually the largest diameter and shortest of all coronary arteries. From its main stem, the left coronary artery divides into its two major branches: the left anterior descending (LAD) coronary artery and the circumflex. The LAD further subdivides into the first diagonal, the first septal, the right ventricular, the minor septals, the second diagonal, and the apical branches. Similarly, the circumflex subdivides into four or five branches, the largest branch being the obtuse marginal.[7]

The right coronary artery (RCA) supplies blood flow to most of the right ventricle as well as the posterior part of the left ventricle. As with the LAD, the RCA branches into major vessels, which supply blood flow to specific areas of the heart. In order of origin, the RCA divides into the conus branch, sinus node branch, right ventricular branches, atrial branch, acute marginal branch, atrioventricular (AV) node branch, posterior descending, LV, and left atrial branches.[7] Because of wide variation in coronary artery distribution and the need to confirm the precise location of atherosclerotic plaques, most patients with angina undergo coronary arteriography. Patients with severe left main CAD are at higher risk because obstruction of this large coronary artery jeopardizes almost the entire left ventricle. Similarly, patients with three-vessel CAD are at higher risk than patients with single-vessel disease (see Chapter 17, Myocardial Infarction).

Pathophysiology

Angina pectoris typically occurs when myocardial oxygen demand exceeds myocardial oxygen supply (perfusion). The underlying pathologic condition of this mismatch invariably is the presence of atherosclerosis in one or more of the epicardial coronary arteries (conductance vessels).[1–3] If the size of the atherosclerotic plaque obscures <50% of the diameter of the vessel, coronary blood flow can be augmented sufficiently during exertion by the intramyocardial arterioles (resistance vessels), and the patient is pain free. In patients with chronic stable angina, most coronary artery stenoses are >70%. A linear decrease in coronary blood flow occurs as the plaque occupies more of the arterial lumen until high-grade (>80%) obstruction develops. At this point, the decrease in blood flow is out of proportion to plaque size.[8] The impaired blood flow with atherosclerotic lesions may be adversely affected by vasomotor dysfunction leading to inappropriate vasoconstriction and further reduction in blood supply.[9] Functionally, coronary blood flow is absent when lesions obstruct >95% of the vessel lumen.[8]

Collateral blood vessels (i.e., side branches of a coronary artery that join one of the three principal arteries or connect two points along the same artery) may offer protection against myocardial ischemia. The distribution and extent of collateral vessels are variable. These usually are very small and have no function in the normal heart. If blood flow is obstructed, however, collateral vessels assume more importance and can restore some myocardial blood flow. When myocardial oxygen demand is increased excessively, however, collateral blood flow usually is insufficient, and angina or other myocardial ischemia syndromes develop.[3,10]

A thorough understanding of the determinants of myocardial oxygen supply and demand is needed to better comprehend the rationale for the use of traditional pharmacotherapeutic agents in the treatment of stable and unstable anginal syndromes.

Myocardial Oxygen Supply and Demand

The oxygen demand of the heart is determined by its work load. The major determinants of myocardial oxygen consumption are heart rate, contractility, and intramyocardial wall tension during systole (Fig. 16-2; also, see Chapter 18, Heart Failure). Intramyocardial wall tension, which is the force the heart is required to develop and sustain during contraction, is affected primarily by changes in ventricular chamber pressures and volume. Both enlargement of the ventricle and increased pressure within the ventricle increase the systolic wall force and consequently myocardial oxygen demand. Increases in contractility and heart rate also result in increased oxygen demand. Pharmacologic control of angina is, in part, directed toward decreasing the myocardial oxygen demand by decreasing heart rate, myocardial contractility, or ventricular volume and pressures.[8]

Of the many factors that affect oxygen supply to the heart (Fig. 16-2), coronary blood flow and oxygen extraction are most important. Oxygen extraction by heart cells is high (~70%–75%) even at rest. When extra demand is placed on the heart, myocardial oxygen extraction increases slightly and

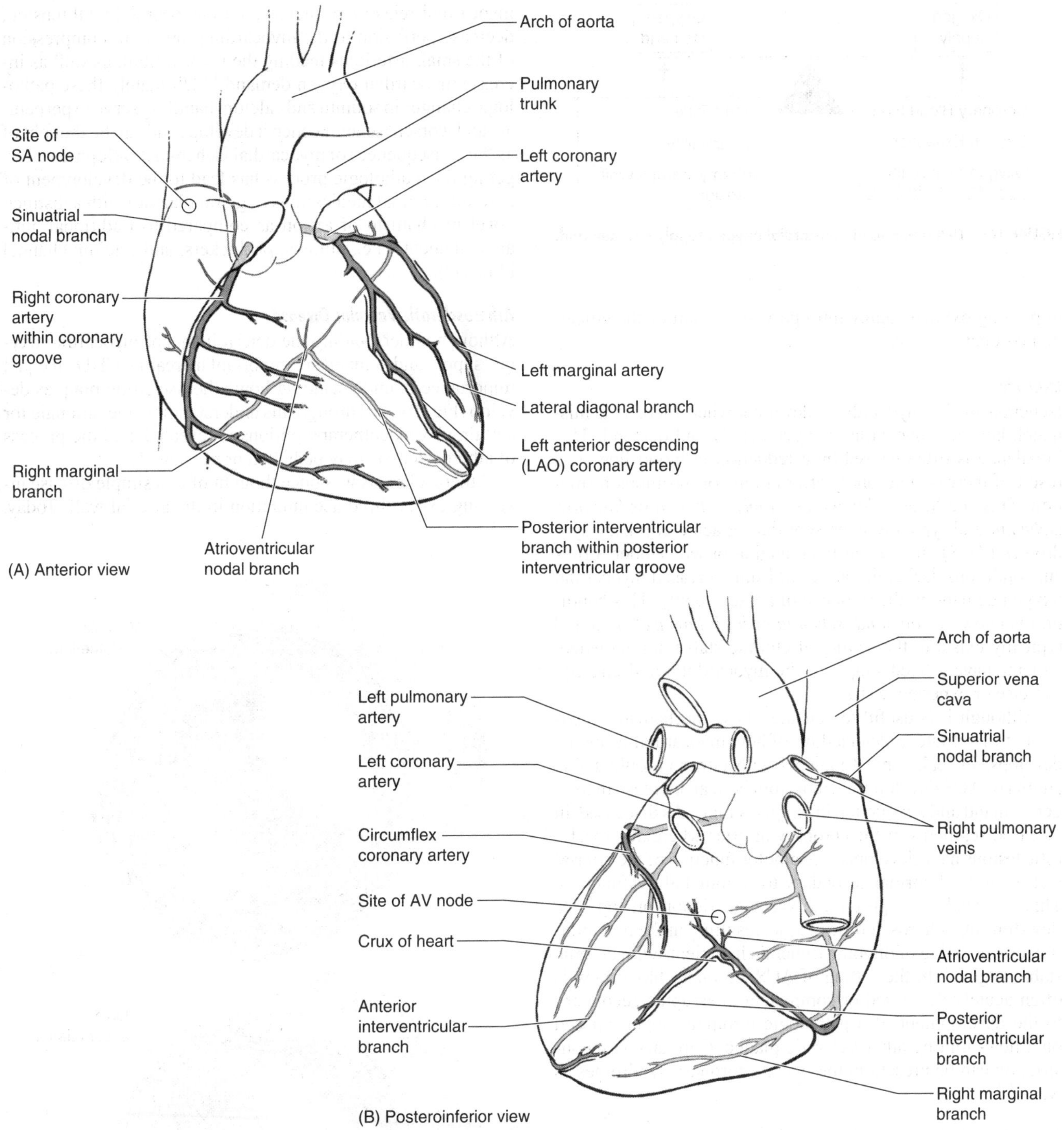

FIGURE 16-1 Coronary arteries. The right coronary artery (RCA) originates from the aorta and courses in the atrioventricular (coronary) groove to reach the posterior surface of the heart. The left coronary artery splits into the circumflex branch that supplies blood to the lateral and posterior walls of the left ventricle, and a left anterior descending (LAD) branch, which supplies blood to the anterior wall of the left ventricle.

plateaus at approximately 80%. Because oxygen extraction is increased only modestly when the heart is heavily stressed, high oxygen demands must be met by increases in coronary blood flow. Sudden increases in oxygen demand lead to a rapid decrease in coronary vascular resistance and an increase in coronary blood flow. The mechanisms by which coronary artery resistance is decreased during increased demand are not completely understood, but likely involve various mediators, such as adenosine and nitric oxide (NO) released from the myocytes and endothelium.[8] The oxygen content of arterial blood also is important. Therefore, the hematocrit (Hct), hemoglobin (Hgb), and arterial blood gases (ABG) should be monitored. In a similar fashion to targeting determinants of myocardial oxygen demand, pharmacologic control of angina is directed at

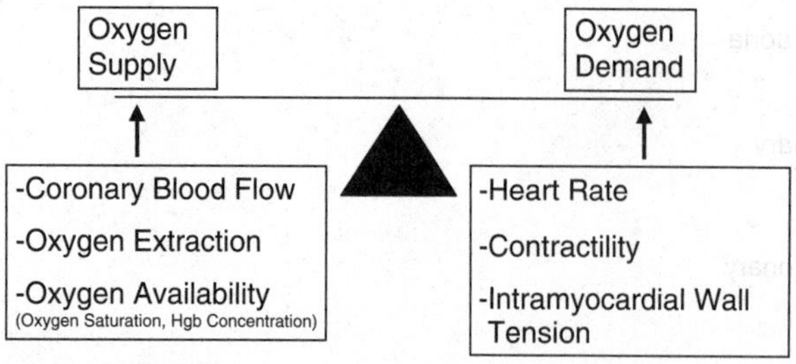

FIGURE 16-2 Determinants of myocardial oxygen supply and demand.

improving oxygen supply through vasodilation of the epicardial coronary arteries.

Ischemia

Ischemia in the myocardium develops when there is a mismatch between myocardial oxygen supply and demand. This imbalance is often caused by a reduction in blood flow as a result of increased coronary arterial tone or thrombus formation. This condition is known as *supply ischemia* or *low-flow ischemia* and typically is present during acute coronary syndromes (ACS) such as unstable angina or MI. Under different conditions, ischemia can result from increased myocardial oxygen demand in the presence of a fixed supply. This condition is known as *demand ischemia* or *high-flow ischemia* and typically exists in the setting of chronic stable angina where patients have a fixed supply to the myocardium and undergo exercise or experience stress.[3,8]

Although it is useful to consider these mechanisms separately to facilitate understanding of how myocardial ischemia develops, in reality most patients with either chronic stable angina or ACS develop ischemia from both an increase in oxygen demand and a reduction in oxygen supply. As discussed, in diseased segments of the coronary arteries where atherosclerotic lesions have developed, vasomotor function of the arterial wall is often abnormal secondary to endothelial dysfunction. This can lead to inappropriate vasoconstriction on top of a flow-limiting atherosclerotic plaque, resulting in the precipitation or worsening of ongoing ischemia in patients with chronic stable angina.[8] In the setting of ACS, coronary blood flow is often acutely decreased or completely interrupted secondary to the development of a pathologic thrombus superimposed on a flow-limiting atherosclerotic plaque. Coronary vasoconstriction can be present in these acute coronary syndromes as well.[11,12]

Intracellular Sodium and Calcium Handling

Recent investigations highlight the role of the late sodium current (I_{Na}) in the development and maintenance of myocardial ischemia. Most sodium enters the myocardium in phase 0 of the action potential. Under normal conditions, however, a small amount of sodium will enter the cell during phase 2 (plateau phase) of the action potential.[13] When ischemia is present, sodium handling is altered such that a substantial increase occurs in the late I_{Na}. The increase in intracellular sodium triggers an increase in the influx of calcium through the reverse mode of the sodium-calcium exchanger. The net result of the alterations in intracellular ion handling is intracellular calcium overload.[14,15] Increases in intracellular calcium impair myocardial relaxation, increase intramyocardial wall tension, decrease perfusion to the myocardium owing to compression of the small arterioles feeding the myocardium, as well as increase myocardial oxygen demand.[16] Ultimately these pathologic changes in sodium and calcium handling serve to perpetuate and worsen ischemia once it develops and can be thought of as the consequences of myocardial ischemia development. Targeting this pathologic process has lead to the development of new anti-anginal medications (e.g., ranolazine) with a distinct, novel mechanism of action as compared to traditional anti-anginal agents (i.e., nitrates, β-blockers, and calcium channel blockers).

Atherosclerotic Vascular Disease

Although understanding the determinants of myocardial oxygen supply and demand are important in treating CHD, of equal importance is understanding how atherosclerotic plaques develop (Fig. 16-3). Through this understanding, the rationale for certain pharmacotherapy options is revealed, and the process of atherosclerosis may be halted or prevented.

Atherosclerosis was once thought of as a simple disease involving excess lipid accumulation in the arterial wall. Today,

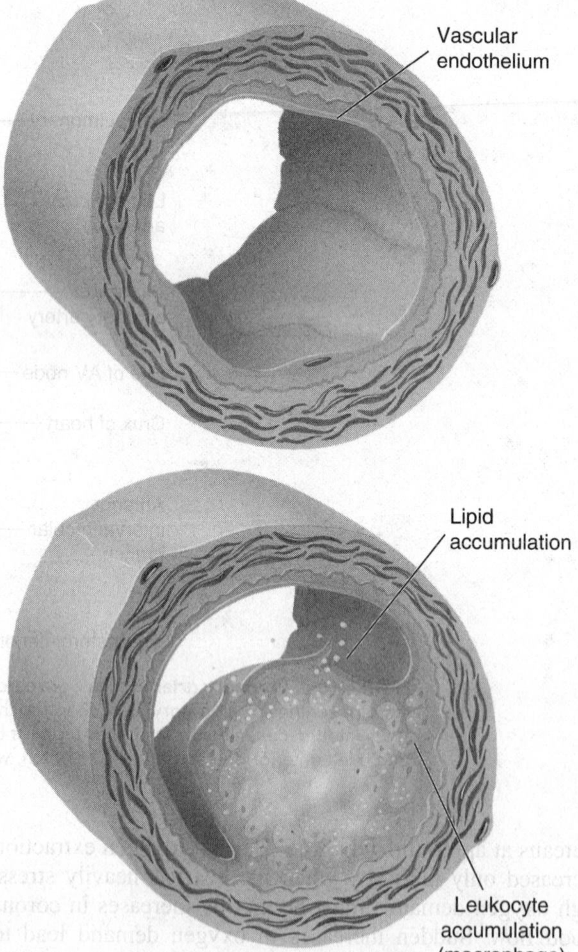

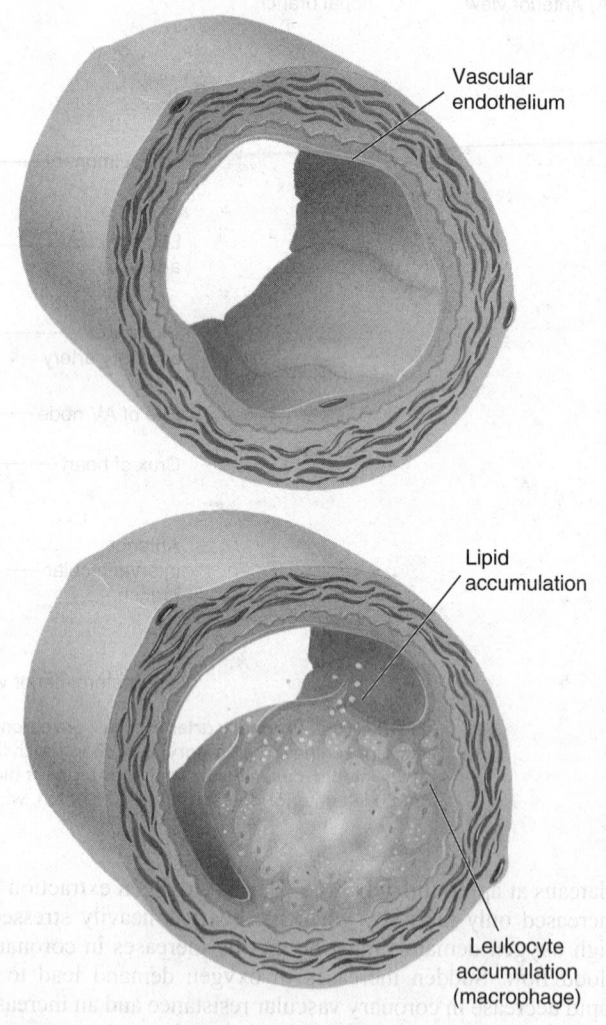

FIGURE 16-3 Process of atherosclerosis. (Copyright © Anatomical Chart Co., Hagerstown, MD.)

atherosclerosis is recognized as a complex and lifelong process. Recent advances in vascular biology demonstrate that inflammation plays a fundamental role in all stages of the atherosclerotic process. Examination of atherosclerotic lesions demonstrates that each plaque contains elements of inflammation and a fibroproliferative response. Although the initial stages of atherosclerosis remain speculative, it is generally thought that the first step is lipid accumulation (primarily low-density lipoprotein cholesterol [LDL-C]) in the vascular wall and subsequent oxidation of LDL lipoproteins. This is followed by leukocyte recruitment and accumulation in the vessel wall. Early lesions (fatty streaks) are present in all people at a young age and primarily consist of activated macrophages and T lymphocytes. Once within the arterial wall, the leukocyte can take up oxidized cholesterol and become a lipid-laden macrophage (foam cell). As lesions progress, smooth muscle cells (SMC) migrate, proliferate, and secrete large amounts of extracellular matrix (collagen), promoted by the release of several proinflammatory cytokines produced by leukocytes. The end result is the presence of an elevated plaque, which occludes the vessel lumen (also see Chapter 12, Dyslipidemias, Atherosclerosis, and Coronary Heart Disease). The inflammatory process is not only involved in the initiation and a development of atherosclerosis, but also is directly involved in the acute thrombotic complications of atherosclerosis, such as MI or unstable angina. Cytokines produced by activated macrophages induce the production of proteolytic enzymes, which break down the extracellular matrix and render the plaque more susceptible to rupture.[17,18]

A key factor in plaque formation is the functional status of the vascular endothelium (Fig. 16-4). Historically, the endothelium was thought to act simply as the inner barrier of blood vessels. This single-cell layer, however, has several functions, including the synthesis and secretion of many different substances and the regulation of the local vascular environment. One of the key substances synthesized is endothelium-derived relaxing factor (EDRF), identified as nitric oxide. Nitric oxide has vasodilatory, antithrombotic, anti-inflammatory, and growth-inhibiting properties. In the response to injury hypothesis, the endothelium is damaged and loses the ability to secrete NO and the ability to regulate the vascular environment. Without NO, the endothelium facilitates inflammation, thromboses, and extracellular growth. In this setting, atherosclerotic plaques can develop.[19,20]

Traditional risk factors, such as smoking, hypertension, hyperlipidemia, diabetes, and obesity, are linked to the process of atherosclerosis through their ability to produce oxidative stress within the vasculature. Increased oxidative stress leads to progressive decreases in NO levels and endothelial dysfunction, providing the substrate for atherosclerosis to develop.[18] In addition, dietary patterns typically seen in western industrialized countries have been linked to increased oxidative stress within the vasculature. This may partially explain the link between dietary patterns and development of atherosclerosis.[21] Recent research provides a more in-depth understanding of the link between obesity and the development of CAD. Adipose tissue, rather than just being a passive storage vehicle, is a metabolically active organ that secretes a number of active cytokines that promote inflammation and oxidative stress within the vasculature.[22] Adiponectin levels are also decreased in obesity, which further serves to promote atherosclerosis development.[23] The role of a healthy lifestyle and dietary pattern are both more crucial than ever in preventing the development or progression of CAD.

Although traditional risk factors have long been appreciated as the underlying cause for the development of CAD, continuing research efforts have attempted to identify novel risk factors to refine risk assessment for the development of CAD. The novel risk factors include C-reactive protein, homocysteine, fibrinogen, and lipoprotein(a), among others.[24] Findings from the INTERHEART study indicate, however that little may be gained from identifying additional risk factors.[25] In this large case-control international study, nine clinical risk factors were strongly associated with the development of first ever MI and accounted for >90% of the risk for developing CAD (Table 16-1). Importantly the results were consistent across gender, geographic regions, and ethnic groups, suggesting strategies to reduce the incidence of CAD can be applied universally.

Platelet Aggregation and the Formation of Thrombi

Although plaque rupture and the formation of a superimposing thrombus are commonly considered in the pathophysiology of ACS,[11] platelet activation and thrombus formation also are integral to the chronic atherosclerotic process. Advances in

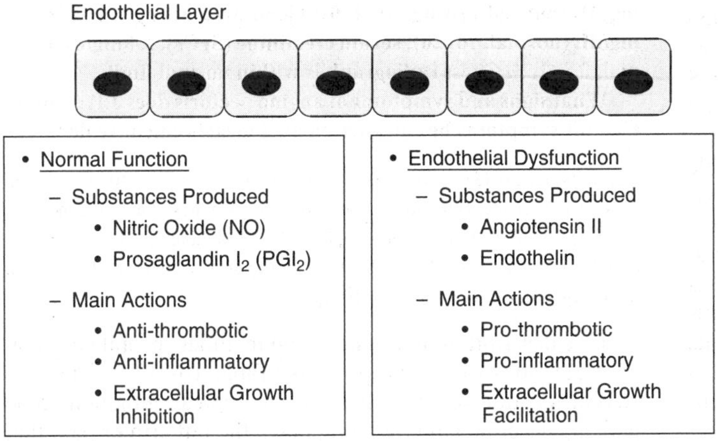
Endothelial Layer
• Normal Function
– Substances Produced
• Nitric Oxide (NO)
• Prosaglandin I_2 (PGI_2)
– Main Actions
• Anti-thrombotic
• Anti-inflammatory
• Extracellular Growth Inhibition
• Endothelial Dysfunction
– Substances Produced
• Angiotensin II
• Endothelin
– Main Actions
• Pro-thrombotic
• Pro-inflammatory
• Extracellular Growth Facilitation

FIGURE 16-4 Endothelial function.

Table 16-1 Risk Factors for First Time Myocardial Iinfarction From the INTERHEART Study[25]

Risk Factor	*Adjusted Odds Ratio (99% CI)*
ApoB–to–Apo A-1 ratio	3.25 (2.81–3.76)
Current smoking	2.87 (2.58–3.19)
Psychosocial	2.67 (2.21–3.22)
Diabetes	2.37 (2.07–2.71)
Hypertension	1.91 (1.74–2.10)
Abdominal obesity	1.62 (1.45–1.80)
Moderate alcohol intake	0.91 (0.82–1.02)
Exercise	0.86 (0.76–0.97)
Vegetable and fruits daily	0.70 (0.62–0.79)
All combined	129.2 (90.2–185.0)

vascular biology have demonstrated that platelets can both be a source of inflammatory mediators, as well as be activated by generalized inflammation within the vasculature.[26] In response to arterial vessel wall injury (e.g., an atherosclerotic lesion), platelets aggregate and release granular contents.[17] These activities further enhance platelet aggregation, vasoconstriction (dynamic obstruction), and in many cases, thrombus formation. Although coronary atherosclerosis is the underlying mechanism for most patients with anginal syndromes, thrombotic factors commonly play a key role in the pathogenesis of myocardial ischemia. Both blood flow turbulence and stasis can cause intermittent platelet aggregation or intermittent coronary artery thrombosis. Thus, platelet-active agents are used in the treatment of chronic stable angina and unstable angina, primary prevention of MI, secondary prevention of myocardial ischemia and acute MI, and in patients after coronary angioplasty or coronary artery bypass grafting (CABG).

Approach to a Patient With Anginal Symptoms

The medical management of anginal syndromes always should be individualized. The first step for any given patient is a detailed history and physical examination. Once this information is available, an estimate can be made of the probability of CAD being present (low, intermediate, high). The probability estimate will often help direct which diagnostic tests are appropriate to perform, as well as the utility of the results obtained (positive predictive value).[1,2] In addition, it is important to discern as soon as possible whether the patient's reported chest discomfort is consistent with chronic stable angina, or represents the presence of ACS. Patients presenting with ACS often are at high short-term risk of MI or death and warrant hospitalization with aggressive treatment strategies.[11,12] Regardless of whether a patient is experiencing chronic stable angina or ACS, patients often receive medications to alleviate or prevent ischemia, medications that prevent pathologic thrombus formation and may alleviate or prevent the progression of atherosclerosis (vasculoprotective agents), as well as undergo revascularization procedures such as percutaneous coronary intervention (PCI) or CABG. In addition, all patients with anginal syndromes should receive instructions on changes to adopt a healthy lifestyle and dietary pattern, as well as appropriate control of risk factors for CAD.

CHRONIC STABLE EXERTIONAL ANGINA

Signs and Symptoms

1. J.P., a 62-year-old retired dairy farmer, is hospitalized for evaluation of chest pain. About 3 weeks before admission, he noted substernal chest pain brought on by lifting heavy objects or walking uphill. He describes a crushing or viselike pain that never occurs at rest and is not associated with meals, emotional stress, or a particular time of day. When J.P. stops working, the pain subsides in about 5 minutes.

J.P.'s mother and brother died of a heart attack at ages 62 and 57, respectively; his father, who is alive at age 86, has survived one heart attack and one stroke. Family history (except for J.P.) is negative for diabetes mellitus. J.P. is 5′10″ tall and weighs 235 lb; he drinks two or three beers per day and does not smoke or chew tobacco.

J.P.'s other medical problems include a 10-year history of hypertension, diabetes for 4 years, and traumatic amputation of the right hand. Until 3 weeks ago, J.P. could perform all his farm chores without difficulty, including heavy labor. He follows a no-added-salt diet, but consistently eats at fast-food establishments with his favorite meal consisting of two cheeseburgers and French fries.

J.P.'s medication history reveals the following: metoprolol (Toprol XL) 100 mg every day, glipizide (Glucotrol) 5 mg twice daily (BID) and losartan (Cozaar) 50 mg every day. He rarely uses over-the-counter medications. He has a history of an allergic reaction to sulfa drugs.

On admission to the cardiac ward, J.P. appears his stated age and is in no apparent distress. Resting vital signs include supine blood pressure (BP), 164/98 mmHg (normal, 120/80); regular pulse, 73 beats/minute (normal, 65–75); and respiratory rate, 12 breaths/minute (normal, 8–14). He has no peripheral edema or neck vein distention, and lung auscultation is within normal limits. Abdominal examination is unremarkable and he is alert and oriented × 3. Cardiac auscultation reveals a regular rate and rhythm with a normal S_1 and S_2; third or fourth heart sounds and murmurs are not noted. A 12-lead ECG reveals normal sinus rhythm at a rate of 75 beats/minute without evidence of previous MI. All intervals are within normal limits.

Admitting laboratory values include the following: Hct, 43.5% (normal, 40%–45%); white blood cell (WBC) count, 5,000/mm^3 (normal, 5,000–10,000); sodium (Na), 140 mEq/L (normal, 136–144); potassium (K), 4.7 mEq/L (normal, 3.5–5.3); magnesium (Mg), 1.9 mEq/L (normal, 1.7–2.7); random blood glucose, 152 mg/dL (normal fasting, 65–110); blood urea nitrogen (BUN), 27 mg/dL (normal, 10–20); serum creatinine (SrCr), 1.4 mg/dL (normal, 0.5–1.2). Chest radiograph is within normal limits.

What signs and symptoms of angina pectoris does J.P. exhibit? Can his symptoms be categorized on a measurement scale?

[SI units: Hct, 0.435 (normal, 0.40–0.45); WBC count, 5 × 10^9/L (normal, 5–10 × 10^9/L); Na, 140 mmol/L (normal, 136–144); K, 4.7 mmol/L (normal, 3.5–5.3); Mg, 0.95 mmol/L (normal, 0.85–1.35); random blood glucose, 6.16 mmol/L (normal, 3.6–6.1); BUN, 9.6 mmol/L of urea (normal, 3.57–7.14); SrCr, 124 μmol/L (normal, 44.2–106)]

J.P.'s description of his chest pain includes several common characteristics of angina pectoris (Table 16-2).[1–3] The substernal location of J.P.'s chest pain is typical, although some patients describe pain radiating down the left arm or pain that

Table 16-2 Characteristics of Angina Pectoris[1–3]

Symptoms	Duration of Symptoms
Sensation of pressure or heavy weight on chest alone or with pain	0.5–30 min
Pain described variably as feeling of tightness, burning, crushing, squeezing, vicelike, aching, or "deep"	**Electrocardiogram**
Gradual increase in intensity followed by gradual fading away (distinguished from esophageal spasm)[a]	ST-segment depression >2 mm
SOB with feeling constriction about the larynx of upper trachea	T-wave inversion
Location of Pain or Discomfort	**Precipitating Factors**
Over the sternum or very near to it	Mild, moderate, or heavy exercise, depending on patient
Anywhere between epigastrium and pharynx	Effort that involves use of arms above the head
Occasionally limited to left shoulder and left arm	Cold environment
Rarely limited to right arm	Walking against the wind
Lower cervical or upper thoracic spine	Walking after a large meal
Left interscapular or suprascapular area	Emotions: fright, anger, or anxiety
Radiation of Pain	Coitus
Medial aspect of left arm	**Nitroglycerin Relief**[a]
Left shoulder	Relief of pain occurring within 45 sec to 5 min of taking nitroglycerin
Jaw	
Occasionally, right arm	

[a] Esophageal spasm and other gastrointestinal disorders occasionally mimic anginal pain and also can be relieved by nitroglycerin.
SOB, shortness of breath.

is referred to the shoulder area or jaw. J.P.'s pain is described as crushing or viselike in quality, which also is common; a fullness in the throat or jaw may occur simultaneously or in lieu of chest pain. In some cases, the patient may not consider these sensations as pain, describing them instead as a sense of pressure or heaviness. Many patients complain of shortness of breath (SOB), J.P.'s symptoms are related to exercise and exertion—both known precipitating factors of angina. Most episodes of exertional angina last several minutes in duration and are relieved with rest. Because J.P. has never sought medical attention for his chest pain, his response to NTG cannot be determined.

After getting a detailed description of J.P.'s symptom complex, his physician can characterize his chest pain and make a global assessment. Initially, the chest pain should be classified as either typical angina, atypical angina, or noncardiac chest pain. Furthermore, angina should also be classified as either stable or unstable. This distinction is important because it indicates whether his short-term risk of an acute coronary event could be life-threatening. Attempts to categorize J.P.'s anginal symptoms on an objective measurement scale (e.g., Canadian Cardiovascular Society Grading Scale) can be misleading.[27] For example, a sedentary 65-year-old patient's class II symptoms may be tolerable, but the same symptoms could significantly disable an active 50-year-old patient.

J.P.'s chest pain is of a quality and duration characteristic of angina, provoked by exertion, and relieved by rest; therefore, J.P.'s constellation of symptoms can be classified as typical chest pain. J.P.'s symptoms do not occur at rest, however, so they can be classified as stable angina.[1–3]

2. Assess J.P.'s physical examination. What signs and symptoms are relevant to the angina?

The physical examination typically provides little information about the presence of CAD. The most useful findings pertain to the cardiovascular system where heart rate and BP can be increased during an acute anginal episode. J.P.'s physical examination is characteristic for a man of his age with angina.[3] He is obese and hypertensive, but his cardiac examination is normal. The presence of murmurs would have required further workup; the absence of a third heart sound suggests that the left ventricle may be functioning normally. (See Chapter 18, Heart Failure, for a description of third heart sounds.) The absence of a fourth heart sound in J.P. is indicative of a low probability of either CHD or a cardiac end-organ damage resulting from systemic hypertension. His chest radiograph, which is normal, does not present evidence of other complications commonly associated with myocardial ischemia (e.g., enlarged heart, heart failure).

J.P.'s physical examination should also evaluate the possibility of peripheral vascular disease and abdominal aortic aneurysm. The presence of xanthomas would suggest severe hypercholesterolemia, but these were not noted in J.P.

Diagnostic Procedures

3. J.P.'s medical history and family history support the diagnosis of chronic stable angina. What other objective diagnostic procedures are helpful to confirm CHD and angina?

A 12-lead ECG reading should be obtained in all patients with symptoms suggestive of angina pectoris, although it will be normal in >50% of patients. Although not useful in establishing a definitive diagnosis of CAD, the ECG will be useful at detecting important information regarding conduction abnormalities, left ventricular hypertrophy, ongoing ischemia, or evidence of a previous myocardial infarction. Chest radiography is typically not useful except in patients with symptoms of heart failure, valvular disease, or pericardial disease. In these selected patients, echocardiography may also be used to better (a) evaluate the structure and function of the cardiac valves,

(b) characterize the extent of ischemia during pain, or (c) assess global left ventricular systolic function.[3] Electron beam computerized tomography (EBCT) is evolving as a potential noninvasive approach to detecting significant CAD through identification of coronary artery calcification. Although an attractive alternative to other invasive diagnostic measures, current information suggest that a sufficient level of variability exists in repeated measure of coronary calcium by EBCT and that the specificity of the procedure remains poor. Current guidelines do not recommend the routine use of EBCT in the diagnosis of chronic stable angina.[28]

Exercise Tolerance Test

An exercise tolerance test or treadmill test would be helpful in the diagnosis of CAD in J.P. Under controlled circumstances, J.P. would exercise to a preset level, and the test would be indicative of CAD on the development of angina, ECG signs of ischemia, arrhythmias, abnormal heart rate, or abnormal BP response. The product of the heart rate and systolic BP (i.e., *the rate–pressure or double product*) correlates well with myocardial oxygen demand. The rate–pressure product normally rises progressively during exercise, with the peak value best describing the cardiovascular response to stress. Often, patients with stable angina experience chest pain at a consistent rate–pressure product.[29]

Abnormal responses of either BP or heart rate may signal CAD. A normal BP response to exercise is a gradual rise in systolic BP with the diastolic BP (DBP) remaining unchanged. A rise or fall of DBP >10 mmHg is considered abnormal. A fall in systemic BP (SBP) during exercise is especially ominous because this indicates that the cardiac output cannot increase sufficiently to overcome the vasodilation in the skeletal muscle vascular bed.

During exercise, the heart rate increases steadily until it reaches a plateau. The maximal heart rate depends on age, drug therapy, and cardiovascular fitness. Some patients exhibit an abnormal slowing of heart rate, especially when taking β-blockers. Therefore, β-blockers should be tapered off (i.e., gradually discontinued) before treadmill testing when the test is being used for diagnosis or risk stratification. Similarly, digoxin can also interfere with the results of exercise testing, and other testing modalities are recommended if digoxin cannot be safely discontinued before treadmill testing. In patients with a history such as J.P.'s, the exercise tolerance test helps to confirm the presence of CAD and provides a risk stratification that may be helpful in determining whether he is a candidate for revascularization therapy.[29]

Myocardial Imaging

Stress imaging studies, either echocardiographic or nuclear, are preferred over the exercise tolerance test in patients with left bundle-branch block, electronically paced ventricular rhythm, prior revascularization (percutaneous coronary intervention or coronary artery bypass surgery), pre-excitation syndrome, >1 mm ST-segment depression at rest, or other ECG conduction abnormalities. In addition, many patients are not able to develop an appropriate level of cardiac stress through exercise; pharmacologic stress testing is preferred in these patients.[1]

Pharmacologic stress may be achieved through the use of dipyridamole, adenosine, or dobutamine. Each of these agents is used to induce changes in the balance between myocardial oxygen supply and demand, similar to walking on a treadmill during the exercise stress test. Vasodilators (dipyridamole and adenosine) promote vasodilation in normal coronary segments, but have no effect in arteries affected by atherosclerosis. The net result is shunting of blood away from diseased coronary arteries and the development of ischemia that may be detected by changes in blood pressure, heart rate, or ECG changes. These agents are typically used in conjunction with myocardial perfusion scintigraphy. Stress thallium-201 myocardial perfusion imaging provides a dynamic picture of the heart. The radionuclide is injected at peak stress and an image is obtained within several minutes. A defect in myocardial uptake of the thallium indicates an area of ischemia or possible infarction.[1]

Dobutamine is a positive inotrope and typically is used with echocardiography. Administration of dobutamine leads to an increase in myocardial oxygen demand secondary to increases in heart rate and contractility. If demand exceeds available oxygen supply, ischemia develops. Subsequent to the infusion of dobutamine, defects or decreases in the wall motion or thickening of the left ventricle are indicative of ischemia.[1]

Cardiac Catheterization

4. Should J.P. undergo cardiac catheterization? How will the results of this invasive procedure influence future therapy?

Coronary artery disease can be diagnosed definitively only by coronary catheterization and subsequent angiography. In addition, angiography is the most accurate means of identifying less common causes of chronic stable angina, such as coronary artery spasm.[1,30] Cardiac catheterization is a procedure used to provide vascular access to the coronary arteries. Once access is gained with an intravascular catheter, a number of procedures (angiography, ventriculography, percutaneous coronary intervention) can be performed. Access to the vasculature is usually obtained percutaneously through the brachial or femoral arteries. From this point, the catheter is advanced through the vasculature until the coronary arteries are accessible. After the tip of the catheter is advanced into the coronary arteries, radiocontrast dye is injected into the coronary arteries and the location and extent of atherosclerosis can be determined. Approximately 75% of patients with chronic stable angina, such as J.P., are noted to have one-, two-, or three-vessel disease by this procedure (approximately equally divided).[3]

The results of angiography will be useful in determining the risk of death or MI in J.P. and, subsequently, the course of needed treatment. For example, patients who have a significant stenosis in the left main coronary artery are at high risk of death and should undergo CABG.[31]

Risk Stratification and Prognosis

5. J.P. is found to have two-vessel CAD with obstructive lesions of 55% and 70%; the LAD coronary artery is not involved. What is his prognosis?

The prognosis of patients with stable angina is variable and dependent on the presence of other factors and comorbid conditions. Developing a level of risk for a particular patient helps determine the appropriate treatment strategy. The extent of CAD, quantification of ventricular function, the response to stress testing, as well as the initial clinical evaluation all help to provide a estimate of risk in a given patient.

J.P.'s history and physical examination suggest he does not have HF; poor LV function would be an ominous concurrent finding. J.P. also does not have three-vessel disease or blockage of the LAD artery.[1] Overall, he probably will do well with medical therapy. His life expectancy depends on progression of the disease and development of other complications of CHD (e.g., HF, MI, sudden cardiac death). Medical therapy is a reasonable treatment strategy for J.P., but revascularization via percutaneous transluminal coronary angioplasty (PTCA) is an equally viable option. Although PTCA with or without stent placement would offer no mortality advantage over medical therapy at this time, it has been shown to decrease the incidence of recurrent symptoms.[1] Both strategies, including both pros and cons, should be offered to J.P. so that an informed decision can be made in accord with his wishes.

Presently, J.P. is not a candidate for CABG because the usual indications for surgical therapy include presence of left main CAD, presence of three-vessel disease (especially if LV function is impaired), or ineffectiveness of medical therapy.[30,31]

Overview of Medical Management

6. After consultation, J.P. and his cardiologist elect to control his angina medically. What are the goals of his therapy and how can they be achieved?

Two major pharmacotherapeutic goals exist for treating all patients with angina. The first goal includes relief of symptoms and reduction of myocardial ischemia to improve quality of life. The second goal, and more important overall, is to prevent major complications of CAD such as acute MI and death. Therapies that prevent death (vasculoprotective agents) should receive priority. As with any chronic disease, education of the patient and his or her family are important objectives. The ultimate goal of patient education is a better quality of life through improved understanding of the disease and its therapy. Every effort should be made to reverse J.P.'s modifiable risk factors (i.e., obesity, hypertension, and diabetes). He also could receive one or more of the following: a nitrate, calcium channel blocker (CCB), β-adrenergic blocker, ranolazine, angiotensin-converting enzyme (ACE) inhibitor, or antiplatelet drug.[1] J.P. should continue metoprolol therapy because it will be helpful in treating both his hypertension and angina. Compliance to metoprolol should be assessed because his BP was elevated on admission. His BUN and creatinine are slightly elevated (probably as a consequence of his hypertension), and he developed angina symptoms despite use of a β-blocker. Reduction of precipitating factors may be difficult, given J.P.'s work. He should be counseled, however, to avoid sudden bursts of physical activity. Moderate exercise should be encouraged, such as a walking program. J.P.'s family members should be screened for smoking because passive (secondhand) smoke can aggravate angina.

GENERAL MANAGEMENT

Patients and family members should receive education regarding the nature of chronic stable angina, the progressive nature of CAD, as well as specific information regarding potential complications and overall prognosis. All patients should be able to recite specific instructions for how to deal with exertional angina attacks. These include immediate cessation of the provoking activity, rest, as well as the use of sublingual (SL) nitroglycerin for immediate relief. All patients with CAD and angina should have a prescription for SL nitroglycerin, as well as receive instructions for the appropriate use and storage of the medication.[32] If rest or SL nitroglycerin does not provide adequate relief from angina after the first dose, patients should be instructed to immediately call for medical assistance.[2,11,12]

Risk Factors and Lifestyle Modifications

7. What independent risk factors for CAD are present in J.P.? Which of these may be altered?

The first step in the treatment of any patient with chronic stable angina, or CAD for that matter, should be the modification of any existing risk factors and the adoption of a healthy lifestyle. By addressing the underlying circumstances which likely led to the development of CAD, a significant impact can be made at halting the progression of the disease and preventing complications of CAD. Current recommendations for the goals for risk factor management are listed in Table 16-3.[33] In addition to specific risk factor goals, attention should be paid to evidence that may favor specific drug therapies that have evidence supporting reductions in morbidity and mortality. Examples would include the use of metformin[34] or pioglitazone[35] in the treatment of type 2 diabetes, the use of 3-hydroxy-3-methylglutaryl co-enzyme A inhibitors (HMG-CoA reductase inhibitors) in the treatment of hyperlipidemia,[1,2,33] as

Table 16-3 AHA/ACC Guidelines for the Secondary Prevention for Patients with Coronary and Other Atherosclerotic Vascular Disease[33]

Risk Factor	*Intervention and Goal*
Smoking	Complete cessation No exposure to environmental tobacco smoke
Blood pressure	<140/90 mmHg <130/80 mmHg if patient has diabetes or chronic kidney disease
Lipid management	LDL-C <100 mg/dL If triglycerides >200 mg/dL, non–HDL-C should be <130 mg/dL
Diabetes	Hemoglobin A_{1C} <7%
Physical activity	At least 30 min of moderate intensity aerobic activity (e.g., brisk walking) for minimum of 5 days/wk
Weight management	BMI between 18.5–24.9 kg/m^2 Waist circumference men <40 in Waist circumference women <35 in
Influenza vaccination	Patients with CAD should have an annual influenza vaccination

BMI, body mass index; CAD, coronary artery disease; HDL-C, high-density lipoprotein cholesterol; LDL-C, low-density lipoprotein cholesterol.

well as the use of ACE inhibitors for the treatment of hypertension.[36]

J.P. has several risk factors for CAD, some of which cannot be altered, such as middle age, male gender, and a strong family history of CAD. Risk factors, such as hypertension, obesity, hypercholesterolemia, smoking, and possibly stress, can potentially be modified to decrease the likelihood of adverse sequelae for J.P. His hypertension should be controlled and his serum cholesterol concentration should be tested and fractionated for LDL, high-density lipoprotein (HDL), and triglycerides (TG) (see Chapter 12, Dyslipidemias, Atherosclerosis, and Coronary Heart Disease). A fasting hemoglobin A_1C should be drawn with a goal of <7% (see Chapter 50, Diabetes Mellitus). Dietary modification and weight reduction for J.P. are mandatory, because they positively influence several risk factors. J.P., however, does not smoke cigarettes, which would significantly increase his cardiovascular risk.[1] J.P.'s active lifestyle may influence his prognosis favorably.[37]

Dietary Interventions

8. J.P. states he had heard that antioxidants such as vitamin E could benefit him along with a daily B vitamin. Are there other dietary changes he could make that would benefit his cardiovascular disease?

Because oxidation of LDL in the arterial wall was identified as a key step in the atherosclerotic process, considerable interest exists in the theory that supplementation with high doses of antioxidants, such as vitamin E, vitamin C, and β-carotene, might mitigate this process and slow the progression of atherosclerosis. Early observational studies of dietary patterns high in these antioxidants seemed to confirm this theory. Multiple large randomized studies, however, have shown no positive effect from supplemental intake of antioxidants, such as vitamin E, on the incidence of cardiovascular outcomes including MI or death. These findings were observed in both primary and secondary prevention of cardiovascular events. J.P. should be informed that supplemental intake of vitamin E will not have any positive effect on his cardiovascular disease. (See Chapter 12 Dyslipidemias, Atherosclerosis, and Coronary Heart Disease, for further discussion.)[38,39]

Interest in the use of supplemental intake of folic acid and B vitamins stems from their ability to lower homocysteine levels. It is well established that elevated levels of homocysteine are associated with a higher incidence of cardiovascular disease.[40,41] Despite this association, the great majority of appropriately designed, randomized, placebo-controlled studies have demonstrated that supplemental ingestion of folic acid and B vitamins has no impact in reducing hard cardiovascular outcomes such as MI or death in patients with CAD.[42] Therefore, similar to the advice for vitamin E, J.P. should be counseled that folic acid and B vitamin supplementation will not provide him any tangible cardiovascular benefit.

In contrast to the data regarding specific dietary interventions, such as vitamin E or folic acid, several healthy dietary patterns have compelling evidence to support their implementation to prevent the development or progression of CAD. These include the substitution of nonhydrogenated saturated fats for saturated fats and trans-fats in the diet; consumption of omega-3 fatty acids (primary source is fish); and consumption of a diet high in fruits, vegetables, nuts, and whole grains.[43] When patients post-MI were randomized to a traditional western diet or a Mediterranean diet high in fruits, vegetables, cereals, beans, nuts, and olive oil as the primary source of fat intake, a 50% to 70% lower risk was seen of recurrent heart disease (which includes cardiac death and nonfatal MI).[44,45] These dietary alterations are in line with the current dietary guidelines from the American Heart Association.[43] Additional trial data have demonstrated a beneficial effect of either increasing weekly fish consumption, or taking omega-3 fatty acid fish oil supplements on reducing cardiovascular morbidity and mortality.[46–48] J.P. can make a number of dietary changes that can significantly benefit his cardiovascular disease, and he should be encouraged to do so. J.P. should be asked if he regularly consumes alcohol and counseled to limit his intake to one to two drinks per day if he does.[43]

ANTI-ISCHEMIC DRUG THERAPY

Organic Nitrates

Nitrates are commonly used in the treatment of all anginal syndromes. They are effective in treating all forms of angina because they decrease venous return to the heart and, therefore, decrease cardiac work load. Nitrates also promote coronary vasodilation, even in the presence of atherosclerosis. Nitrates generally are well tolerated. To prevent loss of effect over time, however, they must be scheduled to provide a nitrate-free interval of 10 to 12 hours. Therefore, nitrates should be combined with a β-blocker or a CCB (e.g., verapamil, diltiazem). The individual nitrate products differ primarily in their onset and duration of action.

Mechanism of Action

9. During the first hospital day, J.P. decides to walk up three flights of stairs when returning to his room from the cafeteria instead of taking the elevator. Midway through the third flight of stairs J.P. develops chest pain. After quickly performing a 12-lead ECG, the physician instructs J.P. to place a 0.4-mg sublingual NTG tablet (Nitrostat) under his tongue. This relieves the pain. J.P.'s physician elects to continue metoprolol and add both short- and long-acting nitrates. What is the mechanism by which NTG relieves angina? Why should J.P. continue his metoprolol therapy?

The mechanism of action of NTG and the other nitrate esters is not completely understood, although they have been used for >100 years. The overall benefits of nitrates result from a reduction in myocardial oxygen demand caused by venodilation and some arteriolar dilation.[1,2,32] Nitrates produce vasodilation by at least two mechanisms: stimulation of cyclic guanosine monophosphate (cGMP) production and inhibition of thromboxane synthetase. Organic nitrates are converted into NO. Nitric oxide is identical to EDRF, an endogenous vasodilator. Nitric oxide reacts with sulfhydryl groups in the vascular smooth muscle to produce S-nitrosothiols, which subsequently activate guanylate cyclase and increase the intracellular concentration of cGMP. cGMP controls the amount of vascular smooth muscle calcium available for muscle contraction by binding to calmodulin and phosphorylating myosin light chain kinase. The cGMP enhances calcium uptake into the sarcoplasmic reticulum, or inhibits its cellular influx. Because less calcium is available, dilation occurs.[32,49]

The peripheral effects of sublingual NTG in J.P. include dilation of both veins and arteries. Venous dilation is more pronounced because relaxation of arterial smooth muscle requires higher plasma NTG levels. By dilating the veins and reducing preload to the heart, filling pressures in the ventricles are reduced. This, in turn, reduces myocardial oxygen demand, thereby relieving J.P.'s angina.[32,49] (See Chapter 18, Heart Failure, for a more detailed discussion of preload.)

Metoprolol should be continued in J.P. because it both lowers BP and exerts antianginal effects. In addition, administration of nitrates must include a daily nitrate-free interval; metoprolol will provide continued protection from ischemia during this time.[49] The addition of long-acting nitrates will provide J.P. additional protection against developing angina, and short-acting NTG will provide J.P. acute relief when an anginal attack occurs.

Short-Acting Preparations

Sublingual Nitroglycerin

DOSING

10. How should J.P.'s dose of sublingual NTG be determined? Can NTG be used prophylactically?

Because sensitivity to NTG varies among patients, the dosage should be individualized (Table 16-4). Most patients, however, use a dose of 0.4 mg. An optimal dosage relieves pain and produces an objective hemodynamic response, such as a 10-mmHg fall in systolic BP or a 10-beat/minute rise in heart rate. High doses can cause intolerable orthostatic hypotension, however.[49]

The administration of sublingual NTG is also useful in patients who have a good understanding of what level of exertion produces their chest pain. About 5 to 10 minutes before J.P. is about to undergo heavy exertion, he can take a sublingual NTG tablet to prevent angina.[1]

Table 16-4 Commonly Prescribed Organic Nitrates

Drug	*Dosage Form*	*Duration*	*Onset (min)*	*Usual Dosage*
Short-acting				
Nitroglycerin (NTG)	Sublingual (SL)	10–30 min	1–3	0.4–0.6 mg[a,b]
NTG	Translingual spray	10–30 min	2–4	0.4 mg/metered spray[a,b]
NTG	Intravenous (IV)	3–5 min[c]	1–2	Initially 5 mcg/min. Increase every (Q) 3–5 min until pain is relieved or hypotension occurs
Long-acting[d]				
NTG	Sustained release (SR) capsule	4–8 hr	30	6.5–9 mg Q 8 hr
NTG	Topical ointment[e]	4–8 hr	30	1–2 inches Q 4–6 hr[f]
NTG	Transdermal patch	4–>8 hr	30–60	0.1–0.2 mg/hr to start; titrate up to 0.8 mg/hr[f]
NTG	Transmucosal	3–6 hr	2–5	1–3 mg Q 3–5 hr[f]
ISDN[g]	SL	2–4 hr	2–5	2.5–10 mg Q 2–4 hr[f]
	Chewable	2–4 hr	2–5	5–10 mg Q 2–4 hr[f]
	Oral	2–6 hr	15–40	10–60 mg every 4–6 hr[f]
	SR	4–8 hr	15–40	40–80 mg Q 6–8 hr[f]
ISMN[h]	Tab (ISMO, Monoket)	7–8 hr	30–60	10–20 mg twice daily (BID) (morning and midday) to start; titrate to 20–40 mg BID[f]
	SR tablet (Imdur)	8–12 hr	30–60	60 mg every day (QD) to start; titrate to 30–120 mg QD

[a] When using sublingual or translingual spray forms of NTG, patients should administer the dose while sitting to minimize tachycardia, hypotension, dizziness, headache, and flushing. The optimal dose relieves symptoms with <10–15 mmHg drop in systolic blood pressure or <10 beat/min rise in pulse. Pain relief is rapid (onset 1–2 min; relief in 3–5 min), but up to three doses at 5-min intervals may be given. After this, medical assistance should be summoned.

[b] Sublingual NTG tablets are degraded rapidly by heat, moisture, and light. They should be stored in a cool, dry place; do not leave the lid open or refrigerate. Tablets should be stored in the original manufacturer's container or a glass vial because the tablets volatilize and bind to many plastic vials and cotton. Previously, stinging of the tongue was an indicator of fresh tablets, but newer formulations only cause stinging in ~75% of patients.

[c] Duration after infusion discontinued.

[d] Longer-acting forms of nitrates are effective drugs, but it is important to understand their limitations to optimize effectiveness. Sublingual isosorbide dinitrate (ISDN) tablets display an onset and duration intermediate between that of sublingual NTG and oral ISDN. Because of high presystemic (1st-pass) metabolism of the oral forms of both NTG and ISDN, very large doses may be required compared with SL or chewable dosage forms. Small oral doses (2.5 mg NTG, 5 mg ISDN) are probably not effective; doses as large as 9 mg NTG and 60 mg ISDN are not uncommon. Despite claims for longer activity, ointments and oral forms are often only effective for 4–8 hr, even when given as SR preparations. Also, continued daily use leads to rapid development of tolerance (see f).

[e] Squeeze 1″ to 2″ of ointment onto the calibrated paper enclosed in the package with tube. Carefully spread the ointment on chest in a thin layer ~2″–2″ in size. Keep area covered with applicator paper. Wipe off previous dose before adding new dose or if hypotensive. If another person applies the ointment, avoid contact with fingers or eyes to prevent headache or hypotension.

[f] Dosage regimens should maintain a nitrate-free interval (e.g., bedtime) to decrease tolerance development. Give last oral dose or remove ointment or transdermal patch at 7 P.M. Give last dose of SR ISDN in early afternoon.

[g] ISDN, isosorbide dinitrate.

[h] ISMN, isosorbide monohydrate, major active metabolite of ISDN; 100% bioavailable; no first-pass metabolism, but tolerance may still occur. Rapid release (ISMO, Monoket) as 10- and 20-mg tablets. SR form (Imdur) as 60-mg tablets. OK to cut Indur in half, do not crush or chew.

PATIENT INSTRUCTIONS

11. What instructions should J.P. receive with regard to the use and storage of sublingual NTG? How rapidly will sublingual NTG relieve J.P.'s chest pain?

When angina occurs, J.P. should sit down immediately and place the NTG tablet under his tongue; he should not swallow it. Many patients experience dizziness and lightheadedness, which is minimized by sitting. The onset of action is within 1 to 2 minutes, and pain usually is relieved within 3 to 5 minutes. If he needs more than one tablet, he can take a maximum of three tablets over 15 minutes. If the pain persists or is unimproved 5 minutes after the first dose of NTG, the patient should call 9-1-1 as they may be experiencing an MI.[11,12]

The tablets should be dispensed in the original, unopened manufacturer's container and stored in the original brown bottle. Because sublingual NTG tablets are degraded by heat, moisture, and light, they should be stored in a cool, dry place, but not refrigerated. The bottle should be closed tightly after each opening. Safety caps are not necessary, although patients should be cautioned to keep all medications out of the reach of children. The cotton plug sometimes is difficult to remove. Therefore, it should be discarded on initial receipt of the prescription and should not be replaced. Use of cotton other than that supplied by the manufacturer should be discouraged because NTG tablets are volatile and are adsorbed by household cotton. This results in a significant loss in tablet effectiveness. Expiration dating should be monitored closely, and tablets should be replaced immediately if they are exposed to excessive light, heat, moisture, or air. Once a container is opened, the tablets should be used for only a limited time—usually from 6 months to 1 year.[49] A tablet left out of the bottle on a table will lose its effectiveness in just a few hours.

Long-Acting Nitrates

12. J.P. does well over the next several months, but he is still bothered by occasional angina episodes, ranging from one to four times per week. He was changed to the translingual spray form of NTG (0.4 mg/spray) because he had difficulty with storage of the tablets. The attacks usually are precipitated by strenuous work and are relieved by rest and two or three NTG sprays. The quality and location of the pain are unchanged, although the duration has increased by 1 or 2 minutes. He follows a low-cholesterol, no-added-salt diet.

Physical examination is unchanged except for a 20-lb weight loss. Vital signs include the following: supine BP, 119/76 mmHg; heart rate, 65 beats/minute; and respiratory rate, 12 breaths/minute. J.P.'s cardiologist elected to start a long-acting prophylactic nitrate (isosorbide mononitrate) as well as continuing his β-blocker and angiotensin-receptor blocker (ARB) therapy. What therapeutic endpoints should be used to evaluate the efficacy of long-acting nitrates? Could a CCB have been used instead of the long-acting nitrate?

Long-acting nitrates occupy a key role in the prevention of angina of all types. Their mechanism of action is the same as that of short-acting NTG. The goals of therapy are to decrease the number, severity, and duration of J.P.'s anginal attacks.

A CCB could be prescribed for J.P. instead of isosorbide mononitrate because he has no contraindications to this class of drugs. A CCB would have been a good alternative if his BP had remained elevated, but for now, J.P.'s BP and pulse are within a desired range. Because sublingual nitrates were well tolerated by J.P., a long-acting nitrate would be acceptable. A CCB (e.g., amlodipine) is an alternative as long as J.P.'s BP is not unduly decreased by this combination of drugs. Ultimately, the decision is based on the prescriber's personal choice and past experience, as well as the entire spectrum of the patient's disease complex.

Nitrate Tolerance

13. Will J.P. develop tolerance to the long-acting nitrate?

Early evidence for the development of nitrate tolerance and dependence came from the munitions industry. Workers in this industry were constantly exposed to NTG and ethylene glycol dinitrate, components of explosives.[50] Tolerance can develop in as few as 24 hours after continuous exposure to nitrate preparations, however, the degree of tolerance may be variable in terms of percentage of efficacy lost. Tolerance can be limited by maintaining a nitrate-free interval of about 10 to 12 hours daily. Nitrate dosing schedules should be arranged to permit a nitrate-free interval during which time the patient may receive angina protection from β-adrenergic blockers or CCB. Most often, this nitrate-free interval is arranged during the night because angina is more likely to occur during the work day. Patients with nocturnal angina should arrange their nitrate-free interval during the day.[51] Because long-acting nitrates must be dosed intermittently to avoid tolerance, metoprolol therapy will provide J.P. with continuous protection, even during the nitrate-free interval. Although J.P. uses a long-acting nitrate, he still will respond favorably to sublingual NTG. No evidence indicates that use of long-acting nitrates leads to resistance or tolerance to the effects of sublingual NTG.

MECHANISM OF ACTION

14. What is the mechanism of action for nitrate tolerance?

Several mechanisms of nitrate tolerance have been proposed, including the depletion of sulfhydryl groups, which are necessary for the biotransformation of nitrate to NO; neurohormonal activation; plasma volume expansion; and abnormalities in NO signal transduction. More recent investigations, however, have identified that chronic nitrate administration produces a state of oxidative stress, leading to dysfunction of mitochondrial aldehyde dehydrogenase, which is the enzyme responsible for biotransformation of nitrates to NO.[52,53]

One potential consequence of this current theory is that long-term administration of organic nitrates, by producing neurohormonal activation and endothelial dysfunction, may have long-term detrimental effects. Further research is needed to confirm this hypothesis for nitrate tolerance and its long-term consequences on patient outcomes.[54]

INTERMITTENT APPLICATION OF TRANSDERMAL NITROGLYCERIN

15. Are all nitrate delivery systems capable of inducing nitrate tolerance? How can tolerance be minimized?

All organic nitrates exhibit similar hemodynamic effects through a common pharmacologic mechanism; yet, the differing pharmacokinetic profiles of the nitrate delivery systems lead to a variation in the development of tolerance.[49]

Short-acting formulations (e.g., sublingual NTG, oral NTG spray, and sublingual isosorbide dinitrate) are not likely to induce tolerance given their rapid onset of action and short duration of effect. Oral nitrates and transdermal products, both having an extended duration of action, are likely to induce tolerance.

Intermittent application of transdermal NTG can limit tolerance development in patients with both chronic stable angina and HF. The effects of continuous (24 hours/day) and intermittent (16 hours/day) transdermal NTG (10 mg/day) were compared in 12 men with chronic stable angina who also were being treated with β-blockers or CCB.[55] Nitrate efficacy was maintained with intermittent treatment and an 8-hour nitrate-free interval. Tolerance to the antianginal effects occurred, however, with continuous transdermal NTG treatment. Twelve-hour intermittent patch therapy also prevents tolerance.[56] The minimal time necessary for a nitrate-free interval is unknown.

Intravenous (IV) NTG, a cornerstone therapy in management of patients with unstable angina and severe HF, is associated with nitrate tolerance if it is administered as a sustained infusion. The immediate hemodynamic benefits observed with NTG infusions in patients with severe chronic heart failure were greatly reduced 24 to 48 hours after continuous IV therapy. Tolerance to IV NTG was prevented by infusing NTG for only 12 hours followed by a 12-hour nitrate-free interval.[57] Intermittent NTG infusions for patients with unstable angina appear reasonable, but have not been fully evaluated.

Isosorbide Dinitrate

16. J.P. ultimately receives a prescription for oral isosorbide dinitrate (Isordil) 30 mg three times daily (TID). How should he be instructed to take his medication so that he is nitrate free for 10 to 12 hours?

Despite the availability of nitrate preparations that can be dosed once or twice a day (isosorbide mononitrate), oral isosorbide dinitrate is still commonly used in the treatment of angina. J.P. should take his oral nitrate at 7 AM, noon, and 5 PM because his exercise-induced angina is likely to occur during daylight hours. He may need to adjust this schedule if he arises earlier than 7 AM because early-morning angina is common. Some physicians prescribe isosorbide dinitrate twice a day at 7 AM and noon for patients with less severe anginal syndrome.

17. Does isosorbide mononitrate offer any distinct advantages over other nitrate preparations for angina prophylaxis?

Isosorbide mononitrate (ISMO, Monoket, and Imdur) is the primary metabolite of isosorbide dinitrate. In fact, most of the clinical activity of isosorbide dinitrate is due to the mononitrate. Therefore, both drugs share a similar pharmacology. Isosorbide mononitrate does not undergo first-pass metabolism and has no active metabolites. Its oral bioavailability is almost 100%, and its overall elimination half-life is about 5 hours.[49] Maximal serum concentrations are observed 30 to 60 minutes after a dose. To minimize the potential development of nitrate tolerance, isosorbide mononitrate should be used in a twice-daily, asymmetric dosing regimen in which the first dose is taken on awakening and the second dose about 7 hours later. Because of this unconventional dosing pattern and the availability of the sustained-release (SR) product, which can be taken once a day, most use of isosorbide mononitrate is in the form of the SR preparation (Imdur).

General precautions and adverse reactions for isosorbide mononitrate are similar to those for the other nitrates. Potential advantages for the clinical use of isosorbide mononitrate are less dosage fluctuation because of the absence of presystemic clearance and an effective once- or twice-daily dosing schedule, which could perhaps lead to improved patient dosing adherence. Nevertheless, isosorbide dinitrate is effective clinically when administered two or three times a day and is a viable alternative.

Transdermal Patches

18. J.P. likes the idea of using topical nitrates instead of an oral agent. Are the transdermal patches a viable alternative?

Transdermal NTG patches originally were designed to provide angina protection with once-daily application. The concept of a compact, easy-to-apply transdermal NTG patch prompted pharmaceutical manufacturers to design a number of products, which the U.S. Food and Drug Administration (FDA) subsequently approved based on plasma level data, not clinical efficacy studies. Subsquently, the shortcomings of plasma level data have become apparent and prompted numerous clinical efficacy studies.

Transdermal NTG therapy has been shown to increase exercise duration and maintain an anti-ischemic effect for 12 hours after patch application. These beneficial responses remained consistent throughout 30 days of therapy. No significant nitrate tolerance or rebound was noted when the patch was applied for not more than 12 of 24 hours.[49]

Although the various patches use different pharmaceutical delivery systems, clear-cut advantages of one over another are not apparent. Despite variations in surface area and NTG content, the most important common denominator of the transdermal NTG systems is the amount of drug released per hour expressed as the release rate (e.g., 0.2 mg/hour). Each product label includes this information. Low dosages (0.2 to 0.4 mg/hour) may not produce sufficient plasma and tissue concentrations to produce a clinically significant effect[3]; however, it is still recommended to start with a low-dose patch and titrate upward as needed. Because the skin is the major factor influencing NTG absorption rate, product release characteristics do not favor one system over another. Contact dermatitis has been reported with the transdermal patches. Patient instructions are included with the patches and should be reviewed with the patient, emphasizing the appropriate time for application and removal of the patch.

Adrenergic Blockers

MECHANISM OF ACTION

19. T.I. has a 5-year history of chronic stable angina. Cardiac catheterization 3 months ago showed two-vessel coronary artery disease with obstructions of 55% and 65% in the right coronary and circumflex coronary arteries, respectively. Despite appropriate use of sublingual NTG tablets (0.4 mg) and oral isosorbide dinitrate (40 mg at 6 AM, noon, and 5 PM), T.I. is having four to five angina attacks per week. His physician writes a prescription

for atenolol (Tenormin) 50 mg every day. How do β-adrenergic blockers prevent angina?

β-Adrenergic blockers reduce myocardial oxygen demand by decreasing catecholamine-mediated increases in heart rate, BP, and, to some extent, myocardial contractility.[58–60] As such, β-blockers have been demonstrated to be very effective at reducing anginal symptoms and ischemia, including silent myocardial ischemia.[1,2] β-Blockers might also favorably affect myocardial metabolism, coronary microvasculature, collateral blood flow, myocardial blood flow, and oxygen-hemoglobin affinity.[61]

In patients with chronic angina, current guidelines recommend β-blockers be administered before a nitrate or a CCB when long-term therapy is indicated.[1,2] Although β-blockers significantly reduce anginal symptoms, increase exercise tolerance, as well as time to ST-segment depression during exercise testing, few randomized controlled trials have assessed the impact of β-blockers on clinical outcomes in patients with chronic stable angina.[60] Several cohort and case-control studies have demonstrated, however, that β-blockers do improve clinical outcomes, including reductions in mortality in patients with chronic stable angina or CAD.[62–66] In addition, recent evidence indicates that β-blockers may also slow the progression of atherosclerosis.[67] In a meta-analysis of clinical trials that compared the three classes of anti-ischemics, differences in long-term mortality were not noted. β-Blockers, however, were more effective in lowering the incidence of anginal episodes.[68] β-Blockers are generally considered the most effective class of agents at preventing silent myocardial ischemia.[3] In addition, β-blockers clearly lower morbidity and mortality in patients with hypertension,[69] acute MI,[11,12] and heart failure.[60] Although mortality benefits have not been demonstrated specifically in patients with chronic angina, the body of literature available supports the recommendation that all patients with angina should receive a β-blocker as initial therapy unless contraindicated.[36] (See Chapter 13, Essential Hypertension, and Chapter 18, Heart Failure, for more in-depth information on β-blocker product availability, dosage forms, pharmacology, and dosing.)

Judging Therapeutic Endpoint

20. How can the efficacy of the atenolol be assessed?

All patients receiving antianginal drugs should be monitored for frequency of angina attacks and NTG consumption. Nevertheless, this provides only an estimate of therapeutic efficacy because the patient's exercise and stress levels change from day to day. Traditionally, clinicians have monitored the reduction in resting heart rate and have progressively increased the β-blocker dose until the resting heart rate was 55 or 60 beats/minute. Heart rates <50 beats/minute may be acceptable, provided the patient is asymptomatic and heart block is not present. This approach does not take into account, however, that although the initial β-blocker dose reduces heart rate, subsequent increases in dose may only slightly reduce the resting heart rate. Variations in resting heart rate are normal and subject to the influence of the endogenous sympathetic nervous system and other exogenous factors, such as drugs, tobacco, and caffeine-containing beverages. β-Blockers with intrinsic sympathomimetic activity (e.g., pindolol) will not reduce the resting heart rate as much as β-blockers lacking this activity.[59]

Exercise testing is probably the most accurate, but least practical method of documenting the adequacy of β-blocker therapy. During an exercise tolerance test, atenolol should substantially increase the time T.I. walks before developing angina. There also may be a reduction in ST-segment depression during exercise, indicating less myocardial ischemia. The heart rate-SBP product probably will be markedly lowered, reflecting a decrease in both heart rate and systolic wall tension.[58] β-Blocker dosages needed to achieve these effects are highly variable. Therefore, therapy should be initiated with the lowest possible effective dosage and titrated upward. Continuous assessment of T.I.'s exercise tolerance is advisable.

Dosing Frequency

21. Is once-daily dosing of atenolol sufficient to provide T.I. with 24-hour protection? How often should immediate-release propranolol be administered?

The pharmacodynamic effects of β-blockers are longer than their plasma half-lives, and β-blockers can be dosed once or twice a day for angina. The half-life of atenolol is about 10 hours during chronic dosing; however, clinical studies support a once-a-day dosing schedule.[61]

Propranolol has a relatively short plasma half-life of 2 to 3 hours, yet clinicians have observed that a single dose lowers the heart rate and BP for at least 12 hours. Subsequent studies have confirmed the efficacy of twice-daily dosing for propranolol in the treatment of angina. (See Chapter 13, Essential Hypertension, for detailed pharmacokinetic and pharmacodynamic discussion of β-blockers.)[61]

β-Blocker Cardioselectivity

Contraindications

22. R.O. is a 65-year-old man with a 40-pack-year smoking history and a 13-year history of insulin-dependent diabetes mellitus. His ability to walk is limited by peripheral vascular disease and claudication, as well as by exertional angina. A β-blocker is to be initiated for treatment of chronic angina. Which β-blocker would be preferable for this patient?

Although all β-blockers are equally effective in the treatment of angina, R.O.'s medical history poses several relative contraindications to the use of some β-blockers. His smoking history may have caused some degree of chronic obstructive pulmonary disease (COPD) with a bronchospastic component despite the absence of a medical history. His history of diabetes and peripheral vascular disease will influence the selection of a β-blocker for management of his angina. A cardioselective β-blocker offers several advantages in R.O.[59] Drugs such as acebutolol (Sectral), atenolol, and metoprolol (Lopressor) primarily inhibit β_1-receptors in the heart and produce less blockade of β_2-receptors in the bronchial and vascular smooth muscle. In patients with asthma and obstructive lung disease, β_2-receptors mediate airway responsiveness and blockade of β_2-receptors can cause severe bronchospasm and respiratory difficulty. In one meta-analysis, cardioselective β-blockers were not found to produce clinically significant adverse respiratory effects in patients who had mild to moderate reactive airway disease.[70]

Cardioselective β-blockers also are less likely to inhibit β_2-mediated vasodilation in the peripheral arterioles. Therefore, cardioselective β-blockers are preferred over nonselective β-blockers for patients with peripheral vascular disease and Raynaud's disease. Blockade of peripheral β_2-receptors would permit unopposed α-mediated vasoconstriction and could decrease R.O.'s walking tolerance markedly.

Although β-blockers can alter glucose metabolism and mask the symptoms of hypoglycemia, their use has clearly been demonstrated to lower overall mortality in diabetic patients after acute MI.[11,12] In addition, diabetic patients in general develop more severe CAD and overall have a worse prognosis than patients without diabetes. Because of the significant beneficial effects on mortality with β-blockers, diabetes should not be considered a contraindication to β-blocker therapy.

Adverse Effects

23. If R.O. receives a cardioselective β-blocker, could he still experience more difficulty breathing or walking?

Cardioselectivity is not an all-or-none response; instead, it is a dose-dependent phenomenon. As the dose is increased, cardioselectivity is lost. The dose at which cardioselectivity will be lost in R.O. cannot be predicted, however; even a very small dose (e.g., metoprolol 37.5 mg) could cause wheezing.[59,61] Some evidence suggests that atenolol may have a larger window of dosing than metoprolol before cardioselectivity is lost. Similarly, a cardioselective drug could worsen R.O.'s claudication. If R.O. experiences worsening control of COPD or peripheral vascular disease, a better alternative may be a CCB either alone or with intermittent nitrate therapy.

Abrupt Withdrawal

24. J.F., a 76-year-old retiree with a long history of chronic stable angina controlled with oral isosorbide mononitrate 90 mg every day, and atenolol 100 mg every day, stopped his atenolol 36 hours ago when he forgot to get his prescriptions refilled. He is transported to the hospital emergency department (ED) for treatment of angina unresponsive to five NTG tablets. How could J.F.'s situation have been avoided?

The β-blocker withdrawal syndrome places patients with CAD at high risk for adverse cardiovascular events, which may include acute MI and sudden cardiac death. After J.F.'s angina has been controlled with medications during this particular hospitalization and before reinstitution of β-blocker therapy, he should be warned not to precipitously discontinue his β-blockers in the future. Failure to renew prescriptions and financial hardship are common reasons for abrupt discontinuation, and clinicians need to have sufficient professional rapport with patients to understand when patients encounter difficulties in obtaining medications.

The β-blocker withdrawal syndrome is a rebound phenomenon resulting from heightened β-receptor density and sensitivity (i.e., upregulation) subsequent to receptor blockade. An "overshoot" in heart rate, as a consequence of sympathoadrenal activity from abrupt β-blocker withdrawal increases myocardial oxygen demand and platelet aggregation. Withdrawal syndromes may be less severe in patients taking β-blockers with partial agonist activity.[56,58]

If β-blockers are to be discontinued, a gradual tapering schedule (preferably over 1 to 2 weeks) should be used. Shorter periods for β-blocker withdrawal (e.g., 2–3 days) have been proposed, although the optimal strategy for discontinuation is not known. Ensuring that β-blockers are tapered and that the patient is reasonably monitored for adverse events for the duration of the taper is imperative. Patients should limit physical activity throughout the β-blocker withdrawal period and seek prompt medical attention when angina symptoms become apparent.

Calcium Channel Blockers

Classification

Calcium channel blockers are highly diverse compounds. They differ markedly in chemical structure as well as specificity for cardiac and peripheral tissue. Using these characteristics, it is possible to classify calcium antagonists into several major types (Table 16-5).[71,72]

Both diltiazem and verapamil exert qualitatively similar effects on myocardial and peripheral tissue. They slow conduction and prolong the refractory period in the AV node. Ventricular refractory period is not affected. Therefore, the antiarrhythmic utility of these drugs is limited to controlling the ventricular rate in supraventricular tachyarrhythmias. Both agents can depress myocardial contractility and should be used with caution in patients with LV dysfunction (heart failure). They are moderate peripheral vasodilators and potent coronary artery vasodilators.[71,72]

Nifedipine is the prototype compound of the dihydropyridine derivatives. Although amlodipine, felodipine, isradipine, and nicardipine are second-generation dihydropyridines, only nicardipine and amlodipine currently are approved for the treatment of chronic stable angina pectoris. In addition, amlodipine is indicated for vasospastic angina. In contrast to diltiazem or verapamil, the dihydropyridines do not slow cardiac conduction and, therefore, have no antiarrhythmic action. They, however, are more potent peripheral vasodilators and are associated with a reflex increase in the heart rate. All dihydropyridines have negative inotropic effects in vitro, but these effects, clinically, are overshadowed by the reflex sympathetic activation and decreased afterload. The net effect of these actions essentially results in no depression of myocardial function (see Chapter 18, Heart Failure).[71,72] The dihydropyridines also can dilate coronary arteries, but vary in their potency.

Pharmacology

Depending on the agent, CCBs decrease myocardial oxygen demand and increase myocardial blood supply.[71,72] By inhibiting smooth muscle contraction, CCBs dilate blood vessels and decrease resistance to blood flow. Dilation of peripheral vessels reduces systemic vascular resistance and BP, thus decreasing the work load of the heart. Coronary artery dilation improves coronary blood flow. Diltiazem and verapamil also decrease the myocardial contractile force (negative inotropic effect) as well as heart rate. All these actions can reduce angina symptoms.

Table 16-5 Calcium Channel Blockers in Anginal Syndromes[a]

Drug Name	*FDA Approved[a]*	*Usual Dose for Chronic Stable Angina[b]*	*Product Availability[c]*
Dihydropyridines			
Amlodipine	Angina, hypertension	2.5–10 mg QD	2.5, 5, 10 mg tab
Felodipine	Hypertension	5–20 mg QD	5, 10 mg ER tab
Isradapine	Hypertension	2.5–10 mg BID 5–10 mg QD	2.5, 5 mg IR cap 5, 10 mg CR tab
Nicardipine	Angina (IR only), Hypertension	20–40 mg TID 30–60 mg BID	20, 30 mg IR cap 30, 45, 60 mg SR cap
Nifedipine	Angina, Hypertension	10–30 mg TID 30–180 mg QD	10, 20 mg IR cap 30, 60, 90 mg ER tab
Nisoldipine (Sular)	Hypertension	20–60 mg QD	10, 20, 30, 40 mg ER tab
Diphenylalkylamines			
Verapamil	Angina, hypertension, SVT	30–120 mgTID/QID 120–240 mg BID 120–480 mg Q HS	40, 80, 120 mg IR tab 120, 180, 240 mg SR tab 180, 240 mg DR, ER tab 120, 180, 240, 360 mg ER cap 100, 200, 300 mg DR, ER tab
Benzothiazepines			
Diltiazem	Angina, hypertension, SVT	30–120 mg TID/QID 60–180 mg BID 120–480 mg QD	30, 60, 90, 120 mg IR tab 60, 90, 120, 180 mg SR cap 120, 180, 240, 300, 360 mg cap 120, 180, 240 mg ER cap 120, 180, 240, 300, 360, 420 mg ER cap

[a] FDA-approved indications vary among IR and ER products. However, most all have been used clinically for both angina and hypertension. Avoid IR release products in hypertension.
[b] Because of short half-lives, most of these drugs are given TID if using IR tabs or caps. Amlodipine has a long half-life and is given PD.
Also see Tables 14-15 and 14-16 in Chapter 14: Essential Hypertension.
Cap, capsules; CD, controlled diffusion; CR, controlled release; DR, delayed release; ER, extended release; FDA, U.S. Food and Drug Administration; HS, bedtime; IR, immediate release; Q, every; QID, four times a day; SR, sustained release; SVT, supraventricular including atrial fibrillation, atrial flutter, and reentry; Tab, tablets; XL and XR, extended release.

Potent arterial (peripheral) vasodilators, such as nifedipine, markedly reduce peripheral vascular resistance,[71] and reflexively stimulate the sympathetic nervous system to cause a slight to moderate increase in heart rate and perhaps increase myocardial oxygen demand (Table 16-6). The cardiodepressant effect of verapamil- and diltiazem-like drugs prevents reflex tachycardia. Verapamil and diltiazem are more likely to worsen ventricular function in patients with HF secondary to systolic dysfunction.[72] Two dihydropyridines, amlodipine and felodipine, have been studied in the setting of LV dysfunction and found to be relatively safer than other calcium blockers in heart failure, but have a negligible effect on mortality.[71] Therefore, these two drugs are available options in patients with HF who have other disease states that would benefit from CCB therapy. Diltiazem and verapamil should be avoided in HF. Individualization of CCB therapy must consider the drug's overall pharmacologic effect and side effect profile.

Indications for Use

25. B.N., a 56-year-old man, has just undergone cardiac catheterization, which showed two-vessel CAD. He refuses to take nitrates because they cause severe headaches. His medical history includes asthma and hyperlipidemia. His physician begins antianginal therapy with oral diltiazem 120 mg every day. Are the calcium channel blockers indicated for all types of angina?

Calcium channel blockers are effective in both vasospastic and classic exertional angina. These drugs relieve vasospasm of the large coronary arteries and, as a result, are effective in treating Prinzmetal's variant angina. Their beneficial effect in chronic stable (effort-induced) angina is the result of multiple factors. Their vasodilatory effects in the coronary circulation increase myocardial oxygen supply, whereas dilation of the peripheral arterioles leads to a reduction in myocardial oxygen demand. Because coronary vasospasm can occur at the site of an atherosclerotic plaque, a CCB is particularly useful in patients who have a vasospastic component to their angina.

Although β-blockers are considered the drugs of choice when instituting antianginal therapy, recent data indicate that the selection of a heart rate-lowering CCB may also be a reasonable first-line choice as well. Calcium channel blockers and β-blockers appear to provide equivalent efficacy in head-to-head trials of chronic stable angina.[73,74] In addition, the available head-to-head trials with sufficient numbers also suggest that CCBs and β-blockers produce similar effects on cardiovascular outcomes and mortality in patients with chronic stable angina.[75,76] In addition, several recent trials in the setting of hypertension have demonstrated that CCBs can produce meaningful reductions in mortality.[77–79] It would appear that either

Table 16-6 Calcium Channel Blockers

Effect	*Dihydropyridine Derivatives*[a]	*Diltiazem*	*Verapamil*
Peripheral vasodilation[b]	+++	++	++
Coronary vasodilation[b]	+++	+++	++
Negative inotropes[c]	±	++	+++
AV node suppression[c]	±	+	++
Heart rate	Increase (reflex)	Decrease or unchanged	Decrease or unchanged
Pharmacokinetics[d]			
Dosing[e]			
Side Effects			
Nausea, vomiting	+ (most)	+/1	±
Constipation	Not observed	±	+
Hypotension, dizziness[g]	++	+	+
Flushing, headache	++	+	+
Bradycardia, heart failure (HF) symptoms	±	+	++
Reflex tachycardia, angina	+[g]	Not observed	Not observed
Peripheral edema	+	±	±
Drug Interactions[h]			

Also see Tables 13-15 and 13-16 in Chapter 13: Essential Hypertension.

[a] Dihydropyridine derivatives U.S. Food and Drug Administration (FDA) approved for angina: amlodipine (Norvasc), nicardipine (Cardene), and nifedipine (Adalat, Procardia). See Table 13–6 for others that are approved for hypertension but have been used clinically for angina. Investigational: nitrendipine (Baypress).

[b] Peripheral and coronary vasodilation helpful for angina, hypertension, and possibly HF, but peripheral dilation is the basis for side effects of flushing, headache, and hypotension.

[c] Atrioventricular (AV) node suppression is helpful for controlling supraventricular arrhythmias, but this property plus the negative inotropic effect may worsen HF. Nifedipine has less negative inotropic effect than verapamil and diltiazem, but still may worsen HF. Amlodipine may have the least negative inotropic effect.

[d] All have poor bioavailability owing to high first-pass metabolism and all are eliminated primarily by hepatic metabolism; intra- and interindividual variability in bioavailability and metabolism is extensive. Diltiazem, nifedipine, nicardipine, and verapamil have short half-life (<5 hr) requiring frequent dosing or use of sustained release (SR) products. Amlodipine, isradipine (8 hr), and felodipine (10–20 hr) have longer half-life.

[e] See Table 13-6 and Tables 13-16 in Chapter 13: Essential Hypertension.

[g] Hypotension and reflex tachycardia most with immediate release nifedipine, occasional with immediate-release diltiazem and verapamil, minimal with sustained release products or intrinsically long-acting agents.

[h] Diltiazem and verapamil, weak CYP 3A4 inhibitors and strong P-glycoprotein inhibitors. Increase cyclosporine and digoxin bioavailability via increased gastrointestinal (GI) transport and possibly less gut metabolism. Case reports of cyclosporine renal toxicity when combined with diltiazem. Bradycardia and heart failure risk with combined verapamil and digoxin via additive AV block and negative inotropic effects. Risk of interaction with drugs metabolized by CYP 3A4 not known.

a heart rate-lowering CCB, or a β-blocker, may be considered relatively equal options and initial therapy for chronic stable angina. The selection of a particular class will likely be dictated by patient characteristics.

In the case of B.N., his asthma may be worsened by the addition of a β-blocker. Although a cardioselective β-blocker could be tried to see if B.N. could tolerate it, a heart rate-lowering CCB is a good alternatives to a β-blocker for the treatment of angina in this situation. The choice of a CCB as initial therapy in this patient is appropriate because of B.N.'s previous intolerance to nitrates and because nitrate therapy requires the scheduling of a nitrate-free period.[1] Patients with significant peripheral arterial disease, or demonstrated exercise intolerance to β-blockers, are also likely good candidates for CCB monotherapy for chronic angina. For patients with a history of MI or who have HF, β-blockers would likely be preferred because of the substantial literature demonstrating improved outcomes in these patient populations. In the absence of any patient-specific characteristics to help guide selection, it is pertinent to recognize that current guidelines still recommend β-blockers as the primary initial antianginal therapy.[1,2]

Although the selection of a heart rate-lowering CCB may be generally preferred, the distinct pharmacologic and adverse event profiles of the various classes may also help dictate agent selection. Some side effects of CCBs reflect an extension of their hemodynamic and electrophysiologic profiles and, therefore, are predictable (Table 16-6). Dihydropyridine-induced hypotension and dizziness occur in approximately 15% of patients. Patients also may complain of light-headedness, facial flushing, headache, and nausea. Swelling of the lower legs and ankles (peripheral edema) is related to the potent peripheral vasodilating effects of these agents. Verapamil and diltiazem have similar side effect profiles, although diltiazem appears to be better tolerated. The lower incidence of side effects reported with diltiazem, compared with verapamil, may reflect a true difference or, perhaps, less aggressive dosing regimens. Both drugs can cause sinus bradycardia and worsen already existing conduction defects and heart block.[65] Neither should be used in patients with sick sinus syndrome or advanced degrees of heart block unless a functioning ventricular pacemaker is present. Patients should be monitored for signs of worsening HF, such as SOB, weight gain, and peripheral edema. Verapamil-induced constipation can be particularly troublesome to the elderly. Rare instances of fecal impaction requiring surgery illustrate the need for the aggressive use of stool-softening agents and, often, bulk-forming laxatives.

Generalized fatigue and nonspecific gastrointestinal (GI) complaints can occur with any of the calcium channel blockers. In rare instances, elevations of hepatic enzymes and acute hepatic injury have occurred with CCBs. Appreciation for the individual side effect profiles helps determine preference for one CCB over another. B.N. is not likely to experience major side effects with either verapamil or diltiazem.

Pharmacokinetics

26. Do any of the calcium channel blockers require dosage adjustment in patients with renal or hepatic disease?

Currently available calcium channel antagonists demonstrate similar pharmacokinetic properties.[71] With the exception of amlodipine and the SR formulations, all are absorbed rapidly after oral administration and generally reach peak concentrations within 1 to 2 hours. Peak concentrations for amlodipine usually are achieved within 6 to 9 hours after administration. Although calcium channel antagonists are well absorbed, bioavailability generally is low owing largely to first-pass metabolism. In addition, calcium channel antagonists tend to have high metabolic clearances; their pharmacokinetic parameters are related to hepatic blood flow and intrinsic clearance, and they are metabolized almost exclusively by the liver. Furthermore, intraindividual and interindividual variations in bioavailability and total body clearance for most calcium channel antagonists are great. Therefore, dosage adjustment probably is necessary in patients with severe hepatic impairment, but not in those with renal disease.

Sustained-Release Calcium Channel Blockers

27. L.M., a 45-year-old female surgeon with a 3-year history of hypertension, recently was switched to sustained release verapamil 240 mg BID. As newly diagnosed with chronic stable angina, she wonders if studies support the use of SR calcium channel blockers in angina.

Nifedipine, diltiazem, and verapamil all were originally introduced into the United States as immediate-release preparations. As a consequence, dosing regimens called for TID or four times daily (QID) administration. SR CCBs are attractive alternatives to immediate-release products. The SR formulations of verapamil, diltiazem, and nifedipine offer promise in improving patient drug adherence and, thereby, better control of anginal episodes. L.M. uses the first SR CCB marketed in the United States. SR verapamil is absorbed more slowly than immediate-release verapamil, thus providing more constant serum levels. The SR formulation, with a bioavailability of 0.9, extends the verapamil elimination half-life to 12 hours compared with about 6 hours observed with the immediate-release product.[80] Although some patients experience adequate control with once-daily SR verapamil, most patients require twice-daily dosing.[67] Another SR verapamil product (Verelan) uses beaded capsules and can be dosed reliably once a day. Therefore, SR verapamil and Verelan should not be interchanged. The side effect profiles for immediate-release and SR verapamil are similar, with constipation being frequent.

Diltiazem SR also exhibits slowed absorption and a prolonged half-life compared with immediate-release diltiazem. As with verapamil SR, twice-daily dosing of diltiazem SR is appropriate for most patients. A newer version of SR diltiazem (Cardizem CD available as 180-, 240-, and 300-mg capsules) may be given once daily. It is important that the Cardizem SR and Cardizem CD products are not confused. Another SR diltiazem product (Dilacor SR) uses yet another delivery system. Although verapamil SR and diltiazem SR and CD are FDA approved for treatment of hypertension only, many clinicians use these drugs to treat angina.

Sustained-release nifedipine (Procardia XL) uses a unique drug delivery system based on the osmotic pump principle. The GITS (GI system) nifedipine tablet consists of a semipermeable membrane that surrounds an active drug core. The core is composed of two layers: an active drug layer and an inert, but osmotically active push layer. Water entering the tablet from the GI tract activates the osmotic pump mechanism and pushes the active nifedipine out through a laser-drilled hole in the tablet's active layer. The inert components eventually are eliminated in the feces as a shell. The tablet should not be crushed, divided, or chewed. It should be taken at the same time each day and may be taken either with food or on an empty stomach.

The GITS nifedipine provides consistent (zero order rate), 24-hour serum nifedipine levels independent of pH or GI motility. Although this formulation decreases the vasodilatory effects observed with immediate-release nifedipine, dose-related edema is a common adverse experience occurring in 10% to 30% of patients. Headache is another common adverse effect. Limited experience suggests that patients switched from immediate-release nifedipine to GITS nifedipine will experience fewer angina episodes and side effects. Another form of extended-release tablets (Adalat CC) can be administered once daily and appears to be therapeutically equivalent to GITS nifedipine. Nevertheless, when patients are converted to any SR CCB, reassessment of therapeutic efficacy is necessary. Because variations in SR products exist, they should not be substituted for one another without prior approval and patient counseling. The cost of the SR CCB is similar to the equivalent immediate-release doses. At one time, the use of generic immediate-release products was considered a cost-saving alternative, but now generic SR products are marketed as well.

Any of the SR preparations of nifedipine, verapamil, or diltiazem are reasonable choices for patients with chronic stable angina. Immediate-release preparations of CCBs should be reserved for situations in which rapid titration of the dose is needed or desired, such as in patients with supraventricular arrhythmias. As stated, use of immediate-release nifedipine should be discouraged in any situation owing to the risk of reflex sympathetic drive and potential precipitation of myocardial ischemia. (See Chapter 13, Essential Hypertension, for further discussion of SR dosage forms of calcium channel blockers.)

Ranolazine

Approved by the FDA in early 2006, ranolazine is the first new antianginal agent marketed in nearly 20 years. The need for additional agents to modify and treat myocardial ischemia is illustrated by the fact that many patients have contraindications to one or more traditional antianginal agents, or may not tolerate larger therapeutic doses of a specific drug used as monotherapy. Others may have intolerance to the additive hemodynamic effects of combination therapy, as well as incomplete relief of symptoms from revascularization therapy. For example, despite the effectiveness of PCI at relieving symptoms of angina, 10% to 25% of patients still have angina and 60% to 80% require antianginal therapy 1 year after the procedure.[81,82] Therefore, a need clearly exists for new antianginal agents to complement existing pharmacologic and revascularization strategies.

Mechanism of Action

Unlike traditional antianginal agents, such as β-blockers, CCBs, and long-acting nitrates, ranolazine does not have any appreciable effects on heart rate, arterial resistance vessels, the inotropic state of the myocardium, or coronary blood flow. When administered clinically, no changes in blood pressure or heart rate are observed.[83] As such, ranolazine does not affect myocardial oxygen supply or demand in the traditional sense. Early preclinical work identified inhibition of fatty acid oxidation as the probable mechanism for antianginal efficacy.[84,85] Subsequent investigations revealed, however, that these effects only occur at plasma concentrations of ranolazine substantially higher than those obtained with current approved doses.[86,87] It is now known that ranolazine's anti-ischemic effects are modulated through inhibition of the late sodium current (I_{Na}).[16,83] By inhibiting late sodium entry, and hence calcium overload during ischemia, ranolazine effectively inhibits the consequences of ischemia such as decreased microvascular perfusion, as well as increased myocardial oxygen demand. This novel mechanism of action offers the possibility of complementary effects when added to more traditional antianginal agents which act through their hemodynamic actions.

Pharmacokinetics and Dosing

Initial investigations of ranolazine involved an immediate-release product that necessitated three times/day dosing. Because of the short half-life of the parent drug, the peak-to-trough ratio in clinical studies were suboptimal, with significant loss of therapeutic efficacy at the end of the dosing interval.[88–91] Consequently, ranolazine is marketed as an extended-release tablet formulation that should be dosed twice daily. Maximal plasma concentrations are observed 4 to 6 hours after administration of the extended-release formulation with a terminal half-life of 7 hours. With twice-daily dosing of the extended-release preparation, a more favorable peak-to-trough fluctuation of 1.6 is observed.[83] Steady-state is typically reached within 3 days and oral bioavailability is in the 30% to 55% range. Ranolazine is primarily metabolized by the liver through cytochrome P450 (CYP) 3A4 (70%–85%), and CYP2D6 (10%–15%). Ranolazine also is a substrate for P-glycoprotein.[16,83] Patients should initially be started at an oral dose of 500 mg twice daily, which can be titrated up to a maximal dose of 1,000 mg twice daily.

Place in Therapy

28. **A.E., a 65-year-old man, has been treated for chronic angina pectoris for 4 years. He refuses cardiac catheterization and revascularization; however, his coronary risk factors include a strong family history of cardiovascular disease and hyperlipoproteinemia. He experienced rheumatic fever at age 12; 5 years ago, his mitral valve was replaced. At that time, he had two-vessel CAD with 80% and 85% occlusion and an LV EF of 30% (normal, 55%). Current medications include a prescription for SL nitroglycerin; warfarin 5 mg for 5 days/week and 2.5 mg for 2 days/week; metoprolol 50 mg every day; enalapril 10 mg every day; digoxin 0.125 mg/day (serum digoxin concentration drawn 18 hours after the last dose is 0.7 ng/mL); oral simvastatin 40 mg every day; and furosemide 40 mg/day. At his regular follow-up visit with his cardiologist, A.E. reports an increase in weekly anginal attacks over the last 2 months during his daily routine of working in his yard. Current vital signs include a blood pressure of 110/60 mmHg and a resting heart rate of 60 beats/minute. What therapeutic options would be available for A.E. for additional control of his chronic stable angina? Would ranolazine be an option?**

As discussed, monotherapy for chronic stable angina typically starts with a β-blocker or, in select patients, a heart rate-lowering CCB. These agents are typically titrated up based on both efficacy and tolerance. Once a maximal dose of the initial agent is reached, additional antianginal agents can be added, if needed, for additional symptom control. The choice of which agent to add on is likely dictated by the specific characteristics of the patient. In a patient on a β-blocker who needs additional blood pressure control, the addition of a dihydropyridine CCB would seem prudent. A nondihydropyridine agent may be an option, however, if additional heart rate control is also needed. Conversely, in a patient maximized on β-blocker therapy, with adequate blood pressure control and also a history of heart failure, the addition of a long-acting nitrate may be preferred. Triple therapy with a β-blocker, a CCB, and a nitrate is also an option in patients whose condition is difficult to control, but careful attention must be paid to the additive hemodynamic effects to minimize intolerance.

In the setting of additional antianginal therapy, ranolazine should be considered. Several large, randomized studies with ranolazine have been conducted, all demonstrating it is effective at reducing ischemia and angina when added on to existing therapy. Although not FDA approved as monotherapy in the treatment of chronic stable angina, the Monotherapy Assessment of Ranolazine in Stable Angina (MARISA) trial randomized patients in a crossover fashion who had met screening exercise treadmill criteria to either escalating doses of ranolazine (500 mg BID, 1,000 mg BID, 1,500 mg BID) or placebo. All other antianginal agents, except for SL nitroglycerin, were discontinued before start of the study. Ranolazine significantly increased exercise duration, time to onset of angina, and to 1 mm ST-segment depression during exercise treadmill testing.[86] Similar results were seen in the Combination Assessment of Ranolazine in Stable Angina (CARISA) trial where ranolazine (500 mg BID, 750 mg BID, 1,000 mg BID) was added onto antianginal monotherapy that consisted of either atenolol 50 mg/day, diltiazem 180 mg/day, or amlodopine 5 mg/day.[87] The Efficacy of Ranolazine in Chronic Angina (ERICA) trial assessed the effects of ranolazine when added to the maximal dose of an existing antianginal agent, in this case amlodopine 10 mg/day. Importantly, up to one-half of the patients enrolled in ERICA were also on a long-acting nitrate. Patients were randomized to either ranolazine 500 mg/day for 1 week and then had their dose increased to 1,000 mg/day for an additional 6 weeks, or placebo. Patients receiving 1,000 mg/day of ranolazine had a significant reduction in both the number of weekly anginal attacks, as well as the number of SL nitroglycerin tablets used on a weekly basis.[92] Ranolazine was well-tolerated in the CARISA, MARISA, and ERICA trials with the most common side effects being dizziness, constipation, nausea, and headache. The incidence of adverse effects increased with increasing doses. No other significant adverse effects were noted, although it is important to note the duration of these trials was limited.[83]

A.E. is at goal heart rate and his blood pressure is well controlled on his current regimen, but he continues to have

Table 16-7 Considerations for the Use of Ranolazine If Patients With Chronic Stable Angina[16,83]

Clinical Issue	Recommended Management Strategy
Renal insufficiency	Ranolazine plasma levels may increase up to 50%. Caution with dose titration to maximal recommended dose.
Hepatic insufficiency	Ranolazine is contraindicated in patients with Child-Pugh Classes A, B, or C hepatic impairment.
Drug interactions: Effects on ranolazine	
CYP 3A4 inhibitors	Plasma concentrations of ranolazine are significantly elevated when combined with potent inhibitors of CYP3A4.
	Ketoconazole, diltiazem, verapamil, and other potent or moderately potent inhibitors of CYP 3A4 should not be coadministered with ranolazine.
CYP 3A4 inducers	Rifampin coadministration should be avoided owing to significant decreases in ranolazine plasma concentrations. Coadministration with other CYP 3A4 inducers should also be avoided.
P-glycoprotein inhibitors	Caution should be exercised when coadministering ranolazine with P-glycoprotein inhibitors.
Drug interactions: effects on other medications	
Simvastatin	Plasma levels of simvastatin are increased twofold with coadministration with ranolazine through CYP 3A4 inhibition by ranolazine. Closely monitor for adverse effects (e.g., myositis) from simvastatin.
Digoxin	Ranolazine coadministration increases plasma concentrations of digoxin by 1.5 times. Adjust dose of digoxin accordingly to maintain desired therapeutic level and response.
CYP 2D6 substrates	Ranolazine can inhibit the activity of CYP 2D6 and thus the metabolism of drugs metabolized by this enzyme may be impaired. The dose of these medications may need to be reduced.
QTc prolongation	Use of ranolazine is contraindicated in patients with pre-existing QTc prolongation.
	Use of ranolazine is contraindicated in patients receiving other QTc prolonging medications.

anginal symptoms. Because of the lack of hemodynamic effects, ranolazine is a reasonable option for A.E., in addition to continuing metoprolol. A long-acting nitrate is also an option, but this could lower his blood pressure more than is desired. A CCB should not be given because A.E. has evidence of poorly controlled heart failure (EF of 30%). His initial dose of ranolazine should be 500 mg orally two times/day and titrated up to 1,000 mg twice daily if needed for additional efficacy.

29. Is ranolazine safe for long-term use in A.E.?

Initial information regarding the safety of ranolazine in patients with longer drug exposure came from the Ranolazine Open Label Experience (ROLE) program,[93] which followed patients from the MARISA and CARISA trials who continued participation in an open-label extension program. A total of 746 patients initially entered the 6-year run-on safety program. At the time of publication, the mean duration of therapy was 2.82 years, with 23.3% of patients discontinuing therapy. One-half of the withdrawals were because of adverse events, but the incidence of common adverse effects did not seem to change from that seen in the randomized portions of the clinical trials. Mortality rates at both 1 year (2.8%) and 2 years (5.6%) indicate no adverse risk of ranolazine on overall mortality.

Additional safety data are now available from the Metabolic Efficiency with Ranolazine for Less Ischemia in Non–ST-Elevation Acute Coronary Syndrome (MERLIN)-TIMI 36 trial.[94] Patients in the MERLIN trial were randomly assigned to ranolazine or placebo in the setting of non–ST-segment ACS. Ranolazine was administered as an IV infusion for 12 to 96 hours, then converted to 1,000 mg twice daily. Patients were assessed for clinical endpoints during the acute hospitalization, then every 4 months thereafter. Treatment was continued for a median of 348 days. The primary endpoint of the trial (cardiovascular death, MI, or recurrent ischemia) trended lower with patients on ranolazine, but was not statistically significant (23.5% placebo, 21.8% ranolazine, $P = 0.11$). The incidence of recurrent ischemia was significantly reduced, however, with ranolazine (4.2% vs. 5.9%, $P = 0.02$), providing additional support for the efficacy of ranolazine in treating chronic stable angina. Although ranolazine appeared to offer no benefit in the setting of ACS, significant long-term safety data were seen in the trial. Importantly, the risk of mortality, sudden cardiac death, or symptomatic arrhythmias was not increased with ranolazine versus placebo. In fact, the incidence of arrhythmias in the first 7 days as documented by Holter monitor was significantly lower with ranolazine than with placebo.[95] This was an important finding given ranolazine produces a dose-dependent increase in the QT interval.[16,83] As QT prolongation activity has been associated with proarrhythmia in other medications, results from the MERLIN trial are reassuring that ranolazine appears to be safe to use for chronic treatment of patients with stable angina.

30. Are there special considerations for the use of ranolazine in A.E.?

Although ranolazine is a promising new option in the treatment of chronic stable angina, careful patient selection is required for the drug to be used safely and effectively. Table 16-7 summarizes significant issues which should be evaluated when the drug is being considered for a patient. For A.E., the main issues are the potential for ranolazine to increase plasma concentrations of both simvastatin (twofold increase) and digoxin (1.5 times increase). A.E. should be monitored closely for possible increased adverse effects from both simvastatin (myalgias, liver toxicity), as well as digoxin (heart block, GI intolerance) after the initiation of ranolazine. The dose of each medication ultimately may need to be decreased.

VASCULOPROTECTIVE DRUG THERAPY

Angiotensin-Converting Enzyme Inhibitors

31. E.R., a 62-year-old woman with a long history of angina pectoris, has survived one out-of-hospital cardiac arrest and two

MIs. She is not considered a surgical candidate for CABG because of severe COPD. Her current medications include oral isosorbide mononitrate 60 mg every day, oral metoprolol 50 mg BID, oral diltiazem CD 240 mg every day, fluticasone two puffs BID, albuterol two puffs as needed (PRN), NTG spray 0.4 mg PRN chest pain, and enteric-coated aspirin 325 mg/day. Would the addition of an ACE inhibitor be beneficial for E.R. at this time?

Historically, ACE inhibitors have not been thought of as having anti-ischemic properties. Recent information indicates, however, that ACE inhibitors have a prominent role in the overall treatment of patients with CAD.

As a class, ACE inhibitors have demonstrated significant benefits on morbidity and mortality in a number of patient groups, such as those with HF, acute MI, and diabetes mellitus.[96] Interest in these agents for the treatment of chronic angina stems from results of studies investigating ACE inhibitors in patients with HF. Overall, ACE inhibitors decreased the risk of MI by approximately 23% in patients with HF.[97,98] This set the stage for the investigation of ACE inhibitors in patients with CAD who do not have LV dysfunction or who are status post MI.

In a large, randomized, placebo-controlled trial of 9,297 patients with chronic CAD and no HF (the HOPE study), ramipril significantly decreased the incidence of death, MI, stroke, need for revascularization, and worsening angina. All patients were on appropriate medical therapy for angina, and the benefit appeared to be independent of any antihypertensive effect of ramipril in the treatment group.[99] Although the direct mechanism of action is unclear, it is thought that ACE inhibitors have a number of beneficial effects relative to the atherosclerosis process. These include antagonizing the growth-mediating properties of angiotensin-2 on smooth muscle cells, preventing the rupture of atherosclerotic plaques by reducing inflammation, reducing LV hypertrophy, and improving endothelial function.[100]

The results of the European trial on reduction of cardiac events with perindopril in stable coronary artery disease (EUROPA) replicated the benefits seen in the HOPE study with the administration of perindopril in 12,218 patients with stable coronary heart disease and no apparent heart failure. Perindopril use (target dose 8 mg every day) for an average of 4.2 years resulted in a 20% relative risk reduction in the combined incidence of cardiovascular death, myocardial infarction, or cardiac arrest.[101] The results of the Prevention of Events with Angiotensin Converting Enzyme Inhibitors (PEACE), however, did not produce similar results as the HOPE and EUROPA trials. In PEACE, the addition of trandolapril 4 mg/day to standard therapy in patients with CAD did not reduce the rate of the primary endpoint, a composite of cardiovascular death, MI, or coronary revascularization.

Several plausible explanations exist for the different results seen in these three trials. The first is that patients in the PEACE trial appeared to be at much lower risk for a cardiovascular event than the patients enrolled in HOPE and EUROPA as evidenced by an event rate in the placebo group in PEACE that was lower than the treatment arm of the HOPE trial. Furthermore, patients in the PEACE trial were in general receiving more intensive risk factor modification as compared with those in the other two trials. Secondly, an inherent difference may exist in the three ACE inhibitors used, or the dosages used in the clinical trials. The results of the PEACE trial call into question whether all patients with CAD should receive an ACE inhibitor. ACE inhibitors are well established in the treatment of patients with HF, MI, and diabetes, however, so it is certainly prudent to treat patients with stable angina and the other compelling indications with an ACE inhibitor.[36]

While in theory angiotensin-receptor blockers (ARBs) should produce the same beneficial effects as ACE inhibitors in patients with atherosclerosis, there are no clinical trials available documenting whether this is indeed true. However, given the similar results ARBs have shown to ACE inhibitors in patients with HF and post-MI, and the significant beneficial effects with ARBs seen in treating patients with hypertension and diabetes, the administration of an ARB in patients with CAD and intolerance to ACE inhibitors seems reasonable.[36]

Antiplatelet Therapy

Aspirin

32. E.R. is taking enteric-coated aspirin every day. She wants advice to why she is being given this drug and if it is safe for her stomach. What is the most appropriate dose?

Platelet activation produces coronary occlusion either by formation of a platelet plug or through release of vasoactive compounds from the platelets. Two indices of platelet activity that have been studied intensely in patients with CAD are thromboxane A_2 and prostacyclin. Thromboxane A_2 is a cyclooxygenase-catalyzed product of arachidonic acid metabolism and a potent vasoconstrictor. Prostacyclin (PGI_2), another arachidonic acid metabolite produced under the influence of cyclooxygenase, counterbalances the effect of thromboxane A_2. It is a potent inhibitor of platelet aggregation and a vasodilator. Although PGI_2's production is increased in USA and acute MI, the amount produced is insufficient to fully offset the effects of elevated thromboxane A_2 levels.[102]

The mechanism of action for aspirin's antiplatelet effect is inhibition of cyclooxygenase (see Chapter 15, Thrombosis). By acetylating the active site of cyclooxygenase, aspirin blocks the formation of prostaglandin endoperoxides from arachidonic acid. This inhibits the formation of both thromboxane and prostacyclin. Researchers have tested various aspirin doses hoping to find a dose that inhibits thromboxane synthesis but does not inhibit formation of prostacyclin. A single 100-mg aspirin dose virtually eliminates thromboxane A_2 production, whereas doses below 100 mg result in a dose-dependent reduction in thromboxane A_2 synthesis. Therapeutic benefit has been demonstrated with doses as low as 30 mg/day.[103]

Recent research has attempted to determine the effect of aspirin doses on the thromboxane A_2 to PGI_2 balance. PGI_2 production recovers within hours of aspirin administration because the endothelial cell can resynthesize cyclooxygenase. In contrast, the inhibition of platelet cyclooxygenase is irreversible. Selective inhibition of platelet-generated thromboxane A_2 synthesis has been shown with 75 mg of controlled-release aspirin daily.[102–104] This aspirin formulation undergoes extensive first-pass metabolism forming salicylic acid, a weak and reversible cyclooxygenase inhibitor. Theoretically, administration of 75 mg aspirin daily in a controlled-release formulation may selectively spare vascular endothelial PGI_2 production, but at the same time still inhibit platelet cyclooxygenase. Controlled clinical trials on this proposed aspirin dosage regimen are lacking, however. Therefore, the proposed biochemical selectivity of aspirin on platelet function versus the vascular endothelium is difficult to achieve clinically.

Because of the lack of precise understanding of the pharmacodynamic effect of aspirin, it is not surprising that controversy exists regarding the optimal dose of aspirin to be used in patients with angina, as well as post-MI and as secondary prevention of stroke. It has been believed that higher doses of aspirin would produce a higher level of efficacy than low doses; however, all available literature indicates that low dosages of aspirin (75–325 mg/day) are as effective as higher dosages (625–1,300 mg/day) in the treatment of patients with angina.[104] Conversely, as the aspirin dosage increases, the incidence of adverse effects, especially GI bleeding, increases as well. Therefore, current guidelines recommend a daily dosage of 75 to 162 mg orally for the prevention of MI and death in patients with CAD.[104] Given this information, E.R. should be advised to lower her daily dose of aspirin to 81 mg/day to maintain efficacy but decrease the risk of adverse effects.

Aspirin remains the most commonly prescribed antiplatelet agent for the treatment of cardiovascular disease. Essentially all patients with a history of angina or CAD, especially if they have also experienced an MI, should take aspirin daily. Further discussions of aspirin use in the secondary prevention of MI, combined therapy with thrombolytics in the treatment of acute MI, atrial fibrillation, prosthetic valves, and postoperative CABG are discussed in Chapter 17, Myocardial Infarction, Chapter 15, Thrombosis, and Chapter 19, Cardiac Arrhythmias. Aspirin also is a key drug in treating cerebrovascular disease as presented in Chapter 51, Cerebrovascular Disorders.

Clopidogrel

33. As noted in Question 31, E.R. was taking 325 mg/day of enteric-coated aspirin. This was later reduced to 81 mg/day based on the discussion above. Last week she was hospitalized for rapidly worsening angina, diagnosed as unstable angina. She is being discharged today with a new prescription for oral clopidogrel 75 mg every day. Is the combined use of aspirin and clopidogrel appropriate? How long should clopidogrel be continued?

Clopidogrel (Plavix), a thienopydridine, inhibits platelet function in vivo. Its mechanism of action has not been identified, although it appears to be a noncompetitive antagonist of the platelet adenosine diphosphate (ADP) receptor. Stimulation of the ADP receptor produces platelet activation similar to thromboxane A_2. Clopidogrel at a dosage of 75 mg orally every day was demonstrated in one study to be slightly more effective than aspirin in the secondary prevention of MI and death in patients with various manifestations of atherosclerotic vascular disease.[105] The magnitude of difference in benefit seen with clopidogrel was quite small and not sufficient to justify its broad scale use in the treatment of CAD. Based on this study, the role of clopidogrel historically was to serve as an alternative antiplatelet agent in patients with a true contraindication to aspirin and it is still used in this fashion.[1,2,33]

The combination of aspirin and clopidogrel was compared with aspirin alone in patients with acute coronary syndromes without ST-segment elevation in the CURE study. Patients received combination antiplatelet therapy acutely while in the hospital and continued it for an average of 9 months. The combination of aspirin and clopidogrel significantly reduced the occurrence of death from cardiovascular causes, nonfatal MI, or stroke.[106] The results of the CURE study were confirmed in the Clopidogrel for Results of Events During Observation (CREDO) trial where patients with acute coronary syndromes who were treated with percutaneous coronary intervention with stent placement received aspirin plus clopidogrel acutely in the hospital and then for 1 year. Patients receiving both aspirin and clopidogrel for 1 year had a lower incidence of death, MI, and stroke in comparison to patients who only received aspirin.[107] Based on the results of these two studies, it appears appropriate for E.R. to receive the combination of aspirin and clopidogrel for up to 1 year after her recent episode of ACS. The occurrence of bleeding should be closely monitored because bleeding events were significantly increased in patients receiving combined antiplatelet therapy in both the CURE and CREDO study.[106,107] Dual therapy with aspirin and clopidogrel has not been investigated beyond 1 year; therefore, the combination should be limited to a duration of 1 year in patients who have experienced an acute coronary event.

Given the beneficial effects seen in patients with recent ACS, as well as data supporting the use of dual antiplatelet therapy in patients with PCI plus stent placement, investigators hypothesized that dual therapy with aspirin plus clopidogrel would be superior to aspirin in the treatment of chronic stable CAD. In the Clopidogrel for High Atherothrombotic Risk and Ischemic Stabilization, Management, and Avoidance (CHARISMA) trial, 15,063 patients with documented vascular disease (CAD, cerebrovascular, peripheral arterial disease), or no documented vascular disease but with multiple cardiovascular risk factors, were assigned to aspirin alone or aspirin plus clopidogrel for an average of 28 months duration.[108,109] Unlike the results from ACS studies, however, the combination of aspirin plus clopidogrel did not reduce the incidence of the primary endpoint (risk of death, MI, stroke, or coronary revascularization) as compared with aspirin alone. In a secondary analysis of patients who entered the trial with documented vascular disease, dual therapy did produce statistically significant reductions in the primary endpoint as compared with aspirin. Further trials should be conducted, however, to further elucidate the role of dual antiplatelet therapy outside the setting of ACS or PCI, and at this time combination therapy cannot be recommended as treatment strategy for patients with chronic stable CAD.

Ticlopidine (Ticlid) is a related thienopyridine antiplatelet agent that is similar to clopidogrel in both structure and mechanism of action and is a potential alternative to aspirin for E.R. Ticlopidine compares unfavorably with clopidogrel, however, because of a lack of any data examining its use in ischemic heart disease (IHD) and its side effect profile. Of particular concern is a roughly 2% incidence of neutropenia, which may be life-threatening.[102] Because of these factors, ticlopidine should not be considered as a potential alternative to aspirin now that clopidogrel is available.

Oral anticoagulation with warfarin represents another alternative to aspirin in patients with angina. Although the efficacy of warfarin (international normalized ratio [INR] 2.0–3.0) appears to be similar to aspirin in the prevention of MI and death, the need for monitoring and the risk of bleeding relegate this mode of therapy as second line behind antiplatelet strategies.[33]

Primary Prevention

34. E.R. returns to the pharmacy 1 week later with her brother who wants to know if he should be taking an aspirin a day to prevent heart disease. His only medical history consists of hypertension for which he is taking oral hydrochlorothiazide 25 mg every day. Is primary prevention of CAD with aspirin appropriate for E.R.'s brother?

The question of whether aspirin is valuable in the primary prevention of cardiovascular events has been debated for more than 20 years. Meta-analyses indicate that aspirin reduces the risk of a serious vascular event (nonfatal MI, nonfatal stroke, or death from vascular causes) by 25%; however, low-dose aspirin also doubles the risk of major extracranial bleeding (mostly GI), including hemorrhagic stroke. As these proportional changes for both efficacy and safety apply to any given category of patients with vascular disease, the absolute risk-to-benefit ratio for aspirin in the primary prevention arena will depend on the overall absolute risk of vascular ischemic events.[110,111]

In 2002, the U.S. Preventative Services Task Force developed guidelines for aspirin use in primary prevention based on the results of five large randomized studies.[112] In patients who have a high risk of developing cardiovascular disease (>1.5% per year), the benefits of aspirin in preventing cardiovascular events far outweigh the bleeding risks. In patients at low risk (<0.6% per year), the risk of bleeding events negates any potential benefit in cardiovascular outcomes. Patients at intermediate risk (0.6%–1.4% per year) derive some benefit in preventing cardiovascular events. The magnitude of benefit is not sufficiently large, however, to recommend routine administration of aspirin for primary prevention. In these circumstances patients should be informed about the risks and benefits of aspirin use to make an informed decision about whether they wish to take aspirin to prevent the occurrence of cardiovascular disease.[112] The recommendations from the U.S. Preventative Services Task Force are consistent with recommendations from the American College of Cardiology (ACC), American Heart Association (AHA), American College of Chest Physicians (ACCP), and the American Diabetes Association (ADA).[111]

Recently, the value of aspirin for primary prevention of CAD in women has come under question owing to the overall results of the Women Health Study which did not find a statistically significant reduction in the composite outcome of nonfatal MI, nonfatal stroke, or death.[113] A statistically significant reduction in the risk of ischemic stroke was found, however. A recent meta-analysis that included 51,342 women and 44,114 men found that low-dose aspirin reduced the risk of a composite of cardiovascular events (MI, stroke, cardiovascular mortality) in both men and women. In men, the primary benefit was a reduction in first time MI, whereas a reduction of first time ischemic stroke was observed in women.[114]

For E.R.'s brother, the first step is to calculate what is his risk of developing cardiovascular disease. This can be done by using a validated risk assessment scoring system, such as the Framingham risk score (see Chapter 12, Dyslipidemias, Atherosclerosis, and Coronary Heart Disease).[111] Once his risk is known, an appropriate recommendation can be made regarding his use of aspirin for primary prevention.

Drug Interactions with Nonsteroidal Anti-Inflammatory Drugs

35. During the discussion with E.R. regarding her brother, she is noticed buying a bottle of over-the-counter ibuprofen. On further questioning, it is learned that E.R. suffers from occasional back and knee pain and uses ibuprofen three to five times a week for pain relief. How should E.R. be educated on regarding the use of ibuprofen and aspirin concomitantly?

In 2006, the FDA released a warning statement on the concomitant use of both aspirin and ibuprofen. The impetus for the statement was the growing recognition that nonsteroidal anti-inflammatory drugs (NSAIDs), in particular ibuprofen, may attenuate the antiplatelet effects of low-dose aspirin. This FDA warning was then followed by an updated scientific statement from the AHA.[115] The mechanism behind this interaction is that both aspirin and nonselective NSAID bind to the same acetylation sites of the cyclo-oxygenase enzyme. Although aspirin does this in a nonreversible fashion, binding by an NSAID occurs in a reversible fashion. If an NSAID, such as ibuprofen, is present, aspirin will be unable to bind to its site of action, and will be rapidly cleared from the plasma. The result is the patient will not receive the antiplatelet benefit of aspirin.

E.R. should be counseled on the nature and consequences of the interaction between her low-dose aspirin and ibuprofen. Additionally, if she can avoid or at least minimize (both dose and duration) the use of ibuprofen, the effect on her cardiovascular health would be optimized. If occasional use of ibuprofen cannot be avoided, it should be administered in such a fashion as to minimize the potential for interacting with her low-dose aspirin. This would include taking ibuprofen at least 2 hours after her daily dose of aspirin, as well as taking her daily aspirin dose at least 8 hours after the last dose of ibuprofen. Although similar concerns exist for other nonselective NSAIDs (naproxen, diclofenac), no formal recommendations exist on how to manage concomitant use of these agents with aspirin.

Hormone Replacement Therapy

36. E.R. returns to the pharmacy 4 months later to obtain refills of her isosorbide mononitrate, metoprolol, diltiazem, albuterol, lisinopril, and clopidogrel. She mentions that a few years back she remembers that her mother was put on estrogen by her doctor to help prevent heart disease and is wondering if she should be on estrogen replacement as well?

Epidemiologic evidence initially supported the notion that hormone replacement therapy (HRT) in postmenopausal women would prevent cardiovascular events. When put to the test of a randomized, placebo-controlled trial, the benefits of HRT on cardiovascular disease, however, were not seen and potential harm was noted.[116,117] One of these studies was the Women's Health Initiative (WHI), which sought to answer the question of whether administering estrogen alone (in women without a uterus) or estrogen plus progesterone (in women with a uterus) would prevent the development of CAD in healthy (without history of CAD) postmenopausal women. Unexpectedly, a 29% increase was found in the incidence of CAD in those women on estrogen plus progesterone compared with placebo after an average treatment duration of 5 years. No increase was noted in women on estrogen alone; that part of the trial is still ongoing.[118] Based on the negative results seen in clinical trials of HRT, the AHA released a specific recommendation in 2001 not to initiate HRT for prevention of cardiovascular disease.[33,119,120]

Recent information indicates, however, that HRT may have varying effects, depending on the age and time from menopause for women.[121] When the WHI trial was analyzed in terms of timing of HRT initiation, women in whom HRT was started in close proximity to menopause actually derived a cardiovascular benefit. If HRT was initiated at a time remote from menopause, an increase in cardiovascular events was noted. The results from this analysis need to be confirmed in an appropriately designed trial, but it may be plausible that HRT is safe to use in the first few years after menopause for other indications without any increased risk of cardiovascular events. In the case of E.R., because she is 62 years of age and likely more then 10 years past menopause, she should be educated that the current body of knowledge does not support the use of HRT in the treatment of cardiovascular disease.

VARIANT ANGINA (CORONARY ARTERY SPASM)

Clinical Presentation

37. A.P., a 35-year-old woman, is hospitalized for evaluation of severe chest pain, which occurs almost daily at about 5 AM. A.P. ranks the severity of pain as 7 to 8 on a scale of 1 to 10. It is associated with diaphoresis and is not relieved by change in position. A.P. has no cardiovascular risk factors, and her hobbies include triathlon competition and rock climbing, neither of which has caused chest pain. She follows a strict vegetarian diet and takes no medications. Admission ECG reveals sinus bradycardia at 56 beats/minute. Serum electrolytes, chemistry panel, and cardiac enzymes are all within normal limits.

At 6 AM the next morning, A.P. is awakened abruptly by severe chest pain. Her vital signs include the following: heart rate, 55 beats/minute; supine BP, 110/64 mmHg; and respiratory rate, 12 breaths/minute. An immediate ECG shows sinus bradycardia with marked ST-segment elevation. The pain is relieved within 60 seconds by one NTG 0.4-mg sublingual tablet. During the day, she completes an exercise tolerance test without complication or evidence of CAD.

On the second day, A.P. undergoes cardiac catheterization, and no coronary atherosclerosis is visualized. An ergonovine provocation test is performed during cardiac catheterization. At 3-minute intervals, escalating IV ergonovine maleate bolus doses are given: 0.05, 0.10, and 0.25 mg. After the 0.25-mg dose, A.P. develops severe chest pain associated with an ST-segment elevation of 0.3 mV. The cardiologist observes almost complete vasospasm of the RCA and immediately injects 200 mcg NTG into the coronary artery along with administering two lingual sprays of NTG. A.P.'s chest pain resolves within 60 seconds, and the ECG normalizes within 3 minutes. A.P. is diagnosed as having Prinzmetal's variant angina. Discharge medications include oral amlodopine 10 mg every day at 11 PM and NTG lingual spray 0.4 mg PRN chest pain. Is A.P.'s presentation typical for Prinzmetal's variant angina?

A.P. presents with a classic picture of variant (Prinzmetal's) angina, with transient total occlusion of a large epicardial coronary artery as a result of severe segmental spasm. Clinical manifestations include chest pain occurring at rest, often in the morning hours. As with A.P., patients with Prinzmetal's variant angina generally are younger than patients with chronic stable angina and do not carry a high-risk profile. Other vasospastic disorders, such as migraine attacks or Raynaud's phenomenon, may be present; smoking and alcohol ingestion can be important contributing factors.[122]

The hallmark of variant angina is ST-segment elevation on the ECG, which denotes rapid and complete occlusion of the coronary artery. Many patients also have asymptomatic episodes of ST-segment elevation. Transient arrhythmias and conduction disturbances may be observed during pain, depending on the severity of the myocardial ischemia. In contrast to chronic stable angina in which the heart rate–BP product often is elevated with pain, no hemodynamic factors appear to contribute to Prinzmetal's variant angina.[122]

As documented by angiography, A.P. has vasospasm of the large RCA. This transient, reversible narrowing probably is caused by increased coronary vascular resistance. It can occur in the absence of atherosclerosis, as illustrated by A.P., or it can occur in the presence of CAD. One possible explanation for vasospasm occurring more commonly at night or during the early morning hours is increased vasomotor tone secondary to diurnal variations in catecholamines.

Ergonovine Stimulation Test

38. Why was the ergonovine test used? Was intracoronary NTG necessary to reverse the effects of ergonovine?

Because Prinzmetal's variant angina does not occur predictably, spasm must be induced under controlled circumstances. Ergonovine maleate, an ergot alkaloid that stimulates α-adrenergic and serotonergic receptors, exerts a direct vasoconstrictive effect on the vascular smooth muscle. The ergonovine maleate provocation test is highly specific and sensitive, especially in patients with normal coronary arteries. The risks of the test, which often discourage some physicians from using ergonovine, include arrhythmias (heart blocks, ventricular tachycardia, ventricular fibrillation) and possible MI.[122]

The vasospasm induced by ergonovine should be reversed promptly. Although sublingual NTG tablets or lingual spray might relieve the episode, the coronary vasospasm could be unresponsive to these agents. Direct injection of NTG into the coronary arteries immediately reverses the vasoconstrictor action of ergonovine.

Therapy

39. Oral amlodopine 10 mg every day was ordered for A.P. Would long-acting nitrates or β-adrenergic blockers be alternatives to amlodopine for A.P.? Is one CCB preferable to another for treatment of Prinzmetal's variant angina?

Because of their antispasmodic effects and low incidence of side effects, CCBs are generally selected over nitrates or β-blockers for nocturnal vasospastic angina. All CCBs appear equally effective in preventing Prinzmetal's variant angina.[122] Intrinsically long-acting or SR forms are preferred, however, and some patients may respond better to one agent than to another.

In patients who continue to experience pain using maximal CCB doses, combination therapy with a nitrate should be tried.[122] Nitrates cause vasodilation by a different mechanism than CCBs and are effective in treating Prinzmetal's variant angina.[122] To avoid tolerance, the nitrate-free interval for A.P. should be scheduled during the day so that the early morning hours when vasospasm occurs are covered by NTG. For example, if needed, A.P. could apply a transdermal NTG patch at bedtime and remove it on awakening. Aspirin therapy is indicated for A.P.

β-Blockers are likely to worsen A.P.'s angina because blockade of the β_2-receptors that mediate vasodilation may allow unopposed α_1-mediated vasoconstriction. A cardioselective β-blocker also could worsen Prinzmetal's variant angina. Therefore, a CCB or nitrate is preferable.

40. Will A.P. require treatment for the remainder of her life?

During the first year of therapy, up to 50% of patients experience spontaneous remission by an unknown mechanism. This occurs most often in patients who have had a short duration of symptoms or who have normal or mildly diseased coronary arteries (i.e., isolated vasospasm without atherosclerosis). If A.P. is pain free and not experiencing significant arrhythmias or silent ischemic episodes of Prinzmetal's angina after 1 year, amlodopine could be tapered and discontinued. It is also possible, however, that she will require treatment indefinitely. Modification of smoking and ethanol ingestion may promote remission of Prinzmetal's angina.[122]

41. Can variant angina lead to acute MI or death?

Variant angina, particularly in patients with multivessel coronary artery spasm, can lead to acute MI or death. In a study of 159 consecutive patients with variant angina in Japan who required hospitalization, 76% of patients experienced a cardiac event (acute MI in 19 patients, sudden death in 5 patients, and coronary artery bypass graft in 1 patient) within 1 month of onset of angina.[122] These patients had greatly improved outcomes if treated aggressively with calcium antagonists, nicorandil, and NTG infusion during the early stages. If variant angina persisted, revascularization of coronary arteries with underlying critical lesions was indicated.

MICROVASCULAR ISCHEMIA (SYNDROME X)

42. K.G., a 50-year-old female executive, has undergone an extensive cardiovascular workup for exertional angina associated with a 3-mm ST-segment depression. A recent cardiac catheterization did not reveal any atherosclerosis, and an ergonovine stimulation test did not produce observable coronary vasospasm. The cardiologists believe K.G. has microvascular ischemia. What drug therapy might be indicated for K.G.?

Syndrome X, increasingly known as *microvascular angina,* is a syndrome of angina or anginalike chest pain in the setting of a normal coronary arteriogram. Several theories exist regarding the mechanism of pain production, including microvascular dysfunction producing ischemia or chest discomfort without ischemia in patients who may have an abnormal perception of pain. Microvascular dysfunction can be the result of either diminished responsiveness to vasodilating stimuli (e.g., endothelia relaxation factor [NO], kinins, atrial natriuretic peptide or prostaglandin I_2) or increased sensitivity to vasoconstricting stimuli (e.g., catecholamines, vasopressin, angiotensin-2 or thromboxane A_2). Patients who display a heightened perception of pain may have an awareness of pain in response to atrial stretch or changes in heart rate. Ischemia is not universally present in patients with syndrome X; therefore, different mechanisms may be responsible for symptoms in different patients.[3,123]

Microvascular angina differs substantially from variant angina. Although spasm-causing variant angina may be visible with coronary angiography, the microvascular coronary circulation is not visible. The changes in coronary artery tone are in the distal coronary arteries and perhaps the collateral vessels. Some patients with microvascular ischemia have other smooth muscle disorders, such as esophageal motility disorders. A definite link is found between coronary vasoconstriction and mental or psychological stress.[3]

By symptoms alone, K.G.'s presentation does not significantly differ from that of a patient with exercise-induced angina secondary to atherosclerosis. Of concern is the finding of a 3-mm ST- segment depression on K.G.'s ECG, which raises concern of severe CAD. The negative findings from her cardiac catheterization and ergonovine stimulation testing, however, rule against both CAD and coronary artery spasm as a cause of her symptoms, and help to confirm the diagnosis of syndrome X. Overall, the prognosis for patients with syndrome X appears to be good. Long-term survival is no different from age-matched controls. Most patients, however, continue to experience symptoms and control of anginal pain is the main goal in therapy.[3]

Treatment with a nitrate, CCB, or β-blocker all appear to offer some relief, but overall the response to therapy in these patients is poor. The choice of agent will likely depend on specific patient characteristics. Sublingual NTG, however, is often ineffective at treating acute attacks, although it should still be prescribed.

SILENT MYOCARDIAL ISCHEMIA

Definition

43. Y.G., a 60-year-old man who has had his first complete physical examination in 12 years, is found to have Q waves on ECG, indicating a previous MI. Physical findings are normal except for borderline LV hypertrophy. Abnormal laboratory studies include moderately elevated total serum cholesterol and TG. His medical history is remarkable for hypertension controlled with oral

hydrochlorothiazide 25 mg every day. Y.G. does not recall ever experiencing angina, nor has he ever been told he had a heart attack. What characteristic syndrome does Y.G. exhibit, and how does it differ from angina pectoris?

Y.G. had a silent MI, often the first indicator of silent myocardial ischemia.[5] Silent myocardial ischemia is unrecognized by the patient because there are no symptoms of angina. It can occur in totally asymptomatic persons (type 1), in asymptomatic postinfarction patients (type 2), and in patients with angina (type 3).[124] The prevalence of silent myocardial ischemia is difficult to estimate because it often is undetected. An estimated 1 to 2 million totally asymptomatic men have silent myocardial ischemia, and approximately 50,000 new cases of postinfarction silent ischemia occur each year. Most patients with angina also appear to have episodes of silent ischemia, with the silent episodes occurring two to three times more often than the anginal episodes. The pathogenesis of silent ischemia is not fully defined. An abnormality in pain threshold may exist so that the anginal warning system is not triggered, or it may represent varying activation of coronary vasomotor tone or platelet activity.[3]

Prognosis

44. What is Y.G.'s prognosis?

Y.G.'s prognosis depends on the extent of his underlying CAD, ventricular function, and arrhythmia status. If Y.G. has multivessel disease, he is more likely to develop adverse cardiac events (reinfarction, unstable angina, sudden death) than if he has single-vessel disease. Silent myocardial ischemia is especially ominous in patients with unstable angina.[124]

Diagnosis

45. What diagnostic tests will be used to evaluate Y.G.'s total ischemic burden both before and after therapy is started?

The total ischemic burden, the sum of painful and painless ischemic episodes that occur, is assessed with exercise testing and 24-hour ambulatory electrocardiographic (Holter) monitoring. Both tests measure ST-segment depression, the usual abnormal ECG response to ischemia. ST-segment depression >2 mm at low levels of exercise or ST-depression with hypotension or arrhythmias is a strong indicator of disease. Radionuclide procedures help confirm ECG responses.[124]

Management

46. What management goals and techniques are likely to apply to Y.G.?

Treatment of patients with silent myocardial ischemia is unresolved, but modification of risk factors is mandatory. Y.G.'s cholesterol and hypertension should be corrected and the aim of pharmacotherapy is to abolish all ECG evidence of ischemia. The same drugs used to treat angina (nitrates, β-blockers, CCBs, and aspirin) also prevent silent myocardial ischemia if used at sufficiently high doses or in appropriate combinations. β-Blockers may be the most effective agents in decreasing the episodes of silent ischemia. Calcium antagonists are useful, but dihydropyridines are less efficacious than verapamil and diltiazem. Aspirin and nitrates also are key therapies in treating silent myocardial ischemia. Each patient requires careful titration to reduce both symptomatic and asymptomatic ischemic episodes. Although many questions remain unanswered about silent myocardial ischemia, it is no longer acceptable to treat painful ischemic episodes only.[3,124]

REVASCULARIZATION

Percutaneous Coronary Intervention

47. T.T., a 54-year-old man, had a recent onset of angina that was precipitated by exertion. His current medications include oral isosorbide mononitrate 30 mg every day, oral atenolol 50 mg every day, NTG SL 0.4 mg PRN for chest pain, and enteric-coated aspirin 81 mg/day. After discussions with his cardiologist, he elects to undergo revascularization with PCI for symptom relief. What is the current standard for prevention of acute complications during PCI?

Percutaneous coronary intervention (PCI), also known as angioplasty, involves the percutaneous insertion of a balloon catheter into the femoral artery in a similar fashion to angiography. The catheter is advanced up the aorta and into the coronary arteries at the coronary sinus. PCI, which was introduced in 1977, initially involved the inflation of a catheter-borne balloon that mechanically dilated a coronary artery obstruction through arterial intimal disruption, plaque fissuring, and stretching of the arterial wall. Balloon inflations were repeated until the plaque was compressed and coronary blood flow resumed. Since then, alternative devices have been developed, including rotational blades designed to remove atheromatous material, lasers to ablate plaques, and intracoronary stents that are designed to maintain the patency of the vessel after it is reopened.[125] Stents can be of the bare metal (BMS) variety, or contain a drug impregnated on the surface of the stent to prevent restenosis (drug-eluting stent or DES). It is estimated that more than 1,265,000 PCI procedures are performed in the United States each year. An overwhelming majority of these procedures involve placement of a BMS or DES (Fig. 16-5). PCI is indicated in patients with single- or multivessel disease and who are either symptomatic or asymptomatic.[125,126]

Because of mechanical disruption of the atherosclerotic plaques and exposure of plaque contents to the bloodstream during PCI, potent antiplatelet and antithrombotic strategies are needed to prevent acute thrombotic events such as MI and death. Initially, strategies involved the use of high-dose unfractionated heparin and aspirin. Current strategies involve the administration of aspirin, clopidogrel, an antithrombin agent, as well as a glycoprotein (Gp) IIb/IIIa receptor antagonist in selected patients. In patients not taking aspirin on a daily basis, 300 to 325 mg of aspirin should be given at least 2 hours before the procedure. Patients currently on daily aspirin therapy should receive 75 to 325 mg of aspirin before PCI is performed. A 600-mg loading dose of clopidogrel on or before the time of the procedure is currently recommended, producing an antiplatelet action within 2 hours.[11,126]

With the development of the Gp IIb/IIIa receptor antagonists, significant improvements were made in patient outcomes during and after PCI.[126] Currently, three agents are available

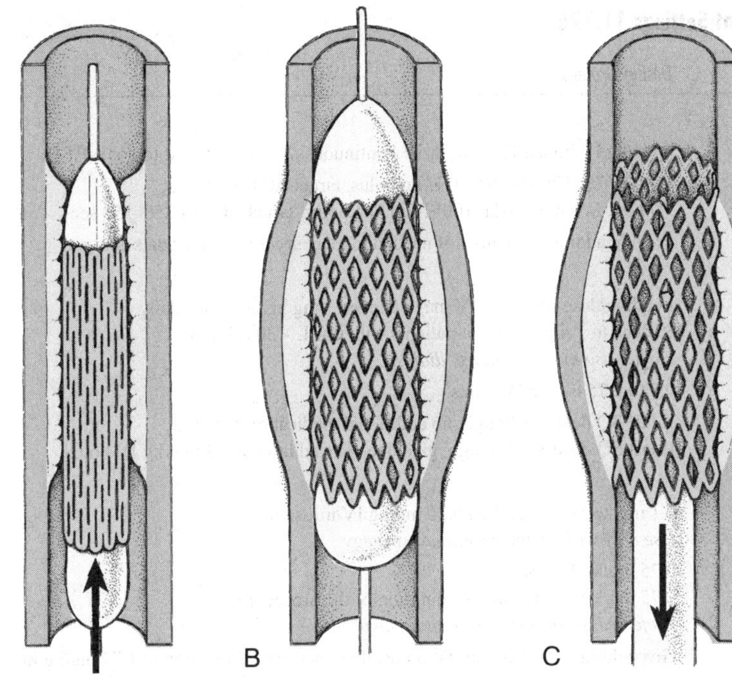

FIGURE 16-5 Vascular stent. A: A balloon catheter positions stent at site of arterial stenosis. **B:** inflation of balloon dilates artery and expands stent. **C:** balloon is collapsed and withdrawn, leaving expanded stent in position. (Illustration by Neil O. Hardy, Westpoint, Conn.)

in the United States (Table 16-8). Abciximab, a human-murine monoclonal antibody fragment, was the first agent available. Subsequently epitifibatide (cyclic heptapeptide) and tirofiban (nonpeptide mimetic) have become available.[126] These agents, when administered IV during PCI and for 12 to 24 hours afterward, significantly decrease the risk of death, acute MI, or need for repeat PCI. Major adverse effects include bleeding and thrombocytopenia. Therefore, hematocrit and platelet counts should be monitored appropriately. Clearance of both eptifibatide and tirofiban is renal, and dose adjustments should take place accordingly.[127]

In addition to appropriate use of the antiplatelet agents (aspirin, clopidogrel and Gp IIb/IIIa inhibitors), patients having PCI should also receive adequate antithrombin therapy during the procedure. Available options include unfractionated heparin (UFH), the low-molecular weight heparin (LMWH) enoxaparin, and the direct thrombin inhibitor bivalirudin. Any of the available agents may be initiated at the time of the procedure, or may be continued with appropriate dose adjustment if administered to the patient before PCI. See Table 16-9 for information regarding appropriate dosing and management strategies for each agent. Current guidelines do not specify a preference for any particular antithrombin agent during the course of PCI. Therefore, the choice of agent will likely depend on local practice variations. Antithrombin agents are typically discontinued immediately after the PCI procedure unless a compelling separate indication exists for therapeutic anticoagulation. Of note, significant interest exists in using direct thrombin inhibitors, such as bivalirudin, in place of heparin during PCI. One advantage for this approach is that most

Table 16-8 Indications and Dosing of Glycoprotein IIb/IIIc Receptor Antagonists

Indication	*Abciximab (ReoPro)*	*Eptifibatide (Integrilin)*	*Tirofiban (Aggrestat)*
Percutaneous transluminal coronary angioplasty (PCTA)	0.25 mg/kg IV bolus, then 0.125 mcg/kg/min IV infusion × 12 hr	180 mcg/kg IV bolus, then 2.0 mcg/kg/min IV × 20–24 hr Repeat 180 mcg/kg IV bolus 10 mins after first bolus	Not approved use
Coronary stent placement	0.25 mg/kg IV bolus, then 0.125 mcg/kg/min IV infusion × 12 hr	Same dose as for PCTA	Not approved use
Acute coronary syndrome (unstable angina and non–Q-wave MI)	Not approved use	180 mcg/kg IV bolus, then 2.0 mcg/kg/min IV × 20–24 hr	0.4 mcg/kg/min IV load × 30 mins, then 0.1 mcg/kg/min IV infusion × 48–102 hr Reduce dose by 50% if CrCl <30 mL/min

CrCl, creatinine clearance; IV, intravenous.

Table 16-9 Dosing of Antithrombin Agents in Different Settings 11,126

Antithrombin Agent	*Dosing Strategy*
Unfractionated Heparin	
Acute coronary syndromes: Medical management	60 U/kg IV bolus, 12 U/kg/hr IV continuous infusion, titrated to goal aPTT
PCI: Therapy initiated at time of procedure	With IV Gp IIb/IIIa: 60–70 U/kg bolus, target ACT of 200 sec Without IV Gp IIb/IIIa: 100–140 U/kg bolus, target ACT of 250–350 sec
PCI: Continuation of prior therapy	Provide additional boluses if needed to meet specified ACT goals above
Enoxaparin	
Acute coronary syndromes: Medical management	Loading dose of 30 mg IV may be given 1 mg/kg SQ twice daily Reduce to 1 mg/kg QD in patients with CrCL <30 mL/min *Do not use in renal failure, dialysis*
PCI: Therapy initiated at time of procedure	0.5 to 0.75 mg/kg IV bolus
PCI: Continuation of prior therapy	If last SQ dose <8 hr ago; no additional medication required If last SQ dose 8–12 hr ago; give one-time additional 0.3 mg /kg IV bolus
Bivalirudin	
Acute coronary syndromes: Medical management	0.1 mg/kg IV bolus, then 0.25 mg/kg IV infusion *Use only with an interventional strategy*
PCI: Therapy initiated at time of procedure	0.75 mg/kg IV bolus 1.75 mg/kg IV infusion for duration of the procedure *Preferred agent if HIT present or suspected*
PCI: Continuation of prior therapy	Give additional 0.5 mg/kg IV bolus, then increase IV infusion to 1.75 mg/kg/hr
Fondaparinux	
Acute coronary syndromes: Medical management	2.5 mg SQ QD *Contraindicated in patients with a CrCL <30 mL/min*
PCI: Therapy initiated at time of procedure	Not recommended
PCI: Continuation of prior therapy	Give 50–60 mg/kg IV bolus of UFH for adequate protection during PCI procedure

ACT, activated clotting factor; HIT, heparin-induced thrombocytopenia; IV, intravenous; PCI, percutaneous coronary intervention; QD, every day; SQ, subcutaneous; UFH, unfractionated heparin.

patients receiving bivalirudin during PCI do not require a Gp IIb/IIIa receptor antagonist. This strategy has the potential to reduce overall medication costs, as well as decrease the incidence of bleeding in association with PCI.[128]

48. T.T. undergoes PCI plus placement of a drug-eluting stent (sirolimus) to address a 75% lesion in his proximal left circumflex artery. What advantages and disadvantages are there in the decision to place a DES versus a BMS in T.T.?

The overall success of any procedure is directly related to the experience of the operator, patient factors (such as LV function or number of vessels treated), and the equipment used. In patients receiving balloon angioplasty alone (without stent placement), repeat revascularization procedures (either repeat angioplasty or surgery) may be required in as many as 32% to 40% of cases because of the reoccurrence of plaque at the angioplasty site. The process is known as *restenosis*.[125] Many pharmacologic strategies have been studied in an attempt to reduce the risk of restenosis. The outcome with most methods has been disappointing. The only strategy that has been associated with a decrease in restenosis is the use of intraluminal stents.[125] Stents are essentially metal scaffolding devices placed into the vessel after balloon inflation has taken place. They provide a physical barrier to the reoccurrence of a significant stenosis at the site. One of the early drawbacks of the use of stents was the need for complicated anticoagulation regimens, including aspirin, heparin, dipyridamole, and warfarin, to prevent in-stent thrombosis. Dual antiplatelet therapy—a combination of clopidogrel and aspirin—is effective at reducing in-stent thrombosis and is now recommended for use after stent placement.[126] The duration of dual antiplatelet therapy will depend on the type of stent used, as well as other clinical characteristics of the patient.

Recently, stents that elute antiproliferative agents such as sirolimus (SES) or paclitaxel (PES) have been shown in clinical trials to reduce the incidence of restenosis compared with BMS.[129,130] Restenosis rates in clinical trials with these DES were in the single digit range, as compared to 15% to 20% with traditional BMS. Soon after their introduction to the U.S. market, DES use grew to the point that >90% of stent use was DES. This trend abruptly halted in the fall of 2006 when several reports indicated a higher than expected incidence of stent thrombosis a year or more after DES placement. Although late stent thrombosis had previously been reported with BMS usage, the incidence was rare.[130] Shortly after these initial reports, an explosion of scientific literature emerged on the topic. Many potential explanations exist for the occurrence of late stent thrombosis in a patient receiving a DES, but perhaps the most relevant from a pharmacotherapy standpoint is the delayed healing response seen with DES compared with BMS. After placement of an intracoronary stent, a healing process typically occurs resulting in growth of a protective layer of endothelial cells over the stent surface, removing the stent surface from blood exposure and drastically reducing the stimulus for thrombosis. In the case of DES coated with paclitaxel or sirolimus, cellular growth may be inhibited, significantly impairing endotheliazation of the stent surface. In a small number of patients, endothelialization does not seem to occur at all. In this scenario, the stent structure remains continually exposed to flowing blood and is a potent stimulus for thrombosis.[131] Because of the concerns of late stent thrombosis, the usage of DES has dramatically decreased. Some use of DES is likely to continue, however owing to the tangible benefits in reduction of revascularization procedures in some patients. Therefore, practitioners will need to continue to stay abreast of evolving information regarding appropriate strategies to prevent late stent thrombosis.

Although there has been speculation to the causes of late stent thrombosis with DES as described above, one critical issue that has been identified is the premature discontinuation of dual antiplatelet therapy consisting of aspirin and clopidogrel. Previous recommendations called for varying durations of combined therapy, depending on the type of stent used. Because of the recognition of a delayed healing response to DES, current guidelines recommend at least 1 year of dual antiplatelet therapy in patients receiving a DES if patients are not at an elevated risk of bleeding. For BMS placement, dual antiplatelet therapy should continue for a minimum of 1 month, and up to 1 year ideally, but this extended duration is not as critical as it is in the setting of DES placement. The dose of aspirin during dual antiplatelet therapy should be 162 to 325 mg/day, and then decreased to 81 mg/day once dual antiplatelet therapy is discontinued. When administered, the dose of clopidogrel should be 75 mg/day.[126]

For T.T. the decision of placing a DES versus a BMS will likely be a lower risk of needing a repeat revascularization for restenosis within 6 to 9 months. He will, however, need to take dual antiplatelet therapy for at least a year, significantly increasing the costs of his prescriptions as well as putting him at an increased risk of bleeding in the long run. Regardless, it is vital that T.T. be educated about the importance of maintaining his therapy with aspirin and clopidogrel is to prevent complications. This discussion should commence before the PCI procedure to assess whether T.T. has the economic resources to comply with the needed therapy, or whether there may be any planned upcoming surgery necessitating the discontinuation of antiplatelet therapy. If these present a problem for T.T., placement of a BMS is a viable option. T.T. should also be counseled to alert his cardiologist if another health care professional wishes to discontinue antiplatelet therapy for any reason.[132]

49. Would revascularization therapy with coronary artery bypass grafting have been a better option for T.T. than PCI and stent placement?

Coronary Artery Bypass Graft Surgery

Coronary artery bypass grafting is a complicated surgical procedure during which an atherosclerotic vessel is "bypassed" using either a patient's saphenous vein or internal mammary artery (IMA; Fig. 16-6). The "graft" (i.e., the saphenous vein or IMA) then allows blood to flow past the obstruction in the native vessel. The goals of antianginal therapy, whether medical (pharmacologic) or revascularization, remain unchanged: (a) to prolong life, (b) to prevent MI, and (c) to improve the quality of life.

The outcomes of medical therapy, PCI, and revascularization with CABG have been compared, and current guidelines are available.[31] Of interest to practitioners and patients are the relative effects of each treatment modality on mortality, occurrence of symptoms, and quality of life. When compared with medical treatment in patients who would not be considered high risk, PCI in general offers no improvement in the long-term incidence of MI or cardiovascular death, but significantly reduces symptoms.[1,126] Because of his escalating symptoms on triple drug therapy, the choice of PCI for T.T. is justified.

Certain high-risk patient subgroups clearly have an improved outcome with CABG. These include (a) patients with significant left main coronary disease; (b) patients who have three-vessel disease, especially with LV dysfunction; (c) patients with two-vessel disease with a significant proximal LAD lesion; (d) patients who have survived sudden cardiac death; and (e) patients who are refractory to medical treatment. In patients who do not meet these criteria, either medical treatment, or PCI is a viable option.[1,31] Because T.T does not fall into one of these categories, PCI is preferable at this time owing to the

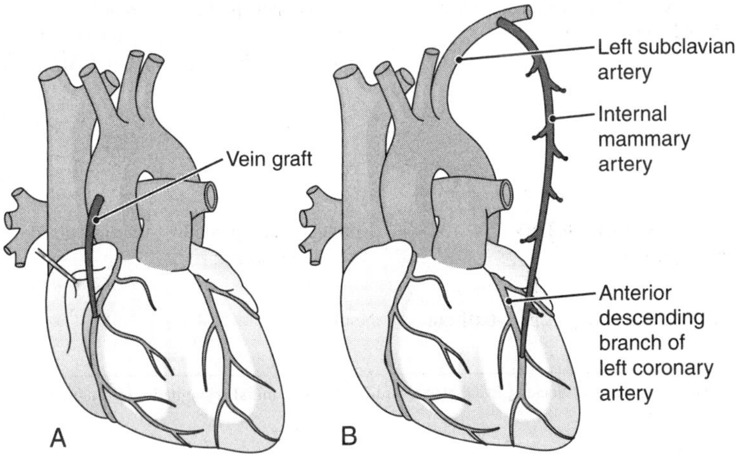

FIGURE 16-6 Coronary artery bypass graft (CABG). A: A segment of the saphenous vein carries blood from the aorta to a part of the right coronary artery that is distal to an occlusion. **B:** The mammary artery is used to bypass an obstruction in the left anterior descending (LAD) coronary artery. (From Cohen BJ. Medical Terminology. 4th ed. Philadelphia: Lippincott Williams & Wilkins; 2003, with permission.)

less invasive nature of the procedure and the equivalent outcomes that are seen in long-term prognosis. These results were recently confirmed in the Clinical Outcomes Utilizing Revascularization and Aggressive Drug Evaluation (COURAGE) trial.[133] Patients with CAD were randomized to aggressive medical treatment with optimization of medical therapy and risk factors, or aggressive medical treatment plus PCI. Over a 4.6-year period, no significant difference was noted between the groups in cardiovascular outcomes (death, MI, stroke, hospitalization for ACS). The only difference noted was better control of anginal symptoms early on with PCI, but that difference was no longer significant at the end of the study. These results highlight the crucial role of optimizing medical therapy (including diet, lifestyle changes, risk factor modification) for patients with CAD, regardless of whether revascularization is performed.

ACUTE CORONARY SYNDROMES: UNSTABLE ANGINA AND NON–ST-SEGMENT ELEVATION MYOCARDIAL INFARCTION

50. F.G., a 54-year-old man, is brought to the ED by helicopter for treatment of severe, unrelenting chest pain of 2 hours' duration. He has no history of CAD, but cardiac risk factors include a strong positive family history of CAD, a 45-pack-year smoking history, and a 5-year history of hypertension. He is taking oral metoprolol 100 mg BID. Physical examination reveals a middle-aged man in obvious distress with the following vital signs: heart rate, 110 beats/minute; BP, 176/108 mmHg; respiratory rate, 18 breaths/minute; and temperature, 37°C. Normal lung and heart sounds are heard, with the exception of an S_4 gallop. Examination of F.G.'s abdomen and extremities is unremarkable, as is the funduscopic examination. F.G. has received 10 mg morphine sulfate IV and three sublingual 0.4 mg NTG tablets and is still experiencing severe pain that is associated with ST-segment depression. He is placed on oxygen (2 L by nasal prongs) and an NTG infusion (5 mcg/minute). Rapid upward titration of the NTG to 60 mcg/minute alleviates the chest pain. His admitting diagnosis is acute coronary syndrome. What general guidelines exist for the treatment of acute coronary syndromes?

Clinical Presentation

Acute coronary syndromes include unstable angina (also known as *preinfarction angina, crescendo angina,* and *angina at rest*), non–ST-segment elevation myocardial infarction (NSTEMI), and ST-segment elevation myocardial infarction (STEMI). On presentation, the ultimate diagnosis usually cannot be determined because the diagnosis of MI requires the presence of biomarkers such as creatinine kinase (CK) or troponin. Often these results are not available for the first 12 to 24 hours. Because of this delay in the determination of the final diagnosis, initial treatment must be driven by other factors. One critical factor during the acute presentation is the initial ECG and, more specifically, whether ST-segment elevation is present on the initial ECG. Patients who have ST-segment elevation acute coronary syndromes (e.g., acute MI) are candidates for immediate reperfusion therapy and are discussed in detail in Chapter 17, Myocardial Infarction. Treatment of patients who present with non–ST-segment elevation acute coronary syndromes (this includes patients presenting with ST-segment depression, T-wave inversions, or no ECG changes) is discussed briefly here.[11]

Unstable angina is a syndrome falling between chronic stable angina and MI. The prognosis of patients with unstable angina is variable, and classification systems have been developed to determine whether a patient is at low, intermediate, or high risk for acute MI and death in the short term (Table 16-10).[11] Patients at intermediate or high risk should be hospitalized for acute treatment and assessment of potential long-term treatment strategies. Patients at low risk may be treated without

Table 16-10 Short-Term Risk of Death or Nonfatal Myocardial Infarction (MI) in Patients With Unstable Angina

Feature	*High Risk (at least one of the following must be present)*	*Intermediate Risk (no high-risk features, but must have one of the following)*	*Low Risk (no high- or intermediate-risk features, but may have any of the following)*
History	Accelerating tempo of ischemic symptoms in preceding 48 hr	Prior MI, peripheral or cerebrovascular disease, or CABG, prior aspirin use	
Character of pain	Prolonged ongoing (>20 min), rest pain	Prolonged (>20 min) rest angina, now resolved, with moderate or high likelihood of CAD	New-onset angina[32] CCS class III or IV angina in the past 2 wk without prolonged (>20 min) rest pain, but with moderate or high likelihood of CAD
Clinical findings	Pulmonary edema New or worsening MR murmur S_3 or new/worsening rales Hypotension, bradycardia, tachycardia Age >75 yr		
ECG	Angina at rest with transient ST-segment changes >0.05 mV Bundle-branch block, new or presumed new	T-wave inversions >0.2 mV Pathologic Q waves	Normal or unchanged ECG during episode of chest discomfort
Cardiac markers	Markedly elevated (e.g., TnT or TnI >0.1 ng/ml)	Slightly elevated (e.g., TnT >0.01 but <0.1 ng/mL)	Normal

CABG, coronary artery bypass graft; CAD, coronary artery disease; CCS, Canadian Cardiovascular Society; ECG, electrocardiogram; MR, mitral regurgitation; S_3, third heart sound; TnI, troponin I; TnT, troponin T.
Adapted from ref. 11, with permission.

admission to the hospital. F.G. is a high-risk patient because he has ST-segment depression at rest or with pain.

Management

Coronary arteriographic studies of patients with USA usually reveal severe atherosclerotic disease complicated by the rupture of an atherosclerotic plaque with the formation of a superimposing thrombus.[11] Therefore, the pathophysiology of USA is closely related to that of MI, and similar treatment strategies are used in both disease states. The treatment of USA in recent years has evolved to include medical therapy as well as revascularization procedures. Typically, revascularization with PCI is reserved for patients who are considered intermediate to high risk for developing adverse cardiovascular outcomes in the next 30 days or whose condition does not stabilize with medical therapy.[11]

The immediate challenge in the treatment of USA is relief of pain and control of all ischemic episodes. Hospitalization, bedrest, diagnosis, and treatment of underlying precipitating factors, such as infection, anemia, hypertension, heart failure, and arrhythmias, are essential. Pharmacologic therapy is targeted at relieving ischemia and at attenuating the thrombotic process.

As with patients experiencing an acute MI, β-blockers should be administered acutely because they have been demonstrated to prevent the progression to MI and death. Nitrates, both sublingually and then intravenously, are effective for relieving pain and acutely treating ischemia. CCBs are effective for treating ischemia in patients with USA, but should be reserved for patients who have ischemia refractory to β-blockade.[11]

A 325-mg dose of chewable aspirin should be administered to all patients because it has been shown to prevent the progression to MI and death. In addition, the combined use of aspirin (81–325 mg daily) and clopidogrel (300 mg load, 75 mg orally every day) acutely and for up to 1 year in patients with USA/NSTEMI has been shown to decrease the risk of cardiovascular death, MI, or stroke at 30 days and up to 1 year.[106,107] Based on these results from the CURE and CREDO studies, aspirin and clopidogrel should be administered to all patients with USA/NSTEMI who are unlikely to undergo PCI acutely. In patients who will undergo emergent PCI for treatment of USA/NSTEMI, clopidgrel administration can be delayed until the procedure is completed and then continued for up to 1 year, depending on the course of events during PCI.

Historically UFH has been the primary antithrombin used in the treatment of ACS. The beneficial effects of UFH are additive to aspirin in the prevention of acute MI and death.[11] Several new antithrombotic strategies have become available, which may improve on the results seen with aspirin and UFH. These include LMWH, the synthetic pentasaccharide fondaparinux, as well as the direct thrombin inhibitor bivalirudin. Each of these agents has demonstrated efficacy in the setting of non–ST-segment ACS and the choice of agent will likely be determined by cost, physician preference, and overall treatment strategy (invasive versus conservative management).

Several LMWHs have been investigated in the setting of USA and non–Q-wave MI and, as a group, are considered at least as effective as UFH at improving clinical outcomes. Results for individual agents have not been uniform, however. Trials comparing enoxaparin with UFH have consistently shown that enoxaparin is superior to UFH in preventing cardiovascular events. Trials investigating other LMWH have only demonstrated equivalency to UFH. Based on these results from clinical trials, the current ACC/AHA guidelines specifically recommend enoxaparin as the LMWH of choice to be used during ACS.[11]

In patients who are at low risk and being treated with a conservative medical strategy, UFH, enoxaparin, and fondaparinux all represent reasonable options for antithrombin therapy. Enoxaparin or fondaparinux are preferred, however, owing to demonstrated superiority for enoxaparin in clinical trials as compared with UFH,[134] as well as equivalence of enoxaparin and fondaparinux in the Organization to Assess Strategies in Acute Ischemic Syndromes (OASIS)-5 study.[135] In the conservative management setting, bivalirudin is not an option because trial data in this setting are lacking, as well as the prohibitive cost associated with a prolonged infusion duration. UFH is typically continued for 48 hours, whereas enoxaparin and fondaparinux can be continued for up to the duration of hospitalization.

In patients who present with non–ST-segment ACS, and who are at high risk requiring aggressive intervention with early angiography (with or without PCI), UFH, bivalirudin, enoxaparin, and fondaparinux all are reasonable options. Support for bivalirudin comes from the ACUITY trial, which demonstrated similar outcomes with a reduced incidence of bleeding for bivalirudin as compared with heparin (UFH or enoxaparin).[136] Although fondaparinux is listed as an option in association with an invasive strategy, the need for an additional antithrombin agent with anti-IIa activity during PCI makes this a less attractive strategy.[11] Dosing strategies for various antithrombin agents can be found in Table 16-9.

The Gp IIb/IIIa receptor antagonists are potent antiplatelet agents that provide significantly improved outcomes in patients with USA/NSTEMI who are being treated medically or who undergo revascularization via PCI.[137] These agents have a unique mechanism of action in that they block the final common pathway in platelet aggregation. Platelets can be stimulated by a number of different agonists (e.g., epinephrine, serotonin, ADP, thromboxane A_2), some of which may be inhibited by aspirin (thromboxane A_2) or clopidogrel. Blockade of one or more of these agonists by aspirin or clopidogrel still leaves the platelet susceptible to stimulation via other agonists. Regardless of the initial stimulus, the end result is the expression of the Gp IIb/IIIa receptor. This receptor is critical because it binds and cross-links fibrin, which stabilizes the clot. This process is blocked with the receptor antagonists. Because of their mechanism of action, the Gp IIb/IIIa antagonists are significantly more potent in terms of their antiplatelet effects than aspirin or clopidogrel.

These agents, in addition to aspirin, clopidogrel, and antithrombin therapy, significantly decrease the composite risk of death, acute MI, and urgent revascularization in patients with USA/NSTEMI. The Gp IIb/IIIa receptor antagonists currently are recommended as options in patients with USA/NSTEMI in one or more of the following groups: (a) in whom catheterization and PCI is planned; (b) who have continuing ischemia despite treatment with aspirin, UFH/LMWH/fondaparinux/bivalirudin, nitrates, β-blockers, and clopidogrel; and/or (c) who have other high risk features, such as elevated troponin or ST-segment changes on the initial ECG.[11]

REFERENCES

1. Fraker TD Jr et al., writing on behalf of the 2002 Chronic Stable Angina Writing Committee. 2007 chronic angina focused update of the ACC/AHA 2002 Guidelines for the Management of Patients With Chronic Stable Angina: a report of the American College of Cardiology/American Heart Association Task Force on Practice Guidelines Writing Group to Develop the Focused Update of the 2002 Guidelines for the Management of Patients With Chronic Stable Angina. *J Am Coll Cardiol* 2007;50:2264.
2. Fox K et al. Guidelines on the management of stable angina pectoris: executive summary. The task force on the management of stable angina pectoris of the European Society of Cardiology. *Eur Heart J* 2006;27:1341.
3. Morrow DA et al. Chronic coronary artery disease. In: Braunwald E, ed. *Heart Disease: A Textbook of Cardiovascular Medicine.* 8th ed. Philadelphia: WB Saunders; 2008.
4. Okumura K et al. Diffuse disorder of coronary artery vasomotility in patients with coronary spastic angina. Hyperreactivity to the constrictor effects of acetylcholine and the dilator effects of nitroglycerin. *J Am Coll Cardiol* 1996;27:45.
5. Cohn PF et al. Silent myocardial ischemia. *Circulation* 2003;108:1263.
6. American Heart Association. *2008 Heart and Stroke Statistical Update.* Dallas: American Heart Association; 2007.
7. Popma JJ. Coronary arteriography and intravascular imaging. In: Braunwald E, ed. *Heart Disease: A Textbook of Cardiovascular Medicine.* 8th ed. Philadelphia: WB Saunders; 2008.
8. Canty JM. Coronary blood flow and myocardial ischemia. In: Braunwald E, ed. *Heart Disease: A Textbook of Cardiovascular Medicine.* 8th ed. Philadelphia: WB Saunders; 2008.
9. Camici PG et al. Coronary microvascular dysfunction. *N Engl J Med* 2007;356:830.
10. Koerselman J et al. Coronary collaterals: an important and underexposed aspect of coronary artery disease. *Circulation* 2003;107:2507.
11. Anderson JL et al. ACC/AHA 2007 guidelines for the management of patients with unstable angina/non-ST-elevation myocardial infarction: a report of the American College of Cardiology/American Heart Association Task Force on Practice Guidelines (Writing Committee to Revise the 2002 Guidelines for the Management of Patients With Unstable Angina/Non-ST-Elevation Myocardial Infarction): developed in collaboration with the American College of Emergency Physicians, American College of Physicians, Society for Academic Emergency Medicine, Society for Cardiovascular Angiography and Interventions, and Society of Thoracic Surgeons. *J Am Coll Cardiol* 2007;50:e1.
12. Antman EM et al. 2007 focused update of the ACC/AHA 2004 Guidelines for the Management of Patients With ST-Elevation Myocardial Infarction: a report of the American College of Cardiology/American Heart Association Task Force on Practice Guidelines (Writing Group to Review New Evidence and Update the ACC/AHA 2004 Guidelines for the Management of Patients With ST-Elevation Myocardial Infarction). *J Am Coll Cardiol* 2008;51:210.
13. Belardinelli L et al. Inhibition of late (sustained/persistent) sodium current: a potential drug target to reduce intracellular sodium-dependent calcium overload and its detrimental effects on cardiomyocyte function. *Eur Heart J* 2004;(Suppl)6:I3.
14. Kusuoka H et al. Role of sodium/calcium exchange in the mechanism of stunning: protective effect of reperfusion with high sodium solution. *J Am Coll Cardiol* 1993;21:240.
15. Imahashi K et al. Intracellular sodium accumulation during ischemia as the substrate for reperfusion injury. *Circ Res* 1999;84:1401.
16. Chaitman BR. Ranolazine for the treatment of chronic angina and potential use in other conditions. *Circulation* 2006;113:2462.
17. Libby P. The vascular biology of atherosclerosis. In: Braunwald E, ed. *Heart Disease: A Textbook of Cardiovascular Medicine.* 8th ed. Philadelphia: WB Saunders; 2008.
18. Hansson GK. Inflammation, atherosclerosis, and coronary artery disease. *N Engl J Med* 2005; 352:1685.
19. Deanfield JE et al. Endothelial function and dysfunction. Testing and clinical relevance. *Circulation* 2007;115:1285.
20. Widlansky ME et al. The clinical implications of endothelial dysfunction. *J Am Coll Cardiol* 2003;42:1149.
21. Zarraga IGE et al. Impact of dietary patterns and interventions on cardiovascular health. *Circulation* 2006;114:961.
22. Berg A et al. Adipose tissue, inflammation, and cardiovascular disease. *Circ Res* 2005;96:939.
23. Han SH et al. Adiponectin and cardiovascular disease. Response to therapeutic interventions. *J Am Coll Cardiol* 2007;49:531.
24. Ridker PM et al. Risk factors for atherosclerotic disease. In: Braunwald E, ed. *Heart Disease: A Textbook of Cardiovascular Medicine.* 8th ed. Philadelphia: WB Saunders; 2008.
25. Yusuf S et al. Effect of potentially modifiable risk factors associated with myocardial infarction in 52 countries (the INTERHEART study). *Lancet* 2004;364:937.
26. Davi G et al. Platelet activation and atherothrombosis. *N Engl J Med* 2007;357:2482.
27. Cox J et al. The Canadian cardiovascular society grading scale for angina pectoris: is it time for refinements? *Ann Intern Med* 1992;117:677.
28. Greenland P et al. ACCF/AHA 2007 clinical expert consensus document on coronary artery calcium scoring by computed tomography in global cardiovascular risk assessment and in evaluation of patients with chest pain: a report of the American College of Cardiology Foundation Clinical Expert Consensus Task Force (ACCF/AHA writing committee to update the 2000 expert consensus document of electron beam computed tomography). *J Am Coll Cardiol* 2007;49:378.
29. Gibbons R et al. ACC/AHA 2002 guideline update for exercise testing: a report of the American College of Cardiology/American Heart Association Task Force on Practice Guidelines (Committee on Exercise Testing), 2002. American College of Cardiology Web site. Available at: www.acc.org/clinical/guidelines/exercise/dirIndex.htm.
30. Scanlon PJ et al. ACC/AHA guidelines for coronary angiography: a report of the American College of Cardiology/American Heart Association Task Force on Practice Guidelines (Committee on Coronary Angiography). *J Am Coll Cardiol* 1999;33:1756.
31. Eagle KA et al. ACC/AHA 2004 guideline update for coronary artery bypass graft surgery: a report of the American College of Cardiology/American Heart Association Task Force on Practice Guidelines (Committee to Update the 1999 Guidelines for Coronary Artery Bypass Graft Surgery). American College of Cardiology Web Site. Available at: http://www.acc.org/clinical/guidelines/cabg/cabg.pdf.
32. Parker JD et al. Nitrate therapy for stable angina pectoris. *N Engl J Med* 1998;338:520.
33. Smith S et al. AHA/ACC guidelines for secondary prevention for patients with coronary and other atherosclerotic vascular disease: 2006 update. *Circulation* 2006;113:2363.
34. UKPDS group. Effect of intensive blood glucose control with metformin on complications in overweight patients with type 2 diabetes (UKPDS 34). *Lancet* 1998;352:854.
35. Dormandy JA et al. Secondary prevention of macrovascular events in patients with type 2 diabetes in the PROactive Study (PROspective pioglitazone clinical trial in macrovascular events): a randomized controlled trial. *Lancet* 2005;366:1279.
36. Rosendorff C et al. Treatment of hypertension in the prevention and management of ischemic heart disease. A scientific statement from the American Heart Association Council for High Blood Pressure Research and the councils on clinical cardiology and epidemiology and prevention. *Circulation* 2007;115:2761.
37. Sui X et al. Cardiorespiratory fitness and adiposity as mortality predictors in older adults. *JAMA* 2007;298(21):2507.
38. Kris-Etherton PM et al. for the Nutrition Committee of the American Heart Association Council on Nutrition, Physical Activity, and Metabolism. Antioxidant vitamin supplements and cardiovascular disease. *Circulation* 2004;110:637.
39. Bjelakovic G et al. Mortality in randomized trials of antioxidant supplements for primary and secondary prevention. *JAMA* 2007;297:842.
40. Wald DS et al. Homocysteine and cardiovascular disease: evidence on causality from a meta-analysis. *BMJ* 2002;325:1202.
41. The Homocysteine Studies Collaboration. Homocysteine and risk of ischemic heart disease and stroke. *JAMA* 2002;288:2015.
42. Bazzano LA et al. Effect of folic acid supplementation on risk of cardiovascular diseases. A meta-analysis of randomized trials. *JAMA* 2006; 296:2720.
43. Lichtenstein AH et al. Diet and lifestyle recommendations revision 2006. A scientific statement from the American Heart Association Nutrition Committee. *Circulation* 2006;114:82.
44. Lorgeril M et al. Mediterranean α-linoleic acid-rich diet in secondary prevention of coronary heart disease. *Lancet* 1994;343:1454.
45. Lorgeril M et al. Mediterranean diet, traditional risk factors, and the rate of cardiovascular complications after myocardial infarction. Final report of the Lyon diet heart study. *Circulation* 1999;99: 779.
46. Singh RB et al. Effect of an Indo-Mediterranean diet on progression of coronary artery disease in high risk patients (Indo-Mediterranean Diet Heart Study): a randomized single-blind trial. *Lancet* 2002;360:1455.
47. Trichopoulou A et al. Mediterranean diet and survival among patients with coronary heart disease in Greece. *Arch Intern Med* 2005;165:929.
48. Parikh P et al. Diets and cardiovascular disease: an evidence-based assessment. *J Am Coll Cardiol* 2005;45:1379.
49. Abrams J et al. The organic nitrates and nitroprusside. In: Frishman WH et al., eds. *Cardiovascular Pharmacotherapeutics.* 2nd ed. New York: McGraw-Hill; 2003.
50. Abrams J. Nitrate tolerance and dependence. *Am Heart J* 1980;99:113.
51. Shaw SV et al. Selection and dosing of nitrates to avoid tolerance during sustained antianginal therapy. *Formulary* 1999;34:590.
52. Munzel T et al. Explaining the phenomenon of nitrate tolerance. *Circ Res* 2005;97:618.
53. Hink U et al. Oxidative inhibition of the mitochondiral aldehyde dehydrogenase promotes nitroglycerin tolerance in human blood vessels. *J Am Coll Cardiol* 2007;50:2226.
54. Thomas GR et al. Once daily therapy with isosorbide-5-mononitrate causes endothelial dysfunction in humans. *J Am Coll Cardiol* 2007;49: 1289.
55. Luke R et al. Transdermal nitroglycerin in angina pectoris: efficacy of intermittent application. *J Am Coll Cardiol* 1987;10:642.
56. Cowan JC et al. Prevention of tolerance to nitroglycerin patches by overnight removal. *Am J Cardiol* 1987;60:271.
57. Packer M et al. Prevention and reversal of nitrate tolerance in patients with congestive heart failure. *N Engl J Med* 1987;317:799.

58. Expert Consensus document on β-adrenergic receptor blockers. The Task Force on β-blockers of the European Society of Cardiology. *Eur Heart J* 2004;25:1341.
59. Reiter MJ. Cardiovascular drug class specificity: β-blockers. *Prog Cardiovasc Dis* 2004;47(1):11.
60. Bangalore S et al. Cardiovascular protection using β-blockers. *J Am Coll Cardiol* 2007;50:563.
61. Goldstein S. β-Blocking drugs and coronary heart disease. *Cardiovasc Drug Ther* 1997;11:219.
62. Hippisley-Cox J et al. Effect of combinations of drugs on all cause mortality in patients with ischemic heart disease: nested case-control analysis. *BMJ* 2005;330:1059.
63. Kernis SJ et al. Does β-blocker therapy improve clinical outcomes of acute myocardial infarction after successful primary angioplasty? *J Am Coll Cardiol* 2004;43:1773.
64. Bunch TJ et al. Effect of β-blocker therapy on mortality rates and future myocardial infarction rates in patients with coronary artery disease but no history of myocardial infarction or congestive heart failure. *Am J Cardiol* 2005;95:827.
65. Go AS et al. Statin and β-blocker therapy and the initial presentation of coronary heart disease. *Ann Intern Med* 2006;144:229.
66. Pepine CJ et al. Effects of treatment on outcome in mildly symptomatic patients with ischemia during daily life. The Atenolol Silent Ischemia Study (ASIST). *Circulation* 1994;90:762.
67. Sipahi I et al. β-blockers and progression of coronary atherosclerosis: pooled analysis of 4 intravascular ultrasonography trials. *Ann Intern Med* 2007;147:10.
68. Heidenreich PA et al. Meta-analysis of trials comparing β-blockers, calcium antagonists, and nitrates for stable angina. *JAMA* 1999;281:1927.
69. Chobanian AV et al. The Seventh Report of the Joint National Committee on Prevention, Detection, Evaluation, and Treatment of High Blood Pressure. The JNC 7 Report. *JAMA* 2003;289:2560.
70. Salpeter S et al. Cardioselective β-blockers in patients with reactive airway disease: a meta-analysis. *Ann Intern Med* 2002;137:715.
71. Frishman WH et al. Calcium channel blockers. In: Frishman WH et al., eds. *Cardiovascular Pharmacotherapeutics.* 2nd ed. New York: McGraw-Hill; 2003.
72. Abernathy DR et al. Calcium antagonist drugs. *N Engl J Med* 1999;341(19):1447.
73. von Arnim T. Medical treatment to reduce total ischemic burden: total ischemic burden bisoprolol study (TIBBS), a multicenter trial comparing bisoprolol and nifedipine. The TIBBS Investigators. *J Am Coll Cardiol* 1995;25:231.
74. Savonitto S et al. Combination therapy with metoprolol and nifedipine versus monotherapy in patients with stable angina pectoris. Results of the International Multicenter Angina Exercise (IMAGE) Study. *J Am Coll Cardiol.* 1996;27:311.
75. Dargie HJ et al. Total Ischaemic Burden European Trial (TIBET). Effects of ischaemia and treatment with atenolol, nifedipine SR and their combination on outcome in patients with chronic stable angina. The TIBET Study Group. *Eur Heart J* 1996;17:104.
76. Rehnqvist et al. Treatment of stable angina pectoris with calcium antagonists and β-blockers. The APSIS study. Angina Prognosis Study in Stockholm. *Cardiologia.* 1995;40(12 Suppl 1):301.
77. Nissen SE et al. Effect of antihypertensive agents on cardiovascular events in patients with coronary disease and normal blood pressure. The CAMELOT study: a randomized controlled trial. *JAMA* 2004:292:2217.
78. Pepine CJ et al. A calcium antagonist vs. a non-calcium antagonist hypertension treatment strategy for patients with coronary artery disease. The international verapamil-trandolapril study (InVEST): a randomized controlled trial. *JAMA* 2003;2805.
79. Poole-Wilson PA et al. Effect of long-acting nifedipine on mortality and cardiovascular morbidity in patients with stable angina requiring treatment (ACTION trial): randomized controlled trial. *Lancet* 2004;364:849.
80. Davidson CL et al. Sustained-release calcium channel blockers. *Hospital Therapy* 1989;Nov:35.
81. Holubkov R et al. Angina 1 year after percutaneous coronary intervention: a report from the NHLBI Dynamic Registry. *Am Heart J* 2002;144:826.
82. Serruys PW et al. for the Arterial Revascularization Therapies Study Group. Comparison of coronary-artery bypass surgery and stenting for the treatment of multivessel disease. *N Engl J Med* 2001;344:1117.
83. Dobesh PP et al. Ranolazine: a new option in the management of chronic stable angina. *Pharmacotherapy* 2007;27(12):1659.
84. Wolff AA et al. Metabolic approaches to the treatment of heart disease: the clinicians' perspective. *Heart Fail Rev* 2002;7:187.
85. Belardinelli L et al. Inhibition of late (sustained/persistent) sodium current: a potential drug target to reduce intracellular sodium-dependent calcium overload and its detrimental effects on cardiomyocyte function. *Eur Heart J* 2004;(Suppl)6:I3.
86. Chaitman BR et al. for the MARISA Investigators. Anti-ischemic effects and long-term survival during ranolazine monotherapy in patients with chronic severe angina. *J Am Coll Cardiol* 2004;43:1375.
87. Chaitman BR et al. for the CARISA Investigators. Effects of ranolazine with atenolol, amlodipine, or diltiazem on exercise tolerance and angina frequency in patients with severe chronic angina. A randomized controlled trial. *JAMA* 2004;291:309.
88. Cocco et al. Effects of a new metabolic modulator, ranolazine, on exercise tolerance in angina pectoris patients treated with β-blocker of diltiazem. *J Cardiovasc Pharmacol* 1992;20:131.
89. Thadani U. Double-blind efficacy and safety study of a novel anti-ischemic agent, ranolazine, versus placebo in patients with chronic stable angina pectoris: Ranolazine Study Group. *Circulation* 1994;90:726.
90. Pepine CJ et al. A controlled trial with a novel anti-ischemic agent, ranolazine, in chronic stable angina pectoris that is responsive to conventional anti-anginal agents. *Am J Cardiol* 1999;84:46.
91. Rousseau MF et al. Comparative efficacy of ranolazine versus atenolol for chronic angina pectoris. *Am J Cardiol* 2005;95:311.
92. Stone PH et al. Antianginal efficacy of ranolazine when added to treatment with amlodipine. The ERICA (Efficacy of Ranolizine in Chronic Angina) Trial. *J Am Coll Cardiol* 2006;48:566.
93. Koren MJ et al. Long-term safety of a novel antianginal agent in patients with severe chronic stable angina. The ranolazine open label experience (ROLE). *J Am Coll Cardiol* 2007;49:1027.
94. Morrow DA et al. Effects of ranolazine on recurrent cardiovascular events in patients with non-ST-elevation acute coronary syndromes. The MERLIN-TIMI 36 Trial. *JAMA* 2007;297:1775.
95. Scirica BM et al. Effect of ranolazine, an antiaginal agent with novel electrophysiologic properties, on incidence of arrhythmias in patients with non–ST-segment elevation acute coronary syndrome. *Circulation* 2007;116:1647.
96. Sica DA et al. The renin-angiotensin axis: angiotensin-converting enzyme inhibitors and angiotensin-receptor blockers. In: Frishman WH et al., eds *Cardiovascular Pharmacotherapeutics.* 2nd ed. New York: McGraw-Hill; 2003.
97. Yusuf S et al. Effect of enalapril on myocardial infarction and unstable angina in patients with low ejection fractions. *Lancet* 1992;340:1173.
98. Pfeffer MA et al. Effect of captopril on mortality and morbidity in patients with left ventricular dysfunction after myocardial infarction: results of the Survival and Ventricular Enlargement Trial. *N Engl J Med* 1992;327:669.
99. The Heart Outcomes Prevention Evaluation Study Investigators. Effects of an angiotensin-converting enzyme inhibitor, ramipril, on cardiovascular events in high-risk patients. *N Engl J Med* 2000;342:145.
100. Al-Mallah MH et al. Angiotensin-converting enzyme inhibitors in coronary artery disease and preserved left ventricular systolic function. A systematic review and meta-analysis of randomized controlled trials. *J Am Coll Cardiol* 2006;47:1576.
101. The European trial on reduction of cardiac events with perindopril in stable coronary artery disease investigators. Efficacy of perindopril in reduction of cardiovascular events among patients with stable coronary artery disease: randomised, double-blind, placebo-controlled, multicentre trial (the EUROPA study). *Lancet* 2003;362:782.
102. Frishman WH et al. Antiplatelet and antithrombotic drugs. In: Frishman WH et al., eds. *Cardiovascular Pharmacotherapeutics.* 2nd ed. New York: McGraw-Hill; 2003
103. Awtry EH et al. Aspirin. *Circulation* 2000;101:1206.
104. Campbell CL et al. Aspirin dose for the prevention of cardiovascular disease: A systemic review. *JAMA* 2007;297:2018.
105. CAPRIE steering committee. A randomized, blinded, trial of clopidogrel versus aspirin in patients at risk for ischemic events (CAPRIE). *Lancet* 1996;348:1329.
106. The Clopidogrel in Unstable Angina to Prevent Recurrent Events Trial Investigators. Effects of clopidogrel in addition to aspirin in patients with acute coronary syndromes without ST-segment elevation. *N Engl J Med* 2001;345:494.
107. Steinhubl SR et al. Early and sustained dual oral antiplatelet therapy following percutaneous coronary intervention. *JAMA* 2002;288:2411.
108. Bhatt DL et al. Clopidogrel and aspirin versus aspirin alone for the prevention of atherothrombotic events. *N Engl J Med* 2006;354:1706.
109. Bhatt DL et al. Patients with prior myocardial infarction, stroke, or symptomatic peripheral disease in the CHARISMA trial. *J Am Coll Cardiol* 2007;49:1982.
110. Patrono C et al. Low-dose aspirin for the prevention of atherothrombosis. *N Engl J Med* 2005;353:2373.
111. Saseen JJ. ASHP Therapeutic Position Statement on the Daily Use of Aspirin for Preventing Cardiovascular Events. *Am J Health Syst Pharm* 2005;62:1398.
112. U.S. Preventative Services Task Force. Aspirin for the primary prevention of cardiovascular events: recommendation and rationale. *Ann Intern Med* 2002;136:157.
113. Ridker PM et al. A randomized trial of low-dose aspirin in the primary prevention of cardiovascular disease in women. *N Engl J Med* 2005;352:1293.
114. Berger JS et al. Aspirin for the primary prevention of cardiovascular events in women and in men. *JAMA* 2006;295:306.
115. Antman EM et al. Use of nonsteroidal antiinflammatory drugs. *Circulation* 2007;115:1634.
116. Michels KB et al. Postmenopausal hormone therapy. A reversal of fortune. *Circulation* 2003;107:1830.
117. Hulley S et al. Randomized trial of estrogen plus progestin for secondary prevention of coronary heart disease in postmenopausal women. Heart and Estrogen/Progestin Replacement Study (HERS) Research Group. *JAMA* 1998;280:605.
118. Writing Group for the Women's Health Initiative Investigators. Risks and benefits of estrogen plus progestin in healthy postmenopausal women: principal results from the Women's Health Initiative Randomized Controlled Trial. *JAMA* 2002;288:321.
119. Mosca L et al. American Heart Association. Hormone replacement therapy and cardiovascular disease: a statement for health care professionals from the American Heart Association. *Circulation* 2001;104:499.
120. U.S. Preventative Services Task Force. Hormone therapy for the prevention of chronic conditions in postmenopausal women: recommendations from the U.S. Preventative Services Task Force. *Ann Intern Med* 2005;142:855.

121. Rossouw JE et al. Postmenopausal hormone therapy and risk of cardiovascular disease by age and years since menopause. *JAMA* 2007;297:1465.
122. Cannon CP et al. Unstable angina and non–ST-elevation myocardial infarction. In: Braunwald E, ed. *Heart Disease: A Textbook of Cardiovascular Medicine.* 8th ed. Philadelphia: WB Saunders; 2008.
123. Camici PG et al. Coronary microvascular dysfunction. *N Engl J Med* 2007;356:830.
124. Cohn PF et al. Silent myocardial ischemia. *Circulation* 2003;108:1263.
125. Popma JJ et al. Percutaneous coronary and valvular intervention. In: Braunwald E, ed. *Heart Disease: A Textbook of Cardiovascular Medicine.* 8th ed. Philadelphia: WB Saunders; 2008.
126. King SB III et al. 2007 focused update of the ACC/AHA/SCAI 2005 Guideline Update for Percutaneous Coronary Intervention: a report of the American College of Cardiology/American Heart Association Task Force on Practice Guidelines: (2007 Writing Group to Review New Evidence and Update the 2005 ACC/AHA/SCAI Guideline Update for Percutaneous Coronary Intervention). *J Am Coll Cardiol* 2008;51:172.
127. Cheng JWM. Efficacy of glycoprotein IIb/IIIa-receptor inhibitors during percutaneous intervention. *Am J Health Syst Pharm* 2002;59(Suppl): S5.
128. Lincoff AM et al. Bivalirudin and provisional glycoprotein IIb/IIIa blockade compared with heparin and planned glycoprotein IIb/IIIa blockade during percutaneous coronary intervention. *JAMA* 2003;289:853.
129. Daemen J et al. Drug eluting stent update 2007. Part I: A survey of current and future generation drug-eluting stents: meaningful advances or more of the same? *Circulation* 2007;116:316.
130. Daemen J et al. Drug-eluting stent update 2007. Part II: Unsettled issues. *Circulation* 2007:116:961.
131. Windecker S et al. Late coronary stent thrombosis. *Circulation* 2007;116:1952.
132. Grines CL et al. Prevention of premature discontinuation of dual antiplatelet therapy in patients with coronary artery stents. *Circulation* 2007;115:813.
133. Boden WE et al. Optimal medical therapy with or without PCI for stable coronary disease. *N Engl J Med* 2007;356:1503.
134. Califf RM et al. A perspective on trials comparing enoxaparin and unfractionated heparin in the treatment of non–ST-segment acute coronary syndromes. *Am Heart J* 2005;149:S91.
135. The Fifth Organization to Assess Strategies in Acute Ischemic Syndromes Investigators. Comparison of fondaparinux and enoxaparin in acute coronary syndromes. *N Engl J Med* 2006;354:1464.
136. Stone GW et al. Bivalirudin for patients with acute coronary syndromes. *N Engl J Med* 2006;355:2203.
137. Boersma E et al. Platelet glycoprotein IIb/IIIa inhibitors in acute coronary syndromes: a meta-analysis of all major randomised clinical trials. *Lancet* 2002;359:189.

CHAPTER 17

Myocardial Infarction

Robert Lee Page II, Jean M Nappi

Acute myocardial infarction (AMI), now referred to as ST segment elevation myocardial infarction (STEMI), is a manifestation of ischemic heart disease characterized by cellular death or necrosis occurring in the setting of severe or prolonged ischemia. STEMI is believed to be the result of complete occlusion in a coronary artery.

STEMI is a medical emergency requiring immediate intervention. Until the 1980s, patients with AMI were treated symptomatically. Their pain was controlled; arrhythmic complications were treated; and bed rest, nitrates, and β-blockers minimized the amount of oxygen required by the heart. In 1980, an angiographic study by DeWood et al. found total occlusion in a coronary artery in 87% of patients who were examined by angiography within the first 4 hours of symptoms.[1] This study stimulated interest in using thrombolytics to interrupt the progression of myocardial necrosis. Thrombolytics and percutaneous coronary intervention (PCI) are now considered first-line therapies unless a contraindication is present. A committee composed of representatives from the American College of Cardiology (ACC) and the American Heart Association (AHA) periodically review the literature and publish practice guidelines to aid health care practitioners in selecting the most effective treatments for patients with STEMI.[2,3]

Epidemiology

The estimated annual incidence of STEMI is 565,000 for new and 300,000 for repeat attacks.[4] Twenty to 30% of patients die before reaching a hospital, presumably as a result of ventricular fibrillation.[4] Prompt recognition and treatment of AMI have dramatically reduced event-related mortality since the 1990s. In-hospital and 30-day mortality rates have been estimated to be 8.8% and 18.4%, respectively.[5] Treatment disparities and access to care exist for women, blacks, and patients who are at least 75 years of age.[6–8]

Pathophysiology

The majority of AMIs results from occlusion of a coronary artery secondary to thrombus formation overlying a lipid-rich atheromatous plaque that has undergone fissuring or rupture. Damage to the plaque results in blood being exposed to collagen and fatty acids; this in turn activates platelets, the first step in thrombosis and formation of a fibrin clot. Rarely, coronary artery spasm may cause an AMI in a patient with normal coronary arteries, particularly in the setting of cocaine abuse. More likely, spasm occurs before, during, or after the AMI and further compromises blood flow in an already stenotic artery.[9]

Most infarctions are located in a specific region of the heart and are described as such (e.g., anterior, lateral, inferior). Some patients develop permanent electrocardiographic abnormalities (Q waves) following an AMI. In the past, patients with Q-wave infarctions were generally believed to have more extensive necrosis and a higher in-hospital mortality rate. Patients with a non–Q-wave infarct were believed to have a greater likelihood of experiencing postinfarction angina and early reinfarction. More recently, however, these distinctions have come into question. Some cardiologists now believe that there is no difference in prognosis. The terminology has changed: Q-wave MI is now called STEMI and non–Q-wave MI is now called non–ST segment elevation MI (NSTEMI) or non–ST segment elevation acute coronary syndrome (NSTE-ACS). An anterior wall infarction carries a worse prognosis than an inferior or lateral wall infarction.[10]

Clinical Presentation

It is important to make the diagnosis of STEMI as quickly as possible so appropriate action may be taken. Patients may complain of prolonged substernal chest pain or pressure, shortness of breath, diaphoresis, nausea, and vomiting. In some patients, the symptoms may be confused with indigestion or other gastrointestinal (GI) complaints. The pain may be atypical in nature and location. The pain might be described as burning, and it may occur in the arms, shoulder, neck, jaw, or back.[2,3] Presentation may differ by gender and age. Men commonly complain of chest pain, whereas women present with nausea and diaphorsis.[11] Elderly patients may present with hypotension or cerebrovascular symptoms rather than chest pain. However, not all STEMIs are symptomatic: An estimated 20% of STEMIs are "silent," and this presentation tends to occur more frequently in the elderly and people with diabetes.

The physical examination is not particularly helpful in making the diagnosis of STEMI, but the findings are important in guiding initial therapy. Signs of severe left ventricular or right ventricular dysfunction may be present (see Chapter 19). The patient may have severe hypertension due to pain or, conversely, may be hypotensive. Significant tachycardia (heart rate >120 beats/minute) suggests a large area of damage. On cardiac auscultation, a fourth heart sound (S_4) may be heard, denoting an ischemia-induced decrease in left ventricular compliance. New cardiac murmurs may be heard, resulting from papillary muscle dysfunction. The cerebral and peripheral vasculature should be assessed. Patients with a history of cerebrovascular disease may not be eligible for thrombolytic therapy. Peripheral pulses should be examined to assess perfusion and to obtain a baseline before invasive procedures are instituted.

Table 17-1 Differential Diagnosis of Acute Myocardial Infarction

Acute cerebrovascular disease
Aortic dissection
Acute anxiety or panic attacks
Esophageal rupture or spasm
Gallbladder disease
Pancreatitis
Peptic ulcer disease
Pericarditis
Pneumothorax
Pulmonary embolism
Spinal or chest wall diseases

Diagnosis

Failure to make the appropriate diagnosis in STEMI can lead to disastrous results. The list of other medical conditions that mimic the presentation of STEMI is extensive (Table 17-1). In addition to the patient's history and presentation, the diagnosis of STEMI is based on the ECG and laboratory results in a cardiac injury profile. Usually two of the three criteria (history, ECG changes, and cardiac injury profile findings) should be consistent with STEMI before the diagnosis is made.[2,3]

The electrocardiogram (ECG) is an indispensable tool in the diagnosis of STEMI and has become the key point in the decision pathway. The presence of ST segment elevation is used to identify patients who will benefit from thrombolytic therapy. The 12-lead ECG is helpful in determining the location of an infarct. The presence of a new Q wave, new bundle branch block, or ST segment elevation is consistent with a STEMI. The electrocardiographic diagnosis of a STEMI is extremely difficult in the presence of a left bundle branch block. Figures 17-1 and 17-2 show the ECG in a patient presenting with STEMI before and after successful thrombolysis.[12]

Patients presenting with ischemic chest pain but without ST segment elevation and without laboratory evidence of

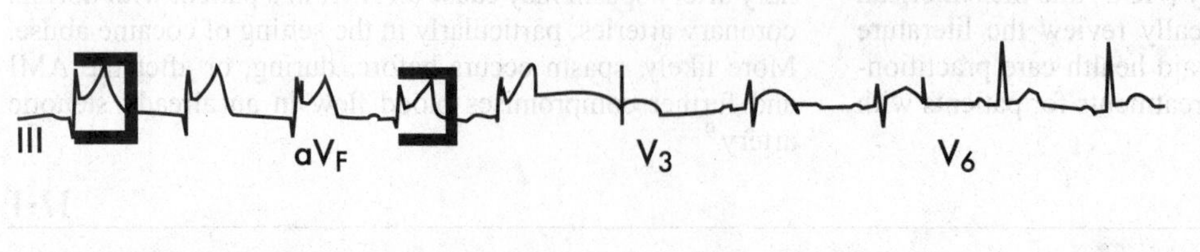

FIGURE 17-1 On this admission electrocardiogram (ECG), note the extensive ST segment elevation in leads II, III, and aV_F (*brackets*), indicating an inferior wall AMI. The patient also displays reciprocal ST segment depression in I and aV_L (*arrows*), which are the lateral ECG leads and are opposite the inferior leads.

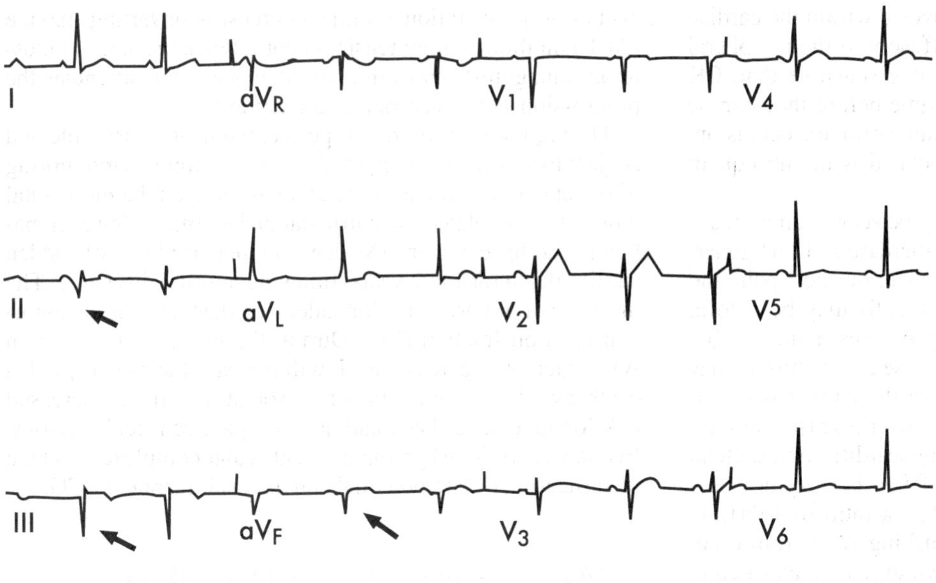

FIGURE 17-2 After successful thrombolysis, the electrocardiogram shows no ST segment changes suggestive of ischemia, but evolution of new Q waves in leads II, III, and aV_F (*arrows*) is apparent.

infarction are classified as having unstable angina, part of the acute coronary syndrome spectrum. Patients with a history consistent with ischemic chest pain, without ST segment elevation, but who develop a positive cardiac injury profile (i.e., elevated troponin) within hours of presentation are also given the diagnosis of AMI (referred to as NSTEMI or NSTE-ACS). Patients with NSTEMI and unstable angina continue to have some blood flow, although limited, through the affected coronary artery. Patients with NSTEMI usually have partial occlusion of the artery and/or thrombi that are comprised largely of platelets and fibrinogen. Thrombolytic therapy is not beneficial in these patients and is a major point of differentiation.[3] Figure 17-3 shows the relationship between different forms of acute coronary syndromes (ACSs).

Laboratory Changes

When a cardiac cell is injured, enzymes are released into the circulation. The measurement of cardiac enzymes is routine in making the diagnosis of AMI. One of the enzymes used for the laboratory diagnosis of AMI is creatine kinase (CK).

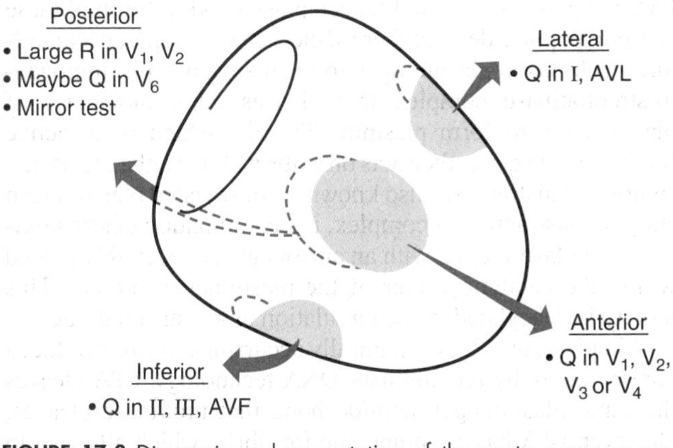

FIGURE 17-3 Diagnosis and presentation of the acute coronary syndromes. *Source:* Reprinted with permission from Dubin D. Infarction. In Dubin D, ed. Rapid Interpretation of EKGs. 6th Ed. Tampa. COVER Publishing Co., 2000:290.

There are three isoenzymes of CK: the BB, MM, and MB bands. Of these, the CK-MB isoenzyme is the most specific for the diagnosis of AMI. It can appear in the serum within 3 to 6 hours after myocardial damage, and levels generally peak in 12 to 24 hours.[2,3] Serum enzymes are normally determined at admission and then repeated at least once 12 hours after the onset of chest pain. The magnitude of rise of peak CK is related to the size of the infarct, but the peak may be missed if admission is delayed. There are several conditions other than AMI in which CK-MB may be elevated (Table 17-2).[13] CK is usually reported as enzymatic activity (U/L), and CK-MB is reported as mass (ng/mL) in either plasma or serum. CK-MB is often reported as percentage of activity.

The most sensitive markers of damage to cardiac muscle are the troponins I and M. The troponins are enzymes that normally

Table 17-2 Conditions Where CK-MB Isoenzyme May Be Elevated

False Elevations	*Myocardial Damage*
Isoenzyme variant	Myocardial infarction
Nonspecific fluorescence	Myocardial puncture/trauma
Spillover of CK-MM	Myocarditis
	Pericarditis
Peripheral Source of CK-MB	**Systemic Disorders With Cardiac Involvement**
Athletic activity (e.g., marathons)	Hyperthermia
Cesarean section	Hypothermia
Surgery (gastrointestinal, prostate)	Muscular dystrophy
Myositis	Reye syndrome
Rhabdomyolysis	
Tumors	
Miscellaneous	
Hypothyroidism	
Renal failure	
Subarachnoid hemorrhage	

CK, creatine kinase.

Adapted with permission from Lee TH, Goldman L. Serum enzyme assays in the diagnosis of acute myocardial infarction. Recommendations based on a quantitative analysis. Ann Intern Med. 1986;105:221.

regulate the interaction of actin and myosin within the cardiac cell. When cell death occurs, they diffuse into the peripheral circulation. Although troponins are more sensitive than CK and CK-MB, they have a similar lag time before they can be detected in the blood following an acute coronary occlusion. Elevation of troponins has been associated with subsequent cardiac events.[13]

Another laboratory change that may be seen is an increase in lactate dehydrogenase (LDH). The increase in LDH generally appears 24 to 48 hours after the onset of chest pain and peaks in 3 to 6 days. Measurement of LDH may be helpful in patients who present with a history of chest pain that began several days before admission. In these cases, the CK may have already returned to normal before the patient is evaluated. Increases in LDH are also seen in liver disease, hemolysis, leukemia, pulmonary embolism, myocarditis, and skeletal muscle disease. LDH is comprised of five isoenzymes. Because the heart muscle contains LDH_1, a ratio of LDH_1 to $LDH_2 > 1$ may be helpful in distinguishing AMI from other disorders. Because troponins are known to remain elevated in patients who have sustained myocardial necrosis, they have replaced the less specific LDH enzyme. Other nonspecific laboratory changes that occur in AMI include hyperglycemia and increases in aspartate aminotransferase, the white blood cell count, and C-reactive protein.[13]

Complications

The primary complications of AMI can be divided into three major groups: pump failure, arrhythmias, and recurrent ischemia and reinfarction. Depression of cardiac function following an AMI is related directly to the extent of left ventricular damage. As a result of decreased cardiac output and decreased perfusion pressure associated with left ventricular dysfunction, a number of compensatory mechanisms become activated. The levels of circulating catecholamines increase in an attempt to increase contractility and restore normal perfusion. In addition, the renin-angiotensin-aldosterone system is enhanced, leading to an increase in systemic vascular resistance and sodium and water retention. These compensatory mechanisms can eventually worsen the imbalance between myocardial oxygen supply and consumption by increasing the myocardial oxygen demand.

Signs and symptoms of heart failure are common in patients who have abnormal wall motion affecting 20% to 25% of the left ventricle. If 40% or more of the left ventricle is damaged, cardiogenic shock and death can occur.[14] In addition to systolic dysfunction, patients who have suffered an AMI may also have diastolic dysfunction. Scar formation following an AMI may lead to a decrease in ventricular compliance, resulting in abnormally high left ventricular filling pressures during diastole. (See Chapter 18 for further discussion on systolic dysfunction versus diastolic dysfunction.)

Decreased contractility and a compensatory increase in left ventricular end-diastolic volume and pressure lead to increased wall stress within the left ventricle. Left ventricular enlargement is an important determinant of mortality after AMI. Over a period of days to months following an AMI, the infarcted area may expand as a result of dilatation and thinning of the left ventricular wall. These changes are known as *ventricular remodeling*. In addition, hypertrophy of the noninfarcted myocardium occurs. Administration of oral angiotensin-converting enzyme (ACE) inhibitors, angiotensin receptor blockers, and/or aldosterone antagonists may limit remodeling and will attenuate the progression of left ventricular dilatation.[15]

During the peri-infarction period, the heart is irritable and subject to ventricular arrhythmias. The continuous monitoring of patients in a coronary care unit has reduced the in-hospital mortality rate related to ventricular arrhythmias. However, patients who have had an AMI have an increased risk of sudden cardiac death for 1 to 2 years following hospital discharge. The most important predictor for sudden cardiac death is an abnormal ejection fraction (EF). During the first 30 days after an AMI, each 5% decrease in EF will increase the risk of sudden death by 21%.[14] Other factors associated with an increased risk for sudden cardiac death are complex ventricular ectopy, frequent (>10/hour) premature ventricular complexes, and the identification of late potentials on a signal-averaged ECG.

OVERVIEW OF DRUG AND NONDRUG THERAPY

Thrombolytics

In the management of patients with AMI, emphasis has shifted from preventing or managing complications (arrhythmias, pain, and blood pressure [BP] control) to limiting the extent of myocardial necrosis and preventing reinfarction. The 2004 update of the ACC/AHA guidelines for the management of patients with STEMI addressed the most significant advances made in the prior 2.5 years and should be used in conjunction with the 1999 guidelines.[2]

Because the majority of STEMI cases result from the sudden occlusion of a coronary artery due to the formation of a thrombus, the therapeutic priority is to open the occluded artery as quickly as possible. This is accomplished by administering a thrombolytic that enhances the body's own fibrinolytic system or by mechanically reducing the obstruction with PCI.

Large clinical trials have proven that administration of a thrombolytic agent reduces mortality. Early mortality from STEMI has been reduced by approximately one-third (from 10%–15% to 6%–10%) with the advent of thrombolytic therapy.[16]

The thrombolytics currently used for STEMI patients in the United States are streptokinase, anistreplase, alteplase (t-PA), reteplase (r-PA), and tenecteplase (TNK). Streptokinase is a polypeptide derived from β-hemolytic streptococcal cultures. It binds to plasminogen to form an active plasminogen-to-streptokinase complex that cleaves other molecules of plasminogen to form plasmin. Plasmin, which is an active fibrinolytic enzyme, then acts on a fibrin clot to enhance its dissolution. Anistreplase, also known as anisoylated plasminogen streptokinase activator complex, is a combination of streptokinase and plasminogen with an anisoyl group reversibly placed within the catalytic center of the plasminogen moiety. This moiety is deacylated in the circulation at a controlled rate.

Alteplase, or t-PA, is a naturally occurring enzyme produced commercially by recombinant DNA technology. t-PA cleaves the same plasminogen peptide bond that urokinase cleaves. However, t-PA has a binding site for fibrin, which allows it to bind to a thrombus and preferentially lyse it over the circulating plasminogen.

Table 17-3 Pharmacologic Comparison of Available Thrombolytic Agents

Drug	Enzymatic Efficiency for Clot Lysis	Fibrin Specificity	Potential Antigenicity	Average Dose	Dosing Administration	Cost
Streptokinase (Streptase)	High	Minimal	Yes	1.5 MU	1 hr IV infusion	Low
Anistreplase (Eminase)	High	Minimal	Yes	30 U	2–5 min IV infusion	Moderate
Alteplase (Activase)	High	Moderate	No	100 mg	15 mg IV bolus, 50 mg over 30 min, then 35 mg over 60 min[a]	High
Reteplase (Retavase)	High	Moderate	No	10+10 U	10 U IV bolus, sec bolus 30 min later	High
Tenecteplase (TNK)	High	High	No	30–50 mg (based on weight)[b]	Bolus over 5–10 sec	High

[a]For patients = 65 kg; reduced doses for patients weighing <65 kg.
[b]For patients <60 kg, 30 mg; 60–69 kg, 35 mg; 70–79 kg, 40 mg; 80–89 kg, 45 mg; 90 kg, 50 mg.
Adapted from references 2, 3, 16, and 17.

Reteplase is a genetically modified plasminogen activator that is similar to t-PA. Reteplase has a longer half-life, allowing it to be administered as two bolus injections 30 minutes apart, rather than as a bolus plus infusion.

TNK is a genetically modified form of t-PA. Compared to t-PA, TNK has a longer plasma half-life, better fibrin specificity, and higher resistance to inhibition by plasminogen-activator inhibitor. The pharmacologic properties of these agents are compared in Table 17-3.[2,3,17]

Urokinase, although available in the United States, has not gained widespread use as a thrombolytic agent for patients with STEMI. The ideal thrombolytic would be thrombus specific, easily administered, highly efficacious, inexpensive, and rapid acting, and the incidence of reocclusion and side effects would be low. Unfortunately, such an ideal thrombolytic does not exist. Three problems common to all thrombolytics are the inability to open 100% of coronary artery occlusions, inconsistent ability to maintain good blood flow in the infarcted artery after it is opened, and bleeding complications. Good blood flow is commonly defined as thrombolysis in myocardial infarction (TIMI) grade 3 flow, which is complete reperfusion of the vessel.

To minimize the risk of bleeding complications, contraindications to the use of thrombolytics must be evaluated prior to administration (Table 17-4).[2,3] There are relatively few absolute contraindications to thrombolytic therapy, but each patient should be assessed carefully to ascertain whether the potential benefit outweighs the potential risk. Because of the serious nature of intracerebral hemorrhage associated with thrombolytic therapy, patients should be selected carefully before receiving these agents.[2] Generally, the diagnosis of STEMI must be ensured, with a history consistent with ischemic heart disease, presence of ST segment elevation in two contiguous leads, or a new left bundle branch block on the ECG. Once the diagnosis is made, the thrombolytic should be administered immediately if there are no contraindications.

The benefit derived from thrombolytic therapy is directly related to the time from the onset of chest pain to the time of administration. The 2004 guidelines recommend initiation of thrombolytic therapy within 12 hours from the onset of chest pain. However, data from clinical trials suggest that mortality reduction is greater when thrombolytic therapy is initiated within 0 to 2 hours of symptom onset compared to treatment begun more than 2 hours after symptoms have begun (44% vs. 20%, respectively, $p = 0.001$).[2,3] The guidelines recommend a "door-to-needle time" of 30 minutes, meaning the diagnosis of STEMI and initiation of thrombolytic therapy should ideally take place within 30 minutes from the time the patient arrives at the hospital door.

Table 17-4 Risk Factors Associated With Bleeding Complications Secondary to Thrombolytic Use

Major (thrombolytics contraindicated)	Intracranial tumor (primary or metastatic)
	Prior intracranial hemorrhage
	Recent head/facial trauma within 3 months
	Suspected aortic dissection
	Ischemic stroke within 3 months, EXCEPT acute ischemic stroke within 3 hr
	Active internal bleeding or bleeding diathesis (excluding menses)
Important (relative contraindication)	Uncontrolled hypertension on presentation (SBP >180 mm, DBP >110 mmHg)
	Chronic, severe, poorly controlled hypertension
	Prior ischemic stroke >3 months, dementia, or known intracranial pathology
	Puncture of a noncompressible vessel
	Cardiopulmonary resuscitation for >10 min
	Major surgery (<3 wk)
	Recent internal bleeding within 24 wk
	Active peptic ulcer
	Current use of anticoagulants (the higher the INR, the greater the risk for bleeding)
	Pregnancy
	For streptokinase or anistreplase: prior exposure (>5 days) or prior allergic reaction

DBP, diastolic blood pressure; INR, international normalized ratio; SBP, systolic blood pressure.
From reference 2.

Antiplatelet and Anticoagulant Drugs

When thrombolysis occurs, whether due to the administration of a thrombolytic agent or through activation of the body's own fibrinolytic system, the fibrin clot begins to disintegrate. As the clot dissolves, there is a paradoxic increase in local thrombin generation and enhanced platelet aggregability, which may lead to rethrombosis. Aspirin, unfractionated heparin (UFH), and low-molecular-weight heparin (LMWH) have been used to minimize repeat thrombosis. LMWH may offer advantages over heparin due to its ease of administration, improved bioavailability, and less need for monitoring. Bivalirudin, lepirudin, and argatroban are thrombin inhibitors that bind directly to thrombin and inactivate it. Unlike UFH, the direct thrombin inhibitors (DTIs) offer better protection against thrombin reactivation after therapy discontinuation. When used with early invasive treatment (<72 hours), DTIs appear to reduce the rate of death or reinfarction to a greater extent than UFH (9.50% vs. 13.86%, respectively, $p < 0.05$).[18] The 2004 ACC/AHA guidelines recommend DITs, specifically bivalirudin, as an alternative to heparin in patients with heparin-induced thrombocytopenia.[2]

Another class of agents being used is the glycoprotein (GP) IIb/IIIa inhibitors. GP IIb/IIIa receptors are abundant on the platelet surface. Platelets become activated when patients are having an acute ischemic coronary event or are undergoing a PCI. With platelet activation, the GP IIb/IIIa receptor undergoes a conformational change that increases its affinity for binding to fibrinogen. The binding of fibrinogen to receptors on platelets results in platelet aggregation, which can lead to thrombus formation. The GP IIb/IIIa receptor inhibitors prevent platelet aggregation by preventing fibrinogen from binding to GP IIb/IIIa receptor sites on activated platelets. The GP IIb/IIIa inhibitors are more often used in conjunction with aspirin and UFH in patients with ischemic chest pain, usually without ST segment elevation (ACS patients) and in patients undergoing PCI. When used in conjunction with thrombolytic agents for patients with STEMI, the dose of thrombolytic drug is reduced by one-half.

β-Blockers

In addition to antiplatelet, antithrombotic, and thrombolytic agents, β-blockers are fundamental in the management of AMI. Before the advent of thrombolytics, β-blockers were shown to decrease infarct-associated morbidity and mortality. These benefits are additive to those of thrombolytics. β-blockers decrease myocardial oxygen consumption, limit the amount of myocardial damage, and reduce some of the complications of MI, specifically sudden death attributed to ventricular fibrillation. During the prethrombolytic era, 28 randomized clinical trials involving more than 27,000 patients with AMI were conducted to evaluate β-blocker use. A retrospective analysis of these studies suggests that β-blockers reduce mortality by 14% with a 19% reduction in nonfatal reinfarction and a 19% reduction in nonfatal cardiac arrest during the first week in hospital. These short-term benefits are also seen with long-term use in the post-MI period. Unless there are contraindications to their use, β-blocking agents should be prescribed for all patients having an AMI, and they should be continued indefinitely.[2,3]

Statins

HMG-CoA reductase inhibitors or statins reduce long-term morbidity and mortality in patients with cardiovascular disease. What is less clear is whether statins provide short-term benefit when started immediately after hospitalization for AMI. Beyond their lipid-lowering properties, statins are believed to exhibit pleiotropic effects, which include plaque stabilization, anti-inflammation, antithrombogenicity, enhancement of arterial compliance, and modulation of endothelial function.[19] Data regarding early intensive statin therapy in patients with STEMI or NSTEMI exist with atorvastatin, simvastatin, pravastatin, and fluvastatin.[20] Debate continues to exist over which statin to initiate, the dosage, and the timing[21] (see Chapter 13).

Vasodilators

Other strategies for minimizing myocardial damage include the use of vasodilators in the peri-infarction period. Progressive left ventricular dilatation ("remodeling") occurs in some patients following an AMI and has become an important marker for prognosis. Vasodilators reduce oxygen demand and myocardial wall stress by reducing afterload and/or preload and can halt the remodeling process. Some vasodilators may increase the blood supply to the myocardium by enhancing coronary vasodilatation.

ACE inhibitors have been assessed in a large number of clinical trials, and all trials using oral agents have demonstrated a benefit in reducing mortality.[2,3] Only one trial has not shown a benefit. Enalapril was studied in the Cooperative New Scandinavian Enalapril Survival Study (CONSENSUS-II) trial. In this study, more than 6,000 patients were randomized to either placebo or enalapril, which was started within 24 hours from the onset of chest pain. Enalapril was initiated by intravenous (IV) administration, followed by oral enalapril administration 6 hours later. In this trial, enalapril did not improve 6-month survival, but this may be because hypotension was more common in the enalapril-treated group. It appears that early IV administration of ACE inhibitors results in excessive hypotension, offsetting their potential benefits. The benefit of ACE inhibitors is greatest in patients with anterior infarction, signs of heart failure, tachycardia, or a history of previous infarction. Ideally, oral ACE inhibitors should be started within 24 hours of diagnosis, after BP has stabilized. Initial doses should be low and then titrated as quickly as possible.[2,3]

The effects of nitrates have been evaluated in AMI patients. Pooled effects from several studies show a small but statistically significant benefit in reducing mortality in patients receiving nitrates. Nitroglycerin (NTG) is more beneficial than nitroprusside in this population. IV NTG is recommended for routine use during the first 24 to 48 hours in most patients with STEMI, particularly those with large anterior wall infarctions.[2,3]

Another class of vasodilators that has been investigated in the treatment of AMI is the calcium channel blockers. There are several proposed mechanisms whereby a calcium channel blocker might be beneficial. As a group, they dilate coronary and peripheral vessels. They could alleviate some of the coronary vasospasm present at the time of coronary thrombosis. In addition, they are effective anti-ischemic agents through their action in improving coronary blood supply and reducing myocardial oxygen demand. Because intracellular calcium overload has been observed in the ischemic myocardium, it was believed that calcium channel blockers would protect cardiac cells during the peri-infarction period. Despite these theoretical benefits, the outcomes of clinical trials have varied, depending on the individual drug used and the timing of administration resulting in a decline in use.[2,3]

There have been two trials evaluating diltiazem in the setting of AMI. The first study evaluated the effect of oral diltiazem, started 24 to 72 hours after the onset of chest pain, on reinfarction rates in patients with non–Q-wave AMI. There was a 51% reduction in the reinfarction rate in the diltiazem group compared to placebo after 14 days of follow-up. Diltiazem also reduced the frequency of postinfarction angina. Another trial initiated oral diltiazem (240 mg daily) 3 to 15 days after infarction in patients with both Q wave and non–Q wave. Diltiazem was continued indefinitely, and patients were followed for 12 to 52 months. Overall, there was no difference in mortality between the two groups. However, patients assigned to diltiazem who did not have pulmonary congestion at the time of randomization had a reduced number of cardiac events compared to placebo patients. In contrast, patients who had signs of pulmonary congestion at the time of randomization had an unfavorable response to diltiazem (i.e., more deaths from cardiac causes or nonfatal reinfarction). Diltiazem may be used to lower the heart rate or decrease angina in patients who cannot tolerate a β-blocker. However, diltiazem should be avoided in patients with signs or symptoms of pulmonary congestion because its negative inotropic properties may worsen systolic function.[2,3]

The Danish Verapamil Infarction Trial (DAVIT-II) study showed a trend toward a reduction in mortality at 18 months in patients receiving verapamil (11.1% vs. 13.8% in the placebo group). In patients who did not have heart failure at the time of randomization, verapamil showed a statistically significant benefit in reducing mortality (7.7% vs. 11.8% in the placebo group). In contrast to the diltiazem trial, verapamil had neither a demonstrable benefit nor a detrimental effect in patients with heart failure. It has been suggested that the use of verapamil and diltiazem should be limited to patients who do not tolerate β-blocker therapy and who do not have systolic dysfunction.[2,3]

Analgesics

It is important to abolish the patient's pain as quickly as possible because the pain and anxiety associated with an AMI will contribute to increased myocardial oxygen demand. If the pain is not relieved by the thrombolytic and anti-ischemic medications (e.g., nitrates, β-blockers), then additional analgesia may be necessary. Morphine and meperidine are the two most commonly prescribed analgesics.

Oxygen

Many patients are modestly hypoxemic during the initial hours of an AMI. Oxygen should be administered via nasal cannula to all patients suspected of having ischemic pain. Patients with severe hypoxemia or pulmonary edema may require intubation and mechanical ventilation.[2,3]

Antiarrhythmics

Ventricular arrhythmias, including ventricular fibrillation, are common complications associated with myocardial ischemia and AMI. Lidocaine, procainamide, and amiodarone are the drugs of choice for the treatment of ventricular arrhythmias in the peri-infarction period. The routine use of prophylactic lidocaine or other antiarrhythmic agents to prevent ventricular tachycardia and ventricular fibrillation is not recommended. Although the routine use of lidocaine may reduce the number of episodes of ventricular fibrillation, it may contribute to an increased number of episodes of asystole (see Chapter 20).[2,3]

Suppression of ventricular ectopy following an AMI with the chronic use of oral antiarrhythmic agents is not recommended. Results of Cardiac Arrhythmia Suppression Trial (CAST)-I and CAST-II demonstrated an increase in mortality in asymptomatic patients with ventricular ectopy following an AMI who were treated with flecainide, encainide, or moricizine.[2,3]

Stool Softeners

It is common to administer agents such as docusate to prevent constipation in AMI patients because straining causes undesirable stress on the cardiovascular system. Table 17-5 summarizes the common adjunctive therapy used in patients with AMI.

Nondrug Therapy

PCI is an attractive alternative to thrombolytic therapy. PCI consists of the insertion of a guidewire though a catheter into the occluded coronary vessel. Using fluoroscopy, the wire is directed and manipulated across the stenosis. A balloon angioplasty catheter is then progressed across the guidewire to the stenosis and inflated, which mechanically compresses the plaque in the vessel to increase lumen size. However, when balloon angioplasty alone is employed, reocclusion (9%–20%), reintervention (10%–20%), and restenosis (31%–45%) of the affected coronary artery occur. To correct these problems, a bare metal or drug-eluting stent may be placed in the coronary lumen (Fig. 17-4).[22] Specific guidelines have been published by the ACC/AHA addressing PCI and stent use in AMI.[23]

PCI is preferred only if a skilled interventional cardiologist and catheterization laboratory are available, if the procedure can be preformed within 90 minutes after initial medical contact, and/or a contraindication for a thrombolytic exists.[23] Thrombolytic therapy is preferred for patients whose first medical contact occurs less than 3 hours after symptom onset but for whom PCI is not immediately available, those who seek medical attention less than 1 hour after onset of symptoms, and those with a history of anaphylaxis to radiographic contrast material.

The disadvantages of PCI include the longer amount of time needed to mobilize the personnel needed to prepare the catheterization laboratory and its initial higher cost. A potential advantage of PCI is the greater ability to achieve TIMI grade 3 flow in the affected vessel (90% vs. 50%–60%, respectively).[22] Pooled data from major trials comparing PCI to thrombolysis have found PCI to be associated with fewer major adverse cardiac events, irrespective of patient presentation time.

Table 17-5 Adjunctive Therapy for Acute Myocardial Infarction

Drug	Indication	Dose and Duration	Therapeutic End Points	Precautions	Comments
ACE inhibitors[a]	AMI with EF <40%	Usual captopril dose 12–50 mg TID; then start longer-acting ACE inhibitor. Duration indefinite.	Titrate to usual doses and maintain systolic BP >90–110 mmHg	Avoid IV therapy within 48 hr of infarct	Oral therapy in patients with EF <40%.
Aldosterone antagonists	AMI with EF <40% with symptomatic HF or DM currently receiving ACE inhibitors	Spironolactone 12.5–50 mg daily or eplerenone 25–50 mg daily.	Titrate to heart failure symptom control without evidence of hyperkalemia	Hyperkalemia	Avoid if potassium ≥5 mEq/L or Scr ≥2.5 mg/dL for men and 2.0 mg/dL for women. Dose can be increased every 4–8 weeks.
Aspirin[a]	AMI and ischemic heart disease	160–325 mg during AMI, then 75–325 mg/day for an indefinite period.	No firm end point	Active bleeding, thrombocytopenia	Unless clear contraindication exists, aspirin should be given to all AMI patients.
β-blockers[a]	General use in all AMI patients to reduce reinfarction and improve survival	Variable; titrate to HR and BP. Immediate IV therapy preferable. Duration indefinite. See Table 17–8 for specific dosing recommendations.	Titrate to resting HR approx. 60 beats/min, maintain systolic BP >100 mmHg	Usual β-blocker contraindications. Observe HR and BP closely when given IV	Unless clear contraindication exists, β_1-selective agents such as metoprolol and atenolol should be given to all AMI patients. In patients with systolic dysfunction, metoprolol or carvedilol can be considered.
Calcium channel blockers	Postinfarction angina, non–Q-wave AMI	Usual doses of calcium channel blockers are used. Duration dictated by clinical scenario (see Chapter 17).	Titrate to usual doses and maintain systolic BP >90 mmHg	Usual calcium channel blocker contraindications. Avoid in patients with pulmonary congestion or EF <40%	a) In patients with good EF, most calcium channel blockers will exert beneficial effects. b) Some data support use of verapamil or diltiazem for non–Q-wave AMI, but not dihydropyridine types.
Clopidogrel[a]	For patients with aspirin allergy	75 mg/day	No firm end point	Active bleeding, thrombotic thrombocytopenia purpura (rare)	
Clopidogrel + aspirin[a]	For STEMI, prior to thrombolytic therapy or PCI	300 mg load 10–45 minutes before thrombolytic therapy, followed by 75 mg daily and continued to the day of angiography; aspirin 150–325 mg on first day, then 75–162 mg daily.	No firm end point	Active bleeding, thrombotic thrombocytopenia purpura (rare)	Whether administered before thrombolytic or PCI, clopidogrel + aspirin reduced CV death, MI, or ischemia at 30 days. The 600 mg load should be considered if a GIIb/IIIa is not used. Aspirin + clopidogrel should be continued for at least 1 month after placement of a BMS and at least 1 year for DES.
	For STEMI	75 mg daily; aspirin 162 mg daily.	No firm end point		Initial clopidogrel dose should be started within 24 hr of symptoms and continued until hospital discharge.
	For NSTEMI and unstable angina patients	300 mg load, followed by 75 mg daily for 1–9 months; aspirin 75–325 mg daily.	No firm end point	Clopidogrel + aspirin reduced death, reinfarction, or stroke through index hospitalization	

Table 17-5 Adjunctive Therapy for Acute Myocardial Infarction *(Continued)*

Drug	*Indication*	*Dose and Duration*	*Therapeutic End Points*	*Precautions*	*Comments*
Factor Xa inhibitor	To replace UFH or LMWH in ACS and STEMI	STEMI Fondaparinux: 2.5 mg SQ daily for 8 days or discharge. ACS Fondaparinux: 2.5 mg SQ daily for 6 days.	No firm end point No firm end point	Active bleeding	In STEMI, fondaparinux reduced mortality and reinfarction without increased bleeds or strokes compared to UFH, but only in patients not undergoing PCI. In ACS, fondaparinux was at least as effective as enoxaparin but exhibited less bleeding. Can possibly be used in HIT.
Heparin[a]	Acute anticoagulation, patients undergoing reperfusion with t-PA	Variable; 60 U/kg loading at initiation of t-PA, then 12 U/kg/hr. Usual duration 24–48 hr.	aPTT ratio 1.5–2.5 patient's control value	Active bleeding, thrombocytopenia	Unless clear contraindication exists, UFH should be given to all AMI patients who do not receive thrombolytic therapy.
Lidocaine	Treatment of VT, VF	Variable, 1.5 mg/kg loading dose, then 14 mg/min. Use for <48 hr.	Cessation of arrhythmia	Bradycardia. Observe for CNS toxicity.	Some data indicate increased mortality with generalized use.
LMWH[a]	To replace UFH in STEMI and ACS	STEMI Enoxaparin: 30 mg IV bolus (optional), then 1 mg/kg SQ twice daily for 7– 8 days Dalteparin: 100 U/kg SQ prior to thrombolytic, then 120 U/kg twice daily. ACS Enoxaparin: 1 mg SQ twice daily for 28 days. Dalteparin: 120 U/kg SQ twice daily for 6 days.	No firm end point	Active bleeding	In ACS, enoxaparin was superior to UFH for reducing mortality and ischemic events. In STEMI, compared to UFH, LMWHs may lower coronary reocclusion with variable effects on mortality.
Morphine	Treatment of severe chest pain; venodilator	2–5 mg IV Q3–5 min PRN.	Decreased chest pain and HR	Bradycardia, right ventricular infarct	Good choice for acute pain relief along with NTG.
Nitrates[a]	General use in most AMI patients	Variable; titrate to pain relief or systolic BP. 5–10–200 mcg/min typical regimen. Usually maintain IV therapy for 24–48 hr after infarct.	Titrate to pain relief or systolic BP > 90 mmHg	Use cautiously in right ventricular infarct or large inferior infarct because of effects on preload	Use acetaminophen, NSAIDs, narcotics for headache. NTG should be tapered gradually in ischemic heart disease patients.
Warfarin	Left ventricular thrombus	Variable; titrate to INR. Duration usually for several months.	INR 2–3 patient's control value	Usual warfarin problems such as noncompliance, bleeding, diatheses	May be useful in the presence of a left ventricular thrombus to prevent embolism.

[a] Indicates specific drug therapies that are known to reduce morbidity and/or mortality.

ACE, angiotensin-converting enzyme; ACS, acute coronary syndrome; AMI, acute myocardial infarction; aPTT, activated partial thromboplastin time; BMS, bare metal stent; BP, blood pressure; CNS, central nervous system; CV, cardiovascular; DES, drug-eluting stent; DM, diabetes mellitus; EF, ejection fraction; GIIb/IIIa, glycoprotein 2b3a inhibitor; HF, heart failure; HIT, heparin-induced thrombocytopenia; HR, heart rate; INR, international normalized ratio; IV, intravenously; LMWH, low-molecular-weight heparin; NSAIDs, nonsteroidal anti-inflammatory drugs; NSTEMI, non–ST segment elevation myocardial infarction; NTG, nitroglycerin; PCI, percutaneous coronary intervention; PRN, as needed; Q, every; Scr, serum creatinine; SQ, subcutaneously; STEMI, ST segment elevation myocardial infarction; TID, three times a day; t-PA, tissue plasminogen activator; UHF, unfractionated heparin; VF, ventricular fibrillation; VT, ventricular tachycardia.

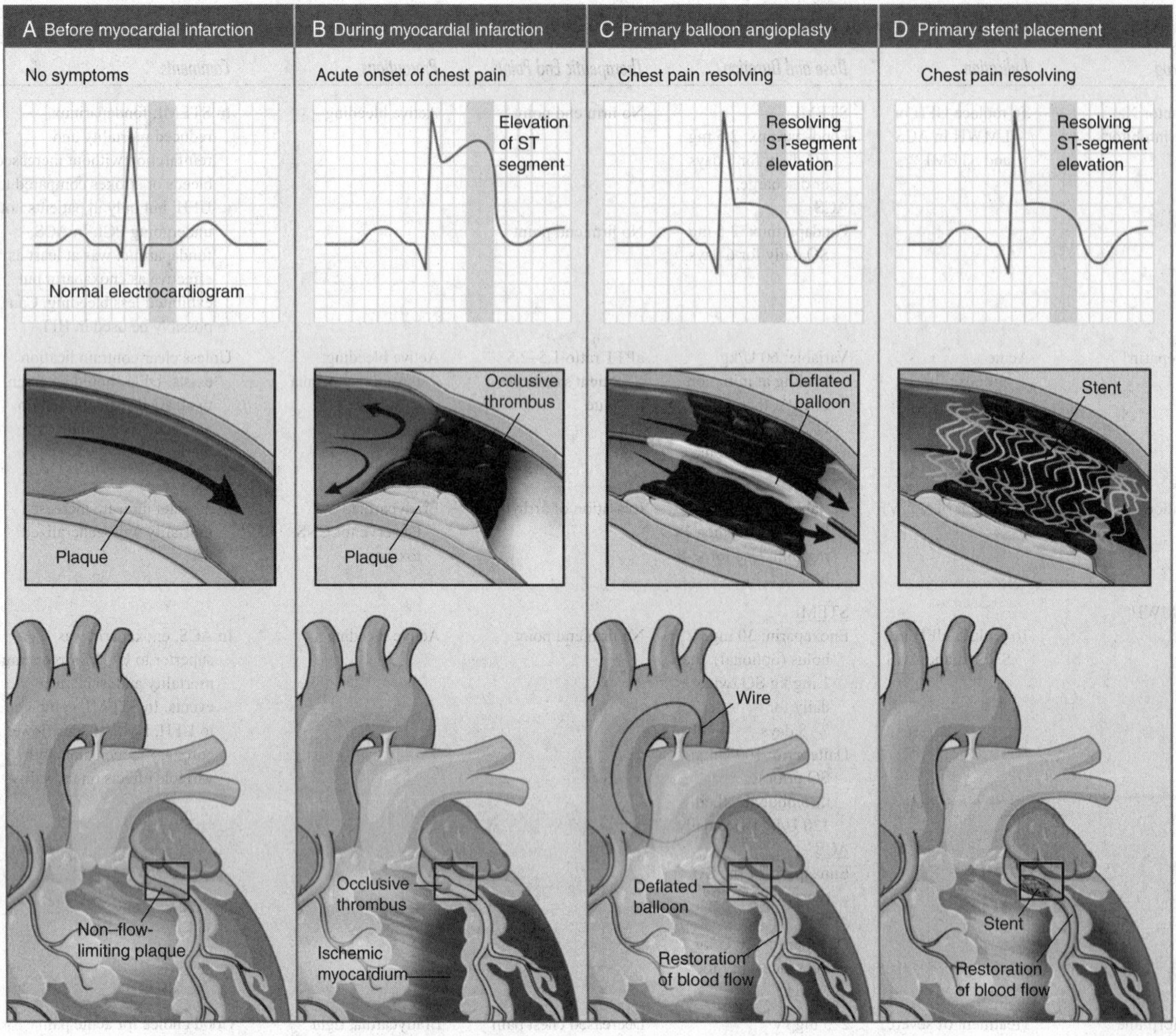

FIGURE 17-4 Myocardial infarction before, during, and after percutaneous coronary intervention. *Source:* Reprinted from reference 22, with permission.

Unfortunately, many hospitals do not have the facilities or skilled personnel to complete this procedure in the necessary time frame.[22]

SIGNS AND SYMPTOMS OF ACUTE MYOCARDIAL INFARCTION

1. P.H., a 65-year-old, 80-kg man, is being admitted to the emergency department (ED) after experiencing an episode of sustained chest pain while mowing his yard. After waiting 5 hours, he called 911 and was transported to the ED. Physical examination reveals a diaphoretic man who appears ashen. Heart rate and rhythm are regular and no S_3 or S_4 sounds are present. Vital signs include BP 180/110 mmHg, heart rate 105 beats/minute, and respiratory rate 32 breaths/minute. P.H.'s chest pain radiates to his left arm and jaw, and he describes the pain as "crushing" and "like an elephant sitting on my chest." He rates it as a "10/10" in intensity. Thus far, his pain has not responded to five sublingual (SL) NTG tablets at home and three more in the ambulance. His ECG reveals a 3-mm ST segment elevation and Q waves in leads I and V_2 to V_4. Based on this, P.H. is diagnosed with an anterior infarction. Laboratory values include sodium (Na), 141 mEq/L (normal, 135–145); potassium (K), 3.9 mEq/L (normal, 3.5–5); chloride (Cl), 100 mEq/L (normal, 100–108); CO_2, 20 mEq/L (normal, 24–30); blood urea nitrogen (BUN), 19 mg/dL (normal, 8–25); serum creatinine (SrCr), 1.2 mg/dL (normal, 0.6–1.5); glucose, 149 mg/dL (normal, 70–110); magnesium (Mg), 1.3 mEq/L (normal, 1.5–2); CK, 1,200 U/L (normal, 60–370), with a 12% CK-MB fraction (normal, 0%–5%); troponin-I, 60 ng/mL (normal, <2); cholesterol, 259 mg/dL (normal, <200); and triglycerides, 300 mg/dL (normal, 40–150). P.H. has a prior history of coronary artery disease (CAD). A previous cardiac catheterization 2 years ago revealed a lesion in his middle left anterior descending coronary artery (75% stenosis) and in the proximal left circumflex artery (30% stenosis). His ventriculogram at the time showed an EF of 58%. These lesions were deemed suitable for medical

management. He also has a history of recurrent bouts of bronchitis with bronchospastic disease for 10 years, diabetes mellitus treated with insulin for 18 years with fair control, and mild hypertension with fair control for 20 years. His father died of an MI at age 70. His mother and siblings are all alive and well. P.H. has smoked one pack of cigarettes a day for 30 years, and he drinks approximately one six-pack of beer a week. He has no history of IV drug use. On admission, P.H.'s medications include insulin glargine 40 U daily; albuterol inhaler, PRN; hydrochlorothiazide, 25 mg daily; NTG patch, 0.2 mg/hour; and NTG SL, 0.4 mg PRN chest pain. What signs and symptoms does P.H. have that are consistent with the diagnosis of AMI?

[SI units: Na, 141 mmol/L (normal, 135–145); K, 3.9 mmol/L (normal, 3.5–5.0); Cl, 100 mmol/L (normal, 100–108); CO_2, 20 mmol/L (normal, 24–30); BUN, 6.8 mmol/L (normal, 2.9–8.9); SrCr, 72 mmol/L (normal, 36–90); glucose, 8.3 mmol/L (normal, 3.9–6.1); Mg, 0.65 mmol/L (normal, 0.75–1.0); CK, 20 and 33.34 kat/L, respectively (normal, 1.0–6.7); cholesterol, 6.7 mmol/L (normal, <5.2); triglycerides, 3.9 mmol/L (normal, 0.45–1.7)]

P.H. described his pain as a pressure sensation, which is common with ischemic heart disease. The chest discomfort associated with AMI is described more often as pressure or as a tight band around the chest rather than pain. Although P.H. was involved in physical exertion when his chest pain began, this is not always the case. It can begin at rest and, frequently, in the early morning hours. At least 20% of patients with AMI have no pain or discomfort; these are described as having "silent" MIs. Presentations range from asymptomatic to shortness of breath, hypotension, heart failure, syncope, or ventricular arrhythmias. Silent or atypical infarctions occur more commonly in people with diabetes or hypertension and in the elderly. P.H. is diaphoretic, a common finding, but other common symptoms such as nausea and anxiety are not present. He also describes his pain as "10/10" in intensity, or perhaps "the worst pain I've ever experienced," which is typical of an AMI. The typical patient with an uncomplicated AMI has few useful physical findings. The diagnosis primarily lies in the symptoms, the ECG, and the laboratory findings.

The history of diabetes, hypertension, smoking, and a positive family history in P.H. are all risk factors for coronary disease. His admission BP is high, which could indicate poor underlying control or anxiety and stress related to his AMI. The blood sugar of 140 mg/dL is high, again indicating either poor control or a stress response. Measurement of glycosylated hemoglobin is indicated during his hospitalization to better assess his diabetes control.[2,3]

Laboratory Abnormalities

2. **What laboratory abnormalities can you expect to see in P.H.?**

P.H. demonstrates several laboratory abnormalities commonly seen in AMI. His CK was high on admission and the CK-MB of 12% (normal, <5%) is indicative of myocardial necrosis. CK-MB rises acutely over the first 12 to 24 hours and returns to normal in 2 to 3 days. The troponin level is also increased, which is consistent with myocardial necrosis. Several other nonspecific laboratory findings should be monitored in P.H. Hyperglycemia may develop because P.H. is a diabetic, but this can also occur in nondiabetic patients. Total cholesterol and HDL cholesterol concentrations may fall dramatically within a few days following an AMI; therefore, it is best to check serum lipid profiles within 24 to 48 hours. Leukocytosis and an increase in the erythrocyte sedimentation rate may also be observed with AMI.[2,3]

ST Segment Elevation Myocardial Infarction versus Non–ST Segment Elevation Myocardial Infarction

3. **P.H. was noted to have "ST segment elevation and Q waves" on the ECG. What are the implications of a ST segment elevation versus non–ST segment elevation MI?**

Perhaps the most important diagnostic test in someone who is suspected to have an AMI is the ECG. The ECG is an important tool because it is noninvasive, can be performed rapidly, is readily available in most clinical settings, and adds valuable clues as to where the AMI is located (i.e., anterior, inferior, lateral) (Fig. 17-4). It is valuable in determining whether a thrombolytic should be administered. Although enzyme profiles are helpful, the results are often not available for hours, or the patient may present to the hospital before the cardiac enzymes are present in the serum. Therefore, enzymes allow one to confirm "retrospectively" the presence of an AMI, but do not necessarily influence the immediate therapeutic course for the patient. P.H. has classic ECG changes such as ST segment elevation and Q waves. Their presence in the anterior ECG leads (V_2–V_4) indicates which part of the heart is affected and also points to the coronary arteries that are likely to be blocked. P.H.'s previous left anterior descending lesion may have had a plaque rupture leading to thrombosis of the vessel.

The presence of ST segment elevation in two contiguous leads indicates severe ischemia and occlusion of the coronary artery. Every effort should be made to open the infarct-related artery as soon as possible. If the ECG showed ST segment depression instead of elevation, P.H. would not be eligible for thrombolytic therapy.

Anterior versus Inferior Infarction

4. **What are the prognostic implications of an anterior versus an inferior MI?**

Damage to the anterior section of the heart is more likely to be associated with increased morbidity (e.g., left ventricular dysfunction) and mortality. The patients at highest risk of death are those with an anterior AMI, left ventricular dysfunction, and complex ventricular ectopy.[10] P.H. is at an increased risk because he has sustained an anterior AMI.

Risk Stratification

5. **What is P.H.'s initial risk of morality based on his presenting signs and symptoms?**

Much of the information used to stratify patients is based on their physical findings, test results, and past medical history. Risk stratification should be conducted on initial diagnosis and repeated or modified as needed based on an initial response to therapy and results of laboratory findings.

The first risk stratification method was introduced in 1967 by Killip et al. and found to be a useful, easy tool for early risk stratification for patients with STEMI.[24,25] Higher Killip class was found to be associated with increased in-hospital and 1-year mortality (Table 17-6). The TIMI risk score was introduced in 2000 and can be used with either STEMI or NSTEMI.[26,27] For STEMI, the higher the risk score, the greater the 30-day mortality rate. In the case of NSTEMI, the higher the risk score, the greater the 14-day risk of death or MI. Table 17-6 describes the various risk factors and corresponding percentage risks.

P.H. has a TIMI risk score of 7 based on his age (2 points); history of angina, hypertension, and diabetes (1 point); heart rate (2 points); location of his MI (1 point); and time to reperfusion therapy (1 point). P.H. has a 30-day mortality rate of 23%, thereby highlighting the serious nature of his heart disease and the importance of adherence to medications.

Table 17-6 Risk Stratifications Tools for Acute Myocardial Infarction

TIMI Risk Score[a]

STEMI Risk Factor	No. of Points	*NSTEMI* Risk Factor	No. of Points
Age 65–75 yr	2	Age ≥65 yr	1
Age ≥75 yr	3	≥3 risk factors for CAD[b]	1
SBP <100 mmHg	3	Prior history of CAD[c]	1
Heart rate >100 beats/min	2	Aspirin use in past 7 days	1
Killip class II–IV	2	≥2 anginal events in past 24 hr	1
Weight <67 kg	1	ST segment deviation ≥0.5 mm	1
History of HTN, diabetes, or angina	1	Elevation of cardiac markers[d]	1
Time to reperfusion therapy >4 hr	1		
Anterior ST segment elevation or left bundle branch block	1		

Killip Class[e]

Class	*Symptoms*	*In-Hospital and 1-yr Mortality (%)*
I	No heart failure	5
II	Mild heart failure, rales, S_3, congestion on chest radiograph	21
III	Pulmonary edema	35
IV	Cardiogenic shock	67

[a]TIMI risk score data from refs. 26 and 27. A risk score is calculated by adding the total number of risk factors. Total points for STEMI are 0–14, in which risk scores of 0, 2, 4, 6, 7, and >8 correspond to a 30-day mortality rate of 0.8%, 2.2%, 7.3%, 16%, 23%, and 36%, respectively. Total points for NSTEMI are 0–7, in which scores of 0 or 1, 3, 5, and 7 correspond to a 3%, 5%, 12%, or 19% risk of death or repeat MI at 14 days, respectively.

[b]Risk factors include smoking, diabetes, hypertension, family history of coronary artery disease, and hypercholesterolemia.

[c]Defined as a prior coronary stenosis ≥50%; history of previous MI, percutaneous coronary intervention, or coronary artery bypass graft; or chronic stable angina pectoris associated with a positive exercise tolerance test or pharmacologically induced nuclear imaging or echocardiographic changes (positive nuclear imaging or echocardiographic changes required if female).

[d]Either troponin I or T or CK-MB.

[e]Killip class data from reference 25.

CAD, coronary artery disease; HTN, hypertension; NSTEMI, non–ST segment elevation myocardial infarction; SBP, systolic blood pressure; STEMI, ST segment elevation myocardial infarction; TIMI, thrombolysis in myocardial infarction.

TREATMENT

Therapeutic Objectives

6. What are the immediate and long-term therapeutic objectives in treating P.H.?

The immediate therapeutic objectives in treating P.H. are to minimize the amount of myocardial necrosis that develops, to alleviate his symptoms, and to prevent his death. These objectives are achieved primarily by restoring coronary blood flow (administering a thrombolytic and/or performing a PCI) and lowering myocardial oxygen demand. Any life-threatening ventricular arrhythmias that develop must be treated. The long-term therapeutic objectives are to prevent or minimize recurrent ischemic symptoms, reinfarction, heart failure, and sudden cardiac death. The specific therapeutic regimens are discussed in the questions that follow.

Thrombolytic Therapy

7. Is P.H. a candidate for thrombolytic therapy? Is any one agent preferred?

AMI is a medical emergency and rapid administration of drug therapy is crucial to save myocardial tissue. The results of several major trials have shown unequivocally that if used appropriately, thrombolytics can reduce the mortality associated with an AMI.[2,3] Because mortality benefit is greatest when thrombolytic therapy is administered within 2 hours of symptom onset, many institutions are employing early prehospital thrombolytic therapy, in which trained paramedics administer the thrombolytic in the field.[16]

Controversy still exists over which thrombolytic should be used, the best dosing regimen, the most appropriate adjunctive therapy, and whether the risk outweighs the benefit in some subpopulations of patients (e.g., those with an inferior AMI). Each issue is discussed in subsequent cases.

P.H. has a history of hypertension, and at presentation, his BP is 180/110 mmHg. A BP this high is a relative contraindication to thrombolytic therapy because of an increased risk of cerebral hemorrhage; however, P.H. has an anterior MI and is likely to benefit from thrombolytic therapy. In this case, he should receive IV NTG immediately because the onset of blood pressure control with this agent usually occurs within minutes. Once his systolic BP is <180 mmHg and the diastolic is <110 mmHg, a thrombolytic can be administered. The NTG will also reduce the workload on his heart and may provide pain relief.

Because P.H. has severe pain and ECG changes consistent with an anterior AMI, he is at great risk for substantial morbidity and/or mortality. Alteplase is more rapid acting and effective in restoring TIMI grade 3 blood flow than streptokinase; however, the slightly increased risk of stroke and the increase in cost with t-PA may outweigh its advantages. The argument for or against a specific thrombolytic is probably less important than the decision to use an agent and to administer the medication as soon as possible after the onset of symptoms. P.H. is fortunate because he has presented within 5 to 6 hours of the onset of chest pain.

Dosage Regimens

8. "Alteplase 100 mg infused over 90 minutes" is ordered for P.H. Is this an appropriate dosage? If streptokinase, anistreplase, reteplase, or tenecteplase had been ordered, what would be an appropriate regimen?

To enhance reperfusion while minimizing bleeding complications, accelerated dosage regimens of t-PA are recommended. The recommended regimen is a 15 mg bolus followed by a 50 mg infusion over 30 minutes and then the remaining 35 mg over 60 minutes. The Global Utilization of Streptokinase and t-PA for Occluded Arteries (GUSTO) trial used this accelerated or front-loaded regimen for administration of t-PA. In this trial, t-PA was compared to streptokinase and a combination of streptokinase and t-PA. The results showed that t-PA alone was the most effective in reducing mortality. The 30-day mortality rate for the accelerated t-PA group was 6.3% compared to 7.3% in the streptokinase group. In GUSTO, the t-PA regimen was also weight adjusted, such that after the 15 mg bolus dose, the infusion was 0.75 mg/kg over 30 minutes followed by 0.5 mg/kg over 60 minutes. The maximum dose received was 100 mg.

Most of the large trials with streptokinase have used an IV infusion of 1.5 MU administered over 60 minutes. There have been some trials in which the infusion was shortened to 30 minutes; however, there have been no large studies that have compared a 30-minute infusion to a 60-minute infusion.

Anistreplase is usually given intravenously as 30 U over 2 to 5 minutes. This convenient dosing schedule is the major advantage of this agent. As mentioned previously, it has been suggested that prehospital administration of anistreplase by emergency services personnel would reduce the amount of time from the onset of chest pain to the administration of this lifesaving drug.

Reteplase was compared to t-PA in the GUSTO-III trial. Reteplase has a slower clearance from the body, allowing the drug to be given as a bolus without the need for a constant infusion. In the GUSTO-III trial, reteplase was administered in two bolus doses of 10 MU, given 30 minutes apart. The mortality rate and incidence of stroke were the same in the two groups of patients.

TNK was compared to t-PA in the Second Assessment of Safety and Efficacy of a New Thrombolytic (ASSENT-2) trial. TNK was administered as a bolus of 30 to 50 mg over 5 to 10 seconds, based on body weight (Table 17-3). No difference existed between TNK and t-PA in 30-day mortality and stroke.

Many institutions have streptokinase in addition to one of the more expensive, fibrin-selective agents (t-PA, reteplase, or TNK) on their formulary. Choice of the later is based on contract pricing, ease of administration, and simplicity of dosing regimen. From GUSTO and GUSTO III, t-PA and reteplase are effective therapies for achieving early coronary reperfusion, providing an advantage over streptokinase. The 2004 ACC/AHA guidelines recommend t-PA or reteplase for patients who present early after onset of chest pain and in those with a large area of injury (e.g., anterior infarction) who have a low risk for an intracranial bleed. However, based on the ASSENT-2 trial, TNK appears to be just as effective as t-PA with fewer bleeding complications. Compared to t-PA, both TNK and reteplase can be administered as bolus doses.[2,3]

Once P.H.'s BP is controlled, he should receive a thrombolytic as quickly as possible. Because he appears to be having a large anterior infarction, the added cost of t-PA, r-PA, or TNK versus streptokinase may be justified. Table 17-7 summarizes the major thrombolytic trials. With regard to medication safety, the thrombolytic dose should always be carefully checked because over- and underdosing of thrombolytics has been associated with higher 30-day mortality.[2,3,28]

Adjunct Therapy

9. Orders are written for UFH 5,000 U IV bolus, followed by 1,000 U/hour by continuous infusion. Also prescribed is aspirin 325 mg STAT. Are both agents necessary?

The Second International Study of Infarct Survival (ISIS-2) trial showed that aspirin 160 mg/day alone and in combination with streptokinase reduced mortality in patients with AMI by 23% and 42%, respectively, when compared to a control group of patients who received neither aspirin nor streptokinase. In doses of 160 mg or more, aspirin generates a prompt clinical antithrombotic effect as a result of its inhibition of thromboxane A_2 production. Thus, immediate administration of 160 to 325 mg of aspirin in patients diagnosed with AMI, regardless of whether they receive thrombolytics, is indicated. In the acute setting, aspirin should be chewed because it is absorbed more quickly. All patients should receive 75 to 325 mg of daily aspirin indefinitely following AMI. If patients have a contraindication to aspirin, clopidogrel can be substituted.[2,3]

The use of UFH as adjunct therapy to prevent reocclusion has been evaluated in many studies (Table 17-7). Overall, it appears that UFH administration offers no benefit to patients receiving streptokinase or anistreplase.[2,3] However, because P.H. will receive t-PA, due to his anterior wall infarct, an IV UFH bolus followed by a continuous infusion should be started before the end of the t-PA infusion. The 2004 ACC/AHA guidelines recommend a 60 U/kg bolus of UFH at the initiation of t-PA, followed by a maintenance infusion of 12 U/kg/hour or a maximum of a 4,000 U bolus, followed by 1,000 U/hour. The target activated partial thromboplastin time should be 1.5 to 2.0 × control (generally 50–75 seconds). UFH should always be considered in patients at high risk for systemic or venous embolism.

10. Would P.H. benefit from the addition of clopidogrel to his current drug regimen?

Recent studies have defined the potential role of in-hospital clopidogrel as an integral part of reperfusion therapy in patients with STEMI. Although the data with clopidogrel are quite promising, the risk and cost of chronic therapy of the drug must be weighed against its benefits.

The Clopidogrel as Adjunctive Reperfusion Therapy-Thrombolysis in Myocardial Infarction 28 (CLARITY-TIMI

Table 17-7 Summary of Major Thrombolytic Trials

Trial	*Thrombolytics*	*Heparin, Aspirin, LMWH*	*Number of Patients*	*Duration of Symptoms*	*Results*
ISIS-2 1988	Streptokinase 1.5 MU over 1 hr vs. placebo	Also randomized to aspirin 160 mg/day or no aspirin. Heparin not specified.	17,187	<24 hr	Streptokinase, aspirin, streptokinase + aspirin all reduced mortality compared to placebo. Most benefit from streptokinase + aspirin. Aspirin alone and in combination with streptokinase reduces mortality. Some benefit from aspirin and/or streptokinase even administered late.
ISG 1990	t-PA 100 mg over 3 hr vs. streptokinase 1.5 MU over 1 hr	Also randomized to heparin SQ or no heparin. All patients received aspirin and atenolol unless contraindicated.	20,891	<6 hr	No significant difference in hospital mortality between streptokinase and t-PA. More episodes of major bleeding with streptokinase and more strokes with t-PA. Results questioned due to the use of SQ heparin.
ISIS-3 1992	t-PA (duteplase) 0.6 MU over 4 hr vs. streptokinase 1.5 MU over 1 hr vs. APSAC 30 U over 3 min	Also randomized to SQ heparin or no heparin. All patients received aspirin 162 mg/day.	41,299	<24 hr	No significant difference in mortality between thrombolytics. More episodes of major bleeding with heparin and more strokes with t-PA. Results questioned due to the use of SQ heparin.
GUSTO 1993	t-PA 1.25 mg/kg (100 mg) over 90 min vs. streptokinase 1.5 MU over 1 hr vs. t-PA 1 mg/kg + streptokinase 1 MU over 1 hr	Aspirin 160–325 mg/day to all patients. Heparin IV with t-PA groups. Heparin IV or SQ in streptokinase groups.	41,021	<6 hr	Statistically significant decrease in 30-day mortality in the t-PA group (6.3%) vs. streptokinase (7.3%). More strokes in t-PA groups.
GUSTO-III 1997	t-PA 100 mg over 90 min vs. r-PA 10 + 10 U	Aspirin 160 mg immediately, then daily. Heparin 5,000 U bolus, 1,000 U/hr.	15,059 No upper age limit	<6 hr	Mortality rate at 30 days was 7.47% in r-PA vs. 7.24% in t-PA (p = NS). Stroke occurred in 1.64% of r-PA patients vs. 1.79% of t-PA patients (p = NS).
ASSENT-2 1999	TNK 30–50 mg over 5–10 sec vs. t-PA 1.25 mg/kg over 90 min	Aspirin 150–325 mg and heparin 4,000 U bolus, 800 U/hr for patients 67 kg or 5,000 U bolus, 1,000 U/hr >67 kg.	16,949	<6 hr	No significant difference in 30-day mortality, death or nonfatal stroke, or intracranial bleeding between thrombolytics. TNK had significantly fewer bleeding complications.
GUSTO-V 2001, 2002	r-PA two 10 U boluses vs. r-PA two 5 U boluses + abciximab 0.25 mg/kg bolus, 0.125 mcg/kg/min for 12 hr	Aspirin 150–325 mg orally or 250–500 mg IV immediately, then 75–325 mg daily. For r-PA alone: heparin 5,000 U bolus, 1,000 U/hr. (≥80 kg) or 800 U bolus, 800 U/hr. (<80 kg). For combination therapy, heparin 60 U/kg bolus, 7 U/kg/hr.	16,588	<6 hr	No significant difference between groups in all-cause mortality at 30 days and 1 year, confirmed cerebrovascular events, or nonfatal disabling strokes. Combination therapy had a statistically significant higher rate of bleeding complications ($p < 0.0001$).
ASSENT-3 2001	TNK 30–50 mg over 5 sec vs.TNK 15–25 mg over 5 sec + abciximab 0.25 mg/kg bolus, 0.125 mcg/kg/min for 12 hr	Aspirin 150–325 mg orally. For full-dose TNK, patients were randomized to either enoxaparin 30 mg bolus, 1 mg/kg Q 12 hr 7 days or IV heparin 60 U bolus, 12 U/kg/hr 48 hr. For combination therapy, 40 U bolus, 7 U/kg/hr.	6,095	<6 hr	For the composite end point of 30-day mortality, reinfarction, or refractory ischemia, event rates were 6.1% for full-dose TNK + enoxaparin, 5.2% for half-dose TNK+ abciximab, 8.8% for full-dose TNK + heparin ($p < 0.0001$). No significant difference in 30-day mortality between groups. More major bleeding ($p = 0.0002$) and transfusions ($p = 0.001$) in the abciximab group compared to heparin.
ASSENT-4 2006	Standard PCI vs. pretreatment with TNK 30–50 mg over 5 sec, 1–3 hr before PCI	Aspirin 150–325 mg orally and single heparin bolus (70 U/kg for PCI group, 60 U/kg for TNK group).	1,667	<6 hr	Study terminated early due to increased in-hospital mortality in the TNK group (6%) compared to standard PCI (3%) ($p = 0.0105$). Patients receiving TNK had more strokes ($p < 0.0001$) and 90-day reinfarction ($p = 0.0279$) and repeat revascularizations ($p = 0.0041$).

APSAC, anisoylated plasminogen streptokinase activator complex; IV, intravenously; LMWH, low-molecular-weight heparin; NS, nonsignificant TNK, tenecteplase; PCI, percutaneous coronary intervention; r-PA, reteplase; SQ, subcutaneously; t-PA, tissue plasminogen activator.
From reference 2, 3, and 28.

28) evaluated 3,497 patients (18–75 years of age) with STEMI who received standard thrombolytic therapy, aspirin, and UFH, and were scheduled for angiography within 2 days. Patients received either clopidogrel (300 mg loading dose, followed by 75 mg daily) or placebo within 10 minutes of thrombolytic administration. Clopidogrel was continued up to and including the day of angiography and stopped. The primary end point was the composite of an occluded infarct-related artery on predischarge angiography or death or an MI up to the start of coronary angiography. Compared to placebo, patients in the clopidogrel group demonstrated a 36% reduction in the primary end point ($p < 0.001$). By 30 days, the clopidogrel treatment group had a 20% reduction in cardiovascular death, recurrent MI, or recurrent ischemia ($p = 0.03$). No difference in the rate of major bleeding was seen between groups.[29]

Similar results were seen in the Adjunctive Reperfusion Therapy (PCI-CLARITY) study in which STEMI patients scheduled for PCI received pretreatment with either placebo or clopidogrel (300–600 mg load, then 75 mg daily) up to and including the day of angiography.[30] Those receiving clopidogrel had a 38% reduction in the MI or stroke prior to PCI ($p = 0.028$), as well as a 46% reduction in the incidence of cardiovascular death, MI, or stroke 30 days following the procedure ($p = 0.008$). No difference in the rate of major bleeding was seen between groups.

Finally, the Clopidogrel and Metoprolol in Myocardial Infarction Trial (COMMIT) evaluated the effect of administrating either clopidogrel 75 mg daily with no loading dose or placebo in 45,852 patients presenting with STEMI.[31] The initial clopidogrel dose was given within 24 hours of symptom onset and continued until hospital discharge or up to 4 weeks in the hospital. Compared to placebo, the allocation to clopidogrel was associated with a 9% reduction in death, reinfarction, or stroke ($p = 0.002$) and a 7% reduction in all-cause mortality ($p = 0.03$). No significant excess in bleeding was noted in the treatment group or in those who received concomitant thrombolytic therapy or who were younger than 70 years.

Based on the data from COMMIT, P.H. could safely receive clopidogrel 75 mg daily as an inpatient. However, long-term clopidogrel use in patients with STEMI remains questionable, unless the patient receives a stent. As discussed later in the chapter, most of the data with maintenance clopidogrel use are documented in patients with acute coronary syndromes (NSTE-ACS) and PCI.

11. Would P.H. benefit from a LMWH, factor Xa inhibitor, or a GP IIb/IIIa inhibitor added to his thrombolytic regimen?

The replacement of UFH with a LMWH, factor Xa inhibitor, or the addition of an antiplatelet agent such as a GP IIb/IIIa inhibitor to thrombolytic therapy has been evaluated in patients with STEMI.

In the Enoxaparin and Thrombolysis Reperfusion for Acute Myocardial Infarction Study-25 (ExTRACT-TIMI 25), 20,506 patients with STEMI scheduled for thrombolytic therapy were randomized to receive either enoxaparin throughout the index hospitalization or continuous infusion UFH for 48 hours.[32] Enoxaparin was dosed according to age and renal function. For patients younger than 75 years, enoxaparin was dosed as a fixed 30 mg bolus followed 15 minutes later by 1 mg/kg subcutaneously (SQ) twice daily. For patients older than 75 years, the bolus was eliminated, and the dose reduced to 0.75 mg/kg SQ twice daily. If the creatinine clearance was <30 mL/minute, the dose was modified to 1.0 mg/kg SQ daily. UFH was dosed according to weight (60 U/kg bolus, followed by 12 U/kg/hour) and adjusted to achieve an aPTT 1.5 to 2.0 × control. The composite end point of death or nonfatal MI through 30 days occurred in 12.0% in the UFH group and 9.9% in the enoxaparin group, representing a 17% risk reduction ($p < 0.001$). Although no difference was noted in mortality between the two groups, treatment with enoxaparin did reduce the 30-day risk of nonfatal reoccurrence of AMI by 33% compared to UFH ($p < 0.001$). However, major bleeding was higher in the enoxaparin group compared to those receiving UFH (2.1% vs. 1.4%, respectively, $p < 0.001$).[2,3]

The TIMI-14 trial demonstrated enhanced reperfusion (TIMI 3 flow) using reduced-dose t-PA combined with abciximab (0.25 mg/kg bolus, then 12-hour infusion of 0.125 mcg/kg/minute) compared to full-dose t-PA alone. This improvement occurred without an increase in the risk of major bleeding.[33] Similar rates of enhanced reperfusion have also been observed with the combination of double-bolus dose eptifibatide (180/90 mcg/kg, 10 minutes apart) with a 48-hour infusion (1.33 mcg/kg/minute) plus half-dose t-PA (50 mg).[2,3]

In the GUSTO-V trial, 16,588 patients with STEMI were randomized to standard-dose reteplase or half-dose reteplase plus full-dose abciximab. There was no difference in death rates between the groups at 30 days or 1 year. The combination group had less reinfarction and recurrent ischemia, but this benefit was offset by more episodes of moderate and severe bleeding, especially in the elderly.[2,3]

The ASSENT-3 trial randomized 6,095 AMI patients to full-dose TNK + enoxaparin, half-dose TNK + UFH, and a 12-hour infusion of abciximab, or full-dose TNK + UFH. The addition of either abciximab or enoxaparin to TNK reduced the composite end point of 30-day mortality, in-hospital reinfarction, or ischemia compared to UFH. More major bleeding complications were seen with abciximab compared to UFH.[2,3]

The Enoxaparin as Adjunctive Antithrombin Therapy for ST-Elevation Myocardial Infarction (ENTIRE-TIMI 23) trial evaluated the use of a thrombolytic in combination with a GP IIb/IIIa inhibitor and either UFH or LMWH. In this trial, 483 AMI patients were randomized to full-dose TNK or half-dose TNK + abciximab. Each group was then randomized to receive either UFH or enoxaparin. Patients receiving full-dose TNK plus enoxaparin exhibited lower 30-day mortality/recurrent MI rates compared to those receiving TNK + UFH. Rates of major bleeding were highest with the TNK, abciximab, and enoxaparin combination.[2,3]

The Organization for the Assessment of Strategies for Ischemic Syndromes (OASIS) 6 was a complex, randomized double-blind trial of 12,092 patients with STEMI designed to assess the effect of early initiation of fondaparinux with primary PCI and medical therapy.[34] The study compared the effects of fondaparinux (2.5 mg/day for up to 8 days) with two different control arms: stratum 1, in which placebo was used if UFH was not indicated; and stratum 2, in which UFH was administered for up to 48 hours followed by placebo for up to 8 days. Each control group included a mix of the different treatment strategies, with essentially all primary PCI patients receiving UFH. Compared to the control group, those receiving fondaparinux had a significant reduction in the composite of death or reinfarction at 30 days (11.2% vs. 9.7%, respectively, $p = 0.008$). Significant reductions in this end point were also observed at 9 days (7.4% for the fondaparinux group vs. 8.9% for the controls, $p = 0.003$), and at the end of the study (13.4% vs. 14.8%, $p = 0.008$). Specifically, in stratum 1, fondaparinux reduced the incidence of death or MI compared to the control group (11.2% vs. 14.0%, $p < 0.05$), but in stratum 2, demonstrated no difference in this end point when compared to UFH. Fondaparinux did not appear to offer benefit in patients who were managed with primary PCI. Although the rates of death, MI, and severe bleeds did not differ in these patients, there was a higher rate of catheter thrombosis with fondaparinux.

In a meta-analysis of 11 trials involving 27,115 STEMI patients who received adjunctive abciximab in addition to either PCI or thrombolytic therapy, use of abciximab was associated with a significant reduction in 30-day ($p = 0.047$) and 6- to 1-month mortality ($p = 0.01$) in patients undergoing PCI but not in those receiving thrombolytic therapy. Although both reperfusion strategies demonstrated a significant reduction in 30-day reinfarction ($p < 0.05$), only those patients receiving abciximab with a thrombolytic had an increased risk in major bleeding ($p < 0.001$).[35]

For P.H., enoxaparin could be substituted for UFH based on the ExTRACT-TIMI 25 trial. However, P.H. will have a higher risk for bleeding and will need to be monitored closely. Because P.H. is not undergoing PCI, he may not benefit from the addition of a GP IIb/III at this time. GP IIb/IIIa inhibitors are used primarily in NSTEMI and PCIs. If a GP IIb/IIIa inhibitor was to be used in conjunction with a thrombolytic agent for patients with STEMI, the dose of the thrombolytic agent is reduced by one-half.

Determination of Reperfusion

12. How can you monitor for successful reperfusion in P.H. after he has received thrombolytic therapy?

Performing coronary angiography following thrombolytic therapy will reveal whether the infarcted artery is open, how vigorous the blood flow is, and the extent of residual stenosis. There are several clinical indicators that correspond with reperfusion, one of which is the resolution of chest pain. Some investigators have found the development of "reperfusion arrhythmias" to be associated with infarct-related artery patency, but neither of these clinical markers is very reliable.

Two other methods used to estimate reperfusion are the ECG and laboratory changes. Because the extent of the reduction of ST segment elevation may be related to the extent of patency, 12-lead ECGs should be obtained frequently. ECGs have the advantage of being readily available and noninvasive.

Early peaking of total CK and the CK-MB isoenzyme levels may also differentiate patients who have achieved reperfusion from those in whom thrombolytic therapy has failed. Lewis et al. found an absolute rise in CK activity of 480 U/L or a relative rise of 34% within the first hour following successful thrombolysis. CK-MB activity was found to have a relative rise of 27% during the first hour. In the absence of reperfusion, CK activity was only increased by 15 U/L or had a relative rise of 3% over the first 2.5-hour period.[2,3]

Some hospitals routinely evaluate regional wall motion using echocardiography. Unfortunately, it may take several days before improvement in wall motion is seen; therefore, it is difficult to use this test to assess the initial success of thrombolysis.

It is important to determine whether thrombolysis has been successful because the prognosis of the patient appears to be related to the presence or absence of an open infarct-related artery. If thrombolytic therapy fails to open the infarct-related artery, then the patient may benefit from mechanical revascularization such as PCI or a coronary artery bypass graft (CABG) surgical procedure.[2,3,22]

Overall, coronary angiography is expensive, and although rare, it does carry the risk of major bleeding, stroke, and renal dysfunction. To minimize expense and complications, P.H. should undergo a 12-lead ECG to evaluate reperfusion.

Time From Onset of Chest Pain

13. If P.H.'s arrival at the hospital had been delayed >6 hours from the onset of his chest pain, should he still have received a thrombolytic?

Although efforts should be directed toward administering a thrombolytic as early as possible, many patients present several hours after the onset of chest pain. There are several theoretical reasons why the late administration of a thrombolytic may be helpful. Some patients present with a "stuttering" MI, which is chest pain that waxes and wanes over a period of hours or days, presumably from recurrent or ongoing ischemia. These patients should be considered candidates for thrombolytic therapy or angiographic evaluation. The magnitude of left ventricular dilatation may be diminished by reperfusion of the infarct-related artery, even if it is late. Another potential advantage of opening an infarct-related artery, even hours after an MI, is that the opened artery could become a source of collateral blood flow in the future. The Gruppo Italiano per lo Studio della Streptochinasi nell'Infarto Miocardico (GISSI)-1 trial enrolled patients within 12 hours from the onset of chest pain. After 12 months of follow-up, the cumulative survival rate showed a statistically significant benefit from the administration of streptokinase compared to placebo. However, a subgroup analysis showed no benefit for the patients who received streptokinase after 6 hours from the onset of chest pain.[2,3]

The ISIS-2 trial expanded patient enrollment to include patients admitted within 24 hours from the onset of chest pain. In that trial, there was a 17% reduction in vascular death at 5 weeks in the streptokinase group treated 5 to 24 hours from the onset of chest pain, compared to a 35% reduction in the group who received streptokinase within 4 hours from the onset of pain. Although the benefit was reduced, a statistically and clinically significant benefit was still present.[2,3]

Overall, there appears to be a statistically significant benefit associated with administering a thrombolytic up to 12 hours from the onset of chest pain and a trend toward benefit when given between 13 and 24 hours. Late administration may be most beneficial in patients at the highest risk for mortality. This would include the elderly, patients with large infarctions, and those with continuing pain or hypotension.[36] P.H. still may benefit from thrombolytic therapy even if he presents beyond the 6-hour time frame. If he is still having symptoms, he probably has viable myocardium at risk that may be salvaged. Streptokinase is the most cost-effective drug and the thrombolytic that has been shown to be effective in this situation.

Readministration of Thrombolytic Agents

14. This is P.H.'s first infarction. If he had a history of a previous MI that was treated with a thrombolytic agent, would he still be eligible for thrombolysis?

The need to administer a thrombolytic for a second infarction is becoming common. Many patients who are admitted to a hospital with AMI have a history of a previous infarction. Both streptokinase and anistreplase are associated with the formation of neutralizing antibodies within several days following administration and up to 4 years with streptokinase. Unfortunately, the clinical significance of these antibodies on thrombolytic efficacy remains unknown. Based on observations made in ISIS-2, repeat doses of streptokinase were associated with allergic reactions (4.4% of individuals) consisting of shivering, pyrexia, or rashes, which were resistant to use of prophylactic corticosteroids.[37] If P.H. was presenting with a second infarction within a year and had received streptokinase for his first infarction, the thrombolytic of choice would be t-PA, TNK, or reteplase.

15. P.H. was stable initially following thrombolysis, but 48 hours later he experienced recurrent chest pain and ECG changes consistent with extension of his infarct. The attending cardiologist would like to readminister t-PA at this time. Is this a reasonable course of therapy?

Reocclusion of the infarct-related artery following initial successful thrombolysis is a major setback for this therapeutic strategy. If reocclusion occurs, mechanical intervention (e.g., PCI) is often attempted. Debate has existed between whether to readminister the thrombolytic or refer the patient for PCI.[38] In a meta-analysis of eight trials composed of 1,177 patients with STEMI who failed thrombolytic therapy, patients receiving rescue PCI showed no significant reduction in all-cause mortality, but had a 27% risk reduction in heart failure ($p = 0.05$) and 42% reduction in reinfarction ($p = 0.04$) when compared with conservative treatment. Repeat fibrinolytic therapy was not associated with significant improvements in all-cause mortality or reinfarction. Both treatment strategies demonstrated a significant increase in minor bleeding, but PCI was associated with an increase in stroke.[39]

In the case of P.H., a repeat infusion with t-PA would probably be safe, but it may not be effective. As discussed in question 12, repeat doses of streptokinase should be avoided. If facilities for either PCI or surgery exist at the institution, many cardiologists would choose an invasive strategy at this time for P.H.

Use in the Elderly

16. B.T., an 85-year-old woman, presents to the ED with a history and examination that are nearly identical to P.H.'s. Should an elderly person (older than 70 years) be treated any differently with regard to thrombolytic therapy?

Some of the early trials with thrombolytic therapy excluded the elderly. Although the elderly may have a higher prevalence of relative contraindications such as severe hypertension or history of stroke at presentation, they also have a higher incidence of mortality following an AMI. The 30-day mortality rate following an AMI is 19.6% for patients between 75 and 85 years of age and 30.3% for those who are 85 years of age.[40] In a trial using streptokinase, a higher incidence of bleeding in patients older than age 70 was reported. However, in the ISIS-2 trial, the greatest reduction in mortality occurred in the elderly subgroup. There are no controlled trials in which thrombolytic therapy has increased mortality in the elderly. If B.T. had no contraindications to thrombolytic therapy, she should receive it. However, in a high-risk cohort of elderly female patients (older than 75 years, <67 kg), the ASSENT investigators demonstrated that, compared with bolus and infusion of t-PA, TNK was associated with lower rates of major bleeding (15.15% vs. 8.33%) and intracerebral hemorrhage (3.02% vs. 1.14%).[2,3,36]

Strokes Associated With Thrombolysis

17. G.M., a 45-year-old man, presents with signs and symptoms consistent with an anterolateral AMI. On admission, he received t-PA (100 mg over 90 minutes). He developed nystagmus, blurred vision, dysarthria, and paresthesias in his right hand 18 hours after the infusion. How often are stroke symptoms observed in patients with AMI? Is there a difference in the risk of stroke among the various thrombolytic agents?

Stroke is a serious but infrequent complication of AMI. In the prethrombolytic era, thrombotic stroke occurred in 3.7% of AMI patients. In recent years, the number of ischemic strokes has diminished to <0.6%, with a 17% mortality rate.[41] The risk factors identified for stroke associated with AMI include large, akinetic segments of myocardium and the presence of a left ventricular mural thrombus. Other comorbid conditions can also increase stroke risk such as atrial fibrillation, hypertension, diabetes, CABG, and previous stroke. An estimated one third of patients with anterior wall infarction who do not receive a thrombolytic will develop a mural thrombus, usually within the first week of the event.[41] Echocardiograms are recommended before discharge in patients who have had an anterior wall infarction to rule out a mural thrombus.

The risk of stroke was analyzed from the GISSI-2 and International Study trials, where streptokinase was compared to t-PA with and without SQ UFH. Of the 20,768 patients who had complete records, 236 had a stroke while in the hospital. Thirty-one percent of the cases were intracerebral hemorrhage, 42% were ischemic stroke, and 26% were not classified. More hemorrhagic and ischemic strokes occurred in patients receiving t-PA (1.33% vs. 0.94% for streptokinase). Elderly patients (older than age 70) had a stroke rate of 2.6% with t-PA and 1.6% with streptokinase. Patients older than age 75 had a higher incidence of death and stroke compared to patients younger than 75 in the GUSTO trial. Patients older than 75 who were randomized to the t-PA group had a higher incidence of hemorrhagic stroke (2.08%) versus those randomized to either streptokinase group (1.23%). This has prompted some to suggest that patients older than age 75 should receive streptokinase rather than t-PA.[40] Furthermore, Van De Graaff et al. suggested that administration of thrombolytic therapy within 15 minutes of hospital arrival is associated with a 42% lower risk of in-hospital stroke ($p < 0.05$).[41]

Risk of Ventricular Fibrillation

18. After thrombolysis, P.H. is in normal sinus rhythm with rare premature ventricular contractions (PVCs). Should he receive prophylactic lidocaine?

Ventricular fibrillation is a major cause of death in patients who are having an AMI. More than half of the episodes of ventricular fibrillation that occur with an AMI are within 1 hour of the onset of symptoms. Because ventricular fibrillation is estimated to occur in 2% to 19% of patients with AMI, prophylactic lidocaine has been used in an attempt to reduce this complication.[42] It was assumed initially that ventricular ectopy such as frequent PVCs or short runs of ventricular tachycardia would precede any episodes of ventricular fibrillation. However, it was noted that not all patients who developed ventricular fibrillation had warning arrhythmias, so it became routine to give all patients with AMI prophylactic infusions of lidocaine. Subsequent meta-analyses of the use of prophylactic lidocaine in AMI found that while lidocaine was associated with a 35% reduction of ventricular fibrillation, no significant reduction in all-cause mortality was noted. In fact, early mortality and asystole, although not significant, were detected in the lidocaine-treated patients.[43] Nonetheless, as ventricular fibrillation is treated readily with defibrillation in an intensive care unit, the risk of prophylactic lidocaine in all patients may exceed the benefit. Because electrical cardioversion is an unpleasant experience, it is reasonable to use prophylactic lidocaine in patients at highest risk for ventricular fibrillation (see Chapter 19).

Risks of Using Lidocaine

19. How should lidocaine be given, and if so, for how long? How should lidocaine be monitored?

Lidocaine should be given as a loading dose followed by a continuous infusion. Loading doses of 1 mg/kg (maximum 100 mg) are used, followed by a constant infusion of 20 to 50 mcg/kg/minute. Patients should be monitored for the side effects of lidocaine; the most common are those associated with central nervous system toxicity. Symptoms may include drowsiness, dizziness, tremor, paresthesias, slurred speech, seizures, and coma. Massive overdoses may cause respiratory depression. Lidocaine may suppress ventricular escape mechanisms, leading to atrioventricular block or asystole. The overall incidence of side effects in studies has been approximately 15%.[42,43]

Plasma Concentrations

20. What factors following an AMI may complicate the measurement of lidocaine plasma concentrations?

The likelihood of developing adverse effects from lidocaine is dose related; however, side effects are frequently reported when plasma concentrations are within the therapeutic range. The elderly and patients with heart failure and hepatic dysfunction have reduced clearance of lidocaine and may be predisposed to lidocaine toxicity. Lidocaine is bound to $alpha_1$-acid glycoprotein (AAG) and albumin in the serum. AAG plasma concentrations have been shown to increase within 36 hours of the time of infarction.[44] Patients with AMI have an increased binding of lidocaine to AAG and a rise in total lidocaine plasma concentrations, but a reduced percentage of free lidocaine. This could result in a patient with a plasma lidocaine concentration that is above the "therapeutic range" without signs of toxicity. Therefore, plasma lidocaine concentrations may be difficult to interpret in the setting of AMI. (See Chapter 19 for a complete discussion of lidocaine dosing and toxicity.)

Magnesium

21. Will the administration of IV magnesium be beneficial for P.H.? How is magnesium administered?

There has been considerable debate regarding the use of magnesium in the setting of AMI. The potential mechanisms by which magnesium may benefit a patient include an antiarrhythmic effect, an antiplatelet effect, reversal of vasoconstriction, reduction of catecholamine secretion, and enhancement of adenosine triphosphate production.

In the Second Leicester Intravenous Magnesium Intervention Trial (LIMIT-2), a randomized, placebo-controlled, double-blind trial of 2,316 patients with suspected AMI, IV magnesium was found to decrease mortality at 28 days by 24%. However, in the Magnesium in Coronaries (MAGIC) trial, 6,213 patients with AMI were randomized to 2 g of IV magnesium sulfate given as a bolus followed by a 17 g infusion over 24 hours or matching placebo. Early administration of magnesium did not reduce 30-day mortality. There was no benefit seen in the ISIS-4 study.[2,3]

At this time, most clinicians do not routinely administer IV magnesium to AMI patients. However, because P.H. has a low serum magnesium concentration (1.3 mEq/L), he could benefit from the drug. Increasing P.H.'s serum magnesium concentration to 2.0 mEq/L could reduce his risk for potential arrhythmias. Based on trials using magnesium in AMI, P.H. should receive 8 mmol over 5 to 15 minutes followed by 65 to 72 mmol, or 8 to 9 g, given as an IV infusion over 24 hours.[2,3]

β-Blockers

22. The physician has written orders for IV metoprolol 5 mg Q 5 minutes for three doses. What are some of the benefits of administering β-blockers to P.H.? Should they be given early in his therapeutic course as IV therapy or simply started as oral therapy a few days after the infarct?

As with thrombolytics, β-blockers offer significant benefits to the MI patient in both the acute infarct period and/or several days later as initial oral therapy. Several large trials were designed to give early IV β-blockers (up to 24 hours after symptom onset), followed by oral therapy; other studies used oral therapy alone beginning days after the infarct. Early IV administration appears to be most beneficial, with a reduction of mortality of around 25% in the first 2 days when the results of these trials are pooled. However, late oral therapy alone, up to 21 days post-MI in the β-Blocker in Heart Attack Trial, was also associated with a substantial reduction in mortality (around 10%).[2,3]

Propranolol, metoprolol, timolol, and atenolol have been studied extensively. All have been given by early IV administration. Typically, metoprolol and atenolol are used in the acute setting due to their β-1 selectivity, ease of dosing and administration, and weight of evidence. Oral carvedilol, a nonselective β- and α-blocker, has been used in the peri-infarction period, specifically in patients with left ventricular dysfunction. In the Carvedilol Post-Infarction Survival Control in Left Ventricular Dysfunction (CAPRICORN) trial, carvedilol reduced all-cause and cardiovascular mortality as well as recurrent nonfatal MI.[2,3]

In general, if a patient has transient cardiac decompensation (e.g., hypotension, bradycardia, or worsening symptoms of heart failure) during the acute infarct period, early IV β-blockers are withheld. The patient's condition is then observed for a few days; if it stabilizes, oral therapy is initiated and titrated slowly. Data from COMMIT highlight the importance of tailored β-blockade therapy.[45] In this study, 45,852 patients were randomized to receive placebo or metoprolol (up to 15 mg IV, then 200 mg orally daily) within 24 hours of AMI. Although metoprolol use reduced reinfarction ($p < 0.001$) and ventricular fibrillation rates ($p < 0.001$) compared to placebo, the drug was also associated with a significant increase in episodes of cardiogenic shock ($p < 0.00001$). In a subgroup analysis, patients with hemodynamic instability at randomization appeared to bear the brunt of early cardiogenic shock associated with metoprolol.

Because P.H. has experienced an uncomplicated MI and is stable, he is a candidate for early IV therapy. Acute and chronic dosing regimens for β-blockers are listed in Table 17-8.[2,3]

Use in Diabetes

23. What are some reasons for concern about the use of a β-blocker in P.H. (refer to the data presented in question 1)? How should this therapy be monitored?

Recall that P.H. has a long-standing history of hypertension and diabetes and that his admission BP was 180/110 mmHg and heart rate was 100 beats/minute. Historically, the presence of diabetes was a relative contraindication for β-blockade due to the adverse effects on insulin release and blunting of the hypoglycemia-associated tachycardia. However, diabetics comprise a large portion of AMI patients, and many β-blocker trials contained diabetic AMI patients. Gottlieb et al. found that post-MI diabetic patients treated with β-blockers experience a 36% reduction in mortality.[46]

Furthermore, data from the Glycemic Effects in Diabetes Mellitus: Carvedilol-Metoprolol Comparison in Hypertensives (GEMINI) trial suggest that in hypertensive, diabetic patients receiving RAS blockade, carvedilol does not affect glycemic control and may improve insulin sensitivity compared to metoprolol.[47] Due to these positive data, β-blockers would have to possess major negative effects on the diabetic condition to be considered contraindicated. Diabetic patients who are given β-blockers should receive nonintrinsic sympathomimetic activity, cardioselective agents (e.g., metoprolol, atenolol) or a more cardioselective α-β blocker (e.g., carvedilol). Patients should be advised to monitor their blood glucose levels carefully for both hypo- and hyperglycemia after the β-blocker is initiated, making adjustments to their insulin or oral hypoglycemic therapy as needed.

In a patient like P.H., a low dose of metoprolol 25 mg twice a day (BID) or carvedilol 3.125 mg BID can be given and titrated to either adequate β-blockade or loss of diabetic control. At these doses, the relative β_1 selectivity will be more likely to remain intact and is less likely than some of the nonspecific β-blockers to affect his diabetes.

Use in Hyperlipidemia

P.H. has elevated serum cholesterol (259 mg/dL) and triglyceride (300 mg/dL) levels. His low-density lipoprotein (LDL) and high-density lipoprotein (HDL) cholesterol levels are unknown. Although β-blockers have undesirable effects on plasma lipids (they decrease HDL and increase total cholesterol and triglycerides), the evidence in support of their use in MI patients is compelling (see Chapter 13). β-blockers have reduced post-MI morbidity and mortality in hyperlipidemic patients. An appropriate lipid-lowering treatment plan should be developed and initiated as soon as possible.

Use in Heart Failure

Years ago, heart failure was considered a contraindication to β-blockade, but that is no longer the case. There are several factors to consider before withholding β-blockers. In general, patients who receive early IV β-blockade will benefit from this therapy. If the patient has a relative contraindication to β-blockade, one could consider using esmolol (500 mcg/kg IV bolus over 1 minute followed by a maintenance infusion of 50 to 300 mcg/kg/minute), which has a short duration of action. IV β-blockade should be withheld only if the patient has signs and symptoms of moderate to severe left ventricular dysfunction. However, chronic, oral therapy should be initiated before discharge (see Chapter 19). β-blockade should be given to P.H. because he has no heart failure symptoms and his previous EF was >50%.

Table 17-8 Dosing Summary of β-Blockers in Acute Myocardial Infarction

β-Blocker	IV Dose	Chronic Dose
Atenolol (Tenormin)	Administer 5 mg IV over 5 min, followed by 5 mg IV 10 min later; after second IV dose, immediately begin 50 mg PO, followed by 50 mg PO 12 hr later.[a]	50–100 mg PO daily[a]
Carvedilol (Coreg)	None	6.25–25 mg PO twice daily[a]
Metoprolol (Toprol)	Administer 5 mg IV over 2 min for three doses; 15 min after the last IV dose, begin 50 mg PO Q 6 hr for eight doses.[a]	50–100 mg PO twice daily[a]
Propranolol (Inderal)	Administer 58 mg IV over 5 min, followed by 40 mg PO 2 hr apart, then Q 4 hr for seven doses.[a]	180–240 mg PO daily in 24 divided doses[a]
Timolol (Blocadren)	Administer 1 mg IV, followed by 1 mg IV 10 min later; 10 min after the second IV dose, begin constant infusion of 0.6 mg/hr for 24 hr; on completion of infusion, begin 10 mg PO twice daily.	10 mg PO twice daily[a]

[a]FDA-approved dose.
IV, intravenously; PO, orally; Q, every.
From references 2 and 3.

Use in Pulmonary Disease

P.H.'s acute situation is complicated by his history of intermittent pulmonary problems. In deciding whether to attempt use of β-blockers in patients with pulmonary disease, one must determine the nature of the pulmonary problem (i.e., reactive airways or restrictive lung disease). It also would be helpful to determine P.H.'s need for routine use of β-agonists to help quantify the severity of his disease. By history, P.H. does not use β-agonist bronchodilators routinely. No history is given regarding his pulmonary function tests or the degree of reversibility of his airway disease with bronchodilators. β_1-selective antagonists are the drugs of choice in these patients, but at higher doses (e.g., metoprolol doses >100 mg/day), the relative β_1 selectivity may be lost. Similar to the argument regarding diabetes, a patient would need to experience significant worsening of the pulmonary disease to justify avoiding β-blockers. A better history of P.H.'s pulmonary problems should be obtained; if they are minor, low doses of metoprolol or atenolol (started in the hospital so he may be monitored closely) should be considered.

Weighing the risk versus benefit of β-blockers, one could make a case for cautiously administering IV agents to him at this time. His dose of IV metoprolol (5 mg Q 5 minutes for three doses) is a typical treatment plan. He must have frequent monitoring of heart rate, BP, and respiratory status. Therapy should be discontinued if P.H.'s heart rate drops below 60 beats/minute, systolic BP falls below 100 mmHg, or any respiratory distress is noted. Oral metoprolol therapy could begin at 25 to 50 mg a few hours after his last IV dose. Substituting the ultra–short-acting agent esmolol for metoprolol is an option for P.H. because any adverse effects would be relatively short lived. Unfortunately, there are no data to support the use of esmolol for an AMI.

Objective evidence of adequate β-blockade consists of a resting heart rate of 50 to 60 beats/minute, an exercise heart rate of <120 beats/minute, and/or a resting systolic BP of 100 to 120 mmHg. Therefore, P.H. needs a significant reduction in heart rate and BP from his admission values (100 beats/minute and 180/110 mmHg, respectively) to be considered as having achieved adequate β-blockade.[48]

24. Several days later, a routine echocardiogram is performed on P.H. that shows hypokinesis of the anterior and lateral left ventricular walls, a slightly enlarged left ventricle, no valvular abnormalities, EF 35% to 40%, and the appearance of a thrombus in the left ventricle. Clinically, he has no signs or symptoms of heart failure. What are the therapeutic and prognostic implications of this echocardiogram?

Hypokinesis of the infarcted areas of the heart is not unusual. P.H. may have an area of "stunned" or "hibernating" myocardium; it could take several weeks to recover some of the wall motion if the area is still viable.[49] Therefore, P.H. may recover some of the wall motion and EF over time.

The presence of a thrombus in the left ventricle is a risk factor for embolization. Several studies have shown that this may increase P.H.'s risk of experiencing a later embolic event. If P.H. is believed to be compliant with his medications, he would be a candidate for warfarin therapy (titrated to an international normalized ratio [INR] of 2 to 3) for 1 to 3 months because of this thrombus. This should be enough time for the thrombus to organize and become less of an embolic threat. Because of his reduced EF, P.H. is an ideal candidate for treatment with an ACE inhibitor and β-blocker.

Nitroglycerin

25. A.J., a 75-year-old man, presents to the ED with complaints of dizziness and chest discomfort. He is a poor historian, but it appears that his symptoms have been ongoing for >12 hours. His physician is concerned that the symptoms represent an STEMI. He had a GI bleed 6 weeks ago and has chronic obstructive pulmonary disease with a bronchospastic component. The ECG is consistent with a new anterolateral AMI. His vital signs are BP, 150/94 mmHg; heart rate, 55 beats/minute; and respiratory rate, 20 breaths/minute. Physical examination reveals wheezing. What is the best treatment strategy for A.J.?

Because of the time delay since symptoms first appeared and his history of recent GI bleeding, A.J. is not a good candidate for thrombolysis. β-blockers also should be avoided in A.J. because of his serious pulmonary disease and current heart rate. Thus, symptomatic management with IV NTG is indicated, and PCI should be considered. NTG lowers the left ventricular filling pressure and systemic vascular resistance, thereby reducing myocardial oxygen consumption and myocardial ischemia. At lower doses (<50 mcg/minute), IV NTG preferentially dilates the venous capacitance vessels, which leads to a decrease in left ventricular filling pressure.[2,3] For patients who have signs of pulmonary congestion, IV NTG is of particular value. (See Chapter 16 for further discussion of NTG pharmacology.)

26. How should IV NTG be administered to A.J.? How should it be monitored?

IV NTG should be initiated with a small bolus dose of 15 mcg. A constant infusion is then delivered by a controlled infusion device, starting with 5 to 10 mcg/minute, which is then increased by an additional 5 to 10 mcg/minute every 5 to 10 minutes.[2,3] Many cardiologists routinely give patients an infusion of NTG for the first 24 to 48 hours following an AMI. Increasing doses may be required over this period to maintain the desired hemodynamic effect due to tolerance that occurs from prolonged nitrate exposure. However, if >200 mcg/minute is needed to achieve the desired response, another vasodilator such as nitroprusside or an ACE inhibitor may be needed. NTG is typically administered in combination with thrombolytics in patients who require relief of myocardial ischemia. Two studies have reported that concurrent administration of NTG may impair the thrombolytic effects of t-PA, but these data have been questioned.[50,51]

Some patients may have a problem with increased sensitivity to NTG, described as development of mean BP <80 mmHg. Of the patients who become hypotensive, many have an inferior AMI. Ferguson et al. noted that hypotension following NTG infusion was a common complication in patients with right ventricular infarction.[52]

NTG readily migrates into many plastics; therefore, manufactured solutions are available only in glass containers. Some filters may absorb NTG, so they should be avoided. Polyvinyl chloride (PVC) tubing may absorb NTG, especially during the early phases of infusion. Some institutions use non-PVC tubing for NTG infusions to minimize this problem. However, if standard PVC tubing is used, the usual starting dose of nitroglycerin is 25 mcg/minute and should be titrated to hemodynamic response.[2,3]

A.J.'s BP should be monitored closely during this infusion. On admission, his BP was elevated at 150/94 mmHg, and his pulse rate was low at 55 beats/minute. After starting NTG, we would expect to see his BP decline; the pulse rate may or may not increase. The NTG dose should be titrated to relieve pain while avoiding hypotension. In patients with evidence of heart failure, NTG can reduce left ventricular filling pressure (preload), as well as improve orthopnea and pulmonary congestion. However, excessive doses of IV NTG can reduce left ventricular filling pressure and potentially decrease cardiac output, especially in patients like A.J. who do not have signs of heart failure. The end points for dose titration include relief of pain or other symptoms. The systolic BP should be kept equal to 90 mmHg. Nitrate tolerance can be minimized by providing a nitratefree interval to the patient. If A.J. later receives chronic nitrate therapy with either an oral agent or a transdermal delivery system, a nitratefree interval should be used (see Chapter 16).

27. Because A.J. has an elevated BP (154/94 mmHg), should he receive nitroprusside instead of NTG?

NTG is preferred over nitroprusside in the setting of an AMI. Although the drugs have similar hemodynamic effects, nitroprusside has been shown to increase ST segment elevation, whereas NTG decreases ST segment elevation.[53] Others have shown similar results and have proposed that nitroprusside may redistribute coronary blood flow away from the ischemic area, causing a worsening of the injury, known as coronary steal.[54]

Analgesic Use

28. A.J.'s chest pain becomes increasingly severe despite NTG, and the physician is considering use of a potent analgesic. Which analgesic would be best for A.J.?

The pain associated with AMI is due to continuing tissue ischemia surrounding the area of infarcted tissue. The relief of pain should involve efforts to optimize the myocardial blood supply and minimize myocardial oxygen demand. Pain is usually relieved with successful thrombolysis. Other interventions can include oxygen, nitroglycerin, and β-blockers. As noted previously, A.J. is not a candidate for either thrombolysis or β-blockade. If his pain continues despite administration of IV NTG, he will need an analgesic. A.J. may also need to undergo emergency revascularization with either PCI or bypass surgery.

Morphine sulfate is usually the analgesic of choice in patients with AMI. In addition to diminishing pain and anxiety, morphine also has beneficial hemodynamic effects. By reducing pain and anxiety, the release of circulating catecholamines is diminished, possibly reducing the associated arrhythmias. Morphine also causes peripheral venous and arterial vasodilatation, which reduces preload and afterload, and consequently, the myocardial oxygen demand. Morphine is administered in small (2- to 4-mg) IV doses as often as every 5 minutes if needed. Cumulative doses of 25 to 30 mg may be required. The risks associated with morphine use include hypotension, bradycardia, and respiratory depression. Because A.J. already has bradycardia, meperidine may be used because it has vagolytic properties.

POSTINFARCTION ARRHYTHMIAS

29. D.T., a 45-year-old man who is recovering from an AMI (onset 12 hours ago), is noted to have sustained ventricular tachycardia on the telemetry monitor in the coronary care unit. During the episode, he was hemodynamically unstable (BP 80/40 mmHg, heart rate >200 beats/minute). The arrhythmia was terminated with a 100-J countershock. He now is in sinus rhythm and clinically stable. Would D.T. be a candidate for further workup of the arrhythmia? If so, what tests are appropriate?

In the past, it was assumed that ventricular ectopy in the immediate post-MI period would be a negative prognostic factor, especially for sudden cardiac death. Overall, ventricular arrhythmias detected during hospitalization have not been helpful in identifying patients at high risk for sudden cardiac death on long-term follow-up.[55] Because D.T.'s arrhythmia occurred within the first 48 hours after the infarct (i.e., the peri-infarct period, when some residual ischemia may be occurring), he is not a candidate for any further specific arrhythmia workup, such as electrophysiologic testing. D.T. should receive a β-blocker and aspirin during hospitalization and after discharge to prevent reinfarction and reduce mortality.

30. Two weeks after D.T.'s AMI, he returns to the clinic for routine follow-up. A Holter monitor (continuous ambulatory ECG monitoring) is ordered for him because he states that he has had several "skipped beats" since the MI. This is a new finding. The results of the Holter indicate that he is having >30 PVCs/hour that are asymptomatic to mildly symptomatic. What is the appropriate antiarrhythmic therapy at this time?

It has been known for some time that frequent PVCs in patients with organic heart disease (e.g., post MI) are indicators for an increased risk of sudden cardiac death. However, the CAST showed that when PVCs were suppressed with flecainide, encainide, or moricizine, survival was significantly worse than in patients treated with placebo. This may be related to the proarrhythmic effects of these drugs (see Chapter 20). Therefore, treatment of asymptomatic or mildly symptomatic PVCs with antiarrhythmics (other than β-blockers) in this type of MI patient is not recommended. A pooled-data analysis of class I antiarrhythmic trials in these patients also supports these conclusions. Therapies should be aimed at correcting the patient's underlying ischemia and/or coexisting heart failure rather than administering antiarrhythmics. D.T. should not be given any of the class I antiarrhythmics.[2,3]

Amiodarone has been extensively studied in post-MI patients. The largest trials to date have been the Canadian Amiodarone Myocardial Infarction Arrhythmia Trial (CAMIAT) and European Myocardial Infarction Amiodarone Trial (EMIAT) studies. CAMIAT enrolled 1,202 patients between 6 and 45 days post MI who had $\geq$10 PVCs/hour. EMIAT enrolled 1,486 patients between 5 and 21 days post MI with a documented EF <40%. CAMIAT found a nonsignificant reduction in total mortality rate but a 38% reduction ($p = 0.03$) in the rate of ventricular fibrillation or arrhythmic death. EMIAT also found no difference in total mortality rate, but a 32% reduction ($p = 0.05$) in arrhythmic death and resuscitated cardiac arrest. The Amiodarone Trials Meta-Analysis Investigators evaluated data from 6,553 post-MI patients enrolled in 13 randomized trials. These investigators found that amiodarone significantly reduced the total mortality rate by 13% and the arrhythmic/sudden death rate by 29%.[2,3]

Outside amiodarone, randomized trials also strongly support implantable cardioverter-defibrillators (ICDs) as an option for secondary prevention in patients with prior life-threatening arrhythmias and as primary prophylaxis for those with a low EF and CAD[56] (see Chapter 20).

At this time, D.T. should not receive empiric amiodarone or an ICD because his symptoms are mild and treatment would not prolong his life.

ACUTE CORONARY SYNDROMES

31. J.W. is a 55-year-old man who presented to the ED with chest tightness and shortness of breath. He gives a history of similar symptoms the prior day that lasted 15 minutes. He was given aspirin 325 mg and started on an IV NTG infusion, which was increased to 80 mcg/minute; at that time, his BP was 100/60 mmHg, and his heart rate was 88. His ECG continued to show ST segment depression in the anterior leads. His shortness of breath was relieved, but he still complained of chest tightness. His past medical history is unremarkable, and he was on no medications prior to admission. He has smoked a pack of cigarettes per day for the past 30 years. Blood is drawn for troponin and CK as well as routine chemistries. Based on his symptoms and ECG, the diagnosis is presumed unstable angina. Should J.W. receive an additional oral antiplatelet agent?

J.W. is presenting with signs and symptoms consistent with ACS. If his cardiac enzymes come back positive, his diagnosis will be NSTEMI. If they remain unchanged, his diagnosis will be unstable angina. Regardless of the diagnosis, clopidogrel should be added to aspirin as soon as possible on admission. It should be administered for 1 month and may be given for up to 9 months in patients who are not at a high risk for bleeding.

In hospitalized patients with unstable angina or NSTEMI who do not require early interventional therapy, clopidogrel may be used in combination with aspirin. In the Clopidogrel in Unstable Angina to Prevent Recurrent Ischemic Events (CURE) trial, 12,562 patients with NSTEMI presenting within 24 hours were randomized to receive placebo + aspirin (75–325 mg) or clopidogrel (300 mg, immediately followed by 75 mg daily) plus aspirin. After 9 months, cardiovascular death, MI, or stroke occurred in 11.5% of patients in the placebo group and 9.3% in those receiving clopidogrel ($p < 0.001$). Clopidogrel was associated with reductions in severe ischemia and revascularization. Compared to placebo, an increase in major and minor bleeding was seen with clopidogrel. Based on these data, clopidogrel with aspirin should be administered immediately on admission and continued for at least 1 month and up to 9 months.[2,3]

In the PCI-CURE study, 2,658 patients from the CURE trial undergoing PCI were randomized to receive clopidogrel or placebo in addition to aspirin. Patients were treated prior to the PCI with aspirin and study medication for a median of 10 days. After the PCI, patients received open-label clopidogrel or ticlopidine for about 2 to 4 weeks, after which the study drug was restarted for a mean of 8 months. In the clopidogrel group, there was a statistically significantly reduction in the composite of cardiovascular deaths, MIs, or urgent target-vessel revascularizations within 30 days of the PCI compared to placebo (4.5% vs. 6.4%, $p = 0.03$). Overall, patients receiving clopidogrel exhibited a 31% reduction in cardiovascular death or MI compared to those receiving placebo ($p = 0.002$).[2,3]

Based on these data, in patients with unstable angina or NSTEMI receiving aspirin and undergoing PCI, clopidogrel should be administered prior to the procedure, followed by 1 month and possibly up to 12 months of additional treatment. In patients undergoing elective CABG or other surgery, clopidogrel should be discontinued for 5 to 7 days prior to the procedure.

32. What other antithrombotic medications should be considered for J.W.?

The ACC/AHA guidelines recommend the use of either LMWH or UFH for the treatment of unstable angina/NSTEMI.[2,3] Enoxaparin is preferred over UFH unless CABG is anticipated within 24 hours. In the Efficacy and Safety of Subcutaneous Enoxaparin (ESSENCE) study, enoxaparin (1 mg/kg SQ twice daily) was compared to UFH (5,000 U IV bolus followed by continued infusion titrated to an activated partial thromboplastin time of 55–86 seconds) administered for 48 hours to 8 days. The composite outcome of death, MI, or recurrent angina at 14 days was 19.8% in the UFH group versus 16.6% in the enoxaparin group, a 20% relative risk reduction. This benefit was maintained over 1 year.

In the TIMI-11B trial, enoxaparin (30 mg IV bolus followed by 1 mg/kg SQ twice daily for 8 days) compared to UFH (70 U/kg bolus followed by 15 U/kg/hour for 3–8 days) reduced the composite end point of death, MI, or need for urgent revascularization at 8 days ($p = 0.048$) and 43 days ($p = 0.048$).

In the Superior Yield of the New Strategy of Enoxaparin, Revascularization and Glycoprotein IIb/IIIa Inhibitors (SYNERGY) trial, 9,978 high-risk NSTEMI patients were randomized to receive either enoxaparin (1 mg/kg SQ twice daily) or weight-based UFH (60 U/kg bolus followed by 12 U/kg/hour adjusted to an aPTT 1.5 to 2 × control) prior to an early invasive strategy. Enoxaparin was found to be as efficacious as UFH in reducing 30-day all-cause mortality or nonfatal MI but was associated with a significant risk of major bleeding ($p = 0.008$).[57] Bleeding was especially problematic in those patients who crossed-over from one treatment to the other during the trial.

Finally, enoxaparin has been compared with the factor Xa inhibitor fondaparinux. In the OASIS-5 trial, 20,078 NSTEMI patients were randomized to receive either fondaparinux (2.5 mg SQ daily) or enoxaparin (1 mg/kg SQ twice daily) for a mean of 6 days and evaluated at 9 days for the primary end point of death, MI, or refractory ischemia. No difference existed between groups for the primary end point; however, compared to enoxaparin, fondaparinux demonstrated a significantly lower incidence of major bleeding at 9 days ($p < 0.001$) and a greater reduction in mortality at 30 days ($p = 0.05$).[58]

The addition of a LMWH with a GP IIb/IIIa inhibitor for the initial management of unstable angina/NSTEMI has been evaluated in small trials. The major finding was that major hemorrhage rarely occurred in the combination arms (0.3%–1.8%). Although not powered to detect a difference, the rates of ischemic events were noted to be similar between the LMWH and UFH groups.[59] Similar findings have also been seen when a DTI, bivalirudin, has been added to a GP IIb/IIIa.[60]

33. What is the role of a GP IIb/IIIa inhibitor in patients with NSTE-ACS or NSTEMI?

The ACC/AHA guidelines recommend that a platelet GP IIb/IIIa inhibitor be administered, in addition to aspirin and/or clopidogrel and UFH or LMWH, to patients in whom PCI is planned.[23] A GP IIb/IIIa inhibitor may also be administered just prior to PCI. Eptifibatide or tirofiban, when used in combination with aspirin and UFH or LMWH, is also approved for the medical management of patients with NSTE-ACS. When used to treat patients medically, the GP IIb/IIIa inhibitors (in combination with the other drugs previously mentioned) are generally given for 2 to 3 days.

The GUSTO-IV-ACS trial enrolled 7,800 patients with unstable angina/NSTEMI in whom early (<48 hours) revascularization was not intended. All patients received aspirin and either UFH or LMWH. They were randomized to placebo, an abciximab bolus and 24-hour infusion, or an abciximab bolus and 48-hour infusion. At 30 days, death or MI occurred in 8.0% of patients taking placebo, 8.2% of patients receiving 24-hour abciximab, and 9.1% of patients receiving 48-hour abciximab ($p = \text{NS}$). At 48 hours, death occurred in 0.3%, 0.7%, and 0.9% of patients in these groups, respectively (placebo vs. abciximab at 48 hours, $p = 0.008$). Abciximab should be used only if a patient is planning to undergo PCI; it should be avoided if only medical management is intended. Major trials have been done with other GP IIb/IIIa inhibitors in patients with ACS, showing them to be useful for the medical management of NSTE-ACS.[61,62]

LONG-TERM THERAPY

Angiotensin-Converting Enzyme Inhibitors

34. A patient with an uncomplicated MI has no signs or symptoms of heart failure. An order is written for captopril 12.5 mg three times a day (TID). Is this appropriate? If so, how should the therapy be monitored?

After an AMI, the heart undergoes processes that initially compensate for the loss of contractile function but may increase the long-term risk for development of heart failure. This is referred to as "remodeling" of the ventricle. (See Chapter 18 for a more detailed description of ventricular remodeling.) The increase in the number of survivors of AMI has increased the number of heart failure patients.

In the SAVE (Survival and Ventricular Enlargement) trial, captopril (up to 50 mg TID) had a statistically significant beneficial effect on mortality when given to asymptomatic patients with an EF <40% who were 3 to 16 days post MI. This 4-year follow-up study also showed significant decreases in morbidity from heart failure and recurrent AMI in the captopril group. Data from the ISIS-4, GISSI-3, Trandolapril cardiac evaluation (TRACE), Infarction Ramipril Efficacy (AIRE), and Second Survival of Myocardial Infarction Long-term Evaluation (SMILE) trials have also shown a benefit with the use of ACE inhibitors post MI.[2,3]

Based on these studies, oral ACE inhibitor therapy should be started within the first 24 hours of an AMI, preferably after completion of thrombolytic therapy and BP stabilization (systolic BP >100 mmHg). ACE inhibitor therapy is particularly beneficial in patients with an anterior infarction and an EF <40% (even if asymptomatic) or clinical evidence of heart failure.[2,3] ACE inhibitors may be used to prevent the occurrence of heart failure symptoms or for treatment of heart failure in the AMI patient. However, unlike β-blockers, the use of IV ACE inhibition therapy is not recommended by the ACC/AHA guidelines.[2,3] Captopril could be given on postinfarct day 2 or 3, beginning with a test dose of 6.25 mg and then titrated to a maintenance dosage of 25 to 50 mg TID. BP should be monitored closely, with the systolic BP maintained above 90 mmHg. Renal function and serum potassium levels should be followed closely during the first few months of therapy. In diabetics, an ACE inhibitor may also benefit long-term renal function.[63] Once it is established that the patient can tolerate an ACE inhibitor, he or she can be switched to a longer-acting agent such as lisinopril or enalapril to simplify the regimen. (See Chapter 18 for ACE inhibitor dosing recommendations.)

If the patient cannot tolerate an ACE inhibitor due to cough, an ARB may be an alternative. In the Optimal Therapy in Myocardial Infarction with the Angiotensin II Antagonist Losartan (OPTIMAAL) Trial and Valsartan in Acute Myocardial Infarction Trial (VALIANT), losartan and valsartan demonstrated similar reductions in all-cause mortality compared to captopril, with a nonsignificant trend in favor of captopril. Dual therapy of captopril with valsartan offered no additional benefits but increased side effects.[2,3]

Aldosterone Antagonists

35. Should this patient receive an aldosterone antagonist?

Like angiotensin II, aldosterone also plays an important role in left ventricular remodeling. (See Chapter 18 for further discussion of aldosterone.) Inhibiting aldosterone directly in addition to ACE inhibitor therapy was first evaluated in the heart failure patients in the Randomized Aldactone Evaluation Study (RALES).[64] Patients who received spironolactone exhibited a 30% reduction in mortality compared to placebo ($p < 0.001$). Another aldosterone antagonist, eplerenone, is a selective inhibitor of the mineralocorticoid receptor with fewer sexual side effects.

In the Eplerenone Post Acute Myocardial Infarction Heart Failure Efficacy and Survival Study (EPHESUS), 6,600 patients with AMI and an EF <40% were allocated to optimal medical therapy with either eplerenone or placebo. After 16 months, a 15% risk reduction in mortality ($p = 0.008$), 13% reduction in sudden death ($p = 0.002$), and 21% reduction in cardiovascular death or hospitalization ($p = 0.02$) was seen in the eplerenone group compared to placebo.[64]

Based on these data, the 2004 ACC/AHA guidelines recommend an aldosterone antagonist in STEMI patients without significant renal dysfunction (creatinine <2.5 mg/dL in men and <2.0 mg/dL in women) or hyperkalemia (potassium <5 mEq/L) who are already receiving therapeutic doses of an ACE inhibitor, have an EF <40%, and have either symptomatic heart failure or diabetes.[2,3]

Because our patient does not have heart failure or diabetes, he is not a candidate for aldosterone antagonism. However, if his EF was <40%, either spironolactone or eplerenone would be an option. Serum potassium and renal function would need to be carefully checked 3 days and at 1 week after therapy initiation and every month for the first 3 months. ACE inhibitor and potassium supplement doses may need to be adjusted.[64]

β-Blockers

36. Should the previous patients receive a β-blocker upon discharge?

The 2004 ACC/AHA guidelines recommend β-blocker therapy indefinitely for all patients following an AMI.[2,3] The benefits of β-blockers in reducing reinfarction and mortality are believed to outweigh the risk, even in patients with asthma, insulin-dependent diabetes, severe peripheral vascular disease, first-degree heart block, and moderate left ventricular dysfunction. Due to his bronchospastic disease, P.H. should be carefully titrated on a β-blocker to see if he can tolerate it. Propranolol, metoprolol, and atenolol are available as generics, making any of them a cost-effective alternative. Metoprolol or carvedilol are considered first-line choices in patients with heart failure, whereas atenolol or metoprolol should be considered in patients with stable asthma or bronchospastic pulmonary disorder.

Lipid-Lowering Agents

37. Should AMI patients be started on a lipid-lowering agent? When should it be initiated?

Although the results of a complete fasting lipid panel were not made available, P.H. had elevated total cholesterol and triglycerides as part of his routine screening laboratory tests. A complete fasting lipid profile would be helpful and should be completed within 24 hours of presenting with an AMI. This is often overlooked or not done because the patient is not fasting. Most patients will require a low-cholesterol, low saturated fat diet in addition to lipid-lowering therapy. The goal for P.H. will be to reduce his LDL to <100 mg/dL, with an ideal goal of <70 mg/dL with a statin (see Chapter 12). When triglycerides are >200 mg/dL, drug therapy with niacin or a fibrate is beneficial.[2,3] Hormone replacement therapy is not beneficial for secondary prevention in postmenopausal women. If a patient is receiving hormone replacement therapy, it should be discontinued during the acute event (see Chapter 12).

The Myocardial Ischemia Reduction with Aggressive Cholesterol Lowering (MIRACL) trial, which enrolled NSTEMI patients, reported a 16% lower rate of death and nonfatal major cardiac events at 4 months follow-up in patients receiving atorvastatin 80 mg/day within 24 to 96 hours of hospitalization when compared with placebo ($p = 0.048$). The A to Z trial, showed a favorable trend toward major cardiovascular event reduction during 624 months follow-up in AMI patients receiving an intensive simvastatin regimen (40 mg/day for 1 month followed by 80 mg/day thereafter) initiated within 12 hours of stabilization when compared with those receiving a less intensive regimen (placebo for 4 months followed by simvastatin 20 mg/day).[2,3,65]

In the case of P.H., a statin should be administered during his hospitalization. Statin choice and dose should be based on current published evidence, cost, and potential drug interactions (see Chapter 12).

Antithrombotic Agents

38. Three days before P.H.'s anticipated discharge, the medical team is discussing the need to administer long-term anticoagulant therapy with warfarin in addition to antiplatelet therapy with aspirin. Is either therapy indicated for P.H. at this time?

In addition to its use in the setting of AMI, aspirin is routinely prescribed for post-MI patients. The prophylactic role of aspirin in asymptomatic patients has also been established by such trials as the Physicians' Health Study as well as in patients with chronic stable angina.[66,67]

Antiplatelet therapy should be lifelong because of its effects on secondary prevention of reinfarction. There appears to be no difference in efficacy over a wide range of aspirin doses (75–1,500 mg/day), although higher doses may increase the incidence of side effects. Much interest exists in using lower doses of aspirin for cardiovascular disease. Most clinicians use dosages of 81 to 325 mg daily or every other day.[68,69]

Long-term warfarin may be beneficial in some patients, but clinical judgment is needed to decide whether the benefit is likely to exceed the risk. Kaplan reviewed data for the development of left ventricular thrombi in AMI and found an incidence of approximately 35% in patients who suffered an anterior infarct.[70] Although anticoagulation will decrease the incidence of stroke, <3% of patients will develop a cerebrovascular accident following an AMI if not anticoagulated. The ACC/AHA guidelines recommend warfarin for post-MI patients unable to take aspirin or clopidogrel, patients with a left ventricular thrombus, and those with persistent atrial fibrillation.[2,3] There is also consensus that post-MI patients with extensive wall motion abnormalities and those with paroxysmal atrial fibrillation will benefit from anticoagulation. Data have suggested that the use of high-intensity warfarin (INR 3–4) or moderate intensity warfarin (INR 2–2.5) with low-dose aspirin (75–100 mg) may significantly reduce subsequent cardiovascular events and death post MI compared to aspirin (100–160 mg).[71]

P.H. is probably a good candidate for 1 to 3 months of warfarin therapy titrated to an INR of 2 to 3 because of his left ventricular thrombus. The use of low-dose aspirin in conjunction with warfarin will probably not increase his risk of bleeding.

39. Is clopidogrel more effective than aspirin in reducing the risk for further cardiovascular events?

In patients with STEMI and NSTEMI, clopidogrel (Plavix) may be used when aspirin is contraindicated or not tolerated; however, it is significantly more expensive than aspirin. In the Clopidogrel Versus Aspirin in Patients at Risk of Ischemic Events (CAPRIE) trial, 19,185 patients with atherosclerotic vascular disease such as ischemic stroke, MI, or peripheral arterial disease were randomized to clopidogrel 75 mg once daily or aspirin 325 mg once daily and followed for 1 to 3 years. On completion of the study, an intention-to-treat analysis demonstrated a lower risk for the combined end points of ischemic stroke, MI, or vascular death in the clopidogrel group compared to aspirin (5.32% vs. 5.83%, $p = 0.043$). A post hoc analysis of these data found a lower rate of AMI in patients receiving clopidogrel compared to aspirin (4.2% vs. 5.04%, $p = 0.008$).[2,3] (See Chapters 16 and 55 for further discussion of anticoagulants and antiplatelet drugs.) However, the 2004 ACC/AHA guidelines still recommend aspirin over clopidogrel, except when aspirin is contraindicated or if a patient is undergoing PCI with stent placement.[2,3]

40. How would you summarize the long-term therapy needed by P.H. on discharge?

Appropriate discharge medications for P.H. include a β-blocker, aspirin 81 mg/day, an ACE inhibitor, and warfarin to achieve an INR of 2 to 3. He also should receive a prescription for sublingual NTG to carry with him for use as needed. Some clinicians also might choose to continue his low-dose chronic nitrate therapy. These agents should be continued long term except for the warfarin, which should be discontinued after a few months. P.H. can be started on a statin drug to reach his LDL goal of <100 mg/dL, ideally 70 mg/dL. Routine liver function tests should be obtained prior to initiation of therapy and periodically thereafter. His previous hydrochlorothiazide may be discontinued because his hypertension will likely be controlled with the β-blocker and ACE inhibitor. His insulin should be continued, and his blood glucose monitored closely. The goal is to achieve a state of β-blockade that will allow P.H. to maintain a systolic BP of >100 mmHg; therefore, the clinician must balance the hypotensive effects of the ACE inhibitor and the β-blocker. If P.H. experiences postinfarction angina, then the addition of a calcium channel blocker such as diltiazem and/or chronic nitrate therapy would be indicated.

LIFESTYLE MODIFICATIONS

41. What types of lifestyle modifications should P.H. be encouraged to pursue to reduce his risk factors?

P.H. must be encouraged to stop smoking; this may be the most important intervention. Rosenburg et al. showed that the risk of AMI in men who quit smoking was reduced to that of nonsmokers within a few years after quitting[72] (see Chapter 85). Weight management, diabetic treatment, and serum lipid control are also important risk factors to address. (See Chapters 13 and 50 for further information on lipid-lowering drugs and diet therapy.)

SUMMARY

The use of thrombolytics and PCI has significantly improved the survival of patients with STEMI. Despite the overwhelming results favoring thrombolytic therapy in all subgroups, it is believed that these agents remain underused in patients with STEMI. The major risk associated with thrombolysis is bleeding, especially within the central nervous system. Another problem associated with thrombolytic therapy is reocclusion of the artery that was initially opened. Coronary angioplasty is more effective than thrombolytic therapy; however, it is available only in hospitals with experienced invasive cardiologists, thereby limiting its availability to many patients.

Aspirin should be given to all patients with AMI; unless there is a contraindication, β-blockers and statins should be administered as well. Clopidogrel is often used in conjunction with aspirin, especially in patients receiving stents. ACE inhibitors and aldosterone antagonists have been shown to be beneficial in patients who have left ventricular dysfunction (EF <40%) and are also recommended for secondary prevention. Nitrates are also useful, but care must be taken to maintain an adequate perfusion pressure. Secondary prevention emphasizing a healthy lifestyle and aggressive lipid lowering are important components to the overall treatment plan.

REFERENCES

1. DeWood MA et al. Prevalence of total coronary occlusion during the early hours of transmural myocardial infarction. *N Engl J Med* 1980;303:897.
2. Antman EM et al. ACC/AHA guidelines for the management of patients with ST-elevation myocardial infarction—executive summary. A report of the American College of Cardiology/American Heart Association Task Force on Practice Guidelines (Writing Committee to Revise the 1999 Guidelines for the Management of Patients With Acute Myocardial Infarction). *J Am Coll Cardiol* 2004;44:671.
3. Braunwald E et al. ACC/AHA guideline update for the management of patients with unstable angina and non-ST-segment elevation myocardial infarction—2002: summary article: a report of the American College of Cardiology/American Heart Association Task Force on Practice Guidelines (Committee on the Management of Patients With Unstable Angina). *Circulation* 2002;106:1893.
4. Rosamond W et al. Heart disease and stroke statistics—2007 update: a report from the American Heart Association Statistics Committee and Stroke Statistics Subcommittee. *Circulation* 2007;115:e69.
5. Bradley EH et al. Hospital quality for acute myocardial infarction: correlation among process measures and relationship with short-term mortality. *JAMA* 2006;296:72.
6. Alexander KP et al. Evolution in cardiovascular care for elderly patients with non-ST-segment elevation acute coronary syndromes: results from the CRUSADE National Quality Improvement Initiative. *J Am Coll Cardiol* 2005;46:1479.
7. Skinner J et al. Mortality after acute myocardial infarction in hospitals that disproportionately treat black patients. *Circulation* 2005;112:2634.
8. Vaccarino V et al. Sex and racial differences in the management of acute myocardial infarction, 1994 through 2002. *N Engl J Med* 2005;353:671.
9. Libby P. Atherosclerosis: disease biology affecting the coronary vasculature. *Am J Cardiol* 2006;98:3Q.
10. Gomez JF et al. Prognostic value of location and type of myocardial infarction in the setting of advanced left ventricular dysfunction. *Am J Cardiol* 2007;99:642.
11. Arslanian-Engoren C et al. Symptoms of men and women presenting with acute coronary syndromes. *Am J Cardiol* 2006;98:1177.
12. Zimetbaum PJ, Josephson ME. Use of the electrocardiogram in acute myocardial infarction. *N Engl J Med* 2003;348:933.
13. Dahdal WY. The heart and myocardial infarction. In: Lee M, ed. *Basic Skills in Interpreting Laboratory Data*. 3rd ed. Bethesda, MD: American Society of Health System Pharmacists; 2004:297.
14. Solomon SD et al. Sudden death in patients with myocardial infarction and left ventricular dysfunction, heart failure, or both. *N Engl J Med* 2005;352:2581.
15. Tiyyagura SR, Pinney SP. Left ventricular remodeling after myocardial infarction: past, present, and future. *Mt Sinai J Med* 2006;73:840.
16. Smalling RW. Role of fibrinolytic therapy in the current era of ST-segment elevation myocardial infarction management. *Am Heart J* 2006;151:S17.
17. Turcasso NM, Nappi JM. Tenecteplase for treatment of acute myocardial infarction. *Ann Pharmacother* 2001;35:1233.
18. Sinnaeve PR et al. Direct thrombin inhibitors in acute coronary syndromes: effect in patients undergoing early percutaneous coronary intervention. *Eur Heart J* 2005;26:2396.
19. Ray KK, Cannon CP. The potential relevance of the multiple lipid-independent (pleiotropic) effects of statins in the management of acute coronary syndromes. *J Am Coll Cardiol* 2005;46:1425.
20. Hulten E et al. The effect of early, intensive statin therapy on acute coronary syndrome: a meta-analysis of randomized controlled trials. *Arch Intern Med* 2006;166:1814.
21. Ray KK et al. Beyond lipid lowering: what have we learned about the benefits of statins from the acute coronary syndromes trials? *Am J Cardiol* 2006;98:18P.
22. Keeley EC, Hillis LD. Primary PCI for myocardial infarction with ST-segment elevation. *N Engl J Med* 2007;356:47.

23. Smith SC, Jr. et al. ACC/AHA/SCAI 2005 guideline update for percutaneous coronary intervention—summary article: a report of the American College of Cardiology/American Heart Association Task Force on Practice Guidelines (ACC/AHA/SCAI Writing Committee to Update the 2001 Guidelines for Percutaneous Coronary Intervention). *J Am Coll Cardiol* 2006;47:216.
24. Killip T, III, Kimball JT. Treatment of myocardial infarction in a coronary care unit. A two year experience with 250 patients. *Am J Cardiol* 1967;20:457.
25. Rott D et al. Usefulness of the Killip classification for early risk stratification of patients with acute myocardial infarction in the 1990s compared with those treated in the 1980s. Israeli Thrombolytic Survey Group and the Secondary Prevention Reinfarction Israeli Nifedipine Trial (SPRINT) Study Group. *Am J Cardiol* 1997;80:859.
26. Antman EM et al. The TIMI risk score for unstable angina/non-ST elevation MI: a method for prognostication and therapeutic decision making. *JAMA* 2000;284:835.
27. Morrow DA et al. Application of the TIMI risk score for ST-elevation MI in the National Registry of Myocardial Infarction 3. *JAMA* 2001;286:1356.
28. Primary versus tenecteplase-facilitated percutaneous coronary intervention in patients with ST-segment elevation acute myocardial infarction (ASSENT-4 PCI): randomised trial. *Lancet* 2006;367:569.
29. Sabatine MS et al. Addition of clopidogrel to aspirin and fibrinolytic therapy for myocardial infarction with ST-segment elevation. *N Engl J Med* 2005;352:1179.
30. Sabatine MS et al. Effect of clopidogrel pretreatment before percutaneous coronary intervention in patients with ST-elevation myocardial infarction treated with fibrinolytics: the PCI-CLARITY study. *JAMA* 2005;294:1224.
31. Chen ZM et al. Addition of clopidogrel to aspirin in 45,852 patients with acute myocardial infarction: randomised placebo-controlled trial. *Lancet* 2005;366:1607.
32. Antman EM et al. Enoxaparin versus unfractionated heparin with fibrinolysis for ST-elevation myocardial infarction. *N Engl J Med* 2006;354:1477.
33. Antman EM et al. Combination reperfusion therapy with abciximab and reduced dose reteplase: results from TIMI 14. The Thrombolysis in Myocardial Infarction (TIMI) 14 investigators. *Eur Heart J* 2000;21:1944.
34. Yusuf S et al. Effects of fondaparinux on mortality and reinfarction in patients with acute ST-segment elevation myocardial infarction: the OASIS-6 randomized trial. *JAMA* 2006;295:1519.
35. De Luca G et al. Abciximab as adjunctive therapy to reperfusion in acute ST-segment elevation myocardial infarction: a meta-analysis of randomized trials. *JAMA* 2005;293:1759.
36. Mehta RH et al. Reperfusion strategies for acute myocardial infarction in the elderly: benefits and risks. *J Am Coll Cardiol* 2005;45:471.
37. Elliott JM et al. Neutralizing antibodies to streptokinase four years after intravenous thrombolytic therapy. *Am J Cardiol* 1993;71:640.
38. Mendoza CE et al. Management of failed thrombolysis after acute myocardial infarction: an overview of current treatment options. *Int J Cardiol* 2007;114:291.
39. Wijeysundera HC et al. Rescue angioplasty or repeat fibrinolysis after failed fibrinolytic therapy for ST-segment myocardial infarction: a meta-analysis of randomized trials. *J Am Coll Cardiol* 2007;49:422.
40. La Manna A et al. Which strategy should be used for acute ST-elevation myocardial infarction in patients aged more than 75 years? *J Cardiovasc Med (Hagerstown)* 2006;7:388.
41. Van de Graaff E et al. Early coronary revascularization diminishes the risk of ischemic stroke with acute myocardial infarction. *Stroke* 2006;37:2546.
42. Wyman MG et al. Prevention of primary ventricular fibrillation in acute myocardial infarction with prophylactic lidocaine. *Am J Cardiol* 2004;94:545.
43. Yadav AV, Zipes DP. Prophylactic lidocaine in acute myocardial infarction: resurface or reburial? *Am J Cardiol* 2004;94:606.
44. Routledge PA et al. Increased alpha-1-acid glycoprotein and lidocaine disposition in myocardial infarction. *Ann Intern Med* 1980;93:701.
45. Chen ZM et al. Early intravenous then oral metoprolol in 45,852 patients with acute myocardial infarction: randomised placebo-controlled trial. *Lancet* 2005;366:1622.
46. Gottlieb SS et al. Effect of beta-blockade on mortality among high-risk and low-risk patients after myocardial infarction. *N Engl J Med* 1998;339:489.
47. Bakris GL et al. Metabolic effects of carvedilol vs metoprolol in patients with type 2 diabetes mellitus and hypertension: a randomized controlled trial. *JAMA* 2004;292:2227.
48. Gibbons RJ et al. ACC/AHA 2002 guideline update for the management of patients with chronic stable angina—summary article: a report of the American College of Cardiology/American Heart Association Task Force on Practice Guidelines (Committee on the Management of Patients With Chronic Stable Angina). *J Am Coll Cardiol* 2003;41:159.
49. Conti CR. The stunned and hibernating myocardium: a brief review. *Clin Cardiol* 1991;14:708.
50. Nicolini FA et al. Concurrent nitroglycerin therapy impairs tissue-type plasminogen activator-induced thrombolysis in patients with acute myocardial infarction. *Am J Cardiol* 1994;74:662.
51. Romeo F et al. Concurrent nitroglycerin administration reduces the efficacy of recombinant tissue-type plasminogen activator in patients with acute anterior wall myocardial infarction. *Am Heart J* 1995;130:692.
52. Ferguson JJ et al. Significance of nitroglycerin-induced hypotension with inferior wall acute myocardial infarction. *Am J Cardiol* 1989;64:311.
53. Chiariello M et al. Comparison between the effects of nitroprusside and nitroglycerin on ischemic injury during acute myocardial infarction. *Circulation* 1976;54:766.
54. Mann T et al. Effect of nitroprusside on regional myocardial blood flow in coronary artery disease. Results in 25 patients and comparison with nitroglycerin. *Circulation* 1978;57:732.
55. Huikuri HV et al. Sudden death due to cardiac arrhythmias. *N Engl J Med* 2001;345:1473.
56. Heidenreich PA et al. Overview of randomized trials of antiarrhythmic drugs and devices for the prevention of sudden cardiac death. *Am Heart J* 2002;144:422.
57. Ferguson JJ et al. Enoxaparin vs unfractionated heparin in high-risk patients with non-ST-segment elevation acute coronary syndromes managed with an intended early invasive strategy: primary results of the SYNERGY randomized trial. *JAMA* 2004;292:45.
58. Yusuf S et al. Comparison of fondaparinux and enoxaparin in acute coronary syndromes. *N Engl J Med* 2006;354:1464.
59. Wong GC et al. Use of low-molecular-weight heparins in the management of acute coronary artery syndromes and percutaneous coronary intervention. *JAMA* 2003;289:331.
60. Stone GW et al. Bivalirudin for patients with acute coronary syndromes. *N Engl J Med* 2006;355:2203.
61. Levine GN et al. Newer pharmacotherapy in patients undergoing percutaneous coronary interventions: a guide for pharmacists and other health care professionals. *Pharmacotherapy* 2006;26:1537.
62. Zimarino M, De Caterina R. Glycoprotein IIb-IIIa antagonists in non-ST elevation acute coronary syndromes and percutaneous interventions: from pharmacology to individual patient's therapy: part 1: the evidence of benefit. *J Cardiovasc Pharmacol* 2004;43:325.
63. Lewis EJ et al. The effect of angiotensin-converting-enzyme inhibition on diabetic nephropathy. The Collaborative Study Group. *N Engl J Med* 1993;329:1456.
64. Hunt SA et al. ACC/AHA 2005 guideline update for the diagnosis and management of chronic heart failure in the adult: a report of the American College of Cardiology/American Heart Association Task Force on Practice Guidelines (Writing Committee to Update the 2001 Guidelines for the Evaluation and Management of Heart Failure): developed in collaboration with the American College of Chest Physicians and the International Society for Heart and Lung Transplantation: endorsed by the Heart Rhythm Society. *Circulation* 2005;112:e154.
65. de Lemos JA et al. Early intensive vs a delayed conservative simvastatin strategy in patients with acute coronary syndromes: phase Z of the A to Z trial. *JAMA* 2004;292:1307.
66. Final report on the aspirin component of the ongoing Physicians' Health Study. Steering Committee of the Physicians' Health Study Research Group. *N Engl J Med* 1989;321:129.
67. Ridker PM et al. Low-dose aspirin therapy for chronic stable angina. A randomized, placebo-controlled clinical trial. *Ann Intern Med* 1991;114:835.
68. Harrington RA et al. Antithrombotic therapy for coronary artery disease: the seventh ACCP conference on antithrombotic and thrombolytic therapy. *Chest* 2004;126:513S.
69. Menon V et al. Thrombolysis and adjunctive therapy in acute myocardial infarction: the seventh ACCP conference on antithrombotic and thrombolytic therapy. *Chest* 2004;126:549S.
70. Kaplan K. Prophylactic anticoagulation following acute myocardial infarction. *Arch Intern Med* 1986;146:593.
71. Andreotti F et al. Aspirin plus warfarin compared to aspirin alone after acute coronary syndromes: an updated and comprehensive meta-analysis of 25,307 patients. *Eur Heart J* 2006;27:519.
72. Rosenberg L et al. The risk of myocardial infarction after quitting smoking in men under 55 years of age. *N Engl J Med* 1985;313:1511.

CHAPTER 18

Heart Failure

Harleen Singh, and Joel C. Marrs

INTRODUCTION

The descriptive terminology, diagnostic techniques, and treatment of heart failure (HF) have undergone significant change in the past 15 to 20 years. Since 1994, a series of consensus and evidence-based practice guidelines have been published in an effort to standardize HF management. The first was from an expert panel appointed by the Agency for Health Care Policy and Research (AHCPR) and the RAND Corporation.[1] At about the same time, the American College of Cardiology (ACC)/American Heart Association (AHA) Task Force on Practice Guidelines published their initial recommendations.[2] The recommendations from both groups were remarkably similar and included three key principles: differentiation of HF into systolic and diastolic dysfunction, recommendation of ejection fraction measurement to determine type of HF, and establishing angiotensin-converting enzyme (ACE) inhibitors as the gold standard for the treatment of HF. The Heart Failure Society of America (HFSA) Guidelines were first released in 1999,[3] and updated in 2006.[4] The European Society of Cardiology (ESC) published updated guidelines in 2005.[5] Important additions from these later guidelines include recommendation of β-adrenergic blockers for all patients with New York Heart Association (NYHA) class II and III HF and use of low-dose spironolactone (Aldactone) in class IV HF. The ACC/AHA guidelines were updated in 2001 and revised again in 2005.[6,7] These revised guidelines continue to adhere to the four disease stages of HF first assigned by the ACC/AHA 2001 guidelines. The guidelines also incorporate the latest clinical trials and continue to emphasize the role of neurohumoral drug therapy. Furthermore, the updated guidelines recognize the large growing geriatric population and end-of-life issues and how these will impact the management of advanced HF. It is highly recommended that practitioners look at least annually for the most recently published guidelines to be aware of the rapidly evolving treatment strategies for HF.

Epidemiology of Heart Failure

Heart failure "is a complex clinical syndrome that can result from any structural or functional cardiac disorder that impairs the ability of the ventricle to fill with or eject blood."[6] As a consequence the heart fails to pump sufficient blood to meet the body's metabolic needs. "The cardinal manifestations of HF are dyspnea (breathlessness) and fatigue, which can limit exercise tolerance; and fluid retention, which can lead to pulmonary congestion and peripheral edema."[6] Congestive heart failure (CHF) is a specific subset of HF characterized by left ventricular systolic dysfunction and volume excess presenting as an enlarged, blood-congested heart. Because of wide variability in the causes and clinical presentation of HF, it is recommended that the term congestive heart failure be abandoned.

It is estimated that 5 million people in the United States (1.5% to 2% of the population) have HF.[7,8] The prevalence continues to increase, with 550,000 new cases diagnosed each year. A recent analysis by an Olmstead county (Minnesota) epidemiologic group showed that, although the prevalence of systolic HF did not change significantly, the recognition of diastolic HF has increased.[9] HF incidence approaches 10 per 1,000 population after age 65 and is the most common cause of hospitalizations in the elderly population in the United States. In 2004, approximately 1 million people were hospitalized for HF. Direct and indirect health care costs of HF in 2007 are estimated to be $33.2 billion. HF is the number one discharge diagnosis in the Medicare population (70,000 hospitalized for HF). In the last 10 years the reported HF visits rose to 3.4 million. In the year 2001, Medicare expended $5,912 per discharge for Medicare beneficiaries with HF.[8] More aggressive treatment of hypertension may have contributed to the lower incidence of HF in some populations, whereas improved survival after myocardial infarction (MI) may leave others at greater risk of developing post-infarction HF. As the size of the geriatric population increases, HF likely will become a more frequently encountered clinical entity.

Quality of life is adversely affected by progressive functional disability. Of greater consequence is the high mortality rate. Of men and women under age 65 who have HF, 80% and 70%, respectively, will die with in 8 years.[8] Despite earlier diagnosis and aggressive medical management, the prognosis is poor.

Etiology

Low-Output Versus High-Output Failure

Traditionally, HF has been described as being either *low-output* or *high-output failure,* with a predominance (>90%) of cases being low-output failure (Table 18-1). In both types, the heart cannot provide adequate blood flow (tissue perfusion) to meet the body's metabolic demands, especially during exercise. The hallmark of classic low-output HF is a diminished volume of blood being pumped by a weakened heart in patients who have otherwise normal metabolic needs.

In high-output failure, the heart itself is healthy and pumps a normal or even higher than normal volume of blood. Because of high metabolic demands caused by other underlying medical disorders (e.g., hyperthyroidism, anemia), the heart becomes exhausted from the increased workload and eventually cannot

Table 18-1 Classification and Etiology of Left Ventricular Dysfunction

Type of Failure	*Characteristics*	*Contributing Factors*	*Etiology*
Low output, systolic dysfunction (dilated cardiomyopathy)[a] (60%–70% of cases)	Hypofunctioning left ventricle; enlarged heart (dilated left ventricle); ↑left ventricular end-diastolic volume; EF <40%; ↓stroke volume; ↓CO; S_3 heart sound present	1. ↑Contractility (cardiomyopathy) 2. ↓Afterload (elevated SVR)	1. Coronary ischemia,[b] MI, mitral valve stenosis or regurgitation, alcoholism, viral syndromes, nutritional deficiency, calcium and potassium depletion, drug induced, idiopathic 2. Hypertension, aortic stenosis, volume overload
Low output, diastolic dysfunction (30%–40% of cases)	Normal left ventricular contractility; normal size heart; stiff left ventricle; impaired left ventricular relaxation; impaired left ventricular filling; ↓left ventricular end-diastolic volume; normal EF; ↓SV; ↓CO; exaggerated S_4 heart sound	1. Thickened left ventricle (hypertrophic cardiomyopathy) 2. Stiff left ventricle (restrictive cardiomyopathy) 3. ↑Preload	1. Coronary ischemia,[b] MI hypertension, aortic stenosis and regurgitation, pericarditis, enlarged left ventricular septum (hypertrophic cardiomyopathy) 2. Amyloidosis, sarcoidosis 3. Sodium and water retention
High-output failure (uncommon)	Normal or ↑contractility; normal size heart; normal left ventricular end-diastolic volume; normal or ↑EF; normal or increased stroke volume; ↑CO	↑Metabolic and oxygen demands	Anemia and hyperthyroidism

[a] Same as congestive heart failure if symptoms also present.
[b] Heart failure caused by coronary artery ischemia or myocardial infarction classified as "ischemic" etiology. All other types combined as "nonischemic."
CO, cardiac output; EF, ejection fraction; K, potassium; MI, myocardial infarction; SV, stroke volume; SVR, systemic vascular resistance.

keep up with demand. The primary treatment of high-output HF is amelioration of the underlying disease. The remainder of this chapter focuses on the treatment of low-output HF.

Left Versus Right Ventricular Dysfunction

Simple classification of HF as being low-output failure does not adequately describe the complex nature of this disorder. Consequently, low-output HF is further divided into left and right ventricular dysfunction, or a combination of the two (biventricular failure). Because the left ventricle is the major pumping chamber of the heart, it is not surprising that *left ventricular dysfunction* is the most common form of low-output HF and the major target for pharmacologic intervention. Right ventricular dysfunction may coexist with left ventricular HF if damage is sustained by both sides of the heart (e.g., after MI) or as a delayed complication of progressive left-sided HF (see Question 1).

Isolated right-sided ventricular dysfunction, which is relatively uncommon, is usually caused by either primary or secondary *pulmonary arterial hypertension* (PAH). In these conditions, elevated pulmonary artery pressure impedes emptying of the right ventricle, thus increasing the workload on the right side of the heart.[10,11] Primary PAH is idiopathic, caused by stenosis or spasm of the pulmonary artery of unknown etiology. Secondary causes include collagen vascular disorders, sarcoidosis, fibrosis, exposure to high altitude, drug and chemical exposure, and cor pulmonale. Drug-induced sources include opioid overdoses (especially heroin), 5 hydoxytryptamine 2B (5HT-2B) agonists (e.g., dexfenfluramine, fenfluramine, and pergolide), and pulmonary fibrosis caused by intravenous (IV) injection of poorly soluble forms of methylphenidate (e.g., IV drug users injecting partially dissolved Ritalin tablets). Cor pulmonale is defined as pulmonary hypertension, and secondary right-sided failure as a complication of chronic obstructive pulmonary disease (COPD).

Systolic Versus Diastolic Dysfunction; Ischemic Versus Nonischemic Heart Failure

Left ventricular dysfunction is further subdivided into systolic and diastolic dysfunction, with mixed disorders also being encountered (Table 18-1). In both forms, the *stroke volume* (SV) (i.e., the volume of blood ejected by the heart with each systolic contraction; normal, 60–130 mL) and the subsequent 1-minute *cardiac output* (CO) (i.e., SV × heart rate; normal, 4 to 7 L/minute) are reduced. In diagnosing HF, a critical marker differentiating systolic from diastolic dysfunction is the *left ventricular ejection fraction* (LVEF), defined as the percentage of left ventricular end-diastolic volume expelled during each systolic contraction (normal, 60%–70%).

In *systolic dysfunction,* the LVEF is <40%, dropping to <20% in advanced HF. Thus, systolic dysfunction is synonymous with low ejection fraction (EF) heart failure and is almost always caused by factors causing the heart to fail as a pump (decreased myocardial muscle contractility). The heart dilates as it becomes congested with retained blood, leading to an enlarged hypokinetic left ventricle.

Heart failure caused by damage to heart muscle or valves because of chronic coronary ischemia or after MI is classified as *ischemic,* with all other types grouped as *nonischemic*. Coronary artery disease is the cause of HF in approximately two thirds of patients with left ventricular systolic dysfunction. Other causes of left ventricular pump failure include persistent arrhythmias, post-streptococcal rheumatic heart disease, chronic alcoholism (alcoholic cardiomyopathy), viral infections, or unidentified etiology (idiopathic dilated cardiomyopathy). Chronic hypertension, and certain cardiac valvular disorders (aortic or mitral stenosis), also precipitate systolic HF by increasing resistance to CO (i.e., a high afterload state).

In contrast, left ventricular diastolic dysfunction refers to impaired relaxation and increased stiffness of the left ventricle; ejection fraction may or may not be abnormal and the patient may or may not be symptomatic. The terms *diastolic dysfunction* and *diastolic heart failure* are not synonymous. Diastolic dysfunction is one diagnostic criterion for diastolic heart failure. Diastolic HF is defined as "a clinical syndrome of HF characterized by a normal ejection fraction and abnormal diastolic function."[12–16] In this form of HF, cardiac muscle function (contractility) is *not* impaired and, most importantly, the EF remains $\geq$45%. The SV and CO, however, are still reduced because the end-diastolic ventricular volume is less than normal. In simple terms, a high fraction of a low volume is ejected. Possible causes for diastolic failure include coronary ischemia, long-standing uncontrolled hypertension, left ventricular wall scarring after an MI, ventricular wall hypertrophy, hypertrophic cardiomyopathy (formerly known as idiopathic hypertrophic subaortic stenosis), constrictive pericarditis, restrictive cardiomyopathy (e.g., amyloidosis and sarcoidosis), and valvular heart disease (mitral stenosis, acute aortic regurgitation, mitral regurgitation). These factors lead to left ventricular stiffness (reduced wall compliance), an inability of the ventricle to relax during diastole, or both, which result in an elevated resting pressure within the ventricle despite a relatively low volume of blood in the chamber. In turn, the elevated pressure impedes left ventricular filling during diastole that would normally occur by passive inflow against a low resistance pressure gradient. Heart size is usually (but not always) normal. To summarize, in diastolic dysfunction regardless of the EF, the SV and CO are deficient because of impaired ventricular filling and a relatively small left ventricular volume. It is estimated that 20% to 60% of patients with HF may have normal LVEF and reduced ventricle compliance.[1,7,12–16] Because coronary ischemia, MI, and hypertension are contributors to both systolic and diastolic failure, many patients have symptoms of a combined disorder.

The pathology of systolic dysfunction most closely resembles what has historically been referred to as "congestive heart failure"; nevertheless, in the strictest sense, CHF only exists if the patient has both systolic dysfunction and the classic symptoms of HF. Tremendous variability exists in the clinical presentation of both systolic and diastolic dysfunction, however, and both disorders can have essentially identical symptoms.[6,12] For example, some patients with either systolic or diastolic dysfunction exhibit exercise intolerance, but have little evidence of fluid retention. Others may have significant edema with few complaints of exercise intolerance or shortness of breath. It is also possible to have no symptoms in the early stages of both forms of HF. For all these reasons, it is best to avoid the abbreviation *CHF*, especially because CHF has also been used to denote *chronic heart failure*. In the meantime, clinicians are strongly encouraged to obtain an EF measurement in all patients with suspected HF to help define the clinical state more fully.[1–6]

Some drugs used to treat systolic dysfunction, such as digoxin, can worsen symptoms in diastolic dysfunction. Conversely, negative inotropes (β-adrenergic blockers and calcium channel blockers) may be beneficial in diastolic dysfunction by slowing the heart and allowing the ventricles to fill more fully at low pressures.

Cardiac Workload

A common factor to all forms of HF is increased cardiac workload. Four major determinants contribute to left ventricular workload: preload, afterload, contractility, and heart rate (HR).

PRELOAD

Preload describes forces acting on the *venous* side of the circulation to affect myocardial wall tension. The relationship is as follows: as venous return (i.e., blood flowing into the heart) increases, the volume of blood in the left ventricle increases. The volume is maximal when filling finishes at the end of diastole (left ventricular end-diastolic volume). This increased volume raises the pressure within the ventricle (left ventricular end-diastolic pressure), which in turn increases the "stretch," or wall tension, of the ventricle. Peripheral venous dilation and decreased peripheral venous volume diminish preload, whereas peripheral venous constriction and increased peripheral venous volume increase preload.

Elevated preload can aggravate HF. For example, rapid administration of blood plasma expanders and osmotic diuretics or administration of large amounts of sodium (Na) or sodium-retaining agents can increase preload. A malfunctioning aortic valve (aortic stenosis, aortic insufficiency), resulting in regurgitation of blood back into the left ventricle, also can increase the volume of blood that must be pumped. A malfunctioning mitral valve (mitral regurgitation) can cause retrograde ejection of blood from the left ventricle back into the left atrium, with a resultant decrease in EF. In patients with systolic failure, ventricular blood is ejected less efficiently because of a hypofunctioning left ventricle; the volume of blood retained in the ventricle is thus increased, and preload becomes elevated. In diastolic failure with a stiffened left ventricle, relatively small increases in end-diastolic volume from sodium and water overload can lead to exaggerated increases in end-diastolic pressure, despite normal or even reduced end-diastolic volumes.

AFTERLOAD

Afterload is the tension developed in the ventricular wall as contraction (systole) occurs. The tension developed during contraction is affected by intraventricular pressure, ventricular diameter, and wall thickness. More simply, afterload is regulated by the systemic vascular resistance (SVR) or impedance against which the ventricle must pump during its ejection and it is chiefly determined by arterial blood pressure (BP). Hypertension, atherosclerotic disease, or a narrowed aortic valve opening increases arterial impedance (afterload), thereby increasing the workload on the heart. Hypertension is a major etiologic factor in the development of both systolic and diastolic HF. The Framingham group found that 75% of patients who developed HF had a history of hypertension.[17,18] The risk of developing HF was six times greater for hypertensive than for normotensive patients.

CARDIAC CONTRACTILITY

The terms *contractility* and *inotropic state* are used synonymously to describe the myocardium's (cardiac muscle's) inherent ability to develop force and shorten its fibers independent of preload or afterload. Myocardial contractility is decreased when myocardial fibers are diminished or poorly functioning as may occur in patients with primary cardiomyopathy, valvular heart disease, coronary artery disease, or following an MI. Defects in contractility play a major role in systolic HF, but are not a component of pure diastolic dysfunction. Occasionally, drugs, such as nonselective β-adrenergic blockers or doxorubicin (Adriamycin), induce HF by decreasing myocardial contractility. (See Questions 4 and 5 for a more complete discussion of drug-induced HF.) As summarized in Table 18-1, the major contributors to systolic failure are decreased contractility and increased afterload, whereas structural abnormalities and increased preload play a greater role in diastolic failure.

HEART RATE

An increased heart rate is a reflex mechanism to improve CO as EF declines. As discussed below, the sympathetic nervous system is the major mediator of this response. The workload and energy demands of a rapid heart rate ultimately place undo strain on the heart, however, and can eventually worsen HF.

Pathogenesis

When the heart begins to fail, the body activates several complex compensatory mechanisms in an attempt to maintain CO and oxygenation of vital organs. These include increased sympathetic tone, activation of the renin-angiotensin-aldosterone system (RAAS), sodium and water retention, other neurohormonal adaptations, and cardiac "remodeling" (ventricular dilation, cardiac hypertrophy, and changes in left ventricular lumen shape). The long-term consequences of these adaptive mechanisms can create more harm than good, however (Fig. 18-1). The relative balance of each of these adaptive processes can vary depending on the type of HF (systolic versus diastolic dysfunction) and even from patient to patient with the same type of disorder. An understanding of the potential benefits and adverse consequences of these compensatory mechanisms is essential to understanding the signs, symptoms, and treatment of HF.[19]

Sympathetic (Adrenergic) Nervous System

Stroke volume, CO, or both are low in both systolic and diastolic left ventricular dysfunction, resulting in decreased tissue perfusion. The body's normal physiologic response to a decreased CO is generalized activation of the adrenergic (sympathetic) nervous system as evidenced by increased circulating levels of norepinephrine (NE) and other catecholamines. The inotropic (increased contractility) and chronotropic (increased HR) effects of NE initially maintain near-normal CO and preserve perfusion of vital organs such as the central nervous system (CNS) and myocardium. Catecholamine-mediated vasoconstriction in the skin, gastrointestinal (GI) tract, and renal circulation, however, decreases perfusion of these organs and ultimately increases the workload on the heart by increasing SVR. Other adverse consequences of NE activation include impaired sodium excretion by the kidneys, restricted ability of coronary arteries to supply blood to the ventricular wall (myocardial ischemia), increased automaticity of cardiac tissue to provoke arrhythmias, hypokalemia, and oxidative stress to trigger programmed cell death (apoptosis).[6]

In the long term, high levels of NE or its metabolites are potentially harmful to heart muscle because they decrease β_1-receptor sensitivity and reduce β_1-receptor density on the surface of myocardial cells by as much as 60% to 70% in severe HF.[20–25] The normal ratio of β_1:β_2 receptors in the heart is 75 to 80:20 to 25. As a negative feedback response to overstimulation, this balance is shifted to a ratio of 60 to 70:30 to 40 in the failing myocardium by downregulation of β_1 subtype receptors. This selective downregulation of β_1-receptors is accompanied by a complex phenomenon of "uncoupling of the

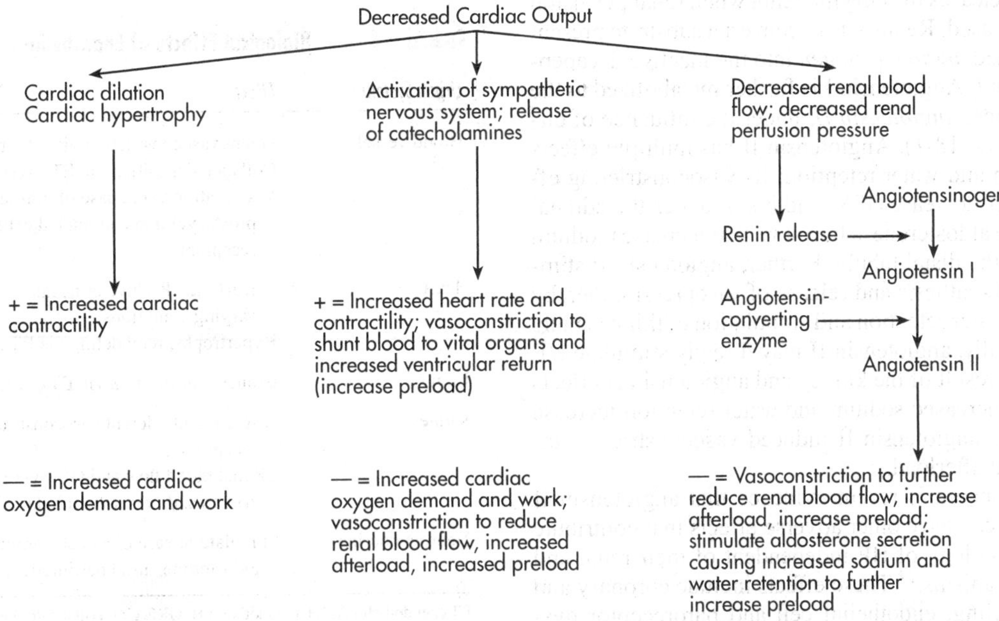

FIGURE 18-1 Adaptive mechanisms in systolic heart failure (HF). +, beneficial results; –, negative (detrimental) effects.

β_1- and β_2-receptor activity," whereby the number of β_2-receptors are unchanged and the responsiveness of these receptors in eliciting a response can be reduced by 30%.[20] Over time this leaves the myocyte less responsive to adrenergic stimuli and further decreases contractile function. At the same time, the postsynaptic β_1 subtype is upregulated in the failing heart resulting in cell growth (hypertrophy) and a positive inotropic effect. β_2 receptors on the presynaptic side of the sympathetic nerve act to suppress NE release, providing a partial protective mechanism from adrenergic overstimulation.

Alterations in sympathetic adrenergic receptors in the heart during HF are complex and partially determined by genetic phenotype. Interestingly, among black patients with HF is seen a disproportionately high incidence of polymorphisms for variants of the β_1-receptor that are associated with increased function. Additionally, a variant of the β_2-receptor with defective response to adrenergic overstimulation is also seen. These combined defects are found less often in whites, perhaps partially explaining a higher incidence of HF in blacks. A better understanding of α and β receptor phenotyping may someday lead to improved prevention and treatment strategies for HF.[26]

Renal Function and the Renin-Angiotensin System

The combined actions of the decreased CO and vasoconstriction secondary to sympathetic tone in HF causes decreased renal blood flow (RBF). This, in turn, sets off a complex chain of events leading to sodium and water retention and, eventually, increased blood volume. Renal vascular resistance is increased and the glomerular filtration rate (GFR) is decreased. As the GFR decreases, more sodium is reabsorbed in the proximal tubule. Additionally, the glomerular filtrate may be preferentially shunted to nephrons with long loops of Henle, increasing the surface area for sodium reabsorption. A diminished effective circulating plasma volume and angiotensin II also stimulate release of antidiuretic hormone (ADH) from the pituitary, resulting in the retention of free water in the renal collecting ducts.

The kidney releases the enzyme renin when renal perfusion pressure is decreased. Renin acts to convert a substrate present in the blood called *angiotensinogen* into the inactive decapeptide, *angiotensin I.* Angiotensin I is further metabolized to the active decapeptide, *angiotensin II,* under the influence of circulating *ACE* (Fig. 18-1). Angiotensin II has multiple effects favoring sodium and water retention: Its vasoconstricting effects may further decrease GFR, and it stimulates the adrenal glands to secrete aldosterone, a hormone that increases sodium reabsorption in the distal tubule. Further, angiotensin II stimulates increased synthesis and release of vasopressin, thereby increasing free water retention and stimulation of thirst centers in the CNS. Finally, angiotensin II may directly stimulate NE release. The net result of the kidney and angiotensin II effects is detrimental. Increased sodium and water retention increase preload, whereas angiotensin II-induced vasoconstriction increases SVR and afterload.

Of further concern is recent evidence that angiotensin II and aldosterone can have other adverse effects that contribute to the pathophysiology of HF independent of their renal and electrolyte mechanisms.[27] These effects include coronary and vascular remodeling, endothelial cell and baroreceptor dysfunction, and inhibition of myocardial NE uptake. Morphologic studies indicate that a chronic excess of aldosterone (plus salt loading), as occurs in HF, can cause fibrosis in the atria and ventricles, kidneys, and other organs in animals and humans.[27] Thus, aldosterone may promote the remodeling of organs and fibrosis, independent of angiotensin II.

Other Hormonal Mediators

ENDOTHELINS

Several other regulatory hormones and cytokines have been identified as playing a role in the pathogenesis and adaptation to HF. The first of these are the endothelins, a family of 21 amino acid peptides.[28,29] Within this family, endothelin-1 (ET-1) is the most active. ET-1 was first isolated from vascular endothelial cells, but it is also synthesized by vascular and airway smooth muscle, cardiomyocytes, leukocytes, and macrophages. Serum concentrations of ET-1 are elevated in HF, pulmonary hypertension, MI, ischemia, and shock and are implicated in causing vasoconstriction, potentiation of cardiac remodeling, and decreased renal blood flow and glomerular filtration. Although these effects of ET-1 are detrimental in HF, its pharmacology is complex and dependent on the relative balance of two distinct G protein-coupled receptor subtypes referred to as ET_A and ET_B. As illustrated in Table 18-2, ET-1 can elicit opposing effects from each receptor, with the net effect being dependent on the relative density of the two receptors.

Synthesis of ET-I begins with a precursor protein called pre-proendothelin (PPET-1) and involves several enzymatic steps and intermediates. Key enzymes in its synthesis are dibasic specific endopeptidase, carboxypeptidase, and endothelin-converting enzyme. Possible therapeutic implications of understanding this synthetic pathway are development of specific inhibitors of one or more of the enzymes to prevent activation of ET-1. Alternatively, selective inhibitors of ET_A receptors could shift responses toward the favorable aspects of ET_B receptor activation. Currently, no such drugs exist, but bosentan (Tracleer) and tezosentan are investigational nonselective dual ET_A/ET_B antagonists. Bosentan has U.S. Food and Drug

Table 18-2 Biological Effects of Endothelin-1

Organ System	*Effect*
Blood vessels	Potent vasoconstriction via ET_A receptors Collagen deposition via ET_A receptors Vasodilation via release of nitrous oxide and prostacyclin in endothelial cells via ET_B receptors
Heart	↑Heart rate. Positive or negative inotropism under varying conditions Hypertrophy, remodeling via ET_A receptors
Lungs	Bronchoconstriction via ET_A receptors
Kidney	Afferent and efferent vasoconstriction via ET_A receptors ↓Renal blood flow and GFR via ET_A receptors Natriuresis, diuresis via tubular ET_B receptors
Neuroendocrine	Stimulate release of catecholamines, renin, aldosterone, atrial natriuretic hormone

ET_A, endothelin A; ET_B, endothelin B; GRF, glomerular filtration rate.
Adapted from Ergul A. Endothelin-1 and endothelin receptor antagonists as potential cardiovascular therapeutic agents. *Pharmacotherapy* 2002;22:54, with permission.

Administration (FDA) approval for the treatment of pulmonary hypertension and is being investigated for use in HF.[10,11]

NATRIURETIC PEPTIDES

Natriuretic peptides are a family of peptides containing a common 17 amino acid ring. A-type natriuretic peptide (ANP), previously referred to as either atrial natriuretic peptide or atrial natriuretic factor, is secreted by the atrial myocardium in response to dilation and stretch. Similarly, B-type natriuretic peptide (BNP), formerly referred to as brain natriuretic peptide, is produced by the ventricular myocardium in response to elevations of end-diastolic pressure and volume. Type-C (CNP) is secreted by lung, kidney, and vascular endothelium in response to shear stress. Collectively, the natriuretic peptides have been referred to as "cardiac neurohormones" and are generally considered to be a favorable form of neurohormonal activation. Among their positive attributes are antagonism of the renin-angiotensin system, inhibition of sympathetic outflow, and endothelin-1 antagonism. The net effect is peripheral and coronary vasodilation to decrease preload and afterload on the heart. As their name implies, they also have diuretic or natriuretic properties with improved renal blood flow and glomerular filtration resulting from afferent arteriolar dilation and possibly efferent arteriolar constriction. Sodium reabsorption is blocked in the collecting duct by virtue of an indirect aldosterone inhibition. Natriuretic peptides also inhibit vasopressin secretion from the pituitary gland and block "salt appetite" and thirst centers in the CNS. Each of these CNS effects contributes further to diuresis. Of note, type-C has minimal diuretic properties.

Earlier research on natriuretic peptides centered on ANP, but BNP is now receiving greater attention both for diagnostic and treatment purposes. BNP precursor is cleaved to produce the biologically active C-terminal fragment (BNP) and an inactive N-terminal fragment (NT-proBNP). Plasma level measurement of either BNP or NT-proBNP can be used as a biologic marker to differentiate HF-induced acute dyspnea from other causes of respiratory distress (e.g., chronic bronchitis).[30–32] BNP levels >200 pcg/L indicate a high probability of HF. Higher concentrations correlate to severity of heart failure, with a mean plasma level of 241 pcg/mL in NYHA class I patients and >800 pcg/mL in NYHA class IV HF. Similarly, clinical resolution of symptoms is often accompanied by a decline in BNP concentration. (Also see Question 9 later in this chapter).

Possible therapeutic implications are synthesis of natriuretic hormone analogs or inhibitors of their metabolism as possible drug therapies. Nesiritide (Natrecor) is a recombinant produced human B-type natriuretic peptide approved by the FDA for IV management of acute HF exacerbations in hospitalized patients.[33,34] Downregulation of natriuretic peptide receptors, however, occurs during chronic HF, reducing the protective benefit of their actions and possibly limiting their usefulness as therapeutic entities.

Metabolism by neutral endopeptidase (NEP) and receptor sequestration are the primary modes of clearance of natriuretic peptides. NEP is a plasma membrane-bound zinc-metalloprotease enzyme found primarily in renal tubular cells, but also in the lung, GI tract, adrenal gland, heart, brain, and peripheral vasculature. This enzyme also assists in the degradation or metabolism of bradykinin and possibly of angiotensin II. It is speculated that drugs formulated to inhibit NEP (and thus maintain protective natriuretic peptide levels) might have additive effects to ACE inhibitors in the treatment of HF and hypertension. On the other hand, administering an NEP inhibitor in the absence of a concurrent ACE inhibitor, theoretically, could be counterproductive by leaving unopposed angiotensin II activity. No selective NEP inhibitors are being actively investigated.

VASOPRESSIN RECEPTOR ANTAGONISTS

To date, all standard therapies to relieve acute decompensated heart failure (ADHF) have had disappointing outcomes. These agents have either caused serious side effects or increased mortality in HF. The potent vasoconstrictor antidiuretic hormone arginine vasopressin, which modulates volume homeostasis, is elevated in HF. Early studies with tolvaptan (selective vasopressin subtype V2 receptor antagonist) demonstrated improvement in congestive symptoms of HF and overall hemodynamic profile.[35]

Recent publication of the findings in the EVERST trial, which studied the efficacy of vasopressin antagonism in heart failure, provides evidence for another possible drug in the war chest of HF.[36,37] Tolvaptan was tested in 4,133 patients with ADHF with NYHA class III-IV and LVEF of <40%. All patients also received standard therapy (ACE inhibitors, angiotensin receptor blockers [ARB], β-blockers, diuretics, nitrates, and hydralazine). The patients were randomized within 48 hours of hospitalization to 30 mg/day tolvaptan or placebo. The trial was a composite of three distinct analyses. The primary endpoint for the two identical short-term trials was to assess the change in global clinical status and body weight at day 7 or the day of discharge, whichever came earlier. The primary outcome for the long-term trial was all cause mortality and cardiovascular (CV) death or HF hospitalizations. The results of the short-term trial showed only modest improvement in the global clinical score compared with placebo. The most clinical benefit was seen in change in body weight. The long-term trial failed to show any statistical significance between the study drug and placebo in achieving the primary endpoints. Common side effects that resulted in the discontinuation of tolvaptan were dry mouth and thirst. In a small number of patients, hyponatremia was corrected. In conclusion, the results of EVERST trials suggest a novel drug with a potential role in ADHF. Because long-term benefits are lacking, the use of tolvaptan should be restricted to patients with similar characteristics as the original study design.

CALCIUM SENSITIZERS

Calcium sensitizers represent another new class of drugs under investigation for the treatment of ADHF. They exert positive inotropic effects by stabilizing the calcium troponin C-complex and facilitating actin-myosin cross-bridging without increasing myocardial consumption of adenosine triphosphate.[38] Levosimendan (Simdax), the prototype for this drug class, has a dual mechanism of action to increase myocardial contractibility and induce vasodilation. Unlike other inotropic agents, it does not affect the intracellular calcium concentrations and, therefore, has a lower potential for inducing proarrhythmias. The safety and efficacy of levosimendan in ADHF has been evaluated in placebo-controlled trials and in comparative trials with dobutamine. In patients with decompensated HF, levosimendan significantly reduced the incidence

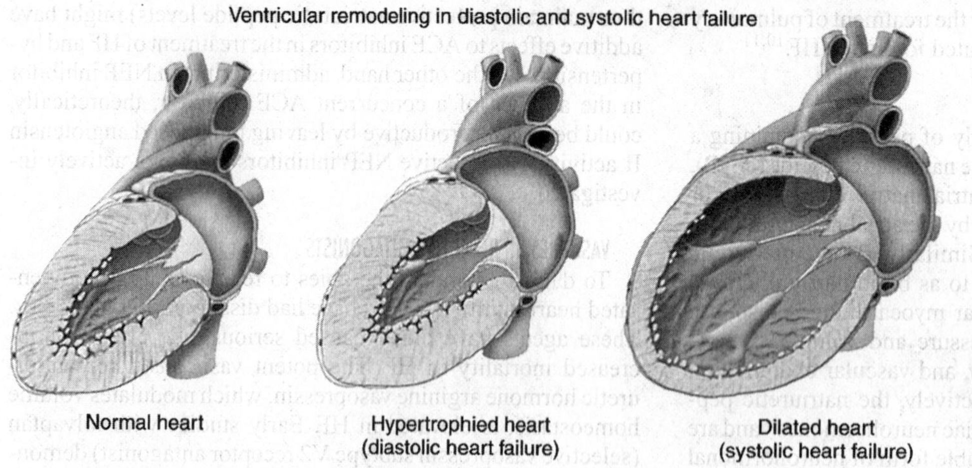

FIGURE 18-2 Cardiac remodeling. (Reprinted with permission from Jessup M, Brozena S. Medical progress: heart failure. *N Engl J Med* 2003;348:2007. Copyright 2003 Massachusetts Medical Society. All rights reserved.)

of worsening HF, and improved hemodynamic indices.[39–41] In addition, mortality was lower in the levosimendan group. These trials, however, were not powered to show a difference in mortality as an endpoint. A recent trial comparing levosimendan with dobutamine in acute HF, designed to confirm the beneficial effects on morbidity and mortality, did not reduce all-cause mortality, which contrasts with earlier studies.[42] The most common adverse effects associated with levosimendan are headache and hypotension. Currently it is only approved in Europe for ADHF.

INFLAMMATORY CYTOKINES, INTERLEUKINS, TISSUE NECROSIS FACTOR, PROSTACYCLIN, AND NITROUS OXIDE

Vascular endothelial cells release various other proinflammatory cytokines, vasodilator, and vasoconstrictor substances, including interleukin cytokines (IL-1β, IL-2, IL-6), tumor necrosis factor (TNF-α), prostacyclin, and nitrous oxide (NO) (also known as endothelium-derived relaxing factor).[43–45] The exact role of these mediators in the pathogenesis of HF is unclear. Recent studies have shown that patients with HF have elevated levels of the proinflammatory cytokines IL-1β, IL-6, and TNF-α that correlate with the severity of disease.[45–47] Initial enthusiasm for use of the TNF-α receptor antagonist etanercept (Enbrel) as a treatment of HF has been abandoned after disappointing results in larger phase 2 and 3 clinical trials.[48] Of even greater concern, at least 47 spontaneous adverse event reports were made to the FDA describing new onset HF or exacerbation of existing HF with etanercept and infliximab in patients being treated for either Crohn disease or rheumatoid arthritis.[49]

Other investigators have tried using either NO or prostacyclin (epoprostenol) as therapeutic vasodilators with mixed success.[50–52] A particular concern with prostacyclin was a trend toward increased death rates despite an improved hemodynamic status in treated patients during the Flolan International Randomized Survival Trial (FIRST).[52]

Cardiac Remodeling

Progression of HF results in a process referred to as *cardiac remodeling*, characterized by changes in the shape and mass of the ventricles in response to tissue injury.[53] The three primary manifestations of cardiac remodeling are chamber dilation, left ventricular cardiac muscle hypertrophy, and a resulting spherical shape of the left ventricular chamber (Fig. 18-2) Cardiac remodeling, which starts months to years before the appearance of clinical symptoms, contributes to the progression of the disease despite treatment.

CARDIAC DILATION

Cardiac dilation results when the ventricles fail to pump an adequate volume of blood with each contraction. This is most evident in systolic dysfunction. If the rate at which blood is delivered to the heart (preload) remains the same, but the rate at which it is pumped to other tissues diminishes, residual blood will begin to accumulate in the ventricles. Thus, end-diastolic volume increases, myocardial fibers are stretched, and the ventricle(s) become dilated. In the healthy heart, the end-diastolic volume is about 180 to 200 mL. With an EF of 60%, the SV is approximately 100 mL, leaving an end-systolic residual volume in the ventricle of 80 to 100 mL. Early in HF, a near normal SV of 100 mL is maintained, although the EF may be low (e.g., 33%). This leaves a 200- to 300-mL end-systolic residual volume in the ventricle. Over time, an enlarged heart will become evident on a chest radiograph, and the body cannot completely compensate. Cardiac dilation is less evident in diastolic dysfunction because normal contractility is maintained and the stiffened left ventricle is resistant to filling and not likely to enlarge (Fig. 18-2).

FRANK–STARLING CURVE

The Frank-Starling ventricular function curve (Fig. 18-3) implies a curvilinear relationship between left ventricular myocardial muscle fiber "stretch" (wall tension) and myocardial work. As stretch increases, the volume of blood ejected with each systolic contraction (stroke volume) increases. In systolic HF, the work capacity for any degree of stretch is diminished. A simple analogy is drawn using a balloon. The greater amount of air blown into a balloon, the more it stretches and, if released, the farther it flies around a room. As the balloon gets old, it loses its elasticity and thus has less recoil when stretched. Similarly, dilation of the ventricles initially may serve as an effective compensating mechanism in systolic failure, but it becomes inadequate as the elastic limits of the myocardial muscle fibers are reached. HR may also increase to maintain CO if SV is low. The downside of cardiac dilation is increased myocardial

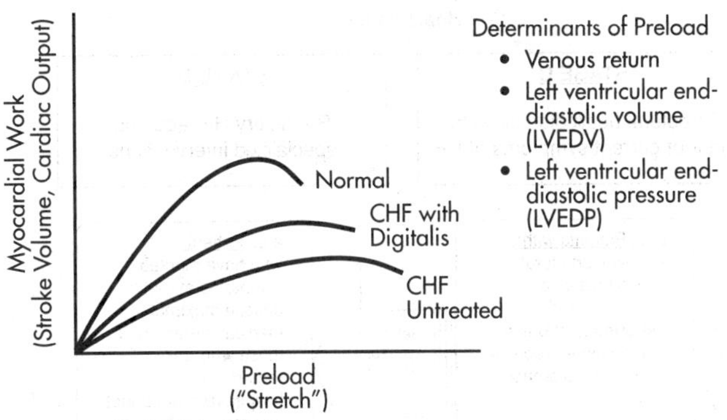

FIGURE 18-3 Representation of Frank-Starling ventricular function curve.

oxygen demand. Theoretically, as cardiac dilation progresses beyond a certain point, CO could decrease (as visualized on the descending limb of the Starling curve), but this rarely is observed clinically.

CARDIAC HYPERTROPHY

Cardiac hypertrophy, a long-term adaptation to increased diastolic volume in systolic failure, represents an absolute increase in myocardial muscle mass and muscle wall thickness (Fig. 18-2). This is somewhat analogous to increased muscle mass in skeletal muscle in response to weight lifting or other forms of exercise. Cardiac hypertrophy should not be confused with cardiac dilation. Of the two, hypertrophy provides more desirable effects, but its absolute benefit is inadequate in severe disease.

Functional Limitation Classification and Stages of Heart Failure

NEW YORK HEART ASSOCIATION CLASSIFICATION

The NYHA classification scheme identifies four categories of functional disability associated with HF. Patients in class I are well compensated with no physical limitations and lack symptoms with ordinary physical activity. In class II, ordinary physical activity results in mild enhancement of symptoms and imparts slight limitations on exercise tolerance. Patients in class III are comfortable only at rest; even less than ordinary physical activity leads to symptoms. In class IV, symptoms of HF are present at rest and no physical activity can be undertaken without symptoms. Determination of class placement for a specific patient is highly subjective and will vary between observers. In some cases, subdivisions such as class III_A or III_B may be used to further individualize grading of severity.

A shortcoming of the NYHA classification scheme is that it does not include asymptomatic individuals who are at high risk for developing HF and who may benefit from preemptive lifestyle changes and drug therapy. The 2001 ACC/AHA Practice Guidelines introduced a new staging algorithm that can be used in conjunction with the NYHA classifications.[6] Patients in stage A have hypertension, coronary artery disease, diabetes mellitus, or other conditions that, if left untreated, can result in the development of overt HF. HF symptoms or identifiable abnormalities of the myocardium or heart valves are absent in stage A. Patients in stage B remain asymptomatic but have structural defects within the heart (e.g., left ventricular hypertrophy, dilation, or valve disease) that indicate the existence of impending HF. Patients in stage C exhibit varying degrees of HF symptoms corresponding to NYHA classes I–III along with structural changes in the heart consistent with systolic or diastolic HF. Stage D in the ACA/AHA scheme roughly correlates to NYHA class IV. Patients in this latter category are frequently hospitalized, dependent on IV therapy, and could be considered to have end-stage disease. Table 18-3 summarizes these two classification schemes and how they overlap.

Treatment Principles

The 2005 ACC/AHA Task Force Practice Guidelines serve as the primary basis for recommendations within this chapter.[7] A clinical algorithm reprinted from the ACC/AHA guidelines is found in Figure 18-4.[7] The ACC/AHA Task Force recommends that most patients with HF should be routinely treated with a combination of the following classes and drugs: a diuretic, an ACE inhibitor, a β-adrenergic blocker, and (usually) digitalis.[7]

Table 18-3 American College of Cardiology-American Heart Association (ACC/AHA) Staging and New York Heart Association (NYHA) Classification of Heart Failure

ACA-AHA Stage	*NYHA Functional Class*
A. At high risk for heart failure, but without structural heart disease (normal heart exam) or symptoms of heart failure (e.g., patients with hypertension, coronary heart disease, diabetes, alcoholism, or strong family history)	No corresponding category
B. Structural heart disease present (e.g., LV hypertrophy, dilation, fibrosis, old MI), but without symptoms of heart failure	I. Asymptomatic or no limitations on normal physical activity, but symptoms with strenuous exercise.
C. Structural heart disease with prior or current symptoms of heart failure	II. Symptoms of heart failure with normal activity or with moderate exertion III. Symptomatic with minimal exertion; marked limitations in physical activity including activities of daily life (e.g., bathing, dressing) (or IIIB). Symptoms of heart failure at rest.
D. Refractory heart failure requiring specialized interventions	IV (or IVB). Symptoms of heart failure at rest and requiring hospitalization or intravenous inotropic support

Adapted from Foody J, et al. β-Blocker therapy in heart failure. Part I: Scientific review. Part II: Clinical applications. *JAMA* 2002;287:883 (part I) and 890 (part II), with permission.

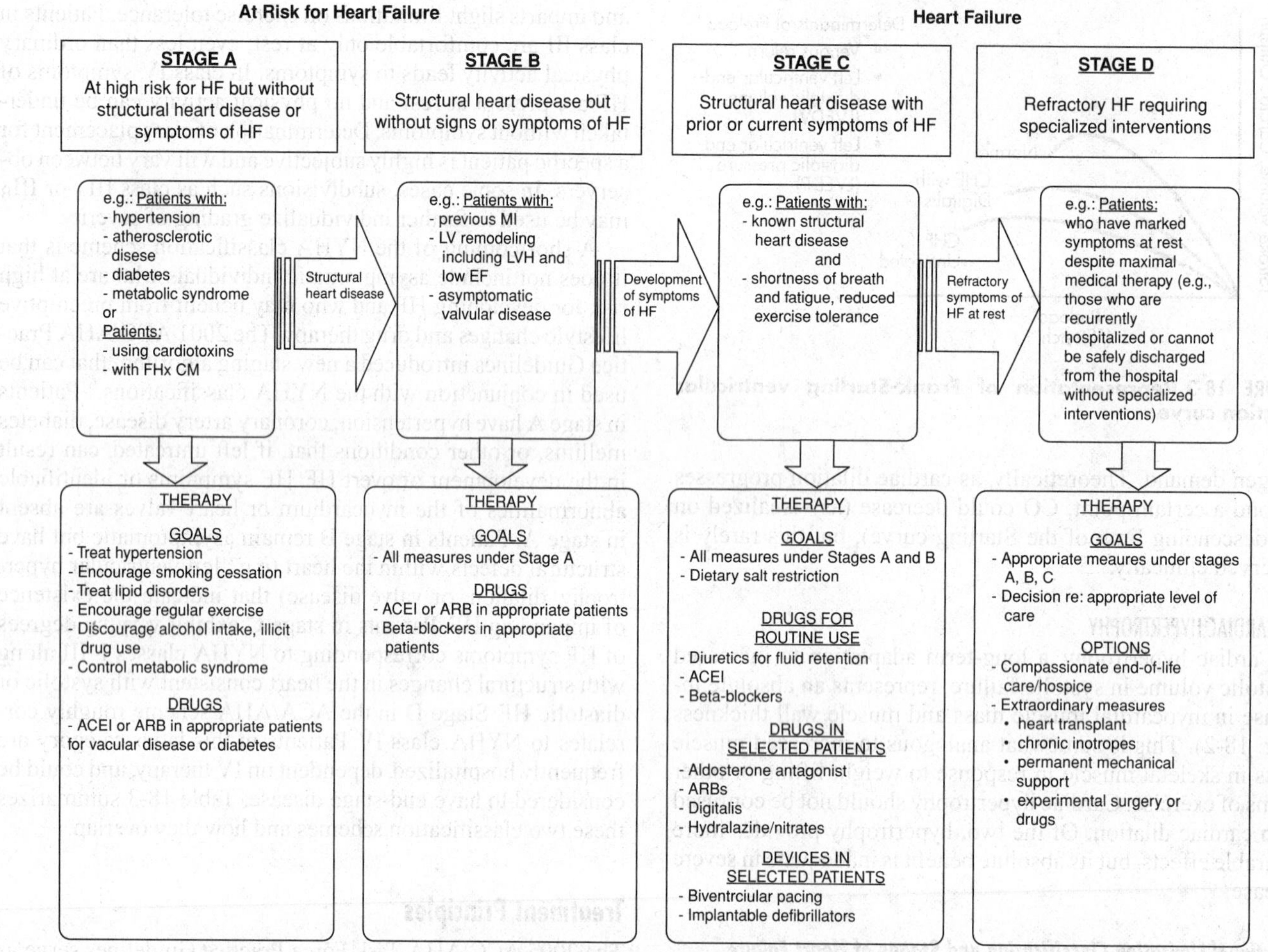

FIGURE 18-4 Stages in the development of heart failure/recommended therapy by stage. FHx CM indicates family history of cardiomyopathy; ACEI, angiotensin converting enzyme inhibitor; ARB, angiotensin receptor blocker. (Reprinted ACC/AHA 2005 guidelines update for the diagnosis and management of chronic heart failure in the adult: a report of the American College of Cardiology, American Heart Association Task Force on Practice Guidelines (Writing Committee) to update the 2001 Guidelines for the Evaluation and Management of Heart Failure. *J Am Coll Cardiol* 2005;46E1, with permission.)

An aldosterone antagonist (e.g., spironolactone) is a fifth class of drug recommended for patients with advanced HF.

The objectives of therapy for all forms of HF are to abolish disabling symptoms, avoid complications such as arrhythmias, and improve the quality of the patient's life. Increased walking distance during a 6-minute treadmill test or transition to a lower NYHA symptom class is used as a rough measure of success for these objectives. Specific quality of life questionnaires are also available. The ultimate goal is to prolong survival in individuals and reduce mortality rates within the population of patients with HF. Short of a heart transplant, none of the treatment measures are curative.

Nonspecific medical management of systolic HF includes addressing CV risk factors, correcting underlying disease states (e.g., hypertension, ischemic heart disease, arrhythmias, lipid disorders, anemia, or hyperthyroidism), moderate physical activity as tolerated, immunization with influenza and pneumococcal vaccines to reduce the risk of respiratory infections, and discontinuing possible drug-induced causes. A sodium-restricted diet and diuretics are required if fluid retention is evident. Pharmacotherapeutic interventions include ACE inhibitors, certain β-blocking drugs (e.g., carvedilol and metoprolol), digoxin, and other vasodilators (nitrates, hydralazine, or angiotensin receptor blockers). Amiodarone is indicated in the treatment of symptomatic ventricular tachycardia and atrial fibrillation (AF) associated with HF. The role of natriuretic peptides, endothelin inhibitors, vasopressin receptor antagonists, and calcium sensitizers continue to be investigated. Nondigitalis inotropic agents and TNF-α inhibitors, although theoretically valuable, have yielded disappointing results and significant complications, including arrhythmias and increased mortality rates.

Treatment of diastolic failure is less well defined.[12–16] The term *heart failure with normal left ventricular ejection fraction* has been proposed instead of diastolic heart failure. A sodium-restricted diet and diuretics are indicated for symptomatic relief of shortness breath or edema. ACE inhibitors are frequently used, although controlled trials of effectiveness are lacking. Negative inotropes such as nonselective β-blockers (e.g., propranolol) and calcium blockers (especially verapamil) are often advocated to slow HR and allow more efficient ventricular filling during diastole. Digitalis is relatively contraindicated, especially in patients with ventricular septal hypertrophy.

Physical Activity

Patients should be encouraged to maximize their activities of daily life and exercise to maintain physical conditioning. Edema can be minimized by use of elastic hosiery, which increases interstitial pressure and helps mobilize fluid into vascular spaces. During acute exacerbations, bed rest and restricted physical activity decrease the metabolic demands of the failing heart and minimize gravitational forces contributing to the formation of edema. Renal perfusion is increased in the prone position, resulting in diuresis and eventual mobilization of edema fluid.

Sodium-Restricted Diet

Reduction of dietary salt is prudent in patients with hypertension or evidence of fluid retention, but is not required in all patients. No evidence indicates that salt restriction in normotensive or asymptomatic patients will prevent the onset of HF. It is convenient to remember that 1 g of sodium (Na) is equivalent to 2.5 g of salt (NaCl), and that one level teaspoon of salt weighs approximately 6 g. Similarly, 1 g Na = 43 mEq Na and 1 g NaCl = 17 mEq Na. In patients with clinically evident HF, moderate sodium restriction (<3 g/day Na) may allow patients to use lower doses of diuretics by decreasing blood volume and offsetting abnormal retention of sodium by the kidneys. If the kidney's ability to excrete sodium is not severely compromised, it is possible to approach normal balance by restricting sodium intake to match excretion. Although <1 g of sodium chloride (NaCl) is required to meet physiologic needs, the average U.S. diet contains 10 g. Dietary sodium can be reduced to 2 to 4 g of NaCl by eliminating cooking salt. This diet is more palatable and leads to better adherence than a severely salt-restricted diet.

Diuretics: Clinical Use and Renal Pharmacology

Only those points salient to the treatment of HF are included in this chapter. Diuretic use also is discussed in Chapter 13, Essential Hypertension. (See Chapter 11, Fluid and Electrolyte Disorders, for a thorough review of kidney physiology and the classification, mechanism of action, and side effects of diuretics.)

Diuretics are indicated in both systolic and diastolic HF for patients with circulatory congestion (pulmonary and peripheral edema) or cardiac distension (enlarged heart on chest radiograph). They produce symptomatic relief more rapidly than other drugs for HF. Monotherapy with diuretics is discouraged, however, even in patients with mild symptoms that respond well to diuretics. Because activation of the renin-angiotensin-aldosterone and sympathetic nervous systems contribute to the progression of HF, diuretics should be combined with an ACE inhibitor and a β-blocker unless contraindications exist. Conversely, continuous treatment with diuretics is not always necessary in patients with little or no evidence of fluid overload, and diuretics are relatively contraindicated in persons who are volume depleted or have compromised renal blood flow.[6,7]

By enhancing renal excretion of sodium and water, diuretics diminish vascular volume, thus relieving ventricular and pulmonary congestion and decreasing peripheral edema. Initially, the goal of diuretic therapy is symptomatic relief of HF by decreasing excess volume without causing intravascular volume depletion. Once excess volume is removed, therapy is aimed at maintaining sodium balance and preventing reaccumulation of new fluid, while avoiding dehydration. The rate at which edema fluid can be removed is limited by its rate of mobilization from the interstitial to the intravascular fluid compartment. If diuresis is too vigorous, intravascular volume depletion, hypotension, and a paradoxical decrease in CO (caused by compromised venous return and inadequate ventricular filling) may result. Weight loss exceeding 1 kg/day is to be avoided except in patients with acute pulmonary edema.

The effectiveness of diuretics depends on the amount of sodium delivered to their site of action in the kidney and the patient's renal function.[54,55] Proximal tubular reabsorption of sodium is increased in patients with severe HF when RBF is compromised, rendering thiazide and potassium sparing diuretics (which act primarily on the distal tubule) minimally effective. Thiazides increase the fractional excretion of sodium no more than 5% and lose their effectiveness when creatinine clearance (Cl_{Cr}) decreases to <30–50 mL/minute. The loop diuretics (furosemide, bumetanide, and torsemide) are more potent and retain their effectiveness until the creatinine clearance is <5 mL/minute. Metolazone has diuretic effects intermediate to that of the thiazide and loop diuretics and may maintain activity in patients with compromised renal function. In most patients with HF, loop diuretics are preferred. In addition to having activity in the ascending limb of the loop of Henle, furosemide has vasodilating properties that decrease renal vascular resistance. It also enhances sodium excretion by shifting RBF from the long juxtamedullary nephrons to shorter superficial nephrons. In pulmonary edema, the initial beneficial effects of furosemide may result more from dilation of venous capacitance vessels (decreasing preload) than from diuresis.[54,55]

The onset of response after an IV injection of loop diuretics is ≤10 minutes, peaking within the first 30 minutes, and usually abating within 2 hours. Natriuresis usually begins 30 to 90 minutes after the oral administration of loop diuretics; it peaks within the first or second hour and lasts for 6 to 8 hours. The usual recommended doses for the loop diuretics are found in Table 18-4.[54]

The concept of ceiling doses for loop diuretics should be understood.[54,55] A key observation is that the effectiveness of diuretics depends on delivery (active secretion) of the drug into the proximal tubule in the kidney. Slow absorption (even if bioavailability is high) or protein binding impair tubular delivery and compromise diuretic response. Once the drug is in the tubule, however, further drug delivery produces no greater diuresis. Increasing single doses beyond the ceiling dose produces no additional diuretic response. As an alternative, improved diuresis may be obtained by giving the drug more frequently.

As discussed later in this chapter, combinations of diuretics with different mechanisms (e.g., a loop diuretic and metolazone) are used in patients whose conditions are refractory to high-dose loop diuretics.[54,55] Because diuresis can lead to

Table 18-4 Loop Diuretic Dosing

	Furosemide	Bumetanide	Torsemide
Usual daily oral dose (mg)	20–160	0.5–4	10–80
Ceiling dose (mg)			
Normal renal function	80–160 (PO/IV)	1–2 (PO/IV)	20–40 (PO/IV)
Cl_{Cr}: 20–50 mL/min	160 mg (PO/IV)	2 (PO/IV)	40 mg (PO/IV)
Cl_{Cr}: <20 mL/min	200 IV, 400 (PO)	8–10 (PO/IV)	100 (PO/IV)
Bioavailability	10%–100% Average 50% Lower with food	80%–90% Lower with food	80%–100% No food effect

IV, intravenous; PO, oral.
Adapted from Kramer BK, et al. Diuretic treatment and diuretic resistance in heart failure. *Am J Med* 1999;106:90, with permission.

compensatory activation of the RAAS, combining a diuretic with an ACE inhibitor or using spironolactone has a theoretic basis (see Question 13).

Diuretics are indicated in diastolic HF, but pose a difficult challenge. This form of HF is highly volume dependent, becoming significantly worse in states of fluid overload, but responding with a rapid reduction in filling pressures and resolution of dyspnea following diuresis. Conversely, chronic diuretic use therapy runs the risk of restricting the end-diastolic volume, resulting in a significant reduction of CO. Thus, elevated filling pressure may be controlled at the expense of a greatly reduced SV such that the symptoms of dyspnea may be traded for those of fatigue and loss of exercise tolerance.[56]

Aldosterone Antagonists

Despite their profound effects on reducing HF symptoms, no data substantiate that loop diuretics counteract the underlying cause of HF or modify mortality rates. The aldosterone antagonists (e.g., eplerenone and spironolactone) exert a mild diuretic effect by competitive binding of the aldosterone receptor site in the distal convoluted renal tubules. They are also referred to as potassium retaining or potassium sparing diuretics because sodium excretion at this level of the kidney is accompanied by an equimolar exchange for potassium. The Randomized Aldactone Evaluation study investigators found that spironolactone substantially reduced both morbidity and mortality in a select group of patients with severe HF (NYHA class III and IV).[57] The authors speculated, however, that the protective effect of spironolactone was related more to a reduction in aldosterone-induced vascular damage and myocardial or vascular fibrosis than to its diuretic effect. Similarly, reduced mortality was observed in patients with left ventricular dysfunction following a recent MI treated with 25 to 50 mg of eplerenone (Inspra)[58] (see Question 14). No evidence indicates that the direct acting potassium sparing diuretics amiloride or triamterene exert a similar protective effect. The 2005 ACC/AHA guidelines recommend initiating aldosterone antagonists in patients with severe HF and in patients immediately post-MI who have LV dysfunction.[7]

Angiotensin-Converting Enzyme Inhibitors and Angiotensin Receptor Inhibitors[59–62]

Drugs with vasodilating properties have become a primary treatment modality of HF. Arterial dilation provides symptomatic relief of HF by decreasing arterial impedance (afterload) to left ventricular outflow. Venous dilation decreases left ventricular congestion (preload). The combination of these two properties provides additive benefits to alleviate the symptoms of HF and increase exercise tolerance. The first vasodilator drugs to be studied were hydralazine (essentially a pure arterial dilator) and nitrates (predominately venous dilators). By combining these two drugs, significant reductions in HF symptoms can be achieved along with a modest reduction in mortality rates. With the advent of ACE inhibitors, the use of hydralazine and nitrates has been relegated to a secondary role.

Angiotensin-converting enzyme inhibitors (e.g., benazepril [Lotensin], captopril [Capoten], enalapril [Vasotec], fosinopril [Monopril], lisinopril [Prinivil, Zestril], moexipril [Univasc], perindopril [Aceon], quinapril [Accupril], ramipril [Altace]), and trandolapril [Mavik]) possess both afterload and preload reducing properties (by blocking angiotensin II-mediated vasoconstriction) and volume-reducing potential (by inhibiting activation of aldosterone). They not only produce similar hemodynamic effects to the hydralazine-nitrate combination as a single agent, but they also favorably modify cardiac remodeling independent of vasodilation and have a more tolerable side effect profile. These advantages, coupled with evidence that ACE inhibitors slow the rate of mortality in HF more than the hydralazine-nitrate combination, led the authors of all the current guidelines to recommend unequivocally that ACE inhibitors are the drugs of choice for initial therapy, even in patients with relatively mild left ventricular systolic dysfunction.[1–3,6]

The 2005 ACC/AHA guidelines state:

ACE inhibitors should be prescribed to all patients with HF due to left ventricular systolic dysfunction (LVEF) unless they have a contradiction to their use or have been shown to be unable to tolerate treatment with these drugs. Because of their favorable effects on survival, treatment with an ACE inhibitor should not be delayed until the patient is found to be resistant to treatment with other drugs. In general, ACE inhibitors are used together with β-blockers. ACE inhibitors should not be prescribed without diuretics in patients with current or recent history of fluid retention, because diuretics are needed to maintain sodium balance and prevent the development of peripheral and pulmonary edema. ACE inhibitors should be initiated at low doses, followed by gradual increments in dose if lower doses have been well tolerated. Fluid retention can blunt the therapeutic effects and fluid depletion can potentiate the adverse effects of ACE, healthcare providers should ensure that the appropriate doses of diuretics are used before and during treatment with these drugs. Clinicians should attempt to use doses that have been shown to reduce CV events in clinical trials, but they should not delay the initiation of β-blockers in patients because of a failure to reach target ACE inhibitor doses.[7]

The pharmacologic actions of all the ACE inhibitors are essentially identical, but some of them have not been extensively studied or received FDA approval for use in HF. Their value in diastolic failure still is being investigated. Expanded discussion of ACE inhibitor use and side effects is found later in this chapter starting with Question 16.

A related class of drugs includes the angiotensin receptor blocker drugs candesartan [Atacand], eprosartan [Teveten], irbesartan [Avapro], losartan [Cozaar], olmesartan [Benicar], telmisartan [Micardis], and valsartan (Diovan).[59,62] The receptor inhibitors offer theoretic advantages over ACE inhibitors by being more specific for angiotensin II blockade and having a lower risk of drug-induced cough. On the other hand, indirect block of bradykinin, NE, or prostaglandins by some or all of the ACE inhibitors may offer an advantage over receptor inhibitors. Before the Candesartan in the Treatment of Heart Failure—Assessment of Reduction in Mortality and Morbidity (CHARM) trial, no convincing evidence showed that angiotensin receptor blockers (ARB) were as effective as ACE inhibitors in reducing morbidity and mortality in patients with HF (see Question 20). According to the 2005 ACC/AHA guidelines, ARB are recommended in patients who are intolerant to ACE inhibitors (e.g., angioedema or intractable cough). Also, ARB can be considered as an add-on therapy in patients who continue to be symptomatic despite optimal conventional therapy. Currently, only candesartan and valsartan have FDA approved labeling for the treatment of HF.

β-Adrenergic Blocking Agents [21–26]

Until the mid 1990s, some variation of the following statement could be found in any standard text on the treatment of HF: "β-blockers and other negative inotropes are contraindicated." This is a logical extension of previously held belief that sympathomimetic agonists and other positive inotropes are the logical choice to counteract the hemodynamic defects of systolic failure and that negative inotropes will exacerbate HF. A better understanding of the pathophysiology of HF led to a rethinking of this logic.[20–25] As discussed, cardiac adrenergic drive initially supports the performance of the failing heart, but long-term activation of the sympathetic nervous system exerts deleterious effects that can be counteracted by the use of β-blockers. Nonetheless, initial trials with propranolol, pindolol, and labetalol in patients with systolic failure were disappointing. Much more favorable results have been achieved with metoprolol (Lopressor, Toprol XL) and bisoprolol, both of which are partially selective β_1-blockers, and carvedilol (Coreg), a mixed α_1- and nonselective β-blocking agent. Extended release metoprolol succinate (Toprol XL) and carvedilol are FDA approved for use in HF. Although some patients can initially have a temporary worsening of symptoms, continued use results in improved quality of life, fewer hospitalizations, and most importantly, longer survival. The 2005 ACC/AHA guidelines state that β-blockers should be prescribed to all patients with stable HF owing to reduced LVEF unless they have a contraindication to their use or have been shown to be unable to tolerate treatment with these drugs. β-Blocker treatment should be initiated as soon as LV dysfunction is diagnosed because of favorable effects that treatment can have on survival and disease progression. Intolerance or resistance to other HF therapies should not precede nor delay the initiation of β-blocker use in patients with HF.[7] β-Blockers are discussed in greater detail in the case study portion of this chapter (see Questions 27–30 and 52).

Digitalis Glycosides (Digoxin)

Digitalis glycosides have several pharmacologic actions on the heart. Digoxin is the only drug from this family still marketed following the withdrawal of digitoxin in the late 1990s. It binds to and inhibits sodium-potassium (Na^+-K^+) adenosine triphosphatase (ATPase) in cardiac cells, decreasing outward transport of sodium and increasing intracellular concentrations of calcium within the cells. Calcium binding to the sarcoplasmic reticulum causes an increase in the contractile state of the heart.

Until recently, the primary benefit of digoxin in systolic HF was assumed to be an increase in the force of contraction (positive inotropic effect) of the failing heart to increase EF and CO. Recent evidence suggests that even at serum concentrations below those associated with positive inotropism, digoxin has beneficial neurohumoral and autonomic effects by reducing sympathetic tone and stimulating parasympathetic (vagal) responses.[6,63–66] Inhibition of (Na^+-K^+) ATPase in vagal afferent fibers sensitizes cardiac baroreceptors to reduce sympathetic outflow from the CNS. Similarly, inhibition of (Na^+-K^+) ATPase in renal cells reduces renal tubular reabsorption of sodium and indirectly suppresses renin secretion. This has led to the suggestion that the positive benefits of digoxin can be obtained with a lower risk of side effects by using smaller than traditional doses.[6]

In addition to effects on contractility, digoxin decreases the conduction velocity and prolongs the refractory period of the atrioventricular (AV) node. This AV node–blocking effect prolongs the PR interval and is the basis for use of digoxin in slowing the ventricular response rate in patients with AF and other supraventricular arrhythmias (see Chapter 19, Cardiac Arrhythmias). At higher serum concentrations, however, digoxin increases cardiac automaticity and irritability and decreases the refractory period of the atrial and ventricular myocardium, all of which predispose the patient to a multitude of unwanted heart rhythm disturbances.

Before the advent of ACE inhibitors, the emphasis of HF management was to stimulate the failing heart with inotropes. Digoxin was considered the obvious drug of choice, particularly for patients with coexistent HF and supraventricular arrhythmias. This was followed by a period when the role of digoxin was challenged, especially in patients with normal sinus rhythm, with critics proclaiming it as being minimally effective and having a high risk for toxicity. As evidence mounted that vasodilators could improve survival rates, no such data existed for digoxin. In the past few years, several studies have confirmed a clinical benefit for digoxin in reducing HF symptoms, independent of rhythm status, but survival data are still not convincing (see Question 15). As a result, the latest clinical guidelines state that digoxin therapy is unlikely to benefit patients with stage A or stage B HF. In these patients, digoxin can be used for symptom management, only if they are treated with drug therapy shown to prolong survival (ACE inhibitors and β-blockers) or have not responded adequately to appropriate therapy. Patients in stage C or stage D HF who are symptomatic, with an enlarged heart and reduced LVEF, digoxin can be beneficial.[7] Monotherapy with digoxin or in combination with only a diuretic is no longer recommended. Digoxin can also be considered in patients with HF who also have chronic AF, although β-blockers may be more effective than digoxin in controlling the ventricular response, especially during exercise. It is also important to document the patient's EF before considering the use of digoxin because the digitalis glycosides are not useful in diastolic HF and, in fact, may worsen this form of left ventricular dysfunction. Further discussions of the controversies surrounding digoxin use and detailed dosing guidelines are found in the case studies.

DIGOXIN PHARMACOKINETICS (TABLE 18-5)

Digoxin is a polar glycoside that is adequately but incompletely absorbed. Studies from the 1970s indicated that the absorption of oral tablets varied between manufacturers and from lot to lot of the same product.[67–71] (See the sixth edition of *Applied Therapeutics: The Clinical Use of Drugs* for the citations and abstracts of older articles.) In some instances, the differences were only in the *rate* of absorption but not necessarily in the *extent* of absorption (i.e., bioavailability) (Table 18-5). At least part of the variability correlated to differences *in vitro* dissolution. For this reason, most clinicians prefer to use the brand name product (Lanoxin), but published data regarding the lack of equivalence of current generic products are lacking. Four manufacturers (Bertek, Caraco, Stevens J, and Actavis Totowa) now market generic versions of digoxin that have been given an AB rating (one under the brand name of Digitek).

Bioavailability of digoxin also depends on the dosage form given. Again, most published information is from the 1970s and is subject to such limitations as differences in methodology between studies (single-dose versus multiple-dose studies) and use of nonspecific assays. The original studies appear to underestimate digoxin bioavailability.[67–71] As summarized by Reuning and others and based on studies using improved assay methods, the bioavailability of conventional tablets ranges from 70% to 80% (mean, 75%), whereas that of the commercially available elixir is slightly greater, ranging from 75% to 85%.[70] Nonetheless, considerable interpatient and intrapatient variability exists. Higher bioavailability of solutions reported in some studies might be of little clinical relevance because the solutions used were prepared extemporaneously from solutions for injection.

Lanoxicaps are a liquid-filled soft gelatin capsule form of digoxin with improved bioavailability averaging 90% to 100%. The digoxin content of these capsules, however, is 80% of the corresponding tablet. Thus, a 0.2-mg Lanoxicaps is approximately equal to a 0.25-mg digoxin tablet. Because of high cost relative to conventional tablets, use of the capsules usually is reserved for those cases when the response achieved with the tablets has been erratic.

Digoxin's rapid onset of action (30–60 minutes) corresponds with peak plasma levels. Maximal effects from a single dose are observed 5 to 6 hours after drug administration, a time at which drug distribution in the body is complete. Digoxin has a steady-state volume of distribution averaging 6.7 L/kg of lean body weight (range, 4–9 L/kg).[67,70,71] Only 23% is protein bound, but the volume of distribution may be decreased significantly in renal failure (see Questions 46 and 47). A serum level of 0.8 to 2 ng/mL was recommended in older guidelines as being the therapeutic target, but new evidence indicates therapeutic benefit and greater safety by targeting serum

Table 18-5 Digoxin Pharmacokinetics

Parameter	Value
Bioavailability (F)	
Tablets	0.75 (0.5–0.9)[a]
Elixir	0.80 (0.65–0.9)
Liquid-filled capsules	0.95 (0.8–1.0)
Half-Life ($t^1/_2$)	
Normal	1.6–2 day
Renal failure	≥4.4 day
Children	0.7–1.5 day
Volume of Distribution (Vd)[b]	
Normal	6.7 (4–9) L/kg
Renal failure	Smaller: 4.7 (1.5–8.5) L/kg
Clearance (Cl)	
Normal	1.02 Cl_{Cr} + 57 mL/min *or* 2.7 L/min/kg
Severe HF	0.88 Cl_{Cr} + 23 mL/min
% Renally Cleared Unchanged	PO: 50–60% IV: 70–75%
% Nonrenal Elimination	40% (20–55%)
% Eliminated/Day	14% + Cl_{Cr}/5
% Enterohepatic Recycling	6.8%
Protein Binding	20–30%
Therapeutic Serum Concentration[c]	0.5–1.2 ng/mL
Digitalizing (loading) dose[d]	0.5–1 mg or 0.01–0.02 mg/kg
Usual Maintenance Dose[e]	0.125–0.25 mg/day
Pediatric Dosing	
Neonate loading	0.01–0.03 mg/kg IV
Infant loading	0.01–0.05 mg/kg PO
>2-year-old load	0.05 mg/kg PO
Premature maintenance	0.001–0.009 mg/kg/day
Neonate maintenance	0.01 mg/kg/day
Infant maintenance	0.015–0.025 mg/kg/day
>2-year-old maintenance	0.01–0.015 mg/kg/day

[a]Mean value with range in parentheses.
[b]Volume of distribution decreases in renal failure, possibly because of change in protein binding.
[c]Digoxin serum concentration and effect are poorly correlated. Levels drawn <6 hours after a dose may be falsely elevated. Spironolactone and endogenous digoxin-like substances in the blood of neonates and renal failure patients can result in falsely elevated levels. Resting concentrations may be higher than those taken after exercise.
[d]Loading doses not recommended except for patients in acute distress, but it takes several days (five half-lives) to reach steady-state with maintenance dose. A more specific loading dose can be calculated by multiplying the desired steady-state concentration by the volume of distribution.
[e]The dosage should be adjusted lower in the elderly or those with renal insufficiency by first estimating Cl_{Cr} to calculate an estimated digoxin clearance. The dosage is estimated by multiplying the target serum concentration times the estimated clearance.
Cl_{Cr}, creatine clearance; HF, heart failure; IV, intravenous; PO, by mouth.

concentrations in the range of 0.5 to 1.2 ng/mL (see Questions 34 and 36).

Digoxin has a half-life ($t_{1/2}$) of 1.6 to 2 days (36–40 hours) and is characterized by first-order pharmacokinetics.[67,69–71] With renal impairment, the half-life of digoxin is prolonged, reaching 4.4 days or more in total anuria.[70–72] The renal clearance of digoxin (1.86 mL/minute/kg) is slightly greater than creatinine clearance, indicating a component of tubular secretion. Many have the erroneous impression that nonrenal excretion of digoxin is unimportant. In fact, anywhere from 20% to 40% of a given digoxin dose is excreted nonrenally, either as metabolites or in the feces,[67,69–71] corresponding to a nonrenal clearance of 40 to 60 mL/minute (0.82 mL/minute/kg). In a few individuals, up to 55% of a dose is eliminated as metabolites, primarily as inactive dihydrodigoxin.[70–72] Little digoxin (6.8%) enters the enterohepatic circulation, and its metabolism is unaltered in patients with cirrhosis.

Digoxin absorption, bioavailability, and elimination are partially mediated by P-glycoprotein (PGP), a multidrug transporter that acts as a drug efflux pump across cell membranes in epithelial and endothelial cells of the intestine, kidney, and liver.[71,73] For drugs and toxins affected by PGP, the net effect is to reduce bioavailability (by transporting drugs from the blood back into the gut lumen) and promote clearance (e.g., by enhancing renal tubular secretion). For digoxin, this system comes into play when certain drugs that block the action of PGP are taken along with digoxin.[73,74] For example, quinidine blocks intestinal and renal PGP, thus increasing digoxin bioavailability and reducing renal clearance. As a result, digoxin serum levels rise. This and other digoxin drug interactions are considered in greater detail in Questions 38–40.

In approximately 10% of patients given digoxin, a substantial portion of the drug can be metabolized by bacteria in the GI tract to cardioinactive reduced metabolites.[71,72,75] In isolated cases, significantly increased requirements for digoxin dosage may be seen in patients who excrete large amounts of digoxin by this route. The resulting reduced bioavailability of digoxin is more of a problem when slowly absorbed generic tablets are used as opposed to rapidly absorbed solutions or Lanoxin brand tablets. In addition, concurrent use of certain oral antibiotics (e.g., erythromycin or clarithromycin) can lead to increased digoxin toxicity. This was initially ascribed to altered intestinal metabolism by the antibiotics, but with better understanding of the role of PGP in digoxin absorption and excretion, a probable explanation is that these antibiotics inhibit renal PGP, thus reducing enhanced digoxin renal clearance (See Question 40).

Jelliffe et al. present digoxin elimination in a slightly different context by describing the percent elimination in 24 hours.[76] By plotting creatinine clearance versus percent of drug eliminated per day (Fig. 18-5), they found a linear relationship between 24-hour drug excretion and renal function. As can be seen from the figure, the best-fit equation of the line ($y = b + mx$) is:

$$\%\ \text{Digoxin eliminated/day} = 14 + \frac{Cl_{cr}}{5} \quad \textbf{(18-1)}$$

where the y intercept (b), representing nonrenal elimination, is 14%, and the slope of the line (m), representing that portion of daily elimination dependent on renal elimination, is one-fifth. At a creatinine clearance of 100 mL/minute, the percent

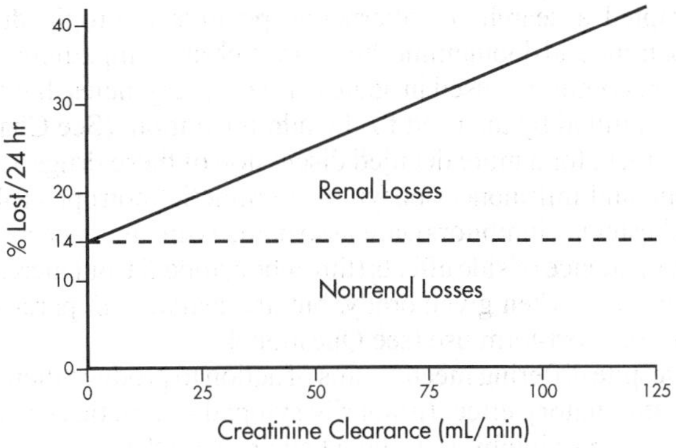

FIGURE 18-5 Relationship of digoxin elimination to renal function.

eliminated per day is 35%, whereas at a creatinine clearance of 0 (i.e., anuria), the percent eliminated per day is 14%, all via nonrenal clearance mechanisms.

Other Vasodilating Drugs: Hydralazine and Nitrates

Although ACE inhibitors have become the vasodilator drug of choice, the first vasodilators used in patients with HF were hydralazine and nitrates. Hydralazine (Apresoline) is a potent arterial dilating agent that provides symptomatic relief of HF by decreasing arterial impedance (afterload) to left ventricular outflow. Nitrates (e.g., nitroglycerin [NTG], isosorbide dinitrate, and isosorbide mononitrate) have venous dilating properties that decrease left ventricular congestion (preload). Used in combination, these two agents have additive benefits in alleviating the symptoms of HF and increasing exercise tolerance. Importantly, the hydralazine-isosorbide dinitrate combination was the first treatment regimen to show improved survival in severe HF compared with placebo (while patients continued their previous diuretic and/or digitalis therapy). In the *post hoc* analysis of the hydralazine-isosorbide dinitrate combination trial, there appeared to be greater efficacy in the cohort of black patients. The African American Heart Failure Trial (AHeFT)[77] has subsequently been performed and confirms the finding that the addition of hydralazine combined with isosorbide dinitrate to standard HF therapy with an ACE inhibitor and/or a β-blocker showed added benefit. Based on the results of AHeFT, the FDA has approved the combination product of hydralazine and isosorbide dinitrate (BiDil) for the treatment of HF as an adjunct to standard HF therapy in black patients. The 2005 ACC/AHA guideline recommendations state that the combination of hydralazine and a nitrate might be reasonable in patients with current or prior HF symptoms and reduced LVEF who cannot tolerate ACE inhibitors or ARB. The guidelines go on to say that the addition of hydralazine and isosorbide dinitrate to patients with HF receiving ACE inhibitors and β-blockers, is reasonable and can be effective in blacks with NYHA functional class III or IV HF.[7] The role of these vasodilators in diastolic failure is not well studied. IV NTG and nitroprusside (a mixed arterial and venous dilator) are also used in hospitalized patients with acute HF exacerbations (see Questions 47).

Other Inotropic Agents

Previous doubt about the clinical effectiveness of digitalis derivatives and concern over their potential for toxicity prompted a search for alternative positive inotropic drugs. Dopamine and dobutamine, both of which are sympathomimetics, are commonly used in acute cardiac emergencies, but their use is limited by the need for IV administration. (See Chapter 21, Shock, for a more detailed discussion of these drugs.) Amrinone and milrinone, nonsympathomimetic inotropes (phosphodiesterase inhibitors), are associated with an unacceptably high incidence of side effects (thrombocytopenia and increased death rates) when given orally, but are available in parenteral form for short-term use (see Question 48).

Despite differing mechanisms of action to produce their cardiac stimulatory effect (primarily sympathomimetics or phosphodiesterase inhibitors), and whether or not the drug also has vasodilating properties (e.g., flosequinan), a disturbing trend emerged: Initial positive hemodynamic effects during the first few weeks to months of therapy with all of these drugs was followed by a trend toward increased mortality compared with placebo with continued therapy. The explanation for these unexpected findings are related to an overall undesirability of further enhancing sympathetic tone, overstimulation of an already fatigued heart, or proarrhythmic effects of some of the drugs. Whatever the mechanism, the enthusiasm for using inotropic therapy has waned. It is important, however, not to extrapolate these results to digoxin in light of the newer findings that digoxin also has neurohumoral modulating effects. All inotropes are relatively contraindicated in diastolic HF.

Calcium Channel Blockers

Amlodipine (Norvasc), felodipine (Plendil), isradipine (DynaCirc), nifedipine (Adalat, Procardia), and nicardipine (Cardene) are examples of calcium antagonists with arterial vasodilating and antispasmodic properties. They offer the theoretic advantage of being afterload-reducing agents in HF, but their applicability in systolic dysfunction is diminished by negative inotropic effects. Among these drugs, only amlodipine[78] and felodipine[79] have been documented to be safe in HF (i.e., do not make HF worse), but only a small subset of patients with nonischemic dilated cardiomyopathy actually had a positive beneficial effect with amlodipine.[78] Until more data are available, calcium channel blockers other than amlodipine and felodipine are contraindicated in patients with systolic dysfunction. On the other hand, the negative inotropic effects of some calcium antagonists, especially that of verapamil (Calan, Isoptin, Verelan), is an indication for use in diastolic HF.

PATIENT EVALUATION

Signs and Symptoms

1. A.J., a 58-year-old man, is admitted with a chief complaint of increasing shortness of breath (SOB) and an 8 kg weight gain. Two weeks before admission, he noted the onset of dyspnea on exertion (DOE) after one flight of stairs, orthopnea, and ankle edema. Since then, his symptoms have increased. He has also noted episodic bouts of paroxysmal nocturnal dyspnea (PND). Since then, he has been able to sleep only in a sitting position. A.J. notes a productive cough, nocturia (two to three times/night), and mild, dependent edema.

A.J.'s other medical problems include a long history of heartburn; a 10-year history of osteoarthritis, managed with various nonsteroidal anti-inflammatory drugs (NSAID); depression, and hypertension, which has been poorly controlled with hydrodiuril (HCTZ). A strong family history of diabetes mellitus is also present.

Physical examination reveals dyspnea, cyanosis, and tachycardia. A.J. has the following vital signs: BP, 160/100 mm Hg; pulse, 90 beats/minute; and respiratory rate, 28 breaths/minute. He is 5 ft 11 in tall and weighs 78 kg. His neck veins are distended. On cardiac examination, an S_3 gallop is heard; point of maximal impulse (PMI) is at the sixth intercostal space (ICS), 12 cm from the midsternal line (MSL). His liver is enlarged and tender to palpation, and a positive hepatojugular reflux (HJR) is observed. He is noted to have 3+ pitting edema of the extremities and sacral edema. Chest examination reveals inspiratory rales and rhonchi bilaterally.

The medication history reveals the following current medications: HCTZ 25 mg QD; ibuprofen (Motrin) 600 mg QID; ranitidine (Zantac) 150 mg QHS; citalopram (Lexapro) 20 mg QD. He has no allergies and no dietary restrictions.

Admitting laboratory values include the following: hematocrit (Hct), 41.1% (normal, 40%–45%); white blood cell (WBC) count, 5,300/mm^3 (normal, 5,000–10,000/mm^3); Na, 132 mEq/L (normal, 136–144 mEq/L); potassium (K), 3.2 mEq/L (normal, 3.5–5.3 mEq/L); chloride (Cl), 100 mEq/L (normal, 96–106 mEq/L); bicarbonate, 30 mEq/L (normal, 22–28 mEq/L); magnesium (Mg), 1.5 mEq/L (normal, 1.7–2.7 mEq/L); fasting blood sugar (FBS), 100 mg/dL (normal, 65–110 mg/dL); uric acid, 8 mg/dL (normal, 3.5–7 mg/dL); blood urea nitrogen (BUN), 40 mg/dL (normal, 10–20 mg/dL); serum creatinine (SrCr), 0.8 mg/dL (normal, 0.5–1.2 mg/dL); alkaline phosphatase, 44 U (normal, 40–80 U/L); aspartate aminotransferase (AST), 30 U/L (normal, 8–42 U/L); BNP 364 pcg/mL (normal <200 pcg/mL); and thyroid-stimulating hormone (TSH) 2.0 μU/mL (0.5–5.0 μU/mL) The chest radiograph shows bilateral pleural effusions and cardiomegaly.

What signs, symptoms, and laboratory abnormalities of HF does A.J. exhibit? Relate these clinical findings to the pathogenesis of the disease and to left-sided or right-sided HF.

[SI units: Hct, 0.411 (normal, 0.4–0.45); WBC count, 5.3 109/L (normal, 5.0–10.0); Na, 132 mmol/L (normal, 136–144); K, 3.2 mmol/L (normal, 3.5–5.3); Cl, 90 mmol/L (normal, 96–106); bicarbonate, 30 mmol/L (normal, 22–28); Mg, 0.1 mmol/L (normal, 0.85–1.35); FBS, 6.661 mmol/L (normal, 3.608–6.106); uric acid, 475.84 mmol/L (normal, 208.18–416.36); BUN, 14.28 mmol/L (normal, 3.57–7.14); SrCr, 70.72 mmol/L (normal, 44.2–106.08); alkaline phosphatase, 120 U (normal, 40–80); and AST, 100 U/L (normal, 8–42 U/L)(normal LFT, Na and Mg, chloride)]

The signs and symptoms of HF observed in A.J. are easily visualized when recalling that the work of the left ventricle is the major determinant of CO and that blood flows from the left ventricle into the arterial system, through capillaries into the venous system, and back into the right side of the heart. From the right side, the blood circulates through the pulmonary tree and back into the left ventricle. Thus, left-sided ventricular dysfunction primarily causes pulmonary symptoms because of back-up of blood into the lungs, whereas right-sided ventricular dysfunction causes mostly signs of systemic venous congestion. Although left ventricular failure usually develops first, most patients, including A.J., present with signs of combined left- and right-sided failure. The signs and symptoms of both left-sided and right-sided ventricular dysfunction are summarized in Table 18-6.

Table 18-6 Signs and Symptoms of Heart Failure

	Left Ventricular Failure	Right Ventricular Failure[a]
Subjective	DOE SOB Orthopnea (two to three pillows) PND, cough Weakness, fatigue, confusion	Peripheral edema Weakness, fatigue
Objective	LVH ↓BP EF <40%[b] Rales, S_3 gallop rhythm Reflex tachycardia ↑BUN (poor renal perfusion)	Weight gain (fluid retention) Neck vein distention Hepatomegaly Hepatojugular reflux

[a] Isolated right-sided failure occurs with long-standing pulmonary disease (cor pulmonale) or after pulmonary hypertension.
[b] Ejection fraction normal in patients with diastolic dysfunction.
BP, Blood pressure, BUN, blood urea nitrogen; DOE, dyspnea on exertion; EF, ejection fraction; LVH, left ventricular hypertrophy; PND, paroxysmal nocturnal dyspnea; SOB, shortness of breath.

Left-Sided Heart Failure (Left Ventricular Dysfunction)

Weakness, fatigue, and cyanosis result from decreased CO and compromised tissue perfusion. If the left ventricle is not emptied completely, blood backs up into the pulmonary circulation. SOB, dyspnea (labored or uncomfortable breathing) on exertion (DOE), a productive cough, rales (crackles in the lung during auscultation), pleural effusions on chest radiograph, and cyanosis all result from pulmonary congestion. Pulmonary symptoms are aggravated in the reclining position, which minimizes the gravitational effects on excess fluids in the extremities and improves venous return to the heart and lungs. SOB in the prone position (orthopnea) is quantified by the number of pillows the patient must lie on to sleep comfortably. A.J., for example, could sleep only sitting upright. PND, also called *cardiac asthma*, is characterized by severe SOB that awakens the patient from sleep and is alleviated by an upright position. PND results from pulmonary vascular congestion that has advanced to pulmonary edema and bronchospasm while the patient sleeps.

Left ventricular hypertrophy (LVH) and cardiac dilation are caused by an increased end-diastolic volume (see section on Pathogenesis). These effects are observed on chest radiography as an enlarged heart silhouette. The PMI corresponds to the apex of the left ventricle and is visualized as an external pulsation on the left side of the chest. It is displaced laterally and downward from its normal location at the fifth intercostal space, <10 cm from the midsternal line. An S_3 gallop rhythm denotes a third heart sound often heard in close time proximity to the second heart sound (closing of the aortic and pulmonary valves) in HF. Rapid filling of the ventricles causes the S_3 sound and, in an adult, usually indicates decreased ventricular compliance. In patients with mitral valve regurgitation, an S_3 heart sound is common and denotes systolic dysfunction and elevated filling pressure. *Tachycardia* is caused by compensatory increases in sympathetic tone.

Weight gain and *edema* reflect sodium and water retention resulting from decreased renal perfusion (see section on Pathogenesis). As RBF and GFR decrease, a disproportionate amount of BUN may be retained. This phenomenon is termed *prerenal azotemia* and may be detected by an elevated BUN-to-serum creatinine ratio of >20:1. A.J. has a ratio of >40:1. Prerenal azotemia also can be caused by dehydration and overuse of diuretics. Frequency of urination at night (*nocturia*) is because of improved perfusion of the kidney when the patient is lying down.

Right-Sided Heart Failure (Right Ventricular Dysfunction)

The signs and symptoms of right ventricular dysfunction are related either to hypervolemia or the back-up of blood from the right ventricle into the peripheral venous circulation. The overall effect is development of *systemic venous hypertension.*

Dependent pitting edema results from increased venous and capillary hydrostatic pressure, causing a redistribution of fluid from the intravascular to interstitial spaces. Ankle and pretibial edema are common findings after prolonged standing or sitting because fluid tends to localize in the dependent portions of the body secondary to gravitational forces. Sacral edema can be present in patients at bed rest. Edema is subjectively quantified on a 1+ (minimal) to 4+ (severe) scale. A.J. has 3+ pitting edema.

Hepatomegaly, hepatic tenderness, and ascites (fluid in the abdomen) arise from hepatic venous congestion and increased portal vein pressure. Metabolism of drugs highly dependent on the liver for body elimination can be notably impaired by both the backward venous congestion of the liver from right-sided heart failure and the decreased arterial perfusion of the liver from left-sided heart failure. Congestion of the GI tract makes the patient *anorectic.*

Neck vein distention, primarily seen as internal jugular venous distention (JVD), denotes an elevated jugular venous pressure (JVP). How high the neck veins are distended while the patient is lying down and how much the patient's head has to be raised before the JVD disappears give the clinician a rough estimate of the patient's central venous pressure (CVP). Jugular distension in centimeters is measured as the vertical distance from the top of the venous pulsation down to the sternal angle. Neck vein distension of <4 cm when the patient is lying with the head elevated at a 45 degree angle is considered normal for an average, healthy adult. Applying pressure to the liver can cause further distention of the neck veins if hepatic venous congestion is present. This phenomenon is termed *hepatojugular reflux.*

Ejection Fraction Measurement

2. Does A.J. have systolic or diastolic HF?

Shortness of breath, crackles on auscultation, neck vein distention, edema, and nearly all of A.J.'s other signs and symptoms are common between either form of left ventricular HF. An enlarged heart on a chest radiograph increases the suspicion of systolic failure, but this finding can be absent in some patients with systolic failure and present in others with diastolic failure.

The only correct way to differentiate systolic from diastolic failure is by measuring the LVEF. Thus, it is imperative that A.J., as with all patients with suspected HF, have an EF measured before beginning therapy because the treatment strategies between the two disorders differ. Two-dimensional echocardiography coupled with Doppler flow studies (Doppler echocardiogram) is the diagnostic test of choice for measuring EF. This procedure uses sound waves, similar to sonar technology, to visualize and measure ventricular wall thickness, chamber size, valvular functioning, and pericardial thickness. EF is visually estimated based on changes in ventricular chamber size between diastole and systole. This method of EF measurement is not as technically accurate as that provided by ventriculography, but the procedure is more comfortable for the patient, and the correlation of the measured EF to that of the other methods is acceptable. The EF results from echocardiography are graded as normal, or mildly, moderately, or severely depressed.

Radionuclide left ventriculography (also called a multiple gated acquisition [MUGA] scan) uses radiolabeled technetium as a tracer to measure left ventricular hemodynamics. Although this method is the most accurate measurement of EF, it is moderately invasive because it requires venipuncture and radiation exposure. In addition, radionuclide scanning does not provide information on the architecture of the left ventricle. Magnetic resonance imaging and computed tomography are useful in evaluating ventricular mass but do not provide EF data.

Subsequently, A.J. underwent an echocardiogram. The results were reported as LVH with mild to moderate depression of EF, correlating approximately to an EF of 30% to 40%. This indicates mild systolic dysfunction. Because he has the combination of systolic dysfunction and classic congestive signs, he fits the criteria for having true CHF.

Stages of Heart Failure and New York Heart Association Classification

3. What stage of HF does A.J. exhibit according the ACA/AHA criteria? How severe is A.J.'s disability according to the NYHA functional classification of HF?

The ACA/AHA staging scheme and the NYHA functional classification are described in the pathogenesis section of this chapter and are summarized in Table 18-3.[6,22]

Because A.J. has active symptoms of HF and structural changes in cardiac architecture, he is in ACA/AHA stage C. On admission, A.J. is in NYHA functional class III_B or IV_A as evidenced by a need to sleep upright and an inability to undertake even minimal physical activity. Two years ago he would have been considered NYHA class II, but 3 weeks ago he was classified class III_A. Because he will not require inotropic support, he is not in ACA/AHA stage D.

Predisposing Factors

4. What factors contributed to the cause of A.J.'s HF?

Age and Hypertension

A.J.'s age of 58 puts him in a high-risk category for development of CV disease. He is especially vulnerable to HF because of his poorly controlled hypertension, which places an increased afterload on his left ventricle.

Nonsteroidal Anti-Inflammatory Drugs and Sodium Content

Ibuprofen used for A.J.'s arthritis could contribute to sodium overload. All NSAID (including COX-2 inhibitors) have well–documented, renally mediated sodium–retaining properties, increasing the blood volume by up to 50% in some individuals (see Chapter 43, Rheumatoid Disorders).[80] Published epidemiologic studies have indicated that NSAID can exacerbate HF symptoms, resulting in hospitalizations for HF.[81–83] This has been reported in patients with or without a previous diagnosis of HF.[84] NSAID exert their anti-inflammatory effects by inhibiting prostaglandins (PG) (prostacyclin and thromboxane). In the presence effective circulating volume depletion (HF or renal insufficiency), renal perfusion depends on prostaglandin synthesis. Blocking PG leads to sodium reabsorption, thus counteracting the beneficial effects of diuretics and ACE inhibitors. Without a compelling reason for their use, NSAID should be avoided in patients with HF.

Another potential source for sodium overload is in IV formulations. Sodium chloride is often used as a diluent for IV drug administration. Selected parenteral antibiotics, particularly nafcillin and ticarcillin, have high sodium content which should not be overlooked. Likewise, many over-the-counter (OTC) products, such as effervescent antacids and headache powders contain sodium bicarbonate (Alka-Seltzer, Bromo-Seltzer, Goody's Headache powder), making these drugs exceptionally high sources of sodium. Most prescription and nonprescription drug labels carry a disclosure of sodium content, however.

A.J.'s hypertension and HF are both poorly controlled and he has gained 8 kg. His clinical presentation (orthopnea, dyspnea, SOB, lower extremity edema, elevated JVP) clearly indicate fluid overload. This could be a result of high-dose ibuprofen use. His HCTZ should be replaced by a loop diuretic to enhance diuresis and resolve signs and symptoms of HF. Also, an ACE inhibitor should be added to the current regimen for BP control. Once he is euvolemic, consider adding a β-blocker before discharge. Lowering the dose or preferably discontinuing all NSAID might reduce sodium retention and edema and allow ACE inhibitor therapy to be more effective. Acetaminophen is an alternative for treating his osteoarthritis, although it lacks anti-inflammatory properties.

Diet

It is possible that A.J.'s diet contains a considerable excess of sodium from foods such as canned soups and vegetables, potato chips, or overuse of salt at mealtime. Dietary supplements (e.g., Ensure and Sustacal) and sports drinks (e.g., Gatorade) can also be rich sources of sodium. He should follow a controlled-sodium (e.g., 2–3 g/day) diet. If salt substitutes are used, he should be warned that they are high in potassium and could cause hyperkalemia if used concurrently with potassium supplements, an aldosterone inhibitor (spironolactone), or other potassium-sparing diuretics (amiloride, triamterene).

Drug-Induced Heart Failure

5. What are the basic mechanisms by which drugs can induce HF, and how can an understanding of these mechanisms be predictive of drugs to avoid in A.J.?

Drug-induced HF is mediated by three basic mechanisms: inhibition of myocardial contractility (negative inotropic agents), proarrhythmic effects, or expansion of plasma volume (Table 18-7). The latter category includes drugs that act primarily on the kidney (to either alter RBF or increase

Table 18-7 Drugs That May Induce Heart Failure

Negative Inotropic Agents	
β-Blockers[a]	Most evident with propranolol or other nonselective agents
	Less with agents with intrinsic sympathomimetic activity (acebutolol, carteolol, pindolol); can also be caused by use of timolol eye drops
Calcium channel blockers[a]	Verapamil has most negative inotropic and AV-blocking effects; amlodipine has least
Antiarrhythmics	Most with disopyramide (Norpace); also quinidine
	Least with amiodarone
Direct Cardiotoxins	
Cocaine, amphetamines	Overdoses and long-term myopathy
Anthracycline cancer chemotherapeutic drugs	Daunomycin and doxorubicin (Adriamycin); dose related; keep total cumulative dose <600 mg/m^2
Proarrhythmic Effects	
Class IA, IB, Class III antiarrhythmic drugs	QT interval widening
	Probable torsade de pointe
	HF develops if disturbed rhythm compromises cardiac functioning
Non-antiarrhythmic drugs	Same mechanism as above
(See reference 87 for a complete list)	Often associated with drug interactions that inhibit metabolism of the offending drug leading to higher than desired plasma levels
Expansion of Plasma Volume	
Antidiabetics	Metformin high dose may increase risk of lactic acidosis.
	Na retention with pioglitazone (Actos) and rosiglitazone (Avandia)
NSAID	Prostaglandin inhibition; Na retention
Glucocorticoids, androgens, estrogens	Mineralocorticoid effect; Na retention
Licorice	Aldosterone-like effect; Na retention
Antihypertensive vasodilators (hydralazine, methyldopa, prazosin, minoxidil)	↓Renal blood flow, activation of renin-angiotensin system
Drugs high in Na$^+$	Selected IV cephalosporins and penicillins
	Effervescent or bicarbonate containing antacids or analgesics
	Also liquid nutrition supplements
Unknown Mechanism	
Tumor necrosis factor antagonists	Multiple case reports of new-onset HF or exacerbation of prior HF with etanercept and infliximab in patients with Crohns disease or rheumatoid arthritis

[a] β-Blockers and verapamil may be beneficial in diastolic HF. Carvedilol and metoprolol counteract autonomic hyperactivity in systolic dysfunction.
AV, atrioventricular; HF, heart failure; IV, intravenous; Na, sodium; NSAID, nonsteroidal anti-inflammatory drugs.

sodium retention) or those that increase total body sodium and water because of their high sodium content.

The most recognized negative inotropic agents are the β-blockers. Nonselective β-adrenergic blockers (e.g., propranolol) decrease myocardial contractility and slow the HR. Both of these factors can compromise the heart's ability to empty effectively. Therefore, these drugs should not be used in systolic HF. Other well-documented negative inotropes include the calcium channel blockers (CCB), most notably verapamil (Calan, Isoptin); various antiarrhythmic agents, especially disopyramide (Norpace), quinidine, and other class IA drugs; and the anthracycline cancer chemotherapeutic agents (daunomycin and doxorubicin [Adriamycin]). The anthracyclines have a direct, dose-related cardiotoxicity that can be minimized by limiting total cumulative doses to 500 to 600 mg/m^2.[85,86] For a more detailed description of anthracycline toxicity (see Chapter 89, Adverse Effects of Chemotherapy). In the final group of drugs gaining increased notoriety as cardiotoxins are the amphetamine-like drugs and cocaine when used chronically in large quantities or after an overdose.

Drugs that increase the QT interval induce proarrhythmic effects in some patients. Worsening of HF occurs if the disturbed rhythm compromises cardiac functioning. Of particular concern is drug-induced torsade de pointes. Paradoxically, class IA (quinidine, disopyramide, and procainamide), class IC (encainide, flecainide, and propafenone), and class III (amiodarone, dofetilide, ibutilide, and sotalol) antiarrhythmics are among the best-documented proarrhythmic drugs. A multitude of noncardiac drugs, however, also are associated with QT interval prolongation and torsade de pointe (see Chapter 19, Cardiac Arrhythmias).[87]

Examples of drugs that induce sodium and water retention are NSAID (via prostaglandin inhibition), certain antihypertensive drugs, glucocorticoids, androgens, estrogens, and licorice. Weight gain accompanied by peripheral and pulmonary edema has been observed in patients with stable HF given the thiazolidinedione antidiabetic drugs pioglitazone and rosiglitazone.[88] Worsening of HF appears to be dose dependent and is presumed to be at least partly caused by fluid retention. As a consequence, the FDA requires that the package insert for these two drugs recommend they not be administered to patients with NYHA class III or IV HF and that they be used cautiously in earlier stages of HF. Antihypertensive drugs either decrease RBF via direct vasodilation (e.g., hydralazine, minoxidil, diazoxide) or via inhibition of the autonomic nervous system (e.g., guanethidine, methyldopa). Glucocorticoids and licorice (glycyrrhizic acid, carbenoxolone) have an aldosterone-like action.

TREATMENT

Therapeutic Objectives

6. What are the therapeutic goals in treating A.J.?

Cure is not a feasible therapeutic objective in patients with any form of HF. Exceptions include patients who are candidates for cardiac transplantation or in certain forms of idiopathic dilated cardiomyopathy (e.g., viral origin). The immediate objective for A.J. is to provide symptomatic relief as assessed by a reduction in his complaints of SOB and PND, improved sleep quality, and increased exercise tolerance. Over the next several days or weeks, the goal will be to get him back to his baseline status of NYHA class II or III HF. Parameters used to measure success in meeting this objective include reduced peripheral and sacral edema, weight loss, slowing of the HR to <90 beats/minute, normalization of BP, reduction of the BUN back to baseline, a smaller heart size on chest radiograph, decreased neck vein distention, loss of the S_3 heart sound, and an improved EF.

Long-range goals are to improve A.J.'s quality of life, including better tolerance of daily life activities, fewer future hospitalizations, avoidance of side effects of his therapy, and ultimately, an increased survival time. The achievement of these goals depends on the severity of A.J.'s disease, his understanding of his disease, and his adherence to prescribed interventions.

Diuretics

7. Bed rest and a 3-g sodium diet were ordered. Why should A.J. continue his diuretic therapy?

Excessive volume increases the workload of a compromised heart, and diuretics are an integral part of therapy. This is especially true if volume overload is symptomatic (e.g., pulmonary congestion) as it is in A.J. Diuretics produce symptomatic improvement more rapidly than any other drug for HF. They can relieve pulmonary and peripheral edema within hours or days, whereas the clinical effects of ACE inhibitors, β-blockers, and digoxin take weeks to months to be fully realized. Diuretics, however, should not be used alone in HF. Even when they are initially successful in controlling symptoms and reducing edema, they are ineffective in maintaining clinical stability for long periods without the addition of other drugs. More importantly, activation of the renin-angiotensin-aldosterone and sympathetic nervous systems in response to diuresis could possibly lead to HF progression.

Current guidelines all recommend diuretic therapy, both acutely and chronically, if clinical volume overload is evident, but further state that patients without peripheral or pulmonary edema can be treated either intermittently or without diuretics.[1–3,6,7] Diuretics used on an intermittent (as-needed) basis are titrated based on changes in weight gain, neck vein distention, peripheral edema, or SOB. Patients with a good understanding of their disease can be instructed to weigh themselves daily and start taking their medicine if they gain more than 1 to 2 pounds in 1 day or 5 pounds over 1 week or have leg swelling. Doses can be withheld as long as patients are at their target weight. In other cases, diuretic-free intervals or weekends can be arranged. Even with these options, if the patient has experienced volume overload at some time during the course of his or her disease, either past or present, a diuretic should always be part of the regimen.[6,7]

Despite their remarkable initial benefits, vigorous diuretic therapy carries the risk of volume depletion and diminished CO. Abrupt worsening of renal function (increased BUN or SrCr) or hypotension indicates the need to consider temporarily discontinuing diuretics.

Essentially, all patients with clinically evident HF require loop diuretics. A.J. has obvious signs of volume overload, indicating a need for more vigorous diuresis with a loop diuretic. His elevated BUN is worrisome and could worsen if he becomes dehydrated. The more likely outcome, however, is improved renal blood flow as his heart failure symptoms resolve, and subsequently improved renal function tests.

Furosemide and Other Loop Diuretics

8. It is decided to begin a combination regimen of furosemide and an ACE inhibitor for A.J. What route, dose, and dosing schedule of furosemide should be used?

ROUTE OF ADMINISTRATION

The pharmacology and dose comparison of loop diuretics is discussed in the Treatment Principles section of this chapter and in Table 18-4. Furosemide is the most commonly used loop diuretic for HF because of greater clinical experience and low cost. Bumetanide and torsemide are preferred in some settings because of more predictable absorption.[54,55,89,90]

According to one group of investigators, patients with HF treated with torsemide fare better than those receiving furosemide.[90] During a 1-year open-label trial of 234 subjects, patients receiving torsemide were less likely to be admitted to the hospital for HF (17% with torsemide versus 32% for furosemide; $p = 0.01$). Admissions for all cardiovascular causes were also lower among patients taking torsemide (44%) than patients taking furosemide (59%). No differences were found in all cause hospital admission between the two groups (71% torsemide, 76% furosemide). Fatigue scores improved better in patients treated with torsemide, but no difference was found between groups in the rate of dyspnea score improvement. Because generic furosemide is much less costly to prescribe, routine switching to torsemide cannot be advocated until these results are verified by a double-blind, placebo-controlled trial.

Erratic responses to furosemide are more prevalent in persons with severe HF or diminished renal function. Some patients respond promptly and vigorously to small oral doses of furosemide, whereas others require large IV doses to achieve only minimal diuresis. Part of these differences can be explained by the drug's pharmacokinetics.[54,91] Oral absorption of furosemide is incomplete, averaging 50% to 60% in healthy subjects and 43% to 46% in those with renal failure. When taken with a meal, absorption is delayed because of slowed gastric emptying, but the total amount absorbed does not differ significantly from that in fasting states. Claims are that the absorption and, therefore, effectiveness of furosemide is further diminished in patients with HF attributable to edema of the bowel and decreased splanchnic blood flow. This has been partially refuted by one investigator, who noted an average furosemide bioavailability of 61% in patients with HF, the same as in normal patients.[92] Total absorption in patients with HF varies widely (34%–80%), however, and both the rate of absorption and time to peak urinary excretion are delayed for furosemide and bumetanide.[54,55,92]

When interpreting these bioavailability data, another important factor must be considered. The rate and extent of absorption are not only different among individuals (as illustrated by the examples already given), but intraindividual variability also exists. Ingestion of the same brand of furosemide by the same individual on multiple occasions can show up to a threefold difference in bioavailability. These differences are evident whether considering the innovator's brand (Lasix) or one of several generic brands.[54,55,93,94] As with digoxin, these data on bioavailability differences are old and have not been verified or refuted by newer studies.

It might inferred that IV therapy is the preferred route, giving a better response for any given dose. Surprisingly, this is not always the case. In both healthy volunteers and patients with HF, total daily fluid and electrolyte loss after oral therapy and parenteral therapy are comparable. The major difference is in the time course of response. During the first 2 hours, diuresis from the IV dose far exceeds that from the oral therapy, but by 4 to 6 hours, the total urinary output is equivalent.[92,95,96] Therefore, considering the significant cost differential between oral and parenteral furosemide, the clinical advantage in using IV therapy is small. Exceptions to the rule are those patients with severe pulmonary edema who need acute symptomatic relief and those patients who have failed to respond to an adequate oral challenge.

DOSING

Typically, a patient's treatment is initiated with 20 to 40 mg of oral or IV furosemide given as a single dose and monitored for responsiveness (Table 18-4). If the desired diuresis is not obtained, the dose can be increased in 40- to 80-mg increments over the next several days to a total daily dose of 160 mg/day, usually divided into two doses. For torsemide, a usual starting dose is 10 to 20 mg/day, but a ceiling effect is noted in patients with HF at a dosage of 100 to 200 mg/day.[54,97] Equivalent doses of bumetanide are 0.5 to 1.0 mg once or twice daily, titrated to a maximum of 10 mg daily. Because A.J. is not in acute distress, it could be argued that oral therapy would suffice. The decision, however, is to give a single 40 mg IV dose of furosemide for immediate symptom control, followed by 40 mg each morning.

Opinions differ to whether furosemide should be given once daily or in multiple doses. The drug's short half-life of 2 to 4 hours implies the need for multiple dosing. Nonetheless, equivalent daily diuresis has been observed following the same dose given in single or divided doses.[98] Another investigator found better effects from divided doses.[99] Because evening and nighttime doses of diuretics often disturb patients' sleep patterns (because of nocturnal diuresis), the total daily dose usually should be given as a single morning dose. For patients with symptomatic nocturnal dyspnea, two-thirds of the dose is given in the morning and one-third in the late afternoon or, if necessary, at night. Torsemide (Demadex) has a slightly longer half-life and generally can be given once daily.

Adverse Effects

9. Examine A.J.'s laboratory values (see Question 1). Does A.J. have any of abnormal values? What is the significance of these abnormalities?

More thorough discussions of diuretic-induced side effects are found in Chapter 11, Fluid and Electrolyte Disorders and Chapter 13, Essential Hypertension. Those findings pertinent to A.J.'s case are discussed below.

AZOTEMIA

A.J. has an elevated BUN (40 mg/dL) but a normal SrCr (0.8 mg/dL). Normally, a BUN-to-creatinine ratio of 10 to 20:1 is seen. Progressive renal failure is characterized by an elevation of both BUN and creatinine. A disproportionately elevated BUN relative to creatinine is indicative of prerenal azotemia, the major cause of which is dehydration (e.g., overdiuresis) or poor renal perfusion (e.g., HF). SCr will also rise in some patients with prerenal azotemia, but will quickly return to normal with rehydration.

A.J.'s laboratory values reflect prerenal azotemia, but his edematous state and elevated BP point to a cause other than dehydration. The most probable cause of his azotemia is decreased RBF secondary to uncompensated HF. Diuretics should not be withheld and, in fact, judicious diuresis should improve his HF and help lower his BUN. Caution must be exercised because prolonged overdiuresis and dehydration can cause renal ischemia, leading to true renal damage. If this happens, the SCr also will begin to rise (see also Question 23).

HYPONATREMIA

A marginally low serum sodium of 132 mEq/L is noted. Low serum sodium, however, is *not* necessarily a sign of overdiuresis. Serum sodium reported by the laboratory is the *concentration* of sodium in the serum. A person may be significantly overdiuresed (dehydrated) with a large body deficit of sodium, but if that sodium is lost isotonically, the serum sodium concentration will be normal. Conversely, a person such as A.J. can be volume overloaded (edema and hypertension), indicating excessive body sodium, but the serum sodium concentration may be normal or even low as explained below.

Hyponatremia (low serum sodium concentration) reflects the dilutional effect of extra free water in the plasma on sodium concentration. The most common causes of dilutional hyponatremia are excess ADH production or excessive water drinking (i.e., electrolyte-free fluids). Following a severely sodium-restricted diets, persons can develop hyponatremia. Likewise, patients given too much diuretic and who are then given salt-free fluids or who have compensatory ADH release by the body can become hyponatremic. Dilutional hyponatremia, resembling the syndrome of inappropriate antidiuretic hormone (SIADH) secretion, has been described following treatment with thiazide and loop diuretics. Patients with HF or hepatic cirrhosis are more likely to develop diuretic-induced dilutional hyponatremia because of preexisting defects in free water clearance. The exact cause of hyponatremia in A.J. is unknown, but his marginally low serum sodium does not contraindicate continued diuretic therapy.

HYPOKALEMIA

A.J. has a serum potassium of 3.2 mEq/L. Hypokalemia reflecting total body potassium depletion is a well-described, but often over emphasized, side effect of thiazide and loop diuretics. Using a definition of hypokalemia as a serum potassium <3.5 mEq/L, the incidence is 15% to 40% in patients receiving 50 to 100 mg/day of HCTZ.[100,101] Lower doses of HCTZ (12.5–25 mg), however, can produce similar antihypertensive effect as higher doses, with little, or no change in plasma concentrations of potassium. Hypokalemia is associated with an increased incidence of ventricular arrhythmias. The development of arrhythmias may not be seen until the plasma concentration falls to 3.0 meq/L or lower.[102] Some studies showed increased ectopic activity in persons with serum levels between 3.0 and 3.5 mEq/L.[103–105] These latter studies have been criticized for including patients at high risk for complications. Mild hypokalemia can escalate into life-threatening hypokalemia, however. Also to be taken into account is the serum potassium concentration in patients before therapy, as well as the actual degree of fall in serum potassium. It is estimated that the risk of arrhythmias increases by 27% with each 0.5 meq/L reduction in the plasma potassium concentration below 3.0 mEq/L.[106]

In chronic HF, potassium abnormalities are commonly seen, which is probably caused by the pathophysiologic alterations (renal dysfunction, activation of RAAS, and enhanced sympathetic tone) coupled with mandated aggressive diuresis. Several investigators have reported sudden cardiac death related to low serum potassium levels.[107,108] Consensus guidelines for potassium replacement recommend that in patients with HF, instead of using higher doses of non–potassium-sparing diuretics it would be beneficial to use low doses in combination with potassium-sparing diuretics. This will prevent the risk of sudden cardiac death. Some experts recommend that the best strategy to avoid arrhythmias in patients with HF is to maintain serum potassium levels between 4.5 and 5.0 mEq/L.[109]

A.J.'s serum potassium is 3.2 mEq/L. Although long-term potassium supplementation is not necessary with concomitant administration of ACE inhibitors. A.J. will be receiving increased doses of diuretics over the next several days and, therefore, may need additional potassium supplementation to prevent life-threatening hypokalemia. In addition, he could start digoxin in the future. Because low serum potassium levels predispose a patient to digitalis toxicity (see Questions 41–43), potassium replacement is warranted for A.J. (see Question 10).

HYPOMAGNESEMIA

A.J.'s serum magnesium level is 1.5 mEq/L. Severe hypomagnesemia can lead to somnolence, muscle spasms, a decreased seizure threshold, and cardiac arrhythmias, effects similar to those seen with hypocalcemia and hyperkalemia. Some investigators have claimed that many of the arrhythmias previously ascribed to diuretic-induced hypokalemia were actually caused by diuretic-induced hypomagnesemia.[110] Concurrent hypokalemia and hypomagnesemia can be especially dangerous. A.J. should be given 1 g of $MgSO_4$ IV and observed for changes in his magnesium level. If needed, he could be given oral supplements of magnesium.

HYPERURICEMIA

Increases of 1 to 2 mg/dL in uric acid levels are common during thiazide administration. Rarely, 4- to 5-mg/dL elevations have been reported. A.J. shows an increase of 1 mg/dL. Most patients who develop elevated uric acid levels during treatment with diuretic agents remain asymptomatic and need not be treated. Only those with uric acid levels persistently >10 mg/dL, as well as those with a history of gout or a familial predisposition, should be considered for treatment with urate-lowering agents (see also Chapter 42, Gout and Hyperuricemia).

BNP

A.J.'s BNP is elevated (365 pcg/mL). Various studies evaluating the diagnostic accuracy of BNP and N-terminal pro-B-type natriuetic peptide (NT-ProBNP) have used different cut-offs to define abnormal values. The most commonly used plasma concentration to define the upper limit of normal for BNP is 100 pcg/mL, with concentrations >200 pcg being considered an indicator of heart failure. Corresponding, concentrations for NT-proBNP are 125 pcg/mL for patients <75 years of age and 450 pcg/mL for patients >75 years of age. In patients with renal impairment, the clearance of these peptides is reduced; therefore, the reference range is 200 pcg/mL for BNP and the corresponding value for NT-proBNP is 1200 pcg/mL.[111] Moreover, concentration of these biomarkers is influenced by other factors such as age, sex, obesity, and other cardiac and noncardiac comorbidities. Asymptomatic patients with HF can also present with elevated BNP or NT-proBNP levels. This confounds the accurate interpretation of these markers and makes it challenging to integrate their usefulness into routine clinical practice. Elevated BNP and NT-ProBNP have an established utility in ruling out HF in patients who present to the emergency department with shortness of breath.[112] Measuring BNP levels for monitoring and guiding titration of drug therapy is still under investigation. According to the ACC/AHA guidelines, the value of serial BNP measurements in guiding therapy for patients with HF is not well established.[7] A.J's elevated BNP levels, along with his clinical presentation, is indicative of HF exacerbation.

Potassium Supplementation

10. The physician gave A.J. one 1-g dose of magnesium sulfate and three 20-mEq doses of potassium chloride IV. This raised his serum magnesium to 2.0 and his potassium to 3.9 mEq/L. Should he receive prophylactic magnesium or potassium supplementation? What is the best drug and appropriate dose?

At this time A.J. does not need further magnesium replacement, but his serum magnesium level should be remeasured after he has received furosemide for a few days. If the level drops again, maintenance therapy with oral magnesium oxide tablets can be started.

A fall in serum potassium concentration can be seen within hours of the first dose of a diuretic, and the maximal fall usually is reached by the end of the first week of treatment. Potassium supplementation is not required in all patients receiving diuretics. They should be monitored frequently in the first few months of diuretic therapy to determine their potassium requirements. Similarly, when diuretics are stopped, it can take several weeks for serum potassium to return to normal. Therefore, it is possible that A.J.'s admitting potassium level of 3.2 mEq/L reflects the nadir of his response to HCTZ. His initial response to potassium supplementation shows that his hypokalemia will be easily controlled. It might be argued that he should be observed for a few days and not given further supplements; however, because his diuresis is to be increased and digitalis therapy may later be considered, potassium supplementation is warranted.

DIETARY SUPPLEMENTS AND DOSAGE FORMS

Potassium replacement can be accomplished by one or more of the following: dietary supplementation with potassium-containing foods, pharmacologic replacement with various oral potassium salts, or use of potassium-sparing diuretics. Table 18-8 lists the potassium content of selected foods. Inclusion of these foods in the patient's diet may be all that is required to maintain potassium balance, especially in the 60% to 90% of people who are not susceptible to hypokalemia in the first place. The food products listed are expensive, however, and many are high in sodium, which makes them difficult to use for people following low-salt diets. Salt substitutes are another exogenous source of potassium. Patients using these products liberally may get adequate potassium replacement; in fact, they can contribute to hyperkalemia. Some patients object to the taste of salt substitutes.

Table 18-8 Potassium Content of Selected Foods (400 mg Potassium is Approximately Equal to 10 mEq K^+)[a]

Food	Quantity	Potassium Content (mg) (Approximate)
Meats		
Beef chuck	3 oz	200–400
Beef round	3 oz	200–400
Hamburger	3 oz	200–400
Rib roast	3 oz	200–400
Chicken fryer	4 oz	>400
Turkey	4 oz	200–400
Vegetables		
Artichoke	1 medium	200–400
Avocado	½ uncooked	200–400
Baked potato	1 medium	>400
Sweet corn	½ cup	200–400
Dried beans	8 oz (1 cup) cooked	>400
Lima beans	½ cup	200–400
Tomato	1 medium raw or 4 oz (½ cup) cooked	200–400
Brussels sprouts	½ cup	200–400
Broccoli	4 oz (½ cup cooked)	200–400
Collard greens	4 oz (½ cup cooked)	200–400
Spinach	4 oz (½ cup cooked)	200–400
Winter squash	4 oz (½ cup cooked)	>400
Fruits		
Banana	1 medium	>400
Orange	1 medium	200–400
Grapefruit	1 cup	200–400
Apricot	3 medium	>400
Peach	1 medium	200–400
Nectarine	1 large	>400
Cantaloupe	8 oz (1 cup)	>400
Honeydew melon	8 oz (1 cup)	>400
Watermelon	8 oz (1 cup)	200–400
Raisins	½ cup	>400
Prunes	4 medium	200–400
Dates	4 oz (½ cup)	>400
Juices and milk		
Orange	8 oz (1 cup)	>400
Grapefruit	8 oz	200–400
Pineapple	8 oz	200–400
Prune	8 oz	>400
Tomato	8 oz	>400
Milk	8 oz (1 cup)	200–400

[a] 39 mg K^+ = 1 mEq.

If potassium replacement is prescribed, only *potassium chloride* (KCl) should be used because potassium-wasting diuretics can cause hypochloremic alkalosis; if the chloride ion is not replaced, alkalosis and hypokalemia will persist, even if large quantities of potassium are given.

Klor-Con and Kaon-Cl are slow-release, solid dosage forms of KCl crystals imbedded in a wax matrix. They are equal to KCl solution in bioavailability and are associated with less GI bleeding, ulceration, and stricture formation than enteric-coated potassium tablets. The major drawback to their use is high cost and the large number of tablets needed per day. Klor-Con has only 600 mg (8 mEq) or 750 mg (10 mEq) per tablet. Kaon-Cl contains 750 mg (10 mEq) per tablet. Slow-release potassium tablets should be avoided in patients with impaired GI motility, and enteric-coated potassium tablets should be avoided at all times.

A slow-release, microencapsulated form of KCl (Micro K, multiple generics) was originally postulated to produce fewer GI mucosal ulcerations than wax matrix slow-release tablets.[113] Other investigators, however, could not detect any difference between the two formulations,[114,115] and the Boston Collaborative Drug Surveillance Program could not find a positive association between wax matrix potassium use and significant upper GI bleeding.[116]

Another sustained-release potassium product, K-Dur, available as either 750 mg (10 mEq) or 1,500 mg (20 mEq) tablets, can either be swallowed whole or dissolved in water. It offers the advantage of being tasteless even when prepared as a solution. The only patient complaint is that the capsules dissolve in the mouth if not swallowed quickly.

DOSE REQUIREMENTS

It is difficult to predict the dose of KCl that will be required to maintain proper potassium balance. Many patients do well with 20 mEq/day, but it is questionable how many of these need any supplement at all. People with well-documented hypokalemia can require anywhere from 20 to 120 mEq of KCl/day.[100,101,117] Those patients with disease states associated with high circulating aldosterone levels require doses of potassium in excess of 60 mEq/day.

POTASSIUM-SPARING DIURETICS

11. Would use of a potassium-sparing diuretic such as triamterene offer any advantage over a potassium supplement to prevent or treat hypokalemia? What dose should be used?

The direct-acting, potassium-sparing diuretics (amiloride and triamterene) may be more effective in preventing or correcting the fall in serum potassium than potassium supplements.[118,119] These agents reduce urinary potassium losses, minimize alkalosis, and mobilize edema. Approximate equivalent doses are amiloride 20 mg and triamterene 200 mg. At these doses, potassium-replenishing capacity is similar to that observed with a 10- to 20-mEq KCl supplement.[118]

Dyazide (or generic equivalent) and Maxzide are popular products that contain a combination of triamterene plus HCTZ. Although these products are effective in most cases, their cost is warranted only in a patient with documented hypokalemia with thiazide use alone. In one study, one full-strength Maxzide tablet (50 mg thiazide; 75 mg triamterene) was equivalent to 20 to 40 mEq of KCl.[119] Moduretic (a combination of amiloride plus a thiazide) could also be used.

Hyperkalemia is the major toxicity from all the potassium-sparing diuretics and could occur even when they are used in combination with potassium-wasting diuretics. As a general rule, direct-acting, potassium-sparing diuretics should not be used together with either KCl, ACE inhibitors, ARB, or aldosterone inhibitors (spironolactone). Their combined use is warranted, however, in those patients requiring >50 mEq/day of KCl. Judicious monitoring is necessary to avoid hyperkalemia. (Also see Question 14 for additional considerations for using spironolactone in patients with severe HF.)

Monitoring

12. After a single 40-mg IV dose of furosemide, A.J. is begun on 40 mg of furosemide each morning and KCl tablets 20 mEq BID. How should his therapy be monitored?

A.J. needs to be monitored for both an improvement in his HF and for side effects (Tables 18-6 and 18-9). Subjectively, the clinician should monitor for decreased pulmonary distress and an increased exercise tolerance, demonstrating control of HF. Objective monitoring parameters for disease control include weight loss (ideal, 0.5–1 kg/day until ideal dry weight is achieved), a decrease in edema, flattening of neck veins, and disappearance of the S_3 gallop and rales. Because A.J. has hypertension, his BP also requires monitoring with a goal to reduce it to <120/80 mm Hg.

Table 18-9 Monitoring Parameters with Diuretics

↓CHF symptoms (see Table 18-6)
Weight loss or gain; goal is 1–2 pound weight loss/day until "ideal weight" achieved[a]
Signs of volume depletion
Weakness
Hypotension, dizziness
Orthostatic changes in BP[b]
↓Urine output
↑BUN[c]
Serum potassium and magnesium (avoid hypokalemia and hypomagnesemia)
↑ Uric acid
↑ Glucose

[a] Weight loss may be greater during first few days when significant edema is present.
[b] A ↓ in systolic BP of 10–15 mm Hg or a ↓ in diastolic BP of 5–10 mm Hg.
[c] A rising BUN can be caused by either volume depletion from diuretics or poor renal flow from poorly controlled HF. Small boluses of 0.9% saline can be given cautiously to differentiate a rising BUN from volume depletion versus poor cardiac output. If volume depletion is present, saline will cause an ↑ in urine output and a ↓ in BUN. However, if the patient has severe HF, the saline could cause pulmonary edema.
BP, blood pressure; BUN, blood urea nitrogen; HF, heart failure; K, potassium; Mg, magnesium.

Patients are sometimes instructed to record their weight each day and are allowed to adjust their diuretic dose based on changes observed. If they are at their ideal "dry weight," they may reduce their dose of diuretic by 50% or even hold one or more doses. If weight increases more than 1 or 2 pounds in a day or 5 pounds per week, edema increases, or SOB returns, the dose of diuretic is temporarily increased.

Dizziness and weakness are subjective indices of volume depletion, hypotension, or potassium loss. Muscle cramps and abdominal pain could indicate rapid changes in electrolyte balance. Objectively, a lowering of BP, especially on standing, and a rising BUN (prerenal azotemia) signify overdiuresis. As discussed in Questions 9 and 10, serum sodium, potassium, and uric acid should be monitored routinely. Questioning the patient with regard to the onset of diuresis (relative to drug ingestion) and the duration of the diuretic effect helps develop the most convenient schedule for the patient.

Refractory Patients: Combination Therapy

13. Another patient presents with an initial history was similar to A.J.'s. After nearly 2 years of relatively good HF control on a regimen of 40 mg furosemide, 20 mg QD lisinopril, 200 mg QD metoprolol succinate, and 0.125 mg QD digoxin, urinary output diminished about 1 week ago and edema increased significantly. Nonadherence to drug therapy and salt restriction was ruled out. The dose of furosemide was increased to 80 mg QD two days ago without much effect. Should the dose of furosemide be increased further? Could another diuretic be added to the therapy?

As described in the discussion of the pharmacology of diuretics earlier in the chapter, all loop and thiazide diuretics must reach the tubular lumen to be effective. Because these drugs are highly bound to serum proteins and endogenous organic acids, they cannot enter the tubular lumen by glomerular filtration. For diuresis to begin, they must be transported into the proximal tubule by active secretion from the blood into the tubule. If this active transport is blocked, diuretics will not reach their site of action. This can lead to a diminished diuretic response in patients with either renal insufficiency or decreased RBF associated with uncompensated HF. In particular, patients with renal insufficiency or poor RBF often require large doses of diuretics to achieve a desired response. Endogenous organic acids also can accumulate during renal insufficiency, avidly binding the drug and preventing its access to the site of action.[54,55]

Both the total amount of drug delivered to the tubule and the rate of delivery of the drug to the tubule determine the magnitude of diuretic response elicited.[54,55] This explains why 80 mg of furosemide yields more diuresis than a 40-mg dose and why an IV injection provides a more rapid and vigorous diuresis than an oral dose. Once a threshold concentration (ceiling dose) is achieved within the tubule, higher concentrations produce no greater intensity of effect, but the duration of action may be prolonged. (See Question 8 for an expanded discussion about loop diuretic bioavailability and the concept of "gut wall edema.")

In addition to these explainable causes, many patients develop a blunted diuretic response with continued therapy for unknown reasons. Generally, alternative treatment plans are pursued when the dose given approaches the ceiling doses for each drug listed in Table 18-4. Continuous infusions of furosemide (2.5–3.3 mg/hour), bumetanide (1 mg/hour), or torsemide (3 mg/hour) can be more efficacious than intermittent bolus doses in patients with severe HF or renal insufficiency.[54,55,120–124] Even higher doses are recommended by one clinician: 0.25 to 1 mg/kg/hour for furosemide, 0.1 mg/kg/hour for bumetanide, and 5 to 20 mg/hour for torsemide.[125] Another institution uses an aggressive protocol of a 100-mg IV bolus of furosemide followed by a continuous IV infusion at a rate of 20 to 40 mg/hr, which is doubled every 12 to 24 hours in nonresponding patients to a maximal infusion rate of 160 mg/hr to attain a diuresis rate of 100 mL/hr or higher.[126]

In some instances, switching from one loop diuretic to another can overcome the problem.[55,58,125] For example, torsemide might work when furosemide fails because of more reliable absorption with torsemide.[89,90] If this maneuver fails, a combination of diuretics can be tried. The most effective regimens combine drugs that work at two different parts of the tubule.[55,58] For example, a loop diuretic that works on the ascending limb of the loop of Henle is added to metolazone that blocks sodium reabsorption in the distal tubule. Various thiazide diuretics, including chlorthalidone (Hygroton), chlorothiazide (Diuril), and HCTZ, have been reported to effectively enhance diuresis when combined with a loop diuretic, but it is unclear if the responses are simply additive or truly synergistic. Rarely, triple therapy regimens of metolazone, loop, and potassium-sparing diuretics are used to optimize diuresis and electrolyte control.

Most clinicians choose a combination of metolazone plus furosemide or bumetanide based on demonstrated value in the literature and clinical experience. A small dose of metolazone (5 mg) is first added to the furosemide therapy, doubling the dose of metolazone every 24 hours until the desired diuretic response is achieved. If the synergism desired is seen with the first dose, the dose of the loop diuretic should be decreased. Metolazone's longer duration of action can cause a greater than predicted diuresis and electrolyte loss when combined with a loop diuretic. Thus, careful monitoring of weight, urine output, BP, and BUN is required. Because no parenteral form of metolazone exists, chlorothiazide, at a dose of 500 to 1,000 mg once or twice daily, is the only option for a non–loop diuretic that can be given intravenously.

Nondiuretic Effect of Spironolactone: Effect on Mortality

14. We return now to A.J. who was treated in Questions 1 to 12. It has been 2 days since he started furosemide, potassium supplements, and an ACE inhibitor. He complains of gastric cramping after each dose of potassium, even when taken with food. It is decided to discontinue the potassium supplement and start spironolactone at a dosage of 25 mg/day. Does this therapy offer any advantages other than diuresis and a source of potassium repletion?

Aldosterone contributes to HF through the increased retention of sodium and the depletion of potassium. Likewise, the diuretic and potassium-sparing actions of spironolactone are attributed to inhibition of aldosterone.[118] Until recently, it was believed that optimal doses of ACE inhibitors fully suppressed the production of aldosterone because angiotensin II is a potent stimulus for aldosterone production. It is now recognized, however, that aldosterone levels can remain elevated through a combination of nonadrenal production and reduced hepatic clearance. In addition, it has become clear that both angiotensin II and aldosterone have other negative effects on the CV system, including myocardial and vascular fibrosis, direct vascular damage, endothelial dysfunction, oxidative stress, and prevention of norepinephrine uptake by the myocardium.[27,127] This led the Randomized Aldactone Evaluation Study (RALES) investigators to test the hypothesis that low doses of spironolactone might impart a cardioprotective effect in patients with severe HF independent of diuresis or potassium retention.[57] In this trial, 1,663 patients with a history of NYHA class IV HF within the previous 6 months (but in class III or IV on study entry), an EF of 35% or less, and continued treatment (unless contraindicated or not tolerated) with a loop diuretic (100%), an ACE inhibitor (94%), and digoxin (74%) were randomized to receive either spironolactone 25 mg ($n = 822$) or placebo ($n = 841$). The dose of spironolactone could be increased to 50 mg if HF worsened without evidence of hyperkalemia.

The study was discontinued prematurely after a mean follow-up of 24 months when a statistically significant reduction in mortality was observed. There were 386 deaths in the placebo group (46%) compared with 284 (35%) in the spironolactone group. These differences were first evident at 2 to 3 months after starting treatment. The greatest risk reduction was in CV deaths. In addition, more subjects had symptomatic improvement (as evidenced by moving to a lower NYHA class) and fewer had symptomatic worsening with the active drug. Hospitalization rates were lower in the patients treated with spironolactone. Serum creatinine and potassium concentrations were somewhat higher with active drug, but the changes were not considered clinically significant. Hyperkalemia developed in 2% of the patient on spironolactone and 1% of those on placebo. Gynecomastia was reported in 10% of men treated with spironolactone compared with only 1% of those receiving placebo.

It is important to emphasize that nearly all subjects had continuing HF symptoms despite maximal drug therapy with multiple drugs, including an ACE inhibitor. Although ACE inhibitors indirectly suppress aldosterone at therapeutic doses, the inhibition is not as complete as with spironolactone. Thus, this study provided the first clinical evidence that spironolactone protects against myocardial and vascular fibrosis and alters hemodynamic or hormonal mediators of HF.

Subsequently, the aldosterone receptor inhibitor eplerenone (Inspra) was studied in 6,632 patients with left ventricular dysfunction following MI. In the EPHESUS study, subjects were randomized to receive either eplerenone 25 mg QD initially, titrated to 50 mg QD, or placebo.[58] Concurrent therapy included diuretics (60%), ACE inhibitors (87%), β-blockers (75%), and aspirin (88%). During a mean follow-up of 16 months, there were 478 deaths (14.4%) in the active treatment group compared with 554 deaths (16.7%) with placebo (relative risk, 0.85; $p = 0.008$). Most deaths were from CV causes. Similar to spironolactone, more subjects experienced hyperkalemia with eplerenone than with placebo. Because eplerenone does not block progesterone and androgen receptors, gynecomastia and sexual dysfunction may be less.[58,127] Eplerenone was initially approved by the FDA for hypertension, and gained labeling for patients after MI in late 2003.

Because A.J. had NYHA class III symptoms when first seen, he fits the profile of the subjects in the RALES study, although he had not been taking his ACE inhibitor sufficiently long to obtain the full therapeutic benefit. Starting A.J. on spironolactone is appropriate because of his intolerance of potassium supplements and it might provide CV protection. The dose of 25 mg was chosen for A.J. This was the dose studied in RALES trial. This dose may or may not be sufficient to normalize his serum potassium. He will need to be followed to determine whether larger doses of spironolactone will be necessary or if a small dose of a potassium supplement might need to be restarted. If gynecomastia develops, eplerenone could replace spironolactone. (Also, see Question 21 regarding risk factors for hyperkalemia with spironolactone.)

Drugs of First Choice After Diuretics

Vasodilators and ACE Inhibitors: Comparison With Digoxin

15. The medical resident on your team asks you if it would be appropriate to add digoxin to A.J's medical treatment of HF. He has been told by a colleague that in clinical trials digoxin reduced both HF symptoms and hospitalizations for HF? What would you recommend?

Debates raged for years about whether digitalis glycosides or vasodilators should be the drug(s) of first choice for treating HF. By the time the AHCPR and first ACC/AHA guidelines were published in 1994 to 1995, a clear consensus was evident.[1,2] Vasodilators are first-line therapy, with digoxin being added for patients with either supraventricular arrhythmias, failure to achieve symptomatic relief with vasodilators alone, or intolerable side effects from vasodilators. ACE inhibitors are preferred over other vasodilators because of proved efficacy, convenience of dosing, and fewer side effects. By 1999, experts also recommended starting β-blocker therapy earlier in the treatment plan.[3] This latter point is discussed later. To understand the reason for the increased emphasis on ACE inhibitors and secondary role of digoxin requires an historical overview. A partial review is given here, but the citations and abstract of older articles are found in the sixth edition of *Applied Therapeutics: The Clinical Use of Drugs.*

CONTROVERSY OVER EFFICACY OF DIGOXIN

Correction of the underlying defect is a rational approach to the treatment of any disease. When considering HF solely as "pump failure" with a weakened myocardial muscle, then digitalis is the logical choice to improve cardiac contractility, CO, and renal perfusion. By focusing on symptom relief and increased exercise tolerance as markers of benefit, digoxin is effective. Critics, however, raised concerns that symptom relief was less in patients with normal sinus rhythm than in those with supraventricular arrhythmias. The most vocal critics claimed that the risk of digitalis toxicity did not warrant using this class of drugs in patients with normal sinus rhythm.

Using multivariate analysis, one group of investigators concluded that a third heart sound (S_3 gallop rhythm), an enlarged heart, and a low EF best predict those patients with normal sinus rhythm who will derive a beneficial response from digoxin.[128] Several other meta-analyses and critical reviews of the literature later concurred that many of the original trials were designed improperly or lacked proper controls and that digoxin therapy provides a beneficial effect, especially in patients with severe symptomatic ventricular systolic dysfunction.[129,130]

VASODILATORS IMPROVE SURVIVAL (TABLE 18-10)

While these debates were ongoing, recognition of the contributions of the RAAS and the sympathetic nervous system in perpetuating the defects of HF brought initial interest in vasodilators. Again, the focus was on symptom relief. First hydralazine and nitrates, then their combination, and finally ACE inhibitors were all shown to be effective in reducing the symptoms of HF. Nonetheless, digitalis was usually used

Table 18-10 Clinical Trials of ACE Inhibitors in Left Ventricular Dysfunction[60]

Study	*Patient Population*	*ACE Inhibitor*	*Time Started After MI*	*Treatment Duration*	*Outcome*
Studies in LV Dysfunction					
CONSENSUS[132]	NYHA IV ($n = 253$)	Enalapril vs. placebo		1 day–20 mos	Decreased mortality and HF
SOLVD-Treatment[134]	NYHA II/III ($n = 2{,}569$)	Enalapril vs. placebo		22–55 mo	Decreased mortality and HF
V-HeFT II[135]	NYHA II/III ($n = 804$)	Enalapril vs. hydralazine, isosorbide		0.5–5.7 yrs	Decreased mortality and sudden death
SOLVD-Prevention	Asymptomatic LV dysfunction ($n = 4{,}228$)	Enalapril vs. placebo		14.6–62 mos	Decreased mortality and HF hospitalizations
Studies in LV Dysfunction after MI					
SAVE[193]	MI, decreased LV function ($n = 2{,}331$)	Captopril vs. placebo	3–16 days	24–60 mos	Decreased mortality
CONSENSUS II[192]	MI ($n = 6{,}090$)	Enalaprilat/enalapril vs. placebo	24 hrs	41–180 days	No change in survival; hypotension with enalaprilat
AIRE[194]	MI and HF ($n = 2{,}006$)	Ramipril vs. placebo	3–10 days	>6 mos	Decreased mortality
ISIS-4[335]	MI ($n = >50{,}000$)	Captopril vs. placebo	24 hrs	28 days	Decreased mortality
GISSI-3[337]	MI ($n = 19{,}394$)	Lisinopril vs. placebo	24 hrs	6 wks	Decreased mortality
TRACE[148]	MI, decreased LV function ($n = 1{,}749$)	Trandolapril vs. placebo	3–7 days	24–50 mos	Decreased mortality
SMILE[336]	MI ($n = 1{,}556$)	Zofenopril vs. placebo	24 hrs	6 wks	Decreased mortality

Adapted from Brown N, Vaughan D. Angiotensin-converting enzyme inhibitors. *Circulation* 1998;97:1411, with permission from reference.

first, especially in those patients with either supraventricular arrhythmias, an S_3 gallop rhythm, or both. Vasodilators were added to those patients failing a combined regimen of a diuretic and digoxin.

Finally, investigators began focusing on the more important issue of improving survival in patients with HF. The first evidence for decreased mortality came from the First Veteran's Administration Cooperative Study (V-HeFT I), which showed combined hydralazine–isosorbide dinitrate (hydralazine isosorbide dinitrate) treatment reduced mortality to a greater extent than placebo in patients with NYHA class III or IV HF.[131] All subjects continued their previously prescribed diuretic and digitalis regimens. Active intervention consisted of combination hydralazine (300 mg/day) plus isosorbide dinitrate (160 mg/day). Cumulative mortality rates over an average of 2.3 years were significantly lower in the combination therapy group (38.7%) than with placebo (44%). Exercise tolerance and LVEF were improved with combination therapy at both the 8-week and 1-year follow-up, but not in the placebo group.

The Cooperative North Scandinavian Enalapril Survival (CONSENSUS) study was the first to show improved survival in patients with HF treated with an ACE inhibitor.[132,133] A total of 253 men and women with severe HF (NYHA class IV) were treated with either enalapril or placebo. Digitalis, diuretics, and other vasodilators were continued. At the end of 6 months, 42% of patients in the enalapril group showed symptomatic improvement compared with 22% of those on placebo. The mortality rate was 26% in patients treated with enalapril compared with 44% in the placebo group, a 40% reduction. Follow-up at 2 years showed a sustained effect, with mortality being 47% with enalapril and 74% with placebo, a 37% reduction. Almost all deaths were cardiac in origin.

Although the results from both studies were encouraging, the high rate of mortality in the vasodilator groups (even when combined with diuretics and digoxin) is evidence of the poor outcome in patients with advanced HF. This is a sobering reminder of the poor prognosis associated with the later stages of HF despite aggressive therapy. In addition, both V-HeFT I and CONSENSUS I left several questions unanswered: Does vasodilator therapy work without digitalis? Would patients with less advanced HF (NYHA class I or II) show similar benefit? Which is the better treatment regimen, hydral-iso or an ACE inhibitor?

The SOLVD study addressed the issue of treating patients with less severe disease.[134] Subjects with NYHA class II or III HF and an EF <35% were treated with either enalapril at a dosage of 2.5 to 20 mg/day (n = 1,284) or placebo (n = 1,285) in addition to conventional therapy over an average of 41.4 months. Mortality rate was 35.2% in the enalapril group compared with 39.7% in the placebo group, with the greatest benefit being a reduction in deaths attributed to progressive HF. Two lessons can be gained from this trial: Patients with less severe disease also experience symptom improvement from vasodilator therapy, as well as experiencing lower mortality rates.

Next, the second Veteran's Administration Cooperative Study (V-HeFT II)[135,136] sought to answer the question of relative benefit of hydral-iso versus enalapril. Patients receiving diuretics and digoxin for HF of varying degrees of severity (primarily functional class II or III) were randomized to either enalapril at a fixed dose of 20 mg/day or the hydralazine isosorbide dinitrate combination at a dosage of 300 mg hydralazine plus 160 mg of isosorbide. Mortality rates were lower in the enalapril group (18%) than with combination therapy (28%), with the greatest benefit in both groups being for patients with less severe disease (functional class I or II). Although a placebo group was not included in this trial, the survival rate with hydralazine isosorbide dinitrate was the same as seen in V-HeFT I,[131] inferring a beneficial effect with hydralazine isosorbide dinitrate in V-HeFT II as well. In addition, treatment with hydralazine isosorbide dinitrate was more effective than enalapril in improving patients' exercise tolerance and body oxygen consumption during peak exercise. EF also increased faster (but not necessarily to a greater extent) with hydralazine isosorbide dinitrate than with enalapril. In both V-HeFT I[131] and V-HeFT II,[136] enalapril was better tolerated than hydralazine isosorbide dinitrate. In summary, a trend toward better symptom control occurred with hydralazine isosorbide dinitrate, but improved survival and fewer side effects were seen with enalapril. Although not specifically studied in this trial, these trends suggest a possible benefit to using all three drugs in combination together.

In all these trials, the investigators were careful to include only patients with systolic failure as evidenced by an EF <40%. Thus taken as a whole, they provide convincing evidence for the value of vasodilators in systolic failure.

DIGOXIN WITHDRAWAL TRIALS

In 1993, two digoxin withdrawal trials, PROVED[137] and RADIANCE,[138] were published. Both attempted to determine whether patients with HF who are already treated with digoxin will show deterioration of control or remain stable after discontinuation of digoxin. In both studies, patients had documented systolic failure (LVEF <35% by radionuclide ventriculography), mild to moderate symptoms (NYHA class II or III); and they were in normal sinus rhythm and were stable for at least 3 months with a treatment regimen of a diuretic and digoxin (baseline digoxin level 0.9–2.9 ng/mL). A significant difference was that patients in the RADIANCE trial were also stabilized on an ACE inhibitor in addition to the diuretic and digoxin.[137] A 12-week, double-blind, placebo-controlled treatment period followed initial stabilization in both studies. Patients in the active treatment groups continued digoxin at their previous dose. Those in the placebo groups were withdrawn from digoxin and given an identical looking placebo.

In PROVED,[137] 42 subjects continued digoxin and 46 were given placebo. There were 29% treatment failures in the withdrawal group compared with only 19% in those still taking digoxin. Treatment failure was defined as worsening HF symptoms requiring a therapeutic intervention (e.g., increased diuretic dosage or addition of a new drug), an emergency department (ED) visit or hospitalization for HF, or death. Exercise tolerance worsened in more patients taking placebo. Those taking digoxin tended to maintain lower body weight and HR as well as higher EF. In the RADIANCE study, 85 subjects continued digoxin therapy and 93 were switched to placebo.[138] Over the 12-week follow-up period, only 4 of the subjects taking digoxin (4.7%) developed worsening symptoms compared with 23 (24.7%) of the placebo-treated patients. More of the placebo-treated patients had worsening of the EF and lower quality of life scores. The finding that deterioration in symptoms after discontinuing digoxin often was delayed for several weeks offers a possible explanation why earlier clinical trials using shorter observation periods failed to establish a benefit from digoxin. When comparing the two trials directly, fewer patients deteriorated in both arms in the RADIANCE study. Whether this is attributed to a greater benefit from combining an ACE inhibitor with a diuretic compared with using a diuretic alone cannot be established.

These studies establish a beneficial effect of digoxin, even in those patients receiving concurrent ACE inhibitors in RADIANCE. At least two factors, however, limit extrapolation to all patients with HF. First, the investigators only assessed the value of therapy indirectly by using a withdrawal design instead of initiating therapy in patients previously untreated with digoxin. Second, the patients had advanced disease as evidenced by NYHA class II or III symptoms despite triple drug therapy. Thus, the benefit of digoxin as initial monotherapy in early disease is still open to debate.

EFFECT OF DIGOXIN ON MORTALITY

An obvious missing link was whether treatment with digoxin improves survival rates. The seminal study to answer this question is the Digitalis Intervention Group (DIG) study.[139] In this study 6,800 patients with HF from 302 centers in the United States and Canada were randomized to receive either digoxin ($n = 3,397$) or placebo ($n = 3,403$). Eligibility requirements included an EF of 45% or less (mean, 28% in both treatment groups), normal sinus rhythm, and clinical evidence of HF. Most subjects were in NYHA class II or III HF, although a small number of both class I and class IV subjects were included. Concurrent therapies were diuretics (82%), ACE inhibitors (94%), and nitrates (42%). Of subjects in both groups, 44% were taking digoxin before randomization. The starting digoxin dose (or matching placebo) was based on age, weight, and renal function, with subsequent adjustments made according to plasma level measurements. Approximately 70% of subjects in both groups ended up taking 0.25 mg/day, compared with 17.5% taking 0.125 mg/day and 11% receiving dosages of 0.375 mg/day or higher. By 1 month, 88.3% of subjects on active drug had serum levels between 0.5 and 2.0 ng/mL, with a mean of 0.88 ng/mL. Patients were followed for an average of 37 months (range, 28 to 58 months).

For the primary outcome of total mortality from any cause, 34.8% of patients on digoxins and 35.1% of those on placebo patients died; corresponding CV deaths were 29.9% and 29.5%, respectively. Although neither of these differences is statistically different, a trend was seen toward fewer HF-associated deaths and statistically fewer hospitalizations (risk ratio, 0.72) with active treatment. As would be expected, cases of suspected digoxin toxicity were greater in the active treatment group (11.9% vs. 7.9%), but the incidence of true toxicity was low. These results can be interpreted either as disappointing in that overall mortality is not reduced, or as positive in that hospitalizations were fewer in the digoxin group and there is no increase in mortality as reported with nondigitalis inotropes.

This study improves on the PROVED and RADIANCE trials because it added digoxin to other therapy as opposed to being a withdrawal study and also because of the larger study population. Because nearly all patients were receiving concurrent vasodilator therapy, the value of digoxin as monotherapy on mortality rates remains unanswered.

DIRECT COMPARISON OF DIGOXIN TO VASODILATORS

Little data are available to directly compare digoxin with an ACE inhibitor.[140–142] Two widely quoted studies are the Captopril-Digoxin Multicenter Research Group Study[141] and the Canadian Enalapril vs. Digoxin Study Group trial.[142] Similarities between these two trials are inclusion of NYHA class II or III patients, all of whom had a reduced EF and were in normal sinus rhythm. All subjects continued to take diuretics, but other vasodilator therapy was discontinued. About half of the patients had an S_3 gallop rhythm, and about 60% were taking digoxin before entry into the studies. After an appropriate run-in period during which time diuretic doses were stabilized and previous digoxin therapy was discontinued, patients were randomized to receive either digoxin or an ACE inhibitor.

In the Captopril-Digoxin study, both drugs were superior to placebo as measured by symptom scores and treadmill exercise time.[141] The trend toward a more favorable functional improvement with captopril (41% improving with captopril, 31% with digoxin, 22% with placebo) was nonsignificant. The increase in the EF in the digoxin group was greater. Six-month mortality was unchanged with either drug compared with placebo. More minor side effects were associated with captopril (44% vs. 30%), but more patients had to discontinue digoxin because of side effects (4.2% vs. 2.9%).

In the Enalapril-Digoxin study, more patients in the enalapril group showed functional improvement at 4 weeks (18% vs. 10%) and fewer showed functional deterioration (12.5% vs. 23%).[142] By the end of 14 weeks, however, an equal number of patients had improved with both drugs (19%), but more patients continued to show deterioration with digoxin (30% vs. 12.5%). No differences in the more objective measurements of exercise time, left ventricular function, BP, pulse, and electrocardiographic (ECG) changes were noted between the two groups. More patients withdrew from the digoxin arm because of side effects.

Taken in the aggregate, these studies show no clear benefit of one class of drug vs. the other; ACE inhibitors may be slightly more rapid in onset of effect and associated with better tolerance of side effects, but digoxin may improve EF to a greater extent. Mortality differences were undetectable in the Captopril-Digoxin study because of the relatively mild disease in the patients at the outset resulting in mortality rates of only 6% to 8% in either study group. A larger sample size and longer duration of observation would be required to detect a significant difference in mortality.

To summarize, based on clinical outcomes (resolution of symptoms and improved cardiac function), both vasodilators and digitalis glycosides are effective in patients with documented systolic dysfunction. The documented improvement in survival rates with both hydralazine isosorbide dinitrate and ACE inhibitors, coupled with the neutral findings of the DIG study, tip the balance in favor of ACE inhibitors as initial therapy in all stages of HF. The use of both classes of drugs, plus diuretics, is indicated for severe HF.

The latest clinical ACC/AHA guidelines state that digoxin therapy is unlikely to benefit patients with stage A or stage B HF[7]. In these patients, digoxin can be used for symptom management, only if they are treated with drug therapy shown to prolong survival (ACEI and β-blockers) or have not responded adequately to appropriate therapy. For patients in stage C or stage D HF who are symptomatic, with enlarged heart and reduced LVEF, digoxin can be beneficial. Monotherapy with digoxin or in combination with only a diuretic is no longer recommended.[5]

In the case of A.J., his physician should be discouraged from starting digoxin at this time. Instead, he should be counseled to continue with the already prescribed ACE inhibitor in addition to continuing the furosemide. A strong argument can be made for starting a β-blocker such as metoprolol or carvedilol now or within the next few days. Based on your advice, A.J.'s doctor has decided to withhold digoxin and assess the response to just one drug (i.e., the ACE inhibitor) for now.

Angiotensin-Converting Enzyme Inhibitors

Agents of Choice

16. The formulary for A.J.'s insurance company only covers four ACE inhibitors: benazepril, captopril, enalapril, and lisinopril. Benazepril is being promoted because the current contract makes it the least expensive of the four drugs. Is there a preference for any specific agent to order for A.J.?

As a general rule, formulary decisions are first based on comparative pharmacologic activity, efficacy, and drug safety. Other factors to consider are labeled (FDA approved) indications, convenience of dosing schedule, and—all else being equal—the cost to the pharmacy (or institution) and the patient (or insurance carrier). A confounding factor is that hypertension is the primary labeled indication for all of the ACE inhibitors and was the initial basis for placing these drugs on formularies. The indication for HF was added after initial marketing and does not appear in the FDA-approved labeling for all of the drugs. Each of these factors is considered below.

The basic mechanism of action of all ACE inhibitors is the same and is described in the pathogenesis section of this chapter.[59–61,143] They inhibit ACE (also called kinase II), thereby reducing the activation of angiotensin II, a major contributor to the undesired hemodynamic responses to HF. Decreased circulating levels of norepinephrine, vasopressin, neurokinins, luteinizing hormone, prostacyclin, and NO also have been noted after administration of ACE inhibitors.

In addition, ACE is responsible for degradation of bradykinin, substance P, and possibly other vasodilatory substances unrelated to angiotensin II. Thus, part of the beneficial effects of ACE inhibitors is caused by the accumulation of bradykinin (Fig. 18-6). After attaching to bradykinin-2 (B_2) receptors, vasodilation is produced by stimulating the production of arachidonic acid metabolites, peroxidases, nitric oxide, and endothelium-derived hyperpolarizing factor in vascular endothelium. In the kidney, bradykinin causes natriuresis through direct tubular effects.

The net effect is that ACE inhibitors regulate the balance between the vasoconstrictive and salt-retentive properties of angiotensin II and the vasodilatory and natriuretic properties of bradykinin. The physiologic consequences of the pharmacologic effects of ACE inhibitors are reduced pulmonary capillary wedge pressure (preload) and lowered systemic vascular resistance and systolic wall stress (afterload). CO increases without an increase in HR. ACE inhibitors promote salt excretion by augmenting RBF and reducing the production of aldosterone and antidiuretic hormone. The beneficial effects on RBF, coupled with the drug's indirect inhibition of aldosterone, lead to a mild diuretic response, a distinct benefit over other vasodilator compounds such as hydralazine.

Vasodilation and diuresis are not the only value of ACE inhibitors in HF. Angiotensin II enhances vascular remodeling

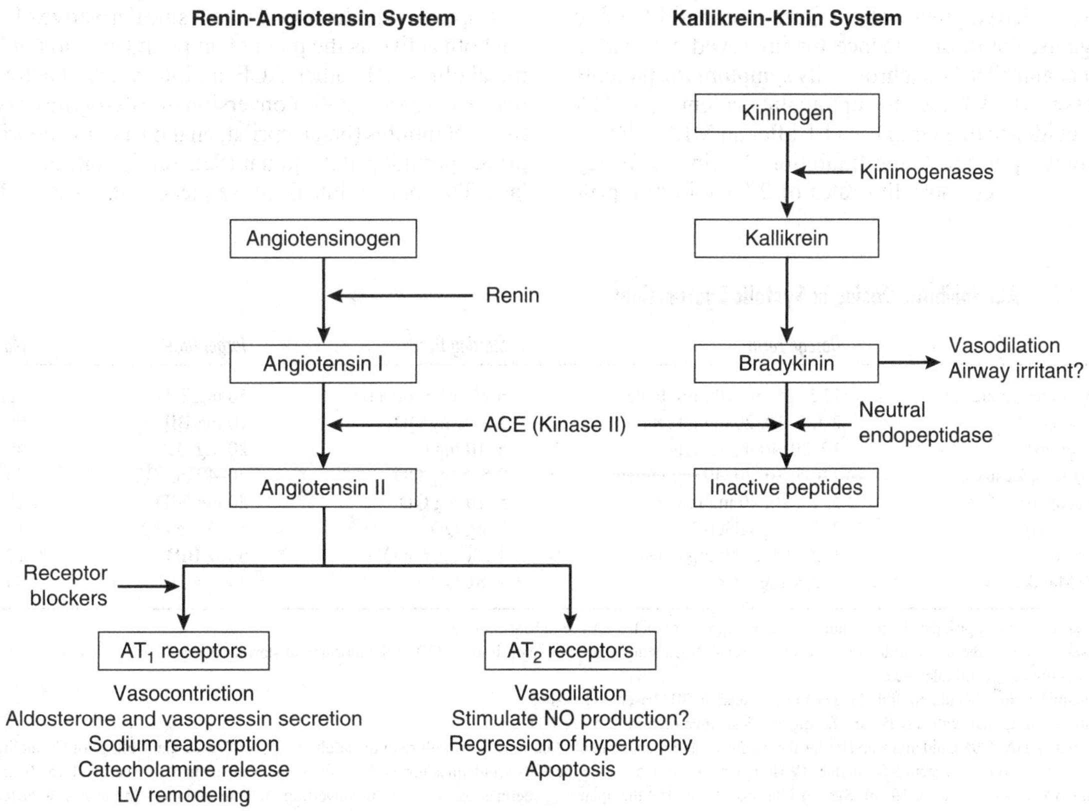

FIGURE 18-6 Angiotensin receptor blocker mechanism. ACE, angiotensin-converting enzyme; LV, left ventricular; NO, nitrous oxide.

(referred to as trophic effects on cardiac myocytes), whereas bradykinin impedes this process.[59,144] In experimental models, ACE inhibitors impede ventricular remodeling by blocking the trophic effects of angiotensin II on cardiac myocytes. Evidence to whether preserving bradykinin levels effects remodeling is inconclusive, although it might attenuate the progressive deposition of collagen during the chronic phase of post-MI cardiac remodeling.

As of this writing, *captopril (Capoten), enalapril (Vasotec), fosinopril (Monopril), lisinopril (Prinivil, Zestril),* and *quinapril (Accupril)* have FDA-labeled approval for symptomatic relief of HF symptoms (Table 18-11). Evidence exists that other agents such as *benazepril (Lotensin)* also increase exercise capacity and quality of life in patients with chronic HF.[145] *Moexipril (Univasc), ramipril (Altace),* and *trandolapril (Mavik)* have FDA-labeled approval for the treatment of left ventricular dysfunction after myocardial infarction. There does not seem to be a significant difference in side effects between agents. Based on these factors, no one drug is preferred over another.

Numerous placebo-controlled trials have documented the favorable effects of ACE inhibitor therapy on hemodynamic variables, clinical status, and symptoms of HF.[143,146] Multiple studies demonstrate a consistent 20% to 30% relative reduction in HF mortality that is superior to other vasodilator regimens including the hydralazine–nitrate combination or angiotensin receptor inhibitors (see Question 15). The benefits of ACE inhibitors are independent of the etiology of HF (ischemic vs. nonischemic) or the severity of symptoms (NYHA class I through class IV).

Table 18-10 provides a brief summary of the results of the key ACE inhibitor HF trials.[59–61,131–134,136,146,335–337] Many of these were reviewed previously in Question 15. Of the five approved agents, the most evidence for improved survival is available for enalapril in both chronically symptomatic patients (NYHA classes II–IV) and asymptomatic patients (NYHA class I) with evidence of an impaired EF after an MI.[131–134,136] A 3-year follow-up to the Acute Infarction Ramipril Efficacy (AIRE) study reported mortality rates of 27.5% in ramipril-treated subjects (target dose, 5 mg twice daily) compared with 38.9% with placebo, a 36% risk reduction.[147] Published data are also available for a positive effect on reducing short-term mortality with captopril, lisinopril, trandolapril, and zofenopril, primarily in relatively small populations of patients with chronic symptoms or in patients with new onset HF symptoms following an MI.[60,148,149]

Direct comparison of different ACE inhibitors is limited to three trials. The first two comparing lisinopril (5 to 20 mg every day) to either captopril (12.5–50 mg daily in two divided doses)[150] or enalapril (5–20 mg daily)[151] were only 12 weeks in duration. Exercise duration improved significantly with all three drugs at weeks 6 and 12. No statistically significant differences were found between drugs for NYHA class changes, HF symptoms, or side effects, although a trend was noted toward greater exercise duration at week 12 with lisinopril compared with enalapril. In the third study, fosinopril (5–20 mg) was compared with enalapril (5–20 mg) daily for 1 year.[152] The fosinopril group had significantly fewer patients who were hospitalized for HF or who died (19.7%) than did the enalapril group (25%; $p = 0.028$). Nearly 60% of patients in the fosinopril group improved their NYHA class. The incidence of orthostatic hypotension was lower in the fosinopril group (1.6% vs. 7.6%, $p = 0.05$). No explanation was provided to why there might be a difference.

Based on the total body of data, it is difficult to designate an agent of choice. The 2005 ACC/AHA guidelines recommend selecting an ACE inhibitor that has shown reductions in both morbidity and mortality in clinical trials in either HF or in populations after MI. The following ACE inhibitors are considered first-line options based on clinical trials: captopril, enalapril, lisinopril, perindopril, ramipril, or trandolapril.[7]

Captopril and lisinopril (the lysine derivative of enalaprilat) are both active as the parent compound and do not have active metabolites. All other ACE inhibitors are inactive prodrugs that require enzymatic conversion by esterolytic enzymes to active metabolites (benazeprilat, enalaprilat, fosinoprilat, moexiprilat, perindoprilat, quinaprilat, ramiprilat, and trandolaprilat). The only clinical consequence of these differences is

Table 18-11 ACE Inhibitor Dosing in Systolic Dysfunction[a]

Drug	Dosage Form	Starting Dose[b]	Target Dose[c]	MaximumalDose
Captopril[d] (Capoten, generic)	12.5, 25, 50, 100 mg tablets	6.25–12.5 mg TID	50 mg TID	100 mg TID
Enalapril (Vasotec)	2.5, 5, 10, 20 mg tablets	2.5–5 mg QD	10 mg BID	20 mg BID
Fosinopril (Monopril)	10, 20, 40 mg tablets	5–10 mg QD	20 mg QD	40 mg QD
Lisinopril (Prinivil, Zestril)	2.5, 5, 10, 20, 40 mg tablets	2.5–5 mg QD	20–40 mg QD	40 mg QD
Quinapril (Accupril)	5, 10, 20, 40 mg tablets	5–10 mg QD	20 mg BID	20 mg BID
Perindopril (Aceon)	2, 4, 8 mg tablets	2 mg QD	8–16 mg QD	16 mg QD
Ramipril (Altace)	1.25, 2.5, 5, 10 mg capsules	1.25–2.5 mg QD	5 mg BID	10 mg BID
Trandolapril (Mavik)	1, 2, 4 mg tablets	1 mg QD	4 mg QD	8 mg QD

[a]Benazepril, cilazapril, moexipril, peridnopril, ramipril, trandolapril not labeled for use in heart failure.

[b]Start with lowest dose to avoid bradycardia, hypotension, or renal dysfunction. All but captopril given QD in the morning at starting doses. Increase dose slowly at 2- to 4-week intervals to assess full effect and tolerance.

[c]Enalapril, quinapril, ramipril could possibly be given QD instead of BID based on half-life.

[d]Captopril is short acting. Start with a 6.25- or 12.5-mg test dose, then 6.25 to 12.5 mg TID.

Adapted from ACC/AHA 2005 Guidelines update for the diagnosis and management of chronic heart failure in the adult: a report of American College of Cardiology, American Heart Association Task Force on Practice Guidelines (Writing Committee) to update the 2001 Guidelines for the Evaluation and Management of Heart Failure. *J Am Coll Cardiol* 2005;46E1; and American Society of Health-System Pharmacists. ASHP therapeutic guidelines on angiotensin-converting-enzyme inhibitors in patients with left ventricular dysfunction. *Am J Health Syst Pharm* 1997;54:2999, with permission.

a slightly delayed onset of effect with the first dose (2–6 hours for captopril, 4–12 hours for the others). Of greater distinction, captopril has a relatively short half-life and duration of action, necessitating three to four times daily administration in most patients. Although this characteristic may be advantageous when initiating therapy by allowing closer assessment of early side effects, for chronic maintenance it is preferred to use a drug that can be given either once or twice daily. All other ACE inhibitors meet this criterion, either as the parent drug (lisinopril) or as the active metabolite (all others). Based solely on half-life data, there would be no expected difference between any of the longer-acting agents. Theoretically, they could all be administered once daily. Package insert labeling and common standards of practice, however, have led to twice daily dosing, especially at higher doses, for enalapril, quinapril, and ramipril.

We can conclude that A.J. should start captopril for 1 to 2 days for initial dosage titration, but then quickly transferred to a longer-acting drug if he has a good response to the captopril. Because of the lack of demonstrated superiority of one agent over another, cost does become a factor in choosing a long-acting ACE inhibitor. Because costs are often site- or agency-specific, reflecting interplay between institutional or managed care purchasing contracts and insurance company or drug benefit manager policies, it is not possible to identify the single less expensive agent. A.J.'s doctor decides not to use benazepril, even though it is the least expensive drug, because it does not have FDA approval for HF. Instead, he chooses to start enalapril based on evidence for clinical efficacy, improved survival, and availability of a reduced-cost generic.

Dosage

17. A captopril dosage of 25 mg TID was ordered for A.J. How will this dosage be titrated in preparation for conversion to enalapril? How should he be monitored?

CAPTOPRIL DOSING

Continued experience with captopril has led to a better understanding of dose-response relationships and more rational therapy. Complete inhibition of ACE is achieved with 10 to 20 mg, but larger doses prolong the duration of action. Early single-dose studies suggested that large doses (25–150 mg) were needed for maximal reduction of HF symptoms. Thus, until a better understanding was gained on how to use the drug, patients often were started on 25 mg every 8 hours and quickly titrated to 150 to 300 mg/day. It is now recommended to start patients on doses as low as 6.25 to 12.5 mg every 8 hours for a few days and then titrate to the desired symptomatic and objective responses. This conservative dosing approach minimizes the bradycardia and hypotension associated with higher doses and also allows better assessment of changes that may occur in the patient's renal function. It is especially important to start with low doses in persons with renal insufficiency or a very low EF. Renal function and serum potassium should be assessed within 1 to 2 weeks of initiation of therapy and periodically thereafter, especially in patients with preexisting hypotension, hyponatremia, diabetes, or azotemia and in those taking potassium supplements or potassium-sparing diuretics.[6,7]

Diuretic therapy must be monitored to prevent volume depletion or azotemia. ACE inhibitors are relatively contraindicated in people who are volume depleted or who have severe renal impairment.

Although symptoms might abate in some patients within the first 48 hours of therapy with an ACE inhibitor, the clinical responses to these drugs are generally delayed and might require several weeks or months to become apparent. The lag period likely results from the time needed for the body to readjust various hormonal responses rather than a pharmacokinetic or pharmacologic phenomenon. Even if symptoms do not abate, long-term treatment with an ACE inhibitor should be maintained because these drugs can reduce the risk of hospitalization or death independent of their effect on symptoms. Abrupt withdrawal can lead to clinical deterioration and should be avoided unless life-threatening side effects (e.g., angioedema or renal failure) are evident.[153]

Reviewing A.J.'s history (Question 1) and repeat vital signs and laboratory values (Question 15), we recall that he was hypertensive and had an elevated BUN at the time of his hospitalization. Both of these problems abated after starting furosemide, but his BUN is now still slightly above normal, although he is not hypotensive. We are, therefore, less concerned about the risk of hypotension, but we are unsure of how the ACE inhibitor will affect his renal function. If CO increases as desired, his renal function should improve; but if he becomes hypotensive, renal function may get worse. The 25-mg dose as currently ordered is probably safe in a stable patient such as A.J. It is prudent, however, to recommend lowering A.J.'s dosage of captopril to 12.5 mg as a single dose on the first morning. For less stable patients, a starting dose of 6.25 mg should be used. If A.J.'s BP and renal function remain stable after the test dose, he can get a total of three doses, approximately 8 hours apart, of 12.5 mg on the first day. On day 2, the dose can be raised to 25 mg three times daily. If he again remains stable on day 3, his regimen can be converted to enalapril, using a single daily dose.

CAPTOPRIL COMPARED WITH ENALAPRIL

18. After 2 days of taking captopril, A.J.'s exercise capacity has improved and his lower extremity edema has abated, but his HF is not optimally controlled. He is assessed to have between NYHA class II and III symptoms. BP values throughout the day have fluctuated in the range of 127–145/80–95 mm Hg and his weight is down to 70 kg. Repeat laboratory measurements include the following: Na, 139 mEq/L; K, 4.7 mEq/L; Cl, 98 mEq/L; CO_2, 27 mEq/L; BUN, 24 mg/dL; and SrCr, 0.6 mg/dL. An order is written to begin 5 mg/day of enalapril. Is this an appropriate choice of therapy? What is the target dose for him?

DOSE-RESPONSE RELATIONSHIPS

Cumulative evidence from all the clinical trials indicates a relationship between the degree of abatement in HF symptoms and the dose of drug given. Larger doses are more likely to improve the patient's quality of life and reduce the incidence of hospital stays, but the impact of larger doses when assessing mortality data is less clear. At the same time, higher doses are associated with a greater risk of side effects. Based on these principles, proposed recommended starting, target, and maximal doses for the ACE inhibitors are listed in Table 18-11.[7,61]

In general, the guidelines conclude that ACE inhibitors should be initiated at low doses, but titrated to the maximal tolerated target dose. Supporting this principle are the results of the ATLAS Trial.[154,155] Lisinopril was given to 3,164 patients hospitalized during the previous 6 months and with NYHA class II–IV HF and an LVEF <30%. Open label lisinopril 2.5 to 5 mg was given for first 2 weeks, then 12.5 to 15 mg for an additional 2 weeks. If the initial doses were tolerated, subjects were randomized to daily therapy with lisinopril 2.5 to 5 mg (low dosage) or 32.5 to 35 mg (high dosage). All-cause mortality did not differ between the two groups (8% lower in the highest dose group compared with the lowest dose; $p = 0.128$). In the high dosage group, hospitalizations and the combined end point of death and hospitalization were reduced by 24% ($p = 0.003$) and 12% ($p = 0.002$), respectively. The higher dosage was tolerated by 90% of patients assigned this dose.

Despite these recommendations for using the highest tolerated doses, evidence also suggests that lower doses are beneficial. For example, the UK Heart Failure Network Study found that 10 mg twice daily enalapril was no more effective than 2.5 mg twice per day.[156] In this study, enalapril was given in low (2.5 mg BID), moderate (5 mg BID), and higher (10 mg BID) dosages to patients with NYHA class II–III HF. The primary combined end point (death, hospitalization from HF, and worsening HF incidence) occurred in 12.3%, 12.9%, and 14.7%, respectively, of patients receiving low, moderate, and higher enalapril dosages. None of the between group differences were statistically different. Mortality, evaluated separately, was 4.2%, 3.3%, and 2.9%, respectively, which were all not significant comparisons. Further information on dosing, pharmacologic, and pharmacokinetic information regarding the ACE inhibitors is found in Chapter 13, Essential Hypertension.

For enalapril, the recommended starting dosage is 2.5 to 5 mg/day. For older patients or those with other risk factors (i.e., systolic BP <100 mm Hg, those taking large doses of either loop diuretics or potassium-sparing diuretics, or those with preexisting hyponatremia, hyperkalemia, or renal insufficiency), the starting dosage of 2.5 mg/day would be more appropriate. This dosage, or an equivalent with one of the other drugs, should also be considered if the patient is being started directly on a long-acting drug without prior titration on captopril. For a patient such as A.J. who has already been treated with captopril for 2 days with no evidence of intolerance, a 5-mg dose is an appropriate recommendation.

The long-term target dosage of enalapril for A.J. is 10 to 20 mg BID. No clear formula exists for deciding how quickly to titrate to this dose. It depends on several factors, including the degree of reduction in his HF symptoms and side effects, and his motivation to take the medicine. Whenever dosage adjustments are made, it may take as few as 24 hours for the patient to perceive symptom reduction, but generally full hemodynamic steady state is not reached for 1 to 2 months. On the other hand, hypotension and other side effects are more immediate. A.J. should have his dose reassessed in 1 to 2 weeks to determine whether he can tolerate a dosage increase to 5 mg BID. Thereafter, an extra 5 mg/day could be added every 2 to 4 weeks. Thus, it could take 6 months or more to titrate upward to 20 mg BID. If the response to his symptoms is not positive and he has no side effects, the rate of titration could be made faster, either by shortening the assessment periods (e.g., every week) or by using larger dosage increments (e.g., 10-mg increase).

One study comparing long-term treatment with 50 mg TID of captopril vs. 20 BID of enalapril showed more hypotensive episodes and compromised cerebral and renal function in the patients treated with enalapril.[157] From this, it was postulated that the more sustained hypotensive effect of enalapril may actually be a disadvantage. A potential confounding variable, however, is that the 40-mg daily dose of enalapril may have been disproportionately high compared with the 150 mg/day dose of captopril.

ACE Inhibitor–Induced Cough

19. M.Y., presents to the outpatient HF clinic with an annoying productive cough after 6 weeks of lisinopril therapy. He has been titrated up to a dose of 20 mg QD. He is also taking 40 mg of furosemide OD, 50 mg metoprolol succinate OD, and 50 mg spironolactone OD. His HF symptoms are much improved. About 2 weeks ago, he developed an annoying nonproductive cough that persisted throughout the day and also made it difficult for him to fall asleep at night. After about 1 week, he went to see his primary care physician who told him that he had bronchitis and recommended that he use a guaifenesin and dextromethorphan containing cough syrup. During a routine clinic visit today, he still is bothered by his "bronchitis." A chest examination reveals no evidence of wheezing, the S_3 heart sound has disappeared, and he still has a few crackles, but much less than when he was first admitted. His neck veins are only minimally elevated over normal, his ankle edema is 1+, and his weight is still 70 kg. BP today is 140/90 mm Hg. All laboratory values are normal except his potassium high at 5.0 mEq/L, BUN and creatinine are 19 mg/dL and 0.6 mEq/dL, respectively. Could the cough and "bronchitis" be a symptom of his HF? What are the recommendations for an ACE-induced cough?

Cough can be a sign of HF in patients with pulmonary congestion. In extreme cases, patients demonstrate "cardiac asthma" with severe air hunger, wheezing, and dyspnea. However, A.J.'s HF is much improved as evidenced by the objective data. The absence of wheezing and no prior history of asthma or smoking make an obstructive airways disease (asthma or COPD) unlikely. It is possible that he does have bronchitis, but he does not recall having a cold or other respiratory illness preceding the cough. Without other causes, a lisinopril-induced cough is suggested.

This side effect occurs with all ACE inhibitors.[158] Case reports indicate a possible lower incidence with fosinopril (Monopril), but this has not been confirmed under controlled conditions.[159] Cough is a well-established complication of lisinopril. ACE inhibitor-induced cough presents as a dry, nonproductive cough sometimes described as a "tickle in the back of the throat." This complication can arise within hours of first dose, or it can present after weeks to months of starting an ACE inhibitor. Although, resolution of the cough can occur within 1 to 4 weeks, in some patients, it can persist up to 3 months after discontinuation of therapy.

Various case reports have found an incidence of cough in 5% to 35% of all patients. The incidence may be even lower, approximately about 3%, and is dose independent.[160] One investigator found a 5% to 10% incidence in white patients of European descent that rose to nearly 50% in Chinese patients.[161] There may also be a higher incidence in women and black populations.[158]

Bradykinin accumulation within the upper airway, decreased metabolism of proinflammatory mediators, such as substance P or prostaglandins, or both are proposed mechanisms of ACE inhibitor-induced cough. These chemicals then act as irritant substances in the airways to increase bronchial reactivity and induce coughing. Bradykinin stimulates unmyelinated afferent sensory C fibers by type J receptors involved in the cough reflex. Bradykinin is also a potent bronchoconstrictor, but pulmonary function remains unchanged, and persons with asthma are no more susceptible to the reaction than those who do not have asthma. Substance P, also degraded by ACE, has been implicated because it is a neurotransmitter for afferent sensory fibers, specifically C fibers. Because this is a pharmacologic effect rather than an allergic reaction, dosage reduction or switching from one ACE inhibitor to another is generally not helpful. Likewise, dosage reduction is often not helpful. The only way to definitively diagnose the drug-induced cough is to discontinue therapy. Even then, false–positive results can occur if the patient had a mild case of bronchitis that spontaneously resolved at about the same time that the ACE inhibitor was discontinued. If the cough persists after drug discontinuation, other causes should be investigated.

The AHA guidelines recommend continuing ACE inhibitors if the cough is not severe even when other causes of cough have been excluded. Arguing in favor of this action is the long-term survival benefits of ACE inhibitors. On the contrary, American College of Chest Physicians (ACCP) evidence-based practice guidelines recommend discontinuation of therapy if ACE inhibitor-induced cough is even suggested.[160] After cessation of therapy, resolution of cough confirms the diagnosis. For patients with persistent cough, ARB or hydralazine-isosorbide are safe alternatives. For now, M.Y. can continue taking lisinopril for another couple of weeks to determine if the cough will resolve on its own. His symptoms of HF have abated since the initiation of ACEI and the cough may be no more than an annoyance. He is not at risk for developing asthma or other airway problems. If his cough persists, an ARB is probably the best alternative.

The ACCP guidelines suggest that in patients for whom continuation of ACE therapy is determined to be medically necessary, either attempt rechallenge with an ACE inhibitor (although only a small subset of patients will tolerate the reintroduction of therapy with no reoccurrence of cough) or use a pharmacologic agent to suppress the cough (e.g., aspirin, amlodipine, ferrous sulfate).

Angiotensin Receptor Blockers

20. M.Y., is sufficiently disturbed by his cough and he has requested discontinuing lisinopril. Because he has had such good success with the ACE inhibitor, his physician wants to replace lisinopril with valsartan 40 mg BID. What evidence indicates that valsartan or other angiotensin-receptor blocking drugs are effective in treating HF? Are these drugs still associated with causing a cough?

Angiotensin II that is normally activated by the renin-angiotensin cascade interacts with several different membrane-bound receptors, two of which include angiotensin type 1 (AT_1) and type 2 (AT_2) receptors (Fig. 18-6).[59,62,162] Attachment to AT_1 is responsible for most of the unwanted CV actions of angiotensin II, including vasoconstriction, activation of aldosterone, and stimulation of norepinephrine release. Angiotensin-receptor antagonists all preferentially bind to AT_1 to competitively inhibit attachment by endogenous angiotensin II, thus blocking angiotensin II activity.

As described above, ACE inhibition both affects angiotensin II production and also impairs the metabolism of bradykinin, substance P, and other vasoactive substances.[59,62,162] These substances do not interact with either of the angiotensin receptors, but may independently be associated with production of the cough and first-dose hypotension seen with ACE inhibitors. By giving an AT_1 receptor antagonist, the positive benefits of blocking the CV effects of angiotensin II are achieved while sparing alteration of the kinin metabolism. Indeed, nearly all trials using various ARB to treat hypertension or HF have shown a reduced incidence of cough relative to the ACE inhibitors, with prevalence no greater than that of placebo. Of further interest is preliminary information that angiotensin II attachment to the AT_2 receptor might actually lead to beneficial effects, including vasodilation and protection of the vascular wall from proliferative atherosclerotic effects. These responses should remain intact with AT_1 receptor antagonists, but are at least partially blunted by ACE inhibitors.

Life-saving drugs (e.g., ACE inhibitors, β-blockers, and spironolactone) have an established role in the management of HF. Despite these therapies, many patients with HF remain at a high risk of CV death. Several clinical trials in HF have shown potential therapeutic benefit of the receptor antagonists in modifying HF symptoms (Table 18-12).[162–169] A meta-analysis combined data on all-cause mortality and HF-related hospitalizations from 17 clinical trials that compared an ARB with either placebo or an ACE inhibitor in patients with HF.[163] Most of the trials also assessed short-term clinical end points such as exercise tolerance and EF. In total, 12,469 patients participated and 5 ARB (candesartan, eprosartan, irbesartan, losartan, and valsartan) were tested, assuming a class effect for all ARB. ARB favorably improved exercise tolerance and EF compared with placebo. They were not superior to ACE inhibitors in reducing all-cause mortality or hospitalizations for HF, however. The combination of an ARB and an ACE inhibitor was superior to ACE inhibitor monotherapy in reducing hospitalizations for HF but not in improving survival. In patients not receiving an ACE inhibitor (but receiving other HF drugs), a nonsignificant trend favored ARB over placebo for both reductions in all-cause mortality and hospitalizations for HF.

The first major clinical trial comparing an ARB with an ACE inhibitor in patients with HF was the Evaluation of Losartan in the Elderly (ELITE) study.[167] Among the strengths of this trial are (*a*) a relatively large population (722 subjects) who were all ACE inhibitor–naive, (*b*) comparison of the receptor antagonist with an ACE inhibitor (captopril), and (*c*) an adequate duration (48 weeks) to allow a preliminary outcome evaluation of frequency of hospitalizations and incidence of death. All subjects were 65 years of age or older with NYHA class II–IV HF, had an EF of 40% or less (mean, 31%), and were not previously treated with either an ACE inhibitor or an ARB. Diuretics were used by 75% of the subjects, with 55% taking digoxin and 40% taking a non–ACE-inhibitor vasodilator. Losartan was started at 12.5 mg/day in 352 patients and titrated to a dose as high as 50 mg/day in 300 of them. The 370 subjects randomized to captopril began therapy at 6.25 mg three times daily and

Table 18-12 Clinical Trials of Angiotensin Receptor Blockers (ARB) in Heart Failure (HF)

Trial	Patient Population	ARB	Treatment Duration	Outcome
ELITE[167]	NYHA II-IV ($N = 722$) EF ≤40%	Losartan (50 mg QD) or Captopril (50 mg TID)	48 wks	No significant difference observed for the primary endpoint (persistent renal dysfunction) or the secondary endpoint (composite of death/HF admissions) Losartan was associated with a lower mortality than Captopril
RESOLVD[169]	NYHA II-IV ($N = 768$) EF ≤ 40%	Candesartan (4, 8 or 16 mg), or Candesartan (4 mg or 8 mg) + 20 mg Enalapril, or 20 mg Enalapril	43 wks	Combination has greater benefits on LV remodeling. No difference in mortality No difference in NYHA class, QOL, 6 min walking distance
ELITEII[168]	NYHA II-IV ($N = 3,152$) EF ≤40%	Losartan (50 mg QD) or Captopril (50 mg TID)	48 wks	Losartan was not superior to Captopril in improving survival, but was significantly better tolerated. A subgroup analysis of ELITE II found a greater risk of death when Losartan was used in addition to β-blockers
Val-Heft[170]	NYHA II-IV ($N = 5,010$) EF < 40%	Valsartan 160 mg bid or placebo bid	23 mos	There was no difference in mortality between the two groups. In patients previously receiving both ACEI and a β-blocker (N = 1,610) the risk of death was increased with the addition of Valsartan
CHARM[172] Alternative	NYHA II-IV ($N = 2,028$) EF ≤40%	Candesartan (32 mg) vs. placebo.	34 mos	23% reduction in CV mortality or HF hospitalization favoring the Candesartan group. More side effects in the Candesartan group (hypotension, hyperkalemia, inc SCr vs placebo
CHARM[173] Added	NYHA II-IV ($N = 2,548$) EF ≤40%	Candesartan (32 mg) + ACEI vs placebo	41 mos	15% risk reduction in CV mortality or HF admissions compared to placebo. However more side effects in the candesartan group (hypotension, hyperkalemia, increased SCr) vs placebo
CHARM[174] Preserved	NYHA II-IV ($N = 3,032$) EF>40%	Candesartan (32 mg) vs placebo	37 mos	Composite endpoint failed to reach significance. More side effects in the Candesartan group (hypotension, hyperkalemia, increased SCr) vs placebo
CHARM[175] Overall	NYHA II-IV ($N = 7,599$)	Candesartan (32 mg) vs placebo	38 mos	There was no overall difference in primary outcome of all cause death.

ACEI, angiotensin converting enzyme inhibitor; EF, Ejection fraction; QOL, quality of life.

were titrated to a maximal dose of 50 mg three times daily (n = 310). For the primary study end point, a sustained increase in renal function decline, the two drugs performed identically with 10.5% of subjects in each group having a >0.3 mg/dL rise in SrCr. Similarly, functional ability increases were equal in both groups, and only 5.7% of both groups were hospitalized for worsening HF. An unexpected finding was a nonsignificant trend toward more deaths from all-causes in the captopril group (n = 32, 8.7%) compared with losartan (n = 17; 4.8%). Also, more subjects discontinued captopril than losartan because of adverse effects (20.8% vs. 12.2%). In particular, 3.8% of patients on captopril stopped the drug because of cough compared with none of those on losartan.

Several limitations of this study should be noted: (*a*) by design, the patients were all elderly; (*b*) 40% of the subjects were taking other vasodilators as a confounding variable; and (*c*) the primary end point was renal function changes, not hospitalization or death. Nonetheless, the study provided evidence that losartan is at least as effective as the reference ACE inhibitor (captopril) and that patients with HF have equal or fewer side effects with losartan, especially less cough.

The follow-up ELITE II Trial was specifically designed to test the hypothesis that losartan is superior to captopril in terms of reduction in mortality and morbidity in patients 60 years of age or older.[168] Inclusion criteria and the dosages of losartan and captopril were identical to the first ELITE Trial. By enrolling a larger number of subjects (N = 3,162), it was powered to assess the primary endpoint of all-cause mortality. The intent was to continue the study until a combined total of 510 deaths occurred between the two treatment groups. After a mean follow-up of 1.5 years, no significance difference was seen in all-cause mortality (17.7% losartan vs. 15.9% captopril), sudden death (9% vs. 7.3%), or all-cause mortality plus hospitalization (47.7% vs. 44.9%) between the two treatment groups. Although ARB treatment was not clinically superior to ACE-inhibitor therapy, it was better tolerated with a withdrawal rate of 9.4%, as compared with 14.5% with ACE-inhibitor therapy ($p = 0.001$). Specifically, significantly fewer patients experienced cough with the ARB.

In the Randomized Evaluation of Strategies for Left Ventricular Dysfunction (RESOLVD)[169] study, 768 subjects were randomized to receive enalapril (up to 20 mg/day), candesartan (up to 16 mg/day), or a combination of both drugs added to diuretics, digoxin, or both for an average of 43 weeks. Inclusion criteria included NYHA class II–IV HF, LVEF <40%, and a 6-minute walking distance <500 meters. As in the ELITE trials, all the subjects were ACE inhibitor-naive. The combination of candesartan and enalapril was more beneficial for preventing left ventricular dilation and suppressing neurohormonal activation than either candesartan or enalapril alone. No differences were found among any of the three treatment groups in either hospitalization or mortality rates. Although not powered as a mortality trial, mortality rates were higher in the subjects receiving candesartan alone (6.1%) or candesartan combined with enalapril (8.7%) than in the group that received enalapril alone (3.7%).

The Val-HeFT trial was a double-blind, placebo-controlled study to measure the morbidity and mortality in NYHA class II–IV HF patients given valsartan.[170] In contrast to the ELITE and RESOLVD studies, 93% of subjects were already taking an ACE inhibitor at the time of randomization, 35% were taking a β-blocker, and 30% were taking both drugs. Patients were randomized to receive valsartan (n = 2,511) or placebo (n = 2,499) twice daily. The starting dose of valsartan was 40 mg BID, which was then titrated up to 160 mg BID by doubling the dose every 2 weeks. The target dose was achieved in 84% of patients taking the active drug. After a mean follow-up of 23 months (range, 0 to 38 months), no significant difference was observed in all-cause mortality between the valsartan group (19.7%) and the control group (19.4%). The combined end point of mortality and morbidity (including hospitalization from HF, cardiac arrest with resuscitation, and need for IV support) was significantly reduced among patients receiving valsartan (723 events, 28.8%) as compared to those receiving placebo (801 events, 32.1%), a 13% reduction ($p = 0.009$). Adverse events were low, leading to discontinuation of valsartan in 9.9% of subjects compared with 7.2% with placebo. Dizziness, hypotension, and renal impairment all occurred more frequently in those treated with valsartan.

Subgroup analysis of the VAL-HeFT study data raises interesting questions. For example, the observed reduction in the combined end point of morbidity and mortality was most pronounced in the small subgroup of only 226 patients (7% of the total study population) not receiving an ACE inhibitor compared with patients on the combination of an ACE inhibitor and valsartan. Further *post hoc* analysis found that within the 35% of subjects (n = 1,610) taking the combination of an ACE inhibitor and a β-blocker at baseline, the addition of valsartan as a third drug was associated with a trend toward increased morbidity and a statistically significant increase in the combined end point of mortality and morbidity. The clinical significance of these findings is unknown.

The overall study results suggest that a combination of valsartan and an ACE inhibitor reduces morbidity, but not mortality. Despite the intriguing results of the subgroup analysis, it is difficult to determine the independent effect of valsartan (i.e., when not combined with an ACE inhibitor or β-blocker) on morbidity or mortality. More worrisome is the implication that the three-drug combination of valsartan, an ACE inhibitor, and a β-blocker adversely affects morbidity and mortality.

Subsequent trials were designed to determine if a combination of neurohumoral agents provided additional benefits without causing harm in patients with HF. The Valsartan in Acute Myocardial Infarction Trial (VALIANT) of stable patients after MI with left-ventricular dysfunction was designed to test the hypothesis that valsartan alone and in combination with captopril (ACE inhibitors) will improve survival. In VALIANT, 70% of the patients were also receiving β-blockers. All-cause mortality, the primary endpoint, was identical in all groups. In addition, an increased rate of side effects was seen in the combination group. The failure to show a statistically significant difference in survival benefits could be owing to the trial design. The patients were simultaneously started on an ACE inhibitor and ARB, which is a variation from typical heart failure trials where patients are entered with an ACE inhibitor before the initiation of an ARB. Interestingly, among the subgroup of patients taking β-blockers, no evidence was found of harmful interaction with triple therapy.[171] As a result of the VALIANT trial, the FDA approved the use of valsartan in patients at high risk following a heart attack and, in those with HF, the drug is no longer only reserved for ACE intolerant patients.

The most evidence addressing the efficacy and safety of ARB in HF comes from a series of three investigations known collectively as the Candesartan in Heart Failure Assessment of Reduction in Morbidity and Mortality (CHARM) trial. The individual components of the CHARM Program are (*a*) CHARM-Alternative, (*b*) CHARM-Added, and (*c*) CHARM-Preserved.[172–174] All three investigations were randomized, double-blind, placebo-controlled trials that enrolled adult patients (>18 years of age) with at least a 4-week history of symptomatic (NYHA class II–IV) heart failure. Subjects randomized to candesartan were started on 4 mg and titrated to 32 mg once daily, as tolerated. Standard therapy (diuretics, β-blockers, digoxin, and spironolactone) was continued. For all three trials, the primary endpoint was the combined incidence of CV death, HF hospitalizations, or both. The differences in admission criteria and outcomes between the individual trials are discussed in the sections below.

CHARM-Alternative enrolled 2,028 subjects who met all of the inclusion criteria defined above plus two additional criteria: an EF of 40% or less (i.e., systolic dysfunction) and intolerance of ACE inhibitors (cough 72%, hypotension 13%, renal dysfunction 12%). Thus, subjects in this group received either an ARB alone (n = 1,013) or placebo (n = 1,015) without an ACE inhibitor, but this was not a head-to-head comparison of an ACE inhibitor with an ARB. After a median follow-up of 33.7 months, a 23% reduction was found in the primary outcome of CV death, hospital admission for HF, or both in the candesartan group (33%) compared with placebo (40%, $p = 0.004$). The overall incidence of drug discontinuations because of adverse events was not statistically different between candesartan (21%) and placebo (19%), but there were significantly more reports of symptomatic hypotension (3.7% vs. 0.9%), increased creatinine levels (6.1% vs. 2.7%), and hyperkalemia (1.9% vs. 0.3%) in those treated with candesartan. Of 39 patients who previously experienced angioedema on an ACE inhibitor, only 1 patient discontinued the study drug because of angioedema (Table 18-13). It is concluded that candesartan was generally well tolerated and reduced cardiovascular morbidity and mortality in patients with symptomatic chronic HF who were not receiving ACE inhibitors because of intolerance.

The CHARM-Added trial attempted to determine if the combination of an ACE-inhibitor plus an ARB offered any clinical advantages compared with an ACE inhibitor alone in patients with symptomatic HF with an ejection fraction of 40% or less (systolic dysfunction). Prior use of an ACE inhibitor was required for the 2,548 patients enrolled in this trial (96% were

Table 18-13 Adverse Events That Lead to Permanent Drug Discontinuation

Trial	*Outcomes*	*Candesartan*	*Placebo*	*P Value*
CHARM-Alternative[172]	Any adverse event or laboratory abnormality	21.5%	19.3%	0.23
	Hypotension	3.7%	0.9%	<0.0001
	Increased creatinine	6.1%	2.7%	<0.0001
	Hyperkalemia	1.9%	0.3%	0.0005
CHARM-Added[173]	Any adverse event or laboratory abnormality			0.0003
	Hypotension	4.5%	3.5%	0.079
	Increased creatinine	7.8%	4.1%	0.0001
	Hyperkalemia	3.4%	0.7%	<0.0001
CHARM-Preserved[174]	Any adverse event or laboratory abnormality	17.8%	13.5%	0.001
	Hypotension	2.4%	1.1%	0.006
	Increased creatinine	4.8%	2.4%	<0.001
	Hyperkalemia	1.5%	0.6%	0.019
CHARM-Overall[174]	Any adverse event or laboratory abnormality	21%	16.7%	<0.001
	Hypotension	3.5%	1.7%	<0.0001
	Increased creatinine	6.2%	3.0%	<0.0001
	Hyperkalemia	2.2%	0.6%	<0.0001

on an ACE inhibitor dose comparable to that used in previous mortality trials). At baseline, 55% of the patients were treated with β-blockers and 17% were on spironolactone. After a median follow-up of 41 months, 483 (38%) of patients in the combination ACE inhibitor-candesartan added group experienced the primary outcome of CV death, hospital admission for HF, or both compared with 538 (42%) in the placebo plus ACE inhibitor group (a 15% relative risk reduction, $p = 0.011$). Overall, the addition of candesartan to an ACE inhibitor and other usual HF treatments leads to a further clinically important reduction in CV events in patients with chronic systolic HF. It is interesting to compare the result of the CHARM-Added trial with those of the Val-HeFT trial. In Val-HeFT, 93% of the subjects receiving the ARB valsartan were concurrently receiving an ACE inhibitor. The combined end point of morbidity and mortality was significantly reduced with combination therapy in Val-HeFT, but not mortality alone. In that trial was also seen a trend toward more deaths in the small subgroup receiving the triple combination of a β-blocker with an ACE inhibitor and ARB. β-Blocker use had no adverse effect in CHARM-Added.

Limited information has been published regarding the role of ARB in patients with HF with preserved LV function (i.e., diastolic dysfunction). CHARM-Preserved enrolled 3,023 subjects who met the overall CHARM trial inclusion criteria defined previously plus one additional criterion: an EF of >40% (mean 54%). Thus, subjects would be classified as having symptomatic HF with normal (preserved) ejection fraction. They received either an ARB alone (n =1,514) or placebo; only 20% of subjects in both groups were taking an ACE inhibitor at randomization, 56% were on a β-blocker, and 11% were on spironolactone.[174] After a median follow-up of 36.6 months, a nonsignificant trend was noted toward reduction in the primary outcome of CV death or hospital admission for HF in the candesartan group (22%) compared with placebo (24.3%, $p = 0.118$). Cardiovascular deaths (170 vs. 170) and all cause mortality (244 vs. 237) were nearly identical in both groups, but the total number of hospitalizations for HF (402 vs. 566) was significantly reduced in the candesartan group ($p = 0.014$). Secondary outcomes consisting of composites of the primary outcomes plus MI, nonfatal stroke, and coronary revascularization also showed a nonsignificant trend in favor of candesartan. The most common side effects with candesartan were hypotension (2.4%), increase in creatinine (4.8%), and hyperkalemia (1.5%). Discontinuation because of an adverse event occurred in 17.8% of those treated with candesartan compared with 13.5% of placebo recipients ($p = 0.001$) (Table 18-13). Overall, the conclusion is that, in symptomatic patients with diastolic HF, no significant improvement in morbidity or mortality occurs with candesartan compared with placebo, other than a significant reduction in HF-related hospitalizations.

The combined results of all three CHARM components (CHARM-Added, CHARM-Alternative and CHARM-Preserved) were reported in the CHARM–Overall trial.[175] This composite analysis evaluates the benefits of candesartan in symptomatic patients with HF, regardless of left ventricular systolic function. Overall, 3,803 patients were assigned to candesartan and 3,796 to placebo. A different primary endpoint was chosen for the CHARM-Overall analysis: all-cause death. Although the combined results failed to detect a clinically significant reduction in all-cause death between candesartan and placebo (9% reduction; $p = 0.32$), significant reductions were seen in CV death (12%), hospital admission for HF (21%), and combined CV death or hospital admission for HF (the primary end point for the individual trials—16%).

The results of the CHARM trial further reinforce the conclusion that ARB can reduce morbidity and mortality in symptomatic patients with systolic HF, and they can be safely used in patients who are intolerant to ACE. Combination therapy (ACE inhibitor plus ARB) with concomitant use of β-blockers appears to be beneficial and safe, as long as patients are closely monitored for adverse effects. For symptomatic patients with HF with normal ejection fraction (diastolic dysfunction), addition of an ARB may be beneficial in reducing hospitalizations; however, the study did not show improved survival.

Based on this information, it is considered that the ARBs cause less cough than ACE-inhibitors and provide survival benefits in systolic HF. Because of his prior use of large doses of lisinopril with no evidence of hypotension, M.Y. should be able to tolerate valsartan (40 mg BID). He should be evaluated in 2 weeks for resolution of his cough. (See Chapter 13, Essential Hypertension, for further information on the mechanisms of action, metabolism, and dosing of ARB.)

Other ACE Inhibitor and Angiotensin Receptor Blocker Side Effects

HYPERKALEMIA

21. Based on the data in Question 19, are there other side effects of M.Y.'s medications that need special monitoring? Will changing from lisinopril to valsartan reduce the risk of these side effects?

The ACE inhibitors, ARB, and β-blockers all have the potential to raise serum potassium concentrations via indirect aldosterone inhibition and other neurohormonal actions.[176,177] For most patients, the magnitude of increase in serum potassium concentration from ACE inhibitors and ARB alone is relatively small, but the risk for developing hyperkalemia is greater if the patient has compromised renal function or advanced HF. Combination therapy of an ACE or ARB with potassium supplements, potassium-sparing diuretics, or β-blockers further accentuates the risk of hyperkalemia, regardless of the sequence of initiation of the individual drugs.

Of greater concern, several case reports and case series have reported hyperkalemia and hospitalizations induced by spironolactone in patients with HF. This became more evident as prescribing patterns for spironolactone dramatically changed after publication of the RALES study.[178] Not only was there a significant increase in the number of prescriptions for spironolactone for patients with HF, but doses higher than recommended by the clinical trials were often used, especially in patients with evidence of preexisting renal dysfunction. In addition, evidence indicated inadequate monitoring of serum potassium, renal function, and concomitant drug therapy (also see Question 14). Although concurrent use of a potassium-losing diuretic (e.g., a thiazide or loop diuretic) may counteract potassium retention from spironolactone or other drugs (ACE inhibitors, ARB, β-blockers), it is nearly impossible to predict who will develop hypo- or hyperkalemia or remain normokalemic.[179,180] Thus, each patient must be assessed individually for personal response to various drug combinations and whether there is a need for potassium supplements or a reduction in their doses (Table 18-14).

M.Y. is concurrently receiving lisinopril and spironolactone. His potassium levels are elevated at 5.0 mEq/L. M.Y.'s dietary potassium intake should be assessed. He should be asked about the use of NSAID as well as herbal remedies, because herbs can be a hidden source of dietary potassium. He is on a combination of lisinopril and spironolactone. If M.Y. had to continue on lisinopril, his dose of lisinopril or spironolactone could be reduced. With the substitution of valsartan for lisinopril, the spironolactone dose will still most likely have to be lowered because ARB can also cause hyperkalemia by blocking the effects of aldosterone in the kidney identical to ACE inhibitors. On the other hand, if he were switched to a hydralazine–nitrate combination in place of the lisinopril, his spironolactone should be continued for its disease-modifying effects.

Table 18-14 Management of Hyperkalemia in Patients Treated With Aldosterone Antagonists

Guidelines for Minimizing the Risk of Hyperkalemia

1. Impaired renal function is a risk factor for hyperkalemia during treatment with aldosterone antagonists. The risk of hyperkalemia increases progressively when serum creatinine >1.6 mg/dL.* In elderly patients or others with low muscle mass in whom serum creatinine does not accurately reflect glomerular filtration rate, determination that glomerular filtration rate of creatinine clearance >30 mL per min is recommended.
2. Aldosterone antagonists should not be administered to patients with baseline serum potassium >5.0 mEq/L.
3. An initial dose of spironolactone 12.5 mg or eplerenone 25 mg is recommended, after which the dose may be increased to spironolactone 25 mg or eplerenone 50 mg if appropriate.
4. The risk of hyperkalemia is increased with concomitant use of higher doses of ACEI (captopril ≥75 mg daily; enalapril or lisinopril ≥10 mg daily).
5. Nonsteroidal anti-inflammatory drugs and cyclo-oxygenase-2 inhibitors should be avoided.
6. Potassium supplements should be discontinued or reduced.
7. Close monitoring of serum potassium is required; potassium levels and renal function should be checked in 3 days and at 1 week after initiation of therapy and at least monthly for the first 3 months.
8. Diarrhea or other causes of dehydration should be addressed emergently.

[a] Although the entry criteria for the trials of aldosterone antagonists included creatinine >2.5 mg/dL, most patients had creatinine much lower; in one trial, 95% of patients had creatinine of ≤1.7 mg/dL.

ACEI, angiotensin converting enzyme inhibitor.

From ACC/AHA 2005 Guidelines update for the diagnosis and management of chronic heart failure in the adult: a report of American College of Cardiology, American Heart Association Task Force on Practice Guidelines (Writing Committee) to update the 2001 Guidelines for the Evaluation and Management of Heart Failure. *J Am Coll Cardiol* 2005;46E1.

ANGIOEDEMA

22. R.S. is a 65-year-old black man who recently experienced new onset HF with presenting symptoms of shortness of breath while playing golf and persistent edema. Until then, he was healthy and taking no medications. He does not smoke, has no history of asthma or COPD, and no known allergies to food or drugs. R.S. has been taking furosemide 40 mg QD and lisinopril 10 mg QD for 3 weeks. He woke up this morning complaining of difficult breathing, neck swelling, and a "thick tongue." Could this be an abnormal presentation of HF? What drug side effect may be occurring?

Angioedema (angioneurotic edema) is a severe, potentially life-threatening complication of ACE inhibitor treatment.[181–183] Characterized by facial and neck swelling with obstruction to air flow by laryngeal and bronchial edema, this reaction resembles anaphylaxis. These symptoms are compatible with those being experienced by R.S. The mechanism of ACE inhibitor induction of angioedema is unknown, but is thought to be related to hypersensitivity to accumulated vasodilating kinins, similar to the cough reaction.

Some, but not all persons with drug-induced angioedema have a history of familial angioedema associated with a genetic defect in their complement system. ACE inhibitors are contraindicated in this population. In one series of case reports, 22% of the reported angioedema reactions occurred within 1 month of starting therapy, with the remaining 77% arising from several months to years later.[182] Blacks and females may have a higher prevalence. The timing of when R.S. started lisinopril and his being black are consistent with the diagnosis of drug-induced angioedema.

Of concern is the observation that ACE inhibitor-induced angioedema is often misdiagnosed.[183] Several of the patients described in one series had been re-treated with the same or a different ACE inhibitor followed by a repeat episode of angioedema. It is prudent to avoid all ACE inhibitors in any patient with a history of angioedema from any cause.

Because the mechanism of ACE-induced angioedema is speculated to be caused by kinin accumulation, changing R.S.

to an ARB might be an option.[184] Several case reports, however, have implicated candesartan, losartan, and valsartan as possible causative agents of angioedema.[181,185–188] In some cases, the subjects had previously experienced angioedema with an ACE inhibitor (indicating possible cross reactivity), whereas others were ACE inhibitor-naive. One author claims that ARB-induced angioedema usually manifests after long-term administration (late onset) and with milder symptoms compared with relatively earlier onset with ACE inhibitors. Similar findings showing a low, but potential risk for ARB-induced angioedema in patients who are ACE inhibitor intolerant comes from the CHARM-Alternative trial.[172] Of 39 patients with a history of angioedema while taking an ACE inhibitor, 3 developed angioedema on candesartan, although only 1 of the 3 actually discontinued taking candesartan. This and other conclusions regarding risk will require further observation. For now, it is prudent not to start an ARB in R.S. Options include starting a β-blocker or hydralazine-isosorbide. As discussed in Case 51, hydralazine-isosorbide might be a better choice for a black man.

EFFECTS OF ACE INHIBITORS AND ARB ON KIDNEY FUNCTION

23. B.N., a 62-year-old man, was admitted to the cardiac care unit (CCU) with a 2-day history of breathlessness causing him to sleep upright in a chair and preventing him from walking to the bathroom. Physical examination showed 4+ pitting edema of the legs, scrotal and sacral edema, and significantly distended neck veins. He had a CVP of 26 mm Hg (normal, 12). Laboratory values were: urine output, <20 mL/hour; BUN, 48 mg/dL; SCr, 2.0 mg/dL; and serum potassium, 3.2 mEq/L. Home medications, faithfully administered by his wife, included furosemide 240 mg/day, KCl 40 mEq/day, hydralazine 75 mg Q 6 hr, isosorbide dinitrate 20 mg Q 6 hr, metoprolol XL 200 mg QD, and digoxin 0.125 mg QD. He was not taking either an ACE inhibitor or an ARB because of a history of fluctuating SCr while taking both of these drugs.

A 100-mg IV bolus of furosemide in the ED resulted in a urine output of 600 mL over 2 hours, but with a subsequent rise of his BUN to 65 mg/dL. Finally, B.N. began captopril 12.5 mg TID. Within 2 days, B.N.'s breathing improved, his CVP was down to 16 mm Hg, and he was diuresing briskly. He was discharged 1 week later with mild SOB on exertion, 2+ ankle edema, and a reduction of his BUN to 28 mg/dL. Discharge medications included furosemide 120 mg/day, lisinopril 10 mg QD, metoprolol XL 200 mg QD, and digoxin 0.125 mg QD.

B.N. had a BUN of 48 mg/dL and a SCr of 2.0 mg/dL when he started captopril. The BUN first went up while he was in the hospital and later declined. Explain why these changes occurred. Are ACE inhibitors contraindicated in patients with renal insufficiency? Can they be used safely with diuretics in patients with renal insufficiency?

[SI units: BUN, 17.14, 23.21, and 9.99 mmol/L, respectively; SCr, 176.9 mmol/L; K, 3.2 mmol/L]

Note: The CVP measurement in this question refers to central venous pressure, an indicator of the right ventricular filling pressure or preload. (Refer to Chapter 21, Shock, and Question 48 in this chapter for a more thorough review of this and other cardiac hemodynamic monitoring parameters.) His initial CVP of 26 mm Hg was significantly elevated and the repeat value of 16 mm Hg was returning toward the normal value of 12 mm Hg.

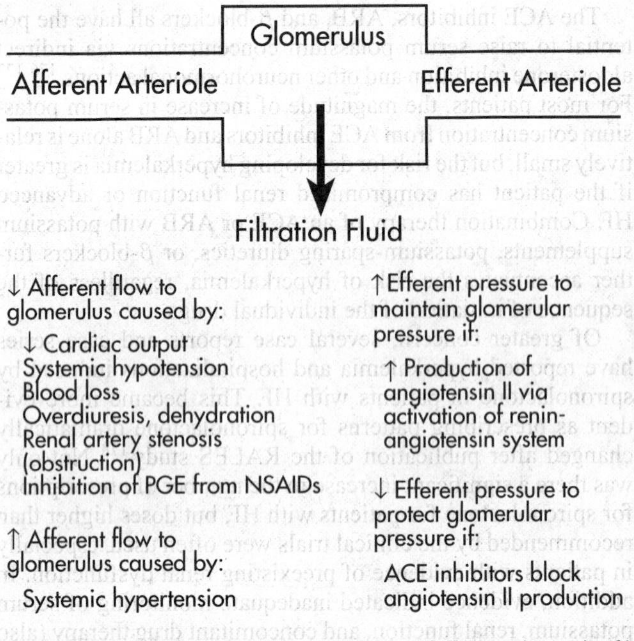

FIGURE 18-7 Factors affecting renal blood flow. Glomerular filtration is optimal when adequate hydrostatic pressure is maintained in the glomerulus. Governing factors include the blood flow rate to the glomerulus and the balance of afferent and efferent arteriole dilation/constriction. ACE, angiotensin-converting enzyme; NSAIDs, nonsteroidal anti-inflammatory drugs; PGE, prostaglandin E.

The effects of ACE inhibitors and ARB on RBF and renal function are complex. As seen in Figure 18-7, glomerular filtration is optimal when intraglomerular pressure is maintained at normal pressures. The balance between afferent flow into the glomerulus and efferent flow exiting the glomerulus determines the intraglomerular pressure. A drop in afferent flow or pressure occurring as a result of hypotension, volume loss (e.g., blood loss or overdiuresis), hypoalbuminemia, decreased CO (e.g., HF), or obstructive lesions such as renal artery stenosis all can significantly lower intraglomerular pressure and lead to impaired renal function. Similarly, long-standing hypertension can damage glomerular basement membrane capillaries and cause renal insufficiency.

In the case of low-pressure or low-flow states, the RAAS is activated to maintain intraglomerular pressure. A key factor in preserving glomerular pressure is *efferent vasoconstriction* mediated by angiotensin II. Increased efferent pressure helps to maintain intraglomerular pressure by impeding blood flow out of the glomerulus. When patients with low-pressure states are given ACE inhibitors or ARB, the protective mechanism of efferent vasoconstriction is inhibited and renal function can significantly and rapidly worsen. Conversely, in patients with hypertensive renal disease, glomerular function actually can improve because the ACE inhibitors lower afferent pressure and help protect the kidney. ACE inhibitors slow the progression of diabetic nephropathy and reduce proteinuria independent of their effect on BP (see Chapter 50, Diabetes Mellitus).

Patients with HF present with a complex picture. By decreasing afterload and preload, hope is that CO will improve after ACE inhibitor or ARB therapy, thus preserving or even enhancing RBF. If, however, starting ACE inhibitors or ARB leads to a rapid decrease in systemic BP that is not followed by an increase in CO, worsening renal function may ensue. It is impossible to predict which event will occur. Therefore, ACE inhibitor or ARB therapy needs to be started with low doses and careful monitoring of the BP and renal function should occur as dosages are increased. Diuretics are not contraindicated, but the diuretic dosage may need to be reduced to avoid volume depletion and hypotension.

These events are illustrated in B.N. When he was first diuresed, the BUN increased. Addition of an ACE inhibitor in combination with furosemide led to significant clinical benefit, including improved renal function. For now, B.N. is tolerating captopril and is obtaining the desired effect. Because he has a history of fluctuating renal function with both ACE inhibitors and ARB, he will require frequent observation. NSAID also must be used with caution because inhibition of vasodilating renal prostaglandins in patients with low afferent flow can worsen renal function (see Question 26).

LESS COMMON SIDE EFFECTS

24. What side effects other than those experienced by M.Y., B.N., and R.J. have been associated with ACE inhibitors? Are any of these unique to a specific drug, or are they all a class effect?

Captopril initially was associated with significant side effects. Of subjects, 10% to 15% of those in early studies developed skin eruptions or fever. These effects were associated primarily with higher dosage (average, 683 mg/day) and are found less frequently when the drug is used in smaller doses (<225 mg/day). Skin reactions may be edematous, urticarial, erythematous, maculopapular, or morbilliform in nature. That the rashes disappear with continued therapy in some patients suggests that they may be caused by potentiation of kinin-mediated skin reactions. Transient loss of taste (ageusia), reflex tachycardia, and hypotension also are common at high doses. None of these have occurred in any of the patients in our cases.

Proteinuria, a transient rise in serum creatinine (independent of the mechanisms described in the previous question), agranulocytosis, neutropenia, and fatal pancytopenia[189] also have been attributed to captopril therapy. The marrow toxicity is minimized by keeping total daily doses below 75 mg and avoiding the use of captopril in patients with advanced renal failure.

A theoretic advantage of the newer ACE inhibitors over captopril is the lack of a sulfhydryl group as part of their clinical structures. The sulfhydryl group (also found in penicillamine) is associated with a high incidence of rashes, ageusia, proteinuria, and neutropenia. The clinical significance of this difference remains to be determined, especially because captopril side effects have declined since clinicians have begun to prescribe lower doses.

All ACE inhibitors are contraindicated in pregnancy.[190] Teratogenic effects, including kidney failure and skull and facial deformities, have been reported when taken during the second or third trimester of pregnancy. Risk of use during the first trimester is less clear.

One report described captopril-induced inhibition of digoxin renal clearance, resulting in increased serum digoxin levels.[191] As with many of the other digoxin interactions described elsewhere in this chapter, the clinical significance of this interaction remains to be defined.

ACE Inhibitors in Asymptomatic Patients

25. W.N. is a 44-year-old white man diagnosed with an acute MI by ECG and cardiac enzyme changes 3 days ago following an episode of acute chest pain while driving his car. He was immediately treated with IV NTG and morphine and underwent thrombolytic therapy with streptokinase within 2 hours of the pain. He has no history of angina or hypertension, but was told that he had a high cholesterol level during a screening program 2 years ago. He was taking no medication before this event. Of note, W.N. has a strong family history of coronary artery disease and hyperlipidemia.

His hospital course has been unremarkable with only one episode of mild chest pain responding to sublingual NTG. BP is 130/83 mm Hg, pulse is 80 beats/minute with a regular rhythm. He has no ectopy, no complaints of SOB, and no evidence of edema. Lung sounds are normal as is his chest radiograph. All laboratory values have been normal except for an elevated creatine kinase (CK) and lactate dehydrogenase (LDH) on the day of admission, a total cholesterol of 245 mg/dL, and an LDL of 180 mg/dL. In preparation for discharge, he underwent repeat angiography and EF was measured by radionuclide ventriculography. His coronary arteries remain patent, but the EF is 35%. Discharge medications include aspirin 82 mg QD and simvastatin 5 mg QHS.

W.N. has evidence of left ventricular dysfunction based on his EF but is asymptomatic. How would his HF be staged in the ACC/AHA scheme and in the NYHA classification? Should he be started on a diuretic, an ACE inhibitor, or both?

This case exemplifies a patient with asymptomatic (NYHA symptom class I) left ventricular dysfunction. An EF <40% indicates systolic dysfunction following heart muscle damage from the MI. These abnormalities would place him in stage B by the ACC/AHA guidelines (Table 18-3). An absence of edema, SOB, or other clinical symptoms argues against the need for diuretics. The ACC/AHA guidelines, however, recommend starting patients such as W.N. on both an ACE inhibitor and a β-blocker.[6,7]

Evidence supports the use of ACE inhibitors in asymptomatic patients with early left ventricular dysfunction to slow the progression of the disease, possibly by retarding the remodeling effects on the cardiac muscle that may otherwise occur. This is best exemplified by the results of the SOLVD prevention trial.[191] Subjects enrolled in this study were actually a subset of the original SOLVD study,[134] with one important difference; although they had an EF of <35%, they were asymptomatic at the time of entry into the trial. Patients received either placebo (2,117 subjects) or enalapril titrated to a dose of 2.5 to 20 mg/day (2,111 subjects). Diuretics and all other active drugs were withheld unless the patient developed overt HF. Over the 37.4-month study period, 20% of the enalapril-treated patients developed symptoms of HF compared with 30% in the placebo group, a 37% reduction. The treatment group also had fewer hospitalizations for anginal symptoms and MI. As would be expected in this relatively low-risk population, mortality rates were low (14.9%–15.8%) and not statistically significant between the two groups. The death rates became more divergent in favor of enalapril late in the study as more patients developed overt HF. Because W.N. has no contraindications to using an ACE inhibitor, he should be started on 5 mg/day of enalapril and titrated to a target dose of 20 to 40 mg/day.

The reader also is referred to Chapter 17, Myocardial Infarction, for a related discussion on the early use of ACE inhibitors in symptomatic patients following infarction (CONSENSUS II, SAVE, and AIRE trials).[192–194] Chapter 17 also thoroughly reviews the rationale for prescribing β-blockers in all patients following an MI unless contraindications exist. W.N.'s physician chose not to use propranolol because of his low LVEF. This is an acceptable choice, but metoprolol should be substituted for propranolol. Metoprolol reduces morbidity and mortality following MI and also slows the onset and progression of HF.

DRUG INTERACTION OF ACE INHIBITORS WITH ASPIRIN

26. Enalapril was started in B.N. for the reasons stated in Question 25. Aspirin, 82 mg QD, has also been prescribed. What are the potential benefits and risks of this combination of drugs?

Aspirin is recommended for all patients following MI (see Chapter 18, Myocardial Infarction). Several studies suggest that aspirin may attenuate the beneficial affects of ACE inhibitors when given together in patients with HF and other cardiovascular disorders. The proposed mechanism is inhibition of prostaglandin formation by aspirin, thus counteracting the clinical effects of ACE inhibitors that rely in part on prostaglandins to elicit their positive hemodynamic effects. The significance of this interaction is still being debated. Two comprehensive reviews of this interaction appear elsewhere.[195,196] Both conclude that insufficient data exist to firmly establish or refute an adverse clinical outcome associated with the combination of aspirin and an ACE inhibitor in patients with HF.

The most widely quoted supporting evidence for a possible adverse effect comes from subgroup analysis of the SOLVD trial that compared enalapril with placebo in patients with HF.[134] Overall, patients taking aspirin and other antiplatelet drugs at the beginning of the trial had lower mortality rates. Antiplatelet drugs, however, were of benefit primarily only in patients taking placebo as opposed to those taking enalapril. The combination of enalapril with an antiplatelet agent was not associated with a mortality benefit, whereas combining placebo with aspirin was associated with reduced mortality (0.68 hazard ratio; 95% confidence interval [CI], 0.58 to 0.80). Similarly, the mortality benefit of enalapril was primarily in patients not taking antiplatelet agents (0.77 hazard ratio; 95% CI, 0.657 –0.87) as opposed to those who were taking them (1.10 hazard ratio; 95% CI, 0.3 to 1.30). These observations are limited because it was a *post hoc*, retrospective analysis of the study data, and continuing use of antiplatelet drugs at the end of the trial was not assessed. Four other small published trials and two abstracts indicate a possible interaction with aspirin, all of which are limited by small sample sizes, short duration of assessment (single dose to several weeks), and reliance on hemodynamic measures, such as peripheral vascular resistance and pulmonary responses, instead of HF clinical outcomes.[195,196] In these trials, the interaction appeared to be limited to aspirin and various ACE inhibitors, but was not observed between aspirin and losartan or between ticlopidine (which does not affect prostaglandins) and ACE inhibitors. Conversely, one published trial and two abstracts cited in the review articles suggest no interaction between aspirin or ifetroban (a thromboxane A_2 receptor antagonist) and an ACE inhibitor.[195,196] In the largest of these trials (317 patients with ischemic cardiomyopathy and LVEF <35%) and with the longest follow-up (mean, 5.7 years), use of aspirin was associated with lowered risk of mortality and hospital readmission, regardless of whether an ACE inhibitor was prescribed. Recently, a retrospective review of aspirin use in combination with ACE inhibitors in patients with HF resulted in no adverse effects seen in regard to the long-term survival.[197] Dosages of aspirin (100 mg/day or less) interact little with ACE inhibitors, whereas higher dosages may carry a greater risk. Some patients, for unknown reasons, are more susceptible to the interaction.

The 2005 ACC/AHA practice guidelines claim that many physicians believe that the data supporting the existence of an adverse interaction between aspirin and ACE inhibitors are not sufficiently compelling to justify altering the current practice of prescribing the two agents together.[7] In contrast, other physicians would consider the withdrawal of aspirin (because no data indicate it can reduce the risk of ischemic events in patients with HF) or use of an alternative antiplatelet agent, such as clopidogrel, which does not interact with ACE inhibitors and which may have superior effects in preventing ischemic events.[7]

Use of β-Blockers in Systolic Heart Failure

27. Returning to the case of AJ: After 3 days of furosemide and an ACE inhibitor, A.J.'s PND has resolved, but he still has difficulty walking without SOB and fatigue. His lower extremity edema has significantly reduced. His current BP is 145/90 mm Hg, pulse 82 beats/minute and his weight has dropped to 73 kg after diuresis. Repeat laboratory measurements include the following: Na, 139 mEq/L; K, 4.3 mEq/L; Cl, 98 mEq/L; CO_2, 27 mEq/L; BUN, 27 mg/dL; and SrCr, 0.6 mg/dL. The medical team has decided to discharge the patient soon. You recommend that the patient should be initiated on a β-blocker before discharge. What is your rationale?

The physiologic basis for the use of β-blockers in HF and the changes observed in receptor sensitivity is described in greater detail in the pathophysiology section of this chapter.[20–25] β-blockers have been evaluated during randomized clinical trials in more than 20,000 patients with varying degrees of systolic HF.[20–25] Five meta-analyses have arrived at the same conclusions: the use of β-blockers is associated with a consistent 30% reduction in mortality and a 40% reduction in hospitalizations in patients with HF.[198–202]

The 2005 ACC/AHA guidelines state that because bisoprolol, metoprolol succinate and carvedilol have been shown to reduce both HF symptoms and mortality, they should be prescribed to all patients with stable HF caused by left ventricular systolic dysfunction, unless there is a contraindication to their use or the patient is unable to tolerate treatment with a β-blocker.[7] They should be a part of the primary treatment plan, usually in combination with a diuretic and an ACE inhibitor. Contrary to the practice of some clinicians, the use of β-blocker drugs should not be delayed until the patient is found to be resistant to treatment with other drugs. Another common misperception is that patients who have mild symptoms or who appear clinically stable on diuretics and ACE inhibitors (with or without digoxin) do not require additional treatment. Even these patients should receive a β-blocker to slow the rate of disease progression and reduce the risk of sudden death. Similarly, patients need not be taking high doses of ACE inhibitors before being considered for treatment with a β-blocker. To the contrary, in patients taking a low dose of an ACE inhibitor, the addition of a β-blocker produces a greater reduction in symptoms and in the risk of death than an increase in the dose of an ACE inhibitor. Only those clinically unstable patients who are hospitalized in an intensive care unit, require IV positive inotropic support, have severe fluid overload or depletion, have symptomatic bradycardia or advanced heart block (unless treated with a pacemaker), or a history of poorly controlled reactive airways disease should not be given a β-blocker.[5] Recent data, show that β-blockers can be initiated prior to discharge in patients hospitalized for HF, if they did not require IV inotropic support for their HF exacerbation.[203]

Based on all these factors, there is no question that A.J. should be started on a β-blocker. Treatment with a β-blocker should be initiated at low doses, followed by gradual increments in dose every 1 to 2 weeks as tolerated by the patient. Transient bradycardia, hypotension, and fatigue are not uncommon during the first 24 to 48 hours when β-blockers are first started or during subsequent incremental increases in dosage. Thus, patients should be monitored daily for changes in vital signs (pulse and blood pressure) and symptoms during this up-titration period. Bradycardia, heart block, and hypotension can be asymptomatic and require no intervention other than instructing the patient not to arise too quickly from a lying position to avoid postural changes. If either of these complications is accompanied by dizziness, lightheadedness, or blurred vision, it may be necessary to reduce the dose β-blocker, the ACE inhibitor, or both or to slow the up titration. The sense of lassitude generally resolves within several weeks without other intervention, but may be a reason to slow up-titration of the dose and rarely to reduce the dose or discontinue therapy. In patients where benefits are especially apparent, but bradycardia or heart block is a concern, insertion of a pacemaker should be considered.

Because initiation of β-blocker therapy can also cause fluid retention, patients should be instructed to weigh themselves daily and to adjust concomitantly administered diuretics as appropriate. Conversely, diuretic doses should be decreased temporarily when patients become hypotensive or their BUN begins to rise. Planned increments in the dose of a β-blocker should be delayed until any side effects observed with lower doses are tolerable or absent. In clinical trials, up to 85% of patients are able to tolerate short- and long-term treatment with these drugs and achieve the maximal planned dose.

Metoprolol and Bisoprolol

28. Metoprolol succinate (12.5 mg) is prescribed for A.J. Is this a good choice of agent and starting dose? What other similar drugs have been used to treat HF?

Several clinical trials substantiate the clinical benefits of metoprolol, a relatively selective β_1-receptor blocker, in HF.[204–207] By blocking β_1 receptors in the myocardium, HR, contractility, and CO are reduced at rest and during exercise, without a compensatory increase in peripheral vascular resistance. The relative sparing of β-receptors in the peripheral vasculature and lungs reduces vasoconstrictive and bronchospastic complications. In contrast to bucindolol and carvedilol, metoprolol has been shown to upregulate myocardial β_2-receptors.[20]

In the Metoprolol in Dilated Cardiomyopathy (MDC) study, 383 patients with nonischemic dilated cardiomyopathy and class II or III HF were randomized to immediate-release metoprolol tartrate (initiated at 5 mg BID and titrated to 100–150 mg/day in divided doses) or placebo.[207] All were continued on standard therapy with diuretics, vasodilators, and digoxin as tolerated. In this trial was noted a nonstatistically significant trend toward both decreased mortality and listing for heart transplantation in the active treatment group.

Of greater interest is the Metoprolol CR/XL Randomized Intervention Trial in Heart Failure (MERIT HF) in which a 35% reduction in all-causes of mortality was observed with sustained-release metoprolol succinate.[207] In this trial, 3,991 patients, most of whom had either NYHA class II or III HF, were randomized to metoprolol succinate controlled-release/extended-release (CR/XL) or placebo. The starting dose of metoprolol was 12.5 to 25 mg/day, which was gradually increased every 2 weeks to the target dose of 200 mg/day. Conventional therapy with diuretics, ACE inhibitors, and digoxin was continued. At the end of the trial, 64% of subjects assigned to active drug had reached the target dose. Planned follow-up was for 2 years, but the study was halted prematurely because of a statistically significant decrease in all-cause mortality in the metoprolol arm. Specifically, there was a 34% reduction in total mortality with a 38% decrease in cardiovascular mortality, a 41% reduction in sudden death, and a 49% reduction from death owing to worsening HF. All-cause hospitalization was also reduced by 18% and hospitalization for worsening HF was decreased by 35%. Although the number of subjects was too small to detect a statistical difference, patients with severe (class IV) HF seemed to benefit as well. Up to 15% of subjects had clinical worsening of HF, even at low metoprolol doses.

Encouraging results have also been seen with another relative β_1-selective drug, bisoprolol fumarate (Zebeta).[208,209] In the first Cardiac Insufficiency Bisoprolol Study (CIBIS I), 641 subjects with moderate to severe HF were randomized to placebo or bisoprolol (starting dose, 1.25 mg/day; maximal dose, 5 mg/day) added to conventional therapy for an average of 23 months.[208] A statistically significant reduction in HF-associated hospitalization with the active drug and a nonsignificant trend toward reduced mortality were noted. In the larger Second Cardiac Insufficiency Bisoprolol Study (CIBIS II), reduction in both hospitalization and mortality in the bisoprolol-treated group was significant.[209] A total of 2,647 patients were included in the second trial and doses were increased to as high as 10 mg/day. The study was stopped prematurely (average follow-up, 1.3 years) because of a 34% reduction in total mortality with bisoprolol. *Post hoc* analysis showed a 44% reduction in sudden death and a 26% reduction in death owing to worsening HF. As in the MERIT HF study, the number of patients with severe (class IV) HF was inadequate to determine the value of β-blocker therapy in this population.

Two dosage forms of metoprolol are marketed: metoprolol succinate extended release (Toprol XL) and metoprolol tartrate immediate release (Lopressor and generic). Only metoprolol succinate form is approved for HF in the United States, indicated for patients with mild to moderate (NYHA class II or III) HF of ischemic, hypertensive, or cardiomyopathic origin. The starting dose of 12.5 mg of metoprolol succinate prescribed for A.J. is consistent with the clinical trials and manufacturer's package insert labeling. If the initial dose is tolerated, the dose can be doubled to 25 mg OD for an additional 2 to 4 weeks. The final target dose is 150 to 200 mg daily either as 100 mg BID or 200 mg QD.

An alternative is to use immediate release metoprolol tartrate (Lopressor) even though it is not approved for this indication in the United States. Following a test dose of 12.5 mg, the starting dose is 12.5 mg twice daily for 1 or 2 weeks. The smallest immediate release tablet size available is 25 mg tablets, therefore during the initial 1 to 2 weeks of treatment, the tablets will have to be split in half to achieve the appropriate dosing regimen. Since the only FDA-approved dosage form of metoprolol is the extended release succinate product, it is prescribed in most cases. Maintenance with a generic form of the immediate release product is less expensive, however, than the brand name extended release product.

When choosing among the various formulations of metoprolol, pharmacokinetic and bioavailability differences should be considered.[204,205] Metoprolol succinate available as 25, 50, 100, and 200 mg tablets. Each tablet contains many tiny metoprolol succinate pellets, each individually coated with an ethylcellulose polymeric membrane. GI fluid penetrates the membrane of each pellet and slowly dissolves the drug. The saturated metoprolol solution is then released at a constant rate over 20 hours, consistent with zero-order kinetics, and provides β-blockade for 24 hours. The extended release formulation retains its release characteristics even if the scored tablet is divided in half, but it should not be crushed or chewed.

Absorption of metoprolol tartrate is approximately 95%, but the bioavailability metoprolol succinate is only 50% because of extensive first pass metabolism.[204,205] Systemic bioavailability of the extended release product is even lower, averaging 70% of the immediate release preparation. This is likely because of the greater opportunity for first pass metabolism during slow absorption and less opportunity to saturate the metabolizing enzyme system. Because metoprolol succinate has consistently reduced bioavailability compared with immediate release metoprolol tartrate there is a concern that if a patient is receiving metoprolol tartrate and is switched to the same dosage of the succinate formulation, the patient, in effect, will receive approximately 25% less drug. Clinical studies, however, indicate that the β-blocking effects are similar, perhaps because of the prolonged action of the succinate product. The higher peak concentrations obtained with the metoprolol tartrate formulation is accompanied by a greater potential for hypotension compared with metoprolol succinate. Because the dosage has to be titrated to an individual patient, these differences may not be relevant unless the patient is being switched from one product to the other.

Metoprolol has several metabolic routes of elimination that can affect dosing and drug interactions. The major routes of elimination are via α-hydroxylation, O-demethylation, and N-dealkylation.[204,205] A smaller portion is metabolized by cytochrome P450 2D6, and drugs that inhibit metabolism of that isoenzyme may affect the drug's plasma levels. Approximately 10% of patients are poor metabolizers, resulting in higher drug plasma concentrations in these patients.

A.J. should be advised that clinical response to metoprolol is usually delayed and may require 2 to 3 months to become apparent. Even if symptoms do not abate, long-term treatment should be maintained to reduce the risk of major clinical events. Abrupt withdrawal of treatment with a β-blocker can lead to clinical deterioration and should be avoided.[210]

Bisoprolol is FDA approved for treatment of HF. Dosage size limitations, however, restrict clinical use of this drug. For example, the starting dose of bisoprolol is 1.25 mg/day, whereas the smallest commercially available dose is a 5-mg scored tablet. Attempting to break the tablet into quarters is not practical.

Carvedilol

29. Might carvedilol be a better alternative than metoprolol for A.J.? What would be an appropriate dose and dosing schedule?

Carvedilol (Coreg), a mixed α- and β-blocker, was the first drug of this class to obtain FDA approval for management of HF.[211] It might also have antioxidant effects to protect against loss of cardiac myocytes and to act as a scavenger of oxygen-free radicals that could potentiate myocardial necrosis. The correlation of these findings to clinical outcome is unknown.

Two pivotal studies support the use of carvedilol. The first was the U.S. Carvedilol Heart Failure Study.[212–216] Subjects were almost equally divided between class II and III HF and all had an EF of 35% or less (mean, 22%) despite diuretics (95%), digoxin (90%), and an ACE inhibitor (95%). Subjects with a major myocardial event in the previous 3 months were excluded. After an initial open-label period when all patients received 6.25 mg twice daily of carvedilol, subjects were stratified based on severity of their HF and then randomized to either placebo (n = 398) or carvedilol (n = 690). The maximal dose given was 50 mg twice daily. Using an intention-to-treat analysis, 7.8% of deaths occurred in the placebo group over an average of 6.5 months compared with only 3.2% in the active treatment group, a statistically significant 65% risk reduction ($p = 0.001$). Most notably, death caused by progressive HF or sudden cardiac death was reduced. The patients treated with carvedilol also had fewer HF-related hospitalizations (19.6% vs. 14.1%). The most common side effect with carvedilol was dizziness, usually during the first few days of therapy, but more patients discontinued placebo for worsening HF or side effects than with carvedilol.

In the Australia/New Zealand Carvedilol Study, 415 patients with chronic, stable HF (NYHA class II or III, 85% taking concurrent ACE inhibitors, and average EF of 28%) were randomized to placebo (n = 208) or carvedilol (n = 207).[217] As in the U.S. study, those with severe symptoms were excluded, although 88% had a history of MI. Maintenance doses in subjects randomized to carvedilol ranged from 6.25 to 25 mg twice daily with an average follow-up of 19 months.

After 12 months, EF had increased by 5.3% and heart size was reduced in the carvedilol group compared with essentially no change in the placebo group. No differences between groups were found in treadmill exercise time, change in NYHA classification, or HF symptom scores, however. Only 26% of patients on carvedilol and 28% of those receiving placebo had improved NYHA symptom scores, with most (58% in both groups) having neither improvement nor worsening of symptoms.

At 19 months, the frequency of episodes of worsening HF was similar in the two groups. Total deaths in the carvedilol group (n = 20) were less than the placebo group (n = 26), but most of the difference in mortality was attributed to noncardiovascular deaths. No difference was found in death from HF, MI, or total cardiac-related deaths. On a more positive note, there were 68% fewer hospital admissions for HF in the carvedilol group (n = 23) than for the placebo group (n = 33). Overall, these findings could be interpreted as being evidence for safety with either no overall benefit or a modest improvement with carvedilol.

The original FDA-approved indication for carvedilol was to reduce the progression of HF in patients with mild to moderate (NYHA class II or III) HF of ischemic or cardiomyopathic origin and whose conditions had been stabilized with other drugs (digitalis, diuretics, and ACE inhibitors). In keeping with the exclusion of patients with an unstable condition from the study protocols, carvedilol was not approved for use in NYHA class IV decompensated cardiac failure. As discussed in the next case, later studies confirmed the value of carvedilol in NYHA class IV HF. As with any β-blocker, carvedilol is not recommended for use in patients with asthma, COPD, or poorly controlled diabetes.

The starting dose of carvedilol is 3.125 mg twice daily, with a doubling of the dose every 2 weeks as needed or tolerated up to a maximum of 25 mg twice daily in patients weighing <85 kg and 50 mg twice daily in larger patients. Hypotension, bradycardia, fluid retention, and worsening HF symptoms can occur in the first few weeks of therapy, necessitating additional diuretics, a reduction of dose, or discontinuation of carvedilol. Taking carvedilol with food slows the rate of absorption and reduces the incidence of orthostatic hypotension, which occurs in up to 10% of patients taking the drug. Carvedilol phosphate (Coreg CR), a once-a-day extended release form of carvedilol, is market in the United States for hypertension treatment, but currently it has not been studied in patients with HF.

Because carvedilol is metabolized by the cytochrome P450 2D6 (CYP2D6) enzyme system, several potential drug interactions should be considered.[211,218] The best documented are inhibition of metabolism by cimetidine and decreased carvedilol serum concentrations when taken with rifampin. Known inhibitors of CYP2D6 (e.g., quinidine, fluoxetine, paroxetine, and propafenone) can increase the risk of toxicity (especially hypotension), but substantiating data are lacking. Carvedilol has also been reported to increase serum digoxin levels by 15% by an unknown mechanism. Other sources of intrasubject variability in carvedilol response may be caused by differences in the extent or rate or absorption, stereospecific metabolism of the two isomers of the drug (carvedilol is a racemic mixture of S[−] and R[+] isomers), and impaired metabolism in the 10% of the population who lack CYP2D6 activity.[218]

Choice of β-Blocker: Metoprolol vs. Carvedilol

No consensus exists regarding the relative superiority of one β-blocker over another. Although the additional properties of carvedilol (e.g., α_1 blockade and antioxidant properties) provide a theoretical basis for selecting carvedilol over metoprolol succinate or bisoprolol, the data from clinical trials provide conflicting conclusions. In one small head-to-head trial, carvedilol showed greater improvement in hemodynamic response during peak exercise and EF but no difference in symptom scores or exercise tolerance.[219] Another reported 30 patients with HF with persistent symptoms, despite at least 1 year of combined metoprolol and an ACE inhibitor.[220] They were enrolled in an open-label, parallel trial and randomized either to continue with metoprolol (mean dose, 142 ± 44 mg/day) or to cross over to maximal tolerated doses of carvedilol (mean dose, 74 ± 23 mg/day). At the end of 12 months, patients randomized to carvedilol showed a greater decrease in end-diastolic volume, more improvement in LVEF, and fewer ectopic beats on electrocardiogram. No significant difference was seen in symptoms or quality of life measures nor a negative effect of carvedilol on peak oxygen consumption.

One meta-analysis attempted a comparison of carvedilol with metoprolol using the surrogate end point of LVEF as a comparator.[221] Nineteen randomized, placebo or concurrent controlled trials involving a total of 2,184 patients with impaired LVEF were reviewed. Patients received a mean dose of 58 mg of carvedilol or the equivalent of 162 mg of extended release metoprolol. Combined results from the placebo controlled trials showed that both drugs significantly improved LVEF, with carvedilol found to be significantly better than metoprolol. Carvedilol increased LVEF 0.065% more than placebo compared with a 0.038% increase with metoprolol. These differences persisted when patients with ischemic HF were compared with those with nonischemic cardiomyopathy. In head-to-head comparative trials, carvedilol once again raised LVEF greater than metoprolol. No apparent difference, however, was noted between the two drugs based on improvements in symptom scores or exercise tolerance. The authors caution that EF is only one of several end points to be measured, and the question of superiority in clinical outcomes, such as mortality rates, remains unanswered.

Since publication of the meta-analysis, the results of the COMET trial became available.[222] In this multicenter, double-blind trial, 3,029 patients with NYHA class II–IV HF and EF <35% were randomized to either carvedilol (target dose, 25 mg BID) or metoprolol tartrate (target dose, 50 mg BID). Diuretics and ACE inhibitors were continued in all subjects if tolerated. All-cause mortality was 34% for carvedilol compared with 40% with metoprolol ($p = 0.0017$). The composite end point of mortality or all-cause hospital admissions was not statistically significant between groups (74% carvedilol and 76% metoprolol). One criticism of this study was use of metoprolol tartrate instead of the FDA-approved metoprolol succinate form. Comparable doses between the two study groups has been questioned because the target dose of carvedilol was 25 mg twice daily compared with the target dose of metoprolol tartrate being 50 mg twice daily. Also, the trial used resting HR to determine comparable β-blockade among study groups rather than HR response to exercise. Exercise-induced HR changes are considered a better indicator of β-blockade.

Side effects and patient tolerance is similar between β-blockers in most trials. One investigator observed that carvedilol caused more hypotension and dizziness than metoprolol or bisoprolol, possibly owing to α_1 blockade or more rapid absorption.[223] Thus, metoprolol or bisoprolol may be preferred in patients with hypotension or with complaints of dizziness. Conversely, carvedilol may be preferred in patients with inadequately controlled hypertension.

Whether carvedilol is a better choice for A.J. cannot be definitely answered. A starting dosage of 3.125 mg twice daily of carvedilol could be used in place of metoprolol. Because of lower cost, it is decided to continue metoprolol and reserve use of carvedilol only if A.J. has difficulty tolerating metoprolol.

β-Blockers in Severe Heart Failure

30. The original clinical trials of β-blockers excluded patients with severe (NYHA class IV) HF at the time of randomization. For this reason the FDA limited the original approval of carvedilol for use in class II–III HF. Likewise, the ACC/AHA guidelines strongly support the use of β-blockers in class II–III HF, but are less definitive about severe HF. What evidence supports or refutes the use of β-blockers in class IV HF?

The COPERNICUS study demonstrated clear benefit of carvedilol without undue side effects in patients with severe HF.[224] Conversely, the BEST Trial reported unimpressive results with another drug, bucindolol.[225] Details of these two trials are provided below.

The COPERNICUS study was a double-blind, placebo-controlled trial assessing the clinical benefits and risks of carvedilol in 2,289 patients with advanced HF (NYHA class IIIB/IV).[224] Subjects had symptoms of HF at rest or with minimal exertion and an EF of 25% or less despite diuretics (99%), ACE inhibitors (97%), and digoxin (67%). Excluded were subjects who required intensive care, had significant fluid retention, were hypotensive, had evidence of renal insufficiency, or were receiving IV vasodilators or positive inotrope drugs. The starting dose of carvedilol or matching placebo was 3.125 mg twice daily, which was increased every 2 weeks to a target dose of 25 mg twice daily. Of those in the carvedilol group, 65% achieved the target dose, with the mean dose being 37 mg at the end of the first 4 months of the trial. The trial was discontinued prematurely after an average patient follow-up of 10.4 months because of a significant survival benefit from carvedilol. There were 130 deaths in the carvedilol group and 190 deaths in the placebo group, with a 35% decrease in the risk of death with carvedilol (95% CI, 19% to 48%; $p = 0.0014$). For the secondary end point of all deaths and hospitalizations combined, there were 425 events with carvedilol compared with 507 in the placebo group, a 24% decrease (95% CI, 13% to 33%, $p = 0.001$). Fewer patients in the carvedilol group (14.8%) than in the placebo group (18.5%) withdrew because of adverse effects at 1 year ($p = 0.02$).

A concern over using β-blockers in patients with class IV HF is that they may be predisposed to more side effects during the initiation phase of therapy. One study retrospectively analyzed the outcomes of 63 patients who were NYHA class IV compared with 167 subjects ranging from class I through III.[226] Adverse events occurred more frequently in the class IV patients (43%) than in the other subjects (24%; $p = 0.0001$) and more often resulted in permanent withdrawal of the drug (25% vs. 13%). Conversely, more class IV patients treated with carvedilol improved by more than one NYHA functional class than in the less symptomatic group (59% vs. 37%). A reanalysis of the COPERNICUS study data did not confirm a higher rate of intolerance over the first 8 to 12 weeks of carvedilol compared with placebo.[227] No difference was found between carvedilol and placebo in terms of death, hospitalizations, or withdrawal because of adverse events during the first 8 weeks of therapy.

The BEST Investigators failed to demonstrate that bucindolol, a nonselective β-blocker with vasodilator properties, improved overall survival in patients with NYHA class III–IV HF.[225] They randomized 2,708 patients to receive either bucindolol or placebo. Although the active drug yielded a significant decrease in norepinephrine levels and improvement in left ventricular function, the study was stopped prematurely because of the low probability of showing any significant cardiovascular mortality benefit over placebo. A possible explanation is that bucindolol has intrinsic sympathomimetic activity (ISA) that may counteract some of the benefits of β-blockade. Moreover, subgroup analysis suggested that black patients might have fared worse with bucindolol, raising concerns that β-blockers may not be effective therapy for black patients with advanced HF (see Question 52 for further discussion of possible racial differences in drug response).

It can be concluded that β-blockers are safe and effective in class IV HF. The best data exist for carvedilol. Bucindolol should be avoided.

Digitalis Glycosides

Preparation for Treatment

31. Over the next 2 months, A.J.'s dose of extended release metoprolol was gradually increased to 200 mg/day. Other than some episodes of fatigue and lassitude during each dosage increment, he tolerated metoprolol well and, over time, he was more functional than he had been for several years. Over the ensuing 9 months, however, he again had several episodes of HF symptoms that necessitated a gradual increase of his furosemide dose to 120 mg in the morning and 40 mg in the mid afternoon. A potassium supplement was reinstituted because his potassium levels were beginning to fluctuate as his furosemide was increased.

Today, his wife brought him to the ED because she could no longer care for him. His chief complaints are weakness, dizziness, extreme SOB, and inability to get out of bed. His weight has increased to 80 kg. His BP is considerably lower at 128/83 mm Hg, with a postural drop to 112/75 mm Hg. Abnormal laboratory values on admission are BUN, 31 mg/dL and serum creatinine, 1.4 mg/dL. His K is 4.3 mEq/dL. An ECG shows a HR of 98 beats/minute, normal sinus rhythm (NSR), and LVH, but no T-wave changes or ectopy. His valsartan is held for 24 hours while he is diuresed with several 40- and 80-mg boluses of IV furosemide and maintained on an NTG drip titrated to lower his pulmonary capillary wedge pressure (PCWP) below 15 and to keep his systolic BP >100 mm Hg. The plan is to reinstitute valsartan and to begin a digitalis glycoside. Is digitalis indicated for A.J.? What digitalis preparation should be prescribed?

Digoxin is the only digitalis glycoside marketed in the United States. The arguments for and against its use are presented in Question 15. Most of the recommendations stem from the Digoxin Intervention Group trial that found, in patients who had primarily class II or III symptoms, treatment with digoxin for 2 to 5 years had little effect on mortality, but modestly reduced the combined risk of death and hospitalization.[139]

As presented earlier in this chapter, the ACC/AHA guidelines indicate that patients with HF are unlikely to benefit from the addition of digoxin in stage A or stage B HF. In these patients, digoxin can be used for symptom management, only if they are treated with drug therapy shown to prolong survival (ACE inhibitors and β-blockers) or have not responded adequately to appropriate therapy. In those patients who are stage C HF with current or prior symptoms of HF, despite receiving optimal doses of ACE inhibitors of β-blockers, digoxin can be beneficial to reduce HF hospitalizations. A.J. fits the latter situation and, thus, is a logical candidate for adding digoxin as a fourth therapeutic intervention.

Digoxin is also prescribed routinely in patients with HF and concurrent chronic AF, but β-blockers may be more effective in controlling the ventricular response, especially during exercise. Digoxin should be avoided if the patient has significant sinus or atrioventricular block, unless the block is treated with a permanent pacemaker. It should be used cautiously in patients taking other drugs that can depress sinus or AV nodal function (e.g., amiodarone or β-blockers), although patients usually will tolerate this combination.

When A.J. entered the hospital today, he initially required IV furosemide and a NTG drip, but quickly stabilized. Digoxin is not indicated as primary therapy for stabilization of patients with acutely decompensated HF. Such patients should first receive appropriate treatment, including IV medications, as A.J. did. Thereafter, digoxin can be started as part of a long-term treatment strategy.

Gender Differences in Response to Digoxin

32. If A.J. had been a woman, would it have made in any difference in the determination to prescribe digoxin?

Until recently, nothing indicated that gender-based differences existed relative to prognosis of HF or in response to drugs such as digoxin. Two interesting reports published in 2002 sparked interest in this topic. The first was an extension of the Framingham Heart Study.[228] It was observed that over the past five decades the incidence of HF has been constant in men, but has declined by 31% to 40% in women during the interval of the last decade. During the last decade, survival rates for patients with HF have improved in both men and women, although the mortality rate is higher in men than in women. The more aggressive use of drugs, such as ACE inhibitors and β-blockers, are likely contributors to the improved outcomes. The authors speculate that the differences observed between men and women may reflect different causes of HF. For example, hypertension is a predominate cause of HF in women, whereas more men have prior MI as a contributor to HF.

The second report (a review article) more directly addresses the question of use of digoxin in men compared with women.[229] As previously discussed, the DIG Trial reported approximately equal mortality rates (35%) in subjects with HF randomized to either placebo or digoxin, while continuing usual doses of diuretics and ACE inhibitors.[139] A 12% reduction was found in the rate of death from HF in the digoxin group, but a corresponding increase was noted in death presumed to be caused by arrhythmias. On retrospective *post hoc* analysis of the DIG study data, it was discovered that women overall had a lower death rate from any cause than men (31.0% vs. 36.1%, $p = 0.001$), an absolute difference of 5.8%.[229] The death rate was also lower among women in the placebo group than among men taking placebo (28.9% vs. 36.9%; $p = <0.001$). Likewise, women taking digoxin had a lower death rate than men taking active drug (33.1% vs. 35.2%), but this difference was not statistically different ($p = 0.034$). A surprising finding was that women taking digoxin had a higher death rate than women taking placebo (33.1% vs. 28.9%), whereas death rates in men where essentially equal in both groups. The authors speculate that a possible mechanism for the increased risk of death among women taking digoxin is an interaction between hormone-replacement therapy and digoxin. Progesterone might increase serum digoxin levels by inhibiting PGP, thus reducing digoxin renal tubular excretion. Consistent with this hypothesis, digoxin serum concentrations after 1 month of digoxin intervention were higher in women than in men. The study investigators, however, did not routinely gather data on estrogen and hormone replacement therapy or consistently measure serum digoxin levels later in the trial. Because these observances are a retrospective, it is difficult to establish the clinical significance of the data and it is premature to argue against the use of digoxin in women. Nonetheless, it is prudent to recommend keeping serum digoxin concentrations <1.0 to 1.2 ng/mL in all patients and avoid hormone replacement therapy in women with HF when taking digoxin.

Loading Dose

33. Can A.J. be started with a properly chosen digoxin maintenance dose, or is a loading (digitalizing) dose necessary?

Loading doses of digoxin are rarely necessary. Slow initiation of therapy with maintenance doses of digoxin in lieu of a loading dose is the method of choice for ambulatory or non-acutely ill patients with normal renal function. Even in the acute care setting, no indication exists for loading doses of digoxin for HF alone. The exception might be if the patient has AF and it is desired to control ventricular response as quickly as possible. Even then, alternative drugs are likely to be used (see Chapter 19, Cardiac Arrhythmias).

The main disadvantage to foregoing a loading dose is the delay in accumulating maximal body glycoside stores and achieving therapeutic effects. The time required to achieve 92% of plateau concentrations of a drug administered on a routine basis at maintenance doses is four half-lives. Thus, a patient with normal renal function ($t^1\!/_2 = 1.8$ days) given a daily dose of 0.125 mg of digoxin will reach peak serum concentration in approximately 7 days. If the same patient was anephric ($t^1\!/_2 = 4.4$ days), it would take 17 days to reach plateau, and the maximal concentration would be approximately 2.5 times that of a healthy subject receiving the same dose. Slow digitalization can delay the onset of toxic signs, which could go unrecognized if the patient is at home.

A further argument against using a loading dose is that no evidence indicates that achieving a steady-state serum concentration quicker has any demonstrable effect on the time to reduction of HF symptoms. In any case, the full benefit of digoxin can be delayed for several days or weeks. Thus, clinicians should avoid rapidly increasing doses. For example, it would be improper to increase a patient's maintenance dose after 3 days if no clinical improvement had been observed.

A.J. is in moderate to severe HF and in the hospital. It could be argued that a loading dose of digoxin would be safe in this environment and possibly could speed his therapeutic response. Nonetheless, the logical decision is to forgo a loading dose.

Serum Level Interpretation

34. What is the target serum digoxin concentration for A.J.?

The target therapeutic serum digoxin concentration is 0.5 to 1.2 ng/mL (mean, 0.75 ng/mL). Many older textbooks, review articles, and clinical trials contain the prior standard of targeting serum digoxin concentrations in the range of 0.8 to 2 ng/mL, or a mean of 1.0 ng/mL. These older recommendations should be abandoned. Factors driving this change are information suggesting that the positive hemodynamic and neurohormonal effects of digoxin can be achieved at lower serum concentrations than those needed to induce a positive inotropic effect (see digoxin pharmacology discussion in the introduction to this chapter),[63–66] use of digoxin as an adjunct to vasodilator therapy instead of as the primary intervention, and allowance for possible overestimation of the patient's renal function because of fluctuating control of HF. The correlation between serum digoxin concentrations and both therapeutic and toxic responses is considered in greater detail in Questions 36 and 41.

Maintenance Dose

35. As predicted, A.J.'s renal function improved with diuresis and IV NTG. The latest values are BUN 24 mg/dL and SrCr 0.8 mg/dL. Determine the appropriate maintenance dose of digoxin for A.J.

The usual maintenance doses of digoxin have traditionally ranged from 0.125 to 0.25 mg/day. With the increased emphasis on targeting lower serum concentrations, more patients are now empirically started at 0.125 mg/day. For example, because A.J. is of average body size, is relatively young, and has essentially normal kidney function, he empirically would have been started on a 0.25 mg/day maintenance dose in the past. A 0.125 mg dose, however, is recommended for him now. It is safest to start with a conservative dose and assess his needs after 1 to 2 weeks.

In all cases, smaller doses of digoxin are given to patients with impaired excretion rates (e.g., those with renal failure, older patients) or small-framed individuals. For example, a totally anuric patient may receive only 0.0625 mg/day. Because of the long half-life of digoxin, all patients are given a single daily dose.

Monitoring Parameters

36. Even after hearing the dosing principles from the prior question, A.J.'s physician decided to use a dose of 0.25 mg/day of digoxin because of his experience in using this size dose previously. How should A.J.'s digitalis therapy be monitored? How useful are digoxin serum levels in monitoring therapy?

No clear therapeutic end point exists for digitalis therapy. Nonspecific ECG changes (ST depression, T-wave abnormalities, and shortening of the QT interval) correlate poorly with both toxic and therapeutic effects of the drug.[70,71] Although digoxin serum levels are readily available from most clinical laboratories, no "therapeutic level" and corresponding "toxic level" are clearly defined.

SERUM LEVEL INTERPRETATION

As stated in Question 34, a serum digoxin concentration of 0.5 to 1.2 ng/mL is now considered therapeutic because the beneficial parasympathomimetic and antiadrenergic effects of digoxin occur at lower concentrations than the inotropic effects. Interestingly, a recent *post hoc* analysis of the DIG trial, found that patients with serum digoxin concentrations in the range of 0.5 to 0.8 ng/mL had lower all-cause mortality rates than patients with serum concentrations in either the 0.9 to 1.1 ng/mL range or >1.2 ng/mL.[139,230] A few patients, especially if they are hypokalemic or hypomagnesemic, will manifest apparent signs of toxicity when serum digoxin concentrations are <1 ng/mL. At the other extreme, some patients tolerate concentrations >2 ng/mL with no signs of overt toxicity. Such overlap between therapeutic concentrations and toxic levels limits the absolute value of serum level monitoring. Serum levels can be used as a guide in confirming suspected toxicity or in explaining a poor therapeutic response, but clinical evaluation ultimately remains the best therapeutic guide. The correlation between serum digoxin concentrations and toxicity is considered in greater detail in Questions 40 and 41.

When interpreting serum digoxin concentrations, several procedural problems and patient characteristics must be taken into account. These include proper timing of sample collection, the effects of exercise, assay technique, and possible interfering substances in the patient's blood. A discussion of each of these factors follows.

Following an IV bolus dose or a single oral dose, equilibration of digoxin between the blood and tissues is slow. Because of this slow distribution phase, digoxin levels obtained <6 to 8 hours after the last dose may be falsely elevated and can lead to a misdiagnosis of toxicity. At steady-state, serum digoxin concentrations obtained after 24 hours (just before the next dose) are considered most reliable. If a sample is obtained randomly, the time of the last dose should be carefully noted.

Physical activity increases binding of digoxin to skeletal muscle; by redistributing the drug from the blood to the tissue, a lower serum digoxin concentration is observed clinically.[231,232] The more strenuous the exertion, the greater the magnitude of effect, but even daily physical activity such as walking can decrease serum digoxin concentration by 20%.[232] About 2 hours of supine rest is required for digoxin levels to reach a new steady state. Clinical consequences of this effect might be the inappropriate increase of the digoxin dose or failure to identify a possible toxic level in a patient who has a serum digoxin concentration drawn soon after walking briskly.

Similarly, a patient's serum digoxin concentration while hospitalized might be higher than serum digoxin concentrations drawn as an outpatient even with no dose change. Conversely, other investigators concluded that the changes in concentration are not clinically relevant during everyday activity and may only be of consequence for patients with large differences in activity level in the time surrounding the blood draws.[232] Obviously, a standardized approach to obtaining blood samples is key to the appropriate interpretation of results.

INTERFERING SUBSTANCES

In addition to the poor correlation between serum digoxin concentration and clinical effect, both endogenous and exogenous substances can interfere with the digoxin assay.[233–235] This is complicated further by the existence of a multitude of different assay methodologies, some of which are more susceptible to interference than others. All the tests are based on immunoassay methods, including several different fluorescence polarization immunoassays (FPIA) and numerous enzymatic immunoassays (e.g., CLIA, EMIT, TDx, ACA, Dimension,

Vitros). Among potential interfering substances are drugs and chemicals that are structurally similar to digoxin, most notably spironolactone (Aldactone) and possibly corticosteroids. Some assays also measure accumulated digoxin metabolites.

Other patient groups may have "endogenous digoxin-like substances" in their blood, imparting falsely elevated measurements. This has been noted in patients with liver and renal failure, pregnant women, and 2- to 6-day-old neonates. One theory is that excess bile acids in neonates or patients with liver or renal disease may be a source of endogenous digoxin-like immunoreactive factors (DLIF).[234] In some of these patient groups, "digoxin levels" as high as 1.4 ng/mL may be measured without any drug in the body. It is essential that anyone monitoring serum digoxin levels be aware of which assay method is used in their laboratory and which substances can cause false–positive reactions. New turbidimetric digoxin immunoassays and enzyme-linked immunosorbent digoxin assays minimize or almost completely eliminate interference with DLIF, but enzymatic immunoassays are still the standard assay being utilized in United States laboratories.[233,235,236]

CLINICAL EVALUATION

As with diuretic and vasodilator therapy, clinical monitoring is the key to evaluating adequacy of digitalis therapy. As A.J. begins to improve, he should have less dyspnea and complain less of orthopnea; venous distention and signs of pulmonary congestion will diminish or disappear; diuresis (monitored through urinary output and weight loss) may increase; and a lower HR may be observed.

The response of HR to digitalis can vary, depending on the patient's underlying disease. Because bradycardia and other rhythm disturbances may herald digitalis toxicity, daily monitoring of A.J.'s pulse will be needed until his condition and serum levels have reached a steady state. Ankle edema does not mobilize immediately and is a poor therapeutic end point.

Factors That Alter Response

37. Two days after starting digoxin, A.J. was discharged from the hospital. After 10 days of taking a maintenance dose of 0.25 mg, a serum digoxin level drawn during a clinic visit was reported as 0.7 ng/mL. Examination in the outpatient clinic 2 weeks later revealed that he had become progressively dyspneic and edematous since his hospital discharge. A STAT serum digoxin level at 3:00 PM was 0.3 ng/mL. A.J. had taken his dose of digoxin at 8:00 AM. What are some possible explanations for these events?

As stated in Question 36, serum levels are not an absolute guide to monitoring digitalis therapy. A partial explanation could be that A.J. was not at rest when the level was drawn. In this case, however, the low serum levels are accompanied by deterioration in his symptoms of HF. We can be reasonably sure of the accuracy of the serum concentration measured because it was drawn at the appropriate time (i.e., at steady-state and at least 6 to 8 hours after the last dose); further, A.J.'s responses were compatible with the reported level. When doubt exists regarding the reliability of a reported serum level, the laboratory should be asked to repeat the measurement.

PATIENT ADHERENCE

Patient adherence must definitely be taken into consideration whenever unusually low serum concentrations are seen or a lack of response to any drug is observed. It is possible that A.J. is a poor complier because his BP was high on his first admission. He should be carefully counseled on the proper use of his medications.

DIGOXIN MALABSORPTION

Alteration of the absorption of digoxin following oral administration in patients with malabsorption syndromes has been studied.[68,237] Finding was that poor and erratic absorption occurred in patients with malabsorption states, such as sprue, short-bowel syndrome, and rapid intestinal transit. Other investigators studied digoxin bioavailability in malabsorptive states, but could not demonstrate large differences in serum digoxin concentrations. They found, however, that use of more soluble forms, such as liquid-filled capsules, gave a better absorption than conventional tablets.[68]

ALTERED DIGOXIN METABOLISM

Altered digoxin metabolism is rare, but should be considered. One patient has been described who required 1 to 2 mg digoxin daily to control AF.[238] Although her half-life for digoxin was the same as control subjects, she metabolized a greater percentage of digoxin to cardioinactive products. Also, as previously stated, approximately 10% of persons given digoxin demonstrate bacterially mediated metabolism of the drug in the GI tract leading to a relative decrease in total amount of drug absorbed.[75]

Concurrent metabolic abnormalities can decrease the responsiveness of digoxin. Hypocalcemia has been reported to cause a digitalis resistance, as has hyperthyroidism[70,71] (see Chapter 49, Thyroid Disorders).

Drug Interactions

QUINIDINE

38. As suspected, A.J. was found to have been taking his digoxin only sporadically. After being counseled on the importance of good adherence, he was restarted on 0.25 mg/day. He did well for the next 6 months until he noted the onset of palpitations, which were diagnosed by ECG as atrial fibrillation. A digoxin level drawn at that time was 1.2 ng/mL, but all other laboratory tests were normal. He began quinidine sulfate at a dosage of 200 mg QID with rapid resolution of the atrial fibrillation. Four days later, during a follow-up clinic visit, he was noted to have bradycardia with a pulse rate of 50 beats/minute. He also complained of nausea, dizziness, and weakness. His digoxin level was 2.0 ng/mL. What factors could be contributing to the apparent digitalis toxicity in A.J.?

In the past, quinidine and digoxin were frequently used adjunctively in the treatment of AF: digoxin to control ventricular response by decreasing AV node conduction, and quinidine to decrease atrial irritability. With the advent of newer drugs, this combination has largely fallen out of favor. Reports show that >90% of patients previously stabilized by digoxin who subsequently begin quinidine experience a 2- to 2.5-fold increase in serum digoxin levels.[239–241] The actual magnitude of effect is highly variable and may depend on the dose of quinidine administered. Little change is seen with quinidine doses of <500 mg/day. Serum digoxin concentrations usually begin to rise within 24 hours of starting quinidine and reach a new steady state in about 5 days. Conversely, when quinidine is discontinued, digoxin concentrations return to prequinidine levels in about 5 days.

Several conflicting effects of quinidine on digoxin pharmacokinetics have been observed.[71,74] The most consistent finding is a 40% to 50% decrease in total body clearance of digoxin; much of this change is accounted for by decreased renal clearance.

The nonrenal clearance of digoxin also is affected by quinidine as evidenced by up to a doubling of digoxin plasma levels after addition of quinidine in patients with chronic renal failure.[242,243] A reduced volume of distribution has been observed in some individuals, but this is not a consistent finding. Digoxin's half-life does not change, probably because the changes in distribution and clearance tend to counterbalance each other. A unifying mechanism to explain all of these observations is the ability of quinidine to inhibit PGP-mediated drug transport in the kidney, intestine, and possibly the liver.[71,73,74] Under usual conditions, digoxin enters the renal tubule via both glomerular filtration and renal tubular secretion, the latter mechanism being under the influence of PGP-mediated transport. Inhibition of PGP by quinidine in the kidney partially blocks the tubular secretion step, thus decreasing renal clearance of the digoxin. In the intestines, PGP facilitates active transport of absorbed digoxin back into the intestinal tract. The net effect of inhibition of gut PGP by quinidine is increased bioavailability of digoxin.

Digoxin is found in only small concentrations in the plasma, with most of the drug being distributed to lean body tissues (e.g., skeletal and cardiac muscle). Despite clear evidence that serum digoxin levels are increased with quinidine, much less is known about the importance of this interaction on the heart and the clinical effects that ensue. Because both of these drugs can individually cause GI intolerance (e.g., nausea, vomiting, diarrhea), AV block, and bradycardia, it is difficult to differentiate simple additive effects from a true drug interaction without measuring serum level changes. One 9-month study of hospital admissions for suspected digitalis toxicity observed that 50% of patients treated with the quinidine–digoxin combination had ECG evidence of digoxin toxicity compared with 5% of patients taking digoxin alone or in combination with verapamil or amiodarone.[244] Conversely, many patients tolerate the increased serum levels of digoxin with no apparent adverse consequences.

Faced with the complexity of this interaction, it is difficult for the clinician to plan a course of action when using these two drugs together. It has been suggested that the dose of digoxin be reduced by 50% when adding quinidine. Although this might minimize bradycardia, ventricular tachyarrhythmias, and GI effects, it also can lead to a loss of desired neurohormonal or positive inotropic effects. A more rational approach is to use smaller doses of digoxin in all patients, whether or not they are taking quinidine. Then, when adding quinidine, patients can maintain their previous digoxin dose with careful clinical monitoring for undesirable side effects. If necessary, a serum digoxin level can be obtained after 5 to 7 days of concurrent therapy. If it exceeds 1.2 ng/mL, the dose can be decreased. Concentrations in excess of 2.0 ng/mL are a definite cause for concern. A.J. should have his digoxin dose reduced to 0.125 mg QD.

Treatment of Supraventricular Arrhythmias in Heart Failure

DIGOXIN DRUG INTERACTION WITH AMIODARONE AND PROPAFENONE

39. Quinidine was started in A.J. because of atrial fibrillation. What alternatives to quinidine and digoxin could be recommended for A.J.? What other potential drug interactions does this present?

Supraventricular arrhythmias are frequently encountered in HF because volume or pressure overload can cause atrial distention and irritability. Specifically, atrial fibrillation is present in 25% to 50% of patients with advanced HF, contributing to reduced exercise capacity, increased risk of pulmonary or systemic emboli, and worse long-term prognosis.[6,245] As in any patient with these arrhythmias, drug therapy should be aimed at controlling ventricular rate and preventing thromboembolic events. Cardioversion to normal sinus rhythm is unlikely to be successful. Left ventricular function and clinical status frequently improve after controlling atrial fibrillation, however, whether or not normal sinus rhythm is restored.

Digoxin slows the ventricular response associated with atrial fibrillation and, thus, is a logical choice in patients with concurrent HF. A potential limiting factor is that digoxin's AV blocking properties are most evident at rest, but are less consistent during exercise. Hence, digoxin may be ineffective at controlling exercise-induced tachycardia that limits the patient's functional capacity. β-Blockers are more effective than digoxin during exercise.[246–248] Propranolol or atenolol are the β-blockers of choice in patients without HF, but metoprolol is a better choice in those with HF because of its proved role in HF management. If digoxin, β-blockers, or both are ineffective, amiodarone is another useful alternative. Verapamil and diltiazem are not appropriative choices for rate control in patients with HF because of their negative inotropic effects.

The benefits of restoring sinus rhythm remain unclear (see Chapter 19, Cardiac Arrhythmias.) Most patients who are electrically cardioverted revert to atrial fibrillation in a short time. The use of most other antiarrhythmic agents (e.g., quinidine, procainamide, propafenone, and other class II antiarrhythmics), except amiodarone, is associated with worse prognosis because of proarrhythmic effects and should be avoided. Warfarin is required for patients with AF, but not for other patients with HF. Finally, atrioventricular nodal ablation may be needed if tachycardia or bothersome symptoms persist despite aggressive pharmacologic intervention.

A.J. developed AF while already taking a relatively high dose of digoxin (0.25 mg/day) and metoprolol. As discussed above, quinidine is not the best choice because of its drug interaction potential and side effects, most notably the potential to cause other life-threatening arrhythmias. One alternative is to discontinue quinidine, keep the digoxin dose at 0.25 mg QD, and continue metoprolol. If his AF-associated palpitations persist, amiodarone should be started. (See Chapter 19, Cardiac Arrhythmias, for dosing of amiodarone in supraventricular tachyarrhythmias.) Because amiodarone is also a PGP inhibitor with a documented ability to reduce digoxin clearance in a manner similar to that described with quinidine, A.J.'s digoxin dose will need to be lowered to 0.125 mg.[71,73] The onset of the interaction may not be apparent for a prolonged time because of the long half-life of amiodarone. As serum concentrations of amiodarone slowly increase, digoxin clearance and bioavailability will be changing simultaneously. The net effect may be easily overlooked, but can result in increased serum concentrations of 30% to 60%. Similarly, propafenone increases digoxin steady-state concentrations by 30% to 60% in a dose-dependent fashion over the range of 450 to 900 mg/day of propafenone.[71,249]

Other Digoxin Drug Interactions

40. What other potential drug interactions with digoxin might affect A.J.'s therapy?

Two comprehensive reviews of cardiac glycoside drug interactions have been compiled.[239,250] Since publication of these earlier reviews, a greater understanding of PGP-mediated drug interactions has evolved.[73,74] A brief summary of all digoxin interactions is found in Table 18-15. Two of the better-documented interactions (quinidine and amiodarone) were discussed in the previous cases. Others drugs recently recognized as raising digoxin serum concentrations through PGP inhibition include atorvastatin (increased intestinal absorption),[251] CCB (especially verapamil and diltiazem),[252] erythromycin and clarithromycin (reduced renal digoxin clearance),[253,254] and cyclosporine. Conversely, rifampin[255] and St. John's Wort[256] reduce oral digoxin bioavailability and serum concentrations via induction of intestinal PGP. Mylanta is the only drug listed in Table 18-15 that A.J. was taking. He should be counseled to avoid antacids within 1 or 2 hours before or 1 hour after a dose of digoxin or to use a nonprescription histamine$_2$ receptor blocker.

Digitalis Toxicity

SIGNS AND SYMPTOMS

41. Digoxin was prescribed for Z.T., a 70-year-old man with mild HF. The label on his prescription bottle instructed him to take one tablet (0.25 mg) BID for 3 days, then one tablet daily thereafter. Ten days later Z.T. returned to the clinic complaining of extreme fatigue, anorexia, nausea, and a "funny" heart beat.

Table 18-15 Digoxin Drug Interactions[a]

Drug[b]	*Effect*
Drugs Lowering Serum Digoxin Concentration	
Antacids	↓Bioavailability via adsorption in gut
Cancer chemotherapy	Possible ↓bioavailability (especially combinations of cyclophosphamide and vincristine)
Cholestyramine (Questran)	↓Bioavailability via adsorption in gut
Colestipol (Colestid)	↓Bioavailability via adsorption in gut
Kaolin-pectin	↓Bioavailability via adsorption in gut
Laxatives	↓Bioavailability via gut hypermotility
Metoclopramide (Reglan)	↓Bioavailability via enhanced gastric emptying (slow-release digoxin only)
Neomycin	Malabsorption of digoxin
Psyllium hydrophilic mucilloid (Metamucil) and dietary bran fiber	Possible ↓bioavailability via adsorption in gut
Rifampin[255]	Probable induction of intestinal P-glycoprotein causing ↓bioavailability. ↓Serum concentration after oral, but not IV digoxin. No change in digoxin renal clearance or half-life.
St. John's Wort[256]	Possible induction of P-glycoprotein
Sulfasalazine (Azulfidine)	Malabsorption of digoxin
Drugs Raising Serum Digoxin Concentration	
Alprazolam[329]	↑Serum digoxin levels by unknown mechanism
Amiodarone (Cordarone)[71,73]	↑Serum digoxin levels by unknown mechanism
Atorvastatin[251]	20% increase in serum digoxin concentration with 80 mg dose, minimal effect with 20 mg dose. Speculated to inhibit intestinal P-glycoprotein, but not proven
Calcium channel blockers[71,73,252] (See Question 56)	Inhibition of P-glycoprotein. Best documented with verapamil.
Captopril[191]	Inhibition of digoxin renal clearance by unknown mechanism
Clarithromycin[253,254]	Inhibition of P-glycoprotein, decreased digoxin renal clearance
Cyclosporine[71,73]	Inhibition of P-glycoprotein, decreased digoxin renal clearance
Erythromycin	↑Bioavailability in persons who normally metabolize digoxin in intestinal tract. May also inhibit P-glycoprotein in gut.
Itraconazole[330]	↑Serum digoxin levels by unknown mechanism
Omeprazole[331,332]	↑Bioavailability (slight) due to altered gut metabolism
Propafenone[71,249]	Inhibition of P-glycoprotein
Quinidine (see Question 38)[71,73,74,239–244]	Inhibition of P-glycoprotein; decreased digoxin renal clearance and increased bioavailability.
Propantheline (Pro-Banthine)	↑Bioavailability via slowed gastric emptying (slow-release digoxin only)
Telmisartan[333]	Unknown mechanism. Increased peak serum concentration 3–4 hr after dose, but only slight increase in 24 hr AUC or trough serum concentration

[a]References 71, 239, and 250 include a discussion of many of these interactions that do not include a specific reference citation.
[b]Reference numbers.
AUC, area under curve.

Close questioning and a "tablet count" disclosed that Z.T. failed to decrease his digoxin to 0.25 mg/day. An ECG revealed multiple premature ventricular contractions (PVC) and second degree AV block. A STAT serum digoxin level was 2.8 ng/mL. What signs and symptoms in Z.T. are consistent with digitalis toxicity? What are some other adverse effects of digitalis?

This case illustrates a risk of using digoxin loading doses and one of several ways that digitalis toxicity might present. The clinical presentation of digitalis toxicity is unpredictable. In some cases, a high serum digoxin level without any appreciable adverse effects is the only clue to possible digitalis toxicity. In other patients, such as Z.T., a multitude of symptoms can be present, including both noncardiac signs (e.g., GI complaints) and rhythm disturbances (e.g., palpitation, heart block, arrhythmias).

The most important adverse effects are those relating to the heart. A common misperception is that GI or other noncardiac signs will precede cardiac toxicity. To the contrary, cardiac symptoms precede noncardiac symptoms of digitalis toxicity in up to 47% of cases. Frequently (26%–66%), nonspecific arrhythmias are the only manifestation of toxicity, with estimates that rhythm disturbances occur in 80% to 90% of all patients with digitalis toxicity.[257] On the other hand, rhythm disturbances in patients taking digitalis are not always related to toxicity. In one study of 100 consecutive patients with suspected digitalis-induced arrhythmias, only 24 were confirmed as being toxic as defined by resolution of cardiac irritability following drug withdrawal. In the other 76 patients, the dysrhythmia persisted long after drug removal.[258]

Most known arrhythmias can occur as a result of digoxin toxicity. Decreased conduction velocity through the AV node presents as a prolonged PR interval (first-degree AV block) and is seen in many patients with therapeutic levels of digitalis. As exemplified in Question 38, however, higher concentrations of digitalis can impair conduction and result in bradycardia or a variable block (second-degree AV block). With severe toxicity, complete (third-degree) AV block results in dissociation of the atrial and ventricular rates with a slow idioventricular rate predominating. AV block also may predispose patients to accelerated junctional rhythms. Increased automaticity of the atria can cause multifocal atrial tachycardia (MAT) with block, paroxysmal atrial tachycardia (PAT) with block, or atrial fibrillation.

Ventricular arrhythmias (as seen in Z.T.) are among the most common rhythm disturbances caused by digitalis toxicity and include unifocal and multifocal PVC, bigeminy (every other beat is a PVC), trigeminy, ventricular tachycardia, and ventricular fibrillation. Comprehensive reviews are available on the topic of digitalis-induced arrhythmias.[257,258]

Hyperkalemia can develop as a consequence of massive digitalis poisoning.[259] Toxic doses of digitalis severely poison the Na^+ -K^+ -ATPase system, causing inhibition of the uptake of potassium by the myocardium, skeletal muscle, and liver cells. The shift of potassium from inside to outside the cell can result in significant hyperkalemia, especially in patients with underlying renal insufficiency. These same patients also are likely to accumulate digoxin in the body because of decreased clearance of the drug. Cardiac ectopy can be potentiated by the increase in serum potassium, especially when the potassium concentration exceeds 5 mEq/L. Paradoxically, in patients with good renal function, hyperkalemia can enhance renal excretion of potassium, resulting in a deficit in total body potassium despite the continued high serum concentration of potassium.

Vague GI symptoms characteristic of digitalis toxicity are difficult to evaluate because anorexia and nausea are also part of H.F.'s clinical picture. During one prospective clinical study, an equal frequency of anorexia and nausea occurred in both toxic and nontoxic patients taking digoxin.[260] Anorexia may be the earliest symptom, followed in 2 to 3 days by nausea. More than 25% of patients have GI symptoms for >3 weeks before diagnosis. Nonspecific abdominal pain and bloating caused by nonocclusive mesenteric ischemia secondary to digitalis-induced vasoconstriction also has occurred.

Central nervous symptoms of digitalis are common, possibly associated with potassium depletion in neural tissue. Chronic digitalis intoxication resulting from misformulation was observed in 179 patients.[260] Acute extreme fatigue or visual disturbances were a complaint in 95% of these patients. Approximately 80% experienced weakness of the arms and legs, and 65% had psychic disturbances in the form of nightmares, agitation, listlessness, and hallucinations. Hazy vision and difficulties in both reading and red-green color perception frequently were present. Other complaints included glitterings, dark or moving spots, photophobia, and yellow-green vision. Disturbances in color vision returned to normal 2 or 3 weeks after discontinuation of digitalis.

Interestingly, six elderly patients had apparent digitalis-induced visual disturbances at serum concentrations below those considered to be toxic (all <1.5 ng/mL; range, 0.2 to 1.5 ng/mL).[261] Five of the reactions were described as photopsia (seeing lights not present in the environment) and one person had decreased visual acuity. Color vision disturbances or seeing color lights, both well-described with digitalis toxicity, were absent. The symptoms went away in all but one subject when digoxin was discontinued.

Some prospective studies showed a good correlation between serum digoxin levels and toxicity,[260,262,263] whereas other investigators found a poor correlation.[264,265] In one study, 87% of digitalis-toxic patients had levels >2 ng/mL and 90% of nontoxic patients had levels <2 ng/mL. Conversely, other investigators found that nearly 50% of subjects with a serum digoxin level >3 ng/mL were clinically stable without signs of digitalis toxicity.[264] In the largest series studied to date, the average serum digoxin concentration in documented toxic patients (i.e., those with a suspected digitalis-induced arrhythmia that disappeared after drug withdrawal) was 2.9 ng/mL compared with 1.0 ng/mL in patients with suspected digitalis toxicity, but in whom the arrhythmia persisted after drug withdrawal.[258] Approximately 38% of documented toxic patients, however, had serum digoxin concentrations <2 ng/mL (false–negative test results). Once levels exceed 6 ng/mL, the risk of mortality greatly increases.[266]

Because a significant overlap between toxic and therapeutic levels exists, serum level determinations are currently most useful as an aid in confirming suspected digitalis toxicity and in individualizing dosing regimens so that toxicity might be avoided. In particular, subjects with low serum potassium concentrations can demonstrate digitalis toxicity at lower serum digoxin concentrations.[267]

Allergic reactions to digitalis are rare. Unilateral or bilateral gynecomastia is observed during chronic digoxin administration and is reversible on withdrawal of the drug. This latter effect may occur in addition to the gynecomastia seen with spironolactone.

PREDISPOSING FACTORS

42. B.V., a 64-year-old alcoholic man, is admitted to the hospital with a 3-day history of epigastric pain radiating to the back and associated with nausea and vomiting. B.V. also has cirrhosis of the liver and mild HF that is well controlled with furosemide 80 mg/day, ramipril 2.5 mg BID, and digoxin 0.25 mg/day. He has a 3-year history of severe rheumatoid arthritis, which is moderately relieved with NSAID and prednisone 15 mg/day. Because the initial impression was acute pancreatitis, B.V. was placed on a nasogastric suction and 3 L of D51/4 NS daily. The next evening, the laboratory report disclosed the following: Na, 136 mEq/L (normal, 136–144 mEq/L); K, 2.3 mEq/L (normal, 3.5–5.3 mEq/L); Cl, 90 mEq/L (normal, 96–106 mEq/L); bicarbonate, 32 mEq/L (normal, 23–28 mEq/L); Mg, 1.3 mEq/L (normal, 1.7–2.7 mEq/L); creatinine, 0.8 mg/dL (normal, 0.5–1.2 mg/dL); AST, 80 U (normal, 40 U); alkaline phosphatase, 130 U (normal, 80 U); amylase, 1,200 U (normal, 4–25 U); digoxin, 1.8 ng/mL; and Cl_{Cr}, 100 mL/minute (normal, 100–125 mL/minute). An ECG showed a HR of 70 beats/minute with occasional PVC and runs of bigeminy. What factors predispose B.V. to digitalis toxicity?

[SI units: Na, 136 mmol/L (normal, 134–144); K, 2.3 mmol/L (normal, 3.5–5.3); Cl, 90 mmol/L (normal, 96–106); bicarbonate, 32 mmol/L (normal, 23–28); Mg, 0.65 mmol/L (normal, 0.85–1.35); creatinine, 70.72 mmol/L (normal, 44.2–106.08); AST, 80 U/L (normal, 40); alkaline phosphatase, 130 U/L (normal, 80); amylase, 1,200 U/L (normal, 4–25); and Cl_{Cr}, 1.67 mL/sec (normal, 1.67–2.08)]

This is an example of a subtle presentation of digitalis toxicity. The serum level is in the high end of the therapeutic range. Nevertheless, B.V. shows clinical signs of digitalis toxicity (e.g., PVC and bigeminy). His renal function is normal, so digoxin renal clearance should not be significantly altered. The major contribution to toxicity in B.V. is hypokalemia.

The association between digitalis toxicity and hypokalemia is well recognized. It has been observed that twice as much digitalis is required to produce toxicity in patients with serum potassium of 5 mEq/L than in those with a serum potassium of 3 mEq/L.[267] A few patients will develop signs of toxicity with serum digitalis concentrations as low as 1.5 ng/mL if hypokalemia is present. Therefore, drugs, diseases, and medical maneuvers that induce hypokalemia or reduce the serum potassium from elevated to normal levels may unmask digitalis toxicity. A low serum potassium has been observed to increase the uptake of digitalis by the myocardial tissue.[268]

B.V. is taking furosemide. All diuretics, with the exception of potassium-sparing diuretics, can cause hypokalemia through kaliuresis. In addition, prednisone in high doses promotes potassium excretion in the distal portion of the renal tubule. B.V.'s prednisone dose should be tapered and eventually discontinued while one of the newer disease-modifying drugs is started (see Chapter 43, Rheumatic Disorders). Similarly, diseases in which mineralocorticoid activity is high (e.g., Cushing's disease, hyperaldosteronism) are associated with low serum potassium levels. B.V.'s history of cirrhosis could lead to development of portal hypertension and ascites, both of which are associated with hyperaldosteronism.

Other causes of hypokalemia in B.V. include vomiting and nasogastric suction. Similarly, hypokalemia can result from diarrheal losses, including drug-induced diarrhea (e.g., amoxicillin, quinidine).

Although the relationship of hypokalemia to digitalis toxicity is stressed, hyperkalemia is also a risk factor.[259] A bimodal effect of potassium on the AV node has been observed, whereby both hypokalemia and hyperkalemia may delay AV nodal conduction resulting in bradycardia and compensatory ventricular ectopy.

B.V. has metabolic alkalosis (HCO_3^-, 32 mEq/L) from the combined effects of diuretic therapy, vomiting, and nasogastric suctioning of hydrogen ion. Alkalosis results in the redistribution of potassium intracellularly and an increased renal excretion of potassium, thereby potentiating effects of hypokalemia (see Chapter 10, Acid-Base Disorders). In addition, alkalosis in and of itself has been associated with an increased incidence of digitalis toxicity. This is attributed to an intracellular depletion of potassium caused by increased urinary excretion and a relative increase in the ratio of extracellular to intracellular potassium.[268] This has the same effect on the membrane potential as digoxin.

Another metabolic problem that could contribute to digitalis toxicity in B.V. is hypomagnesemia. The causes are the same as for hypokalemia, including diuretic therapy, nasogastric suction losses, and chronic alcoholism. The prevalence of hypomagnesemia is higher in digitalis-toxic patients; magnesium sulfate has been used successfully in the treatment of digitalis toxicity.[269]

Although not illustrated by B.V., hypercalcemia theoretically can predispose patients to digitalis toxicity. The electrical and contractile effects of calcium on the myocardium are similar to those of digitalis. For this reason, rapid IV infusions of calcium can facilitate the development of digitalis toxicity, and normal or low doses of digitalis can induce toxicity in patients with hypercalcemia (e.g., hyperparathyroidism or metastatic cancer). The clinical significance of calcium-induced digitalis toxicity is questionable; there have been no reports of digitalis toxicity secondary to oral administration of calcium-containing products.

Age may be an important predisposing factor in the production of digitalis toxicity in B.V. The same IV dose of digoxin administered to elderly and young patients produces higher serum concentrations of digoxin in the elderly. The higher levels and prolonged half-life observed in these patients are likely caused by diminished renal clearance of the drug and this population's smaller body size. It is important to emphasize that, although the serum creatinine of elderly patients may be within normal limits, the mean creatinine clearance is reduced.

The response to digitalis also can be altered in the very young (see Question 45). Lower doses are recommended in premature infants and neonates (<1 month) because of the decreased renal function normally observed in newborns.[270] Although absorption, tissue distribution, and excretion of digoxin in infants are similar to those observed in adults, infants excrete a smaller percentage of digoxin metabolites than adults.

TREATMENT OF DIGITALIS TOXICITY

43. How should B.V.'s digitalis toxicity be treated?

Withholding Digitalis and Electrolyte Replacement

For many patients without life-threatening arrhythmias or major electrolyte imbalances, simple withdrawal of digitalis is the only treatment required. Although it may take five half-lives for the drug to be totally eliminated from the body, the serum concentration will drop to a safe level after one to two half-lives (2 to 3 days for digoxin) in most individuals.

B.V. does not have significantly elevated digoxin levels, so his ectopy should disappear rapidly with drug withdrawal. His major problem is related to hypokalemia that must be corrected. As a general rule, potassium replacement should be considered in any patient with digitalis-induced ectopic beats who has low or normal serum potassium levels. Oral administration is acceptable unless the patient cannot take medication orally or has life-threatening ectopy. If digitalis-induced arrhythmias are sufficiently severe to warrant intravenously administered potassium, the maximal recommended rate of administration is 40 mEq/hour (preferably 10 mEq/hour) at a concentration not exceeding 80 to 100 mEq/L. A total of several hundred milliequivalents of potassium might be required to replete body stores. Potassium should be administered with caution in patients who have conduction disturbances characterized by second-degree or complete AV block because high doses can further depresses conduction velocity in the AV node.

B.V. has a significant potassium deficit with potentially dangerous arrhythmias but no contraindications to potassium therapy. He should receive 80 to 120 mEq of IV potassium over the next 24 hours and then be switched to an appropriate oral dose. He should be monitored for signs and symptoms of potassium toxicity with frequent ECG tracings (look for tall, peaked T waves; prolonged PR interval) and serum potassium determinations.

It is important to obtain a serum magnesium concentration when measuring potassium levels. Patients with a low serum magnesium level (<1.5 mEq/L) or whose condition fails to respond after potassium repletion should receive a 20 mg/kg (2 g in an adult) loading dose of magnesium sulfate administered as a 10% solution over 20 minutes, followed by a continuous infusion at a rate of 0.5 to 2 g/hour to maintain a serum magnesium level of at least 4 to 5 mEq/L. Magnesium is relatively contraindicated in patients with renal failure, hypermagnesemia, or a high-level AV block. The infusion should be discontinued if deep tendon reflexes are diminished or serum concentrations of magnesium exceed 7 mEq/L.

Antiarrhythmic Agents

Patients with bradycardia because of second- or third-degree AV block should be given IV atropine. The usual atropine dose is 0.5 to 1 mg over 1 to 2 minutes with a repeat in 15 to 30 minutes if the patient does not respond. Doses <0.5 mg can paradoxically worsen the AV block. Atropine should be used with caution in patients with prostatic hypertrophy because significant urinary retention and postrenal azotemia can occur. Alternatively, a temporary pacemaker can be placed. Because B.V.'s HR is 70 beats/minute, atropine is not indicated.

Virtually all of the antiarrhythmic agents have been used to treat digitalis-induced arrhythmias. Lidocaine and phenytoin have a theoretic advantage over quinidine-like agents because they do not further depress AV conduction. Phenytoin is particularly efficacious in the suppression of digitalis-induced tachyarrhythmias with or without first- or second-degree AV block. For B.V., potassium replacement will probably be all that is required. Because of his bigeminy, however, lidocaine could be administered for a few hours until he has been given sufficient potassium supplementation. (See Chapter 19, Cardiac Arrhythmias, for dosing guidelines for lidocaine and phenytoin.)

Peritoneal and hemodialysis are ineffective in removing digoxin from the body, but charcoal hemoperfusion is used for life-threatening overdoses in patients with renal failure.[271]

Digoxin Immune Fab

44. All the treatments above are symptomatic. When is a specific antidote such as digoxin immune Fab indicated?

Most treatment regimens for digitalis toxicity are supportive only, either by counteracting the pharmacologic effects of digitalis or by interfering with further absorption of ingested tablets. A more definitive treatment consists of administration of digoxin-specific antibodies that bind digoxin molecules, rendering them unavailable for binding at receptors in the heart and other areas of the body.[272–277] The antibodies bind intravascular digoxin and also diffuse into interstitial spaces to bind free digoxin. As the extracellular unbound (free) digoxin concentration decreases, intracellular digoxin diffuses into extracellular fluid and becomes available to be bound to the antidigoxin antibodies. A concentration gradient is thus created that promotes release of digoxin from binding sites. Ultimately, the digitalis–antibody complex is excreted in the urine. The official name of this product is digoxin immune Fab, ovine sold under the brand names of Digibind and DigiFab.

The use of digoxin Fab products is restricted to potentially life-threatening intoxications (severe arrhythmias or hyperkalemia) that are either refractory to more conservative therapy or associated with extremely high serum concentrations. The major reason for this approach is the high cost of digoxin Fab.

Digoxin immune Fab is supplied as a lyophilized powder (38 mg/vial of Digibind, 40 mg/vial of DigiFab) that, after reconstitution with 4 mL of sterile water for injection, yields a 10 mg/mL solution that should be used within 4 hours. One milligram of digoxin immune Fab binds 12.5 mcg of digoxin. Thus, the contents of one vial will bind approximately 0.5 mg of digoxin. The actual dose administered varies according to the estimated amount of digitalis glycoside in the body. For digoxin, the amount of drug in the body can be estimated by the formula:

$$\text{Body load in mg} = \frac{5.0(\text{SDC})(\text{Weight in kg})}{1{,}000} \qquad \textbf{(18-2)}$$

where 5.0 is the volume of distribution of digoxin in liters per kilogram. An oral absorption of approximately 80% for digoxin is assumed. From this estimate, the total number of vials required for neutralization is calculated by dividing the total body load by 0.5 mg/vial. Patients with renal failure have a smaller volume of distribution of digoxin and thus have higher serum concentrations for any given dose.

In cases of extremely large single-dose ingestions for which the results of digoxin serum concentrations are not available, an empiric dose of 380 to 400 mg (10 vials) is given to an adult. An additional 380 to 400 mg can be given if needed.

For patients with toxicity during chronic therapy, 228 to 240 mg (6 vials) is adequate to treat most adults, whereas 38 to 40 mg (1 vial) is appropriate for children weighing <20 kg. The antibody usually is administered IV over 30 to 45 minutes, but it can be given more rapidly if the patient is in acute distress. It is recommended that the drug be infused through a 0.22-micron filter. Efficacy and safety is the same in children as in adults.[273]

Clinical improvement in the signs and symptoms of digitalis intoxication should occur within 30 minutes of antibody administration, with complete reversal of symptoms in 4 hours. If, after several hours, toxicity has not been adequately reversed or symptoms reappear, an additional dose can be given. In patients with renal insufficiency, the digitalis–antibody complex can be retained in the body for a prolonged time. If retained sufficiently long, Fab fragments could be degraded by the reticuloendothelial system, releasing active digitalis glycosides back into the circulation and necessitating re-treatment. For this reason, it has been proposed to give 50% of the calculated dose immediately over 15 minutes, then the remaining 50% as a continuous infusion over 7 hours.[274]

Immediately after treatment with digoxin-specific Fab, the active (free or unbound) digitalis concentration decreases to nearly undetectable levels, but the total (free plus antibody-bound) digoxin concentration increases. In <1 hour, the total concentration increases by 10- to 20-fold, peaking in about 10 hours at concentrations often exceeding several hundred nanometers per liter. The monitoring of serum digoxin levels following treatment with Digibind is of no value because most clinical laboratories measure only "total" serum concentrations of digitalis glycosides, a composite of both "free" and bound (to protein or Fab) drug.[275,276]

The Fab fragment–digoxin complex is excreted via the kidneys. It takes several days before the entire complex is removed, allowing routine digoxin assays to once again become reliable. In one study of patients with varying degrees of renal function, the half-life of the initial phase of total digoxin decline was 11.6 hours and the half-life of the second, or terminal, elimination phase was 118 ± 57 hours.[276] Unbound digoxin serum levels rebound to a mean maximal free digoxin concentration of 1.7 ± 1.3 mmol/L in 77 ± 46 hours, but are delayed to a greater extent in anephric patients.[275] Paradoxical return of toxicity may be caused either by release of digoxin from the Fab-digoxin complex or late redistribution of digoxin from tissue stores into the plasma.[274,276] As long as antibodies remain in the system, further therapy with digitalis preparations is compromised because of binding of any new doses. Thus, monitoring of unbound concentrations is necessary.

Side effects to digoxin-specific Fab antibodies are uncommon, but several cautions must be heeded.[277] HF or AF can be precipitated by the removal of the pharmacologic effects of the digitalis glycoside. Similarly, as Na^+-K^+-ATPase enzyme activity is restored, hypokalemia can develop. Serum potassium concentrations must be monitored frequently for the first several hours after Fab administration because potassium levels can drop precipitously as potassium shifts back into cells. This may require immediate potassium supplementation.

The incidence of hypersensitivity or other allergic reactions after Fab administration is rare, but the risk after repeated ingestions is unknown.[277] Skin testing according to the directions in the digoxin immune Fab package insert should be followed in individuals at high risk, especially in patients with known allergies to sheep serum or in whom digoxin-specific Fab has been administered previously. If an accelerated allergic reaction occurs, the drug infusion should be discontinued and appropriate therapy initiated, including antihistamines, corticosteroids, and airway management. Epinephrine should be used cautiously in patients with arrhythmias.

Pediatric Dosing

45. H.H., a 3-year-old girl with a congenital heart defect, is displaying increased symptoms of HF. She is awaiting surgery for repair of a ventricular septal defect and a damaged aortic valve. In the meantime, she is to receive digoxin therapy. All laboratory values, including renal function and electrolytes, are within normal limits. She weighs 28 lb (12.7 kg). Should digoxin dosing for H.H. be formulated using the same guidelines as for an adult? What loading dose and maintenance dose should H.H. be given?

Although many of the general principles that apply to use of digoxin in adults also apply to children, certain practical considerations and changes in pharmacokinetic parameters must be considered.[270] Dosing in children is complicated by rapid changes in body size and tissue distribution, GI motility, and maturation of the liver and kidney.

Most children cannot swallow conventional tablets or capsules and must be given the liquid (elixir) dosage form. Although the pediatric population does not differ significantly from adults in their ability to absorb digoxin, large individual variability is noted and the elixir is generally more bioavailable than the tablets (Fig. 18-1).

An important difference is noted between children and adults in regard to tissue uptake and volume of distribution of digoxin. As noted previously, the average adult has a steady-state digoxin volume of distribution of 6.7 L/kg. Greater variability is seen in very young to older children with volume of distribution reported to be 7.5, 16.3, and 16.1 L/kg in neonates, 11-month-old infants, and children, respectively.[270] Children have slightly higher digoxin protein-binding than adults, but neither group has a high enough percentage bound (i.e., <50%) to significantly affect tissue concentrations of the drug.

As in adults, clearance and half-life of digoxin in children are highly dependent on renal function and, to a lesser degree, on metabolism and biliary excretion. Elimination data in children are limited by the small number of available reports and the absence of studies in healthy pediatric subjects; nonetheless, a few generalizations can be made. Total body clearance is significantly impaired in premature and term neonates (with $t_{1/2}$ ranging from 61–170 hours). Older children and adolescents clear the drug at approximately the same rate as adults. These findings are consistent with poorly developed renal function in premature or young newborns, but the kidney becomes highly functional by 1 month of life and function approaches that of an adult by 1 year of age.

From these data, can be surmised that after the first year of life and through early childhood, children will need a *larger* dose on a per-kilogram basis than adults. This is based on a larger apparent volume of distribution, not altered drug clearance. Although no clear consensus is available on dosing of digoxin in children, the following guidelines have been published[270]: premature and term neonates should be digitalized with 0.01 to 0.03 mg/kg IV; infants should be given 0.04 to 0.05 mg/kg orally. For maintenance, the premature neonate can be given 0.001 to 0.009 mg/kg/day, neonates 0.010 mg/kg/day, and infants (1 month to 2 years) 0.015 to 0.025 mg/kg/day. For children older than 2 years of age, the loading dose is 0.05 mg/kg orally followed by a daily maintenance dose of 0.01 to 0.015 mg/kg. As in adults, doses are adjusted based on clinical signs, renal function, and serum levels (Table 18-5).

For H.H., an argument can be made for starting a maintenance dose without a loading dose because she is not in acute distress. If a loading dose is required, an oral elixir could be used at 0.05 mg/kg (0.6–0.65 mg), split into two doses. Maintenance would be started at 0.01 mg/kg or approximately 0.125 mg/day. These doses are surprisingly large and reflect the large volume of distribution in children.

This IV loading dose is considerably smaller than what would be used in a person with normal renal function because of assuming a smaller volume of distribution. A corresponding oral loading dose would be approximately 0.3 mg after correcting for an average bioavailability of 75%. When using larger loading doses, the total dose is often divided into two portions, giving two-thirds of the dose to start and the remaining one-third 6 to 8 hours later. Because the dose for R.D. is small, the entire 0.2 mg can be given at once. If after 8 to 12 hours she is still in atrial fibrillation, an extra 0.1 mg could be given safely because the serum concentration was targeted at only 0.75 ng/mL.

Critical Care Management of Heart Failure

Non-ACE Inhibitor Vasodilator Therapy

46. L.M., a 50-year-old black man, was admitted several days ago with severe, progressive, and debilitating symptoms of HF. Family history is significant in that his father and two brothers died of heart attacks shortly after the age of 40. L.M. has a 12-year history of HF that is symptomatic despite treatment with full therapeutic doses of furosemide, enalapril, carvedilol, and digoxin. He has no history of hypertension, but previous studies suggested a diagnosis of cardiomyopathy with an EF of 18%. Over the previous 8 months, L.M.'s DOE became progressively worse, and for the month before admission he was confined to bed because of extreme fatigue. He awoke once or twice nightly with PND.

Physical examination on this admission revealed a dyspneic, cyanotic man in obvious distress but with no complaints of chest pain. His BP was 100/66 mm Hg and his pulse was 105 beats/minute. Significant JVD, bilateral rales, hepatomegaly, and 3+ peripheral edema also were observed. Chest radiograph revealed cardiomegaly and pulmonary congestion. L.M. was admitted to the CCU where a Swan-Ganz catheter was passed from an antecubital vein to the pulmonary artery.

Before therapy, L.M.'s PCWP was 27 mm Hg (normal, 5 to 12 mm Hg) and his cardiac index (CI) was 1.9 L/minute/m^2 (normal, 2.7 to 4.3 L/minute/m^2). Several doses of IV furosemide were given, and IV nitroprusside was initiated at a dosage of 16 mcg/minute and eventually increased to 200 mcg/minute. At this dose, L.M.'s PCWP decreased to 15 mm Hg and his CI increased to 2.5 L/minute/m^2. He was eventually discharged home with furosemide 80 mg BID, spironolactone 50 mg QD, enalapril 20 mg BID, carvedilol 25 mg BID, digoxin 0.125 mg/day, hydralazine 75 mg QID, and isosorbide dinitrate 40 mg Q 6 hr. Categorize L.M.'s HF by NYHA class and ACC/AHA staging.

On admission L.M. was in NYHA class IV HF despite maximal doses of the recommend four-drug therapy with a loop diuretic, ACE inhibitor, β-blocker, and digoxin. He was approaching ACC/AHA stage D as well. His PCWP was high and his CI was low, reflecting pulmonary vascular congestion (elevated preload) and poor CO, respectively. (See Chapter 21, Shock, for a more thorough review of principles of Swan-Ganz catheterization and hemodynamic monitoring. Also see the introduction to this chapter to review the concepts of afterload, preload, and the relative contributions of arterial and venous dilation to these hemodynamic changes). The immediate objective of therapy is to provide symptomatic relief by decreasing the PCWP and increasing the CO.

Most patients with acute HF can be classified into one of four hemodynamic profiles using relatively simple assessment techniques (Fig. 18-8).[278–281] When using this scheme, patients are assessed for the presence or absence of elevated venous filling pressures (wet vs. dry patients) and adequacy of vital organ perfusion (warm vs. cold patients). Elevated filling pressure can be assessed at the patient's bedside by observing orthopnea, jugular venous distension, the presence of a third heart sound (S_3), peripheral edema, and ascites. Presence or absence of rales on auscultation is not considered a reliable indicator.[281] Hypotension, weak peripheral pulse, a narrow pulse pressure (<25%), cool forearms and legs, decreased mental alertness, and rising BUN and SrCr are indicators of decreased organ perfusion. In one series, 67% of patients admitted to the hospital with a low LVEF and class IV HF symptoms were classified as "wet and warm," with 28% assessed as "cold and wet," and only 5% as "cold and dry."[278] Few if any patients were in the "warm and dry category" because this is the status one is trying to achieve in well-compensated patients. Continuous blood pressure, ECG, urine flow, and pulse oximetry measurements are standard noninvasive monitoring for all patients. Invasive hemodynamic monitoring is used in critically ill patients when more precise measurements of filling pressure (e.g., right atrial or pulmonary artery pressure), systemic vascular resistance, and CO or cardiac index are desired. The goals are to achieve a right atrial pressure of <5 to 8 mm Hg, pulmonary artery pressure of <25/10 mm Hg, pulmonary artery wedge pressure of 12 to 16 mm Hg or less, a systemic vascular resistance of 900 to 1,400 dyn.s.m^{-5}, and a cardiac index of 2.8 to 4.2 L/minute/m^2 (see Chapter 21, Shock, for more detailed discussion of hemodynamic monitoring).

For most patients presenting in the "wet and warm" category, the primary intervention is aggressive diuresis to reduce fluid overload rapidly. This is followed by optimization of the standard three-drug regimen of ACE inhibitors, β-blockers, and digoxin. In more severe cases (e.g., when pulmonary artery wedge pressure is >18 mm Hg), initial use of an IV vasodilator, such as nitroglycerin or nesiritide, to reduce preload may be indicated. Nesiritide offers an advantage of having both natriuretic and vasodilatory properties and can add to the diuretic effect of furosemide in refractory patients.[34] Careful monitoring of pulmonary wedge pressure and cardiac index is necessary to avoid excessive reduction of pulmonary pressure that will then lead to deterioration of CO. In some cases, pulmonary artery pressure must be maintained somewhat above the normal range for optimal balance. Milrinone and other inotropes are not necessary for these patients, and may even cause deterioration of symptoms.[282,283] (See also question 53 for further discussion of dobutamine and milrinone.)

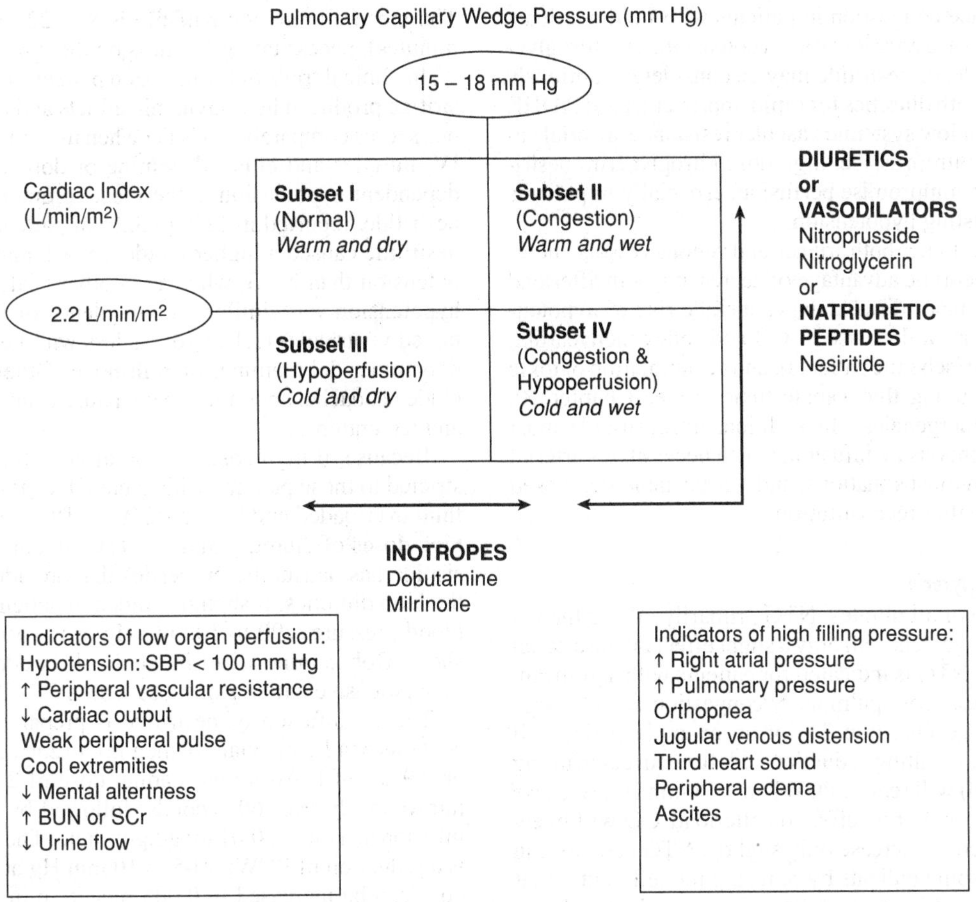

FIGURE 18-8 Hemodynamic profile of acute heart failure. BUN, blood urea nitrogen; SBP, systolic blood pressure; SrCr, serum creatinine. (Adapted with permission. Copyright © 2002 American Medical Association. All rights reserved.)

The "wet and cold" patients, such as L.M., who present with signs of both volume overload and hypoperfusion are more clinically challenging. Pulmonary artery wedge pressure is elevated and cardiac index is <2.2 L/minute/m^2. Immediate attention must be directed toward correcting hypoperfusion followed by aggressive diuretic therapy as in the "wet and warm" patients. β-Blockers and ACE inhibitors should be temporarily withdrawn if symptomatic hypotension is present. Because these patients often have both a low CO and high systemic vascular resistance, both vasodilators (e.g., nitroglycerin and nitroprusside) and an inotropic-vasodilator (e.g., dobutamine, low dose dopamine, or milrinone) might be considered; however, agreement is not unanimous regarding the agent of choice. The desired effect is reduced right-sided filling pressure (reduced preload via venous dilation) and reduced resistance to left ventricular outflow (reduced afterload via arterial dilation), both of which can increase CO and responsiveness to IV diuretics. These patients are generally monitored with pulmonary artery catheterization. The use of nesiritide in place of nitroprusside is possible, although it has not been well studied in this patient type. After stabilization, nitroprusside is slowly withdrawn and ACE inhibitors are reinstituted, sometimes in combination with an oral nitrate, oral hydralazine, or both. Chronic discontinuation of ACE inhibitors with transition to a hydralazine–nitrate combination becomes necessary when SrCr and BUN levels remain chronically elevated or worsen after ACE inhibitor dosage escalation. If inotropes are used, they can be started simultaneously with nitroprusside or reserved for patients not responding to vasodilators. Dobutamine may be preferred to milrinone because it causes less hypotension and is less expensive. Both milrinone and dobutamine are associated with undesirable tachyarrhythmias. Low dose dopamine is indicated if renal function is deteriorating.

The rare patient with low CO without evidence of volume overload ("cold and dry") may be relatively stable and poses less need for immediate intervention. A short course of dobutamine or milrinone can be tried, but ultimately these patients should be placed on an outpatient regimen that includes an oral β-blocker if they are not already on this therapy.

Nitroprusside

47. What is the role of vasodilator therapy in L.M.?

On admission, L.M. had an elevated PCWP and a low CI. The presence of an elevated JVD and peripheral edema indicate volume overload. He is hypotensive, consistent with his low CI. Thus, he fits into the "wet and cold" category described in the previous question. Consistent with this diagnosis, he was given vigorous diuresis and nitroprusside. The HFSA guidelines[4] recommend the addition of vasodilators in conjunction with diuretics to reduce congestion in patients with fluid overload. In the presence of asymptomatic hypotension, IV nitroglycerin, nitroprusside, or nesiritide may be considered cautiously in combination with diuretics for rapid improvement of ADHF. In the presence of low systemic vascular resistance, arterial vasodilators (e.g., nitroprusside, high dose nitroglycerin, nesiritide) can further compromise perfusion, especially in patients who have preexisting hypotension.

Nitroprusside dilates both arterial and venous vessels; therefore, it has the theoretic advantage of decreasing both afterload and preload. Its major disadvantages include risk of hypotension that can cause a decrease in CO and reflex tachycardia; coronary steal (in ischemic patients); and accumulation of toxic metabolites, including thiocyanate toxicity (see Chapter 20, Hypertensive Emergencies). In addition, nitroprusside must be given by continuous IV infusion, which necessitates arterial line placement in most situations, and it is unstable if exposed to heat and light after reconstitution.

Intravenous Nitroglycerin

As the prototype of all nitrates, NTG primarily dilates the venous capacitance vessels with only a slight effect on the arterial bed. Intravenous NTG is indicated for patients with significant respiratory distress from pulmonary congestion despite large diuretic doses (see Question 31 for an example patient). It is hoped that the resulting reduction in left ventricular filling pressure (preload) will reduce PCWP to <18 mm Hg. Because nitrates have minimal or no effect on afterload, CO will likely remain unchanged or increase only slightly. NTG actually can decrease CO in some patients by reducing the left ventricular filling pressure to <15 mm Hg. Nitroprusside is a better choice for patients such as L.M. who have a low CI without evidence of myocardial ischemia. (See Chapter 17, Myocardial Infarction, and Chapter 21, Shock, for more information on dosing and side effects of IV NTG.)

Patients should be initiated on small doses of nitroprusside (6–20 mcg/minute) that are increased slowly to a maximum of 300 to 800 mcg/minute until a decrease in the PCWP or arterial pressure is observed. When stopping nitroprusside therapy, a slow taper is recommended because a rebound increase in HF has been observed 10 to 30 minutes after drug withdrawal. (For a more thorough discussion of nitroprusside use, see Chapters 20, Hypertensive Emergencies and 21, Shock.)

Nesiritide

Nesiritide (Natrecor) is recombinantly produced human B-type natriuretic peptide (hBNP) containing the same 32 amino acids as native hBNP.[33,34] (The pharmacologic activity of the natriuretic peptides was reviewed in the pathogenesis section of this chapter.) BNP binds to guanylate cyclase receptors on vascular smooth muscle (the BNP receptor) leading to expression of cyclic GMP and subsequent vasodilation. Other actions include inhibition of ACE, sympathetic outflow, and endothelin-1. Peripheral and coronary dilation coupled with improved renal blood flow and increased glomerular filtration all contribute to the beneficial effects of nesiritide. Metabolic clearance of nesiritide is by a combination of binding to cell surfaces with subsequent cellular internalization and lyposomal proteolysis as well as proteolytic cleavage by endopeptidase (e.g., neutral endopeptidase). It undergoes only minimal renal clearance. The mean elimination half-life is 8 to 22 minutes (mean, 18 minutes), necessitating IV infusion therapy.

In clinical trials of hospitalized patients with severe HF, nesiritide produced hemodynamic effects and reduction in dyspnea scores comparable to NTG when used in combination with IV diuretics and either dopamine or dobutamine.[33,34] Dose-dependent hypotension is the most common side effect with nesiritide, reported in 11% to 32% of patients. In some trials, nesiritide caused a higher incidence or longer duration of hypotension than NTG, whereas in other trials the incidence of hypotension was similar. The incidence of PVC and nonsustained ventricular tachycardia is less with nesiritide than with dopamine, dobutamine, or milrinone. Other side effects include headache, abdominal pain, nausea, anxiety, bradycardia, and leg cramps.

Because of high cost, the use of nesiritide is generally restricted to those patients with acute HF exacerbations who are fluid overloaded and have a PCWP >18 to 20 mm Hg despite high doses of diuretics and IV NTG. In contrast to NTG, nesiritide has natriuretic properties that are additive to those of the loop diuretics. It should avoided in patients with a systolic blood pressure <90 to 100 mg Hg or in cases of cardiogenic shock. Dobutamine or milrinone should be added or substituted in hypotensive patients or those with a CI <2.2 L/minute/m^2.

The IV infusion of nesiritide is prepared by diluting the contents of a 1.5 mg vial to 6 mcg/mL in 250 mL of 5% dextrose or 0.9% NaCl. An initial loading dose of 2 mcg/kg is given intravenously over 60 seconds, followed by a continuous IV infusion at a rate of 0.01 mcg/kg/minute. The desired response is a reduction of PCWP of 5 to 10 mm Hg at 15 minutes. The dose can be increased in 0.005 mcg/kg/minute increments at 3-hour intervals to a maximum of 0.03 mcg/kg/minute. Dosage should be titrated to a PCWP <18 mm Hg and a systolic BP >90 mm Hg.

Although nesiritide is indicated in the treatment of ADHF, concerns have been raised about its safety. A meta-analysis of randomized, controlled trials of nesiritide in ADHF suggests that nesiritide use may be associated with worsening renal function and increased mortality.[284,285] The conclusions of the meta-analysis have been criticized, however. For example, the Vasodilation in the Management of Acute congestive Heart Failure (VMAC) study that was included in the meta-analysis was not designed to evaluate renal endpoints and, therefore, the inclusion of the renal effects from this study may not be appropriate.[286] Also, differences in baseline characteristics of the treatment groups may have contributed to an increased risk of 30-day mortality seen in those patients treated with nesiritide.

The efficacy and safety of nesiritide have also been evaluated in the outpatient setting. The Follow-up Serial Infusions of Nesiritide (FUSION I) trial[287] was a pilot trial that included 202 patients with NYHA class III–IV who had been hospitalized for ADHF at least twice within the preceding year and once in the preceding month. Patients were randomized to receive usual care with or without open-label nesiritide. A subgroup of patients were identified as high risk if they had at least four of the following: serum creatinine >2.0 mg/dL during the preceding month, NYHA class IV for the preceding 2 months, >65 years of age, a history of sustained ventricular tachycardia, ischemic HF etiology, diabetes, or use of nesiritide or inotropic agents as outpatients within the preceding 6 months. These patients at high risk experienced fewer HF exacerbations and renal adverse effects with nesiritide infusions.

This suggestion of potential benefit and safety in outpatients with severe HF was further explored in the Follow-Up Serial Infusions of Nesiritide for the Management of Patients With Heart Failure (FUSION II) trial.[288] This was a randomized, placebo-controlled, double-blind prospective trial of 911 subjects with advanced HF or chronic decompensated HF. Subjects were randomized to receive a 2 mcg/kg nesiritide bolus followed by a 0.01 mcg/kg/minute infusion for 4 to 6 hours, or a matching placebo regimen, once or twice weekly for 12 weeks. Both groups also received optimal medical therapy and device therapy. Patients were entered only if their creatinine clearance was <60 mL/minute. No outpatient IV inotropic or vasodilator therapy was allowed during the 24-week study. After 24 weeks, no difference was noted in the primary end point of either death or hospitalization for cardiac or renal causes among patients in the nesiritide and placebo groups. Significantly more ($p = 0.79$) drug-related adverse events occurred in those in the nesiritide group (42.0%) compared with the placebo group (27.5%), mainly caused by hypotension. The incidence of worsening renal function, however, was significantly lower ($p = 0.046$) with nesiritide (32% in nesiritide group vs. 39% in the placebo group). There was no evidence that changes in SrCr were associated with renal harm.

The results of these studies alleviate some concerns regarding the safety of nesiritide. Additional data from the Acute Study of Clinical Effectiveness of Nesiritide in Decompensated Heart Failure (ASCEND-HF) study will shed more light on the safety and efficacy of nesiritide in ADHF.[289]

L.M. responded well to nitroprusside and needed no other therapy. However, IV nitroglycerin and IV nesiritide are alternatives to nitroprusside in patients with either "wet and warm" or "wet and cold" acute HF. Nitroglycerin or nesiritide can either be a substitute for nitroprusside or combined with nitroprusside.

Use of Inotropic Drugs

48. B.J. is a 60-year-old man who presents to the emergency department with worsening dyspnea on exertion. He reports increased SOB over the last week. His medical history includes HTN, CAD, hyperlipidemia, and HF (EF 25%). His medications include metoprolol XL 100 mg QD, enalapril 5 mg QD, furosemide 40 mg BID, aspirin 81 mg, and lovastatin 20 mg HS. His vital signs on admission included BP 92/70 mmHg, HR 92 beats/min RR 18 breaths/minute, O_2 saturation 94% on room air. Laboratory values were BUN 20 mg/dL, SrCr 1.4 mg/dL PCWP 21 mm Hg, CI 1.8 L/min/m^2, SVR 580 dyne sec/cm^5. Physical examination reveals pulmonary and peripheral edema. He is given 80 mg IV furosemide and he does not respond adequately. The decision is to admit him to the CCU. His SrCr has increased to 1.8 mg/dL. Is B.J. a candidate for inotrope therapy? Why is milrinone preferred over amrinone?

Dopamine and Dobutamine

The hemodynamic profile of B.J. is category IV (cold and wet) because of hypoperfusion and congestion. According to the HFSA guidelines, IV inotropic agents (dobutamine, dopamine, milrinone, amrinone) are indicated in symptomatic patients with reduced LVEF, low CO, or end-organ dysfunction (i.e., worsening renal function), and in patients who are intolerant to vasodilators.[4] They are also recommended for patients with cardiogenic shock or refractory symptoms, and may be used in patients requiring perioperative support following cardiac and noncardiac surgery or for those awaiting transplantation. Dopamine is more effective as an arterial dilator, especially in the kidney, whereas dobutamine has more potent inotropic properties. (See Chapter 21, Shock, for further information on dopamine and dobutamine dosing.)

Phosphodiesterase Inhibitors: Amrinone and Milrinone

Although β-agonists, such as dobutamine, have been traditionally used in patients with ADHF, the phosphodiesterase inhibitors, amrinone (Inocor) and milrinone (Primacor), are alternatives to the catecholamines and vasodilators for the short-term parenteral treatment of severe congestive failure. These agents selectively inhibit phosphodiesterase F-III, the cyclic-adenosine monophosphate (AMP)-specific cardiac phosphodiesterase. They have direct cardiac-stimulating effects, but they are not sympathomimetics or inhibitors of Na+-K+-dependent ATP. Enzyme inhibition results in increased cyclic AMP levels in myocardial cells and, thus, enhances contractility. Their activity is not blocked by β-blockers. Because they are phosphodiesterase inhibitors, they also act as vasodilators. It has been suggested that at low doses they act more as unloading agents rather than inotropes; others refute this viewpoint. Their overall hemodynamic effect probably results from a combination of positive inotropic action plus preload and afterload reduction.

Amrinone initially was investigated for oral use, but it failed to gain FDA approval because of dose-dependent, reversible thrombocytopenia (up to 20% of patients), drug fever, liver function abnormalities, and possibly drug-induced ventricular arrhythmias. Amrinone remains available in an IV form for short-term use in severe HF. Therapy is initiated with a 0.75 mg/kg bolus over 2 to 3 minutes followed by a maintenance infusion of 5 to 10 mcg/kg/minute. Higher doses occasionally have been given, but doses exceeding 18 mcg/kg/day should be avoided. It has a half-life of approximately 2.5 to 3.5 hours in healthy individuals; this is prolonged to 6 to 12 hours in patients with HF. Lower doses are necessary in patients with renal insufficiency because amrinone is 50% excreted unchanged in the kidney. All dilutions should be made in saline (0.45%–0.9%) because amrinone is incompatible with dextrose-containing solutions.

With IV use, the major side effects to monitor are hypotension and precipitation of arrhythmias. The prevalence of thrombocytopenia is reduced to 2.4% with parenteral use. In summary, amrinone is effective in reducing SVR and PCWP and in increasing cardiac output, but as described below it appears to be less effective than dobutamine.

Milrinone is structurally and pharmacologically similar to amrinone.[290–292] Besides inhibiting phosphodiesterase, it also may increase calcium availability to myocardial muscle. It has both inotropic and vasodilating properties. Heart rate increase and myocardial consumption may be less with milrinone than with dobutamine.[282–283] The half-life of milrinone is short (1.5–2.5 hours) with renal clearance accounting for approximately 80% to 90% of total body elimination. Milrinone is about 15 to 20 times more potent than amrinone on a weight basis. A typical loading dose is 50 mcg/kg administered over 10 minutes followed by a maintenance infusion of 0.5 mcg/kg/minute. The infusion is adjusted according to hemodynamic and clinical responses and should be lowered in patients with renal insufficiency. The primary concern with the use of milrinone is induction of ventricular arrhythmias, reported in up to 12% of patients. Supraventricular arrhythmias, hypotension, headache, and chest pain also have been reported. Thrombocytopenia is rare, a distinct advantage over amrinone. Overall, milrinone has become the drug of choice among the phosphodiesterase inhibitors.

The Outcomes of a Prospective Trial of Intravenous Milrinone for Chronic Heart Failure (OPTIME-CHF) trial assessed the in-hospital management of 951 patients with acute HF exacerbation (NYHA class III or IV, mean LVEF 23%), but not in cardiogenic shock.[282,283] In addition to standard diuretic and ACE inhibitor therapy, subjects were randomized to receive either milrinone or placebo. The initial milrinone infusion rate was 0.5 mcg/kg/minute with no loading dose. For the primary end point of total numbers of days hospitalized for cardiovascular causes from the time of the start of study drug infusion to day 60, no difference was found between active drug and placebo (mean 12.3 days with milrinone and 12.5 days with placebo), nor was any difference seen in the mean number of days of hospitalization during the primary event. Death rates within 60 days were 10.3% with milrinone and 8.9% with placebo (NS, $p = 0.41$).[282] Follow-up analysis categorized subjects by etiology of HF (ischemic vs. nonischemic).[283] Not unexpectedly, those with an ischemic cause did less well with hospital rates of 13.0 days for ischemic patients compared with 11.7 days for those without ischemia ($p = 0.2$). Corresponding death rates over 60 days were 11.6% and 7.5% ($p = 0.03$). Importantly, within the cohort of patients with ischemia ($n = 485$), milrinone-treated patients tended to have worse outcomes than those treated with placebo: 13.6 hospital days with milrinone vs. 12.4 days with placebo. Death occurred in 13.3% of patients on milrinone compared with 10.0% of those on placebo. For the composite of patients dying or being rehospitalized, 42% of milrinone subjects had events compared with 36% with placebo ($p = 0.01$). In contrast, nonischemic patients ($n = 464$) had a trend toward better outcomes with milrinone than with placebo: 10.9 hospital days for milrinone vs. 12.6 days with placebo, 7.3% deaths with milrinone compared with 7.7% with placebo, and the composite of death or hospitalization occurring in 28% of subjects with milrinone vs. 35% with placebo. From these data, the following conclusions can be drawn. The benefits of milrinone in patients with acute exacerbations of HF are minimal and more likely to be seen in patients with a nonischemic etiology of HF. Worse outcomes may be seen in patients with ischemic HF. Milrinone was not associated with excess mortality.

Few trials have yet compared dobutamine with milrinone in ADHF patients. One small retrospective analysis evaluated 329 patients admitted for ADHF with an EF of <20% who either received IV dobutamine or milrinone.[293] Hemodynamic response, need for additional therapies, adverse effects, length of stay, and drug cost were evaluated. Patients in both groups were comparable in clinical presentation. Further, both groups had similar HR, BP, PCWP, and CO at baseline. The milrinone group, however, had higher mean pulmonary arterial pressure. A greater percentage of patients received dobutamine therapy (269, 81.7%) vs. milrinone therapy (60, 18.3%.). Only 19% of patients were taking β-blockers before admission. Clinical outcomes in both groups were similar. There was no significant difference in the in-hospital mortality rate, adverse effects, ventilator use, or length of stay. More patients in the dobutamine group required nitroprusside to achieve optimal hemodynamic response. A slightly better hemodynamic response occurred in the milrinone group, which did not translate into a more beneficial short-term clinical outcome. The study concluded that because both drugs have comparable efficacy, dobutamine may be a better choice than milrinone because it provided more drug cost savings during the hospital stay.

Other factors to consider when deciding which inotropic agent should be used in ADHF are renal function, BP, and concomitant β-blocker use. Milrinone has a longer half-life than dobutamine, and accumulates in cases of renal dysfunction. Milrinone is also a vasodilator, which can limit its use in patients with hypotension. The concomitant use of β-blockers can antagonize the action of dobutamine.

B.J. has responded poorly to IV furosemide, his renal function has deteriorated and his systolic BP is low. Patients with advanced HF, reduced blood pressure, and normal or low systemic vascular resistance often will not tolerate vasodilator therapy. Inotropic agents may be necessary to maintain circulatory function in these patients. According to HFSA guidelines, IV inotropes may be considered for patients who are unresponsive to diuretics or who have worsening renal function, especially if they have marginal systolic BP (<90 mm Hg). Phosphodiesterase inhibitors are preferred over dobutamine for patients who are receiving concomitant β-blockers. For the above-mentioned reasons, B.J. is a candidate for milrinone therapy. Patients must be on telemetry because milrinone has the potential to cause arrhythmias. Vital signs, SrCr, symptom relief, and urine output should be monitored. Once the patient's hemodynamic profile improves, milrinone should be discontinued and oral furosemide therapy can be resumed. At discharge, the outpatient HF medications should be optimized.

Outpatient Inotropic Infusions

49. Are there any indications for using repeated intermittent infusions of inotropes as part of a home care regimen?

It has been proposed to use regularly scheduled (e.g., weekly) intermittent infusions of dobutamine or milrinone in outpatient care centers or at home. The long-term safety and efficacy of inotropic therapy in general is regarded with skepticism, however. Nearly all the data on this therapeutic approach are from open-label and uncontrolled trials or studies that compare two inotropic agents without a placebo group.[294–298] It is unclear if the benefit observed was the result of more intensive patient monitoring or an actual pharmacologic benefit. It also is speculated that long-term therapy actually may be cardiotoxic, as evidenced by an acute worsening of HF on withdrawal of the drug. The only placebo-controlled trial of intermittent infusion dobutamine was terminated because of excess mortality in the treatment group.[295] Death occurred in 32% of 31 patients treated with dobutamine and only 14% of 29 treated with placebo. Whether this phenomenon is was caused by progression of the underlying heart disease, continued drug therapy, or is a true cardiotoxic effect remains unknown. No corresponding data exist for milrinone, although as cited previously, a placebo-controlled trial with milrinone failed to support the routine use of IV milrinone as an adjunct to standard therapy in the treatment of patients hospitalized for an acute exacerbation of chronic HF.[282,283] For this reason, the ACA/AHA guidelines explicitly indicate that intermittent infusions of dobutamine and milrinone in the long-term treatment of HF, even if advanced stages, should be avoided.[6] Dobutamine is sometimes administered as long-term infusions (5–7.5 mcg/kg/minute continuously for 48–72 hours) in patients with refractory HF while awaiting transplant. The infusion is repeated as often as weekly.

Hydralazine

50. After L.M.'s condition was controlled with nitroprusside therapy, he was given his original medications plus spironolactone, hydralazine, and isosorbide dinitrate. Why were hydralazine and isosorbide used? What other forms of nitrates can be used in place of the isosorbide? Is combination therapy rational?

L.M. had already been treated with a loop diuretic, an ACE inhibitor (enalapril), a β-blocker, and digoxin. Despite this therapy, he was still doing poorly. Spironolactone was added for reasons discussed in Question 14. A possible next step in treating a patient with this advanced stage of HF is the addition of a non-ACE inhibitor vasodilator.

Hyralazine's predominate action is as an arteriolar dilator, making hydralazine the prototype afterload-reducing agent. Decreasing aortic impedance (afterload) is of little benefit in a normal or minimally diseased heart, but it may greatly improve severely compromised left ventricular function. SVR is decreased predictably and this, in turn, increases cardiac output (cardiac index).[135,136,299] Hydralazine is also a direct-acting, smooth muscle relaxant with significant arteriolar dilating effects in the kidneys and limbs. It has essentially no effect on the venous system or on hepatic blood flow.

The reflex tachycardia and hypotension that frequently accompany hydralazine therapy when used in treating hypertension are minimal or absent, however, when it is used to treat HF. Increased CO overrides vasodilatory effects in the latter instance. In patients with end-stage cardiomyopathy, however, significant hypotension still can occur if the heart cannot respond appropriately. Another beneficial response to hydralazine is reduction of pulmonary vascular resistance in patients with severe pulmonary hypertension. This pulmonary arteriolar dilating effect of hydralazine is generally less beneficial than the venodilating effects of drugs such as nitrates and nitroprusside. Because hydralazine is devoid of venous dilating properties, CVP and PWCP are unchanged.[136,299]

The effect of a single dose occurs in about 30 minutes and lasts up to 6 hours. Larger doses than typically used for the treatment of hypertension may be required for HF management. The average maintenance dose is 200 to 400 mg/day (50–100 mg every 6 hours). L.M. required 75 mg four times a day. Hydralazine used as monotherapy is not associated with long-term improvement in functional status, however.[299] Combination therapy of hydralazine with either nitrates or ACE inhibitors is highly effective.

Although tachyphylaxis generally is not a significant problem with prolonged courses of hydralazine, some patients require increased diuretic doses to counteract hydralazine-induced fluid retention. This latter response reflects activation of the renin-angiotensin system following vasodilation of the renal vasculature. Other side effects accompanying hydralazine include transient nausea during the first few days of therapy; headache, flushing, or tachycardia; and a lupus syndrome associated with prolonged, high doses. (See Chapter 13, Essential Hypertension, for further discussion of hydralazine side effects and dosing.)

Oral and Topical Nitrates

Nitrates have complementary effects to those of hydralazine.[135,136] They primarily dilate venous capacitance vessels, with minimal effects on selected arterial beds (coronary and pulmonary arteries). Venous dilation reduces preload, resulting in significant reductions in PCWP and right atrial pressure. They are especially effective in reducing the symptoms of pulmonary edema. The lack of significant arterial dilation accounts for the observations that SVR is minimally reduced and CO remains unchanged. Nitrate monotherapy is indicated for HF patients with valvular defects such as mitral or aortic regurgitation. In these patients, reduction of the ventricular filling pressure reduces left ventricular congestion.

ISOSORBIDE DINITRATE

Because sublingual NTG has a short duration of response, more attention has been focused on sublingual and oral isosorbide dinitrate. Sublingual isosorbide is well absorbed and does not undergo first-pass metabolism. Its onset is rapid (approximately 5 minutes), but its effects are relatively short (1–3 hours). The usual starting dosage is 5 mg every 4 to 6 hours, but dosages may be titrated to 20 mg or more every 4 to 6 hours. These larger doses are associated with longer beneficial effects (approximately 3 hours), but also a high frequency of intolerable headaches and hypotension.

Previous claims of a poor response to orally administered isosorbide because of a large first-pass metabolic effect have been refuted. Large oral doses overwhelm the metabolic capacity of the liver and produce beneficial effects. Oral isosorbide has a slow onset (15–30 minutes), but the duration of activity is slightly longer than that associated with sublingual administration (4–6 hours). Oral doses of 5 mg are probably ineffective; 10 mg is the smallest effective starting dose with further titration to dosages as high as 20 to 80 mg every 4 to 6 hours. The best dose for both sublingual and oral nitrates is that which provides the desired beneficial effect with the least side effects.

TRANSDERMAL NITROGLYCERIN

An innovative approach to NTG administration is transdermal patch systems (Minitran, Nitrek, Nitro-Dur). Topical application of these systems is said to provide 24 hours of continuous cutaneous absorption with more convenience and less mess than NTG ointment. Although most published data on these dose forms are in patients with angina, several reports are on their use in HF.

The initial enthusiasm for transdermal NTG has been tempered by the suggestion that tolerance develops quickly, resulting in a benefit for much less than 24 hours following patch application. Considerable debate has arisen over this topic.[300–302] Some reviewers suggest abandoning this form of therapy, whereas others argue that the studies showing negative benefit were flawed. Removal of the patch during the night might lead to restoration of response the following day. It has been suggested that while the antianginal effects of NTG are attenuated with chronic therapy, the beneficial preload-reducing properties for HF are sustained. Large doses (20–40 mg/24 hour), however, may be required, necessitating the use of several patches per day and resulting in significant expense to the patient. (See Chapter 16, Ischemic Heart Disease: Anginal Syndromes, for a more detailed discussion on the application and controversy surrounding NTG transdermal patches.)

Hydralazine–Nitrate Combination

Combined afterload and preload reduction is clearly of benefit both in improving symptoms and in enhancing long-term survival. Compared with ACE inhibitors, the hydralazine–isosorbide combination provides more significant improvement in exercise tolerance, but the side effect profile and survival statistics are better with ACE inhibitors.[131] With combination therapy, CO is greater for any given level of ventricular filling pressure. Generally, the use of the two drugs together is not accompanied by reflex tachycardia or hypotension, but it is important to be careful not to compromise coronary blood flow in patients with coexistent angina.

The most compelling argument for the use of combination hydralazine and nitrate vasodilator therapy comes from the results of the two Veterans Administration Cooperative Studies (V-HeFT I and V-HeFT II).[131,135,136] As discussed in more detail in Question 15, these two studies not only confirmed symptomatic relief and improved exercise tolerance with combination therapy, but they also showed improved survival. Also, see Question 51 for the a discussion of the possible unique place in therapy of the hydralazine–nitrate combination in black patients.

In summary, nitrates alone are indicated for those patients with signs and symptoms of isolated pulmonary and venous congestion (i.e., dyspnea, increased pulmonary pressure, neck vein distention, edema). Conversely, use of an arterial dilator is more appropriate in a patient with high SVR, low CO, and normal PCWP. Most patients, such as L.M., exhibit symptoms of decreased CO and elevated venous pressure, making combination therapy the most attractive option. Although the hydralazine–isosorbide combination actually reduces symptoms slightly better than ACE inhibitors, the data on survival are more impressive with the ACE inhibitors. As illustrated by L.M.'s treatment regimen, a combination of an ACE inhibitor plus hydralazine, a nitrate, or both, is common in patients with far advanced disease.

Role of Race in the Pharmacotherapy of Heart Failure

51. Because L.M. is black, would he be expected to respond any differently to ACE inhibitors or hydralazine–isosorbide dinitrate than a patient who is not black?

In general, black patients develop HF at an earlier age and are more likely to have hypertension as a cause for HF. Conversely, the etiology of HF in non-black patients more often results from ischemic heart disease. The rate of death caused by HF is higher for black patients than for non-black patients.

ACE Inhibitors and Hydralazine–Isosorbide

Racial differences in response to drug therapy have been proposed, although this issue is far from resolved.[303–306] For example, a *post hoc* analysis of the V-HeFT trial data cited previously showed no difference in annual mortality between black (n = 180) and non-black patients (n = 450) in the placebo group (17.3% vs. 18.8%).[131,273] Black patients in the hydralazine-nitrate group had a significantly lower annual mortality rate (9.7%), however, than did black subjects in the placebo group (17.3%), whereas non-black subjects had no survival benefit from the drug combination (16.9% vs. 18.8%). This implies that black patients, but not non-blacks, derive benefit from the treatment with hydralazine–isosorbide. These same investigators then reanalyzed the V-HeFT II trial results for possible racial differences between response to enalapril and the hydralazine–nitrate combination.[136,304] The outcome is difficult to interpret because of the absence of a placebo group. The all-cause annual mortality rate for blacks (n = 215) was identical in the two drug groups (12.8% with enalapril and 12.9% with hydralazine–isosorbide.) In non-blacks (n = 574), the corresponding mortality rates were 11% with enalapril and 14.9% with hydral-iso. These data could be interpreted as either superior response to hydralazine–isosorbide in black subjects or inferior activity of ACE inhibitors in black patients. The latter interpretation is consistent with the hypothesis that ACE inhibitors might have a lesser BP-lowering effect in black patients with hypertension compared with non-blacks. A similar reanalysis of the SOLVD Prevention and Treatment[134] trials, both of which compared enalapril with placebo in patients with recent MI, concluded that enalapril therapy is associated with a significant reduction in the risk for hospitalization for HF among white patients (44% reduction) with left ventricular dysfunction, but not among similar black patients. Confounding variables contributing to all of the analyses presented include disproportionately low numbers of blacks in the trials, and possibly more underlying risk factors (e.g., hypertension) in the black subjects.

To further address the effect of race on response to ACE inhibitors, a meta-analysis of the seven major ACE inhibitor studies, representing a total of 14,752 patients was conducted.[305] The conclusion was that that relative risk for mortality when taking an ACE inhibitor compared with placebo was identical (0.89) for both black and white patients. The authors of the meta-analysis urged that ACE inhibitors not be withheld from black patients. One other consideration with ACE inhibitors is an observed higher rate, although still rare, of angioedema in blacks than in whites. Until more data are available, ACE inhibitors should not be withheld from black patients, but careful monitoring is required to assess response.

The African American Heart Failure Trial (AHeFT) was designed to determine possible superiority of combination hydralazine plus isosorbide dinitrate in black patients.[77] AHeFT was a randomized comparison trial (n = 1050) of hydralazine-isosorbide dinitrate and placebo in black patients with NYHA class III or IV HF who were receiving standard HF therapy (94% diuretics, 87% β-blockers, 93% ACE inhibitors or ARB, 62% digoxin, and 39% aldosterone antagonists). The primary end point was a composite of all-cause death, first hospitalization for HF, and quality of life scores at 6 months with secondary end points being individual components of the primary end point. Reduction in the composite primary end point events was statistically significant in favor of the active drug combination. Importantly, all-cause mortality declined 43% in the hydralazine–isosorbide dinitrate arm vs. placebo ($p = 0.012$). The study also reported a 39% reduction in first hospitalization for HF in the hydralazine–isosorbide dinitrate group vs. placebo ($p < 0.001$). As a result, the 2005 ACC/AHA guideline recommendations state that the addition of hydralazine and isosorbide dinitrate to HF patients receiving ACE inhibitors and β-blockers is effective in blacks with NYHA functional class III or IV HF.[7] The results of AHeFT were also the primary factor leading the FDA to approve the combination product of hydralazine and isosorbide dinitrate (BiDil) for adjunctive treatment of heart failure in self-identified black patients already receiving standard therapy. Advantages of using BiDil in clinical practice include use of the same product studied in the clinical trial and potential improved compliance by using a combination tablet. Cost, however, may be lower when using generic hydralazine and isosorbide as separate drugs.

β-Blockers

A possible racial difference in response to β-blocker drugs has also been hypothesized based on differential effects observed in patients with hypertension.[303,305,306] A *post hoc* analysis of the various U.S. Carvedilol Heart Failure trials[212–216] concluded, however, that the benefit of carvedilol was apparently of similar magnitude in both black ($n = 217$) and non-black ($N = 877$) patients.[306] Using the combined end point of the risk of death from any cause or hospitalization, the risk reduction of β-blockers compared with placebo was 48% in black patients and 30% in non-black patients. Because fewer black patients were studied, these differences did not reach statistical significance. Also seen were a significant improvement in NYHA functional class, EF, and patient global symptom assessment with carvedilol in both black and non-black patients.

Contradictory evidence comes from the β-Blocker Evaluation of Survival Trial (BEST).[225] In this trial (also discussed in Question 30), 2,708 patients with NYHA class III (92%) or IV (8%) HF were randomly assigned to either bucindolol or placebo. Bucindolol is a nonselective β-blocker with partial agonist activity that imparts weak vasodilation. A unique characteristic of this study was that a subgroup analysis for racial differences was planned from the start. Although there was a trend toward reductions in cardiovascular mortality and hospitalization with the active drug, the trial was terminated after 2 years when it was determined that there was no mortality benefit of active drug compared to placebo (33% mortality in placebo group vs. 30% with bucindolol). A subgroup analysis showed a mortality benefit in non-black subjects, but none in black subjects. Subsequently, a meta-analysis of the five major β-blocker in HF studies was conducted, representing a total of 12,727 patients.[305] When the BEST was included in the meta-analysis, the relative risk for mortality when taking an ACE inhibitor compared with placebo was 0.69 in white subjects, but only 0.97 for black patients. When this trial was excluded, the relative risks were reduced in both groups to 0.63 and 0.67 in whites and blacks, respectively. The difference between the two groups was not statistically significant, although the 95% confidence interval for black patients was broader and included 1.0 (0.38–1.16). Based on all of these factors, it is likely that black patients will derive similar benefit from β-blockers as do whites when given carvedilol, metoprolol, or bisoprolol. Bucindolol should be avoided, most likely because of its partial agonist activity.

Left Ventricular Diastolic Dysfunction

52. D.F., a 58-year-old white woman, has a 5-year history of HF symptoms, including decreased exercise capacity, SOB, and distended neck veins. She has minimal peripheral edema. History is suggestive of rheumatic fever as a child, but she does not recall having any cardiac symptoms when she was younger, other than being told she had a murmur. Her symptoms are controlled with diuretics. She has history of hypertension. She has no other medical problems and all laboratory test findings are normal. Her BP is 155/85 and HR 90 beats/minute. Cardiac examination reveals a prominent S_4 heart sound and murmurs consistent with both significant mitral regurgitation and mild aortic regurgitation. Noninvasive echocardiography reveals a normal EF of 50%. Prior treatment included furosemide, most recently at 120 mg/day. The physician is considering adding a β-blocker or CCB to control the BP. Why might this consideration be appropriate?

This case exemplifies a patient with diastolic heart failure (DHF), also referred to as heart failure with preserved LV function. Risk factors for DHF include advanced age, female sex, hypertension, and coronary artery disease. This diagnosis can be made on the basis of LVH, clinical evidence of HF, a normal EF, and Doppler tissue echocardiography findings. The ideal treatment strategies for DHF have not been devised. Also, no drug selectively enhances myocardial relaxation without having associated effects on left ventricular contractility or on the peripheral vasculature.[12–16]

Factors affecting HF control, such as dietary sodium intake, fluid intake, compliance, and NSAID and herbal remedy use, should be appropriately managed along with drug therapy. Symptomatic left ventricular diastolic HF is initially treated similarly to other forms of HF, by slow diuresis. Diuresis decreases preload and lessens passive congestion of the ventricles. Excessive lowering of venous and ventricular filling pressures, however, can worsen cardiac output and hypotension.

The most common cause of DHF is hypertension that leads to left ventricular hypertrophy and decreased cardiac compliance.[307] Recent ACC/AHA guidelines recommend treating associated hypertension in accordance with the national guidelines and suggest considering lower blood pressure targets for patients with DHF (<130/80 mm Hg).[7] Drugs that cause regression of LV hypertrophy (e.g., ACE inhibitor, ARB, β-blockers) may also slow or reverse structural abnormalities associated with DHF.

Although ACE inhibitors have been used with success in some patients with DHF, the role of RAAS inhibition in HF with preserved LV function has not been rigorously studied. Several recent clinical trials have attempted to address this issue. In the Perindopril in Elderly patients with Chronic HF (PEP-CHF) trial,[308] the ACE inhibitor perindopril failed to reduce the incidence of the primary endpoint (all-cause mortality or HF hospitalizations), but did reduce symptoms and improved functional capacity over 2 years in patients with preserved LV function. The CHARM-preserved trial[174] also failed to show any difference in CV mortality, but fewer hospitalizations were seen in the candesartan group (see Question 21).

The Valsartan in Diastolic Dysfunction (VALIDD) trial,[309] the first large-scale, randomized trial comparing the effects of valsartan or placebo added to standard antihypertensive therapy (which included diuretics, β-blockers, CCB or α-blockers) in patients with mild hypertension and diastolic HF. The hypothesis of this trial was that RASS inhibition with an ARB would be associated with greater improvement in diastolic dysfunction, possibly because of a greater regression of LVH or myocardial fibrosis. Patients with a history of stage 1 or 2 essential hypertension were randomized to receive either valsartan 160 mg, up-titrated to 320 mg, or matching placebo. Patients who did not achieve a target blood pressure goal of <135/80 mm Hg received additional therapy starting with a diuretic followed by a CCB or a β-blocker, then an α-blocker (excluding ARB, ACE, and aldosterone blockers). The primary endpoint was the change in diastolic myocardial relaxation velocity from baseline to 9 months with a secondary endpoint of change in LV mass. During the study, the placebo group received more concomitant antihypertensive therapy compared with the valsartan group. A small, but significant, increase was seen in diastolic relaxation velocity in both groups from baseline to follow-up ($p < 0.001$), but no significant difference between the treatment groups ($p = 0.29$). Blood pressure reduction at the end of the trial did not differ significantly between the two treatment groups (13 mm Hg reduction in valsartan vs. 10 mm Hg in placebo), which was associated with significant improvement in diastolic function. Thus, the authors concluded that aggressive BP control—even in mild hypertension—was associated with improvement in diastolic dysfunction, irrespective of whether BP reduction was achieved with a RAAS inhibitor or other antihypertensive agents. Several other trials are in progress that may provide further insight into the role of RAAS inhibitors in preserved LV function HF.

β-blockers or CCB are other classes of drugs of interest in DHF. Part of their value is to control hypertension, a risk factor for all forms of HF. More specific to DHF, β-blockers and CCB (especially verapamil) possess negative inotropic properties that may favorably influence the pathophysiology of diastolic dysfunction by (a) slowing the HR to allow more time for complete ventricular filling (via more complete left atrial emptying), particularly during exercise; (b) reducing myocardial oxygen demand; and (c) controlling BP. In addition, negative inotropic agents decrease myocardial contractility and can assist in overcoming the mechanical obstruction of the aortic and mitral valves during systole in patients with hypertrophic cardiomyopathy. Both agents also are beneficial in decreasing ischemia in patients with coronary artery disease.

Previous HF trials of β-blockers demonstrating decreased morbidity and mortality have mainly focused on patients with reduced LVEF. The Study of the Effects of Nebivolol Intervention on Outcomes and Rehospitalization in Seniors with Heart Failure (SENIORS) study[309] is the first major trial to evaluate β-blocker use in elderly HF patients (70 years or older), irrespective of LV function. The trial randomized patients to Nebivolol (n = 1,067) or placebo (n = 1,061). Nebivolol is a selective β_1-adernergic receptor blocker with vasodilator properties that are mediated through nitric oxide release. This effect may be beneficial in elderly patients, who tend to have low reserves of endothelial vasodilation.

The primary endpoint of the study was the combination of all-cause mortality and cardiovascular hospital admissions. The end point was significantly reduced by 14% in the Nebivolol group, regardless of the ejection fraction. Prospective subgroup analyses of the primary outcome by LVEF (≤35% or >35%), gender, age (≤75 years or >75 years) showed benefits across all subgroups. Patients with EF>35%, however, appeared to benefit a little more than those with low EF%, and all-cause mortality was lower in patients aged >75 years. The study reinforces the current recommendations that all HF patients with reduced EF should receive β-blockers. Only 35% of the patients had preserved LV function, however, and were mostly men. This is not typical of patients with HF, who are generally females and who tend to have greater incidence of diastolic HF.

Further studies are required to define the role of β-blockers in subject groups that are under-represented. On the other hand, no randomized controlled trials have demonstrated mortality benefits with CCB in patients with preserved LV function. CCB can be used in patients who have a contraindication to β-blockers to control BP and HR. Non-dihydropyridine CCB should not be used in patients with impaired LV dysfunction, however.

D.F. fulfills the criteria for having diastolic dysfunction, probably on the basis of mitral and aortic regurgitation as a result of childhood rheumatic fever. Her BP is not at goal and her HR is elevated. As already discussed, uncontrolled hypertension can promote left ventricle hypertrophy and myocardial remodeling, and can adversely affect the diastolic function. Therefore, an additional antihypertensive agent is warranted. Tachycardia alone can compromise the ventricle filling time and cause myocardial ischemia. So far, no data support use of one agent over the other. β-blockers and CCB can each reduce BP and HR. Because more experience has accrued with β-blockers and some mortality data on their use with DHF patients, D.F. can be started on a β-blocker such as metoprolol (25 mg BID).

53. A.F., a 48-year-old man, has a 5-year history of atrial fibrillation and mild HF stabilized with furosemide 40 mg/day and digoxin 0.25 mg/day. His previously well-controlled BP is now rising; the last pressure was 160/100 mm Hg despite good adherence with his diuretic therapy. All laboratory findings are normal. The digoxin level is 1.2 mg/mL. Is there evidence that calcium channel blockers may be helpful in controlling both hypertension and HF? If a calcium channel blocker is prescribed, will any interactions occur with his other drugs?

The arterial vasodilator properties of CCB form the basis for their use in hypertension. A logical extension would suggest a role in HF symptom management via afterload reduction. Use of these drugs, however, is limited by their negative inotropic effect, resulting from inhibition of calcium influx into heart muscle cells. This can result in a worsening of HF.[310–312] Clinically, verapamil elicits the most negative inotropic effect and the dihydropyridine derivatives the least; diltiazem has intermediate effects. It is important not to develop a false sense of security that nifedipine or other dihydropyridines are clinically devoid of negative inotropic effects as demonstrated by the following randomized, crossover trial comparing IV hydralazine (5–30 mg) with oral nifedipine (20–50 mg) in 15 patients.[311] Both drugs were equally effective in reducing BP and SVR (a sign of afterload reduction), but hydralazine was more effective in increasing SV and CI. Four of the patients taking nifedipine experienced deterioration of their HF symptoms. The authors concluded that the vasodilatory properties of nifedipine are partially offset by its negative inotropic effect and that hydralazine is clinically superior.

A follow-up study using a randomized, crossover design challenged 28 patients with class II or III HF with nifedipine, isosorbide, and a combination of the two.[312] Of patients, 24% on nifedipine and 26% on combined therapy had worsening of symptoms and required hospitalization compared with none in the isosorbide treatment arm.

The search for a more vascular selective CCB has focused on the newer agents amlodipine and felodipine. In the Prospective Randomized Amlodipine Survival Evaluation (PRAISE) trial, patients with dyspnea or fatigue at rest or minimal exertion (NYHA class III or IV) and an EF of 30% or less (mean 21%), were randomized to either placebo (n = 582) or amlodipine (n = 571) and followed for a median of 13.8 months (range, 6–33 months).[78] The starting dose of amlodipine (5 mg daily) was titrated to 10 mg daily if tolerated; the average dose at the end of the trial was 8.8 mg daily. Essentially all the patients were taking a combination of a diuretic, an ACE inhibitor, and digoxin. Nitrates were allowed for chest pain management, but hydralazine was excluded. For the combined primary end point of death from any cause, a cardiovascular-related hospitalization, or both, a nonstatistically different 9% risk reduction was noted in events with amlodipine compared with placebo (39% vs. 42%). For death rates alone, 33% of patients on amlodipine died compared with 38% in the placebo group. Again, these differences were not statistically significant ($p = 0.07$). Changes in EF, specific symptom scores, and quality of life measures were not reported, but the frequency of hospitalization for worsening HF was similar in both groups (36% amlodipine, 39% placebo.) Peripheral edema and pulmonary edema were more frequent in the amlodipine group, but hypertension and angina were more evident in the placebo group.

Stratification of the subjects into those with evidence of ischemic heart disease vs. those with nonischemic dilated cardiomyopathy showed a trend toward improved survival with amlodipine in the patients without ischemia. Overall, the results of this trial show a neutral effect of amlodipine, indicating that it could be used safely for concurrent hypertension or angina without making HF worse, but it does not appear to offer a significant advantage in actually treating the HF.

Similar findings have been reported with felodipine in the third report from the Vasodilator-Heart Failure Trial Study Group (V-HeFT III).[79] The primary objectives of this study were to evaluate the effects of extended-release (ER) felodipine (n = 224) compared with placebo (n = 226) on exercise tolerance, clinical symptoms, and clinical signs of HF for up to 39 months. Subjects were all men, with class II–III HF and an EF of <45% (mean, 30%). Before starting the study drug, subjects were optimized with an ACE inhibitor (97% with enalapril), diuretics (87%–90%), and digoxin (75%). The starting dose for felodipine was 2.5 mg twice daily, with a goal dose of 5 mg twice daily (mean dose, 8.6 mg/day after titration). At the 3-month evaluation point, EF increased slightly (2.1 ± 7.0%) with amlodipine, compared with –0.1% ± 6% with placebo. At 12 months, no difference was seen between the two groups (0.6 ± 8.6% with felodipine vs. –0.6 ± 8.6% with placebo).

During the first 12 weeks of evaluation, neither felodipine nor placebo had either a positive or negative effect on time to dyspnea or fatigue on exercise testing; however, thereafter, a trend toward deterioration in exercise capacity was found with placebo, but not with felodipine. In the first 3 months, slightly more patients on felodipine were hospitalized than those on placebo (14.7% vs. 10.6%), but overall the rate of hospitalization was identical in the two groups (42% to 43%). The study was not powered to evaluate the effect of felodipine on mortality, but the observed mortality rates were 13.8% in the felodipine arm and 12.9% in the placebo arm.

In contrast to the PRAISE trial, treatment with felodipine had a more favorable effect in the subgroup of patients with a history of ischemia and CAD. The only adverse effect more common in the patients on felodipine was edema, which was reported at least once in 21% of felodipine subjects and 12.8% of those on placebo. The conclusions are almost identical to those with amlodipine: there does not seem to be any negative consequences to using felodipine, but it has little role in the management of HF. Both the amlodipine and felodipine trials leave unanswered the question of efficacy of CCB in patients not already taking an ACE inhibitor or digoxin.

Based on the previous discussion, nifedipine is not a good choice for A.F. In fact, nifedipine is contraindicated in any patient with systolic dysfunction. Likewise, verapamil is contraindicated even though it would otherwise lower his BP and control his atrial fibrillation by virtue of its AV nodal-blocking effect. Amlodipine and felodipine are safer alternatives for A.F.'s hypertension, but still not preferred. The more logical solution to A.F.'s problem is to add an ACE inhibitor and possibly a β-blocker to get a dual effect of controlling his BP and treating his HF. Digoxin can be continued for rate control of his atrial fibrillation, although as discussed in Question 40, adding a β-blocker can also help in rate control.

Interaction With Digoxin

In the absence of HF, a case could be made for the use of verapamil or diltiazem together with digoxin for additive benefit in the treatment of supraventricular arrhythmias; but, as with the use of digoxin and quinidine, a risk of increased digoxin serum levels exists. The most reproducible interaction is with verapamil.[71,73,252] Steady-state concentrations of digoxin are consistently increased by 44% to 70% after the addition of verapamil. In some instances, the changes are only transient, with digoxin levels returning toward baseline concentrations (but not completely) after several weeks of continued combination therapy. The interaction is more pronounced in patients taking larger doses of verapamil (240–360 mg/day) and in patients taking quinidine as well. Verapamil's primary action is the reduction of nonrenal digoxin clearance, at least partially mediated by increased digoxin bioavailability via inhibition of intestinal PGP by verapamil.

Several investigators also have confirmed an interaction with diltiazem, but the magnitude of the rise in serum digoxin concentrations (20%–35%) is less than that seen with verapamil. One study reported a 45% increase in digoxin concentrations after nifedipine, whereas several other investigators could not detect a change in digoxin clearance. Although not confirmed, the mechanism may involve inhibition of PGP by diltiazem, thus enhancing digoxin bioavailability. In summary, an interaction between CCB and digoxin definitely should be considered when using verapamil; it may be of some concern with diltiazem, and is probably insignificant with nifedipine.

Ventricular Arrhythmias Complicating Heart Failure

Amiodarone

54. B.J. (from Question 48) was stabilized over the next several days and discharged home with furosemide 40 mg QD, enalapril 5 mg QD, metoprolol XL 100 mg QD, aspirin 81 mg QD, and NTG 0.4 mg sublingual (SL) to be used as needed for chest pain. His EF after the infarction was 23%. Laboratory values were all normal. ECG monitoring during B.J.'s hospital stay showed normal sinus rhythm, but he was having 15 to 20 asymptomatic PVC/hour. At that time, it was decided not to treat his arrhythmia other than with metoprolol because he was asymptomatic. Over the next several months, he continued to have frequent PVC during follow-up examinations in the cardiology clinic.

It has now been 5 months since B.J.'s infarction and he is still having up to 12 to 15 PVC/minute. His exercise capacity is limited by SOB after walking about a block despite having his enalapril increased to 20 mg/day, metoprolol XL to 200 mg/day, and adding digoxin 0.25 mg QD. The furosemide is still at 40 mg/day because he has little edema. Is an antiarrhythmic agent indicated for B.J. at this time? What is the agent of choice and what dose should be given?

Premature ventricular contractions and other arrhythmias are a common complication of left ventricular dysfunction and may be present regardless of whether the patient has had an MI. Approximately 50% to 70% of patients with HF have episodes of nonsustained ventricular tachycardia on ambulatory monitoring.[6] This myocardial irritability may be a result of autonomic hyperactivity or ventricular remodeling that can accompany HF. It is not clear, however, if these rhythm disturbances contribute to sudden death or simply reflect the underlying disease process. Recent studies suggest that sudden death in patients with HF is more likely caused by an acute ischemic event in patients with underlying CAD or to a bradyarrhythmia or electromechanical dissociation in patients with nonischemic cardiomyopathy. More importantly, suppression of ventricular ectopy in patients with HF has not been shown to lead to a reduction of sudden death in clinical trials. B.J.'s PVC were first noted after his MI. As discussed in detail in Chapters 17 (Myocardial Infarction) and 19 (Cardiac Arrhythmias), neither prophylactic antiarrhythmic therapy nor treatment of asymptomatic PVC following an MI has been proven to improve outcome or survival. In fact, because of concerns over proarrhythmic effects of most class IA (e.g., quinidine) and class IC (e.g., encainide, flecainide) drugs, as well as sotalol, treatment is considered contraindicated.

It has now been several months since B.J.'s infarct and he continues to have frequent PVC along with HF symptoms that place him in the NYHA class II–III category. It is suggested that amiodarone has value in patients with HF with arrhythmias because it has both antiarrhythmic properties as well as coronary vasodilating effects and α- and β-blocking properties. Thus, it may offer a dual benefit to reduce myocardial irritability and improve the hemodynamics of HF.

One meta-analysis reviewed 13 randomized, controlled trial of prophylactic amiodarone in patients with either recent MI (n = 8) or HF (n = 5).[313] None of the individual trials was powered to detect a mortality reduction of 20%. After loading doses of 400 to 800 mg/day for 2 weeks, maintenance doses ranged from 200 to 400 mg/day. This information taken as a whole, the authors concluded that prophylactic amiodarone reduces the rate of arrhythmic or sudden death in high-risk patients and this effect results in an overall 13% reduction in total mortality. Because this analysis combined trials of both MI and HF patients, it is helpful to look at two of the key HF trials.

In the Grupo de Estudio de la Sobrevida en la Insuficiecia Cardiaca en Argentina (GESICA) study,[314] 516 patients with class II to IV HF symptoms (79% class III or IV), an average EF of 20%, and frequent PVC on cardiac monitoring were randomized to receive either standard treatment (diuretics, vasodilators, digoxin) or a fixed dose of amiodarone plus standard treatment. The dose of amiodarone was 600 mg daily for the first 2 weeks, then 300 mg/day for at least 1 year. Of 260 patients on amiodarone, 87 (33.5%) died during follow-up compared with 106 of 256 (41.4%) receiving standard treatment, a statistically significant difference in favor of amiodarone ($p = 0.02$). Similarly, the number of HF-related hospitalizations was reduced with amiodarone. No data were presented on changes in EF, but a trend toward more patients in the amiodarone group being judged to have a decrease of at least one stage in NYHA class was noted.

Somewhat different outcomes were noted by the investigators in the Veteran's Administration Cooperative Survival Trial of Antiarrhythmic Therapy in Congestive Heart Failure (CHF-STAT) study.[315,316] Entry criteria to this trial were similar to the GESICA study, with a primary indicator being >10 asymptomatic PVC per minute on 24-hour monitoring, but without sustained ventricular tachycardia. A higher dose of amiodarone was used, starting with 800 mg for the first 2 weeks, then 400 mg/day for 1 year. The dose was reduced to 300 mg/day after the first year, with the average follow-up being 45 months (4.5 years maximum). Disappointingly, no difference between groups for either all-cause mortality (39% amiodarone vs. 42% placebo) or sudden cardiac death (15% amiodarone vs. 17% placebo) was found. Similarly, 2-year survival was 69.4% with amiodarone and 70.8% with placebo. Higher survival in the amiodarone group after the first 2 years was a noted trend, but the number of subjects followed for longer periods was not sufficiently large to establish significance. An encouraging finding in this study was that EF improved more in the patients treated with amiodarone, rising from a baseline average of 24.9% to posttreatment values of 33.7%. Corresponding change in the standard treatment group was from a baseline of 25.8% to 29.2% at follow-up. Despite the increase in EF, symptom scores did not differ between the two groups.

Together, these two studies still leave unclear the role of amiodarone in patients with HF with asymptomatic arrhythmias. The encouraging finding is that amiodarone does not seem to have a negative effect on mortality as seen with other antiarrhythmic agents or with inotropic stimulants. On the other hand, the two studies cited have conflicting findings regarding value in improving survival and functional capacity of patients. In comparing the two studies, it has been noted that the patients in the GESICA study had more advanced disease (79% class III or IV; average EF 20%; 55% 2-year placebo mortality) than those in the VA study (43% class III or IV; average EF 25%; 29% 2-year placebo mortality); more patients had nonischemic cardiomyopathy in GESICA (60%) compared with 29% in the VA study; 99% of the VA subjects were men, whereas 19% of GESICA subjects were women; and the dose of amiodarone was lower in GESICA.[317] Further subgroup analysis suggests that those with more advanced disease, nonischemic cardiomyopathy, and female sex have better outcomes. Contradicting this speculation was a trend toward better outcomes in the small number of patients with class II symptoms in GESICA.[314] Other factors to consider are the potential for significant side effects with amiodarone (see Chapter 19, Cardiac Arrhythmias) and the risk that digoxin levels might increase after the addition of amiodarone (see Question 39).

The ACC/AHA guidelines do not recommend routine ambulatory ECG monitoring in to detect asymptomatic ventricular arrhythmias in patients with HF, and also recommend against treatment if such arrhythmias are inadvertently detected.[7] If symptomatic ventricular arrhythmias should arise, or there is determined to be a high risk for sudden death, one of the following should be considered: a β-blocking drug, amiodarone, and/or an implantable cardioverter-defibrillator (ICD). As discussed extensively throughout this chapter, nearly all patients with HF should have a β-blocker as part of their regimen because these drugs reduce all cause mortality, not just sudden death. B.J. was started on metoprolol after his MI, but continued to have ectopy despite continued use of a β-blocker. Nonetheless, it is decided not to use amiodarone because he has ischemic cardiomyopathy and is not bothered by his arrhythmia.

IMPLANTABLE CARDIOVERTER-DEFIBRILLATER

55. Is B.J. a candidate for an implantable cardioverter-defibrillator implantation?

Although amiodarone is the preferred antiarrhythmic agent in patients with HF with reduced EF to prevent reoccurrent atrial fibrillation and symptomatic ventricular arrhythmias, it has not shown survival benefits. Ventricular arrhythmias are associated with high frequency of sudden cardiac death (SCD) in patients with HF. Numerous trials have established the role of ICD in primary and secondary prevention of sudden cardiac death. The most recent trial, the Sudden Cardiac Death in Heart Failure trial (SCD-HeFT) evaluated the efficacy of amiodarone in patients with LV dysfunction.[317] The patients (NYHA class II–III) were randomized to conventional therapy or placebo, conventional therapy plus amiodarone, or conventional therapy plus ICD. Amiodarone was no better than placebo, whereas, ICD decreased mortality by 23%. A subgroup analysis showed that patients with class II HF had a greater drop in mortality with ICD use than class III patients. Also, amiodarone decreased survival in class III HF. The role of amiodarone in patients with NYHA class III needs to be further evaluated before it is routinely used in patients with LV dysfunction.

The 2005 ACC/AHA guidelines recommend the use of ICD in patients after MI with reduced LVEF and who have a history of ventricular arrhythmias. ICD is also recommended for primary prevention in patients with nonischemic cardiomyopathy and ischemic heart disease who have a LVEF ≤30%, with NYHA functional class II or III symptoms while on optimal standard oral therapy, and in patients who have reasonable expected survival with a good functional status of 1 or more years.[7] Patients with ischemic heart disease should be at least 40 days post MI to receive an ICD. B.J. is currently on optimal HF drug regimen. Based on the results of SCD-HeFT trial, he would benefit from ICD implantation.

CARDIA-RESYNCHRONIZATION THERAPY

56. C.M., a 49-year-old woman with a history of cardiomyopathy (EF 25%), presents to the HF clinic with NYHA class III symptoms. She reports increased SOB, chest pain, and fatigue. She has been optimized on drug therapy for 3 months. Her medications include metoprolol 200 mg QD, furosemide 40 mg BID, lisinopril 20 mg QD, spironolactone 25 mg QD, and KCl 40 mEq. An ECG showed sinus rhythm at a rate of 72 beats/minute, QRS duration of 144 millisecond. Is she a candidate for CRT?

Approximately one-third of the patients with advanced systolic HF exhibit intra- or interventricular conduction delays that cause the ventricles to beat asynchronously.[318] This ventricular dyssynchrony, which is often seen on the ECG as a wide QRS complex with a left bundle branch block, can lead to deleterious effects on cardiac function. Patients may present with reduced EF, decreased CO, and presence of NYHA class III–IV HF symptoms. These are all associated with increased mortality.

Cardiac resynchronizathion therapy (CRT) is the use of cardiac pacing to coordinate the contraction of the left and right ventricles.[319] Initial randomized trials of CRT show reduced HF symptoms, and improved exercise tolerance and quality of life; but they have not demonstrated conclusive mortality benefits. The Comparison of Medical Therapy, Pacing, and Defibrillator in Heart Failure (COMPANION) trial[319] enrolled 1,520 patients with NYHA class II or IV(ischemic or non-ischemic cardiomyopathies, QRS interval of at least 120 milliseconds, and LVEF ≤35%) who were treated with optimal drug therapy (ACE, diuretics, β-blockers, and spironolactone). Patients were randomized to receive optimal drug therapy (OPT) alone, OPT and CRT with a pacemaker, or OPT and CRT with ICD (CRT-D). The primary endpoint was a composite of all-cause mortality and hospitalization. Both CRT and CRT-D groups were associated with a decreased risk of primary endpoint, respectively ($p = 0.014$, $p = 0.01$) compared with OPT alone. All-cause mortality at 1 year was decreased by 24% in the CRT group and 43% in the CRT-D group however was not significantly reduced in the CRT group.

The results of the Cardiac Resynchronization in Heart Failure study (CARE-HF)[320] extended the landmark findings of the COMPANION trial. CARE-HF demonstrated a significant all-cause mortality reduction for CRT pacing without defibrillator backup (CRT-P) in patients with HF medically treated similarly. This study was conducted in a total of 813 patients. The inclusion criteria were NYHA class III–IV, EF ≤35%, and QRS duration of ≥120 milliseconds (MS). Approximately 35% of patients had ischemic heart disease. The primary endpoint of all-cause deaths and hospitalizations for a major cardiovascular reason occurred in fewer patients in the CRT group compared with the OPT group (39% vs. 55%; $p < 0.001$). Death or hospitalization for worsening HF was also significantly reduced in the CRT group.

Thus, the combined results of CARE-HF and COMPANION confirm the importance of CRT and CRT-D in improving ventricular function, HF symptoms, and exercise tolerance, while also reducing frequency of HF hospitalizations by 37% and death by 22%.[321] The role of CRT in patients with mild HF symptoms, narrow QRS, chronic atrial fibrillation, and right bundle branch block need to be explored.

According to the 2005 ACC/AHA guidelines,[7] patients with NYHA class III and ambulatory patients with class IV HF should receive CRT (unless contraindicated) if they meet the following criteria: LVEF ≤35%, presence of electric asynchrony as shown by a wide QRS (>120 milliseconds), and receiving optimal HF standard medical therapy. Despite optimal doses of HF medications, C.M. continues to have HF symptoms. CRT could provide incremental benefits beyond what is provided with neurohormonal therapy.

Herbal Products and Nutritional Supplements

57. W.L., a 60-year-old man with HF recently diagnosed by his naturopath, is concerned by his decreasing exercise capacity and increasing SOB during his morning walks in the local mall. His blood pressure is 170/85 mm Hg and he has 1 to 2+ ankle edema. He distrusts medical doctors and wants to treat his HF naturally. One time in the past he was given hydrochlorothiazide for BP reduction, but stopped taking it after a few days because he did not tolerate the urinary urgency it caused. The naturopath has prescribed 200 mg/day of Hawthorn leaf and 50 mg/day of coenzyme Q. How effective is this treatment plan likely to be?

Hawthorn

Hawthorn extracts from the leaves and flowers of *Crataegus monogyna* and *C. oxyacantha* have been reported to have beneficial effects in mild HF.[322,323] Oligomeric procyanids and flavanoids are considered the key active ingredients. Hawthorn extracts have shown positive inotropic action, weak ACE inhibition, vasodilating properties, and increased coronary blood flow *in vitro* and in animal models. In short-term (8 weeks or less), placebo-controlled trials in patients with the equivalent of NYHA class II HF, modest improvements were noted in exercise tolerance and subjective symptoms as well as decreases in HR and BP. Patients with more advanced HF were excluded. A systematic review by Pittler et al. also concluded that hawthorn extract was efficacious in the treatment of HF on top of standard HF therapy.[324] Conversely, the results of the Hawthorne Extract Randomized Blinded Chronic Heart Failure (HERB-CHF) trial failed to provide any evidence that hawthorn was beneficial in patients with HF who were already receiving standard medical therapy.[325] The Commission E monograph lists no side effects or contraindications. In clinical trials, side effects of hawthorn include nausea, vomiting, diarrhea, palpitations, chest pain, and vertigo. These side effects are more common when doses exceed 900 mg/day, but in some trials have not occurred more often than placebo. The risks and benefits of using hawthorn and digoxin together, both of which have positive inotropic effects, is not known.

To further investigate the longer-term benefits of hawthorn, additive effects to conventional therapy, and effect on mortality were tested in the Survival and Prognosis: Investigation of Crataegus Extract WS 1442 in Congestive Heart Failure (SPICE) trial.[326] The trial enrolled 2,681 patients with NYHA class II–III, LVEF ≤35%, who were randomized to hawthorn or placebo for 2 years. Although the study failed to show any clear cardioprotective benefits in the treatment of chronic HF, hawthorn was well tolerated and can be safely added to standard therapy.

Coenzyme Q

Coenzyme Q, also known as ubiquinone and ubidecarenone, is an endogenously synthesized provitamin that is structurally similar to vitamin E and serves as a lipid-soluble electron transport carrier in mitochondria and aids in the synthesis of adenosine triphosphate.[327,328] It might also have membrane-stabilizing properties, enhance the antioxidant effects of vitamin E, and stabilize calcium-dependent slow channels. In animal models, it has positive inotropic effects, although weaker than from digoxin. As has been reviewed, more than 18 open-label and double-blind, randomized clinical trials have been conducted of coenzyme Q in patients with HF ranging from NYHA classes II to IV.[327] Doses varied from 50 to 200 mg/day. In contrast to Hawthorn, the patients in many of these trials were also taking diuretics, ACE inhibitors, and digoxin. Different trials used different end point measurements. Positive effects on subjective symptoms, NYHA class improvement, EF, quality of life and hospitalization rates have all been observed. Two trials, however, failed to demonstrate significant changes in EF, vascular resistance, or exercise tolerance. None of the trials had sufficiently large samples sizes or adequate duration of assessment to detect reduction in mortality. Side effects were consistently minimal, but included nausea, epigastric pain, diarrhea, heartburn, and appetite suppression. Mild increases in lactate dehydrogenase and hepatic enzymes have been rarely reported with coenzyme Q doses in excess of 300 mg/day.

It can be concluded that hawthorn and coenzyme Q are both safe in the treatment of HF and might provide symptomatic improvement, especially in patients with mild HF (NYHA class II). Only coenzyme Q has been shown to be of benefit as an adjunct to conventional therapies. It is unknown if using hawthorn and coenzyme Q together, as prescribed for W.L., will have an additive effect. No conclusion can be drawn about their effects on mortality rates.

W.L. has poorly controlled systolic hypertension and HF that is beginning to interfere with his activities of daily life. Although evidence indicates that patients with NYHA class II HF obtain symptomatic improvement with hawthorn and coenzyme Q, this does not address W.L.'s hypertension. (As reviewed by Tran et al.,[327] conflicting data exist on the value of coenzyme Q in lowering blood pressure.) Also the results of the SPICE trial did not demonstrate any mortality benefits. Also, no incremental benefits were seen when combined with standard therapy. Even if W.L. and his naturopath are both satisfied with his responses to hawthorn and coenzyme Q, significant concern still exists of what will happen when and if his disease progresses. Uncontrolled hypertension in patients with HF can further lead to cardiac remodeling resulting in worsening HF. Currently he is presenting with symptomatic HF, therefore he should be started on a diuretic to alleviate his symptoms. Starting with a 20-mg dose of furosemide and titrating slowly may be one approach. For all of the reasons cited throughout this chapter, one must also argue strongly for starting an ACE inhibitor to control his hypertension. He should be counseled that the urinary frequency he experienced previously should diminish after a few days.

He is being started on both hawthorn and coenzyme Q simultaneously. If he does improve, it will be difficult to assess whether it is because of only one of the agents or the combination. With this in mind, it might be more logical to continue hawthorn alone at a dose of 450 mg BID. If no benefit is derived after 1 month, hawthorn should be stopped and coenzyme Q started at 100 mg/day.

REFERENCES

1. Agency for Health Care Policy and Research. *Heart failure: Evaluation and Care of Patients with Left-ventricular Systolic Dysfunction*. Clinical practice guidelines, no. 11. Public Health Service, US Department of Health and Human Services, 1994. (AHCPR Publication no. 94-0612).
2. American College of Cardiology/American Heart Association Task Force on Practice Guidelines. Guidelines for the evaluation and management of heart failure. *J Am Coll Cardiol* 1995;26:1376 and *Circulation* 1995;92:2764.
3. Adams K et al. for the Heart Failure Society of America (HFSA) Practice Guidelines Committee. HFSA guidelines for the management of patients with heart failure caused by left ventricular systolic dysfunction-pharmacologic approaches. *Pharmacotherapy* 2000;20:495. Also available at www.hfsa.org.
4. Adams KF, Lindenfeld J, Arnold JMO et al. Executive summary: HFSA 2006 comprehensive heart failure practice guideline. *J Card Fail* 2006; 12:10.
5. The task Force for the Diagnosis and Treatment of Chronic Heart Failure of the European Society of Cardiology. Guidelines for The diagnosis and treatment of chronic heart failure: executive summary(update 2005). *Eur Heart J* 2005;26: 1115.
6. Hunt SA et al. ACC/AHA guidelines in the evaluation and management of chronic heart failure in the adult: a report of the American College of Cardiology/American Heart Association Task Force on Practice Guidelines (Committee to Revise the 1995 Guidelines for the Evaluation and Management of Heart Failure). 2001. American College of Cardiology Web Site. Available at http://www.acc.org/clinical/guidelines/failure/hf_index.htm. *Circulation* 2001;104:2996 (executive summary).
7. Hunt SA et al. ACC/AHA 2005 guideline update for the diagnosis and management of chronic heart failure in the adult: a report of American College of Cardiology, American Heart Association Task Force on Practice Guidelines (Writing Committee) to update the 2001 Guidelines for the Evaluation and Management of Heart Failure. *J Am Coll Cardiol* 2005;46:E1.
8. Rosmond W et al. For the American Heart Association statistics Committee and stroke statistics subcommittee, Heart Disease and stroke statistics—2007 update: a report from the American Heart Association statistics committee and stroke subcommittee. *Circulation* 2007;115:69.
9. Redfield MM et al. Burden of systolic and diastolic ventricular dysfunction in the community: appreciating the scope of heart failure epidemic. *JAMA* 2003;289:194.
10. Pass S, Dusing M. Current and emerging therapy for primary pulmonary hypertension. *Ann Pharmacother* 2002;36:1414.
11. Chatterjee K et al. Pulmonary hypertension: hemodynamic diagnosis and management. *Arch Intern Med* 2002;162:1925.
12. Zile M. Heart failure with preserved ejection fraction: is this diastolic heart failure? *J Am Coll Cardiol* 2003;41:1519.
13. Yamamota K et al. Left ventricular diastolic dysfunction in patients with hypertension and preserved systolic dysfunction. *Mayo Clin Proc* 2000;75:148.
14. Gaasch WH. Diagnosis and treatment of heart failure based on left ventricular systolic or diastolic dysfunction. *JAMA* 1994;271:1276.
15. Ramachandran SV et al. Congestive heart failure with normal left ventricular systolic function: clinical approach to the diagnosis and treatment of diastolic heart failure. *Arch Intern Med* 1996;156: 146.
16. Garcia M. Diastolic dysfunction and heart failure: causes and treatment options. *Cleve Clin J Med* 2000;67:727.
17. Ho KK et al. The epidemiology of heart failure: the Framingham Study. *J Am Coll Cardiol* 1993; 22(Suppl 6):6A.
18. Kannel WB, Belanger AJ. Epidemiology of heart failure. *Am Heart J* 1991;121:951.
19. Schreier R, Abraham W. Hormones and hemodynamics in heart failure. *N Engl J Med* 1999;341:577.
20. Hash TW, Prisant M. β-Blocker use in systolic heart failure and dilated cardiomyopathy. *J Clin Pharmacol* 1997;37:7.
21. Patterson JH, Rogers JE. Expanding role of β-blockade in the management of chronic heart failure. *Pharmacotherapy* 2003;23:451.
22. Foody J et al. β-Blocker therapy in heart failure. Part I: Scientific review. Part II: Clinical applications. *JAMA* 2002;287:883 (part I) and 890 (part II).
23. Munger M, Cheang KI. β-Blocker therapy: a standard of care for heart failure. *Pharmacotherapy* 2000;20(Suppl):359S.
24. Goldstein S. Benefits of β-blocker therapy for heart failure. *Arch Intern Med* 2002;162:641.
25. Bristow MR. Mechanistic and clinical rationale for using β-blockers in heart failure. *J Card Fail* 2000;6:8.
26. Small K et al. Synergistic polymorphisms of β1- and alpha2c-adrenergic receptors and the risk of congestive heart failure. *N Engl J Med* 2002;347:1135.
27. Weiber K. Aldosterone in congestive heart failure. *N Engl J Med* 2001;345:1689.
28. Ergul A. Endothelin-1 and endothelin receptor antagonists as potential cardiovascular therapeutic agents. *Pharmacotherapy* 2002;22:54.
29. Nguyen B, Johnson, J. The role of endothelin in heart failure and hypertension. *Pharmacotherapy* 1998;18:706.
30. Maisel A et al. Rapid measurement of the B-type natriuretic peptide in the emergency diagnosis of heart failure. *N Engl J Med* 2002;347:161.
31. Lee C et al. Surrogate endpoints in heart failure. *Ann Pharmacother* 2002;36:479.
32. Troughton RW et al. Treatment of heart failure guided by plasma amino terminal brain natriuretic peptide (N-BNP) concentrations. *Lancet* 2000;355:1126.
33. Vichiendilokkul A et al. Nesiritide: a novel approach for acute heart failure. *Ann Pharmacother* 2003;37:247.
34. Colucci W et al. Intravenous nesiritide, a natriuretic peptide, in the treatment of decompensated heart failure. *N Engl J Med* 2000;343:246.
35. Gheorghiade M et al. Effects of tolvaptan a vasopressin antagonist, in patient hospitalized with worsening heart failure. *JAMA* 2004;291: 1963.
36. Gheorghiade M et al. Short-term clinical effects of tolvaptan, an oral vasopressin antagonist in patients hospitalized for heart failure. The EVEREST Clinical Trials. *JAMA* 2007;297:1332.
37. Konstam MA et al. Effects of oral tolvaptan in patient hospitalized with worsening heart failure. *JAMA* 2007;297:1319.
38. Earl GL et al. Levosimendan: A novel inotropic agent for treatment of acute decompensated heart failure. *Ann Pharmacotherapy* 2005;39:1888.
39. Follath F et al. Efficacy and safety of intravenous levosimendan compared with dobutamine in severe low output heart failure (the LIDO study): a randomized double-blind trial. *Lancet* 2002;360:196.
40. Moiseyev VS et al. Safety and efficacy of novel calcium sensitizer, levosimendan, in patients with left ventricular failure due to an acute myocardial infarction. *Eur Heart J* 2002;23:1422.
41. Packer M. REVIVE II: Multicenter placebo-controlled trial of levosimendan on clinical status in acutely decompensated heart failure. Presented at the American Heart Association Scientific Sessions 2005, Dallas, Texas, November 13–16, 2005.
42. Mebazaa A et al. The SURVIVE Randomized Trial: levosimendan vs dobutamine for patients with acute decompensated heart failure. *JAMA* 2007;297:1883.
43. Shan K et al. The role of cytokines in disease progression in heart failure. *Current Concepts in Cardiology* 1997;12:218.
44. Kapadia S et al. The role of cytokines in the failing human heart. *Cardiol Clin* 1998;16:645.
45. Mabuchi N et al. Relationship between interleukin-6 production in the lungs and pulmonary vascular resistance in patients with congestive heart failure. *Chest* 2002;121:1195.
46. Bolger A, Anker S. Tumour necrosis factor in chronic heart failure. *Drugs* 2000;60:1245.
47. Herrera-Garza E et al. Tumor necrosis factor: a mediator of disease progression in the failing human heart. *Chest* 1999;115:1170.
48. Bozkurt B et al. Results of targeted anti-tumor necrosis factor therapy with etanercept (Enbrel) in patients with advanced heart failure. *Circulation* 2001;103:1044.
49. Kwon H et al. Case reports of heart failure after therapy with tumor necrosis factor antagonist. *Ann Intern Med* 2003;138:807.
50. Vanhoutte PM et al. Endothelium-derived relaxing factors and converting enzyme inhibition. *Am J Cardiol* 1995;76:3E.
51. Sueta CA et al. Safety and efficacy of epoprostenol in patients with severe congestive heart failure. *Am J Cardiol* 1995;75:34A.
52. Califf R et al. A randomized controlled trial of epoprostenol therapy for severe congestive heart failure: the Flolan international randomized survival trial (FIRST). *Am Heart J* 1997;134:44.
53. O'Connell JB, Bristow M. The economic burden of heart failure. *Clin Cardiol* 2000;23(Suppl III):6.
54. Brater DC. Pharmacology of diuretics. *Am J Med Sci* 2000;319:38.
55. Kramer BK et al. Diuretic treatment and diuretic resistance in heart failure. *Am J Med* 1999;106:90.
56. Sharpe N, Doughty R. Epidemiology of heart failure and ventricular dysfunction. *Lancet* 1998;352 (Suppl 1):S13.
57. Pitt B et al. The effect of spironolactone on morbidity and mortality in patients with severe heart failure. *N Engl J Med* 1999;341:709.
58. Pitt B et al. Eplerenone, a selective aldosterone blocker, in patients with left ventricular dysfunction after myocardial infarction. *N Engl J Med* 2003; 348:1309.

59. Rodgers J, Patterson JH. The role of the renin-angiotensin-aldosterone system in the management of heart failure. *Pharmacotherapy* 2002;20(Suppl):368S.
60. Brown N, Vaughan D. Angiotensin-converting enzyme inhibitors. *Circulation* 1998;97:1411.
61. American Society of Health-System Pharmacists. ASHP therapeutic guidelines on angiotensin-converting-enzyme inhibitors in patients with left ventricular dysfunction. *Am J Health Syst Pharm* 1997;54:2999.
62. Patterson JH. Angiotensin II receptor blockers in heart failure. *Pharmacotherapy* 2003;23:173.
63. VanVeldhuisen D et al. Value of digoxin in heart failure and sinus rhythm: new features of an old drug. *J Am Coll Cardiol* 1996;28:813.
64. VanVeldhuisen D et al. Progression of mild untreated heart failure during 6 months follow-up and clinical and neurohumoral effects of ibopamine and digoxin as monotherapy. *Am J Cardiol* 1995;75:796.
65. Krum H et al. Effect of long-term digoxin therapy on autonomic function in patients with chronic heart failure. *J Am Coll Cardiol* 1995;25:289.
66. Gheorghiade M et al. Effects of increasing maintenance doses of digoxin on left ventricular function and neurohormones in patients with chronic heart failure treated with diuretics and angiotensin-converting enzyme inhibitors. *Circulation* 1995;92:1801.
67. Aronson JK. Clinical pharmacokinetics of digoxin therapy 1980. *Clin Pharmacokinet* 1980;5:137.
68. Heizer W et al. Absorption of digoxin from tablets and capsules in subjects with malabsorption syndromes. DICP, *Ann Pharmacother* 1989;23:764.
69. Moordian A. Digitalis: an update of clinical pharmacokinetics, therapeutic monitoring techniques and treatment recommendations. *Clin Pharmacokinet* 1988;15:165.
70. Reuning R et al. Digoxin. In: Evans W et al., eds. *Applied Pharmacokinetics*. 3rd Ed. Vancouver: Applied Therapeutics, 1992:20.
71. Bauer L. Digoxin. In: *Applied Clinical Pharmacokinetics*. New York: McGraw Hill, 2001:265.
72. Aronson JK. Clinical pharmacokinetics of cardiac glycosides in patients with renal dysfunction. *Clin Pharmacokinet* 1983;8:155.
73. Yu D. The contribution of P-glycoprotein to pharmacokinetic drug interactions. *J Clin Pharmacol* 1999;39:1203.
74. Fromm MF et al. Inhibition of P-glycoprotein-mediated drug transport: a unifying mechanism to explain the interaction between digoxin and quinidine. *Circulation* 1999;99:552.
75. Lindebaum J et al. Inactivation of digoxin by the gut flora: reversibility by antibiotic therapy. *N Engl J Med* 1981;305:789.
76. Jelliffe RW et al. A nomogram for digoxin therapy. *Am J Med* 1974;57:63.
77. Taylor AL et al. Combination of isosorbide dinitrate and hydralazine in blacks with heart failure. *N Engl J Med* 2004;351:2049.
78. Packer M et al. for the Prospective Randomized Amlodipine Survival Evaluation Study Group. The effect of amlodipine on morbidity and mortality in severe heart failure. *N Engl J Med* 1996;335:1107.
79. Cohn J et al. for the Vasodilator-Heart Failure Trial Study Group. Effect of the calcium antagonist felodipine as supplemental vasodilator therapy in patients with chronic heart failure treated with enalapril. V-HeFT III. *Circulation* 1997;96:856.
80. Johnson D et al. Effect of cyclooxygenase-2 inhibitors on blood pressure. *Ann Pharmacother* 2003;37:442.
81. Huerta C et al. Non-steroidal anti-inflammatory drugs and risk of first hospitalization admissions for heart failure in the general population. *Heart* 2006;92:610.
82. Heerdink ER et al. NSAIDS associated with increased risk of congestive heart failure in elderly patients taking diuretics. *Arch Intern Med* 1998;158,1108.
83. Page J et al. Consumption of NSAIDS and the development of congestive heart failure in elderly patients: an under-recognized public health problem. *Arch Intern Med* 2000;160:777.
84. Feenstra J et al. Association of non-steroidal anti-inflammatory drugs with first occurrence of heart failure and with relapsing heart failure. *Arch Intern Med* 2002;162:265.
85. Shan K et al. Anthracycline-induced cardiotoxicity. *Ann Intern Med* 1996;125:47.
86. Singal P, Iliskovic N. Doxorubicin-induced cardiomyopathy. *N Engl J Med* 1998;339:900.
87. Crouch M et al. Clinical relevance and management of drug-related QT interval prolongation. *Pharmacotherapy* 2003;23:881.
88. Page RL II et al. Possible heart failure exacerbation associated with rosiglitazone: case report and literature review. *Pharmacotherapy* 2003;23:945.
89. Risler T et al. Comparative pharmacokinetics and pharmacodynamics of loop diuretics in renal failure. *Cardiology* 1994;84(Suppl 2):155.
90. Murray MD et al. Torsemide more effective that furosemide for treatment of heart failure. *Am J Med* 2001;111:513.
91. Cutler R, Blair A. Clinical pharmacokinetics of furosemide. *Clin Pharmacokinet* 1979;4:279.
92. Greither A et al. Pharmacokinetics of furosemide in patients with congestive heart failure. *Pharmacology* 1979;19:121.
93. Straughn A et al. Bioavailability of seven furosemide tablets in man. *Biopharm Drug Dispos* 1986;7:113.
94. McNamara P et al. Influence of tablet dissolution on furosemide bioavailability: a bioequivalence study. *Pharm Res* 1987;4:150.
95. Kelly M et al. Pharmacokinetics of orally administered furosemide. *Clin Pharmacol Ther* 1979;15:1778.
96. Kelly M et al. A comparison of the diuretic response to oral and intravenous furosemide in diuretic resistant patients. *Curr Ther Res Clin Exp* 1977;21:1.
97. Vargo D et al. The pharmacodynamics of torsemide in patients with congestive heart failure. *Clin Pharmacol Ther* 1995;57:601.
98. Stallings S et al. Comparison of natriuretic and diuretic effects of single and divided doses of furosemide. *Am J Hosp Pharm* 1979;36:68.
99. Wilson T et al. Effect of dosage regimen and natriuretic response to furosemide. *Clin Pharmacol Ther* 1976;18:165.
100. Kosman ME. Management of potassium problems during long-term diuretic therapy. *JAMA* 1974;230:743.
101. Davidson C et al. Effect of long-term diuretic treatment on body potassium in heart disease. *Lancet* 1976;2:1044.
102. Siegel D et al. Diuretics serum and intracellular electrolyte levels, and ventricular arrhythmias in hypertensive men. *JAMA* 1992;267:1083.
103. Steiness E et al. Cardiac arrhythmias induced by hypokalemia and potassium loss during maintenance digoxin therapy. *Br Heart J* 1976;38:167.
104. Holland OB et al. Diuretic-induced ventricular ectopic activity. *Am J Med* 1981;770:762.
105. Hollifield JW et al. Thiazide diuretics, hypokalemia and cardiac arrhythmias. *Acta Med Scand* 1981;647:67.
106. Tsuji H et al. The association of levels of serum potassium and magnesium with ventricular premature complexes (the Framingham Heart Study). *Am J Cardiology* 1994;74:237.
107. Nolan J et al. Prospective study of heart rate variability and mortality in chronic heart failure: results of United Kingdom Heart Failure Evaluation and Assessment of Risk Trial (UK-Heart). *Circulation* 1998;98:1510.
108. Grobbee DE et al. Non-potassium sparing diuretics and risk of sudden death. *J Hypertens* 1995;13:1539.
109. Cohn JN et al. New Guidelines for Potassium Replacement in Clinical Practice. *Arch Intern Med* 2000;160:2429.
110. Hollifield JW. Potassium and magnesium abnormalities: diuretics and arrhythmias in hypertension. *Am J Med* 1984;77(5A):28.
111. Felker GM et al. Natriuretic peptides in the diagnosis and management of heart Failure. *CMAJ* 2006;175:611.
112. Maisel AS et al. For the Breathing Not Properly Multinational Study investigators. Rapid measurement of B-type natriuretic peptide in emergency diagnosis of heart failure. *N Engl J Med* 2002;347:161.
113. McMahon FG et al. Effect of potassium chloride supplements on upper gastrointestinal mucosa. *Clin Pharmacol Ther* 1984;38:852.
114. Patterson DJ et al. Endoscopic comparison of solid and liquid potassium chloride supplements. *Lancet* 1983;2:1077.
115. Aselton PJ, Jick H. Short-term follow-up study of wax matrix potassium chloride in relation to gastrointestinal bleeding. *Lancet* 1983;1:184.
116. Jick H et al. A comparison of wax matrix and microencapsulated potassium chloride in relation to upper gastrointestinal illness requiring hospitalization. *Pharmacotherapy* 1989;9:204.
117. Schwartz A et al. Dosage of potassium chloride elixir to correct thiazide-induced hypokalemia. *JAMA* 1974;230:702.
118. Sklath H, Gums J. Spironolactone: a reexamination. Drug Intelligence and Clinical Pharmacy, *Ann Pharmacother* 1990;24:52.
119. Schnaper H et al. Potassium restoration in hypertensive patients made hypokalemic by hydrochlorothiazide. *Arch Intern Med* 1989;149:2677.
120. Lahav M et al. Continuous infusion furosemide in patients with severe CHF. *Chest* 1992;102:725.
121. Rudy D et al. Loop diuretics for chronic renal insufficiency: a continuous infusion is more efficacious than bolus therapy. *Ann Intern Med* 1991;115:360.
122. Van Meyel J et al. Continuous infusion of furosemide in the treatment of patients with congestive heart failure and diuretic resistance. *J Intern Med* 1994;235:329.
123. Dormans T et al. Diuretic efficacy of high-dose furosemide in severe heart failure: bolus injections versus continuous infusion. *J Am Coll Cardiol* 1996;28:376.
124. Kramer W et al. Pharmacodynamics of torsemide as an intravenous injection and as a continuous infusion to patients with congestive heart failure. *J Clin Pharmacol* 1996;36:265.
125. Sica D, Gehr TW. Diuretic combinations in refractory edema states. *Clin Pharmacokinet* 1996; 30:229.
126. Howard P, Dunn M. Aggressive diuresis is safe and cost effective for severe heart failure in the elderly. *Chest* 2001;119:807.
127. Jessup M. Aldosterone blockade and heart failure. *N Engl J Med* 2003;348:1380.
128. Lee DCS et al. Heart failure in outpatients. *N Engl J Med* 1982;306:699.
129. Jaeschke R et al. To what extent do congestive heart failure patients in normal sinus rhythm benefit from digoxin therapy? A systematic overview and meta-analysis. *Am J Med* 1990;88:279.
130. Kulick D, Rahimtoola S. Current role of digitalis therapy in patients with congestive heart failure. *JAMA* 1991;265:2995.
131. Cohn J et al. Effect of vasodilator therapy on mortality in chronic congestive heart failure. *N Engl J Med* 1986;314:1547.
132. The Consensus Trial Study Group. Effects of enalapril on mortality in severe congestive heart failure: results of the Cooperative North Scandinavian Enalapril Survival Group. *N Engl J Med* 1987;316:1429.
133. Kjekshus J et al. Effects of enalapril on long-term mortality in severe congestive heart failure. *Am J Cardiol* 1992;69:103.
134. The SOLVD Investigators. Effect of enalapril on survival in patients with reduced left ventricular ejection fractions and congestive heart failure. *N Engl J Med* 1991;325:295.
135. Rector TS et al. Evaluation by patients with heart failure of the effects of enalapril compared with

hydralazine plus isosorbide dinitrate on quality of life. V-HeFT II. *Circulation* 1993;87(Suppl VI):V171.
136. Cohn J et al. A comparison of enalapril with hydralazine-isosorbide dinitrate in the treatment of chronic congestive heart failure. *N Engl J Med* 1991;325:303.
137. Uretsky B et al. For the PROVED Investigative Group. Randomized study assessing the effect of digoxin withdrawal in patients with mild to moderate chronic congestive heart failure. *J Am Coll Cardiol* 1993;26:93.
138. Packer M et al. Withdrawal of digoxin from patients with chronic heart failure treated with angiotensin-converting-enzyme inhibitors. *N Engl J Med* 1993;329:1.
139. Garg R et al. On behalf of The Digitalis Intervention Group. The effect of digoxin on mortality and morbidity in patients with heart failure. *N Engl J Med* 1997;336:525.
140. Crozier I, Ikram H. Angiotensin converting enzyme inhibitors versus digoxin for the treatment of congestive heart failure. *Drugs* 1992;43:637.
141. The Captopril-Digoxin Multicenter Research Group. Comparative effects of therapy with captopril and digoxin in patients with mild to moderate heart failure. *JAMA* 1988;259:539.
142. Davies R et al. Enalapril versus digoxin in patients with congestive heart failure: a multicenter study. *J Am Coll Cardiol* 1991;18:1602.
143. White CM. Angiotensin-converting-enzyme inhibition in heart failure or after myocardial infarction. *Am J Health Syst Pharm* 2000;57(Suppl 1):S18.
144. Wollert KC, Drexler H. The kallikreins-kinin system in post myocardial infarction cardiac remodeling. *Am J Cardiol* 1997;80(Suppl):158A.
145. Colfer H et al. Effects of once daily benazepril on exercise tolerance and manifestations of chronic congestive heart failure. *Am J Cardiol* 1992;70:354.
146. Garg R et al. Overview of randomized trials on angiotensin-converting enzyme inhibition on mortality and morbidity in patients with heart failure. *JAMA* 1995;273:1450.
147. Hall A et al. on behalf of the AIREX Study Investigators. Follow-up study of patients randomly allocated to ramipril or placebo for heart failure after acute myocardial infarction: AIRE Extension (AIREX) Study. *Lancet* 1997;349:1493.
148. Kober L et al. For the Trandolapril Cardiac Evaluation (TRACE) Study. A clinical trial of the angiotensin-converting-enzyme inhibitor trandolapril in patients with left ventricular dysfunction after myocardial infraction. *N Engl J Med* 1995;333:1670.
149. Amrosioni E et al. The effect of angiotensin-converting-enzyme inhibitor zofenopril on mortality and morbidity after anterior myocardial infarction. *N Engl J Med* 1995;332:80.
150. Bach R, Zardini P. Long acting angiotensin-converting-enzyme inhibition: once daily lisinopril versus twice-daily captopril in mild to moderate heart failure. *Am J Cardiol* 1992;70:70C.
151. Zannad F et al. Comparison of treatment with lisinopril versus enalapril for congestive heart failure. *Am J Cardiol* 1992;70:78C.
152. Zannad F et al. for the Fosinopril in Heart Failure Study Investigators. Differential effects of fosinopril and enalapril in patients with mild to moderate chronic heart failure. *Am Heart J* 1998;136:672.
153. Pflugfelder PW et al. Clinical consequences of angiotensin-converting enzyme inhibitor withdrawal in chronic heart failure: a double-blind, placebo-controlled study of quinapril. The Quinapril Heart Failure Trial Investigators. *J Am Coll Cardiol* 1993;22:1557.
154. Hobbs RE. Results of the ATLAS study. High or low doses of ACE inhibitors for heart failure?. *Cleve Clin J Med* 1998;65:539.
155. Packer M et al. Comparative effects of low and high doses of the angiotensin-converting enzyme inhibitor, lisinopril, on morbidity and mortality in chronic heart failure. *Circulation* 1999;100:2312.
156. The Network Investigators. Clinical outcome with enalapril in symptomatic chronic heart failure; a dosage comparison. *Eur Heart J* 1998;19:481.
157. Packer M et al. Comparison of captopril and enalapril in patients with severe chronic heart failure. *N Engl J Med* 1986;315:847.
158. Luque C, Ortiz M. Treatment of ACE inhibitor induced cough. *Pharmacotherapy* 1999;19:804.
159. Sharif MN et al. Cough induced by quinapril with resolution after changing to fosinopril. *Ann Pharmacol Ther* 1994;28:720.
160. Dicpinigaitis PV. Angiotensin-converting enzyme inhibitor-induced cough: ACCP evidence-based clinical practice guidelines. *Chest* 2006;129:1695.
161. Woo KS, Nicholls MG. High prevalence of persistent cough with angiotensin-converting enzyme inhibitors in Chinese. *Br J Clin Pharmacol* 1995;40:141.
162. Martineau P, Goulet J. New competition in the realm of renin-angiotensin axis inhibition: the angiotensin II receptor antagonists in congestive heart failure. *Ann Pharmacother* 2001;35:71.
163. Jong P et al. Angiotensin receptor blockers in heart failure: a meta-analysis of randomized controlled trials. *J Am Coll Cardiol* 2002;39:463.
164. Riegger GAJ et al. Improvement in exercise tolerance and symptoms of congestive heart during treatment with candesartan cilexetil. *Circulation* 1999;100:2224.
165. Havranek EP et al. Dose-related beneficial long-term hemodynamic and clinical efficacy of irbesartan in heart failure. *J Am Coll Cardiol* 1999; 33:1174.
166. Dickstein K et al. Comparison of the effects of losartan and enalapril on clinical status and exercise performance in patients with moderate to severe heart failure. *J Am Coll Cardiol* 1995;26: 438.
167. Pitt B et al. Randomized trial of losartan versus captopril in patients over 65 with heart failure. *Lancet* 1997;349:747.
168. Pitt B et al. for the ELITE II Investigators. Effect of losartan compared with lisinopril on mortality in patients with symptomatic heart failure: randomized trial—the losartan heart failure survival study ELITE II. *Lancet* 2000;355:1582.
169. McKelvie RS et al. For the RESOLVD Pilot Study Investigators. Comparison of candesartan, enalapril, and their combination in congestive heart failure: randomized evaluation of strategies for left ventricular dysfunction (RESOLVD) pilot study. *Circulation* 1999;100:1056.
170. Cohn J, Tognoni G, for the Valsartan Heart Failure Trial Investigators. A randomized trial of the angiotensin-receptor blocker valsartan in chronic heart failure. *N Engl J Med* 2001;345:1667.
171. Solomon SD et al. The valsartan in acute myocardial infarction trial (VALIANT) investigators. Sudden death in patients with myocardial infarction and left ventricular dysfunction, heart failure, or both. *N Engl J Med* 2005 23;352:2581.
172. Granger CB et al. Effects of candesartan in patients with chronic heart failure and reduced left-ventricular systolic function intolerant to ACEIs: the CHARM-Alternative trial. *Lancet* 2003;362:772.
173. McMurray JJV et al. Effects of candesartan in patients with chronic heart failure and reduced left-ventricular systolic function taking ACEIs: the CHARM-Added trial. *Lancet* 2003;362:767.
174. Yusuf S et al. Effects of candesartan in patients with chronic heart failure and preserved left-ventricular ejection fraction: the CHARM-Preserved Trial. *Lancet* 2003;362:777.
175. Pfeffer MA et al. , for the CHARM Investigators and Committees. Effects of candesartan on mortality and morbidity in patients with chronic heart failure: the CHARM-overall programme. *Lancet* 2003;362:759.
176. Schepkens H et al. Live threatening hyperkalemia during combined therapy with angiotensin-converting enzyme inhibitors and spironolactone: an analysis of 25 cases. *Am J Med* 2001;110:438.
177. Wregner E et al. Interaction of spironolactone with ACE inhibitors or angiotensin receptor blockers: analysis of 44 cases. *BMJ* 2003;327:147.
178. Juurlink DN et al. Rates of hyperkalemia after publication of randomized aldactone evaluation study. *N Engl J Med* 2004:351:543.
179. Palmer BF. Managing hyperkalemia cause by inhibition of renin-angiotensin aldosterone system. *N Engl J Med* 2004;35:585.
180. Shah KB et al. The adequacy of laboratory monitoring in patients treated with spironolactone for congestive heart failure. *J Am Coll Cardiol* 2005;46:845.
181. Vleeming W et al. ACE inhibitor-induced angioedema. Incidence, prevention, and management. *Drug Saf* 1998;18:171.
182. Brown NJ et al. Black Americans have an increased risk of angiotensin converting enzyme inhibitor associated angioedema. *Clin Pharmacol Ther* 1996;60:8.
183. Brown NJ et al. Recurrent angiotensin converting enzyme inhibitor associated angioedema. *JAMA* 1997;278:832.
184. Gavras I, Gavras H. Are patients who develop angioedema with ACE inhibition at risk for the same problem with AT-1 receptor blockade? *Arch Intern Med* 2003;163:240.
185. Abdi R et al. Angiotensin II receptor blocker-associated angioedema. On the heels of ACE inhibitor angioedema. *Pharmacotherapy* 2002;22: 1173.
186. Lo KS. Angioedema associated with candesartan. *Pharmacotherapy* 2002;22:1176.
187. Van Rijnsoever EW et al. Angioneurotic edema attributed to the use of losartan. *Arch Intern Med* 1998;158:2063.
188. Frye C, Pettigrew T. Angioedema and photosensitive rash induced by valsartan. *Pharmacotherapy* 1998;18:866.
189. Gavras I et al. Fatal pancytopenia associated with the use of captopril. *Ann Intern Med* 1981;94:58.
190. Hanssens M et al. Fetal and neonatal effects of treatment with angiotensin-converting enzyme inhibitors in pregnancy. *Obstet Gynecol* 1991;78: 128.
191. Cleland J et al. The effects of captopril on serum digoxin and urinary urea and digoxin clearances in patients with congestive heart failure. *Am Heart J* 1986;112:130.
192. Swedberg K et al. Effects of the early administration of enalapril in mortality in patients with acute myocardial infarction (CONSENSUS II). *N Engl J Med* 1992;327:628.
193. Pfeffer M et al. Effect of captopril on mortality and morbidity in patients with left ventricular dysfunction after myocardial infarction: the Survival and Ventricular Enlargement Trial (SAVE). *N Engl J Med* 1992;327:669.
194. The Acute Infarction Ramipril Efficacy (AIRE) Study Investigators. Effect of ramipril on mortality and morbidity of survivors of acute myocardial infarction with clinical evidence of heart failure. *Lancet* 1993;342:821.
195. Nawarskas J, Spinler S. Update on the interaction between aspirin and angiotensin-converting enzyme inhibitors. *Pharmacotherapy* 2000;20: 698.
196. Olson K. Combined aspirin/ACE inhibitor treatment for HF. *Ann Pharmacother* 2001;35:1653.
197. Harjai KJ et al. Use of aspirin in conjunction with angiotensin-converting enzyme inhibitors does not worsen long-term survival in heart failure. *Int J Cardiol* 2003;88:207.
198. Avezum A et al. Beta-blocker therapy for congestive heart failure. *Can J Cardiol* 1998;14:1045.
199. Lechat P et al. Clinical effects of beta-adrenergic blockade in chronic heart failure. *Circulation* 1998;98:1184.
200. Doughty R et al. Effects of beta-blocker therapy on mortality in patients with heart failure. *Eur Heart J* 1997;18:560.
201. Heidenreich PA et al. Effects of beta-blockade on mortality in patients with heart failure. *J Am Coll Cardiol* 1997;30:27.

202. Brophy J et al. Beta-blockers in congestive heart failure: a Bayesian meta-analysis. *Ann Intern Med* 2001;134:550.
203. Gattis WA et al. Predischarge initiation of carvedilol in patients hospitalized for decompensated heart failure: results of the Initiation Management Predischarge: Process for Assessment of Carvedilol Therapy in Heart Failure (IMPACT-HF) trial. *J Am Coll Cardiol* 2004;43:1534.
204. Gattis W. Metoprolol CR/XL in the treatment of chronic heart failure. *Pharmacotherapy* 2001;21:604.
205. Tangeman H, Patterson JH. Extended-release metoprolol succinate in chronic heart failure. *Ann Pharmacother* 2003;37:701.
206. Waagstein F et al. for the Metoprolol in Dilated Cardiomyopathy (MDC) Trial Study Group. Beneficial effects of metoprolol in idiopathic dilated cardiomyopathy. *Lancet* 1993;342:1441.
207. Merit HF Study Group. Effect of metoprolol CR/XL in chronic heart failure: metoprolol CR/XL randomized intervention trial in congestive heart failure (MERIT HF). *Lancet* 1999;353:2001.
208. CIBIS Investigators and Committees. A randomized trial of β-blockade in heart failure: the cardiac insufficiency bisoprolol study. *Circulation* 1994;90:1765.
209. CIBIS II Investigators and Committees. The cardiac insufficiency bisoprolol study II: a randomized trial. *Lancet* 1999;353:9.
210. Waagstein F et al. Long term beta-blockade in dilated cardiomyopathy: effects of short- and long-term metoprolol treatment followed by withdrawal and readministration of metoprolol. *Circulation* 1989;80:551.
211. Bleske B et al. Carvedilol: therapeutic application and practice guidelines. *Pharmacotherapy* 1998;18:729.
212. Packer M et al. , for the US Carvedilol Heart Failure Study Group. The effect of carvedilol on morbidity and mortality in patients with chronic heart failure. *N Engl J Med* 1996;334:1349.
213. Bristow MR et al. , for the MOCHA Investigators. Carvedilol produces dose related improvements in left ventricular function and survival in subjects with chronic heart failure. *Circulation* 1996;94:2807.
214. Packer M et al. For the PRECISE Group. Double-blind, placebo-controlled study of the effects of carvedilol in patients with moderate to severe heart failure. *Circulation* 1996;94:2793.
215. Colucci WS et al. For the US Carvedilol Heart Failure Study Group. Carvedilol inhibits clinical progression in patients with mild symptoms of heart failure. *Circulation* 1996;94:2800.
216. Conn J et al. For the US Carvedilol Heart Failure Study Group. Safety and efficacy of carvedilol in heart failure. *J Card Fail* 1997;3:173.
217. Australia/New Zealand Heart Failure Research Collaborative Group. Randomised, placebo controlled trial of carvedilol in patients with congestive heart failure due to ischemic heart disease. *Lancet* 1997;349:375.
218. Meadowcroft A et al. Pharmacogenetics and heart failure: a convergence with carvedilol. *Pharmacotherapy* 1997;17:637.
219. Kukin ML et al. Prospective randomized comparison of effect of long-term treatment with metoprolol or carvedilol on symptoms, exercise, ejection fraction, and oxidative stress in heart failure. *Circulation* 1999;99:2645.
220. Di Lenarda A et al. Long-term effects of carvedilol in idiopathic dilated cardiomyopathy with persistent left ventricular dysfunction despite chronic metoprolol. *J Am Coll Cardiol* 1999;33:1926.
221. Packer M et al. Comparative effects of carvedilol and metoprolol on left ventricular ejection fraction: results of a meta-analysis. *Am Heart J* 2001;141:899.
222. Poole-Wilson PA et al. Comparison of carvedilol and metoprolol in clinical outcomes in patients with chronic heart failure in the Carvedilol or Metoprolol European Trial (COMET). *Lancet* 2003;362:7.
223. Metra R et al. A prospective, randomized, double blind comparison of the long-term effects of metoprolol versus carvedilol. *Circulation* 2000;102:546.
224. Packer M et al. , for the Carvedilol Prospective Randomized Cumulative Survival Study Group (COPERNICUS). Effect of carvedilol on survival in chronic severe heart failure. *N Engl J Med* 2001;344:1651.
225. BEST Investigators. A trial of the beta-blocker bucindolol in patients with advanced chronic heart failure. *N Engl J Med* 2001;344:1659.
226. Macdonald P et al. Tolerability and efficacy of carvedilol in patients with New York Heart Association class IV heart failure. *J Am Coll Cardiol* 1999;33:924.
227. Krum H et al. Effects of initiating carvedilol in patients with severe chronic heart failure: results from the COPERNICUS Study. *JAMA* 2003;289:712.
228. Levy D et al. Long term trends in the incidence of and survival with heart failure. *N Engl J Med* 2002;347:1397.
229. Rathorne S et al. Sex-based differences in the effect of digoxin for the treatment of heart failure. *N Engl J Med* 2002;347:1403.
230. Rathore S et al. Association of serum digoxin concentration and outcomes in patients with heart failure. *JAMA* 2003;289:871.
231. Hall P et al. The effect of everyday exercise on steady state digoxin concentrations. *J Clin Pharmacol* 1989;29:1083.
232. Teague AC et al. The effect of age and everyday exercise on steady-state plasma digoxin concentrations. *Pharmacotherapy* 1995;15:502.
233. Karbosk J et al. Marked digoxin-like immunoreactive factor interference with an enzyme immunoassay. *Drug Intelligence and Clinical Pharmacy* 1988;22:703.
234. Toseland P et al. Tentative identification of the digoxin-like immunoreactive substance. *Ther Drug Monit* 1988;10:168.
235. Schrader B et al. Digoxin like immunoreactive substances in renal transplant patients. *J Clin Pharmacol* 1991;313:1126.
236. Dasgupta A. Therapeutic drug monitoring of digoxin. *Toxicol Rev* 2006;25:273.
237. Hall WHC et al. Titrated digoxin XXII. Absorption and excretion in malabsorption syndrome. *Am J Med* 1974;56:437.
238. Luchi RJ et al. Unusually large digitalis requirements: a study of altered digoxin metabolism. *Am J Med* 1968;37:263.
239. Hooymans P, Merkus F. Current status of cardiac glycoside drug interactions. *Clinical Pharmacy* 1985;4:404.
240. Fitchtl B, Doering W. The quinidine-digoxin interaction in perspective. *Clin Pharmacokinet* 1983;8:137.
241. Bigger JT, Leahy E. Quinidine and digoxin: an important interaction. *Drugs* 1982;24:229.
242. Fenster P et al. Digoxin-quinidine interaction in patients with chronic renal failure. *Circulation* 1982;66:1277.
243. Doering W et al. Quinidine-digoxin interaction: evidence for involvement of an extra-renal mechanism. Eur *J Clin Pharmacol* 1982;21:281.
244. Mardel A et al. Quinidine enhances digitalis toxicity at therapeutic serum digoxin levels. *Clin Pharmacol Ther* 1993;53:457.
245. Stevenson WG et al. Improving survival for patients with advanced heart failure. *J Am Coll Cardiol* 1995;26:1417.
246. Matsuda M et al. Effects of digoxin, propranolol and verapamil on exercise in patients with chronic isolated atrial fibrillation. *Cardiovasc Res* 1991; 25:453.
247. David D et al. Inefficacy of digitalis in the control of heart rate in patients with chronic atrial fibrillation: beneficial effects of an added beta-adrenergic blocking agent. *Am J Cardiol* 1979;44:1378.
248. Farshi R et al. Ventricular rate control in chronic atrial fibrillation during daily activity and programmed exercise: a crossover open-label study of five drug regimens. *J Am Coll Cardiol* 1999;33:304.
249. Nolan P et al. Effects of co-administration of propafenone on the pharmacokinetics of digoxin in healthy volunteer subjects. *J Clin Pharmacol* 1989;29:46.
250. Rodin S, Johnson B. Pharmacokinetic interactions with digoxin. *Clin Pharmacokinet* 1988;11:227.
251. Boyd RA et al. Atorvastatin coadministration may increase digoxin concentrations by inhibition of intestinal P-glycoprotein-mediated secretion. *J Clin Pharmacol* 2000;40:91.
252. Verschraagen M et al. P-glycoprotein system as a determinant of drug interactions. The case of digoxin-verapamil. *Pharmacol Res* 1999;40:301.
253. Tanaka H et al. Effect of clarithromycin on steady-state digoxin concentrations. *Ann Pharmacother* 2003;37:178.
254. Wakasugi H et al. Effect of clarithromycin on renal excretion of digoxin: interaction with P-glycoprotein. *Clin Pharmacol Ther* 1998;64:123.
255. Greiner B et al. The role of intestinal P-glycoprotein in the interaction of digoxin and rifampin. *J Clin Invest* 1999;104:147.
256. Johne A et al. Pharmacokinetic interaction of digoxin with an herbal extract from St. John's wort (Hypericum perforatum). *Clin Pharmacol Ther* 1999;66:338.
257. Kelly R, Smith T. Recognition and management of digitalis toxicity. *Am J Cardiol* 1992;69:108G.
258. Bernabei R et al. Digoxin serum concentration measurements in patients with suspected digitalis arrhythmias. *J Cardiovasc Pharmacol* 1980;2:319.
259. Relsdorff E et al. Acute digitalis poisoning: the role of intravenous magnesium sulfate. *J Emerg Med* 1986;4:463.
260. Lely AH et al. Non-cardiac symptoms of digitalis intoxication. *Am Heart J* 1972;83:149.
261. Butler V et al. Digitalis induced visual disturbances with therapeutic digitalis concentrations. *Ann Intern Med* 1995;123:675.
262. Beller GA et al. Digitalis intoxication: a prospective clinical study with serum level correlations. *N Engl J Med* 1971;284:989.
263. Lee T, Smith T. Serum digoxin concentration and diagnosis of digitalis toxicity. *Clin Pharmacokinet* 1983;8:279.
264. Park G et al. Digoxin toxicity in patients with high serum digoxin concentrations. *Am J Med Sci* 1987;30:423.
265. Shapiro W. Correlative studies of serum digitalis levels and the arrhythmias of digitalis intoxication. *Am J Cardiol* 1978;41:852.
266. Ordog G et al. Serum digoxin levels and mortality in 5100 patients. *Ann Emerg Med* 1987;16:32.
267. Jelliffe RW. Factors to consider in planning digoxin therapy. *J Chronic Dis* 1971;24:407.
268. Brater C et al. Digoxin toxicity in patients with normokalemic potassium depletion. *Clin Pharmacol Ther* 1977;22:21.
269. Young IS. Magnesium status and digoxin toxicity. *Br J Clin Pharmacol* 1991;32:717.
270. Bendayan R, McKenzie M. Digoxin pharmacokinetics and dosage requirements in pediatric patients. *Clinical Pharmacy* 1983;2:224.
271. Marbury T et al. Advanced digoxin toxicity in renal failure; treatment with charcoal hemoperfusion. *South Med J* 1979;72:279.
272. Antman E. Treatment of 150 cases of life threatening digitalis toxicity. *Circulation* 1990;81:1744.
273. Woolf A et al. The use of digoxin-specific Fab fragments for severe digitalis intoxication in children. *N Engl J Med* 1992;326:1739.
274. Borron S et al. Advances in the management of digoxin toxicity in the older patient. *Drugs Aging* 1997;10:18.
275. Ujhelyi MR, Robert S. Pharmacokinetic aspects of digoxin-specific FAB therapy in the management of digitalis toxicity. *Clin Pharmacokinet* 1995;28: 483.
276. Ujhelyi MR et al. Influence of digoxin immune Fab therapy and renal dysfunction on the disposition of total and free digoxin. *Ann Intern Med* 1993;119:273.
277. Hickey AR et al. Digoxin immune Fab in the

management of digitalis intoxication: safety and efficacy results of an observational surveillance study. *J Am Coll Cardiol* 1991;17:590.
278. Nohria A et al. Medical management of advanced heart failure. *JAMA* 2002;287:628.
279. Grady KL et al. Team management of patients with heart failure: a statement for healthcare professionals from the Cardiovascular Nursing Council of the American Heart Association. *Circulation* 2000;102:2443.
280. Stevenson LW et al. Optimizing therapy for complex or refractory heart failure: a management algorithm. *Am Heart J* 1998;135(Suppl):S293.
281. Stevenson LW et al. The limited reliability of physical signs for estimating hemodynamics in chronic heart. *JAMA* 1989;261:884.
282. Cuffe M et al. Short term intravenous milrinone for acute exacerbations of chronic heart failure: a randomized controlled trial. *JAMA* 2002;287: 1541.
283. Felker G et al. Heart failure etiology and response to milrinone in decompensated heart failure. Results from the OPTIME-CHF study. *J Am Coll Cardiol* 2003;41:997.
284. Sackner-Bernstein JD, Skopicki HA, Aaronson KD. Risk of worsening renal function with nesiritide in patients with acutely decompensated heart failure. *Circulation* 2005;111:1487.
285. Sackner-Bernstein JD et al. Short-term risk of death after treatment with nesiritide for decompensated heart failure: a pooled analysis of randomized controlled trials. *JAMA* 2005;293:1900.
286. Publication committee for the VMAC investigators (vasodilatation in the management of acute CHF). Intravenous nesiritide vs nitroglycerin for treatment of decompensated congestive heart failure: a randomized controlled trial. *JAMA* 2002;287: 1531.
287. Yancy CW et al. Safety and feasibility of using serial infusions of nesiritide for heart failure in an outpatient setting (from the Fusion I Trial). *Am J Cardiol* 2004;94:595.
288. Yancy CW et al. Results of the follow-up serial infusions of nesiritide for the management of patients with [advanced] heart failure (Fusion II) trial. American College of Cardiology 2007; March 25,2007; New Orleans, Louisiana, Late Breaking Clinical Trials, 56th Annual Scientific Session.
289. Scios. Scios announces international outcomes trial of NATRECOR (nesiritide) [press release]. June 1, 2006. Available at: http://www.sciosinc.com/scios/pr_1149131419.
290. Hillerman D, Forbes W. Role of milrinone in the management of congestive heart failure. Drug Intelligence and Clinical Pharmacy, *Ann Pharmacother* 1989;23:357.
291. DiBianco R et al. A comparison of oral milrinone, digoxin and their combination in the treatment of patients with chronic heart failure. *N Engl J Med* 1989;320:677.
292. Packer M et al. (PROMISE study research group). Effect of milrinone on mortality in severe chronic heart failure. *N Engl J Med* 1991;325:1468.
293. Yamani MH et al. Comparison of dobutamine-based and milrinone-based therapy for advanced decompensated congestive heart failure: hemodynamic efficacy, clinical outcome, and economic impact. *Am Heart J* 2001;142:998
294. Cesario D et al. Beneficial effects of intermittent home administration of the inotrope/vasodilator milrinone in patients with end-stage congestive heart failure: a preliminary study. *Am Heart J* 1998;135:121.
295. Elis A et al. Intermittent dobutamine treatment in patients with chronic refractory heart failure: a randomized, double-blind, placebo-controlled study. *Clin Pharmacol Ther* 1998;63:682.
296. Applefeld NM et al. Outpatient dobutamine and dopamine infusions in the management of chronic heart failure: clinical experience in 21 patients. *Am Heart J* 1987;114:589.
297. Marius-Nunez AL et al. Intermittent inotropic therapy in an outpatient setting: a cost-effective therapeutic modality in patients with refractory heart failure. *Am Heart J* 1996;132:805.
298. Leier CV et al. Parenteral inotropic support for advanced congestive heart failure. *Prog Cardiovasc Dis* 1998;41:207.
299. Mulrowe J, Crawford M. Clinical pharmacokinetics and therapeutic use of hydralazine in congestive heart failure. *Clin Pharmacokinet* 1989;16:86.
300. Roth A et al. Early tolerance to hemodynamic effects of high dose transdermal nitroglycerin in responders with severe chronic heart failure. *J Am Coll Cardiol* 1987;9:858.
301. Jordan RA et al. Rapidly developing tolerance to transdermal nitroglycerin in congestive heart failure. *Ann Intern Med* 1986;104:295.
302. Earle G et al. Intravenous nitroglycerin tolerance in patients with ischemic cardiomyopathy and congestive heart failure. *Pharmacotherapy* 1998;18:203.
303. Kalus J, Nappi J. Role of race in the pharmacotherapy of heart failure. *Ann Pharmacother* 2002;36:471.
304. Carson P et al. Racial differences in response to therapy for heart failure: analysis of the Vasodilator-Heart Failure Trials. *J Card Fail* 1999;5:178.
305. Shekelle P et al. Efficacy of angiotensin-converting enzyme inhibitors and beta-blockers in the management of left ventricular systolic dysfunction according to race, gender and diabetic status: a meta-analysis of major clinical trials. *J Am Coll Cardiol* 2003;41:1529.
306. Yancy C et al. Race and the response to adrenergic blockade with carvedilol in patients with chronic heart failure. *N Engl J Med* 2001;344:1358.
307. Aurigemma GP et al. Diastolic heart failure. *N Engl J Med* 2004;351:1097.
308. Cleland JG et al. The Perindopril in elderly people with Chronic Heart Failure (PEP-CHF) Study. *Eur Heart J* 2006;27:2338.
309. Flather MD et al. Randomized trial to determine the effect of nebivolol on mortality and cardiovascular hospital admission in elderly patients with heart failure (SENIORS). *Eur Heart J* 2005;26:215.
310. Reicher-Reiss H, Barasch E. Calcium antagonists in patients with heart failure, a review. *Drugs* 1991;42:343.
311. Elkayam U et al. Differences in hemodynamic response to vasodilators due to calcium channel antagonism with nifedipine and direct acting antagonism with hydralazine in chronic refractory congestive heart failure. *Am J Cardiol* 1984;54: 126.
312. Elkayam U et al. A prospective randomized, double-blind crossover study to compare the efficacy and safety of chronic nifedipine therapy with that of isosorbide dinitrate and their combination in the treatment of chronic congestive heart failure. *Circulation* 1990;82:1954.
313. Amiodarone Trials Meta-Analysis Investigators. Effect of prophylactic amiodarone on mortality after acute myocardial infarction and in congestive heart failure: a meta-analysis of individual data from 6500 patients in randomized trials. *Lancet* 1997;350:1417.
314. Doval CH et al. Randomized trial of low-dose amiodarone in severe congestive heart failure. Eurupo de Estudio de la Sobreivida en la Insuficiencia Cardiaca en Argentina (GESICA) *Lancet* 1994;344:493.
315. Singh S et al. Amiodarone in patients with congestive heart failure and asymptomatic ventricular arrhythmia. *N Engl J Med* 1995;333:77.
316. Massie B et al., For the CHF-STAT investigators. Effect of amiodarone on clinical status and left ventricular function in patients with congestive heart failure. *Circulation* 1996;93:2128.
317. Bardy GH et al. Sudden Cardiac Death in Heart failure Trial(SCD-HeFT) investigators. Amiodarone or an implantable cardioverter-defibrillator for congestive heart failure. *N Engl J Med.* 2005;352:225.
318. Jarcho JA. Resynchronizing ventricular contraction in heart failure. *N Engl J Med* 2005;352:1594.
319. Bristow MR et al. Cardiac-resynchronization therapy with or without an implantable defibrillator in advanced chronic heart failure. *N Engl J Med* 2004;350:2140.
320. Cleland JGF et al. The effect of cardiac resynchronization on morbidity and mortality in heart failure. *N Engl J Med.* 2005;352:1539.
321. McAlister FA et al. Cardiac resynchronization therapy for patients with left ventricle systolic dysfunction. *JAMA* 2007;297:2502.
322. De Smet P. Herbal remedies. *N Engl J Med* 2002;347:2046.
323. American Botanical Council. Hawthorn leaf with flower. Excerpted from Herbal Medicine: Expanded Commission E Monographs. 2000. http://www.herbalgram.org/).
324. Pittler MH et al. Hawthorn extract for treating chronic heart failure: meta-analysis of randomized trials. *Am J Med* 2003;114:665.
325. Tauchert M. Efficacy and safety of crataegus extract WS 1442 in comparison with placebo in patients with chronic stable New York Heart Association class III heart failure. *Am Heart J* 2002;143:910.
326. Holubarsch CJF, Colucci WS, Meinertz T et al. Crataegus extract WS 1442 postpones cardiac death in patients with congestive heart failure class NYHA II–III: A randomized, placebo-controlled, double-blind trial in 2681 patients. American College of Cardiology 2007 Scientific Sessions March 27, 2007; New Orleans, LA. Late breaking clinical trials-3, Session 414–415
327. Tran MT et al. Role of coenzyme Q_{10} in chronic heart failure, angina, and hypertension. *Pharmacotherapy* 2001;21:797.
328. Pepping J. Alternative therapies: coenzyme Q. *Am J Health Syst Pharm* 1999;56:519.
329. Guven H et al. Age related digoxin alprazolam interaction. *Clin Pharmacol Ther* 1993;54:42.
330. Sachs M et al. Interaction of itraconazole and digoxin. *Clin Infect Dis* 1993;16:400.
331. Cohen AF et al. Effect of omeprazole on digoxin bioavailability [Abstract]. *Br J Clin Pharmacol* 1991;31:656P.
332. Oosterhuis B et al. Minor effect of multiple dose omeprazole in the pharmacokinetics of digoxin after a single oral dose. *Br J Clin Pharmacol* 1991;32:569.
333. Stangier J et al. The effects of telmisartan on the steady-state pharmacokinetics of digoxin in 12 healthy male volunteers. *J Clin Pharmacol* 2000;40:1373.
334. Soloman SD et al. Effect of angiotensin receptor blockade and antihypertensive drugs on diastolic function in patients with hypertension and diastolic dysfunction: a randomized trial. *JAMA* 2007;297:1883.
335. ISIS Collaborative Group. ISIS-4: randomized study of oral captoril in over 50,000 patients with suspected acute myocardial infarction. *Circulation* 1993;88(Suppl 1):I-394.
336. Ambrosion E, Borghi C, Magnani B. The effect of the angiotensin-converting-enzyme inhibitor zofenopril on mortality and morbidity after interior myocardial infarction *N Engl J Med* 1995;332:80.
337. Gruppo Italiano per lo studio della sopra vivenza nell infarto mio-cardico. GISSI-3: effects of lisinopril and transdermal glyceryl (rinitrate singly and together on 6-week mortality and ventricular function after acute myocardial infarction) *Lancet* 1994;343:115.

CHAPTER 19

Cardiac Arrhythmias

C. Michael White, Jessica C. Song, James S. Kalus

Adequate blood pumping depends on a continuous, well-coordinated electrical activity within the heart. This chapter reviews and discusses cardiac electrophysiology, arrhythmogenesis, common arrhythmias, and antiarrhythmic treatment.

Electrophysiology

Cellular Electrophysiology

An electrical potential exists across the cell membrane that changes in a cyclic manner related to the flux of ions across the cell membrane, principally K^+, Na^+, and Ca^{2+}. If the change in the membrane potential is plotted against time in a given cycle of a His-Purkinje fiber, a typical action potential results (Fig. 19-1).

The action potential can be described in five phases. Phase 0 is related to ventricular depolarization resulting from sodium entry into the cell through fast sodium channels. On a surface electrocardiogram (ECG), phase 0 is represented by the QRS complex. Phase 1 is the overshoot phase where calcium enters the cell and contraction occurs. During phase 2, the plateau phase, inward depolarizing currents through slow sodium and calcium channels are counterbalanced by outward repolarizing potassium currents. Phase 3 constitutes repolarization, which on an ECG is represented by the T wave. During phase 4, sodium moves out of the cell and potassium moves into the cell via an active pumping mechanism. During this phase, the action potential remains flat in some cells (e.g., ventricular muscle) and does not change until it receives an impulse from above. In other cells (e.g., sinoatrial [SA] node), the cell slowly depolarizes until it reaches the threshold potential and again spontaneously depolarizes (phase 0). The shape of the action potential depends on the location of the cell (Fig. 19-1). In both

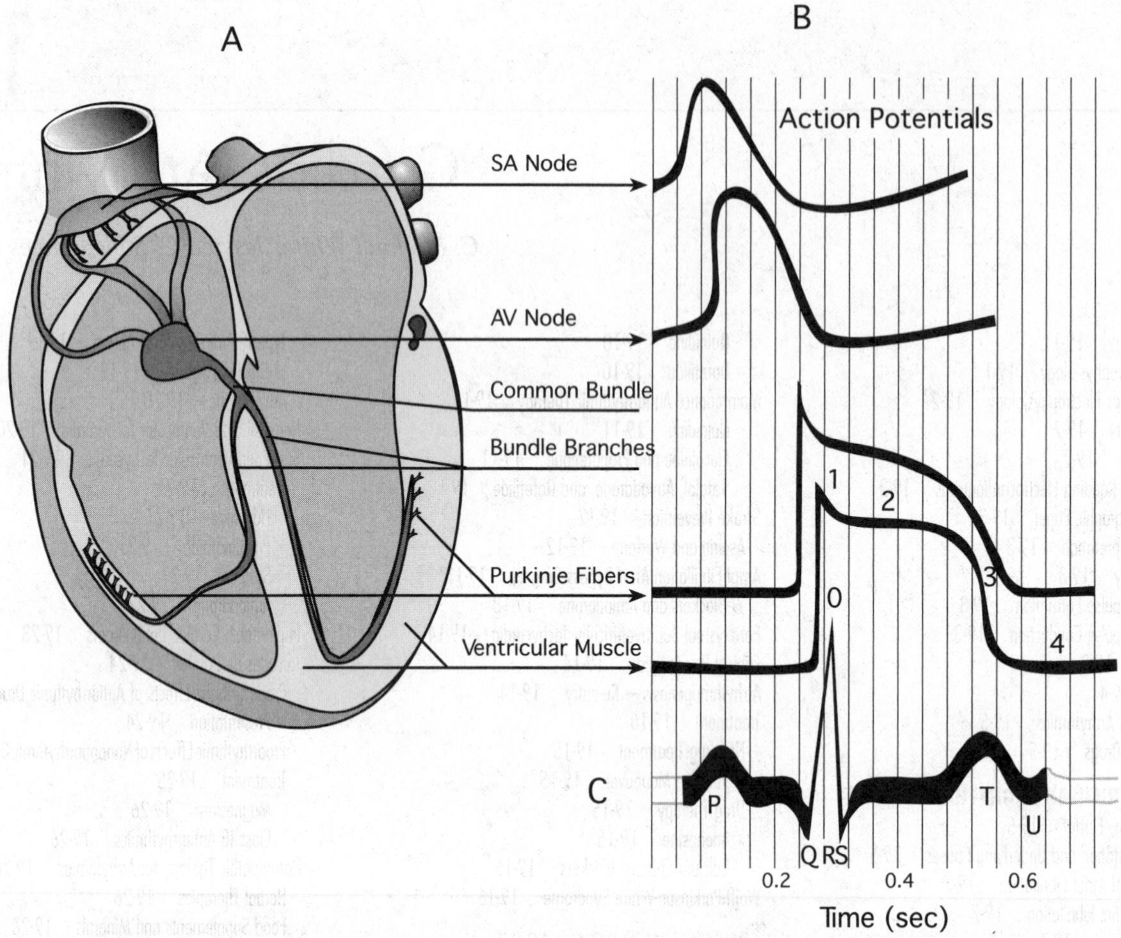

FIGURE 19-1 The cardiac conduction system. **A:** Cardiac conduction system anatomy. **B:** Action potentials of specific cardiac cells. **C:** Relationship of surface electrocardiogram to the action potential. SA, sinoatrial; AV, atrioventricular.

the SA and atrioventricular (AV) nodes, the cells are more dependent on calcium influx than sodium influx, resulting in a less negative resting membrane potential, a slow rise of phase 0, and the capability of spontaneous (automatic) phase 4 depolarization (Fig. 19-1).

The upward slope of phase 0, referred to as V_{max}, is related to the conduction velocity. The steeper the slope, the more rapid is the rate of depolarization. Another influence on V_{max} is the point at which depolarization occurs. The less negative the threshold potential, the slower V_{max} will be, and hence conduction velocity is slowed. Drugs can affect V_{max} and conduction velocity by blocking the fast sodium channels or by making the resting membrane potential less negative (e.g., class I agents).

The action potential duration is the length of time from phase 0 to the end of phase 3. The effective refractory period is the length of time that the cell is refractory and will not propagate another impulse. Both measurements can be obtained from intracardiac recordings of the action potential. Class IA and III agents prolong the refractoriness of the heart.

Normal Cardiac Electrophysiology

Normal cardiac electrical activity begins with automatic impulse generation (automaticity) at the SA node and then normal impulse conduction through the heart.

AUTOMATICITY

Automaticity is the ability of cells (often referred to as pacemaker cells) to depolarize spontaneously. These cells are located in the SA and AV nodes and the His-Purkinje system. The SA node is normally the dominant pacemaker because it reaches the threshold faster than other nodes in a normal heart, resulting in 60 to 100 depolarizations per minute. The innate AV node and Purkinje rate of depolarization is 40 to 60 and 40 depolarizations per minute, respectively. In the healthy heart, the AV node and Purkinje fibers are prevented from spontaneous depolarization (overridden) by the more frequent impulses from the SA node. If the normal conduction system is disrupted (e.g., after a myocardial infarction [MI]), the AV node or Purkinje fibers may temporarily become the dominant pacemaker.

CONDUCTION

An impulse normally originates in the SA node and travels down the specialized intranodal pathways to activate the atrial muscle and the AV node. The AV node holds the impulse briefly before releasing it to the bundle of His. It then travels to the right and left bundle branches and out to the ventricular myocardium via the Purkinje fibers. The ECG tracing consists of a series of complexes that correspond to electrical activity

Table 19-1 Normal Electrophysiological Intervals

Interval	Normal Indices (milliseconds)	Electrical Activity	Measured by
P-R	120–200	Atrial depolarization	Surface ECG
QRS	<140	Ventricular depolarization	Surface ECG
QTc[a]	<400	Ventricular repolarization	Surface ECG
J-T[b]	—	Ventricular repolarization	Surface ECG
A-H[c]	<140	—	Intracardiac lead
H-V[d]	<55	—	Intracardiac lead

[a]QTc interval is the Q-T interval corrected for heart rate. A common method for calculating QTc is the Q-T interval/(R-R interval)$^{1/2}$ (Bazett formula).
[b]J-T interval is obtained by subtracting the QRS interval from the Q-T interval.
[c]A-H interval is the time it takes for an impulse to travel from the sinotrial node to the bundle of his.
[d]H-V interval is the time it takes for an impulse to travel from the bundle of His to the Purkinje fibers.
ECG, electrocardiogram.

in a specific location or anatomic site. By convention, these electrical deflections have been labeled the P wave, QRS complex, and T wave. The P wave represents depolarization of the atria, whereas the QRS complex reflects ventricular depolarization. The T wave reflects repolarization of the ventricles. To evaluate the intact conduction system, conduction intervals at different sites can be obtained. The normal intervals as measured by ECG or intracardiac electrodes are shown in Table 19-1. Drugs and ischemia can alter the conduction and hence the ECG intervals. The effects of antiarrhythmic agents on the ECG are described in Table 19-2.

An Approach to Reading Electrocardiograms

Electrocardiographic Paper

Calculation of the various intervals and widths is facilitated by recording the ECG waveforms on graph paper consisting of large squares defined by heavier lines, which in turn are composed of smaller squares. Each small square is 1 mm long and represents 0.04 seconds. The larger squares are composed of five small squares (5 mm in length) and represent 0.20 seconds (Fig. 19-2).

Table 19-2 Pharmacologic Properties of Antiarrhythmics

Type	Surface ECG: P-R Interval	Surface ECG: QRS Interval	Surface ECG: Q-T Interval	Conduction Velocity	Refractory Period
IA	0/↑	↑	↑↑	↑↓[a]	↑
IB	0	0	0	0/↓	↓
IC	↑	↑↑	↑	↑	0
II	↑↑	0	0	↓[b]	↑[b]
III	0[c]	0	↑↑	0	↑
IV	↑↑	0	0	↓[b]	↑[b]

[a]Conduction increases at low dosages and decreases at higher dosages.
[b]On atrial and atrioventricular nodal tissue.
[c]May cause P-R prolongation independent of class III antiarrhythmic activity.
ECG, electrocardiogram.

Rhythm Interpretation

ECG tracings are evaluated through a systematic review as described:

1. Is the rate fast or slow? A simple method to determine the rate is to count the number of complexes occurring within 6 seconds and multiply by 10. Most ECG recording paper places vertical lines at the top of the grid, 3 seconds apart. Therefore, if eight complexes appear within a 6-second length of strip, the rate is 80 beats/minute.
2. Are there P waves before each QRS complex, and is their configuration normal? Are the P wave–to–P wave and R wave–to–R wave intervals regular or irregular? If the rhythm is irregular, is the pattern of irregularity consistent (regularly irregular) or totally random (irregularly irregular)? P waves appearing before the QRS complex usually indicate that the impulse originated in the SA node and was subsequently conducted to the ventricle. Abnormal-appearing P waves indicate that an atrial site other than the SA node is initiating the beat. Irregular rhythms may be due to an impulse originating from a site other than the SA node before the normal pacemaker can fire (premature beat); they also may result from failure to conduct impulses from the atria.
3. Are the P-R and QRS complexes within normal limits? Is the QRS complex normal in its configuration? Impulses originating above the ventricles with normal conduction through the bundle branches and myocardium produce a normal-appearing, narrow QRS complex. Impulses originating in the ventricle give rise to wide, bizarre-appearing QRS complexes.

Pathophysiology

Abnormal Impulse Formation

Abnormal impulse formation can arise from abnormal automaticity or triggered activity originating from the SA node (e.g., sinus bradycardia) or other sites (e.g., junctional or idioventricular tachycardia). Causes of abnormal automaticity include hypoxia, ischemia, or excess catecholamine activity.

Triggered activity occurs when there is an attempted depolarization before or after the cell is fully repolarized, but not by a pacemaker cell (Fig. 19-3). These after-depolarizations may occur in phase 2 or 3 (early) or phase 4 (delayed) of the action potential. Early after-depolarizations (EADs) arise from a reduced level of membrane potential and may require a bradycardic state. Torsades de pointes (TdP), a form of polymorphic ventricular tachycardia (VT), is believed to be initiated by EADs. Delayed after-depolarizations, often seen with digoxin toxicity, are believed to be secondary to an overload of intracellular free calcium.

Abnormal Impulse Conduction

RE-ENTRY

The most common abnormal conduction leading to arrhythmogenesis is re-entry. A re-entrant circuit is formed as normal conduction occurs down a pathway that bifurcates into two pathways (e.g., AV node or left and right bundle branches). The impulse travels along one pathway (Fig. 19-4, pathway 1) but encounters unidirectional antegrade (forward movement) block in the other pathway (Fig. 19-4, pathway 2). The impulse that passed through the unblocked pathway propagates in a

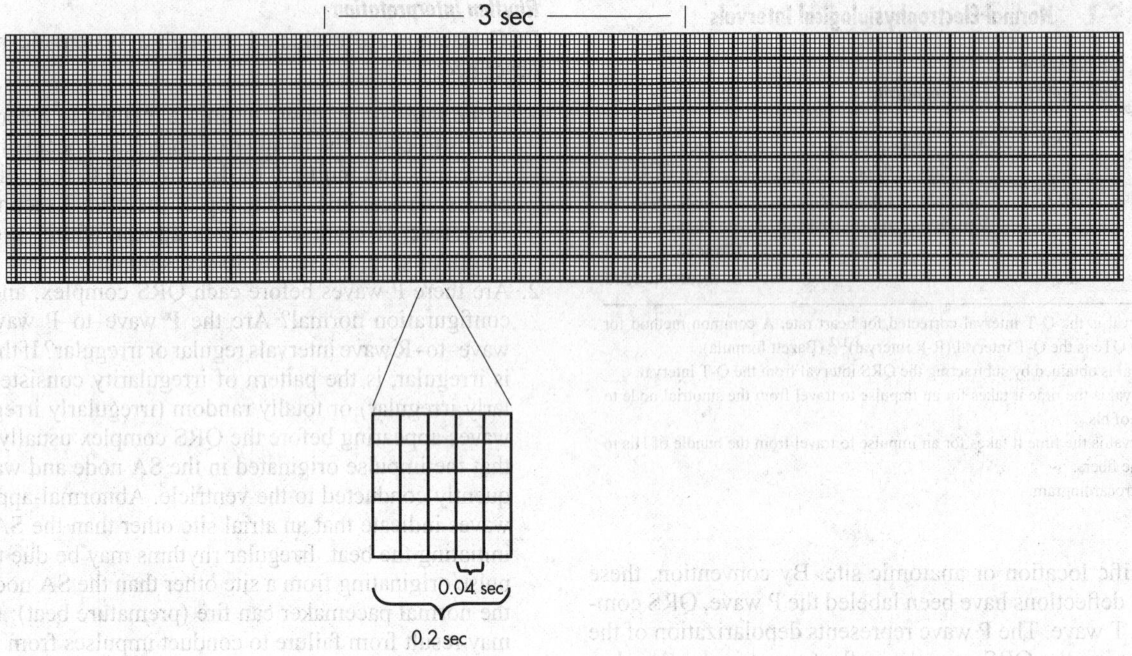

FIGURE 19-2 Electrocardiogram recording paper.

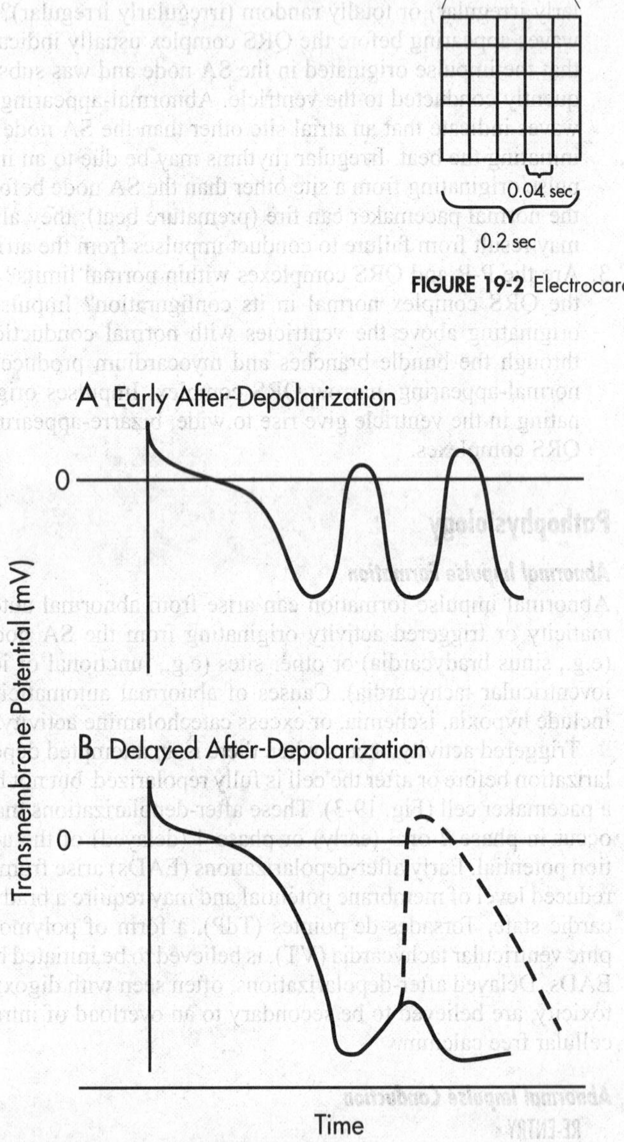

FIGURE 19-3 Triggered activity. **A:** Early after-depolarizations; repolarization is interrupted by secondary depolarization. Such responses may excite neighboring fibers and be propagated. **B:** Delayed after-depolarizations; after full repolarization is achieved, the cell transiently depolarizes. If the delayed after-depolarization reaches threshold, a propagating response can be seen (– – –). *Source:* Reproduced with permission from Bigger JT, Hoffman BF. Antiarrhythmic drugs. In: Goodman AG et al, eds. Goodman and Gilman's The Pharmacologic Basic of Therapeutics. New York: McGraw Hill; 1991:853.

retrograde manner (i.e., moves backward) through the previously blocked pathway. This abnormal impulse can travel down the first pathway again when it is not refractory. Supraventricular and monomorphic VT are both examples of re-entrant arrhythmias (see question 20).

BLOCK

Another form of abnormal impulse conduction occurs when the normal conducting pathway is blocked and the impulse is forced to travel through nonpathway tissues to cause depolarization. Common examples are left bundle branch blocks

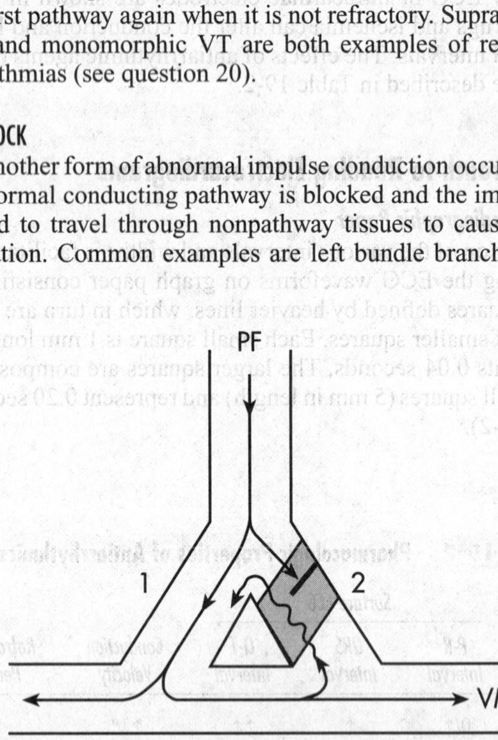

FIGURE 19-4 Re-entrant circuit of the ventricle. A branched Purkinje fiber (PF) terminates on a strip of ventricular muscle (VM). The shaded area in branch 2 represents a depolarized area that is the site of a one-way block; thus, the sinus impulses are blocked in this area, but retrograde impulses are propagated. Retrograde conduction in branch 2 is slow enough for the cells in branch 1 to recover and respond to the re-entry impulse. *Source:* Reproduced with permission from Bigger JT, Hoffman BF. Antiarrhythmic drugs. In: Goodman AG et al, eds. Goodman and Gilman's The Pharmacologic Basic of Therapeutics. New York: McGraw Hill; 1991:853.

(LBBBs) and right bundle branch blocks (RBBBs) in the ventricles. A block in one path necessitates retrograde conduction through the opposite bundle to stimulate both ventricles. Typically, the nonpathway tissue conducts the electrical impulse more slowly than normal conduction tissues.

Classification of Arrhythmias

All arrhythmias originating above the bundle of His are referred to as supraventricular arrhythmias. These may include sinus bradycardia, sinus tachycardia, paroxysmal supraventricular tachycardia, atrial flutter, atrial fibrillation (AF), Wolff-Parkinson-White (WPW) syndrome, and premature atrial contractions (PACs). These arrhythmias are characterized by normal QRS complexes (i.e., normal ventricular depolarization) unless there is a bundle branch block. Not all of these rhythm changes are necessarily a sign of pathology. For example, athletes with a well-conditioned heart and large stroke volume commonly have slow heart rates (sinus bradycardia). Vigorous exercise is commonly accompanied by transient sinus tachycardia.

Arrhythmias originating below the bundle of His are referred to as ventricular arrhythmias. These include premature ventricular contractions (PVCs), VT, and ventricular fibrillation (VF).

Conduction blocks often are categorized separately based on their level or location, which can be a supraventricular site (e.g., first-, second-, or third-degree AV block, see Question 27) or in the ventricle (e.g., RBBB or LBBB). An alternative method of classifying arrhythmias is based on the rate: bradyarrhythmia (<60 beats/minute) or tachyarrhythmia (>100 beats/minute).

Antiarrhythmic Drugs

Based on their electrophysiologic and pharmacologic effects, there are four Vaughn-Williams antiarrhythmic drug classes. Class I drugs, sodium channel blockers, are subdivided further, depending on the duration of channel blockade (class IA is intermediate, IB is quick, and IC is long). Class II drugs are β-adrenergic blockers, class III drugs are potassium channel blockers, and class IV drugs are calcium channel blockers. The classification, pharmacokinetics, and adverse effects of these agents are summarized in Table 19-3.

Class IA and class III antiarrhythmics increase repolarization time, the QTc interval, and the risk of TdP. Class II and IV antiarrhythmics can decrease the heart rate (may cause bradycardia), decrease the force of ventricular contractility (may decrease stroke volume), and prolong the PR interval (may cause second- or third-degree AV block). Class IB antiarrhythmics work only in ventricular tissue, so they cannot be used in AF or atrial flutter. Class IC antiarrhythmic agents are useful, but should never be used after an MI or with heart failure (HF) or severe left ventricular hypertrophy (classified as structural heart diseases) because increased mortality can result. These drugs are discussed in greater detail later.

SUPRAVENTRICULAR ARRHYTHMIAS

The specific arrhythmias include (a) those primarily atrial in origin, such as AF, atrial flutter, paroxysmal sinus tachycardia, ectopic atrial tachycardia, and multifocal atrial tachycardia; and (b) atrioventricular nodal re-entrant tachycardia (AVNRT) and atrioventricular re-entrant tachycardia (AVRT) involving accessory pathways within the atria and/or ventricle. AVNRT and AVRT often self-terminate and are paroxysmal (episodic) in nature; thus, they are commonly referred to as paroxysmal supraventricular tachycardias (PSVTs). The most common supraventricular arrhythmias are AF, atrial flutter, and PSVT.

Atrial Fibrillation/Flutter

AF is characterized by rapid, ineffective writhing of the atrial muscle with a classic "irregularly irregular" ventricular rate. The source of the arrhythmia is one or more ectopic areas (foci) that act as independent pacemakers and fire at such a rate as to suppress normal impulse generation from the SA node. On the ECG, no identifiable P waves are present (Fig. 19-5). In contrast, atrial flutter (Fig. 19-6) is characterized by typical sawtooth atrial waves, at a rate of 280 to 320 beats/minute and a variable ventricular rate, depending on the nature of the AV block present (e.g., 2:1, 3:1, or 4:1 block). In most cases, the ventricular rate is approximately 150 beats/minute. Patients with atrial flutter often progress to AF. The underlying diseases and treatments of atrial flutter and AF are similar. The arrhythmogenic mechanism of AF may be due to multiple re-entrant wavelets, occurring in a paroxysmal, chronic, or acute pattern. The most common presentation is paroxysmal atrial fibrillation (PAF), which can progress to chronic AF; thus, the two overlap. An example of PAF is presented in the following section.

Clinical Manifestation and Underlying Causes

1. J.K., a 66-year-old man, presents with complaints of mild shortness of breath (SOB) and palpitations for the last 2 weeks. He experienced palpitations of shorter duration three times in the last year, but these were not associated with SOB. His medical history includes type II diabetes mellitus for the past 5 years, hypertension, and gout. There is no history of rheumatic heart disease, MI, HF, pulmonary embolism, or thyroid disease. Medications include glyburide (DiaBeta) 5 mg twice a day (BID), hydrochlorothiazide 25 mg/day, and allopurinol (Zyloprim) 300 mg/day. J.K. does not smoke or drink alcohol. Physical examination reveals a blood pressure (BP) of 136/84 mmHg, pulse of 154 beats/minute with an irregularly irregular pattern, respiratory rate (RR) of 16 breaths/minute, and temperature of 98.2°F. He has bilateral rales on chest auscultation. Cardiac examination reveals an irregularly irregular rhythm without murmurs, gallops, or rubs. His jugular vein is distended 4 cm, but no organomegaly is found. His extremities have 1+ pitting edema. The ECG shows AF (Fig. 19-5), and the chest radiograph is compatible with mild HF. A cardiac echocardiogram reveals the atrial size to be <5 cm (normal) and a previously unknown ejection fraction (EF) of 35% (low). In view of his history and previous episodes, J.K. is diagnosed with PAF. Which of J.K.'s other medical problems may predispose him to AF development? What other conditions commonly are associated with AF?

AF is commonly associated with or a manifestation of other diseases or disorders (Table 19-4).[1] When treatable underlying causes are present, they should be corrected because this may resolve the AF. This episode of AF in J.K. could be due to

Table 19-3 Vaughn-Williams Classification of Antiarrhythmic Agents

Drug and Classification	Pharmacokinetics	Indications	Side Effects
Class IA (can cause torsade de pointes similar to class III agents)			
Quinidine sulfate (83% quinidine; SR: Quinidex) Quinidine gluconate (62% quinidine; SR: Quinaglute)	$t_{1/2}$ = 6.2 ± 1.8 hr (affected by age, cirrhosis); Vd = 2.7 L/kg (↓ in HF); liver metabolism, 80%; renal clearance, 20%; Cp = 2–6 mcg/mL, CYP3A4 substrate, CYP2D6 inhibitor, P-glycoprotein inhibitor	AF (conversion or prophylaxis), WPW, PVCs, VT	Diarrhea, hypotension, N/V, cinchonism, fever, thrombocytopenia, proarrhythmia
Procainamide (Pronestyl; Pronestyl SR, Procan SR)	$t_{1/2}$ = 3 ± 0.6 hr; Vd = 1.9 ± 0.3 L/kg; liver metabolism 40%; renal clearance (GFR + possible CTS) 60%; active metabolite (NAPA)[a] Cp = 4–10 mcg/mL	AF (conversion or prophylaxis), WPW, PVCs, VT	Hypotension, fever, agranulocytosis, SLE (joint/muscle pain, rash, pericarditis), headache, proarrhythmia
Disopyramide (Norpace; SR: Norpace CR)	$t_{1/2}$ = 6 ± 1 hr; Vd = 0.59 ± 0.15 L/kg; liver metabolism, 30%; renal clearance, 70%; Cp = 3–6 mcg/mL	AF, WPW, PSVT, PVCs, VT	Anticholinergic (dry mouth, blurred vision, urinary retention), HF, proarrhythmia
Class IB[b] (cannot use to treat atrial arrhythmias)			
Lidocaine (Xylocaine)	$t_{1/2}$ = 1.8 ± 0.4 hr; Vd = 1.1 ± 0.4 L/kg; liver metabolism, 100%; Cp = 1.5–6 mcg/mL	PVCs, VT, VF	Drowsiness, agitation, muscle twitching, seizures, paresthesias, proarrhythmia
Mexiletine (Mexitil)	$t_{1/2}$ = 10.4 ± 2.8 hr; Vd = 9.5 ± 3.4 L/kg; liver metabolism, 35%–80%; Cp = 0.5–2 mcg/mL	PVCs, VT, VF	Drowsiness, agitation, muscle twitching, seizures, paresthesias, proarrhythmia, N/V, diarrhea
Tocainide (Tonocard)	$t_{1/2}$ = 13.5 ± 2.3 hr; Vd = 3 ± 0.2 L/kg; liver metabolism, 60%–65%; Cp = 6–15 mcg/mL	PVCs, VT, VF	Drowsiness, agitation, muscle twitching, seizures, paresthesias, proarrhythmia, N/V, diarrhea, agranulocytosis
Class IC (cannot be used in patients with structural heart disease)			
Flecainide (Tambocor)	$t_{1/2}$ = 12–27 hr; CYP2D6 substrate, 75%; renal clearance, 25%; Cp = 0.4–1 mcg/mL	AF, PSVT, severe ventricular arrhythmias	Dizziness, tremor, lightheadedness, flushing, blurred vision, metallic taste, proarrhythmia
Propafenone (Rythmol)	$t_{1/2}$ = 2 hr (extensive metabolizer); 10 hr (poor metabolizer); Vd = 2.5–4 L/kg, CYP2D6 substrate/inhibitor, P-glycoprotein inhibitor	PAF, WPW, severe ventricular arrhythmias	Dizziness, blurred vision, taste disturbances, nausea, worsening of asthma, proarrhythmia
Moricizine (Ethmozine)	$t_{1/2}$ = 1.3–3.5 hr; Vd >300 L	Severe ventricular arrhythmias	Nausea, dizziness, perioral numbness, euphoria
Class III (can cause torsade de pointes similar to class IA agents)			
Amiodarone (Cordarone)	$t_{1/2}$ = 40–60 days; Vd = 60–100 L/kg; erratic absorption; liver metabolism, 100%; oral F = 50%, Cp = 0.5–2.5 mcg/mL, CYP1A2, 2D6, 2C9, 3A4 inhibitor, P-glycoprotein inhibitor	AF, PAF, PSVT, severe ventricular arrhythmias, VF	Blurred vision, corneal microdeposits, photophobia, skin discoloration, constipation, pulmonary fibrosis, ataxia, hypo/hyperthyroid, hypotension, N/V
Sotalol[c] (Betapace)	$t_{1/2}$ = 10–20 hr; Vd = 1.2–2.4 L/kg; renal clearance, 100%	AF (prophylaxis), PSVT, severe ventricular arrhythmias	Fatigue, dizziness, dyspnea, bradycardia, proarrhythmia
Dofetilide (Tikosyn)	$t_{1/2}$ = 7.5–10 hr; Vd = 3 L/kg; renal elimination, 60% (GFR + CTS), CYP3A4 substrate	AF or atrial flutter conversion and prophylaxis	Chest pain, dizziness, headache, proarrhythmia
Bretylium (Bretylol)	$t_{1/2}$ = 8.9 ± 1.8 hr; Vd = 5.9 ± 0.3 L/kg; renal clearance, 80%–90%	VT, VF	Hypotension, N/V, lightheadedness, dizziness, transitory hypertension, tachycardia
Ibutilide (Corvert)	$t_{1/2}$ = 6 (2–12) hr; Vd = 11 L/kg, Cp = undefined	AF or atrial flutter conversion	Headache, nausea, proarrhythmia

[a] NAPA is 100% renally eliminated and possesses class III antiarrhythmic activity.

[b] Phenytoin is classified as a class IB antiarrhythmic.

[c] Possesses both class II and III antiarrhythmic activity.

AF, atrial fibrillation; AF, atrial flutter; Cp, steady-state plasma concentration; CR, controlled release; CTS, cation tubular secretion; GFR, glomerular filtration rate; HF, heart failure; NAPA, *N*-acetylprocainamide; N/V, nausea and vomiting; PAF, paroxysmal atrial fibrillation; PSVT, paroxysmal supraventricular tachycardia; PVC, premature ventricular contraction; SLE, systemic lupus erythematosus; SR, sustained release; $t_{1/2}$, half-life; Vd, volume of distribution; VF, ventricular fibrillation; VT, ventricular tachycardia; WPW, Wolff-Parkinson-White syndrome.

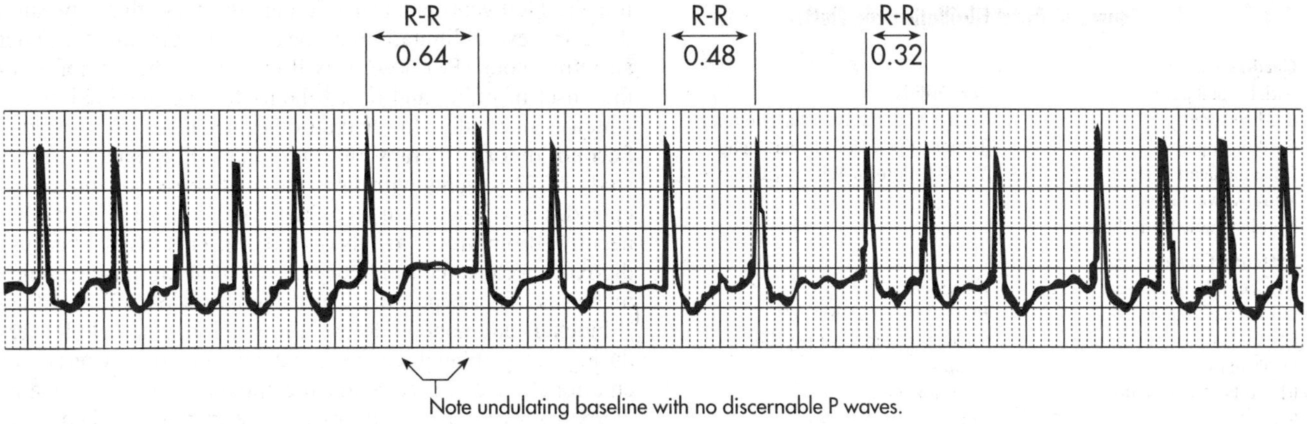

FIGURE 19-5 Atrial fibrillation. Note the irregularly irregular R-R intervals, undulating baseline without definitive P waves, normal width of the QRS complexes, and ventricular rate of 140 beats/minute.

a previously undiagnosed cardiomyopathy (EF = 35%). In a small percentage of patients who do not have underlying heart disease, AF is called "lone" AF, which usually has a more benign course.

Consequences of Atrial Fibrillation

2. What clinical findings demonstrated by J.K. are typically associated with AF? What are the likely consequences of his AF?

The most common complaint in AF, as illustrated by J.K.'s history, is chest palpitations (the sensation of the heart beating rapidly or unusually in the chest). This is a result of the rapid ventricular contraction rate, which typically ranges from 100 to 160 beats/minute. The H-R and R-R interval (time from the R wave in one QRS complex to the R wave in the next complex) is irregularly irregular (random irregularity). During AF, the atrial kick, or the atria's contribution to stroke volume (via the Frank-Starling mechanism), is lost. Because the atrial kick may account for 20% to 30% of the total stroke volume, symptoms of inadequate blood flow such as lightheadedness, dizziness, or reduced exercise tolerance may occur during AF. However, some patients are asymptomatic except for palpitations. Depending on the underlying ventricular function, signs of HF, such as SOB and peripheral edema, may develop, as experienced by J.K. Conversely, AF could have been precipitated by his previously undiagnosed underlying HF.

Patients with AF are at risk for thrombotic stroke.[2] With the chaotic movement of the atria, normal blood flow is disrupted and atrial mural thrombi may form. The risk of stroke increases following restoration of normal sinus rhythm, which allows more efficient cardiac contractility and expulsion of the thrombus. Patients with nonvalvular AF have a fivefold increase in the risk of stroke; this risk increases as patients have an increased number of associated risk factors. Other concurrent diseases that may increase the risk of stroke are HF, cardiomyopathy, thyrotoxicosis, congenital heart disease, and valvular heart disease.

Treatment of Atrial Fibrillation

GOALS OF THERAPY

3. What are the initial therapeutic goals and general approaches used to treat AF in patients like J.K.?

The two initial goals of treatment are to relieve symptoms and reduce the risk of stroke. Slowing the ventricular rate during AF can help accomplish the first goal in most patients; anticoagulation can help achieve the second goal if it is indicated. Cardioversion to normal sinus rhythm can be delayed unless the patient is hemodynamically compromised due to the AF.

VENTRICULAR RATE CONTROL

4. J.K. is given a 1-mg loading dose of digoxin, followed by a 0.25-mg every day (QD) maintenance dose. What is the purpose of administering digoxin? What are the relative advantages and disadvantages of digoxin compared with other agents to control ventricular rate?

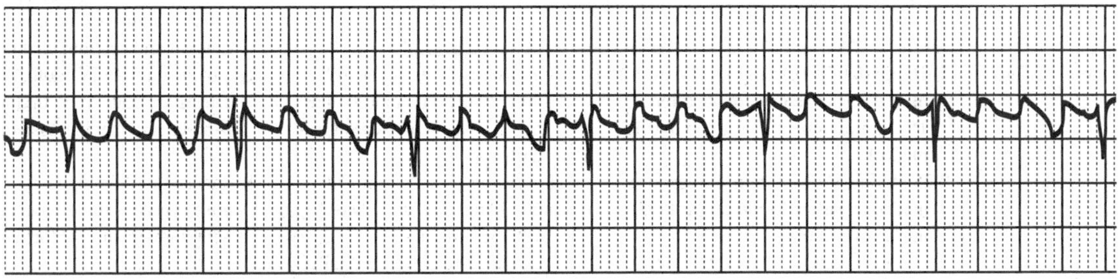

FIGURE 19-6 Atrial flutter. Note the sawtooth appearance of the rhythm strip. *Source:* Reproduced with permission from Stein E. Rapid Analysis of Arrhythmias: A Self-Study Program. 2nd ed. Philadelphia: Lea & Febiger; 1992.

Table 19-4 Causes of Atrial Fibrillation and Flutter

Cardiac Causes	
Atrial septal defect	Pericarditis
Cardiac surgery	Tachycardia-bradycardia syndrome
Cardiomyopathy	Tumors, lipomatous hypertrophy
Ischemic heart disease	Wolff-Parkinson-White syndrome
Mitral valve disease	
Nonrheumatic heart disease	
Systemic Causes	
Alcohol ("holiday heart")	Pneumonia
Cerebrovascular accident	Pulmonary embolism
Chronic pulmonary disease	Sudden emotional or psychological stress
Defibrillation	
Electrolyte abnormalities	Thyrotoxicosis
Fever	Trauma
Hypothermia	

Reproduced with permission from reference 22.

Digoxin

The first treatment goal is to slow the ventricular response rate, which allows better ventricular filling with blood. Table 19-5 displays the agents commonly used to control the ventricular response and provides the loading and maintenance doses. Because of its direct AV node blocking effects and vagomimetic properties, digoxin prolongs the effective refractory period of the AV node and reduces the number of impulses conducted through the AV node (negative dromotropy). Cardioversion to normal sinus rhythm can be delayed unless the patient is hemodynamically compromised due to the AF.

Digoxin should not be regarded as first-line therapy for control of ventricular response rate in AF, except in patients with impaired left ventricular function or HF.[3] First, this is because there are several limitations associated with digoxin use. After an intravenous (IV) dose, it will take more than 2 hours for the onset of effect and 6 to 8 hours for the maximal effect, which is markedly slower than other negative dromotropes.[4] Second, digoxin therapy may prolong AF episodes. In one study of 72 patients with PAF, the relative risk of longer AF episodes associated with digoxin was 4.3 compared with other negative dromotropic agents ($p = 0.01$). This may be because digoxin shortens the refractory period of atrial muscle, which increases AF susceptibility. Third, digoxin is less effective than β-blockers and nondihydropyridine calcium channel blockers during states of heightened sympathetic tone (e.g., exercise or emotional stress), a common precipitant of PAF.[3–6] Finally, digoxin serum concentrations may be increased when combined with P-glycoprotein inhibitors such as verapamil, quinidine, propafenone, flecainide, and amiodarone.[7–10] Normally, P-glycoprotein in the brush border membrane of intestinal enterocytes pumps digoxin into the lumen of the gut and reduces its bioavailability. When digoxin is given with inhibitors, more complete absorption occurs. (See Chapter 18 for further discussion of digoxin and digoxin drug interactions.)

5. What other drugs can be used for ventricular rate control, and what are their relative advantages and disadvantages compared with digoxin?

β-Adrenergic Blocking Agents

β-adrenergic blocking agents are another class of negative dromotropes used in AF. Propranolol, metoprolol, and esmolol are available for IV administration. Each agent rapidly controls the ventricular rate both at rest and during exercise. β-blockers are the first choice in high catecholamine states

Table 19-5 Agents Used for Controlling Ventricular Rate in Supraventricular Tachycardias[a]

Drug	Loading Dose	Usual Maintenance Dose	Comments
Digoxin (Lanoxin)	10–15 mcg/kg LBW up to 1–1.5 mg IV or PO over 24 hr (e.g., 0.5 mg initially, then 0.25 mg Q 6 hr)	*PO:* 0.125–0.5 mg/day; adjust for renal failure (see Chapter 19)	Maximum response may take several hours; use with caution in patients with renal impairment
Esmolol (Brevibloc)	0.5 mg/kg IV over 1 min	50–300 mcg/kg/min continuous infusion with bolus between increases	Hypotension common; effects additive with digoxin and calcium channel blockers
Propranolol (Inderal)	0.5–1.0 mg IV repeated Q 2 min (up to 0.1–0.15 mg/kg)	*IV infusion:* 0.04 mg/kg/min *PO:* 10–120 mg TID	Use with caution in patients with HF or asthma; additive effects seen with digoxin and calcium channel blockers
Metoprolol (Lopressor)	5 mg IV at 1 mg/min	*PO:* 25–100 mg BID	Use with caution in patients with HF or asthma; additive effects seen with digoxin and calcium channel blockers
Verapamil (Isoptin, Calan)	5–10 mg (0.075–0.15 mg/kg) IV over 2 min; if response inadequate after 15–30 min, repeat 10 mg (up to 0.15 mg/kg)	*IV infusion:* 5–10 mg/hr *PO:* 40–120 mg TID or 120–480 mg in sustained-release form daily	Hypotension with IV route; AV blocking effects are additive with digoxin and β-blockers; may increase digoxin levels
Diltiazem (Cardizem)	0.25 mg/kg IV over 2 min; if response inadequate after 15 min, repeat 0.35 mg/kg over 2 min	*IV infusion:* 5–15 mg/hr *PO:* 60–90 mg TID or QID or 180–360 mg in extended-release form daily	Response to IV therapy occurs in 4–5 min; hypotension; effects additive with digoxin and β-blockers

[a] AV nodal ablation is a nonpharmacologic alternative to control the ventricular response, but the effect is permanent and requires chronic ventricular pacing afterward.
AV, atrioventricular; BID; twice a day; HF, heart failure; LBW, lean body weight; PO, orally; IV, intravenously; Q, every; QID, four times a day; TID, three times a day.

such as thyrotoxicosis and postcardiac surgery. However, given their negative inotropic effects, β-blockers should not be used to acutely control the ventricular response in patients with HF. Even though β-blockers are used to treat HF (e.g., bisoprolol, carvedilol, metoprolol), they need to be started at low doses and titrated prudently over several weeks to therapeutic doses[11,12] (see Chapter 18). When trying to achieve rate control, more aggressive dosing may be needed. β-blockers should also be avoided in patients with asthma because of their β_2-blocking properties, and blood sugar levels should be monitored more closely in patients with diabetes mellitus because the signs and symptoms of hypoglycemia (except sweating) can be masked.

Calcium Channel Blockers

Calcium channel blockers are also effective in slowing ventricular rate at rest and during exercise. Both verapamil and diltiazem can be administered IV for a rapid (4–5 minutes) reduction in heart rate.[13] They work through their effect on slow calcium channels within the AV node. Although the duration of action produced by bolus dosing is short, both agents can be administered either as a continuous drip or orally. Given the ability of calcium channel blockers to cause arteriolar dilation, a transient decrease in blood pressure can be expected. IV calcium pretreatment can be used to attenuate the blood pressure decrease among patients with hypotension, near hypotensive blood pressure, or left ventricular dysfunction. Calcium pretreatment does not appear to diminish the negative dromotropic effects of nondihydropyridine calcium channel blockers.[14–16] Verapamil and diltiazem should be used with caution in HF, and verapamil can increase the concentrations of other cardiovascular drugs such as digoxin, dofetilide, simvastatin, and lovastatin.[17] Verapamil and diltiazem are good alternatives to β-blockers in asthmatics.[3]

For chronic therapy, oral negative dromotropes are recommended. A recent study suggests that β-blockers are the most effective rate controlling agents but that many patients require changes from initial therapy before adequate rate control is achieved.[18] If higher-dose monotherapy with one of the negative dromotropes is needed to control symptoms but is associated with intolerable side effects, combining lower-dose digoxin with a β-blocker or calcium channel blocker might be effective.[5,19–21]

J.K. has signs of HF, so digoxin is a reasonable choice. IV verapamil and β-blockers may worsen the signs and symptoms of HF and the β-blockers may mask signs of hypoglycemia in J.K. The goal of rate control should be a resting and an exercising heart rate of <90 and 140 beats/minute, respectively.[21]

LONG-TERM MANAGEMENT STRATEGY

Rate versus Rhythm Control

6. Despite adequate rate control with digoxin (resting heart rate = 75 beats/minute), J.K. still complains of SOB. Would a rhythm or rate control strategy be most appropriate for J.K. at this point?

Several trials have compared rate control to rhythm control as long-term management strategies in AF. The North American Atrial Fibrillation Follow-up Investigation of Rhythm Management (AFFIRM) study was the largest of these. AFFIRM was a randomized, multicenter comparison of rate control and rhythm control, and it enrolled 4,060 patients with AF and a high risk of stroke.[22] The primary end point was all-cause mortality. Antiarrhythmic drugs were chosen at the discretion of the treating physician, but more than 60% of the patients received amiodarone or sotalol as the initial antiarrhythmic agent. Rate control agents included digoxin, β-blockers, and nondihydropyridine calcium channel blockers. After a mean follow-up of 3.5 years, there was a trend toward lower overall mortality ($p = 0.08$), with significant reductions in hospitalizations (10% lower, $p = 0.001$) and TdP (300% lower, $p = 0.007$) in the rate control group. The results of three smaller studies of rate versus rhythm control in AF echo those of AFFIRM.[23–25] Rate control has also been shown to be more favorable from a cost-effectiveness standpoint, and quality of life appears to be the same, regardless of whether a long-term rate or rhythm control strategy is chosen.[26–28]

In conclusion, using rhythm control in patients with AF rather than rate control does not improve outcomes and increases the risk of hospitalizations and TdP. This suggests that a majority of patients can simply be managed with rate control and, if indicated, anticoagulation. However, it should be noted that studies in this area generally included older, less symptomatic patients, and it is unclear whether a rhythm control strategy could be beneficial in younger, highly symptomatic patients.[3]

Conversion to Normal Sinus Rhythm

7. Due to continued bothersome symptoms, J.K. is scheduled for elective cardioversion in 3 weeks. Warfarin treatment is begun, and J.K.'s prothrombin time is to be maintained at an international normalized ratio (INR) of 2 to 3. Why is warfarin therapy being used?

J.K. is to be maintained on warfarin for 3 weeks before cardioversion to prevent the embolization of any atrial clots. These atrial clots form most often in small side pouches on the atria called appendages.[3,29] Because the frequency of right atrial appendage thrombosis is half that of left atrial appendage thrombosis in AF patients, the risk of stroke is enhanced much more than the risk of pulmonary embolism.[29] Studies in patients with AF showed that those who were anticoagulated before cardioversion had a lower incidence (0.8%) of emboli than those who were not anticoagulated (5.3%).[30] Warfarin is recommended during the 3-week period before cardioversion for patients who have been in AF for more than 2 days.[31] The dose should be titrated to produce an INR of 2 to 3. If cardioversion is successful, patients should remain on warfarin for 4 weeks because normal atrial activity/function may not return for up to 3 weeks, and patients may be at risk of late embolization.[32] J.K. has had AF for a minimum of 2 weeks; thus, he should be maintained on warfarin for 3 weeks before he is scheduled for cardioversion.

Cardioversion can be accomplished pharmacologically or with electrical or direct current (DC) cardioversion. DC cardioversion quickly and effectively restores 85% to 90% of patients with AF to normal sinus rhythm.[32] If DC conversion alone is ineffective, it can be repeated in combination with antiarrhythmic drugs.[33] In one study, the success rate of electrical cardioversion was significantly higher in AF patients (duration of AF averaged 119 days) with ibutilide pretreatment (1 mg) compared to those without pretreatment (100% vs. 72%,

$p = 0.001$).[33,34] Other studies have found promising results with class IA antiarrhythmic agents and contradictory data with flecainide. Amiodarone is effective for this purpose, but it may be inconvenient to load patients with amiodarone several days before DC cardioversion.[3]

Although DC cardioversion is highly effective, its use is limited to some degree by the need for general anesthesia (short-acting benzodiazepine, barbiturate, or propofol). Pharmacologic conversion could be used in order to avoid the use of general anesthesia or if a patient wants to avoid DC cardioversion; however, success rates are generally lower with pharmacologic cardioversion than with DC cardioversion. One study suggests that attempting chemical conversion first with ibutilide, with all failures subsequently receiving electrical cardioversion, is more cost effective (saving $138/patient) than using DC cardioversion in all patients.[34] Therefore, many factors must be considered when selecting the optimal method for cardioversion of atrial fibrillation in an individual patient.

Chemical Conversion—Ibutilide, Propafenone, and Flecainide

8. The decision is made to attempt chemical cardioversion with ibutilide. If therapy fails, J.K. will undergo DC cardioversion later in the day. How does ibutilide therapy compare with the other therapeutic choices for chemical cardioversion? What type of patient is likely to remain free of AF recurrence following cardioversion?

Many class I and III antiarrhythmic agents have been evaluated for efficacy in placebo-controlled trials for conversion of AF or atrial flutter to normal sinus rhythm. The best-studied agents include IV ibutilide, oral propafenone, IV or oral flecainide, oral quinidine, oral sotalol, oral and IV amiodarone, and oral dofetilide. This section focuses on ibutilide, propafenone, and flecainide.

IV ibutilide, a class III antiarrhythmic agent with potassium channel–blocking and slow sodium channel–enhancing effects, was the first agent that the U.S. Food and Drug Administration (FDA) approved for the termination of recent onset AF/atrial flutter. Ibutilide is administered as a 1-mg infusion over 10 minutes, followed by another 1-mg infusion over 10 minutes if conversion has not occurred by 10 minutes after the infusion. The conversion rate for recent onset AF is 35% to 50%; the conversion rate is 65% to 80% in atrial flutter. Coadministration of magnesium (1–2.2 g) with ibutilide produced a 20% relative increase in rate of successful conversion.[35]

As is the case with most class III antiarrhythmic agents, the main adverse effect is TdP, which occurred in approximately 4% of patients. Coadministration of ibutilide with magnesium may also reduce the risk for TdP; however, more study is needed in this area.[31] A recent study suggests that the use of ibutilide for acute conversion in patients already taking amiodarone or propafenone does not increase proarrhythmia risk.[36] Aside from the risk of TdP, therapy is well tolerated.[37,38]

Propafenone is a class IC agent with β-blocking properties. When given in doses of 450 to 750 mg orally (600 mg was the most used dose), the initial conversion rate in patients with AF ranged from 41% to 57%. In contrast to ibutilide, no patients experienced ventricular arrhythmias (including TdP), but a risk of hypotension, bradycardia, and QRS prolongation was noted.[39–41]

Oral flecainide is another class IC antiarrhythmic agent. In one study, 300 mg oral flecainide converted 68% of patients to sinus rhythm within 3 hours and 91% of patients by 8 hours. Another study using 2 mg/kg IV flecainide over 10 minutes followed by 200 to 300 mg orally demonstrated a 71% conversion rate. The efficacy in atrial flutter has yet to be established. Sinus node dysfunction; prolongation of intraventricular rhythm; dizziness, weakness, and gastrointestinal (GI) disturbances have been reported.[42,43]

Conversion to and maintenance of normal sinus rhythm is determined by the duration of the arrhythmia, underlying disease processes, and left atrial size. Duration of AF for more than 1 year significantly reduces the chances of maintaining a normal sinus rhythm.[44] When the atrial size exceeds 5 cm, there is a <10% chance of maintaining normal sinus rhythm at 6 months.

J.K.'s chance of being maintained in normal sinus rhythm is good because the duration of his AF is short and the echocardiogram revealed only slight enlargement of his left atrium. Ibutilide is chosen because it has good efficacy and safety, does not interact with digoxin like propafenone can, and is not contraindicated like the class IC agents in patients with heart failure or left ventricular hypertrophy (structural heart disease) like J.K.

Quinidine

9. If an agent like quinidine is used, instead of ibutilide, to convert the patient to normal sinus rhythm, why would it be especially important to attempt ventricular rate control first?

The effects of quinidine and other type IA antiarrhythmic agents on the AV node are bimodal. At low concentrations, AV node conduction may be enhanced by the drug's antivagal properties. If this occurs before normal sinus rhythm is achieved by quinidine, the ventricular rate may actually increase. At higher concentrations, the type IA agents slow AV node conduction. Because it is difficult to predict which effect on the AV node will predominate in a given patient, it is prudent to initiate a rate controlling agent first.

Dofetilide

10. After failing cardioversion with ibutilide, J.K. is converted to normal sinus rhythm using a single 200-J electric shock. He is discharged from the hospital on digoxin and warfarin and advised to follow up with a cardiologist 4 weeks later. Within 2 weeks, J.K. experiences several episodes of brief, symptomatic, and self-terminating palpitations. His physician prescribes oral dofetilide and informs J.K. that he will be admitted to the hospital for the first 3 days of treatment to determine a safe and effective dose. Why is dofetilide unique among the antiarrhythmic drugs used in AF and atrial flutter? What drug interactions limit its use?

Oral dofetilide is a class III antiarrhythmic agent that inhibits the delayed rectifier potassium current (IKr).[45,46] It is the only class III agent indicated for both acute cardioversion of AF/atrial flutter and maintenance of normal sinus rhythm. However, the risk of TdP has prompted its manufacturer to mandate a minimum of 3 days of ECG monitoring in a properly equipped facility during therapy initiation. Two clinical trials, EMERALD (European and Australian Multicenter Evaluative Research on Atrial Fibrillation Dofetilide)[47] and SAFIRE-D (Symptomatic Atrial Fibrillation Investigation and Randomized Evaluation of Dofetilide),[48] have shown AF/atrial flutter patients to have conversion rates of 30% on higher doses of dofetilide. Patients failing chemical conversion received electrical conversion. If this conversion succeeded, they were continued on dofetilide for 1 year. At 1 year, 60% of those converted with the 500-mcg dose were still in sinus rhythm. Also, dofetilide appears to exert neutral effects on mortality rates in HF and post-MI patients.[49,50]

The dofetilide dose is based on the patient's creatinine clearance (Cl_{cr}); the doses are 500, 250, and 125 mcg twice daily with Cl_{cr} above 60 mL/minute, 40 to 60 mL/minute, and 20 to 39 mL/minute, respectively. The QTc interval must be measured (using a 12-lead ECG) 2 to 3 hours after the first dose. If the QTc interval does not increase by >15% or if it does not surpass 500 milliseconds (550 milliseconds in patients with ventricular conduction abnormalities), the QTc interval still needs to be measured 2 to 3 hours after each subsequent dose, but not with a 12-lead ECG. If the QTc interval exceeds the above parameters, the subsequent dose should be reduced by 50%. If the QTc interval measured 2 to 3 hours after the first adjusted dose (using a 12-lead ECG) is still above the acceptable range, dofetilide should be discontinued. If the QTc interval is within an acceptable range following the first adjusted dose, all subsequent postdose QTc intervals do not need to be measured with a 12-lead ECG. All patients must be ECG monitored by at least a single lead for 3 days.[51]

Drug interactions pose a significant problem with dofetilide. Cimetidine, ketoconazole, megestrol, prochlorperazine, and trimethoprim (including in combination with sulfamethoxazole) inhibit active tubular secretion of dofetilide and can elevate dofetilide plasma concentrations.[46,51] Because the incidence of TdP is directly related to dofetilide plasma concentrations, concomitant use with these agents is contraindicated.[51] Concomitant administration of dofetilide with verapamil or hydrochlorothiazide increases the incidence of TdP by an unknown mechanism and is contraindicated as well.[46] Concurrent use of agents that can prolong the QTc interval is not recommended with dofetilide.[51] Dofetilide also undergoes metabolism by the CYP3A4 isoenzyme to a minor extent. Therefore, inhibitors of this isoenzyme (e.g., amiodarone, azole antifungal agents, diltiazem, nefazodone, protease inhibitors, quinine, serotonin reuptake inhibitors, zafirlukast) should be coadministered with caution with dofetilide. Other agents that can potentially increase dofetilide levels (through inhibition of tubular secretion) include amiloride, metformin, and triamterene. Hence, these agents should be cautiously coadministered with dofetilide.[51]

Maintenance Antiarrhythmic Therapy

11. Evaluate the value of using an antiarrhythmic agent to maintain J.K. in normal sinus rhythm. What are the risks and benefits of the different antiarrhythmic agents used for this purpose?

Whether J.K. should be placed on an antiarrhythmic is a judgment of benefit versus risk. There is no doubt that various antiarrhythmics can prevent episodes of AF. However, J.K.'s need for antiarrhythmic therapy should be weighed against the potential for adverse effects. Overall, both rate and rhythm control strategies lead to similar rates of overall mortality, but the risk of hospitalization and TdP and cost is likely higher with rhythm control. Hence, if adequate rate control can eliminate J.K.'s symptoms, that is the preferred strategy. If symptoms are limiting his quality of life or adequate rate control cannot be achieved, rhythm control is a valuable option. In this case, the physician has chosen rhythm control, and there are no compelling reasons to try to persuade him otherwise given the symptomatic nature of the AF episodes. The question now becomes how to choose the best antiarrhythmic agent for J.K. To do this, the efficacy and adverse effect profiles for each agent should be reviewed.

Class IA, IC, and III antiarrhythmics (see Table 19-2 for electrophysiologic and ECG effects and Table 19-3 for pharmacokinetics and side effects) prevent the recurrence of AF. Quinidine, flecainide, sotalol (Betapace AF), and dofetilide are approved by the FDA for maintenance of sinus rhythm; propafenone and amiodarone are commonly used as well.

Quinidine

If quinidine is used, sustained-release (SR) formulations such as quinidine sulfate (Quinidex) or quinidine gluconate (Quinaglute) are preferred because they produce smaller peak-to-trough fluctuations than rapid-release products and can be administered twice daily to enhance compliance. Nausea, vomiting, and diarrhea occurring early in therapy are reported in up to 30% of patients receiving quinidine, requiring 10% to discontinue therapy. A unique symptom complex referred to as cinchonism occurs when quinidine blood levels exceed 5 mcg/mL. This disorder is characterized by disturbed hearing (tinnitus, decreased auditory acuity), visual abnormalities (blurred vision, altered color perception, diplopia), and central nervous system (CNS) alterations (headache, confusion, delirium). Quinidine raises digoxin serum concentrations, which is important in J.K., but it is also a potent inhibitor of the CYP2D6 isoenzyme, which affects the metabolism of carvedilol, codeine, desipramine, and propafenone. HF and older age are additional risk factors that can raise quinidine concentrations, which would be a confounder for J.K. Use of quinidine is limited to third-line therapy for this indication based on a meta-analysis showing improved maintenance of sinus rhythm but nonsignificant increases in mortality (3.2% mortality vs. 0.8%).[52]

Flecainide and Propafenone

The class IC agents flecainide and propafenone are effective in suppressing AF.[53–55] The efficacy rate may be as high as 61% to 92% for flecainide.[56] Flecainide and possibly other class IC agents may cause other arrhythmias, especially in patients with structural heart disease, and they should be avoided in such patients. Propafenone, a class IC agent with β-blocking properties, is as efficacious as flecainide and is relatively safe in patients without ischemic heart disease and an EF above 35%; it may be preferred in patients who require additional AV blockade.[57,58] In comparison with quinidine (average dose 1,067 mg), propafenone (average dose 615 mg) was significantly better at reducing the occurrence of AF and at reducing the ventricular rate when AF occurred. A 75% reduction in symptomatic arrhythmic attacks occurred in 75% of the propafenone group versus 46% of the quinidine group. Both therapies were well tolerated, with 4% of patients in both groups withdrawing. Dizziness was the most common reason for discontinuation in the propafenone group, whereas

GI disturbances were most common in the quinidine group.[59] Propafenone was superior to placebo and sotalol in a study of 254 patients with paroxysmal or persistent AF.[60] In this study, the monthly rate of developing either AF recurrence or an adverse effect was 5.26% with sotalol, 3.13% with propafenone, and 9.19% with placebo. Propafenone was also shown to be superior to amiodarone when both efficacy and adverse effects were considered in another study.[55] Monthly progression to AF recurrence or adverse effects in this study was 3.18% for amiodarone and 3.96% for propafenone.

A novel approach to maintaining sinus rhythm with flecainide and propafenone has been recently reported.[61] In this study, patients with AF and no significant cardiovascular disease self-administered oral propafenone or flecainide on experiencing symptoms of AF recurrence. AF recurrence was experienced on 618 occasions in 165 patients. Patient-initiated therapy was successful in converting 84% of these patients and 7% experienced adverse effects. Use of this strategy (single dose of propafenone or flecainide when AF recurs instead of chronic suppression) also reduced the number of emergency room visits and hospitalizations.

Sotalol, Amiodarone, and Dofetilide

Class III agents (sotalol, dofetilide, and amiodarone) prolong refractoriness in the atria, ventricle, AV node, and accessory pathway tissue, and can prevent recurrence of AF. The efficacy of sotalol in delaying the recurrence of AF was evaluated in a double-blind, placebo-controlled, multicenter, randomized trial that enrolled 253 patients with AF or atrial flutter.[62] The median times to recurrence were 27, 106, 229, and 175 days with placebo, sotalol 160 mg/day (divided in two doses), sotalol 240 mg/day (divided in two doses), and sotalol 320 mg/day (divided in two doses), respectively. In one comparative study, sotalol was as effective as quinidine in maintaining sinus rhythm after cardioversion.[63] The risk of developing TdP with sotalol has prompted its manufacturer to mandate a minimum of 3 days of ECG monitoring in a properly equipped facility during therapy initiation. Furthermore, during initiation and titration, QTc intervals should be monitored 2 to 4 hours after each dose, and sotalol is contraindicated in patients with a Cl_{cr} of less than 40 mL/minute. Bradycardia, dizziness, and GI disturbances are common intolerable side effects of sotalol.[64]

Amiodarone is more effective than quinidine, sotalol, and propafenone.[65–69] The Canadian Trial of Atrial Fibrillation (CTAF) compared the ability of low-dose amiodarone (200 mg/day) versus propafenone (450–600 mg/day) and sotalol (160–320 mg/day) to prevent recurrence of atrial fibrillation in 403 patients with a recent episode of AF (within the preceding 6 months).[67] After a mean follow-up of 16 months, 35% of the amiodarone-treated patients had a recurrence of AF versus 63% in the combined group with sotalol and propafenone ($p = 0.001$). Another more recent study supports the CTAF study results by demonstrating superior efficacy with amiodarone as compared to sotalol and placebo.[68] Low doses of amiodarone (200–400 mg/day) have a high rate of efficacy and a reduced incidence of the serious adverse effects often associated with high doses of this drug.[66] In view of its unusual pharmacokinetics and potential serious adverse effects, however (see Table 19-3 and Questions 30, 36, and 37), amiodarone should be reserved for patients with HF, where it has specific safety data, or when other agents such as sotalol, propafenone, or dofetilide have failed.[3]

Dofetilide is another class III agent that has been shown to be effective for the maintenance of sinus rhythm after conversion and safe in heart failure patients (see question 10 for dosing in renal impairment, critical drug interactions, and monitoring).

In view of J.K.'s new onset of HF and frequent uncomfortable episodes of AF, dofetilide, and amiodarone are logical first choices with proven efficacy and studies in HF patients showing relative safety. Propafenone and flecainide are contraindicated in patients like JK with structural heart disease (heart failure and possible left ventricular hypertrophy due to hypertension).

12. Do any medications without direct effects on cardiac ion channels have a role in maintaining sinus rhythm?

Angiotensin-converting enzyme (ACE) inhibitors, angiotensin receptor blockers (ARBs), and statins may have a potential role in the management of atrial fibrillation. A recent meta-analysis reported that ACE inhibitors or ARBs prevent the development of atrial fibrillation (odds ratio [95% confidence interval (CI)] = 0.51 [0.36–0.72]), prevented failure of DC cardioversion (0.47 [0.24–0.92]), and prevented recurrence of atrial fibrillation after DC cardioversion (0.39 [0.20–0.75]).[70] These agents likely prevent structural remodeling of the atria in patients with or at risk for atrial fibrillation. Therefore, these medications probably prevent the formation of the substrate necessary for atrial fibrillation. Preliminary data suggest that statins may also prevent AF recurrence after DC cardioversion of persistent AF.[71] In this study, 3-month recurrence rate in the control group was 45.8% compared to 12.5% in the statin (atorvastatin) group ($p = 0.02$). The anti-inflammatory properties of atorvastatin were proposed as the reason for less recurrence with statin therapy because C-reactive protein was reduced in the atorvastatin group but not the control group.

13. If J.K. fails trials of multiple antiarrhythmic agents, what nonpharmacologic treatments are available to him for maintenance of sinus rhythm?

A premature stimulus originating from the pulmonary veins is often responsible for initiating atrial fibrillation. As such, a technique in which ablation is used to isolate the pulmonary veins has been developed. At 1 year, this technique prevented AF recurrence in 86% of patients, while antiarrhythmic drugs prevented recurrence in 22% of patients ($p < 0.001$).[72]

Stroke Prevention

ASPIRIN AND WARFARIN

14. J.K. is discharged from the hospital on dofetilide 500 mcg BID, which is appropriate given his Clcr of 92 mL/minute. He has been doing fine for 2 weeks after discharge. Should J.K. remain on warfarin therapy? Should aspirin be added or substituted?

Patients with nonvalvular and valvular AF have a 5- and 17-fold increased risk for stroke compared with patients without AF, respectively.[2] Stroke can lead to death or significant neurologic disability in up to 71% of patients, with an annual recurrence rate as high as 10%.[73] In large, randomized trials, patients with nonvalvular atrial fibrillation benefited from antithrombotic therapy. In the Stroke Prevention in Atrial Fibrillation (SPAF) study, both aspirin 325 mg/day and warfarin (titrated to an INR 2.0–4.5) reduced the risk of stroke significantly with an acceptable level of hemorrhagic complications.[74] In this trial, patients younger than 60 years of age without hypertension, recent heart failure, or prior thromboembolism had a low risk of thromboembolism and did not benefit from warfarin therapy.[74] The results of SPAF II and Copenhagen Atrial Fibrillation, Aspirin and Anticoagulation Trials, both of which were direct comparisons of warfarin and aspirin, indicate that warfarin is more effective than aspirin in preventing stroke.[75,76] Although greater efficacy was derived from warfarin therapy in the SPAF II study, a higher incidence of bleeding complications was noted with warfarin in patients older than 75 years of age, especially those with risk factors for bleeding (previous thromboembolism, GI, or genitourinary bleeding).[75]

Patients younger than 60 years who have "lone" AF should be maintained on aspirin alone because the bleeding risk with warfarin is maintained, but the benefits are reduced in this population. Older patients and those with thromboembolic risk factors should receive warfarin because the benefits of therapy far outweigh the risks, and the patient should maintain an INR of 2.0 to 3.0.[77,78]

A common issue with warfarin therapy is the variability in dosing requirements from patient to patient. Intensive participation in anticoagulation monitoring is necessary to ensure that patients reach a therapeutic range and stay within that range. Recently, a simple blood test has been developed for commercial use called the PGx Predict warfarin test. This test could be used to help predict maintenance warfarin dose requirements by assessment of CYP2C9 genotype and VKORC1 genotype.[79] Certain polymorphisms in CYP2C9 genotype translates into variability in activity of the CYP2C9 enzyme, a principal enzyme in warfarin metabolism. The VKORC1 gene encodes for part of the vitamin K epoxide reductase complex, the target for warfarin therapy. Therefore, VKORC1 genotype polymorphisms lead to variability in sensitivity to the effects of warfarin. Use of this test may become more common in the future and could help simplify the dosing of warfarin in patients with atrial fibrillation.

Because J.K. has a low bleeding risk (no history of thromboembolism, diastolic hypertension, or GI/genitourinary bleeding) and an increased risk of stroke due to his age (66 years), he should continue to receive warfarin therapy without concomitant aspirin. Even though J.K. is in normal sinus rhythm on dofetilide at this time, in the AFFIRM trial, only 73% and 63% of patients remained in sinus rhythm at 3 and 5 years, respectively.[22] These patients did not necessarily know when they went back into AF.

15. M.P. is a 38-year-old woman who has had chronic atrial flutter for the past 2 years. She has no other medical history and is taking metoprolol 50 mg BID. She does not want to take the drug any longer because it reduces her exercise tolerance. Is there a nonpharmacologic therapy for atrial flutter? Does the treatment of atrial flutter differ from the treatment of AF? Is radiofrequency catheter ablation an acceptable nonpharmacologic option for M.P.?

As mentioned previously, atrial flutter is an unstable rhythm that often reverts to sinus rhythm or progresses to AF. If atrial flutter is episodic, its underlying cause should be identified and treated if possible. If a patient remains in atrial flutter, the treatment goals (control of ventricular rate, return to normal sinus rhythm) are the same as those for AF. Similar agents and doses can be used to control the ventricular response. Chemical conversion, low-energy (<50 J) DC cardioversion or rapid atrial pacing may acutely convert atrial flutter back to sinus rhythm, but the recurrence of atrial flutter is high.

Radiofrequency catheter ablation therapy is a nonpharmacologic treatment of atrial flutter. Electrophysiologic studies are performed initially to determine the optimal site for ablation. Various sections of the atria and pulmonary veins (where they intersect with the atria) are probed with a catheter that delivers cardiac pacing. Once an area is stimulated with pacing and an atrial ectopic/re-entrant focus is recognized, the area is ablated. Ablation destroys atrial or pulmonary vein tissue integral to the initiation or maintenance of the atrial flutter by delivering electrical energy over electrodes on the catheter. This procedure is successful in 75% to 90% of cases and can be recommended for patients with atrial flutter who are drug resistant or drug intolerant, or who do not desire long-term therapy.

Radiofrequency ablation therapy may be suitable for M.P. However, if exercise intolerance is her primary complaint, this can be relieved by switching M.P. to another drug such as verapamil.

Atrial Fibrillation After Bypass Surgery

β-BLOCKERS AND AMIODARONE

16. H.L., a 55-year-old woman with triple vessel disease, is scheduled for coronary artery bypass surgery (CABG) in 3 days. Her medical history includes exercise-induced angina treated with nitrates, metoprolol, and diltiazem. What is the incidence of AF after CABG surgery? Should H.L. be treated with a drug to prevent the postoperative occurrence of AF?

More than 750,000 CABG or heart valve surgeries (cardiothoracic surgery) are performed annually in the United States.[80] Without prophylaxis, AF develops in up to 65% of patients, and two-thirds of the cases occur on postoperative day 2 or 3.[81] The underlying mechanism is unknown, but it may be related to sympathetic activation, pericarditis, or atrial dilation from volume overload.[82,83] The arrhythmia usually converts spontaneously but can result in temporary symptomatology (lightheadedness), a higher risk of cerebrovascular accident, and a longer hospital stay.[83]

β-blockers, amiodarone, and sotalol are proven prophylactic strategies to reduce the incidence of postcardiothoracic surgery AF.[83–85] Of these, β-blockers and amiodarone have been shown to reduce other clinical events and shorten length of stay.[80,83–85] In addition, both β-blockers and amiodarone can be used together in the same patient as a prophylactic strategy.[84,85] If a patient is receiving a β-blocker before surgery and cannot receive it after surgery, the risk of postcardiothoracic surgery AF is even higher than if they were never on the β-blocker (due to β-blocker withdrawal). Therefore diligence in trying to assure continued β-blockade in these patients is important.[85]

Although many studies evaluating the use of amiodarone prophylaxis have been conducted, the Atrial Fibrillation Suppression Trial II (AFIST II) had a regimen that allowed for dosing patients with elective and emergent surgery and the beneficial results were in addition to a high baseline utilization of β-blockers.[85] In AFIST II, a hybrid IV and oral amiodarone regimen was evaluated versus placebo. In this study, IV amiodarone (1,050 mg) was given over 24 hours after surgery and then oral drug (400 mg three times daily) was given for 4 postoperative days (equal to 7 g oral drug given over 5 days). In

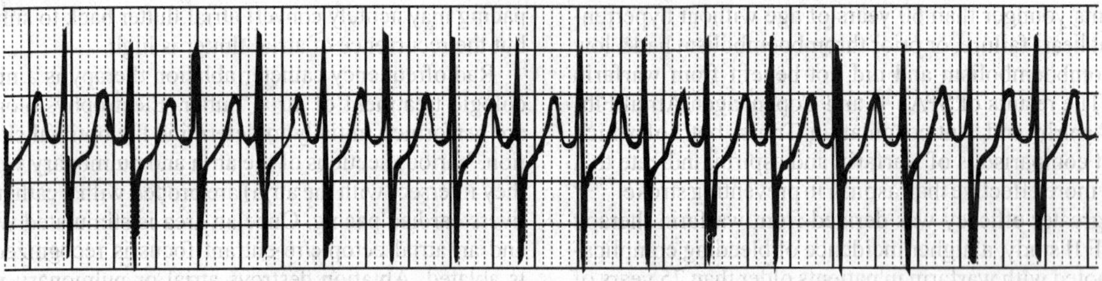

FIGURE 19-7 Supraventricular tachycardia. *Source:* Reproduced with permission from Stein E. Rapid Analysis of Arrhythmias: A Self-Study Program. 2nd ed. Philadelphia: Lea & Febiger; 1992.

this study, amiodarone reduced the 30-day risk of AF by 42.7% and symptomatic AF by 68.3%. Amiodarone regimens using all oral dosing have also been studied and showed similar benefits with similar delivered amiodarone doses.[83,84]

17. H.L.'s metoprolol therapy was discontinued prior to surgery and she was not treated prophylactically. There were no immediate postsurgery complications. On postoperative day 2, she develops AF with a ventricular response rate of 142 beats/minute and a BP of 126/75 mmHg. How should H.L. be managed?

β-blocker withdrawal after surgery is one of the most potent risk factors for developing postcardiac surgery AF. Now that she has AF, the decision to treat H.L.'s AF depends on her heart rate and how well she tolerates the arrhythmia; antiarrhythmics are often not needed in the short-term management of this disorder. For many years, digoxin has been used to control the ventricular response. However, following surgery, patients have a high sympathetic tone, and digoxin is often ineffective. β-blockers are effective and preferred if there are no other contraindications.[86] They are especially preferred in patients such as H.L., who have been taking β-blockers preoperatively because withdrawal of β-blockers can increase the occurrence of postoperative AF.[86,87]

H.L.'s rapid ventricular rate should be controlled. Propranolol 1 mg IV every 5 minutes (up to 0.1 mg/kg), metoprolol 5 mg IV repeated at 2-minute intervals (up to a total dose of 15 mg), esmolol 0.5 mg/kg bolus followed by a continuous infusion at a rate of 50 to 300 mcg/kg/minute, or verapamil 5 to 10 mg IV every 1 to 4 hours are all options for H.L., who appears to be hemodynamically stable. If one of these therapy choices is ineffective, a loading dose of digoxin can be administered IV as adjunctive therapy with a β-blocker or verapamil.

18. Metoprolol is started and ventricular rate control is achieved 4 minutes after administering the second 5-mg dose. The patient receives 50 mg oral metoprolol therapy an hour later, converts to normal sinus rhythm spontaneously the next day, and is prepared for discharge. The metoprolol therapy is discontinued. Should an antiarrhythmic agent be initiated for H.L. to prevent recurrence of AF?

Using prophylactic antiarrhythmic agents after discharge in patients with AF within a few days of CABG surgery does not seem to protect against recurrent AF. In one trial, all patients with AF after CABG surgery were given verapamil, quinidine, amiodarone, or placebo at discharge and were then followed with Holter monitoring for 90 days. There was no difference in the occurrence of AF between the placebo group (3.3% incidence) and the other groups (6.7% incidence for each treatment group).[88] Because H.L. was treated with metoprolol for angina pectoris before the surgery, therapy can be reinitiated if the anginal pain resumes with exercise.

Paroxysmal Supraventricular Tachycardia

Clinical Presentation

19. B.J., a 32-year-old woman, presents to the emergency department (ED) complaining of fatigue and palpitations. She has had similar episodes approximately twice a year for the past 2 years but has not sought medical attention. She is in no apparent distress and has a temperature of 98°F, heart rate of 180–190 beats/minute, BP of 95/60 mmHg, and RR of 12 breaths/minute. Her ECG (Fig. 19-7) shows a heart rate of 185 beats/minute; the P waves cannot be found, and the QRS complex is 110 milliseconds (normal <120). The diagnosis is PSVT. What is the clinical presentation of PSVT, and what are the consequences of this arrhythmia?

PSVT often has a sudden onset and termination. At the time of PSVT, the heart rate is usually 180 to 200 beats/minute. As illustrated by B.J., patients experience palpitations as well as nervousness and anxiety. In patients with a rapid ventricular rate, dizziness and presyncope (near-fainting) can occur, and the rhythm may degenerate to other serious arrhythmias. Depending on the underlying heart function, angina, HF, or shock may be precipitated. It has not been demonstrated that patients with episodes of PSVT are at an increased risk of stroke.

Arrhythmogenesis—Re-entry

20. What is the arrhythmogenic mechanism of PSVT?

AV nodal re-entry is the most common mechanism of paroxysmal supraventricular arrhythmias (Fig. 19-4). Under certain conditions, such as following an acute MI, atrial impulses will be blocked in one of the two AV nodal pathways in a unidirectional manner (antegrade block). After the impulse reaches the distal end of one pathway, it will conduct in a retrograde fashion through the other pathway, setting up a circular movement causing tachycardia.

Reciprocating tachycardias occur when there is an accessory pathway. Orthodromic AV reciprocating tachycardia is a re-entry tachycardia involving antegrade conduction through the AV node and retrograde conduction through a bypass tract. Antidromic AV reciprocating tachycardia is a re-entry tachycardia involving antegrade conduction through an accessory pathway and retrograde conduction via the AV node or

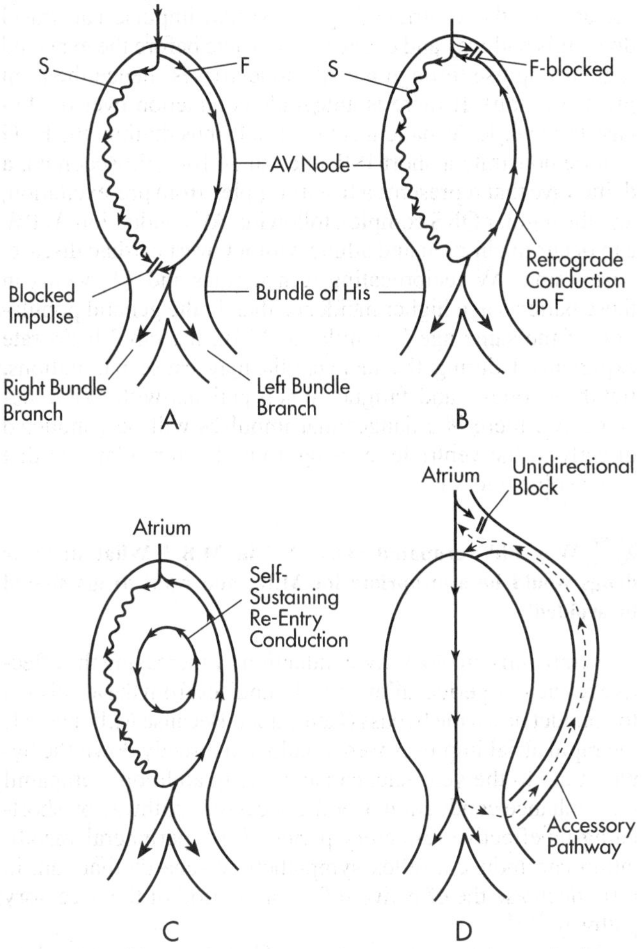

FIGURE 19-8 The atrioventricular (AV) node in paroxysmal supraventricular tachycardia and Wolff-Parkinson-White syndrome. A. A bifurcation of an impulse, one propagated fast and another slow. B. The slow impulse in Figure 19-8A can send impulses in a retrograde fashion. C. The re-entry from Figure 19-8A to Figure 19-8B can be self-sustaining. D. Normal impulse conduction through the AV node, but abnormal retrograde conduction up an accessory pathway, as would be seen in a patient with Wolff-Parkinson-White syndrome.

another accessory pathway (e.g., WPW syndrome) (Fig. 19-8). Antidromic reciprocating tachycardias manifest as wide QRS complexes resembling ventricular arrhythmias.

Treatment

21. B.J. tries the Valsalva maneuver, and her ventricular rate is reduced to 175 beats/minute; the other parameters are unchanged. She is given adenosine 6 mg as an IV bolus, administered over 1 minute, with no effect on the PSVT rate. Another dose of adenosine 12 mg has no effect. No side effects are noted from therapy. What treatment options can be used if B.J. is hemodynamically unstable? What is the Valsalva maneuver? What is a probable reason for B.J.'s unresponsiveness to adenosine? Are there any drug interactions that might diminish adenosine's effect?

NONDRUG TREATMENT

Valsalva Maneuver

Although her BP is low at 95/60 mmHg, B.J. is maintaining an adequate perfusion pressure, so nondrug treatment or vagal maneuvers should be attempted first. Two common vagal techniques are pressure over the bifurcation of the internal and external carotid arteries and the Valsalva maneuver (forcible exhalation against a closed glottis, similar to bearing down to have a bowel movement). The increase in pressure induced by these maneuvers is sensed by the baroreceptors, causing a reflex decrease in sympathetic tone and an increase in vagal tone. The increase in vagal tone will increase refractoriness and slow conduction in the AV node, thereby slowing the heart rate; the arrhythmia will terminate in 10% to 30% of cases.[89] If B.J. is hemodynamically unstable or becomes hemodynamically unstable at any time, she should receive synchronous DC cardioversion.

DRUG THERAPY

Adenosine

Drug therapy involves blocking the AV node because most PSVT rhythms involve a re-entry circuit within this area. Adenosine, a purine nucleoside that exerts a transient negative chronotropic and dromotropic effect on cardiac pacemaker tissue, is considered the drug of choice for the acute treatment of PSVT because of its rapid and brief effect.[90] An initial 6-mg IV bolus is given; if this is unsuccessful within 2 minutes, it can be followed by one or two additional 12-mg IV boluses, up to a maximum of 30 mg. Because of its short half-life (9 seconds), adenosine should be administered as a rapid bolus (over 1–3 seconds), followed immediately by a saline flush. Thus, B.J.'s failure to respond is likely attributed to the prolonged (1-minute) infusion time.

Theoretically, adenosine may be ineffective or higher doses may be required in patients who are receiving theophylline because theophylline is an effective adenosine receptor blocker. Larger doses of other methylxanthines (caffeine or theobromine) may also theoretically interact like theophylline. Conversely, concomitant use of dipyridamole may accentuate adenosine's effects because dipyridamole blocks the adenosine uptake (and subsequent clearance).

22. B.J. is given 12 mg adenosine IV over 2 seconds, followed by a 20-mL normal saline flush. Thirty seconds later, she complains of chest tightness and pressure. Is B.J. experiencing a heart attack? Is this response a result of a drug interaction between adenosine and another medication?

B.J. is experiencing a common side effect of adenosine. Patients receiving adenosine should be warned that they may experience transient chest heaviness, flushing, or feelings of anxiety. SOB and wheezing may be observed in patients with asthma. Lower doses are usually required in heart transplant patients, and caution should be observed when administering adenosine to these patients.

Calcium Channel Blockers

23. B.J. is still in PSVT. What other acute therapeutic options should be considered at this time?

Nondihydropyridine calcium channel blockers, verapamil and diltiazem, can be used in patients with PSVT. Verapamil (2.5–5 mg IV given over 2 minutes) achieves peak therapeutic effects in 3 to 5 minutes after dosing and can be repeated at 10- to 15-minute intervals to a maximum dose of 20 mg if needed. The elderly should receive the verapamil infusion over 3 minutes. Patients ages 8 to 15 years should receive 0.1 to 0.3 mg/kg as an IV bolus over 1 minute. A repeat dose of 0.1 to 0.2 mg/kg can be administered 15 to 30 minutes later if the effect was inadequate. Diltiazem is given as a 0.25-mg/kg IV bolus over 2 minutes, and a second bolus of 0.35 mg/kg can be given 15 minutes later if the effect is inadequate. Both calcium channel blockers have an 85% conversion rate.[91] However, verapamil should not be used in patients with wide complex tachycardia of unknown origin because it may lead to hemodynamic compromise and, potentially, VF.

β-blockers and digoxin can be used if calcium channel blockers or adenosine fail.

24. B.J. is given 5 mg IV verapamil over 1 minute, followed by an additional 5 mg 10 minutes later. She converts to normal sinus rhythm 3 minutes after the second dose. Because she has experienced symptoms that could be attributed to PSVT in the past, she may be a candidate for chronic therapy to slow conduction and increase refractoriness at the AV node. Which agents have been evaluated for this indication? Is there a role for radiofrequency catheter ablation therapy for PSVT like there is for atrial flutter?

On a long-term basis, PSVT is managed with agents that slow conduction and increase refractoriness in the AV node, thereby preventing a rapid ventricular response. These include oral verapamil, diltiazem, β-blockers, or digoxin. Class IA, IC, and III agents are used occasionally to slow conduction and increase refractoriness of the fast bypass tract to prevent triggering impulses such as premature atrial and ventricular contractions. Radiofrequency catheter ablation is indicated if drug therapy cannot be administered safely (e.g., in a pregnant woman), managed conveniently (e.g., in noncompliant patient), or tolerated (because of side effects).

Electrophysiologic testing is used to determine the location of the re-entrant tract, which then can be abolished, thereby interrupting accessory pathways. This treatment approach potentially is curative and is used increasingly in medical centers under the direction of a specially trained electrophysiologist.

B.J. has had a few episodes of PSVT in the past but has not been on any suppressive therapy. This history suggests that chronic suppressive therapy should be tried first. Because she responded to IV verapamil, oral SR verapamil (Isoptin SR) was prescribed at a dosage of 240 mg/day.

Wolff-Parkinson-White Syndrome

25. M.B., a 35-year-old man, presents to the ED with a chief complaint of chest palpitations for 4 hours. He relates a history of many similar self-terminating episodes since he was a teenager. He took an unknown medication 5 years ago that decreased the occurrence of the palpitations, but he stopped taking it due to side effects. M.B.'s vital signs are BP 96/68 mmHg; pulse 226 beats/minute, irregular; RR 15 breaths/minute; and temperature 98.7°F. A rhythm strip confirms AF, with a QRS width varying from 0.08 to 0.14 seconds. To control the ventricular rate, 10 mg IV verapamil is administered over 2 minutes. Within 2 minutes, VF is noted on the monitor. M.B. is defibrillated to normal sinus rhythm. A subsequent ECG demonstrates a P-R interval of 100 milliseconds (normal 120–200) and delta waves compatible with WPW. What is WPW syndrome?

WPW is a pre-excitation syndrome in which there is an accessory bypass tract (known as a Kent bundle) connecting the atria to the ventricle (Fig. 19-8). An impulse can travel down this pathway and excite the ventricle before the expected regular impulse through the AV node arrives (hence the term pre-excitation). If there is antegrade conduction over the bypass tract while the patient is in normal sinus rhythm, the ECG will demonstrate a short P-R interval ($<$100 milliseconds), a delta wave that represents a fused complex from pre-excitation, and the regular QRS complex following AV conduction. WPW can occur in children and adults without overt cardiac disease. Paroxysmal AV reciprocating tachycardias and AF occurs in these patients at a higher incidence than in the general population of the same age.[92] Similar to M.B., the rapid heart rate experienced during the tachycardia may cause palpitations, lightheadedness, and fatigue. When patients with WPW develop AF, there is a danger that impulses will be conducted directly to the ventricle, causing a rapid ventricular rate that may evolve into VF.

26. Why did verapamil cause VF in M.B.? What drug or drugs would be appropriate for M.B., and what drugs should be avoided?

Verapamil can block AV conduction by increasing the effective refractory period, allowing all impulses from the atrial area to conduct down the bypass (Kent) tract. Because M.B. had AF, the rapid atrial impulses were conducted directly down the bypass tract to the ventricle, causing VF. In addition, verapamil may enhance conduction over the accessory pathway by shortening its effective refractory period. Also, peripheral vasodilation can induce a reflex sympathetic discharge that can, in turn, decrease the effective refractory period of the accessory pathway.[93,94]

The most common presentation of WPW syndrome involves normal antegrade conduction down the AV node and retrograde conduction back up through the accessory pathway. This will manifest as orthodromic reciprocating re-entrant tachycardia. Thus, drugs that inhibit antegrade impulse conduction through the AV node (e.g., verapamil, digoxin) will terminate the re-entrant tachycardia and can be suitable in the absence of AF. The less common variety of WPW is antegrade conduction through the accessory pathway with retrograde transmission up through the AV node, resulting in an antidromic re-entrant tachycardia. Similarly, AV nodal blocking agents will terminate this type of re-entrant tachycardia. In some situations, such as experienced by M.B., rapid AF with an accessory pathway occurs, which can lead to VF and cardiac arrest.

The antiarrhythmic drugs used to treat patients with AF who have an accessory pathway, such as M.B., include those that depress conduction and increase the effective refractory period of the fast sodium channel–dependent tissue of the accessory pathway. This includes most class I antiarrhythmics, with the class IB agents being least effective. Procainamide, an FDA-approved drug for this indication, is a reasonable first choice.[95] Propafenone and flecainide are also effective and may be preferred over procainamide.[96–99] Amiodarone and sotalol may also be effective, but clinical experience is limited.[100–102] Radiofrequency ablation of the bypass tract is used more frequently for these patients to prevent VF.

Further therapy for M.B. may not be useful at this time. However, if he has recurrent AF or other symptomatology associated with WPW, radiofrequency catheter ablation or drug therapy as outlined previously could be indicated.

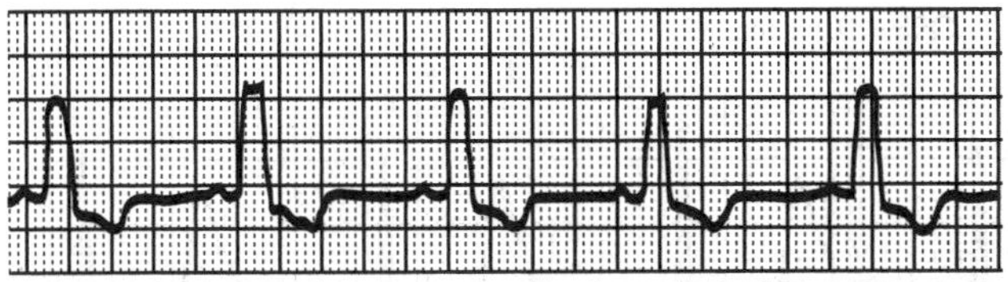

FIGURE 19-9 Bundle branch block. Note that the QRS interval is prolonged. A 12-lead electrocardiogram is required to make the diagnosis of left bundle branch block. *Source:* Reproduced with permission from Stein E. Rapid Analysis of Arrhythmias: A Self-Study Program. 2nd ed. Philadelphia: Lea & Febiger; 1992.

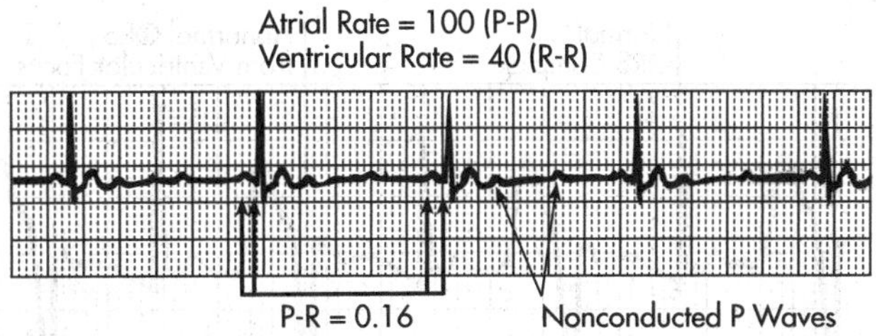

FIGURE 19-11 Second-degree atrioventricular block type II (3:1 fixed block).

CONDUCTION BLOCKS

Various arrhythmias can result from blockage of impulse conduction. These can occur above the ventricle, such as first-, second-, and third-degree (complete) AV block. Others, such as RBBB or LBBB and trifascicular block, originate below the bifurcation of the His bundle. Although conduction blocks can be classified as either supraventricular or ventricular arrhythmias, they are discussed as a separate group because their mechanism of arrhythmogenesis is similar and their treatment is different from other arrhythmias.

27. H.T., a 63-year-old man, was admitted to the coronary care unit (CCU) 12 hours ago with an acute inferior wall MI. He has remained stable. On admission, he had the rhythm strip shown in Figure 19-9 (LBBB). Twelve hours later, it has changed to the rhythm strip shown in Figure 19-10 (Wenckebach or type I, second-degree AV block). Are these rhythms potentially hazardous to H.T.? How is second-degree AV block different from first- or third-degree AV block?

H.T.'s rhythm strip revealed a diagnosis of LBBB. Bundle branch block occurs when the electrical impulse cannot be conducted along the left or right fascicle of the His-Purkinje system (Fig. 19-1). In H.T., the impulse travels down the right bundle normally, and the right ventricle contracts at the normal time. The left bundle is blocked and, therefore, the left side is depolarized from an impulse conducted from the right ventricle. This impulse must travel through atypical conduction tissues (with slower conduction), and hence the left side depolarizes later. This is revealed on the ECG by a widened QRS complex. Bundle branch blocks, particularly in the left fascicle, are associated with coronary artery disease, systemic hypertension, aortic valve stenosis, and cardiomyopathy.[103] Typically, they do not lead to clinical cardiac dysfunction on their own. Because H.T. has LBBB, he can develop complete heart block (third-degree block) if for any reason his right fascicle is damaged.

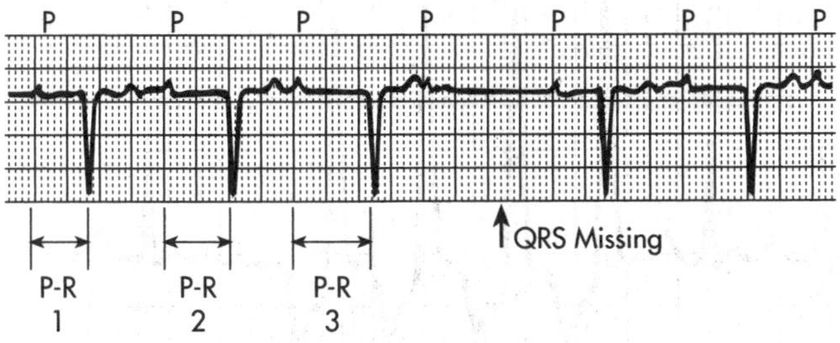

FIGURE 19-10 Second-degree atrioventricular block type I (Wenckebach). The P-R interval progressively prolongs until, after the third complex, a QRS complex is not conducted. *Source:* Reproduced with permission from Stein E. Rapid Analysis of Arrhythmias: A Self-Study Program. 2nd ed. Philadelphia: Lea & Febiger; 1992.

First-degree AV block is usually asymptomatic. The ECG will show P waves with a prolonged P-R interval (normal >200 milliseconds), but each wave is followed by a normal QRS complex. First-degree AV block is a common finding in patients taking digoxin, verapamil, or other drugs that slow AV conduction.

Second-degree heart block consists of two types. Mobitz type I (Wenckebach) is characterized by progressive lengthening of the P-R interval with each beat and a corresponding shortening of the R-R interval until finally an impulse is not conducted; the cycle then starts over again. Mobitz type II (Fig. 19-11) impulse conduction is blocked in a fixed, regular pattern (e.g., 3:1 block, where for every three P waves, only one is conducted).

Third-degree heart block (complete heart block) occurs when none of the impulses from the SA node are conducted to the ventricles. During third-degree block, the ventricle must develop its own pacemaker (escape rhythm), which may be too slow to provide adequate cardiac output, causing the patient to become symptomatic. A mechanical pacemaker is needed for treatment of third-degree AV block. AV blocks can be caused by drugs, acute MI, amyloidosis, and congenital abnormalities.[104]

Atropine

28. How should H.T.'s heart block be treated?

H.T. is experiencing a Wenckebach rhythm, which is often transient following an inferior wall MI. As long as he is hemodynamically stable, he should be monitored closely. If his heart rate and BP drop, atropine 0.5 mg IV bolus (maximum 2 mg) can increase the heart rate. This is only a short-term therapy; if the hemodynamic compromise persists, a pacemaker must be inserted to initiate the impulse to control the heart rate.

VENTRICULAR ARRHYTHMIAS

Recognition and Definition

Ventricular arrhythmias arise from irritable ectopic foci within the ventricular myocardium. Impulses from these ectopic foci generate wide, bizarre-looking QRS complexes leading to PVCs (Fig. 19-12). PVCs can arise from the same ectopic site (unifocal) or can be multifocal in origin. They can be simple (e.g., isolated or infrequent) or complex (e.g., R on T, in which

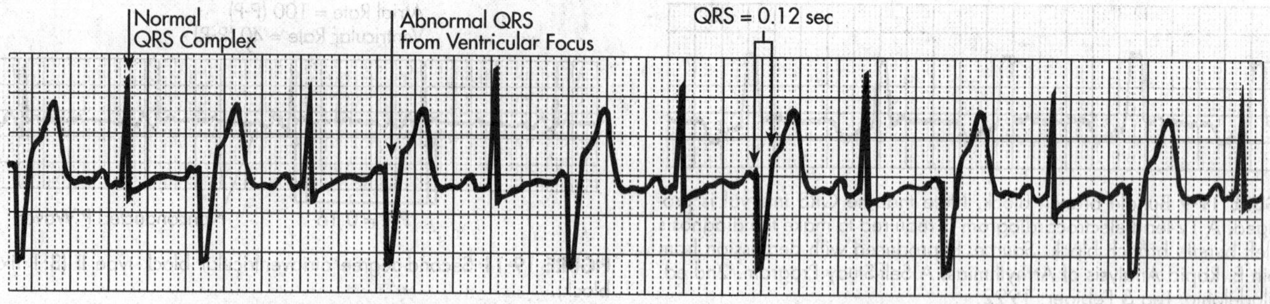

FIGURE 19-12 Premature ventricular contraction. Every other beat is a premature ventricular (ectopic) contraction.

the R wave of a PVC falls on top of a normal T wave). Other presentations include runs of two or more beats, bigeminy (every other beat is a PVC), or trigeminy (every third beat is a PVC). Three consecutive PVCs are usually defined as VT, which can be nonsustained or sustained. Ventricular flutter, VF, and TdP are other serious forms of ventricular arrhythmias (Figs. 19-13 to 19-16). The presentation, etiology, treatment, and ion channels associated with TdP are discussed separately.

Nonsustained ventricular tachycardia (NSVT) (Fig. 19-13) commonly is defined as three or more consecutive PVCs lasting <30 seconds and terminating spontaneously. Sustained VT (SuVT) is defined as consecutive PVCs lasting >30 seconds, with a rate usually in the range of 150 to 200 beats/minute. P waves are lost in the QRS complex and are indiscernible. SuVT (Fig. 19-15) is a serious development because it can degenerate into VF. Ventricular flutter is characterized by sustained, rapid, regular ventricular beats (normal >250/minute) and usually degenerates into VF. VF (Fig. 19-14) is characterized by irregular, disorganized, rapid beats with no identifiable P waves or QRS complexes. It is believed to be triggered by multiple reentrant wavelets in the ventricle. There is no effective cardiac output in patients with VF.[103,104]

Etiology

Common factors that cause ventricular arrhythmias are ischemia, the presence of organic heart disease, exercise, metabolic or electrolyte imbalance (e.g., acidosis, hypokalemia or hyperkalemia, hypomagnesemia), or drugs (digitalis, sympathomimetic amines, antiarrhythmics). It is essential to identify and remove any treatable cause (e.g., metabolic or electrolyte imbalance and proarrhythmic drugs) before initiating antiarrhythmic drug therapy.

Evaluation of Life-Threatening Ventricular Arrhythmias

An episode of life-threatening ventricular arrhythmia (i.e., SuVT, TdP, VF) carries a significant risk of morbidity and mortality. Adequate documentation of the arrhythmia and its suppression by either drugs or a mechanical device are essential. Patients suspected of having or documented to have symptoms of a life-threatening arrhythmia (e.g., syncope, out-of-hospital cardiac arrest) should be admitted to the hospital and evaluated. At present, two approaches are used to evaluate the arrhythmia and the effectiveness of therapy: ambulatory (Holter) monitoring and electrophysiologic studies.[103,104]

Holter Monitoring

Holter monitoring is continuous ECG monitoring, usually for 24 to 48 hours, with or without exercise (e.g., treadmill exercise). The patient wears a portable ECG monitoring device in a purselike carrier and maintains a written log of daily activities and possible arrhythmia symptoms. The ECG is then played back in the laboratory, correlating the presence of arrhythmias with patient activity and symptoms. Monitoring should be implemented before and after drug intervention. One criterion clinically used in judging efficacy is that a drug is considered effective if it suppresses 100% of runs of VT longer than 15 beats, 90% of shorter runs, 80% of paired PVCs, or 70% of all PVCs, and there is an absence of exercise-induced VT.[105]

Electrophysiologic Studies

Electrophysiologic studies are the second approach in evaluating the efficacy of antiarrhythmic drugs. This approach is especially useful in patients with sporadic ventricular arrhythmias that may be missed by short-term monitoring. This procedure involves right ventricular catheterization and introduction

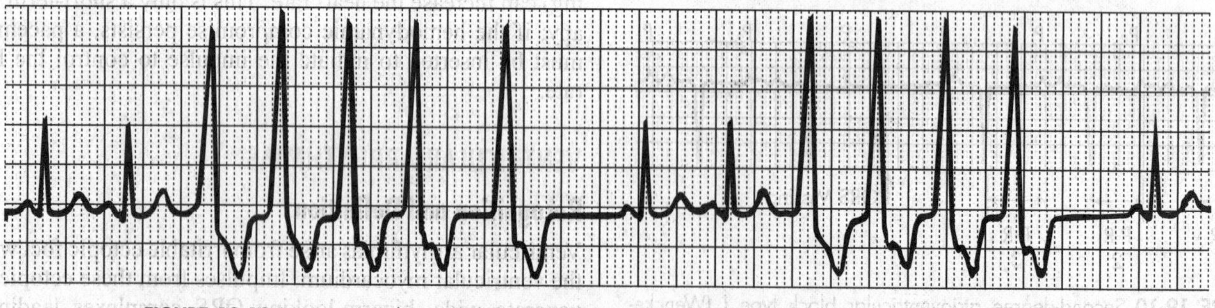

FIGURE 19-13 Nonsustained ventricular tachycardia. *Source:* Reproduced with permission from Goldberger AI, Goldberger E. Clinical Electrocardiology: A Simplified Approach. 4th ed. St. Louis, MO: Mosby–Year Book; 1990.

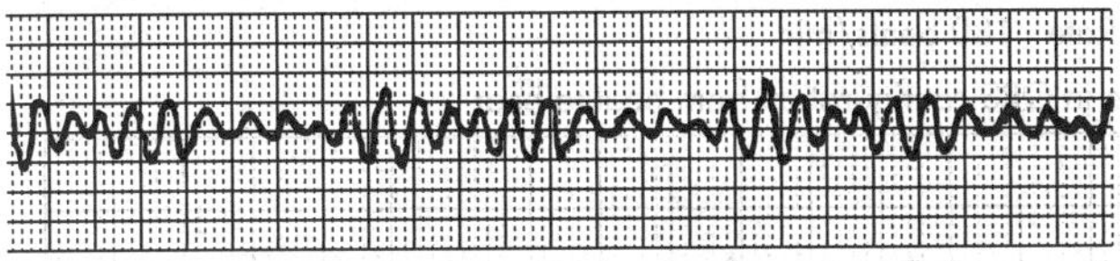

FIGURE 19-14 Ventricular fibrillation.

of up to three electrical stimuli at the right ventricular apex of the heart to induce baseline VT.[106] If the arrhythmia is not reproducibly induced, repeated stimulation with up to three extra stimuli is usually performed at the right ventricular outflow tract. Once VT is reproducibly induced at baseline, drug therapy is started. The drug is considered effective if the SuVT is rendered noninducible or occurs in runs of less than six beats. A partial response to drug therapy is obtained if the drug converts SuVT to NSVT or decreases the VT rate (e.g., increases VT cycle length by 100 milliseconds), with elimination of symptoms.[107]

Drugs that achieve satisfactory response by Holter technique or complete suppression by the electrophysiologic technique have been shown to improve long-term survival in uncontrolled trials.[108–110] Similarly, a partial response by the electrophysiologic method has also improved long-term outcome.[111] In a randomized, comparative study of Holter monitoring versus electrophysiologic study, Holter monitoring led to a prediction of efficacy more often than electrophysiologic study, although there was no difference in the success of drug therapy as selected by either method.[110]

Premature Ventricular Contractions

29. **A.S., a 56-year-old woman, is admitted to the CCU with a diagnosis of acute anterior wall MI. Her vital signs are BP 115/75 mmHg, pulse 85 beats/minute, and RR 15 breaths/minute. Auscultation of the heart reveals an S_3 gallop. Her electrolytes include potassium (K) 3.8 mEq/L (normal 3.5–5.0) and magnesium (Mg) 1.4 mEq/L (normal 1.6–2.4). Otherwise, her examination is within normal limits. Two days later, an echocardiogram estimates her EF to be 35% (normal >50%). During her stay in the CCU and in the step-down unit, multiple PVCs (15/minute) were noted on the bedside monitor. No antiarrhythmic agent was ordered. Should A.S.'s multiple PVCs be treated with a class I antiarrhythmic drug?**

[SI units: K, 3.8 mmol/L (normal 3.5–5.0); Mg, 0.72mmol/L (normal 0.8–1.2)]

Occasional PVCs are a benign, natural occurrence, even in a healthy heart, and are not an indication for drug therapy. Similarly, asymptomatic simple forms of PVCs, even in patients with other cardiac disease, are usually not an indication for treatment. However, the presence of frequent PVCs is a well-described risk factor for sudden cardiac death (SCD).[112] In patients with a low EF induced by the PVCs or NSVT, the risk for sudden cardiac death can increase 13-fold. Suppressing PVCs under these conditions may reduce the risk of SCD.

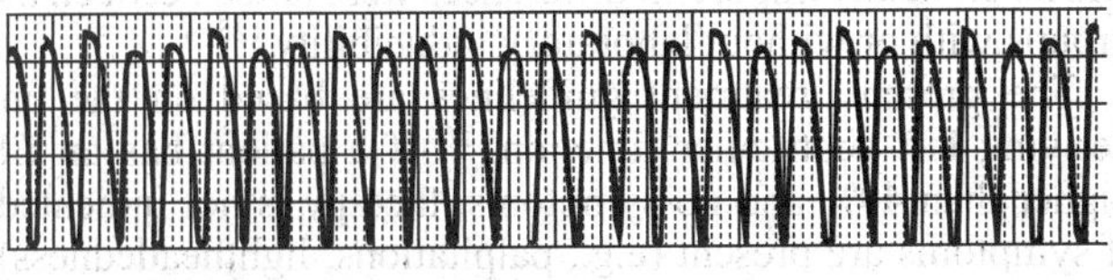

FIGURE 19-15 Sustained ventricular tachycardia.

Type IC Antiarrhythmic Agents

Because PVCs are a risk factor for SCD, the National Institutes of Health launched the Cardiac Arrhythmia Suppression Trial (CAST)[113,114] to assess the benefit of PVC suppression in survivors of MI. CAST was a prospective, randomized, placebo-controlled trial that evaluated three antiarrhythmic agents: flecainide, encainide, and moricizine (all class IC agents). The choice of these drugs was based on results of a pilot study of 1,498 patients that showed adequate suppression of arrhythmia (PVCs) in the target population. Ten months after initiation of the study, CAST was discontinued because of excess total mortality and cardiac arrests in patients receiving flecainide and encainide. Forty-three of 755 patients in the flecainide/encainide group died of arrhythmia or cardiac arrest versus 16 of the 743 patients taking placebo. Furthermore, total mortality in the flecainide/encainide group was 8.3% (63/755) compared with 3.5% (26/743) in the placebo group.[113] In the moricizine group, which was reported separately in CAST II, 16 of 660 patients in the drug group died compared with 3 of 668 patients in the placebo group in the initial 2 weeks. Subsequent long-term follow-up did not show a difference between moricizine and placebo.[114] It is generally believed that the excessive death rate in the drug-treated groups was due to the proarrhythmic effect of the drugs. Because the patients enrolled in CAST were asymptomatic and at low risk for the development of arrhythmias, they were at greater risk for drug toxicity (relative to benefit). Although many issues have been raised concerning CAST, one conclusion is that patients with a recent MI and the presence of asymptomatic PVCs should not be treated with encainide, flecainide, or moricizine. Whether other class I antiarrhythmics will produce similar results is unknown. Thus, the decision not to treat A.S.'s PVCs with class I antiarrhythmic medications was a sound one. The proarrhythmic effects of the drug may outweigh the potential danger of PVCs at this time.

30. **What alternatives to class I antiarrhythmics should be considered for A.S.?**

β-Blocking Agents

A β-blocker should be considered in this patient and in all patients with an acute MI unless specific contraindications exist. β-blocking drugs have been shown to reduce the risk of reinfarction and cardiac arrest when started early in the course of an MI and continued for more than 7 to 14 days. In pooled analyses from 28 clinical trials on β-blockers, the mortality rate was decreased by 28% at 1 week, with most of the benefit obtained within the first 48 hours. An 18% reduction in reinfarction and a 15% reduction in cardiac arrest were also documented.[115–117] A recent substudy looking specifically at patients with new signs of mild to moderate HF and acute MI determined that IV metoprolol (5-mg bolus every 5 minutes repeated three times to deliver 15 mg over 15 minutes) followed by 200 mg/day of oral metoprolol reduced overall mortality significantly at 3 months and 1 year.[118] This suggests that a

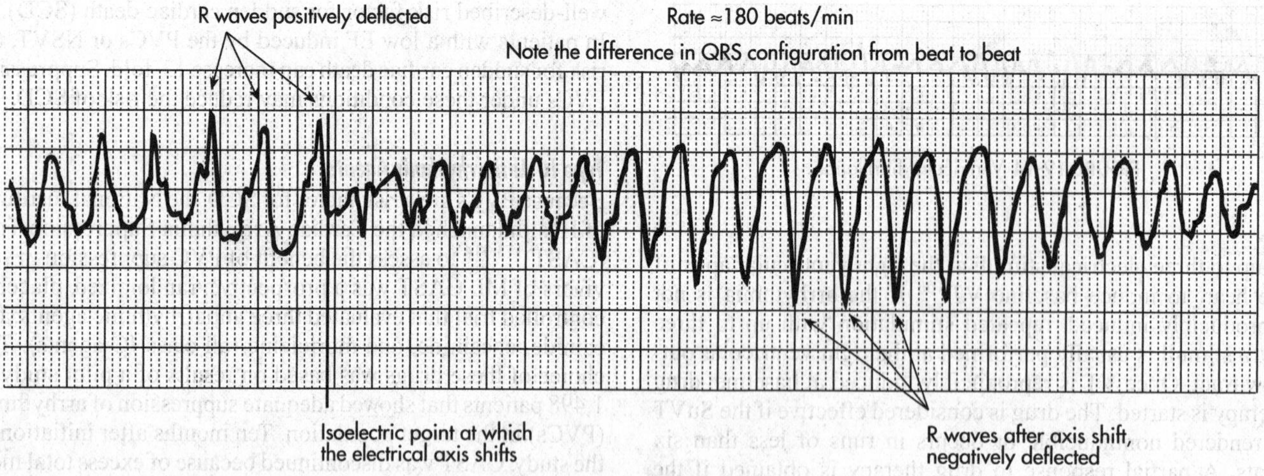

FIGURE 19-16 Torsades de pointes.

reduced EF after MI (as in A.S.) or a large MI is not a contraindication to β-blocker therapy.

The importance of the β-blocking effect after MI is further illustrated by the results of two MI sotalol trials. The first trial of sotalol, a class III antiarrhythmic agent with β-blocking properties, showed an 18% reduction in overall mortality, which was similar to that seen in other β-blocking trials.[119] The second trial, the Survival With Oral D-Sotalol (SWORD) trial, evaluated the d-isomer of sotalol only. This isomer does not have β-blocking properties, and this trial was stopped early because the mortality rate was significantly increased.[120] The American Heart Association and the American College of Cardiology recommend the routine use of IV β-blockers (followed by oral therapy) to prevent the early occurrence of VF[121] (see Chapter 17).

Amiodarone

In high-risk patients with MI who are not candidates for β-blockade, alternative antiarrhythmic therapy with amiodarone can be considered. Amiodarone is a class III antiarrhythmic agent but also has antiadrenergic, class I, and class IV activity. The first trial evaluating the use of amiodarone in patients who had specific contraindications for β-blockade was conducted in Poland. Treatment with amiodarone (800 mg/day for 7 days followed by 400 mg/day for 6 days of the week for 1 year) was associated with a significant reduction in cardiac mortality and significant ventricular arrhythmias. Overall mortality showed a trend toward benefit, but statistical significance was not achieved.[122] An evaluation of amiodarone in post-MI patients with frequent PVCs (>10/hour) or at least one run of VT was conducted in the Canadian Amiodarone Myocardial Infarction Arrhythmia Trial (CAMIAT).[123] In this trial, amiodarone (10 mg/kg/day for 14 days, then 300–400 mg/day for 16 months) significantly reduced the incidence of VF or arrhythmic death by 48.5% compared with placebo. Arrhythmic death alone was reduced by 32.6%, and all-cause mortality was reduced by 21.2%, but statistical significance was not achieved for these end points. Patients with heart failure or a previous MI had a majority of the benefit from amiodarone therapy.

A complementary study, the European Myocardial Infarct Amiodarone Trial (EMIAT), evaluated MI survivors with a reduced EF (<40%).[124] Based on the results of this study, amiodarone (800 mg for 14 days, then 400 mg for 14 weeks, and then 200 mg for the rest of the study) significantly reduced arrhythmic deaths by 35% compared with placebo. However, this study did not demonstrate any trend toward reduced mortality (mortality was 13.86% with amiodarone vs. 13.72% with placebo). This suggests that amiodarone should not be used in all patients with a reduced EF after an MI, but that it could benefit patients in whom antiarrhythmic therapy is indicated. Hence, if A.S. reports problematic symptoms associated with the PVCs or develops additional risk factors for arrhythmia while on β-blockade, antiarrhythmic therapy with amiodarone can be given without an increased risk of overall mortality[122–124] (see Chapter 17).

Nonsustained Ventricular Tachycardia

31. D.S., a 62-year-old man, was admitted recently for an inferior wall MI. Following the infarction, he has been free of further pain and does not exhibit signs of HF. An echocardiogram shows an EF of 48%, but D.S. does experience runs of VT (Fig. 19-13) lasting from three beats to 20 seconds in length. D.S. states that he feels his heart racing during the longer episodes. Should D.S.'s VT be treated? If so, what are the treatment options?

D.S. is experiencing NSVT, which can occur in patients with underlying heart disease, both ischemic and nonischemic (idiopathic dilated cardiomyopathy, hypertrophic cardiomyopathy). It is not clear which of these patients is at highest risk for SCD. The Multicenter Unsustained Tachycardia Trial (MUSTT) used electrophysiologic testing to see if laboratory inducibility of sustained monomorphic VT could predict the duration or frequency of NSVT in patients with NSVT, coronary artery disease, and a reduced EF. No significant difference in the frequency or duration of spontaneous NSVT was noted, and no clinically important differences were noted between the groups with or without laboratory inducibility.[125]

The present treatment guidelines are based on the underlying left ventricular function.[126] If a patient has an EF higher than 40% and no symptoms, therapy is not indicated. If symptoms are present (e.g., palpitations, lightheadedness), a β-blocker is preferred unless it is contraindicated by the presence of uncompensated HF or asthma/chronic obstructive pulmonary disease. In addition to controlling symptoms, β-blockers reduce the incidence of cardiac death in post-MI patients with and without PVCs.[127] If the patient has a reduced EF (<40%), it is uncertain what the best treatment should be. However, oral β-blocker therapy, with careful titration of dosage, may be considered because β-blockade is now an approved therapeutic approach in HF patients.

Because D.S. is symptomatic but has preserved ventricular function, he should certainly be started on a β-blocker. Pindolol or any other β-blocker with intrinsic sympathomimetic activity should be avoided because they have not been shown to be "cardioprotective" following an MI. The results from the CAMIAT study suggest a role for amiodarone in this patient if β-blockers are contraindicated or inadequate.[123]

Sustained Ventricular Tachycardia

Treatment

32. S.L., a 64-year-old woman, presents to the ED with a chief complaint of palpitations. Her medical history includes hypertension controlled with a diuretic and an inferior wall MI 6 months ago. She is pale and diaphoretic but able to respond to commands. Her vital signs are BP 95/70 mmHg, pulse 145 beats/minute, and RR 10 breaths/minute. When telemetry monitoring is established, S.L. is found to be in SuVT (Fig. 19-15). S.L. states that she has a history of allergy to Novocain. How should she be treated?

The acute treatment of patients with SuVT depends on their hemodynamic stability. If unstable, patients should receive synchronous cardioversion, which will decrease the chance of triggering VF. If the patient is conscious, a short-acting benzodiazepine (e.g., midazolam) should be administered before the procedure.

LIDOCAINE

In patients with stable BP, IV agents such as lidocaine or procainamide are used to abolish the tachycardia. Lidocaine can be administered as a 1-mg/kg bolus, no faster than 50 mg/minute. More rapid rates can cause hypotension and asystole. If the initial bolus does not "break" the tachycardia, additional boluses of 0.5 mg/kg are administered 8 to 10 minutes apart until a total dose of 3 mg/kg is given. The need for a supplemental bolus dose at 8 to 10 minutes is based on the rapid distribution half-life (8 minutes) of lidocaine. At one distribution half-life, the plasma concentration is reduced by 50%, and the concentration at the effective site (the central compartment) is also reduced by 50%.[128]

PROCAINAMIDE

Procainamide is an alternative agent if lidocaine is ineffective or is not tolerated. The efficacy of lidocaine is low (11%–25% success) if it is being used to convert VT not arising during ischemia or within 72 hours of an MI, while the efficacy of procainamide is similar, regardless of the presence of baseline ischemia or infarction.[129] A loading dose of 12 mg/kg is administered at a rate of 50 mg/minute. Hypotension is often the rate-limiting factor and can be minimized by administering the drug at a slower rate (20–35 mg/minute). Once the patient has converted to normal sinus rhythm, a continuous infusion (dosage, 1–4 mg/minute) can be started. The infusion should be reduced in renal failure because the parent drug and the active metabolite, *N*-acetyl procainamide (NAPA), can accumulate. NAPA itself has class III antiarrhythmic activity and is eliminated entirely by the kidneys.

S.L. is hemodynamically stable at this time, so lidocaine should be given in an attempt to abolish the tachycardia. Lidocaine can be used even though S.L. reports an allergy to procaine (Novocain). Procaine is an ester-type local anesthetic, whereas lidocaine and procainamide are amide-type local anesthetics; thus, there is no cross-reactivity between the two types.

33. A 1-mg/kg lidocaine bolus is given at 50 mg/minute, and two additional boluses of 0.5 mg/kg are given at 10-minute intervals before normal sinus rhythm is restored. A continuous infusion of lidocaine is started at 4 mg/minute and continued for 48 hours. How should lidocaine concentrations be monitored over the next 12 to 24 hours?

Once converted to normal sinus rhythm, S.L. can be maintained on a continuous lidocaine infusion at a rate based on the estimated clearance of the drug (1–4 mg/minute). Lidocaine clearance can be reduced by HF, acute MI, advanced age, significant liver disease, and drugs such as propranolol or cimetidine.[128,130,131] Under these conditions, a lower infusion rate should be used and the plasma lidocaine concentration determined in 12 to 24 hours (see average therapeutic concentration in Table 19-3). The lidocaine concentration also should be obtained after 24 hours if a prolonged infusion is anticipated because lidocaine clearance decreases in this situation. Phenobarbital and phenytoin may increase lidocaine clearance, thereby lowering the plasma concentration.[132]

34. After 17 hours of the lidocaine infusion, S.L. is having difficulty manipulating a spoon to eat her Jell-O. She is becoming increasingly agitated and is inaccurately saying that people keep coming into her room and taking her things. Could these side effects be a result of lidocaine toxicity?

S.L. is probably exhibiting CNS side effects from lidocaine. If longer-term antiarrhythmic therapy is needed, it should be with another agent that is administered orally.

Lidocaine toxicity typically presents as alterations in the CNS such as dizziness, drowsiness, paresthesias, visual disturbances, tinnitus, slurred speech, trembling, loss of coordination, confusion, somnolence, hallucinations, unresponsiveness, seizures, or agitation. Cardiovascular toxicity (conduction disturbances, bradyarrhythmias, and hypotension) is rare and usually occurs when serum concentrations exceed 9 mcg/mL. Lidocaine also possesses weak negative inotropic activity, which is clinically most evident during prolonged infusions or in patients with a pre-existing depressed myocardium (e.g., acute MI).[133] In those at-risk individuals, negative inotropy could reduce cardiac output and cause or worsen HF symptoms. It is likely that S.L. is experiencing lidocaine toxicity, and her infusion should be reduced to 2 mg/minute or lidocaine therapy discontinued.

SOTALOL

35. S.L.'s attending physician believes that she should undergo further testing, and an electrophysiologist is consulted. It is determined that electrophysiologic testing is necessary because S.L. has a history of SuVT. On baseline testing, SuVT at a rate of 220 beats/minute was induced twice with the catheter placed at the

right ventricular apex. Sotalol 80 mg BID is prescribed. Describe the properties of sotalol and its adverse effects. How effective is sotalol in this situation? Is it the right choice for S.L.?

Sotalol is a unique agent that possesses nonselective β-blocking activity (class II) and prolongs repolarization (class III activity).[134] The immediate effect of sotalol in suppression of inducible VT or fibrillation is modest, generally averaging response rates of 30% to 35% using Holter monitoring, but as high as 56% in one report.[110] However, a randomized, comparative trial called the Electrophysiologic Study Versus Electrocardiographic Monitoring (ESVEM) study, using both Holter monitoring and electrophysiologic testing, demonstrated that sotalol treatment produced a significantly lower probability of recurrence of arrhythmia, death from any cause, death from a cardiac cause, and death from arrhythmia compared with other drugs.[110] Thus, the initial or acute efficacy of sotalol, although not impressive, can lead to better long-term results than many other drugs. The adverse effects associated with sotalol (e.g., fatigue, bradycardia, hypotension, TdP) are covered in the AF and TdP sections, respectively.

Because S.L. has no contraindications and had an MI 6 months ago, sotalol is a suitable initial choice. Sotalol can be initiated at 80 mg twice daily and advanced to a maximum recommended dose of 640 mg/day. The half-life of sotalol is 8 to 18 hours. Because it is cleared by the kidneys, its clearance is reduced and its half-life prolonged in patients with renal dysfunction. S.L.'s BP, heart rate, and ECG should be monitored. If her rate-related ("corrected") Q-T (QTc) interval becomes prolonged (see section on TdP), the dose should be reduced or the drug discontinued.

AMIODARONE

36. Sotalol is discontinued because S.L. developed a QTc interval above 500 milliseconds. What is the role of amiodarone for S.L.'s arrhythmia based on its efficacy and safety? If S.L. is to be treated with amiodarone, how should it be initiated and monitored?

Amiodarone exhibits properties of classes I, II, III, and IV antiarrhythmic agents. Although it has class II effects on the heart, amiodarone is virtually devoid of antiadrenergic effects outside the heart and is not contraindicated in patients with asthma. The antiadrenergic effects arise from inhibition of adenylate cyclase, the enzyme that catalyzes production of the second-messenger product cyclic adenosine monophosphate. Amiodarone can also cause a reduction in ß-1 receptor density.[129,135]

This drug has unique pharmacokinetic properties. Its apparent volume of distribution is 5,000 L. Because it is extensively bound to tissue and is lipophilic, its half-life after long-term administration is 14 to 53 days. The main metabolite of amiodarone is desethylamiodarone. Although this metabolite is active, its contribution to the overall antiarrhythmic activity is not clearly delineated.

Because of the extremely long half-life of amiodarone, loading doses are used to accelerate the onset of drug effect. One to 2 g/day (200–500 mg four times daily) is given over a 1-week period; after that time, a maintenance dose can be established. Typically, for treating ventricular arrhythmias, 300 to 400 mg/day is used for maintenance, but doses may range from 100 to 800 mg/day. Although a concentration–effect relationship is hard to determine for amiodarone, levels above 2.5 mg/L are associated with an increased incidence of adverse effects.[135]

Amiodarone has many serious adverse effects involving a variety of organ systems, the most serious and life-threatening of which is pulmonary fibrosis. This historically occurred in 5% to 10% of the population given chronic doses of 600 to 1,200 mg QD for amiodarone, with a 5% to 10% mortality rate for those who developed it.[136] Large-scale, multicenter, double-blind, placebo-controlled clinical trials in HF and after MI have provided much information on the safety of amiodarone using new and lower dosages (e.g., maintenance doses of 300–400 mg QD). From these trials, comprising 2,250 patients who received amiodarone for 1 or 2 years, there were three deaths from pulmonary fibrosis in the EMIAT study (0.4% incidence in this study), and no deaths were reported in the other studies.[67,122–124,129,137] Severe pulmonary fibrosis was reported in 0.3% of patients in a Polish study and in 1.2% of patients in the CHF STAT trial (compared with 0.9% in the placebo group).[67,122] Unspecified pulmonary disorders were reported in 5.2% of patients in the EMIAT study (compared with 4% in the placebo group) and in 3.8% of patients in the CAMIAT study (compared with 1.2% in the placebo group). The dosage regimens and beneficial effects of therapy from the Polish, EMIAT, and CAMIAT studies were reported in the section on the treatment of PVCs. Briefly, the dosage for all studies ranged from 600 to 800 mg/day for 7 to 14 days as a loading dose followed by maintenance regimens of 300 to 400 mg/day.

Despite the lower incidence of adverse pulmonary events observed in these studies, it is still necessary to monitor for the development of pulmonary fibrosis. A baseline chest radiograph and pulmonary function tests (diffusion capacity in particular) are recommended. The chest radiograph should be repeated at 6- to 12-month intervals, but pulmonary function tests need be repeated only if symptoms (dyspnea, nonproductive cough, weight loss) occur. Patients should be specifically questioned about these symptoms because early detection can decrease the extent of lung damage[67,122–124,138] (see Chapter 25).

Liver toxicity can range from an asymptomatic elevation of transaminases (two to four times normal) to fulminant hepatitis. Thus, liver enzymes should be monitored at baseline and every 6 months (see Chapter 29). The most common GI complaints are nausea, anorexia, and constipation.

Both hypothyroidism and hyperthyroidism have been reported, although hypothyroidism is more common. The thyroid complications are a consequence of amiodarone's large iodine content and its ability to block the peripheral conversion of thyroxine (T_4) to triiodothyronine (T_3).

Other bothersome side effects are corneal deposits (usually asymptomatic); blue-gray skin discoloration in sun-exposed areas; photosensitivity; exacerbation of HF; and CNS effects that include ataxia, tremor, dizziness, and peripheral neuropathy. Other than an eye examination and pulmonary function tests, which should be repeated when the patient is symptomatic, all other blood tests should be repeated every 6 months for routine monitoring.[136]

37. S.L. is placed on amiodarone 400 mg BID for 7 days. On day 2 of amiodarone therapy, her INR is 2.5. On day 8, she is switched

to 400 mg/day of amiodarone for maintenance therapy. Her INR on day 16 of amiodarone therapy is 4.2, and warfarin is held. Why is her INR above normal?

Amiodarone is a potent enzyme inhibitor of the cytochrome P450 enzyme system. Two of the most significant interactions associated with amiodarone are with warfarin and digoxin. Warfarin is composed of two isomers, R and S. The R-isomer is eliminated through the cytochrome P450 1A2 system, whereas the S-isomer is eliminated through the cytochrome P450 2C9 system. The S-isomer is five times more potent than the R-isomer. Amiodarone inhibits the elimination of warfarin's isomers through both enzyme sites. However, the time course of the interaction is somewhat different than other enzyme inhibitors due to amiodarone's long half-life. When amiodarone is added to stable warfarin therapy, close monitoring (at least weekly) is needed for up to 4 weeks.[139] Usually, dosages of warfarin are reduced by 30% to 50% after amiodarone is instituted.[139]

Amiodarone inhibits the elimination of digoxin as well. Digoxin levels increase approximately 50% by day 5 and 100% by day 14[140] (see Chapter 18). Close monitoring is required for 2 weeks after digoxin initiation.[140] Even if amiodarone is discontinued, it can continue to interact with other drugs for more than a month (depending on the dose delivered) due to its long half-life.[9] Amiodarone may substantially increase the levels of quinidine, whereas ritonavir (Norvir) may potently inhibit the elimination of amiodarone.[139]

Implantable Cardiac Defibrillators

38. After 2 weeks on amiodarone, S.L. develops a run of VT lasting about 2 minutes. She is admitted for placement of an implantable cardioverter-defibrillator (ICD). What is an ICD, and how does it work?

ICDs are devices implanted under the skin with wires or patches that are advanced or attached so they are in direct contact with the ventricular myocardium. The ICD has sensing, pacing, and defibrillation capabilities. When an arrhythmia is sensed, the ICD will first try to pace the heart out of the arrhythmia. This is most effective (80% successful) when the VT rate before pacing is below 180 beats/minute. If pacing fails to terminate the arrhythmia, a generator will turn on and create a certain number of joules (J) of energy. Unlike external paddle defibrillators, which deliver 100 to 360 J of energy, the energy delivered by an ICD to defibrillate the heart is usually 5 to 30 J. This is adequate for two main reasons. The ICD delivers energy directly to the heart rather than having to pass the energy through skin, bone, and other organs. The use of a biphasic waveform in an ICD rather than a monophasic waveform also reduces the energy needed to defibrillate.

As the energy needed to defibrillate the heart with an ICD is increased, the amount of time the generator needs to create the energy is also increased. This is problematic because long charge times leave the patient in the arrhythmia for a longer period of time and may cause syncope. As such, the lowest energy needed to defibrillate the patient (the defibrillation threshold) is determined experimentally. To do this, the patient has an arrhythmia started by the electrophysiologist, and the device is set to shock at different energies to determine the lowest successful defibrillation energy. The electrophysiologist then sets the energy output at 10 J above that level (a safety margin).[141] Using the "DFT 10-J" rule prolongs battery life and reduces syncopal episodes associated with arrhythmia recurrence versus always using the ICD's maximal energy output.

However, the impact of drugs, herbals, and endogenous substances on the DFT are not well described. If a drug significantly increases the DFT, then it may reduce the effectiveness of a 10-J safety margin.

The first major results from a randomized trial came in 1996 with the publication of the MADIT (Multicenter Automatic Defibrillator Implantation Trial) study.[142] This study enrolled 196 patients with prior MI; left ventricular EF 35% or below; documented asymptomatic NSVT; and inducible, nonsuppressible, ventricular tachyarrhythmia on electrophysiologic testing. The effect of ICDs versus conventional medical therapy (the majority of patients received amiodarone) on the primary end point, all-cause mortality, was followed for an average of 27 months. There were 39 deaths in the conventional medical therapy group and 15 deaths in the ICD group (hazard ratio for the ICD was 0.46; 95% CI, 0.26–0.82; $p = 0.009$).

A few years later, the results from the MUSTT extended the evidence that ICD therapy may have beneficial effects on mortality in patients at high risk for sudden death.[143] This larger study ($n = 704$) had similar inclusion criteria to the MADIT trial with the exception of a slightly higher EF cut-off (>40%). The primary end point was cardiac arrest or death due to arrhythmia. Patients were randomized to electrophysiologically guided therapy or no antiarrhythmic therapy. Of the patients who received electrophysiologically guided therapy, nearly half received antiarrhythmic drugs (mostly class I agents), and the remainder were given ICDs. The primary end point was achieved in 25% of patients receiving electrophysiologically guided therapy and in 32% of patients who did not receive antiarrhythmic therapy (relative risk, 0.73; 95% CI, 0.53–0.99).

The Antiarrhythmics Versus Implantable Defibrillators (AVID) study compared ICDs to therapy with amiodarone or sotalol. This study investigated a population at high risk (they had already experienced VF and been cardioverted previously, or they had documented VT with syncope or another serious complication and an EF <40%). Overall, 1,016 patients were randomly assigned to either antiarrhythmics or ICDs. This study was stopped early (after 18 months) because the incidence of overall mortality was significantly lower in the ICD group (15.8%) than in the antiarrhythmic group (24.0%).[144]

Patients with ICDs who have frequent bouts of ventricular arrhythmogenesis are at high risk of developing ICD anxiety (known as ICD psychosis). They live in fear of their ICD going off again because it causes pain and they are forced to think of their own mortality. Use of antiarrhythmic agents to reduce the number of times the ICD goes off per month usually helps alleviate this anxiety.

Whether ICDs could be used in patients at high risk of arrhythmia (post-MI with a left ventricular EF <30%) but without past ventricular arrhythmic events was investigated in the Multicenter Automatic Defibrillator Implantation Trial II (MADIT II). ICD implantation plus conventional therapy was compared with conventional therapy alone. Conventional therapy consisted of β-blockers, ACE inhibitors, lipid-lowering drugs, diuretics, and digoxin in approximately 60% to 80% of patients in both groups. The ICD group had a 31% lower overall mortality rate than the conventional therapy group. If this therapy becomes standard of care for this population, approximately 3 to 4 million patients will be eligible, and 400,000 new patients will be eligible each year.[145]

Clearly, S.L. should have the device placed: It is her best chance for prolonging long-term survival. Depending on the number of times the machine discharges per month and the patient's response, adjunctive antiarrhythmics may be needed.

Torsades de Pointes

Proarrhythmic Effects of Antiarrhythmic Drugs and Clinical Presentation

39. G.G. is a 71-year-old woman who is taking sotalol 80 mg BID for a previous episode of SuVT. At baseline, her QTc interval was 445 milliseconds, and her Cl_{cr} was 52 mL/minute. Four weeks after therapy was initiated, she complained of bouts of dizziness. She went to her cardiologist's office earlier today, and an ECG was performed by the ECG technician. She was released and told that the cardiologist would call her later in the day after she read the ECG. While driving home 10 minutes ago, she passed out and hit a parked car. When the paramedics arrived, the ECG strip showed TdP with a ventricular rate of 110 beats/minute. She is now awake and alert. The ECG taken in the physician's office shows a QTc interval prolonged at 540 milliseconds. What is QTc interval prolongation? Why does QTc interval prolongation indicate an increased risk of TdP? Could an antiarrhythmic agent such as sotalol cause this arrhythmia? How does Cl_{cr} factor into this?

The QT interval denotes ventricular depolarization (the QRS complex in the cardiac cycle) and repolarization (from the end of the QRS complex to the end of the T wave). Certain ion channels in phases 2 and 3 of the action potential are vital in determining the QT interval (Fig. 19-1). An abnormal increase in ventricular repolarization increases the risk of TdP. TdP is defined as a rapid polymorphic VT preceded by QTc interval prolongation. TdP can degenerate into VF and as such can be life threatening (Fig. 19-16).[146]

Because there is tremendous variability in the QT interval resulting from changes in heart rate, the QT is frequently corrected for heart rate (QTc interval). Several correction formulas for the QT interval exist and give similar results at most heart rates. The most common correction formula uses QT and RR intervals measured in seconds as follows: [$QTc = QT/(RR^{0.5})$].

The Committee for Proprietary Medicinal Products suggests that a QTc interval over 500 milliseconds or a level that has increased as a result of medications by more than 60 milliseconds from baseline is a cause for concern of enhanced risk of TdP. Increases of 30 to 60 milliseconds from baseline are a potential concern.[146] The American College of Cardiology, American Heart Association, and European Society of Cardiology produced combined guidelines that address this issue as well. They suggest that agents prolonging the QTc interval through potassium channel blockade, with the possible exception of amiodarone, should be dosed to keep the QTc in sinus rhythm below 520 milliseconds.[3] As an aside, amiodarone is unique among class III antiarrhythmic agents in that it blocks both IKr and the slow IK channel (IKs). This provides less heterogeneity in ventricular repolarization and reduces the risk of TdP over agents that prolong the QTc interval solely by IKr blockade.

G.G. was in excess of the acceptable QTc interval of 500 milliseconds shortly before the time when TdP occurred. This QTc interval is much higher than would be expected in a subject without drug therapy or other risks of TdP. In a 150-subject trial, the average QTc interval of patients without comorbid diseases or concurrent medications was 403 ± 28 milliseconds. The QTc interval was 13 milliseconds lower in men than women (397 ± 27 and 410 ± 28 milliseconds, respectively). This is backed up by epidemiologic studies where 70% of TdP was found to occur in women. The QTc interval also increases with aging. Within the age categories of 20 to 40 years, 41 to 69 years, and >69 years, the QTc intervals were 397 ± 27, 401 ± 28, and 412 ± 28 milliseconds, respectively.[147] Hence, G.G.'s increased age and female gender probably contributed to her higher baseline QTc interval of 445 milliseconds, but this is still below the baseline 450 milliseconds cut-off for using sotalol.

Sotalol is known to cause QTc interval prolongation in a dose-dependent manner. Total daily doses of 160, 320, 480, and >640 mg gave patients a steady-state QTc interval of 463, 467, 483, and 512 milliseconds, and the incidence of TdP was 0.5%, 1.6%, 4.4%, and 5.8%, respectively.

It is likely that G.G.'s reduced renal function put her at high risk for sotalol accumulation and accentuated QTc interval prolongation. In patients with a Cl_{cr} above 60 mL/minute, the sotalol dose of 80 mg BID is appropriate, but in patients like G.G. with a Cl_{cr} <40 to 60 mL/minute, the starting dose should be 80 mg daily owing to sotalol's predominant renal clearance.

40. What transient conditions or other disorders can increase the risk of TdP in patients on class IA or III antiarrhythmics?

Hypokalemia, hypomagnesemia, and hypocalcemia are important transient causes of QTc interval prolongation. Follow-up ECG monitoring is advised if a patient on a class IA or III antiarrhythmic has a disorder that radically alters electrolytes, such as severe diarrhea, metabolic acidosis, or ketoacidosis. Also, patients with renal failure have dramatic electrolyte shifts occurring during dialysis that may cause QTc interval changes. As such, avoidance of these antiarrhythmics or close ECG monitoring is warranted.

All class III and class IA antiarrhythmic agents except amiodarone and ibutilide exhibit IKr potassium channel reverse use dependence: This means that they block IKr potassium channels when the channels are in their inactive state. As such, the QTc interval will tend to shorten at faster heart rates and lengthen at slower heart rates. Hence, patients with an acceptable QTc interval while in AF may have an elevated QTc interval after they convert back to sinus rhythm if the ventricular rate markedly slows. A second ECG should be taken once sinus rhythm is restored to avoid this complication. Proper ventricular rate control with class II or IV antiarrhythmics before using chemical cardioversion can reduce the chances of dramatic heart rate reductions after conversion to sinus rhythm. In addition, patients who develop a bradycardic disorder should be monitored very closely. Finally, patients with vasovagal syncope usually experience transient vagally mediated bradycardia during a syncopal episode. This can increase the QTc interval and may make therapy more dangerous.

Investigators have discovered gene mutations responsible for hereditary long QTc interval syndrome,[148] an inherited cardiac disorder that predisposes patients to syncope, seizures, and sudden death. Sudden death in long QTc interval syndrome is usually secondary to TdP, which degenerates into VF.[148,167] Drug therapy with QTc-prolonging agents would be risky in this population.

Because G.G. did not have a family history of hereditary long QT syndrome, but was being treated with sotalol (an agent known to be associated with TdP) in renal dysfunction, it can be assumed that sotalol therapy was responsible for her arrhythmia.

Proarrhythmic Effects of Nonantiarrhythmic Drugs

41. Which nonantiarrhythmic drugs cause TdP? What is the mechanism of TdP initiation in this situation?

Nonantiarrhythmic agents can also exhibit potassium channel inhibition and can prolong the QTc interval. Most of these drugs, including erythromycin, fluoroquinolones, and antipsychotics cause QTc interval prolongation by inhibiting the IKr ion channel, just like quinidine and sotalol.[146,149–151] Ranolazine, however, inhibits IKr, IKs, calcium, and sodium channels, and given its unique pharmacologic profile, the relationship between QTc interval prolongation and TdP is not established.[152]

In general, nonantiarrhythmic agents increase the QTc interval in relation to the dosage administered and the blood concentration attained.[150,151] However, antipsychotics such as ziprasidone seems to have a plateau effect for QTc prolongation. The placebo group had a 2.6-millisecond reduction in the QTc interval, compared to increases of 0.6 to 9.7 milliseconds over the range of approved doses of ziprasidone (<80–160 mg/day). When doses >200 mg/day were given, the QTc interval increases were 6.4 milliseconds on average, suggesting a plateau effect. This is underscored by the experience with the drug to date, where 10 cases of overdose (>300 mg single dose) were reported, with no QTc interval exceeding 500 milliseconds.[153]

In most subjects, the QTc interval prolongation for nonantiarrhythmic agents is less than the 30-millisecond increase from baseline that consensus groups have defined as being a potential concern for TdP. The lack of concern for a general population receiving normal doses of antiarrhythmics is underscored by data on terfenadine that led to its eventual removal from the market. It increased random ECG QTc intervals by 4 to 18 milliseconds in most studies. In addition, when its metabolism is blocked via CYP3A4 enzyme inhibitors such as itraconazole and ketoconazole, QTc interval increases of 41 and 82 milliseconds resulted, respectively.[146] Terfenadine underwent the largest evaluation of the risk of life-threatening ventricular arrhythmias to date in the COMPASS study. This cohort trial compared the incidence of life-threatening arrhythmic events in 597,189 patients from four medicaid databases. Terfenadine was compared to two other over-the-counter (OTC) antihistamines (diphenhydramine and clemastine—the active ingredient in Tavist) and ibuprofen. In this trial, terfenadine was shown to have significantly fewer life-threatening arrhythmic events (0.037%) than the other OTC antihistamines (0.085%, $p = 0.05$) and ibuprofen (0.057%, $p = 0.05$), and similar events to clemastine (0.021%). However, when the subgroup of patients receiving ketoconazole with terfenadine was evaluated, the adjusted relative risk was 23.55 times that of terfenadine alone ($p = 0.001$), a substantial risk.[154] Hence, the risk of arrhythmogenesis was not realized before taking into account the pharmacokinetic drug interaction, which in previous studies had been shown to increase the QTc interval into the zone for concern. Patient with renal failure (including those on dialysis), severe electrolyte disturbances, or hereditary long QTc interval syndrome were not rigorously studied but would theoretically also be at greater baseline risk.

Drug interactions accentuating the blood concentrations and subsequently the risk of TdP led to the withdrawal of terfenadine, astemizole, and cisapride from the U.S. market.[155,156]

Interestingly, erythromycin is not only metabolized through the cytochrome P450 3A4 system, but its active metabolite can also inhibit the cytochrome P450 3A4 system. Because the metabolite of erythromycin must be enzymatically activated and accumulate in the plasma before inhibiting the 3A4 system, it does not usually affect its own elimination (autoinhibition), but it can affect other drugs eliminated through this metabolic route.[156]

The antipsychotics are unique in that inhibitors of their metabolism do not result in appreciable increase in the QTc interval. This is likely because of the aforementioned QTc interval plateau effect. This was clearly demonstrated in Study 054, where several atypical antipsychotics (ziprasidone, risperidone, olanzapine, and quetiapine) and two typical antipsychotics (thioridazine and haloperidol) were evaluated. Therapy was given for more than 21 days to allow steady state to occur, and maximal doses in the package inserts were used for all drugs except thioridazine, for which half the maximum dose was given. In the second phase of the study, a CYP metabolic inhibitor was added to assess the impact of drug interactions on the QTc interval. In phase I of the trial, only thioridazine had QTc interval increases above 30 milliseconds (average 35.6 milliseconds; 95% CI, 30.5–40.7 milliseconds). None of the other agents had an average or an upper limit of the 95% CI for the QTc interval change exceeding 30 milliseconds. In phase II, the use of a specific CYP enzyme inhibitor did not cause a significant increase in the QTc interval for any agent compared to phase I.[157]

A list of nonantiarrhythmic agents implicated in causing QTc interval prolongation and known pharmacokinetic drug interaction increasing the blood concentrations of these drugs is given in Table 19-6.

Because G.G. was not taking nonantiarrhythmic agents that are associated with TdP, sotalol is still the most likely culprit.

Treatment

42. How should TdP be treated? What treatments should be considered for L.S.?

If the patient is significantly hemodynamically compromised (frequently associated with a ventricular rate >150 beats/minute and unconsciousness) while in TdP, electrical cardioversion is the therapy of choice and should be given immediately. Stepwise increasing shocks of 100 to 200, 300, and 360 J (monophasic energy) can be tried if earlier shocks are unsuccessful.

Table 19-6 Nonantiarrhythmic Agents Implicated in QTc Interval Prolongation or Torsades de Pointes[a]

Drug Class	Agent	Drugs That Increase Blood Concentrations of These QTc Interval Prolonging Drugs
Antianginal	Ranolazine	CYP3A4 inhibitors
Antibiotics: macrolides	Erythromycin (lactobionate and base)	CYP3A4 inhibitors
Antibiotics: fluoroquinolones	Gatifloxacin, grepafloxacin, lomefloxacin, moxifloxacin, sparfloxacin	
Antibiotics: other	Trimethoprim-sulfamethoxazole, pentamidine isethionate	
Antidepressants	Tricyclics, maprotiline	CYP1A2, 2D6, or 2C9 inhibitors
Antiemetics	Dolasetron	
Antimalarials	Mefloquine, quinine	Sodium bicarbonate, acetazolamide, cimetidine
Antipsychotics	Atypicals, butyrophenones, typicals	CYP1A2, 2D6, 2C9, 3A4 inhibitors
Calcium channel blockers	Bepridil	
Dopaminergics	Amantadine	Hydrochlorothiazide, quinidine, quinine, trimethoprim-sulfamethoxazole
Narcotics	Methadone	CYP3A4 and 1A2 inhibitors
Sympathomimetics	Albuterol, ephedra, epinephrine, metaproterenol, terbutaline, salmeterol	Monoamine oxidase inhibitors
Other	Arsenic, organophosphates	

[a] An up-to-date list can be found at www.torsade.org.

MAGNESIUM

In a hemodynamically stable patient, magnesium is frequently considered the drug of choice to restore normal sinus rhythm. It benefits patients whether they have hypomagnesemia or normal serum magnesium levels. However, magnesium is not effective for patients with polymorphic VT without TdP and with normal QT intervals. A common magnesium regimen is 1 to 2 g given over 5 to 10 minutes (in 50 mL D5W) as a loading dose and then 1 g/hour for up to 24 hours. However, loading doses of 1 to 6 g given over several minutes followed by an IV infusion for 5 to 48 hours at a rate of 3 to 20 mg/minute have also been used. The exact mechanism of action for magnesium in TdP is not known, but it reduces the occurrence of triggered activity such as early after-depolarizations and has L-type calcium channel and IK1 blockade during phase 3 of the action potential.

CLASS IB ANTIARRHYTHMICS

The second class of drugs commonly used to abolish TdP is the class IB antiarrhythmic agents (e.g., mexiletine, lidocaine, tocainide). Unlike quinidine and the class III antiarrhythmic agents, the class IB agents do not inhibit potassium outflow during phases 2 and 3.[150,158] In addition, blockade of inward sodium channels causes a shortening of the QT interval in some patients. Preliminary data suggest that class IB antiarrhythmic agents have considerable benefit in patients with sodium channel–activated QT prolongation, but virtually no effect on patients with potassium channel blockade–induced QT prolongation.[159,160] In a landmark trial, mexiletine was given to patients who had hereditary long QT syndrome,[159] and the patients were analyzed by their genetic etiology of long QT. The group with a deficient gene for the potassium channel had no QT shortening, whereas those with a defective sodium gene had significant shortening of the QT interval. These divergent responses were confirmed in an in vitro study using mexiletine with either clofilium, a potassium channel blocker, or almokalant, a pure sodium channel activator.[160]

Cardioacceleration with isoproterenol (1–4 mcg/minute) or cardiac pacing has also been shown to be beneficial.[161,162] As previously described, sotalol, quinidine, and *N*-acetyl procainamide's ability to prolong the action potential duration is diminished at faster heart rates (reverse use dependence).[163] The more the IKr potassium channels are activated, the less susceptible the channels are to inhibition by potassium channel–blocking drugs.

Because G.G. has regained consciousness and is hemodynamically stable, a bolus injection of 2 g magnesium should be administered over 10 minutes. If it is successful, a continuous infusion of magnesium (1 g/hour for up to 24 hours) should be given, and the serum potassium level should be determined. If hypokalemia is present, it should be corrected. If the arrhythmia recurs, cardiac pacing should be used. If the patient becomes hemodynamically unstable again, electrical cardioversion with 200 J is warranted. Future drug therapy with appropriately dosed sotalol, amiodarone, or ICD therapy will need to be determined subsequently.

Naturopathic Therapy for Arrhythmias

43. D.B. is interested in natural products to replace his antiarrhythmic therapy, which he says is too expensive. Are there any herbal or natural agents that can prevent or treat arrhythmias?

Herbal Therapies

Many herbal remedies have been touted as beneficial in "normalizing heart rhythm," but in vivo supportive data are lacking for most agents. Avoid using herbal products that contain cardiac glycosides such as lily of the valley, oleander, strophantus, hispidus seeds, squill, dogbane, *Adonis vernalis*, ouabain, and *Thevetia peruviana*. Although the effects can mimic those of digoxin, there is no way to monitor blood concentrations so they cannot be used safely.

Food Supplements and Minerals

Omega-3 fatty acids and magnesium are the best-studied alternative and complementary therapies for arrhythmias and are described as follows. In addition, dietary deficiencies of taurine

Table 19-7 Commonly Used Drugs in Cardiac Arrest

Drug	Formulation	Dosage/Administration[a]	Rationale/Indications	Comments
Amiodarone	50 mg/mL Vials: 3, 9, 18 mL	300 mg diluted in 20–30 mL D5W or NS; additional 150 mg (diluted solution) can be given for recurrent or refractory VT or VF.	Exhibits antiadrenergic properties and blocks sodium, potassium, and calcium channels. First-line antiarrhythmic pulseless VT and VF.	Excipients (polysorbate 80 and benzyl alcohol) can induce hypotension. Failing to dilute can induce phlebitis.
Atropine Sulfate	0.05, 0.1, 0.4, 0.5, and 1 mg/mL	1 mg IV, repeated every 3–5 minutes (maximum of 3 mg) for persistent asystole.	Blocks parasympathetic activity due to excessive vagal activity. Indicated in asystole, or slow PEA.	Must be given rapidly to avoid paradoxical vagal activity.
Epinephrine	0.1 mg/mL (1:10,000) or 1 mg/mL (1:1,000)	10 mL of a 1:10,000 solution of epinephrine (1 mg; dilute 1:1,000 solution in 0.9% sodium chloride) every 3–5 minutes.	Increases coronary sinus perfusion pressure through α-1 stimulation. Indicated in pulseless VT, VF, asystole, and PEA.	Epinephrine or vasopressin can be used for these indications.

PEA, pulseless electrical activity; VF, ventricular fibrillation; VT, ventricular tachycardia.

and selenium may predispose to arrhythmias. If deficiencies are found, supplementation seems promising.[164,165]

The largest prospective randomized controlled trial to test the efficacy of omega-3 fatty acids for secondary prevention of coronary heart disease was the Grupo Italiano per lo Studio della Spravvivenza nell'Infarcto Miocardico (GISSI) prevention study.[166] In this trial, 11,324 patients with coronary heart disease were randomized to 300 mg vitamin E, 850 mg omega-3 fatty acids (given as eicosapentaenoic acid [EPA] and docosahexanoic acid [DHA] ethyl esters), both, or neither. After 3.5 years, the group given omega-3 fatty acids had a 20% reduction in overall mortality and a 45% reduction in sudden death. Vitamin E was ineffective. Limitations to this study were that it was not placebo controlled, and the dropout rate was 25%. However, a prospective cohort study, a case-control study, and four prospective dietary intervention trials also demonstrated a reduction in sudden cardiac death from increases in sources high in omega-3 fatty acids (e.g., fatty fish). A nested case-control study showed that patients with MI and subsequent sudden death had lower levels of both EPA and DHA in their blood than MI patients without sudden death.[167]

Animal and in vitro studies suggest that omega-3 fatty acids may prevent arrhythmias by reducing the amount of scar tissue formation after an MI, and prevent calcium overload by maintaining the activity of L-type calcium channels and by inhibiting voltage-gated sodium channels.[168]

In addition to its beneficial effects in AF and TdP chemical conversion, magnesium has been evaluated as a ventricular rate controller in AF. In a small study, IV magnesium ($MgSO_4$, 2 g over 1 minute then 1 g/hour for 4 hours) reduced the heart rate by 16% within 5 minutes and then maintained the heart rate. No heart rate change occurred in the placebo group.[169] In a direct comparative trial versus verapamil (5 mg plus 5 mg IV followed by an infusion of 0.1 mg/minute), verapamil was significantly better as a rate controller (28% of patients had a heart rate <100 beats/minute with magnesium vs. 48% for verapamil). However, the magnesium group had significantly better conversion to normal sinus rhythm (58% in the magnesium group vs. 23% in the verapamil group).[170] Combination therapy with digoxin and magnesium versus digoxin alone was investigated in a small study. Digoxin use alone resulted in 50% of patients achieving a ventricular rate of <90 beats/minute at 24 hours. However, combination therapy with $MgSO_4$ (2 g over 15 minutes, then 8 g $MgSO_4$ over 6 hours) and digoxin resulted in 100% of patients achieving the ventricular rate goal.[171] There is some indication that magnesium can also benefit patients on digoxin chronically for AF who have frequent PVCs. Magnesium glycerophosphate 570 mg daily (23.4 mmol elemental magnesium) or placebo was given over the course of 4 weeks. The use of magnesium reduced the incidence of PVCs by 56%. No difference was noted for the patients randomized to placebo over the 4 weeks.[172] Future studies should be conducted to further evaluate this potentially cost-effective therapy.

In summary, omega-3 fatty acids may provide protection against ventricular arrhythmias in patients with ischemic heart disease. How it interacts with other antiarrhythmic agents is not well studied. In AF, magnesium can improve the rate-controlling effects of digoxin, but it should be used only when digoxin alone cannot adequately control the ventricular response. Magnesium does not seem to inhibit spontaneous cardioversion and may have some efficacy in chemical cardioversion.

CARDIOPULMONARY ARREST

Cardiopulmonary Resuscitation

Cardiac arrest from VF, pulseless VT, pulseless electrical activity (PEA), and asystole are life-threatening emergencies. Table 19-7[173] reviews commonly used drugs for these indications, and Figure 19-17 highlights key features of the management of pulseless arrest. This section reviews important aspects of therapy and provides clinical pearls, but the reader should also review the national consensus source document for these disorders, which includes more detail than can be given here.[173]

Treatment

44. M.N., a 52-year-old man, is visiting his wife, who is hospitalized for pneumonia. He goes into the bathroom and 2 minutes later his wife hears a dull thud. She calls out for her husband, but he does not respond. After an additional 2 minutes, health care

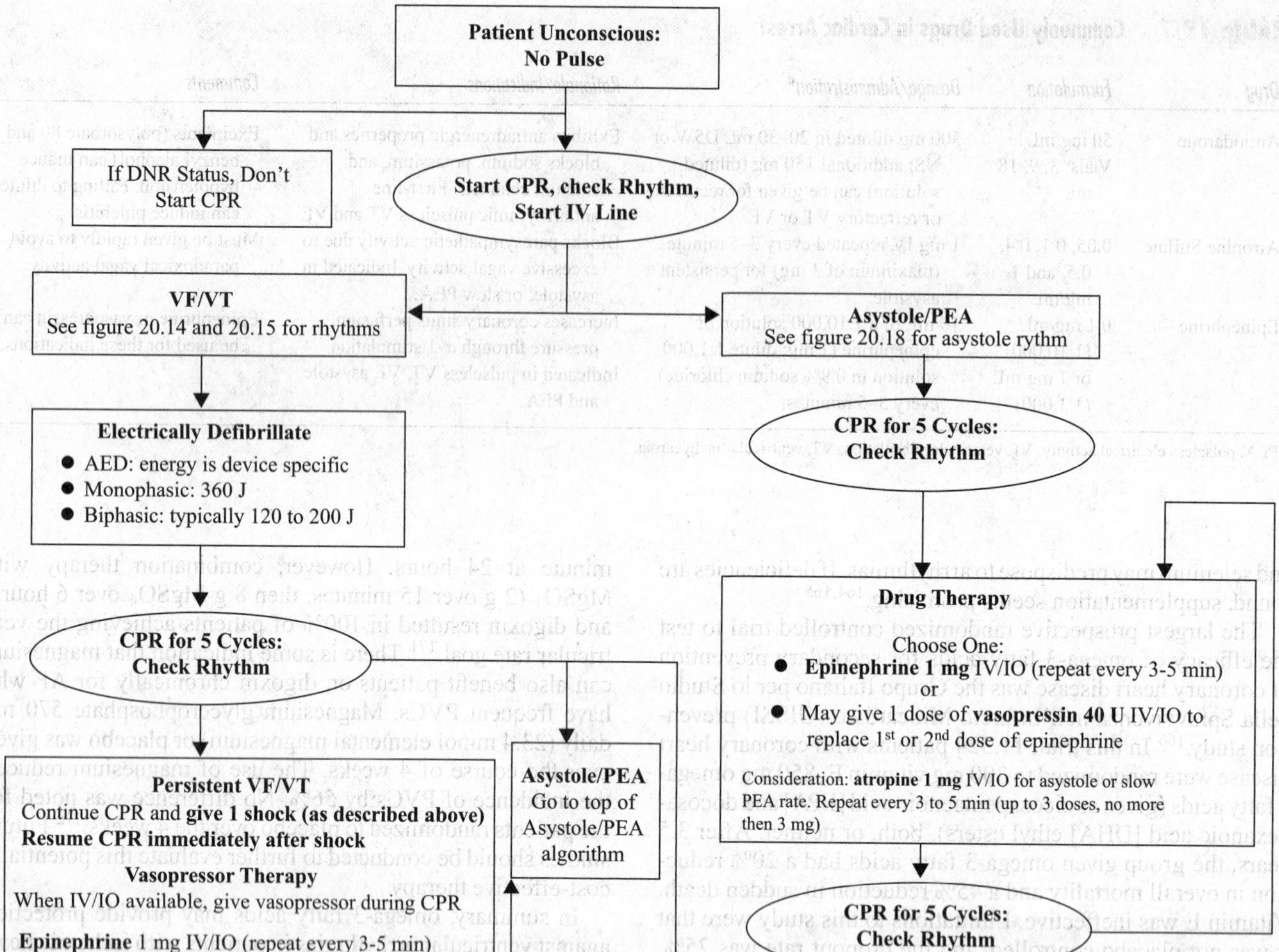

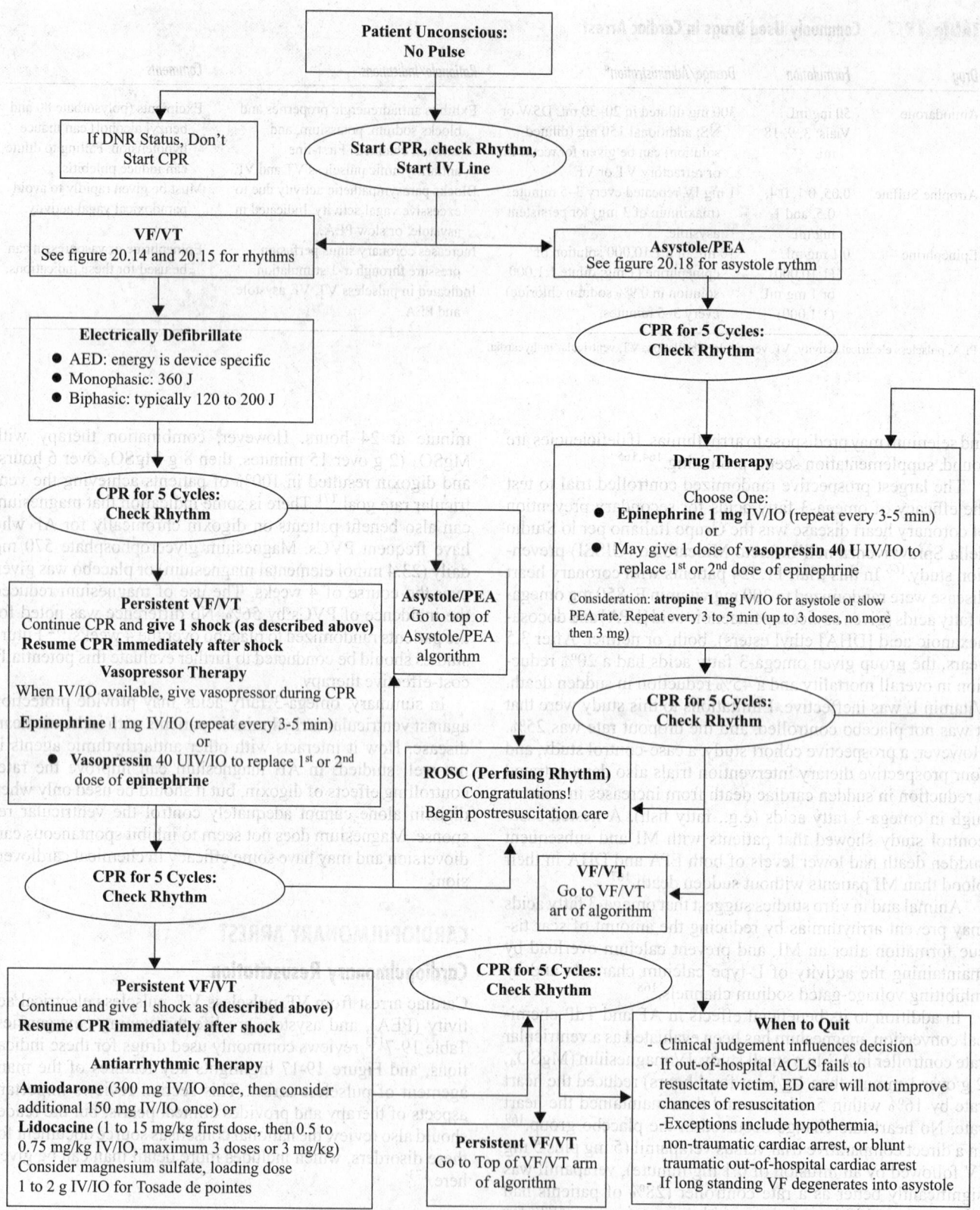

FIGURE 19-17 Cardiac arrest treatment algorithm. AED, automated external defibrillator; CPR, cardiopulmonary resuscitation; DNR, do not resuscitate; ED, emergency department. IO, intraosseous; IV, intravenous; PEA, pulseless electrical activity; ROSC, restoration of spontaneous circulation; VF, ventricular fibrillation; VT, ventricular tachycardia. *Source:* Adapted from reference 173.

workers open the bathroom door and find M.N. unresponsive and pulseless. Cardiopulmonary resuscitation (CPR) is initiated and a Code Blue is called. The ECG shows VF (Fig. 19-14), and there is no BP. In addition to CPR, what initial therapy is available?

Determining the underlying rhythm disturbance is important because it directs health care workers to follow the advanced cardiac life support (ACLS) algorithm for pulseless VT or VF (Fig. 20.17). This algorithm calls for electrical defibrillation first, but other clinicians should work to establish IV access in case defibrillation fails.[173]

External Defibrillation

Although commercially available manual defibrillators provide monophasic or biphasic waveform shocks, the biphasic defibrillator has become the preferred device due to its high first-shock efficacy (>90% termination of VF at 5 seconds post-shock). Biphasic defibrillators deliver one of two waveforms, a truncated exponential waveform or a rectilinear waveform. Most commercially available biphasic defibrillators display the device-specific energy dose range that should be used. Respective initial selected energies of 150 to 200 J and 120 J are reasonable choices for initial shocks delivered by truncated exponential waveform and rectilinear waveform defibrillators, respectively. However, if a health care provider operating a manual biphasic defibrillator is uncertain of the effective energy dose to terminate VF, an initial 200 J shock can be employed. For second and subsequent shocks delivered by manual biphasic defibrillators, the same or higher energies should be used. For first and subsequent shocks, a shock of 360 J should be delivered if a monophasic defibrillator is used to terminate VF.[173]

45. The initial shock fails to cause a return of spontaneous circulation in M.N. An IV line is established in a peripheral arm vein. The algorithm now calls for epinephrine or vasopressin, but which one should be used?

Epinephrine/Vasopressin

Although epinephrine stimulates β-1, β-2, and α-1 adrenoreceptors, it is the α-1 adrenoceptor effects that are most closely associated with efficacy in VF or pulseless VT.[173] Applying α-1 adrenoceptor stimulation increases systemic vascular resistance (via vasoconstriction), which elevates coronary perfusion pressure. This increase in coronary perfusion pressure is most likely the key to enhancing the return of spontaneous circulation after subsequent electrical defibrillation. Epinephrine may convert fine VF to a coarse variety that may be more amenable to defibrillation.

The recommended dose of epinephrine is 1 mg (10 mL of a 1:10,000 dilution; refer to Table 19-7) given by IV push. The dosage can be repeated at 3- to 5-minute intervals during resuscitation. If the drug is given IV via a peripheral line, which in this case includes a peripherally inserted central catheter, then a 20-mL flush with normal saline is recommended to ensure delivery into the central compartment. Only chest compressions cause blood circulation in VF or pulseless VT, so movement of drugs from the periphery to the heart (where the benefit will occur) is severely impaired.

If intravenous access is unavailable, health care providers may attempt to establish intraosseous (IO) access in the patient. For IO injection of drugs, a cannula should be placed in a noncollapsible venous plexus; the onset and systemic drug concentrations achieved with IO administration are similar to that achieved by central venous access. Typical sites of IO needle insertion include the anterior tibial bone marrow, distal femur, medial malleolus, or anterior superior iliac spine.

Vasopressin is an exogenously administered antidiuretic hormone. In supraphysiological doses, vasopressin stimulates V1 receptors and causes peripheral vasoconstriction. Vasopressin use during CPR causes intense vasoconstriction to the skin, skeletal muscle, intestine, and fat, with much less constriction of coronary vascular beds. Cerebral and renal vasodilation occurs as well.[173]

The results of a prospective, randomized, controlled, multicenter study ($n = 1,186$) that enrolled out-of-hospital cardiac arrest patients who presented with VF, PEA, or asystole, showed that administration of vasopressin as adjunctive therapy resulted in similar survival to hospital admission rates compared with adjunctive epinephrine therapy.[174] Patients were randomized to receive two ampules of 40 IU vasopressin or two ampules of 1 mg epinephrine. The second dose of vasopressor was injected if spontaneous restoration of circulation did not occur within 3 minutes after the first injection of the drug. If the absence of spontaneous circulation persisted, the physician administering CPR had the option of injecting epinephrine. The primary outcome measure of the study was overall survival to hospital admission. The reported survival rates were similar between the two treatment groups for both patients with PEA and those with VF. Of note, a post-hoc analysis showed that survival to hospital admission rates were 29% and 20%, respectively, for vasopressin- and epinephrine-treated patients who presented with asystole requiring CPR ($p = 0.02$).

An in-hospital study of 200 cardiac arrest patients (initial rhythm: 16%–20% VF, 3% VT, 41%–54% PEA, 27%–34% asystole) showed no difference in 1-hour or hospital discharge survival for vasopressin 40 IU versus epinephrine 1 mg.[175] Similarly, a recent meta-analysis of five randomized trials showed no survival advantage of vasopressin treatment over epinephrine treatment at the times of hospital discharge or 24 hours posttreatment.[176]

Based on these trials, it would be reasonable to use a single dose of vasopressin 40 IU as an alternative to either the first or second dose of epinephrine 1 mg in the treatment of VF (or pulseless VT).

ENDOTRACHEAL ADMINISTRATION

If IV access is not available, endotracheal administration of epinephrine is acceptable. Many agents (lidocaine, epinephrine, atropine, or naloxone [LEAN]) can be delivered via this route.[173,177] The patient should be horizontal rather than in the Trendelenburg position. A catheter should be passed beyond the tip of the endotracheal tube, at which point chest compressions should be stopped. The drug solution should be sprayed quickly down the endotracheal tube, followed by 5 to 10 rapid ventilations with a respirator bag. Medications should be diluted in 10 mL of normal saline or distilled water. Endotracheal absorption is greater with distilled water than with normal saline, but distilled water has a more negative effect on Pa_{O_2}. In general, the total bioavailability by the endotracheal route is reduced compared with the direct IV route; therefore, 2 to 2.5 times the usual dose should be given.

If IV or endotracheal routes are not available, then intracardiac injection could be used. Potential problems with the intracardiac route include pneumothorax, inability to perform chest compressions while the intracardiac drugs are being given, and coronary artery laceration. Intramuscular or subcutaneous administration is not appropriate because poor peripheral perfusion leads to unpredictable absorption.

46. Because M.N. has an IV site and the time from cardiac arrest to ACLS was brief, epinephrine was chosen and a 1-mg bolus was given, followed with a 20-mL normal saline flush. The arm was elevated for 20 seconds to ensure adequate delivery. Thirty seconds after administration, a 200-J shock is given (via biphasic manual defibrillator), but it fails to convert VF. What can be done now?

The most recently updated ACLS guideline calls for the use of amiodarone in cases of VF or pulseless VT that do not respond to CPR, a minimum of two shocks, and a vasopressor.[173]

Intravenous Amiodarone/Lidocaine

The effect of amiodarone in VF or pulseless VT was studied in the ARREST (Amiodarone for Resuscitation of Refractory Sustained Ventricular Tachyarrhythmias) trial.[178] This study was conducted in patients who experienced cardiac arrest in an out-of-hospital situation with therapy given by paramedics in the field. Patients who failed three stacked shocks and one dose of epinephrine with an electrical countershock were randomized to amiodarone 300 mg IV bolus or placebo. This was followed by other antiarrhythmics used in ACLS (2000 guidelines; lidocaine, procainamide, or bretylium) if the clinicians desired. Amiodarone significantly increased the chance of survival to hospital admission (44% vs. 34% of placebo group, $p = 0.03$), but survival to hospital discharge was not changed. Of note, 66% of patients received antiarrhythmic drug treatment for pulseless VT or VF after amiodarone administration. In addition, recipients of amiodarone were more likely to experience hypotension (59% vs. 48% of placebo, $p = 0.04$) or bradycardia (41% vs. 25% of placebo group, $p = 0.004$).

The occurrence of hypotension among amiodarone recipients has been attributed to the presence of two excipients, polysorbate 80 and benzyl alcohol. Of interest, a recent study conducted by Somberg et al.[179] showed that a new formulation of amiodarone (Amio-Aqueous; Academic Pharmaceuticals, Lake Bluff, IL) had a similar risk of hypotension as lidocaine after VT termination (1% in both groups).

The ALIVE (Amiodarone Versus Lidocaine in Ventricular Ectopy, $n = 347$) trial directly compared IV amiodarone 300 mg to lidocaine 1- to 1.5-mg/kg bolus.[180] In this trial, patients needed to fail three stacked shocks and epinephrine plus an additional shock to be eligible for randomization to either amiodarone or lidocaine. Amiodarone was given as an initial dose of 5 mg/kg followed by a shock. If unsuccessful, a dose of 2.5 mg/kg was given followed by a subsequent shock. Lidocaine was given as a 1.5-mg/kg bolus followed by a shock. If therapy failed, then a second bolus of 1.5 mg/kg was used with a subsequent shock. If the first antiarrhythmic drug failed, other routine antiarrhythmic drugs for cardiac arrest (per 2000 ACLS guidelines; e.g., procainamide, bretylium) could be tried. Patients given amiodarone were 90% more likely to experience the primary outcome, survival to hospital admission, than those given lidocaine ($p = 0.009$). Unfortunately, no significant advantage to hospital discharge occurred (5% vs. 3%).

On the basis of these findings, amiodarone is the only antiarrhythmic agent with proven ability to improve return of spontaneous circulation and short-term survival versus other antiarrhythmic therapy. However, it has not yet been shown to improve survival to hospital discharge.[178,180] Lidocaine should be considered as an alternative to amiodarone for VF or pulseless VT patients who remain unresponsive to multiple shocks, epinephrine/vasopressin, and CPR. The dosing regimens of amiodarone and lidocaine for the treatment of VT or pulseless VF are highlighted in Table 19-7.

47. Amiodarone 300 mg followed by electrical defibrillation fails to cause a return of spontaneous circulation in M.N. A subsequent 150-mg dose also fails. However, M.N. did convert to normal sinus rhythm for 9 seconds before going back into VF. Should resuscitation be discontinued?

M.N. is at serious risk of death due to VF. However, as long as M.N. remains in VF, it is appropriate to continue active therapy. If M.N. degenerates into asystole after this long period of VF, then resuscitation efforts should be discontinued. However, if a patient only had a brief period of VF before having asystole, it is prudent to use the asystole algorithm and apply active therapy.

48. Because the patient is still in VF and had a brief period in sinus rhythm, a 1.5-mg/kg bolus of lidocaine is given. Is it necessary to give additional bolus doses or start a lidocaine infusion at this time?

In cardiac arrest, the movement of lidocaine from the initial volume of distribution to the total body volume of distribution is attenuated, and with a cardiac output of only 15% of normal with chest compressions, there is not enough liver perfusion to clear the lidocaine, making supplemental boluses or continuous infusion unnecessary while cardiac arrest continues. M.N. converts to sinus rhythm, and the rhythm holds. He is unconscious and has three broken ribs, and his mental functioning or long-term survival is not known at this time. M.N. is a candidate for two supplemental bolus doses (0.75 mg/kg) at 10-minute intervals now and for a continuous infusion of lidocaine at 30 to 50 mcg/kg/minute.

Pulseless Electrical Activity

49. J.D. is an 80-year-old woman who experiences cardiac arrest in the hospital. A rhythm is noted on the monitor, but no femoral pulse is felt. M.N. is in PEA. How should she be treated?

PEA is the clinical situation in which there is organized electrical activity on the monitor without a palpable pulse. Although electrical activity is present, it fails to stimulate the

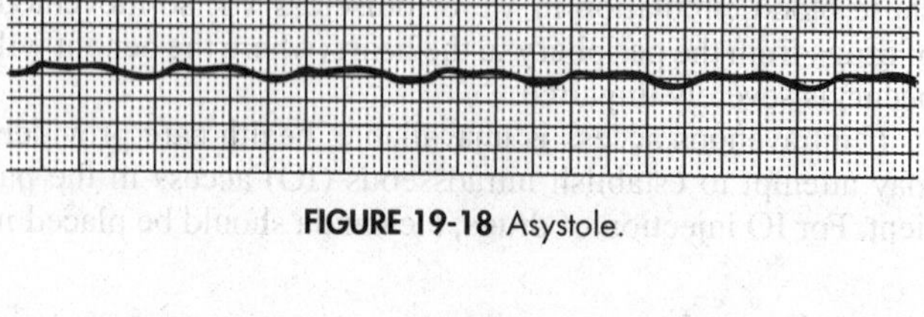

FIGURE 19-18 Asystole.

contractile process. Virtually all patients in true PEA die. However, not all patients who present with a rhythm and no pulse are in true PEA. Therefore, it is important to rule out treatable causes in patients who appear to be in PEA. The major treatable causes are hypovolemia, hypoxia, acidosis, hyperkalemia, hypokalemia, hypothermia, cardiac tamponade, pulmonary embolism, acute coronary syndrome, trauma, and drug overdose. In the absence of an identifiable cause, the focus of resuscitation is to administer high-quality CPR, and after the initial rhythm check, resume CPR during the establishment of IV/IO access.[173]

Once IV/IO access becomes available, administer epinephrine 1 mg every 3 to 5 minutes or give one dose of vasopressin 40 U in place of the first or second dose of epinephrine, because published studies have failed to demonstrate a survival advantage of either vasopressor for patients experiencing PEA.[173,175,176] In addition, although its efficacy has not been validated by prospective controlled studies, the current ACLS guidelines recommend the consideration of atropine as an adjunct to vasopressor treatment for patients in PEA. Atropine 1 g can be given every 3 to 5 minutes up to a maximum dose of 3 mg for persistent PEA. Figure 19-17 summarizes the sequence of interventions in PEA.

In establishing the diagnosis of PEA, two points should be made. First, the carotid artery is the preferred site to check for a pulse. A systolic pressure of 80 mmHg is required to generate a radial pulse, 70 mmHg for a femoral pulse, and 60 mmHg for a carotid pulse. A Doppler ultrasound can be used to more accurately determine if blood flow is present. Second, it may be useful to interrupt CPR and listen for heart sounds. The presence of sounds indicates that the heart valves are opening and closing and that contraction is occurring. Thus, one should intensify the search for a treatable cause. The absence of heart sounds does not confirm a lack of contraction.

Asystole

50. K.K. is a 73-year-old man who experiences cardiac arrest. The ECG shows a flat line, and the patient is determined to be in asystole (Fig. 19-18). Is this rhythm treatable?

Lack of electrical activity or asystole, such as PEA, carries a grave prognosis. Its development usually indicates a prolonged arrest, which may explain its poor response to treatment. However, a few patients will go directly from a sinus rhythm into asystole and may be resuscitated. Enhanced parasympathetic tone, possibly due to a vagal reaction, manipulation of the airway from intubation, suctioning or insertion of an oral airway, or chest compression, may play a role in inhibiting supraventricular and ventricular pacemakers. Therefore, anticholinergic or parasympathetic drugs that block vagal activity may be beneficial.

As described in case 45, a post-hoc analysis performed by Wenzel et al.[205] demonstrated superior survival rates at the time of hospital admission in vasopressin-treated patients, compared to epinephrine-treated patients. However, no difference in intact neurologic survival was noted between the two vasopressor treatment groups. Consequently providers may choose to administer vasopressin 40 IU IV (in place of a first or second dose of epinephrine) or epinephrine 1 mg IV every 3 to 5 minutes. Because of its vagolytic effects, atropine 1 mg IV may be repeated every 3 to 5 minutes or until a total of 3 mg has been administered. Figure 19-17 summarizes the sequence of interventions in patients with asystole.

The patient should be evaluated for adequate oxygenation and ventilation or the presence of severe metabolic imbalances. Electrical defibrillation to rule out fine VF may be attempted, but defibrillation of asystole is of no benefit. When VF and asystole are terminated, it is common for the patient to become hypotensive. Fluids and inotropic and vasopressor support are then warranted.

REFERENCES

1. Gereats PR, Kienzie MG. Atrial fibrillation and atrial flutter. *Clin Pharm* 1993;12:121.
2. Albers GW et al. Stroke prevention in nonvalvular atrial fibrillation. *Ann Intern Med* 1991;115:727.
3. Fuster V et al. ACC/AHA/ESC 2006 guidelines for the management of patients with atrial fibrillation: a report of the American College of Cardiology/American Heart Association Task Force on Practice Guidelines and the European Society of Cardiology Committee for Practice Guidelines (Writing Committee to Revise the 2001 Guidelines for the Management of Patients With Atrial Fibrillation). *Circulation* 2006;114:e257.
4. Roberts SA et al. Effectiveness and costs of digoxin treatment for atrial fibrillation and flutter. *Am J Cardiol* 1993;72:567.
5. Beasley R et al. Exercise heart rates at different serum digoxin concentrations in patients with atrial fibrillation. *Br Med J* 1985;290:9.
6. Farshi R et al. Ventricular rate control in chronic atrial fibrillation during daily activity and programmed exercise: a crossover open-label study of five drug regimens. *J Am Coll Cardiol* 1999;33:304.
7. Woodland C et al. The digoxin–propafenone interaction: characteristics of a mechanism using renal tubular cell monolayers. *J Pharmacol Exp Ther* 1997;283:39.
8. Fenster PE et al. Pharmacokinetic evaluation of the digoxin–amiodarone interaction. *J Am Coll Cardiol* 1985;5:108.
9. Freitag D et al. Digoxin–quinidine and digoxin–amiodarone interactions: frequency of occurrence and monitoring in Australian repatriation hospitals. *J Clin Pharm Ther* 1995;20:179.
10. Weiner P et al. Clinical course of acute atrial fibrillation treated with rapid digitalization. *Am Heart J* 1983;105:223.
11. White CM. Catecholamines and their blockade in congestive heart failure. *Am J Health Syst Pharm* 1998;55:676.
12. Ikram H et al. Therapeutic controversies with use of beta-adrenoceptor blockade in heart failure. *Am J Cardiol* 1993;71(Suppl C):54c.
13. Waxman HL et al. Verapamil for control of ventricular rate in paroxysmal supraventricular tachycardia and atrial fibrillation or flutter: a double-blind randomized cross-over study. *Ann Intern Med* 1981;94:1.
14. Hariman RJ et al. Reversal of the cardiovascular effects of verapamil by calcium and sodium: differences between electrophysiologic and hemodynamic response. *Circulation* 1979;59:797.
15. Lang J et al. Effect of gradual rise in plasma calcium concentration on the impairment of atrioventricular nodal conduction due to verapamil. *J Cardiovasc Pharmacol* 1986;8:6.
16. Salerno DM et al. Intravenous verapamil for treatment of multifocal atrial tachycardia with and without calcium pretreatment. *Ann Intern Med* 1987;107:623.
17. Pauli-Magnus C et al. Characterization of the major metabolites of verapamil as substrates and inhibitors of p-glycoprotein. *J Pharmacol Exp Ther* 2000;293:376.
18. Olshansky B et al. The atrial fibrillation follow-up investigation of rhythm management (AFFIRM) study. *J Am Coll Cardiol* 2004;43:1201.
19. Falk RH, Leavitt JF. Digoxin for atrial fibrillation: a drug whose time has gone? *Ann Intern Med* 1991;114:573.
20. Zarowitz BJ, Gheorghiade M. Optimal heart rate control for patients with chronic atrial fibrillation: are pharmacologic choices truly changing? *Am Heart J* 1992;123:1401.
21. Rawes JM. What is meant by a "controlled" ventricular rate in atrial fibrillation? *Br Heart J* 1990;63:157.
22. The Atrial Fibrillation Follow-up Investigation of Rhythm Management (AFFIRM) Investigators. A comparison of rate control and rhythm control in patients with atrial fibrillation. *N Engl J Med* 2002;347:1825.
23. Hohnloser SH et al. Rhythm versus rate control in atrial fibrillation—pharmacological intervention in atrial fibrillation (PIAF): a randomised trial. *Lancet* 2000;356:1789.

24. Van Gelder IC et al. Rate control vs. electrical cardioversion for persistent atrial fibrillation (RACE) study group. *N Engl J Med* 2002;347:1834.
25. Opolski G et al. Rate control vs rhythm control in patients with nonvalvular persistent atrial fibrillation: the results of the polish how to treat chronic atrial fibrillation (HOT CAFE) study. *Chest* 2004;126:476.
26. Marshall DA et al. Cost-effectiveness of rhythm versus rate control in atrial fibrillation. *Ann Intern Med* 2004;141:653.
27. Hagens VE et al. Effect of rate or rhythm control on quality of life in persistent atrial fibrillation: results from the RAte Control versus Electrical cardioversion (RACE) study. *J Am Coll Cardiol* 2004;43:241.
28. Hagens VE et al. Rate control is more cost-effective than rhythm control for patients with persistent atrial fibrillation—results from the RAte Control versus Electrical cardioversion (RACE) study. *Eur Heart J* 2004;25:1542.
29. de Divitiis et al. Right atrial appendage thrombosis in atrial fibrillation: its frequency and its clinical predictors. *J Am Coll Cardiol* 1999;34:1867.
30. Bjerkelund CJ, Oining OM. The efficacy of anticoagulant therapy in preventing embolism related to DC electrical conversion of atrial fibrillation. *Am J Cardiol* 1969;23:208.
31. Laupacis A et al. Antithrombotic therapy in atrial fibrillation. *Chest* 1992;102(suppl):426S.
32. Falk RH, Podrid PJ. Electrical cardioversion of atrial fibrillation. In: Falk RH, Podrid PJ, eds. *Atrial Fibrillation: Mechanisms and Management*. New York: Raven Press; 1992:181.
33. Oral H et al. Facilitating transthoracic cardioversion of atrial fibrillation with ibutilide pretreatment. *N Engl J Med* 1999;340:1849.
34. Dunn A et al. Efficacy and cost-analysis of ibutilide. *Ann Pharmacother* 2000;34:1233.
35. Kalus JS et al. Impact of prophylactic i.v. magnesium on the efficacy of ibutilide for conversion of atrial fibrillation or flutter. *Am J Health Syst Pharm* 2003;60:2308.
36. Fragakis N et al. Efficacy and safety of ibutilide for cardioversion of atrial flutter and fibrillation in patients receiving amiodarone or propafenone. *PACE* 2005;28:954.
37. Naccarelli GV et al. Electrophysiology and pharmacology of ibutilide. *Am J Cardiol* 1996;78(Suppl 8A):12.
38. Kowey PR, VanderLugt JR. Safety and risk/ benefit analysis of ibutilide for acute conversion of atrial fibrillation/flutter. *Am J Cardiol* 1996;78(Suppl 8A):46.
39. Boriani G et al. Oral propafenone to convert recent-onset atrial fibrillation in patients with and without underlying heart disease: a randomized, controlled trial. *Ann Intern Med* 1997;126:621.
40. Azpitarte J et al. Value of single oral loading dose of propafenone in converting recent-onset atrial fibrillation: results of a randomized, double-blind, controlled study. *Eur Heart J* 1997;18:1649.
41. Botto GL et al. Conversion of recent onset atrial fibrillation with single loading dose of propafenone: is hospital admission absolutely necessary? *PACE* 1996;19(pt II):1939.
42. Capucci A et al. Effectiveness of loading oral flecainide for converting recent onset atrial fibrillation to sinus rhythm in patients without organic heart disease or with only systemic hypertension. *Am J Cardiol* 1992;70:69.
43. Goy JJ et al. Restoration of sinus rhythm with flecainide in patients with atrial fibrillation. *Am J Cardiol* 1988;62:38D.
44. Keefe DL et al. Supraventricular tachyarrhythmias: their evaluation and therapy. *Am Heart J* 1986;111:1150.
45. Singh BN. Current antiarrhythmic drugs: an overview of mechanisms of action and potential clinical utility. *J Cardiovasc Electrophysiol* 1999;10:283.
46. Kalus JS, Mauro VF. Dofetilide: a class III–specific antiarrhythmic agent. *Ann Pharmacother* 2000;34:44.
47. Greenbaum RA et al. Conversion of atrial fibrillation and maintenance of sinus rhythm by dofetilide. The EMERALD (European and Australian Multicenter Evaluative Research on Atrial Fibrillation Dofetilide) study [abstract]. *Circulation* 1998;98(Suppl):I-633.
48. Singh S et al. Efficacy and safety of oral dofetilide in converting to and maintaining sinus rhythm in patients with chronic atrial fibrillation or atrial flutter. The Symptomatic Atrial Fibrillation Investigative REsearch on Dofetilide (SAFIRE-D) study. *Circulation* 2000;102:2385.
49. Torp-Pedersen C et al. Dofetilide in patients with congestive heart failure and left ventricular dysfunction. *N Engl J Med* 1999;341:857.
50. Kober L et al. Effect of dofetilide in patients with recent myocardial infarction and left ventricular dysfunction: a randomised trial. *Lancet* 2000;356:2052.
51. Song JC, White CM. Dofetilide (Tikosyn). *Conn Med* 2000;64:601.
52. Coplen SE et al. Efficacy and safety of quinidine therapy for maintenance of sinus rhythm after cardioversion: a meta-analysis of randomized control trials. *Circulation* 1990;82:1106.
53. Pietersen A et al. Usefulness of flecainide for prevention of paroxysmal atrial fibrillation and flutter. *Am J Cardiol* 1991;67:713.
54. Pritchett EL et al. Propafenone treatment of symptomatic paroxysmal supraventricular arrhythmias: a randomized placebo-controlled, crossover trial in patients tolerating oral therapy. *Ann Intern Med* 1990;114:539.
55. Porterfield JG, Porterfield JM. Therapeutic efficacy and safety of oral propafenone for atrial fibrillation. *Am J Cardiol* 1989;63:114.
56. Bolognesi R. The pharmacologic treatment of atrial fibrillation. *Cardiovasc Drug Ther* 1991;5:617.
57. The Flecainide And Propafenone Italian Study (FAPIS) Investigators. Safety of long-term flecainide and propafenone in the management of patients with symptomatic paroxysmal atrial fibrillation: report from the Flecainide And Propafenone Italian Study investigators. *Am J Cardiol* 1996; 77:60A.
58. Aliot E et al. Comparison of the safety and efficacy of flecainide versus propafenone in hospital outpatients with symptomatic paroxysmal atrial fibrillation/flutter. *Am J Cardiol* 1996;77:66A.
59. Lee SH et al. Comparisons of oral propafenone and quinidine as an initial treatment option in patients with symptomatic paroxysmal atrial fibrillation: a double-blind, randomized trial. *J Intern Med* 1996;239:253.
60. Kochiadakis GE et al. Sotalol versus propafenone for long-term maintenance of normal sinus rhythm in patients with recurrent symptomatic atrial fibrillation. *Am J Cardiol* 2004;94:1563.
61. Alboni P et al. Outpatient treatment of recent-onset atrial fibrillation with the "pill-in-the-pocket" approach. *N Engl J Med* 2004;351:2384.
62. Benditt DG et al. Maintenance of sinus rhythm with oral d,l-sotalol therapy in patients with symptomatic atrial fibrillation and/or atrial flutter. *Am J Cardiol* 1999;84:270.
63. Juul-Moller S et al. Sotalol vs. quinidine for the maintenance of sinus rhythm after direct current conversion of atrial fibrillation. *Circulation* 1990;82:1932.
64. Lee SH et al. Comparison of oral propafenone and sotalol as an initial treatment in patients with paroxysmal atrial fibrillation. *Am J Cardiol* 1997;79:905.
65. Vitolo E et al. Amiodarone vs quinidine in the prophylaxis of atrial fibrillation. *Acta Cardiol* 1981;26:431.
66. Gosselink ATM et al. Low-dose amiodarone for maintenance of sinus rhythm after cardioversion of atrial fibrillation or flutter. *JAMA* 1992;267: 3289.
67. Singh SN et al. Amiodarone in patients with congestive heart failure and symptomatic ventricular arrhythmia: survival trial of antiarrhythmic therapy in congestive heart failure. *N Engl J Med* 1995;333:77.
68. Singh BN et al, for the Sotalol Amiodarone Atrial Fibrillation Efficacy Trial (SAFE-T) Investigators. Amiodarone versus sotalol for atrial fibrillation. *N Engl J Med* 2005;352:1861.
69. Kochiadakis GE et al. Long-term maintenance of normal sinus rhythm in patients with current symptomatic atrial fibrillation: amiodarone vs propafenone, both in low doses. *Chest* 2004;125: 377.
70. Kalus JS et al. The impact of suppressing the renin-angiotensin system on atrial fibrillation. *J Clin Pharmacol* 2006;46:21.
71. Ozaydin M et al. Effect of atorvastatin on the recurrence rates of atrial fibrillation after electrical cardioversion. *Am J Cardiol* 2006;97:1490.
72. Pappone C et al. A randomized trial of circumferential pulmonary vein ablation versus antiarrhythmic drug therapy in paroxysmal atrial fibrillation. The APAF study. *J Am Coll Cardiol* 2006;48:2340.
73. Brass LM et al. Warfarin use among patients with atrial fibrillation. *Stroke* 1997;28:2382.
74. Stroke Prevention in Atrial Fibrillation (SPAF) Investigators. SPAF study: final results. *Circulation* 1991;84:527.
75. Stroke Prevention in Atrial Fibrillation Investigators. Warfarin vs. aspirin for prevention of thromboembolism in atrial fibrillation: Stroke Prevention in Atrial Fibrillation II study. *Lancet* 1994;343:687.
76. Petersen P et al. Placebo-controlled, randomized trial of warfarin and aspirin for prevention of thromboembolic complications in chronic atrial fibrillation. *Lancet* 1989;1:175.
77. Boston Area Anti-Coagulation Trial for Atrial Fibrillation Investigators. The effect of low-dose warfarin on the risk of stroke in patients with nonrheumatic atrial fibrillation. *N Engl J Med* 1990;323:1505.
78. Stroke Prevention in Atrial Fibrillation Investigators. Adjusted-dose warfarin versus low-intensity, fixed-dose warfarin plus aspirin for high-risk patients with atrial fibrillation: Stroke Prevention in Atrial Fibrillation III randomized clinical trial. *Lancet* 1996;348:633.
79. Sconce EA et al. The impact of CYP2C9 and VKORC1 genetic polymorphism and patient characteristics upon warfarin dose requirements: proposal for a new dosing regimen. *Blood* 2005;106: 2329.
80. Coleman CI et al. Impact of prophylactic postoperative beta-blockade on post-cardiothoracic surgery length of stay and atrial fibrillation. *Ann Pharmacother* 2004;38:2012.
81. Maisel WH et al. Atrial fibrillation after cardiac surgery. *Ann Intern Med* 2001;135:1061.
82. Kalus JS et al. Impact of fluid balance on incidence of atrial fibrillation after cardiothoracic surgery. *Am J Cardiol* 2004;94:1423.
83. DiDomenico RJ et al. Pharmacologic strategies for prevention of atrial fibrillation after open heart surgery. *Ann Thorac Surg* 2005;79:728.
84. Giri S et al. Oral amiodarone for the prevention of atrial fibrillation after open heart surgery, the Atrial Fibrillation Suppression Trial (AFIST): a randomized placebo-controlled trial. *Lancet* 2001;357: 830.
85. White CM et al. Intravenous plus oral amiodarone, atrial septal pacing, or both strategies to prevent post-cardiothoracic surgery atrial fibrillation: the Atrial Fibrillation Suppression Trial II (AFIST II) Circulation 2003;108[Suppl II]:200.
86. Rubin DA et al. Predictors, prevention and long-term prognosis of atrial fibrillation after CABG operation. *J Thorac Cardiovasc Surg* 1987;94: 331.
87. Salazar C et al. Beta-blockade therapy for supraventricular tachyarrhythmias after coronary surgery: a propranolol withdrawal syndrome? *Angiology* 1979;30:816.
88. Yilmaz AT et al. Long-term prevention of atrial fibrillation after coronary artery bypass surgery: comparison of quinidine, verapamil, and amiodarone in maintaining sinus rhythm. *J Cardiac Surg* 1996;11:61.

89. Sager PT. Narrow complex tachycardias: differential diagnosis and management. *Cardiol Clin* 1991;9:619.
90. Faulds D. Adenosine: an evaluation of its use in cardiac diagnostic procedures, and in the treatment of PSVT. *Drugs* 1991;41:596.
91. Garrat C et al. Comparison of adenosine and verapamil for termination of paroxysmal junctional tachycardia. *Am J Cardiol* 1989;64:1310.
92. Sung RJ et al. Mechanism of spontaneous alternation between reciprocating tachycardia and atrial flutter/fibrillation in the Wolff-Parkinson-White syndrome. *Circulation* 1977;56:409.
93. Gulamhusein S et al. Acceleration of the ventricular response during atrial fibrillation in the WPW syndrome after verapamil. *Circulation* 1982;65:348.
94. Falk RH. Proarrhythmia in patients treated for atrial fibrillation or flutter. *Ann Intern Med* 1992;117:141.
95. Gaita F et al. Wolff-Parkinson-White syndrome: identification and management. *Drugs* 1992;43:185.
96. Camm AJ et al. Effects of flecainide on atrial electrophysiology in the Wolff-Parkinson-White syndrome. *Am J Cardiol* 1992;70:33A.
97. O'Nunain S et al. A comparison of intravenous propafenone and flecainide in the treatment of tachycardias associated with the Wolff-Parkinson-White syndrome. *PACE* 1991;14(pt II):2028.
98. Chen X et al. Efficacy of ajmaline and propafenone in patients with accessory pathways: a prospective randomized study. *J Cardiovasc Pharmacol* 1994;24:664.
99. Auricchio A. Reversible protective effect of propafenone or flecainide during atrial fibrillation in patients with an accessory atrioventricular connection. *Am Heart J* 1992;124:932.
100. Mitchell LB et al. Electropharmacology of sotalol in patients with Wolff-Parkinson-White syndrome. *Circulation* 1987;76:810.
101. Feld GK et al. Clinical and electrophysiologic effects of amiodarone in patients with atrial fibrillation complicating the Wolff-Parkinson-White syndrome. *Am Heart J* 1988;115:102.
102. Kunze KP et al. Sotalol in patients with Wolff-Parkinson-White syndrome. *Circulation* 1987;75:1050.
103. Goldschlager N, Goldman MJ. Principles of Clinical Electrocardiography. Norwalk, CT: Appleton & Lange; 1989:74.
104. Zipes DP. Specific arrhythmias: diagnosis and treatment. In: Braunwald E, ed. *Heart Disease*. Philadelphia: WB Saunders; 1992:714.
105. The ESVEM Investigators. Determinants of predicted efficacy of antiarrhythmic drugs in the electrophysiologic study vs. electrocardiographic monitoring trial. *Circulation* 1993;87:323.
106. Tisdale JE et al. Efficacy of class 1C antiarrhythmic agents in patients with inducible ventricular tachycardia refractory to therapy with class 1A antiarrhythmic drugs. *J Clin Pharmacol* 1993;33:623.
107. Bleske BE et al. Acute effects of combination of 1B and 1C antiarrhythmics for the treatment of ventricular tachycardia. *J Clin Pharmacol* 1989;29:998.
108. Graboys TB et al. Long-term survival of patients with malignant ventricular arrhythmia treated with antiarrhythmic drugs. *Am J Cardiol* 1982;50:477.
109. Wilber DJ et al. Out-of-hospital cardiac arrest: use of electrophysiologic testing in the prediction of long-term outcome. *N Engl J Med* 1988;318:19.
110. Mason JW et al. A comparison of electrophysiologic testing with Holter monitoring to predict antiarrhythmic-drug efficacy for ventricular tachyarrhythmias. *N Engl J Med* 1993;329:445.
111. Waller TJ. Reduction in sudden death and total mortality by antiarrhythmic therapy evaluated by electrophysiologic drug testing: criteria of efficacy in patients with sustained ventricular tachyarrhythmia. *J Am Coll Cardiol* 1987;10:83.
112. Bigger JT et al. The relationships among ventricular arrhythmias, left ventricular dysfunction, and mortality in the 2 years after myocardial infarction. *Circulation* 1984;69:250.
113. Echt DS et al. Mortality and morbidity in patients receiving encainide, flecainide, or placebo. *N Engl J Med* 1991;324:781.
114. The Cardiac Arrhythmia Suppression Trial II Investigators. Effect of the antiarrhythmic agent moricizine on survival after myocardial infarction. *N Engl J Med* 1992;327:227.
115. β-blocker Heart Attack Research Group. A randomized trial of propranolol in patients with acute myocardial infarction. *JAMA* 1982;247:1707.
116. Lau J et al. Cumulative meta-analysis of therapeutic trials for myocardial infarction. *N Engl J Med* 1992;327:248.
117. Rogers WJ. Contemporary management of acute myocardial infarction. *Am J Med* 1995;99:195.
118. Herlitz J et al. Effect of metoprolol on the prognosis for patients with suspected acute myocardial infarction and indirect signs of congestive heart failure (a subgroup analysis of the Goteberg Metoprolol Trial). *Am J Cardiol* 1997;80:40J.
119. Julian DG et al. Controlled trial of sotalol for 1 year after myocardial infarction. *Lancet* 1982;82:1142.
120. Waldo AL et al. Preliminary mortality results from the Survival With ORal d-sotalol (SWORD) trial [abstract]. *J Am Coll Cardiol* 1995;20:15A.
121. Antman EM et al. ACC/AHA guidelines for the management of patients with ST-segment elevation myocardial infarction. *J Am Coll Cardiol* 2004;75:3.
122. Ceremuzynski L et al. Effect of amiodarone on mortality after myocardial infarction: a double-blind, placebo-controlled, pilot study. *J Am Coll Cardiol* 1992;20:1056.
123. Caims JA, for the Canadian Amiodarone Myocardial Infarction Arrhythmia Trial. Randomised trial of outcome after myocardial infarction in patients with frequent or repetitive ventricular premature depolarisations: CAMIAT. *Lancet* 1997;349:675.
124. Julian DG, for the European Myocardial Infarction Amiodarone Trial. Randomised trial of effect of amiodarone on mortality in patients with left-ventricular dysfunction after recent myocardial infarction: EMIAT. *Lancet* 1997;349:667.
125. Buxton AE, for the MUSTT Investigators. Nonsustained ventricular tachycardia in coronary artery disease: relation to inducible sustained ventricular tachycardia. *Ann Intern Med* 1996;125:35.
126. Pires LA, Huang SKS. Nonsustained ventricular tachycardia: identification and management of high-risk patients. *Am Heart J* 1993;126:189.
127. Friedman CM et al. Effect of propranolol in patients with myocardial infarction and ventricular arrhythmias. *J Am Coll Cardiol* 1986;7:1.
128. Winter ME. Lidocaine. In: Koda-Kimble MA, ed. *Basic Clinical Pharmacokinetics*. 3rd ed. Vancouver, WA: Applied Therapeutics; 1994:242.
129. Caron MF et al. Amiodarone in the new AHA guidelines for ventricular arrhythmias. *Ann Pharmacother* 2001;35:1248.
130. Lalka D et al. Lidocaine pharmacokinetics and metabolism in acute myocardial infarction patients. *Clin Res* 1980;28:329A.
131. Abernathy DR et al. Impairment of lidocaine clearance in elderly male subjects. *J Cardiovasc Pharmacol* 1983;5:1093.
132. Conrad KA et al. Lidocaine elimination: effects of metoprolol and of propranolol. *Clin Pharmacol Ther* 1983;33:133.
133. Pharand C et al. Prophylactic lidocaine for lethal ventricular arrhythmias following acute myocardial infarction: 8- vs. 48-hour infusion [abstract]. *J Am Coll Cardiol* 1993;21:451A.
134. Singh B. Electrophysiologic basis for the antiarrhythmic actions of sotalol and comparison with other agents. *Am J Cardiol* 1993;72:8A.
135. Gagnol JP et al. Amiodarone: biochemical aspects and haemodynamic effects. *Drugs* 1985;(suppl 3):1.
136. Wilson JS, Podrid PJ. Side effects from amiodarone. *Am Heart J* 1991;121:158.
137. Doval HC, for the Grupo de Estudio de la Sobrevida en la Insufficiencia en Argentina (GESICA). Randomised trial of low-dose amiodarone in severe congestive heart failure. *Lancet* 1994;344:493.
138. Burkart F et al. Effect of antiarrhythmic therapy on mortality in survivors of myocardial infarction with asymptomatic complex ventricular arrhythmias: Basel Antiarrhythmic Study of Infarct Survival (BASIS). *J Am Coll Cardiol* 1990;16:1711.
139. Tatro DS, ed. *Drug Interaction Facts*. St. Louis, MO: Facts and Comparisons, Inc.; 2003.
140. Nademanee K et al. Amiodarone–digoxin interaction: clinical significance, time course of development, potential pharmacokinetic mechanisms and therapeutic implications. *J Am Coll Cardiol* 1984;4:111.
141. Saksena S, Madan N. Management of the patient with an implantable cardioverter-defibrillator in the third millennium. *Circulation* 2002;106:2642.
142. Moss AJ et al. Improved survival with an implanted defibrillator in patients with coronary disease at high risk for ventricular arrhythmia. *N Engl J Med* 1996;335:1933.
143. Buxton AE et al. A randomized study of the prevention of sudden death in patients with coronary artery disease. *N Engl J Med* 1999;341:1882.
144. The Antiarrhythmics Versus Implantable Defibrillators (AVID) Investigators. A comparison of antiarrhythmic drug therapy with implantable defibrillators in patients resuscitated from near-fatal ventricular arrhythmias. *N Engl J Med* 1997;337:1576.
145. Moss AJ et al. Prophylactic implantation of a defibrillator in patients with myocardial infarction and reduced ejection fraction. *N Engl J Med* 2002;346:877.
146. Bednar MM et al. The QT interval. *Prog Cardiovasc Dis* 2001;43:1.
147. Tran H et al. An evaluation of the impact of gender and age on QT and QTc dispersion among normal individuals. *Ann Noninvasive Electrocardiol* 2001;6:129.
148. Darbar D et al. Pharmacogenetics of antiarrhythmic therapy. *Expert Opin Pharmacother* 2006;7:1583.
149. Daleau P et al. Erythromycin inhibition of potassium channels. *Circulation* 1992;86:1276.
150. Goodman JS, Peter CT. Proarrhythmia: primum non nocere. In: Mandel WJ, ed. *Cardiac Arrhythmias: Their Mechanisms, Diagnosis, and Management*. 3rd ed. Philadelphia: JB Lippincott; 1995:173.
151. Tran HT. Torsades de pointes induced by nonantiarrhythmic drugs. *Conn Med* 1994;58:291.
152. McBride BF. Focus on ranolazine. *Formulary* 2003;38:461.
153. Weiden PJ et al. Best clinical practice with ziprasidone: update after one year of clinical experience. *J Psych Pract* 2002;8:81.
154. Pratt CM et al. Risk of developing life-threatening ventricular arrhythmias associated with terfenadine in comparison with over-the-counter antihistamines, ibuprofen and clemastine. *Am J Cardiol* 1994;73:346.
155. Landrum-Michalets E. Update: clinically significant cytochrome P-450 drug interactions. *Pharmacotherapy* 1998;18:84.
156. Cupp MJ, Tracy TS. Role of the cytochrome P450 3A subfamily in drug interactions. *US Pharmacist* 1997;22:HS9.
157. Glassman AH, Bigger JT. Antipsychotic drugs: prolonged QTc interval, torsades de pointes, and sudden death. *Am J Psychiatry* 2001;158:1774.
158. Symanski JD, Gettes LS. Drug effects on the electrocardiogram: a review of their clinical importance. *Drugs* 1993;46:219.
159. Priori SG et al. Differential response to Na^+ channel blockade, beta-adrenergic stimulation, and rapid pacing in a cellular model mimicking the SCN5A and HERG defects in the long QT syndrome. *Circ Res* 1996;78:1009.
160. Napolitano C et al. Torsades de pointes: mechanisms and management. *Drugs* 1994;47:51.
161. Schwartz PJ et al. Long QT syndrome patients with mutations of the SCN5A and HERG genes have differential responses to Na^+ channel blockade and to increases in heart rate: implications for gene specific therapy. *Circulation* 1995;92:3381.

162. Miwa S et al. Monophasic action potentials in patients with torsades de pointes. *Jpn Circ J* 1994; 58:248.
163. Whalley DW et al. Basic concepts in cellular cardiac electrophysiology: part II: block of ion channels by antiarrhythmic drugs. *PACE* 1995;18: 1686.
164. Wang GX et al. Antiarrhythmic actions of taurine. *Adv Exp Med Biol* 1992;315:187.
165. Lehr D. A possible beneficial effect of selenium administration in antiarrhythmic therapy. *J Am Coll Nutr* 1994;13:496.
166. Grupo Italiano per lo Studio della Spravvivenza nell'Infarcto Miocardico Investigators. Dietary supplementation with omega-3 polyunsaturated fatty acids and vitamin E after myocardial infarction. *Lancet* 1999;354:447.
167. Albert CM et al. Blood levels of long-chain omega-3 fatty acids and the risk of sudden death. *N Engl J Med* 2002;346:1113.
168. Kris-Etherton PM et al. Fish consumption, fish oil, omega-3 fatty acids, and cardiovascular disease. *Circulation* 2002;106:2747.
169. Hays JV et al. Effect of magnesium sulfate on ventricular rate control in atrial fibrillation. *Ann Emerg Med* 1994;24:61.
170. Gullestad L et al. The effect of magnesium versus verapamil on supraventricular arrhythmias. *Clin Cardiol* 1993;16:429.
171. Brodsky MA et al. Magnesium therapy in new-onset atrial fibrillation. *Am J Cardiol* 1994;73: 1227.
172. Lewis RV et al. Oral magnesium reduces ventricular ectopy in digitalised patients with chronic atrial fibrillation. *Eur J Clin Pharmacol* 1990;38: 107.
173. Hazinski MF, et al. 2005 American Heart Association guidelines for cardiopulmonary resuscitation and emergency cardiovascular care. *Circulation* 2005;112:(24 Suppl 1).
174. Wenzel V et al. A comparison of vasopressin and epinephrine for out-of-hospital cardiopulmonary resuscitation. *N Engl J Med* 2004;350: 105.
175. Stiell IG et al. Vasopressin versus epinephrine for inhospital cardiac arrest: a randomized controlled trial. *Lancet* 2001;358:105.
176. Aung K et al. Vasopressin for cardiac arrest: a systematic review and meta-analysis. *Arch Intern Med* 2005;165:17.
177. Raehl CL. Endotracheal drug therapy in cardiopulmonary resuscitation. *Clin Pharm* 1986;5: 572.
178. Kudenchuk PJ et al. Amiodarone for resuscitation in out-of-hospital cardiac arrest due to ventricular fibrillation. *N Engl J Med* 1999;341:871.
179. Somberg JC et al. Lack of a hypotensive effect with rapid administration of a new aqueous formulation of intravenous amiodarone. *Am J Cardiol* 2004;93:576.
180. Dorian P et al. Amiodarone as compared with lidocaine for shock-resistant ventricular fibrillation. *N Engl J Med* 2002;346:884.

CHAPTER 20

Hypertensive Crises

Kelly Summers, Kristin Watson, Robert Michocki

The term *hypertensive crisis* is arbitrarily defined as a severe elevation in blood pressure (BP), generally considered to be a diastolic pressure >120 mmHg.[1] If these disorders are not treated promptly, a high rate of morbidity and mortality will ensue.[2] These disorders are divided into two general categories: *hypertensive emergencies* and *hypertensive urgencies* (Table 20-1).[3,4] Signs and symptoms of these disorders are nonspecific and may overlap. The distinction usually depends on the clinical assessment of the life-threatening nature of each episode. The term *hypertensive emergency* describes a clinical situation in which the elevated BP is immediately life threatening and needs to be lowered to a safe level (not necessarily to normal) within a matter of minutes to hours.[1,3] The level to which the BP is elevated does not in itself represent a true emergency. A *hypertensive urgency* is less acute and can be accelerated or even malignant. It is not immediately life threatening, and a reduction of BP to a safe level can occur more slowly over 24 to 48 hours.[1,5]

Hypertensive crises are usually characterized by an acute and marked elevation of arterial pressure, arteriolar spasm, necrotizing arteriolitis (necrosis in the media of the arterioles), and secondary organ damage. Hypertensive emergencies generally occur in patients with catecholamine producing adrenal tumors (pheochromocytoma), renal vascular disease, or accelerated essential hypertension. Acute life-threatening elevations of BP can also occur in previously normotensive individuals with acute glomerulonephritis, head injury, or severe burns; during pregnancy (eclampsia); and with use of recreational drugs such as cocaine, as well as from abrupt drug withdrawal, drug–drug interactions (including herbal medications), erythropoietin administration, or drug–food interactions (i.e., patients receiving monoamine oxidase inhibitors who ingest foods rich in tyramine).[6–8]

Rapid, severe BP elevation is not always the hallmark of a hypertensive emergency. Indeed, even moderate elevations of arterial pressure in the context of multiple disease states demand prompt treatment. Examples include acute left ventricular failure, intracranial hemorrhage, eclampsia, dissecting aortic aneurysm, and postoperative bleeding at suture sites.

Hypertensive emergencies rarely develop in previously normotensive patients.[9] Most commonly, they complicate the accelerated phase of poorly controlled, chronic hypertension.[1] In several studies of patients with hypertensive emergency, a history of hypertension was previously diagnosed in >90% of the patients, suggesting that hypertensive emergencies are almost entirely preventable.[9,10] Effective management of chronic hypertension has lowered the number of patients who present with hypertensive emergencies to <1%.[11] In a study on the prevalence of end organ complications in hypertensive crisis, central nervous system (CNS) abnormalities were the most frequently reported. Cerebral infarctions were noted in 24%, encephalopathy in 16%, and intracranial or subarachnoid hemorrhage in 4% of patients. CNS abnormalities were followed in incidence by cardiovascular complications, such as acute heart

Table 20-1 Hypertensive Emergencies Versus Urgencies

Emergencies	*Urgencies*
Severely elevated blood pressure (diastolic >120 mmHg)[a]	Severely elevated blood pressure (diastolic >120 mmHg)[a]
Potentially life threatening	Not life threatening
End organ damage present or high risk:	Minimal end-organ damage with no pending complications
CNS (dizziness, N/V, encephalopathy, confusion, weakness, intracranial or subarachnoid hemorrhage, stroke)	Accelerated malignant hypertension
Eyes (ocular hemorrhage or funduscopic changes, blurred vision, loss of sight)	Optic disc edema
Heart (left ventricular failure, pulmonary edema, MI, angina, aortic dissection)	Coronary artery disease
Renal failure/insufficiency	Post- or perioperative hypertension Pre- or post-kidney transplant
Pheochromocytoma crisis	
Drug-induced hypertensive crisis	
MAOI–tyramine interactions	
Overdose with PCP, cocaine, or LSD	
Drug interaction–induced hypertension	
Clonidine withdrawal	
Cocaine use	
Eclampsia (complicated pregnancy)	
Requires immediate pressure reduction	Treated over several h to d
Requires IV therapy (Table 20-2)	Oral therapy or slower-acting parenteral drugs preferred (Table 20-3)

[a]Degree of blood pressure elevation less diagnostic than rate of pressure rise and presence of concurrent diseases or end organ damage. See Chapter 13 for staging of hypertension.
CNS, central nervous system; IV, intravenous; LSD, lysergic acid diethylamide; MAOI, monoamine oxidase inhibitor; MI, myocardial infarction; N/V, nausea and vomiting; PCP, phencyclidine.

failure and pulmonary edema, which were seen in 36% of patients and acute myocardial infarction and unstable angina in 12% of patients. Acute dissection was noted in 2% and eclampsia in 4.5% of patients.[9]

However, even with effective therapy, the mortality for patients with a history of hypertensive crisis continues to be significant. Hypertensive emergencies occur more often in African Americans than in Caucasians, among patients who have no primary care physician, and among those who do not adhere to their treatment regimens.[9,12] In addition, systolic blood pressure control has been identified as an independent risk factor for the development of hypertensive crisis.[13]

ACCELERATED AND MALIGNANT HYPERTENSION

The terms *accelerated* and *malignant hypertension* have been used to describe severe hypertension accompanied by specific funduscopic changes.[4,14] Accelerated hypertension is characterized by the presence of retinal hemorrhages, exudates (yellow deposits within the retina due to leaks from capillaries and microaneurysms), and arteriolar narrowing and spasm. The incidence of accelerated hypertension among ambulatory patients is diminishing, and mortality from it is declining.[15] Malignant hypertension, an extension of the accelerated form, is remarkable for the presence of papilledema (edema of the optic nerve).[11] It occurs more commonly in middle-age hypertensive patients, with peak prevalence in the 40- to 60-year age range. If malignant hypertension occurs with no previous history of hypertension or in a patient who is younger than 30 or older than 60, a secondary cause should be suspected. Despite the funduscopic changes, the terms *accelerated* and *malignant* are often used synonymously. It is now also known that the clinical outcomes do not differ on the basis of funduscopic findings, suggesting that they are part of the same process.[15] Currently, these terms are used infrequently and have been replaced by terms such as "hypertensive crisis," "hypertensive emergency," and "hypertensive urgency."[16] Although hypertensive emergencies are much less common than hypertensive urgencies, without a thorough patient history it is often difficult to know whether end organ dysfunction is new or has progressed.

Signs and Symptoms

Symptoms associated with hypertensive crisis are highly variable and reflect the degree of damage to specific organ systems. The primary sites of damage are the CNS, heart, kidneys, and eyes.

Central Nervous System

CNS damage can present solely as a severe headache or may be accompanied by dizziness, nausea, vomiting, and anorexia. Headache (42%) and dizziness (30%) were the most frequently reported symptoms for emergency room patients diagnosed with hypertensive urgency.[17] Mental confusion with apprehension indicates more severe disease, as does nystagmus, localized weakness, or a positive Babinski sign (i.e., upward extension of the great toe and spreading of the smaller toes when moderate pressure is applied along a curve from the sole to the ball of the foot). CNS damage may be rapidly progressive, resulting in coma or death. If a cerebrovascular accident has occurred, slurred speech or motor paralysis may be present.

Other Complications

Cardiac complications of hypertensive crisis include heart failure (HF), acute pulmonary edema, angina pectoris, and acute coronary syndrome. Myocardial infarction (MI) can also be precipitated. Ocular symptoms of hypertensive crisis usually are related to changes in visual acuity. Complaints of blurred vision or loss of eyesight are often associated with funduscopic findings of hemorrhages, exudates, and occasionally papilledema. Renal complications include hematuria, proteinuria, pyelonephritis, and elevated serum blood urea nitrogen (BUN) and creatinine levels.

Principles of Treatment

Oral Versus Parenteral Therapy

An elevated BP in the absence of life-threatening signs or symptoms is not an indication for parenteral treatment. Oral antihypertensive regimens are more appropriate for the management of these urgent cases. Practitioners should exercise caution in the treatment of patients with elevated blood pressures in the absence of target organ damage. Aggressive dosing with oral medications to rapidly lower blood pressure is not without risk and can lead to hypotension and subsequent morbidity. Some have suggested that the term "hypertensive urgency" leads to overly aggressive treatment and should be discarded in favor of a less ominous term such as "uncontrolled" blood pressure.[5] In contrast, hypertensive emergencies require immediate hospitalization, generally in an intensive care unit, and the administration of parenteral antihypertensive medications to reduce arterial pressure.[18] Effective therapy greatly improves the prognosis, reverses symptoms, and arrests the progression of end organ damage. Treatment reverses the vascular changes in the eyes and slows or arrests the progressive deterioration in renal function. Treatment of malignant hypertension can transiently worsen renal function. However, after 2 to 3 months of adequate medical therapy, renal function may gradually improve to the premalignant level of renal insufficiency or to a new, slightly deteriorated level. The time required for recovery of renal function ranges from 2 weeks to 2 years. A low serum creatinine level, in the absence of marked cardiomegaly or renal shrinkage, has been associated with a good chance for recovery of renal function.[19] In patients with mild encephalopathy, neurologic symptoms resolve within 24 hours after treatment.[20] Resolution of papilledema occurs in 2 to 3 weeks, whereas funduscopic exudates can require up to 12 weeks for complete resolution.[21] Whether treatment can completely reverse end organ damage is related to two factors: how soon treatment is begun, and the extent of damage at the initiation of therapy.

There are two fundamental concepts in the management of hypertensive emergencies. First, immediate and intensive therapy is required and takes precedence over time-consuming diagnostic procedures. Second, the choice of drugs will depend on how their time course of action and hemodynamic and metabolic effects meet the needs of a crisis situation. If encephalopathy, acute left ventricular failure, dissecting aortic aneurysm, eclampsia, or other serious conditions are present, the BP should be lowered promptly with rapid-acting, parenteral antihypertensive medications such as diazoxide (Hyperstat), esmolol (Brevibloc), enalaprilat (Vasotec IV), fenoldopam (Corlopam), hydralazine (Apresoline), labetalol (Normodyne, Trandate), nicardipine (Cardene IV), nitroglycerin (Tridil, Nitrostat IV, Nitro-Bid IV), nitroprusside (Nipride), or trimethaphan (Arfonad) [1,3,4,11,22–24] (Table 20-2). If a slower BP reduction over several hours or days is acceptable, rapid-acting oral therapy using captopril (Capoten), clonidine (Catapres), prazosin (Minipress), labetalol, or minoxidil (Loniten) may be used [4,11,24–26] (Table 20-3). A summary of treatment recommendations for acutely lowering blood pressure for selected indications are listed in Table 20.4.

Goals of Therapy

The rate of BP lowering must be individualized because ischemic damage to the heart and brain can be provoked by a precipitous fall in BP.[26–30] Antihypertensive drugs should be used cautiously in patient groups at high risk for developing hypotensive complications, such as the elderly and patients with severely defective autoregulatory mechanisms. The latter group includes those with autonomic dysfunction or fixed sclerotic stenosis of cerebral or neck arteries.[31] In addition, patients who have chronically elevated BP are less likely to tolerate abrupt reductions in their BP, and the amount of reduction appropriate for those patients is somewhat less than for those whose BP is acutely elevated. In patients with hypertensive encephalopathy, cerebral hypoperfusion may occur if the mean BP is reduced by >40%.[32] Thus, it has been suggested that the mean pressure be lowered by no more than 20% to 30%.[32,33] For hypertensive emergencies, it is recommended that the mean arterial pressure be reduced initially by no more than 25% (within minutes to 1 hour), then if stable, this should be followed by further reduction toward a goal of 160/100 mmHg within 2 to 6 hours and gradual reduction to normal over the next 8 to 24 hours.[3] A diastolic pressure of 100 to 110 mmHg is an appropriate initial therapeutic goal.[1] Lower pressures may be indicated for patients with aortic dissection. Another exception to this rule applies in patients with acute cerebrovascular accidents. Cerebral autoregulation is disrupted in this setting and the use of antihypertensives may cause a reduction in cerebral blood flow and increasing morbidity. Current guidelines recommend lowering blood pressure following acute ischemic stroke in the presence of end organ damage if the blood pressure is >220/120 mmHg in patients ineligible for thrombolytic therapy or >185/110 mmHg in those who are candidates for thrombolytics.[34,35] Lower blood pressure in patients undergoing thrombolytic therapy reduces the risk of intracerebral bleeding.

HYPERTENSIVE URGENCIES

Patient Assessment

1. M.M. is a 60-year-old African American male with a long history of heart failure, poorly controlled hypertension believed to be due to nonadherence, and a history of MI. He was referred from a community health center this morning for a thorough evaluation of his elevated BP. He has not taken his captopril (Capoten), amlodipine (Norvasc), or hydrochlorothiazide for the past 7 days. M.M. is completely asymptomatic. Physical examination reveals a BP of 180/120 mmHg and a pulse of 92 beats/minute. Funduscopic examination is pertinent for mild arteriolar narrowing, without hemorrhages or exudates. The discs are flat. His lungs are clear, and the cardiac examination is unremarkable. The electrocardiogram (ECG) indicates normal sinus rhythm (NSR) at a rate of 90 beats/minute with first-degree atrioventricular (AV) block. The chest radiograph is interpreted as mild cardiomegaly. Serum electrolytes, BUN, and serum creatinine (SrCr) are within normal limits. A urinalysis (UA) is significant for 2+ proteinuria. What is the therapeutic objective in treating M.M.? How quickly should his BP be lowered, and what therapeutic options are available?

M.M. has stage II hypertension with a BP of 180/120 mmHg.[3] However, the absolute magnitude of BP elevation does not in itself constitute a medical emergency requiring an acute reduction in BP. There is no evidence of encephalopathy, cardiac decompensation, chest pain, or rapid change in renal function. Therefore, no evidence exists to indicate a rapid deterioration in the function of target organs.

As is often the case, M.M.'s lack of BP control is related to medication nonadherence. M.M.'s clinical presentation requires that his BP be lowered over the next several hours, while being careful not to induce hypotension. Rapid-acting oral agents can be used for this purpose; parenteral therapy is not warranted. A number of different oral regimens using clonidine, captopril, labetalol, prazosin, or minoxidil are available.

Table 20-2 Parenteral Drugs Commonly Used in the Treatment of Hypertensive Emergencies

Drug (Brand Name)	*Dose/Route*	*Onset of Action*	*Duration of Action*
Nitroprusside[a] (Nitropress) 50 mg/2 mL (most commonly used)	IV infusion[a] Start: 0.5 mcg/kg/min Usual: 2–5 mcg/kg/min Max: 8 mcg/kg/min	Sec	3–5 min after D/C infusion
Diazoxide (Hyperstat IV) 300 mg/20 mL	50–150 mg IV Q 5 min or as infusion of 7.5–30 mg/min[d]	1–5 min	4–12 hr
Enalaprilat[e] (Vasotec IV) 1.25 mg/mL 2.5 mg/2 mL	0.625–1.25 mg IV Q 6 hr	15 min (max, 1–4 hr)	6–12 hr
Esmolol[f] (Brevibloc) 100 mg/10 mL 2,500 mg/10 mL concentrate	250–500 mcg/kg over 1 minute then 50–300 mcg/kg/min	1–2 min	10–20 min
Fenoldopam (Corlopam) 10 mg/mL 20 mg/2 mL 50 mg/5 mL	0.1–0.3 mcg/kg/min	<5 min	30 min
Hydralazine[g] (generic) 20 mg/mL	10–20 mg IV	5–20 min	2–6 hr
Labetalol[h] (Normodyne) 20 mg/4 mL 40 mg/8 mL 100 mg/20 mL 200 mg/20 mL	2 mg/min IV or 20–80 mg Q 10 min up to 300 mg total dose	2–5 min	3–6 hr
Nicardipine[i] (Cardene IV) 25 mg/10 mL	IV loading dose 5 mg/hr increased by 2.5 mg/hr Q 5 min to desired BP or a max of 15 mg/hr Q 15 min, followed by maintenance infusion of 3 mg/hr	2–10 min (max, 8–12 hr)	40–60 min after D/C infusion
Nitroglycerin[j] (Tridil, Nitro-Bid IV, Nitro-Stat IV) 5 mg/mL 5 mg/10 mL 25 mg/5 mL 50 mg/10 mL 100 mg/20 mL	IV infusion pump 5–100 mcg/min	2–5 min	5–10 min after D/C infusion
Trimethaphan (Arfonad) 500 mg/10 mL	IV infusion pump 0.5–5 mg/min	1–5 min	10 min after D/C infusion
Phentolamine (Regitine)	1–5 mg IV initially, repeat as needed	Immediate	10–15 min

[a]Nitroprusside is the drug of choice for acute hypertensive emergencies. It is supplied as 50 mg of lyophilized powder that is reconstituted with 2–3 mL of 5% dextrose in water (D_5W), yielding a red-brown solution. The contents of the vial are added to 250, 500, or 1,000 mL of D_5W to produce a solution for IV administration at a concentration of 200, 100, or 50 mcg/mL, respectively. The container should be wrapped with metal foil to prevent light-induced decompensation. Under these conditions, the solution is stable for 4 to 24 hr. A rising BP may indicate loss of potency. A change in color to yellow does not indicate effectiveness. The appearance of a dark brown, green, or blue color indicates loss in activity. The drug is more effective if the head of the bed is slightly raised. When changing to a new bag, the administration rate may require adjustment.

[b]Thiocyanate levels rise gradually in proportion to the dose and duration of administration. The $t_{1/2}$ of thiocyanate is 2.7 days with normal renal function and 9 days in patients with renal failure. Toxicity occurs after 7–14 days in patients with normal renal function and 3–6 days in renal failure patients. Thiocyanate serum levels should be measured after 3–4 days of therapy, and the drug should be discontinued if levels exceed 10–12 mg/dL. Thiocyanate toxicity causes a neurotoxic syndrome of toxic psychosis, hyperreflexia, confusion, weakness, tinnitus, seizures, and coma.

[c]Signs of cyanide toxicity include lactic acidosis, hypoxemia, tachycardia, altered consciousness, seizures, and the smell of almonds on the breath. Concurrent administration of sodium thiosulfate or hydroxocobalamin may reduce the risk of cyanide toxicity in high-risk patients.

[d]Diazoxide is administered as a bolus dose (13 mg/kg Q 5 min to a max of 150 mg/injection) or as a slow infusion (15–20 mg/min) until a diastolic pressure of 100 mmHg is reached. Significant fluid retention following diazoxide can cause HF and pulmonary edema. Concurrent loop diuretics are recommended (e.g., furosemide 40 mg IV) if diazoxide is given by rapid IV bolus. Reflex in heart rate and stroke volume are potentially dangerous in patients with angina or MI. Concurrent β-blockers may be protective.

[e]Not approved by the U.S. Food and Drug Administration for treatment of acute hypertension.

[f]Approved for intraoperative and postoperative treatment of hypertension.

[g]Parenteral hydralazine is an intermediate treatment between oral agents and more aggressive therapies such as nitroprusside or diazoxide. It can be given IV or intramuscularly, but there is no appreciable difference in onset of action (20–40 min) between the two routes. This slow onset minimizes hypotension.

[h]Labetalol is contraindicated in acute decompensated HF due to its β-blocking properties. A solution for continuous infusion is prepared by adding two 100-mg ampules to 160 mL of IV fluid to give a final concentration of 1 mg/mL. Infusions start at 2 mg/min and are titrated until a satisfactory response or a cumulative dose of 300 mg is achieved.

[i]Indicated for short-term treatment of hypertension when the oral route is not feasible or desirable.

[j]Requires special delivery system due to drug binding to PVC tubing. Also see Chapters 16 and 17 for further information regarding nitroglycerin.

ACE, angiotensin-converting enzyme; BP, blood pressure; Ca, calcium; D/C, discontinued; HF, heart failure; IV, intravenous; MI, myocardial infarction; Na, sodium; Q, every.

Major Side Effects (All Can Cause Hypotension)	Mechanism of Action	Avoid or Use Cautiously in Patients with These Conditions
Nausea, vomiting, diaphoresis, weakness, thiocyanate toxicity,[b] cyanide toxicity (rare)[c]	Arterial and venous vasodilator	Renal failure (thiocyanate accumulation), pregnancy, increased intracranial pressure
Hyperglycemia, Na retention,[d] tachycardia, painful extravasation	Arterial vasodilator	Angina pectoris, MI, aortic dissection, pulmonary edema, intracranial hemorrhage
Hyperkalemia	ACE inhibitor	Hyperkalemia, renal failure in patients with dehydration or bilateral renal artery stenosis, pregnancy (teratogenic)
Nausea, thrombophlebitis, painful extravasation	β-adrenergic blocker	Asthma, bradycardia, decompensated HF, advanced heart block
Tachycardia, headache, nausea, flushing	Dopamine-1 agonist	Glaucoma
Tachycardia, headache, angina	Arterial vasodilator	Angina pectoris, MI, aortic dissection
Abdominal pain, nausea, vomiting, diarrhea	α- and β-adrenergic blocker	Asthma, bradycardia, decompensated HF
Headache, flushing, nausea, vomiting, dizziness, tachycardia; local thrombophlebitis change infusion site after 12 hr	Arterial vasodilator (Ca channel blocker)	Angina, decompensated HF, increased intracranial pressure
Methemoglobinemia, headache, tachycardia, nausea, vomiting, flushing, tolerance with prolonged use	Arterial and venous vasodilator	Pericardial tamponade, constrictive pericarditis, or increased intracranial pressure
Tachyphylaxis, ileus, constipation, urinary retention, pupillary dilation	Ganglionic blocker	Postoperative glaucoma
Chest pain, nausea, vomiting, dizziness, headache, nasal congestion, arrhythmia	α-adrenergic blocker	Angina, coronary insufficiency, MI or history of MI, hypersensitivity to mannitol

In M.M., restarting his medications in a controlled manner so as not to drop his BP too rapidly may also be a reasonable option for treatment. Later, he can be converted to a regimen designed to enhance outpatient compliance by selecting medications with once-daily dosing. For example, lisinopril or another long-acting angiotensin-converting enzyme (ACE) inhibitor would be preferred for outpatient maintenance instead of the captopril previously prescribed. Good patient counseling will help M.M. better understand the severity of his disease and the need to take his medications. Timely follow-up within several days following treatment of hypertensive urgency is of paramount importance for the appropriate management of these patients.

Oral Drug Therapy

Rapidly Acting Calcium Channel Blockers

2. M.M.'s physician has ordered nifedipine to be given 10 mg sublingually. Is this appropriate therapy to acutely lower his BP?

Clonidine, labetalol, prazosin, minoxidil, and captopril have all been used to lower BP acutely. These oral agents take several hours to adequately lower pressure and are therefore useful in treating hypertensive urgencies but not emergencies. Oral ACE inhibitors, other than captopril, are not useful for acutely lowering BP because their onset of action is too slow. The immediate-release calcium channel blockers, including diltiazem, verapamil, and nicardipine, can rapidly lower BP; however, the most extensive experience is with nifedipine. Nifedipine, when given orally or by the "bite and swallow" method, was previously recommended as a rapid-acting alternative to parenteral therapy in the acute management of hypertension. However, its use has been associated with life-threatening adverse events due to ischemia, MI, and stroke.[26–30] The prompt absorption of rapidly acting calcium channel blockers is followed by a sudden and precipitous decrease in BP as a result of peripheral vasodilation. This reduces coronary perfusion, induces a reflex tachycardia, and increases myocardial oxygen consumption.[28,36] Decreased cerebral blood flow with sublingual nifedipine has also been reported.[37] Elderly patients with underlying coronary or

Table 20-3 Oral Drugs Commonly Used in the Treatment of Hypertensive Urgencies

Drug (Brand Name)	Dose/Route	Onset of Action	Duration of Action	Major Side Effects[a]	Mechanism of Action	Avoid or Use Cautiously in Patients With These Conditions
Captopril[b] (Capoten) 12.5-, 25-, 50-, 100-mg tablets	6.5–50 mg PO	15 min	4–6 hr	Hyperkalemia, angioedema, BUN if dehydrated, rash, pruritus, proteinuria, loss of taste	ACE inhibitor	Renal artery stenosis, hyperkalemia, dehydration, renal failure, pregnancy
Clonidine (Catapres) 0.1-, 0.2-, 0.3-mg tablets	0.1–0.2 mg PO initially, then 0.1 mg/hr up to 0.8 mg total	0.5–2 hr	6–8 hr	Sedation, dry mouth, constipation	Central α-2-agonist	Altered mental status, severe carotid artery stenosis
Labetalol (Normodyne, Trandate) 100-, 200-, 300-mg tablets	200–400 mg PO repeated Q 2–3 hr	30 min –2 hr	4 hr	Orthostatic hypotension, nausea, vomiting	α- and β-adrenergic blocker	Heart failure, asthma, bradycardia
Minoxidil (Loniten) 2.5-, 10-mg tablets	5–20 mg PO	30–60 min; maximum response in 2–4 hr	12–16 hr	Tachycardia, fluid retention	Arterial and venous vasodilator	Angina, heart failure

[a] All may cause hypotension, dizziness, and flushing.
[b] Other oral ACE inhibitors too slow in onset to be useful but can be used for maintenance.
ACE, angiotensin-converting enzyme; ↑BUN, blood urea nitrogen; PO, orally.

cerebrovascular disease, volume depletion, or concurrent use of other antihypertensive drugs are at increased risk for significant adverse events. In addition, no outcome data are currently available to critically assess the efficacy of this therapeutic intervention. Therefore, until more data become available, administration of immediate-release nifedipine capsules or other rapidly acting calcium channel blockers sublingually, by the "bite and chew" method, or by swallowing intact is not recommended.

The cavalier use of rapid-release nifedipine to acutely lower BP is potentially dangerous and should be discouraged in M.M. His age, history of MI, absence of symptoms, and lack of new or progressive target organ damage do not warrant the acute and potentially dangerous drop in BP. M.M.'s BP can be managed

Table 20-4 Treatment Recommendations for Hypertensive Crises

Clinical Presentation	Recommendation	Rationale
Aortic dissection	Nitroprusside, nicardipine, or fenoldopam plus esmolol or IV metoprolol; labetalol; trimethaphan. Avoid inotropic therapy.	Vasodilator will decrease pulsatile stress in aortic vessel to prevent further dissection expansion. β-blockers will prevent vasodilator-induced reflex tachycardia.
Angina, myocardial infarction	Nitroglycerin plus esmolol or metoprolol; labetalol. Avoid nitroprusside.	Coronary vasodilation, decreased cardiac output, myocardial workload, and oxygen demand. Nitroprusside may cause coronary steal.
Acute pulmonary edema, left ventricular failure	Nitroprusside, nicardipine, or fenoldopam plus nitroglycerin and a loop diuretic. Alternative: enalaprilat. Avoid nondihydropyridines, β-blockers.	Promotion of diuresis with venous dilatation to decrease preload. Nitroprusside, enalaprilat decrease afterload. Nicardipine may increase stroke volume.
Acute renal failure	Nicardipine or fenoldopam. Avoid nitroprusside, enalaprilat.	Peripheral vasodilation without renal clearance. Fenoldopam shown to increase renal blood flow.
Cocaine overdose	Nicardipine, fenoldopam, verapamil, or nitroglycerin. Alternative: labetalol. Avoid β-selective blockers.	Vasodilation effects without potential unopposed α-adrenergic receptor stimulation. CCBs control overdose-induced vasospasm.
Pheochromocytoma	Nicardipine, fenoldopam, or verapamil. Alternatives: phentolamine, labetalol. Avoid β-selective blockers.	Vasodilation effects without potential unopposed α-adrenergic receptor stimulation.
Hypertensive encephalopathy, intracranial hemorrhage, subarachnoid hemorrhage, thrombotic stroke	Nicardipine, fenoldopam, or labetalol. Avoid nitroprusside, nitroglycerin, enalaprilat, hydralazine.	Vasodilation effects without compromised CBF induced by nitroprusside and nitroglycerin. Enalaprilat and hydralazine may lead to unpredictable BP changes when carefully controlled BP management is required.

BP, blood pressure; CBF, cerebral blood flow; CCB, calcium channel blocker; IV, intravenous.

safely using other oral medications. Captopril, labetalol, or clonidine can be used to lower his BP, and he can be restarted on his oral maintenance regimen with appropriate follow-up care.

Clonidine

3. A decision is made not to use nifedipine, but rather to give M.M. oral clonidine. What is an appropriate starting dose? What is the correlation between the loading dose and the maintenance dose?

Clonidine is considered a safe, effective first-line therapy for hypertensive urgency. It is a centrally acting, α_2-adrenergic agonist that inhibits sympathetic outflow from the CNS. After acute administration, clonidine reduces mean arterial pressure, cardiac output, stroke volume, and cardiac rate. There is little change in the total peripheral resistance or renal plasma flow. The initial reduction in cardiac output is caused by decreased venous return to the right side of the heart secondary to venodilation and bradycardia, not secondary to decreased contractility. Guanabenz (Wytensin) has a similar mechanism of action, but documented efficacy in the acute treatment of hypertension is lacking.

BP can be lowered gradually over several hours using oral clonidine. Traditional dosing regimens have included an initial oral loading dose (0.1–0.2 mg) followed by repeated doses of 0.1 mg/hour until the desired response is achieved or until a cumulative dose of 0.5 to 0.8 mg is reached.[38] A significant reduction in BP is first seen within 1 hour, and the mean arterial pressure decreases by 25% in most patients after several hours. Anderson et al. reported a 94% response rate to an oral loading dose.[38] Patients required a mean total dose of 0.45 mg, and the maximum response occurred 5 to 6 hours after the start of therapy. Some authors, however, have cautioned against the use of sequential loading doses, citing lack of benefit over placebo and the potential for unpredictable adverse effects, particularly abrupt occurrences of hypotension.[39] If loading doses are to be used, it is especially important to reduce doses in patients with volume depletion, those who have recently used other antihypertensive drugs, and the elderly.[1,23,40]

The acute response to oral clonidine loading is not predictive of the daily dose required to maintain acceptable BP control. Maintenance oral therapy with clonidine is somewhat empiric; however, total daily doses should be spread between twice and three times daily dosing due to the drug's short half-life. The major portion of the total daily dose can be given at bedtime to minimize daytime sedation.

ADVERSE EFFECTS AND PRECAUTIONS

4. What precautions should be exercised when using the oral clonidine loading regimen?

Oral clonidine is generally well tolerated. Adverse effects include orthostatic hypotension, bradycardia, sedation, dry mouth, and dizziness. Sedation is a particularly troublesome side effect, and because of this, clonidine should not be used in patients in whom mental status is an important monitoring parameter. Because clonidine can decrease cerebral blood flow by up to 28%, it should not be used in patients with severe cerebrovascular disease.[22,41] Clonidine also should be avoided in patients with HF, bradycardia, sick sinus syndrome, or cardiac conduction defects,[23] as well as patients at risk for medication nonadherence because of the rapid rise in BP that can occur with sudden drug withdrawal.[42,43]

Other Oral Drugs

CAPTOPRIL

5. M.M. has a history of heart failure and normal renal function on admission. Based on these findings, would captopril be a reasonable choice for initial treatment? How should it be given? What if his BUN or SrCr were elevated?

Captopril, an orally active ACE inhibitor, has been used both orally and sublingually to acutely lower BP.[44,45] Captopril decreases both afterload and preload, increases regional blood flow, and lowers total peripheral vascular resistance.[23] For this reason, captopril and other ACE inhibitors are often considered the drugs of choice in patients with heart failure. (See Chapter 18 for a discussion of the use of ACE inhibitors in heart failure.) Given that M.M. appeared to be well controlled on his ACE inhibitor prior to arbitrarily stopping his medications, it is reasonable to restart an ACE inhibitor and reinforce medication adherence issues.

After oral administration, the onset of action of captopril occurs within minutes and peaks 30 to 90 minutes after ingestion. Sublingual captopril (25 mg) significantly reduces angiotensin II levels within 24 hours.[46] Sublingual captopril also has been recently reported to increase cerebral blood flow to a greater extent in patients with BP >180/120 mmHg compared to nifedipine.[37] Clinically, it reduces BP within 10 to 15 minutes, with effects persisting for 2 to 6 hours. Sublingual captopril is as effective as nifedipine in acutely reducing mean arterial pressure in both urgent and emergent conditions.[45,47,48]

Despite these beneficial effects, captopril, as well as all other ACE inhibitors, must be used with caution in patients with renal insufficiency or volume depletion. In most cases, an elevated BUN or SrCr will provide a clue to the existence of these conditions; however, captopril can also induce severe renal failure in patients with bilateral renal artery stenosis or renal artery stenosis in a solitary kidney. Such conditions may not be easy to detect in the context of an acute hypertensive emergency. Therefore, in patients in whom these conditions can be excluded, captopril can be considered for therapy. First-dose hypotension is a common limiting factor with captopril use. This complication is most likely to occur in patients with high renin levels, such as those who are volume depleted or those receiving diuretics. Under these circumstances, initial doses should not exceed 12.5 mg, with repeat doses an hour or more later if necessary. Although he was not taking his diuretic, M.M. is still likely to have high renin levels due to his history of HF. Therefore, captopril would be a reasonable choice as initial therapy in M.M., which can later be replaced by a longer-acting ACE inhibitor.

MINOXIDIL, PRAZOSIN, AND LABETALOL

6. What other oral agents are used to acutely lower BP?

Minoxidil, a potent oral vasodilator, has been used successfully in the treatment of severe hypertension.[49,50] An oral loading dose of 10 to 20 mg produces a maximal BP response in 2 to 4 hours and can be followed by a dose of 5 to 20 mg every 4 hours if necessary. Unfortunately, its onset of action is slower than that of clonidine or captopril. Another complicating factor is that β-blockers and loop diuretics generally must be used concomitantly to counteract minoxidil-induced reflex tachycardia and fluid retention.[50] Therefore, minoxidil should be used only in patients who are refractory to other forms of therapy or who have previously been taking this agent.

Prazosin has been used to a limited degree to treat hypertensive urgencies. An oral loading dose of 5 mg maximally reduced BP within 60 to 120 minutes.[51] However, hypotension can be a significant limiting factor. More controlled studies are required before this drug can be recommended.

Oral labetalol, a combined α- and β-receptor antagonist, is an alternative to oral clonidine or captopril for the treatment of severe hypertension, but the most appropriate dosing regimen remains to be determined.[52–55] Initial doses of 100 to 300 mg may provide a sustained response for up to 4 hours.[53] Labetalol (200 mg given at hourly intervals to a maximum dose of 1,200 mg) was comparable to oral clonidine in reducing mean arterial pressure.[55] An alternative regimen using 300 mg initially followed by 100 mg at 2-hour intervals to a maximum of 500 mg was also successful in acutely lowering BP.[54] However, Wright et al.[56] were unable to achieve an adequate BP response in a small series of patients using a single loading dose of 200 to 400 mg. Because labetalol can cause profound orthostatic hypotension, patients should remain in the supine position and should be checked for orthostasis before ambulation. In addition, labetalol should be avoided in patients with asthma, bradycardia, or advanced heart block.

Following initial treatment with oral captopril, M.M.'s BP was reduced to 150/100 mmHg. His oral medications were then restarted, captopril was switched to lisinopril, and he was scheduled for follow-up in 1 week.

HYPERTENSIVE EMERGENCIES

Patient Assessment

7. M.R., a 55-year-old African American male, presents to the emergency department (ED) with a 3-day history of progressively increasing shortness of breath (SOB). Over the past 2 days, he developed a severe headache unrelieved by ibuprofen (Advil), as well as substernal chest pain, anorexia, and nausea. His medical history includes asthma and a 5-year history of angina, which resulted in hospitalization for an acute inferior MI 2 months before admission. He has been taking albuterol via metered-dose inhaler (MDI; Proventil, Ventolin), furosemide (Lasix), isosorbide dinitrate (Isordil Titradose, Sorbitrate), felodipine (Plendil), and lisinopril (Prinivil, Zestril), but discontinued these medications on his own 3 weeks ago.

Physical examination reveals an anxious-appearing man who is alert, oriented, and in moderate respiratory distress. His vital signs include a pulse of 125 beats/minute, respiratory rate of 36 breaths/minute, BP of 220/145 mmHg without orthostasis, and a normal body temperature. Funduscopic examination shows arteriolar narrowing and AV nicking without hemorrhages, exudates, or papilledema. There is no jugular venous distention, but bilateral carotid bruits are present. Chest examination reveals decreased breath sounds with bilateral rales extending to the tip of the scapula. M.R.'s heart is displaced 2 cm left of the midclavicular line with no thrills or heaves. The rhythm is regular with an S_3 and an S_4 gallop; no murmurs are noted. The remainder of M.R.'s examination is within normal limits.

Significant laboratory values include sodium (Na), 142 mEq/L (normal 136–144); potassium (K), 4.9 mEq/L (normal 3.5–5.5); chloride (Cl), 101 mEq/L (normal 96–106); bicarbonate, 23 mEq/L (normal 23–28); BUN, 30 mg/dL (normal 10–20); creatinine, 1.2 mg/dL (normal 0.5–1.2); hematocrit (Hct), 38% (normal 40%–45%); hemoglobin (Hgb), 13 g/dL (normal 14–18); and white blood cell (WBC) count and differential, within normal limits. UA shows 1+ hemoglobin and 1+ protein. Microscopic examination of the urine reveals 5 to 10 red blood cells (RBCs) per high-power field (HPF) and no casts. Pulse oximetry reveals an oxygen saturation of 88%. An ECG demonstrates sinus tachycardia and left ventricular hypertrophy. The chest radiograph shows moderate cardiomegaly and bilateral fluffy infiltrates.

What aspects of M.R.'s history and physical examination are characteristic of an emergent need to immediately lower his BP?

[SI units: Na, 142 mmol/L (normal 136–144); K, 4.9 mmol/L (normal 3.5–5.5); Cl, 101 mmol/L (normal 96–106); bicarbonate, 23 mmol/L (normal 23–28); BUN, 10.71 mmol/L urea (normal 3.57–7.14); creatinine, 106 mmol/L (normal 44.2–106.08); Hct, 0.38 (normal 0.40–0.45); Hgb, 130 g/L (normal 140–180)]

As discussed previously, hypertensive crisis occurs most often in African American men and individuals between the ages of 40 and 60. M.R. meets all characteristics of this population. Furthermore, many patients who present with hypertensive emergencies have a recent history of discontinuing the use of their antihypertensives,[9,12] as is the case with M.R and M.M. in case 1.

Recent-onset severe headache, nausea, and vomiting are consistent with CNS signs of severe hypertension, as are the acute onset of angina (substernal pain) and HF (SOB, increased pulse and respiratory rate, cardiomegaly, S_3, and chest x-ray findings of pulmonary edema). The absence of signs of right-sided HF such as jugular venous distention or hepatomegaly suggests an acute onset of HF caused by hypertension as opposed to a gradual worsening of chronic HF. M.R.'s urinary sediment is relatively unimpressive at this time, especially in light of his history, and his ocular complications are minimal.

Parenteral Drug Therapy

Nitroprusside

8. M.R. is to be started on nitroprusside. Is this an appropriate choice of drug? What alternatives to nitroprusside are available?

M.R.'s arterial pressure should be lowered with parenteral medications, which have a rapid onset of action. Nitroprusside, fenoldopam, intravenous (IV) nitroglycerin, and trimethaphan all decrease total peripheral resistance rapidly with minimal effect on myocardial oxygen consumption and heart rate. Of these agents, either nitroprusside or fenoldopam would be preferred in patients with hypertension accompanied by acute left ventricular failure in the absence of MI. Parenteral nitroglycerin is similar to nitroprusside except that it has relatively greater effect on venous circulation and less effect on arterioles. It is most useful in patients with coronary insufficiency, ischemic heart disease, MI, or hypertension following coronary bypass surgery (also see question 24). In addition, nitroprusside and IV nitroglycerin may both improve elevated left ventricular diastolic pressures in patients presenting with hypertensive urgency. Trimethaphan is not an acceptable choice because rapid tolerance develops to its hypotensive action and its use is associated with many side effects (see Question 29). Fenoldopam and nitroprusside are equally efficacious in acutely lowering BP.[57–60] Both drugs have an immediate onset, are easily titratable, have a short duration of action, and are relatively well tolerated. Fenoldopam may also increase renal blood flow, thereby reducing the risk for worsening renal function.[61–64] Unlike nitroprusside, fenoldopam does not cause cyanide or thiocyanate toxicity, but it is considerably more expensive than nitroprusside.

Therefore, in the absence of any significant renal or liver disease, nitroprusside is the preferred treatment for M.R.

HEMODYNAMIC EFFECTS

Nitroprusside has many pharmacologic effects that should improve M.R.'s condition. It dilates both venous and arterial vessels, thereby increasing venous capacitance and decreasing the venous return or preload on the heart (see Chapters 18 and 21). A decrease in the pulmonary capillary wedge pressure and ventricular filling pressure will ultimately improve M.R.'s pulmonary edema. Afterload is also decreased as a result of arterial dilation. This action increases cardiac output, reduces arterial pressure, and increases tissue perfusion.

CONCURRENT USE OF DIURETICS

9. Should M.R. be given a diuretic before nitroprusside therapy is begun?

Administration of potent IV diuretics is relatively ineffective in the acute treatment of hypertension except in patients with concomitant volume overload or HF. Many patients with hypertensive emergencies are vasoconstricted and have normal or reduced plasma volumes; therefore, diuretics have little effect and may actually aggravate renal failure or cause other adverse effects.[19,65] Furthermore, when diuretics are given acutely in combination with other antihypertensive agents, profound hypotension can occur.

The immediate value of diuretics in acute HF is related more to their hemodynamic effects (venodilation) than to diuresis. Venodilation following IV diuretic administration decreases right-sided cardiac filling pressures, decreases pulmonary artery and wedge pressures, and increases cardiac output before diuresis occurs.[66] The presence of HF and severely elevated BP in M.R. warrants the IV administration of either furosemide 20 to 40 mg or bumetanide (Bumex) 1 mg.

DOSING AND ADMINISTRATION

10. How should nitroprusside be prepared and administered? What dose should be used initially?

Because of its extreme potency, sodium nitroprusside must be prepared in exact concentrations and administered at precisely calculated rates using a controlled infusion device, and BP must be closely monitored. Sodium nitroprusside is supplied in units of 50 mg of lyophilized powder. The powder is reconstituted with 2 to 3 mL of 5% dextrose in water (D_5W), shaking gently to dissolve.[67] The contents of the vial are then added to 250, 500, or 1,000 mL of D_5W to produce a solution for IV administration with a drug concentration containing 200, 100, or 50 mcg/mL. This solution should have a slight brownish tint.

Nitroprusside decomposes on exposure to light, so the solution should be shielded with an opaque sleeve. It is not necessary to protect the tubing from light. Reconstituted solutions are stable for 24 hours at room temperature. A change in the solution's color from light brown to dark brown, green, orange, or blue indicates a loss in activity, and the solution should be discarded.

Effective infusion rates range from 0.25 to 10 mcg/kg/minute. Cyanide toxicity may occur with prolonged administration or with infusion rates >2 to 3 mcg/kg/minute.[68,69] For M.R., an infusion of nitroprusside should be initiated at a rate of 0.25 mcg/kg/minute, using a microdrip regulator or an infusion pump. The dose should be increased slowly by 0.25 mcg/kg/minute every 5 minutes until the desired pressure is achieved. A maximum infusion rate of 10 mcg/kg/minute has been recommended. If adequate BP reduction is not achieved within 10 minutes following maximum dose infusion, nitroprusside should be discontinued.[3] The dosage must be individualized according to patient response using continuous intra-arterial BP recording and observing for signs or symptoms of toxicity.

THERAPEUTIC END POINT

11. A nitroprusside infusion of 0.25 mcg/kg/minute is started. What is the goal of therapy?

M.R.'s arterial pressure should be reduced to near-normal levels; however, because he has cerebral occlusive disease (carotid bruits), excessive reduction of his BP should be avoided. Overly aggressive reduction of BP in the presence of major cerebral vessel stenosis may decrease cerebral blood flow and produce strokes or other neurologic complications.

Normal cerebral blood flow remains relatively constant over a wide range of systemic BP measurements through autoregulatory mechanisms.[41,70] The autoregulatory effects can prevent gross alterations in cerebral blood flow from either slow or rapid changes in systemic arterial pressures. In addition, the BP required to maintain cerebral perfusion is higher in hypertensive patients than in normotensive individuals. If M.R.'s BP is reduced excessively, cerebral blood flow may decrease sharply. Therefore, a diastolic BP of 100 to 105 mmHg would be a reasonable initial therapeutic goal for him. If hypotension occurs, nitroprusside should be discontinued and M.R. should be placed in the Trendelenburg position, where the head is kept lower than the trunk.

CYANIDE TOXICITY

12. M.R. is being treated with nitroprusside. However, over the last 36 hours, dose titration to 7 mcg/kg/minute has been necessary to control his BP. Is he at risk for developing cyanide toxicity? What indices of toxicity should be monitored? Should thiosulfate or hydroxocobalamin be given to prevent toxicity?

A major concern when using sodium nitroprusside is toxicity secondary to the accumulation of its metabolic byproducts, cyanide and thiocyanate. Sodium nitroprusside decomposes within a few minutes after IV infusion. Free cyanide, which represents 44% of nitroprusside by weight, is released into the bloodstream, producing prussic acid (hydrogen cyanide), which is responsible for the acute toxicity.[71] The amount of hydrogen cyanide released is directly proportional to the size of the dose.[72] Endogenous detoxification of cyanide occurs through a mitochondrial rhodanese system, which, in the presence of a sulfur donor such as thiosulfate, converts cyanide to thiocyanate.[71] This enzymatic detoxification of cyanide exhibits zero-order pharmacokinetics and is dependent on the enzyme rhodanese and an adequate supply of thiosulfate. A healthy person can eliminate cyanide hepatically at a rate equivalent to the cyanide production during a nitroprusside infusion of up to approximately 2 mcg/kg/minute.[73] Theoretically, cyanide can be expected to accumulate in the body when the rate of the sodium nitroprusside infusion exceeds 2 mcg/kg/minute for a prolonged period. This rise can be prevented by administering sodium thiosulfate simultaneously.[74,75] A mixture of 0.1% sodium nitroprusside plus 1% sodium thiosulfate is as effective as sodium nitroprusside alone and is substantially less toxic.[74] For this reason, some clinicians have recommended that all patients receiving nitroprusside receive concomitant thiosulfate infusions.[76,77] IV boluses of thiosulfate may be effective, but they require frequent dosing. Rindone and Sloane[72] noted that 10 mg of sodium thiosulfate for every 1 mg of nitroprusside should be considered in high-risk patients (e.g., those with malnutrition) or when large doses of nitroprusside are administered (>3 mcg/kg/minute). The presence of hepatic or renal failure may also predispose the patient to cyanide toxicity.[73,78] However, no studies have assessed the chemical compatibility of nitroprusside and sodium thiosulfate.

It is generally stated that symptomatic cyanide toxicity occurs infrequently, although several deaths have been reported after the use of sodium nitroprusside.[77] Cyanide toxicity occurs most commonly when large doses (total dose 1.5 mg/kg) of nitroprusside are administered rapidly to patients undergoing a surgical procedure that requires induction of hypotension. However, cyanide toxicity and mortality associated with nitroprusside exceed 3,000 and 1,000 cases per year, respectively, according to two sources.[77,79] The increasing concern about cyanide toxicity has resulted in a revision of the product label, which warns that sodium nitroprusside administration increases the body's concentration of cyanide ion to toxic and potentially fatal levels, even when given within the range of recommended doses. The revised labeling further states that infusions at the maximum recommended dose can overwhelm the body's ability to buffer the cyanide within 1 hour.

Although concurrent sodium thiosulfate administration has been recommended in high-risk patients, no clinical data are available to indicate that it reduces overall mortality. Furthermore, this intervention may result in the accumulation of thiocyanate, particularly if sodium thiosulfate is given at high infusion rates or to patients with renal insufficiency. A 1-year retrospective review at a tertiary care teaching hospital with a level 1 trauma center found that none of the patients receiving nitroprusside at infusion rates >2 mcg/kg/minute were concurrently treated with sodium thiosulfate.[80]

Hydroxocobalamin has also been used to reduce cyanide toxicity secondary to nitroprusside infusions.[78] The concurrent administration of a continuous infusion of hydroxocobalamin (25 mg/hour) lowers RBC and plasma cyanide concentrations.[81] Hydroxocobalamin combines with cyanide to form cyanocobalamin, which is nontoxic and excreted in the urine. Approximately 2.4 g of hydroxocobalamin is required to neutralize the cyanide released from 100 mg of nitroprusside. Therefore, its use is limited due to poor availability and cost considerations. Importantly, unlike hydroxocobalamin, cyanocobalamin is not effective in reducing or preventing cyanide toxicity.

To summarize, the use of hydroxocobalamin or sodium thiosulfate is likely to be of greatest value in patients receiving large doses of sodium nitroprusside acutely or in patients receiving high infusion rates for an extended period. However, with the availability of safer alternatives (e.g., fenoldopam, IV labetalol, IV nicardipine) for use in high-risk patients, the use of hydroxocobalamin or thiosulfate is rarely required.

Cyanide toxicity can be detected early by monitoring M.R.'s metabolic status. Lactic acidosis is an early indicator of toxicity because the progressive inactivation of cytochrome oxidase by cyanide results in increased anaerobic glycolysis.[81] A low plasma bicarbonate concentration and low pH, accompanied by an increase in the blood lactate or lactate-to-pyruvate ratio, and an increase in the mixed venous blood oxygen tension could indicate cyanide toxicity.[82] Additional signs of cyanide intoxication include tachycardia, altered consciousness, coma, convulsions, and the occasional smell of almonds on the breath.[72,82] Hypoxemia resulting from pulmonary arterial shunting has also been reported during nitroprusside therapy. Measuring serum thiocyanate levels is of no value in detecting the onset of cyanide toxicity. If toxicity develops, the infusion should be stopped and appropriate therapy for cyanide intoxication instituted. The need for such a high-dose infusion of nitroprusside to maintain M.R.'s pressure may increase his risk for cyanide toxicity, warranting close monitoring of his acid–base balance.

THIOCYANATE TOXICITY

13. Explain the difference between cyanide toxicity and thiocyanate toxicity. What is M.R.'s risk for thiocyanate toxicity if he is continued on a dose of 7 mcg/kg/minute? Is monitoring of serum thiocyanate concentrations necessary?

Sodium nitroprusside is more likely to produce thiocyanate toxicity. Although this complication is also rare, patients with renal failure who receive prolonged infusions are particularly susceptible. The cyanide released from nitroprusside is normally metabolized by thiosulfate in the liver to thiocyanate via sulfation. This conversion of cyanide to thiocyanate proceeds relatively slowly, and thiocyanate levels rise gradually in proportion to the dose and duration of sodium nitroprusside administration. The half-life of thiocyanate is 2.7 days with normal renal function and 9 days in patients with renal failure.[76] When sodium nitroprusside is infused for several days at moderate dosages (2–5 mcg/kg/minute), toxic levels of thiocyanate can occur within 7 to 14 days in patients with normal renal function and 3 to 6 days in patients with severe renal disease.[71] A total daily dose of up to 125 mg is nontoxic in patients with normal renal function, whereas 1,000 mg/day may produce toxicity within 24 to 48 hours. Unfortunately, infusion of sodium thiosulfate, which helps reduce cyanide toxicity, can cause accumulation of thiocyanate, resulting in clinical toxicity, especially in patients with renal failure.[78]

Thiocyanate causes a neurotoxic syndrome manifested by psychosis, hyperreflexia, confusion, weakness, tinnitus, seizures, and coma.[73,76] Prolonged exposure to thiocyanate can suppress thyroid function through inhibition of iodine uptake and binding by the thyroid.[76] Routine measurement of blood levels of thiocyanate is unnecessary and is recommended only in patients with renal disease or when the duration of the nitroprusside infusion exceeds 3 or 4 days. Nitroprusside should be discontinued if serum thiocyanate levels exceed 10 to 12 mg/dL.[83,84] Life-threatening toxicity is of concern when blood thiocyanate levels exceed 20 mg/dL. In emergency cases, thiocyanate can be readily removed by hemodialysis.[76]

For M.R., the potential for thiocyanate toxicity is low because his renal function is normal and the anticipated infusion duration is relatively short. Therefore, measurement of thiocyanate levels is not indicated at this time.

Other side effects associated with nitroprusside therapy include nausea, vomiting, diaphoresis, nasal stuffiness, muscular twitching, dizziness, and weakness. These effects are usually acute and occur when nitroprusside is administered too rapidly. They can be reversed by decreasing the infusion rate.

14. M.R.'s serum chemistries and arterial blood gas values indicate a metabolic acidosis. Should the nitroprusside infusion be continued at 7 mcg/kg/minute? What alternative is available?

Although the duration of M.R.'s nitroprusside therapy has been short, tolerance to the antihypertensive effect requires the use of a high-dose infusion to maintain BP control. Thus, acidosis may represent toxicity as a result of cyanide accumulation. The nitroprusside infusion should be discontinued at this time, and another rapidly acting, easily titratable parenteral antihypertensive such as fenoldopam or IV nicardipine should be initiated.

Fenoldopam

15. What are the advantages and disadvantages of fenoldopam compared with sodium nitroprusside?

HEMODYNAMIC EFFECTS

Fenoldopam is a parenteral, rapidly acting, peripheral dopamine-1 agonist used to manage severe hypertension when a rapid reduction of BP is required.[85–88] Stimulation of the dopamine-1 receptors vasodilates coronary, renal, mesenteric, and peripheral arteries.[89] Vasodilation of the renal vasculature increases renal blood flow in hypertensive patients,[61,62,64] a property that may be particularly advantageous in patients with impaired renal function.[63,90] However, no outcome data are available to document that this effect reduces morbidity and mortality in patients with severe hypertension. Fenoldopam has also been used to control perioperative hypertension in patients undergoing cardiac bypass surgery because, relative to nitroprusside, it either maintains or increases urinary output.[91,92] Fenoldopam is as effective as sodium nitroprusside for the acute treatment of hypertension and does not cause either cyanide or thiocyanate toxicity.[58–60] Fenoldopam is as efficacious as, but considerably more expensive than, sodium nitroprusside.[57] Outcome studies will be required to assess the impact of fenoldopam on increasing renal blood flow and urine output in the management of patients with hypertensive emergencies. Until such time, it should be used only as an alternative to nitroprusside in patients such as M.R., who are at high risk for cyanide or thiocyanate toxicity.

DOSING AND ADMINISTRATION

16. How should fenoldopam be administered?

Fenoldopam is administered as a continuous infusion (without a bolus dose) beginning at a rate of 0.1 mcg/kg/minute. It is then titrated upward, according to BP control, in increments of 0.05 to 0.1 mcg/kg/minute at 15-minute intervals. The maximum dose is 1.6 mcg/kg/minute, and its use has been studied for up to 48 hours of therapy. Clearance of fenoldopam is not altered by renal or liver disease. Like nitroprusside, fenoldopam also has a short duration of action, with an elimination half-life of approximately 5 minutes, thus allowing for easy titration. Once the target blood pressure is achieved, fenoldopam can be gradually tapered as oral therapy is initiated, if rebound hypertension has not occurred.[87,93]

ADVERSE EFFECTS

17. M.R. is converted to a continuous infusion of fenoldopam, and his BP is well controlled on 0.3 mcg/kg/minute. What monitoring parameters should be followed?

Fenoldopam is well tolerated and relatively free of side effects. BP and heart rate should be followed closely to avoid hypotension and dose-related tachycardia. The vasodilating effect may also cause flushing, dizziness, and headache. Serum electrolytes should be monitored, and in some cases, potassium supplementation is required. Fenoldopam should be used cautiously in patients with glaucoma or intraocular hypertension due to a dose-dependent increase in intraocular pressure.[94,95]

18. Which antihypertensive agents should be avoided in M.R.? Why?

Labetalol, a potent, rapidly acting antihypertensive with both α- and β-blocking activity, is very effective in the treatment of various hypertensive emergencies,[96–102] but it should not be used in M.R. (see Question 19). Hemodynamically, labetalol reduces peripheral vascular resistance (afterload), BP, and heart rate, with almost no change in the resting cardiac output or stroke volume.[103]

M.R. is experiencing chest pain, and he is tachycardic; these signs and symptoms are most likely caused by his severely uncontrolled hypertension and the presence of acute left ventricular failure. Even though labetalol might improve M.R.'s angina, the negative inotropic action could acutely compromise his left ventricular dysfunction, an effect that outweighs the potential benefit of afterload reduction. In addition, even though labetalol is one of the safest β-blocking drugs when used in patients with asthma,[104] no β-blocker should be used as initial treatment in patients with asthma. Labetalol should be used only if alternative methods of reducing M.R.'s pressure fail.

Diazoxide, a potent, rapidly acting hypotensive agent closely related to the thiazide group of drugs, should also be avoided in M.R. for several reasons (see Question 25). The hypotensive action is caused by a reduction in peripheral vascular resistance through direct relaxation of arterioles. As arterial pressure is lowered, baroreceptor reflexes are activated, leading to cardiac stimulation with increased heart rate, stroke volume, and cardiac output. The cardiostimulating effect of diazoxide could be potentially dangerous in patients such as M.R., who have ischemic heart disease and a recent history of MI.[105] Neurologic and cardiovascular symptoms may occur with rapid administration of diazoxide.

There are other reasons why diazoxide should be avoided or used cautiously in M.R. Although diazoxide has a thiazide-like structure, it causes significant sodium and water retention, which could be deleterious in a patient such as M.R. with severe HF and pulmonary edema.[106,107] The exact mechanism for this effect is unknown, but it may be through an activation of the renin system or a direct antinatriuretic effect on the renal tubules.

Labetalol

19. C.M., a 52-year-old Caucasian male, is admitted to the hospital with a 3-day history of increasing exertional substernal chest pain (without SOB), diaphoresis, nausea, and vomiting. His history is significant for poorly controlled hypertension, glaucoma, and angina pectoris. Prior medications include dorzolamide ophthalmic drops (Trusopt), atenolol (Tenormin), hydrochlorothiazide, and oral nitrates. Physical examination reveals an anxious man who is alert and oriented. He has a BP of 210/146 mmHg without orthostasis and a regular pulse of 115 beats/minute. Bilateral hemorrhages and exudates are present on funduscopic examination. The lungs are clear and the heart is enlarged, but there are no murmurs or gallops. Examination of the abdomen is unremarkable, and there is no peripheral edema. The neurologic examination is normal.

Significant laboratory values include the following: Na, 140 mEq/L (normal 136–144); Cl, 109 mEq/L (normal 96–106); bicarbonate, 18 mEq/L (normal 23–28); BUN, 49 mg/dL (normal 10–20); and creatinine, 2.8 mg/dL (renal function previously noted to be within normal limits). UA shows proteinuria and hematuria. The ECG demonstrates sinus tachycardia with left axis deviation, left ventricular hypertrophy, and nonspecific ST-T wave changes. The chest radiograph reveals mild cardiomegaly.

C.M. is given nitroglycerin sublingually (Nitrostat), and 1 inch of nitroglycerin ointment (Nitrol Paste) is applied topically. He is started on IV labetalol. Is this choice of treatment reasonable, considering C.M.'s angina and acute renal failure?

[SI units: Na, 140 mmol/L (normal 136–144); Cl, 109 mmol/L (normal 96–106); bicarbonate, 18 mmol/L (normal 23–28); BUN, 17.493 mmol/L urea (normal 3.57–7.14); creatinine, 247.52 mmol/L (normal 44.2–106.08)]

The presence of chest pain, retinopathy, and new onset renal disease, as well as the magnitude of the BP elevation in C.M., warrant a prompt reduction in BP. The combination of sublingual and topical nitroglycerin may help in acutely lowering his BP and relieving his chest pain while waiting for more definitive treatment to be implemented.

IV labetalol is a potent antihypertensive drug that has been used successfully in various hypertensive emergencies.[96–102] Labetalol blocks both β- and α-adrenergic receptors and also may exert a direct vasodilator effect. The β-blockade is nonselective with α to β potency of 3:1 for oral and 7:1 for IV labetalol. Labetalol is particularly advantageous in C.M. because the immediate onset of action will reduce peripheral vascular resistance without causing reflex tachycardia. Myocardial oxygen demand will be reduced and coronary hemodynamics will be improved, making this agent an excellent choice for patients such as C.M., who have coronary artery disease or MI. In addition, IV labetalol does not significantly reduce cerebral blood flow; therefore, it may be useful in patients with cerebrovascular disease.[1,23]

Fenoldopam or nitroprusside could also be used to treat C.M. Fenoldopam could potentially benefit renal function by increasing renal blood flow, but C.M.'s history of glaucoma would preclude its use. In addition, equally effective but less costly alternatives are available. Treatment with nitroprusside would expose C.M. to the potential risk of cyanide and thiocyanate toxicity with his new onset renal failure. In contrast, labetalol has been used successfully in patients with renal disease without deleterious side effects.[108,109] Labetalol is eliminated by glucuronidation in the liver, with <5% of the dose being excreted unchanged in the urine. Therefore, labetalol may be better tolerated than nitroprusside by patients with hepatic failure because toxic nitroprusside metabolites also accumulate in this situation. The presence of renal disease in C.M. will not necessitate an alteration in the dose of labetalol.

CONTRAINDICATIONS

20. What cautions should be exercised when using labetalol in C.M.?

Labetalol's disadvantages are primarily related to its β-blocking effects, which predominate over its α-blocking effects. Therefore, it should not be used in patients with asthma, heart block greater than first degree, or sinus bradycardia, and it should be used with caution in patients with severe uncontrolled HF[97,101,110] (see Question 18). None of these is present in C.M. Like other β-blockers, labetalol may mask the symptoms of hypoglycemia in insulin-dependent diabetic patients; it should also be used with caution in patients with Raynaud's syndrome.[110] Labetalol has been effective in the treatment of hypertension associated with pheochromocytoma and excess catecholamine states.[111] However, because labetalol is primarily a β-blocker, paradoxic hypertension may occur in patients with pheochromocytoma. These individuals have adrenal tumors that excrete high amounts of norepinephrine, which results in relatively unopposed α-receptor stimulation.[112] More clinical experience is required before labetalol can be recommended in patients with pheochromocytoma.[5,96] Labetalol may also be particularly useful for the treatment of antihypertensive withdrawal syndromes.[11]

21. Will C.M.'s age or prior use of antihypertensives affect his response to labetalol?

There appears to be a positive correlation between age and response to labetalol. Older patients achieve a greater reduction in BP and, therefore, require smaller doses.[113,114] Failure to lower BP has also been observed.[115–117] This phenomenon was believed to be related to single-bolus administration or prior treatment with α- and β-blocking drugs.[110] However, subsequent studies have confirmed the effectiveness of labetalol in patients pretreated with antihypertensives, including β-blockers.[118]

22. How should parenteral labetalol be given to C.M.?

For acute BP reduction, C.M. should be placed in the supine position. IV labetalol can be given by pulse administration or continuous infusion.[96–101] Small incremental bolus injections are administered, beginning with 20 mg given over 2 minutes, followed by 40 to 80 mg every 10 to 15 minutes until the desired response is achieved or a cumulative dose of 300 mg is reached. The desired response is usually achieved with a mean dose of 200 mg in 90% of patients.[97] Following IV injection, the maximal effect occurs within 5 to 10 minutes,[99] and the antihypertensive response may persist for >6 hours.[118] Because the rate of BP reduction is accelerated with an increase in infusion rate,[99] a controlled continuous infusion may provide a more gradual reduction in arterial pressure with less frequent adverse effects.[101,119] A solution for continuous infusion (0.5–2.0 mg/minute) is prepared by adding two ampules (200 mg total) to 160 mL of IV fluid to give a final concentration of 1 mg/mL. The infusion can then be started at a rate of 2 mg/minute and titrated until a satisfactory response is achieved or until a cumulative dose of 300 mg is reached.

PARENTERAL/ORAL CONVERSION

23. C.M. was treated with a labetalol infusion and required a cumulative dose of 180 mg to achieve a diastolic pressure of 100 mmHg. His anginal symptoms resolved almost immediately, but 3 hours after the infusion, C.M. became faint and dizzy while ambulating. Should oral labetalol be withheld? When oral labetalol is given, what adverse effects can be expected?

Postural hypotension and dizziness are dose related and more commonly associated with the IV route of administration.[103,110] C.M. should remain in a supine position following the IV administration of labetalol, and his ability to tolerate an upright position should be established before permitting ambulation. Oral labetalol can be given to C.M. when his supine diastolic BP increases by 10 mmHg. There is no correlation between the oral maintenance dose and the total initial IV dose. C.M. should be started on an empirical dose of 100 to 200 mg oral labetalol twice daily, and this should be titrated as necessary. Other side effects commonly associated with labetalol include nausea, vomiting, abdominal pain, and diarrhea in up to 15% of the patients.[110] Scalp tingling is an unusual side effect that has been reported in a few patients after IV administration; it tends to disappear with continued treatment. Other side effects include tiredness, weakness, muscle cramps, headache, ejaculation failure, and various skin rashes.

Nitroglycerin

24. Would parenteral nitroglycerin be an acceptable alternative to labetalol for C.M.?

Severe, uncontrolled hypertension in the setting of unstable angina or MI requires an immediate reduction in BP. Nitroprusside has been used successfully, but IV nitroglycerin can have more favorable effects on collateral coronary flow in patients with ischemic heart disease.[120] By diminishing preload, nitroglycerin decreases left ventricular diastolic volume, diastolic pressure, and myocardial wall tension, thus reducing myocardial oxygen consumption.[121] These changes favor redistribution of coronary blood flow to the subendocardium, which is more vulnerable to ischemia. At high dosages, nitroglycerin dilates arteriolar smooth muscles, and this reduction in afterload also decreases myocardial wall tension and oxygen consumption.[122]

IV nitroglycerin has a rapid onset of action and a short duration, and is easily titratable. It is generally appropriate to begin IV nitroglycerin at dosages in the range of 5 to 10 mcg/minute, increased as needed to control pressure and symptoms. The usual dose is in the range of 40 to 100 mcg/minute. The major limiting side effects are headache and the development of tolerance. In general, IV nitroglycerin is well suited for use in patients such as C.M. who have unstable angina or in patients who have hypertension associated with MI or coronary bypass surgery.

Diazoxide

25. R.N., a 32-year-old African American female, is admitted to the hospital with a 2-day history of nausea, blurred vision, confusion, and an intractable generalized headache. Her medical history is remarkable for asthma and diet-controlled diabetes mellitus. Physical examination reveals an alert but disoriented woman with a BP of 220/160 mmHg (without orthostasis) and a pulse of 110 beats/minute. There is no evidence of heart failure, but the neurologic examination reveals an altered mental status. Serum electrolytes, BUN, creatinine, UA, chest x-ray, and ECG are within normal limits. R.N.'s plasma glucose level is 275 mg/dL. The assessment at this time is hypertensive encephalopathy. Diazoxide is ordered. How should diazoxide be administered to R.N. to achieve an optimal hypotensive response? Under what circumstances is diazoxide preferred over other agents?

Diazoxide should be administered as a small bolus or by slow infusion because larger doses cause cerebral and cardiovascular hypoperfusion due to an abrupt decline in blood pressure. Studies confirm that diazoxide can be administered safely and effectively as a minibolus (1–3 mg/kg every 5–15 minutes to a maximum of 150 mg in a single injection) or by slow infusion (15–30 mg/minute)[123,124] until a diastolic BP of 100 mmHg is achieved. Single-dose injections of >150 mg should not be used. Diazoxide can also be given by repetitive infusions according to the following schedule: loading dose of 7.5 mg/kg IV over 1.5 hours (which usually decreases mean arterial pressure by 25%), followed by 10% of the loading dose every 6 hours for maintenance.[125] In general, diazoxide should be used only in patients who (a) cannot tolerate labetalol (e.g., asthma or advanced heart block), (b) require a more gradual lowering of BP than that produced by nitroprusside, and (c) require a more rapid and certain drop in BP than that which can be produced by oral antihypertensive agents.[126]

Diazoxide should be used with caution in patients with diabetes mellitus because it can increase blood glucose. Blood glucose needs to be monitored during therapy and treated accordingly.[127]

The hypotensive effects of diazoxide begin within 1 minute, and maximum effects occur within 2 to 5 minutes. The patient should remain recumbent for 15 to 30 minutes after the injection of each dose of diazoxide, and the BP should be monitored every 5 minutes for the first 30 minutes. The duration of action is variable in that the BP gradually increases to the pretreatment level in 3 to 15 hours. Diazoxide, when given by slow infusion, produces a maximum reduction in mean arterial pressure of 25% in 25 to 30 minutes, which lasts up to 8 hours.[124,126] If R.N. fails to respond to the first dose, repeated doses should be given at 10-minute intervals until a cumulative dose of 600 mg is reached.

A major disadvantage of diazoxide is the occurrence of reflex tachycardia, which can precipitate or worsen angina in patients with coronary artery disease. Small IV doses of propranolol (0.2 mg/kg) can be used in situations in which tachycardia is dangerous.[126]

Hydralazine

26. T.M., a 30-year-old Caucasian male with a history of chronic glomerulonephritis and poorly controlled hypertension, came to the ED complaining of early morning occipital headaches during the past week. He has no other complaints. He has not taken any BP medication in a month. Physical examination revealed an afebrile male in no acute distress with a BP of 160/120 mmHg without orthostasis and a regular pulse of 90 beats/minute. Funduscopic examination revealed bilateral exudates without hemorrhages or papilledema. The lungs were clear. Cardiac examination was pertinent for cardiomegaly and an S_4 gallop. The remainder of the physical workup was normal.

Laboratory results include Hct, 32%; BUN, 40 mg/dL; creatinine, 2.5 mg/dL; and bicarbonate, 18 mEq/L. UA reveals 2+ protein, 2+ hemoglobin with 4 to 10 RBCs/HPF. The ECG demonstrates NSR with left ventricular hypertrophy. The chest radiograph is unremarkable.

T.M. was given 20 mg hydralazine IV, and a repeat BP after 1 hour was 150/100 mmHg. What are the advantages and disadvantages of parenteral hydralazine, and when should it be used to acutely lower BP?

[SI units: Hct, 0.32; BUN, 14.28 mmol/L urea; creatinine, 221 mmol/L; bicarbonate, 18 mmol/L]

Hydralazine is a direct vasodilator that reduces total peripheral resistance through relaxation of arterial smooth muscle. It is rarely used to treat hypertensive emergencies, excluding eclampsia, because its antihypertensive response is less predictable than that of other parenteral agents. It is not consistently effective in controlling crises associated with essential hypertension.

Contraindications

Hydralazine should not be used in patients with coronary heart disease because the reflex tachycardia causes an increase in myocardial oxygen demand, which may result in the development or worsening of ischemic symptoms. In addition, hydralazine should be avoided in patients with aortic dissection because of its reflex cardiostimulating effect. In contrast, hydralazine can be useful in patients such as T.M., who have chronic renal failure because the reflex increase in cardiac output is accompanied by an increase in organ perfusion. In addition, there is considerable experience with the use of hydralazine in patients with eclampsia who are less likely to have underlying coronary artery disease (see Chapter 47).

DOSING AND ADMINISTRATION

Parenteral hydralazine should be considered an intermediate treatment between oral agents and more aggressive therapy with such agents as fenoldopam or nitroprusside. It can be given IV or intramuscularly. The onset of action develops slowly over 20 to 40 minutes, thus minimizing the risk of acute hypotension. Parenteral doses are considerably lower than oral doses because of increased bioavailability.

Other Parenteral Drugs

27. Are there alternatives to hydralazine for parenteral treatment of hypertensive urgencies?

INTRAVENOUS ENALAPRILAT

Enalaprilat, the active metabolite of the oral prodrug enalapril (Vasotec), is approved by the U.S. Food and Drug Administration for the treatment of hypertension when oral therapy is not feasible. Although not approved for the treatment of hypertensive crisis, enalaprilat has been used to treat severe hypertension.[128–133] The initial dose is 0.625 to 1.25 mg IV and can be repeated every 6 hours, if necessary. Initial doses should not exceed 0.625 mg in patients receiving diuretics or in patients with clinical evidence of hypovolemia. The onset of action is within 15 minutes, but the maximum effect may take several hours. Because only 60% of the patients respond to BP reduction within 30 minutes, it cannot be reliably used to acutely lower pressure in emergent cases.[131] Although higher initial doses have been successfully used to achieve BP control,[132] some evidence indicates that doses >0.625 mg do not significantly alter the magnitude of enalaprilat's antihypertensive effect.[130] Because ACE inhibitors do not impair cerebral blood flow, enalaprilat may be useful for the hypertensive patient at risk for cerebral hypoperfusion. Enalaprilat also is beneficial in patients with HF. Precautions for the use of enalaprilat are similar to those of captopril (see question 5). Because of the prolonged time required to achieve an adequate response, limited clinical experience, and variable response rates (especially in African Americans), enalaprilat cannot be recommended for the routine treatment of patients with hypertensive emergencies.[131,133]

INTRAVENOUS ESMOLOL

Esmolol is a parenteral cardioselective β_1-blocker with a rapid onset and short duration of action. It has been used primarily in perioperative settings to control tachycardia induced by various surgical stimuli, including endotracheal intubation.[134] Esmolol has also been used to manage supraventricular tachyarrhythmias.[135,136] It has been particularly useful in treating postoperative hypertension, especially if associated with tachycardia. In a small series of patients undergoing cardiac bypass surgery, the antihypertensive effect of esmolol was comparable to that of nitroprusside.[137]

Hypotension is the most commonly reported adverse event and is directly related to the duration of esmolol administration.[138] However, because of the short half-life, resolution of hypotension occurs within 30 minutes of discontinuing the infusion. Like other β-blockers, esmolol is contraindicated in patients with asthma, advanced heart block, or severe HF.

For the management of hypertension, esmolol should be given as a loading dose of 250 to 500 mcg/kg over 1 minute, followed by a maintenance infusion of 50 to 300 mcg/kg/minute. Irritation, inflammation, and induration at the infusion site occur in 5% to 10% of patients.

INTRAVENOUS CALCIUM CHANNEL BLOCKERS

Parenteral verapamil (Isoptin) and diltiazem (Cardizem), although clinically effective for prompt lowering of blood pressure, have not been extensively studied in patients with hypertensive emergencies. In addition, they should be used with extreme caution when acutely treating any hypertensive patient with concomitant systolic HF due to their negative inotropic effects. Nicardipine (Cardene IV), in contrast, has been proven effective in multiple studies of populations with hypertensive emergencies, and, as a dihydropyridine, has less negative inotropic activity compared to nondihydropyridines.

Intravenous Verapamil

IV verapamil (5–10 mg) produces a significant reduction in BP, which occurs within 15 minutes and persists for 6 to 8 hours. As a cardiovascular drug, it is primarily used as a rate-controlling agent in the treatment of supraventricular tachycardias.

Intravenous Diltiazem

IV diltiazem is approved for temporary control of the ventricular rate in atrial fibrillation or atrial flutter and for rapid conversion of paroxysmal supraventricular tachycardia.[139–141] Parenteral diltiazem has also been used to control hypertension that occurs intraoperatively and postoperatively[142,143] and in patients with acute coronary artery disease.[144,145] However, published experience with the use of IV diltiazem for the treatment of severe hypertension is limited. Onoyama et al.[146] administered a continuous infusion of diltiazem at a dosage of 5 to 40 mcg/kg/minute to a small group of patients with hypertensive crisis. A normotensive level was achieved within 6 hours without any signs of organ ischemia. In a follow-up study,[147] a continuous infusion of diltiazem averaging 11 mcg/kg/minute resulted in a 25% reduction in both systolic and diastolic BP measurements within 30 minutes. The magnitude of the decrease was directly correlated with the pretreatment BP level. Atrioventricular nodal conduction abnormalities were noted in both studies during drug infusion. Patients receiving IV diltiazem require continuous monitoring by ECG and frequent BP checks. This form of therapy should be avoided in patients with sick sinus syndrome or advanced degrees of heart block. Until additional information is available, caution should be exercised in using parenteral diltiazem to lower BP acutely.

Intravenous Nicardipine

Nicardipine is a potent cerebral and systemic vasodilator and a useful therapeutic option in the management of severe hypertension. Unlike other dihydropyridines, nicardipine is photo resistant, water soluble, and available intravenously. Its onset of action is within 1 to 2 minutes, and its elimination half-life is 40 minutes.[148] Hemodynamic evaluations demonstrated that IV nicardipine significantly decreased mean arterial pressure and systemic vascular resistance and significantly increased cardiac index with little or no change in heart rate.[149] Titratable IV nicardipine has been studied extensively for use in controlling postoperative hypertension,[149–153] severe hypertension,[154,155] and acute hypertension in patients with hemorrhagic or ischemic stroke.[156,157]

In the treatment of postoperative hypertension,[149] IV nicardipine was administered as an infusion titrated in the following manner: 10 mg/hour for 5 minutes, 12.5 mg/hour for 5 minutes, and 15 mg/hour for 15 minutes, followed by a maintenance infusion of 3 mg/hour thereafter. The mean response time and infusion rate were 11.5 minutes and 12.8 mg/hour, respectively. Ninety-four percent of the patients responded, and adverse effects included hypotension (4.5%), tachycardia (2.7%), and nausea and vomiting (4.5%).

The efficacy and safety of IV nicardipine for the treatment of severe hypertension were documented in a double-blind, placebo-controlled multicenter trial of 123 patients.[154] Therapy of IV nicardipine was begun with dosages of 5 mg/hour and titrated up to 15 mg/hour as indicated until the therapeutic end point was achieved. The mean dosage of IV nicardipine at the end of maintenance therapy was 8.7 mg/hour. Ninety-one percent of patients on nicardipine achieved the prespecified BP target within a mean administration time of 77 minutes. In an open-label trial,[155] patients receiving nicardipine required significantly fewer dose adjustments per hour than patients receiving nitroprusside (1.7 vs. 3.3, respectively). Serious adverse effects reported in these trials were uncommon. The most commonly reported adverse effects included headache, hypotension, tachycardia, dizziness, and nausea.

When compared with sodium nitroprusside for patients with severe hypertension, IV nicardipine was as effective with fewer adverse effects.[155] In studies of patients receiving nicardipine versus nitroprusside for postoperative hypertension following cardiac endarterectomy and coronary artery bypass grafting, breakthrough BP was controlled more rapidly with nicardipine and required fewer overall dose titrations. In addition, nicardipine was well tolerated and did not lead to an increased risk of complications.[158,159]

In summary, IV nicardipine is an alternative to sodium nitroprusside for the immediate treatment of severe and postoperative hypertension.[40,160] It has a rapid onset of action, with sustained BP control over the infusion period. It is easily titratable, with a predictable response, and is relatively free of severe adverse effects. It may be useful in patients with cerebral insufficiency or peripheral vascular disease. Because of the potential for reflex tachycardia, it should be used with caution in patients with coronary ischemia.

INTRAVENOUS PHENTOLAMINE (REGITINE)

IV phentolamine is primarily used in the management of hypertensive emergencies induced by catecholamine excess, as seen in pheochromocytoma. The mechanism of action is through nonselective competitive antagonist at α-adrenergic receptors. Phentolamine is dosed in 1- to 5-mg boluses and should be given cautiously due to the risk of causing hypotension. The onset of action is almost immediate and the duration of action is short (<15 minutes). IV infusions are not recommended due to unpredictable drops in BP. As BP control is achieved, an oral α-adrenergic blocking agent such as phenoxybenzamine (Dibenzyline) can be given if needed. β_1- and β_2-selective antagonists are not recommended for BP control in cases of pheochromocytoma.[161]

Aortic Dissection

Treatment

28. B.S., a 68-year-old Caucasian male with a long history of hypertension, asthma, and noncompliance, presents to the local ED complaining of the sudden onset of severe, sharp, diffuse chest pain that radiates to his back between his shoulder blades. Significant findings on physical examination include a pulse of 100 beats/minute, BP of 200/120 mmHg, clear lungs, and an S_4 without murmurs. The laboratory data are unremarkable. The ECG results are interpreted as sinus tachycardia with left ventricular hypertrophy, but no acute changes are noted. The chest radiograph is significant for widening of the mediastinum. An emergency chest computed tomography scan reveals a dissection

at the arch of the aorta. What antihypertensive medication would be most appropriate for B.S., and why?

Dissection of the aorta occurs when the innermost layer of the aorta (the intima) is torn such that blood enters and separates its layers. The ultimate treatment for dissection of the aorta depends on its location and severity; however, the first principle of therapy is to control any existing hypertension with agents that do not increase the force of cardiac contraction. This lessens the force that the cardiac impulse transmits to the dissecting aneurysm.

THERAPEUTIC CONSIDERATIONS

The aim of antihypertensive therapy in aortic dissection is to lessen the pulsatile load or aortic stress by lowering the BP. Reducing the force of left ventricular contractions, and consequently the rate of rise of aortic pressure, retards the propagation of the dissection and aortic rupture.[162] The treatment of choice for aortic dissection has classically been a vasodilatory agent such as sodium nitroprusside, fenoldopam, or nicardipine in combination with a β-blocker titrated to a heart rate of 55 to 65 beats/minute.[162,164] Labetalol monotherapy has been used as an alternative.[165] These drugs decrease BP, venous return, and cardiac contractility.

One common regimen is a combination of IV sodium nitroprusside (0.5–2 mcg/kg/minute) plus IV esmolol (25–200 mcg/kg/minute).[160] The concurrent administration of a β-blocking agent with a vasodilator is desirable because the latter may induce reflex tachycardia in response to vasodilation.

Trimethaphan can also be used in aortic dissection. Its advantage over sodium nitroprusside is that it reduces both arterial pressure and its rate of increase; therefore, it does not require concurrent administration of β-blockers. However, the major disadvantages are tachyphylaxis, urinary retention, and ileus. Direct vasodilators such as diazoxide and hydralazine should be avoided because they increase stroke volume and left ventricular ejection rate. These effects augment the pulsatile flow and accentuate the sharpness of the pulse wave. This increases mechanical stress on the aortic wall and may lead to further dissection.[161]

Depending on the location of the dissection, surgical intervention may be required.[164,166] However, until a definitive diagnosis is made, the primary goal is to reduce the BP and myocardial contractility to the lowest level compatible with the maintenance of adequate renal, cerebral, and cardiac perfusion.[161] In aortic dissection, the systolic BP should be lowered to 100 to 120 mmHg or a mean arterial pressure <80 mmHg.[166]

The first choice of drug for B.S. is trimethaphan. Although labetalol or a combination of nitroprusside with esmolol has been used successfully in the antihypertensive treatment of dissecting aortic aneurysms, B.S.'s medical history of asthma precludes the use of β-blockers.

TRIMETHAPHAN

29. How should trimethaphan be administered, and what indices of toxicity should be monitored?

Trimethaphan is a ganglionic blocking drug that inhibits sympathetic nervous effects on the arterioles, veins, and heart. Its hypotensive effect is immediate. Severe hypotension after administration of trimethaphan may last for 10 to 15 minutes. The hypotensive effect is most pronounced when the patient is upright, and it is often necessary to elevate the head of the bed to achieve an optimal effect. To correct hypotension, trimethaphan should be discontinued and the patient should be placed in the Trendelenburg position.

The drug is usually prepared in a concentration of 500 mg/L of D_5W. The infusion is initiated at 0.5 to 1 mg/minute, and the rate is increased every 3 to 5 minutes until the desired response is obtained. Because minor changes in the infusion rate can produce dramatic changes in BP, the rate must be carefully regulated (preferably by a constant infusion pump), and the BP must be monitored continuously. Therapy with oral antihypertensive agents should begin simultaneously, and an attempt should be made to discontinue the ganglionic blocker within 48 hours before significant tolerance renders the patient resistant to its action.

The prolonged use of trimethaphan is limited by its important sympathoplegic side effects and the rapid development of tachyphylaxis. Urinary retention often occurs with prolonged therapy, necessitating insertion of an indwelling catheter. Constipation and paralytic ileus may occur, as well as paralysis of visual accommodation.

Cocaine-induced Hypertension

Treatment

30. B.K. is a 54-year-old Caucasian male who presents to the ED complaining of 8/10 chest pain associated with diaphoresis and nausea that began 2 hours ago. BK reports using cocaine about 1 hour before his chest pain began. His medical and social histories include hypertension for which he takes hydrochlorothiazide 25 mg daily. He also admits to using cocaine five to seven times per week for the past 21 years and smoking one and a half packs per day for the past 35 years. An ECG reveals ST segment elevations <1 mm in leads V_2 and V_3 and sinus tachycardia. Cardiac enzymes are drawn, and the first set is negative. His cardiac exam was unremarkable. His vital signs include a blood pressure of 205/162 mmHg; heart rate of 132 beats/minute, regular rate and rhythm; and respiratory rate of 24 breaths/minute, and he is afebrile. All laboratory values are within normal limits. Chest x-ray is unremarkable. What agents should be used to manage cocaine-induced hypertension? What agents should be avoided?

Cocaine, a sympathomimetic, can induce severe hypertension by inhibiting the reuptake of norepinephrine and dopamine and thereby increasing neurotransmitter concentrations in the synaptic cleft. This leads to pronounced vasoconstriction and tachycardia. This increase in heart rate and/or BP increases cardiac oxygen demand leading to coronary vasospasm. Cocaine exerts its onset of action within seconds to minutes and has a serum half-life of 30 to 90 minutes.[167,168]

Management of cocaine-associated hypertensive crisis should be controlled with nicardipine, verapamil, or nitroglycerin. Calcium channels blockers and IV nitroglycerin are preferred in patients with active myocardial ischemia because they have both been shown to reverse cocaine-induced hypertension and vasoconstriction.[169,170] Benzodiazepines can also be used because they can attenuate the effect of cocaine on the cardiac system, decrease chest pain, and reduce heart rate.[167,171] Fenoldopam and nitroprusside can be used as alternative agents.[172,173]

The use of β-blockers should be avoided in patients who present with hypertension or myocardial ischemia/MI with recent cocaine use. β-blockers will result in unopposed α-adrenergic vasoconstriction, leading to further elevation in BP and heart rate.[172,173] Labetalol possesses both α- and β-blockade, and its use has been reported in cocaine-intoxicated patients.[174] Labetalol has been shown to increase seizure activity and mortality in animals with cocaine intoxication and does not alleviate cocaine-induced coronary vasoconstriction.[175,176] Labetalol has also been shown to worsen BP when α-stimulation has been left unopposed in patients with pheochromocytoma.[112,177] Therefore, caution should be used if labetalol is used in patients with recent cocaine use.

REFERENCES

1. Calhoun DA, Oparil S. Treatment of hypertensive crisis. *N Engl J Med* 1990;323:1177.
2. Ault MJ, Ellrodt AG. Pathophysiologic events leading to the end organ effects of acute hypertension. *J Emerg Med* 1985;3(Suppl 2):10.
3. The Seventh Report of the Joint National Committee on Prevention, Detection, Evaluation and Treatment of High Blood Pressure. NIH Publication 04–5230. Bethesda, MD: National Institutes of Health; 2004.
4. Bales A. Hypertensive crisis: how to tell if it's an emergency or an urgency. *Postgrad Med* 1999;105:119.
5. Vidt DG. Hypertensive crises: emergencies and urgencies. *J Clin Hypertens* 2004;6:520.
6. Abo-Zena RA et al. Hypertensive urgency induced by an interaction of mirtazapine and clonidine. *Pharmacotherapy* 2000;20:476.
7. Patel S et al. Hypertensive crisis associated with St. John's wort. *Am J Med* 2002;112:507.
8. Novac BL et al. Erythropoietin-induced hypertensive urgency in a patient with chronic renal insufficiency: case report and review of the literature. *Pharmacotherapy* 2003;23:265.
9. Zampaglione B et al. Hypertensive urgencies and emergencies: prevalence and clinical presentation. *Hypertension* 1996;27:144.
10. Bennett NM, Shea S. Hypertensive emergency: case scenarios, sociodemographic profile, and previous care of 100 cases. *Am J Public Health* 1988;78:636.
11. Ram CV. Immediate management of severe hypertension. *Cardiol Clin* 1995;13:579.
12. Shea S et al. Predisposing factors for severe uncontrolled hypertension in an inner-city minority population. *N Engl J Med* 1992;327:776.
13. Tisdale JE et al. Risk factors for hypertensive crisis: importance of out-patient blood pressure control. *Fam Prac* 2004;21:420.
14. Hammond S et al. Ophthalmoscopic findings in malignant hypertension. *J Clin Hypertens* 2006;8:221.
15. Webster J et al. Accelerated hypertension: patterns of mortality and clinical factors affecting outcomes in treated patients. *Q J Med* 1993;86:485.
16. Aggarwal M, Khan IA. Hypertensive crisis: hypertensive emergencies and urgencies. *Cardiol Clin* 2006;24:135.
17. Bender SR et al. Characteristics and management of patients presenting to the emergency department with hypertensive urgency. *J Clin Hypertens* 2006;8:12.
18. McRae RP et al. Hypertensive crisis. *Med Clin North Am* 1986;70:749.
19. Bakir A, Dunea G. Accelerated and malignant hypertension: experience from a large American inner city hospital. *Int J Artif Organs* 1989;12:675.
20. McNair A et al. Reversibility of cerebral symptoms in severe hypertension in relation to acute antihypertensive therapy. *Acta Med Scand* 1984;6935:107.
21. Winer N. Hypertensive crisis. *Crit Care Nurs Q* 1990;13:23.
22. Hirschl MM. Guidelines for the drug treatment of hypertensive crisis. *Drugs* 1995;50:991.
23. Murphy C. Hypertensive emergencies. *Emerg Med Clin North Am* 1995;13:973.
24. McKindley DS, Boucher BA. Advances in pharmacotherapy: treatment of hypertensive crisis. *J Clin Pharm Ther* 1994;19:163.
25. Gales MA. Oral antihypertensives for hypertensive urgencies. *Ann Pharmacother* 1994;28:352.
26. Psaty BM et al. The risk of myocardial infarction associated with antihypertensive drug therapies. *JAMA* 1995;274:620.
27. Leavitt AD, Zweifler AJ. Nifedipine, hypotension, and myocardial injury. *Ann Intern Med* 1988;108:305.
28. O'Mailia JJ et al. Nifedipine-associated myocardial ischemia or infarction in the treatment of hypertensive urgencies. *Ann Intern Med* 1987;107:185.
29. Schwartz M et al. Oral nifedipine in the treatment of hypertensive urgency: cerebrovascular accident following a single dose. *Arch Intern Med* 1990;150:686.
30. Fami MJ et al. Another report of adverse reactions to immediate-release nifedipine. *Pharmacotherapy* 1998;18:1133.
31. Bertel O et al. Effects of antihypertensive treatment on cerebral perfusion. *Am J Med* 1987;82(Suppl 3B):29.
32. Dinsdale HB. Hypertensive encephalopathy. *Neurol Clin* 1983;1:3.
33. Waldman R et al. Treatment of hypertensive encephalopathy. *Neurology* 1983;33:118.
34. Talbert RL. The challenge of blood management in neurologic emergencies. *Pharmacotherapy* 2006;26(8 pt 2):123S.
35. Adams H et al. Guidelines for the early management of patients with ischemic stroke: 2005 guideline update. *Stroke* 2005;36:916.
36. Grossman E et al. Should a moratorium be placed on sublingual nifedipine capsules given for hypertensive emergencies and pseudoemergencies? *JAMA* 1996;276:1328.
37. Gemici K et al. Evaluation of the effect of sublingually administered nifedipine and captopril via transcranial Doppler ultrasonography during hypertensive crisis. *Blood Press* 2003;12:46.
38. Anderson RJ et al. Oral clonidine loading in hypertensive urgencies. *JAMA* 1981;246:848.
39. Handler J. Case studies in hypertension: hypertensive urgency. *J Clin Hypertens* 2006;8:61.
40. Varon J. Clinical review: the management of hypertensive crises. *Crit Care* 2003;7:374.
41. Reed WG et al. Effects of rapid blood pressure reduction on cerebral blood flow. *Am Heart J* 1986;111:226.
42. Stewart M, Burris JF. Rebound hypertension during initiation of transdermal clonidine. *Drug Intell Clin Pharm* 1988;22:573.
43. Vernon C, Sakula A. Fatal rebound hypertension after abrupt withdrawal of clonidine and propanolol. *Br J Clin Pract* 1979;33:1112.
44. Damasceno A et al. Efficacy of captopril and nifedipine in black and white patients with hypertensive crisis. *J Hum Hypertens* 1997;11:471.
45. Misra A et al. Sublingual captopril in hypertensive urgencies. *Postgrad Med J* 1993;69:498.
46. van Onzenoort HA et al. The effect of sublingual captopril versus intravenous enalaprilat on angiotensin II plasma levels. *Pharm World Sci* 2006;28:131.
47. Komsuoglu B et al. Treatment of hypertensive urgencies with oral nifedipine, nicardipine, and captopril. *Angiology* 1991;42:447.
48. Angeli P et al. Comparison of sublingual captopril and nifedipine in immediate treatment of hypertensive emergencies. *Arch Intern Med* 1991;151:678.
49. Wood BC et al. Oral minoxidil in the treatment of hypertensive crisis. *JAMA* 1979;241:163.
50. Alpert MA, Bauer JH. Rapid control of severe hypertension with minoxidil. *Arch Intern Med* 1982;142:2099.
51. Hayes JM. Prazosin in severe hypertension. *Med J Aust* 1977;2(Suppl 2):30.
52. McDonald AJ, Yealy DM. Oral labetalol versus oral nifedipine in hypertensive urgencies. *Ann Emerg Med* 1989;18:461.
53. Gonzalez ER et al. Dose response evaluation of oral labetalol in patients presenting to the emergency department with accelerated hypertension. *Ann Emerg Med* 1991;20:333.
54. Zell-Kanter M, Leikin JB. Oral labetalol in hypertensive urgencies. *Am J Emerg Med* 1991;9:136.
55. Atkin S et al. Oral labetalol versus oral clonidine in the emergency treatment of severe hypertension. *Am J Med Sci* 1992;303:9.
56. Wright SW et al. Ineffectiveness of oral labetalol for hypertensive urgency. *Am J Emerg Med* 1990;8:472.
57. Devlin JW, Seta ML, Kanji S, Somerville AL. Fenoldopam versus nitroprusside for the treatment of hypertensive emergency. *Ann Pharmacother* 2004;38:755.
58. Panacek E et al. Randomized, prospective trial of fenoldopam vs. sodium nitroprusside in the treatment of acute severe hypertension. *Acad Emerg Med* 1995;2:959.
59. Pilmer B et al. Fenoldopam mesylate versus sodium nitroprusside in the acute management of severe systemic hypertension. *J Clin Pharmacol* 1993;33:549.
60. Reisin E et al. Intravenous fenoldopam versus sodium nitroprusside in patients with severe hypertension. *Hypertension* 1990;15(Suppl 1):159.
61. Garwood S, Hines R. Perioperative renal preservation: dopexamine, and fenoldopam: new agents to augment renal performance. *Semin Anesth Periop Med Pain* 1998;17:308.
62. Murphy M et al. Augmentation of renal blood flow and sodium excretion in hypertensive patients during blood pressure reduction by intravenous administration of the dopamine-1 agonist, fenoldopam. *Circulation* 1987;6:1312.
63. Shusterman N et al. Fenoldopam but not nitroprusside improves renal function in severely hypertensive patients with impaired renal function. *Am J Med* 1993;95:161.
64. Elliott W et al. Renal and hemodynamic effects of intravenous fenoldopam versus nitroprusside in severe hypertension. *Circulation* 1990;81:970.
65. McKinney TD. Management of hypertensive crisis. *Hosp Pract* 1992;27:133.
66. Brater DC et al. Prolonged hemodynamic effect of furosemide in congestive heart failure. *Am Heart J* 1984;4:1031.
67. *United States Pharmacopeia Drug Information: Nipride*. Greenwood Village, CO: Thomson Micromedex; 2003.

68. Hirschl M. Guidelines for the drug treatment of hypertensive crises. *Drugs* 1995;50:991.
69. Nightingale S. New labeling for sodium nitroprusside emphasizes risk of cyanide toxicity. *JAMA* 1991;265:847.
70. Lavin P. Management of hypertension in patients with acute stroke. *Arch Intern Med* 1986;146:66.
71. Schultz V. Clinical pharmacokinetics of nitroprusside, cyanide, thiosulphate and thiocyanate. *Clin Pharmacokinet* 1984;9:239.
72. Rindone JP, Sloane EP. Cyanide toxicity from sodium nitroprusside: risks and management. *Ann Pharmacother* 1992;26:515.
73. Friederich J, Butterworth J. Sodium nitroprusside: twenty years and counting. *Anesth Analg* 1995;81:152.
74. Schultz V et al. Hypotensive efficacy of a mixed solution of 0.1% sodium nitroprusside and 1% sodium thiosulphate. *J Hypertens* 1985;3:485.
75. Baskin S et al. The antidotal action of sodium nitrite and sodium thiosulfate against cyanide poisoning. *J Clin Pharmacol* 1992;32:368.
76. Curry SC, Capell-Arnold P. Toxic effects of drugs used in the ICU: nitroprusside, nitroglycerin, and angiotensin converting enzyme inhibitors. *Crit Care Clin* 1991;7:555.
77. Robin E, McCauley R. Nitroprusside-related cyanide poisoning: time (long past due) for urgent, effective interventions. *Chest* 1992;102:1842.
78. Zerbe NF, Wagner BK. Use of vitamin B_{12} in the treatment and prevention of nitroprusside-induced cyanide toxicity. *Crit Care Med* 1993;21:465.
79. Sarvotham S. Nitroprusside therapy in post-open heart hypertensives: a ritual tryst with cyanide death. *Chest* 1987;91:796.
80. Johanning R et al. A retrospective study of sodium nitroprusside use and assessment of the potential risk of cyanide poisoning. *Pharmacotherapy* 1995;15:773.
81. Cottrell JE et al. Prevention of nitroprusside-induced cyanide toxicity with hydroxocobalamin. *N Engl J Med* 1978;298:809.
82. Kayser SR et al. Hydroxocobalamin in nitroprusside-induced cyanide toxicity. *Drug Intell Clin Pharm* 1986;20:365.
83. Stumpf JL. Drug therapy in hypertensive crises. *Clin Pharm* 1988;7:582.
84. Dwyer M, Morris C. Toxicity of sodium nitroprusside. *Conn Med* 1993;57:489.
85. Fenoldopam. *Med Lett Drug Ther* 1998;40:57.
86. Ellis D et al. Treatment of hypertensive emergencies with fenoldopam, a peripherally acting dopamine (DA_1) receptor agonist. *Crit Care Med* 1998;26(1 Suppl):A23.
87. Brogden R, Markham A. Fenoldopam: a review of its pharmacodynamic and pharmacokinetic properties and intravenous clinical potential in the management of hypertensive urgencies and emergencies. *Drugs* 1997;54:634.
88. Murphy MB et al. Fenoldopam—a selective peripheral dopamine-receptor agonist for the treatment of severe hypertension. *N Engl J Med* 2001;345:1548.
89. Nichols A et al. The pharmacology of fenoldopam. *Am J Hypertens* 1990;3:116S.
90. White W, Halley S. Comparative renal effects of intravenous administration of fenoldopam mesylate and sodium nitroprusside in patients with severe hypertension. *Arch Intern Med* 1989;149:870.
91. Oparil S et al. A new parenteral antihypertensive: consensus roundtable on the management of perioperative hypertension and hypertensive crises. *Am J Hypertens* 1999;12:653.
92. Goldberg M, Larijani G. Perioperative hypertension. *Pharmacotherapy* 1998;18:911.
93. Yakazu Y et al. Hemodynamic and sympathetic effects of fenoldopam and sodium nitroprusside. *Acta Anaesthesiol Scand* 2001;45:1176.
94. Everitt D et al. Effect of intravenous fenoldopam on intraocular pressure in ocular hypertension. *J Clin Pharmacol* 1997;37:312.
95. Piltz J et al. Fenoldopam, a selective dopamine-1 receptor agonist, raises intraocular pressure in males with normal intraocular pressure. *J Ocul Pharmacol Ther* 1998;14:203.
96. Cressman MD et al. Intravenous labetalol in the management of severe hypertension and hypertensive emergencies. *Am Heart J* 1984;107:980.
97. Wilson DJ et al. Intravenous labetalol in the treatment of severe hypertension and hypertensive emergencies. *Am J Med* 1983;75(Suppl):95.
98. Smith WB et al. Antihypertensive effectiveness of intravenous labetalol in accelerated hypertension. *Hypertension* 1983;5:579.
99. Dal Palu C et al. Intravenous labetalol in severe hypertension. *Br J Clin Pharmacol* 1982;13(Suppl 1):97S.
100. Lebel M et al. Labetalol infusion in hypertensive emergencies. *Clin Pharmacol Ther* 1985;37:615.
101. Vidt DG. Intravenous labetalol in the emergency treatment of hypertension. *J Clin Hypertens* 1985;2:179.
102. Patel RV et al. Labetalol: response and safety in critically ill hemorrhagic stroke patients. *Ann Pharmacother* 1993;27:180.
103. Kanto JH. Current status of labetalol, the first alpha- and beta-blocking agent. *Int J Clin Pharmacol Ther Toxicol* 1985;23:617.
104. George RB et al. Comparison of the effects of labetalol and hydrochlorothiazide on the ventilatory function of hypertensive patients with asthma and propranolol sensitivity. *Chest* 1985;88:815.
105. Kanada S et al. Angina-like syndrome with diazoxide therapy for hypertensive crisis. *Ann Intern Med* 1976;84:696.
106. Vidt DG et al. Safety of diazoxide administration in antihypertensive therapy: an analysis of 1,268 injections in 423 patients [abstract]. *Clin Pharmacol Ther* 1977;21:120.
107. Moser M. Diazoxide: an effective vasodilator in accelerated hypertension. *Am Heart J* 1974;87:791.
108. Walstad RA et al. Labetalol in the treatment of hypertension in patients with normal and impaired renal function. *Acta Med Scand* 1982;212(Suppl 665):135.
109. Wood AJ et al. Elimination kinetics of labetalol in severe renal failure. *Br J Clin Pharmacol* 1982;13(Suppl):81.
110. MacCarthy EP et al. Labetalol: a review of its pharmacology pharmacokinetics, clinical uses and adverse effects. *Pharmacotherapy* 1983;3:193.
111. Abrams JH et al. Successful treatment of a monoamine oxidase inhibitor-tyramine hypertensive emergency with intravenous labetalol. *N Engl J Med* 1985;313:52.
112. Navaratnarajah M et al. Labetalol and phaeochromocytoma. *Br J Anaesth* 1984;56:1179.
113. Kelly JG et al. Bioavailability of labetalol increases with age. *Br J Clin Pharmacol* 1982;14:304.
114. Eisalo A et al. Treatment of hypertension in the elderly with labetalol. *Acta Med Scand* 1982;665(Suppl):129.
115. McGrath BP et al. Emergency treatment of severe hypertension with intravenous labetalol. *Med J Aust* 1978;2:410.
116. Anderson CC et al. Poor hypotensive response and tachyphylaxis following intravenous labetalol. *Curr Med Res Opin* 1978;5:424.
117. Yeung CK et al. Comparison of labetalol, clonidine and diazoxide intravenously administered in severe hypertension. *Med J Aust* 1979;2:499.
118. Pearson RM et al. Intravenous labetalol in hypertensive patients treated with β-adrenoceptor blocking drugs. *Br J Clin Pharmacol* 1976;3(Suppl 3):795.
119. Cumming AM et al. Intravenous labetalol in the treatment of severe hypertension. *Br J Clin Pharmacol* 1982;13(Suppl 1):93S.
120. Flaherty JT et al. Comparison of intravenous nitroglycerin and sodium nitroprusside for treatment of acute hypertension developing after coronary artery bypass surgery. *Circulation* 1982;65:1072.
121. Chun G, Frishman WH. Rapid-acting parenteral antihypertensive agents. *J Clin Pharmacol* 1990;30:195.
122. Francis GS. Vasodilators in the intensive care unit. *Am Heart J* 1991;121:1875.
123. Huysmans FT et al. Combined intravenous administration of diazoxide and beta-blocking agent in acute treatment of severe hypertension or hypertensive crisis. *Am Heart J* 1982;103:395.
124. Ram CV et al. Individual titration of diazoxide dosage in the treatment of severe hypertension. *Am J Cardiol* 1979;43:627.
125. Ogilvie RI et al. Diazoxide concentration–response relation in hypertension. *Hypertension* 1982;4:167.
126. Garrett BN et al. Efficacy of slow infusion of diazoxide in the treatment of severe hypertension without organ hypoperfusion. *Am Heart J* 1982;103:390.
127. Finnerty F. Hyperglycemia after diazoxide administration. *N Engl J Med* 1971;285:1487.
128. Rutledge J et al. Effect of intravenous enalaprilat in moderate and severe hypertension. *Am J Cardiol* 1988;62:1062.
129. Evans RR et al. The effect of intravenous enalaprilat (MK-422) administration in patients with mild to moderate essential hypertension. *J Clin Pharmacol* 1987;27:415.
130. Hirschl M et al. Clinical evaluation of different doses of intravenous enalaprilat in patients with hypertensive crises. *Arch Intern Med* 1995;155:2217.
131. White C. Pharmacologic, pharmacokinetic, and therapeutic differences among ACE inhibitors. *Pharmacotherapy* 1998;18:588.
132. Misra M et al. Evaluation of the efficacy, safety, and tolerability of intravenous enalaprilat in the treatment of grade III essential hypertension in Indian patients. *Indian Heart J* 2004;56:67.
133. DiPette DJ et al. Enalaprilat, an intravenous angiotensin-converting enzyme inhibitor, in hypertensive crises. *Clin Pharmacol Ther* 1985;38:199.
134. Menkhaus P et al. Cardiovascular effects of esmolol in anesthetised humans. *Anesth Analg* 1985;64:327.
135. Allin D et al. Intravenous esmolol for the treatment of supraventricular tachyarrhythmia: results of a multicenter, baseline-controlled safety and efficacy study in 160 patients. *Am Heart J* 1986;112:498.
136. Anderson S et al. Comparison of the efficacy and safety of esmolol, a short-acting beta-blocker, with placebo in the treatment of supraventricular tachyarrhythmias. *Am Heart J* 1986;111:42.
137. Gray R et al. Use of esmolol in hypertension after cardiac surgery. *Am J Cardiol* 1985;56:49F.
138. Benfield P, Sorkin E. Esmolol: a preliminary review of its pharmacodynamic and pharmacokinetic properties, and therapeutic efficacy. *Drugs* 1987;33:392.
139. Salerno DM et al. Efficacy and safety of intravenous diltiazem for treatment of atrial fibrillation and atrial flutter. *Am J Cardiol* 1989;63:1046.
140. Ellenbogen KA et al. A placebo-controlled trial of continuous intravenous diltiazem infusion for 24-hour heart rate control during atrial fibrillation and atrial flutter: a multicenter study. *J Am Coll Cardiol* 1991;18:891.
141. Dougherty AH et al. Acute conversion of paroxysmal supraventricular tachycardia with intravenous diltiazem. *Am J Cardiol* 1992;79:587.
142. Koh H et al. Clinical study of total intravenous anesthesia with droperidol, fentanyl, and ketamine: control of intraoperative hypertension with diltiazem. *Jpn J Anesth* 1991;40:1376.
143. Boylan JF et al. A comparison of diltiazem, esmolol, nifedipine, and nitroprusside therapy of post-CABG hypertension. *Can J Anaesth* 1990;37:S156.
144. Jaffe AS. Use of intravenous diltiazem in patients with acute coronary artery disease. *Am J Cardiol* 1992;69:25B.
145. Fang ZY et al. Intravenous diltiazem versus nitroglycerin for silent and symptomatic myocardial ischemia in unstable angina pectoris. *Am J Cardiol* 1991;68:42C.
146. Onoyama K et al. Effect of drug infusion or a bolus injection of intravenous diltiazem on hypertensive crisis. *Curr Ther Res* 1987;42:1223.
147. Onoyama K et al. Effect of a drip infusion of diltiazem on severe systemic hypertension. *Curr Ther Res* 1988;43:361.

148. Cheung D et al. Acute pharmacokinetic and hemodynamic effects of intravenous bolus dosing of nicardipine. *Am Heart J* 1990;119:438.
149. IV Nicardipine Study Group. Efficacy and safety of intravenous nicardipine in the control of postoperative hypertension. *Chest* 1991;99:393.
150. Halpern NA et al. Nicardipine infusion for postoperative hypertension after surgery of the head and neck. *Crit Care Med* 1990;18:950.
151. Halpern NA et al. Postoperative hypertension: a prospective placebo controlled, randomized, double-blind trial with intravenous nicardipine hydrochloride. *Angiology* 1990;41:992.
152. Kaplan JA. Clinical considerations for the use of intravenous nicardipine in the treatment of postoperative hypertension. *Am Heart J* 1990;119:443.
153. Halpern NA et al. Postoperative hypertension: a prospective, placebo controlled, randomized, double-blind trial with intravenous nicardipine hydrochloride. *Angiology* 1990;41:992.
154. Wallin JD et al. Intravenous nicardipine for treatment of severe hypertension. *Arch Intern Med* 1989;149:2662.
155. Neutel J et al. A comparison of intravenous nicardipine and sodium nitroprusside in the immediate treatment of severe hypertension. *Am J Hypertens* 1994;7:623.
156. Qureshi AI et al. Treatment of acute hypertension in patients with intracerebral hemorrhage using American Heart Association guidelines. *Crit Care Med* 2006;34:1975.
157. Curran MP et al. Intravenous nicardipine. *Drugs* 2006;66:1755.
158. Kwak YL et al. Comparison of the effects of nicardipine and sodium nitroprusside for control of increased blood pressure after coronary artery bypass graft surgery. *J Int Med Res* 2004;32:342.
159. Dorman T et al. Nicardipine versus nitroprusside for breakthrough hypertension following carotid endarterectomy. *J Clin Anesth* 2001;13:16.
160. Haas AR et al. Current diagnosis and management of hypertensive emergency. *Semin Dial* 2006;19:502.
161. Varon J, Marik PE. The diagnosis and management of hypertensive crises. *Chest* 2000;118:214.
162. Chen K et al. Acute thoracic aortic dissection: the basics. *J Emerg Med* 1997;15:859.
163. Khoynezhad A et al. Managing emergency hypertension in aortic dissection and aortic aneurysm surgery. *J Card Surg* 2006;21:S3.
164. DeSanctis RW et al. Aortic dissection. *N Engl J Med* 1987;317:1060.
165. Lindsay J. Aortic dissection. *Heart Dis Stroke* 1992;2:69.
166. Gupta R et al. Cardiovascular emergencies in the elderly. *Emerg Med Clin North Am* 2006;24:339.
167. Lange RA, Hillis LD. Cardiovascular complications of cocaine use. *N Engl J Med* 2001;345:351.
168. Shanti CM, Lucas CE. Cocaine and the critical challenge. *Crit Care Med* 2003;31:1851.
169. Brogan WC III et al. Alleviation of cocaine-induced coronary vasoconstriction by nitroglycerin. *J Am Coll Cardiol* 1991;18:581.
170. Negus BH et al. Alleviation of cocaine-induced coronary vasoconstriction with intravenous verapamil. *Am J Cardiol* 1994;73:510.
171. Honderick T. A prospective, randomized, controlled trial of benzodiazepines and nitroglycerine or nitroglycerine alone in the treatment of cocaine-associated acute coronary syndromes. *Am J Emerg Med* 2003;21:39.
172. Ramoska E, Sacchetti AD. Propranolol-induced hypertension in treatment of cocaine intoxication. *Ann Emerg Med* 1985;14:1112.
173. Lange RA et al. Potentiation of cocaine-induced coronary vasoconstriction by beta-adrenergic blockade. *Ann Intern Med* 1990;112:897.
174. Gay GR, Loper KA. The use of labetalol in the management of cocaine crisis. *Ann Emerg Med* 1998;17:282.
175. Boehrer JD et al. Influence of labetalol on cocaine-induced coronary vasoconstriction in humans. *Am J Med* 1993;94:608.
176. Spivey WH et al. Comparison of labetalol, diazepam, and haloperidol for the treatment of cocaine toxicity in a swine model. *Ann Emerg Med* 1990;19:467.
177. Chung PCH et al. Elevated vascular resistance after labetalol during resection of a pheochromocytoma. *Can J Anaesth* 2002;49:148.

CHAPTER 21

Shock

Andrew D. Barnes and Susan H. Lee

INTRODUCTION

Shock is defined in simple terms as a syndrome of impaired tissue perfusion usually, but not always, accompanied by hypotension. This impairment of tissue perfusion eventually leads to cellular dysfunction, followed by organ damage and death if untreated. The most common causes of shock are situations that result in a reduction of intravascular volume (hypovolemic shock), myocardial pump failure (cardiogenic shock), or increased vascular capacitance (distributive shock, sepsis). The type of treatment required depends on the etiology.

In recent years, medical support of patients with shock has improved because of better technologies for hemodynamic monitoring, recognition of the value of vigorous volume replacement, appropriate use of inotropic and vasoconstrictive agents, and the development of better ways to treat the underlying cause of the shock syndrome. Understanding the principles of shock should further enhance prompt recognition

Table 21-1 Classification of Shock and Precipitating Events

Hypovolemic Shock
- Hemorrhagic
  - Gastrointestinal bleeding
  - Trauma
  - Internal bleeding: ruptured aortic aneurysm, retroperitoneal bleeding
- *Nonhemorrhagic*
  - Dehydration: vomiting, diarrhea, diabetes mellitus, diabetes insipidus, overuse of diuretics
  - Sequestration: ascites, third-space accumulation
  - Cutaneous: burns, nonreplaced perspiration and insensible water losses

Cardiogenic Shock
- *Nonmechanical Causes*
  - Acute myocardial infarction
  - Low cardiac output syndrome
  - Right ventricular infarction
  - End-stage cardiomyopathy
- *Mechanical Causes*
  - Rupture of septum or free wall
  - Mitral or aortic insufficiency
  - Papillary muscle rupture or dysfunction
  - Critical aortic stenosis
  - Pericardial tamponade

Distributive Shock
- *Septic Shock*
  - Anaphylaxis
- *Neurogenic*
  - Spinal injury, cerebral damage, severe dysautonomia
- *Drug-Induced*
  - Anesthesia, ganglionic and adrenergic blockers, and over-doses of barbiturates, narcotics
- *Acute Adrenal Insufficiency*

of patients at risk, rapid initiation of corrective measures, and development of innovative treatment regimens.

CAUSES

Table 21-1 outlines the classification of shock and precipitating events.[1] Recognition of the etiology and underlying pathology of the various forms of shock is essential for managing this condition. The distinctions among subtypes of shock only apply, however, in the relatively early stages. As the syndrome evolves and compensatory mechanisms are overwhelmed, it becomes increasingly difficult to determine the subtypes because the clinical and pathophysiologic features of advanced shock are the same for all. Also, different types of shock can occur at the same time (e.g., a patient with septic shock who is also hypovolemic).

PATHOPHYSIOLOGY

Tissue perfusion is a complex process of oxygen and nutrient delivery as well as waste removal. When perfusion is impaired, it sets up a cascade of events that can eventually end in death. Although the etiology of shock is varied, the eventual progression (if untreated) to cell death and subsequent organ dysfunction results from a common pathway of ischemia, endogenous inflammatory cytokine release, and the generation of oxygen radicals. When cells are subjected to a prolonged period of ischemia, anaerobic metabolism begins. This inefficient process results in a decrease of adenosine triphosphate (ATP) stores and causes the buildup of lactic acid and other toxic substances that can alter the cellular machinery and eventually result in cell death. In the advanced stages of shock, irreversible cellular damage leads to multiple organ system failure (MOSF), also known as multiple organ dysfunction syndrome (MODS).

Inflammatory cytokines are produced by the body in response to ischemia, injury, or infection. The phrase *systemic inflammatory response syndrome* (SIRS) is the recommended umbrella term to describe any acute, overwhelming inflammatory response, independent of the cause.[2] This syndrome can occur after a wide variety of insults, including hemorrhagic shock, infection (septic shock), pancreatitis, ischemia, multitrauma and tissue injury, and immune-mediated organ injury. SIRS is usually a late manifestation of hypovolemic forms of shock. It is uncommon in cardiogenic shock, but is the hallmark of septic shock. SIRS is clinically characterized by profound vasodilation, which impairs perfusion, and increased capillary permeability, which can lead to reduced intravascular volume.

The following mediators have been identified as possible causes of the proinflammatory reaction underlying sepsis and multiple organ failure[3]:

- Macrophages and their products
- Cytokines: tumor necrosis factor (TNF), interleukin-1(IL-1), interleukin-6 (IL-6), and interleukin-8 (IL-8)
- Neutrophils and products of degranulation
- Platelets and the coagulation factors formed on their surfaces
- Derivatives of arachidonic acid
- T and B lymphocytes and their products

CLINICAL PRESENTATION

Independent of the pathophysiologic cause, the clinical syndrome of shock progresses through several stages. During each step, the body uses and exhausts various compensatory mechanisms to balance oxygen delivery (Do_2) and oxygen consumption (Vo_2) in an effort to maintain perfusion of vital organs. A major determinant of tissue perfusion is the systemic or mean arterial pressure. Mean arterial pressure (MAP) is a function of the product of blood flow (cardiac output [CO]) and systemic vascular resistance (SVR). Cardiac output is the product of heart rate (HR) and stroke volume (SV) (Fig. 21-1). Vascular resistance is determined primarily by vascular smooth muscle tone, modulated by the sympathoadrenal system and by circulating humoral and local metabolic factors. These interacting factors are what contribute to the clinical syndrome seen in patients with shock.

The classic findings observed with shock include the following:

- Systolic blood pressure (SBP) <90 mmHg (or >60 mmHg decrease from baseline in a hypertensive patient)
- Tachycardia (HR >90 beats/minute)
- Tachypnea (respiratory rate [RR] >20 breaths/minute)
- Cutaneous vasoconstriction: cold, clammy, mottled skin (although not typical of distributive shock)

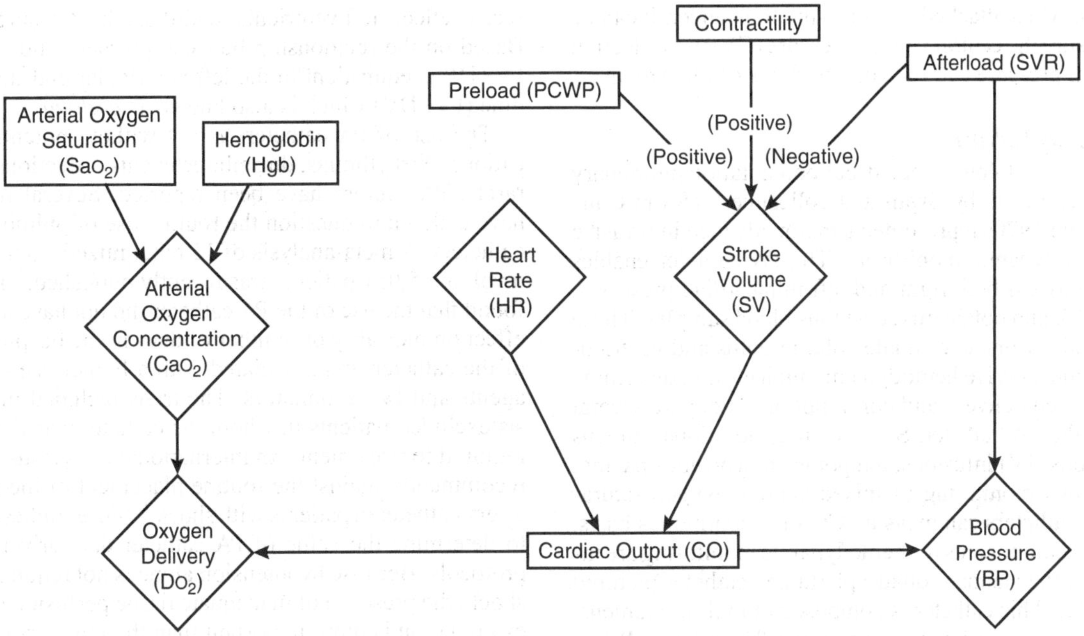

FIGURE 21-1 Determinants of blood pressure, cardiac output, and oxygen delivery.

- Mental confusion (agitation, stupor, or coma)
- Oliguria: urine output <20 mL/hour
- Metabolic acidosis (lactic acidosis secondary to anaerobic glycolysis)

Not all these described findings are encountered in every patient with shock, and considerable variability exists in both the rapidity and sequence of onset. This depends on the severity of the initiating event, the underlying mechanism, and the baseline condition of the patient, including medications that may alter the clinical presentation. Therefore, it is important to consider the patient's medical and pharmacologic history while closely monitoring for subtle clinical changes that may signal impending deterioration and necessitate immediate intervention.

HEMODYNAMIC MONITORING

Hemodynamic monitoring in the critically ill patient is mandatory to properly assess and manage various shock states. Both noninvasive and invasive monitoring techniques can be used to measure cardiovascular performance in patients and to differentiate the causes of various conditions that result in hypoperfusion and organ dysfunction. The values obtained with hemodynamic monitoring should always be used in conjunction with clinical judgment.

Noninvasive Monitoring

An important part of hemodynamic monitoring in the critically ill patient involves noninvasive measures. Clinical examination and vital signs (temperature, HR, BP, RR) provide valuable information regarding the cardiovascular system and organ perfusion. Other well-established noninvasive techniques for monitoring the hemodynamic status of patients include pulse oximetry (for measuring arterial oxygen saturation [Sao_2]) and transthoracic echocardiography, which can estimate the functional status of the heart and heart valves.

New noninvasive technologies are being developed. End tidal carbon dioxide ($EtCO_2$) monitors are used to determine oxygen consumption and help guide therapies designed to improve oxygen delivery and consumption. New devices that can measure CO and tissue perfusion noninvasively (or minimally invasively), such as gastric tonometry, esophageal Doppler monitoring, thoracic bioimpedance, and others have been developed,[4,5] but are not used routinely in most intensive care units (ICU). Although important, noninvasive measures have limitations, and certain hemodynamic values must be measured invasively at the present time.

Invasive Monitoring

The evaluation of critically ill patients is a complicated matter, and data that can be important in the diagnosis and assessment of illness as well as the patient's response to therapy must occasionally be obtained by invasive techniques.

Arterial Pressure Line

The arterial line is a common tool in the ICU. It consists of a small catheter placed into an artery (usually the radial or femoral artery) and attached to a pressure transducer. This allows for continuous measurement of BP and also provides for easy access for arterial blood gas (ABG) samples to be drawn and analyzed. Arterial lines should never be used for medication administration.

Central Venous Catheter

Common in the ICU, the central venous catheter consists of a large-bore catheter usually inserted into either a subclavian or jugular vein. It can be used for infusion of fluid and medications; when attached to a pressure transducer, it can be used to measure the central venous pressure (CVP), a reflection of right atrial pressure and the volume status of the patient.

Pulmonary Artery Catheter

The introduction of flow-directed, balloon flotation pulmonary artery (PA) catheters by Swan and colleagues[6] (Swan-Ganz catheter) in the 1970s represented a major advance in invasive bedside hemodynamic monitoring. The PA catheter enables clinicians to assess both right and left intracardiac pressures, determine CO, and obtain mixed venous blood samples. These capabilities allow one to evaluate volume status and ventricular performance, derive hemodynamic indices, and determine systemic oxygen delivery and consumption. There are several versions of the PA catheter. Some include additional lumens for intravenous (IV) infusions, temporary transvenous pacing, and continuous monitoring of mixed venous oxygen saturation. Newer catheters can measure CO on a continuous basis. The essential components for hemodynamic monitoring are incorporated in the standard quadruple lumen catheter pictured in Figure 21-2. This catheter is composed of multiple lumens, each terminating at different points along the catheter. When properly positioned, the proximal port (C) terminates in the right atrium is used to measure right atrial pressure, to inject fluid for CO determination, and to administer IV fluids. The distal port (B), which terminates at the tip of the catheter (E), is positioned in the pulmonary artery beyond the pulmonary valve and is used to measure pulmonary artery and pulmonary capillary wedge pressure (PCWP; described below) and to obtain mixed venous blood samples. Intermittent inflation of the balloon is accomplished by inserting 1.5 mL of air into the balloon inflation valve (D). The thermistor (A) contains a temperature probe and electrical leads that connect to a computer, which calculates CO by the thermodilution technique.

Although the pulmonary artery catheter is confined to the pulmonary vasculature, left ventricular (LV) pressure can be ascertained from the PCWP. When the balloon is inflated, the PA catheter advances to a pulmonary artery branch of equal diameter and becomes lodged or "wedged" in this position. Because forward flow from the right ventricle ceases beyond the wedged PA segment, a static fluid column exists between the LV and PA catheter tip during diastole when the mitral valve is open. If no pressure gradients are in the pulmonary vasculature beyond the balloon and if mitral valve function is normal, the PCWP then equilibrates with all distal pressures and thus indirectly reflects left ventricular end-diastolic pressure (LVEDP). Based on the relationship between pressure and volume, the LVEDP is equivalent to the left ventricular end-diastolic volume (LVEDV) which is also known as *preload.*

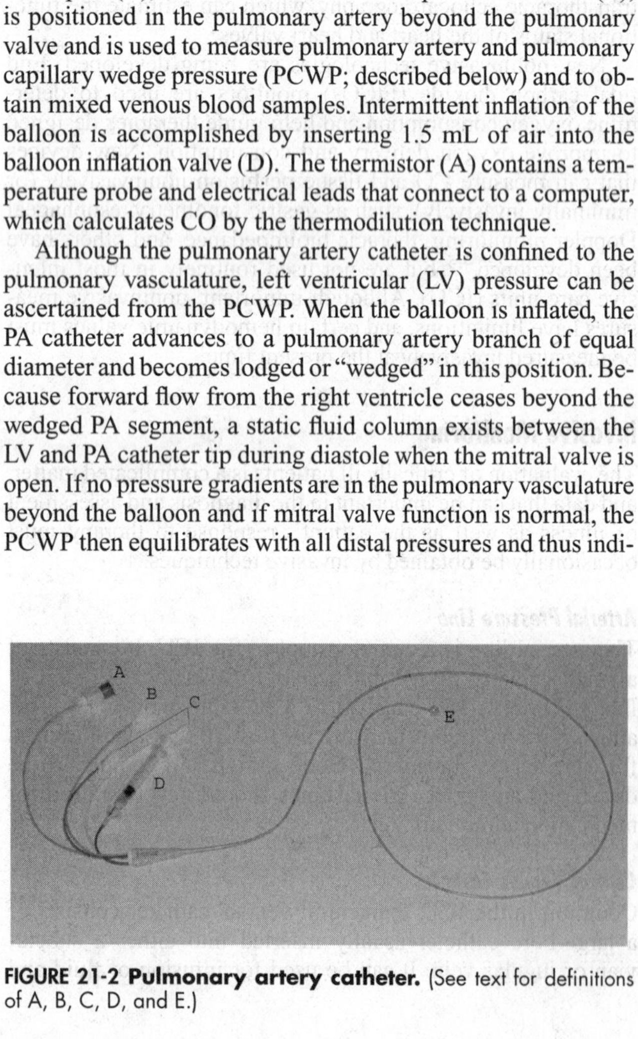

FIGURE 21-2 Pulmonary artery catheter. (See text for definitions of A, B, C, D, and E.)

The use of PA catheters is not without potential complications. Arrhythmias, thrombotic events, infections, and, very rarely, PA rupture have been reported. Several recent trials have called into question the routine use of pulmonary artery catheters. A meta-analysis of 13 randomized, controlled trials involving 5,051 patients was recently published.[7] The authors found that the use of the PA catheter did not have a significant effect on mortality or number of days in the hospital. The use of the catheter was associated with a higher use of inotropic agents and IV vasodilators. The trials included in the analysis excluded patients in whom the catheter was thought to be required for treatment. An international consensus conference recommends against the routine placement of the pulmonary artery catheter in patients with shock.[8] More studies are needed to determine the value of PA catheter data-driven treatment protocols. Because hypotension alone is not required to define shock, the presence of inadequate tissue perfusion on physical examination is more important than the numbers obtained by invasive monitoring.[8]

DETERMINANTS OF CARDIAC FUNCTION AND HEMODYNAMIC INDICES

The effective interpretation and management of hemodynamic parameters requires a thorough understanding of the physiologic determinants of CO and arterial pressure. Assuming oxygen content of blood is adequate, CO and SVR are the ultimate determinants of oxygen delivery and adequate arterial pressure, and thus overall tissue perfusion. As outlined in Figure 21-1, cardiac output may be quantified as the product of SV and HR. SV is determined by preload, afterload, and contractility. The effects of these factors on hemodynamic parameters are interrelated and complex and must be assessed carefully when selecting therapeutic interventions that will produce the desired response. A good review of the determinants of cardiac performance is found in Chapter 18, Heart Failure. Table 21-2 and the Glossary provide definitions of terms and normal hemodynamic indices, which are discussed in the following section.

Measured Hemodynamic Indices

Right Atrial Pressure and Central Venous Pressure

The right atrial pressure (RAP), as measured by a PA catheter, reflects the filling pressure or end-diastolic pressure of the right ventricle (RV) and is used as an index of RV preload. Central venous pressure, as determined by a catheter advanced to the superior vena cava or right atrium, is another means of measuring RV filling pressure and is considered equivalent to the RAP. Vascular capacitance, circulating blood volume, and myocardial contractility maintain RAP. A low RAP usually reflects hypovolemia or vasodilation. An elevated RAP can signify increased intravascular volume, right ventricular heart failure, tricuspid regurgitation, pulmonary embolus, pulmonary hypertension, obstructive airway disease with cor pulmonale, or pericardial tamponade. In tamponade, the LV filling pressure also is elevated to the same degree as the RAP.

Table 21-2 Normal Hemodynamic Values and Derived Indices

	Equation	Normal Value	Units
Directly Measured			
Blood pressure (BP) (systolic/diastolic)		120–140/80–90	mmHg
Cardiac output (CO)	$CO = SV \times HR$	4–7	L/min
Central venous pressure (CVP)[a]		2–6	mmHg[b]
Heart rate (HR) (pulse)		60–80	beats/min
Mean pulmonary artery pressure (MPAP)		12–15	mmHg
Pulmonary artery pressure (PAP) (systolic/diastolic)		20–30/8–12	mmHg
Pulmonary capillary wedge pressure (PCWP)		5–12[c]	mmHg
Derived Indices			
Cardiac index (CI)	$CI = \frac{CO}{BSA}$[d]	2.5–4.2	L/min/m^2
Left ventricular stroke work index (LVSWI)	$LVSWI = (MAP - PCWP)(SVI)(0.0136)$	35–85	g/m^2/beat
Mean arterial pressure (MAP)	$MAP = \frac{2(\text{Diastolic BP}) + \text{Systolic BP}}{3}$	80–100	mmHg
Perfusion pressure (PP)	$PP = MAP - PCWP$	50	mmHg
Pulmonary vascular resistance (PVR)	$PVR = \frac{(MPAP - PCWP)}{CO}$ (74)	20–120	dynes.sec.cm^{-5}
Stroke volume (SV)	$SV = \frac{CO}{HR}$	60–130	mL/beat
Stroke volume index (SVI)	$SVI = \frac{SV}{BSA}$	30–75	mL/beat/m^2
Systemic vascular resistance (SVR)[e]	$SVR = \frac{(MAP - CVP)}{CO}$ (74)	800–1,440	dyne.sec.cm^{-5}
Systemic vascular resistance index (SVRI)	$SVRI = SVR \times BSA$	1,680–2,580	dyne.sec.cm^{-5}.m^2
Oxygen delivery (Do_2)	$Do_2 = CO - Cao_2$ $[Cao_2 = (Hgb - Sao_2 - 13.9)]$	700–1,200	mL/min
Oxygen consumption (Vo_2)	$Vo_2 = Co - Hgb - 13.9 - (Sao_2 - Svo_2)$	200–400	mL/min

[a] CVP is essentially synonymous with RAP.
[b] 2–6 mmHg = 3–6 cm H_2O (conversion: 1 mm = 1.34 cm H_2O).
[c] May optimally ↑ PCWP to 16–18 mmHg in critically ill patients.
[d] BSA, body surface area = 1.7 m^2 (average male).
[e] SVR is synonymous with total peripheral resistance (TPR).

Right-sided heart pressures are unreliable indicators of concurrent LV function.[9] In patients with cardiac or pulmonary disease or on mechanical ventilation, RAP or CVP measurements actually may vary inversely with the PCWP. Therefore, reliance on right-sided heart pressures from CVP catheters alone is adequate only in select patients.

Pulmonary Artery Systolic Pressure

Pulmonary artery systolic (PAS) pressure is obtained during systole after the opening of the pulmonic valve when blood is ejected from the right ventricle into the pulmonary artery. It measures the pressure generated by the RV during contraction. Elevations in PAS pressure occur when pulmonary vascular resistance is increased. This occurs in patients with acute or chronic parenchymal pulmonary disease, pulmonary embolus, hypoxemia, or acidosis, as well as in those receiving vasoactive drugs. A low PAS pressure usually results from a reduced circulating blood volume.

Pulmonary Artery Diastolic Pressure

Pulmonary artery diastolic (PAD) pressure is measured during diastole after the closure of the pulmonic valve when the blood moves from the pulmonary artery into the pulmonary capillaries. As previously described with respect to the PCWP, the PAD pressure also may reflect LVEDP. Under normal circumstances, the PAD pressure is approximately equal (within 1–3 mmHg) to the PCWP and can be used in place of the latter as an indication of LVEDP. Because the catheter is more proximally located and is not in a "wedged" position, the PAD pressure may not correlate as well as the PCWP with the LVEDP. In conditions that increase pulmonary vascular resistance, such as those mentioned for pulmonary artery systolic pressure, the PAD may be substantially greater than the PCWP. Also, when heart rates are >120 beats/minute, PAD pressure exceeds PCWP. This is because diastole is shortened and reduces the time necessary for equilibrium of blood flow.

Pulmonary Capillary Wedge Pressure

Pulmonary capillary wedge pressure is the most reliable reflection of LVEDP measured with the pulmonary artery catheter. LVEDP, in turn, provides the closest approximation of preload, the initial end-diastolic fiber length, which is determined clinically by LVEDV. Because neither LVEDV nor LVEDP are readily measurable, PCWP is used as an indicator of preload.

Preload is an important determinant of stroke volume. The relationship between preload and stroke volume is illustrated in Figure 21-3, the Frank-Starling curve. According to this mechanism, the degree of myocardial fiber shortening, and hence SV, is proportional to the initial myocardial fiber length, or ventricular volume, at the onset of contraction. As shown in Figure 21-1, if HR remains the same, SV is proportional to cardiac output. Initially, for any given state of contractility, an increase in preload generates a contraction that results in a corresponding increase in SV. Once an optimal preload is attained, as indicated by the flat portion of the curve, further elevations in ventricular filling pressure will not enhance SV and, in fact, can result in a decline in contractility and a decrease in SV. Significant increases or decreases in the level of ventricular contractility (inotropy), independent of alterations in preload or afterload, result in shifts in the ventricular function curve, with corresponding changes in SV. As shown in Figure 21-3, enhanced myocardial contractility caused by such

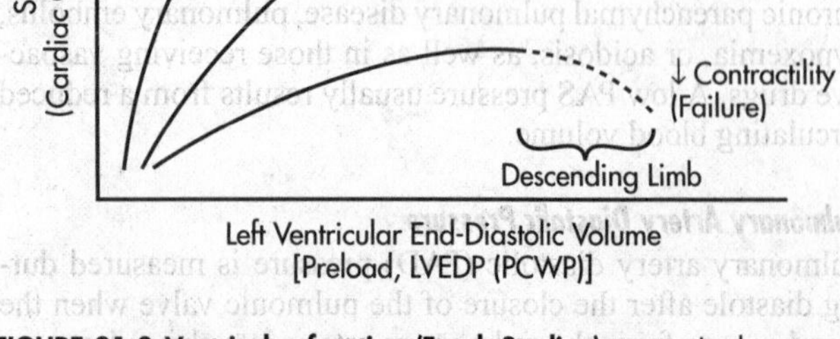

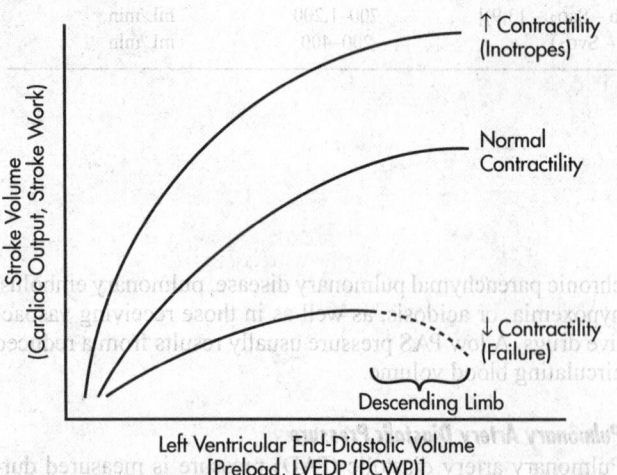

FIGURE 21-3 Ventricular function (Frank-Starling) curve. In the normal heart, as preload (LVEDP), measured clinically by PCWP, increases, stroke volume (cardiac output, stroke work) increases, until the contractile fibers reach their capacity, at which point the curve flattens. A change in contractility causes the heart to perform on a different curve. If the contractile fibers exceed their capacity, as with severe heart failure, the heart will operate on the descending limb of the curve.

factors as increased sympathetic nerve activity, endogenous catecholamines, or exogenous inotropic agents, shifts the ventricular function curve upward and to the left, thus augmenting SV for a given preload. Conditions that reduce contractility, such as loss of contractile mass, use of pharmacologic depressants, systemic hypoxia, local ischemia, or acidosis, shift the curve downward and to the right, thereby diminishing SV.

Although LVEDP or PCWP can generally be substituted for LVEDV when evaluating cardiac function, the use of PCWP as a reflection of LVEDV has limitations. In patients with mitral stenosis, pulmonary veno-occlusive disease, or high levels of positive end-expiratory pressure (PEEP) with mechanical ventilation, PCWP will exceed LVEDV and inaccurately reflect LVEDV.

The relationship between LVEDP and LVEDV is curvilinear and is determined by compliance. In conditions in which ventricular compliance is abnormal, the correlation between LVEDP and LVEDV is altered, and PCWP cannot be assumed to accurately reflect preload. Therefore, it is important to be aware that certain conditions or interventions can result in potential alterations in ventricular compliance and PCWP and interpret measurements accordingly.

The PCWP also is a useful measure of pulmonary capillary hydrostatic pressure, the major driving force for the development of pulmonary congestion. Thus, the PCWP helps the clinician determine whether pulmonary edema is cardiogenic or noncardiogenic in origin. PCWP is higher than pulmonary hydrostatic pressure with adult respiratory distress syndrome (ARDS) or elevated pulmonary vascular resistance.

Cardiac Output

Cardiac output determination involves injecting a 10-mL bolus of cold crystalloid solution through the PA catheter and measuring the temperature at the tip of the catheter via the thermistor. The relationship between the temperature change over time and blood flow allows calculation of the CO.[10] PA catheters are available that use a small heat generator and a heat sink in the catheter itself, which allows the continuous determination of CO with the same concept of thermodilution. Some conditions may make measurement of CO less reliable. Tricuspid valve regurgitation and intracardiac shunts, such as ventricular septal defects, affect the way blood flows past the tip of the thermistor and, thus, may give erroneous values.

Mixed Venous Oxygen Saturation

Mixed venous oxygen saturation (SvO_2) can be measured with fiberoptic sensors in newer versions of the PA catheter, or it can be measured directly from blood drawn from the catheter before oxygenation in the lungs. It can be used as an indicator of the global adequacy of perfusion and can be used to calculate the body's consumption of oxygen (VO_2, see later section). The SvO_2 may be particularly useful in situations in which CO measurements are unreliable (e.g., tricuspid valve regurgitation) or in clinical situations in which oxygen consumption is increased despite normal oxygen delivery (e.g., septic shock).

Derived Hemodynamic Indices

Parameters that reflect cardiovascular function can be derived from the hemodynamic measurements obtained from the Swan-Ganz catheter (Table 21-2 and Glossary).

Stroke Volume

Stroke volume is the amount of blood ejected by the ventricle with each systolic contraction, and it is directly proportional to the contractile state of the myocardium. When CO is increased by therapeutic maneuvers, it is important to know whether the increase is caused by an inotropic (SV) or a chronotropic response (HR).

Cardiac Index

Cardiac index is the CO adjusted for body surface area (BSA). Because CO is a relative measure based on size, cardiac index provides a more meaningful assessment of a person's output.

Pulmonary Vascular Resistance and Systemic Vascular Resistance

Pulmonary vascular resistance (PVR) and systemic vascular resistance (SVR, afterload) are determined by dividing the change in pressure by the flow (pressure change/cardiac output = resistance). Therapeutic maneuvers that alter SVR do not indicate a change in any specific vascular bed, such as the renal or splanchnic vascular beds; changes in SVR reflect the overall change. The systemic vascular resistance index (SVRI) is a normalized SVR for body surface area.

Left Ventricular Stroke Work Index

Left ventricular stroke work index (LVSWI) is an indication of LV contractility that takes into account preload, afterload, and CO. The constant 0.0136 is the conversion factor that changes millimeters of mercury per liter (mmHg/mL) into gram-meters. Elevation in LVSWI can be achieved by changing preload, afterload, or contractility.

Oxygen Transport Variables

Hypoperfusion associated with shock is not as readily detectable as hypotension. An imbalance between oxygen supply and demand may not be recognized until irreversible organ dysfunction has begun. Thus, it can be valuable in some patients to monitor oxygen transport variables and use these values to guide therapy.

Oxygen Delivery

Oxygen delivery (Do_2) can be calculated as the product of CO and the arterial concentration of oxygen (Cao_2). Hemoglobin concentration (Hgb) and arterial oxygen saturation (Sao_2) are the primary determinants of Cao_2. A smaller contribution to the equation is the amount of oxygen dissolved in the blood, determined by the arterial pressure of oxygen (Pao_2), which can be left out to simplify calculations:

$$Do_2 = (CO)(Cao_2)$$

where

$$Cao_2 = (Hgb)(Sao_2)(13.9)$$

Oxygen Consumption

Oxygen consumption (Vo_2) estimates the oxygen demand of the body and can be calculated as the product of CO and the difference between the arterial and venous concentrations of oxygen ($Cao_2 - CVo_2$). Rearranged and simplified, the equation can be represented as follows:

$$Vo_2 = (CO)(Hgb)(13.9)(Sao_2 - Svo_2)$$

Normally, consumption is independent of supply, except at low rates of Do_2. In some critically ill patients, however, consumption can depend on supply even in what would be considered "normal" Do_2 ranges. In these patients, it may be appropriate to increase the delivery of oxygen until the increase in consumption has reached a plateau.[11] This may help to "repay" some of the oxygen debt induced by hypoperfusion. Further increases in Do_2 to supranormal ranges with inotropic drugs, such as dobutamine, have not been conclusively shown to benefit patients and may have a detrimental effect.[12,13] A factor to consider in evaluating these values and the studies that use them is the potential for mathematic coupling of data. CO, hemoglobin, and arterial oxygen saturation are common components of both equations. Errors in the measurement of these parameters lead to errors in the calculation of both delivery and consumption of oxygen.

ETIOLOGIC CLASSIFICATION OF SHOCK AND COMMON MECHANISMS

The most common clinical conditions associated with the major forms of shock are reviewed in the following sections and detailed in Table 21-1. The pathogenesis, epidemiology, clinical, and hemodynamic manifestations for each classification are briefly discussed and further illustrated in case studies throughout the chapter. Table 21-3 describes the common hemodynamic findings for the various forms of shock.

Hypovolemic Shock

Shock secondary to a reduction in intravascular volume is referred to as *hypovolemic shock*. Whether the primary insult is the external loss of fluid volume (e.g., blood, plasma, or free water) or the internal sequestration of these fluids into body cavities (third spacing), the overall result is reduced venous return (decreases in CVP and PCWP) and decreased CO (Table 21-3). The severity of hypovolemic shock depends on the amount and rate of intravascular volume loss and each person's capacity for compensation. Although responses vary,

Table 21-3 Hemodynamic Findings in Various Shock States

	Hypovolemic	*Cardiogenic*	*Distributive (Septic)*
Heart Rate	↑	↑	↑
Blood Pressure[a]	↓	↑/↓	↓
Cardiac Output	↓	↓	↓[b]
Preload (PCWP)	↓	↑	↑/↓
Afterload (SVR)	↑	↑	↓

[a]Patients may be in a state of compensated shock in which BP is normal but clinical signs of hypoperfusion are evident.
[b]Cardiac output is increased early in sepsis but can be decreased in late, severe.

a healthy person may tolerate an acute loss of as much as 30% of his or her intravascular volume with minimal clinical signs and symptoms.[14] Compensatory mechanisms such as increases in HR, myocardial contractility, and SVR, are sufficiently effective for this loss in volume such that measurable falls in systolic BP are not detected. Losses in excess of 80% generally overwhelm compensatory mechanisms and the patient's condition can deteriorate to overt shock with hypotension and signs of hypoperfusion. If restorative measures are not taken immediately, irreversible shock and death may result. The most common and dramatic cause of hypovolemic shock is hemorrhagic shock in which intravascular volume depletion occurs as a result of bleeding. Trauma is responsible for most cases of acute hemorrhagic shock; other significant causes are rupture of vascular aneurysms, acute gastrointestinal bleeding, ruptured ectopic pregnancy, and postoperative bleeding. Other mechanisms for hypovolemic shock are conditions associated with either (*a*) excess fluid losses from gastrointestinal or renal sources or (*b*) plasma loss caused by burns or sequestration (also known as *third-space accumulation*).

Cardiogenic Shock

A shock state arising primarily from an abnormality of cardiac function constitutes cardiogenic shock. The causes of cardiogenic shock can be separated largely into mechanical and nonmechanical (Table 21-1), although occasionally, patients may have a combination of causes. Regardless of the source, the underlying problem in cardiogenic shock is a decrease in CO that is not caused by a reduction in circulating blood volume. This decrease in CO results in the syndrome of shock: hypotension with a decrease in arterial BP, and hypoperfusion as the delivery of oxygenated blood to the tissues is reduced. Eventually, organ dysfunction and death result if measures to restore perfusion are not successful.

The most common cause of cardiogenic shock is LV dysfunction and necrosis as a result of acute myocardial infarction (AMI) (see Chapter 17, Myocardial Infarction). Necrosis of the left ventricle can be the result of a single massive myocardial infarction (MI), or it may follow numerous smaller events. Increases in sympathetic tone—seen clinically as increased HR and peripheral vasoconstriction—initially serve to increase CO and maintain central arterial pressure. When LV necrosis exceeds approximately 40% of the contractile mass of the heart, normal compensatory responses can no longer maintain CO, and hypotension and hypoperfusion result. In addition to decreased perfusion to vital tissues and organs, the decrease in CO leads to a reduction in the flow of blood through the coronary arteries, which can lead to infarct extension and a further worsening of cardiac performance.

The incidence of cardiogenic shock after AMI has remained relatively stable over the past 20 years. A recent study found an average incidence of 7.1% from 1975 to 1997.[15] The in-hospital mortality for those patients developing shock has decreased somewhat over this time frame, most likely because of coronary reperfusion strategies. The overall mortality rate, however, has remained high, with most series reporting an average of 60% to 80%.[15,16]

Cardiogenic shock caused by mechanical problems occurs relatively infrequently. In this setting, the systolic function (contractile ability) of the heart may be normal, but other defects render the heart unable to eject a normal volume of blood. Pericardial tamponade (bleeding into the pericardial sac) and tension pneumothorax (air leakage from the lung into the chest) cause cardiogenic shock by compressing the heart and decreasing the diastolic filling. Acute valvular insufficiency or stenosis prevents the normal ejection of blood. Ventricular septal or free wall rupture can occur, often in the setting of AMI, with the reduction in CO related to the inability of the LV to eject a normal volume of blood during systole.

Nonmechanical origins of cardiogenic shock involve a decrease in the function of the heart muscle itself. Myocardial infarction involving the RV can cause cardiogenic shock, even with normal LV systolic function. In this situation, the volume of blood reaching the LV (preload) is reduced because of the right ventricle's inability to move blood to the left side of the heart. In most patients with cardiogenic shock and RV infarction, significant LV dysfunction is present as well.

Patients with chronic heart failure (HF) (see Chapter 18, Heart Failure) usually can compensate for their poor cardiac function, but acute exacerbations can cause cardiogenic shock with hypotension, hypoperfusion, and organ dysfunction. Cardiac dysfunction occasionally can be seen with severe sepsis because of increases in the production of inflammatory cytokines that have a depressant effect on the myocardium. A similar picture also can be seen following cardiopulmonary bypass during heart surgery, which activates the inflammatory cascade.

The symptoms of cardiogenic shock are largely the same as for other types of shock. Hypotension and signs of inadequate tissue perfusion, such as confusion, oliguria, tachycardia, and cutaneous vasoconstriction, are present in many patients. Differentiating cardiogenic shock from distributive or hypovolemic shock requires further examination. A history of coronary artery disease or symptoms of MI are important findings. Hypovolemia occurs in up to 20% of patients in cardiogenic shock, but patients frequently have signs of volume overload because the heart cannot move blood through the circulation. Peripheral edema can be seen in the extremities; lung sounds are diminished and rales may be present as pulmonary edema develops. These findings are particularly evident in patients with severe HF.

Because the distinction between cardiogenic and other forms of shock can be difficult to make based on physical examination alone, further testing with invasive hemodynamic monitoring may be required to establish the diagnosis and guide therapy. Table 21-4 lists the common laboratory, electrocardiogram (ECG), chest radiograph findings, and Table 21-3 lists the common hemodynamic findings in cardiogenic shock.

Distributive Shock

Distributive shock is characterized by an overt loss of vascular tone, causing acute tissue hypoperfusion. Although numerous events can initiate distributive shock, most cases are readily reversed by supportive measures and treatment or elimination of the underlying cause.

Septic Shock

Distributive shock secondary to sepsis, or septic shock, is associated with a high mortality rate, reflecting the limited therapeutic options available at this time. Approximately

Table 21-4 Typical Findings of Early Cardiogenic Shock

- Arterial blood gas (ABG)
  - Hypoxemia secondary to pulmonary congestion with ventilation-perfusion abnormalities
  - Metabolic acidosis with a compensatory respiratory alkalosis
- Elevated blood lactate levels (which contributes to the acidosis)
- Complete blood count (CBC)
  - Leukocytosis
  - Thrombocytopenia (if disseminated intravascular coagulation is present)
- Elevated cardiac enzymes if myocardial infarction is present
- Electrocardiogram (ECG)–one or more of the following
  - T-wave changes indicating infarction
  - Left bundle-branch block
  - Sinus tachycardia
  - Arrhythmia
- Chest radiograph
  - Pulmonary edema or evidence of adult respiratory distress syndrome (ARDS)
- Echocardiography
  - Valvular or mechanical problems if present
  - Normal or decreased ejection fraction
- Hemodynamic monitoring–one or more of the following
  - Reduced cardiac output
  - Arterial hypotension
  - Elevated pulmonary capillary wedge pressure (PCWP) and pulmonary artery pressure (PAP)
  - Elevated systemic vascular resistance (SVR)

500,000 cases of sepsis syndrome are seen annually, with mortality rates ranging from about 30% at 1 month to 50% at 5 months. Epidemiology studies show that approximately 25% of cases of sepsis syndrome eventually result in septic shock. Septic shock is the number one cause of death in the noncoronary ICU and the 13th most common cause of death in the United States. It has been projected that the incidence of sepsis will increase 1.5% per year mainly because of the disproportionate growth of the elderly in the U.S. population.[17–20]

The consensus conference of the American College of Chest Physicians (ACCP) and the Society of Critical Care Medicine (SCCM) defines sepsis syndrome as a systemic inflammatory response resulting from infection.[2] When associated organ dysfunction, hypoperfusion, or hypotension is present, it is termed *severe sepsis;* when hypotension persists despite adequate fluid resuscitation and requires inotropic or vasopressor support, it is termed *septic shock* (see Table 21-5 for definitions). More than half the cases of septic syndrome occur in the ICU, one-third occur in other currently hospitalized patients, and 10% to 15% of cases are present on admission to the emergency department (ED).[19] Progression to septic shock occurs in about half of patients who have septic syndrome within 1 month of onset, as defined by hypotension. Persons most at risk for septic shock are those who are immunocompromised or have underlying conditions that render them susceptible to bloodstream invasion. Groups at risk include neonates, the elderly, patients with acquired immune deficiency syndrome (AIDS), alcoholics, childbearing women, and those undergoing surgery or who have experienced trauma. Other predisposing factors include coexisting diseases such as diabetes mellitus, malignancies, chronic hepatic or renal failure, and hyposplenism; exposure to immunosuppressant drugs and cancer chemotherapy; and procedures such as insertion of urinary catheters, endotracheal tubes, and IV lines.

Septic shock is characterized initially by a normal or high cardiac output and a low systemic vascular resistance (Table 21-3). Hypotension is caused by the low SVR as well as alterations in macrovascular and microvascular tone, which result in maldistribution of blood flow and volume. Changes in the microvasculature can lead to loss of normal microvascular autoregulatory mechanisms resulting in constriction of capillaries, changes in cellular rheology, fibrin deposition, and neutrophil adherence. This causes vascular "sludging" and, in some cases, arteriovenous shunts that bypass capillary beds. Loss of intravascular fluid caused by increased vascular permeability and third spacing of fluid further adds to hypovolemia. In an effort to compensate for the changes in volume and SVR, the body goes into a hyperdynamic state and increases CO. Most patients develop myocardial dysfunction as manifested by decreased myocardial compliance, reduced contractility, and ventricular dilation, but maintain a normal CO because of tachycardia and cardiac dilatation. Although the cause of, and mechanism for, this abnormality are not fully understood, it is not believed to be caused by myocardial ischemia. Rather, it is thought to be caused by one or more circulating inflammatory mediators, such as cytokines, tumor necrosis factor-α (TNF-α), platelet activating factor (PAF), arachidonic acid, nitric oxide (NO), and reactive oxygen species. In late septic shock, the body is no longer able to compensate because of the cardiac effects of the inflammatory mediators and myocardial edema, therefore resulting in a decreased CO. The end product of this complicated pathway is cellular ischemia, dysfunction, and eventually cellular death unless the chain of events is interrupted.

The pathogenesis of sepsis is more fully understood now, but the exact mechanisms are still not completely clear. It is known that the changes that take place during sepsis are caused by the immunologic host response to infection which involves inflammatory and immunodepressive (anti-inflammatory) phases. It is unknown, however, whether these phases are sequential (inflammatory then immunodepressive) or whether immunosuppression is a primary response to sepsis rather than a compensatory response.

The inflammatory stage of sepsis is initiated by an infection with a microorganism, most commonly bacterial. Organisms can either enter the bloodstream directly (producing positive blood cultures) or may indirectly elicit a systemic inflammatory response by locally releasing their toxins or structural components at the site of infection. The lipopolysaccharide endotoxin of gram-negative bacteria is the most potent soluble product of bacteria that can initiate a response and is the most studied, but other bacterial products can initiate the response, including exotoxins, enterotoxins, peptidoglycans, and lipoteichoic acid from gram-positive organisms. The binding of these toxins to cell receptors promotes proinflammatory cytokine production, primarily TNF-α and IL-1. These toxins stimulate the production and release of numerous endogenous mediators that are responsible for the inflammatory consequences of sepsis.

Table 21-5 ACCP/SCCM Consensus Conference Definitions

Infection	Microbial phenomenon characterized by an inflammatory response to the presence of microorganisms or the invasion of normally sterile host tissue by those organisms.
Bacteremia	The presence of viable bacteria in the blood.
Systemic inflammatory response syndrome (SIRS)	The systemic inflammatory response to a variety of severe clinical insults. The response is manifested by two or more of the following conditions: Temperature >38°C or <36°C Heart rate >90 beats/min Respiratory rate >20 breaths/min or $Paco_2$ <32 mmHg (<4.3 kPa) WBC >12,000 cells/mm^3, <4,000 cell/mm^3, or >10% immature (bands) forms
Sepsis	The systemic response to infection. The systemic response is manifested by two or more of the following conditions as a result of infection: Temperature >38°C or <36°C Heart rate >90 beats/min Respiratory rate >20 breaths/min or $Paco_2$ <32 mmHg (<4.3 kPa) WBC >12,000 cells/mm^3, <4,000 cell/mm^3, or >10% immature (band) forms
Severe sepsis	Sepsis associated with organ dysfunction, hypoperfusion, or hypotension. Hypoperfusion and perfusion abnormalities may include, but are not limited to, lactic acidosis, oliguria, or an acute alteration in mental status.
Septic shock	Sepsis with hypotension, despite adequate fluid resuscitation, along with perfusion abnormalities that may include, but are not limited to, lactic acidosis, oliguria, or an acute alteration in mental status. Patients who are on inotropic or vasopressor agents may not be hypotensive at the time that perfusion abnormalities are measured.
Hypotension	A systolic BP of <90 mmHg or a reduction of >40 mmHg from baseline in the absence of other causes for hypotension.
Multiple organ dysfunction syndrome	Presence of altered organ function in an acutely ill patient such that homeostasis cannot be maintained without intervention.

Reprinted with permission from American College of Chest Physicians (ACCP)/Society of Critical Care Medicine (SCCM) Consensus Conference. Definitions for sepsis and organ failure and guidelines for the use of innovative therapies in sepsis. *Crit Care Med* 1992;20:864, with permission.

The cytokines act synergistically to directly affect organ function and stimulate the release of other proinflammatory cytokines, such as IL-6, IL-8, PAF, complement, thromboxanes, leukotrienes, prostaglandins, NO, and others.

The presence of these cytokines promotes inflammation and vascular endothelial injury, but also causes an overwhelming activation in coagulation. Thrombin has potent proinflammatory and procoagulant activities and its production is increased in sepsis. The human body normally counteracts these effects by increasing fibrinolysis, but the homeostatic mechanisms in the septic patient are dysfunctional. There are decreases in the levels of protein C, plasminogen, and antithrombin III as well as increased activity of plasminogen activator inhibitor-1 (PAI-1) and thrombin activatable fibrinolysis inhibitor (TAFI), endogenous agents that inhibit fibrinolysis.[21] The patient is in a coagulopathic state, which promotes formation of microvascular thrombi leading to hypoperfusion, ischemia, and ultimately, organ failure. Multiple organ failure is responsible for about half the deaths caused by septic shock.[22]

The clinical features of septic shock are fever, chills, nausea, vomiting, and diarrhea. Characteristic laboratory findings include leukocytosis or leukopenia; thrombocytopenia with or without coagulation abnormalities; and often, hyperbilirubinemia. These features are usually readily detectable and occur within 24 hours after bacteremia develops, particularly if the bacteremia is caused by gram-negative organisms. In the extremes of age (very young or very old) or in debilitated patients, hypothermia can be present, however, and positive findings may be limited to unexplained hypotension, mental confusion, and hyperventilation.

In contrast to the classic progression of shock, persons dying from septic shock often have a normal or elevated CO. Death within the first week after the onset of sepsis occurs as a result of intractable arterial hypotension that is secondary to a significantly depressed SVR. This causes extensive maldistribution of blood flow in the microvasculature, with subsequent tissue hypoxia and the development of lactic acidosis. Death occurring beyond the first week usually is caused by multiple organ failure that began during the acute circulatory failure. Severe, unresponsive hypotension as a result of a decreased CO does occur in a subpopulation of patients with septic shock; cardiogenic shock becomes superimposed on the distributive shock of sepsis, but this is not the most common cause of death.[23]

HYPOVOLEMIC SHOCK

Acute Hemorrhagic Shock

1. B.A. is a 55-year-old man brought to the ED after being stabbed in the abdomen; he had significant blood loss at the

scene. On arrival, he is confused and oriented only to person. His skin is pale and cool, with vital signs showing a HR of 125 beats/minute, SBP of 85 mmHg, and a RR of 30 breaths/minute. Describe the physiologic changes in B.A. in response to his injury. What are the goals of resuscitation in patients with hemorrhagic shock?

B.A. has lost a significant amount of intravascular fluid directly from his stab wound and also from traumatic tissue edema. He is hypotensive with a compensatory increase in both HR and respiratory rate (RR). His pale, cool skin indicates shunting of blood from the periphery to maintain perfusion of vital organs. Based on his clinical presentation, B.A. is in decompensated shock.

The major hemodynamic abnormality in hypovolemic shock is decreased venous return (preload) to the heart, resulting in a decrease in CO. Oxygen delivery to the tissues is reduced from this and from the loss of oxygen-carrying hemoglobin. The physiologic response of the body to a sudden decrease in volume (preload) is a release of catecholamines (epinephrine, norepinephrine). The subsequent increase in HR and contractility help maintain CO. The peripheral vasoconstriction caused by the sympathomimetic response serves to maintain arterial pressure. In addition, fluid shifts from the interstitial spaces into the vasculature to increase preload. These responses are effective at maintaining BP in patients with a loss of up to approximately 30% of the total blood volume. B.A.'s increased HR and signs of peripheral vasoconstriction are consistent with these compensatory changes. His SBP is still low, however, and he has signs of decreased perfusion to his brain, manifested by confusion and disorientation. Given the severity of his condition, if intravascular losses are not rapidly replaced, myocardial dysfunction may ensue and lead to irreversible shock.

The goals of resuscitation of patients in hypovolemic shock are the correction of inadequate tissue perfusion and oxygenation, and limiting secondary insults, such as reperfusion injury or compartment syndrome. HR, BP, and urine output have been traditional markers for the adequacy of resuscitation, but reliance on these end points alone is acceptable only in the initial management of hemorrhagic shock. One concern is that patients may persist in a state of compensated shock even after these parameters are normalized.[24,25] Ongoing deficiencies in oxygen delivery to vital organs may progress and, if left untreated, organ dysfunction and death may result. Measurement of base (bicarbonate) deficit and lactate levels can be used to assess the global adequacy of perfusion. Metabolic acidosis can signal that resuscitation is incomplete despite normal vital signs.

Treatment

CHOICE OF FLUID IN HYPOVOLEMIC SHOCK

2. Is an IV saline solution adequate to compensate for BA's blood loss? What other type of fluid might be better to resuscitate this patient?

Once an adequate airway is established and initial vital signs are obtained, the most important therapeutic intervention in hypovolemic shock is the infusion of IV fluids. Initially, crystalloids or colloids are used to restore blood volume as blood products may not be immediately available and are frequently unnecessary to manage mild shock (10%–20% blood loss).[14]

CRYSTALLOIDS VERSUS COLLOIDS

Crystalloids are isotonic solutions that contain either saline (0.9% sodium chloride; "normal saline") or a saline equivalent (lactated Ringer's [LR] solution). *Colloidal solutions* contain large oncotically active molecules that are derived from natural products such as proteins (albumin), carbohydrates (dextrans, starches), and animal collagen (gelatin) (Table 21-6).

The choice of a crystalloid versus a colloid solution to restore blood volume in hemorrhagic shock is controversial. The controversy primarily involves the ultimate distribution of these fluids in the extracellular compartment, which, in turn, depends on their composition. Isotonic solutions (normal saline or RL solution) freely distribute within the extracellular fluid compartment, which is divided between the interstitial and intravascular spaces at a ratio of 3:1. This distribution is determined by the net forces of colloid oncotic pressure (COP) and hydrostatic pressure, both inside and outside the capillary vascular space. Consequently, large volumes of crystalloid fluid are required to expand the intravascular space during resuscitation. In contrast, intact capillary membranes are relatively impermeable to colloids and, therefore, colloids effectively expand the intravascular space with little loss into the interstitium. Comparatively smaller volumes of colloids than of crystalloids are thus required for resuscitation, and because these large molecules persist intravascularly, their duration of action is longer. It is often thought that three to four times as much volume of crystalloid is necessary to provide the same degree of volume expansion as obtained from a colloid. Many of the colloidal agents, however, can cause allergic or hypersensitivity reactions as well as coagulopathic effects and colloids are much more expensive than crystalloids.

Proponents of crystalloids argue that both intravascular and interstitial fluids are depleted in hypovolemic shock because of the rapid shifts between the extracellular compartments. Volume replacement of both fluid spaces is best accomplished

Table 21-6 Composition and Properties of Crystalloids

Solution	Sodium (mEq/L)	Chloride (mEq/L)	Potassium (mEq/L)	Calcium (mEq/L)	Magnesium (mEq/L)	Lactate (mEq/L)	Tonicity Relative to Plasma	Osmolarity (mosm/l)
5% Dextrose	0	0	0	0	0	0	Isotonic	253
0.9% Sodium Chloride	154	154	0	0	0	0	Isotonic	308
Plasma-Lyte (Baxter)	140	103	10	5	3	8	Isotonic	312
Lactated Ringer's	130	109	4	3	0	28	Isotonic	273
7.5% Sodium Chloride	1,283	1,283	0	0	0	0	Hypertonic	2,567

by using crystalloids. In addition, loss of capillary integrity in shock can cause the leak of larger molecules (e.g., the colloidal proteins) into the interstitium. This increase in the oncotic pressure in the interstitium would favor fluid movement out of the vascular space into the tissues, with resultant edema.

Proponents of colloids contend that resuscitation with these solutions more rapidly and effectively restores intravascular volume following acute hemorrhage. For a given infusion volume, colloidal solutions (e.g., albumin) will expand the intravascular space two to four times more than crystalloids. Because a larger volume of crystalloid would have to be infused to restore the vascular space, the risk of developing pulmonary edema may be higher. It is also argued that large volumes of crystalloids will further dilute the plasma proteins, resulting in a decrease in the COP, which can also promote the development of pulmonary edema. This concept is based on Starling's law of capillary forces governing fluid movement, which in the pulmonary vessel wall is determined by the COP-PCWP gradient (i.e., the net force generated by the colloid oncotic pressure minus the pulmonary hydrostatic pressure [PCWP]). The normal colloid oncotic pressure is 25 mmHg and an average PCWP is 12 mmHg; thus, a net intravascular force of 13 mmHg favors fluid retention in the vascular space. In critically ill patients, a COP-PCWP gradient <6 mmHg is thought to be associated with a higher incidence of pulmonary edema. Despite these theoretic differences, clinical studies comparing colloids with crystalloids have failed to show any differences in the development of pulmonary edema. Research suggests that certain subgroups may be at greater risk for the development of pulmonary edema, but considerable variance remains because of differences in physiologic end points, criteria for assessing pulmonary edema, and the extent of shock.

In an effort to find a consensus among the results of divergent clinical trials, numerous meta-analyses have been performed comparing resuscitation with crystalloids or colloids. Two earlier meta-analyses concluded that resuscitation of burn and trauma patients with colloids results in increased mortality.[26,27] The explanation offered for the detrimental effect of colloids is that trauma and burns cause an increase in pulmonary capillary and vascular permeability resulting in extravasation of the colloid into the interstitium, which further worsens the effective vascular volume and pulmonary edema. The Cochrane Database analysis found that albumin was associated with an overall higher risk of death, whereas the most recent meta-analysis funded by the Plasma Protein Therapeutics Association did not find an increase in mortality in any patient groups including trauma.[28,29] It is important to recognize that several limitations to these meta-analyses exist because of differences in study inclusion criteria (heterogeneity), differences in fluid management, and dosages of albumin used. What is known is the difference in cost per therapy. One study determined the secondary cost-effectiveness analysis per therapy, which revealed that the cost of using crystalloids was $43.13 per life saved, as opposed to $1,493.60 per life saved with colloid.[28] These estimates were based on an average per-patient intake of 6.57 L of fluid for the crystalloid group, at a cost of $5.95/L, and an average of 230 g of albumin in the colloid group, at a cost of $5.00/g.

Recent evidence supports the idea that albumin may not be as detrimental as once thought. The SAFE trial is the largest randomized, prospective trial to evaluate albumin versus normal saline (NS) resuscitation in the critically ill.[30] The primary end point was 28-day mortality, which was not statistically different for albumin compared with NS. Also no statistical differences were identified in any of the preidentified subgroups (trauma, ARDS, severe sepsis), although a trend was seen toward increased mortality in the trauma patients who received albumin, most specifically in patients with head trauma. Because resuscitation with albumin was not found to be better than saline, this landmark trial will most likely alter perceptions of albumin; whether or not this trial will have an impact on albumin prescribing practices remains to be determined.

Given the lack of evidence for a significant clinical difference between crystalloids and colloids and the greater expense of using albumin, the guidelines for the use of resuscitation fluids developed by the University Hospital Consortium (UHC), a nonprofit alliance of U.S. academic medical centers, remain unchanged.[31] For the resuscitation of hemorrhagic shock, crystalloids should be the initial fluid of choice. The American College of Surgeons Advanced Trauma Life Support course[14] also recommends the rapid infusion of isotonic crystalloids for the initial fluid resuscitation of trauma patients. Thus, use of either normal saline or LR solution would be appropriate for B.A. Albumin and blood are not needed.

CRYSTALLOIDS

3. A large-bore IV catheter is inserted into B.A.'s arm and STAT blood samples are sent for type and crossmatch, complete blood count (CBC), prothrombin time (PT), partial thromboplastin time (PTT), and serum chemistry (BUN, creatinine, Na, K, Cl, and bicarbonate). Warmed LR solution (2 L) is infused rapidly, and the operating room is notified. B.A.'s systolic BP has increased to 90 mmHg, but the bleeding has not stopped. A Foley catheter is inserted to measure urine output. LR is continued, with 500 to 1,000 mL boluses ordered to be given to maintain hemodynamic stability while waiting for fully crossmatched blood. Are the doses of LR given to B.A. appropriate? What clinical and objective parameters should be monitored to determine the success of fluid replacement?

Volume Requirements

Isotonic crystalloids equilibrate rapidly between the interstitial and intravascular spaces at a ratio of 3:1. For every liter of fluid infused, approximately 750 mL will pass into the interstitium, whereas 250 mL will remain in the plasma. Based on estimated blood loss, the "three-to-one rule" may be applied as a general guideline: for each 1 mL of blood loss, 3 mL of crystalloid is infused. Because this determination of blood loss is based solely on clinical assessment and not on quantitative measurements, treatment is best directed by the response to initial therapy rather than the initial classification. Close observation of hemodynamic status with consideration of the patient's age, particular injury, and prehospital fluid therapy is essential to avoid inadequate or excessive fluid administration.

A safe and effective approach for using crystalloids in the resuscitation of patients in hemorrhagic shock is to give 1 to 2 L of fluid as an initial bolus as rapidly as possible for an adult or 20 mL/kg for a pediatric patient.[14] Additional fluid boluses may be necessary, depending on the patient's response. Between boluses, fluids are slowed to maintenance rates

(150–200 mL/hour), with ongoing evaluation of the patient's physiologic response for signs of continued blood loss or inadequate perfusion that would indicate the need for additional volume replacement.

Indications that circulation is improving include normalization of BP, pulse pressure, and HR. Signs that actual organ perfusion is normalizing and that fluid resuscitation is adequate include improvements in mental status, warmth and color of skin, improved acid-base balance, and increased urinary output. The minimal acceptable urine output for a patient is 0.5 mL/kg. Persistent metabolic acidosis in a normothermic shock patient usually indicates the need for additional fluid resuscitation; sodium bicarbonate is not recommended unless the pH is <7.2.[14] The serum lactate and base deficit are important values to track to determine that the patient is receiving adequate resuscitation. It is important to note that resuscitation is not defined by just one value or number, such as BP, but the constellation of indicators of overall perfusion.

LACTATED RINGER'S VERSUS NORMAL SALINE

4. Is there an advantage to using LR solution over normal saline?

The American College of Surgeons Committee on Trauma recommends lactated Ringer's solution as the fluid of choice for the initial resuscitation of trauma patients and normal saline as the second choice.[14] Because normal saline has a high chloride content (45 mEq more than LR), it can cause hyperchloremic acidosis, thereby worsening the tissue acidosis that occurs in the setting of hypovolemic shock. This likelihood is increased with impaired renal function. LR, in contrast, is a buffered solution designed to simulate the intravascular plasma electrolyte concentration. It contains 28 mEq/L of lactate, which is metabolized to bicarbonate in patients with normal circulation and intact liver function.[32] In situations in which hepatic perfusion is reduced (20% of normal) or hepatocellular damage is present, lactate clearance may be significantly decreased, particularly in combination with hypoxia (O_2 saturation 50% of normal).[33] In patients with shock and those having cardiopulmonary bypass during surgery, the half-life of lactate, normally 20 minutes, increases to 4 to 6 hours and 8 hours, respectively. Because unmetabolized lactate can be converted to lactic acid, prolonged infusion of LR could cause tissue acidosis in predisposed patients. In actuality, however, no differences in serum pH, electrolytes, lactate, or survival have been found in patients with hemorrhagic trauma who have received either LR or normal saline. In practice, normal saline and LR typically are used interchangeably because neither solution appears to be superior to the other.

HYPERTONIC SALINE

5. What is the role of hypertonic saline (HS) in the setting of hemorrhagic shock?

The use of HS (with and without dextran) for resuscitation in hemorrhagic shock has been studied extensively in animal models,[34–36] and more recently has been the focus of clinical research.[37–39] The advantage of HS as a resuscitative fluid is the smaller volume of fluid required to expand the intravascular compartment as compared with isotonic solutions. This could be a particular advantage in the prehospital setting (e.g., field rescue by emergency medical technicians) given the large volumes of fluids necessary to keep up with ongoing blood loss.

With a high concentration of sodium, HS exerts an osmotic effect, translocating fluid from the interstitial and cellular compartments to the intravascular space. Consequently, plasma volume is rapidly expanded to a greater extent than similar volumes of crystalloid solutions, and systemic BP, CO, and oxygen transport are readily increased. HS also improves myocardial contractility, causes peripheral vasodilation, and redistributes blood flow preferentially to the splanchnic and renal circulation. In addition, intracranial pressure is reduced, which may be a potential advantage in trauma patients with concomitant head injury.[34–39]

Hypertonic saline-dextran (7.5% sodium chloride in 6% dextran 70 [HSD]) was compared with isotonic crystalloid solution for prehospital resuscitation in a multicenter trial of hypotensive trauma patients.[38] Patients were randomly assigned to receive 250 mL of either HSD or a standard isotonic solution, after which fluids were given as necessary to achieve stabilization. No differences in overall survival were noted; however, a significant survival advantage was seen in the HSD group requiring surgery. Fewer complications occurred in the HSD group, including a lower incidence of ARDS, renal failure, and coagulopathy. Although serum sodium levels were significantly higher in the HSD group, no adverse clinical symptoms of hypernatremia were seen.

In a similar trial, the effects of resuscitation with 250-mL volumes of HS (7.5%), HSD, or normal saline were compared in trauma patients admitted to the ED in hypovolemic shock.[39] Differences in overall mortality or complication rates in the three groups were not significant. In comparison to isotonic saline, however, the hypertonic solutions significantly improved MAP and significantly decreased the volume of fluid required to restore systolic pressure.

Recent studies with HS suggest that it may help to reduce multiple organ system failure and infections following traumatic injury. The mechanism has yet to be fully elucidated, but in animal models, HS reduces neutrophil margination,[40] which may play a role in the development of lung injury, ARDS, and reperfusion injury. In another study the use of HS resulted in a decreased susceptibility to sepsis and improved survival in a murine model of hemorrhagic shock.[41]

These clinical trials suggest that HS may be safe and effective for the initial resuscitation of hemorrhagic shock and may help prevent the development of posttraumatic multiple organ system failure and sepsis. Despite these positive findings, hypertonic saline solutions are not widely used.

BLOOD REPLACEMENT

6. B.A. has received 3 L of LR solution to maintain hemodynamic stability. His current vital signs are BP, 92/60 mmHg; HR, 115 breaths/minute; and RR, 28 breaths/minute. He is still confused and is becoming more agitated and combative. Urine output has been only 10 mL in the past 30 minutes. Laboratory results include the following: hematocrit, 23% down from 27% (normal, 40%–54%); hemoglobin, 7.6 g/dL down from 9 g/dL (normal, 14–18 g/dL); ABG pH, 7.18 (normal, 7.35–7.45); Pco_2, 35 mmHg (normal, 35–45 mmHg); Po_2, 110 mmHg (normal, 75–100 mmHg); and HCO_3^-, 17 mEq/L (normal, 23–29 mEq/L). Two

units of packed red blood cells (PRBC) are now available, and B.A. is being prepared for the operating room. Describe the current status of B.A.'s resuscitation and the need for blood products.

[SI units: Hct, 0.23 (normal, 0.40–0.54); hemoglobin, 1.18 mmol/L (normal, 2.17–2.79 mmol/L); HCO_3^-, 17 mmol/L (normal, 23–29 mmol/L)]

B.A. is still exhibiting signs of inadequate tissue perfusion. Although his BP has improved and his HR has decreased, his mental status has declined, urine output has been negligible, and his blood gas indicates metabolic acidosis. B.A. has not been adequately resuscitated from his hemorrhage, is still actively bleeding, and should receive the available blood at this point.

The prior conventional approach to the transfusion of critically ill patients was to maintain the hemoglobin above 10 g/dL or the hematocrit above 30%. This transfusion trigger was found to be detrimental in a population of mixed medical-surgical ICU patients compared with a group of patients who were maintained at a lower hemoglobin of 7 g/dL and therefore received fewer transfusions. This lower hemoglobin level may be appropriate for critically ill patients who are in an ICU and have decreased hematocrit values because of fluid resuscitation and daily blood draws, but not for a patient who is actively bleeding as evidenced by the falling hemoglobin and hematocrit and signs of underperfusion. In acute hemorrhage, the actual degree of blood loss is not accurately reflected by the hemoglobin and hematocrit values, and it also does not take into account the body's ability to compensate for the loss of oxygen-carrying capacity. Because it takes at least 24 hours for all fluid compartments to come to equilibrium, a normal hematocrit (or Hgb concentration) in the setting of hemorrhagic shock does not rule out significant blood loss or indicate adequacy of transfusion. Only when equilibrium has been reached can these measures be used reliably to gauge blood loss. On the other hand, if cardiopulmonary function is normal and if volume status is maintained, an increase in CO can compensate for a reduction in hemoglobin (O_2 content) to a certain degree (Fig. 21-1).

Because inadequacy of tissue perfusion, and hence oxygen delivery, is the primary abnormality in shock, the need for transfusion therapy is more accurately determined by the patient's oxygen demand, rather than an arbitrary hematocrit or hemoglobin value. Calculation of Do_2 and Vo_2 can be used to determine the adequacy of perfusion. Although these values can be determined by use of a pulmonary artery catheter and arterial and venous blood samples, for practical purposes, the patient's response to initial fluid resuscitation and clinical signs of inadequate tissue perfusion are the primary determinants for blood transfusion. Patients who are not acutely bleeding and who do not respond to initial volume resuscitation or who transiently respond but remain tachycardic, tachypneic, and oliguric, clearly are underperfused and will likely require blood transfusion. Trauma patients who have acute bleeding issues or who demonstrate signs of underperfusion should be considered for transfusion much sooner, thus B.A. should receive a transfusion.

ADVERSE EFFECTS OF TRANSFUSION

7. After the transfusion, B.A. has a serum potassium concentration of 4.8 mEq/L (normal, 3.7–5.2 mEq/L) compared with 4.5 mEq/L before the transfusion. Could this be a result of the blood product? Is B.A. also at risk for contracting human immunodeficiency virus (HIV) or viral hepatitis from his transfusion of PRBC? Would whole blood be a better choice than packed cells?

Possible risks of blood transfusions include electrolyte abnormalities, hemolytic reactions, transmission of infectious disease, coagulopathies, and immunosuppression. Banked blood is stored with citrate anticoagulant additive. With multiple transfusions, the large amount of citrate can cause hypocalcemia and acid-base abnormalities. Hyperkalemia also can occur because transfusion of stored blood causes the release of potassium from hemolyzed (ruptured) red blood cells (RBC). Hemolytic transfusion reactions are the most common cause of acute fatalities from blood transfusions. Astute recognition of the signs and symptoms of a transfusion reaction, such as anxiety, pain at infusion site, fever, hypotension, tachycardia, hemolysis, and hemoglobinuria, can prevent unnecessary morbidity and mortality. Transfusions can also cause acute lung injury owing to recipient neutrophil priming by reactive lipid products from the red blood cell membrane, which causes capillary endothelial damage in the lungs. The increase in serum potassium observed in B.A. may be from the blood product or it may simply reflect hemolysis of blood cells in the test tube after the blood draw. In either case, the measured serum concentration of 4.8 mEq/L is not sufficiently high to be of concern. It is unlikely that a true hemolytic reaction is occurring.

Blood products and donors are screened for disease, thus transmission of viral illness is a small risk. It is estimated that the transmission of hepatitis B is 1 case for every 63,000 units transfused, hepatitis C is 1:103,000, and HIV is 1:676,000.[42]

Hemostatic abnormalities, specifically coagulopathies and thrombocytopenia, may be transiently related to dilution from administration of large volumes of crystalloids, colloids, or banked blood, but are more likely caused by the extent of injury and the development of disseminated intravascular coagulopathy. Banked whole blood contains sufficient coagulation factors (including labile factors V and VIII) to maintain hemostasis during the life span of the unit; however, it does not contain platelets because they do not survive the temperatures required for RBC storage.

Immunosuppression has also been associated with blood transfusions as evidenced by enhanced graft survival in renal transplant recipients, tumor recurrence in patients with colorectal carcinoma, and in postoperative infections. The immunosuppression from transfusion is multifactorial, but it is most likely caused by the infusion of donor white cells, which create a competition between the donor and recipient leukocytes. This mechanism is not, however, the only cause because immunosuppression is associated with autologous blood transfusions as well as the infusion of plasma alone.

Whole blood offers no significant advantage over packed red cells as long as other less-expensive fluids (crystalloids) are used for volume expansion. After extracting the red cells to provide oxygen-carrying capacity, other blood elements (e.g., fresh frozen plasma and platelets, clotting factors) can be used for other patients with specialty needs. Thus, packed RBC are an appropriate blood replacement product for B.A. His PT, PTT, platelets, electrolytes, and mixed venous blood gases, if available, should be monitored frequently. These tests enable correction of any coagulopathy or electrolyte abnormality and assist in the assessment of the adequacy of tissue oxygenation. This information, in addition to the aforementioned factors, can be used to gauge his response to therapy and his need for supplemental blood products such as platelets and frozen fresh plasma.

Because of the limited supply and potential adverse effects associated with blood, research is under way to develop blood substitutes. The ideal agent would have a longer shelf life, a reduced risk of disease transmission, and less risk of transfusion reactions. The agents in various stages of clinical research include the modified hemoglobins and the perfluorocarbons. The exact role the blood substitutes would play in transfusions is unclear, and problems have occurred, such as short half-life and vasoconstriction associated with some of the products thus far. No agents have yet been approved, but research is continuing.

Postoperative Hypovolemia

Hypovolemia versus Pump Failure

8. B.A. goes to the operating room and they find several colonic tears that require a colon resection. He has been admitted to the ICU following surgery, intubated and receiving 60% oxygen. His ABG are adequate and he is receiving 150 mL/hour of LR solution intravenously. His initial post-operative and 2-hour postoperative hemodynamic profiles are as follows (initial parameters in parentheses): BP (S/D/M), 90/50/63 (110/70/68) mmHg; pulse, 90 beats/min (84); CO, 3 L/min (4.5); CVP, 6 (10); PCWP, 8 mmHg (12); SVR, 1,200 dyne.sec.cm^{-5} (950); urine output, 25 mL/hour (70); temperature, 37.9°C (35); Hct, 32% (30%). Based on the hemodynamic profile, determine whether B.A. is hypovolemic or experiencing pump failure following his surgery.

[SI unit: Hct, 0.32 (normal, 0.40–0.54)]

Most of B.A.'s hemodynamic changes are consistent with hypovolemia. These include a drop in BP, CVP, CO, PCWP, and urine output. The decrease in PCWP suggests that preload is reduced, resulting in a lower CO. Urine output has declined and probably reflects a compensatory drop in renal perfusion to preserve intravascular volume. The pulse pressure is narrowed, suggesting blood flow has decreased. (Changes in pulse pressure correlate with changes in SV in individual patients; that is, as pulse pressure narrows, SV decreases.) B.A.'s HR did not increase by that much, but it is unclear if he was taking any medications before his injury, such as a β-blocker. As the body temperature rises postoperatively, vasodilation decreases SVR and increases the intravascular space. If intravascular volume is inadequate and increased sympathetic tone cannot generate a sufficient CO, mean BP falls. The most likely explanation for the hemodynamic change in B.A. is hypovolemia, although he also should be evaluated for the occurrence of a perioperative cardiac event. His ABG should be checked to assess oxygen requirements.

Causes

9. What are the most likely causes of hypovolemia in B.A.?

Common causes of hypovolemia in surgical patients are postoperative bleeding, third spacing, and temperature-related vasodilation. Postoperative bleeding can produce hypovolemia; however, B.A.'s initial and 2-hour postoperative hematocrit of 30% and 32%, respectively, do not support bleeding as a cause.

Following major vascular or bowel surgery, it is not unusual for patients to "third space" significant amounts of intravascular volume. The bowel walls and interstitial space can sequester large amounts of fluids, and this can produce a state of relative hypovolemia as is occurring with B.A. This is especially apparent for the first 12 to 24 hours after the surgical procedure. B.A. is receiving 150 mL/hour of LR solution, but this is apparently not sufficient to maintain his intravascular volume.

Mild hypothermia is common during operative procedures. As patients warm up postoperatively, vasodilation occurs, expanding the intravascular space. If the amounts of IV fluids administered are insufficient to compensate for the increased venous capacitance, BP and CO will decline during the rewarming phase, which can range from 1 to 6 hours. B.A. has rewarmed from 34°C to 37°C in 2 hours, which is not unusual after a major operative procedure. His temperature could conceivably rise to as high as 38°C to 38.5°C during the first 12 to 24 hours after surgery.

Other considerations include inadequate fluid administration during the operative procedure and the effects of drugs given in the operating room or in the immediate postoperative period (e.g., morphine sulfate and other narcotics) that have systemic vasodilatory properties.

Volume Replacement and Ventricular Function

10. How will volume replacement improve B.A.'s CO and perfusion pressure?

Starling's mechanism indicates that the volume of blood returned to the heart is the main determinant of volume pumped by the heart. Therefore, as venous return is increased, the CO also will increase within physiologic limits (Fig. 21-1). The PCWP, which approximates LV end-diastolic volume, can be used to assess venous return or preload to the left ventricle.

A ventricular function curve can be constructed by plotting a measure of cardiac pumping action (CO, SV, or LVWSI) against a measure of preload (PCWP). A change in preload moves the ventricular output upward or downward along a given curve (Fig. 21-3). Two hours after surgery, B.A.'s PCWP has fallen from 12 to 8 mmHg and his CO has fallen from 4.5 to 3 L/minute. Therefore, additional volume replacement is warranted.

11. B.A. is given a 500-mL bolus of NS over 10 minutes and this results in the following hemodynamic profile: BP (S/D/M), 96/60/71 mmHg; pulse, 84 beats/minute; CO, 3.5 L/minute; PCWP, 10 mmHg; SVR, 1,170 dyne.sec.cm^{-5}. Assess B.A.'s response to the fluid challenge (see Table 21-2 for normal values).

According to the Starling curve, a small change in PCWP in response to a volume challenge with a minimal change in CO, represents a ventricle on the flat portion of the ventricular function curve (Fig. 21-3). Additional fluid therapy given to these patients can increase their risk for pulmonary edema without improving CO. In contrast, a large change in PCWP in response to a fluid challenge with a significant increase in CO represents a ventricle on the steep portion of the curve. In B.A., the change in PCWP from 8 to 10 mmHg and the increase in CO show that he is still responsive to fluid; thus, it is reasonable to administer more fluid to enhance CO and renal perfusion.

Fluid Challenge

12. One hour after the 500-mL NS bolus, B.A.'s hemodynamic profile returns to his postoperative state. ABG are acceptable and LR solution is infusing at 200 mL/hour. B.A. is continuing to "third-space" intravascular volume. Based on this information, develop guidelines for additional fluid challenges in B.A.

Acceptable guidelines for administering additional fluid challenges to hypovolemic patients are based on the direction and degree of change in the various hemodynamic parameters in response to a fluid load rather than to their absolute values. These include the right atrial pressure, PCWP, CO, and BP. Using the PCWP as a guide, an increase in the PCWP of 5 mmHg after a 250- to 500-mL fluid challenge over 10 minutes implies the LV is still functioning on the steep portion of the volume-pressure curve. If the PCWP rises abruptly as fluid is given, with a small change in CO, the flat portion of the ventricular function curve has been reached and the IV infusion rate should be slowed. If signs and symptoms of inadequate tissue perfusion fail to improve or worsen and if the PCWP remains >16 to 18 mmHg, fluid challenges should be stopped and inotropic therapy initiated.

Generally, most critically ill patients require a CI >2.5 L/minute/m^2 and a PCWP of 10 to 18 mmHg to maintain acceptable MAP of 65 to 75 mmHg. A downward trend in the lactate and base deficit, the change in hemodynamic parameters as well as vital signs and urine output should serve as appropriate indicators for additional fluid.

13. B.A. has received a total of 3.5 L normal saline in boluses over the past 6 hours and remains hemodynamically unchanged. His urine output has averaged 25 mL/hour for the past 4 hours, indicating volume replacement is inadequate. Given his age and the lack of response to initial crystalloid administration, the decision is made to infuse 500 mL of 6% hetastarch over the next 30 minutes. How does hetastarch compare with human serum albumin as a volume expander for B.A.?

Albumin and Hetastarch

Albumin, the predominant protein in the plasma, accounts for approximately 80% of the colloid oncotic pressure,[43] the force that maintains fluid in the intravascular space. Human serum albumin is the colloidal agent against which all others are compared for volume-expanding properties. It is prepared commercially from pooled donor plasma that is heat-treated to eliminate the potential for disease transmission. On infusion, 5% albumin increases plasma volume by approximately half the volume infused, or 18 mL/g, with an initial duration of action of 16 hours.[43] Substantial side effects primarily involve transient clotting abnormalities and anaphylactic reactions (0.5%), both of which are rare.[35] The anaphylactoid reaction is caused by the pasteurization process, causing albumin to polymerize, which produces an antigenic macromolecule. Albumin solutions also contain citrate, which can lower serum calcium concentrations, and which in turn could theoretically lead to decreased LV function.[32] It is now generally believed that the effects on coagulation and serum calcium are related to the volume of fluid infused rather than albumin administration.[43] Albumin is available as a 5% solution that is isotonic with the plasma and a 25% solution that is hypertonic. The 5% solution is generally preferred for routine volume expansion, whereas the 25% solution is most useful in correcting hypoproteinemia or intravascular hypovolemia in patients with excess interstitial water.

Hetastarch or hydroxyethyl starch (HES) is a synthetic colloid made from amylopectin, which closely resembles human serum albumin, but is considerably less expensive. Available as a 6% solution in normal saline, HES expands the plasma volume by an amount greater than the volume infused because the high oncotic pressure draws water from the interstitial spaces. HES solutions are composed of a wide range of molecular weights which explains its complex pharmacokinetics. It has an average molecular weight of 69,000 units with a range of 10,000 units to greater than 1 million units. Smaller molecular weights are excreted more quickly in the urine, whereas larger particles remain in the circulation longer and are slowly taken up by tissues or the reticuloendothelial system. The clinical effects of HES last up to 24 hours. Hetastarch generally is well tolerated with a low incidence of side effects and allergic reactions. Dose-related reductions in platelet count and transient increases in PT and PTT have been reported with moderate infusions of HES (<1,500 mL/day) and are significant with larger volumes.[44] HES causes factor VIII levels to be lowered beyond that which can be attributed to hemodilution and also increases fibrinolysis. This places patients with von Willebrand's disease at greater risk of bleeding. There have not been any direct accounts of HES causing bleeding, but it is recommended that a maximum of 20 mL/kg/day (or 1,500 mL) be used to prevent alterations in coagulation parameters. Most patients respond to 500 to 1,000 mL so this limit does not usually impede treatment. HES can also cause elevation in serum amylase levels up to three times the normal level. This is because hetastarch binds to amylase and thus delays its excretion. HES does not actually interfere with pancreatic function.

Numerous clinical studies have compared albumin and hetastarch for fluid resuscitation in patients with and without shock. One study reported that HES was as effective as albumin in restoring hemodynamic stability and improving oxygen delivery in patients who were given comparable amounts of either fluid over 24 hours.[45] Other studies in hypovolemic patients have reported no difference in hemodynamic parameters when similar volumes of either HES or albumin were given as serial boluses to maintain CO and ventricular filling pressures.[46,47] In postoperative cardiac surgery patients, HES and albumin were found to be equally efficacious in restoring volume status and maintaining hemodynamic stability.[48,49]

In summary, resuscitation with moderate volumes of hetastarch is safe and hemodynamically equivalent to albumin. Either 5% albumin or 6% HES would be acceptable for intravascular volume expansion in B.A.

CARDIOGENIC SHOCK

Postoperative Cardiac Failure

Assessment by Hemodynamic Profile

14. R.G. is a 68-year-old man who is admitted to the ICU following coronary artery bypass grafting. He has a long history of ischemic heart disease with two previous myocardial infarctions. His preoperative ejection fraction was 45%. He also has a history of hypertension and hypercholesterolemia. His home medications

are aspirin, lisinopril, metoprolol, and simvastatin. He is sedated, intubated, and on mechanical ventilation with 60% inspired oxygen. One hour after admission to the ICU, his blood pressure and urine output have fallen. Urine output has dropped from 80 mL/hour initially to 15 mL/hour. Chest tube output has been stable at 40 mL/hour. His ECG shows no signs of ischemia. Laboratory values show pH 7.32 (normal, 7.36–7.44); $Paco_2$ 28 mmHg (normal, 35–45); Pao_2 110 mmHg (normal, 80–100); HCO_3^- 20 mEq/L (normal, 23–29); Hct 34% (normal, 39%–49%). His current hemodynamic profile shows: BP (S/D/M) 92/45/61; pulse 105 beats/min; CO 2.8 L/minute (normal, 4–7) CI 1.4 L/minute/m^2 (normal, 2.5–4.2); CVP 12 mmHg (normal, 2–6); PA pressure (S/D) 35/22 mmHg (normal, 20–30/8–12); PCWP 22 mmHg (normal, 5–12) SVR 1400 dyne.sec.cm^{-5} (normal, 800–1,440). What is your assessment of R.G.'s clinical status and hemodynamics?

[SI units: HCO_3^-, 20 mmol/L (normal, 23–29 mmol/L); Hct, 0.34 (normal, 0.39–0.49)]

Clinically, R.G. has signs of hypoperfusion manifested by low urine output and metabolic acidosis. Evaluation of his hemodynamics will help determine a potential cause for his hypoperfusion and decide on appropriate therapeutic interventions to prevent his condition to worsen to serious organ dysfunction and death.

Possible causes of hypoproliferative shock or shock in cardiac surgery patients include hypovolemia from operative and postoperative bleeding; excessive vasodilation from medications; the effects of cardiopulmonary bypass on the inflammatory cascade; tamponade; or perioperative MI. Another concern is "stunning" of the myocardium caused by surgical trauma, which can take from hours to days to resolve.

Hypovolemia should always be evaluated first when assessing hemodynamic profiles. Using pressor or inotropic agents in the setting of hypovolemia is rarely effective and can lead to serious adverse effects (e.g., cardiac arrhythmias). Also, correction of hypovolemia is relatively straightforward and can be accomplished rapidly. R.G.'s tachycardia, low urine output, low blood pressure, and low cardiac output could indicate volume depletion. His hematocrit is adequate, however, and the data from his PA catheter show an elevated CVP and PCWP, suggesting that preload is not the problem.

Excessive vasodilation is also unlikely in R.G., given that his calculated SVR (afterload) is in the high normal range. Cardiac tamponade should always be considered after cardiac surgery, and is usually manifested by very high CVP, PCWP and PA pressures, with significant decreases in CO and BP. R.G.'s CVP and PCWP are not as high as would be expected in pericardial tamponade, and his chest tube output has remained consistent, suggesting that blood is not accumulating.

Based on this hemodynamic profile, it appears that R.G. is in shock because of acute heart failure, most likely from postoperative myocardial dysfunction, although he should also be evaluated for myocardial ischemia or infarction and to rule out early cardiac tamponade. This evaluation should not delay the initiation of therapy. His severely depressed CO should be treated immediately to prevent further decompensation.

Therapeutic Interventions

15. The chest radiograph shows mild pulmonary edema, and fine rales were heard throughout the lower half of lung fields on auscultation. Tamponade is not evident on the radiograph. The ECG shows ST-T wave changes, but no indication is seen of an acute MI. Cardiac enzymes are pending. BP and CO need to be improved to increase perfusion to vital organs. Three therapeutic interventions are available: fluid challenge, vasodilators, and inotropic agents. How would these choices affect R.G.'s ventricular function?

FLUID CHALLENGE (PRELOAD INCREASE)

Augmentation of preload with a fluid challenge to improve CO is the first option. However, R.G.'s PCWP is already 22 mmHg and increasing this value above 18 to 20 mmHg usually does not result in further benefit.[50] Furthermore, R.G. has signs of pulmonary edema on chest radiograph and his Pao_2 is 110 mmHg on 60% inspired oxygen (Fio_2). Therefore, elevation of intravascular volume might increase the pulmonary vascular hydrostatic pressure and worsen his pulmonary edema. If a fluid challenge is attempted to enhance preload, no more than 100 mL of normal saline should be given without repeating the hemodynamic measurements. If the PCWP rises, but the CO does not improve, fluid challenges should be discontinued. Elevating the preload without appreciably improving CO also can increase LV wall tension, which is a major determinant of myocardial oxygen consumption; consequently, myocardial ischemia could develop. Although R.G. has signs of pulmonary edema, diuretics to reduce his volume overload can be detrimental to his cardiac output and should not be used until R.G.'s hemodynamics and signs of hypoperfusion have improved.

VASODILATORS (AFTERLOAD REDUCTION)

A peripheral vasodilator also could be used. This will decrease pulmonary venous congestion by reducing preload (PCWP), and thus pulmonary vascular hydrostatic pressure. It will improve CO by decreasing the resistance to ventricular ejection (afterload) as well. With myocardial ischemia, a reduction of the LV filling pressure may improve subendocardial blood flow, reduce the myocardial wall tension, and reduce the LV radius. The resultant decrease in myocardial oxygen consumption will help prevent further depression of cardiac function. In patients with LV failure, arterial resistance is elevated because of a reflex increase in sympathetic tone in response to a fall in systemic arterial pressure. In LV failure, CO becomes increasingly dependent on resistance to outflow from the left ventricle. Lowering the SVR will shift the ventricular function curve up and to the left, depending on whether an arterial, venous, or mixed vasodilator is used, thereby improving cardiac performance at a lower filling pressure (Fig. 21-4).

R.G. appears to have LV failure with elevations in PCWP and SVR. Vasodilator therapy in this setting will likely improve his CO and, therefore, increase the delivery of oxygen to the tissues and prevent organ dysfunction. The major risk of vasodilator therapy in R.G., however, is further reduction of an already low MAP. Although the reduction in BP may be offset by an increase in CO, a significant drop in arterial BP could occur, which could reduce coronary pressure and thereby exacerbate or produce myocardial ischemia in addition to decreasing perfusion to other vital organ systems. Vasodilator therapy should be reserved for situations in which hemodynamic monitoring shows the patient to have LV failure with elevations in PCWP, SVR, and a systolic BP >90 mmHg.

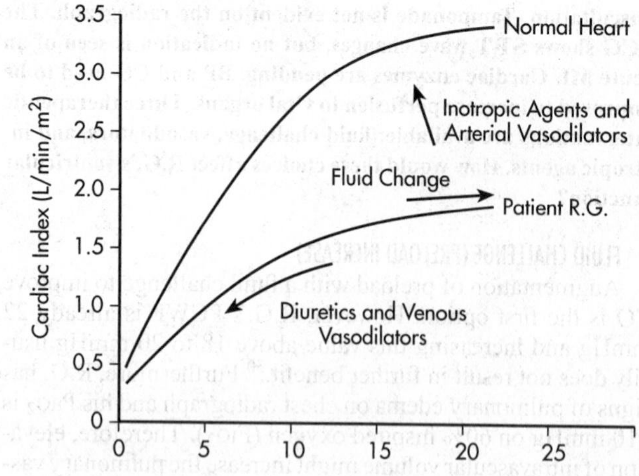

FIGURE 21-4 Ventricular function curve for R.G. PCWP, pulmonary capillary wedge pressure.

INOTROPIC SUPPORT

A rapid-acting inotropic agent (e.g., dopamine, dobutamine, epinephrine) also can be used to increase myocardial contractility and CO. This intervention shifts the ventricular function curve upward and slightly to the left (Fig. 21-4). The disadvantage of this intervention is that improved CO is accompanied by an increased myocardial oxygen demand. Depending on the agent selected, three of the determinants of myocardial oxygen consumption could be elevated: HR, contractility, and ventricular wall tension. Therefore, inotropic support is directed at establishing or maintaining a reasonable arterial pressure and ensuring adequate tissue perfusion by improving the CO.

In summary, the most appropriate therapeutic intervention for R.G. at this time would be inotropic support. The PCWP is elevated, suggesting that the preload has been maximized; therefore, fluid boluses may worsen R.G.'s pulmonary edema. Although R.G.'s SVR is slightly elevated (1,400 $dyne.sec.cm^{-5}$), his BP is low; therefore, initial use of a peripheral vasodilator could jeopardize perfusion. Thus, an acceptable initial therapeutic intervention to improve CO and tissue perfusion is inotropic support. After a reasonable BP has been established, addition of a peripheral vasodilator could be considered to further enhance CO if needed, and diuretics added to reduce his pulmonary edema.

Inotropic Agents

16. Which inotropic agent is the best choice for R.G.?

DOPAMINE

Dopamine, a precursor of norepinephrine, has inotropic, chronotropic, and vasoactive properties, all of which are dose dependent (Table 21-7). At 0.5 to 2 mcg/kg/minute, dopamine stimulates dopaminergic receptors primarily in the splanchnic, renal, and coronary vascular beds, which may produce vasodilation, improve renal blood flow (controversial), and maintain natriuresis. The effect on dopaminergic receptors is not blocked by β-blockers, but is antagonized by dopaminergic-blocking agents such as the butyrophenones and phenothiazines.

Table 21-7 Inotropic Agents and Vasopressors

		Receptor Sensitivity			Pharmacologic Effect			
Drug	*Usual Dose*	α	β_1	β_2	*VD*	*VC*	*INT*	*CHT*
Dobutamine	2.5–15 mcg/kg/min	+	+++	++	++	– –	+++[a]	+
Dopamine	0.5–2 mcg/kg/min[b] (renal)	– –	– –	– –	– –[b]	+	+	+
	2–5 mcg/kg/min	– –	+	– –	– –[b]	+	+	+
	5–10 mcg/kg/min	+	++	– –	++	++	++	++
	15–20 mcg/kg/min	+++	++	– –	– –[b]	+++	++	++
Epinephrine[c]	0.01–0.1 mcg/kg/min	+	+++	++	+	–	+++	++
	0.1 mcg/kg/min	+++	++	++	– –	+++	++	++
Isoproterenol	0.01–0.1 mcg/kg/min	– –	++++	+++	+++	– –	+++	+++
Milrinone	50 mcg/kg bolus, then 0.375–0.75 mcg/kg/min	– –	– –	– –	+++	– –	++	– –
Norepinephrine	0.05–0.5 mcg/kg/min Highly variable, titrate to desired MAP	++++	++	– –	– –	+++	+[d]	+
Phenylephrine	0.5–5 mcg/kg/min Highly variable, titrate to desired MAP	+++	– –	– –	– –	+++	– –	– –
Vasopressin[e]	0.04 units/min[f]	– –	– –	– –	– –	+++	– –	– –

[a] Dobutamine, amrinone, and milrinone have more inotropic effect than dopamine.
[b] Dopamine at 0.5–2 mcg/kg/min stimulates dopaminergic receptors, causing vasodilation in the splanchnic and renal vasculature.
[c] Epinephrine has predominant inotropic effects; norepinephrine has predominant vasoconstrictive effect. Epinephrine may vasodilate at low dosages, vasoconstrict at high dosages.
[d] Cardiac output unchanged or may decline because of vagal reflex responses that slow the heart.
[e] Vasopressin stimulates V_1 receptors to cause vasoconstriction in the periphery.
[f] Dosing for sepsis; in other vasodilatory conditions, may be titrated from 0.01 to 0.1 U/min.
CHT, chronotropic; INT, inotropic; MAP, mean arterial pressure; SBP, systolic blood pressure; VC, peripheral vascular vasoconstriction; VD, peripheral vascular vasodilation.

Depending on the clinical state of the patient, low dosages of dopamine may slightly increase myocardial contractility, but usually will not alter HR or SVR significantly.

At 2 to 5 mcg/kg/minute, the improved cardiac performance produced by dopamine is through direct stimulation of β_1-adrenergic receptors and indirectly through release of norepinephrine from nerve terminals. Increased β_1-adrenergic receptor stimulation increases stroke volume (inotropic effect), HR (chronotropic effect), and consequently CO. These cardiac effects can be blocked by β-blockers.

At infusion rates of 5 to 10 mcg/kg/minute, the α-adrenergic receptors are activated. At this dosage, the vasoactive effects on peripheral blood vessels are unpredictable and depend on the net effect of β_1-adrenergic stimulation, α-adrenergic stimulation, and reflex mechanisms. MAP and PCWP usually will rise.

At doses >15 to 20 mcg/kg/minute, dopamine primarily stimulates peripheral α-adrenergic receptors. SVR increases, splanchnic and renal blood flow decreases, and LV filling pressure is raised. Cardiac irritability is a potential complication and the overall myocardial oxygen consumption is increased. The increase in SVR limits CO; thus, infusion rates should be limited to <10 to 15 mcg/kg/minute in patients with cardiac failure.

DOBUTAMINE

Dobutamine, a synthetic catecholamine, is a potent positive inotropic agent with predominant direct β_1-agonist effects and weak β_2- and α_1-effects. With greater β_2-vasodilatory than α_1-vasoconstrictive actions, dobutamine can produce reductions in systemic and pulmonary vascular resistance. The reduction in SVR also may be caused by a reflex decrease in vasoconstriction secondary to enhanced CO. Phenoxybenzamine blocks the α-adrenergic response and propranolol blocks the β-adrenergic response. Unlike dopamine, dobutamine does not release endogenous norepinephrine or stimulate renal dopaminergic receptors.[51]

Studies assessing dobutamine in cardiac failure demonstrate consistent increases in CO and stroke volume, with reductions in PCWP and SVR. The reduction in filling pressures, as indicated by a lowered PCWP, results in a decrease in LV wall tension and oxygen consumption. Consequently, coronary perfusion pressure, a major determinant of coronary blood flow, improves and, thus, the oxygen supply to the heart is improved (see Glossary for the definition of perfusion pressure). In comparison to dopamine, dobutamine tends to induce less tachycardia. This feature, combined with the reductions in PCWP and systemic vascular pressure, in addition to the increased perfusion pressure, tends to reduce overall myocardial oxygen consumption.

Compared with dopamine, dobutamine has equal or greater inotropic action. Dobutamine lowers PCWP and SVR with increasing doses, whereas dopamine may increase PCWP and SVR with increasing doses.[52] The effect on HR is variable; however, evidence suggests that dobutamine is less chronotropic than dopamine at lower infusion rates. In the clinical setting, dobutamine may be preferred in patients with depressed CO, elevated PCWP, and increased SVR with mild hypotension. The increase in CO may not be sufficient to raise the BP in a patient who initially is moderately to severely hypotensive. Thus, dopamine may be preferred in patients with depressed CO, normal or moderately elevated PCWP, and moderate or severe hypotension.

EPINEPHRINE

Similar to dopamine, epinephrine has dose-dependent hemodynamic effects (Table 21-7). At lower infusion ranges (0.01–0.1 mcg/kg/minute) epinephrine stimulates β_1-adrenergic receptors, causing increases in HR and contractility. As the dose increases, more α_1-receptor stimulation occurs, resulting in vasocontriction and corresponding increases in SVR.

Epinephrine is frequently used in the cardiac surgery setting, despite a lack of comparative evidence. A survey from Germany found that epinephrine was the first agent chosen for low cardiac output by 41.8% of physicians, compared with dobuatmine by 30.9%.[53] The favorable hemodynamic effects (increased CO and BP) make it an attractive option for R.G.; however, epinephrine can induce hyperglycemia through gluconeogenesis and has been shown to increase lactate levels compared with other pressors and inotropes.[54] R.G. already has signs of acidosis (pH 7.32, HCO_3^- 20 mEq/L) and increased lactic acid production by epinephrine could be detrimental to his organ function. Epinephrine should be reserved for patients with a markedly depressed cardiac output in conjunction with severe hypotension.

In summary, very few comparable studies of inotropic agents in this setting have been conducted and, thus, the selection of agent is often based on the expected clinical benefit as well as individual experience with the drugs. R.G. would benefit from an increase in his CO, as well as in his MAP. The clinician elects to start R.G. on a dopamine infusion.

Selection and Initiation of Therapy

17. Based on the hemodynamic dose effects described in the previous question, at what dose would you initiate a dopamine infusion in R.G.? What therapeutic outcomes are anticipated at this dose and over what time? What adverse effects may be encountered with this dose of dopamine?

R.G. has a MAP of 61 mmHg, a CI of 1.4 L/minute/m^2, a PCWP of 22 mmHg, and an HR of 105 beats/minute. The goal of therapy is to increase the CI to at least 2.5 L/minute/m^2, maintain a MAP of at least 70 mmHg (preferably closer to 80 mmHg, depending on clinical signs of hypoperfusion), reduce the PCWP, and maintain a HR <125 beats/minute. A urine output of at least 0.5 mL/kg/hour (37 mL/hour in R.G.) is desirable. A reasonable initial infusion rate would be 3 mcg/kg/minute. This dose should increase cardiac contraction and CO, resulting in an increase in renal blood flow. Because the onset of action is within minutes, the patient can be re-evaluated and the infusion rate can be titrated upward by 1 to 2 mcg/kg/minute every 10 minutes, depending on the hemodynamic data obtained. The hemodynamic response to dopamine is highly variable among patients; thus, careful titration to lowest effective infusion rate is advised.

Adverse effects encountered with dopamine infusion include increased HR, anginal pain, arrhythmias, headache, hypertension, vasoconstriction, nausea, and vomiting. Extravasation of large amounts of dopamine during infusion can cause ischemic necrosis and sloughing. At higher dosages, α_1-adrenergic effects are more prominent, causing peripheral arterial vasoconstriction and an increase in venous pressure that leads to increases in afterload, preload, and myocardial oxygen demand as well as ischemia.

18. Dopamine is initiated at 3 mcg/kg/minute in R.G. and titrated to 8 mcg/kg/minute over the next 2 hours. A repeat chest radiograph shows slight worsening of pulmonary edema. The following hemodynamic profile is obtained (previous values are in parentheses): BP (S/D/M), 115/62/80 mmHg (92/45/61); pulse, 140 beats/minute (105); CO, 3.8 L/minute (2.8); CI, 2.2 L/minute/m^2 (1.4); RAP, 10 mmHg (12); PCWP, 20 mmHg (22); SVR, 1,473 dyne.sec.cm^{-5} (1,400); urine output, 30 mL/hour (15); and Hct, 36% (34). Do these data indicate a favorable or adverse hemodynamic effect from dopamine in R.G.?

Dopamine at 8 mcg/kg/minute has established a trend in the desired direction for CI; however, the HR has increased significantly. The SVR and PCWP have not changed appreciably, and the urine flow has increased. Further analysis reveals that the stroke volume (CO/HR) has only increased from 25 mL/beat to 27 mL/beat; thus, the major increase in CO has resulted from the chronotropic rather than the inotropic effect of dopamine. As a net response, the dopamine has most likely affected the myocardial oxygen supply-to-demand ratio adversely; however, this cannot be established definitively. R.G. should be monitored closely for signs of myocardial ischemia.

Changing Therapy

19. The clinician decides that a HR of 140 beats/minute is unacceptable in R.G., who has a history of MI. Subsequent attempts to taper the dopamine to lessen the induced tachycardia without dropping the CI and perfusion pressure are unsuccessful. Dobutamine is suggested as an alternative to dopamine. What hemodynamic changes would you expect with dobutamine in R.G.? Does dobutamine offer any advantages over dopamine?

As mentioned above, dobutamine has equivalent or greater inotropic action than dopamine and can cause less tachycardia. The major difference between the two agents is the effect of dopamine on α_1-receptors. With dobutamine's absence of clinical effect on α_1, patients may experience a decrease in the SVR resulting from the unopposed β_2-receptor effects. In R.G., we should see an increase in CI from the inotropic effect and perhaps a decrease in SVR which would further improve his CI. We will have to monitor R.G. carefully as his MAP is still relatively low, and any major reduction in vascular resistance could adversely affect this.

20. How would you initiate therapy with dobutamine and reduce the dopamine?

Dobutamine should be started at a low dosage (i.e., 2.5 mcg/kg/minute). The onset of effect is rapid and the half-life short (approximately 2 minutes), with steady-state conditions generally achieved within 10 minutes of initiation of therapy. This allows dose titration every 10 minutes based on patient tolerance. The rate of infusion required to increase CO typically is between 2.5 and 10 mcg/kg/minute, although higher infusion rates are sometimes rarely required (up to 20 mcg/kg/minute). Once the dobutamine has been started, a reduction in the dose of dopamine should be attempted. A decrease of 20% of the current infusion rate every 10 to 15 minutes is reasonable.

21. What are the adverse effects associated with dobutamine?

Adverse effects that can occur during dobutamine administration are arrhythmias, nausea, anxiety, and tremors. The increases in contractility and HR caused by dobutamine can cause an increase in myocardial oxygen consumption and can lead to ischemia in patients with coronary artery disease. Another limiting factor to dobutamine is tolerance to its hemodynamic effects with long-term continuous use. A decline in CO and HR has been seen after prolonged infusion and is most likely caused by downregulation of β_1-receptors. Of concern, evidence suggests that inotropic agents can be associated with an increased risk of mortality in patients with heart failure despite the improvement of symptoms and hemodynamic indices.[55]

EFFECTS ON HEMODYNAMICS

22. Dobutamine is initiated and titrated up to 7.5 mcg/kg/minute. Concurrently, the dopamine is tapered down to 2.0 mcg/kg/minute, resulting in the following hemodynamic profile (previous values in parentheses): BP (S/D/M), 122/60/80 mmHg (115/62/80); pulse, 115 beats/minute (140); CO, 4.2 L/minute (3.8); CI, 2.5 L/minute (2.2); RAP, 10 mmHg (10); PCWP, 16 mmHg (20); SVR, 1,333 dyne.sec.cm^{-5} (1,473); Pao_2, 115 (110) mmHg; $Paco_2$, 38 (28) mmHg; pH, 7.41 (7.32); HCO_3^-, 24 mEq/L (20); and urine output, 60 mL/hour (30). Assess the improvement in hemodynamic change and urine output with the addition of dobutamine and decreased infusion rate of dopamine.

The CI has continued to increase and the PCWP and SVR have fallen. The increase in perfusion pressure in conjunction with the fall in afterload, preload, and HR will favorably affect the myocardial oxygen supply:demand ratio. The fall in HR with the increase in CO indicates that the stroke volume has increased significantly from 27 to 36 mL/beat. Other signs of improved systemic perfusion include the reversal of the acidosis observed initially and improved urine output.

The improved urine output can be attributed to the combined effects of dobutamine on the CO and subsequent improvement in the perfusion to the kidney and perhaps to the renal effects of dopamine, although the latter effects are controversial and have been debated vigorously. Traditionally, it was thought that the effects of low-dose dopamine on the dopaminergic receptors in the renal vasculature improves kidney blood flow and, consequently, renal function. Randomized, controlled trials have demonstrated increases in urine output with low-dose dopamine,[56] but have not been able to show a reduction in incidence or degree of renal dysfunction.[57,58] Despite the lack of convincing evidence for benefit, low-dose dopamine is widely used in critical care units. The use of low-dose dopamine often does not produce any hemodynamic changes, and adverse effects are rare.[59] Thus, its use can be considered in patients with oliguria, with the understanding that it may only have a diuretic action.

Tapering Inotropic Support

23. R.G. has remained stable with dobutamine 7.5 mcg/kg/minute and dopamine 2.0 mcg/kg/minute for the past 4 hours. Urine output continues to be adequate. How would you taper the inotropic agents and what parameters would you monitor?

An acceptable method is to taper dobutamine by 2 mcg/kg/minute every 30 to 60 minutes and discontinue the dopamine. At such a low infusion rate, the effect of dopamine on R.G.'s hemodynamics is probably negligible and there is no need to titrate down at this level. Dobutamine has an elimination half-life of approximately 2.5 minutes; thus, steady-state plasma levels will occur in a short period. When tapering vasoactive agents, it is prudent, however, to let the patient stabilize hemodynamically at new infusion rates for a period that exceeds the time to achieve a new steady-state plasma concentration. After each reduction in the infusion rate, hemodynamic data can be assessed. Reasonable guidelines would be to keep the mean arterial pressure at 75 to 80 mmHg, HR at <110 beats/minute, PCWP at 12 to 18 mmHg, and CI at >2.5 L/minute/m^2. After the dobutamine is discontinued, the dopamine can be discontinued as well. R.G. should be evaluated for reinstitution of the medications he was receiving before surgery.

Severe Heart Failure

Assessment by Hemodynamic Profile

24. A.R. is a 65-year-old woman admitted to the ICU in acute respiratory distress. She has a medical history of coronary artery disease, an MI 4 years ago, hypertension, HF, and renal insufficiency. A.R. has a history of poor compliance with her medications and admits to discontinuing her usual medications (furosemide, enalapril, metoprolol, and digoxin) 5 days ago.

A.R. is confused, in obvious distress, and cannot catch her breath. Her extremities are pale and slightly cool. Her vital signs are as follows: temperature, 36.8°C; HR, 124 beats/minute; RR, 35 breaths/minute; BP, 104/65; and Sao_2, 85% on 6 L/minute of O_2 via a face mask. Her admission weight is 95 kg (stated home weight, 87 kg). A Foley catheter and peripheral IV are placed, and samples are sent to the laboratory for analysis. ABG values include the following: pH, 7.33 (normal, 7.35–7.45); $Paco_2$, 28 mmHg (normal, 35–45 mmHg); Pao_2, 57 mmHg (normal, 75–100 mmHg); and HCO_3^-, 20 mEq/L (normal, 23–29 mEq/L). Other laboratory results are sodium, 130 mEq/L (normal, 136–145 mEq/L); potassium, 5.2 mEq/L (normal, 3.5–5.0 mEq/L); and creatinine, 1.9 mg/dL (normal, 0.2–0.8 mg/dL). A pulmonary artery catheter is placed and initial hemodynamic values are RAP, 15 mmHg (normal, 2–6 mmHg); PCWP, 30 mmHg (normal, 5–12 mmHg); pulmonary artery pressure (PAP), 45/28 mmHg (S/D); CO, 3.5 L/minute (normal, 4–7 L/minute); CI, 1.6 L/minute (2.5–4.2 L/min) (BSA, 2.2 m^2); and SVR, 1,440 dyne.sec.m^{-5} (normal, 800–1,440 dyne.sec.m^{-5}). Chest radiograph shows pulmonary edema with no signs of pneumonia. ECG shows sinus tachycardia with nonspecific T-wave changes and LV hypertrophy.

Describe A.R.'s clinical situation and assess her hemodynamic variables. What initial therapies should be instituted? (Also see Chapter 19, Heart Failure.)

[SI units: sodium, 130 mmol/L (normal, 136–145); potassium, 5.2 mmol/L (normal, 3.5–5); creatinine, 168 μmol/L (normal, 18–71 μmol/L)]

A.R. is in respiratory distress because of pulmonary edema and acute heart failure. Her vital signs show a decreased BP and poor oxygenation. Her CO is low with high preload (PCWP, 30 mmHg) and she has increased SVR. She has some signs of inadequate perfusion manifested by her confusion and cool skin. As described in Chapter 18, patients can be classified into four different hemodynamic categories based on volume status (wet versus dry) and organ perfusion status (cold vs. warm) with subsequent treatment strategies based on which category the patients fits.[60,61] A.R would best be described as wet and warm, although she does have some early evidence of inadequate perfusion as well.

A.R.'s laboratory values (potassium, 5.2 mEq/L; creatinine, 1.9 mg/dL) show renal insufficiency, and the low serum sodium (130 mEq/L) most likely represents volume overload and hemodilution because total body sodium load in patients with HF is usually high. A.R.'s high RAP and PCWP are consistent with volume overload as well and probable cardiogenic pulmonary edema. In many patients, the onset of pulmonary congestion occurs when the PCWP is 18 to 20 mmHg, and overt pulmonary edema can occur when the PCWP exceeds 30 mmHg. Filling pressures are elevated secondary to activation of the renin-angiotensin system with subsequent sodium and water retention by the kidney in response to the low CO. Patients with chronic HF often can tolerate higher filling pressures (PCWP) than patients who acutely develop HF because the change is gradual. It is, therefore, important to follow the clinical signs, rather than treat a specific number for patients in pulmonary edema.

Improvement of A.R.'s respiratory status is the initial priority, and she should be intubated if attempts to provide supplemental oxygen via face mask are not successful in elevating her Po_2. An MI should be ruled out, although the probable precipitating event is the noncompliance with her medication regimen. In the "wet and warm" patient, diuretics should be given to reduce volume overload and pulmonary edema. (See Chapter 18, Heart failure for a discussion of diuretic use in patients with heart failure.)

Therapeutic Interventions

VASODILATORS

25. Sixty minutes after a 40-mg IV furosemide dose, A.R. is now more confused, and her urine output has declined after an initial good response to the furosemide. A.R.'s vital signs are HR, 110 beats/minute; BP, 110/50 mmHg; RR 20 breaths/minute; and Sao_2 93% on 100% face mask O_2. The PA catheter shows a RAP of 16 mmHg; PAP, 38/24 mmHg; PCWP, 24 mmHg; CO, 4.2 L/min; CI, 1.9 L/min/m^2; and SVR, 1,028 dyne.sec.m^{-5}. Laboratory results show the following: Po_2, 79; Hct, 34%; Hgb, 11.2; and Svo_2, 54%. What other therapeutic options are available for treatment of A.R.'s acute HF and pulmonary edema given the current hemodynamic values and clinical situation?

A.R.'s condition has deteriorated clinically; her calculated oxygen delivery is low (Do_2 608 mL/minute) and her mixed venous oxygen saturation (Svo_2) is decreased, suggesting hypoperfusion. Improvement in A.R.'s CO is needed to increase perfusion and prevent organ dysfunction. A.R. is now best classified as "wet and cold." Vasodilators have become an accepted part of treatment for HF based on the following underlying pathophysiology (also see Chapter 18, Heart Failure). As CO falls, the sympathetic nervous system and renin-angiotensin system are activated to maintain circulatory stability. Arterial pressure is maintained by the excessive increase in SVR (afterload), which increases the resistance to ejection of blood from the LV. Venoconstriction shifts some of the blood volume from the peripheral veins to the central circulation, which contributes to an elevation of right and left atrial pressures (preload). A normal heart responds to the increase in preload and afterload by increasing contractility, but in HF, the heart's intrinsic capacity to increase contractility has been lost. As a result, the neurohormonal compensatory mechanism activated to maintain arterial pressure increases the work load on the heart and this leads to a further decrease in CO. Patients tend to spiral down this vicious cycle until the CO is lower and the SVR is higher than optimal to maintain perfusion pressure. Vasodilators disrupt the compensatory mechanisms that elevate preload and afterload and shift the ventricular function curve upward, which allows a greater CO at a lower LV filling pressure.

Three categories of vasodilators are available. Arterial vasodilators (e.g., hydralazine) decrease afterload, thus reducing impedance to LV outflow. Venous vasodilators (e.g., nitroglycerin [NTG]) primarily decrease venous return (preload), thus improving ventricular compliance, subendocardial coronary perfusion, and pulmonary hydrostatic pressure. Finally, mixed arterial and venous vasodilators have balanced effects on both preload and afterload reduction (e.g., nitroprusside, nesiritide, angiotensin-converting enzyme inhibitors). The fall in SVR from arterial vasodilation can potentially cause hypotension and a reflex increase in HR; however, this is infrequently seen in patients with HF because the decrease in SVR is counterbalanced by an increase in CO, which tends to maintain arterial pressure. Excessive preload reduction can cause deficient ventricular filling, thereby reducing the CO. The overall response in any given patient depends on that patient's baseline hemodynamic and volume status. At this time, A.R.'s BP has normalized, but she still has signs of inadequate perfusion. A trial of a vasodilator therapy for afterload and preload reduction may improve A.R.'s clinical status.

Nitroprusside

26. The clinician decides to begin an infusion of nitroprusside for afterload and preload reduction in A.R. How should therapy be initiated? What are the end points of therapy? What adverse effects are associated with nitroprusside infusion?

The initial infusion rate of nitroprusside should be no greater than 0.5 mcg/kg/minute. The infusion rate can be titrated upward by 0.25 mcg/kg/minute every 5 minutes until the mean arterial pressure falls 5 to 10 mmHg. Nitroprusside will lower SVR through arterial vasodilation and will decrease PCWP through venodilation. Cardiac output will increase as the afterload is reduced. Reasonable goals of therapy in A.R. are a cardiac index of >2.5 L/minute. A mean arterial pressure above 70 mmHg will ensure adequate organ perfusion, but BP should be kept as low as A.R. tolerates clinically, because this will reflect maximal afterload reduction. A reduction in PCWP to a level that maintains CO without causing pulmonary edema is also desirable. In A.R., a goal PCWP of 16 to 18 mmHg is reasonable.

Adverse effects associated with nitroprusside administration include excessive hypotension, reflex tachycardia, potential worsening of myocardial ischemia, thiocyanate toxicity (especially with renal dysfunction, prolonged infusions, and high infusion rates), accumulation of cyanide with subsequent cyanide toxicity, worsening arterial hypoxemia from increases in ventilation–perfusion mismatch, and, rarely, methemoglobinemia and hypothyroidism. (Also see Chapter 20, Hypertensive Emergencies, for a discussion of nitroprusside.)

27. Over the next 2 hours, A.R. received two doses of IV furosemide (40 mg). Nitroprusside was titrated to 1.2 g/kg/minute resulting in the following hemodynamic profile (previous values in parentheses): BP (S/D/M), 100/50/66 mmHg (110/50/70); pulse, 94 beats/minute (110); CI, 2.8 L/minute/m^2 (1.9); PCWP, 22 mmHg (24); SVR, 906 dyne.sec.cm^{-5} (1,028); urine output, 50 mL/hour (10); PaO_2, 80 mmHg (70); $PaCO_2$, 46 mmHg (46); pH, 7.32 (7.26); and HCO_3^-, 24 mEq/L (21). Cardiopulmonary examination reveals an S_3 gallop and bibasilar rales are present, but diminished from previous examination. The ECG shows a sinus rhythm. Evaluate the effect that nitroprusside and furosemide have had on A.R.'s hemodynamic profile and clinical status.

The CI has improved significantly (1.9 to 2.8 L/minute/m^2) and the stroke volume has increased from 27 to 48 mL/beat. The improved stroke volume has decreased endogenous catecholamine levels, which, in turn, has decreased the HR (110–94 beats/minute) and SVR. A.R. has improved clinically and her ABG indicate improvement of the metabolic acidosis. The increased urine output can be attributed to the combined effects of the diuretic and increased CO. Overall, A.R. has improved substantially. Supplemental oxygen still is required, but the oxygen concentration needed to maintain an adequate arterial oxygen content has been lowered.

At this point, a further reduction in preload may benefit A.R.'s respiratory function because the PCWP still is elevated at 22 mmHg. The mean arterial pressure is slightly lower than acceptable, however, and a further increase in the nitroprusside dose to reduce preload further may lower the MAP to a level that would compromise coronary and cerebral perfusion, as well as perfusion to other vital organs.

CHOICE OF ADDITIONAL THERAPY

28. What therapeutic interventions are available to further reduce A.R.'s preload and improve her status?

Four options are available. The first is to continue current therapy (nitroprusside and furosemide) and wait for the diuresis to continue to reduce preload. However, because her MAP is slightly lower than desired, signs of inadequate systemic perfusion must be monitored closely as a guide to additional or reduced diuretic therapy. The goal is to find the filling pressure (PCWP) that maximizes SV without causing pulmonary edema.

The second option to reduce preload would be the addition of IV NTG. An initial dose of 0.25 mcg/kg/minute is reasonable. Initial titration should be in 0.25 mcg/kg/minute increments at intervals of 3 to 5 minutes guided by patient's clinical response. If no response is seen at 1 mcg/kg/minute, titration increments of 0.5 to 1 mcg/kg/minute may be used. (See Chapter 17, Myocardial Infarction, and Chapter 18, Heart Failure, for additional discussion of intravenous nitroglycerin.)

The third option is to continue the nitroprusside and add dobutamine to improve CO through inotropic support. A dobutamine infusion of 3 mcg/kg/minute is a reasonable initial dose. Either choice is acceptable as long as A.R. is monitored closely.

A fourth option would be the use of an agent, such as nesiritide (see below), to reduce preload and potentially augment diuresis, although A.R.'s blood pressure may not tolerate the hemodynamic effects of this agent.

Transition to Oral Vasodilators

29. After 48 hours of nitroprusside, intermittent furosemide, and low-dose dobutamine, A.R. has remained hemodynamically stable. The decision is made to reinstitute A.R.'s previous medications (furosemide, enalapril, metoprolol, and digoxin). No evidence supports a new MI. How would you reinstitute the enalapril (10 mg BID) and taper the nitroprusside in A.R.?

Guidelines for tapering short-acting vasodilators when substituting long-acting oral agents are not strict. In this case, a reasonable approach would be to give the enalapril (Vasotec) at a lower dosage than A.R. was taking previously (e.g., 5 mg BID) and reduce the nitroprusside infusion rate by 25%. Then, obtain a CO and PCWP every 2 to 4 hours to assess the contribution of the enalapril to the afterload and preload reduction. If the MAP declines excessively after the addition of enalapril, the nitroprusside dose will have to be reduced further. A smooth transition from IV therapy to oral therapy often depends on the skill of the nursing staff and their familiarity with the hemodynamic effects of the drugs. In addition, A.R. will have to be monitored for signs of renal insufficiency, a potential adverse effect of angiotensin-converting enzyme (ACE) inhibitors. If she develops worsening renal function, an alternative vasodilator strategy, such as hydralazine and nitrate therapy, may be necessary (see Chapter 18, Heart Failure).

Other Therapies

PHOSPHODIESTERASE INHIBITORS

30. Milrinone is a noncatecholamine inotropic agent with vasodilator activity. If A.R.'s condition had failed to respond to nitroprusside and furosemide, this drug would have been a potential therapeutic option for treatment of her acute cardiac failure. What are the considerations in choosing which agent to use? How would you dose milrinone and what adverse effects would you expect with its administration? Does milrinone offer any advantage over catecholamine inotropic agents (e.g., dobutamine, dopamine) or a pure vasodilator such as nitroprusside?

The phosphodiesterase (PDE) inhibitors (also referred to as inodilators) are a class of drugs that have combined inotropic and vasodilator effects. All agents in this class have basically the same mechanism of action: they inhibit intracellular phosphodiesterase, the enzyme responsible for metabolic inactivation of cyclic adenosine monophosphate (cAMP). The resulting increased concentration of cAMP enhances sympathetic nervous system activity that produces positive inotropic effects. Increased cAMP also causes relaxation of vascular smooth muscle and, therefore, decreases SVR.

The hemodynamic effects seen with PDE inhibitors include increased inotropy, reduced SVR, and improved LV diastolic compliance. These changes result in an increase in CI and a decrease in LV afterload and filling pressures. Almost all the phosphodiesterase inhibitors have been shown to elevate CI and stroke volume index. Myocardial oxygen demand is increased by the increase in myocardial contractility and HR. On the other hand, LV filling pressures and SVR are decreased, leading to a decrease in myocardial oxygen demand. The net effect depends on the balance of the opposing forces.

Milrinone

Milrinone is the phosphodiesterase inhibitor most often used in clinical practice. It is primarily cleared by the kidneys, and has an elimination half-life from 1 to 3 hours in patients with normal renal function. In patients with severe heart failure, or in patients with renal failure, an increase in the elimination half-life can be seen. The onset of action occurs within minutes following a loading dose.

The long half-life of milrinone compared with the catecholamine agents makes a loading dose necessary before an infusion can be started. IV milrinone usually is initiated with a 50 mcg/kg loading dose administered over 10 minutes, followed by a maintenance infusion of 0.25 to 0.75 mcg/kg/minute. The loading dose is frequently skipped in patients at risk for hypotension. Patients with HF or renal insufficiency will have a reduced elimination rate and require dose adjustment.

Intravenous administration of milrinone in patients with severe heart failure results in a significant increase in CO, while decreasing PVR and SVR through vasodilation. HR usually remains unaltered, although hypotension can occur when vasodilation exceeds the increase in CO and in hypovolemic patients. Theoretically, the effect of milrinone on myocardial oxygen consumption should be favorable because it does not substantially alter HR while lowering LV filling pressure. A recent placebo-controlled study of the short-term use (48-hour infusion) of milrinone in patients with acute exacerbations of heart failure found no significant differences in mortality, length of hospitalization, or readmission, and found significant increases in arrhythmias and hypotension in the milrinone group.[62] Although patients were excluded from this trial if their treating physician felt that inotropic therapy was essential, it is important to recognize that the improvement of hemodynamic variables does not necessarily imply improved outcome.

Milrinone therapy has few serious side effects, the most significant being hypotension and arrhythmias. Because milrinone may increase arrhythmia frequency and cause sudden death, it should be used cautiously in patients with severe ventricular arrhythmias. Thrombocytopenia has also been reported with milrinone use.

Compared with pure vasodilators such as nitroprusside, milrinone offers the advantage of positive inotropic action, which can increase CO to a greater degree. The increased inotropy comes at a cost of increased myocardial work, or oxygen consumption, which is a potential disadvantage of PDE inhibitors.

Comparisons of the hemodynamic effects of milrinone, dobutamine, and dopamine show that milrinone is more similar to dobutamine than to dopamine. Therefore, the advantage of milrinone over dopamine would be the same as that of dobutamine over dopamine (see Question 19). In contrast to dobutamine, milrinone is a less potent inotropic agent and a more potent vasodilator. In a comparison of these agents, patients receiving dobutamine had a higher BP and PCWP compared with those on milrinone, reflecting the increased vasodilation with milrinone.[63] The longer duration of action poses a problem if an undesirable effect occurs, although the lack of a chronotropic effect with a resultant increase in myocardial oxygen consumption may be beneficial in A.R., who has a history of MI. Trials evaluating milrinone-based versus dobutamine-based therapy have found similar outcomes in patients with decompensated heart failure and in patients awaiting heart transplantation, with increased cost associated with milrinone.[64,65] The current cost of milrinone has decreased with the arrival of a generic product.

Because the inotropic mechanism of milrinone is independent of β-receptors, it may be of value in patients who do not respond to catecholamine inotropic agents because of β-receptor blockade or downregulation of β-receptors.[66] This may be an important consideration, as β-blocker therapy is becoming standard in the treatment of heart failure as evidenced by the use of metoprolol in A.R. In addition, milrinone has a different mechanism of action and, therefore, it may have synergistic inotropic effects with catecholamines.

NESIRITIDE

31. Nesiritide is a new agent approved for the treatment of decompensated heart failure. What are the hemodynamic effects of nesiritide and how does it compare with other agents used in the treatment of advanced heart failure?

Human brain, or B-type, natriuretic peptide (BNP) is produced by the ventricle in response to increased filling pressures. The endogenous protein has several important actions on hemodynamics as described in Chapter 18, Heart Failure. Nesiritide is a recombinant form that is identical to endogenous BNP. The actions of nesiritide include mixed arterial and venous dilation, increased sodium excretion, and suppression of the deleterious effects of the renin-angiotensin-aldosterone and sympathetic nervous system.[67–69] Compared with placebo, the effects on hemodynamics are a decrease in PCWP, PA pressures, and SVR, and an increase in CO.[69] Nesiritide does not possess direct inotropic activity; the increase in CO is a result of the decrease in afterload.

The Vasodilation in the Management of Acute CHF (VMAC) study evaluated nesiritide compared with nitroglycerin in the treatment of heart failure.[70] The investigators found that nesiritide improved PCWP better than nitroglycerin, and was more effective at reducing the symptoms of dyspnea with fewer adverse effects. Compared with dobutamine in a randomized, open-label trial, nesiritide caused less tachyarrhythmias and more hypotension, with similar effects on the signs and symptoms of CHF.[70] Nesiritide is dosed as a 2 mcg/kg load, followed by an infusion of 0.01 mcg/kg/minute. The infusion may be titrated up to a maximum of 0.03 mcg/kg/minute. Few data are available concerning infusions of nesiritide for longer than 48 hours. The balanced vasodilation and increased sodium excretion with nesiritide makes it an attractive option in the treatment of advanced heart failure, particularly in diuretic-resistant patients with elevated filling pressures and dyspnea. Hypotension is the most common adverse effect, occurring in up to 35% of patients.[70]

The use of nesiritide has generated controversy. A meta-analysis of three randomized, controlled trials suggested that nesiritide use may be associated with worsening renal function and an increased risk of short-term mortality.[71] These findings have been debated considerably with other analyses failing to confirm the increased mortality risk.[72] Until more conclusive outcome data are available, the use of nesiritide should be reserved for those patients with acutely decompensated heart failure who are not responding to more conventional strategies, and should be limited to no more than 48 hours of therapy. (See Chapter 18, Heart Failure, for additional information about the clinical use of nesiritide.)

Acute Myocardial Infarction

Immediate Goals of Therapy and General Considerations

32. M.J., a 57-year-old man, is brought to the ED complaining of severe chest pain and difficulty breathing. On physical examination, M.J. has a BP of 80/40 mmHg (normal, 120/80 mmHg) (by cuff) with a weak pulse of 115 beats/minute (normal, 60–80 beats/minute). His RR is 24 breaths/minute (normal, 18 breaths/minute) and his breathing is shallow. Heart sounds include S_3/S_4 gallops, but no murmurs are heard. The jugular venous pulse is normal. He has diffuse rales over the lower lung fields with moderate wheezing. M.J. is cold and clammy to touch; however, his temperature is normal. He is restless, anxious, and confused about time and date. Arterial blood gas (ABG) measurements on 2 L/minute oxygen via nasal prongs are PaO_2, 65 mmHg (normal, 75–100 mmHg); $PaCO_2$, 44 mmHg (normal, 35–45 mmHg); pH, 7.22 (normal, 7.35–7.45); and HCO_3^-, 18 mEq/L (normal, 23–29 mEq/L). The ECG shows ST segment elevation in the anterior lateral leads and 6 to 10 premature ventricular contractions (PVC) per minute. Serum potassium is normal. A Foley catheter is inserted to monitor urine output. Cardiac enzymes are pending. M.J. has no known history of cardiac disease and takes no medication. What immediate goals of therapy are necessary to stabilize and treat M.J.?

[SI unit: HCO_3^-, 18 mmol/L (normal, 23–29)]

M.J. has signs of cardiogenic shock with decreased systemic perfusion. His BP is low, his HR is elevated, and his respiratory status is compromised. M.J. is restless, anxious, and confused, indicating poor cerebral perfusion. His ABG results indicate a component of metabolic acidosis secondary to poor systemic perfusion. The ST elevation on the ECG is consistent with an acute anterior MI.

As discussed in Chapter 17, Myocardial Infarction, most patients presenting with MI are routinely treated with aspirin, a β-blocker, and a thrombolytic (unless contraindicated) or immediate percutaneous coronary intervention (PCI). The presence of cardiogenic shock can alter the interventional strategy, however. Patients presenting in cardiogenic shock after MI may progress rapidly to irreversible organ system dysfunction as the compensatory mechanisms fail to maintain tissue perfusion. Treatment of these critically ill patients involves two components: (*a*) stabilization and (*b*) definitive treatment. Initial stabilization of the patient must be attained before further evaluation and treatment of the cause of cardiogenic shock can proceed. The goals are to maintain adequate oxygen delivery to the tissues and to prevent further hemodynamic compromise. Stabilization includes (*a*) establishing ventilation and oxygenation (arterial PO_2 should be >70 mmHg); (*b*) restoring central arterial BP and CO with vasopressors and inotropic agents, if needed; (*c*) infusing fluids, if hypovolemic; and (*d*) treating pain, arrhythmias, and acid-base abnormalities, if present.

Administration of oxygen by mechanical ventilation enhances the myocardial oxygen supply and may contribute to improved ventricular performance. Mechanical ventilation is indicated when arterial oxygen saturation cannot be maintained above 85% to 90% despite 100% oxygen per face mask. Once the patient is intubated, maximal sedation should be provided to alleviate anxiety and discomfort.

The arterial pressure must be increased to provide adequate coronary and systemic perfusion to meet oxygen requirements. Some areas of ischemia in the infarct zone may be depressed but viable, provided myocardial oxygen supply exceeds demand. If the myocardial oxygen demands are not met, however, myocardial tissue necrosis will expand into the area of ischemia. This results in further hemodynamic impairment and initiates a vicious feedback cycle that can lead to intractable pump failure and irreversible shock. To be effective, treatment of cardiogenic shock should favorably influence the balance between oxygen supply and demand in the ischemic zone.

Optimizing preload to improve CO and systemic perfusion is crucial, especially in patients with RV infarction. In patients with severe LV impairment caused by cardiogenic shock, increasing intravascular volume can worsen pulmonary congestion. M.J. currently has signs of pulmonary congestion and RV infarction is not immediately evident; thus, a fluid challenge must be administered cautiously or withheld until hemodynamic monitoring can be established.

Inotropic agents or vasopressors should be used to increase systemic BP and re-establish coronary perfusion in patients with cardiogenic shock and hypotension. The use of vasoactive agents is not without risk, however, because they can exacerbate ventricular arrhythmias and increase oxygen consumption in ischemic myocardium. Therefore, the minimal dose that will provide adequate perfusion pressure should be used. Achieving a MAP of 65 to 70 mmHg is the immediate goal of therapy. Elevation of the MAP above 80 mmHg is unnecessary because at this level, coronary blood flow is not significantly changed, but energy expenditure is high.

Correction of metabolic acidosis is best accomplished by treating the underlying cause. Improving tissue perfusion by optimizing oxygen content and increasing CO can eventually restore aerobic metabolism and eliminate lactic acid production. The use of sodium bicarbonate to correct lactic acidosis in cardiogenic shock and other critically ill patients is controversial. Sodium bicarbonate can have numerous adverse effects, such as hypernatremia, paradoxical intracellular acidosis, and hypercapnia; conclusive data on its efficacy are lacking. Bicarbonate therapy, therefore, warrants caution and is recommended only, if at all, when severe acidemia (pH <7.2 or HCO_3^- <10 to 12 mEq/L) is present.

Because inotropic agents and vasoconstrictors can increase myocardial oxygen consumption and potentially extend the area of necrosis in patients with infarct-induced cardiogenic shock, the careful selection and titration of agents that will best preserve myocardium while sustaining systemic arterial pressure and tissue perfusion is essential. Although correction of volume deficits and early pharmacologic support may prevent the extension of myocardial damage, it must be emphasized that exclusive use of these measures does not improve survival. Therefore, drug therapy must be considered only an interim maneuver to preserve myocardial and systemic integrity while further therapeutic interventions and definitive therapy are being considered.

As mentioned, cardiogenic shock following AMI occurs in only a small percentage of patients, but carries a high mortality rate. Reperfusion of the occluded artery is of paramount importance in these patients. Two options are available for restoring patency of the artery. Thrombolytic therapy and percutaneous transluminal coronary angioplasty, with or without stenting (see Chapter 17, Myocardial Infarction).

Thrombolytic therapy in acute MI may reduce the incidence of subsequent cardiogenic shock, but its value may be limited in patients who have already developed shock.[73] The effectiveness of thrombolytics is reduced in this setting, possibly because of reduced delivery of the agent to the coronary artery thrombus as a result of hypotension.[74] The use of an intra-aortic balloon pump (IABP) to augment coronary artery blood flow may improve the efficacy of thrombolytics.[75] In settings when interventional cardiac procedures such as percutaneous transluminal coronary angioplasty (PTCA) or stenting are not readily available, insertion of an IABP and thrombolytics should not be delayed if indicated.

Early PTCA may be of more benefit than thrombolytics in patients with cardiogenic shock complicating acute MI. In a subset of patients with cardiogenic shock in the GUSTO-1 trial, angioplasty resulted in a reduction in 30-day mortality rate from 61% to 43%.[76] Numerous other trials have demonstrated improved outcomes with PTCA in patients with shock compared with historical controls. However, problems with subgroup analysis and nonrandomized trials include the potential for selection bias. Operator skill also is a consideration in this setting, and larger centers with greater experience may have better outcomes than smaller centers.

An early revascularization strategy with angioplasty or bypass surgery was recently compared with medical management of these patients, including thrombolytics and intra-aortic balloon counterpulsation.[77] No significant difference was found in mortality rate at 30 days; however, at 6 months, the mortality rate in the revascularization group was 50.3% versus 63.1% for the medical therapy group. Follow-up at 1 year also demonstrated a significant increase in survival.[78]

Assessment by Hemodynamic Profile

33. M.J. has a history of cerebrovascular disease and is thus ineligible for thrombolytic therapy. Therefore, he will require revascularization in the form of balloon angioplasty or coronary artery bypass surgery to improve his chances of survival. Meanwhile, he is given dopamine at 5 mcg/kg/minute to stabilize him hemodynamically before revascularization procedures are initiated. Lidocaine (100-mg IV bolus plus a 2-mg/minute infusion) also is instituted to correct the PVCs. Oxygen administration is changed to 100% via face mask. Morphine sulfate, 2 mg IV, is given for chest pain. IV NTG was initiated at 0.25 mc/kg/minute for myocardial ischemia, but had to be discontinued because intolerable hypotension developed. M.J. is admitted to the ICU where an arterial line and pulmonary artery line are placed, revealing the following hemodynamic profile (previous values in parentheses): BP (S/D/M), 92/46/61 mmHg (80/40 by cuff); pulse, 122 beats/min (115); CO, 2.8 L/minute; CI, 1.5 L/minute/m^2; RAP, 16 mmHg; PCWP, 26 mmHg; SVR, 1,314 dyne.sec.cm^{-5}; PaO_2, 70 mmHg (65); $PaCO_2$, 48 mmHg (44); pH, 7.24 (7.22); HCO_3^-, 21 mEq/L (18); and urine output, 10 mL/hour. (M.J. weighs 82 kg and has a BSA of 1.9 m^2.) The chest radiograph shows evidence of pulmonary edema. Assess M.J.'s hemodynamic profile and response to dopamine therapy.

M.J.'s clinical and hemodynamic parameters confirm the diagnosis of cardiogenic shock. He is clearly not hypovolemic, as manifested by an elevated RAP and PCWP. Although his SBP is slightly improved, his CI (<1.8 L/minute/m^2), PCWP (>18 mmHg), and low urine output (<25 mL/hour) are all characteristic findings with this form of shock. Patients with cardiogenic shock from an acute event (such as an MI) are usually in a much more critical clinical situation than patients who have an acute exacerbation of chronic heart failure. Patients with HF have compensated over time for the increases in preload and reduced CO, but patients such as M.J. have not had time to develop compensatory mechanisms.

Dopamine, at an infusion rate of 5 to 10 mcg/kg/minute, has made M.J. more tachycardic, has not substantially enhanced CO, and the MAP is less than optimal for coronary perfusion. M.J. has signs of pulmonary edema that are consistent with the elevated pulmonary wedge pressure. The Pao_2 of 70 mmHg is marginally acceptable considering he is on 100% oxygen per face mask.

Therapeutic Interventions

FLUID THERAPY VERSUS INOTROPIC SUPPORT

34. The decision is made to intubate M.J. Would a fluid challenge or additional doses of dopamine improve M.J.'s status?

In M.J., a fluid challenge could exacerbate the pulmonary edema because after an AMI, ventricular compliance is decreased and a small change in LVEDV could result in a disproportionately large increase in PCWP. Thus, in patients with an AMI, the benefits of a fluid challenge must be balanced against the risk of aggravating pulmonary edema. M.J. has an elevated RAP and PCWP, indicating that he has at least adequate, if not excessive, preload. If a fluid challenge is going to be administered, no >100 mL of normal saline should be infused without further evaluation of hemodynamic and clinical data.

Increasing the dopamine infusion rate might improve CO and perfusion pressure, but at the expense of increasing the HR even further. The increased HR, along with the elevated PCWP, could adversely affect the myocardial oxygen supply-to-demand ratio. However, the increase in coronary blood flow (caused by the rise in arterial pressure) and the decrease in LV chamber size (associated with the increase in contractility), it is hoped would tend to offset the increase in myocardial oxygen requirements.

It is not entirely clear which patients in cardiogenic shock will respond to dopamine. One trial of 24 patients in cardiogenic shock found that a mean infusion rate of 9.1 mcg/kg/minute was required to produce beneficial effects on CO, urine output, HR, and PCWP in survivors.[79] Nonsurvivors had no change in MAP, PCWP, or HR at an average infusion rate of 17.1 mcg/kg/minute.

COMBINATION INOTROPIC THERAPY

35. Occasionally, a patient's hemodynamic status improves with the combined use of inotropic agents. Would the addition of dobutamine or a phosphodiesterase inhibitor to treat M.J.'s cardiogenic shock be beneficial?

The combination of dobutamine and dopamine was studied in eight cardiogenic shock patients requiring mechanical ventilation.[80] None of the patients had experienced an MI within the preceding 7 days. Each patient received three infusions in a randomly assigned order: dopamine at 15 mcg/kg/minute; dobutamine at 15 mcg/kg/minute; and a combination of dopamine and dobutamine each at 7.5 mcg/kg/minute. All three regimens increased CI, stroke index, LVSWI, and HR similarly. MAP increased with the dopamine and the dobutamine–dopamine combination, but did not change with dobutamine alone. SVR was significantly lower with dobutamine alone compared with the other two regimens. PCWP was elevated most with the dopamine infusion alone as was myocardial oxygen consumption. The combination regimen offered hemodynamic superiority over either agent alone in this group of patients.

Given M.J.'s significantly low arterial BP, the addition of a PDE inhibitor, such as milrinone, could be problematic. These agents tend to have more vasodilating properties than dobutamine, and their long-half lives can present difficulties in management if hypotension does develop. Until M.J.'s BP is improved, PDE inhibitors should be avoided.

In summary, further inotropic support with dopamine or the addition of dobutamine would be indicated in M.J. at this time. The dopamine could be increased to 12.5 mcg/kg/minute or dobutamine could be initiated at 5 mcg/kg/minute. Neither maneuver is without risk. Dobutamine could lower the MAP, adversely affecting coronary perfusion pressure. Dopamine might elevate the PCWP. The addition of dobutamine or an increase in dopamine dose could increase HR even more. Any of these would adversely affect the myocardial oxygen supply-to-demand ratio and could further extend the area of ischemia or necrosis.

36. Despite the addition of dobutamine at a rate of 5 to 7.5 mcg/kg/minute and initiation of ventilatory support via tracheal intubation, M.J. continues to show signs of deterioration, with progressive obtundation and loss of bowel sounds. His systemic arterial pressure has continued to decline, and his dopamine is now up to 18 mcg/kg/minute. Preload reduction was attempted previously with NTG; however, the drop in BP was intolerable. A repeat hemodynamic profile shows the following (previous values in parentheses): BP (S/D/M), 86/40/55 (92/46/61); pulse, 132 beats/minute (122); CO, 3.0 L/minute (2.8); CI, 1.6 L/minute/m^2 (1.5); RAP, 18 mmHg (16); PCWP, 24 mmHg (26); SVR, 986 dyne.sec.cm^{-5} (1,314); urine output, 8 mL/hour (10); Pao_2, 75 mmHg (70); $Paco_2$, 42 mmHg (48); pH, 7.26 (7.24); and HCO_3^-, 19 mEq/L (21). The ECG shows atrial tachycardia with occasional PVC. What therapeutic alternatives can be considered at this time?

M.J. is still in severe cardiogenic shock and his tissue perfusion continues to deteriorate as evidenced by a further reduction in urine output, a loss in bowel sounds, continuing acidosis, and central nervous system (CNS) obtundation. Because his systemic arterial pressure and tissue perfusion have declined despite the addition of dobutamine and maximal doses of dopamine, additional support with a potent vasopressor and the insertion of an IABP are indicated.

NOREPINEPHRINE

Norepinephrine is a potent α-adrenergic agonist that vasoconstricts arterioles at all infusion rates, thereby increasing SVR. Thus, systemic arterial and coronary perfusion pressures both rise. Norepinephrine also stimulates β_1-adrenergic receptors to a lesser extent, resulting in increased contractility and stroke volume. However, HR and CO usually remain constant, or may even decrease secondary to the increased afterload and reflex baroreceptor activation. Although coronary perfusion pressure is enhanced as a result of the elevation in diastolic pressure, myocardial oxygen consumption also is increased. Consequently, myocardial ischemia and arrhythmias may be exacerbated and LV function further compromised.

Infusions of norepinephrine are begun at 0.01 to 0.05 mcg/kg/minute and titrated upward to achieve a SBP of 90 to 100 mmHg. Administration should be through a central IV line because local subcutaneous necrosis can result from peripheral IV extravasation. Prolonged infusion of larger doses will transiently exert a beneficial effect by diverting blood flow from the peripheral and splanchnic vasculature to the heart and brain; however, this ultimately can compromise capillary perfusion to the extent that end-organ failure, particularly renal failure, ensues.

To reduce the potential risk of end-organ damage, a reasonable approach is to add norepinephrine to the infusion of dobutamine, and reduce the dopamine infusion rate to 0.5 to 2 mcg/kg/minute. This will theoretically support renal and splanchnic perfusion, although this effect is controversial, as discussed above. In addition, any deficits in plasma volume should be corrected when identified by hemodynamic monitoring.

Adverse effects of norepinephrine are related mostly to excessive vasoconstriction and compromise of organ perfusion. Worsening of ventricular function can occur because of increased afterload and tissue necrosis and sloughing can develop if extravasation occurs. Cardiac arrhythmias can emerge and HR can increase; however, in some cases the HR may slow secondary to baroreceptor-mediated reflex increases in vagal tone.

Again, it must be emphasized that pharmacologic support for M.J., particularly the use of norepinephrine, is only an interim maneuver to temporarily maintain hemodynamic function while revascularization procedures are being considered. Patients who cannot be stabilized with pharmacologic intervention, and in whom systemic or myocardial perfusion is becoming compromised, may require further support through insertion of a mechanical circulatory assist device (e.g., intra-aortic balloon pump).

INTRA-AORTIC BALLOON PUMP

When drug therapy is ineffective at stabilizing patients in cardiogenic shock, mechanical intervention should be considered. Mechanical interventions such as intra-aortic balloon counterpulsation can rapidly stabilize patients with cardiogenic shock, especially those with global myocardial ischemia or infarction complicated by mechanical defects, such as papillary muscle rupture or ventricular septal rupture. Intra-aortic balloon counterpulsation augments coronary arterial perfusion pressure during diastole and reduces LV impedance during systole. Sometimes combined inotropic support and intra-aortic balloon counterpulsation are required to maintain an acceptable BP (SBP >90 mmHg) and CI (>2.2 L/minute/m^2).

The IABP or intra-aortic counterpulsation has been in use for more than 15 years and remains the most commonly used mechanical assist device. It is designed to improve coronary perfusion and reduce afterload, thus providing short-term reperfusion of the ischemic myocardium. A 30- to 40-mL balloon catheter is inserted into an artery (usually femoral) and advanced to just below the arch of the aorta. Balloon inflation and deflation are synchronized with the ECG to inflate during diastole (after the aortic valve closes) and deflate at the onset of systole. The inflated balloon in diastole increases coronary perfusion by elevating the mean aortic pressure. The rapid deflation of the balloon at the onset of systole decreases SBP, thus reducing afterload and improving cardiac ejection. The enhanced myocardial perfusion provided by IABP may reduce vasopressor requirements, thereby further decreasing myocardial oxygen consumption. Occasionally, IABP augmentation is sufficient to allow the institution of vasodilators (e.g., nitroprusside) or inodilators (e.g., milrinone). Complications of IABP include thrombocytopenia from the mechanical destruction of platelets and the potential for limb ischemia because of reduced blood flow in the artery into which the IABP catheter is inserted. Heparin anticoagulation is usually used with IABP because the device has a large surface area that can be thrombogenic.

Recently, more advanced circulatory-assist devices (HeartMate, Novacor, Abiomed) have been developed. Mechanical assistance with these devices is used for patients with cardiogenic shock who need support while awaiting definitive, corrective therapy or as a bridging mechanism before cardiac transplantation.[81] Long-term use of some of these devices has been investigated in patients with severe cardiac failure who are not transplant candidates.[82] Implantation of a left ventricular assist device (LVAD) was compared with medical management in patients with severe heart failure. Survival at 1 year was 52% in the LVAD group, compared with 25% in the medical management group. The high cost of these devices will undoubtedly limit their use to only the most severely ill patients.

In summary, M.J.'s condition has continued to deteriorate since his admission to the ICU. Attempts at stabilizing his hemodynamic parameters with dopamine, dobutamine, and norepinephrine have failed. This is evidenced by inadequate tissue perfusion, which is reflected clinically by his continued lactic acidosis, decreased urine output, reduced bowel sounds, and CNS obtundation. M.J.'s best chance of survival is to have early revascularization of his ischemic myocardium with either coronary bypass surgery or PTCA. Meanwhile, the addition of norepinephrine and intra-aortic counterpulsation can provide temporary support for M.J. before his procedure.

SEPTIC SHOCK

Clinical and Hemodynamic Features

37. M.K., a 56-year-old man, was admitted 5 days ago with a chief complaint of acute abdominal pain of 3 days' duration associated with bloody diarrhea, fever, tachypnea, and hypotension. A diagnosis was superior mesenteric artery occlusion with necrotic bowel, leading to surgery for removal of necrotic bowel tissue. During postoperative days 1 through 4, his serum creatinine (SrCr) increased to 1.5, and he could not be completely weaned from ventilatory support. Vital signs were stable. Antibiotic therapy included clindamycin and gentamicin in appropriate doses.

M.K. has a history of coronary artery disease with stable angina pectoris that has been treated with lisinopril, simvastatin and NTG. He had no other medical problems before admission.

On the morning of postoperative day 5, M.K. complains of chills and has a spiking fever to 39.4°C. Physical findings include a BP of 98/60 mmHg, pulse 128 beats/minute, and a RR of

28 breaths/minute. His urine output has dropped to 25 mL/hour and bowel sounds are absent. The chest radiograph shows an enlarged heart with bilateral pulmonary infiltrates and right lower lobe atelectasis. M.K. has become confused and disoriented. ABG on an inspiratory oxygen concentration (FiO_2) of 40% are as follows: PaO_2, 76 mmHg (normal, 75–100 mmHg); $PaCO_2$, 34 mmHg (normal, 35–45 mmHg); HCO_3^-, 15 mEq/L (normal, 23–29 mEq/L); and pH, 7.31 (normal, 7.35–7.45). M.K. has had increased bronchial secretions over the past 2 days. Pertinent laboratory values are SrCr, 1.8 mg/dL (normal, 0.2–0.8 mg/dL); BUN, 32 mg/dL (normal, 10–20 mg/dL); and WBC count, 18,000 cells/mm^3 (normal, 4,500–11,000 cells/mm^3).

Urine, sputum, and blood samples are sent for culture and sensitivity. A fluid bolus of 1,000 mL normal saline is given. Arterial and pulmonary artery catheters are inserted revealing the following hemodynamic profile M.K. weighs 70 kg and has a BSA of 1.7 m^2): BP (S/D/M), 90/50/63 mmHg; pulse, 122 beats/minute; CO, 6 L/minute (normal, 4–7 L/min); CI, 3.5 L/minute/m^2 (normal, 2.5–4.2 L/minute/m^2); PCWP, 12 mmHg (normal, 5–12 mmHg); SVR, 720 dyne.sec.cm^{-5} (normal, 800–1,440 dyne.sec.cm^{-5}). What hemodynamic and clinical features of M.K. are consistent with septic shock?

[SI units: SrCr, 135 μmol/L (normal, 15–61); BUN, 22.72 mmol/L (normal, 7.1 to 14.3); WBC count, 18 10^9/L (normal, 4.5–11); HCO_3^-, 15 mmol/L (normal, 23–29)]

Hemodynamic signs consistent with septic shock include hypotension, tachycardia, elevated CO, low SVR, and a low PCWP. Although the absolute value for CO is high or at the upper limits of the normal range in septic shock, it is inadequate to maintain a BP that will perfuse the essential organs in the face of a decreased SVR, evidenced by the low oxygen delivery and consumption. M.K. has a metabolic acidosis (pH 7.31 with a $PaCO_2$ 30 mmHg, HCO_3^- 15 mEq/L), indicating anaerobic metabolism most likely caused by decreased perfusion causing lactic acidosis, and a CO that is inadequate to meet the oxygen requirements of the tissues.

Other features consistent with septic shock in M.K. include worsening pulmonary function as indicated by his ABG measurement; declining urine output and altered sensorium, indicating decreased renal and cerebral perfusion; a rising WBC count; and a spiking fever.

Therapeutic Approach

The management of septic shock is directed toward three primary areas: (*a*) eradication of the source of infection, (*b*) hemodynamic support and control of tissue hypoxia, and (*c*) inhibition or attenuation of the initiators and mediators of sepsis.

Eradicating the Source of Infection

38. What factors should be considered in determining antimicrobial therapy in septic shock? What are the potential sources of infection in M.K.?

Systemic infection caused by either aerobic or anaerobic bacteria is the leading cause of septic shock. Fungal, mycobacterial, rickettsial, protozoal, or viral infections can also be encountered. Among sepsis syndromes caused by aerobic bacteria, gram-negative organisms (e.g., *Enterobacteriaceae, Pseudomonas,* and *Haemophilus,* in decreasing order of frequency) are implicated slightly more often than gram-positive bacteria (e.g., *Staphylococcus aureus, Staphylococcus* coagulase negative, *Streptococcus,* and *Enterococcus,* from highest to lowest frequency). Even these trends vary, however, depending on the infection site. For example, when an organism can actually be cultured in the blood, slightly more gram-positive infections (35%–40%) than gram-negative infections (30%–35%) are found. In non-bloodstream infections (e.g., respiratory tract, genitourinary system, and the abdomen, in descending order of frequency) 40% to 45% can be attributed to gram-negative organisms and 20% to 25% are caused by gram-positive organisms.[19] Polymicrobial infections make up the next largest group, followed by fungi, anaerobes, and others. In 10% to 30% of sepsis syndrome cases, no organisms can be isolated. Careful consideration of the patient's history and clinical presentation often reveals the most likely cause.

Eradicating the source of infection involves the early administration of antimicrobial therapy, and, if indicated, surgical drainage. The use of an appropriate antibiotic regimen is associated with a significant increase in survival. In one large retrospective study, shock and mortality rates were reduced by 50%.[83] The selection of antibiotics should take into account the presumed site of infection; whether the infection is community- or hospital-acquired; recent invasive procedures, manipulations, or surgery; any predisposing conditions; and the likelihood of drug resistance. Ideally, the primary source of the infection can be determined and therapy specifically tailored to the most likely organisms. If the source of infection is unclear, however, early institution of broad-spectrum antibiotics is generally recommended while awaiting culture results. Empiric therapy is indicated, given a >50% mortality rate caused by gram-negative sepsis within the first 2 days of illness and the increasing frequency of polymicrobial infections.[83] Recommended empiric regimens typically include an aminoglycoside plus a third-generation cephalosporin or a similar broad-spectrum agent to cover for gram-positive cocci, aerobic gram-negative bacilli, and anaerobes (Also see Chapter 56, Principles of Infectious Diseases.)

M.K. has several potential sources of sepsis. The first is hospital-acquired pneumonia. M.K. has been intubated for 5 days, infiltrates appear on chest radiograph, and sputum production has increased over the past 2 days. Abdominal abscess or recurrent bowel ischemia also should be considered because bowel sounds are absent. Although no complaints of abdominal tenderness have been elicited, surgical exploration may be necessary. Other potential sources for infection include the urinary tract because M.K. has had an indwelling Foley catheter in place since admission. All IV catheters should be changed if possible.

Clindamycin is discontinued and imipenem and vancomycin are added to broaden M.K.'s antibiotic coverage. Imipenem should adequately cover nosocomial gram-negative pathogens such as *Pseudomonas aeruginosa* and *Acinetobacter baumannii* as well as abdominal anaerobic organisms. Vancomycin will cover *S. aureus* from possible IV contamination as well as potential staphylococcal pneumonia. Antimicrobial therapy is adjusted once cultures are finalized.

Initial Stabilization

39. What are the immediate goals of therapy in M.K.? How can they be achieved and assessed?

The goals in treating septic shock, in addition to eradicating the precipitating infection, are to optimize the delivery of oxygen to the tissues and to control abnormal use of oxygen and anaerobic metabolism by reducing the tissue oxygen demand. Tissue injury is widespread during sepsis, most likely because of vascular endothelial injury with fluid extravasation and microthromboses, which decrease oxygen and substrate utilization by the affected tissues. The mainstay of therapy is volume expansion to increase intravascular volume, enhance CO, and ultimately delay associated development of refractory tissue hypoxia. The therapeutic goals used for hemodynamic resuscitation are controversial. The issue is whether therapy should be directed to physiologic end points of tissue perfusion or clinical end points, such as BP and urine output. The physiologic end points include clearance of blood lactate concentrations, base deficit, mixed venous oxygen saturation (Svo_2), and increased CO. Although definitive evidence is lacking, a combination of these physiologic and clinical end points should be used to guide therapy.

Fluids are the mainstay of treatment because increasing CO will improve capillary circulation and tissue oxygenation by maintaining sufficient intravascular volume. If fluids do not correct the hypoxia or if filling pressures are increased, the sequential addition of inotropes and vasopressors is indicated. Blood transfusions should be used if the hematocrit is below 21% unless there is an active source of bleeding or a history of cardiac disease, in which case the hematocrit value would be maintained at a higher value. Crystalloids (with electrolytes to correct imbalances) should be initiated to maintain the CI goal as well as a MAP of 65 mmHg or a SBP of 90 mmHg. The MAP is a better reflection of systemic arterial pressure because it considers the diastolic pressure, which is an essential component of blood flow. Although MAP and BP are not absolute measures of blood flow to all vital organs, these pressures are considered the therapeutic end points that will sustain myocardial and cerebral perfusion. After optimization with fluid therapy, inotropic and vasopressor agents are indicated if the patient remains hypotensive with a low CI and if signs of inadequate tissue perfusion persist.

One study has shown that early goal-directed therapy in the treatment of severe sepsis and septic shock leads to improved survival.[84] This approach to patient care integrates both physiologic and clinical end points of resuscitation as early as possible to maintain perfusion during the early stages of sepsis. This study randomized patients admitted to an ED to standard therapy versus goal-directed therapy, which consisted of at least 6 hours of continuous care in the ED where they received a central venous catheter capable of measuring central venous oxygen saturation ($Scvo_2$). The treatment group maintained a CVP of 8 to 12 mmHg with continued fluid boluses and a MAP >65 mmHg with vasopressor treatment initiated if necessary. If the $Scvo_2$ was <70%, red cells were transfused to achieve a hematocrit of at least 30%. If the CVP, MAP, and HCT were optimized and the $Scvo_2$ was still <70%, dobutamine was administered to improve the delivery of oxygen to the tissues. The primary efficacy end point was in-hospital mortality, which was statistically significantly lower in the early goal-directed group. The results of this study have prompted many institutions to develop sepsis bundles that incorporate the same variables and end points of therapy as early as possible in the treatment of sepsis. Sepsis bundles often incorporate the many issues addressed in the Surviving Sepsis Campaign Guidelines, such as ventilatory support, initial choice of antibiotics, glucose control, and stress ulcer prophylaxis.[85]

M.K should receive fluid boluses to maintain perfusion with a MAP >65 mmHg and a CVP in the 8 to 12 mmHg region, and ideally receive a central line to monitor his mixed venous oxygen saturation. Continued, excessive fluid challenges to increase preload in M.K. must be approached cautiously, however, because he has a history of ischemic heart disease and ongoing evidence suggestive of pneumonia, both of which could be made worse by overly aggressive fluid boluses. In addition, patients in septic shock are susceptible to developing noncardiogenic pulmonary edema or ARDS, which can cause severe deterioration in pulmonary function. Therefore, fluid boluses should be given with ongoing monitoring to determine the CVP and PCWP at which CO is maximal. This approach will avoid excessive CVP and PCWP beyond which CO is no longer increased, thereby reducing the potential formation of pulmonary edema.

In summary, the immediate goal of therapy is to maximize oxygen delivery to the tissues. Fluid resuscitation is the mainstay of therapy and improves oxygen delivery by increasing CO; however, inotropic and vasopressor agents are often required for additional cardiovascular support. A favorable response to immediate resuscitative efforts will be reflected by a reversal or halt in the progression of the metabolic acidosis, improved sensorium, and increased urine output. In M.K., surgical evaluation for an ongoing or new abdominal process and selection of appropriate antibiotics while maintaining hemodynamic support are the clinical goals of therapy.

Hemodynamic Management

FLUID THERAPY VERSUS INOTROPIC SUPPORT

40. M.K. is given two 1,000-mL fluid boluses, and norepinephrine is begun at a rate of 0.02 mcg/kg/minute. Over the next 2 hours, he receives 3 L of fluid in boluses and the norepinephrine is increased to 0.15 mcg/kg/minute to maintain his BP. Signs of pulmonary edema have become more prominent. M.K. has the following hemodynamic profile (previous values in parentheses): BP (S/D/M), 94/46/62 mmHg (90/50/63); pulse, 124 beats/minute (122); CO, 7.0 L/minute (6); CI, 3.2 L/minute/m^2 (3.5); RAP, 13 mmHg (8); PCWP, 18 mmHg (12); SVR, 560 dyne.sec.cm^{-5} (733); urine output, 15 mL/hour; Pao_2, 62 mmHg (76); $Paco_2$, 38 mmHg (34); HCO_3^-, 19 mEq/L (15); pH, 7.30 (7.31); Do_2, 445 mL/minute (438); Vo_2, 118 mL/minute (114); and PEEP, 5 cm H_2O. Which of the following therapeutic considerations would be reasonable for M.K. at this time: additional fluid boluses, an increase in the norepinephrine infusion rate, or initiation of a different vasopressor?

M.K. continues to be hypotensive despite a PCWP of 18 mmHg and a norepinephrine infusion rate of 0.15 mcg/kg/minute. The goals of therapy remain the same (i.e., maximize arterial oxygen content and oxygen delivery to reverse cellular anaerobic metabolism).

M.K.'s Pao_2 of 62 mmHg correlates with an oxygen-hemoglobin saturation of approximately 90%, which should provide an adequate arterial oxygen content. However, oxygen delivery still may be inadequate because the CI is <3.5 L/minute/m^2, and Do_2 and Vo_2 have not reached normal levels. In addition, decreased oxygen use can contribute to the continued acidosis. Thus, further attempts to enhance the CI and hence, oxygen delivery, are appropriate. However, M.K. has worsening signs of pulmonary edema and a history of cardiovascular disease that will influence the choice of therapeutic options.

Although fluid administration is the mainstay of therapy in septic shock, the elevation of M.K.'s PCWP to 18 mmHg without a significant increase in CO suggests that an optimal PCWP has been reached. Therefore, additional fluid therapy to maintain his BP may worsen his pulmonary edema and further compromise his pulmonary gas exchange. A plot of CO versus the PCWP (ventricular function curve) would provide a more accurate assessment of the PCWP at which CO is maximal. Additional fluid boluses at this time should be used only to maintain the current level of intravascular volume status.

Vasopressors

NOREPINEPHRINE

When fluid therapy fails to maintain a satisfactory MAP despite an elevated CO, the use of a vasopressor should be considered. Norepinephrine is predominantly an α-adrenergic agonist (Table 21-7) and is frequently used as an adjunct to therapy when inotropic agents alone are unsuccessful. Because concern exists that excessive vasoconstriction might cause reflex decreases in CO and hypoperfusion of vital organs, the use of norepinephrine has often been limited to end-stage shock. However, studies indicate that norepinephrine alone, or in combination with inotropic agents can be beneficial in the management of septic shock.[86]

Martin et al. compared the ability of dopamine and norepinephrine to reverse hemodynamic and metabolic abnormalities of hyperdynamic shock.[87] They prospectively randomized 32 volume-resuscitated patients with hyperdynamic sepsis to receive either dopamine or norepinephrine with the goal of achieving and maintaining normal hemodynamic and oxygen transport parameters for at least 6 hours. If goals were not achieved with one agent, the other agent was added. With the use of dopamine, 31% of patients met the predefined therapeutic goals. In contrast, 93% of patients treated with norepinephrine met the predefined goals. Of the patients who did not respond to dopamine, 91% achieved the goals with the addition of norepinephrine. In this study, norepinephrine was found to be superior to dopamine, with improvement in arterial BP, urine flow, oxygen delivery and consumption, and lactate levels.

In a similar study of patients in whom previous therapy with plasma volume expansion and dopamine or dobutamine had failed, norepinephrine reversed hypotension and significantly increased MAP, SVR, and urine output.[86] The CI was increased, albeit insignificantly, in 7 of 10 patients, presumably because of stimulation of cardiac β-receptors. By limiting the SVRI to 700 dyne.sec.cm^{-5}/m^2, the investigators were able to prevent excessive vasoconstriction and promote an increased perfusion pressure to vital organs as reflected by an improved urine flow. Oxygen delivery and consumption were measured in 6 of 10 patients with variable results. Although no patient died of refractory hypotension, 4 of 10 patients died of progressive hypoxia, leading the authors to conclude that regardless of the catecholamines used, the ultimate goal of therapy should be to maximize oxygen delivery and consumption.

PHENYLEPHRINE

Occasionally, patients will respond to epinephrine or phenylephrine when other catecholamines have failed, although neither of these agents is considered to be first-line therapy. Epinephrine stimulates α-, β_1-, and β_2-adrenergic receptors (Table 21-7). CO is augmented via increased contractility and HR, with the contribution of each being highly variable. Blood vessels in the kidney, skin, and mucosa constrict in response to α-adrenergic stimulation, while vessels in the skeletal muscle vasodilate because of β_2 effects. A biphasic response in SVR is observed with increasing doses as β_2-receptors are activated at the lower range, while α_1-receptors are stimulated at higher levels. The improvement in CO, therefore, may be negated by an increase in afterload at higher dosages.

Phenylephrine is a pure α-adrenergic agonist (Table 21-7) and, thus, increases systolic, diastolic, and mean arterial pressures through vasoconstriction. Reflex bradycardia can occur secondarily because of the absence of β-adrenergic effects. The increase in afterload, while increasing myocardial oxygen consumption, correspondingly increases coronary blood flow because of increased perfusion pressure and autoregulation. Therefore, in patients with myocardial hypoxia, or in those experiencing atrial or ventricular arrhythmias, phenylephrine can be beneficial because it has minimal direct cardiac effects. In situations in which the CO is decreased, however, phenylephrine can be detrimental. This occurs because preload is reduced from interstitial fluid losses as a result of increased capillary hydrostatic pressure effects. This response, in addition to the reflex bradycardia may significantly impair CO (Table 21-7).

VASOPRESSIN

Catecholamines have been the mainstay of treatment to support BP in septic patients once adequate fluid resuscitation has been achieved. Sepsis, however, can cause a decrease in responsiveness to catecholamines resulting in refractory hypotension, possibly because of downregulation of adrenergic receptors. Thus, other avenues of supportive treatment have been researched. Septic patients exhibit an increased sensitivity to vasopressin. Vasopressin is an endogenous hormone that has very little effect on BP under normal conditions, but becomes very important in maintaining BP when the baroreflex is impaired, such as in shock states. Vasopressin's direct vasoconstricting actions are mediated by the vascular V_1-receptors coupled to phospholipase C.[88,89] When these receptors are activated, calcium is released from the sarcoplasmic reticulum in smooth muscle cells leading to vasoconstriction. One study found that vasopressin levels were very low in septic patients, whereas patients in cardiogenic shock displayed an appropriate increase in vasopressin release for the degree of hypotension.[90] The same investigators showed that a low-dose, continuous IV infusion of vasopressin at 0.04 U/minute in 19 patients with septic shock caused a statistically significant increase in vasopressin levels, systolic arterial pressure, and systemic vascular resistance when added to pre-existing catecholamine treatment. Six of ten patients were able to maintain BP on vasopressin alone. Stopping the vasopressin infusion resulted in decreases of BP to pretreatment levels, and reinstitution of the infusion increased BP within minutes. It is presumed that vasopressin secretion is impaired as opposed to enhanced vasopressin metabolism, but it is not entirely clear why this occurs. Most likely it is a combination of a deficient baroreflex-mediated secretion of vasopressin, impaired sympathetic function, and potentially depletion of the secretory stores of vasopressin.

Other studies support the vasopressor effects of vasopressin in septic patients already on catecholamines with persistent hypotension and also show a vasopressor-sparing effect on catecholamines. The most recent double-blind, randomized trial showed that norepinephrine infusion could be decreased by the addition of vasopressin administration.[91] Another statistically significant finding from this study was that urine output and creatinine clearance both increased more in the vasopressin group than in the norepinephrine group. It seems reasonable at this point to use vasopressin in patients with septic shock who are on high doses of catecholamines or those who need further vasopressor support. Further studies are needed to determine if treatment with vasopressin confers a mortality benefit.

M.K. has decreased MAP despite the addition and increased titration of norepinephrine. Because it has been found that patients in septic shock have decreased endogenous levels of vasopressin, it would be reasonable to add vasopressin at 0.04 U/minute to the prior norepinephrine infusion to increase the MAP and renal perfusion.

Inotropic Agents

Although the use of inotropic agents is well established, controlled comparative studies have not clearly determined which agent, or combination of agents, is most useful in the management of septic shock. Because differences among the inotropic agents are significant, however, selection of the most appropriate drug should be guided by careful consideration of the patient's hemodynamic status.

DOPAMINE

Dopamine has frequently been the initial pharmacologic agent chosen for the treatment of septic shock. If the MAP is low with a depressed CO and a low SVR, dopamine is an appropriate choice because its combined α-adrenergic vasoconstrictive actions and β-adrenergic inotropic effects will increase SVR and CO, thereby effectively raising it. In situations in which the PCWP is elevated or in patients with decreased ventricular compliance, the use of dopamine may be limited because it significantly increases venous return and ventricular filling pressure. In addition, dopamine increases shunting of pulmonary blood flow, leading to a decline in Pa_{O_2}. This effect may worsen hypoxemia in patients with pneumonia or ARDS.

DOBUTAMINE

Dobutamine is often advocated as the secondary inotropic agent in the management of septic shock, particularly in patients with low CO and high filling pressures. Dobutamine produces a greater increase in CO than dopamine, but also lowers SVR. In contrast to dopamine, dobutamine lowers PCWP, decreases myocardial oxygen consumption, and causes less pulmonary shunting. Because dobutamine can lower ventricular filling pressure, volume status must be monitored closely to avoid the development of hypotension and reduced MAP. Fluids should be administered as needed to maintain the PCWP at maximal tolerated levels of 16 to 18 mmHg. With the administration of greater amounts of fluid, CO, oxygen delivery, and systemic oxygen consumption are significantly increased. Dobutamine does increase D_{O_2} and CI when given concurrently with or after volume resuscitation. Decreases in Pa_{O_2} and increases in venous P_{O_2}, as well as adverse effects on myocardium, may be evident at higher dosages (>6 mcg/kg/minute).[92]

Combinations of vasopressors and inotropes can also be used to achieve desired hemodynamic parameters. Because gastrointestinal perfusion can be compromised owing to the vasoconstricting effects of catecholamines and may play a role in the pathogenesis of multiple organ dysfunction, the combination of norepinephrine and dobutamine has been studied to determine if an advantage exists to using norepinephrine alone, epinephrine alone, or a combination.[54,93] One prospective study randomized patients with a MAP <60 mmHg despite adequate fluid resuscitation and treatment with high dose dopamine to either dobutamine plus norepinephrine or epinephrine monotherapy titrated to a MAP >80 mmHg.[54] The variables were the MAP, metabolic effects as evidenced by lactate and pyruvate concentrations, and splanchnic perfusion measured by gastric pH (pH_i) and partial pressure of carbon dioxide (P_{CO_2}) gap. This study showed that both therapies, norepinephrine plus dobutamine and epinephrine monotherapy, were equally effective at achieving hemodynamic goals, but that treatment with epinephrine alone could worsen splanchnic oxygen utilization and potentially lead to ischemic injury. Currently, it is unknown whether a specific catecholamine regimen provides a significant benefit over others. There is conflicting data about which vasopressor can increase gastric perfusion and whether this increase can alter progression to organ dysfunction.

41. Given M.K.'s history of cardiovascular disease, what considerations must be accounted for before initiating a vasopressor agent? Outline an overall approach to maintaining adequate hemodynamic status.

M.K. has a history of coronary artery disease and is susceptible to myocardial ischemia. Therefore, a careful balance must be achieved between myocardial oxygen consumption and coronary perfusion pressure. Further attempts to optimize MAP and CI with norepinephrine alone could increase myocardial oxygen consumption and precipitate ischemia. Evidence suggests that the goal of therapy in treating patients with septic shock, or any form of shock for that matter, is not to simply normalize BP, but to optimize oxygen delivery and consumption. Once anemia and hypoxia have been corrected, CO becomes the remaining parameter that can be adjusted to increase oxygen supply, but raising arterial BP and CO with inotropic agents or vasopressors before restoring adequate blood volume actually can worsen tissue perfusion. Therefore, the selection of an inotropic agent must take into consideration the patient's current hemodynamic status and the individual properties of those agents that will most effectively maintain or increase the MAP and CO. In many instances, because of individual variability and response, more than one inotropic agent or addition of a vasopressor is required to achieve these end points. These interventions must be made with strict follow up of the patients' response to the interventions to prevent any adverse consequences, especially in those patients who are predisposed to an adverse event such as M.K.

It is important to realize that the response to exogenous catecholamines in patients with septic shock is highly variable and a successful regimen in one patient may be unsuccessful in another. In addition, septic patients often require infusion rates in the moderate-to-high range. Therefore, the goal is to use one or more agents at the dosages necessary to achieve the desired end points without unduly compromising the patient's status. The use of catecholamines, however, is only a stabilizing measure. Strict attention to all other physiologic parameters—as well as nutritional support, antibiotic modification, and ongoing surgical intervention—cannot be overemphasized.

Other Therapies

Therapies directed against the initiators and mediators of sepsis are currently the focus of intense investigation. As previously discussed, numerous exogenous and endogenous substances are involved in the pathogenesis of sepsis. Strategies under development include antioxidants and free radical scavengers, antiendotoxin therapy, inhibition of leukocytes, secondary mediators (i.e., TNF-α, IL-1, cytokine pathway), coagulation and arachidonic acid metabolites, complement, and NO. Although several experimental therapies hold considerable promise for the future, controlled human data are still lacking.

CORTICOSTEROIDS

42. What is the rationale for the use of glucocorticosteroids in the treatment of septic shock, and is there evidence to support their use for this indication?

The use of corticosteroids in sepsis and septic shock has been a controversial topic for many years. Corticosteroids were originally proposed as a treatment option because of their anti-inflammatory properties with the hope of attenuating the body's response to infection. More recently it has been shown that critically ill patients exhibit impaired cortisol secretion because of a relative adrenocortical insufficiency, and it is suspected that these patients display a glucocorticoid peripheral resistance syndrome. Almost 50% of patients with septic shock exhibit relative adrenal insufficiency defined as a maximal change in cortisol level of <9 mcg/dL after a 250 mcg IV dose of corticotropin.[94]

Several clinical trials have been performed over the past few decades with varying results and meta-analyses have recommended discontinuation of high-dose corticosteroid therapy because of detrimental outcomes.[95,96] End points that have been studied include time to reversal of septic shock (defined by cessation of vasopressor support) and mortality. Older trials used different definitions of septic shock, however, and the timing and dosing of steroids were highly variable. Most recently, the randomized, double-blind, placebo-controlled trial by Annane et al.[97] showed a mortality benefit after 28 days associated with the use of low doses of hydrocortisone and fludrocortisone in patients with relative adrenocortical insufficiency (nonresponders to corticotropin) and septic shock. All patients received a corticotropin stimulation test and relative adrenocortical insufficiency was defined as a response of 9 mcg/dL or less (nonresponders). It was found that in nonresponders, 63% of the placebo group died, whereas 53% of the corticosteroid group died ($p = 0.02$). Time to cessation of vasopressor support was also shortened by the use of steroids in the treatment group compared with placebo in the nonresponders. Responders did not show any benefit from the use of corticosteroids, and actually had slightly worse outcomes when they did receive steroids. This study suggests the use of corticosteroids in vasopressor-dependent septic shock *only* in those patients who exhibit relative adrenal insufficiency. The outcomes of this trial are controversial and some evidence that is not yet published indicates that steroids may not be as beneficial in every patient with septic shock, but possibly only for those with severe sepsis with refractory hypotension.

Because M.K. is refractory to increasing doses of norepinephrine and is in severe sepsis, a corticotropin stimulation test should be administered and hydrocortisone 50 mg IV every 6 hours plus fludrocortisone 50 mcg/feeding tube every 24 hours should be started after the stimulation test. Treatment can be discontinued if the results of the stimulation test show that M.K. is not adrenally insufficient.

STATINS

43. Is there any significance to the fact that M.K. was on statin therapy before his episode of sepsis? Should his statin therapy be continued?

Aside from their well-described lipid-lowering effects, statins appear to have immunomodulatory and anti-inflammatory effects. Statin therapy lowers C-reactive protein levels, inhibits endothelial cell dysfunction, causes upregulation of endothelial NO synthase, and blocks immune cell receptors.[98] A growing body of evidence shows that patients who are on a statin before the inciting septic event may have a decreased likelihood of developing sepsis, and a mortality benefit may exist for those with sepsis or multiple organ dysfunction. All studies in humans thus far have been retrospective and in patients who were previously on a statin. One trial showed a significant survival benefit associated with continuing statin therapy in patients who were bacteremic compared with those who were never on statin therapy.[99] Potentially more important is that the highest mortality was seen in those patients who had been on statin therapy, but had been discontinued (result not statistically significant). These results may lend credence to the idea of a rebound phenomenon that could be detrimental if statins are not continued. Statins are often discontinued in septic patients because of concern for adverse effects and further organ dysfunction. Presently, it is not clear whether statins should always be continued in septic patients, and it is unknown whether statins should be initiated in patients who develop sepsis. Further evidence by means of prospective, randomized trials is needed to further define the role of statins in sepsis.

DROTECOGIN ALFA

44. Is M.K. a candidate for recombinant activated protein C? Is there any evidence to support its use in septic shock, and what are the major risks associated with its use?

Activated protein C (APC) is an endogenous protein that acts as one of the regulators of the coagulation cascade and also interrupts the amplification cycle of inflammation.[21] Protein C is the inactive precursor to APC, and conversion to the active form requires thrombin to complex with thrombomodulin. APC enhances fibrinolysis and has potent inhibitory effects on thrombin, which possesses thrombotic as well as inflammatory effects. Other anti-inflammatory effects of APC stem from suppression of TNF-α, IL-6, and IL-1production.

Patients in septic shock develop microvascular thrombosis, which leads to organ hypoperfusion, cell dysfunction, multiple organ dysfunction, and death. The systemic response to infection activates the coagulation pathway leading to the generation of thrombin and deposition of fibrin as well as initiating an inflammatory reaction via activation of cytokines.

Adult and pediatric septic patients have low levels of protein C and a poor outcome is expected for those patients with the lowest levels.[100] The deficiency in protein C is probably due to enhanced degradation as well as impaired synthesis of protein C. It is also apparent that patients in septic shock exhibit lower levels of thrombomodulin, the protein necessary for the conversion of protein C to activated protein C. Thus, the use of APC would counter the anticoagulant deficiency as well as suppress the inflammatory reaction that would normally take place due to the infection.

The Protein C Worldwide Evaluation in Severe Sepsis (PROWESS)[101] trial is the only published phase III clinical trial reporting the safety and efficacy of drotecogin-α (recombinant APC). It was a randomized, double-blind, placebo-controlled, multicenter trial that was stopped early because of the statistically significant difference in the primary end point, 28-day all-cause mortality, before enrollment was complete. Included in the study were patients with a known or suspected infection plus three or more signs of systemic inflammation and at least one organ system dysfunction caused by sepsis. Patients also had to begin treatment of drotecogin-α at 24 mcg/kg/hour for 96 hours within 24 hours of meeting inclusion criteria. The list of exclusion criteria was extensive to ensure that patients who were at higher risk for bleeding did not participate in the trial. No standardized protocol was established for the critical care provided to the patient (e.g., antibiotics, vasopressors, inotropes). Treatment with APC reduced D-dimer and IL-6 levels, indicating attenuation of the procoagulant and inflammatory effects of sepsis. Treatment with drotecogin-α was associated with a 6.1% absolute reduction in mortality at 28 days after the start of infusion. The incidence of serious bleeding was higher in the APC group, almost reaching statistical significance ($p = 0.06$). A subgroup analysis showed that patients with higher Acute Physiology and Chronic Health Evaluation (APACHE) II scores (>25) benefited the most from treatment with APC. A follow-up study mandated by the U.S. Food and Drug Administration (FDA) showed that APC use in septic patients with single organ failure or an APACHE II score <25 was not effective in achieving a decrease in mortality at 28 days and was actually associated with an increase in bleeding complications.[102] Based on the results of these studies, APC should be used only in patients with sepsis with an APACHE II score >25 or with two or more organ systems in failure.

M.K. meets the criteria for severe sepsis because he meets three of the requirements for SIRS (white blood cell count [WBC] = 18,000 cells/mm^3; use of mechanical ventilation; HR >90 beats/minute) and has three dysfunctional organ systems. He requires vasopressor support, is on a ventilator, and has an increase in his SrCr. He also has several potential sources of infection with pulmonary infiltrates and increased secretions, and the formation of an abdominal abscess is a possibility. His surgery was 5 days before his decompensation, so his bleeding risk should be minimal; however, the patient should be closely monitored. The cost of APC is substantial: approximately $7,000 for a 70-kg person for 96 hours. M.K. is a candidate for APC use; however, the risks of bleeding need to be carefully assessed because the use of APC could lead to devastating adverse events. Because of this, the formation of institutional guidelines to determine the patient population in which this drug can be more safely administered is highly recommended.

45. What other treatment options are under research for septic shock?

Because endotoxin is the initiator of the inflammatory cascade of gram-negative sepsis, extensive research has been devoted to development and study of antibodies against the core lipid-A portion of endotoxin, which possesses most of the biologic activity. To date no antiendotoxin therapies have shown any benefit.

Monoclonal antibodies to TNF-α (anti-TNF-Mab) confer significant protection in various animal models of septic shock induced by endotoxin, gram-negative, or gram-positive bacteremia. Investigations into anti-TNF antibodies prompted a large controlled clinical trial, by the INTERSEPT study group.[103] The results showed no difference in 28-day mortality rates between groups, and patients in the nonshock group derived no benefit. One recent study testing anti-TNF antibody fragments was terminated early because of funding issues; however, a trend was noted toward more shock-free and ventilator-free days.[104] More interesting is the observation that patients without a detectable baseline TNF-α level did worse than those with an elevated baseline level. Some evidence supports a biphasic immunologic pattern with an initial hyperinflammatory phase that is counterbalanced by an anti-inflammatory response, which may lead to a hypoinflammatory state (immunoparalysis). It is possible that tailoring therapy by providing anticytokine therapy to only those patients who are in the proinflammatory state may be beneficial versus providing it to all patients who are in septic shock. More studies are in progress.

Another approach to blocking the effects of TNF involves the use of soluble TNF receptors, which bind to, and inactivate, TNF before it interacts with its cellular receptor. Although effective in primate models of sepsis, a clinical trial examining escalating doses of soluble TNF receptor in patients with sepsis syndrome revealed an increase in mortality in patients receiving higher dosages of the receptor as compared with lower-dose therapy and placebo.[105]

Ethyl pyruvate has recently been identified as an experimental anti-inflammatory agent that also has anticoagulant effects.[106] This is currently the only other agent with a dual immunomodulatory and anticoagulant effect such as drotecogin-α. Clinical studies are needed to determine whether this therapy will have beneficial effects in the treatment of sepsis.

Continuous hemofiltration is a technique that removes proinflammatory mediators, and has potential for treatment of septic patients. The use of adsorbents in hemoperfusion columns aids in the removal of toxic compounds from the circulatory system. Experimental data show that TNF-α, IL-1, IL-6, IL-8, and endotoxin can be removed from the circulation of septic patients by continuous hemofiltration.[107,108] Many animal studies show that hemofiltration improves hemodynamic indices and human data are promising. No controlled, randomized clinical trials have evaluated continuous hemofiltration, however.

GLOSSARY

Afterload: Ventricular wall tension developed during contraction. Determined by the resistance or impedance the ventricle must overcome to eject end-diastolic volume. Left ventricular afterload is determined primarily by systemic vascular resistance; right ventricular afterload is determined primarily by pulmonary vascular resistance.

Arterial pressure (AP): Pressure in the central arterial bed; determined by cardiac output and systemic vascular resistance.

Body surface area (BSA): Average = 1.7 m^2.

Cardiac index (CI): Cardiac output per square meter of body surface area (BSA).

Cardiac output (CO): Amount of blood ejected from the left ventricle per minute; determined by stroke volume and heart rate. CO = SV × HR.

Central venous pressure (CVP)–also called right atrial pressure (RAP): Measures mean pressure in right atrium and reflects right ventricular filling pressure. Primarily determined by venous return to the heart.

Compliance: Distensibility of the relaxed ventricle or stiffness of the myocardial wall.

Contractility: The inotropic state of the myocardium; affects stroke volume and cardiac output independently of preload and afterload.

Heart rate (HR): Number of myocardial contractions per minute; regulated by autonomic nervous system. An increase or decrease alters cardiac output in same direction.

Left ventricular stroke work index (LVSWI): Amount of work the left ventricle exerts during systole; adjusted for body surface area (BSA).

Oxygen consumption (VO_2): The amount of oxygen consumed by the body per unit time. The product of cardiac output and the difference between the arterial and venous concentrations of oxygen.

Oxygen delivery (DO_2): The amount of oxygen delivered by the body per unit time, the product of cardiac output and arterial oxygen concentration.

Perfusion pressure: The pressure gradient between the coronary arteries and the pressure in either the right atrium or left ventricle during diastole. A major determinant of coronary blood flow and oxygen supply to the heart.

Preload: End-diastolic fiber length before contraction; represented by left ventricular end-diastolic volume (LVEDV); approximated by left ventricular end-diastolic pressure (LVEDP) and pulmonary capillary wedge pressure (PCWP). Right ventricular preload is reflected by central venous pressure (CVP) or right arterial pressure (RAP).

Positive end-expiratory pressure (PEEP): The application of positive pressure at the end of the expiratory phase of respiration to improve oxygenation.

Pulmonary artery pressure (PAP): *Systolic* (PAS): Measures pulmonary artery pressure during systole; reflects pressure generated by the contraction of the right ventricle. *Pulmonary artery diastolic* (PAD): Measures pulmonary artery pressure during diastole; reflects diastolic filling pressure in the left ventricle. May approximate pulmonary capillary wedge pressure (PCWP); normal gradient <5 mmHg between PAD and PCWP.

Pulmonary capillary wedge pressure (PCWP): Measures pressure distal to the pulmonary artery; reflects left ventricular filling pressures. May optimally increase to 16 to 18 mmHg in critically ill patients. Usually lower than or within 5 mmHg of *pulmonary artery diastolic* (PAD).

Pulmonary vascular resistance (PVR): Measure of impedance or resistance within the pulmonary vasculature that the right ventricle must overcome during contraction; determines right ventricular afterload.

Stroke volume (SV): Amount of blood ejected from the ventricle with each systolic contraction. SV = CO/HR.

Stroke volume index (SVI): Stroke volume per square meter of body surface area (BSA).

Systemic vascular resistance (SVR): Measure of impedance applied by systemic vascular system to systolic effort of left ventricle; determined by autonomic nervous system and condition of vessels. Determinant of left ventricular afterload.

Systemic vascular resistance index (SVRI): Systemic vascular resistance adjusted for body surface area (BSA).

REFERENCES

1. Parillo JE. Approach to the patient with shock. In: Goldman L, Bennett JC, eds. *Cecil Textbook of Medicine*. Philadelphia: WB Saunders; 2000:496. Edit to reference one made by Paul Montgomery May 15, 2007.
2. ACCP-SCCM Consensus Conference: definitions for sepsis and organ failure and guidelines for the use of innovative therapies in sepsis. *Chest* 1992;101:1644.
3. Bone RC. The pathogenesis of sepsis. *Ann Intern Med* 1991;115:457.
4. Chaney JC et al. Minimally invasive hemodynamic monitoring for the intensivist: current and emerging technology. *Crit Care Med* 2002;30:2338.
5. Cotter G et al. Accurate, noninvasive continuous monitoring of cardiac output by whole-body electrical bioimpedance. *Chest* 2004;125:1431
6. Swan HJC et al. Catheterization of the heart in man with the use of a flow-directed balloon-tipped catheter. *N Engl J Med* 1970;283:447.
7. Shah MR et al. Impact of the pulmonary artery catheter in critically ill patients. *JAMA* 2005;294:1664.
8. Antonelli M et al. Hemodynamic monitoring in shock and implications for management: International Consensus Conference, Paris, France, 27–28 April 2006. *Intensive Care Med* 2007;33:575.
9. Boldt J. Clinical review: hemodynamic monitoring in the intensive care unit. *Crit Care* 2002;6:52.
10. Ganz W et al. A new technique for measurement of cardiac output by thermodilution in man. *Am J Cardiol* 1971;27:392.
11. Shoemaker WC. Oxygen transport and oxygen metabolism in shock and critical illness. *Crit Care Clin* 1996;12:939.
12. Hayes MA et al. Elevation of systemic oxygen delivery in the treatment of critically ill patients. *N Engl J Med* 1994;330:1717.
13. Gattinoni L et al. A trial of goal-oriented hemodynamic therapy in critically ill patients. *N Engl J Med* 1995;333:1025.
14. Shock. In: *Advanced Trauma Life Support Program for Physicians*, Instructor's Manual. Chicago: American College of Surgeons; 1997:101.
15. Goldberg RJ et al. Temporal trends in cardiogenic shock complicating acute myocardial infarction. *N Engl J Med* 1999;340:1162.
16. Barry WL et al. Cardiogenic shock: therapy and prevention. *Clin Cardiol* 1998;21:72.
17. Rangel-Frausto MS et al. The natural history of the systemic inflammatory response syndrome (SIRS): a prospective study. *JAMA* 1995;273;117.
18. Centers for Disease Control and Prevention, National Center for Health Statistics. Mortality patterns–United States, 1990. *Monthly Vital Stat Rep* 1993;41:5.
19. Sands KE et al. Epidemiology of sepsis syndrome in 8 academic medical centers. *JAMA* 1997;278:234.
20. Angus D et al. Epidemiology of severe sepsis in the United States: analysis of incidence, outcome and associated costs of care. *Crit Care Med* 2001;29:1303.
21. Healy D. New and emerging therapies for sepsis. *Ann Pharmacother* 2002;36:648.
22. Hollenberg A et al. Practice parameters for hemodynamic support of sepsis in adult patients in sepsis. *Crit Care Med* 1999;27(3):639.
23. Cunnion RE et al. Myocardial dysfunction in sepsis. *Crit Care Clin* 1989;5:99.

24. Scalea TM et al. Resuscitation of multiple trauma and head injury: role of crystalloid fluids and inotropes. *Crit Care Med* 1994;20:1610.
25. Abou-Khalil B et al. Hemodynamic responses to shock in young trauma patients: need for invasive monitoring. *Crit Care Med* 1994;22:633.
26. Velanovich V. Crystalloids versus colloid fluid resuscitation: a meta-analysis of mortality. *Surgery* 1989;105:65.
27. Choi PT et al. Crystalloids versus colloids in fluid resuscitation: a systematic review. *Crit Care Med* 1999;27:200.
28. Alderson P, et al. Human albumin solution for resuscitation and volume expansion in critically ill patients. *Cochrane Database Syst Rev* 2001: Issue 1.
29. Wilkes M et al. Patient survival after human albumin administration. *Ann Intern Med* 2001;135:149.
30. Finfer S, et al (The SAFE Study Investigators). A comparison of albumin and saline for fluid resuscitation in the intensive care unit. *N Engl J Med* 2004;350:2247.
31. Vermeulen LC et al. A paradigm for consensus. The University Hospital Consortium guidelines for the use of albumin, nonprotein colloid, and crystalloid solutions. *Arch Intern Med* 1995;155:373.
32. Wagner BK et al. Pharmacologic and clinical considerations in selecting crystalloid, colloidal, and oxygen-carrying resuscitation fluids, part 1. *Clin Pharm* 1993;12:335.
33. Almenoff PL et al. Prolongation of the half-life of lactate after maximal exercise in patients with hepatic dysfunction. *Crit Care Med* 1989;17:870.
34. Falk JL et al. Fluid resuscitation in traumatic hemorrhagic shock. *Crit Care Clin* 1992;8:323.
35. Imm A et al. Fluid resuscitation in circulatory shock. *Crit Care Clin* 1993;9:313.
36. Gould SA et al. Hypovolemic shock. *Crit Care Clin* 1993;2:239.
37. Holcroft JW et al. 3 per cent NaCl and 7. 5 per cent NaCl/dextran 70 in the resuscitation of severely injured patients. *Ann Surg* 1987;206:279.
38. Mattox KL et al. Pre-hospital hypertonic saline-dextran infusion for post-traumatic hypotension: the USA multicenter trial. *Ann Surg* 1991;213:482.
39. Younes RN et al. Hypertonic solutions in the treatment of hypovolemic shock: a prospective, randomized study in patients admitted to the emergency room. *Surgery* 1992;111:380.
40. Angle N et al. Hypertonic saline resuscitation diminishes lung injury by suppressing neutrophil activation after hemorrhagic shock. *Shock* 1998;9:164.
41. Coimbra R et al. Hypertonic saline resuscitation decreases susceptibility to sepsis after hemorrhagic shock. *J Trauma* 1997;42:602.
42. Goodnough LT et al. Transfusion medicine. First of two parts-blood transfusion. *N Engl J Med* 1999;340:438.
43. Griffel MI et al. Pharmacology of colloids and crystalloids. *Crit Care Clin* 1992;8:235.
44. Strauss RG. Review of the effects of hydroxyethyl starch on the blood coagulation system. *Transfusion* 1981;21:299.
45. Puri VK et al. Resuscitation in hypovolemia and shock: a prospective study of hydroxyethyl starch and albumin. *Crit Care Med* 1983;11:518.
46. Haupt MT et al. Colloid osmotic pressure and fluid resuscitation with hetastarch, albumin, and saline solutions. *Crit Care Med* 1982;10:159.
47. Lazrove S et al. Hemodynamic, blood volume and oxygen transport responses to albumin and hydroxyethyl starch infusions in critically ill postoperative patients. *Crit Care Med* 1980;8:302.
48. Thompson WL. Hydroxyethyl starch. *Dev Biol Stand* 1980;48:259.
49. Yacobi A et al. Pharmacokinetics of hydroxyethyl starch in normal subjects. *J Clin Pharmacol* 1982;22:206.
50. Forrester JS et al. Medical therapy of acute, myocardial infarction by application of hemodynamic subsets. *N Engl J Med* 1976;295(Pt 1,2):1356.
51. McGhie AI et al. Pathogenesis and management of acute heart failure and cardiogenic shock: role of inotropic therapy. *Chest* 1992;102(5 Suppl 2):626S.
52. Loeb HS et al. Superiority of dobutamine over dopamine for augmentation of cardiac output in patients with chronic low output cardiac failure. *Circulation* 1977;55:375.
53. Kastrup M et al. Current practice of hemodynamic monitoring and vasopressor and inotropic therapy in post-operative cardiac surgery patient in Germany: results from a postal survey. *Acta Anaestheiol Scand* 2007;51:347.
54. Levy B et al. Comparison of norepinephrine and dobutamine to epinephrine for hemodynamics, lactate metabolism, and gastric tonometric variables in septic shock: a prospective, randomized study. *Intensive Care Med* 1997;23:282.
55. Thackray S et al. The effectiveness and relative effectiveness of intravenous inotropic drugs acting through the adrenergic pathway in patients with heart failure—a meta-regression analysis. *Eur J Heart Fail* 2002;4:515.
56. Flancbaum L et al. Quantitative effects of low dose dopamine on urine output in oliguric surgical intensive care unit patients. *Crit Care Med* 1994;22:61.
57. Cotte DB et al. Is renal dose dopamine protective or therapeutic? No. *Crit Care Clin* 1996;12:687.
58. Myles PS et al. Effect of "renal-dose" dopamine on renal function following cardiac surgery. *Anaesth Intensive Care* 1993;21:56.
59. Carcoana OV et al. Is renal dose dopamine protective or therapeutic? Yes. *Crit Care Clin* 1996; 12:677.
60. Grady K et al. Team management of patients with heart failure: a statement for healthcare professionals from the Cardiovascular Nursing Council of the American Heart Association. *Circulation* 2000;102:2443.
61. Nohria A et al. Medical management of advanced heart failure. *JAMA* 2002;287:628.
62. Cuffe MS et al. Short term intravenous milrinone for acute exacerbations of chronic heart failure: a randomized controlled trial. *JAMA* 2002;287:1541.
63. Feneck RO et al. Comparison of the hemodynamic effects of milrinone with dobutamine in patients after cardiac surgery. *J Cardiothorac Vasc Anesth* 2001;15:306.
64. Yamani MH et al. Comparison of dobutamine-based and milrinone-based therapy for advanced decompensated congestive heart failure: hemodynamic efficacy, clinical outcome, and economic impact. *Am Heart J* 2001;142:998.
65. Aranda JM et al. Comparison of dobutamine versus milrinone therapy in hospitalized patients awaiting cardiac transplantation: a prospective randomized trial. *Am Heart J* 2003;145:324.
66. Lowes BD et al. Milrinone versus dobutamine in heart failure subjects treated chronically with carvedilol. *Int J Cardiol* 2001;81:141.
67. Marcus LS et al. Hemodynamic and renal excretory effects of human brain natriuretic peptide infusion in patients with congestive heart failure: a double-blind, placebo-controlled, randomized cross-over trial. *Circulation* 1996;76:91.
68. Abraham WT et al. Systemic hemodynamic, neurohormonal, and renal effects of a steady-state infusion of human brain natriuretic peptide in patients with hemodynamically decompensated heart failure. *J Card Fail* 1998;4:37.
69. Colucci WS et al. Intravenous nesiritide, a natriuretic peptide, in the treatment of decompensated congestive heart failure. *N Engl J Med* 2000;343:246.
70. Publication Committee for the VMAC Investigators. Intravenous nesiritide vs. nitroglycerin for treatment of decompensated congestive heart failure: a randomized controlled trial. *JAMA* 2002;287:1531.
71. Sackner-Bernstein JD et al. Short-term risk of death after treatment with nesiritide for decompensated heart failure: a pooled analysis of randomized controlled trials. *JAMA* 2005;293:1900.
72. Arora RR et al. Short and long term mortality with nesiritide. *Am Heart J* 2006;152:1084.
73. Webb JG. Interventional management of cardiogenic shock. *Can J Cardiol* 1998;14:233.
74. Becker RC. Hemodynamic, mechanical, and metabolic determinants of thrombolytic efficacy: a theoretical framework for assessing the limitations of thrombolysis in patients with cardiogenic shock. *Am Heart J* 1993;125:919.
75. Prewitt RM et al. Intraaortic balloon counterpulsation enhances coronary thrombolysis induced by intravenous administration of a thrombolytic agent. *J Am Coll Cardiol* 1994;23:794.
76. Holmes D et al. Contemporary reperfusion therapy for cardiogenic shock: the GUSTO-I trial experience. *J Am Coll Cardiol* 1995;26:288.
77. Hochman JS et al. Early revascularization in acute myocardial infarction complicated by cardiogenic shock. *N Engl J Med* 1999;341:625.
78. Hochman JS et al. One year survival following early revascularization for cardiogenic shock. *JAMA* 2001;285:190.
79. Holzer J et al. Effectiveness of dopamine in patients with cardiogenic shock. *Am J Cardiol* 1973; 32:79.
80. Richard C et al. Combined hemodynamic effects of dopamine and dobutamine in cardiogenic shock. *Circulation* 1983;67:620.
81. Frazier OH et al. Multicenter clinical evaluation of the HeartMate vented electric left ventricular assist system in patients awaiting heart transplantation. *J Thorac Cardiovasc Surg* 2001;122:1186.
82. Rose EA et al. Long-term mechanical left ventricular assistance for end-stage heart failure. *N Engl J Med* 2001;345:1435.
83. Kreger BE et al. Gram-negative bacteremia IV: reevaluation of clinical features and treatment in 612 patients. *Am J Med* 1980;68:344.
84. Rivers E et al. Early goal-directed therapy in the treatment of severe sepsis and septic shock. *N Engl J Med* 2001;345:1368.
85. Dellinger R et al. Surviving sepsis campaign guidelines for management of severe sepsis and septic shock. *Crit Care Med* 2004;32:858.
86. Meadows D et al. Reversal of intractable septic shock with norepinephrine therapy. *Crit Care Med* 1988;16:663.
87. Martin C et al. Norepinephrine or dopamine for the treatment of hyperdynamic septic shock? *Chest* 1993;103:1826.
88. Holmes C et al. Physiology of vasopressin relevant to management of septic shock. *Chest* 2001; 120:989.
89. Rozenfeld V et al. The role of vasopressin in the treatment of vasodilation in shock states. *Ann Pharmacother* 2000;34:250.
90. Landry D et al. Vasopressin deficiency contributes to the vasodilation of septic shock. *Circulation* 1997;95:1122.
91. Patel B et al. Beneficial effects of short-term vasopressin infusion during severe septic shock. *Anesthesiology* 2002;96:576.
92. Rudis MI et al. Is it time to reposition vasopressors and inotropes in sepsis? *Crit Care Med* 1996; 24:525.
93. Seguin P et al. Effects of epinephrine compared with the combination of dobutamine and norepinephrine on gastric perfusion in septic shock. *Clin Pharmacol Ther* 2002;71:381.
94. Annane D. Resurrection of steroids for sepsis resuscitation. *Minerva Anesthesiology* 2002;68:127.
95. Lefering R et al. Steroid controversy in sepsis and septic shock: a meta-analysis. *Crit Care Med* 1995;23:1294.
96. Cronin I et al. Corticosteroid treatment for sepsis: a critical appraisal and meta-analysis of the literature. *Crit Care Med* 1995;23:1430.
97. Annane D et al. Effect of treatment with low doses of hydrocortisone and fludrocortisone on mortality in patients with septic shock. *JAMA* 2002;288:862.
98. Thomsen R et al. Statin use and mortality within 180 days after bacteremia: a population-based cohort study. *Crit Care Med* 2006;34:1080.
99. Kruger P et al. Statin therapy is associated with fewer deaths in patients with bacteremia. *Intensive Care Med* 2006;32:75.
100. Dhainaut JF et al. Soluble thrombomodulin,

plasma-derived unactivated protein C, and recombinant human activated protein C in sepsis. *Crit Care Med* 2002;30(Suppl 5):S318.
101. Bernard G et al. Efficacy and safety of recombinant human activated protein C for severe sepsis. *N Engl J Med* 2001;344:699.
102. Abraham E et al. Drotecogin alfa (activated) for adults with severe sepsis and a low risk of death. *N Engl J Med* 2005;353:1332.
103. Cohen J et al. An international, multicenter, placebo-controlled trial of monoclonal antibody to human tumor necrosis factor–a patients with sepsis. *Crit Care Med* 1996;24:1431.
104. Rice T et al. Safety and efficacy of affinity-purified, anti-tumor necrosis factor-alpha, ovine fab for injection (CytoFab) in severe sepsis. *Crit Care Med* 2006;34:2271.
105. Fisher CJ et al. Treatment of septic shock with the tumor necrosis factor receptor: Fc fusion protein. *N Engl J Med* 1996;334:1697.
106. Van Zoelen M et al. Ethyl pyruvate exerts combined anti-inflammatory and anticoagulant effects on human monocyte cells. *Thromb and Haemost* 2006;96:789.
107. Bellomo R et al. Continuous hemofiltration as blood purification in sepsis. *New Horizons* 1995;3:732.
108. Jaber BL et al. Extracorporeal adsorbent-based strategies in sepsis. *Am J Kidney Dis* 1997;30(Suppl 4):S44.

PULMONARY DISORDERS

Robin L. Corelli
SECTION EDITOR

CHAPTER 22

Asthma

Timothy H. Self, Cary R. Chrisman, and Christopher K. Finch

ASTHMA

According to the National Institutes of Health (NIH) Expert Panel Report 3 (EPR-3): Guidelines for the Diagnosis and Management of Asthma,[1] *asthma* is defined as a chronic inflammatory disorder of the airways in which many cells and cellular elements play a role, in particular, mast cells, eosinophils, T lymphocytes, neutrophils, and epithelial cells. In susceptible persons, this inflammation causes recurrent episodes of wheezing, breathlessness, chest tightness, and cough, particularly at night and in the early morning. These episodes are usually associated with widespread but variable airflow obstruction that is often reversible either spontaneously or with treatment. The inflammation also causes an increase in the existing bronchial hyperresponsiveness to a variety of stimuli.[2] This definition of asthma is the same as the 1997 NIH guidelines[2] and has evolved from earlier national/international guidelines.[3–6]

At least 22 million Americans have asthma.[1] It is an underdiagnosed and undertreated condition that is estimated to have overall costs exceeding $12 billion annually in the United States.[7] Asthma is the leading cause of lost school days in children and is a common cause of lost workdays among adults.

Mortality from asthma has decreased in the 21st century, from 4,657 deaths in 1999 to 3,816 deaths in 2004 in the United States according to the Centers for Disease Control and Prevention,[8,9] but morbidity and mortality are still unacceptably high, especially in inner-city minority populations. This chapter emphasizes the 2007 NIH EPR-3 guidelines.[1] Application of the principles of these recent guidelines by clinicians and patients is vital to further reducing asthma morbidity and mortality.

Etiology

Childhood-onset asthma is usually associated with atopy, which is the genetic predisposition for the development of immunoglobulin E (IgE)-mediated response to common aeroallergens. Atopy is the strongest predisposing factor in the development of asthma.[1] A very common presentation of asthma is a child with a positive family history of asthma and allergy to tree and grass pollen, house dust mites, household pets, and molds.

Adult-onset asthma may also be associated with atopy, but many adults with asthma have a negative family history and negative skin tests to common aeroallergens. Some of these patients may have nasal polyps, aspirin sensitivity, and sinusitis. In the British 1958 birth cohort study, participants were monitored for wheezing and asthma at periodic intervals from birth into their mid-forties.[10] In the subset of patients who were seemingly asymptomatic during late adolescence and early adulthood, the presence of asthma at 42 years of age was significantly higher in those patients who had a history of wheezing in childhood. Exposure to factors (e.g., wood dusts, chemicals) at the workplace that may cause airway inflammation is also important in many adults. Inflammatory mechanisms are similar, but not the same, as in atopic asthma. Some clinicians may still refer to *intrinsic asthma* when referring to these patients and *extrinsic asthma* when discussing atopic asthma.

In addition to atopy and exposure to occupational chemical sensitizers being major risk factors for the development of asthma, several contributing factors may increase the susceptibility to the development of the disease in predisposed individuals.[1,5] These factors include viral infections, small size at birth, diet, exposure to tobacco smoke, and environmental pollutants.[1,5]

Recent literature has focused on the "hygiene hypothesis," an imbalance of TH2- and TH1-type T lymphocytes, to explain the marked increase in asthma in westernized countries.[1,5,8] Infants who have older siblings, early exposure to day care, and typical childhood infections are more likely to activate TH1 responses (protective immunity), resulting in an appropriate balance of TH1/TH2 cells and the cytokines that they produce. On the other hand, if the immune response is predominately from TH2 cells (which produce cytokines that mediate allergic inflammation), development of diseases such as asthma is more likely. Examples of factors favoring this imbalance include the common use of antimicrobial agents, urban environment, and Western lifestyle. Further insights into the pathogenesis of asthma continue to be discovered.[1,7,11,12]

Pathophysiology

Asthma is caused by a complex interaction between inflammatory cells and mediators. As noted in the definition of asthma, mast cells, eosinophils, T lymphocytes, neutrophils, and epithelial cells are of central importance. The bronchial epithelium in asthmatics has been described as fragile, with various abnormalities including destruction of ciliated cells and overexpression of epidermal growth factors.[13] Figure 22-1 depicts the complex interaction of cells and mediators associated with airway inflammation.

After exposure to an asthma-precipitating factor (e.g., aeroallergen), inflammatory mediators are released from bronchial mast cells, macrophages, T lymphocytes, and epithelial cells. These mediators direct the migration and activation of other inflammatory cells, most notably eosinophils, to the airways.[1,11,12] Eosinophils release biochemicals (e.g., major basic protein and eosinophil cationic protein) that cause airway injury, including epithelial damage, mucus hypersecretion, and increased reactivity of smooth muscle.[1,7,11]

Research continues to determine the role of a subpopulation of T lymphocytes (TH2) in asthmatic airway inflammation.[1,11] TH2 lymphocytes release cytokines (e.g., interleukin [IL]-4 and IL-5) that at least partially control the activation and enhanced survival of eosinophils.[1,4,11] The complexity of airway inflammation is indicated by the fact that at least 27 cytokines may have a role in the pathophysiology of asthma.[11] In addition, at least 18 chemokines (e.g., eotaxins) have been identified that are important in delivery of eosinophils to the airways.[11] One biomarker of airway inflammation is exhaled nitric oxide (NO), which has been used as a treatment guide in chronic asthma.[1] Bronchial NO has been found to be elevated during periods of exacerbations and is measurably decreased with administration of inhaled steroids but not β_2-agonists.[14,15] Failure to adequately minimize severe and long-term airway inflammation in asthma may result in airway remodeling in some patients. Airway remodeling refers to structural changes, including an alteration in the amount and composition of the extracellular matrix in the airway wall leading to airflow obstruction that eventually may become only partially reversible.[1,16]

Hyperreactivity (defined as an exaggerated response of bronchial smooth muscles to trigger stimuli) of the airways to physical, chemical, immunologic, and pharmacologic stimuli is pathognomonic of asthma.[2] Examples of these stimuli include inhaled allergens, respiratory viral infection, cold, dry air, smoke, other pollutants, and methacholine. Endogenous stimuli that can worsen asthma include poorly controlled rhinitis, sinusitis, and gastroesophageal reflux disease.[1] In addition, premenstrual asthma has been reported, but the exact hormonal mechanism is not known.[17]

Although patients with allergic rhinitis, chronic bronchitis, and cystic fibrosis also experience bronchial hyperreactivity, these patients do not experience bronchiolar constriction as severely as do patients with asthma. The degree of bronchial hyperreactivity of asthmatics correlates with the clinical course of their disease, which is characterized by periods of remissions and exacerbations. During times of remission, a more intense stimulus is required to produce bronchospasm than during times of increased symptoms. Numerous theories have been proposed to explain the bronchial hyperreactivity found in asthma, yet none fully explains the phenomenon. Inflammation appears to be the primary process in the pathogenesis of bronchial hyperreactivity; however, neurogenic imbalances in the airways also may play a significant role.[5] Inflamed airways are hyperreactive (i.e., irritable). Hyperreactivity can be measured in the physician's office by having the patient inhale small concentrations of nebulized methacholine or histamine or by exercise (e.g., treadmill). The concentration of aerosolized

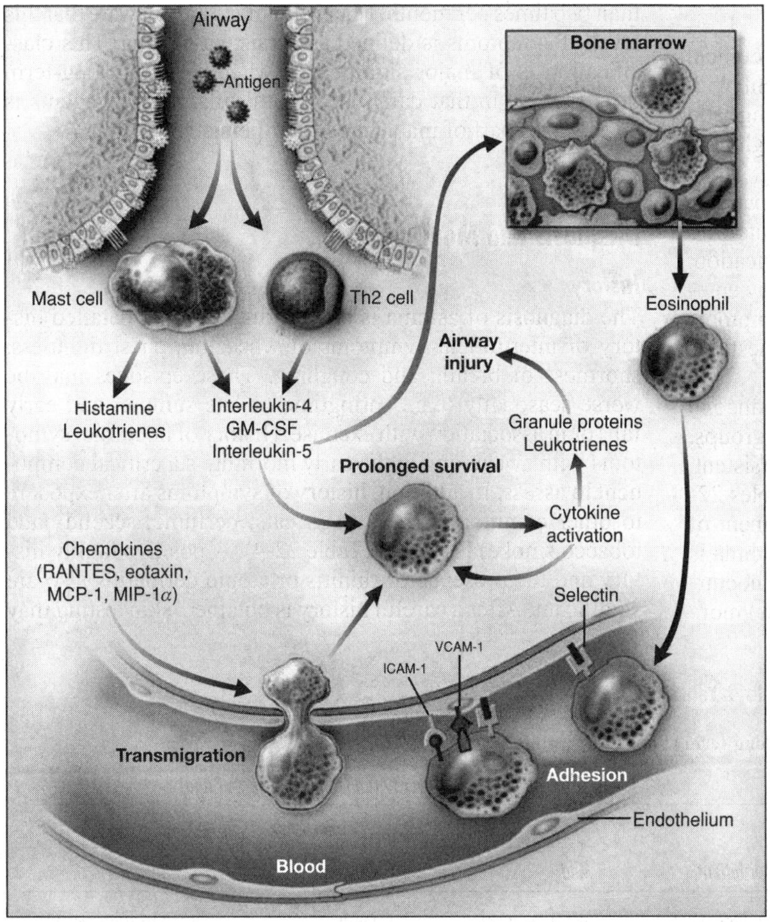

FIGURE 22-1 Airway inflammation. Inhaled antigen activates mast cells and Th2 cells in the airway. They in turn induce the production of mediators of inflammation (such as histamine and leukotrienes) and cytokines including interleukin-4 and interleukin-5. Interleukin-5 travels to the bone marrow and causes terminal differentiation of eosinophils. Circulating eosinophils enter the area of allergic inflammation and begin migrating to the lung by rolling, through interactions with selectins, and eventually adhering to endothelium through the binding of integrins to members of the immunoglobulin superfamily of adhesion proteins: vascular-cell adhesion molecule 1 (VCAM-1) and intercellular adhesion molecule 1 (ICAM-1). As the eosinophils enter the matrix of the airway through the influence of various chemokines and cytokines, their survival is prolonged by interleukin-4 and granulocyte-macrophage colony-stimulating factor (GM-CSF). On activation, the eosinophil releases inflammatory mediators, such as leukotrienes and granule proteins, to injure airway tissues. In addition, eosinophils can generate GM-CSF to prolong and potentiate their survival and contribution to persistent airway inflammation. MCP-1, monocyte chemotactic protein; and MIP-1α, macrophage inflammatory protein. (Reprinted with permission from Busse WW, Lemanske RF. Advances in Immunology. *N Engl J Med* 2001; 344:350–62.)

methacholine or histamine that decreases the forced expiratory volume in 1 second (FEV_1) by 20% is referred to as the PD_{20} or the PC_{20} (provocative dose or concentration that decreases the FEV_1 by 20%).[2] An indicator of optimal anti-inflammatory therapy is an increase in the PD_{20} over time as the airways become less inflamed and therefore less hyperreactive.

Another concept related to inflammation is "late-phase" versus "early-phase" asthma (Fig. 22-2). The inhalation of specific allergens in atopic asthmatics produces immediate bronchoconstriction (measured by a drop in peak expiratory flow [PEF] or FEV_1) that spontaneously improves over an hour or is reversed easily by inhalation of a β_2-agonist. Although this early asthmatic response (EAR) is blocked by the preadministration of β_2-agonists, cromolyn, or theophylline, a second bronchoconstrictive response often occurs 4 to 12 hours later. This late asthmatic response (LAR) often is more severe, more prolonged, and more difficult to reverse with bronchodilators than is the EAR. The LAR is associated with the influx of inflammatory cells and mediators as described previously. Bronchodilators do not block the LAR to allergen challenge; corticosteroids block the LAR but do not affect the EAR; and cromolyn blocks both.[2]

Pathologic changes in asthmatics found at autopsy include (a) marked hypertrophy and hyperplasia of the bronchial smooth muscle, (b) mucous gland hypertrophy and excessive mucous secretion, and (c) denuded epithelium and mucosal edema due to an exudative inflammatory reaction and inflammatory cell infiltration.[1] Hyperinflation of the lungs from air trapping with extensive mucous plugging is found at autopsy in patients who have died from acute asthma attacks, but these changes also are seen at autopsy in asthmatics dying from other causes. The bronchial smooth muscle hypertrophy and mucus hypersecretion are secondary to the chronic inflammatory response.

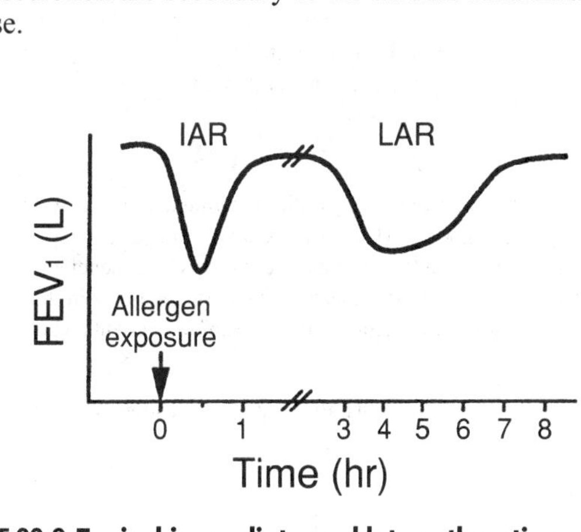

FIGURE 22-2 Typical immediate and late asthmatic responses seen after exposure to relevant allergen. Immediate asthmatic response (IAR) occurs within minutes, whereas late asthmatic response (LAR) occurs several hours after exposure. Patients may demonstrate isolated IAR, isolated LAR, or dual responses. (Reproduced with permission from Herfindal ET, Gourley DR. Textbook of Therapeutics Drug and Disease Management. 7th ed. Baltimore: Williams & Wilkins, 1996.)

Symptoms

The heterogeneity of asthma is reflected best in its clinical presentation. Classically, patients with asthma present with intermittent episodes of expiratory wheezing, coughing, and dyspnea. Some patients, however, experience chest tightness or a chronic cough that is not associated with wheezing. There is a wide spectrum of disease severity, ranging from patients with occasional, mild bouts of breathlessness to patients who wheeze daily despite continuous high dosages of medication. In addition, the severity of asthma may be influenced by environmental factors (e.g., specific seasonal allergens). Symptoms often are associated with exercise and sleep (refer to Questions 43 and 48).

Classification of asthma severity is of major importance in defining initial long-term treatment. Based on three age groups, EPR-3 uses the classifications of intermittent, mild persistent, moderate persistent, and severe persistent asthma (Tables 22-1–22-3). The frequency of symptoms is a key component of asthma classification.[1] For example, mild persistent asthma is defined as symptoms more than two times per week or nocturnal symptoms (including early morning chest tightness) more than two times per month. Many clinicians are unaware that this level of symptoms is defined as persistent asthma. This classification is of major significance when selecting long-term drug therapy in that daily use of anti-inflammatory agents is an essential part of management for persistent asthma.[1]

Diagnosis and Monitoring

History

The diagnosis of asthma is based primarily on a detailed history of intermittent symptoms of wheezing, chest tightness, shortness of breath, and coughing. These episodes may be worse seasonally (e.g., springtime or late summer and early fall) or in association with exercise. History of nocturnal symptoms with awakening in the early morning is a critical component to assess. In addition, history of symptoms after exposure to other common triggers (e.g., cats, perfume, second-hand tobacco smoke) is typical (Table 22-4). A positive family history and the presence of rhinitis or atopic dermatitis also are significant. After a careful history is obtained, skin testing may

Table 22-1 Classifying Asthma Severity in Children 0 to 4 Years of Age

Classifying severity in children who are not currently taking long-term control medication.[a]

			Classification of Asthma Severity (Children 0–4 Years of Age)		
			Persistent		
Components of Severity		Intermittent	Mild	Moderate	Severe
Impairment	Symptoms	≤2 days/week	>2 days/week but not daily	Daily	Throughout the day
	Nighttime awakenings	0	1–2x/mo	3–4x/month	>1x/week
	SABA use for symptom control (not prevention of EIB)	≤2 days/week	>2 days/week but not daily	Daily	Several times per day
	Interference with normal activity	None	Minor limitation	Some limitation	Extremely limited
Risk	Exacerbations requiring oral systemic corticosteroids	0–1/yr	≥2 exacerbation in 6 months requiring oral corticosteroids or ≥4 wheezing episodes in 1 year lasting >1 day AND risk factors for persistent asthma		
			Consider severity and interval since last exacerbation. ← Frequency and severity may fluctuate over time. → Exacerbations of any severity may occur in patients in any severity category.		

Level of severity is determined by both impairment and risk. Assess impairment domain by caregiver's recall of previous 2–4 weeks. Assign severity to the most severe category in which any feature occurs.

At present, there are inadequate data to correspond frequencies of exacerbations with different levels of asthma severity. For treatment purposes, patients who had ≥2 exacerbations requiring oral corticosteroids in the past 6 months, or ≥4 wheezing episodes in the past year, and who have risk factors for persistent asthma may be considered the same as patients who have persistent asthma, even in the absence of impairment levels consistent with persistent asthma.

Classifying severity in patients after asthma becomes well controlled, by lowest level of treatment required to maintain control.[a]

		Classification of Asthma Severity		
		Persistent		
	Intermittent	Mild	Moderate	Severe
Lowest level of treatment required to maintain control (See Fig. 23-7 for treatment steps.)	Step 1	Step 2	Step 3 or 4	Step 5 or 6

[a]EIB, exercise-induced bronchospasm; SABA, short-acting inhaled β_2-agonist.
Reprinted from reference 1.

Table 22-2 Classifying Asthma Severity in Children 5 to 11 Years of Age

Classifying severity in children who are not currently taking long-term control medication.[a]

		Classification of Asthma Severity (Children 5–11 Years of Age)			
			Persistent		
	Components of Severity	*Intermittent*	*Mild*	*Moderate*	*Severe*
Impairment	Symptoms	≤2 days/week	>2 days/week but not daily	Daily	Throughout the day
	Nighttime awakenings	≤2x/month	3–4x/month	>1x/week but not nightly	Often 7x/week
	SABA use for symptom control (not prevention of EIB)	≤2 days/week	>2 days/week but not daily	Daily	Several times per day
	Interference with normal activity	None	Minor limitation	Some limitation	Extremely limited
	Lung function	• Normal FEV_1 between exacerbations • FEV_1 >80% predicted • FEV_1/FVC >85%	• FEV_1 >80% predicted • FEV_1/FVC >80%	• FEV_1 = 60%–80% predicted • FEV_1/FVC 75%–80%	• FEV_1 <60% predicted • FEV_1/FVC <75%
Risk	Exacerbations requiring oral systemic corticosteroids	0–1 in 1 year (see note)	≥2 in 1 year (see note) →		
		← Consider severity and interval since last exacerbation. Frequency and severity may fluctuate over time for patients any severity category. Relative annual risk of exacerbations may be related to FEV_1. →			

Level of severity is determined by both impairment and risk, Assess impairment domain by patient/caregiver's recall of the previous 2–4 weeks and spirometry. Assign severity to the most severe category in which any feature occurs.

At present, there are inadequate data to correspond frequencies of exacerbations with different levels of asthma severity. In general, more frequent and intense exacerbations (e.g., requiring urgent, unscheduled care, hospitalization, or ICU admission indicate greater underlying disease severity. For treatment purposes, patients who had ≥2 exacerbations requiring oral systemic corticosteroids in the past year may be considered the same as patients who have persistent asthma, even in the absence of impairment levels consistent with persistent asthma.

Classifying severity in patients after asthma becomes well controlled, by lowest level of treatment required to maintain control.[a]

	Classification of Asthma Severity			
		Persistent		
Lowest level of treatment required to maintain control	*Intermittent*	*Mild*	*Moderate*	*Severe*
(See Fig. 23-8 for treatment steps.)	Step 1	Step 2	Step 3 or 4	Step 5 or 6

[a]EIB, exercise-induced bronchospasm; FEV_1, forced expiratory volume in 1 second; FVC, forced vital capacity; ICU, intensive care unit; SABA, short-acting β_2-agonist.
Reprinted from reference 1.

be useful in identifying triggering allergens, but it is only of supportive value in the diagnosis of asthma.

Pulmonary Function Tests

The diagnosis of asthma is based in part on demonstration of reversible airway obstruction. A brief discussion of tests to detect reversibility of airway obstruction is important. Furthermore, a short summary of arterial blood gases (ABGs) is pertinent here in assessing the severity of asthma exacerbations.

SPIROMETRY

Lung volumes often are measured to obtain information about the size of the patient's lungs, because pulmonary diseases can affect the volume of air that can be inhaled and exhaled. The tidal volume is the volume of air inspired or expired during normal breathing. The volume of air blown off after maximal inspiration to full expiration is defined as the vital capacity (VC). The residual volume (RV) is the volume of air left in the lung after maximal expiration. The volume of air left after a normal expiration is the functional residual capacity (FRC). Total lung capacity (TLC) is the VC plus the RV. Patients with obstructive lung disease have difficulty with expiration; therefore, they tend to have a decreased VC, an increased RV, and a normal TLC. Classic restrictive lung diseases (e.g., sarcoidosis, idiopathic pulmonary fibrosis) present with decrements in all lung volumes.[18] Patients also may have mixed lesion diseases, in which case the classic findings are not apparent until the disease has advanced considerably.

The spirometer also can be used to evaluate the performance of the patient's lungs, thorax, and respiratory muscles in moving air into and out of the lungs. Forced expiratory maneuvers amplify the ventilation abnormalities produced. The single

Table 22-3 Classifying Asthma Severity in Youths ≥12 Years of Age and Adults

Classifying severity in patients who are not currently taking long-term control medication.[a]

	Components of Severity	Intermittent	Persistent: Mild	Persistent: Moderate	Persistent: Severe
Impairment	Symptoms	≤2 days/week	>2 days/week but not daily	Daily	Throughout the day
	Nighttime awakenings	≤2x/month	3–4x/month	>1x/week but not nightly	Often 7x/week
	SABA use for symptom control (not prevention of EIB)	≤2 days/week	>2 days/week but not >1x/day	Daily	Several times per day
Normal FEV_1/FVC: 8–19 years, 85%; 20–39 years, 80%; 40–59 years, 75%; 60–80 years, 70%	Interference with normal activity	None	Minor limitation	Some limitation	Extremely limited
	Lung function	• Normal FEV_1 between exacerbations • FEV_1 >80% predicted • FEV_1/FVC normal	• FEV_1 ≥80% predicted • FEV_1/FVC normal	• FEV_1 >60% but <80% predicted • FEV_1/FVC reduced 5%	• FEV_1 <60% predicted • FEV_1/FVC reduced >5%
Risk	Exacerbations requiring oral systemic corticosteroids	0–1 in 1 year (see note)	≥ 2 in 1 year (see note) →		
		Consider severity and interval since last exacerbation. Frequency and severity may fluctuate over time for patients any severity category. Relative annual risk of exacerbations may be related to FEV_1.			

Level of severity is determined by assessment of both impairment and risk. Assess impairment domain by patient/caregiver's recall of previous 2–4 weeks and spirometry. Assign severity to the most severe category in which any feature occurs.

At present, there are inadequate data to correspond frequencies of exacerbations with different levels of asthma severity. In general, more frequent and intense exacerbations (e.g., requiring urgent, unscheduled care, hospitalization, or ICU admission) indicate greater underlying disease severity. For treatment purposes, patients who had ≥2 exacerbations requiring oral systemic corticosteroids in the past year may be considered the same as patients who have persistent asthma, even in the absence of impairment levels consistent with persistent asthma.

Classifying severity in patients after asthma becomes well controlled, by lowest level of treatment required to maintain control.[a]

	Intermittent	Persistent: Mild	Persistent: Moderate	Persistent: Severe
Lowest level of treatment required to maintain control (See Fig. 23-9 for treatment steps.)	Step 1	Step 2	Step 3 or 4	Step 5 or 6

[a]EIB, exercise-induced bronchospasm; FEV_1, forced expiratory volume in 1 second: FVC, forced vital capacity; ICU, intensive care unit; SABA, short-acting β_2-agonist.
Reprinted from reference 1.

most useful test for ventilatory dysfunction is the FEV. The FEV is measured by having the patient exhale into the spirometer as forcefully and completely as possible after maximal inspiration. The resulting volume curve is plotted against time (Fig. 22-3) so that expiratory flow can be estimated.

Standard spirometers contain pneumotachographs in the mouthpieces that can measure airflow directly. A number of important measures of lung function are made from the resulting flow-volume curves (Fig. 22-4). The advantages of this technique include a display of simultaneous flows at any lung volume, visual estimation of patient effort and cooperation, high reproducibility within as well as across individuals, and an analysis of the distribution of flow limitation.[18,19] The FEV_1 of the forced vital capacity (FVC, the maximum volume of air exhaled with maximally forced effort from a position of maximal inspiration) commonly is measured to determine the dynamic performance of the lung in moving air. The FEV_1 usually is expressed as a percentage of the total volume of air exhaled and is reported as the FEV_1 to FVC ratio. Healthy persons generally can exhale at least 75% to 80% of their VC in 1 second and almost all of it in 3 seconds. Thus, the FEV_1 normally is 80% of the FVC. The patient's breathing ability is compared against "predicted normal" values for patients with similar physiologic characteristics, because lung volumes depend on age, race, gender, height, and weight. For example, an average-sized young adult male may have an FVC of 4 to

Table 22-4 Sample Questions for the Diagnosis and Initial Assessment of Asthma[a]

A "yes" answer to any question suggests that an asthma diagnosis is likely.

In the past 12 months . . .

- Have you had a sudden severe episode or recurrent episodes of coughing, wheezing (high-pitched whistling sounds when breathing out), chest tightness, or shortness of breath?
- Have you had colds that "go to the chest" or take more than 10 days to get over?
- Have you had coughing, wheezing, or shortness of breath during a particular season or time of the year?
- Have you had coughing, wheezing, or shortness of breath in certain places or when exposed to certain things (e.g., animals, tobacco smoke, perfumes)?
- Have you used any medications that help you breathe better? How often?
- Are your symptoms relieved when the medications are used?

In the past 4 weeks, have you had coughing, wheezing, or shortness of breath . . .

- At night that has awakened you?
- On awakening?
- After running, moderate exercise, or other physical activity?

[a] These questions are examples and do not represent a standardized assessment or diagnostic instrument. The validity and reliability of these questions have not been assessed.

Reprinted from reference 1.

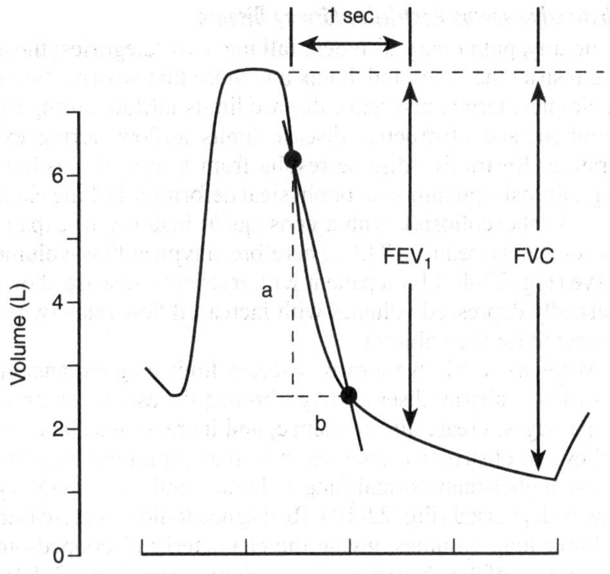

FIGURE 22-3 Volume-time curve from a forced expiratory maneuver.

5 L and a corresponding FEV_1 of 3.2 to 4 L. The FEV_1 and the FVC are the most reproducible of the pulmonary function tests.

PEAK EXPIRATORY FLOW

The PEF is the maximal flow that can be produced during the forced expiration. The PEF can be measured easily with various handheld peak flow meters and commonly is used in emergency departments (EDs) and clinics to quickly and objectively assess the effectiveness of bronchodilators in the treatment of acute asthma attacks. Peak flow meters also can be used at home by patients with asthma to assess chronic therapy. The changes in PEF generally parallel those of the FEV_1; however, the PEF is a less reproducible measure than the FEV_1.[5] A healthy, average-sized young adult male typically has a PEF of 550 to 700 L/minute. Commercial peak flow meters come with a chart for patients to determine their predicted normal PEFs based on their gender, age, and height.

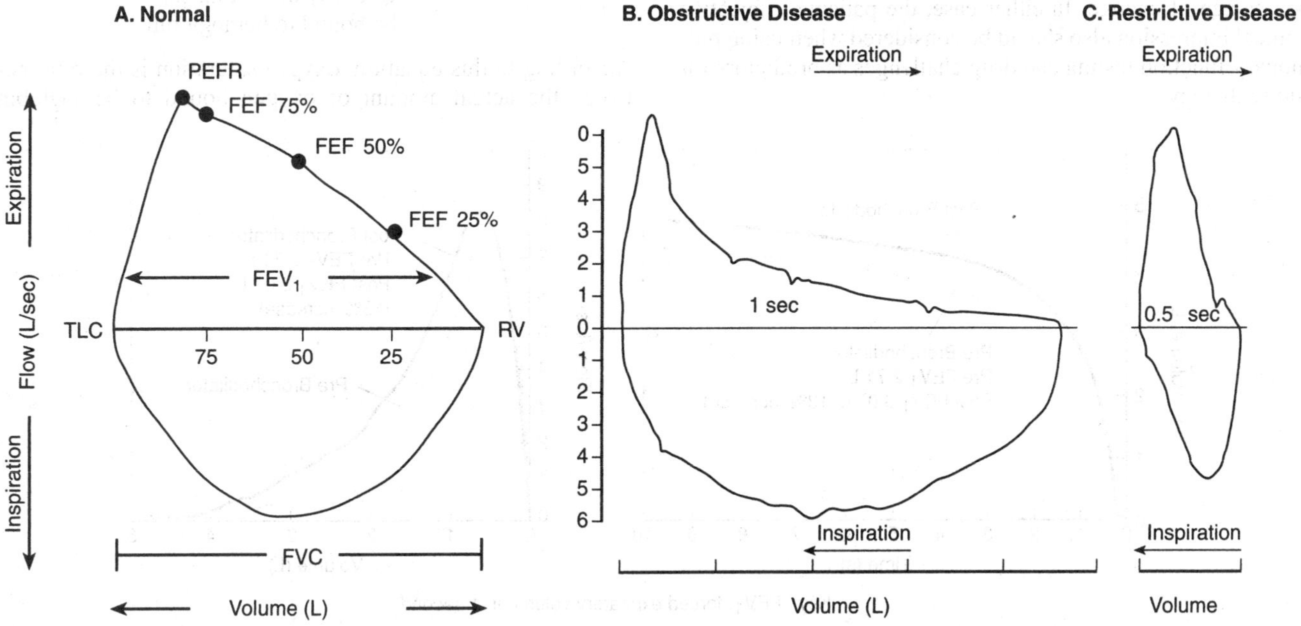

FIGURE 22-4 Flow-volume curves resulting from a forced expiratory maneuver. A: Normal flow-volume curve. **B:** Typical pattern for obstructive disease. **C:** Typical pattern for restrictive disease.

Obstructive versus Restrictive Airway Disease

Generally, pulmonary disorders fall into two categories: those that restrict the lungs and thorax and those that obstruct them. In simplest terms, restrictive disease limits airflow during inspiration, and obstructive disease limits airflow during expiration. Restrictive disease results from a loss of elasticity (e.g., fibrosis, pneumonia) or physical deformities of the chest (e.g., kyphoscoliosis), with a consequent inability to expand the lung and a reduced TLC. Therefore, a typical flow-volume curve (Fig. 22-4C) for a patient with restrictive disease shows markedly depressed volumes with increased flow rates (when corrected for the volume).

Whereas restrictive airway diseases limit lung expansion, obstructive airway diseases (e.g., bronchitis, asthma) narrow air passages, create air turbulence, and increase resistance to airflow. In obstructive diseases, maximal expiration may begin at higher-than-normal lung volumes, and the expiratory flow is depressed (Fig. 22-4B). Resistance to flow is increased at lower lung volumes, giving the characteristic scooped-out appearance of the obstructive flow-volume curve (Fig. 22-4B).

Reversible Airway Obstruction

Spirometry often is used to determine the reversibility of airway disease. Although many generally associate reversibility with bronchospasm, therapy can improve airflow by reversing any of the causative pathologic processes of asthma described previously. Significant clinical reversibility produced from bronchodilators is determined by the tests outlined in Figure 22-5. The FEV_1 is considered the gold standard test for determining reversibility of airway disease and bronchodilator efficacy. Significant clinical reversibility is defined as a 12% improvement in FEV_1 following administration of a short-acting bronchodilator.[1] An improvement of 20% in FEV_1 provides noticeable subjective relief of respiratory symptoms in most patients. For patients with a very low baseline FEV_1 (e.g., <1 L), an absolute improvement of 250 mL sometimes is considered a better indicator of therapeutic benefit than assessing percentage of change. In either case, the patient's subjective clinical impression also should be considered when using pulmonary function testing and drug challenges as predictors for future therapy.

LIMITATIONS OF SPIROMETRY

Because the FEV_1 and the PEF are both highly effort dependent, complete patient cooperation is required for reliable results. Therefore, spirometric tests often are unobtainable in patients who are severely ill as well as in patients who are very old or very young. The FEV_1 and PEF also are relatively insensitive to small airway changes and are therefore unable to detect early mucous plugging and inflammation in small bronchioles. Although the forced expiratory flow $(FEF)_{25\%-75\%}$ is a more sensitive test of small airway obstruction, it is also much more variable, requiring larger changes (30%–40%) to be clinically significant.

Spirometric pulmonary function tests before and after administration of an inhaled bronchodilator can be useful in assessing the reversibility of airway obstruction. If significantly depressed pulmonary function tests are not reversed by the administration of a bronchodilator acutely, a 2- to 3-week trial of oral corticosteroid treatment followed by retesting might detect reversibility.[1]

If pulmonary function is normal or near normal at the time of spirometric assessment, the patient can be challenged by exercise or drugs that are known to produce bronchospasm in asthmatics (e.g., aerosolized methacholine).

Blood Gas Measurements

The best indicators of overall lung function (ventilation and diffusion) are the ABGs (i.e., PaO_2, $PaCO_2$, and pH). Although ABG measurements also are dependent on the patient's cardiovascular status, they are indispensable in assessing both acute and chronic changes in pulmonary patients. (See Chapter 10 Acid-Base Disorders for a review of ABGs.) Another means of assessing the patient's ability to oxygenate tissues adequately is to measure oxygen saturation, which is described by the following equation:

$$O_2 \text{ saturation} = \frac{\text{Quantity of } O_2 \text{ actually bound to hemoglobin}}{\text{Quantity of } O_2 \text{ that can be bound to hemoglobin}} \times 100$$

According to this equation, oxygen saturation is the ratio between the actual amount of oxygen bound to hemoglobin

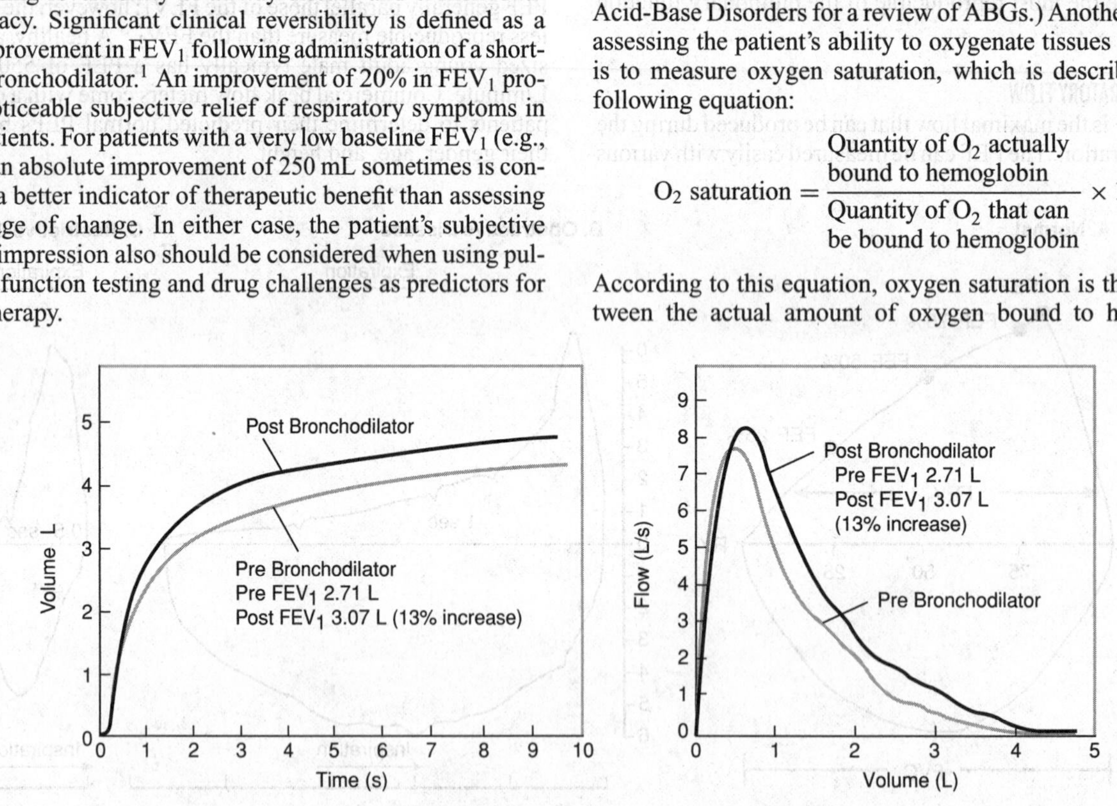

FIGURE 22-5 Interpretation of results of spirometry. The graphs depicted are for illustration only. The Interpretation of flow rates may vary with the age of the patient. (Reprinted with permission from reference 2.)

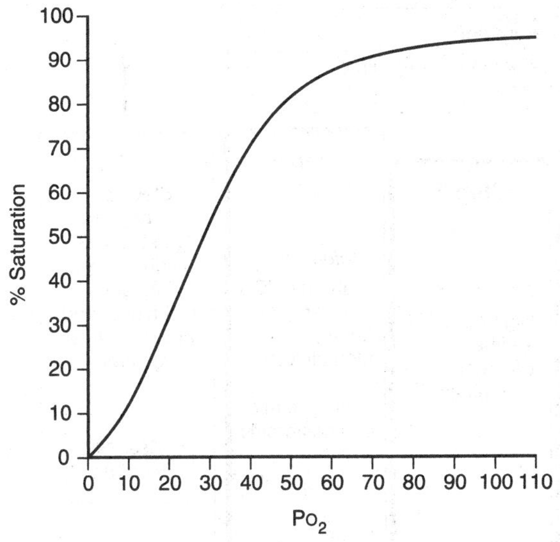

FIGURE 22-6 The oxygen dissociation curve reveals that the percent saturation of hemoglobin increases almost linearly with increases in the arterial O_2 tension until a PaO_2 of 55 to 65 mmHg is reached. At PaO_2 values above this, the increase in hemoglobin saturation becomes proportionately less and relatively little additional oxygen is added to the hemoglobin despite large increases in PaO_2. (Reproduced with permission from Guenther CA, Welch MH. *Pulmonary Medicine.* 2nd ed. Philadelphia: JB Lippincott; 1982.)

and the potential amount of oxygen that could be bound to hemoglobin at a given pressure. The denominator in the preceding equation is the oxygen capacity. The normal oxygen saturation of arterial blood at a PaO_2 of 100 mmHg is 97.5%; that of mixed venous blood at a PO_2 of 40 mmHg is about 75%.[18]

Oxygen saturations can be measured continuously with transcutaneous monitors. This type of monitoring (pulse oximetry) is extremely helpful in determining whether supplemental oxygen therapy is indicated in patients with various chronic respiratory diseases. At a PaO_2 of <60 mmHg, oxygen saturation begins to drop precipitously (Fig. 22-6)

Goals of Therapy

The EPR-3[1] established the following goals of therapy to achieve control of asthma:

Reduce Impairment: (a) Prevent chronic and troublesome symptoms (e.g., coughing or breathlessness in the night, in the early morning, or after exertion), (b) maintain (near) "normal" pulmonary function, (c) maintain normal activity levels (including exercise, other physical activities, and attendance at work or school), (d) require infrequent use of short-acting inhaled β_2-agonist ([SABAs], ≤2 days a week for quick relief of symptoms), and (e) meet patients' and families' expectations of and satisfaction with asthma care.

Reduce Risk: (a) Prevent recurrent exacerbations of asthma and minimize the need for ED visits or hospitalizations; (b) prevent progressive loss of lung function—for children, prevent reduced lung growth; and (c) provide optimal pharmacotherapy with minimal or no adverse effects.

Major Components of Long-Term Management

To achieve these goals of therapy, EPR-3[1] also outlines some general treatment principles. Asthma management has four major components, including (a) measures of asthma assessment and monitoring, (b) education for a partnership in asthma care, (c) control of environmental factors and comorbid conditions that affect asthma, and (d) medications. Optimal long-term management requires a continuous care approach, including each of these four major components, to prevent exacerbations and decrease airway inflammation. Early therapeutic interventions in managing acute exacerbations are very important in decreasing the chance of severe narrowing of the airways. Achieving the goals of asthma therapy also involves individualizing each patient's therapy. In addition, optimal care involves establishing a "partnership" between the patient, the patient's family, and the clinician.

For most patients with asthma, the condition can be extremely well controlled by using the step-care approach recommended by EPR-3[1] (Figs. 22-7–22-9). A concerted effort in patient education as an integral part of state-of-the-art long-term management has been demonstrated to improve outcomes, including quality of life in patients with asthma. Because of the excellent outcomes associated with optimal long-term management, if a patient requires an ED visit or hospitalization, great care should be given to determining how the acute-care visit could have been prevented.

ACUTE ASTHMA

Assessment

Signs and Symptoms

1. Q.C., a 6-year-old, 20-kg girl, presents to the ED with complaints of dyspnea and coughing that have progressively worsened over the past 2 days. These symptoms were preceded by 3 days of symptoms of a viral upper respiratory tract infection (sore throat, rhinorrhea, and coughing). She has experienced several bouts of bronchitis in the last 2 years and was hospitalized for pneumonia 3 months ago. Q.C. is not being treated with any medications at present. Physical examination reveals an anxious-appearing young girl in moderate respiratory distress with audible expiratory wheezes; occasional coughing; a prolonged expiratory phase; a hyperinflated chest; and suprasternal, supraclavicular, and intercostal retractions. Bilateral inspiratory and expiratory wheezes with decreased breath sounds on the left side are heard on auscultation. Q.C.'s vital signs are as follows: respiratory rate (RR), 30 breaths/minute; blood pressure (BP), 110/83 mmHg; heart rate, 130 beats/minute; temperature, 37.8°C; and pulsus paradoxus, 18 mmHg. Her arterial oxygen saturation (SaO_2) by pulse oximetry is 90%. Q.C. is given O_2 to maintain SaO_2 >90% and 2.5 mg of albuterol by nebulizer Q 20 minutes for three doses. After the initial treatment, Q.C. claims some subjective improvement and appears to be more comfortable; however, wheezing on auscultation becomes louder. What signs and symptoms in Q.C. are consistent with acute bronchial obstruction? Does increased wheezing after albuterol indicate failure of the medication?

Asthma is an obstructive lung disease; therefore, the primary limitation to airflow occurs during expiration. This outflow obstruction leads to the classic findings of dyspnea, expiratory wheezes, and a prolonged expiratory phase during the

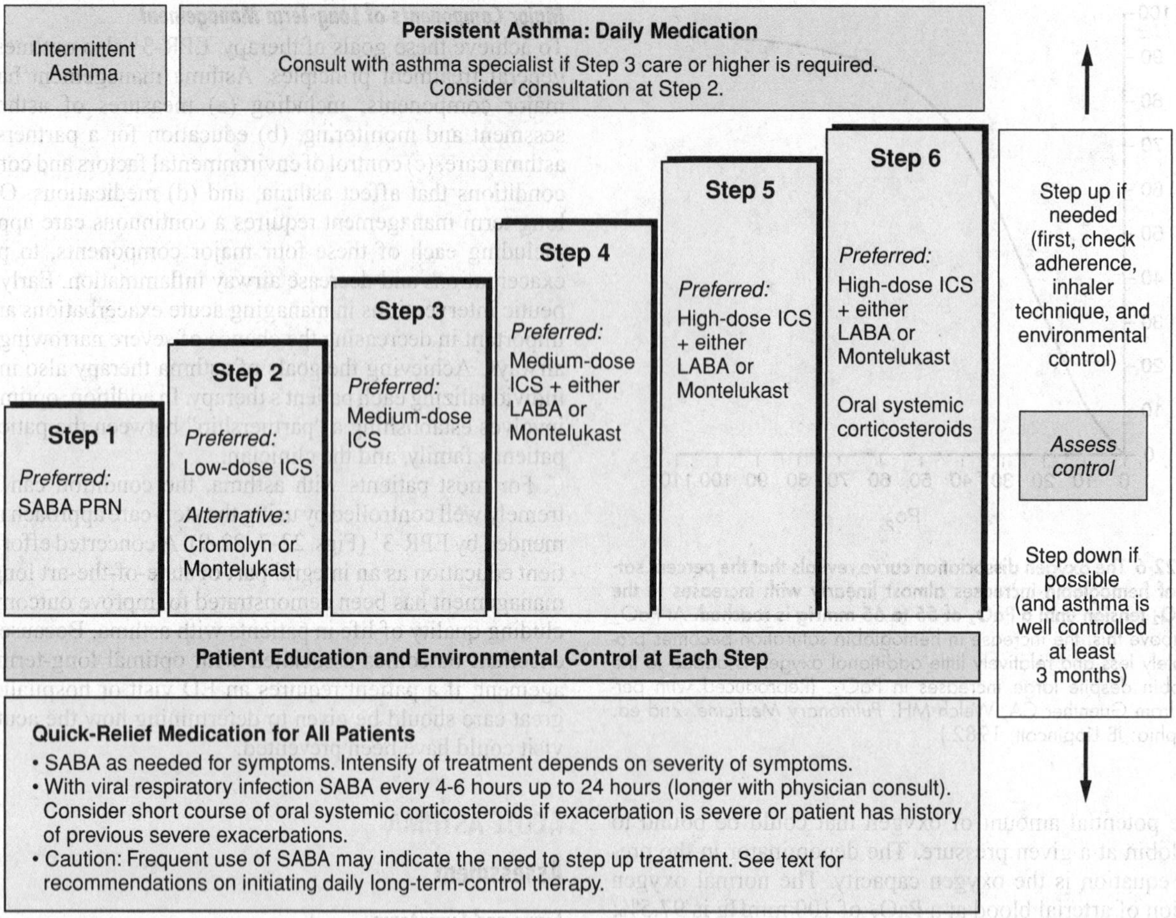

Intermittent Asthma
Persistent Asthma: Daily Medication
Consult with asthma specialist if Step 3 care or higher is required.
Consider consultation at Step 2.
Step 1
Preferred:
SABA PRN
Step 2
Preferred:
Low-dose ICS
Alternative:
Cromolyn or Montelukast
Step 3
Preferred:
Medium-dose ICS
Step 4
Preferred:
Medium-dose ICS + either LABA or Montelukast
Step 5
Preferred:
High-dose ICS + either LABA or Montelukast
Step 6
Preferred:
High-dose ICS + either LABA or Montelukast
Oral systemic corticosteroids
Step up if needed (first, check adherence, inhaler technique, and environmental control)
Assess control
Step down if possible (and asthma is well controlled at least 3 months)
Patient Education and Environmental Control at Each Step
Quick-Relief Medication for All Patients
• SABA as needed for symptoms. Intensify of treatment depends on severity of symptoms.
• With viral respiratory infection SABA every 4-6 hours up to 24 hours (longer with physician consult). Consider short course of oral systemic corticosteroids if exacerbation is severe or patient has history of previous severe exacerbations.
• Caution: Frequent use of SABA may indicate the need to step up treatment. See text for recommendations on initiating daily long-term-control therapy.

Key: **Alphabetical order is used when more than one treatment option is listed within either preferred or alternative therapy.** ICS, inhaled corticosteroid; LABA, inhaled long-acting β_2-agonist; SABA, inhaled short-acting β_2-agonist.

Notes:

- The stepwise approach is meant to assist, not replace, the clinical decisionmaking required to meet individual patient needs.
- If alternative treatment is used and response is inadequate, discontinue it and use the preferred treatment before stepping up.
- If clear benefit is not observed within 4–6 weeks and patient/family medication technique and adherence are satisfactory, consider adjusting therapy or alternative diagnosis.
- Studies on children 0–4 years of age are limited. Step 2 preferred therapy is based on Evidence A. All other recommendations are based on expert opinion and extrapolation from studies in older children.

FIGURE 22-7 Stepwise approach for managing asthma in children 0–4 years of age. (Reproduced with permission from reference 1.)

ventilatory cycle.[1] Wheezing is a whistling sound produced by turbulent airflow through a constricted opening and usually is more prominent on expiration. Thus, the audible expiratory wheezing in Q.C. is compatible with bronchial obstruction. In fact, Q.C.'s obstruction is so severe that even inspiratory wheezes and decreased air movement were detected on auscultation. It is important to realize that the classic symptom of wheezing requires turbulent airflow; therefore, effective therapy of acute asthma actually may result in increased wheezing initially as airflow increases throughout the lung. As a result, Q.C.'s increased wheezing on auscultation is compatible with her clinical improvement following the albuterol nebulizer treatments.

The coughing experienced by Q.C. is another common finding associated with acute asthma attacks. The coughing may be due to stimulation of "irritant receptors" in the bronchi by the chemical mediators of inflammation (e.g., leukotrienes) that are released from mast cells or to the mechanics of smooth muscle contraction.

In the progression of an asthma attack, the small airways become completely occluded during expiration, and air can be trapped behind the occlusion; therefore, the patient has to breathe at higher-than-normal lung volumes.[1] Consequently, the thoracic cavity becomes hyperexpanded, and the diaphragm is lowered. As a result, the patient must use the accessory muscles of respiration to expand the chest wall. Q.C.'s hyperinflated chest and her use of suprasternal, supraclavicular, and intercostal muscles to assist in breathing also are compatible with obstructive airway diseases.

Occlusion of the small airways, air trapping, and resorption of air distal to the obstruction can lead to atelectasis (incomplete expansion or collapse of pulmonary alveoli or

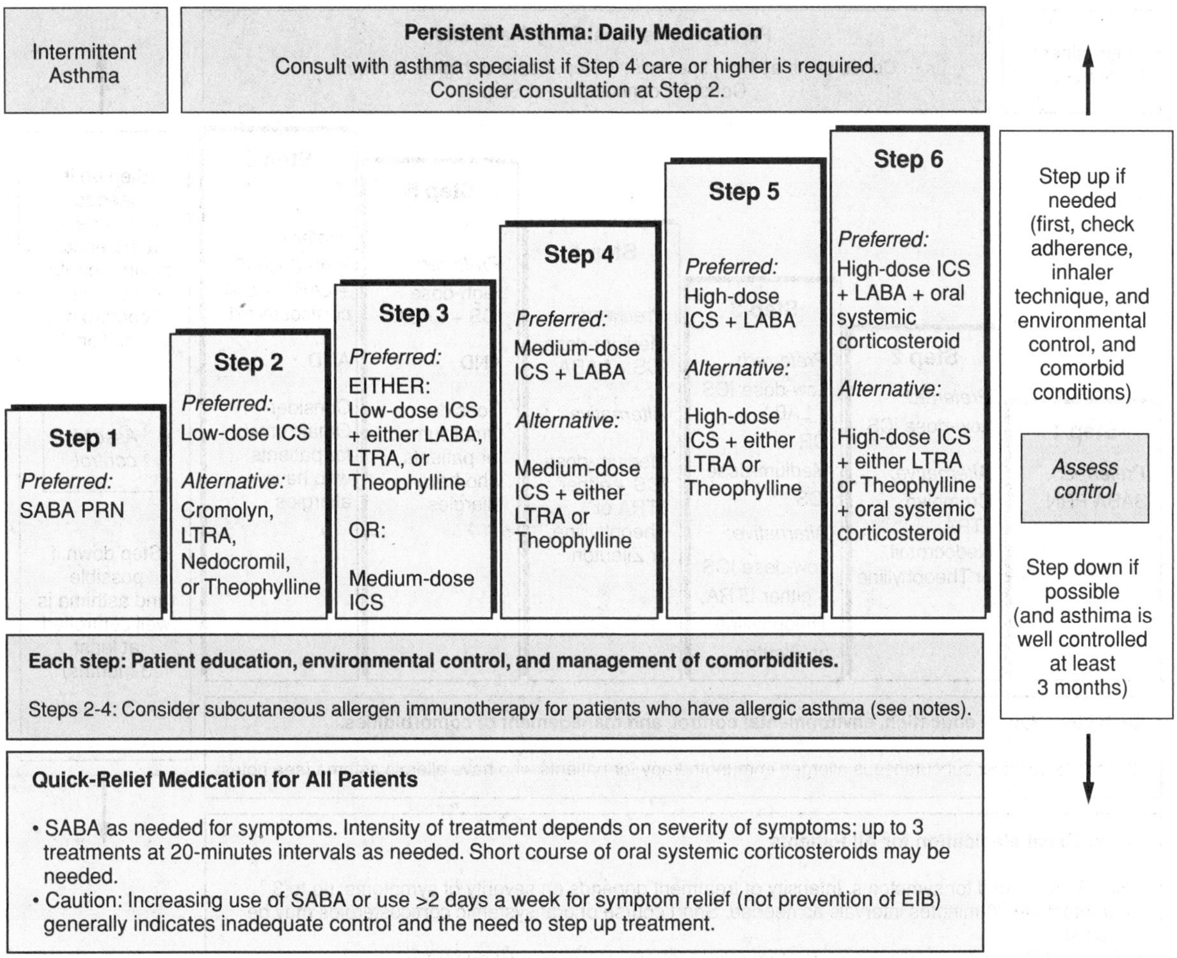
Intermittent Asthma
Persistent Asthma: Daily Medication
Consult with asthma specialist if Step 4 care or higher is required. Consider consultation at Step 2.
Step 1
Preferred: SABA PRN
Step 2
Preferred: Low-dose ICS
Alternative: Cromolyn, LTRA, Nedocromil, or Theophylline
Step 3
Preferred: EITHER: Low-dose ICS + either LABA, LTRA, or Theophylline
OR: Medium-dose ICS
Step 4
Preferred: Medium-dose ICS + LABA
Alternative: Medium-dose ICS + either LTRA or Theophylline
Step 5
Preferred: High-dose ICS + LABA
Alternative: High-dose ICS + either LTRA or Theophylline
Step 6
Preferred: High-dose ICS + LABA + oral systemic corticosteroid
Alternative: High-dose ICS + either LTRA or Theophylline + oral systemic corticosteroid
Step up if needed (first, check adherence, inhaler technique, and environmental control, and comorbid conditions)
Assess control
Step down if possible (and asthima is well controlled at least 3 months)
Each step: Patient education, environmental control, and management of comorbidities.
Steps 2-4: Consider subcutaneous allergen immunotherapy for patients who have allergic asthma (see notes).
Quick-Relief Medication for All Patients
• SABA as needed for symptoms. Intensity of treatment depends on severity of symptoms: up to 3 treatments at 20-minutes intervals as needed. Short course of oral systemic corticosteroids may be needed.
• Caution: Increasing use of SABA or use >2 days a week for symptom relief (not prevention of EIB) generally indicates inadequate control and the need to step up treatment.

Key: **Alphabetical order is used when more than one treatment option is listed within either preferred or alternative therapy.** ICS, inhaled corticosteroid; LABA, inhaled long-acting β_2-agonist, LTRA, leukotriene receptor antagonist; SABA, inhaled short-acting β_2-agonist

Notes:

- The stepwise approach is meant to assist, not replace, the clinical decisionmaking required to meet individual patient needs.
- If alternative treatment is used and response is inadequate, discontinue it and use the preferred treatment before stepping up.
- Theophylline is a less desirable alternative due to the need to monitor serum concentration levels.

FIGURE 22-8 Stepwise approach for managing asthma in children 5–11 years of age. (Reproduced with permission from reference 1.)

of a segment of lobe of the lung). Localized areas of atelectasis often are difficult to distinguish from infiltrates on a chest radiograph, and atelectasis can be mistaken for pneumonia.

Q.C.'s history of multiple bouts of "bronchitis" is significant and typical of many young asthmatics. In any patient with recurring episodes of bronchial symptoms (i.e., bronchitis, pneumonia), the possible diagnosis of asthma should be investigated.

The increased pulse, RR, and anxiety experienced by Q.C. can be attributed both to hypoxemia and the feeling of suffocation. The hypoxemia in acute asthma is due principally to an imbalance between alveolar ventilation and pulmonary capillary blood flow, also know as ventilation-perfusion ($\dot{V}/\dot{Q}$) mismatching.[20] Each alveolus of the lung is supplied with capillaries from the pulmonary artery for gas exchange. When ventilation is decreased to an area of the lung, the alveoli in that area become hypoxic, and the pulmonary artery to that region constricts as a normal physiologic response. As a result, blood flow is shunted to the well-ventilated portions of the lung because of the need to preserve adequate oxygenation of the blood. The pulmonary arteries, however, are not constricted completely, and when a small amount of blood flows to the poorly ventilated alveoli, mismatching is the result. Conditions of diffuse bronchial obstruction (i.e., acute asthma) increase the amount of mismatching. In addition, some mediators of acute bronchospasm (e.g., histamine) further worsen mismatching by constricting bronchial smooth muscle while concurrently relaxing vascular smooth muscle.

Q.C. also demonstrated a significant pulsus paradoxus. *Pulsus paradoxus* is defined as a drop in systolic BP of > 10 mmHg with inspiration. In general, pulsus paradoxus correlates with the severity of bronchial obstruction; however, it is not always present.[20]

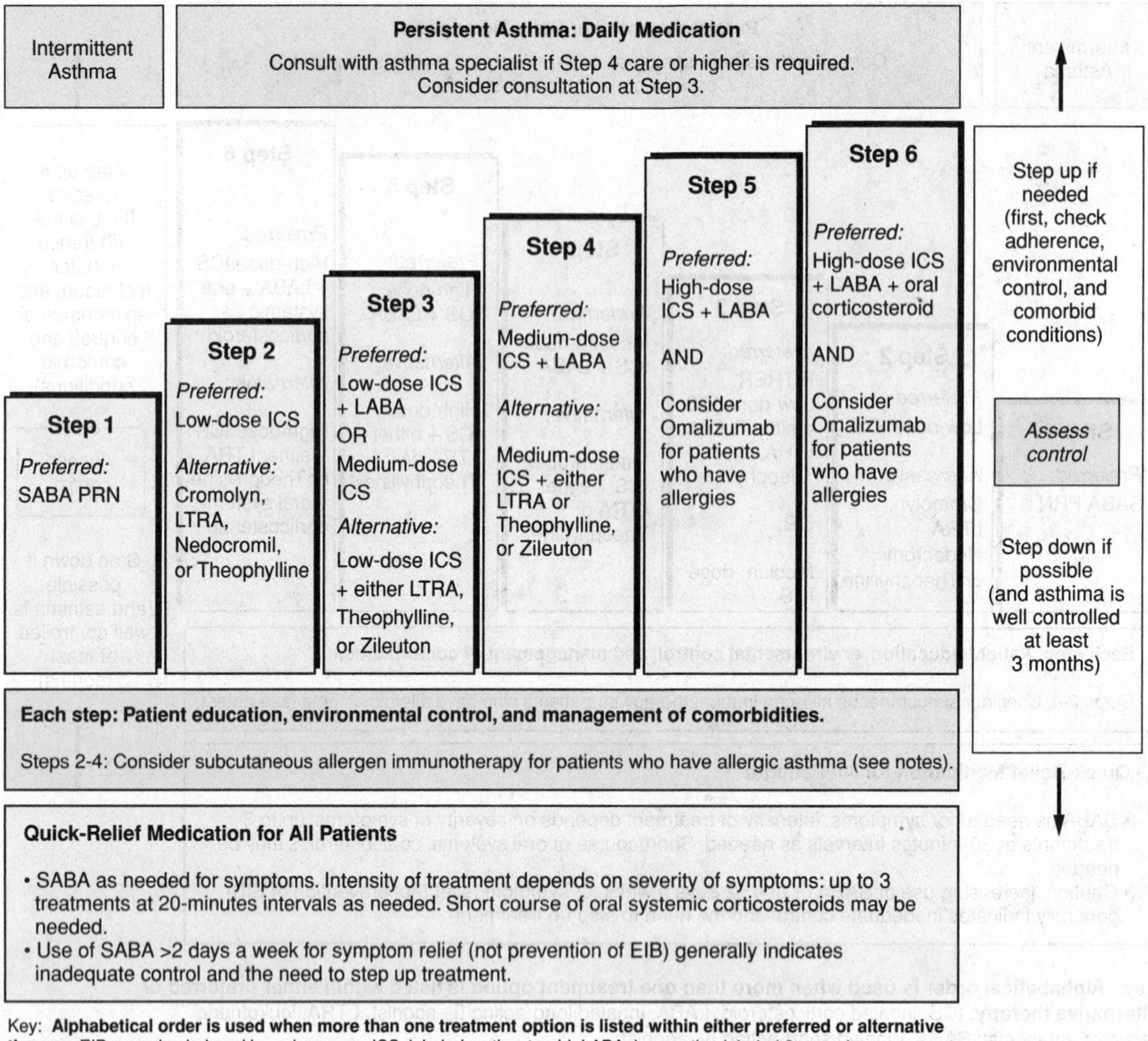
Intermittent Asthma
Persistent Asthma: Daily Medication
Consult with asthma specialist if Step 4 care or higher is required.
Consider consultation at Step 3.
Step 1
Preferred:
SABA PRN
Step 2
Preferred:
Low-dose ICS
Alternative:
Cromolyn, LTRA, Nedocromil, or Theophylline
Step 3
Preferred:
Low-dose ICS + LABA
OR
Medium-dose ICS
Alternative:
Low-dose ICS + either LTRA, Theophylline, or Zileuton
Step 4
Preferred:
Medium-dose ICS + LABA
Alternative:
Medium-dose ICS + either LTRA or Theophylline, or Zileuton
Step 5
Preferred:
High-dose ICS + LABA
AND
Consider Omalizumab for patients who have allergies
Step 6
Preferred:
High-dose ICS + LABA + oral corticosteroid
AND
Consider Omalizumab for patients who have allergies
Step up if needed (first, check adherence, environmental control, and comorbid conditions)
Assess control
Step down if possible (and asthma is well controlled at least 3 months)
Each step: Patient education, environmental control, and management of comorbidities.
Steps 2-4: Consider subcutaneous allergen immunotherapy for patients who have allergic asthma (see notes).
Quick-Relief Medication for All Patients
• SABA as needed for symptoms. Intensity of treatment depends on severity of symptoms: up to 3 treatments at 20-minutes intervals as needed. Short course of oral systemic corticosteroids may be needed.
• Use of SABA >2 days a week for symptom relief (not prevention of EIB) generally indicates inadequate control and the need to step up treatment.

Key: **Alphabetical order is used when more than one treatment option is listed within either preferred or alternative therapy.** EIB, exercise-induced bronchospasm; ICS, inhaled corticosteroid; LABA, long-acting inhaled β_2-agonist; LTRA, leukotriene receptor antagonist; SABA, inhaled short-acting β_2-agonist

Notes:

- The stepwise approach is meant to assist, not replace, the clinical decisionmaking required to meet individual patient needs.
- If alternative treatment is used and response is inadequate, discontinue it and use the preferred treatment before stepping up.
- Zileuton is a less desirable alternative due to limited studies as adjunctive therapy and the need to monitor liver function. Theophylline requires monitoring of serum concentration levels.
- In step 6, before oral systemic corticosteroids are introduced, a trial of high-dose ICS + LABA + either LTRA, theophylline, or zileuton may be considered, although this approach has not been studied in clinical trials.

FIGURE 22-9 Stepwise approach for managing asthma in youth ≥12 years of age and adults. (Reproduced with permission from reference 1.)

Extent of Obstruction

2. What additional tests would be helpful in assessing the extent of pulmonary obstruction in Q.C.?

Chest radiographs are not recommended routinely but should be obtained in patients who are suspected of a complication (e.g., pneumonia).[1] Hyperinflated lungs and areas of atelectasis can be seen on a chest x-ray film; however, chest x-ray studies usually are negative and of little value in evaluating acute asthma attacks. The finding of a local decrease in breath sounds in Q.C.'s left lung may justify the need for a chest x-ray study, particularly if a significant differential in air movement persists after initial therapy. A local decrease in breath sounds may indicate pneumonia, aspiration of a foreign object, pneumothorax, or merely thickened mucous plugging of a large bronchus.

Pulmonary function testing (e.g., FEV_1, PEF) provides objective measurement of the degree of airway obstruction. Peak flow meters are helpful in the ED for assessing both the severity of airway obstruction and the response to bronchodilator therapy. Unfortunately, infants and many young children do not have the cognitive or motor skills necessary to perform pulmonary function tests. EPR-3 points out that in one study, only 65% of children 5 to 16 years of age could complete either FEV_1 or PEF during an acute exacerbation. Because of Q.C.'s initial anxiety, the PEF should be measured after bronchodilator therapy has been initiated when she may be calmer. One disadvantage of pulmonary function tests in acute asthma is that the forced expiratory maneuver commonly triggers coughing. ABG measurements are the gold standard for assessing very severe airway obstruction.[21] EPR-3[1] suggests ABGs for evaluation of PCO_2 in patients who have suspected hypoventilation, severe distress, or FEV_1 or PEF <25% of predicted after initial treatment. However, in less severe exacerbations, ABG measurements are unnecessary if other objective measures of airway obstruction (e.g., pulmonary function tests) have been monitored.[1] In acute asthma, ABG determinations usually indicate hypoxemia because of mismatching and hypocapnia with respiratory alkalosis because of hyperventilation.[21] The degree of hypoxemia correlates with the severity of obstruction. Severe hypoxemia (PO_2 <50 mmHg) that is associated with an FEV_1 <15% of predicted represents very severe airway obstruction.[20,21] Likewise, when the FEV_1 is <25% of the predicted value, carbon dioxide increasingly is retained and the PCO_2 begins to rise into the usual normal range.[1] Because of mismatching and the ease of correction of hypoxemia with oxygen therapy, the PCO_2 is the more sensitive indicator of ventilation abnormalities in acute asthma with prolonged or chronic airway obstruction; carbon dioxide retention (hypercapnia) and respiratory acidosis are prominent. ABG measurements are indicated in patients who fail to respond adequately to initial therapy or in patients requiring hospitalization; they are not indicated at this time for Q.C. A repeat pulse oximetry at 1 hour after treatment initiation is warranted in Q.C. to ensure adequate arterial oxygen saturation.

Need for Hospitalization

3. Q.C. may require hospitalization. Which clinical test is predictive of the need for admission or whether Q.C. will relapse if sent home from the ED? Are Q.C.'s signs and symptoms predictive of whether she will relapse and return to the ED if not hospitalized?

The most useful predictive tool is the FEV_1 or PEF response to initial treatment. Patients who do not improve to at least 40% of predicted FEV_1 or PEF after initial intensive therapy are more likely to require hospitalization.[1] Although Q.C. is not able to perform spirometry, she is able to execute the PEF maneuver, and the plan is to check her PEF after 1 hour of therapy. Signs and symptom scores alone are not adequate to predict outcome of ED treatment of asthma, but scores along with pulse oximetry and PEF or FEV_1 are helpful predictors.[1]

Short-Acting Inhaled β-Adrenergic Agonist Therapy

Short-Acting Inhaled β-Agonists Compared With Other Bronchodilators

4. Why was a SABA selected as the bronchodilator of first choice in preference to other bronchodilators such as aminophylline or ipratropium for Q.C.?

Because of their potency and rapidity of action, inhaled β_2-agonists are considered the first choice for the treatment of acute asthma.[1–5] The bronchodilatory properties of SABAs are particularly effective in reversing early-phase asthma responses. Aminophylline (a theophylline salt) is not as efficacious and has more risks for serious adverse effects than inhaled albuterol.[1–5] Similarly, the bronchodilation from the anticholinergic drug ipratropium is of smaller magnitude than with short-acting inhaled β_2-agonists.[1–5] However, two double-blind pediatric trials found that the sickest children had a reduced rate of hospitalization if given ipratropium with albuterol in the ED.[22,23] In one trial,[22] children with baseline FEV_1 <30% of predicted value had a reduced rate of admission with ipratropium, and in the other trial,[23] children with baseline PEF <50% had a reduced rate of hospital admission. Consequently, although early addition of inhaled ipratropium in adequate doses to SABAs will improve pulmonary function tests and reduce the rate of hospitalization in severely ill patients, Q.C.'s physician chose to use only inhaled short-acting β_2-agonists initially because Q.C. was not severely ill.

Preferred Routes of Administration

5. What is the preferred route of administration for short-acting bronchodilators?

It is well documented that SABAs administered by the inhaled route provide as great or greater bronchodilation with fewer systemic side effects than either the parenteral or oral routes.[1–6] In situations of acute bronchospasm, concerns over adequate penetration of aerosols into the bronchial tree led many clinicians to believe that the parenteral route of administration would be more effective than the inhaled route of administration. In clinical trials, however, SABAs were as effective as the standard treatment of subcutaneous epinephrine for ED treatment of acute asthma in adults and children.[1–6,24] Therefore, short-acting aerosolized β_2-agonists now are considered the agents of choice for ED or hospital management of asthma.[1] β_2-Agonists should not be administered orally to treat acute episodes of severe asthma because of the slow onset of action, lower efficacy, and erratic absorption.[1]

6. Q.C. received albuterol by nebulization. Would intermittent positive-pressure breathing (IPPB) or metered-dose aerosol administration of the SABA have been preferred? Is the dose given by nebulization the same as that given by a metered-dose inhaler (MDI)?

Aerosols are mixtures of particles (e.g., a drug–lipid mixture) suspended in a gas. An MDI consists of an aerosol canister and an actuation device (valve). The drug in the canister is a suspension or solution mixed with propellant. The valve controls the delivery of drug and allows the precise release of a premeasured amount of the product (Fig. 22-10). A second aerosol device, the air jet nebulizer, mechanically produces a mist of drug. The drug is placed in a small volume of solute (typically 3 mL of saline) and then placed in a small reservoir (nebulizer) connected to an air source such as a small compressor pump, oxygen tank, or wall air hose. Air travels from the relatively large-diameter tubing of the air source into a pinhole-sized opening in the nebulizer. This creates a negative pressure at the site of the air entry and causes the drug solution in the bottom of the nebulizer reservoir to be drawn up through a small capillary tube where it then encounters the rapid airflow. The drug solution is forced against a small baffle that causes mechanical formation of a mist (Fig. 22-11). IPPB devices aerosolize drugs in a similar manner as air jet nebulizers except that the airflow that exits the nebulizer in an IPPB device is enhanced to exceed atmospheric pressure. An ultrasonic nebulizer is a type of nebulizer that uses sound waves to generate the aerosol.

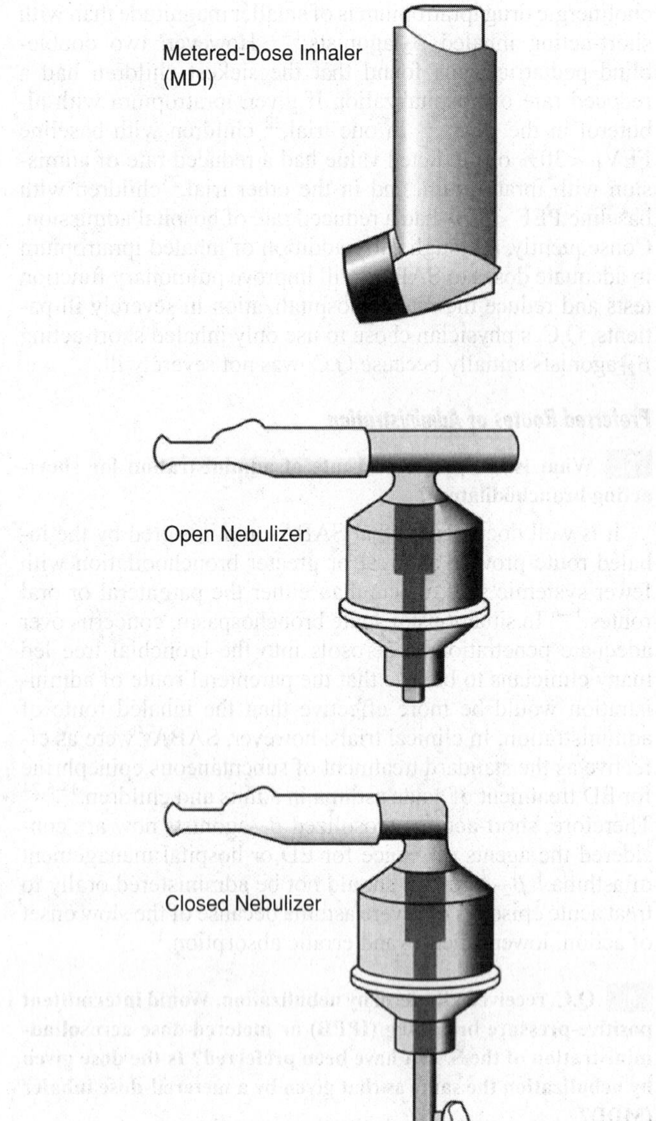

FIGURE 22-10 Metered-dose inhaler and nebulizer.

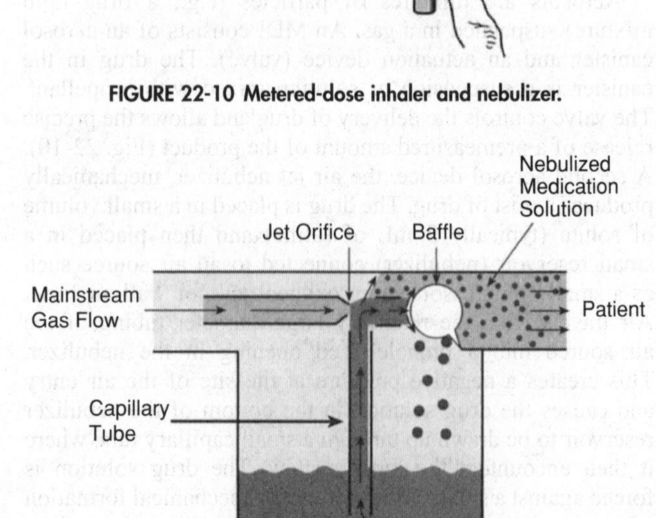

FIGURE 22-11 Air jet nebulizer.

Studies comparing responses to SABAs administered by nebulization versus IPPB have shown no significant advantages for the IPPB method of administration.[5] Furthermore, dose-response studies that compared nebulization with IPPB and pressurized metered-dose aerosols in stable chronic asthma patients have shown no advantage among these methods of administration when equivalent doses are administered.[5,25,26] Each method delivers approximately 10% of the beginning dose to the patient's airways.[27] Trials comparing metered-dose aerosols of short-acting inhaled β_2-agonists with the nebulization of those same drugs in acute asthma also have shown no significant advantage for the nebulization method of administration when the metered-dose aerosolized administration was carefully supervised by experienced personnel and a spacer device was used.[28,29] However, in some younger acutely ill children, it is difficult (even with supervision) to administer an effective SABA with a metered-dose canister. Because many patients and clinicians *perceive* that nebulizers provide more intensive therapy, it often is important psychologically to give at least the first dose of a SABA via a nebulizer. Thereafter, it is more cost-effective to use the therapeutically equivalent MDI plus spacer.[30]

The dose ratio for SABAs delivered by MDI plus spacer versus nebulizer has varied in the literature. For children with mild acute asthma, 2 puffs of albuterol MDI attached to a spacer were not different from 6 to 10 puffs of albuterol or via nebulizer 0.15 mg/kg.[31] In one double-blind trial in children with a severe exacerbation, investigators used a dose ratio of 1:5 (i.e., albuterol MDI-spacer 1 mg [10 puffs]: nebulized albuterol 5 mg).[32] Nebulization of albuterol with compressed air or, preferably, oxygen was the preferred method of administration for Q.C. initially.

DOSING

7. Starting 20 minutes after the first albuterol dose, two more doses of 2.5 mg of albuterol were administered by nebulizer Q 20 minutes over the next 40 minutes. After three treatments, Q.C.'s breath sounds became increasingly clear. She was no longer in distress and could speak in complete sentences. Her PEF was now 70% of predicted, her SaO_2 was 97% on room air, and discharge to home was planned. Were the dose and dosing interval of albuterol appropriate for Q.C.?

Schuh et al.[33] demonstrated that a higher-dose albuterol regimen (0.15 mg/kg vs. 0.05 mg/kg every 20 minutes) produced significantly greater improvement with no greater incidence of adverse effects. Schuh et al.[34] subsequently reported greater efficacy of albuterol in a dose of 0.3 mg/kg (up to 10 mg) hourly over a dose of 0.15 mg/kg (up to 5 mg) hourly in children. The larger dose was tolerated as well as the 0.15 mg/kg dose. Therefore, Q.C.'s albuterol regimen of 2.5 mg (0.13 mg/kg) nebulized every 20 minutes for 40 minutes subsequent to her first dose of aerosolized albuterol could have been even more aggressive but was appropriate. Figure 22-12 and Table 22-5 list the doses for inhaled β-agonists for acute asthma as well as doses of other medications.[1]

COMPARISON OF SHORT-ACTING INHALED β_2-AGONISTS

8. Would another SABA have been more effective in the initial therapy of Q.C.?

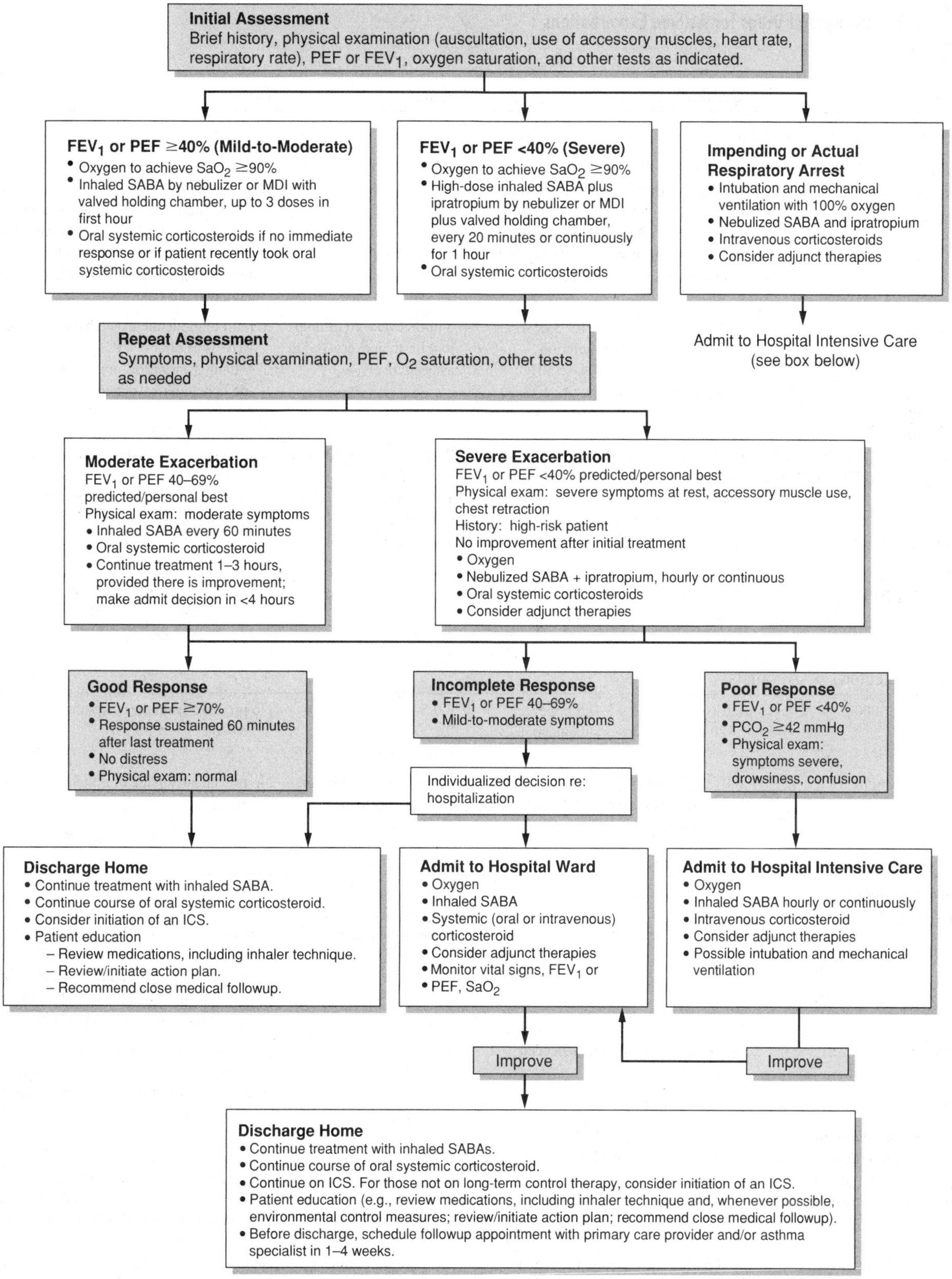

Initial Assessment
Brief history, physical examination (auscultation, use of accessory muscles, heart rate, respiratory rate), PEF or FEV_1, oxygen saturation, and other tests as indicated.
FEV_1 or PEF ≥40% (Mild-to-Moderate)
• Oxygen to achieve SaO_2 ≥90%
• Inhaled SABA by nebulizer or MDI with valved holding chamber, up to 3 doses in first hour
• Oral systemic corticosteroids if no immediate response or if patient recently took oral systemic corticosteroids
FEV_1 or PEF <40% (Severe)
• Oxygen to achieve SaO_2 ≥90%
• High-dose inhaled SABA plus ipratropium by nebulizer or MDI plus valved holding chamber, every 20 minutes or continuously for 1 hour
• Oral systemic corticosteroids
Impending or Actual Respiratory Arrest
• Intubation and mechanical ventilation with 100% oxygen
• Nebulized SABA and ipratropium
• Intravenous corticosteroids
• Consider adjunct therapies
Admit to Hospital Intensive Care (see box below)
Repeat Assessment
Symptoms, physical examination, PEF, O_2 saturation, other tests as needed
Moderate Exacerbation
FEV_1 or PEF 40–69% predicted/personal best
Physical exam: moderate symptoms
• Inhaled SABA every 60 minutes
• Oral systemic corticosteroid
• Continue treatment 1–3 hours, provided there is improvement; make admit decision in <4 hours
Severe Exacerbation
FEV_1 or PEF <40% predicted/personal best
Physical exam: severe symptoms at rest, accessory muscle use, chest retraction
History: high-risk patient
No improvement after initial treatment
• Oxygen
• Nebulized SABA + ipratropium, hourly or continuous
• Oral systemic corticosteroids
• Consider adjunct therapies
Good Response
• FEV_1 or PEF ≥70%
• Response sustained 60 minutes after last treatment
• No distress
• Physical exam: normal
Incomplete Response
• FEV_1 or PEF 40–69%
• Mild-to-moderate symptoms
Individualized decision re: hospitalization
Poor Response
• FEV_1 or PEF <40%
• PCO_2 ≥42 mmHg
• Physical exam: symptoms severe, drowsiness, confusion
Discharge Home
• Continue treatment with inhaled SABA.
• Continue course of oral systemic corticosteroid.
• Consider initiation of an ICS.
• Patient education
– Review medications, including inhaler technique.
– Review/initiate action plan.
– Recommend close medical followup.
Admit to Hospital Ward
• Oxygen
• Inhaled SABA
• Systemic (oral or intravenous) corticosteroid
• Consider adjunct therapies
• Monitor vital signs, FEV_1 or
• PEF, SaO_2
Admit to Hospital Intensive Care
• Oxygen
• Inhaled SABA hourly or continuously
• Intravenous corticosteroid
• Consider adjunct therapies
• Possible intubation and mechanical ventilation
Improve
Improve
Discharge Home
• Continue treatment with inhaled SABAs.
• Continue course of oral systemic corticosteroid.
• Continue on ICS. For those not on long-term control therapy, consider initiation of an ICS.
• Patient education (e.g., review medications, including inhaler technique and, whenever possible, environmental control measures; review/initiate action plan; recommend close medical followup).
• Before discharge, schedule followup appointment with primary care provider and/or asthma specialist in 1–4 weeks.

Key: FEV_1, forced expiratory volume in 1 second; ICS, inhaled corticosteroid; MDI, metered dose inhaler; PCO_2, partial pressure carbon dioxide; PEF, peak expiratory flow; SABA, short-acting β_2-agonist; SaO_2, oxygen saturation

FIGURE 22-12 Management of asthma exacerbations: emergency department and hospital-based care. (Reprinted with permission from reference 1.)

Table 22-5 Dosages of Drugs for Asthma Exacerbations

	Dosages		
Medication	***Child Dose[a]***	***Adult Dose***	***Comments***
Inhaled Short-Acting β_2-Agonists			
Albuterol			
Nebulizer solution (0.63 mg/3 mL, 1.25 mg/3 mL, 2.5 mg/3 mL, 5.0 mg/mL)	0.15 mg/kg (minimum dose 2.5 mg) every 20 min for 3 doses, then 0.15–0.3 mg/kg up to 10 mg every 1–4 hr as needed or 0.5 mg/kg/hr by continuous nebulization.	2.5–5 mg every 20 min for 3 doses, then 2.5–10 mg every 1–4 hr as needed or 10–15 mg/hr continuously.	Only selective β_2-agonists are recommended. For optimal delivery, dilute aerosols to minimum of 3 mL at gas flow of 6–8 L/min. Use large volume nebulizers for continuous administration. May mix with ipratropium nebulizer solution.
MDI (90 mcg/puff)	4–8 puffs every 20 min for 3 doses, then every 1–4 hr inhalation maneuver as needed. Use VHC; add mask in children <4 yr.	4–8 puffs every 20 min up to 4 hr, then every 1–4 hr as needed.	In mild to moderate exacerbations, MDI plus VHC is as effective as nebulized therapy with appropriate administration technique and coaching by trained personnel.
***Levalbuterol* (R-albuterol)**			
Nebulizer solution (0.63 mg/3 mL, 1.25 mg/0.5 mL, 1.25 mg/3 mL)	0.075 mg/kg (minimum dose 1.25 mg) every 20 min for 3 doses, then 0.075–0.15 mg/kg up to 5 mg every 1–4 hr as needed.	1.25–2.5 mg every 20 min for 3 doses, then 1.25–5 mg every 1–4 hr as needed.	Levalbuterol administered in one half the mg dose of albuterol provides comparable efficacy and safety. Has not been evaluated by continuous nebulization.
MDI (45 mcg/puff)	See albuterol MDI dose.	See albuterol MDI dose.	
Pirbuterol			
MDI (200 mcg/puff)	See albuterol MDI dose; thought to be half as potent as albuterol on a milligram basis.	See albuterol MDI dose.	Has not been studied in severe asthma exacerbations.
Systemic (Injected) β_2-Agonists			
***Epinephrine* 1:1,000 (1 mg/mL)**	0.01 mg/kg up to 0.3–0.5 mg every 20 min for 3 doses subcutaneously	0.3–0.5 mg every 20 min for 3 doses subcutaneously	No proven advantage of systemic therapy over aerosol.
***Terbutaline* (1 mg/mL)**	0.01 mg/kg every 20 min for 3 doses, then every 2–6 hr as needed subcutaneously	0.25 mg every 20 min for 3 doses subcutaneously	No proven advantage of systemic therapy over aerosol.
Anticholinergics			
Ipratropium bromide			
Nebulizer solution (0.25 mg/mL)	0.25–0.5 mg every 20 min for 3 doses, then as needed.	0.5 mg every 20 min for 3 doses, then as needed.	May mix in same nebulizer with albuterol. Should not be used as first-line therapy; should be added to SABA therapy for severe exacerbations. The addition of ipratropium has not been shown to provide further benefit once the patient is hospitalized.
MDI (18 mcg/puff)	4–8 puffs every 20 min as needed up to 3 hr.	8 puffs every 20 min as needed up to 3 hr.	Should use with VHC and face mask for children <4 yr. Studies have examined ipratropium bromide MDI for up to 3 hr.
Ipratropium with albuterol			
Nebulizer solution (Each 3 mL vial contains 0.5 mg ipratropium bromide and 2.5 mg albuterol.)	1.5 mL every 20 min for 3 doses, then as needed.	3 ml every 20 min for 3 doses, then as needed.	May be used for up to 3 hr in the initial management of severe exacerbations. The addition of ipratropium to albuterol has not been shown to provide further benefit once the patient is hospitalized.
MDI (Each puff contains 18 mcg ipratropium bromide and 90 mcg albuterol.)	4–8 puffs every 20 min as needed up to 3 hr.	8 puffs every 20 min as needed up to 3 hr.	Should use with VHC and face mask for children <4 yr.

(continued)

Table 22-5 Dosages of Drugs for Asthma Exacerbations (*Continued*)

Medication	*Child Dose*[a]	*Adult Dose*	*Comments*
Systemic Corticosteroids			
	(Applies to all three corticosteroids.)		
Prednisone ***Methyl prednisolone*** ***Prednisolone***	1 mg/kg in 2 divided doses (maximum = 60 mg/day) until PEF is 70% of predicted or personal best.	40–80 mg/day in 1 or 2 divided doses until PEF reaches 70% of predicted or personal best.	For outpatient "burst," use 40–60 mg in single or 2 divided doses for total of 5–10 days in adults (children: 1–2 mg/kg/day maximum 60 mg/day for 3–10 days).

[a]Children, 12 yr of age.
MDI, metered-dose inhaler; PEF, peak expiratory flow; SABA, short-acting β_2-agonist; VHC, valved holding chamber
Reprinted from reference 1.

Short-acting β_2-specific agonists (e.g., albuterol) are preferred over nonspecific agonists (e.g., isoproterenol). Long-acting β_2-agonists (e.g., salmeterol) are not indicated for treatment of asthma in the ED. Levalbuterol (R-albuterol) became available in the late 1990s, but further study is needed to determine whether this single isomer, higher-potency drug offers any clinically significant advantages (i.e., improved outcomes) over racemic albuterol to justify its higher cost.[1,35]

Systemic Corticosteroids in the Emergency Department for Children

9. Should Q.C. receive corticosteroid therapy as part of her ED management?

Yes. Because asthma is primarily an inflammatory airway disease, the degree of inflammation associated with Q.C.'s current exacerbation should be considered. Per EPR-3[1] (Fig. 22-12), if there is not an immediate response to inhaled β_2-agonist therapy, oral systemic corticosteroids should be administered (refer to further discussion of this subject in Questions 14 and 15). Furthermore, if Q.C. had a peak flow meter at home, earlier objective detection of the development of this exacerbation might have prevented an ED visit. When the PEF is in the red zone (<50% of personal best) and poorly responsive to SABAs, early intervention with oral corticosteroids is associated with a reduction in ED visits[1] (Fig. 22-13; refer to the Outcomes section at the end of the chapter). Q.C. and her parents should also understand that if respiratory distress is severe and nonresponsive to treatment, they should proceed to an ED or call 911. Finally, before going home from the ED, Q.C. and her parents should receive some basic education regarding asthma and its acute and long-term management. It is important to follow-up with more detailed education during future clinic visits. Based on EPR-3,[1] Q.C. should receive a short course of systemic corticosteroids as part of her discharge plan, thereby reducing her risk of re-exacerbation. Typically, oral prednisolone solution at a dose of 1 to 2 mg/kg in daily or divided doses twice daily is given for approximately 5 to 7 days. While this regimen is very effective, to improve compliance, several studies have examined shorter (1–2 day) courses of oral or intramuscular dexamethasone and have found similar results when compared with usual regimens of oral prednisone/prednisolone.[36–38]

ADVERSE EFFECTS

10. H.T., a 45-year-old, 91-kg man with a long history of severe persistent asthma, presents to the ED with severe dyspnea and wheezing. He is able to say only two or three words without taking a breath. He has been taking four inhalations of beclomethasone HFA (80 mcg/puff) BID and two inhalations of albuterol MDI QID PRN on a chronic basis. H.T. ran out of beclomethasone a week ago; since then, he has been using his albuterol MDI with increasing frequency up to Q 3 hr on the day before admission. He is a lifelong nonsmoker. His FEV_1 was 25% of the predicted value for his age and height, and his SaO_2 was 82%. Vital signs are as follows: heart rate, 130 beats/minute; RR, 30/minute; pulsus paradoxus, 18 mmHg; and BP, 130/90 mmHg. ABGs on room air were as follows: pH, 7.40; PaO_2, 55 mmHg; and $PaCO_2$, 40 mmHg. Serum electrolyte concentrations were sodium (Na), 140 mEq/L; potassium (K), 4.1 mEq/L; and chloride (Cl), 105 mEq/L. Because of the severity of the obstruction, H.T. was monitored with an electrocardiogram (ECG) that showed sinus tachycardia with occasional premature ventricular contractions (PVCs). Terbutaline 0.5 mg SC was administered with minimal improvement. H.T. then was started on O_2 at 4 L/minute by nasal cannula, followed by another injection of 0.5 mg terbutaline SC. Subsequently, H.T.'s heart rate increased to 145 beats/minute, more PVCs appeared on the ECG, and he complained of palpitations and shakiness. His PEF was now 25% of personal best. Laboratory values were pH, 7.39; PaO_2, 60 mmHg; $PaCO_2$, 42 mmHg; Na, 138 mEq/L; and K, 3.5 mEq/L. What adverse effects experienced by H.T. are consistent with systemic β_2-agonist administration?

H.T. experienced palpitations, which may have been due to the widening of his pulse pressure from vasodilation or the PVCs.[3] Albuterol, terbutaline, and all other β–agonists are cardiac stimulants that may cause tachycardia and, very rarely, arrhythmias. Because they are relatively β_2-specific, the cardiac effects are more prominent with systemic administration (as opposed to inhalation) and at higher dosages. However, other causes of cardiac effects must also be considered, such as hypoxemia, which is also a potent stimulus for cardiac arrhythmias Therefore, H.T.'s tachycardia and PVCs may have been caused by the β_2-agonist, by the worsening of his airway obstruction (as reflected in the increase in $PaCO_2$), or by both of these variables.

The decrease in the serum potassium concentration from 4.1 mEq/L to 3.5 mEq/L could be attributed to β_2-adrenergic activation of the Na^+-K^+ pump and subsequent transport of potassium intracellularly.[39,40] However, at usual doses, aerosolized albuterol and terbutaline cause relatively little effect on serum potassium. The effects may be more noticeable with systemic (oral or injectable) administration. A β_2-adrenergic–mediated increase in glucose and insulin secretion also can contribute to the intracellular shift of potassium.[39]

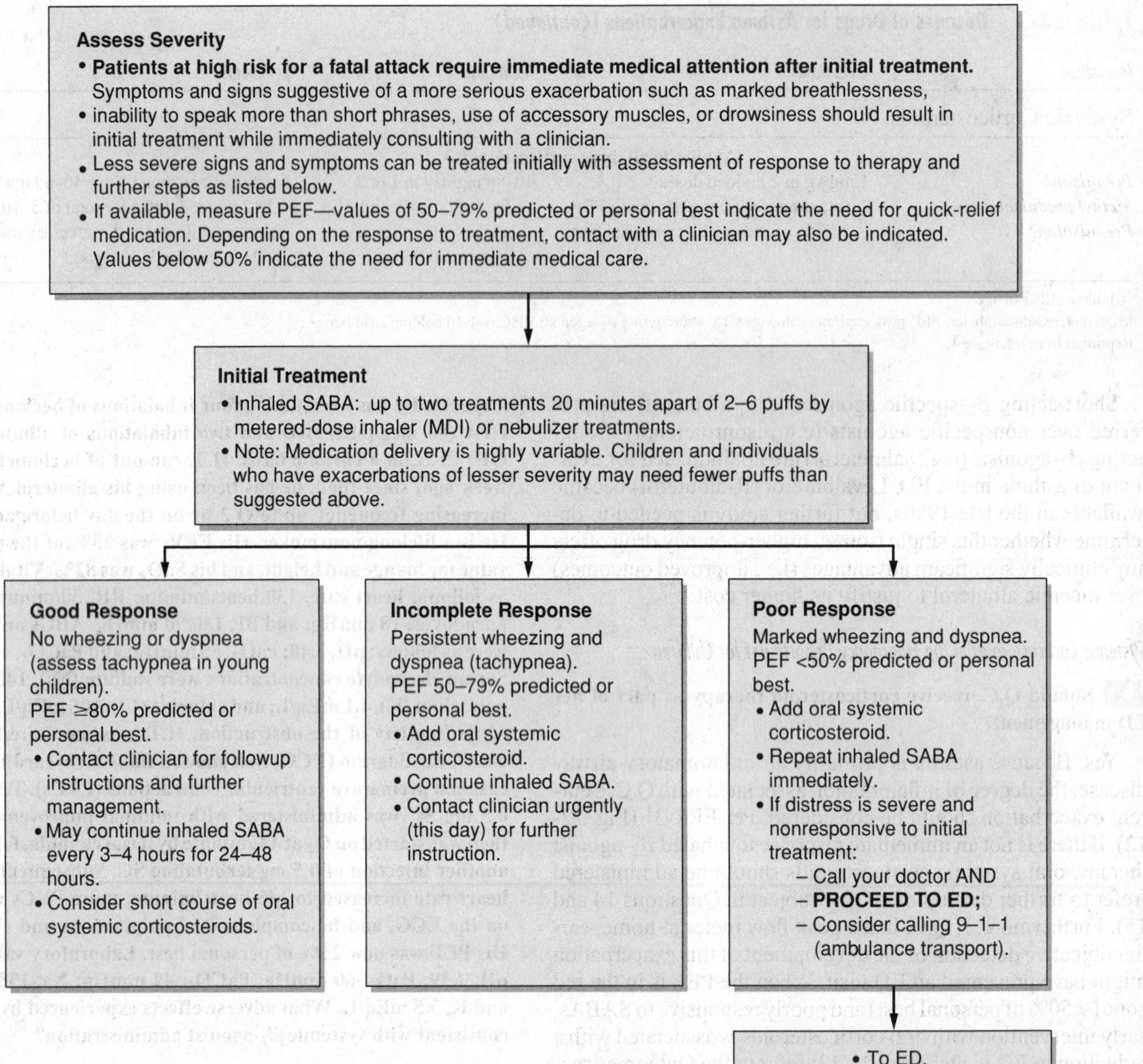
Assess Severity
• Patients at high risk for a fatal attack require immediate medical attention after initial treatment.
Symptoms and signs suggestive of a more serious exacerbation such as marked breathlessness,
• inability to speak more than short phrases, use of accessory muscles, or drowsiness should result in initial treatment while immediately consulting with a clinician.
• Less severe signs and symptoms can be treated initially with assessment of response to therapy and further steps as listed below.
• If available, measure PEF—values of 50–79% predicted or personal best indicate the need for quick-relief medication. Depending on the response to treatment, contact with a clinician may also be indicated. Values below 50% indicate the need for immediate medical care.
Initial Treatment
• Inhaled SABA: up to two treatments 20 minutes apart of 2–6 puffs by metered-dose inhaler (MDI) or nebulizer treatments.
• Note: Medication delivery is highly variable. Children and individuals who have exacerbations of lesser severity may need fewer puffs than suggested above.
Good Response
No wheezing or dyspnea (assess tachypnea in young children).
PEF ≥80% predicted or personal best.
• Contact clinician for followup instructions and further management.
• May continue inhaled SABA every 3–4 hours for 24–48 hours.
• Consider short course of oral systemic corticosteroids.
Incomplete Response
Persistent wheezing and dyspnea (tachypnea).
PEF 50–79% predicted or personal best.
• Add oral systemic corticosteroid.
• Continue inhaled SABA.
• Contact clinician urgently (this day) for further instruction.
Poor Response
Marked wheezing and dyspnea.
PEF <50% predicted or personal best.
• Add oral systemic corticosteroid.
• Repeat inhaled SABA immediately.
• If distress is severe and nonresponsive to initial treatment:
– Call your doctor AND
– PROCEED TO ED;
– Consider calling 9–1–1 (ambulance transport).
• To ED.

Key: ED, emergency department; MDI, metered-dose inhaler; PEF, peak expiratory flow; SABA, short-acting β_2-agonist (quick-relief inhaler)

FIGURE 22-13 Management of asthma exacerbations: home treatment. (Reproduced with permission from reference 1.)

H.T.'s potassium dropped from 4.1 to 3.5 mEq/L. Part of this drop may have been due to the terbutaline injections.

The shakiness (tremors) experienced by H.T. probably can be attributed to β_2-receptor stimulation of skeletal muscle. Again, this effect is most prominent with oral or parenteral administration, but some patients are very sensitive to even small doses of SABAs. To minimize adverse effects, H.T. should have been given frequent high doses of inhaled albuterol rather than SC terbutaline on admission to the ED. He should have also initially been given nebulized ipratropium in addition to albuterol because his FEV_1 was <30% predicted.

β-Adrenergic Agonist Subsensitivity

11. Why did H.T. fail to respond to the initial therapy? Could tolerance to the β_2-agonists have contributed?

Although tolerance to systemic effects of β_2-agonists (e.g., tremor, sleep disturbances) is documented, tolerance to the airway response does not occur to a clinically significant extent.[41] Even with long-term use, the intensity of response to β_2-agonists is retained (i.e., the maximal percent increase in pulmonary function), but the duration of response with each dose may shorten. Such an effect is unlikely with intermittent use but may occur in patients who routinely use large, multiple doses daily. Possible explanations for this variability include downregulation of receptors, disease progression, or true drug tolerance. The exact contribution of each is not known. Therefore, H.T.'s failure to respond to the initial therapy most likely is due to the severity of his airway obstruction. H.T.'s history of severe chronic asthma, the slow progression of this attack, and the lack of response to his inhaled β_2-agonist also are largely due to a significant inflammatory component to this attack.

Thus, bronchodilators would not be expected to immediately reverse the airway obstruction in H.T. It would be difficult to attribute his lack of initial response to therapy to β_2-adrenergic subsensitivity. In addition, it is not likely that β_2-adrenergic receptor polymorphisms could account for H.T.'s initial lack of response.[42]

Although polymorphic variations are documented to be relevant in some stable patients,[1] further study is needed to establish clinical relevance.

Short-Acting Inhaled β-Agonists in Combination With Theophylline

12. When would the addition of theophylline to H.T.'s therapy be indicated?

Studies on the treatment of acute asthma in the ED have failed to demonstrate any benefit of adding theophylline to optimal, inhaled β-agonist therapy,[1,43] and the NIH guidelines do not recommended this practice.[1–6] Further evidence of the lack of value of theophylline in the acute-care setting emerged in the 1990s. Several double-blind, randomized, placebo-controlled studies have demonstrated that theophylline does not add benefit to intensive therapy with inhaled β_2-agonists and systemic corticosteroids in hospitalized adults[44] or children[45–48] who fail to respond to aggressive ED therapy with SABAs. Note in Figure 22-12 from EPR-3[1] that theophylline is not recommended for routine management of hospitalized patients with asthma. Although one study[49] has shown a slight benefit of theophylline in hospitalized adult asthmatics, one of the authors of that study has since noted that if adequate doses of SABAs and systemic corticosteroids are used, theophylline is probably not routinely indicated.[50] While further research is needed to establish whether theophylline may add benefit to hospitalized patients who have impending respiratory failure, routine use of theophylline in hospitalized asthmatics no longer is justified.

13. Repeat measurements of PEF and ABGs indicate continued significant bronchial obstruction. What should be the next step in H.T.'s therapy?

H.T. should have had therapy initiated with inhaled SABAs and certainly now should be changed from systemic to an aerosolized β-agonist. Because of the concern for cardiac toxicity, a β_2-selective agent such as albuterol should be selected. Three or four doses of albuterol, 5 mg by nebulizer administered every 20 minutes, should be started immediately with continuous monitoring of H.T.'s cardiac status. H.T.'s PEF (or preferably FEV_1) also should be monitored.

Short-Acting Inhaled β-Agonists in Combination With Corticosteroids

14. Are systemic corticosteroids appropriate for H.T.? When can a response be expected?

Corticosteroids have potent anti-inflammatory activity and are definitely indicated in H.T.[1–6] In patients like H.T. with acute asthma, corticosteroids decrease airway inflammation[51–54] and increase the response to β_2-selective agonists.[1,51]

Corticosteroids are not smooth muscle relaxants (i.e., not bronchodilators); however, they can relieve bronchial obstruction by improving the responsiveness of β_2-receptors and by inhibiting numerous phases of the inflammatory response (e.g., cytokine production, neutrophil and eosinophil chemotaxis and migration, and release of inflammatory mediators).[1–6]

The anti-inflammatory activity of corticosteroids is delayed for about 4 to 6 hours after the dose has been administered. Corticosteroid-induced restoration of responsiveness to endogenous catecholamines and exogenous β_2-agonists, however, occurs within 1 hour of administration of the corticosteroid in severe, chronic, stable asthmatics.[51] Significant improvement in objective measures (e.g., FEV_1) generally occurs 12 hours after administration.[53] Consequently, EPR-3[1] advocates early initiation of corticosteroids in cases of acute severe asthma. Corticosteroids also hasten the recovery of acute exacerbations of asthma[55–59] and decrease the need for hospitalization if given early in the initial management of acute asthma in the ED.[54]

Based on his initial presentation, H.T. should be started on systemic corticosteroid therapy immediately in the ED (Fig. 22-12). Preferably, oral corticosteroids would have been started at home before H.T.'s exacerbation escalated to this degree of severity (Fig. 22-13).

15. What would be an appropriate dosing regimen of corticosteroids for H.T. in the ED? Would the dose and route be the same if he were hospitalized?

Doses of corticosteroids used to treat acute asthma are largely empiric. Studies comparing very high dosages (e.g., intravenous [IV] methylprednisolone 125 mg every 6 hours in an adult) versus moderate dosages (40 mg every 6 hours) have shown no advantage with very high dosages.[1,60,61] In addition, oral therapy is as efficacious as the IV route.[1,60,61] Dosing recommendations for systemic corticosteroids in the management of asthma exacerbations in the ED or hospital are shown in Table 22-5. Higher corticosteroid dosages may be considered in patients with impending respiratory failure. When patients cannot take oral medication, IV methylprednisolone is preferred over hydrocortisone in patients with heart disease or fluid retention or when high dosages of corticosteroids are used; this is because it has less mineralocorticoid activity.

For patients who require IV corticosteroid therapy, the dosage can usually be reduced rapidly to 60 to 80 mg/day for adults (1–2 mg/kg/day for children) as the condition improves (usually after 48–72 hours). On discharge from the hospital, EPR-3 recommends, for example, prednisone 40 to 80 mg/day in one or two doses for 3 to 10 days. Although some clinicians may prescribe a tapering regimen, no taper is necessary in this situation. On the other hand, if the patient required long-term oral corticosteroid therapy before hospitalization, tapering the dose to the preadmission dosage is prudent. For patients who are discharged from the ED, ≤7 days of prednisone therapy usually is sufficient.

16. H.T. was given one dose of 60 mg methylprednisolone (Solu-Medrol) IV and three doses of albuterol 5 mg/ipratropium 0.5 mg by nebulizer Q 20 minutes in the ED (after the two initial doses of SC terbutaline). H.T. claimed slight subjective improvement after this therapy; yet, expiratory wheezes still were audible, and he still was using his accessory muscles for ventilatory efforts. His PEF improved only to 35% of predicted, and a repeat ABG measurement showed a $PaCO_2$ of 40 mmHg. What should be done at this time?

H.T. still is significantly obstructed despite intensive therapy in the ED. As a result, he should be admitted to the intensive care unit (ICU), where he can be monitored closely.

Respiratory Failure

Signs and Symptoms

17. What would be the best method of assessing the adequacy of therapy in H.T.? What are the signs of impending respiratory failure?

When patients continually must expand their chest wall with high lung volumes over a prolonged period, respiratory muscle fatigue may ensue, resulting in a decreased ventilatory effort. Clinical signs of impending respiratory failure include increased heart rate, decreased breath sounds, agitation from worsening hypoxia, or lethargy from increased CO_2 retention. These clinical signs and symptoms are relatively nonspecific and are affected by many variables. Thus, they should not be used to detect impending respiratory failure.

The best way to assess therapy is to monitor ABGs. The PaO_2 component of an ABG determination is not very helpful because of $\dot{V}/\dot{Q}$ mismatching and the administration of oxygen. The $PaCO_2$ is the best indicator of hypoventilation in acute asthma[1]; however, there is no single value for $PaCO_2$ that indicates impending respiratory failure, because different $PaCO_2$ values are acceptable under different clinical circumstances. A $PaCO_2$ of 55 mmHg 1 to 2 hours after intensive bronchodilator therapy or an increase in $PaCO_2$ of 5 to 10 mmHg/hour during aggressive therapy is an ominous sign. The fact that H.T.'s $PaCO_2$ is not rising with therapy is a good sign.

β_2-Agonists and Other Potential Therapies

18. H.T. initially received two doses of terbutaline 0.5 mg SC and subsequently three doses of albuterol 5 mg/ipratropium 0.5 mg by nebulizer Q 20 minutes in the ED. He has also received IV methylprednisolone 60 mg. Would the IV administration of a β-agonist be indicated in H.T. at this time? What are other potential therapies in H.T.?

Although the use of IV β-agonists for asthmatics in the ICU formerly was advocated, current standards of care discourage the use of these agents.[1] H.T.'s history of PVCs and response to inhaled albuterol also suggest that IV β-agonists are inappropriate at this time. Since standard therapies already administered were not sufficient, IV magnesium sulfate may benefit severely ill patients like H.T.[1,62] Recent research suggests that nebulized isotonic magnesium sulfate is a valuable adjunctive therapy to inhaled albuterol in the treatment of severe asthma exacerbations.[63] Further, heliox (a mixture of helium and oxygen) may also add benefit.[1,64]

Theophylline

19. Intravenous theophylline is being considered for H.T. Is theophylline likely to be of benefit in impending respiratory failure?

It was stated previously that there is no role for theophylline in ED treatment, and its use is not justified for routine hospital admissions for asthma.[1] However, two studies suggest a potential benefit of theophylline for some patients in the ICU who have impending respiratory failure.[65,66] The authors of these studies point out that if theophylline is used, clinicians must be competent in dosing and monitoring serum concentrations. Based on a lack of evidence in several trials in hospitalized asthmatics,[54–58] more trials are needed to evaluate if possible benefits outweigh risks of this drug for impending respiratory failure. Based on inconclusive evidence of improved patient response but documented increased risks, EPR-3 does not recommend the use of theophylline in the hospital.[1] H.T.'s clinicians decide not to use theophylline. If a clinician decides to use theophylline in this setting, a current pharmacokinetics text should be consulted to help ensure safe and effective dosing and monitoring.[67]

RESPONSE TO THERAPY

20. H.T. has continued to improve slowly over the last 72 hours. The nebulizer treatments with albuterol are now administered Q 4 hr, and he is taking oral prednisone 80 mg/day in two divided doses. PEF measurements taken before and after the last albuterol treatment were 65% of predicted and 80% of predicted, respectively. Is H.T.'s long duration of recovery unusual?

No. In a patient such as H.T., whose condition progressively deteriorated over a long period, a slow reversal should be expected. The prolonged deterioration reflects an increasing inflammatory response in the lung. These patients require prolonged, intensive bronchodilator and anti-inflammatory therapy before maximal improvement is noted in pulmonary function tests. Thus, H.T. should continue to receive systemic corticosteroids for approximately 10 days after such a severe acute exacerbation of asthma.[1]

Adverse Effects of Short-Term Corticosteroid Therapy

21. H.T. has been taking corticosteroids for a total of 6 days. Long-term corticosteroid use is associated with many adverse effects (e.g., adrenal suppression, osteoporosis, cataracts). What adverse effects are related to short-term corticosteroid use?

Short courses of daily corticosteroids are usually associated with minor side effects.[55–59] Facial flushing, appetite stimulation, gastrointestinal irritation, headache, and mood changes ranging from a mere sense of well-being to overt toxic psychosis are the most commonly encountered adverse effects of short-term corticosteroid therapy. Acne can be exacerbated in patients susceptible to this skin problem, and weight gain also can occur because of sodium and fluid retention. In addition, hyperglycemia, leukocytosis, and hypokalemia are possible. All of these problems are transient and will disappear over time after the corticosteroids are discontinued. These short-term adverse effects are less common when small corticosteroid doses are used; however, corticosteroid doses must be adequate to prevent disease exacerbation. The minor risks of short-term use are far outweighed by the marked benefits.

Overuse of Short-Acting Inhaled β-Agonists

22. H.T.'s history of increased use of his SABA inhaler during the early stages of this asthma attack and the cardiac irregularities noted during admission suggest improper use of this medication. What are the risks from overuse of β_2-agonists?

The overuse of SABAs as a possible risk factor for asthma death has been debated for decades, and this debate was revived in the early 1990s.[68] Because most deaths from asthma occur outside the hospital setting before the patient can reach medical assistance, the primary cause of death in asthma most probably is due to underestimation of the severity of the asthma attack by the patient and delay in seeking medical help. Overuse of quick reliever medication suggests inadequate asthma control and can lead to fatal asthma.[1,68]

The frequency of as-needed doses of albuterol is a good marker of the adequacy of inhaled anti-inflammatory therapy and environmental control measures. For example, if the patient needs the SABA more than two or three times a day, the clinician should reassess environmental control, increase the dose of inhaled anti-inflammatory therapy, or add other controller agents per the NIH guidelines.[1–6]

Patients should be instructed verbally and in writing regarding the proper use of their inhalers during acute attacks and in recognizing when it is necessary to seek medical assistance (Fig. 22-13). Patients can continue using their short-acting β-agonist inhalers on an as-needed basis until they reach medical care. H.T. should be considered at high risk because of the severity of his latest attack and should be given oral corticosteroids to self-administer at the first sign of significant deterioration.[1] In addition, H.T. should have a home peak flow meter so that he can objectively determine the severity of his attacks. Finally, the β_2-agonist controversy does not extend to use of high dosages in the acute-care setting. High dosages are essential in the ED and hospital and, as discussed previously, usually are tolerated very well.

CHRONIC ASTHMA

Classification of Severity

23. **B.C. is a 3-year-old, 16-kg boy with a 1.5-year history of recurrent wheezing 3 days per week and nocturnal awakenings four times per month.**

The following medications had been prescribed for B.C. by the primary care clinician: albuterol syrup (2 mg/5 mL) 1 teaspoonful TID and albuterol metered-dose aerosol inhalation QID PRN for wheezing. B.C. demonstrates the use of the inhaler with his mother's assistance. The mother holds the inhaler in B.C.'s mouth and actuates it at the end of a deep inhalation. B.C.'s mother tells the clinician that he appears "jittery" after taking albuterol syrup. What is the first step in deciding how to improve B.C.'s long-term drug therapy?

While keeping in mind the goals of therapy defined by the NIH guidelines (EPR-3),[1] the first step here is to classify B.C.'s asthma severity (refer to Table 22-1 for infants to age 4 years). Because B.C. has symptoms 3 days per week and 4 nights per month, he should be classified as "moderate persistent." Note that the presence of even one of the features of severity places the patient in that category.

Selection of Appropriate Initial Long-Term Therapy

24. **What would be a reasonable initial regimen for B.C.?**

Because B.C.'s asthma is classified as moderate persistent, the clinician is now in a position to select appropriate long-term therapy. Using EPR-3[1] for very young children (Fig. 22-7), low- or medium-dose inhaled corticosteroids (ICS) with an as-needed SABA would be the choice for B.C.[1] EPR-3 suggests an initial trial of low dose ICS in very young children who have not previously been treated with ICS. B.C. could receive ICS treatments via nebulizer (budesonide) or MDI + spacer. Most children aged 3 years or younger cannot use dry powder inhalers because of inability to generate sufficient peak inspiratory flow (PIF). As B.C. matures, he may be able to use some dry powder inhalers (e.g. Diskus). Because oral β_2-agonists are not recommended by EPR-3 and since the albuterol syrup was not well tolerated, they should not be used. If concurrent inhaled albuterol is administered correctly, PO albuterol is not needed and would only be expected to add adverse effects. B.C.'s mother must be educated about asthma, its treatment, and the appropriate use of medications (e.g., proper use of inhaler devices; refer to Questions 45 and 46).

25. **It is anticipated that because of his young age, B.C. will find it difficult to use an MDI. What alternative inhalation devices are reasonable?**

Children younger than 5 five years of age generally have a difficult time coordinating the use of standard MDIs; therefore, the ICS and short-acting β_2-agonist should be administered by another mode of delivery. For example, the as-needed β_2-agonist and scheduled ICS could be administered with an inhalational aid such as a spacer or valved holding chamber, which is connected to an MDI. A nebulized corticosteroid preparation (budesonide) is available for very young children.[69] Inhalation aids (also called *spacers*) significantly improve the efficacy of medications that are administered by MDI in very young children or other patients who are unable to coordinate the plain inhalers correctly.[70] The AeroChamber is a widely used valved holding chamber (the medication stays in the chamber for a few seconds until the patient inhales slowly and the inhalation valve opens). An example of a simple open tube device (i.e., without an inhalation valve) is the integrated spacer with the triamcinolone MDI (Azmacort). Studies have shown that many children as young as 2 and 3 years of age can use MDIs with spacer devices by modeling after a parent.[71,72] Spacer devices with face masks are required for some young children. Extender device-assisted delivery of aerosolized medications is as effective as nebulization in the home management of chronic severe asthma[73] and even in the ED treatment of asthma in children.[30–32,73] The InspirEase and AeroChamber are examples of devices that contain a flow indicator whistle that sounds if the patient inhales rapidly. This whistle is particularly effective in teaching the patient the appropriate slow inhalation technique. As a 3-year-old, B.C. may not need a spacer with a face mask, but the clinician should verify correct use of the device by observation of the patient and/or caregiver's administration technique.

Alternatively, the ICS could be administered to selected children by using a breath-activated dry powder inhaler (e.g., budesonide [Pulmicort Flexhaler] or fluticasone [combined with salmeterol in Advair Diskus]). In young children, Diskus has the advantage of requiring lower PIF than Flexhaler, and it has been used successfully in children as young as 4 years of age.[74] Another option is the Twisthaler used for delivery of mometasone (Asmanex), but it is only approved for children $\geq$12 years of age.

Many pediatricians may choose a nebulizer to administer short-acting β_2-agonists to a 3-year-old child. This method is certainly acceptable and very common, but it takes longer to administer the medication (about 15 minutes), and the device must be properly cleaned and maintained. Because B.C. recently turned 3 years old, therapy should be initiated with nebulized budesonide (Pulmicort Respules) in a low dose of 0.25 mg BID. As mentioned previously, EPR-3[1] suggests an initial trial of low-dose ICS in very young children who have not previously been treated with ICS. The plan is to switch B.C. to a dry powder inhaler or MDI-spacer in 12 months, as soon as he and his caregiver can demonstrate correct use. B.C.'s clinician should assess the response to low-dose budesonide in 4 weeks. Therapy can be stepped up if necessary and subsequently stepped down over the coming months, if possible, so that optimal asthma control is achieved at the lowest ICS dose possible.

26. B.C.'s parents are wary of their son taking corticosteroids on a continual basis after having read about serious side effects attributed to corticosteroids on the Internet. How should the parents be counseled?

Corticosteroids reach the systemic circulation minimally via inhalation in part because they are largely inactivated through first-pass hepatic metabolism. However, a dose-dependent response is evident, and clinically significant adverse events resulting from systemic exposure can occur, albeit more commonly with doses at the high end of the range. Long-term studies in pediatric patients have examined the effects of ICS on growth reduction, bone density, and adrenal suppression.

Although ICS can cause a mild and temporary reduction in growth velocity, final height attained in adulthood appears to be within normal limits.[75] Bone density and risk of fractures have not been found in the vast majority of investigations to be affected by ICS.[75] While a measurable reduction in serum and urinary cortisol levels is not an uncommon finding in studies of ICS, clinically significant adrenal insufficiency solely due to ICS is rare, although again it is more likely to occur with high doses.[75] In summary, these adverse effects are generally of minimal clinical significance, with the benefits of well-controlled asthma far outweighing the risks.

The most common local side effect with ICS therapy is oropharyngeal candidiasis (thrush), but this problem is rare with any delivery system. With MDIs, it can be further minimized by use of a spacer device. Rinsing the mouth with water after use of any ICS is also recommended. Another possible local side effect is hoarseness (dysphonia), and spacers may not effectively reduce this problem.[76] Dry powder devices (e.g., Flexhaler) may have less dysphonia associated with their use, but further study is required to verify this.[76]

Seasonal Asthma

27. C.V., a 33-year-old woman, presents to the clinic with a history of asthma and seasonal allergic rhinitis ("hay fever") each spring but not the rest of the year. She describes her asthma as "mild" and intermittent. Except during springtime, her daytime symptoms occur less than once per week, and she does not have nocturnal symptoms. Each spring, however, these symptoms worsen, and she requires her albuterol inhaler (her only asthma medication) TID or QID every day. During springtime, she takes a nonprescription antihistamine, which offers some relief. How can C.V.'s management be improved?

C.V. appears to have intermittent asthma during most of the year but converts to moderate persistent asthma combined with worsening rhinitis symptoms in the springtime. This syndrome is consistent with a diagnosis of seasonal asthma and allergic rhinitis. Although as-needed albuterol is appropriate for most of the year for C.V., she needs anti-inflammatory therapy during the spring.[1] Therapy to reduce airway inflammation should begin before the onset of tree and grass pollen season and continue throughout the spring (e.g., 3 months). Per the NIH guidelines, an excellent treatment option for C.V. is low-dose ICS combined with a long-acting inhaled β_2-agonist (LABA). Monotherapy with medium-dose ICS would also be an acceptable therapy. Not only are the causes and pathophysiology of allergic rhinitis and allergic asthma similar, poorly controlled rhinitis serves as a major asthma trigger. In addition, C.V. should also ideally receive an intranasal corticosteroid if antihistamines (preferably nonsedating) do not provide optimal relief of her allergic rhinitis. Intranasal corticosteroid therapy not only offers excellent relief of nasal symptoms but also improves asthma control.[6] Good control of rhinitis is helpful in maintaining optimal asthma control[1,2] (see Chapter 24, Acute and Chronic Rhinitis). Despite precautions listed in manufacturer literature that older (sedating) antihistamines should be avoided in asthma, these agents are safe in patients with asthma.[1,2]

Corticosteroids

28. S.T., a 12-year-old girl with severe persistent asthma, has not been well controlled on mometasone (Asmanex) one inhalation daily (she admits to using it only when she feels as if she needs it) and uses as-needed inhaled albuterol MDI five or six times every day. When her symptoms worsen, she uses her "breathing machine" (nebulizer) at home. S.T. awakens most nights with wheezing. She has been hospitalized four times in the last 2 years and has required "bursts" of prednisone with increasing frequency. S.T. has missed many days of school in the past year and has withdrawn from physical education classes and her extracurricular sports activity after school. Her parents are concerned about her increased use of prednisone now that she is approaching puberty. S.T. is just finishing a 2-week course of prednisone 20 mg/day and has a round facies appearance typical of chronic oral corticosteroid use. On physical examination, S.T. has diffuse expiratory wheezes, and pulmonary function testing reveals significant reversibility. Her FEV_1 is only 60% predicted before use of albuterol in the physician's office and improves to 75% predicted 15 minutes after use of the SABA. What actions are needed to improve S.T.'s care?

Because S.T. is suffering needlessly and requiring frequent systemic corticosteroids, all efforts must be made to optimize other therapies and to minimize systemic corticosteroid toxicities. Although S.T. is receiving an ICS, she admits to poor adherence. Therefore, with her severe persistent asthma, she initially needs higher-dose ICS therapy. Per EPR-3,[1] she should also receive a LABA. Although short "bursts" of prednisone (e.g., 40 mg/day for 3 days) are very helpful occasionally, frequent short courses often indicate the need to optimize other therapies. Some patients require courses of 1 to 2 weeks. S.T. is requiring longer frequent bursts and is showing signs of adverse effects. Obviously, S.T. and her parents also need a concerted

Table 22-6 Estimated Comparative Daily Dosages for Inhaled Corticosteroids in Children

	Low Daily Dose		Medium Daily Dose		High Daily Dose	
Drug	Child 0–4 Years	Child 5–11 Years	Child 0–4 Years	Child 5–11 Years	Child 0–4 Years	Child 5–11 Years
Beclomethasone HFA						
40 or 80 mcg/puff	NA	80–160 mcg	NA	>160–320 mcg	NA	>320 mcg
Budesonide DPI						
90, 180, or 200 mcg/inhalation	NA	180–400 mcg	NA	>400–800 mcg	NA	>800 mcg
Budesonide inhaled						
Inhalation suspension for nebulization	0.25–0.5 mg	0.5 mg	>0.5–1 mg	1 mg	>1 mg	2 mg
Flunisolide						
250 mcg/puff	NA	500–750 mcg	NA	1,000–1,250 mcg	NA	>1,250 mcg
Flunisolide HFA						
80 mcg/puff	NA	160 mcg	NA	320 mcg	NA	>640 mcg
Fluticasone						
HFA/MDI: 44, 110, or 220 mcg/puff	176 mcg	88–176 mcg	>176–352 mcg	>176–352 mcg	>352 mcg	>352 mcg
DPI: 50, 100, or 250 mcg/inhalation	NA	100–200 mcg	NA	>200–400 mcg	NA	>400 mcg
Mometasone DPI						
200 mcg/inhalation	NA	NA	NA	NA	NA	NA
Triamcinolone acetonide						
75 mcg/puff	NA	300–600 mcg	NA	>600–900 mcg	NA	>900 mcg

DPI, dry powder inhaler; HFA, hydrofluoroalkane; MDI, metered-dose inhaler; NA, not approved and no data available for this age group.
Reprinted from reference 1.

and persistent effort in patient education as a partnership (refer to Patient Education and Outcomes section).

ICS are chemically modified to maximize topical effectiveness while minimizing systemic toxicities. Tables 22-6 and 22-7 are taken from EPR-3[1–5] and compare the dosages of ICS products. These differences in dosages (low, medium, and high) reflect differences among ICS in receptor-binding affinity and topical potency. There are also differences among these agents in oral bioavailability (i.e., absorption of drug that is swallowed after inhalation) and systemic availability via absorption from the lungs. Of these two variables, absorption from the lungs is the most likely contributor to possible hypothalamic-pituitary-adrenal (HPA) suppression or other systemic effects. Fortunately, the total absorption has not been shown to be clinically important except at the higher recommended dosages. Although the various ICS are not equipotent on a microgram-per-microgram basis, major differences in efficacy or adverse effects are not firmly established.[1,75,77] For patients with severe

Table 22-7 Estimated Comparative Daily Dosages for Inhaled Corticosteroids for Youths ≥12 Years of Age and Adults

Drug	Low Daily Dose Adult	Medium Daily Dose Adult	High Daily Dose Adult
Beclomethasone HFA			
40 or 80 mcg/puff	80–240 mcg	>240–480 mcg	>480 mcg
Budesonide DPI			
90, 180, or 200 mcg/inhalation	180–600 mcg	>600–1,200 mcg	>1,200 mcg
Flunisolide			
250 mcg/puff	500–1,000 mcg	>1,000–2,000 mcg	>2,000 mcg
Flunisolide HFA			
80 mcg/puff	320 mcg	>320–640 mcg	>640 mcg
Fluticasone			
HFA/MDI: 44, 110, or 220 mcg/puff	88–264 mcg	>264–440 mcg	>440 mcg
DPI: 50, 100, or 250 mcg/inhalation	100–300 mcg	>300–500 mcg	>500 mcg
Mometasone DPI			
200 mcg/inhalation	200 mcg	400 mcg	>400 mcg
Triamcinolone acetonide			
75 mcg/puff	300–750 mcg	>750–1,500 mcg	>1,500 mcg

DPI, dry powder inhaler; HFA, hydrofluoroalkane: MDI, metered-dose inhaler.
Reprinted from reference 1.

persistent asthma, a logical choice would be a high-potency agent that would allow for a minimum number of inhalations per day, potentially improving treatment adherence. Furthermore, the delivery system used affects pulmonary deposition. For example, the Turbuhaler delivers about twice the dose of budesonide versus an MDI and is associated with excellent efficacy if used correctly.[78] Clinical trials evaluating fluticasone efficacy administered via the Diskus have likewise shown excellent efficacy.[79] The differences between the various dry powder inhalers is discussed later in this chapter. Addition of a spacer device to an MDI also enhances pulmonary deposition. In very high dosages (the equivalent of 1,600 mcg/day of beclomethasone dipropionate), all ICS produce some degree of HPA-axis suppression.[75] The clinical significance of this suppression has yet to be firmly established.

Although low to moderate dosages of ICS are accepted as being quite safe, very high dosages continue to be scrutinized regarding the potential adverse effects.[80] Clearly, for patients who require high dosages for optimal control of asthma, the benefits of therapy with these agents far outweigh the risks.[1,75] A possible association between prolonged, very high dosages of ICS and cataracts[81] and glaucoma[82] has been reported. EPR-3 has summarized recent research that has allayed concerns regarding use of ICS therapy and growth suppression in children (i.e., the decrease in growth velocity is small, not progressive, and appears to be reversible).[1,83,84]

29. How should S.T. be managed?

In the treatment of S.T., most clinicians would begin with a short course (e.g., 1 week) of systemic corticosteroids to maximally improve her pulmonary function. This approach is consistent with EPR-3[1], which recommends gaining quick control. Using short-course systemic therapy is logical because it is inexpensive, efficacious, and associated with low risk. While gaining quick control with a short course of oral corticosteroids, it is logical to start ICS in many patients at a low[1,85] to moderate dosage (as defined in Tables 22-6 and 22-7). The evidence that ICS are highly effective in persistent asthma is unequivocal. Patients in this category who consistently take ICS are at a lower risk of hospitalization and death, and one study found an increased risk of death after discontinuation of ICS compared with patients who remained on these drugs.[86,87] ICS therapy should be initiated concomitantly with a short course of systemic corticosteroid therapy. Patient education at this time may have greater effectiveness, because some patients are more attentive after having just experienced an exacerbation, and they know that change is needed to improve their health. Because S.T.'s asthma is classified as *severe* persistent, it is reasonable to start her on a moderate to high dosage of an ICS in combination with a LABA (Fig. 22-9 and Table 22-3). More aggressive therapy initially is especially important in S.T. because of her four hospitalizations in the last 2 years. In partnership with S.T. and her parents, her preference should be determined as to the delivery method (i.e., discuss options with her regarding breath-activated devices or MDI and spacer, including which spacer). Ideally, the clinician should recognize her emerging independence as a 12 year old and talk with her alone and then with her parents. After S.T. is stabilized for 3 months, attempts should be made to slowly decrease the ICS dosage every 3 months until the lowest-effective dosage is achieved. Administration of the total daily ICS dose is preferred twice daily or in many patients, with mild to moderate persistent asthma, once daily.[1] Since adherence is a major determinant of success or failure with ICS and other therapies, simplified regimens and continued patient education and contact are essential.[1]

Combination of Inhaled Corticosteroids and Long-Acting Inhaled β_2-Agonists

30. Because S.T. is 12 years old, what options are appropriate to minimize the ICS dosage, realizing that aggressive therapy is needed? What are the risks associated with LABAs? Clinicians should monitor for which local side effects in S.T. with ICS therapy?

LABAs have been very successful in prevention of "stepping up" the dose of ICS while markedly enhancing overall asthma control,[78,79,88–90] and this fact is reflected in EPR-3[1]. A reasonable therapeutic option for S.T. would be the combination of fluticasone 500 mcg and salmeterol 50 mcg via Diskus (Advair 500) 1 inhalation BID or the budesonide/formoterol (Symbicort) combination inhaler (160 mcg/4.5 mcg; 2 inhalations BID). S.T. should be reevaluated in 2 weeks. The plan is to "step down" the dose of fluticasone after excellent asthma control is achieved.

ADVERSE EFFECTS ASSOCIATED WITH LONG-ACTING INHALED β_2-AGONISTS

31. S.T.'s parents recently discovered an article in a national newspaper that addressed concerns of using LABAs due to an increased risk of death. Since S.T.'s parents have called and left a message for the clinician, what would be important information to share with her family regarding this issue? What other side effects should S.T. and her family be aware of?

Several randomized trials for over a decade have demonstrated that LABAs have minimal adverse effects (e.g., tachycardia, tremor).[1,78,79,88–90] Although there are limited data, based primarily on one study (SMART),[91] there may be a very small increased risk of asthma-related death and asthma exacerbation in patients receiving LABAs. This small risk is likely due to patients receiving LABAs without concomitant ICS. In fact, EPR-3[1] recommends against the use of LABAs as monotherapy for long-term control of persistent asthma. SMART[91] data suggested that blacks may be at greater risk, but much more study is needed to confirm these data. LABA therapy should *only* be used in combination with ICS in patients with asthma. Combination ICS/LABA therapy for asthma is safe and effective.[1,92] EPR-3[1] suggests giving equal consideration to moderate dose of ICS alone or low-dose ICS combined with LABA for patients with moderate persistent asthma. For S.T., she has severe persistent asthma, and ICS/LABA combination therapy is preferred.[1]

STEP-DOWN TREATMENT

32. After being adherent to her new therapy (fluticasone 500 mcg/salmeterol 50 mcg BID) for 1 month, S.T.'s asthma control has markedly improved. She required no ED visits or hospitalizations, was sleeping through the night, and began to exercise again. Her personal best PEF was 320 L/minute, and she was staying in her green zone (260–320 L/minute), requiring PRN albuterol no more than once per week. After 2 more months, S.T. continues to do well. Although S.T. clearly needs long-term ICS therapy, after 3 months of excellent response, her clinician is now

ready to step down from high-dose fluticasone. What is a prudent approach to dosage reduction?

EPR-3[1] suggests stepping down the dose at a rate of 25% to 50% every 3 months to the lowest dose that maintains control. A step down to fluticasone 250 mcg/salmeterol 50 mcg (Advair 250) BID would be a reasonable reduction in therapy for S.T. If a single ICS product had been started in S.T. initially (e.g., budesonide, beclomethasone, fluticasone), the dosage reduction would normally proceed at a slower pace. However, fluticasone 500 mcg daily, especially in combination with salmeterol, will likely be an adequate dose for S.T. After S.T.'s dose of fluticasone was stepped down to 500 mcg/day, she started requiring only slightly more PRN albuterol (but still was symptom free most days).

33. If symptoms recur during step-down, what management could possibly facilitate dosage reduction of the ICS in S.T.?

During follow-up evaluations, clinicians should carefully investigate factors that may contribute to poor asthma control, including exposure to inhalant allergens, indoor/outdoor irritants, medications, and tobacco smoke. Secondhand smoke exposure has been demonstrated to negate the benefit of ICS in children, and asthma patients who smoke have reduced response to ICS therapy.[93,94]

Leukotriene Modifiers

34. P.W. is a 52-year-old man with mild persistent asthma. His asthma symptoms began when he was 2 years of age, and he has never smoked. P.W. has had numerous drug regimens for his asthma over the years, but he tells his physician that he wants the simplest regimen possible and that he prefers oral medication if at all possible. What is a good choice for controller therapy in P.W.?

In patients of any age with mild persistent asthma, and certainly in children or adolescents, an oral agent such as montelukast with once-daily dosing at bedtime (or zafirlukast with twice-daily dosing) has obvious advantages. An ICS is the preferred treatment for mild persistent asthma. Studies comparing ICS with LTRA have consistently demonstrated the superiority of ICS for most asthma outcome measures,[1] but in patients (adults or children) who much prefer oral therapy to inhaling medication every day, leukotriene modifiers are a reasonable option. The simplest and safest possible oral controller regimen for P.W. is montelukast 10 mg HS (with PRN inhaled albuterol). Bedtime dosing with montelukast is recommended because it will have peak activity late at night and in the early morning hours, when asthma symptoms tend to be more frequent. It is likely that this regimen will result in very good asthma control. If P.W. does not have good control of his asthma when he returns to the clinic in a few weeks, switching to a low-dose ICS in the evening only would keep the regimen simple while enhancing efficacy.

Cromolyn and Nedocromil

35. E.G. is a 7-year-old boy with mild persistent asthma. His family has just moved from the northeastern United States to the Midwest. E.G.'s new pediatrician notes that he has been previously managed only by "as-needed" inhaled albuterol. E.G.'s pediatrician is aware of the NIH guidelines[1] recommendation for ICS in mild persistent asthma, even in small children. However, despite recent evidence in the literature regarding the safety of ICS, she is concerned about the risks of these agents in children and is considering a trial of cromolyn or nedocromil therapy combined with strict environmental control. If the trial fails, she plans to switch to the lowest possible dosage of ICS. Should cromolyn (Intal) or nedocromil (Tilade) be added to E.G.'s β_2-agonist therapy? Is either agent preferred over theophylline or a leukotriene modifier in E.G.?

In studies of childhood asthma, cromolyn has been found to reduce symptoms and the need for acute-care visits, and this drug has an excellent safety profile.[1–6,95] Although theophylline is a relatively weak bronchodilator, it also may have very modest anti-inflammatory effects.[1,50] Note in Figure 22-8 from EPR-3[1] that theophylline, cromolyn, and nedocromil are *alternatives* as controller medications in mild persistent asthma (children 5–11 years of age). Nedocromil is an effective anti-inflammatory agent, especially for mild persistent asthma,[1] and is similar to cromolyn in efficacy and tolerability.[1] Cromolyn and nedocromil have similar mechanisms of action as anti-inflammatory agents, and their mechanisms are compared with other agents in Table 22-8.

Based on efficacy and safety concerns and the need to monitor serum theophylline concentrations, either cromolyn or nedocromil is a better option for E.G.'s controller therapy. E.G. can learn to use an MDI plus spacer device with proper teaching, but the concern is adherence to therapy with the required QID or TID dosing schedule. Cromolyn MDI two puffs QID would be an appropriate regimen here. Therapy should be continued for at least 4 weeks to determine response.

A simpler approach to managing mild persistent asthma in a young child whose physician does not choose the preferred low-dose ICS therapy is once-daily montelukast.[1] Taking a 5-mg cherry chewable montelukast tablet at bedtime is preferred as an option in E.G. over cromolyn, nedocromil, or theophylline.

Theophylline

Dosing

36. K.J., a 14-year-old, 40-kg girl, has a history of recurring cough and wheezing. These symptoms worsen on vigorous running or when she has an upper respiratory infection. She has not required hospitalization for these symptoms but has missed a few school days. She has symptoms daily and uses her pirbuterol inhaler more than two times daily. K.J. has a family history of asthma. A diagnosis of moderate persistent asthma is made. How should K.J. be managed?

Because K.J. has moderate persistent asthma, treatment with an anti-inflammatory agent is indicated. Low to moderate–dose ICS in combination with a LABA is the preferred treatment in a 14-year-old child with moderate persistent asthma.[1] However, K.J.'s clinician opts to prescribe theophylline in combination with a low dose of budesonide via the Flexhaler.

37. What dosage of theophylline is appropriate for K.J.?

Low doses of budesonide combined with twice-daily theophylline that resulted in a median serum theophylline concentration of 8.7 mcg/mL was superior in efficacy to high-dose budesonide as single controller therapy.[96] Thus, it is wise to give a therapeutic trial with low-dose theophylline initially, aiming for serum concentrations between 5 and 10 mcg/mL.

Table 22-8 Long-Term Control Medications

Name/Products (Listed Alphabetically)	*Indications/Mechanisms*	*Potential Adverse Effects*	*Therapeutic Issues (Not All Inclusive)*
Corticosteroids (Glucocorticoids) ***Inhaled (ICS):*** Beclomethasone dipropionate Budesonide Flunisolide Fluticasone propionate Mometasone furoate Triamcinolone acetonide	*Indications* • Long-term prevention of symptoms: suppression, control, and reversal of inflammation. • Reduce need for oral corticosteroid. *Mechanisms* • Anti-inflammatory. Block late reaction to allergen and reduce airway hyperresponsiveness. Inhibit cytokine production, adhesion protein activation, and inflammatory cell migration and activation. • Reverse β_2-receptor downregulation. Inhibit microvascular leakage.	• Cough, dysphonia, oral thrush (candidiasis). • In high doses (Tables 22-6, 22-7), systemic effects may occur, although studies are not conclusive, and clinical significance of these effects has not been established (e.g., adrenal suppression, osteoporosis, skin thinning, and easy bruising). In low to medium doses, suppression of growth velocity has been observed in children, but this effect may be transient, and the clinical significance has not been established.	• Spacer/holding chamber devices with nonbreath-activated MDIs and mouth washing after inhalation decrease local side effects. • Preparations are not absolutely interchangeable on a mcg or per puff basis (Tables 22-6, 22-7 for estimated clinical comparability). New delivery devices may provide greater delivery to airways; this change may affect dose. • The risks of uncontrolled asthma should be weighed against the limited risks of ICS therapy. The potential but small risk of adverse events is well balanced by their efficacy. • "Adjustable dose" approach to treatment may enable reduction in cumulative dose of ICS treatment over time without sacrificing maintenance of asthma control. • Dexamethasone is not included as an ICS for long-term control, because it is highly absorbed and has long-term suppressive side effects.
Systemic: Methylprednisolone Prednisolone Prednisone	*Indications* • For short-term (3–10 days) "burst": to gain prompt control of inadequately controlled persistent asthma. • For long-term prevention of symptoms in severe persistent asthma. suppression, control, and reversal of inflammation. *Mechanisms* • Same as inhaled.	• Short-term use: Reversible abnormalities in glucose metabolism, increased appetite, fluid retention, weight gain, mood alteration, hypertension, peptic ulcer, and rarely aseptic necrosis. • Long-term use: Adrenal axis suppression, growth suppression, dermal thinning, hypertension, diabetes, Cushing's syndrome, cataracts, muscle weakness; in rare instances, impaired immune function. • Consideration should be given to coexisting conditions that could be worsened by systemic corticosteroids, such as herpes virus infections, varicella, tuberculosis, hypertension, peptic ulcer, diabetes mellitus, osteoporosis, and *Strongyloides*.	• Use at lowest effective dose. For long-term use, alternate-day am dosing produces the least toxicity. If daily doses are required, one study shows improved efficacy with no increase in adrenal suppression when administered at 3 PM rather than in the morning.
Cromolyn Sodium and Nedocromil	*Indications* • Long-term prevention of symptoms in mild persistent asthma may modify inflammation. • Preventive treatment prior to exposure to exercise or known allergen. *Mechanisms* • **Anti-inflammatory**. Blocks early and late reaction to allergen. Interferes with chloride channel function. Stabilizes mast cell membranes and inhibits activation and release of mediators from eosinophils and epithelial cells. • Inhibits acute response to exercise, cold dry air, and SO_2.	• Cough and irritation. • 15%–20% of patients complain of an unpleasant taste from nedocromil.	• Therapeutic response to cromolyn and nedocromil often occurs within 2 wk, but a 4- to 6-wk trial may be needed to determine maximum benefit. • Dose of cromolyn by MDI (1 mg/puff) may be inadequate to affect airway hyperresponsiveness. Nebulizer delivery (20 mg/ampule) may be preferred for some patients. • Safety is the primary advantage of these agents.

(continued)

Table 22-8 Long-Term Control Medications (*Continued*)

Name/Products (Listed Alphabetically)	*Indications/Mechanisms*	*Potential Adverse Effects*	*Therapeutic Issues (Not All Inclusive)*
Immunomodulators			
Omalizumab (anti-IgE) For subcutaneous use	*Indications* • Long-term control and prevention of symptoms in adults (≥12 yr old) who have moderate or severe persistent allergic asthma inadequately controlled with ICS. *Mechanisms* • Binds to circulating IgE, preventing it from binding to the high-affinity ($F_{CE}RI$) receptors on basophils and mast cells. • Decreases mast cell mediator release from allergen exposure. • Decreases the number of $F_{CE}RIs$ in basophils and submucosal cells.	• Pain and bruising of injection sites has been reported in 5%–20% of patients. • Anaphylaxis has been reported in 0.2% percent of treated patients. • Malignant neoplasms were reported in 0.5% of patients compared with 0.2% receiving placebo; relationship to drug is unclear.	• Monitor patients following injection. Be prepared and equipped to identify and treat anaphylaxis that may occur. • The dose is administered either every 2 or 4 wk and is dependent on the patient's body weight and IgE level before therapy. • A maximum of 150 mg can be administered in one injection. • Needs to be stored under refrigeration at 2°–8°C. • Whether patients will develop significant antibody titers to the drug with long-term administration is unknown.
Leukotriene Receptor Antagonists	*Mechanisms* • Leukotriene receptor antagonist; selective competitive inhibitor of $CysLT_1$ receptor.		• May attenuate EIB in some patients, but less effective than ICS therapy. • Do not use LTRA + LABA as a substitute for ICS + LABA.
Montelukast tablets and granules	*Indications* • Long-term control and prevention of symptoms in mild persistent asthma for patients ≥1 yr of age. May also be used with ICS as combination therapy in moderate persistent asthma.	• No specific adverse effects have been identified. • Rare cases of Churg-Strauss have occurred, but the association is unclear.	• A flat dose-response curve, without further benefit, if dose is increased above those recommended.
Zafirlukast tablets	• Long-term control and prevention of symptoms in mild persistent asthma for patients ≥7 yr of age. May also be used with ICS as combination therapy in moderate persistent asthma.	• Postmarketing surveillance has reported cases of reversible hepatitis and, rarely, irreversible hepatic failure resulting in death and liver transplantation.	• Administration with meals decreases bioavailability; take at least 1 hr before or 2 hr after meals. • Zafirlukast is a microsomal P450 enzyme inhibitor that can inhibit the metabolism of warfarin. INRs should be monitored during coadministration. • Patients should be warned to discontinue use if they experience signs and symptoms of liver dysfunction (right upper quadrant pain, pruritis, lethargy, jaundice, nausea), and serum ALTs should be monitored.
5-Lipoxygenase Inhibitor	*Mechanisms* • Inhibits the production of leukotrienes from arachidonic acid, both LTB_4 and the cysteinyl leukotrienes.		
Zileuton tablets	*Indications* • Long-term control and prevention of symptoms in mild persistent asthma for patients ≥12 yr of age. • May be used with ICS as combination therapy in moderate persistent asthma in patients ≥12 yr of age.	• Elevation of liver enzymes has been reported. Limited case reports of reversible hepatitis and hyperbilirubinemia.	• Zileuton is microsomal P450 enzyme inhibitor that can inhibit the metabolism of warfarin and theophylline. Doses of these drugs should be monitored accordingly. • Monitor hepatic enzymes (ALT).

(continued)

Table 22-8 Long-Term Control Medications (*Continued*)

Name/Products (Listed Alphabetically)	*Indications/Mechanisms*	*Potential Adverse Effects*	*Therapeutic Issues (Not All Inclusive)*
Long-Acting β_2-Agonists (LABA) *Inhaled LABA:* Formoterol Salmeterol	*Indications* • Long-term prevention of symptoms added to ICS. • Prevention of EIB. • *Not to be used to treat acute symptoms or exacerbations.* *Mechanisms* • **Bronchodilation**. Smooth muscle relaxation following adenylate cyclase activation and increase in cyclic AMP, producing functional antagonism of bronchoconstriction. • Compared with SABA, salmeterol (but not formoterol) has slower onset of action (15–30 min). Both salmeterol and formoterol have longer duration (>12 hr) compared with SABA.	• Tachycardia, skeletal muscle tremor, hypokalemia, prolongation of QTc interval in overdose. • A diminished bronchoprotective effect may occur within 1 week of chronic therapy. Clinical significance has not been established. • Potential risk of uncommon, severe, life-threatening or fatal exacerbation: see text for additional discussion regarding safety of LABAs.	• Not to be used to treat acute symptoms or exacerbations. • Should not be used as monotherapy for long-term control of asthma or as anti-inflammatory therapy. • May provide more effective symptom control when added to standard doses of ICS compared with increasing the ICS dosage. • Clinical significance of potentially developing tolerance is uncertain, because studies show that symptom control and bronchodilation are maintained. • Decreased duration of protection against EIB may occur with regular use.
Oral: Albuterol, sustained-release			• Inhaled route is preferred because LABAs are longer acting and have fewer side effects than oral sustained-release agents. Oral agents have not been adequately studied as adjunctive therapy with ICS.
Methylxanthines Theophylline, sustained-release tablets and capsules	*Indications* • Long-term control and prevention of symptoms in mild persistent asthma or as adjunctive with ICS in moderate or persistent asthma. *Mechanisms* • Bronchodilation. Smooth muscle relaxation from phosphodiesterase inhibition and possibly adenosine antagonism. • May affect eosinophilic infiltration into bronchial mucosa as well as decreases T-lymphocyte numbers in epithelium. • Increases diaphragm contractility and mucociliary clearance.	• Dose-related acute toxicities include tachycardia, nausea and vomiting, tachyarrhythmias (SVT), central nervous system stimulation, headache, seizures, hematemesis, hyperglycemia, and hypokalemia. • Adverse effects at usual therapeutic doses include insomnia, gastric upset, aggravation of ulcer or reflux, increase in hyperactivity in some children, and difficulty in urination in elderly males who have prostatism.	• Maintain steady-state serum concentrations between 5 and 15 mcg/mL. Routine serum concentration monitoring is essential due to significant toxicities, narrow therapeutic range, and individual differences in metabolic clearance. Absorption and metabolism may be affected by numerous factors that can produce significant changes in steady-state serum theophylline concentrations. • Patients should be told to discontinue if they experience toxicity. • Not generally recommended for exacerbations. There is minimal evidence for added benefit to optimal doses of SABA. Serum concentration monitoring is mandatory.

ALT, alanine aminotransferase; Anti-IgE, anti-immunoglobulin E; EIB, exercise-induced bronchospasm; ICS, inhaled corticosteroids; IGS, inhaled glucocorticoids; INR, International Normalized Ratio; LABA, long-acting inhaled β_2-agonist, LTRA, leukotriene receptor agonist; MDI, metered-dose inhaler; SABA, short-acting inhaled β_2-agonist; SVT, supraventricular tachycardia.

Reprinted from reference 1.

In the nonacute asthma patient in whom the theophylline dose requirement is unknown, dosages suggested for ages >1 year are listed in Table 22-9; infant dosing is listed in Table 22-10. Accordingly, the initial dosage in K.J. would be 300 mg/day in divided doses (i.e., 150 mg Q 12 hr). If tolerated, the dosage is increased at 3-day intervals by about 25% to the mean dose that usually is needed to produce a peak theophylline serum concentration between 5 and 10 mcg/mL. The final dosage can be adjusted by using the guidelines listed in Table 22-11. Serum theophylline concentrations should be obtained at steady state (i.e., when there have been no missed doses and no extra doses have been taken for at least 48 hours).

Toxicity

38. M.M., a 14-year-old boy who has been treated with theophylline SR 300 mg BID, now complains of headache and difficulty in getting to sleep. Why should a theophylline serum concentration be evaluated?

Table 22-9 Theophylline Dosing Guide for Chronic Use[a,b]

Starting dose for children 1–15 yr <45 kg: 12–14 mg/kg/day to maximum of 300 mg/day
Starting dose for adults and children 1–15 yr >45 kg: 300 mg/day
Titrate dose upward after 3 days if necessary and if tolerated to:

- 16 mg/kg/day to maximum of 400 mg/day in children 1–15 yr <45 kg
- 400 mg/day in adults and children >45 kg

Titrate dose upward after 3 more days if necessary and if tolerated to:

- 20 mg/kg/day to a maximum of 600 mg/day in children 1–15 yr <45 kg
- 600 mg/day in adults and in children >45 kg

[a] Dose using ideal body weight or actual body weight, whichever is less. These dosages do not apply if liver disease, heart failure, or other factors documented to affect theophylline clearance are present. Doses must be guided by monitoring serum concentrations to ensure optimal safety and efficacy.
[b] Dosing schedule dependent on product selected; sustained-release products are much preferred, if at all possible.
Adapted from reference 98.

Table 22-10 Food and Drug Administration Guidelines for Theophylline Dosing in Infants[a]

Premature Neonates

<24 days postnatal age: 1.0 mg/kg Q 12 hr
≥24 days postnatal age: 1.5 mg/kg Q 12 hr

Term Infants and Infants Up to 52 Wk of Age

Total daily dose (mg) = [(0.2 × age in weeks) + 5.0] × (kg body weight)

- Up to age 26 weeks; divide dose into 3 equal amounts administered at 8-hr intervals
- >26 weeks of age; divide dose into 4 equal amounts administered at 6-hr intervals

[a] Final doses adjusted to a peak steady-state serum theophylline concentration of 5–10 mcg/mL in neonates and 10–15 mcg/mL in older infants.
Adapted from reference 98.

Theophylline side effects can be related to excessive serum concentrations, or adverse effects can be transient and unrelated to the amount in serum. Unfortunately, it is not always possible to determine which it might be. Side effects can include headache, nausea, vomiting, irritability or hyperactivity, insomnia, and diarrhea. With higher serum theophylline levels, cardiac arrhythmias, seizures, and death can occur.[97] Less severe symptoms may not be present before the onset of cardiac arrhythmias or seizures and cannot be relied on as a forewarning of these more serious adverse theophylline effects. It is important not to ignore any symptom consistent with theophylline toxicity. The insomnia and headaches experienced by M.M. may not be associated with excessive (i.e., out of the usual therapeutic range) serum theophylline concentrations, but a reduction in dosage should be contemplated because some patients experience toxicity when serum theophylline concentrations are within the therapeutic range. Guidelines for managing toxicity have been revised.[98]

Drug Interactions

39. T.R., a 55-year-old woman with asthma, is well controlled on theophylline SR 300 mg BID, albuterol two puffs QID PRN, and mometasone (Asmanex) one inhalation at bedtime. A peak theophylline serum concentration obtained 3 months ago was 14 mcg/mL. Six months ago, on the same dose of theophylline, her serum concentration was 15 mcg/mL. M.M. presents with an upper respiratory tract infection, and clarithromycin 500 mg BID is prescribed. Is this antibiotic appropriate?

A large number of medications inhibit cytochrome P450 isoenzymes and are capable of inhibiting the metabolism of theophylline. Because theophylline is metabolized by CYP 1A2, 3A3, and 2E1, inhibitors of these isoenzymes can cause clinically significant interactions.[50,98] Cimetidine, clarithromycin, and some (but not all) of the quinolone antibiotics (e.g., enoxacin, ciprofloxacin) are well documented to inhibit theophylline metabolism.[1,50,98] Because numerous other drugs inhibit the metabolism of theophylline, all patients receiving this agent should be screened carefully for potential interactions. As with any drug interaction, mechanism, time course, management, and clinical significance should be assessed

Table 22-11 Adjusting Doses of Theophylline Based on Serum Concentrations

Peak Theophylline Concentration (mcg/mL)[a]	*Approximate Adjustment in Daily Dose*	*Comment*
<5.0	↑ by 25%	Recheck serum theophylline concentration.
5–10	↑ by 25% if clinically indicated	Recheck serum concentration; ↑ dose only if poor response to therapy.
10–12	Cautious 10% ↑ if clinically indicated	If asymptomatic, no ↑ needed. Recheck serum theophylline concentration before further dose changes.
12–15	Occasional intolerance requires a 10% ↓	If asymptomatic, no dose change needed unless side effects present.
16–20	↓ by 10%–25%	Even if asymptomatic and side effects absent, a dose ↓ is prudent.
20–24.9	↓ by 50%	Omit 1 dose even if asymptomatic and side effects absent, a dose ↓ is indicated.
25–29.9	↓ by >50%	Omit next doses even if asymptomatic and side effects absent; a dose ↓ indicated; repeat serum theophylline concentration after dose adjustment.
>30	Omit next doses; ↓ by 60%–75%	Seek medical attention and consult regional poison center even if not symptomatic; if >60 years of age, anticipate need for treatment of seizures.

[a] It is important that levels are obtained at steady state. If laboratory results appear questionable, suggest repeat measurements.

Table 22-12 Factors Affecting Serum Theophylline Concentrations[a]

Factor	Decreases Theophylline Concentrations	Increases Theophylline Concentrations	Recommended Action
Food	↓ or delays absorption of some sustained-release theophylline (SR) products	↑ rate of absorption (fatty foods)	Select theophylline preparation that is not affected by food.
Diet	↑ metabolism (high protein)	↓ metabolism (high carbohydrate)	Inform patients that major changes in diet are not recommended while taking theophylline.
Systemic, febrile viral illness (e.g., influenza)		↓ metabolism	Decrease theophylline dose according to serum concentration level. Decrease dose by 50% if serum concentration measurement is not available.
Hypoxia, cor pulmonale, and decompensated congestive heart failure, cirrhosis		↓ metabolism	Decrease dose according to serum concentration level.
Age	↑ metabolism (1–9 yr)	↓ metabolism (<6 mon, elderly)	Adjust dose according to serum concentration level.
Phenobarbital, phenytoin, carbamazepine	↑ metabolism		Increase dose according to serum concentration level.
Cimetidine		↓ metabolism	Use alternative H_2-antagonist (e.g., famotidine or ranitidine).
Macrolides: TAO, erythromycin, clarithromycin		↓ metabolism	Use alternative antibiotic or adjust theophylline dose.
Quinolones: ciprofloxacin, enoxacin, pefloxacin		↓ metabolism	Use alternative antibiotic or adjust theophylline dose.
Rifampin	↑ metabolism		Increase dose according to serum concentration level.
Ticlopidine		↓ metabolism	Decrease dose according to serum concentration level.
Smoking	↑ metabolism		Advise patient to stop smoking; increase dose according to serum concentration level.

[a]This list is not all-inclusive; for discussion of other factors, see package inserts.
Modified from reference 1.

before any interventions. For example, cimetidine decreases theophylline clearance within 24 hours, and this interaction should be circumvented by using another H_2-blocker or a proton pump inhibitor (Table 22-12). Classic inducers (e.g., rifampin) of cytochrome P450 also affect theophylline clearance, and patients should be monitored for decreased serum concentrations. In T.R., the interaction with clarithromycin can easily be circumvented by using azithromycin, which does not affect theophylline metabolism.

Anticholinergics

40. R.K. is a 24-year-old graduate student with moderate persistent asthma, which has been well controlled for 10 years with ICS therapy and albuterol PRN. Recently, he has noticed that his asthma symptoms tend to worsen when he has anxiety over major examinations. What drug therapy might be helpful in R.K.?

One of the myths related to asthma is that it is an emotional illness. It is true, however, that among many typical triggers (e.g., aeroallergens, exercise), emotional upset can be a precipitating factor in some asthmatics,[1] and it has been shown that inhaled anticholinergic bronchodilators can block this response.[99] Although it is not an established therapy in this situation, a therapeutic trial of ipratropium given by an MDI is warranted in R.K. He probably only needs to use ipratropium a day or so before major examinations and on the day of the examination (i.e., he is well controlled all other times).

Anticholinergic bronchodilators also are useful in patients with asthma who are intolerant of the side effects of SABAs. For example, a patient who experiences nervousness or tremor with SABAs could use an ipratropium MDI as an alternative. Ipratropium is slower in onset (up to 30 minutes) but may be slightly longer acting than albuterol. As a general rule, anticholinergics are inferior to β_2-agonists in patients with asthma and should not be used as a rescue drug. These agents also benefit some patients who have asthma and then, very unfortunately, smoke for several years and develop chronic obstructive pulmonary disease (COPD). Tiotropium (Spiriva) is an important agent in the treatment of COPD; further research is needed to determine if it has a role in the management of some patients with asthma.[100]

ANTI-IMMUNOGLOBULIN E THERAPY

41. M.M. is a 30-year-old female with severe persistent asthma. Despite optimal assessment, drug therapy, environmental control,

and patient education per the principles of management detailed in EPR-3, she has had two recent hospitalizations due to asthma. Her allergist is considering anti-IgE therapy. Is M.M. a good candidate for such therapy? How would it be given? M.M. has a pretreatment IgE level of 90 IU/mL, and she weighs 55 kg.

Omalizumab (Xolair) is a humanized monoclonal anti-IgE antibody that binds to free IgE in serum. Thus, binding of IgE to high-affinity receptors on mast cells is subsequently inhibited, and the initiation of the allergic inflammatory cascade is blocked.[1,101–105] Omalizumab is effective in reducing oral and ICS dose requirements in patients with severe asthma and in reducing exacerbations.[101,102,105–107] This novel therapy is administered as a 150- to 375-mg subcutaneous injection every 2 or 4 weeks. The dose and frequency of administration are based on the serum total IgE level (IU/mL) and the patient's body weight. Therefore, M.M.'s omalizumab dose is 150 mg SC every 4 weeks.

Common side effects associated with omalizumab include injection site reactions, upper respiratory tract infections, sinusitis, and headache. Less common but potentially serious adverse effects include anaphylaxis (0.2% in postmarketing spontaneous reports), which can occur after any dose even if previous doses have been well tolerated and 24 or more hours after administration, and the development of malignant neoplasms (0.5% of omalizumab-treated patients compared with 0.2% in controls).

Because omalizumab is expensive and must be administered as a subcutaneous injection, it should be reserved for patients with severe asthma who are not adequately controlled with standard therapies. Despite the high cost, anti-IgE therapy might be cost-effective in selected patients with severe disease (e.g., those with frequent ED visits and hospitalizations), because an estimated <5% of asthma patients (severe disease) account for >50% of the dollars spent for asthma care.[108]

42. As the nurse prepares the dose of omalizumab for M.M., what are some special considerations regarding administering and monitoring this drug?

Following reconstitution of omalizumab, the drug must be administered within 4 hours if stored at room temperature and within 8 hours when refrigerated. Due to its viscosity, the injection may take 5 to 10 seconds. No more than 150 mg is injected at each site. While the risk of anaphylaxis is rare, patients should stay in the physician's office for at least 30 minutes after injection of omalizumab and be educated regarding the signs and symptoms of anaphylaxis. After leaving the physician's office, patients should seek emergency medical treatment at the first sign of anaphylaxis. Despite the low risk of severe allergic reactions, the manufacturer recently added a black box warning regarding this risk.

EXERCISE-INDUCED ASTHMA

43. T.W., a 33-year-old woman, presents to the clinic with a history of severe coughing and chest tightness after exercise. She recently joined an exercise club to lose weight but is unable to keep up with others of her own age and relative condition when jogging outside. She recalls having mild respiratory problems as a young child but has never taken any asthma medications. She has a positive treadmill test for exercise-induced asthma (EIA). How should T.W. be treated?

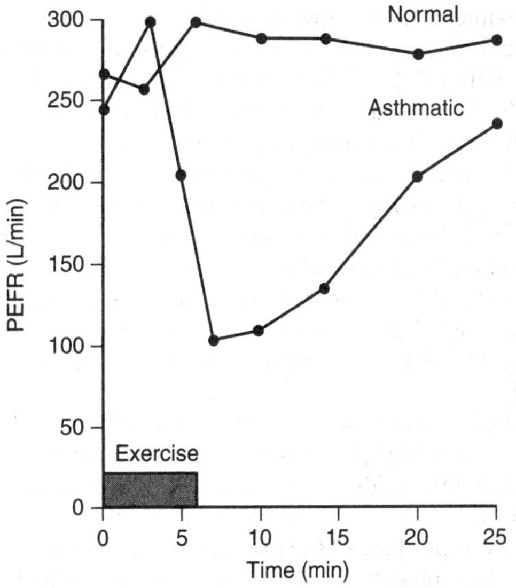

FIGURE 22-14 Changes in peak expiratory flow rate with exercise in an asthmatic and normal subject. PEFR, peak expiratory flow rate.

During sustained exercise, at least 90% of patients with asthma experience an initial improvement in pulmonary functions quickly followed by a significant decline (Fig. 22-14). This phenomenon may be the only symptom of subclinical asthma.[1,109] Patients can be diagnosed by measuring the FEV_1 or PEF before and after exercise (6–8-minute treadmill or bicycle exercise test). A reduction of FEV_1 by >15% of the baseline value is a positive test.

Hyperventilation of cold, dry air increases the sensitivity to EIA and induces bronchospasm.[109] The main stimulus for EIA is respiratory heat loss, water loss, or both,[109] while breathing heated, humidified air completely blocks EIA in many patients.[109] Masks are indicated for patients with EIA in the wintertime, and patients with severe asthma accompanied by EIA also should be encouraged to swim or engage in other indoor exercise that does not promote EIA. A warm-up period before strenuous exercise is helpful in some patients. With appropriate premedication, most EIA can be prevented, so virtually all patients with stable asthma should be encouraged to exercise. The mechanism of bronchoconstriction after airway heat and water loss is still incompletely understood.[109]

Although several drugs inhibit EIA, SABAs are generally the agents of choice for prophylaxis.[1–6,109,110] Inhaled β_2-agonists are superior to cromolyn.[110] For typical periods of exercise (e.g., <3 hours), pretreatment with agents such as albuterol 5 to 15 minutes before exercise usually provides excellent protection from EIA.

For prolonged periods of exercise, LABAs (formoterol, salmeterol) provide several hours of protection.[111] Two differences in formoterol and salmeterol include the delivery systems for inhalation and the onset of action. If either of these agents is to be used to prevent EIA, it is important for the patient to inhale the medication at the proper time before exercise. Formoterol should be inhaled at least 15 minutes before exercise, and salmeterol administration should occur at least 30 minutes before vigorous activity. Patients who are receiving Q 12 hr therapy with either drug concomitantly with ICS for long-term control of asthma, should already be protected and therfore only use albuterol if symptoms occur after exercise.

With maintenance therapy, as opposed to single doses before exercise, bronchoprotection from exercise may be reduced to 5 hours with LABAs.[1] Formoterol is inhaled via the Aerolizer (a single dose is loaded each time), and salmeterol is inhaled through the Diskus (multiple-dose inhaler).

Leukotriene receptor antagonists (e.g., montelukast once-daily chronic therapy) have also been demonstrated to prevent EIA.[112] Finally, it is important to point out that in persistent asthma, long-term anti-inflammatory therapy is helpful in reducing the response to most asthma triggers, including exercise.[1] For most patients who have EIA only, use of a SABA 15 minutes before exercise is the only therapy needed.

Because of the hyperventilation of relatively cool, dry air, jogging is a potent stimulus for EIA. A number of possible therapeutic interventions exist for T.W. She could be encouraged to swim, because the inhalation of humidified warm air is less likely to produce EIA. However, if she wishes to continue jogging, two inhalations of a short-acting β_2-agonist (e.g., albuterol) from a metered-dose aerosol 15 minutes before exercise should provide adequate protection for 2 to 3 hours. If outdoor temperatures are quite cool or cold, T.W. should jog indoors. T.W. also should be counseled to take two additional inhalations if she "breaks through" the initial protection and experiences tightness.

44. W.L., a 17-year-old boy, presents to the clinic with a complaint of dyspnea and coughing that has limited his ability to keep up with his basketball teammates. He states that it is worse when playing outdoors unless the gym is cold and that it seems to be worse (occurring sooner during exercise) than a month ago. W.L. experienced several bouts of bronchitis as a young child but has not had any problems for the past 6 years. His symptoms are consistent with EIA. How should his EIA be treated?

W.L. presents a special problem in that he is a teenager. Both for adolescents and children, peer pressure usually is extremely significant. Optimal prophylaxis is important to allow W.L. to compete at his best level. Embarrassment over not keeping up with teammates can be very hurtful now, and it has implications for setting habits of exercise into adulthood. Many adults with asthma do not exercise because they think they cannot do so based on childhood experiences. Lack of exercise can have a negative impact on physiologic and psychologic well-being. W.L. should receive preventive treatment with an inhaled β_2-agonist. The question is whether he should receive a short-acting or a long-acting agent. The clinician should probe as to the duration of exercise. If W.L. exercises for >3 hours, formoterol or salmeterol administered 15 to 30 minutes before exercise would be a logical choice. Finally, the clinician should verify that exercise is the only factor that precipitates asthma symptoms. It could be that further questioning of W.L. will reveal persistent asthma or mild intermittent asthma beyond EIA only. If that is the case, long-term ICS or montelukast therapy should be started to reduce overall airway hyperresponsiveness.

PATIENT EDUCATION

45. A.B., a 26-year-old woman, calls her clinician and states that she has run out of her albuterol MDI. She has a prescription for a budesonide dry powder inhaler but admits that she does not use this medication "because it doesn't seem to work as well as her albuterol MDI." A.B. has had asthma all of her life. She complains of symptoms most days but has not required visits to the ED or hospitalizations. The provider determines that A.B. is bothered most about daily shortness of breath and worries that her condition may get worse. What should the provider do in this situation?

If optimal long-term drug therapy of asthma is prescribed, treatment may still fail or be suboptimal if the patient does not receive adequate education. Patients with asthma require special educational efforts because of the use of inhalation devices and peak flow meters. In addition, it often is a major challenge to have patients and parents understand the critical importance of long-term daily controller therapy and environmental control. Of course, an important first step in educating asthmatics is to be caring and a good listener. Rather than sharing your knowledge initially, it is important to help establish a "partnership" with the patient by first asking the following question: "What is bothering you the most about your asthma?" Really listening to the patient and then addressing patient concerns is extremely important to successful education and long-term management. EPR-3 lists several patient education activities in Table 22-13.[1]

Table 22-13 Key Educational Messages: Teach and Reinforce at every Opportunity

Basic Facts About Asthma
- The contrast between airways of a person who has and a person who does not have asthma; the role of inflammation
- What happens to the airways in an asthma attack

Roles of Medications—Understanding the Difference Between the Following:
- Long-term-control medications: prevent symptoms, often by reducing inflammation. Must be taken daily. Do not expect them to give quick relief.
- Quick-relief medications: short-acting β_2-agonists relax muscles around the airway and provide prompt relief of symptoms. Do not expect them to provide long-term asthma control. Using quick-relief medication on a daily basis indicates the need for starting or increasing long-term control medications.

Patient Skills
- Taking medications correctly
  - Inhaler technique (demonstrate to patient and have the patient return the demonstration)
  - Use of devices, such as prescribed valved holding chamber, spacer, nebulizer
- Identifying and avoiding environmental exposures that worsen the patient's asthma (e.g., allergens, irritants, tobacco smoke)
- Self-monitoring to:
  - Assess level of asthma control
  - Monitor symptoms and, if prescribed, peak flow
  - Recognize early signs and symptoms of worsening asthmas
- Using written asthma action plan to know when and how to:
  - Take daily actions to control asthma
  - Adjust medication in response to signs of worsening asthma
  - Seek medical care as appropriate

Reprinted from reference 1.

Clinicians can be of invaluable assistance to the patient by repeatedly reinforcing education on the necessity to use anti-inflammatory (and LABA) therapies on a regular schedule. Many patients underuse long-term preventive therapy because no health professional took the time to adequately instruct them that most asthma symptoms are preventable. While underusing the most important medicines for long-term control, many patients overuse "quick relievers" (i.e., SABAs). Health care providers must be able to detect these problems and intervene to enhance patient care.

Because a large percentage of patients have difficulty using MDIs, teaching patients the correct use of MDIs (alone, or in combination with spacers) and dry powder inhalers is absolutely essential.[1,113] In one study, 89% of patients could not perform all of the steps for MDI use correctly.[1,114] Competent teaching requires *observation* of the patient using the devices initially and again on repeat visits to the clinic, hospital, or community pharmacy. Telling the patient about correct use is inadequate. Health professionals must demonstrate use of the devices (live or with videotapes) for patients who cannot use the devices correctly. Although there is more than one correct way to use an MDI, Table 22-14 summarizes two commonly accepted approaches.[1,113] Many asthma experts prefer to use spacers to help ensure optimal efficacy. Spacers should be used in virtually all patients receiving ICS via an MDI, even those with perfect MDI technique, because spacers enhance efficacy and greatly reduce the risk of oropharyngeal candidiasis.[115–117] On the other hand, spacers do not add efficacy to *correct* use of a β_2-agonist MDI.[118] Although any spacer can be helpful, marketed devices that have a flow indicator whistle when inhalation is fast may be preferred (e.g., AeroChamber, InspirEase).

Table 22-14 Steps to Correct Use of Metered-Dose Inhalers[a]

1. Shake the inhaler well and remove the dust cap.
2. Exhale *slowly* through pursed lips.[b]
3. If using the "closed-mouth" technique, hold the inhaler upright and place the mouthpiece between your lips. Be careful not to block the opening with your tongue or teeth.
4. If using the "open-mouth" technique, open your mouth wide and hold the inhaler upright 1–2 inches from your mouth, making sure the inhaler is properly aimed.
5. Press down on the inhaler *once* as you start a *slow*, deep inhalation.
6. Continue to inhale slowly and deeply through your mouth. Try to inhale for at least 5 seconds.
7. Hold your breath for 10 seconds (use your fingers to count to 10 slowly). If 10 seconds makes you feel uncomfortable, try to hold your breath for at least 4 seconds.
8. Exhale *slowly*.[c]
9. Wait at least 30–60 seconds before inhaling the next puff of medicine.

[a]If using a spacer, see manufacturer's instructions. Same basic principles of slow, deep inhalation with adequate breath hold apply. With spacers, put mouthpiece on top of your tongue to ensure that tongue does not block aerosol.

[b]As long as exhalation is slow, exhale can take place over several seconds. Some experts insist on exhaling only a tidal volume, but the key is to exhale *slowly*.

[c]If patient has concomitant rhinitis, exhaling through the *nose* may be of benefit when using corticosteroids, cromolyn, or ipratropium (i.e., some medication may deposit in nose).

Studies have shown that health professionals, like some patients, generally are not competent in using MDIs.[119–121] Obviously, the clinician should practice with a placebo inhaler and gain competence before teaching a patient. Among clinicians who educate asthmatics, pharmacists can be very helpful in teaching correct use of MDIs.[122] Unfortunately, one study showed that community pharmacists commonly are not providing such teaching.[123]

In addition to teaching the correct use of MDIs and spacers, clinicians should help patients via education regarding the correct use of breath-activated dry powder inhalers (e.g., Turbuhaler, Diskus, Aerolizer), breath-activated MDIs (e.g., Autohaler), and nebulizing machines.[1] When using the Flexhaler, for example, patients must clearly understand the need for a rapid (preferably 60 L/minute), deep inhalation (not slow as with an MDI).[124] Such rapid PIF is achievable by some young children, but many children <8 years of age have difficulty reaching PIF >60 L/minute.[124] With the Diskus, PIF does not have to be as rapid as with Flexhaler, but it should be >30 L/minute.[125] In addition, patients need to breath-hold 10 seconds if possible, as with an MDI.

Asthma Self-Management Plans

Objective monitoring of lung function at home with the use of peak flow meters can be very helpful to patients and health care professionals. EPR-3 discusses the debates about PEF versus symptom-based action plans.[1] Use of peak flow meters may be valuable in patients who have had severe exacerbations and those who are "poor perceivers" of deteriorating asthma control. Instructing patients on the correct use of the devices, including use of the green, yellow, and red zones is essential.[1] After establishing that optimal therapy has maintained the PEF in the "green zone" in the early morning, most patients can simply verify their values once daily in the early morning. Analogous to a traffic light, green, yellow, and red zones have been established to guide the patient and clinician. The *green zone* refers to a PEF that is 80% to 100% of "personal best" and generally indicates that therapy is providing good control. Before a course of optimal therapy to attain a personal best, the zones are set based on predicted values found in each peak flow meter package insert. The *yellow zone* indicates a PEF that is 50% to 79% of personal best. Patients should be instructed to call their physician or other health care provider for adjustment in preventive medication if the PEF stays in yellow zone after using two puffs of a β-agonist. The *red zone* indicates a PEF that is <50% of personal best. The patient should know to call his or her health care provider immediately if the use of an inhaled β-agonist does not bring the PEF to the yellow zone or green zone. Figure 22-15 gives an example of PEF monitoring, and Figure 22-16 gives an example of a written action plan.

Correct use of the peak flow meter includes standing, inhaling completely, forming a tight seal with the lips around the mouthpiece, exhaling as hard and fast as possible (blast!), and repeating this maneuver twice. The best of three attempts should be recorded. Beyond giving maximal effort when using peak flow meters, patients should be instructed to place the instrument well into the mouth on top of the tongue to avoid acceleration of air in the mouth with the tongue and buccal musculature. In essence, "spitting" into the peak flow meter causes a dramatic "false" elevation in PEF.[126] Some data

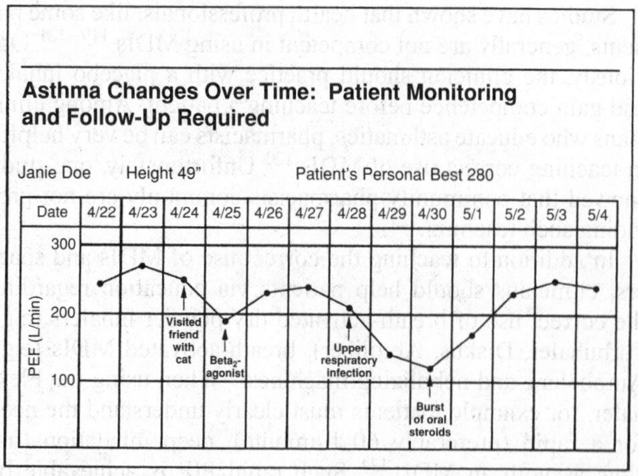

FIGURE 22-15 Asthma changes over time: patient monitoring and follow-up required. (Reproduced with permission from National Institutes of Health. Practical guide for the diagnosis and management of asthma 1997; NIH publication No. 97-4053.)

suggest that females need more initial coaching than men in giving maximum effort when using peak flow meters to ensure accurate assessments of PEF.[127]

A.B. needs education regarding the benefits of long-term inhaled anti-inflammatory therapy. The clinician should explain with enthusiasm that A.B.'s budesonide is an extremely effective medicine and that it is the cornerstone of her asthma management. The delayed onset and safety of ICS must be stressed as well as the requirement of regular use every day. Teaching A.B. the differences between "preventers" and "quick relievers" is essential. Showing her colored pictures, models, or a video of inflamed airways can be very helpful—these teaching aids are available from several pharmaceutical manufacturers. Likewise, a peak flow meter should be given to A.B. and correct use ensured by observing her use of it along with establishment of green, yellow, and red zones, coupled with a written action plan developed by her asthma care provider.[1] A.B. needs to hear from the clinicians treating her that asthma is preventable, and in the words of a title to an NIH booklet for patients, "Your asthma can be controlled: Expect nothing less." As part of comprehensive education, such a positive message from all of her caregivers, as well as carefully listening to A.B.'s concerns, can have a major impact on A.B., who has not been managing her asthma optimally.

46. A.B. tells the provider that she was previously instructed to place the albuterol MDI in front of her open mouth and spray rather than put the MDI in her mouth. She says she is confused because the package insert shows placement of the inhaler in the mouth. Finally, she is concerned that her albuterol was changed to "HFA." What should the clinician tell A.B.?

A.B. is correct that this is a confusing issue to many patients and health professionals. A small number of studies show that the "open-mouth" technique is better, but several other studies with SABAs show that the "closed-mouth" technique is as good as or better than putting the MDI in front of the open mouth.[1,113] In addition, the correctly performed closed-mouth technique is as efficacious with a β_2-agonist as with a spacer[118] or nebulizer.[128] Thus, the closed-mouth technique is perfectly acceptable, as is the open-mouth technique with SABAs or LABAs. One caution with the open-mouth technique is that incorrect aiming of the MDI may result in the aerosol being sprayed onto the face or into the eyes. Finally, due to the phasing out of chlorofluorocarbon (CFC) propellants (prohibited after December 31, 2008), increasing numbers of patients are already using albuterol MDIs with non-CFC propellants (e.g., HFA [tetrafluoroethane]). A.B. should be reassured that albuterol-HFA MDIs have been tested extensively and work as well as her former MDI (but with a less forceful spray).[129]

47. For patients who are using both a bronchodilator and an anti-inflammatory inhaler, is there a preferred sequencing of the inhalers?

For patients who have several inhalers, questions regarding sequencing of the inhalers are frequently asked. First, there is no well-documented evidence that outcomes are better using, for instance, a bronchodilator or an anti-inflammatory agent first. A commonsense approach is that using a rapid-onset bronchodilator such as a β_2-agonist first and then an anti-inflammatory second has some appeal (i.e., quick relief and theoretically enhanced penetration of the anti-inflammatory). However, as discussed previously, short-acting β_2-agonists are preferred for *as-needed use* (and before exercise) and are not generally used on a scheduled basis. Thus, if a patient is not symptomatic at the time the anti-inflammatory is scheduled, current literature suggests that the patient inhales only the anti-inflammatory agent. Therefore, it is usually *not* necessary to counsel patients regarding sequencing of inhaled medications. Because time is limited in counseling patients, teaching them correct inhalation technique, the purpose of each medication (controllers vs. quick relievers), and the need for strict adherence with controller therapies is far more important than spending precious time on the sequencing of inhalers.

NOCTURNAL ASTHMA

48. R.R., a 41-year-old man, presents to the clinic with a history of coughing and shortness of breath that awakens him at least two nights a week. Most mornings on awakening, he complains of chest tightness. He has a history of asthma since childhood and currently is managed with beclomethasone HFA 160 mcg BID via a spacer and albuterol (90 mcg/puff) two puffs Q 6 hr PRN, and before exercise. R.R.'s morning PEF is consistently in the yellow zone, usually at about 400 L/minute (personal best, 600 L/minute), whereas the evening PEF is consistently 550 to 600 L/minute. What treatment should be recommended?

Many patients with asthma complain of symptoms that awaken them in the night or occur on awakening in the morning. Morning cough with or without bronchospasm may be a clue to nocturnal asthma. Although nocturnal asthma may be appropriately viewed as simply another manifestation of airway inflammation, it is so common and troublesome among asthmatics that it deserves special note. Circadian rhythm in PEF is exaggerated in patients with asthma. The difference in PEF in nonasthmatics averages about 8% between 4 PM (maximal airflow) and 4 AM (minimal airflow), but in patients with asthma, the average variation can be as high as about 50%.[130,131] Several mechanisms account for this diurnal variation in PEF. The following are examples of factors that contribute to nocturnal

Asthma Action Plan

For: ________ Doctor: ________ Date: ________

Doctor's Phone Number ________ Hospital/Emergency Department Phone Number ________

GREEN ZONE

Doing Well

- No cough, wheeze, chest tightness, or shortness of breath during the day or night
- Can do usual activities

And, if a peak flow meter is used,

Peak flow: more than ________
(80 percent or more of my best peak flow)

My best peak flow is: ________

Take these long-term control medicines each day (include an anti-inflammatory).

Medicine	How much to take	When to take it
________	________	________
________	________	________

Identify and avoid and control the things that make your asthma worse, like (list here):

________ ________ ________

________ ________ ________

Before exercise, if prescribed, take: ❒ 2 or ❒ 4 puffs ________ 5 to 60 minutes before exercise

YELLOW ZONE

Asthma Is Getting Worse

- Cough, wheeze, chest tightness, or shortness of breath, or
- Waking at night due to asthma, or
- Can do some, but not all, usual activities

-Or-

Peak flow: ________ to ________
(50 to 79 percent of my best peak flow)

First Add: quick-relief medicine—and keep taking your GREEN ZONE medicine.

________ (short-acting β_2-agonist) ❒ 2 or ❒ 4 puffs, every 20 minutes for up to 1 hour
❒ Nebulizer, once

Second **If your symptoms (and peak flow, if used) return to GREEN ZONE after 1 hour of above treatment:**
❒ Continue monitoring to be sure you stay in the green zone.

-Or-

If your symptoms (and peak flow, if used) do not return to GREEN ZONE after 1 hour of above treatment:

❒ Take: ________ (short-acting β_2-agonist) ❒ 2 or ❒ 4 puffs or ❒ Nebulizer

❒ Add: ________ (oral corticosteroid) mg per day For ________ (3–10) days

❒ Call the doctor ❒ before/ ❒ within ________ hours after taking the oral steroid.

RED ZONE

Medical Alert!

- Very short of breath, or
- Quick-relief medicines have not helped, or
- Cannot do usual activities, or
- Symptoms are same or get worse after 24 hours in Yellow Zone

-Or-

Peak flow: less than ________
(50 percent of my best peak flow)

Take this medicine:

❒ ________ (short-acting β_2-agonist) ❒ 4 or ❒ 6 puffs or ❒ Nebulizer

❒ ________ (oral corticosteroid) mg

Then call your doctor NOW. Go to the hospital or call an ambulance if:

- You are still in the red zone after 15 minutes AND
- You have not reached your doctor.

DANGER SIGNS

- **Trouble walking and talking due to shortness of breath**
- **Lips or fingernails are blue**

- **Take ❒ 4 or ❒ 6 puffs of your quick-relief medicine AND**
- **Go to the hospital or call for an ambulance** ________ (phone) **NOW!**

FIGURE 22-16 Sample asthma action plan. (Reproduced from reference 1.)

asthma: increased release of inflammatory mediators,[130,131] increased activity of the parasympathetic nervous system, lower circulating levels of epinephrine, and lower levels of serum cortisol (lowest at about midnight). In addition, for patients whose asthma is triggered by gastroesophageal reflux, this problem is worse at night and is another factor to consider.

The initial approach to managing nocturnal symptoms is the same as that for overall long-term therapy of persistent asthma, including adequate anti-inflammatory agents.[1,131] ICS are often effective in eliminating or reducing nocturnal asthma, including symptoms and the drop in PEF.[131] If low to moderate dosages (i.e., correctly inhaled every day) do not eliminate symptoms, a LABA (salmeterol, formoterol) is indicated. Also, the basic asthma treatment principle of good control of concomitant rhinitis and environmental control, especially in the bedroom (e.g., house dust mites, household pets), should be considered in the patient with nocturnal asthma symptoms.

Bedtime doses of SABAs do not have sufficient duration of action to prevent early morning symptoms. Salmeterol or formoterol, both of which have a 12-hour duration of action, are preferred. Before the advent of LABAs, long-acting oral agents such as SR theophylline often were indicated.[131] Although SR theophylline is helpful, it has the potential to cause more adverse effects than inhaled agents, may interfere with sleep, and is less efficacious.[131] Before a long-acting oral agent is prescribed, adequate inhaled anti-inflammatory therapy should be ensured and then LABAs should be used.

Because asthma is primarily an inflammatory disease and nocturnal symptoms are due largely to airway inflammation, the first drug therapy concern in R.R. is to ensure that he is strictly adhering to his beclomethasone therapy, and demonstrating excellent inhalation technique. If his use of the medication is optimal, a reasonable approach would be to add LABA therapy, because he is already at a moderate ICS dosage.

As part of optimal management of nocturnal asthma, R.R. also should be asked about avoiding or minimizing exposure to his asthma triggers (e.g., if he is allergic to cats, is there a cat in the bedroom?). Follow-up visits for R.R. should verify that the early morning and evening PEF are staying in the green zone and that symptoms, both during the night and on awakening in the morning, have been eliminated.

DRUG-INDUCED ASTHMA

49. M.B., 32-year-old woman with asthma, asks her clinician which over-the-counter medications would be preferred for minor aches and pains. M.B. says that she is very sensitive to aspirin (causes severe wheezing).

The clinician should counsel the patient regarding the fact that patients with asthma who are aspirin sensitive often react to other nonsteroidal anti-inflammatory drugs (NSAIDs) such as ibuprofen by developing asthma symptoms with the first dose. The health care professional should suggest acetaminophen. If M.B. says that acetaminophen does not give adequate relief of her pain, other options are salsalate[2] or consultation with a board-certified allergist with experience in aspirin and NSAID desensitization.[132] The clinician should also suggest consultation with an allergist regarding a recent study that gives strong evidence that cyclo-oxygenase-2 (COX-2) inhibitors are safe in aspirin-sensitive asthma.[133] This case also points out the need for health professionals to pay attention to patient use of nonprescription medications. Although drug-induced asthma may present as relatively mild symptoms in some patients, fatal asthma caused by medicinal agents has been reported numerous times. The most extensive literature on drug-induced asthma involves NSAIDs and β-blockers. Other drugs and drug preservatives also can induce symptoms of asthma, but because the topic is beyond the scope of this chapter, the reader is referred to other sources[134,135] for further discussion.

The percentage of asthmatics reported to be aspirin sensitive ranges from 4% to 28%. Clinical manifestations of aspirin sensitivity include rhinorrhea; mild wheezing; or severe, life-threatening shortness of breath. Once the reaction has occurred, there is a refractory period of 2 to 5 days.[136] If an asthmatic is aspirin sensitive, it is likely that the patient also will react to most other NSAIDs. Aspirin and other NSAIDs share common mechanisms involving the arachidonic acid pathways, including inhibition of cyclo-oxygenase, which results in more rapid synthesis and overproduction of leukotrienes.[136] Not surprisingly, because leukotrienes are an important part of the mechanism of NSAID-induced asthma, inhibitors of 5-lipoxygenase such as zileuton are generally effective in blocking this response.[137] Similarly, leukotriene receptor antagonists such as zafirlukast and montelukast are generally effective in blocking aspirin-induced asthma.[138] Because most patients with asthma do not react to aspirin and other NSAIDs, the NIH guidelines recommend avoiding these agents only in patients with known sensitivity.[1] In addition, patients with severe persistent asthma or nasal polyps should be counseled regarding the risks associated with these drugs. In patients with known sensitivity, acetaminophen or salsalate are recommended for headaches and relatively minor pain.[1] For patients who are sensitive but who need to take aspirin (e.g., post myocardial infarction [MI]) or an NSAID [(e.g., arthritis]), it is possible to desensitize the patient, and daily use then prevents further reaction.[132]

When discussing drug-induced asthma, the other major consideration is β-blockers. These agents should be used with great caution in patients with asthma. Because even β_1-adrenergic blockers lose selectivity as dosages are increased, they, as well as nonselective β-blockers, should be avoided in most patients. Furthermore, ophthalmic timolol has been reported several times to cause fatal asthma and should absolutely be avoided in patients with a history of asthma.[139] Other β-blocker eye drops (e.g., betaxolol) have been reported to have less propensity to induce asthma, but all have some risk.[134,140]

Two notable exceptions to using β-blockers in patients with asthma are patients who are post MI and patients with heart failure.[141] Because β-blockers prolong life post MI and improve the care of patients with heart failure, benefits versus risks should be weighed. Risks outweigh benefits if a patient has severe persistent asthma.[141,142] If a post-MI patient has mild intermittent asthma or well-controlled mild persistent (and possibly moderate persistent[141]) asthma with optimal management, a low dosage of atenolol 50 mg/day is a reasonable consideration where benefits may outweigh risks.[142] Asthma patients have been shown to respond to inhaled β_2-agonists when receiving this dosage of atenolol.[142] While low dosages of β-blockers are not proven to prolong life after an MI, some studies suggest efficacy of lower dosages. For patients with heart failure, metoprolol CR/XL is the cardioselective β-blocker approved in the United States, while carvedilol, which has nonselective β-blocker as well as α-blocking properties, can worsen asthma symptoms.[142]

If a patient with asthma is given a β-blocker and initially reports no symptoms, subsequent exacerbations may not respond well to administration of usual doses of a β-agonist. The drug of choice for β-blocker–induced bronchospasm is ipratropium.[142] A more subtle risk with β-blockers involves the adult with allergic rhinitis and a family history of asthma. If this individual is given a β-blocker for hypertension, symptoms of asthma could be induced, especially if another trigger is introduced such as running in cold, dry air.

OUTCOMES

50. C.C. is a 36-year-old woman admitted to the hospital for asthma. This is her second hospitalization in the past 2 years, and she has had three ED visits during the same period. She also complains of nocturnal awakenings at least 4 nights per week and is bothered that she is gaining weight, because she cannot exercise. Lack of exercise is also troubling her because her 5-year-old daughter wants her to go outside and play with her. C.C. has been taking flunisolide one puff BID without a spacer for years along with frequent PRN albuterol. C.C. carefully controls her home environment. What could her clinicians do to improve her outcomes, including quality of life?

C.C. needs a reassessment of her long-term management considering her very poor outcomes over the past 2 years. First, her clinicians need to establish a partnership with her in education regarding asthma and its management. Clearly, she needs dosage adjustment with her anti-inflammatory therapy. Her dosage is too low, plus she is receiving a low-potency corticosteroid. Based on her recent history, she should be treated initially with high-dose ICS and a LABA, preferably with a more potent ICS product that would require fewer inhalations per day (e.g., combination budesonide-formoterol or combination fluticasone-salmeterol). C.C. should have the importance of daily controller therapy stressed, including the need for strict adherence and proper inhalation technique. C.C. needs a written asthma action plan and an emergency supply of prednisone (i.e., to use when her PEF is in the red zone and unresponsive to albuterol). C.C. should be told to expect a reduced need for albuterol.

Numerous studies have documented that applying the principles of the NIH guidelines[1–6] results in improved clinical outcomes, and many of these studies have been summarized in EPR-3.[1] Several studies have documented that pharmacists who are highly knowledgeable of the NIH guidelines and who work closely with patients and physicians improve outcomes, including reduced ED visits and hospitalizations.[143–148] These successful studies involved highly motivated pharmacists, who were asthma experts based in university-affiliated clinics or in large private HMOs.

A recent randomized controlled trial based in community pharmacies with specially trained pharmacists has also shown very positive outcomes for patients with asthma.[148] Another randomized controlled trial based in chain drug stores with staff pharmacists did not show a benefit related to attempts at asthma care.[149] Unfortunately, the level of training and incentives did not appear optimal, and the authors pointed out that the staff pharmacists were "not universally enthusiastic" about the program. The authors also described their intervention as "cumbersome" for the pharmacists. Further study is needed to assess asthma care in this setting when pharmacists are optimally trained, given appropriate incentives, and enthusiastic about the program.

When assessing the effect of comprehensive management on clinical outcomes, quality-of-life measures should be assessed as well as reduction in ED visits and hospitalizations.[1] To achieve optimal outcomes, attention to each of the four major components of management is required (objective assessment, environmental control, pharmacologic therapy, and patient education as a partnership). Examples of areas that pose special challenges for inner-city patients include psychosocial factors, underuse of controller medications, and passive cigarette smoke.[150–153] As part of overall management to improve outcomes, recent studies have emphasized again the importance of good inhalation technique with ICS and education in use of peak flow meters.[154,155]

51. C.C. returns to the clinic in 2 months and is elated because she is sleeping through the night and not waking up short of breath. In addition, she is beginning to exercise again, which makes her and her child very happy. C.C. has had no further ED visits. What should the clinician do at this point?

Optimal asthma management that improves outcomes is a continuous process of education and reassessment of the overall therapy. Observation of C.C. using her peak flow meter and inhalation devices on each clinic visit is important and should be routine. Having C.C. verbalize her understanding of the role of the ICS plus LABA versus albuterol and the action plan with "crisis" prednisone is important. Despite her current optimism, asking C.C. about her current asthma concerns is important. Over the next month or two, a trial of slowly stepping down the ICS dosage to a medium dose should be attempted. Finally, C.C. needs continued partnership with her clinician.

52. C.C. is in the clinic 2 years later, reflecting with her clinician over her total elimination of ED visits and hospitalizations as well as her improved quality of life. Her management initiated 24 months ago has continued, including environmental control, controller therapy tailored for her, PRN albuterol and early morning PEF monitoring, and partnership with her clinician. Unfortunately, C.C. forgot to get an influenza vaccine last October and became ill with influenza in early March. Although this episode only slightly worsened her asthma symptoms, when she was almost recovered from the flu, she went to the grocery store and breathed secondhand smoke unexpectedly. In addition, early spring tree and grass pollen was affecting her allergic rhinitis. By the time she got back to her house, she was wheezing and her PEF was in the yellow zone, but it responded to three puffs of albuterol. C.C. asks what she should have done if this series of events had resulted in her PEF decreasing to the red zone.

C.C. needs to be re-educated regarding the action plan based on symptoms and PEF values. Referring back to the written plan for doses of albuterol and, if needed, oral corticosteroid therapy is important. Emphasizing the need for annual influenza vaccination in October is important. Reinforcement of the importance of continued preventive therapy that has given such remarkable success is appropriate for C.C. and reassuring her that despite this minor setback, she is in control of her asthma. The clinician should continue to work with her to further tailor the therapy, including control of rhinitis, to maintain optimal outcomes at the lowest dosages and the simplest possible regimen. Recent research has further emphasized the goal of simplified regimens and achieving the lowest effective doses of anti-inflammatory therapy.[156,157]

COMPLEMENTARY ALTERNATIVE THERAPIES

53. C.C. is in the clinic a few months later. She is continuing to have excellent control of her asthma and allergic rhinitis. C.C. asks her health care professional for her opinion of herbal remedies for asthma as well as other nontraditional approaches to treatment.

Complementary and alternative approaches that have been used in the treatment of asthma include black tea, coffee, ephedra, marijuana, dried ivy leaf extract, acupuncture, meditation, and yoga.[1,158,159] Despite the widespread use of alternative medications for chronic conditions, the clinician should discuss with C.C. that there is no established scientific basis for their use in the management of asthma.[1] Complementary alternative medicine cannot be recommended as a substitute for the drug therapy recommended by EPR-3 and other medical literature based on randomized controlled studies.

USE OF VALIDATED QUESTIONNAIRES FOR PATIENT SELF-ASSESSMENT OF ASTHMA CONTROL

54. A multidisciplinary group of health science center students have been invited to present a program on asthma at a local inner-city high school. The small group of nursing, pharmacy, and medical students are discussing the materials they want to use in the program. What would be some key points to cover, and are there validated instruments to assess asthma control that may be helpful?

Volunteer service to help educate patients with asthma is encouraged and has the potential to make a positive difference in the lives of patients and health science center students.[160] Examples of key points to cover at schools, churches, health fairs, or other venues include showing pictures and models of normal versus inflamed airways, avoidance of common asthma triggers, discussion of "preventer" versus "quick-reliever" medications, demonstrations of inhalers and peak flow meters, and written action plans. Discussion of prevention of EIA and showing pictures of famous athletes is of obvious importance. EPR-3 recommends that clinicians encourage patients to use self-assessment tools to determine whether asthma is well controlled.[1] Consequently, the health science center students also decide to use one of those validated questionnaires shown in EPR-3, the Asthma Control Test.[161] The high school students will be told to take the brief test and give it to the clinicians caring for them. For patients whose asthma is not well controlled, the test scores can be a helpful tool in initiating or modifying long-term treatment.

REFERENCES

1. National Institutes of Health. Expert Panel Report 3. Guidelines for the Diagnosis and Management of Asthma. NIH Publication No. 08-4051.0; 2007.
2. National Institutes of Health. Expert Panel Report 2. Guidelines for the Diagnosis and Management of Asthma. NIH Publication No. 97-4051; 1997.
3. National Institutes of Health. Guidelines for the Diagnosis and Management of Asthma. National Asthma Education Program Expert Panel Report. NIH Publication No. 91-3042; 1991.
4. National Institutes of Health. International Consensus Report on Diagnosis and Treatment of Asthma. NIH Publication No. 92-3091; 1992.
5. National Institutes of Health. Global Initiative for Asthma. NIH Publication No. 95-3659; 1995.
6. National Institutes of Health. Guidelines for the diagnosis and management of asthma-update on selected topics 2002. NIH Publication No. 02-5075. *J Allergy Clin Immunol* 2002;110:S1.
7. Weiss KB, Sullivan SD. The health economics of asthma and rhinitis. I. Assessing the economic impact. *J Allergy Clin Immunol* 2001;107:38.
8. Surveillance for Asthma—United States 1980–1999. *MMWR* 2002;51(SS-1):13; Table 10.
9. Moorman J et al. National Surveillance for asthma—United States 1980–2004. *MMWR* 2007; 56:1.
10. Butland BK, Strachan DP. Asthma onset and relapse in adult life: the British 1958 birth cohort study. *Ann Allergy Asthma Immunol* 2007;98:337.
11. Busse WW, Lemanske RF. Asthma. *N Engl J Med* 2001;344:350.
12. Holgate ST, Polosa R. The mechanisms, diagnosis, and management of severe asthma in adults. *Lancet* 2006;368:780.
13. Chanez P et al. Effects of inhaled corticosteroids on pathology in asthma and chronic obstructive pulmonary disease. *Proc Am Thorac Soc* 2004;1:184.
14. Kharitonov SA, Barnes PJ. Effects of corticosteroids on noninvasive biomarkers of inflammation in asthma and chronic obstructive pulmonary disease. *Proc Am Thorac Soc* 2004;1:191.
15. Kharitonov SA et al. Inhaled glucocorticoids decrease nitric oxide in exhaled air of asthmatic patients. *Am J Respir Crit Care Med* 1996;153:454.
16. Davies DE et al. Airway remodeling in asthma: new insights. *J Allergy Clin Immunol* 2003;111:215.
17. Skobeloff EM et al. The effect of the menstrual cycle on asthma presentations in the emergency department. *Arch Intern Med* 1996;156:1837.
18. West JB. *Respiratory Physiology: The Essentials.* 6th ed. Baltimore: Williams & Wilkins; 1999.
19. American Thoracic Society. Standardization of spirometry. *Am J Respir Crit Care Med* 1995;152: 1107.
20. McFadden ER. Clinical physiologic correlates in asthma. *J Allergy Clin Immunol* 1986;77:1.
21. McFadden ER, Lyons HA. Arterial blood gas tension in asthma. *N Engl J Med* 1968;278:1027.
22. Schuh S et al. Efficacy of frequent nebulized ipratropium bromide added to frequent high-dose albuterol therapy in severe childhood asthma. *J Pediatr* 1995;126:639.
23. Qureshi F et al. Effect of nebulized ipratropium on the hospitalization rates of children with asthma. *N Engl J Med* 1998;339:1030.
24. Becker AB et al. Inhaled salbutamol (albuterol) vs. injected epinephrine in the treatment of acute asthma in children. *J Pediatr* 1983;102:465.
25. Shim CS, Williams MH. Effect of bronchodilator therapy administered by canister versus jet nebulizer. *J Allergy Clin Immunol* 1984;73:387.
26. Newman SP. Aerosol deposition considerations in inhalation therapy. *Chest* 1985;88(Suppl): 152.
27. Lewis RA, Fleming JS. Fractional deposition from a jet nebulizer: how it differs from a metered dose inhaler. *Br J Dis Chest* 1985;79:361.
28. Dolovich et al. Device selection and outcomes of aerosol treatment: evidence-based guidelines. *Chest* 2005;121:335.
29. Cates CJ et al. Holding chambers (spacers) versus nebulisers for beta-agonist treatment of acute asthma. *Cochrane Database Syst Rev* 1996;19: CD000052.
30. Leversha AM et al. Costs and effectiveness of spacer versus nebulizer in young children with moderate and severe acute asthma. *J Pediatr* 2000; 136:497.
31. Schuh S et al. Comparison of albuterol delivered by a metered dose inhaler with spacer versus a nebulizer in children with mild acute asthma. *J Pediatr* 1999;135:22.
32. Kerem E et al. Efficacy of albuterol administered by nebulizer versus spacer device in children with acute asthma. *J Pediatr* 1993;123:313.
33. Schuh S et al. High-versus low-dose frequently administered nebulized albuterol in children with severe acute asthma. *Pediatrics* 1989;83:513.
34. Schuh S et al. Nebulized albuterol in acute childhood asthma: comparison of two doses. *Pediatrics* 1990;86:509.
35. Nelson HS. Clinical experience with levalbuterol. *J Allergy Clin Immunol* 1999;104:S77.
36. Gries DM et al. A single dose of intramuscularly administered dexamethasone acetate is as effective as oral prednisone to treat asthma exacerbations in young children. *J Pediatr* 2000;136: 298.

37. Qureshi F et al. Comparative efficacy of oral dexamethasone versus oral prednisolone in acute pediatric asthma. *J Pediatr* 2001;139:20.
38. Altamimi S et al. Single-dose oral dexamethasone in the emergency management of children with exacerbations of mild to moderate asthma. *Pediatr Emerg Care* 2006;22:786.
39. Rohr AS et al. Efficacy of parenteral albuterol in the treatment of asthma: comparison of its metabolic side effects with subcutaneous epinephrine. *Chest* 1986;89:348.
40. Brown MJ et al. Hypokalemia from beta$_2$-receptor stimulation by circulating epinephrine. *N Engl J Med* 1983;309:1414.
41. Lipworth BJ et al. Tachyphylaxis to systemic but not to airway responses during prolonged therapy with high dose inhaled salbutamol in asthmatics. *Am Rev Respir Dis* 1989;140:586.
42. Hall IP. Beta$_2$-adrenoceptor agonists. In Barnes P et al., eds. *Asthma and COPD. Basic Mechanisms and Clinical Management*. Amsterdam: Academic Press; 2002:521.
43. Siegel D et al. Aminophylline increases the toxicity but not the efficacy of an inhaled beta-adrenergic agonist in the treatment of acute exacerbation of asthma. *Am Rev Respir Dis* 1985;132:283.
44. Self TH et al. Inhaled albuterol and oral prednisone therapy in hospitalized adult asthmatics: does aminophylline add any benefit? *Chest* 1990;98:1317.
45. Strauss RE et al. Aminophylline therapy does not improve outcome and increases adverse effects in children hospitalized with acute asthmatic exacerbations. *Pediatrics* 1994;93:205.
46. DiGuiulio GA et al. Hospital treatment of asthma: lack of benefit from theophylline given in addition to nebulized albuterol and intravenously administered corticosteroid. *J Pediatr* 1993;122:464.
47. Carter E et al. Efficacy of intravenously administered theophylline in children hospitalized with severe asthma. *J Pediatr* 1993;122:470.
48. Nuhoglu Y et al. Efficacy of aminophylline in the treatment of acute asthma exacerbation in children. *Ann Allergy Asthma Immunol* 1998;80:395.
49. Huang D et al. Does aminophylline benefit adults admitted to the hospital for an acute exacerbation of asthma? *Ann Intern Med* 1993;119:1155.
50. Weinberger M, Hendeles L. Theophylline in asthma *N Engl J Med* 1996;334:1380.
51. Ellul-Micallef R, Fenech FF. Effect of intravenous prednisolone in asthmatics with diminished adrenergic responsiveness. *Lancet* 1975;2:1269.
52. Shapiro G et al. Double-blind evaluation of methylprednisolone versus placebo for acute asthma episodes. *Pediatrics* 1983;71:510.
53. Fanta CH et al. Glucocorticoids in acute asthma. *Am J Med* 1983;74:845.
54. Littenberg B, Gluck E. A controlled trial of methylprednisolone in the emergency treatment of acute asthma. *N Engl J Med* 1986;314:150.
55. Fiel SB et al. Efficacy of short-term corticosteroid therapy in outpatient treatment of acute bronchial asthma. *Am J Med* 1983;75:259.
56. Harris JB et al. Early intervention with short courses of prednisone to prevent progression of asthma in ambulatory patients incompletely responsive to bronchodilators. *J Pediatr* 1987;110:627.
57. Chapman KR et al. Effect of a short course of prednisone in the prevention of early relapse after the emergency room treatment of acute asthma. *N Engl J Med* 1991;324:788.
58. Lahn M et al. Randomized clinical trial of intramuscular vs. oral methylprednisolone in the treatment of asthma exacerbations following discharge from an emergency department. *Chest* 2004;126:362.
59. Brunette MG et al. Childhood asthma: prevention of attacks with short-term corticosteroid treatment of upper respiratory tract infection. *Pediatrics* 1988;81:624.
60. Connett GJ et al. Prednisolone and salbutamol in the hospital treatment of acute asthma. *Arch Dis Child* 1994;70:170.
61. Harrison BDW et al. Need for intravenous hydrocortisone in addition to oral prednisolone in patients admitted to hospital with severe asthma without ventilatory failure. *Lancet* 1986;1:181.
62. Rowe BH et al. Intravenous magnesium sulfate treatment for acute asthma in the emergency department: a systematic review of the literature. *Ann Emerg Med* 2000;36:181.
63. Hughes R et al. Use of isotonic nebulised magnesium sulphate as an adjuvant to salbutamol in treatment of severe asthma in adults: randomised placebo-controlled trial. *Lancet* 2003;361:2114.
64. Kress JP et al. The utility of albuterol nebulized with heliox during acute asthma exacerbations. *Am J Respir Crit Care Med* 2002;165:1317.
65. Yung M, South M. Randomized controlled trial of aminophylline for severe acute asthma. *Arch Dis Child* 1998;79:405.
66. Ream RS et al. Efficacy of IV theophylline in children with severe status asthmaticus. *Chest* 2001;119:1480.
67. Winter ME. *Basic Clinical Pharmacokinetics*. 4th ed. Baltimore: Lippincott Williams & Wilkins; 2004.
68. Spitzer WO et al. The use of beta agonists and the risk of death and near death from asthma. *N Engl J Med* 1992;326:501.
69. Mellon M et al. Comparable efficacy of administration with face mask or mouthpiece of nebulized budesonide inhalation suspension for infants and young children with persistent asthma. *Am J Crit Care Med* 2000;162(2 Pt 1):593.
70. Pedersen S. Aerosol treatment of bronchoconstriction in children with or without a tube spacer. *N Engl J Med* 1983;308:1328.
71. Croft RD. 2 year old asthmatics can learn to operate a tube spacer by copying their mothers. *Arch Dis Child* 1989;64:742.
72. Sly MR et al. Delivery of albuterol aerosol by AeroChamber to young children. *Ann Allergy* 1988;60:403.
73. Castro-Redriguez JA et al. Beta-agonists through metered dose inhaler with valved holding chamber versus nebulizer for acute exacerbation of wheezing or asthma in children under 5 years of age: a systematic review with meta-analysis. *J Pediatr* 2004;145:172.
74. Van den Berg NJ et al. Salmeterol/fluticasone propionate (50/100 microg) in combination in a Diskus inhaler (Seretide) is effective and safe in children with asthma. *Pediatr Pulmonol* 2000;30:97.
75. Pedersen S. Clinical safety of inhaled corticosteroids for asthma in children. *Drug Saf* 2006;29: 599.
76. Crompton GK et al. Comparison of Pulmicort pMDI plus Nebuhaler and Pulmicort Turbuhaler in asthmatic patients with dysphonia. *Respir Med* 2000;94:448.
77. Kelly HW. Comparison of inhaled corticosteroids. *Ann Pharmacother* 1998;32:220.
78. Pauwels R et al. Effect of inhaled formoterol and budesonide on exacerbations of asthma. *N Engl J Med* 1997;337:1405.
79. Shapiro G et al. Combined salmeterol 50 mcg and fluticasone propionate 250 mcg in the Diskus device for the treatment of asthma. *Am J Respir Crit Care Med* 2000;161:527.
80. Lipworth BJ. Systemic adverse effects of inhaled corticosteroid therapy. *Arch Intern Med* 1999;159:941.
81. Cumming RG et al. Use of inhaled corticosteroids and the risk of cataracts. *N Engl J Med* 1997;337:8.
82. Garbe E et al. Inhaled and nasal glucocorticoids and the risks of ocular hypertension or open-angle glaucoma. *JAMA* 1997;277:722.
83. The Childhood Asthma Management Program Research Group. Long term effects of budesonide or nedocromil in children with asthma. *N Engl J Med* 2000;343:1054.
84. Agertoft L, Pedersen S. Effect of long-term treatment with inhaled budesonide on adult height in children with asthma. *N Engl J Med* 2000;343: 1064.
85. Molen TVD et al. Starting with a higher dose of inhaled corticosteroids in primary care asthma treatment. *Am J Respir Crit Care Med* 1998;158: 121.
86. Suissa S et al. Low-dose inhaled corticosteroids and the prevention of death from asthma. *New Engl J Med* 2000;343:332.
87. Ambikaipakan S et al. Regular use of corticosteroids and low use of short-acting beta-2 agonists can reduce asthma hospitalization. *Chest* 2005;127:1242.
88. Greening AP et al. Added salmeterol versus higher dose corticosteroid in asthma patients with symptoms on existing inhaled corticosteroid. *Lancet* 1994;344:219.
89. Woolcock A et al. Comparison of addition of salmeterol to inhaled steroids with doubling of the dose of inhaled steroids. *Am J Respir Crit Care Med* 1996;153:1481.
90. Bateman ED et al. Can guideline defined asthma control be achieved? The Gaining Optimal Asthma Control Study. *Am J Respir Crit Care Med* 2004;170:836.
91. Nelson HS et al. The Salmeterol Multicenter Asthma Research Trial: a comparison of usual pharmacotherapy for asthma or usual pharmacotherapy plus salmeterol. *Chest* 2006;129:15.
92. Ernst P et al. Safety and effectiveness of long-acting inhaled beta-agonist bronchodilators when taken with inhaled corticosteroids. *Ann Intern Med* 2006;145:692.
93. Halterman JS et al. Benefits of a school-based asthma treatment program in the absence of second-hand smoke exposure. *Arch Pediatr Adolesc Med* 2004;158:460.
94. Tomlinson JEM et al. Efficacy of low and high dose inhaled corticosteroid in smokers versus nonsmokers with mild asthma. *Thorax* 2005;60:282.
95. Adams RJ et al. Impact of inhaled anti-inflammatory therapy on hospitalizations and emergency department visits for children with asthma. *Pediatrics* 2001;107:706.
96. Evans DJ et al. A comparison of low-dose inhaled budesonide plus theophylline and high-dose inhaled budesonide for moderate asthma. *N Engl J Med* 1997;337:1412.
97. Kelly HW. Theophylline toxicity. In: Jenne JW, Murphy S, eds. *Asthma Drugs: Theory and Practice*. New York: Marcel Dekker; 1987:925.
98. Hendeles L et al. Revised FDA labeling guidelines for theophylline oral dosage forms. *Pharmacotherapy* 1995;15:409.
99. Neild JE, Cameron IR. Bronchoconstriction in response to suggestion: its prevention by an inhaled anticholinergic agent. *BMJ* 1985;290:674.
100. Kanazawa H. Anticholinergic agents in asthma: chronic bronchodilator therapy, relief of acute severe asthma, reduction of chronic viral inflammation and prevention of airway remodeling. *Curr Opin Pulm Med* 2006;12:60.
101. Strunk RC, Bloomberg GR. Omalizumab for asthma. *N Engl J Med* 2006;354:2689.
102. Milgrom H et al. Treatment of allergic asthma with monoclonal anti-IgE antibody. *N Engl J Med* 1999;341:1666.
103. Lemanske RF et al. Omalizumab improves asthma-related quality of life in children with allergic asthma. *Pediatrics* 2002;110:e55.
104. Kay AB. Allergic diseases and their treatment. *N Engl J Med* 2001;344:109.
105. Barnes PJ. Therapeutic strategies for allergic diseases. *Nature* 1999;402(6760 Suppl):B31.
106. Busse W et al. Omalizumab, anti-IgE recombinant humanized monoclonal antibody, for the treatment of severe allergic asthma. *J Allergy Clin Immunol* 2001;108:184.
107. Soler M et al. The anti-IgE antibody omalizumab reduces exacerbations and steroid requirement in allergic asthmatics. *Eur Respir J* 2001;18:254.
108. Barnes PJ. Anti-IgE antibody therapy for asthma. *N Engl J Med* 1999;341:2006.
109. Tan RA, Spector SL. Exercise-induced asthma: diagnosis and management. *Ann Allergy Asthma Immunol* 2002;89:226.

110. Godfrey S, Konig P. Suppression of exercise-induced asthma by salbutamol, theophylline, atropine, cromolyn, and placebo in a group of asthmatic children. *Pediatrics* 1975;56:930.
111. Nelson JA et al. Effect of long term salmeterol treatment on exercise induced asthma. *N Engl J Med* 1998;339:141.
112. Leff JA et al. Montelukast, a leukotriene-receptor antagonist for the treatment of mild and exercise-induced bronchoconstriction. *N Engl J Med* 1998;339:147.
113. Newman SP et al. How should a pressurized beta-adrenergic bronchodilator be inhaled? *Eur J Respir Dis* 1981;62:3.
114. Epstein SW et al. Survey of the clinical use of pressurized aerosol inhalers. *Can Med Assoc J* 1979;120:813.
115. Toogood JH et al. Use of spacers to facilitate inhaled corticosteroid treatment of asthma. *Am Rev Respir Dis* 1984;129:723.
116. Salzman GA, Pyszczynski DR. Oropharyngeal candidiasis in patients treated with beclomethasone dipropionate delivered by metered dose inhaler alone and with AeroChamber. *J Allergy Clin Immunol* 1988;81:424.
117. Newman SP. Spacer devices for metered dose inhalers. *Clin Pharmacokinet* 2004;43:349.
118. Rachelefsky GS et al. Use of a tube spacer to improve the efficacy of a metered dose inhaler in asthmatic children. *Am J Dis Child* 1986;140:1191.
119. Self TH et al. Nurses' performance of inhalation technique with metered-dose inhaler plus spacer device. *Ann Pharmacother* 1993;27:185.
120. Interiano B, Guntupalli KK. Metered-dose inhalers: do health care providers know what to teach? *Arch Intern Med* 1993;153:81.
121. Chafin CC et al. Effect of a brief educational intervention on medical students' use of asthma devices. *J Asthma* 2000;37:585.
122. Self TH et al. The value of demonstration and role of the pharmacist in teaching the correct use of pressurized bronchodilators. *Can Med Assoc J* 1983;128:129.
123. Mickle TR et al. Evaluation of pharmacists' practice in patient education when dispensing a metered dose inhaler. *Drug Intell Clin Pharm* 1990;24:927.
124. Toogood JH et al. Comparison of the antiasthmatic, oropharyngeal, and systemic glucocorticoid effects of budesonide administered through a pressurized aerosol plus spacer or the Turbuhaler dry powder inhaler. *J Allergy Clin Immunol* 1997;99:186.
125. Nielsen KG et al. Clinical effect of Diskus dry powder inhaler at low and high inspiratory flow-rates in asthmatic children. *Eur Respir J* 1998;11:350.
126. Strayhorn et al. Elevation of peak expiratory flow by a "spitting" maneuver: measured with five peak flow meters. *Chest* 1998;113:1134.
127. Self TH et al. Gender differences in the use of peak flow meters and their effect on peak expiratory flow. *Pharmacotherapy* 2005;25:526.
128. Mestitz H et al. Comparison of outpatient nebulized vs. metered dose inhaler terbutaline in chronic airflow obstruction. *Chest* 1989;96:1237.
129. Hendeles L et al. Withdrawal of albuterol inhalers containing chlorofluorocarbon propellants. *N Engl J Med* 2007;356:1344.
130. Silkoff PE, Martin RJ. Pathophysiology of nocturnal asthma. *Ann Allergy Asthma Immunol* 1998; 81:378.
131. Holimon TD et al. Nocturnal asthma uncontrolled by inhaled corticosteroids: theophylline or long acting inhaled beta$_2$-agonists. *Drugs* 2001;61: 391.
132. Bernstein ME et al. Aspirin challenge and desensitization for aspirin-exacerbated respiratory disease: a practice paper. *Ann Allergy Asthma Immunol* 2007;98:172.
133. Martin-Garcia C et al. Celecoxib, a highly selective COX-2 inhibitor, is safe in aspirin-induced asthma patients. *J Investig Allergol Clin Immunol* 2003;13:20.
134. Hunt LW, Rosenow EC. Drug-induced asthma. In: Weiss EB, Stein M, eds. *Bronchial Asthma: Mechanisms and Therapeutics*. Boston: Little, Brown; 1993:621.
135. Meeker DP et al. Drug-induced bronchospasm. *Clin Chest Med* 1990;11:163.
136. Szczeklik A, Stevenson DD. Aspirin-induced asthma: advances in pathogenesis, diagnosis, and management. *J Allergy Clin Immunol* 2003;111: 913.
137. Israel E et al. The pivotal role of 5-lipoxygenase products in the reaction of aspirin-sensitive asthmatics to aspirin. *Am Rev Respir Dis* 1993;148: 1447.
138. Holgate ST et al. Leukotriene antagonists and synthesis inhibitors: new directions in asthma therapy. *J Allergy Clin Immunol* 1996;98:1.
139. Odeh M. Timolol eyedrop-induced fatal bronchospasm in an asthmatic patient. *J Fam Pract* 1991;32:97.
140. Dunn TL et al. The effect of topical ophthalmic instillation of timolol and betaxolol on lung function in asthmatic subjects. *Am Rev Respir Dis* 1986;133:264.
141. Salpeter SR et al. Cardioselective beta blockers in patients with reactive airway disease: a meta-analysis. *Ann Intern Med* 2002;137:715.
142. Self TH et al. Cardioselective beta-blockers in patients with asthma and concomitant heart failure or history of myocardial infarction: when do benefits outweigh risks? *J Asthma* 2003;40:839.
143. Cheng B et al. Evaluation of the long term outcome of adult patients managed by the pharmacist-run asthma program in a health maintenance organization. *J Allergy Clin Immunol* 1999;103:51.
144. Pauley T et al. Results of a pharmacy managed, physician directed program to reduce ED visits in a group of inner city adult asthmatic patients. *Ann Pharmacother* 1995;29:5.
145. Kelso T et al. Educational and long term therapeutic intervention in the ED in adult indigent minority patients: effect on clinical outcomes. *Am J Emerg Med* 1995;13:632.
146. Kelso T et al. Comprehensive long term management program for asthma: effect on outcomes in adult African Americans. *Am J Med Sci* 1996; 311:272.
147. McGill KA et al. Improved asthma outcomes in Head Start children using pharmacist asthma counselors. *Am J Respir Crit Care Med* 1997;155: A202.
148. McLean W et al. The BC community pharmacy asthma study: a study of clinical, economic and holistic outcomes influenced by an asthma care protocol provided by specially trained community pharmacists in British Columbia. *Can Respir J* 2003;10:195.
149. Weinberger M et al. Effectiveness of pharmacist care for patients with reactive airway disease. *JAMA* 2002;288:1594.
150. Weil CM et al. The relationship between psychosocial factors and asthma morbidity in inner-city children with asthma. *Pediatrics* 1999;104:1274.
151. Finkelstein JA et al. Underuse of controller medications among Medicaid-insured children with asthma. *Arch Pediatr Adolesc Med* 2002;156: 562.
152. Evans D et al. The impact of passive smoking on emergency room visits of urban children with asthma. *Am Rev Respir Dis* 1987;135:567.
153. Self TH et al. Reducing emergency department visits and hospitalizations in African Americans and Hispanic patients with asthma: a 15-year review. *J Asthma* 2005;42:807.
154. Giraud V, Roche N. Misuse of corticosteroid metered-dose inhaler is associated with decreased asthma stability. *Eur Respir J* 2002;19:246.
155. Finch CK et al. Gender differences in peak flow meter use. *Nurse Pract* 2007;32:46.
156. The American Lung Association Asthma Clinical Research Centers. Randomized comparison of strategies for reducing treatment in mild persistent asthma. *N Engl J Med* 2007;356:2027.
157. Papi A et al. Rescue use of beclomethasone and albuterol in a single inhaler for mild asthma. *N Engl J Med* 2007;356:2040.
158. Blanc PD et al. Use of herbal products, coffee or black tea, and over the counter medications as self-treatments among adults with asthma. *J Allergy Clin Immunol* 1997;100:789.
159. Huntley A, Ernst E. Herbal medicines for asthma: a systematic review. *Thorax* 2000;55:925.
160. Self TH et al. Educating inner-city patients with asthma: a compelling opportunity for volunteer service by health science center students. *J Asthma* 2004;41:1.
161. Nathan RA et al. Development of the asthma control test: a survey for assessing asthma control. *J Allergy Clin Immunol* 2004;113:59.

CHAPTER 23

Chronic Obstructive Pulmonary Disease

Philip T. Diaz and Daren L. Knoell

Definitions

In 2001, the National Institutes of Health (NIH) and the World Health Organization (WHO) collaborated to develop the Global Initiative for Chronic Obstructive Lung Disease (GOLD) guidelines.[1] These guidelines address a wide variety of topics related to chronic obstructive pulmonary disease (COPD), including current concepts of pathophysiology, and recommendations regarding diagnosis and treatment. The guidelines are updated yearly, represent an international effort, and are based on the strength of the evidence supporting them. The most recent definition of COPD according to GOLD is as follows: "Chronic obstructive pulmonary disease (COPD) is characterized by chronic airflow limitation and a range of pathological changes in the lung, some significant extra-pulmonary effects, and important comorbidities which may contribute to the severity of the disease in individual patients. Thus, COPD should be regarded as a pulmonary disease, but these significant comorbidities must be taken into account in a comprehensive diagnostic assessment of severity and in determining appropriate treatment."[1]

Chronic obstructive pulmonary disease generally refers to emphysema or chronic bronchitis. Emphysema is pathologically defined and characterized by alveolar wall destruction and air–space enlargement. Chronic bronchitis is clinically defined as a chronic cough for at least 3 months for 2 consecutive years. Its pathologic hallmark involves inflammation and fibrosis of the small airways.[2]

Clearly, much overlap exists between these two conditions because both are primarily caused by cigarette smoking. It should also be pointed out that small airway inflammation is an important characteristic of COPD, which appears to correlate with the more severe stages of the disease whether or not the patient has "chronic bronchitis."[3] Asthma, the other major disease entity characterized by airflow limitation, can clearly coexist in patients with COPD. Nevertheless, the pattern of airway inflammation in asthma differs significantly from that which occurs in COPD and asthma is not generally considered part of the spectrum of COPD.[4]

Epidemiology

Chronic obstructive pulmonary disease is an extremely important cause of morbidity and mortality. For example, the prevalence of COPD more than doubled between 1990 and 2002, making it the fourth leading cause of death in the United States.[5] Furthermore, it is projected to be the third leading cause of death by the year 2020.[1] This increase in prevalence of COPD is felt to be related to the aging of the population and past smoking behavior, because COPD death rates and prevalence lag behind smoking rates by several decades. Because the smoking rates for women peaked later than rates for men, the increase in COPD prevalence in the United States is related primarily to an increase in COPD among women.[6]

The economic impact of COPD is also significant, with estimated annual treatment costs exceeding $30 billion. This includes health care expenditures of $18 billion and indirect costs of $14 billion (e.g., lost earnings because of illness or early death).[5]

A major cause of disability, COPD currently is considered the 11th leading cause of disability worldwide. Current projections suggest that by the year 2020, COPD will be the 5th leading cause of disability worldwide, behind only ischemic heart disease, major depression, traffic accidents, and cerebrovascular disease.[1]

Risk Factors

Clearly, cigarette smoking is the major risk factor for COPD. Most cases of COPD are attributed to a current or past history of cigarette smoking.[1] Importantly, with more severe disease, the relevance of cigarette smoking as a risk factor becomes even more pronounced. Evidence exists that among patients with severe emphysema ~99% have a history of regular cigarette smoking.[7] It should be noted that only a few smokers develop clinically significant COPD, suggesting that other risk factors may be important cofactors with smoking in COPD development. Such factors include occupational dusts and chemicals,[8–11] indoor and outdoor air pollution,[12–14] and certain infections, including respiratory viruses[15] as well as infection with human immunodeficiency virus (HIV).[16] It is possible that such factors may upregulate the inflammatory response of the lungs to cigarette smoke.[15,16] Genetic factors are also likely to be important, although precise genetic characteristics have not yet been elucidated.[17–19] One exception is α_1-antitrypsin deficiency, which affects <2% of patients with emphysema. Affected individuals have an inherited deficiency of this protective antiprotease and are at much greater risk of developing emphysema than the general population.[20]

The risk of COPD from cigarette smoking is related to an accelerated loss of lung function. After age 35, nonsmokers experience a decline in forced expiratory volume in the first second of expiration (FEV_1) of about 20 to 30 mL/year. In smokers, the decline may be 50 to 120 mL/year[21] A model of the annual decline in lung function in nonsmokers, smokers, and susceptible smokers is illustrated in Figure 23-1.

Pathogenesis

The exact mechanisms responsible for the pathogenesis of COPD are not entirely clear, but likely involve activation of the innate and adaptive immune system leading to chronic inflammation. In general, inhalation of noxious agents, such as cigarette smoke, leads to the activation of resident immune and parenchymal cells, which in turn, recruit additional inflammatory cells from the systemic compartment into the resident tissue and airway (Fig. 23-2). The activation and recruitment of immune cells is largely mediated through the production and release of cytokines and chemokines (Table 23-1). Recent evidence also supports a role for oxidant stress as a disease mediator.[22,23] The consequences of an oxidant-rich environment include the activation of inflammatory genes, inactivation of antiproteases, stimulation of mucous secretion, and increases in plasma exudate.

The most well studied cause of COPD, and particularly emphysema, relates to protease–antiprotease imbalance. In this setting, inflammation promotes the production and release of proteases from inflammatory and parenchymal cells. When the local concentration of antiproteases becomes overwhelmed, proteases go unchecked and destroy the major connective tissue components in the lung, such as elastin, leading to the irreversible loss of alveoli (Table 23-2). The classic example of this occurs in patients with α_1-antitrypsin deficiency.

Although the traditional idea of disease pathogenesis focuses on smoking-related lung *injury*, more recent hypotheses suggest that another important component of disease pathogenesis may involve inadequate lung *repair*. Indeed, recent studies demonstrate that normal lung homeostatic mechanisms are altered in COPD. This may involve inadequate production of growth factors as well as altered regulation of apoptosis, or programmed cell death.[24]

Pathophysiology

The airflow obstruction caused by COPD is usually progressive and attributed to pathologic changes in the lung that affect the proximal airways, peripheral airways, lung parenchyma, and pulmonary vasculature.[3] Alterations in tissue structure are caused by chronic inflammation that involves recruitment of inflammatory cells into the lung, as well as structural changes that result from repeated injury and tissue remodeling. The

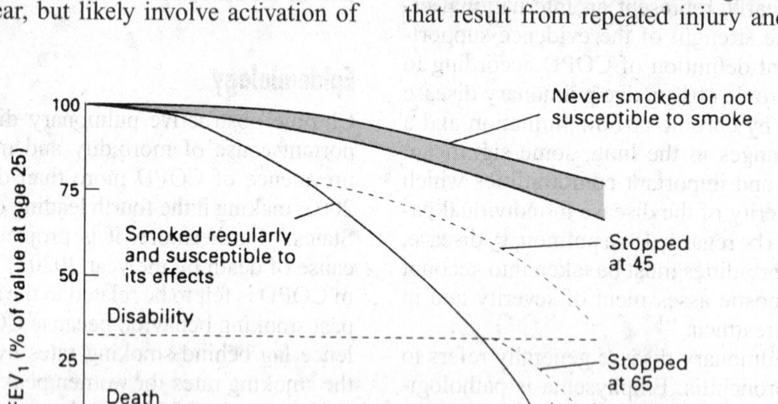

FIGURE 23-1 Model of annual decline in FEV_1 with accelerated decline in susceptible smokers. On stopping smoking subsequent loss is similar to that in healthy nonsmokers. (Modified from Fletcher C, Peto R. The natural history of chronic airflow obstruction. *BMJ* 1977;1:1645.)

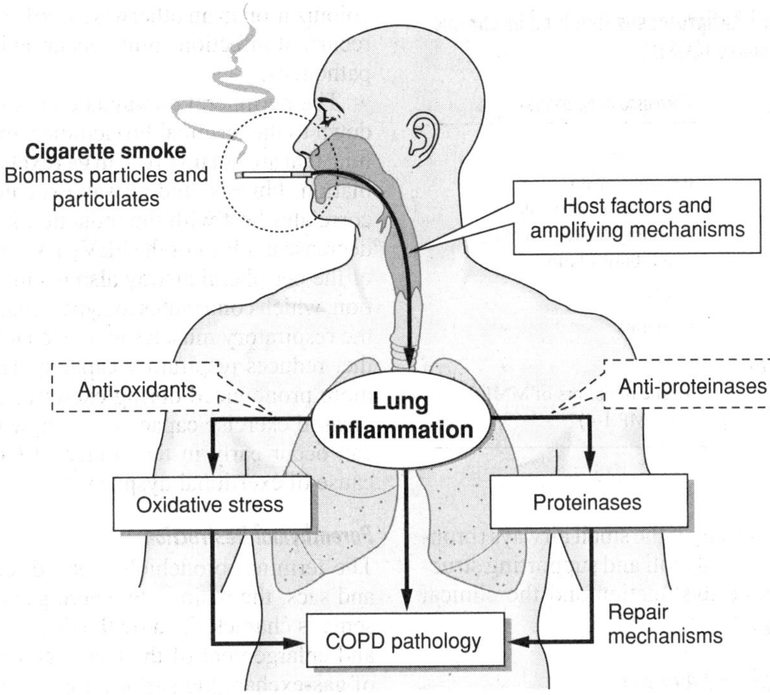

FIGURE 23-2 Pathogenesis of COPD. (Reprinted with permission from reference 1.)

magnitude of structural changes and tissue dysfunction varies among patients and is often distinguished by two major phenotypes that include chronic bronchitis and emphysema. Chronic airflow limitation can result from both of these processes. The GOLD or most recent American Thoracic Society (ATS) and European Thoracic Society guidelines[25] do not distinguish between these two entities; however, the classic definitions and pathophysiologic features are described here to aid in a better understanding of the disease process.

In the simplest view, *bronchitis* is inflammation of the bronchioles. The clinical definition from the ATS for *chronic bronchitis* is "the presence of chronic productive cough for 3 months in each of 2 consecutive years in a patient in whom other causes of chronic cough (e.g., asthma, congestive heart failure, gastroesophageal reflux) have been excluded."[26] *Emphysema* is described as "abnormal permanent enlargement of the airspaces distal to the terminal bronchioles, accompanied by destruction of their walls and without obvious

Table 23-1 Inflammatory Cells and Mediators in Chronic Obstructive Pulmonary Disease (COPD)

Cell	
Neutrophils	↑ in sputum of normal smokers. Further ↑ in COPD and related to disease severity. Few neutrophils are seen in tissue. May be important in mucus hypersecretion and through release of proteases.
Macrophages	Greatly ↑ numbers in airway lumen, lung parenchyma, and bronchoalveolar lavage fluid. Derived from blood monocytes that differentiate within lung tissue. Produce increased inflammatory mediators and proteases in patients with COPD in response to cigarette smoke and may show defective phagocytosis.
T lymphocytes	Both CD4+ and CD8+ cells are increased in the airway wall and lung parenchyma, with ↑ CD8+:CD4+ ratio. ↑ CD8+ T cells (Tc1) and Th1 cells which secrete interferon-γ and express the chemokine receptor CXCR3. CD8+ cells may be cytotoxic to alveolar cells, contributing to their destruction.
B lymphocytes	↑ in peripheral airways and within lymphoid follicles, possibly as a response to chronic colonization and infection of the airways.
Eosinophils	↑ eosinophil proteins in sputum and ↑ eosinophils in airway wall during exacerbations.
Epithelial cells	May be activated by cigarette smoke to produce inflammatory mediators.
Mediators	
Chemotactic factors	• Lipid mediators: e.g., leukotriene B_4 (LTB_4) attracts neutrophils and T lymphocytes. • Chemokines: e.g., interleukin-8 (IL-8) attracts neutrophils and monocytes.
Proinflammatory cytokines	Cytokines, including tumor necrosis factor-α (TNF-α), IL-1β, and IL-6 amplify the inflammatory process and may contribute to some of the systemic effects of COPD.
Growth factors	e.g., transforming growth factor-β (TGF-β) may induce fibrosis in small airways.

Adapted from reference 1, with permission.

Table 23-2 Proteases and Antiproteases Involved in Chronic Obstructive Pulmonary Disease (COPD)

Increased Proteases	*Decreased Antiproteases*
Serine proteases	
Neutrophil elastase	α-1 antitrypsin
Cathepsin G	α-1 antichymotrypsin
Proteinase 3	Secretory leukoprotease inhibitor Elafin
Cysteine proteinases	
Cathepsins B, K, L, S	Cystatins
Matrix metalloproteinases (MMP)	
MMP-8, MMP-9, MMP-12	Tissue inhibitors of MMP 1-4 (TIMP 1-4)

From reference 1, with permission.

fibrosis." The degree of impairment of the small airways (bronchioles) or the lung parenchyma (alveoli and supporting structures) directly influences tissue dysfunction and the clinical symptoms of the patient (Fig. 23-3).

Large (Central) and Small (Peripheral) Airways

The large airways, which include the trachea and first generations of the bronchi, are a major site of inflammation and mucus hypersecretion. This results from an increase in numbers (hyperplasia) and enlargement (hypertrophy) of the submucosal glands and mucus-producing goblet cells within the surface epithelium.[27,28] Overproduction of mucus in the large airways results in a chronic productive cough, as observed in chronic bronchitis, but this does not have a major impact on airflow limitation. Mucus hypersecretion coupled with impaired ciliary function, reduces mucociliary clearance, increases the accumulation of secretions, and enhances the risk of bacteria colonization in an otherwise sterile environment.[29] As a result, recurrent infections often occur owing to the inability to clear pathogens.

The peripheral airway is composed of the smaller bronchi down to the terminal bronchioles, the smallest branches in the lung that are not involved in gas exchange. The extent of inflammation, fibrosis, and airway exudate in the peripheral airway correlates best with the reduction in airflow as measured by a decrease in FEV_1 or the FEV_1/FVC ratio.[3] Chronic obstruction of the peripheral airway also results in air trapping on expiration, which contributes to hyperinflation. Hyperinflation places the respiratory muscles at a mechanical disadvantage and further reduces respiratory capacity. Hyperinflation can become more pronounced during exercise, leading to dyspea and decreased exercise capacity. It is now known that hyperinflation can occur early in the course of COPD and is an important cause of exertional dyspnea.[30]

Parenchymal Destruction

The terminal bronchioles lead directly to the alveolar ducts and sacs, the major site where gas exchange occurs. Emphysema is characterized by the destructive loss of alveolar walls and enlargement of the terminal airspaces resulting in a loss of gas-exchanging surface area.[29,31] In advanced cases, large, balloon-shaped bullous lesions may develop. Rupture of these bullae can lead to collapse of lung segments (pneumothorax). *Panacinar emphysema* is a term used to describe when enlargement of the airspaces is relatively uniform throughout the entire acinus, and involves the respiratory bronchioles and alveoli. The lower lobes are most commonly involved. This is the pattern associated with α_1-antitrypsin deficiency.[26] In centrilobular (centriacinar) emphysema, the primary lesions occur in the respiratory bronchioles, alveolar ducts, and central alveoli, with sparing of the peripheral acini. This is the most common pattern of emphysema and primarily involves

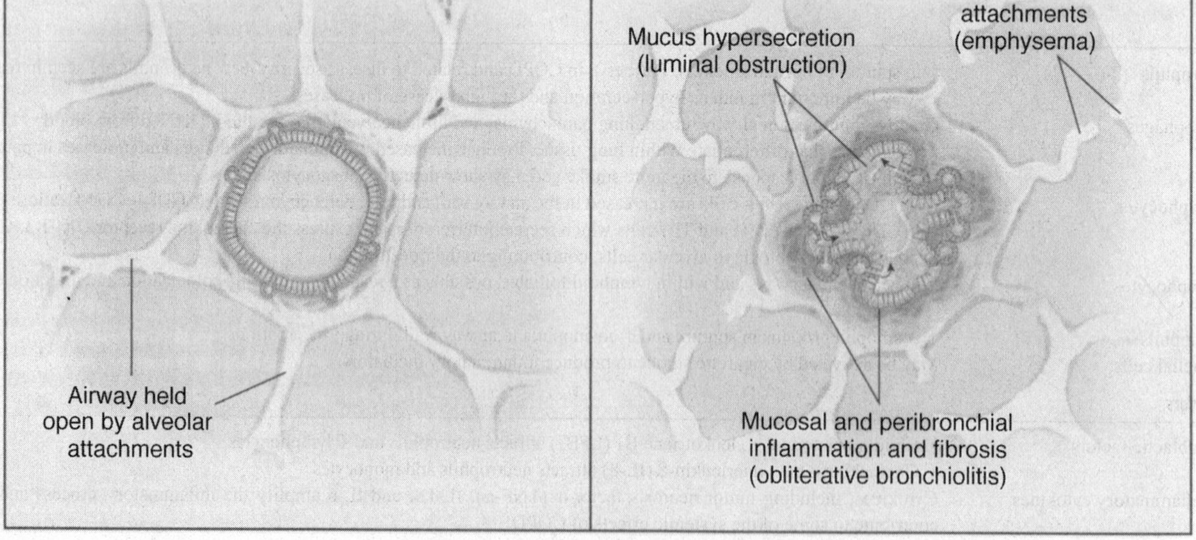

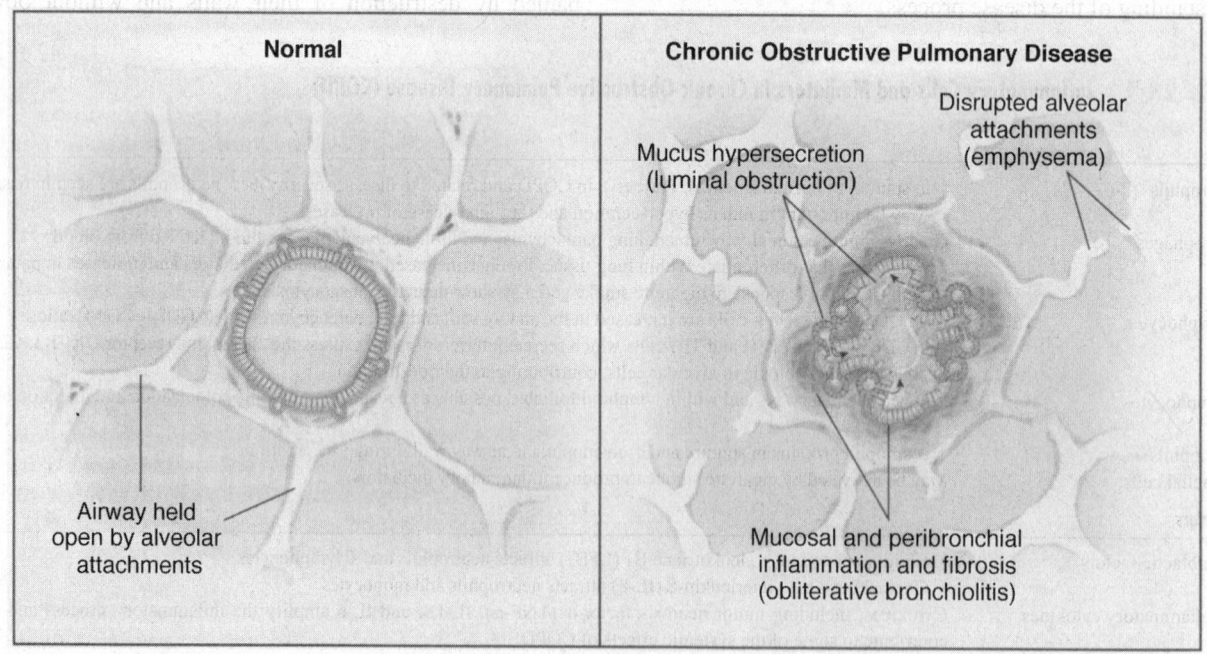

FIGURE 23-3 Inflammatory mechanisms in chronic obstructive pulmonary disease. (From Barnes PJ, Chronic obstructive pulmonary disease. *N Engl J Med* 200;343(4):269. Copyright © Massachusetts Medical Society, 2000.)

the upper lobes of the lung. The distinction between *panlobular* and *centrilobular* emphysema may be relevant with regard to disease pathogenesis and pathophysiology, but is generally not important clinically. Both phenotypes lead to gas exchange abnormalities and loss of lung elastic recoil and structural support. Abnormalities in gas exchange ultimately leads to hypoxemia, hypercarbia, or both. Loss of lung recoil and structural support promotes collapse of small airways during expiration and progressive airflow limitation.

Significant Comorbid Illness

In the later stages of disease, chronic hypoxemia causes persistent vasoconstriction in the lung vascular bed, particularly the small pulmonary arteries. This can result in permanent structural alteration of the blood vessels causing intimal hyperplasia and smooth muscle hypertrophy.[32] The loss of pulmonary capillaries in emphysema can also contribute to increased pulmonary vasculature pressures. The cumulative impact of vascular changes can result in progressive pulmonary hypertension and eventually, right-sided cardiac failure (cor pulmonale).

As COPD progresses, additional systemic consequences can arise, including cachexia, skeletal muscle dysfunction, osteoporosis, depression, and anemia. The cause of these additional systemic disease processes is not entirely clear but likely involves the dynamic interplay of progressive respiratory dysfunction, lung and systemic inflammation, side effects from medication use, and physical debilitation.

In summary, although COPD is primarily a disease of the large and small airways and adjacent alveolar structures, it also includes important systemic consequences. The clinical consequences of the morphologic and pathophysiologic alterations include progressive dyspnea on exertion, chronic cough and sputum production, increased risk for respiratory infections, deconditioning, and an overall reduction in quality of life.

Comparison With Asthma

Because COPD and asthma are both common diseases, both illnesses can coexist in the same patient. Nevertheless, these conditions should be considered as separate and distinct entities (Fig. 23-4). For example, although inflammation is a key component of both conditions, the pattern of inflammation

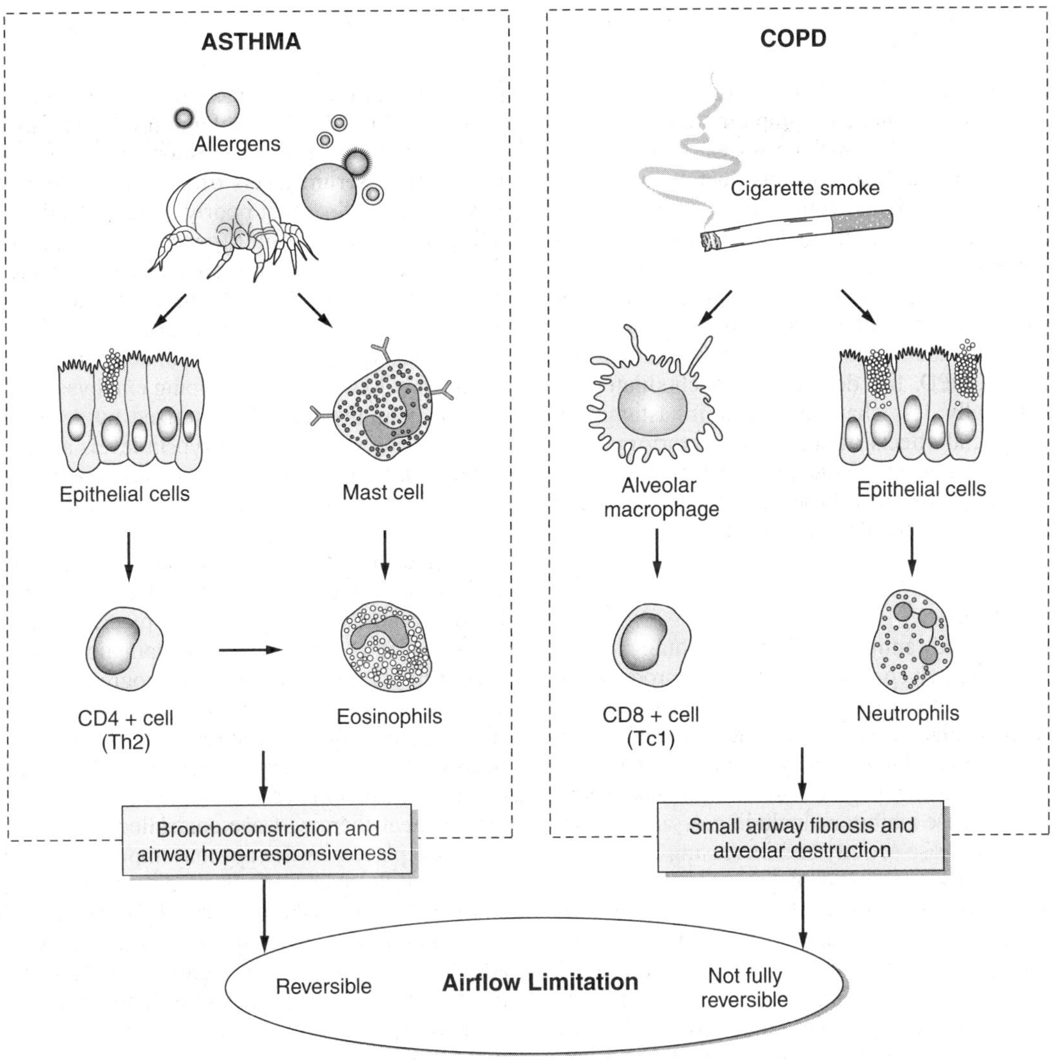

FIGURE 23-4 Inflammatory cascade in COPD and asthma. (Reprinted with permission from reference 1.)

Table 23-3 Differences in Pulmonary Inflammation Between Asthma and Chronic Obstructive Pulmonary Disease (COPD)

	COPD	Asthma	Severe Asthma
Cells	Neutrophils ++ Macrophages +++ CD8+ T cells (Tc1)	Eosinophils ++ Macrophages + CD4+ T cells (Th2)	Neutrophils+ Macrophages CD4+ T cells (Th2) CD8+ T cells (Tc1)
Key Mediators	IL-8, TNF-α, IL-1β, IL-6, NO+	Eotaxin IL-4, IL-5, IL-13 NO+++	IL-8 IL-5, IL-13 NO ++
Oxidative stress	+++	+	+++
Site of disease	Peripheral airways Lung parenchyma Pulmonary vessels	Proximal airways	Proximal airways Peripheral airways
Consequences	Squamous metaplasia Mucous metaplasia Small airway fibrosis Parenchymal destruction Pulmonary vascular remodeling	Fragile epithelium, Mucous metaplasia ↑ Basement membrane Bronchoconstriction	
Response to therapy	Small bronchodilator response Poor response to steroids	Large bronchodilator response Good response to steroids	Smaller bronchodilator response Reduced response to steroids

NO, nitric oxide.
From reference 1, with permission.

differs significantly (Table 23-3). As a result, the pathophysiologic consequences, patient symptoms and response to medications typically differ. Asthma is generally not progressive and symptoms and airflow obstruction are often completely reversible. Patients with asthma respond well to anti-inflammatory medication, including inhaled glucocorticoids. Furthermore, in the absence of an acute exacerbation, significant gas exchange abnormalities are uncommon. COPD, on the other hand, is a progressive and often fatal disorder. Although bronchodilators are clearly helpful in COPD, the degree of bronchodilator reversibility is typically less than that seen in asthma. In addition, the beneficial effects of anti-inflammatory medication, including inhaled glucocorticoids, are much more modest. Patients with COPD, particularly those with emphysema, have substantial derangements in pulmonary gas exchange even at baseline.

α_1-Antitrypsin Deficiency

The best characterized antiprotease in the lung is α_1-antitrypsin. This serum glycoprotein is primarily produced in the liver and works by binding to and neutralizing proteases. As previously described, cigarette smoke can activate and attract inflammatory cells into the lung, thereby promoting the release of proteases such as elastase. Cigarette smoke can also inactivate endogenous protease inhibitors, including α_1-antitrypsin, further supporting protease activity and increasing the risk of tissue damage. This risk of tissue damage is greatly accentuated in patients with α_1-antitrypsin deficiency.

α_1-Antitrypsin deficiency occurs in <2% of all COPD cases. Clinically significant disease is usually associated only with severe deficiency (i.e., serum α_1 levels <45 mg/dL; normal >150 mg/dL). The diagnosis of α_1-antitrypsin deficiency is made by measuring circulating serum α_1-antitrypsin levels, followed by phenotype analysis.[33] The PiM allele confers production of the fully functional protein. Accordingly, a homozygous PiMM individual will produce a functional protein with normal plasma concentrations. Other gene types include PiS (normal serum levels of a poorly functioning enzyme), PiZ (an active form but poorly secreted leading to low circulating levels), and Pi null (gene polymorphism leads to production of a truncated protein and undetectable serum levels of functional protein). Different allele pairs can exist. PiMZ and PiSZ are heterozygous disorders, and PiSS is a homozygous phenotype, all with >35% of normal enzyme activity and a relatively low risk of developing emphysema. PiZZ is a rare homozygous disorder characterized by accelerated lung destruction and serum α_1-antitrypsin levels approximately 15% of normal. In these rare patients, the disease develops as early as age 20, but more typically in the fourth to fifth decade of life.

Replacement therapy is available for patients with COPD with documented α_1-antitrypsin deficiency and emphysema. Patients who do qualify typically receive weekly intravenous infusions of α_1-antitrypsin to maintain acceptable antiprotease activity and minimize the progression of lung disease. This therapy is very expensive, not well tolerated by some (fever, chills, allergic reactions, flu-like symptoms), and has been hampered by supply problems. Currently, no placebo-controlled, randomized trials have documented the efficacy of replacement therapy. Case-controlled studies, however, suggest the replacement therapy may improve outcomes in patients with α_1-antitrypsin deficiency, documented emphysema and an FEV_1 between 35% and 60% of predicted.[20] Three different formulations of α_1-antitrypsin are available: Aralast, Prolastin, and Zemaira. No clinically significant differences exist among these preparations. Because the α_1-antitrypsin products are derived from pooled human plasma, there are also associated risks for the transmission of infectious diseases (e.g., viral infections and Creutzfeldt-Jakob disease).

DIAGNOSIS AND PATIENT ASSESSMENT

The diagnosis of COPD is based on the presence of risk factors (generally smoking), clinical symptoms, and airflow obstruction on spirometric testing.[1] Generally, individuals with COPD present in the sixth decade of life (or later) with symptoms of cough, wheeze, or dyspnea on exertion.[25] Patients usually have at least a 20-pack/year history (e.g. averaging one pack of cigarettes a day for 20 years) history of cigarette smoking. Because the severity of COPD is related to the cumulative exposure to cigarette smoke, patients with more severe disease are likely to be older with a heavier smoking history. Cough and sputum production may be present for many years before airflow limitation develops, but not everyone with those symptoms will develop COPD. Dyspnea on exertion may not be present until the sixth or seventh decade.

On physical examination, patients with early COPD may not exhibit any changes.[25] Later, objective findings include the presence of a barrel chest (defined as an increase in the anteroposterior diameter of the chest), rales (defined as intermittent, nonmusical, brief crackle sounds), rhonchi (defined as continuous, musical high of low pitched sounds), prolonged expiratory phase, and cyanosis.[1] Symptomatic patients may present with decreased breath sounds, wheezes, or slight rales on auscultation. In advanced disease, cyanosis, edema, intercostal retractions, and pursed lip breathing may be present.[1]

Spirometry Testing

Spirometry is the gold standard measurement in assessing and monitoring obstructive lung disease.[1,25] In the evaluation of COPD, spirometry testing should be performed according to published guidelines, when the patient's condition is stable and after administration of two to four puffs of albuterol by metered dose inhaler. During spriometry, a full breath is taken, followed by a forceful exhalation of all the air that can be exhaled (forced vital capacity [FVC]). Flow rates and volumes of air that are expired at different time intervals can be recorded. The FEV_1 is the volume of air that can be expired within the first second of an FVC maneuver. A decrease in the FEV_1/FVC ratio indicates airflow obstruction. Although the range of normal for FEV_1/FVC depends on the age, sex, and height of the patient, a value of <0.70 indicates airflow obstruction that is compatible with COPD.[1,25] Also, patients with COPD may have some improvement in spirometry testing with an acute bronchodilator challenge. The degree of reversibility is typically less than that seen with asthma, although up to 50% of patients with moderate to severe emphysema will have an increase in FVC with acute bronchodilator challenge that meets ATS criteria as significant. It is important to point out that, although a decrease in the FEV_1/FVC ratio categorizes the patient as having airflow obstruction, the disease severity is best assessed by examining the FEV_1 as a percent of predicted. Indeed, most major organizations that have provided recommendations regarding the clinical management of COPD use the percent of predicted FEV_1 to determine the disease severity.[1,25] In addition to being critical for making the diagnosis of COPD, spirometry also affords the best objective way to monitor disease progression. Although optimal frequency of spirometric testing for patients with COPD is not known, spirometry should be considered if there has been a persistent change in clinical symptoms (e.g., worsened dyspnea).

Other pulmonary function testing is sometimes used to assess patients with COPD. The determination of lung volumes, including the total lung capacity (TLC) and residual volume (RV) as well as measurements of the diffusing capacity for carbon monoxide may provide more detail regarding lung physiology. For example, a reduction in diffusing capacity of the lung for carbon monoxide (DL_{CO}) indicates disruption or destruction of the alveolar capillary interface and correlates with the degree of emphysema. Determination of lung volumes may be used to assess the presence of concomitant restrictive lung disease (e.g., idiopathic pulmonary fibrosis) in the case of diagnostic uncertainty. Patients with COPD typically have normal or increased lung volumes; a reduction in total lung capacity may indicate a superimposed restrictive process. Furthermore, lung volumes and diffusion capacity are used to assess patients for surgical procedures, such as lung volume reduction surgery.[7] In general however, spirometric testing is adequate to make the diagnosis of COPD and follow the course of disease.[1,25]

A chest x-ray (CXR) study is often performed during the initial assessment of patients with COPD. Because the CXR lacks sensitivity and demonstrates minimal changes until COPD is moderately severe, its main utility is in ruling out other disease processes that may be contributing to the patients symptoms. In severe disease, the chest radiograph may indicate hyperinflation manifested by a flattened diaphragm or evidence of pulmonary arterial hypertension characterized by enlarged pulmonary arteries.

Assessing the oxygen status of a patient with COPD can be done by pulse oximetry. This should be considered in patients with dyspnea and advanced disease, and patients with evidence of right ventricular pressure overload (e.g., peripheral edema, or jugular venous distension). Although a decrease in pulse oximetry (normal, $\geq$97%) is common in COPD, values of $\leq$88% are consistent with chronic respiratory failure and qualify the patient for supplemental oxygen. Arterial blood gas (ABG) determination is generally reserved for patients with severe disease (i.e., an FEV_1 <50% of predicted). ABG can more precisely define the oxygen status of a patient and can be used to assess whether the patient has carbon dioxide retention (normal PCO_2 = 40 mm Hg). Determining the α_1-antitrypsin concentration is indicated for patients developing COPD before age 45, and for patients who have emphysema without a significant history of cigarette smoking or who have a family history of emphysema.

Classification of Severity and Clinical Presentation

A number of staging systems have been proposed to categorize the severity of COPD. All are based primarily on the degree of airflow obstruction as assessed by the FEV_1.[1,25,26] The staging system recommended by the most recent GOLD guideline is demonstrated in Table 23-4. The GOLD expert panel classifies disease severity into four stages based on spirometric measurements, symptoms, and complications.[1] This staging is intended to serve as an educational and research tool and to guide management strategies. It should be noted that, although FEV_1-based staging systems can provide important prognostic information, more comprehensive scoring systems may provide more discriminating information with regard to survival

Table 23-4 Spirometric Classification of Chronic Obstructive Pulmonary Disease (COPD) Severity Based on Post-Bronchodilator FEV_1

Stage	Classification	Spirometry Results
I	Mild	$FEV_1/FVC < 0.70$ $FEV_1 \geq 80\%$ predicted
II	Moderate	$FEV_1/FVC < 0.70$ $50\% \leq FEV_1 < 80\%$ predicted
III	Severe	$FEV_1/FVC < 0.70$ $30\% \leq FEV_1 < 50\%$ predicted
IV	Very Severe	$FEV_1/FVC < 0.70$ $FEV_1 < 30\%$ predicted or $FEV_1 < 50\%$ predicted plus chronic respiratory failure

FEV_1: forced expiratory volume in one second; FVC: forced vital capacity; respiratory failure: arterial partial pressure of oxygen (Pa_{O_2}) <8.0 kPa (60 mm Hg) with or without arterial partial pressure of CO_2 (Pa_{CO_2}) >6.7 kPa (50 mm Hg) while breathing air at sea level.

in COPD. For example, a scoring system based on body mass index, obstruction on spirometry, dyspnea level, and exercise capacity (BODE) can predict survival in COPD far better than the FEV_1 alone[34] (Table 23-5).

Natural Course

The natural course of COPD is highly variable, generally spanning 20 to 40 years and influenced by numerous factors, including genetic predisposition, exposure to inhaled irritants (tobacco smoke, workplace, or environmental pollutants), and repeated infections. The typical smoker who develops COPD remains asymptomatic for the first two decades of smoking, except for more frequent viral or bacterial upper respiratory tract infections. Clinical symptoms appear after significant irreversible lung damage occurs. After 25 to 30 years of smoking, mild dyspnea on exertion is commonly noted and can be accompanied by a morning cough; however, physical examination and chest radiograph are often unremarkable.[25] With continued exposure to risks (e.g., cigarette smoking), the disease progresses and patients develop increased airflow limitation and worsened dyspnea on exertion, and increased cough and sputum production. Ultimately, structural changes result in alveolar hypoxia and the secondary problems of pulmonary hypertension and cor pulmonale.

Exacerbations, or flares, of COPD are common and can be infectious or noninfectious. Moderate to severe exacerbations may require hospitalization. Acute or chronic respiratory failure can develop secondary to an acute infection, or other factors, including oversedation, heart failure, or pulmonary embolism.[35,36]

GENERAL MANAGEMENT CONSIDERATIONS

The overall goals for treatment of the patient with COPD are depicted in Figure 23-5.[25] The only interventions that have proved to reduce mortality in COPD are smoking cessation, oxygen therapy for patients with severe hypoxemia at rest, and lung volume reduction surgery for very select patients with advanced emphysema.[7,37–39] As such, many of the interventions are aimed at alleviating symptoms and maximizing quality of life.

Because, continued cigarette smoking is associated with accelerated progression of disease in susceptible smokers, smoking cessation is critical to disease treatment. Strategies for smoking cessation are detailed in Chapter 85, Tobacco Use and Dependence. The benefits of smoking cessation in COPD include decreases in respiratory symptoms, exacerbation rate, and lung function decline.[21,40] It should also be noted that cardiovascular complications, including coronary artery disease, are more common in patients with COPD and that smoking cessation may attenuate morbidity and mortality from this complication.

Immunizations provide protection against serious illness and death in patients with COPD.[41] The efficacy, benefit, and cost-effectiveness of vaccination against influenza among this population are significant.[42] Data concerning the value of vaccinating against pneumococcal pneumonia are lacking, but it is

Table 23-5 Variables and Point Values Used for the Computation of the Body-Mass Index, Degree of Airflow Obstruction and Dyspnea, and Exercise Capacity (BODE) Index

Variable	Points 0	1	2	3
Body Mass Index (kg/m²)	≥21	<21		
Obstruction of airflow (FEV1% predicted)	≥65	50–64	36–49	≤35
Dyspnea?	None or only with strenuous exertion	Walking up a slight hill	Walking on the level	Getting dressed
Exercise capacity (6 min walk distance, feet)	> 1,148	820–1,149	492–819	<492

Approximate 4-year survival based on total BODE score:
- 0–2 points: 80%
- 3–4 points: 70%
- 5–6 points: 60%
- 7–10 points: 20%

From reference 25, with permission.

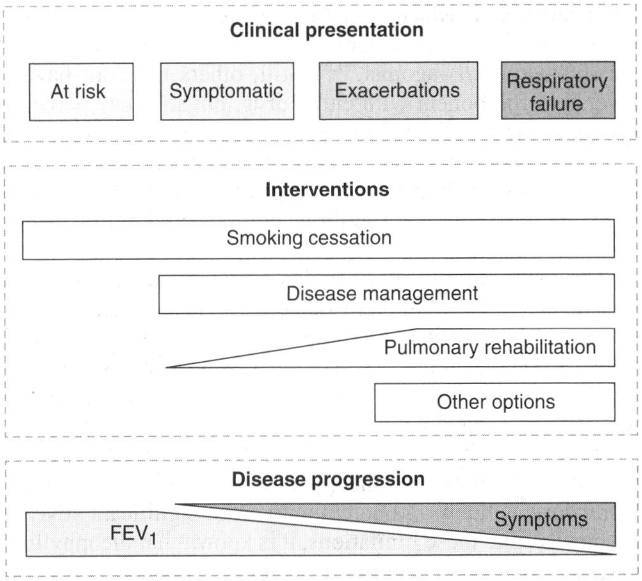

FIGURE 23-5 Continuum of care for chronic obstructive pulmonary disease (COPD). (Reprinted with permission from reference 25)

recommended in the GOLD guidelines because of a favorable risk:benefit ratio.[1]

Pulmonary rehabilitation is an exercise-based program aimed at maximizing the patient's functional status and quality of life. Multiple studies have now documented the beneficial effects of pulmonary rehabilitation, particularly with respect to improved exercise tolerance and alleviation of dyspnea.[43] In addition, cost-effective analysis suggests that pulmonary rehabilitation programs are very cost-effective.[44] Pulmonary rehabilitation programs are multidisciplinary programs typically running for 6 to 12 weeks, two to three sessions per week. A number of interventions are used, including breathing retraining, psychosocial counseling, education, dietary counseling, and airway clearance techniques for patients with chronic sputum production. Arm strengthening and arm endurance exercises are important because patients with COPD commonly have excessive dyspnea when utilizing their upper extremities.[43] The most important component of a pulmonary rehabilitation program is lower extremity endurance training, often utilizing a treadmill or bicycle ergometer. Because the large muscle groups have diminished oxidative capacity,[45–47] likely related to deconditioning and chronic inflammation,[48,49] patients with COPD convert to anaerobic metabolism, leading to increased lactate production for a given level of activity[50] and, subsequently, increased CO_2 production. Lower extremity endurance training can significantly improve mitochondrial oxidative capacity in patients with COPD.[45,51] This physiologic benefit is felt to be an important mechanism whereby pulmonary rehabilitation exerts its effect. Other important effects, such as alleviation of depression and anxiety, may be important as well.[43]

As mentioned, patients with severe resting hypoxemia have improved mortality with supplemental oxygen treatment. Based on studies published in the 1980s, it has been found that patients with a Po_2 $\leq$55 mm Hg (corresponding to an oxygen saturation of ~88%), have decreased mortality and evidence of better end-organ function when treated with supplemental oxygen.[38,39] Whether supplemental oxygen benefits subjects with moderate hypoxemia, corresponding to an oxygen saturation of 89% to 93%, is the objective of an ongoing, randomized, multicenter study, the Long-Term Oxygen Treatment Trial (LOTT).

PHARMACOTHERAPY

The fundamental goals of medication use are to prevent or control symptoms, reduce the frequency and severity of exacerbations, and improve both health status and exercise tolerance. The currently available medications used to treat COPD, however, do not alter the natural course of this condition; therefore, pharmacotherapy should be individualized for each patient and focused on the management of symptoms to improve quality of life.[21,52–54] Because of the potential for limited benefit with therapy, a specific set of desired goals must be defined for each patient before therapy is initiated. The initial outcomes should be realistic and developed jointly by the caregiver and the patient. In general, COPD is a progressive disease and general guidelines will apply to most patients with COPD as they begin to require pharmacologic management.

- The number of medications will cumulatively increase as disease worsens.
- Patients will eventually require daily maintenance therapy for sustained periods unless adverse effects of the medication(s) preclude further use.
- Interindividual variability in medication response is expected and requires careful monitoring over a continuum of time to ensure an acceptable benefit:risk ratio is achieved.

When medications are initiated or modified, a minimal trial period of several weeks to a few months is usually recommended before determining their full benefit. Single-dose challenges and frequent alterations in therapy do not allow adequate assessment and can compromise patient compliance. No consensus currently exists on the most appropriate outcome measure or degree of improvement needed to be determined clinically significant.

Although the standard for assessing benefit from treatment has been to measure spirometric improvement in FEV_1, many patients will not demonstrate noticeable changes following either an acute or extended therapeutic trial of any therapy. Increasingly, clinicians are considering other measures to determine the benefit of therapy. These include measuring improvements in quality of life, dyspnea, and exercise tolerance.[55] Other appropriate measures may include COPD exacerbation rates, utilization of health care resources, and mortality. In most patients, it is important to consider the use of multiple outcome measures, both objective and subjective, to guide the therapeutic decision-making process.

Bronchodilators

Bronchodilators are central to the symptomatic management of COPD and include short-acting and long-acting β_2-agonists, short-acting and long-acting anticholinergic agents, and theophylline. These medications, although pharmacologically distinct, improve airflow primarily by reducing bronchial airway smooth muscle tone. In COPD, the spirometric response, as measured by FEV_1, can be variable and, in many cases, will demonstrate no change, although the patient subjectively feels better. This can be attributed to treatment facilitating emptying of the lungs and a reduction in thoracic hyperinflation at rest and during exercise. No clear evidence exists for benefit of one bronchodilator over another in the chronic management of COPD, although inhaled therapy is generally preferred over oral therapy to achieve a more rapid onset of action and to minimize the risk of systemic exposure and adverse events. A short-acting, selective β_2-agonist or short-acting anticholinergic (ipratropium) are rational first-line treatments for patients with mild disease. Initially, medication should be given for symptomatic relief on an as-needed (PRN) basis. As disease progresses and the frequency of symptoms increases along with medication requirement, the patient should be transitioned onto daily maintenance bronchodilator therapy.[31] At this point, substitution of a short-acting agent with a long-acting agent of the same class is recommended because the bronchodilatory effect will be sustained over a longer duration and reduce the number of daily inhalations. This strategy will also enhance patient compliance. The use of short-acting agents should still be recommended for acute symptomatic relief, especially because the long-acting inhaled agents take a significantly longer period of time for onset of effect following inhalation. The side effects of bronchodilators, particularly β_2-agonists, are predictable and dose dependent, even with excessive use of inhaled agents. The most common adverse effects are an extension of stimulation of β_2-adrenergic receptors that can produce resting sinus tachycardia or provoke cardiac dysrhythmias in predisposed individuals, especially the elderly. Precipitation of somatic tremors and hypokalemia can also occur with excessive use.

The relationship between β_2-agonist use and cardiovascular complications remains somewhat controversial. It is recognized that albuterol and long-acting inhaled β_2-sympathetic agents can induce systemic sympathetic states, hypokalemia, and other metabolic derangements that can contribute to cardiac rhythm disturbances. This has led to speculation that these abnormalities could contribute to an increase in cardiovascular death among patients with COPD using β_2-agonist inhalers.[56] Nevertheless, this speculation has been largely refuted by the recently published TORCH (Towards a Revolution in COPD Health) study, in which >6,000 patients with COPD were randomized to salmeterol, fluticasone, combination salmeterol–fluticasone, or placebo.[57] Overall mortality, cardiovascular mortality, and cardiovascular-related adverse events were no greater in the salmeterol group compared with any of the other groups.

Inhaled anticholinergic agents have less potential to cause adverse events by virtue of their positive charge at physiologic pH leading to negligible systemic absorption. Excessive dry mouth is the most common complaint from patients who use inhaled anticholinergic agents, both short- and long-acting. Cardiovascular complications have been reported with regularly scheduled use of ipratropium bromide, but this association requires further investigation.[58]

It is not unusual to find reports in the literature that suggest superiority of one bronchodilator class over another for COPD treatment. It is difficult, however, to predict individual responses to treatment. For some patients, β_2-agonist bronchodilators will increase airflow, improve pulmonary function test results, and reduce symptoms of dyspnea.[59] Others may achieve greater improvement with an anticholinergic in comparison with a β_2-agonist.[60,61] Still, others may not have a reversible component with either drug, but still may perceive symptomatic benefit.[62,63] Because single-dose trials of inhaled bronchodilators are usually inadequate in predicting long-term response to bronchodilator therapy, a minimum of a 1- to 2-week course of therapy should be administered before evaluating the response.[59,64]

The risks and potential benefits of theophylline have been long debated.[65,66] Although objective evidence demonstrating a patient benefit is often absent, patients with advanced stage COPD may report a worsening of symptoms when theophylline is withdrawn.[66] Currently, theophylline is reserved for patients who do not tolerate, or fail to adequately respond, to a combination of first-line inhaled bronchodilators. The major limitation of theophylline is its relatively narrow therapeutic window and potential to cause significant adverse events. Despite these limitations, it is known that theophylline may positively contribute to a favorable patient response, in the absence of improved pulmonary function, through other mechanisms that include stimulation of diaphragmatic contractility and anti-inflammatory effects. Based on these positive attributes, a more specific class of phosphodiesterase-4 (PDE-4) inhibitors has recently been developed. Cilomast is an orally active, potent, selective PDE-4 inhibitor that has shown benefit in phase III clinical trials involving patients with COPD by maintaining pulmonary function, reducing exacerbations, and improving health status.[67] In comparison with theophylline, cilomast has much less potential for drug–drug interactions and should not require drug level monitoring, thereby making it an attractive alternative pending further clinical study.

Glucocorticoids

Historically, initiation of a short (2-week) course of oral glucocorticoids was often advocated to identify patients with COPD who might benefit from long-term treatment. Recent evidence however, indicates that a short course challenge is a poor method to predict patients who will benefit from long-term inhaled corticosteroid use.[54,68] Based on the lack of evidence and risk for significant side effects that include steroid myopathy and loss of bone density, chronic systemic corticosteroid therapy is not generally recommended. For patients with COPD experiencing an acute exacerbation of their disease, the short-term use of systemic corticosteroids has proven efficacy.

In contrast, inhalation of glucocorticoids leads to substantially less systemic absorption, thereby minimizing many of the risks associated with systemic corticosteroid therapy. Based on this, several national and international studies have been conducted to evaluate the potential benefit of inhaled corticosteroid maintenance therapy.[52–54,69] Well-conducted clinical trials have revealed that daily treatment with inhaled glucocorticoseriods does not delay the long-term decline in FEV_1 in patients with COPD. Daily use can result, however, in a reduction in the frequency of exacerbations and an improvement in overall health status, particularly in patients with more advanced disease.[70–73] Recently, it has been shown that inhaled glucocorticoid use in combination with a long-acting β_2-agonist is more effective than either agent alone or placebo in patients with advanced COPD.[59] Specifically, patients using combination therapy (one inhalation twice daily) experienced decreased exacerbations, improved spirometric values, and increased health status. Although no difference was seen in mortality or disease progression among treatment groups, some advocate maintenance therapy with inhaled glucocorticoids in symptomatic patients with COPD with an FEV_1 <60% predicted.[74] The safety of chronic inhaled glucocorticoids beyond 3 years use is unknown. Safety concerns include decreased bone density, ocular changes, and increased risk of pneumonia. Until definitive trials are completed, long-term patient safety must be taken into consideration and weighed with the beneficial effects of the medication.

PHARMACOLOGIC THERAPY BY DISEASE SEVERITY

As described, it is expected that patients with COPD will require an increase in the dose and number of medications to effectively manage their disease over time. Figure 23-6 provides a summary of the recommended strategy for pharmacologic therapy. Patients with infrequent or intermittent symptoms (stage I: mild COPD) will initially require use of one short-acting bronchodilator on an as-needed basis. As disease progresses beyond this stage (stage II: moderate to stage IV: very severe COPD), PRN use of bronchodilators alone will not maintain adequate relief from these symptoms. Patients will begin to manifest daily symptoms that require maintenance therapy. At this point, regular treatment with one or more long-acting bronchodilator agents is recommended. Patients should also continue to use a short-acting bronchodilator PRN for additional symptomatic relief. In patients with a postbronchodilator FEV_1 of <50% predicted (stage III to stage IV COPD) and a history of repeated exacerbations, maintenance therapy with an inhaled glucocorticosteroid should be added to the long-acting bronchodilators.

In general, nebulization of bronchodilators is primarily reserved for the acute care setting for quick symptomatic relief and is not advocated routinely for home use. In select patients who are not achieving maximal benefit with standard inhalation delivery devices, a 2-week trial with nebulized therapy can be considered and then continued if a clear benefit is observed.[75]

COPD EXACERBATION

An acute exacerbation of COPD is defined as an acute worsening of a patient's chronic symptoms (dyspnea, cough, sputum production) necessitating treatment. Acute exacerbations of COPD are important events in the natural history of this disease.[76,77] They are associated with considerable morbidity; severe exacerbations are associated with an increased mortality.[77] Furthermore, acute exacerbations are responsible

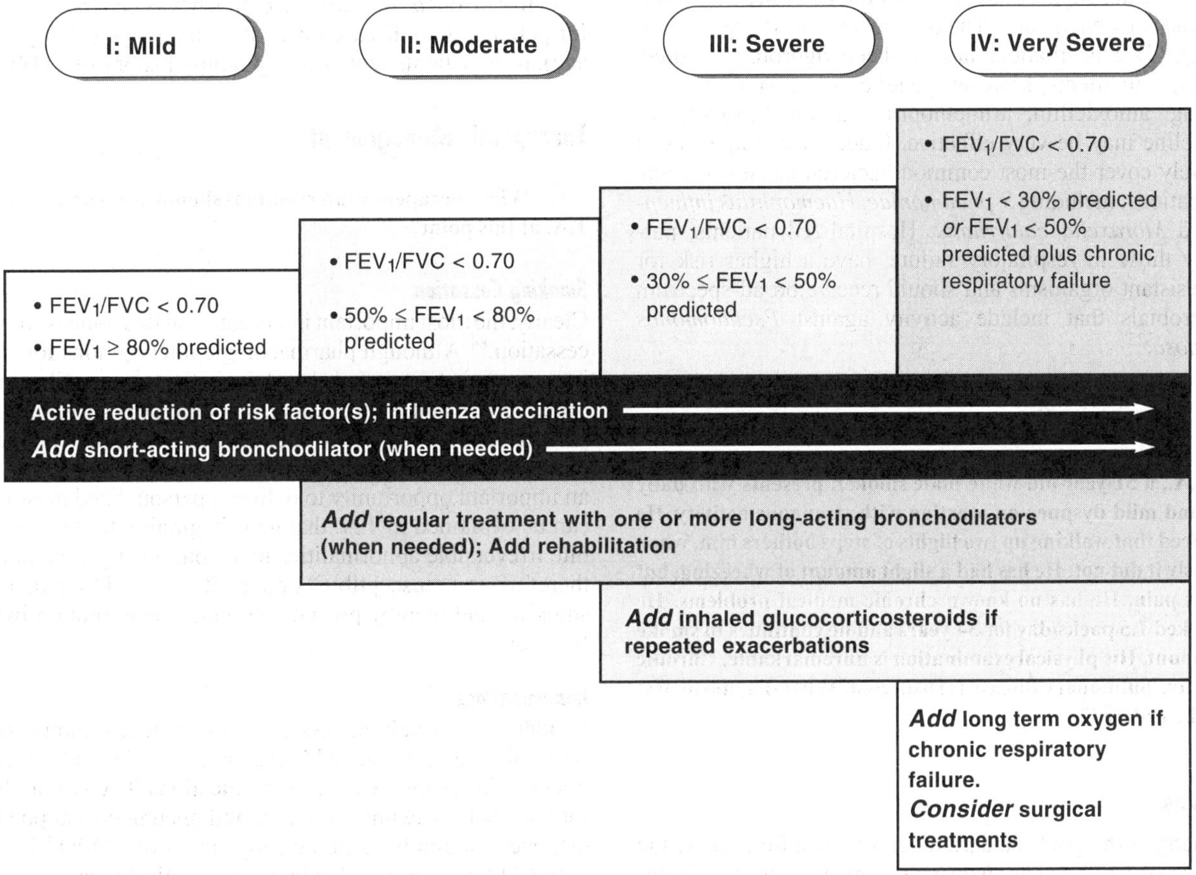

****Postbronchodilator FEV_1 is recommended for the diagnosis and assessment of severity of COPD.***

FIGURE 23-6 Therapy at each stage of COPD. (Reprinted with permission from reference 1.)

for a high percentage of health care costs associated with COPD.[78]

The cause of acute exacerbations is believed to be a result of respiratory tract infections, either viral or bacterial, air-pollution, or other environmental exposures.[79,80] These triggers can initiate increased bronchospasm and airway resistance in an individual with already compromised lung function. Although mild exacerbations may be readily managed with outpatient therapy, severe exacerbations can result in respiratory failure and death, particularly if they occur in a patient with severe COPD.

Key therapeutic interventions for acute COPD exacerbations include regular bronchodilator therapy, a short course of systemic corticosteroid therapy, and antibiotics. Bronchodilator therapy is given PRN by metered dose inhaler (MDI) or nebulizer every 3 to 4 hours. Systemic corticosteroids are commonly given for a 7- to 10-day course. Although 30 to 40 mg/day for 7 to 10 days is commonly used, the optimal dose is not known,[81] High-dose intravenous corticosteroids (methylprednisolone 125 mg every 6 hours) have been shown to be effective in hospitalized patients.[82] Such large doses, however, are associated with an increased risk of hyperglycemia and it is not known whether this regimen is superior to lower dose oral regimens.

Antibiotic use in the setting of an acute exacerbation should be made based on the presence of the following respiratory symptoms: increased dyspnea, sputum volume, and sputum purulence. Data suggest that if two of the three are increased, antibiotics are beneficial.[83] The optimal antibiotic regimen for acute COPD exacerbations has not been rigorously studied. For many outpatients, however, generic, low-cost antibiotics, including amoxicillin, trimethoprim–sulfamethoxazole or doxycycline may be very effective. Indeed, these agents can effectively cover the most common bacterial causes of acute exacerbations, including *S. pneumoniae*, *Haemophilus influenzae*, and *Moraxella catarrhalis*. Hospitalized patients, particularly those in respiratory failure, have a higher risk for more resistant organisms and should receive broad-spectrum antimicrobials that include activity against *Pseudomonos aeruginosa*.[25]

STAGE I (MILD) COPD

1. T.A., a 51-year-old white male smoker, presents with daily cough and mild dyspnea on exertion with strenuous activity. He has noticed that walking up two flights of steps bothers him, when previously it did not. He has had a slight amount of wheezing, but no chest pain. He has no known chronic medical problems. He has smoked 1.5 packs/day for 34 years and he continues to smoke that amount. His physical examination is unremarkable. Chronic obstructive pulmonary disease is suspected. What diagnostic test should be ordered?

Diagnosis

Spirometry is the gold standard diagnostic test for making the diagnosis of COPD. The main values gleaned from spirometry will include the FVC, FEV_1, and the FEV_1/FVC ratio. An FEV_1/FVC <0.70 indicates obstruction to expiratory flow consistent with COPD. The severity of disease is best assessed by the FEV_1 as a percent of predicted. The diagnosis of COPD can be made based on the presence of symptoms (dyspnea, cough, wheeze), risk factors (most often associated with a history of regular cigarette smoking), and airflow obstruction on spirometry.[1]

2. Office spirometry demonstrates an FEV_1/FVC of 0.69 and an absolute FEV_1 of 81% of predicted. At what GOLD stage of COPD is this patient? What other diagnostic tests would be necessary before initiating therapy?

Based on GOLD guidelines, this patient would be considered to have mild COPD (GOLD stage I). A CXR study is often performed to exclude other respiratory diagnoses contributing to the patient's symptoms; however, the abnormal spirometry is sufficient to make the diagnosis of COPD and to initiate therapy.

In certain cases of diagnostic uncertainty or in patients with severe disease being considered for surgical intervention, such as lung volume reduction surgery, a complete set of pulmonary function tests, including the determination of lung volumes and DL_{CO} may be performed. Complete pulmonary function testing, however, is not necessary to make the diagnosis of COPD.

In patients with more severe symptoms or airflow obstruction, assessment of oxygen status by means of pulse oximetry or ABG may be necessary. For example, ABGs are recommended if the FEV_1 is <50% of predicted.[1] An α_1-antitrypsin level to rule out α_1-antitrypsin deficiency is generally reserved for patients with disease onset at a young age (<50 years of age), or in patients with a strong family history of COPD.[1]

Therapeutic Management

3. What therapeutic interventions should be recommended for T.A. at this point?

Smoking Cessation

Clearly, the most important intervention at this point is smoking cessation.[84] Although pharmacologic interventions for smoking cessation are covered elsewhere in the text (see Chapter 85, Tobacco Use and Dependence), it should be pointed out that a personalized message may be beneficial for this patient. Indeed, discussion of spirometry results with the patient can provide an important opportunity to deliver a personalized message. It can be explained to T.A. that he is beginning to develop definite irreversible abnormalities in his pulmonary function and, therefore, is a "susceptible" smoker. It is critical for him to stop smoking and thereby prevent continued deterioration in lung function.

Immunizations

In addition to smoking cessation, this patient's immunization status should be evaluated.[84] According to the GOLD guidelines and in the absence of contraindications, T.A. is a candidate for vaccination against influenza and pneumococcal pneumonia, even though he is in the early stages of COPD.[1] Patients with COPD are at risk for increased morbidity and mortality if they develop either of these infectious complications.

Individuals at greatest risk for significant morbidity and mortality from influenza pneumonia are those with chronic disease, including lung disease. Optimally, the influenza vaccine should be administered between October and January. This allows an adequate antibody response before the peak influenza season, which typically occurs within the first quarter of the year. Annual immunization is required to ensure adequate antibody protection against influenza virus and is effective in reducing morbidity and mortality from influenza.[85] The influenza vaccine is administered intramuscularly; the live attenuated intranasal preparation is not recommended for patients with COPD.

Pneumococcal polysaccharide vaccine (Pneumovax 23) is also recommended for patients with COPD.[1] This vaccine consists of antigen that provides protection against 23 common strains of *Streptococcus pneumoniae.* Candidates for this vaccine include individuals at risk for significant morbidity and mortality if they develop a pneumococcal infection, including patients with chronic lung disease and even those potentially immunocompromised following prolonged use of systemic corticosteroids. Data concerning efficacy of the vaccine in this population are limited, but the GOLD guidelines recommend its use based on expert opinion and a favorable risk:benefit ratio.[1,86] Pneumococcal polysaccharide vaccine is recommended to be administered subcutaneously or intramuscularly as a one-time dose. In some cases, patients require a second dose after 5 years, commonly when the initial dose was administered before age 65.[87] Pneumococcal polysaccharide vaccine used for this purpose should be differentiated from the conjugated, 7-valent pneumococcal vaccine (Prevnar) that is used as a primary immunizing series for infants to provide protection against invasive pneumococcal disease.

To manage T.A.'s symptoms, treatment with a PRN bronchodilator may be reasonable to start. Bronchodilators are the primary pharmacologic therapy used in the management of COPD.[1,25]

Available bronchodilator therapies include β_2-agonists, anticholinergics, and methylxanthines (theophylline). For initial treatment, the most common choice for T.A. would be a short-acting, inhaled β_2-agonist, (e.g., albuterol), an inhaled anticholinergic (e.g., ipratropium), or the combination of these two agents. Any of these therapies has a relatively short onset of action and is effective in relieving symptoms.

β_2-Agonists

β_2-Agonists produce bronchodilation by relaxing bronchial smooth muscle through activation of cyclic adenosine monophosphate (cAMP).[88] The inhalation route of delivery for bronchodilators is recommended over oral therapy based on safety and efficacy. The dose response curve among all available bronchodilators is relatively flat and similar. No evidence suggests that one agent is superior to another.

Albuterol is the most frequently used agent in this class. It is available as a MDI 90 mcg/inhalation and a solution for nebulization (2.5 mg/0.5 mL). The onset of action of short-acting β_2-agonists (e.g., albuterol, pirbuterol) is rapid (within 5 minutes) and generally reaches maximal effect in 15 to 30 minutes. The duration of action is approximately 4 hours. Although inhaled β_2-agonists are usually well tolerated, some patients experience adverse effects (tremors, tachycardia, or nervousness) with even low dosages. Although concern has been expressed about the safety of short-acting, inhaled β_2-agonists in patients with cardiac disease, a cohort study using the Saskatchewan Health Services database concluded that there was no increased risk for fatal or nonfatal myocardial infarction in patients using these agents.[89]

Anticholinergics

The parasympathetic (cholinergic) nervous system plays a primary role in the control of bronchomotor tone in COPD. By inhibiting cyclic guanosine monophosphate (cGMP) in the lung, aerosolized anticholinergic drugs are effective bronchodilators. The bronchodilation produced by anticholinergics in patients with stable COPD is equal or superior to that achieved by inhaled β_2-agonists.

Ipratropium bromide is the primary short-acting anticholinergic agent used in COPD. It is marketed as both an MDI (18 mcg ipratropium per puff) and as a solution for nebulization (0.5 mg ipratropium/2.5 mL). Anticholinergics have an average onset of effect within 15 minutes, with a maximal bronchodilator effect in 60 to 90 minutes, although some patients may experience more rapid symptom relief. The duration of action is 6 hours. Although some reports suggest a quicker onset of action, patients should be advised that the relief of acute symptoms will be slower compared with an inhaled β_2-agonist. A typical dose of ipratropium is two to four inhalations three (TID) to four times (QID) daily. Although well tolerated, some patients experience dry mouth, nausea, and blurred vision with use of ipratropium.

Ipratropium's anticholinergic actions are localized predominantly in the lungs, with an apparent specificity of action in the larger airways. Because it has minimal effects on sputum viscosity, there is little problem with drying of airway secretions. In addition, ipratropium's structure as a quaternary amine increases its polarity, thereby minimizing absorption from the lung and systemic side effects. These structural properties also reduce penetration across the blood–brain barrier, reducing the incidence of confusion and other central nervous system (CNS) side effects.

Combination β_2-Agonists–Anticholinergics

Combination therapy with two different classes of bronchodilators is appealing, because it may decrease the cumulative dose of individual agents, thereby decreasing the risk of side effects while maintaining the benefits of each medication. In addition, anticholinergics and β-agonists have different mechanisms of action, and combining the two classes may provide additional benefit. Indeed, it has been demonstrated that combination therapy results in significantly greater increases in FEV_1 compared with use of either albuterol or ipratropium alone.[90]

STAGE II (MODERATE) COPD

4. J.O., a 46-year-old woman with a 32-pack/year history of cigarette smoking, presents with increasing shortness of breath. She gets winded walking on level ground after about 100 yards. She quit smoking 2 years ago. The chronic cough that she previously had lessened after smoking cessation but the dyspnea is now somewhat worse, despite use of an albuterol inhaler on a PRN basis. On examination, mild wheezing is noted. A CXR is unremarkable. Office spirometry demonstrates an FEV_1/FVC of 0.54 and an absolute FEV_1 of 2.0 L or 60% of predicted.

Postbronchodilator treatment demonstrated an FEV_1 increase by 100 mL, a 5% increase. How should J.O. be treated?

Therapeutic Management

This patient would be considered to have moderate COPD or GOLD stage II. She has had progression of dyspnea despite smoking cessation and the addition of a short-acting β_2-agonist. Because pharmacologic management of COPD involves a step-wise approach, regular use of a long-acting bronchodilator would be the next step in treatment.

The main classes of long-acting bronchodilators currently available include β_2-agonists and anticholinergics. Both classes have been shown to improve quality of life and reduce dyspnea in patients with COPD.

Long-Acting β_2-Agonist

The role of inhaled, long-acting β_2-agonists in the chronic management of COPD has become well established in recent years. Available evidence with both salmeterol and formoterol shows improved pulmonary function, reduced dyspnea, and enhanced quality of life in patients with COPD.[1,25] Additionally, these agents offer the convenience of a long duration of action allowing twice daily dosing. A plateau in bronchodilation is achieved for most patients at the recommended dose for each agent, so no benefits exist in exceeding the recommended dose. In addition, higher doses will increase the risk of adverse events associated with β_2-agonist excess. Therefore, salmeterol should be prescribed as 42 mcg (50 mcg in a dry powder device) twice daily and formoterol at 12 mcg twice daily.

Inhaled, long-acting β_2-agonists relieve symptoms, and improve exercise tolerance and health status for patients with COPD. Several recent studies reported the value of these agents in improving spirometry and overall quality of life.[91–93] Clinical evidence suggests that long-acting β_2-agonists are equally or more effective than short-acting β_2-agonists or ipratropium. Based on these results and the convenience of twice daily dosing, these agents are reasonable options for bronchodilator therapy in patients experiencing chronic persistent symptoms.[1,25]

Tiotropium

Vagal cholinergic tone is a reversible component of the airway limitation in COPD. Stimulation of the vagal parasympathetic nerves causes the release of acetylcholine, which then binds to muscarinic receptors to produce bronchoconstriction and secretion of mucus. Three muscarinic subtypes have been identified in human airways: the M1, M2, and M3 receptors. Tiotropium is a long-acting anticholinergic that binds to the M1, M2, and M3 muscarinic receptors of bronchial smooth muscle.[94] Although tiotropium dissociates rapidly from the M2 receptor, it dissociates much more slowly from the M1 and M3 receptors. In fact, its dissociation from the M1 and M3 receptors is 100 times slower than that of ipratropium. M1 receptors are located on parasympathetic ganglia, where they facilitate postganglionic transmission, thus enhancing cholinergic tone. M3 receptors are found on airway smooth muscle and mucous glands, where activation leads to bronchoconstriction and mucus secretion. Conversely, M2 receptors are located on postganglionic nerve endings, where they serve as autoreceptors regulating acetylcholine release and, thereby, cholinergic tone. Thus, anticholinergics, by virtue of antagonizing M1 and M3, relax airway smooth muscle and can reduce mucus secretion. M2 blockade, however, augments acetylcholine release and thus enhances cholinergic tone. Therefore, the slower dissociation rate from both the M1 and M3 receptors enhances bronchodilation and allows the convenience of once-daily dosing.

This agent has a very long duration of action and can provide effective bronchodilation with once daily dosing. Numerous studies have documented its beneficial effect on pulmonary function and quality of life. An ongoing clinical trial is being performed to see whether tiotropium improves the natural history of disease (i.e., alters the slope of FEV_1 decline over time). Tiotropium is also a quaternary amine with limited systemic absorption; therefore, the agent is well tolerated with dry mouth being the major side effect.

J.O. should be started on a long-acting bronchodilator, such as salmeterol, formoterol, or tiotropium. It should be noted that the tolerability and efficacy of the available long-acting bronchodilators are comparable. The choice of agent is largely based on considerations, such as the frequency of drug administration, the patient's ability to use the inhalation device correctly, and any out-of-pocket costs incurred by the patient. J.O. should also be instructed to continue her albuterol two puffs every 4 hours PRN. A 3-month follow-up visit should be scheduled to assess her response.

5. J.O. is started on tiotropium one puff (18 mcg) daily and returns to the office for a check-up in 3 months as recommended. She has had significant benefit from the medication and has had decreased wheezing and a noticeable improvement in her exercise tolerance. She asks to have spirometry repeated to see if her lung function has improved on the new medication. Spirometry is repeated and no significant improvement noted in her FEV_1. She wonders how she can feel better, with improved exercise tolerance without an improvement in her lung function.

Increasing evidence suggests that bronchodilators, including long-acting β_2-agonists and anticholinergics, may reduce exercise-related dyspnea in patients with COPD by decreasing dynamic hyperinflation.[95] This improvement may be independent of marked changes in spirometry performed at rest. Indeed, because of flow limitation, these patients who exercise can have significant worsening of air-trapping, which can worsen lung compliance and adversely affect respiratory muscle mechanics. A number of studies have shown that alleviation of such "dynamic hyperinflation" may be an important mechanism whereby bronchodilators improve exercise tolerance in patients with obstructive lung disease.[95]

6. J.O. seemed to do reasonably well for a number of years, but now, 5 years later, she has noticed progressive dyspnea on exertion. She is now having difficulty carrying laundry up from her basement and she has noticed that her overall activity level has been curtailed. Repeat office spirometry now shows an FEV_1/FVC of 0.49 and an absolute FEV_1 of 49% of predicted. J.O. has been compliant with her tiotropium regimen and has had no other significant changes to her medical history. She remains smoke free and is not exposed to second-hand smoke in her home and work environments. What therapeutic intervention(s) should be considered at this point?

At this point, J.O would be considered to have severe COPD, or GOLD stage III. She is symptomatic now, despite the regular use of a long-acting bronchodilator. To continue with the stepwise approach, addition of another long-acting bronchodilator with a different mechanism of action would be reasonable. Evidence suggests that the combination of a long-acting anticholinergic and a long-acting β_2-agonist can increase lung function compared with either agent used alone.[96,97] Salmeterol and formoterol have a similar side-effect profile and have similar effectiveness. Either salmeterol one inhalation (50 mcg) every 12 hours or formoterol, one inhalation (12 mcg) twice daily would be reasonable options for J.O.

Safety of Long-Acting Bronchodilators

7. J.O. calls the next day, having read something on the internet regarding possible increased risk of death in people with obstructive lung disease who take long-acting bronchodilators. She is reluctant to take it. What should you tell her?

Although some evidence in asthma indicates that use of long-acting bronchodilators may be associated with an increased risk of death; such evidence does not exist in patients with COPD. In fact, the TORCH study demonstrated no increased risk of death or adverse events among patients prescribed salmeterol compared with placebo.[59] The patient should be reassured that long-acting bronchodilators are safe in COPD.

8. J.O. also wonders if anything else other than her medication can be done for her. What advice might be given?

Pulmonary Rehabilitation

At this point, pulmonary rehabilitation should be strongly considered. In fact, a comprehensive multidisciplinary pulmonary rehabilitation program should be considered in any patient with COPD experiencing persistent shortness of breath despite pharmacologic management.[43]

Increasing evidence points to COPD as a systemic process,[98] and pulmonary rehabilitation addresses the systemic nature of the disease. Figure 23-7 illustrates the cycle that occurs in COPD. Although the proximate cause of disability involves the respiratory system, leading to dyspnea on exertion, this in turn has systemic consequences. Although the changes may be fairly subtle to start, most patients will gradually manifest increasing limitations in their activity. This results in substantial deconditioning. It is likely that this deconditioning, in addition to other factors such as systemic inflammation, adversely affect skeletal muscle function. Indeed, evidence is clear that oxidative capacity is diminished in patients with COPD,[45–47] which results in overall decreased aerobic capacity and results in increased lactic acid production for a given level of activity.[50] The increased acid load will lead to a greater requirement for ventilation, which makes dyspnea more severe. The more dyspneic the patient is, the less activity he or she will do, leading to more deconditioning and recapitulation of the downward spiral.

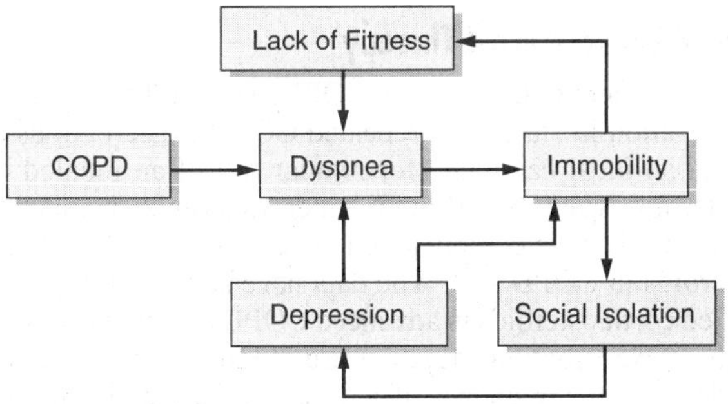

FIGURE 23-7 The Cycle of Physical, Social and Psychosocial Consequences of COPD. (Reprinted with permission from reference 1.)

Pulmonary rehabilitation is an exercise-based, multidisciplinary program that seeks to address this cycle.[43] Most programs generally last 8 to 12 weeks and involve two to three sessions per week. Education, particularly about medication use, as well as psychosocial counseling and breathing retraining are important components of the program. An important component of breathing retraining involves coaching patients how to use pursed lip breathing effectively. Pursed lip breathing involves pursing the lips together (as in whistling) during exhalation. This helps to slow down respirations and also provides a back pressure in the small airways, preventing dynamic airway collapse and exercise-induced hyperinflation. The major intervention, however, is exercise training, especially endurance training of the lower extremities (e.g., using a treadmill or bicycle ergometer). Numerous studies have demonstrated that a rehabilitation program can significantly improve exercise capacity and quality of life, as well as decrease health care utilization.[43] This may partly be related to the beneficial effects of exercise on the oxidative capacity of the skeletal muscles.

J.O. should be referred to a local outpatient pulmonary rehabilitation program. A typical program involves 2-hour sessions, three times per week for 10 weeks. The sessions will involve education, breathing retraining, and strength and endurance exercise training.

STAGE III (SEVERE) COPD

9. R.L., a 66-year-old man with diabetes mellitus and severe (stage III) COPD, presents with increased cough with productive discolored sputum following a "cold." He had been hospitalized 6 weeks earlier with community-acquired pneumonia. He is a former smoker (quit 10 years ago); current medications includes formoterol inhalation powder (12 mcg twice daily [BID]), albuterol MDI two puffs every 4 hours PRN and theophylline 200 mg BID. He also has increased dyspnea and chest tightness. On examination, he is in no acute distress and vital signs are stable. There is increased wheezing on chest examination and the rest of the examination is unchanged. Room air pulse oximetry is 90% and a CXR in the office shows no infiltrates. How should this patient be treated?

Acute Exacerbation of COPD

Antimicrobial Therapy

This patient has increased sputum purulence and increased dyspnea consistent with an exacerbation of COPD. It is not uncommon for such an exacerbation to be triggered by an upper respiratory viral infection. Given that the patient has increased dyspnea and purulent sputum production, a course of systemic corticosteroids (e.g., 30 to 40 mg of prednisone daily for 7 to 10 days) and a course of antibiotics is warranted. In outpatients with low risk factors, a low-cost antibiotic regimen is a reasonable option. Amoxicillin, trimethoprim–sulfamethoxazole or doxycycline could be used. Although other antibiotics are commonly given, no data support that they are superior in this setting when compared with these conventional, less-expensive agents. An acute exacerbation of COPD is one of the few instances where antibiotic therapy is warranted to treat a respiratory infection in the absence of evidence of lower respiratory tract involvement (i.e., pneumonia).

Patients with COPD and risk factors for poor outcome (severe COPD, comorbid conditions, history of frequent exacerbations) may be more susceptible to resistant pathogens. As such, guidelines recommend that a broader spectrum antibiotic regimen be considered, including β-lactam/β-lactamase inhibitor combinations, quinolone antibiotics, or second- or third-generation cephalosporins.[1,25]

Because of his recent hospitalization, R.L. is at increased risk for resistant pathogens, including *P. aeruginosa*. A broad-spectrum antimicrobial regimen, such as oral ciprofloxacin, 750 mg BID or oral levofloxacin 750 mg every day for 7 to 14 days would be appropriate. A course of oral prednisone, 30 mg daily for 7 to 10 days is also indicated to improve R.L.'s lung function, reduce his hypoxemia, and hasten his recovery time.

10. R.L. was treated with oral ciprofloxacin 750 mg BID and demonstrated a decrease in sputum volume and purulence with less dyspnea after 3 days of therapy. However, 5 days later he is feeling palpitations and has become nauseous. What laboratory value should be checked?

This patient has clinical evidence of theophylline toxicity. Both gastrointestinal complaints (e.g., nausea) and CNS symptoms, including sleep difficulty and nervousness, are consistent with theophylline toxicity. Other adverse reactions associated with methylxanthines are cardiac irritability (tachycardia or arrhythmias) and seizures. All these side effects are dose related. Gastrointestinal intolerance, nervousness, and insomnia can occur at any serum concentration, but increase in frequency when serum concentrations are >15 mcg/mL.

In R.L., the addition of the antibiotic ciprofloxacin to his regimen most likely resulted in a drug interaction causing a rise in his theophylline concentration. The potential for an interaction with theophylline varies among the available fluoroquinolone antibiotics. Drug interactions are dependent on several factors, including the dose of each agent and the baseline serum theophylline concentration. Elevations in the theophylline concentration of 25% are typical with ciprofloxacin interactions, although elevations of 50% have been observed. In R.L., a theophylline concentration should be obtained and further doses withheld until results are known.

In general, theophylline metabolism is associated with significant interpatient and intrapatient variability. Patients should be monitored closely for early signs of toxicity as well as for the initiation of drugs that potentially may interact. Understanding and recognizing the potential for drug interactions can allow safe and effective therapy with theophylline.

11. A theophylline serum concentration is measured for R.L. It is reported as 21 mcg/mL. What action should be taken?

The serum concentration is consistent with the interaction between theophylline and ciprofloxacin reported in the literature. His symptoms do not appear life-threatening at this point, so a conservative approach to treatment is appropriate. Theophylline should be withheld for one dose and then restarted at a lower dose (100 mg BID) until the ciprofloxacin therapy is completed. Alternatively, theophylline could be withheld until the antibiotic treatment is finished or discontinued. As mentioned, theophylline has a narrow therapeutic window and has the potential for serious toxicity as is evidenced by the current case. If the patient is unclear how beneficial the theophylline has been, a trial off of the medication is reasonable. After approximately 2 to 4 weeks, R.L. should be reassessed. If he feels that his chronic symptoms are no different without the drug, it should be withheld. On the other hand, his symptoms may become more pronounced without the theophylline and it could then be restarted. Alternatively, it would be reasonable to replace theophylline with an additional long-acting bronchodilator from a different class, in this case, tiotropium.

Chronic obstructive pulmonary disease has a progressive course, highlighted by a worsening of symptoms over time. Because step-wise therapy is recommended, it is not uncommon to find patients on multiple medications "added-on" in an attempt to alleviate symptoms. Nevertheless, it is important periodically to assess the patient to determine if all the medications are continuing to provide symptomatic benefit and are still needed. This may result in a "step-down" approach.

STAGE IV (VERY SEVERE) COPD

12. K.K., a 57year-old woman with a long history of COPD presents to establish care. She is concerned about her recurring hospitalizations because of lung problems. She has been to the emergency department five times in the last year and admitted twice because of episodes of worsening cough, sputum production and dyspnea. Her most recent FEV_1/FVC was 0.46 and her absolute FEV_1 was 45% of predicted. She is currently taking tiotropium one puff (18 mcg) as well as albuterol inhaler PRN for shortness of breath (SOB). She uses oxygen at 2 L/minute when sleeping (~8 hours/night). She is a former smoker, 50 pack years, but quit 2 years ago. What change in treatment would you recommend?

Inhaled Corticosteroid Therapy

This is a patient with advanced COPD, who has had significant deterioration in status and repeated COPD exacerbations and who is an ideal candidate for regular use of an inhaled corticosteroid. A number of multicenter, randomized, controlled clinical trials have demonstrated the efficacy of inhaled corticosteroids in COPD.[70–73] The data have supported the use of inhaled corticosteroids in advanced COPD and in patients with frequent exacerbations. Regular use of inhaled corticosteroids can decrease the frequency of acute exacerbations and improve health-related quality of life.

The recently published TORCH study has defined the benefits and potential side effects of inhaled corticosteroids in a broader patient population of COPD.[57] In this multicenter, randomized, placebo-controlled study, mean FEV_1 was 50% predicted, but entry criteria did not require a history of repeated exacerbations. More than 6,000 patients were randomized to either an inhaled corticosteroid (fluticasone 500 mcg BID), inhaled salmeterol (50 mcg BID), combination fluticasone 500 mcg/salmeterol 50 mcg BID, or placebo. Subjects were followed for approximately 3 years. A significant benefit was seen as measured by decreased exacerbation rates in subjects taking either inhaled fluticasone or a combination of fluticasone–salmeterol therapy. Also, an improvement was found in mortality with combination therapy that approached, but did not reach statistical significance. Overall adverse side effects with inhaled corticosteroids were similar to placebo. An increased risk, however, was seen of lower respiratory tract infections with inhaled fluticasone or fluticasone–salmeterol. Of note, patients did not experience an increased risk of ocular manifestations or decreased bone density with inhaled corticosteroid treatment.

K.K. is already taking tiotropium so a decision must be made regarding step-up therapy. A number of potential interventions exist at this point. The first would be to discontinue the tiotropium and initiate a combination inhaled corticosteroid–long-acting β_2-agonist. Secondly, an inhaled corticosteroid could be added to the tiotropium. Finally, recent data suggest that inhaled tiotropium and combination inhaled corticosteroid–long-acting β_2-agonist therapy may have significant benefits.[99] Currently, any of these three choices is reasonable provided no other major contraindications in doing so exist. It should be noted that currently two corticosteroid–long-acting β_2-agonist inhalers are available: Advair (fluticasone–salmeterol) and Symbicort (budesonide–formoterol). No data suggest that one preparation is superior to the other in the treatment of COPD.

The exact duration of treatment that inhaled glucocorticoids should be given before making an assessment of their benefit is not clear. Generally, an adequate trial is at least 4 to 6 weeks. One rationale for the use of inhaled glucocorticoids in COPD is, however, the prevention of acute exacerbations. As such, it can be very difficult to measure objectively the clinical benefit of the medication in individual patients.

Oxygen Therapy

13. P.J., a 62-year-old man with long-standing COPD, presents with worsening dyspnea on exertion. He is currently prescribed combination fluticasone–salmeterol (Advair 250/50 one puff BID), tiotropium (Spiriva 18 mcg one puff every day), and PRN albuterol (two to four puffs every 4 to 6 hours PRN). P.J. reports excellent compliance with his medications and an evaluation of his inhaler technique reveals he is able to use all three devices correctly. He has undergone pulmonary rehabilitation in the past with some benefit. He is no longer exercising, however. He has smoked 1.5 packs of cigarettes a day for 40 years (60 pack years), but quit 1 year previously. His most recent FEV_1/FVC is 0.41 and his FEV_1 is 1.25 L, or 38% of predicted. His room air oxygen saturation at rest is 85%. On examination, reduced breath sounds are noted in his chest and he has lower extremity edema. His physician recommended supplemental oxygen; however, he is resistant and wonders what kind of benefit he might receive.

The Nocturnal Oxygen Treatment Trial, a randomized controlled study, studied patients with COPD and severe hypoxemia Pao_2 ≤55 mm Hg, or Pao_2 ≤59 mm Hg associated with polycythemia, or peripheral edema.[38] Patients were randomized to continuous oxygen or nocturnal oxygen. The primary outcome variable was mortality. Subjects using continuous oxygen had a significantly greater survival and improved end-organ function, including improved cognitive function. The Medical Research Council Study published in 1981, using similar entry criteria, demonstrated a significant survival benefit with continuous supplemental oxygen compared with no oxygen.[39]

Based on these studies, supplemental oxygen is currently recommended for severe hypoxemia currently defined as an oxygen saturation <88% or Pao_2 ≤55 mm Hg (oxygen saturation <90% or Pao_2 ≤59 mm Hg in the presence of polycythemia or clinical evidence of pulmonary hypertension; e.g., peripheral edema). These guidelines (Table 23-6) are used by Medicare and most insurance companies as criteria to determine coverage for supplemental oxygen. This patient should be encouraged to use supplemental oxygen because it is one of the few available interventions that has been associated with improved survival in COPD.

In addition to supplemental oxygen, the patient should be re-enrolled in pulmonary rehabilitation. As mentioned, existing data suggest that this intervention can improve quality of life and exercise tolerance and decrease health care utilization.

Surgical Treatments for COPD

14. The patient is prescribed supplemental oxygen and enrolls in a pulmonary rehabilitation program. These interventions are successful in improving exercise tolerance; however, he presents 12 months later complaining of worsening dyspnea. In addition, although he is compliant with the oxygen, he is wondering if any other interventions available might improve his lung function and allow him to "get off" of oxygen.

He is re-evaluated with pulmonary function studies, which demonstrate a reduced FEV_1/FVC ratio of 0.38 and an absolute FEV_1 of 29% of predicted. In addition, lung volume

Table 23-6 Guidelines for Insurance Reimbursement of Oxygen Therapy in Chronic Obstructive Pulmonary Disease (COPD)

1. Severe hypoxemia at rest[a]:
   Pao_2 ≤55 mm Hg
   Or
   Pao_2 ≤59 mm Hg, with polycythemia and/or evidence of cor pulmonale
   Or
   Oxygen saturation ≤88%
2. Oxygen desaturation ≤88% with activity or during sleep[b]

[a] Proven to improve survival.
[b] Efficacy not proven.

determinations show severe hyperinflation (TLC = 135% of predicted and air-trapping RV = 292% of predicted). His CXR shows marked decrease in lung markings in the upper lung zones with vascular crowding in the lower lung fields. What therapeutic options are available for P.J.?

Lung volume reduction surgery, which involves the surgical removal of approximately 30% of the volume of each lung, can significantly improve quality of life, exercise tolerance, and mortality in selected patients with COPD. The National Emphysema Treatment Trial (NETT) demonstrated that patients with severe, upper lobe predominant emphysema who have lung volume reduction surgery have significant benefits in health-related quality of life as well as exercise tolerance.[7] Subjects who also had persistently poor exercise tolerance before surgery appeared to have the most benefit compared with control subjects with similar impairment. These patients also had a mortality benefit.[7] The rationale for the surgery is that removing the areas of the lung most involved with emphysema can improve the physiology of the remaining lung. This includes improvement in expiratory airflow and improved lung elastic recoil as well as improved ventilation perfusion matching. The major patient selection criteria for lung volume reduction surgery are depicted in Table 23-7. Following a successful surgery, patients can have improved gas exchange and may no longer require supplemental oxygen.

The CXR for this patient suggests upper lobe predominant emphysema. This would need to be confirmed with a high resolution computed tomography (CT) scan of the chest. Furthermore, the patient would need to complete a comprehensive pulmonary rehabilitation program before surgery. Only few centers within the United States are certified by Medicare to perform lung volume surgery and this could be an important issue for P.J., depending on where he lives. It should be stressed that lung reduction surgery is only appropriate for a select group of patients with advanced emphysema.

Recent studies utilizing bronchoscopic lung volume reduction are currently being evaluated and may prove to be a less invasive option to perform lung reduction in patients with severe emphysema.[100]

In patients with severe emphysema, another option is lung transplantation. This intervention has not been shown to decrease mortality, but can improve quality of life and exercise tolerance in carefully selected candidates.[101] Patients considered are those with severe disease, whose life expectancy is <5 years and individuals with an FEV_1 <25% of predicted.

Table 23-7 Major Selection Criteria for Lung Volume Reduction Surgery

Moderate to severe airflow obstruction
Hyperinflation
Upper lobe predominant emphysema
Nonsmoker
Rehabilitation potential

REFERENCES

1. Buists et al. From the Global Strategy for the Diagnosis, Management and Prevention of COPD, Global Initiative for Chronic Obstructive Lung Disease (GOLD) 2006. Available from: http://www.goldcopd.org. Accessed June 2, 2008.
2. Lamb D. Chronic bronchitis, emphysema and the pathologic basis of chronic obstructive pulmonary disease. In: Hasleton PS, ed. *Spencer's Pathology of the Lung.* 5th ed. New York: McGraw-Hill; 1996: 597.
3. Hogg JC et al. The nature of small-airway obstruction in chronic obstructive pulmonary disease. *N Engl J Med* 2004;350:2645.
4. Barnes PJ. Against the Dutch hypothesis: asthma and chronic obstructive pulmonary disease are distinct diseases. *Am J Respir Crit Care Med* 2006; 174:240.
5. Jemal A. Trends in the leading causes of death in the United States, 1970–2002. *JAMA* 2005;294:1255.
6. Mannino DM. Chronic obstructive pulmonary disease surveillance—United States, 1971–2000. *MMWR Surveill Summ* 2002;51(SS06):1.
7. National Emphysema Treatment Trial Research Group. A randomized trial comparing lung-volume–reduction surgery with medical therapy for severe emphysema. *N Engl J Med* 2003: 348:2059.
8. Trupin L et al. The occupational burden of chronic obstructive pulmonary disease. *Eur Respir J* 2003;22:462.
9. Matheson MC et al. Biological dust exposure in the workplace is a risk factor for chronic obstructive pulmonary disease. *Thorax* 2005;60:645–651.
10. Hnizdo E et al. Association between chronic obstructive pulmonary disease and employment by industry and occupation in the US population: a study of data from the Third National Health and Nutrition Examination Survey. *Am J Epidemiol* 2002; 156:738.
11. Silva GE et al. Asthma as a risk factor for COPD in a longitudinal study. *Chest* 2004;126:59.
12. Orozco-Levi M et al. Wood smoke exposure and risk of chronic obstructive pulmonary disease. European Respiratory Standards for the diagnosis and treatment of patients with COPD: a summary of the ATS/ERS position paper. *Eur Respir J* 2006;27:542.
13. Sezer H et al. A case-control study on the effect of exposure to different substances on the development of COPD. *Ann Epidemiol* 2006;16: 59.
14. Abbey DE et al. Long-term particulate and other air pollutants and lung function in nonsmokers. *Am J Respir Crit Care Med* 1998;158:289.
15. Retamales I et al. Amplification of inflammation in emphysema and its association with latent adenoviral infection. *Am J Respir Crit Care Med* 2001;164: 469.
16. Diaz PT et al. Increased susceptibility to pulmonary emphysema among HIV-seropositive smokers. *Ann Intern Med* 2000;132:369.
17. Zhu G et al. The *SERPINE2* gene is associated with chronic obstructive pulmonary disease in two large populations. *Am J Resp Crit Care Med.* 2007;176:167.
18. Demeo DL et al. Genetic determinants of emphysema distribution in the National Emphysema Treatment Trial. *Am J Respir Crit Care Med* 2007; 176:42.
19. Silverman EK. Progress in chronic obstructive pulmonary disease genetics. *Proc Am Thorac Soc* 2006;3:405.
20. Stoller JK et al. α1-antitrypsin deficiency. *Lancet* 2005;265:2225.
21. Anthonisen MR et al. Effects of smoking intervention and the use of an inhaled anticholinergic bronchodilator on the rate of decline of FEV1. The Lung Health Study. *JAMA* 1994;272:1497.
22. Rahman I. Oxidative stress in pathogenesis of chronic obstructive pulmonary disease. *Cell Biochem Biophys* 2005;43:167.
23. Ito K et al. Decreased histone deacetylase activity in chronic obstructive pulmonary disease. *N Engl J Med* 2005;352:1967.
24. Henson PM et al. Cell death, remodeling, and repair in chronic obstructive pulmonary disease? *Proc Am Thorac Soc* 2006;3:713.
25. Celli BR et al. Standards for the diagnosis and treatment of patients with COPD: a summary of the ATS/ERS position paper. ATS/ERS Task Force Report. *Eur Respir J* 2004;23:932.
26. American Thoracic Society. Standards for the diagnosis and care of patients with chronic obstructive pulmonary disease. *Am J Respir Crit Care Med* 1995;152:S77.
27. Siafakas NM et al. Optimal assessment and management of chronic obstructive pulmonary disease (COPD). The European Respiratory Society Task Force. *Eur Respir J* 1995;8:1398.
28. Madison JM et al. Chronic obstructive pulmonary disease. *Lancet* 1998;352:467.
29. Jeffery PK. Structural and inflammatory changes in COPD: a comparison with asthma. *Thorax* 1998;53:129.
30. O'Donnell DE et al. Dynamic hyperinflation and exercise intolerance in chronic obstructive pulmonary disease. *Am J Respir Crit Care Med* 2001; 164:770.
31. Fabbri LM et al. Global strategy for the diagnosis, management and prevention of COPD: 2003 update [Editorial]. *Eur Respir J* 2003;22:1.
32. Barbera JA et al. Pulmonary hypertension in chronic obstructive pulmonary disease. *Eur Respir J* 2003;21:892.
33. American Thoracic Society/European Respiratory Society Statement: standards for the diagnosis and management of individuals with alpha-1 antitrypsin deficiency. *Am J Respir Crit Care Med* 2003;168: 818.
34. Celli BR et al. The body-mass index, airflow obstruction, dyspnea, and exercise capacity index in

chronic obstructive pulmonary disease. *N Eng J Med* 2004;350:1005.
35. Currie GP et al. ABC of chronic obstructive pulmonary disease. Acute exacerbations. *BMJ* 2006;333:87.
36. Carr SJ et al. Acute exacerbations of COPD in subjects completing pulmonary rehabilitation. *Chest* 2007;132:127.
37. Anthonisen NR et al. The effects of a smoking cessation intervention on 14.5-year mortality. A randomized clinical trial. *Ann Intern Med* 2005;142:233.
38. Nocturnal Oxygen Therapy Trial Group. Continuous or nocturnal oxygen therapy in hypoxemic chronic obstructive lung disease. A clinical trial. *Ann Intern Med* 1980;93:391.
39. Long term domiciliary oxygen therapy in chronic hypoxic cor pulmonale complicating chronic bronchitis and emphysema. Report of the Medical Research Council Working Party. *Lancet* 1981;1:681.
40. Anthonisen NR. The benefits of smoking cessation. *Can Respir J* 2003;10:422.
41. Wongsurakiat P et al. Acute respiratory illness in patients with COPD and the effectiveness of influenza vaccination. A randomized controlled study. *Chest* 2004;125:2011.
42. Wongsurakiat P et al. Economic evaluation of influenza vaccine in Thai chronic obstructive pulmonary disease patients. *J Med Assoc Thai* 2003; 86:497.
43. Nici L et al. American Thoracic Society/European Respiratory Society Statement on Pulmonary Rehabilitation. *Am J Respir Crit Care Med* 2006; 173:1390.
44. Griffiths TL et al. Cost effectiveness of an outpatient multidisciplinary pulmonary rehabilitation programme. *Thorax* 2001;56:779.
45. Maltais AA et al. Oxidative capacity of the skeletal muscle and lactic acid kinetics during exercise in normal subjects and in patients with COPD. *Am J Respir Crit Care Med* 1996;153:288.
46. Jakobsson P et al. Metabolic enzyme activity in the quadriceps femoris muscle in patients with severe chronic obstructive pulmonary disease. *Am J Respir Crit Care Med* 1995;151:374.
47. Sauleda J et al. Cytochrome oxidase activity and mitochondrial gene expression in skeletal muscle of patients with chronic obstructive pulmonary disease. *Am J Respir Crit Care Med* 1998;157:1413.
48. Couillard A et al. Exercise-induced quadriceps oxidative stress and peripheral muscle dysfunction in patients with chronic obstructive pulmonary disease. *Am J Respir Crit Care Med* 2003;167: 1664.
49. Rabinovich RA et al. Increased tumour necrosis factor- plasma levels during moderate-intensity exercise in COPD patients. *Eur Respir J* 2003;21: 789.
50. Casaburi R et al. Reductions in exercise lactic acidosis and ventilation as a result of exercise training in patients with obstructive lung disease. *Am Rev Respir Dis* 1991;143:9.
51. Whittom F et al. Histochemical and morphological characteristics of the vastus lateralis muscle in patients with chronic obstructive pulmonary disease. *Med Sci Sports Exerc* 1998;30:1467.
52. Pauwels RA et al. Long-term treatment with inhaled budesonide in persons with mild chronic obstructive pulmonary disease who continue smoking. *N Engl J Med* 1999;340:1948.
53. Vestbo J et al. Long-term effect of inhaled budesonide in mild and moderate chronic obstructive pulmonary disease: a randomised controlled trial. *Lancet* 1999;353:1819.
54. Burge PS et al. Randomised, double blind, placebo controlled study of fluticasone propionate in patients with moderate to severe chronic obstructive pulmonary disease: the ISOLDE trial. *BMJ* 2000;320:1297.
55. Gross NJ. Outcome measurements in COPD. Are we schizophrenic? *Chest* 2003;123:1325.
56. Salpeter SR et al. Cardiovascular effects of β-agonists in patients with asthma and COPD. A meta-analysis. *Chest* 2004;125:2309.
57. Calverly PMA et al. Salmeterol and fluticasone propionate and survival in chronic obstructive pulmonary disease. *N Engl J Med* 2007;356:775.
58. Anthonisen NR et al. Hospitalizations and mortality in the Lung Health Study. *Am J Respir Crit Care Med* 2002;166:333.
59. Anthonisen NR. Bronchodilator response in chronic obstructive pulmonary disease. *Am Rev Respir Dis* 1986;133:814.
60. Gross NJ. The influence of anticholinergic agents on treatment for bronchitis and emphysema. *Am J Med* 1991;91(Supple 4A):11S.
61. Lakshminarayan S. Ipratropium bromide in chronic bronchitis/emphysema. A review of the literature. *Am J Med* 1986;(Suppl 5A)81:76.
62. O'Donnell DE, Webb FA. Breathlessness in patients with severe chronic airflow limitation. Physiologic correlations. *Chest* 1992;102:824.
63. Belman MJ et al. Variability of breathlessness measurement in patients with chronic obstructive pulmonary disease. *Chest* 1991;99:566.
64. Nisar M et al. Acute bronchodilator trials in chronic obstructive pulmonary disease. *American Review of Respiratory Disease* 1992;146:555.
65. Ramsdell J. Use of theophylline in the treatment of COPD. *Chest* 1995;107:206S.
66. Barnes PJ. Theophylline: new perspectives for an old drug. *Am J Respir Crit Care Med* 2003;167: 813.
67. Rennard SI et al. Cilomilast for COPD: results of a 6-month, placebo-controlled study of a potent, selective inhibitor of phosphodiesterase 4. *Chest* 2006;129:56.
68. Burge PS et al. Prednisolone response in patients with chronic obstructive pulmonary disease: results from the ISOLDE study. *Thorax* 2003;58:654.
69. The Lung Health Study Research Group. Effect of inhaled triamcinolone on the decline in pulmonary function in chronic obstructive pulmonary disease. *N Eng J Med* 200;343:1902.
70. Mahler DA et al. Effectiveness of fluticasone propionate and salmeterol combination delivered via the Diskus device in the treatment of chronic obstructive pulmonary disease. *Am J Respir Crit Care Med* 2002;166:1084.
71. Jones PW et al. Disease severity and the effect of fluticasone propionate on chronic obstructive pulmonary disease exacerbations. *Eur Respir J* 2003;21:68.
72. Calverly P et al. Combined salmeterol and fluticasone in the treatment of chronic obstructive pulmonary disease: a randomised controlled trial. *Lancet* 2003;361:449.
73. Szafranski W et al. Efficacy and safety of budesonide/formoterol in the management of chronic obstructive pulmonary disease. *Eur Respir J* 2003; 21:74.
74. Wilt TJ. Added management of stable chronic obstructive pulmonary disease: a systematic review for a clinical practice guideline. *Ann Intern Med* 2007;147:639.
75. Boe J et al. European Respiratory Society Guidelines on the use of nebulizers. Guidelines prepared by a European Respiratory Society Task Force on the Use of Nebulizers. *Eur Respir J* 2001;18: 228.
76. Cote CG et al. Impact of COPD exacerbations on patient-centered outcomes. *Chest* 2007;131:696.
77. Rivera-Fernandez R et al. Six-year mortality and quality of life in critically ill patients with chronic obstructive pulmonary disease. *Crit Care Med* 2006;34:2317.
78. Jansson S et al. Costs of COPD in Sweden according to disease severity. *Chest* 2002;122:1994.
79. Ko FWS et al. A 1-year prospective study of the infectious etiology in patients hospitalized with acute exacerbations of COPD. *Chest* 2007;131:44.
80. White AJ et al. Chronic obstructive pulmonary disease 6: The aetiology of exacerbations of chronic obstructive pulmonary disease. *Thorax* 2003;58:73.
81. Wood-Baker R et al. Evidence-based review. Systemic corticosteroids in chronic obstructive pulmonary disease: an overview of Cochrane systematic reviews. *Respir Med* 2007;101:371.
82. Niewoehner DE et al. Effect of systemic glucocorticoids on exacerbations of chronic obstructive pulmonary disease. *N Engl J Med* 1999;340:1941.
83. Anthonisen NR. Antibiotic therapy in exacerbations of chronic obstructive pulmonary disease. *Ann Intern Med* 1987;106:196.
84. McIvor A et al. Chronic obstructive pulmonary disease. *BMJ* 2007;334:798.
85. Woodhead M. Guidelines for the management of adult lower respiratory tract infections. *Eur Respir J* 2005;26:1138.
86. Alfageme I et al. Clinical efficacy of anti-pneumococcal vaccination in patients with COPD. *Thorax.* 2006;61:189.
87. Pneumococcal Disease. CDC Pink Book: http://www.cdc.gov/vaccines/pubs/pinkbook/downloads/pneumo.pdf.
88. Giembycz MA et al. Beyond the dogma: novel β2-adrenoceptor signalling in the airways. *Eur Respir J* 2006;27:1286.
89. Suissa S et al. Chronic obstructive pulmonary disease. Inhaled short acting β-agonist use in COPD and the risk of acute myocardial infarction. *Thorax.* 2003;58:43.
90. COMBIVENT Inhalation Aerosol Study Group. In chronic obstructive pulmonary disease, a combination of ipratropium and albuterol is more effective than either agent alone. An 85–day multicenter trial. *Chest* 1994;105:1411.
91. Tashkin DP et al. The role of long-acting bronchodilators in the management of stable COPD. *Chest* 2004;125:249.
92. Mahler DA et al. Efficacy of salmeterol xinafoate in the treatment of COPD. *Chest* 1999;115:957.
93. Aalbers R et al. Formoterol in patients with chronic obstructive pulmonary disease: a randomized, controlled, 3-month trial. *Eur Respir J* 2002;19:936.
94. Barnes PJ. The pharmacological properties of tiotropium. *Chest* 2000;117:63S.
95. O'Donnell DE et al. The clinical importance of dynamic lung hyperinflation in COPD. *COPD: Journal of Chronic Obstructive Pulmonary Disease* 2006;3:219.
96. Cazzola M et al. The functional impact of adding salmeterol and tiotropium in patients with stable COPD. *Respir Med* 2004;98:1214.
97. van Noord JA et al. Effects of tiotropium with and without formoterol on airflow obstruction and resting hyperinflation in patients with COPD. *Chest* 2006;129:509.
98. Wouters EFM. Local and systemic inflammation in chronic obstructive pulmonary disease. *Proc Am Thorac Soc* 2005;2:26 Symposium.
99. Aaron SD et al. Tiotropium in combination with placebo, salmeterol, or fluticasone-salmeterol for treatment of chronic obstructive pulmonary disease: a randomized trial. *Ann Intern Med* 2007;146:545.
100. Hopkinson NR. Bronchoscopic lung volume reduction: indications, effects and prospects. *Curr Opin Pulm Med* 2007;13:125.
101. Patel N et al. Transplantation in chronic obstructive pulmonary disease. *COPD* 2006;3:149.

CHAPTER 24

Acute and Chronic Rhinitis

Tina Penick Brock and Dennis M. Williams

Definitions

Rhinitis is an inflammatory condition affecting the mucous membranes of the nose and upper respiratory system. The term is used broadly to encompass a syndrome of nasal symptoms characterized by periods of rhinorrhea (nasal discharge), pruritus (itching), sneezing, congestion, and postnasal drainage (postnasal drip). These nasal symptoms can be accompanied by ocular redness, itching, and discharge. Rhinitis can be exacerbated by the development or presence of sinusitis. The most common form of rhinitis occurs in response to an allergen, although a variety of other causes have been demonstrated.[1,2]

Practice parameters for the diagnosis and management of allergic and nonallergic rhinitis were published in 1998 by a Joint Task Force representing the American Academy of Allergy, Asthma and Immunology (AAAAI), the American College of Allergy, Asthma and Immunology (ACAAI), and the Joint Council on Allergy, Asthma and Immunology.[1] Following this, the European Academy of Allergology and Clinical Immunology published a consensus statement on the treatment of allergic rhinitis in 2000.[2] More recently, evidence linking asthma and allergic rhinitis epidemiologically, pathologically, and physiologically was published.[3] These data support the tenet that upper respiratory allergic disorders and asthma represent components of a single inflammatory airway syndrome.[4] The resulting guidance, known as *Allergic Rhinitis and Its Impact on Asthma* (ARIA), was adapted for use specifically by pharmacists.[5] An updated version of ARIA has now been published, with the goal of extending the knowledge of allergic rhinitis and filling gaps in areas such as the use of complementary and alternative therapies, rhinitis in developing countries, and rhinitis in athletes.[6]

Prevalence and Impact

Prevalence rates for rhinitis are difficult to quantify because the condition is often undiagnosed, different definitions have been used, and the data collection methods vary.[7,8] In addition, because rhinitis in its mildest form is largely self-managed, it is likely that health statistics under represent the actual scope of the problem[9] and that the prevalence of rhinitis is increasing.[10] Despite these confounders, a conservative estimate suggests that up to 30% of adults (and even more children) are affected by allergic rhinitis (representing the greatest proportion of this family of diagnoses), making it the sixth most common chronic illness in the United States.[11,12]

Rhinitis can lead to sleep disorders, loss of appetite, general weakness, fatigue, mood disorders, decreased concentration, and difficulty learning.[1,9,13] Despite the impact of symptoms and the burden of disease, less than half (47%) of nasal allergy sufferers reported seeing a health care practitioner about their symptoms in the last 12 months.[8] Although symptom severity is associated positively with seeking treatment, 41% of patients who reported several nasal allergy symptoms in the past week had not seen a doctor about this within the last year.[8] Most nasal allergy sufferers report taking medication for their condition; with more than half (53%) reporting that they have used a non-prescription medication and more than a third (36%) reporting that they have used a prescription nasal spray in the past 4 weeks.[8] Most patients taking medications for their symptoms, however, report that they are less than very satisfied with the products they use.[8]

Although rhinitis does not lead to the mortality associated with some illnesses, its prevalence and negative health impact make it an important health problem in the United States. Allergic diseases are the most frequent contributor to the total cost of health-related absenteeism and presenteeism (i.e., being physically present at the workplace, but not being fully functional because of disruptive medical symptoms), with allergic rhinitis being the most prevalent of the allergic diseases. Most employees report annual allergic symptoms on average of 52.5 days, absence 3.6 days, and lack of productivity 2.5 hrs/day when experiencing symptoms.[12] The most recent estimates of the annual cost of allergic rhinitis range from $2 to $5 billion.[14] The total cost of allergic rhinitis in 2002 was estimated to be $4.86 billion, including $4.2 billion in direct costs (e.g., emergency department visits, clinic visits, prescription medications) and $666 million in indirect costs.[15] Clearly, acute and chronic rhinitis has a great impact on the physical and economic health of Americans.

Applied Anatomy and Physiology of the Nose

An understanding of the anatomy and physiology of the nose is helpful in understanding the pathophysiology and presentation of rhinitis, as well as the rationale for various pharmacotherapeutic approaches. The primary functions of the nose are smell, speech, and conditioning of inspired air. Related to the latter, the nose and upper airway warm, humidify, and filter air for delivery to the lungs.[16]

The external nose is pyramidal and consists of paired nasal bones and associated cartilage. Its base has two elliptical-shaped openings called nares, or nostrils. Internally, a septum separates the nasal cavity into two halves and consists of bone and cartilage covered by a mucosal membrane.[17] The lateral walls of the internal cavity contain the conchae, or turbinates. These bony projections increase surface area substantially and contribute to turbulence of airflow, which is useful in filtering and conditioning inspired air. Sinuses and eustachian tubes open into the nasal cavity near the turbinates, as do the lacrimal drainage ducts.[17] Figure 24-1 shows a lateral view of the head with the nasal anatomy labeled.

The membranes of the nasal cavity consist primarily of ciliated columnar epithelial cells with mucus-producing goblet cells interspersed among them. The tiny cilia beat rhythmically to transport mucus across the upper airway membrane to the nasopharynx. The cilia-lined mucous membranes of the nose provide a physical barrier of defense to microorganisms and other particles in the inspired air.[16] In addition, respiratory secretions residing on these mucous membranes contain immunoglobulin A (IgA), which serves as an immunologic defense.[17]

The autonomic nervous system controls the vascular supply and the secretion of mucus to the nasal membrane. Sympathetic activation results in vasoconstriction, which decreases nasal airway resistance. Parasympathetic stimulation results in glandular secretion and nasal congestion.[18] The mucosa is also innervated by the nonadrenergic–noncholinergic system (NANC). Neuropeptides from these nerves (e.g., substance P and neurokinins) play a role in vasodilation, mucus production and inflammation, although their significance is unclear. The trigeminal nerve also provides sensory innervation; the stimulation of which can result in sneezing and itching.[18]

During normal breathing, inspired air flows through the external nose before turning posteriorly almost 90 degrees into the nasopharynx. The airstream then makes another right angle

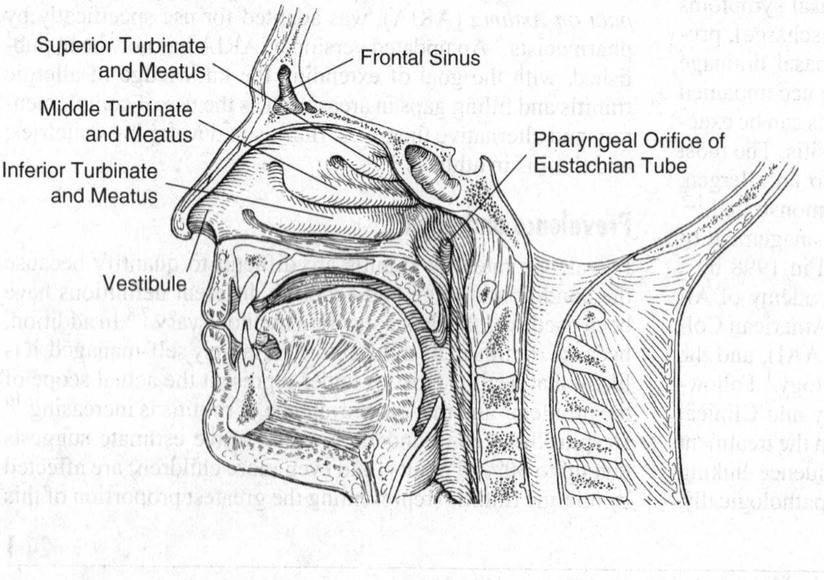

FIGURE 24-1 Lateral view of the head with nasal anatomy. (Reprinted with permission from the LifeArt Human Anatomy II collection.)

turn through the pharynx and larynx toward the lower airway. The upper airway diameter is extremely narrow in places, allowing for close contact between inhaled air and mucosal surfaces. Under normal conditions, turbinates in either side of the nasal cavity swell or contract alternately, resulting in preferential airflow through the right or left nasal cavity. This process is disrupted in the presence of inflammation and congestion. Normal nasal physiology is also affected by the presence of anatomic deformities including septal deviation, nasal polyps, or both.[17]

CLASSIFICATION OF RHINITIS

Rhinitis is not a single disease but rather has multiple causes and underlying pathophysiologic mechanisms.[1,19] Figure 24-2 depicts the common causes of acute and chronic rhinitis symptoms. Strictly speaking, some of these are not causes of rhinitis, but rather disorders (e.g., nasal septal deviation, foreign body) with symptoms that mimic inflammatory conditions of the nose. These conditions are considered in the differential diagnosis of allergic rhinitis.

Acute

The most common cause of acute rhinitis is a viral upper respiratory infection or the common cold. In most patients, these viral infections are self-limited and require only symptomatic treatment.[19] Nasal foreign bodies, especially in young children, are a common cause of acute rhinitis and should be suspected when a pediatric patient presents with acute unilateral symptoms.[16] Hormonal causes of acute rhinitis, usually associated with a clear, watery discharge without other symptoms, include hypothyroidism and pregnancy.[18,20] Finally, the development of acute rhinitis-like symptoms has been attributed to some medications. Angiotensin-converting enzyme inhibitors (ACEI), β-blockers, reserpine, nonsteroidal anti-inflammatory drugs (NSAID), oral contraceptives, phosphodiesterase type 5 inhibitors, and over use of topical decongestants all have been associated with nasal effects.[21,22]

Chronic

Chronic rhinitis can be classified as allergic or nonallergic. Allergic causes are typically associated with atopy, an inherited tendency to develop a clinical hypersensitivity condition.[2] The current guidelines classify allergic rhinitis as either intermittent or persistent based on frequency of symptoms.[6] This has replaced the earlier classification system (seasonal or perennial), which was based on both frequency of symptoms and the allergen responsible.[1] Patients with any form of allergic rhinitis can experience symptoms ranging from mild to severe. This classification system is summarized in Figure 24-3.

Nonallergic causes of chronic rhinitis symptoms include idiopathic rhinitis, nonallergic rhinitis with eosinophilia syndrome (NARES) and anatomic abnormalities.[19] Idiopathic rhinitis, also called *vasomotor rhinitis*, refers to symptoms associated with environmental stimuli, including temperature changes, strong odors, tobacco smoke, stress, or emotional factors.[23] NARES occurs frequently in middle-aged patients who have no evidence of allergic disease excepting the presence of eosinophils in the nasal smear. In these cases, increased permeability of the nasal mucosa is likely caused by non–IgE-mediated inflammation, and neurogenic mechanisms may play a role in membrane hyperreactivity.[19]

Common anatomic causes of chronic rhinitis include nasal septum deviation, nasal polyps, tumors, choanal atresia (a congenital condition where the mouth and nose are not connected), and enlarged adenoids and tonsils. Often these anatomic abnormalities require surgical intervention.[18]

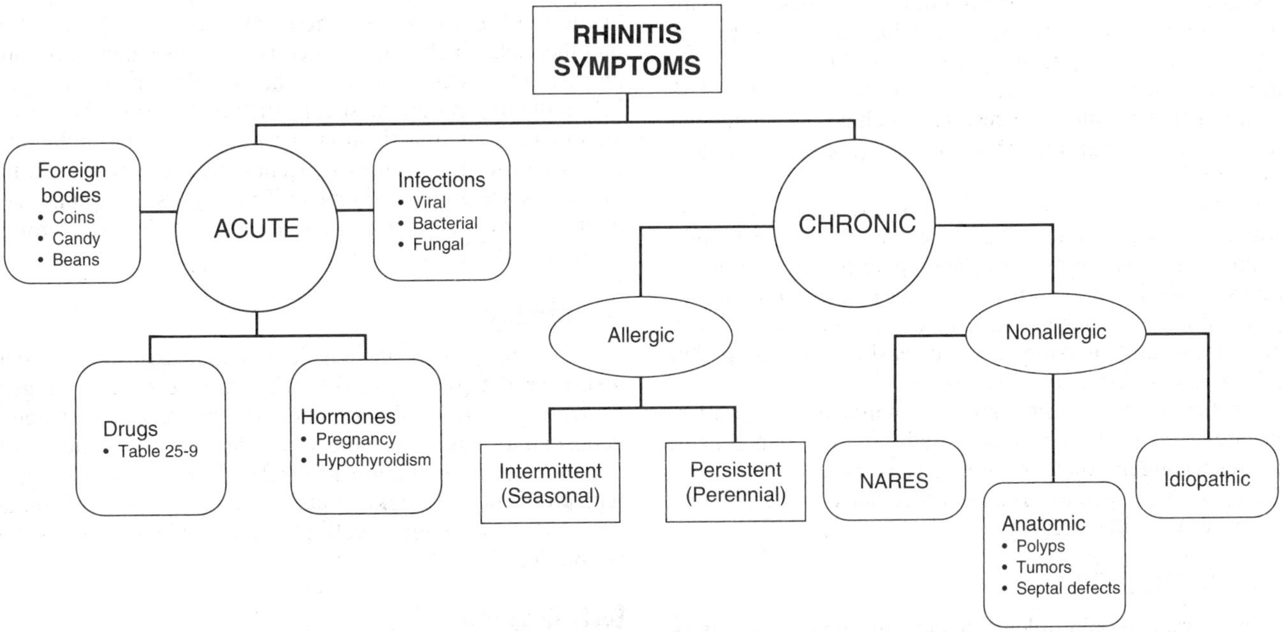

FIGURE 24-2 Possible causes of acute and chronic rhinitis symptoms NARES, nonallergic rhinitis with eosinophilia syndrome.

Intermittent[a] Disease	Persistent[b] Disease
Symptoms occur: Fewer than 4 days/week *or* for fewer than 4 weeks	**Symptoms occur**: At least 4 days/week *and* for at least 4 weeks

Mild	Moderate-Severe
All of the following:	At least *one* of the following:
• Normal sleep	• Impaired sleep
• No impairment of usual daily activities, sport & leisure	• Impairment of daily activities, sports & leisure
• No interference with work or school	• Interference at work or school
• No troublesome symptoms	• Troublesome symptoms

[a]Formerly "seasonal" symptoms.
[b]Formerly "perennial" symptoms.
ARIA, Allergic Rhinitis and its Impact on Asthma

FIGURE 24-3 ARIA classification of allergic rhinitis. (Adapted from references 4,6.)

ETIOLOGY OF ALLERGIC RHINITIS

Genetic, environmental, and lifestyle influences are associated with the development of allergic rhinitis.[6] Problems with methodology and sample size in genome-wide screening studies preclude any definitive conclusions about candidate genes for allergic rhinitis[6]; however, atopy is a significant inheritable factor, and the risk of a child developing allergic symptoms is 50% with one atopic parent and 66% with two atopic parents.[24] Environmental exposures, particularly early in life are also important in the development of symptoms.[25] In addition, lower socioeconomic status may be a risk factor for development of allergic rhinitis.[26]

One theory, referred to as the *hygiene hypothesis*, is that the initial differentiation of lymphocytes early in life has either positive or negative influences on the development of subsequent allergies. In the normal development of the immune system, the lymphocytes differentiate into either Th1 or Th2 cells based on environmental stimuli. Factors associated with a Th1 (allergy protective) response include exposures to various bacteria and viruses, the presence of older siblings, and early attendance in day care. Factors associated with a Th2 (predisposition to allergies) response include environmental exposures to house dust mites, cockroaches, or early, frequent antimicrobial use.[24,27]

In patients with intermittent allergic rhinitis, pollens and airborne mold spores are the most common allergens. Although the pollen season varies with geographic location, grasses, trees, and weeds can be problematic for many people during active pollination. In the United States, ragweed is a primary cause of intermittent symptoms and sensitivity to this pollen is historically referred to as "hay fever."[19]

In patients with persistent allergic rhinitis, the major allergens are house dust mites, indoor molds, animal dander, and cockroach antigen. Another common cause is occupational exposure, in which symptoms can be precipitated by agents such as flour, wood, and detergents.[19]

PATHOPHYSIOLOGY

The primary pathophysiologic feature in allergic rhinitis is inflammation of mucous membranes of the nose. Common symptoms include sneezing, watery discharge, itching of the nose and eyes, nasal obstruction, and postnasal dripping of secretions.[1,6]

The pathogenesis of allergic rhinitis and asthma includes numerous areas of commonality. Inflammation is a central mechanism and the role of cytokines in this process is similar. This has led many scientists and clinicians to adopt the concept of "one airway, one disease."[6] Further evidence for this association includes that rhinitis is a known risk factor for asthma, some patients with rhinitis exhibit bronchial hyperresponsiveness, viral upper respiratory tract infections are a common cause of asthma exacerbations, and sinusitis can worsen asthma.[6] Some treatment strategies, including pharmacotherapy, have a role in both rhinitis and asthma.

Allergic rhinitis is characterized by an immunoglobulin E (IgE)-mediated response that involves three primary steps: sensitization, early-phase events, and late-phase events. This process is depicted in Figure 24-4. Sensitization occurs after initial allergen exposure in a susceptible patient and involves the production of IgE antibodies. These antibodies bind to receptors on other cells, including mast cells. On subsequent exposure, an interaction occurs between the complex of the allergen, IgE antibody, and the mast cell, such that a cross-linking occurs that results in activation and initiation of the inflammatory response. The events can occur early after exposure if the mediators are preformed or late if mediators are synthesized after the process begins or are attracted to the area through chemotaxis.[28]

Sensitization

In an atopic patient, the result of initial exposure to allergens is production of IgE. Following initial exposure, antigen-presenting cells of the immune system react to allergens deposited on the nasal mucosa. This results in helper T-lymphocyte differentiation into Th2 cells, which are associated with production of cytokines and other mediators of inflammation. As a result, memory cells programmed for IgE production are produced.[6,24,28]

Early Response

When a susceptible patient is exposed to an allergen to which previous sensitization has occurred, an early-phase allergic

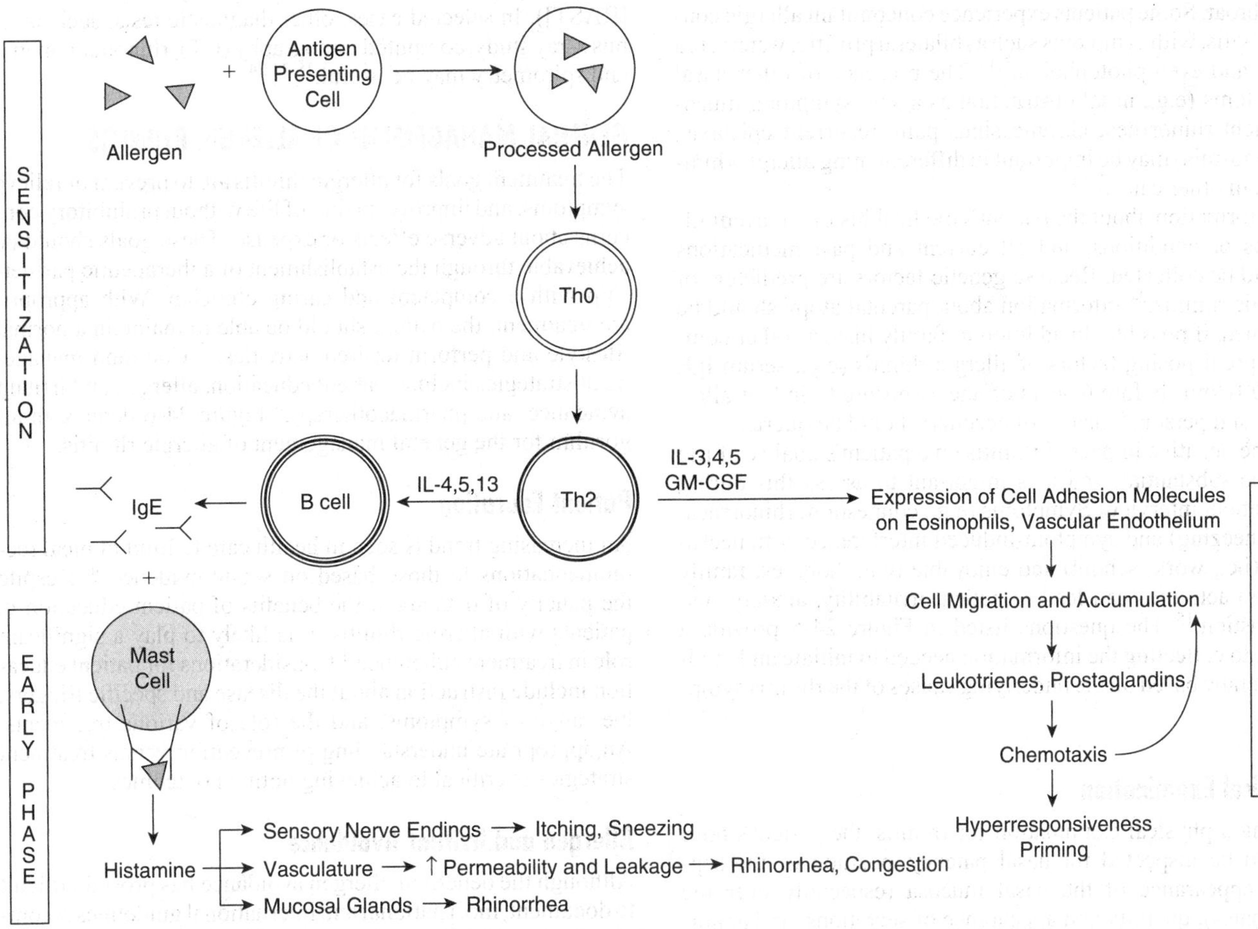

FIGURE 24-4 Pathophysiology of allergic rhinitis.

response generally occurs. This reaction is attributed largely to the interaction between the allergen, IgE, and the sensitized mast cell, resulting in mast cell degranulation. Other cells, including basophils, play an important role as well. As a result, mediators of the allergic response, including histamine, are released along with various chemotactic factors, which amplify and perpetuate the allergic response. Because these mediators are already present in the mast cell, they act within minutes to cause the common symptoms of allergic rhinitis, including itching, sneezing, and congestion.[28,29,30]

Histamine receptors (H_1) are present throughout the nasal mucosa and their activation results in vascular engorgement, leading to nasal congestion, direct stimulation of mucus secretion, and increased glandular secretion.[30] In addition, parasympathetic nervous system stimulation results in cholinergically mediated nasal secretions. Finally, stimulation of peripheral nerve receptors results in itching and sneezing reflexes.[19]

Late Response

Up to one-third of patients with allergic rhinitis also experience a late response that develops approximately 8 hours after initial exposure and may persist for up to 4 hours. In this phase, the nature of inflammation is even more complex, and nasal congestion is a prominent feature. Numerous cells and mediators, including T lymphocytes, cytokines, eosinophils, neutrophils, macrophages, mast cells, and leukotrienes, play important roles. These additional mediators, attracted to the area through chemotaxis, sustain the inflammatory response. This response is also perpetuated through continued exposure to the offending allergen.[31]

DIAGNOSIS AND ASSESSMENT OF RHINITIS

The diagnosis of rhinitis is not defined by one specific laboratory test; rather, it is related to the coordinated results of a thorough patient interview, including medication history, pertinent physical examination, and a limited number of relevant laboratory assessments.[32] Because both allergic and nonallergic stimuli are common; health care practitioners must be able to distinguish these to develop effective management strategies.[19]

History, Signs, and Symptoms

The patient history for rhinitis should include a discussion of the onset, character, frequency, duration, and severity of the patient's symptoms and any identifiable factors that provoke or relieve these symptoms.[1,19,32] Common nasal symptoms suggestive of allergic rhinitis include watery rhinorrhea, nasal pruritis, sneezing, and nasal congestion. Sneezing can occur paroxysmally or be preceded by itching of the nose, ears, eyes, and throat. Some patients experience concomitant allergic conjunctivitis, with symptoms such as bilateral pruritic; watery, red eyes; and even photophobia.[5,19] The presence of other nasal symptoms (e.g., nasal obstruction as a sole symptom, mucopurulent rhinorrhea, chronic sinus pain, recurrent epistaxis, and anosmia) may be important in differentiating allergic rhinitis from other causes.[18]

Information about the patient's medical history, current illnesses or conditions, and all current and past medications should be collected. Because genetic factors are predictors of allergic rhinitis,[24] information about parental atopy should be obtained, if possible. In addition to family history, other common predisposing factors of allergic rhinitis (e.g., serum IgE >100 IU/mL before 6 years of age, exposure to indoor allergens, and personal history of eczema) should be queried.

The negative impact of rhinitis on a patient's quality of life can be substantial, and it is important to assess this during the patient interview. Symptoms (e.g., congestion, rhinorrhea, and sneezing) and symptom-induced interference with necessary (i.e., work, school) and enjoyable (e.g., hobbies, family events) activities can lead to patient irritability, anxiety, and exhaustion.[15] The questions listed in Figure 24-5 provide a guide to collecting the information needed to initiate and modify therapy based on the underlying causes of the rhinitis symptoms.

Physical Examination

During a physical examination for rhinitis, the patient's nose should be inspected for nasal patency, position of the septum, appearance of the nasal mucosa (especially over the turbinates), quantity and appearance of secretions, and abnormal growths.[1,19,32] If the nasal passage is extremely occluded, application of a topical vasoconstrictor (e.g., oxymetazoline 0.025%) allows better visualization. Common physical characteristics of patients with allergic rhinitis are clear nasal discharge and pale, boggy, swollen nasal mucosa.[18,19,32]

The patient's eyes, ears, pharynx, sinuses, and chest should also be examined.[1,19,31] Chronic mouth breathing because of nasal obstruction can cause recognizable facial characteristics or dental abnormalities, such as allergic shiners and nasal crease.[32]

Laboratory Tests

Several diagnostic tests are available for confirming a diagnosis of allergic rhinitis in patients who present with a suggestive history and symptoms. Microscopic examination of nasal secretions can be performed, but current recommendations suggest that this is more commonly used by subspecialists or in research.[19] In allergic conditions, the clinician would expect numerous eosinophils to be present in the sample; however, this could also be true of NARES or nasal polyps.[1]

Immediate hypersensitivity skin tests are used to demonstrate an IgE-mediated response of the skin. This provides confirmatory evidence for a specific allergy.[33] A variety of skin test methods are available; however, the prick and puncture test (in which the wheal and flare reaction is evaluated 15 minutes after allergen administration) is the preferred technique.[6,33] Another method of assessing specific allergens is serum-specific IgE sensitivity via in vitro testing (e.g., radioallergosorbent testing [RAST]). In selected cases, other diagnostic tests, such as sinus x-ray study, computed tomography (CT), rhinomanometry, and spirometry may be useful.[18,33,34]

GENERAL MANAGEMENT OF ALLERGIC RHINITIS

The treatment goals for allergic rhinitis are to prevent or relieve symptoms, and improve quality of life without prohibitory concerns about adverse effects or expense. These goals should be achievable through the establishment of a therapeutic partnership with a competent and caring clinician. With appropriate treatment, the patient should be able to maintain a normal lifestyle and perform desired activities.[35] Common management strategies include patient education, allergen and irritant avoidance, and pharmacotherapy.[6] Figure 24-6 depicts an algorithm for the general management of allergic rhinitis.

Patient Education

An increasing trend is seen in health care to limit clinical recommendations to those based on sound evidence.[36] Despite the paucity of data about the benefits of patient education in patients with allergic rhinitis, it is likely to play a significant role in treatment adherence.[1] Considerations for patient education include instruction about the disease and specific triggers, the range of symptoms, and the role of various treatments. An appropriate understanding of prevention versus treatment strategies is critical to achieving optimal outcomes.

Allergen and Irritant Avoidance

Although the benefit of allergen avoidance has proved difficult to document, most national and international guidelines recommend using this strategy in a comprehensive management plan for allergic rhinitis.[37] Various strategies for minimizing exposure to known allergens (e.g., pollens, house dust mites, molds, animal dander, and cockroaches) are commonly employed for prevention. Because little evidence supports a single physical or chemical intervention to reduce allergen exposure, a multifaceted approach should be used.[6] Efforts to reduce exposure to irritants (e.g., tobacco smoke, indoor or outdoor pollutants) should also be recommended.[38]

Pharmacotherapy

Several classes of medications are used in the management of allergic rhinitis.[38,39] Choices should be based on goals of treatment, safety, efficacy, cost-effectiveness, adherence, severity, comorbidity, and patient preferences.[35] Therapy can be administered orally, topically, or systemically and medications may be used on a regular schedule or an as needed basis.[1] Few cost-effectiveness data exist comparing the classes of therapy, excepting the second generation antihistamines and nasal corticosteroids, which have both been shown to be cost-effective.[40] Table 24-1 summarizes the effectiveness of agents for specific symptoms used in the treatment of allergic rhinitis.

Antihistamines

Antihistamines are most effective for reducing sneezing, itching, and rhinorrhea. They also diminish eye symptoms, but have minimal effects on nasal congestion.[1,4] Although first generation antihistamines (FGA) are efficacious, their use is limited by anticholinergic and sedative effects which challenge

1. Which of the common symptoms of rhinitis is the patient experiencing?
   - Sneezing, nasal itching, runny nose, nasal congestion, postnasal drip, altered sense of smell, watery eyes, itching eyes, ear "popping"
2. What color are the nasal secretions?
   - Clear, white, yellow, green, blood-streaked, rusty brown
3. When did the symptoms first appear?
   - Infancy, childhood, adulthood
4. Where the symptoms associated with a change in state/environment?
   - After a viral upper respiratory infection, after a traumatic blow to the head or face, upon moving into/visiting a new dwelling, after obtaining a new pet
5. How often do the symptoms occur?
   - Daily, episodically, seasonally, constantly
6. For how long has this symptom pattern persisted?
   - Days, weeks, months, years
7. Which factors or conditions precipitate symptoms?
   - Specific allergens, inhaled irritants, climatic conditions, food, drinks
8. Which specific activities precipitate symptoms?
   - Dusting, vacuuming, mowing grass, raking leaves
9. Are other members of the family experiencing similar symptoms?
10. Which of the following are prevalent in the household?
    - Carpeting heavy drapes, foam or feather pillows, stuffed toys, areas of high moisture (basements, bathrooms), tobacco use (by patient or others)
11. Does the patient have other medical conditions that can cause similar symptoms?
12. Is the patient taking any medications that might cause or aggravate these symptoms?
13. What prescription and nonprescription medications have been used for these symptoms in the past? Were they effective? Did they cause any unwanted effects?
14. What is the patient's occupation?
15. What are the patient's typical leisure activities?
16. To what extent have the symptoms interfered with the patient's lifestyle (i.e., are they disabling or merely annoying)?
    - Greatly, somewhat, not much

FIGURE 24-5 Patient history interview.

their cost-effectiveness.[41] The magnitude of these effects is a subject of debate; nonetheless, newer antihistamines (second generation antihistamines, SGA) are recommended as first-line therapy for mild allergic rhinitis.[1,2,34] Antihistamines are available in oral, ophthalmic, and nasal formulations and can also be found in combinations with oral decongestants. They are most effective when administered before allergen exposure.

Nasal Corticosteroid Agents

Nasal corticosteroids, which are recognized as the most effective medication class for the treatment of allergic rhinitis, are particularly useful for more severe or persistent symptoms.[18,34] Although achieving optimal outcomes depends on the patient's ability to use the device correctly, if administered as intended, these agents are appropriate for all symptoms, are generally

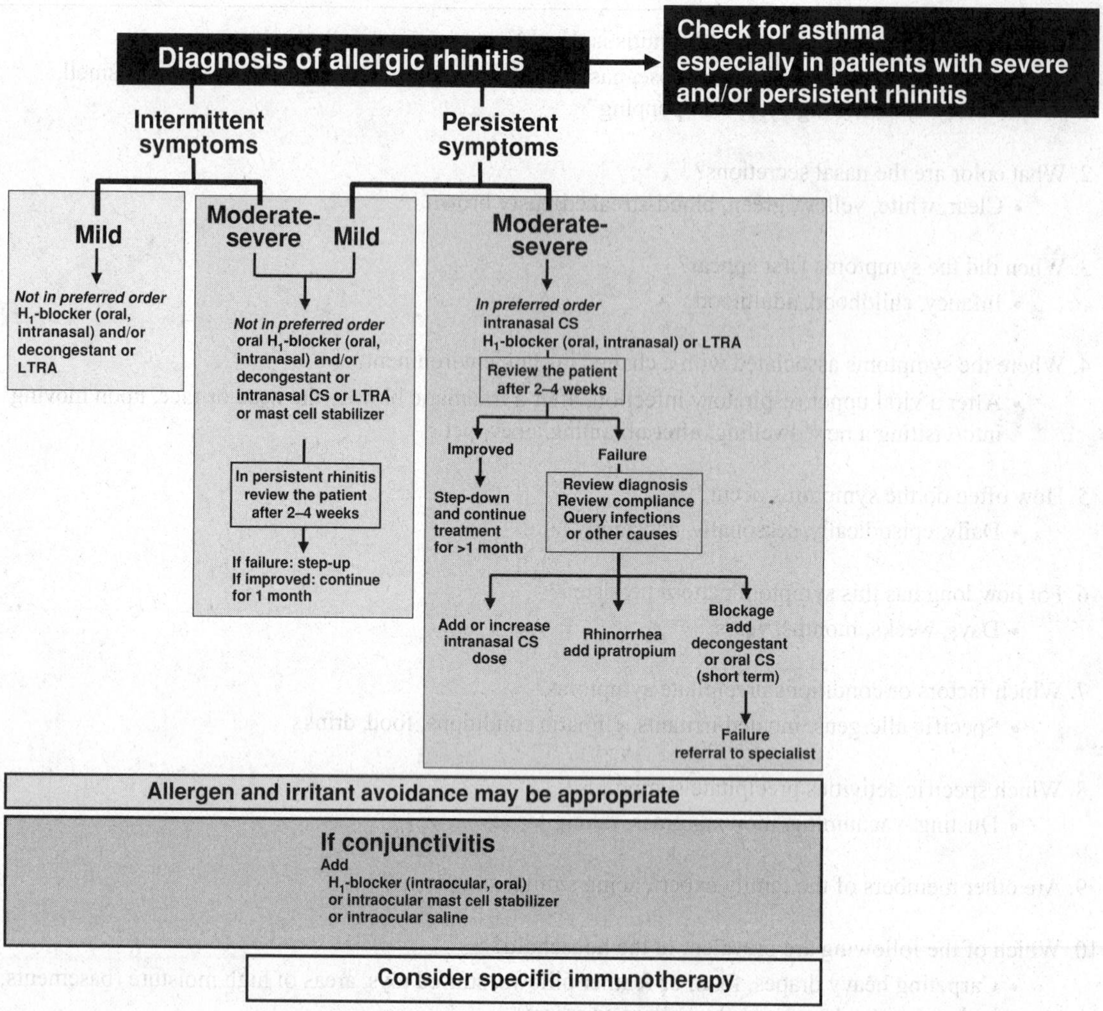

FIGURE 24-6 Treatment algorithm for allergic rhinitis. Treatment should be directed at predominant symptoms (i.e., for eye symptoms in absence of other symptoms use ophthalmic preparation). Prevention strategies are more effective than treatment strategies. For intermittent symptoms, begin treatment several weeks before antigen exposure and discontinue when no longer needed. CS, corticosteroid; LTRA, leukotriene receptor antagonist (leukotriene modifier). (Adapted from reference 6.)

well tolerated, and have few adverse effects.[34] They are most beneficial when dosed on a regular schedule; some evidence indicates, however, that they are effective when used on an as needed basis.[42] Nasal corticosteroids are also useful for some forms of nonallergic rhinitis.

Leukotriene Modifiers

Leukotriene modifiers are effective in relieving many of the nasal symptoms of allergic rhinitis.[43,44] In some studies, the efficacy of leukotriene modifiers is comparable to antihistamines[44]; however, they are generally recommended as adjunct treatment as opposed to monotherapy. These agents may have a role in concomitant asthma and allergic rhinitis, particularly, if both diseases are relatively mild.[45]

Cromolyn

Intranasal cromolyn, a nonsteroidal agent, acts as a mast cell stabilizer and, although safe, it is generally less efficacious than other therapies. Because it is administered four to six times daily and requires several weeks to be effective, it is best reserved for acute prophylaxis before exposure to a known allergen and for use by children or in pregnancy.[46]

Decongestants

Oral and nasal decongestants can effectively reduce nasal congestion produced by allergic and nonallergic forms of rhinitis.[1] Oral agents are often combined with antihistamines, but they can lead to profound side effects (e.g., insomnia, nervousness, urinary retention) and should be used with caution in elderly patients and in those with arrhythmias, hypertension, and hyperthyroidism. Nasal agents are not typically associated with these effects, but should be limited to short-term use to avoid rebound nasal congestion.[2] Recent restrictions on the sale of nonprescription formulations containing pseudoephedrine and questions regarding the efficacy of phenylephrine have resulted in challenges to the optimal use of oral decongestants.

Anticholinergic Agents

Intranasal ipratropium bromide is an anticholinergic agent effective in reducing watery, nasal secretions in allergic rhinitis,

Table 24-1 Effectiveness of Agents[a] Used in Management of Allergic Rhinitis

	Rhinorrhea	Nasal Pruritus	Sneezing	Nasal Congestion	Eye Symptoms	Onset
Antihistamines						
Nasal	Moderate	High	High	0/Low	0	Rapid
Ophthalmic	0	0	0	0	Moderate	Rapid
Oral	Moderate	High	High	0/Low	Low	Rapid
Decongestants						
Nasal	0	0	0	High	0	Rapid
Ophthalmic	0	0	0	0	Moderate	Rapid
Oral	0	0	0	High	0	Rapid
Corticosteroids						
Nasal	High	High	High	High	High	Slow (days)
Ophthalmic	0	0	0	0	High	Slow (days)
Mast Cell Stabilizers						
Nasal	Low	Low	Low	0/Low	Low	Slow (weeks)
Ophthalmic	Low	Low	Low	Low	Moderate	Slow (weeks)
Anticholinergics						
Nasal	High	0	0	0	0	Rapid
Leukotriene Modifiers						
Oral	Low	0/Low	Low	Moderate	Low	Rapid

[a] Immunotherapy can lead to significant responses in all symptom categories; however, onset of action is delayed (months).
High, significant effect; moderate, moderate effect; low, low effect; 0, no effect.
Adapted from references 2, 43.

nonallergic rhinitis, and viral upper respiratory infections.[1,4] Anticholinergic agents have no significant effects on other symptoms.

Ophthalmic Therapies

Ophthalmic products used to treat symptoms of allergic conjunctivitis include antihistamines, mast cell stabilizers, decongestants and nonsteroidal anti-inflammatory agents. These agents are effective in reducing ocular symptoms and may be used in combination with oral and intranasal agents.

Immunotherapy

Allergen immunotherapy should be considered for patients who have severe symptoms despite optimal pharmacotherapy, require systemic corticosteroids, or have coexisting conditions such as sinusitis and asthma.[1] The clinical efficacy of immunotherapy by subcutaneous injection (SIT), sometimes called "allergy shots," is well established.[47] A recent meta-analysis of sublingual immunotherapy (SLIT) showed a reduction in symptoms and medication requirements.[48] Studies involving nasal immunotherapy (NIT) are ongoing.

Anti-IgE Therapy

Omalizumab is a recombinant humanized monoclonal anti-IgE antibody that complexes free circulating IgE in the body. The complex cannot interact with mast cells and basophils and, thus, reduces IgE-mediated allergic reactions. When administered as a subcutaneous injection once or twice monthly, omalizumab has been shown to decrease all nasal symptoms and improve quality of life in patients with allergic rhinitis.[49] Currently, this therapy is approved only for people 12 years of age and older with moderate to severe allergy-related asthma inadequately controlled with inhaled corticosteroids. Recently, the U.S. Food and Drug Administration (FDA) called for a black box label warning to alert users that omalizumab can cause potentially life-threatening allergic reactions after any dose, up to 24 hours after the dose is given and even if there was no reaction to the first dose.[50]

Nondrug Therapies

Supportive care is the foundation of treatment for patients with symptoms of allergic rhinitis.[1] These strategies can be helpful during an acute worsening of symptoms as well as for the patient who suffers chronically. Supportive care can ameliorate discomfort, relieve mild symptoms, and assist with side effects from pharmacotherapies. Examples include the application of compresses to the sinuses or external nasal passages and humidification of mucous membranes with artificial tears or nasal saline solutions.

Recently, the effectiveness of irradiation as a nondrug treatment option for allergic rhinitis has been explored.[51] To date, these studies have shown modest improvement in nasal symptom scores, with mild side effects in small numbers of participants; although larger, controlled trials are needed before safety, efficacy, and cost-effectiveness can be established.

SPECIFIC THERAPEUTIC OPTIONS

Antihistamine Therapy

1. L.B. is a 57-year-old man with a history of controlled hypertension for 10 years and intermittent allergic rhinitis since childhood (confirmed sensitivity to birch tree pollen via skin testing). L.B. presents with complaints of nasal itching, sneezing, clear rhinorrhea, and stuffiness. He usually experiences similar symptoms with added ocular itching every spring, but has noticed that the problem has become persistent since he moved into an older home in the historic district of town. In the past, L.B. has successfully self-medicated his seasonal symptoms with an over-the-counter (OTC) antihistamine and decongestant (diphenhydramine 50 mg and pseudoephedrine 60 mg TID to QID as needed for symptoms), although "nothing seems to help much with the itchy eyes." L.B.'s chronic medications are hydrochlorothiazide 25 mg every morning and amlodipine 10 mg every day. He denies any other medical problems, is afebrile, and his blood pressure is 128/82 mm Hg. He has no history of adverse drug reactions or drug allergies. He does not smoke, but drinks alcohol socially.

Diagnosis of Allergic Rhinitis

2. What elements of L.B.'s presentation indicate a probable diagnosis of allergic rhinitis?

L.B. is exhibiting the classic symptoms of persistent (perennial) allergic rhinitis with intermittent (seasonal) exacerbations: nasal itching, sneezing, watery (often profuse) rhinorrhea, and congestion.[19] His history of positive skin tests and that his symptoms previously responded to antihistamine or decongestant also support the diagnosis. In the past, L.B. has experienced symptoms predictably at the onset of the tree pollination season, with only minimal symptoms during the remainder of the year. Moving into an older home, however, has likely triggered latent sensitivities to dust mite allergens and mold spores.

Allergen Avoidance Measures

3. What allergen avoidance strategies could L.B. use to minimize his exposure to triggers?

Allergen avoidance is commonly used to reduce symptoms in sensitized patients. General agreement is that allergen avoidance should lead to an improvement of symptoms; however, little evidence supports the use of a single physical or chemical method.[37,52] A need exists for well-controlled studies to assess the effects of multiple approaches to allergen avoidance.[53] Although total allergen avoidance is often impractical to implement, simple changes that can reduce exposure to many perennial triggers, such as house dust mites, animal dander, and mold, can assist with symptom control.[1]

Dust mite avoidance (e.g., the use of impermeable covers on box springs, mattresses, and pillows) has traditionally been used as a method of reducing allergen exposure. Although this practice continues to be recommended frequently, a recent study demonstrated despite reduced exposure to antigen, this strategy alone did not reduce symptoms in patients with allergic rhinitis.[54] Other methods of reducing antigen exposure include washing bedding at least weekly in hot water (>130°F) and reducing humidity in the home to below 50%. In addition, replacing carpets with linoleum, tile, or wood floors and replacing curtains and heavy draperies with blinds that can be wiped clean has been recommended.[1]

Mold avoidance is difficult when outdoor humidity levels are high, but removing carpeting may be effective in reducing buildup. Live plants should be removed from the home to reduce mold contamination from the soil. Air conditioners should be used, and filters should be changed frequently to reduce humidity and assist with air filtration.[1]

Because L.B. has recently moved into an older home, he may not have used these avoidance strategies. These should be recommended and explained during the initial clinical consultation.

Therapeutic Objectives for Allergic Rhinitis

4. What are the therapeutic objectives in treating L.B.?

The therapeutic objectives for the treatment of allergic rhinitis are to control symptoms and permit all usual daily activities with no adverse effects of therapy. In patients with seasonal exacerbations, another objective is to prevent the onset of symptoms by anticipating the patient's season of sensitivity. In L.B.'s case, he should use environmental measures to reduce exposure and then begin chronic treatment with possible add-on therapy instituted 2 weeks before the start of pollen season.

5. L.B. has used diphenhydramine for many years with good symptom relief and, as he recalls, only minimal daytime sedation. He asks your opinion regarding whether this is the best treatment for his allergic symptoms. He specifically requests the most cost-effective treatment available because he must pay cash out-of-pocket for any medications.

Choice of Therapeutic Agent

6. What therapy do you recommend and how should it be initiated?

Because of their convenience, oral antihistamines are recommended as initial therapy in patients with allergic rhinitis, particularly those with mild symptoms.[55] They reduce symptoms of nasal itching, sneezing, and rhinorrhea, with variable effectiveness on ocular symptoms but no efficacy for nasal congestion. FGA (e.g., diphenhydramine, brompheniramine, chlorpheniramine, and clemastine) can cause significant side effects because of their sedative and anticholinergic properties. Their use has been supplanted by the SGA (e.g., loratadine, desloratadine, fexofenadine, cetirizine, and levocetirizine), which are equally effective with fewer side effects.[6,56]

In general, SGA include agents marketed after 1980 with one or more of the following properties: (*a*) improved H_1-receptor selectivity, (*b*) absent or reduced sedative effects, and (*c*) antiallergic properties separate from antihistamine effects.[55] The first SGA, astemizole and terfenadine, were withdrawn from the market because of potential cardiovascular toxicity, usually related to higher doses and interactions with agents metabolized via the cytochrome P450 system.[55] This is not a significant concern with currently available SGA; however, many of the current agents undergo substantial hepatic metabolism and some evidence exists of potential drug interactions or variability in metabolic capacity associated with this.[56] Some references have begun referring to the most recently approved agents (i.e., fexofenadine, desloratadine, and levocetirizine) as third generation agents (TGA) to highlight that they are active metabolites of other products. The Consensus Group on New Generation Antihistamines concluded, however, that on the basis of evidence, these agents do not merit a new class title because they do not demonstrate distinct clinical advantages over the SGA.[57,58] For this reason, they will be discussed as SGA in this chapter.

Antihistamines block the effects of histamine by one of two mechanisms: (*a*) as an H_1-receptor antagonist and (*b*) as an inverse agonist of the H_1-receptor.[59] Whereas all marketed antihistamines have sufficient effects on the histamine receptor to provide clinical benefits, the SGA are more specific for the peripheral histamine receptor than are the FGA[60] and, for this reason, they present a lower risk for adverse effects, such as sedation.

L.B. has experienced a good response to an FGA without complaints of excessive drowsiness. However, sedation includes both drowsiness (i.e., the subjective state of sleepiness or lethargy) and impairment (i.e., an objective decrease of absence of specific physical or mental abilities)[61] and evidence indicates that cognitive impairment can occur, even in the absence of overt drowsiness.[61,62]

In light of these findings, the Joint Task Force on Practice Parameters in Allergy, Asthma and Immunology has stated "many patients may not perceive performance impairment that is associated with FGAs. Consequently, SGAs that are associated with less risk or no risk for these side effects should usually be considered."[1] In another expert consensus statement on the use of antihistamines in the treatment of allergic rhinitis, experts agreed that many of the FGA produce sedation, impairment, and reduced quality of life. They acknowledge that allergic rhinitis is more appropriately treated with SGA in all patients.[62] One exception to this is pregnant women in whom there is more long-term data on the use of FGA and, thus, they are preferred by the American College of Obstetrics and Gynecology.[63] If these drugs are not tolerated, cetirizine or loratadine may be considered, ideally after the first trimester.

Second generation agents prevent the onset of symptoms better than they reverse symptoms that are already present. Also, the maximal antihistamine effects occur several hours after the drug's serum concentration peaks.[58] For maximal effect, therefore, the SGA should be administered before allergen exposure, whenever possible. For the same reason, chronic dosing is preferred to intermittent dosing.

Essentially, all the antihistamines listed in Table 24-2 are equally effective.[58,60] Therefore, the choice of agent is based on duration of action, side-effect profile (especially drowsiness and anticholinergic effects), risk of drug interactions, and cost.[64] Some patients claim that one product is more helpful in relieving their symptoms than another; however, for many years there have been reports that tolerance to specific agents can occur after consistent use. Although no pharmacologic explanation exists for these observations,[64] patients may experience benefit from switching therapies if the perception of tolerance occurs.

The major advantages of SGA are their selectivity to the H_1-receptor and their reduced central nervous system (CNS) sedative effects.[58] Desloratadine, fexofenadine, loratadine, and levocetirizine—at prescribed doses—are reported to have an incidence of sedation that does not differ from placebo for both somnolence and performance impairment.[65] Cetirizine and intranasal azelastine are not considered to be entirely nonsedating, although the incidence of sedation is less than with FGA.[58,66] Another advantage of SGA is that most products can be dosed once daily to improve patient adherence to therapy. Specific antihistamines are compared in Table 24-2. In the case of L.B., it would be reasonable to begin therapy with loratadine 10 mg daily, because as an SGA, it has demonstrated efficacy with minimal side effects and is also available without a prescription.

Nasal Antihistamines

7. L.B. has a friend who had side effects from antihistamines and had been given a nasal spray instead. Is it possible to give antihistamines by this route, or is L.B. confusing this with other topical therapies, such as decongestants or corticosteroids?

An aqueous intranasal solution (125 mcg/spray) of azelastine is approved for the treatment of allergic rhinitis. This drug has an objectionable taste, making it unsuitable for oral administration, but the nasal and ophthalmic formulations have been shown beneficial in allergic rhinitis and conjunctivitis.[67–69] In studies comparing intranasal azelastine with oral antihistamines and placebo, azelastine has been found to be equal to the oral antihistamines,[66] although a meta-analysis comparing azelastine with nasal corticosteroids suggests that nasal corticosteroids were superior in efficacy in all but ophthalmic symptoms.[67] As with the oral agents, the intranasal formulation is less effective for nasal congestion than it is for nasal itching, sneezing, and rhinorrhea.[67] Dosing recommendations for azelastine (for adults and children >12 years of age) are two sprays in each nostril twice a day. Before the first use and anytime when the product has not been used for 3 days or more, the dosage form must be primed. This is accomplished by pumping the spray mechanism two to four times until a consistent mist is expelled.

The side effects of azelastine are comparable to the FGA in terms of somnolence (10%–15%) and headache (15% to 30%).[70] Intranasal azelastine can also cause local side effects, including nasal irritation, dry mouth, sore throat, and mild epistaxis. Bad aftertaste remains a significant problem, occurring in up to 20% of patients, even those using the ophthalmic formulations. A potential role for intranasal antihistamines is for patients who do not respond adequately to oral antihistamines.[67] In addition, some patients may prefer the intranasal route of administration or benefit from concomitant therapy with nasal antihistamines and nasal corticosteroids. As a prescription-only product, a nasal antihistamine would be more expensive than many oral alternatives.

Decongestant Therapy

8. What role do decongestants have in L.B.'s treatment?

Nasal congestion is often much less severe in patients who experience only intermittent symptoms, but as L.B.'s symptoms have become persistent since his move, the exact frequency and severity of his nasal congestion should be assessed before recommending drug therapy. In patients with only mild, intermittent symptoms, saline irrigation (administered as

Table 24-2 Oral Antihistamines[a,b] Commonly Used in Allergic Rhinitis

Generic Name (Example Brand Product)	Adult Dose	Pediatric Dose[c]	Other Effects		
First Generation			*Sedative*	*Antiemetic*	*Anticholinergic*
Brompheniramine (*Dimetane*)	4 mg every 4–6 hrs	*Children 6–12 yrs:* 2 mg every 4–6 hrs *Children 2–5 yrs:* 1 mg every 4–6 hrs	+	0	++
Chlorpheniramine (*Chlor-Trimeton*)	4 mg every 4–6 hrs	*Children 6–12 yrs:* 2 mg every 4–6 hrs *Children 2–5 yrs:* 1 mg every 4–6 hrs	+	0	++
Clemastine (*Tavist*)	1.34–2.68 mg every 8–12 hrs	*Children 6–12 yrs:* 0.67–1.34 mg every 12 hrs	++	++	+++
Diphenhydramine (*Benadryl*)	25–50 mg every 4–6 hrs	*Children 6–12 yrs:* 12.5–25 mg every 4–6 hrs *Children 2–5 yrs:* 6.25–12.5 mg every 4–6 hrs	+++	++	+++
Second Generation			*Sedative*	*Antiemetic*	*Anticholinergic*
Cetirizine (*Zyrtec*)	5–10 mg once daily	*Children 6–12 yrs:* 5–10 mg once daily *Children 2–5 yrs:* 2.5–5 mg once daily or 2.5 mg every 12 hrs	+	0	±
Desloratadine[d] (*Clarinex*)	5 mg once daily	*Children 6–11 yrs:* 2.5 mg once daily *Children 1–5 yrs:* 1.25 mg once daily *Children 6–11 mos:* 1 mg once daily	±	0	±
Fexofenadine[d] (*Allegra*)	60 mg every 12 hrs or 180 mg once daily	*Children 6–11 yrs:* 30 mg every 12 hrs (tablets) *Children 2–11 yrs:* 30 mg every 12 hrs (oral suspension)	±	0	±
Levocetirizine[d] (*Xyzal*)	5 mg once daily	*Children 6–11 yrs:* 2.5 mg once daily	±	0	±
Loratadine (*Claritin*)	10 mg once daily	*Children 6–12 yrs:* 10 mg once daily *Children 2–5 yrs:* 5 mg once daily	±	0	±

[a]Many oral antihistamines are sold as combination products with the oral decongestants pseudoephedrine and phenylephrine. The addition of the decongestant may alter the dosing scheme for the product. As of 2005, pseudoephedrine products have been placed behind the pharmacy counter in the United States. Federal law limits the quantity available for purchase to 9 g/mo, 3.6 g/day with signature and photo identification. Individual states may have additional restrictions regarding the sale of pseudoephedrine, consult local boards of pharmacy for details.

[b]Some oral antihistamines are available in both short-acting and extended or sustained release formulations. Refer to package insert for specific dosing instructions for long-acting products.

[c]The Centers for Disease Control and Prevention has released a report concerning the use of antihistamines and decongestants in infants less than 2 years of age. In October 2007, The Consumer Healthcare Products Association on behalf of the makers of over-the-counter (OTC) cough and cold medicines announced voluntary market withdrawals of oral cough and cold medicines that refer to "infants". Although these medicines are safe and effective when used as directed, rare patterns of misuse leading to overdose have been identified, particularly in infants. The voluntary withdrawal does not affect medicines intended for children age 2 and older; however, clinicians are reminded always to ask caregivers about the use of OTC products in order to avoid exposure to multiple medications containing the same or similar ingredients.

[d]Currently available by prescription only.

Adapted from references 57, 64, 98.

frequently as needed) is helpful in soothing and moisturizing irritated nasal mucosa. Antihistamines do little to relieve nasal congestion; therefore, patients with moderate to severe congestion may require a combination of an antihistamine with a decongestant. The combination of an antihistamine and an oral decongestant is more effective than either component alone in the treatment of allergic rhinitis.[56]

Both the topical (nasal) and the oral decongestants are sympathomimetics that directly stimulate α_1-adrenergic receptors, resulting in vasoconstriction. Local effects on the nasal mucosa include decreased tissue hyperemia, decreased tissue swelling, decreased nasal congestion, and improved nasal airway patency.[56] The primary oral decongestants are phenylephrine and pseudoephedrine. Until 2005, pseudoephedrine was the more popular agent; however, because of the potential to use it in the manufacturer of illicit substances (e.g., methamphetamine), restrictions on the allowable quantity and methods for purchasing pseudoephedrine-containing products have been implemented at both the state and federal levels. These restrictions have resulted in the reformulation of many oral decongestant products to include phenylephrine as an alternative decongestant. A recent meta-analysis has questioned the

Table 24-3 Decongestants[a,b] Commonly Used in Allergic Rhinitis

Generic Name (Example Brand Product)	Adult Dose	Pediatric Dose[c]
Oral[a]		
Pseudoephedrine *(Sudafed)*	60 mg every 4–6 hrs (MAX 240 mg/day)	*Children 6–12 yrs*: 30 mg every 4–6 hrs (MAX 120 mg/day) *Children 2–5 yrs*: 15 mg every 4–6 hrs (MAX 60 mg/day)
Phenylephrine *(Sudafed PE)*	10–20 mg every 4 hrs (MAX 120 mg/day)	*Children 6–11 yrs*: 10 mg every 4 hrs (MAX 60 mg/day).
Topical[d]		
Naphazoline *(Privine)*	1–2 drops or sprays/nostril every 6 hrs	*Children <12 yrs*: Avoid, unless under physician direction
Phenylephrine *(Neo-Synephrine)*	0.25–0.5% solution: 2–3 sprays or drops/nostril every 3–4 hrs	*Children 6–11 yrs*: 2–3 sprays or drops (0.25% solution)/nostril every 4 hrs *Children 2–5 yrs*: 2–3 drops (0.125% solution) into each nostril not more than every 4 hrs
Oxymetazoline *(Afrin)*	0.05% solution: 2–3 sprays or drops/nostril every 10–12 hrs	*Children 6–12 yrs*: 2–3 sprays or drops/nostril every 12 hrs
Xylometazoline *(Otrivin)*	0.1% solution: 1–3 sprays or 2–3 drops/ nostril every 8–10 hrs	*Children 2–12 yrs*: 2–3 drops (0.05% solution) into each nostril every 8–10 hrs

[a] Many oral decongestants are sold as combination products with the oral antihistamines. The addition of the antihistamine may alter the dosing scheme for the product. As of 2005, pseudoephedrine products have been placed behind the pharmacy counter in the United States. Federal law limits the quantity available for purchase to 9 grams in a month, 3.6 grams in a day with signature and photo identification. Individual states may have additional restrictions regarding the sale of pseudoephedrine, consult local boards of pharmacy for details.

[b] Some oral decongestants are available in both short-acting and extended/sustained release formulations. Refer to package insert for specific dosing instructions for long-acting products. Note that some extended release formulations are not recommended for children less than 12 yrs of age.

[c] The Centers for Disease Control and Prevention has released a report concerning the use of decongestants and antihistamines in infants less than 2 years of age. In October 2007, The Consumer Healthcare Products Association on behalf of the makers of over-the-counter (OTC) cough and cold medicines announced voluntary market withdrawals of oral cough and cold medicines that refer to "infants". Although these medicines are safe and effective when used as directed, rare patterns of misuse leading to overdose have been identified, particularly in infants. The voluntary withdrawal does not affect medicines intended for children age 2 and older; however, clinicians are reminded always to ask caregivers about the use of OTC products in order to avoid exposure to multiple medications containing the same or similar ingredients.

[d] Limit duration of treatment to <10 days (preferably, <5 days) to minimize risk of rebound congestion.

Adapted from reference 98.

efficacy of phenylephrine as a decongestant in doses approved for nonprescription use and further study is needed before it should be routinely recommended.[71] The available oral and topical decongestants, all of which are available without prescription, are compared in Table 24-3.

Oral decongestants can cause systemic side effects, particularly those associated with CNS stimulation (e.g., nervousness, restlessness, insomnia, tremor, dizziness, and headache).[18] Cardiovascular stimulation (e.g., tachycardia, palpitations, increased blood pressure) also can occur, so patients with hypertension should be monitored carefully while taking oral decongestants.[72] Because oral decongestants are not associated with the development of rebound congestion, in most patients, they are appropriate for chronic use. They are not recommended, however, for use during pregnancy.[63] Topical administration of decongestants generally does not lead to systemic side effects; however, these agents are not appropriate for chronic use in rhinitis because of their potential for causing rebound congestion (see Question 33).

Because L.B. is complaining of nasal congestion, he will require a decongestant in addition to the loratadine. He may choose to use a fixed-dose combination product (e.g., loratadine + pseudoephedrine) or to supplement the daily loratadine with pseudoephedrine as needed. Although L.B. has used pseudoephedrine in the past without a problem, he may require education regarding the new procedures for purchasing this product while assuring him that the new restrictions are not related to the drug's safety as a decongestant. In addition, although his hypertension is controlled, his blood pressure should be monitored regularly to detect any deterioration.

Ocular Therapies

9. L.B.'s new therapies are effective for his persistent nasal symptoms; however, in the spring he complains that his eyes are itchy and watery and that the loratadine and pseudoephedrine do not seem to be helping. How are L.B.'s ocular symptoms related to his allergic rhinitis?

Relationship between Ocular and Nasal Symptoms

Allergic ocular disease is part of the full range of allergic diseases, including rhinitis, eczema, and asthma, which share a common pathophysiology and inflammatory presentation.[73] The most common of the allergic ocular diagnoses is seasonal (intermittent) allergic conjunctivitis, which accounts for up to 50% of all ocular allergy cases. The symptoms of both intermittent and persistent allergic conjunctivitis are identical in that they are caused by allergic response in the conjunctiva to airborne allergens. Seasonal symptoms commonly occur in response to pollens, whereas perennial symptoms are more often associated with house dust mites. The symptoms of allergic conjunctivitis are itchy eyes, with or without a burning sensation, and a watery discharge or tearing. Physical examination reveals conjunctival surfaces that are mildly injected (reddened) with varying degrees of conjunctival edema.

Swelling of the eyelids can also occur. The symptoms are usually bilateral, but not always symmetric.[73]

Because of the potential for long-term damage to vision, persistent ocular conditions should always be assessed by an eye care professional. Other ocular problems that can be confused with allergic conjunctivitis include atopic keratoconjunctivitis, keratopathy, and giant papillary conjunctivitis (see Chapter 51, Eye Disorders).

Choice of Therapeutic Agent

10. What are the treatment options for L.B.'s allergic conjunctivitis, and how does the clinician choose between the available options?

Seasonal and perennial allergic conjunctivitis are treated similarly with only the duration of the treatment course differing (i.e., intermittent versus persistent treatment). Nonpharmacologic treatment includes avoidance of aeroallergens to the extent possible, cold compresses or the use of refrigerated eye drops, and lubrication with frequent application of saline or tear substitutes. Part of the effectiveness of all of the ocular preparations, including lubricating eye drops, is attributable to physical dilution and irrigation of aeroallergens from the eye.[73]

The available therapeutic options for management of allergic conjunctivitis include topical ocular administration of antihistamines, vasoconstrictors, mast cell stabilizers, and NSAID (Table 24-4). Randomized, controlled trials have demonstrated that these agents significantly reduce ocular symptoms, including itching, and improve sleep.[73–77] These ocular medications act by the same mechanisms as their nasal counterparts. In addition, topical ophthalmic corticosteroids have a limited role in the acute management of allergic conjunctivitis; however, they are not indicated for prolonged use because of the risk of serious infectious complications in the eye.

In the case of L.B., a trial of antihistamine + vasoconstrictor combination eye drops (e.g., pheniramine maleate + naphazoline hydrochloride) for management of acute symptoms is an appropriate recommendation for short-term use. Note that the overuse of ocular vasoconstrictors can lead to rebound conjunctivitis, similar to that occurring with nasal decongestants (see section, Drug-Induced Nasal Congestion). If the patient exhibits chronic symptoms, consider a switch to a nasal corticosteroid (which may have better efficacy for combination symptoms[78]) or refer to specialist care.

Cromolyn Therapy

11. J.C. is a 10-year-old girl who recently began experiencing rhinorrhea and sneezing when visiting her father in another state a couple of times each year. On questioning, J.C.'s mother reveals that, although J.C. has not complained of symptoms previously, her father adopted a puppy from the local animal shelter about a year ago and the symptoms correspond to the times that the child spends with the dog. J.C. will be visiting her father again next month, and she is hoping to purchase something without a prescription to prevent her from "getting sick and missing out on her summer vacation." What options are available to treat J.C.'s intermittent symptoms of allergic rhinitis?

J.C. appears to have mild allergic rhinitis triggered by exposure to animal dander. When it is possible to anticipate symptoms, as in J.C.'s case, initiating prophylactic therapy can help lessen the impact of allergen exposure.[1] J.C. appears to be a good candidate for treatment with intranasal corticosteroids or cromolyn sodium, administered regularly beginning several weeks before each trip. Because the mother indicates that she wants to select an OTC product, allergen avoidance strategies plus cromolyn nasal spray would be a reasonable choice for initial therapy. The drawbacks to this are its out-of-pocket cost, its technique-dependent administration, its multiple daily dosing requirements (up to six times daily), and its reduced effectiveness compared with other treatments.[40]

12. What strategies should J.C.'s father use to minimize exposure to the allergic triggers?

To minimize J.C.'s exposure to allergens, the dog should be kept out of the child's bedroom at all times and, when possible, kept outside or confined to an uncarpeted area of the home. J.C.'s father should use a high-quality air filter and should vacuum the home with a double-filter system while J.C. is out of the house. Although evidence is unclear on this topic, it may be helpful to wash the dog weekly while the child visits. The additional expense of regular, commercial cleaning of air ducts is not cost justified.[1]

Instructions for Use

13. How should J.C. be advised to use cromolyn nasal spray to prevent her symptoms?

To be effective, cromolyn nasal spray must be dosed several times each day, which can have a detrimental effect on adherence.[46] The initial dose for the 4% cromolyn sodium nasal spray is one spray in each nostril four to six times daily. In some patients, symptom control can be maintained with dosing two to three times per day. J.C. should be instructed to begin therapy at least two weeks before her planned visit because of the delay in the onset of action for this agent.

The clinician should ensure that both parent and child can demonstrate appropriate administration technique before therapy is initiated. On first use, the device should be primed until a consistent spray is achieved. J.C. should be instructed to gently blow her nose and then spray the cromolyn sodium solution into each nostril in a slightly upward direction, parallel to the nasal septum.

Topical nasal cromolyn has an excellent safety profile, including minimal incidence of adverse effects. Local irritation occurs in <10% of patients, with burning, stinging, and sneezing being the most common manifestations. The safety of cromolyn has made it a popular choice as initial therapy for children with allergic rhinitis and for treating rhinitis during pregnancy.[63] Table 24-5 includes information about intranasal cromolyn dosing and availability.

Intranasal Corticosteroid Therapy

14. A.C. is an 8-year-old boy with allergic rhinitis and asthma. He has been treated with a budesonide Flexhaler for asthma and loratadine for rhinitis. His mother reports that he frequently sneezes, complains of an itchy nose and eyes, and does not sleep well at night because of nasal congestion. She also reports that

Table 24-4 Topical Ophthalmic Medications Commonly Used for Allergic Conjunctivitis

Generic Name (Example Brand Product)	*Available Dosage Forms/Strength*	*Dose*
Antihistamines		
Azelastine (*Optivar*)	Ophthalmic solution: 0.05%	*Adults and children ≥3 yrs:* 1 drop into each affected eye(s) every 12 hrs
Emedastine (*Emadine*)	Ophthalmic solution: 0.05%	*Adults and children ≥3 yrs:* 1 drop in the affected eye(s) up to 4 times daily
Antihistamine/Decongestant Combinations		
Antazoline + Naphazoline (*Vasocon-A*)[a]	Ophthalmic solution: antazoline phosphate 0.5% naphazoline HCl 0.05%	*Adults and children ≥6 yrs:* 1–2 drops in the affected eye(s) every 6 hrs for up to 3 days
Pheniramine + Naphazoline (*Naphcon-A*)[a]	Ophthalmic solution: naphazoline HCl 0.025% pheniramine maleate 0.3%	*Adults and children ≥6 yrs:* 1–2 drops in the affected eye(s) every 6 hrs for up to 3 days
Antihistamine/Mast Cell Stabilizers		
Ketotifen (*Zaditor*)[a]	Ophthalmic solution: 0.025%	*Adults and children ≥3 yrs:* 1 drop in the affected eye(s) every 8–12 hrs
Olopatadine (*Patanol*)	Ophthalmic solution: 0.1%	*Adults and children ≥3 yrs:* 1–2 drops in the affected eye(s) 2 times daily at an interval of 6–8 hrs
Mast Cell Stabilizers		
Cromolyn Sodium (*Crolom*)	Ophthalmic solution: 4%	*Adults and children ≥4 yrs:* 1–2 drops in the affected eye(s) 4–6 times daily
Lodoxamide (*Alomide*)	Ophthalmic solution: 0.1%	*Adults and children ≥2 yrs:* 1–2 drops in affected eye(s) 4 times daily for up to 3 mos
Nedocromil (*Alocril*)	Ophthalmic solution: 2%	*Adults and children ≥3 yrs:* 1–2 drops in the affected eye(s) every 12 hrs
Pemirolast (*Alamast*)	Ophthalmic solution: 0.1%	*Adults and children ≥3 yrs:* 1–2 drops in each affected eye(s) every 6 hrs
Nonsteroidal Anti-Inflammatory Drugs (NSAID)[b]		
Ketorolac (*Acular*)	Ophthalmic solution: 0.5%	*Adults and children ≥3 yrs:* 1 drop into the affected eye(s) 4 times daily.
Corticosteroids		
Loteprednol (*Alrex*)	Ophthalmic suspension 0.2%	*Adults:* 1 drop into the affected eye(s) 4 times daily

[a] Available without a prescription.
[b] Other ophthalmic NSAID (diclofenac, flurbiprofen, suprofen) indicated for intraoperative miosis and for postcataract surgery, but not approved for allergic conjunctivitis.
Adapted from reference 98.

she usually cannot give him loratadine on a daily basis because it makes him drowsy at school. His asthma has been well controlled in the past; however, she is concerned that he is experiencing some shortness of breath and that this might be related to his allergies. While you are talking to him, you note that A.C. breathes exclusively through his mouth, sniffs frequently, and rubs his nose. You also notice dark circles under his eyes. What signs and symptoms of allergic rhinitis is A.C. displaying?

A.C. is displaying the classic signs of allergic airways disease in children. He is sniffing and snorting in response to nasal itching and discharge. The frequent upward rubbing of the nose (generally with the palm of the hand) is known as the "allergic salute" and is caused by nasal itching. Long-standing symptoms can lead to facial abnormalities, including the formation of a transverse crease across the bridge of the nose. Infraorbital discoloration can develop with frequent rubbing of the eyes in patients with severe ocular itching and the resultant dark circles under the eyes are commonly known as "allergic shiners."[32]

Role in Therapy

15. What would be the role of intranasal corticosteroids for this patient?

Intranasal corticosteroids are the most effective therapy available for the treatment of allergic rhinitis. They are safe, well tolerated, and are highly effective in reducing itching, sneezing, rhinorrhea, and congestion.[79] Nasal corticosteroids may also be beneficial in relieving cough associated with postnasal drip in patients with allergic rhinitis.[80] In addition to improving all nasal symptoms, evidence also suggests that intranasal administration of corticosteroids effectively relieves

Table 24-5 Additional Oral and Topical Agents for Rhinitis

Generic (Brand Product)	Available Dosage Forms/Strength	Adult Dose	Pediatric Dose
Oral			
Leukotriene Modifiers Montelukast (*Singulair*)	Tablets: 10 mg Tablets, chewable: 4 mg, 5 mg Oral granules: 4 mg	10 mg once daily	*Children 6–14 yrs:* 5 mg once daily *Children 2–5 yrs:* 4 mg once daily *Children 6–23 mos:* 4 mg once daily
Topical			
Antihistamine Azelastine (*Astelin*)	Nasal spray: 137 mcg/spray	2 sprays/nostril every 12 hrs	*Children 5–11 yrs:* 1 spray/nostril every 12 hrs
Mast cell stabilizer Cromolyn Sodium (*Nasalcrom*)[a]	Nasal spray: 5.2 mg/spray	1 spray/nostril every 4–6 hrs	*Children ≥2 yrs:* 1 spray/nostril every 4–6 hrs
Anticholinergic Ipratropium (*Atrovent*)[b]	Nasal spray: 21 mcg/spray (for perennial symptoms), 42 mcg/spray (for seasonal symptoms)	2 sprays/nostril up to 4 times daily (MAX = 672 mcg/day)	*Children ≥5 yrs:* 2 sprays/nostril up to 4 times daily (MAX = 672 mcg/day)

[a] Available without a prescription

[b] Optimum dosage varies with the response of the individual patient, however; it is always desirable to titrate an individual to the minimum effective dose to reduce the risk of side effects. In addition, the safety and efficacy of the use of ipratropium 42 mcg nasal spray beyond 3 weeks in patients with seasonal allergic rhinitis has not been established.

Adapted from reference 98.

ocular symptoms.[81] These agents also have demonstrated efficacy for nonallergic rhinitis, rhinitis medicamentosa, and nasal polyposis.[22,23] The currently available nasal corticosteroids are listed in Table 24-6.

Intranasal corticosteroids perform well in clinical trials when compared with other therapeutic options. They are frequently rated as more effective than antihistamines, although their effects are technique-dependent.[82,83] In a systematic review of the medical literature performed by the Agency for Healthcare Research and Quality, nasal corticosteroids provided significantly greater relief of symptoms compared with antihistamines for various nasal symptoms and total nasal symptom scores.[84]

Mechanism of Action

16. How do intranasal corticosteroids work to reduce symptoms?

Corticosteroids interact with a specific steroid receptor in the cytoplasm of a cell, and the steroid receptor complex then moves into the cell nucleus where it influences protein synthesis.[85] Among the proteins synthesized is lipocortin,

Table 24-6 Intranasal Corticosteroids[a] Commonly Used for Rhinitis

Generic Name (Example Branded Product)	Available Dosage Forms/Strengths	Adult Dose[a]	Pediatric Dose[a]
Beclomethasone (*Beconase AQ*)	42 mcg/spray	1–2 sprays/nostril twice daily	*Children 6–12 yrs*: 1–2 sprays/nostril twice daily
Budesonide (*Rhinocort Aqua*)	32 mcg/spray	1 spray/nostril once daily (MAX 4 sprays/nostril daily)	*Children 6–12 years:* 1 spray/nostril once daily (MAX 2 sprays/nostril daily)
Fluticasone propionate (*Flonase*)	50 mcg/spray	2 sprays/nostril once daily or 1 spray/nostril twice daily	*Children 4–17 yrs*: 1–2 sprays/nostril once daily
Fluticasone furoate (*Veramyst*)	27.5 mcg/spray	2 sprays/nostril once daily	*Children 2–11 years*: 1–2 sprays/nostril daily
Flunisolide (*Nasarel*)	29 mcg/spray	2 sprays/nostril twice daily (MAX 8 sprays/nostril daily)	*Children 6–14 years:* 1 spray/nostril three times daily or 2 sprays/nostril twice daily (MAX 4 sprays/nostril daily)
Mometasone (*Nasonex*)	50 mcg/spray	2 sprays/nostril once daily	*Children 2–11 yrs:* 1 spray/nostril once daily
Triamcinolone (*Nasacort AQ*)	55 mcg/spray	2 sprays/nostril once daily	*Children 6–11 yrs:* 1–2 sprays/nostril once daily

[a] It is always desirable to titrate an individual patient to the minimum effective steroid dose to reduce the risk of side effects. When the maximum benefit has been achieved and symptoms have been controlled, reducing the steroid dose might be effective in maintaining control of rhinitis symptoms.

Adapted from reference 98.

which inhibits the breakdown of phospholipids to arachidonic acid; this, in turn, inhibits the formation of prostaglandins and leukotrienes. Topical corticosteroids reduce the number of eosinophils, basophils, and mast cells in the nasal mucosa and epithelium; directly inhibit the release of mediators from mast cells and basophils; reduce mucosal edema and vasodilation; stabilize the endothelium and epithelium, resulting in decreased exudation; and reduce the sensitivity of irritant receptors, resulting in decreased itching and sneezing.[33] Topical corticosteroids inhibit both the early- and late-phase reactions to antigen challenge, in contrast to systemic corticosteroids, which inhibit only the late-phase reaction in allergic rhinitis.[86]

17. Are there any specific considerations related to the use of intranasal corticosteroids in treating allergic rhinitis in a patient with concomitant asthma?

Based on the relationship between inflammation in the upper and lower airways, and the similar immunologic mechanisms involved in allergic rhinitis and asthma, it is a reasonable assumption that poor control of upper airway allergies can have a negative impact on asthma control.[87–89] In fact, rhinitis is a risk factor for asthma development,[90] and poorly controlled rhinitis can aggravate asthma control.[91] In a patient with asthma, treatment of allergic rhinitis with nasal corticosteroids can reduce airway hyperresponsiveness and symptoms of asthma.[92]

Historically, the use of antihistamines was considered problematic for patients with asthma because of a theoretic concern about excessive drying of airway secretions caused by the anticholinergic properties of these agents. It is now clear that most patients with asthma can take any of the antihistamines without adverse pulmonary effects.

Choice of Therapeutic Agent

18. What are considerations in selecting among the various nasal corticosteroid products?

Currently marketed intranasal corticosteroid products vary in the pharmacologic characteristics that can influence patient acceptance and adherence; however, there do not appear to be significant advantages with regard to efficacy among them.[93] Topical application is very effective in controlling nasal symptoms with minimal risks of systemic effects.[94] Primary differences among products include potency, dosing regimens, delivery systems, spray volume, and patient preference.[95]

The method to determine potency among topical corticosteroids is to measure topical vasoconstrictive activity on the skin. Cutaneous vasoconstriction may not consistently correlate with anti-inflammatory potency in the nasal mucosa, however.[96] Potency can also be described as a measure of lipophilicity because agents that are highly lipophilic may have faster absorption and longer residence at the receptor in the mucosa. The lipophilicity from highest to lowest among current products is flunisolide, triamcinolone, budesonide, beclomethasone, fluticasone, and mometasone.[96]

The topical-to-systemic potency relationship should also be considered as the ideal agent should exhibit high topical potency and low systemic activity. After topical administration, the corticosteroid may reach the systemic circulation by absorption across the nasal mucosa or through gastrointestinal absorption of the swallowed portion of the dose.[96] Among the available agents, mometasone and fluticasone have the lowest systemic bioavailability, ranging from 0.1% to <2%. Beclomethasone may exert greater systemic effects owing to its metabolism to an active metabolite (beclomethasone 17-monopropionate). For this reason, newer agents are often favored over beclomethasone.[97]

Studies have shown that varying sensory attributes (e.g., taste, smell, aftertaste, throat rundown, nose runout, and feel of spray in nose and throat) affect acceptability of, and preference for, particular nasal corticosteroid products.[93,95] Although more patients rated aftertaste as the most important feature determining their preference,[93] no head-to-head trials have directly compared the available products and, thus, some degree of experimentation may be required in individual patients.

Safety

19. How safe are intranasal corticosteroids in this situation?

The corticosteroids currently available for intranasal administration are listed in Table 24-6. Among available products, intranasal corticosteroids have similar efficacy in clinical trials.[81] Budesonide, flunisolide, triamcinolone, and beclomethasone are indicated for ages 6 years or older. Fluticasone and mometasone are labeled for ages 4 years and older and 2 years and older, respectively.[98]

A common concern regarding the use of corticosteroids in children is the risk of growth suppression. In 1998, the FDA required new labeling on inhaled and intranasal corticosteroid preparations to alert heath care providers that use of these products in children may reduce their rate of growth. Although beclomethasone may be associated with reduced growth velocity,[99] numerous studies have shown no growth delay in children treated long term with newer intranasal steroids.[100–102]

In 2003, the FDA approved revised labeling for fluticasone nasal spray, indicating no adverse effect on growth even with use for up to 1 year. Data are lacking, however, about the potential risk of reduced growth velocity associated with a combination of intranasal and orally inhaled corticosteroids. With this in mind, it is appropriate to recommend agents with low systemic bioavailability and to utilize the lowest effective dose.

Other potential adverse effects of chronic nasal corticosteroids have been investigated. Prolonged topical use of intranasal corticosteroids does not impose a significant risk for mucosal atrophy, histologic changes in nasal mucosa have not been demonstrated, and intranasal candidiasis has never been documented.[103] Although the effects of systemic steroids on the eyes are well-established, nasal steroids have not been shown to increase intraocular pressure.[104] A report from the National Registry of Drug-Induced Ocular Side Effects linked 21 cases of bilateral posterior subcapsular cataracts to the use of intranasal or inhaled corticosteroids[105]; however, several of these patients were also on systemic corticosteroids or had used high-dose beclomethasone for more than 5 years. The risk of cataracts with the newer agents has not been established.[105]

It may be important for the clinician to consider the total corticosteroid load in atopic patients who may be treated with an inhaled or systemic preparation for asthma, intranasal preparation for rhinitis, and dermatologic preparation for eczema, although no guidelines to follow exist in this area. Although nasal steroids are considered safe and are sometimes available without a prescription from pharmacies outside the United States, recently a Joint Taskforce for the American Academy of Allergy, Asthma and Immunology issued a position statement recommending that these agents remain prescription-only and prescribed under the direct supervision of a physician.[106]

Instructions for Use

20. A.C. is given a prescription for budesonide, two actuations in each nostril twice daily. How should he be counseled to use this drug?

Although nasal corticosteroids have an excellent safety profile, some local adverse effects can occur. The currently available products are all aqueous solutions delivered via a manual spray pump; these are much less drying than the original propellant-based aerosol formulations of the same products. The most commonly reported side effect is epistaxis, with excessive nasal dryness and crusting also reported.[32] A more serious concern is the risk for nasal septal perforation. Proper technique in using the nasal corticosteroid products can reduce the risks for these side effects.[1]

Patient education is important to ensure proper use of, and response to, the intranasal corticosteroids. A.C. should be instructed to blow his nose gently before using the nasal inhaler as severe blockage of the nasal passage may prevent deposition of the drug at the intended site of action. If the patient is severely congested, a short course (up to 3 days) of topical decongestant used just before the intranasal corticosteroid may be indicated. The patient should be instructed to direct the spray away from the nasal septum. This is accomplished by pointing the applicator nozzle straight and back using the contralateral hand to ensure application is parallel to the septum.[32]

Therapeutic benefit to nasal steroids is generally appreciated in as few as 2 days, although some newer agents (e.g., budesonide, mometasone, and fluticasone) may begin to relieve symptoms within hours.[81] Fluticasone has been effective when used on an as-needed basis.[42] Nonetheless, it is reasonable to advise patients that full benefit may not be realized for up to 3 weeks.

Systemic Corticosteroids

21. What is the role of systemic corticosteroid therapy for allergic rhinitis?

In contrast to the minimal side effects of the topical corticosteroids, systemic administration of these drugs can cause numerous, and at times serious, side effects. Systemic administration, therefore, must be reserved for only short-term, adjunctive therapy in cases of severe, debilitating rhinitis. In such cases, a short course of relatively high-dose corticosteroid, so-called "burst" therapy, can be administered. Prednisone 40 mg/day for adults or 1 to 2 mg/kg/day for children (or an equivalent dose of a comparable compound) every morning for up to 7 days effectively relieves acute, severe rhinitis symptoms. If A.C. were to have a particularly severe exacerbation of his allergic rhinitis such that it interfered with sleep or ability to attend school, an oral corticosteroid burst would be indicated. More likely, A.C. would require a short course of systemic corticosteroids for an acute asthma exacerbation, but despite the stimulus, short course oral steroids should result in improved nasal symptoms.

Combination Therapy

22. Would there be an advantage in combining various therapies for allergic rhinitis in this patient?

The rationale for combining agents to treat allergic rhinitis is based on the theoretic benefit of additive or synergistic reactions. Various combinations have been studied. Concomitant use of antihistamines and decongestants has been shown to relieve individual nasal symptoms as well as the total symptom score as compared with either agent alone. When combinations of antihistamines and nasal corticosteroids were compared with either agent alone, the combination was superior to antihistamine monotherapy but not to treatment with nasal corticosteroids alone.[107] In one study using an algorithm for treatment, this combination, however, was the standard for severe rhinitis.[108] Studies evaluating the combination of antihistamines and leukotriene modifier therapies have yielded inconsistent results.[109,110] Therefore, it is unclear that the combination is superior to monotherapy with either agent alone and it is likely less effective than treatment with nasal steroids alone.[83] When combination therapy of any kind is used, once symptoms are controlled, one agent should undergo a trial for discontinuation.

Leukotriene-Modifying Agent Therapy

23. K.H. is a 58-year-old man with allergic rhinitis. He has experienced symptoms during ragweed pollen season for several years. He has used various antihistamines for his symptoms during this time with moderate success. At times, K.H. has self-medicated with nonprescription medications, including clemastine and diphenhydramine. This year, he initiated therapy with diphenhydramine 1 week before the pollen season, but began experiencing symptoms of urinary retention after 10 days. His physician advised him that this might be related to the antihistamine aggravating his enlarged prostate and he was given a prescription for fexofenadine. After 1 week, K.H. complains that the medication is not working. After seeing an advertisement on television, he inquires about the use of a leukotriene modifier for his allergic rhinitis. What is the mechanism for the K.H.'s urinary discomfort attributed to the diphenhydramine?

K.H. is exhibiting symptoms of urinary outflow obstruction or prostatism. Common features of this are frequency, hesitancy, slow urine stream, dribbling, and bladder fullness after voiding. The most common cause of obstruction is benign prostatic hyperplasia (BPH). Because the prostate is located anatomically around the urethra, enlargement of the gland can obstruct urine flow.[111]

The bladder and urethra are made up of smooth muscle tissue that is innervated by the sympathetic and parasympathetic divisions of the autonomic nervous system. The detrusor musculature is predominantly innervated by β-adrenergic and cholinergic receptors, whereas the bladder neck (or outlet) is innervated predominately by α-adrenergic receptors. Sympathetic stimulation causes relaxation of the detrusor muscle to allow bladder filling, closure of the urethra, and decreased bladder emptying. Cholinergic stimulation of the detrusor causes contraction of the detrusor to cause bladder emptying. Initially, the detrusor musculature can compensate for the urethral obstruction in BPH. Eventually, however, the detrusor muscle fibers hypertrophy and decompensate, resulting in urinary retention and detrusor hyperreflexia manifesting as urinary frequency, urgency, urge incontinence, and nocturia.[111]

When K.H. took diphenhydramine, the anticholinergic properties of the drug blocked detrusor contraction and precipitated acute urinary retention.[112] In this case, therapy with a SGA (i.e., fexofenadine) is more appropriate because these agents have little to no anticholinergic side effects.

Efficacy

24. What is the rationale and evidence that a leukotriene modifier might be beneficial in this case of allergic rhinitis?

Leukotrienes are important inflammatory mediators in the upper and lower airways and are present in nasal secretions of patients with allergic rhinitis. They serve as inflammatory mediators that result in increased vascular permeability, tissue edema, mucus secretion, and increased eosinophils. These actions lead to the symptoms of allergic rhinitis, as well as those of asthma.[43] In clinical trials, leukotriene modifiers relieve nasal symptoms in patients with allergic rhinitis[44] with similar efficacy to SGA[45] and less efficacy than nasal corticosteroids.[113]

In actual use, the benefit of leukotriene modifiers has been modest; therefore, their role is typically adjunctive to the use of first-line agents for allergic rhinitis.[114] Clinical decisions about the value of combining treatments should be based on the specific clinical situation. Because K.H. has experienced intolerance to first-generation antihistamines and a lack of efficacy with second-generation antihistamines, a trial with a leukotriene-modifying agent is appropriate. Note that a patient with mild asthma and allergic rhinitis may benefit from therapy with a leukotriene modifier with or without an antihistamine. If used, however, a risk exists of a rare complication known as *Churg-Strauss syndrome*, which is characterized by eosinophilia, vasculitic rash, worsening pulmonary symptoms, cardiac complications, and neuropathy.[98] Table 24-5 includes information about the use and availability of montelukast, which is currently the only leukotriene modifier approved for allergic rhinitis.

Complementary and Alternative Therapies

25. C.L., a 25-year-old woman presents in mid-August complaining that her allergies are worsening daily. Symptoms are nasal discharge and obstruction, repetitive sneezing, and itching of the nose, eyes, and throat. She is fatigued and has difficulty concentrating. Her symptoms have been occurring in late spring and summer since high school, and she has used a variety of medications intermittently over the years. C.L. is a competitive runner but has been unable to run as far or as often as usual owing to symptoms. She is also reluctant to use medications as they may be prohibited by her race sponsors. A running partner mentioned that she could control her allergy symptoms with diet, exercise, and herbal remedies purchased at a local nutritional supplement shop. She asks your advice about this. What, if any, alternative treatments have been shown to be efficacious in allergic rhinitis?

Alternative treatments are common among adults with rhinitis and should be taken into account by health care providers. A survey of 300 adults indicated that herbal agents, caffeine-containing products, homeopathy, acupuncture, aromatherapy, reflexology, and massage were common alternative treatments for respiratory conditions.[115] Still, because allergic rhinitis is largely a self-managed disease, it is likely that reported use of these agents is underestimated. For these reasons, patients should always be questioned specifically about the use of alternative therapies during the patient interview. Although some alternative approaches have been deemed to be safe, efficacy for many modalities has not been clearly established.[39] In addition, some complementary therapies have been associated with side effects and potential drug interactions.[116,117]

Some reports have indicated that patients with allergic rhinitis may benefit from hydration and a diet low in sodium, omega-6 fatty acids, and transfatty acids, but high in omega-3 fatty acids (e.g., fish, almonds, walnuts, pumpkin, and flax seeds), and at least five servings of fruits and vegetables per day.[118] These recommendations are not without merit, because they may be beneficial for the population at large, but insufficient evidence exists to support specific value for allergic rhinitis symptoms.

No good clinical data are available on the efficacy of supplements containing vitamin C, grapeseed extract, bee pollen and honey, burdock, ginger, freeze-dried stinging nettle leaves, or quercetin (a bioflavonoid found in apples, buckwheat, grapes, red onions, red wine, and white grapefruit).[39,119] Further studies are needed to assess the efficacy of these supplements and herbs.

Menthol delivered in lozenges and rubs has been shown to have an ameliorating effect on nasal congestion; however, the effects are short-lived.[120] Other forms of aromatherapy suggested to relieve nasal congestion include massaging the essential oils of lavender and niaouli around the sinuses, or inhaling eucalyptus and peppermint oils.[121]

For the motivated patient, mind-body interventions, such as yoga, hypnosis, and biofeedback-assisted relaxation and breathing exercises, are beneficial for stress reduction, in general, which may improve the quality of life associated with rhinitis symptoms and treatment.[116] Acupuncture has been shown to have an attributive effect in inflammatory diseases such as rhinitis; however, not sufficient data are found to recommend this therapy at this time.[122] Although some studies have shown that patients with allergic rhinitis who received homeopathic dilutions of allergens had significantly better nasal air flow than those in the placebo group, overall no difference was seen in subjective measurement on a visual analog scale.[123]

A recent study reported that butterbur extract was as effective as cetirizine for symptoms of hay fever[124]; however, these results have been challenged on methodological concerns.[125] Further investigation is required to determine the role of butterbur extract in the management of rhinitis.[126]

Reports regarding the use of intranasal zinc for upper respiratory symptoms, particularly those associated with the common cold, have been conflicting. Although zinc gels and sprays are popular OTC products, they have been shown to be ineffective in a double-blind, placebo-controlled clinical trial[127] and have been associated in zinc-induced anosmia syndrome, particularly when the products are sniffed deeply.[128]

It has been suggested that herbs that support improved immune function could theoretically also help to ease symptoms of allergy.[129] With this in mind, echinacea has become one of the top-selling herbal products in the United States. Echinacea, however, is closely related to sunflowers, daisies, and ragweed—all members of the Compositae (Asteraceae) family.[130] The possibility that cross-sensitivity between echinacea and other environmental allergens may trigger allergic reactions is supported by an Australian review of all adverse drug reports, including cases of anaphylaxis, associated with echinacea.[131] Patients with known allergy to these plants should be cautioned regarding the use of echinacea products.

Although a variety of alternative remedies are widely available and used frequently in self-treatment, based on evaluation of these data, there is no firm recommendation for C.L. regarding the use of alternative therapies in allergic rhinitis.[39]

Immunotherapy

26. R.C. is a 25-year-old schoolteacher who has experienced allergic symptoms since childhood, but noticed a worsening after she graduated from college and moved to a new area of the country. Although she has mild symptoms year-round, she has severe exacerbations during April through–June and August through October each year. During these periods, she feels that exposure to cut grass and weeds provoke profound nasal symptoms. She also notes that when she spends more time outdoors in spring and early fall, her regular therapy, fluticasone nasal spray, is less effective. She has added loratadine during this time, but is frustrated by having to take so many medications while continuing to experience symptoms. R.C. asks your opinion about allergy shots, remarking that she started them as a child with some relief, but moved after a year and never resumed treatment. Is allergen immunotherapy effective for reducing symptoms of allergic rhinitis?

Efficacy

Allergen-specific immunotherapy has long-term efficacy, induces clinical and immunologic tolerance, and may prevent progression of allergic disease.[132,133] This process usually involves subcutaneous injection (sometimes called "allergy shots") of dilute solutions of allergen extracts to increase tolerance to allergens so that the threshold for symptoms is increased (i.e., subsequent exposure elicits no or mild symptoms).

Immunotherapy administered via SIT has been used empirically since the early 1900s, and its efficacy has been documented in many controlled trials.[134] A meta-analysis of 51 published studies involving 2,871 patients concluded that SIT is effective in the treatment of allergic rhinitis.[47] In addition, studies of immunotherapy for allergic rhinitis in children suggest that immunotherapy may prevent the onset of asthma.[135,136] Taken together, these studies show that SIT should be considered a supplement to drug therapy in specific patients and possibly be used earlier in the course of allergic disease to achieve maximal benefit.[2]

Allergen Testing

27. How can the clinician determine R.C.'s specific sensitivities?

Skin testing using the modified prick test method or a prick-puncture method is used to confirm the diagnosis of allergic rhinitis and to determine specific allergen sensitivities. Skin testing is a highly sensitive and relatively inexpensive objective measurement of allergen sensitivity. Small quantities of allergen are introduced into the skin by pricking or puncturing the skin in the immediate presence of the diluted allergen extract. Fifteen to 35 tests are placed on the upper portion of the back or the palmar surface of the forearms. A positive skin test produces a wheal and flare at the site within 15 to 30 minutes of application. An experienced clinician, usually an allergist, should conduct skin testing using high-quality allergen extracts and should interpret the results.[137]

The allergens tested vary with geographic location, emphasizing the most common offending plant species that generate airborne particles. Pollen, the primary particle, is produced by trees, grasses, and weeds. Each of these plant groups generally pollinate at about the same time each year: trees in the spring, grasses from early to midsummer, and weeds from late summer into fall before the first killing frost. The onset and potency of the pollen season varies with geographic location and weather, particularly with respect to temperature and moisture. Seasonality can be misleading, however, because settled pollen particles from a previous season may be resuspended in the air following the spring snow melt or periods of heavy winds.

Mold spores also are common airborne allergens. The outdoor molds release their spores from early spring through late fall. Within this long season, spore counts increase and decrease, depending on the presence of local flora on which these molds grow (e.g., grain and other crops, forests, and orchards). Some perennial allergens (e.g., house dust mites, insect and animal dander, and some indoor molds) occur consistently across all geographic distributions. In each case, skin test results must be correlated with the patient's clinical history.[132]

R.C.'s perennial symptoms with seasonal exacerbations indicate sensitivity to the common perennial allergens with a particular sensitivity to seasonal allergens such as tree, grass, and weed pollen, but these subjective relationships should be confirmed with skin testing.

An alternative to skin testing is the radioallergosorbent test, in which the patient's serum is tested for allergen-specific IgE antibodies. However, this test is less sensitive and more expensive than skin testing.[138] It is indicated only in selected clinical situations: when a patient consistently reacts positively to the negative control skin test (dermatographism), when antihistamine therapy cannot be discontinued, or when the patient has extensive atopic dermatitis or other skin lesions. Blood eosinophil counts and total serum IgE antibody measurements are neither sensitive nor sufficiently specific to be useful in the diagnosis of allergic rhinitis.[1]

28. Because R.C. is currently using medications (fluticasone nasal spray and loratadine) for her symptoms, should these be discontinued before skin testing?

Antihistamines blunt the wheal-and-flare reaction by blocking the effects of histamine on capillaries. Different antihistamines vary in the extent to which they can inhibit wheal formation and in the duration of the inhibitory effect (Table 24-7). Depending on the agent selected, antihistamines must be discontinued from 24 hours to 10 days before skin testing and even then, considerable interpatient variability exists in blocking effects.[139] For best results, R.C.'s loratadine should be discontinued 10 days before her skin testing.

Other allergy medications, including cromolyn and nasal corticosteroids, have no effect on skin tests. Likewise, most asthma medications, including leukotriene modifiers, inhaled β_2-agonists, cromolyn, theophylline, and inhaled and

Table 24-7 Effects of Antihistamines on Allergen Skin Tests

Drug	Extent of Suppression[a]	Half-life (hr)[b]	Duration of Suppression (day)
Brompheniramine	+	24.9	1–4
Cetirizine	+++	7.4–11 (7)	3–10
Chlorpheniramine	+	24.4 (11)	1–4
Clemastine	++	21.3	1–10
Cyproheptadine	+/–	16	1–4
Desloratadine	+/++	27 (27)	3–10
Diphenhydramine	+/–	4–9	1–4
Fexofenadine	++	14 (18)	3–10
Hydroxyzine	++	20 (7.1)	1–10
Loratadine	+/++	11–24 (3.1)	3–10
Promethazine	+	12	1–4

[a]+++, extensive; ++ moderate; +, mild; +/– minimal to none, – unknown.
[b]Parenthetical numbers indicate half-life in children.
Adapted from references 1, 98, 140.

short-course systemic (burst) corticosteroids have no effect on skin tests.[137,140,141] R.C. can continue the use of fluticasone nasal spray while she waits to be skin tested.

Oral β_2-agonists, long-term systemic corticosteroids, and high-potency topical corticosteroids (applied to the skin testing sites) may block cutaneous wheal-and-flare reactions. Tricyclic antidepressants are potent inhibitors of the wheal-and-flare reaction, and their effects can last up to 10 days. Phenothiazine-type antipsychotics and antiemetics (e.g., chlorpromazine, prochlorperazine) also can block cutaneous reactions to allergens. β_2-blockers can increase skin reactivity.[137] Depending on the indication for drug therapy, however, discontinuation of these drugs before skin testing is not always advisable. Recommendations for discontinuing antihistamines before allergen skin testing are listed in Table 24-8.

29. Is R.C. a candidate for immunotherapy injections?

Immunotherapy via SIT is indicated for patients with evidence of sustained, clinically relevant IgE-mediated disease and a limited spectrum of allergies (i.e., one or two clinically relevant allergens) and in whom pharmacotherapy and avoidance measures are insufficient.[142] Further considerations are the patient's attitude to available treatment modalities, costs of treatment, and the quality of allergen vaccines available for treatment.[132] In the case of R.C., she has year-round symptoms with seasonal exacerbations, she has not experienced symptom relief when using appropriate therapies, and she is motivated to try immunotherapy. In addition, a previous trial in childhood was beneficial. For these reasons, skin testing and a trial of immunotherapy with specific allergens are reasonable.

Other Forms

30. Are there alternatives to injectable delivery of immunotherapy?

Traditional subcutaneous immunotherapy presents some disadvantages, such as costs, adherence, and rare systemic reactions. Because regular injections can be unacceptable to some patients, alternative methods of delivering antigens, such as SLIT and NIT, have been investigated.[143–145] A recent review of sublingual therapy for allergic rhinitis determined that SLIT is a safe treatment that significantly reduces symptoms and medication requirements in allergic rhinitis.[48] Less evidence is found about the efficacy of NIT, but a recent multicenter trial in children suggests improvement in nasal symptom scores as compared with placebo.[145] Neither SLIT nor NIT is currently available in the United States and, although both have shown potential, SIT is still optimal in severe allergic rhinitis with signs of bronchial hyperreactivity.[47]

Length of Therapy

31. If R.C. decides to proceed with immunotherapy, how long should her therapy continue and how long will the effects last?

After identifying the offending allergens via skin testing, subcutaneous immunotherapy is generally administered in two phases. During the build-up phase, increasing doses of allergen are given once or twice a week until a predetermined target or maintenance dose is achieved. This usually takes 3 to 4 months (e.g., 16–18 injections). Once this maintenance dose is reached, shots are usually administered every 2 to

Table 24-8 General Recommendations for Discontinuation of Antihistamines before Allergen Skin Testing

1. Remind patient that allergic symptoms may return during the antihistamine-free period, but that reliable skin tests cannot be performed in a patient taking antihistamines.
2. Discontinue any short-acting antihistamine (i.e., those in Table 24-7 with a duration of suppression ≤4 days) 4 days before skin testing.
3. Discontinue longer-acting antihistamines (i.e., those in Table 24-7 with a duration of suppression >4 days) at an interval appropriate to their duration of effect (e.g., hydroxyzine should be discontinued 10 days before skin testing)
4. Before applying the full battery of skin tests, apply histamine (positive) control and glycerinated diluent (negative) control tests. Application of a 1 mg/mL histamine base equivalent should yield wheal-and-flare diameters of 2–7 mm and 4.5–32.5 mm, respectively, to be considered a normal histamine reaction. A normal cutaneous reaction to histamine control suggests that accurate skin testing can be performed.

Adapted from reference 140.

3 weeks over the ensuing several years of treatment. Clinical improvement with immunotherapy usually occurs in the first year. In a small percentage of patients, there is no improvement and immunotherapy is discontinued. If symptoms are reduced, however, injections are usually continued for 4 to 5 years of maintenance therapy.[132]

Although immunotherapy can lead to long-term remission of symptoms, one drawback is the lengthy treatment period. Preliminary data involving a 2-year study of 19 patients allergic to ragweed who underwent one allergy shot per week for 6 weeks before the ragweed season suggest that significant relief can be obtained from a shorter term of treatment.[144] SIT alters the natural course of disease and evidence suggests that efficacy persists long after therapy ends.[146]

Risks

32. What are the risks associated with immunotherapy?

Local adverse reactions (i.e., redness, swelling) to immunotherapy can be common, but the risk of severe reaction (i.e., anaphylaxis) is low. A new classification system for grading systemic reactions has been proposed, which categorizes these into immediate (occurring within 30 minutes) and late (developing after 30 minutes).[132] In addition, pretreatment with antihistamines during immunotherapy induction has been shown to reduce the incidence of such adverse events. In view of the occasional occurrence of systemic side effects following injections, it is important that SIT be performed by personnel who are fully trained and experienced in the early recognition and treatment of such reactions.[47]

DRUG-INDUCED NASAL CONGESTION

33. L.K. is a 27-year-old man who has suffered intermittent symptoms of allergic rhinitis. He reports that his symptoms are most bothersome in the spring and associated with blooming of various grasses. During these periods, he typically uses chlorpheniramine, which relieves his symptoms adequately. This season, he reports that his symptoms have been more severe, with sneezing, runny nose, and extreme itching in his nose. He has tried chlorpheniramine and recently switched to loratadine, with partial relief of symptoms. He also states that nasal congestion has been more of an issue with this episode and to address this he has used xylometazoline nasal spray for the past 3 weeks. Despite increasing the use of nasal spray from two to four times a day, however, he reports that the congestion is getting worse. What might be an explanation for L.K.'s increasing need for nasal decongestant?

L.K. may be experiencing rhinitis medicamentosa (RM) or rebound congestion, a condition characterized by nasal congestion without rhinorrhea, postnasal drip, or sneezing and is associated with overuse of topical nasal decongestants.[22] For this reason, topical decongestant therapy should be limited to no more than 10 days, but because the time course can vary among patients, preferably fewer than 5 days.[147]

Etiology

34. Why does rhinitis medicamentosa occur?

Sympathomimetic, or adrenergic, agents stimulate α-adrenergic receptors on blood vessels, resulting in vasoconstriction. In the nasal mucosa, the therapeutic effect is relief of nasal congestion associated with edematous, congested blood vessels as a result of the allergic response. Rhinitis medicamentosa occurs as a result of a rebound phenomenon where the vessels in the nasal mucosa become more engorged and edematous as a result of overstimulation of α-adrenergic receptors.[148] As a result, patients use the decongestant more frequently and may increase the dose for relief, creating a vicious cycle. This problem is commonly reported with topical decongestants, but is uncommon with oral agents. Note that topical decongestants should never be used in infants younger than 6 months of age because they are obligate nose breathers and the resulting rebound congestion could cause obstructive apnea.

The precise mechanism of rhinitis medicamentosa is unknown, but theories suggest it may be secondary to the decreased production of endogenous sympathetic norepinephrine through a negative feedback mechanism. With prolonged use or following discontinuation of topical decongestants, the sympathetic nerves may be unable to maintain vasocontriction because norepinephrine release is suppressed.[147] It has also been suggested that benzalkonium chloride (BKC), used in topical decongestant products as a preservative, worsens rhinitis medicamentosa; therefore, some authors recommend using BKC-free products, even though no evidence exists of worsening congestion in subjects who use nasal glucocorticoids containing BKC.[22] In addition to rhinitis medicamentosa, systemic medications and some drugs of abuse can cause nasal congestion or other nasal symptoms.[22] Table 24-9 lists drugs capable of causing rhinitis symptoms.

Strategies for Resolution

35. What are possible strategies to recommend to L.K. to address this problem?

The best strategy for managing rhinitis medicamentosa is prevention, but when that fails, several options for treatment exist.[147] Patients must be educated about the effects and potential complications of topical decongestants whenever they are prescribed or purchased without a prescription. Ideally, topical decongestant use should be limited to fewer than 5 days. If longer treatment is required, the patient should take a 1- to 2-day holiday during which the topical agent is not used before resuming treatment.

In any case of drug-induced nasal congestion, the most important intervention is to discontinue the offending agent and, if necessary, substitute another therapy that will not cause nasal symptoms.[22] In the case of topical decongestants, discontinuation of the nasal spray can be difficult for the patient and presents the clinician with a therapeutic challenge. It also is important to appropriately treat the underlying cause of the nasal congestion that led to the overuse of the topical decongestant.

A simple strategy is to discontinue the topical decongestant spray. This can be done abruptly, but is likely to cause the patient considerable discomfort for the first 4 to 7 days after discontinuation.[147] There are also strategies to ameliorate the uncomfortable symptoms for the patient. The use of saline

Table 24-9 Drugs Capable of Causing Nasal Symptoms

Antihypertensives
Amiloride
Angiotensin converting enzyme (ACE) inhibitor class
β-blocker class
Chlorothiazide
Clonidine
Doxazosin
Guanethidine
Hydralazine
Hydrochlorothiazide
Methyldopa
Phentolamine
Prazosin
Reserpine
Phosphodiesterase type 5 inhibitors
Sildenafil
Tadalafil
Vardenafil
Hormonal products
Estrogens
Oral contraceptives
Pain relievers
Aspirin
Nonsteroidal anti-inflammatory drugs (NSAIDs)
Neuropsychotherapeutic agents
Alprazolam
Amitriptyline
Chlordiazepoxide
Gabapentin
Risperidone
Perphenazine
Thioridazine

Adapted from references 21, 22.

nose drops or spray can moisturize and alleviate nasal irritation. Intranasal corticosteroids often help decrease the tissue inflammation associated with rhinitis medicamentosa and can help patients in the immediate period after discontinuing the topical decongestant. Oral decongestants can also be used for the recovery period. In refractory cases, a short course of systemic corticosteroids may be necessary.[22] Note that if the patient has used the topical decongestant continuously for many months or even years, the nasal mucosa can be damaged irreversibly.

An alternative to abrupt cessation of the topical decongestant is to recommend that the patient discontinue use of the topical decongestant one nostril at a time. In this case, the patient can continue using the topical agent in one nostril while waiting for resolution of the condition in the other nostril. When the drug is withdrawn completely from one nostril, begin decreasing the amount of drug used in the other nostril. For example, have the patient substitute normal saline nasal spray for decongestant spray in the right nostril every other dose. Later, use saline twice for each decongestant dose. Eventually, the decongestant is discontinued totally in the right nostril and saline is substituted. Repeat the process for the left nostril. Saline can be used as often as needed throughout this process and after the topical decongestant is completely withdrawn. This method has been suggested in several reviews, although no prospective trial results are available to support it.[22] Thus, this method should be combined with careful patient education, support, and frequent follow-up.

IDIOPATHIC RHINITIS

36. M.S., a 29-year-old man, complains of profuse watery rhinorrhea that has been a chronic and progressively worsening problem for the past 5 years. He also experiences some nasal congestion with the rhinorrhea, but denies nasal itching or sneezing. Although the symptoms tend to remit and exacerbate, they do not occur in any definable seasonal pattern. His symptoms are worsened by exposure to tobacco smoke, strong fumes such as paint or ammonia, and hot coffee, and they often are associated with headaches. Also, the rhinorrhea is substantially worse on exposure to cold air. M.S. has no other medical problems and no family history for allergies. He does not smoke and drinks only occasionally. His only medication, beclomethasone dipropionate (42 mcg/spray), two sprays in each nostril twice daily as needed, only partially relieves the symptoms. M.S. sniffs and blows his nose several times during the medical history taking. Physical examination reveals a mildly erythematous nasal mucosa and a minimally edematous inferior turbinate. Copious nasal discharge is clear and watery and air movement through the nose is relatively good. There is no sinus tenderness. The remainder of his physical examination is normal. Microscopic examination of a nasal smear demonstrates only a few neutrophils and no eosinophils. What information about M.S. supports the diagnosis of idiopathic rhinitis?

Diagnosis

Idiopathic rhinitis is a diagnosis of exclusion encompassing those patients with nasal mucous membrane inflammation with no proved immunologic, microbiologic, pharmacologic, hormonal, or occupational cause.[23] The syndrome is sometimes called "vasomotor rhinitis," but using this terminology can be confusing because the cause of the symptoms has still not been clearly identified.[1,19] The prevailing theory holds that an imbalance in the autonomic nervous system exists in which the cholinergic parasympathetic activity exceeds the α-adrenergic activity in the nasal mucosa.[23] Theoretically, this is the reason that stimuli that normally increase parasympathetic activity in the nose, such as cold air and inhaled irritants, aggravate symptoms.[149] Still, substantial debate exists over whether idiopathic rhinitis represents a *localized* allergic response in the absence of systemic atopic markers[150] as well as the evidence for inflammatory pathophysiology in the disease.[151]

The symptoms of idiopathic rhinitis are variable. Most patients experience perennial nasal obstruction accompanied by profuse, watery nasal and postnasal discharge. Many patients complain of nasal obstruction as the primary symptom, whereas for others it is rhinorrhea. Sneezing is usually not a prominent symptom and nasal itching is uncommon.[1,19,23] Headache may occur and usually is frontal or localized over the bridge of the nose. In patients with chronic nasal obstruction, chronic sinusitis and significant morbidity can result. In contrast to allergic rhinitis, the onset of symptoms in patients with idiopathic rhinitis usually occurs in adulthood, but before 40 years of age.[19]

Patients report worsening of their symptoms when exposed to nonspecific irritants, including tobacco smoke, industrial pollutants, strong odors and perfumes, newsprint, chemical fumes; cold, dry air; changes in humidity; and ingestion of very cold or very hot beverages or spicy foods. Most patients have no history or evidence of atopy.[19]

The appearance of the nasal mucosa also is variable. The turbinates are usually erythematous and, during an exacerbation, considerable quantities of nasal secretions usually are present. Mast cells may be present in the nasal smear; however, by definition, nasal eosinophilia is not present. Skin tests are usually negative.[23]

37. M.S.'s symptoms of bothersome watery rhinorrhea, nasal congestion, and headache without itching or sneezing are typical. His complaint of worsening symptoms with exposure to noxious inhalants, cold air, and hot beverages supports the diagnosis of idiopathic rhinitis. The nasal smear, which notably lacks large numbers of eosinophils, initially differentiates this disease from NARES. M.S. asks what causes idiopathic rhinitis and what can be done to alleviate his symptoms. What are the available nonpharmacologic and pharmacologic treatments for idiopathic rhinitis?

Choice of Therapeutic Agent

Nasal symptoms in patients with idiopathic rhinitis have been shown to be influenced by psychological factors. Some therapeutic benefit may be realized by establishing an ongoing, trusting relationship between the health care provider and the patient. This should include a thorough explanation of the disease state and the realistic outcomes of therapy for most patients. Psychotherapy is helpful in some cases. In addition, patients should be instructed to avoid as many aggravating factors as possible, such as smoking, exposure to smoke or other irritants, and very cold or very hot beverages. Saline irrigation is valuable as a general soothing and moisturizing treatment. Exercise may be particularly helpful for patients with idiopathic rhinitis because it increases sympathetic tone.[23]

Pharmacotherapy for idiopathic rhinitis should be directed toward the predominant symptoms of the individual patient.[23] For patients with predominant nasal congestion and minimal rhinorrhea, the intranasal corticosteroids may be helpful. The addition of oral decongestants may improve nasal obstruction in some patients with idiopathic rhinitis, but objective measures of improvement are affected variably and side effects can be problematic.

M.S.'s case is typical of the often frustrating course in treating idiopathic rhinitis.[23] Commonly, multiple therapeutic plans fail, and M.S. has responded incompletely and unsatisfactorily to intranasal corticosteroids. Surgical treatments have been attempted for patients in whom medical management fails, although recent clinical evidence is limited primarily to case reports.[152]

In patients such as M.S., who have rhinorrhea as their predominant symptom, nasal ipratropium bromide, a topically active congener of atropine, may decrease nasal secretions.[23] Also, FGA may be helpful because of their anticholinergic drying effects. In general, however, FGA are less effective in the treatment of idiopathic rhinitis than for allergic rhinitis, and patients may have difficulty complying with therapy because of side effects. Of note, the nonsedating SGA have little value in idiopathic rhinitis because they lack anticholinergic properties.

38. How does ipratropium bromide work for idiopathic rhinitis and how effective is it?

Ipratropium bromide's quaternary ammonium structure makes it lipophobic; therefore, it is absorbed poorly from the nasal mucosa and gastrointestinal tract and does not cross the blood–brain barrier. It significantly reduces rhinorrhea (as measured by the number of nose-blowing episodes or daily number of tissues used), but has no effect on sneezing or nasal obstruction.[153]

The recommended dose of ipratropium bromide is two sprays of the 0.03% nasal solution (42 mcg) in each nostril two to three times per day, but dosage individualization (from 168 to 1,600 mcg/ day) is often required to achieve symptomatic relief.[98] A 0.06% nasal formulation is also available, but its use is typically reserved for short-term treatment of common cold symptoms. Table 24-5 includes information about intranasal ipratropium dosing and availability.

In general, intranasal ipratropium bromide is well tolerated, although its use is associated with dose-related side effects.[1] The most common side effects are nasal dryness, nasal burning, bloody nasal discharge (epistaxis), dry or sore throat, and dry mouth.[1] Theoretically, elderly men with BPH may experience difficulty in urinating, but the risk is low because of negligible systemic absorption. No significant adverse cardiovascular or blood pressure effects have been observed.

CONCLUSIONS

The initial management of acute and chronic rhinitis should be directed at preventing symptoms, which can be achieved through a variety of pharmacologic and nonpharmacologic methods. Plans for allergic rhinitis, the most common form, should include patient education, allergen or irritant avoidance and the appropriate medications, including immunotherapy, if indicated. Control of the disease process is the expected outcome—in which patients are able to live their lives comfortably without symptoms or impairment. Customizing therapy for each patient based on symptom history and response to treatments is important. Rhinitis can be controlled and effective management can greatly improve the quality of patients' lives.

ACKNOWLEDGMENTS

The authors acknowledge the assistance of Bridget Audu, Emily Brouwer, Andreia Bruno and Fatima Jeragh Alhaddad in the preparation of this chapter.

REFERENCES

1. Dykewicz MS et al. Diagnosis and management of rhinitis: complete guidelines of the Joint Task Force on Practice Parameters in Allergy, Asthma and Immunology. American Academy of Allergy, Asthma, and Immunology. *Ann Allergy Asthma Immunol* 1998;81(5 Pt 2):478.
2. van Cauwenberge P et al. Consensus statement on the treatment of allergic rhinitis. European Academy of Allergology and Clinical Immunology. *Allergy* 2000;55:116.
3. Vinuya RZ. Upper airway disorders and asthma: a syndrome of airway inflammation. *Ann Allergy Asthma Immunol* 2002;88(4 Suppl 1):8.
4. Bousquet J et al. Allergic rhinitis and its impact on asthma. *J Allergy Clin Immunol* 2001;108(5 Suppl):S147.
5. ARIA in the pharmacy: management of allergic rhinitis symptoms in the pharmacy. Allergic rhinitis and its impact on asthma. *Allergy* 2004;59: 373.
6. Bousquet J et al. Allergic rhinitis and its impact on asthma (ARIA) 2008 update (in collaboration with the World Health Organization, GA(2)LEN and AllerGen). *Allergy* 2008;63(Suppl 86):8
7. Summary of health statistics for U.S. adults: National Health Interview Survey, 2005. http://www.cdc.gov/nchs/fastats/allergies.htm. Accessed August 3, 2007.
8. ALTANA Pharma U.S., Inc. Allergies in America Executive Summary. March 1, 2006.
9. Leger D, et al. Allergic rhinitis and its consequences on the quality of sleep: an unexplored area. *Arch Intern Med* 2006;166:1744.
10. Verlato G et al. Is the prevalence of adult asthma and allergic rhinitis still increasing? Results of an Italian study. *J Allergy Clin Immunol* 2003; 111:1232.
11. Arbes SJ et al. Prevalences of positive skin test results to 10 common allergens in the U.S. population: Results of the Third National Health and Nutrition Examination Survey. *J Asthma Clinical Immunol* 2005;116:377.
12. *Management of Allergic Rhinitis in the Working Age Populations, Evidence Report/Technology Assessment*, Number 67 AHRQ No 03-E013, January 2003.
13. Blaiss MS. Allergic rhinitis and its impairment issues in schoolchildren: a consensus report. *Curr Med Res Opin* 2004;20:1937.
14. Reed SD et al. The economic burden of allergic rhinitis: a critical evaluation of the literature. *Pharmacoeconomics* 2004;22:345.
15. Schoenwetter WF et al. Economic impact and quality of life burden of allergic rhinitis. *Curr Med Res Opin* 2004;20:305.
16. Ricketti AJ. Allergic rhinitis. In: Grammer LC, et al., eds. *Patterson's Allergic Diseases*. Philadelphia: Lippincott Williams & Wilkins, 2002:159.
17. Van Cauwenberge P et al. Anatomy and physiology of the nose and the paranasal sinuses. *Immunol Allergy Clin North Am* 2004 Feb;24:1.
18. Dykewicz MS. Rhinitis and sinusitis. *J Allergy Clin Immunol* 2003;111(2 Suppl):S520.
19. Quillen DM et al. Diagnosing rhinitis: allergic vs. nonallergic. *Am Fam Physician* 2006;73:1583.
20. Ellegard EK. Clinical and pathogenetic characteristics of pregnancy rhinitis. *Clin Rev Allergy Immunol* 2004;26:149.
21. Basu A et al. New treatment options for erectile dysfunction in patients with diabetes mellitus. *Drugs* 2004;64:2667.
22. Ramey JT et al. Rhinitis medicamentosa. *J Investig Allergol Clin Immunol* 2006;16:148.
23. van Rijswijk JB et al. Idiopathic rhinitis, the ongoing quest. *Allergy* 2005;60:1471.
24. Finkelman FD et al. Advances in asthma, allergy mechanisms, and genetics in 2006. *J Allergy Clin Immunol* July 2, 2007. E-pub ahead of print.
25. Marogna M, et al. The type of sensitizing allergen can affect the evolution of respiratory allergy. *Allergy* 2006;611209.
26. Braback L et al. Social class in asthma and allergic rhinitis: a national cohort study over three decades. *Eur Respir J* 2005;26:1064.
27. Bach JF. Six questions about the hygiene hypothesis. *Cell Immunol* 2005;233:158.
28. Rosenwasser L. New insights into the pathophysiology of allergic rhinitis. *Allergy Asthma Proc* 2007;28:10.
29. Theoharides TC et al. Differential release of mast cell mediators and the pathogenesis of inflammation. *Immunol Rev* 2007;217:65.
30. Parsons ME et al. Histamine and its receptors. *Br J Pharmacol* 2006;147(Suppl 1):S127.
31. Kim D et al. Neural aspects of allergic rhinitis. *Curr Opin Otolaryngol Head Neck Surg* 2007; 15:268.
32. Lehman JM et al. Office-based management of allergic rhinitis in adults. *Am J Med* 2007;120:659.
33. Demoly P et al. In vivo methods for study of allergy. In: Adkinson NF Jr et al, eds. *Middleton's Allergy: Principles and Practice.* Philadelphia: Mosby;2003:631.
34. Plaut M et al. Allergic rhinitis. *N Engl J Med* 2005;353;1934.
35. Prenner BM et al. Allergic rhinitis: treatment based on patient profiles. *Am J Med* 2006;119:230.
36. Bousquet J et al. A critical appraisal of 'evidence-based medicine' in allergy and asthma. *Allergy* 2004;59(Suppl 78):12.
37. Custovic A et al. The effectiveness of measures to change the indoor environment in the treatment of allergic rhinitis and asthma. ARIA update (in collaboration with GA(1)LEN). *Allergy* 2005;60:1112.
38. Price D et al. International Primary Care Respiratory Group (IPCRG) Guidelines: management of allergic rhinitis. *Primary Care Respiratory Journal* 2006;15:58.
39. Passalacqua G et al. ARIA Update: I. Systematic review of complementary and alternative medicine for rhinitis and asthma. *J Allergy Clin Immunol* 2006;117:1054.
40. Lange B et al. Efficacy, cost-effectiveness and tolerability of mometasone furoate, levocabastine and disodium cromoglycate nasal sprays in the treatment of seasonal allergic rhinitis. *Ann Allergy Asthma Immunol* 2005;95:272.
41. Sullivan PW et al. Cost-benefit analysis of first generation antihistamines in the treatment of allergic rhinitis. *Pharmacoeconomics* 2004;22:929.
42. Dykewicz MS et al. Fluticasone propionate aqueous nasal spray improves nasal symptoms of seasonal allergic rhinitis when used as needed (prn). *Ann Allergy Asthma Immunol* 2003;91:44.
43. Scow DT et al. Leukotriene inhibitors in the treatment of allergy and asthma. *Am Fam Physician* 2007;75:65.
44. Wilson AM et al. Leukotriene receptor antagonists for allergic rhinitis: a systematic review and meta-analysis. *Am J Med* 2004;116:338.
45. Rodrigo GJ et al. The role of antileukotriene therapy in seasonal allergic rhinitis: a systematic review of randomized trials. *Ann Allergy Asthma Immunol* 2006;96:779.
46. Meltzer EO. Efficacy and patient satisfaction with cromolyn sodium nasal solution in the treatment of seasonal allergic rhinitis: a placebo-controlled study. *Clin Ther* 2002;24:942.
47. Calderon MA et al. Allergen injection immunotherapy for seasonal allergic rhinitis [Review]. *Cochrane Database Syst Rev* 2007 Jan 24; CD001936.
48. Wilson DR et al. Sublingual immunotherapy for allergic rhinitis: systematic review and meta analysis. *Allergy* 2005;60:4.
49. Chervinsky P et al. Omalizumab, an anti-IgE antibody, in the treatment of adults and adolescents with perennial allergic rhinitis. *Ann Allergy Asthma Immunol* 2003;91:160.
50. Press release, FDA. FDA Alert: FDA Proposes to Strengthen Label Warning for Xolair. February 21, 2007. Accessed November 25, 2007 via the web at http://www.fda.gov/bbs/topics/NEWS/2007/NEW01567.html
51. Koreck AI et al. Rhinophototherapy: a new therapeutic tool for the management of allergic rhinitis. *J Allergy Clin Immunol* 2005;115:541.
52. Schmidt LM et al. Of mites and men: reference bias in narrative review articles: a systematics review. *J Fam Pract* 2005;54:334.
53. Marinho S et al. Allergen avoidance in the secondary and tertiary prevention of allergic diseases: does it work? *Primary Care Respiratory Journal* 2006;15:152.
54. Terreehorst I et al. Evaluation of impermeable covers for bedding in patients with allergic rhinitis. *N Engl J Med* 2003;349:237.
55. Bousquet J et al. Requirement for medications commonly used in the treatment of allergic rhinitis. European Academy of Allergy and Clinical Immunology (EAACI), Allergic Rhinitis and Its Impact on Asthma (ARIA). *Allergy* 2003;58:192.
56. Greiner AN et al. Pharmacologic rationale for treating allergic and nonallergic rhinitis. *J Allergy Clin Immunol* 2006;118:985.
57. Holgate ST et al. Consensus group on new generation antihistamines (CONGA): present status and recommendations. *Clin Exp Allergy* 2003;33:1305.
58. Camelo-Nunes IC. New antihistamines: a critical review. *J Pediatr (Rio J)* 2006;82(5 Suppl):S173.
59. Leurs R et al. H1-antihistamines: inverse agonism, anti-inflammatory actions and cardiac effects. *Clin Exp Allergy* 2002;32:489.
60. Passalacqua G et al. Structure and classification of H1-antihistamines and overview of their activities. *Clin Allergy Immunol* 2002;17:65.
61. Casale TB et al. First do no harm: managing antihistamine impairment in patients with allergic rhinitis. *J Allergy Clin Immunol* 2003;111:S835.
62. Bender BG et al. Sedation and performance impairment of diphenhydramine and second-generation antihistamines: a meta-analysis. *J Allergy Clin Immunol* 2003;111:770.
63. Blaiss MS; Food and Drug Administration (U.S.); ACAAI-ACOG (American College of Allergy, Asthma, and Immunology and American College of Obstetricians and Gynecologists.). Management of rhinitis and asthma in pregnancy. *Ann Allergy Asthma Immunol* 2003;90(6 Suppl 3):16.
64. Lehman JM et al. Selecting the optimal oral antihistamine for patients with allergic rhinitis. *Drugs* 2006;66:2309.
65. Limon L et al. Desloratadine: a nonsedating antihistamine. *Ann Pharmacother* 2003;37:237; quiz 313.
66. Corren J et al. Effectiveness of azelastine nasal spray compared with oral cetirizine in patients with seasonal allergic rhinitis. *Clin Ther* 2005;27: 543.
67. Lee TA et al. Meta-analysis of azelastine nasal spray for the treatment of allergic rhinitis. *Pharmacotherapy* 2007;27:852.
68. LaForce CF et al. Efficacy of azelastine nasal spray in seasonal allergic rhinitis patients who remain symptomatic after treatment with fexofenadine. *Ann Allergy Asthma Immunol* 2004;93:154.
69. Canonica GW et al. Topical azelastine in perennial allergic conjunctivitis. *Curr Med Res Opin* 2003;19:321.
70. Lieberman PL et al. Azelastine nasal spray: a review of pharmacology and clinical efficacy in allergic and nonallergic rhinitis. *Allergy Asthma Proc* 2003;24:95.
71. Hatton RC et al. Efficacy and safety of oral phenylephrine: systematic review and meta-analysis. *Ann Pharmacother* 2007;41: 381.
72. Salerno SM et al. Effect of oral pseudoephedrine on blood pressure and heart rate: a meta-analysis. *Arch Intern Med* 2005;165:1686.
73. Abelson MB et al. Ocular allergic disease: mechanisms, disease sub-types, treatment. *Ocul Surf* 2003;1:127.

74. Bielory L et al. Efficacy and tolerability of newer antihistamines in the treatment of allergic conjunctivitis. *Drugs* 2005;65:215.
75. Alexander M et al. Supplementation of fexofenadine therapy with nedocromil sodium 2% ophthalmic solution to treat ocular symptoms of seasonal allergic conjunctivitis. *Clinical and Experimental Ophthalmology* 2003;31:206.
76. Lanier BQ et al. Comparison of the efficacy of combined fluticasone propionate and olopatadine versus combined fluticasone propionate and fexofenadine for the treatment of allergic rhinoconjunctivitis induced by conjunctival allergen challenge. *Clin Ther* 2002;24:1161.
77. Ganz M et al. Ketotifen fumarate and olopatadine hydrochloride in the treatment of allergic conjunctivitis: a real-world comparison of efficacy and ocular comfort. *Adv Ther* 2003;20:79.
78. Bernstein DI et al. Treatment with intra nasal fluticasone propionate significantly improves ocular symptoms in patients with seasonal allergic rhinitis. *Clin Exp Allergy* 2004;34:952.
79. Berger WE et al. Mometasone furoate improves congestion in patients with moderate-to-severe seasonal allergic rhinitis. *Ann Pharmacother* 2005; 39:1984.
80. Gawchik S et al. Relief of cough and nasal symptoms associated with allergic rhinitis by mometasone furoate nasal spray. *Ann Allergy Asthma Immunol* 2003;90:416.
81. Kaiser HB et al. Fluticasone furoate nasal spray: a single treatment option for the symptoms of seasonal allergic rhinitis. *J Allergy Clin Immunol* 2007;119:1430. Epub 2007 April 5.
82. Yanez A et al. Intranasal corticosteroids versus topical H1 receptor antagonists for the treatment of allergic rhinitis: a systematic review with meta analysis. *Ann Allergy Asthma Immunol* 2002;89: 479.
83. Di Lorenzo G et al. Randomized placebo-controlled trial comparing fluticasone aqueous nasal spray in mono-therapy, fluticasone plus cetirizine, fluticasone plus montelukast and cetirizine plus montelukast for seasonal allergic rhinitis. *Clin Exp Allergy* 2004;34:259.
84. Management of allergic rhinitis in the working-age population. Evidence Report/Technology Assessment. Agency for Healthcare Research and Quality Publication No. 02-E013. Vol. 67, 2003:1.
85. Meltzer EO. The pharmacological basis for the treatment of perennial allergic rhinitis and non-allergic rhinitis with topical corticosteroids. *Allergy* 1997;52(Suppl 1):33.
86. Management of allergic and nonallergic rhinitis. Evidence Report/Technology Assessment. Agency for Healthcare Research and Quality Publication No. 02-E023. Vol. 54, 2002:1.
87. Togias A. Rhinitis and asthma: evidence for respiratory system integration. *J Allergy Clin Immunol* 2003;111:1171.
88. Bachert C et al. Allergic rhinitis, rhinosinusitis, and asthma: one airway disease. *Immunology and Allergy Clinics of North America* 2004;24:19.
89. Cruz AA. The 'united airways' require an holistic approach to management. *Allergy* 2005;60:871.
90. Bousquet J et al. Increased risk of asthma attacks and emergency visits among asthma patients with allergic rhinitis: a subgroup analysis of the improving asthma control trial. *Clin Exp Allergy* 2005;35:723.
91. Price D et al. Effect of concomitant diagnosis of allergic rhinitis on asthma-related health care use by adults. *Clin Exp Allergy* 2005;35:282.
92. Sandrini A et al. Effect of nasal triamcinolone acetonide on lower airway inflammatory markers in patients with allergic rhinitis. *J Allergy Clin Immunol* 2003;111:313.
93. Mahadevia PJ et al. Patient preferences for sensory attributes of intranasal corticosteroids and willingness to adhere to prescribed therapy for allergic rhinitis: a conjoint analysis. *Annals of Allergy, Asthma and Immunology* 2004;93:345.
94. Blaiss MS. Safety considerations of intranasal corticosteroids for the treatment of allergic rhinitis. *Allergy and Asthma Proceedings* 2007;28:145.
95. Stokes M et al. Evaluation of patients' preferences for triamcinolone acetonide aqueous, fluticasone propionate, and mometasone furoate nasal sprays in patients with allergic rhinitis. *Otolaryngol Head Neck Surg* 2004;131:225.
96. Trangsrud AJ et al. Intranasal corticosteroids for allergic rhinitis. *Pharmacotherapy* 2002;22: 1458.
97. Zitt M et al. Mometasone furoate nasal spray: a review of safety and systemic effects. *Drug Saf* 2007;30:317.
98. *Drug Facts and Comparisons*. Drug Facts and Comparisons 4. 0 [online] 2008. Available from Wolters Kluwer Health, Inc. Accessed April 20, 2008.
99. Skoner D et al. Detection of growth suppression in children during treatment with intranasal beclomethasone dipropionate. *Pediatrics* 2000;105:e23.
100. Allen DB et al. No growth suppression in children treated with the maximum recommended dose of fluticasone propionate aqueous nasal spray for one year. *Allergy Asthma Proc* 2002;105:E22.
101. Murphy KR et al. Recommended once-daily dose of budesonide aqueous nasal spray does not suppress growth velocity in pediatric patients with perennial allergic rhinitis. *J Allergy Clin Immunol* 2004;113(Suppl):S175.
102. Daley-Yates PT et al. Relationship between systemic corticosteroid exposure and growth velocity: development and validation. *Clin Ther* 2004;26:1905.
103. Laliberte F et al. Clinical and pathologic methods to assess the long-term safety of nasal corticosteroids. French Triamcinolone Acetonide Study Group. *Allergy* 2000;55:718.
104. Spiliotopoulos C et al. The effect of nasal steroid administration on intraocular pressure. *Ear Nose Throat J* 2007;86:394.
105. Bielory L. Ocular toxicity of systemic asthma and allergy treatments. *Curr Allergy Asthma Rep* 200; 6:299.
106. Bielory L et al. ; Joint Task Force of the American Academy of Allergy, Asthma and Immunology; American College of Allergy, Asthma and Immunology. Concerns about intranasal corticosteroids for over-the-counter use: position statement of the Joint Task Force for the American Academy of Allergy, Asthma and Immunology and the American College of Allergy, Asthma and Immunology. *Ann Allergy Asthma Immunol* 2006;96:514.
107. Barnes ML et al. Effects of levocetirizine as add-on therapy to fluticasone in seasonal allergic rhinitis. *Clin Exp Allergy* 2006;36:676.
108. Bousquet J et al. Implementation of guidelines for seasonal allergic rhinitis: a randomized controlled trial. *Allergy* 2003;58:733.
109. Pullerits T et al. Comparison of a nasal glucocorticoid, antileukotriene, and a combination of antileukotriene and antihistamine in the treatment of seasonal allergic rhinitis. *J Allergy Clin Immunol* 2002;109:949.
110. Saengpanich S et al. Fluticasone nasal spray and the combination of loratadine and montelukast in seasonal allergic rhinitis. *Arch Otolaryngol Head Neck Surg* 2003;129:557.
111. McVary KT. A review of combination therapy in patients with benign prostatic hyperplasia. *Clin Ther* 2007;29:387.
112. Blake-James BT et al. The role of anticholinergics in men with lower urinary tract symptoms suggestive of benign prostatic hyperplasia: a systematic review and meta-analysis. *BJU Int* 2007;99: 85.
113. Nathan RA et al. Fluticasone priopionate nasal spray is superior to montelukast for allergic rhinitis while neither affects overall asthma control. *Chest* 2005;128:1910.
114. Kurowski M et al. Montelukast plus cetirizine in the prophylactic treatment of seasonal allergic rhinitis: influence on clinical symptoms and nasal allergic inflammation. *Allergy* 2004;59:280.
115. Blanc PD et al. Alternative therapies among adults with a reported diagnosis of asthma or rhinosinusitis: data from a population-based survey. *Chest* 2001;120:1461.
116. Bielory L. Complementary and alternative interventions in asthma, allergy and immunology. *Ann Allergy Asthma Immunol* 2004;93(2 Suppl 1):S45.
117. Niggemann B et al. Side-effects of complementary and alternative medicine. *Allergy* 2003;58:707.
118. Miyake Y et al. ; Osaka Maternal and Child Health Study Group. Fish and fat intake and prevalence of allergic rhinitis in Japanese females: the Osaka Maternal and Child Health Study. *J Am Coll Nutr* 2007;26:279.
119. Bernstein DI et al. Evaluation of the clinical efficacy and safety of grapeseed extract in the treatment of fall seasonal allergic rhinitis: a pilot study. *Ann Allergy Asthma Immunol* 2002;88:272.
120. Eccles R. Menthol: effects on nasal sensation of airflow and the drive to breathe. *Curr Allergy Asthma Rep* 2003;3:210.
121. Hochwald L. Natural allergy remedies. *New Age* 2001;March/April:36.
122. Zijlstra FJ et al. Anti-inflammatory actions of acupuncture. *Mediators Inflamm* 2003;12:59.
123. Taylor MA et al. Randomised controlled trial of homoeopathy versus placebo in perennial allergic rhinitis with overview of four trial series. *BMJ* 2000;321:471.
124. Schapowal A. Randomised controlled trial of butterbur and cetirizine for treating seasonal allergic rhinitis. *BMJ* 2002;324:144.
125. McArthur CA. Trial does not show that there is no difference between butterbur and cetirizine [Letter]. *BMJ* 2002;324:1277.
126. Shapowal A. Treating intermittent allergic rhinitis: a prospective, randomized, placebo and antihistamine-controlled study of Butterbur extract Ze 339. *Phytother Res Int* 2005;19:530.
127. Eby GA et al. Ineffectiveness of zinc gluconate nasal spray and zinc orotate lozenges in common-cold treatment: a double-blind, placebo-controlled clinical trial. *Altern Ther Health Med* 2006;12:34.
128. Alexander TH et al. Intranasal zinc and anosmia: the zinc-induced anosmia syndrome. *Layngoscope* 2006;116:217.
129. Xue CC et al. Does acupuncture or Chinese herbal medicine have a role in the treatment of allergic rhinitis? *Curr Opin Allergy Clin Immunol* 2006; 6:175.
130. Gunning K. Echinacea in the treatment and prevention of upper respiratory tract infections. *West J Med* 1999;171:1.
131. Mullins RJ et al. Adverse reactions associated with echinacea: the Australian experience. *Ann Allergy Asthma Immunol* 2002;88:42.
132. Alvarez-Cuesta E et al. EAACI, Immunotherapy Task Force. Standards for practical allergen-specific immunotherapy. *Allergy* 2006;61(Suppl)82:1.
133. Frew AJ et al. Efficacy and safety of specific immunotherapy with SQ allergen extract in treatment-resistant seasonal allergic rhinoconjunctivitis. *J Allergy Clin Immunol* 2006;117:319.
134. Malling HJ. Immunotherapy for rhinitis. *Curr Allergy Asthma Rep* 2003;3:204.
135. Moller C et al. Pollen immunotherapy reduces the development of asthma in children with seasonal rhinoconjunctivitis (the PAT-study) *J Allergy Clin Immunol* 2002;109:251.
136. Niggemann B et al. Five year follow-up on the PAT study: specific immunotherapy and long-term prevention of asthma in children. *Allergy* 2006;61:855.
137. Oppenheimer J et al. Skin testing. *Ann Allergy Asthma Immunol* 2006;96(2 Suppl 1):S6.
138. Chinoy B et al. Skin testing versus radioallergosorbent testing for indoor allergens. *Clin Mol Allergy* 2005 Apr 15;3:4.
139. Simons FE. Advances in H1-antihistamines. *N Engl J Med* 2004;351:2203.
140. Sekerel BE et al. The effect of montelukast on allergen-induced cutaneous responses in house dust

mite allergic children. *Pediatr Allergy Immunol* 2003;14:212.
141. Hill SL, 3rd et al. The effects of montelukast on intradermal wheal and flare. *Otolaryngol Head Neck Surg* 2003;129:199.
142. Abramson MJ et al. Allergen immunotherapy for asthma. *Cochrane Database Syst Rev* 2003: CD001186.
143. Andre C et al. A double-blind placebo-controlled evaluation of sublingual immunotherapy with a standardized ragweed extract in patients with seasonal rhinitis. Evidence for a dose-response relationship. *Int Arch Allergy Immunol* 2003;131:111.
144. Nelson HS. Advances in upper airway diseases and allergen immunotherapy. *J Allergy Clin Immunol* 2007;119:872.
145. Marcucci F et al. Low-dose local nasal immunotherapy in children with perennial allergic rhinitis due to dermatophagoides. *Allergy* 2002;57:23.
146. Eng PA et al. Twelve-year follow-up after discontinuation of preseasonal grass pollen immunotherapy in childhood. *Allergy* 2006;61:198.
147. Graf P. Rhinitis medicamentosa: a review of causes and treatment. *Treatment in Respiratory Medicine* 2005;4:21.
148. Lockey RF. Rhinitis medicamentosa and the stuffy nose. *J Allergy Clin Immunol* 2006;118:1017.
149. Fokkens WJ. Thoughts on the pathophysiology of nonallergic rhinitis. *Curr Allergy Asthma Rep* 2002;2:203.
150. van Rijswijk JB et al. Inflammatory cells seem not to be involved in idiopathic rhinitis. *Rhinology* 2003;41:25.
151. Powe DG et al. Evidence for an inflammatory pathophysiology in idiopathic rhinitis. *Clin Exp Allergy* 2001;31:864.
152. Ang YY et al. Treatment of idiopathic gustatory rhinorrhea by resection of the posterior nasal nerve. *Tohoku J Exp Med* 2006;210:165.
153. Meltzer EO et al. Ipratropium bromide aqueous nasal spray for patients with perennial allergic rhinitis: a study of its effect on their symptoms, quality of life, and nasal cytology. *J Allergy Clin Immunol* 1992;90:242.
154. Borum P et al. Ipratropium nasal spray: a new treatment for rhinorrhea in the common cold. *Am Rev Respir Dis* 1981;123(4 Pt 1):418.

CHAPTER 25

Drug-Induced Pulmonary Disorders

Deborah Sako Kubota and James Chan

Because the lungs are exposed directly to the atmospheric environment and whole circulating blood across an enormous surface area, they are uniquely susceptible to the effects of air- and blood-borne toxins. More than 350 drugs and diagnostic agents are known to cause pulmonary injuries of varying pathophysiological patterns, degrees of severity, and pathogenic mechanisms that involve the airways, lung parenchyma, pulmonary vasculature, pleura, and neuromuscular system.[1,2]

The resolution of acute drug-induced pulmonary disorders is dependent on early recognition and identification of the offending agent, its prompt withdrawal, and the initiation of management strategies. The diagnosis of drug-induced pulmonary toxicity generally rests on the exclusion of other causes or disorders with similar presentation. Therefore, it is incumbent on health care providers to have an awareness of the clinical findings consistent with drug-induced pulmonary disorders. An understanding of the mechanism of reaction and possible risk factors for adverse reactions is invaluable in the selection of alternative therapies to avoid or minimize toxicities.[3]

Drug-induced pulmonary disorders can be subdivided into categories based on the pathophysiological patterns of involvement. Some drugs can produce more than one pattern. Tables 25-1 and 25-2 include some commonly encountered pathology and implicated drugs with clinical details of the pulmonary reactions. This is not a complete listing of pathophysiological patterns or drugs reported to cause pulmonary disorders. For more comprehensive drug lists and greater detail, the reader is referred to several general reviews on this topic, including an online database.[2–9]

Generally, the initial step in the management of drug-induced pulmonary disorders is the discontinuation of the offending agent, where possible. Some management strategies include the use of corticosteroids. However, the potential benefit of corticosteroid therapy for the treatment of the serious acute respiratory distress syndrome (ARDS) remains controversial and appears to vary with the drug involved, the extent and type of toxicity elicited, the dosage of corticosteroid, and the time of the administration of corticosteroid therapy during the course of the reaction.[10–12]

PULMONARY FIBROSIS

1. A.E., a 35-year-old man with recently diagnosed Stage IIIB non-seminoma testicular cancer, has completed four cycles of bleomycin, etoposide, and cisplatin (BEP) therapy. A residual retroperitoneal mass is identified, and surgical resection under general anesthesia is scheduled. What is A.E.'s total lifetime dose of bleomycin, and how is this information relevant to his scheduled surgical procedure?

BEP administered every 3 weeks for four cycles is the recommended treatment of Stage IIIB non-seminoma testicular cancer. Bleomycin 30 units is administered weekly for three doses per cycle, for a cumulative dose of 360 units.[13]

Pulmonary toxicity is present in 10% of patients receiving bleomycin, and although it rarely progresses to pulmonary fibrosis, it can lead to death in 1% of all patients who receive this drug. Pulmonary fibrosis is the dose-limiting toxicity of bleomycin. It is recommended that the cumulative lifetime dose of bleomycin be restricted to <400 units, because pulmonary toxicity is rarely fatal at total cumulative doses of <400 units. The incidence increases appreciably if >450 units are given, and approaches a 10% fatality rate when patients receive cumulative doses >550 units. Additional risk factors include older age (increases with every decade over 30 years), renal insufficiency (creatinine clearance <35 mL/minute), and concomitant use of cisplatin.[14–18]

There have been reports of postoperative deaths attributed to the use of supplemental oxygen in patients given bleomycin. This combination may be synergistic for pulmonary toxicity. Although there have been data indicating that restricting inspired oxygen concentration (fraction of inspired oxygen [FiO_2]) to 22% to 25% mitigates the toxicity of combination use, there have also been data showing that the use of higher concentrations (37%–45% FiO_2) may not lead to respiratory failure. As data to support all practices of oxygen administration to patients receiving bleomycin are currently available, it has been recommended that inspired oxygen concentrations be kept at the lowest level that provides adequate tissue oxygenation (oxyhemoglobin saturation by pulse oximetry, SpO_2 >90%), particularly in patients with other risk factors.[15,19]

Table 25-1 Drugs Associated with Pulmonary Disorders[a]

Drugs	Pulmonary Reactions[b]	Drugs	Pulmonary Reactions[b]
Acebutolol	IVc	Inhaled pentamidine	I
Adenosine	I	Interferon-α	IVb, IVc, VIII
Allopurinol	IX	Interferon-β	IIb, VI
Amiodarone	IVb, IVc	Interleukin-2	IIb, VI, VIII
Amphetamine derivatives	III	Intravenous (IV) fluids	IIa
Amphotericin B	I, IVc	Irinotecan	VIII
Angiotensin-converting enzyme inhibitors	I	Isotretinoin	V
Anticoagulants	VII	Isoxsuprine (IV)	IIb
Asparaginase	I	Labetalol	I
Aspirin	I, VIII	Magnesium sulfate (IV)	IIa
Atenolol	I	Melphalan	VIII
Benzalkonium chloride	I	Mesalamine	IVc
Bleomycin	IVb, IVc, VII	Methadone	IIb
Bromocriptine	IVb, VI	Methotrexate	IVa, VIII
Busulfan	IVb, VIII	Minocycline	IVc, V
Cabergoline	IVb, VI	Mitomycin	IIb, IVb, VII
Carbamazepine	IVc, VIII, IX	Morphine	IIb
Carmustine	IVb, VII, VIII	Muromonab CD3	IIb
Cephalosporins	I, IVc	Naloxone	IIb
Chlorambucil	VIII	Nitrofurantoin	IVa, IVb, IVc, V, VI, VII, VIII
Cocaine	IIb, IVc, VII, VIII	Nitrosoureas	IVb, VII, VIII
Contrast media	I, IIa	Nonsteroidal anti-inflammatory drugs	I, V
Corticosteroids	I	Opiates	IIb, VIII
Cromolyn	I	Paclitaxel	I, VIII
Cyclophosphamide	IVb, VIII	Penicillamine	IVc, VIII
Cytarabine	IIb	Penicillins	I, VII
Cytosine-arabinoside	VIII	Phenytoin	VII, IX
Dantrolene	VI	Platelet aggregation inhibitors	VII
Dextran 70	VII	Platelet glycoprotein IIb/IIIa inhibitors	VII
Docetaxel	I, VIII	Propoxyphene	IIb
Doxorubicin	IVc	Propranolol	I
Ergot derivatives	IVb, VI	Propylthiouracil	VII
Erlotinib	IVa	Ritodrine (IV)	IIb
EDTA	I	Salicylates	IIb
Etoposide	VIII	Serotonin-specific reuptake inhibitors	III
Fenfluramine	III	Simvastatin	IVc, VIII
Fentanyl (IV)	I	Sirolimus	IVa, VIII
Fludarabine	VIII	Sulfasalazine	IVc
Gefitinib	IVa, VIII	Sulfites, metabisulfites	I
Gemcitabine	IIb, IVa	Sulfonamides	I, IX
Gold	IVc	Talc (IV)	IVb
Heroin	IIb, III, IVb	Terbutaline (IV)	IIb
HMG Co-A reductase inhibitors	IVc	Thrombolytic agents	VII
Hydralazine	VII	Ticlopidine	IVc, VII
Hydrochlorothiazide	IIb, VIII	Timolol	I
Imatinib	IVa, VIII	Zafirlukast	V
Inhalants/nebulized agents/preservatives	I	Zileuton	V
Inhaled human insulin	I		

[a]This is not a complete listing of all drugs that have been associated with pulmonary disorders or a complete listing of all types of pulmonary disorders reported with the drugs listed. Readers are advised to consult manufacturer labeling and/or general references such as Micromedex[38] for adverse event profiles of individual agents and references and databases specific to drug-induced toxicities such as Pneumotox at http://www.pneumotox.com.[4,8,9,43]

[b] I. Bronchospasm, wheezing, and cough
II. Pulmonary edema: a. Cardiogenic, b. Noncardiogenic
III. Pulmonary hypertension
IV. Interstitial lung disease: a. Infiltrates/pneumonia, b. Pulmonary fibrosis, c. Bronchiolitis obliterans organizing pneumonia
V. Pulmonary eosinophilia
VI. Pleural inflammation
VII. Diffuse alveolar hemorrhage/vasculitis
VIII. Diffuse alveolar damage
IX. Drug hypersensitivity syndrome

Table 25-2 Drug-Induced Pulmonary Disorders

Reaction/Drugs	*Clinical Remarks*
I. Bronchospasm, wheezing, and cough	• Bronchospasm is the most common drug-induced pulmonary adverse event. Many drugs cause bronchospasm via different pathophysiological mechanisms, including extension of pharmacologic effect, direct airway irritation, sensitization with subsequent anaphylactic reactions (IgE-mediated), and anaphylactoid (non–IgE-mediated) reactions.[8,9,43] • Clinical presentation is the same as with nondrug-induced bronchospasms (asthma, COPD; i.e., cough, shortness of breath, wheezing, chest tightness). Risk factors include pre-existing hyperreactive lung disease, smoking, advanced age, and respiratory infections.[8,9] • General management consists of withdrawal and avoidance of the causative agent and potential cross-reactive agents. Treat acute anaphylaxis with small doses of injectable epinephrine: in adults, administer 0.3 to 0.5 mL of a 1:1,000 dilution intramuscularly in the lateral thigh and supplementary treatment, including oxygen, corticosteroids, and parenteral antihistamines.[44] Inhaled β_2-agonists are useful for persistent bronchospasm.[8,9,44]
Adenosine	• IV **adenosine** is associated with a 12% to 28% incidence of dyspnea, which is generally transient.[45] Although there have been reports of bronchospasm when administered to patients with asthma or COPD, recent data indicate that adenosine does not cause bronchospasm as measured by spirometry, but can cause dyspnea, with an increased intensity in asthmatics.[43,46]
Amphotericin B	• Pulmonary reactions (bronchospasm and dyspnea) to **amphotericin B** infusions may be chemical, not allergic. Risk is related to rate of infusion, rather than to dose. This has been reported for both conventional and liposomal formulations.[47] Although generally rapid in onset, there have been delayed reactions for up to several weeks. May involve direct injury of endothelial cells, enhanced pulmonary leukostasis, and release of cyclo-oxygenase (COX) products from the metabolism of arachidonic acid. Characteristic infusion-related chills and fever are related to amphotericin-induced tumor necrosis factor-alpha (TNF-α) and interleukin (IL)-1 production. Pulmonary infiltrates consistent with acute pulmonary edema are common. The drug should be withdrawn, and corticosteroids, nonsteroidal anti-inflammatory drugs (NSAIDs), epinephrine, or aminophylline may be administered. Cautious re-exposure with a slowed rate of infusion and premedication could allow for treatment continuation with the same drug. True allergic reactions to amphotericin are extremely rare. Desensitization in an intensive care unit can be considered in a patient with previous anaphylactic reaction who requires amphotericin therapy.[47–49]
Angiotensin-converting enzyme inhibitors (ACEIs)	• Incidence of **ACEI**-induced cough is 5% to 35% and is twice as likely in women. Likely mediated by bradykinin and substance P normally degraded by angiotensin-converting enzyme, prostaglandins stimulated by bradykinin, or activation of bradykinin receptors. Can occur in the absence of pre-existing hyperreactivity. Characterized by dry, persistent cough, and tickling sensation in the throat, without changes in pulmonary function. Onset from 24 hours to 1 year after start of drug (average 14.5 weeks). Not dose dependent. Cough resolves in 1 to 4 weeks after drug discontinuation (up to 3 months in some patients). In a minority of patients, cough will not recur on rechallenge. Switching therapy to an angiotensin-receptor blocker or agent of another drug class is an option.[8,9,43,50]
Antibiotics cephalosporins penicillins sulfonamides	• **Cephalosporins, penicillins, and sulfonamides** are commonly involved in IgE-mediated bronchospasm. For some compounds, desensitization protocols have been developed.[9,51]
Antineoplastic agents asparaginase taxanes paclitaxel docetaxel	• **Asparaginase** is the most common cause of antineoplastic-induced hypersensitivity reactions (increases from 3%–32% after fourth weekly IV dose). Reactions can be immediate type I IgE-mediated or delayed type II IgM- and IgG-mediated, with symptoms ranging from transient rash to moderate bronchospasm and severe hypotension with or without anaphylaxis. Risk factors include the number of previously administered doses, previous reaction to asparaginase, IV route of administration and higher doses ($\geq$25,000 U/m^2). PEG-asparaginase is tolerated in the majority of patients with hypersensitivity to asparaginase.[52] • Hypersensitivity reactions occur in up to 42% of patients receiving **paclitaxel** (2% serious)[9] and in 25% to 50% of patients receiving **docetaxel**.[53] Symptoms include dyspnea and bronchospasm, as well as urticaria, angioedema, and hypotension. Most reactions occur with the first exposure. To prevent severe hypersensitivity reactions, patients should be premedicated. Regimens typically include a steroid and histamine H_1- and H_2-blocker. In cases of severe reactions, rechallenge should not be attempted.[9,53,54]
β-adrenergic receptor blockers (β-blockers) acebutolol, metipranolol atenolol, metoprolol betaxolol, nadolol bisoprolol, penbutolol carteolol, pindolol carvedilol, propranolol labetalol, sotalol levobunolol, timolol	• Noncardioselective **β-blockers** cause bronchoconstriction in almost all asthmatics by antagonizing the maintenance of normal airway tone by the sympathetic nervous system. They also compromise the bronchodilator effect of inhaled β-adrenergic treatment. Oral, intravenous (IV), and ophthalmic formulations have been implicated. Inhaled anticholinergic agents (e.g., ipratropium bromide) are indicated for β-blocker–induced bronchoconstriction. β_2-agonists will not be effective. Use of cardioselective β-blockers in the lowest dose possible can be considered for chronic obstructive pulmonary disease (COPD) patients who would benefit from β-blocker therapy. However, cardioselectivity is compromised with increasing doses, potentially resulting in β_2 antagonism and bronchoconstriction.[8,9,55,56]

(continued)

Table 25-2 Drug-Induced Pulmonary Disorders (*Continued*)

Reaction/Drugs	*Clinical Remarks*
Contrast media	• Acute life-threatening reactions to **iodinated contrast media** are rare (1.4%) and have decreased with the introduction of nonionic, low-osmolality contrast agents. Iodinated agents can illicit the release of histamines and other mediators via direct degranulation of mast cells. Pretesting for reactions is not useful. Premedication in at-risk patients with corticosteroids, antihistamines, or combinations thereof is not universally supported.[57,58]
Fentanyl	• IV **fentanyl**-induced cough can be explosive and ranges in frequency from 28% to 65%. It appears to increase with rapid injection. Fentanyl cough is attenuated by pretreatment with inhaled cromolyn sodium and corticosteroids. IV ketamine and lidocaine have decreased the frequency, but not the severity of cough.[9,59,60]
Inhalants/nebulized agents and preservatives benzalkonium chloride (BAC) corticosteroids cromolyn desflurane ethylenediamine tetra-acetic acid (EDTA) inhaled human insulin inhaled pentamidine sulfites	• Carrier agents (particles, propellants, and dispersants), pH, osmolality, or temperature of inhalational and nebulized agents used in the treatment of asthma may cause bronchial irritation. Propellants comprise 58% to 99% of metered-dose inhaler products. If there is no response or a history of increased wheezing after inhaled treatment, a change in specific product should be considered.[9,20] • **Inhaled corticosteroids, N-acetylcysteine, pentamidine, and desflurane** are known airway irritants. Preservatives (e.g., **sulfites, metabisulfites, benzalkonium chloride, EDTA**) found in some nebulized solutions can provoke reactions. Inhaled sulfites may stimulate afferent parasympathetic receptors on the lung surface. BAC directly stimulants airway irritant C fibers and causes mast cell degranulation. EDTA potentiates histamine-induced bronchoconstriction.[8,9,61] • **Human insulin inhalation powder (Exubera)** has been associated with a nearly 30% incidence of mild, rarely productive cough, which occurred within seconds to minutes after administration and decreased with continued use. The manufacturer discontinued marketing this product in January 2007.[95–97] • **Inhaled pentamidine** has been associated with cough (38% incidence) and bronchospasm (15% incidence). Prior treatment with an inhaled bronchodilator may help prevent these effects.[9,98]
Nonsteroidal Anti-Inflammatory Drugs (NSAIDs) aspirin	• **NSAIDs** and **Aspirin** have the highest incidence of drug-induced bronchospasm (6%–34%). May be due to inhibition of COX with resultant ↑ synthesis of proinflammatory leukotrienes and ↓ synthesis of anti-inflammatory prostaglandin, PGE_2. Rapid and often life-threatening reaction. Primary therapy is avoidance of NSAIDs that inhibit COX, including selective COX-2 inhibitors. The degree of cross-reactivity is dependent on the potency of inhibition. Sodium salicylate, salicylamide, and choline magnesium trisalicylate can be taken safely. Acetaminophen is a very weak COX inhibitor; on average, <5% of this population will react to acetaminophen, but the incidence increases (34%) with high doses (>1,000 mg). Pretreatment with leukotriene receptor antagonists (LTAs) does not provide consistent prophylaxis. Desensitization to aspirin under medical supervision is an option and will confer protection to cross-reacting NSAIDs.[8,9,43]
Sulfites	• Ingestion of **sulfites** used as preservatives in food and wine can elicit bronchoconstriction (5% incidence), particularly in patients with corticosteroid-dependent asthma.[8]
II. Acute pulmonary edema	• Typical symptoms include dyspnea, chest discomfort, tachypnea, and hypoxemia with crackles on auscultation. Foamy tracheal exudates may develop with alveolar flooding. May be associated with fever and lead to acute respiratory distress syndrome (ARDS).[2,62] • Management focuses on adequate life support, then specific therapy that targets the causes of the accumulation of extravascular water in the lungs. Useful strategies would limit further accumulation of fluid and favor its removal from the lungs.[63]
II. a. Cardiogenic	• Cardiogenic (increased pressure) pulmonary edema can have an insidious onset, as the barriers to fluid and protein that flow into the lungs remain intact. Symptoms may be only vague fatigue, mild pedal edema, and exertional dyspnea. Iatrogenic causes include **IV fluids** with resultant cardiovascular fluid overload.[63]
IV fluids contrast media magnesium sulfate	• The amount of **Contrast media** infused, irrespective of the osmolality, may be a major cause of contrast media–induced pulmonary edema. Risks may reduced by decreasing the volume injected and ensuring a normal state of hydration prior to infusion. Can also cause anaphylactoid reactions. However, pathogenesis may not be related to anaphylaxis or fluid overload, but may involve the chemical irritation of the pulmonary endothelium via formation of endothelium-derived prostacyclin.[3,57,58] • **IV Magnesium sulfate** tocolysis-induced pulmonary edema appears to be due to the delivery vehicle, rather than to the drug itself because higher risk is associated with higher infusion rates and lower drug concentrations. Incidence of pulmonary edema is significantly increased when given with β_2-agonists.[64]
II. b. Noncardiogenic pulmonary edema (NCPE)	• NCPE comprises most cases of drug-induced pulmonary edema via drug-related increases in capillary pulmonary permeability. Can develop within a few days after exposure or immediately after drug administration with rapid alveolar flooding. Fluid in alveolar spaces will contain high concentrations of protein. In addition to drug discontinuation, treatment may require mechanical ventilatory support with positive pressure. Corticosteroid treatment (methylprednisolone 1 mg/kg) started early in the course of ARDS has been shown to be beneficial, but remains controversial.[65] Condition will recur with drug rechallenge.[2,3,10]

Table 25-2 Drug-Induced Pulmonary Disorders *(Continued)*

Reaction/Drugs	*Clinical Remarks*
Antineoplastic agents cytarabine gemcitabine interleukin-2 (IL-2) mitomycin muromonab CD3 vinca alkaloids	• Rare reaction with **antineoplastic** agents. Likely due to due to a cytokine-mediated inflammatory response. High incidence of **cytarabine**-induced NCPE noted with moderate or high doses in patients with leukemia. Although rarely seen with **gemcitabine** (0.1% incidence), NCPE may occur after a single dose, but is generally seen after repeated administration. **IL-2**–induced NCPE is dose related, with an estimated incidence of 3% to 20%. Although severe, it is reversible on discontinuation of IL-2. The combination **mitomycin/vinblastine** is associated with an estimated 2% incidence of NCPE. A cytokine release syndrome (CRS) commonly occurs with initial doses of **muromonab CD3** and may result in serious, potentially fatal cardiorespiratory effects, including pulmonary edema (cardiogenic and noncardiogenic). Overhydration increases the risk of pulmonary edema. Pretreatment with methylprednisolone may reduce cytokine levels and incidence of CRS.[3,62]
IV β_2-agonists ritodrine terbutaline isoxsuprine	• **IV tocolytic β_2-agonists** may cause peripheral vasodilation (with rapid reversal on discontinuation) and resultant large shift of intravascular volume into tissues, including the lungs. Incidence is 0.5% to 5%. It is not clear whether the pathogenic mechanism is cardiogenic or noncardiogenic based on conflicting reports of left ventricular function. Risk factors include excessive administration, infusions >24 hours, anemia, twin or multiple gestations, corticosteroid use, low serum K^+, sustained tachycardia (>140 beats/min). In addition to drug withdrawal, treatment should include oxygen supplementation, fluid restriction with diuretic therapy, and acid–base management.[3,66]
Cocaine	• **Cocaine** abuse is associated with numerous patterns of pulmonary reactions, including pulmonary edema. Whether the mechanism is cardiogenic or noncardiogenic remains speculative.[20]
Hydrochlorothiazide (HCTZ)	• **HCTZ**-induced NCPE is rare, but has occurred within one hour of the first oral dose of HCTZ. Can also develop unexpectedly later in treatment. Usually a history of previous thiazide exposure with mild reaction. More commonly reported in women. May be an idiosyncratic reaction or direct toxic effect. Clinical recovery is rapid, usually within 1 to 2 days. Avoid thiazide diuretics. Other sulfonamide nonantibiotics (e.g., furosemide or glyburide) and antibiotics are not expected to cross-react.[2,3,67]
Naloxone	• High-dose or rapidly infused **naloxone** may cause pulmonary edema.[68]
Opiates heroin methadone morphine propoxyphene	• Common complication of intoxication with **opiates, including morphine, heroin, methadone, and propoxyphene**.[64] • Heroin-induced pulmonary edema is common after IV use. Heroin via injection or inhalation can cause other acute reactions, including bronchospasm. Secondary bacterial and aspiration pneumonias are frequent complications. Treatment consists of naloxone, in addition to respiratory support.[69]
Salicylates	• Risk factors for **salicylate** reaction include serum levels >40 mg/dL, neurologic abnormalities, and proteinuria.[3]
III. Pulmonary hypertension	• Drug-induced primary (idiopathic) pulmonary hypertension (PPH) is rare, but life threatening. Early stages may be asymptomatic. The most frequent presenting symptom is exertional dyspnea, which may be present at rest as the disease progresses. Fatigue, weakness, chest pain, or syncope may also be reported. In addition to supplemental oxygen, management may include diuretics, inotropic agents, anticoagulants, prostacyclin analogues (e.g., epoprostenol), an endothelin receptor antagonist (e.g., bosentan), and calcium channel blockers (nifedipine, amlodipine, and diltiazem have been used most frequently) in patients with proven acute vasoreactivity.[70,102]
Appetite suppressants fenfluramine derivatives amphetamine derivatives	• The widely implicated **anorectic agents** are no longer marketed, but stimulants, in particular **methamphetamine**, have also been strongly associated with the development of PPH. Patients with idiopathic PPH were approximately ten times more likely to have had stimulant use than those with PPH and known risk factors.[71]
Serotonin-specific reuptake inhibitors (SSRIs)	• The risk of persistent pulmonary hypertension of the newborn (PPHN) in mothers taking **SSRI** antidepressants in the second half of their pregnancy is increased from 0.1% in the general population to 0.6%.[72]
IV. Interstitial lung disease (ILD)	• ILD is the most common drug-induced lung disease and can lead to respiratory failure. Presentation may be acute, subacute, or chronic. Symptoms include nonproductive cough, dyspnea, low-grade fever, and diffuse reticular infiltrate on chest x-ray. Diagnosis is based on temporal association between exposure and development of pulmonary infiltrate with meticulous exclusion of other potential causative factors. Types of ILD include interstitial pneumonia, pulmonary eosinophilia, bronchiolitis obliterans organizing pneumonia (BOOP), pulmonary fibrosis, and diffuse alveolar damage (DAD). Oxidant injury, either through the increased production of oxidants (e.g., **bleomycin, cyclophosphamide, nitrofurantoin**) or the inhibition of the antioxidant system (e.g., **carmustine, cyclophosphamide, nitrofurantoin**) accounts for the majority of drug-induced ILD.[2,7,73] • Management tends to be empirical. Following drug withdrawal, respiratory failure is commonly treated with high-dose methylprednisolone, with dose reduction and gradual taper after response. Respiratory distress is commonly treated with low-dose methylprednisolone (1 mg/kg or 60 mg/day) with gradual dose reduction. Immunosuppressants have been used for patients who cannot tolerate corticosteroids or who are unable to taper corticosteroids.[21]

(continued)

Table 25-2 Drug-Induced Pulmonary Disorders *(Continued)*

Reaction/Drugs	*Clinical Remarks*
IV. a. Interstitial infiltrates/pneumonia	• Interstitial infiltrates represent changes on the chest x-ray that occur from diseases involving the space between the alveolus and capillary. The infiltrates consist of fluid and/or cells that gather in this area of the lung.
Epidermal growth factor receptor (EGFR) antagonists/ tyrosine kinase inhibitors (TKIs) cetuximab erlotinib gefitinib imatinib	• **EGFR antagonist/TKIs** have been rarely associated with ILD. **Gefitinib** has been available longer, and there is more information available regarding gefitinib-induced ILD. The worldwide incidence of gefitinib-induced ILD is 1%, with a higher percentage noted in Japan (2%). It may be fatal in one-third to 40% of cases. There are also reports of ILD associated with **erlotinib**, and, rarely, **cetuximab** and **imatinib**. Because epidermal growth factor signaling may play an important role in the coordination of recovery from lung injury, EGFR inhibition may reduce the ability of pneumocytes to respond to lung injury.[23,31]
Gemcitabine	• Relatively uncommon reaction to **gemcitabine**. Risk factors include concomitant administration of bleomycin, vinorelbine, paclitaxel, docetaxel, or chest radiotherapy. The rate could be as high as 48% in patients with Hodgkin's disease who received a combination of gemcitabine and bleomycin. Median time to diagnosis was 48 days after initiation of gemcitabine. May be related to release of proinflammatory cytokines such as TNF-α.[42,74]
Methotrexate	• Pulmonary infiltrate is the most common form of lung toxicity with **methotrexate** (1%–10%). Serum surfactant protein (SP-D) and protein KL-6 levels are related to the severity of the pneumonitis.[75,76]
Nitrofurantoin	• **Nitrofurantoin**-induced acute pneumonitis may be one of the most common of the drug-induced diseases. In a series of patients reporting adverse effects from this drug, 43% reported acute pulmonary reactions. It does not appear to be dose related. Onset of symptoms, fever, dyspnea, and cough occurs within 1 month. Characterized by alveolar interstitial infiltrates, often without pleural involvement. In one series of cases, 52% of patients had infiltrates alone, 15% had infiltrates and effusions, and only 3% had only effusions.[6,66]
Sirolimus	• **Sirolimus** has about an 8% incidence of pulmonary reaction. The major risk factors appear to be high dose (>5 mg/day) and high trough level (>15 ng/mL). Other potential risk factors include use of a loading dose, late exposure compared with de novo treatment, allograft dysfunction, hypervolemia, older age, and male gender.[77]
IV. b. Pulmonary fibrosis	• Pulmonary fibrosis is characterized by accumulation of excessive connective tissue in the lung caused by prolonged exposure to certain drugs. It may or may not be preceded by inflammation (pneumonitis). Evidence suggests that activation of the coagulation cascade and generation of coagulation proteases play a key role. The mean survival time for patients with pulmonary fibrosis has been estimated at five months, but earlier diagnosis and cessation of causative agent may have decreased mortality rates.[7,78]
Cytotoxic drugs bleomycin busulfan carmustine cyclophosphamide interferon-α, -β mitomycin	• **Bleomycin** is the cytotoxic agent with the highest incidence of pulmonary toxicity (3%–40%). Risk factors include cumulative dose (threshold 400–450 U), older age (increases with each decade over 30 years), and radiation therapy. Pneumonitis rarely progresses to fibrosis, but can be fatal (1%). High concentrations of oxygen ($FiO_2 \geq 25\%$) should be avoided when possible due to the possible enhancement of pulmonary toxicity. Bleomycin should be immediately stopped at finding a decrease ≥15% in pulmonary function tests (diffusing capacity for carbon monoxide [DLCO] and vital capacity). Although response to corticosteroids is highly variable, prednisone 60–100 mg/day is recommended.[7,14,17,79] • **Busulfan** pulmonary fibrosis ("busulfan lung") is rare (1%–4%), but usually progressive and fatal. It can occur 1 to 10 years after drug discontinuation. Risk factors include cumulative dose (threshold 500 mg), radiation therapy, and length of therapy.[7,14,20,66,79] • **Carmustine** risk factors include cumulative dose, young age (<7 years), oxygen therapy, and prior lung disease. In one study, 10% of patients receiving 1,000 mg/m^2 of carmustine and 100% of those receiving 1,400 mg/m^2 experienced pulmonary toxicity; overall incidence is approximately 30%–40%. The onset may be very delayed, with a reported occurrence 17 years after treatment. Nitrosourea-induced pulmonary fibrosis may not respond to corticosteroids.[7,14,20,79] • The incidence of **cyclophosphamide**-induced pneumonitis is unknown, but may be largely underestimated. An early onset pneumonitis, occurring within 1 to 6 months of the start of therapy, generally responds to drug withdrawal. However, a delayed pneumonitis, developing after months or years of therapy, can result in progressive fibrosis and pleural thickening, with minimal response to drug withdrawal or corticosteroid therapy.[66] • **Interferon-α, -β** may include or exacerbate sarcoidosis. Sarcoidosis most often (90%) manifests in the lungs and can lead to pulmonary fibrosis.[103] • **Mitomycin** is associated with many types of pulmonary toxicities, including pneumonitis, NCPE, and pleural effusions. Incidence ranges from 10% (monotherapy) to 35% (combined with vinca alkaloids). Risk factors include radiation or oxygen therapy. In patients receiving mitomycin with other anticancer drugs, the FiO_2 concentration perioperatively should be maintained at <50%. Toxicity is not clearly dose dependent. A favorable response to corticosteroid therapy, possibly greater than for other chemotherapy-induced pulmonary injuries, has been reported.[7,66,79]

Table 25-2 Drug-Induced Pulmonary Disorders *(Continued)*

Reaction/Drugs	*Clinical Remarks*
Non-cytotoxic agents amiodarone bromocriptine cabergoline ergot derivatives heroin (IV) methysergide nitrofurantoin pergolide IV abuse of oral drugs	• The incidence of **amiodarone**-induced pulmonary toxicity is dose related: 0.1%–0.5%, up to 200 mg/day; 5%–15%, up to 500 mg/day; and as high as 50%, in doses of 1,200 mg/day. Can occur within 2 weeks or up to more than a decade into treatment. Amiodarone therapy may enhance drug-induced pulmonary toxicity with **cyclophosphamide**. Length of recovery time or recurrence may be correlated with high body mass index.[2,32,80–82] • Pulmonary fibrosis appears to be a class effect of ergot-derived dopamine agonists (**pergolide, bromocriptine, cabergoline, methysergide**). Condition is often irreversible. Pergolide was recently withdrawn from the U.S. market due to the potential for valvulopathy.[99–101] • **Nitrofurantoin** is involved in several forms of pulmonary injury. Most common are an acute hypersensitivity pneumonitis and a chronic alveolitis/fibrosis (nitrofurantoin lung), which do not overlap clinically (see interstitial infiltrates, BOOP, pulmonary eosinophilia, and pleural effusions). Overall estimated incidence of pulmonary injury is <0.01%, with chronic reactions occurring far less commonly than acute. The chronic form is related to dose and duration of therapy, and is commonly found in patients on long-term therapy for persistent bacteriuria. It is characterized by insidious, progressive dyspnea, nonproductive cough, interstitial pneumonitis, and fibrosis, which may impair pulmonary function permanently and may continue to deteriorate. Onset may occur 6 months to many years after either continuous or intermittent use. The utility of corticosteroids in the management of nitrofurantoin pulmonary fibrosis is unclear.[6,7,66,83] • The use of **IV heroin** and of drugs intended for oral use (e.g., crushed methylphenidate pills) can lead to the development of interstitial or vascular foreign body granulomas (talcosis) from the injection of filler materials used as tablet binders or used to cut heroin. Symptoms range from dyspnea and cough to pulmonary hypertension, right-sided heart failure, and sudden death. Radiographs may be normal or show diffuse micronodular densities. Bronchoalveolar lavage (BAL) contains increased lymphocytes and intracellular and free talc. Corticosteroids do not provide consistent improvement.[66,69]
IV. c. Bronchiolitis obliterans organizing pneumonia (BOOP)/cryptogenic organizing pneumonia	• BOOP is an inflammation of the lungs characterized by alveolar fibrosis. The clinician needs to distinguish between underlying connective tissue disease (e.g., polymyalgia) and drug-induced disease. Clinical signs and symptoms include dyspnea, low-grade fever, and, occasionally, acute pleuritic chest pain. Typically, chest films show migratory opacities if taken over a period of weeks or months. There may be occasional "normal" chest x-rays even with continued exposure. The pattern of the opacities may be suggestive of the causative agent. Although resolution of symptoms and radiographic abnormalities generally respond to the discontinuation of medication or corticosteroid therapy, in rare cases, the outcome is fatal.[2,5]
Antimicrobials amphotericin B cephalosporins minocycline nitrofurantoin Cytotoxic drugs bleomycin doxorubicin Cardiovascular drugs acebutolol amiodarone HMG CoA reductase inhibitors (statins) Anti-inflammatory drugs gold mesalamine sulfasalazine Miscellaneous carbamazepine cocaine interferon-α, -β penicillamine ticlopidine	• More than 20 medications are associated with BOOP[5] • Radiographic patterns: Patchy, stellate shadows or diffuse infiltrates may suggest **nitrofurantoin**. Multiple shaggy nodules may suggest **bleomycin, carbamazepine, minocycline, or statins**. Biapical masses have been associated with **mesalamine or sulfasalazine**.[2]
V. Pulmonary eosinophilia	• Pulmonary eosinophilia is characterized by pulmonary infiltration of eosinophils in alveolar spaces, the interstitium, or both. When found with peripheral eosinophilia, it is often called PIE (pulmonary infiltrates with eosinophilia) syndrome. Diagnosis is confirmed by demonstration of an excess of eosinophilia either in lung biopsy or in BAL. Loeffler syndrome is an acute eosinophilic pneumonia with transient pulmonary infiltrates and peripheral blood eosinophilia, characterized by mild or absent respiratory symptoms. Churg-Strauss syndrome (CSS) is a systemic, multiorgan necrotizing vasculitis that includes pulmonary eosinophilia. Drug-induced cases of pulmonary eosinophilia typically show ground-glass opacities in a peripheral and upper lobe distribution.[84–86]

(continued)

Table 25-2 Drug-Induced Pulmonary Disorders *(Continued)*

Reaction/Drugs	*Clinical Remarks*
V. Pulmonary eosinophilia *(Cont'd)*	• Corticosteroids are indicated in severe cases; however, because eosinophils are very sensitive to corticosteroids, their complete disappearance from the bloodstream within hours of administration may obscure the diagnosis.[84,86] • Many drugs have been implicated in causing pulmonary eosinophilia, but the number with established causality with multiple case reports is much less. The drugs most commonly causing pulmonary eosinophilia are **antimicrobial agents (penicillins, clarithromycin, and levofloxacin)** and **NSAIDs.**[86]
Isotretinoin	• **Isotretinoin**-induced PIE is rare, but in one case showed >20% pleural fluid eosinophilia (>10% of nucleated cells).[6]
Leukotriene antagonists (LTAs) zafirlukast zileuton	• Cases of **LTA**-induced CSS are suggested by case reports and postmarketing surveillance. It is not clear if this rare disorder is a direct drug effect or an unmasking of a pre-existing condition on withdrawal of corticosteroids for asthma on initiation of LTA therapy.[43,85]
Minocycline	• **Minocycline** has been associated with pulmonary lupus, hypersensitivity pneumonitis, pleural effusions, and eosinophilic pneumonia. Several cases of respiratory distress have also been reported, including one of a relapsing form of hypersensitivity eosinophilic pneumonia that required mechanical ventilation.[86,87]
Nitrofurantoin	• Most cases of **nitrofurantoin**-induced acute pneumonitis have peripheral eosinophilia (in 83% of patients) and lymphopenia. Pleural eosinophilia has been described (see pulmonary fibrosis, interstitial pneumonia, BOOP, and pleural effusions). The acute effects may be observed within 1 month.[6,66,83]
NSAIDs	• There have been case reports of NSAIDs (**ibuprofen, naproxen, diclofenac, indomethacin, sulindac, and meloxicam**) causing PIE. Prevalence of NSAID-induced PIE is likely underestimated.[88–90]
VI. Pleural inflammation	• Drug-induced pleural reactions are rare compared with those affecting the parenchyma. Pleural reactions range in presentation from asymptomatic effusion to acute pleuritis to symptomatic pleural thickening. Common symptoms of pleural effusion are pleuritic chest pain, dyspnea, and cough. Suggested mechanisms for the development of drug-induced pleural disease include hypersensitivity or allergic reaction, direct toxicity, increased production of oxygen-free radicals, suppression of antioxidant defenses, and chemically-induced inflammation.[6]
Dantrolene	• The incidence of **dantrolene**-induced pleural effusion is rare, but likely underestimated. Onset has occurred from 2 months to 12 years of initial administration. Effusion is usually unilateral, with peripheral and pleural fluid eosinophilia. Fever may be present. Structural similarity to nitrofurantoin suggests an immunologic basis for this reaction. Drug withdrawal results in rapid symptomatic recovery; however, it may take several months for complete resolution of the effusion.[6,91,92]
Ergot alkaloids bromocriptine cabergoline methysergide pergolide	• Pleural effusions or thickening can result from the chronic administration of **ergot alkaloids**, including **bromocriptine, cabergoline**, and **pergolide**. Approximately 6% of patients receiving bromocriptine develop pleuropulmonary complications. Fibrosis typically occurs 12 to 48 months after initiation of therapy and appears to be dose related. Pleural lymphocytosis or eosinophilia may occur. Pleural effusion responds to drug withdrawal; however, fibrosis may not completely resolve.[6,91] • Less than 1% of patients taking methysergide experience pleuropulmonary reactions (pleural effusions and fibrosis). Symptoms occur 1 month to 3 years after initiation of therapy. Increased stimulation of fibroblast activity via increased levels of serotonin is a proposed pathogenic mechanism. Symptoms improve on discontinuation; however, pleural thickening may persist.[6,91]
IL-2	• **IL-2**–induced pleuropulmonary complications occur in approximately 75% of patients, with pleural effusions in approximately 50% of patients receiving IL-2. Capillary leak results in effusions and noncardiogenic pulmonary edema. Pleural effusions may persist in 17% of patients at 4 weeks after drug discontinuation.[6]
Nitrofurantoin	• Up to one-third of acute **nitrofurantoin**-induced pleuropulmonary reactions may include pulmonary effusions, rarely without concomitant parenchymal involvement. In contrast, pleural effusions are rare with the chronic nitrofurantoin syndrome. Effusions are usually bilateral and responsive to prompt drug withdrawal. Severe symptoms can be treated with corticosteroids.[6]
VII. Diffuse alveolar hemorrhage (DAH) and vasculitis	• DAH is characterized by bleeding from pulmonary capillaries, leading to the accumulation of red blood cells in the alveolar spaces. Symptoms include varying degrees of hemoptysis (may be absent in up to 33% of cases), cough, and progressive dyspnea. Hematocrit is reduced with hemorrhagic BAL. Presentation is usually acute, often resulting in respiratory failure by intra-alveolar clotting. DAH can develop in many systemic conditions, and it is difficult to prove drug causality. Drug-related pathogenic mechanisms include hypersensitivity reaction, direct toxicity diffuse alveolar damage (DAD), and coagulation defects. Pulmonary capillaritis, the most frequent underlying histology, and pulmonary veno-occlusive disease (PVOD), a fibrous obliteration of pulmonary venules and small veins, are considered autoimmune reactions.[2,93]

Table 25-2 Drug-Induced Pulmonary Disorders *(Continued)*

Reaction/Drugs	*Clinical Remarks*
Anticoagulants Dextran 70 Platelet aggregation inhibitors Platelet glycoprotein IIb/IIIa inhibitors Thrombolytic agents	• **Anticoagulant and thrombolytic** agents cause pulmonary hemorrhage without damage to the interstitial compartment. Anticoagulant-related bleeding is generally managed by withdrawal of the drug. In addition to drug withdrawal, the addition of corticosteroids may be indicated in other forms or significant cases of DAH.[2,93]
Chemotherapeutic agents bleomycin carmustine gemcitabine mitomycin vinca alkaloids	• **Chemotherapeutic agents** cause direct epithelial injury and damage to the alveolar capillary basement membrane, which can result in DAH. Outcomes are poor (50%–100% mortality), and although high-dose corticosteroid therapy is the only recommended treatment, effectiveness is questionable.[93] • **Bleomycin, carmustine, gemcitabine, mitomycin, and vinca alkaloids** have been associated with the development of PVOD.[93]
Cocaine Hydralazine Mitomycin Nitrofurantoin Penicillin Phenytoin Propylthiouracil	• Pulmonary capillaritis has occurred with **phenytoin** and **propylthiouracil.**[93] • Other drugs associated with hypersensitivity reactions with concomitant DAH include **penicillin, sulfasalazine,** and **hydralazine.**[93] • Smoking crack cocaine, either due to cocaine or the residual solvents, may cause hemoptysis and pulmonary infiltrates due to DAH. Onset is usually within hours and is reversible on discontinuation. There is also a possible relationship between IV cocaine and alveolar hemorrhage.[69,93]
VIII. Diffuse alveolar damage (DAD)	• In DAD, the alveolar epithelial cells are sloughed, and the lung interstitium becomes edematous. Chronic inflammation and fibroproliferation of the alveolar walls can present early in the process. The histopathological basis for ARDS is DAD. In severe cases, DAH can develop with resultant hemoptysis. DAD presents with dyspnea, diffuse pulmonary infiltrates, and ARDS unresponsive to conventional therapy. DAD of recent onset may respond to corticosteroid therapy; however, chemotherapeutic agent-induced DAD carries a poor prognosis.[2,93]
Alkylating agents Antibiotics Antimetabolites Aspirin Carbamazepine Chemotherapeutic agents Cocaine Epidermal growth factor receptor (EGFR) antagonists Hydrochlorothiazide Interferon-α IL-2 Irinotecan Narcotics Nitrofurantoin Nitrosoureas Penicillamine Podophyllotoxins Simvastatin Sirolimus	• Chemotherapeutic agents associated with the development of DAD, which may be accompanied by DAH, include **antibiotics, alkylating agents, antimetabolites, nitrosoureas, podophyllotoxins, tretinoin, gefitinib, imatinib, irinotecan, interferon-α, IL-2, and sirolimus**. The reaction is more severe and frequent with multiple drug treatments or with concurrent radiation therapy or oxygen.[2] • Noncytotoxic drug-induced DAD is unusual, but has been associated with **aspirin, narcotics, crack cocaine, nitrofurantoin, carbamazepine, penicillamine, hydrochlorothiazide, and simvastatin.**[2]
IX. Drug hypersensitivity syndrome (DHS)	• DHS is a systemic idiosyncratic reaction defined by the presence of fever, rash, and organ involvement, including pneumonitis or pulmonary infiltrates. It is associated with aromatic anticonvulsants **(phenytoin, carbamazepine, phenobarbital, felbamate, lamotrigine, oxcarbazepine, and zonisamide)**, and is most commonly reported with phenytoin, carbamazepine, and phenobarbital. DHS develops within 8 weeks of treatment, with a 1 in 1,000 to 10,000 incidence.[2,94] Clinical presentations may involve dermatologic, hematologic, lymphatic, or internal organ systems. Pulmonary reactions include lymphoid interstitial pneumonia, interstitial lung disease, eosinophilic pneumonia, and pleural effusion. Management involves drug withdrawal, supportive care and corticosteroid therapy. Although improvement occurs in a few days after drug discontinuation for most patients, a few experience acceleration of the disease. Continued corticosteroid therapy may be necessary to avoid relapse. There is a mortality rate of up to 10% for DHS. Rechallenge with the drug or related drugs results in relapse of increased severity.[2]
Allopurinol Anticonvulsants carbamazepine phenytoin Sulfonamides	• Drugs known to cause DHS include **allopurinol, anticonvulsants (particularly carbamazepine, phenytoin, and phenobarbital), and sulfonamides**. Other drugs less commonly associated with DHS include **abacavir, atenolol, azathioprine, bupropion, captopril, diltiazem, gold, leflunomide, minocycline, nevirapine, NSAIDs, sulfasalazine, and trimethoprim.**[2,94]

2. What is the postulated mechanism for bleomycin toxicity?

Bleomycin toxicity is attributed to direct cytotoxic injury to the lung epithelium, likely caused by free radical generation following binding of the drug to DNA. It is postulated that the relative lack of hydrolase (an enzyme necessary for degradation of bleomycin) in the lung may contribute to increased pulmonary levels of the drug with resultant toxicity. Studies in animals have confirmed that bleomycin is concentrated in the lungs and skin.[16]

3. How can A.E. be monitored for pulmonary toxicity?

There are no pathognomonic signs or symptoms of bleomycin-related pulmonary damage. Patients usually present with dyspnea, tachypnea, and a nonproductive cough, which can develop from days to weeks. Rales, initially at the bases and then throughout the lungs, may be present on physical examination. Signs and symptoms usually precede changes on the chest radiograph. The utility of pulmonary function tests as an indicator for the extent of the pulmonary damage produced by bleomycin is controversial. Spirometry usually shows a restrictive pattern in the presence of cytotoxic drug-induced pulmonary damage; however, such changes may not always be present in patients with subclinical bleomycin-induced pulmonary fibrosis. For this reason, pulmonary function tests are of questionable predictive value.[16,20]

4. How should A.E. be managed?

Because A.E.'s total cumulative dose of bleomycin is 360 U, he should not receive further treatments of bleomycin to avoid exceeding the recommended total cumulative dose of 400 U. His treatment team should be apprised of A.E.'s treatment with bleomycin to ensure management of the oxygen concentration as recommended in bleomycin-exposed patients.[13,15]

TYROSINE KINASE INHIBITOR-INDUCED INTERSTITIAL LUNG DISEASE

5. J.T., a 55-year-old male with Stage IV, performance status 1, non-small cell lung cancer (NSCLC), adenocarcinoma, completed four cycles of cisplatin/etoposide with disease stabilization. Prior to chemotherapy, he had undergone radiotherapy with 20 treatments of 200 centigray (cGy) per treatment, for a total of 4,000 radiation doses (rads). On return from visiting his family in Japan, 5 months after completing therapy, treatment with erlotinib 150 mg orally was initiated due to disease progression. After 1 month of erlotinib therapy, J.T. was admitted to the hospital due to complaints of increasing cough and dyspnea at rest. He denied resumption of smoking, which he had quit on diagnosis of lung cancer. He was afebrile. Crackles were audible bilaterally. His pulmonary function test results were indicative of a restrictive condition: forced vital capacity (FVC) 61.5% of predicted, forced expiratory volume in 1 second (FEV_1) 69.5% of predicted, FEV_1/FVC ratio 87.7%, 110% predicted, and diffusion capacity for carbon monoxide (DLCO) 48.6% of predicted. Parenchymal shadows were present on his initial chest radiograph. The subsequent high-resolution computed tomography (HRCT) revealed bilateral diffuse ground-glass infiltrates and interlobular septal thickening of the lower lung fields. Lab results included white blood cell count 6,600/mm^3, erythrocyte sedimentation rate (ESR) 30 mm/hour (normal, ≤10 mm/hour in males), and normal electrolyte panel. Electrocardiogram and echocardiogram were normal. Blood and sputum were negative for culture and various infectious pathogen antibody titers. What causes of dyspnea should be investigated in this patient?

The potential causes of dyspnea in a patient with NSCLC include infection, cancer progression, pulmonary embolism (may develop in up to 20% of lung cancer patients), fluid overload, and drug-induced pulmonary disorder. His laboratory and blood culture results argue against the presence of infection. Findings are not suggestive of heart failure or pulmonary embolus. The chest radiograph is not suggestive of disease progression; however, bronchoscopy and bronchoalveolar lavage (BAL) may be useful in some cases of dyspnea in patients with NSCLC to assess for cancer progression versus opportunistic infections.[21]

6. What findings would be suggestive of a tyrosine kinase (TNK) inhibitor-induced interstitial lung disease (ILD)?

A definitive diagnosis depends on the rigorous elimination of other potential etiologies. Other possible causes can be ruled out based on clinical criteria. The short interval between the initiation of erlotinib therapy and the onset of symptoms should raise suspicion that these events are related. The onset of symptoms with erlotinib-induced lung injury has been reported as early as 5 days after start of therapy, but has also been reported after 9 months (median 39 days). Symptoms have typically appeared in the first 1 to 2 months of gefitinib treatment. The presence of bilateral diffuse ground-glass opacities on HRCT is a characteristic finding of drug-induced ILD, although it may not be definitive.[21–23]

7. Why might J.T. have been at greater risk for TNK-inhibitor ILD?

TNK-inhibitors gefitinib and erlotinib are rarely associated with the development of ILD. In the data reviewed by the U.S. Food and Drug Administration (FDA), ILD occurred in ≤1% of patients receiving either agent. The global incidence of gefitinib-induced ILD is about 1%, with a higher incidence in Japan (2%). Several smaller studies in Japan have reported incidences ranging from 4% to 6%. Reasons for higher incidences in Japan may be due to genetic differences involving polymorphisms of transporter genes and drug-metabolizing enzyme genes.[24] Risk factors identified for gefitinib-induced ILD are male gender, history of smoking, pre-existing pulmonary fibrosis, or other pulmonary comorbidities and radiotherapy.[24,25]

8. J.T.'s physician decides to treat J.T. for TNK-inhibitor ILD. How should be proceed, and what recovery might be expected for J.T.?

There is no treatment specific to TNK-inhibitor–induced ILD. Although the discontinuation alone of the TNK-inhibitor may result in symptom resolution, corticosteroids can be used to treat respiratory symptoms.[26] The treatment of drug-induced ILD tends to be empirical, and the optimal dose and duration of corticosteroids for the treatment of most ILDs is not known.[21,27] For patients with severe symptoms of drug-induced ILD, high-dose intravenous (IV) methylprednisolone (e.g., 250 mg four times daily for 3 days) is commonly used. The dose is reduced to a maintenance oral dose (e.g., 0.5–1 mg/kg/day) for several weeks before a gradual dose reduction.[21,29] One of many suggested regimens for the tapering of oral corticosteroids (not specific to ILD treatment) recommends decreasing by ≤2.5 mg prednisone equivalents (e.g., 2 mg methylprednisolone) every 1 to 2 weeks.[28] For less severe symptoms, initiation with oral methylprednisolone (1 mg/kg/day or 60 mg/day) is commonly used to treat drug-induced ILD.[21]

In a retrospective review of four patients diagnosed with gefitinib-induced ILD, all patients discontinued gefitinib and responded favorably to IV methylprednisolone up to 1 g/day. Therapy was reduced to oral maintenance doses of 20 mg to 30 mg/day of oral prednisone.[24] Two case reports of erlotinib-induced ILD reported response to oral steroids (doses not specified). A third case report described the successful resolution of symptoms following a course of 250 mg of IV methylprednisolone given every 6 hours for 3 days, followed by oral prednisone 60 mg daily, with tapering of dose after 2 weeks. Several of these patients also required supplemental oxygen.[23,29,30] Not all reported cases of TNK-inhibitor–induced ILD have noted successful resolution with corticosteroid therapy.[24] Although immunosuppressive agents (azathioprine and cyclophosphamide 1–2 mg/kg/day) with or without corticosteroids have been tried in the treatment of ILDs with variable success, their role remains to be determined.[27] Prognosis can vary significantly from complete resolution to death. Cessation of therapy can result in spontaneous resolution after 2 weeks, or the patient may respond to corticosteroid therapy. If diagnosed early, prognosis with treatment is good. However, permanent and irreversible loss of lung function may result once fibrosis has occurred. Some patients may require supplemental oxygen.[29] Gefitinib-induced ILD has been associated with high mortality rates (i.e., one-third in one report and 40% in another small study).[23,26,31]

Based on available evidence from case reports, J.T.'s physician decided to discontinue erlotinib and administer IV methylprednisolone 250 mg every 6 hours for 3 days. Thereafter, oral prednisone 60 mg daily was given for 2 weeks, with rapid reduction of lung opacities. Dosage was then tapered.

AMIODARONE-INDUCED PULMONARY TOXICITY

9. R.W., a 55-year-old man admitted with a 5-day history of fatigue, exertional dyspnea, and tachypnea, reports that his symptoms have progressively worsened to the point at which he can no longer walk his dog around the neighborhood without feeling "out of breath." He denies experiencing coughing or chest pain. He has a medical history of recurrent ventricular tachycardia and a 10-year history of hypertension controlled with benazepril. Physical examination reveals a tachypneic, tired-looking man with no signs of congestive heart failure evident on physical examination. Diffuse inspiratory crackles are audible on lung auscultation. His blood pressure and temperature are unremarkable. A chest radiograph shows patchy interstitial infiltrates, and HRCT reveals diffuse ground-glass opacities. BAL reveals the appearance of foamy alveolar macrophages and lamellated inclusion bodies. All laboratory tests are within normal limits, except for an elevated ESR. His medications on admission include amiodarone 400 mg every day (QD; initiated 12 months previously) and benazepril 40 mg QD. What signs and symptoms are consistent with a diagnosis of amiodarone-induced pulmonary toxicity in R.W.?

Amiodarone-induced pulmonary toxicity (APT) is one of the leading causes of amiodarone discontinuation. The estimated risks of APT from clinical trials range from 1% to 5%; however, risk appears to be linked to indexes of exposure (a composite of daily dosage and duration of treatment).[2,26] APT can appear within a few days following an initial loading dose or after more than a decade of treatment, with an average onset of 18 to 24 months into treatment. APT is not a single clinical entity and can present as various patterns of pulmonary toxicity, including interstitial pneumonitis, organizing pneumonia, ARDS, pulmonary nodules, and pulmonary fibrosis. Patients commonly present with an insidious progression of symptoms. Fatigue and progressive dyspnea often present for several weeks to months prior to diagnosis. Nonproductive cough, pleuritic chest pain, crackles, weight loss, and hypoalbuminemia can also be present. APT is characterized by alveolar, interstitial, or mixed alveolar interstitial shadows on imaging, and commonly presents with an asymmetric pattern of involvement (in contrast to other drug-induced pulmonary disorders). Differential diagnosis includes left ventricular dysfunction, pulmonary infarction, bronchoalveolar carcinoma or lymphoma, and pulmonary toxicity caused by other commonly prescribed cardiovascular drugs. A thorough physical examination is vital to exclude a diagnosis of congestive heart failure because this population is at high risk for this disorder.[2,32,33]

The earliest sign of APT is typically a precipitous decrease in DLCO. However, this finding alone does not establish a diagnosis. Conversely, a lack of clinically meaningful APT is indicated by the presence of a stable diffusing capacity. Leukocytosis, increased circulating lactate dehydrogenase levels, and an elevated ESR are often noted in patients with APT. Histologic appearances of the lung include septal thickening; interstitial edema; nonspecific inflammation; fibrosis; and lipids within the interstitial, endothelial cells, and alveolar spaces. A large number of free foamy intra-alveolar macrophages support a diagnosis of APT. The role of BAL in the diagnosis of APT is controversial, as a wide range of abnormalities can be found in the BAL of patients with APT. Foam cells with lamellar inclusions in BAL of patients chronically exposed to amiodarone is a routine finding, not necessarily indicative of drug toxicity. However, the diagnosis of classic APT is unlikely in the absence of foam cells. R.W.'s pulmonary complaints, radiographic findings, elevated ESR, and BAL results are all consistent with a diagnosis of APT.[2,32,33]

10. What are risk factors that predispose patients to developing amiodarone-induced pulmonary toxicity?

Risk factors include a higher drug dosage and longer duration of therapy. Prevalence increases from 0.1% to 0.5% with doses up to 200 mg/day to 5% to 15% with doses up to 500 mg/day, and up to 50% with doses of 1,200 mg/day. A review of pulmonary toxicity associated with low-dose amiodarone reported the average age of affected patients was 77 years; the elderly may be at higher risk for APT. Other risk factors include pre-existing lung disease, male gender, and exposure to high concentrations of oxygen, as during surgical procedures.[2,32] R.W.'s overall exposure to amiodarone (dose and duration) may have increased his risk of developing pulmonary toxicity.[2,32,33]

11. What is the likely mechanism of APT in R.W.?

During chronic therapy, amiodarone and its metabolite desethyl-amiodarone (DEAm) accumulate extensively in the tissue of the lung, as well as liver, skin, thyroid, and eye. At therapeutic serum concentrations, both agents are toxic to lung cells, and this toxicity is likely increased by the 100-fold and 500-fold concentration ratio of amiodarone and DEAm in lung tissue. The localization of amiodarone and DEAm, respectively, in cell lysosomes leads to blockage of the turnover of endogenous phospholipids, which then also accumulate in the lung and lead to the characteristic finding of foamy lipid-laden macrophages in BAL or lung tissue of patients receiving chronic amiodarone therapy. Efflux from tissues is slow, and significant amounts of both compounds have been found in the lungs of patients on autopsy 1 year after treatment cessation.[2,32,33]

12. How should R.W. be managed?

Due to the persistence of significant levels of amiodarone and DEAm in lung tissues, the sole withdrawal of amiodarone may not result in improvements in symptoms or imaging. Patients showing substantial involvement on imaging or hypoxemia should be given corticosteroids to try to hasten recovery and possibly minimize the likelihood of lung fibrosis. Continued exposure to amiodarone after discontinuation of the drug necessitates the administration of corticosteroid therapy for extended periods of time to prevent recurrences of symptoms during tapering, which have been reported up to 8 months after the discontinuation of amiodarone. Recurrences may be more severe than the initial episode of APT and may lead to respiratory failure or death. Six months, and more often 1 year, is a reasonable estimate for duration of corticosteroid therapy. Although no data from controlled studies are available, accumulated clinical evidence supports the use of corticosteroids when there are potentially life-threatening signs due to APT. Good data on the dosing and duration of corticosteroid therapy are lacking. However, one suggested regimen is to initiate with a sufficient dosage (e.g., 0.75–1 mg/kg of oral prednisolone or equivalent, or 40–60 mg daily) and maintain pending clinical and radiographic response.[32,34,35] The long-term use of corticosteroids requires monitoring for adverse effects, including opportunistic infections. Following tapering over at least 2 to 6 months and discontinuation of corticosteroid therapy, patients should be monitored for recurrence of APT.[2,32,33,35]

Clinical symptoms may resolve within 2 to 4 weeks; however, chest radiographic findings usually clear over 3 months or more. In some cases, pulmonary toxicity may actually progress before it begins to resolve. However, there is a 10% mortality rate from APT, which increases to 21% to 33% for patients admitted to the hospital for amiodarone pneumonitis. The mortality rate is 50% for those who develop ARDS, even if the drug is discontinued and IV corticosteroid therapy is given.[2,32,33] The routine use of corticosteroids in patients with persistent ARDS (>14 days) is currently not recommended, although the place of corticosteroid therapy in the treatment of acute ARDS remains controversial.[36,37] Other pharmacotherapies (e.g., beta-adrenergic agonists, prostaglandin E1, indomethacin) have not shown any survival benefit.[37]

It was decided that R.W. would likely respond to the discontinuation of amiodarone, followed by treatment with oral corticosteroids. He was started on 40 mg of prednisone with radiologic improvement noted after 2 weeks. The prednisone was then tapered gradually over 6 months. Sotalol treatment was initiated to address R.W.'s ventricular tachycardia.

13. What steps could possibly lead to the prevention or earlier detection of APT?

Given the potential for severe consequences of APT, the early detection of the APT is desirable. However, it has not been proved that earlier diagnosis necessarily improves prognosis. There are currently no evidence-based standards for screening for APT in patients receiving amiodarone. Candidates for amiodarone therapy should be carefully selected, and amiodarone should be titrated to the lowest possible effective dose. The 2007 Heart Rhythm Society guide for clinicians treating patients with amiodarone recommends that chest x-ray and pulmonary function tests, including DLCO, be obtained at baseline and on clinical suspicion of pulmonary toxicity. A pulmonologist should be consulted for patients with abnormal chest x-ray, abnormal pulmonary function test, or unexplained new cough or dyspnea.[34] The optimal frequency of monitoring has not been determined; however, more frequent monitoring of pulmonary function and/or imaging every 3 to 6 months should be undertaken in patients with the greatest risk of developing APT (e.g., those with poor lung function or previous pneumonectomy). Although yearly serial pulmonary function testing in patients receiving conventional doses of amiodarone is likely unrewarding because APT is uncommon in this subset of patients, such patients should be instructed to contact their physicians if they experience symptoms indicative of pulmonary toxicity (e.g., cough, shortness of breath).[32,38]

GEMCITABINE-INDUCED PULMONARY TOXICITY

14. C.B. is a 66-year-old man with NSCLC. One year previously, he had a right upper lobe (RUL) wedge resection and radiation therapy. He now presents with a large local recurrence and enlarged bilateral mediastinal lymph nodes. Weekly IV gemcitabine treatment is initiated. He receives gemcitabine 1 g/m^2 on days 1, 8, and 15, followed by a 2-week rest period. After the second cycle, he presents to the emergency department with complaints of dyspnea on exertion. Physical examination reveals that he has significant peripheral edema, and his vital signs are notable for an O_2 saturation of 82% on room air. C.B. has maintained good room air saturations at all times, despite a 100 pack-year history of smoking and a history of RUL wedge resection. A chest radiograph shows increased interstitial markings. C.B. is admitted to the hospital for further workup of his dyspnea.

How do patients with gemcitabine-induced pulmonary toxicity usually present?

Different terms have been used to describe gemcitabine-associated lung injuries with similar presentations (i.e., capillary leak syndrome, noncardiogenic pulmonary edema, interstitial pneumonitis, acute pneumonitis, ARDS, acute pulmonary toxicity, or acute lung injury). Mild dyspnea occurs in 25% of patients receiving gemcitabine, but there have been only occasional reports of severe lung injury from initial clinical trials or reports to the FDA or manufacturer. Although most cases of gemcitabine-induced pulmonary toxicity are mild and self-limiting, severe lung injury (22%–42%) was recently reported as the dose-limiting toxicity when combination gemcitabine regimens were administered to patients with Hodgkin disease.[41] The most common clinical findings in a review of severe gemcitabine-associated lung injury reports were dyspnea (70%), fever (35%), pulmonary infiltrates (22%), cough (19%), respiratory distress (18%), and hypoxia (14%). The median time to diagnosis was 48 days (range, 1–529 days). Pulmonary toxicity may develop with the first dose of gemcitabine, but more commonly develops after multiple cycles; however, it is not clear whether this is dose related.[39–42]

15. How is gemcitabine-induced pulmonary toxicity diagnosed?

As with other drug-induced pulmonary toxicities, this is a diagnosis of exclusion. Temporal association is important, as is ruling out other causes such as infection, metabolic causes, cardiac compromise, lymphangitic spread, and disease progression. Typical radiologic features include diffuse interstitial and alveolar changes on chest radiograph. Computed tomography shows a ground-glass appearance in conjunction with increased interstitial markings.[42]

16. What is the mechanism of gemcitabine-induced pulmonary toxicity?

The mechanism of gemcitabine-induced lung toxicity is unknown. Cytarabine, another pyrimidine analog, has been known to cause a syndrome of noncardiogenic pulmonary edema in 13% to 28% of patients and develops after treatment with conventional and high-dose regimens. Histopathological studies of these patients show interstitial and intra-alveolar proteinaceous edema consistent with ARDS. It is postulated that damage to the capillary endothelial cells causes the leakage of the fluid resulting in pulmonary edema. In view of the structural and metabolic similarities between the two drugs, it is likely that they share the same mechanism of pulmonary injury.[42]

17. What risk factors that predispose C.B. to the development of gemcitabine-associated pulmonary toxicity?

There is a subset of patients that appears to be more prone to developing pulmonary symptoms, including men, age older than 65 years, significant smoking history, concomitant administration of bleomycin, chemotherapeutic agents known to release cytokine mediators of inflammation (e.g., paclitaxel, docetaxel, or vinorelbine), concomitant or prior radiotherapy, and primary lung neoplasm. C.B. has four such risk factors, including age, a 100 pack-year smoking history, and NSCLC treated with radiation therapy.[39,41,42]

18. How should C.B. be managed?

It has been reported that gemcitabine-associated pulmonary toxicity is generally self-limiting on discontinuation and is often responsive to glucocorticoid therapy alone or plus a diuretic. However, fatal outcomes have resulted from high-risk combinations of chemotherapeutic agents. Gemcitabine should be discontinued, and C.B. should be started on oral corticosteroid therapy (prednisone 40–100 mg has been used) and low-dose furosemide (20–40 mg has been used).[39,41,42]

ACKNOWLEDGMENTS

We want to thank Randolph H. Noble, MD, FCCP, and Mary E. White, MLS, for their invaluable assistance in the preparation of this chapter.

REFERENCES

1. Higenbottam T et al. Understanding the mechanisms of drug-associated interstitial lung disease. *Br J Cancer* 2004;91(Suppl 2):S31.
2. Camus P et al. Drug-induced and iatrogenic infiltrative lung disease. *Clin Chest Med* 2004;25:479.
3. Lee-Chiong T Jr, Matthay RA. Drug-induced pulmonary edema and acute respiratory distress syndrome. *Clin Chest Med* 2004;25:95.
4. Foucher P, Camus P. *Pneumotox On Line: The Drug-induced Lung Diseases* Available at http://pneumotox.com. Accessed June 20, 2008.
5. Epler GR. Drug-induced bronchiolitis obliterans organizing pneumonia. *Clin Chest Med* 2004;25:89.
6. Huggins T, Sahn S. Drug-induced pleural disease. *Clin Chest Med* 2004;25:141.
7. Kelly HW. Pulmonary fibrosis/interstitial pneumonitis. In: Tinsdale J et al., eds. *Drug Induced Diseases*. Bethesda, MD: American Society of Health-System Pharmacists; 2005:241.
8. Raissy H. Asthma and bronchospasm. In: Tinsdale J et al., eds. *Drug-Induced Diseases*. Bethesda, MD: American Society of Health-System Pharmacists; 2005:249.
9. Babu KS, Marshall BG. Drug-induced airway diseases. *Clin Chest Med* 2004;25:113.
10. Meduri G et al. Methylprednisolone infusion in early severe ARDS: results of a randomized controlled trial. *Chest* 2007;131:954.
11. Annane D. Glucocorticoids for ARDS just do it! *Chest* 2007;131:945.
12. Steinberg KP et al. Efficacy and safety of corticosteroids for persistent acute respiratory distress syndrome. *N Engl J Med* 2006;354:1671.
13. National Comprehensive Cancer Network (NCCN). NCCN Clinical Practice Guidelines in Oncology: Testicular Cancer V.2.2008. Available at: http://www.nccn.org/professionals/physician_gls/PDF/testicular.pdf.page 11. Accessed February 18, 2008.
14. Chu E et al., eds. *Physicians' Cancer Chemotherapy Drug Manual*. Boston: Jones and Barlett; 2004.
15. Frerk C. With bleomycin, that's too much oxygen. *Eur J Anaesthesiol* 2006;24:205.
16. O'Sullivan J et al. Predicting the risk of bleomycin lung toxicity in patients with germ-cell tumours. *Ann Oncol* 2003;14:91.
17. Uzel I et al. Delayed onset bleomycin-induced pneumonitis. *Urology* 2005;66:195.
18. National Cancer Institute. Testicular Cancer Treatment (PDQ). Health Professional Version. Available at: http://www.cancer.gov/cancertopics/pdf/treatment/testicular/HealthProfessional/page2. Accessed February 18, 2008.
19. Roizen M, Fleisher L. *Anesthetic implications of concurrent diseases*. In: Miller R, ed. *Miller's Anesthesia 6th ed.* Philadelphia, PA: Elsevier, Churchill Livingstone; 2005.
20. Ben-Noun L. Drug-induced respiratory disorders. *Drug Saf* 2000;23:143.
21. Muller NL et al. Diagnosis and management of drug-associated interstitial lung disease. *Br J Cancer* 2004;91(Suppl 2):S24.
22. *Tarceva (erlotinib) Tablet Prescribing Information*. Melville, NY. OSI Pharmaceuticals, Inc. March 2007.
23. Sandler AB. Nondermatologic adverse events associated with anti-EGFR therapy. *Oncology (Hungtingt)* 2006;20(5 Suppl 2):35.
24. Kataoka K et al. Interstitial lung disease associated with gefitinib. *Respir Med* 2006;100:698.
25. Tammaro K et al. Interstitial lung disease following erlotinib (Tarceva) in a patient who previously tolerated gefitinib (Iressa). *J Oncol Pharm Pract* 2005;11:127.
26. Kitajima H et al. Gefitinib-induced interstitial lung disease showing improvement after cessation: disassociation of serum markers. *Respirology* 2006;11:217.
27. King T. *Interstitial lung disease*. In: Kasper D et al., eds. *Harrison's Principles of Internal Medicine. 16th ed.* New York, NY: McGraw-Hill; 2005: 1557.
28. *AHFS Drug Information*. Bethesda, MD: American Society of Health-system Pharmacists, Inc.; 2008:3088.
29. Vahid B et al. Erlotinib-associated acute pneumonitis: report of two cases. *Can Respir J* 2007;14:167.
30. Bach J et al. Pulmonary fibrosis in a patient treated with erlotinib. *Onkologie* 2006;29:342.
31. Tsuboi M, Le CT. Interstitial lung disease in patients with non-small-cell lung cancer treated with epidermal growth factor receptor inhibitors. *Med Oncol* 2006;23.

32. Camus P et al. Amiodarone pulmonary toxicity. *Clin Chest Med* 2004;25:65.
33. Wang T et al. An unintended consequence: fatal amiodarone pulmonary toxicity in an older woman. *J Am Med Dir Assoc* 2006;7:510.
34. Goldschlager N et al. A practical guide for clinicians who treat patients with amiodarone: 2007. *Heart Rhythm* 2007;4:1250.
35. Silva C et al. The importance of amiodarone pulmonary toxicity in the differential diagnosis of a patient with dyspnea awaiting a heart transplant. *Arq Bras Cardiol* 2006;87:e4.
36. National Heart, Lung, and Blood Institute Acute Respiratory Distress Syndrome (ARDS) Clinical Trials Network. Efficacy and safety of corticosteroids for persistent acute respiratory distress syndrome. *N Engl J Med* 2006;354:1671.
37. Leaver SK, Evans TW. Acute respiratory distress syndrome. *BMJ* 2007;335:389.
38. Amiodarone. Drugdex® Evaluations. Micromedex® Healthcare Series. Thomson Healthcare 1974–2008. http://www.thomsonhc.com Accessed February 2008.
39. Joerger M et al. Gemcitabine-related pulmonary toxicity. *Swiss Med Wkly* 2002;132:17.
40. Kouroussis C et al. High incidence of pulmonary toxicity of weekly docetaxel and gemcitabine in patients with non-small cell lung cancer: results of a dose-finding study. *Lung Cancer* 2004;44:363.
41. Belknap S et al. Clinical features and correlates of gemcitabine-associated lung injury. *Cancer* 2006;106:2051.
42. Gupta N et al. Gemcitabine-induced pulmonary toxicity: case report and review of the literature. *Am J Clin Oncol* 2002;25:96.
43. Raissy HH et al. Drug-induced pulmonary diseases. In: DiPiro JT et al., eds. *Pharmacotherapy: A Pathophysiologic Approach*. New York: McGraw-Hill; 2005:577.
44. Lima MT, Marshall GD. Diseases of allergy: anaphylaxis and serum sickness. In: Rakel RE, Bope ET, eds. *Conn's Current Therapy 2006*. Philadelphia: Elsevier Saunders; 2006:915.
45. Adenosine. Drugdex® Evaluations. Micromedex Healthcare Series. Thomson Healthcare 1974–2008. http://www.thomsonhc.com Accessed February 2008.
46. Burki N et al. the pulmonary effects of intravenous adenosine in asthmatic subjects. *Respir Res* 2006;7:139.
47. Collazos J et al. Pulmonary reactions during treatment with amphotericin B: review of published cases and guidelines for management. *Clin Infect Dis* 2001;33:e75.
48. Lowery MM, Greenberger PA. Amphotericin-induced stridor: a review of stridor, amphotericin preparations, and their immunoregulatory effects. *Ann Allergy Asthma Immunol* 2003;91:460.
49. Rex JH, Stevens DA. Systemic antifungal agents. In: Mandell GL et al., eds. *Mandell, Douglas, and Bennett's Principles and Practice of Infectious Diseases*. Philadelphia: Elsevier Churchill Livingstone; 2005:502.
50. Dicipinigaitis PV. Angiotensin-converting enzyme inhibitor-induced cough: ACCP evidence-based clinical practice guidelines. *Chest* 2006;129 (1 Suppl):169S.
51. Solensky R. Drug desensitization. *Immunol Allergy Clin North Am* 2004;24:425.
52. Bryant R. Use of a protocol to minimize hypersensitivity reactions with asparaginase administration. *J Intraven Nurs* 2001;24:169.
53. Zanotti K, Markham M. Prevention and management of antineoplastic-induced hypersensitivity reactions. *Drug Saf* 2001;24:767.
54. *Taxol (paclitaxel) Prescribing Information*. Princeton, NJ: Bristol-Myers Squibb; July 2007.
55. Salpeter S et al. Cardioselective beta-blockers for chronic obstructive pulmonary disease. *Cochrane Database of Systematic Reviews* 2005, Issue 4. Art No.:CD003566. DIO:10.1002/14651858. CD003566.pub2.
56. Covar R et al. Medications as asthma triggers. *Immunol Allergy Clin North Am* 2005;25:169.
57. Dawson P. Adverse reactions to intravascular contrast agents. *BMJ* 2006;333:663.
58. Tramer MR et al. Pharmacological prevention of serious anaphylactic reactions due to iodinated contrast media: systematic review. *BMJ* 2006;333:675.
59. Pandey C et al. Intravenous lidocaine suppresses fentanyl-induced coughing: a double-blind, prospective, randomized placebo-controlled study. *Anesth Analg* 2004;99:1696.
60. Yeh C et al. Premedication with intravenous low-dose ketamine suppresses fentanyl-induced cough. *J Clin Anesth* 2007;19:53.
61. Toronto Aerosolized Pentamidine Study (TAPS) Group. Acute pulmonary effects of aerosolized pentamidine: a randomized controlled study. *Chest* 1990;96:907.
62. Briasoulis E, Pavlidis N. Noncardiogenic pulmonary edema: an unusual and serious complication of anticancer therapy. *Oncologist* 2001;6:153.
63. Matthay M, Martin T. *Pulmonary edema and acute lung injury*. In: Mason RJ et al., eds. *Mason: Murray & Nadel's Textbook of Respiratory Medicine. 4th ed.* Philadelphia, PA: Elsevier, 2005.
64. Samol JM, Lambers DS. Magnesium sulfate tocolysis and pulmonary edema: the drug or the vehicle? *Am J Obstet Gynecol* 2005;192:1430.
65. Salluh J, Soares M. Methylprednisolone infusion in early severe ARDS. It is pretty, but is it art? *Chest* 2007;132:1096.
66. Limper AH. *Drug-induced pulmonary disease*. In: Mason RJ et al., eds. *Mason: Murray & Nadel's Textbook of Respiratory Medicine*. Philadelphia, PA: Elsevier Saunders, 2005.
67. Knowles SR et al. Hydrochlorothiazide-induced noncardiogenic pulmonary edema: an under recognized yet serious adverse drug reaction. *Pharmacotherapy* 2005;25:1258
68. van Dorp E. Naloxone treatment in opioid addiction: the risks and benefits. *Expert Opin Drug Metab Toxicol* 2006;6:125.
69. Wolff AJ, O'Donnell AE. Pulmonary effects of illicit drug use. *Clin Chest Med* 2004;25:203.
70. McGoon M et al. Screening, early detection, and diagnosis of pulmonary arterial hypertension: ACCP evidence-based clinical practice guidelines. *Chest* 2004;126(Suppl 1):14S.
71. Chin KM et al. Is methamphetamine use associated with idiopathic pulmonary arterial hypertension? *Chest* 2006;130:1657.
72. Wooltorton E. Persistent pulmonary hypertension of the newborn and maternal use of SSRIs. *CMAJ* 2006;174:1555.
73. Takafuji S, Nakagawa T. Drug-induced pulmonary disorders. *Intern Med* 2004;43:169.
74. Rube CE et al. Increased expression of proinflammatory cytokines as a cause of lung toxicity after combined treatment with gemcitabine and thoracic irradiation. *Radiother Oncol* 2004;72:231.
75. Lateef O et al. Methotrexate pulmonary toxicity. *Expert Opin Drug Saf* 2005;4:723.
76. Miyata M et al. Detection and monitoring of methotrexate-associated lung injury using serum markers KL-6 and SP-D in rheumatoid arthritis. *Intern Med* 2002;41:467.
77. Morath C et al. Four cases of sirolimus-associated interstitial pneumonitis: identification of risk factors. *Transplant Proc* 2007;39:99.
78. Howell DC et al. Role of thrombin and its major cellular receptor, protease-activated receptor-1, in pulmonary fibrosis. *Biochem Soc Trans* 2002;30:211.
79. Machtay M. *Pulmonary Complications of Anticancer Treatment*. In: Abeloff M et al., eds. *Abeloff: Clinical Oncology. 3rd ed.* Philadelphia, PA: Elsevier Churchill Livingstone; 2004.
80. Bhagat R et al. Amiodarone and cyclophosphamide: potential for enhanced lung toxicity. *Bone Marrow Transplant* 2001;27:1109.
81. Kharabsheh S et al. Fatal pulmonary toxicity occurring within two weeks of initiation of amiodarone. *Am J Cardiol* 2002; 89:896.
82. Okayasu K et al. Amiodarone pulmonary toxicity: a patient with three recurrences of pulmonary toxicity and consideration of the probable risk for relapse. *Intern Med* 2006;45:1303.
83. Liesching T, O'Brien A. Dyspnea, chest pain, and cough: the lurking culprit. *Postgrad Med* 2002; 112:19.
84. King T. *Interstitial Lung Diseases*. In: Beers M et al., eds. *The Merck Manual of Diagnosis and Therapy*. Whitehouse Station, NJ: Merck Research Station Laboratories, 2006.
85. Jamaleddine G et al. Leukotriene antagonists and the Churg-Strauss syndrome. *Semin Arthritis Rheum* 2002;31:218.
86. Solomon J, Schwarz M. Drug-, toxin-, and radiation therapy-induced eosinophilic pneumonia. *Semin Respir Crit Care Med* 2006;27:192.
87. Oddo M et al. Relapsing acute respiratory failure induced by minocycline. *Chest* 2003;123:2146.
88. Chroneou A et al. Meloxicam-induced pulmonary infiltrates with eosinophilia: a case report. *Rheumatology (Oxford)* 2003;42:1112.
89. Lee Y et al. Ibuprofen-induced eosinophilic pneumonia. *Hosp Med* 2004;65:241.
90. Perng D et al. Pulmonary infiltrates with eosinophilia induced by nimesulide in an asthmatic patients. *Respiration* 2005;72:651.
91. Broaddus C, Light R. Pleural effusion. In: Mason R et al., eds. *Murray & Nadel's Textbook of Respiratory Medicine*. 4th ed. Philadelphia: Elsevier; 2005.
92. Le-Quang B et al. Dantrolene and pleural effusion: case report and review of literature. *Spinal Cord* 2004;42:317.
93. Schwarz M, Fontenot A. Drug-induced diffuse alveolar hemorrhage syndromes and vasculitis. *Clin Chest Med* 2004;25:133.
94. Bohan K, Mansuri T. Anticonvulsant hypersensitivity syndrome: implications for pharmaceutical care. *Pharmacotherapy* 2007;27:1425.
95. *Exubera (insulin human [rDNA origin] Inhalation Powder Prescribing Information*. New York, NY. Pfizer Labs; May 2008.
96. Skyler J et al. Two-year safety and efficacy of inhaled human insulin (Exubura) in adult patients with type 1 diabetes. *Diabetes Care* 2007;30: 579.
97. Exubera website. Available at: http://www.exubera.com/content/con_index.jsp?setShowOn=../content/con_index.jsp&setShowHighlightOn=../content/con_index.jsp Accessed February 2008.
98. Pentamidine. Drugdex® Evaluations. Micromedex® Healthcare Series. Thomson Healthcare 1974–2008. http://www.thomsonhc.com. Accessed February 2008.
99. Bleumink GS et al. Pergolide-induced pleuropulmonary fibrosis. *Clin Neuropharmacol* 2002;25: 290.
100. Kvernmo T et al. A review of the receptor-binding and pharmacokinetic properties of dopamine agonists. *Clin Ther* 2006;28:1065.
101. FDA Public Health Advisory; Pergolide (marketed as Permax), October 6, 2007. http://www.fda.gov/cder/drug/advisory/pergolide.htm. Accessed February 2008.
102. Badesch DB et al. Medical therapy for pulmonary arterial hypertension: ACCP evidence-based clinical practice guidelines. *Chest* 2004;126:35.
103. Marzouk K et al. Interferon-induced granulomatous lung disease. *Curr Opin Pulm Med* 2004;10:435.

GASTROINTESTINAL DISORDERS

CHAPTER 26

Upper Gastrointestinal Disorders

Randolph V. Fugit and Rosemary R. Berardi

Upper gastrointestinal (GI) disorders include a wide spectrum of maladies that range in importance from simple discomfort to life-threatening illness and include dyspepsia, peptic ulcer disease (PUD), gastroesophageal reflux disease (GERD), and upper GI bleeding. The majority of upper GI disorders are acid-related diseases in which gastric acid plays an important role in their development, progression, and treatment. In the United States, over 40 billion dollars is spent yearly treating GI disorders, with over 10 billion dollars of this amount spent on proton pump inhibitors (PPIs), a primary pharmacotherapeutic option used to reduce gastric acid secretion.[1,2] These diseases place a substantial burden on both patients and the health care system. It has been estimated that in 2002, over 5.5 million outpatient clinic visits were for patients evaluated for a diagnosis of GERD, and an additional 2.3 million were seen for dyspepsia or gastritis complaints.[1] Between 250,000 and 300,000 patients are hospitalized each year for upper GI bleeding, and despite numerous advances in diagnostic techniques and management strategies, mortality rates of approximately 9% are reported with more than 2.5 billion dollars spent each year to manage these patients.[3–6]

The introductory section of this chapter includes a brief discussion of the physiology of the upper GI tract and the pharmacotherapy of drugs used to treat upper GI disorders. This section highlights the most important aspects associated with these topics. A more in-depth and comprehensive review can be found in GI textbooks or journal articles that discuss upper GI physiology and the pharmacology, pharmacokinetics, interactions, and side effects of the drugs.

PHYSIOLOGY OF THE UPPER GASTROINTESTINAL TRACT

The upper GI tract consists of the mouth, esophagus, stomach, and the duodenum (Fig. 26-1). Ingested food or liquids pass from the mouth through the esophagus and into the stomach. As these substances enter into the esophagus, the lower esophageal sphincter (LES), an area of smooth muscle near the distal end of the esophagus, relaxes to allow their entry into the stomach. The LES usually remains contracted to prevent the reflux of gastric contents into the esophagus. However, peristaltic contractions of the esophageal muscles allows the LES to remain open until all food has entered the stomach.[7] Although the LES is the primary barrier for the prevention of gastric refluxate entering the esophagus, healthy individuals reflux throughout the day and night without clinical consequences.[8]

The stomach consists of three distinct anatomical regions, each of which possesses specialized functional processes (Fig. 26-1). The cardia, which is the uppermost portion of the stomach at the junction between the esophagus and stomach, is responsible for the mucus secretion that protects against the acid milieu of the stomach. The body, which makes up the majority of the surface area (80%–90%) of the stomach, contains the parietal cells, which are responsible for gastric acid and intrinsic factor (required for vitamin B_{12} absorption) secretion. The body also contains the peptic (chief) cells, which secrete pepsinogen (a precursor to pepsin). Pepsinogen, under acidic conditions in the stomach, is converted to pepsin (a proteolytic enzyme), which is responsible for breaking down protein. The antrum makes up the final 10% to 20% of the stomach. It contains the G cells, which secrete the hormone gastrin, which through a feedback mechanism stimulates acid secretion by the parietal cell. The final portion of the upper GI tract is the duodenum, which begins just after the pylorus and extends to ligament of Trietz. At this point, the jejunum begins the first portion of the lower GI tract.

The parietal cell is responsible for secreting gastric acid (Fig. 26-2). Three stimuli (neurologic, physical, and hormonal) trigger the parietal cell to secrete acid. Neurologic impulses, from the central nervous system (CNS) and initiated by the sight, smell, and taste of food, travel along cholinergic pathways to stimulate the release of acetylcholine, which arrives via nerve endings and activates the muscarinic receptor on the parietal cell.[9] Ingested food causes gastric distention, which triggers the release of acetylcholine and also stimulates G cells within the antrum to produce gastrin. Elevated intragastric pH also stimulates the production of gastrin. Gastrin works via a feedback mechanism which, although produced in response to elevated pH, can be inhibited by low gastric pH. The stomach is protected from overproduction of gastric acid by the release of somatostatin from antral D cells, which signal the G cell to

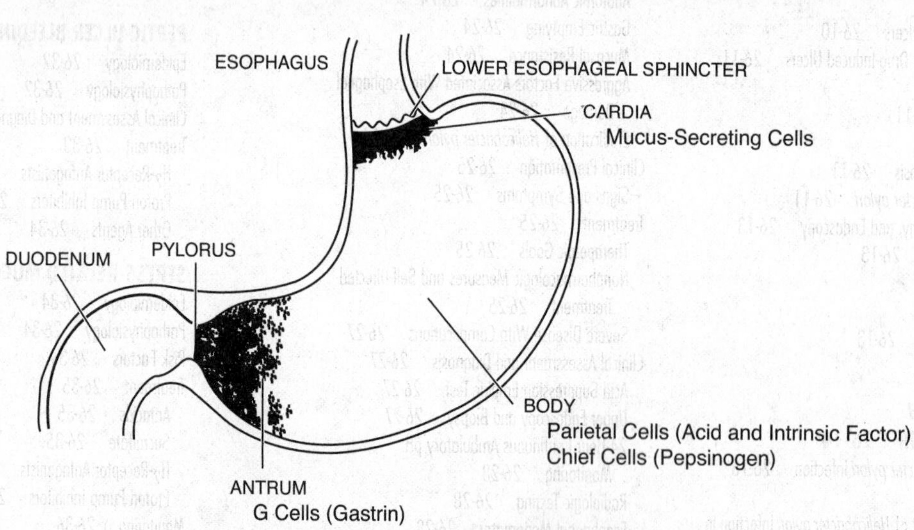

FIGURE 26-1 Gastrointestinal anatomic regions.

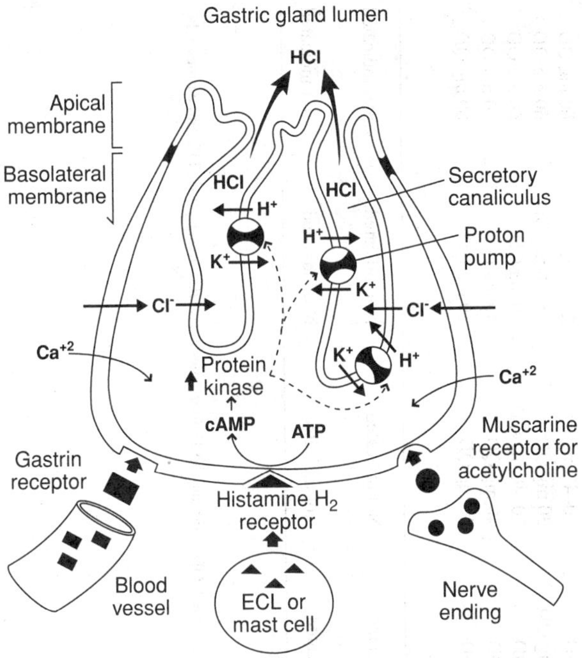

FIGURE 26-2 Parietal cell. *Source:* Used with permission from the APhA Special Report "The Use of Proton Pump Inhibitors in Acid-Peptic Disorders," copyright 1999 by the American Pharmaceutical Association.

stop producing gastrin.[10] Gastrin enters the blood and arrives at the parietal cell, where it binds to the gastrin receptor. Acetylcholine and gastrin promote the release of histamine from the mast cell or enterochromaffinlike (ECL) cells, which then bind to the histamine H_2-receptor on the parietal cell. Histamine release is associated with both postprandial and nocturnal acid secretion. The gastrin, histamine H_2, and muscarinic receptors are located on the basolateral membrane of the parietal cell (Fig. 26-2). Binding of any of these receptors leads to a cascade of events that stimulates gastric acid secretion. Calcium influxes into the parietal cell, leading to increased intracellular levels of calcium. Levels of cyclic adenosine monophosphate (cAMP) also increase and activate intracellular protein phosphokinases. This activates the hydrogen-potassium adenosine triphosphatase (H^+/K^+-ATPase) or proton pump to move into position in the secretory canaliculus located in the apical membrane of the parietal cell. The proton pump is an ion transport pathway that transports hydrogen ions out of the cytoplasm and into the secretory canaliculus, where they are exchanged for potassium ions that enter the parietal cell via the opposite ion channel. In the secretory canaliculus, the hydrogen ion combines with chloride from the blood to form hydrochloric acid (HCl), which is then released from the secretory canaliculus into the gastric acid lumen.[11] The proton pump is the final common pathway for gastric acid secretion.[9,11]

PHARMACOTHERAPY OF DRUGS USED TO TREAT ACID-RELATED DISORDERS

The following section briefly reviews the pharmacotherapy of drugs used to treat acid-related disorders (Table 26-1). Their therapeutic use is discussed under each specific GI disorder.

Antacids and Alginic Acid

Antacids are widely used to relieve mild and infrequent symptoms associated with acid-related diseases. They act by neutralizing gastric acid and thus increasing intragastric pH.[12] The elevation of intragastric pH is dose dependent and usually requires a substantial dose to raise the intragastric pH above 4 or 5.[12,13] Antacids are very quick acting and modestly elevate intragastric pH within minutes, but their duration of action is short (about 30 minutes on an empty stomach). The duration of action can be extended to 3 hours when given with or within 1 hour after a meal).[12] Antacids are available as individual salts or as combination of salts of magnesium, aluminum, calcium, or sodium. Aluminum- and magnesium-containing salts are also able to bind bile salts.[12] Aluminum salts may enhance mucosal protection by increasing mucosal prostaglandins, stimulating mucus and bicarbonate secretion and enhancing microvascular blood flow. Antacids also inhibit the action of pepsin. These findings suggest that in addition to their neutralizing capacity, antacids have other mechanisms by which they act. This helps to explain their many pharmacotherapeutic benefits.[9,12] A review of specific antacid products and their acid-neutralizing capacity is discussed elsewhere.[12] Antacids can also be combined with alginic acid. Alginic acid, however, is not an acid-neutralizing agent. It acts by forming a viscous solution that floats on top of the gastric contents and theoretically protects the esophageal mucosa from the potent acid refluxate.[14]

Antacids are generally well tolerated. The magnesium-containing antacids may cause a dose-related osmotic diarrhea, but combining it with aluminum salts (which can cause constipation when used alone) can offset this side effect. When higher doses of combination magnesium/aluminum antacids are used, the predominating side effect is diarrhea.[12,15] Small amounts of aluminum and magnesium are absorbed systemically and have the potential to accumulate in patients with renal insufficiency and lead to toxicity. Thus, magnesium-containing antacids should be avoided in patients with a creatinine clearance <30 mL/minute, and chronic use of aluminum-containing antacids in patients with renal failure should be avoided.[12,15] Hypercalcemia has been described in patients taking prolonged courses of large doses of calcium carbonate (>20 g/day in patients with normal renal function and >4 g/day in patients with renal failure).[9,12] High-dose regimens of calcium (4–8 g/day) in combination with alkalinizing agents (sodium bicarbonate) can produce the milk-alkali syndrome (i.e., hypercalcemic nephropathy with alkalosis).[9,12,15] Aluminum-containing antacids (with the exception of aluminum phosphate) binds to dietary phosphate within the GI tract to form insoluble salts that are excreted in feces. High-dose or frequent administration may lead to hypophosphatemia.[9,12,15] Sodium bicarbonate should not be used for long periods of time (especially in the renally impaired patient) because systemic alkalosis can result from the accumulation of bicarbonate. Additionally, the high sodium content (274 mg sodium/g sodium bicarbonate) has been associated with sodium retention and may pose a problem in patients with hypertension, ascites, severe renal dysfunction, or congestive heart failure.[9,12,15]

Antacids may interfere with the absorption of many orally administered drugs (e.g., digoxin, phenytoin, isoniazid, ketoconazole, itraconazole, iron preparations) that require an acidic

Table 26-1 Oral Medications Used to Treat Upper Gastrointestinal Disorders

	Gastric and Duodenal Ulcer Healing	Maintenance of Gastric and Duodenal Ulcer Healing	Reduction of Gastric Ulcer Risk Associated With NSAIDs	Relief of Heartburn and Indigestion (OTC Use)	Relief of GERD Symptoms (Rx Use)	Esophageal Healing[a]	Maintenance of Esophageal Healing[a]	Hypersecretory Diseases[a,b]
H_2-Receptor Antagonists								
Cimetidine	300 mg QID 400 mg BID 800 mg QD	400–800 mg HS	Not indicated	200 mg BID PRN	300 mg QID	400 mg QID 800 mg BID	400–800 mg HS	*a*
Famotidine	20 mg BID 40 mg HS	20–40 mg HS	Not indicated	10 mg BID PRN 20 mg BID PRN	20 mg BID	40 mg BID	20–40 mg BID	*a*
Nizatidine	150 mg BID 300 mg HS	150–300 mg HS	Not indicated	75 mg BID PRN	150 mg BID	300 mg BID	150–300 mg BID	*a*
Ranitidine	150 mg BID 300 mg HS	150–300 mg HS	Not indicated	75 mg BID PRN 150 mg BID PRN	150 mg BID	300 mg BID	150–300 mg BID	*a*
Proton Pump Inhibitors								
Esomeprazole	20–40 mg QD	20 mg QD	20 mg QD	Not indicated	20 mg QD	20–40 mg QD	20 mg QD	60 mg QD
Lansoprazole	15–30 mg QD	15–30 mg QD	15–30 mg QD	Not indicated	15–30 mg QD	30 mg QD	15–30 mg QD	60 mg QD
Omeprazole	20 mg QD	20 mg QD	20 mg QD	20 mg QD[c]	20 mg QD	20–40 mg QD	20 mg QD	60 mg QD
Pantoprazole	40 mg QD	40 mg QD	40 mg QD	Not indicated	20 mg QD	40 mg QD	40 mg QD	80 mg QD
Rabeprazole	20 mg QD	20 mg QD	20 mg QD	Not indicated	20 mg QD	20 mg QD	20 mg QD	60 mg QD
Other Agents								
Sucralfate	1 g QID 2 g BID	Not indicated	Not indicated	Not indicated	Not indicated	Not indicated	Not indicated	Not indicated
Misoprostol	Not indicated	Not indicated	200 mcg TID-QID	Not indicated	Not indicated	Not indicated	Not indicated	Not indicated

[a] Although FDA-labeled for this indication, H_2RAs are not recommended even in higher dosages because they are not as effective as the PPIs.
[b] Initial starting dose; daily dosage must be titrated to gastric acid secretory response.
[c] Duration of treatment should not exceed 14 consecutive days; if needed, repeat 14-day treatment every 4 months.
BID twice a day; GERD, gastroesophageal reflux disease; HS, at bedtime; NSAID, nonsteroidal anti-inflammatory drug; OTC, over-the counter; PRN, as needed; QD, every day; QID, four times a day; Rx, prescription; TID, three times a day.

environment for dissolution and absorption.[12,14,16] This may lead to potential therapeutic failures with these medications. Calcium-, aluminum-, or magnesium-containing antacids can bind to concomitantly administered drugs and interfere with the absorption of drugs that are susceptible to complexation with these salts. Tetracyclines and the fluoroquinolones are susceptible to this interaction, as they bind to divalent and trivalent cations.[15] The bioavailability of ciprofloxacin for example is reduced by >50% when concomitantly administered with an antacid, because aluminum and magnesium ions chelate with the antibiotic to form an insoluble and inactive complex. The administration of ciprofloxacin 2 hours before an antacid increases ciprofloxacin bioavailability more than when administered 2 hours after the antacid.[17] An increase in gastric pH may also result in the premature dissolution and altered absorption of enteric-coated dosage forms as the enteric coating is usually designed to dissolve at a pH >6.0.[16] Urinary alkalinization may result in increased urinary excretion (salicylates) or decreased excretion (amphetamines and quinidine) leading to decreased or increased blood concentrations, respectively.[12,15] The majority of these drug interactions can be avoided by separating the antacid from the interacting drug by a minimum of 2 hours.[15]

H_2-Receptor Antagonists

There are currently four H_2-receptor antagonists (H_2RAs) approved for use in the United States. These include cimetidine, ranitidine, famotidine, and nizatidine. All four agents are available in prescription and over-the-counter (OTC) dosage forms as well as oral and parenteral formulations (nizatidine is not available parenterally in the United States). H_2RAs competitively and selectively inhibit the action of histamine on the H_2 receptors of the parietal cells, thus reducing both basal and stimulated gastric acid secretion (Fig. 26-2). Although the relative antisecretory potency on a milligram-per-milligram basis differs (famotidine has the greatest potency followed by nizatidine, ranitidine, and cimetidine), this is not an important factor, as standard oral dosages of the four H_2RAs have been adjusted accordingly to have an equipotent antisecretory effect (Table 26-1).[18] Oral absorption from the small intestine is rapid, and peak drug concentrations usually are achieved within 1 to 3 hours after administration.[18] The bioavailability is lower for cimetidine, famotidine, and ranitidine because they are absorbed incompletely and undergo first-pass metabolism resulting in 40% to 65% bioavailability. The bioavailability of nizatidine is considered near 100% since this agent does not undergo first-pass metabolism.[9,18,19] Parenteral H_2RAs given by the intravenous (IV) route have 90% to 100% bioavailability. All four drugs are eliminated by a combination of hepatic metabolism, glomerular filtration, and tubular secretion.[18] Hepatic metabolism is the principal pathway for the elimination of cimetidine, famotidine, and ranitidine, whereas renal excretion is the major route for elimination of nizatidine.[9,18–22] For each of these agents, the elimination half-life is increased, the total body clearance is decreased, and dosage reduction is recommended for patients with moderate to severe renal insufficiency. The pharmacokinetics appear to be unaffected by hepatic dysfunction; however, in patients with combined hepatic failure and renal insufficiency, dosage reduction is likely necessary.[20]

The H_2RAs are remarkably safe, and the frequency of severe adverse effects is low for all four drugs.[9,23] A meta-analysis of randomized placebo-controlled trials reported no difference in the incidence of adverse events of cimetidine versus placebo.[24] The most common adverse effects include GI discomfort (e.g., diarrhea, constipation), CNS effects (e.g., headache, dizziness, drowsiness, lethargy, confusion, psychosis, and hallucinations), and dermatologic effects (e.g., rashes).[9,23] The most frequent hematologic adverse effect is thrombocytopenia, which occurs in about 1% of patients but is reversible on discontinuation of the H_2RA.[25] Although thrombocytopenia is more commonly reported with IV administration, it is likely that the overall incidence of H_2RA-associated thrombocytopenia is overestimated.[26] Hepatotoxicity, although uncommon, has been described primarily in patients receiving IV H_2RAs.[27] Cimetidine has demonstrated weak antiandrogenic effects, and its use in high doses (hypersecretory conditions) has been associated with gynecomastia and impotence in men. This effect is reversible with discontinuation of the medication or by switching to another H_2RA.[23,28] Patients at highest risk of developing any of these adverse effects include the elderly, those requiring higher doses (usually parenteral), and those with altered renal function.[9]

All four H_2RAs can potentially alter the absorption and reduce the bioavailability of drugs that require an acidic environment for absorption. The most important of these interactions is with ketoconazole, which requires an acidic pH for dissolution and absorption. Concomitant administration of a H_2RA and ketoconazole may lead to therapeutic failure of the antifungal.[9,16] Cimetidine has the greatest potential to cause drug interactions because of its ability to inhibit several hepatic CYP450 isoenzymes. The greatest concern is with those agents that have a relatively narrow therapeutic window (e.g., theophylline, lidocaine, phenytoin, quinidine, and warfarin).[16] Although ranitidine is more potent on a molar basis, it binds less intensely to the CYP450 isoenzyme system than cimetidine. Thus, when used in equipotent doses, there is less potential for interactions. Famotidine and nizatidine do not bind appreciably to the CYP450 system and do not interact with drugs that are metabolized through this hepatic system.[16] Since the H_2RAs undergo renal tubular excretion, there is a potential for competition with other medications.[29] Cimetidine and ranitidine inhibit the tubular secretion of procainamide by as much as 44%, but famotidine does not have this effect.[30] Tachyphylaxis or tolerance has been described with all H_2RAs because of up-regulation of the H_2-receptor site. It appears to occur more frequently with high-dose parenteral formulations but has also been described with oral therapy.[31,32] Tolerance to the antisecretory effect may develop after several days of regularly scheduled (continuous) use but can be avoided by taking the H_2RA only when needed.

Proton Pump Inhibitors

PPIs are highly specific inhibitors of gastric acid secretion and include omeprazole, lansoprazole, rabeprazole, pantoprazole, and esomeprazole. These agents are substituted benzimidazoles and act by irreversibly binding to the H^+/K^+-ATPase (proton pump). The PPIs are the most potent inhibitors of gastric acid secretion in that they inhibit the terminal step in the acid production cycle.[9,33–35] They inhibit both basal and stimulated gastric acid secretion in a dose-dependent and sustained fashion.[34] The PPIs are prodrugs and require an acidic environment for conversion to the active sulfonamide. They are absorbed in the small intestine (protected from the acidic milieu of the stomach by enteric coating) and taken via the bloodstream to the acidic secretory canaliculus of the parietal cell for protonation to the active form (Fig. 26-2).[9,33,35] This conversion requires an actively secreting proton pump, and hence, these agents are most efficacious when taken 30 to 60 minutes prior to a meal on an empty stomach.[35] Despite the short plasma elimination half-lives of these agents (~ 1–2 hours), the duration of the antisecretory effect is considerably longer (48–72 hours depending on the agent used) because of covalent (irreversible) binding to the proton pump.[9,35,36] The PPIs have similar acid-inhibitory effects and healing rates when used in equivalent doses (Table 26-1).[37–42] The PPIs are superior to the H_2RAs in terms of acid reduction and mucosal healing.[37,43] A dosage reduction is not required in patients with renal insufficiency; however a dosage reduction is recommended for patients with severe hepatic impairment.[9,44]

The oral PPIs are formulated as delayed-release enteric-coated granules within capsules (omeprazole, lansoprazole, esomeprazole), delayed-release enteric-coated tablets (pantoprazole, rabeprazole, OTC omeprazole), a rapidly disintegrating tablet (lansoprazole), delayed-release oral suspension (lansoprazole), and an immediate release formulation (omeprazole and sodium bicarbonate capsules and powder for oral suspension). IV formulations in the United States include pantoprazole and esomeprazole. Various methods of administration, specific dosage forms, and compounding options for patients with special needs (e.g., dysphagia, gastric tubes) will be discussed later in this chapter (see Upper Gastrointestinal Bleeding section).

The short-term adverse effects of PPIs are relatively infrequent and comparable to the H_2RAs or placebo. The most common side effects include GI discomfort (e.g., nausea, diarrhea, abdominal pain), CNS effects (e.g., headache, dizziness), and rare isolated reactions (e.g., skin rash, increased liver enzymes).[9,45] The immediate-release formulation of omeprazole contains sodium bicarbonate, and care should be taken in sodium-restricted patient populations, as discussed in the Antacids section. All PPIs are metabolized by the hepatic cytochrome P450 microenzyme system. Omeprazole and esomeprazole have been described as inhibiting CYP2C19 and decreasing the clearance of diazepam, phenytoin, and R-warfarin, while lansoprazole increases the metabolism of theophylline by inducing CYP1A.[35,46] Although the clinical importance of these interactions is thought to be negligible, care should be taken when combining these agents to prevent possible toxicity or therapeutic failure. An increase in intragastric pH may increase the bioavailability of orally administered medications (e.g., digoxin, nifedipine) or decrease the absorption of ketoconazole and cefpodoxime.[35,47]

The PPIs have been associated with a number of adverse effects when used long term and in high dosages. However, in most cases, there is insufficient evidence to support a causal relationship between the PPI and the effect. There is evidence to suggest a relationship between elevated serum gastrin concentrations and ECL hyperplasia as a result of the PPI's profound ability to inhibit gastric acid secretion. It has been hypothesized that this can progress to gastric carcinoid tumors (a precursor of gastric cancer). Although ECL hyperplasia has been described with the use of PPIs, there is no clinical evidence to suggest that long-term (>10 years) therapy progresses to a higher grade of hyperplasia or gastric ECL carcinoid.[9,48,49] Atrophic gastritis has been observed in gastric corpus biopsies from patients treated long term with omeprazole and positive for *Helicobacter pylori*. However, review of the data by the Food and Drug Administration (FDA) has been inconclusive and not able to show causality between long-term use of PPIs, *H. pylori*, and atrophic gastritis.[9,49,50]

PPIs have been associated with an increased risk of infections (e.g., pneumonias, enteric infections) possibly due to the ability of the microorganisms ability to survive in a less acidic environment.[49,51–53] Acute nosocomial infections (pneumonia) associated with critically ill patients will be described later when discussing high-dose oral and parenteral PPI therapy (see Upper Gastrointestinal Bleeding section). Enteric infections and cancer have also been described due to potential bacterial overgrowth. The most common pathogens are *Clostridium difficile*, *Salmonella typhimurium*, and *Campylobacter jejuni*; however, data suggest that they rarely lead to illness.[51,52] A retrospective database study of PPI use describes a near threefold increase in the risk of *C. difficile*–associated diarrhea in patients receiving PPIs versus patients not on a PPI, but the overall risk remains low and should not be considered a contraindication to therapy.[52] Bacterial overgrowth (secondary to PPI treatment) has been hypothesized to increase the risk of gastric cancer, because bacteria in the stomach responsible for conversion of dietary nitrates to nitrites can flourish at a higher pH and increase the development of N-nitrosamines (a carcinogenic by-product). Presently, there are no convincing studies to support the increased production of N-nitrosamines in humans with prolonged PPI therapy.[49,51] Long-term PPI use in older patients on high dosages has also been associated with an increased risk of hip fractures through the presumed inhibition of calcium absorption by PPI-induced hypochlorhydia.[54] Although the overall risk was low and was statistically significant, data from previous studies reported normal calcium absorption in patients on PPIs for at least 4 years.[55] Additional studies are required to confirm a causal relationship.

A decrease in vitamin B_{12} (cyanocobalamin) has been described in patients with long-term PPI use and may occur because gastric acid is required to liberate the vitamin from dietary sources.[49,55] This may only be problematic in the elderly, vegetarians, and patients with chronic alcohol ingestion. PPIs have been associated with interstitial nephritis, but this is an extremely rare finding.[56] Although the long-term effects associated with PPIs appear to be rare, the benefit of long-term use must always be weighed against potential risks for the patient.

Sucralfate

Sucralfate (an aluminum salt of a sulfated dissacharide) promotes gastric mucosal protection by shielding ulcerated tissue from aggressive factors such as acid, pepsin, and bile salts.[57] At a pH of 2.0 to 2.5, sucralfate binds to damaged and ulcerated mucosa, forming a physical barrier against injury from these aggressive factors. The drug has minimal systemic absorption and does not possess antisecretory activity. Sucralfate may also have other protective actions related to the stimulation of mucosal prostaglandins.[9] The most common side effect associated with sucralfate is constipation, which occurs in about 3% of patients. This is most likely due to the aluminum content of the compound. Because aluminum toxicity has occurred secondary to accumulation in patients with renal insufficiency, long-term use should be avoided.[9] Since aluminum salts can bind with dietary phosphate in the GI tract, the potential for hypophosphatemia exists (see Antacids section). Sucralfate tablets are large, and some patients, particularly the elderly, may have difficult swallowing them. Gastric bezoar formation has also been described.[58] A liquid formulation is available for patients with swallowing difficulties. The bioavailability of oral fluoroquinolones, warfarin, phenytoin, levothyroxine, quinidine, ketoconazole, amitriptyline, and theophylline may be reduced when concomitantly administered with sucralfate.[9,16] The mechanism of these interactions is thought to be caused by binding of the medication with sucralfate in the GI tract, thus limiting their absorption. Because of these interactions, sucralfate should be given at least 2 hours after these medications.

Misoprostol

Misoprostol, a synthetic prostaglandin E_1 analog, is the only prostaglandin analog approved for use in the United States. Misoprostol acts primarily by enhancing mucosal defense mechanisms.[9] It produces cytoprotective effects by stimulating the production of mucus and bicarbonate, improving mucosal blood flow, and reducing mucosal cell turnover similar to the effects of endogenous prostaglandin.[9] Misoprostol also produces a dose-dependent inhibition of gastric acid, but even at high doses, it is less than that of the H_2RAs. The use of misoprostol is limited because of its potential to cause a dose-dependent diarrhea (in up to 30% of patients) and abdominal cramping.[9] Taking the drug with meals may help to reduce the diarrhea. Decreasing the daily dose may reduce the diarrhea, but efficacy may be compromised[59] (see Peptic Ulcer Disease section). Other troublesome side effects include nausea, flatulence, and headaches.[9] Misoprostol is excreted primarily as metabolites in the urine, but a dose reduction is not required in patients with renal insufficiency. Misoprostol is an abortifacient because of its uterotrophic effects. Thus, it is contraindicated in women who are pregnant who take it for a GI indication.[9,60] Use in women in their childbearing years requires a negative serum pregnancy test and adequate contraception.

Bismuth Salts

Bismuth subsalicylate has been used for years as an OTC option for many GI aliments. Although its mechanism of action is not completely understood, bismuth is thought to work by binding to and protecting mucosal lesions and enhancing cellular protective mechanisms. Bismuth also has an antimicrobial effect, primarily against *H. pylori*.[9] Bismuth salts have no acid-inhibitory effects. Bismuth-containing products have few side effects, but patients with renal impairment may have a decreased elimination of the bismuth. Bismuth subsalicylate should be used with caution in patients on concomitant salicylates, as the potential exists for salicylate toxicity or increased risk of bleeding. Patients with salicylate allergies or sensitivities should also be warned of the salicylate component. Long-term use is also not advised. Bismuth salts are associated with a harmless black coloring of the stools due to colonic conversion of bismuth to bismuth sulfide and a potential black discoloration of the tongue with liquid dosage forms.[9] Bismuth subcitrate potassium (biskalcitrate) is only available as a combination product with metronidazole and tetracycline for the treatment of *H. pylori*[61] (see Peptic Ulcer Disease section). Although side effects are similar to bismuth subsalicylate, it has the advantage of not containing salicylate.

DYSPEPSIA

The term *dyspepsia* is derived from the Greek words that mean "hard or difficult digestion" and refers to a subjective feeling of pain or discomfort located primarily in the upper abdomen.[62–63] Although the symptom complex and duration may vary, most patients complain of acute dyspeptic symptoms (indigestion) that are often but not necessarily restricted to food or alcohol consumption; medications such as nonsteroidal anti-inflammatory drugs (NSAIDs), antibiotics such as erythromycin, digoxin, theophylline, and bisphosphonates; and smoking or a stressful lifestyle (Fig. 26-3). Chronic dyspepsia is defined as recurrent symptoms that may include epigastric pain, abdominal boating, belching, nausea, vomiting, and early satiety (early sense of fullness with meals). Clinicians consider heartburn an accompanying symptom, but regulatory agencies in the United States and Rome II diagnostic criteria have adopted a definition of chronic dyspepsia for clinical research purposes that excludes heartburn.[63,64] For some individuals, dyspepsia occurs regularly and may indicate a serious underlying medical problem.

Patients who have not undergone diagnostic testing are referred to as having "uninvestigated" dyspepsia, while those who have undergone testing (usually upper endoscopy) are said to have "investigated" dyspepsia (Fig. 26-3). The four major causes of investigated dyspepsia include chronic PUD, GERD with or without esophagitis, malignancy, and functional or idiopathic dyspepsia. Functional dyspepsia is a clinical syndrome in which there is no evidence of mucosal damage related to PUD, GERD, or malignancy found at endoscopy. Specific types of functional dyspepsia include nonulcer dyspepsia (NUD), which describes "ulcer-like" symptoms, and nonerosive reflux disease (NERD), which describes "GERD-like" symptoms in an endoscopy-negative patient.

Epidemiology

Dyspepsia is a common problem that occurs in about 25% of the U.S. population when patients with typical GERD symptoms are excluded.[62] When all patients with heartburn or regurgitation are excluded, the prevalence is lower. The prevalence remains stable, as the number who develop dyspepsia is similar to the number who no longer complain of symptoms.

Pathophysiology

Acute, infrequent dyspepsia is most often related to food, alcohol, smoking, or stress. Chronic dyspepsia may be related to an underlying cause such as PUD, GERD, or malignancy or may not have any known cause (endoscopy-negative, functional, idiopathic dyspepsia). About 40% of patients with functional

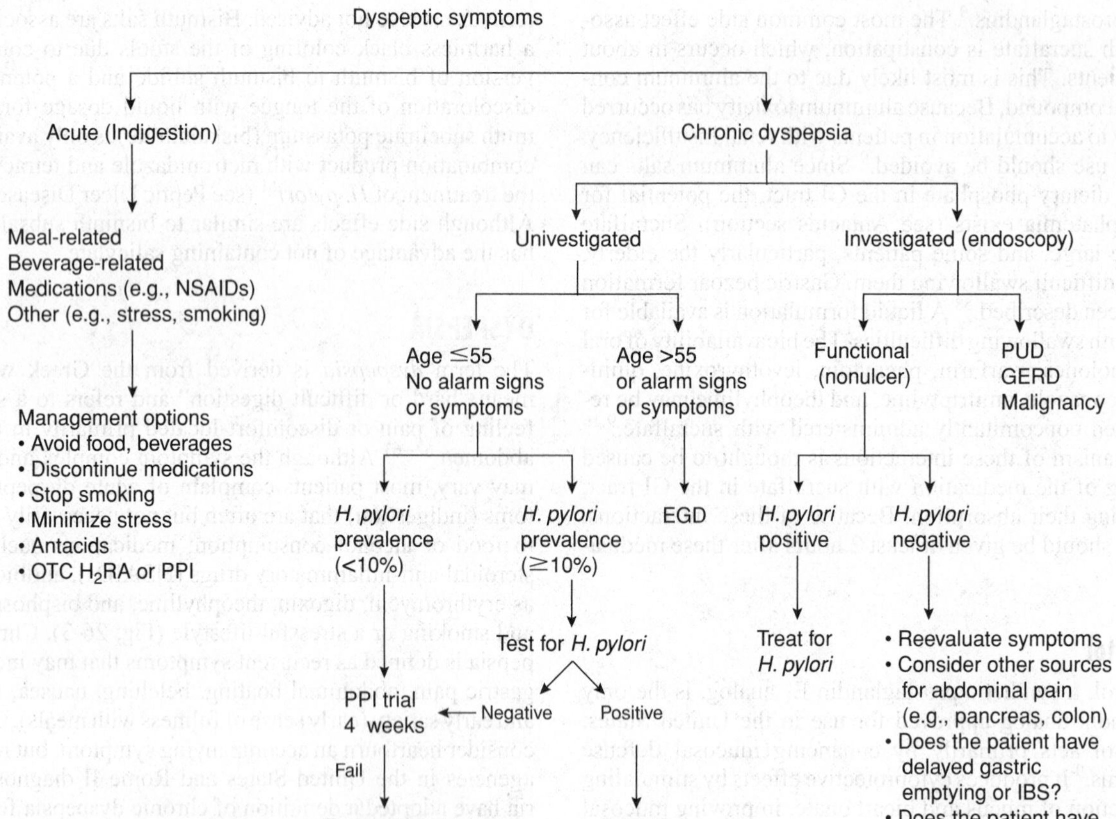

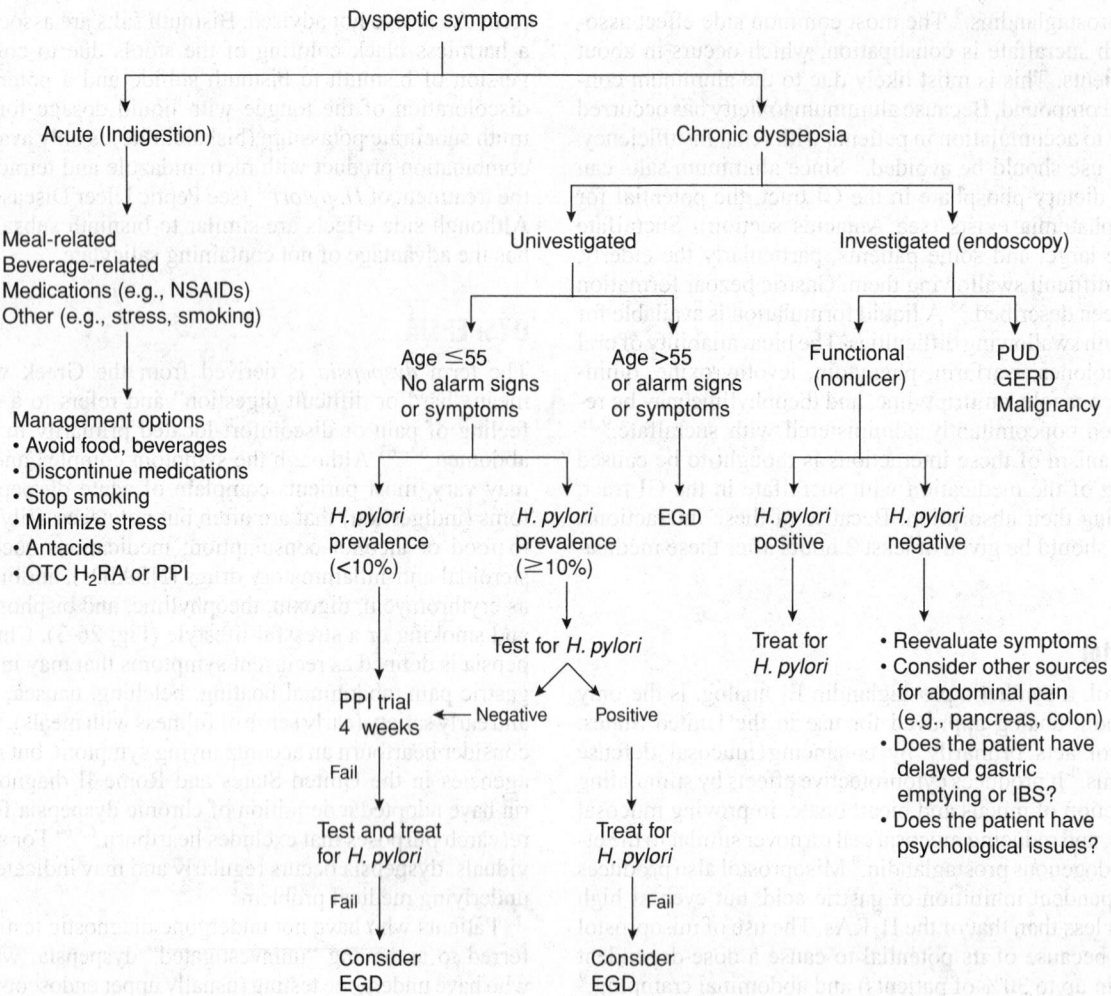

FIGURE 26-3 Management of dyspeptic symptoms. GERD, gastroesophageal reflux disease; *H. pylori*, *Helicobacter pylori*; H_2RA, H_2-receptor antagonist; OTC, over-the-counter; PPI, proton pump inhibitor; PUD, peptic ulcer disease.

dyspepsia have pathophysiological disturbances that involve delayed gastric emptying.[63] There is also evidence that the esophagus, stomach, duodenum, and other regions of the GI tract are hypersensitive and may be associated with irritable bowel syndrome, especially in women.[63] Others have failed to find a pathological association between functional dyspepsia and gastroduodenal motility, hypersensitivity, or any other GI abnormality and suggest that psychologic disturbances are an important contributing factor. Although *H. pylori* infection has been identified in 20% to 60% of patients with functional dyspepsia, its pathophysiological relevance remains uncertain.[62]

Clinical Assessment and Diagnosis

Acute, infrequent dyspepsia is usually self-limiting and generally requires no further investigation. Chronic dyspeptic symptoms cannot be used to predict endoscopic findings of PUD, GERD, or malignancy in patients with uninvestigated dyspepsia.[63,65,66] In addition, individual symptoms or symptom subgroups such as PUD-like, GERD-like, or dysmotility-like dyspepsia are not useful in distinguishing organic disease from functional dyspepsia, nor does it appear to aid in management. This is because there is considerable overlap of symptoms among patients with PUD, GERD, malignancy, and functional dyspepsia.

The clinical assessment of uninvestigated dyspeptic in patients ≤55 years of age with no alarm signs or symptoms includes a test-and-treat *H. pylori* option, which is preferable in geographic areas of moderate to high prevalence of *H. pylori* infection ≥10%)[63] (Fig. 26-3). *H. pylori* testing should be conducted by using a nonendoscopic validated test (see Tests for Detecting *Helicobacter pylori* section). New-onset dyspepsia in an older individual is considered an independent risk factor for an underlying malignancy such as gastric cancer.[63] Dyspeptic patients >55 years of age or those with alarm signs or symptoms should undergo upper endoscopy (Fig. 26-3). Other alarm features that assist in identifying serious underlying diseases, especially malignancy, include early satiety, anorexia, worsening dysphagia or odynophagia, unexplained weight loss (>10% body weight), vomiting, anemia, GI bleeding, lymphadenopathy, jaundice, a history of PUD, a family history of upper GI tract cancer, previous gastric surgery, or malignancy.[63] Although a symptom duration threshold has not been established, a long history of symptoms or antisecretory drug use may suggest a serious underlying condition.

Treatment

The recommended strategies for managing dyspepsia are presented in Figure 26-3. Individuals with acute dyspepsia (indigestion) can be effectively treated with self-directed therapy using antacids or OTC antisecretory drugs if they are unable or unwilling to avoid offending foods and beverages, stop smoking, or discontinue troublesome medications. The initial management of patients ≤55 years of age with uninvestigated dyspepsia and no alarm features depends on the prevalence of *H. pylori* and whether the patient is *H. pylori* positive or negative (Table 26-2). Empiric therapy with a PPI for 4 weeks is considered first line and cost effective in areas with a low prevalence of *H. pylori* and in patients who are *H. pylori* negative.[63] One meta-analysis reports better symptomatic outcomes with a short course of a PPI when compared with H_2RAs, alginate, or placebo.[67] The PPI should be stopped after 1 month if the patient's symptoms respond to treatment. If symptoms recur, then longer-term PPI treatment may be considered, but the need for a PPI should be evaluated every 6 to 12 months.[62] If standard doses of a PPI fail, a short course of doubling the PPI dose may be considered.[62] Prokinetics are not recommended as first-line therapy for uninvestigated dyspepsia in the United States.[62,63] Patients who are *H. pylori* positive should receive a PPI-based eradication regimen[62,65] (see *Helicobacter pylori*–Related Ulcers section).

Early endoscopy with biopsy for *H. pylori* is recommended for patients >55 years of age and those with alarm features. In the event that an abnormality is found, such as PUD, GERD, or malignancy, it should be treated accordingly. The management of NUD is challenging and should take into consideration the cost-effectiveness of treatment.[2] Analyses of trials evaluating H_2RAs and PPIs show that less than one-third of patients become asymptomatic and that PPIs may be marginally superior to H_2RAs.[63] An economic review, however, suggests that PPIs are cost-effective for NUD in the United States.[68] There is no evidence to support the use of antacids or sucralfate,[69] but simethicone may be of benefit.[70] The effectiveness of *H. pylori* eradication in NUD remains controversial, as some meta-analyses show a beneficial effect[71] while others fail to confirm such benefits[72] (Table 26-2). An update of these meta-analyses, however, reports a small therapeutic gain with eradication.[73] The beneficial effects of eradication may last for up to 5 years.[74] Although the benefit of prokinetics have been reported, most studies were conducted with cisapride, which was withdrawn from the U.S. market.[69] The use of available prokinetics (metoclopramide, erythromycin) should be reserved for difficult-to-treat patients because of their limited efficacy and side effects.[63] Antidepressants are often prescribed in NUD but are of uncertain efficacy.[63] Alternative therapies, including herbal products, remain unproven.[63] Patients with persistent dyspepia despite a negative endoscopy in whom PPI therapy and *H. pylori* eradication fails should have their diagnosis reevaluated.

Table 26-2 Indications for Testing and Treating *Helicobacter pylori* Infection

Recommended (evidence established)

- Uninvestigated dyspepsia (depending on *H. pylori* prevalence)
- PUD (active gastric or duodenal ulcer)
- History of PUD (confirmed ulcer not previously treated for *H. pylori*)
- Gastric MALT lymphoma
- Following resection of early gastric cancer
- Reduce the risk of recurrent bleeding from gastroduodenal ulcer

Controversial (evidence not well established)

- NUD
- Individuals using NSAIDs (no signs/symptoms of peptic ulcer)
- GERD
- Individuals at risk for gastric cancer
- Individuals with unexplained iron deficiency anemia

GERD, gastroesophageal reflux disease; MALT, mucosa-associated lymphoid tissue; NUD, nonulcer dyspepsia; NSAID, nonsteroidal anti-inflammatory drug; PUD, peptic ulcer disease.
Adapted from references 63, 78, and 80, with permission.

PEPTIC ULCER DISEASE

PUD is one of the most common gastroenterologic diseases affecting the upper GI tract.[9] Chronic peptic ulcers are defects in the gastric (gastric ulcer) or duodenal (duodenal ulcer) mucosa that require gastric acid for their formation. Chronic peptic ulcers differ from erosions and gastritis in that the ulcer extends deeper into the muscularis mucosa. Stress ulcer is an acute form of peptic ulcer, but it occurs primarily in critically ill patients and differs in its underlying pathogenesis (see Stress-Related Mucosal Bleeding section).

Epidemiology

Peptic ulcers develop in 10% of Americans during their lifetime and result in impaired quality of life, work loss, and high-cost medical care.[9] A declining ulcer rate for younger men and an increasing rate for older women has shifted the prevalence of PUD in the United States from predominantly men to a comparable rate in men and women.[9] Hospitalizations, operations, physician visits, and deaths in the United States have declined by >50% during the last four decades.[9] While hospital admissions for uncomplicated duodenal ulcer have decreased, admissions for ulcer-related complications (bleeding and perforation) have increased.[9] Although the overall mortality from PUD has decreased, death rates have increased among older patients (>75 years) and are most likely related to the use of NSAIDs.

Etiology and Risk Factors

H. pylori and NSAIDs are the two most common causes of chronic PUD and influence the chronicity of the disease.[9] Less common causes include hypersecretory states such as Zollinger-Ellison syndrome (ZES) (see Zollinger-Ellison Syndrome section), viral infections (e.g., cytomegalovirus), radiation, and chemotherapy (e.g., hepatic artery infusion).[9] Factors that may increase the risk of a peptic ulcer include alcohol ingestion, cigarette smoking, diet, and psychologic stress; corticosteroids; and chronic diseases such as chronic renal failure, hepatic cirrhosis, chronic pancreatitis, chronic pulmonary disease, and Crohn's disease.[9]

Helicobacter pylori–Related Ulcers

H. pylori infection is causally linked to chronic gastritis, PUD, mucosa-associated lymphoid tissue (MALT) lymphoma, and gastric cancer (Table 26-2), but only 20% of infected individuals develop symptomatic ulcers and <1% develop gastric cancer.[9,75,76] Differences in strains account for the variable pathogenesis of the organism.[75,76] Evidence is lacking to support a causal role for *H. pylori* and GERD,[77,78] extragastric manifestations (e.g., cardiovascular disease),[79] or iron deficiency anemia.[80]

The prevalence of *H. pylori* varies by geographic location, socioeconomic environment, ethnicity, and age.[75] The infection is more common in developing countries than in industrialized countries. Prevalence in the United States is estimated to be 30% to 40%[80] but is higher in older individuals and in African and Latin Americans.[81] The higher prevalence among older individuals reflects acquisition during infancy and early childhood.[9] However, infection rates in the United States have been declining in children because of improved socioeconomic conditions.[80,81] Prevalence is not affected by gender or smoking. Transmission occurs by the fecal–oral route from an infected person or from fecal-contaminated water or food.[9] Individuals living in the same household are at risk for infection.[9,81] *H. pylori* can also be transmitted through vomitus or the use of inadequately sterilized endoscopes.[9] Transmission by the oral-oral route has been postulated, but it is unlikely.

Nonsteroidal Anti-inflammatory Drug-Induced Ulcers

There is considerable evidence linking the chronic use of NSAIDs with injury to the GI tract.[9,82–84] Gastric and duodenal ulcers develop in 15% to 30% of chronic NSAID users, whereas 1% to 2% experience serious ulcer-related complications.[82,83] Gastric ulcer is most common and develops primarily in the antrum.[75] NSAIDs may cause ulcers in the esophagus and the colon, but these ulcers occur less frequently.[9,84] It has been estimated that about 16,500 NSAID-related deaths and 107,000 hospitalizations occur annually in the United States,[82,83] but the death rates may be overstated because of the recent decline in hospitalizations.[84] Over 111 million NSAID prescriptions are filled each year in the United States at a cost of about 5 billion dollars.[82] Additionally, about 2 million dollars is spent annually on OTC NSAIDs.[82] The risk factors for NSAID-induced ulcers and upper GI complications are listed in Table 26-3. Combinations of factors confer an additive risk.

Table 26-3 Risk Factors for Nonsteroidal Anti-inflammatory Drug-Induced Ulcer and Ulcer-Related Upper Gastrointestinal Complications

Established

- Confirmed prior ulcer or ulcer-related complication
- Age >65 years
- Multiple or high-dose NSAID use
- Concomitant use of aspirin (including cardioprotective dosages)
- Concomitant use of an anticoagulant, corticosteroid, bisphosphonate, clopidogrel, or SSRI
- Selection of NSAID (selectivity of COX-1 vs. COX-2)

Controversial

- *H. pylori*
- Alcohol consumption
- Cigarette smoking

COX-1, cyclo-oxygenase-1; COX-2. cyclo-oxygenase-2; NSAID, nonsteroidal anti-inflammatory drug; SSRI, selective serotonin reuptake inhibitor.
Adapted from references 9, 80, 82–84, 122, and 125, with permission.

Pathophysiology

A physiological balance exists in healthy individuals between gastric acid secretion and gastroduodenal mucosal defense. Peptic ulcers occur when the balance between aggressive factors (gastric acid, pepsin, bile salts, *H. pylori*, and NSAIDs) and mucosal defensive mechanisms (mucosal blood flow, mucus, mucosal bicarbonate secretion, mucosal cell restitution, and epithelial cell renewal) are disrupted.[9] Increased acid secretion may occur in patients with duodenal ulcer, but most patients with gastric ulcer have normal or reduced rates of acid secretion.[11] Pepsin is an important cofactor that plays a role in the proteolytic activity involved in ulcer formation. Mucosal defense and repair mechanisms protect the gastroduodenal mucosa from noxious endogenous and exogenous substances.[9] The viscous nature and near-neutral pH of the mucus-bicarbonate barrier protect the stomach from the acidic contents in the gastric lumen. The maintenance of mucosal integrity and repair is mediated by the production of endogenous prostaglandins. When aggressive factors alter mucosal defense mechanisms, back diffusion of hydrogen ions occurs with subsequent mucosal injury. *H. pylori* and NSAIDs cause alterations in mucosal defense by different mechanisms and are important factors in the formation of peptic ulcers.

Helicobacter pylori–Related Ulcers

H. pylori is a gram-negative, spiral-shaped bacillus that thrives in a microaerophilic environment. The bacterium resides between the mucus layer and surface epithelial cells in the stomach or any location where gastric-type epithelium is found.[9,75] Flagella enable it to move from the lumen of the stomach, where the pH is low, to the mucus layer, where the pH is neutral. The acute infection is accompanied by transient hypochlorhydria, which enables the organism to survive the acidic gastric juice.[85] Although the exact method by which *H. pylori* induces hypochlorhydria is uncertain, it is hypothesized that its urease-producing ability hydrolyzes urea in the gastric juice and converts it to ammonia and carbon dioxide, which creates a neutral microenvironment that surrounds the bacterium.[75] Adherence pedestals permit the bacterium to attach to gastric-type epithelium and prevent it from being shed during cell turnover and mucus secretion. Colonization of the body of the stomach is associated with gastric ulcer. Duodenal ulcers are thought to arise from colonization by antral organisms of gastric-type epithelium that develops in the duodenum in response to changes in duodenal pH.[9,75]

The exact mechanism by which *H. pylori* infection leads to ulceration is not yet known. Direct mucosal damage is produced by virulence factors (e.g., vacuolating cytotoxin, elaborating bacterial enzymes) and adherence.[86,87] Approximately 50% of *H. pylori* strains produce vacuolating cytotoxin (VacA), which leads to cell death and possibly gastric cancer.[87] Strains with cytotoxin-associated gene (CagA) protein are associated with duodenal ulcer, atrophic gastritis, and gastric cancer.[75,76,86] *H. pylori* infection also causes alterations in the host immune response,[9,75] hypergastrinemia leading to increased acid secretion,[9,75] and carcinogenic conversion of susceptible gastric epithelial cells.[76,86,87]

Nonsteroidal Anti-inflammatory Drug-Induced Ulcers

Nonselective NSAIDs (Table 26-4), including aspirin, cause peptic ulcers and upper GI complications by systemically inhibiting protective prostaglandins in the gastric mucosa.[9] NSAIDs inhibit cyclo-oxygenase (COX), the rate-limiting enzyme in the conversion of arachidonic acid to prostaglandins. There are two COX isoforms: cyclo-oxygenase-1 (COX-1), which is found in the stomach, kidney, intestine, and platelets, and cyclo-oxygenase-2 (COX-2), which is induced with acute inflammation.[9] The inhibition of COX-1 is associated with upper GI and renal toxicity, while the inhibition of COX-2 is related to anti-inflammatory effects.[9,88] Nonselective NSAIDs, including aspirin, inhibit both COX-1 and COX-2 to varying degrees and decrease platelet aggregation, which may increase the risk for upper GI bleeding.[9] The partially selective NSAIDs may be associated with less GI toxicity.[9,88–90] Selective COX-2 inhibitors have a similar efficacy to the nonselective NSAIDs but with fewer harmful GI effects.[9,90] In contrast to the nonselective NSAIDs, the COX-2 inhibitors do not possess antiplatelet effects. Two selective COX-2 inhibitors, rofecoxib and valdecoxib (Table 26-4), were withdrawn from the U.S. market in 2004 because of concerns about cardiovascular safety. Celecoxib, a NSAID initially marketed as a COX-2 inhibitor, is now considered a partially selective agent.

Aspirin and nonselective NSAIDs also have a topical (direct) irritating effect on the gastric mucosa, but the resulting inflammation and erosion usually heals within a few days.[63] Formulations such as enteric-coated aspirin, buffered aspirin, NSAID prodrugs, and parenteral or rectal preparations may spare topical effects on the gastric mucosa, but all have the potential to cause a gastric ulcer because of their systemic inhibition of endogenous prostaglandins.[9,91]

Table 26-4 Selected Nonsteroidal Anti-inflammatory Drugs

Salicylates
Acetylated: aspirin
Nonacetylated: trisalicylate, salsalate
Nonsalicylates[a]
Nonselective (traditional) NSAIDs: ibuprofen, naproxen, tolmetin, fenoprofen, sulindac, indomethacin, ketoprofen, ketorolac, flurbiprofen, piroxicam
Partially selective NSAIDs: etodolac, diclofenac, meloxicam, nabumetone
Selective COX-2 inhibitors: celecoxib, rofecoxib[b], valdecoxib[b]

[a]Based on COX-1/COX-2 selectivity ratio *in vitro*.
[b]Withdrawn from U.S. market.
COX-2, cyclo-oxygenase-2; NSAIDs, nonsteroidal anti-inflammatory drugs.

Clinical Presentation

Signs and Symptoms

The signs and symptoms associated with a peptic ulcer range from mild epigastric pain to life-threatening upper GI complications.[9] A change in the character of the pain may indicate an ulcer-related complication. The absence of epigastric pain, especially in the elderly who are taking NSAIDs, does not exclude the presence of an ulcer or related complications. Although the reasons for this are unclear, they may be related to the analgesic effect of the NSAID. There is no one sign or symptom that differentiates a *H. pylori*–related ulcer from a NSAID-induced ulcer. Ulcer-like symptoms may occur in the absence of peptic ulceration in association with *H. pylori*–related gastritis or duodenitis.

Complications

The most serious life-threatening complications associated with chronic PUD are upper GI bleeding (10%–15%), perforation into the abdominal cavity (7%), and gastric obstruction (2%).[9] The incidence of ulcer-related upper GI bleeding and perforation is increased in older patients taking NSAIDs. The bleeding may be occult (hidden), present as melena (black-colored stools), or hematemesis (vomiting of blood). Mortality is high in patients who continue to bleed or who rebleed after the initial bleeding has stopped (see Upper Gastrointestinal Bleeding section) and in patients with a perforated ulcer. The pain associated with perforation is typically sudden, sharp, and severe, beginning initially in the epigastric area but quickly spreading throughout the upper abdominal area. Gastric outlet obstruction is caused by previous ulcer healing and then scarring or edema of the pylorus or duodenal bulb and can lead to symptoms of gastric retention, including early satiety, bloating, anorexia, nausea, vomiting, and weight loss.

Clinical Assessment and Diagnosis

Tests for Detecting *Helicobacter pylori*

The detection of *H. pylori* infection can be made by using gastric mucosal biopsies in patients undergoing upper endoscopy or by nonendoscopic tests[9,80,92] (Table 26-5). The selection of a specific method is influenced by the clinical circumstance and the availability and cost of the individual test. The endoscopic tests require a mucosal biopsy for the rapid urease test, histology, or culture. Medications that reduce urease activity or the density of *H. pylori* may decrease the sensitivity of the rapid urease test by up to 25%.[80] When possible, antibiotics and bismuth salts should be withheld for 4 weeks and H_2RAs and PPIs for 1 to 2 weeks prior to endoscopic testing. Patients who are taking these medications at endoscopy will require histology in addition to the rapid urease test. Two biopsies are taken from different areas of the stomach because patchy distribution of *H. pylori* can result in false-negative results. Acute ulcer bleeding at the time of testing is likely to decrease the sensitivity of the rapid urease test and histology and increase the likelihood of false-negative results.[80,93]

Table 26-5 Diagnostic Tests for *Helicobacter pylori* Infection

Tests Utilizing Gastric Mucosal Biopsy in Patients Undergoing Endoscopy

Rapid Urease Test

- Tests for active *H. pylori* infection; >90% sensitivity and >95% specificity.
- Withhold H_2RAs and PPIs 1 to 2 weeks prior to testing and antibiotics and bismuth salts 4 weeks prior to testing to reduce the risk of false negatives.
- In the presence of *H.pylori* urease, urea is metabolized to ammonia and bicarbonate resulting in an increase in pH, which changes the color of a pH-sensitive indicator.
- Results are rapid (usually within a few hours), and test is less expensive than histology or culture.

Histology

- Considered "gold standard" for detection of *H. pylori* infection; >95% sensitivity and >95% specificity.
- Permits further histologic analysis and evaluation of infected tissue (e.g., gastritis, ulceration, adenocarcinoma); tests for active *H. pylori* infection.
- Results are not immediate; not recommended for intitial diagnosis; more expensive than rapid urease test.

Culture

- Permits sensitivity testing to determine antibiotic choice or resistance; 100% specific.
- Use usually limited to patients who fail several courses of eradication therapy; tests for active *H. pylori* infection.
- Results are not immediate; not recommended for initial diagnosis; more expensive than rapid urease test.

Tests That do not Utilize Gastric Mucosal Biopsy

Urea Breath Test

- Tests for active *H. pylori* infection; >95% sensitivity and >95% specificity.
- Radiolabeled urea with either C^{13} or C^{14} is given orally; urease secreted by *H. pylori* in the stomach (if present) hydrolyzes radiolabed urea to produce radiolabled CO_2, which is exhaled and then quantified from the expired breath; radiation exposure is minimal.
- Withhold H_2RAs and PPIs 1 to 2 weeks prior to testing and antibiotics and bismuth salts 4 weeks prior to testing to reduce the risk of false negatives.
- Used to detect *H. pylori* prior to treatment and to document posttreatment eradicaton.
- Results usually take about 2 days; less expensive than tests that utilize gastric mucosal biopsy but more expensive than serologic tests.
- Availability and reimbursement is inconsistent.

Serologic Antibody Tests

- Detects IgG antibodies to *H. pylori* in serum, whole blood or urine; quantitative serologic tests have a sensitivity of about 85% and specificity of about 79%.
- Qualitative in office tests; provide results quickly (usually within 15 minutes) but yield more variable results.
- Tests are widely available and inexpensive.
- Not of benefit in documenting eradication, because antibodies to *H. pylori* remain positive for years following successful eradication of the infection.
- Results not affected by H_2RAs, PPIs, antibiotics, or bismuth.

Fecal Antigen Test

- Identifies *H. pylori* antigen in stool; sensitivity and specificity comparable to the UBT for initial diagnosis.
- H_2RAs, PPIs, antibiotics, and bismuth may cause false-negative results but to a lesser exent than the UBT.
- Considered an alterative to detecting *H. pylori* prior to treatment and documenting posttreatment eradicaton.

H_2RA, H_2-receptor antagonist; IgG, immunoglobulin G; PPI, proton pump inhibitor; UBT, urea breath test.
Adapted from references 9, 80, and 92, with permission.

Three nonendoscopic tests are available to detect *H. pylori* infection and include the urea breath test (UBT), serologic antibody detection tests, and the fecal antigen test[9,80,92] (Table 26-5). If endoscopy is not planned, these tests are a reasonable choice to determine *H. pylori* status, as they are noninvasive, more convenient, and less expensive than the endoscopic tests. However, testing should only be undertaken if eradication therapy is planned for positive results. The UBT tests for active *H. pylori* infection and is the most accurate noninvasive test.[80,92] The ^{13}carbon (nonradioactive isotope) and ^{14}carbon (radioactive isotope) tests require that the patient ingest radiolabeled urea, which is then hydrolyzed by *H. pylori* (if present in the stomach) to ammonia and radiolabeled bicarbonate. The radiolabeled bicarbonate is absorbed in the blood and excreted in the breath. A mass spectrometer is used to quantitative ^{13}carbon, whereas ^{14}carbon is measured by using a scintillation counter. The serologic antibody tests are a cost-effective alternative for the initial diagnosis of *H. pylori* infection. Antibodies to *H. pylori* can be assessed quantitatively by using the laboratory-based enzyme-linked immunosorbent assay (ELISA) or qualitatively by using the office-based kits. Because the antibody tests do not differentiate between active infection and previously eradicated *H. pylori*, they should not be used to confirm eradication.[9,80,92] The fecal antigen test identifies *H. pylori* antigens in the stool by enzyme immunoassay.[80,92] It is less expensive and easier to perform than the UBT and may be useful in children. Although comparable to the UBT in the initial detection of *H. pylori*, the fecal antigen test may be less accurate when used to document eradication post treatment. Salivary and urine antibody tests are under investigation.[92]

Laboratory Tests, Radiography, and Endoscopy

Generally, laboratory tests are not helpful in the diagnosis of PUD. Fasting serum gastrin concentrations are only recommended for patients unresponsive to therapy or those suspected of having a hypersecretory disease. Serum hematocrit (Hct) and hemoglobin (Hgb) and stool hemoccult tests assist in the evaluation of ulcer-related bleeding.

Gastric acid secretory studies are not routinely performed for patients suspected of having an uncomplicated peptic ulcer. However, measurements of acid secretion are instrumental in the evaluation of patients with severe, recurrent PUD that is unresponsive to standard drug therapy. Acid secretion is expressed as basal acid output (BAO), in response to a meal (meal-stimulated acid secretion), or as maximal acid output (MAO).[11] The BAO, meal-stimulated acid secretion, and MAO varies according to age, gender, health, and time of day. The BAO follows a circadian rhythm, with the highest acid secretion occurring at night and the lowest in the morning. An increase in the BAO:MAO ratio suggests a basal hypersecretory state such as ZES.

Confirmation of a peptic ulcer requires visualizing the ulcer either by GI radiography or upper endoscopy.[9] Radiography is often the initial diagnostic procedure because is less expensive than endoscopy and more widely available. Double-contrast radiography is preferred because it detects 60% to 80% of ulcers, while tests using single-barium contrast detect 30% of peptic ulcers.[9] Fiberoptic upper endoscopy (esophagogastroduodenoscopy [EGD]) is the gold standard, as it detects >90% of peptic ulcers and permits direct inspection, biopsy, visualization of superficial erosions, and sites of active bleeding. Upper endoscopy is preferred if complications are suspected or if an accurate diagnosis is required. If a gastric ulcer is found on radiography, malignancy should be excluded by direct endoscopic visualization and histology.

Clinical Course and Prognosis

The clinical course of PUD is characterized by periods of exacerbations and remissions unless the underlying cause is removed.[9] Eradication of *H. pylori* decreases ulcer recurrence and complications. Prophylactic cotherapy or the use of a selective COX-2 inhibitor decreases the risk for ulcers and related complications in high-risk patients taking NSAIDs. It is estimated that about 20% of patients with chronic PUD experience ulcer-related complications. Mortality is highest in patients with gastric ulcer. Adenocarcinoma in *H. pylori*-infected patients occurs over 20 to 40 years and is associated with a lifetime risk <1%.[9,76]

Treatment

Therapeutic Goals

The therapeutic goals for treating PUD depend on whether the ulcer is related to *H. pylori* or associated with a NSAID. Treatment goals may differ depending on whether the ulcer is initial or recurrent and whether complications have occurred. Treatment is aimed at relieving ulcer symptoms, healing the ulcer, preventing ulcer recurrence, and reducing ulcer-related complications. When possible, the most cost-effective drug regimen should be utilized.

Nonpharmacologic Therapy

Patients with PUD should discontinue NSAIDs (including aspirin) if possible. Patients unable to tolerate certain foods and beverages (e.g., spicy foods, caffeine, and alcohol) may benefit from dietary modifications. Lifestyle modifications including reducing stress and decreasing or stopping cigarette smoking is encouraged.

Probiotics containing strains of *Lactobacillus* and *Bifidobacterium* and foodstuffs (e.g., cranberry juice and some milk proteins) with bioactive components have been studied in at-risk individuals to proactively control colonization of *H. pylori*. When combined with eradication regimens, the same probiotic strains have been reported to augment *H. pylori* eradication by possibly by decreasing mucosal inflammation.[94] The regular intake of probiotics may eventually become a low-cost alternative for individuals at risk for *H. pylori* infection and may enhance eradication in conjunction with drug treatment regimens.

Patients with ulcer-related complications may require surgery for bleeding, perforation, or obstruction. Surgery for medical treatment failures (e.g., vagotomy with pyloroplasty or vagotomy with antrectomy) are rarely performed because of effective medical management. However, patients may present with postoperative consequences (e.g., postvagotomy diarrhea, dumping syndrome, anemia) associated with these procedures.

Pharmacotherapy

Drug regimens used to eradicate *H. pylori* are identified in Table 26-6. First-line therapy should be initiated with a PPI-based three-drug regimen (Fig. 26-4). If a second course of treatment is required, the PPI-based three-drug regimen should contain different antibiotics or a four-drug regimen with a bismuth salt, metronidazole, tetracycline, and a PPI should be used. Successful treatment will heal the ulcer and eradicate the infection (cure the disease). Treatment of *H. pylori*–positive patients with a conventional antiulcer drug is not recommended because of the high rate of ulcer recurrence and complications. Combining a PPI and H_2RA or sucralfate and either a H_2RA or PPI is not recommended, because it adds to drug costs without improving efficacy. Maintenance therapy with a PPI or H_2RA (Table 26-1) should only be necessary in high-risk patients with a history of ulcer complications, those with *H. pylori*–negative ulcers, and patients with other concomitant acid-related diseases (e.g., GERD).

Drug regimens used to treat and prevent NSAID-induced ulcers are identified in Table 26-1. Patients with NSAID-induced ulcers should be tested to determine their *H. pylori* status. *H. pylori*–positive patients should be initially treated with a PPI-based three-drug eradication regimen (Fig. 26-4). If the patient is *H. pylori*–negative, the NSAID should be discontinued and treatment should be initiated with antiulcer medications. The duration of treatment should be extended if the NSAID is continued. Prophylactic cotherapy with a PPI or misoprostol or switching to an NSAID with greater COX-2 selectivity is recommended for patients at risk of developing ulcer-related upper GI complications.

Table 26-6 Oral Drug Regimens Used to Eradicate *Helicobacter pylori* Infection

Drug Regimen	*Dose*	*Frequency*	*Duration*
Proton Pump Inhibitor–Based Three-Drug Regimens			
PPI	Standard dose[a]	BID[a]	10–14 days[b]
Clarithromycin	500 mg	BID	10–14 days[b]
Amoxicillin[c]	1 g	BID	10–14 days[b]
or			
PPI	Standard dose[a]	BID[a]	10–14 days[b]
Clarithromycin	500 mg	BID	10–14 days[b]
Metronidazole[c]	500 mg	BID	10–14 days[b]
Bismuth-Based Four-Drug Regimens			
Bismuth subsalicylate[d]	525 mg	QID	10–14 days
Metronidazole	250–500 mg	QID	10–14 days
Tetracycline	500 mg	QID	10–14 days
plus			
PPI	Standard dose[a]	QD or BID[a]	10–14 days
or			
H_2RA[e]	Standard dose[e]	BID[e]	4–6 wks
Sequential Therapy[f]			
PPI	Standard dose[a]	BID[a]	Days 1–10
Amoxicillin	1 g	BID	Days 1–5
Clarithromycin	250–500 mg	BID	Days 6–10
Metronidazole	250–500 mg	BID	Days 6–10
Salvage or Rescue Therapy			
Bismuth subsalicylate[d]	525 mg	QID	10–14 days
Metronidazole	250–500 mg	QID	10–14 days
Tetracycline	500 mg	QID	10–14 days
PPI	Standard dose[a]	QD or BID[a]	10–14 days
or			
PPI	Standard dose[a]	BID[a]	10–14 days
Amoxicillin	1 g	BID	10–14 days
Levofloxacin	500 mg	QD	10–14 days

[a] Omeprazole 20 mg BID; lansoprazole 30 mg BID; pantoprazole 40 mg BID; rabeprazole 20 mg BID or QD; esomeprazole 20 mg BID or 40 mg QD.
[b] Although 7-day regimens provide acceptable eradication rates, the preferred treatment duration in the United States is 10 to 14 days.
[c] Use amoxicillin in nonpenicillin-allergic individuals; substitute metronidazole for amoxicillin in penicillin-allergic patients.
[d] Pylera, a prepackaged *H. pylori* regimen, contains bismuth subcitrate potassium (biskalcitrate) 140 mg as the bismuth salt in place of bismuth subsalicylate, metronidazole 125 mg and tetracycline 125 mg per capsule. The patient is directed to take three capsules/dose with each meal and at bedtime. A standard dose of a PPI is added to the regimen and taken twice daily. All medications are taken for a 10-day period.
[e] See Table 26-1 for standard peptic ulcer healing dosage regimens.
[f] Requires validation in the United States.
BID, twice a day; H_2RA, H_2-receptor antagonist; PPI, proton pump inhibitor; QID, four times a day; QD, every day.
Adapted from references 9, 75, 80, 96, and 107, with permission.

HELICOBACTER PYLORI–RELATED PEPTIC ULCER

1. R.L. is an otherwise healthy 45-year-old man who works in a high-stress job as an air traffic controller at a major airport. He complains of a 2-week history of "burning stomach pain" sometimes accompanied by "indigestion and bloating." The pain initially occurred several times a day, usually between meals, and sometimes awakened him at night, but it has increased in frequency over the last week. Initially, the pain was temporarily reduced by food or antacids. Last week, R.L. tried an OTC H_2-receptor antagonist that "lasted longer" but did not provide adequate symptom relief. R.L. indicates that he experienced a similar type of pain about 10 years ago when he was treated with omeprazole for a suspected peptic ulcer. He has smoked one pack of cigarettes daily for the past 20 years, has an occasional glass of red wine with dinner, and usually drinks 4 to 6 cups of caffeinated coffee throughout the day. R.L. takes acetaminophen for occasional headaches and a multivitamin but denies the use of any other OTC or prescription medications, including NSAIDs. He denies nausea, vomiting, anorexia, weight loss, and any changes in stool consistency or color. A review of other body systems is noncontributory. There are no known food or drug allergies.

Physical examination is normal except for epigastric tenderness on palpation of the upper abdomen. Vital signs include a temperature of 98.8°F, blood pressure of 132/80, and a heart rate

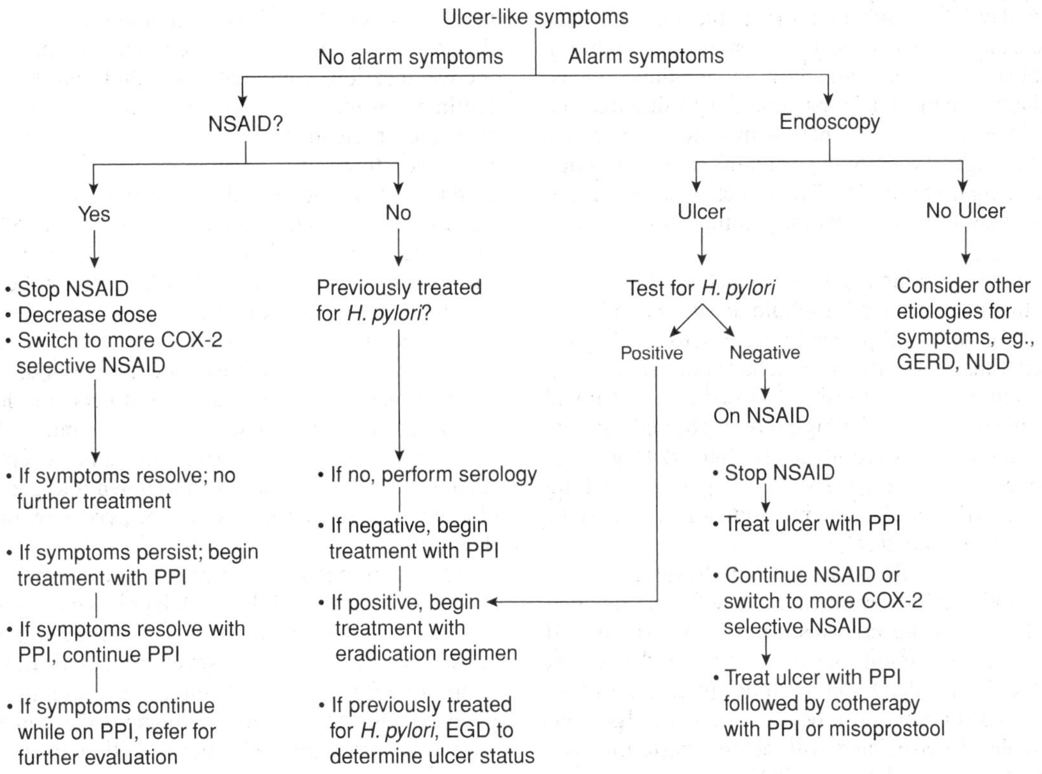

FIGURE 26-4 Management of peptic ulcer disease. *H. pylori, Helicobacter pylori*; H_2RA, H_2-receptor antagonist; NSAID, nonsteroidal anti-inflammatory drug; NUD, nonulcer dyspepsia; PPI, proton pump inhibitor.

of 78 beats/minute. Pertinent laboratory values include Hgb of 14.0 g/dL, Hct of 44%, and a negative stool guiaic test. All other laboratory values are within normal limits. What signs and symptoms are suggestive of a recurrent peptic ulcer?

Most patients with PUD present with abdominal pain that is epigastric and often described as burning or gnawing, while others complain of abdominal discomfort, fullness, or cramping. Epigastric pain, however, does not necessarily correlate with an ulcer, as patients with ulcer-like symptoms may have NUD and asymptomatic patients may have an NSAID-induced ulcer. Heartburn, bloating, and belching may accompany the pain. Ulcer pain typically occurs during the day but can also awaken the patient from sleep (nocturnal pain). In patients with a duodenal ulcer, epigastric pain frequently occurs between meals and is often relieved by food, but this varies from patient to patient. Alternatively, food may precipitate or accentuate pain in patients with a gastric ulcer.

The severity of ulcer pain varies from patient to patient. The pain may be seasonal, occurring more frequently in the spring or fall and occurring in clusters lasting up to a few weeks followed by a pain-free period or remission lasting from weeks to years. Antacids and antisecretory medications usually provide relief of ulcer pain in most patients. Pain usually diminishes or disappears during treatment, but epigastric pain after healing often suggests an unhealed or recurrent ulcer. Changes in the character of the pain may suggest the presence of complications. Nausea, vomiting, anorexia, and weight loss are more common with gastric ulcer but may also be suggestive of ulcer-related complication. The diagnosis of PUD cannot be made on symptoms alone and requires visualization of the ulcer crater.

2. R.L. underwent upper endoscopy (EGD), which revealed a single 0.5-cm ulcer in the duodenal bulb. The ulcer base was clear without evidence of active bleeding. Antral gastritis was biopsy positive for *H. pylori*. What risk factors may have contributed to ulcer recurrence in this patient?

R.L. indicates that he had a similar type of abdominal pain about 10 years ago, when he was treated with omeprazole for a suspected peptic ulcer. When conventional antiulcer therapy (e.g., PPI) is discontinued after ulcer healing, 60% to 100% of patients develop a recurrent ulcer within 1 year.[9,75] The most important factors that influence ulcer recurrence are *H. pylori* infection and NSAID use. It is not known whether R.L. underwent testing for *H. pylori* 10 years ago. The patient denies the use of OTC and prescription NSAIDs. The long-term use of maintenance therapy with conventional antiucler medications (Table 26-1) may have been an option for this patient at the time he was treated for a suspected peptic ulcer, because it reduces ulcer recurrence to 20% to 40% at 1 year.[9] However, the eradication of *H. pylori* (in a *H. pylori*–positive patient) decreases ulcer recurrence to $<$10% at 1 year, cures the disease, and eliminates the need for long-term maintenance therapy in most patients.[9,75]

Other factors such as cigarette smoking, psychologic stress, and diet may have contributed to ulcer recurrence in this patient. There is epidemiologic evidence linking cigarette smoking to PUD. The risk appears proportional to the number of cigarettes smoked per day and is greatest when $>$10 cigarettes are smoked per day.[9] Although a number of mechanisms have been postulated, including delayed gastric emptying, inhibition of pancreatic bicarbonate secretion, promotion of duodenogastric reflux, reduction in mucosal prostaglandin production, and increases gastric acid secretion. There is insufficient evidence to conclude that cigarette smoking actually causes a peptic ulcer.[9] However, cigarette smoking, nicotine, or other components of smoke may provide a favorable milieu for *H. pylori* infection.

R.L. works as an air traffic controller, which is a high-stress job. However, the importance of psychologic stress and how it affects PUD is complex and probably multifactorial. Results from controlled trials are conflicting and have failed to demonstrate a cause-and-effect relationship.[9] However, the clinical observation of ulcer patients with high-stress jobs and a stressful lifestyle suggest that they are adversely affected. Emotional stress may induce behavioral risks such as cigarette smoking and the use of NSAIDs or alter the inflammatory response or resistance to *H. pylori* infection.

Caffeine-containing coffee, tea, and cola beverages, constituents in decaffeinated coffee or tea, caffeinefree carbonated beverages, and alcoholic beverages such as beer and wine all increase gastric acid secretion, but there is no evidence that they increase the risk for PUD. Certain foods (e.g., spicy) may cause dyspepsia but do not cause peptic ulcers. In high concentrations, alcohol is associated with acute gastric mucosal damage and upper GI bleeding, but there is insufficient evidence to confirm that alcohol causes ulcers.[9] Dietary restrictions and bland diets do not alter the frequency of ulcer recurrence. Because certain foods and beverages may exacerbate or worsen ulcer symptoms, the patient may decide to avoid them. R.L. is otherwise healthy and does not have any other medical conditions (e.g., chronic renal failure) that are associated with an increased risk of PUD (see Etiology and Risk Factors section).

3. What are the goals of therapy when treating this patient?

The goals of therapy in a *H. pylori*–positive patient with an active ulcer, a previously documented ulcer, or a history of an ulcer-related complication is to render the patient asymptomatic, heal the ulcer, eradicate the infection, and cure the disease. Treatment should be effective, well-tolerated, easy to comply with, and cost-effective. Drug regimens should have an eradication rate of at least 70% (intention-to-treat) and should minimize the potential for antimicrobial resistance.[75,80,95,96] The use of a single antibiotic, bismuth salt, or antiulcer drug does not achieve this goal.[75] Two drug regimens (PPI and amoxicillin or clarithromycin) are not recommended in the United States because of marginal eradication rates and because the use of only one antibiotic increases the risk for antibiotic resistance[9,75]

Primary Treatment of *Helicobacter pylori* Infection

4. What is the preferred *H. pylori* eradication regimen for this patient? Which factors should be taken into consideration when selecting an eradication regimen?

The selection of a first-line eradication regimen should include an antibiotic combination that permits second-line treatment (if necessary) with different antibiotics. The antibiotics that have been most extensively studied and found to be effective in various combinations include clarithromycin, amoxicillin, metronidazole, and tetracycline.[9,75] The recommended first-line eradication therapies in the United States are the PPI-based three-drug regimens[75,80,95,96] (Table 26-6). When given in recommended dosages, most recent studies report intention-to-treat eradication rates of 70% to 80%.[80] Increasing the antibiotic daily dose usually does not improve eradication rates. When combined with a PPI and clarithromycin, the inclusion of amoxicillin or metronidazole provides similar eradication rates.[97] However, amoxicillin is usually preferred initially because it is associated with little or no bacterial resistance, has fewer adverse effects, and leaves metronidazole as an option for second-line therapies.[9] Thus, the PPI-amoxicillin-clarithromycin regimen is an acceptable first-line regimen for R.L., as he has no known allergies to drugs (including penicillin) and has not received previous eradication therapy.

The recommended duration of treatment in the United States is 14 days, even though 10 to 14 days is typically used and international guidelines recommend a treatment duration of 7 to 10 days.[80] A meta-analysis of seven trials indicates that a 14-day course of a PPI-based triple therapy containing clarithromycin yielded better eradication rates than a 7-day course and showed a trend toward improved efficacy with a 10-day course when compared with 7 days.[98] A large randomized trial also reports the superiority of a 14-day eradication regimen over a 7-day regimen.[99] A longer treatment duration favors a higher eradication rate and is less likely to be associated with antimicrobial resistance.[75,80] A treatment duration <7 days is not recommended and is associated with unsatisfactory eradication rates. A meta-analysis of 13 studies indicates that twice-daily dosing of the PPI in the PPI-based regimens containing clarithromycin may be superior to a single daily dose.[100] Pretreatment with a PPI dose prior to initiating *H. pylori* eradication does not appear to decrease eradication rates.[101] Prolonged treatment with the PPI beyond 14 days is not necessary for ulcer healing in most patients.

A 14-day bismuth-based four-drug regimen that contains a H_2RA (Table 26-6) yields eradication rates similar to those achieved with a PPI-based three-drug regimen containing clarithromycin.[75,80] A meta-analysis of five randomized trials reports eradication rates of 79% for PPI-based clarithromycin triple therapy and 80% for bismuth-based quadruple therapy when using intention to-treat analysis.[102] Quadruple therapy (bismuth, metronidazole, and tetracycline) using a PPI instead of a H_2RA permits a shorter duration of treatment (10 days vs. 14 days) and may provide increased efficacy in patients with metronidazole-resistant strains of *H. pylori*.[102,103] Comparable eradication rates have been achieved by using a novel bismuth-based quadruple therapy containing bismuth subcitrate potassium (biskalcitrate) in place of bismuth subsalicylate and a twice-daily PPI[104] (Table 26-6). Increasing the duration of quadruple therapy to 1 month does not substantially increase eradication. The bismuth-based four-drug regimens are as effective as the PPI-based three-drug regimens containing clarithromycin and are indicated as first-line therapy. However, the complexity of these regimens often relegates them to second-line status in clinical practice.

Alternative first-line therapies are needed because of the declining eradication rates reported with the PPI-based three-drug regimens containing clarithromycin and the bismuth-based four-drug regimens.[80] These lower eradication rates have been attributed to an increase in clarithromycin and metronidazole resistance. Sequential therapy with a PPI and amoxicillin for 5 days followed by a PPI, clarithromycin, and an imidazole for an additional 5 days (Table 26-6) has achieved eradication rates that are superior to the PPI-based three-drug regimens containing clarithromycin.[80,105] An increased efficacy has also been reported with sequential therapy in patients with clarithromycin-resistant *H. pylori* strains.[106] The rationale for sequential eradication therapy is to initially treat the patient with antibiotics that rarely promote resistance (e.g., amoxicillin) in order to reduce the bacterial load and preexisting resistant organisms and then to follow with different antibiotics to kill the remaining organisms. Although the precise mechanism for the success of sequential therapy is uncertain, the higher efficacy may be related to the increased number of antibiotics (amoxicillin, metronidazole, and clarithromycin) to which the organism is exposed. Although sequential therapy looks promising, it must be validated in the United States before it can be recommended as first-line eradication therapy.

Patient Education

5. R.L. is prescribed a 14-day PPI-based three-drug eradication containing amoxicillin and clarithromycin. What instructions would you provide R.L. regarding his medications?

R.L. should be informed of the importance of taking his medications as prescribed in order to minimize treatment failure and the development of antibiotic resistance. He should be advised that the PPI is an integral part of the three-drug regimen and should be taken twice daily 30 to 60 minutes before breakfast and dinner (see Pharmacotherapy Proton Pump Inhibitor section) along with the amoxicillin and clarithromycin (Table 26-6). If he were taking a bismuth-based four-drug regimen containing a PPI, all medications except the PPI should be taken four times a day with meals and at bedtime. If the PPI is to be taken once daily, it should be taken 30 to 60 minutes prior to breakfast; if twice daily, the second dose should be taken 30 to 60 minutes prior to dinner.

R.L. should also be informed of the most common side effects associated with his treatment regimen. All antibiotics included in the *H. pylori* eradication regimens are usually associated with mild side effects, including nausea, abdominal pain, and diarrhea. *C. difficile*–associated diarrhea, a serious antibiotic-related complication, occurs occasionally. Oral thrush and vaginal candidiasis (in women) may also occur. Clarithromycin and metronidazole may cause taste disturbances. If R.L.'s medications included metronidazole, tetracycline, or a bismuth salt, he should be provided additional information on these medications. Metronidazole-containing regimens increase the frequency of side effects (especially when the dose is >1 g/day) and may be associated with a disulfiramlike reaction in patients who consume alcohol. Tetracycline may cause photosensitivity and should not be used in children because it may cause tooth discoloration. Bismuth salts may cause darkening of the tongue and stool.

Regimens for the Management of *Helicobacter pylori* Infection in Patients With Penicillin Allergies

6. What would have been the preferred initial *H. pylori* eradication regimen if R.L. had a documented allergy to penicillin?

There are two first-line treatment options if R.L. had a documented allergy to penicillin. Metronidazole can be substituted for amoxicillin in the PPI-based three-drug regimen, as similar eradication rates are achieved[97,107] (Table 26-6). Alternatively, the bismuth-based four-drug regimens may also be used, as they provide similar eradication rates to the PPI-based three-drug regimens.

7. What drug substitutions are acceptable in the PPI-based three-drug and bismuth-based four-drug eradiation regimens?

Substitution of one PPI for another is acceptable and does not enhance or diminish eradication rates in either the three- or four-drug regimens.[80,108] A PPI may be substituted for a H_2RA in the bismuth-based four-drug regimen (Table 26-6). However, a H_2RA should not be substituted for a PPI in the three-drug regimens[109] unless the patient is unable to tolerate the PPI.[110] There are insufficient data to support the substitution of ampicillin for amoxicillin, doxycycline for tetracycline, and azithromycin or erythromycin for clarithromycin.

Substitution of clarithromycin 250 to 500 mg four times a day for tetracycline in the bismuth-based four-drug regimen yields similar results, but substitution of amoxicillin for tetracycline lowers the eradication rate and is not recommended.[9,102]

8. What are the most important predictors of *H. pylori* treatment outcomes, and how may they alter R.L.'s response to treatment?

The two most important factors in predicting a favorable response to *H. pylori* eradication are medication adherence and antibiotic resistance.[75,80,96,111,112] Medication adherence decreases with multiple medications, increased frequency of administration, increased duration of treatment, intolerable adverse effects, and costly drug regimens. Although a longer treatment duration may contribute to nonadherence, missed doses in a 7-day regimen may also lead to failed eradication.[111] The bismuth-based four-drug regimen requires the patient to take medications four times a day and as many as 18 tablet/capsules per day. The complexity of this regimen explains why many consider it second-line even though it is similar in efficacy to the PPI-based three-drug regimens that are taken twice daily. While mild side effects are common with all of the eradication regimens, some patients will experience clinically important effects that lead to discontinuation of a specific drug or of the entire regimen. There are limited data to suggest that smoking, alcohol consumption, and diet may negatively impact eradication.[111]

Antibiotic resistance is an important determinant of successful *H. pylori* eradication.[80,87,96,111] Antibiotic resistance rates among *H. pylori* strains in the United States from 1993 to 1999 were reported to be 37.0% for metronidazole, 10.0%

for clarithromycin, and 1.4% for amoxicillin.[113] More recent data collected from 1998 to 2002 reveal resistance rates of 25.0% for metronidazole, 13.0% for clarithromycin, and 0.9% for amoxicillin.[114] Although difficult to compare, it appears that clarithromycin rates have increased, while metronidazole and amoxicillin have remained relatively stable. It is likely that the increase in clarithromycin resistance may explain, in part, the decreasing efficacy of clarithromycin-containing eradication regimens.[80] The clinical importance of metronidazole resistance is uncertain, as higher metronidazole doses and the synergistic effect of combining metronidazole with other antibiotics appears to render resistance to metronidazole more relative. Alternatively, even though resistance to clarithromycin is lower, it is more likely to affect the clinical outcome.[80,111] Resistance to amoxicillin and tetracycline is uncommon. Resistance to bismuth has not been reported. Other factors that may contribute to treatment failure include the specific *H. pylori* strain and CYP2C19 polymorphism when PPIs are used as part of the eradication regimen.[80]

9. What parameters should be monitored to determine R.L.'s response to treatment?

Posttreatment testing to confirm eradication is recommended for patients with a *H. pylori*–related ulcer, persistent dyspeptic symptoms, MALT lymphoma, or early gastric cancer.[80]

However, posttreatment testing is neither practical nor cost-effective for all patients with a *H. pylori*–positive peptic ulcer.[80] When endoscopy follow-up is not necessary, the UBT (Table 26-5) is the preferred test to confirm eradication of *H. pylori*. To avoid confusing bacterial suppression with eradication, the UBT must be delayed at least 4 weeks after the completion of treatment. The term *eradication* or *cure* is used when posttreatment tests conducted 4 weeks after the end of treatment do not detect the organism. Antibody tests should be avoided post treatment, because antibody titers remain elevated for a long period of time (up to 1 year) before they return to the uninfected range following successful eradication.[9,80,92] If performed post treatment, only a negative test is considered to be reliable.

Upper endoscopy should only be used to confirm eradication and ulcer healing if indicated (e.g., severe or frequent recurrent symptoms, current or previous ulcer complication), as the procedure is costly and invasive. When endoscopic follow-up is necessary, testing to prove eradication includes a biopsy for the rapid urease test and histology (Table 26-5). Ulcer healing can also be confirmed at that time.

In clinical practice, the need for confirmation of ulcer healing and eradication must be weighed against the need, feasibility, availability and cost of tests and procedures. Although posttreatment testing to confirm *H. pylori* eradication is recommended, patients like R.L., who present with an uncomplicated *H. pylori*–positive ulcer, are usually monitored for symptomatic recurrence 1 to 2 weeks post completion of drug therapy.[80] The absence of symptoms is considered a surrogate marker for successful ulcer healing and eradication. The persistence, or recurrence, of symptoms within 2 weeks after the end of treatment suggests failure of ulcer healing or eradication or an alternative diagnosis such as GERD.

Therapy for Refractory *Helicobacter pylori* Infection

10. What other drug regimens can be used if R.L. fails initial eradication therapy with a PPI-amoxicillin-clarithromycin regimen?

Eradicating *H. pylori* is more difficult after initial treatment fails, as attempts to eradicate the organism are extremely variable.[75,96] Second-line regimens should (a) avoid using antibiotics that were used during initial therapy, (b) use antibiotics that have less problems with resistance, (c) use drugs that have a topical effect (e.g., bismuth), and (d) employ a 10- to 14-day treatment regimen.[111] If R.L. was not successfully eradicated initially with omeprazole-amoxicillin-clarithromycin, he should receive second-line therapy with bismuth subsalicylate, metronidazole, tetracycline, and a PPI for 10 to 14 days[75,80,111,115] (Table 26-6). An eradication rate of 76% has been reported in the pooled analysis of 16 studies and 24 abstracts when bismuth quadruple therapy is used as second-line therapy after initial treatment failure.[116]

A PPI-based triple therapy containing levofloxacin and amoxicillin (Table 26-6) has been evaluated as second-line therapy in patients with persistent infection. The results of a meta-analysis containing four randomized trials indicates that a 10-day PPI-based three-drug regimen containing levofloxacin was superior to a 7-day bismuth-based four-drug regimen and was associated with fewer side effects.[117] Although the results from the levofloxacin-based regimens look promising, they require validation. A PPI-based three-drug regimen containing rifabutin and amoxcillin reported a 91% eradication rate, but side effects were common.[118] Regimens using furazolidone (100 mg four times a day) in place of metronidazole in either the PPI-based three-drug regimens or the bismuth-based four-drug regimen have been studied and yield variable eradication rates.[111] However, furazolidone is not available in the United States.

NONSTEROIDAL ANTI-INFLAMMATORY DRUG-INDUCED PEPTIC ULCER

11. A.D. is a 70-year-old woman who retired from teaching about 5 years ago. Several days ago, she noticed black "tarry" stools and was hospitalized for an upper GI bleed most likely secondary to NSAID use. She complains of "feeling tired" and occasionally dizzy for about 1 week. A.D. presents with a 5-year history of rheumatoid arthritis for which she takes naproxen 250 mg in the morning and 500 mg in the evening. She states that prior to admission, she was also taking prednisone 10 mg daily about a week for her arthritic pain that was not controlled with naproxen. She denies any history of previous ulcer or ulcer-related complication. Other prescription medications include hydrochlorothiazide 25 mg daily for hypertension. OTC self-directed medications include enteric-coated aspirin 81 mg daily, calcium carbonate, and a multivitamin. A.D. does not use tobacco or drink caffeinated beverages but does have an occasional beer with friends. She denies epigastric pain, nausea, vomiting, anorexia, and weight loss but notes a recent change in stool color. A review of other body systems are noncontributory other than previously indicated. There are no known food or drug allergies.

Physical examination reveals a well-developed weak woman in no acute distress. The abdomen was normal with no pain on

palpation. Bowel sounds were normal with no guarding, masses, hepatomegaly, or spleenomegaly. The rectum was normal but with guiaic-positive stool. Vital signs include a temperature of 98.9°F, blood pressure of 100/65, and a heart rate of 90 beats/minute. Pertinent laboratory values include Hgb of 11.0 g/dL, Hct of 35%, blood urea nitrogen (BUN) 40, and serum creatinine (SrCr) 1.5 mg/dL. All other laboratory values are within normal limits. What factors place A.D. at increased risk for developing an NSAID-induced ulcer and related upper GI bleeding?

The use of a nonselective NSAIDs (e.g., naproxen) is linked to a three- to fourfold increase in upper GI complications while there is a two- to threefold increase with COX-2 inhibitors when partially and highly selective agents are evaluated as a group[90] (Table 26-4). The risk for NSAID-induced ulcer and related complications is dose related, but ulcers can occur at any dosage, including low doses of OTC NSAIDs.[119] Upper GI events can occur at any time during treatment with an NSAID, as the risk for complications is similar throughout treatment. The use of cardioprotective dosages (81–325 mg/day) of aspirin in combination with another NSAID increases the risk of upper GI complications to a greater extent than the use of either drug alone.[82,84,89] The use of buffered or enteric-coated aspirin confers no added protection from ulcer or GI complications.[89,91] Corticosteroids do not increase the ulcer risk when used alone, but the risk is increased twofold in corticosteroid users such as A.D. who are also taking concurrent NSAIDs.[120] A.D.'s age (70 years) is an independent risk factor for NSAID-induced ulcers, as risk increases linearly with the age of the patient[120] (Table 26-3). The increased incidence in older patients may be explained by age-related changes in gastric mucosal defense. The combined risk factors greatly increase A.D.'s risk for an NSAID-related upper GI event, as ulcer risk is additive.

A.D. did not have a history of an ulcer or ulcer-related complication. However, the risk of a NSAID ulcer or complication increases 14-fold in a patient with a previous ulcer or complication.[9] The risk of upper GI bleeding is also markedly increased when NSAIDs are taken with anticoagulants or medications such as clopidogrel.[90] Selective serotonin reuptake inhibitors (SSRIs) have been reported to independently increase the risk of upper GI bleeding,[121] although more recent data suggest the increased bleeding risk may be less than that initially reported.[122] Whether *H. pylori* is a risk factor for NSAID-induced ulcers is uncertain.[89,123] Because the incidence of PUD is higher in a *H. pylori*–positive patient taking NSAIDs, it is possible that they have additive effects.[124]

12. **A.D. was admitted for further evaluation and treatment. An upper endoscopy (EGD) revealed two bleeding antral ulcers (0.2 and 0.4 cm). An antral biopsy was reported to be *H. pylori* negative. All medications were discontinued. Oral oxycodone was instituted at 5 mg every 6 hours when needed to control A.D.'s arthritic pain while she was hospitalized. Consideration was given to decreasing the naproxen dose and switching to acetaminophen, a nonacetylated salicylate, or a partially selective NSAID (Table 26-4), but none of these options were satisfactory for this patient. Treatment was initiated with a continuous infusion of IV pantoprazole for 3 days and then she was switched to oral pantoprazole 40 mg BID. A.D. was discharged on pantoprazole 40 mg QD and naproxen 250 mg in the morning and 500 mg in the evening. All other oral medications were reinstituted except for the prednisone. Will A.D.'s gastric ulcer heal if she continues to take the naproxen?**

The naproxen should be discontinued, if possible, in the presence of an active ulcer.[82,120] If A.D. were able to discontinue the naproxen permanently, a PPI would be preferred, as it provides a more rapid rate of ulcer healing (4 weeks) and symptom relief than H_2RAs or sucralfate (6–8 weeks).[9] Because the naproxen was reinstituted at discharge in the presence of an active ulcer, a PPI is the drug of choice, as potent acid suppression is required to heal the ulcer and relieve the symptoms.[82,120] However, the duration of PPI therapy should be extended from 4 weeks to 8 to 12 weeks.

13. **Which ulcer-healing regimen would you have recommended if A.D. was reported to be *H. pylori* positive?**

All patients with PUD should be tested for *H. pylori*. If positive, patients should be treated with an eradication regimen. A PPI-based eradication regimen is recommended in a *H. pylori*–positive patient with an active ulcer who is also taking an NSAID. One reason for this is that it is not possible to determine whether the *H. pylori*, the NSAID, or both actually caused the ulcer. In addition, if an individual is tested and found to be *H. pylori* positive, he or she should be offered eradication therapy whether or not there is a documented ulcer. The selection of a specific regimen (Table 26-6) depends on a number of factors, including whether the individual is penicillin allergic.

Strategies to Reduce the Risk of NSAID-Induced Peptic Ulcers

14. **Three months later, A.D. returned to her gastroenterologist for a follow-up EGD, which confirmed that the gastric ulcers were healed. On return to her primary care physician, the pantoprazole was changed to ranitidine 150 mg BID. Other medications at this time include naproxen 250 mg in the morning and 500 mg in the evening, enteric-coated aspirin 81 mg QD, calcium carbonate, and multivitamins. What pharmacological options are available to reduce the risk of a NSAID ulcer now that A.D.'s initial ulcer is healed and she continues to take the naproxen and aspirin?**

Strategies to reduce the risk of NSAID ulcers and upper GI complications in a patient taking a nonselective NSAID include cotherapy with a PPI or misoprostol or the use of a selective COX-2 inhibitor in place of the nonselective NSAID.[82,88,89,120,125,126] All PPIs, when used in standard dosages (Table 26-1), are effective for this indication. A reduction in upper GI complications in high-risk patients receiving PPI cotherapy has been reported in two small studies.[127,128]

The H_2RAs should not be recommended as prophylactic cotherapy to reduce the risk of NSAID ulcers. Although standard H_2RA dosages (Table 26-1) are effective in reducing the risk of a duodenal ulcer, they are not effective in reducing the risk of gastric ulcer, which is the most common ulcer associated with NSAIDs.[82,88,89,120] Higher H_2RA dosages (e.g., famotidine 40 mg twice daily) reduce the risk of gastric and duodenal ulcer but are less effective than a PPI.[88,89] There are no studies that have evaluated the use of H_2RAs in reducing the risk of ulcer-related upper GI complications. The H_2RAs may be used when necessary to relieve NSAID-related dyspepsia.

Misoprostol reduces the risk of NSAID-induced gastric and duodenal ulcers.[82,88,89,120] An important trial in rheumatoid arthritis patients indicates that misoprostol also reduces the risk of upper GI complications in high-risk patients.[129] Initially, the recommended dosage was 200 mcg four times a day, but diarrhea and abdominal cramping limited its use. A dosage of 200 mcg three times a day is comparable in efficacy to 800 mcg/day and should be used in patients unable to tolerate the higher dose.[82,88,89] When misoprostol 800 mcg/day was compared with lansoprazole (15 mg/day or 30 mg/day) or placebo, misoprostol and both dosages of lansoprazole reduced the risk of ulcer recurrence, although the PPI was better tolerated.[130] A misoprostol dosage of ≤400 mcg/day reduces the incidence of diarrhea but is less efficacious. A fixed dosage form containing misoprostol 200 mcg and diclofenac (50 mg or 75 mg) is available, but flexibility to individualize dosage is lost.

Two large multicenter clinical trials evaluated the GI safety of COX-2 inhibitors, one using celecoxib (CLASS)[131] and the other rofecoxib (VIGOR).[132] Their trials reported a reduction of 50% to 60% in upper GI events with the COX-2 inhibitors when compared with non- and partially selective NSAIDs. The initial 6-month analysis of celecoxib in the CLASS trial revealed a lower rate of ulcer complications, but evaluation of the data at 13 months indicated that celecoxib did not have a GI safety advantage over ibuprofen or diclofenac.[88,133] The most likely explanation for these results is that celecoxib is not as highly a selective COX-2 inhibitor as was originally anticipated.[134] Thus, its improved GI safety when compared with nonselective NSAIDs has not been established. Further analysis of the results indicated that patients taking cardioprotective doses of aspirin had a similar rate of upper GI events as those taking either diclofenac or ibuprofen.[131] Thus, the gastroprotective benefits of celecoxib may be negated in patients taking low-dose aspirin. Aspirin appears to have similar effects on other COX-2 inhibitors. Unlike the CLASS study, the VIGOR trial excluded aspirin users. Results from this trial indicated that ulcers and related complications were lower with rofecoxib than with naproxen.[132]

Cyclo-oxygenase-2 Inhibitors and Cardiovascular Toxicity

15. What is the concern regarding the use of COX-2 inhibitors and the risk for cardiovascular toxicity?

The risk for cardiovascular events in patients taking COX-2 inhibitors increases with a number of factors, including increased COX-2 selectivity, higher dosages, a longer duration of treatment, and preexisting cardiovascular risk.[133–136] Although ulcers and ulcer-related complications were less likely with rofecoxib than with naproxen in the VIGOR trial, there was an increased number of myocardial infarctions and thrombotic strokes observed with rofecoxib.[132] Similar cardiothrombolic events were observed in other rofecoxib studies of longer duration.[137] In 2004, rofecoxib was withdrawn from the U.S. market. Soon thereafter, valdecoxib was also taken off the market amid concerns about cardiovascular risk.

The cardiovascular safety of celecoxib has also been evaluated, but the risk of myocardial infarction and thrombotic stroke is less certain. Although there appeared to be no difference in cardiovascular risk when celecoxib was compared with diclofenac and ibuprofen in the CLASS trial,[131] a dose-related increase was reported in one large trial.[138] Celecoxib remains available in the United States, but cardiovascular risk must be evaluated in each patient when considering the use of this drug. Patients with cardiovascular disease or risk factors for cardiovascular disease are at greatest risk for cardiovascular events with celecoxib. The lowest effective dose should always be used for the shortest duration of time.

There is increasing evidence that certain non- and partially selective NSAIDs (e.g., ibuprofen, diclofenac, and meloxicam) may also increase the risk of myocardial infarction and thrombotic stroke.[139] The American Heart Association has published recommendations for NSAID use in persons with confirmed cardiovascular disease or risk factors.[140] Recommendations include initiating short-term treatment with less risky options such as acetaminophen or aspirin, tramadol, or narcotics. A NSAID should be considered if these medications are either inappropriate or not effective. The preferred nonselective NSAID is naproxen, because it does not appear to increase cardiovascular risk. NSAIDs with increasing COX-2 selectivity (Table 26-4) may be tried if symptoms are not relieved. However, selective COX-2 inhibitors should be reserved for those patients in whom there are no other alternatives and should be used in the lowest effective dose for the shortest period of time. Thus, GI safety of NSAIDs and selective COX-2 inhibitors must be weighed against the potential increase in cardiovascular risk.

16. How does a COX-2 inhibitor compare with a PPI and a non- or partially selective NSAID when used to decrease ulcer risk and related complications? Have any studies evaluated GI safety in patients taking a COX-2 inhibitor plus a PPI?

Two small nonplacebo controlled trials in *H. pylori*–negative patients at high risk for NSAID-related complications compared celecoxib versus a PPI plus a nonselective or partially selective NSAID.[141,142] These trials were undertaken before the GI and cardiovascular safety of celecoxib was questioned. In the first trial, celecoxib was compared with lansoprazole plus naproxen,[141] while in the second, celecoxib was compared with omeprazole plus diclofenac.[142] The results of these two studies indicate that when celecoxib was compared with a PPI plus a NSAID in high-risk patients, ulcer complications rates were similar but fairly high in both groups.[141,142] Cotherapy using a COX-2 inhibitor plus a PPI in high-risk patients should be considered, but this regimen is reported to have a very modest benefit when compared with a nonselective NSAID plus a PPI.[143]

17. What factors should be considered when evaluating management strategies for patients at risk of a developing a NSAID-induced ulcer? What risk reduction strategies are considered acceptable for A.D.?

Strategies to reduce the risk of NSAID-induced ulcers and related complications depend on the assessment of risk for each patient (Table 26-3). Although some have attempted to define levels of risk, there are no universally accepted definition.[82,88,125,126,144] In general, individuals with no risk factors, most individuals <65 years of age, and those taking NSAIDs in the short term are considered to be at low risk and usually do not require risk-reduction cotherapy. Some patients may benefit from a partially selective NSAID (Table 26-4). Patients at moderate risk include those >65 years of age with one or two risk factors, excluding a history of a prior ulcer or ulcer-related complication. The preferred risk reduction strategy in this group is cotherapy with a PPI. Although cotherapy with misoprotol is also effective, it is used as a second-line therapy because of frequent daily dosing and a dose-dependent diarrhea. When indicated, the patient may be switched to a selective COX-2 inhibitor. The use of a nonselective or partially selective NSAID and a PPI is most likely as effective as a selective COX-2 inhibitor.[125]

Patients like A.D., who have a history of a prior ulcer and ulcer-related upper GI bleed, are at high-risk for future NSAID-related ulcers and complications and require an effective risk-reduction strategy. Additionally, A.D. has other factors that contribute to her high-risk status, including her age (70 years), concurrent use of a nonselective NSAID (naproxen) and enteric-coated aspirin, and the use of corticosteroids. Ranitidine should be discontinued, and A.D. should be switched to an evidence-based risk-reduction regimen. Although the optimal strategy for a high-risk patient like A.D. is unknown, the preferred strategy should take into consideration the risks, benefits, and cost of treatment. High-risk patients may benefit from several strategies, including PPI or misoprostol cotherapy with a nonselective or partially selective NSAID or a selective COX-2 inhibitor. If celecoxib is used, the risk of cardiovascular effects must be weighed against the gastroprotective benefits, especially since A.D. has a history of hypertension. Patients at very high risk, including those with a prior ulcer or complication, renal dysfunction (creatinine clearance <30 mL/minute) and cardiovascular disease should avoid NSAIDs and selective COX-2 inhibitors and should be treated with other analgesics (e.g., tramadol, narcotics), keeping in mind that NSAIDs and selective COX-2 inhibitors are also associated with fluid retention, hypertension, and renal failure.[133,134] The recommended risk-reduction strategy for A.D. is cotherapy with a PPI or misoprostol.

18. What information should be conveyed to A.D. regarding the combined use of OTC aspirin and NSAIDs?

Counsel A.D. to discuss the use of enteric-coated aspirin with her physician to be certain that the benefit of taking cardioprotective aspirin outweighs the risk for an ulcer-related complication. A.D. should be advised that enteric-coated aspirin may protect against the topical mucosal damage in the stomach and minimize dyspepsia, but the enteric coating does not prevent an ulcer from forming. Even low-dose aspirin (e.g., 81 mg/day) remains capable of causing an ulcer, especially when used in conjunction with a NSAID (naproxen). Buffered aspirin may cause less dyspepsia, but buffering does not prevent ulcers. Taking food, milk, or an antacid with aspirin or NSAIDs may minimize dyspepsia but does not prevent an ulcer.

Inform A.D. that she should not take OTC NSAIDs in conjunction with her naproxen unless advised to do so by her physician, as combining NSAIDs use will the risk for ulcers and upper GI bleeding. Advise A.D. that even though NSAIDs available for self-treatment may have different generic names (e.g., ibuprofen, naproxen) or brand names (e.g., Advil, Aleve), they all belong to the same drug class and have similar side effects.

19. A.D.'s physician decides to maintain her on naproxen and enteric-coated aspirin but changes the ranitidine to lansoprazole 30 mg QD. What instructions should you provide A.D. regarding her medications?

A.D. should be advised of the major signs and symptoms of upper GI bleeding and cardiovascular disease and what action should be taken if these signs or symptoms develop. She should be instructed to take the lansoprazole every day 30 to 60 minutes prior to breakfast and continue taking naproxen twice daily. The importance of adhering to PPI cotherapy must be stressed, especially since A.D. may not have accompanying dyspeptic or ulcerlike symptoms. There is a strong relationship between the level of adherence to gastroprotective medication and the risk for ulcers and serious GI complications in patients like A.D. who are high-risk NSAID users.[145] Older patients, like A.D., who are at risk for osteoporosis and hip fractures and who require long-term PPI therapy should be counseled to take recommended dosages of a calcium salt and vitamin D and have periodic bone density examinations.[54]

20. What parameters should be monitored to determine A.D.'s response to treatment?

High-risk patients like A.D. who continue to take a NSAID should be closely monitored for upper abdominal pain and signs or symptoms associated with bleeding, obstruction, or perforation. The presence of upper abdominal pain or a change in the severity of the pain may suggest an upper GI complication. Every effort should be made to monitor A.D.'s compliance to her PPI regimen because of the strong relationship between nonadherence and the risk of upper GI complications in high-risk NSAID users.

ZOLLINGER-ELLISON SYNDROME

ZES is an uncommon gastric acid hypersecretory disease characterized by severe recurrent peptic ulcers that result from a gastrin-producing tumor (gastrinoma).[146–148] The primary tumor is usually located in the duodenum or pancreas, but other locations (e.g., mesenteric lymph nodes, spleen, stomach, liver) have been described.[147] Although most gastrinomas occur sporadically, about 20% occur in association with multiple endocrine neoplasia type 1 (MEN I), which is an autosomal dominant inherited syndrome.[146,147] Most gastrinomas are malignant and tend to be slow growing, but a small number grow and metastasize rapidly to the regional lymph nodes, liver, and bone. Abdominal pain is the most predominant symptom and is usually related to persistent peptic ulcers, which are less responsive to antisecretory therapy. Duodenal ulcers occur most often, but ulcers may also occur in the stomach or jejunum. Diarrhea, which is present in more than half of patients, may precede ulcer symptoms and results from massive gastric acid hypersecretion, which activates pepsinogen and contributes to mucosal damage.[146,147] Steatorrhea may also occur and results from inactivation of pancreatic lipase by intraluminal acid. This leads to the precipitation of bile acids, which in turn reduces micelle formation necessary for fatty acid absorption. Vitamin B_{12} deficiency may develop secondary to malabsorption related to reduced intrinsic factor activity. GERD often occurs and is complicated by esophageal ulcers and strictures. Other symptoms include nausea, vomiting, upper GI bleeding, and weight loss. Bleeding is related to duodenal ulceration and is the presenting symptom in about 25% of patients.

Epidemiology

The incidence of ZES in the United States is 0.1% to 1.0% among patients with duodenal ulcer.[146,148] The average age at presentation is between 45 and 50 years, with men being slightly more affected than women. The morbidity and mortality of ZES is low because of improved medical and surgical management.

Pathophysiology

The pathophysiology of ZES is related to a nonbeta islet cell gastrin-secreting tumor that stimulates the parietal cells of the stomach to hypersecrete gastric acid.[146,147] Large amounts of gastrin are produced by the gastrinoma cells, usually resulting in a profound hypergastrinemia. The gastric parietal cell mass is expanded in response to the trophic effects of hypergastrinemia and causes an increase in basal and stimulated acid output. Hypersecretion of gastric acid results in severe mucosal ulceration, diarrhea, and malabsorption and is responsible for the signs and symptoms associated with ZES.

Clinical Assessment and Diagnosis

The diagnosis of ZES is established when the fasting serum gastrin is >1,000 pg/mL and the BAO is >15 mEq/hour in patients with an intact stomach (or >5 mEq/hour in the postgastric surgery patient) or when hypergastrinemia is associated with a gastric pH value <2.[146,147] When serum gastrin is between 100 and 1,000 pg/mL and gastric pH is <2, a provocative test (secretin or calcium) is recommended to assist in the diagnosis.[147] Imaging techniques are performed to localize the tumor and are useful in evaluating metastatic disease. Upper endoscopy is performed to confirm mucosal ulcerations. The use of PPIs may mask the clinical presentation and complicate the diagnosis.[149]

Treatment

The goal of treatment for ZES is to pharmacologically control gastric acid secretion and to surgically resect the tumor, if possible. The oral PPIs are the drugs of choice for controlling acid secretion. Treatment should be initiated with omeprazole 60 mg/day or an equivalent oral dose of lansoprazole, pantoprazole, esomeprazole or rabeprazole (Table 26-1) and should be titrated to maintain a BAO <10 mEq/hour (1 hour prior to next dose) in uncomplicated patients or <5 mEq/hour in patients with complicated disease.[146–148] Once adequate control of acid secretion has been achieved, the daily PPI dose should be gradually reduced and administered every 8 to 12 hours. In most patients, an omeprazole dose of 60 to 80 mg/day reduces the BAO to target levels, but doses as high as 360 mg/day have been required.[147,148] IV PPIs should be reserved for those patients who are not able to take oral medications.[147] The H_2RAs are no longer used to treat ZES, even though they were initially proven to be effective (Table 26-1). Results of long-term studies indicate that the use of H_2RAs in treating ZES is limited by poor control of gastric acid hypersecretion and the need for high and frequent doses.[147]

Octreotide, a synthetic somatostatin analogue, also inhibits gastric acid secretion and decreases serum gastrin concentrations, but its subcutaneous route of administration, frequent dosing (100–250 mcg three times a day), and side effects (abdominal pain, diarrhea, gallstones, and pain at the injection site) make it less desirable for use in treating ZES.[147] Slow-release formulations of octreotide (Sandostatin LAR) can be administered less frequently (at 4-week intervals) and may be useful in controlling temporal growth.[147] Patients with metastatic gastrinomas can be treated with chemotherapeutic agents to inhibit tumor growth or may require resection of the tumor. Localization and surgical removal of the gastrinoma should be considered in all patients unless widespread metastases exist.

GASTROESOPHAGEAL REFLUX DISEASE

GERD is a common acid-related GI disorder associated with a wide array of symptoms, the most frequent of which is heartburn, and acid regurgitation. Gastroesophageal reflux (GER) is defined as the retrograde passage of gastric contents from the stomach into the esophagus. It is primarily the result of transient relaxation of the LES. When the LES is relaxed, the esophagus is exposed to small amounts of acidic stomach contents. This normal physiological event occurs many times throughout the day in healthy individuals.[8,150] Protective mechanisms such as esophageal peristalsis and bicarbonate-rich saliva quickly return the acidic pH to normal. GERD develops when alterations in reflux result in symptoms, mucosal injury, or both.[151] Esophageal injury occurs with continued exposure of the mucosa to gastric acid and results in inflammation that can progress to ulceration (erosive esophagitis).[8,152] Complications associated with long-standing GERD include esophageal strictures, Barrett's metaplasia (replacement of normal esophageal squamous epithelium by specialized intestinal-like columnar epithelium), and adenocarcinoma of the esophagus.[8]

Epidemiology

GERD is a chronic disease that affects patients across all age groups with equal distribution between men and women.[8] The prevalence of GERD appears to be greater in the Western population with patients presenting with more clinically important disease and complications than in Eastern countries (especially Asian populations) where GERD is uncommon. However, recent studies suggest that GERD may be emerging in the Eastern populations and that its increasing prevalence may someday match Western populations.[153] When considering the symptoms of GERD, such as heartburn and acid regurgitation, the overall prevalence in the United States is approximately 45%.[8] In Western populations, 25% of patients report heartburn monthly, 12% weekly, and 5% describe daily symptoms.[154] It has also been estimated that 7% of the U.S. population have complicated GERD associated with erosive esophagitis; however, this finding is difficult to validate, as most patients do not undergo diagnostic esophageal endoscopy.[8] Many patients with erosive esophagitis are asymptomatic on diagnosis, which suggests that symptoms do not correlate with the degree of esophageal injury. Up to 75% of patients who undergo endoscopic procedures due to symptoms associated with GERD have normal esophageal findings.[155] These patients are identified as having functional heartburn, NERD, or endoscopy-negative reflux disease (ENRD). Other patients with GERD have symptoms that occur outside of the esophagus which are considered atypical or extraesophageal manifestations of GERD. Extraesophageal manifestations may be present with or without accompanying typical symptoms (e.g., heartburn). Extraesophageal manifestations have been estimated to occur in about 80% of patients with at least weekly symptoms of GERD (see Extraesophageal GERD section).[156]

Childhood GERD appears to continue into adolescence and adulthood. Although most infants develop physiological regurgitation, or spitting up, the majority (95%) will have abatement of symptoms by 1.0 to 1.5 years of age.[157,158] However, infants with persisting symptoms beyond 2 years of age are at risk of developing complicated GERD.[159,160] One prospective study evaluated children with a prior diagnosis of complicated GERD (erosive esophagitis) made at about 5 years of age and then reevaluated the subjects 15 years later. This study revealed that 80% of the children reported monthly symptoms of heartburn and regurgitation, while 23% described weekly symptoms. In addition, 30% still required antisecretory therapy, and 24% underwent antireflux surgery[161] (see Chapter 93, Pediatric Considerations). Pregnancy has also been associated with an increased incidence of GERD with 30% to 50% of pregnant women complaining of heartburn; however, in patients without a previous diagnosis of GERD, the symptoms resolve when the child is born.[8] The mechanisms for GERD in pregnancy are related to (a) the hormonal effects of progesterone and estrogen, which lower LES pressure, and (b) increasing intra-abdominal pressure[8,162] (see Chapter 46, Obstetric Drug Therapy).

Complications associated with GERD include esophageal erosions (5%), strictures (4%–20%), and Barrett's metaplasia (8%–20%).[8] Male gender and advancing age (men and women) are associated with an increase in the prevalence of esophageal complications, presumably due to refluxed acidic contents damaging the mucosa over time.[8] Patients with GERD may have a decrease in quality of life. When comparing quality of life in patients with GERD to those with other chronic medical diseases, the quality of life in GERD patients was between patients with psychiatric disorders and patients with mild heart failure.[163]

Etiology and Risk Factors

The causes of GERD are associated with factors that increase the frequency or duration of GER leading to increased contact of the acidic refluxate with the esophageal mucosa. Risk factors associated with GERD include dietary and lifestyle factors, drugs, and certain medical and surgical conditions[8,15,150–152,164–166] (Table 26-7). These factors may precipitate or worsen GERD symptoms by lowering the LES pressure (e.g., nitrates, progesterone, foods high in fat, mint, chocolate) or having a direct irritating effect on the esophageal mucosa (e.g., citrus, tomatoes, bisphosphonates). Stress reflux from increased intra-abdominal pressure has been associated with overeating, coughing, and bending or straining to lift heavy objects as well as tight-fitting clothing.[8,15] Certain

Table 26-7 Risk Factors Associated With Gastroesophageal Reflux Disease

Drugs	***Dietary***
α-adrenergic agonists	Foods high in fat
Anticholinergics	Spicy foods
Aspirin	Carminatives (peppermint, spearmint)
Barbiturates	Chocolate
Benzodiazepines	Caffeine (coffee, tea, colas)
β_2-adrenergic agonists	Garlic or onions
Bisphosphonates	Citrus fruits and juices
Calcium channel blockers	Tomatoes and juice
Dopamine	Carbonated beverages
Estrogen	
Isoproterenol	**Lifestyle**
Iron	Cigarette/Cigar smoke
Narcotics	Obesity
Nitrates	Supine body position
NSAIDs	Tight-fitting clothing
Progesterone	Heavy exercise
Potassium	
Prostaglandins	**Medical/Surgical Conditions**
Quinidine	Pregnancy
Tetracycline	Scleroderma
Theophylline	ZES
Tricyclic antidepressants	Gastroparesis
Zidovudine	Nasogastric tube intubation

NSAID, nonsteroidal anti-inflammatory drug; ZES, Zollinger-Ellison syndrome.
Adapted from references 8, 15, 150–152, and 164–166, with permission.

medical and surgical conditions such as gastroparesis, scleroderma, ZES, and long-term placement of nasogastric tubes may also be associated with GERD.[8] Although it has been suggested that the eradication of *H. pylori* infection may increase the risk of GERD symptoms and esophagitis, additional information is needed to confirm this association.[80,167,168]

Pathophysiology

The pathophysiology of GERD is associated with defects in transient relaxations of the LES, esophageal acid clearance and buffering capabilities, anatomy, gastric emptying, mucosal resistance and with exposure of the esophageal mucosa to aggressive factors (gastric acid, pepsin, and bile salts) leading to esophageal damage.

Transient Relaxations of the Lower Esophageal Sphincter

The LES, when in a resting state, remains at a high pressure (10–30 mmHg) to prevent the gastric contents from entering into the esophagus.[8] Pressures are lowest during the day and with meals and highest at night.[8] Transient relaxations of the LES are short periods of sphincter relaxation that are different from those that occur with swallowing or peristalsis.[8,169,170] They occur due to vagal stimulation in response to gastric distension from meals (most common), gas, stress, vomiting, or coughing and can persist >10 seconds.[8] These transient relaxations of the LES are associated with virtually all GER events in healthy individuals but account for 50% to 80% of occurrences in patients with pathogenic GERD.[8] Thus, not all transient relaxations of the LES are associated with GERD.

A small percentage of patients may also have a continuously weak and hypotensive LES (decreased LES resting tone). Stress reflux increases intra-abdominal pressure and may blow open the hypotensive LES.[8] When LES pressures remain constantly low, the risk for serious complications (e.g., erosive esophagitis) increase dramatically. Scleroderma, which is related to fibrosis of smooth muscle, may reduce LES tone and increase the potential for GERD.[171]

Esophageal Acid Clearance and Buffering Capabilities

Although the number of reflux events and quantity of refluxate are notable, it is the duration of time the mucosa is in contact with these noxious substances that determines esophageal damage and complications. More than 50% of patients diagnosed with severe esophagitis have decreased acid clearance from the esophagus.[8] Peristalsis is the primary mechanism by which acid refluxate is removed from the esophagus. Other mechanisms include swallowing, esophageal distension in response to refluxate, and gravity (which is only effective when the patient is in an upright position).

Saliva plays an important role in the neutralization of gastric acid within the esophagus. Its bicarbonate-rich content buffers the residual acid that remains in the esophagus after peristalsis.[8] However, saliva is only effective on small amounts of gastric acid, as patients with larger volumes of acid refluxate may not have the neutralizing capacity in saliva necessary to protect the esophagus.[8] Swallowing increases the rate of saliva production and esophageal acid clearance. The reduction of swallowing that occurs during sleep is associated with nocturnal GERD. Patients with decreased saliva production (e.g., elderly, patients taking medication with anticholinergic effects, and those with certain medication conditions such as xerostomia or Sjogren's syndrome) may also be at increased risk of developing GERD.[172]

Anatomic Abnormalities

Hiatal hernia (protrusion of the upper portion of the stomach into the thoracic cavity due to weakening in the diaphragmatic muscles) is frequently described as a cause of GERD, but its causal relationship remains uncertain.[8] Although hiatal hernia is associated with a greater degree of esophagitis, strictures, and Barrett's metaplasia, not all patients with hiatal hernia develop symptoms or complications. This may be related to the size of the hiatal hernia and its effect on LES pressure.[8] An increase in the size of the hernia may decrease its ability to remain below the diaphragm during swallowing and thus reduces LES pressure. Hypotensive LES in combination with hiatal hernia increases the likelihood of reflux and complicated disease.[8]

Gastric Emptying

Delayed gastric emptying increases the volume of gastric fluid remaining within the stomach that is available for reflux and is associated with gastric distension.[8] Although delayed gastric emptying is present in up to 15% of patients with GERD, a causal relationship has not been established.[8,173] Because some patients such as those with diabetic gastroparesis also have GERD, the association between delayed gastric emptying and GERD cannot be overlooked.[8]

Mucosal Resistance

The capability of the esophageal mucosa to endure contact with and withstand injury from gastric refluxate (acid and pepsin) is a substantial determinate for the development of GERD. When considering the mucosal resistance within the esophagus compared with that of the stomach and duodenum, the esophagus is less resistant to damage from gastric acid.[8] However, mucosal resistance in the esophagus is composed of many defensive factors working in tandem to prevent esophageal injury. An increase in mucosal cell thickness and intracellular junctional complexes prevents the diffusion of hydrogen ions from penetrating into the esophageal epithelium and leading to cell death.[8] The esophagus also secretes a protective mucous layer and bicarbonate.[174] Enhanced blood flow in response to an acidic environment within the esophagus improves tissue oxygenation, provides nutrients, and helps to maintain a normal acid–base balance.[8] Esophageal injury also occurs when the concentration of acid and pepsin exceed the protection afforded by mucosal resistance mechanisms.

Aggressive Factors Associated With Esophageal Damage

The gastric refluxate, which is composed primarily of gastric acid and pepsin, is the primary aggressive factor associated with GERD. The development and degree of mucosal damage is dependent on the pH and contents of the refluxate as well as the total exposure time of refluxate with the esophageal mucosa. A pH <4 is usually required to produce injury to the esophageal mucosa, but as the refluxate becomes more acidic, the mucosal damage is accelerated.[8] The addition of pepsin (which is converted from secreted pepsinogen in an acidic pH) to the acidic refluxate will markedly increase the propensity of the refluxate to compromise mucosal resistance and increases the potential for esophageal bleeding.[8,173,175] Duodenogastric reflux or alkaline reflux containing bile acids and pancreatic juices may also contribute to esophagitis. Because gastric and duodenogastric reflux are often concomitantly present, their actions may be additive in causing esophageal damage. The duration of total exposure time of the esophagus to the refluxate is the primary mechanism involved in the development of GERD and its complications. The longer the duration of exposure time, the greater the possibility of severe disease, including progression to Barrett's metaplasia.

Eradication of Helicobacter pylori

The relationship between *H. pylori* infection and GERD remains controversial.[167] Early studies suggest that *H. pylori* eradication is associated with increased gastric acidity and subsequent development of erosive esophagitis.[80,167] In contrast, it appears that *H. pylori* may be protective against GERD symptoms and related complications.[80,166,167] This is presumably due to the microorganisms ability to decrease the acidity of the refluxate, as it does not appear to affect the functional defense mechanisms of the esophagus.[167,168] Although *H. pylori* testing in patients with GERD is not standard practice, if the patient is tested and found to be *H. pylori* positive, eradication is recommended[80] (see Primary Treatment of *Helicobacter pylori* section).

Clinical Presentation

Signs and Symptoms

21. W.J. is a 39-year-old, 130-kg, 67-inch-tall man who presents with complaints of indigestion. He describes a burning sensation behind his breastbone and some belching that is often associated with an acid taste in the back of his mouth. He indicates that his symptoms began a few months ago, and they only occur a few times a month, especially after eating large or spicy meals. Also, if he eats too close to his bedtime, the burning keeps him up at night. He has used liquid antacids in the past for these symptoms and states they work fairly well, but he has to take frequent doses, as the symptoms return quickly. He asks if there is something that he could take to prevent his symptoms. He does not take any other medications. Which of W.J.'s symptoms are consistent with GERD?

Symptoms that are typically associated with GERD include heartburn, or pyrosis (a retrosternal burning that occurs in the upper esophagus and travels up through the throat), regurgitation of gastric contents into the throat, or in many patients, the presence of both.[8,176] These symptoms may be episodic or meal related and are often alleviated by antacids.[8,176] Heartburn, the most frequent typical symptom, is caused by the contact of acidic refluxate with nerve endings within esophageal mucosa.[8] Other symptoms include water brash (salty or sour fluid occurring abruptly within the mouth), early satiety, belching, hiccups, nausea, and vomiting.[8] Worrisome symptoms (alarm signs or symptoms) include dysphagia (trouble swallowing), odynophagia (painful swallowing), vomiting of blood, bloody or tarry stools, unexplained weight loss, and anemia.[8,176] These symptoms suggest complicated disease such as erosive esophagitis, esophageal stricture, malignancy, or GI bleeding and require immediate evaluation by a health care professional. Some patients, such as the elderly, may not have typical GERD symptoms, but present initially with alarm symptoms.[8,177] This is due in part to older patients having a reduced pain perception and a possible reduction in the acidity of the refluxate.[8] Other patients may present with only extraesophageal or atypical symptoms (see Treatment of the Extraesophageal Manifestations of GERD section). Despite the lack of esophageal symptoms, the potential for serious esophageal damage exists, as there is no correlation between symptoms and the degree of esophageal injury.[8] W.J.'s symptoms of a burning sensation (heartburn), regurgitation soon after eating spicy or large meals, and the association of symptoms with eating a meal near his bedtime are all consistent with GERD. The fact that his symptoms are relieved by his use of antacids is also suggestive of GERD.

Treatment

Therapeutic Goals

22. What are the therapeutic goals for the treatment of W.J.'s GERD?

The therapeutic goals for the management of GERD are to alleviate symptoms, promote esophageal healing, prevent recurrence, provide cost-effective pharmacotherapy, and avoid long-term complications.[8] One long-term consequence is Barrett's esophagus, or Barrett's metaplasia, which is identified in 10% to 15% of GERD patients on endoscopic evaluation.[8] This premalignant condition may predispose the patient to esophageal adenocarcinoma. Patients with Barrett's esophagus have a 30- to 125-fold greater risk of developing esophageal cancer than an age-matched population.[178] GERD is a chronic disease that carries the potential for serious complications.

Nonpharmacologic Measures and Self-Directed Treatment

23. What lifestyle and dietary changes may potentially reduce W.J.'s GERD symptoms?

Lifestyle and dietary modifications comprise the initial step in managing patients with GERD[15,166,176,179] (Table 26-8). Strategies should be discussed with the patient and tailored to his or her specific needs. The paucity of evidence to date suggests that although many patients may benefit from these modifications, they are unlikely to completely alleviate symptoms in most patients.[176,179] Lifestyle modifications are aimed at reducing acid exposure within the esophagus by increasing LES pressure, decreasing intragastric pressure, improving esophageal acid clearance, and avoiding specific agents that irritate the esophageal mucosa. There is evidence to support several modifications that reduce esophageal gastric acid exposure and symptoms.[179] These include raising the head of the bed 6 to 8 inches by using blocks underneath the legs of the bed or using a foam wedge instead of traditional pillows; sleeping in a left lateral decubitus position; and weight loss, which also decreases intra-gastric pressure.[179] Avoiding large meals within 3 hours of bedtime or lying down in the supine position may also decrease symptoms.

Patients with GERD symptoms should avoid troublesome foods and beverages (Table 26-7). However, the evidence suggesting benefit is absent or unclear.[176,179] When possible, appropriate alternative OTC or prescription medications that do not exacerbate GERD symptoms should be recommended. It is likely that most GERD patients have tried many of the dietary and lifestyle modifications without obtaining satisfactory relief of their symptoms and that others will not be amenable to making these changes in their life. However, appropriate lifestyle and dietary modifications should be recommended to all patients with GERD symptoms.

W.J. should be counseled to lose weight, wear loose-fitting clothing, and avoid eating spicy meals that he knows will exacerbate his symptoms. Recommend that he avoids eating at least 3 hours before bedtime and that he considers raising the head of his bed 6 to 8 inches with wooden blocks. W.J. should be asked to keep a journal in order to track symptoms in relationship to diet and lifestyle and to record the effect of any lifestyle and dietary modifications. The health care practitioner should review the journal and discuss with W.J. which dietary and lifestyle factors trigger symptoms and which measures are most effective in relieving his symptoms.

24. Which OTC treatment options (if any) would you recommend for W.J.?

Many patients with mild, infrequent symptoms can be managed with OTC medications[8,15,176,180–182] (Fig. 26-5). First, a determination must be made as to the suitability of the patient for self-treatment. If the patient does not meet the criteria for

Table 26-8 Dietary and Lifestyle Modifications Used to Manage Gastroesophageal Reflux Symptoms

Dietary	*Medication*	*Lifestyle*
Avoid foods listed in Table 26-7	Avoid medications with a potential to relax the lower esophageal sphincter or have a direct irritant effect on the esophageal mucosa (Table 26-7)	Stop or decrease smoking/tobacco
Avoid eating large meals	Medications with the potential to irritate the esophagus should be taken with a full glass of water	Avoid alcohol
Avoid eating within 3 hours of bedtime		Weight loss[a]
		Elevate the head of bed 6–8 inches or use a foam wedge[a]
		Sleep in the left lateral decubitus position[a]

[a] Sufficient evidence exists to support lifestyle modification.
Adapted from references 8, 15, 166, 176, and 179, with permission.

self-treatment as described below, he or she should be referred for further medical evaluation.[15,176] It is important to ensure that the following are not present: alarm signs or symptoms, severe or frequent (2 or more days a week) heartburn lasting >3 months, presence of extraesophageal manifestations (see Question 28), or symptoms that persist despite appropriate drug therapy. OTC antacids and H_2RAs are the drugs of choice for patients with mild, infrequent heartburn. The nonprescription PPI (omeprazole) should be reserved for patients who experience frequent heartburn.[15]

Antacids remain an effective option for treating mild, infrequent heartburn, as they rapidly (within minutes) relieve symptoms, but the duration of symptom relief only lasts about 30 minutes when taken on an empty stomach.[8,15,176] The duration can be extended for several hours if taken within 1 hour after a meal.[15] Antacids are available in tablet and liquid form and are usually interchangeable when used in recommended dosages.[15] The dose can be repeated every 1 to 2 hours as needed, but the maximum recommended daily dose should not be exceeded. The addition of alginic acid to the antacid may improve symptom relief for some patients.[8,180] Patients requiring frequent or regular antacid use for more than 2 weeks should be reevaluated, as an OTC H_2RA or PPI may be needed.[15] About 20% of patients will achieve symptom relief with the use of antacids.[8,176] Antacids are not effective in healing erosive esophagitis.[8]

The OTC H_2RAs are indicated for mild to moderate infrequent GERD symptoms.[15,176] When compared with antacids, their onset of symptom relief occurs within 30 to 45 minutes, and they have a longer duration of action (up to 10 hours).[8,15] One benefit of the H_2RAs is that they can be taken prior to eating a heavy or spicy meal as prophylaxis for postprandial

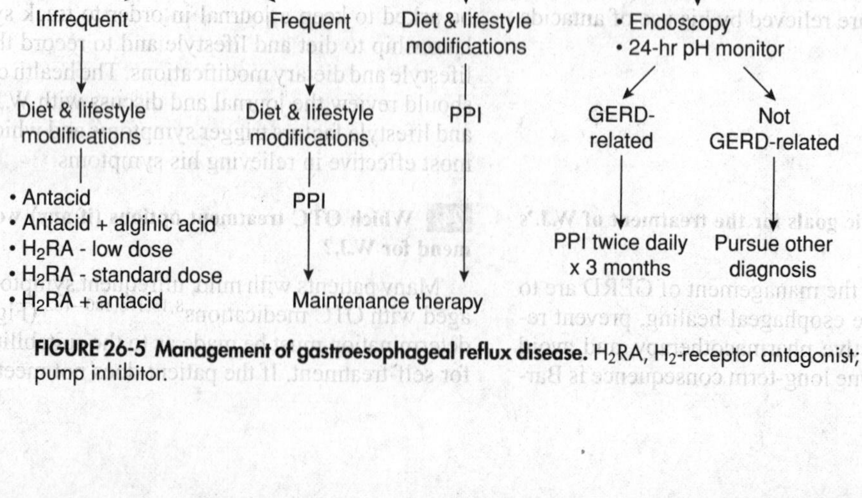

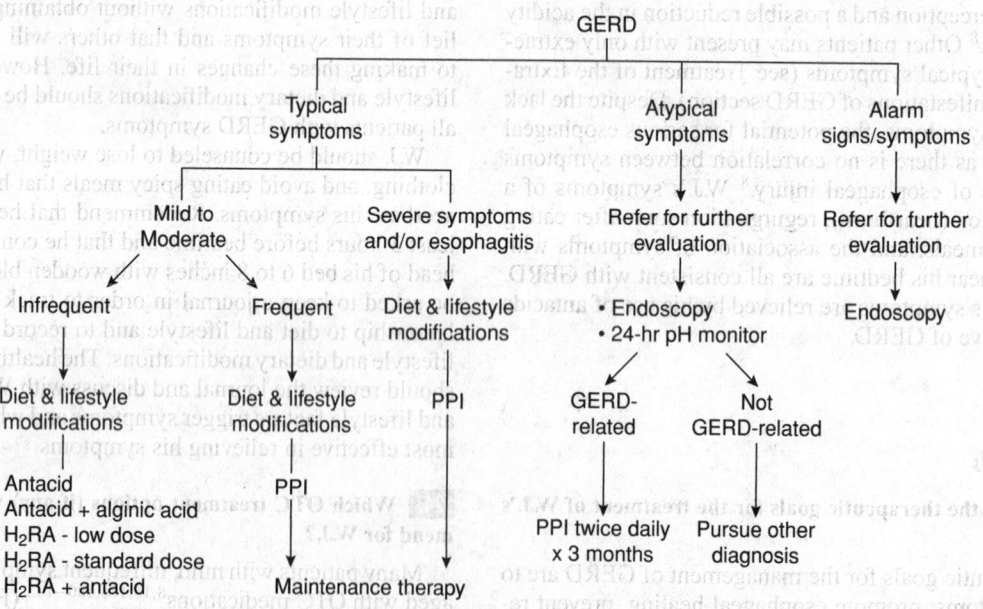

FIGURE 26-5 Management of gastroesophageal reflux disease. H_2RA, H_2-receptor antagonist; PPI, proton pump inhibitor.

GERD symptoms.[8,15,175] They also have a beneficial effect on reducing nocturnal acid secretion.[15] Tachyphylaxis (tolerance) has been reported with continued use of H_2RAs, but this effect can be overcome with intermittent or as-needed use.[15] OTC H_2RAs are available in one-half the original prescription low dose and as the full prescription doses. Patients should use the lower OTC dose twice daily for mild, intermittent symptoms and the higher dose twice daily for moderate symptoms[15] (Table 26-1). The four OTC H_2RAs (cimetidine, famotidine, ranitidine, nizatidine) are interchangeable when used in recommended dosages.[15,175] Patients should avoid cimetidine if the potential for a clinically important drug interaction exists with drugs metabolized by the hepatic CYP P450 enzyme system. When used for self-treatment, the H_2RA dose should not exceed two doses per day, and the treatment duration should not exceed 2 weeks. Use beyond 2 weeks should be under the care of a health care provider.[8,15]

Omeprazole is available OTC in the original prescription strength of 20 mg. A potent inhibitor of gastric acid, it is indicated for use in patients with frequent heartburn (2 or more days a week).[15] The onset of symptom relief is slower (2 to 3 hours) than with the H_2RAs, and complete relief may require up to 4 days after initiating therapy. The PPIs are superior to the H_2RAs with regard to symptom relief and duration of acid suppression.[15] Patients should take omeprazole 30 to 60 minutes prior to a meal (breakfast is preferable) and not take more than 20 mg daily for up to 2 weeks. Another course of therapy should not be taken more then every 4 months unless directed by a health care provider, as this may indicate more serious disease.[15,176]

W.J. is an appropriate candidate for self-treatment because his symptoms are mild and occur infrequently, and he has no alarm symptoms. Although antacids are an acceptable option for W.J., he has tried these and is unhappy with the frequency of dosing needed to relieve his heartburn. Because W.J. has requested a medication to specifically "prevent" meal-related symptoms, he should take a H_2RA 30 to 60 minutes prior to eating or drinking. If symptoms remain infrequent but are unrelated to meals, the use of an OTC H_2RA as needed for symptoms may be required. He can increase the dose to twice daily if symptom relief is not optimal and may consider OTC omeprazole if symptoms occur more than 2 days a week. If he continues to have symptoms beyond 2 weeks, the symptoms become more severe, or they are accompanied by alarm symptoms, he should be referred for further evaluation.

Severe Disease With Complications

25. L.F. is a 48-year-old woman who presents to her primary care provider complaining of recurrent heartburn occurring daily for the past 6 weeks. She states that the heartburn occurs frequently after meals and often wakens her at night. Lately, she has been experiencing difficulty swallowing solid foods. L.F. currently smokes two packs of cigarettes per day and likes to have a glass of wine each night before bedtime. She states that she occasionally uses OTC ranitidine 150 mg orally up to twice daily, which temporarily relieves her symptoms. What diagnostic modalities are available for the evaluation of her GERD?

Clinical Assessment and Diagnosis

Numerous diagnostic options exist for the evaluation of the patient with presumed GERD. The medical history should include the identification of specific symptoms and an assessment of symptom frequency, severity, and duration as well as risk factors or triggers. An empiric diagnosis can be made in the majority of patients based on the symptoms of heartburn and regurgitation. However, patients who present with severe symptoms, alarm symptoms, or long-standing GERD or who do not respond to empiric therapy warrant further diagnostic evaluation.

Acid Suppression Empiric Test

A trial of a PPI is commonly used to empirically diagnose typical GERD-like symptoms in patients without alarm symptoms or symptoms of complicated disease. Doses used in clinical trials range from 20 mg to 60 mg omeprazole (or equivalent) once daily for up to 4 weeks.[1,183] If symptoms are relieved after a short trial of a PPI, an empiric diagnosis of GERD may be made and other invasive and costly diagnostic methods may be avoided.[8,150,176,180,184] However, this methodology is not without its limitations. The test cannot differentiate between other acid-related disorders such as PUD, and studies evaluating its ability to detect GERD versus other diagnostic options have been equivocal.[8,183,184] Despite these shortcomings, guidelines suggest that an empiric trial of a PPIs is appropriate in selected patients given its ease of use and reduced cost.[176] The empiric use of a PPI may also be beneficial in identifying patients with extraesophageal manifestations of GERD[8] (see Treatment of Extraesophageal Manifestations of GERD section). Further diagnostic evaluation is warranted in patients who do not respond to acid suppressive therapy, who present with alarm symptoms or symptoms suggestive of complicated disease, or who have long-standing GERD where the possibility of Barrett's esophagus exists.

Upper Endoscopy and Biopsy

Upper endoscopy is the primary diagnostic method for evaluating the esophageal mucosa for injury or cellular changes. This test is highly specific yet only moderately sensitive for the diagnosis of GERD, since many patients present with nonerosive disease. There are four primary reasons why endoscopy is performed in patients suspected of having GERD.[8,185] The first is to rule out significant disease (e.g., adenocarcinoma of the esophagus) or complications (e.g., stricture); the second is to screen for Barrett's metaplasia; the third is the ability to evaluate and grade the severity of esophagitis; and the fourth is to allow the provider to optimize treatment and predict the long-term course of the disease. The endoscope can be fitted with surgical instruments to allow the operator to perform procedures or obtain tissue specimens for biopsy. Endoscopic grading of the esophagus is based on the level of inflammation and mucosal damage. Two endoscopic classification systems are used for the grading of esophagitis[186,187] (Table 26-9). The Savary-Miller classification categorizes patients from grade 0 to grade 4 based on the severity of mucosal erosions of the esophagus.[186] The addition of a grade 5 was added to include the diagnosis of Barrett's esophagus.[188] Although this classification system is no longer recommended in the United States,

Table 26-9 Classification Systems for Endoscopically Determined Esophagitis

The Savary-Miller Classification System of Esophagitis

Grade 0	Normal esophageal mucosa
Grade 1	Erythema or diffusely red mucosa, edema causing accentuated folds
Grade 2	Isolated round or linear erosions extending from the gastroesophageal junction upward, not involving entire circumference
Grade 3	Confluent erosions extending around entire circumference or superficial ulceration without erosions
Grade 4	Complicated cases; erosions as in grade 3 plus deep ulcerations, strictures, or columnar epithelium-lined esophagus
Grade 5	Presence of Barrett's metaplasia

The Los Angeles Classification System of Esophagitis

Grade A	One (or more) mucosal break no longer that 5 mm that does not extend between the tops of two mucosal folds
Grade B	One (or more) mucosal break more that 5 mm long that does not extend between the tops of two mucosal folds
Grade C	One (or more) mucosal break that is continuous between the tops of two or more mucosal folds but that involves <75% of the circumference
Grade D	One (or more) mucosal break which involves at least 75% of the esophageal circumference

Adapted from references 186–188, with permission.

it is still used in many practices. The Los Angeles classification is preferred because it is more specific and categorizes patients from A to D based on the number of mucosal breaks, their size, and the amount of surface area with esophagitis involvement.[187] There is no classification for normal esophagus with this system and symptomatic patients are often classified with NERD.

Biopsy of the esophageal mucosa is performed during endoscopy, and tissue samples are evaluated by microscopy for evidence of Barrett's metaplasia or neoplastic disease.[8] In patients with suspected Barrett's metaplasia, the biopsy is obtained after the esophagus has healed to prevent misinterpretation of the inflammatory markers for dysplastic syndrome. Mucosal biopsy for inflammatory markers in nonerosive disease remains debatable.

24-Hour Continuous Ambulatory pH Monitoring

Ambulatory pH monitoring is a valuable diagnostic test for evaluating GERD. It is especially helpful in patients who have not responded adequately to reasonable pharmacotherapy, in patients with nonerosive disease, and when there is the need to correlate reflux events with symptoms. A small (2–3 mm diameter) pH electrode is threaded through the patient's nostril (similar to placing a nasogastric tube), past the patient's larynx, to approximately 5 cm above the LES in the distal esophagus.[1,8] Once it is connected to a logging device, which documents pH measurements every few seconds, it allows for the determination of reflux events (defined as esophageal pH <4), duration of reflux events, and percentage of time within a 24-hour period that the patient's pH is <4. The patient is asked to keep a diary to record symptomatic events that can be correlated with a decrease in esophageal pH. This is especially important when correlating extraesophageal manifestations with reflux events.

Radiologic Testing

The barium esophagram (barium swallow) is used primarily to identify suspected esophageal abnormalities such as strictures, narrowing, and hiatal hernia and to determine peristalsis disorders.[8] The procedure is relatively noninvasive and inexpensive when compared with endoscopy.

Esophageal Manometry

Esophageal manometry is used to evaluate the patients LES pressure and esophageal peristalsis.[8] This procedure does not have a specific role in the diagnosis of GERD, as it does not detect the presence of acid within the esophagus. It is used primarily to evaluate patients prior to 24-hour continuous ambulatory pH monitoring and antireflux surgical procedures (e.g., Nissen fundoplication) to determine the location of the LES.[8,189]

26. L.F.'s frequent severe symptoms continue despite full-dose OTC H_2RA therapy and the presence of warning signs warranted that she undergo endoscopy, which revealed moderate esophagitis (Los Angeles grade C), the presence of an esophageal stricture, and no evidence of Barrett's metaplasia. Esophageal dilation was performed during the procedure to widen the lumen of the esophagus. What treatment options exist for L.F.?

Pharmacotherapy

Antacids

Antacids are useful only in the relief of mild symptoms associated with GERD (see Nonpharmacologic Measures and Self-Directed Treatment section). Because of their short duration of action and inability to heal erosive esophagitis, they are not an option for treating moderate to severe GERD.[8]

H_2-Receptor Antagonists

The H_2RAs are effective in treating patients with mild to moderate GERD, but response rates vary with the severity of disease, the dose of the drug, and the duration of therapy. The H_2RAs are considered equally effective when used in equipotent doses for symptomatic relief and esophageal healing (Table 26-1). They are effective in reducing nocturnal symptoms but only modestly effective in relieving meal-related symptoms, as they only block one mechanism of parietal cell activation (the H2 receptor).[8] The H_2RAs relieve symptoms in about 50% to 60% of patients treated after 12 weeks of continuous therapy and are superior to placebo.[176,190] Increasing the H_2RA dose may not improve symptoms in some patients.[191] Esophageal healing requires higher doses (e.g., famotidine 40 mg BID) compared with those used for symptom relief (Table 26-1). Esophageal healing rates with the H_2RAs are reported to be about 50% after 8 to 12 weeks of treatment, but rates will vary depending on the degree of esophagitis.[176,190] For example, endoscopic healing rates in trials with high-dose H_2RAs were approximately 60% to 90% in patients with grades I and II esophagitis but were only 30% to 50% in patients with more severe disease (grades III and IV esophagitis).[8,190] When a H_2RA is used to heal the esophagus, higher daily dosages and prolonged treatment (8–12 weeks) are required.[176] Some investigators have attributed inadequate esophageal healing to the development of tachyphylaxis.[180]

Proton Pump Inhibitors

The PPIs are the drugs of choice for patients with frequent moderate to severe GERD symptoms and esophagitis because they provide more rapid relief of symptoms and esophageal healing than do the H_2RAs. When used in recommended dosages, all of the PPIs provide similar rates of symptom relief and esophageal healing (Table 26-1). Their superior efficacy, when compared with the H_2RAs, is related to their ability to maintain an intragastric pH >4 for a long duration time (up to 24 hours/day vs. up to 10 hours with a H_2RA).[15,192] Typically, PPIs are taken once daily 30 to 60 minutes before breakfast, but if a second dose is required, it should be taken prior to the evening meal.

A large meta-analysis of 16 trials confirms that PPIs are superior to the H_2RAs for achieving rapid and complete relief of GERD symptoms. Complete symptom relief (within 4–12 weeks) was achieved in 77.4% of patients taking a PPI versus 47.6% of those taking and H_2RA ($p < 0.0001$).[190] PPIs have also been shown to heal esophagitis more quickly and effectively than the H_2RAs. In the same meta-analysis, which evaluated 43 double or single blinded, randomized studies (including patients with severe esophagitis), the PPIs (83.6%) were more effective than H_2RAs (51.9%) at healing erosive esophagitis at 12 weeks.[190] Healing also occurred more quickly with PPI therapy in that by week two, 63.4% of patients had healed with the PPI, while it took 12 weeks with the H_2RAs for 60.2% of patients to heal.[190] Another large meta-analysis, which evaluated over 33 randomized trials, demonstrated similar results with 81.7% of patients healed at 8 weeks with a PPI versus 52.0% with a H_2RA.[193]

Esophageal healing among the five PPIs appears to be equivalent, as about 85% to 90% of patients achieve complete healing at 8 weeks in numerous head-to-head trials with equivalent doses.[38–41] One meta-analysis, which compared esophageal healing rates among omeprazole 20 mg, lansoprazole 30 mg, pantoprazole 40 mg, and rabeprazole 20 mg (each given once daily), reported no statistical difference.[37] However, all of the PPIs were superior to ranitidine 300 to 600 mg/day. Esomeprazole 40 mg once daily has been reported to be superior to omeprazole 20 mg once daily, both at 4 and 8 weeks, when used to heal erosive esophagitis.[194] However, the esomeprazole 40 mg and omeprazole 20 mg dosages are not equipotent, and this study has been heavily criticized based on this fact. Another study, which compared equipotent doses of esomeprazole (40 mg) and lansoprazole (30 mg), also suggests that esomeprazole has superior healing rates (92.6% vs. 88.8%, respectively).[40] In contrast, a similar study comparing lansoprazole 30 mg with esomeprazole 40 mg showed no statistical difference in esophageal healing, albeit with a smaller population.[41] Given the disparity in the results of these comparative trials, some clinicians prefer esomeprazole 40 mg/day as a better option, especially for those patients with severe erosive esophagitis. However, clinical evidence to support this practice is minimal.

The ability of a high-dose PPI to reverse Barrett's metaplasia remains controversial.[8] Although studies have demonstrated islands of normal squamous epithelium returning, no data have determined that this is associated with a risk reduction in adenocarcinoma.[8] In fact, others have suggested that this return of normal mucosa may actually mask carcinogenic changes occurring deeper in the gastric mucosa.[195]

Improvement of quality of life has also been evaluated in patients receiving PPI therapy in the management of GERD. A recent study comparing esomeprazole with ranitidine over a period of 6 months showed a significant improvement in both physical functioning and sleep with the PPI therapy.[196]

Prokinetic Agents

Two prokinetic agents, metoclopramide and bethanechol, may be effective in the management of GERD. Both drugs stimulate the motility of the upper GI tract without altering gastric acid secretion and increase LES pressure.[8] Although these drugs may provide relief of symptoms, they are ineffective in healing erosive esophagitis unless they are combined with a H_2RA or PPI. Prokinetics are not widely used to treat GERD, because they are not as effective as other treatments and are associated with numerous side effects. Prokinetics are reserved for patients who are refractory to other available treatment options or who have delayed gastric emptying.

Sucralfate

Sucralfate appears to be effective in treating mild cases of GERD and possibly mild esophagitis but is not effective in the management of severe disease.[197] Given better options at this time, sucralfate is rarely used in the management of GERD.

The PPIs are considered the drugs of choice for patients with frequent or severe GERD symptoms, or who have complicated disease, because of their potent inhibition of gastric acid secretion[176,180–182] (Fig. 26-5). In this case, L.F., who presents with severe esophagitis (Los Angeles grade C), will require a PPI taken once daily in order to relieve her symptoms and heal the esophagus (Table 26-1). A reasonable option for L.F. would be lansoprazole 30 mg daily to be taken 30 to 60 minutes prior to breakfast each morning for the next 8 weeks; however, if the cost of pharmaceuticals is a issue for L.F., generic omeprazole 40 mg daily would also be appropriate. L.F. should also be counseled regarding lifestyle and dietary modifications, including smoking cessation and abstinence from alcohol. She should avoid eating large meals prior to bedtime and may wish to elevate the head of her bed by 6 to 8 inches with wooden blocks.

Maintenance Therapy

27. L.F.'s symptoms resolved in about 2 weeks after starting PPI therapy, and she remained asymptomatic after 8 weeks. She then underwent endoscopy again, which revealed that the esophagus had healed completely. Her primary care physician then stopped

the PPI. Now, 2 weeks later, she is experiencing mild heartburn. Is L.F. a candidate for long-term maintenance therapy?

GERD is chronic disease. Up to 80% of patients with severe esophagitis and 15% to 30% with less severe disease have a symptomatic relapse within 6 months after discontinuing treatment.[8] The goal of maintenance therapy is to keep the patient symptom-free and prevent potentially life-threatening complications. Continuous maintenance therapy with a daily PPI is more effective than a H_2RA, with reported relapse rates of 25% and 50%, respectively.[8] Thus, PPIs are the drugs of choice for maintaining remission in patients with healed esophagitis. A H_2RA may be considered for patients with mild nonerosive disease. Although one-half of the PPI dose used for esophageal healing has been suggested, guidelines indicate that the recommended maintenance dose should be the dose that is required to render the patient asymptomatic.[176,180] Maintenance therapy with lansoprazole 15 mg to 30 mg once daily should be initiated in L.F., given the level of her esophagitis and recurrence of symptoms after the PPI was discontinued, to reduce the risk of morbidity associated with this chronic, relapsing disease.

On-Demand Pharmacotherapy

The use of intermittent (on-demand) courses of PPI therapy (2–4 weeks) have been suggested as being potentially beneficial in patients with GERD.[198–203] One trial, which compared continuous maintenance therapy with esomeprazole 20 mg daily versus on-demand therapy with the same drug and dose in patients with healed erosive esophagitis, reported that continuous therapy was superior to on-demand therapy (81% vs. 58%, respectively) in maintaining endoscopic remission at 6 months.[203] The ability to maintain remission with on-demand therapy was reduced as the severity in esophagitis increased. Although numerous studies with a variety of PPIs have demonstrated patient satisfaction with on-demand therapy,[199–202] a systemic review of 17 trials evaluating the use of on-demand therapy indicates that intermittent therapy should only be considered in patients with mild, nonerosive disease.[198]

Combination of a Proton Pump Inhibitor and H_2-Receptor Antagonists

The addition of a H_2RA at bedtime to a once or twice daily PPI regimen is sometimes used for patients who continue to have nocturnal symptoms, although the evidence to support this combination remains inconclusive. The rational for this practice is based on evidence that suggests a period of nocturnal acid breakthrough (defined as intragastric pH <4 for longer than 1 hour during the night) in a significant number of patients despite twice-daily PPI therapy, suggesting that histamine release may have an important function in nocturnal acid secretion.[204] One study suggests that the addition of a H_2RA to a twice-daily PPI regimen resulted in a statistically significant reduction in nocturnal acid breakthrough during the sleeping hours.[204] This trial, however, evaluated only a single bedtime dose of a H_2RA and did not consider the tachyphylaxis that can occur with continuous use. A more recent trial using a twice-daily PPI regimen with continuous use of a H_2RA for 4 weeks demonstrated no difference in nocturnal acid suppression, suggesting that tolerance does play an important role in the use of H_2RAs for this indication.[32] It has been theorized that one way to possibly avoid this occurrence is to use the H_2RA on only an as-needed basis when lifestyle and dietary modifications are not effective for preventing nocturnal symptoms.[8]

Nonerosive Reflux Disease

Up to 75% patients with typical GERD symptoms who undergo endoscopy will not have evidence of esophagitis or complicated disease.[205] These patients are described as having functional heartburn, NERD or ENRD and usually undergo 24-hour ambulatory pH monitoring to determine whether abnormal reflux is present despite a negative endoscopy. A trial of a PPI is usually indicated despite no esophageal findings, as many patients will respond to this therapy.[205] Further medical evaluation is usually required if a patient does not respond to PPI therapy despite a doubling of the daily dose.

Extraesophageal Manifestations

28. S.P. is a 71-year-old retired gentleman who was eating dinner with his wife when he experienced a sudden onset of chest pain described as crushing, burning, and squeezing. His wife notified emergency personnel, who transported S.P. to the emergency department. His past medical history reveals some cardiovascular risk factors, including age, hypertension, hyperlipidemia, and a sedentary lifestyle. His medications prior to admission include aspirin 81 mg daily, hydrochlorothiazide 25 mg daily, and atorvastatin 40 mg at bedtime. He also takes OTC famotidine 20 mg daily as needed for dyspepsia. On examination, he complains of substernal crushing chest pain that has lasted over 1 hour. He is diaphoretic and extremely anxious. He denies any shortness of breath, pain radiating to upper extremities or jaw, or cough. His vital signs include a temperature of 99.1°F, blood pressure 155/95 mmHg and heart rate of 115 beats/minute. Pertinent laboratory results at this time are white blood cell (WBC) count 7,700/mm^3, Hgb 14.2 g/dL, Hct 45%, platelets 270,000/mm^3, SrCr 1.1 mg/dL, BUN 11 mg/dL, total cholesterol 161 mg/dL, low-density lipoprotein 96 mg/dL, high-density lipoprotein 30 mg/dL, triglycerides 190 mg/dL, sodium (Na) 141 mEq/L, potassium (K) 4.1 mEq/L, and troponin I 0.3 ng/mL. Electrocardiogram reveals sinus tachycardia with no evidence of ST-segment elevation, depression, or T-wave inversion or new left bundle branch block. Because of S.P.'s cardiovascular risk factors and indeterminate troponin, he underwent immediate diagnostic cardiac catheterization, which showed normal coronary angiography and an ejection fraction of 65%. S.P. was diagnosed with noncardiac chest pain (NCCP). Could S.P.'s chest pain be associated with an extraesophageal manifestation of GERD?

Extraesophageal (atypical) manifestations of GERD are those signs and symptoms that occur outside of the esophagus yet are presumed to be associated with GERD. The extraesophageal manifestations of GERD include NCCP; pulmonary symptoms; and complaints related to the ear, nose, and throat; as well as hypersalivation and dental erosions (Table 26-10). Interestingly, these symptoms are often the only complaint that a patient has when he or she presents to the health care provider.[206,207]

Table 26-10 Atypical Manifestations of Gastroesophageal Reflux Disease

Noncardiac Chest Pain	*Pulmonary*
Ear, nose, and throat	Chronic cough
Laryngitis/Pharyngitis	Nonallergic, nonseasonal asthma
Hoarseness	Aspiration
Globus sensation	Bronchiectasis/Bronchitis
Laryngeal cancer	Sleep apnea
Sinusitis	Idiopathic pulmonary fibrosis
Otitis	Pneumonia
Other	
Hypersalivation	
Dental erosions	

Adapted from references 207 and 208, with permission.

Noncardiac Chest Pain

About 30% of patients with anginalike chest pain have normal coronary arteries or minimal microvascular disease as demonstrated by cardiac angiography.[208] About 40% to 50% of these patients will have concomitant GERD as demonstrated by an abnormal esophageal endoscopy or ambulatory pH monitoring.[209,210] The symptoms associated with NCCP are very similar to those associated with cardiac angina. The chest pain is usually described as crushing, squeezing, or burning; retrosternal in location; and with or without lateral radiation to the upper extremities, back, neck, or jaw. The pain is often temporally related to a meal or occurs nocturnally, usually awakening the patient and continuing for hours. The onset of pain may coincide with a reflux episode, and symptoms are often relieved by oral antacid therapy.[211] Numerous trials have evaluated the use of acid suppression as a means to treat NCCP once cardiac etiology has been ruled out through appropriate evaluation.[212–216] The PPI test, in which a short course (1–8 weeks) of high-dose (twice-daily) PPI is used, is an effective diagnostic tool and is associated with a reduction in costs compared with other diagnostic methods of GERD. An appropriate workup for coronary artery disease must be performed in all patients presenting with chest pain *prior* to considering a GI cause or trial of antireflux therapy. This is especially important in women, the elderly, and diabetic patients, as their initial presentation may be similar to GI complaints when in fact an acute coronary syndrome is present.

Asthma and Gastroesophageal Reflux Disease

GERD may play a role in the pathophysiology of asthma. Reports suggest that concomitant GERD occurs in 34% to 89% of the asthmatic population.[217] Two theoretical mechanisms exist as to how GERD can potentially exacerbate asthma symptoms. The reflex theory proposes that symptoms result from the direct irritation of the vagus nerve when refluxate comes into contact with the esophageal mucosa, resulting in reflex bronchospasm.[218] In contrast, the reflux theory proposes that aspiration of refluxed acid into the lungs causes caustic injury of tissue within the bronchial tree, resulting in asthmatic symptoms.[219] An important meta-analysis of trials that evaluated the effects of antireflux therapy on patients with asthma indicates that asthma symptoms improved in 69% of patients, that the use of asthma medications was reduced by 62%, and that only 26% of the subjects showed improvement in evening peak expiratory flow rate. All other pulmonary function tests (PFTs) showed little or no change with antireflux therapy.[220] However, this meta-analysis only evaluated studies of up to 8 weeks in duration. A recent trial with esomeprazole 40 mg daily for 3 months demonstrated improvements in PFTs and a decreased use of short-acting rescue bronchodilators in asthmatics with GERD compared with asthmatics without GERD.[221] One-third of the patients in the GERD group were also able reduce their dose of inhaled corticosteroid and remained stable.

Otolaryngology Symptoms and Gastroesophageal Reflux Disease

GERD is the most common etiologic factor in 80% of patients with chronic hoarseness[222] and in 25% to 50% of patients with a globus sensation (the feeling that something is caught in the throat).[223–226] Symptoms relating to GERD are responsible for up to 10% of the patients seen by otolaryngologists.[227] The most likely mechanism for the pathophysiology of GERD-related laryngitis is that damage and inflammation occurs at night while the patient is sleeping. It is during this time when upper esophageal sphincter pressures are especially low and the protective or neutralizing mechanisms of cough and salivation are suppressed.[228] This damage may be in addition to injury or laryngeal inflammation sustained from other causes such as excessive voice usage, chronic throat clearing or cough, vomiting, or injury from endotracheal tubes.[229] The extent of injury in GERD-related hoarseness is directly related to the exposure time of the pharyngeal mucosa to the refluxate as well as the pH. Patients with GERD-related hoarseness usually do not have any other GERD-related symptoms. The diagnostic procedure of choice is laryngoscopy and should be considered in all patients presenting with GERD-related hoarseness. Once the diagnosis of GERD-related hoarseness or laryngitis is established, the patient will likely require extended high-dose PPI therapy with the realization that the majority of patients will relapse within 6 weeks once therapy is discontinued.[230]

S.P.'s chest pain is not of cardiac origin based on angiographic findings. Therefore, it is reasonable to presume that he having an extraesophageal manifestation of GERD. S.P.'s symptoms were meal related, and he has a history of dyspepsia for which he takes an OTC H_2RA. The H_2RA should be discontinued, and S.P. should be given a trial of empiric twice-daily PPI therapy for a 2 to 4 week period. If symptoms are severe, the use of endoscopy (to determine if esophageal damage is present) or 24-hour esophageal pH monitoring (to correlate reflux events with symptomatic chest pain) is appropriate.

Treatment of the Extraesophageal Manifestations of Gastroesophageal Reflux Disease

Treatment should be initiated with a high-dose (twice-daily) PPI for at least 3 months before considering drug therapy to be ineffective.[208] Alternatively, it is possible that GERD may not be the cause of the patient's symptoms.

29. S.P. responded well to the trial of omeprazole 40 mg orally twice daily and has not had chest pain in 2 months. He has heard that surgical options exist that may eliminate his need for

medications, as they are very expensive for him. Is S.P. a candidate for antireflux surgery?

Antireflux Surgery

Numerous surgical and endoscopic procedures exist for patients with GERD. These include, but are not limited to, Nissen fundoplication, Toupet partial fundoplication, Belsey Mark IV repair, and the Hill posterior gastroplexy repair, as well as newer endoscopic techniques.[8] The primary goal of these procedures is to restore LES pressure by repairing a hiatal hernia or diaphragmatic hiatus. Appropriate candidates include patients who are in a good health and request another treatment option due to poor medication adherence, patients who are unable to afford their medication, patients who suffer from side effects or worry about risks with long-term therapy, patients with extraesophageal symptoms who have responded well to antireflux therapy, or patients experiencing volume regurgitation and aspiration of gastric contents who have not responded to PPI therapy.[8,209] Despite the availability of these surgical options, the consideration of antireflux surgery is one in which the benefits should be heavily weighed against the risks of such an invasive approach, as these procedures are not without potential complications. The effectiveness of these procedures has been questioned, as many patients will still require drug therapy.[209] S.P. has responded well to high-dose PPI therapy for his NCCP, but he describes some financial difficulties with affording his medications. Alternatively, he is 64 years of age, which may increase the risk associated with surgery. S.P. should be referred for further medical evaluation to determine whether he is a candidate for antireflux surgery.

UPPER GASTROINTESTINAL BLEEDING

Upper GI bleeding is a common medical emergency that occurs in about 170 cases per 100,000 adults annually and is associated with increased morbidity and mortality as well as substantial costs to the health care system.[231,232] Despite advances in endoscopic hemostatic therapy and pharmacotherapy, the mortality rate associated with upper GI bleeding remains at 7% to 10%, which is the same as it has been for the last 30 to 40 years. However, mortality is higher in hospitalized patients.[3,231,233–235] Upper GI bleeding can be categorized as either variceal or nonvariceal bleeding (see Chapter 28, Complications of End-Stage Liver Disease). Nonvariceal bleeding describes bleeding associated with PUD or stress-related mucosal bleeding (SRMB). Other causes include erosive esophagitis, Mallory-Weiss tear (a tear near the gastroesophageal junction associated with retching or coughing), and malignancy.[235] Although PUD and SRMB are both acid-related disorders, their presentation and pathophysiology differ.

PEPTIC ULCER BLEEDING

Epidemiology

About 50% of all upper, nonvariceal GI bleeding is due to PUD.[4,233,234] Bleeding ulcers account for approximately 150,000 hospitalizations in the United States each year.[233,234] The mortality rate for peptic ulcer bleeding can be as high as 10%. It has been suggested that an older presenting patient population (>60 years of age) with a greater number of comorbidies may account for this continued high mortality rate.[3,231,233,234] Fortunately, the vast majority (80%) of upper GI bleeding events are self-limited and require only minimal intervention.[3,234–236] Length of stay has been dramatically reduced due to a majority of patients who receive early endoscopy (within 24 hours of admission) and up to 35% who undergo endoscopic hemostatis procedures.[4] However, in the 20% of patients who continue to bleed or rebleed after appropriate intervention, mortality increases to nearly 40%.[4,232]

Pathophysiology

The most common causes of upper GI bleeding in patients with PUD are NSAID use and *H. pylori* infection. Bleeding occurs when an ulcer extends deeper into the mucosa and erodes the wall of a blood vessel.[234,235] The incidence of *H. pylori* infection in bleeding ulcers is 15% to 20% lower than in patients with nonbleeding ulcers.[9,234] Bleeding associated with PUD is generally not caused by the hypersecretion of gastric acid, with the exception of patients with ZES.[234] The pathophysiology and risk factors associated with PUD are described earlier in this chapter (see Peptic Ulcer Disease section).

Clinical Assessment and Diagnosis

The clinical presentation of a patient with a bleeding peptic ulcer usually includes the presence of melena (dark, tarry stools), which occurs in 20% of patients, hematemesis (vomiting of blood) in 30%, and both in about 50% of patients. Up to 5% of patients present with hematochezia (bloody diarrhea) indicative of rapid and substantial blood loss.[234] The primary step in evaluating the patient is to assess the degree of urgency for rapid medical management.[235] Hypovolemia due to substantial blood loss can rapidly lead to shock. The initial management of these patients should focus on volume resuscitation and improving the patient's hemodynamic status. Clinical features suggestive of high-risk for rebleeding or mortality include patients >60 years of age, serious comorbidities (e.g., hepatic or renal dysfunction, cardiac or pulmonary disease), hemodynamic instability (e.g., hypotension, tachycardia), shock, poor health, continued bleeding, mental status changes, and prolonged prothrombin/activated partial thromboplastin time (aPTT) (or elevated international normalized ratio [INR]).[3,231,234–237] These patients should immediately be transferred to an intensive care setting.

Most patients should receive early diagnostic endoscopic evaluation within 24 hours of presentation to determine the source of the bleeding, to predict the risk for rebleeding, and, when required, to perform endoscopic interventions directed at stopping the bleeding ulcer and restoring hemostasis.[231,235] Risk of rebleeding may be predicted based on the presenting lesion(s) identified on endoscopy.[234] The most common ulcer identified on endoscopy is a clean-base ulcer found in about 42% of patients. This ulcer has a very low risk of rebleeding (5%), and the patient can usually be discharged immediately after recovery from the endoscopy and managed with appropriate antisecretory therapy. Intermediate stigmata of bleeding include lesions identified as flat-spot ulcers and/or adherent clots, which have a risk of rebleeding of 10% and 22%, respectively. Although endoscopic procedures are not usually necessary with flat-spot ulcers, adherent clots remain an area of controversy and usually require the endoscopist to attempt to remove the clot and manage the underlying lesion as appropriate.[235] Patients identified with high-risk ulceration (nonbleeding visible vessel or active bleeding) will require endoscopic intervention and have a high risk of rebleeding (43% and 55%, respectively) despite intervention. Nonbleeding visible vessel and active bleeding are associated with an 11% mortality on initial presentation.[234] Ulcer size is also predictive of mortality and rebleeding, as ulcers >1 or 2 cm in diameter confer greater risk.[233,234] Despite appropriate endoscopic hemostasis, 10% to 30% will rebleed within 48 to 72 hours following treatment.[231,233,235] Mortality associated with rebleeding is about 25% to 37%.[232,235] Patients undergoing endoscopy should be tested for *H. pylori* infection with biopsy (rapid urease test), as infection with this organism is associated with an increased risk of rebleeding.[4,231] Because false negatives can occur in the presence of active bleeding, all *H. pylori*–negative patients should have a confirmatory follow-up test with serologic antibody testing on discharge to ensure that the patient is not infected.[231]

Treatment

Patients with upper GI bleeding require rapid risk stratification based on the presenting signs and symptoms. Patients with hemodynamic instability require immediate institution of resuscitative measures.[235,238] IV access should be obtained with a large-bore catheter to facilitate the administration of fluids and blood products.[4] Intravascular volume should initially be repleted with normal saline to prevent the patient from going into hypovolemic shock. During this time, blood can be typed and crossed in the event a transfusion is required.[325] A nasogastric tube should be placed to allow for lavage and determination of the upper GI tract as the source of the bleed and evaluation of continued bleeding.[4,231,238]

Endoscopic evaluation with hemostatic techniques (when required) should be performed as soon as safely possible.[231,235] Endoscopic hemostasis is the cornerstone of management for patients with serious bleeding ulcers, as it reduces the incidence of rebleeding, the need for surgery, and mortality when compared with placebo or drug therapy.[231] Endoscopic procedures include thermocoagulation, laser therapy, injection therapy (epinephrine, ethanol, or saline), injection with sclerosing agent, or placement of endoscopic clips. Combining thermocoagulation with injection therapy is superior to either therapy alone and hemoclipping alone in patients with serious ulcer bleeding.[231,233] Despite initial hemostasis, however, the potential for rebleeding remains high, especially in patients with high-risk lesions.[234,235]

Improvements in hemostatic parameters (e.g., platelet aggregation, inactivation of pepsin, and correction of coagulation) leading to clot stabilization correlate directly with an intragastric pH >6).[232,233,236] Therefore, treatment with an antisecretory drug is beneficial in patients after endoscopy to promote healing of the lesion. After the acute phase, the patient should be placed on appropriate drug therapy to continue healing and prevent ulcer recurrence (see Peptic Ulcer Disease section). Patients who are *H. pylori* positive should receive appropriate eradication therapy.[4,231]

H_2-Receptor Antagonists

Once widely used to manage upper GI bleeding, the H_2RAs are now considered inferior to the PPIs for reducing the incidence of rebleeding and the need for surgery.[231,233] This is likely due to the inability of the H_2RAs to achieve an intragastric pH $\geq$6 (even with continuous IV administration) and the rapid development of tachyphylaxis (especially with high IV doses).[231–233,236,239] Thus, the H_2RAs are no longer recommended for the prevention of rebleeding associated with a peptic ulcer.[231]

Proton Pump Inhibitors

The PPIs are the drugs of choice to reduce the incidence of PUD-related rebleeding and the need for surgical intervention.[240–244] However, no clinical trials were able to show a mortality benefit when entire treatment cohorts were evaluated. A Cochrane Collaboration meta-analysis of 24 studies evaluating randomized, controlled trials that compared IV or orally administered PPIs with H_2RAs or placebo showed similar results with a reduction in rebleeding, surgery, and repeat endoscopic treatment.[240] Although no reduction in the number of deaths were identified when all patients were considered, PPI treatment of patients at the highest risk of mortality, as evidenced by endoscopically determined active bleeding or nonbleeding visible vessel, did impart a mortality benefit. All-cause mortality was also reduced in Asian trials, with a concomitant greater reduction in the incidence of rebleeding and need for surgery than in trials performed elsewhere in the world. This may be explained by the inclusion of a younger patient population, more potent acid suppression because of genetic polymorphism in P450 metabolism leading to a slower clearance of PPIs, a lower parietal cell mass, and a greater incidence of *H. pylori* infection.[240]

Despite the data, important questions remain as to the most appropriate dose and route of administration for PPIs in patients with peptic ulcer bleeding. Evidence suggests that patients with low-risk lesions (clear-base or flat-spot ulcers) may be treated with oral PPIs and immediately discharged after endoscopy, as rebleeding is infrequent in this population.[231,240,245] However, in patients with higher-risk endoscopic stigmata, a parenteral PPI should be administered and titrated to an intragastric pH >6 after the endoscopic procedure.[231,240] Current guidelines suggest an initial IV bolus equivalent to 80 mg of omeprazole followed by a continuous IV infusion of 8 mg/hour of the omeprazole equivalent for 72 hours (although no head-to-head trials of omeprazole equivalence have been performed with pantoprazole or esomeprazole, most clinicians consider them equivalent on a milligram-per-milligram basis).[231,232,233,236,240] Rebleeding is highest during this first 72 hours and is the reason for such high-dose therapy.[233,235] This strategy has been compared with standard-dose therapy with IV omeprazole 40 mg/day in a retrospective analysis that found the high-dose therapy to be superior with respect to rebleeding, surgical requirement, and mortality.[246] One meta-analysis has also suggested that PPI therapy is associated with reduced blood transfusion requirements.[247] Some patients may be switched to an oral PPI if rapid stabilization occurs, but careful clinical assessment should be performed to ensure the patient is stable.[245] Early initiation of a PPI bolus infusion prior to endoscopy has been shown to reduce the proportion of patients with active bleeding once endoscopy is performed, reduce the requirements for endoscopy, and reduce hospital stay.[248] However, this strategy should not replace early endoscopic management in high-risk patients, as combination PPI therapy with endoscopic maneuvers have been proven to be better than monotherapy with an IV PPI.[231,249] High-dose oral PPI therapy after endoscopic treatment may also be efficacious in patients with peptic ulcer bleeding.[236,240] However, one trial evaluating the use of high-dose esomeprazole (40 mg orally twice daily for 3 days) versus placebo after endoscopic hemostasis failed to show a reduction in rebleeding, transfusions, surgery, or mortality.[250]

Other Agents

The use of somatostatin or octreotide is not recommended for the treatment of patients with nonvariceal upper GI bleeding, as there is no evidence of benefit to support their use.[231] However, these agents are commonly used in the management of variceal bleeding (see Chapter 28, Complications of End-Stage Liver Disease).

STRESS-RELATED MUCOSAL BLEEDING

Acute stress-related mucosal damage (SRMD) is a type of erosive gastritis that occurs in critically ill patients with severe physiological stress (e.g., surgery, trauma, organ failure, sepsis, severe burns, neurologic injuries).[236,251–253] The term *stress ulcer* is a misnomer in that SRMD may range from numerous diffuse superficial erosive mucosal lesions (those that do not penetrate the muscularis mucosa) to major deep ulceration (penetration of the muscularis mucosa and potentially submucosa).[254,255] Initial lesions occur early (<24 hours) and appear as subepithelial petechiae that can develop into superficial erosions and ulcerations.[253,254] Early stress-related mucosal lesions are multiple, usually asymptomatic, without perforation, and commonly bleed from superficial mucosal capillaries.[252,254] The gastric fundus is the most likely anatomical region of the stomach to be involved. Distal lesions involving the gastric antrum and duodenum have also been described, but tend to appear later in the hospital course and are often deeper and associated with a greater probability for bleeding.[254] SRMB from these lesions may be categorized into three distinct types based on clinical presentation.[252–255] Occult bleeding is defined as aspirated gastric fluid or stool that is guaiac-positive for the presence of occult blood and without other signs or symptoms. Overt bleeding, defined as frank hemorrhage identified by hematemesis (bloody vomitus or the appearance of coffee grounds in gastric aspirates or vomitus), hematochezia (bloody diarrhea), or melenic stools. Clinically important bleeding or life-threatening bleeding is the presence of overt bleeding that is associated with hemodynamic changes (tachycardia, hypotension, orthostatic changes, or hemoglobin concentration decline of >2 g/dL) and the requirement of transfusion of blood products. Endoscopic therapy is generally not a viable option because of the extensive distribution of lesions associated with SMBD.[235]

Epidemiology

The majority (>75%) of critically ill patients admitted to intensive care units (ICUs) will develop mucosal lesions consistent with SRMD within 24 hours of admission.[252–255] Only a small percentage (up to 6%) of these patients will progress to clinically important GI bleeding.[252–255] Clinically important SRMB has been associated with an increased length of stay in the ICU by up to 11 days and results in substantial increases in the cost of health care.[252–254,256] The mortality of clinically important SRMB approaches 50%, but mortality may also be associated with underlying comorbidities related to the critical illness.[236,253]

Pathophysiology

Numerous factors have been identified in the pathogenesis of SRMD and resultant bleeding. These include gastric acid and pepsin secretion, disruptions to the normal homeostatic mechanisms that protect the gastric mucosa against the highly acidic environment (decreases in prostaglandin, bicarbonate, and GI mucus formation as well as impaired turnover of gastric epithelium), GI motility disturbances, and mucosal ischemia resulting from decreased blood flow.[252,253,255] Gastric acid is likely the central factor associated with development of SRMD.[254] Because of the absence of protective defenses, substantial amounts of acid are not required for the formation of lesions, but some acid is required for damage to occur.[255] Although some patients may have increased acid secretion (e.g., sepsis, CNS injuries, small bowel resections), the majority of critically ill patients have normal or decreased acid secretion.[251,254,255] Pepsin secretion is associated with the lysis of clots due to its protolytic action on fibrin.[250] Gastric prostaglandins play a key role in the cellular defense against gastric acid.[255] These prostaglandins are responsible for maintaining the integrity of the mucosal barrier by stimulating mucus and bicarbonate production; regulating blood flow; and to some degree, inhibition of acid production. Mucosal ischemia secondary to splanchnic hypoperfusion also plays a large role in the pathogenesis of SRMD.[252,255] Mucosal ischemia is associated with reduced ability to neutralize hydrogen ions leading to intracellular acidosis within the mucosa and subsequent cell death. These factors all contribute to an imbalance by increasing injurious factors and reducing the protective mechanisms within the gastric fundus.

Risk Factors

30. J.S., a 58-year-old, 110-kg male was admitted to the medical ICU for severe necrotizing pancreatitis identified on abdominal computed tomography. The patient was immediately made "nothing by mouth" (NPO) and started on imipenem/cilastatin 1,000 mg IV Q 8 hr. He was given meperidine 50 mg intramuscularly Q 6 hr for pain. He subsequently developed shortness of breath on his third day after admission. He required intubation and was placed on a ventilator. A chest x-ray showed a left lower lobe infiltrate suggestive of hospital-acquired pneumonia. Antibiotic coverage was increased with the addition of ciprofloxacin 400 mg IV q12h and linezolid 600 mg IV Q 12 hr. He has a temperature of 103.5°F, heart rate of 115 beats/minute, and blood pressure of 70/40 mmHg. Pertinent laboratory results at this time are WBC count 38,000/mm^3, Hgb 13.6 g/dL, Hct 40%, platelets 150,000/mm^3, SrCr 1.3 mg/dL, BUN 24 mg/dL, INR 1.0, aPTT 39 seconds, aspartate aminotransferase (AST) 292 Units/L, alanine aminotransferase (ALT) 305 Units/L, amylase 508 Units/L, and lipase 624 Units/L. In addition to the antimicrobials and initiation

Table 26-11 Risk Factors for Stress-Related Mucosal Bleeding

- Respiratory failure
- Coagulopathy
- Hypotension
- Sepsis
- Hepatic failure
- Acute renal failure
- Enteral feeding
- High-dose corticosteroids[a]
- Organ transplant
- Anticoagulants
- Severe burns (>35% of body surface area)
- Head injury
- Intensive care unit stay >7 days
- History of previous GI hemorrhage

[a]Greater than 250 mg/day hydrocortisone or equivalent.
Adapted from references 251–254, with permission.

of fluid resuscitation, the critical care team is considering stress ulcer prophylaxis. What risk factors does J.S. have (if any) for SRMB, and is he a candidate for stress ulcer prophylaxis?

Numerous risk factors have been associated with SRMB[251–254] (Table 26-11). However, a large landmark, multicenter, prospective study involving more than 2,200 critically ill patients admitted to a medical ICU identified only the requirement of mechanical ventilation (respiratory failure) or coagulopathy as independent risk factors for development of clinically important bleeding.[257] Considering the cost associated with the redution of risk related to SRMB, the authors concluded that only these two risk factors warrant the use of prophylactic therapy. Because not all risk factors impose the same level of risk, clinical guidelines and most practitioners recommend prophylaxis only when the patient is mechanically ventilated, has a coagulopathy, or when two or more of the remaining risk factors are present[251,253] (Table 26-11). J.S.'s risk factors include septic shock as evidenced by hemodynamic instability and mechanical ventilation. Therefore, a prophylactic regimen to reduce the risk of SRMB is appropriate.

Treatment

31. What options exist to prevent SRMB in J.S.?

Not all patients admitted to the critical care unit will require prophylaxis for SRMB. However, since mortality can be high in patients when bleeding occurs, evaluation of risk is of absolute importance to ensure that protective pharmacotherapy is initiated in appropriate patients.[251–253] Because acid is required for mucosal injury, the inhibition of gastric acid is the primary target when pharmacotherapy is used to reduce the risk of SRMB. An intragastric pH >4 is the recommended goal of therapy.[233,236,251–255] Therapeutic options include the use of antacids, sucralfate, H_2RAs, and PPIs (Table 26-12).

Antacids

The use of aggressive antacid therapy is superior to placebo in reducing clinically important SRMB when an intragastric pH >3.5 is maintained.[252,253] Although antacids are effective in preventing SRMB, their use has fallen out of favor due to difficult administration regimens (every 1–2 hours) with the continuous requirement of intragastric pH monitoring for dose titration, electrolyte abnormalities (especially in patients with renal dysfunction), diarrhea, constipation, and the potential risk of aspiration pneumonia.[252–254] In addition, an elevated intragastric pH can lead to the proliferation of bacteria within the stomach, and aspiration of these microbes may be associated with nosocomial pneumonia.[252]

Sucralfate

Sucralfate is effective in preventing SRMB but does not have an important effect on intragastric pH.[258,259] Despite the fact that antisectory therapy is preferred, sucralfate remains an available therapeutic option. Early studies suggested a reduction in nosocomial pneumonia with sucralfate when compared with ranitidine or antacids. However, a more recent randomized trial involving 1,200 mechanically ventilated patients revealed no increase in pneumonia with the H_2RAs when compared with sucralfate or antacids.[260] The usual dose of 1 g four times daily can present problems within the critical care setting because of multiple daily dosing, binding of other drugs, and occlusion of nasogastric tubes (may be reduced with available suspension). Other potential issues include the potential for aluminum toxicity in patients with renal failure, constipation, and electrolyte imbalances. The concomitant use of sucralfate with antisecretory therapy may reduce the effectiveness of sucralfate as an intragastric pH <4 is needed for conversion to its active form, which binds to the gastric mucosa.[253]

H_2-Receptor Antagonists

The H_2RAs are effective in preventing SRMB and are the most widely used for this indication.[261,262] Although only cimetidine

Table 26-12 Stress-Related Mucosal Bleeding Prevention: Regimens and Doses

Agent	Dose and Frequency of Administration	FDA Approval[a]
Antacid	30 mL PO/NG Q 1–2 hr	No
Cimetidine	300 mg IV Q 6–8 hr or	No
	300 mg IV loading dose, then 50 mg/hr continuous IV infusion	Yes
Famotidine	20 mg IV Q 12 hr or	No
	1.7 mg/hr continuous infusion	No
Ranitidine	50 mg IV Q 6–8 hr or	No
	6.25 mg/hr continuous infusion	No
Sucralfate	1 g PO/NG Q 6 hr	No
Omeprazole	20–40 mg PO/NG[b] Q 12–24 hr	No
Omeprazole/ Sodium bicarbonate powder for oral suspension	40 mg PO/NG initially, followed by 40 mg in 6–8 hr as a loading dose, then 40 mg PO/NG Q 24 hr	Yes
Lansoprazole	30 mg PO/NG[b,c] Q 12–24 hr	No
Pantoprazole	40 mg IV/PO/NG[b] Q12–24 hr	No
Esomeprazole	40 mg IV Q 12–24 hr	No

[a]For prevention of stress-related mucosal bleeding.
[b]Extemporaneously compounded in sodium bicarbonate.
[c]Oral disintegrating tablet.
IV, intravenous; NG, by nasogastric tube; PO, by mouth; Q, every.

continuous infusion has been FDA-labeled for the prevention of SRMB, continuous or intermittent infusions of ranitidine and famotidine are most often used for this indication.[236,252] Continuous infusions have been suggested as being more effective in maintaining a pH >4, but there are no data comparing these two treatment options with respect to clinical outcomes.[254] Despite this, intermittent dosing is used more commonly than continuous infusions for the prophylaxis of SRMB.[236,252,261,262]

Numerous meta-analyses have evaluated the effectiveness of H_2RAs for prophylaxis of SRMB.[263,264] Cook et al. reviewed 63 randomized trials and determined that prophylaxis with the H_2RAs was associated with a statistically significant reduction in overt and clinically important upper GI bleeding when compared with no therapy and a significant reduction in overt bleeding when compared with antacids.[263] A trend toward reduced clinically important bleeding was identified when H_2RAs were compared with sucralfate, but this was not statistically significant. In another meta-analysis, ranitidine was shown to be of no benefit in preventing SRMB and increased the risk of pneumonia.[264] However, neither of these meta-analyses included the large study involving 1,200 mechanically ventilated patients that compared sucralfate, ranitidine, and placebo.[260] Despite these conflicting results, the H_2RAs remain a recommended option for the prophylaxis of SMRB.[261,262] One shortcoming of H_2RAs is that tolerance may develop (within 72 hours) and thus theoretically lead to potential prophylaxis failure.[239] The H_2RAs are eliminated renally, and dosage reductions may be required in patients with renal failure.

Proton Pump Inhibitors

The PPIs, because of their profound ability to inhibit gastric acid secretion and lack of tolerance to their antisecretory effect, would appear to be the preferred option for preventing SRMB. However, there is very little evidence to confirm their clinical superiority to the H_2RAs for this indication. Observational studies have compared the PPIs with H_2RAs or placebo in critically ill patients in small populations using varied predetermined end points.[253] These studies suggest that the PPIs provide greater acid suppression compared with the H_2RAs and are likely to be as effective in preventing SRMB.[265–267] One study in 359 critically ill patients evaluated the use of immediate-release omeprazole suspension in bicarbonate given via nasogastric tube at a dose of 40 mg for two doses, then 40 mg/day versus IV cimetidine given as a 300 mg bolus and then infused at 50 mg/hour (dosing was adjusted for patients with renal dysfunction).[268] The results indicate that the PPI-bicarbonate suspension was associated with a greater mean time of intragastric pH >4 than the cimetidine infusion but that the rate of clinically important bleeding did not differ between cimetidine (6.8%) and omeprazole (4.5%). The FDA considered the immediate-release omeprazole-bicarbonate suspension to be noninferior to cimetidine for the prevention of SRMB.[269]

The incidence of nosocomial pneumonia in patients receiving PPI therapy in the critical care setting has been evaluated. A 22-month observational study in 80 patients receiving either omeprazole or ranitidine did not find a difference in the rates of nosocomial pneumonia between the two groups, thus suggesting rates may be equivalent.[270] Numerous alternative administration options exist for patients in the critical care setting who cannot take medications by mouth, have nasogastric tubes in place, or have difficulty swallowing[253,269,271] (Table 26-13). The PPIs are becoming first-line therapy for the prevention of SRMB, but additional studies are needed to confirm the most effective dose and route of administration in order to obtain optimal clinical outcomes in patients at risk of SRMB.[252,261]

Monitoring

32. J.S. has been started on famotidine 20 mg IV every 12 hours. How should this pharmacotherapy be monitored for safety and efficacy?

The famotidine dose should be adjusted to maintain an intragastric pH >4 and should be based on severity of the patient's illness, renal function, and intragastric pH measurements. The intragastric pH can be determined with an indwelling probe or by measuring the pH of nasogastric aspirates. The patient

Table 26-13 Alternative Proton Pump Inhibitor Administration Options

	Omeprazole	*Lansoprazole*	*Pantoprazole*	*Esomeprazole*	*Rabeprazole*
Capsule granules sprinkled on selected soft foods (i.e., applesauce)		√[a]		√[a]	
Capsule granules mixed in water and flushed down NG tube				√	
Capsule granules mixed in juice (can be administered via NG tube if required)	√	√[a]		√[a]	
Extemporaneous compound of PPI in bicarbonate for NG tube	√	√	√		
Package for oral suspension	√[a,b]	√[a,c]			
Oral disintegrating tablet		√[a]			
IV formulation	Not available in the United States	Removed from U.S. market	√[a]	√[a]	

[a]Labeled by the Food and Drug Administration for this administration option.
[b]Omeprazole suspensions available in 20-mg and 40-mg packets with bicarbonate (1,680 mg); both contain same amount of bicarbonate, and two 20-mg packets cannot be substituted for one 40-mg packet.
[c]Not to be administered via NG tube, as occlusion of tube is possible.
IV, intravenous; NG, nasogastric; PPI, proton pump inhibitor.
Adapted from references 253, 269 and 271, with permission.

should be monitored for signs of bleeding (e.g., presence of blood or coffee ground material in nasogastric aspirates, hematemesis, hematochezia, or melena), hypotension, reductions in hemoglobin or hematocrit, and thrombocytopenia.

33. Over the next 6 days, J.S. improves and is subsequently removed from mechanical ventilation and transferred to the medical ward. He is now able to eat normally. Should J.S. be continued on SRMD prophylaxis?

Patients receiving prophylaxis for SRMB should be evaluated for the continued presence of risk factors. As the patient improves, the risk factors should in turn be reversed, and the need for SMRB prophylaxis should diminish. Factors such as extubation, correction of coagulopathies, discharge from the intensive care setting, and the ability to take oral feeding advocate the discontinuation of prophylaxis. Erstad et al. surveyed 153 institutions with the United States and found that in 65% of the hospitals, >25% of patients remained on SRMB prophylaxis after discharge from the ICU.[272] This can lead to increased costs, the potential of the patient being discharged on medication for which there is no indication, and future potential adverse effects from the medication. Since J.S. does not possess any risk factors for SRMB, the famotidine should be discontinued at this time.

REFERENCES

1. Shaheen NJ et al. The burden of gastrointestinal and liver diseases. *Am J Gasterenterol* 2006;101:1.
2. Sandler RS et al. The burden of selected digestive diseases in the United States. *Gastroenterology* 2002;122:1500.
3. Imperiale TF et al. Predicting poor outcome from acute upper gastrointestinal hemorrhage. *Arch Intern Med* 2007;167:1291.
4. Conrad SA. Acute upper gastrointestinal bleeding in critically ill patients: causes and treatment modalities. *Crit Care Med* 2002;30(Suppl):S365.
5. Johanson JF. Curbing the costs of GI bleeding. *Am J Gastroenterol* 1998;93:1384.
6. Gilbert DA. Epidemiology of upper gastrointestinal bleeding. *Gastrointestinal Endosc* 1990; 36(Suppl):8.
7. Biancani P et al. Esophageal motor function. In: Yamada T et al., eds. *Textbook of Gastroenterology.* 4th ed. Philadelphia: Lippincott Williams & Wilkins; 2003:166.
8. Richter JE. Gatroesophageal reflux disease. In: Yamada T et al., eds. *Textbook of Gastroenterology.* 4th ed. Philadelphia: Lippincott Williams & Wilkins; 2003:1196.
9. Del Valle J et al. Acid peptic disorders. In: Yamada T et al., eds. *Textbook of Gastroenterology.* 4th ed. Philadelphia: Lippincott Williams & Wilkins; 2003:1321.
10. Freston JW et al. Effects of hypochlorhydria and hypergastrinemia on structure and function of gastrointestinal cells: a review and analysis. *Dig Dis Sci* 1995;40(Suppl):50S.
11. Del Valle J et al. Gastric secretion. In: Yamada T et al., eds. *Textbook of Gastroenterology.* 4th ed. Philadelphia: Lippincott Williams & Wilkins; 2003:266.
12. Maton PN et al. Antacids revisited: a review of their clinical pharmacology and recommended therapeutic use. *Drugs* 1999;57:855.
13. Fordtran JS et al. *In vivo* and *in vitro* evaluation of liquid antacids. *N Engl J Med* 1973;288:923.
14. Washington N et al. Patterns of food and acid reflux in patients with low-grade oesophagitis: the role of an antireflux agent. *Aliment Pharmacol Ther* 1998;12:53.
15. Zweber A, Berardi RR. Heartburn and dyspepsia. In: *Handbook of Nonprescription Drugs.* 15th ed. Washington, DC: American Pharmaceutical Association; 2006:265.
16. Welage LS, Berardi RR. Drug interactions with antiulcer agents: considerations in the treatment of acid-peptic disease. *J Pharm Pract* 1994;VII:177.
17. Nix DE et al. Effects of aluminum and magnesium antacids and ranitidine on the absorption of ciprofloxacin. *Clin Pharmacol Ther* 1989;46:700.
18. Lin JH. Pharmacokinetic and pharmacodynamic properties of histamine H_2-receptor antagonist. *Clin Pharmacokinet* 1991;20:218.
19. Feldman M, Burton ME. Histamine-receptor antagonists: standard therapy for acid-peptic diseases. Part 1. *N Engl J Med* 1990;323:1672.
20. Feldman M, Burton ME. Histamine-receptor antagonists: standard therapy for acid-peptic diseases. Part 2. *N Engl J Med* 1990;323:1749.
21. Schunack W. What are the differences between the H_2-receptor antagonists? *Alimentary Pharmcol Ther* 1987;1(Suppl 1):493S.
22. Price AH, Brogden RN. Nizatidine: a preliminary review of its pharmacodynamic and pharmacokinetic properties and therapeutic use in peptic ulcer disease. *Drugs* 1988;36:521.
23. Sax MJ. Clinically important adverse effects and drug interactions with H_2-receptor antagonists: an update. *Pharmacotherapy* 1987;7:110S.
24. Richter JM et al. Cimetidine and adverse reactions: a meta-analysis of randomized clinical trials of short-term therapy. *Am J Med* 1989;87:278.
25. Aymard JP et al. Haematological adverse effects of histamine H_2-receptor antagonists. *Med Toxicol Adverse Drug Exp* 1988;3:430.
26. Wade EE et al. H_2-antagonist-induced thrombocytopenia: is this a real phenomenon? *Intensive Care Med* 2002;28:459.
27. Lewis H. Hepatic effects of drugs used in the treatment of peptic ulcer disease. *Am J Gastroenterol* 1987;82:987.
28. Jenson RT et al. Cimetidine-induced impotence and breast changes in patients with gastric hypersecretory states. *N Engl J Med* 1983;308:883.
29. Nazario M. The hepatic and renal mechanisms of drug interactions with cimetidine. *Drug Intell Clin Pharm* 1986;20:342.
30. Kosoglou T, Vlasses PH. Drug interactions involving renal transport mechanisms: an overview. *Ann Pharmacother* 1989;23:116.
31. Merki HS, Wilder-Smith CH. Do continuous infusions of omeprazole and ranitidine retain their effect with prolonged dosing. *Gastroenterology* 1994;106:60.
32. Fackler WK et al. Long-term effect of H_2RA therapy on nocturnal gastric acid breakthrough. *Gastroenterology* 2002;122:625.
33. Welage LS, Berardi RR. Evaluation of omeprazole, lansoprazole, pantoprazole, and rebeprazole in the treatment of acid-related diseases. *J Am Pharm Assoc* 2000;40:52.
34. Jones R, Bytzer P. Acid suppression in the management of gastro oesophageal reflux disease: an appraisal of treatment in primary care. *Aliment Pharmacol Ther* 2001;15:765.
35. Welage LS. Pharmacologic properties of proton pump inhibitors. *Pharmacotherapy* 2003;23:74S.
36. Hatelbakk JG. Review article: gastric activity comparison of esomeprazole with other proton pump inhibitors. *Aliment Pharmacol Ther* 2003;17(Suppl 1):10.
37. Caro JJ et al. Healing and relapse rates in gastroesophageal reflux disease treated with the newer proton-pump inhibitors lansoprazole, rabeprazole, and pantoprazole compared to with omeprazole, ranitidine, and placebo: evidence from randomized clinical trails. *Clin Ther* 2001;23:998.
38. Dekkers CP et al. Double-blind, placebo-controlled comparison of rabeprazole 20 mg vs. omeprazole 20 mg in the treatment of erosive or ulcerative gastro-oesophageal reflux disease. *Aliment Pharmacol Ther* 1999;13:49.
39. Mossner J et al. A double-blind study of pantoprazole and omeprazole in the treatment of reflux oesophagitis: a multicentre trial. *Aliment Pharmacol Ther* 1995;9:321.
40. Castell DO et al. Esomeprazole (40 mg) compared with lansoprazole (30 mg) in the treatment of erosive esophagitis. *Am J Gastroenterol* 2002;97: 575.
41. Howden CW et al. Evidence for therapeutic equivalence of lansoprazole 30 mg and esomeprazole 40mg in the treatment of erosive oesophagitis. *Clin Drug Invest* 2002;22:99.
42. Horn JR, Howden CW. Review article: similarities and differences among delayed-release proton-pump inhibitor formulations. *Aliment Pharmacol Ther* 2005;22:20.
43. Wang WH et al. Head-to-head comparison of H2-receptor antagonists and proton pump inhibitors in the treatment of erosive esophagitis: a meta-analysis. *World J Gastroenterol* 2005;11:4067.
44. Stedman CAM, Barclay ML. Review article: Comparison of the pharmacokinetics, acid suppression and efficacy of proton pump inhibitors. *Aliment Pharmacol Ther* 2000;14:963.
45. Ramakrishnan A, Katz PO. Overview of therapy for gastroesophageal reflux disease. *Gastrointest Clin North Am* 2003;13:57.
46. Anderson T. Pharmacokinetics, metabolism and interactions of acid pump inhibitors: focus on omeprazole, lansoprazole, and pantoprazole. *Clin Pharmcokinet* 1996;31:9.
47. Reilly JP. Safety of proton-pump inhibitors. *Am J Health Syst Pharm* 1999;56(Suppl 4):S11.
48. Rindi G et al. Effects of 5 years of treatment with rabeprazole or omeprazole on the gastric mucosa. *Eur J Gastroenterol Hepatol* 2005;17:559.
49. Laine L et al. Review article: potential gastrointestinal effects of long term acid suppression with proton pump inhibitors. *Aliment Pharmacol Ther* 2000;14:651.
50. Kuipers EJ et al. Atrophic gastritis and Helicobacter pylori infection in patients with reflux esophagitis treated with omeprazole or fundoplication. *N Engl J Med* 1996;334:1018.
51. Williams C, McColl KEL. Review article: proton pump inhibitors and bacterial overgrowth. *Aliment Pharmacol Ther* 2006;23:3.
52. Dial S et al. Use of gastric acid-suppressive agents and the risk of community-acquired *Clostridium difficile*-associated disease. *JAMA* 2005;294:2989.
53. Laheij RJF et al. Risk of Community-acquired pneumonia and use of gastric acid-suppressive drugs. *JAMA* 2004;292:1955.
54. Yang Y-X et al. Long-term proton pump inhibitor therapy and risk of hip fracture. *JAMA* 2006; 296:2947.

55. Koop H. Review article: metabolic consequences of long-term inhibition of acid secretion by omeprazole. *Aliment Pharmacol Ther* 1992;6:399.
56. Sierra F et al. Systematic review: proton pump inhibitor-associated acute interstitial nephritis. *Aliment Pharmacol Ther* 2007;26:545.
57. Shorrock CJ, Rees WDW. Effect of sucralfate on human gastric bicarbonate secretion and local prostaglandin E_2 metabolism. *Am J Med* 1989; 86(Suppl 6A):2.
58. McCarthy DM. Sucralfate. *N Engl J Med* 1991;325: 1017.
59. Graham DY et al. Prevention of NSAID-induced gastric ulcer with misoprostol: multicentre, double-blind, placebo-controlled trial. *Lancet* 1988;2:1277.
60. Wolfe MM et al. Gastrointestinal toxicity of nonsteroidal antiinflammatory drugs. *N Engl J Med* 1999;340:1888.
61. Hussar DA. New drugs: retapamulin, bismuth subcitrate potassium, and rotigotine. *J Am Pharm Assoc* 2007;47:539.
62. Talley NJ et al. American Gastroenterological Association technical review on the evaluation of dyspepsia. *Gastroenterology* 2005;129:1756.
63. Talley NJ, Vakil N. Practice Parameters Committee of the American College of Gastroenterology. Guidelines for the management of dyspepsia. *Am J Gastroenterol* 2005;100:2324.
64. Vakil N. Dyspepsia and GERD: breaking the rules. *Am J Gastroenterol* 2005;100:1489.
65. American Gastroenterological Association medical position statement: evaluation of dyspepsia. *Gastroenterology* 2005;129:1753.
66. Erstad BL. Dyspepsia: initial evaluation and treatment. *J Am Pharm Assoc* 2002;42:460.
67. Delaney BC et al. Initial management strategies for dyspepsia. *Cochrane Database Syst Rev* 2003;2:CD001961.
68. Moayyedi P et al. The efficacy of proton pump inhibitors in non-ulcer dyspepsia: a systematic review and economic analysis. *Gastroenterology* 2004;127:1329.
69. Moayyedi P et al. Pharmacological interventions for non-ulcer dyspepsia. *Cochrane Database Syst Rev* 2003;1:CD001960.
70. Holtmann G et al. A randomized placebo-controlled trial of simethicone and cisapride for the treatment of patients with functional dyspepsia. *Aliment Pharmacol Ther* 2002;16:1641.
71. Moayyedi P et al. Eradication of *Helicobacter pylori* for non-ulcer dyspepsia. *Cochrane Database Syst Rev* 2003;1:CD002096.
72. Laine L et al. Therapy for *Helicobacter pylori* in patients with nonulcer dyspepsia. A meta-analysis of randomized controlled trails. *Ann Intern Med* 2001;134:361.
73. Moayyedi P et al. An update of the Cochrane systematic review of *Helicobacter pylori* eradication therapy in nonulcer dyspepsia: resolving the discrepancy between systematic reviews. *Am J Gastroenterol* 2003;98:2621.
74. McNamara D et al. Does *Helicobacter pylori* eradication affect symptoms in nonulcer dyspepsia: a 5-year follow-up study. *Helicobacter* 2002;7:317.
75. Suerbaum S, Michetti P. *Helicobacter pylori* infection. *N Engl J Med* 2002;347:1175.
76. Starzynska T, Malfertheiner P. *Helicobacter* and digestive malignancies. *Helicobacter* 2006;11(Suppl 1):32.
77. Matysiak-Budnik T et al. *Helicobacter pylori* and non-malignant diseases. *Helicobacter* 2006; 11(Suppl 1):27.
78. Delaney B, McColl K. Review article: *Helicobacter pylori* and gastro-oesophageal reflux disease. *Aliment Pharmacol Ther* 2005;22(Suppl 1):32.
79. Solnick JV et al. Extragastric manifestations of *Helicobacter pylori* infection—other *Helicobacter* species. *Helicobacter* 2006;11(Suppl 1):46.
80. Chey WD, Wong BCY. Practice Parameters Committee of American College of Gastroenterology. Guideline on the management of *Helicobacter pylori* infection. *Am J Gastroenterol* 2007;102:1808.
81. Queiroz DMM, Luzza F. Epidemiology of *Helicobacter pylori* infection. *Helicobacter* 2006; 11(Suppl 1):1.
82. Laine L. Approaches to nonsteroidal anti-inflammatory drug use in the high-risk patient. *Gastroenterology* 2001;120:594.
83. Cryer B. NSAID-associated deaths: the rise and fall of NSAID-associated GI mortality. *Am J Gastroenterol* 2005;100:1694.
84. Lanas A et al. A nationwide study of mortality associated with hospital admission due to severe gastrointestinal events and those associated with nonsteroidal antiinflammatory drug use. *Am J Gastroenterol* 2005;100:1685.
85. Sachs G et al. The control of gastric acid and *Helicobacter pylori* eradication. *Aliment Pharmacol Ther* 2000;14:1383.
86. Hatakeyama M, Brzozowski T. Pathogenesis of *Helicobacter pylori* infection. *Helicobacter* 2006;11 (Suppl 1):14.
87. Basset C et al. *Helicobacter pylori* infection: anything new should we know? *Aliment Pharmacol Ther* 2004;20(Suppl 2):31.
88. Micklewright R et al. Review article: NSAIDs, gastroprotection and cyclo-oxygenase-II-selective inhibitors. *Aliment Pharmacol Ther* 2003;17:321.
89. Naesdal J, Brown K. NSAID-associated adverse effects and acid control aids to prevent them: a review of current treatment options. *Drug Safety* 2006;29:119.
90. Garcia Rodriguez LA et al. Risk of upper gastrointestinal complications among users of traditional NSAIDs and COXIBs in the general population. *Gastroenterology* 2007;132:498.
91. Kelly JP et al. Risk of aspirin-associated major upper gastrointestinal bleeding with enteric-coated or buffered product. *Lancet* 1996;348:1413.
92. Dzierzanowska-Fangrat K et al. Diagnosis of *Helicobacter pylori* infection. *Helicobacter* 2006; 11(Suppl 1):6.
93. Gisbert JP, Abraiira V. Accuracy of *Helicobacter pylori* diagnostic tests in patients with bleeding peptic ulcer: a systematic review and meta-analysis. *Am J Gastroenterol* 2006;101:848.
94. Gotteland M et al. Systematic review: are probiotics useful in controlling gastric colonization by *Helicobacter pylori*. *Aliment Pharmacol Ther* 2006;23:1077.
95. Malfertheiner P et al. Current concepts in the management of *Helicobacter pylori* infection. The Maastricht III Consensus Report. *Gut* 2007;56: 772.
96. Qasim A, O'Morain CA. Review article: treatment of *Helicobacter pylori* infection and factors influencing eradication. *Aliment Pharmacol Ther* 2002;16(Suppl 1):24.
97. Bochenek WL et al. Eradication of *Helicobacter pylori* by 7-day triple-therapy regimens combining pantoprazole with clarithromycin, metronidazole or amoxcillin in patients with peptic ulcer disease; results of two double-blind, randomized studies. *Helicobacter* 2003;8:626.
98. Calvet X et al. A meta-analysis of short versus long therapy with a proton pump inhibitor, clarithromycin and either metronidazole or amoxycillin for treating *Helicobacter pylori* infection. *Aliment Pharmacol Ther* 2000;14:603.
99. Paoluzi P et al. 2-week triple therapy for *Helicobacter pylori* infection is better than 1-week in clinical practice: a large prospective single-center randomized study. *Helicobacter* 2006;11:562.
100. Vallve M et al. Single vs. double dose of a proton pump inhibitor in triple therapy for *Helicobacter pylori* eradication: a meta-analysis. *Aliment Pharmacol Ther* 2002;16:1149.
101. Janssen MJR et al. Meta-analysis: the influence of pre-treatment with a proton pump inhibitor on *Helicobacter pylori* eradication. *Aliment Pharmacol Ther* 2005;21:341.
102. Gene E et al. Triple vs quadruple therapy for treating *Helicobacter pylori* infection: a meta-analysis. *Aliment Pharmacol Ther* 2003;17:1137.
103. Fischback LA et al. Meta-analysis: the efficacy, adverse events, and adherence related to first-line anti-*Helicobacter pylori* quadruple therapies. *Aliment Pharmacol Ther* 2004;20:1071.
104. Laine L et al. Bismuth-based quadruple therapy using a single capsule of bismuth biskalcitrate, metronidazole, and tetracycline given with omeprazole versus omeprazole, amoxicillin, and clarithromycin for eradication of *Helicobacter pyori* in duodenal ulcer patients: a prospective, randomized, multicenter, North American trial. *Am J Gastroenterol* 2003;98:562.
105. Varia D et al. Sequential therapy versus standard triple-drug therapy for *Helicobacter pylori* eradication. *Ann Intern Med* 2007;146:556.
106. De Francesco V et al. Clarithromycin-resistant genotypes and eradication of *Helicobacter pylori*. *Ann Intern Med* 2006;144:94.
107. Gisbert JP et al. *Helicobacter pylori* first-line treatment and rescue options in patients allergic to penicillin. *Aliment Pharmacol Ther* 2005;22:1041.
108. Vergara M et al. Meta-analysis: comparative efficacy of different proton-pump inhibitors in triple therapy for *Helicobacter pylori* eradication. *Aliment Pharmacol Ther* 2003;18:647.
109. Gisbert JP et al. Meta-analysis: proton pump inhibitors vs. H_2-receptor antagonists—their efficacy with antibiotics in *Helicobacter pylori* eradication. *Aliment Pharmacol Ther* 2003;18:757.
110. Graham DY et al. Meta-analysis: proton pump inhibitor or H2-receptor antagonist for *Helicobacter pylori* eradication. *Aliment Pharmacol Ther* 2003;17:1229.
111. Megraud F, Lamouliatte H. Review article: the treatment of refractory *Helicobacter pylori* infection. *Aliment Pharmacol Ther* 2003;17:1333.
112. Lee M et al. A randomized controlled trial of an enhanced patient compliance program for *Helicobacter pylori* therapy. *Arch Intern Med* 1999;159:2312.
113. Meyer JM et al. Risk factors for *Helicobacter pylori* resistance in the United States: the surveillance of *H. pylori* antimicrobial resistance partnership (SHARP) study, 1993–1999. *Ann Intern Med* 2002; 136:13.
114. Duck WM et al. Antimicrobial resistance incidence and risk factors among *Helicobacter pylori*-infected persons in the United States. *Emerg Infect Dis* 2004;10:1088.
115. Gisbert JP, Pajares JM. Review article: *Helicobacter pylori* rescue regimen when proton pump inhibitor-based triple therapies fail. *Aliment Pharmacol Ther* 2002;16:1047.
116. Hojo M et al. Pooled analysis on the efficacy of the second-line treatment regimens for *Helicobacter pylori* infection. *Scand J Gastroneterol* 2001;36:690.
117. Saad R et al. Levofloxacin triple or PPI quadruple salvage therapy for persistent *Helicobacter pylori* infection: results of a meta-analysis. *Am J Gastroenterol* 2006;101:488.
118. Borody TJ et al. Efficacy and safety of rifabutin-containing "rescue-therapy" for Helicobacter pylori infection. *Aliment Pharmacol Ther* 2006;23: 481.
119. Thomas J et al. Over-the-counter nonsteroidal anti-inflammatory drugs and risk of gastrointestinal symptoms. *Am J Gastroenterol* 2002;97:2215.
120. Yuan Y et al. Peptic ulcer disease today. *Nat Clin Pract Gastroenterol Hepatol* 2006;3:80.
121. Dalton SO et al. Use of SSRIs and risk of upper gastrointestinal tract bleeding: a propulation-based cohort study. *Arch Intern Med* 2003;163:59.
122. Tata LJ et al. Does concurrent prescription of selective serotonin reuptake inhibitors and non-steroidal anti-inflammatory drugs substantially increase the risk of upper gastrointestinal bleeding? *Aliment Pharmacol Ther* 2005;22:175.
123. Laine L. Review article: the effect of *Helicobacter pylori* infection on nonsteroidal anti-inflammatory drug-induced upper gastrointestinal tract injury. *Aliment Phamacol Ther* 2002;16(Suppl 1):34.
124. Huang JQ et al. Role of *Helicobacter pylori* infection and nonsteroidal anti-inflammatory drugs in peptic ulcer disease: a meta-analysis. *Lancet* 2002;369:14.

125. Chan FKL, Graham DY. Review article: prevention of non-steroidal anti-inflammatory drug gastrointestinal complications—review and recommendations based on risk assessment. *Aliment Pharmacol Ther* 2004;19:1051.
126. Dubois RW et al. Guidelines for the appropriate use of non-steroidal anti-inflammatory drugs, cyclo-oxygenase-2-specific inhibitors and proton pump inhibitors in patients requiring chronic anti-inflammaotry therapy. *Aliment Pharmacol Ther* 2004;19:197.
127. Chan PKI et al. Preventing recurrence of upper gastrointestinal bleeding in patients with *Helicobacter pylori* infection who are taking low-dose aspirin or naproxen. *N Engl J Med* 2001;344:967.
128. Lai KC et al. Lansoprazole for the prevention of recurrences of upper gastrointestinal complications from long-term low-dose aspirin use. *N Engl J Med* 2002;346:2033.
129. Silverstein FE et al. Misoprostol reduces serious gastrointestinal complications in patients with rheumatoid arthritis receiving nonsteroidal anti-inflammatory drugs: a randomized, double-blind, placebo-controlled trial. *Ann Intern Med* 1995;123:241.
130. Graham DY et al. Ulcer prevention in long-term users of nonsteroidal anti-inflammatory drugs: results of a double-blind, randomized, multicenter, active- and placebo-controlled study of misoprostol vs lansoprazole. *Arch Intern Med* 2002;152:169.
131. Silverstein F et al. Gastrointestinal toxicity with celecoxib vs nonsteroidal antiinflammatory drugs for osteoarthritis and rheumatoid arthritis. The CLASS study: a randomized controlled trial. *JAMA* 2000;284:1247.
132. Bombardier C et al. Comparison of upper intestinal toxicity of rofecoxib and naproxen in patients with rheumatoid arthritis. VIGOR Study Group. *N Engl J Med* 2000;343:1520.
133. Fitzgerald GA. Coxibs and cardiovascular disease. *N Engl J Med* 2004;351:1709.
134. Cryer B. Gastrointestinal effects of NSAIDs and COX-2 specific inhibitors. Available at: http://www.fda.gov/ohrms/dockets/ac/05/slides/2005--4090S1_02_FDA-Cryer.ppt#624,26,Slide%2026. Accessed February 24, 2008.
135. White WB. Cardiovascular effects of the cyclooxygenase inhibitors. *Hypertension* 2007;49:408.
136. Abraham NS et al. Cyclooxygenase-2 selectivity of non-steroidal anti-inflammatory drugs and the risk of mycardial infarction and cerebrovascular accident. *Aliment Pharmacol Ther* 2007;25:913.
137. Bresalier RS et al. Cardiovascular events associated with rofecoxib in colorectal adenoma chemoprevention trial. *N Engl J Med* 2005;352:1092.
138. Bertagnolli MM et al. Celecoxib for the prevention of sporadic colorectal adenomas. *N Engl J Med* 2006;355:873.
139. Kearney PM et al. Do selective cyclooxygenase-2 inhibitors and traditional non-steroidal antiinflammatory drugs increase the risk of atherothrombosis? Meta-analysis of randomized trials. *BMJ* 2006; 322:1302.
140. Antman EM et al. Use of nonsteroidal antiinflammatory drugs: an update for clinicians. A scientific statement from the American Heart Association. *Circulation* 2007;115:1634.
141. Lai KC et al. COX-2 inhibitor compared with proton pump inhibitor in the prevention of recurrent ulcer complications in high-risk patients taking NSAIDs. *Gastroenterology* 2001;120:A104. Abstract.
142. Chan FD et al. Celecoxib versus diclofenac and omeprazole in reducing the risk of recurrent ulcer bleeding in patients with arthritis. *N Engl J Med* 2002;347:2104.
143. Scheiman JM et al. Prevention of ulcers by esomeprazole in at-risk patients using nonselective NSAIDs and COX-2 inhibitors. *Am J Gastroenterol* 2006;101:701.
144. Laine L et al. Stratifying the risk of NSAID-related upper gastrointestinal clinical events; results of a double-blind outcomes study in patients with rheumatoid arthritis. *Gastroenterology* 2002;123:1006.
145. Van Soest EM et al. Adherence to gastroprotection and the risk of NSAID-related upper gastrointestinal ulcers and haemorrhage. *Aliment Pharmacol Ther* 2007;26:265.
146. Del Valle J, Scheiman JM. Zollinger-Ellison syndrome. In: Yamada T et al., eds. *Textbook of Gastroenterology.* 4th ed. Philadelphia: Lippincott Williams & Wilkins; 2003:1377.
147. Tomassetti P et al. Treatment of Zollinger Ellison syndrome. *World J Gastroenterol* 2005;11:5423.
148. Campana D et al. Zollinger-Ellison syndrome. *Minerva Med* 2005;96:187.
149. Corleto VD et al. Does the widespread use of proton pump inhibitors mask, complicate and/or delay the diagnosis of Zollinger-Ellison syndrome? *Aliment Pharmacol Ther* 2001;15:1555.
150. Moayyedi P, Talley NJ. Gastro-oesophageal disease. 2006;367:2086.
151. DeVault KR, Castell DO. Updated guidelines for the diagnosis and treatment of gastroesophageal reflux disease. *Am J Gastroentrol* 2005;100:190.
152. Storr M et al. Pharmacologic management and treatment of gastroesophageal reflux disease. *Dis Esophagus* 2004;17:197.
153. Goh K-L. Gastroesophageal reflux disease (GERD) in the East same as the West. *J Clin Gastroenterol* 2007;41(Suppl 2):S54.
154. Moayyedi P, Axon ATR. Gastro-oesophageal reflux disease: the extent of the problem. *Aliment Pharmacol Ther* 2005;22(Suppl 1):11.
155. Devault KR. Review article: the role of acid suppression in patients with non-erosive reflux disease or functional heartburn. *Aliment Pharmacol Ther* 2006;23(Suppl 1):33.
156. Locke GR et al. Prevalence and clinical spectrums of gastroesophageal reflux: a population based study in Olmstead County Minnesota. *Gastroenterology* 1997;112:1448.
157. Nelson SP et al. Prevalence of symptoms of gastroesophageal reflux during infancy: a pediatric practice-based survey. Pediatric Practice Research Group. *Arch Pediatr Adolesc Med* 1997;151:569.
158. Faubion WA, Zein NN. Gastroesophageal reflux in infants and children. *Mayo Clin Proc* 1998;73:166.
159. Shepherd RW et al. Gastroesophageal reflux in children: clinical profile, course and outcome with active therapy in 126 cases. *Clin Pediatr* 1987;26: 55.
160. Treem WR et al. Gastroesophageal reflux in the older child: presentation response to treatment and long-term follow-up. *Clin Pediatr* 1991;30:435.
161. El-Serag HB et al. Childhood GERD is a risk factor for GERD in adolescents and young adults. *Am J Gastroenterol* 2004;99:806.
162. Richter JE. Review article: the management of heartburn in pregnancy. *Aliment Pharmacol Ther* 2005;22:749.
163. Enck P et al. Quality of life in patients with upper gastrointestinal symptoms: results from the Domestic/International Gastroenterology Surveillance Study (DIGEST). *Scand J Gasteroenterol* 1999;34(Suppl):48.
164. Weinberg DS, Kadish SL. The diagnosis and management of gastroesophageal disease. *Med Clin North Am* 1996;80:411.
165. Gelfand MD. Gastroesophageal reflux disease. *Med Clin North Am* 1991;75:923.
166. Benamouzig R, Airinei G. Diet and reflux. *J Clin Gasteroenterol* 2007;41(Suppl 2):S64.
167. Makola D et al. *Helicobacter pylori* infection and related gastrointestinal disease. *J Clin Gastroenterol* 2007;41:548.
168. Delaney B, McColl K. Review article: *Helicobacter pylori* and gastro-oesophageal reflux disease. *Aliment Pharmacol Ther* 2005;22(Suppl 1):32.
169. Holloway R, Dent J. Pathophysiology of gastroesophageal reflux disease: lower esophageal sphincter dysfunction in gastroesophageal reflux disease. *Gastroenterol Clin North Am* 1990;19:517.
170. Dent J et al. Mechanisms of lower oesophageal sphincter incompetence in patients with symptomatic gastrooesophageal reflux. *Gut* 1988;29: 1020.
171. Zamost BJ et al. Esophagitis in scleroderma: prevalence and risk factors. *Gasteroenterology* 1987;92:421.
172. Bozymski EM. Pathophysiology and diagnosis of gastroesophageal reflux disease. *Am J Hosp Pharm* 1993;50(Suppl 1):S4.
173. Richter JE. Do we know the cause of reflux disease? *Eur J Gastroenterol Hepatol* 1999;1(Suppl 1):S3.
174. Goldman JL et al. Esophageal mucosal resistance: a factor in esophagitis. *Gastroenterol Clin North Am.* 1990;19:565.
175. Kahrilas PJ. GERD pathogenesis, pathophysiology, and clinical manifestations. *Cleve Clin Med J* 2003;70(Suppl 5):S4.
176. DeVault KR et al. Updated guidelines for the diagnosis and treatment of gastroesophageal reflux disease. *Am J Gastroenterol* 2005;100:190.
177. Pilotto A et al. Clinical features of reflux esophagitis in older people: a study of 840 consecutive patients. *J Am Geriatr Soc* 2006;54:1537.
178. Reynolds JC. Barrett's esophagus: reducing the risk of progression to adenocarcinoma. *Gastroenterol Clin North Am* 1999;28:917.
179. Kaltenbach T et al. Are lifestyle measures effective in patients with gastroesophageal reflux disease? *Arch Intern Med* 2006;166:965.
180. Tytgat GNJ. Review article: treatment of mild and severe cases of GERD. *Aliment Pharmacol Ther* 2002;16(Suppl 4):73.
181. Vivian EM, Thompson MA. Pharmacologic strategies for treating gastroesophageal reflux disease. *Clin Ther* 2000;22:654.
182. Fendrick AM. Management of patients with symptomatic gastroesophageal reflux disease: a primary care perspective. *Am J Gastroenterol* 2001; 96(Suppl):S29.
183. Numans ME et al. Short-term treatment with proton-pump inhibitors as a test for gastroesophageal reflux disease. *Ann Intern Med* 2004;140: 518.
184. Vakil N. Review article: how valuable are proton-pump inhibitors in establishing a diagnosis of gastro-esophageal reflux disease? *Aliment Pharmacol Ther* 2005;22(Suppl 1):64.
185. Younes Z, Johnson DA. Diagnostic evaluation in gastroesophageal reflux disease. *Gastroentrol Clin North Am* 1999;28:809.
186. Savary M, Miller G. The Esophagus. *Handbook and Atlas of Endoscopy.* Solothurn, Switzerland: Gassman AG; 1978.
187. Lundell LR et al. Endoscopic assessment of oesophagitis: clinical and functional correlates and further validation of the Los Angeles classification. *Gut* 1999;45:172.
188. Armstrong D et al. Endoscopic assessment of oesophagitis. *Gullet* 1991;1:63.
189. Waring JP et al. The preoperative evaluation of patients considered for laparoscopic antireflux surgery. *Am J Gastroenter* 1995;90:35.
190. Chiba N et al. Speed of healing and symptom relief in grade II to IV gastroesophageal reflux disease: a meta-analysis. *Gastroenterology* 1997;112: 1798.
191. Kahrilas PJ et al. High- versus standard-dose ranitidine for control of heartburn in poorly responsive acid reflux disease: a prospective, controlled trial. *Am J Gastroenterol* 1999;94:92.
192. Hunt RH. Importance of pH control in the management of GERD. *Arch Intern Med* 1999;159:649.
193. Wang WH et al. Head-to-head comparison of H2-receptor antagonists and proton pump inhibitors in the treatment of erosive esophagitis: a meta-analysis. *World J Gastroenterol* 2005;11:4067.
194. Richter JE et al. Efficacy and safety of esomeprazole compared with omeprazole in GERD patients with erosive esophagitis: a randomized controlled trial. *Am J Gastroenterol* 2001;96:656.
195. Sampliner RE, Carmargo E. Normalization of esophageal pH with high-dose proton pump inhibitor therapy does not result in regression of Barrett esophagus. *Am J Gastroenterol* 1997;92:582.

196. Hansen AN et al. Long-term management of patients with symptoms of gastro-oesophageal reflux disease—a Norwegian randomised prospective study comparing the effects of esomeprazole and ranitidine treatment strategies on health-related quality of life in a general practitioners setting. *Int J Clin Pract* 2006;60:15.
197. Ros J et al. Healing of erosive esophagitis with sucralfate and cimetidine: influence of pretreatment lower esophageal sphincter pressure and serum pepsinogen I levels. *Am J Med* 1991;91(Suppl 2A):107S.
198. Pace F. Systematic review: maintenance treatment of gastro-oesophageal reflux disease with proton pump inhibitors taken on-demand. *Aliment Pharmacol Ther* 2007;26:195.
199. Bytzer P et al. Six-month trial of on-demand rabeprazole 10 mg maintains symptom relief in patients with non-erosive reflux disease. *Aliment Pharmacol Ther* 2004;20:181.
200. Talley NJ et al. Esomeprazole 40 mg and 20 mg is efficacious in the long-term management of patients with endoscopy-negative gastro-oesophageal reflux disease: a placebo-controlled trial of on-demand therapy for 6 months. *Eur J Gastroenterol Hepatol* 2002;14:857.
201. Scholten T et al. On-demand therapy with pantoprazole 20 mg as effective long-term management of reflux disease in patients with mild GERD: the ORION trial. *Digestion* 2005;72:76.
202. Bigard MA, Genestin E. Treatment of patients with heartburn without endoscopic evaluation: on-demand treatment after effective continuous administration of lansoprazole 15 mg. *Aliment Pharmacol Ther* 2005;22:635.
203. Sjostedt S et al. Daily treatment with esomeprazole is superior to that taken on-demand for maintenance of healed erosive oesophagitis. *Aliment Pharmacol Ther* 2005;22:183.
204. Peghini PL et al. Ranitidine controls nocturnal gastric acid breakthrough on omeprazole: a controlled study in normal subjects. *Gastroenterology* 1998;115:1335.
205. DeVault KR. Review article: the role of acid suppression in patients with non-erosive reflux disease or functional heartburn. *Aliment Pharmacol Ther* 2006;23(Suppl 1):33.
206. Richter JE. Extraesophageal presentations of gastroesophageal reflux disease: an overview. *Am J Gastroenterol* 2000;95(Suppl):S1.
207. Richter JE. Review article: extraesophageal manifestations of gastro-oesophageal reflux disease. *Aliment Pharmacol Ther* 2005;22(Suppl 1):70.
208. Ockene IS et al. Unexplained chest pain in patients with normal coronary arteriograms: a follow-up study of functional status. *N Engl J Med* 1980;303:1249.
209. Demeester TR et al. Esophageal function in patients with angina-type chest pain and normal coronary angiograms. *Ann Surg* 1982;196:488.
210. Kline M et al. Esophageal disease in patients with angina-like chest pain. *Am J Gastroenterol* 1981;75:116.
211. Katz PO et al. Esophageal testing of patients with noncardiac chest pain or dysphagia: results of three years experience with 1161 patients. *Ann Intern Med* 1987;106:593.
212. Richter JE. Chest pain and gastroesophageal disease. *J Clin Gastroenterol* 2000;30(Suppl):S39.
213. Stahl WG et al. Diagnosis and treatment of patients with gastroesophageal reflux and noncardiac chest pain. *South Med J* 1994;87:739.
214. Achem SR et al. Effects of omeprazole versus placebo in treatment of noncardiac chest pain and gastroesophageal reflux. *Dig Dis Sci* 1997;42:2138.
215. Fass R et al. The clinical and economic value of a short course of omeprazole in patients with noncardiac chest pain. *Gastroenterology* 1998;115:42.
216. Pandek WM et al. Short course of omeprazole: a better first diagnostic approach to noncardiac chest pain than endoscopy, manometry, or 24-hour esophageal pH monitoring. *J Clin Gastroenterol* 2002;35:307.
217. Harding SM, Richter JE. Gastoesophageal reflux disease and asthma. *Sem Gastrointest Dis* 1992;3:139.
218. Mansfield LE et al. The role of the vagus nerve in airway narrowing caused by intraesophageal hydrochloric acid provocation and esophageal distension. *Ann Allergy* 1981;47:431.
219. Bretza J, Novey HS. Gastroesophageal reflux and asthma. *West J Med* 1979;131:320.
220. Field SK, Sutherland LR. Does medical antireflux therapy improve asthma in asthmatics with gastroesophageal reflux?: a critical review of the literature. *Chest* 1998;114:275.
221. Bocskei C et al. The influence of gastroesophageal reflux disease and its treatment on asthmatic cough. *Lung* 2005;183:53.
222. Wiener GJ et al. Chronic hoarseness secondary to gastroesophageal reflux disease: documentation with 24-h ambulatory pH monitoring. *Am J Gastroenterol* 1989;84:1503.
223. Richter JE. Extraesophgeal presentations of gastroesophageal reflux disease. *Semin Gastrointest Dis* 1997;8:75.
224. Ohman L et al. Esophageal dysfunction in patients with contact ulcer of the larynx. *Ann Otol Rhinol Laryngol* 1983;92:228.
225. Gaynor EB. Otolaryngologic manifestations of gastroesophageal reflux. *Am J Gastroenterol* 1991;86:801.
226. Champion GL, Richter JE. Atypical presentations of gastroesophageal reflux disease: chest pain, pulmonary, and ear, nose, throat manifestations. *Gastroenterologist* 1993;1:18.
227. Gaynor EB. Laryngeal complications of GERD. *J Clin Gastroenterol* 2000;30(Suppl):S31.
228. Klinkenberg-Knol EC. Otolaryngologic manifestations of gastroesophageal reflux disease. *Scand J Gastroenterol* 1998;33(Suppl):24.
229. Wong RKH et al. ENT Manifestations of gastroesophageal reflux. *Am J Gastroenterol* 2000;95(Suppl):S15.
230. Kamel PL et al. Omeprazole for the treatment of posterior laryngitis. *Am J Med* 1994;96:321.
231. Barkun A et al. Consensus recommendations for managing patients with nonvariceal upper gastrointestinal bleeding. *Ann Intern Med* 2003;139:843.
232. van Leerdam ME, Rauws EAJ. The role of acid suppression in upper gastrointestinal ulcer bleeding. *Best Pract Res Clin Gastroenterol* 2001;15:463.
233. Sung JJY. The role of acid suppression in the management and prevention of gastrointestinal hemorrhage associated with gastroduodenal ulcers. *Gastroenterol Clin North Am* 2003;32:S11.
234. Laine L, Peterson WL. Bleeding peptic ulcer. *N Engl J Med* 1994;331:717.
235. Elta GH. Approach to the patient with gross gastrointestinal bleeding. In: Yamada T et al., eds. *Textbook of Gastroenterology*. 4th ed. Philadelphia: Lippincott Williams & Wilkins; 2003:698.
236. Devlin JW et al. Proton pump inhibitor formulary considerations in the acutely ill. Part 2: clinical efficacy, safety, and economics. *Ann Pharmacother* 2005;39:1844.
237. Elmunzer BJ et al. Risk stratification in upper gastrointestinal bleeding. *J Clin Gastroenterol* 2007;41:559.
238. Pisegna JR. Treatment patients with acute gastrointestinal bleeding. *Pharmacotherapy* 2003;23:81S.
239. Merki HS, Wilder-Smith CH. Do continuous infusions of omeprazole and ranitidine retain their effect with prolonged dosing. *Gastroenterology* 1994;106:60.
240. Leotiadis GI et al. Proton pump inhibitor therapy for peptic ulcer bleeding: Cochrane Collaboration meta-analysis of randomized controlled trials. *Mayo Clin Proc* 2007;82:286.
241. Bardou M et al. Meta-analysis: proton-pump inhibition in high-risk patients with acute peptic ulcer bleeding. *Aliment Pharmacol Ther* 2005;21:677.
242. Lau JY et al. Effect of intravenous omeprazole on recurrent bleeding after endoscopic treatment of bleeding peptic ulcers. *N Engl J Med* 2000;343:310.
243. Lin HJ et al. A prospective randomized comparative trial showing that omeprazole prevents rebleeding in patients with peptic ulcer after successful endoscopic therapy. *Arch Intern Med* 1998;158:54.
244. Barkun A et al. Prevention of peptic ulcer rebleeding using continuous infusion of pantoprazole vs. ranitidine: a multicenter, multinational, randomized, double-blind, parallel-group comparison. *Gastroenterology* 2004;126(Suppl 2):A78. Abstract 609.
245. Leontiadis GI, Howden CW. Pharmacologic treatment of peptic ulcer bleeding. *Curr Treat Options Gastroenterol* 2007;10:134.
246. Simon-Rudler M et al. Continuous infusion of high-dose omeprazole is more effective than standard-dose omeprazole in patients with high-risk peptic ulcer bleeding: a retrospective study. *Aliment Pharmacol Ther* 2007;25:949.
247. Leontiadis GI et al. Systematic review and meta-analysis: proton-pump inhibitor treatment for ulcer bleeding reduces transfusion requirements and hospital stay results form the Cochrane Collaboration. *Aliment Pharmacol Ther* 2005;22:169.
248. Lau JY et al. Omeprazole before endoscopy in patients with gastrointestinal bleeding. *N Engl J Med* 2007;356:1631.
249. Sung JJY et al. The effect of endoscopic therapy in patients receiving omeprazole for bleeding ulcers with nonbleeding visible vessel or adherent clots. *Ann Intern Med* 2003;139:237.
250. Wei K-L et al. Effect of oral esomeprazole on recurrent bleeding after endoscopic treatment of bleeding ulcers. *J Gastroenterol Hepatol* 2007;22:43.
251. American Society of Health-System Pharmacists. ASHP therapeutic guidelines on stress ulcer prophylaxis. *Am J Health Syst Pharm* 1999;56:347.
252. Stollman N, Metz DC. Pathophysiology and prophylaxis of stress ulcer in intensive care unit patients. *J Crit Care* 2005;20:35.
253. Jung R, MacLaren R. Proton-pump inhibitors for stress ulcer prophylaxis in critically ill patients. *Ann Pharmacother* 2002;36:1929.
254. Mutlu GM et al. GI complications in patients receiving mechanical ventilation. *Chest* 2001;119:1222.
255. Fennerty MB. Pathophysiology of upper gastrointestinal tract in the critically ill patient: rationale for the therapeutic benefits of acid suppression. *Crit Care Med* 2002;30(Suppl):S351.
256. Cook DJ et al. The attributable mortality and length of intensive are unit stay of clinically important gastrointestinal bleeding in critically ill patients. *Crit Care* 2001;5:368.
257. Cook DJ et al. Risk factors for gastrointestinal bleeding in critically ill patients. *N Engl J Med* 1994;330:377.
258. Tryba M. Risk of acute stress bleeding and nosocomial pneumonia in ventilated intensive care unit patients: sucralfate versus antacids. *Am J Med* 1987;83(Suppl 3B):117.
259. Bresalier RS et al. Sucralfate suspension versus titrated antacid for the prevention of acute stress related gastrointestinal hemorrhage in critically ill patients. *Am J Med* 1987;83(Suppl 3B):110.
260. Cook D et al. A comparison of sucralfate and ranitidine for the prevention of upper gastrointestinal bleeding in patients requiring mechanical ventilation. *N Engl J Med* 1998;338:791.
261. Daley RJ et al. Prevention of stress ulceration: current trends in critical care. *Crit Care Med* 2004;32:2008.
262. Lam NP et al. National survey of stress ulcer prophylaxis. *Crit Care Med* 1999;27:98.
263. Cook DJ et al. Stress ulcer prophylaxis in critically ill patients. Resolving discordant meta-analyses. *JAMA* 1996;275:308.
264. Messori A et al. Bleeding and pneumonia in intensive care patients given ranitidine and sucralfate for prevention of stress ulcer: meta-analysis of randomized controlled trials. *BMJ* 2000;321:1.
265. Levy MJ et al. Comparison of omeprazole and ranitidine for stress ulcer prophylaxis. *Dig Dis Sci* 1997;42:1255.

266. Phillips JO et al. A multicenter, prospective, randomized clinical trial of continuous I.V. ranitidine vs. omeprazole suspension in the prophylaxis of stress ulcer. *Crit Care Med* 1998;26:A101. Abstract.
267. Roberts KW et al. Effect of lansoprazole suspension versus continuous intravenous ranitidine on gastric pH of mechanically ventilated intensive care unit patients. *Crit Care Med* 2000;28:A185. Abstract.
268. Conrad SA et al. Randomized, double-blind comparison of immediate-release omeprazole oral suspension versus intravenous cimetidine for the prevention of upper gastrointestinal bleeding in critically ill patients. *Crit Care Med* 2005;33: 760.
269. Package insert. Zegerid (omeprazole/sodium bicarbonate). San Diego, CA: Santarus, Inc. Available at: http://www.zegerid.com/assets/pdfs/prescribing_information.pdf. Accessed June 12, 2008.
270. Mallow S et al. Do proton pump inhibitors increase the incidence of nosocomial pneumonia and related infectious complications when compared with histamine-2 receptor antagonists in critically ill trauma patients? *Curr Surg* 2004;61:452.
271. Devlin JW et al. Proton pump inhibitor formulary considerations in the acutely ill. Part 1: pharmacology, pharmacodynamics, and available formulations. *Ann Pharmacother* 2005;39:1667.
272. Erstad BL et al. Survey of stress ulcer prophylaxis. *Crit Care* 1999;3:145.

CHAPTER 27

Lower Gastrointestinal Disorders

Geoffrey C. Wall

OVERVIEW OF INFLAMMATORY BOWEL DISEASE

Definition and Epidemiology

Inflammatory bowel disease (IBD) is a generic classification for a group of chronic, idiopathic, relapsing inflammatory disorders of the gastrointestinal (GI) tract. IBD is common in developed countries.[1] It is estimated that more than 600,000 persons in the United States have IBD, and the prevalence of these disorders ranges from 20 to 200 per 100,000 people; however, the prevalence of IBD may actually be greater because many affected patients may be asymptomatic or have mild symptoms for which they do not seek medical attention.[2,3] By convention, IBD is divided into two major disorders: ulcerative colitis (UC) and Crohn's disease (CD).[2,4] However, approximately 10% to 15% of patients with IBD have symptoms that defy this schema.[5] Both UC and CD frequently affect a similar group of patients (Table 27-1). Whites appear to have the higher incidence of IBD compared with Asians or blacks.[6] In particular, Jews of European descent may have up to a fourfold increase in the incidence of IBD. Studies have found trends toward an increased incidence of IBD in urban compared with rural communities. Hypotheses for this trend include overcrowding, exposure to infectious agents, and lifestyle differences. Although both UC and CD are generally considered diseases of the young, with peak incidences from ages 20 to 40 years, about 15% of IBD cases are diagnosed in patients older than 60 years.[7] There seems to be no significant gender preference for IBD.

Etiology

The true cause of IBD is unclear; however, hypotheses for these disorders include a combination of genetic abnormalities, chronic infection, environmental factors (bacterial, viral, and dietary antigens), autoimmunity, and other abnormalities of immunoregulatory mechanisms.[1] Whatever the mechanism, it is now generally agreed that the symptoms of IBD result from dysregulation of the mucosal immune system. The role of genetics has been strongly supported by epidemiologic studies, showing familial aggregation, consistent ethnic differences, and an increased concordance rate in monozygotic twins. Patients with a first-degree relative with IBD are at an

Table 27-1 Population Characteristics of Patients at High Risk for Inflammatory Bowel Disease Development

No sexual predilection
Peaks between ages of 15 and 30 years
European ancestry
Urban greater than rural dwellers
Whites greater than non-whites
Jews living in Europe and North America greater than non-Jews
Occurs in familial clusters

Reprinted from reference 3, with permission.

increased risk of developing the disorder, with a frequency of up to 40%.[8] Detailed mapping of chromosome 16 in the Human Genome Project found a strong association with the *NOD2* (also termed *CARD15*) gene and increased susceptibility to CD, particularly ileal and ileocolonic disease.[9] Evidence exists that patients with an *NOD2* polymorphism have a weakened mucosal immune response to bowel flora, which may cause chronic inflammation.[9] Smoking has been the most consistent and most studied environmental factor associated with IBD. Interestingly, the effects of smoking are different between UC and CD, with smokers having a decreased risk of developing UC but an increased risk for CD.[3] Use of nonsteroidal anti-inflammatory drugs (NSAIDs) has been associated with exacerbation of IBD.[10]

Although emotional stress has long been believed to play a role in IBD flares, objective evidence to support this notion remains scant. Debated for decades, the theory of an infectious etiology for IBD remains appealing.[8] Murine models of colitis have shown a decreased development of IBD in a microbefree environment. Repeated exposure of the GI tract to a particular micro-organism may trigger the immune dysregulation evident in this disease. However, some investigators believe that normal intestinal flora may be a catalyst for IBD. As mentioned previously, patients may be genetically predisposed to mucosal immune dysregulation, and either normal flora or bacterial pathogens may trigger the inflammatory response that leads to IBD. At various times, common intestinal organisms such as *Escherichia coli* and unusual bacteria such as *Mycobacterium paratuberculosis* have been investigated as causes of IBD, although no definitive conclusions regarding their etiologic role have been reached.[11]

Pathogenesis

Under normal conditions, the mucosal immune system interacts with luminal antigens and mucosal bacteria on a continuous basis to maintain a state of controlled inflammation. As might be expected, the GI tract is exposed to an extremely high number of antigenic substances daily, and a delicate balance must exist for the system to operate properly. Several immune-specific genes partially determine the type of antigens that will trigger the immune response. In IBD, this immune response is perpetuated and an autoimmune cascade occurs. Thus, proinflammatory cytokines in the gut trigger an "attack" on the colonic mucosa by leukocytes and other factors leading to edema, ulceration, and destruction of the tissue. Normal immune regulators fail to halt this process and the disease progresses. This can be due to a lack of regulatory or suppressor cells, an enhanced numbers of T cells, or both. The T-cell immune response is Th1 dominated, which is manifested by an increased production of interferon and tumor necrosis factor which promotes macrophage activation and development of delayed-type hypersensitivity response. In UC, Th2 response dominates with an increased production of interleukin (supports humoral-mediated immunity).[12] Studies have demonstrated that this increase of proinflammatory cytokines, chemokines, prostaglandin, and reactive oxygen species leads to increased inflammation and tissue destruction.[5]

Clinical Presentation

UC usually presents as shallow, continuous inflammation of the colon ranging from limited forms of proctitis (rectal involvement only) to disease involving the entire colon. Crypt abscesses consisting of accumulations of polymorphonuclear neutrophil (PMN) cells, necrosis of the epithelium, edema, hemorrhage, and surrounding accumulations of chronic inflammatory cells are typical in UC.[13] Fistulas, fissures, abscesses, and small bowel involvement are not present. The inflammation is limited to the mucosa, which presents as friable, granular, and erythematous, with or without ulceration. Most patients with UC experience a chronic, intermittent course of disease. Chronic, loose, bloody stools are the most common symptom of UC.[2,4] Other common complaints include tenesmus (urge to defecate) and abdominal pain. Patients with pancolitis usually have more severe symptoms than those with disease limited to the rectum. Mild UC is defined as fewer than four stools a day, no systemic signs of toxicity, and a normal erythrocyte sedimentation rate (ESR). Moderate disease is characterized by more than four stools a day but minimal evidence of systemic toxicity. Severe disease is defined as more than six bloody stools a day, fever, tachycardia, anemia, and/or an ESR >30.[14,15] Proctitis is usually considered a separate type of UC for treatment purposes. Relapses and remissions are common in UC, with up to 70% of patients with active disease relapsing within 1 year after induction treatment.[16,17]

CD is a chronic, transmural, patchy, granulomatous, inflammatory disease that can involve the entire GI tract, from mouth to anus, with discontinuous ulceration (so-called "skip lesions"), fistula formation, and perianal involvement. The degree of colonic involvement is variable; however, the terminal ileum is most commonly affected. Intestinal involvement is characteristically segmented and can be interrupted by areas of normal tissue. Unlike UC, the severity of the disease does not correlate directly with the extent of bowel involvement. Patients usually present with one of three patterns of disease: predominantly inflammatory, stricturing, or fistulizing. These patterns are the primary determinants of the disease course and the nature of complications.[3] The inflammatory infiltrate is made up of T and B lymphocytes, macrophages, and plasma cells.

The disease course of CD is variable. Years of frequent relapses may be followed by complete remission. Patients with IBD often require surgery to control symptoms. For patients with UC, surgery is often curative. In contrast, in patients with CD, the frequency of recurrent disease after surgery is high and anatomically correlates with the original pattern of the disease.[18]

Table 27-2 Pathophysiological Differences Between Ulcerative Colitis and Crohn's Disease

Characteristic	*Ulcerative Colitis*	*Crohn's Disease*
Incidence (per year)	6–12/100,000	5–7/100,000
Anatomical location	Colon and rectum	Mouth to anus
Distribution	Continuous, diffuse, mucosal	Segmental, focal, transmural, rigid, thick, edematous, and fibrotic
Bowel wall	Shortened, loss of haustral markings, generally not thickened	
Gross rectal bleeding	Common	Infrequent
Crypt abscesses	Common	Infrequent
Fissuring with sinus formation	Absent	Common
Noncaseating granulomas	Absent	Common
Strictures	Absent	Common
Abdominal mass	Absent	Common
Abdominal pain	Infrequent	Common
Toxic megacolon	Occasional	Rare
Bowel carcinoma	Greatly increased	Slightly increased

Adapted from references 1–4, 17, and 18.

Table 27-3 Extraintestinal Complications of Ulcerative Colitis and Crohn's Disease

Manifestation	*Ulcerative Colitis (%)*	*Crohn's Disease (%)*
Acute arthropathy	10–15	15–20
Erythema nodosum	10–15	15
Pyoderma gangrenosum	1–2	1–2
Iritis/uveitis	5–15	5–15
Ankylosing spondylitis	1–3	3–5
Sacroiliitis	9–11	9–11
Primary sclerosing cholangitis	2–7	1
Choledocholithiasis	<1	15–30
Nephrolithiasis	<1	5–10
Amyloidosis	<1	Rare

Reprinted from reference 3, with permission.

Patients usually present with abdominal pain and chronic, often nocturnal, diarrhea.[2,4,18] Weight loss, low-grade fever, and fatigue are also common. Features such as abdominal masses or abscesses and fistula (an abnormal communication between two organs) can make management of CD difficult and often require surgical intervention. Fistulizing disease is particularly difficult to treat and is the source of significant morbidity in CD patients. Enterocutaneous and enterorectal fistula are common, but other types, such as enterovaginal, can occur. Fistula can be excruciatingly painful, can be a source of infection, and can also exert significant psychosocial distress. Other similarities and differences in the pathophysiology of these disease states are outlined in Table 27-2.[2,3,17,18] Extraintestinal manifestations of IBD that can cause significant morbidity include reactive arthritis, uveitis, ankylosing spondylitis, pyoderma gangrenosum, and primary biliary cirrhosis. Although their incidence varies, many of the manifestations of UC and CD are similar, as summarized in Table 27-3.[5,17,18]

A careful patient history, physical examination, and endoscopic and radiologic studies are necessary to determine the severity of IBD. Laboratory studies such as an increased ESR can also aid in the diagnosis, but no single marker is pathognomic. Defining the severity of CD is a difficult, yet important step in successful treatment.[19] Current guidelines from the American College of Gastroenterology define mild-to-moderate CD as ambulatory patients who are able to tolerate oral feeding without signs of systemic toxicity. Moderate-to-severe disease is defined as patients with symptoms of fever, weight loss, abdominal pain, nausea and vomiting, and/or significant anemia. Severe fulminant disease refers to patients with persistent symptoms despite standard induction regimens or those with signs of severe systemic toxicity.[19]

Treatment

When considering IBD therapy, one must appreciate that the cause of the disease is unknown and, therefore, precludes definitive therapy. In addition, specific therapy depends on the anatomical location of the disease. Other factors to take into consideration are coexisting medical conditions, patient perception of quality of life, medication adherence behavior, lifestyle (e.g., smoking), dietary factors, and patient's knowledge of the disease.[4]

With the advent of newer treatments for IBD, aggressive goals of therapy should be considered. These would include (a) complete relief from symptoms (induction and maintenance of remission); (b) improving quality of life; (c) maintaining adequate nutritional status; (d) relieving intestinal inflammation, dysfunction, and the development of cancer; and (e) reducing the need for surgery or chronic corticosteroid use.[20] The ideal medications should be effective, easy to administer with few side effects, and cost effective.[14,15,19]

Most drug therapies for IBD have been tested for both UC and CD (Table 27-4). It is important to differentiate therapy used for acute exacerbations from those used to maintain remission.[14]

Aminosalicylates

Aminosalicylates were the first class of drugs to show benefits in IBD. The prototypical agent is sulfasalazine, which is composed of sulfapyridine (a sulfonamide antibiotic) linked by an azo bond to 5-aminosalicylic acid (5-ASA). The former moiety acts as a carrier to transport 5-ASA past its primary absorption site in the upper intestine. Later, cleavage of the azo bond by lower intestinal bacteria releases 5-ASA (the active moiety) for localized action in the colon. Systemic absorption of the sulfapyridine is responsible for most of the drug's adverse effects, but contributes nothing to the therapeutic benefit.

A significant number of patients discontinue this medication because of dose-dependent adverse effects, including nausea, vomiting, headache, alopecia, and anorexia. Other idiosyncratic adverse effects include hypersensitivity rash, hemolytic anemia, hepatitis, agranulocytosis, pancreatitis, and male infertility. This poor adverse effect profile has led to the development of safer sulfa free compounds that contain only 5-ASA.

Table 27-4 Pharmacotherapy for Inflammatory Bowel Disease

Drug	*Indication*	*Dose*	*Adverse Reactions*	*Comment*
Sulfasalazine	UC: mild-to-moderate maintenance CD: limited role	See Table 27-5	N/V, diarrhea, HA, rash, myelosuppression	High ADR rate has caused use to decline
Mesalamine	UC: mild-to-moderate induction/maintenance CD: limited role	See Table 27-5	N/V, diarrhea, HA, abdominal pain	Topical forms effective for proctitis and distal UC
Olsalazine	As above	See Table 27-5	As above, diarrhea common	
Balsalazide	As above	See Table 27-5	As above	
Corticosteroids	UC: mild-to-severe induction CD: mild-to-severe induction	Various	Hyperglycemia, CNS excitation, immunosuppression, osteoporosis, cataracts	Goal should be avoiding chronic use in UC and CD
Budesonide	UC: limited role CD: mild-to-moderate induction/maintenance	9 mg daily	As above for corticosteroids, probably less short-term effects	Long-term use may still cause chronic corticosteroid ADRs
6-MP/azathioprine	UC: mild-to-severe maintenance CD: mild-to-severe maintenance	6-MP: 0.75–1.5 mg/kg/day Azathioprine: 1.5–2.5 mg/kg/day	N/V, diarrhea, HA, rash, myelosuppression (esp. neutropenia), pancreatitis	
Methotrexate	UC: limited role CD: mild-to-moderate induction/maintenance	25 mg IM/SQ weekly induction dose, then 15 mg weekly for maintenance	N/V, stomatitis, hepatoxicity, pulmonary fibrosis	Usually reserved for patients who have failed 6-MP/azathioprine
Infliximab	UC: moderate-to-severe induction/maintenance CD: moderate-to-severe induction/maintenance (fistulizing disease)	5 mg/kg IV at weeks 0, 2, and 6, then Q 8 weeks thereafter	Infusion reactions (acute and delayed), immunosuppression, reactivation of latent infection (TB, hepatitis B, histoplasmosis), may worsen neuromuscular disease and congestive heart failure	Probable small increase in lymphoma Scheduled treatment preferred to episodic treatment to maintain response and decrease delayed infusion reactions

UC, ulcerative colitis; CD, Crohn's disease; N/V, nausea/vomiting; HA, headache; ADR, adverse drug reaction; CNS, central nervous system; 6-MP, 6-mercaptopurine; IM, intramuscularly; SQ, subcutaneously; IV, intravenously; TB, tuberculosis.
Adapted from refreances 15 and 35.

Techniques to decrease systemic absorption and maximize local delivery of 5-ASA to the lower bowel include creating pH-dependent materials to delay drug dissolution and developing hybrid or dimer molecules of 5-ASA that are activated by gut bacteria (Fig. 27-1). Various synonyms and generic names have been assigned to these 5-ASA derivatives, including aminosalicylate, mesalamine, and mesalazine (in Europe). Up to 90% of sulfasalazine-intolerant patients are able to tolerate these newer agents, and use of sulfasalazine has largely fallen out of favor for the treatment of IBD.[21] Various

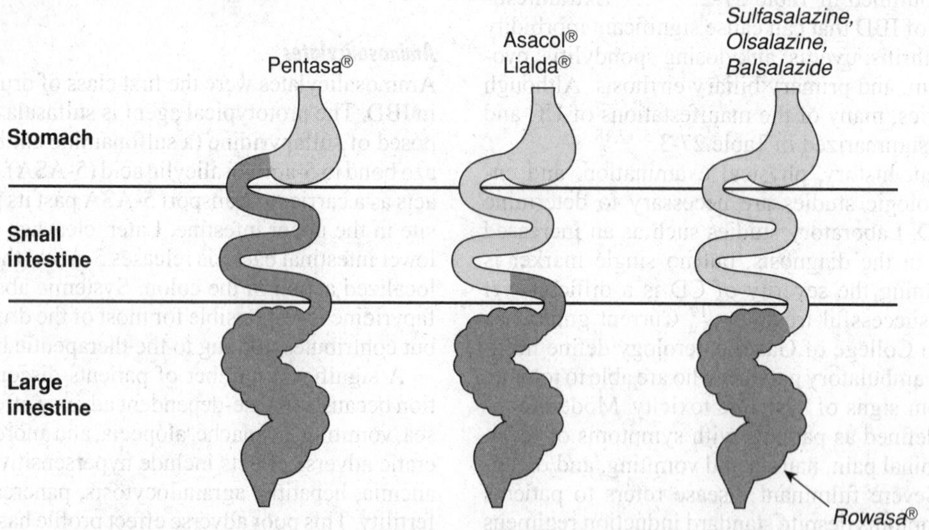

FIGURE 27-1 Sites of action of the 5-ASA compounds. Adapted from Gary Lichtenstein, MD, Professor of Medicine, University of Pennsylvania, Philadelphia.

mesalamine products have been developed for oral or rectal administration. Administration of mesalamine by retention enemas or suppositories is significantly more effective in the treatment of active distal colitis than placebo and at least as effective as sulfasalazine given rectally or orally.[22] Olsalazine consists of two 5-ASA molecules connected by a diazo bond that is cleaved in the gut to release both active moieties. The newest 5-ASA agent to be approved for UC is balsalazide.[23] Similar to olsalazine, balsalazide is a 5-ASA dimer that is cleaved by gut bacteria to its active form. Significant efficacy advantages of any 5-ASA drug over another have not been demonstrated.[23,24] Combination oral and rectal therapy for ulcerative proctitis may be superior to either modality alone.[25] 5-ASA suppositories are indicated for proctitis, whereas enema formulations can be useful in IBD confined to the distal colon. With the exception of abdominal pain, cramps, and discomfort (8.1%), rectally administered mesalamine is well tolerated.[22,26] Enemas or suppositories should be administered in the evening. Mesalamine enemas are significantly more expensive than oral forms of 5-ASA. The oral 5-ASA agents are effective in inducing remission in mild-to-moderate UC and for maintaining remission in UC and perhaps for mild CD confined to the colon. Recent studies, some using newer formulations of 5-ASA, have evaluated the use of higher doses of these drugs for UC. Two trials examined a 6-week course of high-dose (4.8 g daily) Asacol© tablets versus standard-dose therapy (2.4 g daily).[27] A pooled analysis of these trials demonstrated that patients receiving higher doses of 5-ASA were more likely to achieve treatment success than those in the standard-dose group (72% vs. 58%, $p < 0.05$). Adverse effects of the oral 5-ASA compounds include diarrhea (especially with olsalazine), headache, arthralgias, abdominal pain, and nausea. Interstitial nephritis has rarely been reported with chronic use of mesalamine, but the association remains controversial. Cross-reactive allergic reactions to mesalamine in patients with a previous reaction to sulfasalazine have also been documented. An important drug interaction is the possibility of increasing 6-mercaptopurine levels in patients receiving balsalazide.[28]

Corticosteroids

Corticosteroids are the most commonly used agents in the treatment of acute flares in patients with moderate-to-severe IBD.[5,15,19] The anti-inflammatory actions of corticosteroids are well known, but how these translate into their full mechanism of controlling IBD is not completely understood. First-line treatment for moderate-to-severe active UC includes doses of corticosteroid equivalent to 40 to 60 mg of prednisone. Data are insufficient to demonstrate any difference between single versus divided oral doses or continuous versus intermittent bolus intravenous (IV) administration. IV doses should be equivalent to hydrocortisone 300 mg/day or methylprednisolone 40 to 60 mg/day.[15] Although corticosteroids are effective for inducing remission in most cases of IBD, up to 30% of patients may not respond. Corticosteroids are not effective and should be avoided for maintenance therapy of CD and UC.[2,19]

Topical steroids (enemas, foams, and suppositories) are beneficial for distal colitis and can serve as an adjunct in patients with rectal disease that also have more proximal disease and have failed topical 5-ASA therapy.[15,29] Steroids are absorbed to a significant extent from the rectum and, with long-term use, can cause adrenal suppression.[30] Oral enteric-coated budesonide is approved for the treatment of CD. Budesonide possesses a high degree of topical anti-inflammatory activity with low systemic bioavailability.[31] The Entocort EC formulation of budesonide delivers drug primarily to the ileum and ascending colon.[32] It was believed that these factors would make budesonide more effective than traditional corticosteroids, while decreasing systemic side effects. Current data suggest that budesonide may be as effective or slightly less effective than traditional corticosteroids in active CD. Short-term corticosteroid-associated adverse effects may be less than with traditional agents, but adrenal suppression has been detected in study patients receiving budesonide, and its long-term safety profile remains to be determined.[33] The use of budesonide to maintain remission in patients with CD remains uncertain.[34] European guidelines for CD consider budesonide the preferred treatment for mild ileocolonic disease.[35]

Immunomodulators

Azathioprine and 6-mercaptopurine (6-MP) are commonly used for the management of steroid-dependent and quiescent IBD. Azathioprine is converted to 6-MP, which is then metabolized to thioinosinic acid, the active agent that inhibits purine ribonucleotide synthesis and cell proliferation. It also alters the immune response by inhibiting natural killer cell activity and suppressing cytotoxic T-cell function.[30] Azathioprine (2–2.5 mg/kg/day) and 6-MP (1–1.5 mg/kg/day) are used in the treatment of active UC and CD in patients whose conditions have not responded to systemic steroids.[5,15,36] These agents are also used as maintenance therapy for both UC and CD and may be used as "steroid-sparing" agents in patients unable to be weaned from corticosteroids.[37] Because of the long onset of action of 6-MP and azathioprine, many clinicians prefer to induce remission with either corticosteroids or infliximab and use these agents for maintaining remission. Adverse effects of 6-MP/azathioprine include rash, nausea, pancreatitis, and diarrhea. Myelosuppression, especially neutropenia, may have a delayed onset, and clinicians should monitor the complete blood count monthly for the first 3 months of treatment, then every 3 months thereafter.[19] Neutropenia necessitating discontinuation of therapy occurs in approximately 10% of patients. Despite previous concerns, it appears these agents do not increase the risk of developing lymphoma.

Methotrexate (MTX), a folate antagonist, impairs DNA synthesis. It may also reduce interleukin-1 (IL-1) production or induce apoptosis of selected T-cell populations.[26,30] MTX appears to be ineffective for induction or maintenance of UC.[38] However, data suggest that MTX (15–25 mg IM weekly) may have a role for both initial and chronic treatment of CD.[39,40] The onset of effect often takes weeks to months with MTX. Most experts and recent guidelines suggest reserving MTX use for patients with CD intolerant of, or refractory to, 6-MP/azathioprine treatment.[35] Adverse effects with MTX include stomatitis, neutropenia, nausea, hypersensitivity pneumonitis, alopecia, and hepatotoxicity. MTX-induced nausea and stomatitis may be prevented by the addition of folic acid 1 mg PO daily. Some data suggest that even the risk of hepatotoxicity may be ameliorated by folate use.[41]

Cyclosporine (CSA), which selectively inhibits T-cell–mediated responses, has advantages over azathioprine, 6-MP, and MTX because of its more rapid onset of action.[37] Both oral and IV forms have been used to manage severe UC.[42] Due to serious adverse effects, CSA is usually reserved for patients with severe UC refractory to corticosteroids. CSA 4 mg/kg IV daily has been used in severe steroid-refractory UC.[15] A recent randomized controlled trial found equal efficacy (about 85% response) with a 2-mg/kg dose compared to the standard 4-mg/kg dose.[43] The role of CSA therapeutic drug monitoring for this indication has not been firmly established but may be beneficial for toxicity monitoring.[43] The use of CSA for maintenance therapy or nonfistulizing disease is uncertain.

Infliximab

Early research indicating an increase in the amount of tumor necrosis factor-alpha (TNF-α) in the stool of patients with active CD, as well as an increase in the amount of lamina propria cells in the gut, led investigators to target this cytokine for treatment of CD.[44] Infliximab is a recombinant chimeric monoclonal antibody that binds to human TNF-α and neutralizes its biological activity by binding with high affinity to both soluble cell receptors and free TNF-α in the blood. Infliximab is indicated for a broad spectrum of IBD patients. This includes inducing and maintaining remission in patients with moderate-to-severe active CD who have had an inadequate response to conventional treatment.[45,46] It is also effective for healing CD fistula, with data showing that chronic treatment can maintain fistula closure and decrease the need for surgery.[47,48] Most recently, infliximab received an indication for the induction and maintenance of moderate-to-severe UC refractory to other treatment.[49] For all indications, infliximab is given as a 5 mg/kg IV infusion over 2 hours. An induction regimen, administered at 0, 2, and 6 weeks is followed by a maintenance infusion every 8 weeks. Some clinicians will increase the dose to 10 mg/kg in patients experiencing a loss of response. The response to infliximab is usually rapid, often occurring within several days, and can be dramatic in up to 60% of patents. Recent European guidelines for CD outline the importance of this therapy, especially in patients with corticosteroid intolerance or dependence.[35] Because infliximab is a monoclonal antibody, a number of immunologic-mediated adverse effects are associated with therapy. Antibodies to infliximab have been detected in up to 60% of CD patients using the drug,[50] and although a causative relationship remains unclear, patients who develop these antibodies may be at more risk not only for infusion reactions but also for reduced efficacy over time. Immediate infusion-related reactions such as fever, chills, pruritus, urticaria, and (rarely) severe cardiopulmonary symptoms can occur in about 1% of patients. Delayed hypersensitivity reactions resembling serum sickness and severe pulmonary symptoms are rarely reported and are more common in patients receiving episodic (rather than scheduled maintenance) treatment.[51] Use of infliximab with concomitant immunosuppressives, such as azathioprine, decreases the development of these antibodies. Infectious complications, including pneumonia, cellulitis, sepsis, cholecystitis, endophthalmitis, furunculosis, and reactivation of tuberculosis and histoplasmosis, have also been reported in 2% to 6% of patients.[52,53] Tubercular infections, including reactivation of latent disease are a particular concern with infliximab, and patients should be appropriately screened for latent disease before starting infliximab treatment.[54] Patients who have latent tuberculosis (usually identified by a positive tuberculin test) must start antitubercular treatment before use of infliximab can be considered. Patients with active tuberculosis should not receive the drug. Numerous case reports of reactivation of hepatitis B have also been published, and some experts recommend a serum hepatitis screen before therapy with infliximab begins.[55] Lupuslike symptoms, such as arthralgias, have been seen rarely and usually resolve after discontinuation of the drug. Patients with serious active infections, a history of chronic infections, a history of a neural demyelinating disorder, or severe heart failure should avoid infliximab treatment.[52] The latter two cautions are due to previous reports of exacerbations of multiple sclerosis and heart failure when patients with those diseases received anti–TNF-α therapy.

Other Biological Therapies

Success with infliximab in IBD has led scientists to develop and test other biological therapies designed to either block proinflammatory mediators or enhance anti-inflammatory mediators in the gut. Therapies, such as onercept and interleukins-10 and -11, have been examined or are undergoing investigation for CD.[56] To date, three other biologic agents are approved in the United States for the treatment of moderate-to-severe CD: the humanized α4-integrin antibody natalizumab, the fully humanized anti-TNF-α antibody adalimumab, and, most recently, pegylated humanized Fab' fragments against TNF-α (certolizumab pegol). Two randomized controlled trials have found that natalizumab may be beneficial for induction and maintenance of remission in a small subset of patients, but at the increased risk of developing progressive multifocal leukoencephalopathy, a potentially fatal adverse effect.[57] Natalizumab is approved for inducing and maintaining remission in adults with moderate-to-severe CD who have had an inadequate response to or are unable to tolerate conventional therapies. Adalimumab is approved for the treatment of moderate-to-severe CD and may be particularly useful in patients with an attenuated response to infliximab.[58] Clinical studies have suggested a roughly equivalent symptom response between adalimumab and infliximab, and because the former drug is also a potent TNF-α blocker, similar safety concerns and adverse effects have been shown between the two agents.[59–60] Certolizumab contains only the antibody receptor for TNF-α bound to polyethylene glycol to increase its duration in the body. Like the other biologic agents discussed it is effective in both inducing and maintaining remission in CD.[61] Infectious and other adverse effects have been reported in clinical trials that are similar to other TNF-α blockers. The precise place in therapy of the newer biologic agents for CD is controversial. Most experts consider infliximab the biologic agent of first choice with the other agents reserved for a loss/lack of efficacy or adverse effects. Some experts are also advocating the earlier use of these agents in an attempt to forestall or prevent CD complications such as fistula development, but this topic is also controversial.[62]

Antibiotics

Because an infectious etiology has been proposed for IBD, it stands to reason that antibiotics may have some utility.[5,11,14] All studies showing benefit of antibiotics have been in patients with CD; no consistent benefit has been demonstrated for patients with UC.[15,19,63] Metronidazole, which also has immunosuppressive properties, is the best studied antibiotic. It is especially effective in patients with perianal and postoperative CD, with benefits improving as the dosage is increased up to a maximum of 2 g/day.[64] Adverse effects with chronic, high-dose metronidazole include metallic taste and peripheral neuropathy, which is common. The European guidelines for

CD relegate the use of metronidazole to active gut infection, bacterial overgrowth, or perianal CD for a maximum duration of 6 months.[35]

Nutritional Therapies

Nutritional therapies for IBD have been used because dietary intraluminal antigens may stimulate a mucosal immune response.[8] Patients with active CD respond to bowel rest, total parenteral nutrition (TPN), or total enteral nutrition. Bowel rest and TPN are as effective as corticosteroids for inducing remission in patients with active CD in the short term.[65] Enteral nutrition, with elemental or peptide-based preparation, appears to be as efficacious as TPN, without its associated complications. Unfortunately, poor compliance often limits this modality. Neither enteral nor parenteral nutrition is effective treatment for the maintenance of remission.[18] UC is not effectively treated with either TPN or enteral nutrition.

Supportive Therapy

Symptomatic management of IBD is important to the patient's quality of life. This includes pain relief and diarrhea control. Loperamide or diphenoxylate-atropine may be used to treat mild symptoms provided obstruction or toxicity is not evident.[26] Severe worsening of symptoms and abdominal distention may indicate toxic megacolon caused by the inability to empty rapidly produced secretory products of the bowel. Patients should be monitored for iron and vitamin B_{12} deficiencies, especially if ileal involvement is extensive or resection has been performed.

Surgery

Surgery is indicated in the treatment of UC when the patient (a) fails to respond to medical management acutely or chronically, (b) develops uncontrollable drug-related complications, (c) experiences impaired quality of life from the disease or its drug therapy, (d) develops complications of a severe attack (perforation, acute dilation), (e) fails to grow and develop at a normal rate, or (f) develops carcinoma of the rectum or colon.[17] In addition, patients who have had UC for longer than 10 years or who demonstrate premalignant changes on rectal biopsy may be managed surgically as a prophylactic measure against colonic carcinoma.[66]

Generally accepted indications for surgical intervention in patients with CD include failure of medical management, incapacitation because of the disease or its drug therapy, retarded growth and development in children, intestinal obstruction, fistula formation, abscess formation, toxic megacolon, perforation and hemorrhage, and carcinoma.[19] Despite advances in medical treatment of CD, surgical intervention is common in these patients.

ULCERATIVE COLITIS

Pathophysiology and Clinical Presentation

1. C.M., a 25-year-old female college student, has had episodic, watery diarrhea and colicky abdominal pain relieved by defecation for the past 9 months. Eight weeks before admission, the diarrhea increased to 3 to 5 semiformed stools daily. The frequency of the stools gradually increased to 5 to 10 times a day 1 week ago. At that time, C.M. noted bright red blood in the stools. Stool frequency has now increased to 10 to 15 per day, although the volume of each stool is estimated to be only "one-half cupful." She feels a great urgency to defecate, even though the volume is small. She has not traveled outside the United States, has not been camping, and has not taken any antibiotics within the past 6 months.

C.M. complains of anorexia and a 10-lb weight loss over the past 2 months. For the past 4 months, she has had intermittent swelling, warmth, and tenderness of the left knee, which is unassociated with trauma. She denies any skin rashes or any difficulties with her vision. A review of other body systems and social and family history are noncontributory.

C.M. appears to be a slightly anxious and tired young woman of normal body habitus. Her temperature is 100°F; her pulse rate is 100 beats/minute and regular. Physical examination is normal, except for evidence of acute arthritis of the left knee and tenderness of the left lower abdomen to palpation.

Stool examination shows a watery effluent that contains numerous red and white cells with no trophozoites. Stool cultures and an amebiasis indirect hemagglutination test are negative. Other laboratory values include hematocrit (Hct), 32% (normal, 33%–43%); hemoglobin (Hgb), 8.5 g/dL (normal, 12.3–15.3 g/dL); white blood cell (WBC) count, 15,000/mm^3 (normal, 4.4–11.3/mm^3) with 82% PMNs (normal, 50%–70%); ESR, 70 mm/hour (normal, <20 mm/hour); serum albumin, 2.4 g/dL (normal, 3.5–5.0 g/dL); and alanine aminotransferase (ALT), 35 U/mL (normal, 8–20 U/mL).

Sigmoidoscopy showed evidence of granular, edematous, and friable mucosa with continuous ulcerations extending from the anus throughout the colon.

What is the most likely cause of C.M.'s diarrheal illness, and what is the evidence for this? How should the signs and symptoms be managed and monitored?

C.M.'s presentation is typical of a patient with new onset UC. Drug-induced (pseudomembranous colitis) and infectious (parasitic) causes of diarrhea have been ruled out by history (no travel outside the United States, no recent camping, no antibiotic use) and stool examination. As discussed previously, UC is an inflammation of the mucosal layer of the colon and rectum.[17] Characteristically, the inflammation does not extend beyond the submucosa, and transmural ulcers are rare. On examination, the mucosa appears erythematous and is friable. Differentiation from CD is made by sigmoidoscopic and radiologic evidence of continuous distribution of pathology (as opposed to segmental), as well as the anatomical location (confined to colon and rectum).

C.M. presents with the classic triad of UC clinical symptoms: chronic diarrhea, rectal bleeding, and abdominal pain. The diarrhea is secondary to the decreased colonic absorption of water and electrolytes and diminished colonic segmental contractions that normally serve to decrease the flow of bowel content. A good indication of the severity of the patient's disease is the volume of stool passed per day.[15,17] C.M.'s disease would be classified as severe. As the severity of the disease increases, incontinence and nocturnal diarrhea commonly occur. Diarrhea can vary in severity from three to four bowel movements daily to one to two bowel movements per hour. The stools are usually soft, mushy, formed, and often contain small amounts of mucus mixed with blood, although in patients with mild, early involvement, blood and mucus may be totally absent. In addition to the diarrhea, the malabsorption of water and electrolytes causes dehydration, weight loss (as observed in C.M.), and electrolyte disturbances.

C.M.'s rectal bleeding is secondary to colonic mucosal erosions and occurs in most patients with UC.[17] Generally, bright red blood mixed in the stools indicates a colonic origin, whereas blood-streaked stools indicate an anal or rectal origin. The anemia associated with UC is generally secondary to this rectal bleeding. It presents as a hemorrhagic or iron-deficiency anemia, depending on the acuteness of the bleeding. Hemoglobin and hematocrit laboratory values often are decreased as in C.M.'s case. Chronic inflammatory disease–induced hypoalbuminemia is often exacerbated by malnutrition.

C.M.'s abdominal pain and cramping are caused by spasm of the irritated and inflamed colon. This abdominal pain is commonly associated with urgency to defecate. As illustrated by C.M., the pain is usually relieved with defecation, even though the stool volume may be small.

C.M.'s arthritis and elevated liver enzymes (alkaline phosphatase and ALT) are indicative of the extraintestinal manifestations that occur in IBD (Table 27-3). Her nonspecific symptoms (i.e., anorexia, fatigue, weight loss, anxiety, tachycardia) could become profound during an exacerbation of UC.[23] Fever, leukocytosis, and increased ESR are also systemic manifestations of an inflammatory disease. Rehydration is important to assure fluid balance and maintain good renal function.

2. Would it be safe to administer loperamide to C.M.?

Treatment of the diarrhea associated with UC is often difficult. In patients with mild-to-moderate disease, antidiarrheals, such as loperamide or diphenoxylate with atropine, may help minimize chronic diarrhea. Extreme caution must be used, however, especially in patients with severe disease because of the chance of inducing toxic megacolon (see question 13). For this reason, antidiarrheals are best avoided in patients with severe active disease and, if used, should be titrated according to the volume of stool produced. Bulk-forming agents, such as psyllium, may be helpful for patients suffering from constipation caused by ulcerative proctitis.[67]

Remission Induction

Corticosteroids

3. What agents can be used to induce disease remission in C.M.?

Corticosteroids are the most effective agents to induce remission of acute, severe exacerbations of UC.[15] Clinical improvement or remission occurs in 45% to 90% of patients taking 15 to 60 mg/day of prednisone, with an increased response at 40 to 60 mg/day. However, corticosteroids are not beneficial for maintaining remission. One strategy to minimize adverse effects of therapy with corticosteroids includes well-defined tapering regimens. Once improvement has occurred, prednisone is tapered by 5 to 10 mg/week until the dose is 15 to 20 mg/day. The dosage is then tapered by 2.5 to 5 mg/week until the drug is discontinued. Unfortunately, a subset of patients will experience a disease flare if the steroid dosage is decreased or tapered too quickly. IV corticosteroids are an important option, especially in patients who have poor oral intake. Patients with active distal disease can be treated with hydrocortisone enemas; however, 5-ASA topical therapy is as or more effective. Other medications that could be considered for induction of remission would include cyclosporine and infliximab. Due to cost and safety issues with these agents, they should probably be considered only in fulminant disease or in those who have failed corticosteroids.[68]

4. Methylprednisolone at a dosage of 40 mg IV Q 6 hr is ordered. What are the treatment goals for C.M.?

The goal of parenteral corticosteroid therapy for C.M. should be to achieve a rapid therapeutic response as measured by decreased frequency of stools, decreased pain, and decreased fever and heart rate. This goal may be attained with a high initial dose followed by a gradual dosage reduction to minimize the development of corticosteroid adverse reactions. The initial dose, as well as the rate of a subsequent dosage reduction, should be individualized based on the severity of the patient's signs, symptoms, and disease course.

Poorly nourished patients in whom oral intake is expected to be absent for more than 7 days should receive parenteral nutrition, and treatment should be continued until oral feeding is tolerated.[69] An adequate response is defined as resolution of fever, improved patient well-being, no tachycardia, and less abdominal tenderness on palpation. Diarrhea is usually considered to be resolved with four or fewer bowel movements daily. Stools are rarely formed at this stage, but macroscopic bleeding has stopped. Patients can then receive oral prednisone, a 5-ASA drug, and a light diet. If the patient does not respond within 72 hours of starting high-dose corticosteroids, cyclosporine, infliximab, or surgery may be indicated (see question 16). Once C.M.'s symptoms are controlled, the goal should be to switch to oral corticosteroids and discharge her from the hospital.

ORAL ADMINISTRATION

5. C.M. is responding well to methylprednisolone. She is afebrile, her abdominal pain is reduced (to a score of 5 on a 1–10 scale), and her diarrhea is decreasing. When is the oral route of corticosteroid administration indicated in UC? What are the most appropriate dosages?

Oral corticosteroids are effective for the initial treatment of mild-to-moderate acute UC.[26] In addition, they should be substituted for parenteral corticosteroids once a satisfactory initial response of more severe exacerbations has been achieved. In one controlled trial, 40 mg/day of prednisone was significantly more efficacious than 20 mg/day in controlling ambulatory patients with moderately severe acute UC.[30] Prednisone doses of 60 mg/day had no additional therapeutic value, but caused more adverse effects. In addition, a single 40-mg morning dose of prednisone was as effective as and more convenient than an equivalent divided dose (10 mg QID). Therefore, the initial dose of corticosteroid for a patient with moderately severe acute UC is 40 mg of prednisone or its equivalent administered once daily in the morning.

TOPICAL ADMINISTRATION

6. What if C.M.'s UC was limited to the distal colon or rectum? Would topical corticosteroids be indicated? When should other topical agents be used (e.g., 5-ASA)?

Topically administered 5-ASA and corticosteroids, in the form of suppositories, foams, and retention enemas, are effective in the management of acute, mild-to-moderate UC that is limited to the distal colon and rectum.[22,70,71] To justify the use of such a difficult route of administration, a clear-cut advantage of either increased efficacy or decreased side effects over other administration routes for these agents must be demonstrated.

Theoretically, 5-ASA and corticosteroids administered via this topical route provide a higher concentration of drug to the diseased mucosal area, exerting a local anti-inflammatory effect while minimizing systemic side effects. Unfortunately, variable but significant systemic absorption (up to 90%) and adrenal suppression occur from the topical administration of corticosteroid to the rectum and distal colon.[31] Therefore, the beneficial effects produced by topical use of these agents may accrue from both systemic and local effects. The apparent and relatively low incidence of corticosteroid side effects associated with topical administration may be related to the low doses used and to the infrequent administration (daily to twice daily) needed to control mild acute UC. When prednisolone is given in equivalent doses orally and rectally, the incidence of side effects and therapeutic effects are similar.[72]

5-ASA suppositories and enemas are preferred over topical corticosteroids for the treatment of distal UC and proctitis because they produce higher remission rates in proctitis and effectively maintain remission of distal UC.[71,73,74] For distal UC, therapy is initiated with a nightly enema (4 g mesalamine), and the response should be evaluated in 3 to 4 weeks. If remission is attained, therapy can be tapered to one enema every third night. Simultaneous therapy with oral plus topical mesalamine showed greater efficacy than either alone in achieving remission of distal UC.[15,23] Administrating one suppository twice daily for 3 to 6 weeks of 5-ASA is generally sufficient to induce disease remission in patients with mild acute proctitis. Improvement should be seen in 2 to 3 weeks, and therapy should be maintained until complete remission is achieved. Therapy can then be tapered to one suppository or enema, two to three times weekly. If topical corticosteroids are to be used to manage mild, acute UC, the corticosteroid of choice would be the one with the lowest absorptive characteristics. Unfortunately, no trials have compared the absorption characteristics of all corticosteroids available for administration by this route. The available evidence indicates that, of the hydrocortisone salts, the acetate is the least absorbed.[75]

ADVERSE EFFECTS

7. What particular corticosteroid adverse effects are of importance in patients with IBD?

Corticosteroid side effects and precautions for use often limit the therapeutic effectiveness of these agents and should never be overlooked[76] (see Chapter 44, Connective Tissue Disorders: The Clinical Use of Corticosteroids, for a detailed discussion of these effects). Certain glucocorticoid adverse effects are of particular importance in patients with IBD in that they may mimic, mask, or intensify symptoms and complications of this disease. For example, the symptoms of one of the major complications of intestinal perforation, peritonitis, may be masked by corticosteroids. Other deleterious effects of corticosteroids include hyperglycemia, avascular necrosis, cataract formation, and central nervous system effects, including mood disorders, insomnia, psychoses, and euphoria.

Corticosteroids have been noted to mask the clinical signs of abdominal and pelvic abscess in IBD patients, resulting in septic complications. Other corticosteroid adverse effects that may be secondary to either the drug and/or IBD include retardation of growth and development in prepubescent patients, osteoporosis with secondary pathological fractures and spinal column decompression, and hypokalemic alkalosis.[76] Patients with IBD may have decreased bone mineral density, especially with prolonged use of corticosteroids. This is an often overlooked side effect of these drugs. One study suggested that even budesonide, with its low overall bioavailability causes this adverse effect.[77] Thus, calcium, vitamin D supplements, and possibly bisphosphonates (e.g., alendronate 5 mg daily) are recommended to minimize metabolic demineralization in all IBD patients taking corticosteroids for longer than 3 months.[78]

8. C.M. is still responding well to oral prednisone; however, her blood glucose concentrations have ranged from 250 to 450 mg/dL (normal, 70–110 mg/dL). Her physician would like to try another modality for active treatment. What other drugs could be used for remission induction?

Sulfasalazine and 5-ASA

Previously, sulfasalazine was considered the drug of choice in UC exacerbation because of its demonstrated efficacy and reduced toxicity when compared to corticosteroids.[30] However, controlled trials have shown that corticosteroids may act more promptly than sulfasalazine alone for severe acute UC.[5,30] Sulfasalazine use has declined significantly since the availability of better tolerated 5-ASA formulations (Table 27-5). Clinical

Table 27-5 Comparison of Aminosalicylate Compounds

Generic (Trade)	*Delivery System*	*Intestinal Site of Release*	*Usual Dose and Frequency*
Balsalazide (Colazal)	Bacterial cleavage of azo bond	Colon	750 mg PO TID
Mesalamine (Asacol)	pH-dependent coating (Eudragit S) dissolves at pH ≥7	Ileum (distal), colon	800 mg PO TID
Mesalamine (Lialda)	Multi-matrix (pH-sensitive coating and delayed-release)	Ileum (distal), colon	2.4–4.8 g PO QD
Mesalamine (Pentasa)	Controlled-release microspheres	Duodenum, jejunum, ileum, colon	1 g PO QID
Mesalamine (Rowasa)	Direct topical therapy	Rectum (supp) Descending colon/rectum (enema)	500 mg PR QD-BID 4 g/60mL enema PR QHS
Olsalazine (Dipentum)	Bacterial cleavage of azo bond	Colon	500 mg PO BID
Sulfasalazine (Azulfidine)	Bacterial cleavage of azo bond	Colon	Initially 500 mg PO BID; increase to 1g PO TID-QID

BID, twice daily; PO, orally; PR, per rectum; QHS, at bedtime; QID, four times daily; TID, three times daily; supp, suppository

From Fernandez-Becker NQ, Moss AC. Improving delivery of aminosalicylates in ulcerative colitis: effect on patient outcomes. Drugs 2008;68:1089. *Drug Facts and Comparisons* Drug Facts and Comparisons 4.0 [on-line] 2008. Available from Wolters Kluwer Health Inc. Accessed June 17, 2008.

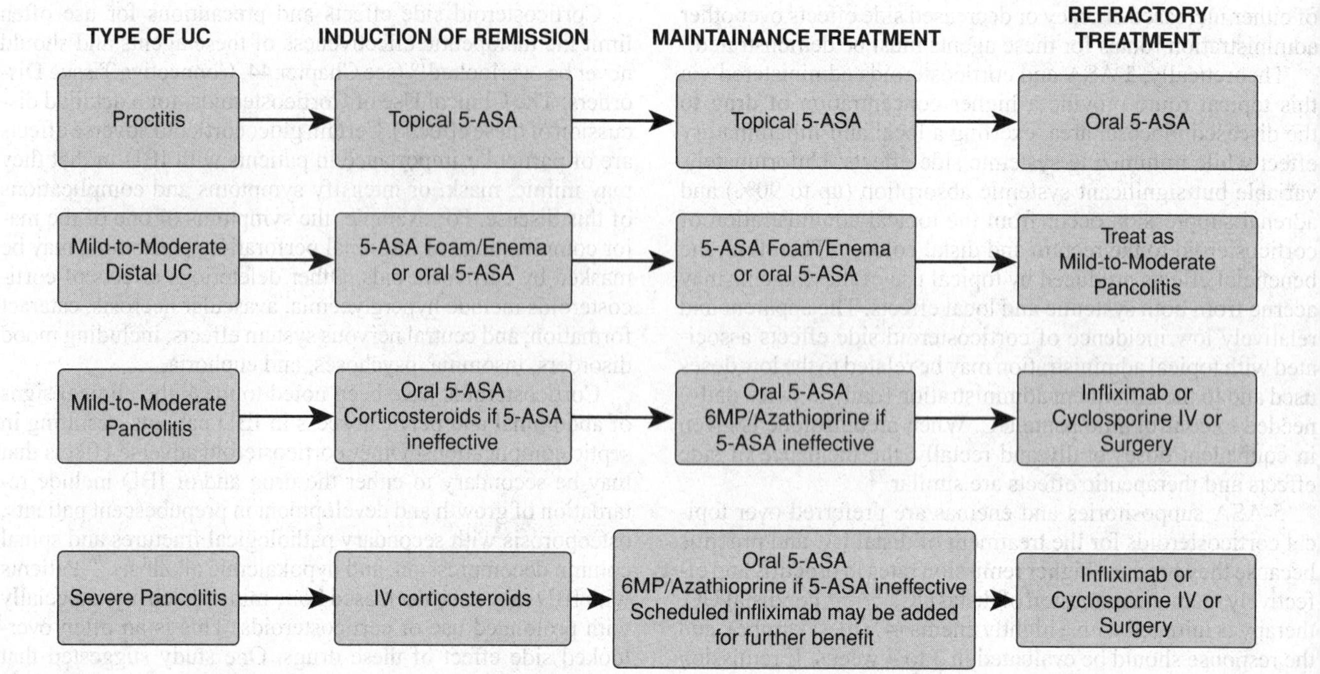

FIGURE 27-2 Treatment algorithm for ulcerative colitis. 5-ASA, mesalamine products, including mesalamine (e.g., Asacol, Pentasa, Rowasa), olsalazine, and balsalazide (see text for selection guidelines); UC, ulcerative colitis; pancolitis, extensive ulcerative colitis; 6MP, 6-mercaptopurine; IV, intravenous. *Source:* Adapted from references 15 and 76.

improvement or remission of mild-to-moderate UC can be attained in 40% to 74% of patients treated with oral 5-ASA in doses ranging from 1.5 to 4.8 g/day with further improved response at dosages >2 g/day.[23,79] For mild-to-moderate proctitis or proctosigmoiditis, topical 5-ASA has been effective in 60% to 89% of patients. Both suppositories (0.5–2 g/day) and enemas (1–4 g/day) have been used.[73] In summary, oral 5-ASA compounds are usually considered first-line therapy for mild-to-moderate exacerbations of UC, with systemic corticosteroids reserved for more severe active UC or milder disease that has failed 5-ASA treatment. Even though sulfasalazine is less expensive than mesalamine compounds, the latter drugs are usually chosen because of their superior tolerability. Figure 27-2 describes a treatment approach to UC.

Remission Maintenance

Mesalamine

9. C.M. feels much better and claims to be "back to normal." Her abdominal pain is gone, and she currently has two formed, nonbloody stools daily. Most of her laboratory parameters have returned to normal (ESR, 25 mm/hour; blood glucose, 80 mg/dL; WBC, 8,000/mm³). She is currently taking mesalamine (Asacol®) 400 mg PO TID. What drug regimen should be used to maintain disease remission in C.M.?

5-ASA agents significantly reduce the incidence of relapse in UC patients who are in remission.[15,23] At 12 months, about 65% to 70% of patients remain relatively symptom free compared to placebo.[80] As discussed previously, the anatomical site of disease is an important consideration in the selection of a 5-ASA preparation. Data also suggest that, if tolerated, a higher dosing strategy has a higher treatment success rate and should be the goal for most patients. In contrast, oral and topical corticosteroids do not prevent relapse of UC once remission has occurred.

On the basis of this information, C.M.'s mesalamine should be titrated to a total dose of 4.8 g in divided doses. If she experiences a relapse, a course of oral corticosteroids may be needed to reachieve remission. Prophylactic therapy should be continued indefinitely unless intolerable adverse effects develop.[26]

ADVERSE EFFECTS

10. C.M.'s mesalamine has been increased to 1,200 mg QID for UC maintenance therapy. Several days after starting this higher dose of mesalamine, C.M. developed anorexia, nausea, and epigastric pain. What is the possible cause of C.M.'s symptoms? How can they be minimized?

C.M. appears to be experiencing adverse effects of mesalamine. Although usually better tolerated than sulfasalazine, unwanted adverse effects occur in 10% to 45% of patients.[30] Most 5-ASA adverse reactions are dose related and tend to occur early in the course of therapy.

Dose-related 5-ASA adverse effects can be minimized by initiating the patient on a low dosage (1–2 g/day) and gradually increasing the amount to tolerated therapeutic levels of 2.4 to 4.8 g/day.[81] If dose-related reactions do occur, the drug should be discontinued until the symptoms subside, then it may be reinstituted at a lower dosage. C.M.'s symptoms are probably dose-related adverse reactions to the mesalamine. The dosage should be decreased, or the drug temporarily withheld. If tolerated, the dosage can be increased slowly as necessary, or she can be switched to another agent to maintain disease remission such as an immunomodulator.

TERATOGENICITY

11. C.M. would like to have a baby. What are the fertility and pregnancy concerns in a patient with IBD? Should she receive 5-ASA maintenance therapy if she becomes pregnant and plans to breast-feed her baby?

Fertility concerns are common in patients with IBD because many of these patients are of child-bearing age. Fertility is generally normal in patients with IBD, with the exception of active CD.[82] In males, fertility may be reduced due to azoospermia if they are using sulfasalazine. Pregnant women with UC tend to have normal outcomes, but some evidence suggests that patients with CD have an increased risk for preterm delivery and babies with lower birth weights. Pregnancy itself does not seem to activate quiescent disease. Because active disease increases the chances of a complicated pregnancy, efforts to control IBD are critical. Increases in congenital defects or newborn toxicity have not been attributed to sulfasalazine or standard-dose mesalamine use during pregnancy.[83] Thus, UC patients being maintained on these agents can be continued on the drug during pregnancy.[84] The supplemental dose of folate recommended for most pregnant women may need to be increased whenever sulfasalazine therapy is prescribed.[81] Little data on olsalazine or balsalazide use in pregnancy exist.

Although sulfasalazine and sulfapyridine do appear in breast milk, the actual concentrations are estimated to be low.[85] In addition, the ability of sulfapyridine and sulfasalazine to displace bilirubin is minimal, which probably explains why the literature has no reports of jaundice in breastfed babies whose mothers take sulfasalazine. Conservatively, it is appropriate to monitor bilirubin concentrations in infants nursing from mothers taking this drug. The American Academy of Pediatrics classifies mesalamine and sulfasalazine as agents that have produced adverse effects in a nursing infant and advises cautious use during breast-feeding because of possible allergic reactions. Thus, C.M. may continue her mesalamine therapy during conception and pregnancy, but she and her providers will have to weigh the risks of potential toxicity versus the benefits of breast-feeding. If C.M. decides to breast-feed, she should carefully monitor the infant for signs of diarrhea.

Other agents may be used in pregnant patients with IBD. Human studies suggest that prednisone and prednisolone are well tolerated and appear to pose a small risk to the fetus in utero. In fact, IBD is more detrimental to the fetus than corticosteroids, thus warranting continued use when necessary during pregnancy.[82] The American Academy of Pediatrics considers prednisone to be compatible with breast-feeding. The studies of metronidazole have arrived at conflicting conclusions. Several studies, case reports, and reviews have described the use of metronidazole as safe for use during pregnancy,[86] whereas others have shown possible associations with malformations.[87] These malformations include, but are not limited to, hydrocele (two cases), congenital dislocated hip (one case), metatarsus varus (one case), mental retardation (one case), and midline facial defects (two cases). The long-term risks from metronidazole exposure have not been fully elucidated. The Centers for Disease Control and Prevention recommends that metronidazole be considered contraindicated during the first trimester. Using the drug for trichomoniasis in the second and third trimesters may be acceptable if other therapies have failed. For other indications, the risk–benefit ratio must be considered.

Immunosuppressants are alternatives for patients with refractory IBD. These agents can cause low fetal birth weight and congenital abnormalities, but they have been used safely in pregnant transplant patients.[82] Due to a paucity of objective information concerning 6-MP/azathioprine use in pregnancy, these agents should only be used if absolutely necessary to maintain quiescent disease activity. Due to possible maternal toxicity, the role of CSA is limited. Methotrexate is contraindicated during pregnancy[86] (see Chapter 46, Obstetric Drug Therapy).

12. C.M.'s dose of mesalamine was decreased to 800 mg BID. After 2 weeks, C.M. continued to have nausea, diarrhea, and headache severe enough to cause her to miss classes and call in sick from her part-time job. What types of therapy should be considered at this point?

Immunosuppressive and Biological Agents

The results of several trials suggest azathioprine and 6-MP are appropriate alternatives for patients with active UC that has not responded to systemic steroids.[15,37] These drugs are also used to maintain remission, although they are probably used more in CD than UC for this purpose (see Question 20).

Infliximab is now approved in the United States for moderate-to-severe UC (both for induction therapy and to maintain remission) that is refractory to other modalities. Due to the cost and adverse effects of the drug, it should probably be reserved for patients with severe symptoms or patients who cannot tolerate other treatments.

CSA has also been used to treat active UC. In one clinical trial, an 82% response rate was achieved using IV CSA 4 mg/kg/day for severe steroid-refractory UC.[88] CSA blood levels should be obtained, although correlation of clinical response and toxicity to blood levels has not been consistent. Many drug interactions and adverse effects are associated with CSA. Hypertension, gingival hyperplasia, hypertrichosis, paresthesias, tremors, headaches, electrolyte disturbances, and nephrotoxicity are common.[26] Studies using oral CSA for maintenance of remission in UC have been disappointing.[42] In C.M., a reasonable choice would be azathioprine 2.5 mg/kg/day. Monthly monitoring of WBC counts and periodic assessment for any signs and symptoms of pancreatitis would be appropriate.

Toxic Megacolon

Signs and Symptoms

13. One year has passed since C.M. last had an acute attack of UC. She has been taking azathioprine 2.5 mg/kg/day. Now she presents with a fever of 104°F, a heart rate of 110 beats/minute, abdominal pain, weakness, and a sudden decrease in frequency of bowel movements. Physical examination discloses abdominal distention with nonlocalized rebound tenderness, tympany, and no bowel sounds. Abnormal laboratory values include a leukocytosis of 15,000 WBC/mm^3 and serum potassium of 3.0 mEq/L (normal, 3.5–5.0 mEq/L). Other laboratory parameters, including serum

amylase and lipase, are within normal limits. Radiographic examination of the abdomen shows the transverse colon dilated to 9 cm. What is the most probable cause of C.M.'s symptoms? What are potential sequelae of this complication of IBD?

C.M.'s signs and symptoms are consistent with an acute dilation of the colon associated with systemic toxemia. This complication of UC, commonly referred to as toxic megacolon, occurs in about 5% of patients at some time during their disease course.[17] Toxic megacolon is also a complication of Crohn's colitis and ileocolitis.

Toxic megacolon represents the most life-threatening complication of IBD and has an overall mortality rate of up to 16% with perforation. It is defined as a severe attack of colitis with total or segmental colonic dilation.[17] A patient is considered toxic if colonic dilation is present with two or more of the following symptoms: temperature >101.5°F, tachycardia with a pulse rate >100 beats/minute, leukocytosis with a WBC count >10,000 cells/mm^3, or hypoalbuminemia with an albumin <3.0 g/dL. Other symptoms include abdominal distention and tenderness, anemia, hypotension, and electrolyte imbalance. Signs and symptoms present in C.M. that are consistent with toxic megacolon include prostration, fever, tachycardia, electrolyte imbalance, abdominal pain and tenderness, leukocytosis, dilation of the colon to a diameter >6 cm, signs of diminished colonic peristalsis as evidenced by decreased stool frequency, and absence of bowel sounds. Other signs consistent with this diagnosis include dehydration, anemia, and hypoalbuminemia.[15] Colonic perforation followed by peritonitis and hemorrhage is the major complication of toxic megacolon. C.M.'s condition should be considered a medical emergency.

PREDISPOSING FACTORS

14. What factors does C.M. have that predispose her to toxic megacolon? What drugs should be avoided in C.M.?

A contributing factor that predisposes C.M. to the development of toxic megacolon is hypokalemia, which decreases bowel wall muscular tone.[17,89] Other predisposing factors include the use of antispasmodics, such as the opiates or anticholinergic agents, and irritant cathartics, such as castor oil, barium enemas, and hypoproteinemia, which produces bowel wall edema.[17,89] Although corticosteroids may be necessary for the treatment of IBD, they may mask signs of peritonitis, a precursor to toxic megacolon.

MEDICAL MANAGEMENT

15. What medical therapeutic modalities should be considered for the treatment of C.M.'s toxic megacolon?

General supportive measures are used to arrest the necrotic process taking place in the colon. C.M.'s bowel should be allowed to rest. Nothing should be taken by mouth, and nasogastric suction should be initiated to prevent passage of swallowed air and fluid into the colon. Fluid and electrolyte imbalances must be addressed, and C.M.'s hypokalemia should be corrected as quickly as safely possible. She should also be given adequate nutritional support, including TPN, if a prolonged recovery is anticipated. High doses of IV corticosteroids should be initiated. C.M. is not currently taking steroids, but if she were, the dose would need to be increased to prevent adrenal insufficiency. A blood sample should be sent for culture and sensitivity, and C.M. should begin empiric antibiotic therapy because she exhibits signs and symptoms of systemic bacteremia and sepsis (e.g., leukocytosis, fever, tachycardia). The antibiotic regimen chosen should include an agent effective against anaerobes and *Enterobacteriaceae* because both types of organisms occur in large numbers in the colon.

Other measures that may be appropriate in patients with toxic megacolon would include discontinuance of any drugs (e.g., opiates, anticholinergic agents) that decrease intestinal peristalsis and might predispose the patient to this condition. C.M. must be monitored carefully for signs of improvement or persistent dilation, perforation, peritonitis, and hemorrhage.

SURGICAL INTERVENTION

16. C.M. has been treated as previously described for 3 days. Nevertheless, her abdominal radiologic examination indicates no diminution in the caliber of the distended bowel, her temperature continues to spike to 103°F with negative blood cultures, and the abdomen remains distended and silent. Fluid and electrolyte imbalances have been restored. How should C.M. be managed at this point?

Within the first 72 hours of therapy and observation, the need for corrective surgery will be determined.[15,89] The three general patterns of response are improvement, no change, and deterioration. Those who improve with medical therapy demonstrate decreased colonic distention, a return of bowel sounds, and a decreased pulse and temperature. Medical management should be continued in these patients as long as they continue to show progress. Unfortunately, only 50% of toxic megacolon patients respond satisfactorily to medical therapy.[17]

C.M.'s course is illustrative of most patients with toxic megacolon who show fluctuating degrees of response to medical management. These patients may appear to respond initially with decreased tachycardia and fever but become toxic again in 2 to 3 days. Despite signs of improvement, change in bowel sounds or a decrease in colonic size may be variable. If these objective parameters do not improve, perforation of the colon may occur unless they are managed surgically (subtotal colectomy and ileostomy). Early surgery reduces the overall mortality rate in patients such as C.M.

17. J.K. is a 49-year-old man who has had UC for 22 years. His disease is fairly well controlled with mesalamine tablets 800 mg PO TID. He has not had any UC flares for more than 5 years. He underwent a colonoscopy 1 week ago for routine cancer screening. Pathology results from this procedure indicate premetaplastic lesions in several areas of his colon. What are C.K.'s medical and surgical options for treatment of these lesions?

Of the various therapeutic modalities available for the management of UC, surgery is the most definitive form of therapy in that it is curative in most instances.[90] Because the lesions in UC are generally localized and continuous, colectomy will remove the primary focus of the disease. It will also eliminate both extraintestinal and local complications of UC in most patients. In addition, patients may require further surgery for anastomotic leaks, intraperitoneal abscesses, adhesions, obstruction, stomal ileitis, and mechanical problems associated with the ileostomy. Patient acceptability of ileostomies is poor, and major psychological adjustments are required of patients and their families.[81] Patients must be given support and educated with regard to the care of their ileostomies; this includes the prevention and management of common skin problems as well as control of odor and leakage of the effluent. Therefore, even though UC can be cured by surgery, it is indicated only after all reasonable nonsurgical forms of therapy have been exhausted. Considering the degree of inflammatory damage that occurs in colonic tissue, it is probably not surprising that the risk for colon cancer is elevated in patients with UC. Interestingly, at least one study has suggested that chronic 5-ASA therapy may be protective against colon cancer.[92] Surveillance colonoscopies are recommended on a regular basis (usually every 1–2 years after the patient has had the disease 10 years) to screen for precancerous lesions.[66] If dysplastic lesions are detected, as they have been in J.K., surgical resection is usually considered the treatment of choice. Thus, even in patients with well-controlled UC, surgery may be required for cancer prevention.

CROHN'S DISEASE

Pathophysiology and Clinical Presentation

18. J.P., a 30-year-old man, was well until 18 days ago when he developed crampy right lower quadrant abdominal pain associated with an increased frequency of semiformed stools (four to five per day). The pain was episodic at first, exacerbated by meals, and somewhat relieved by defecation. During this time, J.P. experienced anorexia and a 15-lb weight loss. He denied any change in vision, joint pain, or the appearance of skin rashes. He has not traveled outside the United States or taken antibiotics recently.

Physical examination is essentially normal, except for soft, loose, watery stools that are streaked with fat and positive for occult blood. The abdomen is tender on palpation of the right lower quadrant. Pertinent laboratory values include Hct, 28% (normal, 39%–49%); Hgb, 9 g/dL (normal, 14.0–17.5 g/dL); WBC count, 14.0 × 10^9/L (normal, 4.4–11.3 × 10^9 /L); and ESR, 60 mm/hour (normal, <20 mm/hour).

Results of sigmoidoscopy and rectal biopsy are negative. Stool cultures and toxin studies for *Clostridium difficile* are negative, as is the examination for signs of trophozoites. A barium enema shows an edematous ileocecal valve and a terminal ileum that has a nodular irregularity of the mucosa. Follow-up endoscopy reveals a cobblestone-appearing terminal ileum with areas of normal tissue separated by diseased mucosa.

Which of J.P.'s signs, symptoms, and laboratory data are consistent with CD? Describe the pathophysiological basis for J.P.'s clinical presentation.

J.P., like most patients with CD, presents with the classic symptom triad of abdominal pain, diarrhea, and weight loss.[18] His most frequent symptom is right lower quadrant abdominal pain, which is secondary to an indolent inflammatory process in the ileocecal area. Diarrhea is also a characteristic symptom; however, in contrast to UC, the stools are usually partly formed, and gross blood is generally not visible. If the disease is limited to the colon, the diarrhea may be of the same quality and quantity as that associated with UC. If the disease is limited to the ileum, as it appears to be with J.P., the diarrhea is generally moderate, with four to six stools daily. If ileal involvement is significant, bile salt malabsorption may occur, resulting in steatorrhea. Weight loss may be pronounced in patients with long-standing CD[2,18] because of anorexia and malabsorption.

Rectal bleeding often occurs in patients with CD, particularly those with colonic involvement, although it is not as common as that associated with UC. Slow blood loss may occur in patients with disease limited to the small intestine, which may cause occult blood-positive feces and, eventually, anemia, as illustrated by J.P. Massive hemorrhage is usually a late complication of CD and is generally due to transmural ulceration and subsequent erosion into a major blood vessel.

J.P.'s leukocytosis and increased ESR demonstrate that, like UC, CD is a systemic disease. Extraintestinal manifestations such as arthritis, liver disease, and skin rash occur in CD with the same frequency as UC (Table 27-3).[3] However, some types of extraintestinal disease appear to be more common in UC (e.g., primary biliary cirrhosis) than CD (e.g., pyoderma gangrenosum).[94]

Most patients with CD have recurrent, symptomatic episodes of pain and diarrhea with gradual progression of their disease to shorter and shorter asymptomatic periods. Although the clinical course is generally progressive, 10% of patients will remain essentially asymptomatic after a few acute episodes.[5] Other patients may only manifest a slight fever for years until a late complication of the disease, such as fistula formation, develops. Alternatively, CD may be rapidly progressive.

Remission Induction

19. What agents can be used to induce a remission of J.P.'s CD?

Because the clinical course of CD varies among patients, the management of this disease must be individualized. The anatomical location of the disease is also an important determinant of therapy. Most investigations evaluating the treatment of acute symptomatic CD have ignored this factor and are therefore difficult to assess or compare.[26]

Corticosteroids

Corticosteroids are the most widely used therapeutic agents for the treatment of active, symptomatic CD.[19,95] A systematic review of the literature confirms that steroids have a valuable role in remission induction.[31] Landmark studies have demonstrated that approximately 60% to 80% of patients with active CD will respond to a course of steroids. These agents seem to be particularly effective in ileal and ileal-colonic disease and can induce remission in even moderate-to-severe CD. Budesonide is recommended in the European CD guidelines for active mild-to-moderate ileocolonic CD.[35]

5-ASA

Although previously used extensively for mild to moderate CD, current trial data and expert opinion have limited the role of 5-ASA drugs to mild active colonic CD. A large meta-analysis comparing 5-ASA (Pentasa) versus placebo found a small and probably clinically insignificant treatment benefit.[96] Some experts still argue in favor of chronic 5-ASA treatment, especially in light of the possible role of these agents in colon cancer protection, as mentioned previously. Recent European guidelines suggest that sulfasalazine is an option only in mild active colonic CD.[35]

Other Induction Agents

The immunomodulators azathioprine, 6-MP, and MTX have onset action of weeks to months and are not usually appropriate therapy alone for treatment of a CD flare. Infliximab is effective as a treatment for both active and quiescent disease. It can be

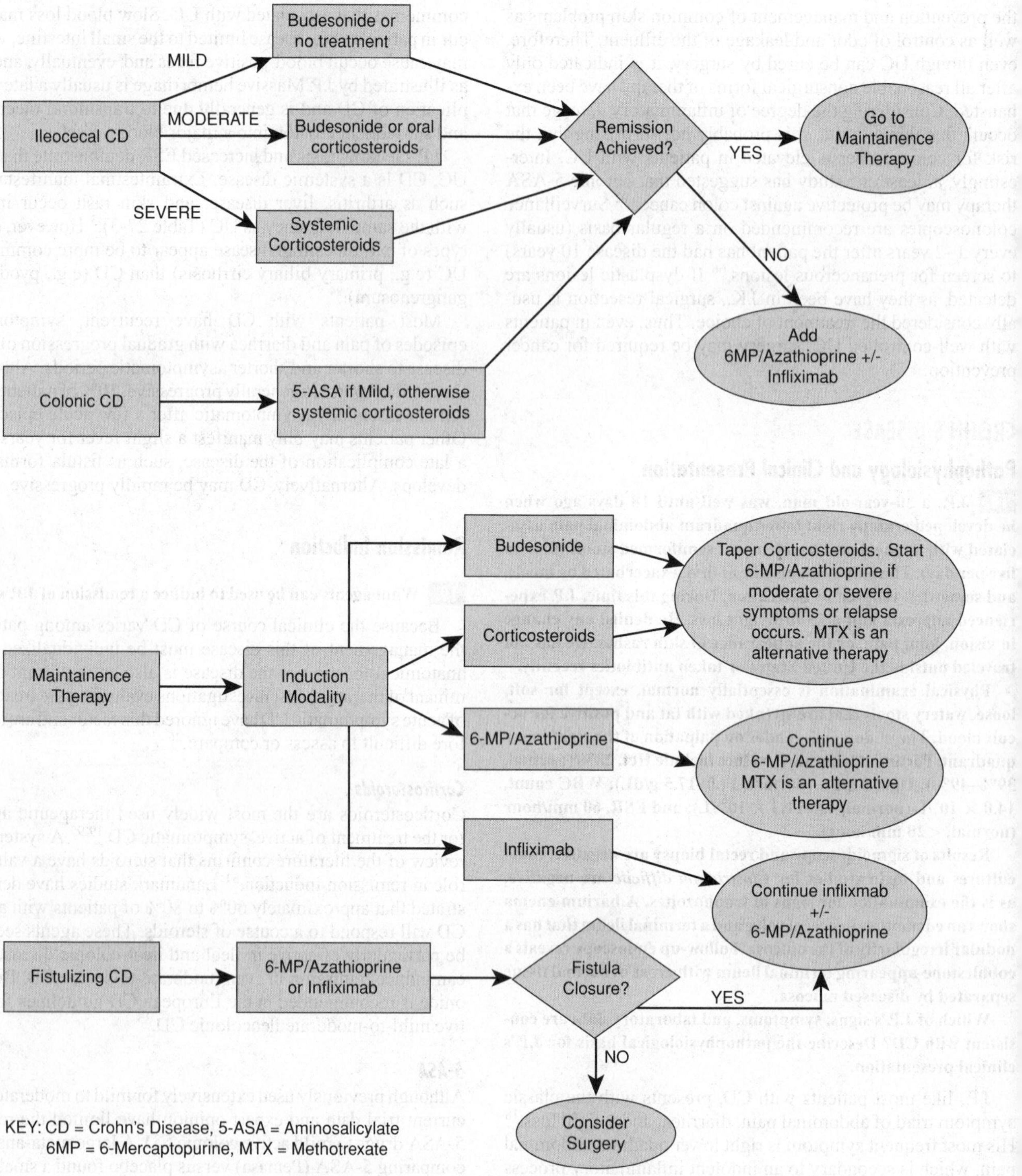

FIGURE 27-3 Treatment algorithm for Crohn's disease.

used alone due to its rapid onset; however, many experts elect to have patients on concomitant immunomodulator therapy, based on the theory that this decreases the development of anti-infliximab antibodies. Due to its expense and concerns of safety, use of infliximab is often reserved for severe disease, as a steroid-sparing strategy, or in patients who do not tolerate other modalities. A treatment algorithm based on guidelines[19,35] for the treatment of CD is depicted in Figure 27-3.

Remission Maintenance

20. After 4 weeks of prednisone 40 mg daily, J.P. experienced fewer symptoms of CD; he has one to two well-formed stools a day, increased appetite and weight, decreased abdominal pain and tenderness, and normal body temperatures. Should prednisone be discontinued? What agents are effective in maintaining remission of symptoms in patients with CD?

Corticosteroids

Once prednisone has induced remission of active symptomatic CD, attempts should be made to taper the drug.[19] The tapering schedule is usually fairly slow (typically, a dose reduction of 5%–10% per week), taking several weeks to months to complete. Several studies have demonstrated that corticosteroids are ineffective in maintaining remission in CD, and many patients continue to have active disease while receiving therapy. However, a significant subset of patients (25%) with CD requires chronic administration of corticosteroids to prevent recurrence of symptoms (termed steroid-dependent CD).[97] Given the poor long-term adverse effect profile of steroids, many clinicians attempt treatment with other modalities to maintain remission.

Sulfasalazine

Large long-term studies have shown that the continued use of sulfasalazine or mesalamine in patients with symptomatic CD is not significantly more effective in preventing recurrence of symptoms than placebo, irrespective of original disease location.[98] An exception to this may be the maintenance of postsurgical CD.[99]

6-Mercaptopurine/Azathioprine

Evidence suggests that both 6-MP and azathioprine have a major role in maintenance treatment of CD.[100] In addition, these agents are often used as a "steroid-sparing" strategy. Recent guidelines recommend the use of 6-MP and azathioprine in most relapsing cases of CD, regardless of anatomical site, and for both severe and steroid-dependant disease.[35] Provided patients are appropriately monitored, these agents are safe with a favorable risk–benefit ratio. Both 6-MP and azathioprine are the first-line immunomodulators used in CD. Should these agents be ineffective or not tolerated, either MTX or infliximab can be used to maintain remission.[22] Some experts believe that infliximab should be used earlier in the course of relapsing disease, especially in patients with fistula.[101]

In summary, J.P.'s prednisone should be tapered as suggested previously and then discontinued if possible. As the tapering regimen is begun, J.P. should start 6-MP 1.5 mg/kg/day or azathioprine 2.5 mg/kg/day. This is due to the long onset of effect for the latter drugs (usually 3–6 months). J.P.'s WBC counts should be monitored regularly and he should be counseled regarding the signs and symptoms of severe infection (e.g., fever, sore throat, or chills) and pancreatitis (e.g., severe epigastric pain and nausea).

ADVERSE EFFECTS

21. Six weeks after starting to taper J.P.'s prednisone dosage (currently, 10 mg/day) and the initiation of azathioprine, he returns to the clinic for routine laboratory monitoring. His WBC count is 1,800/mm^3 with an absolute neutrophil count of 1,100/mm^3. He is afebrile and without complaint. His physical examination is negative for any sign of infection. Why is J.P. experiencing leukopenia? What is the treatment for this side effect?

6-MERCAPTOPURINE/AZATHIOPRINE MONITORING

Azathioprine is a prodrug that is converted to the active moiety, 6-MP, in the liver. 6-MP is then metabolized by xanthine oxidase, hypoxanthine-guanine-phosphoribosyltransferase, or thiopurine-S-methyltransferase (TPMT). Genetic polymorphism determines the extent of TPMT activity. In approximately 90% of whites, TPMT activity is considered high, but the remainder of the population have either intermediate or low TPMT activity.[100] These patients are predisposed to 6-MP/azathioprine myelosuppression because diminished TPMT activity leads to the metabolism of these compounds being shunted to the other enzymatic pathways. Accumulation of the 6-thioguanine byproducts is correlated with leukopenia. Recently, a laboratory test to assess TPMT activity has been developed and found to be effective in guiding therapy with azathioprine or 6-MP, while minimizing the incidence of bone marrow suppression.[102] Some data even suggest that patients with a high TPMT level may be less likely to respond to these drugs.[103] Still, the optimal role for this test remains to be fully determined, and although some experts are screening patients before initiating therapy with azathioprine or 6-MP, routine use cannot be recommended at this time.

In patients who have developed neutropenia from azathioprine therapy, as J.P. has, the primary treatment is to discontinue azathioprine. In most cases, the WBC count will normalize over several days to weeks. In extreme cases, the use of granulocyte colony-stimulating factor may be considered.[104] J.P. should be monitored for signs and symptoms of infection, and the azathioprine should be held. Frequent, probably daily, WBC determinations should be made until the count is above 3,000/mm^3.

Other Agents

22. J.P.'s leukocyte count returns to normal after 2 weeks. Unfortunately, he experiences a flare of his CD symptoms; specifically, an increase in diarrhea and abdominal pain that J.P. has noted over the past 5 days. What other agents should be considered to maintain remission in J.P.?

A number of other immunosuppressive drugs have been examined in CD. Methotrexate produces and maintains remission in patients with refractory disease. Clinical improvement or reduction in corticosteroid dosages have been observed with 15 mg/week oral methotrexate or 25 mg/week of intramuscular or subcutaneous methotrexate in 39% to 54% of patients who had active bowel disease or fistulas.[105] In clinical studies, GI toxicity was the most common reason for discontinuing treatment, but neutropenia and liver enzyme elevations were also reported.[106] European guidelines recommend reserving methotrexate for patients who have failed or are intolerant of 6-MP/azathioprine. Some experts consider MTX to be inferior to 6-MP/azathioprine in CD, but no comparison studies have been published to date.

CSA has a limited role for remission induction treatment in patients with severe, refractory CD. It has no role in maintaining remission.

METRONIDAZOLE

Metronidazole has been advocated for the treatment of active CD, especially that involving fistulas or the perineal area. Earlier controlled trials demonstrated that 800 mg/day of metronidazole is at least as effective as sulfasalazine (3,000 mg/day) in treating active CD and that it was more effective than placebo in patients with disease relapse.[18,107] In contrast to these positive reports, Ambrose and others demonstrated in a prospective, randomized trial that although metronidazole was more effective than placebo in improving symptoms after 2 weeks of therapy (67% vs. 35%) for patients with relapse of their disease, no difference was noted at the end of 4 weeks of therapy.[108] Recent guidelines recommend that antibiotics have little role in the maintenance of remission in CD, but may be helpful in fistulizing disease or in patients with abscesses. Taste disturbances and peripheral neuropathy are the most commonly reported adverse effects associated with metronidazole treatment. The long-held dogma that ethanol causes a disulfiramlike reaction with metronidazole has been questioned.[109]

INFLIXIMAB

23. J.P. has developed an enterocutaneous fistula with his latest disease exacerbation, and nothing is helping him achieve remission. What alternatives exist?

Infliximab is now firmly established as an important therapy in the treatment of CD, especially fistulizing disease. However, a number of concerns regarding this agent must be discussed with the patient before initiation of therapy. It is an expensive therapy (about $15,000/year), and a full pharmacoeconomic analysis of this agent in CD has not yet been published.[110] Infliximab should be considered for moderate-to-severe disease that does not respond to other therapies. Fistulizing disease seems to respond particularly well to infliximab, and its use may avert the need for surgery.[111] Acute and delayed hypersensitivity reactions can occur and are occasionally life threatening. Some clinicians premedicate patients with a combination of diphenhydramine, acetaminophen, or corticosteroids before an infusion; however, the most effective strategy to avoid a serious reaction is to regularly monitor vital signs during infliximab infusion and slow the rate or stop the infusion if any symptoms develop. The majority of reactions consist of headache, flushing, itching, and dizziness, with anaphylactic reactions rarely occurring. It is hypothesized that patients who receive regular infliximab therapy or are taking concomitant immunosuppressive drugs are at a decreased risk for these reactions.[112] Also of concern is the development of human antichimeric antibodies in some patients receiving infliximab.

Infliximab should be avoided in patients who have a serious active infection. Due to reports that infliximab treatment may reactivate tuberculosis, all patients considered for treatment must receive a tuberculin skin test to rule out the disease (see Chapter 61, Tuberculosis). If this test is negative and, because J.P. does not appear to have any other contraindications, he would seem to be an appropriate candidate for infliximab. If latent tuberculosis is found, antitubercular treatment must be initiated before infliximab can be considered.[52] In addition, screening for hepatitis B (and probably C) is reasonable due to the number of cases describing reactivation of these viral infections. Concern that use of infliximab may increase the risk of malignancies is currently under investigation. Studies examining this issue may be difficult to interpret because CD itself may cause an increase in lymphoproliferative cancers.[44] Also, other immunosuppressant agents commonly used for CD (e.g., MTX, CSA) may increase the risk of developing cancer.[37] Current data concerning a link between infliximab use and malignancy are conflicting.[109] To date, the balance of data suggests a small but real risk of developing lymphoma in CD patients using infliximab, but despite this, its use is associated with an increase in quality adjusted years of life.[114–116]

24. J.P. consents to the use of infliximab, and it is successful at keeping him symptom free. However, after 2 years of remission, J.P. is hospitalized for an acute exacerbation of right lower quadrant pain associated with abdominal distention, lack of bowel movements, and vomiting over the past 24 hours. Radiographic studies indicate partial small bowel obstruction at the terminal ileum. Is surgery indicated at this time?

SURGERY IN CROHN'S DISEASE

Because medical therapy of CD is often inadequate, 78% of patients with this disease will require surgery within 20 years of symptom onset.[6] In contrast to UC, surgical removal of the involved bowel in CD is not a definitive form of therapy. CD can recur even after extensive resections.[18] Various investigations have determined that cumulative recurrence rates after surgery for this disease are as high as 80%, depending on the surgical procedure and disease location. Therefore, multiple operations and their attendant risks are often necessary over the life span of the CD patient. Depending on the amount and site of the bowel removed during surgery, specific malabsorption syndromes can occur (e.g., vitamin B_{12} malabsorption with removal of the terminal ileum). If an ileostomy is part of the surgical procedure, the patient will have to undergo significant psychological adjustments. Therefore, surgery is indicated only for specific complications that are unresponsive to medical therapy and should be avoided if possible.[86]

OVERVIEW OF IRRITABLE BOWEL SYNDROME

Irritable bowel syndrome (IBS) is one of the most common chronic disorders causing patients to seek medical treatment. It exerts a significant economic burden and is responsible for considerable morbidity in Western countries. Until recently, little was understood about the pathophysiology or etiology of this disorder. Indeed, some controversy exists today as to whether IBS is a distinct syndrome or a grouping of several chronic GI disorders. Still, investigators have made strides in understanding IBS, particularly the role of the enteric nervous system in the etiology of this disorder. As a result, new pharmacotherapeutic options are emerging for patients suffering from this often bewildering condition.

IBS can be defined as "a functional bowel disorder in which abdominal pain is associated with defecation or a change in bowel habit with features of disordered defecation and distension."[117,118] The incidence of IBS has been reported to be 15% to 20% in Western countries.[119] It is the most common disorder seen by gastroenterologists and is commonly seen by primary care clinicians as well.[120,121] Prevalence rates are dependent on IBS diagnostic criteria, which have varied over the years. A female gender predominance of about 3:1 is evident in most epidemiologic studies of IBS.[122] Some studies have demonstrated a white predominance in IBS, whereas other studies have found no such association.[123] Many patients with IBS never seek medical attention, and those who do tend to see their physician frequently.[124] Many of these patients also suffer from other functional disorders, such as fibromyalgia and interstitial cystitis, and psychiatric disorders, such as major depression and generalized anxiety disorder.[125] As mentioned previously, the economic costs associated with IBS are considerable; it is estimated that IBS accounts for $33 billion in direct and indirect costs in the United States annually.[126]

Pathophysiology

Although knowledge of the cause of IBS remains incomplete, several theories have emerged to explain the underlying pathophysiology of this disorder. Previously, the primary cause of IBS was believed to be psychiatric or psychosomatic. This picture was at least partially validated by the finding that many IBS patients had psychiatric comorbidities. More recently, it is believed that factors such as psychological stress may exacerbate the disease, but they are not the sole cause of IBS.[127] It has long been known that IBS patients tend to exhibit visceral hypersensitivity to colonic stimulation or manipulation. Although concomitant anxiety and hypervigilance undoubtedly played a role in such observations, it is now believed that the reaction to visceral stimuli in these patients results in the perception of abdominal pain, whereas patients without IBS would have no symptoms. The etiology of this hypersensitivity is the focus of intense research efforts. Theories have emerged suggesting that the activation of silent gut nociceptors due to ischemia or infection may lead to increased abdominal pain in IBS.[127] Other experts propose that an increase in the excitability of neurons in the dorsal horn of the spinal cord lead to gut hyperalgesia. An abnormality in the processing of ascending signals from the dorsal horn may be responsible for a lower pain threshold in IBS patients. Similarly, findings suggest that neurotransmitter abnormalities may cause the symptoms of IBS. Of particular interest is the role of serotonin (5-HT) in the etiology of this disorder. Greater than 95% of the body's 5-HT is located in the GI tract and is stored in many cells, such as enterochromaffin cells, neurons, and smooth muscle cells. When released, this 5-HT can trigger both GI smooth muscle contraction and relaxation, as well as mediate GI sensory function.[128] Different 5-HT receptor subtypes may be responsible for these differing actions. A study examining rectal biopsy specimens in patients with IBS found defects in 5-HT signaling, supporting the theory of neurotransmitter abnormalities.[129] The primary 5-HT subtypes in the GI tract are 5-HT_3 and 5-HT_4. Some data suggest that IBS patients may have higher levels of 5-HT in the colon compared with control subjects.[130] Thus, these receptors have become the target of pharmacotherapeutic manipulation for IBS.

Another proposed pathological mechanism of IBS is altered colonic motility. Diarrhea, constipation, and abdominal bloating are common features of IBS. Patients with IBS are often categorized as having either diarrhea-predominant or constipation-predominant disease.[131] About one-half of patients with IBS report increased symptoms postprandially, and patients with diarrhea-predominant IBS (DP-IBS) have been shown to have an exaggerated response to cholecystokinin after eating, leading to increased colonic propulsions.[132] However, constipation-predominant IBS (CP-IBS) patients tend to have fewer colonic propulsions postprandially. Patients in whom bloating is the primary symptom of IBS may have gas production from poor fermentation of carbohydrates.[133] This has led investigators to search for a link between food intolerance and IBS.

Etiology

The pathogenesis of IBS is poorly understood, although consensus theories are emerging. Some investigators believe that inflammation of the GI mucosa associated with infection may be the triggering factor that results in IBS, although this notion is controversial.[134,135] The fact that symptoms associated with IBS can appear in up to 30% of patients who had an episode of bacterial gastroenteritis in the recent past lend credence to an infectious etiology.[136] Also controversial is the possible association of a history of physical or sexual abuse and the development of IBS.[127] Most IBS patients under emotional or psychological stress will report an exacerbation of their symptoms, but this is not surprising considering that such stressors affect non-IBS patients' GI function as well.[135] Familial clustering of IBS patients suggests that both genetics and formative environments may play a role in the pathogenesis of this disorder.[137] Finally, food intolerances (e.g., lactose intolerance) may be involved in the etiology of IBS or may be misdiagnosed as IBS.

Diagnosis

One of the more challenging and frustrating aspects of IBS is its lack of biochemical or physical markers that are pathognomic for the disorder. Thus, the diagnosis of IBS is usually symptom based.[138] Unfortunately, this lack of "objective" criteria for diagnosis can propagate the notion that IBS is a psychological or psychosomatic disorder. Many patients express frustration with the traditional medical establishment and individual providers.[139] In addition, the lack of a definitive marker for diagnosis may lead clinicians to order excessive testing and procedures in patients with suspected IBS. To address these issues, guidelines for the diagnosis and management of IBS have been published in the United States and Canada.[138,140] Both guidelines suggest that extensive testing in IBS patients is usually unnecessary provided that patients are younger than 50 years and do not present with any so-called "alarm symptoms" (Table 27-6). Several symptom-driven criteria have been published, including the recently proposed Rome III criteria (Table 27-7). Both consensus panels agree that once IBS is diagnosed, it should be further differentiated by symptom pattern into DP-IBS, CP-IBS, or pain-predominant IBS (PP-IBS). Because there is no known cure for IBS, it is logical to use these subgroups to help direct symptomatic therapy. In most cases, the primary clinician can successfully manage the IBS patient

Table 27-6 Alarm Symptoms Requiring Gastroenterology Consultation

Weight loss
Gastrointestinal bleeding
Anemia
Fever
Frequent nocturnal symptoms

From reference 137.

Table 27-7 Rome III Criteria—Diagnostic Criteria for Irritable Bowel Syndrome

- More than 3 months of symptoms
- Abdominal pain at least 3 days per month relieved with defecation *and/or* associated with a change of stool consistency or frequency

From Drossman et al. Rome III: The Functional Gastrointestinal Disorders. McLean, VA: Degnon Associates; 2006.

using the treatment algorithm depicted in Figure 27-4. However, the presence of alarm symptoms or an unusual finding on routine examination (e.g., thyroid abnormality) may prompt further referrals and testing.

There are limited data concerning the natural history of IBS.[127] IBS is generally considered a benign disease with a good prognosis.[137] Patients' symptoms often wax and wane, and, in some cases, the syndrome resolves spontaneously.[138]

Management

25. V.H. is a 33-year-old woman who presents with complaints of severe abdominal pain (rated 6 on a scale of 1–10), bloating, and the passage of hard pelletlike stools about every 3 days. This has gone on for about 6 months, and V.H. notices that an "attack" occurs usually after a large meal. Her past medical history is significant for a generalized anxiety disorder. Her current medications include buspirone and YAZ©(drospirenone and ethinyl estradiol). Her immediate family is alive and well, except for a brother with depression. She drinks socially and does not smoke or use illicit drugs. V.H. is concerned that her symptoms are indicative of cancer. How should the clinician respond to V.H.'s concerns?

Patient Education

Clinicians must reassure patients with IBS that their symptoms are real. Furthermore, patients should be thoroughly counseled concerning the prognosis of IBS. Many patients are fearful that their symptoms are indicative of severe pathology such as cancer. Reassurance and education are vital to assuage fears and to reinforce the generally benign nature of this disorder. Involving patients at the earliest stages in their treatment plan is vital for patient acceptance and to avoid "doctor shopping."[124] Helping patients discover triggers that may exacerbate IBS symptoms is an effective strategy for treating the disorder and empowering the patient. This may include having the patient keep a food diary and attending IBS educational classes.[124,133] As noted previously, psychological disorders are present in a large segment of IBS patients. The clinician should again reinforce the notion that IBS is not "all in the patient's head." However, treatment of comorbid disorders, including the discovery of a history of physical or sexual abuse (and possible posttraumatic stress disorder), is an important component in successfully treating IBS.[125,144]

26. After a discussion concerning IBS, V.H. seems less worried. She relates her concern that her dietary habits are responsible for the symptoms she is experiencing. She wonders if changing her diet will "cure" her of IBS. What is the role of diet in the treatment of IBS? Will V.H. be relieved of her IBS symptoms if she changes her diet?

Diet

As mentioned previously, food intolerance may cause symptoms similar to those associated with IBS. Patients with lactose intolerance can experience pain, bloating, and diarrhea after ingesting milk-based products. A dietary and symptom diary may reveal such an intolerance, and avoidance of the implicated foods would constitute effective treatment.[124] Unfortunately, most patients with IBS have difficulty complying with exclusion diets or will not achieve significant relief with them. Patients with CP-IBS may benefit from increased dietary consumption of fiber.[145] Both U.S. and Canadian IBS guidelines state that an increase in dietary fiber (e.g., wheat bran up to 20 g daily) is a reasonable first-line treatment for CP-IBS.[137,140] However, large doses of fiber can lead to abdominal gas and bloating, and overall objective long-term evidence of benefit in IBS is lacking.[146,148]

27. V.H. has gradually increased her dietary fiber over the past 6 weeks. The frequency of her stools has improved slightly, but she often still feels constipated. In addition, new symptoms of abdominal bloating have occurred in the past week. What is a reasonable strategy to treat V.H.'s CP-IBS?

Pharmacotherapy for Constipation-Predominant IBS

In patients with CP-IBS in whom fiber therapy fails, other standard laxatives may be tried for symptomatic relief.[140] Few well-designed trials looking at any laxative for IBS have been published. The Canadian IBS guidelines recommend occasional use of osmotic laxatives such as citrate of magnesia or lactulose. These agents are usually well tolerated, although they can occasionally cause abdominal bloating. Other adverse effects of the osmotic laxatives include diarrhea, taste disturbances, and hypermagnesemia (especially in patients with renal impairment). Some experts believe that newer laxatives containing propylene glycol may be better tolerated, but no data in IBS patients exist to support this.[127] Although laxatives may provide relief of constipation, they will not effectively treat abdominal pain. Thus, other treatments will be required in many patients.

28. Several months have passed since V.H. was first diagnosed with CP-IBS. She has had therapeutic trials of several agents that were either poorly tolerated (poor palatability of propylene glycol) or lacked effectiveness. What other options are available for treating V.H.'s CP-IBS?

Tegaserod

Stimulation of the 5-HT_4 receptor accelerates colonic transit and has been exploited as a target for pharmacotherapy of CP-IBS. The first of these agents, tegaserod, was approved in the United States for women with CP-IBS. Tegaserod is a specific 5-HT_4 partial agonist that has been evaluated in several 12-week trials. These studies evaluated tegaserod 6 mg PO BID versus placebo in women with at least a 3-month history of CP-IBS symptoms.[148,149] The primary outcome measures were patient-assessed global improvement of IBS symptoms and specific improvement in abdominal pain and bloating. The studies demonstrated a modest but significant benefit with tegaserod. Unfortunately post-marketing analysis by the FDA found an increase incidence of heart attack, stroke, and unstable angina in patients receving the drug and in April 2008, the

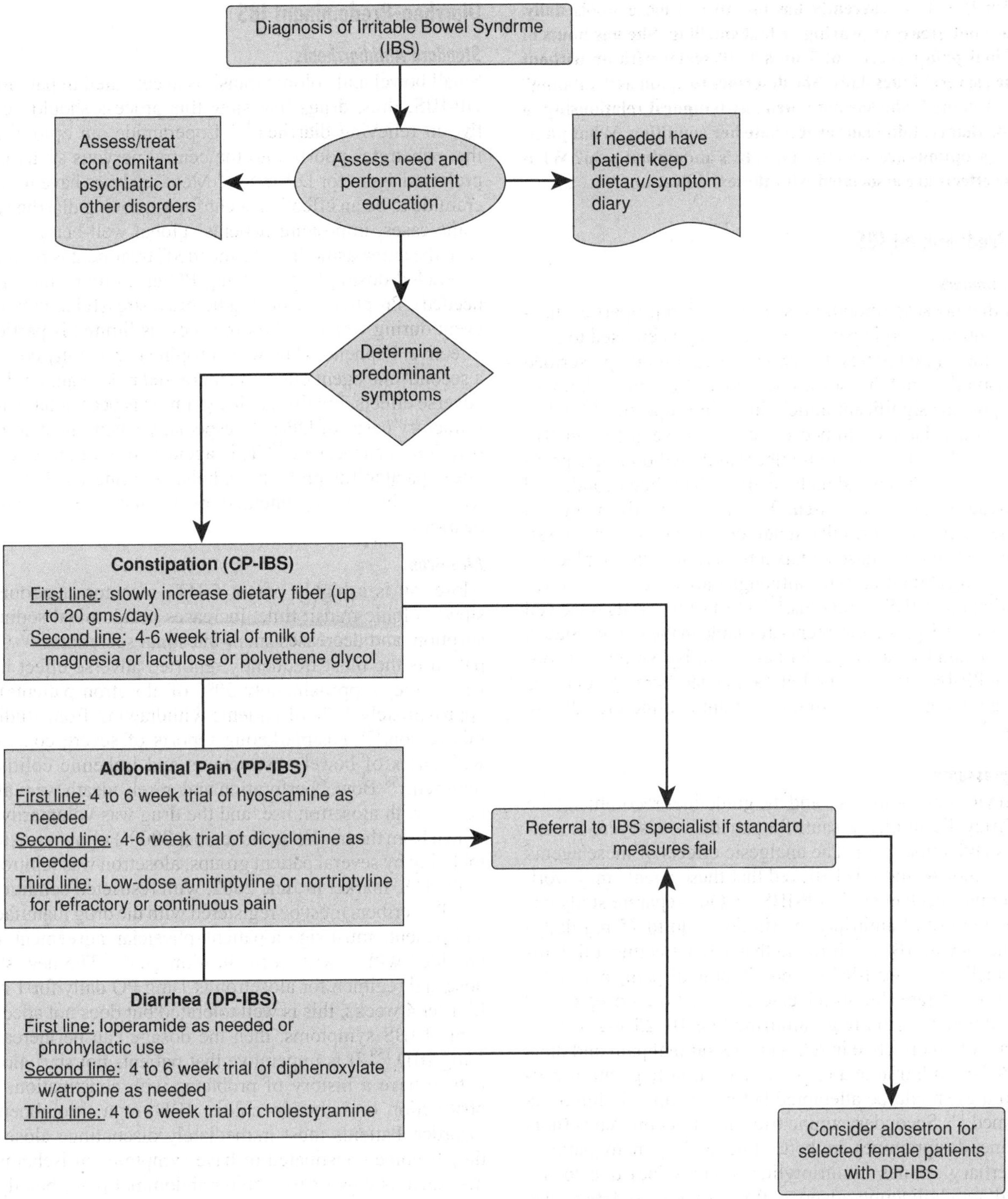

FIGURE 27-4 Treatment algorithm for irritable bowel syndrome. *Source:* Adapted from references 135, 138, and 140.

manufacturer of tegaserod halted all sales and marketing of this agent.[150]

29. **L.K. is a 38-year-old woman who has a long history of abdominal pain and episodic diarrhea. L.K. works as a sales representative for a major software vendor and is called on periodically to make formal presentations. She finds that just before these presentations she develops "attacks" of abdominal pain and diarrhea. Her past medical history is significant for fibromyalgia, which manifests as chronic tiredness and fatigue. She has no other medical problems and takes no medications. She does not drink, smoke, or use illicit drugs. She has undergone an extensive workup, including colonoscopy, upper GI endoscopy with small bowel follow-through, CT abdominal scans, serum electrolytes, thyroid function tests, and stool studies. These procedures and tests were negative, and L.K.'s gastroenterologist has diagnosed**

her with IBS. L.K. currently has one to two loose stools daily. They are not greasy appearing or foul smelling. She has bouts of abdominal pain (severity of 7 on a 1–10 scale) with or without diarrhea several times daily. She describes the pain as "stabbing" and "cramping." She has not noted any temporal relationship to meals or that certain foods exacerbate her condition. What pharmacologic options are available for L.K.'s abdominal pain? What adverse effects are associated with these medications?

Pain-Predominant IBS

Antispasmodics

Drugs that possess smooth muscle relaxation properties, usually by anticholinergic pathways, have long been used to treat IBS. In the United States, the two most commonly prescribed antispasmodics are hyoscyamine and dicyclomine, both of which possess significant anticholinergic properties.[124] Clinical trials that have examined the use of these agents in IBS have been plagued by small numbers and methodologic problems, and recently several meta-analyses have been conducted to provide insight in this area. The most recently published of these analyses had results in agreement with older studies, namely, that smooth muscle relaxants were superior to placebo in improving abdominal pain, although they were less effective at treating other IBS symptoms.[151] Most of the trials reviewed did not use antispasmodic agents available in the United States. Both U.S. and Canadian guidelines list antispasmodics as options for PP-IBS. If prescribed, an "as needed" strategy of use is preferred to continuous dosing due to anticholinergic adverse effects.[135]

Antidepressants

The previous meta-analysis and the guidelines recommend the use of tricyclic antidepressants for patients with severe or continuous abdominal pain. The analgesic effects of these agents are well known, and it is believed that these agents may work by a similar mechanism in PP-IBS.[152] One separate study examined the use of amitriptyline (in doses up to 75 mg daily) for patients with IBS.[153] It found that active treatment did improve feelings of well-being and abdominal pain, but had a large dropout rate due to adverse effects. Low doses of tricyclic antidepressants (e.g., amitriptyline 10–25 mg at bedtime) are often effective in relieving abdominal pain and diarrhea. A 3-month trial at a target dose of drug (e.g., amitriptyline 50 mg) should be attempted before therapeutic failure is confirmed.[135] Secondary amine tricyclic antidepressants (nortriptyline, desipramine) are better tolerated by many patients than tertiary amines (amitriptyline, imipramine) due to decreased anticholinergic adverse effects such as sedation, dry mouth and eyes, urinary retention, and weight gain. The evidence supporting the use of other antidepressants is limited; however, a small controlled study with fluoxetine in CP-IBS (with pain) did show some benefit.[154]

30. Two weeks after L.K. starts nortriptyline 25 mg Q HS, she reports significant relief from both her abdominal pain and fatigue. She reports that she is sleeping better, and she now rates her pain as a 2 on a 1-to-10 scale. Her diarrhea has improved somewhat; however, she still suffers from a "diarrhea attack" before each presentation. What other treatments are available for DP-IBS? What are the risks and benefits of these treatments?

Diarrhea-Predominant IBS

Standard Antidiarrheals

Small bowel and colonic transit is accelerated in patients with DP-IBS; thus, drugs that slow this process should be effective in relieving diarrhea.[135] Loperamide, an opioid agonist that penetrates poorly into the central nervous system, is the preferred agent for DP-IBS.[124] Meta-analyses have found loperamide to be an effective agent for improving diarrhea and, in some cases, improving patients' global well-being.[147,155] As with the antispasmodics, "as-needed" treatment is preferred to scheduled dosing (e.g., 2–4 mg PO up to four times daily as needed). Prophylactic dosing before a stressful situation or an event during which bathroom access is limited is particularly effective. Diphenoxylate with atropine is generally considered a second-line agent due to its increased risk of anticholinergic adverse effects. Finally, cholestyramine is occasionally used in refractory cases of DP-IBS, especially when bile acid malabsorption is suspected.[156] This agent is often poorly tolerated due to palatability problems. Cholestyramine also has a significant number of drug interactions of which the clinician must be aware.

Alosetron

Alosetron is a highly potent 5-HT_3 receptor antagonist that slows colonic transit time, increases intraluminal sodium absorption, and decreases small intestinal secretions.[157] Constipation is the most frequently reported adverse effect in clinical studies (approximately 30% of alosetron patients), with approximately 10% of patients withdrawing from studies for this reason.[157] Postmarketing reports of severe constipation with cases of bowel obstructions and ischemic colitis were reported.[158] Bowel perforation and, rarely, death were also reported with alosetron use, and the drug was voluntarily withdrawn from the market in November 2000. Following extensive lobbying by several patient groups, alosetron was reintroduced to the U.S. market in June 2002, with restricted conditions for use. Prescribers must be registered with the drug manufacturer, and patients must sign a patient–physician agreement and be provided with a written medication guide. The new starting dose and regimen for alosetron is 1 mg PO daily for 1 month. If, after 4 weeks, this is well tolerated but does not adequately control IBS symptoms, then the dosage can be increased to 1 mg BID.[159] It is imperative that patients not start alosetron if they have a history of problems with constipation, bowel obstruction or ischemic colitis, IBD, or a thromboembolic disorder. Patients must immediately discontinue alosetron if they become constipated or have symptoms of ischemic colitis, such as new or worsening abdominal pain, bloody diarrhea, or blood in the stool. A recent review of the mandatory postmarketing surveillance system designed to monitor the safety of the drug found an overall low rate of ischemic colitis.[160]

Emerging Therapies

Currently, numerous agents are being investigated for all types of IBS.[161] Several serotonergic agonists and antagonists, including cilansetron and renzapride, have shown some efficacy in small trials and are undergoing further examination. Alvimopan, a peripheral μ-opioid antagonist designed for opioid-induced constipation may have utility in CP-IBS;

however, formal studies are needed to delineate its role. The possible association of bacterial GI infection and IBS have prompted some investigators to postulate that small bowel flora overgrowth may be responsible for the symptoms of IBS.[162] The nonabsorbable antibiotic rifaximin (indicated for treatment of traveler's diarrhea) was shown in a small study to improve global symptoms in IBS for up to 10 weeks, so further study of this modality is warranted.[163] Probiotic agents such as *Lactobacillus plantarum and Bifidobacterium infantis,* which may alter colonic inflammation, have shown some efficacy in a small study.[164] Most recently lubiprostone, a gastrointestinal chloride channel activator that enhances intestinal fluid secretion and acts as a laxative, was approved in the United States for CP-IBS in women over age 18. Published data to date suggest that 8 mcg orally twice daily is effective in improving constipation and abdominal pain in CP-IBS, but nausea and diarrhea are limiting adverse effects.[162] Lubiprostone's role in CP-IBS is yet to be fully defined.

REFERENCES

1. Papadakis KA, Targan SR. Current theories on the causes of inflammatory bowel disease. *Gastroenterol Clin North Am* 1999;28:283.
2. Botoman VA et al. Management of inflammatory bowel disease. *Am Fam Physician* 1998;57:57.
3. Andres PG, Friedman S. Epidemiology and the natural course of inflammatory bowel disease. *Gastroenterol Clin North Am* 1999;28:255.
4. Bickston SJ, Cominelli F. Inflammatory bowel disease: short and long-term treatments. In: Schrier RW et al., eds. *Advances in Internal Medicine.* St. Louis, MO: Mosby; 1998:143.
5. Podolsky DK. Inflammatory bowel disease. *N Engl J Med* 2002;347:417.
6. Loftus EV et al. The epidemiology and natural history of Crohn's disease in population-based patient cohorts from North America: a systematic review. *Aliment Pharmacol Ther* 2002;16:51.
7. Pardi DS et al. Treatment of inflammatory bowel disease in the elderly: an update. *Drugs Aging* 2002;19:355.
8. Fiocchi C. Inflammatory bowel disease: etiology and pathogenesis. *Gastroenterology* 1998;115:182.
9. Marks DJ et al. Defective acute inflammation in Crohn's disease: a clinical investigation. *Lancet* 2006;367:668.
10. Evans JM et al. Non-steroidal anti-inflammatories are associated with emergence admission to hospital for colitis due to inflammatory bowel disease. *Gut* 1997;40:619.
11. Swidsinski A et al. Mucosal flora in inflammatory bowel disease. *Gastroenterology* 2002;122:44.
12. Targan SR et al. Immunologic mechanisms intestinal diseases. *Ann Intern Med* 1987;106:853.
13. Konstantinos A et al. Current theories on the causes of inflammatory bowel disease. *Gastroenterol Clin North Am* 1999;28:283.
14. Carter MJ et al. Guidelines for the management of inflammatory bowel disease in adults. *Gut* 2004;53(Suppl 5):V1.
15. Kornbluth A, Sachar DB. Ulcerative colitis practice guidelines in adults (update): American College of Gastroenterology Practice Parameters Committee. *Am J Gastroenterol* 2004;99:1371.
16. Langholtz E et al. Incidence and prevalence of ulcerative colitis in Copenhagen County from 1962–1987. *Scand J Gastroenterol* 1991;26:1247.
17. Jewell DP. Ulcerative colitis. In: Feldman M et al., eds. *Gastrointestinal and Liver Disease.* 6th ed. Philadelphia: WB Saunders; 1998:1735.
18. Kornbluth A et al. Crohn's disease. In: Feldman M et al., eds. *Gastrointestinal and Liver Disease.* 6th ed. Philadelphia: WB Saunders; 1998:1708.
19. Hanauer SB, Sandborn W. Management of Crohn's disease in adults. *Am J Gastroenterol* 2001;96:635.
20. Sandborn WJ. What's new: innovative concepts in inflammatory bowel disease. *Colorectal Dis* 2006;8(Suppl 1):3(9.
21. Collins P, Rhodes J. Ulcerative colitis: diagnosis and management. *BMJ* 2006;333:340.
22. Bitton A. Medical management of ulcerative proctitis, proctosigmoiditis, and left-sided colitis. *Semin Gastrointest Dis* 2001;12:263.
23. Katz S. Update in medical therapy of ulcerative colitis. *J Clin Gastroenterol* 2002;34:397.
24. Greeen JEB et al. Balsalazide is more effective and better tolerated than mesalamine in ulcerative colitis. *Gastroenterology* 1998;114:15.
25. Safdi M et al. A double-blind comparison of oral versus rectal mesalamine versus combination therapy in the treatment of distal ulcerative colitis. *Am J Gastroenterol* 1997;92:1867.
26. Stein RB, Hanauer SB. Medical therapy for inflammatory bowel disease. *Gastroenterol Clin North Am* 1999;2:297.
27. Hanauer SB et al. Delayed-release oral mesalamine 4.8 g/day (800 mg tablet) versus 2.4 g/day (400 mg tablet) for treatment of moderately active ulcerative colitis: combined analysis of two randomized, double-blind, controlled trials. *Gastroenterology* 2005;125:A74.
28. Lowry PW et al. Balsalazide and azathioprine or 6-mercaptopurine: evidence for a potentially serious drug interaction. *Gastroenterology* 1999;116:1505.
29. Marshall JK, Irvine EJ. Rectal corticosteroids versus alternative treatments in ulcerative colitis: a meta-analysis. *Gut* 1997;40:775.
30. Hanauer SB et al. The pharmacology of anti-inflammatory drugs in inflammatory bowel disease. In: Kirsner JB, Shorter RP, eds. *Inflammatory Bowel Disease.* Baltimore: Williams & Wilkins; 1995:643.
31. Sang YX, Lichtenstein GR. Corticosteroids in Crohn's disease. *Am J Gastroenterol* 2002;97:803.
32. Entocort product information, AstraZeneca, Inc., Sodertalje, Sweden, 2005.
33. Rutgeerts P et al. A comparison of budesonide with prednisolone for active Crohn's disease. *N Engl J Med* 1994;331:842.
34. Sandborn WJ et al. Budesonide for maintenance of remission in patients with Crohn's disease in medically induced remission: a predetermined pooled analysis of four randomized, double-blind, placebo-controlled trials. *Am J Gastroenterol* 2005;100:1780.
35. Travis SPL et al. European evidence based consensus on the diagnosis and management of Crohn's disease: current management. *Gut* 2006;55(Suppl 1):i16.
36. Hanauer SB. Drug therapy: inflammatory bowel disease. *N Engl J Med* 1996;334:841.
37. Sandborn WJ. A review of immune modifier therapy for inflammatory bowel disease: azathioprine, 6-mercaptopurine, cyclosporin and methotrexate. *Am J Gastroenterol* 1996;91:423.
38. Oren R et al. Methotrexate in ulcerative colitis: a double blind, randomized Israeli multicenter trial. *Gastroenterology* 1996;110:1416.
39. Feagen BG et al. Methotrexate for the treatment of Crohn's disease. *N Engl J Med* 1995;332:292.
40. Feagan BG et al. A comparison of methotrexate with placebo for the maintenance of remission in Crohn's disease. *N Engl J Med* 2000;342:1627.
41. van Ede AE et al. Effect of folic or folinic acid supplementation on the toxicity and efficacy of methotrexate in rheumatoid arthritis: a forty-eight week, multicenter, randomized, double-blind, placebo-controlled study. *Arthritis Rheum* 2001;44:1515.
42. Farrell RJ, Peppercorn MA. Ulcerative colitis. *Lancet* 2002;359:331.
43. Van Assche G et al. Randomized, double-blind comparison of 4 mg/kg versus 2 mg/kg intravenous cyclosporine in severe ulcerative colitis. *Gastroenterology* 2003;125:1025.
44. Blam ME et al. Integrating anti-tumor necrosis factor therapy in inflammatory bowel disease: current and future perspectives. *Am J Gastroenterol* 2001;96:1977.
45. Targan SR et al. A short-term study of chimeric monoclonal antibody cA2 to tumor necrosis factor alpha for Crohn's disease. *N Engl J Med* 1997;337:1145.
46. Hanauer SB et al. Maintenance infliximab for Crohn's disease: the ACCENT I randomised trial. *Lancet* 2002;359:1541.
47. Sands BE et al. Infliximab maintenance therapy for fistulizing Crohn's disease. *N Engl J Med* 2004;350:876.
48. Lichtenstein GR et al. Infliximab maintenance treatment reduces hospitalizations, surgeries, and procedures in fistulizing Crohn's disease. *Gastroenterology* 2005;128:862.
49. Rutgeerts P et al. Infliximab for induction and maintenance therapy for ulcerative colitis. *N Engl J Med* 2005;353:2462.
50. Baert F et al. Influence of immunogenicity on the long term efficacy of infliximab in Crohn's disease. *N Engl J Med* 2003;348:601.
51. Riegart-Johnson DL et al. Delayed hypersensitivity reaction and acute respiratory distress syndrome following infliximab infusion. *Inflamm Bowel Dis* 2002;8:186.
52. Remecade package insert, Centocor, Inc., Malvern, PA, April 2007.
53. Keane J et al. Tuberculosis associated with infliximab a tumor necrosis factor alpha-neutralizing agent. *N Engl J Med* 2001;345:1098.
54. Van Assche GV. Safety issues with biological therapies for inflammatory bowel disease. *Curr Opin Gastroenterol* 2006;22:370.
55. Esteve M et al. Chronic hepatitis B reactivation following infliximab therapy in Crohn's disease patients: need for primary prophylaxis. *Gut* 2004;53:1363.
56. Wilhelm SM et al. Novel therapies for Crohn's disease: focus on immunomodulators and antibiotics. *Ann Pharmacother* 2006;40:1804.
57. Sandborn WJ et al. Natalizumab induction and maintenance therapy for Crohn's disease. *N Engl J Med* 2005;353:1912.
58. Papadakis KA et al. Safety and efficacy of adalimumab (D2E7) in Crohn's disease patients with an attenuated response to infliximab. *Am J Gastroenterol* 2005;100:75.
59. Sandborn WJ et al. Adalimumab for maintenance treatment of Crohn's disease: results of the CLASSIC II trial. *Gut.* 2007;56:1232.
60. Ho GT et al. The use of adalimumab in the management of refractory Crohn's disease. *Aliment Pharmacol Ther.* 2008;27:308.
61. Schreiber S et al. Maintenance therapy with certolizumab pegol for Crohn's disease. *N Engl J Med.* 2007;357:239.

62. Velayos FS, Sandborn WJ. Positioning biologic therapy for Crohn's disease and ulcerative colitis. *Curr Gastroenterol Rep.* 2007;9:521.
63. Turunen U et al. A double-blind, placebo controlled six-month trial of ciprofloxacin treatment improved prognosis in UC. *Gastroenterology* 1994;106:A786.
64. Achkar JP, Hanauer SB. Medical therapy to reduce postoperative Crohn's disease recurrence. *Am J Gastroenterol* 2000;95:1139.
65. O'Keefe SJ, Rooser BG. Nutrition and inflammatory bowel disease. In: Targan SR, Shanahan F, eds. *Inflammatory Bowel Disease: From Bench to Bedside.* Baltimore: Williams & Wilkins; 1994: 461.
66. Eaden JA, Mayberry JF. Colorectal cancer complicating ulcerative colitis: a review. *Am J Gastroenterol* 2000; 95:2710.
67. Myers S. Medical management and prognosis. In: Haubrich W, Schaffner F, eds. *Gastroenterology.* Philadelphia: WB Saunders; 1995:1498.
68. Bocker U. Infliximab in ulcerative colitis. *Scand J Gastroenterol* 2006;41:997.
69. Aspen Board of Directors and the Clinical Guidelines Task Force. Guidelines for the use of parenteral and enteral nutrition in adult and pediatric patients. *JPEN* 2002;26(1 Suppl):1SA.
70. Marshall JK, Irvine EJ. Topical aminosalicylate (ASA) therapy for distal ulcerative colitis: a meta-analysis. *Gastroenterology* 1994;106:A1037.
71. Marshall JK, Irvine EJ. Rectal corticosteroids versus alternative treatments in UC: a meta-analysis. *Gut* 1997;40:775.
72. Peppercorn MA. Advances in drug therapy for inflammatory bowel disease. *Ann Intern Med* 1990;112:50.
73. Marshall JK, Irvine EJ. Putting rectal 5-aminosalicylic acid in its place: the role in distal ulcerative colitis. *Am J Gastroenterol* 2000;95:1628.
74. Hanauer SB. Dose-ranging study of mesalamine (Pentasa) enemas in the treatment of acute ulcerative proctosigmoiditis: results of a multi-centered placebo-controlled trial. The US Pentasa Enema Study Group. *Inflamm Bowel Dis* 1998;4:79.
75. Lima JJ et al. Bioavailability of hydrocortisone retention enemas in normal subjects. *Am J Gastroenterol* 1980;73:232.
76. Ardizzone S, Porro GB. Comparative tolerability of therapies for ulcerative colitis. *Drug Saf* 2002;25:561.
77. Cino M, Greenberg GR. Bone mineral density in Crohn's disease: a longitudinal study of budesonide, prednisone and non-steroid therapy. *Am J Gastroenterol* 2002;97:915.
78. Anonymous. Recommendations for the prevention and treatment of glucocorticoid-induced osteoporosis: 2001 update. *Arthritis Rheum* 2001;44:1496.
79. Hanauer S et al. Mesalamine capsules for treatment of active ulcerative colitis. *Am J Gastroenterol* 1993;88:1188.
80. Nayar M, Rhodes JM. Management of inflammatory bowel disease. *Postgrad Med J* 2004;80:206.
81. Kastrup EK, ed. Sulfasalazine. In: *Drug Facts and Comparisons.* St. Louis, MO: Facts and Comparisons; 2000:1162.
82. Alstead EM. Inflammatory bowel disease in pregnancy. *Postgrad Med J* 2002;78:23.
83. Diav-Citrin O. The safety of mesalazine in human pregnancy: a prospective controlled cohort study. *Gastroenterology* 1998;114:23.
84. Hanan IM. Inflammatory bowel disease in the pregnant woman. *Comp Ther* 1998;24(9):409.
85. Briggs GG et al., eds. Sulfasalazine. In: *Drugs in Pregnancy and Lactation.* 7th ed. Baltimore: Williams & Wilkins; 2005:1506.
86. Korelitz BI. Inflammatory bowel disease and pregnancy. *Gastroenterol Clin North Am* 1998;27:213.
87. Briggs GG et al., eds. Metronidazole. In: *Drugs in Pregnancy and Lactation.* 7th Ed. Baltimore: Williams & Wilkins; 2005:1066.
88. Lichtiger S et al. Cyclosporin in severe ulcerative colitis refractory to steroid therapy. *N Engl J Med* 1994;330:1841.
89. Berg DF et al. Acute surgical emergencies in inflammatory bowel disease. *Am J Surg* 2002;184:45.
90. Becker JM. Surgical therapy for ulcerative colitis and Crohn's disease. *Gastroenterol Clin North Am* 1999;28:371.
91. Robb B, Pritts T. Quality of life in patients undergoing ileal pouch-anal anastomosis at the University of Cincinnati. *Am J Surg* 2002;183:353.
92. Eaden J et al. Colorectal cancer prevention in ulcerative colitis: a case-control study. *Aliment Pharmacol Ther* 2000;14:145.
93. Cho JH. The *Nod2* gene in Crohn's disease: implications for future research into the genetics and immunology of Crohn's disease. *Inflamm Bowel Dis* 2001;7:271.
94. Gasche C. Complications of inflammatory bowel disease. *Hepatogastroenterology* 2000;47:49.
95. Saloman P et al. How effective are current drugs for Crohn's disease? A meta-analysis. *J Clin Gastroenterol* 1992;14:211.
96. Hanauer SB, Stromberg U. Oral Pentasa in the treatment of active Crohn's disease: a meta-analysis of double-blind, placebo-controlled trials. *Clin Gastroenterol Hepatol* 2004;2:379.
97. Faubion WA et al. The natural history of corticosteroid therapy for inflammatory bowel disease: a population-based study. *Gastroenterology* 2001;121:255.
98. Gisbert JP et al. Role of 5-aminosalicylic acid (5-ASA) in treatment of inflammatory bowel disease: a systematic review. *Dig Dis Sci* 2002;47:471.
99. Achkar JP, Hanauer SB. Medical therapy to reduce postoperative Crohn's disease recurrence. *Am J Gastroenterol* 2000;95:1139.
100. Nielsen OH et al. Review article: the treatment of inflammatory bowel disease with 6-mercaptopurine or azathioprine. *Aliment Pharmacol Ther* 2001;15:1699.
101. Travis SPL. Infliximab and azathioprine: bridge or parachute? *Gastroenterology* 2006;130:1354.
102. Cuffari et al. Use of erythrocyte 6-thioguanine metabolite levels to optimize azathioprine therapy in patients with inflammatory bowel disease. *Gut* 2001;48:642.
103. Cuffari C et al. Thiopurine methyltransferase activity influences clinical response to azathioprine in inflammatory bowel disease. *Clin Gastroenterol Hepatol* 2004;2:410.
104. Turgeon N et al. Safety and efficacy of granulocyte colony-stimulating factor in kidney and liver transplant recipients. *Transpl Infect Dis* 2000;2:15.
105. Arora S et al. A double-blind, randomized, placebo-controlled trial of methotrexate in CD. *Gastroenterology* 1993;102:A591.
106. Fraser AG et al. The efficacy of methotrexate for maintaining remission in inflammatory bowel disease. *Aliment Pharmacol Ther* 2002;16:693.
107. Ursling B et al. A comparative study of metronidazole and sulfasalazine for active Crohn's disease: the cooperative Crohn's disease study in Sweden. II. Results. *Gastroenterology* 1982;83:550.
108. Ambrose NS et al. Antibiotic therapy for treatment in relapse of intestinal Crohn's disease. *Dis Colon Rectum* 1985;28:81.
109. Visapaa JP et al. Lack of disulfiram-like reaction with metronidazole and ethanol. *Ann Pharmacother* 2002;36:971.
110. Lombardi DA et al. Medical management of inflammatory bowel disease in the new millennium. *Compr Ther* 2002;28:39.
111. Lichtenstein GR et al. Infliximab maintenance treatment reduces hospitalizations, surgeries, and procedures in fistulizing Crohn's disease. *Gastroenterology* 2005;128:862.
112. Panaccione R. Infliximab for the treatment of Crohn's disease: review and indications for clinical use in Canada. *Can J Gastroenterol* 2001;15:371.
113. Bickston SJ et al. The relationship between infliximab treatment and lymphoma in Crohn's disease. *Gastroenterology* 1999;117:1433.
114. Sandborn WJ, Loftus EV. Balancing the risks and benefits of infliximab in the treatment of inflammatory bowel disease. *Gut* 2004;53:780.
115. Siegel CA et al. Risks and benefits of infliximab for the treatment of Crohn's disease. *Clin Gastroenterol Hepatol* 2006;4:1017.
116. Rutgeerts P et al. Review article: infliximab therapy for inflammatory bowel disease—seven years on. *Aliment Pharmacol Ther* 2006;23:451.
117. Drossmen DA et al. Rome II: a multinational consensus document on functional gastrointestinal disorders. *Gut* 1999;45(Suppl 2):1.
118. Talley NJ. Serotoninergic neuroenteric modulators. *Lancet* 2001;358:2061.
119. Drossman DA et al. Irritable bowel syndrome: a technical review for practice guideline development. *Gastroenterology* 1997;112:2120.
120. Everheart JE et al. Irritable bowel syndrome in office-based practice in the United States. *Gastroenterology* 1991;100:998.
121. Mirchell CM et al. Survey of the AGA membership relating to patients with functional gastrointestinal disorders. *Gastroenterology* 1987;92:121.
122. Sandler R. Epidemiology of irritable bowel syndrome in the United States. *Gastroenterology* 1990;99:409.
123. Olden KW. Diagnosis of irritable bowel syndrome. *Gastroenterology* 2002;122:1701.
124. Horwitz BJ et al. The irritable bowel syndrome. *N Engl J Med* 2001;344:1846.
125. Ballenger JC et al. Consensus statement on depression, anxiety, and functional gastrointestinal disorders. *J Clin Psychiatry* 2001;62(Suppl 8):48.
126. Talley NJ. Medical costs in community subjects with irritable bowel syndrome. *Gastroenterology* 1995;109:1736.
127. Talley NJ. Irritable bowel syndrome: a little understood organic bowel disease? *Lancet* 2002;360:555.
128. Kim DY et al. Serotonin: a mediator of the brain-gut connection. *Gastroenterology* 2000;95:2698.
129. Coates MD et al. Molecular defects in mucosal serotonin content and decreased serotonin reuptake transporter in ulcerative colitis and irritable bowel syndrome. *Gastroenterology* 2004;126:1657.
130. Bearcroft CP et al. Postprandial plasma 5-hydroxytryptamine in diarrhoea predominant irritable bowel syndrome: a pilot study. *Gut* 1998;42:42.
131. Ragnarsson G et al. Division of the irritable bowel syndrome into subgroups on the basis of recorded symptoms in two outpatient samples. *Scand J Gastroenterol* 1999;34:993.
132. Chey WY et al. Colonic motility abnormality in patients with irritable bowel syndrome exhibiting abdominal pain and diarrhea. *Am J Gastroenterol* 2001;96:1499.
133. King TS et al. Abnormal colonic fermentation in irritable bowel syndrome. *Lancet* 1998;352:1187.
134. Gwee KA et al. The role of psychological and biological factors in postinfective gut dysfunction. *Gut* 1999;44:400.
135. Camilleri M. Management of the irritable bowel syndrome. *Gastroenterology* 2001;120:652.
136. Neal KR et al. Prevalence of gastrointestinal symptoms six months after bacterial gastroenteritis and risk factors for development of the irritable bowel syndrome: postal survey of patients. *BMJ* 1997;314:779.
137. Morris-Yates AD et al. Evidence of a genetic contribution to functional bowel disorder. *Am J Gastroenterol* 1998;93:1311.
138. Fass R et al. Evidence- and consensus-based practice guidelines for the diagnosis of irritable bowel syndrome. *Arch Intern Med* 2001;161:2081.
139. Bertram S et al. The patient's perspective of irritable bowel syndrome. *J Fam Pract* 2001;50:521.
140. Paterson WG et al. Recommendations for the management of irritable bowel syndrome in family practice. *Can Med Assoc J* 1999;161:154.
141. Owens DM et al. The irritable bowel syndrome: long-term prognosis and the physician(patient interaction. *Ann Intern Med* 1995;122:107.
142. Janssen HA et al. The clinical course and prognostic determinants of the irritable bowel syndrome: a literature review. *Scand J Gastroenterol* 1998;33:561.
143. Colwell LJ et al. Effects of an irritable bowel syndrome educational class on health-promoting

behaviors and symptoms. *Am J Gastroenterol* 1998;93:901.
144. Drossman DA. Diagnosing and treating patients with refractory functional gastrointestinal disorders. *Ann Intern Med* 1995;122:107.
145. Cann PA et al. What is the benefit of coarse wheat bran in patients with irritable bowel syndrome? *Gut* 1984;25:168.
146. Voderholzer WA et al. Clinical response to dietary fiber treatment of chronic constipation. *Am J Gatroenterol* 1997;92:95.
147. Jailwala J et al. Pharmacologic treatment of the irritable bowel syndrome: a systemic review of randomized, controlled trials. *Ann Intern Med* 2000;133:136.
148. Muller-Lissner SA et al. Tegaserod, a 5-HT_4 receptor partial agonist, relieves symptoms in irritable bowel syndrome patients, with abdominal pain, bloating, and constipation. *Aliment Pharmacol Ther* 2001;15:1655.
149. Novick J et al. A randomized, double-blind, placebo-controlled trial of tegaserod in female patients suffering from irritable bowel syndrome with constipation. *Aliment Pharmacol Ther* 2002;16: 1877.
150. Zelnorm (tagaserod maleate) information, FDA CDER website. http://www.fda.gov/cder/drug/infopage/zelnorm/default.htm. Accessed June 1, 2008.
151. Tack J et al. Systematic review: the efficacy of treatments for irritable bowel syndrome—a European perspective. *Aliment Pharmacol Ther* 2006;24:183.
152. Clouse RE. Antidepressants for functional intestinal syndromes. *Dig Dis Sci* 1994;39:2352.
153. Rajagopalan M et al. Symptom relief with amitriptyline in the irritable bowel syndrome. *J Gastroenterol Hepatol* 1998;13:738.
154. Vahedi H et al. The effect of fluoxetine in patients with pain and constipation-predominant irritable bowel syndrome: a double-blind randomized-controlled study. *Aliment Pharmacol Ther* 2005; 22:381.
155. Akehurst R et al. Treatment of irritable bowel syndrome: a review of randomized controlled trials. *Gut* 2001;48:272.
156. Wilkliams AJK et al. Idiopathic bile acid malabsorption—a review of clinical presentation, diagnosis, and response to treatment. *Gut* 1991;32:1004.
157. Talley N. Serotonergic neuroenteric modulators. *Lancet* 2001;358:2061.
158. Moynihan R. Alosetron: a case study in regulatory capture, or a victory for patients' rights. *BMJ* 2002;325:592.
159. Lotronex prescribing information, GlaxoSmithKline, Inc., September 2002.
160. Chang L et al. Incidence of ischemic colitis and serious complications of constipation among patients using alosetron: systematic review of clinical trials and post-marketing surveillance data. *Am J Gastroenterol* 2006;101:1069.
161. Andresen V, Camilleri M. Irritable bowel syndrome recent and novel therapeutic approaches. *Drugs* 2006;66:1073.
162. Talley NJ. Irritable bowel syndrome. *Intern Med J* 2006;36:724.
163. Pimentel M et al. The effect of a nonabsorbed oral antibiotic (rifaximin) on the symptoms of the irritable bowel syndrome: a randomized trial. *Ann Intern Med* 2006;145:557.
164. O'Mahony L et al. *Lactobacillus* and *Bifidobacterium* in irritable bowel syndrome: symptom responses and relationship to cytokine profiles. *Gastroenterology* 2005;128:541.
165. Johanson JF et al. Clinical trial: phase 2 study of lubiprostone for irritable bowel syndrome with constipation. *Aliment Pharmacol Ther*. 2008;27:685.

CHAPTER 28

Complications of End-Stage Liver Disease

Yasar O. Tasnif and Mary F. Hebert

OVERVIEW

According to the National Vital Statistics Report published by the Center for Disease Control and Prevention, chronic liver disease and cirrhosis is the 12th leading cause of death in the United States accounting for approximately 26,000 deaths each year.[1] Cirrhosis, or end-stage liver disease, can be defined as fibrosis of the hepatic parenchyma resulting in nodule formation and altered hepatic function, which results from a sustained wound healing response to chronic or acute liver injury from a variety of causes. Although there are other common causes of cirrhosis, most cases of cirrhosis worldwide result from chronic viral hepatitis, or liver injury associated with chronic alcohol consumption.[2] This chapter describes the pathogenesis of cirrhosis and the associated complications of portal hypertension (esophageal varices, gastric varices, ascites, spontaneous bacterial peritonitis, hepatic encephalopathy, and hepatorenal syndrome), the clinical symptoms of these complications, and the pharmacologic approach to their treatment.

PATHOGENESIS OF CIRRHOSIS

The liver consists of the hepatic parenchyma (hepatocytes) and a large proportion of nonparenchymal cells, including sinusoidal endothelial cells, Ito cells, and macrophages also known as Kupffer cells. Most of the liver's role in detoxification (phase I and II metabolism) takes place within the hepatocytes, whereas the nonparenchymal cell population provides physical and biochemical structure to the liver as well as active transport of substances into the bile.[3] Although the liver has a strong capacity to regenerate, this ability can be impaired by toxic or viral agents, such as ethanol and hepatitis viruses.[4]

Stress on the liver, such as chronic ethanol abuse in humans, leads to liver injury and over time cirrhosis and a disruption of hepatic function. Fatty liver or steatosis from ethanol, the first stage of liver injury, is characterized by lipid deposition in the hepatocytes. Steatosis is followed by liver inflammation (steatohepatitis), hepatocyte death, and collagen deposition leading to fibrosis. The specific mechanisms by which chronic ethanol-induced liver injury is initiated and progresses are not completely understood.[5] Research into the causes of alcohol-related liver injury has primarily focused on the role of ethanol-induced oxidative stress on the liver. Multiple pathways leading to oxidative stress have been described, and many systems likely contribute to the ability of ethanol to induce a state of oxidative stress. It is important to note that not all heavy drinkers develop liver cirrhosis.[6] Factors such as gender, genetic predisposition, and chronic viral infection play a role in the development and progression of ethanol-induced liver disease.[7]

Hepatitis C virus (HCV) affects millions of people worldwide, with approximately 20% of infections progressing to cirrhosis.[8] The progression of liver disease in patients with HCV is dependent on both patient and viral factors. Although the mechanisms by which HCV causes liver damage are not well known, a few proposed mechanisms for liver injury associated with HCV infection include diminished immune clearance of HCV, oxidative stress, hepatic steatosis, increased iron stores, and increased rate of hepatocyte apoptosis.[9] Because only a small percentage of patients infected with HCV develop cirrhosis, factors other than viral clearance, such as the individual's immune response to the virus, age at the time of infection, gender, hepatic iron content, and HCV genotype are all implicated as cofactors in the development of cirrhosis.[10]

Among other causes, autoimmune hepatitis, primary biliary cirrhosis, primary sclerosing cholangitis, biliary atresia, metabolic disorders (e.g., Wilson's disease and hemochromatosis), chronic inflammatory conditions (e.g., sarcoidosis), and vascular derangements can lead to hepatic fibrosis and cirrhosis.[2] Although not common, end-stage liver disease can also stem from problems related to obesity. An estimated 20% of Americans have nonalcoholic fatty liver disease (NAFLD), a condition that in most cases has no symptoms, but is occasionally characterized by symptoms of upper abdominal discomfort and right upper quadrant fullness. The most common physical examination findings are obesity and occasionally hepatomegaly, with biopsy results showing macrovesicular steatosis or fatty liver. Risk factors commonly associated with the development of NAFLD include obesity, hyperlipidemia, and diabetes. Although corticosteroids cause fatty liver, NAFLD diagnosis excludes corticosteroids and other causes of fatty liver such as hepatitis B, hepatitis C, autoimmune hepatitis, and Wilson's disease. Nonalcoholic steatohepatitis (NASH) is a more serious form of NAFLD. Most patients generally tolerate NAFLD well, whereas NASH can lead to cirrhosis. Current evidence suggests that insulin resistance and lipid peroxidation play a role in the pathogenesis of this condition.[11,12] Regardless of the cause of end-stage liver disease, the most frequent complications of portal hypertension are esophageal or gastric varices, ascites with or without spontaneous bacterial peritonitis, hepatic encephalopathy, and hepatorenal syndrome.[13]

COMPLICATIONS OF CIRRHOSIS

Portal Hypertension

The portal vein begins as a confluence of the splenic, superior mesenteric, inferior mesenteric, and gastric veins, and ends in the sinusoids of the liver (Fig. 28-1). Blood in the portal vein contains substances absorbed from the intestine, and delivers these substances to the liver to be metabolized before entering the systemic circulation.[14,15] Once the portal blood reaches the liver, it crosses through a high-resistance capillary system within the hepatic sinusoids.

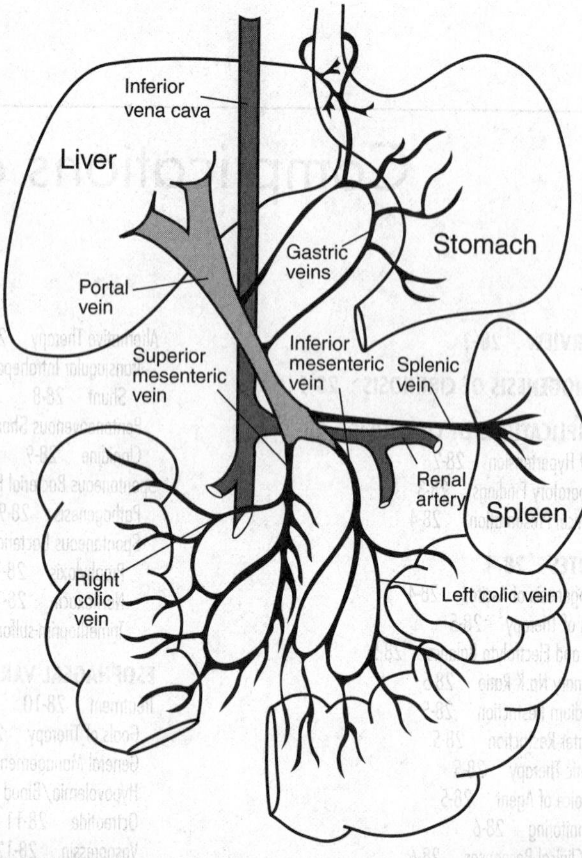

FIGURE 28-1 Schematic diagram of portal venous system.

Portal pressure is a function of flow and resistance to that flow across the hepatic vasculature, and described mathematically by Ohm's law (Pressure = Flow × Resistance).[16] In cirrhosis, increased intrahepatic resistance results from intrahepatic vasoconstriction that is hypothesized to be caused by a deficiency in intrahepatic nitric oxide (NO). Increased intrahepatic resistance also results from an enhanced activity of vasoconstrictors, and by structural changes within the liver owing to liver regeneration, sinusoidal compression, and fibrosis. Portal hypertension results from both an increase in resistance to portal flow and also an increase in portal venous inflow, which is hypothesized to be caused by splanchnic vasodilatation that, in turn, is secondary to increase NO production in the extrahepatic circulation leading to vasodilation and increased in-flow.[17]

Portal pressure can be assessed by the use of surgical procedures which are invasive and not routinely performed. The hepatic venous pressure gradient (HVPG), which reflects the gradient between the portal vein and vena cava pressure, is another accurate, safe, and less invasive procedure that has been widely accepted as a measurement of the portal venous pressure gradient.[18–20] Normal portal pressure is generally below 6 mmHg, and in cirrhotic patients may increase to 7 to 9 mmHg. Clinically significant portal hypertension develops, however, when the portal pressure increases above 10 to 12 mmHg, the threshold for complications of portal hypertension, such as

Table 28-1 Classification and Etiologies of Portal Hypertension

Classification	*Prehepatic*	*Intrahepatic*	*Posthepatic*
Etiologies	Splenic vein thrombosis	Hepatic cirrhosis	Hepatic vein obstruction (Budd-Chiari syndrome)
	Portal vein thrombosis	Hepatic fibrosis	Inferior vena cava obstruction
		Nodular regeneration (with distortion of hepatic veins)	Right-sided heart failure

esophageal varices and ascites.[19,21] Portal hypertension can be further classified as prehepatic, intrahepatic, or posthepatic portal hypertension (Table 28-1).[22–24] Persistent portal hypertension may (a) change both blood flow as well as the lymphatic circulation and lead to ascites formation; (b) increase pressure in the vessels that branch off the portal vein, such as the coronary veins, leading to the formation of esophageal varices; and (c) lead to the development of increased abdominal collateral circulation. Hepatic encephalopathy and hepatorenal syndrome are other complications associated with advanced cirrhosis and portal hypertension.[22–24]

Laboratory Findings

Laboratory evaluations may not reflect the extent of the parenchymal necrosis, cellular regeneration, and fibrotic nodular scarring in cirrhotic liver disease. Conventional liver "function" tests, such as the serum aminotransferases (aspartate aminotransferases [AST, formerly known as SGOT], alanine aminotransferases [ALT, formerly known as SGPT]), and alkaline phosphatase, are actually better characterized as liver "injury" tests and are modestly helpful to the clinician for screening hepatobiliary disease and following liver injury progression. These tests, however, do not quantitatively measure the functional capacity of the liver. The aminotransferases are released during the normal turnover of liver cells (see Chapter 2, Interpretation of Clinical Laboratory Tests). High serum concentrations of aminotransferases suggest release of these enzymes from injured hepatocytes. The serum concentrations of AST and ALT may initially rise very high with acute liver injury and then fall when the cause for liver injury is removed or when necrosis is so severe, that few hepatocytes remain.

Because alkaline phosphatase is present in high concentrations in biliary canaliculi (as well as bone, intestines, kidneys, and white blood cells [WBC]), an increase in the serum concentration of alkaline phosphatase is greater with biliary injury rather than during a parenchymal injury. High serum concentrations of gamma glutamyl transpeptidase and bilirubin are also suggestive of biliary injury. Increases in alkaline phosphatase, and AST, ALT, or both serum concentrations may suggest hepatic injury, but because they are also found intracellularly in other places in the body, their elevation is not diagnostic for liver disease.[25,26]

Serum concentrations of proteins such as albumin, or factor V and VIII, as well as coagulation tests such as the prothrombin time (PT) and international normalized ratio (INR), can provide insight into the functional capacity of the liver. The hepatic parenchymal cells exclusively synthesize albumin, therefore albumin concentrations can provide some indication of hepatocellular function. Changes in albumin concentration are nonspecific, however, and can be influenced by other factors, including poor nutrition, renal wasting (proteinuria), and gastrointestinal (GI) losses. Prolongation of PT owing to vitamin K deficiency often caused by cholestasis, usually improves within 24 hours after a 10-mg subcutaneous or oral dose of vitamin K. A prolonged PT owing to poor hepatic synthetic function is not responsive, however, to the administration of vitamin K. If the INR requires rapid correction because of bleeding or a planned invasive procedure, fresh frozen plasma should be transfused.[27]

A number of the factors described above have been incorporated into the Child-Turcotte-Pugh classification of liver disease severity (Table 28-2).[22–24,28,29] This classification yields a scoring system to help clinicians grade disease severity, and predict the long-term risk of mortality and quality of life. A person with Child-Turcotte-Pugh class A cirrhosis may survive as long as 15 to 20 years, whereas those with class C cirrhosis may survive only 1 to 3 years.[30] The main limitation of the Child-Turcotte-Pugh classification is the use of subjective measures, such as ascites and hepatic encephalopathy, which are subject to clinical interpretation and may be altered by therapy.[31,32]

An alternative method for assessing short-term survival in patients with liver disease is the Model for End-Stage Liver

Table 28-2 Child-Turcotte-Pugh Classification of Severity of Liver Disease[a]

Score	*1 Point*	*2 Points*	*3 Points*
Bilirubin (mg/dL)	<2	2–3	>3
Albumin (mg/dL)	>3.5	3–3.5	<3
Prothrombin time (sec)[b]	<4	4–6	>6
Ascites	None	Easily controlled (mild)	Poorly controlled (moderate)
Encephalopathy (grade)	None	Mild (1 and 2)	Advanced (3 and 4)

[a]Class A, <7 points; class B, 7–9 points; class C, 10–15 points.
[b]Seconds prolonged.

Disease (MELD) score that utilizes laboratory values, and is used to predict short-term (3 month) mortality associated with liver disease. The MELD score is calculated by the formula[32]:

$$\text{MELD score} = (0.957 \times \ln[\text{creatinine mg/dL}] + 0.378 \times \ln[\text{total bilirubin mg/dL}] + 1.120 \times \ln[\text{INR}] + 0.643) \times 10$$

Because of the good correlation between the MELD score and short-term mortality as well as the objective nature of the MELD scoring system, it has replaced the Child-Turcotte-Pugh score in the United Network for Organ Sharing (UNOS) prioritization of organ allocation of cadaveric livers for transplantation.[33–35] MELD scores range from 6 (less ill) to 40 (gravely ill).[36] A high MELD score is strongly associated with early pretransplantation wait-list mortality. Therefore a patient with a higher MELD score is given priority by UNOS in terms of organ allocation.

1. R.W. is a 54-year-old man with a 2-week history of nausea, vomiting, and lower abdominal cramps without diarrhea. Despite chronic anorexia, he has managed to drink a fifth of vodka (750 mL) and eat about two meals a day for the past 2 years. During this time, he experienced a 30-lb weight loss. He began drinking 9 years ago when his wife became disabled following diagnosis of a brain tumor. Two years ago, his alcohol consumption increased from one pint to a fifth daily. Recently, he has noted bilateral edema of his legs, an increased tenseness and girth of his abdomen, jaundice and scleral icterus. His medical history is noncontributory, other than a history of spontaneous bacterial peritonitis (SBP).

Physical examination reveals an afebrile, jaundiced, and cachectic male in moderate distress. Spider angiomas were found on his face and upper chest. In addition, palmar erythema was noted. Abdominal examination reveals prominent veins on a very tense abdomen. The liver edge is percussed below the right costal margin and ascites is noted by shifting dullness and a fluid wave. The spleen is not palpable. On neurologic examination, R.W. is awake and oriented to person, place, and time. Cranial nerves II to XII are grossly intact, but a decrease in vibratory sensation of the lower extremities is noted bilaterally. Admission laboratory data are as follows: sodium 135 mEq/L; chloride 95 mEq/L; potassium 3.8 mEq/L; bicarbonate 25 mEq/L; blood urea nitrogen (BUN) 15 mg/dL; serum creatinine (SrCr) 1.4 mg/dL; glucose 136 mg/dL; hemoglobin 11.2 g/dL; hematocrits (Hct) 33.4%; AST 212 IU (normal, 0–35 IU); alkaline phosphatase 954 IU (normal, 30–120 IU); PT 13.5 seconds with a control of 12 seconds (INR 1.1); total/direct bilirubin 18.8/10.7 mg/dL (normal, 1.0/<0.5 mg/dL); albumin 2.3 g/dL (normal, 3.5–4.0); and guaiac positive stools. On admission to the hospital, the impression is alcoholic cirrhosis, ascites, and heme-positive stools.

What subjective and objective evidence are compatible with alcoholic cirrhosis in R.W.?

Clinical Presentation

R.W.'s liver function tests (elevated AST, alkaline phosphatase, and bilirubin) and physical findings (an enlarged, palpable liver edge; jaundice; spider angiomas on his face and upper chest; palmar erythema; and cachexia) are all consistent with advanced alcoholic cirrhosis in a patient with a history of chronic alcohol abuse. The prolonged PT and hypoalbuminemia suggest impaired hepatic synthesis of both albumin and vitamin K-dependent clotting factors. The low albumin contributes to both the ascites and edema. The bilirubin of 18.8 mg/dL suggests that vitamin K absorption may be a factor in the prolonged PT. The presence of ascites (an enlarged fluid-filled abdomen) and prominent abdominal veins are suggestive of portal hypertension. A biopsy of the liver may confirm or establish the presence and severity of cirrhosis. R.W.'s prolonged PT, however, will increase the risk of bleeding from a liver biopsy. R.W.'s positive guaiac finding could be indicative of bleeding esophageal varices but could also be explained by bleeding from another GI source. This needs to be confirmed by endoscopy. He is oriented to person, place and time, but needs to be fully tested for hepatic encephalopathy. R.W.'s MELD score is 22 which predicts a 90-day mortality of approximately 20%.[33] A patient's MELD score may increase or decrease over a period of time depending on the patient's clinical status and treatment. A number of MELD scores will be calculated over the course of R.W.'s treatment if the patient is listed as a transplantation candidate to determine his status for organ allocation.[36] Muscle wasting and poor nutrition are the most common causes of weight loss in patients with alcoholic cirrhosis (see Chapter 84, Alcohol Use Disorders).

ASCITES

Pathogenesis of Ascites

2. What physiologic mechanism predisposes R.W. to fluid accumulation in the peritoneal cavity?

Ascites, or accumulation of fluid in the peritoneal cavity, is the most commonly encountered clinical symptom of cirrhosis.[37] This complication can be detected during the physical examination when >3 L of fluid has accumulated. In addition to an obviously enlarged abdomen, R.W. was found to have a positive fluid wave and shifting dullness, indicating that the abdominal enlargement is not simply obesity. The fluid wave can be observed by having the patient lie on his or her back. While supporting one side of the abdomen with one hand, use the second hand to tap the opposite side of the abdomen. A wave of fluid moving across the abdomen can be felt by the hand on the opposite side. If the diagnosis is in doubt, ascites is confirmed with ultrasound. Once ascites develops, the 1-year survival rate decreases to about 50%.[37]

In cirrhosis, hepatic venous outflow is restricted, resulting in an increase in the portal vein back-pressure. High hepatic venous pressure leads to high intrasinusoidal pressure and development of ascites across the hepatic capsule. Portal hypertension from cirrhosis is associated with splanchnic dilatation and increased splanchnic blood flow. This increase in splanchnic blood flow is associated with an upregulation of endothelial nitric oxide synthase (eNOS) and increased production of a potent vasodilator, NO. This increase in NO has been proposed as a major mediator of the arterial dilatation and hyperdynamic circulation in cirrhosis.[38] NO leads to an overall vasodilated state. The systemic compensation to this vasodilation is an increase in cardiac output and sodium and water retention in the kidneys as a result of activation of the renin-angiotensin aldosterone system (RAAS).[39] The activation of RAAS, in addition to R.W.'s hypoalbuminemia (2.3 g/dL) leads to worsening of the ascites. Exudation of fluid from the splanchnic capillary bed and the liver surface when the drainage capacity of the lymphatic system is exceeded, and decreased ability of fluid to be contained within the vascular space owing to impaired hepatic albumin synthesis, contributes to the development of ascites.

Goals of Therapy

3. What are the therapeutic goals in the treatment of R.W.'s ascites?

The goals of treatment for R.W.'s ascites are to mobilize ascitic fluid; to diminish abdominal discomfort, back pain, and difficulty in ambulation; as well as to prevent complications (e.g., bacterial peritonitis, hernias, pleural effusions, hepatorenal syndrome, and respiratory distress). The goal is a weight loss of 0.5 to 1 kg/day, which corresponds to a net fluid volume loss of about 0.5 to 1 L/day. Treatment of ascites in R.W. should be undertaken cautiously and gradually because acid-base imbalances, hypokalemia, or intravascular volume depletion caused by overly aggressive therapy can lead to compromised renal function, hepatic encephalopathy, and death.[40–42] The initial medical management of ascites involves restriction of sodium intake and the use of diuretics to promote salt and water excretion.[40,42]

Fluid and Electrolyte Balance

4. The 24-hour urinary electrolytes for R.W. were Na, 10 mEq/L and K, 28 mEq/L. Why would sodium or water restriction be appropriate (or inappropriate) for R.W.?

Urinary Na:K Ratio

Normally, the urine concentration of electrolytes mirrors the serum concentration of electrolytes (i.e., sodium concentration is greater than that of potassium). A reversal of this pattern (i.e., potassium excretion exceeding sodium excretion) may indicate a relative hyperaldosteronism secondary to diminished renal blood flow and low oncotic pressure. A study by Trevisani et al.[43] evaluated renal sodium and potassium handling, and plasma aldosterone in a 24-hour period in cirrhotic patients without ascites (n = 7), with ascites (n = 8), and healthy controls (n = 7). Plasma aldosterone was significantly higher in patients with ascites, resulting in reduced renal sodium excretion, and more than doubling of renal potassium excretion in comparison to healthy controls.[43] For urine electrolyte monitoring to be meaningful, the first sample must be obtained before initiating diuretic therapy.[44,45]

Sodium Restriction

Although serum sodium in patients with ascites is often low, they are total body sodium overloaded. Sodium restriction has been shown to enhance mobilization of ascites, because fluid loss and weight change are directly related to sodium balance in patients with portal-hypertension–related ascites.[46] This finding has been incorporated into the American Association for the Study of Liver Diseases (AASLD) guidelines for the treatment of ascites. The AASLD recommends that dietary sodium should be restricted to ≤ 2,000 mg/day [88 mmol/day].[42] Although bedrest has been advocated in the past, no controlled trials support this practice. R.W. should benefit from sodium restriction of ≤2 g/day.

Water Restriction

A large prospective, observational study (n = 997) by Angeli et al.[47] evaluated the prevalence of low serum sodium concentration and the association between serum sodium levels with severity of ascites and complications of cirrhosis. The results indicated that low serum sodium levels are a common feature in patients with cirrhosis, and that serum sodium concentrations <135 mEq/L are associated with a poor control of ascites as well as a greater frequency of hepatic encephalopathy, hepatorenal syndrome, and spontaneous bacterial peritonitis compared with patients with serum sodium concentrations within the normal range (135–145 mEq/L).[47] In addition, very low serum sodium concentrations (<120 mEq/L) are independent predictors of 3- to 6-month mortality from the MELD score in patients with end-stage liver disease. The AASLD recommends that water restriction should be implemented in cirrhotic patients who have severe dilutional hyponatremia (serum Na <120–125 mEq/L).[42] For R.W., water restriction is not indicated at this time because his serum sodium concentration is within normal limits (135 mEq/L).

Diuretic Therapy

Choice of Agent

5. R.W. was prescribed sodium restriction after initial evaluation. Spironolactone 100 mg/day and furosemide 40 mg/day were ordered to induce diuresis. Why is spironolactone preferred over other diuretics in the treatment of ascites?

Most patients with advanced liver disease have high circulating levels of aldosterone.[48] High serum concentrations of aldosterone may be attributed to both increased production and decreased excretion of the hormone. Increased portal pressure, ascites, depletion of intravascular volume, and decreased renal perfusion can lead to activation of the RAAS.[49] In addition, hepatic shunting also increases aldosterone production by decreasing renal blood flow.[50] The liver metabolizes aldosterone, and hepatic impairment prolongs the physiologic half-life of aldosterone.[51] The AASLD consensus guidelines recommend the use of spironolactone as the initial diuretic of choice in the treatment of ascites.[42] Although no large comparative studies have evaluated different diuretics as first-line treatment of ascites, spironolactone is a rational diuretic choice for R.W. based on its aldosterone antagonist activity. Perez-Ayuso et al.[52] conducted a small randomized trial to study the efficacy of furosemide versus spironolactone in nonazotemic cirrhotic patients (n = 40) with ascites. They found that spironolactone was more effective than furosemide, and that the activity of the renin-aldosterone system influences the diuretic response to furosemide and spironolactone in patients with cirrhosis. In the study, patients were treated with furosemide (initial doses of 80 mg/day, maximal dose of 160 mg/day) or spironolactone (initial dose 150 mg/day, maximal dose of 300 mg/day). Patients not responding to furosemide or spironolactone were later converted to the alternate therapy. The results showed a higher response to spironolactone than furosemide (18/19 vs. 11/21; p <0.01). Of the 10 non-responders to furosemide, 9 responded to spironolactone when therapy was switched. The authors also found that patients with higher renin and aldosterone levels did not respond to furosemide and required higher doses of spironolactone to achieve a diuretic response.[52]

Some clinicians may initiate spironolactone at a dose of 25 mg once or BID; however, much larger doses (100–400 mg/day) are generally necessary to antagonize the high circulating levels of aldosterone present in patients with ascites.[42] The diuretic effect is enhanced when spironolactone is combined with sodium restriction (0.5–2 g/day).[41] In addition, furosemide can be started to minimize the risk of hyperkalemia and enhance diuresis. The AASLD guidelines recommend starting spironolactone 100 mg and furosemide 40 mg simultaneously and maintaining a 100:40 mg ratio. The doses of both oral diuretics can be increased simultaneously every 3 to 5 days (maintaining the ratio) to achieve adequate response. Usual maximal doses are 400 mg/day of spironolactone and 160 mg/day of furosemide.[42] In controlled clinical trials, sodium restriction and diuretic therapy are effective in 90% of patients without renal failure.[53–55]

Triamterene and amiloride can be used as alternatives to spironolactone if intolerable side effects (e.g., gynecomastia) occur with spironolactone.[42,57] In a small trial conducted by Angeli et al.,[58] cirrhotic patients were randomized to receive amiloride (n = 20) or potassium canrenoate (an active metabolite of spironolactone not available in the United States; n = 20), to study the efficacy of each drug in nonazotemic cirrhotic patients with ascites. The initial doses of amiloride and potassium canrenoate were 20 and 150 mg, respectively, and were increased (up to 60 and 500 mg/day) if no response occurred. Nonresponders to the highest doses of each drug were later converted to the alternate agent. A higher response rate was seen in the canrenoate group versus the amiloride group (14/20 vs. 7/20; $p < 0.025$). The authors also assessed plasma aldosterone activity and found that all responders to amiloride had normal plasma aldosterone concentrations, and all nonresponders to amiloride who later responded to potassium canrenoate had increased levels of plasma aldosterone.[58]

Eplerenone (a selective aldosterone blocker, more specific for the aldosterone receptor with a lower affinity for progesterone and androgen receptors than spironolactone) has been studied in patients with heart failure, hypertension, and renal disease.[59,60] The usual dose for eplerenone is 25 to 50 mg/day.[61] No dosage adjustment is needed with mild to moderate liver disease, but severe liver disease has not been studied.[62] Approximately 10% of patients treated with spironolactone develop gynecomastia or breast pain, with 2% requiring drug discontinuation.[63] In contrast, gynecomastia occurs at a similar rate with eplerenone as with placebo (0.5%).[64,65] Eplerenone is also much more expensive than spironolactone.[65] The lower risk of gynecomastia with eplerenone may make it a useful alternative to spironolactone. However, given its higher cost and the lack of data in the treatment of ascites and patients with severe liver disease, its eventual role in ascites treatment remains unclear.

R.W. should receive spironolactone 100 mg and furosemide 40 mg simultaneously (and maintaining a 100:40 mg ratio) as recommended by the AASLD.[42] This approach to therapy may be taken, as long as the patient is carefully monitored for diuretic complications and a clinical response to diuresis (see Questions 6, 7, and 8).

Monitoring

CLINICAL RESPONSES

6. What clinical responses should be monitored to ensure the therapeutic effectiveness of spironolactone therapy for R.W.?

Because ascitic fluid is slow to re-equilibrate with vascular fluid, diuresis >0.5 to 1 kg/day (0.5–1 L) may be associated with volume depletion, hypotension, and compromised renal function.[42] Patients may tolerate a faster diuresis if peripheral edema is present. Once edema has resolved, a scaled back weight loss, not to exceed 0.5 kg/day, can be used as a rule of thumb to minimize the risk of renal insufficiency induced by plasma volume contraction and other diuretic-induced complications.[42,66] Monitoring body weight and abdominal girth are routinely performed in both the inpatient and outpatient settings. Monitoring fluid intake and urine output are performed primarily for inpatients, owing to practical constraints in the outpatient setting. Ideally, urine output should exceed fluid intake by about 300 to 1,000 mL/day. These measurements do not account for nonrenal fluid losses; therefore, total fluid loss will be somewhat higher. Abdominal girth measurement (circumference around the abdomen) is subject to error, because of its dependence on patient position and measurement location on the abdomen.[56] Attempts should be made to standardize patient position (e.g., sitting at a 45-degree angle) and location of measurement (level of umbilicus) to minimize variability in abdominal girth measurements.

LABORATORY PARAMETERS

7. What laboratory parameters could be monitored to assess the therapeutic efficacy of R.W.'s spironolactone treatment?

Serum concentrations of creatinine and urine chemistries (sodium and potassium) can be monitored to define and guide the need for increasing dosage of spironolactone. A low baseline urine Na:K ratio (<1.0) suggests high intrinsic aldosterone activity and that larger dosages of spironolactone may be needed, as is the case for R.W. If necessary, the dosage of adjunctive diuretic therapy may be doubled after a few days.[49] AASLD recommends increasing both spironolactone and furosemide simultaneously every 3 to 5 days (maintaining a 100:40 mg ratio) to achieve adequate diuresis and maintain a normal serum potassium.[42]

Diuretic Complications and Management

8. The spironolactone dosage was increased to 200 mg/day and 80 mg/day (maintaining a 100:40 mg ratio). What potential complications from the diuretic therapy might arise in R.W. and how can they be minimized?

ELECTROLYTE AND ACID-BASE DISTURBANCES

Hyponatremia, hyperkalemia, metabolic alkalosis, and uncommonly hypokalemia occur as side effects of diuretic therapy in patients with ascites. Hyponatremia results from a reduction in filtered sodium, an increase in sodium reabsorption and a reduction in free water clearance (dilutional hyponatremia). Diuresis exacerbates hyponatremia by causing volume depletion and antidiuretic hormone (ADH) release. Hyponatremia, if present, usually can be corrected by temporary withdrawal of diuretics and free water restriction.[53,67–69] Although serum sodium may be low, these patients are total body sodium overloaded. Hyperkalemia is common in patients with refractory ascites and impaired renal function requiring high doses of diuretics such as spironolactone. Hyperkalemia can be approached in multiple ways, depending on the clinical situation (see Chapter 12, Fluid and Electrolyte Disorders). Furosemide is added to the therapeutic regimen to maintain normal serum potassium. Decreasing or holding spironolactone may be appropriate depending on the patient's renal function and serum potassium.[42] Metabolic alkalosis, another acid-base disorder found in cirrhotic patients as a result of loop diuretics, occurs because of increased urinary hydrogen loss from enhanced distal hydrogen secretion. Hypokalemia often accompanies metabolic alkalosis owing to loop diuretics.[42,68] Furosemide can be temporarily withheld in patients presenting with hypokalemia.[42] R.W. has some degree of renal impairment (SrCr 1.4 mg/dL) and is receiving spironolactone and furosemide. Therefore, his electrolytes and renal function tests should be monitored daily while hospitalized. After hospital discharge, monitoring will be dictated by the stability of the patient and need for diuretic dosage adjustments. For example, outpatients may need electrolytes and renal function monitoring once or twice weekly early after hospital discharge to as infrequently as every 3 months for the very stable patient.

PRERENAL AZOTEMIA

Prerenal azotemia usually results from over diuresis with subsequent compromise of intravascular volume and decreased renal perfusion. In addition to looking for clinical signs of hypovolemia, such as dizziness, orthostatic hypotension, and increased heart rate, frequent measurements of BUN and serum creatinine concentrations provide a relatively simple means of assessing the intravascular volume. A gradual rise in serum creatinine, BUN as well as the BUN:serum creatinine ratio can serve as a warning to slow the rate of diuresis.[70] In a small study conducted by Pockros et al.,[66] serial measurements of plasma volume and ascites volume were made during treatment with diuretics in patients with cirrhosis (n = 14). Patients with ascites and no edema were able to mobilize >1 L/day during rapid diuresis, but at the expense of plasma volume contraction and renal insufficiency. Patients with peripheral edema appear to be somewhat protected from these effects and may safely undergo diuresis at a more rapid rate (>2 kg/day) until edema resolves.[66] Others suggest, however, that the maximal daily fluid loss should not exceed >0.5 L/day (>0.5 kg/day) for patients with ascites alone or >1 L/day (>1 kg/day) for those with both ascites and edema to prevent plasma volume depletion and decreased renal perfusion. If faster removal of ascites is required because of respiratory distress, large-volume paracentesis may be more effective than rapid diuresis (see Question 9).[42,45,71,72]

Because R.W. presented with both edema and ascites, an initial fluid loss of up to 1 L/day would be reasonable. The rate of weight loss should be slowed not to exceed >0.5 L/day when the edema resolves. Gradual diuresis avoids diuretic-induced depletion of intravascular fluid volume by permitting ascitic fluid to equilibrate with intravascular fluid. Long-term management of ascites is done in the outpatient setting. Severe cases with respiratory distress or impaired ambulation as well as patients with spontaneous bacterial peritonitis require hospitalization. If outpatient therapy is an option, a weekly evaluation initially would be prudent to prevent over diuresis and electrolyte disturbances.[53]

Refractory Ascites

9. Over the next several days, R.W.'s spironolactone dosage was increased to 400 mg/day. Furosemide was simultaneously increased to 80 mg twice daily (BID) without major improvement in his diuresis. Laboratory data revealed that R.W.'s SrCr had increased to 3.2 mg/dL (calculated creatinine clearance: 26 mL/minute) and his BUN had increased to 45 mg/dL. Serum electrolytes were as follows: K, 3.1 mEq/L; Na, 130 mEq/L; Cl, 88 mEq/L; and bicarbonate, 32 mEq/L. R.W. became progressively short of breath because of restricted diaphragmatic movement secondary to his significantly enlarged abdomen. What therapeutic measures are appropriate for refractory (diuretic-resistant) ascites?

Because of the increase in SrCr and respiratory distress, R.W.'s ascites treatment needs modification. Patients with cirrhosis experiencing respiratory distress despite diuretic and sodium restriction warrant more aggressive second-line treatment, including large volume paracentesis, shunting procedures, or both.[42] Paracentesis involves the removal of ascitic fluid from the abdominal cavity with a needle or a catheter. Although paracentesis can remove large amounts of ascitic fluid (e.g., 10 L), removal of as little as 1 L of fluid may provide considerable relief from the painful stretching of skin and the respiratory distress that occurs with massive ascites. The ascitic fluid often reaccumulates rapidly after paracentesis owing to transudation of fluid from the interstitial and plasma compartments into the peritoneal cavity. The major complications of overly aggressive, large-volume paracentesis include hypotension, shock, oliguria, encephalopathy, and renal insufficiency. Other potential complications of paracentesis are hemorrhage, perforation of the abdominal viscera, infection, and protein depletion.[42]

Albumin

10. R.W. continues to reaccumulate ascitic fluid and is exhibiting signs of declining renal function. A 6-L paracentesis coupled with a 50-g albumin infusion is ordered. Why are albumin infusions used in conjunction with paracentesis?

Large volume (>4 L) paracentesis should be performed for patients with tense ascites resulting in respiratory distress or impaired ambulation. Large volume paracentesis alone is associated, however, with paracentesis-induced circulatory dysfunction (PICD). PICD is characterized by a reduction in systemic vascular resistance and significant increase in plasma renin activity and plasma norepinephrine.[73] Following paracentesis, a period of impaired circulatory function occurs, which manifests as worsening renal function 24 to 48 hours after the procedure.[74] Intravenous (IV) albumin infusions are commonly administered to prevent PICD following large volume paracentesis.[42]

Although albumin is costly and sometimes in short supply, for some patients, it is an appropriate treatment in conjunction with paracentesis.[75] Patients treated with large volume paracentesis (≥6 L/day) and IV albumin (40 g after each tap) were compared with patients treated with paracentesis and saline solution. The incidence of PICD was significantly higher in the saline-treated group versus the albumin-treated group (33.3% vs. 11.4%, respectively). The prevalence of PICD following paracentesis depends on the volume of ascites removed.[75] For large volume paracentesis ≥6 L, 8 to 10 g of albumin is typically administered for each liter of ascites removed.[42] Post-paracentesis albumin infusion may not be necessary for a single paracentesis of <4 to 5 L.[42] Use of albumin in combination with large volume paracentesis produces an expansion of circulating blood volume, increases cardiac output, and suppresses release of renin and norepinephrine.[74]

The effects of albumin administration for a variety of indications on patient mortality have also been evaluated. Wilkes et al.[76] conducted a meta-analysis of 55 randomized, controlled trials comparing albumin therapy with crystalloid therapy, no albumin, or lower doses of albumin on patient mortality (27 involved surgery or trauma; 4 involved burns; 5 involved hypoalbuminemia; 6 involved high-risk neonates; 5 involved ascites; and 8 involved other indications). For all trials, the relative risk for death was 1.11 (95% confidence interval [CI], 0.95–1.28). For ascites, in particular, the relative risk for death was 0.93 (95% CI, 0.67–1.28). Overall, albumin did not affect mortality.[76] In a study by Sort et al.,[77] patients with SBP (n = 126) were randomized to receive IV antibiotics alone (n = 63) or IV antibiotics and albumin (n = 63). Albumin (1.5 g/kg) was administered at the time of SBP diagnosis, and again on day 3 (1 g/kg). The albumin group had a lower incidence of renal impairment (10% vs. 33%; $p = 0.002$), overall mortality at 3 months (22% vs. 41%; $p = 0.03$) and hospital mortality (10% vs. 29%; $p = 0.01$) than the group that did not receive albumin.[77]

Dextran 70 and Other Plasma Expanders

The use of synthetic plasma expanders in combination with large volume paracentesis has been explored as a therapeutic option for patients with ascites refractory to diuretics and fluid restriction.[78,79] Gines et al.[79] studied patients with ascites refractory to diuretic therapy. Patients were randomized to paracentesis plus albumin (n = 97), dextran 70 (n = 93), or polygeline (n = 99). More patients treated with dextran 70 (34.4%) or polygeline (37.8%) versus those receiving albumin (18.5%) experienced PICD. In addition, during follow-up, patients who experienced PICD versus those who did not, had a shorter time to first readmission (1.3 vs. 3.5 months; $p = 0.03$) and a shorter survival (9.3 vs. 16.9 months; $p = 0.01$).[79] Hydroxyethyl starch, an effective colloid agent for intravascular volume expansion, should not be used in patients with chronic liver disease, because repeated administration of this agent to patients with cirrhosis has been reported to accumulate in the hepatocytes, causing severe portal hypertension and acute liver failure.[80] R.W. should be given 50 g of 25% albumin administered at a rate of 3 mL/minute, for the 6 L of ascitic fluid removed. More rapid administration than 3 mL/minute in hypoproteinemic patients can cause circulatory overload and pulmonary edema. R.W. should be monitored for anaphylactic reactions (rare), hypo- and hypertension, and signs of pulmonary edema.[81–83]

Alternative Therapy

11. What alternative treatments are available for management of refractory ascites? How would these alternatives be applied in R.W.'s case?

Transjugular Intrahepatic Portosystemic Shunt

Transjugular intrahepatic portosystemic shunt (TIPS) is another option for patients who are refractory to the pharmacologic interventions described above. It is an interventional (nonsurgical) technique for establishing a shunt in patients with portal hypertension (Fig. 28-2).[84] The TIPS procedure involves opening a conduit between the hepatic vein and intrahepatic segment of the portal vein with an expandable metal stent placed during an angiographic procedure. This

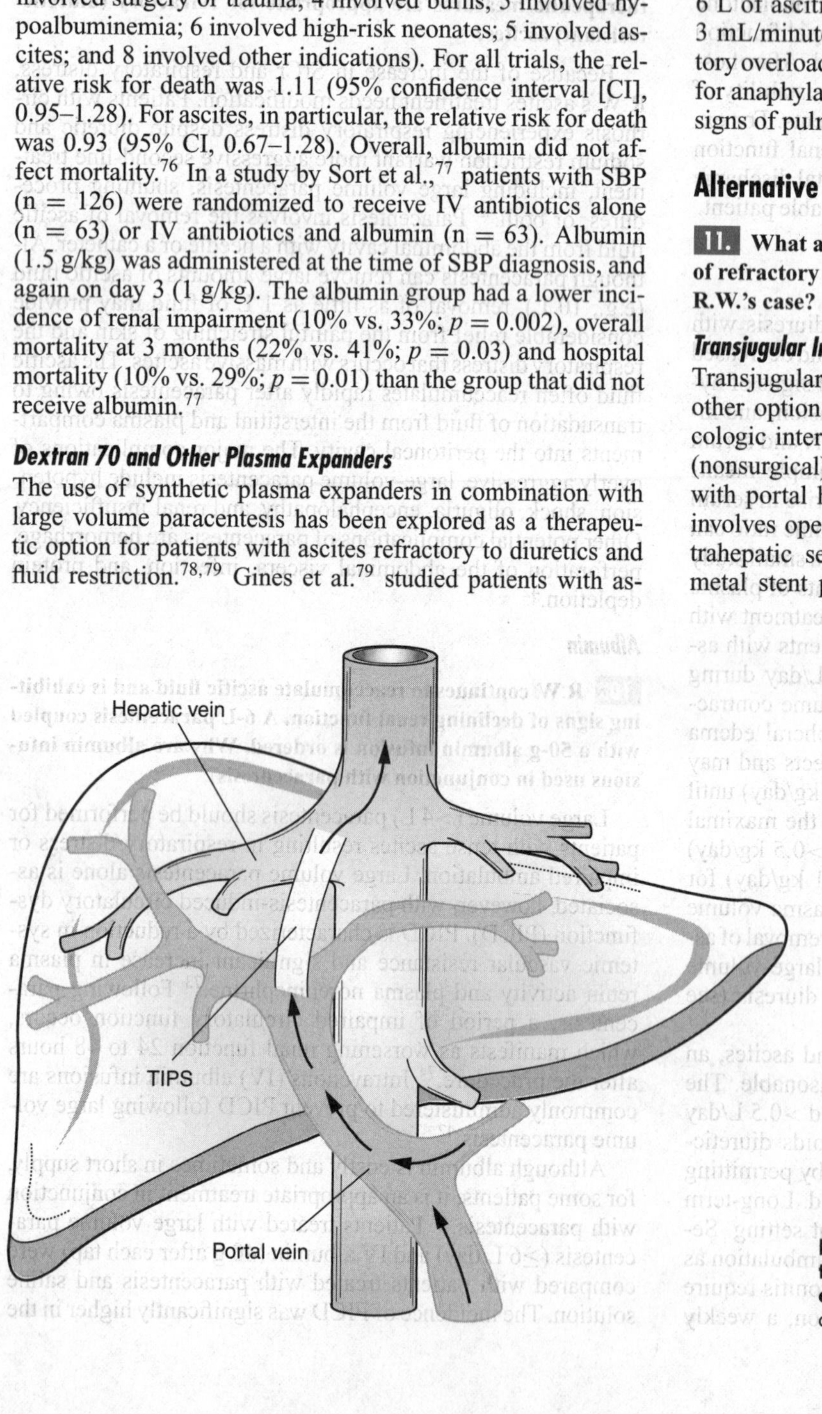

FIGURE 28-2 Transjugular intrahepatic portosystemic shunt (TIPS) decompressing the portal circulation into the systemic circulation. (Reproduced with permission from reference 84.)

low-resistance channel allows blood to return to the systemic circulation and reduces portal pressure. In addition, TIPS may improve urinary sodium excretion. The major complications of TIPS include severe encephalopathy, and shunt occlusion. Hepatic encephalopathy (see Question 19) occurs in approximately 20% of patients following TIPS.[84] Because of poor prognosis, liver transplantation should be considered for appropriate candidates refractory to pharmacologic treatment and or shunt placement.[42] Selection of surgical shunt procedures may include evaluation of liver transplantation candidacy as some procedures may complicate the feasibility of a future liver transplantation procedure.

A study by Gines et al.[85] evaluated TIPS versus large volume paracentesis plus albumin in the control of refractory ascites. Patients with cirrhosis and refractory ascites were randomly assigned to TIPS (n = 35) or repeated paracentesis plus IV albumin (n = 35). The probability of survival without liver transplantation was 41% at 1 year and 26% at 2 years in the TIPS group, as compared with 35% and 30%, respectively in the paracentesis group not significant (NS). Recurrence of ascites and development of hepatorenal syndrome (49% and 9%, respectively) were lower in the TIPS group compared with the paracentesis group (83% and 31%, respectively; $p = 0.003$ and $p = 0.03$) whereas the frequency of severe hepatic encephalopathy was greater in the TIPS group ($p = 0.03$). The calculated costs of procedures performed per patient in the TIPS group were 103% greater than those in the paracentesis and albumin group.[85]

Treatment guidelines recommend TIPS for the treatment of refractory ascites in patients for whom paracentesis is contraindicated, ineffective as determined by the frequency of repeated paracentesis (more than three times per month), or intolerant of repeated large volume paracentesis.[42,86]

Peritoneovenous Shunt

A peritoneovenous shunt consists of a surgically implanted valve in the abdominal wall, an intra-abdominal cannula, and an outflow tube tunneled subcutaneously from the valve to a vein that empties directly into the superior vena cava. In this manner, ascitic fluid can be withdrawn from the abdominal cavity and be returned to the vascular space. Multiple contraindications exist to surgical shunts and significant surgical risks that increase with worsening hepatic function.[87] Gines et al.[88] compared peritoneovenous shunting (LaVeen Shunt) with paracentesis plus albumin infusions, and found shunting to be more effective in the long-term management of ascites as reflected by a longer period before readmission, a lower number of readmissions for ascites, and lower diuretic requirements. Peritoneovenous shunting did not improve survival over paracentesis, and the probability of shunt occlusion was 52% after 2 years.[88] In summary, the lack of survival benefit, surgical complications, including fibrous adhesions complicating future liver transplantation, and high risk of shunt occlusion have led to the reserving of peritoneovenous shunt procedures for patients with ascites and fairly well-preserved renal and hepatic function and are not candidates for liver transplantation, in whom more standard therapies fail.[42]

Clonidine

It has been shown that the activation of the sympathetic nervous system leads to renal hypoperfusion and sodium retention. The activated sympathetic nervous system stimulates renal α_1-adrenoreceptors and causes decreases in renal blood flow and glomerular filtration rate. Additionally, norepinephrine increases proximal tubular reabsorption of sodium and enhances renin, aldosterone, and vasopressin secretions.[89–91] Preliminary evidence has suggested that clonidine may be of benefit in refractory ascites and those with an activated sympathetic nervous system. Lenaerts et al.[92] conducted a very small study comparing repeated large volume paracentesis with the combination of clonidine–spironolactone in the treatment of patient with refractory ascites. Study patients (n = 20) were randomly assigned to receive repeated large volume paracentesis (4–5 L every 48 hours) plus IV albumin (7 g/L of ascites) until ascites disappeared, or a combination of clonidine 0.075 mg BID for 8 days and then clonidine 0.075 mg BID with spironolactone 200 to 400 mg daily for 10 days. Both groups were discharged with spironolactone adjusted according to individual response (maximal dose of 400 mg/day). During the first hospitalization, the mean weight loss in the paracentesis group was higher than in the clonidine group, but the mean hospital stay was shorter in the clonidine group ($p \leq 0.01$). Clonidine decreased sympathetic activity and increased glomerular filtration rate. During the follow-up, the number of rehospitalizations for ascites was higher and the mean time to the first readmission was shorter in the paracentesis group than in the clonidine group ($p \leq 0.01$).[92]

Lenaerts et al.[91] also studied the effects of clonidine on ascites treatment in patients with cirrhosis and an activated sympathetic nervous system (plasma norepinephrine concentration >300 picogram/mL). Patients were randomized to receive placebo (n = 32) or clonidine 0.075 mg BID (n = 32) for 3 months, as well as spironolactone 200 mg/day (furosemide 40 mg/day was added for insufficient response). Diuretics were individually titrated to response. The time needed for diuretic response was shorter and diuretic dosage lower in the clonidine group than placebo. In addition, the diuretic complications (hyperkalemia and renal impairment) were significantly lower in the clonidine group ($p < 0.01$). The time to the first readmission for tense ascites was shorter in the placebo group than in the clonidine group.[91] The addition of clonidine to diuretic therapy may be an effective therapeutic modality; however, a large randomized trial is needed to establish the role of clonidine in the treatment of ascites.

In consideration of R.W.'s increasing serum creatinine concentration, rising BUN, and the grave prognosis of hepatorenal syndrome, TIPS is a reasonable therapeutic alternative if R.W. cannot tolerate or requires frequent large volume paracentesis.

Spontaneous Bacterial Peritonitis

Pathogenesis

12. Should R.W. receive spontaneous bacterial peritonitis prophylaxis?

Spontaneous bacterial peritonitis is an infection that occurs in cirrhotic patients and accounts for about 25% of the infections in this population. SBP is defined as the spontaneous infection of the ascitic fluid in the absence of an identified intra-abdominal source of infection or inflammation. This condition has a mortality rate of about 30% to 50%.[93,94] The diagnosis of SBP is defined by a polymorphonuclear cell count (PMN) of $\geq$250 cells/mm^3 or a positive bacterial culture of the ascitic fluid. Patients with ascites caused by cirrhosis, with overlapping complications such as prior episodes of SBP and upper GI bleeding, and patients with low-protein (≤1 g/dL) ascites are at an increased risk for the development of SBP. Gram-negative enteric bacilli account for most SBP episodes (most commonly by *Escherichia coli* and *Klebsiella* species).[95,96] The primary mechanism for SBP is bacterial translocation from the gut, although multiple mechanisms have been proposed. Other factors in the pathogenesis of SBP may include the inability of the gut to contain bacteria and the failure of the immune system to clear the organisms once they have translocated. Cirrhosis can lead to intestinal bacterial overgrowth, and the intestinal permeability may be enhanced in cirrhotic patients with portal hypertension and bowel edema favoring bacterial translocation into the portal vein or lymphatics. Organisms may reach the systemic circulation from the mesenteric lymph nodes causing bacteremia. Deficiencies in the reticuloendothelial system in cirrhotic patients can lead to bacteria not being cleared from the circulation, which eventually leads to colonization of the ascitic fluid. Endogenous antimicrobial activity is diminished or nonexistent in patients with low-protein ascites, and if the immune system fails to destroy the bacteria, bacterascites (cultures from ascitic fluid are positive but the number of PMN is <250 cells/mm^3), in some cases, may progress to SBP (culture positive and PMN ≥250 cells/mm^3).[95,96]

Spontaneous Bacterial Peritonitis Prophylaxis

NORFLOXACIN

Because of its activity against aerobic enteric gram-negative bacilli and poor oral absorption, norfloxacin has been utilized for prophylaxis in patients at increased risk for SBP.[97] A multicenter, double-blind trial was conducted comparing norfloxacin 400 mg/day versus placebo in the prevention of SBP recurrence in cirrhotic patients (n = 80) with a prior episode of SBP. The results of the trial showed that the overall probability of SBP recurrence at 1 year of follow-up was 20% in the norfloxacin group and 68% in the placebo group ($p = 0.006$). Of note, in a small subset of patients (n = 6) who had stool cultures, norfloxacin administration produced a selective intestinal decontamination of aerobic gram-negative bacilli from the fecal flora without significant changes in other microorganisms.[98] In a prospective randomized study, selective intestinal decontamination with norfloxacin (n = 32) was compared with untreated controls (n = 31) in cirrhotic patients with low ascitic fluid total protein levels. A significantly lower incidence of infections and SBP were found (0% vs. 22.5%; $p < 0.05$) in patients receiving norfloxacin, but no significant change in mortality.[97,99] In a randomized controlled trial conducted by Fernandez et al.,[100] cirrhotic patients with low-protein ascitic levels (<1.5 g/dL) and with advanced liver failure (Child-Turcotte-Pugh score >9, serum bilirubin level >3 mg/dL), or impaired renal function (serum creatinine level >1.2 mg/dL, BUN >25 mg/dL, or serum sodium level <130 mEq/L) were included to compare norfloxacin (n = 35; 400 mg/day) with placebo (n = 33) in the primary prophylaxis of SBP. The trial showed a reduced incidence of SBP (7% vs. 61%; $p < 0.001$), and hepatorenal syndrome (28% vs. 41%; $p = 0.02$) in the norfloxacin group compared with placebo. There was also an improved 3-month (94% vs. 62%, $p = 0.003$) and 1-year (60% vs. 48%; $p = 0.05$) probability of survival in the norfloxacin group compared with placebo.[100]

One concern regarding norfloxacin prophylaxis is the emergence of infections caused by *E. coli* resistant to quinolones in cirrhotic patients undergoing prophylaxis with norfloxacin. Not surprisingly, a study by Ortiz et al.[101] showed that in cirrhotic patients with infections caused by norfloxacin-resistant *E. coli* as compared with those with norfloxacin-sensitive *E. coli*, were more likely to have received norfloxacin previously (82% vs. 22%; $p < 0.0001$).[101]

TRIMETHOPRIM-SULFAMETHOXAZOLE

Trimethoprim-sulfamethoxazole (n = 25; 160/800 mg/day given 5 days a week) has been compared with norfloxacin (n = 32; 400 mg/day) for SBP prophylaxis in patients with prior SBP and low-protein ascites. No significant difference in SBP recurrence was seen between the two groups (9.4% in the norfloxacin group and 16% in the trimethoprim-sulfamethoxazole; $p = 0.68$). Trimethoprim-sulfamethoxazole may be a reasonable alternative to norfloxacin, although the study was small. The incidences of side effects (skin rash, epigastric pain, and worsening of renal function) were higher in the trimethoprim-sulfamethoxazole group.[102] A meta-analysis was conducted to assess the effect of antibiotic prophylaxis (long-term administration of quinolones or trimethoprim-sulfamethoxazole) on prevention of infections and survival rate in cirrhotic patients with GI bleeding. Antibiotic prophylaxis significantly increased the mean survival rate by 9.1%.[103] Patients with a history of SBP and those with low-protein ascites with advanced liver failure or renal impairment appear to benefit from SBP prophylaxis.[42,97] Further studies are needed to evaluate the effectiveness of SBP prophylaxis for other subgroups of patients with low-protein ascites.[93,104] R.W. would benefit from the addition of SBP prophylaxis because he has had a prior episode of SBP. A reasonable prophylactic regimen would be long-term administration of norfloxacin 400 mg/day to prevent recurrence of SBP. This dosage is acceptable based on his renal function (estimated CrCl 26 mL/minute).[105]

ESOPHAGEAL VARICES

Treatment

13. C.V., a 55-year-old, pale-looking woman with known primary alcoholic cirrhosis, was admitted for a chief complaint of hematemesis. C.V. has a history of recurrent upper GI bleeding and documented esophageal varices. She has no other significant medical history. On examination, her blood pressure (BP) was 78/40 mmHg, pulse rate was 110 beats/minute, and respiratory rate was 22 breaths/minute. Her skin was cold; chest and cardiac examinations were within normal limits and abdominal examination revealed ascites and a palpable spleen. Bowel sounds were normal. Laboratory values included the following: Hgb 7 g/dL (normal, 11.5–15.5 g/dL); Hct 22% (normal, 33%–43%); albumin 3.0 g/dL (normal, 4–6 g/dL); AST 160 IU (normal, 0–35 IU); ALT 250 IU (normal, 0–35 IU); alkaline phosphatase 40 IU (normal, 30–120 IU); and creatinine 2.0 mg/dL (normal, 0.6–1.2 mg/dL; calculated creatinine clearance: 30 mL/minute). The PT was 18 seconds with a control of 12 secs (INR 1.5). Serum electrolytes were all within normal limits. An electrocardiogram (ECG) revealed sinus tachycardia. What are the immediate goals of therapy and treatment measures of the highest priority in managing C.V.'s hematemesis?

Goals of Therapy

Most patients with cirrhosis develop portal hypertension, which in turn can progress to bleeding varices (dilated veins in the upper GI tract that protrude into the esophageal or gastric lumens). Of patients with Child-Turcotte-Pugh A cirrhosis, 40% develop esophageal varices, as compared with 85% of those with Child-Turcotte-Pugh C.[106] Unless varices bleed, they do not cause significant complications or symptoms.

The progression and severity of varices is directly related to the severity of portal hypertension. The major sites of concern in portal hypertension are the coronary vein, draining the bottom of the esophagus and upper stomach, and the veins draining the spleen and lower GI tract. The scarring and fibrosis associated with cirrhosis initially leads to an increase in portal vein pressure (PVP). The PVP may eventually rise, causing backflow of blood supply and subsequent pressure in the veins coming off the portal vein. Hyperkinetic circulation in the branches of the portal vein raises the esophageal transmural pressure and increases the risk of upper GI bleeding. Because the veins are designed for low-pressure circulation (5–8 mmHg) and generally cannot tolerate a sustained hyperdynamic circulation, the shunting of high portal pressure blood results in gastric and esophageal varices. When PVP exceeds 12 mmHg, patients are at increased risk of variceal hemorrhage.[107]

Varices can be visualized only during a diagnostic endoscopy. Esophageal varices are graded as small or large (>5 mm). The presence or absence of red signs (red wale marks or red spots) on varices is also noted.[106]

Despite improvement in the management of portal hypertension, massive bleeding from esophageal or gastric varices is the leading cause of death in patients with cirrhosis.[108] Prevention of variceal bleeding is critical because the mortality rate remains at 32% in Child-Turcotte-Pugh classification C patients.[109] New varices develop at a rate of 5% to 10% per year in cirrhotic patients. Once varices develop, they enlarge by 4% to 10% each year.[110] Acute variceal bleeding is considered a medical emergency and should be treated immediately. Treatment goals include volume resuscitation, acute treatment of bleeding, and prevention of recurrence of variceal bleeding. Approximately 10% of patients are refractory to endoscopic and medical intervention and may require life-saving portal decompressive shunt surgery or TIPS.[111]

General Management

Resuscitation is the first priority in patients with acute bleeding episodes. An indwelling nasogastric tube (NG) should be placed, then saline or tap water lavage of the stomach, with suctioning of the gastric contents, should be initiated promptly to prevent airway complications such as aspiration pneumonia.[84,112] Obtunded or unconscious patients should be intubated to maintain and protect the airway. Pharmacologic treatment should be initiated immediately to reduce bleeding and the risk of hypotension-induced renal failure. The patient should also be monitored for any abnormal electrolyte and metabolic chemistries (e.g., potassium, sodium, bicarbonate), hypoxia (e.g., PO_2, pH), serum creatinine, and decreased urinary output.[112]

Rebleeding is most likely to occur within the first 48 hours in patients with large varices and in patients with advanced liver disease (i.e., Child-Turcotte-Pugh class C (Table 28-2). Factors associated with early rebleeding include age >60 years, acute renal failure, and severe initial bleeding defined by hemoglobin <8 g/dL at presentation. Risk factors for late rebleeding are severe liver failure, continued alcohol abuse, large variceal size, renal failure, and hepatocellular carcinoma.[113]

Hypovolemia/Blood Loss

Care should be taken when correcting hypovolemia so as not to increase the degree of portal hypertension by overtransfusion, which can increase the risk of further bleeding. Hypovolemia should be immediately managed to maintain mean arterial pressure at 80 mmHg and the hemoglobin at approximately 8 g/dL.[106,114] C.V.'s pallor, cold and clammy skin, rapid pulse, and a systolic BP <80 mmHg suggest significant hypotension and hypovolemia needing correction with whole blood or packed red cell transfusion along with fresh frozen plasma.[113,115]

Patients with liver disease and elevated bilirubin frequently develop some level of vitamin K deficiency because of fat malabsorption. Prolongation of the PT owing to vitamin K deficiency usually improves within 24 hours after a 10-mg subcutaneous or oral dose of vitamin K. A prolonged PT owing to poor hepatic synthetic function is not responsive to the administration of vitamin K, because the PT prolongation results from poor synthetic function rather than vitamin K deficiency. If the INR requires rapid correction because of bleeding or a planned invasive procedure, fresh frozen plasma should be transfused. Although vitamin K is often administered in the treatment of acute variceal bleeding, there is no data to support this practice.[116]

14. Three units of whole blood and two units of fresh frozen plasma were transfused initially. C.V.'s stomach was lavaged with saline, and the gastric aspirate from the NG tube continued to be strongly positive for blood. Four hours later, her bleeding still persisted. What other pharmacologic interventions can be used to control C.V.'s bleeding esophageal varices?

Several vasoconstricting drugs have been used to control variceal bleeding. The first, and at one time the gold standard, was vasopressin (Pitressin).[117,118] This naturally occurring hormone (also known as 8-arginine vasopressin, ADH) is produced by the posterior pituitary and was originally derived for the treatment of diabetes insipidus in persons with pituitary insufficiency. Its use to control variceal bleeding is a non–U.S. Food and Drug Administration (FDA)-labeled use that takes advantage of its intense smooth muscle and vasoconstrictive properties. Because efficacy of vasopressin for treatment of esophageal bleeding is limited and adverse effects (e.g., abdominal cramping, arrhythmias, and gangrene) are of great concern (Table 28-3), it has largely been replaced by octreotide. Nonetheless, some clinicians still prescribe vasopressin.

Octreotide

Octreotide (Sandostatin) is a synthetic analog of the somatostatin, with similar pharmacologic properties and a slightly longer half-life. Somatostatin is available in Europe, but is substituted with octreotide or vapreotide (orphan drug status) in the United States (Table 28-3).[117,119,120] Octreotide is shown to be effective for controlling acute variceal bleeding and appears comparable in efficacy to vasopressin and balloon tamponade, with fewer side effects. Octreotide is administered as a 50- to

Table 28-3 Treatment of Acute Bleeding

Therapy	*Mechanism*	*Side Effects and Risks*
Octreotide	Selective and potent vasoconstrictor that reduces portal and collateral blood flow by constricting splanchnic vessels	Diarrhea, hyperglycemia, hypoglycemia, constipation, rectal spasms, abnormal stools, headache, dizziness, and fat malabsorption
Vasopressin	Nonspecific vasoconstrictor of all parts of the vascular bed	Abdominal cramping, nausea, tremor, skin blanching, phlebitis, hematoma at the site of the infusion, worsening of hypertension, angina, arrhythmias, myocardial infarction, bowel necrosis, gangrene, and dilutional hyponatremia
Endoscopic band ligation (EBL) or endoscopic variceal ligation (EVL)	An elastic band is placed around the mucosa and submucosa of the esophageal area containing the varix, leading to strangulation, fibrosis, and ideally obliteration of the varix	Moderate bleeding, hypotension, gastrointestinal discomfort, esophageal ulceration, and perforation
Sclerotherapy	Injection of 0.5 to 5 mL of a sclerosing agent (e.g., concentrated saline: 11.5% NaCl or ethanolamine oleate [Ethamolin]) into each varix at points about 2 cm apart to induce immediate hemostasis (cessation of bleeding within 2 to 5 min)	Esophageal ulceration, stricture formation, esophageal perforation, retrosternal chest pain, and temporary dysphagia
Balloon tamponade	Bleeding is controlled by direct compression of the varices at the gastroesophageal junction or at the bleeding site by a Sengstaken-Blakemore tube or Lintern tube (gastric varices only). The tube is passed through the mouth and into the stomach. A balloon is then inflated, which applies direct compression to the varices.	Aspiration (>10% incidence), pressure necrosis, pneumonitis, esophageal ulceration and rupture, bleeding on balloon deflation, chest pain, asphyxia (aspiration may be minimized by endotracheal intubation and continued aspiration of oropharyngeal secretions)
Transjugular intrahepatic portal systemic shunt (TIPS)	A conduit between the hepatic vein and intrahepatic segment of the portal vein with an expandable metal stent is placed during an angiographic procedure. This channel allows blood to return to the systemic circulation and reduces portal pressure.	Bleeding, thrombosis, stenosis, severe encephalopathy, hepatic failure, shunt occlusion and shunt migration

100-mcg bolus followed by an infusion of 25 to 50 mcg/hour for 18 hours to 5 days. In one study, patients ($n = 68$) with portal hypertension and upper GI bleed were randomized to receive octreotide ($n = 24$), vasopressin ($n = 22$), or omeprazole ($n = 22$). Complete bleeding control was achieved in all patients receiving octreotide after 48 hours of therapy compared with 64% of vasopressin-treated patients, and 59% in the omeprazole groups ($p < 0.005$). Patients receiving vasopressin also experienced more side effects (abdominal cramps, nausea, tremor, decreased cardiac output, myocardial ischemia, and bronchial constriction) than those receiving octreotide or omeprazole ($p < 0.01$). In the patients with bleeding not controlled within 48 hours in the vasopressin and omeprazole groups, complete bleeding control was subsequently achieved by octreotide.[121] In a meta-analysis of octreotide and somatostatin versus vasopressin in the management of acute esophageal variceal bleeds (6 trials; $n = 275$), octreotide and somatostatin appeared to be more effective in controlling acute bleeding (82% vs. 55%; p = NS) and had less adverse effects requiring discontinuation than vasopressin (0 vs. 10%; $p = 0.00007$).[122] In general, both octreotide and somatostatin are fairly well tolerated.[121] Although some centers may still initiate therapy with vasopressin, most will use octreotide as first-line therapy and reserve vasopressin for treatment failures.

Vasopressin

Vasopressin (Table 28-3) is effective in reducing or terminating bleeding in approximately 60% of patients with variceal hemorrhage.[117,118] Of concern are reports of patients developing hypertension, angina, arrhythmias, and rarely, myocardial infarction while receiving vasopressin. Vasopressin is given as a continuous IV infusion because of its short half-life. To minimize dose-related adverse effects, the lowest effective dosage should be used. Vasopressin may be administered by peripheral IV infusion, but use of a central vein is preferred because of the risk of tissue necrosis if extravasation occurs. Most commonly, vasopressin is initiated as a continuous IV infusion of 0.2 to 0.4 unit/minute, and increased every hour by 0.2 unit/minute until control of bleeding is obtained (maximal dose 0.9 unit/minute). Approximately 12 hours after the control of bleeding, the infusion rate can be decreased by half. Higher doses should be avoided because dosages exceeding 1 unit/minute fail to control hemorrhage in patients who are unresponsive to lower dosages.[123] When the bleeding is controlled, it is customary to taper vasopressin over 24 to 48 hours, but tapering does not appear to decrease the incidence of rebleeding or side effects.[117] Because of the potential for serious cardiovascular and dermatologic complications caused by nonspecific vasoconstriction, vasopressin should be used only when necessary and for a duration necessary to control bleeding. The duration of infusion should not exceed 72 hours.

Nitroglycerin can help to minimize the side effects of vasopressin. Nitroglycerin administration may also enhance the reduction in portal pressure and reduce the adverse vascular and cardiac effects. When given by IV infusion, the nitroglycerin dosage is 40 to 200 mcg/min.[117,119,124] A randomized trial by Gimson et al.[125] was conducted to determine the efficacy of nitroglycerin when added to a vasopressin. The results of the trial found a lower rate of complications in the vasopressin and nitroglycerin group compared with vasopressin alone. Combination therapy was also more effective in controlling variceal hemorrhage. A total of 57 patients received either vasopressin or vasopressin plus nitroglycerin, for an infusion period of 12 hours. At the end of the 12-hour period, hemorrhage was controlled in 68% receiving combined therapy versus 44% in those given vasopressin alone ($p < 0.05$). Major complications requiring cessation of therapy were less common in those given nitroglycerin compared with those given vasopressin alone ($p < 0.02$).[125] Interestingly, a meta-analysis of four randomized controlled trials ($n = 157$) comparing vasopressin for the acute treatment of variceal bleeding with nonactive treatment or placebo found no difference in mortality.[117]

Terlipressin

Terlipressin (Glypressin), a synthetic analog of vasopressin and a prodrug of lypressin (currently not available in the United States), effectively controls acute bleeding from esophageal varices in 80% of patients. Fewer cardiovascular side effects have been associated with terlipressin than with vasopressin.[126] Octreotide, vapreotide, vasopressin, and terlipressin have been shown to have efficacy in the control of acute variceal hemorrhage.[127,128] Terlipressin, however, is the only medication for the acute treatment of variceal hemorrhage that has been shown to improve patient survival. In a meta-analysis of seven randomized, placebo-controlled trials ($n = 443$), terlipressin led to significant reductions in mortality as compared with placebo (relative risk [RR] of 0.66; 95% CI 0.49–0.88).[129]

Pharmacologic therapy (somatostatin or its analogues [octreotide or vapreotide] or terlipressin) should be initiated as soon as variceal hemorrhage is suspected and continued for 3 to 5 days after diagnosis is confirmed.[106]

Endoscopic Variceal Ligation and Sclerotherapy

15. Vasopressin and octreotide are nonspecific vasoconstrictors that require continuous IV infusion and carry a risk of systemic side effects. What are endoscopic variceal ligation, sclerotherapy, and balloon tamponade?

After successful resuscitation, endoscopy should be performed within 12 hours to establish the cause of bleeding. Fiberoptic endoscopy allows direct visualization of the esophagus and location of the bleeding sites. Those with actively bleeding varices can be treated with endoscopic variceal ligation (EVL), sclerotherapy, or balloon tamponade. EVL is a well-tolerated procedure (Table 28-3).[127,130–134] Villanueva et al.[135] conducted a randomized, controlled trial comparing variceal ligation and sclerotherapy as an emergency endoscopic treatment added to somatostatin infusion in acute variceal bleeding. Patients admitted with acute GI bleeding and with suspected cirrhosis received somatostatin infusion (for 5 days). Endoscopy was performed within 6 hours and those with esophageal variceal bleeding were randomized to receive either sclerotherapy ($n = 89$) or ligation ($n = 90$). The authors found that the use of variceal ligation instead of sclerotherapy had a lower failure rate (4% vs. 15%; $p = 0.02$), and a lower transfusion requirement ($p = 0.05$). No statistically significant differences were found in mortality. Adverse effects (e.g., aspiration pneumonia, esophageal bleeding, ulceration, and chest pain) occurred in 28% of patients receiving sclerotherapy and 14% with ligation (RR = 1.9, 95% CI = 1.1 to 3.5; $p = 0.03$).[135] In another similar but smaller study, Sarin et al.[136] found that the rate of rebleeding was lower in the EVL group ($n = 47$) than in the sclerotherapy group ($n = 48$) (6.4% vs. 20.8%; $p < 0.05$). EVL is the recommended form of therapy for acute esophageal variceal bleeding, although sclerotherapy may be used in the acute setting if ligation is technically difficult. Endoscopic treatments are best used in combination with pharmacologic therapy, which preferably should be started before endoscopy.[128] The AASLD Practice Guidelines Committee and the Practice Parameters Committee of the American College of Gastroenterology (ACG) on the Prevention and Management of Gastroesophageal Varices and Variceal Hemorrhage in Cirrhosis recommend that for the control and management of acute hemorrhage, the combination of vasoconstrictive pharmacologic therapy and variceal ligation is the preferred approach.[106]

Balloon Tamponade

Balloon tamponade controls bleeding by direct compression at the bleeding site (Table 28-3). It is important to remember that balloon tamponade is only a temporary measure and can cause pressure necrosis after 48 to 72 hours. Thus, the balloon should be deflated after 12 to 24 hours. Balloon tamponade will achieve temporary control of the bleeding and allow time for other measures (e.g., EVL or sclerotherapy) to be undertaken. Also, deflation and removal of the tube can result in removal of the fibrin scab at the bleeding site, resulting in rebleeding. Balloon tamponade is only used in massive bleeding and for a maximum of 24 hours, as a temporary 'bridge' until definitive treatment can be instituted.[106,127,137,138]

Alternative Treatment Modalities

16. C.V. was immediately treated with octreotide and EVL. Although the procedure was transiently successful, variceal bleeding has developed again. What alternative treatment modalities could be used?

Although the combination of pharmacotherapy (somatostatin, terlipressin, or octreotide) in combination with endoscopic procedures (EVL or sclerotherapy) has been shown to be beneficial in controlling acute bleeding, a chance exists for variceal rebleeding episodes.[106,127] Poor responders to initial therapy may require surgical correction of the underlying portal hypertension to control the bleeding.

TRANSJUGULAR INTRAHEPATIC PORTAL SYSTEMIC SHUNT

Henderson et al.[139] conducted a prospective, randomized, multicenter trial comparing distal splenorenal shunts (DSRS) or TIPS for variceal bleeding refractory to medical treatment with β-blockers and endoscopic therapy. Patients with Child-Turcotte-Pugh class A and B cirrhosis ($n = 140$) and refractory variceal bleeding were enrolled and randomized to DSRS or TIPS with a follow-up for 2 to 8 years. No significant differences were found in survival at 2 and 5 years (DSRS, 81% and 62%; TIPS, 88% and 61%, respectively). Thrombosis, stenosis, and reintervention rates were significantly higher in the TIPS group (DSRS, 11%; TIPS, 82%; $p < 0.001$). Rebleeding, encephalopathy, ascites, need for transplantation, quality of life, and costs did not significantly differ between groups. DSRS and TIPS had similar efficacy in the control of refractory variceal bleeding in Child-Turcotte-Pugh class A and B patients, although reintervention rates were significantly greater for TIPS compared with DSRS.[139] TIPS has the advantage of being less invasive and faster than surgical portal systemic shunts. Long-term patency of the TIPS remains problematic (Table 28-3).[130] TIPS can be used as a bridge to liver transplantation, and may be an effective option for nonsurgical patients or those with advanced cirrhosis (Child-Turcotte-Pugh Score C) with recurrent bleeding, uncontrolled by pharmacologic and endoscopic therapy.[106,127,140,141]

SURGERY

Surgical creation of a portacaval shunt has been effective in reducing portal pressure and in preventing recurrent bleeding. These shunts, however, are associated with a high incidence of hepatic encephalopathy and may exacerbate hepatic parenchymal dysfunction by shunting blood away from the liver. Mesocaval shunts and distal splenorenal shunts are also effective in preventing variceal rebleeding and may be associated with a lower incidence of hepatic encephalopathy.[142]

Infection Prophylaxis—Short-Term Antibiotics

Short-term administration of antibiotics for the prevention of bacterial infections in patients with variceal hemorrhage has shown favorable results.[93,143,144] In a prospective, randomized trial comparing norfloxacin 400 mg BID for 7 days (n = 60) with no treatment controls (n = 59), the norfloxacin group had a significantly lower incidence of SBP (3.3% vs. 16.9%; $p < 0.05$); although, the decrease in mortality (6.6% vs. 11.8%) did not reach statistical significance.[143] Because of the emergence of infections caused by quinolone-resistant bacteria, Fernandez et al.[144] compared oral norfloxacin versus IV ceftriaxone in the prophylaxis of bacterial infection in cirrhotic patients with GI hemorrhage. Patients were randomly assigned to oral norfloxacin 400 mg BID (n = 57) or IV ceftriaxone 1 g/day (n = 54) for 7 days. Antibiotics were initiated following emergency endoscopy and within 12 hours of hospital admission. The probability of developing proved infections (26% vs. 11%; $p < 0.03$), and bacteremia or spontaneous bacterial peritonitis (12% vs. 2%, $p < 0.03$) was significantly higher in patients receiving norfloxacin as compared with ceftriaxone. No significant difference was seen in mortality, within the 10 days after inclusion, between treatment groups.[144]

The AASLD and ACG consensus guidelines recommend 7 days of antibiotic prophylaxis for prevention of SBP in patients with variceal hemorrhage with oral norfloxacin (400 mg BID) or ciprofloxacin IV (400 mg BID) when oral administration is not possible. Ceftriaxone IV (1 g/day) may be a preferable option in centers with a high prevalence of quinolone-resistant organisms.[106] C.V. should be treated with norfloxacin 400 mg orally once daily (dose adjusted for creatinine clearance of 30 mL/minute), or ceftriaxone 1 g/day for 7 days to prevent SBP.

Primary Prophylaxis

17. All variceal hemorrhage interventions up to this point were aimed at terminating the acute bleeding episode. Could drug therapy have helped prevent the first episode of bleeding from C.V.'s esophageal varices?

Preventing the initial occurrence of variceal bleeding is referred to as *primary prevention* or *primary prophylaxis*. Pharmacologic prophylaxis is aimed at reducing the HVPG to ≤12 mmHg, or a decrease in baseline of ≥20%.[145,146] In a small study by Vorobioff et al.,[145] none of the patients with HVPG ≤12 mmHg (n = 6) bled from portal hypertensive-related causes as compared to 42% in the HVPG >12 mmHg group (n = 24). In addition, only 1 of the 6 patients with a HVPG ≤12 mmHg as compared with 16 in the HVPG >12 mmHg group died during the study period ($p < 0.06$). This study suggests that patients with an HVPG ≤12 mmHg may have a better prognosis than those with HVPG >12 mmHg. Escorsell et al.[146] has shown that a fall of HVPG by ≥20% from baseline was associated with a decreased risk of variceal bleeding (6% vs. 45%; $p = 0.004$).

β-BLOCKERS

Nonselective β-adrenergic blockers decrease portal pressure through a reduction in portal venous inflow as a result of a decrease in cardiac output (β_1-adrenergic blockade) and splanchnic blood flow (β_2-adrenergic blockade). They are the most frequently studied drug class for primary prevention of bleeding. Only nonselective β-blockers have an adrenergic dilatory effect in mesenteric arterioles resulting in a decrease in portal blood circulation and pressure. Nonselective β-blockers have been studied in comparison with other modalities of treatment, such as endoscopic variceal ligation, for the primary prevention of variceal hemorrhage in patients with existing varices in a number of randomized trials.[147,148] Usual starting dosages of propranolol are 10 mg three times a day, or nadolol 20 mg daily. Selective β-blockers (e.g., atenolol and metoprolol) have little effect on mesenteric arterioles and have not been shown to be effective in primary prophylaxis.[149]

Propranolol or nadolol, given in dosages to reduce the resting heart rate to 55 to 60 beats/minute or by 25%, have been shown to prevent or delay the first episode of variceal bleeding.[17] Nonselective β-blockers are considered first-line therapy in the prevention of variceal hemorrhage based on numerous randomized, placebo-controlled trials and meta-analyses.[127,150] For example, Pascal et al.[151] conducted a prospective, randomized, multicenter, single-blind trial of propranolol compared with placebo in the prevention of bleeding in patients with large esophageal varices without previous bleeding. Patients received either propranolol (n = 118) or placebo (n = 112), with the endpoints of the study being bleeding and death. The dosage of propranolol was progressively increased to decrease the heart rate by 20% to 25%. The cumulative percentages of patients free of bleeding 2 years after inclusion in the study (74% vs. 39%; $p < 0.05$) and cumulative 2-year survival (72% vs. 51%; $p < 0.05$) were higher in the propranolol group versus the placebo group.

The role of propranolol added to EVL in the prevention of first variceal bleeding has also been compared with EVL alone as primary prophylaxis. Sarin et al.[152] conducted a prospective, randomized, controlled trial comparing EVL with propranolol (n = 72) with EVL alone (n = 72) in the prevention of first variceal bleeding among patients with high-risk varices. EVL was performed at 2-week intervals until obliteration of varices. Propranolol was administered at a dosage sufficient to reduce heart rate to 55 beats/minute or 25% reduction from baseline, and continued after obliteration of varices. No significant differences were seen in the rates of bleeding and survival between groups, although more patients in the EVL alone group had recurrence of varices ($p = 0.03$).[152]

Treatment with a β-blocker must be continued indefinitely. A study by Abraczinskas et al.[153] reported the outcomes of patients in whom β-blocker therapy was discontinued. Patients completing a prospective, randomized, double-blind, placebo-controlled trial of propranolol for the primary prevention of variceal hemorrhage were tapered off of propranolol and placebo and followed prospectively for subsequent events. The authors found that when propranolol was withdrawn, the risk of variceal hemorrhage increased from 4% (while on propranolol therapy) to 24% (after propranolol withdrawal), and was comparable to the risk of bleeding in an untreated population (22% in the placebo group from the previous study). The authors suggested that the protective effect of propranolol against variceal hemorrhage was no longer present. Also, patients who discontinued β-blockers experienced increased mortality compared with the untreated population (48% vs. 21%; $p < 0.05$).[153] Therefore, avoiding sudden discontinuation of β-blockers in this population is essential.

The AASLD/ACG guidelines recommend nonselective β-blockers for primary prophylaxis in patients with small varices that have not bled but are at increased risk of hemorrhage (Child B or C or presence of red wale marks on varices). Patients with medium or large varices that have not bled but are at a high risk of hemorrhage (Child B or C or variceal red wale markings on endoscopy), nonselective β-blockers or EVL may be recommended. In contrast, patients with medium or large varices that have not bled and are not at the highest risk of hemorrhage (Child A patients and no red signs), nonselective β-blockers are preferred and EVL should be considered in patients with contraindications or intolerance or noncompliance to β-blockers. The β-blocker should be titrated to the maximal tolerated dose.[106]

ISOSORBIDE-5-MONONITRATE

Isosorbide-5-mononitrate has been evaluated as primary prophylaxis for variceal hemorrhage as monotherapy in patients intolerant or refractory to β-blockers and in combination with β-blockers in a number of trials and in prior consensus conferences.[154] Isosorbide-5-mononitrate in combination with β-blockers has had mixed success, however, when studied for primary prevention of bleeding in patients with cirrhosis. Also, its use as monotherapy has not proved to be effective.[154,155] Garcia-Pagan et al.[155] conducted a multicenter, prospective, double-blind randomized controlled trial evaluating whether isosorbide-5-mononitrate prevented variceal bleeding in cirrhotic patients (n = 133) with gastroesophageal varices, who had contraindications or could not tolerate β-blockers. Patient received isosorbide-5-mononitrate (n = 67) or placebo (n = 66). No significant differences were noted in the 1- and 2-year actuarial probability of bleeding or survival between the two treatment groups.[155]

When combined with a β-blocker, isosorbide-5-mononitrate causes a greater reduction in the hepatic venous pressure gradient than propranolol alone.[156] Merkel et al.[157] examined the value of combining nadolol and isosorbide-5-mononitrate for primary prevention of variceal bleeding. Patients in the nadolol monotherapy group (n = 74) received between 40 and 160 mg/day titrated to achieve a 20% to 25% decrease in resting heart rate. Patients receiving both drugs (n = 72) received nadolol and isosorbide-5-mononitrate 10 to 20 mg orally BID. The overall risk of variceal bleeding was 18% in the nadolol group compared with 7.5% in the combined treatment group ($p = 0.03$). A higher number of patients had to be withdrawn from the study owing to side effects in the group receiving combination therapy compared with the nadolol monotherapy group (8 vs. 4 patients).[157] The AASLD and ACG guidelines suggest that nitrates (either alone or in combination with β-blockers), shunt therapy, or sclerotherapy should not be used in the primary prophylaxis of variceal hemorrhage.[106]

Secondary Prophylaxis

18. C.V.'s hepatologist would like to start treatment to prevent further variceal hemorrhage. What are the long-term objectives for the treatment of C.V.? What treatment approaches can be used to prevent a recurrence of bleeding (secondary prevention)?

Secondary prevention or *secondary prophylaxis* is the terminology used to describe therapy to prevent rebleeding once it has occurred. All patients who survive a variceal bleeding episode should receive therapy to prevent recurrent episodes. It is important that the initiation of β-blockers be delayed until after recovery of the initial variceal hemorrhage. Initiation of a β-blocker during the treatment of an acute bleed would block the patient's acute tachycardia in response to his or her hypotension, which may adversely impact survival. The benefit of nonselective β-blockers in the prevention of rebleeding episodes has been demonstrated by a number of trials.[130,158,159] For example, a trial by Colombo et al.[158] studied the efficacy of β-blockers in preventing rebleeding in cirrhotic patients. Patients were randomly assigned to propranolol (n = 32), atenolol (n = 32), or placebo (n = 30). Randomization was made at least 15 days after the bleeding episode. Propranolol was given orally and titrated until the resting pulse rate was reduced by approximately 25%, and atenolol was given at a fixed dose of 100 mg daily. The incidence of rebleeding was significantly lower in patients receiving propranolol than in those on placebo ($p = 0.01$). Bleeding-free survival was better for patients on active drugs than for those on placebo (propranolol vs. placebo, $p = 0.01$; atenolol versus placebo, $p = 0.05$).[158]

Eradication of varices by endoscopic procedures is also effective in preventing recurrent variceal bleeding.[17,159] A study by de la Pena et al.[159] showed that nadolol plus EVL (n = 43) reduced the incidence of variceal rebleeding compared with EVL alone (n = 37). Variceal bleeding recurrence rate was 14% in the EVL plus nadolol group and 38% in the EVL group ($p = 0.006$). Mortality was similar in both groups and the actuarial probability of variceal recurrence at 1 year was lower in the EVL plus nadolol group than in the EVL alone group (54% vs. 77%; $p = 0.06$). The adverse effects in the β-blocker group were high, and led to the withdrawal of 20% to 30% of patients.[159] Interestingly, Gonzalez-Suarez et al.[160] conducted a study to compare the occurrence of SBP in cirrhotic patients treated with nadolol plus isosorbide mononitrate (n = 115) versus sclerotherapy or endoscopic variceal ligation (n = 115) for the prevention of rebleeding. They found that the probability of SBP was lower in the medication group at 1 year (6% vs. 12%; $p = 0.08$) and at 5 years (22% vs. 36%; $p = 0.08$). The probability of survival was similar in both groups.[160]

TIPS may be an option for those patients who fail both EVL and prophylaxis with β-blocker therapy. Escorsell et al.[161] studied 91 Child-Turcotte-Pugh class B or C cirrhotic patients surviving their first episode of variceal bleeding. Subjects were randomized to TIPS ($n = 47$) or combination therapy with propranolol and isosorbide-5-mononitrate ($n = 44$) to prevent variceal rebleeding. Rebleeding occurred in a lower percentage of patients treated with TIPS versus those treated with drug (13% vs. 39%; $p = 0.007$). The 2-year rebleeding probability was lower in the TIPS group (13% vs. 49%; $p = 0.01$). Encephalopathy was more frequent in TIPS than in patients treated with drug (38% vs. 14%, $p = 0.007$). Child-Turcotte-Pugh class improved more frequently in those treated with drug than with TIPS (72% vs. 45%; $p = 0.04$). The 2-year survival probability was identical (72%). The cost of therapy was double for TIPS treatment. Drug therapy was less effective than TIPS in preventing rebleeding; however, drug therapy caused less encephalopathy, had identical survival, and more frequent improvement in Child-Turcotte-Pugh class with lower costs than TIPS in high-risk cirrhotic patients.[161]

The AASLD/ACG guidelines suggest the use of a combination of nonselective β-blockers plus EVL for secondary prophylaxis. TIPS should be considered in patients who are Child A or B who experience recurrent variceal hemorrhage despite combination pharmacological and endoscopic therapy.[106]

Depending on the size of C.V.'s varices on endoscopy and the risk of hemorrhage, C.V. should have been given nonselective β-blockers (propranolol or nadolol) or EVL to prevent or delay the first episode of variceal bleeding. Because C.V. has a history of recurrent upper GI bleeding, the best option to prevent further bleeding is to initiate a nonselective β-blocker and begin EVL. The β-blocker should be titrated to reduce the resting heart rate to 55 to 60 beats/minute or by 25%. EVL should be repeated every 1 to 2 weeks until obliteration with a repeat endoscopy performed 1 to 3 months after obliteration and then every 6 to 12 months to check for variceal recurrence.[106] If this combination fails to prevent variceal hemorrhage, then TIPS would be considered as a therapeutic option.

HEPATIC ENCEPHALOPATHY

19. R.C., a 57-year-old man, was admitted to the hospital because of nausea, vomiting, and abdominal pain. He had a long history of alcohol abuse, with multiple hospital admissions for alcoholic gastritis and alcohol withdrawal. Physical examination revealed a cachectic male patient with clouded mentation who was not responsive to questions about name and place. Tense ascites and edema were noted, and the liver was percussed at 9 cm below the right costal margin. The spleen was not palpated, and no active bowel sounds were heard. Laboratory results on admission included the following: Na 132 mEq/L; K 3.7 mEq/L; Cl 98 mEq/L; bicarbonate 27 mEq/L; BUN 24 mg/dL; SrCr 1.4 mg/dL; Hgb 9.2 g/dL; Hct 24.1%; AST 520 IU (normal, 0–35 IU); alkaline phosphatase 218 IU (normal, 30–120 IU); lactate dehydrogenase (LDH) 305 IU (normal, 82–226); and total bilirubin 3.5 mg/dL. PT was 22 seconds with a control of 12 seconds (INR 1.8).

A 60-g protein, 2,000-kcal diet was ordered. Furosemide 40 mg IV every 12 hours was ordered in an attempt to reduce the edema and ascites. Morphine sulfate and prochlorperazine (Compazine) were ordered for his abdominal pain and nausea, respectively. Two days after admission, R.C. had an episode of hematemesis. He became mentally confused and at times nonresponsive to verbal command. An NG tube was inserted and coffee ground material was produced on continuous suctioning. Saline lavage was continued until the aspirate became clear. The next morning, R.C. was still in a confused mental state. He demonstrated prominent asterixis, and fetor hepaticus was noted in his breath. On the second day of his hospitalization, laboratory data were as follows: Hgb 7.4 g/dL; Hct 21.2%; K 3.1 mEq/L; SrCr 1.4 mg/dL; BUN 36 mg/dL; PT 22 seconds with a control of 12 seconds (INR 1.8); and guaiac positive stool. Hepatic encephalopathy and upper GI bleeding were added to the problem list.

What aspects of R.C.'s history are compatible with a diagnosis of hepatic encephalopathy?

Hepatic coma or encephalopathy is a metabolic disorder of the central nervous system (CNS), which occurs in patients with either advanced cirrhosis or fulminate hepatic failure. It is commonly accompanied by portal systemic shunting of blood. The clinical features (as seen in R.C.) include altered mental state, asterixis, and fetor hepaticus. During the early phase of encephalopathy, the altered mental state may present as a slight derangement of judgment and personality, and change in sleep pattern or mood. Drowsiness and confusion become more prominent as the encephalopathy progresses. Finally, unresponsiveness to arousal and deep coma ensue.

Asterixis, or flapping tremor, is the most characteristic neurologic abnormality in hepatic encephalopathy. This tremor can be demonstrated by having the patient hyperextend his or her wrist with the forearms outstretched and fingers separated. It is characterized by bilateral, but synchronous, repetitive arrhythmic motions occurring in bursts of one flap (twitch) every 1 to 2 seconds. Asterixis is not specific for hepatic encephalopathy and may also be present in uremia, hypokalemia, heart failure, ketoacidosis, respiratory failure, and sedative overdose.

Fetor hepaticus, a peculiar sweetish, musty, pungent odor to the breath, is believed to be caused by circulating unmetabolized mercaptans. A staging scheme for grading the severity of hepatic encephalopathy is found in Table 28-4.[162,163] As discussed in the questions that follow, the pharmacologic management of encephalopathy is guided by both an understanding of the pathogenesis of this disorder and the stage of severity demonstrated by the individual patient. In most cases, hepatic encephalopathy is fully reversible; therefore, it is likely a metabolic or neurophysiologic rather than an organic disorder.[162] Progressive hepatic encephalopathy (a plasma ammonia level >150 μmol/L), however, can lead to irreversible brain damage caused by increased intracranial pressure, brain herniations, and death.[164,165]

Pathogenesis

20. What is the pathogenesis of hepatic encephalopathy?

Several theories exist about the pathogenesis of hepatic encephalopathy. The most widely referenced theories involve abnormal ammonia metabolism, altered ratio of branched chain to aromatic amino acids, imbalance in brain neurotransmitters, such as γ-aminobutyric acid (GABA) and serotonin,

Table 28-4 Stages of Encephalopathy

Physical Sign	Stage I Prodrome	Stage II Impending Coma	Stage III Stupor	Stage IV Coma	Stage V Coma
Mental status	Alert; slow mentation; euphoria, occasional depression, confusion; sleep pattern reversal	Stage I signs amplified; lethargic, sleepy	Arousable, but generally asleep; significant confusion	Unarousable or responds only to pain	Unarousable
Behavior	Restless, irritable, disordered speech	Combative, sullen, loss of sphincter control	Sleeping, confusion, incoherent speech	None	None
Spontaneous motor activity	Uncoordinated with tremor	Yawning, grimacing, blinking	Decreased, severe tremor	Absent	None
Asterixis	Absent	Present	Present	Absent	Absent
Reflexes	Normal	Hyperactive	Hyperactive + Babinski	Hyperactive + Babinski	Absent

derangement in the blood brain–barrier, and exposure of the brain to accumulated "toxins".[166] None of these are considered to be a single cause, and the pathogenesis of hepatic encephalopathy is likely to be multifactorial.

Ammonia

Ammonia is a byproduct of protein metabolism, and a large portion is derived from dietary ingestion of proteins or presentation of protein-rich blood into the GI tract (e.g., from bleeding esophageal varices). Bacteria present in the GI tract digest protein into polypeptides, amino acids, and ammonia. These substances are then absorbed across the intestinal mucosa, where they are either further metabolized, stored for later use, or used for production of new proteins. Ammonia is readily metabolized in the liver to urea, which is then renally eliminated. When blood flow and hepatic metabolism are impaired by cirrhosis, serum and CNS concentrations of ammonia are increased. The ammonia that enters the CNS combines with α-ketoglutarate to form glutamine, an aromatic amino acid. Ammonia has been considered central to the pathogenesis of hepatic encephalopathy. An increased ammonia level raises the amount of glutamine within astrocytes, causing an osmotic imbalance resulting in cell swelling and ultimately brain edema. Although high serum ammonia and cerebrospinal glutamine concentrations are characteristic of encephalopathy, they may not be the actual cause of this syndrome.[165,167]

Amino Acid Balance

Body stores of branched chain and aromatic amino acids are affected by their rate of synthesis from protein metabolism (both in the GI tract and in the liver), their utilization in the resynthesis of new proteins within the liver, and their utilization by various tissues for energy. In both acute and chronic liver failure, the serum concentrations of aromatic amino acids significantly increase and the ratio of the branched chain to aromatic amino acids is altered as a result. The utilization of branched chain amino acids for skeletal muscle metabolism during liver failure can decrease branched chain amino acids.[166] At the same time, the blood–brain barrier appears to be more permeable to aromatic amino acid uptake into the cerebrospinal fluid (CSF). Once in the CSF, some aromatic compounds can be metabolized to produce "false neurotransmitters" (e.g., tyrosine conversion to octopamine) that disrupt normal CSF neurotransmitter balance, and compete with norepinephrine for normal CNS function.[167]

γ-Aminobutyric Acid

Schafer et al.[168] proposed that, in liver disease, gut-derived GABA escapes hepatic metabolism, crosses the blood–brain barrier, binds to its postsynaptic receptor sites, and causes the neurologic abnormalities associated with hepatic encephalopathy. Others hypothesize that endogenous benzodiazepinelike substances, via their agonist properties, contribute to the pathogenesis of hepatic encephalopathy by enhancing GABA-ergic neurotransmission. The role of GABA and endogenous benzodiazepines in hepatic encephalopathy is still not clearly defined and requires further clarification.[169,170]

Of all the toxins suspected to cause hepatic coma, ammonia and certain aromatic amino acids are those most commonly studied. Other precipitating factors (Table 28-5) increase the serum ammonia or produce excessive somnolence in patients with impending hepatic coma. Excess nitrogen load and metabolic abnormalities may increase ammonia levels and precipitate an exacerbation of hepatic encephalopathy.[171,172]

21. What are the probable precipitating causes of hepatic encephalopathy in R.C.?

The main precipitating cause of the encephalopathy in R.C. was the sudden onset of upper GI bleeding. The bacterial degradation of blood in the gut results in absorption of large amounts of ammonia and possibly other toxins into the portal system. Other important contributory factors in this case are diuretic-induced hypovolemia (BUN:Serum creatinine ratio, >20), hypokalemia (potassium, 3.1 mEq/L), and potentially metabolic alkalosis (continuous NG suctioning and furosemide). Overzealous diuretic therapy enhances hepatic encephalopathy by inducing prerenal azotemia, hypokalemia, and metabolic alkalosis. Alkalosis promotes diffusion of nonionic ammonia and other amines into the CNS. The associated intracellular acidosis "traps" the ammonia by converting it back to ammonium ion (NH_4^+).[173,174]

Table 28-5 Factors That May Precipitate Hepatic Encephalopathy

Excess Nitrogen Load	Fluid and Electrolyte Abnormalities	Drug-Induced Central Nervous System Depression
Bleeding from gastric and esophageal varices	Hypokalemia	Sedatives
Peptic ulcer	Alkalosis	Tranquilizers
Excess dietary protein	Hypovolemia	Narcotic analgesics
Azotemia or kidney failure	Excessive diarrhea	
Deteriorating hepatic function	Over diuresis	
Infection: tissue catabolism		
Constipation	Excessive vomiting	

Sedating drugs can also precipitate hepatic encephalopathy. Drugs that have been associated with hepatic encephalopathy are opioids (e.g., morphine, methadone, meperidine, codeine), sedatives (e.g., benzodiazepines, barbiturates, chloral hydrate), and tranquilizers (e.g., phenothiazines). Encephalopathy precipitated by most drugs can be explained by increased CNS sensitivity and decreased hepatic clearance with subsequent drug and, in some cases, active metabolite accumulation. In addition, the effects of morphine, chlorpromazine, and diazepam may be increased in liver disease because of decreased plasma protein binding. Thus, the morphine and prochlorperazine that were prescribed for R.C. also may have contributed to the worsening of his hepatic encephalopathy. Although not applicable to this case, excessive dietary protein, infections, and constipation can contribute to excess nitrogen load and the genesis of hepatic coma as well (Table 28-5).

Treatment and General Management

22. What steps should be taken to manage R.C.'s hepatic encephalopathy?

After identifying and removing precipitating causes of hepatic coma, therapeutic management is aimed primarily at reducing the amount of ammonia or nitrogenous products in the circulatory system. In general, the 2006 European Society for Clinical Nutrition and Metabolism (ESPEN) recommends an energy intake of 35 to 40 kcal/kg of body weight/day and a protein intake of 1.2 to 1.5 g/kg of body weight/day is recommended for cirrhotic patients and those awaiting liver transplantation surgeries.[175–178] A study conducted by Cordoba et al.[179] assessed the effects of the amount of protein in the diet on the evolution of hepatic encephalopathy. Cirrhotic patients admitted to the hospital for encephalopathy ($n = 30$) were randomized to two dietary groups, in addition to standard measures to treat hepatic encephalopathy, for 14 days. The first group followed a progressive increase in the dose of protein in the diet, and received 0 g of protein for the first 3 days, then the amount of protein was increased progressively every 3 days (12, 24, and 48 g) up to 1.2 g/kg/day for the last 2 days. The second group received 1.2 g/kg/day from the first day. Results showed that the course of hepatic encephalopathy was not significantly different between both dietary protein restriction groups. The patients in the first group, however, experienced a higher degree of protein breakdown.[179]

23. How are lactulose and neomycin used in hepatic encephalopathy? Which agent would be more appropriate for R.C.?

Lactulose

Lactulose is broken down by GI bacteria to form lactic, acetic, and formic acids. It is believed that acidification of colonic contents converts ammonia into the less readily absorbed ammonium ion. Back diffusion of ammonia from the plasma into the GI tract may also occur. The net result is a lower plasma ammonia concentration. The absorption of other protein breakdown products (e.g., aromatic amino acids) may also be reduced. Lactulose-induced osmotic diarrhea may also decrease the intestinal transit time available for ammonia production and absorption, and may help clear the GI tract of blood. Lactulose syrup (10 g/15 mL) has been used successfully in both acute and chronic hepatic encephalopathy. For acute encephalopathy, lactulose 30 to 45 mL is administered every hour until evacuation occurs. Then, the dosage is titrated to two to four soft bowel movements per day and clear mentation. When the oral route of administration is not possible, as in the treatment of a comatose patient, it may be necessary to administer the drug through an NG tube. Alternatively, a rectal retention enema compounded with 300 mL of lactulose in 700 mL water can be prepared. The lactulose water mixture (125 mL) is retained for 30 to 60 minutes, although this may be difficult in patients with altered mental status. The beneficial clinical effect of lactulose occurs within 12 to 48 hours. Patients may need long-term administration of lactulose as maintenance therapy, especially in patients with recurring encephalopathy. For chronic encephalopathy, oral dosing of lactulose should be administered daily to four times daily titrating to two to four soft stools per day and clear mentation. The chronic administration of lactulose permits better dietary protein tolerance and is well tolerated if dosages are kept sufficiently low to avoid diarrhea.[180]

Very limited data exist evaluating the efficacy of lactulose for the treatment of hepatic encephalopathy. Care should be taken not to induce excessive diarrhea that could lead to dehydration and hypokalemia, both of which have been associated with exacerbation of hepatic encephalopathy. Although lactulose is generally well tolerated, 20% of patients may complain of gaseous distention, flatulence, or belching. Diluting it with fruit juice, carbonated beverages, or water can reduce the excessive sweetness of the syrup.[163]

Neomycin

Neomycin, at dosages of 500 mg to 1 g orally four times daily, or as a 1% solution (125 mL) given as a retention enema (retained for 30–60 minutes) four times daily, is effective in reducing plasma ammonia concentrations (presumably by decreasing protein-metabolizing bacteria in the GI tract). Approximately 1% to 3% of the neomycin dose is absorbed. Chronic use in patients with severe renal insufficiency can cause ototoxicity or nephrotoxicity. Routine monitoring of the serum creatinine, the presence of protein in the urine, and estimation of creatinine clearance are advisable for patients receiving high dosages for more than 2 weeks.[180] Neomycin therapy can also produce a reversible malabsorption syndrome that not only suppresses the absorption of fat, nitrogen, carotene, iron, vitamin B_{12}, xylose, and glucose, but also decreases the absorption of some drugs, such as digoxin, penicillin, and vitamin K.[163]

Comparison With Lactulose

Lactulose and neomycin appear to have similar efficacy for the acute treatment of hepatic encephalopathy.[181] In the treatment of an acute exacerbation, particularly in an acute GI bleed, lactulose may, however, produce a faster response than neomycin. Neomycin may be used in patients who do not respond to lactulose.[180]

Interestingly, while lactose therapy is considered the standard of practice in both acute and chronic hepatic encephalopathy, a meta-analysis evaluating the efficacy of lactulose in patients with hepatic encephalopathy questions its benefit.[182] Large randomized, controlled trials are needed to determine the optimal treatment for hepatic encephalopathy management.[165]

Neomycin in Combination With Lactulose

24. Would the combined use of neomycin and lactulose have any additive beneficial effect for R.C.?

The ACG guidelines state that combination therapy of lactulose and neomycin may be reasonable in patients who do not respond to monotherapy. Although the mechanism of additive effects is unclear, theoretically it may be that either degradation of lactulose may not be essential for reduction of ammonia level or there are other unknown mechanisms for the activity of lactulose. Lactulose should be tried first, and if satisfactory results do not occur, neomycin alone should be given a trial. If both agents fail when used as monotherapy, the two agents can then be tried in combination.[180] Although the combined use of lactulose and neomycin may be beneficial, lactulose alone may be more desirable for long-term use because it is potentially less toxic in patient with renal impairment. Further research is needed evaluating the efficacy of combination therapy.

25. Are there other potential treatments for hepatic encephalopathy?

Rifaximin

Rifaximin is a synthetic antibiotic structurally related to rifamycin. It displays a wide spectrum of antibacterial activity against gram-negative and gram-positive bacteria, both aerobic and anaerobic, and has a very low rate of systemic absorption.[183] It has been available for enteric bacterial conditions for more than a decade in several countries outside the United States, and was recently introduced in the United States for the treatment of travelers' diarrhea.[184] Miglio et al.[185] conducted a randomized, controlled, double-blind study to evaluate the efficacy and tolerability of rifaximin (400 mg three times daily) in comparison to neomycin (1 g three times daily) treatment for 14 days each month over 6 months (n = 49). During the study, blood ammonia concentrations in both the rifaximin and in the neomycin groups decreased a similar amount. The advantage of rifaximin over neomycin for the treatment of hepatic encephalopathy is for patients intolerant to neomycin or those with renal insufficiency.[185] Bucci et al.[186] evaluated the use of rifaximin in a double-blind study comparing rifaximin and lactulose in patients (n = 58) with moderate to severe hepatic encephalopathy. Rifaximin was administered at a dose of 1,200 mg/day, and lactulose was administered at a dose of 30 g/day, both for 15 days. At the end of the treatment period, cognitive function test scores improved in both groups. Also, concentrations of ammonia normalized after 7 days of treatment in both groups. Rifaximin therapy was better tolerated.[186] Although the data reported from these and other trials suggest a benefit with rifaximin for the treatment of hepatic encephalopathy, larger trials must be conducted to determine its eventual place in therapy.

Flumazenil

Based on the theory of increased GABA-ergic neurotransmission in hepatic encephalopathy, flumazenil, a benzodiazepine antagonist, has been evaluated for its role in the treatment of hepatic encephalopathy. Several trials have demonstrated both clinical and electrophysiologic improvement in patients with hepatic encephalopathy.[187] In one study, 60% of patients had transient neurologic improvement after the administration of IV flumazenil 0.5 mg.[188] However an IV product with modest benefits in the treatment of hepatic encephalopathy is not an ideal treatment option.

Lactulose would be the preferred option to treat R.C.'s encephalopathy because it would shorten the time to clear the blood from his GI tract and, it is hoped, lead to a rapid resolution of his encephalopathy. Although neomycin is not contraindicated for R.C., the potential for worsening of his coagulopathy (by interfering with vitamin K absorption) and risk of nephrotoxicity (SrCr 1.4 mg/dL) make this a less optimal choice. If R.C.'s renal function continues to decline, neomycin may become contraindicated. Lactulose can be initiated at 30 mL every hour until diarrhea occurs; the dose can then be reduced to maintain two to four soft stools per day and improved mental status. R.C. may receive lactulose by NG tube if necessary in the early treatment period. Rifaximin 400 mg three times daily may be an option if lactulose therapy fails, because it can be used in renal insufficiency. Finally, flumazenil would not be recommended owing to its lack of evidence as a beneficial chronic therapy.

HEPATORENAL SYNDROME

26. Lactulose treatment was initiated at 30 mL every hour and titrated to effect with some improvement in R.C.'s mental status. A few days after resolution of his GI bleeding, his serum creatinine increased from 1.4 to 2.7 mg/dL and he became progressively oliguric. His BP was 85/65 mmHg, pulse rate was 70 beats/minute,

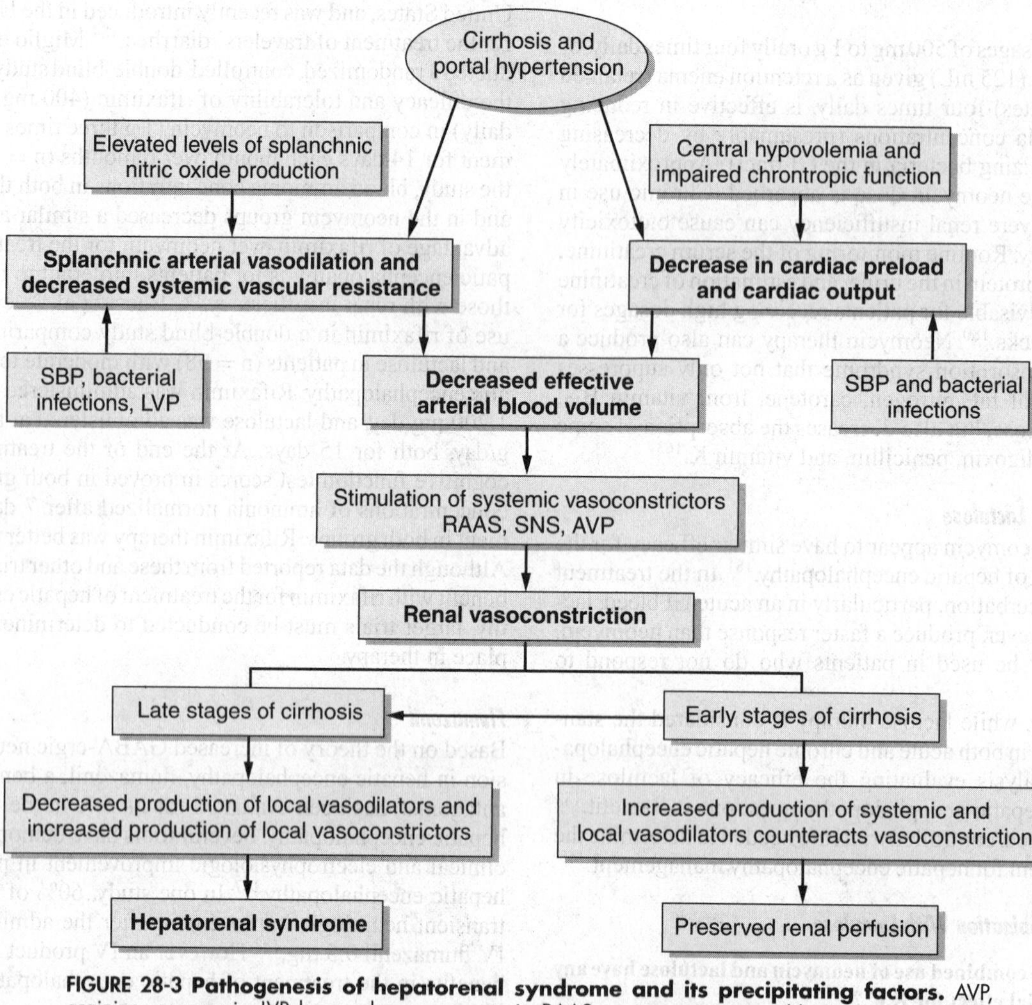

FIGURE 28-3 Pathogenesis of hepatorenal syndrome and its precipitating factors. AVP, arginine vasopressin; LVP, large-volume paracentesis; RAAS, renin–angiotensin–aldosterone system; SBP, spontaneous bacterial peritonitis; SNS, sympathetic nervous system. (Reproduced with permission from reference 190.)

and respiratory rate was 16 breaths/minute. Furosemide was discontinued, and R.C. was treated with albumin infusions to allow volume expansion and improve urine output. A renal ultrasound did not reveal any specific abnormalities. Minimal improvement occurred in his blood pressure and urine output. Laboratory results included the following: Na 123 mEq/L; K 3.6 mEq/L; Cl 98 mEq/L; bicarbonate 25 mEq/L; BUN 96 mg/dL; SrCr 2.7 mg/dL; Hgb 8.4 g/dL; Hct 27.1%; AST 640 IU (normal, 0–35 IU); alkaline phosphatase 304 IU (normal, 30–120 IU); LDH 315 IU (normal, 82–226 IU); and total bilirubin 4.1 mg/dL. PT was 22 seconds with a control of 12 seconds (INR 1.8). A 24-hour urinalysis showed protein 50 mg/day; RBC 1 to 2 per high power field (HPF); negative for WBC, glucose, and ketones. After exclusion of other possible causes of kidney disease, R.C. is diagnosed with hepatorenal syndrome.

Pathogenesis

Hepatorenal syndrome (HRS) is a complication of advanced cirrhosis. It is characterized by an intense renal vasoconstriction, which leads to a very low renal perfusion and glomerular filtration rate, as well as a severe reduction in the ability to excrete sodium and free water.[189] Cardenas et al.[190] have summarized the pathogenesis and the precipitating factors of HRS (Fig. 28-3). HRS is diagnosed by exclusion of other known causes of kidney disease in the absence of parenchymal disease. The revised criteria for the diagnosis of HRS as defined by the International Ascites Club are listed in Table 28-6.[191,192]

Table 28-6 Diagnostic Criteria for Hepatorenal Syndrome in Cirrhosis

1. Cirrhotic patients with ascites
2. Serum creatinine >133 μmol/L (1.5 mg/dL)
3. No improvement of serum creatinine (↓ to a level of ≤133 μmol/L) after at least two days along with
   a. Diuretic withdrawal and
   b. Volume expansion with albumin (1 g/kg of body weight per day up to a maximum of 100 g/day)
4. The absence of shock
5. No current or recent treatment with nephrotoxic drugs
6. The absence of parenchymal kidney disease as indicated by
   a. Proteinuria >500 mg/day,
   b. Microhematuria (>50 red blood cells per high power field),
   c. And/or abnormal renal ultrasonography

From reference 192, with permission.

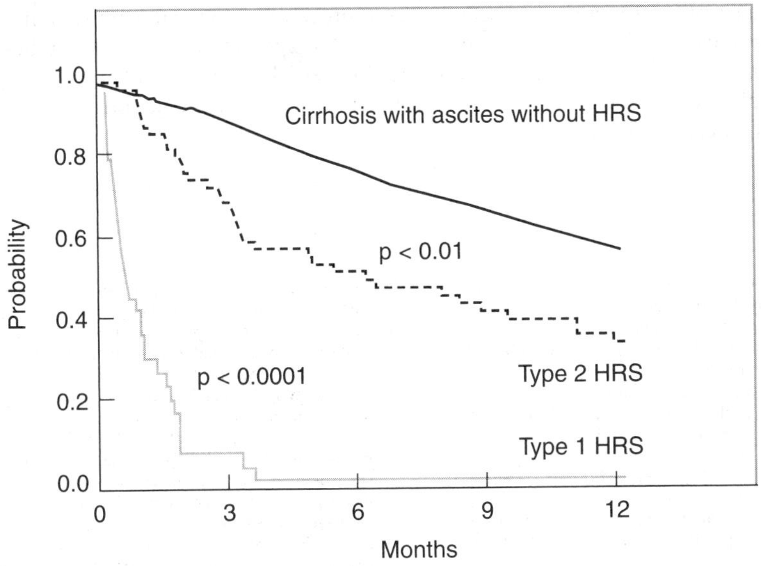

FIGURE 28-4 Actuarial probability to survive in cirrhotic patients with different renal impairments: nonazotemic patients (continuous line); patients with HRS type-2 (dotted line) and patients with HRS type-1 (red line). (Reproduced with permission from reference 192.)

Hepatorenal syndrome can be classified into two categories. Type-1 HRS is characterized by an acute and progressive kidney failure defined by doubling of the initial serum creatinine concentrations to a level >2.5 mg/dL in <2 weeks. Type-1 HRS is precipitated by factors such as SBP or large volume paracentesis, but can occur without a precipitating event. This usually occurs within the setting of an acute deterioration of circulatory function characterized by hypotension and activation of endogenous vasoconstrictor systems. It may be associated with impaired cardiac and liver functions as well as encephalopathy. The prognosis of patients exhibiting type-1 HRS is very poor (Fig. 28-4).[192,193] In contrast, type-2 HRS is a progressive deterioration of kidney function with a serum creatinine from 1.5 to 2.5 mg/dL. It is often associated with refractory ascites, and has a better survival rate than that of patients with type-1 HRS.[190–192]

Treatment

Treatments for HRS are still investigational. HRS is associated with a high mortality rate (within 2 weeks of diagnosis of type-1 HRS and within 6 months of type-2 HRS). The definitive treatment for type-1 and type 2 HRS is liver transplantation, which is the only treatment that assures long-term survival.[69] The main goal of pharmacologic therapy is to reverse HRS sufficiently so that appropriate candidates for liver transplantation can survive until suitable donor organs can be procured.[191,192] Diuretics therapy must be stopped because this can worsen the kidney disease.[190]

A small randomized study by Solanki et al.[194] showed that vasoconstrictor therapy using terlipressin, in conjunction with albumin, was an effective treatment for patients with type-1 HRS. Patients were randomly assigned to treatment with IV terlipressin 1 mg at 12-hour intervals (n = 12) or placebo at 12-hour intervals (n = 12). Urine output, creatinine clearance, and mean arterial pressures significantly increased in patients treated with terlipressin compared with the placebo group ($p < 0.05$). Survival was significantly higher in the terlipressin group compared with placebo (42% vs. 0%; $p < 0.05$). All survivors in the terlipressin group had a reversal of HRS.[194]

Other nonrandomized studies suggest that vasoconstrictor therapy with norepinephrine (combined with albumin and furosemide) or midodrine (combined with octreotide and albumin), improve renal function in patients with type 1 HRS. The impact of vasoconstrictor therapy in terms of efficacy (i.e., improvement of kidney function and survival) and safety should be evaluated in large, randomized clinical trials.[195–197] Duvoux et al.[197] conducted a pilot study describing the efficacy and safety of norepinephrine in combination with IV albumin and furosemide in patients (n = 12) with type-1 HRS. Norepinephrine was given for 10 ± 3 days, at a mean dosage of 0.8 ± 0.3 mg/hour. Reversal of HRS was observed in 83% of patients after a median of 7 days, with a reduction in serum creatinine (358 ± 161 to 145 ± 78 μmol/L; $p < 0.001$), a rise in creatinine clearance (13 ± 9 to 40 ± 15 mL/minute; $p = 0.003$), an increase in mean arterial pressure (65 ± 7 to 73 ± 9 mmHg, $p = 0.01$) and a marked reduction in active renin and aldosterone plasma concentrations ($p < 0.05$).[197]

Type-2 HRS manifests itself as a progressive disease and, therefore, patients do not present acutely with deterioration in kidney function. No particular treatment exists for type-2 HRS. The main clinical problem in type-2 HRS is refractory ascites, which can be controlled by large volume paracentesis along with IV albumin or TIPS.[190,195,198] Studies are needed to determine the place in therapy for vasoconstrictors and other potential treatments (e.g. TIPS) in patients with type-2 HRS.[192]

Because of the poor prognosis associated with hepatorenal syndrome, R.C. should be evaluated for transplantation. It may be beneficial to enroll R.C. in investigational research studies evaluating the use of vasoconstrictor therapy in conjunction with albumin while awaiting transplantation.

27. When should liver transplantation be considered in patients with end-stage liver disease?

Liver transplantation for appropriate candidates may be the best option for end-stage liver disease and its complications. Transplantation is generally considered in patients with refractory ascites, severe hepatic encephalopathy, esophageal or gastric varices and hepatorenal syndrome.[199] Because of the shortage of organs available and significant complications associated with transplantation, therapeutic alternatives should be considered to avoid the necessity for transplantation. For those patients who are transplantation candidates, therapeutic strategies to improve outcomes after transplantation should be considered in therapeutic decision-making before transplantation (see Chapter 34, Kidney and Liver Transplantation, for further information on the indications for liver transplantation).[198]

REFERENCES

1. Minino AM et al. Deaths: preliminary data for 2004. *Natl Vital Stat Rep* 2006;54:1.
2. Friedman SL. Liver fibrosis—from bench to bedside. *J Hepatol* 2003;38(Suppl 1):S38.
3. Roberts RA et al. Role of the Kupffer cell in mediating hepatic toxicity and carcinogenesis. *Toxicol Sci* 2007;96:2.
4. Tarla MR et al. Cellular aspects of liver regeneration. *Acta Cirúrgica Brasileira* 2006;21(Suppl 1):63.
5. Pritchard MT et al. Ethanol-induced liver injury: potential roles for egr-1. *Alcohol Clin Exp Res* 2005;29(Suppl 11):S146.
6. Dey A et al. Alcohol and oxidative liver injury. *Hepatology* 2006;43(Suppl 1):S63.
7. Tome S et al. Current management of alcoholic liver disease. *Aliment Pharmacol Ther* 2004;19:707.
8. Falcon V et al. HCV core protein localizes in the nuclei of nonparenchymal liver cells from chronically HCV-infected patients. *Biochem Biophys Res Commun* 2005;329:1320.
9. Safdar K et al. Alcohol and hepatitis C. *Semin Liver Dis* 2004;24:305.
10. Ramalho F. Hepatitis C virus infection and liver steatosis. *Antiviral Res* 2003;60:125.
11. Liangpunsakul S et al. Treatment of nonalcoholic fatty liver disease. *Current Treatment Options in Gastroenterology* 2003;6:455.
12. Cave M et al. Nonalcoholic fatty liver disease: predisposing factors and the role of nutrition. *Journal of Nutritional Biochemistry* 2007;18:184.
13. Heidelbaugh JJ et al. Cirrhosis and chronic liver failure: part II. Complications and treatment. *Am Fam Physician* 2006;74:767.
14. Gallego C et al. Congenital and acquired anomalies of the portal venous system. *Radiographics* 2002;22:141.
15. Wachsberg RH et al. Hepatofugal flow in the portal venous system: pathophysiology, imaging findings, and diagnostic pitfalls. *Radiographics* 2002;22:123.
16. Langer DA et al. Nitric oxide and portal hypertension: interface of vasoreactivity and angiogenesis. *J Hepatol* 2006;44:209.
17. Garcia-Tsao G. Portal hypertension. *Current Opinion in Gastroenterology* 2006;22:254.
18. Groszmann R et al. Measurement of portal pressure: when, how, and why to do it. *Clin Liver Dis* 2006;10:499.
19. Wadhawan M et al. Hepatic venous pressure gradient in cirrhosis: correlation with the size of varices, bleeding, ascites, and child's status. *Dig Dis Sci* 2006;51:2264.
20. Laleman W et al. Portal hypertension: from pathophysiology to clinical practice. *Liver International* 2005;25:1079.
21. Rodriguez-Vilarrupla A et al. Current concepts on the pathophysiology of portal hypertension. *Annals of Hepatology* 2007;6:28.
22. Lata J et al. Management of acute variceal bleeding. *Dig Dis* 2003;21:6.
23. Yeung E et al. The management of cirrhotic ascites. *Medscape General Medicine* 2002;4:8.
24. Sherman DS et al. Assessing renal function in cirrhotic patients: problems and pitfalls. *Am J Kidney Dis* 2003;41:269.
25. Dufour DR et al. Diagnosis and monitoring of hepatic injury. II. Recommendations for use of laboratory tests in screening, diagnosis, and monitoring. *Clin Chem* 2000;46:2050.
26. Dufour DR et al. Diagnosis and monitoring of hepatic injury. I. Performance characteristics of laboratory tests. *Clin Chem* 2000;46:2027.
27. Henderson JM et al. Portal hypertension. *Curr Prob Surg* 1998;35:379.
28. Friedman SL. Efficacy of abstinence and specific therapy in alcoholic liver disease. In: Rose BD, ed. *UpToDate.* Wellesley, MA; 2003.
29. Durand F et al. Assessment of the prognosis of cirrhosis: Child-Pugh versus MELD. *J Hepatol* 2005;42(Suppl 1):S100.
30. Riley TR 3rd et al. Preventive strategies in chronic liver disease: part II. Cirrhosis. *Am Fam Physician* 2001;64:1735.
31. Dangleben DA et al. Impact of cirrhosis on outcomes in trauma. *J Am Coll Surg* 2006;203:908.
32. Freeman RB Jr et al. The new liver allocation system: moving toward evidence-based transplantation policy. *Liver Transpl* 2002;8:851.
33. Dunn W et al. MELD accurately predicts mortality in patients with alcoholic hepatitis. *Hepatology* 2005;41:353.
34. Kamath PS et al. A model to predict survival in patients with end-stage liver disease. *Hepatology* 2001;33:464.
35. Heuman DM et al. MELD-XI: a rational approach to "sickest first" liver transplantation in cirrhotic patients requiring anticoagulant therapy. *Liver Transpl* 2007;13:30.
36. Talking about Transplantation: Questions and Answers for Patients and Families About MELD and PELD (Online Brochure). Retrieved November 12, 2007 from the United Network of Organ Sharing Web site: http://www.unos.org/.
37. Krige JE et al. ABC of diseases of liver, pancreas, and biliary system: portal hypertension-2. Ascites, encephalopathy, and other conditions. *BMJ* 2001;322:416.
38. Bekheirnia MR et al. Pathophysiology of water and sodium retention: edematous states with normal kidney function. *Curr Opin Pharmacol* 2006;6:202.
39. Jalan R et al. Hepatic encephalopathy and ascites. *Lancet* 1997;350:1309.
40. Suzuki H et al. Current management and novel therapeutic strategies for refractory ascites and hepatorenal syndrome. *QJM* 2001;94:293.
41. Moore KP et al. The management of ascites in cirrhosis: report on the consensus conference of the International Ascites Club. *Hepatology* 2003;38:258.
42. Runyon BA. Practice Guidelines Committee, American Association for the Study of Liver Diseases (AASLD). Management of adult patients with ascites due to cirrhosis. *Hepatology* 2004;39:841.
43. Trevisani F et al. Circadian variation in renal sodium and potassium handling in cirrhosis. The role of aldosterone, cortisol, sympathoadrenergic tone, and intratubular factors. *Gastroenterology* 1989;96:1187.
44. Biswas KD et al. Hepatorenal syndrome. *Trop Gastroenterol* 2002;23:113.
45. Gentilini P et al. Update on ascites and hepatorenal syndrome. *Dig Liver Dis* 2002;34:592.
46. Eisenmenger WJ et al. The effect of rigid sodium restriction in patients with cirrhosis of the liver and ascites. *J Lab Clin Med* 1949;34:1029.
47. Angeli P et al. Hyponatremia in cirrhosis: results of a patient population survey. *Hepatology* 2006;44:1535.
48. Asbert M et al. Circulating levels of endothelin in cirrhosis. *Gastroenterology* 1993;104:1485.
49. Runyon BA. Albumin infusion for spontaneous bacterial peritonitis. *Lancet* 1999;354:1838.
50. Javle P et al. Hepatosplanchnic haemodynamics and renal blood flow and function in rats with liver failure. *Gut* 1998;43:272.
51. Coppage WS, Jr. et al. The metabolism of aldosterone in normal subjects and in patients with hepatic cirrhosis. *J Clin Invest* 1962;41:1672.
52. Perez-Ayuso RM et al. Randomized comparative study of efficacy of furosemide versus spironolactone in patients with liver cirrhosis and ascites. *Gastroenterology* 1983;84:961.
53. Runyon BA. Treatment of patients with cirrhosis and ascites. *Semin Liver Dis* 1997;17:249.
54. Bernardi M et al. Efficacy and safety of the stepped care medical treatment of ascites in liver cirrhosis: a randomized controlled clinical trial comparing two diets with different sodium content. *Liver* 1993;13:156.
55. Gatta A et al. A pathophysiological interpretation of unresponsiveness to spironolactone in a stepped care approach to the diuretic treatment of ascites in nonazotemic cirrhotic patients with ascites. *Hepatology* 1991;14:231.
56. Runyon BA. Management of adult patients with ascites caused by cirrhosis. *Hepatology* 1998;27:264.
57. Yamamoto S. Disappearance of spironolactone-induced gynecomastia with triamterene. *Intern Med* 2001;40:550.
58. Angeli P et al. Randomized clinical study of the efficacy of amiloride and potassium canrenoate in nonazotemic cirrhotic patients with ascites. *Hepatology* 1994;19:72.
59. Delyani JA et al. Eplerenone: a selective aldosterone receptor antagonist (SARA). *Cardiovasc Drug Rev* 2001;19:185.
60. Zillich AJ et al. Eplerenone—a novel selective aldosterone blocker. *Ann Pharmacother* 2002;36:1567.
61. Pitt B et al. Eplerenone, a selective aldosterone blocker, in patients with left ventricular dysfunction after myocardial infarction. *N Engl J Med* 2003;348:1309.
62. Inspra Product Information. Pfizer Inc. New York; New York, 2005.
63. Pitt B et al. Randomized Aldactone Evaluation Study Investigators. The effect of spironolactone on morbidity and mortality in patients with severe heart failure. *N Engl J Med* 1999;341:709.
64. Pitt B et al. The EPHESUS trial: eplerenone in patients with heart failure due to systolic dysfunction complicating acute myocardial infarction. Eplerenone Post-AMI Heart Failure Efficacy and Survival Study. *Cardiovasc Drugs Ther* 2001;15:79.
65. Tang WH et al. Aldosterone receptor antagonists in the medical management of chronic heart failure. *Mayo Clin Proc* 2005;80:1623.
66. Pockros PJ et al. Rapid diuresis in patients with ascites from chronic liver disease: the importance of peripheral edema. *Gastroenterology* 1986;90:1827.
67. Runyon BA. Historical aspects of treatment of patients with cirrhosis and ascites. *Semin Liver Dis* 1997;17:163.
68. Ahya SN et al. Acid-base and potassium disorders in liver disease. *Semin Nephrol* 2006;26:466.
69. Gines A et al. Incidence, predictive factors, and prognosis of the hepatorenal syndrome in cirrhosis with ascites. *Gastroenterology* 1993;105:229.
70. Antes LM et al. Principles of diuretic therapy. *Dis Mon* 1998;44:254.

71. Wong F. Liver and kidney diseases. *Clin Liver Dis* 2002;6:981.
72. Wong F et al. New challenge of hepatorenal syndrome: prevention and treatment. *Hepatology* 2001;34:1242.
73. Ruiz-del-Arbol L et al. Paracentesis-induced circulatory dysfunction: mechanism and effect on hepatic hemodynamics in cirrhosis. *Gastroenterology* 1997;113:579.
74. Arroyo V et al. Ascites and hepatorenal syndrome in cirrhosis: pathophysiology basis of therapy and current management. *J Hepatol* 2003;38(Suppl 1):S69.
75. Sola-Vera J et al. Randomized trial comparing albumin and saline in the prevention of paracentesis-induced circulatory dysfunction in cirrhotic patients with ascites. *Hepatology* 2003;37:1147.
76. Wilkes MM et al. Patient survival after human albumin administration. A meta-analysis of randomized, controlled trials. *Ann Intern Med* 2001;135:149.
77. Sort P et al. Effect of intravenous albumin on renal impairment and mortality in patients with cirrhosis and spontaneous bacterial peritonitis [Comment]. *N Engl J Med* 1999;341:403.
78. Terg R et al. Dextran administration avoids hemodynamic changes following paracentesis in cirrhotic patients. *Dig Dis Sci* 1992;37:79.
79. Gines A et al. Randomized trial comparing albumin, dextran 70, and polygeline in cirrhotic patients with ascites treated by paracentesis. *Gastroenterology* 1996;111:1002.
80. Christidis C et al. Worsening of hepatic dysfunction as a consequence of repeated hydroxyethyl starch infusions. *J Hepatol* 2001;35:726.
81. Buminate 25% Product information. Baxter Healthcare Corp. Glendale CA 2002.
82. Plasbumin-25. Product information. Talecris Biotherapeutics Inc. Glendale CA 2005.
83. Lexi-Comp Online TM. Lexi-Drugs Online TM. Hudson, Ohio: Lexi-Comp, Inc.; 2007; September 22, 2007.
84. Therapondos G et al. Management of gastroesophageal varices. *Clin Med* 2002;2:297.
85. Gines P et al. Transjugular intrahepatic portosystemic shunting versus paracentesis plus albumin for refractory ascites in cirrhosis. *Gastroenterology* 2002;123:1839.
86. Boyer TD et al. American Association for the Study of Liver Diseases Practice Guidelines: the role of transjugular intrahepatic portosystemic shunt creation in the management of portal hypertension. *J Vasc Interv Radiol* 2005;16:615.
87. Tueche SG et al. Peritoneovenous shunt in malignant ascites. The Bordet Institute experience from 1975-1998. *Hepatogastroenterology* 2000;47:1322.
88. Gines P et al. Paracentesis with intravenous infusion of albumin as compared with peritoneovenous shunting in cirrhosis with refractory ascites. *N Engl J Med* 1991;325:829.
89. Arroyo V et al. Sympathetic nervous activity, renin-angiotensin system and renal excretion of prostaglandin E2 in cirrhosis. Relationship to functional renal failure and sodium and water retention. *Eur J Clin Invest* 1983;13:271.
90. Henriksen JH et al. Hepatorenal disorders. Role of the sympathetic nervous system. *Semin Liver Dis* 1994;14:35.
91. Lenaerts A et al. Effects of clonidine on diuretic response in ascitic patients with cirrhosis and activation of sympathetic nervous system. *Hepatology* 2006;44:844.
92. Lenaerts A et al. Comparative pilot study of repeated large volume paracentesis vs. the combination on clonidine-spironolactone in the treatment of cirrhosis-associated refractory ascites. *Gastroenterol Clin Biol* 2005;29:1137.
93. Ghassemi S et al. Prevention and treatment of infections in patients with cirrhosis. *Best Pract Res Clin Gastroenterol* 2007;21:77.
94. Filik L et al. Clinical and laboratory features of spontaneous bacterial peritonitis. *East Afr Med J* 2004;81:474.
95. Caruntu FA et al. Spontaneous bacterial peritonitis: pathogenesis, diagnosis, treatment. *Journal of Gastrointestinal and Liver Disease* 2006;15:51.
96. Sheer TA et al. Spontaneous bacterial peritonitis. *Dig Dis* 2005;23:39.
97. Frazee LA et al. Long-term prophylaxis of spontaneous bacterial peritonitis in patients with cirrhosis. *Ann Pharmacother* 2005;39:908.
98. Gines P et al. Norfloxacin prevents spontaneous bacterial peritonitis recurrence in cirrhosis: results of a double-blind, placebo-controlled trial. *Hepatology* 1990;12:716.
99. Soriano G et al. Selective intestinal decontamination prevents spontaneous bacterial peritonitis. *Gastroenterology* 1991;100:477.
100. Fernández J et al. Primary prophylaxis of spontaneous bacterial peritonitis delays hepatorenal syndrome and improves survival in cirrhosis. *Gastroenterology* 2007;133:818.
101. Ortiz J et al. Infections caused by *Escherichia coli* resistant to norfloxacin in hospitalized cirrhotic patients. *Hepatology* 1999;29:1064.
102. Alvarez RF et al. Trimethoprim-sulfamethoxazole versus norfloxacin in the prophylaxis of spontaneous bacterial peritonitis in cirrhosis. *Arq Gastroenterol* 2005;42:256.
103. Bernard B et al. Antibiotic prophylaxis for the prevention of bacterial infections in cirrhotic patients with gastrointestinal bleeding: a meta-analysis. *Hepatology* 1999;29:1655.
104. Rimola A et al. Diagnosis, treatment and prophylaxis of spontaneous bacterial peritonitis: a consensus document. International Ascites Club. *J Hepatol* 2000;32:142.
105. Noroxin. Product information. Merck & Co. Inc. Whitehouse Station, NJ; 2004.
106. Garcia-Tsao G et al. Prevention and management of gastroesophageal varices and variceal hemorrhage in cirrhosis. Practice Guidelines Committee of the American Association for the Study of Liver Diseases (AASLD); Practice Parameters Committee of the American College of Gastroenterology (ACG). *Am J Gastroenterol* 2007;102:2086.
107. Sarin SK et al. Gastric varices and portal hypertensive gastropathy. *Clin Liver Dis* 2001;5:727.
108. Graham DY et al. The course of patients after variceal hemorrhage. *Gastroenterology* 1981;80:800.
109. Carbonell N et al. Improved survival after variceal bleeding in patients with cirrhosis over the past two decades. *Hepatology* 2004;40:652.
110. de Franchis R et al. Natural history of portal hypertension in patients with cirrhosis. *Clin Liver Dis* 2001;5:645.
111. Wu JC et al. Update on treatment of variceal hemorrhage. *Dig Dis* 2002;20:134.
112. Chung S. Management of bleeding in the cirrhotic patient. *J Gastroenterol Hepatol* 2002;17:355.
113. Bhasin DK et al. Variceal bleeding and portal hypertension: much to learn, much to explore. *Endoscopy* 2002;34:119.
114. Thabut D et al. Management of acute bleeding from portal hypertension. *Best Pract Res Clin Gastroenterol* 2007;21:19.
115. McKiernan PJ. Treatment of variceal bleeding. *Gastrointest Endosc Clin North Am* 2001;11:789.
116. Martí-Carvajal AJ et al. Vitamin K for upper gastrointestinal bleeding in patients with liver diseases. *Cochrane Database Syst Rev* 2005;(3):CD004792.
117. Goulis J et al. Role of vasoactive drugs in the treatment of bleeding oesophageal varices. *Digestion* 1999;60(Suppl 3):25.
118. Iwao T et al. Effect of vasopressin on esophageal varices blood flow in patients with cirrhosis: comparisons with the effects on portal vein and superior mesenteric artery blood flow. *J Hepatol* 1996;25:491.
119. Law AW et al. Octreotide or vasopressin for bleeding esophageal varices. *Ann Pharmacother* 1997;31:237.
120. de Franchis R. Longer treatment with vasoactive drugs to prevent early variceal re-bleeding in cirrhosis. *Eur J Gastroenterol Hepatol* 1998;10:1041.
121. Zhou Y. Comparison of the efficacy of octreotide, vasopressin, and omeprazole in the control of acute bleeding in patients with portal hypertensive gastropathy: a controlled study. *J Gastroenterol Hepatol* 2002;17:973.
122. Imperiale TF. A meta-analysis of somatostatin versus vasopressin in the management of acute esophageal variceal hemorrhage. *Gastroenterology* 1995;109:1289.
123. Stump DL et al. The use of vasopressin in the treatment of upper gastrointestinal haemorrhage. *Drugs* 1990;39:38.
124. Anderson JR et al. Development of cutaneous gangrene during continuous peripheral infusion of vasopressin. *BMJ (Clin Res Ed)* 1983;287:1657.
125. Gimson AE et al. A randomized trial of vasopressin and vasopressin plus nitroglycerin in the control of acute variceal hemorrhage. *Hepatology* 1986;6:410.
126. Bruha R et al. Double-blind randomized, comparative multicenter study of the effect of terlipressin in the treatment of acute esophageal variceal and/or hypertensive gastropathy bleeding. *Hepatogastroenterology* 2002;49:1161.
127. de Franchis R. Evolving consensus in portal hypertension. Report of the Baveno IV consensus workshop on methodology of diagnosis and therapy in portal hypertension. *J Hepatol* 2005;43:167.
128. Calès P et al. Early administration of vapreotide for variceal bleeding in patients with cirrhosis. French Club for the Study of Portal Hypertension. *N Engl J Med* 2001;344:23.
129. Ioannou GN et al. Systematic review: terlipressin in acute oesophageal variceal haemorrhage. *Aliment Pharmacol Ther* 2003;17:53.
130. Dib N et al. Current management of the complications of portal hypertension: variceal bleeding and ascites. *CMAJ* 2006;174:1433.
131. Lay CS et al. Endoscopic variceal ligation versus propranolol in prophylaxis of first variceal bleeding in patients with cirrhosis. *J Gastroenterol Hepatol* 2006;21:413.
132. Tatemichi M et al. Differences in hemostasis among sclerosing agents in endoscopic injection sclerotherapy. *Dig Dis Sci* 1996;41:562.
133. Dagher L et al. Variceal bleeding and portal hypertensive gastropathy. *Eur J Gastroenterol Hepatol* 2001;13:81.
134. Goff JS. Endoscopic variceal ligation. In: Rose BD, ed. *UpToDate Inc.* Waltham, MA; 2007.
135. Villanueva C et al. A randomized controlled trial comparing ligation and sclerotherapy as emergency endoscopic treatment added to somatostatin in acute variceal bleeding. *J Hepatol* 2006;45:560.
136. Sarin SK et al. Prospective randomized trial of endoscopic sclerotherapy versus variceal band ligation for esophageal varices: influence on gastropathy, gastric varices and variceal recurrence. *J Hepatol* 1997;26:826.
137. Helmy A et al. Review article: current endoscopic therapeutic options in the management of variceal bleeding. *Aliment Pharmacol Ther* 2001;15:575.
138. Gow PJ et al. Modern management of esophageal varices. *Postgrad Med J* 2001;77:75.
139. Henderson JM et al. Distal splenorenal shunt versus transjugular intrahepatic portal systematic shunt for variceal bleeding: a randomized trial. *Gastroenterology* 2006;130:1643.
140. Tripathi D et al. The role of the transjugular intrahepatic portosystemic stent shunt (TIPSS) in the management of bleeding gastric varices: clinical and haemodynamic correlations. *Gut* 2002;51:270.
141. Hidajat N et al. Transjugular intrahepatic portosystemic shunt and transjugular embolization of bleeding rectal varices in portal hypertension. *AJR Am J Roentgenol* 2002;178:362.
142. Jovine E et al. Splenoadrenal shunt. An original portosystemic decompressive technique. *Hepatogastroenterology* 2001;48:107.
143. Soriano G et al. Norfloxacin prevents bacterial infection in cirrhotics with gastrointestinal hemorrhage. *Gastroenterology* 1992;103:1267.

144. Fernandez J et al. Norfloxacin vs ceftriaxone in the prophylaxis of infections in patients with advanced cirrhosis and hemorrhage. *Gastroenterology* 2006;131:1049.
145. Vorobioff J et al. Prognostic value of hepatic venous pressure gradient measurements in alcoholic cirrhosis: a 10-year prospective study. *Gastroenterology* 1996;111:701.
146. Escorsell A et al. Predictive value of the variceal pressure response to continued pharmacological therapy in patients with cirrhosis and portal hypertension. *Hepatology* 2000;31:1061.
147. Brett BT et al. Primary prophylaxis of variceal bleeding in cirrhosis. *Eur J Gastroenterol Hepatol* 2001;13:349.
148. Groszmann RJ et al. Beta-blockers to prevent gastroesophageal varices in patients with cirrhosis. *N Engl J Med* 2005;353:2254.
149. Uribe M et al. Portal-systemic encephalopathy and gastrointestinal bleeding after cardioselective beta-blocker (metoprolol) administration to patients with portal hypertension. *Arch Med Res* 1995;26:221.
150. Talwalkar JA et al. An evidence-based medicine approach to beta-blocker therapy in patients with cirrhosis. *Am J Med* 2004;116:759.
151. Pascal JP et al. Propranolol in the prevention of first upper gastrointestinal tract hemorrhage in patients with cirrhosis of the liver and esophageal varices. *N Engl J Med* 1987;317:856.
152. Sarin SK et al. Endoscopic variceal ligation plus propranolol versus endoscopic variceal ligation alone in primary prophylaxis of variceal bleeding. *Am J Gastroenterol* 2005;100:797.
153. Abraczinskas DR et al. Propranolol for the prevention of first esophageal variceal hemorrhage: a lifetime commitment? *Hepatology* 2001;34:1096.
154. Angelico M et al. Effects of isosorbide-5-mononitrate compared with propranolol on first bleeding and long-term survival in cirrhosis. *Gastroenterology* 1997;113:1632.
155. Garcia-Pagan JC et al. Isosorbide mononitrate in the prevention of first variceal bleed in patients who cannot receive beta-blockers. *Gastroenterology* 2001;121:908.
156. Vorobioff J et al. Propranolol compared with propranolol plus isosorbide dinitrate in portal-hypertensive patients: long-term hemodynamic and renal effects. *Hepatology* 1993;18:477.
157. Merkel C et al. Randomised trial of nadolol alone or with isosorbide mononitrate for primary prophylaxis of variceal bleeding in cirrhosis. Gruppo-Triveneto per L'ipertensione portale (GTIP). *Lancet* 1996;348:1677.
158. Colombo M et al. Beta-blockade prevents recurrent gastrointestinal bleeding in well-compensated patients with alcoholic cirrhosis: a multicenter randomized controlled trial. *Hepatology* 1989;9:433.
159. de la Pena J et al. Variceal ligation plus nadolol compared with ligation for prophylaxis of variceal re-bleeding: a multicenter trial. *Hepatology* 2005;41:572.
160. Gonzalez-Suarez B et al. Pharmacologic treatment of portal hypertension in the prevention of community-acquired spontaneous bacterial peritonitis. *Eur J Gastroenterol Hepatol* 2006;18:49.
161. Escorsell A. TIPS versus drug therapy in preventing variceal rebleeding in advanced cirrhosis: a randomized controlled trial. *Hepatology* 2002;35:385.
162. Ong JP et al. Hepatic encephalopathy. *Eur J Gastroenterol Hepatol* 2001;13:325.
163. Abou-Assi S et al. Hepatic encephalopathy. Metabolic consequence of cirrhosis often is reversible. *Postgrad Med* 2001;109:52.
164. Clemmesen JO et al. Cerebral herniation in patients with acute liver failure is correlated with arterial ammonia concentration. *Hepatology* 1999;29:648.
165. Wright G et al. Management of hepatic encephalopathy in patients with cirrhosis. *Best Pract Res Clin Gastroenterol* 2007;21:95.
166. Als-Nielsen B et al. Branched-chain amino acids for hepatic encephalopathy. *Cochrane Database Syst Rev* 2003;(2):CD001939.
167. James JH. Branched chain amino acids in hepatic encephalopathy. *Am J Surg* 2002;183:424.
168. Schafer DF et al. Potential neural mechanisms in the pathogenesis of hepatic encephalopathy. *Prog Liver Dis* 1982;7:615.
169. Jones EA et al. The involvement of ammonia with the mechanisms that enhance GABA-ergic neurotransmission in hepatic failure. *Adv Exp Med Biol* 1997;420:75.
170. Basile AS et al. Ammonia and GABA-ergic neurotransmission: interrelated factors in the pathogenesis of hepatic encephalopathy. *Hepatology* 1997;25:1303.
171. Butterworth RF. Hepatic encephalopathy: a neuropsychiatric disorder involving multiple neurotransmitter systems. *Curr Opin Neurol* 2000;13:721.
172. Haussinger D et al. Hepatic encephalopathy in chronic liver disease: a clinical manifestation of astrocyte swelling and low-grade cerebral edema? *J Hepatol* 2000;32:1035.
173. Gerber T et al. Hepatic encephalopathy in liver cirrhosis: pathogenesis, diagnosis and management. *Drugs* 2000;60:1353.
174. Blei AT. Diagnosis and treatment of hepatic encephalopathy. *Baillieres Best Pract Res Clin Gastroenterol* 2000;14:959.
175. Plauth M et al. ESPEN Guidelines on Enteral Nutrition: liver disease. *Clin Nutr* 2006;25:285.
176. Plauth M et al. ESPEN guidelines for nutrition in liver disease and transplantation. *Clin Nutr* 1997;16:43.
177. Marsano LS et al. Current nutrition in liver disease. *Curr Opin Gastroenterol* 2002;18:246.
178. Heyman JK et al. Dietary protein intakes in patients with hepatic encephalopathy and cirrhosis: current practice in NSW and ACT. *Med J Aust* 2006;185:542.
179. Cordoba J et al. Normal protein diet for episodic hepatic encephalopathy: results of a randomized study. *J Hepatol* 2004;41:38.
180. Blei AT et al. Practice Parameters Committee of the American College of Gastroenterology. *Am J Gastroenterol* 2001;96:1968.
181. Orlandi F et al. Comparison between neomycin and lactulose in 173 patients with hepatic encephalopathy: a randomized clinical study. *Dig Dis Sci* 1981;26:498.
182. Als-Nielsen B et al. Non-absorbable disaccharides for hepatic encephalopathy: systematic review of randomised trials. *BMJ* 2004;328:1046.
183. Festi D et al. Management of hepatic encephalopathy: focus on antibiotic therapy. *Digestion* 2006;73(Suppl 1):94.
184. Williams R et al. Rifaximin, a nonabsorbed oral antibiotic, in the treatment of hepatic encephalopathy: antimicrobial activity, efficacy, and safety. *Rev Gastroenterol Disord* 2005;5(Suppl 1):S10.
185. Miglio F et al. Rifaximin, a non-absorbable rifamycin, for the treatment of hepatic encephalopathy. A double-blind, randomised trial. *Curr Med Res Opin* 1997;13:593.
186. Bucci L et al. Double-blind, double-dummy comparison between treatment with rifaximin and lactulose in patients with medium to severe degree hepatic encephalopathy. *Curr Med Res Opin* 1993;13:109.
187. Als-Nielsen B et al. Benzodiazepine receptor antagonists for acute and chronic hepatic encephalopathy. *Cochrane Database of Systematic Reviews* 2001;CD002798.
188. Laccetti M et al. Flumazenil in the treatment of acute hepatic encephalopathy in cirrhotic patients: a double blind randomized placebo controlled study. *Dig Liver Dis* 2000;32:335.
189. Arroyo V et al. Advances in the pathogenesis and treatment of type-1 and type-2 hepatorenal syndrome. *J Hepatol* 2007;46:935.
190. Cardenas A et al. Therapy insight: management of hepatorenal syndrome. *Nature Clinical Practice Gastroenterology & Hepatology* 2006;3:338.
191. Arroyo V et al. New treatments of hepatorenal syndrome. *Semin Liver Dis* 2006;26:254.
192. Salerno F et al. Diagnosis, prevention and treatment of the hepatorenal syndrome in cirrhosis. A consensus workshop of the international ascites club. *Gut* 2007;56:1310.
193. Alessandria C et al. MELD score and clinical type predict prognosis in hepatorenal syndrome: relevance to liver transplantation. *Hepatology* 2005;41:1282.
194. Solanki P et al. Beneficial effects of terlipressin in hepatorenal syndrome: a prospective, randomized placebo-controlled clinical trial. *J Gastroenterol Hepatol* 2003;18:152.
195. Moreau R et al. Diagnosis and treatment of acute renal failure in patients with cirrhosis. *Best Pract Res Clin Gastroenterol* 2007;21:111.
196. Angeli P et al. Reversal of type 1 hepatorenal syndrome with the administration of midodrine and octreotide. *Hepatology* 1999;29:1690.
197. Duvoux C et al. Effects of noradrenalin and albumin in patients with type I hepatorenal syndrome: a pilot study. *Hepatology* 2002;36:374.
198. Gines P et al. Hepatorenal syndrome. *Lancet* 2003;362:1819.
199. Francoz C et al. Indications of liver transplantation in patients with complications of cirrhosis. *Best Pract Res Clin Gastroenterol* 2007;21:175.

CHAPTER 29

Adverse Effects of Drugs on the Liver

Curtis D. Holt

INTRODUCTION

Drug-induced liver injury (DILI) is a term that is used to describe abnormalities in liver function following exposure to a drug or noninfectious agent.[1,2] Generally, a distinction should be made between hepatic injury and function, because when function is impaired, clinically significant liver disease usually follows. The loss of hepatic function often leads to a compromised ability to perform activities of daily living, hospitalization, or life threatening events. Before World War II, DILI was an issue of minor proportions, but with the introduction of a large number of new drugs during the ensuing 25 years, a notable increase in the instances of DILI was observed. Over the past few years, there has been a heightened awareness of DILI in the United States. DILI has been associated with nearly 1,000 agents and is the single most common reason for drug withdrawal from the market by the Food and Drug Administration (FDA). Furthermore, DILI is responsible for more than 50% of all cases of acute liver failure with acetaminophen being the principal offending agent (28% of cases in 1998, increasing to 51% of cases in 2003), accounting for 15% of all liver transplants in the United States.[1–3] Additional causative agents of DILI include antibacterials (especially antitubercular agents), nonsteroidal anti-inflammatory drugs (NSAIDs), and antiepileptic drugs. Thus, the widespread risk of DILI imparts a challenging task for health care professionals.

Hepatotoxicity appears to be responsible for 2% to 5% of the cases of jaundice or acute hepatitis and for even fewer cases of chronic liver disease [1,4–23] but the true incidence is difficult to determine. The exact incidence may be much greater due to under reporting, complexities in diagnosis and detection, and limited follow-up of exposed persons. Other data suggest that adverse drug reactions cause a larger number of liver diseases than previously reported.[1,2,6–8] However, certain patient populations may have a greater incidence of DILI.[9–16] For example, in a population-based study conducted in France from 1997 to 2000, researchers found that the crude incidence of hepatotoxicity was 13.9 cases per 100,000 patients per year; 12% of the patients were hospitalized, and 6% died.[10] The agents most often responsible for hepatotoxicity in this report included antimicrobials (25%), psychotropic agents (22.5%), lipid lowering agents (12.5%), and NSAIDs (10%). The authors noted that the observed frequency of hepatotoxicity was 16 times greater than that typically reported to the drug regulatory authorities as part of the postmarketing surveillance system. Based on these findings, the authors speculated that the incidence and severity of drug-induced liver dysfunction is grossly underestimated in the general population. Additionally, investigators from a Swedish University hospital reported that DILI cases occurred more often in females and accounted for 77/1,164 (6.6%) of all referrals to an outpatient hepatology clinic.[11]

Until recently, a paucity of data has existed with respect to the incidence and outcome of DILI or acute liver failure in the United States. This was due to the relatively rare occurrence of the condition, the variability among patient referral systems in North America, and the lack of an organized data registry.[1,2,8,9,17] Subsequently, a consortium of liver centers was developed to prospectively define the etiologies and outcomes of patients with acute liver failure.[1,2,5,12] This organization, known as the Drug-induced Liver Injury Network (DILIN), was challenged with the specific aim of studying the problem of hepatotoxicity (http://dilin.dcri.duke.edu). Over a 41-month period beginning in 1998, 308 patients (≥15 years) with acute liver failure from 17 tertiary care liver centers were studied.[12] Results showed that most of these patients were women (73%) with a median age of 38 years. The primary cause of acute liver failure was acetaminophen overdose (39% of cases), followed by idiosyncratic drug reactions (13%). Short-term transplant-free survival was 68% and 25% for patients with acute liver failure secondary to acetaminophen ingestion or an idiosyncratic drug reaction, respectively. Additionally, a comprehensive summary of their findings with respect to DILI was published.[12] Other data also suggest that in cases of acute liver failure, fatality rates are high and range from 10% to 50%.[24–27]

EPIDEMIOLOGY AND RISK FACTORS

Epidemiologic reports suggest the overall prevalence of DILI is low.[28–37] For example, the risk of liver injury secondary to NSAIDs use is 1 to 10/100,000 exposed individuals,[20–22,28,29,37] and the combination of amoxicillin with clavulanic acid has been associated with hepatitis in 1 to 5 per 1 million exposed individuals.[1,18,22,32,33] Isoniazid-induced liver injury may occur in as many as 100/100,000 exposed persons, possibly because of its ability to exert a metabolic type of hepatotoxicity,[1,7,21–23] whereas the rate of acute liver failure with lovastatin is 1/1.14 million patient-treated years.[34] Furthermore, the incidence of significant elevation in ALT or AST associated with the use of protease inhibitors (PIs) in combination with other antiretroviral agents has been reported to be up to 9.5% in the randomized controlled registration trials.[1,22,35,36] However, the reported rate of ADRs may be a poor indicator of risk, because it depends on case recognition and definition as well as the motivation of observers to report ADRs.

Recent methodology, such as prescription event monitoring, medical record linkage, and case-controlled studies, have better defined the true risk of an agent's association with DILI.[2,7,31] In many circumstances, drugs are the only cause of liver injury, whereas in other cases, they may augment the relative risk for types of liver injury that could potentially occur even without drug exposure. For example, salicylates are associated with Reye's syndrome, oral contraceptives have been linked to hepatic veno-occlusive disease, and methotrexate may exacerbate hepatic fibrosis in patients with coexisting alcoholic and diabetic types of fatty liver disease.[5,14,38]

1. C.W. is a 63-year-old female, 61 inches tall, and weighs 75 kg with a history of chronic urinary tract infections for which she had previously taken prophylactic trimethoprim-sulfamethoxazole. C.W. also has a history of generalized tonic-clonic seizures following an automobile accident 7 years ago. For the previous 18 months, her seizures have been well controlled on valproic acid 1 g Q 8 hr. Of note, C.W. has recently been initiated on venlafaxine 50 mg twice daily (BID) for treatment of depression. On a routine visit to the neurology clinic, she was noted to have ALT, 66 U/L (normal, 5–40); AST, 88 U/L (normal, 5–40); alkaline phosphatase, 85 U/L (normal, 21–91); and total bilirubin, 0.8 mg/dL (normal, 0.1–1.2). What nonpharmacologic risk factors does C.W. have for DILI?

Several host factors affect the risk of DILI (Table 29-1). As previously described, most hepatic adverse drug reactions occur in adults rather than in children.[1,2,6,22,38] In the adult population, the relative risk of hepatotoxicity induced by isoniazid,[23,39] halothane,[40] erythromycin estolate and its analogues,[5,7,22,41–43] and diclofenac[44] is greater in patients older than 40 years of age. Generally, the increased frequency of adverse reactions observed in adults may correspond with an increased exposure, ingestion of multiple agents, or altered drug disposition. Exceptions to these findings include valproic acid- or salicylate-induced hepatotoxicity, which occurs most commonly in children younger than 3 years of age.[1,2,45,46] Although DILI is uncommon in children, it accounts for about 25% of childhood acute liver failure. Causative agents include acetaminophen, antiepileptic drugs, antineoplastic drugs, herbal supplements, and recreational drug use. Gender may also be related to risks for DILI. For example, female gender has been associated with an increased risk of hepatotoxicity, especially from agents such as halothane,[40] nitrofurantoin,[47] methyldopa,[6,7] and sulfonamides.[9,48]

In addition to age and gender, genetic factors may also have an impact on the ability to metabolize or eliminate drugs, encode pathways of bile excretion, and modulate the immune response. Although rarely encountered, a familial predisposition to hepatic ADRs from agents, such as halothane[40,49] and phenytoin,[50] has been shown. Other factors that have an impact on DILI risk include a previous history of ADRs and ingestion of multiple drugs. The mechanism of DILI in the latter appears to be enhanced cytochrome P450-mediated metabolism of the second agent to toxic intermediates (i.e., acetaminophen, isoniazid, and valproic acid). Chronic excessive ingestion of alcohol may also enhance the risk of DILI from agents, such as acetaminophen, by reducing the body's stores of glutathione, which essentially lowers the dose threshold for hepatotoxicity. Other concomitant diseases or conditions, such as rheumatoid arthritis, diabetes, hyperthyroidism, obesity, pregnancy, infection with human immunodeficiency virus, hepatitis B or hepatitis C virus, or renal dysfunction, may also place patients at risk for DILI.[1,2,22,51–60] Furthermore, drug dose, concentration, and duration of intake may be additional determinants in DILI. Environmental risk factors, such as malnutrition may also enhance the risk of DILI.[22]

Thus, C.W.'s age, gender, and obesity appear to be nonpharmacologic risk factors for developing DILI. However, because C.W. is asymptomatic and does not have manifestations of DILI, her baseline laboratory values are not reported, and the current hepatic enzyme elevation is less than three times normal, she should undergo close monitoring of her liver function tests within the next 2 to 4 weeks and return to the clinic for a follow-up.

PATHOPHYSIOLOGY OF HEPATIC INJURY

Because the hepatotoxicity of drugs is often related to reactive metabolites and exposure to these intermediates is determined by genetic and environmental factors, having a general

Table 29-1 Risk Factors for Developing Drug-induced Liver Disease[1,5,7,22,28]

Factor	*Examples of Drugs Affected*	*Comments*
Age	Isoniazid, nitrofurantoin, halothane	Increased incidence/severity with age >60 year
	Valproic acid, salicylates	Higher incidence in children
Sex	Halothane, methyldopa, nitrofurantoin	Higher incidence in females
	Flucloxacillin, azathioprine	Higher incidence in males
Dose	Acetaminophen, aspirin	Higher-blood concentrations associated with risk of hepatotoxicity
	Methotrexate, vitamin A	Total dose, frequency, and duration associated with hepatotoxic risk
Genetic factors	Halothane, phenytoin, sulfonamides, isoniazid	Numerous familial cases; defective epoxide hydrolases increase susceptibility to phenytoin and halothane associated injury; acetylator phenotype may predispose to isoniazid hepatotoxicity
	Valproic acid	Familial cases, correlation with mitochondrial enzyme abnormalities
History of other drug reactions	Halothane, enflurane; erythromycins; diclofenac, ibuprofen	Rare incidence of cross-sensitivity reported between drug classes
Concomitant drug therapy	Acetaminophen	Isoniazid, zidovudine may lower toxic dose threshold for hepatotoxicity
	Busulfan, azathioprine	Increased risk of hepatic veno-occlusive disease
	Valproic acid	Other anti-epileptic drugs increase risk of hepatotoxicity
Excessive alcohol use	Acetaminophen	Lowered dosage threshold
	Isoniazid, methotrexate	Increased liver injury and enhanced fibrosis
Other diseases		
Obesity	Halothane hepatitis, methotrexate	Increased liver injury and enhanced fibrosis
Fasting	Acetaminophen	Increased risk of hepatotoxicity
Renal failure	Tetracycline, methotrexate	Increased liver injury and enhanced fibrosis
Preexisting liver disease	Niacin (nicotinamide), methotrexate	Increased risk of liver injury
Organ transplantation	Azathioprine, busulfan	Increased risk of vascular toxicity
AIDS	Dapsone, trimethoprim-sulfamethoxazole, oxacillin	Increased risk of liver injury; hypersensitivity
Diabetes	Methotrexate	Increased risk of hepatic fibrosis

understanding of the pathophysiology and pathways is important. Thus, hepatic injury secondary to phase I mediated cytochrome P450 (toxification), phase II (detoxification) conjugation reactions, and phase III (excretion/transport), as well as biochemical mechanisms of cellular injury or death, will be reviewed in the following section.[1,2,18,22]

The liver is an extremely resilient organ and is well equipped to resist toxic insults because of its unique cellular attributes (e.g., cell cooperation, acute-phase response, synthesis of hepatoprotective substances). Despite this resiliency, the liver is vulnerable to injury because it is frequently exposed to agents in their most reactive, thus toxic, forms. Because the liver is located between the absorptive lining of the gastrointestinal tract and drug targets within the body, orally administered drugs enter the portal circulation and undergo "first-pass metabolism," leading to significant exposure of the drug or its metabolites to the hepatocytes. Several factors promote the close contact between hepatocytes, blood, and drugs, including (a) the structure of the hepatic sinusoids; (b) the fenestrated hepatic endothelium; and (c) the enhanced overall surface area of the hepatocytes.[6,22,61,62] The liver may also be rapidly exposed to intravenously administered drugs because it receives approximately 25% of the cardiac output.

Hepatic uptake of drugs is thought to occur through passive diffusion, carrier-mediated uptake, facilitated transport, or active transport. After drugs have entered the hepatocytes, back diffusion out of the cells may be minimized through cytosolic transfer proteins, such as glutathione S-transferase, fatty acid–binding proteins, and 3–hydroxysteroid dehydrogenase.[61,62] Drugs are, thereby, transferred to either the endoplasmic reticulum, where they are metabolized, or to the canalicular membrane, where transporters actively secrete endogenous or exogenous substances into the bile. Because most drugs are primarily lipophilic, they are not readily excreted in the urine or bile and must be converted to a more excretable hydrophilic form. The liver is responsible for this biotransformation either through phase I mediated cytochrome P450 oxidative metabolism and formation of potentially hepatotoxic metabolites (toxification)[62,63] or through phase II conjugation (detoxification)[62,63] reactions.

In drugs undergoing oxidative metabolism, an activated oxygen molecule is integrated into lipophilic substrates resulting in the formation of reactive electrophiles, free radicals, and reduced oxygen compounds.[62,63] Reactive electrophiles can bind to cellular membranes, disrupt their function, and subsequently lead to hepatocellular necrosis.[6,63,64] Examples of causes of this type of liver injury include isoniazid and acetaminophen. Free radical formation from agents, such as carbon tetrachloride (CCl_4), may lead to peroxidative injury of membrane lipids and necrosis,[7,62,63] whereas activated oxygen appears to be primarily associated with pulmonary injury rather than with DILI.[62,63] Several cytochrome P450 isoenzymes exist that have different substrates and can be expressed differently based on increasing age, genetic polymorphisms, and environmental conditions.

Because cellular function is overwhelmingly disrupted through these cytochrome P450-mediated mechanisms, cellular death is a common result. This process occurs through the following mechanisms: (a) plasma membrane alteration and disruption of the cytoskeleton (e.g., loss of ionic gradients);

(b) mitochondrial dysfunction (e.g., decline in adenosine triphosphate levels and disrupting fatty acid oxidation); (c) loss of intracellular homeostasis; and (d) activation of degradative enzymes.[62,62] Additional mechanisms causing hepatocellular death are immunoallergenic (antibody-mediated cytotoxicity or induction of direct cytolytic T-cell responses). Another response involving cytokines (e.g., interferon, tumor necrosis factor, and Fas pathways), nitric oxide, complement activation, and other immune cells (e.g., Kupffer's, thymus, sinusoidal endothelial cells) has also been postulated, which results in inflammation and neutrophil-mediated hepatotoxicity.[5,62,63,65,66] Finally, apoptosis (programmed cellular death) may occur simultaneously with immune-mediated injury.

A second means of drug metabolism is by phase II (detoxification) conjugation reactions. Phase II reactions occur through binding drug metabolites to glutathione, glucuronate, or sulfate, which leads to the formation of nontoxic, readily excretable hydrophilic products.[62,63,66] Subsequently, these compounds are excreted from the body in bile or urine through excretory transporters in the hepatocyte canalicular and sinusoidal membrane (phase III elimination). Inadequate detoxification due to reduced binding substance concentrations (e.g., inadequate glutathione stores) may lead to a greater concentration of a reactive metabolite. An example of phase II-induced liver injury may arise from the inability to detoxify phenytoin metabolites. In addition, the combination of phase I- and phase II-induced liver injury may occur in situations resulting in both formation of toxic metabolites and inadequate detoxification (e.g., acetaminophen).

Overall, the pathogenesis of hepatotoxic drug reactions is likely a result of a "multi-hit" process.[5,62] Several genetic P 450 isoenzyme variants that result in toxic metabolites, the involvement of suppressor and attenuator pathways modulating the hepatotoxic effects, cell-mediated and antibody-induced immune responses, cell surface neoantigens and cytokine expression (interleukin-10 and tumor necrosis factor), inadequate detoxification pathways and individual genetic predisposition all may contribute to DILI. Ultimately, a series of events beginning with intracellular hepatocyte disruption, cellular necrosis, and apoptosis, followed by an immune inflammatory response have been proposed to cause DILI. The actual incidence and resolution of a DILI event may rely on the adaptive phenotypes of the host, which likely is a function of a genetic predisposition. The emerging field of pharmacogenomics could help predict and identify patients with aberrant gene polymorphisms or P450 alleles that affect drug concentrations leading to DILI.

Histopathologically, there are no absolute definitive features of DILI. However, certain patterns suggest a drug etiology. These include (a) zonal necrosis or fatty changes that are associated with mitochondrial injury and (b) mixed histologic manifestations of necrosis and cholestasis. The presence of neutrophils and/or eosinophils within destructive bile duct lesions is suggestive of DILI.[5,62]

Classification of Drug-induced Liver Injury

The nature of drug-induced liver injury may mimic several known liver diseases, but classification is challenging due to overlap between categories and the fact that some drugs may be associated with more than one syndrome. Often there is discordance between the clinical and laboratory features of the liver disease and hepatic histology. Identification of specific patterns or syndromes provides only a clue to the diagnosis of DILI; more important is the temporal relationship between drug administration and liver injury or exclusion of other causes of liver disease. Therefore, drugs are often classified as predictable or unpredictable hepatotoxins, and as a result, the terms *intrinsic hepatotoxicity* and *idiosyncrasy* have evolved to help clinically characterize the proposed drug-induced mechanism of hepatic injury. Briefly, intrinsic hepatotoxicity generally is dose dependent and has a short and consistent latency period between drug exposure and liver injury, whereas idiosyncratic reactions occur without warning, are unrelated to dose and may have a latency period from a few days to 12 months. Idiosyncratic reactions often result from a hypersensitivity reaction (immunologic) or metabolic aberration (altered drug metabolism).

However, because the aforementioned terms may not fully elucidate all forms of DILI, the nature of the hepatic injury has been further delineated based on the time frame in which it occurs (i.e., acute vs. chronic), or it may be classified based on whether the drug-induced liver insult is confined to the hepatocytes (hepatocellular injury) or involves areas such as the biliary tract, liver parenchyma, or hepatic vasculature. Finally, several types of drug-induced lesions resulting from acute or chronic administration of drugs are recognized histologically. Along with the proposed mechanism for liver injury and the time frame of occurrence, the histologic characterization of hepatic lesions is also useful in describing DILI and is reviewed next.

Intrinsic and Idiopathic Reactions to Drugs as Causes of Hepatic Injury

From a clinical perspective, the terms used for identifying and describing drug-induced hepatic injury are *intrinsic hepatotoxicity* and *idiosyncrasy* (Table 29-2). Intrinsic or true hepatotoxins (e.g., chloroform) have the inherent property of predictably injuring the liver. Idiosyncratic or unpredictable hepatotoxins (e.g., halothane) cause hepatic damage only in a small number of uniquely susceptible individuals. The major differences between these two types of drug-induced hepatic injury are listed in Table 29-3.

Table 29-2 Mechanisms of Drug-induced Hepatotoxicity[1,2,15,22,28]

Classification	Lesion	Incidence
Intrinsic Hepatotoxicity		
Direct hepatotoxins	Necrosis or steatosis	High
Indirect hepatotoxins		
Cytotoxic	Steatosis or necrosis	High
Cholestasis	Bile casts	High
Host Idiosyncrasy		
Hypersensitivity	Hepatocellular or cholestatic	Low
Metabolic abnormality	Hepatocellular or cholestatic	Low

Table 29-3 Characteristics of Intrinsic versus Idiosyncratic Hepatotoxins

Intrinsic	*Idiosyncratic*
Distinctive histologic pattern observed for any given drug	Variable histologic pattern of lesions
Dose-dependent hepatotoxicity	Dose-independent hepatotoxicity
Elicited in all individuals	Only a small fraction of exposed individuals affected
Reproducible in experimental animals	Cannot be reproduced in experimental animals
Predictable appearance of lesions and usually a brief latent period following exposure	Appearance of lesions bears no temporal relationship to the institution of drug therapy
No extrahepatic manifestations of hypersensitivity	Lesions often accompanied by extrahepatic manifestations of hypersensitivity (e.g., fever, rash, eosinophilia)

Intrinsic Hepatotoxicity

Intrinsic hepatotoxins can be subdivided into direct and indirect toxins. Direct intrinsic hepatotoxins (e.g., carbon tetrachloride) destroy hepatocytes by a physicochemical attack, mostly through the toxic effects of their metabolites. There are no known direct hepatotoxins that are used as therapeutic agents.[5,7]

In contrast, indirect hepatotoxins (e.g., antimetabolites) induce structural changes in the hepatocytes by competitive inhibition of essential metabolites or by interference with selective metabolic or secretory processes of the hepatocytes. These changes in the hepatocytes can be due to either cytotoxic or cholestatic mechanisms. Indirect intrinsic hepatotoxins that produce cytotoxic changes include tetracycline, mechlorethamine, alcohol, acetaminophen, and mercaptopurine.[13–15,22,28] Indirect intrinsic cholestatic hepatotoxins produce jaundice and hepatic dysfunction by interfering with mechanisms for the excretion of bile from the liver (e.g., C-17 alkylated anabolic steroids, C-17 ethinylated contraceptive steroids).[7,22,62,63]

2. One month after her initial visit, C.W. returns to the clinic with a 1-week history of jaundice, anorexia, fever, and nausea while continuing to take her valproic acid (well-controlled seizures with no change in pattern). Upon obtaining an additional medication history, C.W. states that she briefly reinitiated her trimethoprim-sulfamethoxazole for a couple of days during the last 4 weeks for a recurrence of her urinary tract infection, and increased her venlafaxine dose to 100 mg BID. Laboratory values are as follows: ALT, 164 U/L (normal, 5–40); AST, 177 U/L (normal, 5–40); alkaline phosphatase, 105 U/L (normal, 21–91); and total bilirubin, 2.3 mg/dL (normal, 0.1–1.2). What type of liver injury could C.W. have and what is the clinical significance of her elevated liver function tests?

Idiosyncrasy

Like intrinsic hepatic injuries, idiosyncratic injuries may be cytotoxic, cholestatic, or mixed.[7,22,62,63] Most idiosyncratic drug reactions cause damage to hepatocytes throughout the hepatic lobule with various degrees of necrosis and apoptosis. Hepatic injury due to host idiosyncrasy can be caused by hypersensitivity reactions or by other mechanisms (e.g., an aberrant metabolic pathway for the drug in the susceptible patient). The liver injury may be tentatively attributed to hypersensitivity when it develops after a "sensitization" period of 1 to 5 weeks and is accompanied by systemic characteristics of rash, fever, and eosinophilia.[7,22,62,63] These hallmarks of an immunological reaction suggest that the hepatic injury is caused by drug allergy, especially when they reappear in response to a subsequent challenge dose of the drug. Examples of drugs causing allergic hepatic dysfunctions are methyldopa, phenytoin, *para*-aminosalicylic acid, chlorpromazine, erythromycin estolate, rarely clarithromycin, and sulfonamides.[1,5,14,22,41] Thus, C.W.'s recent elevation of liver function tests could be explained as an apparent "idiosyncratic" reaction to her trimethoprim-sulfamethoxazole (Table 29-4). Furthermore, the second-generation nonselective serotonin reuptake inhibitor venlafaxine has also been identified as a possible cause of hepatic injury. Two cases of venlafaxine-associated "hepatitis" have been reported in the literature.[1,22,69] The first case occurred in a 44-year-old woman receiving 150 mg/day within 7 months of initiating therapy, whereas the second case was reported in a 78-year-old man within 1 month of a dosage increase from 37.5 mg/day to 150 mg/day. In both cases, discontinuation of venlafaxine resulted in resolution of

Table 29-4 Drug-induced Hepatotoxicity[a]

Drug	*Clinical Remarks*
I = Incidence H = Hepatocellular (elevated ALT) M = Mixed (elevated ALP + elevated ALT) C = Cholestatic (elevated ALP + TBL)	
Acarbose I: Low H[138]	Mild ALT elevation, diabetic patients receiving long-term therapy should be monitored closely.
Acetaminophen	See Chapter 5: Managing Acute Drug Toxicity
Alcohol	See Chapter 28: Complications of End-Stage Liver Disease
Allopurinol I: Occasional H[1,139]	Onset of symptoms varies from 7 days to 6 weeks, but mostly during the first month. Mild to moderate increases in alkaline phosphatase and AST have been reported in most cases. Hepatic granulomas are observed in about half the cases. Fever, rash, and eosinophilia are frequent. Incidence may be increased in those on diuretics or with decreased renal function. Death from hepatic failure occurs rarely.

(continued)

Table 29-4 Drug-induced Hepatotoxicity[a] *(Continued)*

Drug	*Clinical Remarks*
Amiodarone I: Uncommon H[93,94,140–143]	Phospholipidosis is a frequent hallmark of amiodarone therapy. Serum transferase levels modestly increase in about 40% of patients. Liver disease is frequently associated with peripheral neuropathy, corneal deposits, a bluish skin discoloration, or thyroid dysfunction. Incidence and severity of these adverse effects appear to be dose and duration related. Due to the long half-life of amiodarone, liver injury may persist for months even after the drug is discontinued. In severe hepatitis, jaundice, hepatomegaly, ascites, and encephalopathy can develop. Fatal cases of amiodarone-induced hepatitis have been reported after IV loading doses. Polysorbate 80, an organic surfactant that is added to the IV solution of amiodarone, may be responsible for hepatotoxicity.
Amoxicillin-clavulanic acid (Augmentin) I: Low C[32,33,131–134]	More than 100 cases of cholestatic jaundice have been reported with this combination. Onset of symptoms range from 2–45 days. Common clinical features include jaundice, pruritus, GI distress, and eosinophilia. Although 40% of this combination is used in pediatric patients, hepatic dysfunction has largely been observed in adults >30 years, suggesting advancing age as a risk factor; male to female ratio was about 2:1. Because some patients had previous or later exposure to amoxicillin without complications, it has been suggested that clavulanic acid or the combination is the cause.
Androgenic steroids I: High incidence of hepatic dysfunction; cholestatic jaundice dose related C[1,6,144,145]	Anabolic steroids with an alkyl group in the C-17 position are more likely to cause hepatic dysfunction and jaundice than testosterone and 19-nortestosterone. Although hepatic enzymes can be increased by 10%–20%, many patients might not have clinical symptoms. However, cholestatic jaundice can develop in patients taking the drug for 1–10 months. The onset of cholestatic jaundice and the severity of hepatic dysfunction are dose dependent. The larger the daily dose, the more likely is the development of jaundice. Individual susceptibility and preexisting liver disease enhance the potential for hepatic damage. Jaundice may be preceded by nonspecific prodromal symptoms such as malaise, mild anorexia, and nausea. Pruritus may be present in about 10% of patients. Serum transferase levels usually <150 U/mL. Values for alkaline phosphatase are normal or modestly increased in most patients. Serum bilirubin levels are usually <170 mmol/L (9.9 mg/dL), but occasionally patients may reach up to 800 mmol/L (46.8 mg/dL). Recovery is prompt after cessation of the drug, but may take up to 6 months in severe cases Anabolic-androgenic steroids have been associated with a number of cases of peliosis hepatis. Peliosis hepatis is a vascular lesion that may rupture and lead to hemoperitoneum in some patients. Hepatic adenoma and carcinoma also have been ascribed to the taking of androgens. Anabolic steroids are more likely incriminated in causing hepatic carcinoma than estrogens. The degree of risk probably relates to the type of anabolic steroid, dose, and duration of therapy. Clinically, patients with hepatocellular carcinoma may present with hepatomegaly, abdominal discomfort, pain, or jaundice. In some cases, the patients are asymptomatic with normal biochemical tests.
Aspirin and other salicylates I: 0.1%–0.5% C[1,6,146,147]	Anicteric injury may occur in 5%–50% of patients with high salicylate blood levels (>15 mg/dL). Most patients who have developed hepatic injury have had levels >25 mg/dL, although a few instances have been noted at levels as low as 10 mg/dL. The injury is manifested by increased serum transferases (10- to 40-fold) and is reversible upon withdrawal of the drug. Fatal hepatitis is very rare. Bilirubin levels are normal or moderately elevated. Children with juvenile rheumatoid arthritis or acute rheumatic fever, and adults with active RA or SLE seem to be more vulnerable. Recently, cholestatic hepatitis during low-dose (250 mg/day) aspirin therapy has been reported. Use of salicylates in children with varicella or influenza-like illnesses is reported to be strongly associated with an increased risk of Reye's syndrome, which includes liver failure as part of the syndrome.
Azathioprine I: Rare M[1,148–151]	Only a few isolated instances of cholestatic jaundice have been attributed to azathioprine. Jaundice starts 3 weeks to 6 months after initiation of therapy. Generalized pruritus, widespread abdominal pain, and hypochromic greasy diarrhea may be present. Although azathioprine has been used in the treatment of chronic active hepatitis, worsening of the hepatic disease also may occur. Azathioprine is the most common drug in the United States implicated in causing VOD. Approximately 20% of bone marrow and renal transplant patients may be affected with a mortality rate of 50%. VOD results from a nonthrombotic concentric occlusion of the lumen of small intrahepatic veins, also known as "bush tea" disease.
Bupropion I: Rare H, C[1,6,152,153]	Laboratory findings primarily show increase in ALT within 6 months of initiation of therapy. Fatal cases with autoimmune characteristics have been reported.
Calcium channel blockers I: Rare H[178–183]	Mild to marked elevations in liver function test results have been reported in <1% of patients taking diltiazem, and drug discontinuation was not required. Six case reports of hepatocellular injury, usually early in the therapy (1–8 weeks), have been published. Eight reported cases of hepatic injury have been associated with nifedipine, each producing acute hepatocellular, cholestatic, or a mixed hepatocellular picture. Three additional chronic cases have been documented beginning 9–72 months after initiation of therapy. Cases were characterized by steatosis and the presence of Mallory-like bodies. Nicardipine, a similar agent, has also been associated with hepatocellular injury. Verapamil-induced hepatocellular injury has been reported in about 6 cases. Hypersensitivity was the proposed mechanism of the injury.

Table 29-4 Drug-induced Hepatotoxicity[a] *(Continued)*

Drug	*Clinical Remarks*
Captopril I: Rare M[1,119–122]	Hepatotoxicity, usually cholestatic in nature, has been reported with captopril, enalapril, and lisinopril use. Cross-sensitivity also has been reported. Jaundice was the most common finding, followed by pruritus, nausea, other GI symptoms, fever, rash, and confusion. Onset of symptoms varied from 5 days to 12 months (mean: 14 weeks; median: 1 month). Doses employed were variable. Hepatotoxicity usually resolves in 2 weeks to 9 months after ACE inhibitors are stopped, but may progress to liver failure and death if therapy is continued.
Carbamazepine I: <1% M[55,56,83,154–156]	Hepatotoxic syndrome resembles that observed with phenytoin. Onset of injury is usually within the first 8 weeks of therapy in 80% of cases. Hepatic injury is associated with modest hyperbilirubinemia, fever, rash, and eosinophilia. Morphologic features are hepatocellular, cholestatic or mixed. Fatality rates are less than those reported with phenytoin and range from 7%–12%.
Chlorpromazine (CPZ) I: 0.1%–0.2% C[157,158]	The effect of age, gender, race, or other predisposing factors has not been established. In approximately 80% of cases, icterus develops between 1–5 weeks of CPZ treatment. In rare instances, jaundice has developed after the first dose. Prodromal symptoms consist of fever, itching, abdominal pain, anorexia, and nausea. Skin rash is observed only in about 5% of reported cases. CPZ jaundice often resembles extrahepatic obstructive jaundice. Severe pruritus is common and may be the first evidence of hepatic injury in some patients. Serum alkaline phosphatase and cholesterol levels are often markedly elevated. Serum transferase levels are increased slightly to moderately in almost all patients. Eosinophilia has been noted in 25%–50% of cases reported. The outlook for CPZ-induced jaundice is good. Cholestatic jaundice associated with CPZ often resolves within 8 weeks but occasionally may continue for a year or longer. Some of the patients with prolonged cholestasis have developed a syndrome resembling that of primary biliary cirrhosis. The clinical syndrome is characterized by itching, xanthoma, hepatomegaly, and splenomegaly. Although it has been suggested that this syndrome is frequently benign and reversible, at least two cases of irreversible cirrhosis and fatality due to CPZ have been described. Other phenothiazines also have been reported to cause cholestatic jaundice, but no reliable estimate of the incidence is available. Because there is a potential for cross-sensitivity between chlorpromazine and other phenothiazines, it is best to avoid using any agent in this class for patients who have had CPZ-induced jaundice. Cholestasis also has been associated with almost all other phenothiazines, and the clinical manifestations reported are similar to chlorpromazine.
Chlorpropamide (and other sulfonylurea oral hypoglycemics) I: Rare M[159–163]	Host factors that modify the susceptibility to hepatic injury are unknown. Onset of jaundice usually occurs between 2–6 weeks of chlorpropamide therapy. Initial symptoms are anorexia, nausea, and vomiting. Soon thereafter, dark urine, jaundice, and clay-colored stools appear. Pruritus and hepatomegaly are common. Fever, rash, and eosinophilia occur frequently but not in all cases. Complete recovery generally occurs within 1–3 months after chlorpropamide is stopped. Patients who recover from chlorpropamide-induced jaundice apparently do not relapse when given tolbutamide. Other sulfonylureas in clinical use (i.e., acetohexamide, tolbutamide, glibenclamide, and tolazamide) also have been reported to cause jaundice, but the incidence appears to be very low.
Clindamycin I: Rare M[6,131,164]	Patients present with elevated ALP and ALT. Rarely fatal; resolution follows discontinuation of the drug.
Clopidogrel I: Rare C[1,165]	Rapid onset of elevation in ALP and TBL. Monitoring of liver function tests may be warranted.
Contraceptive steroids (OCs) I: Dose related 1:10,000 in Europe and North America; 1:4000 in Chile and Scandinavia 1) M[1,6,166–175]	1) Estrogens can selectively interfere with bilirubin excretion by the liver. The importance of structural specificity of the estrogen molecule in causing hepatic dysfunction has been established. The phenolic character of ring A and the addition of an alkyl group at the C-17 position of the estrogen molecule seem to be responsible for the injury. Progesterone has little or no demonstrable adverse effect on hepatic function by itself, but may enhance the hepatic injury produced by the estrogens. Transient hepatic dysfunction occurs much more frequently and may be as high as 40%–50% of patients taking these agents but the overall incidence of jaundice appears to be much lower (i.e., 1 per 4,000–10,000). Postmenopausal women appear to be more susceptible to hepatic dysfunction induced by estrogen than younger women. Certain ethnic groups (Swedes, Chileans) seem to be more prone to develop anicteric dysfunction than others. Susceptibility to estrogen-induced cholestasis probably is related to a genetic factor because of the strong link with recurrent cholestasis of pregnancy. The jaundice usually is noted during the first 6 months of therapy and often during the first cycle. Jaundice is preceded by nonspecific symptoms including malaise, anorexia, nausea, and pruritus. Splenomegaly is not seen and hepatomegaly is infrequent. Serum concentrations of bilirubin levels are increased moderately in most cases (≥10 mg/dL) but values >20 mg/dL have been described. Other biochemical features resemble the jaundice produced by the C-17 alkylated anabolic steroids. Prognosis of the cholestatic jaundice is good. In most individuals, the clinical syndrome resolves completely within 1 month of discontinuation.

(continued)

Table 29-4 Drug-induced Hepatotoxicity[a] (Continued)

Drug	Clinical Remarks
2) Adenoma, peliosis hepatis	2) Hepatic adenoma was a very rare tumor before the widespread use of contraceptive steroids. Since then, the increase in incidence of adenoma seems to have paralleled the increased use of OCs. Women taking contraceptive steroids for periods >5 years appear to be at higher risk of developing an adenoma than those who have taken the drug <3 years. One-third to one-half of patients found to have adenoma remain asymptomatic. Approximately one-third may present with a painful, tender mass. The remaining one-fourth to one-third of reported patients often present with a sudden life-threatening intra-abdominal hemorrhage secondary to rupture of the adenoma. Prognosis is good if the adenoma can be resected before the rupture. For patients with hemoperitoneum, the outlook is fair if the diagnosis is made promptly and the tumor resected. Otherwise, death may result from hemorrhagic shock, coagulation abnormalities, and related complications. Peliosis hepatis is a rare complication from contraceptive steroids and often occurs along with the adenoma.
3) Budd-Chiari syndrome	3) Budd-Chiari syndrome is characterized by acute or subacute development of abdominal pain, hepatomegaly, portal hypertension, ascites, edema, and moderate jaundice. This syndrome is caused by thrombosis and subsequent occlusion of the hepatic veins. Although this complication is very rare, an extremely high mortality rate clearly makes it an important consideration in the use of estrogens.
4) Carcinoma	4) Several types of malignant tumors have been associated with the use of OCs. Over 100 cases have been reported, but the incidence is low when compared to the widespread use of OCs. Hepatic carcinoma may be more likely in women who have used the OCs for >8 years.
Cyclosporine I: Uncommon M[6,176,177]	Increased serum transferase, gamma-glutamyl transferase, and serum bilirubin concentrations are signs of cyclosporine hepatotoxicity. Elevated LFTs have been observed in about 4% of renal transplant, 7% of heart allograft, and 4% of liver transplant recipients, usually during the first month of cyclosporine therapy. Reduction of cyclosporine dosage usually reverses hepatotoxic effects. Several cases of cholestasis have been reported. There was a significant increased incidence of VOD among patients who received cyclosporine and methotrexate (CYC-MTX) versus those who received cyclosporine and methylprednisolone (70% vs. 18%) as prophylaxis against graft-versus-host disease for allogenic bone marrow transplantation. Incidence of early deaths due to VOD was significantly higher in the CYC-MTX group (25% vs. 4.5%).
Erythromycin M[1,41–43,131]	Erythromycin-associated cholestasis is primarily associated with the estolate salt; less common with the ethylsuccinate and propionate derivatives. Children may be less susceptible than adults. Onset of cholestatic jaundice usually occurs 1–3 weeks after exposure; however, patients previously exposed may exhibit symptoms within 2 days. Abdominal pain occurs in about 75% of the cases. Icterus may precede or accompany GI complaints, such as anorexia, nausea, and vomiting. Fever occurs in about 60% of patients, and rash is often absent. Eosinophilia occurs frequently (45%–80%). Serum bilirubin values are generally <100 mmol/L (5.8 mg/dL). Response to a challenge dose of the same erythromycin derivative is usually prompt. The hepatic injury is reversible, and jaundice often subsides within 2–5 weeks after the drug is discontinued. Cholestatic jaundice has also been reported with clarithromycin and in seven cases of patients receiving roxithromycin.
Felbamate I: <1% C[57,184]	Twenty-three cases of hepatic failure have been reported following the use of felbamate, 13 of these were not clearly related to felbamate therapy. Of the remaining 10 cases, 5 deaths were attributable to felbamate. The overall incidence appears to be 1 per 26,000–34,000 exposed. The drug remains available; close biochemical and hematologic monitoring has been recommended.
Fluoroquinolones I: Rare H[131,185–189]	Elevations in aminotransferase, bilirubin, and alkaline phosphatase levels were observed in 1.8%–2.5% of patients who received fluoroquinolones. Sporadic cases of drug-induced hepatitis had appeared in the literature for ciprofloxacin, enoxacin, ofloxacin, and norfloxacin. Hepatic injury due to fluoroquinolones apparently is not dose related and generally is reversible when the drug is stopped. However, one fatal case of hepatic failure, apparently due to oral ciprofloxacin, was reported. The broad spectrum fluoroquinolone trovafloxacin has also been associated with more than 100 cases of hepatotoxicity, fourteen of which involved acute liver failure, with liver transplantation required in four of these. An immuno-allergenic mechanism has been suggested as an etiology. The drug remains available in the United States for very restricted indications.
Fluoxetine (paroxetine) I: Very low H[1,6,190,191]	According to three published reports of fluoxetine-induced liver disease, patients generally presented with elevated bilirubin, ALT, and AST. Patients generally required from several weeks to months before liver function tests normalized.
Haloperidol I: Low C[6,192]	Incidence has been estimated to be between 0.2% and 3% of recipients. Most reported cases of jaundice appear to be cholestatic.

Table 29-4 Drug-induced Hepatotoxicity[a] *(Continued)*

Drug	*Clinical Remarks*
Halothane I: 1) Mild form >25% 2) Severe 1:35,000 to 1:3,500 C[40,49,52,54,81,193–196]	Halothane exposure may be followed by two distinct types of hepatotoxicity: asymptomatic with abnormal laboratory values only or severe acute hepatitis with massive hepatic necrosis. The incidence and severity appear to be greater in females and enhanced by obesity and previous exposure to halothane or irradiation. Jaundice is rare in children and young adults <30 years. The clinical syndrome of halothane-induced liver disease often consists of a history of unexplained delayed fever postoperatively (>3 days) after halothane anesthesia. There is usually a latent period of 5–14 days between the anesthetic episode and the appearance of hepatic injury, but it may appear as early as 1 day after the operation in patients who have had multiple prior exposures to halothane. Fever with or without chills, aching, anorexia, nausea, and abdominal distress preceded jaundice in 75% of the patients. After jaundice appears, other manifestations of serious hepatocellular damage often develop rapidly. Coagulation abnormalities, ascites, renal insufficiency, GI bleeding, and encephalopathy may follow. Values for serum transferases are markedly elevated (≥3000 U/L), whereas alkaline phosphatase is increased only modestly. Eosinophilia has been observed in 20%–50% of reported cases. Rash is uncommon. Mortality rate for halothane hepatitis ranges from 14%–67%. Serological testing for antibodies specific to halothane-altered antigens is positive in about 75% of patients and can be used as a diagnostic aid along with the drug history and clinical presentation.
Isoniazid (INH)[1,39,131,197,198]	See Chapter 61: Tuberculosis. Fast and slow acetylators may be equally susceptible to the hepatotoxic effects of INH. It appears that specific P450 isoenzymes may be involved because of the enhanced hepatotoxicity by alcohol, other drugs (rifampicin), and advancing age.
Irbesartan/Losartan I: Rare C (irbesartan)[199] H (losartan)[200]	Eight cases of hepatotoxicity due to angiotensin II antagonist are reported in the literature. General presentation following initiation of therapy (1 week to 5 months) includes anorexia, and abdominal pain. Age of patients range from 41–77 years with female predominance.
Ketoconazole I: 0.03%–0.1% H[1,6,131,201–206]	Serum transferase concentrations can be increased in 8%–12% of patients without overt clinical symptoms. Symptomatic hepatic injury is infrequent and often presents as a mixed or cholestatic jaundice. Fulminant hepatitis is also possible. Hepatitis is more common in females, especially those over 40 years of age, and usually occurs after 10 days to 26 weeks of therapy. Hypersensitivity manifestations are usually absent. Fluconazole, itraconazole, and voriconazole have also been implicated in cases of hepatic injury, but the overall incidence is extremely low.
Lovastatin I: Very rare H[1,34,207–211]	In 613 patients who received lovastatin during controlled trials, the most common laboratory abnormalities were elevations in hepatic enzymes. Serum concentrations of ALT, AST, and CPK were increased by 7.3%, 5.9%, and 5.1%, respectively. Serum aminotransferase concentrations were increased by more than threefold in about 1.9% of all patients in this study. Increased transferase levels have been reported in patients with the homozygous form of familial hypercholesterolemia and may be dose related. Hepatitis, fatty change in the liver, cholestatic jaundice, and chronic active hepatitis have been reported rarely. Liver function tests are usually reversible after a few weeks upon discontinuation, but recovery may be delayed for up to 21 months. Rechallenge can result in elevations of aminotransferases in about 50% of patients. Lovastatin should be avoided in patients who have liver disease or a history of alcohol abuse. Pravastatin and simvastatin also have been reported to cause increases in aminotransferases that may lead to cessation of therapy. Simvastatin has been associated with at least five cases of presumed hepatitis.
Methotrexate (MTX) I: Dose, frequency, and duration related H[1,6,212,213]	MTX frequently causes steatosis and portal inflammation in the liver when it is used in the acute treatment of leukemia, choriocarcinoma, and other neoplastic diseases. Overt clinical symptoms occasionally accompany these lesions. Prolonged use of MTX in patients with psoriasis may lead to hepatic fibrosis and cirrhosis but apparently not in those with RA. The likelihood of hepatic injury probably is directly related to the total dose and duration of therapy; it is inversely related to the time interval between doses. Other risk factors include age, obesity, diabetes, alcoholism, and perhaps severity of psoriasis. Biochemical changes provide insensitive reflections of MTX-induced hepatic injury. Serum concentrations of AST and ALT are usually increased for 1–2 days after a single dose of MTX; however, cirrhosis can develop insidiously without increases in the liver enzyme concentrations. Serial liver biopsies at yearly intervals are highly recommended for patients with psoriasis to facilitate the discovery of cirrhosis and its complications which can progress without overt clinical symptoms. Some of these patients may progress to hepatic failure and death. Early recognition of this syndrome can minimize irreversible hepatic damage and improve long-term survival. Preventative measures include giving intermittent rather than small daily doses of MTX. Single weekly dosing regimens of <15 mg have been successful in reducing the incidence of significant hepatic injury.

(continued)

Table 29-4 Drug-induced Hepatotoxicity[a] (Continued)

Drug	Clinical Remarks
Nonsteroidal anti-inflammatory drugs (NSAIDs) I: 1:100,000 recipients H[1,6,37,214–221]	Two-thirds of the cases of sulindac-induced hepatic injury had clinical hallmarks of hypersensitivity. Ratio of females to males was 3.5:1 with 69% of patients >50 years. Most commonly reported clinical features of sulindac-induced hepatitis were jaundice (67%), nausea (67%), fever (55%), rash (48%), pruritus (40%), and eosinophilia (35%). Onset ranged from 1 day to 3 years, but mostly <8 weeks. Rechallenge leads to recurrence in a few days, thus suggesting an allergic mechanism. Complete recovery occurred in all patients 2–3 weeks after drug discontinuation. Severe cholestatic hepatitis, which can progress to subacute hepatic necrosis, has been reported with piroxicam. Elderly patients >60 years seem to be more prone to piroxicam-induced cholestasis. Liver enzymes may take 3–4 months to return to normal levels after piroxicam is discontinued. Other NSAIDs, such as naproxen, diclofenac, ketoprofen, and ibuprofen, also have been implicated. Although cases of NSAID-induced hepatitis are rare, they can be fatal; serious hepatoxicity resulted in the removal of benoxaprofen and bromfenac from the U.S. market. The majority of cases of hepatitis secondary to NSAIDs occur within the first few months of treatment.
Nitrofurantoin I: Rare M[1,91,131,222–224]	Symptoms of hepatic injury are usually abrupt with fever (60%), rash (30%), and eosinophilia (70%). Approximately two-thirds of the patients have had previous exposure to nitrofurantoin. The latent period before the development of symptoms ranges from 2 days to 5 months, but is usually within the first 5 weeks. Cholestatic jaundice is the most common acute injury observed with nitrofurantoin. Biochemical abnormalities and jaundice are generally reversible when the drug is discontinued. CAH of the "lupoid" type is rare and may be accompanied by pulmonary lesions. Most patients have a low serum albumin concentration and a high gamma globulin serum concentration. Antinuclear and/or antismooth muscle autoantibodies are found in most patients. Few cases of cirrhosis have been reported.
Oxacillin and its derivatives I: Low C[131,225–227]	Oxacillin has been associated with rare cholestatic jaundice and numerous cases of anicteric hepatic dysfunction. Liver transferase levels can be as high as 1,000 U/L in some cases. Alkaline phosphatase levels are only modestly elevated and serum bilirubin remains normal in most patients. Eosinophilia accompanies only about 25% of cases. Upon cessation of oxacillin, liver enzyme values generally return to normal within 2 weeks. Apparently there is no cross hepatotoxicity between oxacillin and other penicillins. Nafcillin or penicillin G often can be substituted without recurrence of liver injury. Cloxacillin and flucloxacillin also have been associated with severe cholestatic jaundice. Occasionally, the cholestatic injury may last for months to years even after the drug is stopped. Estimated incidence of flucloxacillin-induced liver dysfunction ranged from 1:11,000–1:30,000 prescriptions. Higher risk was associated with female sex, age, high daily doses, and duration of >2 weeks.
Phenytoin I: <1% M[1,58,59,154]	Subclinical hepatic enzyme elevation is common with phenytoin but overt hepatitis is much less common. Children seem to be less vulnerable to hepatic injury from phenytoin. Almost 80% of cases involved adults >20 years. Symptoms generally occur after 1–5 weeks of therapy. Fever, rash, lymphadenopathy, and eosinophilia followed by jaundice appear in most patients. Leukocytosis with lymphocytosis and atypical lymphocytes is common. The syndrome resembles that of serum sickness or infectious mononucleosis. Biochemical features are similar to those of severe viral hepatitis. Values for AST and ALT are very high (200–4,000 U/L), and the serum concentrations of alkaline phosphatase usually is only modestly increased. A case mortality rate of about 30% is due partly to accompanying severe hypersensitivity reactions (e.g., exfoliative dermatitis) and partly to resulting hepatic failure. A single case of phenytoin-induced chronic persistent hepatitis which was verified by histology and rechallenge was reported.
Propylthiouracil (PTU) I: Rare H, C[6,228,229]	Asymptomatic and transient elevations of liver enzymes are common in patients receiving PTU (up to 28% in one study). However, ALT levels decrease after dosage reduction and normalize in most cases. Signs and symptoms of hepatocellular damage usually appear within 2–4 weeks after initiation of the drug and often are accompanied by rash, fever, and lymphadenopathy. CAH and cholestatic jaundice secondary to PTU have been described. Fatal cases of PTU-induced jaundice have been attributed to hepatic necrosis or accompanying granulocytosis.
Quinidine I: Rare M[5,6,20]	Mild hepatic injury induced by quinidine most commonly occurs within 6–12 days of initiation of treatment and is usually anicteric. Quinidine-induced hepatitis is usually heralded by fever in association with increased AST, ALT, LDH, and ALP levels. Discontinuation of the drug usually results in rapid resolution of fever and laboratory abnormalities. Upon rechallenge with a single dose of quinidine, most patients have promptly developed fever and increased concentrations of serum transferases, thereby supporting hypersensitivity as a mechanism.
Risperidone I: Very rare H[1,230]	Atypical presentation; hepatocellular damage occurs weeks to months following exposure. Reverses upon discontinuation of therapy.
Rifampin[1,39,131]	See Chapter 61: Tuberculosis
Sertraline I: Very rare H[1,231]	The primary presentation is increased ALT levels between 1 and 5 months after exposure. It is likely to be an idiosyncratic mechanism.

Table 29-4 Drug-induced Hepatotoxicity[a] *(Continued)*

Drug	*Clinical Remarks*
Sulfamethoxazole-trimethoprim (Co-Trimoxazole) I: Very low M[1,6,43,70–73,131,232,234]	Twelve cases of cotrimoxazole-induced liver injury (including fatality) have been reported. The cholestasis can be severe and might last for >12 months, even after the drug was stopped. Prominent features are pruritus, fever, skin rash, arthralgias, and eosinophilia.
Sulfonamides I: 0.5%–1% cholestatic jaundice M[1,6,131]	Clinical presentation of hepatic injury often occurs within 5–14 days, but occasionally presents as late as several months. About 25% of the patients with hepatic dysfunction have had prior exposure to sulfonamides. The reaction is characterized by fever, rash, and signs of visceral and bone marrow injury. The clinical and morphologic features of such reactions resemble those of serum sickness. Usually, the onset of symptoms is sudden, with fever, anorexia, nausea, vomiting, and sometimes rash. Jaundice appears on the third to sixth day after the onset of fever, but may be delayed for as long as 2 weeks. Dark urine and acholic stools are frequent, and hepatomegaly may be noted. Prognosis depends on the extent of cytotoxic injury. Case fatality rate is reportedly above 10%. Patients who survive generally recover slowly over a period of several weeks to months. Fatal massive necrosis has been described with pyrimethamine-sulfadoxine (Fansidar). Slow acetylators are more susceptible to sulfonamide-included hepatic injury.
Tetracyclines I: Low H[1,6,131,235,236]	Tetracycline has been reported to produce hepatic steatosis. The development of clinically significant fatty liver appears to depend on the presence of high blood levels of the drug. Large doses (>1.5 g/day) of tetracycline, especially when given IV to pregnant women or individuals with renal disease, may give rise to severe hepatic injury. Clinical manifestations usually appear 4–10 days after initiation of tetracycline therapy. Early symptoms include nausea, vomiting, abdominal pain, hematemesis, and headache. Mild jaundice then follows. Hemorrhagic complications, azotemia, hypotension, shock, and coma may develop subsequently. Tetracycline-induced massive steatosis does not differ clinically or morphologically from the spontaneous form of fatty liver of pregnancy. Mortality rate from this syndrome is 80%. This serious untoward reaction can be avoided by using safer alternative antibiotics whenever possible.
Tricyclic antidepressants (TCAs) (amitriptyline, imipramine, desipramine) I: Rare to infrequent C[1,6,237–242]	TCAs usually cause a mixed hepatitis with either the necrotic or the cholestatic component predominating depending on the agent. Jaundice appears within 1 week to 4 months. Hypersensitivity manifestations are seen in some patients. Severe hepatic necrosis and death are rare. Prolonged cholestasis and progressive hepatic fibrosis have been reported in a few cases.
Troglitazone I: Very low C[1,6,123–130]	Reports of troglitazone-associated liver failure led to the removal of this agent from the U.S. market by the FDA in 2000. However, the clinical presentation of thiazolidinedione DILI is significant because this class of agents is still routinely administered to manage type II diabetes. The clinical presentation of thiazolidinedione DILI includes significant increases in ALT (>20× upper limit of normal) between the third and several months (mean 147 days; range 17–287) following initiation of therapy. In patients who had therapy discontinued, ALT usually returned to baseline (mean, 55 days; range 8–142). Patients may not have symptoms of liver dysfunction (e.g., fatigue, nausea, and abdominal pain), yet jaundice may be present in some instances. Liver transplantation was required in some cases. Additional thiazolidinediones, such as rosiglitazone and pioglitazone, may also be associated with idiosyncratic hepatotoxicity. Two case reports describe ALT and AST elevations following initiation of rosiglitazone therapy with rapid normalization following discontinuation.
Valproic acid I: 0.05%–0.1% H[1,6,74–78,154,243]	Valproate can increase the serum transferase concentration in 6%–44% of patients without overt clinical symptoms. Numerous cases of fatal and nonfatal liver disease due to valproate have been reported. Infants and young children (<2 years) are at much higher risk than adults. Lethargy, lassitude, anorexia, nausea, vomiting, edema, facial puffiness, and a frequent change in the pattern of convulsions may precede jaundice, ascites, and hemorrhage. Severe hepatic necrosis can result in coma and azotemia. Prothrombin time is prolonged, serum ammonia concentrations are increased, and hypoglycemia may occur. The hepatotoxicity is thought to be related to an inherited or acquired deficiency in the beta oxidation of valproate resulting in increased formation of a toxic metabolite (4-envalproate). This toxic metabolic pathway seems to be cytochrome P450 enzyme-dependent and is inducible by other drugs such as phenobarbital and phenytoin.
Zidovudine (HAART) I: Very low H[1,6,35,36,244–247]	See Chapter 69: Pharmacotherapy of Human Immunodeficiency Virus Infection Patients generally present with weakness, malaise, abdominal discomfort, prolonged coagulation time, acidosis, an increase in ALT, hyperbilirubinemia, and hepatomegaly following several months of therapy. The primary injury is macrovesicular steatosis, but cholestasis has also been seen. Discontinuation of therapy may only reverse acidosis. Didanosine and nevirapine have also caused macrovesicular steatosis and have lead to several cases of fulminant hepatic failure. Of the PIs, indinavir has been reported to produce hepatic injury.

[a]ACE = Angiotensin converting enzyme; ALP = Alkaline phosphatase; ALT = Alanine aminotransferase; AST = Aspartate aminotransferase; CAH = Chronic active hepatitis; GI = Gastrointestinal; IV = Intravenous; LDH = Lactate dehydrogenase; LFTs = Liver function tests; OCs = Oral contraceptives; PIs = Protease inhibitors; RA = Rheumatoid arthritis; SLE = Systemic lupus erythematosus; SR = Sustained-release; TBL = Total bilirubin; VOD= Veno-occlusive disease.

liver function tests within 5 weeks, and 4 months, respectively. Thus, C.W. should be advised to discontinue trimethoprim-sulfamethoxazole and venlafaxine, and the clinician should monitor her liver function tests closely for the next several weeks to months. Generally, the recovery from a sulfonamide-induced injury depends on the extent of the cytotoxic injury but usually occurs over a period of weeks to months.[70–73]

Idiosyncratic hepatic injury also can be caused by toxic metabolites (e.g., isoniazid, halothane, valproate, ketoconazole, methyldopa).[1,7,13,22] The idiosyncratic or unpredictable hepatic injury that results from a metabolic aberration rather than hypersensitivity usually develops after variable latent periods of 1 week to 12 months and usually is not accompanied by fever, rash, eosinophilia, or histologic findings of eosinophilic or granulomatous inflammation in the liver. In addition, reproduction of the hepatic injury requires administration of the drug for a period of days or weeks, rather than for only one or two doses, presumably to allow for accumulation of toxic metabolites.

Furthermore, C.W.'s clinical presentation could also be explained by her chronic ingestion of valproic acid (Table 29-4). The hepatotoxicity associated with valproic acid is thought to be related to an inherent or acquired deficiency in the β-oxidation of valproic acid, resulting in formation of a toxic metabolite (4-envalproate).[7,22,46,74–78] However, infants and children younger than 2 years of age are at much higher risk than adults for valproic acid-induced liver disease. In addition, there appears to be a change in the pattern of the seizure frequency, which generally precedes clinical manifestations (jaundice, anorexia, fever, nausea) of valproic acid-induced liver disease. Although possible, it is unlikely that C.W.'s DILI is from valproic acid because of her age (>2 years). Thus, it should be continued with close monitoring for resolution of clinical symptoms and liver function tests as described previously.

The classification of the mechanism of hepatic injury by an individual drug into either intrinsic, predictable hepatotoxicity, or unpredictable idiosyncrasy can sometimes be impossible, and in many instances, both major types of mechanisms may have a role. Thus, toxic hepatitis may occur after large overdoses of an intrinsically hepatotoxic drug or in an idiosyncratic manner after therapeutic doses. The reasons for the unique susceptibility of some patients are still poorly understood, and both genetic and acquired factors are likely to be involved.[5,9,18,19,22]

FORMS OF DRUG-INDUCED LIVER DISEASE

In addition to classifying DILI as a result of intrinsic hepatotoxicity or idiosyncratic reactions, the nature of the hepatic lesion can be used to categorize a specific type of liver injury. However, there are several limitations to fully differentiating the number and forms of DILI based on the nature of the hepatic lesion. These limitations may include an inability to completely analyze the histologic, clinical, and biochemical characteristics of the offending agent or the lack of recognition and confidence in implicating a potentially hepatotoxic agent due to the sporadic nature of ADR reporting. Other limitations may include the concomitant use of additional hepatotoxic agents, pre-existing hepatic diseases, and the inability to rechallenge a patient with the agent in question. Despite these concerns, drug-induced hepatic injury continues to be classified according to the morphology of the liver injury, the presumed mechanism, or the circumstances of drug-induced damages.

Drug-induced hepatic lesions can also generally be characterized as either acute (clinical or histologic evidence present for <3 months) or chronic (clinical or histologic evidence present for >3 months). Although acute injuries have received the most attention, chronic DILI has become increasingly prevalent. Both types of injury (acute and chronic), along with the characteristic clinical patterns and lesion(s), are discussed in the following sections.

Acute Drug-induced Liver Disease

The FDA, American Pharmaceutical Manufacturers, and selected members of the American Association of the Study of Liver Diseases (AASLD) have adopted guidelines that recommend that an alanine aminotransferase level of more than three times the upper limit of normal and a total bilirubin level of more than twice the upper limit be used as a combined test to define clinically relevant abnormalities on liver tests with additional verification through analysis of available clinical data. Elevations in serum enzyme levels, including alanine aminotransferase, aspartate aminotransferase, and alkaline phosphatase, are to be considered as indicators of liver injury as opposed to increases in both total and conjugated bilirubin levels, which should be considered measures of overall liver function. Furthermore, the pattern of liver injury is important to recognize, because specific drugs elicit an injury according to one pattern or another. Thus, the pattern of DILI can be hepatocellular, mixed, or cholestatic (Table 29-5). Clinically, hepatocellular injury pertains to elevations of alanine aminotransferase, mixed patterns are manifested by an elevated alkaline phosphatase, and the cholestatic pattern in defined by an increase in both alkaline phosphatase and total bilirubin levels. Hepatocellular injury can be either cytotoxic or cytolytic, and it results in damage to the liver parenchyma. The lesions responsible for hepatocellular injury can be due to necrosis, steatosis, or a combination thereof. Most cases of DILI have a "mixed" pattern with features of both hepatocellular and cholestatic injury. Cholestatic injury depicts arrested bile flow with jaundice and is associated with minimal or no parenchymal injury.[5,7,22,79]

Precise measures of conjugated bilirubin are infrequently obtained and the direct reacting bilirubin fraction overestimates bilirubin elevations. Thus, a concept of combining the measures of liver injury and function were developed from a clinical observation (referred to as Hy's law) that states that "drug-induced hepatocellular jaundice is a serious lesion."[1,2,22] Furthermore mortality rates are approximately 10% in patients who have both hepatocellular injuries with jaundice, even if the offending agent is discontinued.[1,2,22] Two surveys have supported the assertion that drug-induced hepatocellular injury with jaundice results in greater mortality or the need for liver transplantation than is cholestatic or mixed injury.[1,2] Because C.W. has evidence of hepatic injury and compromised function, she is more likely to have a greater risk of mortality and require liver transplantation. Thus, she should be referred to an inpatient setting for additional evaluation of her liver disease.

Table 29-5 Features of Acute Drug-induced Acute Hepatic Injury [1,5–6,7,15,22,28]

			Biochemical Markers		
Lesion	*Syndrome*	*Clinical Presentation*	*ALT/AST*	*ALK/Phos*	*Examples of Offending Agents*
Hepatocellular					
Necrosis	Acute hepatitis	A, N, V	8–200×	3×	Isóniazid, diclofenac, halothane
Sinusoidal beading	Pseudomononucleosis	A, N, V, L, S	8–200×	Variable	Phenytoin, dapsone
Massive	Acute liver failure	A, N, V, L, S, C, E	25–200×	<3×	Phenytoin, dapsone
Subacute	Prolonged hepatitis	A, N, V, J, FG	8–25×	<3×	Propylthiouracil, diclofenac
Spotty	Subclinical	None	2–5×	<3×	Isoniazid, diclofenac
Steatosis, microvesicular	Reye-like	N, V, E	2–15×	<3×	Tetracycline
Cholestatic Injury					
Hepatocanalicular					
Bile casts + spotty necrosis					
Portal inflammation	Obstructive jaundice	A, N, J, PR, FV, R, P	8×	>3×	Carbamazepine, erythromycin estolate, sulfonylureas
Canalicular	Obstructive jaundice	PR, J, P	<5×	<3×	Anabolic steroids
Bile casts					Oral contraceptives

A, anorexia; ALKPhos, alkaline phosphatase; ALT, alanine aminotransaminase; AST, aspartate aminotransaminase; C, coagulopathy; E, encephalopathy; FG, fatigue; FV, fever; J, jaundice; L, lymphadenopathy; N, nausea; P, pain; PR, pruritus; R, rash; S, splenomegaly; V, vomiting.

Hepatocellular Injury

NECROSIS

Drug-induced hepatocellular necrosis may primarily involve cells in a centrilobular (zonal) pattern (e.g., acetaminophen, CCl_4, enflurane, ferrous sulfate, halothane), a diffuse (nonzonal) pattern, or hepatocytes similar to that of viral hepatitis (e.g., methyldopa), or it may affect significant portions of the entire liver (e.g., valproic acid).[5,7,22,28] Additional agents reported to cause hepatocellular injury include trazodone, diclofenac, nefazodone, venlafaxine, and lovastatin.[5,7,22] Serum aminotransferases are the hallmark of hepatic damage. The serum AST and ALT in patients with hepatic necrosis are elevated from 8 to 500 times the upper limit of normal, whereas values for alkaline phosphatase are usually increased modestly to no more than three times normal.[5,13,15,22,80] Blood cholesterol concentrations are often normal or sometimes low. These biochemical patterns resemble those observed in acute viral hepatitis; thus, hepatocellular necrosis is often referred to as *drug-induced* or *toxic hepatitis*.[1,5,7,22] Clinical features include fatigue, anorexia, nausea, and jaundice. With increasing degrees of liver cell necrosis, patients may experience manifestations of acute liver failure, such as deep jaundice, coagulopathy, ascites, hepatic encephalopathy, coma, and death.[7,24,26,27] A final clinical presentation of drug-induced acute hepatitis may mimic infectious mononucleosis.[6,7,22,28] In addition to hepatocellular injury, lymphadenopathy, lymphocytosis, and circulating lymphocytes may be present. This presentation has been associated with the use of phenytoin, dapsone, sulfonamides, and *para*-aminosalicylic acid.[6,7,22,28]

STEATOSIS

A second type of acute drug-induced lesion is steatosis, which can be microvesicular or macrovesicular. In microvesicular steatosis, the hepatocytes are filled with many tiny droplets of fat that do not displace the nucleus (e.g., valproic acid, tetracycline, aspirin overdose).[22,37,46,81–83] In macrovesicular steatosis, the hepatocyte contains a large fat droplet that displaces the nucleus to the periphery (e.g., ethanol, glucocorticoids, methotrexate). Generally, acute toxic steatosis is likely to be microvesicular, whereas chronic steatosis is usually macrovesicular (e.g., amiodarone, tamoxifen). Although microvesicular steatosis results in enlargement of the liver, routine liver function tests often remain normal. In contrast, fatty degeneration caused by drugs such as valproic acid may result in irreversible cell damage reflected by increased AST and ALT serum concentrations of 100 to 500 U/L.[7,22,46] Elevations in aminotransferase levels in patients with drug-induced hepatic steatosis are not as high as those reported with hepatocellular necrosis. The histologic picture of drug-induced fatty degeneration is similar to that observed with fatty liver of pregnancy or Reye's syndrome[1,5,6,22,28] Certain drugs (e.g., high dosages of estrogens) also can induce a form of degenerative, necrotizing liver damage known as *fatty liver hepatitis,* which can eventually result in micronodular cirrhosis.[1,5–7,22] Fatty liver hepatitis is often asymptomatic, and the appearance of malaise, diarrhea, fever, jaundice, leukocytosis, ascites, or edema may indicate that the damage is already irreversible with a poor prognosis.

Cholestatic Injury

CANALICULAR AND HEPATOCANALICULAR

Cholestatic injury has been associated with two prominent types of lesions.[1,5–7,22,28] These are manifested by bile stasis without inflammation and with minimal parenchymal injury (i.e., bland, pure, or steroid cholestasis) or by cholestasis with inflammation and slight parenchymal injury (i.e., cholestatic hepatitis, pericholangitis, cholangiolitic cholestasis, or sensitivity cholestasis). The former can be characterized as *hepatocanalicular* (i.e., combined with hepatocyte injury), whereas the latter is referred to as *canalicular* (i.e., portal inflammation).

Canalicular cholestasis is characterized by AST and/or ALT elevations less than eightfold above normal, normal cholesterol, alkaline phosphatase elevations less than threefold above normal, in a patient who is jaundiced or has a serum bilirubin level >42 mmol/L. In contrast, hepatocanalicular cholestasis usually presents with AST and/or ALT levels less than eightfold elevated, increased cholesterol, and alkaline phosphatase 3- to 10-fold above normal. Patients with AST, ALT, and alkaline phosphatase levels in the canalicular range but with a serum bilirubin level <42 mmol/L are categorized as having an "indeterminate type," because these values could reflect either minor hepatocellular injury or anicteric injury of the cholestatic type. Hepatocanalicular injury is typically seen in chlorpromazine-induced jaundice, and the canalicular type usually is observed in cases resulting from anabolic or contraceptive steroids.[1,2,5,7,22]

Drug-induced canalicular and hepatocanalicular cholestatic injury often resembles extrahepatic obstructive jaundice both clinically and biochemically.[1,5,13,22,28] Pruritus, jaundice, pale stools, and dark urine are the primary clinical manifestations. Other patient complaints may include upper abdominal pain or dull abdominal aching. The serum bilirubin level is increased in all cases of drug-induced cholestasis, but it usually is <170 mmol/L (normal, 2–17), although on occasion, it can be >800 mmol/L.[1,4,5,15,22,28] The serum aminotransferase concentrations are generally only moderately increased. The serum concentrations of alkaline phosphatase are usually increased more than threefold when cholestasis is caused by oral hypoglycemic agents, some antithyroid drugs, erythromycin estolate and its derivatives, or chlorpromazine (hepatocanalicular), but they do not increase as much when the cholestasis is not accompanied by cellular injury (e.g., anabolic, contraceptive steroids).[5,13,15,22,28]

The immediate prognosis in patients with either hepatocanalicular or canalicular injury is good. The mortality rate for pure cholestasis is much lower than when the cholestasis is accompanied by cytotoxic damage and is believed to be <1%.[5,13,22,28] However, a syndrome of chronic intrahepatic cholestasis with clinical, biochemical, and histologic features that resemble primary biliary cirrhosis (PBC) has been observed following acute drug-induced cholestasis[22,82,83] (Table 29-6). These cases of PBC-like disease are likely to resolve, yet a permanent and fatal PBC-like syndrome (vanishing bile duct syndrome) has been identified.[5,7,22,82,83]

Mixed Injury

Mixed forms of drug-induced injury can be primarily hepatocellular with significant cholestatic characteristics, or primarily cholestatic with significant hepatocellular features. They appear to be more consistent with a drug-induced etiology rather than with viral hepatitis. Biochemical markers for mixed cholestatic injury may be defined by elevations in ALT, AST (values more than eight times the upper level of normal), and alkaline phosphatase levels (values more than three times the upper level of normal).

Several drugs appear to exhibit a distinct relationship between their therapeutic class and the type of injury they elucidate.[5,7,15,22,28] For example, some anti-epileptic drugs (e.g., phenytoin, carbamazepine) tend to produce hepatocellular or mixed hepatocellular jaundice. Most neuroleptic agents tend to produce cholestatic (hepatocanalicular) jaundice, whereas hydrazide antidepressants cause hepatocellular jaundice, and tricyclic antidepressants primarily cause cholestatic injury.

Nevertheless, most drugs do not exhibit a distinct relationship between their therapeutic class and the type of injury they induce. Specifically, some oral hypoglycemic agents such as acetohexamide produce mixed hepatocellular injury, whereas others, such as chlorpropamide, tolbutamide, and tolazamide, cause cholestatic jaundice.[5,7,15,22,28] Second-generation hypoglycemic agents, such as glyburide and glipizide, have rarely been associated with causing cholestatic jaundice. Also, the antimicrobial agent nitrofurantoin and the NSAID sulindac may cause either cholestatic or hepatocellular injury.[22,37] Gold compounds appear to be associated with cholestatic rather than hepatocellular jaundice, but this relationship is not consistent. Other agents that lead to mixed injury include *para*-aminosalicylic acid, sulfonamides, amoxicillin-clavulanate, cyclosporine, methimazole, carbamazepine, troglitazone (no longer available), and herbal supplements.[5,7,22,28] The mortality rate of the mixed form seems to depend on the extent of cytotoxic injury.

Table 29-6 Drug-induced Chronic Cholestasis Compared With Primary Biliary Cirrhosis[7,15,22,28]

Characteristics	*Drug-induced Chronic Cholestasis*	*Primary Biliary Cirrhosis*
Associated disease	Irrelevant	Sicca syndrome
Drug intake	Phenothiazines, organic arsenicals	None
Clinical symptoms	Pruritus, early severe jaundice, xanthomas, hepatomegaly, splenomegaly, cirrhosis	Pruritus, latent mild jaundice, xanthomas, hepatomegaly splenomegaly, meloderma, cirrhosis
Laboratory Markers		
Bilirubin	1–20 mg/dL	1–5 mg/dL
ALT/AST	2–8×	2–8×
Alkaline phosphatase	3–10×	3–10×
Histologic Markers		
Ductopenia	Slight	Remarkable
Nonsuppurative cholangitis	Absent	Present
Hepatic granulomas	Absent	Present

ALT, alanine aminotransaminase; AST, aspartate aminotransaminase.

Table 29-7 Features of Drug-Induced Chronic Hepatic Injury[5–7,15,22,28]

Lesion	Associated Syndrome	Biochemical Markers ALT/AST	ALK Phos	Examples of Offending Agents
Hepatocellular				
Necroinflammatory	Chronic hepatitis	3–50×	1–3×	Nitrofurantoin, minocycline, methyldopa
Steatosis	Alcoholic steatosis	1–3×	1–3×	Methotrexate, glucocorticoids
Phospholipidosis	Alcoholic hepatitis	1–5×	Variable	Amphophilic agents
Pseudoalcoholic	Alcoholic hepatitis	1–5×	Variable	Amiodarone, perhexiline
Cholestatic Injury				
Cholangiodestructive	Primary biliary cirrhosis	1–3×	3–20×	Carbamazepine, haloperidol
Biliary sclerosis	Sclerosing cholangitis	1–5×	3–20×	Floxuridine
Granulomatous	Hepatomegaly; hepatitis	1–3×	3–20×	Allopurinol, carbamazepine, hydralazine, quinine
Vascular Lesions				
Peliosis	Hepatomegaly	1–3×	<3×	Anabolic steroids, oral contraceptives
Budd-Chiari syndrome	Congestive hepatopathy	2–20×	Variable	Oral contraceptives
Veno-occlusive	Congestive hepatopathy	2–20×	Variable	Pyrrolizidine alkaloids, azathioprine
Sinusoidal dilation	Hepatomegaly	3×	Variable	Oral contraceptives
Pericellular/sinusoidal fibrosis	Noncirrhotic portal HTN	1–3×	Variable	Vitamin A
Neoplasm				
Adenoma, carcinoma	Asymptomatic hepatic mass	Variable	Variable	Oral contraceptives, anabolic steroids

ALK Phos, alkaline phosphatase; ALT, alanine aminotransaminase; AST, aspartate aminotransaminase; HTN, hypertension.

Chronic Drug-induced Liver Disease

Chronic adverse effects of drugs on the liver generally can be categorized based on the type of lesion or on similarity to clinical syndromes (Table 29-7). These categories include parenchymal lesions secondary to chronic hepatitis, subacute hepatic necrosis, chronic steatosis, phospholipidosis (PL), or fibrosis and cirrhosis. Also included are two forms of cholestatic lesions either from chronic intrahepatic cholestasis or biliary sclerosis. In addition, vascular, granulomatous, and neoplastic lesions may also lead to chronic hepatic disease.[5,7,22,28]

Parenchymal Disease

CHRONIC HEPATITIS

Formerly categorized as chronic active or persistent hepatitis, all chronic necroinflammatory disease of the liver is now referred to as *chronic hepatitis* (CH).[84] In addition to viral etiologies (e.g., hepatitis B virus, hepatitis C virus), autoimmune hepatitis (AIH), Wilson's disease, and cryptogenic cirrhosis, drug-induced hepatic parenchymal lesions have been reported. Drug-induced lesions appear to mimic AIH because they predominantly affect females and are accompanied by hyperglobulinemia, antinuclear antibodies, anti–single-strand DNA, and other serologic autoimmune markers.[5,7,22,28] Drugs associated with this syndrome include dantrolene, diclofenac, fenofibrate, methyldopa, minocycline, nitrofurantoin, sulfonamides, and drugs of abuse such as ecstasy. Acetaminophen and isoniazid also have been incriminated in causing chronic active viral hepatitis-like disease, perhaps owing to continued toxic injury rather than an autoimmune response.[5,7,13,22] To date, at least 24 drugs have been associated with CH, and although the overall presentation is not homogeneous, they have been categorized into four separate types of injury.[13,22]

The first group (type 1) consists of drugs that induce liver injury that resembles autoimmune hepatitis.[6] Drugs associated with this from of injury are often taken for prolonged periods and are continued beyond the initial liver insult. The overall incidence of this "type" appears to be <5%. Unique clinical features in this group includes a high incidence in women (>90% of cases reported), hypergammaglobulinemia, autoantibodies, and a chronic necroinflammation rich in plasma cells.

Type 2 drug-induced chronic hepatitis is characterized by antibody formation against isoforms of cytochrome P450 or other microsomal proteins, which apparently leads to "neoantigen" production during biotransformation.[5,13,22,85–87] Compared with type 1, hyperglobulinemia is not a prominent feature of this entity. Only two drugs (dihydralazine and tienlic acid) have led to this type of drug-induced CH.

Drugs such as etretinate, lisinopril, sulfonamide, and trazodone make up a third form of drug-induced CH, but the serologic markers of autoimmune disease are absent.[6,7,22] Patients with type 3 injury often have elevations in their aminotransferases with histologic evidence of chronic hepatitis.

Type 4 of drug-induced CH consists of agents, such as acetaminophen, aspirin, and dantrolene, which produce chronic toxicity rather than the chronic necroinflammatory disease that resembles chronic hepatitis.[22,28,88,89]

Overall, the clinical picture of drug-induced CH has mixed characteristics, with features of both acute and chronic hepatic injury. Patients may first present with either features of acute hepatocellular injury or clinical evidence of cirrhosis. Physical examination often reveals a firm, enlarged liver, splenomegaly, and spider angiomas with or without ascites,

Jaundice, anorexia, and fatigue are common. Arthralgias or "arthritis" may occur. Serum transferase levels are usually moderately increased; hypoalbuminemia and coagulopathy are common.[90,91] Recognition of drug-induced CH is extremely important because withdrawal of the responsible drug may lead to marked improvement and complete resolution of the injury within 4 weeks. However, continuation of these agents may lead to cirrhosis, fulminant hepatic failure and death.

SUBACUTE HEPATIC NECROSIS

Subacute hepatic necrosis (toxic cirrhosis) is different from acute necrosis and CH in that the clinical deterioration is slower than that seen in acute injury, yet it progresses faster than that associated with CH. Manifestations include a progressive, serious liver disease with deep jaundice and evidence of cirrhosis. Drugs that have been associated with this type of presentation include isoniazid,[28,39] methyldopa,[6,90] nitrofurantoin,[91] and propylthiouracil.[92]

CHRONIC STEATOSIS

Compared with the acute microvesicular type of drug-induced steatosis, chronic steatosis is usually macrovascular and has minimal clinical manifestations. Ethanol, glucocorticoids, and a number of antineoplastic agents such as methotrexate (which all primarily lead to hepatomegaly) are agents associated with this type of insult.[7,22] Glucocorticoid-induced steatosis appears to be benign, whereas methotrexate-induced steatosis can progress to cirrhosis. However, in some instances, the lesions seen in chronic steatosis may be microvesicular and lead to prominent hepatic disease (i.e., necrosis). This presentation has been reported with asparaginase and valproic acid. Valproic acid not only can induce microvesicular lipid deposits in the liver, but also causes fatty degeneration that can result in chronic liver failure with encephalopathy and a fatal outcome.[7,22,74–79]

PHOSPHOLIPIDOSIS

PL occurs frequently and is caused by an amphophilic drug (i.e., a drug that is both lipophilic and hydrophilic) that accumulates within the lysosomes. PL is usually clinically silent or causes only mild liver dysfunction. Hepatomegaly is the predominant feature of PL with or without other organ injury (e.g., PL of peripheral nerves, lungs, thyroid, and skin). Pseudoalcoholic liver disease (PALD) or nonalcoholic steatohepatitis (NASH) consisting of steatosis, focal necrosis, inflammatory aggregates, and Mallory bodies in association with PL have also been reported. These lesions have progressed to cirrhosis in several instances after long-term administration of amiodarone[5,6,82,93,94] This clinical presentation of PALD or NASH can include hepatomegaly, ascites, spider angiomas, wasting syndrome, neuropathy, and moderate increase in aminotransferases (less than five times the upper limit of normal).

FIBROSIS AND CIRRHOSIS

CH, PL-associated PALD, chronic cholestatic injury, lesions affecting hepatic outflow, and chronic injury from methotrexate and etretinate can all lead to hepatic fibrosis and cirrhosis. Portal hypertension and its associated complications are the main characteristics in advanced cases.

Cholestatic Lesions

CHRONIC INTRAHEPATIC CHOLESTASIS

One form of drug-induced chronic intrahepatic cholestasis has features that resemble PBC, but it does not have some of the defining characteristics of PBC such as late-onset jaundice or antimitochondrial antibodies.[5,7,82,83] Common clinical findings associated with this form of lesion are pruritus, early-onset jaundice, and elevated serum bilirubin and alkaline phosphatase levels, but only moderately increased AST and ALT levels. In advanced stages, xanthomatosis, ascites, edema, and portal hypertension may occur. Bile duct destruction and portal inflammation are less significant from chronic cholestatic-associated drug-induced injury compared with PBC, and it may lead to a unique form of the vanishing bile duct syndrome. Drugs reported to cause this syndrome include carbamazepine, haloperidol, imipramine, phenothiazines (chlorpromazine, prochlorperazine), sulfamethoxazole-trimethoprim, thiabendazole, and tolbutamide.[5,7,82,83]

BILIARY SCLEROSIS

A second form of cholestatic cholestasis is biliary sclerosis, which has been observed in cases of bile duct injury produced by intrahepatic arterial infusion of floxuridine.[95] The incidence of injury due to floxuridine appears to be high. Clinical features include upper abdominal pain, anorexia, weight loss, and jaundice. Alkaline phosphatase levels are more than three times normal, whereas the aminotransferases are less than five times the normal limit.

Vascular Lesions

Four significant drug-induced vascular lesions have been reported, including hepatic vein thrombosis, hepatic venule occlusion, peliosis hepatitis, and hepatoportal sclerosis. Vascular injury that affects efferent blood flow (e.g., portal blood flow) to the liver leads to hepatic vein thrombosis. Budd-Chiari syndrome can be manifested by symptoms such as hepatomegaly, abdominal pain, ascites, moderate elevations in serum aminotransferases, and occasionally, jaundice.[38] Rapid deterioration and death may soon follow. This type of injury can be caused by oral contraceptives (OCs), and although the incidence remains low relative to the large number of women taking OCs, case-controlled studies demonstrate that women taking these agents have greater than double the risk compared with other women of developing this lesion.

Veno-occlusive disease as a result of injury and fibrotic occlusion of the terminal hepatic venules has clinical symptoms similar to those of Budd-Chiari syndrome and may result in death or can be followed by complete recovery. This type of hepatic injury has historically been associated with alkaloid derivatives (e.g., etoposide, vincristine, vinblastine), but agents such as thioguanine, azathioprine, chemotherapeutic agents (e.g., busulfan, cyclophosphamide, dactinomycin, methotrexate, mitomycin) and radiation injury serve as common etiologies.[5,7,98] Additional etiologies of this type of injury include herbal medications or dietary supplements that are often obtained in natural food stores.[99]

Peliosis Hepatitis

Peliosis hepatis, a rarely encountered blood-filled cyst in the liver, can be caused by anabolic or contraceptive steroids, as well as related agents such as danazol.[5,7,100] Most cases with this type of injury are often associated with hepatic tumors or with cholestatic jaundice induced by the offending drug. Clinical manifestations include hepatomegaly, jaundice, or liver failure.[100] Occasionally, the cyst may rupture and result in a syndrome of hemoperitoneum.

Drug-induced portal hypertension may occur without evidence of cirrhosis.[5,7,28] An example is hepatoportal sclerosis after chemotherapeutic or immunosuppressive therapy.[5,7,101] Additional causes of this lesion include chronic exposure to inorganic arsenicals, copper sulfate, and vinyl chloride, as well as vitamin A intoxication.[5,7,13,22] Clinically, splenomegaly, leukopenia, thrombocytopenia, pancytopenia, or esophageal varices may be present.

Granulomatous Hepatitis (Drug-Induced)

Granulomatous reactions are a common presentation of DILI and account for 2% to 29% of cases of granulomatous hepatitis. The clinical presentation includes fever, malaise, headache, and myalgia between 10 days and 4 months after the initiation of treatment, with splenomegaly present in up to 15% of cases. Hepatic granulomas are always noncaseating and can be surrounded by eosinophils. The granulomas can be accompanied by cytotoxic or cholestatic injury as part of a hypersensitivity reaction (e.g., allopurinol, methyldopa, penicillin, phenytoin, quinidine, sulfonamides) or without any clinical evidence of hepatic injury (e.g., gold salts).[7,13,22,28,102] Up to 60 drugs have been associated with hepatic granulomas.[5,7,22]

Neoplastic Lesions

Several associations between pharmacologic agents and liver tumors have been reported, but causality has been difficult to prove because of the infrequent nature of these events. Hepatocellular adenoma and carcinoma, although rare, are clearly associated with the use of OCs and anabolic (C-17 alkylated) steroids.[5,7,103–107] Several cases of hepatic adenomas have involved women, virtually all of whom had a history of OC use. The results of two large, case-controlled studies suggest that the incidence is between 3 and 4 per 100,000 exposed persons annually. This represents a relative risk (compared with patients not receiving OCs) of approximately 20-fold in those patients ingesting OCs for <10 years and more than 100-fold in those exposed for >10 years.[5,103] Similarly, some cases have been associated with anabolic steroid use in men.[104] Danazol has been associated with causing hepatocellular adenoma and carcinoma in humans, whereas griseofulvin, hycanthone, and isoniazid have been known to produce hepatocellular carcinoma in experimental animals.[5,7,22] OCs have also been associated with causing hepatocellular carcinomas [7,105] and possibly focal nodular hyperplasia.[6,7,106,107]

In general, prognosis of DILI is good when the offending agent is withdrawn; however, the prognosis clearly is affected by the type of liver damage (injury vs. function as described earlier), the duration of the insult, and whether the hepatic damage is irreversible.[5,13,14,22]

HERBAL SUPPLEMENT-INDUCED HEPATOTOXICITY

3. H.D. is a 48-year-old female with a history of chronic back pain secondary to an auto accident 3 years ago. She previously had taken oral Vicodin (hydrocodone 5 mg/acetaminophen 500 mg), 1 to 2 tablets Q 6 hr for pain relief, but recently, she discontinued the drug because of constipation; subsequently, the pain became worse. After several months of acupuncture as primary therapy, H.D. began taking the herbal supplement Jin Bu Huan per her mother's recommendation. However, after taking the herbal remedy for 2 months, H.D. began experiencing fever, fatigue, and mild abdominal pain. Her husband noticed that H.D. had also become "jaundiced" around that time; as a result, he brought her to the emergency department for treatment. Upon obtaining a careful medication history, laboratory tests revealed that H.D.'s ALT, AST, and total bilirubin were 1,378 U/L, 1,333 U/L, and 3.9 mg/dL, respectively. A biopsy was also obtained, and the results are pending. What is the association between herbal medications and hepatotoxicity?

Previous reports indicated that 3% of the population of the United States had taken herbal medications for a variety of reasons (e.g., analgesia, sedation, nutrition, weight reduction, skin disorders).[99,108–118] Herbals used for treating these diseases can be derived from the root, stem, leaf, or seed of a plant and are available as crude and commercial products. Recent studies show that 42% of Americans take some form of complementary and alternative medicine, and that herbal medicine use is now estimated to be 12.5%. In the United States, herbal products are labeled as dietary supplements, which are not expected to meet the standards for drugs specified in the Federal Food, Drug, and Cosmetic act. Because they are exempt from the rigorous regulations that are required for drug approval in the United States, there are considerable disparities in the composition of these agents. In addition, 20% to 30% of patients attending hepatology clinics use herbal remedies on the erroneous assumption that these agents are "natural" and, therefore, safe.[111,113] Although herbal remedies have historically been considered benign, a plethora of information has suggested that many agents are associated with toxic effects and they are not safe (Table 29-8). Some include asafetida, chaparral leaf, camphor, carp capsules, comfrey, dai-saiko-to (TJ-9), gentian, germander, greater celandine, hops, impila, isabgol, kava, mistletoe, mother wart, pennyroyal oil, senna fruit extract, skullcap, and valerian.[99,111,113,117] Adverse effects usually manifest when the recommended threshold for toxic doses are surpassed, although the duration of therapy may also be a factor. The range of herbal-induced liver injury includes minor transaminase elevations, acute and chronic hepatitis, steatosis, cholestasis, zonal or diffuse hepatic necrosis, hepatic fibrosis and cirrhosis, veno-occlusive disease, and acute liver failure requiring liver transplantation.[99]

In one representative report, seven adult patients ingesting Jin Bu Huan, a traditional herbal remedy used primarily as a sedative and analgesic, presented with fever, fatigue, nausea, pruritus, abdominal pain, jaundice, and hepatomegaly at a mean time of 20 weeks (range, 7–52 weeks) after ingestion of normal doses of this agent.[111,113,118] Serum transaminases were increased 20- to 50-fold in most cases. One patient who had taken the agent for 12 months underwent a liver biopsy, which showed lobular hepatitis with microvesicular steatosis. Resolution of liver injury occurred within 8 weeks after the cessation of therapy. Other than a female predominance, no predisposing risk factors for developing liver disease were evident in this case series. However, it appears that concomitant agents that induce cytochrome P450 enzymes may also increase

Table 29-8 Selected Herbal Medications/Remedies Associated With Hepatic Injury[108–118]

Herb	Proposed Use	Toxic Ingredient	Feature of Hepatic Injury
Comfrey Gordolobo yerba tea Mate tea	Health tonic	Pyrrolizidine alkaloids	Veno-occlusive disease
Chinese medicinal tea	Health tonic	T'u-san-chi'i (Compositae)	Veno-occlusive disease
Jin bu huan	Sedative, analgesic	*Lycopodium serratum*	Hepatocellular injury: hepatitis, fibrosis, steatosis
Chinese herbs	Eczema, psoriasis	Many	Nonspecific hepatic injury
Germander (tea, capsules)	Weight reduction, health tonic	*Teucrium chamaedrys*	Hepatitis: necrosis, fibrosis
Chaparral leaf	Herbal remedy	*Larrea tridenta*	Hepatic necrosis
Mistletoe/skullcap/valerian	Herbal tonic, cathartic	Senna, podophyllin, aloin	Elevated liver function tests
Margosa oil	Tonic	*Melia azadirachta indica*	Reye's syndrome
Pennyroyal oil (squaw mint)	Abortifacient, herbal remedy	Labiatae plants (possibly diterpenes)	Elevated liver function tests
Oil of cloves	Dental pain	Unknown	Dose-dependent hepatotoxin

susceptibility to developing liver disease. In summary, because herbal agents are readily available, are not subject to rigorous purity testing or regulation, and may often contain small amounts of arsenic or cadmium, it is critical for clinicians to obtain a detailed medication use history when evaluating atypical cases of liver injury. H.D. should discontinue this agent and, pending the biopsy results, be followed closely for the next few weeks for resolution of her liver injury. However, if her symptoms worsen, liver transplantation may be necessary.

PATIENT ASSESSMENT

4. K.V., a 52-year-old female with a 12-year history of type 2 diabetes is admitted with a 2-week history of nausea, anorexia, fatigue, and intense generalized pruritus. She noted dark urine, light-colored stools, and yellow pigmentation of the skin about 10 days ago, which has progressively worsened. She reports no history of fever, rash, vomiting, abdominal pain, or fatty food intolerance. She denies use of alcohol or recreational drugs and has never had a blood transfusion nor has she recently traveled to a foreign country. Her medical history includes diabetes controlled by diet and pioglitazone (for the past 18 months) and hypertension treated with hydrochlorothiazide (HCTZ) and lisinopril for the past 4 years. One month ago, K.V. was treated with a 10-day course of amoxicillin-clavulanic acid (Augmentin) for sinusitis, but her symptoms remained throughout therapy. Subsequently, she was placed on a 5-day course of telithromycin.

On admission, K.V. appears weak and icteric. Other significant findings include scratch marks and a slightly tender, but normal-sized, liver. Vital signs are all within normal limits. Laboratory findings show the following: serum AST, 430 U/L; serum ALT, 294 U/L; alkaline phosphatase, 1,230 U/L; conjugated bilirubin 0.8 mg/dL (range 0.0–0.2 mg/dL); total bilirubin 3.8 mg/dL (range 0.2–1.1 mg/dL); and albumin, 4.1 g/dL. All other chemistry data are within normal limits. Complete blood count (CBC) and differential count are normal. Serologic tests for hepatitis A, B, and C all are negative. Ultrasound with a subsequent magnetic resonance image (MRI) shows a normal biliary tract system with no obstruction in the bile ducts or gallbladder or near the end of the pancreas. Liver biopsy showed preserved normal liver architecture, marked centrilobular cholestasis with bile pigment in hepatocytes and canaliculi, and a mild portal inflammatory infiltrate with an excess of eosinophils.

K.V. is placed on a 1,200-calorie daily diet with no added salt and regular insulin before meals titrated to a premeal glucose level of 100 to 150 mg/dL. All other drugs are discontinued. Cholestyramine (Questran) 4 g PO TID is started for itching. By the fifth day of hospitalization, her laboratory values are as follows: AST, 85 U/L; ALT, 214 U/L; alkaline phosphatase, 288 U/L; and conjugated/total bilirubin 0.3 mg/dL and 1.8 mg/dL, respectively. Her blood pressure increased to 190/105 mmHg and HCTZ 25 mg/day is restarted with a plan to add a calcium channel blocker if this does not adequately control her blood pressure. What signs and symptoms are suggestive of DILI in K.V.?

Diagnosis

There is no single test, including a liver biopsy that can be used to diagnose DILI.[1,2,22] Routine screening of serum aminotransferases in patients taking potentially hepatotoxic drugs generally is not recommended because the changes in laboratory tests often are delayed or erratic in onset, making detection of abnormalities difficult. Elevations of less than three times normal may reflect normal variations or spurious laboratory results. However, minor elevations that continue to trend upward on repeat evaluations or that are more than three times normal are cause for concern, especially in the presence of increased bilirubin levels. The presence of nonspecific symptoms ranging from anorexia, nausea, and fatigue to more specific symptoms, such as jaundice, in the setting of the administration of prescription or nonprescription medications or dietary supplements should direct suspicion toward drug-related hepatic injury. Other potential causes of liver injury in the diagnostic workup must also be ruled out including: (a) hepatitis A, B, and C (or hepatitis E with a history of recent travel to a developing country); (b) alcoholic or autoimmune hepatitis; (c) biliary tract disease; (d) hemodynamic insults; and (e) genetic and metabolic disorders (e.g., hemochromatosis α_1-antitrypsin deficiency or Wilson's disease)[1,2,22] (see Fig. 1). Thus, liver injury in the absence of another etiology could be drug-induced, but a meticulous drug history in relation to the onset of the injury is mandatory. The clinical presentation of hepatotoxicity is most evident with acute hepatocellular injury and cholestatic liver disease.

In K.V., weakness, anorexia, dark urine, light-colored stools, icterus, pruritus, hyperbilirubinemia, and a high-serum alkaline phosphatase concentration suggest cholestatic jaundice.

Table 29-9 Components and Caveats in Assessing Cause in the Diagnosis of Drug-related Hepatic Injury[1,2]

1. Exposure to a drug must precede the onset of liver injury for diagnosis as drug-induced.
   Caveat: The latent period for the onset of injury after drug use is highly variable.
2. Disease as a cause of liver injury should be ruled out before concluding that hepatotoxicity is drug related.
   Caveat: Drugs taken concurrently should also be evaluated.
3. Injury may prove when administration of a drug is stopped (dechallange).
   Caveat: Liver injury may initially worsen for days or weeks. In severe cases, falling enzyme levels may indicate impending liver failure, not improvement, especially if accompanied by worsening function.
4. Liver injury may recur more rapidly and severely on repeated exposure, especially if immunological in nature. (rechallenge)
   Caveat: Worsening on rechallenge may not occur if adaptive tolerance has occurred.

The slightly tender liver and the high-serum concentrations of AST and ALT suggest hepatocellular damage. K.V.'s clinical presentation is consistent with that of a mixed cholestatic-cytotoxic hepatic injury.

Etiology

5. How can the potential etiology of DILI be determined, and what was the most likely etiology in K.V.?

Drug-induced liver injury should be suspected in every patient with jaundice. Relevant elements and caveats in assessing the cause of DILI are outlined in Table 29-9. A negative history of fever, abdominal pain, and fatty food intolerance rule out gallbladder disease in K.V. She has no history of alcoholism and her viral hepatitis serologic tests are negative. In addition, negative ultrasound studies rule out the possibility of extrahepatic obstructive jaundice.

The presence of dark urine rules out unconjugated hyperbilirubinemia, which may be associated with hemolysis. AST elevations alone may be seen in injury to cardiac and skeletal muscles, but together with increased ALT, as in K.V., usually indicate hepatic origin. The presence of eosinophils in the liver biopsy, together with the rapid decline of serum aminotransferases, alkaline phosphatase, and bilirubin concentrations toward normal when all drugs are withdrawn, supports the assessment of drug-induced hepatitis in K.V.

There are several possible causes for K.V.'s drug-induced hepatitis, including telithromycin, amoxicillin-clavulanic acid, pioglitazone, hydrochlorothiazide, and lisinopril. Hydrochlorothiazide is an unlikely candidate because allergic cholestatic jaundice is very rarely associated with thiazide diuretics, and K.V. has taken the drug for 4 years. Lisinopril, like other angiotensin-converting enzyme inhibitors, can cause acute hepatocellular injury with mostly mixed hepatocellular and cholestatic injury; pure hepatocellular injury is rare. Furthermore, most cases of lisinopril-induced hepatic injury occur within the first 14 weeks of exposure.[119–137] Thus, lisinopril, which is known to cause mixed hepatocellular injury, is probably not the causative agent in K.V. based on the time frame of the presentation of hepatic injury. Pioglitazone, on the other hand, has been reported to cause a mixed cholestatic-cytotoxic injury, but not to the same degree as its predecessor, troglitazone, which was previously withdrawn from the market due to over 90 cases of hepatotoxic effects (68 fatalities and 10 required liver transplantation).[123–130] There are few reports of pioglitazone-associated hepatotoxicity. In one case, a 49-year-old male taking 30 mg/day for 6 months was found to have an ALT level three times the upper limit of normal, and a serum bilirubin concentration five times the upper limit of normal.[1,22,129] Therefore, it is unlikely in K.V. because she had been taking pioglitazone for 18 months and her ALT elevation is not consistent with those previously reported. Amoxicillin-clavulanic acid, a semisynthetic penicillin–lactamase inhibitor combination drug, has been reported to cause hepatic dysfunction and jaundice in a number of patients.[131–134] The latent period between the initiation of the drug and onset of jaundice or hepatic dysfunction ranged from 2 to 45 days with a mean of 27 days. In review of K.V.'s recent history of amoxicillin-clavulanic acid intake and the physical and laboratory findings, amoxicillin-clavulanic acid is a probable cause of DILI.

Additionally, telithromycin, the first ketolide agent approved by the FDA, was designed to have improved antimicrobial activity and pharmacokinetics compared to macrolide antimicrobials. Although the occurrence of telithromycin related hepatotoxicity is rare (1.6%) based on clinical trials, the precise incidence is unknown. The FDA Adverse Reporting System described 10 postmarketing cases of hepatic adverse events associated with telithromycin use.[131,135–137] The severity of the reactions ranged from serious to fatal (two deaths) and was associated with cholestatic hepatitis, abnormal aminotransferase levels, increased bilirubin levels, liver disorder, cholestatic jaundice, and hepatocellular damage. The duration of administration of telithromycin ranged from 1 to 30 days, and patients were from 35 to 85 years of age. In 2006, the FDA announced changes to the product labeling for telithromycin to warn healthcare practitioners and patients about the risk of liver injury. This was based on several reports of serious liver injury and liver failure, along with four deaths and one liver transplant. Furthermore, another case series describe similar cases of severe DILI secondary to telithromycin use resulting in death or liver transplantation. Thus, K.V.'s recent exposure to telithromycin and her laboratory and physical findings are consistent with telithromycin-induced liver injury. Nevertheless, the possibility of hydrochlorothiazide- or pioglitazone-induced hepatic injury cannot be ruled out without an inadvisable rechallenge test with one or both of these drugs.

Procedure to Determine

To determine the cause of DILI, a detailed drug history should be obtained for all patients with jaundice (Table 29.10). Special attention should be paid to the duration of exposure to a specific drug and its relationship to the onset of symptoms. A history of taking OCs, nonprescription drugs such as laxatives and vitamins, and illicit drug use should not be overlooked and obtained. Predisposing factors to drug-induced hepatitis, if any, should be noted (Table 29-1). The presumptive diagnosis of DILI requires a history of exposure to a drug, awareness of the characteristic syndromes produced by various agents, and a search for supportive evidence. If the liver injury is accompanied by fever, rash, and eosinophilia, the likelihood of drug-induced disease increases. In some instances, these features may be associated with lymph node enlargement, lymphocytosis, and atypical circulating lymphocytes, leading to a syndrome that mimics infectious mononucleosis and serum sickness. Additional plausible systemic manifestations are listed in Table 29-7. Lack of these features, however, does not exclude the possibility of drug-induced disease.[2,7,222,224] As described previously, differentiation of DILI from viral hepatitis involves evaluation of the epidemiologic circumstances; serologic studies to detect hepatitis A, B, or C antigens or antibodies; and determination of whether a history of receiving blood transfusions or injection with a contaminated syringe exists. Distinction between drug-induced cholestatic jaundice and extrahepatic obstructive jaundice often requires radiographic or ultrasonic studies. If liver biopsy reveals cholestasis with an eosinophil-rich portal inflammation, as observed in K.V., drug-induced causes are more likely.

Rechallenge With Offending Agent

6. Should K.V. be given a challenge dose of amoxicillin-clavulanic acid or telithromycin to confirm the cause of her DILI?

Confirmation of the cause may be obtained by giving a rechallenge dose of the incriminated drug. Recurrence of hepatic dysfunction or hyperbilirubinemia after a test dose offers valuable support for the diagnosis. Failure to develop abnormalities, however, does not preclude drug-induced dysfunction, because only 40% to 60% of patients show a recurrence of hepatic injury after a test dose.[1,2,5,7,20] Furthermore, some drugs will produce the hepatic injury only after an extended period (1 to 12 weeks) of readministration. Testing for the effect of a challenge dose can be potentially dangerous if the drug is known to cause hepatocellular injury, whereas rechallenge is considered safe if the drug usually leads to cholestasis alone. Therefore, risk must be weighed against benefit before giving a challenge dose of an incriminated drug to a patient.

Rechallenge of K.V. with amoxicillin-clavulanic acid or telithromycin is potentially dangerous given her clinical picture consistent with hepatocellular injury. Rapid occurrence of jaundice and liver enzyme abnormalities following rechallenge with amoxicillin-clavulanic acid or telithromycin suggests an immunoallergic type of idiosyncrasy.[1,5,7,20,22,28] Since alternative antibiotics can be used to manage K.V.'s infection, rechallenging with amoxicillin-clavulanic acid or telithromycin is not recommended, because a recurrent injury may be more severe than the initial insult.

Management

7. Was K.V. treated appropriately for her suspected drug-induced hepatic injury?

If patients present with symptoms, especially jaundice and signs of acute liver failure (e.g., encephalopathy) the administration of any potential hepatotoxic agent should be discontinued. To assess liver injury, biochemical tests should be obtained at baseline and serially; consultation with a gastroenterologist or hepatologist is recommended. In most cases of DILI improvement occurs, but at variable rates. Worsening of DILI may occur followed by a long protracted course of recovery (weeks to months), and may be seen following discontinuation of the suspected offending agents. In K.V.'s case, all medications taken before admission were discontinued and an atypical rapid recovery was observed. The management of drug-induced jaundice is similar to the treatment of other hepatic diseases. Treatment usually includes a diet high in carbohydrates, moderately high in protein, and adequate in calories (e.g., 2,000–3,000 calories/day). However, a lower caloric diet was prescribed for K.V. because of her diabetes. Treatment of jaundice is mainly supportive. If itching is severe, the use of cholestyramine to enhance the rate of bile acid excretion may alleviate the symptoms. If possible, the use of amoxicillin-clavulanic or telithromycin acid should be avoided in K.V., and appropriate alternative drugs should be used instead. If present, ascites, esophageal variceal bleeding, and other complications are treated accordingly. The use of large doses of glucocorticoids (e.g., 1,000 mg hydrocortisone/day) in acute hepatic failure is largely empirical and may have a role in hypersensitivity related cases, but otherwise is not recommended.[13,25–27] There was no indication of these complications in K.V.

8. What preventative measures can be taken to minimize the risk of DILI in patients like K.V.?

During the stages of drug development, opportunities to prevent hepatotoxicity occur.[1,19,22] Preclinical animal data can help detect dose-related, predictable hepatotoxicity rather than unpredictable hepatotoxicity in humans. Phase 1 drug trials provide the initial opportunity to assess the hepatotoxic risk of drugs in humans. Generally, these trials have a small number of subjects and the duration of exposure of an agent is short at relatively low dosages. As a drug enters phase 2 trials, exposure to higher dosages occurs, but the relatively small number of patients still limits the determination of hepatotoxic risk. During phase 3 efficacy trials, more patients can be exposed to a drug and the relative likelihood of hepatotoxicity is increased. However, there are still relatively low numbers of patients enrolled in clinical trials, and to predict a true incidence of hepatotoxicity in 1 in 1,000 patients requires at least 3,000 be studied. Thus, phase 3 clinical trials may underpredict the true risk of a drug's hepatotoxic potential.

Perhaps the most significant time period for recognizing drug-induced liver injury is in the postmarketing time period.[1,19,22] During this time, several thousand patients may be exposed to an agent and surveillance programs such as the FDA MedWatch program may help elucidate and report drug-related hepatotoxicity. This type of program is voluntary, and probably underreports the frequency and severity of DILI. Clinicians should also rely on case reports that appear in the medical literature to help guide or confirm suspicion of the risk of drug-related hepatotoxicity from prescription drugs, over the counter drugs, herbal (dietary) supplements, or other alternative medications. Additionally, patients should be educated on the recognition and symptoms of DILI and instructed to report any perceived adverse events promptly (Table 29-10). Finally, the evolving science of pharmacogenomics may help clinicians predict those at greatest risk of DILI, but currently genetic testing has not been added to

Table 29-10 Essential Guidelines in the Recognition and Prevention of Hepatotoxicity in Clinical Practice[1,2]

Do not ignore symptoms	When a drug is being used, even vague symptoms such as nausea, anorexia, malaise, fatigue, and right upper quadrant pain as well as specific symptoms such as itching or jaundice should prompt consideration of hepatotoxicity. Testing for liver injury and abnormal function should be performed.
Take a careful history	Elicit a detailed history of prescribed and nonprescribed over-the-counter herbal and other medications or remedies with dates and amounts.
Remove the causative agent	Discontinue the causative agent or agents, especially if symptoms have occurred or abnormal liver function (e.g., increased bilirubin level or prothrombin time) exists. Watch closely over time for changes and consult a hepatologist or gastroenterologist.
Pay attention to "Hys" Law	Jaundice that appears after drug-induced hepatocellular liver injury suggests a serious and potentially fatal liver problem, consult a specialist at once.
Report the injury	1-800-332-1088 (telephone) 1-800-332-4178 (fax) http//www.fda.gov/medwatch Provide information for differential diagnosis and assessment of cause, time course of the reaction, and normal ranges of laboratory tests.

routine patient management strategies. The ability to implement novel fields, such as proteonomics and metabonomics, may also provide insight into establishing the mechanisms of DILI.

DRUGS REPORTED TO CAUSE CLINICALLY SIGNIFICANT HEPATIC DYSFUNCTION

There are many reports of drug-related hepatitis in the literature. Most of these are reports of single cases involving one drug and are difficult to evaluate. Furthermore, hepatic drug effects that occurred early after exposure may differ in character from those that occurred later (e.g., chlorpromazine). In addition, certain drugs may cause various types of morphologic responses via different mechanisms (i.e., hepatotoxic vs. idiosyncratic). In an attempt to summarize and facilitate discussion of the vast amount of information on this subject, selected drugs that have been implicated in causing significant liver dysfunction are listed in Table 29-4. The hepatotoxicity of acetaminophen (see Chapter 5, Managing Acute Drug Toxicity), antituberculous agents (see Chapter 61, Tuberculosis) and certain antiretrovirals (see Chapter 69, Pharmacotherapy of Human Immunodeficiency Virus Infection) are included in other chapters. The types of morphologic findings and presumed mechanisms of hepatotoxicity for each drug are presented in Table 29-4. References are listed so that more detailed information may be obtained if desired. In the column labeled "Clinical Remarks," prominent clinical features, such as clinical presentation, dose, and duration of therapy associated with the adverse effect, pertinent laboratory data, and prognosis are summarized.

ACKNOWLEDGMENT

The author would like to acknowledge Amy Choi for her contribution to this chapter.

REFERENCES

1. Navarro VJ et al. Drug-related hepatotoxicity. *N Engl J Med* 2006;354:731.
2. Watkins PB et al. Drug induced liver injury: summary of a single topic clinical research conference. *Hepatology* 2006;43:618.
3. Russo MW et al. Liver transplantation for acute liver failure from drug induced liver injury in the United States. *Liver Transplant* 2004;10:1018.
4. Pratt DS et al. Evaluation of abnormal liver-enzyme results in symptomatic patients. *N Engl J Med* 2000;342:1266.
5. Lee WM. Drug-induced hepatotoxicity. *N Engl J Med* 2003;349:474.
6. Kaplowitz N. *Drug Induced Liver Disease*. 2nd ed. New York: Informa; 2007.
7. Andrade RJ et al. Outcome of acute idiosyncratic drug-induced liver injury: long-term follow-up in a hepatotoxicity registry. *Hepatology* 2006;44:1581.
8. Lazarou J et al. Incidence of adverse drug reactions in hospitalized patients. *JAMA* 1998;279:1200.
9. Friis H et al. Drug-induced hepatic injury: an analysis of 1100 cases reported to the Danish Committee on Adverse Drug Reactions between 1978 and 1987. *J Intern Med* 1992;232:133.
10. Sgro C et al. Incidence of drug-induced hepatic injuries: a French population-based study. *Hepatology* 2002;36:451.
11. De Valle MB et al. Drug-induced liver injury in a Swedish University hospital out-patient hepatology clinic. *Alim Pharmacol Ther* 2006;24:1187.
12. Ostapowicz G et al. Results of a prospective study of acute liver failure at 17 tertiary care centers in the United States. *Ann Intern Med* 2002;137:947.
13. Zimmerman HJ. *Hepatotoxicity: Adverse Effects of Drugs and Other Chemicals on the Liver*. 2nd ed. Philadelphia: Lippincott Williams & Wilkins; 1999.
14. Zimmerman HJ. Drug-induced liver disease. *Clin Liver Dis* 2000;473.
15. Kaplowitz N. Drug-induced liver disorders. *Drug Safety* 2001;24:483.
16. Clarkson A et al. Surveillance for fatal suspected adverse drug reactions in the UK. *Arch Dis Child* 2002;87:462.
17. Etwel FA et al. A surveillance method for the early identification of idiosyncratic adverse drug reactions. *Drug Safety* 2008;31:169.
18. Kaplowitz N. Idiosyncratic drug hepatotoxicity. *Nature* 2005;4:489.
19. Castell JV et al. Allergic hepatitis induced by drugs. *Curr Opin Allergy Clin Immunol* 2006;6:258.
20. Arrundel C et al. Drug induced liver disease 2006. *Curr Opin Gastroenterol* 2006;23:244.
21. Andrade RJ et al. Assessment of drug-induced hepatotoxicity in clinical practice: a challenge for gastroenterologists. *World J Gastroenterol* 2007; 13:329.
22. Abboud G et al. Drug-induced liver injury. *Drug Safety* 2007;30:277.
23. Durand F et al. Hepatotoxicity of antitubercular treatments. *Drug Safety* 1996;15:394.
24. Hoofnagle JH et al. Fulminant hepatic failure: summary of a workshop. *Hepatology* 1995;21:240.
25. O'Grady J. Modern management of acute liver failure. *Clin Liver Dis* 2007;11:291.
26. Lee WM. Acute liver failure. *N Engl J Med* 1993; 329:1862.
27. Shakil AO et al. Fulminant hepatic failure. *Surg Clin North Am* 1999;79:77.
28. Larrey D. Drug-induced liver disease. *J Hepatology* 2000;32(Suppl 1):77.
29. Manoukian AV et al. Nonsteroidal anti-inflammatory drug-induced hepatic disorders. *Drug Safety* 1996;15:64.
30. Garcia-Rodriguez LA et al. The risk of acute liver injury associated with cimetidine and other acid-suppressing anti-ulcer drugs. *Br J Pharmacol* 1997;43:183.
31. Garcia-Rodriguez LA et al. A review of the epidemiologic research on drug-induced acute liver injury using the general practice research data base in the United Kingdom. *Pharmacotherapy* 1997;17:721.
32. Larey D et al. Hepatitis associated with amoxicillin-clavulanic acid combination: report of 15 cases. *Gut* 2002;33:368.
33. Nathani MG et al. An unusual case of amoxicillin/clavulanic acid-related hepatotoxicity. *Am J Gastroenterol* 1998;93:1363.
34. Tolman KG. The liver and lovastatin. *Am J Cardiol* 2002;89:1374.

35. Jain MK et al. Drug-induced liver injury associated with HIV medications. *Clin Liver Dis* 2007;11:615.
36. Nunez M. Hepatotoxicity of antiretrovirals: incidence, mechanisms, and management. *J Hepatol* 2006;44:S132.
37. Aithal GP et al. Nonsteroidal anti-inflammatory drug-induced hepatotoxicity. *Clin Liver Dis* 2007;11:563.
38. Valla D et al. Drug-induced vascular and sinusoidal lesions of the liver. *Baillere's Clin Gastroenterol* 1998;2:481.
39. Saukkomen JJ et al. An official ATS statement: hepatotoxicity of antitubercular therapy. *Mer J Resp Crit Care Med* 2006;174:935.
40. Stock JGL et al. Unexplained hepatitis following halothane. *Anesthesiology* 1985;63:424.
41. Braun P. Hepatotoxicity of erythromycin. *J Infect Dis* 1973;119:300.
42. Fox JC et al. Progressive cholestatic liver disease associated with clarithromycin treatment. *J Clin Pharmacol* 2002;42:676.
43. Brown BA et al. Clarithromycin-induced hepatotoxicity. *Clin Infect Dis* 1995;20:1073.
44. Banks AT et al. Diclofenac-associated hepatotoxicity: analysis of 180 cases reported to the Food and Drug Administration as adverse reactions. *Hepatology* 1995;22:820.
45. Zimmerman HJ. Effects of aspirin and acetaminophen on the liver. *Arch Intern Med* 1981; 141:333.
46. Dreifuss FE et al. Valproic acid hepatic fatalities: analysis of United States cases. *Neurology* 1986;36(Suppl 1):133.
47. Stricker BC et al. Hepatic injury associated with the use of nitrofurans: a clinicopathological study of 52 reported cases. *Hepatology* 1988;8:599.
48. Lindgren A et al. Liver reactions from trimethoprim. *J Int Med* 1994;236:281.
49. Hoft RH et al. Halothane hepatitis in three pairs of closely related women. *N Engl J Med* 1981;304:1023.
50. Gennis M et al. Familial occurrence of hypersensitivity to phenytoin. *Am J Med* 1991;91:631.
51. O'shea D et al. Effect of fasting and obesity in humans on the 6-hydroxylation of chlorzoxazone: a putative probe of CYP2E1 activity. *Clin Pharmacol Ther* 1994;56:35a.
52. Spracklin DK et al. Cytochrome P-4502E1 is the principal catalyst of human oxidative halothane metabolism *in vitro*. *J Pharmacol Exp Ther* 1997;281:400.
53. Frank AK et al. Isoniazid hepatitis among pregnant and postpartum Hispanic patients. *Publ Health Rep* 1989;104:151.
54. Smith AC et al. Characterization of hyperthyroidism enhancement of halothane-induced hepatotoxicity. *Biochem Pharmacol* 1983;32: 3531.
55. Rodriguiz EA et al. Cancer chemotherapy I: hepatocellular injury. *Clin Liver Dis* 2007;11:641.
56. Wang T et al. Mechanisms and outcomes of drug-and toxicant-induced liver toxicity in diabetes. *Crit Rev Toxicol* 2007;37:413.
57. Huang MJ et al. Clinical interactions between thyroid and liver diseases. *Gastroenterol Hepatol* 1995;10:344.
58. Levin MD et al. Hepatotoxicity of oral and intravenous voriconazole in relation to cytochrome P450 polymorphisms. *J Antimicrob Chemother* 2007;60:1104.
59. Krahenbuhl S et al. Acute liver failure in two patients with regular alcohol consumption ingesting paracetamol at therapeutic dosage. *Digestion* 2007;75:232.
60. McDonald GB et al. Veno-occlusive disease of the liver after bone marrow transplantation: diagnosis, incidence, and predisposing factors. *Hepatology* 1994;4:116.
61. LeBlanc GA. Hepatic vectorial transport of xenobiotics. *Chem Biol Interact* 1994;90:101.
62. Schwabe RF et al. Mechanisms of liver injury. *Amer J Physiol Gastrointest Liver Physiol* 2006;290:G583.
63. Losser MR et al. Mechanisms of liver damage. *Semin Liver Dis* 1996;16:357.
64. Mitchell JR et al. Acetaminophen-induced hepatic injury: protective effect of glutathione in man and rationale for therapy. *Clin Pharmacol Ther* 1974;16:676.
65. Luster MI et al. The role of tumor necrosis factor in chemical induced hepatotoxicity. *Ann New York Acad Sci* 2002;220.
66. Jaeschke H et al. Mechanisms of hepatotoxicity. *Toxicol Sci* 2002;65:166.
67. Cardona X et al. Venlafaxine associated hepatitis. *Ann Intern Med* 2000;132:417.
68. Horsmans Y et al. Venlafaxine-associated hepatitis. *Ann Intern Med* 1999;130:994.
69. Spigset O et al. Hepatic injury and pancreatitis during treatment with serotonin reuptake inhibitors: data from the World Health Organization (WHO) database of adverse drug reactions. *Int Clin Psychopharmacol* 2003;18:157.
70. Sotolongo RP et al. Hypersensitivity reaction to sulfasalazine with severe hepatotoxicity. *Gastroenterology* 1978;75:95.
71. Abi-Mansur P et al. Trimethoprim-sulfamethoxazole induced cholestasis. *Am J Gastroenterol* 1981; 76:356.
72. Thies PW, Dull WL. Trimethoprim-sulfamethoxazole-induced cholestatic hepatitis. Inadvertent rechallenge. *Arch Intern Med* 1984;144:1691.
73. Zitelli BN et al. Fatal hepatic necrosis due to pyrimethamine-sulfadoxine (Fansidar). *Ann Intern Med* 1987;106:393.
74. Zimmerman HJ, Ishak KG. Valproate-induced hepatic injury. Analysis of 23 fatal cases. *Hepatology* 1982;2:591.
75. Suchy FJ et al. Acute hepatic failure associated with the use of sodium valproate. *N Engl J Med* 1979;300:962.
76. Young RSK et al. Reye-like syndrome associated with valproic acid. *Ann Neurol* 1980;7:389.
77. Levin TL et al. Valproic-acid-associated pancreatitis and hepatic toxicity in children with endstage renal disease. *Pediatr Radiol* 1997;27:192.
78. Konig SA et al. Fatal liver failure associated with valproate therapy in a patient with Freidreich's disease: review of valproate hepatotoxicity in adults. *Epilepsia* 1999;40:1036.
79. Mohi-ud-din R et al. Drug and chemical induced cholestasis. *Clin Liver Dis* 2004;8:95.
80. Amacher DE. Serum transaminase elevations as indicators of hepatic injury following administration of drugs. *Reg Toxicol Pharmacol* 1998;27:119.
81. Nomura F et al. Effects of anticonvulsant agents on halothane induced liver injury in human subjects and experimental animals. *Hepatology* 1986;6:952.
82. Desmet VJ. Vanishing bile duct syndrome in drug-induced liver disease. *J Hepatol* 1997;26(Suppl 1):31.
83. Forbes GM et al. Carbamazepine hepatotoxicity: another cause of the vanishing bile duct syndrome. *Gastroenterology* 1992;102:1385.
84. Ishak KG. Chronic hepatitis: morphology and nomenclature. *Mod Pathol* 1994;7:690.
85. Homberg JC et al. Drug-induced hepatitis associated with anticytoplasmic organelle autoantibodies. *Hepatology* 1985;5:722.
86. Beaune PH et al. Human endoplasmic reticulum autoantibodies appearing in a drug-induced hepatitis are directed against a human liver cytochrome P450 that hydroxylates the drug. *Proc Natl Acad Sci USA* 1987;84:551.
87. Bourdi M et al. Anti-liver endoplasmic reticulum autoantibodies are directed against human cytochrome P450 I A2. *J Clin Invest* 1990;85: 1967.
88. Utili R et al. Dantrolene-associated hepatic injury. *Gastroenterology* 1977;72:610.
89. Seaman WE et al. Aspirin-induced hepatotoxicity in patients with systemic lupus erythematous. *Ann Intern Med* 1974;80:1.
90. Rodman JS et al. Methyldopa hepatitis. A report of six cases and review of the literature. *Am J Med* 1976;60:941.
91. Black M et al. Nitrofurantoin-induced chronic active hepatitis. *Ann Intern Med* 1980;92:62.
92. Mihas AA et al. Fulminant hepatitis and lymphocyte sensitization due to propylthiouracil. *Gastroenterology* 1976;70:770.
93. Simon EB et al. Amiodarone hepatotoxicity simulating alcoholic liver disease. *N Engl J Med* 1984;311:167.
94. Harris L et al. Side effects of long-term amiodarone therapy. *Circulation* 1983;67:45.
95. Ludwig J et al. Floxuridine-induced sclerosing cholangitis: an ischemic cholangiopathy? *Hepatology* 1989;9:215.
96. Valla D et al. Risk of hepatic vein thrombosis in relationship to recent use of oral contraceptives: a case control study. *Gastroenterology* 1986;90: 807.
97. Maddrey WC et al. Hepatic vein thrombosis (Budd-Chiari syndrome): possible association with the use of oral contraceptives. *Semin Liver Dis* 1987;7:32.
98. McDonald GB et al. Veno-occlusive disease following bone marrow transplantation: a cohort of 355 patients. *Ann Intern Med* 1993;118:255.
99. Stedman C. Herbal toxicity. *Semin Liver Dis* 2003;22:195.
100. Bagheri SA et al. Peliosis hepatis associated with androgenic-anabolic steroid therapy: a severe form of injury. *Ann Intern Med* 1974;81:610.
101. Shepard P et al. Idiopathic portal hypertension associated with cytotoxic drugs. *J Clin Oncol* 1990;43:206.
102. Ishak KG, Zimmerman HJ. Drug-induced and toxic granulomatous hepatitis. *Clin Gastroenterol* 1988;2:463.
103. Edmondson HA et al. Liver-cell adenomas associated with the use of oral contraceptives. *N Engl J Med* 1976;294:470.
104. Mays ET et al. Hepatic tumors induced by sex steroids. *Semin Liv Dis* 1994;4:147.
105. Neuberger J et al. Oral contraceptive and hepatocellular carcinoma. *Br Med J* 1987;292:1355.
106. Kerlin P et al. Hepatic adenoma and focal nodular hyperplasia: clinical, pathologic and radiologic features. *Gastroenterology* 1983;84:994.
107. Zafrani ES et al. Drug-induced vascular lesions of the liver. *Arch Intern Med* 1983;143:495.
108. Verma S et al. Complementary and alternative medicine in hepatology: review of the evidence of efficacy. *Clin Gastroent Hepatol* 2007;5:408.
109. Simanto L et al. A collaborative study of cancer incidence and mortality among vinyl chloride workers. *Scand J Work Environ Health* 1991;17:159.
110. Kane JA et al. Hepatitis caused by traditional Chinese herbs: possible toxic components. *Gut* 1995;36:146.
111. Stickel F et al. Herbal hepatotoxicity. *J Hepatol* 2005;43:901.
112. Seef LB et al. Complementary and alternative medicine in chronic liver disease. *Hepatology* 2001;34:595.
113. Furbee BR et al. Hepatotoxicity associated with herbal products. *Clin Lab Med* 2006;26:227.
114. Seeff LB. Herbal hepatotoxicity. *Clin Liver Dis* 2007;11:577.
115. Ridker PM et al. Hepatic veno-occlusive disease associated with the consumption of pyrrolizidine-containing dietary supplements. *Gastroenterology* 1985;88;1050.
116. Larrey D et al. Hepatitis after germander (Teucrium chamaedrys) administration: another instance of herbal medication hepatotoxicity. *Ann Intern Med* 1992;117:129.
117. Beuers U et al. Hepatitis after chronic abuse of senna [letter]. *Lancet* 1991;1:372.
118. Woolf GM et al. Acute hepatitis associated with the Chinese herbal product Jin Bu Huan. *Ann Intern Med* 1994;121:729.
119. Rahmat J et al. Captopril-associated cholestatic jaundice. *Ann Intern Med* 1985;102:56.
120. Schattner A et al. Captopril-induced jaundice: report of 2 cases and review of 13 additional reports in the literature. *Am J Med Sci* 2001;322: 236.

121. Hagley MT et al. Hepatotoxicity associated with angiotensin-converting enzyme inhibitors. *Ann Pharmacother* 1993;27:228.
122. Larrey D et al. Fulminant hepatitis after lisinopril administration. *Gastroenterology* 1990;99:1832.
123. Murphy EJ et al. Troglitazone-induced fulminant hepatic failure. *Acute liver failure study group. Dig Dis Sci* 2000;45:549.
124. Kohlroser J et al. Hepatotoxicity due to troglitazone: report of two cases and review of the literature. *Am J Gastroenterol* 2000;95:272.
125. Gitlin N et al. Two cases of severe clinical and histologic hepatotoxicity associated with troglitazone. *Ann Intern Med* 1998;129:36.
126. Forman LM et al. Hepatic failure in a patient taking rosiglitazone. *Ann Intern Med* 2000;132:118.
127. Al-Salman J et al. Hepatocellular injury in a patient receiving rosiglitazone. *Ann Intern Med* 2000;132:121.
128. Isley WL et al. Hepatotoxicity of the thiazolidinediones. *Diabetes Obes Metab* 2001;3:389.
129. Gale EA. Lessons from the glitazones: a story of drug development. *Lancet* 2001;357:1870.
130. May LD et al. Mixed hepatocellular-cholestatic liver injury after pioglitazone therapy. *Ann Intern Med* 2002;136:449.
131. Polson JE. Hepatotoxicity due to antibiotics. *Clin Liver Dis* 2007;11:549.
132. Limauro DL et al. Amoxicillin/clavulanate-associated hepatic failure with progression to Stevens-Johnson syndrome. *Ann Pharmacother* 1999;3:560.
133. Silvain C et al. Granulomatous hepatitis due to combination of amoxicillin and clavulanic acid. *Dig Dis Sci* 1992;37:150.
134. Hebbard GS et al. Augmentin-induced jaundice with a fatal outcome. *Med J Aust* 1992;156:285.
135. Bolesta S et al. Elevated hepatic transaminases associated with telithromycin therapy: a case report and literature review. *Am J Health Syst Pharm* 2008;65:37.
136. Dore DD et al. Telithromycin use and spontaneous reports of hepatotoxicity. *Drug Safety* 2007;30:697.
137. Clay KD et al. Severe hepatotoxicity of telithromycin: tree case reports and literature review. *Ann Intern Med* 2006;144:E1.
138. Hsiaso SH et al. Hepatotoxicity with acarbose therapy. *Ann Pharmacother* 2006;40:151.
139. Butler RC et al. Acute massive hepatic necrosis in a patient receiving allopurinol. *JAMA* 1977;237:437.
140. Chan AL et al. Fatal amiodarone-induced hepatotoxicity: a case report and literature review. *Int J Clin Pharmacol Ther* 2008;46:96.
141. Simon JB et al. Amiodarone hepatotoxicity simulating alcoholic liver disease. *N Engl J Med* 1984;311:167.
142. Kalantzis N et al. Acute amiodarone-induced hepatitis. *Hepatogastroenterology* 1991;38:71.
143. Snir Y et al. Fatal hepatic failure due to prolonged amiodarone treatment. *J Clin Gastroenterology* 1995;20:265.
144. Nadell J et al. Peliosis hepatis. Twelve cases associated with oral androgen therapy. *Arch Pathol Lab Med* 1977;101:405.
145. Bagheri SA et al. Peliosis hepatis associated with androgenic-anabolic steroid therapy. A severe form of hepatic injury. *Ann Intern Med* 1974;81:610.
146. Seaman WE et al. Aspirin-induced hepatotoxicity in patients with systemic lupus erythematosus. *Ann Intern Med* 1974;80:1.
147. Lopez-Morante AJ et al. Aspirin-induced cholestatic hepatitis. *J Clin Gastroenterol* 1993;16:270.
148. Aguilar HI et al. Azathioprine-induced lymphoma manifesting as fulminant hepatic failure. *Mayo Clin Proc* 1997;72:643.
149. Read AE et al. Hepatic veno-occlusive disease associated with renal transplantation and azathioprine therapy. *Ann Intern Med* 1986;104:651.
150. Perini GP et al. Azathioprine-related cholestatic jaundice in heart transplant patients. *J Heart Transplant* 1990;9:577.
151. Meys E et al. Fever, hepatitis and acute interstitial nephritis in a patient with rheumatoid arthritis. Concurrent manifestations of azathioprine hypersensitivity. *J Rheumatol* 1992;19:807.
152. Humayun F et al. A fatal case of bupropion (Zyban) hepatotoxicity with autoimmune features. *J Med Case Reports* 2007;1:88.
153. Khoo AL et al. Acute liver failure with concurrent bupropion and carbimazole therapy. *Ann Pharmacother* 2003;37:220.
154. Ahmed SN et al. Antiepileptic drugs and liver disease. *Seizure* 2006;15:156.
155. Hazdie N et al. Acute liver failure induced by carbamazepine. *Arch Dis Child Mar* 1990;65:315.
156. Luke DR et al. Acute hepatotoxicity after excessively high doses of carbamazepine on two occasions. *Pharmacotherapy* 1986;6:108.
157. Ishak KG et al. Hepatic injury associated with the phenothiazines. Clinicopathologic and follow-up study of 36 patients. *Arch Pathol Lab Med* 1972;93:283.
158. Derby LE et al. Liver disorders in patients receiving chlorpromazine or isoniazid. *Pharmacotherapy* 1993;13:353.
159. Goldstein MJ et al. Jaundice in a patient receiving acetohexamide. *N Engl J Med* 1966;275:97.
160. Baird RW et al. Cholestatic jaundice from tolbutamide. *Ann Intern Med* 1960;53:194.
161. Van Thiel DH et al. Tolazamide hepatotoxicity. *Gastroenterology* 1974;67:506.
162. Rigberg LA et al. Chlorpropamide-induced granulomas. *JAMA* 1976;235:409.
163. Van Basten JP et al. Glyburide-induced cholestatic hepatitis and liver failure. Case-report and review of the literature. *Neth J Med* 1992;40:305.
164. Aygun C et al. Clindamycin-induced acute cholestatic hepatitis. *World J Gastroenterol* 2007;28:5408.
165. NG JA et al. Clopidogrel-induced hepatotoxicity and fever. *Pharmacotherapy* 2006;26:1023.
166. Reyes H. The enigma of intrahepatic cholestasis of pregnancy. *Hepatology* 1982;2:87.
167. Kreek MJ. Female sex steroids and cholestasis. *Semin Liver Dis* 1987;7:8.
168. Lindberg MC. Hepatobiliary complications of oral contraceptives. *J Gen Intern Med* 1992;7:199.
169. Berg JW et al. Hepatomas and oral contraceptives. *Lancet* 1974;2:349.
170. Edmondson HA et al. Liver cell adenomas associated with the use of oral contraceptives. *N Engl J Med* 1976;294:470.
171. Klatskin G. Hepatic tumors. Possible relationship to use of oral contraceptives. *Gastroenterology* 1977;73:386.
172. Kerlin P et al. Hepatic adenoma and focal nodular hyperplasia: clinical, pathologic and radiologic features. *Gastroenterology* 1983;84:994.
173. Van Erpecum KJ et al. Pelio hepatis and cirrhosis after long term use of oral contraceptives: case report. *Am J Gastroenterol* 1988;83:572.
174. Goodman ZD, Ishak KG. Hepatocellular carcinoma in women: probable lack of etiologic association with oral contraceptive steroids. *Hepatology* 1982;2:440.
175. Forman D et al. Cancer of the liver and the use of oral contraceptives. *Br Med J* 1986;292:1357.
176. Klintmalm GBG et al. Cyclosporin A hepatotoxicity in 66 renal allograft recipients. *Transplantation* 1981;32:488.
177. Kassianides C et al. Liver injury from cyclosporine A. *Dig Dis Sci* 1990;35:693.
178. Sarachek NS et al. Diltiazem and granulomatous hepatitis. *Gastroenterology* 1985;88:1260.
179. Shallcross H et al. Fatal renal and hepatic toxicity after treatment with diltiazem. *Br Med J* 1987;295:1236.
180. Richter WO et al. Serious side effect of nifedipine. *Arch Int Med* 1987;147:1850.
181. Isoard B et al. Pseudoalcoholic hepatitis during treatment with nicardipine. *Presse Med* 1988;17:647.
182. Stern EH et al. Possible hepatitis from verapamil. *N Engl J Med* 1982;306:612.
183. Brodsky SJ et al. Hepatotoxicity due to treatment with verapamil. *Ann Intern Med* 1981;94:490.
184. French J et al. Practice advisory: the use of felbamate in the treatment of patients with intractable epilepsy. *Neurology* 1999;52:1540.
185. Halkin H. Adverse effects of the fluoroquinolones. *Rev Infect Dis* 1988;10(Suppl 1):S258.
186. Blum A. Ofloxacin-induced acute severe hepatitis. *South Med J* 1991;84:1158.
187. Villeneuve JP et al. Suspected ciprofloxacin-induced hepatotoxicity. *Ann Pharmacother* 1995;29:257.
188. Chen JL et al. Acute eosinophilic hepatitis from trovafloxacin. *N Engl J Med* 2000;342:359.
189. Spahr L et al. A fatal hepatitis related to levofloxacin. *J Hepatol* 2001;35:308.
190. DeSanty KP et al. Antidepressant-induced liver injury. *Ann Pharmacother* 2007;41:1201.
191. Qiang C et al. Acute hepatitis due to fluoxetine therapy. *Mayo Clin Proc* 1999;74:692.
192. Crane GE et al. A review of clinical literature on haloperidol. *Int J Neuropsychiatry* 1967;3(Suppl 1):5111.
193. Neuberger JM. Halothane and hepatitis. Incidence, predisposing factors and exposure guidelines. *Drug Safety* 1990;5:28.
194. Shipton EA. Halothane hepatitis revisited. *S Afr Med J* 1991;80:261.
195. Gunza JT et al. Postoperative elevation of serum transaminases following isoflurane anesthesia. *J Clin Anesth* 1992;4:336.
196. Slayter KL et al. Halothane hepatitis in a renal transplant patient previously exposed to isoflurane. *Ann Pharmacother* 1993;27:101.
197. Tostmann A et al. Antituberculosis drug-induced hepatotoxicity: concise up to date review. *J Gastroenterol Hepatol* 2007;1440.
198. Yee WW et al. Antitubercular drugs and hepatotoxicity. *Respirology* 2006;11:699.
199. Andrade RJ et al. Cholestatic hepatitis related to use of irbesartan: a case report and a literature review of angiotensinsin II antagonist-associated hepatotoxicity. *Eur J Gastroenterol Hepatology* 2002;14:887.
200. Tabak F et al. Losartan induced hepatic injury. *J Clin Gastroenterol* 2002;34:585.
201. Lewis JH et al. Hepatic injury associated with ketoconazole therapy. Analysis of 33 cases. *Gastroenterology* 1984;86:503.
202. Findor JA et al. Ketoconazole-induced liver damage. *Medicine* 1998;58:277.
203. Samonis G et al. Prophylaxis of oropharyngeal candidiasis with fluconazole. *Rev Infect Dis* 1990;12(Suppl 3):S364.
204. Mann SK et al. Itraconazole-induced acute hepatitis [letter]. *Br J Dermatol* 1993;129:500.
205. Potoski B et al. The safety of voriconazole. *Clin Infect Dis* 2002;35:1273.
206. Lustar I et al. Safety of voriconazole and dose individualization. *Clin infect Dis* 2003;36:1087.
207. Bhardwaj SS et al. Lipid-lowering agents that cause drug-induced hepatotoxicity. *Clin Liver Dis* 2007;11:597.
208. Grimbert S et al. Acute hepatitis induced by HMG-CoA reductase inhibitors. *Dig Dis Sci* 1994;39:2032.
209. Haria M et al. Pravastatin: a reappraisal of its pharmacological properties and clinical effectiveness in the management of coronary heart disease. *Drugs* 1997;53:299.
210. Roblin X et al. Simvastatin-induced hepatitis. *Gastroenterol Clin Biol* 1992;16:101.
211. Boccuzzi SJ et al. Long-term experience with simvastatin. *Drug Invest* 1993;5:135.
212. Shergy WJ et al. Methotrexate-associated hepatotoxicity: retrospective analysis of 210 patients with rheumatoid arthritis. *Am J Med* 1988;85:771.
213. Lewis JH, Schiff ER. Methotrexate-induced chronic liver injury: guidelines for detection and prevention. *Am J Gastroenterol* 1988;83:1337.
214. Daniele B et al. Sulindac-induced severe hepatitis. *Am J Gastroenterol* 1988;83:1429.

215. Wood LJ et al. Sulindac hepatotoxicity: effects of acute and chronic exposure. *Aust NZ J Med* 1985;15:397.
216. Jick H et al. Liver disease associated with diclofenac, naproxen, and piroxicam. *Pharmacotherapy* 1992;12:207.
217. Hepps KS et al. Severe cholestatic jaundice associated with piroxicam. *Gastroenterology* 1991;101:1737.
218. Ouellette GS et al. Reversible hepatitis associated with diclofenac. *J Clin Gastroenterol* 1991;13:205.
219. Nores JM et al. Acute hepatitis due to ketoprofen. *Clin Rheumatol* 1991;10:215.
220. Tarazi EM et al. Sulindac-associated hepatic injury: analysis of 91 cases reported to the Food and Drug Administration. *Gastroenterology* 1993;104:569.
221. Rabkin JM et al. Fatal fulminant hepatitis associated with bromfenac use. *Ann Pharmacother* 1999;33:945.
222. Koulaouzidis A et al. Nitrofurantoin-induced lung- and hepatotoxicity. *Ann Hepatol* 2007;6:119.
223. Paiva LA et al. Long-term hepatic memory for hypersensitivity to nitrofurantoin. *Am J Gastroenterol* 1992;87:891.
224. Schattner A et al. Nitrofurantoin-induced immune-mediated lung and liver disease. *Am J Med Sci* 1999;317:336.
225. Taylor C et al. Oxacillin and hepatitis. *Ann Intern Med* 1979;90:857.
226. Olsson R et al. Liver damage from flucloxacillin, cloxacillin and dicloxacillin. *J Hepatol* 1992;15:154.
227. Maraqa NF et al. Higher occurrence of hepatotoxicity and rash in patients treated with oxacillin compared with those treated with nafcillin and other commonly used antimicrobials. *Clin Infect Dis* 2002;34:50.
228. Ozenirler S et al. Propylthiouracil-induced hepatic damage. *Ann Pharmacother* 1996;30:960.
229. Liaw YF et al. Hepatic injury during propyl thiouracil therapy in patients with hyperthyroidism. *A cohort study. Ann Intern Med* 1993;118:424.
230. Wright TM et al. Resperidone and quetiapine induced cholestasis. *Ann Pharmacother* 2007;41:1518.
231. Persky S et al. Sertraline hepatotoxicity. *Dig Dis Sci* 2003;48:939.
232. Burkhard S et al. Fulminant hepatic failure in a child as a potential adverse effect of trimethoprim-sulfamethoxazole. *Eur J Pediatr* 1995;154:530.
233. Munoz SJ et al. Intrahepatic cholestasis and phospholipidosis associated with the use of trimethoprim-sulfamethoxazole. *Hepatology* 1990;12:342.
234. Kowdley KV et al. Prolonged cholestasis due to trimethoprim-sulfamethoxazole. *Gastroenterology* 1992;102:2148.
235. Heaton PC et al. Association between tetracycline or doxycycline and hepatotoxicity: a population based case control study. *J Clin Pharm Ther* 2007;32:483.
236. Schultz JC et al. Fatal liver disease after intravenous administration of tetracycline in high dosage. *N Engl J Med* 1963;269:999.
237. Lucena MI et al. Antidepressant induced hepatotoxicity. *Expert Opin Drug Safety* 2003;2:249.
238. Ilan Y et al. Hepatic failure associated with imipramine therapy. *Pharmacopsychiatry* 1996;29:79.
239. Horst DA et al. Prolonged cholestasis and progressive hepatic fibrosis following imipramine therapy. *Gastroenterology* 1980;79:550.
240. Powell WJ et al. Lethal hepatic necrosis after therapy with imipramine and desipramine. *JAMA* 1968;206:642.
241. Yon J et al. Hepatitis caused by amitriptyline therapy. *JAMA* 1975;232:833.
242. Warning on Serzone. *JAMA* 2002;287:1102.
243. Sztajnkrycer MD. Valrpoic acid toxicity: overview and management. *J Clin Toxicol* 2002;40:789.
244. Sidiq H et al. HIV-related liver disease: infections versus drugs. *Gastroenerol Clin North Amer* 2006;35:487.
245. Acosta BS et al. Zidovudine-associated type B lactic acidosis and hepatic steatosis in an HIV-infected patient. *South Med J* 1999;92:421.
246. Cattelan AM et al. Severe hepatic failure related to nevirapine treatment. *Clin Infect Dis* 1999;29:455.
247. Brau N et al. Severe hepatitis in three AIDS patients treated with indinavir. *Lancet* 1997;349:924.

RENAL DISORDERS

Myrna Munar
SECTION EDITOR

CHAPTER 30

Acute Renal Failure

Donald F. Brophy

DEFINITION

Acute renal failure (ARF) is characterized clinically by an abrupt decrease in renal function over a period of hours to days, resulting in the accumulation of nitrogenous waste products *(azotemia)* and the inability to maintain and regulate fluid, electrolyte, and acid–base balance.[1] Many attempts have been made to objectively quantify ARF based on laboratory data, daily urine output, or the need for renal replacement therapy (RRT), but a consensus using these parameters has not been attained. Traditionally, ARF has been defined as an increase in serum creatinine (SrCr) of >0.5 mg/dL when the baseline SrCr is <2.5 mg/dL, and an increase in SrCr of >1.0 mg/dL when the baseline SrCr is >2.5 mg/dL.[1] These criteria are often inaccurate because SrCr and glomerular filtration rate (GFR) do not follow a linear relationship. Diagnosing ARF solely on creatinine concentration is problematic because many patients are in a high catabolic state as a result of their critical illness. Catabolism leads to the accumulation of creatinine and noncreatinine waste products (urea nitrogen), organic acids, water, and electrolytes. To help clarify much of this confusion, the Acute Dialysis Quality Initiative created an international expert panel, which has proposed a new classification system named "RIFLE."[2] This system represents various stages of ARF, including risk, injury, failure, loss (defined as the need for dialysis at least 1 month following failure), and finally "end-stage renal disease." Although it is too early to tell if this new classification system will provide advantages over traditional definitions, it represents a significant step forward to detect and prevent ARF. Regardless of the definitions used, the clinician should suspect ARF when the kidney is unable to regulate fluid, electrolyte, acid–base, or nitrogen balance, even in the presence of a normal SrCr concentration.

EPIDEMIOLOGY

Acute renal failure occurs almost exclusively in hospitalized patients; hallmark studies conducted in the United States and abroad indicate the incidence of *community-acquired ARF* (development of ARF before hospitalization) is just 1%; approximately 75% of these admissions result from decreased kidney blood flow, termed *prerenal azotemia.* Other less-common causes include obstructive uropathy (17%) and intrinsic renal disease (11%).[3] Community-acquired ARF can usually be reversed by correcting the underlying problems of volume status or obstruction. Hospital-acquired ARF is much more common, and the incidence and severity vary based on intensive care unit (ICU) or non-ICU setting.[4] The incidence of ARF in general medicine patients is approximately 2% to 5%, with the most common causes being prerenal azotemia, postoperative complications, or nephrotoxin exposure. These patients can experience one or more of these renal insults throughout their hospitalization. Conversely, ICU-acquired ARF is more prevalent and severe. Data suggest the incidence of ARF in patients in the ICU approaches 25%, stemming from multiple risk factors, including older age, infection, nephrotoxin exposure, male gender, multiorgan dysfunction, and the need for mechanical ventilation.[5] Although many patients with ARF will initially require dialysis, a small percentage will devlop end-stage renal disease requiring long-term dialysis.

PROGNOSIS

Despite recent advances in dialysis delivery and the development of sophisticated continuous RRT, ARF continues to have a grim prognosis. Indeed, the occurrence of ARF in critically ill patients carries at least a 50% mortality rate.[6] Worse yet, the mortality rate increases correspondingly by 10% with each additional failed organ system. The mortality rate of ARF has declined minimally during the last 50 years. This slow decline may be explained in part by three important factors. First, patients are older when they develop ARF. Second, patients are often afflicted with serious underlying medical illnesses beyond ARF. Third, the clinical severity status of the patient is much higher now than ever before. Before the widespread availability of RRT, the most common causes of death in patients with ARF were fluid and electrolyte disorders and advanced uremia. Today, the most common causes of death are infection, bleeding, cardiopulmonary failure, and withdrawal of life support.[7,8]

CLINICAL COURSE

Three distinct phases of ARF exist. The *oliguric phase* generally occurs over 1 to 2 days and is characterized by a progressive decrease in urine production. Urine production of <400 mL/day is termed *oliguria,* and urine production of <50 mL/day is termed *anuria.* The oliguric stage may last from days to several weeks. *Nonoliguric renal failure* (>400 mL/day of urine output) carries a better prognosis compared with oliguric renal failure, although the exact reason remains unknown. Similarly, the shorter the duration of oliguria, the higher the likelihood of successful recovery. This is probably because the renal insults in these cases are less severe (e.g., dehydration, nephrotoxin exposure, postrenal obstruction). Strict fluid and electrolyte monitoring and management are required during this phase until renal function normalizes.

After the oliguric phase, a period of increased urine production occurs over several days; this is called the *diuretic phase.* This phase signals the initial repair of the kidney insult. The diuretic phase can result, in part, from a return to normal GFR before tubular reabsorptive capacity has fully recovered. The elevated osmotic load from uremic toxins and the increased fluid volume retained during the oliguric phase may also contribute to the diuretic phase. Despite the increased urine production, patients may remain markedly azotemic for several days. Daily modifications in the fluid and electrolyte requirements are necessary based on urine output.

The *recovery phase* occurs over several weeks to months, depending on the severity of the patient's ARF. This phase signals the return to the patient's baseline kidney function, normalization of urine production, and the return of the diluting and concentrating abilities of the kidneys.

PATHOGENESIS

The production and elimination of urine requires three basic physiologic events.

- Blood flow to the glomeruli
- The formation and processing of ultrafiltrate by the glomeruli and tubular cells
- Urine excretion through the ureters, bladder, and urethra

Many conditions can alter the above physiologic events leading to ARF. These are classified as *prerenal azotemia, functional, intrinsic,* and *postrenal* ARF (Table 30-1). It is possible for more than one of these categories to coexist.

Normal renal function depends on adequate renal perfusion. The kidneys receive up to 25% of cardiac output, which is >1 L/minute of blood flow. Prerenal azotemia occurs when blood flow to the kidneys is reduced. Major causes include decreased intravascular volume (e.g., hemorrhage, dehydration, including overdiuresis), decreased effective circulating volume states (e.g., cirrhosis or chronic heart failure [CHF]), hypotensive events (e.g., shock or medication-related hypotension), and renovascular occlusion or vasoconstriction. Because no structural damage occurs to the kidney parenchyma per se, correcting the underlying cause rapidly restores GFR. Sustained prerenal conditions can result, however, in glomerular ischemia causing acute tubular necrosis (ATN).

Functional ARF results when medical conditions or drugs impair glomerular ultrafiltrate production or intraglomerular hydrostatic pressure. Blood travels through the afferent arteriole and enters the glomerulus, where it is filtered, and exits through the efferent arteriole (Fig. 30-1). The afferent and efferent arterioles work in concert to maintain adequate glomerular capillary hydrostatic pressure to form ultrafiltrate. Many medications can drastically reduce intraglomerular hydrostatic pressure and GFR by producing afferent arteriolar vasoconstriction or efferent arteriolar vasodilation (Fig. 30-2).

Intrinsic ARF can occur at the microvascular level of the nephron, glomeruli, renal tubules, or interstitium. Vasculitic diseases (e.g., Wegener's granulomatosis, cryoglobulinemic

Table 30-1 Causes of Acute Renal Failure

Classification	*Common Clinical Disorders*
Prerenal Azotemia	**Intravascular Volume Depletion**
	Hemorrhage (surgery, trauma)
	Dehydration (gastrointestinal losses, aggressive diuretic administration)
	Severe burns
	Hypovolemic shock
	Sequestration (peritonitis, pancreatitis)
	Decreased Effective Circulating Volume
	Cirrhosis with ascites
	Congestive heart failure
	Hypotension, Shock Syndromes
	Antihypertensive vasodilating medications
	Septic shock
	Cardiomyopathy
	Increased Renal Vascular Occlusion or Constriction
	Bilateral renal artery stenosis
	Unilateral renal stenosis in solitary kidney
	Renal artery or vein thrombosis (embolism, atherosclerosis)
	Vasopressor medications (phenylephrine, norepinephrine)
Functional Acute Renal Failure	**Afferent Arteriole Vasoconstrictors**
	Cyclosporine
	Nonsteroidal anti-inflammatory drugs
	Efferent Arteriole Vasodilators
	Angiotensin-converting enzyme inhibitors
	Angiotensin II–receptor antagonists
Intrinsic Acute Renal Failure	**Glomerular Disorders**
	Glomerulonephritis
	Systemic lupus erythematosus
	Malignant hypertension
	Vasculitic disorders (Wegener's granulomatosis)
	Acute Tubular Necrosis
	Prolonged prerenal states
	Drug induced (contrast media, aminoglycosides, amphotericin B)
	Acute Interstitial Nephritis
	Drug induced (quinolones, penicillins, sulfa drugs)
Postrenal Acute Renal Failure	**Ureter Obstruction (Bilateral or Unilateral in Solitary Kidney)**
	Malignancy (prostate or cervical cancer)
	Prostate hypertrophy Anticholinergic drugs (affect bladder outlet muscles)
	Renal calculi

vasculitis) involve the small vessels of the kidney. Glomerulonephritis and systemic lupus erythematosus, although relatively uncommon, result in glomerular damage. ATN is by far the most common cause of intrinsic ARF. In fact, the term *acute tubular necrosis* is often used interchangeably with *ARF.* ATN occurs in part because the renal tubules require high oxygen delivery to maintain their metabolic activity. Consequently, any condition that causes ischemia to the tubules (e.g., hypotension, decreased blood flow) can induce ATN. Moreover, the tubules may be exposed to exceedingly high concentrations of nephrotoxic drugs (e.g., aminoglycosides). Interstitial nephritis or inflammation within the renal parenchyma, is most often associated with drug administration (e.g., penicillins).

Postrenal ARF occurs when there is an outflow obstruction in the upper or lower urinary tract. Lower tract obstruction is most common and can be caused by prostatic hypertrophy, prostate or cervical cancer, anticholinergic drugs that cause bladder sphincter spasm, or renal calculi. Upper tract obstruction is less common and occurs when both ureters are obstructed or when one is obstructed in a patient with a single

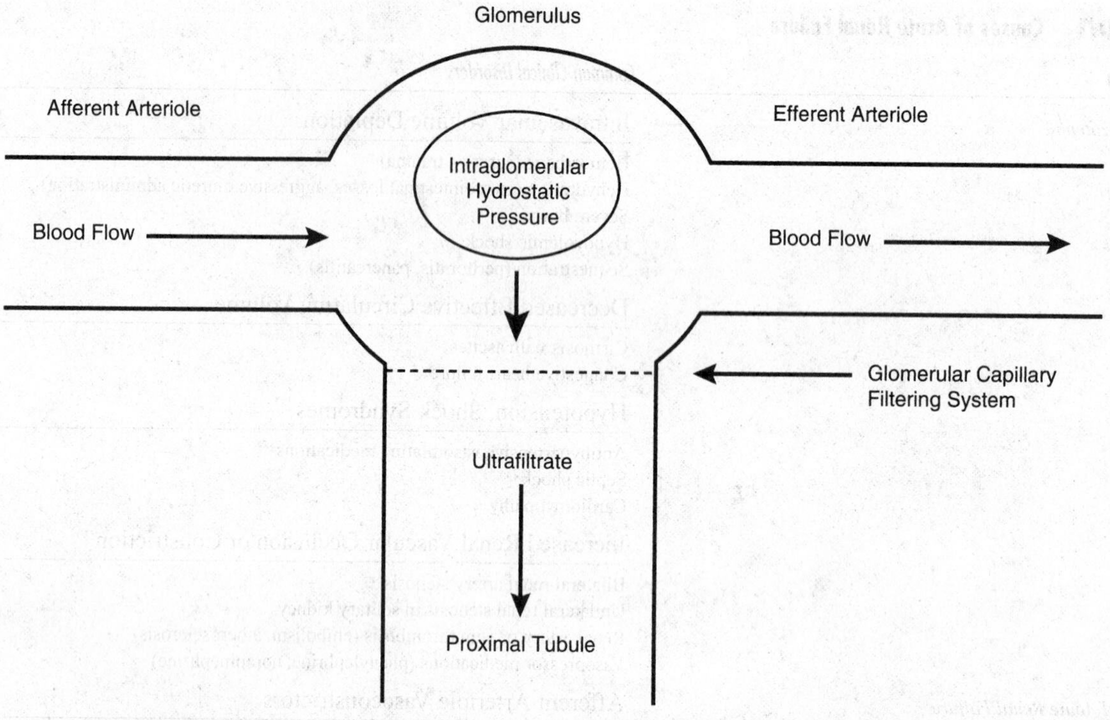

FIGURE 30-1 Schematic of renal blood flow. Blood enters the glomerulus via the afferent arteriole. The intraglomerular hydrostatic pressure leads to ultrafiltration across the glomerular into the proximal tubule. The unfiltered blood leaves the glomerulus via the efferent arteriole. In conditions of decreased renal perfusion, efferent arteriolar vasoconstriction occurs to increase intraglomerular hydrostatic pressure and maintain ultrafiltrate production. Afferent arteriolar vasodilation also occurs to improve blood flow into the glomerulus.

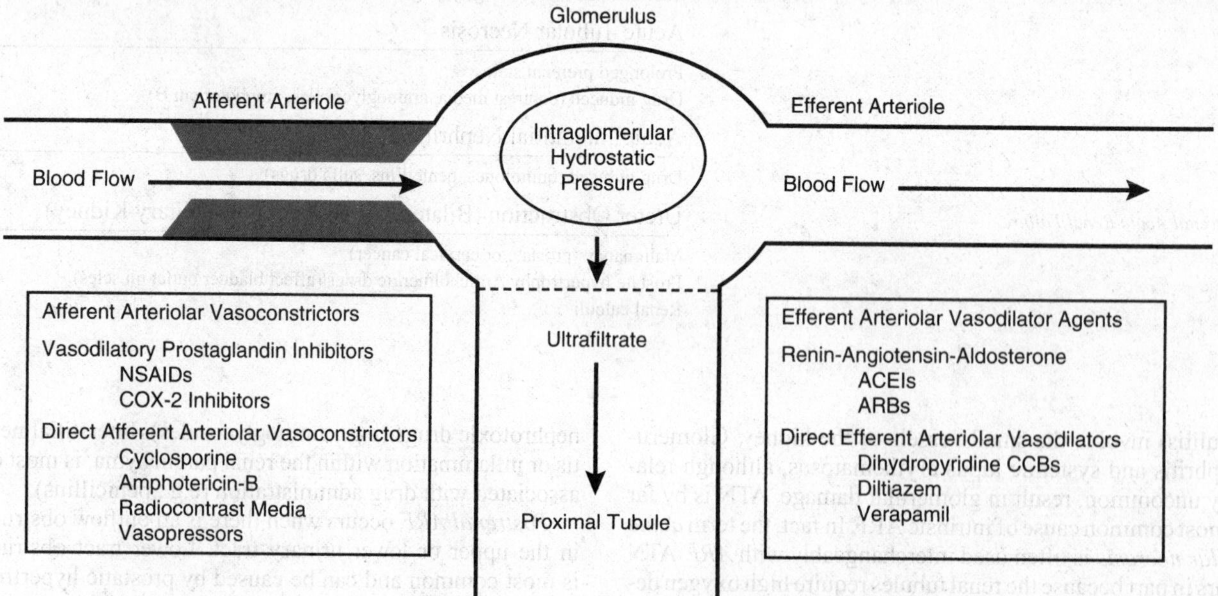

FIGURE 30-2 Drugs that alter renal hemodynamics by causing afferent arteriole vasoconstriction or efferent arteriole vasodilation. ACEIs, angiotensin-converting enzyme inhibitors; ARBs, angiotensin II-receptor blockers; CCBs, calcium channel blockers; COX-2, cyclooxygenase-2; NSAIDs, nonsteroidal anti-inflammatory drugs.

functioning kidney. Postrenal ARF usually resolves rapidly after the obstruction has been removed. Postobstructive diuresis can be dramatic (e.g., 3–5 L/day).

CLINICAL EVALUATION

History and Physical Examination

A detailed history and physical examination often reveal the cause(s) of ARF. The clinician's responsibility is to ask specific, open-ended questions regarding the patient's chief complaint; history of present illness; medical history; family, social, and allergy history; and current prescription and nonprescription medication use. Probing for pertinent information regarding recent surgery, nephrotoxin exposure, or concurrent medical conditions can aid in rapidly determining the etiology of ARF. For example, does the patient have pre-existing conditions that point toward prerenal azotemia, such as CHF or liver disease? Did the patient receive prophylactic antibiotics before surgery? Did the patient hemorrhage or have protracted hypotension during surgery? Furthermore, assessment of the vital sign flowchart for documented weight loss, hypotensive events, fluid intake, and urine output may also prove useful.

A thorough physical examination, when used in conjunction with the history, can be invaluable in confirming the cause of ARF. The patient's volume status should be evaluated first. Evidence of dehydration (e.g., syncope, weight loss, orthostatic hypotension) or decreased effective circulating volume (e.g., ascites, pulmonary edema, peripheral edema, jugular venous distention) usually indicates prerenal azotemia. The presence of edema in a patient with normal cardiac function can, however, signal the early signs of nephrotic syndrome. Concurrent rash and ARF associated with recent antibiotic exposure suggest drug-induced allergic interstitial nephritis. The clinician should suspect rhabdomyolysis in a patient with trauma or crush injuries and ARF. An enlarged prostate, painful urination, or wide deviations in urine volume can suggest obstructive ARF causes. Flank and lower abdominal pain suggest upper obstruction, whereas urinary frequency, hesitancy, dribbling, and abdominal fullness indicate lower obstruction.

Laboratory Evaluation

Quantifying Glomerular Filtration Rate

Because of the dynamic changes that occur in ARF, it is difficult to quantify renal function accurately in this population. Although equations were created decades ago to address the dynamic changes in SrCr during ARF, none have proved helpful. One of the most widely used clinical measures for estimating GFR is determination of creatinine clearance (ClCr). Creatinine is produced at a relatively constant rate by nonenzymatic hydrolysis of muscle stores of creatine and phosphocreatine. An individual's muscle mass, age, and sex are predictors of creatinine production. Under steady-state conditions, the urinary excretion of creatinine equals the creatinine production rate, and the SrCr concentration remains relatively stable. Creatinine is freely filtered at the glomerulus, with about 10% to 20% eliminated by active tubular secretion. Consequently, the ClCr overestimates the true GFR by 10% to 20%. As GFR declines further, tubular creatinine secretion can account for up to 50% of creatinine elimination, which may overestimate actual GFR by as much as 100%. Commonly used drugs, such as trimethoprim, can inhibit the secretion of creatinine. Accordingly, administration of these agents can increase the SrCr and decrease ClCr without affecting GFR.[9] Various methods for determining ClCr have been developed, including urine and nonurine methods. All these methods have potential limitations and pitfalls when used in patients with ARF. Clinicians commonly use nonurine methods for estimating kidney function. The Cockcroft-Gault (CG) equation is one method commonly used to estimate ClCr[10]:

$$\mathrm{Cl_{Cr}} = \frac{(140 - \mathrm{Age})\,(\mathrm{IBW})}{(72)\,(\mathrm{SrCr})} \qquad \textbf{30-1}$$

where age is in years, *IBW* is ideal body weight in kilograms [male IBW $= 50 + (2.3$ height $\times >60$ inches); female IBW $= 45 + (2.3 \times$ height >60 inches)], and *SrCr* is the serum creatinine concentration (mg/dL).

For women, the CG equation is multiplied by 0.85 to account for decreased muscle mass. The CG equation should not be used to estimate GFR in patients with rapidly changing SrCr concentrations because it was derived from normal, healthy subjects with stable renal function. The CG equation produces falsely high ClCr estimates in the early stages of ARF and falsely low ClCr estimates when ARF is resolving. An example of this is a patient who develops ATN and anuria. Within the first few days, the creatinine level may increase slightly because it takes time for the serum creatinine concentration to achieve a new steady state. In fact, the calculated ClCr may even remain in the normal range, although the true GFR is substantially lower. The converse is true with patients recovering from ATN. As the diuretic phase of ATN begins, urine output can be dramatic, but patients may remain markedly azotemic for several days. Using the CG equation in this setting will produce a falsely low ClCr estimate. The CG equation is also inaccurate in populations that have little muscle mass, such as elderly, obese, or cachectic patients.

A more recent development is the acceptance of the abbreviated Modification of Diet in Renal Disease (MDRD) equation for quantifying GFR in most clinical laboratories.[11,12] As such, clinicians are routinely provided the estimated GFR (eGFR) for their respective patients. An important point is that the results from the MDRD and CG equation are not interchangeable. For example, the MDRD equation should only be used to quantify GFR and to detect or stage the degree of chronic kidney disease; the CG equation should be used simply as a guideline for drug dosing adjustment in patients with ARF. No published data using the MDRD in cases of ARF exist.

In the past, many clinicians advocated the collection of timed urine specimens to calculate creatinine clearance in ARF. Although this may seem relatively easy, it is susceptible to serious errors, particularly the timing of the collection and assuring the patient has not voided urine in the commode. For these reasons, the practice of collecting timed urine specimens is not routinely performed.

Blood Tests

Assessment of the blood urea nitrogen (BUN) and creatinine concentrations is crucial for guiding the diagnosis, treatment, and monitoring of ARF. The BUN:SrCr ratio can delineate prerenal causes from intrinsic and postrenal causes. Urea reabsorption is inversely proportional to the urine flow rate. The

Table 30-2 Urinary Indices in Acute Renal Failure

Component	*Prerenal Azotemia*	*Acute Tubular Necrosis*	*Postrenal Obstruction*
Urine Na^+ (mEq/L)	<20	>40	>40
FE_{Na^+}	<1%	>2%	>1%
Urine/plasma creatinine	>40	<20	<20
Specific gravity	>1.010	<1.010	Variable
Urine osmolality (mOsm/kg)	Up to 1,200	<300	<300

normal steady-state BUN:SrCr ratio is approximately 10:1. In prerenal conditions, the BUN:SrCr ratio is >20:1 because sodium and water are actively reabsorbed in the renal tubules to expand the effective circulating volume. Urea, an ineffective osmole, is reabsorbed as a result of increased water reabsorption, while creatinine is not reabsorbed. Whereas the SrCr may increase owing to decreased glomerular filtration, BUN increases to a greater degree as a result of increased proximal reabsorption.

The presence of hypercalcemia or hyperuricemia can indicate a hematologic malignancy. *Tumor lysis syndrome* is a condition that occurs in patients with leukemia after chemotherapy induction. The destruction of cancerous cells results in the release of large quantities of cellular contents (e.g., potassium, uric acid) into the bloodstream, which can overwhelm the kidney's functional ability, especially in dehydrated states.

Other elevated enzymes may also aid in the diagnosis of ARF. An increased level of creatine kinase or myoglobin in the face of ARF usually indicates rhabdomyolysis. Eosinophilia may suggest acute allergic interstitial nephritis from drug exposure. High levels of circulating immune complexes in the presence of ARF suggest glomerulopathies.[1]

Urinalysis

The urinalysis is an important diagnostic tool for differentiating ARF into prerenal azotemia, intrinsic, or obstructive ARF (Table 30-2). The presence of highly concentrated urine, as determined by elevated urine osmolality and specific gravity, suggests prerenal azotemia. During dehydrated states, *vasopressin (antidiuretic hormone [ADH])* is secreted, and the *renin-angiotensin-aldosterone (RAA) system* is activated. These mechanisms promote the reabsorption of water and sodium at the collecting duct of the nephron, which serves to expand the effective circulating volume in an attempt to restore renal perfusion. As a result of diminished urine volume, the urine osmolality and specific gravity increase dramatically. Patients with prerenal azotemia and oliguria often have a urine osmolality >500 mOsm/kg. The maximal urine osmolality can exceed 1,200 mOsm/kg.

The presence of proteinuria or hematuria can indicate glomerular damage. Nephrotic syndrome is characterized by urinary protein losses >3.5 g/1.73 m^2/day. Proteinuria can also result from tubular damage; however, the protein loss is rarely >2 g/day. The protein content can be used to differentiate glomerular versus tubular damage. The low-molecular-weight protein, 2-microglobulin is freely filtered at the glomerulus and reabsorbed at the proximal tubule. Therefore, the presence of excessive β_2-microglobulin in the urine suggests a tubular source of ARF, such as ATN. Conversely, albumin is not readily filtered at the glomerulus; hence, the presence of heavy albuminuria suggests a glomerular source of ARF.

Microscopic examination of the urine provides helpful clues for determining the source of ARF (Table 30-3). Pigmented granular casts are generally seen with ischemic or nephrotoxin-induced ARF. White blood cells (WBC) and WBC casts can indicate an inflammatory process in the glomerulus, such as acute interstitial nephritis (AIN) or pyelonephritis. Red blood cells (RBC) and RBC casts can result from strenuous exercise or can indicate glomerulonephritis. Allergic interstitial nephritis can be detected by the presence of urinary eosinophils. Obstructive ARF causes, such as nephrolithiasis, can be identified by the presence of crystals in the urine. Cystine, leucine, and tyrosine crystals are considered pathologic. The presence of calcium oxalate crystals may suggest toxic ingestion of ethylene glycol.

Urinary Chemistries

Analyzing urine electrolyte concentrations and simultaneously comparing them with serum sodium and creatinine concentrations is useful for differentiating between prerenal azotemia and ATN (Table 30-2). The fractional excretion of sodium (FE_{Na^+}) is a measurement of how actively the kidney is reabsorbing sodium, and it is calculated as the fraction of filtered

Table 30-3 Clinical Significance of Urinary Sediment in Acute Renal Failure

Cellular Debris	*Clinical Significance*
Red blood cells	Glomerulonephritis IgA nephropathy Lupus nephritis
White blood cells	Infection (pyelonephritis) Glomerulonephritis Acute tubular necrosis
Eosinophils	Drug-induced acute interstitial nephritis Pyelonephritis Renal transplant rejection
Hyaline casts	Glomerulonephritis Pyelonephritis Congestive heart failure
Red blood cell casts	Acute tubular necrosis Glomerulonephritis Interstitial nephritis
White blood cell casts	Pyelonephritis Interstitial nephritis
Granular casts	Dehydration Interstitial nephritis Glomerulonephritis Acute tubular necrosis
Tubular cell casts	Acute tubular necrosis
Fatty casts	Nephrotic syndrome
Myoglobin	Rhabdomyolysis
Crystals	Nonspecific

sodium excreted in the urine using creatinine as a measure of GFR. In normal conditions, the proximal tubule reabsorbs 99% of filtered sodium. The FE_{Na^+} formula is listed as follows: (Eq. 30-2)

$$FE_{Na^+}(\%) = \frac{(UNa)\ (SrCr)}{(U_{Cr})\ (SNa)} \times 100\% \qquad \textbf{30-2}$$

where *UNa* is the urine sodium concentration (mEq/L), *SrCr* is the serum creatinine concentration (mg/dL), *UCr* is the urine creatinine concentration (mg/dL), and *SNa* is the serum sodium concentration (mEq/L).

In prerenal azotemia, the functional ability of the proximal renal tubule remains intact. In fact, its sodium-reabsorbing abilities are markedly enhanced because of the effects of circulating vasopressin and activation of the RAA system. Both the FE_{Na^+} and urinary sodium concentration become markedly low ($<1\%$ and <20 mEq/L, respectively) in prerenal conditions. In contrast, these indices are elevated in ATN because the renal tubules lose their ability to reabsorb sodium; the FE_{Na^+} is $>2\%$, and the urine sodium is >40 mEq/L. FE_{Na^+} values between 1% and 2% are generally inconclusive. The clinician should ensure that the patient is not receiving scheduled thiazide or loop diuretic therapy when the FE_{Na^+} is calculated. These diuretics increase natriuresis, thereby making the results difficult to interpret.

PRERENAL AND FUNCTIONAL ACUTE RENAL FAILURE

Congestive Heart Failure and Nonsteroidal Anti-Inflammatory Drug Use

1. A.W. is a 71-year-old white man who had a ST-segment elevation myocardial infarction (STEMI) 2 months ago. His ejection fraction is currently 15% (normal, 50%–60%). He presents today for his 2-month follow-up clinic appointment complaining of shortness of breath, dyspnea on exertion, and inability to produce much urine. His medical history is significant for long-standing hypertension, coronary artery disease, osteoarthritis, and recent-onset heart failure (HF) after his MI. His home medications include furosemide 40 mg every day, enalapril 5 mg daily, metoprolol XL 100 mg daily, digoxin 0.125 mg daily, atorvastatin 40 mg QD, and naproxen sodium 550 mg twice daily (BID), all of which are taken orally (PO). With the exception of naproxen, A.W. often forgets to take his medications. Physical examination reveals lower leg 3+ pitting edema, pulmonary crackles and wheezes, positive jugular venous distention, and an S_3 heart sound. His vital signs are significant for a blood pressure (BP) of 198/97 mm Hg and a weight gain of 4 kg since his last visit 2 months ago. Last month, his BUN and SrCr were 23 (normal, 5–20) and 1.2 mg/dL (normal, 0.5–1.2), respectively. What are A.W.'s risk factors for ARF?

[SI units: BUN, 8.2 mmol/L (normal, 1.8–7.1); SrCr, 106 mol/L (normal, 44.2–106)]

A.W.'s risk factors for ARF are CHF with poor cardiac output (ejection fraction, 15%) that resulted from his STEMI and his medication, naproxen sodium. CHF is a major cause of functional ARF.[13] A.W.'s diminished cardiac output has resulted in decreased effective circulating volume and activation of the RAA system, which are impairing his renal perfusion. In states of decreased renal perfusion, prostaglandins E_2 and I_2 compensate for the afferent arteriole vasoconstriction by stimulating afferent arteriole vasodilation, and thereby enhancing renal blood flow. Prostaglandin synthesis is mediated predominantly by cyclooxygenase-1 (COX-1) and perhaps cyclooxygenase-2 (COX-2). Nonsteroidal anti-inflammatory drugs (NSAID), such as naproxen, are often overlooked as causes of ARF.[14,15] NSAID exert their pharmacologic effect by inhibiting prostaglandin synthesis, thereby negating compensatory vasodilation. NSAIDs induce abrupt decreases in GFR in at-risk patient populations, specifically those with CHF, liver disease, the elderly, or dehydrated patients. Indomethacin is associated with the highest risk of NSAIDs-induced renal ischemia, whereas aspirin appears to have the lowest risk. Naproxen, ibuprofen, piroxicam, and diclofenac are considered intermediate in their relative capacities to acutely compromise renal perfusion.[15,16] Sulindac may offer a "renal-sparing" effect. Sulindac is a prodrug that is converted to its active sulfide metabolite by the liver and then becomes reversibly oxidized back to its parent compound in the kidney; renal prostaglandin synthesis is essentially unaltered by sulindac. Cases of sulindac-induced renal dysfunction have been reported when the drug was administered to patients with cirrhosis and ascites.

COX-2 inhibitors also inhibit prostaglandin synthesis. A study comparing the effects of rofecoxib and celecoxib to nonselective NSAIDs demonstrated similar renovascular effects.[16] These data suggest that COX-2 selective agents do not offer any benefit over nonselective NSAID with regard to renovascular effects. Figure 30-2 illustrates common medications that alter renal hemodynamics by causing either afferent arteriole vasoconstriction or efferent arteriole vasodilation.

2. A.W.'s cardiologist obtains a stat digoxin level, electrolyte panel, urinalysis, and urine electrolyte panel. The digoxin level is reported as "not detectable" (target, 0.5–0.8 ng/mL). Other significant serum laboratory values include Na^+ of 140 mEq/L (normal, 135–145), BUN 56 mg/dL (normal, 5–20), and creatinine of 1.5 mg/dL (normal, 0.5–1.2). The urinalysis is significant for a urinary osmolality of 622 mOsm/kg (normal, 300–500 mOsm/kg), and specific gravity of 1.092 (normal, 1.010–1.020). The urine electrolytes are significant for Na^+ of 12 mEq/L (normal, 20–40) and creatinine of 87 mg/dL. What laboratory findings suggest functional ARF?

[SI units: sodium, 140 mmol/L(normal, 135–145); BUN, 20 mmol/L (normal, 1.8–7.1); SrCr, 132.6 mol/L (normal, 44.2–106); urine Cr, 7691 mol/L]

A.W. has classic laboratory findings associated with poor renal perfusion (Table 30-2). It is important to compare the current and previous laboratory data to assess acute changes in renal function. Compared with last month, A.W.'s renal function has deteriorated based on substantial increases in BUN and SrCr concentrations; BUN has increased nearly twofold and creatinine by 25%. The BUN:SrCr ratio is $>20:1$, suggesting poor renal blood flow, which is corroborated by other urinary indices such as the urinary Na^+ 12 mEq/L; specific gravity (elevated), 1.090; urine osmolality, 622 mOsm/kg; and the calculated FE_{Na^+}, 0.14%. These values reflect the ability of the renal tubules to respond to vasopressin and aldosterone in an attempt to expand effective circulating volume and restore renal perfusion.

Another consideration is furosemide-induced volume depletion; however, the nondetectable serum digoxin level

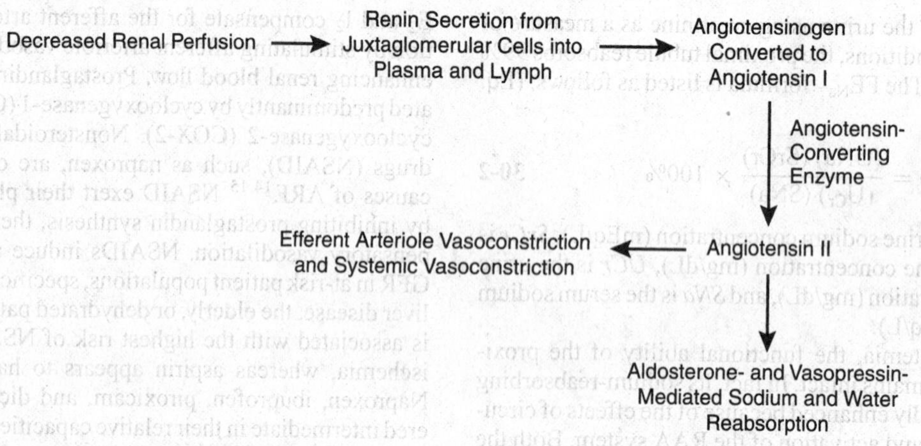

FIGURE 30-3 Compensatory hormonal mechanisms of decreased renal perfusion.

indicates likely noncompliance with his medications. A more likely explanation is poor renal perfusion because of his heart failure (i.e., low cardiac output).

3. How should A.W.'s prerenal azotemia be treated?

The presence of volume overload in the face of prerenal azotemia suggests a decreased effective circulating volume, most likely from poorly controlled HF. Restoring and improving A.W.'s cardiac output and renal perfusion will rapidly correct the prerenal azotemia. This can be achieved by (a) assuring adherence to his heart failure medications (furosemide, enalapril, metoprolol XL, and digoxin), (b) controlling BP to a goal of <135/85 mm Hg by decreasing both preload and afterload, and (*c*) modifying any drug therapy that has deleterious effects on the renal hemodynamics (e.g., NSAID). The specific therapies for controlling hypertension and improving cardiac output are presented in Chapter 14, Essential Hypertension, and Chapter 19, Heart Failure. Naproxen should be discontinued and substituted with acetaminophen to treat his osteoarthritis. Normal renal function should return in a few days after correction of the underlying causes.

Angiotensin-Converting Enzyme Inhibitor- and Angiotensin Receptor Blocker-Induced Acute Renal Failure

4. G.B. is a 53-year-old white woman with hypertension, coronary artery disease, peripheral vascular disease, and diabetes, for which she had been taking hydrochlorothiazide 25 mg PO daily, atorvastatin 10 mg PO daily, aspirin 81 mg PO daily, and NPH insulin 30 U subcutaneously Q morning and 15 U subcutaneously Q evening. At last week's clinic visit, she had two consecutive BP readings of 187/96 and 193/95 mm Hg, respectively, measured 20 minutes apart. At that time, G.B.'s primary care physician discontinued her hydrochlorothiazide and started her on lisinopril 5 mg PO daily. She returns to the clinic today for her 1-week follow-up appointment complaining of dizziness, very little urine production over the past week, and swelling in her ankles. Her BP is 98/43 mm Hg. A stat serum electrolyte panel is significant for a BUN of 62 mg/dL (normal, 5–20) and an SrCr of 6.1 mg/dL (normal, 0.5–1.2). Why is G.B. experiencing ARF?

[SI units: BUN, 22.1 mmol/L (normal, 1.8–7.1); SrCr, 539 mol/L (normal, 44.2–106)]

Inhibition of the RAA system in patients with compromised renal blood flow is a common cause of functional ARF. A basic understanding of the effects of the RAA system on renal hemodynamics is necessary in this situation (Fig. 30-3). When renal perfusion is impaired, the juxtaglomerular cells of the kidney secrete renin into the plasma and lymph. Renin cleaves circulating angiotensinogen to form angiotensin I (AT I), which is further cleaved by angiotensin-converting enzyme (ACE), to form angiotensin II (AT II). AT II induces two physiologic events to improve renal perfusion. First, it directly causes systemic vasoconstriction, which shunts blood to the major organs, and indirectly increases intravascular volume through aldosterone- and vasopressin-mediated activity. Second, it preferentially vasoconstricts the efferent renal arteriole to maintain adequate intraglomerular hydrostatic pressure. Under conditions of decreased arterial pressure or effective circulating volume, the RAA system is activated and plasma renin and AT II activity are increased.[17]

G.B. has extensive atherosclerotic disease indicated by the presence of coronary artery and peripheral vascular disease. Atherosclerosis not only affects major blood vessels, but also the macro- and microvasculature of the kidney; indeed, atherosclerosis is a major cause of renal artery occlusion and decreased renal perfusion. This activates the RAA system, which causes sodium and water reabsorption and AT II-mediated efferent arteriole vasoconstriction, in an attempt to restore normal renal perfusion and intraglomerular hydrostatic pressure.

The administration of ACE inhibitors directly inhibits the formation of AT II, which is necessary for efferent arteriole vasoconstriction. Consequently, the compensatory physiologic event that maintains G.B.'s renal blood flow is inhibited, thereby reducing her intraglomerular hydrostatic pressure and GFR. ACE inhibitors are contraindicated in patients with bilateral renal artery stenosis or unilateral stenosis in patients with a single functioning kidney.[17]

5. Are there other factors that predispose patients to ACE inhibitor-induced ARF?

In addition to the above situation, three other general scenarios will result in the development of ARF with ACE inhibitors. First, conditions of sodium and water depletion (e.g., dehydration, overdiuresis, poor fluid intake, low-sodium diet) can increase the dependency of the efferent arteriole on AT II. When ACE inhibitors are given in these situations, GFR can fall dramatically, and SrCr rises. ARF can be averted by withholding the ACE inhibitor (or diuretic, or both) for a day and repleting the intravascular fluid volume with a saline-containing fluid (e.g., normal saline or 0.45% saline). The ACE inhibitor can be restarted at the same dose after adequate hydration. Second, ACE inhibitors can decrease the mean arterial pressure to such a degree that renal perfusion cannot be sustained. This is more likely to occur with long-acting agents or in situations in which the pharmacologic half-life of the ACE inhibitor is prolonged (e.g., pre-existing renal disease). Finally, ACE inhibitors may precipitate ARF in patients who are taking concomitant drugs with renal afferent arteriole vasoconstricting effects, most notably cyclosporine and NSAIDs.

6. How is ACE inhibitor-induced ARF managed?

Patients who are receiving ACE inhibitors should be monitored judiciously with regard to their serum creatinine and electrolyte concentrations. Once an ACE inhibitor is initiated, an increase in SrCr of 20% to 30% can be expected.[17] This slight increase should not worry clinicians, because it typically normalizes within 2 to 3 months. SrCr rises greater than this along with reduced urine output signal ARF, however. ARF related to ACE inhibitors is usually reversible, principally because the ARF is caused by inadequate glomerular capillary pressure, which is restored as soon as sufficient AT II is produced. This normally takes 2 to 3 days to re-equilibrate. Anecdotally, ARF appears to develop more commonly in hypotensive patients or in those with intravascular volume depletion (e.g., patients with HF receiving high-dose diuretics). In these conditions, it is prudent to replete the intravascular fluid volume or temporarily discontinue diuretic therapy. ACE inhibitor therapy should be temporarily discontinued and reinstituted when the patient has a normalized intravascular volume and is hemodynamically stable.

7. Do angiotensin II–receptor blockers (ARB) cause less ARF compared with ACE inhibitors?

The ARBs competitively inhibit the angiotensin II receptor. At least two subtypes of the angiotensin II receptors exist: AT I and AT II. The ARBs exert their pharmacologic effect at the AT I receptor subtype, which is responsible for most, if not all, of the cardiovascular effects of angiotensin II, such as vasoconstriction, aldosterone release, and β-adrenergic stimulation. Few differences are seen in the incidence of ARF between ACE inhibitors and ARBs,[18] and one should not be interchanged with the other in an attempt to decrease ARF risk.

INTRINSIC ACUTE RENAL FAILURE

Intrinsic ARF is a general term that connotes damage at the parenchymal level of the kidney. The term *acute tubular necrosis* is often used to describe this type of ARF, but this is a histologic diagnosis that describes only one of several intrinsic disorders. Pragmatically, intrinsic ARF can be subdivided into vascular, glomerular, or tubular disorders.

Disorders involving the large renal vessels are relatively uncommon. Acute renal artery or vein occlusion can be caused by vasculitis, atheroembolism, thromboembolism, dissection, or clamping of the ascending aorta during surgery. To affect serum BUN and creatinine, occlusion must be bilateral, or it can be unilateral in patients with concomitant renal insufficiency or one functioning kidney. Reduced blood flow to the renal microvasculature and glomeruli also can result in ARF. Common examples are rapidly progressing glomerulonephritis (RPGN) and vasculitis. If these conditions become sufficiently severe, they can cause ischemia, resulting in superimposed ATN. Any disorder that produces tubular ischemia, such as prolonged hypotension or shock syndromes, can result in ATN.

Nephrotoxic drugs are a common cause of ATN, especially when given in septic or volume-contracted patients. The various mechanisms by which drugs can cause ATN, are explained in detail later in this chapter. Although relatively uncommon, drug-induced acute interstitial nephritis (AIN) is another type of intrinsic ARF. This is a hypersensitivity reaction that results from the formation of drug–antibody complexes that subsequently deposit in the glomerular membrane.

Acute Glomerulopathies

Poststreptococcal Glomerulonephritis

8. B.M. is an 18-year-old male college freshman in otherwise good health who recently developed strep throat. He received a 10-day course of amoxicillin, which cleared the infection. He returns to the student health center after completing his 10-day course complaining of "puffy eyes," swelling in his legs, a cough productive of clear sputum, and decreased urine output that appears "tea-colored." Other than the amoxicillin, he is not on any medication. Baseline records from a routine physical examination 2 months ago revealed a serum BUN and creatinine of 10 mg/dL and 0.8 mg/dL (normal, 5–20 and 0.5–1.2), respectively, and a BP of 120/80 mm Hg. Today, the physical examination is significant for a BP of 176/95 mm Hg, 2+ peripheral edema, and bilateral pulmonary rales. The urinalysis is significant for gross hematuria, nephritic-range proteinuria, RBC and WBC casts, and epithelial cells. B.M.'s SrCr has increased to 7.1 mg/dL. Based on the history, physical examination, and laboratory findings, what is the most likely cause of ARF in this patient?

[SI units: BUN, 3.6 mmol/L (normal, 1.8–7.1); SrCr, 70.7 and 627.6 mol/L, respectively (normal, 44.2–106)]

B.M.'s recent history of a streptococcal infection with the development of ARF suggests poststreptococcal glomerulonephritis (PSGN), which results from the formation of antibodies against streptococcal antigens. The streptococcal–antigen immune complexes are deposited in the glomerulus, resulting in complement, cytokine, and clotting cascade activation; neutrophils and monocytes attack the glomerulus causing glomerulonephritis. The onset of PSGN is usually 7 to 21 days after the start of the pharyngeal infection. PSGN is the most common acute-onset, immune-mediated, diffuse glomerulopathy. It primarily affects children, although it can affect any age group and is more prevalent in males than in females. Only certain serologic subtypes of group A hemolytic streptococci, known as *nephritogenic* strains, cause PSGN. Strains that follow pharyngeal infections (e.g., strep throat) include types 1, 3, 4, 6, 12, 25, and 49. Type 49 is the most prevalent strain worldwide. Positive diagnosis of PSGN requires identification of a nephritogenic group A hemolytic streptococcal strain;

objective urinalysis findings suggestive of glomerular damage, such as proteinuria, hematuria, and casts; and elevated streptococcal antibody titers.

B.M. exhibits the classic physical and laboratory findings associated with PSGN. The pertinent positive physical findings include periorbital, pulmonary, and peripheral edema; tea-colored urine, hypertension, and decreased urine output. Edema is a common manifestation, with periorbital edema typically being the first to appear. Reduced GFR, proteinuria, and sodium retention by the kidney all contribute to edema formation. When protein, principally albumin, is lost in the urine, the intravascular oncotic pressure declines, causing a shift of fluid into the extravascular space. The loss of intravascular volume stimulates sodium and water reabsorption by the kidney via aldosterone and vasopressin, which often produces stage 1 to 2 hypertension.

Pertinent laboratory data in B.M. include elevated SrCr, and urinalysis positive for hematuria, proteinuria, WBC casts, and epithelial cells. Hematuria, which is found in almost all patients with PSGN, accounts for the reddish-brown, tea-colored urine. Other commonly found urine sediments include cellular casts and hyaline and granular casts. Oliguria is common in PSGN, but anuria is rare.

9. Are there other tests that can be used to confirm this diagnosis?

Given that B.M. has received a 10-day course of amoxicillin, it is unlikely that throat cultures for the nephritogenic group A hemolytic streptococcal strain will be positive. Cultures of close contacts may, however, be positive for the streptococcal strain, even if they are asymptomatic. The presence of circulating antibodies to the nephritogenic streptococcal strains indicates recent exposure. The antistreptolysin O (ASO), antihyaluronidase (AHase), antideoxyribonuclease B (ADNase B), and antinicotyladenine dinucleotidase (NADase) antibody titers can be measured clinically. ASO titers begin to rise 2 weeks after pharyngeal infection, peak at 4 weeks, and slowly decline over 1 to 6 months. No correlation exists between degree of ASO rise and nephrogenicity. In fact, ASO titers may not be elevated at all if early antibiotic treatment is initiated or in cases of streptococcal skin infections. The use of ADNase and AHase titers is more specific to detect recent infection in these situations.

The streptozyme test, which can be used clinically for rapid screening purposes, uses several antistreptococcal antibody assays. False–positive and false–negative results are common, however, because of cross-reactivity between the antibody and normal collagen.

Serial complement determinations may be of value in diagnosing PSGN. Decreased levels of C3 protein and hemolytic complement activity (CH50) are observed in nearly all patients with active PSGN. Serum C3 levels can fall by nearly 50% of normal in the first weeks of infection and return to normal within 8 weeks after infection. No correlation, however, exists between the degree of C3 depression and severity of nephritis. Circulating antibody complexes of C3 can be found in patients with acute infection.

Rarely, is renal biopsy needed, but it may be prudent in patients who present with atypical symptoms, such as anuria, prolonged oliguria, marked azotemia, hematuria for >3 weeks, or in those who have no streptococcal antibody titers.

10. What are the therapeutic goals and treatment options for PSGN?

The therapeutic goals are to minimize further kidney damage and to provide symptomatic relief for B.M. The underlying streptococcal infection should be treated with appropriate antibiotics, but as illustrated by B.M., this has no effect in preventing PSGN. Family members and close contacts of the infected patient should receive antibiotic prophylaxis as well. Restriction of protein to 0.8 g/kg/day may be beneficial in patients with marked proteinuria, and antihypertensive drugs can be used on a short-term basis to control BP. Sodium and water restriction is beneficial in reducing edema, and loop diuretics may be used as needed for symptomatic pulmonary or peripheral edema. Close monitoring of electrolytes is warranted if diuretics are used. Dialysis is rarely required.

Rapidly Progressive Glomenularnephritis

11. Are there other glomerulopathies that cause ARF?

Yes. RPGN, also called *crescentic glomerulonephritis,* is a clinical syndrome of rapid decline in renal function (from days to weeks) combined with the hallmark findings of gross hematuria, proteinuria, and the presence of extensive glomerular crescents (>50% of glomeruli) on renal biopsy. It is not uncommon for patients with RPGN to have a 50% decline in GFR in only a few weeks. RPGN is a medical emergency, and treatment success depends on how early therapy is initiated. If left untreated, progression to end-stage renal disease or death is almost certain.

Idiopathic RPGN is divided into three categories based on immunofluorescence microscopy. Type I idiopathic RPGN is characterized by linear deposition of immunoglobulins, primarily IgG, along the glomerular basement membrane (GBM) indicating anti-GBM antibodies. Type II idiopathic RPGN is identified by granular immunoglobulin and complement depositions in the glomerular microvasculature and mesangium suggesting immune complex deposition. Type III idiopathic RPGN is also called *pauci-immune* because there are no hallmark immunoglobulin or complement findings on immunofluorescence microscopy. Type III idiopathic RPGN is identified by the presence of circulating antineutrophil cytoplasmic antibodies.

Multisystem vasculitic disorders that result in glomerular capillary inflammation are the most common cause of RPGN.[19] Many of these patients present with nonspecific flu-like symptoms such as fever, weight loss, myalgia, and malaise with proteinuria and hematuria.[20] Uremic symptoms can occur with severe disease. The presence of ARF with pulmonary congestion, cough, hemoptysis, or dyspnea suggests *Wegener's granulomatosis.* The treatment for autoimmune RPGN generally involves immunosuppressive agents, such as prednisone, azathioprine, or cyclophosphamide. A more detailed discussion of glomerulonephritis is presented in Chapter 31, Chronic Kidney Disease.

Nonsteroidal Anti-Inflammatory Drug-Induced Glomerulopathy

12. What drugs cause glomerulonephropathy?

Minimal-change disease and *membranous nephropathy* have been associated with NSAID use.[21] The mechanism is probably related to NSAID-induced inhibition of the cyclooxygenase pathway, which leads to increased arachidonate

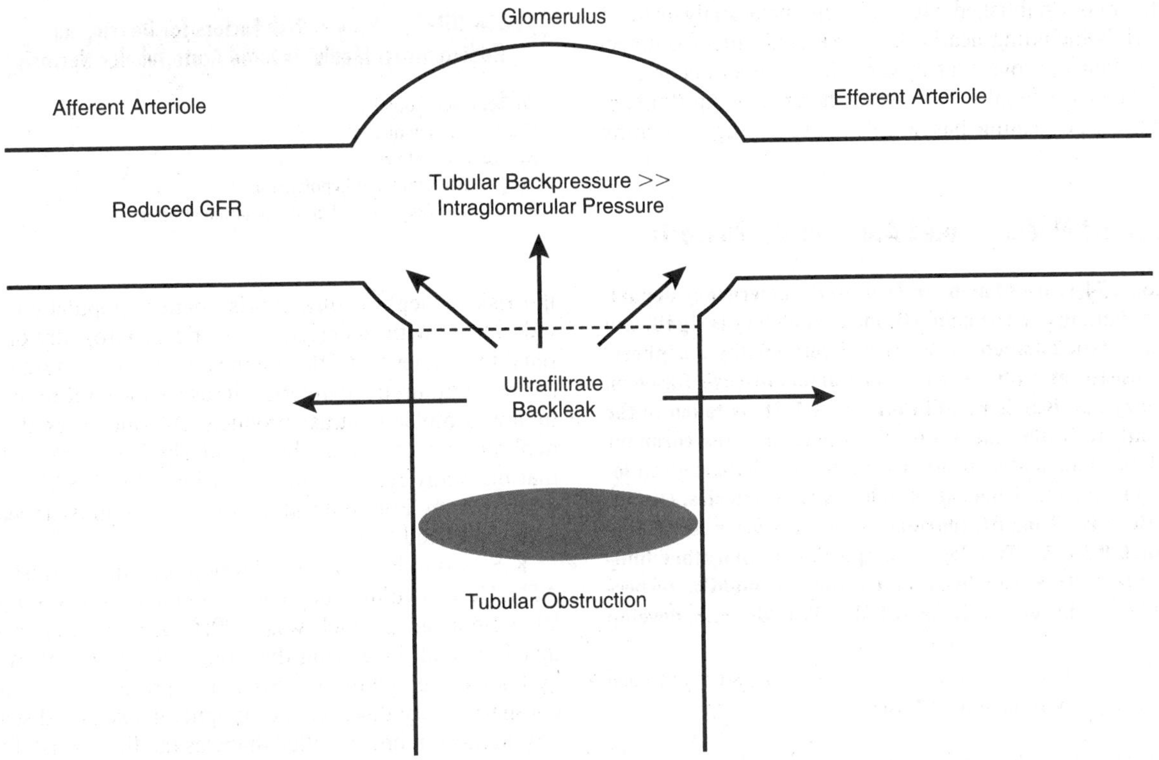

FIGURE 30-4 Schematic of acute tubular necrosis (ATN). The process is initiated by ischemia or nephrotoxin exposure that leads to tubular cell death. The cellular debris sloughs off and obstructs the proximal tubule lumen. Once the nephron is obstructed, a backleak of the glomerular ultrafiltrate occurs across the tubular basement membrane and impairment of glomerular filtration. During the recovery phase of ATN, the obstructive cellular casts are released into the urine and filtration begins to normalize. GFR, glomerular filtration rate.

catabolism and increased proinflammatory leukotriene production. The hallmark feature of NSAID-induced nephropathy is nephrotic-range proteinuria. The nephropathy resolves slowly over several months once the NSAID is discontinued.

TUBULOINTERSTITIAL DISEASES

Acute Tubular Necrosis

Acute tubular necrosis arises most often from ischemia or drug-induced causes.[1,22] Prolonged prerenal conditions, such as hypotension, surgery, overwhelming sepsis, or major burns, can lead to ischemic ATN. Unlike prerenal azotemia, tubular cell death occurs in ATN, and immediate volume resuscitation will not reverse the damage. The pathophysiology of ATN is complex and remains unclear. It is currently thought that when tubular cells die, they slough off into the tubule lumen and contribute to cast formation. The casts completely obstruct the tubule lumen and increase intratubular pressure, which causes a back leak of ultrafiltrate across the tubular basement membrane (Fig. 30-4). The aforementioned processes are mediated by a variety of substances, including calcium, phospholipases, and perhaps growth factors as well as free radical and protease activation.

Treatment With Diuretics and Dopamine

13. Do diuretics and dopamine have a role in treating established ATN?

It is well documented that patients with nonoliguric renal failure have significantly better outcomes compared with those with oliguria. This is probably because patients who are nonoliguric have less extensive renal damage and are better able to maintain fluid and electrolyte balance. Loop diuretics are commonly used in established ATN in an attempt to convert patients with oliguria to a nonoliguric state. Numerous clinical trials, however, have failed to demonstrate improved mortality or duration of azotemia in oliguric patients who receive loop diuretics, despite improved urine output. Two large systematic reviews of the primary literature convincingly showed that diuretic therapy plays little role in altering the course of ARF, decreasing length of hospitalization, or helping recover renal function.[23,24] These data suggest that, although patients who are nonoliguric generally have better outcomes, converting a patient from oliguria to nonoliguria through pharmacologic intervention does not improve patient outcomes. Currently, the only role that diuretic administration has in patients with established ATN is to increase urine output, which facilitates fluid, electrolyte, and nutritional support.

Another controversy that has been debated extensively in the literature is the use of dopamine in patients with established ATN. Dopamine is a catecholamine that stimulates dopaminergic receptors at low dosages (1–3 mcg/kg/minute), and α- and β-receptors at higher dosages (5–20 mcg/kg/minute). Animal and human studies have demonstrated that low-dose dopamine improves renal blood flow by inducing afferent arteriolar vasodilation. No data, however, support the use of dopamine in the treatment of established ARF. A recent meta-analysis of 61 clinical trials including nearly 3,500 patients failed to detect any significant improvement in variables such as occurrence of ARF, need for renal replacement therapy, or mortality.[25] Unequivocally, dopamine has no role in preventing or treating ARF.

Radiocontrast Media–Induced Acute Tubular Necrosis

14. K.S., a 74-year-old man, presents to the emergency department complaining of chest pain. His medical history is significant for advanced type 2 diabetes mellitus, with retinopathy, peripheral vascular disease, and advanced coronary artery disease. Based on cardiac enzymes, K.S. is ruled in for STEMI. He is taken to the cardiac catheterization laboratory for a percutaneous coronary intervention. Immediately before the procedure, K.S. is given iohexol PO to enhance visualization of his cardiac arteries. His admission BUN is 37 mg/dL (normal, 5–20) and SrCr is 1.5 mg/dL (normal, 0.5–1.2). Two days later, pertinent laboratory findings include a BUN and SrCr of 60 and 2.0 mg/dL, respectively, and his urine output is 700 mL/day. Why did K.S. develop ARF?

[SI units: BUN, 13.1 and 21.3 mmol/L (normal, 1.8–7.1); SrCr, 132.6 and 176.8 mol/L, respectively (normal, 44.2–106)]

Radiocontrast media administration is one of the most common causes of drug-induced ATN. Although no set criteria exist for its diagnosis, it is generally considered when the SrCr increases by >0.5 g/dL over 2 to 5 days. Contrast-induced nephropathy (CIN) usually presents as a nonoliguric ATN. It is also differentiated from other forms of ATN in that the FE_{Na^+} is usually <1% (vs. the typical >2%). Nephropathy is indicated by a progressive rise in creatinine 24 to 48 hours after contrast administration, which usually peaks within 5 days. The degree of creatinine rise and the presence of oliguria are widely variable. Because of the lack of an accepted CIN definition and differences in both clinical trial design and populations studied, estimating the true prevalence of CIN is daunting. Nevertheless, patients without risk factors prevalence have a relatively minute risk of developing CIN; for those with recognized risk factors prevalence may approach 50%.[26]

The mechanisms by which radiocontrast media induce ARF are complex. Initially, the radiocontrast medium produces renal vasodilation and an osmotic diuresis. This, however, is followed by intense vasoconstriction in the medullary portion of the kidney, which has been demonstrated by significant decreases in medullary Po_2 after contrast administration.[27] The ischemia is compounded by the increased medullary O_2 consumption because of the osmotic diuresis. Consequently, disequilibrium exists between O_2 supply and demand creating ischemic ATN. Various vasoactive substances are suspected of decreasing medullary blood flow, including oxygen-free radicals, prostaglandins, endothelin, nitric oxide, angiotensin II, and adenosine. Endothelin and adenosine are potent vasoconstrictors that are directly released from endothelial cells on exposure to radiocontrast media.

15. What are the risk factors for CIN?

The documented risk factors for CIN are listed in Table 30-4. Any condition that decreases renal blood flow increases the risk of nephropathy. At-risk patient populations include individuals with underlying diabetic nephropathy or chronic renal insufficiency, CHF, volume depletion, or those receiving aggressive diuretic regimens. The use of the ionic high-osmolar or low-osmolar contrast products also increases the risk of nephropathy, as well as the previously discussed medications that markedly reduce renal perfusion (e.g., NSAIDs, COX-2 inhibitors, ACE inhibitors). Iso-osmolar contrast appears to be better tolerated.

Table 30-4 Proven Risk Factors for Developing Radiocontrast Media–Induced Acute Tubular Necrosis

Diabetic nephropathy
Chronic kidney disease
Severe heart failure
Volume depletion and hypotension
Dosage and frequency of contrast administration

K.S. was at high risk for developing radiocontrast-induced ATN. He was volume depleted, as evidenced by his admission BUN:SrCr ratio, which was >20:1. Second, it is very likely that K.S. had underlying diabetic nephropathy, as evidenced by his elevated admission SrCr. The presence of retinopathy, coronary artery disease, and peripheral vascular disease suggest long-term uncontrolled diabetes mellitus, a risk factor for nephropathy.

Prevention

16. What strategies can be performed to prevent the occurrence of CIN?

Attempts have been made to minimize or prevent CIN using a variety of approaches. Medullary vasodilation with dopamine infusions have generally had disappointing results. Volume expansion, mannitol, and furosemide have been tried as a means of "flushing" radiocontrast from the kidney. *Volume expansion* is a rational approach to prevent renal dysfunction in this population because human and animal data have revealed dehydration as a major risk factor for developing CIN. Hydration with normal saline, hypotonic saline (0.45% sodium chloride), and sodium bicarbonate in dextrose have all shown benefits in preventing CIN. Notably, sodium bicarbonate may be more beneficial in decreasing the incidence of radiocontrast nephropathy relative to other fluids because it reduces oxygen-free radicals in the renal medulla and, therefore, increases the medullary pH. Whatever fluid is given, data suggest it should be infused before and after the procedure to adequately reduce the risk of developing nephropathy. Another important point is that the administration of diuretics such as mannitol and furosemide should be avoided. These diuretics result in volume depletion and increase oxygen demand in the medullary portion of the kidney when diuresis occurs, thereby counteracting the benefits of hydration. Other therapeutic modalities for the prevention of CIN have been studied. A systematic review and meta-analysis of *aminophylline* and *theophylline* have affirmed a renoprotective effect in patients who have underlying chronic kidney disease; however, large-scale clinical trials are lacking.[28] Although the use of calcium channel blockers theoretically seems rational to prevent contrast-induced ATN, limited clinical data exist. Other emerging data suggest that *ascorbic acid* may be

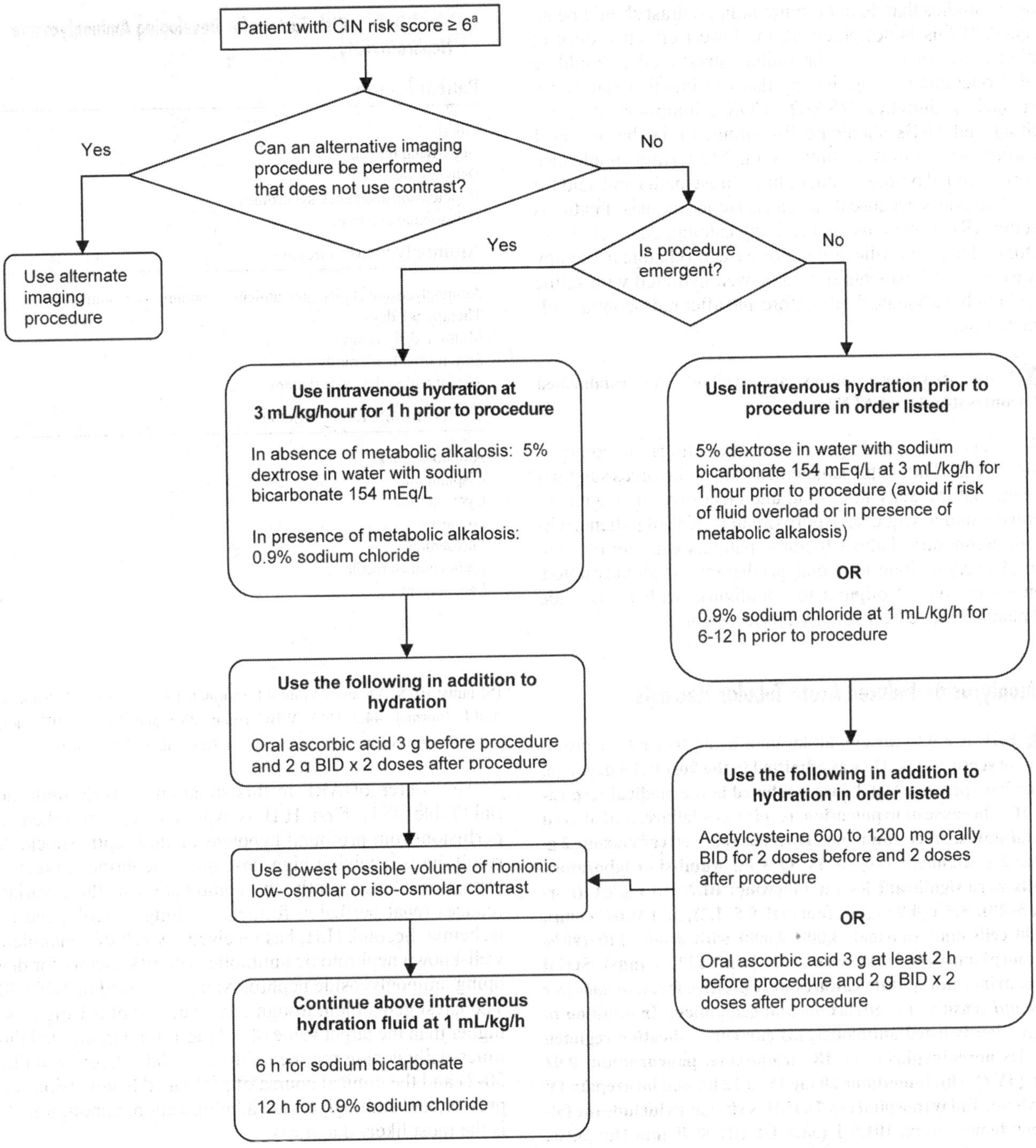

FIGURE 30-5 Preventing contrast-induced nephropathy (CIN) in high-risk populations. (From reference 26, with permission.)

beneficial in preventing contrast nephropathy given its antioxidant effects; however, large-scale prospective trials are lacking.[29]

N-acetylcysteine (NAC) has received the most attention for its renal-sparing effects relative to radiocontrast media. Indeed, since 2001, nearly 30 primary studies and more than 10 meta-analyses have been conducted to assess its prophylactic effects.[26] Although much data have been generated with NAC, many of these studies have significant pitfalls, including relatively small sample size; single-center design; heterogeneity of patient populations; differing doses, dosage forms, and schedules of NAC therapy; and differing hydration regimens. Therefore, trying to delineate meaningful conclusions from this body of literature is daunting. At this time, recommending a specific dose of NAC is difficult. The commonly accepted regimen at many institutions is 600 mg orally twice daily pre- and postprocedure for a total of four doses along with concomitant hydration therapy.

Figure 30-5 summarizes one possible strategy to prevent CIN in high-risk populations. When possible, alternative imaging studies that do not require radiocontrast should be attempted. If this is not practical, the lowest effective dose of nonionic, iso- or low-osmolar radiocontrast media should be used. Concomitant drug therapy that can impair renal perfusion, such as diuretics, NSAIDs, COX-2 inhibitors, ACE inhibitors, and ARBs, should be discontinued 1 day before and 1 day after radiocontrast administration. Metformin should also be discontinued before giving radiocontrast media and held for at least 48 hours because it can cause lactic acidosis if patients develop ARF. If patients are receiving calcium channel blockers for underlying cardiovascular disease, no change in therapy is warranted. All patients should be well hydrated with saline or sodium bicarbonate fluids before and after radiocontrast administration.

17. What treatment options are available for established radiocontrast-induced ATN?

Few data exist regarding treatment of existing radiocontrast-induced ATN. The acute management largely involves supportive care that includes strict fluid and electrolyte management to prevent undue sequelae. Approximately 25% of patients will require temporary dialysis therapy; patients who are oliguric generally require long-term dialysis therapy. As already noted, attempts to convert oliguria to nonoliguria with furosemide and mannitol have been largely unsuccessful.

Table 30-5 Risk Factors for Developing Aminoglycoside Nephrotoxicity

Patient Factors
Elderly
Underlying renal disease
Dehydration
Hypotension and shock syndromes
Hepatorenal syndrome
Aminoglycoside Factors
Aminoglycoside choice: gentamicin > tobramycin > amikacin
Therapy >3 days
Multiple daily dosing
Serum trough >2 mg/L
Recent aminoglycoside therapy
Concomitant Drug Therapy
Amphotericin B
Cisplatinum
Cyclosporine
Foscarnet
Furosemide
Radiocontrast media
Vancomycin

Aminoglycoside-Induced Acute Tubular Necrosis

18. H.H. is a 43-year-old, 80-kg man being treated for gram-negative septic shock. He was admitted to the hospital 6 days ago, but he has spent the last 3 days intubated in the medical respiratory ICU because of hypotension, respiratory failure, and altered mental status. Since admission, H.H. has received ceftriaxone 2 g/day and gentamicin 140 mg IV Q 8 hr. Admission laboratory results were significant for the following: BUN, 13 mg/dL (normal, 5–20); SrCr, 0.9 mg/dL (normal, 0.5–1.2); and WBC count, 23,500 cells/mm^3 (normal, 4,000–9,000) with a left shift (90% polymorphonuclear leukocytes [PMN] and 12% bands). Serial blood, urine, and sputum cultures were positive for *Acinetobacter baumanii* sensitive to ceftriaxone and gentamicin. In addition to the previously listed antibiotics, his current medication regimen includes norepinephrine IV 18 mcg/minute, pancuronium 0.02 mg/kg IV Q 3 hr, famotidine 20 mg IV Q 12 hr, and lorazepam IV 2 mg/hour. Today (hospital day 7), H.H.'s vital signs include the following: temperature, 101.5°F (38.6°C); BP, 90/40 mm Hg; pulse, 135 beats/minute; and respirations, 20 breaths/minute. Significant laboratory values are as follows: BUN, 67 mg/dL; SrCr, 5.4 mg/dL; and WBC count, 16,700 cells/mm^3 with continued left shift. Over the last 2 days, H.H.'s urine output has steadily declined, and today it is 700 mL/24 hours (normal, 1,500–2,500). Urine electrolytes were obtained and reveal Na$^+$, 55 mEq/L (normal, 20–40) and creatinine, 26 mg/dL (normal, 50–100). A urinalysis revealed many WBC (normal, 0–5), 3% RBC casts (normal, 0%–1%), brush-border cells (normal, negative), and granular casts (normal, negative) with an osmolality of 250 mOsm/kg (normal, 400–600). Serum gentamicin concentrations obtained with the last dose reveal a peak of 15 mg/dL (target, 6–10) and a trough of 9.1 mg/dL (target, <2.0). Given the history and laboratory data, what is the likely source of H.H.'s ARF?

[SI units: BUN, 4.6 and 24 mmol/L (normal, 1.8–7.1); SrCr, 79.6 and 477.4 mol/L (normal, 44.2–106); WBC count, 23.5 and 16.7 × 10^6 (normal, 4.0–9.0); urine creatinine, 2,298 μmol/L (normal, 4,419–8,838)]

The source of ARF in this situation is likely multifactorial (Table 30-1). First, H.H. is experiencing diminished renal perfusion from profound hypotension and septic shock. As a result, he is receiving high-dose norepinephrine, a potent vasopressor. Consequently, the combination of these variables reduces renal perfusion further, resulting in prolonged renal ischemia. Second, H.H. has received 1 week of gentamicin, a well-known nephrotoxic antibiotic. The risk factors for developing aminoglycoside nephrotoxicity are listed in Table 30-5. The latest gentamicin trough concentration of 9.1 mg/L is far higher than the target value of <2 mg/L for a traditional three-times-daily dosing regimen. Given the laboratory data (Table 30-2) and the clinical course of prolonged hypotension, vasopressor, and aminoglycoside administration, nonoliguric ATN is the most likely diagnosis.

Presentation

19. How does aminoglycoside-induced ATN present, and what are the mechanisms of toxicity?

H.H. illustrates the typical presentation of aminoglycoside-induced nephrotoxicity. Generally, the onset occurs after 5 to 7 days of treatment and presents as a hypo-osmolar, nonoliguric renal failure with a slow rise in SrCr.[30] Because of the tubular necrosis that occurs, the urinalysis is often positive for low-molecular-weight proteins, tubular cellular casts, epithelial cells, WBC, and brush-border cells.[31] H.H.'s plasma and urinary laboratory indices are consistent with those listed for ATN in Table 30-2.

The mechanism of aminoglycoside-induced ATN is complex. Approximately 5% of filtered aminoglycoside is actively reabsorbed by the proximal tubule cells. These agents are polycationic and bind to the negatively charged brush-border cells within the tubule lumen. Once attached, these agents undergo pinocytosis and enter the intracellular space, setting off complex biochemical events that result in the formation of myeloid bodies. With continued formation of myeloid bodies, the brush-border cells swell and burst, releasing large concentrations of aminoglycoside and lysosomal enzymes into the tubule lumen, thereby beginning a cascade of further tubular destruction.[30,32] The following rank order of nephrotoxicity has been collated from human and animal data: neomycin > gentamicin = tobramycin = amikacin = netilmicin > streptomycin.[31]

Extended-Interval Dosing

20. Is "extended-interval" aminoglycoside dosing less nephrotoxic than multiple daily dosing regimens?

Extended-interval aminoglycoside dosing entails the administration of one large daily aminoglycoside dose. This dosing scheme takes advantage of the concentration-dependent killing activity and postantibiotic effect observed with aminoglycosides while minimizing time-dependent toxicity. The net effect of this dosing scheme, purportedly, is greater efficacy with reduced toxicity. Aminoglycoside nephrotoxicity is a function of drug exposure, and it might be minimized with extended-interval dosing because of saturable uptake kinetics in the proximal tubule. That is, only a maximal amount of aminoglycoside is transported into the tubule cell, no matter how much aminoglycoside is present in the tubule. Consequently, once saturation occurs, the remaining aminoglycoside concentration passes through the proximal tubule without being absorbed, and is excreted in the urine. Accumulation is therefore averted.[33] This concept is supported by studies demonstrating that continuous-rate gentamicin infusions, which produce sustained low plasma concentrations, result in greater proximal tubule uptake and nephrotoxicity than extended-interval regimens. This is probably because the achieved drug concentrations are well below those required to saturate the uptake mechanism. Extended-interval dosing results in very high peak concentrations to improve efficacy and generally undetectable trough concentrations before the next dose, thus minimizing accumulation.

Numerous clinical trials and meta-analyses have compared the efficacy and toxicity of extended-interval aminoglycoside dosing with conventional multiple daily dosing regimens. Many of these meta-analyses concluded that less nephrotoxicity was associated with extended-interval aminoglycoside dosing. Given the inherent biases of meta-analyses, these results, however, must be interpreted cautiously. For example, meta-analyses combine results from different clinical trials, which can differ in patient population, severity of illness scores, degree of underlying renal dysfunction, and dosing regimen and duration of therapy. Most of the clinical trials did not show a clinically or statistically significant difference in efficacy or toxicity between regimens. Contemporary practice suggests that patients should receive extended-interval aminoglycoside dosing unless they have specific contraindications.

In summary, extended-interval aminoglycoside dosing appears to result in similar or greater efficacy, with similar or reduced toxicity. This dosing schedule is also less costly when considering therapeutic drug monitoring, preparation, and administration costs. Although the typical extended interval in patients with normal renal function is dosing every 24 hours, the interval may have to be prolonged to several days in patients with renal failure.

Drug-Induced Acute Interstitial Nephritis (AIN)

Drug-induced AIN accounts for approximately 1% to 3% of all ARF cases. A variety of antibiotics, such as penicillins, cephalosporins, quinolones, sulfonamides, and rifampin, as well as NSAID have been implicated as major causes of drug-induced AIN. The pathophysiology of this reaction is not well understood; however, it is suspected that either humoral or cell-mediated immune mechanisms or both are involved.[34] Humoral immune reactions occur within minutes to hours of drug exposure and involve the drug or its metabolite acting as a hapten that binds to host proteins, making them antigenic. The drug-protein antigens become lodged in the renal tubules, which initiate the inflammatory cascade. Cell-mediated injury can occur days to weeks after drug exposure and is identified by the presence of mononuclear inflammation and the lack of detectable immune complexes. This suggests a delayed hypersensitivity rather than a direct cytotoxic effect from a given drug. Both immune mechanisms probably contribute to the development of drug-induced AIN.

Penicillin-Induced AIN

21. J.S. is a 50-year-old woman who developed a cellulitis 3 days after a car door was closed on her right hand. She was admitted to the hospital, where blood and wound cultures were found to be positive for methicillin-sensitive *Staphylococcus aureus.* She received two full days of nafcillin 2 g IV Q 4 hr before being discharged to complete a 14-day course with dicloxacillin 500 mg PO four times daily (QID). Ten days after discharge, J.S. returned to the emergency department complaining of malaise, fever, diffuse rash, hematuria, and reduced urine output. The following laboratory values were significant: BUN, 39 mg/dL (normal, 5–20); SrCr, 2.3 mg/dL (normal, 0.5–1.2); and WBC count, 18,500 cells/mm^3 (normal, 4,000–9,000) with 18% eosinophils. The urinalysis was positive for elevated specific gravity, WBC, RBC, eosinophiluria, and a FE_{Na^+} of 3%. What objective data suggest drug-induced AIN?

[SI units: BUN, 13.9 mmol/L (normal, 1.8–7.1); SrCr, 203.3 mol/L (normal, 44.2–106); WBC count, 18.5 × 10^6 (normal, 4.0–9.0)]

J.S.'s onset of symptoms suggests drug-induced AIN. As illustrated by this case, the median onset of penicillin-induced AIN generally occurs 6 to 10 days after drug exposure. Hallmark symptoms of AIN include fever, macular rash, and malaise. Fever is present in nearly all patients with AIN, whereas rash occurs in 25% to 50% of patients. J.S.'s objective laboratory data that suggest AIN include azotemia, elevated SrCr, proteinuria, cellular urinary sediment, eosinophilia, and eosinophiluria. Her FE_{Na^+} of 3% suggests intrinsic renal disease and her eosinophiluria and eosinophilia indicate an immune-mediated allergic reaction. Drug-induced AIN is generally nonoliguric, but oliguria can develop in severe cases of AIN.

22. How should J.S.'s drug-induced AIN be treated?

The dicloxacillin should be stopped immediately because most patients recover normal kidney function once the offending agent is discontinued. General supportive measures that maintain fluid and electrolyte balance are necessary. Corticosteroids have been used with variable results to shorten the duration of ARF, but no clinical guidelines have been developed to delineate when to administer them and for how long. Some administer prednisone 1 mg/kg for 7 days and then gradually taper the dose over the next several weeks. The response to corticosteroids may be delayed or absent in some patients. Dialysis may be needed in patients who are oliguric, but it is usually not required for those who are nonoliguric. The clinician should document J.S.'s allergic reaction to penicillins because repeated exposure is likely to result in similar reactions.

POSTRENAL ACUTE RENAL FAILURE

Any condition that results in the obstruction of urine flow at any level of the urinary tract is termed *postrenal ARF*. Common causes of postrenal ARF are stone formation, underlying malignancies of the prostate or cervix, prostatic hypertrophy, or bilateral ureter strictures. Conditions that result in bladder outlet obstruction (e.g., prostatic hypertrophy) are the most common causes of postrenal ARF. The onset of signs and symptoms is generally gradual; it often presents as decreased force of urine stream, dribbling, or polyuria. Drugs can also result in insoluble crystal formation in the urine and should be included in the differential diagnosis.

Nephrolithiasis

Kidney stones are relatively common and affect approximately 10% of all people at least once in their lifetime.[35] A strong genetic predisposition appears to exist in this population. Epidemiologic data have found that men with stones were three times more likely to have parents or siblings with a history significant for stones.[36] In addition to genetics, other underlying risk factors exist for stone development (Table 30-6). Nephrolithiasis has a male:female incidence of 3:1, and whites are twice as likely as blacks to develop stones. Kidney stones generally consist of uric acid, cystine, struvite (also called magnesium ammonium phosphate or triple phosphate nephrolithiasis), and calcium salts. Of these, calcium stones are by far the most prevalent.

Calcium Stones

Calcium nephrolithiasis constitutes approximately 70% to 80% of all kidney stones,[36] with calcium oxalate and calcium phosphate stones making up most of these. Genetic factors appear to play an important role in the development of calcium nephrolithiasis; the stereotypical patient is a man in his third to fifth decade of life. Other risk factors for developing calcium nephrolithiasis are low urine output, inadequate hydration (e.g., living in a hot climate and not drinking adequate fluids), hypercalciuria, hyperoxaluria, hypocitraturia, hyperuricosuria, and distal renal tubular acidosis. Generally, more than one of these conditions is present simultaneously.

Table 30-6 Risk Factors for Nephrolithiasis

Low urine volume
Hypercalciuria
Hyperoxaluria
Hyperuricosuria
Hypercitruria
Chronically low or high urinary pH

Struvite Stones

Magnesium ammonium phosphate crystallization, termed *struvite stones*, represents the second most common type of nephrolithiasis (~2%–20% of cases). Struvite stones can result in significantly high morbidity and mortality because they tend to recur and can result in irreversible kidney damage.[37] These stones often fill the renal collecting ducts and assume a "staghorn" appearance. Struvite stones generally result when existing stones are colonized with *Proteus,* a bacterium that produces urease, an enzyme that hydrolyzes urea and alkalinizes the urine. The alkaline environment promotes the formation of insoluble crystals of ammonium, calcium, and phosphate. *In vitro*, simply alkalinizing the urine results in the immediate precipitation of amorphous struvite stones. Populations at risk for developing struvite stones include obese women, patients with frequent urinary tract infections or pyelonephritis, and patients with genitourinary tract abnormalities that promote bacterial colonization or make eradication of infection difficult. The most problematic form of stone disease develops in paralyzed patients with indwelling Foley catheters. Recurrent nephrolithiasis is one of the most common causes of death in patients with spinal cord injury. Treatment of struvite stones can consist of surgical intervention; prolonged courses of broad-spectrum antibiotics; administration of acetohydroxamic acid, which inhibits bacterial urease; or shock-wave lithotripsy.[37]

Uric Acid Stones

Uric acid stones commonly occur in patients whose uric acid metabolism is altered because of various medical conditions. In particular, patients with gout and those receiving chemotherapy are susceptible to these stones. This topic is discussed further in Chapter 43, Gout and Hyperuricemia.

Cystine Stones

Cystinuria is a rare autosomal-recessive hereditary disorder of amino acid transport in the renal tubules that results in the urinary excretion of large amounts of cystine. These stones form when the cystine excretion rate exceeds the urinary solubility limit. The calculi form staghorns in the renal tubules and can cause urinary obstruction, infection, and ARF. Therapy of cystine stones is targeted at reducing the urinary cystine excretion while increasing its urinary solubility. This can be accomplished by diet modification, increased fluid intake, urine alkalization, and drug therapy. Low-sodium diets decrease cystine excretion, and restriction of methionine, a cystine precursor, may reduce cystine excretion. It may also result in depletion of other important amino acids, however. To decrease the urinary cystine concentrations, urine volume should be increased by maintaining a fluid intake of >4 L/day. The solubility of cystine in urine also can be increased by alkalinizing the urine. Pharmacologic therapy is indicated when the above nondrug measures have failed. Drug therapy is targeted at increasing the urinary solubility of cystine, which can be achieved by forming a thiol-cysteine disulfide bond. D-Penicillamine and tiopronin are the most commonly used drugs, although tiopronin appears to be better tolerated than D-penicillamine.

Presentation and Treatment

23. T.C., a 48-year-old man, presents to the emergency department complaining of sharp flank pain radiating to the groin, gross hematuria, and dysuria. He states that these symptoms have been present for 4 hours and that they are similar to previous episodes of calcium nephrolithiasis he has experienced. Serum chemistries are ordered and are significant only for a BUN of 34 mg/dL (normal, 5–20) and an SrCr of 1.5 mg/dL (normal, 0.5–1.2), which are up from his baseline values of 15 and 0.9 mg/dL, respectively. A urine sample was obtained and visualized with microscopy. It was determined that T.C. passed a kidney stone, based on the large amount of calcium oxalate crystals found in the urinary sediment. On questioning, he admits that he has not been drinking much fluid over the past week owing to a busy work schedule, and his urine volume has been markedly lower than usual. What are the common subjective and objective data that suggest nephrolithiasis, and how can this be prevented from occurring in the future?

[SI units: BUN, 12.1 and 5.3 mmol/L (normal, 1.8–7.1); SrCr, 132.6 and 79.5 mol/L, respectively (normal, 44.2–106)]

T.C. illustrates the classic presentation of nephrolithiasis: acute, severe flank pain that radiates to the groin. It is usually accompanied by gross or microscopic hematuria, dysuria, or frequency. Of symptomatic calculi, 90% pass spontaneously, as in T.C.'s case, and invasive surgical treatment is rarely necessary.[38] The risk factors that predispose T.C. to stone recurrence include a previous episode of nephrolithiasis, age within the fourth decade, and decreased fluid intake and urine output.

T.C. should take preventive measures to reduce the likelihood of stone recurrence. Many randomized trials have demonstrated that nondrug and pharmacologic mechanisms can prevent stone formation. The most cost-effective way to prevent stone formation is to increase fluid intake. A classic 5-year randomized study compared a high fluid intake group (>2 L/day) with one that had normal daily fluid intake (~1 L/day). The results demonstrated a significantly longer time to stone recurrence (39 vs. 25 months) in the high fluid intake group.[39] Dietary modifications remain controversial. Although it appears that limiting protein, calcium, and sodium intake should decrease the likelihood of recurrent nephrolithiasis, the data are conflicting.[40] In summary, a high calcium intake probably increases the risk of nephrolithiasis but only in patients with absorptive hypercalciuria and not in normal subjects.

Pharmacologic control of calcium oxalate stones has been tried with thiazide diuretics.[41] Thiazide diuretics promote calcium reabsorption in the distal tubule, which decreases the concentration in the lumen. Thiazides also may decrease intestinal calcium absorption in patients with absorptive hypercalciuria, although this remains unclear. Patients receiving thiazide diuretics should be sodium restricted because excessive sodium intake negates their hypocalciuric effect. Allopurinol has been used successfully to prevent recurrent calcium oxalate nephrolithiasis, presumably by inhibiting purine and uric acid metabolism.[41] Alkalization of the urine with potassium citrate and potassium-magnesium citrate also prevents recurrent calcium oxalate nephrolithiasis.

Table 30-7 Commonly Used Drugs That Cause Crystal-Induced Acute Renal Failure

Acyclovir
Indinavir
Methotrexate
Sulfonamides
Triamterene

T.C. should be instructed to drink at least 2 L of fluid (~eight 8-ounce glasses) daily. Given his busy work schedule, a thiazide diuretic probably is not the most convenient option for T.C., and noncompliance is likely. Allopurinol 200 mg orally once daily is probably the most convenient preventive strategy for T.C., and data suggest it is effective in preventing recurrent nephrolithiasis. Alternatively, urinary alkalinization with potassium citrate or potassium-magnesium citrate is likely to benefit T.C., but it may be less convenient because it needs to be administered two to four times daily.

Drug-Induced Nephrolithiasis

24. Can drugs crystallize in the urine and cause ARF?

Many commonly prescribed drugs are insoluble in urine and crystallize in the distal tubule (Table 30-7). Risk factors that predispose patients to crystalluria include severe volume contraction, underlying renal dysfunction, or acidotic or alkalotic urinary pH. In conditions of renal hypoperfusion, high concentrations of drug become stagnant in the tubule lumen. Drugs that are weak acids (e.g., methotrexate, sulfonamides) precipitate in acidic urine; drugs that are weak bases (e.g., indinavir, other protease inhibitors) precipitate in alkaline urine. Prevention of crystal-induced ARF is targeted at dosage adjustment for patients with underlying renal dysfunction, volume expansion to increase urinary output, and urine alkalization. Similarly, for established crystal-induced ARF, the above general supportive measures of urinary alkalization and volume expansion should be performed. Dialysis may be necessary in a small percentage of patients. With appropriate pharmacotherapy, crystal-induced ARF is usually reversible without long-term complications.

SUPPORTIVE MANAGEMENT OF ACUTE RENAL FAILURE

25. What is the supportive management of ARF?

Despite years of study, no pharmacologic "cure" for ARF exists. Therefore, supportive therapy is directed at preventing its morbidity and mortality. This is achieved by close patient monitoring; strict fluid, electrolyte, and nutritional management; treatment of life-threatening conditions, such as pulmonary edema, hyperkalemia, and metabolic acidosis; avoidance of nephrotoxic drugs; and the initiation of dialysis or continuous renal replacement therapies (CRRT).

Clinicians should closely monitor patient vital signs (e.g., weight, temperature, BP, pulse, respirations, and fluid intake and output) at least once every shift. Daily weights can forewarn the clinician of edematous weight gain. The patient's medication profile should be reviewed daily to assess for appropriate dosage adjustment in renal dysfunction. Because estimation of ClCr is difficult in patients with rapidly changing renal function, therapeutic drug monitoring should be performed when using drugs with narrow therapeutic indices. When possible, nephrotoxic drugs should be avoided, but this may be difficult in patients who are septic or hypotensive and require nephrotoxic antibiotics and vasopressors. Preventive measures to reduce the likelihood of ARF should be used, such as ensuring adequate hydration, using dosing strategies or products that are associated with less nephrotoxicity, and avoiding drug therapy combinations that enhance nephrotoxicity (e.g., NSAID, aminoglycosides). If patients with ARF are receiving total parenteral nutrition, close monitoring of serum chemistries is needed to identify fluid and electrolyte abnormalities.

Supportive drug therapy may be used to reduce ARF symptoms. As discussed, diuretics currently have no role in preventing ARF progression or reducing mortality, but they can prevent complications, such as pulmonary and peripheral edema, and they may prevent tubular obstruction from ATN. The patient's volume status should be assessed daily, and fluids should be adjusted based on laboratory chemistries, urine output, and gastrointestinal and insensible losses. Dietary sodium restriction of 2 to 2.5 g/day should be instituted to prevent edema formation.

Diuretics for Edema in Acute Renal Failure

If edema occurs, intravenous (IV) furosemide is preferred because of its potency and pulmonary vasodilation properties. Oral furosemide therapy should be avoided because gut edema may limit its bioavailability. *Torsemide,* another loop diuretic, has excellent oral bioavailability and is unaffected by gut edema. Previously, torsemide was reserved for patients with demonstrated bioavailability problems with furosemide because of cost concerns, but a generic version of torsemide is now available. The dosage of diuretic needed is highly patient specific, especially in those with frank proteinuria, glomerulonephritis, or the nephrotic syndrome. Furosemide is highly protein bound, and thus binds to filtered protein, which negates its pharmacologic effect on the kidneys. Combinations of loop and thiazide diuretics may be needed in patients with ARF if they become diuretic resistant. This combination acts synergistically to block sodium and water reabsorption in both Henle's loop and the distal convoluted tubule. Other alternatives include continuous loop diuretic infusions, such as furosemide 1 mg/kg/hour. The infusion rate should not exceed 4 mg/minute because these rates are associated with ototoxicity, especially when given in combination with aminoglycoside antibiotics. Close monitoring of potassium, magnesium, and calcium is necessary when giving large doses of loop diuretics.

Hyperkalemia commonly occurs in patients with ARF because the kidneys regulate potassium homeostasis. Acute therapy of hyperkalemia is discussed in Chapter 12, Fluid and Electrolyte Disorders. In cases in which conventional pharmacologic treatment is not feasible, emergency hemodialysis should be performed.

Metabolic acidosis is a common manifestation of ARF because the kidneys are responsible for excreting organic acids. As GFR declines to <30 mL/minute, organic acids accumulate and clinical symptoms can occur. Severe metabolic acidosis should be corrected with dialysis, but early initiation of oral sodium bicarbonate may prolong or obviate the need for dialysis.

Extracorporeal Continuous Renal Replacement Therapy

Renal replacement therapy is not always indicated in ARF. It is reserved for patients with severe acid-base disorders, fluid overload, hyperkalemia, symptomatic uremia, or drug intoxications. RRT can be divided into intermittent hemodialysis or CRRT, such as continuous peritoneal dialysis or extracorporeal CRRT. The decision to use one over the other is most often decided by the nephrologist's experience and comfort level. Extracorporeal CRRT differs from peritoneal and hemodialysis in its mechanism of solute removal; dialysis modalities rely primarily on solute diffusion across a semipermeable membrane, whereas CRRT relies primarily on convective ultrafiltrate production. This discussion will be limited to extracorporeal CRRT therapies. (See Chapter 33, Renal Dialysis, for a complete overview of peritoneal and hemodialysis.)

Not all *extracorporeal CRRT* is alike[42]; many variations exist and include modalities such as continuous arteriovenous hemofiltration (CAVH), continuous venovenous hemofiltration (CVVH), continuous venovenous hemodialysis (CVVHD), and continuous venovenous hemodiafiltration (CVVHDF). Differences between these modalities are illustrated in Table 30-8. Drug dosing can be difficult in patients receiving these therapies, especially in those who are undergoing both dialysis and hemofiltration modalities (i.e., CVVHDF).

Table 30-8 Comparison of Extracorporeal Continuous Renal Replacement Therapies

Parameter	*Continuous Venovenous Hemofiltration (CVVH)*	*Continuous Arteriovenous Hemofiltration (CAVH)*	*Continuous Venovenous Hemodialysis (CVVHD)*	*Continuous Venovenous Hemodiafiltration (CVVHDF)*
Volume control in hypotensive patients	Good	Variable	Good	Good
Solute control in highly catabolic patients	Adequate	Inadequate	Adequate	Adequate
Blood flow rates in hypotensive patients	Adequate	Poor	Adequate	Adequate
Ease of drug dosing	Published recommendations	Difficult	Difficult	Difficult
Dialytic solute clearance	None	None	Moderate	Moderate
Convective solute clearance	Good	Good	Minimal	Moderate
Corresponding GFR (mL/min)	15–17	10–15	17–21	25–26
Blood pump required	Yes	No	Yes	Yes
Replacement fluid required	Yes	Yes	Yes	Yes
Pharmacy expense	High	High	High	High

GFR, glomerular filtration rate.

Both CAVH and CVVH are modalities that rely solely on convective solute removal. Convection is simply the movement of water and solutes across a high-flux dialyzer or hemofilter. Because it does not depend on the molecular weight (MW) of a given solute, small solutes (MW, <500 D) and middle MW solutes (MW, 500–15,000 D) are removed to the same extent if they fit through the membrane pore. Drugs and solutes <15,000 D are removed very well. Most penicillin, cephalosporin, and aminoglycoside antibiotics have MW <500 D, and vancomycin's MW is 1,450 D. Continuous convective modalities are much better than dialysis for middle molecule and low–molecular-weight protein removal. CRRT is also better able to maintain a constant total body water volume. These therapies allow for a more gradual removal of large fluid volumes (3–5 L/day), which is not possible with conventional dialysis therapies.

Continuous Arteriovenous Hemofiltration)

The first extracorporeal therapy, CAVH, was developed in the late 1970s. In this technique, a patient's blood is accessed through an artery and systemic BP and cardiac output are used as the driving forces to pump it through a high-flux hemofilter. Heparin is infused prefilter to prevent clot formation within the hemofilter. Blood flow rates are modest at 90 to 150 mL/minute. The mean arterial pressure (MAP) generates a transmembrane pressure (TMP) that filters plasma water and dissolved solutes (urea, creatinine, and drugs) across the hemofilter membrane.[43] Most of the filtered solution, or ultrafiltrate, is replaced by a solution that contains normal electrolyte concentrations. In volume-overloaded patients, a desired volume of plasma can be maintained by adjusting the volume of replacement fluid returned to the patient. The primary disadvantage of CAVH is that arterial access is often complicated by bleeding, aneurysm, ischemia, or embolism. Second, because blood flow and ultrafiltration depend on the MAP, volume and solute control becomes difficult in patients who become hypotensive or hypercatabolic.[44] These disadvantages have been averted to a degree through the introduction of venovenous access and the addition of blood roller pumps.

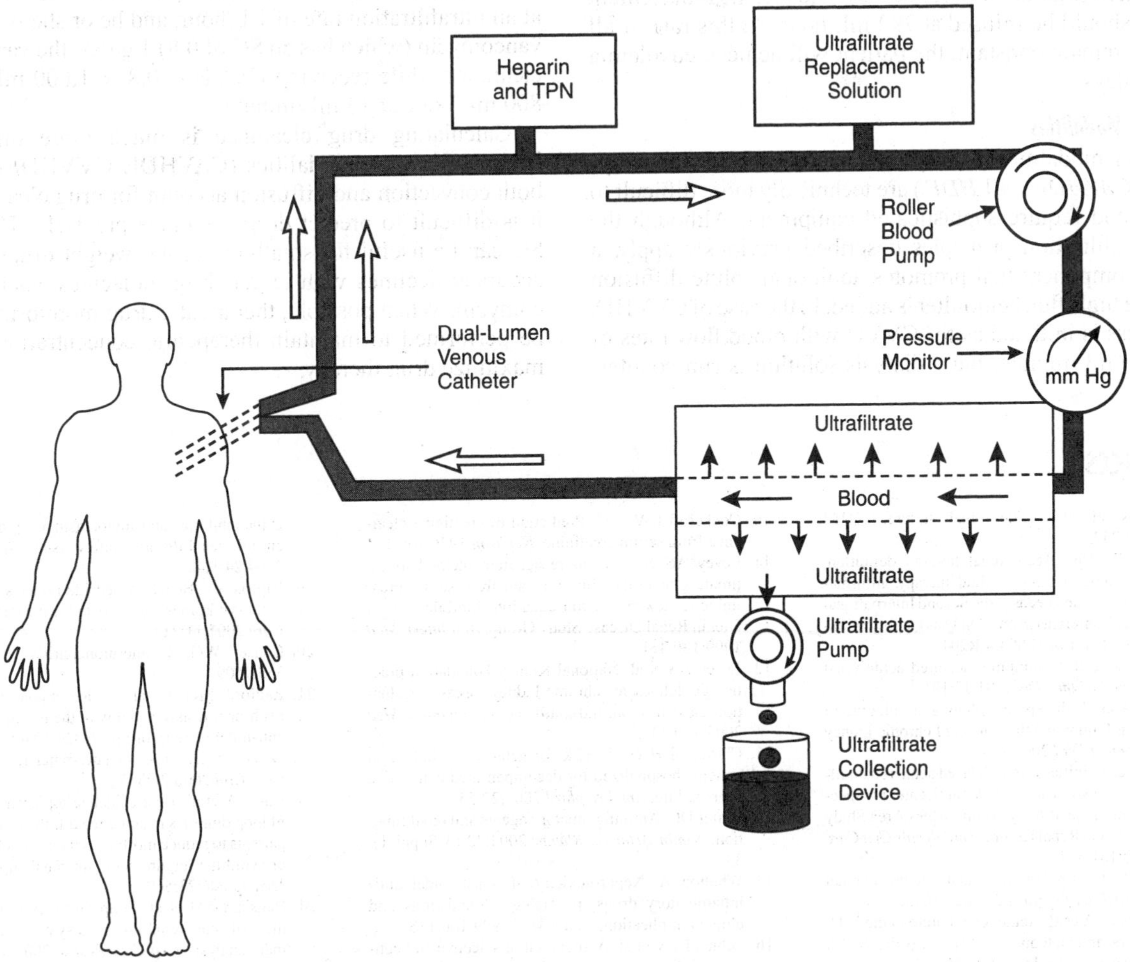

FIGURE 30-6 Schematic of continuous venovenous hemofiltration (CVVH). Blood is accessed by a dual-lumen catheter in a central vein and is pumped through the extracorporeal circuit by a roller blood pump. The blood pump maintains a constant hydrostatic pressure to create ultrafiltration, even in hypotensive conditions. Patients receiving CVVH are most often in the intensive care unit and often receive concomitant parenteral nutrition. Heparin is infused prefilter to prevent clot formation within the circuit. The ultrafiltrate replacement solution is provided back to the patient through a second venous catheter port at a rate that achieves a desired total body water volume. (From reference 45, with permission.)

Continuous Venovenous Hemofiltration

A major advancement in extracorporeal CRRT is CVVH. Venous access is obtained by inserting a dual-lumen catheter into a central vein (e.g., internal jugular or subclavian), and a roller pump provides a constant driving force for the blood to enter the hemofilter (Fig. 30-6).[45] The pressure generated by the roller pump results in continuous ultrafiltrate production. The blood flow rate is considerably increased by the roller pump, achieving rates of 100 to 200 mL/minute, which provides adequate ultrafiltrate, even in patients who are hypotensive or hypercatabolic. The ultrafiltrate production rate is generally started at 1 L/hour, which corresponds to a GFR of approximately 16 mL/minute. On exiting the hemofilter, the blood is returned through the second lumen of the venous access; a replacement solution containing normal electrolyte concentrations is also infused. As with CAVH, the patient's volume status can be controlled by adjusting the volume of replacement solution. A common example is a patient with volume overload of 20 L after surgery who develops ARF. A reasonable goal in such a patient is a net fluid loss of 5 L/day. If the CVVH ultrafiltration rate is 1 L/hour, the total daily volume of fluid removal will be 24 L/day. To achieve a net loss of 5 L/day, the volume of replacement solution needs to be 19 L. Hence, the replacement solution should be infused at 792 mL/hour. At this rate, if all variables remain constant, the patient will achieve euvolemia within 4 days.

Combined Modalities

The CRRT modalities that combine hemofiltration with dialysis (e.g., *CAVHDF, CVVHDF*) are technically more difficult to perform and require sophisticated equipment. Although the same ultrafiltration principles described previously apply, a dialysis component that promotes additional solute diffusion across the high-flux hemofilter is added. In the case of CVVHD, the process is initiated as for CVVH with blood flow rates of 50 to 200 mL/minute, but a dialysis solution is run countercurrent along the hemofilter at 10 to 35 mL/minute, resulting in diffusion of solutes. This makes drug dosing extremely difficult because clinicians must account for both diffusive and convective drug removal.

Estimating Drug Removal

26. Are there ways to calculate drug removal in extracorporeal CRRT modalities?

Two recent reviews provide an excellent background on dosing drugs in patients receiving CRRT.[45,46] The principles for drug removal in hemofiltration are basically identical with those for removal in hemodialysis. For example, drugs with a small volume of distribution and low protein binding are removed readily by these modalities. The *sieving coefficient* (SC) of a drug is the non–protein-bound fraction of the drug that is in plasma. For example, an SC of 0.8 means that 80% of the drug is unbound in plasma. Drug SC can be obtained from the literature or by measuring concentrations simultaneously in the prefilter blood and ultrafiltrate. The ratio of the ultrafiltrate concentration to plasma concentration is the SC. Drug clearance can be calculated by multiplying the SC by the ultrafiltration rate. For example, if a patient is receiving CVVH at an ultrafiltration rate of 1 L/hour, and he or she is receiving vancomycin (which has an SC of 0.8) 1 g/day, the vancomycin clearance while receiving CVVH is $0.8 \times 1{,}000$ mL/hour = 800 mL/hour or 13 mL/minute.

Calculating drug clearance is much more difficult in hemodiafiltration modalities (CAVHDF, CVVHDF) because both convection and diffusion account for drug clearance and it is difficult to predict drug clearance precisely. The use of SC can be useful for small–molecular-weight drugs, but the accuracy declines with larger drug molecules, such as vancomycin. When possible, therapeutic drug monitoring should be performed to maintain therapeutic concentrations and to maximize drug therapy.

REFERENCES

1. Singri N et al. Acute renal failure. *JAMA* 2003;289:747.
2. Bellomo R et al. Acute renal failure—definition, outcomes, animal models, fluid therapy, information technology and needs—the Second International Consensus Conference Acute Dialysis Quality Initiative Group. *Crit Care* 2004;4:R204.
3. Kaufman J et al. Community-acquired acute renal failure. *Am J Kidney Dis* 1991;17:191.
4. Block CA et al. the epidemiology and outcome of acute renal failure and the impact of chronic kidney disease. *Semin Dial* 2006;19:450.
5. Guerin C et al. Initial versus delayed acute renal failure in the intensive care unit. A multicenter prospective epidemiological study. Rhone-Alpes Area Study Group on Acute Renal Failure. *Am J Respir Crit Care Med* 2000;161:872.
6. Vincent JL et al. Epidemiology and outcome in renal failure. *Intl J Artif Organs* 2004;27:1013.
7. de Mendonca A et al. Acute renal failure in the ICU: risk factors and outcome evaluated by the SOFA score. *Intensive Care Med* 2000;26:915.
8. Pruchnicki MC et al. Acute renal failure in hospitalized patients: Part I. *Ann Pharmacother* 2002;36:1261.
9. Andreev E et al. A rise in plasma creatinine that is not a sign of renal failure: which drugs can be responsible? *J Intern Med* 1999;246:247.
10. Cockcroft DW et al. Prediction of creatinine clearance from serum creatinine. *Nephron* 1976;16:31.
11. Levey AS et al. A more accurate method to estimate glomerular filtration rate from serum creatinine: a new prediction equation. Modification of Diet in Renal Disease Study Group. *Ann Intern Med* 1999;130:461.
12. Levey AS et al. National Kidney Foundation practice guidelines for chronic kidney disease: evaluation, classification, and stratification. *Ann Intern Med* 2003;139:137.
13. Chittineni H et al. Risk for acute renal failure in patients hospitalized for decompensated congestive heart failure. *Am J Nephrol* 2007;27:55.
14. Brater DC. Antiinflammatory agents and renal function. *Semin Arthritis Rheum* 2002;32 (3 Suppl 1): 33.
15. Whelton A. Nephrotoxicity of nonsteroidal anti-inflammatory drugs: physiologic foundations and clinical implications. *Am J Med* 1999;106:13S.
16. Schneider V et al. Association of selective and conventional nonsteroidal antiinflammatory drugs with acute renal failure: a population based, nested case-control analysis. *Am J Epidemiol* 2006;164:881.
17. Schoolwerth AC et al. Renal considerations in angiotensin converting enzyme inhibitor therapy: AHA Scientific Statement. *Circulation* 2001;104:1985.
18. Mangrum AJ et al. Angiotensin converting enzyme inhibitors and angiotensin receptor blockers in chronic renal disease: safety issues. *Semin Nephrol* 2004;24:168.
19. Papiris SA. Bench-to-bedside reviews: pulmonary-renal syndromes—an update for the intensivist. *Crit Care* 2007;11:213.
20. Couser WG. Glomerulonephritis. *Lancet* 1999; 353:1509.
21. Radford MG Jr. et al. Reversible membranous nephropathy associated with the use of nonsteroidal anti-inflammatory drugs. *JAMA* 1996;276:466.
22. Taber S et al. Drug-associated renal dysfunction. *Crit Care Clin* 2006;22:357.
23. Davis A et al. Best evidence topic report. The use of loop diuretics in acute renal failure in critically ill patients to reduce mortality, maintain renal function, or avoid the requirements for renal support. *Emerg Med J* 2006;23:569.
24. Bagshaw SM et al. Loop diuretics in the management of acute renal failure: a systematic review and meta-analysis. *Crit Care Resusc* 2007;9:60.
25. Friedrich JO et al. Meta-analysis: low-dose dopamine increases urine output but does not prevent renal dysfunction or death. *Ann Intern Med* 2005;142:510.
26. Bolesta SB et al. Contrast-induced nephropathy. In: Dunsworth TS et al., eds. *Pharmacotherapy Self-Assessment Program.* 6th ed. Nephrology Module.

Lenexa, KS: American College of Clinical Pharmacy; 2007:73.
27. Sanaei-Ardekani M. Contrast-induced nephropathy: a review. *Cardiovasc Revasc Med* 2005;6:82.
28. Bagshaw SM. Theophylline for prevention of contrast induced nephropathy: a systematic review and meta-analysis. *Arch Intern Med* 2005;165: 1087.
29. Spargias K. Ascorbic acid prevents contrast-mediated nephropathy in patients with renal dysfunction undergoing coronary angiography or intervention. *Circulation* 2004;110:2837.
30. Mingeot-Leclercq M et al. Aminoglycosides: nephrotoxicity. *Antimicrob Agents Chemother* 1999;43:1003.
31. Barclay ML et al. Once daily aminoglycoside therapy: is it less toxic than multiple daily doses and how should it be monitored? *Clin Pharmacokinet* 1999;36:89.
32. Swan SK. Aminoglycoside nephrotoxicity. *Semin Nephrol* 1997;17:27.
33. Rybak MJ et al. Prospective evaluation of the effect of an aminoglycoside dosing regimen on rates of observed nephrotoxicity and ototoxicity. *Antimicrob Agents Chemother* 1999;43:1549.
34. Alexopolous E. Drug-induced acute interstitial nephritis. *Ren Fail* 1998; 20:809.
35. Park S. Medical management of urinary stone disease. *Expert Opin Pharmacother* 2007;8:1117.
36. Manthey DE et al. Nephrolithiasis. *Emerg Med Clin North Am* 2001;39:383.
37. Rodman JS. Struvite stones. *Nephron* 1999;81(Suppl 1):50.
38. Borghi L et al. Urine volume: stone risk factor and preventative measure. *Nephron* 1999;81(Suppl 1):31.
39. Borghi L et al. Urinary volume, water, and recurrences in idiopathic calcium nephrolithiasis: a 5-year randomized prospective study. *J Urol* 1996;155: 839.
40. Grases F. Renal lithiasis and nutrition. *Nutrition Journal* 2006;5:23.
41. Pearle MS. Prevention of nephrolithiasis. *Curr Opin Nephrol Hypertens* 2001;10:203.
42. Joy MS. A primer on continuous renal replacement therapy for critically ill patients. *Ann Pharmacother* 1998;32:362.
43. Palevsky PM et al. The Acute Dialysis Quality Initiative–part V: operational characteristics of CRRT. *Adv Ren Replace Ther* 2002;9:268.
44. Bellomo R et al. The Acute Dialysis Quality Initiative–part V: operational characteristics of CRRT. *Adv Ren Replace Ther* 2002;9:255.
45. Mueller BA. Acute renal failure. In: DiPiro JT et al., eds. *Pharmacotherapy: A Pathophysiologic Approach.* 5th ed. New York, NY: McGraw-Hill; 2002:771.
46. Kuang D et al. Pharmacokinetics and antimicrobial dosing adjustment in critically ill patients during continuous renal replacement therapy. *Clin Nephrol* 2007;67:267.
47. Palevsky PM. Dialysis modality and dosing strategy in acute renal failure. *Semin Dial* 2006;19:165.

CHAPTER 31

Chronic Kidney Disease

Amy Barton Pai and Todd A. Conner

INTRODUCTION

Chronic kidney disease (CKD) describes the continuum of kidney dysfunction from early to late-stage disease. Estimated glomerular filtration rates (eGFR) range from 90 mL/minute/1.73 m^2 in the early stages to 15 mL/minute/1.73 m^2 in the late stages of disease. The most severe stage occurs when the eGFR is less than 15 mL/minute/1.73 m^2 and is known as end-stage renal disease (ESRD).[1] Patients with ESRD require renal replacement therapy in the form of dialysis or transplantation to sustain life. Complications associated with CKD that increase the complexity of the condition and include fluid and electrolyte abnormalities, anemia, cardiovascular disease, hyperparathyroidism, bone disease, and malnutrition. Optimal treatment of patients with CKD is best achieved using a multidisciplinary approach to address the concurrent medical problems and complex pharmacotherapeutic regimens. Alterations in drug disposition that occur with kidney impairment and the subsequent need for dosage

Table 31-1 Staging of Chronic Kidney Disease Based on eGFR

Stage	Description	eGFR (mL/min/1.73 m²)
	At increased risk	≥90 (with CKD risk factors)
1	Kidney damage with normal or ↑ eGFR	≥90
2	Kidney damage with mild ↓ eGFR	60–89
3	Moderate ↓ eGFR	30–59
4	Severe ↓ eGFR	15–29
5	Kidney failure	<15 (or need for renal replacement therapy)

Adapted with permission from the National Kidney Foundation. NKF-K/DOQI Clinical Practice Guidelines for Chronic Kidney Disease: Evaluation, Classification, and Stratification. *Am J Kidney Dis* 2002;39:S1.

adjustments are additional considerations when determining rational pharmacotherapy in this population.

Definitions

Chronic kidney disease is characterized by a progressive deterioration in kidney function ultimately leading to irreversible structural damage to existing nephrons. Based on the progressive nature of this condition, a staging system has been established to classify kidney disease according to the eGFR, which is estimated clinically using creatinine clearance (Cl_{Cr}) (Table 31-1).[1] Specifically, CKD is defined as kidney damage with a normal or a mildly decreased eGFR (stages 1 and 2) or a eGFR <60 mL/minute/1.73 m² for at least 3 months with or without evidence of kidney damage (stages 3 to 5). Kidney damage is indicated by pathologic abnormalities or markers of injury, including abnormalities in blood or urine tests and imaging studies.[1] The presence of protein in the urine (defined as *proteinuria, albuminuria,* or *microalbuminuria* based on protein type and amount) is an early and sensitive marker of kidney damage.

A substantial decline in kidney function also leads to *azotemia,* the condition resulting from accumulation of nitrogenous wastes such as urea (blood urea nitrogen [BUN]), and an increased risk for developing complications of CKD. Uremic signs and symptoms from accumulation of nitrogenous wastes and other toxins lead to a myriad of complications affecting most major organ systems. Laboratory abnormalities include azotemia, hyperphosphatemia, hypocalcemia, hyperkalemia, metabolic acidosis, and worsening anemia. Clinical signs of CKD and its associated complications, including hypertension and uremic symptoms (e.g., nausea, anorexia), and bleeding are observed as the disease advances to stages 3 through 5. Interventions to slow the progression of kidney disease and potentially reverse the disease process are critical, because patients with a decline in eGFR to <30 mL/minute/1.73 m² (stage 4), in general, will ultimately have ESRD.

Epidemiology of Chronic Kidney Disease

Incidence and Prevalence

The Third National Health and Nutrition Examination Survey (NHANES III), a national study of more than 18,000 persons 20 years of age or older conducted from 1988 through 1994, provides information on the stages of CKD in the U.S. population.[2] From these data, it is estimated that 8.3 million Americans have CKD stages 3 to 5. They also reported that 11.3 million Americans are at risk for developing or have mild decrease in kidney function (CKD stage 1 and 2).[1]

Data describing the ESRD population are made available annually by the U.S. Renal Data System (USRDS). The reports characterize the development, treatment, morbidity, and mortality associated with ESRD in the United States and include data from patients with kidney transplants. Based on the most recent data from the USRDS, more than 472,000 patients were receiving renal replacement therapy for ESRD at the end of 2004, with approximately 104,000 new patients starting treatment during that year.[3] A continued increase in incidence rates of ESRD has been observed over the past decade, although this rate has decreased to approximately 1.5% to 5% per year over the past 5 years.[3] The continued increase in incidence rates of ESRD, in conjunction with a relatively stable death rate for this population, accounts for the overall increase in the prevalence of ESRD. CKD has been identified as one of the focus areas for the Healthy People 2010 national health initiative; one of the specific objectives is to reduce the number of new cases of ESRD.[4]

Populations at increased risk for developing ESRD include males and the older population, particularly patients 65 years of age and older. More than 49% of incident hemodialysis patients in 2004 were age 65 or older, a much larger percentage than for the peritoneal dialysis and transplant populations.[3] Racial distribution of the dialysis population shows that the prevalence is greatest in whites (61%) and blacks (32%), followed by Hispanics (14%) and Asians (4%). Blacks and Native Americans have a three to four times greater incident rate of kidney failure than white individuals.[3]

Etiology

Chronic kidney disease most often results from a progressive loss of functioning nephrons caused by a primary kidney disease or as a secondary complication of certain systemic diseases, but it can also result from an acute event causing irreversible damage to the kidneys. The leading causes of ESRD in patients newly diagnosed in 2004 were diabetes mellitus (44%), hypertension (27%), and chronic glomerulonephritis (8%).[3] Among Native Americans, diabetes is the predominant etiology, accounting for nearly two-thirds of the ESRD cases. Diabetes also accounts for higher rates of ESRD in blacks and Hispanics than in whites. Another of the Healthy People 2010 national health objectives for CKD is to focus on efforts to reduce the incidence of ESRD in blacks, Hispanics, and Native Americans.[4] Hypertension remains the most common cause of ESRD among blacks, with approximately one-third of cases attributed to this disease. A variety of causes are responsible for the remaining cases of ESRD, among which are cystic kidney disease, other urologic causes, and acquired immunodeficiency syndrome (AIDS) nephropathy.

Mortality

Advances in dialysis and transplantation have improved patient care; however, mortality rates during the first year of ESRD have not improved over the past decade (first-year adjusted death rate is 234/1,000 patient-years in the year 2003 for prevalent ESRD patients).[3] Patients with cardiovascular disease on dialysis have a fivefold greater risk of all-cause mortality when compared with the general Medicare population and with patients with CKD not yet requiring renal replacement therapy. Comorbid conditions, low albumin, malnutrition, and anemia at initiation of dialysis are strong predictors of mortality. Life expectancy is 20% to 25% of that of the general population. Cardiovascular-related events, particularly cardiac arrest and myocardial infarction, are the leading causes of death in the ESRD population. This is not surprising given the high prevalence of coexisting cardiac disorders in patients with ESRD and the elevated risk for mortality associated with these conditions. The Healthy People 2010 initiative for CKD will also focus on decreasing deaths from cardiovascular disease.[4] Infection (predominantly septicemia) and cerebrovascular disease are also substantial contributors to overall mortality in patients with ESRD.[3]

Drug-Induced Causes of Chronic Kidney Disease

Analgesic Nephropathy

Analgesic nephropathy is a form of tubulointerstitial kidney disease characterized by renal papillary necrosis as a primary lesion and chronic interstitial nephritis as a secondary lesion resulting from habitual ingestion of a mixture of two antipyretic analgesics and usually caffeine, codeine, or both.[5] Analgesic nephropathy is part of the *analgesic syndrome,* including such nonrenal complications as anemia, peptic ulcer disease, urinary tract infection, and atherosclerosis.[5] Phenacetin, an acetaminophen prodrug, was the first agent to be identified as causing this syndrome. Currently in the United States, most cases are caused by long-term use or misuse of compound analgesics containing acetaminophen and aspirin along with caffeine or codeine.[5] Similar findings in terms of the effect on kidney function have also been observed with nonsteroidal anti-inflammatory drugs (NSAID), with both acute and chronic manifestations associated with long-term use.[6] The cumulative amount (at least 1 to 2 kg of acetaminophen), rather than the duration of analgesic intake, is the primary risk factor for developing chronic analgesic nephropathy.[7] Recommendations made by the National Kidney Foundation (NKF) on analgesic use have been published.[5]

Analgesic nephropathy is more prevalent in female patients, with a female-to-male ratio of 5 to 7:1. The peak incidence occurs between the fourth and the fifth decades of life.[5,7] Patients usually complain of chronic pain syndromes and, in most cases, psychiatric manifestations indicative of an addictive behavior are observed. At presentation, patients may have a reduced eGFR and findings consistent with CKD. During acute necrosis, patients may experience flank pain, pyuria, and hematuria. As necrosis progresses, cellular debris can cause ureteral obstruction. Kidney dysfunction is characterized as a salt-wasting nephropathy, with a substantial reduction in urine-concentrating and urine-acidifying capabilities. The exact mechanism for kidney damage is uncertain; however, it is thought that because acetaminophen accumulates in the renal medulla, its oxidative metabolite produced by the medullary cytochrome P450 enzyme system may bind to macromolecules causing cellular necrosis. Although the reduced form of glutathione in the medulla can prevent this process, agents that reduce medullary glutathione content (e.g., aspirin) may promote kidney damage. This mechanism may explain a lack of analgesic nephropathy associated with acetaminophen alone. NSAID, which attenuate prostaglandin-mediated vasodilation, may induce an ischemic state within the renal medulla, leading to papillary necrosis.[6]

Data on the adverse renal effects of selective cyclooxygenase 2 (COX-2) inhibitors is less clear. Recently, a meta-anlaysis of 114 randomized, double-blind clinical trials evaluated the adverse renal events of COX-2 inhibitors. The authors reported that, of the six agents evaluated, only rofecoxib was associated with adverse renal effects, defined as significant changes in urea or creatinine levels, clinically diagnosed kidney disease, or renal failure. Higher doses and longer duration of therapy were associated with higher rates of renal dysfunction.[8] Rofecoxib was voluntarily withdrawn from the market in 2004 because of increased concern about cardiovascular events.

The long-term management of analgesic nephropathy primarily involves strict abstinence from use of NSAID and combination analgesics. If possible, patients should be encouraged to maintain a high fluid intake to prevent obstruction of the tubules with necrotic debris and to reduce the risk of urinary tract infection. If such patients develop ESRD, treatment is similar to that for those with kidney disease from other causes. For patients requiring analgesics, aspirin or propoxyphene taken alone may be reasonable alternatives. Acetaminophen as a single agent may be safe, although habitual use can contribute to progression of kidney disease as well as to liver toxicity.[7] Patients requiring chronic analgesic therapy should use the lowest dose to control pain, avoid combination products when possible, and maintain adequate hydration.

Lithium Nephropathy

Although lithium use has been associated with alterations in kidney function secondary to acute functional and histologic changes, its role in the development of chronic changes (i.e., chronic interstitial nephritis) is less clear. Both the concentrating ability within the kidney and the eGFR may decline with long-term lithium use.[9] In addition, chronic interstitial changes may develop in patients receiving lithium, particularly those with high serum lithium concentrations. Despite these findings, however, others have failed to implicate lithium as a chronic nephrotoxic agent.[10] In patients taking lithium chronically, close monitoring of serum lithium concentrations is advised, and serum creatinine (SrCr) measurements should be obtained annually to detect changes in kidney function.

Progressive Kidney Disease Treatment Options

Treatment of patients with stage 1 to 4 CKD focuses on reducing risk factors for progression of CKD (e.g., uncontrolled hypertension and diabetes) and providing interventions that delay progression. Management of complications of CKD, including fluid and electrolyte abnormalities, anemia, hyperphosphatemia, secondary hyperparathyroidism, metabolic acidosis, and malnutrition, is necessary once patients were in stage 3 CKD and beyond. Renal replacement therapies including hemodialysis (HD), peritoneal dialysis (PD), and kidney transplantation are treatment options for patients with ESRD. In the 1950s, a patient diagnosed with ESRD faced unavoidable death with a life expectancy of days to weeks. Continued development of treatment options for ESRD introduced in the 1960s dramatically reduced ESRD-related morbidity and mortality. At the end of 2004, 66% of patients with ESRD were undergoing HD, 29% had a functioning transplant, and 5% were receiving PD.[3]

Medication Use

Data regarding medication use in dialysis patients, including those having HD and PD, reveal that these patients are prescribed a total of 8 to 11 medications per patient.[11,12] According to the USRDS, antihypertensive agents were prescribed for 75% of patients, with calcium channel blockers and angiotensin-converting enzyme (ACE) inhibitors as the most common agents. Approximately 80% of patients on dialysis were prescribed phosphate-binding agents with a similar percentage of patients requiring erythropoietin. These patterns of medication use are reflective of the prevalence of complications in the latter stages of CKD. The extent of medication use and the complexity of prescribed drug regimens contribute to nonadherence and medication-related problems (MRP) in the ESRD population. To manage MRP, some dialysis facilities have utilized a clinical pharmacist, which has been shown to be cost-effective and is associated with maintenance of health-related quality of life in patients on HD.[13,14]

Economics

The cost of treating patients with ESRD is substantial, with most of this cost paid by the federal government. In 2004, the cost was $18.5 billion dollars, 6.7% of the Medicare budget.[3] This amount reflects a consistent increase from prior years and an increase in the percentage of the Medicare budget dedicated to ESRD care. The increase is most likely associated with the higher prevalence of ESRD, changes in the standard of care, reimbursement structure, and types of patients being treated (e.g., diabetic patients versus nondiabetic patients). Higher costs of treatment were associated with diabetes and patients with low hemoglobin values at initiation of dialysis. Outpatient pharmacy-related costs accounted for approximately $60.1 million of the ESRD Medicare budget for 2004.[3]

Pathophysiology

Progression of kidney disease to ESRD generally occurs over months to years and is assessed by the rate of decline in eGFR. There are approximately 1 million nephrons per kidney, each maintaining its own single nephron eGFR. Progressive loss of nephron function results in adaptive changes in remaining nephrons to increase single nephron eGFR.[15] Over time, the compensatory increase in single nephron eGFR leads to hypertrophy and an irreversible loss of nephron function from sustained increases in glomerular pressure. Glomerulosclerosis (glomerular arteriolar damage) develops from prolonged elevation of glomerular capillary pressure and increased glomerular plasma flow leading to a continuous cycle of nephron destruction. Regardless of the cause, a predictable and continuous decrease in kidney function occurs in patients when the eGFR drops below a "critical" value, to approximately one-half of normal.[16] The rate of decline remains fairly constant for an individual, but can vary substantially among patients and disease states. A more rapid rate of decline in kidney function has been associated with black race, lower baseline eGFR, male gender, older age, and smoking. Compared with hypertensive kidney disease, conditions associated with a faster decline include diabetic kidney disease, glomerular diseases, and polycystic kidney disease.[1] Progressive disease is typically identified by persistent proteinuria, decreasing kidney function, and the development of glomerulosclerosis. Although early changes in kidney function can be detected through routine laboratory monitoring, most patients do not develop symptoms of uremia until they have reached the more severe stages (stage 4 CKD and ESRD).

As the leading causes of ESRD in the United States, diabetes, hypertension, and glomerular diseases have been the focus of research to identify their associated mechanisms of kidney damage. Diabetes accounts for most cases of ESRD, which are caused not only by poor glycemic control, but also by concurrent hypertension.[3] Excess filtration of glucose and contact with glomerular and tubular cells result in increased cellular osmotic pressure and thickening of the capillary basement membrane. The resulting glomerulopathy may or may not result in proteinuria. Systemic hypertension is a potent stimulus for the progression of kidney disease because of its association with increased single nephron eGFR.[15,17] Coexistent diabetes and hypertension increase the risk of developing ESRD by five- to sixfold compared with persons with hypertension alone. Proteinuria, one of the initial diagnostic signs, may also contribute to the progressive decline in kidney function, with a more rapid rate of progression associated with higher protein excretion.[18] Immunologic and hemodynamic mechanisms have been identified to explain the glomerular injury and increase in renal plasma flow associated with proteinuria and high protein intake. Inflammatory cytokines may be responsible for fibrosis and renal scarring ultimately resulting in loss of nephron function.

Dyslipidemias, which are common in patients with CKD, are often observed concurrently with proteinuria. Increased low-density lipoprotein (LDL) cholesterol, total cholesterol, and apolipoprotein B, as well as decreased high-density lipoprotein (HDL) cholesterol, have been observed in patients with progressive kidney disease.[19] Hypercholesterolemia has been associated with loss of kidney function in patients with and without diabetes.[20,21] Accumulation of apolipoproteins in glomerular mesangial cells contributes to cytokine production and infiltration of macrophages and has been implicated in the progression of CKD, primarily in the presence of previous kidney disease or other risk factors such as hypertension.[22] LDL is thought to promote glomerular damage by initiating a series of cellular events in mesangial cells and through oxidation to a more cytotoxic derivative once within these cells. Although serum total cholesterol, triglycerides, and apolipoprotein B all correlate with the rate of decline in eGFR, it is not clear that they directly increase the rate of progression of kidney disease, particularly when present with concomitant conditions that also cause kidney damage. Some evidence, however, suggests that treatment of hypercholesterolemia with statin therapy in patients with CKD may reduce proteinuria and progression of CKD.[23]

Clinical Assessment

Evaluation of Kidney Function

The most reliable and practical means available to determine baseline kidney function and monitor progression of kidney disease over time is eGFR. The ideal marker of eGFR should be a nontoxic substance that is freely filtered at the glomerulus and not secreted, reabsorbed, or metabolized by the kidney. Inulin and exogenous radioactive markers have been used to assess eGFR because they meet these criteria; however, they are not readily available to clinicians, require intravenous (IV) administration, and are costly. Creatinine is an endogenous substance that is derived from the breakdown of muscle creatine phosphate. It is excreted primarily by glomerular filtration; thus, creatinine clearance (Cl_{Cr}) has been used as a reasonable surrogate for eGFR. There are limitations to consider when using methods to assess eGFR that incorporate creatinine. Creatinine is eliminated not only through glomerular filtration, but also via tubular secretion. As nephron function declines, tubular secretion of creatinine contributes more substantially to overall elimination of creatinine such that Cl_{Cr} overestimates true eGFR. As a result, disease progression may be underestimated. Administration of cimetidine to patients before measurement of Cl_{Cr} may provide a more accurate assessment because cimetidine blocks tubular secretion of creatinine.[24]

Serum creatinine (SrCr) alone is used clinically as an index of kidney function; however, multiple limitations to this practice exist. In the initial stages of kidney disease, SrCr may remain within the normal range. Consequently, SrCr may be relatively insensitive in detecting early kidney disease and is not accurate for estimating the progression of the disease. Because generation of creatinine is proportional to total muscle mass, it is affected by diet (notably by the ingestion of meats), age, and gender. Generally, muscle mass declines with age and is smaller in women. Thus, a SrCr that is in the upper limit of normal (e.g., 1.2 mg/dL) for a young athletic male is likely to be associated with a high creatinine clearance, whereas the same SrCr in a 70-year-old woman could indicate compromised renal function. Use of creatinine to assess kidney function in patients with liver disease may also lead to overestimation of eGFR.[25] This may be attributed to decreased production of creatine, the precursor to creatinine, by the liver or increased tubular secretion of creatinine by the kidney. Also, substantial variation is seen in the calibration of SrCr among laboratories that can result in differences in measured SrCr. Although SrCr can provide a rough estimate of kidney function, other means of assessing eGFR should be used when a more accurate determination is necessary. Other markers of early kidney damage, such as proteinuria, should also be evaluated in patients at risk for kidney disease.

Several equations have been developed to calculate eGFR that incorporate SrCr and other variables (especially age and gender) for reasons described above. The most commonly used equation is the Cockcroft-Gault equation, which provides an estimate of Cl_{Cr} in patients with stable kidney function[26] (see Chapter 31, Acute Renal Failure). More recently a prediction equation was developed using data from the Modification of Diet in Renal Disease (MDRD) study, a multicenter trial that evaluated the effects of dietary protein restriction and blood pressure (BP) control on progression of kidney disease.[27] This equation, referred to as the *MDRD equation*, may provide a better estimate of GFR based on the fact that the equation was derived using eGFR measured directly by urinary clearance of a radiolabeled marker (^{125}I-Iothalamate) as opposed to creatinine, and included a relatively large and diverse population (>500 white and black individuals with varying degrees of kidney disease) for derivation and validation of the equation. The MDRD equation[27] is as follows:

$$\text{Estimated GFR (mL/minute/1.73 m}^2) = 170 \times (\text{SrCr})^{-0.999} \times (\text{Age})^{-0.176} \times (\text{BUN})^{-0.170} \times (\text{Alb})^{+0.318} \times (0.762 \text{ if female}) \times (1.18 \text{ if African American}) \qquad \textbf{(31-1)}$$

An abbreviated version has also been developed[1]:

$$\text{Estimated GFR (mL/minute/1.73 m}^2) = 186 \times (\text{SrCr})^{-1.154} \times (\text{Age})^{-0.203} \times (0.742 \text{ if female}) \times (1.21 \text{ if African American}) \qquad \textbf{(31-2)}$$

The Schwartz[28] equation is used to assess eGFR in children as follows:

$$\text{Creatinine clearance (mL/minute)} = [k \times \text{length (in cm)}]/\text{SrCr}$$

where k is dependent on age: infant (1 to 52 weeks) k = 0.45; child (1 to 13 years) k = 0.55; adolescent male k = 0.7; and adolescent female k = 0.55. **(31-3)**

Although historically accepted as a more accurate method, calculation of Cl_{Cr} using 24-hour urine collection methods has not been proved to be more reliable than use of the Cockcroft-Gault or MDRD equations. Problems with urine collection methods include incomplete urine collection, diurnal variation in eGFR, and variation in creatinine excretion. Despite these limitations, shorter collection times or spot untimed urine samples may be useful to determine creatinine excretion. Populations in whom estimation of GFR using a 24-hour urine collection is more reasonable include patients with variation in dietary intake of creatine sources, such as vegetarians, or persons with poor muscle mass (e.g., malnourished individuals or amputees).[1]

Estimation of GFR by the MDRD equation is used to follow the progression of kidney disease. Frequent assessment of drug selection and dosage regimen design should be integral to the evaluation of a patient with progressive kidney disease. The Cockcroft-Gault equation is most commonly used to evaluate the appropriate doses of drugs that are eliminated by the kidney.

Proteinuria

In patients who have (or are at risk for) kidney disease, additional assessment of kidney function should include evaluation of urinary protein excretion, which has been shown to be predictive of disease progression. Protein is not normally filtered at the glomerulus and is present only in trace amounts in the

Table 31-2 Diagnostic Criteria for Proteinuria and Albuminuria

	Total Protein			Albumin		
	24-hr Collection (mg/day)	Spot Urine Dipstick (mg/dL)	Spot Urine Protein-SrCr Ratio (mg/g)	24-hr Collection (mg/day)	Spot Urine Dipstick (mg/dL)	Spot Urine Albumin-SrCr Ratio (mg/g)
Normal	<300	<30	<200	<30	<3	<17 (men) <25 (women)
Microalbuminuria	NA	NA	NA	30–300	>3	17–250 (men) 25–355 (women)
Albuminuria or clinical proteinuria	>300	>30	>200	>300	NA	>250 (men) >355 (women)

SrCr, serum creatinine.
Adapted from National Kidney Foundation. NKF-K/DOQI Clinical Practice Guidelines for Chronic Kidney Disease: Evaluation, Classification, and Stratification. *Am J Kidney Dis* 2002;39:S1, with permission.

urine. With glomerular damage, proteinuria is commonly observed. Proteinuria may precede elevations in SrCr and should be considered as an early marker of kidney damage. *Microalbuminuria* is defined as an albumin excretion rate of 20 to 200 mcg/minute or 30 to 300 mg/24 hour. Specific assays with increased sensitivity relative to standard assays are required for detecting quantities of protein in the range defined as microalbuminuria. *Proteinuria* is defined as a total protein excretion rate >200 mcg/minute or >300 mg/24 hour (referred to as *albuminuria* if albumin is the only protein measured). Total protein includes albumin and other proteins, such as low molecular weight globulins and apoproteins. Assessment of albuminuria is a better indicator of early kidney disease because it is primarily indicative of glomerular damage as opposed to total protein, which is not as specific for glomerular damage. Other tests, including urinalysis, radiographic procedures, and biopsy, may also be valuable in further assessing kidney function.

Quantification of albumin can be done using timed urine samples. Typically, a 24-hour collection period is used, although a timed sample collected overnight may be more reliable because protein excretion can vary throughout the day and with postural changes (i.e., orthostatic proteinuria). Untimed or "spot" urine samples for measurement of protein- or albumin-to-creatinine ratios are often more convenient. As opposed to measuring protein or albumin in a timed collection, this method corrects for variations in hydration status and may be more accurate because protein excretion is normalized to glomerular filtration. The albumin and creatinine concentrations in the urine are measured from a spot urine sample, preferably from a first-morning urine sample, because it correlates best with 24-hour protein excretion. If a first morning urine sample is not available, a random sample is acceptable. Factors associated with proteinuria, such as ingestion of a high-protein meal and vigorous exercise, must be considered when evaluating urinary protein. Measuring urinary protein postexercise will result in a falsely elevated urine protein level as a consequence of an increase in the membrane permeability of the glomeruli to protein and a saturation of the tubular reabsorption process of filtered protein. To minimize this risk, it is recommended to wait approximately 4 hours postexercise to test for proteinuria.[29] Screening for albuminuria can also be done using urine dipstick testing of a spot urine sample. Reagent strips are available from several commercial test products and differ with regard to the specified testing procedure and the sensitivity and specificity for detecting albuminuria. Patients with a positive dipstick screening test should have a subsequent quantitative assessment of the protein- or albumin-to-creatinine ratio to confirm proteinuria.

According to the NKF-Kidney Disease Outcomes Quality Initiative (K/DOQI) Clinical Practice Guidelines for CKD, persistent proteinuria is diagnosed by at least two positive quantitative tests spaced by at least 1 to 2 weeks. The American Diabetes Association (ADA) defines microalbuminuria as a positive test on at least two of three quantitative measurements performed within a 3- to 6-month period. ADA criteria specify albumin-to-creatinine ratios of 30 to 300 mcg/mg as consistent with microalbuminuria, whereas higher values are indicative of albuminuria.[30] The NKF-K/DOQI Guidelines for CKD provide criteria for diagnosis of proteinuria and albuminuria based on testing method and gender (Table 31-2).[1]

Staging of Chronic Kidney Disease

Historically the term *chronic renal insufficiency* was used to describe patients with decreased kidney function not requiring dialysis. This included a broad range of patients from the earlier stages of the disease, with eGFR >60 mL/minute/1.73 m^2, as well as those patients with more severe disease, with eGFR <30 mL/minute/1.73 m^2. Failure to distinguish patients at these differing levels of kidney function also resulted in failure to recognize differences in management approaches required at varying levels of eGFR. Only recently has a uniform classification system been adopted to describe the various stages of kidney dysfunction, similar to the rationale for staging or classifying other chronic disease (e.g., hypertension). This staging system was developed to promote a more consistent dialogue when referring to patients with kidney dysfunction and use of terminology associated with a more objective description. Kidney disease is classified into five stages based on the eGFR (Table 31-1).[1] A patient with stage 1 or 2 CKD would have some pathologic abnormality indicative of kidney damage (See *Definitions* above), although their eGFR is relatively normal. Continued screening and interventions to delay progression are essential at these stages. Patients with stages 3 to 5 CKD are diagnosed with the disease based on eGFR alone (eGFR

<60 mL/minute/1.73 m^2). At these stages, management of complications becomes a standard of care. Stage 5 is the most severe stage when the eGFR is <15 mL/minute/1.73 m^2 and dialysis or transplantation is necessary.

Complications

Complications begin to develop as kidney disease progresses, most often when patients reach to stage 3 CKD and the eGFR is <60 mL/minute/1.73 m^2. Among these complications are fluid and electrolyte abnormalities, anemia, hyperphosphatemia, hyperparathyroidism, metabolic acidosis, cardiovascular complications, and poor nutritional status. Often, these complications go unrecognized or are inadequately managed during the earlier stages of CKD, leading to poor outcomes by the time a patient is in need of dialysis therapy. Hypoalbuminemia and anemia were identified in more than 50% of a population of patients new to dialysis therapy, and these findings were associated with a decreased quality of life.[31] Late referral to a nephrologist to manage specific kidney disorders and associated complications has also been associated with increased mortality in the ESRD population.[32] These and similar reports underscore the need for early and aggressive therapy to manage complications of CKD. These complications will be presented in more detail throughout this chapter. Complications associated with dialysis therapy are discussed in Chapter 32, Renal Dialysis.

Prevention

Appropriate management of CKD includes measures to prevent or slow progression of the disease and regular evaluation of kidney function to assess changes in disease severity and to monitor therapy. This includes aggressive strategies to manage the disorders that cause kidney disease or are known to accelerate the disease process, such as diabetes, hypertension, high protein intake, and dyslipidemias (see Chapter 12, Dyslipidemias, Athrosclerosis and Coronary Heart Disease; Chapter 13, Essential Hypertension; and Chapter 50, Diabetes Mellitus).

Antihypertensive Therapy

The association between BP and kidney disease is difficult to establish because hypertension is both a cause and a result of kidney failure. Hypertension, whether the primary cause of kidney disease or a coexisting disease in the presence of other etiologies, can promote kidney damage through transmission of elevated systemic pressure to glomeruli. The result is glomerular capillary hyperperfusion and hypertension leading to progressive kidney damage as nephron destruction continues. Glomerular ischemia induced by damage to preglomerular arteries and arterioles can also occur. Antihypertensive therapy prevents kidney damage and slows the rate of progression of CKD in both diabetic and nondiabetic patients.[30,33] The added benefit of reduced cardiovascular mortality further supports the use of antihypertensive therapy in patients at risk for progressive CKD. Despite what is known about the beneficial effects of BP control in patients with CKD, data from NHANES III indicate that only 11% of individuals with hypertension and elevated SrCr had BP measurements below 130/85 mmHg (the previous goal BP in patients with CKD) and just 27% had BP less than 140/90 mmHg.[1,2]

The target BP for patients with or at risk for kidney disease differs from that recommended for the general population with hypertension. Evidence now exists to support lowering BP beyond the generally advocated target of <140/90 mmHg. According to the Seventh Report of the Joint National Committee on Prevention, Detection, Evaluation, and Treatment of High Blood Pressure (JNC-7) and recommendations from the NKF-K/DOQI Hypertension and Diabetes Executive Committee, the goal BP for individuals with CKD or diabetes is <130/80 mmHg.[34,35] Results from the MDRD study showed that further lowering of BP to <125/75 mmHg (or a mean arterial pressure <92 mmHg) was more beneficial than usual BP control in patients with higher rates of urinary protein excretion (>1 g proteinuria/day).[18,30] The benefit seen in the low-target-BP group was maintained for 7 years after the end of randomization.[30] The effects of more aggressive BP lowering on progression of kidney disease were also studied in the African American Study of Kidney Disease and Hypertension (AASK) trial.[36] In this population, some evidence was seen in support of a lower BP goal in patients with higher baseline proteinuria; however, the effect on eGFR did not reach statistical significance. Changes in eGFR over a 4-year evaluation period did not differ significantly between patients with a mean BP of 141/85 mmHg and those with stricter control to a mean BP of 128/78 mmHg.[36] A *post hoc* analysis of the AASK trial found that patients with proteinuria >1 g/day assigned to the low-target BP group slowed progression to ESRD.[37] Clearly, BP control is important to delay progression of kidney disease, and with the expanding data supporting more aggressive BP lowering in patients with more severe proteinuria, the importance of BP control in this patient population is pivotal in slowing progression of CKD.

Blood pressure reduction with any agent or combination of agents is reasonable in patients with CKD. Among the available classes of antihypertensive agents, ACE inhibitors (e.g., enalapril, captopril, lisinopril) and angiotensin receptor blockers (ARB; e.g., losartan, irbesartan, candesartan) may afford additional benefits in preserving kidney function. In conditions of decreased kidney function and eGFR, angiotensin II primarily causes compensatory vasoconstriction of the efferent arteriole, thereby increasing glomerular capillary pressure (P_{GC}) and eGFR (Fig. 31-1). This effect is beneficial in conditions of acute renal failure; however, sustained increases in P_{GC} cause hypertrophy of individual nephrons and progressive kidney disease. ACE inhibitor and ARB therapy prevents this chronic increase in glomerular pressure mediated by angiotensin II. Benefits of ACE inhibitors have been demonstrated in patients with diabetes who had some degree of proteinuria, suggesting that use of ACE inhibitors be considered in this population regardless of BP.[33,38–40] In patients without diabetes, ACE inhibitors have been shown to reduce BP, decrease proteinuria, and slow the progression of kidney disease when compared with other agents.[36,41–43] An initial and mild decrease in eGFR is expected with ACE inhibitor therapy; therefore, an increase in SrCr of approximately 30% within the first 2 months of therapy is acceptable.[44] Hypotension, acute kidney failure, and severe hyperkalemia are reasons to consider discontinuing therapy (also, see Chapter 18, Heart Failure.)

Angiotensin II receptor blockers offer similar benefits to ACE inhibitors based on their ability to decrease efferent arteriolar resistance by blockade of the angiotensin type 1 (AT_1)

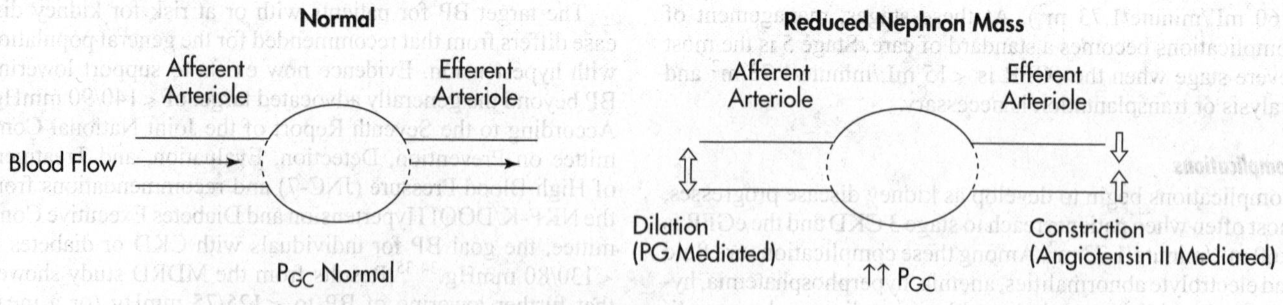

FIGURE 31-1 Renal hemodynamics are dependent on afferent and efferent arteriolar tone and glomerular capillary pressure (P_{GC}). With reduced nephron mass, afferent arteriolar vasodilation (mediated primarily by prostaglandins PGI_2 and PGE_2) and efferent arteriolar constriction (mediated primarily by angiotensin II) occur within remaining functioning nephrons to compensate. This leads to an increase in blood flow, intraglomerular capillary filtration pressure (P_{GC}), and hyperfiltration (increased single-nephron eGFR). Sustained increases in plasma flow and hydrostatic pressure lead to hyperfiltration injury and glomerular sclerosis. Over time, these changes contribute to continued loss of nephron function (i.e., progression of kidney disease). Angiotensin-converting enzymes (ACE) inhibitors and angiotensin receptor blockers (ARB) prevent vasoconstriction of the efferent arteriole and reduce the P_{GC}.

receptor. In patients with type 2 diabetes mellitus, losartan decreased the incidence of a doubling of SrCr by 25% and of ESRD by 28% when compared with placebo after a mean of 3.4 years of therapy.[45,46] Similar effects were observed in the Irbesartan Diabetic Nephropathy Trial (IDNT) with a 23% decreased risk of ESRD observed in patients treated with irbesartan.[47] In both studies, these beneficial effects were independent of reduction in BP. Reduction in the degree of proteinuria has also been demonstrated with candesartan and valsartan.[48,49] Combination therapy with an ARB and an ACE inhibitor may confer additional benefits than either therapy used alone, but larger clinical trials are needed to further ascertain the effect combination therapy will have on proteinuria and reducing time to HD.[50]

Aliskiren is the first available agent in a new class of antihypertensives that targets the renin-angiotensin-aldosterone system (RAS) by inhibiting renin. The advantages of renin inhibition include inhibition of the rate-limiting step of angiotensin II formation, preventing compensatory RAS activation by ACE inhibitor or ARB therapy, and possible synergistic effects with other antihypertensive regimens. Potential additional advantages in the CKD population include nonrenal elimination and possible antiproteinuric effects. Clinical trials evaluating the use of aliskiren in the CKD population are lacking, therefore, its role remains undefined until further data are available.[51]

Calcium channel blockers have been considered for preventing progression of kidney disease because of their effects on renal hemodynamics and cytoprotective and antiproliferative properties, which prevent mesangial expansion and renal scarring. The nondihydropyridine agents (i.e., diltiazem and verapamil) have been beneficial in reducing proteinuria when compared with dihydropyridines (e.g., amlodipine), which have been found to worsen proteinuria.[52] The NKF-K/DOQI guidelines suggest that dihydropyridine calcium channel blockers should not be used alone in nondiabetic or diabetic kidney disease with proteinuria, but can be used safely in combination with an ACE inhibitor or ARB. Combination therapy with an ACE inhibitor and nondihydropyridine agents has resulted in greater reductions in proteinuria in patients with diabetes than with either agent alone, suggesting that it may be rational to use multiple agents in this population.[53]

β-Blockers may offer benefits in the treatment of diabetic nephropathy as demonstrated by the United Kingdom Prospective Diabetes Study, which showed similar effects of atenolol and captopril on decreasing the incidence of albuminuria in patients with diabetes.[54]

Dietary Protein Restriction

Proteinuria was identified as the most significant predictor of ESRD in patients with type 2 diabetes and early CKD.[46] Evidence such as this has led to investigation of measures to decrease the degree of proteinuria. In addition to controlling the primary causes of kidney disease (e.g., diabetes, hypertension, and glomerulopathies) and using ACE inhibitor and ARB therapy, dietary protein restriction has been evaluated as a strategy for reducing proteinuria and delaying progression of kidney disease. Increases in protein ingestion are associated with a rise in eGFR, potentially because of structural changes of the glomerulus and changes in renal plasma flow with increased protein load.[55]

A number of studies have investigated the effect of protein restriction on disease progression with varying results.[56–58] These conflicting conclusions may result from differences in study design, patient populations, methods to assess kidney function, degrees of protein restriction, and dietary compliance. Evidence of the beneficial effects of protein restriction is primarily from nondiabetic patients and individuals with type 1 diabetes with protein restricted to approximately 0.6 to 0.8 g/kg of body weight per day.

In the MDRD study, the effects of protein and phosphorus restriction on progression of kidney disease were evaluated.[56] Nondiabetic patients with what is now considered stage 3 to 4 CKD (eGFR 25 to 55 mL/minute/1.73 m^2) received either a normal protein (1.3 g/kg/day) or low-protein (0.58 g/kg/day) diet, whereas those with more severe kidney disease (eGFR 13 to 24 mL/minute/1.73 m^2) were randomized to a low-protein or very-low-protein diet (0.28 g/kg/day). Within each protein category, patients were either maintained at a normal or low mean arterial pressure. A secondary analysis of the MDRD study, which accounted for dietary compliance, suggested that patients with severe kidney disease (eGFR <25 mL/minute/1.73 m^2) could benefit from protein restriction to 0.6 g/kg/day.[57]

Recently, a follow-up analysis of the above trial was published, which found that after a mean follow-up of 7.3 years, no significant difference was seen in decline in eGFR for each group.[59]

The potential benefits of protein restriction in patients with CKD must be weighed against the potentially adverse effect on overall nutritional status. Malnutrition is prevalent in patients with CKD starting dialysis and is a predictor of mortality in this population.[60] The decision to restrict protein should be done with referral to a dietitian and frequent monitoring of nutritional status.

Treatment of Dyslipidemia

Lipoprotein metabolism is altered early in the course of kidney disease and becomes pronounced with more advanced disease, making hyperlipidemia common in patients with CKD. Elevated triglyceride, total cholesterol, LDL cholesterol, and decreased HDL cholesterol levels are generally observed. The predominance of triglyceride-rich apo-B lipoproteins may contribute to the progression of kidney disease and is also a risk factor for the development of cardiovascular morbidity and mortality.[61]

The role of antihyperlipidemic drug therapy in preventing progression of CKD is uncertain. Use of statin therapy has been associated with decreased proteinuria and preservation of eGFR in a small number of patients with CKD.[23,62] A meta-analysis of trials, predominantly in patients with diabetes and CKD, showed that lipid-lowering therapy slowed the rate of decline in eGFR.[63] Despite uncertainty of therapy to delay progression, treatment of dyslipidemia should be considered, because abnormal lipid metabolism predisposes patients to cardiovascular disease. The question of whether strategies used to prevent and treat hyperlipidemia in the general population should be extrapolated to the population with kidney disease was addressed by the NKF Task Force on Cardiovascular Disease.[61] This group supported application of the National Cholesterol Education Program (NCEP ATP III) guidelines to the population with kidney disease and classified these patients in the highest risk group.[64] Guidelines for management of dyslipidemias in patients with CKD have recently been made available (NKF-K/DOQI guidelines).[65] These guidelines also support classifying patients with CKD in the highest risk category for cardiovascular disease, equivalent to the risk for patients with coronary artery disease. The choice of the specific antihyperlipidemic agent should be based on the individual lipid profile. In general, NCEP guidelines should be followed, with particular consideration of the effect of such interventions on patients with CKD, such as dietary restrictions and use of agents that are renally eliminated. Hydroxymethylglutaryl-coenzyme A (HMG-CoA) reductase inhibitors, which are necessary to lower LDL cholesterol, may have added cardiovascular benefits. Fibrates should be used cautiously in patients with CKD, because all agents in this class are renally metabolized, and all are eliminated primarily via the renal route leading to a possible increase risk of myositis and increase in SrCr. Small studies have shown that excretion of gemfibrozil in renal insufficiency to be less severely compromised, therefore the NKF-K/DOQI recommends gemfibrozil as the fibrate of choice in patients with CKD and hypertriglyceridemia (see Chapter 12, Dyslipidemias, Athrosclerosis and Coronary Heart Disease).

END-STAGE RENAL DISEASE (STAGE 5 CHRONIC KIDNEY DISEASE)

Clinical Signs and Symptoms

During stages 4 and 5, patients may develop the more severe signs and symptoms associated with advanced kidney disease, often referred to as the *uremic syndrome*. The manifestations and metabolic consequences of advanced kidney disease are listed in Table 31-3. These manifestations certainly may develop in the earlier stages of CKD, underscoring the importance of early intervention, but become more prominent as the disease worsens. The pathogenesis of these disorders has been attributed, in part, to the accumulation of uremic toxins. The search for uremic toxins has led to the identification of nitrogenous compounds that are consistently observed in the serum of patients with kidney disease. A cause-and-effect relationship between these compounds and the clinical manifestations of uremia has not been clearly established, however.

Treatment

Dialysis and Transplantation

As ESRD becomes inevitable, the appropriate dialysis modality must be selected based on patient preference and options

Table 31-3 Metabolic Effects of Progressive Kidney Disease

Cardiovascular	**Hematologic**
Hypertension	Anemia
Congestive heart failure	Bleeding complications
Pericarditis	Immune suppression
Atherosclerosis	**Musculoskeletal**
Arrhythmias	Renal bone disease
Metastatic calcifications	Amyloidosis
Dermatologic	**Neurologic**
Altered pigmentation	Lethargy
Pruritus	Depressed sensorium
Endocrine	Tremor
Calcium-phosphorous imbalances	Asterixis
Hyperparathyroidism	Muscular irritability and cramps (i.e., restless legs syndrome)
Metabolic bone disease	Seizures
Altered thyroid function	Motor weakness
Altered carbohydrate metabolism	Peripheral neuropathy
Hypophyseal-gonadal dysfunction	Coma
Decreased insulin metabolism	**Psychological**
Erythropoietin deficiency	Depression
Fluid, Electrolyte, and Acid-Base Effects	Anxiety
Fluid retention	Psychosis
Hyperkalemia	**Miscellaneous**
Hypermagnesemia	Reduced exercise tolerance
Hyperphosphatemia	
Hypocalcemia	
Metabolic acidosis	
Gastrointestinal	
Anorexia	
Nausea, vomiting	
Delayed gastric emptying	
GI bleeding	
Ulcers	

GI, gastrointestinal.

for vascular access for HD or peritoneal access for PD. Early planning for dialysis therapy and timely initiation may lower patient morbidity and mortality. (Indications for dialysis and considerations in selection of modality are discussed in Chapter 33, Renal Dialysis.) Kidney transplantation is an option for all patients with ESRD without specified contraindications if a suitable organ match is available (see Chapter 34, Kidney, Liver, and Pancreas Transplantation).

Pharmacotherapy

Pharmacotherapy in patients with ESRD involves interventions to manage comorbid conditions and complications. The extent of medication use, including medications administered during dialysis therapy, contributes to the potential for drug interactions, adverse reactions, and nonadherence to therapy.[12] The effect of decreased kidney function on absorption, distribution, metabolism, and elimination of pharmacologic agents, in addition to the contribution of dialysis to drug removal, further complicates pharmacotherapy in this population (see Chapter 33, Dosing of Drugs in Renal Failure). Appropriate pharmacotherapeutic management includes choice of rational agents based on the indication, a regular comprehensive review of all medications, and frequent re-evaluation to adjust regimens relative to kidney function.

DIABETIC NEPHROPATHY

1. M.R. is a 32-year-old, Native American woman (weight, 63 kg; height, 5′8″) with a 15-year history of type 1 diabetes mellitus. She presents to the diabetes clinic with a 1-week history of nausea, vomiting, and general malaise. She has been noncompliant with regular appointments and her blood glucose has generally remained >200 mg/dL on prior evaluations, with a hemoglobin A1C of 9.1% (goal, <7%) 2 months ago. M.R. has been treated for peptic ulcer disease for the past 6 months. The workup reveals the following pertinent laboratory values: serum sodium (Na), 143 mEq/L (normal, 135–147 mEq/L); potassium (K), 5.3 mEq/L (normal, 3.5–5.0 mEq/L); chloride (Cl), 106 mEq/L (normal, 95–105 mEq/L); CO_2 content, 18 mEq/L (normal, 22–28 mEq/L); SrCr, 2.9 mg/dL (normal, 0.6–1.2 mg/dL); BUN, 63 mg/dL (normal, 8–18 mg/dL); and random blood glucose, 220 mg/dL (normal, 140 mg/dL). Physical examination revealed a BP of 155/102 mmHg, mild pulmonary congestion, and 2+ pedal edema. Additional laboratory studies show serum phosphate, 7.6 mg/dL (goal, 3.5–4.6 mg/dL); calcium (Ca), 8.8 mg/dL (goal, 8.4–9.5 mg/dL); magnesium (Mg), 2.8 mEq/L (normal, 1.6–2.4 mEq/L); and uric acid, 8.8 mg/dL (normal, 2.0–7.0 mg/dL). Hematologic studies show hematocrit (Hct), 26% (normal, 36%–46%); hemoglobin (Hgb), 8.7 g/dL (normal, 12–16 mg/dL); and white blood cell (WBC) count, 9,600/mm³ (normal, 3,200–9,800/mm³). Red blood cell (RBC) indices are normal. Platelet count is 175,000/mm³ (normal, 130,000–400,000/mm³). M.R.'s reticulocyte count is 2.0% (normal, 0.1%–2.4%). Her urinalysis (UA) showed 4+ proteinuria, later quantified as a urinary albumin of 700 mg/24 hrs (normal, <30 mg/day). What subjective and objective data in M.R. are consistent with a diagnosis of advanced kidney disease?

[SI units: Na, 143 mmol/L (normal, 135–147); K, 5.3 mmol/L (normal, 3.5–5.0); Cl, 106 mmol/L (normal, 95–105); CO_2, 18 mmol/L (normal, 22–28); SrCr, 256 μmol/L (normal, 50–110); BUN, 22 mmol/L of urea (normal, 3.0–6.5); glucose, 12.2 mmol/L (normal, <11 mmol/L); phosphate, 2.45 mmol/L (normal, 1.13–1.48); Ca, 2.2 mmol/L (normal, 2.1–2.38); Mg, 1.4 mmol/L (normal, 0.8–1.20); uric acid, 524 μmol/L (normal, 120–420); Hct, 0.26 (normal, 0.36–0.46); Hgb, 87 g/L (normal, 120–160); WBC count, 9,600 × 10^6 /L (normal, 3,200–9,800); platelet count, 175 × 10^9/L (normal, 130–400); reticulocyte count, 0.02 (normal, 0.001–0.024), urinary albumin, 0.7 g/day (normal, <0.03)]

M.R.'s abnormal values for SrCr, BUN, serum potassium, magnesium, phosphate, uric acid, CO_2 content, hemoglobin, and hematocrit are all consistent with kidney disease and its associated complications. Assuming relatively stable kidney function (i.e., no acute changes in kidney function), her eGFR is approximately 24 mL/minute/1.73 m² based on the MDRD equation, placing her in stage 4 CKD (eGFR 15–29 mL/minute/1.73 m²). As the eGFR declines to the degree observed in M.R., normal regulation of fluids and electrolytes is impaired. Elevations in SrCr, BUN, sodium, potassium, magnesium, phosphate, and uric acid as well as signs of fluid accumulation are observed. Although potassium is mildly elevated in M.R., overall potassium balance is usually maintained within the normal range until more severe kidney disease develops (i.e., eGFR <10 mL/minute/1.73 m²). The substantial degree of proteinuria observed in M.R. is consistent with more advanced glomerular damage. Volume overload from continued intake and decreased sodium and water excretion leads to weight gain (although likely not observed in M.R. because of her recent onset of nausea and vomiting), hypertension, congestive pulmonary disease, and edema. Metabolic acidosis results from impaired synthesis of ammonia by the kidney, which normally buffers hydrogen ions and facilitates acid excretion. Anemia associated with CKD is caused primarily by decreased erythropoietin production by the kidneys, but it also can be caused by increased bleeding from uremia and her peptic ulcer disease. M.R.'s recent onset of nausea, vomiting, and malaise may be a consequence of the accumulation of uremic toxins (azotemia) from the decline in kidney function, although such symptoms are generally associated with BUN values greater than that observed in M.R.

2. What is the cause of M.R.'s advanced kidney disease?

Based on M.R.'s presentation, her kidney disease is most likely caused by diabetic nephropathy from her 15-year history of type 1 diabetes mellitus. Her history of noncompliance with regular appointments, elevated blood glucose concentration, and high hemoglobin A1C values support poor control of diabetes and diabetic nephropathy as the primary etiology. Diabetic nephropathy rarely develops within the first 10 years after onset of type 1 diabetes. The annual incidence is greatest after approximately 20 years' duration of diabetes and declines thereafter.[66] ESRD develops in 50% of patients with type 1 diabetic within 10 years and in >75% of patients within 20 years.[66] M.R. fits this pattern in that she has diabetic nephropathy after a 15-year history of diabetes, although her nephropathy was likely evident several years previously. M.R. may also be at increased risk for developing ESRD because Native Americans have a higher risk of ESRD relative to non-Hispanic whites.[3]

Diabetic nephropathy is a microvascular complication of diabetes resulting in albuminuria and a progressive decline in kidney function. Diabetic nephropathy develops in approximately one-third of all patients with type 1 and type 2 diabetes, with a larger percentage of patients with type 1 diabetes developing ESRD. Because type 2 diabetes is more prevalent, however, these patients account for most of diabetic patients starting dialysis.[66] With the increased prevalence of diabetes and the increase in life expectancy of this population, it is likely that diabetic nephropathy will remain the leading cause of ESRD in the United States.[3,4] Whereas most research has focused on the pathophysiology, prevention, and treatment of diabetic nephropathy in type 1 diabetes, it is reasonable to extrapolate available evidence on prevention of diabetic nephropathy to the population with type 2 diabetes.

The exact mechanisms leading to the development of diabetic nephropathy are not clearly defined; however, several predictive factors for the development and progression of kidney damage have been identified. These include elevated BP, plasma glucose, glycosylated hemoglobin, and cholesterol; smoking; advanced age; male gender; and potentially, high protein intake.[67,68] Insulin deficiency and increased ketone bodies have also been proposed as contributors to the pathogenesis. Advanced glycosylation end products (AGE) that form in conditions of hyperglycemia have also been implicated as a cause of end organ damage. The accumulation of multiple AGE is associated with the severity of kidney disease in patients with diabetic nephropathy.[69] A genetic predisposition exists in that higher rates of diabetes and nephropathy, hypertension, cardiovascular events, albuminuria, and elevated BP have been observed in relatives of patients with type 2 diabetes.[67,70] Certain genes and polymorphisms have also been associated with the development of diabetic nephropathy, and further exploration into this area may prove beneficial in identifying high-risk patients.[71]

3. What is the significance of M.R.'s albuminuria?

Albuminuria, the earliest sign of kidney involvement in patients with diabetes mellitus, correlates with the rate of progression of kidney disease. For most patients, eGFR begins to decline once proteinuria is established. Because of this association, annual testing for the presence of microalbuminuria is indicated in patients who have had type 1 diabetes for more than 5 years and in all patients with type 2 diabetes starting at diagnosis.[72] The presence of albuminuria indicates irreversible kidney damage. M.R. has likely reached the point at which such damage is inevitable, because her urinary protein exceeds ranges normally observed at the earlier stages of kidney disease. M.R.'s current laboratory data suggest that she has substantial kidney disease and has developed associated complications of the disease. Although progression to ESRD is generally beyond prevention at this stage, appropriate intervention can extend the time period until M.R. will require dialysis therapy.

Management

4. How should M.R.'s kidney disease be managed?

Because reversal of M.R.'s kidney disease is unlikely, the primary goals are to delay the need for dialysis therapy as long as possible and to manage complications. The three main risk factors for the progression of incipient nephropathy to clinical diabetic nephropathy are poor glycemic control, systemic hypertension, and high dietary protein intake (>1.5 g/kg/day). M.R.'s current random blood glucose concentration of 220 mg/dL, history of elevated glucose on prior visits, and increased hemoglobin A1C indicate poorly controlled diabetes, which will accelerate progression of her diabetic nephropathy. Thus, her blood glucose concentrations need to be maintained within target concentrations while avoiding hypoglycemia. M.R.'s elevated BP is likely the result of kidney disease and changes in intravascular volume; reduction of BP may prevent further damage to functioning nephrons. Similarly, protein intake should be less liberal in an attempt to reduce the rate of further progression, although this needs to be evaluated in the context of her overall nutritional status.

Intensive Glucose Control

Strict glycemic control is clearly indicated to reduce proteinuria and to slow the rate of decline in eGFR.[66] The Diabetes Control and Complications Trial (DCCT) was a multicenter trial in 1,441 patients, which was designed to address how rigidly blood glucose concentrations should be controlled to reduce diabetic complications.[73] The DCCT evaluated the effect of intensive insulin treatment for type 1 diabetes on the development and progression of long-term complications, including diabetic nephropathy. Patients were randomized to receive either conventional insulin treatment (one to two insulin doses a day) or intensive treatment (three or more insulin doses a day). The goal of the intensive regimen was to maintain fasting blood glucose concentrations between 70 and 120 mg/dL, with postprandial blood glucose concentrations <180 mg/dL. After a mean follow-up of 6.5 years, the intensive insulin regimen reduced the overall risk of microalbuminuria (defined as urine albumin ≥40 mg/24 hours) by 39%, and albuminuria (defined as urine albumin ≥300 mg/24 hours) by 54%. Stricter glycemic control was associated with an increased incidence of hypoglycemic episodes, however.[73] The effect of intensive glycemic control has also been studied in patients with type 2 diabetes. Over a 10-year treatment period, glucose control with either insulin or an oral sulfonylurea reduced microvascular complications, including albuminuria, when compared with conventional dietary therapy.[74]

Based on this information and the need to minimize risk of hypoglycemia, the recommended goals in the adult diabetic population are a preprandial plasma glucose of 90 to 130 mg/dL, peak postprandial plasma glucose of <180 mg/dL, and an A1C <7%.[72] M.R. will benefit from intensive insulin therapy and achievement of these goals despite her advanced kidney disease. M.R. should be counseled on appropriate techniques for insulin administration and home glucose monitoring, particularly given her history of noncompliance. Compliance with this regimen will require motivation as well as encouragement from M.R.'s family and health care providers. (See Chapter 50, Diabetes Mellitus, for a more complete discussion of intensive insulin therapy and counseling.)

Antihypertensive Therapy

Systemic hypertension usually occurs with the development of microalbuminuria in patients with type 1 diabetes and is present in about one-third of patients at the time of diagnosis of type 2 diabetes. The coexistence of these disorders further increases the risk of cardiovascular events. Hypertension may be a result of underlying diabetic nephropathy and increased plasma volume or increased peripheral vascular resistance. Regardless of the etiology, virtually any level of untreated hypertension (either systemic or intraglomerular) is associated with a reduction in eGFR. As such, the control of systemic and intraglomerular BP is perhaps the single most important factor for retarding the progression of kidney disease and has been shown to increase life expectancy in patients with type 1 diabetes.[33]

Patients with diabetes and hypertension develop elevated systemic vascular resistance and increased vasoconstriction from angiotensin II, which are in large part responsible for the glomerular damage characteristic of diabetic nephropathy. Although the management of hypertension with virtually any agent can attenuate the progression of kidney disease, ACE inhibitors, which inhibit the synthesis of angiotensin II, and ARB, which block angiotensin II AT_1 receptors, are preferred owing, in part, to the effects of these agents on renal hemodynamics (Fig. 31-1). Reductions in proteinuria and a decreased rate of decline in eGFR have been observed with ACE inhibitors and ARB in patients with type 1 and type 2 diabetes (see also the Prevention section in Progressive Kidney Disease in this chapter).[33,38–40,45–50] As a result of these and other studies, ACE inhibitors or ARB should be considered for all patients with diabetes and microalbuminuria, even if their BP is normal.[66] Data comparing these two classes of agent are lacking. A recent trial compared the effects of the ARB, telmisartan, with the ACE inhibitor, enalapril, in patients with type 2 diabetes over 5 years. Conclusion was that the renoprotective effects of telmisartan were not inferior to enalapril, but a large dropout rate limits interpretation of the results. Additional trials may help clarify if one class of agents is superior to the other.[75]

The primary goal in M.R. is to delay development of ESRD and to reduce the risk of cardiovascular complications and death. Treatment with an ACE inhibitor, such as enalapril, should be initiated, because she has substantial albuminuria (700 mg/day) and an elevated BP. An ARB (e.g., losartan) is a reasonable alternative to an ACE inhibitor in patients with ACE inhibitor-induced cough or other adverse effects that do not cross-react with an ARB. The initial product selected is generally based on tolerance to therapy and cost. A goal BP for M.R., based on the fact that she has type 1 diabetes and kidney disease, is a BP $<130/80$ mmHg.[34,35] Because the beneficial effects of ACE inhibitor therapy occur over months to years, M.R. must be monitored on a long-term basis for changes in kidney function and albuminuria and for side effects of therapy, such as hyperkalemia. An increase in SrCr of up to 30% is acceptable with initiation of therapy with ACE inhibitors or ARB.[44] Contraindications for the use of ACE inhibitors and ARB include bilateral renal artery stenosis and pregnancy. The risk of hyperkalemia must also be weighed against the potential beneficial effects of these agents.

Some evidence suggests that a nondihydropyridine calcium channel blocker (e.g., diltiazem, verapamil) may be beneficial alone or in combination with an ACE inhibitor.[52,76,77] Diuretics may be considered for patients with diabetic nephropathy and edema, depending on their degree of kidney function. For patients with kidney disease as extensive as that observed in M.R. (eGFR <30 mL/minute/1.73 m^2), loop diuretics are generally preferred because, unlike thiazide diuretics, they may retain their effect at this reduced eGFR level (see Chapter 12, Fluid and Electrolyte Disorders and Chapter 13, Essential Hypertension). Other antihypertensive agents may be considered based on response to initial therapy and changes in kidney function. Currently, clinical studies are examining the use of the aldosterone blocker, spironolactone, and the selective aldosterone blocker, eplerenone, for use in patients with diabetic nephropathy and overt proteinuria on maximal doses of both an ACE inhibitor and an ARB. These agents have antiproteinuric effects, but the potential increase risk for hyperkalemia when adding these agents to patients already as an ACE inhibitor and ARB warrants further evaluated of their use. The effect on slowing of progression of kidney disease has not been evaluated with these agents.[78]

Dietary Protein Restriction

High protein consumption accelerates the progression of diabetic nephropathy, presumably because of increased glomerular hyperfiltration and intraglomerular pressure. In patients with overt albuminuria, some evidence indicates that the rate of decline in eGFR, as well as urinary albumin excretion, can be blunted by restricting protein intake to 0.6 to 0.8 g/kg/day and maintaining an isocaloric diet.[30,57] Limited evidence indicates, however, a beneficial role of dietary protein restriction in diabetic patients with microalbuminuria. Nonetheless, given the potential benefits to delay progression of kidney disease, M.R. should be advised to maintain an isocaloric diet with a protein intake of 0.8 g/kg/day ($\sim$10% of daily calories).[66] The decision to decrease this intake even further to 0.6 g/kg/day must be based on the rate of decline in eGFR and her nutritional status. Because the typical Western diet is high in protein, some patients may have difficulty complying with such a low-protein diet because of its perceived unpalatability. Intervention by a dietitian is recommended to design a feasible dietary regimen limited in protein, yet consistent with nutritional requirements in a diabetic patient.

FLUID AND ELECTROLYTE COMPLICATIONS

Sodium and Water Retention

5. Assess M.R.'s sodium and water balance. What interventions may be used to address this problem?

As illustrated in M.R., patients in the latter stages of CKD commonly retain sodium and water. This is supported by M.R.'s elevated BP, 2+ pedal edema, and mild pulmonary congestion. Sodium and water retention also lead to weight gain, although this may not be evident in M.R. because of volume loss from her recent onset of nausea and vomiting. Early in the course of CKD, glomerular and tubular adaptive processes develop, such as an increase in the fractional excretion of sodium (FE_{Na}). These mechanisms enable patients to maintain relatively normal sodium and water homeostasis. As M.R.'s normal serum sodium concentration indicates, this value is of little use in establishing the diagnosis of total body sodium and fluid excess because retention of sodium and water usually occurs in an isotonic fashion, leaving the serum sodium concentration relatively normal. Eventually, however, patients with advanced kidney dysfunction exhibit signs of sodium and fluid retention, because sodium balance is maintained at the expense of increased extracellular volume, which results in hypertension. Expansion of blood volume, if not controlled, can cause peripheral edema, heart failure, and pulmonary edema. Thus, management of sodium and water retention is essential. To achieve control, most patients with more advanced kidney disease will be placed on sodium restriction (~2 to 4 g/day) and fluid restriction (~2 L/day). These restrictions will depend on the current dietary intake, extent of volume overload, and urine output and should be altered according to the special needs of the patient. The primary consideration in CKD is that the kidney cannot adjust quickly to changes in sodium intake; therefore, any dietary intervention should be initiated gradually. Because M.R. has edema and hypertension, initial restriction of salt to 4 g/day, which is essentially a no-added-salt diet, is reasonable at this stage.

Because some patients with more advanced kidney disease produce normal amounts of urine, whereas others may produce less (or no urine if the patient has ESRD), fluid restrictions must be based on urine output. Diuretic therapy, usually with loop diuretics (e.g., furosemide, bumetanide, torsemide), is often required. Combination therapy with two different types of diuretics (i.e., loop and thiazide) may be successful in patients resistant to a single agent; however, limitations in efficacy of diuretics exist under certain conditions (e.g., a reduced eGFR and hypoalbuminemia), and these situations must be considered when designing a diuretic regimen. Thiazide diuretics as single agents are generally not effective when the eGFR is <30 mL/minute/1.73 m^2, as in M.R. The possible exception is use of the thiazidelike diuretic, metolazone, which may retain its effect at reduced eGFRs.[79] As kidney failure progresses, manifestations of excess fluid accumulation develop that are resistant to more conventional interventions, and dialysis will be required to control volume status.

Hyperkalemia

6. M.R. has a serum potassium concentration of 5.3 mEq/L. Describe the mechanisms by which potassium imbalance occurs in patients such as M.R. who have progressive CKD.

[SI unit: K, 5.3 mmol/L]

Hyperkalemia can result from a combination of factors, including diminished renal potassium excretion, redistribution of potassium into the extracellular fluid owing to metabolic acidosis, and excessive potassium intake. In M.R., all these mechanisms are likely to be contributing to hyperkalemia, although in the short-term dietary intake of potassium may not be substantial because of her recent onset of nausea and vomiting.

Potassium normally is filtered at the glomerulus and undergoes nearly complete reabsorption throughout the renal tubule. Distal tubular secretion is the primary mechanism by which potassium is excreted in the urine. A variety of factors affect this distal secretion of potassium, including aldosterone, sodium load presented to the distal reabsorptive site, hydrogen ion secretion, the amount of nonresorbable anions, urinary flow rate, diuretics, mineralocorticoids, and potassium intake.[80] Serum potassium concentrations are relatively well maintained within normal limits in patients with CKD. At eGFR >10 mL/minute/1.73m^2 hyperkalemia is rare without an endogenous or exogenous load of potassium. This balance is maintained despite a decreasing nephron population and an overall drop in eGFR, because the remaining nephrons undergo adaptive changes to enhance the distal tubular secretion of potassium per nephron (i.e., increased fractional excretion of potassium, FE_K).[81] Gastrointestinal (GI) excretion of potassium is also important because increased GI excretion and fecal losses may account for up to 50% of the daily potassium loss in patients with severe kidney disease. M.R.'s eGFR of 24 mL/minute/1.73 m^2 is above the "threshold" value for adequate potassium homeostasis. M.R. should be carefully observed for manifestations of hyperkalemia as her kidney disease progresses.

Additional factors that alter potassium homeostasis include metabolic or respiratory acidosis. Acidotic conditions can cause a redistribution of intracellular potassium to the extracellular fluid. M.R. has metabolic acidosis as indicated by a serum bicarbonate of 18 mEq/L. This condition may account for her mildly elevated potassium concentration. Correction of metabolic acidosis could lower her potassium concentration. For each 0.1-unit change in blood pH, an average corresponding opposite change of approximately 0.6 mEq/L in the serum potassium concentration occurs (see Chapter 10, Acid-Base Disorders).

M.R. is not taking any drugs that could contribute to hyperkalemia, although the influence of ACE inhibitors and ARB must be considered because they are now advocated for M.R. to delay progression of kidney disease. Potassium-sparing diuretics, such as spironolactone (Aldactone), triamterene (Dyrenium), and amiloride (Midamor), should be avoided in patients with severe CKD because they decrease tubular secretion of potassium. Some diabetic patients with only mild degrees of kidney disease develop hyperkalemia from these diuretics because they have low plasma renin activity and, as a result, lower aldosterone concentrations.

7. Is treatment of M.R.'s potassium indicated? How should severe hyperkalemia be managed?

Treatment of hyperkalemia depends on the serum concentration of potassium as well as the presence or absence of symptoms and electrocardiographic (ECG) changes. Manifestations of hyperkalemia include weakness, confusion, and muscular or respiratory paralysis. These symptoms may be absent, however, especially if hyperkalemia develops rapidly. Early ECG changes include peaked T waves, followed by a decreased R-wave amplitude, widened QRS complex, and a prolonged PR interval. These changes may progress to complete heart block with absent P waves and, finally, a sine wave. Ventricular arrhythmias or cardiac arrest may ensue if no effort to lower serum potassium is initiated. Hyperkalemic ECG changes are uncommon at potassium concentrations of <7 mEq/L, but occur regularly at concentrations >8 mEq/L.

M.R. has a mild elevation in potassium to 5.3 mEq/L; therefore, no specific treatment is required. Generally, treatment is unnecessary if the potassium concentration is <6.5 mEq/L and there are no ECG changes. Although this serum potassium concentration does not require immediate intervention, close monitoring for hyperkalemia and its manifestations is necessary. This would be particularly important after starting ACE inhibitor therapy, which can contribute to development of hyperkalemia by decreasing aldosterone production. If potassium concentrations rise above 6.5 mEq/L, and especially if they are accompanied by neuromuscular symptoms or changes in the ECG, treatment should be instituted.

Goals of therapy include prevention of adverse events related to excessive potassium and reduction of serum potassium concentrations to a relatively normal range (4.5–5.5 mEq/L). Chronic management involves prevention of hyperkalemia by limiting potassium intake and avoiding the use of agents that could elevate potassium levels. This requires regular monitoring of potassium concentrations. Acute management involves reversal of cardiac effects with calcium administration and reduction of serum potassium. The latter can be achieved by shifting potassium intracellularly with administration of glucose and insulin, β-adrenergic agonists, or alkali therapy (if metabolic acidosis is a contributing factor) and by removing potassium using exchange resins or dialysis (see Chapter 11, Fluid and Electrolyte Disorders).

Metabolic Acidosis

8. Assess M.R.'s acid-base status. How should her acid-base disorder be managed?

M.R.'s low blood CO_2 content and high chloride concentration are consistent with metabolic acidosis. Normal buffering of hydrogen ions by the bicarbonate and carbonic acid system as well as other extracellular and intracellular buffers, including proteins, phosphates, and hemoglobin, is essential for maintaining normal acid-base balance (i.e., normal pH). Normal metabolism of ingested food produces approximately 1 mEq/kg of metabolic acid daily, which must be excreted by the kidneys (primarily as ammonium ion) to maintain acid-base balance. The kidney is responsible for reabsorption of bicarbonate and excretion of hydrogen ions through buffering by ammonia (produced by the kidney) and filtered phosphates. Reduced bicarbonate reabsorption and impaired production of ammonia by the kidneys are the major factors responsible for development of metabolic acidosis in advanced kidney disease. As nephron function declines, production of ammonia is increased to compensate for a decrease in secretion of hydrogen ions; however, once the maximal capacity for ammonia production is reached, acidosis develops. Mild hyperchloremia is generally observed in the earlier stages. As kidney disease progresses, metabolic acidosis with an elevated anion gap is observed owing to accumulation of organic acids (see Chapter 10, Acid-Base Disorders). Bone carbonate stores serve as a source of alkali, but over time cannot compensate for changes in acid-base balance. Metabolic acidosis can contribute to bone disease by promoting bone resorption, and it may also influence nutritional status by decreasing albumin synthesis and promoting a negative nitrogen balance.[82]

M.R.'s mild acidosis should be treated with a goal of normalizing the plasma bicarbonate concentration or at least achieving bicarbonate levels near $\geq$ 22 mEq/L. Treatment includes use of preparations containing sodium bicarbonate or sodium citrate. Each 650-mg tablet of sodium bicarbonate provides 8 mEq of sodium and 8 mEq of bicarbonate. Shohl's solution and Bicitra contain 1 mEq of sodium and the amount of citrate or citric acid to provide 1 mEq of bicarbonate/mL. These latter agents may be used in patients who experience excessive GI distress with sodium bicarbonate from production and elimination of carbon dioxide. If a patient such as M.R. is sodium and fluid overloaded, it is important to consider that sodium bicarbonate can exacerbate this problem. Polycitra, or potassium citrate, is a possible alternative; however, the potassium content limits its use in patients with more severe kidney disease. Citrate also promotes aluminum absorption and should not be used in patients taking aluminum-containing agents. The NKF-K/DOQI guidelines do not give an exact recommendation of the amount of bicarbonate supplementation to achieve a bicarbonate $\geq$22 mEq/L. The use of two to four 650-mg sodium bicarbonate tablets per day, usually divided into two to three doses, is a typical regimen used to correct metabolic acidosis. Equations based on the serum bicarbonate level are available if an immediate correction of the metabolic acidosis is warranted.[83]

Once dialysis therapy is initiated in patients with kidney disease, IV and oral supplementation with bicarbonate or citrate or citric acid preparations is generally not required. At this point, dialysis therapy is used to chronically manage metabolic acidosis through use of dialysate baths containing bicarbonate. Bicarbonate is added to the dialysate solution and is delivered through the process of diffusion from the dialysate bath into the plasma (see Chapter 32, Renal Dialysis). If dialysis therapy is initiated in M.R., the continued need for oral bicarbonate supplementation should be reassessed.

Other Electrolyte and Metabolic Disturbances of Chronic Kidney Disease

9. What other electrolyte and metabolic disturbances are exhibited by M.R.?

The mild degree of hypermagnesemia seen in M.R. is a common finding in patients with CKD owing to decreased elimination of magnesium by the kidney. Magnesium is eliminated by the kidney to the extent required to achieve normal serum magnesium concentrations until eGFR is $<$30 mL/minute/1.73 m^2. Serum magnesium concentrations $<$5 mEq/L rarely cause symptoms. Higher concentrations can lead to nausea, vomiting, lethargy, confusion, and diminished tendon reflexes, whereas severe hypermagnesemia may depress cardiac conduction. The risk of hypermagnesemia can be reduced by avoiding magnesium-containing antacids and laxatives and by use of magnesium-free dialysate in patients with stage 5 CKD requiring dialysis.

M.R.'s hyperphosphatemia is a result of decreased phosphorus elimination by the kidneys (see Question 17 for a more detailed discussion of hyperphosphatemia). Based on the NKF-K/DOQI guidelines for bone metabolism, patients should reduce dietary phosphorus to 800 to 1,000 mg/day while maintaining adequate nutritional needs.[84] Phosphorus-containing laxatives and enemas should also be avoided. Hyperphosphatemia is associated with low serum calcium concentrations, not a current finding in M.R.

M.R. also has mild hyperuricemia. Asymptomatic hyperuricemia frequently develops in patients with kidney disease owing to diminished urinary excretion of uric acid. In the absence of a history of gout or urate nephropathy, asymptomatic hyperuricemia does not require treatment.

ANEMIA OF CHRONIC KIDNEY DISEASE

10. What findings in M.R. are consistent with the diagnosis of anemia of CKD, and what is the etiology of this disorder?

M.R.'s hemoglobin of 8.7 g/dL and hematocrit of 26% are substantially lower than the normal range for premenopausal females (hemoglobin, 12–16 g/dL; hematocrit, 36%–46%) indicating that she has anemia.[85] Her normal RBC indices suggest her red cells are of normal size, but the absence of an elevated reticulocyte count suggests an impaired bone marrow response for her degree of anemia. Her recent history of peptic ulcer disease may also have contributed to the observed drop in hemoglobin and hematocrit as a result of blood loss. Her complaint of general malaise is consistent with the symptoms of anemia.

Characteristics and Etiology

Anemia, which affects most patients with CKD, is caused by a decreased production of erythropoietin (EPO), a glycoprotein that stimulates red blood cell production in the bone marrow and is released in response to hypoxia. Approximately 90% of the total EPO is produced in the peritubular cells of the kidney; the remainder is produced by the liver. EPO concentrations in patients with kidney failure are lower than in individuals with normal kidney function who have the same degree of anemia and, therefore, the same stimulus for EPO production and release.[86]

Anemia appears as early as stage 3 CKD and is characterized by normochromic (normal color) and normocytic (normal size) red blood cells unless a concomitant iron, folate, or B_{12} deficiency exists. A direct correlation between eGFR and hematocrit has been demonstrated with a 3.1% decrease in hematocrit for every 10 mL/minute/1.73 m^2 decline in eGFR.[87] A higher prevalence of anemia occurs in the population with an eGFR <60 mL/minute/1.73 m^2.[1] Pallor and fatigue are the earliest clinical signs, with other manifestations developing as anemia worsens progressively with declining kidney function. A significant consequence of anemia is development of left ventricular hypertrophy (LVH), further contributing to cardiovascular complications and mortality in patients with CKD. LVH has been observed in approximately 30% of patients with eGFR 50 to 75 mL/minute/1.73 m^2 (stages 2 and 3 CKD) and in up to 74% of patients at the start of dialysis (stage 5 CKD).[88,89] These findings support the need for early and aggressive treatment of anemia of CKD before the development of stage 5 CKD.

A more complete workup for anemia of CKD is recommended for patients with an eGFR of <60 mL/minute/1.73 m^2.[1,85] This workup includes monitoring of hemoglobin and hematocrit, assessment of iron indices with correction if iron deficiency is present, and evaluation for sources of blood loss, such as bleeding from the GI tract. This workup should be done regularly as CKD progresses because of the association between anemia and the progressive decline in eGFR.

As discussed later in this chapter (see Question 12), the availability of recombinant human EPO to directly stimulate erythrocyte production revolutionized the treatment of CKD-associated anemia. However, iron deficiency is the leading cause of erythropoiesis stimulating agent (ESA) hyporesponsiveness and must be corrected before ESA therapy is initiated (see Question 12 for Iron Therapy). Iron deficiency can develop as a result of increased requirements for RBC production with ESA administration and from chronic blood loss owing to bleeding or hemodialysis. Identification and management of iron deficiency through regular follow-up testing and iron supplementation is essential for adequate RBC production (see Question 12 for Iron Therapy and also Chapter 86, Anemias).[85] M.R.'s iron status should be assessed at this time to determine if iron supplementation is needed.

Other factors that contribute to anemia include a shortened RBC life span secondary to uremia, blood loss from frequent phlebotomy and HD, GI bleeding, severe hyperparathyroidism, protein malnutrition, accumulation of aluminum, severe infections, and inflammatory conditions.[85] Substances present in the plasma of patients with CKD, collectively termed "uremic toxins," may inhibit the production of EPO, the bone marrow response to EPO, and the synthesis of heme. The negative effects of these substances on RBC production are supported by improvement in erythropoiesis with dialysis, which removes these uremic toxins. This uremic environment also causes a decrease in the RBC life span, from a normal life span of 120 days to approximately 60 days in patients with severe CKD. A shortened RBC life span has been observed in uremic patients transfused with RBC from individuals with normal kidney function, whereas RBC from uremic individuals have a normal survival time when transfused into patients without kidney failure.[90]

Blood loss also contributes to anemia of CKD, particularly in patients requiring HD. With each HD session, generally performed three times per week, blood loss occurs. In addition, these patients are usually administered heparin during dialysis or antiplatelet drugs to prevent vascular access clotting, which further increases the risk of bleeding. Although a stool guaiac test was not performed in M.R., many patients with uremia and CKD will have a positive guaiac reaction because of the risk of bleeding from uremia itself. M.R. also has a peptic ulcer, which increases her potential for blood loss.

Other deficiencies can contribute to anemia of CKD. Deficiency of folic acid, as evidenced by low serum folate concentrations and macrocytosis, is relatively uncommon in patients with early kidney disease, but occurs most often in patients on dialysis, because folic acid is removed by dialysis. Therefore, the daily prophylactic administration of the water-soluble vitamins, including 1 mg of folic acid, is recommended. Routine use of the fat-soluble vitamin A is discouraged, because hypervitaminosis A may develop, contributing to anemia.[91] Several multivitamin preparations devoid of vitamin A (e.g., Nephrocaps) are available for patients with kidney failure. Pyridoxine (vitamin B_6) deficiency can also occur in both dialyzed and nondialyzed patients with CKD. Significant similarities are seen between this deficiency and the symptoms of uremia, which include skin hyperpigmentation and peripheral neuropathy. Current multivitamin products for patients with stage 5 CKD contain adequate amounts of pyridoxine to prevent deficiency.

Goals of Therapy

11. What are the goals of therapy for anemia of CKD in M.R.?

Target Hemoglobin and Hematocrit

NKF-K/DOQI guidelines recommend a target of ≥11 g/dL for hemoglobin (≥33% for hematocrit) in patients with CKD receiving ESA therapy.[85] It is at these targets that benefits such as increased survival, exercise capacity, quality of life, cardiac output, cognitive function, and decreased risk of LVH were observed in the CKD population.[85] Routine maintenance of hemoglobin levels ≥13 g/dL (≥39% for hematocrit) is not recommended for patients being treated with ESA secondary to increased risk for mortality and for serious cardiovascular and thromboembolic events. Two recent trials evaluated the efficacy and safety of hemoglobin targets in patients with CKD not on HD. These trials showed no benefit on left ventricular mass index. In one study, increased mortality rates were observed in the high target hemoglobin group. Likely this is based on these recent data that the target hemoglobin will be restricted to a more narrow range in the future.[92,93]

Hemoglobin, rather than hematocrits, should be used to evaluate anemia in this population for several reasons. Hematocrit is dependent on volume status, which can be problematic for patients with fluctuations in plasma water (e.g., dialysis, volume overload). In addition, a number of variables can affect the hematocrit value, including temperature, hyperglycemia, the size of the red blood cell, and the counters used for the test. These variables do not significantly affect hemoglobin, making it the preferred test for anemia.[85]

Once M.R.'s iron status is evaluated, and corrected if necessary, ESA therapy may be started (see Treatment below).

Iron Status

Because iron deficiency is the primary cause of ESA-hyporesponsiveness, assessment of iron status is essential before initiating erythropoietic therapy. The two tests that best evaluate iron status are the transferrin saturation percent (TSAT), a measure of iron immediately available for erythropoiesis, and serum ferritin, a measure of storage iron.[85] Transferrin is a carrier protein and its concentration depends on nutritional status. The TSAT indicates the saturation of the protein transferrin with iron and is determined as:

$$\frac{\%\,\text{TSat} = \text{serum iron (mcg/dL)}}{\text{TIBC (mcg/dL)}} \times 100 \qquad \textbf{(31-4)}$$

where TIBC is the total iron-binding capacity of the transferrin protein. Serum ferritin is a marker for iron reserves, which are stored primarily in the reticuloendothelial system (e.g., liver, spleen). The goal of iron replacement therapy is to maintain the TSAT >20% and a serum ferritin >100 ng/mL for CKD stages 2 through 4 and >200 ng/mL for CKD stage 5 to provide sufficient iron for erythrocyte production.[85] Values below these targets are indicative of absolute iron deficiency. A functional iron deficiency may exist when ferritin is >500 ng/mL, TSAT is <20%, and anemia persists despite appropriate ESA therapy. In these cases, iron supplementation may lead to improved erythropoiesis. Other tests, including the percentage of hypochromic red cells, reticulocyte hemoglobin content, serum transferrin receptor, red cell ferritin, and zinc protoporphyrin, have been proposed as indicators of iron status.[85] Although some of these markers have demonstrated predictive value in assessing iron status, either alone or in conjunction with other laboratory data, further investigation is warranted to determine their utility and to make such testing procedures readily available.

Treatment

12. Describe the options available to treat anemia of CKD and achieve the goals of therapy in M.R.

Iron Therapy

Before initiating ESA therapy, M.R.'s iron indices should be determined. If M.R. is iron deficient, as indicated by the TSAT and serum ferritin and other supporting laboratory data (see Chapter 86, Anemias), supplemental iron therapy should be administered. If iron deficiency is the cause of anemia, M.R. may benefit from iron supplementation alone (i.e., without erythropoietic therapy) to increase hemoglobin and hematocrit. Peptic ulcer disease will need to be evaluated as a source of blood loss. Given the poor bioavailability of oral iron and patient noncompliance, oral iron is usually inadequate for repletion of iron in patients receiving HD who experience chronic blood loss.[94] For the population with early CKD and for patients receiving peritoneal dialysis, an initial trial of oral iron may correct the deficiency because these patients do not have the same degree of blood loss. For some patients, however, IV therapy will be required to replete iron and meet the increased demands once erythropoiesis is stimulated with ESA therapy. Administration of IV iron requires IV access and frequent outpatient visits, which are drawbacks to therapy with IV iron in CKD stage 3 and 4. A recent trial examined an accelerated dosing regimen (500 mg given on two consecutive days) of IV iron sucrose to address these issues. This regimen was adequate to restore iron stores with only two patients experiencing hypotension related to iron therapy.[95]

Common infusion-related effects associated with IV iron include hypotension, myalgias, and arthralgias. Despite the controversy over the best strategy for iron supplementation in patients with early CKD, current recommendations support reserving IV iron for patients in whom oral iron has failed.[96] Therefore, a trial of oral iron is reasonable for M.R. Oral iron supplementation with 200 mg/day of elemental iron should be started to address iron deficiency, if present, and this regimen should be continued to maintain sufficient iron status while receiving ESA therapy. Many oral iron preparations are available, and their iron content varies as will the number of tablets or capsules that must be taken per day to provide the required elemental iron (Table 31-4). Some oral formulations include

Table 31-4 Oral Iron Preparations

Preparation	*Common Brand Names*	*Commonly Prescribed Unit Size (Amount Elemental Iron in mg)*	*Number of Units/Day to Yield 200 mg Elemental Iron*
Ferrous sulfate	Slow FE, Fer-In-Sol	325 (65)	3 tablets
Ferrous gluconate	Feratab	325 (36)	5 tablets
Ferrous fumarate	Femiron, Feostat	200 (66)	3 capsules
Iron polysaccharide	Niferex, Nu-Iron	150 (150)	2 capsules
Heme iron polypeptide	Proferrin-ES Proferrin-Forte	12 (12)	17 tablets

[a] Unit size reflects common tablet/capsule sizes prescribed and not necessarily that of the brand names listed.

ascorbic acid to enhance iron absorption. A heme iron product, Proferrin-ES, has recently been approved. Heme iron is more readily absorbed; however, a large number of tablets are required to supply the 200 mg elemental iron (Table 31-4). M.R. should be advised to take oral iron on an empty stomach to maximize absorption, unless side effects prevent this strategy. She also should be counseled on potential drug interactions with oral iron (e.g., antacids, quinolones) and GI side effects (e.g., nausea, abdominal pain, diarrhea, constipation, dark stools). Noncompliance with therapy is a primary cause of therapeutic failure with oral iron.

If M.R.'s condition does not respond to oral therapy, as indicated by either persistent iron deficiency based on iron indices, or inadequate response to what is considered an adequate dose and duration of erythropoietic therapy, IV iron is necessary. The IV iron preparations currently available are iron dextran (InFeD, DexFerrum), sodium ferric gluconate complex in sucrose (Ferrlecit), and iron sucrose (Venofer). The dextran products have caused anaphylactic reactions and, as a result, have a FDA mandated black box warning that requires administration of a 25 mg test dose followed by a 1-hour observation period before the total dose of iron is infused.[97] The dextran component is believed to be the cause of such reactions. The dose of IV iron recommended to correct absolute iron deficiency is a total dose of 1 g administered in divided doses or over a prolonged period to minimize the risk of adverse effects.[85] For iron dextran, the approved dose is 100 mg increments, administered over 10 dialysis sessions for patients on HD to provide a total of 1 g.[97] Larger doses of 500 mg up to the total 1-g dose have been safely administered over a longer infusion period of 4 to 6 hours.[85,96]

Sodium ferric gluconate and iron sucrose are the most widely used iron products in the CKD population. Both the ferric gluconate and iron sucrose products have been used successfully in patients who have experienced allergic reactions to the dextran products and evidence indicates that they are safer: 8.7 adverse events per million doses for dextran versus 3.3 adverse events for gluconate.[98] To provide the recommended total dose of 1 g, ferric gluconate is administered as 125 mg (10 mL) over eight consecutive dialysis sessions for patients on HD. The dose can be administered as a slow IV injection at a rate of up to 12.5 mg/minute or diluted in 100 mL of normal saline and infused over 1 hour.[99] Administration of 125 mg over 10 minutes (without a test dose) was determined to be a safer alternative to dextran preparations in patients on HD and is an approved dosing strategy.[99,100] Doses up to 250 mg over 1 hour have been administered safely.[101] The flexibility of administering larger doses of iron is an important factor in achieving efficiencies in the outpatient setting for patients with early CKD and those receiving PD.

Iron sucrose (Venofer) is a polynuclear iron hydroxide sucrose complex. The recommended dose of iron sucrose is 100 mg (5 mL) over 10 consecutive HD sessions to provide the total dose of 1 g.[102] The dose can be administered by a slow IV injection over 5 minutes or diluted in 100 mL of normal saline and infused over at least 15 minutes. As with sodium ferric gluconate, a test dose is not required. Iron sucrose doses of 250 to 300 mg have been safely administered over 1 hour and found to be as effective as sodium ferric gluconate administration in maintaining hemoglobin in patients receiving epoetin.[103]

Smaller doses of IV iron, in increments of 25 to 200 mg, can be administered on a weekly, every 2 week, or a monthly basis, to patients without absolute iron deficiency. These doses will sustain adequate iron stores, maintain target hemoglobin values, and potentially reduce the required dose of the erythropoietic agent.[85,104] This regimen is most convenient for patients on HD who have regular IV access and increased iron needs because of chronic blood loss. Maintenance iron therapy replaces these losses and minimizes the need for the more aggressive 1-g total doses of IV iron required for absolute iron deficiency. If HD is started in M.R. in the future, regular dosing of IV iron during dialysis is the most reasonable way to maintain adequate iron required for sustained erythropoiesis. Iron indices should be monitored at least every 3 months to guide IV iron therapy. Targeting a ferritin of $\geq$500 ng/mL is not routinely recommended because of the lack of evidence available.[85] A recent study evaluated the response to iron therapy in patients with elevated ferritin (500–1,200 ng/mL) and a low TSAT ($\leq$25%) found that administration of IV iron resulted in a statistically significant increase in Hgb levels and a faster Hgb response in patients receiving ESA therapy.[105] This strategy, however, could lead to increased exposure to free iron, which may place the patient at an increase risk of adverse effects (e.g., inflammation, oxidative stress).[106]

Ferumoxytol, a semisynthetic carbohyrdrate-coated, magnetic iron oxide preparation, is in phase III clinical trials for use in patients with CKD requiring iron supplementation. A potential advantage of ferumoxytol is that higher doses can be safely administered over a shorter period (17 seconds). There is also a proposed reduced immunologic sensitivity, resulting in less risk for anaphylactic type reactions compared with the other available high molecular weight IV iron products (e.g., iron dextran).[107]

Erythropoiesis Stimulating Agent (ESA) Therapy

Recombinant human EPO is the primary treatment option for patients such as M.R. with anemia of CKD. Regular dialysis may improve an anemic condition, but it will not restore the hemoglobin and hematocrit concentrations to normal because the primary cause of anemia is reduced EPO production by the kidneys. Although blood transfusions were once the mainstay of treatment, they are now avoided, if possible, because they are associated with a risk for viral diseases (hepatitis, human immunodeficiency virus [HIV]), iron overload, and further suppression of erythropoiesis. Transfusions may be required in certain patients with substantially low oxygen-carrying capacity, substantial blood loss, and in those patients exhibiting persistent symptoms of anemia (fatigue, dyspnea on exertion, tachycardia). M.R. is currently not a candidate for transfusions based on her hemoglobin of 8.7 g/dL (hematocrit 26%) and the absence of significant symptoms on presentation. Androgens were previously used to treat the anemia of CKD because they directly or indirectly raise EPO concentrations. Their routine use is not recommended, however, because the erythropoietic response is inconsistent, they cause many adverse effects, and recombinant EPO is now available.

HUMAN ERYTHROPOETIN-EPOETIN ALFA

Human erythropoietin or epoetin, the exogenous form of EPO, is produced using recombinant technology. Epoetin alfa is available in the United States, whereas epoetin beta is available primarily outside the United States. Since it became available in 1989, epoetin alfa (Epogen, Procrit) has provided an effective treatment option for anemia and has substantially decreased the need for RBC transfusions. Epoetin alfa stimulates the proliferation and differentiation of erythroid progenitor cells, increases hemoglobin synthesis, and accelerates the release of reticulocytes from the bone marrow.

For patients such as M.R. who do not yet require dialysis and for patients receiving PD, epoetin alfa is generally administered by subcutaneous (SC) injection. However, patients on HD often receive epoetin alfa by IV administration because easy IV access is established. According to the NKF-K/DOQI guidelines for anemia management, SC administration is preferred because lower doses can be administered less frequently and cost is lower than with IV administration.[85,108] Starting doses for SC administration are 80 to 120 U/kg/wk (~6,000 U/wk), whereas IV starting doses are 120 to 180 U/kg/wk (~9,000 U/wk). Based on the half-life of epoetin alfa (8.5 hours IV, 24.4 hours SC), the total weekly dose is usually divided into smaller doses, administered one to three times per week with SC administration and three times per week for IV administration in patients on HD.[109] For patients being converted from IV to SC administration whose hemoglobin is within the target range, the SC dose is usually two-thirds the IV dose.[85] For patients not yet at the target hemoglobin, a SC dose equivalent to the IV dose is recommended. Patients receiving epoetin alfa SC should be instructed on the appropriate administration technique, which includes rotating the sites for injection (e.g., upper arm, thigh, abdomen).

Extended dosing intervals for SC administration of epoetin alfa have been evaluated in patients with CKD who are not having dialysis.[108,109] Doses of 10,000 U once weekly to 40,000 U once every 4 weeks have been shown to maintain target hemoglobin values for those patients with CKD not on dialysis.[110,111] Such dosing strategies may provide more convenient therapy for these patients who are not yet on dialysis, but must come to the clinic for erythropoietic therapy.

DARBEPOETIN ALFA

Darbepoetin alfa (Aranesp) was approved in 2001 for the treatment of anemia of CKD, whether or not the patient requires dialysis. Darbepoetin is a hyperglycosylated analog of epoetin alfa that stimulates erythropoiesis by the same mechanism. Instead of the three N-linked carbohydrate chains on epoetin alfa, darbepoetin has five, which increase the capacity for sialic acid residue binding on the protein. The increased protein binding slows total body clearance and increases the terminal half-life to 25.3 hours and 48.8 hours following IV and SC administration, respectively. Darbepoetin alfa's longer half-life relative to epoetin alfa offers the potential advantage of less frequent dosing to maintain target hemoglobin values.

Studies in patients with early CKD (stages 3 and 4) determined that starting SC doses of 0.45 mcg/kg administered once per week and 0.75 mcg/kg once every other week were effective in achieving target hemoglobin and hematocrit values in patients who had not previously received erythropoietic therapy.[112] In patients on dialysis converted from epoetin alfa to darbepoetin alfa (IV and SC), darbepoetin maintained target hemoglobin values when administered less frequently (i.e., one dose every week in patients previously receiving epoetin alfa three times per week and one dose every other week in patients previously receiving epoetin once weekly).[113,114]

Table 31-5 Estimated Darbepoetin Alfa Starting Doses Based on Previous Epoetin Alfa Dose

Previous Weekly Epoetin Alfa Dose[a,b] *(<2,500 U/wk)*	*Weekly Darbepoetin Alfa Dose (6.25 –mcg/wk)*
2,500–4,999	12.5
5,000–10,999	25
11,000–17,999	40
18,000–33,999	60
34,000–89,999	100
≥90,000	200

[a] Darbepoetin alfa should be administered weekly for patients receiving epoetin alfa two or three times per week and every other week for patients receiving epoetin alfa once per week.

[b] For patients requiring darbepoetin alfa every other week, the weekly dose of epoetin alfa should be multiplied by 2 and this dose used in the conversion chart to determine the appropriate darbepoetin alfa dose.

Adapted from Aranesp [darbepoetin alfa] package insert. Thousand Oaks, CA: Amgen Inc.; July 19, 2002, with permission.

The approved starting dose of darbepoetin alfa in patients who have not previously received epoetin therapy is 0.45 mcg/kg given either IV or SC once weekly.[115] Patients who are already receiving epoetin therapy may be converted to darbepoetin alfa based on the current total weekly epoetin dose (Table 31-5).[115] For patients currently receiving epoetin alfa two to three times per week, darbepoetin alfa may be administered once weekly. Patients who are receiving epoetin alfa once weekly should receive darbepoetin alfa once every 2 weeks. To calculate the once every 2-week darbepoetin dose, the weekly epoetin alfa dose should be multiplied by 2 and that value used in column 1 of Table 31-5 to find the corresponding darbopoetin dose from column two in Table 31-5. For example, a patient receiving epoetin 6,000 U/wk should receive 40 mcg of darbepoetin alfa once every 2 weeks (6,000 U epoetin × 2 = 12,000 U, which corresponds to a weekly darbepoetin dose of 40 mcg).[115]

Epoetin alfa and darbepoetin alfa are generally well tolerated, with hypertension being the most common adverse event reported. Although elevated BP is not uniformly considered a contraindication to therapy, BP should be monitored closely so that changes in antihypertensive therapy and the dialysis prescription are made, if justified. Failure to elicit a response to erythropoietic therapy requires evaluation of factors that cause resistance, such as iron deficiency, infection, inflammation, chronic blood loss, aluminum toxicity, malnutrition, and hyperparathyroidism. Resistance to erythropoietic therapy has been observed in patients receiving ACE inhibitors, although data are conflicting.[116,117] Rare cases of antibody formation to epoetin therapy have been reported.[118] Neutralizing anti-EPO antibodies were identified in 13 patients with pure red-cell aplasia who required blood transfusions after a course of therapy with epoetin alfa or beta.[118] Similar cases have been reported, primarily with one epoetin alfa product manufactured outside the United States, Eprex. Some evidence supports cross-reactivity of these antibodies with darbepoetin, although the information is currently limited.[119] Although the clinical implications of antibody formation in patients receiving erythropoietic therapy are uncertain, clinicians should be aware of these reports when evaluating response to therapy.

Treatment of M.R.'s anemia must be initiated, given the chronic nature of her kidney disease and her current hemoglobin and hematocrit. Patients with hemoglobin values <11 g/dL (hematocrit, <33%), such as M.R., are the best candidates for erythropoietic therapy. It is also important to identify and correct any iron or folate deficiency and perform a stool guaiac test to rule out active GI bleeding. Iron supplementation is indicated, not only if M.R. is iron deficient, but also to maintain iron status while receiving erythropoietic therapy (see section on iron therapy). Although administration of iron alone may improve her anemia, epoetin alfa or darbepoetin alfa will likely be required, based on the severity of her anemia and the progressive nature of her kidney disease. M.R. may start epoetin alfa at a dose of 6,000 U (~100 units/kg) administered SC once per week or divided into two weekly doses of 3,000 U, assuming her iron status is appropriate (see section on iron status). Another option would be darbepoetin alfa administered at a dose of 25 mcg (0.45 mcg/kg) SC once per week. She also should be instructed on how to administer SC epoetin alfa or darbepoetin alfa. Dose adjustments should not be made more frequently than once every 4 to 6 weeks for either agent because of the time course for response (i.e., the pharmacodynamic effects on RBC homeostasis). The time it takes to reach a new steady-state, when RBC production is equal to RBC destruction, depends on the life span of the red cell, which is approximately 60 days in patients with kidney failure. Therefore, it will take approximately 2 to 3 months to reach a plateau in measured hemoglobin/hematocrit. Dose adjustments should be made based on M.R.'s hemoglobin and hematocrit, which should be monitored every 1 to 2 weeks after initiation of therapy or following a dose change. If a rapid increase in hemoglobin/hematocrit is observed (hemoglobin >1.0 g/dL, hematocrit >3%–4%, over a 1- to 2-week period) or the target hemoglobin/hematocrit is exceeded, then doses of either agent should be decreased by approximately 25%. If response is inadequate (hemoglobin increase <1 g/dL, hematocrit increase <2%–3%, in 2 to 4 weeks), then the doses should be increased by approximately 50% for epoetin alfa and 25% for darbepoetin alfa.[85,115] Once stable, the hemoglobin/hematocrit should be monitored every 2 to 4 weeks. If a response is not observed despite appropriate dose titration, M.R. should be evaluated for possible reasons for nonresponse (i.e., iron deficiency, bleeding, aluminum intoxication, hyperparathyroidism, infection).

In early 2007, a FDA mandated black-box warning was added to the safety labeling for all ESA products, which states that use of ESA therapy may increase the risk for death and for serious cardiovascular events when administered to achieve a hemoglobin >12 g/dL. This came as a result of four recently completed cancer trials that evaluated new dosing regimens, use of ESA in a new patient population, and use of new unapproved ESA. Since then, two trials in patients with CKD have shown that targeting Hgb levels >13 g/dL results in increase mortality and morbidity, thus observing these black-box warnings in CKD is warranted.[92,93]

CONTINUOUS ERYTHROPOIETIN RECEPTOR ACTIVATOR (CERA)

Continuous erythropoietin receptor activator (Mircera) has completed phase III of its clinical development program and has received an approval letter from the FDA for use in patients with CKD with anemia. CERA is twice the molecular weight of EPO because of the addition of a single 30-kd polymer chain into the erythropoietin molecule resulting in a considerably longer elimination half-life compared with EPO (130 hours vs. 4–28 hours). This allows for extended interval dosing of biweekly and once monthly. It has an efficacy and safety profile comparable to available ESA. The approved dosing of CERA is pending the release of the FDA-approved package insert. Extended interval dosing agents, such as CERA, have several advantages in patients with CKD stage 3 and 4, including improved patient compliance, less administration costs, reduced burden on patient from fewer injections given, and less outpatient visits to receive IV administration.[120]

Other novel molecules that promote erythropoiesis are in phase II and III clinical trials. These include hematide (an erythropoietin-mimetic peptide) and the hypoxia-inducible factor (HIF) stabilizers. The latter are orally active agents that induce both renal and extrarenal erythropoietin production. If these investigational agents are approved, they will provide health care professionals new options to correct anemia in CKD.

CARDIOVASCULAR COMPLICATIONS

13. **H.B. is a 65-year-old white man with stage 5 CKD who has just started chronic HD. He comes in today for his third HD session (dialysis scheduled three times per week, 4-hour duration). He has a history of hypertension, which has been poorly controlled over the past 4 months (BP ranges 150–190/85–105 mmHg), and he has experienced shortness of breath and a significant weight gain over the past month. His pertinent medical history includes hypertension for the past 14 years. H.B.'s current medications include metoprolol 50 mg BID, furosemide 80 mg BID, calcium carbonate 500 mg TID with meals, and Nephrocaps 1 PO QD. H.B.'s most recent predialysis BP was 175/98 mmHg, and his postdialysis BP was 158/90 mmHg. A recent ECG showed evidence of LVH.**

Predialysis laboratory values were as follows: serum sodium (Na), 140 mEq/L (normal, 135–147 mEq/L); potassium (K), 5.1 mEq/L (normal, 3.5–5.0 mEq/L); chloride (Cl), 101 mEq/L (normal, 95–105 mEq/L); CO_2 content, 23 mEq/L (normal, 22–28 mEq/L); SrCr, 8.8 mg/dL (normal, 0.6–1.2 mg/dL); BUN, 84 mg/dL (normal, 8–18 mg/dL); phosphate, 5.2 mg/dL (normal, 2.5–5.0 mg/dL); Ca, 8.6 mg/dL (normal, 8.8–10.4 mg/dL); serum albumin, 3.0 g/dL (normal, 4.0–6.0 g/dL); cholesterol (nonfasting), 345 mg/dL (normal, <200 mg/dL); triglycerides, 285 mg/dL (normal, <200 mg/dL); Hct, 27% (normal, 39%–49%); and Hgb, 9.0 g/dL (normal, 13–16 g/dL). H.B. has a urine output of 50 mL/day. What conditions evident in H.B. put him at increased risk of cardiovascular complications and mortality?

[SI units: Na, 140 mmol/L (normal, 135–147); K, 5.1 mmol/L (normal, 3.5–5.0); Cl, 101 mmol/L (normal, 95–105); CO_2, 23 mmol/L (normal, 22–28); SrCr, 778 μmol/L (normal, 50–110); BUN, 30 mmol/L of urea (normal, 3.0–6.5); phosphate, 1.68 mmol/L (normal, 0.8–1.60); Ca, 2.15 mmol/L (normal, 2.2–2.6); serum albumin, 30 g/L (normal, 40–60 g/L); cholesterol, 8.9 (normal, <5.2); triglycerides, 3.2 (normal, <2.3); Hct, 0.27 (normal, 0.39–0.49); and Hgb, 90 g/L (normal, 130–160 for male patients)]

H.B. has uncontrolled hypertension that is not being adequately managed with his current drug therapy or HD.

Hypertension is associated with LVH, ischemic heart disease, and heart failure, all of which are contributing factors to overall mortality in patients with stage 5 CKD who are undergoing dialysis.[3] H.B.'s ECG evidence of LVH should trigger additional evaluation to determine the extent of cardiac involvement and diagnosis of heart failure, which is associated with increased mortality in both diabetic and nondiabetic patients (see Chapter 18, Heart Failure). LVH develops early in the course of CKD and progresses as kidney disease progresses.[88,89] H.B. is in the most severe stage of CKD and has greatest likelihood of developing LVH. Anemia contributes substantially to the development of LVH and heart failure as well. H.B.'s hemoglobin of 9.0 g/dL (hematocrit 27%) is below the target value and requires treatment with erythropoietic therapy and iron supplementation based on evaluation of his iron indices (see section on anemia).

Additional factors that increase the risk of cardiovascular complications and mortality in H.B. include the elevated cholesterol and triglycerides levels as well as hypoalbuminemia (serum albumin, 3.0 g/dL). Increased levels of homocysteine are common in patients with kidney failure and have been associated with increased risk of coronary artery disease (CAD).[121] Because elevated concentrations of homocysteine have been observed in conjunction with decreased folate and vitamin B_{12} levels, more aggressive supplementation of these vitamins in this population has been suggested. Because H.B.'s total corrected calcium (corrected for hypoalbuminemia; see Question 17 for an explanation of this correction) is 9.4 mg/dL, his calcium, calcium-phosphorus product, and use of a calcium-containing phosphate binder will need to be monitored frequently. Cardiac calcification is common in patients with kidney disease and also is associated with cardiovascular complications. It has been reported that up to 80% of patients with ESRD have detectable coronary artery calcification.[122]

Cardiovascular disease and complications continue to be the leading cause of mortality in patients with kidney failure. According to data from a large population of patients on dialysis, cardiovascular disease increases the risk of all-cause mortality fivefold when compared with the general Medicare population without kidney disease.[3] All-cause death rates are almost four times greater in patients on dialysis age 65 and older, such as H.B., than in the general Medicare population.[3] For these reasons, the risk of CAD should be evaluated regularly in patients with ESRD (see Chapter 32, Renal Dialysis).

Hypertension

14. What options are available to treat H.B.'s hypertension considering his other cardiac complications and BP goal?

Dialysis

Hypertension is common in patients with CKD with a prevalence that varies depending on the cause of CKD and residual kidney function. Prevalence of hypertension has been estimated to be 80% in HD and 50% in PD populations.[79] Multiple factors are involved in the development of hypertension in the CKD population, including extracellular volume expansion from salt and water retention and activation of the renin-angiotensin-aldosterone system.[123] Increased sympathetic tone also has been observed with an increase in norepinephrine activity.

Because H.B. is just beginning dialysis therapy, it is difficult to assess the degree to which volume removal will ultimately affect his BP. To control BP related to volume changes, dialysis therapy should be adjusted as needed to achieve H.B.'s *dry weight,* the postdialysis weight at which symptoms of hypervolemia and hypovolemia are absent. H.B. has had recent findings consistent with worsening volume status (shortness of breath, weight gain) that should be considered when modifying his dialysis prescription; further workup is needed to determine if H.B. has systolic or diastolic heart failure. It is also important to counsel H.B. on the importance of salt and fluid intake restriction between HD sessions to minimize weight gain, volume expansion, and hypertension. Restriction of salt intake to 2 to 3 g/day and fluid to 1 L/day is appropriate and will require regular follow up by a dietitian.

Antihypertensive Therapy

Antihypertensive therapy should be used in conjunction with dialysis therapy in H.B. to target a BP $<$140/90 mmHg pre-HD and $<$130/80 mmHg post-HD.[79] For some patients, initiation of dialysis alone may achieve this goal and antihypertensive therapy may be withdrawn. The BP goal in patients with stage 5 CKD should minimize cardiovascular complications, but it should not increase the risk for hypotension and its associated complications during dialysis. The choice of an agent is based on the patient's comorbid conditions, because no single agent has a proven mortality benefit in patients on HD. The complexity of managing hypertension in patients on HD is enhanced by the apparent "U"-shaped relationship between BP and mortality. A study of patients on HD found an increased risk of cardiac-related death at systolic BP $<$110 mmHg and at systolic BP $>$180 mmHg.[124] The mortality risk with a low pre-HD BP may be indicative of severe cardiac disease at the initiation of HD. If patients experience hypotensive symptoms during HD, the goal BP can be increased, but they also should be evaluated for other cardiovascular disorders. Because the BP between dialysis sessions varies owing to volume changes, the ideal time to measure BP relative to dialysis (i.e., predialysis versus postdialysis) is unclear, but predialysis BP has been favored.

Diuretics are commonly used in patients in the early stages of CKD. As previously discussed, the effectiveness of diuretics depends on the amount of sodium delivered to their site of action in the renal tubule and on the patient's kidney function. For example, a decrease in the eGFR from 125 to 25 mL/minute/1.73 m^2, theoretically, could result in an approximate 80% decrease in the amount of sodium filtered. Early in the course of kidney failure, thiazides or thiazidelike diuretics are effective antihypertensive agents. As eGFR is further reduced (eGFR $<$30 mL/minute/1.73 m^2), the thiazide diuretics become essentially ineffective. Potassium-sparing diuretics are also ineffective and may increase the risk of hyperkalemia in this population. Loop diuretics (e.g., furosemide), which function more proximally, are indicated in patients with stage 4 CKD (eGFR 15–29 mL/minute/1.73 m^2).[125] These drugs can be effective for BP and volume control in patients with advanced kidney disease if residual kidney function is substantial (urine output $>$100 mL/day). Their effect must be frequently reevaluated based on urine output and any effect on volume control.

H.B.'s urine output should be assessed to determine the rationale for continued use of furosemide and the current dose should be assessed, because doses higher than his current dose of 80 mg BID are often required in patients with this degree of kidney dysfunction. It is likely that furosemide will need to be discontinued as H.B.'s residual renal function declines.

Given the role of the renin-angiotensin system in the development of hypertension in patients with CKD, ACE inhibitors are a logical choice for antihypertensive therapy. ACE inhibitors are effective antihypertensive agents in patients with CKD and have been shown to reverse LVH.[126] They are underused in this population, however. Response must be assessed individually to determine if renin-angiotensin-aldosterone activity is a predominant etiology of hypertension. Initiating therapy with low doses is prudent to evaluate patient response and tolerance. Use of these agents in combination with other antihypertensives is often required for adequate BP control. Most of these agents can be administered once daily; however, because of the renal elimination of the parent drug or active metabolite, dosage adjustments are necessary in patients with CKD. Fosinopril is the exception, because it undergoes substantial hepatic elimination. ACE inhibitors should also be used cautiously in patients dialyzed with the polyacrylonitrile (AN69) membrane. This is because ACE inhibitors decrease the breakdown of bradykinin. Bradykinin production is increased in patients who experience systemic or immune-mediated reactions when blood comes in contact with the dialyzer, which can lead to anaphylactic reactions. Such reactions are common with AN69 because of its composition; therefore, ACE inhibitor use in combination with this dialyzer should be avoided.

Although ARB effectively lower BP in patients without kidney disease,[127] less is known about their effectiveness in patients with kidney failure. These agents may offer an alternative to ACE inhibitors in patients experiencing kinin-mediated adverse effects; however, similar side effects have been reported with ARB. The combined use of ARB with other antihypertensive agents may be rational when patients are unresponsive to other regimens. One ARB, valsartan, has been approved for use in heart failure and this may offer an advantage in patients with concurrent heart failure[128]; however, this concept must be studied in a CKD population.

Calcium channel blockers are effective antihypertensives in patients with CKD. Because the nondihydropyridine agents (i.e., diltiazem, verapamil) have negative chronotropic and inotropic effects, they should be used with care in patients with heart disease. Generally, dosage adjustment is not required in patients with kidney disease.

Other agents used to treat hypertension in the CKD population include β-blockers, centrally acting agents (e.g., clonidine, methyldopa), vasodilators (e.g., minoxidil, hydralazine), and α_1-adrenergic blockers (prazosin, terazosin, doxazosin). β-Blockers inhibit release of renin and may be useful in hypertension associated with CKD. Risk versus benefit should be evaluated when β-blockade is considered in conjunction with other comorbid conditions such as asthma, heart failure, and lipid abnormalities. Dosage adjustment is required for the less lipophilic agents (i.e., atenolol, acebutolol, nadolol).

H.B. is currently taking the β-blocker, metoprolol, and the loop diuretic, furosemide. It is likely that his diuretic will need to be discontinued as his residual kidney function decreases and response to therapy is inadequate. Although an effective antihypertensive, metoprolol may not be the best single agent for H.B. and its use must be reassessed based on the recent evidence of LVH and whether systolic or diastolic dysfunction is diagnosed on further workup. If changes in H.B.'s HD prescription to improve volume control and achieve his dry weight do not reduce his BP, another antihypertensive regimen should be selected. A reasonable antihypertensive regimen would include an ACE inhibitor (e.g., enalapril) with or without β-blocker therapy or a calcium channel blocker based on cardiac findings. The selection will depend substantially on follow-up results of his cardiac disease, BP control with HD, and the development of adverse effects (see Chapter 13, Essential Hypertension, and Chapter 18, Heart Failure).

Dyslipidemia

15. How should H.B.'s lipid abnormalities be treated?

H.B. has elevated serum cholesterol and triglyceride concentrations, a common finding in patients with CKD. Dyslipidemia and increased oxidative stress contribute to premature atherogenesis in these patients. Several atherogenic factors in patients with CKD have been postulated, including arterial wall injury, platelet activation and adherence, smooth muscle cell proliferation, and intra-arterial accumulation of cholesterol. Whether lowering of serum lipids will improve long-term morbidity and mortality remains to be determined, but treatment should be consistent with NCEP ATP III guidelines and the NKF-K/DOQI guidelines for treatment of dyslipidemias.[64,65] Dietary intervention successfully reduces triglyceride and cholesterol concentrations, and many drugs are available to treat lipid abnormalities in patients with stage 5 CKD (see Chapter 12, Dyslipidemias, Athrosclerosis and Coronary Heart Disease). Statin use has been supported by recent evidence associating these agents with a decrease in cardiovascular mortality and all-cause mortality in patients on dialysis.[129] Because many β-adrenergic blocking drugs might elevate triglyceride concentrations, antihypertensive drugs with insignificant or beneficial effects on serum lipids (e.g., ACE inhibitors, calcium channel blockers, clonidine, prazosin) may be preferable.

SECONDARY HYPERPARATHYROIDISM AND RENAL OSTEODYSTROPHY

16. D.B. is a 42-year-old white woman who has a 24-year history of type 1 diabetes mellitus with complications of diabetic nephropathy, retinopathy, and neuropathy. She has hypothyroidism and was diagnosed with stage 5 CKD 4 years ago. She started HD three times weekly at that time. Her current medications include levothyroxine 0.1 mg/day, metoclopramide (Reglan) 10 mg TID before meals, insulin aspart 10 U with meals, insulin glargine 25 U QHS, docusate 100 mg QD, OsCal 500 mg PO TID with meals, EPO 5,000 U IV twice weekly, iron sucrose 100 mg IV (TIW), paricalcitol 1 mcg IV three times per week (TIW), and Nephrocaps 1 capsule QD. At a recent clinic visit, findings on physical examination included a BP of 128/84 mmHg, diabetic retinopathic changes with laser scars bilaterally, and diminished sensation bilaterally below the knees. Her laboratory values were as follows: normal serum electrolytes; a random blood glucose

of 175 mg/dL (normal, 140 mg/dL); BUN, 45 mg/dL (normal, 8–18 mg/dL); SrCr, 8.9 mg/dL (normal, 0.6–1.2 mg/dL), Hgb, 10 g/dL (goal, >11 g/dL); WBC count, 6,200/mm^3 (normal, 3,200–9,800/mm^3); Ca, 8.5 mg/dL (normal, 8.4–9.5 mg/dL); phosphate, 6.8 mg/dL (normal, 2.5–5.0 mg/dL); intact parathyroid hormone (iPTH), 450 pg/mL (normal, 5–65 pg/mL); total serum protein, 5.0 g/dL (normal, 6.0–8.0 g/dL); serum albumin, 3.1 g/dL (normal, 4.0–6.0 g/dL); and uric acid, 8.9 mg/dL (normal, 2.0–7.0 mg/dL). Describe the etiology of D.B.'s abnormal bone, calcium, phosphorus, and PTH findings.

[SI units: blood glucose, 9.7 mmol/L (normal, <11 mmol/L); BUN, 16.1 mmol/L of urea (normal, 3.0–6.5); SrCr, 787 μmol/L (normal, 50–110); Hgb, 100 g/L (goal, 110 g/L); WBC count, 6,200 × 10^6 /L (normal, 3,200–9,800); Ca, 2 mmol/L (normal, 2.1–2.36); phosphate, 2.19 mmol/L (normal, 0.8–1.60); total serum protein, 50 g/L (normal, 60–80); serum albumin, 31 g/L (normal, 40–60 g/L); uric acid, 529 μmol/L (normal, 120–420)]

Etiology

Renal osteodystrophy (ROD) is the term used to describe the skeletal manifestations that occur as kidney function declines. Collectively, ROD refers to specific bone abnormalities that include osteitis fibrosa (most common pattern), osteomalacia, osteosclerosis, and osteopenia. Hyperphosphatemia, hypocalcemia, hyperparathyroidism, decreased production of active vitamin D, and resistance to vitamin D therapy are all frequent problems in CKD that can lead to the secondary complication of ROD.

The interrelationships between phosphorus, calcium, vitamin D, and PTH have been reviewed extensively.[130,131] Retention of phosphorus and secondary hyperparathyroidism (sHPT) play a major role in the development of osteitis fibrosa or high-turnover bone disease. The "trade-off" hypothesis best describes the events leading to changes in bone metabolism.[130] As eGFR decreases, phosphorus excretion by the kidney decreases, resulting in hyperphosphatemia. Hyperphosphatemic conditions lead to a corresponding decrease in ionized calcium concentration, a primary stimulus for release of PTH from the parathyroid gland. Higher concentrations of PTH decrease renal tubular reabsorption of phosphorus and promote its excretion. Both serum phosphorus and calcium concentrations are corrected depending on the degree of remaining kidney function, but this occurs at the expense of an elevated PTH concentration (the "trade off"). As kidney disease becomes more severe (eGFR <30 mL/minute/1.73 m^2), the phosphaturic response to PTH diminishes and sustained hyperphosphatemia and hypocalcemia develop. In response to hypocalcemia, calcium is mobilized from the bone, a mechanism largely controlled by PTH. Virtually all patients with kidney failure develop sHPT. Decreased PTH degradation by the kidney may also contribute to the hyperparathyroid state in patients with kidney disease.

The kidney is the principal organ responsible for vitamin D production and, as such, vitamin D metabolism is altered in the presence of uremia. Persistent hyperphosphatemia inhibits the normal conversion of 25-hydroxyvitamin D_3 to its biologically active metabolite, 1,25-dihydroxyvitamin D_3, by the enzyme 1-α-hydroxylase. This enzyme is present in proximal tubular cells of the kidney and is necessary for conversion of vitamin D to the active form. This active form of vitamin D, also known as *calcitriol*, increases gut absorption of calcium and interacts with vitamin D receptors on the parathyroid gland to suppress PTH release. As a result of decreased calcitriol production, the absorption of dietary calcium in the gut is diminished, contributing to hypocalcemia. Decreased suppression of PTH release by vitamin D in conjunction with hypocalcemia promotes continued stimulus for mobilization of calcium from bone. Furthermore, uremic patients require a higher extracellular calcium concentration to suppress secretion of PTH. This is also described as an increase in the calcium "set point" or the concentration of calcium required to inhibit 50% of maximal PTH secretion.[130]

The chronic effects of hyperparathyroidism on the skeleton lead to bone pain, fractures, and myopathy. In children, these effects may be particularly severe and usually retard growth. The metabolic acidosis of kidney disease also contributes to a negative calcium balance in the bone.

D.B.'s presentation is consistent with ROD based on the observed changes in bone architecture and abnormalities in serum phosphorus, calcium, and PTH; all can be attributed to her kidney disease.

Treatment

17. What are the goals of therapy for D.B.'s calcium, phosphorus, and PTH abnormalities? What options are available to treat these disorders?

The management objectives for D.B. are to (*a*) maintain near-normal serum calcium and phosphorus concentrations, (*b*) prevent secondary hyperparathyroidism, and (*c*) restore normal skeletal development without inducing adynamic bone disease (or low bone turnover). The NKF-K/DOQI guidelines for bone metabolism and disease suggest target levels for serum calcium and phosphorus, the calcium and phosphorus product (Ca-P), and intact PTH for each stage of CKD.[84,131] These goals are best achieved with dietary phosphorus restriction, appropriate use of phosphate-binding agents, vitamin D therapy, calcimimetics, and dialysis.

Dietary Restriction of Phosphorus

In general, serum phosphorus should be maintained at near normal levels in the earlier stages of CKD (~2.7–4.6 mg/dL), with a higher range (3.5–5.5) accepted in patients with stage 5 CKD.[84] Dietary phosphorus restriction can prevent hyperphosphatemia and maintain target phosphorus concentrations. Protein restriction will also limit phosphorus intake, because high-protein foods tend to contain high amounts of phosphorus (Table 31-6).[132] The challenge is in tailoring a diet that fulfills these criteria while providing adequate nutrition. During the early stages of kidney disease (eGFR <60 mL/minute/1.73 m^2), dietary phosphorus should be reduced to 800 to 1,000 mg/day (~60% of normal) through restriction of meat, milk, legumes, and carbonated beverages to achieve normal phosphorus concentrations.[84,133] Patients requiring dialysis have less dietary phosphorus restriction with a recommended phosphorus intake of approximately 800 to 1,200 mg/day.[133] While phosphorus is removed to some extent by dialysis, neither HD nor PD removes adequate amounts to warrant complete liberalization of phosphorus in the diet. Regular dietary counseling

Table 31-6 Phosphorus Content of Select High-Protein Foods

Food	Portion Size	Phosphorus Content (mg)
Black-eyed peas, cooked	1 cup	288
Cheese, American	4 ounces	1,200
Cheese, cheddar	4 ounces	545
Cheese creamed cottage	4 ounces	150
Cheese, Swiss	4 ounces	800
Chicken, cooked	3.5 ounces	190
Chocolate candy	2 ounces	130
Egg	1 large	100
Fish, cooked	4 ounces	400
Hamburger, ground sirloin	3.5 ounces	186
Ice cream	8 ounces	163
Kidney beans, cooked	1 cup	278
Lamb	3.5 ounces	200
Liver, chicken	3.5. ounces	312
Milk, whole or skim	8 ounces (1 cup)	278
Peanut butter	2 tablespoons	118
Peanuts	3.5 ounces	466
Pork tenderloin	3.5 ounces	301
Salmon, canned	3.5 ounces	344
Sardines, canned in oil	3.5 ounces	434
Shrimp	3.5 ounces	156
Soybeans	1 cup	322
Steak, sirloin	4 ounces	282
Tofu	3.5 ounces	128
Tuna fish, canned	3.5 ounces	250
Turkey	3.5 ounces	200
Yogurt, plain	8 ounces	270

Data from Bowes AP, Church HN. *Bowes & Church's Food Values of Portions Commonly Used*. Philadelphia: Lippincott-Raven; 1998.

by a renal dietitian is necessary to reinforce the importance of phosphorus restriction and other dietary recommendations.

Phosphate-Binding Agents

Significant reduction of serum phosphorus may be difficult to achieve with dietary intervention alone, particularly in patients with more advanced kidney disease (eGFR <30 mL/minute/1.73 m^2). For these patients, phosphate-binding agents used in conjunction with dietary restriction are necessary. Phosphate-binding agents limit phosphorus absorption from the GI tract by binding with the phosphorus present from dietary sources. Therefore, these agents must be administered with meals. Available binders include products that contain calcium, lanthanum, aluminum, or magnesium cations or the polymer-based agent, sevelamer hydrochloride (Renagel).

CALCIUM-CONTAINING PREPARATIONS

Calcium-containing preparations, especially calcium carbonate and calcium acetate, are frequently used to prevent hyperphosphatemia in patients with kidney disease. The many preparations available vary in their calcium content (Table 31-7). Correction of hypocalcemia is an added beneficial effect of the calcium-containing preparations; however, a risk exists of hypercalcemia and cardiac calcification associated with the prolonged use of these agents.[134] Compared with calcium carbonate, calcium acetate binds about twice the amount of phosphorus for the same amount of calcium salts, which may be owing to the increased solubility of calcium acetate in both acidic and alkaline environments.[135] Despite the reduction in the dose of elemental calcium required with the acetate product, the incidence of hypercalcemia does not differ.[135] Calcium citrate is a calcium salt with a phosphate-binding capacity

Table 31-7 Phosphate-Binding Agents

Product	Select Available Agents[a]	Content of Compound	Starting Dose
Calcium carbonate (40% calcium)	Tums	200, 300, 400 mg	0.8–2 g elemental Ca with meals
	Os-Cal-500	500 mg	
	Nephro-Calci	600 mg	
	Caltrate 600	600 mg	
	Calcarb HD (powder)	2,400 mg/packet	
	$CaCO_3$ (multiple preparations)	200–600 mg	
Calcium acetate (25% calcium)	Phos-Lo 667 mg	169 mg	2–3 tablets with meals
Sevelamer hydrochloride (polymer-based)	Renagel (tablet, capsule)	400, 800 mg (tablet)	800–1,600 mg with meals
Lanthanum carbonate	Fosrenol	250, 500, 750, 1,000 mg	250–500 mg with meals
Aluminum hydroxide[b]	AlternaGel (suspension)	600 mg/5 mL	300–600 mg with meals
	Amphojel (tablet and suspension)	300, 600 mg (tablet) 320 mg/5 mL (suspension)	
	Alu-Cap (capsule)	400 mg	
	Alu-Tab	500 mg	
	Basaljel (tablet, capsule, and suspension)	500 mg (tablet, capsule) 400 mg/mL (suspension)	
Magnesium carbonate[b]	Mag-Carb (capsule)	70 mg	70 mg with meals
Magnesium hydroxide[b]	Milk of Magnesia (tablet and suspension)	300, 600 mg (tablet) 400, 800 mg/5 mL (suspension)	300–400 mg with meals

[a] Tablet unless noted otherwise.
[b] Not first-line choice as a phosphate binder for chronic use.

similar to that of calcium carbonate; however, because it also increases aluminum absorption from the GI tract, its use is not recommended in patients with kidney disease.

Although calcium-containing binders have an added benefit of correcting hypocalcemia, the potential for hypercalcemia must be frequently evaluated in patients receiving these agents chronically. Simultaneous administration of vitamin D preparations and calcium also increases the risk of hypercalcemia. A "corrected" serum calcium and the "Ca-P product" (defined below) should be determined before therapy is started and at regular intervals thereafter.

Serum calcium should be maintained at near normal levels in the earlier stages of CKD. Calculating corrected calcium adjusts for the change in the ratio of free (unbound) versus protein bound calcium owing to reduced serum albumin concentrations. A narrower range is recommended in patients with stage 5 CKD (upper range of ~9.5 mg/dL) to prevent both hypocalcemia and hypercalcemia.[84]

$$\text{Corrected total calcium (mg/dL)} = \text{Total calcium (mg/dL)} + 0.8 \times [4\text{-Serum albumin (g/dL)}] \qquad \textbf{(31-5)}$$

The calculation for Ca-P is as follows:

$$\text{Ca-P} = \text{Corrected calcium (mg/dL)} \times \text{serum phosphorus (mg/dL)} \qquad \textbf{(31-6)}$$

The calculated Ca-P value gives some indication to when calcium and phosphate may precipitate and be deposited into soft tissue (e.g., coronary vasculature). Based on the increased risk of mortality associated with an elevated Ca-P product and the potential for cardiac calcification, the ideal Ca-P product target has been decreased to $<55\ mg^2/dL^2$.[84] This is much lower than the former recommendation of <65 to $70\ mg^2/dL^2$ and more difficult to achieve. When the Ca-P product exceeds the target value, the patient should be switched to a non–calcium-based phosphate binder. Alternatives include sevelamer and cations, such as lanthanum carbonate, aluminum, or magnesium preparations. For patients requiring dialysis, reducing the calcium concentration of the dialysate bath may decrease the risk of hypercalcemia. Although avoiding hypercalcemia should reduce the risk of cardiac calcification, calcifications still can occur because of other contributing factors in the CKD population (e.g., hyperphosphatemia).

Nausea, diarrhea, and constipation are other side effects of calcium-containing products. Because calcium-containing binders may interact with other drugs, timing of their administration relative to other agents must be considered. Fluoroquinolones and oral iron, for example, should be taken at least 1 or 2 hours before calcium-containing phosphate binders. Importantly, if the calcium products are being used as supplementation to treat hypocalcemia or osteoporosis, they should be taken between meals to enhance intestinal absorption. This is in contrast to their administration with meals if they are being used as phosphate binders. Starting doses of common calcium-containing phosphate binders are listed in Table 31-7.

SEVELAMER HYDROCHLORIDE

Sevelamer hydrochloride (Renagel) is a nonabsorbed, polymer-based product that binds phosphorus in the GI tract.[136] The benefit of lowering phosphorus without significantly affecting serum calcium has led to the increased use of sevelamer in patients with CKD, and it is now considered a first-line agent in patients with stage 5 CKD.[84] Sevelamer also lowers LDL and total serum cholesterol, a substantial benefit considering the increased risk of cardiovascular events in this population.[137] The combined use of sevelamer and calcium supplementation has been evaluated. Coadministration of calcium (900 mg/day elemental calcium) with sevelamer resulted in greater decreases in both phosphorus and PTH than either agent alone without significant increases in serum calcium.[138] This may prove to be a useful way to control phosphorus and PTH, while avoiding both hypocalcemia and hypercalcemia.

Sevelamer has a potential benefit of attenuating the progression of coronary calcification, which may be related to its LDL and total serum cholesterol-lowering effects and a benefit from reduced calcium loading. The actual benefit of sevelamer on mortality is controversial. The *post hoc* analysis of the Renagel in New Dialysis (RIND) trial showed a survival advantage with sevelamer compared with calcium acetate, however, the Dialysis Clinical Outcomes Revisited (DCOR) trial failed to show a difference in mortality between the two agents.[139] One explanation for the disparity in these results may be the difference in the population of patients on HD between the two trials. The RIND included incident patients on HD, whereas the DCOR included prevalent patients who likely would have advanced cardiovascular disease.

Sevelamer is available as a 403-mg capsule and as 400-mg and 800-mg tablets. The starting dose is variable and depends on the baseline serum phosphorus concentration (800 mg TID with meals if serum phosphorus is <7.5 mg/dL; 1,600 mg TID with meals if serum phosphorus is >7.5 mg/dL).[136] Gradual adjustments can be made at 2-week intervals, based on serum phosphorus levels. Dosing guidelines for sevelamer are also available for patients being converted from calcium acetate. Based on studies showing similar reductions in serum phosphorus, 800 mg of sevelamer is considered equivalent to 667 mg of calcium acetate (169 mg elemental calcium).[136]

Data regarding drug interactions with sevelamer are limited; however, in recent evaluations, no drug interactions with digoxin, warfarin, metoprolol, and enalapril were observed.[136] The current prescribing information recommends administering sevelamer 1 hour before or 3 hours after administration of other agents with narrow therapeutic indices.[136] The administration of sevelamer to patients on HD has been associated with a lowering of serum bicarbonate. Several studies have confirmed this effect and it should be taken into account when using this agent.[140]

LANTHANUM CARBONATE

Lanthanum carbonate (Fosrenol) is a newly approved phosphate binder that offers another option for a noncalcium, nonaluminum preparation. When ingested, it dissociates into a trivalent cation with similar binding capacity as aluminum salts, and lanthanum also has been found to be as effective and tolerable as standard treatment. Both calcium and iPTH were lower in the lanthanum group.[141] Lanthanum is mainly excreted via the biliary route, with minimal renal elimination.

Studies have evaluated the deposition and toxicity of lanthanum in the bone, liver, and brain because of concerns of lanthanum accumulation. Although lanthanum accumulates in lysosomes in the liver, this has not been correlated with increased liver enzymes or hepatobiliary adverse events in patients receiving lanthanum 3.75 g/day for up to 3 years.[142] This is likely an excretory process through the biliary tract similar to iron and copper. A prospective trial of patients on HD receiving lanthanum for 1 year found minimal deposition of lanthanum within the bone and less likelihood of adynamic bone histology compared with patients receiving calcium carbonate.[143] Over a 2-year period, patients receiving lanthanum were not found to accelerate the natural deterioration in cognitive function seen in patients on HD.[144]

Lanthanum is supplied as chewable tablets for oral administration in four strengths: 250, 500, 750, and 1,000 mg. The recommended initial total daily dose is 750 to 1,500 mg given with meals and dosage titration up to a maximal dosage of 3,000 mg daily should be based on serum phosphate levels. The most frequent adverse events reported in clinical trials are nausea and vomiting.[145]

OTHER PHOSPHATE BINDERS

Aluminum preparations bind dietary phosphorus in the GI tract from both dietary sources and enterohepatic secretions and form an insoluble aluminum–phosphate complex that is excreted in the stool. Although these products were once used as first-line agents to decrease phosphorus, their use lost favor because of accumulation of aluminum in patients with CKD. Elevated serum aluminum concentrations and aluminum deposition in bone and other tissues of patients with kidney disease have been associated with osteomalacia, microcytic anemia, and a fatal neurologic syndrome, referred to as *dialysis encephalopathy*.[146] Treatment of aluminum toxicity requires chelation with deferoxamine. Aluminum-containing agents should only be considered on a short-term basis (up to 4 weeks) for patients with an elevated Ca-P product; however, sevelamer is generally preferred in these situations. Sucralfate, used primarily for the treatment of ulcers, also contains aluminum and should be used cautiously in patients with kidney disease.

Magnesium agents (magnesium hydroxide, magnesium carbonate) may be beneficial, but as with aluminum, their use should be limited, because at the high doses required to control serum phosphorus concentrations, severe diarrhea and hypermagnesemia invariably result. Magnesium might, however, be considered in patients whose serum phosphorus concentrations cannot be controlled adequately by other phosphate-binding agents. In this instance, a magnesium-containing phosphate binder may be added in conjunction with a reduction in the dialysate magnesium concentration (in the dialysis population). These agents should not be considered first-line therapy for control of phosphorus and careful monitoring of magnesium is warranted if therapy is started.

D.B.'s corrected calcium is approximately 9.2 mg/dL and the Ca-P product is 66 mg^2/dL^2. More aggressive control of serum phosphorus is needed to achieve a phosphorus level <5.5 mg/dL. Currently she is receiving 1,500 mg of elemental calcium. Although presumably much of this calcium will be bound to phosphorus in the GI tract, a potential exists for calcium absorption. Because her Ca-P product is above the threshold of 55 mg/dL, she is at increased risk for cardiac calcification and adverse outcomes. The total dose of elemental calcium provided by binders should not exceed 1,500 mg/day (or 2,000 mg/day from binders and diet).[84] Sevelamer should be started to limit her calcium exposure and decrease her phosphorus levels. The recommended starting dose is 800 mg TID with meals and titrated based on follow up of calcium, phosphorus, and Ca-P values. Adjustments should also be considered in conjunction with vitamin D therapy (see section on vitamin D below). D.B. should be instructed to take her phosphate binder with meals. This regimen should be implemented in conjunction with a restricted-phosphorus diet. Regular reinforcement of the importance of compliance is necessary, because nonadherence with prescribed dietary phosphorus restriction and drug therapy is one of the most significant factors associated with treatment failure. Use of a low-calcium dialysate may also help decrease her risk of hypercalcemia.

Vitamin D

CALCITRIOL

Vitamin D occurs naturally as ergocalciferol (vitamin D_2) and cholecalciferol (vitamin D_3), both of which are inactive precursors of active forms of vitamin D. An intermediate activation step (25-hydroxylation) occurs in the liver to produce 25-hydroxy vitamin D (25-hydroxycalciferol), which is also relatively inactive. Final activation (1-hydroxylation) occurs in the kidney, yielding calcitriol (1,25-dihydroxycholecalciferol), the active form of vitamin D. Thus, the response to vitamins D_2 and D_3 in patients with compromised renal function can vary, depending on the degree of kidney dysfunction and the ability of the kidney to metabolize 25-hydroxyvitamin D to calcitriol. For unexplained reasons, some patients in the early stages of CKD can also have decreased levels of 25-hydroxyvitamin D, reducing substrate for producing calcitriol.[147] Altered vitamin D metabolism that occurs in this population may warrant measurement of 25-hydroxyvitamin D and supplementation with vitamin D precursors, such as ergocalciferol.[84] Oral therapy with active vitamin D (oral calcitriol) or an analog (oral doxercalciferol) is likely warranted only when PTH remains elevated despite normal 25-hydroxyvitamin D levels.[84,147] As the final, active metabolite of vitamin D, calcitriol is required in patients with more severe kidney disease (stage 5 CKD).

Administration of active vitamin D, in conjunction with control of serum phosphorus and calcium, is necessary in many patients with CKD to control PTH and prevent ROD. Calcitriol interacts with the vitamin D receptor (VDR) located in the parathyroid gland, intestines, bone, and kidney. It is thought to decrease PTH messenger RNA (mRNA) resulting in decreased PTH secretion. It also lowers the calcium set point for PTH release in patients with CKD with sHPT, most likely through a direct effect on calcium receptors within the parathyroid gland.[130] In addition, calcitriol stimulates calcium absorption from the GI tract to correct hypocalcemia and prevent sHPT. To avoid hypercalcemia, the lowest-effective dose should be used and the patient's serum calcium and the Ca-P product should be monitored at least every 2 weeks for 1 month and then monthly thereafter. Furthermore, control of serum phosphorus is critical before calcitriol is initiated, because this agent also increases GI phosphorus absorption.

Calcitriol is available as an oral formulation (Rocaltrol) or IV formulation (Calcijex). Administration of calcitriol by either the oral or IV route may be based on conventional dosing (usually 0.25–0.5 mcg/day) or pulse dosing (intermittent dosing of 0.5 to 2.0 mcg two to three times per week). Higher doses (e.g., 4 mcg three times per week) are generally required to reduce PTH secretion in more severe sHPT (PTH >1,000 pg/mL). Daily dosing of 0.25 to 0.5 mcg may be preferred in patients with hypocalcemia, because this regimen primarily works to stimulate calcium absorption from the GI tract. Intermittent dosing of IV calcitriol is more routine in the HD population, because administration is coordinated with dialysis. In contrast, oral dosing is more convenient in patients with CKD who are not having dialysis and the PD population. Intact PTH and serum calcium concentrations are used to determine starting doses and dosing adjustments for calcitriol. Acceptable iPTH ranges of three to four times normal have been proposed in patients with stage 5 CKD to prevent sHPT while avoiding adynamic bone disease.[131,147] Lower iPTH ranges of one to two times normal may be more reasonable in patients with stage 4 CKD.[84]

Intact PTH (1–84 PTH) is the 84 amino acid biologically active form of this hormone. It is metabolized into smaller, less active fragments (e.g., 7-84 PTH) with activity that is not well characterized. These fragments are cleared from the circulation by the kidney and may accumulate in patients with CKD. Assays used for iPTH measure the intact structure as well as the biologically active and inactive PTH fragments. Thus, proposed ranges for iPTH in current guidelines are based on these assays. Recently, assays that measure only the biologically active form (1-84 PTH) have become available. When iPTH is measured using both methods, there is roughly a 2:1 ratio between the nonspecific and specific assay results. For example, the current guidelines for iPTH in patients with stage 5 CKD state a value of 150 to 300 pg/mL (i.e., three to four times normal); this would correspond to a 1-84 PTH concentration of approximately 75 to 150 pg/mL measured by the new methods.[148] These newer assays have not yet been adopted for most of the CKD population; however, they are being used in some clinical settings. Clearly, the clinician must know which assay has been used to appropriately interpret the results, establish the desired PTH range, and correctly adjust therapy.

Dose adjustments of calcitriol are generally made in 0.5- to 1.0-mcg increments every 2 to 4 weeks in the early stages of therapy until iPTH and serum calcium are maintained at target levels. If hypercalcemia develops, the decision to withhold therapy or to switch to a vitamin D analog (see section on vitamin D analogs) must be made. Serum iPTH should be monitored every 3 to 6 months, and adjustments of calcitriol doses made to maintain the goal iPTH and to prevent hypercalcemia and hyperphosphatemia.

VITAMIN D ANALOGS

The unique interactions of vitamin D with the VDR have led to the development of vitamin D analogs, which vary in their affinity for the VDR. In the case of treatment for sHPT, some were developed to retain the suppressive effect on PTH release while decreasing the potential for hypercalcemia relative to calcitriol. Currently approved agents for managing sHPT in the United States are paricalcitol (Zemplar), also referred to as 19-nor-1,25-dihydroxyvitamin D_2, and doxercalciferol (Hectorol), or 1-α-hydroxyvitamin D_2. Doxercalciferol requires conversion to the active form (1-α-,25-dihydroxyvitamin D_2) by the liver.

In patients with sHPT, paricalcitol significantly decreases iPTH without significantly increasing calcium, phosphorus, or Ca-P product.[149,150] In one such study, a significant rise in calcium concentration (within the normal range) was observed after 12 weeks of paricalcitol therapy at a maximal dose of 0.12 mcg/kg. Patients experiencing transient episodes of hypercalcemia (calcium >11 mg/dL) were evaluated with regard to their corresponding iPTH levels. An iPTH level <100 pg/mL was associated with an increase in serum calcium concentration equal to or beyond the upper limits of normal, indicating that these events were caused by inappropriate dosing and oversuppression of PTH.[149] Based on these data, the recommended initial dose of paricalcitol is 0.04 mcg/kg to 0.1 mcg/kg IV administered with each dialysis session or every other day.[151] Doses can be titrated by 2- to 4-mcg increments every 2 to 4 weeks based on iPTH values. Some data have also suggested paricalcitol dosing based on initial PTH levels (paricalcitol dose = PTH/80), rather than weight, as a reasonable dosing strategy.[151] Oral paricalcitol capsules are now available for use in CKD stages 3 and 4, and are available in three strengths (1, 2, and 4 mcg) administered daily or TIW. The starting dose should be 1 mcg daily or 2 mcg TIW if the baseline iPTH level is ≤500 pg/mL and 2 mcg daily or 4 mcg TIW if the iPTH is >500 pg/mL. Dosage adjustments based on change in iPTH levels should occur every 2 to 4 weeks.[152]

The recommended conversion ratio for calcitriol to paricalcitol is 1:4 (i.e., for every 1 mcg of calcitriol, 4 mcg of paricalcitol should be administered). This information is based on similar efficacy observed when patients treated for secondary hyperparathyroidism with calcitriol were switched to paricalcitol using this dosing strategy.[149] A lower ratio of 1:3 also has been proposed in patients resistant to therapy with calcitriol.[153] Although data comparing paricalcitol with calcitriol are currently limited, one study reported fewer cases of hyperphosphatemia with paricalcitol at doses that had equivalent efficacy with regard to PTH suppression. A trend was also seen toward more rapid suppression of PTH in patients treated with paricalcitol.[154]

Doxercalciferol is another vitamin D analog that has provided an alternative to the active form of vitamin D and has been studied in patients with stage 5 CKD on dialysis.[155,156] Intermittent oral therapy was administered to patients on HD with hyperparathyroidism (iPTH, >400 pg/mL) in a multicenter trial. In this study, 10 mcg of oral doxercalciferol was administered three times per week with HD.[155] Of the 99 patients completing the study, 83% achieved the target iPTH; higher doses and longer therapy was required for patients with more severe sHPT (PTH, 1,200 pg/mL). Hypercalcemia occurred in a larger percent of patients in the doxercalciferol group compared with placebo, and this was corrected by lowering the doxercalciferol dose or by reducing calcium-containing phosphate binders. In another study, intermittent IV therapy was compared with intermittent oral administration.[156] The doses were 4 mcg IV or 10 mcg orally three times per week with HD. Oral and IV therapy were both effective in reducing iPTH levels in patients with sHPT; however, some evidence indicated that intermittent IV therapy may result in less hypercalcemia and hyperphosphatemia than oral intermittent therapy. Comparisons with calcitriol have not been reported. The recommended starting dose of doxercalciferol for patients on dialysis is 4 mcg IV or 10 mcg orally administered three times per week with dosing titration based on changes in iPTH.[157]

Vitamin D analogs offer an alternative for patients in whom persistent hypercalcemia develops with calcitriol therapy. Use of these agents is increasing in clinical practice because of the concerns of hypercalcemia and its adverse consequences. Recent retrospective reports indicate a mortality benefit with vitamin D therapy. A historical cohort study of patients on HD, found that patients receiving either calcitriol or paricalcitol had lower overall and cardiovascular-related mortality rates than those not receiving vitamin D therapy.[158] Two trials also examined the survival advantages among the different forms of vitamin D in patients on HD.[159,160] One report indicated that receiving paricalcitol for 36 months conferred a survival advantage starting at 12 months from initiation of therapy and increased over time compared with those receiving calcitriol.[159] Another study reported that patients taking either paricalcitol or doxercalciferol had a significantly lower mortality rate than patients receiving calcitriol, although when adjusted for laboratory values and clinic standardized mortality, no difference was found between the products.[160]

Possible biologic reasons for vitamin D improving outcomes include its role downregulating the RAS and immunomodulatory properties. A prospective trial would be required to confirm a survival advantage associated with vitamin D therapy.

Calcimimetics

The discovery of extracellular calcium-sensing receptors (CaSR) has prompted research with calcimimetic agents that allosterically modulate CaSR. CaSR have been identified in the parathyroid gland, thyroid, nephron, brain, intestine, bone, lung, and other tissues. Calcimimetic agents increase the sensitivity of the CaSR to extracellular calcium ions, inhibit the release of PTH, lowering PTH levels within hours after administration. The calcimimetic cinacalcet is the first agent in this class to be approved by the FDA. Pooled data from two phase III trials of this agent demonstrated efficacy in lowering PTH concentrations and Ca-P product in patients on HD with sHPT and a higher proportion of patients achieved NKF-K/DOQI recommended targets for PTH, calcium, phosphorus, and Ca-P product.[161] No data are found on survival rates for patients receiving cinacalcet versus those treated with vitamin D. Cinacalcet, however, offers an additional choice of agent to lower PTH when vitamin D cannot be increased because of elevated calcium, phosphorus, or calcium-phosphorus product. Current studies are also examining the role of combined therapy with cinacalcet and vitamin D therapy to improve achievement of bone metabolism and disease targets.[162]

Appropriate treatment for D.B. should be based on assessment of her serum calcium, phosphorus, and PTH values. She currently has an elevated PTH, phosphorus, and calcium-phosphorus product; therefore, cinacalcet should be started in conjunction with her dietary phosphorus restriction, phosphate-binder regimen, and vitamin D therapy. Cinacalcet should be initiated at a dose of 30 mg daily with dosage titrations occurring every 2 to 4 weeks to 60, 90, 120 or a maximum of 180 mg daily to achieve target iPTH levels. Serum calcium and phosphorous levels should be drawn within 1 week after initiation or dosage increase, and plasma PTH levels drawn within 4 weeks after initiation of therapy or dosage adjustment. Nausea and vomiting are the most common adverse events associated with cinacalcet. In phase III trials, 66% of patients receiving cinacalcet experienced at least one episode of hypocalcemia (serum calcium <8.4 mg/dL), although, <1% of patients discontinued treatment.[163] The high incidence of hyocalcemia is not solely caused by lowered PTH activity, but is also attributed to the mechanism of action of cinacalcet. It is thought that activation of CaSR in bone, intestine, and other tissues may contribute to hypocalemia.[164,165] Most episodes of hypocalemia occur during the initiation of cinacalcet therapy and slowly titrating the dose reduces the risk. Seizures caused by hypocalcemia have been reported, however. Vitamin D or calcium-based binders can be increased to manage serum calcium levels between 7.5 and 8.4 mg/dL. If serum calcium falls below 7.5 mg/dL and is associated with symptoms of hypocalcemia and vitamin D cannot be increased further, cinacalcet should be withheld until serum calcium is 8.0 mg/dL or the patient is asymptomatic. Cinacalcet is a strong in vitro inhibitor of CYP2D6, therefore, dose adjustments of concomitant medications that are predominantly metabolized by CYP2D6 may be required. Ketoconazole has also been documented to interact with cinacalcet. Cinacalcet is a substrate of CYP3A4, and ketaconazole, a potent inhibitor of CYP3A4, has been shown to increase the area under the curve (AUC) of cinacalcet 2.3 times. Thus, other inhibitors of the CYP3A4 isoenzyme should be used in caution in patients receiving cinacalcet.[163] Short-term aluminum hydroxide may be another alternative if more aggressive lowering of phosphorus is necessary.

Parathyroidectomy

The parathyroid glands enlarge as a compensatory response to disturbances of phosphorus, calcium, and calcitriol metabolism in patients with CKD. Timely administration of vitamin D therapy to prevent parathyroid hyperplasia is crucial, because treatment with vitamin D cannot adequately reverse established hyperplasia.[133] Under circumstances in which severe sHPT cannot be controlled by dietary phosphorus restriction and drug therapy, parathyroidectomy is considered. Parathyroidectomy can be subtotal, total, or total with autotransplantation. One of the major complications of parathyroidectomy is the early development of postsurgical hypocalcemia. Clinical symptoms of hypocalcemia include muscle irritability, fatigue, depression, and memory loss. Patients should be monitored closely following parathyroidectomy, and all patients with signs or symptoms of hypocalcemia should be treated with calcium supplementation (see Chapter 11, Fluid and Electrolyte Disorders). In patients who have had subtotal parathyroidectomy, the remaining parathyroid tissues will start functioning adequately, so that the acute hypocalcemia is only transient, lasting only a few days. With total parathyroidectomy, however, hypocalcemia is permanent, necessitating long-term treatment with calcitriol and oral calcium supplements (1–1.5 g/day of elemental calcium).

OTHER COMPLICATIONS OF CKD

Endocrine Abnormalities Caused by Uremia

18. Does D.B.'s hypothyroidism have any relationship to her CKD? What other endocrine abnormalities are associated with uremia?

Disturbances in thyroid function are frequently encountered in patients with CKD because the kidney is involved in all aspects of peripheral thyroid hormone metabolism. Common laboratory abnormalities include reduced serum concentrations of total thyroxine (T_4) and 3,5,3′-triiodothyronine (T_3) and a low free thyroxine index (FTI). The thyroid-stimulating hormone (TSH) concentration is usually normal, but peripheral conversion of T_4 to T_3 is reduced in uremic patients.[166] Despite these abnormalities, clinical hypothyroidism does not occur solely as a result of kidney disease, probably because the amount of free (unbound to protein) thyroid hormone in serum remains normal. Hypothyroidism in patients with kidney failure should be confirmed by the presence of an elevated serum TSH concentration and a low serum concentration of free T_4.

Other endocrine abnormalities that have been observed in patients with CKD include gonadal dysfunction leading to impotence, diminished testicular size, menstrual abnormalities, and cessation of ovulation.[167] Decreased libido and infertility occur in both sexes. Uremic women should avoid becoming pregnant, because there is a low likelihood of successful delivery. In children with kidney disease, growth retardation occurs despite normal or elevated growth hormone. Hyperprolactinemia and altered vasoactive hormone activity are other endocrine disturbances that can occur in patients with CKD.[166]

Altered Glucose and Insulin Metabolism

19. Other than the obvious effect of D.B.'s diabetes mellitus on blood glucose, are there any effects of kidney disease itself on glucose metabolism?

Uremia often is associated with glucose intolerance early in the course of kidney disease in nondiabetic patients and this may be referred to as "pseudodiabetes." Specifically, patients with CKD often exhibit an abnormal response to an oral glucose challenge and have sustained hyperinsulinemia.[168] The fasting blood glucose is typically within normal limits. Diminished tissue sensitivity to the action of insulin is also observed. Although their exact role is unclear, several uremic toxins, including urea, creatinine, guanidinosuccinic acid, and methylguanidine, have been implicated as causes for insulin resistance. Elevated concentrations of growth hormone, PTH, and glucagon also may contribute to glucose intolerance. Most nondiabetic patients with kidney disease do not require therapy for hyperglycemia, and dialysis can correct these abnormalities in glucose metabolism.[166]

Patients with diabetes mellitus and advanced kidney disease may experience improved glucose control and decreased insulin requirements. This is because the kidney is responsible for a substantial amount of daily insulin degradation and, as the disease progresses, less insulin is cleared, and its metabolic half-life is increased.[166] A decreased clearance of insulin by muscle tissue also can occur in patients with uremia. Thus, in diabetic patients with progressive kidney disease, blood glucose concentrations should be monitored and insulin doses adjusted to avoid hypoglycemia. D.B. has stage 5 CKD and is receiving her insulin in the peritoneal dialysate solution. Hyperglycemia is also a concern in D.B. because the glucose present in her continuous ambulatory peritoneal dialysis (CAPD) fluid to promote fluid removal will be absorbed systemically. Insulin dosage adjustments should be made on the basis of repeated home blood glucose measurements, changes in the CAPD prescription, and glycosylated hemoglobin determinations.

Gastrointestinal Complications

20. One month before her current clinic visit, D.B. complained of nausea and vomiting of partially digested food. Metoclopramide (Reglan) was begun at that time. Could D.B.'s nausea and vomiting have been caused by her kidney failure? Was the appropriate therapy selected?

Gastrointestinal abnormalities are extremely common in patients with CKD and include anorexia, nausea, vomiting, hiccups, abdominal pain, GI bleeding, diarrhea, and constipation.[169] Diminished gastric motility can occur from uremia; however, this problem may improve with adequate HD. Dyspeptic complaints and gastroparesis may be more prevalent in the PD population than in the HD population and in the earlier stages of CKD.[170] D.B has diabetes and diabetic neuropathy, which also contributes to the delayed gastric emptying (diabetic gastroparesis) and retention of food in the upper intestinal tract. This frequently causes distention, nausea, and vomiting. Metoclopramide is recommended to relieve these symptoms, although the risk for extrapyramidal side effects should be considered. A lower dose of 5 mg before meals may be warranted for D.B. Cisapride (Propulsid), a prokinetic agent that has restricted access, is contraindicated in patients with kidney disease because its use is associated with the development of arrhythmias in this population.

Severe uremia also causes nausea and vomiting, and these can be initial presenting symptoms of kidney failure. Although antiemetics, such as prochlorperazine (Compazine), are used, dialysis is the preferred therapy. Drug-induced nausea and vomiting always should be considered, because patients with CKD often take multiple drugs and are at risk for drug toxicity because of diminished kidney function (e.g., digitalis intoxication).

Bleeding

21. During her clinic visit, D.B. reports that her bowel movements have become black and tarry in appearance. A rectal examination reveals guaiac-positive stools. Is GI bleeding related to kidney failure?

D.B. should be evaluated for peptic ulcer disease and lower GI bleeding. Uremic patients are at risk for bleeding from mucosal surfaces such as the stomach. D.B.'s hemoglobin and hematocrit are below the target values (11–12 g/dL for hemoglobin, 33% to 36% for hematocrit), despite therapy with epoetin, and it is likely that bleeding is contributing to poor responsiveness to therapy. Angiodysplasia of the stomach and duodenum, as well as erosive esophagitis, are the most common causes of bleeding in patients with CKD.[171] Treatment of upper GI bleeding in uremic patients usually consists of cautious use of antacid therapy and H_2-receptor antagonists, which should be given in reduced doses according to the degree of kidney function. Proton pump inhibitors are primarily eliminated by nonrenal routes and can be administered at standard doses (see Chapter 26, Upper Gastrointestinal Disorders). Use of H_2-receptor antagonists has generally replaced chronic antacid use for treatment of dyspepsia in patients with CKD.

Neurologic Complications

22. S.H., a 64-year-old, 72-kg, black man, went to his primary care physician because of weakness, nausea, lethargy, decreased exercise tolerance, and general malaise that has developed over the past few weeks. S.H. had not been seen by a physician for >10 years. His medical history was unremarkable, except he recalls being told approximately 5 years ago that he had borderline hypertension. He was taking no medications. The physician's examination revealed a BP of 168/92 mmHg, and funduscopic examination showed grade III hypertensive changes. On neurologic examination, S.H. was slightly confused, appeared somnolent, and had diminished sensation to pinprick in both lower extremities; asterixis was present. Examination of the skin showed pallor and excoriations across the abdomen, legs, and arms. Pertinent laboratory values were as follows: Hct, 20% (normal, 39%–49%); Hgb, 6.7 g/dL (normal, 13–16 g/dL); WBC count, 9,100/mm^3 (normal, 3,200–9,800/mm^3); serum Na, 135 mEq/L (normal, 135–147 mEq/L); K, 5.8 mEq/L (normal, 3.5–5.0 mEq/L); Cl, 109 mEq/L (normal, 95–105 mEq/L); CO_2 content, 16 mEq/L (normal, 22–28 mEq/L); random blood glucose, 121 mg/dL (normal, <140 mg/dL); BUN, 199 mg/dL (normal, 8–18 mg/dL); SrCr, 19.8 mg/dL (normal, 0.6–1.2 mg/dL); Ca, 8.5 mg/dL (normal, 8.8–10.4 mg/dL); phosphate, 11.1 mg/dL (normal, 2.5–5.0 mg/dL); intact PTH, 830 pg/mL (normal, 5–65 pg/mL); uric acid, 11.9 mg/dL (normal, 2.0–7.0 mg/dL); and albumin, 3.0 g/dL (normal, 4.0–6.0 g/dL).

Renal ultrasonography revealed no obstruction and small kidneys bilaterally. Subsequent kidney biopsy showed chronic glomerular scarring. S.H. was diagnosed with stage 5 CKD, likely caused by chronic, untreated hypertension. What is the likely explanation for S.H.'s altered mental status? What treatment, if any, is indicated for his neurologic findings?

[SI units: Hct, 0.20 (normal, 0.39–0.49); Hgb, 67 g/L (normal, 130–160); WBC, 9,100 × 10^6/L (normal, 3,200–9,800); Na, 135 mmol/L (normal, 135–147); K, 5.8 mmol/L (normal, 3.5–5.0); Cl, 109 mmol/L (normal, 95–105); CO_2, 16 mmol/L (normal, 22–28); blood glucose, 6.7 mmol/L (normal, <11 mmol/L); BUN, 71.0 mmol/L of urea (normal, 3.0–6.5); SrCr, 1,750 μmol/L (normal, 50–110); Ca, 2.12 mmol/L (normal, 2.2–2.6); phosphate, 3.58 mmol/L (normal, 0.8–1.60); uric acid, 708 μmol/L (normal, 120–420); and albumin, 30 g/L (normal, 40–60)]

Disorders of the central nervous system (CNS) that occur in patients with untreated kidney disease and in those receiving dialysis are referred to collectively as *uremic encephalopathy*. Symptoms generally occur when the eGFR is <10% of normal. Although S.H.'s altered neurologic function is most likely caused by uremia, a careful drug history should exclude the possibility of drug effects. Symptoms of uremic encephalopathy include alterations in consciousness, thinking, memory, speech, psychomotor behavior, and emotion. Patients or their family members may note fatigue, daytime drowsiness, insomnia, diminished cognitive abilities, slurred speech, vomiting, and emotional volatility. The patient also may complain of being cold, having "restless legs," or "burning feet." The encephalopathy may progress to ataxia, vertigo, nystagmus, coma, and convulsions. Electroencephalograms (EEG) of patients with CKD usually show diffuse abnormalities.

Evidence supports PTH as a major contributing factor to the altered neurologic status of patients with ESRD; however, other uremic toxins can play a role in this disorder. PTH may enhance the entry of calcium into the brain and peripheral nerves, but it also may be directly neurotoxic. In all likelihood, S.H.'s altered mental status will improve with dialysis and correction of his hyperparathyroidism, although additional factors, such as his advanced age, must be considered.

The peripheral nervous system also shows abnormal function in many patients with advanced CKD, as illustrated by S.H., who has loss of sensation in his legs by pinprick examination. Typically, the peripheral neuropathy will be slowly progressive, distal, and symmetric, usually first involving sensory function. The abnormalities seen usually are indistinguishable from other types of neuropathy, especially diabetic neuropathy. Nerve conduction studies often reveal abnormalities preceding clinical symptoms. Treatment generally consists of measures to alleviate symptoms with agents, such as tricyclic antidepressants (e.g., amitriptyline) and anticonvulsants (e.g., phenytoin, gabapentin). Increasing the intensity of dialysis does not seem to affect the neuropathy; however, successful renal transplantation may ameliorate nerve dysfunction.

Abnormalities of the autonomic nervous system also have been observed in patients with kidney failure and present as postural hypotension, impotence, impaired sweating, and alterations in gastric motility. HD may be more likely to correct autonomic dysfunction in nondiabetic patients.

Dermatologic Complications

23. Why does S.H. have excoriations on his skin? What therapy would be useful?

Several dermal abnormalities have been observed in patients with CKD, including hyperpigmentation, abnormal perspiration, skin dryness, and persistent pruritus. Of these, *uremic pruritus* can be the most bothersome for the patient and may lead to repeated scratching and skin excoriation. Hyperparathyroidism, hypervitaminosis A, and dermal mast cell proliferation with subsequent histamine release have been suggested as causes of pruritus.[172]

Treatment of pruritus often is a frustrating experience for the patient and clinician. Although many therapies have been advocated, few have provided sustained benefit. A trial-and-error approach is recommended. Efficient dialysis therapy relieves pruritus in some patients and pharmacologic therapy may be avoided.[173] When necessary, initial pharmacologic treatment usually consists of oral antihistamines (e.g., hydroxyzine). Topical emollients or topical steroids may provide benefit if antihistamine therapy is not completely successful. If pruritus is still present, other treatment options can be tried. These include cholestyramine, ultraviolet B (UVB) phototherapy, and oral administration of activated charcoal. Control of calcium and phosphorus concentrations and prevention of secondary hyperparathyroidism are also advocated to reduce pruritus in patients with CKD.

GLOMERULAR DISEASE

Glomerular diseases lead to many complications that result from disruption of normal glomerular structure and function.

Several clinical syndromes of glomerular disease exist; however, glomerulonephritis, characterized as proliferation and inflammation of the glomerulus, is observed most frequently. According to the most recent USRDS report, glomerulonephritis as a broad category remains the third leading cause of ESRD in the United States, accounting for approximately 8.4% of new cases and a higher proportion of the PD population (14.6%) when compared with the HD population (8%).[3] In developing countries, glomerulonephritis is more common as a cause of kidney failure because various infectious processes responsible for glomerulonephritis are more common.

Nephrotic Syndrome

Nephrotic syndrome is characterized by proteinuria >3.5g/day, hypoalbuminemia, edema, and hyperlipidemia. In more severe conditions, hypercoagulable conditions may be present because of loss of hemostasis control proteins, including antithrombin III, protein S, and protein C. This syndrome can occur with or without a change in glomerular filtration rate. Nephrotic syndrome may be caused by a primary disease, such as membranous glomerulopathy, which is characterized by deposition of immune complexes, or other systemic diseases including diabetic glomerulosclerosis and amyloidosis. Elevated serum cholesterol and triglycerides are observed in patients with this degree of proteinuria (>3.5 g/day). This hyperlipidemic condition also predisposes patients with nephrotic syndrome to accelerated atherosclerosis. Hyperlipidemia itself can also contribute to progression of kidney disease. Because nephrotic syndrome is associated with numerous causes, further evaluation of the patient for systemic causes is required to then determine the course of therapy and prognosis.

Chronic Glomerulopathies

Glomerulonephritis can occur as a primary disease that is idiopathic in origin (focal segmental glomerulosclerosis [FSGS]) or as a secondary manifestation of other systemic disease (lupus nephritis [LN]), Wegener's granulomatosis). Renal biopsy is often required for definitive diagnosis. Glomerular lesions associated with glomerulopathies are characterized as diffuse, focal, or segmental, depending on the extent of involvement of individual glomeruli. Pathologic changes are characterized as proliferative, membranous, and sclerotic based on the pattern observed. Proliferative changes usually involve an overgrowth of the epithelium or mesangium, whereas membranous changes are typically described as a thickening of the glomerular basement membrane. Signs and symptoms of glomerulonephritis include hematuria, proteinuria, and decreased kidney function. An autoimmune reaction is the predominant pathogenic process leading to most forms of primary and secondary glomerulonephritis. Although a number of autoantibodies are associated with glomerulonephritis, their exact role in the pathogenesis of glomerulonephritis is still unclear. Nonetheless, analysis of autoantibodies in the clinical setting can aid in early diagnosis of glomerulonephritis.[174]

Glomerular damage generally occurs in two phases: acute and chronic. During the acute phase, immune reactions occur within glomeruli that stimulate the complement cascade, ultimately resulting in glomerular damage. Nonimmune mechanisms that occur in response to loss of nephron function and hyperfiltration of remaining nephrons are characteristic of the chronic phase.

Glomerulonephritis often causes acute renal failure. Patients with damage to >50% of glomeruli in the presence of rapid loss in kidney function (over days to weeks) are classified as having *rapidly progressive glomerulonephritis* (RPGN).[174] If kidney involvement is severe, signs and symptoms of uremia may develop. RPGN may be classified based on the immunopathogenic etiology of the glomerular damage: (*a*) immune complex deposition (e.g., LN), (*b*) nonimmune deposit-mediated mechanism (e.g., Wegener's granulomatosis), and (*c*) sclerotic lesions of the glomerulus (e.g., FSGS).[174] This chapter focuses on the treatment of the more common forms of chronic glomerulonephritis (i.e., LN, Wegener's granulomatosis, FSGS).

Lupus Nephritis

Systemic lupus erythematosus (SLE) is a multisystem autoimmune disease characterized by abnormalities in cell-mediated immunity, such as B-cell hyperresponsiveness and defective T-cell–mediated suppressor activity. In certain predisposed individuals, SLE can lead to the development of LN, a secondary form of glomerulonephritis. LN is the prototypical immune complex-mediated kidney disease, characterized by deposition or in situ formation of autoantibody–antigen complexes along the glomerular capillary network. LN remains an important cause of mortality. Up to 60% of adults with SLE have some degree of kidney involvement later in the course of their disease, discernible from clinical evidence of kidney damage: heavy proteinuria, hematuria, decreased eGFR, and hypertension. Early in the disease, laboratory abnormalities indicative of kidney involvement are seen in approximately 25% to 50% of patients.

24. C.W., a 34-year-old black woman with a 7-year history of SLE, presents to the nephrology clinic for follow up of her LN. Pertinent laboratory values are as follows: serum Na, 146 mEq/L (normal, 135–147 mEq/L); K, 4.2 mEq/L (normal, 3.5–5.0 mEq/L); Cl, 100 mEq/L (normal, 95–105 mEq/L); CO_2 content, 25 mEq/L (normal, 22–28 mEq/L); SrCr, 2.0 mg/dL (normal, 0.6–1.2 mg/dL); BUN, 20 mg/dL (normal, 8–18 mg/dL); and WBC count, 9,600/mm^3 (normal, 3,200–9,800/mm^3). RBC indices were normal. Platelet count is 175,000/mm^3 (normal, 130,000–400,000/mm^3). Her 24-hour urine contained 2.3 g of albumin (normal, <30 mg/day), and her urine analysis shows 12 RBC/high-power field (HPF) (normal, 0–3). Compared with her visit of a week ago, C.W.'s kidney function and urinary indices (proteinuria, hematuria) show substantial worsening of her nephritis. C.W. was hospitalized, and a kidney biopsy showed inflammation of 40% of the glomeruli. What subjective and objective data in C.W. are consistent with a diagnosis of LN, and what is the stage of her nephritis?

[SI units: Na, 146 mmol/L (normal, 135–147); K, 4.2 mmol/L (normal, 3.5–5.0); Cl, 100 mmol/L (normal, 95–105); CO_2, 25 mmol/L (normal, 22–28); SrCr, 177 μmol/L (normal, 50–110); BUN, 7.14 mmol/L of urea (normal, 3.0–6.5); WBC, 9,600 × 10^6/L (normal, 3,200–9,800); platelet count, 175 × 10^9/L (normal, 130–400); urinary albumin, 2.3 g/day (normal, <0.03)]

C.W. has clinical evidence of kidney damage as demonstrated by her proteinuria, hematuria, and increased SrCr

Table 31-8 2003 International Society of Nephrology/Renal Pathology Society Classification of Lupus Nephritis

Class	*Histologic Characterization*	*Usual Clinical Presentation*
I	Minimal mesangial lupus nephritis	Mild proteinuria
II	Mesangial proliferative glomerulonephritis	Mild proteinuria and urine sediment abnormalities
III	Focal and segmental proliferative glomerulonephritis A: Active lesions; A/C: active and chronic lesions; C: chronic lesions	Proteinuria and hematuria
IV	Diffuse proliferative segmental (S) or global (G) glomerulonephritis A: Active lesions; A/C: active and chronic lesions; C: chronic lesions	Heavy proteinuria; active sediment; hypertension; renal failure
V	Membranous glomerulonephritis	Proteinuria; often nephrotic syndrome
VI	Advanced sclerosing glomerulonephritis	Proteinuria; renal failure; nephrotic syndrome

Data from reference 175.

concentration. Glomerular damage is most evident by the presence of RBC or red cell casts in the urine, a finding observed in C.W.

CLASSIFICATIONS

The International Society of Nephrology and the Renal Pathology Society (ISN/RPS) classification system was developed in 2003 to replace the previous classification system published by the World Health Organization. (Table 31-8).[175] This classification scheme provides a reasonable correlation among histopathology, outcome, and response to treatment. C.W. has proteinuria, hematuria, and inflammation of <50% of her glomeruli, and she is diagnosed as having class III/A (focal proliferative) glomerulonephritis.

TREATMENT

25. Should C.W.'s LN be treated?

Unlike nonrenal manifestations of SLE, serologic markers of disease correlate poorly with LN. Therefore, elevations in SrCr and worsening of proteinuria and hematuria, as seen in C.W., are used as primary markers of disease activity.

Treatment of LN must address both management of the acute disease process and maintenance therapy for the more stable chronic disease process. A general consensus is that patients, such as C.W., who present with focal or diffuse proliferative glomerulonephritis (class III or IV), should be treated aggressively, with the primary goal of preventing irreversible kidney damage. The prognosis of kidney function in patients with SLE has improved. The likelihood of developing ESRD or dying within 10 years of diagnosis has decreased from >80% to <20%; however, the prognosis is worse in blacks when compared with the white population treated for SLE.[176] Elevated serum creatinine, heavy proteinuria, anemia, and disease onset during childhood or in those >60 years of age are other predictors of a worse prognosis. Advances in pharmacologic therapy (i.e., safer immunosuppressive regimens, and antihypertensives) have improved the prognosis for the population as a whole.

The treatment of LN is primarily empiric but is based, to some extent, on histologic findings. Although appropriate treatment can improve patient outcomes, vigorous attempts to suppress SLE activity may lead to serious drug-related complications. Because the primary strategy in the treatment of LN involves suppression of the immune system with corticosteroids and cytotoxic agents, such as cyclophosphamide (CYC), azathioprine (AZA), and mycophenolate mofetil (MMF), clinicians need to be aware of the potential complications associated with therapy. Therefore, careful monitoring of patients is essential in determining the indication for treatment and improving prognosis. Toxicities associated with immunosuppressive agents depend on both the dose and the duration of therapy. Abnormalities in hematopoiesis, such as neutropenia and thrombocytopenia, are the most common adverse effects associated with cytotoxic agents. Immunosuppression, in general, increases a patient's susceptibility to a vast array of infections and to lymphocytic malignancies. In addition, the alkylating agent CYC can cause nausea and vomiting, gonadal toxicity, hemorrhagic cystitis, and alopecia. The antimetabolite azathioprine AZA can cause pancreatitis and abnormalities in liver function. The selective inhibitor of inosine-monophosphate-dehydrogenase MMF, although relatively benign compared with the other agents, can cause GI disturbances.

Induction Therapy

Therapy for LN is usually not indicated in patients with normal renal function and proteinuria <2 g, regardless of class, because these patients have a good prognosis. Corticosteroids represent the cornerstone of therapy in patients with a mild form of LN. Low-dose prednisone should be initiated for patients with stable LN. In patients with a more severe form (class III and IV), prednisone 1 to 2 mg/kg/day for 4 to 8 weeks, as a single morning dose, may be initiated. Gradual tapering of prednisone to a low-dose regimen of 0.2 to 0.4 mg/kg/day must be attempted once glomerulonephritis has stabilized. For the treatment of acute exacerbations of LN, high-dose pulse therapy with methylprednisolone may be warranted. Given that C.W.'s LN has worsened, she should receive 3 days of therapy with pulse methylprednisolone (0.5 to 1 g IV, not to exceed 1 g) for 3 days in an attempt to reduce the degree of proteinuria and improve kidney function.[176] Although generally well tolerated, rapid methylprednisolone injections can cause transient tremor, flushing, and altered taste sensation. To reduce the risk of adverse effects associated with the rate of injection, C.W. should receive methylprednisolone over 30 minutes. After a course of pulse methylprednisolone therapy, oral prednisone at a dose 10 to 20 mg daily may be initiated.[176] Suppression of C.W.'s active LN should be demonstrated by a reduction in proteinuria and hematuria and an increase in her eGFR.

The addition of cytotoxic agents is reserved for patients who do not respond to corticosteroids alone, or those who have unacceptable toxicity to corticosteroids, worsening renal function, severe proliferative lesions, or evidence of sclerosis on renal biopsy. Induction therapy with six monthly pulse doses of IV CYC (0.5–1 g/m^2) or six doses of CYC given every 2 weeks at a dose of 0.5 g/m^2 along with steroid therapy was shown to have improved renal outcomes with less flares and relapses.[177,178] Before, and for 24 hours after initiating IV CYC, the patient must be well hydrated to prevent bladder toxicity. Recently, MMF (2,000–3,000 mg/day times 6 months) has been proven to be as effective as CYC in the induction treatment for LN.[179] Given the significant toxicities associated with CYC (e.g. gonadal toxicity, hemorrhagic cystitis), the anti-inflammatory properties of MMF resulting in a possible retardation of atherosclerosis and the lower side effect profile with MMF, the option to use MMF as an alternative agent in LN seems promising, but its use in LN is still unclear. Studies are currently ongoing to determine the optimal dosing and duration of therapy with MMF, as well as, which patient population would benefit the most from this therapy in the induction therapy for LN.

Maintenance Therapy

Once the acute flare resolves (generally in up to 12 weeks), low-dose, maintenance steroid therapy with 5 to 15 mg/day of prednisone can be initiated in combination with cytotoxic therapy, if indicated, based on severity of LN. In a meta-analysis assessing the efficacy of therapeutic agents used to treat LN, improved outcomes (total mortality and ESRD) were associated with use of oral prednisone in combination with IV CYC. As a result, the National Institutes of Health (NIH) recommends the use of IV CYC pulse therapy (0.5 to 1 g/m^2) every 3 months for up to 2 years for maintenance therapy of LN.[180] An additional benefit of combination therapy with immunosuppressive agents is their steroid-sparing effect and, potentially, lower risk of steroid toxicity.

Studies have evaluated other immunosuppressive agents (AZA, MMF) for maintenance therapy in light of the toxicities associated with CYC. The most recent trial compared maintenance therapy with AZA (1 to 3 mg/day) and MMF (500–3,000 mg/day) with CYC along with steroids after induction with CYC in patients with severe LN. Patients receiving AZA had a lower mortality rate than with CYC and the MMF treatment group had fewer relapses than the CYC treatment group.[181] Until results from long-term trials with AZA and MMF are available, CYC is still considered first-line therapy for most classes of LN. MMF and AZA may be indicated in patients resistant to CYC therapy or with a more severe type of LN (class III and IV). The addition of CYC, AZA, and MMF, along with corticosteroid therapy, should be considered in C.W. once the acute lupus flare resolves. Once suppression of C.W.'s LN is documented, initiation of either AZA or MMF and steroids are indicated because of the severity of her LN (class III). The duration of therapy is dictated by the individual's response, but typically patients will require up to 2 years of maintenance therapy.

Alternative Agents

Exploration of alternative therapies for LN are also being studied. Rituximab, a monoclonal antibody that inhibits B-cell production, is being studied because B-cell hyperactivity is one of the major pathophysiologic mechanisms of LN. Small studies in patients with LH resistant to therapy have shown rituximab to be of benefit.[180] Cyclosporine, in doses of 5 mg/kg/day, may also provide an alternative therapy to treat lupus in the maintenance phase in patients unresponsive to treatment.[176]

Wegener's Granulomatosis

26. J.M. is a 42-year-old white man who presents to the clinic with a 1-month history of cough, nasal congestion, facial pain with headache, fever, and lethargy. Over the past week, he has noted bright red blood in his phlegm, which has worsened in the past 3 days. Pertinent laboratory values are as follows: serum Na, 143 mEq/L (normal, 135–147 mEq/L); K, 5.1 mEq/L (normal, 3.5–5.0 mEq/L); Cl, 102 mEq/L (normal, 95–105 mEq/L); CO_2 content, 24 mEq/L (normal, 22–28 mEq/L); SrCr, 2.8 mg/dL (normal, 0.6–1.2 mg/dL); BUN, 41 mg/dL (normal, 8–18 mg/dL). This compares with last year's physical checkup visit when his SrCr and BUN were within the normal range. Hematologic studies reveal an Hct of 35% (normal, 8–18 mg/dL); an Hgb of 11.7 g/dL (normal, 13–16 g/dL); mean corpuscular volume (MCV) 69 mm^3 (normal, 76–100 mm^3); mean corpuscular Hgb (MCH) concentration 24% (normal, 33%–37%); and reticulocyte count 1.8% (normal, 0.1% –2.4%). RBC indices are normal. Platelet count was 175,000/mm^3 (normal, 130,000–400,000/mm^3). His 24-hour urine contains 3.8 g of albumin (normal, <30 mg) and his eGFR is calculated to be 27 mL/minute/1.73 m^2. His urine also contains many RBC casts and 16 RBC/HPF (normal, 0–3 RBC/HPF). Chest radiograph shows alveolar shadowing spreading from the hilar region. The result of J.M.'s cytoplasmic-staining, antineutrophil cytoplasmic antibody (c-ANCA) is positive. Based on his subjective and objective data, which of the chronic glomerulopathies is J.M. likely to have?

[SI units: Na, 143 mmol/L (normal, 135–147); K, 5.1 mmol/L (normal, 3.5–5.0); Cl, 102 mmol/L (normal, 95–105); CO_2, 24 mmol/L (normal, 22–28); SrCr, 247 μmol/L (normal, 50–110); BUN, 14.6 mmol/L of urea (normal, 3.0–6.5); Hct, 0.35 (normal, 0.39–0.49); Hgb, 117 g/L (normal, 130–160); MCV, 69 fL (normal, 76–100); MCH, 0.24 (normal, 0.33–0.37); reticulocyte count, 0.019 (normal, 0.001–0.024); eGFR, 0.40 mL/second]

Wegener's granulomatosis is a primary systemic vasculitis characterized by granulomatous inflammation of the upper and lower respiratory tract and secondary glomerulonephritis. Primary systemic vasculitic syndromes, such as Wegener's granulomatosis, often cause glomerulonephritis. Although vasculitis involves inflammation of blood vessels of any size, the small- and medium-size vessels are most commonly affected.[182] The etiology of Wegener's granulomatosis is unclear; however, an autoimmune response is suspected for two reasons. First, Wegener's granulomatosis is a systemic inflammatory disease without a known infectious etiology. Second, good treatment response can be obtained with immunosuppressive therapy.

The clinical features of Wegener's granulomatosis include upper airway disease, such as sinusitis, epistaxis, and nasopharyngitis, as well as otitis media caused by blockage of the eustachian tube. Constitutional symptoms include fever, night sweats, arthralgia, anorexia, and malaise. After a few months, weakness may progress, severely limiting physical activity. Although the lungs are invariably affected, most patients remain asymptomatic; however, cough and hemoptysis may be present. J.M.'s presenting symptoms are consistent with the above clinical features. The laboratory signs also are nonspecific and indicate the presence of a systemic inflammatory process. They include an elevated erythrocyte sedimentation rate in virtually all patients, anemia of chronic disease, and thrombocytosis.[182] Hematuria and proteinuria can be prominent features of Wegener's granulomatosis and are present on initial presentation in 80% of patients. The presence of severely diminished kidney function, seen in approximately 10% of patients, is an ominous sign, with nearly one-third of these patients progressing to ESRD. All patients with Wegener's granulomatosis are at risk for developing irreversible, rapidly progressive kidney failure. Renal histologic findings are nonspecific, with most patients exhibiting necrotizing crescentic glomerulonephritis.[182]

Wegener's granulomatosis is diagnosed primarily by the presenting signs and symptoms. According to the American College of Rheumatology 1990 classification, a person is diagnosed with Wegener's granulomatosis if any two of the following four criteria are present: (a) nasal or oral inflammation, (b) abnormal chest radiograph, (c) microhematuria (>5 RBC/HPF) or RBC casts in the urine sediment, or (d) granulomatous inflammation on biopsy.[182] J.M. has satisfied three of the four criteria for diagnosing Wegener's granulomatosis.

TREATMENT

27. How should J.M.'s Wegener's granulomatosis be treated?

The discovery of c-ANCA and its strong association with Wegener's granulomatosis has permitted a more certain diagnosis. Because of the substantial rise in titer that commonly precedes relapse of Wegener's granulomatosis, the c-ANCA test is best used to follow the course of disease activity and guide induction of therapy. Treatment with CYC and corticosteroids results in improvement in kidney function in approximately 80% to 85% of patients, versus 75% with pulse steroids alone.[183] The main predictive factors for treatment success are the extent of kidney damage before therapy starts and how long therapy is delayed after symptoms develop.

Cyclophosphamide

Because Wegener's granulomatosis is considered an autoimmune inflammatory disease, immunosuppressive therapy is the mainstay of treatment. Therapy is generally indicated for 6 months if remission occurs and up to 12 months in resistant cases.[183] J.M. should be initiated on oral CYC 2 mg/kg/day, as a single morning dose to prevent irreversible glomerular scarring. With a more fulminate form of the disease, higher doses (4–5 mg/kg/day) may be used, although the potential for toxicities must be carefully considered. High fluid intake (>3 L/day) reduces the risk of hemorrhagic cystitis. Regular urinalysis should be performed (every 3–6 months) to detect hematuria caused by hemorrhagic cystitis.

Induction treatment with pulse IV boluses of CYC is not satisfactory because of high relapse rates and increased toxicity. However, the two conditions for which IV CYC may be considered are (a) patients whose conditions have not responded to conventional treatment and (b) patients in whom severe kidney dysfunction developed initially, including those requiring dialysis. In the former, IV CYC 1 g/m^2 in 150 mL of saline can be administered over 60 minutes. The dose must be reduced by 25% in patients with a eGFR <10 mL/minute/1.73 m^2. This regimen may be administered monthly for 6 months, after which a dosage reduction may be attempted.[184]

Corticosteroids

The main role of corticosteroids is to induce remission of the disease. J.M. should receive prednisone 1 mg/kg/day in addition to cyclophosphamide. The combined regimen should be continued for 2 to 4 weeks until the immunosuppressive effect of CYC becomes evident. Then, over the next 2 months, the prednisone dose can be tapered to 60 mg every other day to reduce the risk of infection. Then, the dose can be tapered by 5 mg/week to discontinue prednisone over 3 to 6 months. For patients with a more fulminate form of the disease, pulse methylprednisolone 1 g/m^2/day for three doses is administered. The dose can be repeated in 1 to 2 weeks if disease progression is uncontrolled.

Azathioprine

Because of its poor efficacy, AZA should not be used as a first-line agent to treat active Wegener's granulomatosis. If remission is induced with CYC and the patient cannot tolerate long-term treatment with that agent, AZA 2 mg/kg/day may be substituted.

Alternative Agents

Other agents have been studied as alternatives to CYC. Use of trimethoprim-sulfamethoxazole over 1 year was evaluated for patients in remission or after treatment with CYC and prednisolone.[185] A reduction in relapse rate was demonstrated compared with placebo. Subgroup analysis indicates, however, that only patients with upper respiratory tract disease had a lower relapse rate, but not in those with renal or lung involvment.[185] Methotrexate may be beneficial for patients with milder disease, although one study demonstrated high relapse rates in patients treated initially with weekly methotrexate and daily prednisone; disease was controlled in only select patients.[186]

Focal Segmental Glomerulosclerosis

28. A.G. is a 37-year-old morbidly obese (BMI 40 kg/m^2), black woman who presents to the clinic with complaints of increased swelling in her extremities over the last 2 weeks, decreased urine output, and pink-colored urine. Her medical history is significant only for hypertension, which is well controlled with amlodipine 5 mg PO QD. She takes no other prescription or over-the-counter (OTC) medications. Pertinent laboratory values are as follows: SrCr 2.1 mg/dL (normal, 0.6–1.2 mg/dL), a spot albumin-to-creatinine ratio of 1,200 mg/g (normal, <30 mg/g), her UA showed 18 RBC/ HPF (normal, 0–3), and eGFR of 34 mL/minute/1.73 m^2. The nephrologist schedules a biopsy to obtain a definitive diagnosis for her new onset kidney disease. Biopsy results are as follows: light micrograph shows a moderately large segmental area of sclerosis with capillary collapse on the upper left side of the glomerular tuft; the lower right segment is relatively normal. Electron micrograph shows diffuse epithelial cell foot process fusion with occasional loss of the epithelial cells. The other major finding is massive subendothelial hyaline deposits under the glomerular basement membrane. The pathologist's impression is FSGS. What is the relevance of FSGS and what are the management strategies for FSGS?

[SI units: SrCr, 185 μmol/L (normal, 50–110)]

Focal segmental glomerulosclerosis is characterized by sclerotic lesions of the glomerulus, which can be either focal or segmental in nature. The development of FSGS may be idiopathic (primary) or secondary to other diseases (i.e., morbid obesity, sickle cell disease, congenital heart disease, AIDS). Currently, FSGS is the leading cause of idiopathic nephrotic syndrome and accounts for 15% to 20% of the cases. Black patients are two to four times more likely to develop idiopathic FSGS than white patients and they have a higher incidence of ESRD caused by FSGS.[187]

Most all patients with FSGS will present with proteinuria, but only about half of them will initially present with nephrotic syndrome. Patients with nephrotic sydrome will also likely present with hypertension, increased serum creatinine levels, and hematuria. During the early stages of FSGS, the symptoms may be indistinguishable from minimal-change nephropathy, a glomerulopathy characterized by similar lesions within the glomeruli. A renal biopsy is necessary for diagnosis. Predictors of increased risk of progression to ESRD include massive proteinuria (>10 g/day), higher serum creatinine level (>1.3 mg/dL), and black race.[187]

TREATMENT

Corticosteroids

A.G. should be placed on steroids, in addition to an ACE inhibitor or ARB and a loop diuretic, because she has FSGS and nephrotic syndrome.[188] A course of high-dose steroids (1–2 mg/kg) over 3 to 4 months with tapering of the dose over 3 months is recommended. The higher remission rates associated with this high-dose regimen compared with low-dose regimens have led to this regimen. The median time to remission is 3 to 4 months, with most patients achieving complete remission by 5 to 9 months. Patients whose proteinuria does not respond after a 4-month trial of therapy should be considered resistant to steroids and be rapidly tapered off over 4 weeks.[187]

Cytotoxic Agents

The addition of cytotoxic agents (CYC, AZA, chlorambucil) may be considered for A.G. if she is steroid resistant, intolerant of long-term steroid therapy, severely nephrotic, frequently relapsing, or steroid dependent. The data supporting the use of these agents in FSGS are limited. Retrospective studies have shown that use of cytotoxic drugs can produce complete remission in 50% of cases. Length of therapy of these agents may predict the remission rates of FSGS. Recent prospective studies are supporting a longer duration of therapy. Patients who received either chlorambucil or CYC up to 75 weeks obtained a higher complete remission rate (30%–47%). The duration of use of these agents is limited by their toxicities (gonadal toxicity, malignancies). Cumulative doses of 300 mg/kg of CYC and 10 mg/kg of chlorambucil have been shown to increase the risk of developing these toxicities, thus limiting the exposure to these agents is important.[187]

Cyclosporine

Evidence supporting the efficacy and safety of cyclosporine in FSGS is minimal, but therapy with doses of 5 mg/kg/day for 6 to 12 months has been found to be effective and can result in remission rates of up to 69% in patients resistant to steroid and cytotoxic therapy.[189,190] Limitations of cyclosporine therapy include high relapse rate (23%–100%), side-effect profile (nephrotoxicity, hypertension), and resistance to therapy. The former two limitations may be overcome by prolonged treatment with a slow tapering and targeting lower doses of cyclosporine. The exact dose and duration of cyclosporine therapy should be determined by the response of the patient's proteinuria and serum creatinine. Further studies will determine the role cyclosporine therapy has in certain types of patients with FSGS.

Mycophenolate Mofetil

Mycophenolate mofetil has the least available studies evaluating its use in FSGS. Recently, a small study of patients with FSGS resistant to steroids, cytotoxic agents, or both and cyclosporine received MMF for 6 months. At the end of 6 months, 44% of patients had improved proteinuria, but no patient achieved complete remission.[191] Other studies examining MMF therapy at doses of 1,500 to 2,000 mg/day have found no clinically significant reduction in proteinuria or have little effect on remission rates.[189] Treatment with MMF in FSGS is very limited and well-designed, prospective, randomized trials are necessary to determine its role, if any, in FSGS.

REFERENCES

1. NKF-K/DOQI Clinical Practice Guidelines for Chronic Kidney Disease: Evaluation, Classification, and Stratification. *Am J Kidney Dis* 2002;39:S1.
2. Coresh J et al. Prevalence of chronic kidney disease and decreased kidney function in the adult U.S. population: third national health and nutrition examination survey. *Am J kidney Dis* 2003;41:1.
3. U.S. Renal Data System, USRDS 2006 Annual Data Report: Atlas of End-Stage Renal Disease in the United States, National Institutes of Health, National Institute of Diabetes and Digestive and Kidney Diseases, Bethesda, MD; 2006.
4. U.S. Department of Health and Human Services. *Healthy People 2010.* 2nd ed. *With Understanding and Improving Health and Objectives for Improving Health.* 2 vols. Washington, DC: U.S. Government Printing Office; November 2000.
5. Henrich WL et al. Analgesics and the kidney: summary and recommendations to the Scientific Advisory Board of the National Kidney Foundation from an Ad Hoc Committee of the National Kidney Foundation. *Am J Kidney Dis* 1996;27:162.
6. Bennett WM et al. The renal effects of nonsteroidal anti-inflammatory drugs: summary and recommendations. *Am J Kidney Dis* 1996;28 (Suppl 1):S56.
7. Perneger TV et al. Risk of kidney failure associated with the use of acetaminophen, aspirin, and nonsteroidal antiinflammatory drugs. *N Engl J Med* 1994;331:675.
8. Zhang J et al. Adverse effects of cyclooxygenase 2 inhibitors on renal and arrhythmia events: meta-analysis of randomized trials. *JAMA* 2006;296:1619.
9. Bendz H et al. Kidney damage in long-term lithium patients: a cross-sectional study of patients with 15 years or more on lithium. *Nephrol Dial Transplant* 1994;9:1250.
10. Kallner G et al. Renal, thyroid and parathyroid function during lithium treatment: laboratory tests in 207 people treated for 1–30 years. *Acta Psychiatr Scand* 1995;91:48.
11. U.S. Renal Data System, USRDS 1998 Annual Data Report. National Institutes of Health, National Institute of Diabetes and Digestive and Kidney Diseases, Bethesda, MD; 1998.
12. Manley HJ et al. Factors associated with medication-related problems in ambulatory hemodialysis patients. *Am J Kidney Dis* 2003;41: 386.
13. Manley HJ et al. The clinical and economic impact of pharmaceutical care in end-stage renal disease patients. *Semin Dial* 2002;15:45.
14. Pai AB et al. Assessment of quality of life in hemodialysis patients receiving pharmaceutical care. *Pharmacotherapy* 2005;25:1465.
15. Kriz W et al. Pathways to nephron loss starting from glomerular diseases-insights from animal models. *Kidney Int* 2005;67:404.
16. Zandi-Nejad K et al. Strategies to retard the progression of chronic kidney disease. *Med Clin North Am* 2005;89:489.
17. Klag MJ et al. Blood pressure and end-stage renal disease in men. *N Engl J Med* 1996;334:13.
18. Peterson JC et al. Blood pressure control, proteinuria, and the progression of renal disease. The Modification of Diet in Renal Disease Study. *Ann Intern Med* 1995;123:754.
19. Attman PO et al. Abnormal lipid and apolipoprotein

composition of major lipoprotein density classes in patients with chronic renal failure. *Nephrol Dial Transplant* 1996;11:63.
20. Appel G et al. Analysis of metabolic parameters as predictors of risk in the RENAAL study. *Diabetes Care* 2003;26:1402.
21. Schaeffner ES et al. Cholesterol and the risk of renal dysfunction in apparently healthy men. *J Am Soc Nephrol* 2003;14:2084.
22. Boes A et al. Apolipoprotein A-IV predicts progression of chronic kidney disease: the mild to moderate kidney disease study. *J Am Soc Nephrol* 2006;17:528.
23. Bianchi S et al. A controlled, prospective study of the effects of atorvastatin on proteinuria and progression of kidney disease. *Am J Kidney Dis* 2003;41:565.
24. Hellerstein S et al. Creatinine clearance following cimetidine for estimation of glomerular filtration rate. *Pediatr Nephrol* 1998;12:49.
25. Caregaro L et al. Limitations of serum creatinine level and creatinine clearance as filtration markers in cirrhosis. *Arch Intern Med* 1994;154:201.
26. Cockcroft DW et al. Prediction of creatinine clearance from serum creatinine. *Nephron* 1976;16:31.
27. Levey AS et al. A more accurate method to estimate glomerular filtration rate from serum creatinine: a new prediction equation. Modification of Diet in Renal Disease Study Group. *Ann Intern Med* 1999;130:461.
28. Schwartz GJ et al. The use of plasma creatinine concentration for estimating glomerular filtration rate in infants, children, and adolescents. *Pediatr Clin North Am* 1987;34:571.
29. Poortmans JR et al. Renal protein excretion after exercise in man. *Eur J Appl Physiol Occup Physiol* 1989;58:476.
30. Walters BA et al. Health-related quality of life, depressive symptoms, anemia, and malnutrition at hemodialysis initiation. *Am J Kidney Dis* 2002;40:1185.
31. Stack AG. Impact of timing of nephrology referral and pre-ESRD care on mortality risk among new ESRD patients in the United States. *Am J Kidney Dis* 2003;41:310.
32. Sarnak MJ et al. The effect of lower target blood pressure on the progression of kidney disease: long-term follow-up of the modification of diet in renal disease study. *Ann Intern Med.* 2005;142:342.
33. Strippoli GFM et al. Role of blood pressure targets and specific antihypertensive agents used to prevent diabetic nephropathy and delay its progression. *J Am Soc Nephrol.* 2006;17:S153.
34. Chobanian AV el al. The Seventh Report of the Joint National Committee on Prevention, Detection, Evaluation, and Treatment of High Blood Pressure. *JAMA* 2003;289:2560.
35. Bakris GL et al. National Kidney Foundation Hypertension and Diabetes Executive Committee Working Group. Preserving renal function in adults with hypertension and diabetes. *Am J Kidney Dis* 2000;36:646.
36. Wright JT et al. Effect of blood pressure lowering and antihypertensive drug class on progression of hypertensive kidney disease: results from the AASK trial. *JAMA* 2002;288:2421.
37. Lea J et al. The relationship between magnitude of proteinuria reduction and risk of end-stage renal disease: results of the African American study of kidney disease and hypertension. *Arch Intern Med* 2005;165:947.
38. Laffel LM et al. The beneficial effect of angiotensin-converting enzyme inhibition with captopril on diabetic nephropathy in normotensive IDDM patients with microalbuminuria. North American Microalbuminuria Study Group. *Am J Med* 1995;99:497.
39. Parving HH et al. Long-term beneficial effect of ACE inhibition on diabetic nephropathy in normotensive type 1 diabetic patients. *Kidney Int* 2001;60:228.
40. Vijan S et al. Treatment of hypertension in type 2 diabetes mellitus: blood pressure goals, choice of agents, and setting priorities in diabetes care. *Ann Intern Med* 2003;138:593.
41. Maschio G et al. Effect of the angiotensin-converting-enzyme inhibitor benazepril on the progression of chronic renal insufficiency. *N Engl J Med* 1996;334:939.
42. Giatras I et al. Effect of angiotensin-converting enzyme inhibitors on the progression of nondiabetic renal disease: a meta-analysis of randomized trials. *Ann Intern Med* 1997;127:337.
43. Agadoa LY et al. Effect of ramipril on renal outcomes in hypertensive nephrosclerosis. *JAMA* 2001;285:2719.
44. Bakris GL et al. Angiotensin-converting enzyme inhibitor-associated elevations in serum creatinine: is this a cause for concern? *Arch Intern Med* 2000;160:685.
45. Brenner BM et al. Effects of losartan on renal and cardiovascular outcomes in patients with type 2 diabetes and nephropathy. *N Engl J Med* 2001;345:861.
46. Keane WF. Recent advances in management of type 2 diabetes and nephropathy: lessons from the RENAAL study. *Am J Kidney Dis* 2003;41(Suppl 2):S22.
47. Lewis EJ et al. Renoprotective effect of the angiotensin-receptor antagonist irbesartan in patients with nephropathy due to type 2 diabetes. *N Engl J Med* 2001;345:851.
48. Kurokawa K. Effects of candesartan on the proteinuria of chronic glomerulonephritis. *J Hum Hypertens* 1999;13(Suppl 1):S57.
49. Suzuki, et al. Renoprotective effects of low-dose valsartan in type 2 diabetic patients with diabetic nephropathy. *Diabetes Res Clin Pract* 2002;57:179.
50. MacKinnon M et al. Combination therapy with an angiotensin receptor blocker and an ACE inhibitor in proteinuric renal disease: a systematic review of the efficacy and safety data. *Am J Kidney Dis* 2006;48:8.
51. Van Tassell BW et al. Aliskiren for renin inhibition: a new class of antihypertensives. *Ann Pharmacother* 2007;41:456.
52. Smith AC et al. Differential effects of calcium channel blockers on size selectivity of proteinuria in diabetic glomerulopathy. *Kidney Int* 1998;54:889.
53. Ritz E et al. Angiotensin converting enzyme inhibitors, calcium channel blockers, and their combination in the treatment of glomerular disease. *J Hypertens Suppl* 1997;15:S21.
54. UK Prospective Diabetes Study Group. Efficacy of atenolol and captopril in reducing risk of macrovascular and microvascular complications in type 2 diabetes: UKPDS 39. *BMJ* 1998;317:713.
55. Brandle E et al. Effect of chronic dietary protein intake on the renal function in healthy subjects. *Eur J Clin Nutr* 1996;50:734.
56. Klahr S et al. The effects of dietary protein restriction and blood-pressure control on the progression of chronic renal disease. Modification of Diet in Renal Disease Study Group. *N Engl J Med* 1994;330:877.
57. Levey AS et al. Effects of dietary protein restriction on the progression of advanced renal disease in the Modification of Diet in Renal Disease Study. *Am J Kidney Dis* 1996;27:652.
58. Kasiske BL et al. A meta-analysis of the effects of dietary protein restriction on the rate of decline in renal function. *Am J Kidney Dis* 1998;31:954.
59. Levey AS et al. Effect of dietary protein restriction on the progression of kidney disease: long-term follow-up of the Modification of Diet in Renal Disease (MDRD) study. *Am J Kidney Dis* 2006;48:879.
60. Pupim LB et al. Nutrition and metabolism in kidney disease. *Semin Nephrol* 2006;26:134.
61. Levey AS et al. Controlling the epidemic of cardiovascular disease in chronic renal disease: what do we know? What do we need to learn? Where do we go from here? National Kidney Foundation Task Force on Cardiovascular Disease. *Am J Kidney Dis* 1998;32:853.
62. Lam KS et al. Cholesterol-lowering therapy may retard the progression of diabetic nephropathy. *Diabetologia* 1995;38:604.
63. Sandhu S et al. Statins for improving renal outcomes: a meta-analysis. *J Am Soc Nephrol* 2006;17:2006.
64. Third Report of the National Cholesterol Education Program (NCEP) Expert Panel on Detection, Evaluation, and Treatment of High Blood Cholesterol in Adults (Adult Treatment Panel III) final report. *Circulation* 2002;106:3143.
65. DOQI clinical practice guidelines on managing dyslipidemias in chronic kidney disease. *Am J Kidney Dis* 2003;41(4 Suppl 3):S1.
66. NKF-K/DOQI Clinical Practice Guidelines and Clinical Practice Recommendations for Diabetes for Chronic Kidney Disease. *Am J Kidney Dis* 2007;49(Suppl 2):S1.
67. Keller CK et al. Renal findings in patients with short-term type 2 diabetes. *J Am Soc Nephrol* 1996;7:2627.
68. Ravid M et al. Main risk factors for nephropathy in type 2 diabetes mellitus are plasma cholesterol levels, mean blood pressure, and hyperglycemia. *Arch Intern Med* 1998;158:998.
69. Vlassara H et al. Diabetes and advanced glycation endproducts. *J Intern Med* 2002;251:87.
70. Agius E et al. Familial factors in diabetic nephropathy: an offspring study. *Diabetic Medicine* 2006;23:331.
71. Breyer MD et al. Genetics of diabetic nephropathy: lessons from mice. *Semin Nephrol* 2007;27:237.
72. American Diabetes Association: Standards of Medical Care in Diabetes 2007. *Diabetes Care* 2007;30(Suppl 1):S4.
73. The Diabetes Control and Complications Trial Research Group. The effect of intensive treatment of diabetes on the development and progression of long-term complications in insulin-dependent diabetes mellitus. *N Engl J Med* 1993;329:977.
74. UK Prospective Diabetes Study (UKPDS) Group. Intensive blood-glucose control with sulphonylureas or insulin compared with conventional treatment and risk of complications in patients with type 2 diabetes (UKPDS 33). *Lancet* 1998;352:837.
75. Barnett AH et al. Diabetics Exposed to Telmisartan and Enalapril Study Group. Angiotensin-receptor blockade versus converting-enzyme inhibition in type 2 diabetes and nephropathy. *N Engl J Med* 2004;351:1952.
76. Bakris GL et al. Calcium channel blockers versus other antihypertensive therapies on progression of NIDDM associated nephropathy. *Kidney Int* 1996;50:1641.
77. Bakris G et al. Effects of an ACE inhibitor combined with a calcium channel blocker on progression of diabetic nephropathy. *J Hum Hypertens* 1997;11:35.
78. Epstein M. Aldosterone blockade: an emerging strategy for abrogating progressive renal disease. *Am J Med* 2006;119:912.
79. NKF-K/DOQI clinical practice guidelines on hypertension and antihypertensive agents in chronic kidney disease. *Am J Kidney Dis* 2004;43(Suppl 1):S1.
80. Schaefer TJ et al. Disorders of potassium. *Emerg Med Clin N Am* 2005;23:723.
81. Gennari FJ et al. Hyperkalemia: an adaptive response in chronic renal insufficiency. *Kidney Int* 2002;62:1.
82. Ballmer PE et al. Chronic metabolic acidosis decreases albumin synthesis and induces negative nitrogen balance in humans. *J Clin Invest* 1995;95:39.
83. Adrogue HJ. Metabolic acidosis: pathophysiology, diagnosis and management. *J Nephrol* 2006;19:S62.
84. Eknoyan G et al. Bone metabolism and disease in chronic kidney disease. *Am J Kidney Dis* 2003;42(Suppl 3):1.
85. National Kidney Foundation. K/DOQI Clinical Practice Guidelines for Anemia of Chronic Kidney Disease. Update 2006. *Am J Kidney Dis* 2006;47(Suppl 3):S11.

86. Erslev AJ. Erythropoietin. *N Engl J Med* 1991;324:1339.
87. Kazmi WH et al. Anemia: an early complication of chronic renal insufficiency. *Am J Kidney Dis* 2001;38:803.
88. Levin A et al. Left ventricular mass index increase in early renal disease: impact of decline in hemoglobin. *Am J Kidney Dis* 1999;34:125.
89. Foley RN et al. Clinical and echocardiographic disease in patients starting end-stage renal disease therapy. *Kidney Int* 1995;47:186.
90. Himmelfarb J. Hematologic manifestations of renal failure. In: Greenberg A, ed. *Primer on Kidney Diseases.* 4th ed. Philadelphia: Elsevier Saunders; 2005:465.
91. Fishbane S et al. Hypervitaminosis A in two hemodialysis patients. *Am J Kidney Dis* 1995;25:346.
92. Singh AK et al. Correction of anemia with epoetin alfa in chronic kidney disease. *N Engl J Med* 2006;355:2085.
93. Drueke TB et al. Normalization of hemoglobin level in patients with chronic kidney disease and anemia. *N Engl J Med* 2006;355:2071.
94. Markowitz GS et al. An evaluation of the effectiveness of oral iron therapy in hemodialysis patients receiving recombinant human erythropoietin. *Clin Nephrol* 1997;48:34.
95. Blaustein DA et al. The safety and efficacy of an accelerated iron sucrose dosing regimen in patients with chronic kidney disease. *Kidney Int Suppl* 2003;87:72.
96. Ahsan N. Infusion of total dose iron versus oral iron supplementation in ambulatory peritoneal dialysis patients: a prospective, cross-over trial. *Adv Perit Dial* 2000;16:80.
97. Schein Pharmaceutical, Inc; INFeD (iron dextran injection, USP) package insert. Sorham Park, NJ: Schein Pharmaceutical, Inc; March 2006.
98. Chertow GM et al. Update on adverse drug events associated with parenteral iron. *Nephrol Dial Transplant* 2006;21:378.
99. Watson Pharmaceuticals, Inc; Ferrlecit (sodium ferric gluconate complex in sucrose injection) package insert. Corona, CA: Watson Pharmaceuticals, Inc; September 2006.
100. Michael B. Sodium ferric gluconate complex in hemodialysis patients: adverse reactions compared to placebo and iron dextran. *Kidney Int* 2002;61:1830.
101. Folkert VW et al. Chronic use of sodium ferric gluconate complex in hemodialysis patients: safety of higher-dose (> or = 250 mg) administration. *Am J Kidney Dis* 2003;41:651.
102. American Reagent Laboratories, Inc; Venofer (iron sucrose injection) package insert. Shirley, NY: American Reagent Laboratories, Inc; October 2006.
103. Chandler G et al. Intravenous iron sucrose: establishing a safe dose. *Am J Kidney Dis* 2001;38:988.
104. Fishbane S et al. Reduction in recombinant human erythropoietin doses by the use of chronic intravenous iron supplementation. *Am J Kidney Dis* 1995;26:41.
105. Coyne DW et al. Ferric gluconate is highly efficacious in anemic hemodialysis patients with high serum ferritin and low transferrin saturation: results of the Dialysis Patients' Response to IV Iron with Elevated Ferritin (DRIVE) study. *J Am Soc Nephrol* 2007;18:975.
106. Lim PS et al. Enhanced oxidative stress in haemodialysis patients receiving intravenous iron therapy. *Nephrol Dial Transplant* 1999;14:2680.
107. Spinowitz BS et al. The safety and efficacy of ferumoxytol therapy in anemic chronic kidney disease patients. *Kidney Int* 2005;68:1801.
108. Besarab A et al. Meta-analysis of subcutaneous versus intravenous epoetin in maintenance treatment of anemia in hemodialysis patients. *Am J Kidney Dis* 2002;40:439.
109. Ateshkadi A et al. Pharmacokinetics of intraperitoneal, intravenous, and subcutaneous recombinant human erythropoietin in patients on continuous ambulatory peritoneal dialysis. *Am J Kidney Dis* 1993;21:635.
110. Provenzano R et al. Extended epoetin alfa dosing as maintenance treatment for the anemia of chronic kidney disease: the PROMPT study. *Clin Nephrol* 2005;64:113.
111. Provenzano R et al. Once-weekly Procrit is effective in treating the anemia of chronic kidney disease: final results from the POWER study [Abstract]. *J Am Soc Nephrol* 2002:13:641A.
112. Suranyi MG et al. Treatment of anemia with darbepoetin alfa administered de novo once every other week in chronic kidney disease. *Am J Nephrol* 2003;23:106.
113. Nissenson AR et al. Randomized, controlled trial of darbepoetin alfa for the treatment of anemia in hemodialysis patients. *Am J Kidney Dis* 2002;40:110.
114. Locatelli F et al. Treatment of anaemia in dialysis patients with unit dosing of darbepoetin alfa at a reduced dose frequency relative to recombinant human erythropoietin (rHuEpo). *Nephrol Dial Transplant* 2003;18:362.
115. Aranesp (darbepoetin alfa) package insert. Thousand Oaks, CA: Amgen Inc; April 2007.
116. Onoyama K et al. Worsening of anemia by angiotensin converting enzyme inhibitors and its prevention by antiestrogenic steroid in chronic hemodialysis patients. *J Cardiovasc Pharmacol* 1989;13(Suppl 3):S27.
117. Abu-Alfa AK et al. ACE inhibitors do not induce recombinant human erythropoietin resistance in hemodialysis patients. *Am J Kidney Dis* 2000;35:1076.
118. Casadevall N et al. Pure red-cell aplasia and antierythropoietin antibodies in patients treated with recombinant erythropoietin. *N Engl J Med* 2002;346:469.
119. Weber G et al. Allergic skin and systemic reactions in a patient with pure red cell aplasia and anti-erythropoietin antibodies challenged with different epoetins. *J Am Soc Nephrol* 2002;13:2381.
120. Macdougall IC. CERA (continuous erythropoietin receptor activator): a new erythropoiesis-stimulating agent for the treatment of anemia. *Current Hematology Reports* 2005;4:436.
121. Prichard S. Risk factors for coronary artery disease in patients with renal failure. *Am J Med Sci* 2003;325:209.
122. Kalpakian MA et al. Vascular calcification and disordered mineral metabolism in dialysis patients. *Semin Dial* 2007;20:139.
123. Rosenberg ME et al. The paradox of the renin-angiotensin system in chronic renal disease. *Kidney Int* 1994;45:403.
124. Zager PG et al. "U" curve association of blood pressure and mortality in hemodialysis patients. *Kidney Int* 1998;54:561.
125. Suki WN. Use of diuretics in chronic renal failure. *Kidney Int Suppl* 1997;59:S33.
126. Cannella G et al. Prolonged therapy with ACE inhibitors induces a regression of left ventricular hypertrophy of dialyzed uremic patients independently from hypotensive effects. *Am J Kidney Dis* 1997;30:659.
127. Burnier M et al. Comparative antihypertensive effects of angiotensin II receptor antagonists. *J Am Soc Nephrol* 1999;10(Suppl 12):S278.
128. Cohn JN. Improving outcomes in congestive heart failure: Val-HeFT. Valsartan in heart failure trial. *Cardiology* 1999;(Suppl 1):19.
129. Seliger SL et al. HMG-CoA reductase inhibitors are associated with reduced mortality in ESRD patients. *Kidney Int* 2002;61:297.
130. Llach F. Secondary hyperparathyroidism in renal failure: the trade-off hypothesis revisited. *Am J Kidney Dis* 1995;25:63.
131. Martin KJ et al. Diagnosis, assessment, and treatment of bone turnover abnormalities in renal osteodystrophy. *Am J Kidney Dis* 2004;43:558.
132. Bowes AP et al. *Bowes & Church's Food Values of Portions Commonly Used.* Philadelphia: Lippincott-Raven; 1998.
133. Delmez JA. Renal osteodystrophy and other musculoskeletal complications of chronic renal failure. In: Greenberg A, ed. *Primer on Kidney Diseases.* 4th ed. Philadelphia: Elsevier Saunders; 2005: 448.
134. Goodman WG et al. Coronary-artery calcification in young adults with end-stage renal disease who are undergoing dialysis. *N Engl J Med* 2000;342:1478.
135. Almirall J et al. Calcium acetate versus calcium carbonate for the control of serum phosphorus in hemodialysis patients. *Am J Nephrol* 1994;14:192.
136. Renagel package insert. Geltex Pharmaceuticals; October 2004.
137. Chertow GM et al. Long-term effects of sevelamer hydrochloride on the calcium phosphate product and lipid profile of haemodialysis patients. *Nephrol Dial Transplant* 1999;14:2907.
138. Chertow GM et al. A randomized trial of sevelamer hydrochloride (RenaGel) with and without supplemental calcium. Strategies for the control of hyperphosphatemia and hyperparathyroidism in hemodialysis patients. *Clin Nephrol* 1999;51:18.
139. Block GA et al. Mortality effect of coronary calcification and phosphate binder choice in incident hemodialysis patients. *Kidney Int* 2007;71: 438.
140. Marco MP et al. Treatment with sevelamer decreases bicarbonate levels in hemodialysis patients. *Nephron* 2002;92:499.
141. Finn WF. Lanthanum carbonate versus standard therapy for the treatment of hyperphosphatemia: safety and efficacy in chronic maintenance hemodialysis patients. *Clin Nephrol* 2006;65:191.
142. Hutchison AJ et al. Long-term efficacy and tolerability of lanthanum carbonate: results from a 3-year study. *Nephron Clinical Practice* 2006;102:61.
143. D'Haese PC et al. A multicenter study on the effects of lanthanum carbonate (Fosrenol) and calcium carbonate on renal bone disease in dialysis patients. *Kidney Int Suppl* 2003;85:73.
144. Altmann P et al. Cognitive function in stage 5 chronic kidney disease patients on hemodialysis: no adverse effects of lanthanum carbonate compared with standard phosphate-binder therapy. *Kidney Int* 2007;71:252.
145. Shire US, Inc. Fosrenol package insert. Wayne, PA; November 2005.
146. Malluche HH. Aluminum and bone disease in chronic renal failure. *Nephrol Dial Transplant* 2002;17(Suppl 85):21.
147. Levin A et al. Prevalence of abnormal serum vitamin D, PTH, calcium and phosphorus in patients with chronic kidney disease: results of the study to evaluate early kidney disease. *Kidney Int* 2007;71:31.
148. Goodman WG et al. Parathyroid hormone (PTH), PTH-derived peptides, and new PTH assays in renal osteodystrophy. *Kidney Int* 2003;63:1.
149. Martin KJ et al. Therapy of secondary hyperparathyroidism with 19-nor-1alpha,25-dihydroxyvitamin D2. *Am J Kidney Dis* 1998;32(Suppl 2):S61.
150. Lindberg J et al. A long-term, multicenter study of the efficacy and safety of paricalcitol in end-stage renal disease. *Clin Nephrol* 2001;56:315.
151. Zemplar Package Insert. Abbott Laboratories Inc, Abbott Park, IL. [Oral May 2005, Intravenous September 2005.
152. Martin KJ et al. Paricalcitol dosing according to body weight or severity of hyperparathyroidism: a double-blind, multicenter, randomized study. *Am J Kidney Dis* 2001;38(Suppl 5):S57.
153. Llach F et al. Paricalcitol in dialysis patients with calcitriol-resistant secondary hyperparathyroidism. *Am J Kidney Dis* 2001;38(Suppl 5):S45.
154. Sprague SM et al. Suppression of parathyroid hormone secretion in hemodialysis patients: comparison of paricalcitol with calcitriol. *Am J Kidney Dis* 2001;38:S51.
155. Frazao JM et al. Intermittent doxercalciferol (1alpha-hydroxyvitamin D(2)) therapy for secondary hyperparathyroidism. *Am J Kidney Dis* 2000;36:550.

156. Maung HM et al. Efficacy and side effects of intermittent intravenous and oral doxercalciferol (1–hydroxyvitamin D_2) in dialysis patients with secondary hyperparathyroidism: a sequential comparison. *Am J Kidney Dis* 2001;37:532.
157. Genzyme Corp. Hectorol package insert. Cambridge, MA. [Oral June 2006, Intravenous January 2006].
158. Teng M et al. Activated injectable vitamin D and hemodialysis survival: a historical cohort study. *J Am Soc Nephrol* 2005;16:1115.
159. Teng M et al. Survival of patients undergoing hemodialysis with paricalcitol or calcitriol therapy. *N Engl J Med* 2003;349:446.
160. Tentori F et al. Mortality risk among hemodialysis patients receiving different vitamin D analogs. *Kidney Int* 2006;70:1858.
161. Moe SM et al. Achieving NKF-K/DOQI bone metabolism and disease treatment goals with cinacalcet HCl. *Kidney Int* 2005;67:760.
162. Lazar E et al. Long-term outcomes of cinacalcet and paricalcitol titration protocol for treatment of secondary hyperparathyroidism. *Am J Nephrol* 2007;27:274.
163. Amgen Inc. Sensipar package insert. Thousand Oaks, CA; 2007.
164. Van Abel M et al. Down-regulation of Ca2+ transporters in kidney and duodenum by the calcimimetic compound NPS R-467. *J Am Soc Nephrol* 2003;14[abstract].
165. Yamaguchi T et al. Expression of extracellular calcium-sensing receptor in human osteoblastic MG-63 cell line. *Am J Physiol Cell Physiol* 2001;280:C382.
166. Kovalik EC. Endocrine manifestations of renal failure. In: Greenberg A, ed. *Primer on Kidney Diseases.* 2nd ed. San Diego: Academic Press; 1998:472.
167. Palmer BF. Sexual dysfunction in uremia. *J Am Soc Nephrol* 1999;10:1381.
168. Fliser D et al. Insulin resistance and hyperinsulinemia are already present in patients with incipient renal disease. *Kidney Int* 1998;53:1343.
169. Etemad B. Gastrointestinal complications of renal failure. *Gastroenterol Clin North Am* 1998;27:875.
170. Schoonjans R et al. Dyspepsia and gastroparesis in chronic renal failure: the role of Helicobacter pylori. *Clin Nephrol* 2002;57:201.
171. Tsai CJ et al. Investigation of upper gastrointestinal hemorrhage in chronic renal failure. *J Clin Gastroenterol* 1996;22:2.
172. Robertson KE et al. Uremic pruritus. *Am J Health Syst Pharm* 1996;53:2159.
173. Hiroshige K et al. Optimal dialysis improves uremic pruritus. *Am J Kidney Dis* 1995;25:413.
174. Little MA et al. Rapidly progressive glomerulonephritis: current and evolving treatment strategies. *J Nephrol* 2004;17(Suppl 8):S10.
175. Weening JJ et al. The classification of glomerulonephritis in systemic lupus erythematosus revisited. *Kidney Int* 2004;65:521. Erratum in: *Kidney Int* 2004;65:1132.
176. Hejaili FF et al. Treatment of lupus nephritis. *Drugs* 2003;63:257.
177. Gourley MF et al. Methylprednisolone and cyclophosphamide, alone or in combination, in patients with lupus nephritis: a randomized, controlled trial. *Ann Intern Med* 1996;125:549.
178. Houssiau FA et al. Immunosuppressive therapy in lupus nephritis: the Euro-Lupus Nephritis Trial, a randomized trial of low-dose versus high-dose intravenous cyclophosphamide. *Arthritis Rheum* 2002;46:2121.
179. Ginzler EM et al. Mycophenolate mofetil or intravenous cyclophosphamide for lupus nephritis. *N Engl J Med* 2005;353:2219.
180. Waldman M et al. Update on the treatment of lupus nephritis. *Kidney Int* 2006;70:1403.
181. Contreras G et al. Sequential therapies for proliferative lupus nephritis. *N Engl J Med* 2004;350: 971.
182. Leavitt RY et al. The American College of Rheumatology 1990 Criteria for the Classification of Wegener's Granulomatosis. *Arthritis Rheum* 1990;33:11.
183. White ES et al. Pharmacological therapy for Wegener's granulomatosis. *Drugs* 2006;66:1209.
184. Specks U et al. Granulomatous vasculitis: Wegener's granulomatosis and Churg-Strauss syndrome. *Rheum Dis Clin North Am* 1990;16: 377.
185. Stegeman CA. Trimethoprim-sulfamethoxazole (Co-Trimoxazole) for the prevention of relapses of Wegener's granulomatosis. *N Engl J Med* 1996;335:16.
186. Stone JH et al. Treatment of non-life threatening Wegener's granulomatosis with methotrexate and daily prednisone as the initial therapy of choice. *J Rheumatol* 1999;26:1134.
187. Korbet, SM. The treatment of primary focal segmental glomerulosclerosis. *Ren Fail* 2000;22: 685.
188. Korbet SM. Angiotensin antagonists and steroids in the treatment of focal segmental glomerulosclerosis. *Semin Nephrol* 2003;23:219.
189. Ponticelli C et al. Other immunosuppressive agents for focal segmental glomerulosclerosis. *Semin Nephrol* 2003;23:242.
190. Cattran DC. Cyclosporine in the treatment of idiopathic focal segmental glomerulosclerosis. *Semin Nephrol* 2003;23:234.
191. Cattran DC et al. Mycophenolate mofetil in the treatment of focal segmental glomerulosclerosis. *Clin Nephrol* 2004;62:405.

CHAPTER 32

Renal Dialysis

Myrna Y. Munar

The prevalence of end-stage renal disease (ESRD) in the United States at the end of 2004 was nearly 472,000 people. Of these, 71.2% (336,000) were treated by dialysis (3.4% greater than in 2003) and the remainder had received a kidney transplant.[1] Prevalence in both populations has more than doubled since 1988, with the rate of growth slightly higher in the transplant group. Although the incidence of ESRD continues to increase each year, the rate of increase has fallen from approximately 10% to less than 2% over the past 20 years. The reasons for this decline are unknown but may be owing to reporting or to a true change in the incidence rate. Patients age 45 to 64 years account for the largest segment of the ESRD population. In 2004, 94,891 new patients with ESRD began therapy with hemodialysis, 6,686 were placed on peritoneal dialysis, and 2,200 received a transplant. The shortage of donor kidneys and the existence of patients with ESRD who are unacceptable transplant recipients sustain the demand for dialysis. Kidney transplantation is further discussed in Chapter 34, Kidney, Liver, and Pancreas Transplantation.

The two primary modes of dialysis therapy are *hemodialysis* (HD) and *peritoneal dialysis* (PD). Variations of PD include *continuous ambulatory peritoneal dialysis* (CAPD) and *automated peritoneal dialysis* (APD), an increasingly common modality that permits greater patient flexibility with dialysis. Among the nearly 335,000 dialysis patients in the United States, 92% undergo HD.[1] Most of these patients receive dialysis three times a week in a center designed primarily for stable, ambulatory patients at either a hospital-based or a free-standing dialysis facility. Home HD accounts for <1% of dialysis patients. Patients having PD also are managed through dialysis centers for routine care, although less often than patients on HD. Several factors are considered in the selection of the type of dialysis for each patient. Often, the overriding consideration is the suitability of the procedure for the patient's lifestyle. A patient who needs flexibility and freedom from a rigid schedule may prefer PD over HD to avoid the necessity of being at a dialysis center three times weekly for a 3- to 4-hour dialysis treatment. Other considerations include the availability of a vascular access site for HD, or a patient's ability to perform self-care for dialysate exchanges with PD.

Without dialysis or transplantation, patients with ESRD will die of the metabolic complications of their renal failure. Overall morbidity and mortality are generally similar for both HD and PD; however, the first-year death rate is higher for HD than PD, and is reported to be 280 versus 249 deaths per 1,000 patient years. Second-year death rates are similar, at 268 and 286 deaths per 1,000 patient years for HD and PD, respectively.[2] The length of time on dialysis (HD and PD) influences the mortality rate. Since 1985, the mortality rate for patients who have been on dialysis less than 2 years has fallen 25%, from 289 deaths per 1,000 patient years to 216. In patients on dialysis 5 or more years, however, the mortality rate has risen to a plateau of 8% since 2001.[1]

Patient characteristics and comorbid conditions influence the death rate, including age (increased with increased age), race (increased in white patients), and primary cause of ESRD (increased with diabetes and hypertension compared with glomerulonephritis).[3] The expected survival of a patient having chronic dialysis compared with the average life expectancy in the United States is significantly reduced. For example, at 60 years of age, the average survival is approximately 4 years for a patient on dialysis compared with 21 years for the average population. Among patients on dialysis, those with diabetes (the most common cause of ESRD) or hypertension have a higher mortality rate than patients without these conditions. The all-cause mortality rates are 370 and 382 deaths per 1,000 patient years, for diabetes and hypertension, respectively, compared with 311 and 215 for patients with chronic nephritis and cystic kidney disease.[2] Over the past 15 years, however, deaths caused by heart disease, cerebrovascular disease, or septicemia, have fallen most dramatically among dialysis patients with diabetes from a peak of 36% to 7.5% in 2004.[1] Other factors associated with mortality include body mass index (BMI) (decreased with increased BMI) and serum albumin (decreased with increased albumin).[2] Summary reports and analysis of survival and mortality are included as part of the annual report of the United States Renal Data System (USRDS).[1]

The demographic characteristics of the ESRD population are based primarily on data from the Centers for Medicare and Medicaid Services (CMS), because patients with ESRD are eligible for Medicare benefits. Coverage for ESRD began in 1973, when Congress enacted the End-Stage Renal Disease Program as an amendment to Medicare.[4] Total Medicare expenditures in 2004 were $299.6 billion, of which $20.1 billion, or 6.7%, were for the ESRD program. This represents an increase in the fraction expended for ESRD from 4.5% in 1991. The total per person per month (PPPM) costs for dialysis fell 2.1% from 2003 and 2004 to $1,135.80; however, the costs for erythropoiesis stimulating agents (ESA), parenteral (intravenous [IV]) iron, and IV vitamin D rose 11% to 13%.[1]

The rapid growth of the number of patients having dialysis calls attention to the need for practitioners who understand the processes and therapies for these patients. Both HD and PD were developed as methods for the removal of metabolic waste products across a semipermeable membrane. HD is an extracorporeal (dialysis membrane is outside of the body) process, whereas PD uses the patient's peritoneal membrane for the clearance of water and solutes. This chapter addresses the fundamental clinical aspects of both HD and PD, including principles, complications, and management. Throughout the chapter, reference will be made, when appropriate, to the clinical practice guidelines developed by the National Kidney Foundation, originally published in 1997, and updated in 2000 and 2006.[5–8] The initial guidelines focused on dialysis issues, the Dialysis Outcomes Quality Initiative (DOQI), and included four workgroups: Hemodialysis Adequacy,[9] Peritoneal Dialysis Adequacy,[10] Vascular Access,[11] and Anemia.[12] The updated clinical practice guidelines have been renamed the Kidney Disease Outcomes Quality Initiative (K/DOQI) to reflect the broader nature and impact of renal impairment. Additional clinical practice guidelines developed under K/DOQI include Nutrition of Chronic Renal Failure[13] and Chronic Kidney Disease: Evaluation, Classification, and Stratification.[14] The latter guideline is addressed in Chapter 31, Chronic Kidney Disease.

HEMODIALYSIS

Principles and Transport Processes

Dialysis is a process that facilitates the removal of excess water and toxins from the body, both of which accumulate as a result of inadequate kidney function. During HD, a patient's anticoagulated blood (circulated to the dialyzer from a vein in the arm) and an electrolyte solution that simulates plasma (dialysate) are simultaneously perfused through a dialyzer (artificial kidney) on opposite sides of a semipermeable membrane. Solutes (e.g., metabolic waste products, toxins, potassium, and other electrolytes) are removed from the patient's blood by diffusing across concentration gradients into the dialysate. The rate of removal (flux) of various solutes from the blood is a function of blood and dialysate flow rates through the dialyzer, relative concentration of each solute in the blood and dialysis solution (thus determining their concentration gradients across the membrane), physical characteristics of the dialysis membrane (e.g., total available surface area, thickness, and pore size), and properties (e.g., molecular size in daltons, molecular weight, volume of distribution, and protein binding) of the solute being removed. Because blood and dialysate flow in opposite directions through the dialyzer, the concentration gradient for each solute across the membrane is amplified (Fig. 32-1). This principle is defined in greater detail in the section labeled "dialyzer characteristics."

Solutes from the blood are removed through diffusion and convection. *Diffusion* is the process whereby the molecule moves across its concentration gradient by passing through pores in the dialysis membrane.[15,16] Once the concentration of a solute reaches equilibrium on both sides of the membrane, the net movement is zero because the rate of movement from the blood to dialysate compartment is equal to the rate from the dialysate to the blood compartment. For most substances, equilibrium is not achieved, either because the blood and dialysate flow rates are too rapid, or the molecule is too large to easily move through the pores.

Convection is the process that removes toxins during dialysis through the ultrafiltration of plasma water from the blood compartment.[15,16] A controlled pressure difference across the semipermeable membrane permits water movement through the membrane pores, which carries with it solute into the dialysate, thereby further enhancing solute removal. The removal of solutes by convection during ultrafiltration generally is small relative to their elimination through diffusion.

Dialyzer Characteristics

Dialyzers are characterized by many factors, such as membrane composition, size, and ability to clear solutes. Their primary component is the dialysis membrane, made of cellulose (e.g., cuprammonium cellulose), substituted cellulose (e.g., cellulose acetate, cellulose triacetate), cellulosynthetic (e.g., Hemophan), or synthetic polymer (e.g., polysulfone, polyacrylonitrile [PAN], polymethylmethacrylate [PMMA]).[17] Membranes differ not only by composition, but also by surface area, thickness, and configuration within the dialyzer. The most common configuration is the hollow fiber dialyzer, whereby the membrane is formed as thousands of hollow fibers that run the length of the dialyzer. Blood flows through the fibers and the dialysate flows in the space surrounding the fibers within the dialyzer cartridge. The result is an extremely large surface area for diffusion, which is functionally increased further by the movement of blood and dialysate in opposite directions so that equilibrium is never fully achieved. Another, less common design is the parallel-plate configuration, whereby blood and dialysate flow between alternating sheets of the membrane.

Functionally, dialysis filters can be differentiated based on their ability to remove solutes and water. Dialyzers are characterized as low-flux or high-flux based on pore size and ability to remove small versus large molecules. One method of categorizing and comparing efficiency (flux) of dialyzer units is their relative in vitro and in vivo clearance rates of marker solutes of varying molecular size. This information is usually printed on the outside of the dialyzer or in the package insert (specification chart) for the dialyzer. For example, urea (molecular size 60 Da) is a marker of small-molecule transport

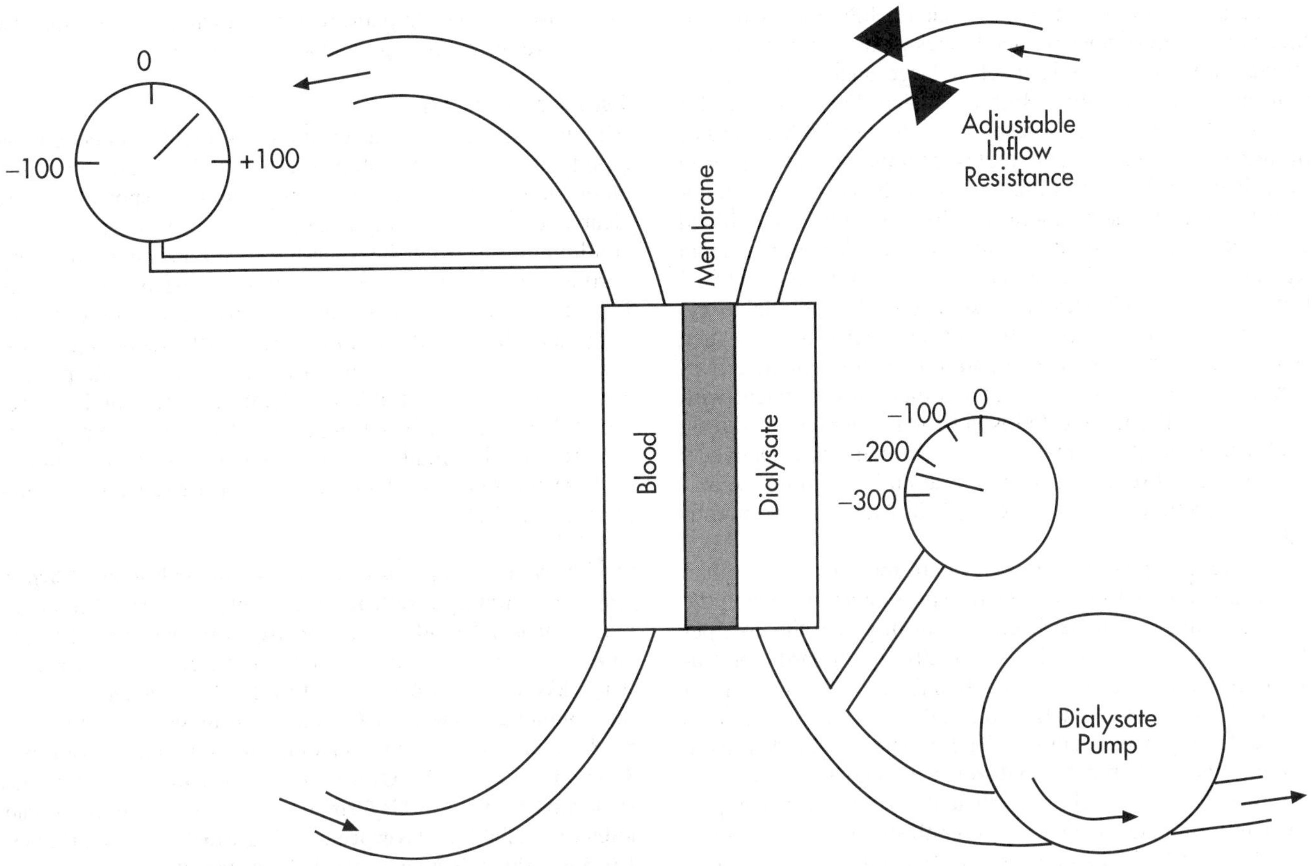

FIGURE 32-1 Representation of hemodialysis with blood flowing in one direction and dialysate in the opposite, separated by a semipermeable membrane. Note pressure monitors and dialysate pump with variable inflow resistance to create negative pressure for ultrafiltration from the blood compartment. (Reproduced from reference 18.)

across the dialysis membrane. Urea (found in the blood as blood urea nitrogen [BUN]) distributes freely throughout body water and is cleared rapidly by HD, even when using standard low flux dialyzers.[18–21] Because the pore size of most dialyzer membranes is large enough to allow this small molecule to freely diffuse, the rate-limiting step for the removal of urea is blood flow through the dialyzer. A larger-molecule, vitamin B_{12} (1,355 Da), also has been used as a measure of dialysis efficiency. Because vitamin B_{12} is too large to easily cross through the pores of conventional dialysis membranes, its dialysis clearance is less dependent on blood flow than on urea. Instead, the overall removal of vitamin B_{12} depends more on the type of membrane (i.e. thickness and pore size) and the duration of dialysis. More recently, the clearance of β_2-microglobulin, an even larger molecule than vitamin B_{12} (11,800 Da), has been used to characterize the flux of a dialyzer.[5,17] High-flux dialyzers are defined as providing β_2-microglobulin clearances of at least 20 mL/minute.[5] High-flux membranes have larger pores and are able to clear larger molecules (e.g., middle molecules such as β_2-microglobulin and leptin) and drugs (e.g., vancomycin or vitamin B_{12}, with molecular weights in the range of 1,000–5,000) more effectively than low-flux membranes with smaller pores. High-flux membranes also have a greater permeability to water, as reflected in a KUf value (to be defined later) of >10 mL/hour/mmHg. Importantly, β_2-microglobulin is not only a surrogate marker for middle molecule dialysis clearance, but it has also been found to be predictive of mortality.[22] It also plays a role in the pathogenesis of amyloidosis (see section on Amyloidosis, for further discussion). β_2 -microglobulin clearance, however, is not consistently reported in all dialyzer specification charts.

Similarly, molecular weight of drugs is a predictor of dialysis clearance. At a molecular weight of <500 (e.g., aminoglycosides and theophylline) dialyzability is expected to be high. For these drugs, the actual amount dialyzed will vary based on protein binding (i.e., amount of unbound drug available to cross the dialysis membrane), volume of distribution (Vd) (i.e., a large Vd indicates a relatively small amount of drug will be available in the blood for dialysis), blood flow rate through the dialyzer, dialysis flow rate, and dialyzer surface area. Drugs with a molecular weight between 500 and 100 (e.g., morphine and digoxin) are less well dialyzed. For digoxin, a greater problem is its large Vd and relatively low serum concentrations. Even if the drug in the blood is effectively removed, tissue-bound drug will quickly redistribute back into the blood as soon as dialysis is completed, a phenomenon known as *rebound*. Finally, large molecular weight drugs, such as vancomycin, are poorly dialyzed by conventional dialyzers, but may be removed using high-flux techniques described later in this chapter.

The efficiency of a dialyzer is also a function of its surface area. High-efficiency membranes generally have a large surface area and are able to clear large quantities of small molecules, such as urea. High-efficiency dialyzers can also have small or large pores resulting in low or high clearance of larger molecular weight solutes. Membranes also differ in their degree of biocompatibility. Free hydroxyl groups on unsubstituted cellulose membranes when in contact with blood evoke complement response and cytokine release, which can lead to hypotension, fever, and platelet activation in patients.[23] Use of these membranes is discouraged.[5] The free hydroxyl groups can be substituted with other chemical structures, such as acetate, to improve biocompatibility. Complement activation and cytokine release occur to a much lesser extent with substituted cellulose or cellulosynthetic membranes, and least of all with synthetic membranes made from plastics. Dialyzers coated with antioxidants, such as vitamin E, to minimize oxidant stress and to improve biocompatibility, are under investigation.[24]

Synthetic, high-flux membranes are more expensive than conventional cellulose, but when reuse systems in which the filter is cleansed and sterilized are put in place, the cost per dialysis session is reduced substantially.[25] Standards for dialyzer reuse are set by the Association for the Advancement of Medical Instrumentation. Both manual and automated systems are used to reprocess dialyzers. These systems include rinsing of blood and clots from the dialyzer, cleaning with agents such as dilute sodium hypochlorite (bleach), testing of dialyzer performance, and sterilization. Among all membranes, reuse of high-flux synthetic membranes is associated with a lower risk of mortality, particularly when exposed to bleach.[26] The average number of times a dialyzer is reused depends on quality control standards within the dialysis center, but generally it is 10 or more times for a patient. Universal precautions should be used to handle dialyzers. Controversial issues regarding reuse programs include safety of disinfectants, dialyzer efficiency after processing, contamination and risk of infection, and pyrogenic reactions. The potential benefits and risks of dialyzer reuse have not adversely affected morbidity or mortality.[25,26] One study, however, reported a survival advantage when patients were switched from reuse to single use dialyzers.[27] As a result of declining prices and the decision of a major dialysis manufacturer to discontinue reuse, single use dialyzers may become more commonplace.[5]

A typical package insert for a dialyzer will provide information on the clearance of various molecules (e.g., urea, creatinine, phosphate, and vitamin B_{12}). Urea clearance has become a common measure of comparison for membranes; however, clearance also depends on other factors, such as blood and dialysate flow rates.[15,16] A more standard measure for comparison is KoA urea, the mass transfer area coefficient for urea. Based on the urea clearance data from the package insert, KoA urea can be estimated based on blood flow. Using this information, the dialysis prescription can be individualized to provide a specified dose of dialysis for the patient.

Patients having chronic HD typically are dialyzed for 3 to 4 hours, three times a week, either Monday-Wednesday-Friday or Tuesday-Thursday-Saturday. During the interdialytic period, fluids ingested and produced through metabolic processes are retained in the patient. Although patients generally are on fluid-restricted diets, accumulation of 1 to 5 L of fluid (translating into 1- to 5-kg weight gain) between sessions is common and must be removed during the dialysis treatment.

Blood and Dialysate Flow

Although small-molecule clearance is highly dependent on blood flow, the relationship is not strictly linear. Increased blood flow yields a less than proportional response in urea clearance.[18] This is likely because of an insufficient time for equilibration to occur between the blood and dialysate compartments as well as a greater membrane resistance to diffusion from an increased stagnant layer. A typical blood flow rate for dialysis is 400 to 500 mL/minute but is dependent on the vascular access site and the cardiovascular status of the patient. Some patients are not able to tolerate this rate, and a lower blood flow rate may be necessary. Dialysate flow rates generally are 500 mL/minute and can be increased to 800 mL/minute for high-flux dialysis, which will increase urea clearance by approximately 10%.[28]

1. R.W., a 55-year-old man with a 25-year history of hypertension and kidney insufficiency, presents to the renal clinic for reassessment of his kidney function. He is 70 inches tall and weighs 70 kg. Since his last visit 3 months ago, his creatinine clearance (Cl_{Cr}) has decreased from 22 to 12 mL/minute (normal, 75–125 mL/minute) and the BUN has increased to 89 mg/dL (normal, 8–18 mg/dL). The serum potassium (K) is 4.5 mEq/L (normal, 3.5–5.0 mEq/L) and HCO_3 is 17 mEq/L (normal, 24–30 mEq/L). He has selected HD as his form of therapy until a suitable donor kidney is available and is expected to begin dialysis within the next 1 to 3 months. When he begins dialysis, he will be dialyzed three times a week for 4 hours each treatment, using a Fresenius F-60S dialyzer, with blood and dialysate flows of 400 and 500 mL/minute, respectively, and bicarbonate-containing dialysate. What characteristics of the Fresenius F-60S dialyzer make it a good choice for R.W.? What determines the composition of the dialysate?

[SI units: Cl_{Cr}, 0.37 and 0.2 mL/second, respectively (normal, 1.24–2.08); BUN, 31.8 mmol/L (normal, 3–6.5); K, 4.5 mmol/L (normal, 3.5–5)]

The Fresenius dialyzer is a high-flux dialyzer as described in the introduction.[17] This polysulfone membrane is a synthetic membrane with larger pore sizes than conventional cellulose membranes. The F-60S has a KUf, the ultrafiltration coefficient (volume of water removed/mmHg across the membrane per hour of dialysis), of 40 mL/mmHg/hour, indicating a high ultrafiltration capability; an in vitro KoA_{urea} (the urea mass transfer area coefficient) of 709, a measure of dialyzer efficiency for urea removal; urea clearance of 185 mL/minute at a blood flow of 200 mL/minute; and a surface area of 1.3 m^2. This information can be located in the product literature from the manufacturer or summary tables from common dialysis references.[17] These data are used to individualize the dialysis prescription for a patient.

Dialysate Composition

Dialysate composition usually is standardized within certain limits of electrolyte content, yet allows for individualization as necessary. Water is obtained through the public water system, which then undergoes treatment by reverse osmosis, followed by ion exchange with activated charcoal to remove contaminants, such as aluminum, copper, and chloramines, as well as bacteria and endotoxins.[29] The dialysate solution does not

Table 32-1 Electrolyte Composition of Hemodialysis and CAPD Dialysate Solutions

Solute	Hemodialysis (mEq/L)	CAPD (mEq/L)
Sodium	135–145	132
Potassium	0–4	0
Calcium	2.5–3.5	3.5
Magnesium	0.5–1.0	1.5
Chloride	100–124	102
Bicarbonate	30–38	
Lactate		35
pH	7.1–7.3	5.5

CAPD, continuous ambulatory peritoneal dialysis.

require sterilization because the dialysis membrane separates the blood and dialysate compartments. Nevertheless, pyrogen reactions may occur, and a greater risk may exist with high-flux membranes because of the increased pore size.

The final dialysate solution is prepared in the dialysis machine by proportioning a dialysate concentrate with the purified water, resulting in a final product, which typically contains those elements listed in Table 32-1. By adjusting electrolyte concentration in the dialysate, the efficiency of dialysis for particular chemicals can be manipulated. For example, if the patient is hyperkalemic, the dialysate contains a low concentration of potassium. On the other hand, if the patient is normokalemic at the start of dialysis, the potassium concentration of the dialysate is set at a normal physiologic concentration to minimize flux of this electrolyte across the membrane. If the concentration of a solute is higher in the dialysate than in the blood, the net movement will be into the blood, not out.

Before delivery, the dialysate is heated to 37°C to maintain body temperature and avoid hemolysis, which can occur with excessive heating. Metabolic acidosis, which is associated with ESRD because of an inability to excrete the daily obligatory load of acid, is controlled with the addition of bicarbonate buffer to the dialysate solution.[17] Precipitation of calcium carbonate previously was a problem with the addition of bicarbonate to the dialysate, which led to the use of acetate to control acidemia instead. Acetate enters the blood compartment by diffusion from the dialysate and is metabolized to bicarbonate in vivo. Acetate, however, is associated with hypotension and cardiac instability during HD and is no longer used.[30] Improvements in delivery systems that provide for special mixing methods prevent precipitation and allow for the resumption of bicarbonate dialysis. Liquid bicarbonate concentrate and reconstituted bicarbonate-containing dialysate, however, can support the growth of gram-negative bacteria, filamentous fungi, and yeast.[15] Use of dry bicarbonate cartridges or membrane filters at the point where the dialysate leaves the machine before entering the patient's dialyzer obviates the problem of bacterial growth and contamination of the final dialysate solutions.[15,31]

Vascular Access

2. To achieve a sufficient blood flow for dialysis, R.W. must have a vascular site for chronic access. What are the options for chronic vascular access in R.W.?

A permanent vascular access site provides easy access to high blood flow, which cannot be achieved through routine venipuncture of superficial veins. Different types of vascular access are available: arteriovenous (AV) fistula, AV graft composed of expanded polytetrafluoroethylene (PTFE), double-lumen or tunneled catheters, and catheters with subcutaneously implanted access ports. AV fistulas and grafts are placed in the nondominant arm. Ideal vascular access delivers blood flow rates necessary for chronic HD, has a long period of use, and has a low rate of complications (e.g.,. infection, stenosis, thrombosis, aneurysm, and limb ischemia).

An AV fistula is preferred because of its longer survival of approximately 75% at 3 years (compared with 30% for the AV graft) and low rates of complications.[32] An AV fistula is created surgically by subcutaneous anastomosis of an artery to an adjacent vein. The K/DOQI guidelines for vascular access advocate placement of a fistula at the location of the wrist (radial-cephalic), or secondarily the elbow (brachial-cephalic), as the preferred vascular access sites. If neither of these is feasible for the patient, insertion of an arteriovenous graft or creation of a transposed brachial basilica vein fistula is recommended. During the dialysis procedure, one needle or catheter is placed into the fistula site to deliver blood to the dialyzer. This is often referred to as the "arterial line" to the dialyzer. Blood exiting the dialyzer is returned back to the patient's fistula site through a second catheter and needle, referred to as the "venous line" from the dialyzer.

Central venous catheters are discouraged for chronic vascular access. Although preferred, the AV fistula may not be suitable for patients with poor vasculature, such as elderly patients or those with diabetes, atherosclerosis, or small vessels. The fistula should preferably be created 3 to 4 months before its intended use to allow the vein to mature. The graft can be used soon after insertion, although 2 weeks will allow for healing at the anastomosis sites and may prolong patency. If R.W. has adequate vasculature, a fistula should be created for chronic access based on the higher long-term graft survival. Vascular access is critical for chronic HD and often has been labeled the "Achilles' heel" of dialysis therapy. Complications associated with vascular access are a significant problem in patients having chronic HD. The most common is thrombosis, usually the result of venous stenosis.[7] If not treated, thromboses will result in loss of the access. Access-related complications are a major cause of hospitalization and, therefore, attention to these problems is important clinically and economically.

Anticoagulation

3. Recommend a reasonable anticoagulation regimen for R.W. with the initiation of his HD. What are alternatives for patients at high risk for bleeding?

Most patients having HD are anticoagulated with IV heparin during the dialysis treatment. Anticoagulation is necessary to prevent blood from clotting in the extracorporeal circuit for patients having HD. Several methods have been used in an attempt to provide adequate anticoagulation without increasing the risk of bleeding. Approaches include the administration of heparin in adequate quantities to anticoagulate the patient during the dialysis procedure either by intermittent bolus injections or an initial bolus followed by a continuous infusion.[33] Modern HD delivery systems have incorporated heparin infusion devices that can be programmed to provide the desired infusion rate during dialysis.

With no evidence of a bleeding disorder, recent surgery, or other risk factors for heparin anticoagulation, therapy should be initiated with a 2,000-unit bolus of IV heparin 3 to 5 minutes before initiation of dialysis, followed by an infusion of 1,200 units/hour.[33] The target activated clotting time (ACT) is 40% to 80% above the average baseline for the dialysis unit (e.g., 200–250 seconds, for normal values of 120–150 seconds). The clinician should monitor for signs of bleeding and measure the ACT at 1-hour intervals during dialysis. Heparin should be discontinued 1 hour before the end of dialysis to prevent excessive bleeding following dialysis. Using these standard doses, the estimated elimination half-life for heparin is approximately 50 minutes and it should have a linear dose-response relationship within the target ACT.[33]

Patients at increased risk of bleeding include those who have had recent surgery, retinopathy, gastrointestinal (GI) bleeding, and cerebrovascular bleeding. For these patients, the goal is to prevent clot formation within the dialysis circuit as well as to minimize the risk of active bleeding. This may be accomplished by using "minimal-dose" heparin (tight ACT control), or even heparin-free anticoagulation. The minimal dose heparin approach individualizes therapy to achieve ACT values 40% above baseline following an initial bolus of 750 units.[33,34] The ACT is measured 3 minutes after the bolus dose, which should allow for vascular distribution of the heparin to be complete. If the goal ACT level is not achieved, repeat bolus doses of heparin can be administered at a dose that is adjusted based on the expectation of a linear response. For example, if the first dose of 750 units reaches 75% of the ACT goal, an additional 250 units would be appropriate for the second dose. Similarly, the initial heparin maintenance infusion rate of 600 units/hour can be modified by monitoring the ACT at 30-minute intervals. Adjustments in the infusion rate should be proportionate to the bolus dose needed to maintain the ACT at 40% above baseline. Samples collected for determination of ACT should be obtained from the arterial line into the dialyzer, before the infusion of heparin, to reflect systemic anticoagulation effects.

An alternative to heparinization for patients having dialysis with high blood flow rates is heparin-free dialysis.[33,35] This approach requires priming the hemodialysis circuit and dialyzer with heparin 3,000 units/L in normal saline to coat the extracorporeal surfaces. The heparin-containing priming fluid is allowed to drain by filling the circuit with either the patient's blood or normal saline alone at the outset of dialysis. Next, hemodialysis is set at a high blood flow rate of 400 mL/minute, if tolerated. During dialysis, the dialyzer is flushed with normal saline every 15 to 30 minutes to rinse away microclots that may have formed. The incidence of clotting with this approach is approximately 5%.

Enoxaparin and dalteparin are two low-molecular-weight heparins (LMWH) that are commercially available, but not yet approved by the U.S. Food and Drug Administration (FDA) for hemodialysis. In a randomized, crossover study comparing the safety and efficacy of enoxaparin with standard heparin, a dose of 1.0-mg/kg body weight of enoxaparin produced less minor fibrin or clot formation in the dialyzer, but more frequent minor hemorrhage between dialyses. Dosage reduction of enoxaparin to 0.75 mg/kg body weight resulted in similar efficacy and eliminated the minor hemorrhage.[36] Differences in body weight were found to influence maximal concentrations of dalteparin. Therefore, weight-based dosing of dalteparin in patients having hemodialysis is under investigation.[37] Tinzaparin also has been shown to be effective as an anticoagulant during HD, using an IV dose of 75 IU/kg just before dialysis.[38]

Because LMWH undergo renal elimination, dose adjustments are necessary in patients with ESRD, accompanied by careful patient monitoring. While LMWH inhibit factor Xa, factor XIIa, and kallikrein, measurement of antifactor Xa activity is the only available laboratory monitoring parameter for these factors. Because active heparin metabolites that are not detected by the factor Xa assay can accumulate in dialysis patients, the clinical utility of this test is unclear.[39–41]

Another concern with LMWH is that patients on dialysis exhibit greater sensitivity to their effect than healthy volunteers.[41] Furthermore, LMWH administered at fixed-weight doses and without monitoring show unpredictable anticoagulant effects in patients with stage 4 and 5 chronic kidney disease. In a case series of patients on HD treated with LMWH for acute coronary syndrome, two patients who received as few as two to three doses of LMWH developed dialysis access site bleeding, hematuria, and massive melena. Another subject who received 10 doses developed hemorrhagic pericardial effusion resulting in death. Only one patient in the series, who received a total of five doses, did not develop hemorrhagic complications.[42] Based on these findings, it is recommended that unfractionated heparin, rather than LMWH, should be used in patients on dialysis for prophylaxis and treatment of thromboembolic disease.[43]

Another class of agents with potential use in patients requiring anticoagulation during HD are the direct thrombin inhibitors, argatroban and lepirudin (Refludan). Their use is especially attractive in individuals who experience heparin-induced thrombocytopenia (HIT). This complication is reported to occur in 0% to 12% of patients on HD receiving heparin for anticoagulation. Argatroban is a synthetic derivative of L-arginine, which is approved by the FDA for use in patients susceptible to thrombosis who also have a history of HIT. Most dosage regimens for argatroban consist of an initial bolus dose followed by a continuous infusion during dialysis. Because it is eliminated by nonrenal routes, argatroban dosing in patients with renal failure is the same as for patients with normal kidney function.[44] Similarly, dialysis clearance of argatroban during high-flux hemodialysis is clinically insignificant, making dose adjustments in patients on dialysis unnecessary.[45,46] Murray et al.[45] evaluated three argatroban regimens in patients having high-flux hemodialysis. Anticoagulation was more consistently achieved (ACT >140% of baseline) when a continuous infusion of 2 mcg/kg/minute with or without a bolus of 250 mcg/kg was used. The infusion was discontinued 1 hour before the end of the HD session. Argatroban therapy provided adequate, safe anticoagulation throughout HD. No thrombosis, bleeding, or other serious adverse events occurred.[45]

Another antithrombin product, lepirudin, is produced through recombinant DNA technology. It is biologically similar to hirudin, which is isolated from the saliva of leeches. Unlike argatroban, lepirudin is significantly cleared by the kidneys and requires individualized dosage adjustment based on the patient's residual renal function.[44,47] No established dosage regimens exist, because elimination is substantially delayed; monitoring should be performed using a target activated partial thromboplastin time (aPTT) of 2.0 to 2.5 times baseline. Further studies are necessary to define the role of these newer agents in patients having chronic HD.

The regional administration of trisodium citrate through the arterial line is an alternative to systemic anticoagulation. It binds free calcium, which is necessary for the coagulation process. The calcium citrate complex is removed by the dialysate and, based on plasma calcium values, calcium chloride is administered on the venous side to replace the citrate-bound calcium to prevent hypocalcemia or hypercalcemia. Some of the administered citrate is returned to the patient and is metabolized to bicarbonate, leading to metabolic alkalosis in some cases. Regional citrate anticoagulation is reserved for patients who are at risk for bleeding and requires additional monitoring to adjust the dual infusions.[33] In a prospective study of 1,009 consecutive high-flux dialysis procedures in 59 patients, long-term citrate anticoagulation achieved excellent anticoagulation (99.6%) with rare (0.2%) adverse effects on ionized calcium levels, electrolytes, and acid-base balance.[48]

Dialysis Prescription

Individualization of the "prescription" to quantify the desired "dose" of dialysis to be delivered to a particular patient on any given day has undergone several advances during the past decade. In 1981, the report of the National Cooperative Dialysis Study (NCDS) showed a relationship between the degree of dialysis delivered to the patient and morbidity.[19,20,49] Average serum urea concentrations during hemodialysis, expressed as time-averaged serum urea concentrations (TAC), were determined as an index of dialysis adequacy. Four groups of patients were randomized to different combinations of time-averaged serum urea concentrations (low TAC (50 mg/dL) or high TAC (100 mg/dL)) and length of dialysis (2.5–3.5, or 4.5–5.0 hours). No differences were found in mortality during the 1-year study; however, patients with higher urea exposure (high TAC) experienced a greater withdrawal rate from the study and more hospitalizations compared with patients with lower urea concentrations. These data suggested that urea kinetics could be used to model dialysis therapy and that urea could be used as a surrogate marker for the adequacy of dialysis. Because it is well recognized that other uremic toxins also contribute to the overall morbidity among these patients, surrogate markers of their removal by dialysis have been used in an attempt to better define the adequacy of dialysis. For example, creatinine (MW 113 D), which is slightly larger than urea, has been explored as a marker, but it offers no additional predictive benefit. As described in the introduction to this chapter, vitamin B_{12} is a marker for the class of "middle molecules" that are thought to be responsible for many of the complications of uremia. Because vitamin B_{12} is a larger molecule than urea or creatinine, it is not easily cleared by membranes with smaller pores, although it is more effectively cleared by high-flux membranes. Nonetheless, the utility of vitamin B_{12} as a surrogate for dialysis adequacy has not been established.[15]

Further analysis of the NCDS data by Gotch et al.[20] using a pharmacokineticlike term, Kt/V, demonstrated a relationship between morbidity and Kt/V. The Kt/V term is based on the predialysis and postdialysis BUN values, distribution of urea, and duration of dialysis. K is the urea clearance (mL/minute), t is time (minutes), and V is distribution volume for urea (mL). The term has no units and represents the quantity of dialysis delivered to the patient, or the total volume of blood cleared of urea, relative to the urea distribution volume in a given patient. Its basic relationship depends on the first-order elimination of urea, as seen in the following general equations:

$$BUN_{post} = BUN_{pre}\,(e^{-Kt/V})$$
$$Kt/V = -\ln(BUN_{post}/BUN_{pre})$$

Patients with a Kt/V <0.9 had a 54% failure rate, defined as death, hospitalization, or withdrawal from the study for medical reasons, whereas those with a Kt/V >0.9 had a 13% failure rate on dialysis. Based on these data, it was recommended that patients receive a dialysis "dose" of Kt/V >1.0 when having dialysis three times weekly.

Several refinements of the Kt/V relationship have been made to better approximate the actual observations in patients on HD. These include corrections for ultrafiltration of fluid during dialysis; access and cardiopulmonary recirculation, which result in dilution of the arterial urea concentration in vivo; single-pool, variable volume model for urea (spKt/V); using body water volume in the denominator, so the clearance expression is reduced from a flow to a fractional removal rate (rate constant), and adding residual renal urea clearance to compute an "adjusted" or "total" Kt/V. Failure to account for residual renal clearance could lead to excessive dialysis that would compromise quality of life. On the other hand, omission will protect patients from underdialysis when residual kidney function is lost.[5] Timing of blood sample collection is very important to avoid diluted samples and postdialysis rebound of the plasma urea concentration.[18] Redistribution of urea can occur for 30 to 60 minutes after dialysis treatment, and the greatest change will be evident in the first few minutes following dialysis. The effect of redistribution on Kt/V is a reduction in the apparent dose of dialysis provided to the patient.[5]

Observations after the NCDS were implemented suggest a discrepancy between the prescribed dialysis and actual delivered dialysis, with conclusions that some patients are not receiving adequate dialysis.[50] The K/DOQI clinical practice guidelines for HD adequacy address the issue in detail and recommend formal urea kinetic modeling to determine the appropriateness of the patient's dialysis prescription. The minimal delivered dose of dialysis should be a Kt/V of at least 1.2 per dialysis, which corresponds to an average urea reduction ratio (URR, the percent reduction of plasma urea following an HD treatment) of 65%. To achieve this delivered dose, the guidelines further recommend that the prescribed dose be based on a Kt/V of 1.4 per dialysis or a URR of 70%.[5]

The National Institutes of Health supported the HEMO study, a multicenter, prospective, randomized trial to assess the impact of the dialysis prescription on morbidity and mortality in hemodialysis patients.[51] In this study (N = 1,846), subjects were randomized to standard-dose hemodialysis with a goal Kt/V of 1.3 or to high-dose hemodialysis with a goal Kt/V of 1.7. Patients were also randomized to dialysis with either a low-flux or high-flux filter. Neither a higher dose of dialysis or use of high-flux filters significantly improved survival or reduced morbidity. No major benefit in the primary outcome of mortality or in secondary outcomes relating to various causes of hospitalizations (e.g., cardiac causes, infection) combined with mortality was observed in the high-dose group. The results of the HEMO study provided little evidence to support increasing the dialysis prescription beyond the K/DOQI recommendations.

4. What are the variables that determine the Kt/V for R.W.?

Based on a target Kt/V of 1.4 and known characteristics of the dialysis system, it is possible to develop a dialysis prescription to achieve that value.[5,17] The operative variables include the type and size of dialysis membrane with known urea removal characteristics, blood and dialysate flow rates, and duration of treatment. The membrane usually is determined based on the type of dialysis delivery equipment in the facility and economic factors. The size of the filter to be used is determined by the size of the patient, with larger patients generally being dialyzed using membranes with larger surface area. Blood flow rate is maximized based on the type of equipment and pump capability, as well as the ability of the patient's cardiovascular system to tolerate a high blood flow. High-flux dialysis usually is carried out with a blood flow rate of 400 to 500 mL/minute and rapid- and high-efficiency dialysis blood flow rates of 300 to 500 mL/minute.[15,16] The last variable—time—is important to consider in providing adequate dialysis therapy to the patient. Longer dialysis sessions allow for greater Kt/V values, and it is unknown whether an upper limit exists for ideal therapy. With the introduction of high-flux membranes, dialysis treatment times were initially reduced to provide therapy to patients in a more cost-efficient manner. The total removal of urea was considered to be similar with higher urea clearance and shorter dialysis sessions, thereby allowing for reductions in personnel to manage the center and the ability to dialyze more patients.

Concern regarding increased morbidity and mortality in the United States in the early 1990s, compared with other industrialized nations, resulted in an examination of dialysis practices. Many factors were thought to contribute to this situation, including an older dialysis population, patients with more comorbid conditions being accepted to dialysis programs, and a shorter dialysis duration. Independent of the use of high-flux membranes and higher blood flow rates, the duration of dialysis appears to be a very important factor. This may be related to the clearance of uremic toxins other than urea and the removal of fluid which, if not removed, contributes to hypertension. An international study of 22,000 patients on HD in the Dialysis Outcomes and Practice Patterns Study (DOPPS) found that longer treatment time (>240 minutes) and higher Kt/V were independently and synergistically associated with lower mortality.[52] Every 30 minutes longer on HD was associated with a 7% lower relative risk of mortality (RR = 0.93; P <0.0001). One dialysis center in Tassin, France, reported improved patient survival with dialysis sessions of 8 hour/day, three times weekly. The mean Kt/V was 1.67, and the survival rate was 87% at 5 years, 75% at 10 years, and 55% at 15 years.[53] Although these data are promising, a major dilemma in U.S. centers is insufficient funding for prolonged dialysis and the unwillingness of many patients to commit the time required for more prolonged dialysis treatment on a chronic basis. Newer approaches for longer, slow dialysis are under investigation, including overnight HD in the home.[54] A systematic review of available evidence revealed improvements in blood pressure control and hemoglobin levels after conversion from traditional intermittent hemodialysis to nocturnal hemodialysis (defined as dialysis occurring at least 5 nights per week and at least 6 hour/night).[55] No differences in these values, however, were noted when compared with controls. Moreover, the impact of nocturnal hemodialysis on mortality is not yet known.

Fluid Removal

In addition to solute removal, the artificial kidney must be used to maintain fluid balance in the patient without renal function. Most patients will become anuric once stabilized on HD, requiring control of ingested fluids between treatment sessions. Fluid removal during dialysis then is necessary to achieve the "dry weight," or weight below which the patient could become symptomatic from volume depletion. The dry weight for R.W. has been set at 69.1 kg. Below this weight, R.W. exhibited symptoms of orthostasis. Achieving the dry weight is accomplished by ultrafiltration, through adjustment of the transmembrane pressure. Negative pressure on the dialysate side of the membrane results in movement of fluid across the membrane from the blood compartment.[15,16] Dialysate membranes are characterized by their water permeability, or KUf. Most membranes have values in the range of 2.0 to 8.0 mL/mmHg/hour, although high-flux membranes may have values as high as 60 mL/mmHg/hour. Adjustment of the transmembrane pressure will provide the desired ultrafiltration rate, based on the amount of fluid to be removed (predialysis weight + IV saline + ingested fluids during dialysis – dry weight). For patients undergoing dialysis three times weekly, weight gains of 1 to 5 kg are common between sessions. For membranes with KUf values >10 mL/mmHg/hour, volumetric circuitry in newer dialysis machines should be used to avoid errors in rates of fluid removal based on transmembrane pressure. Modern hemodialyzers have built-in functions to adjust the transmembrane pressure and remove fluid at a predetermined rate.

Complications

Hypotension

5. The dry weight for R.W. is 69.1 kg. During his most recent dialysis session, he complained of nausea and light-headedness 3 hours into the procedure. His diastolic pressure had dropped from 85 to 60 mmHg. Ultrafiltration was discontinued, and he recovered without further event. His postdialysis weight was 69.9 kg. What are possible etiologies for his hypotension?

Many complications can occur in patients having HD. The most common is intradialytic hypotension (IDH), which can produce a variety of clinical signs and symptoms, including nausea and vomiting, dizziness, muscle cramps, and headache. The reported incidence of hypotension is 10% to 30%, and even higher in patients with specific risk factors, such as autonomic dysfunction with diabetes and cardiac disease. It primarily is caused by excessive fluid removal from the vascular compartment at a rate exceeding mobilization of fluid stores.[56] As a consequence, patients with an inadequate hemodynamic response to intravascular volume depletion will develop a decrease in blood pressure and other symptoms. An ultrafiltration rate >10 mL/hour/kg was found to be associated with higher odds of IDH (odds ratio = 1.30; P = 0.045) and a higher risk of mortality (RR 1.02; P = 0.02).[52] It may be necessary to adjust the dry weight upward if the patient is volume depleted and symptomatic following dialysis. Another cause of hypotension is related to excessive heating of the dialysate, which can produce vasodilation. Cooling of the dialysate to slightly below body temperature may correct this problem, although many patients are uncomfortable and do not tolerate the cooling effect. The use of acetate as the buffer in the dialysate has been associated with hypotension because of its direct vasodilating effects, but it is no longer used. Antihypertensive therapy before dialysis may exacerbate hypotensive episodes as well; in some patients, these drugs may need to be withheld until after the dialysis session. Immediate treatment of the hypotensive episode can be accomplished by placing the patient in the Trendelenburg position (bed positioned with legs raised and head lowered), administering a small (100 mL) bolus of normal saline into the venous blood line, and reducing the ultrafiltration rate.

Several pharmacologic agents have been proposed for the management of IDH, including ephedrine, fludrocortisone, caffeine, vasopressin, L-carnitine, sertraline, and midodrine. Perazella[57] reviewed these agents for their potential use in the treatment of IDH and concluded that only midodrine, sertraline and L-carnitine have shown potential benefit in patients. Midodrine is an oral prodrug that is converted to desglymidodrine, a selective α_1-agonist. Doses of 10 to 20 mg, 30 minutes before dialysis are effective for most patients, but the presence of active myocardial ischemia is a major contraindication.[57] Sertraline is a selective serotonin reuptake inhibitor that has shown promise in IDH at daily doses of 50 to 100 mg/day. The mechanism is proposed to be through attenuation of paradoxical sympathetic withdrawal. L-carnitine has also been shown to have potential benefit for treatment of IDH with IV doses of 20 mg/kg at dialysis. Its mechanism of action is not known but it may be related to improvements in vascular smooth muscle and cardiac functioning.[57]

Because the volume status of R.W. is associated with his weight, another consideration is a change in his lean mass. R.W. has noted an improvement in his appetite lately and, as a result, added a few extra pounds. It is important to consider "real" weight changes when assessing the dry weight and volume status. Without appropriately increasing the dry weight goal to compensate for his real weight gain, R.W. became volume depleted and hypotensive. His dry weight should be adjusted upward to the point at which he no longer is symptomatic (to ~70 kg).

6. What other hemodialysis related complications must be watched for and how can they be treated?

Muscle Cramps

Perhaps also related to fluid shifts, muscle cramps developing during dialysis may be induced by excessive ultrafiltration resulting in altered perfusion of the affected tissues. Several treatments have been attempted, including reduced ultrafiltration and infusion of hypertonic saline or glucose to improve circulation.[58,59] Exercise and stretching of the affected limbs also may be beneficial. Long-term therapy may be directed at prevention with the use of vitamin E 400 IU at bedtime.[60] Vitamin E in combination with vitamin C 250 mg daily has been found to be more effective than either therapy alone.[61] Vitamin C therapy, however, is known to produce hyperoxaluria, oxalate-containing urinary stones, and renal damage. Therefore, the-long term safety of vitamin C in hemodialysis patients needs to be evaluated. Quinine sulfate is no longer available for use in leg cramps. It is associated with a number of serious adverse events, some of which are potentially fatal. In February 2007, the FDA ordered the manufacturing of unapproved quinine to cease.

Hypersensitivity

Reports of anaphylactic reactions to dialyzer membranes, particularly on initial exposure, may be directly related to the membrane itself, or to ethylene oxide, which is commonly used to sterilize the dialyzer.[62,63] Membranes most commonly responsible for reactions are unsubstituted cellulose membranes (bioincompatible) or the high-flux polyacrylonitrile membrane when used in conjunction with angiotensin-converting enzyme (ACE) inhibitors.[64] This latter reaction is thought to be related to the inhibition of bradykinin metabolism by ACE inhibitors, resulting in an anaphylactoid reaction.

Dialysis Disequilibrium

Dialysis disequilibrium is a syndrome that has been recognized since the initiation of HD more than 30 years ago. Its etiology is related to cerebral edema, and patients new to HD are at a greater risk because of the accumulation of urea.[65] Rapid removal of urea from the extracellular space lowers the plasma osmolality, thereby leading to a shift of free water into the brain. Lowering of intracellular pH, as can occur during dialysis, has also been suggested as a cause. Clinical manifestations occur during or shortly after dialysis and include central nervous system (CNS) effects, such as headache, nausea, altered vision, and in some cases, seizures and coma. Treatment is aimed at prevention by initiating dialysis gradually by using shorter treatment times at lower blood flow rates in new patients. Direct therapy can be provided in the form of IV hypertonic saline or mannitol.[65]

Some of the long-term complications associated with HD include thrombosis or infection of the access site, aluminum toxicity, and amyloidosis.

Thrombosis

Access loss is most often the result of thrombosis, which is usually a consequence of venous stenosis. Prospective monitoring of access function (e.g., intra-access flow; static or dynamic venous pressures; measurement of access recirculation; and physical findings, such as swelling of the arm, clotting of the graft, prolonged bleeding after needle removal, or altered character of the pulse or thrill) is paramount to the prevention of thrombosis. Fistula patency generally is much greater than synthetic graft patency; yet, thrombosis and loss of function may occur in both.[7,66] The stenosis may be corrected by percutaneous transluminal angioplasty (PCTA) or, if necessary, surgical revision of the access site. Successful correction is effective as a means to prevent thrombosis. Once it occurs, thrombosis is managed by surgical thrombectomy or with pharmacomechanical or mechanical thrombolysis. Thrombolytic therapy, administered by pulse spray technique of urokinase or streptokinase, combined with mechanical thrombectomy is as effective as surgical thrombectomy.[67] The pulse spray technique involves rapid pulse injections of small aliquots of highly concentrated thrombolytics directly into the clot. More recently, because of the potentially life-threatening adverse events associated with streptokinase and the nonavailability of urokinase, clinicians have evaluated the use of alteplase as an alternative thrombolytic agent.[68] Alteplase and reteplase appear to be effective for thrombomechanical lysis of the vascular access site.[68,69] Thrombolytic therapy should be avoided in those patients with an increased risk of bleeding.

Anticoagulants and antiplatelet agents have been evaluated in the prevention of graft thrombosis. In two separate randomized, placebo-controlled trials, therapy with low-dose warfarin to achieve a target international normalized ratio (INR) of 1.4 to 1.9 or combination therapy with clopidogrel and aspirin in patients with PTFE grafts showed no benefit in the prevention of thrombosis or prolongation of graft survival.[70,71] In both studies, patients receiving active treatment experienced a significantly increased risk of bleeding.

Infection

Access infections, usually involving grafts to a greater extent than a native fistula, are predominantly caused by *Staphylococcus aureus* or *S. epidermidis*. Infections with gram-negative organisms as well as Enterococcus occur with a lower frequency.[7] Access infections can lead to bacteremia and sepsis with or without local signs of infection. Treatment usually is initiated with vancomycin, administered as a single, 1-g dose, repeated as necessary, depending on the type of dialysis being used, or cefazolin 20 mg/kg three times weekly, and gentamicin 2 mg/kg with appropriate serum concentration monitoring.[72] High-flux dialysis results in greater removal of vancomycin than conventional dialysis and, therefore, more than a single dose may be necessary for adequate treatment.[73,74] Vancomycin can be given either during or after high-flux dialysis. A vancomycin postdialysis dosing algorithm using fewer vancomycin concentrations for patients receiving thrice-weekly high-flux dialysis was developed by Pai et al.[75] The algorithm achieved predialysis vancomycin concentrations comparable to those found with more frequent monitoring. Cost savings was realized because of a 70% reduction in the number of drug concentrations. Intradialytic dosing of vancomycin is a convenient mode of drug administration in patients receiving high-flux dialysis. It avoids the need for additional intravenous access, longer stays in the hemodialysis unit, or home antibiotic administration. Two studies have shown that vancomycin dosing in the last 1 to 2 hours of high-flux hemodialysis achieves adequate predialysis plasma concentrations of 5 to 20 mcg/mL depending on the administered dose.[76,77] K/DOQI clinical practice guidelines for vascular access also advocate surgical incision and resection of infected grafts. Fistula infections are rare and should be treated as subacute bacterial endocarditis with 6 weeks of antibiotic therapy.[7]

Aluminum Toxicity

Aluminum accumulation in patients having HD was a significant problem before water sources were adequately treated to remove aluminum.[29] Major complications of aluminum toxicity include dementia, aluminum bone disease, and anemia. Aluminum accumulation still occurs in patients treated with aluminum-containing antacids as binding agents for phosphate in the GI tract, although not to the degree associated with water supplies.[78] Aluminum toxicity is diagnosed by clinical signs and symptoms associated with the aforementioned conditions, and a serum aluminum concentration of >200 ng/mL or a deferoxamine-stimulated serum aluminum concentration increase of >200 ng/mL.[79] Deferoxamine chelates with serum aluminum and the shift in equilibrium results in movement of aluminum from tissue storage sites. The complex can be removed by dialysis (600 Da), and high-flux membranes are capable of removing the complexed aluminum in a single dialysis session, minimizing systemic exposure to deferoxamine and its potential adverse effects. The latter include mucormycosis, a fungal infection caused by a rhizopus that grows avidly in iron media, as well as ocular, auditory, and neurologic toxicity.[80,81] Deferoxamine generally is continued until the stimulated aluminum concentration is <50 ng/mL, which may require 1 year of therapy.[82]

Amyloidosis

Amyloidosis is caused by the deposition of β_2-microglobulin–containing amyloid in joints and soft tissues over prolonged periods.[83] The incidence of amyloidosis is approximately 50% after 12 years of dialysis and nearly 100% after 20 years. β_2-Microglobulin (MW 11,800 Da) normally is eliminated by filtration and metabolism in the intact nephron. Renal failure leads to reduced elimination and accumulation of this substance even during dialysis. High-flux membranes are more effective than conventional membranes for the removal of β_2–microglobulin, but they have not been in use long enough to evaluate their role in preventing amyloidosis. Carpal tunnel syndrome, manifested as weakness and soreness in the thumb from pressure on the median nerve, is the most common symptom. Bone cysts also appear along with joint deposition of amyloid, which can impair mobility.[83] The type of membrane used for dialysis also has been implicated in increasing the rate of production of β_2-microglobulin, in that some types seem to cause more rapid amyloid deposition. Biocompatible membranes are proposed to stimulate production to a lesser degree, but prospective studies demonstrating their long-term benefit have not been conducted.[84]

Malnutrition

Chronic kidney disease produces a catabolic state in patients and, along with the multifactorial complications of ESRD, leads to malnutrition. Serum albumin concentrations <3.0 g/dL are associated with an increased mortality rate compared with higher values. Inadequate dietary intake and losses of amino acids by dialysis contribute to protein malnutrition, which in turn can lead to additional complications, such as impaired wound healing, susceptibility to infection, and others (see Chapter 31, Chronic Kidney Disease, for further discussion).

L-CARNITINE

L-Carnitine supplementation has been advocated in patients with ESRD to relieve intradialytic symptoms. It is a metabolic cofactor that facilitates transport of long-chain fatty acids into the mitochondria for energy production. This cofactor is found in both plasma and tissue as free carnitine, the active component, or bound to fatty acids as acylcarnitine. The primary source of carnitine is dietary intake, primarily from red meat and dairy products. Patients with renal failure may have what appear to be normal or elevated total carnitine concentrations but low levels of free carnitine. Accumulation of acylcarnitine, decreased carnitine synthesis, reduced dietary intake, and dialytic losses may account for the normal to elevated total concentrations in this population.[85,86]

Carnitine is a small water-soluble molecule that is freely dialyzed, thus its levels are reduced in hemodialysis. The potential benefits of correcting this relative carnitine deficiency have been primarily studied in patients having chronic HD. Recommended doses of carnitine are 10 to 20 mg/kg IV after each HD treatment. Although some have suggested that carnitine supplementation benefits muscle cramps and hypotension during dialysis, as well as minimizing fatigue, skeletal muscle weakness, cardiomyopathy, and anemia resistant to large does of erythropoietic therapy, no evidence supports its routine use in patients undergoing chronic HD.[13]

PERITONEAL DIALYSIS

Peritoneal dialysis is performed using several different modalities, including the most common, continuous ambulatory peritoneal dialysis. Development of specialized devices to facilitate the exchange process and improve patient convenience has led to processes referred to as automated peritoneal dialysis, including continuous cycling peritoneal dialysis (CCPD) and nocturnal intermittent dialysis (NIPD). CAPD is the most common method for chronic PD, but the APD methods are rapidly growing. The number of patients with ESRD having treatment with PD in the United States increased from approximately 10,000 in 1985 to a peak of about 32,000 in 1995 and has been on the decline, with 27,000 in 2000 and 25,765 in 2005.[1,2]

Principles and Transport Processes

Continuous ambulatory peritoneal dialysis is performed by the instillation of 2 to 3 L of sterile dialysate solution into the peritoneal cavity through a surgically placed resident catheter. The solution dwells within the cavity for 4 to 8 hours, and then is drained and replaced with a fresh solution. This process of fill, dwell, and drain is performed three to four times during the day, with an overnight dwell by the patient in his or her normal home or work environment[87–89] (Fig. 32-2). Conceptually, the process is similar to HD in that uremic toxins are removed by diffusion down a concentration gradient across a membrane into the dialysate solution. In this case, the peritoneal membrane covering the abdominal contents serves as an endogenous dialysis membrane, and the vasculature embedded in the peritoneum serves as the blood supply to equilibrate with the dialysate. A primary difference is that because the dialysate solution is resident, the result is a very slow dialysate flow rate of approximately 7 mL/minute when 10 L of fluid is drained per day. Solute loss occurs by diffusion for small molecules, and through convection for larger, middle molecules.

Blood and Dialysate Flow

Hemodialysis provides constant perfusion of fresh dialysate, thereby maintaining a large concentration gradient across the dialysis membrane throughout the dialysis treatment. During a typical dwell period for CAPD, urea and other substances increase in the dialysate relative to unbound plasma concentrations. For a daytime dwell period of 4 hours, urea achieves nearly equal concentrations with plasma; therefore, the rate of elimination can become very small (Fig. 32-3). Instillation of fresh dialysate solution will re-establish the diffusion gradient leading to an increased rate of urea removal. For a patient making four exchanges of 2 L each per day, assuming the urea

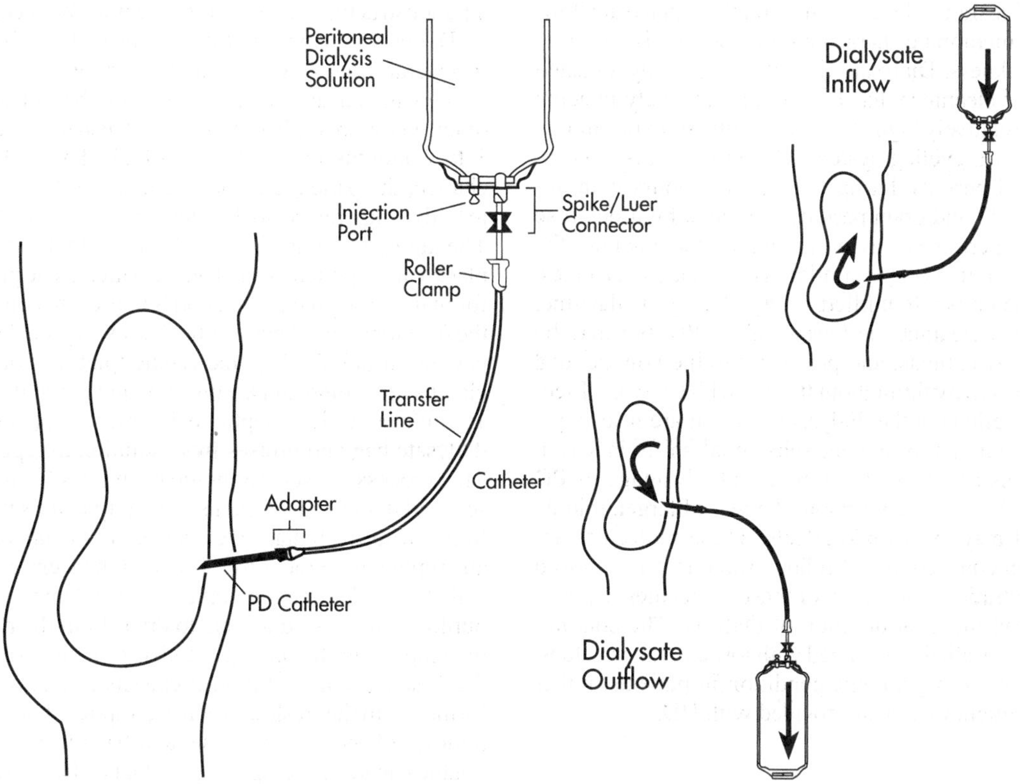

FIGURE 32-2 Schematic representation of CAPD components and techniques of inflow and outflow. (From Schoenfeld P. Care of the patient on peritoneal dialysis. In: Cogan MG, et al., eds. *Introduction to Dialysis.* 2nd ed. New York: Churchill Livingstone; 1991:200, with permission.)

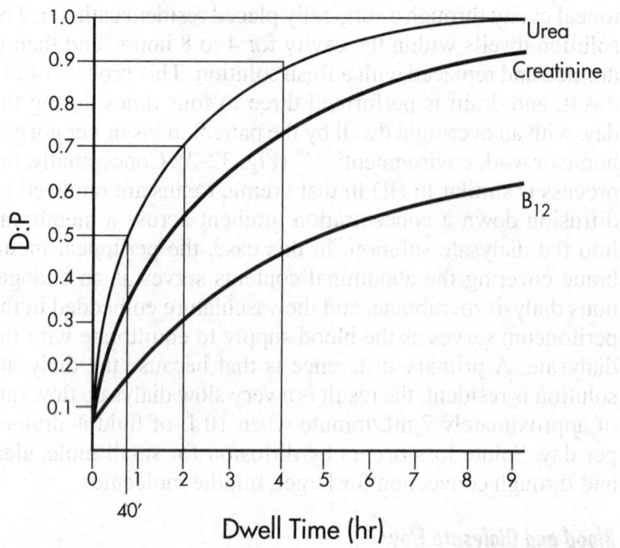

FIGURE 32-3 Rate of entry into peritoneal dialysate of urea, creatinine, and vitamin B_{12}. The y-axis indicates the ratio of dialysate to plasma concentration (D:P). (From Blake PG et al. Physiology of peritoneal dialysis. In: Daugirdas JT et al., eds. *Handbook of Dialysis*. 4th ed. Philadelphia: Lippincott Williams & Wilkins; 2007:332, with permission.)

dialysate concentration equals the plasma concentration, and 2 L are removed by ultrafiltration, the urea clearance would be approximately 7 mL/minute. This is substantially lower than urea clearances achieved with HD; therefore, CAPD must be performed continually throughout the week to achieve adequate urea removal. Clearance depends on blood flow; dialysate flow; and peritoneal membrane characteristics, such as size, permeability, and thickness. Dialysate flow, the only easily adjusted variable to alter clearance, has been used effectively in acute PD to achieve relatively high clearances with 30- to 60-minute dwell periods in a cycling system. CCPD uses this concept of shorter dwell periods during the sleeping hours with automatic fill, dwell, and drain periods, leaving a high-dextrose dialysate in the peritoneal cavity throughout the day until the next cycling session. NIPD is similar, with nightly exchanges, but the peritoneum is left unfilled, or dry, during the daytime. As a result, urea clearance is lower with NIPD, but may be suitable for many patients, and preferable to the volume load in the peritoneal cavity throughout the day with CCPD.[87] Electrolyte concentrations in the dialysate solution are near physiologic concentrations to prevent substantial shifts in serum electrolyte levels (Table 32-1). A potential advantage of PD compared with HD is the continuous dialysis of larger, middle molecules that may exert toxic effects. These molecules are cleared through convection and follow water as it is removed through ultrafiltration. Clearance of these molecules depends less on flow and more on duration of dialysis. The continuous process of PD, albeit associated with low clearance values, provides for a more physiologic condition in patients, rather than the intermittent treatment provided with HD.

Fluid Removal

Fluid is removed by ultrafiltration through adjustment of the transmembrane pressure during HD. Because this pressure is not easily adjusted in PD, fluid is removed by altering the osmotic pressure within the dialysate. This is accomplished by the addition of dextrose monohydrate to the dialysate in varying concentrations, depending on the degree of fluid removal necessary in the patient. Concentrations of dextrose in commercially available solutions include 1.5%, 2.5%, and 4.25%, with net fluid losses during a 4-hour dwell period of 200 and 400 mL for the 1.5% and 2.5% solutions, respectively, and approximately 700 mL for the 4.25% solution following an overnight dwell.[90] As the dwell time persists, the dextrose is absorbed and is diluted by the movement of fluid from the vascular space, so that most ultrafiltration occurs early during the dwell period.

Acid-base balance is achieved through the absorption of lactate from the dialysate, which subsequently is metabolized to bicarbonate in vivo. Bicarbonate is not compatible with the calcium and magnesium in the dialysate and can lead to precipitation.

Access

Delivery of dialysate into the peritoneal cavity is accomplished through an indwelling catheter inserted through the abdominal wall. The most common design is the Tenckhoff catheter, made of silicone rubber or polyurethane; it consists of a tube, straight or curled, with many holes in the distal end for fluid inflow and outflow.[91] The catheter also has a single or double cuff, which serves to anchor it to the internal and external attachment sites by promoting fibrous tissue growth; this also serves as a barrier to bacterial migration. Several modifications to the original catheter have appeared on the market, mostly in an attempt to overcome problems related to outflow of dialysate. Maintaining an unobstructed outlet port is essential for successful PD.

Delivery of dialysate through the catheter is accomplished in several modes. A straight transfer set uses tubing attached to the catheter at one end, and to the bag of dialysate at the other, via a spike. The transfer set usually is changed every 1 to 2 months in the dialysis clinic. For each dialysate exchange, the patient attaches a bag of fresh dialysate, warmed to body temperature, to the transfer set and infuses the solution. The tubing is clamped and rolled up with the attached bag and placed into a pouch carried on the patient. The primary purpose for maintaining the connection is to prevent contamination and the development of peritonitis. Following the dwell period, the patient unrolls the bag and tubing, places it on the floor, unclamps the tubing and awaits drainage of the fluid, usually 5 to 15 minutes. Using aseptic technique, the patient changes the dialysate bag and infuses fresh solution to repeat the process. This process is used rarely today and has been replaced by Y sets and double bag systems. The Y transfer set employs three limbs, with fresh dialysate attached to the upper arm of the Y, an empty bag to the lower arm, and the stem connected to the catheter.[91] Clamping the inflow arm and opening the stem and outflow arm allow dialysate to drain from the peritoneum into the empty bag. Reversing the clamps then permits infusion of the fresh dialysate solution after a small rinse of the line is performed with the fresh solution. Clamping of the catheter allows removal of the Y transfer set and bags from the patient. The double bag system employs preattached bags to both limbs and the patient and makes only a single connection to the catheter. Use of the Y transfer set has reduced episodes of peritonitis from approximately 1 for every 9 to 12 patient-months to 1 for every 24 to 36 patient-months.[92] PD performed with the cycler involves only two disconnections of the system, compared with four for CAPD.

Dialysis Prescription

The initial CAPD prescription for most patients consists of three exchanges during the day with 1.5% dextrose and a fourth, overnight exchange with 4.25% dextrose. This would be expected to achieve fluid removal of approximately 1,300 mL, based on 200 mL from each daytime exchange and 700 mL overnight. Based on assessment of the patient's fluid status, it may be necessary to increase or decrease the dialysate prescription to achieve fluid balance. Fluid retention is solved by increasing the dextrose content of the daytime exchanges, beginning with 2.5% in place of one of the 1.5% solutions. This is expected to result in an additional removal of 200 mL, and therapy can be further adjusted as necessary. For patients with excessive fluid removal, it may be possible to decrease the number of exchanges per day as long as adequate solute removal is present. If four exchanges are needed, the fluid intake can be liberalized to maintain adequate hydration.

Cycler machines automatically cycle dialysate into and out of the peritoneal cavity. Patients having CCPD will generally need three to five exchanges, each lasting approximately 2 hours, using a cycler while the patient sleeps. During the daytime hours, the patient maintains a reservoir of dialysate in the peritoneal cavity resulting in a long dwell. The cycler process repeats at night. Six to eight exchanges are performed every night for patients having NIPD. The peritoneum is left dry and patients do not continue dialysis during the day. Nightly dwell times are generally 1 to 2 hours for each exchange, resulting in a higher clearance for small molecules because of the increased dialysate flow rate.[87]

Dextrose is the dextrorotatory form of glucose. Glucose is a small molecule that rapidly diffuses across the peritoneal membrane. As glucose is absorbed, the osmotic gradient of the dwell progressively dissipates reducing ultrafiltration. Toward the end of the long dwell, more dialysate fluid may be absorbed than ultrafiltered, resulting in a negative net ultrafiltration volume where the drained volume is less than the infused volume. A negative net ultrafiltration volume is undesirable. Greater ultrafiltration and fluid management are predictors of survival.[93] An alternative to dextrose as the osmotic agent in the dialysate solution is icodextrin (Extraneal). It is approved for use in the United States in patients having CAPD or APD during the long dwell period. It is a starch-derived, water-soluble, glucose polymer that is approximately 40% absorbed and subsequently metabolized to maltose oligosaccharides. Unlike glucose, icodextrin does not readily diffuse across the peritoneal membrane, but is slowly removed from the peritoneal cavity via convective uptake into the peritoneal lymphatics.[94] It is superior to 1.5%, 2.5%, and 4.15% dextrose solutions for ultrafiltration.[95,96] Its use may be most beneficial in those patients characterized as high average to high transporters.

7. M.J., a 27-year-old woman, has a 14-year history of insulin-dependent diabetes mellitus. She is 5 feet 5 inches tall and weighs 60 kg. One complication of her diabetes is ESRD necessitating dialysis. She has been undergoing CAPD for 1 year and, until now, has done well without any complications. Her dialysis prescription consists of three exchanges with 1.5% dextrose during the day and a fourth, overnight exchange with 4.25% dextrose. She has a double-cuff Tenckhoff catheter and uses a Y transfer set for her exchanges. Her blood pressure is controlled and she shows no evidence of edema. She has no residual renal function. Her most recent serum laboratory results showed the following: calcium (Ca) 10.9 mg/dL (normal, 8.8–10.2 mg/dL) and K 3.2 mEq/L (normal, 3.5–5.0 mEq/L). Calculate the prescribed amount of dialysis for M.J.

[SI units: Ca, 2.7 mmol/L (normal, 2.2–2.6); K, 3.2 mmol/L (normal, 3.5–5)]

Residual renal clearance and greater urine volume, rather than peritoneal clearance, have been shown to be significant and important predictors of patient survival.[97,98] The 2006 K/DOQI clinical practice guidelines for PD adequacy recommend that total small-molecule clearance should be measured as Kt/V_{urea} and is based on a 24-hour collection of urine (kidney Kt/V_{urea}) and a 24-hour collection of effluent for CAPD and APD (peritoneal Kt/V_{urea}).[6] In the new guidelines, the target Kt/V_{urea} has been revised downward to at least 1.7 week from the previous Kt/V_{urea} of 2.0/wk because levels above this range have not been shown to improve outcomes. Renal and peritoneal Kt/V can be added to achieve the target.

Determining the number of exchanges needed for solute removal is based on the clearance of urea as a surrogate for uremia. Based on dialysate urea achieving 90% of plasma urea at the end of the dwell period, and four exchanges per day, the fluid removal would be approximately 9,300 mL/day, or a urea clearance of 59 L/week. For M.J., body water content (urea distribution volume) is approximately 33 L (0.55 L/kg); therefore, the dialysis prescription would provide a weekly Kt/V of 1.79. Based on her dialysis prescription, M.J. should achieve the target dose. The evidence for a Kt/V 1.79 is based on the assumptions that the patient has no residual renal function, there is full equilibration between dialysate and plasma with respect to urea, the target urea concentration is 60 mg/dL, and the normalized protein catabolic rate (nPCR) is between 1.0 and 1.2 g/kg/day, indicating adequate nutrition. Larger patients may need a larger volume for each exchange (up to 3 L) or an additional exchange per day to achieve the target Kt/V. The increased volume is preferable because of the inconvenience of an additional exchange.

M.J. also is noted to have an elevated serum calcium concentration of 10.9 mg/dL, probably as a result of her calcium carbonate requirements to serve as a binder of dietary phosphate. Dialysate preparations with a low calcium concentration (2.5 mEq/L) compared with the standard concentration of 3.5 mEq/L can help control hypercalcemia associated with increased oral calcium intake. Potassium is not present in the dialysate solution but can be supplemented in patients who are not able to maintain potassium within the normal range. M.J. has a somewhat low serum potassium concentration of 3.2 mEq/L. Therefore, providing a dialysate concentration of 4 mEq/L will sustain normal concentrations and prevent hypokalemia. This is particularly important for patients receiving digitalis preparations.

Assessment of Dialysis Adequacy

8. Assess the actual dialysis provided to M.J., based on a 24-hour collection of 9,130 mL dialysate with a urea concentration of 54 mg/dL and serum urea concentration of 60 mg/dL.

Following stabilization of the patient on the new dialysis prescription, it is necessary to assess the adequacy of the delivered dialysis dose. According to the 2006 K/DOQI clinical practice guidelines for PD adequacy, Kt/V should be measured within 1 month of initiating peritoneal dialysis and every 4 months thereafter.[6] This is accomplished by taking into account both the peritoneal and residual renal clearance of urea, and comparing these with the target Kt/V. Dialysis urea clearance is determined by collecting and measuring the dialysate, as well as urine output, for a 24-hour period.[10,99] Clearance is calculated by standard methods: rate of elimination divided by average plasma concentration. The sum of the two urea clearances then is multiplied by 7 to determine the volume cleared per week, and then it is divided by the urea distribution volume (estimated from total body water content). This value then is compared with the target weekly Kt/V value for assessment and adjustment of the prescription. For M.J., the urea clearance was 5.7 mL/minute, or 57.5 L/week. Based on her estimated urea distribution volume of 33 L, her weekly Kt/V is approximately 1.74, near the target of 1.7, not accounting for any residual renal function that may be present.

Another test of peritoneal function is the peritoneal equilibration test (PET).[100] It is a standardized semiquantitative test of peritoneal membrane transport function, and is useful to assess membrane function over time as well as to provide guidance for the appropriate mode of PD for a patient. Based on the ratio of dialysate to plasma concentration of a solute at 2 hours into a 4-hour dwell, the patient is characterized as a high, high-average, low-average, or low transporter. Glucose absorption also is assessed by comparing the dialysate concentration at 2 hours with the baseline. High transporters are those who equilibrate rapidly, and would benefit from NIPD therapy with rapid overnight exchanges. Low transporters can be treated with standard CAPD, as long as the Kt/V is sufficient to meet their needs.

Complications

9. M.J. now presents to the dialysis clinic with complaints of abdominal tenderness and cloudy effluent. Examination of the dialysate reveals a white blood cell (WBC) count of 330 cells/mm^3 with 62% neutrophils. Gram stain is positive for gram-positive cocci. Her diabetes has been controlled by the addition of 10 units of regular insulin to each daytime bag and 15 units to the overnight bag. How should M.J.'s infection be treated?

[SI unit: WBC, 0.33 × 10^9 cells/L (normal, <0.05 × 10^9)]

Peritonitis

The most significant complication among patients having PD is peritonitis, which is frequently caused by coagulase-negative staphylococci, including *S. epidermidis* (30.6%) or *S. aureus* (17.5%).[71,101] The patient usually presents with abdominal pain, nausea and vomiting, and fever with or without a cloudy effluent. Bacterial peritonitis generally is accompanied by an elevated dialysate WBC count >100/mm^3 with >50% neutrophils. A positive Gram stain should be followed by culture, with therapy initiated in the interim. For lower cell counts or negative Gram stain, a culture should be obtained followed by treatment for positive cultures and continued observation for negative results. Specific consensus recommendations of the Advisory Committee on Peritonitis Management of the International Society for Peritoneal Dialysis (ISPD) are located at http://www.ispd.org.[102] These guidelines were first published in 1983 and revised in 1989, 1993, 1996, 2000, and 2005. The initial focus of the ISPD recommendations was the treatment of peritonitis and exit-site infections. The most recent guidelines stress the importance of prevention.

Empiric antibiotics must cover both gram-positive and gram-negative organisms.[102] The increasing prevalence of vancomycin-resistant organisms has resulted in a shift in empiric therapy away from vancomycin, toward first-generation cephalosporins: cefazolin or cephalothin. Without a Gram stain, therapy should be initiated with a combination of cefazolin or cephalothin (to cover gram-positive organisms) and ceftazidime (to cover gram-negative organisms), coadministered in the same dialysate solution at a dose of 1 g/bag for both drugs, once daily, given intraperitoneally.[103] Separate syringes must be used to add the antibiotics to dialysis solutions. An aminoglycoside can be used in place of ceftazidime, but it is not recommended initially, in an attempt to preserve residual renal function. Gentamicin, tobramycin, or netilmicin are given at doses of 0.6 mg/kg/bag, once daily, and for amikacin, 2 mg/kg/bag once daily. Antibiotics should be allowed to dwell for at least 6 hours.[102] In addition to antibiotics, heparin 500 to 1,000 units/L may be added to each exchange to prevent the formation of fibrin clots, which can result in catheter failure.[103] Subsequent antibiotic therapy should be based on culture and sensitivity results, incorporating specific dosage regimens based on the treatment guidelines.[103]

This is M.J.'s first episode of peritonitis. The most likely pathogen, a Staphylococcus species, is consistent with the positive Gram stain. Her treatment should consist of cefazolin or cephalothin alone. Vancomycin should not be used for empiric therapy. Instead, it should be reserved for methicillin-resistant *Staphylococcus aureus* (MRSA) infections or methicillin-resistant *S. epidermidis* (MRSE) if M.J. does not respond to empiric therapy. Heparin 1,000 units/L should be added to the dialysate to prevent fibrin clots from forming and obstructing outflow from the peritoneal cavity. Her blood glucose should be monitored, because infection causes insulin resistance and peritonitis will increase glucose and insulin absorption. Inability to control the blood glucose concentration may require temporary discontinuation of the intraperitoneal (IP) insulin and administration by another route.

For patients having APD, the choice of first-line antibiotics is the same as for CAPD because the likely organisms are similar. Drug dosage regimens, however, can differ because patients having CCPD or NIPD undergo PD only during the night-time hours, and those having NIPD do not have residual peritoneal fluid during the day. For aminoglycoside antibiotics, once daily dosing is preferred for the foregoing reasons, as well as their longer duration of action because of the post-antibiotic effect (see Chapter 32, Chronic Kidney Disease). Vancomycin and other glycopeptides can be administered intermittently because of their prolonged elimination half-life in patients with ESRD. Because of the lack of clinical trials with other antibiotics in patients having APD, extrapolation from the CAPD literature may be necessary. A review addresses the current knowledge and issues surrounding the pharmacokinetics of antibiotics in patients with peritonitis undergoing APD.[104]

Exit-Site Infection

Prevention of catheter exit-site infections (and thus peritonitis) is the primary goal of exit-site care.[102] Several preventative measures are important: adequate catheter placement, dedicated postoperative catheter care, and routine daily care of the exit site. Dressing changes of a newly placed catheter are done by a dialysis nurse using sterile technique until the exit site is well healed, which can take up to 2 weeks. Once the exit site is well healed, the patient is educated and trained to do routine exit-site care. Routine care consists of thorough handwashing with antibacterial soap before touching the exit site. Antiseptics that contain at least 60% ethanol or isopropyl alcohol can be used to augment handwashing.[105] The exit site is then washed daily with antibacterial soap, although use of an antiseptic (e.g., povidone iodine or chlorhexidine) is a reasonable option.[102] Hydrogen peroxide should be avoided as a routine antiseptic because it causes drying. After daily cleansing, antimicrobial creams (e.g., mupirocin, gentamicin) are applied around the catheter exit site using a cotton swab. Mupirocin ointment, not the cream, can cause structural damage to polyurethane catheters, and should be avoided in patients with these catheters.[102] Catheter exit-site infections are most often caused by *S. aureus* and Pseudomonas species.[99] In a randomized, double-blind trial, gentamicin sulfate 0.1% cream was found to be as effective as mupirocin 2% cream in preventing *S. aureus* infections.[106] Gentamicin cream was also highly effective in reducing *P. aeruginosa* and other gram-negative catheter infections, whereas mupirocin cream was not. A longer time to first catheter infection and a reduction in peritonitis, particularly gram-negative organisms, was also seen with gentamicin use. For these reasons, daily gentamicin cream at the exit site is considered to be the prophylaxis of choice in patients having PD.[106] Finally, the catheter should be immobilized with a small gauze dressing and tape to prevent pulling and trauma to the exit site, which may lead to infection.

Empiric therapy for exit-site infections may be started immediately, and should always cover *S. aureus*. Oral antibiotic therapy has been shown to be as effective as IP therapy.[102] Local erythema alone can be treated with topical agents, whereas purulent drainage indicates more significant infection and the need for systemic antibiotics.[103] Hypertonic saline dressings, as well as oral antibiotic therapy, can be used for especially severe exit-site infections.[102] Hypertonic saline is prepared by adding 1 tablespoon of salt to 1 pint (500 mL) of sterile water. The solution is then applied to gauze and wrapped around the catheter exit site for 15 minutes, once or twice a day. Gram-positive organisms are treated with first-generation oral cephalosporins, a penicillinase-resistant penicillin, or trimethoprim-sulfamethoxazole (TMP-SMX). A 1-week course of rifampin may be added at 600 mg/day orally (in single or split dose) for nonresponding infections with positive cultures after 1 week of appropriate therapy. Rifampin monotherapy treatment of *S. aureus* should be avoided. In areas where tuberculosis is endemic, rifampin should also be avoided in the treatment of *S. aureus* to reserve this drug for treatment of tuberculosis.[102] Oral quinolone antibiotics are recommended as first-line agents in the treatment of *P. aeruginosa* exit-site infections. *P. aeruginosa* infections are difficult to treat and often require prolonged therapy with two antibiotics.[102] If the infection is slow to resolve or if in cases of a recurrence, a second antipseudomonal drug can be added (e.g., ceftazidime IP). Gram-negative organisms can be treated with ciprofloxacin 500 mg orally twice daily.[103] Scheduling of the quinolone dose is important so that coadministration with foods or other drug therapies that may chelate the quinolone in the gut is avoided. Potentially chelating agents include calcium products, iron, multivitamins, antacids, zinc, sucralfate, and dairy products. Antibiotic therapy should be continued for a minimum of 2 weeks until the exit site appears entirely normal.

Weight Gain

Dextrose is present in dialysate solutions primarily to serve as an osmotic agent for the removal of fluid during each exchange. Higher concentrations are expected to result in greater fluid removal. Approximately 500 to 1,000 kcal/day are absorbed as glucose from PD solutions, which can lead to weight gain in patients. Some patients may require modification of oral caloric intake to avoid excessive weight gain. Insulin requirements generally are increased in patients with diabetes as a result of the additional calories and, when administered IP, usually are two to three times the normal subcutaneous dose because of their reduced bioavailability of 20% to 50% by this route.

REFERENCES

1. U.S. Renal Data System, USRDS 2006 Annual Data Report. National Institutes of Health, National Institute of Diabetes and Digestive and Kidney Diseases, Bethesda, MD; 2006.
2. U.S. Renal Data System, USRDS 2002 Annual Data Report. National Institutes of Health, National Institute of Diabetes and Digestive and Kidney Diseases, Bethesda, MD; 2002.
3. U.S. Renal Data System, USRDS 2001 Annual Data Report. National Institutes of Health, National Institute of Diabetes and Digestive and Kidney Diseases, Bethesda, MD; 2001.
4. Pastan S et al. Dialysis therapy. *N Engl J Med* 1998;338:1428.
5. NKF-K/DOQI Clinical Practice Guidelines for Hemodialysis Adequacy: Update 2006. *Am J Kidney Dis* 2006;48(Suppl1):S2.
6. NKF-K/DOQI Clinical Practice Guidelines for Peritoneal Dialysis Adequacy: Update 2006. *Am J Kidney Dis* 2006;48(Suppl1):S91.
7. NKF-K/DOQI Clinical Practice Guidelines for Vascular Access. *Am J Kidney Dis* 2006;48(Suppl1): S176.
8. NKF-K/DOQI Clinical Practice Guidelines and Clinical Practice Recommendations for Anemia of Chronic Kidney Disease. *Am J Kidney Dis* 2006;47(5Suppl3):S11.
9. I. NKF-K/DOQI Clinical Practice Guidelines for Hemodialysis Adequacy: Update 2000. *Am J Kidney Dis* 2001;37(Suppl 1):7.
10. II. NKF-K/DOQI Clinical Practice Guidelines for Peritoneal Dialysis Adequacy: Update 2000. *Am J Kidney Dis* 2001;37(Suppl 1):65.
11. III. NKF-K/DOQI Clinical Practice Guidelines for Vascular Access: Update 2000. *Am J Kidney Dis* 2001;37(Suppl 1):137.
12. IV. NKF-K/DOQI Clinical Practice Guidelines for Anemia of Chronic Kidney Disease: Update 2000. *Am J Kidney Dis* 2001;37(Suppl 1):182.
13. NKF-K/DOQI Clinical Practice Guidelines for Nutrition of Chronic Renal Failure. I. Adult Guidelines. *Am J Kidney Dis* 2000;35(Suppl 2):S17.
14. NKF-K/DOQI Clinical Practice Guidelines for Chronic Kidney Disease: Evaluation, Classification, and Stratification. *Am J Kidney Dis* 2002; 39:S1.
15. Schulman G et al. Hemodialysis. In: Brenner BM, ed. *Brenner and Rector's the Kidney.* 7th ed. Philadelphia: Saunders; 2004.
16. Daugirdas JT. Physiologic principles and urea kinetic modeling. In: Daugirdas JT, et al., eds. *Handbook of Dialysis.* 4th ed. Philadelphia: Lippincott, Williams & Wilkins; 2007:25.
17. Ahmad S et al. Hemodialysis apparatus. In: Daugirdas JT et al., eds. *Handbook of Dialysis.* 4th ed. Philadelphia: Lippincott, Williams & Wilkins; 2007:59.
18. Daugirdas JT et al. A nomogram approach to hemodialysis urea modeling. *Am J Kidney Dis* 1994;23:33.
19. Laird NM et al. Modeling success or failure of dialysis therapy. The National Cooperative Dialysis Study. *Kidney Int* 1983;13(Suppl):S101.

20. Gotch FA et al. A mechanistic analysis of the National Cooperative Dialysis Study (NCDS). *Kidney Int* 1985;28:526.
21. Shinaberger JH. Quantitation of dialysis: historical perspective. *Semin Dial* 2001;14:238.
22. Cheung AK et al. Serum B-2 microglobulin levels predict mortality in dialysis patients: results of the HEMO study. *J Am Soc Nephrol* 2006;17:546.
23. van Ypersele de Strihou C. Are biocompatible membranes superior for hemodialysis therapy? *Kidney Int* 1997;52(Suppl 62):S101.
24. Libetta C et al. Vitamin E-loaded dialyzer resets PBMC-operated cytokine network in dialysis patients. *Kidney Int* 2004;65:1473–81.
25. National Kidney Foundation Report on Dialyzer Reuse. Task Force on Reuse of Dialyzers, Council on Dialysis, National Kidney Foundation. *Am J Kidney Dis* 1997;30:859.
26. Port FK et al. Mortality risk by hemodialyzer reuse practice and dialyzer membrane characteristics: results from the USRDS dialysis morbidity and mortality study. *Am J Kidney Dis* 2001;37:276.
27. Lowrie EG et al. Reprocessing dialysers for multiple uses: recent analysis of death risks for patients. *Nephrol Dial Transplant* 2004;19:2823.
28. Hauck M et al. In vivo effects of dialysate flow rate on Kt/V in maintenance hemodialysis patients. *Am J Kidney Dis* 2000;35:105.
29. Wathen RL et al. Water treatment for hemodialysis. In: Cogan MG et al., eds. *Introduction to Dialysis.* 2nd ed. New York: Churchill Livingstone; 1991:45.
30. Daugirdas JT et al. Hemodialysis apparatus. In: Daugirdas JT et al., eds. *Handbook of Dialysis.* 3rd ed. Philadelphia: Lippincott, Williams & Wilkins; 2001:46.
31. Ward RA et al. Product water and hemodialysis solution preparation. In: Daugirdas JT et al., eds. *Handbook of Dialysis.* 4th ed. Philadelphia: Lippincott, Williams & Wilkins; 2007:79.
32. Churchill DN et al. Canadian hemodialysis morbidity study. *Am J Kidney Dis* 1992;18:214.
33. Davenport A et al. Anticoagulation. In: Daugirdas JT et al., eds. *Handbook of Dialysis.* 4th ed. Philadelphia: Lippincott, Williams & Wilkins; 2007:204.
34. Lohr JW et al. Minimizing hemorrhagic complications in dialysis patients. *J Am Soc Nephrol* 1991;2:961.
35. Schwab SJ et al. Hemodialysis without anticoagulation. One-year prospective trial in hospitalized patients at risk for bleeding. *Am J Med* 1987;83:405.
36. Saltissi D et al. Comparison of low-molecular-weight heparin (enoxaparin sodium) and standard unfractionated heparin for hemodialysis anticoagulation. *Nephrol Dial Transplant* 1999;14:2698.
37. Perry SL et al. A multi-dose pharmacokinetic study of dalteparin in haemodialysis patients. *Thromb Haemost* 2006;96:750.
38. Hainer JW et al. Intravenous and subcutaneous weight-based dosing of the low molecular weight heparin tinzaparin (Innohep) in end-stage renal disease patients undergoing chronic hemodialysis. *Am J Kidney Dis* 2002;40:531.
39. Harenberg J. Is laboratory monitoring of low-molecular weight heparin therapy necessary? Yes. *J Thromb Haemost* 2004;2:547.
40. Bounameaux H et al. Is laboratory monitoring of low-molecular weight heparin therapy necessary? No. *J Thromb Haemost* 2004;2:551.
41. Brophy DF et al. The pharmacokinetics of enoxaparin do not correlate with its pharmacodynamic effect in patients receiving dialysis therapies. *J Clin Pharmacol* 2006;46:887.
42. Farooq V et al. Serious adverse incidents with the usage of low molecular weight heparins in patients with chronic kidney disease. *Am J Kidney Dis* 2004;43:531.
43. Hirsh J et al. Heparin and low-molecular weight heparin: the Seventh ACCP Conference on Antithrombotic and Thrombolytic Therapy. *Chest* 2004;126:188S.
44. O'Shea SI et al. Alternative methods of anticoagulation for dialysis-dependent patients with heparin-induced thrombocytopenia. *Semin Dial* 2003;16:61.
45. Murray PT et al. A prospective comparison of three argatroban treatment regimens during hemodialysis in end-stage renal disease. *Kidney Int* 2004;66:2446.
46. Tang IY et al. Argatroban and renal replacement therapy in patients with heparin-induced thrombocytopenia. *Ann Pharmacother* 2005;39:231.
47. Bucha E et al. R-hirudin as anticoagulant in regular hemodialysis therapy: finding of therapeutic R-hirudin blood/plasma concentrations and respective dosages. *Clin Appl Thromb Hemost* 1999;5:164.
48. Apsner R et al. Citrate for long-term hemodialysis: prospective study of 1,009 consecutive high-flux treatments in 59 patients. *Am J Kidney Dis* 2005;45:557.
49. Lowrie EG et al. Effect of the hemodialysis prescription on patient morbidity: report from the National Cooperative Dialysis Study. *N Engl J Med* 1981;305:1176.
50. Delmez JA et al. Hemodialysis prescription and delivery in a metropolitan area. The St. Louis Nephrology Study Group. *Kidney Int* 1992;41:1023.
51. Eknoyan G et al. Effect of dialysis dose and membrane flux in maintenance hemodialysis. *N Engl J Med* 2002;347:2010.
52. Saran R et al. Longer treatment time and slower ultrafiltration in hemodialysis: associations with reduced mortality in the DOPPS. *Kidney Int* 2006;69:1222.
53. Charra B et al. Survival as an index of adequacy of dialysis. *Kidney Int* 1992;41:1286.
54. Pierratos A. Nocturnal home hemodialysis: an update on a 5-year experience. *Nephrol Dial Transplant* 1999;14:2835.
55. Walsh M et al. A systematic review of the effect of nocturnal hemodialysis on blood pressure, left ventricular hypertrophy, anemia, mineral metabolism, and health-related quality of life. *Kidney Int* 2005;67:1500.
56. Daugirdas JT. Dialysis hypotension: a hemodynamic analysis. *Kidney Int* 1991;39:233.
57. Perazella MA. Pharmacologic options available to treat symptomatic intradialytic hypotension. *Am J Kidney Dis* 2001;38(Suppl 4):S26.
58. Canzanello VJ et al. Hemodialysis-associated muscle cramps. *Semin Dial* 1992;5:299.
59. Sherman RA. Acute therapy of hemodialysis-related muscle cramps. *Am J Kidney Dis* 1982;2:287.
60. Roca AO et al. Dialysis leg cramps : efficacy of quinine vs. vitamin E. *ASAIO J* 1992;38:M481.
61. Khajehdehi P et al. A randomized, double-blind, placebo-controlled trial of supplementary vitamins E, C and their combination for treatment of haemodialysis cramps. *Nephrol Dial Transplant* 2001;16:1448.
62. Tielemans C. Immediate hypersensitivity reactions and hemodialysis. *Adv Nephrol* 1993;22:401.
63. Lemke H-D et al. Hypersensitivity reactions during hemodialysis: role of complement fragments and ethylene oxide antibodies. *Nephrol Dial Transplant* 1990;5:264.
64. Pegues DA. Anaphylactoid reactions associated with reuse of hollow-fiber hemodialyzers and ACE inhibitors. *Kidney Int* 1992;42:1232.
65. Arieff AI. Dialysis disequilibrium syndrome: current concepts on pathogenesis and prevention. *Kidney Int* 1994;45:629.
66. Hakim R et al. Hemodialysis access failure: a call to action. *Kidney Int* 1998;54:1029.
67. Valji K et al. Pulse-spray pharmacomechanical thrombolysis of thrombosed hemodialysis access grafts: long-term experience and comparison of original and current techniques. *Am J Roentgenol* 1995;164:1495.
68. Cooper SG. Pulse-spray thrombolysis of thrombosed hemodialysis grafts with tissue plasminogen activator. *Am J Roentgenol* 2003;180:1063.
69. Falk A et al. Reteplase in the treatment of thrombosed hemodialysis grafts. *J Vasc Interv Radiol* 2001;12:1257.
70. Crowther MA et al. Low-intensity warfarin is ineffective for the prevention of PTFE graft failure in patients on hemodialysis: a randomized controlled trial. *J Am Soc Nephrol* 2002;13:2331.
71. Kaufman JS et al. Randomized controlled trial of clopidogrel plus aspirin to prevent hemodialysis access graft thrombosis. *J Am Soc Nephrol* 2003;14:2313.
72. Leehey DJ et al. Infections. In: Daugirdas JT et al., eds. *Handbook of Dialysis.* 4th ed. Philadelphia: Lippincott, Williams & Wilkins; 2007:542.
73. DeSoi CA et al. Vancomycin elimination during high-flux hemodialysis: kinetic model and comparison of four membranes. *Am J Kidney Dis* 1992;20:354.
74. Pollard TA et al. Vancomycin redistribution: dosing recommendations following high-flux hemodialysis. *Kidney Int* 1994;45:232.
75. Pai AB et al. Vancomycin dosing in high flux hemodialysis: a limited sampling algorithm. *Am J Health-Syst Pharm* 2004;61:181.
76. Mason NA et al. Comparison of 3 vancomycin dosage regimens during hemodialysis with cellulose triacetate dialyzers: post-dialysis versus intradialytic administration. *Clin Nephrol* 2003;60:96.
77. Ariano RE et al. Adequacy of a vancomycin dosing regimen in patients receiving high-flux hemodialysis. *Am J Kidney Dis* 2005;46:681.
78. DeBroe ME et al. New insights and strategies in the diagnosis and treatment of aluminum overload in dialysis patients. *Nephrol Dial Transplant* 1993;8(Suppl 1):47.
79. Chazan JA et al. Plasma aluminum levels (unstimulated and stimulated): clinical and biochemical findings in 185 patients undergoing chronic hemodialysis for 4 to 95 months. *Am J Kidney Dis* 1989;13:284.
80. Boelaert JR et al. Mucormycosis during deferoxamine therapy is a siderophore-mediated infection: in-vitro and in-vivo studies. *J Clin Invest* 1993;91:1979.
81. Olivieri NF et al. Visual and auditory neurotoxicity in patients receiving subcutaneous deferoxamine infusion. *N Engl J Med* 1986:314:869.
82. Felsenfeld AJ et al. Deferoxamine therapy in hemodialysis patients with aluminum-associated bone disease. *Kidney Int* 1989;35:1371.
83. Koch KM. Dialysis-related amyloidosis. *Kidney Int* 1992;41:1416.
84. Diaz RJ et al. The effect of dialyzer reprocessing on performance and –2 microglobulin removal using polysulfone membranes. *Am J Kidney Dis* 1993;21:405.
85. Hurot J et al. Effects of L-carnitine supplementation in maintenance hemodialysis patients. *J Am Soc Nephrol* 2002;13:708.
86. Bellinghieri G et al. Carnitine and hemodialysis. *Am J Kidney Dis* 2003;41(Suppl 1):S116.
87. Brophy DF et al. Automated peritoneal dialysis: new implications for pharmacists. *Ann Pharmacother* 1997;31:756.
88. Gokal R et al. Peritoneal dialysis. *Lancet* 1999;353:823.
89. Burkart JM et al. Peritoneal dialysis. In: Brenner BM, Rector FC, eds. *The Kidney.* 5th Ed. Philadelphia: WB Saunders, 1996:2507.
90. Blake PG. Adequacy of peritoneal dialysis and chronic peritoneal dialysis prescription. In: Daugirdas JT et al., eds. *Handbook of Dialysis.* 4th ed. Philadelphia: Lippincott, Williams & Wilkins; 2007:387.
91. Gokal R et al. Peritoneal catheters and exit-site practices toward optimal peritoneal access: 1998 update. *Perit Dial Int* 1998;18:11.
92. Port FK et al. Risk of peritonitis and technique failure by CAPD connection technique: a national study. *Kidney Int* 1992;42:967.
93. Brown EA et al. Survival of functionally anuric patients on automated peritoneal dialysis: The

European APD Outcome Study. *J Am Soc Nephrol* 2003;14:2948.
94. Moberly JB et al. Pharmacokinetics of icodextrin in peritoneal dialysis patients. *Kidney Int* 2002;62(Suppl 81):S23.
95. Wolfson M et al. Review of clinical trial experience with icodextrin. *Kidney Int* 2002;62(Suppl 81):S46.
96. Finkelstein F et al. Superiority of icodextrin compared to 4.25% dextrose for peritoneal ultrafiltration. *J Am Soc Nephrol* 2005;16:546.
97. Bargman JM et al. Relative contribution of residual renal function and peritoneal clearance to adequacy of dialysis: A reanalysis of the CANUSA Study. *J Am Soc Nephrol* 2001;12:2158.
98. Paniagua R et al. Effects of increased peritoneal clearances on mortality in peritoneal dialysis: ADEMEX, a prospective, randomized, controlled trial. *J Am Soc Nephrol* 2002;13:1307.
99. Chatoth DK et al. Morbidity and mortality in redefining adequacy of peritoneal dialysis: a step beyond the National Kidney Foundation-Dialysis Outcomes Quality Initiative. *Am J Kidney Dis* 1999;33:617.
100. Twardowski ZJ. Peritoneal equilibration test. *Perit Dial Bull* 1987;7:138.
101. Burkart JM et al. Peritoneal dailysis. In: Brenner BM, ed. *Brenner and Rector's the Kidney.* 7th ed. Philadelphia: Saunders; 2004.
102. Piraino B et al. ISPD Guidelines/recommendations. Peritoneal dialysis-related infections recommendations: 2005 update. *Perit Dial Int* 2005; 25:107.
103. Keane WF et al. Adult peritoneal dialysis-related peritonitis treatment recommendations: 2000 update. *Perit Dial Int* 2000;20:396.
104. Manley HJ et al. Treatment of peritonitis in APD: pharmacokinetic principles. *Semin Dial* 2002;15:418.
105. Bender FH et al. Prevention of infectious complications in peritoneal dialysis: best demonstrated practices. *Kidney Int* 2006;70:S44.
106. Bernardini J et al. Randomized, double-blind trial of antibiotic exit site cream for prevention of exit site infection in peritoneal dialysis patients. *J Am Soc Nephrol* 2005;116:539.

CHAPTER 33

Dosing of Drugs in Renal Failure

David J. Quan and Francesca T. Aweeka

BASIC PRINCIPLES

An increasing amount of information is available on the disposition of drugs in renal disease. It is important to design specific pharmacotherapeutic regimens for patients with renal impairment. Many patients are treated with multiple medications, which may require dosage adjustment. Without careful dosing and therapeutic drug monitoring for select agents in these patients, accumulation of drugs or toxic metabolites can occur, resulting in serious adverse effects.

In addition to altered drug elimination, a number of factors associated with kidney disease predispose patients to the potential for drug toxicity. Renal disease can affect the pharmacokinetic disposition as well as the pharmacodynamic effect of drugs. For example, the physiologic changes associated with uremia can alter drug absorption, protein binding, distribution, or elimination. These physiologic changes can alter drug concentrations in the plasma or blood, and at the targeted tissue site of activity, thereby affecting drug efficacy and toxicity.

Little is known about the effect of renal disease on drug pharmacodynamics. Pharmacodynamics (or "what the drug does to the body") quantitatively describes the pharmacologic or toxicologic effects of drugs relative to the drug concentration. Patients with renal disease may have a different response to a given drug concentration than a patient with normal renal function. Data in the area of pharmacodynamics and renal disease are limited. Patients with renal disease can be more sensitive to some drugs, and can experience an increased frequency of adverse drug reactions, with or without dosing modifications.

Figure 33-1 illustrates the relationship between pharmacokinetics and pharmacodynamics. The dose of drug produces a drug concentration, which results in a pharmacologic or toxic effect. Figure 33-2 illustrates how different components of drug disposition influence the ability of a drug to exert its pharmacologic effect at the site of action.

Effect of Renal Failure on Drug Disposition

Bioavailability

Although several factors can affect drug absorption in patients with kidney disease, only limited data are available that definitively document altered bioavailability. The absorption of drugs in patients with renal disorders could be inhibited by gastrointestinal (GI) disturbances present with uremia (e.g., nausea, vomiting, diarrhea), uremic gastritis, and pancreatitis. Edema of the GI tract, which can occur in patients with nephrotic syndrome, can cause impaired absorption. Gastric and intestinal motility as well as gastric emptying time can be

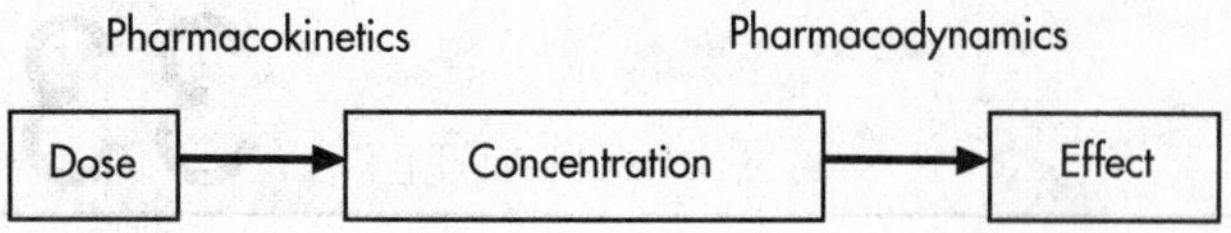

FIGURE 33-1 Relationship between pharmacokinetics and pharmacodynamics and the relationship of these two scientific principles to drug dose and concentration, and drug concentration and effect.

altered by the neuropathy that is commonly associated with uremia. Uremia also can increase gastric ammonia, leading to an increased gastric pH. Drugs that require an acidic environment for absorption, such as ferrous sulfate, may be less bioavailable.[1] Calcium-containing antacids that often are used by patients with renal failure for GI symptoms and hyperphosphatemia will neutralize hydrochloric acid in the stomach and increase gastric pH. Patients with end-stage renal disease often take oral phosphate binders, such as sevelamer, which can impair the absorption of other medications.

The bioavailability of orally administered drugs also depends on the extent to which the drug is eliminated by first-pass (presystemic) metabolism. In an early study, the first-pass hepatic metabolism of oral propranolol was found to be reduced in patients with renal disease, leading to increased bioavailability.[2] Subsequent studies, however, have attributed these observed increased concentrations of propranolol in renal failure to a significant increase in the blood-to-plasma ratio.[3] Not only can decreased first-pass metabolism contribute to increased bioavailability, but intestinal P-glycoprotein activity may be decreased as well.[4] Additional drugs exhibiting increased bioavailability in renal disease include cloxacillin, propoxyphene, dihydrocodeine, encainide, and zidovudine (AZT). For example, the area under the curve (AUC) of dihydrocodeine is increased by 70% in those patients with impaired renal function.[5]

Protein Binding and Volume of Distribution

The extent to which a drug exerts its pharmacologic effects is related to the amount of free or unbound drug available for distribution to the target tissues. Patients with renal failure often have alterations in plasma protein binding, which can increase the amount of unbound drug.[6] Although this generally is true for acidic drugs, the binding of basic drugs is usually unchanged or possibly decreased in renal disease. Clinically, this is most important for highly protein-bound drugs (>80%). Decreased protein binding of these drugs results in increases in the free fraction of drug. This leads to an increase in the apparent volume of distribution (Vd), and plasma clearance for drugs with a low-extraction ratio. A simultaneous increase in both the Vd and clearance results, however, in little or no change in the elimination half-life ($t_{1/2}$) of these drugs. Alternatively, the Vd of high-extraction ratio drugs can increase without a concomitant change in clearance. In this situation, the elimination half-life would increase, based on the relationships:

$$Kd = Cl/Vd$$
$$t_{1/2} = 0.693 \times Vd/Cl$$

In patients with renal failure, the accumulation of uremic toxins may alter protein binding. When the free fraction of drugs that are highly protein bound changes, the interpretation of the total drug concentration must also be considered. That is, with increasing free fraction, the total drug concentration necessary to exert the desired pharmacologic effect is lower than that needed under normal conditions.

Hypoalbuminemia is a common complication of renal failure. Because acidic rather than basic drugs are bound to albumin, their protein binding tends to be altered in patients with renal failure (Table 33-1).[7] Patients with uremia accumulate acidic by products that may inhibit binding, or displace acidic drugs from albumin binding sites. This is supported by the observed improvement in protein binding following removal of uremic byproducts by hemodialysis. Finally, the conformation or structural arrangement of albumin is altered in renal disease, which may reduce the number and affinity of binding sites for drugs. Studies have demonstrated differences in the amino acid composition of albumin between healthy people and patients with uremia.[8]

The anticonvulsant, phenytoin, is a classic example of a drug whose protein binding is altered in renal disease.[9] This is discussed in more detail later in this chapter.

Renal disease can change the Vd of various drugs. The Vd or "apparent volume of distribution" is the "volume" or size of a compartment necessary to account for the total amount of drug in the body if it were present throughout the body at the same concentration as that found in plasma. A decrease in the plasma protein binding of highly protein-bound drugs, such as phenytoin, leads to an increase in the apparent Vd.

Drugs that are not highly protein bound (e.g., gentamicin, isoniazid) have little change in their Vd in renal disease. Digoxin is a unique exception in that its Vd is decreased in renal disease. This is attributed to a decrease in myocardial tissue uptake of digoxin, leading to a decrease in the myocardial- or tissue-to-serum concentration ratio.[10]

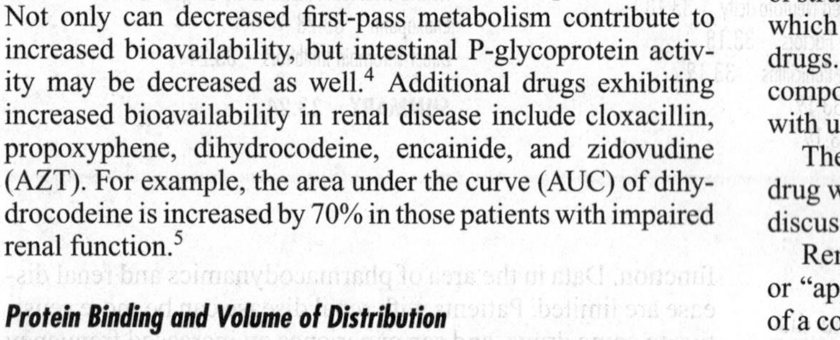

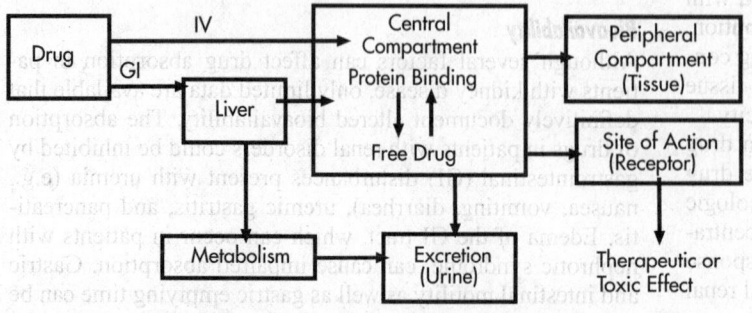

FIGURE 33-2 Factors influencing drug disposition and therapeutic or toxic effects. Following drug administration, a number of factors can influence pharmacokinetic parameters, such as bioavailability, volume of distribution, clearance, and target tissue binding. These factors may include first-pass metabolism, protein binding, and renal and liver function.

Table 33-1 Plasma Protein Binding (%) of Acidic Drugs in Renal Failure

Drug	Normal	Renal Failure
Cefazolin	85	69
Cefoxitin	73	25
Clofibrate	97	91
Diazoxide	94	84
Furosemide	96	94
Pentobarbital	66	59
Phenytoin	88–93	74–84
Salicylate	87–97	74–84
Sulfamethoxazole	66	42
Valproic acid	92	77
Warfarin	99	98

Elimination

The extent to which renal disease affects the elimination of a drug depends on the amount of drug normally excreted unchanged in the urine and the degree of renal impairment. As kidney disease progresses, the kidney's ability to excrete uremic toxins diminishes. Consequently, the ability to eliminate certain drugs that are renally excreted also decreases. If the dose of these drugs is not modified for patients with renal dysfunction, these drugs will accumulate, leading to an increase in the pharmacologic effect and the potential for toxicity.

The kidney eliminates drugs primarily by filtration or active secretion. Characteristics of a drug that determine its ability to be filtered include its affinity for protein binding and its molecular weight. Drugs with low protein binding or those that are displaced from proteins in the setting of renal disease (e.g., phenytoin) are filtered more readily. Molecules with a high molecular weight (>20,000 Da) are not readily filtered because of their large size. The reasons for how renal disease selectively alters the process of glomerular filtration or tubular secretion of specific drugs are not well understood. The renal elimination of drugs in patients with renal disease usually is estimated by measuring the ability of the kidney to eliminate substances such as creatinine (i.e., creatinine clearance [Cl_{Cr}]) (see Chapter 31, Acute Renal Failure).

Renal disease can also have an important impact on the elimination of drugs that are primarily metabolized by the liver.[11] Metabolic processes, such as hydroxylation and glucuronidation, often produce inactive, more polar compounds that can be eliminated by the kidney. The metabolites of some drugs (e.g., meperidine, morphine, procainamide) are pharmacologically active or toxic. In patients with renal disease, these metabolites may accumulate, leading to an increase in pharmacologic activity and adverse effects.[12,13] For example, the central nervous system (CNS) toxicity observed in renal disease has been attributed to accumulation of the morphine metabolite, morphine-6-glucuronide. Therefore, careful dosing modifications or avoidance of these drugs are warranted in patients with renal impairment. Metabolic enzymes have been found within renal tissue, and may play a role in the metabolism of some of these drugs.[14,15] For example, the nonrenal clearance of drugs (e.g., acyclovir) decreases in patients with renal impairment, and is believed to be caused by a decrease in "renal" metabolism.[16]

Although renal and hepatic dysfunction may alter the metabolism and excretion of many drugs, the disposition of excipients used to formulate medications should also be considered. The pharmacokinetics of itraconazole and voriconazole are not significantly altered in the setting of renal dysfunction. The parenteral formulations of itraconazole and voriconazole contain the solubilizing agent, β-cyclodextrin. Cyclodextrin is rapidly eliminated by glomerular filtration, but can accumulate in patients with renal impairment, causing GI disturbances.[17]

Drug Removal by Dialysis

The effect of dialysis on the removal of a specific drug must be considered when using medications in patients undergoing dialysis. Patients may need supplemental doses of a medication after a dialysis session or alteration in their dosage to maintain therapeutic drug concentrations. Dialysis also can be initiated to hasten drug removal from the body in some cases of drug overdose.

When using dialysis to manage a drug overdose, patients may respond clinically to factors unrelated to dialysis of the drug. For example, declining plasma concentrations may be caused by concurrent drug elimination by hepatic metabolism or renal excretion, which is independent of the dialysis procedure itself. Furthermore, clinical improvement may result from removal of active metabolites by dialysis rather than the parent compound.

The primary literature should be used to determine if any information is available about the ability of dialysis to remove drug. The application of data from the literature to a specific clinical situation often is difficult, however, and information pertaining to the dialysis of a specific drug may be limited. Anecdotal case reports in the primary literature seldom provide quantitative information. The effectiveness of dialysis is often based on a positive clinical outcome rather than on objective measurements of drug concentrations in the plasma and dialysate.

When applying information from the primary literature to a specific patient, the specifics of the dialyzer (e.g., type of machine, membrane surface area, pore size, and blood and dialysis flow rates) must be considered (see Chapter 32, Renal Dialysis). Furthermore, patient-specific information (e.g., time of drug ingestion, liver and renal function) from case reports in the literature also should be evaluated appropriately. The method used to calculate dialysis clearance also should be considered. In addition, clinical investigators often use predialysis and postdialysis serum drug concentrations for estimating drug dialyzability without considering the contributing effects of drug metabolism and excretion on drug elimination.

Drug-Specific Properties

The physical and chemical characteristics of drugs can be used to predict the effectiveness of dialysis on drug removal.[18–20] Low-molecular-weight (MW) compounds are more readily dialyzed by conventional hemodialysis procedures because they can pass with greater ease across the dialysis membrane. Using cuprophane dialysis membranes, compounds with a MW $\leq$500 are more likely to be significantly dialyzed than compounds with a high MW (e.g., vancomycin, MW $\approx$ 1,400). Newer high-flux dialyzers using polysulfone membranes more effectively remove large chemical compounds (see High-Flux

Hemodialysis below and Chapter 32, Renal Dialysis). In addition, the water solubility of a compound can also help predict drug dialyzability because water-soluble drugs are removed more readily than lipid-soluble compounds.

Pharmacokinetic characteristics (e.g., Vd, protein binding) also can affect drug dialyzability. A drug with a large Vd that distributes widely into the peripheral tissues resides minimally in the plasma and therefore is not substantially removed by dialysis. This is particularly true for highly lipid-soluble drugs such as digoxin (Vd = 300–500 L), and amiodarone (Vd = 60 L/kg). In addition, drugs that are highly protein bound, such as warfarin (99%) and ceftriaxone (83%–96%), are not significantly removed by dialysis because the large protein–drug complex is unable to pass through the dialysis membrane.

The plasma clearance of a drug should also be compared with the dialysis clearance. Clearance values are additive. Dialysis clearance must contribute substantially to the patient's own clearance to enhance drug elimination. For example, zidovudine (AZT) has a large plasma clearance in patients with severe renal disease (≈1,200 mL/minute). Therefore, despite a hemodialysis clearance of 63 mL/minute, the contribution of dialysis to AZT removal is negligible.

High-Flux Hemodialysis

High-flux hemodialysis utilizes higher blood and dialysate flow rates compared with conventional methods. The enhanced efficiency of high-flux dialysis and the larger pore size of the polysulfone membranes allow for small- and mid-MW compounds (e.g., vancomycin) to be partially removed. Drugs such as gentamicin and foscarnet, which are removed by conventional dialysis, are also efficiently removed by high-flux hemodialysis.[21,22] In many cases, the net amount of drug removed during a high-flux dialysis session is greater than the amount removed during conventional dialysis because of the use of higher blood flow rates. The principal difference is the greater efficiency and the ability to clear drugs of larger MW compared with conventional dialysis.

Continuous Ambulatory Peritoneal Dialysis

Continuous ambulatory peritoneal dialysis (CAPD) uses the patient's peritoneum as the dialysis membrane. Patients maintained with CAPD undergo infusion of a dialysate solution via a catheter inserted into the peritoneal cavity; the solution is allowed to dwell in the cavity for several hours. The accumulated fluid and uremic byproducts diffuse from the blood into the dialysate solution, which is exchanged every 4 to 8 hours (see Chapter 32, Renal Dialysis).

Some drugs, such as antibiotics, can be administered intraperitoneally in patients on CAPD by directly adding it to the dialysate solution. This is particularly useful for patients with peritonitis who require high intraperitoneal concentrations of antimicrobial agents to treat this infection. Following intraperitoneal administration of drugs, such as the aminoglycosides, plasma and intraperitoneal drug concentrations will eventually reach equilibrium. Despite systemic absorption of these drugs from the peritoneal fluid, peritoneal dialysis usually is inefficient at removing drugs from the plasma.[23] Because CAPD contributes little to the overall elimination of most drugs, dosage modifications are not always necessary in patients having this procedure.

Continuous Renal Replacement Therapies

Continuous arteriovenous hemofiltration (CAVH) and continuous venovenous hemofiltration (CVVH) are forms of continuous renal replacement therapy (CRRT) used in the critically ill patient with acute renal failure. These therapies are typically reserved for patients who are unable to tolerate hemodialysis because of hemodynamic instability. As with hemodialysis, this procedure removes fluid, electrolytes, and low- and mid-MW molecules from the blood. Using a hollow fiber that is made of a semipermeable membrane, water and solutes are filtered by hydrostatic pressure. A countercurrent dialysate can be added to the circuit to improve solute removal (CAVHD or CVVHD).

Limited data are available on the effect of CAVH or CVVH on the removal of drugs. Drugs that have a high sieving coefficient (permeability of a drug through a semipermeable membrane), such as the aminoglycosides, ceftazidime, vancomycin, and procainamide, are readily removed by CAVH or CVVH.[24–26] Data concerning the removal of drugs by hemodialysis cannot be extrapolated to CAVH or CVVH because of differences in the membranes used, blood flow rates, ultrafiltration rate, dialysate flow rate, and the continuous nature of the procedure compared with intermittent hemodialysis. A way does exist to estimate CVVH clearance and determine the appropriate dosage regimen based on the pharmacologic characteristics of a specific drug (see Question 8).

Hemoperfusion

Hemoperfusion is another method of drug removal that may be used to facilitate the elimination of a drug in the setting of an overdose.[27,28] During the hemoperfusion procedure, blood is passed through a column of adsorbent material (e.g., activated charcoal or resin) to bind toxins and drugs. Hemoperfusion can be particularly useful for removing large-MW compounds or highly protein-bound drugs that are not removed efficiently by hemodialysis. Large compounds and drug–protein complexes are adsorbed onto the high-surface-area resin as blood passes through the adsorbent column. Hemoperfusion can also be used to remove lipid-soluble drugs not easily removed by hemodialysis. Lipid-soluble drugs often have a large Vd. Removal of drugs by hemoperfusion is of limited value because a significant amount of these lipophilic compounds reside in peripheral tissues.

Pharmacodynamics and Renal Disease

Few studies have investigated the pharmacodynamics of drugs in patients with renal disease. Clinical observations report that patients with renal disease are more sensitive to various drugs. For example, morphine has been associated with increased neurologic depression in patients with renal failure.[29,30] The ability of morphine to potentiate the CNS depressant effects of uremia may result from an alteration in the permeability of the blood–brain barrier that results in higher CNS levels of morphine and morphine-6-glucuronide.

Another example of altered drug response in uremia is that of nifedipine, which, at similar unbound plasma concentrations, has an increased antihypertensive effect in patients with renal disease.[31] The mean maximal effect change in diastolic blood pressure (E_{max}) values in the control group and in patients with severe renal failure were 12% and 29%, respectively.

Therefore, the dose of nifedipine needs to be adjusted in patients with renal disease because of changes in drug effects rather than pharmacokinetic alterations.

The pharmacokinetics of warfarin is not significantly altered in renal failure. Patients with renal failure who are prescribed warfarin have a higher incidence of hemorrhagic complications, likely because of platelet dysfunction from uremia, and drug–drug interactions from concomitant medications.[32,33]

PHARMACOKINETICS AND PHARMACODYNAMICS OF SPECIFIC DRUGS IN RENAL FAILURE

Ceftazidime

Dosage Modification: Factors to Consider

1. G.G., a 31-year-old, 70-kg woman with a 3-year history of systemic lupus erythematosus (SLE), presents to the emergency department (ED) with a 5-day history of fatigue, weakness, and nausea as well as worsening of her facial rash and a fever of 40°C. Her SLE had been moderately controlled until this acute flare. Her admission laboratory workup now reveals the following pertinent values: potassium (K), 6.0 mEq/L (normal, 3.6–4.8 mEq/L); sodium (Na), 142 mEq/L (normal, 135–144 mEq/L); serum creatinine (SrCr), 3.4 mg/dL (normal, 0.6–1.3 mg/dL); and blood urea nitrogen (BUN), 38 mg/dL (normal, 7–20 mg/dL). Complete blood count (CBC) reveals a hematocrit (Hct) of 32% (normal, 35%–45% [females]) and a hemoglobin (Hgb) of 9.2 g/dL (normal, 11.8–15.4 g/dL [females]). The platelet count is 50,000/mm^3 (normal, 140,000–300,000) and her erythrocyte sedimentation rate (ESR) is 35 mm/hr (normal, 0–20). Physical examination is significant for a blood pressure (BP) of 136/92 mm Hg and 2+ pedal edema. Prednisone is started at a dose of 1.5 mg/kg/day.

Two weeks into her hospital course, G.G.'s condition worsens and signs of sepsis develop. *Pseudomonas aeruginosa* is cultured from her urine. Therapy with ceftazidime is initiated at a dose of 1 g Q 8 hr, a dose commonly used for patients with good renal function. Considering that G.G.'s renal function has remained stable and that she has an estimated Cl_{Cr} of 27 mL/minute, what factors should be considered before modifying her dose? What would be an appropriate dose of ceftazidime for G.G.?

[SI units: K, 6.0 mmol/L (normal, 3.6–4.8); Na, 142 mmol/L (normal, 135–144); SrCr, 300.56 μmol/L (normal, 53.04–114.92); BUN, 13.57 mmol/L urea (normal, 2.5–7.14); Hct, 0.32 (normal, 0.35–0.45); Hgb, 92 g/L (normal, 118–154); platelet count, 50 × 10^9/L (normal, 140–300); ESR, 35 mm/hour (normal, 0–20)]

Before modifying the dose of any drug, its route of elimination should be established. The elimination of most drugs that primarily are cleared by the kidneys will be decreased in the setting of renal impairment. The degree to which renal impairment affects elimination depends on the percentage of unchanged drug that is excreted by the kidney. For many drugs that are cleared by the kidneys, relationships between some measurement of renal function (e.g., Cl_{Cr}) and some parameter of drug elimination (e.g., plasma clearance or half-life) have been established to help the clinician determine the appropriate dosing modifications in patients with renal disease.

In contrast, the clearance of drugs that are eliminated primarily by nonrenal mechanisms (e.g., hepatic metabolism) is not altered significantly in patients with renal disease. Limited data indicate, however, that the kidney may play a role in drug metabolism. Enzymes with metabolic capacity have been found within renal tissue (see Question 12). The clinical importance of this elimination pathway is unclear.

Of clinical significance is the role of the kidney in eliminating pharmacologically active or toxic metabolites. Despite the metabolism of the parent drug and the lack of renal elimination of unchanged drug, the formation of active, more water-soluble metabolites that may accumulate with renal dysfunction warrants dosage adjustment or avoidance of the drug entirely (e.g., meperidine; see Question 22).

Another factor important to consider is the "therapeutic window" for a given drug. The therapeutic window is the range of drug concentrations thought to be most effective. Drug concentrations below this range are usually subtherapeutic, whereas concentrations above this range can lead to a greater incidence of adverse effects. For drugs with a wide therapeutic window, the difference between toxic and therapeutic concentrations is large. Drugs that are cleared primarily by the kidney may require dosing modifications in patients with renal dysfunction. Aggressive dose reduction may not be necessary, however, for drugs with a large therapeutic window, particularly if the adverse effects of the drug (e.g., fluconazole) are relatively mild. This is in contrast to drugs (e.g., aminoglycosides, vancomycin, or foscarnet), which are eliminated primarily by the kidney and have narrow therapeutic windows. For these drugs, the toxic plasma concentrations are very close to the therapeutic drug concentrations, with little room for dosing error. Table 33-2 summarizes the pharmacokinetics and dosing guidelines for drugs commonly used in patients with renal failure.

Ceftazidime is a cephalosporin that has excellent activity against most strains of *Pseudomonas* sp. As with most cephalosporins, ceftazidime primarily is cleared by the kidneys, with little nonrenal or hepatic elimination. The correlation between the clearance of ceftazidime and Cl_{Cr} in mL/minute is represented by the following equation[34]:

$$Cl_{ceftaz}\,(mL/min) = (0.95)(Cl_{cr}) + 6.59 \qquad \textbf{(33-1)}$$

Using Equation 33-1, the clearance of ceftazidime in G.G. is estimated to be 32 mL/minute compared with an average normal clearance of approximately 100 mL/minute. Because her drug clearance is approximately one-third of normal, she would require about one-third of the normal daily dose (i.e., 1 g every 24 hours). As with other cephalosporins, ceftazidime has a large therapeutic window.[37] Failure to reduce the dose from a normal dose of 1 g every 8 hours might, however, lead to accumulation of ceftazidime, predisposing G.G. to seizures and other adverse effects associated with toxic β-lactam antibiotic plasma levels.[35,36] This is in contrast to the aminoglycosides, which must be dosed based on specific pharmacokinetic calculations. Therefore, more generalized or empirical dosage modifications can be made with ceftazidime.

Aminoglycosides

2. G.G.'s medical team decides that the addition of an aminoglycoside antibiotic is now necessary to treat her infection. Considering that her renal function has remained stable, how should the gentamicin be dosed in G.G.? Is it best to alter the dose or the dosing interval for this drug?

Table 33-2 Pharmacokinetics and Dosing Guidelines for Drugs Commonly Used in Renal Failure[152]

Drug	Oral Availability (%)	Protein Binding (%)	Vd (L/kg)	Metabolism and Excretion	$t_{1/2}$ (hr)	Normal Dose Cl_{Cr} > 50 mL/min	Dose Change With Renal Failure Cl_{Cr} (mL/min)	Effect of Dialysis
Acyclovir	15–30	15	0.7	76%–82% excreted renally; 14% hepatic	Normal: 2.1–3.2 Anephric: 20	5 mg/kg Q 8 hr	10–50: 5 mg/kg Q 12–24 hr <10: 2.5 mg/kg Q 24 hr	Dialyzed; 80 mL/min
Adefovir	59	<4	0.35–0.39	45% excreted in urine	5–7	10 mg QD	20–49: 10 mg Q 48 hr 10–19: 10 mg Q 72 hr HD: 10 mg Q 7 days	Moderately dialyzed
Allopurinol	90	0	0.6	Metabolized to active oxypurinol metabolite, which is excreted renally; 6%–12% excreted unchanged renally	Normal: 1.1–1.6 Anephric: No change; 7 days oxypurinol	300 mg QD	10–50: 200 mg QD <10: 100 mg QD	Oxypurinol; moderately dialyzed
Amikacin	Parenteral	<5	0.2–0.3	94%–99% excreted renally	Normal: 2–3 Anephric: 36–82	See section on aminoglycoside pharmacokinetics	See section on aminoglycoside pharmacokinetics	Dialyzed; 22–38 mL/min
Amphotericin B	Parenteral	90–95	4	95%–97% hepatic metabolism or inactivation in body tissue; 3.5%–5.5% excreted unchanged renally	Normal: Initial: 24–48; Terminal: 15 days Anephric: No change	0.3–1 mg/kg Q 24 hr	10–50: 100% Q 24 hr <10: 100% Q 24–48 hr (to minimize azotemia)	Not dialyzed: large Vd
Ampicillin	32–76	29	0.3	73%–92% excreted renally; 12%–24% hepatic metabolism or biliary elimination	Normal: 0.8–1.5 Anephric: 20	1–2 g Q 4–6 hr	10–50: 1–1.5 g Q 6 hr <10: 50% 1 g Q 8–12 hr	Moderately dialyzed
Argatroban	Parenteral	54	0.174	16% excreted in urine	0.65–0.85	2 mcg/kg/min adjusted to appropriate aPTT	No change	20% removed by dialysis
Atenolol	50	<5	1.2	75% excreted renally; 10% hepatic; 10% feces	Normal: 5–6 Anephric: 42–73	50–100 mg QD	10–50: ↓ 50% and titrate <10: ↓ 50% and titrate	Moderately dialyzed
Aztreonam	Parenteral	50–60	0.15–0.38	60%–70% excreted renally; 12% hepatic	Normal: 1.3–2.2 Anephric: 6–9	1–2 g Q 6–8 hr	10–50: 1–2 g Q 8–12 hr <10: 1 g Q 12–24 hr	Moderately dialyzed
Captopril	65	30 (↓ R)	0.7	36%–42% excreted renally; 50% hepatic	Normal: 1.7–1.9 Anephric: 21–32	6.25–12.5 mg Q 8–12 hr	10–50: No change <10: ↓ 25% and titrate	Moderately dialyzed; 80–120 mL/min
Cefazolin	Parenteral	84–92	0.2	>95% excreted renally; 3–5% hepatic	Normal: 1.8–2.6 Anephric: 12–40	1–2 g Q 8 hr	10–50: 0.5–1.5 g Q 12 hr <10: 0.5–1 g Q 24 hr	Moderately dialyzed

Cefepime	Parenteral	20	0.23	>80% renally excreted	Normal = 2 Anephric = 13–18	1–2 g Q 8–12 hr	30–60 mL/min = 1–2 g Q 12–24 hr 10–29 mL/min = 0.5–2 g Q 24 hr <10 mL/min = 0.25–1 g Q 24 hr	Moderately dialyzed
Cefixime	50	69	0.1–1.0	20%–40% excreted renally; 50% excreted by nonrenal mechanisms	Normal: 3.5 Anephric: 12–15	200–400 mg Q 12–24 hr	10–50: No change <10: 50% Q 12–24 hr	Not dialyzed
Cefoperazone	Parenteral	87–93	0.16	70%–85% excreted unchanged in bile; 15–30% excreted renally	Normal: 1.6–2.6 Anephric: 2.5	1–2 g Q 8–12 hr	10–50: No change <10: ↓ with concurrent hepatic disease	Slightly dialyzed
Cefotaxime	Parenteral	38	0.22–0.36	40%–60% hepatic (desacetyl active metabolite; 25% activity of parent compound); 40%–65% excreted renally	Normal: 0.9–1.1 Anephric: 2.3–3.5, 12–20 (metabolite)	1–2 g Q –12 hr	10–50: 1–2 g Q 12 hr	Moderately dialyzed
Cefotetan	Parenteral	75–91	0.13	50%–88% excreted renally; 12% excreted in bile	Normal: 3–4.2 Anephric: 13	1–2 g Q 12 hr	10–50: 1–2 g Q 24 hr <10: 0.5–1 g Q 24 hr	Slightly/moderately dialyzed
Cefoxitin	Parenteral	65–79	0.27	85% excreted renally; up to 15% biliary and/or hepatic	Normal: 0.7–0.8 Anephric: 12–24	1–2 g Q 6–8 hr	10–50: 1–2 g Q 12–24 hr <10: 0.5–1 g Q 24 hr	Moderately dialyzed
Ceftazidime	Parenteral	20–30	0.2–0.3	73%–84% excreted renally	Normal: 1.6–2 Anephric: 13–25	1–2 g Q 8 hr	10–50: 1–2 g Q 12–24 hr <10: 0.5 g Q 24 hr	Dialyzed
Ceftizoxime	Parenteral	17–25	0.2–0.4	78%–92% excreted renally	Normal: 1.4–1.7 Anephric: 19–30	1–2 g Q 8–12 hr	10–50: 1–2 g Q 12–24 hr <10: 0.5 g Q 24 hr	Moderately dialyzed
Ceftriaxone	Parenteral	83–96 (concentration dependent)	0.1	40%–67% excreted renally; 40% excreted in bile	Normal: 6.5–8.9 Anephric: 12	1–2 g Q 12–24 hr	10–50: 1–2 g Q 24 hr <10: 1–2 g Q 24 hr	Not dialyzed
Cefuroxime	Parenteral and 40–50 (as axetil salt)	33	0.19	90%–95% excreted renally	Normal: 1.1–1.7 Anephric: 15–17	0.75–1.5 g Q 6–8 hr	10–50: 50 –75% Q 8–12 hr <10: 25–50% Q 24 hr	Moderately dialyzed
Cephradine	90–100	6–20	0.25–0.33	80%–95% excreted renally; 5%–20% hepatic metabolism or biliary/fecal elimination	Normal: 0.7–0.9 Anephric: 8–15	250–500 mg Q 6 hr	10–50: 250–500 mg Q 12 hr <10: 250–500 mg Q 24 hr	Moderately dialyzed
Cimetidine	62	20	0.9–1.1	40%–80% excreted renally; some metabolism	Normal: 1.5 Anephric: 3.3–4.6	PO: 400 mg Q 12 hr IV: 300 mg Q 8 hr	10–50: ↓ 25% <10: ↓ 50%	Slightly dialyzed

Table 33-2 Pharmacokinetics and Dosing Guidelines for Drugs Commonly Used in Renal Failure[152] —cont'd

Drug	Oral Availability (%)	Protein Binding (%)	Vd (L/kg)	Metabolism and Excretion	$t_{1/2}$ (hr)	Normal Dose $Cl_{Cr} > 50$ mL/min	Dose Change With Renal Failure Cl_{Cr} (mL/min)	Effect of Dialysis
Ciprofloxacin	50–85	22	2.2	62% excreted renally; the rest cleared hepatically, in the bile and via intestinal mucosa	Normal: 4 Anephric: 8.5	250–750 mg Q 12 hr (PO)	10–50: 250–500 mg Q 12 hr <10: 250–750 mg Q 24 hr	Slightly dialyzed
Clindamycin	50	94	0.6	85% hepatic to active and inactive metabolites; 10% excreted renally; 5% feces	Normal: 2–4 Anephric: 1.6–3.4	600–900 mg Q 6–8 hr	10–50: No change <10: No change	Not dialyzed
Codeine	40–70	7	3–4	Hepatic with some active metabolites; little renal elimination (5%–17%)	Normal: 2.9–4 Anephric: 19	No change	10–50: ↓ 25% and titrate <10: ↓ 50% and titrate	?
Cyclosporine	<5–89	>96	3.5	Extensively metabolized to active and inactive metabolites; <1% excreted renally	Normal: 6–13 Anephric: 16	No change	10–50: No change <10: No change	Not dialyzed
Daptomycin	Parenteral	90–93	0.1	78% renally eliminated	Normal: 9 Anephric: 29	4–6 mg/kg Q 24 hr depending on indication	4–6 mg/kg Q 48 hr depending on indication	Minimally dialyzed
Digoxin	70	25 (↓ R)	5–8 (↓ R)	70% excreted renally	Normal: 36–44 Anephric: 80–120	No change	10–50: ↓ 50% <10: ↓ 75%	Not dialyzed
Emtricitabine	93	<4	N.D.	86% excreted in urine	10	200 mg QD	30–49: 200 mg Q 48 hr 15–29: 200 mg Q 72 hr <15 or HD: 200 mg Q 96 hr	Moderately dialyzed
Enalapril[a]	36–44	<50	1	61% excreted renally; 33% excreted in feces	Normal: 5–11 Anephric: 36	No change	10–50: ↓ 50% and titrate <10: ↓ 50% and titrate	Slightly/moderately dialyzed
Ertapenem	Parenteral	85–95	0.12	80% excreted in urine	4	1 g QD	<30: 500 mg QD	Moderately dialyzed
Erythromycin	30–65 (varies with salt)	84–90	0.9	85%–95% hepatic to inactive metabolites; 5–15% excreted renally	Normal: 1.4–2 Anephric: 4	0.25–1 g Q 6 hr	10–50: No change <10: No change	Slightly dialyzed
Ethambutol	75–80	<5	1.6	65%–80% excreted renally and 20% in feces; 8–15% hepatic	Normal: 3.1 Anephric: 18–20	15 mg/kg Q 24 hr	10–50: 7.5–10 mg/kg Q 24 hr <10: 5 mg/kg Q 24 hr	Slightly dialyzed

Fluconazole	>85	11–12	0.8	70% excreted renally; some hepatic metabolism	Normal: 20–50 Anephric: 98	100–200 mg Q 24 hr	10–50: 50–200 mg Q 24 hr <10: 50–100 mg Q 24 hr	Moderately dialyzed
Foscarnet	Parenteral	14–17	0.4–0.7	>80% excreted renally	Normal: 2–3 Anephric: >100	>80 mL/min: 60 mg/kg Q 8 hr 50–80 mL/min: 60 mg/kg Q 12 hr	10–50 mL/min: 60 mg/kg Q 24–48 hr <10 mL/min: 60 mg/kg Q 48 hr	Moderately dialyzed
Ganciclovir	5–9	1–2	0.5	>90% excreted renally	Normal: 2.5–3.6 Anephric: 11.5–28	>80 mL/min: 5 mg/kg Q 12 hr 50–80 mL/min: 2.5 mg/kg Q 12 hr	10–50: 1.25–2.5 mg/kg Q 24 hr <10: 1.25 mg/kg Q 24 hr	Dialyzed
Gentamicin	Parenteral	5–10	0.31	90%–97% excreted renally	Normal: 1.5–3 Anephric: 20–54	See section on aminoglycoside pharmacokinetics	See section on aminoglycoside pharmacokinetics	Dialyzed; 24–50 mL/min
Ibuprofen	>80	99	0.15	Primarily metabolized; 45%–60% excreted unchanged and as metabolites	Normal: 2 Anephric: No change	200–600 mg Q 4–6 hr	10–50: No change <10: No change	Not dialyzed
Imipenem	Parenteral	10–20	0.23–0.42	60%–75% excreted renally; 22% hepatic to inactive metabolites	Normal: 0.8–1.3 Anephric: 2.9–3.7	5–10 mg/kg Q 6–8 hr	10–50: 5–10 mg/kg Q 8–12 hr <10: 5–10 mg/kg Q 12 hr	Moderately dialyzed
Indomethacin	98	90	0.26	Hepatic metabolism to inactive metabolites; <15% excreted unchanged	Normal: 2.6 Anephric: No change	25–50 mg Q 8–12 hr	10–50: No change <10: No change	?
Ketoconazole	50–76	99	0.36	51% hepatic; 45% excreted unchanged in feces; 3% renally	Normal: 3–8 Anephric: No change	200–400 mg Q 24 hr (depends on infection severity)	10–50: No change <10: No change	Not dialyzed
Labetalol	20–38	50	8–10	5% excreted renally; 95% hepatic	Normal: 5 Anephric: ? prolonged	No change	10–50: No change <10: No change	Not dialyzed
Lamivudine	86	<36	1.3	70% excreted in urine	5–7	HIV infection: 300 mg QD or 150 mg BID	HIV infection: 30–49: 150 mg QD 15–29: 150 mg × 1, then 100 mg QD 5–14: 150 mg × 1, then 50 mg QD <5: 150 mg × 1, then 25 mg QD	Slightly dialyzed

Table 33-2 Pharmacokinetics and Dosing Guidelines for Drugs Commonly Used in Renal Failure[152]—cont'd

Drug	Oral Availability (%)	Protein Binding (%)	Vd (L/kg)	Metabolism and Excretion	$t_{1/2}$ (hr)	Normal Dose $Cl_{Cr} > 50$ mL/min	Dose Change With Renal Failure Cl_{Cr} (mL/min)	Effect of Dialysis
Lepirudin	Parenteral	<10	12 L	35% excreted unchanged in urine	1.3	LD = 0.4 mg/kg MD = 0.15 mg/kg/hr adjusted to appropriate aPTT	LD = 0.2 mg/kg MD: 45–60: 0.075 mg/kg/hr 30–44: 0.045 mg/kg/hr 15–30: 0.0225 mg/kg/hr <15: Do not use	Unknown
Levetiracetam	100	<10	1	66% excreted in urine	7	500–1500 mg BID	50–80: 500–1,000 mg BID 30–50: 250–750 mg BID <30: 250–500 mg BID HD: 500–1,000 mg 24 hr	Dialyzed
Levofloxacin	99	24–38	0.92–1.36	60%–87% renally excreted	Normal: 6–8 Anephric: 76	250–750 mg QD	20–49 mL/min: 500–750 mg ×1, then 250–750 mg Q 24–48 hr <20 mL/min; 500 to 750 mg ×1, then 250–500 mg Q 48 hr	Not dialyzed
Lidocaine	Parenteral	50–70	1.7 (↑ H)	Hepatic metabolism to inactive and active metabolites (glycyl xylidide)	Normal: 1.5–1.8 Anephric: No change	Maintenance dose: 2–4 mg/min	10–50: No change <10: No change	Not dialyzed
Linezolid	100	31%	0.64–0.96	30% renally excreted	Normal: 5 Anephric: No change	600 mg BID	No change	30% removed by hemodialysis, give dose after dialysis
Lithium	100	0	0.5–0.8	95% excreted renally	Normal: 22–29 Anephric: Prolonged	Variable (titrate with Cl_{Cr} to therapeutic levels of 0.4–0.8)	10–50: ↓ 25–50% <10: 50–75%	Moderately dialyzed/ dialyzed
Meperidine	48–53	58	4.4	Hepatic hydrolysis and conjugation, active normeperidine metabolites; 10% excreted renally	Normal: 3–7 Anephric: ?	50–100 mg Q 3–4 hr (IV, IM)	10–50: 75–100% Q 6 hr <10: 50% Q 6–8 hr (use cautiously)	?
Meropenem	Parenteral	2	0.26	70% renally excreted	Normal: 1 Anephric: 15.7	1 g Q 8 hr	26–50 mL/min: 1 g Q 12 hr 10–25 mL/min: 1 g Q 24 hr <10 mL/min: 500 mg Q 24 hr	Moderately dialyzed

Methotrexate	16–95 (dose dependent)	50	0.4–0.8	>90% cleared renally; 10% metabolized to 7-OH-MTX	Normal: $\alpha = 1.5–3.5$; $\beta = 8–15$ Anephric: Prolonged	No change	10–50: Adjust according to serum concentration <10: Avoid	Not/slightly dialyzed
Metoprolol	38	13	4	90% hepatic; 10% excreted renally	Normal: 3–4 Anephric: No change	50–200 mg QD	10–50: No change <10: No change	Metabolites dialyzed
Mezlocillin	Parenteral	26–42	0.2	45–65% excreted renally; 35–55% excreted hepatobiliary	Normal: 0.8–1.2 Anephric: 3–6	50 mg/kg Q 4–6 hr	10–50: 100% Q 6–8 hr <10: 50% Q 8 hr	Slightly/moderately dialyzed; 29 mL/min
Moxifloxacin	90	50	1.7–2.7	20% renally excreted	Normal: 12 Anephric: 14.5	400 mg QD	No change	Unknown
Nadolol	34	20	2	75% excreted renally; 25% hepatic	Normal: 15–20 Anephric: 45	40–80 mg QD	10–50: ↓ 50% and titrate <10: ↓ 50% and titrate	Moderately dialyzed
Nafcillin	50	85–90	0.35	Up to 70% hepatic; 25–30% excreted renally	Normal: 1–1.5 Anephric: 1.9	1–2 g Q 4–6 hr	10–50: No change <10: No change	Not dialyzed
Nifedipine	45	98	0.8–1.1	100% hepatic	Normal: 2–4 Anephric: 3.8	No change	10–50: No change <10: No change (? response in renal failure patients)	?
Penicillin G	15–30	60	0.9–2.1	50% excreted renally; 19% hepatic	Normal: 0.4–0.9 Anephric: 4–10	2–3 MU Q 4 hr	10–50: Dose (MU/D) = 3.2 + Cl_{Cr}/7 <10: Dose (MU/D) = 3.2 + Cl_{Cr}/7	Moderately dialyzed; 46 mL/min
Pentamidine	Parenteral	69	12	<5% eliminated renally over 24 hr	Normal: 6 (5–9 days, urine data) Anephric: ?	4 mg/kg/day (IV)	10–50: No change <10:100% QD–QOD	Probably not dialyzed
Phenobarbital	100	48–59	0.6	Hepatic metabolism; renal excretion: 10%–40% unchanged and active metabolites	Normal: 100 Anephric: ?	No change	10–50: No change <10: Slight ↓	Moderately dialyzed/ dialyzed
Phenytoin	>90	85–95 (↓ R, H)	0.5–0.7 (↑ R)	Hepatic metabolism; <5% excreted unchanged; 75% as inactive p-HPPH metabolites; concentration-dependent kinetics	Normal: 10–30 Anephric: 6–10	300–400 mg QD (titrate)	10–50: No change <10: No change (lower therapeutic level)	Not dialyzed
Piperacillin	Parenteral	16–22	0.2–0.47	50%–60% excreted renally; up to 30%–40% excreted in bile	Normal: 0.8–1.4 Anephric: 4–6	50 mg/kg Q 4–6 hr	10–50: 100% Q 6 hr <10: 50–75% Q 8 hr	Moderately dialyzed

Table 33-2 Pharmacokinetics and Dosing Guidelines for Drugs Commonly Used in Renal Failure[152] —cont'd

Drug	Oral Availability (%)	Protein Binding (%)	Vd (L/kg)	Metabolism and Excretion	$t_{1/2}$ (hr)	Normal Dose Cl_{Cr} > 50 mL/min	Dose Change With Renal Failure Cl_{Cr} (mL/min)	Effect of Dialysis
Procainamide	75–95	15	1.7–2.3	Hepatic metabolism to active NAPA; 50%–60% excreted renally	Normal: 2.5–4.7 (NAPA: 6) Anephric: 11–16 (NAPA: 42)	0.5–1.5 g Q 4–6 hr	10–50: 100% Q 6–12 hr <10: 100% Q 12–24 hr	Moderately dialyzed
Propranolol	36–40	88–94	2.9	Primarily hepatic; <1% excreted renally	Normal: 3–5 Anephric: No change	10–40 mg Q 6 hr (PO) and titrate	10–50: No change <10: No change	Not dialyzed
Ranitidine	52	15	0.8–1.1	70% excreted renally; some hepatic	Normal: 1.4–2.4 Anephric: 5–10	300 mg Q HS	10–50: ↓ 25% <10: ↓ 50%	Slightly dialyzed
Sulfamethoxazole	90–100	50–70 (↓ R)	0.14–0.36 (↑ R)	65%–80% hepatic to inactive compounds; 20%–30% excreted renally	Normal: 7–12 Anephric: 10–50	Q 6–12 hr	10–50: Q 12–24 hr <10: Q 24 hr	Slightly/moderately dialyzed
Tenofovir	25–40	7.2	1.3	70%–80% excreted in urine	17	300 mg QD	30–49: 300 mg Q 48 hr 10–29: 300 mg twice a week HD: 300 mg Q 7 days or after 12 hr of HD	Dialyzed
Tobramycin	Parenteral	<10	0.33	90%–97% excreted renally	Normal: 2.5 Anephric: 33–70	See section on aminoglycoside pharmacokinetics	See section on aminoglycoside pharmacokinetics	Dialyzed; 50–60 mL/min
Trimethoprim	85–90	40–70	1–2	53%–80% excreted renally; 20%–35% hepatic	Normal: 8–16 Anephric: 24–62	Q 6–12 hr	10–50: Q 12–24 hr	Slightly/moderately dialyzed
Valganciclovir (prodrug converted to ganciclovir)	60 (converted to ganciclovir)	1–2	0.7	>90% excreted renally	4	Induction: 900 mg BID Maintenance: 900 mg QD	Induction: 40–59: 450 mg BID 25–39: 450 mg QD 10–24: 450 mg Q 48 hr Maintenance: 40–50: 450 mg QD 25–39: 450 mg Q 48 hr 10–24: 450 mg twice a week	Dialyzed
Vancomycin	<10	10–55	0.5–0.7	80%–90% excreted renally; 10%–20% hepatic metabolism	Normal: 4–9 Anephric: 129–190	See section on vancomycin pharmacokinetics	See section on vancomycin pharmacokinetics	Conventional: not dialyzed; high flux: moderately dialyzed
Zidovudine	64	34–38	1.4	Primarily hepatic to inactive GAZT metabolite; 18% excreted renally	Normal: 0.8–2.9 Anephric: No change	100–200 mg Q 8 hr	10–50: No change <10: Possible ↓	Not dialyzed

[a]Pharmacokinetic values are for the active enalaprilat metabolite.
QD, every day; PO, orally; BID, twice a day; LD, loading dose; MD, maintenance dose; QHS, at bedtime; IV, intravenously; IM, intramuscularly

Table 33-3 Advantages and Disadvantages of General Approaches to Dosing Adjustments in Renal Disease

Method	Advantages	Disadvantages
Variable Frequency		
Use the same dose but ↑ the dosing interval	Same Cp_{ave}, Cp_{max}, Cp_{min} Normal dose	Levels may remain subtherapeutic for prolonged periods in patients requiring dosing intervals >24 hr
Variable Dose With Fixed Cp_{ave}		
↓ dose to maintain a target Cp_{ave}; keep the dosing interval the same	Same Cp_{ave} Normal dosing interval	↓ peak levels, which may ↑ be subtherapeutic; ↑ trough levels, which may ↑ potential for toxicity

Cp_{ave}, average plasma concentration; Cp_{max}, maximum plasma concentration; Cp_{min}, minimum plasma concentration.

Alteration of Dose versus Dosing Interval

The aminoglycosides (e.g., tobramycin, gentamicin, amikacin) are effective in the treatment of serious systemic infections caused by gram-negative organisms such as *Pseudomonas* sp. Unlike the cephalosporins and penicillins, however, the aminoglycosides have a relatively narrow therapeutic window. Using pharmacokinetic principles, a dose regimen can be designed to produce specific peak and trough serum concentrations. Peak serum concentrations (Cp_{peak}) (e.g., gentamicin or tobramycin 5–8 mg/L) correlate best with therapeutic efficacy, whereas toxicity tends to correlate with elevated trough levels (Cp_{trough}), which reflects prolonged exposure to high drug concentrations. To minimize the risk of toxicity, trough levels of <2 mg/L should be maintained. In patients with normal renal function, these target serum aminoglycoside concentrations are usually obtained following standard doses (e.g., 1.5 mg/kg) administered every 8 hours. For most patients, peak and trough levels are usually measured once steady state is achieved, which is typically within 24 hours.[38–41]

Many clinicians now utilize once-daily dosing of the aminoglycosides (e.g., 5 mg/kg every 24 hours) for patients with normal renal function in an attempt to minimize aminoglycoside accumulation and nephrotoxicity. The rationale for this regimen is based on the aminoglycosides' concentration-dependent killing and post-antibiotic effect. This approach is not recommended for patients with renal impairment, however. When once-daily dosing is used, peak concentrations are less helpful; however, trough concentrations should be monitored, and are usually below the limit of analytic detection (<1 mg/L). The discussion regarding aminoglycoside dosing in renal impairment that follows is based on the traditional an every 8-hour dosing regimen.

Aminoglycosides are almost completely eliminated by the kidneys; thus, the clearance of these drugs essentially is equal to the glomerular filtration rate (GFR). The pharmacokinetic properties of gentamicin and tobramycin are similar. A close correlation exists between Cl_{Cr} and gentamicin total body clearance. As renal function deteriorates, aminoglycoside doses must be modified to maintain the desired peak and trough plasma concentrations. Failure to appropriately adjust the dosage of aminoglycosides in renal insufficiency can lead to high drug plasma levels that can result in ototoxicity and nephrotoxicity.

In many cases, the aminoglycoside dose can be modified by extending the dosing interval rather than simply reducing the dose. This permits maintenance of adequate peak plasma concentrations to ensure efficacy, while allowing for sufficient elimination between doses to produce trough levels <2 mg/L. The advantages and disadvantages of adjusting the dosing interval versus reducing the dose are summarized in Table 33-3.

Figure 33-3 illustrates the effect of increasing the dosing interval in a patient such as G.G. with renal function that is 30% of normal. Although this is the preferred method for adjusting the dose of aminoglycosides, for many other drugs requiring dose adjustments in renal disease, simple dosage reduction is sufficient (Table 33-2).

Determination of Appropriate Dose

A number of methods have been developed to determine the appropriate aminoglycoside dose for patients.[42] One method is Bayesian forecasting, in which pharmacokinetic data obtained in the individual patient are integrated with population parameters. Initially, a dose is used that is based on population parameter values adjusted for characteristics such as increased SrCr. Drug concentrations for the individual patient are measured at specific times (e.g., peak and trough measurements) and these are compared with the expected values from the population data. Individualized pharmacokinetic parameter estimates are

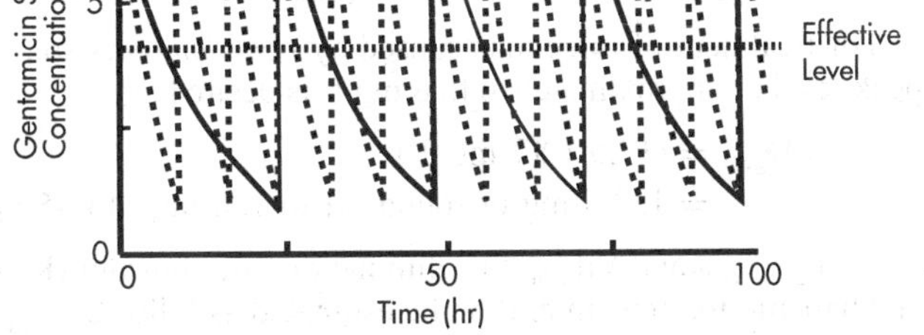

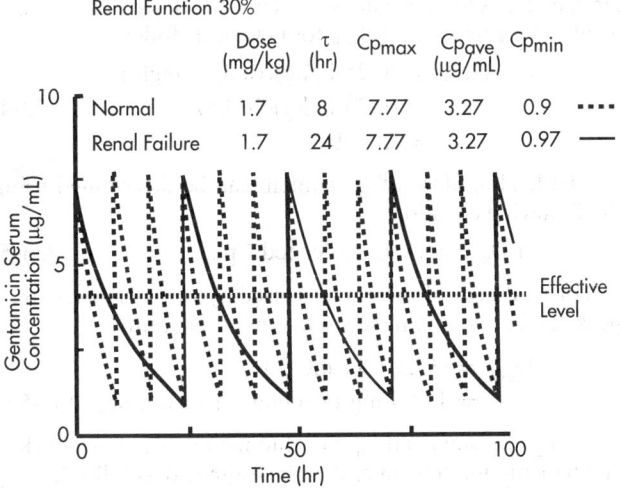

FIGURE 33-3 Serum concentration versus time profile for a patient with renal function 30% of normal in whom the interval of drug administration has been extended for dose adjustment. Advantages to this method are summarized in Table 33-3. (From Brater DC. *Drug Use in Renal Disease.* Sydney: ADIS Health Science Press; 1983, with permission.[153])

subsequently derived using Bayes' theorem to calculate a more patient-specific dosing regimen.[43]

Because of the wide interpatient variability in aminoglycoside pharmacokinetic parameters and the therapeutic index for these drugs is narrow, doses should be adjusted based on pharmacokinetic principles (e.g., Bayesian calculations or methods described later in this chapter) and plasma concentrations that are specific for this patient.

PATIENT-SPECIFIC METHODS

Sawchuk and Zaske developed a method to derive patient-specific estimates of Vd and clearance (Cl) based on the patient's size and estimated Cl_{Cr}.[40] These parameters can be used to calculate a specific dose for G.G. that will produce the desired gentamicin peak and trough concentrations. If steady-state serum concentrations of gentamicin are known, they can be used to calculate even more specific parameters. To initiate gentamicin therapy, pharmacokinetic parameters should first be estimated from population values.

The clearance of gentamicin (Cl_{gent}) can be calculated based on G.G.'s Cl_{Cr}. Using the Cockroft and Gault equation,[44] the Cl_{Cr} can be estimated as follows:

$$Cl_{cr}\ (\text{males}) = \frac{(140 - \text{age})(\text{IBW})}{(\text{SrCr})(72)} \quad \textbf{(33-2)}$$

$$Cl_{cr}\ (\text{females}) = \frac{(140 - \text{age})(\text{IBW})}{(\text{SrCr})(72)}(0.85) \quad \textbf{(33-3)}$$

where IBW is ideal body weight in kg, age in years, and SrCr is serum creatinine in mg/dL.

With a SrCr of 3.4 mg/dL, an ideal body weight of 70 kg, and an age of 31, G.G.'s estimated Cl_{Cr}, is 27 mL/minute.

For practical purposes, Cl_{gent} is usually considered equivalent to Cl_{Cr}. Therefore, Cl_{gent} also is approximately 27 mL/minute or 1.6 L/hour. The Vd of gentamicin (Vd_{gent}) is approximately 0.25 L/kg in patients with normal or impaired renal function.[40,44,45]

The Vd_{gent} will be different in obese patients or those who with fluid overload. Although G.G. does have some fluid retention, this is minimal and should not affect her Vd_{gent} significantly. Therefore, the Vd_{gent} for G.G. is as follows:

$$\begin{aligned} Vd_{gent} &= (0.25\ \text{L/kg})(\text{Body Weight}) \\ &= (0.25\ \text{L/kg})(70\ \text{kg}) \\ &= 17.5\ \text{L} \end{aligned} \quad \textbf{(33-4)}$$

The loading dose of gentamicin can be determined using the following equation:

$$LD_{gent} = (Vd_{gent})(\text{desired } Cp_{peak}) \quad \textbf{(33-5)}$$

For treatment of infections caused by *Pseudomonas* sp., a peak level of approximately 6 to 8 mg/L is desired:

$$\begin{aligned} LD_{gent} &= (17.5\ \text{L})(7\ \text{mg/L}) \\ &= 122.5\ \text{mg or round off to 120 mg} \end{aligned} \quad \textbf{(33-5A)}$$

Using Cl_{gent} and Vd_{gent}, the elimination rate constant (Kd) and half-life for gentamicin can be estimated as follows:

$$\begin{aligned} Kd &= \frac{Cl_{gent}}{Vd_{gent}} \\ &= \frac{1.6\ \text{L/hr}}{17.5\ \text{L}} \\ &= 0.091\ \text{hr}^{-1} \end{aligned} \quad \textbf{(33-6)}$$

$$\begin{aligned} t_{1/2} &= \frac{0.693}{Kd} \\ &= \frac{0.693}{0.091\ \text{hr}^{-1}} \\ &= 7.6\ \text{hr} \end{aligned}$$

For the aminoglycosides, the dosing interval (τ) is determined by doubling the half-life because by the end of two half-lives, 75% of the drug will have been eliminated. This will usually lead to a desired trough level of <2 mg/L. Therefore, gentamicin should be administered at least every 16 hours. For convenience, an interval of 24 hours can be used, which also will achieve the desired trough concentration.

Gentamicin is usually infused over 30 minutes. To determine the peak gentamicin concentration, serum samples are drawn 30 minutes after the infusion has been completed. Because the estimated elimination half-life of gentamicin in G.G. (7.6 hours) is much longer than the infusion time (0.5 hours), the intravenous bolus model can be used to calculate an appropriate maintenance dose.

To achieve the peak concentration of 7 mg/L, the following equation can be used:

$$\begin{aligned} \text{Dose} &= \frac{(Cp_{peak})(1 - e^{-Kdt})(Vd_{gent})}{(e^{-Kdt_{sample}})} \\ &= \frac{(7\ \text{mg/L})(1 - e^{-(0.091\ \text{hr}^{-1})(24\ \text{hr})})(17.5\ \text{L})}{(e^{-(0.091\ \text{hr}^{-1})(1\ \text{hr})})} \\ &= 119.2\ \text{mg} \\ &= \text{or round off to 120 mg} \end{aligned} \quad \textbf{(33-7)}$$

where t_{sample} usually equals 1 hour (30 minutes following a 30-minute infusion).

The expected trough level in G.G. can now be estimated by the following equation:

$$\begin{aligned} Cp_{trough} &= (Cp_{peak})(e^{-Kdt_{sample}}) \\ &= (7\ \text{mg/L})(e^{-(0.091\ \text{hr}^{-1})(24\ \text{hr})}) \\ &= 0.8\ \text{mg/L} \end{aligned} \quad \textbf{(33-8)}$$

Although not the case for G.G., patients with normal renal function may eliminate a significant amount of gentamicin during the 30-minute infusion. In these patients, the intermittent infusion model should be used to account for this loss of drug, where t_{in} is the duration of the infusion:

$$\text{Dose} = \frac{(Cl_{gent})(Cp_{peak})(1 - e^{-Kdt})(t_{in})}{(1 - e^{-Kdt_{in}})(e^{-Kd\tau})} \quad \textbf{(33-9)}$$

Revised Parameters

3. After 72 hours of gentamicin therapy, G.G.'s peak and trough levels are 7.6 and 2.6 mg/L, respectively. Her physician attributes this to a gradual decline in renal function. (Her most recent SrCr is 4.8 mg/dL.) How would you revise G.G.'s dosing regimen based on these levels?

A gentamicin trough level of >2 mg/L suggests that G.G.'s dosing interval is too short. Although her peak concentration is within the normal range of 5 to 8 mg/L, her trough concentration indicates that she is at a potentially toxic level. Her pharmacokinetic parameters can be revised based on these values, and a new Kd can be estimated from the equation:

$$\text{Kd} = \frac{\ln\left(\frac{Cp_1}{Cp_2}\right)}{\Delta t} = \frac{\ln\left(\frac{7.6\ \text{mg/L}}{2.6\ \text{mg/L}}\right)}{23\ \text{hr}} = 0.047\ \text{hr}^{-1} \quad \textbf{(33-10)}$$

Because little change in G.G.'s Vd_{gent} is expected, a new Cl_{gent} ($Cl_{revised}$) can be estimated from her revised elimination constant (if necessary, a revised Vd_{gent} could be calculated, keeping Cl_{gent} constant, although the clearance is more likely to change than the volume of distribution):

$$\begin{aligned} Cl_{revised} &= (Vd_{gent})(\text{Kd}) \\ &= (17.5\ \text{L})(0.047\ \text{hr}^{-1}) \quad \textbf{(33-11)} \\ &= 0.82\ \text{L/hr} \end{aligned}$$

These revised values for Kd and Cl can now be used to calculate a revised maintenance dose to maintain the Cp_{trough} at <2 mg/L using Equation 33-7:

$$\begin{aligned} \text{Dose} &= \frac{(7\ \text{mg/L})(1 - e^{-(0.047\ \text{hr}^{-1})(48\ \text{hr})})(17.5\ \text{L})}{e^{-(0.047\ \text{hr}^{-1})(1\ \text{hr})}} \\ &= 115\ \text{mg} \quad \textbf{(33-11A)} \\ Cp_{trough} &= (7\ \text{mg/L})(e^{-(0.047\ \text{hr}^{-1})(48\ \text{hr})}) \\ &= 0.73\ \text{mg/L} \end{aligned}$$

The revised dose is now 115 mg (or ~110 mg) every 48 hours.

4. What are some limitations in calculating G.G.'s Cl_{Cr} based on her SrCr? Can this estimate safely be used to predict gentamicin clearance?

The level of kidney function is best estimated by the glomerular filtration rate (GFR). The GFR cannot be directly measured. Prediction equations such as the Modification of Diet in Renal Disease (MDRD) study include variables, such as serum creatinine, age, body weight, race, and gender, in the estimation of GFR.[46] Although the MDRD equations are a good measure of GFR, they have not been validated for the dosing of drugs in the setting of renal dysfunction.[47,48]

The creatinine clearance is a widely used estimation of renal function in patient care settings. The creatinine clearance is often used to assess the degree of renal impairment and develop rational drug dosing recommendations.[49] For patients with stable renal function, Cl_{Cr} can be estimated from SrCr using the Cockroft and Gault equation (see Equations 33-2 and 33-3). In a patient such as G.G., however, whose renal function has diminished during the hospital course, estimation of renal function based on her increasing SrCr becomes more difficult. Because her SrCr does not reflect a steady-state level, the previous equations can no longer be used to accurately estimate her renal function. Because G.G.'s SrCr has increased rapidly from 3.4 to 4.8 mg/dL over the past few days, her Cl_{Cr} is probably much lower than that estimated using the Cockroft and Gault method. A rising SrCr may represent a decline in renal function manifesting as an accumulation of creatinine.

Effect of Hemodialysis

Conventional Dialysis

GENTAMICIN

5. G.G.'s renal function continues to deteriorate to the extent that she requires hemodialysis. What additional alterations in her gentamicin dosing regimen are necessary when she is having dialysis?

Gentamicin has a molecular weight of about 500 and is significantly removed by conventional hemodialysis.[41] Gentamicin has a relatively low Vd, averaging 0.25 L/kg, and is about 10% bound to proteins. The dialysis clearance of gentamicin using conventional methods depends on the actual filter used as well as the blood and dialysate flow rates. Dialysis clearance averages 45 mL/minute compared with an average plasma clearance of 5 mL/minute in patients with end-stage renal disease (ESRD).[50,51] Therefore, G.G.'s gentamicin dose must be adjusted to compensate for the amount of drug that will be removed by dialysis. Because drug removal represents a combination of drug elimination by the body and dialysis, the following equation can be used:

$$Cl_{total} = Cl_{dial} + Cl \quad \textbf{(33-12)}$$

where Cl_{total} is the total clearance of the drug during dialysis, Cl_{dial} is the clearance by dialysis, and *Cl* is plasma clearance. If dialysis clearance is high relative to plasma clearance, drug removal will be enhanced by the dialysis procedure. The total clearance of gentamicin in a patient with severe renal dysfunction during dialysis is 50 mL/minute (45 mL/minute + 5 mL/minute) or 10 times the clearance while off dialysis. Plasma clearance and dialysis clearance are related to the elimination half-life by the following equation:

$$t_{1/2} = \frac{(0.693)(\text{Vd})}{Cl_{dial} + Cl} \quad \textbf{(33-13)}$$

Thus, assuming a constant Vd of 17.5 L (i.e., 0.25 L/kg × 70 kg), the elimination half-life on dialysis is approximately 4 hours compared with 40 hours off dialysis. In addition, the extent (fraction) of drug removal (FD) during a timed dialysis run can be predicted from the following equation:

$$\text{FD} = 1 - e^{-(Cl + Cl_{dial})(t/\text{Vd})} \quad \textbf{(33-14)}$$

where t is the duration of dialysis. Therefore, the fraction of gentamicin removed (FD) during a 4-hour conventional dialysis procedure is approximately 50%. If specific data are not available for dialysis and plasma clearance, the following equation will predict fraction removed using the elimination half-life data alone obtained during dialysis:

$$\text{FD} = 1 - e^{-(0.693/t_{1/2on})(t)} \quad \textbf{(33-15)}$$

The estimated value of 50% removal is consistent with literature values indicating that 50% to 70% of a dose of gentamicin is removed during a 4-hour dialysis procedure. A limitation of this equation, however, is that it does not consider the redistribution of drug from the tissues back into the plasma following the dialysis procedure.

These data suggest that one-half the dose of gentamicin should be given to G.G. following each dialysis session.

It generally is difficult to calculate an appropriate maintenance dose for patients having hemodialysis that will maintain peak and trough concentrations similar to patients with normal renal function, in part because of the large variability found in aminoglycoside pharmacokinetic parameters.[51,52] Sustained plasma concentrations >2 mg/L can increase the risk of toxicity; however, dosing gentamicin to achieve trough concentrations of <2 mg/L may lead to prolonged periods of subtherapeutic concentrations. Therefore, in patients receiving hemodialysis, gentamicin doses are given to achieve a predialysis trough concentration of approximately 3 mg/L. A maintenance gentamicin dose of 1 mg/kg after each dialysis session commonly is used to achieve this desired concentration.

CEFTAZIDIME

6. Why does the dose of ceftazidime in G.G. have to be adjusted because of her hemodialysis when this drug has such a large therapeutic window?

Because only 21% of ceftazidime is protein bound and its Vd is 0.2 L/kg, it should be readily removed by hemodialysis. The mean dialysis clearance of ceftazidime is 55 mL/minute, with 55% of the drug removed during 4 hours of conventional hemodialysis.[53] A supplemental dose of ceftazidime should be given to G.G. following each hemodialysis session to maintain a therapeutic concentration. Half of the daily ceftazidime dose should be administered after each dialysis session.

High-Flux Hemodialysis

7. G.G.'s physician is considering changing her from a conventional dialysis system to a high-flux system that uses high efficiency polysulfone membranes. How does the dialyzability of gentamicin and ceftazidime differ with high-flux hemodialysis compared with conventional hemodialysis?

High-flux hemodialysis is more effective than conventional dialysis at removing certain pharmacologic agents (see Chapter 32, Renal Dialysis) because the membranes are more efficient and the blood flow through the dialyzer is increased. Although limited data are available, a greater fraction of drugs, such as aminoglycosides, ceftazidime, and vancomycin, are removed by high-flux versus conventional hemodialysis.[54,55] Approximately 50% to 70% of gentamicin is removed during a 2.5-hour, high-flux dialysis session.[56,57] The clearance of ceftazidime by high-flux dialysis is 75 to 240 mL/minute compared with 55 mL/minute for conventional hemodialysis.[54] Thus, further dosage adjustments for gentamicin and ceftazidime may be necessary if she is converted from conventional hemodialysis to high-flux hemodialysis.

Continuous Venovenous Hemofiltration

8. What changes would be necessary in G.G.'s gentamicin dosing if she were to start a continuous renal replacement therapy such as CVVH?

Because of the continuous nature of CVVH and CAVH, the extent of drug eliminated by continuous renal replacement therapies will differ from intermittent modes such as hemodialysis. The clearance of a drug in a patient receiving CVVH can be described in a fashion similar to Equation 33-12, where Cl_{dial} is replaced with Cl_{cvvh}.

$$Cl_{total} = Cl + Cl_{cvvh} \qquad \textbf{(33-16)}$$

In G.G., the $Cl_{revised}$ from Equation 33-11 can be used for the plasma clearance (Cl). The clearance by CVVH can be described by Equation 33-17:

$$Cl_{cvvh} = Fu \times UFR \qquad \textbf{(33-17)}$$

where Fu is the fraction of drug unbound, and UFR is the ultrafiltration rate. Gentamicin exhibits low plasma protein binding (Fu = 0.95). Typical ultrafiltration rates for CVVH are approximately 1 L/hour, but can vary.

$$\begin{aligned} Cl_{cvvh} &= Fu \times UFR \\ &= 0.95 \times 1\ L/hr \\ &= 0.95\ L/hr \end{aligned} \qquad \textbf{(33-17A)}$$

$$\begin{aligned} Cl_{total} &= Cl_{revised} + Cl_{cvvh} \\ &= 0.82\ L/hr + 0.95\ L/hr \\ &= 1.77\ L/hr \\ &= 29.5\ ml/min \end{aligned} \qquad \textbf{(33-17B)}$$

Because the clearance of gentamicin approximates that of creatinine clearance, G.G.'s total clearance is approximately one-third the normal clearance of 100 mL/minute. Therefore, the gentamicin dose should be approximately one-third of the normal dose. G.G. should be given 1.5 mg/kg/day or 100 mg of gentamicin as a single daily dose (normal dose is ~5 mg/kg/day). Gentamicin trough concentrations should be monitored, and her dose adjusted to maintain a trough concentration of <2 mg/L.

Continuous Ambulatory Peritoneal Dialysis

9. J.J., a 24-year-old man with ESRD, is maintained with CAPD. He presents to the ED with a fever of 38.2°C and complains of severe abdominal pain. He also reports that his peritoneal dialysate has become cloudy over the past few days. All these symptoms are consistent with peritonitis, a frequent complication of CAPD. His culture results reveal *Escherichia coli*, sensitive to gentamicin. How should gentamicin be dosed in this patient?

Management of dialysis-related peritonitis can vary from one institution to another. Antibiotics often are administered intraperitoneally with or without systemic antibiotic therapy. For less severe cases, intraperitoneal (IP) administration is often considered sufficient. With IP administration, the goal is to deliver a concentration of drug similar to the desired plasma concentration for the treatment of systemic infections. Therefore, 8 mg of gentamicin into each liter of dialysate (or 16 mg into a 2-L bag of dialysate) is recommended. Once equilibrium or steady state is achieved, the dialysate concentration will be comparable to the concentration of gentamicin in the plasma. Despite a more rapid transfer of drug into the plasma because of increased permeability of the peritoneal membrane in patients with peritonitis, there will still be a substantial lag time before steady state is reached. For more serious cases of peritonitis, concomitant systemic antibiotics should be given.

10. Is gentamicin eliminated by CAPD?

In general, most drugs are not well removed via CAPD. This is particularly true for drugs that are highly protein bound or for drugs with a large Vd. Gentamicin and other aminoglycosides, on the other hand, are effectively removed by CAPD because they have low protein binding and a small Vd. It is estimated that 10% to 50% of gentamicin is removed by CAPD.[58]

Acyclovir

Renal Clearance

11. D.M., a 28-year-old man with acquired immune deficiency syndrome (AIDS), presents with a severe herpetic infection requiring intravenous (IV) acyclovir. Because of other complications associated with his human immunodeficiency virus (HIV) infection, D.M. has developed renal insufficiency during his hospital course. His SrCr is 4.5 mg/dL (normal, 0.6–1.4 mg/dL), and his Cl_{Cr} is 20 mL/minute (normal, 80–110 mL/minute). What are important considerations for dosing acyclovir in D.M. now, and if he requires dialysis?

[SI units: SrCr, 397.8 μmol/L (normal, 53.04–123.76); ClCr, 0.33 mL/sec (normal, 1.33–1.83)]

Acyclovir is used to prevent or treat a variety of viral infections, such as those caused by herpes simplex and varicella zoster viruses.[59] Acyclovir is cleared primarily by the kidneys, with approximately 70% to 80% excreted unchanged in the urine. Dosage adjustment is necessary in patients with renal disease.[16,60] Renal tubular secretion in addition to filtration contributes to the elimination of acyclovir, which explains why the renal clearance of acyclovir is about three times greater than the estimated Cl_{Cr}.

Acyclovir also can precipitate in the renal tubules and exacerbate D.M.'s renal failure. This is more likely to occur when high doses are infused too rapidly to patients with renal dysfunction.[60] To minimize nephrotoxicity, the patient should be adequately hydrated to maintain good urine flow, and the acyclovir dose should be infused over 1 hour. Nephrotoxicity is usually reversible on discontinuation of the drug or reduction of the dose.

In addition, acyclovir-associated neurotoxicity correlates with elevated plasma concentrations, and further underscores the need for adequate dosage adjustments in patients with renal dysfunction.[61]

The clearance of acyclovir correlates with the Cl_{Cr} according to the following relationship:

$$\begin{aligned} &Cl_{acyclovir} \text{ in mL/min/1.73 m}^2 \qquad (33\text{-}18) \\ &= (3.4)(Cl_{cr} \text{ in mL/min/1.73 m}^2) + 28.7) \end{aligned}$$

In patients with normal renal function, the clearance of acyclovir ranges from 210 to 330 mL/minute; in patients with ESRD, the clearance is 29 to 34 mL/minute.[16,60,62] Although this change in clearance primarily results from decreased renal clearance of the drug, nonrenal clearance of acyclovir also decreases in these patients.[16,62] As a result, the elimination half-life increases significantly from approximately 3 hours in patients with normal kidney function to 20 hours in patients with ESRD. Therefore, doses should be reduced proportionately from a normal daily dose of 15 mg/kg body weight (5 mg/kg given every 8 hours) for serious herpes simplex infections to doses as low as 2.5 mg/kg/day (given as a single daily dose) in patients with ESRD.[63] Because D.M. has a Cl_{Cr} of 20 mL/minute and an estimated $Cl_{acyclovir}$ of 97 mL/minute (approximately one-third of normal), a single daily dose of 5 mg/kg (one-third of normal) would be appropriate to treat this infection (see Table 33-2).

Dialysis

Acyclovir is moderately removed by conventional hemodialysis, with plasma concentrations decreasing by 60% after 6 hours of dialysis.[64] The elimination half-life on and off dialysis is 6 and 20 hours, respectively, whereas the dialysis clearance averages 80 mL/minute. Therefore, a supplemental dose of 2.5 mg/kg following dialysis is recommended to replace the amount of drug removed by hemodialysis. No data are available on the removal of acyclovir by high-flux hemodialysis.

Effect of Renal Dysfunction on Metabolism

12. Does D.M.'s renal dysfunction affect the metabolism of acyclovir? Are there other drugs that are affected similarly?

Approximately 20% of acyclovir is cleared by nonrenal mechanisms.[16,62] The only significant metabolite that has been isolated is 9-carboxymethoxymethylguanine, which accounts for 9% to 14% of an administered dose. It is believed that this metabolite is a product of hepatic metabolism; however, the kidney may also play an important role.[16] Whether renal dysfunction alters hepatic metabolism or metabolic enzymes are present within the kidney is unclear. Studies have shown that renal tissue contains many of the same metabolic enzymes found in the liver. Mixed-function oxidases have been found in segments of the proximal tubule, whereas other metabolic processes, such as glucuronidation, acetylation, and hydrolysis, also occur within the kidney.[14,15]

Several studies have examined the effect of renal failure on hepatic metabolic enzyme activity.[65,66] Most of these investigations were carried out in animals that had diminished microsomal, mitochondrial, and cytosolic enzyme activities. Renal dysfunction substantially alters the nonrenal clearance of certain cephalosporins, such as ceftizoxime and cefotaxime,[67–69,70] as well as the benzodiazepines, diazepam, and desmethyldiazepam.[71,72]

Zidovudine (AZT)

Dosage Adjustment

13. D.M. also is being treated with AZT for his HIV disease. Will his AZT doses need to be adjusted?

Zidovudine was the first drug approved for treatment of HIV infection and is still used as part of combination antiretroviral regimens. Because it has potent bone marrow-suppressive effects,[73] the dose of AZT may require adjustment based on the patient's clinical response and the development of toxicity.

AZT is metabolized primarily by the liver to the inactive glucuronide metabolite, GAZT, which is eliminated by the kidneys. Only 18% of AZT is eliminated unchanged by the kidneys. Little change in AZT clearance and elimination half-life occurs in patients with renal failure. Two studies report only slight increases in the elimination half-life (from 1.0–1.4 hours, and from 1.4–1.9 hours in patients with renal failure),[74,75] whereas another case report measured a half-life of 2.9 hours in a single patient with renal impairment.[76]

Although GAZT accumulates in renal disease, this is not clinically important.[74]

Despite little change in AZT plasma levels, patients with renal failure are predisposed to bone marrow suppression because their kidneys produce less erythropoietin. In addition, their white blood cell (WBC) counts are also decreased. Therefore, AZT should be used more cautiously in these patients (see chapter 69, Pharmacotherapy of Human Immunodeficiency Virus Infection).

Hemodialysis

14. Is AZT significantly removed by dialysis?

A number of reports describe the removal of AZT by dialysis.[74–76] Based on the chemical characteristics, AZT would be expected to be dialyzable: it has a low MW of 267, a relatively small Vd (1–2.2 L/kg), and low protein binding (34%–38%). The dialysis clearance of AZT is minimal, however, when compared with its plasma clearance in patients with renal failure. Clearance by dialysis averages 63 mL/minute compared with a plasma clearance (following oral administration) of approximately 1,200 mL/minute. Little change occurs in the AZT plasma levels during dialysis; however, the elimination of GAZT may be enhanced.[74]

Penicillin

Dosage Adjustment

15. T.H., a 57-year-old, 85-kg man with chronic renal failure secondary to poorly controlled hypertension, presents to the ED with a 24-hour history of fever (39°C), altered mental status, nausea, and vomiting. On physical examination he was found to have nuchal rigidity and a positive Brudzinski sign. Laboratory analysis revealed the following: WBC count, 22,000/mm^3 with 89% neutrophils; BUN, 45 mg/dL; and SrCr, 4.4 mg/dL. A lumbar puncture revealed cerebrospinal fluid (CSF) with a WBC count of 2,000/mm^3 (90% polymorphonuclear neutrophils), a glucose concentration of 36 mg/dL, and a protein concentration of 280 mg/dL. Gram-positive diplococci were seen on CSF smear. A diagnosis of meningococcal meningitis was made, and potassium penicillin G was ordered. What dose should be used?

[SI units: count, 2.2×10^9/L and 0.2×10^9/L, respectively; BUN, 16.065 mmol/L urea; SrCr, 388.96 μmol/L; glucose, 1.998 mmol/L; protein, 2.8 g/L]

Meningococcal meningitis can be treated with 20 to 24 MU (million units) of IV penicillin G in patients with normal renal function. As with many β-lactam antibiotics, penicillin is primarily excreted unchanged in the urine with little or no evidence of hepatic metabolism. Thus, the elimination half-life, which averages <1 hour in patients with normal kidney function, increases to 4 to 10 hours in patients with ESRD.[77–79]

Methods to modify the dose of penicillin in renal insufficiency have been developed by numerous investigators. The clearance of penicillin correlates closely to Cl_{Cr} according to the following equation [79]:

$$Cl_{pen} \text{ in mL/min} = 35.5 + 3.35\ Cl_{cr} \text{ in mL/min} \quad (33\text{-}19)$$

This correlation is based on data from patients with varying degrees of renal impairment.

An equation to estimate the total daily dose for patients with renal failure to achieve serum levels similar to those produced by high-dose penicillin (20–24 MU/day) in patients with normal renal function has been developed for patients with an estimated Cl_{Cr} of <40 mL/minute. The dose for T.H. should be given in equal divided doses at 6- or 8-hour intervals:

$$Dose_{pen} \text{ in MU/day} = 3.2 + (Cl_{cr}/7) \quad (33\text{-}20)$$

Using the Cockroft and Gault method, T.H.'s Cl_{Cr} is approximately 20 mL/minute. Therefore, his daily dose of penicillin should be 6 MU. A dose of 2 MU every 8 hours would be appropriate for T.H.

As is true for many agents, these dosing recommendations are empiric and based on pharmacokinetic principles for patients in renal failure. These recommendations have not been subjected to carefully designed clinical trials that establish therapeutic efficacy. Therefore, other factors that can influence host response also should be considered when designing an individualized therapeutic regimen. These include the host's immune status, the presence of other medical conditions, microbial sensitivity patterns, and changes in pharmacokinetic disposition (e.g., concomitant liver disease, fluid overload, dehydration).

Penicillin-Induced Neurotoxicity

16. The medical intern fails to consider T.H.'s renal dysfunction when he prescribes penicillin, and begins a dose of 4 MU Q 4 hours. Four days later, T.H. is encephalopathic (confused, disoriented, and difficult to arouse), with some twitching that is noted on the right side of his face. Are these toxic symptoms associated with high-dose penicillin? What predisposing factors may contribute to this neurotoxicity?

T.H. is experiencing signs of neurotoxicity that are consistent with elevated penicillin concentrations in the plasma and CSF. Penicillin usually produces few serious adverse effects. When large doses are used in patients with renal impairment, toxic symptoms such as those exhibited by T.H. can result. Signs and symptoms of penicillin-induced CNS toxicity include myoclonus, complex or generalized seizure activity, and encephalopathy progressing to coma.[35,36]

PREDISPOSING FACTORS

T.H.'s renal dysfunction predisposes him to penicillin-induced neurotoxicity. In a review of 46 cases of penicillin-associated neurotoxicity, decreased renal function was present in 35 patients.[36] Several possible explanations for this observation exist. First, penicillin accumulates in patients with renal failure. Second, the binding of acidic drugs (such as penicillin) to albumin is decreased, resulting in an increased fraction of "free" or active drug that can pass into the CSF. Third, an alteration in the blood–brain barrier has been observed in uremic patients, which can lead to further increases in CSF drug levels.[35] Finally, high plasma concentrations of penicillin *per se* may contribute to changes in the blood–brain barrier permeability of this drug.[35] All these factors, together with the increased sensitivity of patients with renal failure to centrally acting agents, make CNS toxicity more likely. As with penicillin, the carbapenem antibiotic combination, imipenem–cilastatin, is associated with a higher incidence of seizures in patients with renal dysfunction.[80,81]

Antipseudomonal Penicillins

Piperacillin

17. M.H., a 44-year-old, 70-kg woman with acute nonlymphocytic leukemia, is admitted to the oncology ward for placement of a Hickman catheter for her chemotherapy. Seven days following treatment with cytarabine (Ara-C) and daunorubicin, her temperature spiked to 39.4°C. Other physical findings consistent with sepsis included a BP of 109/70 mm Hg, pulse rate of 102 beats/min, and a respiratory rate of 27 breaths/minute. M.H. is neutropenic with a WBC count of 1,400/mm^3 (3% polymorphonuclear leukocytes, 70% lymphocytes, and 22% monocytes). Her platelet count is 16,000/mm^3. M.H. also has renal dysfunction as reflected by an SrCr and BUN of 2.6 and 38 mg/dL, respectively. Empiric therapy for sepsis is started with tobramycin, piperacillin/tazobactam, and vancomycin. How should piperacillin/tazobactam be dosed in M.H.?

[SI units: platelet count, 16 × 10^9/L; SrCr, 229.84 μmol/L; BUN, 13.566 mmol/L urea]

Piperacillin is an antipseudomonal penicillin that is often used with an aminoglycoside to treat serious infections caused by gram-negative organisms.[82] Piperacillin is commonly given as a combination with tazobactam, a β-lactamase inhibitor.[83] In patients with normal renal function, piperacillin is primarily excreted unchanged by the kidney with a clearance of 2.6 mL/minute/kg, and a half-life of approximately 1 hour.[84,85] Doses of piperacillin/tazobactam can be as high as 4.5 g every 6 hours for the treatment of serious *Pseudomonal* sp. infections. In patients with ESRD, mean piperacillin clearance and half-life values are 0.7 mL/minute/kg and 3.3 hours, respectively.[84–86] Although these parameters are significantly different, they are less than those expected for a drug primarily cleared by the kidneys, suggesting that some other compensatory mechanism for elimination must be present. Piperacillin is partially cleared by biliary excretion, a route of elimination that is increased in patients with renal failure.[86,87] Therefore, aggressive dosage reductions in M.H. are unnecessary. An appropriate dose of piperacillin/tazobactam for M.H. would be 3.375 g every 8 hours (Table 33-2).

Vancomycin

Pharmacokinetic Dosage Calculations

18. In addition to the aforementioned regimen, vancomycin therapy is initiated at 500 mg Q 24 hr to cover the possibility of an infection resistant to antistaphylococcal penicillins, such as nafcillin. Is this an appropriate dosing regimen for M.H.?

Vancomycin is a bactericidal antibiotic with excellent activity against most gram-positive organisms such as methicillin-resistant *Staphylococcus aureus* (MRSA) and *Streptococcus* sp., including some isolates of *Enterococcus faecalis*. It is used empirically in the febrile neutropenic patient, because the incidence of infection secondary to resistant organisms is much greater in this patient population. However, cases of vancomycin-resistant enterococci (VRE) have emerged at rates as high as 50%, raising concern and reducing its empiric use.[88]

Vancomycin is poorly absorbed by the oral route and must be administered intravenously when used to treat systemic infections. As with many other antibiotics, vancomycin primarily is cleared by the kidneys.[89] Significant toxicities have been associated with elevated serum concentrations, making careful dosing modification in renal failure necessary.[90]

As with the aminoglycosides, pharmacokinetic calculations can be used to individualize a dosing regimen to produce the desired peak and trough plasma levels. Unlike the aminoglycosides, the therapeutic range for vancomycin is less clear. Normally, doses are designed to achieve peak levels of 25 to 40 mg/L and trough levels of 10 to 15 mg/L.[91,92] The correlation between vancomycin toxicity (e.g., ototoxicity) and plasma levels is not well defined. Some clinicians have suggested, however, that plasma levels ≥80 mg/L may correlate with auditory dysfunction.

Vancomycin has an elimination half-life of 3 to 9 hours in patients with normal renal function.[93] This increases to 129 to 189 hours in patients with ESRD.[94–96] Using pharmacokinetic principles and considering that the plasma clearance of vancomycin is approximately 60% to 70% of Cl_{Cr}[91] and the Vd averages 0.7 L/kg,[91,93,97] the estimated Vd_{vanco} and Cl_{vanco} can be calculated using the following equation:

$$Cl_{cr} = 30.5 \text{ mL/min (calculated from Eq. 34-3)}$$

$$\begin{aligned} Cl_{vanco} &= (0.65)(Cl_{cr}) \\ &= (0.65)(30.5 \text{ mL/min}) \\ &= 19.8 \text{ mL/min } \textit{or} \text{ rounded off to } 1.2 \text{ L/hr} \end{aligned} \quad \textbf{(33-21)}$$

$$\begin{aligned} Vd_{vanco} &= (0.7 \text{ L/kg})(\text{Body Weight}) \\ &= (0.7 \text{ L/kg})(70 \text{ kg}) \\ &= 49 \text{ L} \end{aligned} \quad \textbf{(33-22)}$$

Based on estimated values for Cl_{vanco} and Vd_{vanco}, the elimination rate constant can be calculated using the following equation:

$$\begin{aligned} Kd &= \frac{Cl_{vanco}}{Vd_{vanco}} \\ &= \frac{1.2 \text{ L/hr}}{49 \text{ L}} \\ &= 0.024 \text{ hr}^{-1} \end{aligned} \quad \textbf{(33-23)}$$

$$\begin{aligned} Cp_{peak} &= \frac{\frac{Dose}{Vd_{vanco}}}{1 - e^{-Kd\tau}} \\ &= \frac{\frac{500 \text{ mg}}{49 \text{ L}}}{1 - e^{-(0.024 \text{ hr}^{-1})(24 \text{ hr})}} \\ &= 23 \text{ mg/L} \end{aligned} \quad \textbf{(33-24)}$$

$$\begin{aligned} Cp_{trough} &= Cp_{peak}(e^{-Kd\tau}) \\ &= 23 \text{ mg/L}(e^{-(0.024/\text{hr}^{-1})(24 \text{ hr})}) \\ &= 13 \text{ mg/L} \end{aligned} \quad \textbf{(33-25)}$$

Because M.H.'s estimated peak concentration is <40 mg/L and her trough falls within the range of 10 to 15 mg/L, the starting dose of 500 mg every 24 hours is appropriate for M.H.

Routine monitoring of plasma vancomycin concentrations in patients with normal renal function is controversial because the likelihood that toxicity will develop in this group is relatively low. However, in patients with renal failure, such as M.H., it is advisable to measure vancomycin levels several days after initiation of therapy to ensure that they are within an acceptable range.[93,95,96,98] This is prudent if an extended course of therapy is anticipated. Vancomycin is usually infused over 60 minutes. Because there is a distribution phase, plasma samples should be drawn at least 30 minutes after the end of the infusion.

Hemodialysis

19. M.H.'s renal function begins to deteriorate, however, so that she requires hemodialysis. How should her regimen now be altered?

Patients with ESRD may have measurable vancomycin levels for up to 3 weeks following a single dose despite conventional hemodialysis.[96] This suggests that the ability of these patients to eliminate vancomycin is minimal and that little of the drug is removed by conventional hemodialysis. The elimination half-life for vancomycin in these individuals averages 5 to 7 days, which is consistent with a residual vancomycin clearance of 3 to 4 mL/minute.[94–96] Only about 5% of vancomycin is metabolized hepatically in patients with normal renal function.

Conventional hemodialysis removes about 7% of vancomycin during a typical 4-hour dialysis run.[99] The elimination half-life on and off dialysis, and plasma levels of the drug before and after hemodialysis do not differ significantly. The poor removal of vancomycin by conventional hemodialysis is owing to its large MW of 1,400.

Patients receiving conventional hemodialysis are typically given a single, 1-g dose every 7 to 10 days.[93,96,98] Based on M.H.'s estimated Vd of 49 L, this dose will produce an initial peak plasma level of ~20 mg/L. If vancomycin is administered weekly, steady-state peak and trough levels of 40 and 16 mg/L, respectively, would be predicted.

Vancomycin is removed to a greater extent by high-flux hemodialysis than by conventional hemodialysis. As a result, more frequent dosing is necessary to maintain therapeutic vancomycin concentrations. High-flux dialysis clearance of vancomycin using the Fresenius polysulfone dialyzer is 45 to 160 mL/minute and varies with membrane surface area.[55,100] Up to 50% of a dose of vancomycin is removed over 4 hours by high-flux hemodialysis compared with 6.9% using conventional dialysis. A rebound phenomenon following dialysis suggests that the total amount of drug removed may be less than initially reported.[101,102] In any case, the efficiency of high-flux procedures in removing vancomycin is greater than that of conventional dialysis. Therefore, plasma levels should be monitored carefully in these patients, and the necessity for postdialysis replacement doses of around 500 mg (~10–15 mg/kg) should be anticipated.

Amphotericin

Dosing

20. M.H. continues to be febrile despite her triple antimicrobial regimen. Amphotericin therapy is started empirically for a potential fungal infection. In addition, pentamidine is begun to cover *Pneumocystis carinii* pneumonia. How should amphotericin be administered in patients such as M.H. with renal dysfunction?

Amphotericin is an antifungal agent used to treat serious infections, such as invasive Aspergillosis and cryptococcal meningitis. The exact mechanism of elimination for this drug is unclear, but it may involve hepatic metabolism or inactivation in body tissues. Small amounts of amphotericin are gradually excreted in the urine for several weeks following its discontinuation.[103] This slow elimination may be owing to the extensive distribution of amphotericin into peripheral tissue and its large Vd (4 L/kg).[103,104] The drug appears to bind to cholesterol-containing cytoplasmic membranes of various tissues, resulting in a very long elimination half-life of 15 days. Pharmacokinetic studies report no significant change in the disposition of amphotericin in patients with renal or liver disease. Therefore, no dosage adjustments are required in patients with renal dysfunction.

Amphotericin is associated with acute tubular necrosis (ATN), which is believed to be dose dependent.[105–107] To prevent exacerbation of nephrotoxicity, lower doses often are administered to patients with decreased renal function. Administration of amphotericin every other day often is suggested for patients with renal failure. In addition to conventional amphotericin, a liposomal (liposomal amphotericin) or lipid-based formulation is available.[18] Lipid-based formulations have reduced distribution to the kidneys, and they are associated with a lower incidence of nephrotoxicity.[108] Triazole antifungal agents (e.g. fluconazole, voriconazole) or an echinocandin class (e.g. anidulafungin, caspofungin, micafungin) are alternative choices that are not potentially nephrotoxic, nor do they need to be dose adjusted in the setting of renal dysfunction (with the exception of fluconazole). The oral formulation of voriconzole should be used in renal dysfunction or for patients with a Cl_{Cr} <50 mL/minute to prevent accumulation of SBECD (sulfphobutylether beta cyclodextrin), the solvent vehicle found in the IV formulation.[109]

Hemodialysis

Amphotericin is not removed significantly by hemodialysis because it is a very large compound and distributes widely into peripheral tissues. Therefore, little drug remains in the plasma to be removed by dialysis. Studies have found that <5% of amphotericin is removed during a 4-hour conventional hemodialysis period.

Phenytoin

Protein Binding

21. R.S., a 24-year-old man with ESRD from rapidly progressive glomerulonephritis, is treated by hemodialysis three times weekly. He has a 7-year history of generalized tonic–clonic seizures and has been treated with phenytoin. He presents to the ED after having had a seizure lasting about 5 minutes. His mother states that he ran out of phenytoin 4 weeks ago. Because his plasma phenytoin concentration on admission was <2.5 mg/L, R.S. is given an IV loading dose of phenytoin: 15 mg/kg over 30 minutes. Additional admission laboratory work includes the following: SrCr, 8.6 mg/dL (normal, 0.6–1.4); BUN, 110 mg/dL (normal, 7–20); potassium, 5.4 mEq/L; calcium, 9 mg/dL; and albumin,

2.9 g/dL. Eight hours after administration of phenytoin, his level is 5 mg/L. Is this level subtherapeutic?

[SI units: phenytoin, <10 and 19.82 μmol/L, respectively; SrCr, 760.24 μmol/L (normal, 53.04–123.76); BUN, 39.27 mmol/L urea (normal, 2.5–7.14); potassium, 5.4 mmol/L; calcium, 2.24 mmol/L; albumin, 29 g/L]

R.S. has severe renal disease, which will affect how the total (bound plus free) phenytoin concentrations are measured. Decreased plasma protein binding will result in lower measured total phenytoin concentrations, and the calculated apparent volume of distribution may increase. In patients with normal renal function, approximately 90% of the measured phenytoin is bound to albumin, and 10% is free. The free fraction of phenytoin is increased to about 20% to 25% in patients with uremia.[9,110–114] Because the free fraction for phenytoin is increased in patients with uremia, lower plasma concentrations will produce therapeutic effects that will be equivalent to those produced by higher phenytoin concentrations in patients with normal renal function.[6,115] Phenytoin is an acidic drug that is bound primarily to albumin. A number of mechanisms have been proposed that account for the decreased binding, including (*a*) decreased albumin concentration, (*b*) accumulation of uremic byproducts that displace acidic drugs from their binding sites, and (*c*) alteration in the conformation or structure of albumin in uremic patients, resulting in a reduced number of binding sites or decreased affinity for drugs (see Chapter 54, Seizure Disorders). Other acidic drugs with altered protein binding in renal disease are listed in Table 33-1.

Figure 33-4 illustrates changes in phenytoin levels when uremic and nonuremic patients are given equivalent doses.[116]

The following equation should be used to correct for R.S.'s altered binding owing to his renal dysfunction and hypoalbuminemia.[113]

$$Cp_{\text{Normal Binding}} = \frac{Cp'}{(0.48)(1-\alpha)\left(\frac{P'}{P_{NL}}\right)+\alpha} \qquad \textbf{(33-26)}$$

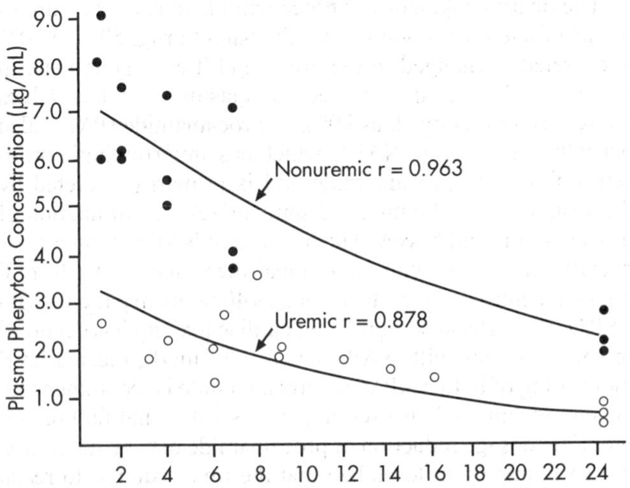

FIGURE 33-4 Plasma phenytoin concentrations in uremic (○) and nonuremic (•) patients following 250 mg of intravenous (IV) phenytoin. (From Letteri JM, et al. Diphenylhydantoin metabolism in uremia. *N Engl J Med* 1971;285:648, with permission.[116])

where Cp′ is the measured plasma concentration reported by the laboratory, and $Cp_{\text{Normal Binding}}$ is the corrected plasma concentration that would be seen if the patient had normal renal function and normal albumin. Alpha (α) is the normal free fraction (0.1), P' is the patient's serum albumin, and P_{NL} is normal albumin (4.4 g/dL). The factor 0.48 was derived from patients on hemodialysis and represents the decreased affinity of phenytoin for albumin.

For R.S., 5 mg/L is comparable to 12 mg/L in a patient without renal failure. Because this falls within the phenytoin's therapeutic range of 10 to 20 mg/L, his measured level is not subtherapeutic.

The factor 0.48 should be used only to estimate changes in protein binding for patients with ESRD receiving hemodialysis. Data for patients with moderate renal disease are limited, and it is unclear what changes exist in the binding of phenytoin to albumin.[111] For patients with normal or moderate renal impairment, the following equation should be used only if the serum albumin is low; the factor 0.48 should be omitted:

$$Cp_{\text{Normal Binding}} = \frac{Cp'}{(1-\alpha)\left(\frac{P'}{P_{NL}}\right)+\alpha} \qquad \textbf{(33-27)}$$

EFFECT OF RENAL FAILURE ON METABOLIZED DRUGS

Meperidine

22. F.G., a 56-year-old woman, is admitted for a cervical laminectomy. She has a history of chronic renal insufficiency (Cl_{Cr} = 20 mL/minute) and arrhythmias that are treated with procainamide. Her admission laboratory values are as follows: SrCr, 4.4 mg/dL (normal, 0.6–1.3 mg/dL); BUN, 66 mg/dL (normal, 7–20 mg/dL); Hct, 34%; and Hgb, 12.6 g/dL.

Following surgery, she complains of severe pain and is treated with meperidine 50 to 100 mg IM Q 3 to 4 hr. Three days postoperatively, F.G. experiences a generalized tonic–clonic seizure. She has no history of seizures. What might be responsible for this sudden event?

[SI units: SrCr, 388.96 μmol/L (normal, 53–114.92); BUN, 23.6 mmol/L urea (normal, 2.5–7.14); Hct, 0.34 1; Hgb, 126 g/L]

Meperidine is a narcotic analgesic commonly used to control acute pain. It is metabolized hepatically via *N*-demethylation to normeperidine, a metabolite known to accumulate in renal insufficiency.[12,117] Although meperidine has both CNS excitatory and depressant properties, normeperidine is a very potent CNS stimulant that can cause seizures in patients with renal failure who are receiving multiple doses of the parent drug.[118] In a study of 67 cancer patients treated with meperidine, 48 developed neurologic adverse effects; 14 of these 48 patients had renal dysfunction defined as a BUN >20 mg/dL.[118] Because the renal clearance of normeperidine correlates significantly with Cl_{Cr}, renal dysfunction can lead to its accumulation, resulting in neurologic toxicity. In another study, the normeperidine-to-meperidine plasma concentration ratio was consistently higher in patients with renal failure, averaging 2.0 compared with a mean of 0.6 for patients with good renal function.[118] Table 33-4 lists examples of additional drugs

Table 33-4 Drugs With Active or Toxic Metabolites Excreted by the Kidney

Drug	*Metabolite*
Acetohexamide	Hydroxyhexamide
Allopurinol	Oxypurinol
Cefotaxime	Desacetylcefotaxime
Chlorpropamide	Hydroxy metabolites
Clofibrate	Chlorphenoxyisobutyrate
Cyclophosphamide	4-Ketocyclophosphamide
Daunorubicin	Daunorubicinol
Meperidine	Normeperidine
Methyldopa	Methyl-o-sulfate-α-methyldopamine
Midazolam	Alpha-hydroxymidazolam
Morphine	Morphine-3-glucuronide Morphine-6-glucuronide
Phenylbutazone	Oxyphenbutazone
Primidone	Phenobarbital
Procainamide	*N*-acetylprocainamide (NAPA)
Propoxyphene	Norpropoxyphene
Rifampicin	Desacetylated metabolites
Sodium nitroprusside	Thiocyanate
Sulfonamides	Acetylated metabolites

that have active or toxic metabolites that may accumulate in renal disease.

Narcotic Analgesics

23. Are the pharmacokinetics or pharmacodynamics of other narcotic analgesics altered in patients with renal insufficiency?

Morphine

The pharmacokinetic disposition of morphine does not appear to be altered in patients with renal failure[119]; however, its active metabolite, morphine-6-glucuronide as well as its principal metabolite, morphine-3-glucuronide, do accumulate in renal disease. The elimination half-life of morphine-6-glucuronide increases from 3 to 4 hours in normal subjects to 89 to 136 hours in subjects with renal failure.[120] This metabolite penetrates the blood–brain barrier more readily, has a greater affinity for CNS receptors, and has analgesic activity that is 3.7 times greater than morphine.[121] Therefore, accumulation of morphine-6-glucuronide may be responsible for the morphine-induced narcosis reported in patients with severe renal disease.[29,30]

Codeine

Other analgesics that have been associated with CNS toxicity in patients with renal failure include codeine, propoxyphene, and dihydrocodeine.[117] The disposition of orally administered codeine does not appear to be altered in renal failure; however, two cases of codeine-induced narcosis have been reported.[122] Although the dose of codeine did not exceed 120 mg/day, CNS and respiratory depression persisted for up to 4 days after discontinuation of codeine, and naloxone administration.

Guay et al.[123] reported a prolonged terminal elimination half-life for intravenous codeine in patients on chronic hemodialysis of 18.7 ± 9 hours versus 4 ± 0.6 hours in subjects with normal renal function. Although the total body clearance was not significantly decreased, the Vd for codeine was approximately twice as large in the dialysis group. The clinical significance of these alterations is not known.

Propoxyphene

Propoxyphene and its metabolite, norpropoxyphene accumulate in renal insufficiency. Norpropoxyphene is eliminated by the kidneys, and its elimination half-life is prolonged in patients with renal failure; however, the half-life of propoxyphene remains unchanged. Accumulation of propoxyphene is thought to result from decreased first-pass metabolism or systemic clearance. Similar pharmacokinetic changes have been observed in patients experiencing dihydrocodeine-associated narcosis.[124,125] The accumulation of these compounds may be associated with CNS and cardiac toxicities in subjects with renal failure, especially after multiple doses.[121] Therefore, these drugs also should be avoided in patients with renal failure.

Hydromorphone

Hydromorphone is metabolized in the liver to hydromorphone-3-glucuronide, dihydroisomorphone, dihydromorphine, and small amounts of hydromorphone-3-sulfate, norhydromorphone, and nordihydroisomorphone.[126] All metabolites that are eliminated are excreted by the kidneys. Hydromorphone can be used in patients with renal failure, however, smaller initial doses may be warranted.[127]

Procainamide

24. F.G.'s procainamide level is 9 mg/L (normal, 4–8 mg/L) and her *N*-acetylprocainamide (NAPA) level is 34 mg/L (normal, 10–20 mg/L). How is the disposition of procainamide affected in patients with renal disease?

[SI units: procainamide level 38.24 mmol/L (normal, 17–34)]

The pharmacokinetics of procainamide in patients with renal insufficiency is complex. Of the parent drug, 50% to 70% is excreted unchanged in the urine, and it can accumulate in patients with renal disease because plasma clearance values are reduced by as much as 70%.[128] Procainamide (PA) is also partially acetylated to NAPA, which has antiarrhythmic properties similar to procainamide and is primarily excreted by the kidneys.[129,130] Figure 33-5 summarizes the elimination of procainamide and NAPA. The half-life of NAPA is longer, especially in patients with renal impairment, increasing from 6 hours in control subjects to as long as 40 hours in patients with ESRD.[128,129] Because significant cardiac toxicity has occurred in some patients with NAPA levels >30 mg/L, plasma level monitoring of both NAPA and procainamide is recommended. When procainamide is used in patients with renal failure, appropriate dosage reduction of procainamide may be necessary. It also is important to realize that the time required to reach steady state for NAPA in patients with renal failure may be as long as 5 days. Therefore, plasma levels measured early in therapy must be interpreted carefully, because these concentrations may be considerably lower than those that will be achieved under steady-state conditions.

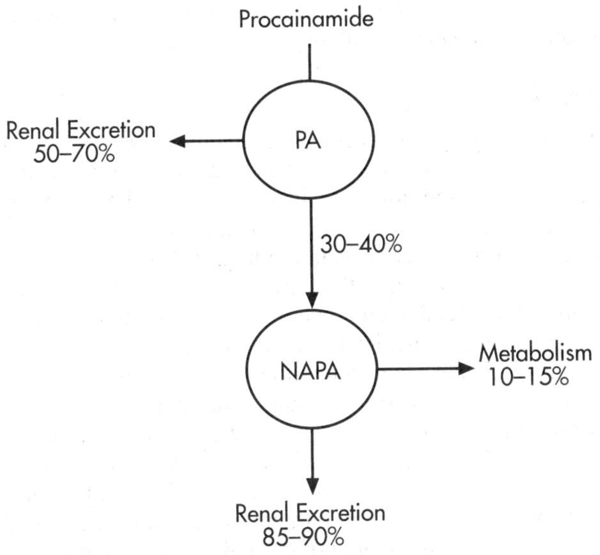

FIGURE 33-5 Elimination of procainamide (PA) and N-acetylprocainamide (NAPA) in subjects with normal renal and liver function.

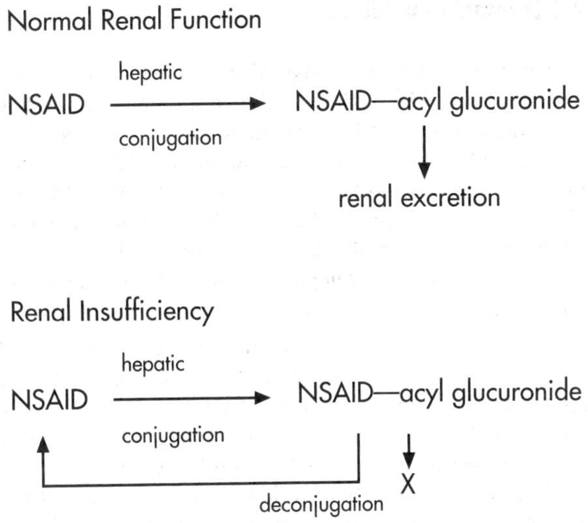

FIGURE 33-6 Schematic representation of pathways of elimination of acyl-glucuronide metabolites or arylpropionic nonsteroidal anti-inflammatory drugs. (From Brater DC. Renal disease. In: Williams R, et al., eds. *Rational Therapeutics*. New York: Marcel Dekker; 1990, with permission.[154] Copyright © 2001 Massachusetts Medical Society. All rights reserved.)

Nonsteroidal Anti-Inflammatory Drugs

25. F.G.'s physician would like to manage her pain with ibuprofen 400 mg Q 6 hours PRN. What factors should be considered when treating renal failure patients with nonsteroidal anti-inflammatory drugs (NSAID)?

Because NSAID have been associated with nephrotoxicity, they should be used cautiously in patients with renal disease.[131] The clinical features of nephrotoxicity are variable, and can present acutely or chronically with or without oliguria. Pathologic changes caused by these drugs also are variable and range from interstitial nephritis to acute tubular necrosis.[131,132] Mechanisms for NSAID-induced nephrotoxicity include inhibition of renal prostaglandin synthesis, leading to altered renal blood flow and ischemia.[133,134] Renal impairment may more likely occur in patients who have abnormally high plasma levels of vasoconstrictor hormones (e.g., angiotensin II and catecholamines).[132] Because a compensatory increase in the synthesis of vasodilatory renal prostaglandins to counteract the vasoconstriction occurs, blockade of this increase by an NSAID can lead to ischemic changes and acute renal failure (see Chapter 30, Acute Renal Failure).

A second proposed mechanism involves an autoimmune response that is triggered by changes in cell-mediated immunity.[135,136] These changes are caused by similar alterations in prostaglandin synthesis by NSAID. Although data are limited, sulindac is an NSAID believed to have renal-sparing effects. Unlike other NSAID, studies suggest that this drug does not inhibit synthesis of renal prostaglandins.[137]

The NSAID accumulate in renal insufficiency, an interesting finding because renal elimination is negligible for these drugs.[138] These compounds primarily are metabolized to an acyl-glucuronide metabolite that accumulates in patients with renal failure. This metabolite is unstable, and can deconjugate, leading to increased levels of parent drug. This phenomenon is represented in Figure 33-6. Of additional importance is fact that many of the NSAID are available as racemic mixtures, with the pharmacologic activity residing primarily with the S-enantiomer. The R-enantiomer can convert selectively to the S-enantiomer, particularly at elevated levels, leading to even greater pharmacologic activity in patients with renal dysfunction.[139,140] This reconversion phenomenon also has been reported for clofibric acid.[141]

Enoxaparin

26. Because F.G. is not ambulating well after her surgery, her physician would like to initiate deep vein thrombosis prophylaxis with enoxaparin. Are there any dosing considerations for enoxaparin in this patient?

Enoxaparin is a low-molecular weight heparin (LMWH) that is used to prevent and treat various thromboembolic disorders, such as deep venous thrombosis, unstable angina, and non–Q-wave myocardial infarction. The kidneys play a major role in the clearance of enoxaparin,[142] and a higher incidence of bleeding complications is associated with the use of enoxaparin in patients with renal dysfunction.[143] The elimination half-life of enoxaparin is prolonged in patients with ESRD, although the other pharmacokinetic parameters are similar to those in healthy subjects.[144,145] The increased incidence of bleeding complications cannot be completely attributed to pharmacokinetic changes, but may also be related to the effects of enoxaparin on anti-factor IIa and antithrombin III, as well as the effects of uremia on hemostasis.[146]

Enoxaparin should be used cautiously in patients with a Cl_{Cr} <30 mL/minute. Although monitoring the anticoagulant effect by anti-Xa activity is not necessary in clinically stable patients, it may be warranted in patients with renal dysfunction as well as those who have other factors that may increase the risk of bleeding complications.

Direct Thrombin Inhibitors

27. A.H. is a 55-year-old woman with a history of chronic renal failure (SrCr 3.7) who is diagnosed with a pulmonary embolus. While being administered anticoagulation with a heparin infusion, her platelet count drops from a baseline of 135 × 10^3 /mm^3 to 40 × 10^3 /mm^3. A positive heparin-platelet factor 4 antibody result confirms the diagnosis of heparin-induced thrombocytopenia. What options are available for the therapeutic anticoagulation of A.H. in the setting of heparin-induced thrombocytopenia?

Argatroban and lepirudin are direct thrombin inhibitors that are U.S. Food and Drug Administration (FDA) approved for the management of heparin-induced thrombocytopenia.[147] Lepirudin is a recombinant hirudin that inhibits the catalytic site of thrombin. The primary route of elimination of lepirudin is by the kidneys, with about 35% excreted unchanged in the urine. The dose of lepirudin should be reduced in the setting of renal dysfunction, and its use should be avoided when the creatinine clearance is <15 mL/minute.[148] Argatroban is primarily removed by the liver, with about 15% eliminated unchanged by the kidneys. Argatroban is preferred in patients with renal dysfunction.[149,150] The dose of argatroban, however, needs to be adjusted in patients with hepatic dysfunction.[151]

SUMMARY

The kidneys play a vital role in maintaining homeostasis by regulating the excretion of water, electrolytes, and metabolic byproducts. In addition, the kidneys are the primary route of elimination for many drugs. Pharmacokinetic changes, such as altered bioavailability, protein binding, drug distribution, and elimination, can occur with many drugs in patients with renal failure. Pharmacodynamic changes, such as altered sensitivity or response to medications, can also occur in this patient population. Renal replacement therapies, such as hemodialysis, continuous ambulatory peritoneal dialysis, and continuous arteriovenous hemofiltration, will aid both in the removal of fluid, electrolytes, and metabolic byproducts in drugs as well. Data from clinical trials provide valuable information about the disposition of drugs in patients with renal failure. Pharmacokinetic principles should be applied when appropriate to determine the optimal dose of drugs for patients with renal failure.

REFERENCES

1. Gambertoglio JG. Effects of renal disease: altered pharmacokinetics. In: Benet LZ et al., eds. *Pharmacokinetic Basis for Drug Treatment.* New York: Raven Press; 1984.
2. Bianchetti GM et al. Pharmacokinetics and effects of propranolol in terminal uremic patients and patients undergoing regular dialysis treatment. *Clin Pharmacokinet* 1978;1:373.
3. Wood AJ et al. Propranolol disposition in renal failure. *Br J Clin Pharmacol* 1980;10:562.
4. Pichette V et al. Drug metabolism in chronic renal failure. *Curr Drug Metab* 2003;4:91.
5. Barnes JN et al. Dihydrocodeine in renal insufficiency: further evidence for an important role of the kidney in handling of opioid drugs. *BMJ* 1985;290:740.
6. Reidenberg MM. The binding of drugs to plasma proteins and the interpretation of measurements of plasma concentrations of drugs in patients with poor renal function. *Am J Med* 1977;62:466.
7. Lam FYW et al. Principles of drug administration in renal insufficiency. *Clin Pharmacokinet* 1997;32:30.
8. Boobis SW. Alteration of plasma albumin in relation to decreased drug binding in uremia. *Clin Pharmacol Ther* 1977;22:147.
9. Reidenberg MM et al. Protein binding of diphenylhydantoin and desmethylimipramine in plasma from patients with poor renal function. *N Engl J Med* 1971;285:264.
10. Jusko WJ et al. Myocardial distribution of digoxin and renal function. *Clin Pharmacol Ther* 1977;16:448.
11. Verbeeck RK et al. Drug metabolites in renal failure. *Clin Pharmacokinet* 1981;6:329.
12. Szeto HH et al. Accumulation of normeperidine, an active metabolite of meperidine, in patients with renal failure or cancer. *Ann Intern Med* 1977;86:738.
13. Gibson TP et al. *N*-acetylprocainamide levels in patients with end-stage renal disease. *Clin Pharmacol Ther* 1976;19:206.
14. Gibson TP. Renal disease and drug metabolism: an overview. *Am J Kidney Dis* 1986;8:7.
15. Gibson TP. The kidney and drug metabolism. *Int J Artif Organs* 1985;8:237.
16. Laskin OL et al. Acyclovir kinetics in end-stage renal disease. *Clin Pharmacol Ther* 1982;31:594.
17. Willems L et al. Itraconazole oral solution and intravenous formulations: a review of pharmacokinetics and pharmacodynamics. *J Clin Pharmacol Ther* 2001;26:159.
18. Boswell GW et al. AmBisome (liposomal amphotericin B): a comparative review. *J Clin Pharmacol* 1998;38:583.
19. Gibson TP et al. Drug kinetics and artificial kidneys. *Clin Pharmacokinet* 1977;2:403.
20. Gwilt PR et al. Plasma protein binding and distribution characteristics of drugs as indices of their hemodialyzability. *Clin Pharmacol Ther* 1978;24:154.
21. Amin NB et al. Characterization of gentamicin pharmacokinetics in patients hemodialyzed with high-flux polysulfone membranes. *Am J Kidney Dis* 1999;34:222.
22. Aweeka FT et al. Effect of renal disease and hemodialysis on foscarnet pharmacokinetics and dosing recommendations. *J AIDS Retrovirol* 1999;20:350.
23. Keller E et al. Drug therapy in patients undergoing continuous ambulatory peritoneal dialysis: clinical pharmacokinetic considerations. *Clin Pharmacokinet* 1990;18:104.
24. Bickley SK. Drug dosing during continuous arteriovenous hemofiltration. *Clin Pharm* 1988;7:198.
25. Golper TA et al. Removal of therapeutic drugs by continuous arteriovenous hemofiltration. *Arch Intern Med* 1985;145:1651.
26. Trotman RL et al. Antibiotic dosing in critically ill adult patients receiving continuous renal replacement therapy. *Clin Infect Dis.* 2005;41:1159.
27. Pond S et al. Pharmacokinetics of hemoperfusion for drug overdose. *Clin Pharmacokinet* 1979;4:329.
28. Panzarino VM et al. Charcoal hemoperfusion in a child with vancomycin overdose and chronic renal failure. *Pediatr Nephrol* 1998;12(1):63.
29. Bigler D et al. Prolonged respiratory depression caused by slow release morphine. *Lancet* 1984;1:1477.
30. Shelly MP et al. Morphine toxicity with dilated pupils. *BMJ* (Clinical Research ed.) 1984;289:1071.
31. Kleinbloesem CH et al. Nifedipine: influence of renal function on pharmacokinetic/hemodynamic relationship. *Clin Pharmacol Ther* 1985;37:563.
32. Levine MN et al. Hemorrhagic complications of anticoagulant treatment. *Chest* 2001;119(Suppl 1):108S.
33. Brinkman WT et al. Valve replacement in patients on chronic renal dialysis: implications for valve prosthesis selection. *Ann Thorac Surg* 2002;74:37.
34. Welage LS et al. Pharmacokinetics of ceftazidime in patients with renal insufficiency. *Antimicrob Agents Chemother* 1984;25:201.
35. Nicholls PJ. Neurotoxicity of penicillin. *J Antimicrob Chemother* 1980;6:161.
36. Fossieck B et al. Neurotoxicity during intravenous infusion of penicillin: a review. *J Clin Pharmacol* 1974;14:504.
37. Gentry LO. Antimicrobial activity, pharmacokinetics, therapeutic indications and adverse reactions of ceftazidime. *Pharmacotherapy* 1985;5:254.
38. Dahlgre JG et al. Gentamicin blood levels: a guide to nephrotoxicity. *Antimicrob Agents Chemother* 1975;8:58.
39. Goodman EI et al. Prospective comparative study of variable dosage and variable frequency regimens for administration of gentamicin. *Antimicrob Agents Chemother* 1975;8:434.
40. Sawchuk RJ et al. Kinetic model for gentamicin dosing with the use of individual patient parameters. *Clin Pharmacol Ther* 1977;21:362.
41. Zaske DE et al. Gentamicin pharmacokinetics in 1,640 patients: method for control of serum concentrations. *Antimicrob Agents Chemother* 1982;21:407.
42. McHenry MC et al. Gentamicin dosages for renal insufficiency. *Ann Intern Med* 1971;74:192.
43. Sheiner LB et al. Forecasting individual pharmacokinetics. *Clin Pharmacol Ther* 1979;26:294.
44. Cockroft DW et al. Prediction of creatinine clearance from serum creatinine. *Nephron* 1976;16:31.
45. Bennett WM et al. Drug prescribing in renal failure: dosing guidelines for adults. *Am J Kidney Dis* 1983;3:155.
46. Levy AS et al. A more accurate method to estimate glomerular filtration rate from serum creatinine: a new prediction equation. *Ann Intern Med* 1999;130:461.
47. Bailie GR et al. Clinical practice guidelines in nephrology: evaluation, classification, and stratification of chronic kidney disease. *Pharmacotherapy.* 2005;25:491.

48. Kuan Y et al. GFR prediction using the MDRD and Cockroft and Gault equations in patients with end-stage renal disease. *Nephrol Dial Transplant* 2005;20:2394.
49. U.S. Food and Drug Administration. Guidance for industry: pharmacokinetics in patients with impaired renal function-study design, data analysis, and impact on dosing and labeling. U.S. Department of Health and Human Services, 1998. Available from http://www.fda.gov/cder/guidance/1449fnl.pdf. Accessed May 24, 2007.
50. Danish M et al. Pharmacokinetics of gentamicin and kanamycin during hemodialysis. *Antimicrob Agents Chemother* 1974;6:841.
51. Halpren BA et al. Clearance of gentamicin during hemodialysis: comparison of four artificial kidneys. *J Infect Dis* 1976;133:627.
52. Dager WE et al. Aminoglycosides in intermittent hemodialysis: Pharmacokinetics with individual dosing. *Ann Pharmacother* 2006;40:9.
53. Nikolaidis P et al. Effect of hemodialysis on ceftazidime pharmacokinetics. *Clin Nephrol* 1985; 24:142.
54. Toffelmire EB et al. Dialysis clearance in high flux hemodialysis with reuse using ceftazidime as the model drug [abstract]. *Clin Pharmacol Ther* 1989;45:160.
55. Lanese DM et al. Markedly increased clearance of vancomycin during hemodialysis using polysulfone dialyzers. *Kidney Int* 1989;35:1409.
56. O'Hara K et al. Removal of gentamicin using polysulfone dialyzers. Unpublished data. 1991.
57. Amin NB et al. Characterization of gentamicin pharmacokinetics in patients hemodialyzed with high-flux polysulfone membranes. *Am J Kidney Dis* 1999;34:222.
58. Somani P et al. Unidirectional absorption of gentamicin from the peritoneum during continuous ambulatory peritoneal dialysis. *Clin Pharmacol Ther* 1982;32:113.
59. Richards DM et al. Acyclovir: a review of its pharmacodynamic properties and therapeutic efficacy. *Drugs* 1983;26:378.
60. Blum MR et al. Overview of acyclovir pharmacokinetic disposition in adults and children (Acyclovir Symposium). *Am J Med* 1982;73:186.
61. Almond MK et al. Avoiding acyclovir neurotoxicity in patients with chronic renal failure undergoing hemodialysis. *Nephron* 1995;69:428.
62. Laskin OL et al. Effect of renal failure on the pharmacokinetics of acyclovir (Acyclovir Symposium). *Am J Med* 1982;73:197.
63. Jayasekara D et al. Antiviral therapy for HIV patients with renal insufficiency. *J AIDS Hum Retrovirol* 1999;21:384.
64. Krasny HC et al. Influence of hemodialysis on acyclovir pharmacokinetics in patients with chronic renal failure (Acyclovir Symposium). *Am J Med* 1982;73:202.
65. Patterson SE et al. Hepatic drug metabolism in rats with experimental chronic renal failure. *Biochem Pharmacol* 1984;33:711.
66. Van Peer AP et al. Hepatic oxidative drug metabolism in rats with experimental renal failure. *Arch Intern Pharmacodyn Ther* 1977;228:180.
67. Ings RMJ et al. The pharmacokinetics of cefotaxime and its metabolites in subjects with normal and impaired renal function. *Rev Infect Dis* 1982;4(Suppl):S379.
68. Fillastre JP et al. Pharmacokinetics of cefotaxime in subjects with normal and impaired renal function. *J Antimicrob Chemother* 1980;6(Suppl): S103.
69. Cuttler RE et al. Pharmacokinetics of ceftizoxime. *J Antimicrob Chemother* 1982;10(Suppl):S91.
70. Gibson TP et al. Imipenem/cilastatin: pharmacokinetics profile in renal insufficiency. *Am J Med* 1985;78:54.
71. Ochs HR et al. Clorazepate dipotassium and diazepam in renal insufficiency: serum concentrations and protein binding of diazepam and desmethyldiazepam. *Nephron* 1984;37:100.
72. Ochs HR et al. Diazepam kinetics in patients with renal insufficiency or hyperthyroidism. *Br J Clin Pharmacol* 1981;12:829.
73. Richman DD et al. The toxicity of azidothymidine (AZT) in the treatment of patients with AIDS and AIDS-related complex: a double-blind, placebo-controlled trial. *N Engl J Med* 1987;317:192.
74. Singlas E et al. Zidovudine disposition in patients with renal impairment: influence of hemodialysis. *Clin Pharmacol Ther* 1989;46:190.
75. Garraffo R et al. Influence of hemodialysis on zidovudine (AZT) and its glucuronide (GAZT) pharmacokinetics: two case reports. *Int J Clin Pharmacol Ther Toxicol* 1989;27:535.
76. Tartaglione TA et al. Zidovudine disposition during hemodialysis with acquired immunodeficiency syndrome. *J AIDS Hum Retrovirol* 1990;3:32.
77. Barza M et al. Pharmacokinetics of the penicillins in man. *Clin Pharmacokinet* 1976;1:297.
78. Gambertoglio J et al. Use of drugs in patients with renal failure. In: Schrrew RW et al., eds. *Diseases of the Kidney*. 5th ed. Boston: Little, Brown; 1993:3211.
79. Bryan CS et al. "Comparably massive" penicillin gm therapy in renal failure. *Ann Intern Med* 1975;82:189.
80. Calandra G et al. Factors predisposing to seizures in seriously ill infected patients receiving antibiotics: experience with imipenem/cilastatin. *Am J Med* 1988;84:911.
81. Norby SR. Carbapenems in serious infections: a risk-benefit assessment. *Drug Saf* 2000;22: 191.
82. Reyes MP et al. Current problems in the treatment of infective endocarditis due to Pseudomonas aeruginosa. *Rev Infect Dis* 1983;5:314.
83. Perry CM et al. Piperacillin/tazobactam: an updated review of its use in the treatment of bacterial infections. *Drugs* 1999;57(5):805.
84. Aronoff GR et al. The effect of piperacillin dose on elimination kinetics in renal impairment. *Eur J Clin Pharmacol* 1983;24:453.
85. Welling PG et al. Pharmacokinetics of piperacillin in subjects with various degrees of renal function. *Antimicrob Agents Chemother* 1983;23:881.
86. Thompson MI et al. Piperacillin pharmacokinetics in subjects with chronic renal failure. *Antimicrob Agents Chemother* 1981;19:450.
87. Giron JA et al. Biliary concentrations of piperacillin in patients undergoing cholecystectomy. *Antimicrob Agents Chemother* 1981;19:309.
88. Austin DJ et al. Vancomycin-resistant enterococci in intensive-care hospital setting; transmission dynamics, persistence, and the impact of infection control programs. *Proc Natl Acad Sci U S A* 1999;96(12):6908.
89. Moellering RC et al. Pharmacokinetics of vancomycin in normal subjects and in patients with reduced renal function. *Rev Infect Dis* 1981;3(Suppl):S230.
90. Farber BF, Moellering RC Jr. Retrospective study of the toxicity of preparations of vancomycin from 1974 to 1981. *Antimicrob Agents Chemother* 1983;23:138.
91. Rotschafer JC et al. Pharmacokinetics of vancomycin: observations in 28 patients and dosage recommendations. *Antimicrob Agents Chemother* 1982;22:391.
92. MacGowan AP. Pharmacodynamics, pharmacokinetics, and therapeutic drug monitoring of glycopeptides. *Ther Drug Monit* 1998;20(5):473.
93. Matzke GR et al. Clinical pharmacokinetics of vancomycin. *Clin Pharmacokinet* 1986;11:257.
94. Tan CC et al. Pharmacokinetics of intravenous vancomycin in patients with end-stage renal failure. *Ther Drug Monit* 1990;12:29.
95. Golper TA et al. Vancomycin pharmacokinetics, renal handling and non-renal clearances in normal human subjects. *Clin Pharmacol Ther* 1988;43:565.
96. Cunha BA et al. Pharmacokinetics of vancomycin in anuria. *Rev Infect Dis* 1981;3(Suppl):S269.
97. Krogstad DJ et al. Single-dose kinetics of intravenous vancomycin. *J Clin Pharmacol* 1980; 20:197.
98. Masur H et al. Vancomycin serum levels and toxicity in chronic hemodialysis patients with staphylococcus aureus bacteremia. *Clin Nephrol* 1983; 20:85.
99. Lanese DM et al. Removal of vancomycin by hemodialysis: a significant and overlooked consideration. *Semin Dialys* 1989;2:73.
100. Foote EF et al. Pharmacokinetics of vancomycin when administered during high flux hemodialysis. *Clin Nephrol* 1998;50:51.
101. Torras J et al. Pharmacokinetics of vancomycin in patients undergoing hemodialysis with polyacrylonitrile. *Clin Nephrol* 1991;36:35.
102. Quale JM et al. Removal of vancomycin by high-flux hemodialysis membranes. *Antimicrob Agents Chemother* 1992;36:1424.
103. Daneshmend TK et al. Clinical pharmacokinetics of systemic antifungal drugs. *Clin Pharmacokinet* 1983;8:17.
104. Starke JR et al. Pharmacokinetics of amphotericin B in infants and children. *J Infect Dis* 1987;155:766.
105. Stamm AM et al. Toxicity of amphotericin B plus flucytosine in 194 patients with cryptococcal meningitis. *Am J Med* 1987;83:236.
106. Sacks P et al. Recurrent reversible acute renal failure from amphotericin. *Arch Intern Med* 1987;147:593.
107. Antoniskis D et al. Acute, rapidly progressive renal failure with simultaneous use of Amphotericin B and pentamidine. *Antimicrob Agents Chemother* 1990;34:470.
108. Brogden RN et al. Amphotericin-B colloidal dispersion. A review of its use against systemic fungal infections and visceral leishmaniasis. *Drugs* 1998;56:365.
109. von Mach MA et al. Accumulation of the solvent vehicle sulphobutylether beta cyclodextrin sodium in critically ill patients treated with intravenous voriconazole under renal replacement therapy. *BMC Clin Pharmacol* 2006;6:6.
110. Tiula E et al. Serum protein binding of phenytoin and propranolol in chronic renal disease. *Intern J Pharmacol Ther Toxic* 1987;23:545.
111. Allison TB et al. Temperature dependence of phenytoin-protein binding in serum: effects of uremia and hypoalbuminemia. *Ther Drug Monit* 1988;10:376.
112. Asconape JJ et al. Use of antiepileptic drugs in the presence of liver and kidney disease: a review. *Epilepsia* 1982;23(Suppl 1):S65.
113. Liponi DF et al. Renal function and therapeutic concentrations of phenytoin. *Neurology* 1984;34:395.
114. Osar-Cederlof I et al. Kinetics of diphenylhydantoin in uremic patients: consequence of decreased protein binding. *Eur J Clin Pharmacol* 1974;7:31.
115. Browne TR. Pharmacokinetics of antiepileptic drugs. *Neurology* 1998;51(5 Suppl 4):S2.
116. Letteri JM et al. Diphenylhydantoin metabolism in uremia. *N Engl J Med* 1971;285:648.
117. Davies G et al. Pharmacokinetics of opioids in renal dysfunction. *Clin Pharmacokinet* 1996;31: 410.
118. Kaiko RE et al. Central nervous system excitatory effects of meperidine in cancer patients. *Ann Neurol* 1982;13:180.
119. Chan GLC et al. The effects of renal insufficiency on the pharmacokinetics and pharmacodynamics of opioid analgesics. *Drug Intell Clin Pharm* 1987;21:773.
120. Osborne RJ et al. Morphine intoxication in renal failure: the role of morphine-6-glucuronide. *BMJ* (Clinical Research ed.) 1986;292:1548.
121. Shimomura K et al. Analgesic effects of morphine glucuronides. *Tohoku J Exp Med* 1971;105:45.
122. Matzke GR et al. Codeine dosage in renal failure. *Clin Pharm* 1986;5:15.
123. Guay DRP et al. Pharmacokinetics and pharmacodynamics of codeine in end-stage renal disease. *Clin Pharmacol Ther* 1987;43:63.
124. Barnes JN et al. Dihydrocodeine narcosis in renal failure. *BMJ* (Clinical Research ed.) 1983;286: 438.
125. Redfern N. Dihydrocodeine overdose treated with

naloxone infusion. *BMJ* (Clinical Research ed.) 1983;287:751.
126. Zheng M et al. Hydromorphone metabolites: isolation and identification from pool urine samples of a cancer patient. *Xenobiotica*. 2002;32:427.
127. Dean M. Opioids in renal failure and dialysis patients. *J Pain Symptom Manage* 2004;28:497.
128. Gibson TP et al. Kinetics of procainamide and NAPA in renal failure. *Kidney Int* 1977;12:422.
129. Stec GP et al. *N*-acetylprocainamide pharmacokinetics in functionally anephric patients before and after perturbation by hemodialysis. *Clin Pharmacol Ther* 1979;26:618.
130. Winkle RA et al. Clinical pharmacology and antiarrhythmic efficacy of *N*-acetylprocainamide. *Am J Cardiol* 1981;47:123.
131. Pirson Y et al. Renal side effects of nonsteroidal anti-inflammatory drugs: clinical relevance. *Am J Kidney Dis* 1986;8:338.
132. Clive DM et al. Renal syndromes associated with nonsteroidal anti-inflammatory drugs. *N Engl J Med* 1984;310:563.
133. Whelton A. Nephrotoxicity of nonsteroidal anti-inflammatory drugs: physiologic foundations and clinical implications. *Am J Med* 1999;106:13S.
134. Delmas PD. Non-steroidal anti-inflammatory drugs and renal function. *Br J Rheumatol* 1995;34(Suppl 1):25.
135. Bender WL et al. Interstitial nephritis, proteinuria and renal failure caused by nonsteroidal anti-inflammatory drugs. *Am J Med* 1984;76:1006.
136. Esteve JB et al. COX-2 inhibitors and acute interstitial nephritis: case report and review of the literature. *Clin Nephrol* 2005;63:385.
137. Davies NM et al. Clinical pharmacokinetics of sulindac; a dynamic old drug. *Clin Pharmacokinet* 1997;32:437.
138. Meffin PJ et al. Enantio-selective disposition of 2-arylpropionic acid non-steroidal anti-inflammatory drugs. I. 2-phenylpropionic acid disposition. *J Pharmacol Exp Ther* 1986;238:280.
139. Evans AM. Comparative pharmacology of S(+)-ibuprofen and RS-ibuprofen. *Clin Rheumatol* 2001;20(Suppl 1):S9.
140. Grubb NG et al. Stereoselective pharmacokinetics of ketoprofen and ketoprofen glucuronide in end-stage renal disease: evidence for a "futile" cycle of elimination. *Br J Clin Pharmacol* 1999;48:494.
141. Gugler R et al. Clofibrate disposition in renal failure and acute and chronic liver disease. *Eur J Clin Pharmacol* 1979;15:341.
142. Buckley MM et al. Enoxaparin: a review of its pharmacology and clinical applications in the prevention of treatment of thromboembolic disorders. *Drugs* 1992;44:465.
143. Gerlach AT et al. Enoxaparin and bleeding complications: a review in patients with and without renal insufficiency. *Pharmacotherapy* 2000;20:771.
144. Cadroy Y et al. Delayed elimination of enoxaparine in patients with chronic renal insufficiency. *Thromb Res* 1991;63:385.
145. Brophy DF et al. The pharmacokinetics of subcutaneous enoxaparin in end-stage renal disease. *Pharmacotherapy* 2001;21:169.
146. Norris M et al. Uremic bleeding: closing the circle after 30 years of controversies? *Blood* 1999;94:2569.
147. Dager WE et al. Heparin-induced thrombocytopenia: treatment options and special considerations. *Pharmacotherapy*. 2007;27:564.
148. Refludan prescribing information. Bayer Health-Care Pharmaceuticals. Wayne, NJ. November 2006.
149. Koster A et al. Argatroban anticoagulation for renal replacement therapy in patients with heparin-induced thrombocytopenia after cardiovascular surgery. *J Thorac Cardiovasc Surg* 2007;133:1376.
150. Reddy BV et al. Argatroban anticoagulation in patients with heparin-induced thrombocytopenia requiring renal replacement therapy. *Ann Pharmacother* 2005;39:1601.
151. Levine RL et al. Argatroban therapy in heparin-induced thrombocytopenia with hepatic dysfunction. *Chest* 2006;129:1167.
152. Schrier RW et al., eds. *Handbook of Drug Therapy in Liver and Kidney Disease*. Boston: Little, Brown; 1990.
153. Brater DC. *Drug Use in Renal Disease*. Sydney: ADIS Health Science Press; 1983.
154. Brater DC. Renal disease. In: Williams R et al., eds. *Rational Therapeutics*. New York: Marcel Dekker; 1990.

SOLID ORGAN TRANSPLANTATION

Marcus Ferrone
SECTION EDITOR

CHAPTER 34

Kidney and Liver Transplantation

David J. Taber and Robert E. Dupuis

Solid organ transplantation is a well accepted therapeutic option for patients with end-stage kidney, liver, heart, and lung disease. For many of these patients, it is the only option. One-year patient survival for these major organs is between 85% and 98%. One-year graft survival approaches these figures as well.[1] Pancreas or combined pancreas–kidney transplantation is available as a treatment for diabetic patients with end-stage renal failure. Intestinal transplantation is performed but in a limited number of patients. Pediatric and elderly patients are transplant candidates, increasing the pool of potential recipients. Surgical techniques involving multiorgan transplantation (e.g., heart with lung, liver, kidney), pancreatic islet cell and liver cell transplantation, intestinal transplantation, living-related and unrelated and segmental human organ transplantation (e.g., kidney, liver, lung, pancreas), domino heart and heart–lung transplantation, along with improvements in mechanical assist devices (e.g., for heart transplant candidates), have made the transplantation of organs an increasingly viable treatment option. Research continues in overcoming the immunologic barriers associated with xenotransplantation (animal to human).

Despite these approaches, many more patients are in need of transplantation than there are organs available. In 2005, about 27,000 organ transplants were performed, whereas 90,000 people were waiting for organs. Consequently, a significant number of candidates die while waiting for a transplant.[1]

During the 1960s, drugs such as azathioprine, prednisone, antilymphocyte serum, and antilymphocyte globulin (ALG) made possible the success of kidney transplantation. In the late 1970s, the introduction of cyclosporine created a new era in solid organ transplantation, and in the 1980s the first monoclonal antibody approved for human use, OKT3, was introduced.

Since the mid-1990s a number of new agents have been approved. These include tacrolimus, mycophenolate mofetil, mycophenolate sodium, sirolimus (formerly rapamycin); monoclonal antibodies, such as daclizumab and basiliximab; and a polyclonal antibody, anti-thymocyte globulin (rabbit). More recently, several agents, such as intravenous immunoglobulins (IVIG), alemtuzumab, and rituximab have also been incorporated into transplant protocols. Several new agents are undergoing investigation. These provide more individualized, specific, and selective therapies for solid organ transplant recipients.

Although transplantation has had a significant positive impact on the quality of life in most patients with end-stage disease, issues such as retransplantation because of graft failure or recurrence of disease, donation source (living-related and unrelated-neonatal organs, animal organs), and costs to individuals, insurers, and society continue to be discussed vigorously. Costs during the initial transplantation period range from $30,000 for kidney transplants up to $250,000 for heart, liver, or lung transplants. In addition, routine follow-up monitoring and drug therapy for the first year can cost $5,000 to $60,000. The ability of transplant recipients, particularly those who are years out from their transplant, to pay for their medications is a major issue. Also, the cost-effectiveness and adverse effects of new immunosuppressive agents are important issues.

The goal of immunosuppressive therapy is to prevent organ rejection, prolong graft and patient survival, and improve quality of life. Short-term (i.e., 1–2-year) survival after transplantation has improved dramatically. Long-term survival also has improved, but not to the same degree.[2] The current immunosuppressive regimens have not produced a permanent state of tolerance (i.e., when the transplanted organ is seen as "self"). Limited data suggest that some selected patients may not require lifetime immunosuppression; these are in a minority, and more definitive studies must be done. As patients live longer after transplantation, the focus of therapy has shifted toward survival and management of long-term complications. Current immunosuppressive drug therapies are associated with significant long-term complications. These include nephrotoxicity, hypertension, hyperlipidemia, osteoporosis, and diabetes, as well as graft loss secondary to infection, malignancy, recurrence of primary disease, and nonadherence. Although rates of acute rejection are significantly lower, this remains a problem, along with chronic rejection. The search for safer and more effective immunosuppressive regimens continues, along with a better understanding of long-term immunosuppression. This chapter addresses the immunology of transplantation and rejection, indications for solid organ transplantation, appropriate use of immunosuppressive agents, and the management of postoperative and long-term complications in the patient who receives a solid organ transplant. Many of these issues are similar for the various types of solid organ transplantations, but there can be significant differences. This chapter addresses some of these issues as they relate to kidney and liver transplantation.

TRANSPLANTATION IMMUNOLOGY

Successful organ transplantation has come from a greater understanding and application of pharmacology, microbiology, molecular and cellular biochemistry and biology, genetics, and immunology. Suppression of the host's immune system and prevention of rejection are vital for host acceptance of the transplanted organ. The ultimate goal is permanent acceptance or tolerance, a situation in which the new organ is seen as "self" by the host's immune system. In general, the currently used immunosuppressive drugs provide a nonpermanent form of tolerance. A basic understanding of the immune system and the mechanisms of rejection is key to the effective use of immunosuppressive drugs in organ transplantation.

Major Histocompatibility Complex and Human Leukocyte Antigen

The degree to which allogeneic grafting (i.e., a transplanted organ from a genetically different donor of the same species) is successful depends on the genetic similarities or differences between the organ of the donor and the immune system of the recipient. The recipient recognizes the transplanted graft as either self or foreign. This recognition is based on the host's reaction to alloantigens or antigens (i.e., substances that initiate an immune response that can lead to rejection of the transplanted organ). These substances, also known as histocompatibility antigens, play a very important role in organ transplantation. Another group of substances that also plays an important role is the ABO blood group system of red blood cells. In general, the donor and recipient must be ABO compatible; otherwise, immediate graft destruction occurs because of antibodies directed against the ABO antigens.

Histocompatibility antigens are glycoproteins that are located on the surface of cell membranes. These are encoded by the major histocompatibility complex (MHC) genes located on the short arm of chromosome 6. In humans, the MHC is called the *human leukocyte antigen* (HLA). The gene products encoded on the HLA are divided into classes I, II, and III based on their tissue distribution, antigen structure, and function. Class I antigens (HLA-A, HLA-B, and HLA-C) are present on all nucleated cell surfaces and are the primary targets for cytotoxic T-lymphocyte reactions against transplanted cells and tissues. The three class II antigens (HLA-DR, HLA-DQ, HLA-DP) have a more limited distribution and are found on macrophages, B lymphocytes, monocytes, activated T lymphocytes, dendritic cells, and some endothelial cells, all of which can act as antigen-presenting cells (APC). Individual HLA loci are extensively polymorphic. Each one possesses two A, B, and DR antigens, one from each parent. This is called a *haplotype.* Recognition of these polymorphic loci by host T lymphocytes appears to account for rejection events seen in vivo. Class III antigens (C4, C2, and Bf) are part of the complement system and do not play a specific role in the graft rejection process.

Rejection of a transplanted organ is the outcome of the natural response of the immune system to a foreign substance, or antigen, and is a complex process, the understanding of which continues to evolve. This process, in some cases segmental and simultaneous, involves an array of interactions between foreign antigens, T lymphocytes, macrophages, cytokines (soluble mediators secreted by lymphocytes, also called *lymphokines, interleukins*), adhesion molecules (also referred to as *costimulatory molecules*), and membrane proteins expressed on a wide variety of cells that enhance binding of T cells, and B lymphocytes. This process of organ rejection ultimately can involve all elements of the immune response, but it is predominantly T-cell–mediated. This process can be divided into several important steps, which include antigen presentation as well as T-cell recognition, activation, proliferation, and differentiation of the various components of the immune response (Fig. 34-1).

For foreign antigens to interact with recipient T cells and B cells, they must be prepared for presentation by APC. These APC (Fig. 34-1) usually are recipient macrophages (indirect pathway of allorecognition), although donor cells—referred to as *dendritic cells* or *passenger leukocytes* and *graft endothelial cells*—also can serve as APC (direct pathway of allorecognition). This phase takes place within the blood, lymph nodes, spleen, and the transplanted organ (Fig. 34-2).

The next step (signal one) involves T-cell recognition of the HLA molecules presented on the surface of the APC. The primary site for this to occur is at the CD3–T-cell receptor complex (TCR) on recipient T lymphocytes. This step involves the binding of the antigen, MHC, and TCR for T-cell activation. These T lymphocytes also express other molecules (clusters of differentiation [CD]) on their surfaces that, along with CD3, recognize and respond to different types of antigens. These T cells are known as *CD4+ cells* (T_H, helper or inducer T cells) and *CD8+ cells* (T_C, cytotoxic or suppressor T cells). CD4+ cells interact with class II antigens. CD8+ cells interact with class I antigens.

In addition, proteins known as adhesion molecules or costimulatory molecules promote T-cell signaling and activation (signal two). For T-cell activation to occur, binding of these costimulatory molecules as well as binding of the TCR with the presented antigen and MHC is required. Examples of these molecules include intercellular adhesion molecule (ICAM)-1 on APC, which bind with lymphocyte function-associated antigen (LFA) expressed on the surface of T cells; ICAM-1 and -3 on APC with CD2 on T cells; B7 (now called CD80 and CD86) on APC with either CD28 or CTLA4 on T cells; CD40 on APC with CD40 ligand (now called *CD154*) on T cells.

The binding of these molecules are critical to T-cell activation. Without this costimulation, T cells undergo abortive activation or programmed T-cell death (apoptosis). These costimulatory molecules have become important targets for investigational drugs (e.g., CTLA4Ig, anti-CD40, anti-CD154) designed to try to prevent acute and chronic rejection and to promote long-term tolerance with minimal immunosuppression or none at all.

Once recognition occurs, T-cell activation and proliferation are initiated. After interacting with class II antigens and stimulation from IL-1 secreted from macrophages, T_H cells produce and secrete cytokines (e.g., interleukin [IL]-2 and interferon-γ. T_H cells are classified according to their cytokine-secretion pattern into either T_{H1} or T_{H2} cells. T_{H1} cells secrete IL-2, interferon (IFN), and tumor necrosis factor (TNF), which stimulate T_C cells. T_{H2} cells secrete IL-4, IL-5, IL-6, IL-10, and IL-13, which stimulate B cells. T_H cells, along with T_C cells, are stimulated to express cell-surface receptors specific for IL-2 (IL-2R) and other cytokines. Once the T_C cells express IL-2R, they bind to IL-2 and other cytokines, which leads to signal transduction that results in proliferation, division and stimulation of T cells (signal 3). These committed T_C cells bind directly to allogeneic cells and produce cell lysis. T_H-secreted cytokines recruit other T cells, which results in further cytotoxicity. During this process, T_H cells also produce cytokines that trigger a cascade of events involving B cells and antibody production, complement fixation, increased macrophage infiltration, neutrophil involvement, fibrin deposition, platelet activation and release, prostaglandin release, and inflammatory response at the graft site. These delayed-type hypersensitivity and humoral responses occur in conjunction with one another and are not mutually exclusive. This results in cellular and tissue graft destruction (Fig. 34-1).

The antibodies produced by plasma cells, which are transformed B cells under the influence of cytokines, bind to the target antigenic cells. This leads to local deposition of complement and results in immune complexation and injury to the graft (complement-mediated cell lysis). The newly formed antibodies cause a series of interactions to occur with T cells, which lead to cytotoxicity (antibody-dependent, cell-mediated cytotoxicity). These cell-mediated and humoral immunologic events can impair organ function so significantly that without therapeutic intervention, complete organ graft dysfunction may occur. Under certain circumstances, which are not clear, the T_C cells can actually downregulate the immune response to alloantigen. These cells are known as *suppressor T cells,* which express CD8+.[3]

Human Leukocyte Antigen Typing

The genetic compatibility between donor and recipient can have an impact on graft survival. For example, in kidney transplantation, the closer the HLA matching is between recipient and donor, the better the outcome, particularly over the long term. To determine this compatibility, a number of laboratory tests, including serologic, flow cytometric, genetic DNA based, and cellular assessments of donor and recipient serum and lymphocytes, are performed before organ transplantation. This process is referred to as *tissue typing*.[4] Lymphocytes are typed for HLA-A, HLA-B, and HLA-DR. Typing for HLA is performed using the donor and recipient lymphocytes for serology-based techniques and any tissue or fluid containing nucleated cells.

The panel reactive antibodies (PRA) test is commonly used to assess organ compatibility because recipients may have HLA

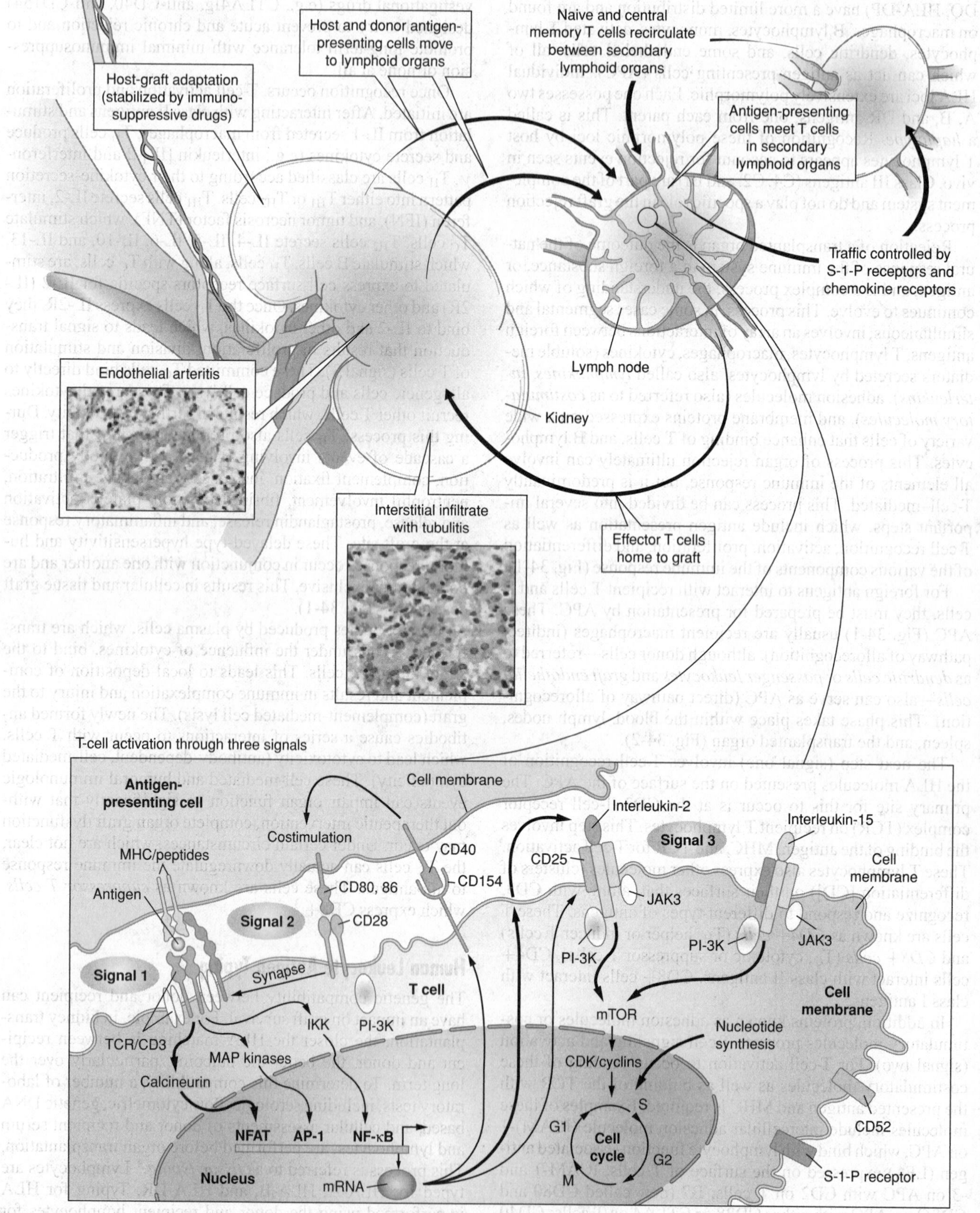

Host-graft adaptation (stabilized by immuno-suppressive drugs)
Host and donor antigen-presenting cells move to lymphoid organs
Naive and central memory T cells recirculate between secondary lymphoid organs
Antigen-presenting cells meet T cells in secondary lymphoid organs
Traffic controlled by S-1-P receptors and chemokine receptors
Lymph node
Endothelial arteritis
Kidney
Interstitial infiltrate with tubulitis
Effector T cells home to graft
T-cell activation through three signals
Antigen-presenting cell
Cell membrane
Interleukin-2
Interleukin-15
Signal 3
Costimulation
CD40
CD154
CD25
Cell membrane
MHC/peptides
CD80, 86
JAK3
Antigen
Signal 2
CD28
JAK3
PI-3K
PI-3K
Signal 1
Synapse
T cell
Cell membrane
IKK
PI-3K
mTOR
TCR/CD3
MAP kinases
Nucleotide synthesis
Calcineurin
CDK/cyclins
S
G1
Cell cycle
G2
M
CD52
NFAT
AP-1
NF-κB
Nucleus
mRNA
S-1-P receptor

FIGURE 34-1 T-Cell activation.

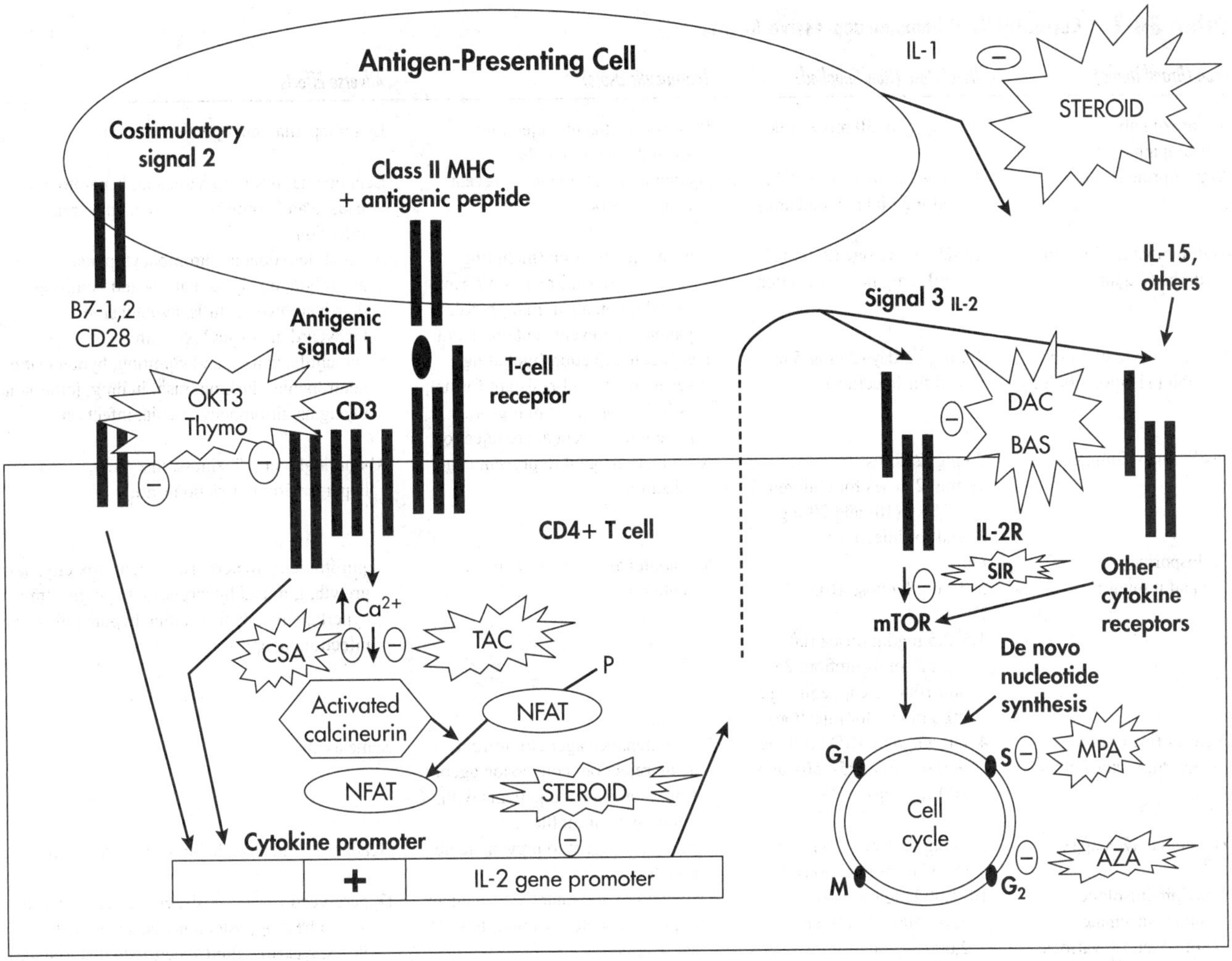

FIGURE 34-2 Schematic representation summarizing the mechanisms of action of approved and investigational immunosuppressive agents. AZA, azathioprine; BAS, basiliximab; CSA, cyclosporine; DAC, daclizumab; TAC, tacrolimus; IL, interleukin; MPA, mycophenolic acid; SIR, sirolimus.

antibodies from previous exposure to antigenic stimuli (e.g., blood transfusions, previous transplantation, pregnancy). In this test, the recipient's serum is tested against a cell panel of known HLA specificities that are representative of possible donors in the general population. The percentage of cell reactions (recipient with donor) determines a recipient's PRA.[4] It is done periodically on patients on the waiting list to determine their immunologic reactivity. The potential recipient with a higher percentage of PRA (>20%–>50%) is at higher risk for rejection.

A lymphocyte cross-match is also performed. In this case, the potential recipient's serum is cross-matched to determine whether preformed antibodies to the donor's lymphocytes are present. A positive cross-match indicates the presence of recipient cytotoxic IgG antibodies to the donor. In solid organ transplantation, this positive cross-match is often considered a strong contraindication, although in some kidney transplants therapeutic approaches involving the use of IVIG, plasmapheresis and rituximab before and after transplant appear to be successful.[5] In liver transplantation, a positive cross-match is not an absolute contraindication because the need is urgent and because the liver appears to be more resistant immunologically to this type of reaction. These liver transplant recipients can, however, develop significant complications and experience early acute rejection.

ABO blood typing is one of the most critical of all evaluations when determining the genetic compatibility for all solid organ transplants. Transplantation of an organ with ABO incompatibility would result in a hyperacute rejection and destruction of the graft, although in kidney transplant therapeutic approaches are being studied to minimize this outcome.[6]

IMMUNOSUPPRESSIVE AGENTS

Improvements in surgical techniques, better postoperative care and monitoring, and more effective immunosuppressive agents have all played significant roles in the success of solid organ transplantation. The use of these immunosuppressives, based on an improved understanding of their mechanisms of action and the mechanisms of rejection, has had the most significant impact on patient and graft survival. The number of currently approved immunosuppressives has significantly increased (Table 34-1), and a significant number of newly developed, more selective and potentially less toxic immunosuppressive

Table 34-1 Currently Used Immunosuppressive Agents

Drug (Brand Name)	*Usual Dose (How Supplied)*	*Therapeutic Use(s)*	*Adverse Effects*
Alemtuzumab (Campath-H1)	0.3 mg/kg or 30 mg × 1 dose	Prevention of acute rejection; steroid-free protocols	Lymphopenia, leukopenia, infection
Azathioprine (Imuran)	1–3 mg/kg/day (50-mg tab; 100-mg vial for injection)	As maintenance agent to prevent acute rejection	Leukopenia, thrombocytopenia, hepatotoxicity, nausea and vomiting, diarrhea, pancreatitis, infection
Antithymocyte globulin, equine (Atgam)	10–20 mg/kg/day (250 mg/5 mL ampule for injection)	Treat acute rejection (including severe or steroid-resistant forms); as induction agent in high-risk patient to prevent acute rejection	Anemia, leukopenia, thrombocytopenia, arthralgia, myalgias, nausea and vomiting, diarrhea, fevers, chills, hypotension, tachycardia, anaphylaxis, infection
Antithymocyte globulin, rabbit (Thymoglobulin)	1.5 mg/kg/day (25 mg/5 mL vial for injection)	Treat acute rejection (including severe or steroid-resistant forms); as induction agent in high-risk patient to prevent acute rejection	Fever, chills, nausea and vomiting, hypotension, neutropenia, flushing, rash, itching, joint pain, myalgias, thrombocytopenia, infection
Basiliximab (Simulect)	20 mg; 2 doses 10 mg; 2 doses for children if <35 kg (10- and 20-mg vial for injection)	As induction agent to prevent acute rejection	Abdominal pain, dizziness, insomnia, hypersensitivity reaction (rare)
Cyclosporine (Sandimmune)	Oral 5–10 mg/kg/dose BID IV 1.5–2.5 mg/kg/dose (100 mg/mL oral solution; 25- and 100-mg cap; 250 mg/5 mL ampule for injection)	As maintenance agent to prevent acute rejection	Nephrotoxicity, hypertension, neurotoxicity, hair growth, gingival hyperplasia, hyperglycemia, hyperkalemia, dyslipidemia, hypomagnesemia, infection, neoplasm
Cyclosporine (Neoral, Gengraf, various others)	4–8 mg/kg/day BID (100 mg oral solution; 25-, 50-, and 100-mg cap)	As maintenance agent to prevent acute rejection; conversion agent from tacrolimus in patients with intolerance or inefficacy	Same as above
Daclizumab (Zenapax)	1 mg/kg; 5 doses (25 mg/5 mL vial for injection)	As induction agent to prevent acute rejection	Headache, infection, hypo- or hypertension
Methylprednisolone sodium succinate (Solu-Medrol, various others)	10–1,000 mg/dose (40-, 125-, 250-, 500-, 1,000- and 2,000-mg vial for injection)	As induction and maintenance agent to prevent acute rejection; to treat acute rejection	Hyperglycemia, psychosis, euphoria, impaired wound healing, osteoporosis, acne, peptic ulcers, gastritis, fluid, electrolyte disturbances, leukocytosis, cataracts, cushingoid state, infection, insomnia, irritability
Mycophenolate mofetil (CellCept)	1.5–3.0 g/day BID (250-mg cap; 500-mg tab; 200 mg/mL oral suspension; 500-mg vial for injection)	As maintenance agent to prevent acute rejection; conversion agent from azathioprine and sirolimus in patients with intolerance or poor response	Diarrhea, nausea and vomiting, neutropenia, dyspepsia, ulcers, infection, thrombocytopenia
Mycophenolate sodium (Myfortic)	360–720 mg BID	As maintenance agent to prevent acute rejection. Alternative to MMF	Similar side effect profile as MMF
OKT3 (Orthoclone)	2.5–5 mg/dose (5 mg/5 mL ampule for injection)	Treat acute rejection (including severe or steroid-resistant forms); as induction agent in high-risk patients to prevent acute rejection	Pulmonary edema, fever, chills, hypotension, weakness, fatigue, muscle, joint pain, aseptic meningitis, altered mental status, infection
Prednisone (Deltasone, others)	5–20 mg/day (1-, 2.5-, 5-, 10-, 20-, 50-, and 100-mg tab)	As maintenance agent to prevent acute rejection	See methylprednisolone
Sirolimus (Rapamune)	2–10 mg/day (1- and 2-mg tab; 1 mg/mL oral solution)	As maintenance agent to prevent acute rejection; conversion agent from CNI or mycophenolate or azathioprine in patients with intolerance or poor response	Dyslipidemia, thrombocytopenia, neutropenia, anemia, diarrhea, impaired healing, mouth ulcers, hypokalemia, arthralgias, infection
Tacrolimus (Prograf)	Oral 0.15–0.3 mg/kg/day BID IV 0.025–0.05 mg/kg/day as continuous infusion (0.5-, 1-, and 5-mg cap; 5 mg/mL ampule for injection)	As maintenance agent to prevent acute rejection; conversion agent from cyclosporine in patients with intolerance	Nephrotoxicity, hypertension, neurotoxicity, alopecia, hyperglycemia, hyperkalemia, dyslipidemia, hypomagnesemia, infection, neoplasm

BID, twice daily; CNI, calcineurin inhibitor; IV, intravenous; MMF, mycophenolate mofetil.

agents are under investigation. Sites of action of the currently used agents, along with some of the investigational agents, are represented in Figure 34-2.

Azathioprine

Azathioprine is a prodrug of 6-mercaptopurine (6-MP). Azathioprine and 6-MP are purine antagonist antimetabolites. The introduction of cyclosporine, tacrolimus, mycophenolate, and sirolimus has led to a significant reduction of azathioprine use or its elimination altogether in immunosuppressive protocols, especially in the United States. It may, however, be useful in some cases because it is available generically, or in patients who cannot tolerate other agents. It continues to be used in other countries.

Azathioprine, a nonspecific immunosuppressive agent, affects both cell-mediated (i.e., T cell) and antibody-mediated (i.e., B cell) immune responses. Because it inhibits the early stages of cell differentiation and proliferation, azathioprine is useful for preventing rejection, but it is ineffective for the treatment of acute rejection. Active metabolites of 6-MP are incorporated into DNA and RNA, thereby interfering with the intracellular formation of thioguanine nucleotides (TGN). 6-MP is intracellularly converted by hypoxanthine phosphoribosyl transferase (HPRT) to thioinosinic acid and then to thioguanine nucleotides. 6-MP may have two separate immunosuppressive effects: inhibition of cellular proliferation and cytotoxicity. A decrease in the levels of intracellular purine ribonucleotides decreases cellular proliferation, and incorporation of TGN into DNA mediates cytotoxicity.[7]

Azathioprine can be given intravenously (IV) or orally. Oral absorption is rapid but incomplete. The usual dose is 1 to 3 mg/kg/day. Although the mean bioavailability of azathioprine in renal transplant recipients is approximately 50%, oral doses usually are not doubled when converting from IV to oral route.

The half-lives for azathioprine and 6-MP are estimated to be 10 to 12 minutes and 40 to 60 minutes, respectively. Major metabolic conversion of azathioprine to 6-MP is via nucleophilic attack by glutathione. The liver and red blood cells are thought to be major tissue sites for this metabolic conversion. The 6-MP formed by this reaction can be metabolized further to thiopurine ribonucleosides and ribonucleotides. Azathioprine pharmacokinetics are not affected by renal dysfunction, but there are higher 6-TGN metabolite concentrations. In contrast, azathioprine's immunosuppressive activity is absent in patients with severe hepatic dysfunction.[8]

The most common adverse effect of azathioprine is bone marrow suppression, which presents as leukopenia or, less commonly, as thrombocytopenia and megaloblastic anemia. Myelosuppression is dose dependent and typically observed after 7 to 14 days of therapy. Bone marrow suppression may be related to a genetic deficiency of the enzyme, thiopurine methyltransferase (TPMT). Low activity of this enzyme is rare but does lead to greater availability of 6-MP, elevated 6-thioguanine levels, and susceptibility to myelosuppression. Low levels of TPMT and specific genetic polymorphisms of this enzyme have been associated with severe azathioprine myelotoxicity and reduced efficacy in some transplant recipients and testing for this polymorphsim has been advocated.[9] Hepatitis, cholestasis, and reversible and irreversible liver damage have been reported with azathioprine use. The irreversible liver damage appears histologically compatible with central vein phlebitis and occlusion, fibrosis, lobular necrosis, and biliary stasis.[10]

The white blood cell (WBC) count should be maintained at $>5{,}000/mm^3$. If it decreases to 3,000 to $5{,}000/mm^3$, the azathioprine dosage should be reduced by 50%. If the dose reduction fails to keep the WBC count above $3{,}000/mm^3$, azathioprine should be discontinued and reinstituted at the lower dose when the leukopenia is resolved, if needed. A similar approach should be taken if thrombocytopenia occurs. If hepatotoxicity or other serious side effects occur, azathioprine is discontinued.

Pancreatitis has been associated with azathioprine. Long-term azathioprine administration also has been associated with the occurrence of non-Hodgkin's lymphoma, squamous cell skin cancer, primary hepatic tumors, fever, rigors, rash, headache, myalgia, tachycardia, hypotension, polyarthritis, and acute hypersensitivity reactions. Anorexia, nausea, and vomiting also occur.

Mycophenolate Mofetil and Mycophenolate Sodium

As a result of several comparative trials in kidney transplant recipients, mycophenolate mofetil (MMF) has replaced azathioprine in many transplantation protocols, especially in the United States. Studies in other transplantation populations have shown positive results as well. MMF is used as adjunctive therapy in combination with cyclosporine or tacrolimus, prednisone, sirolimus, and monoclonal and polyclonal antibodies to prevent acute rejection. It is also used as rescue therapy when patients have not responded to, or cannot tolerate, the side effects of other immunosuppressive agents.[11]

Mycophenolate mofetil, as with azathioprine, can be classified as an antiproliferative antimetabolite in that it also inhibits purine synthesis, but in a more selective manner. Unlike azathioprine, MMF interferes with the *de novo* pathway for purine synthesis. MMF is the morpholinoethyl ester prodrug of mycophenolic acid (MPA), which is the active component. MPA selectively, noncompetitively, and reversibly blocks an enzyme known as inosine monophosphate dehydrogenase (IMPDH) found primarily in actively proliferating T and B lymphocytes. T and B lymphocytes rely on this enzyme and the *de novo* purine pathway to produce purine nucleotides for DNA and RNA synthesis. Thus, MPA interferes with T- and B-cell proliferation. MPA also may affect cytokine production. Other secondary effects include inhibition of B-lymphocyte antibody production, decreased adhesion molecule expression, decreased smooth muscle proliferation and recruitment, and infiltration of neutrophils.[12]

Mycophenolate mofetil is rapidly converted to MPA on IV or oral administration. It is well absorbed. MPA is metabolized almost entirely by the liver to MPA-glucuronide (MPAG), which undergoes enterohepatic recirculation and is ultimately excreted renally as MPAG. MPA is highly protein bound to albumin and renal dysfunction can lead to an increase in free fraction.[13]

A new formulation of MPA, enteric-coated mycophenolate sodium (Myfortic), has been FDA approved to prevent rejection in kidney transplantation, when used in combination with a calcineurin inhibitor (CNI) and corticosteroids. The original purpose of designing the enteric-coated formulation was to reduce or prevent the gastrointestinal side effects commonly seen with MMF. All the compelling data currently published indicates, however, that the efficacy rates and side effect profiles of MMF and mycophenolate sodium are nearly identical. These two agents are *not* bioequivalent; because a 1-g dose of MMF is equivalent to 720 mg of mycophenolate sodium[14] (see Question 35).

Corticosteroids

Prednisone, methylprednisolone, and prednisolone—all synthetic analogs of hydrocortisone—are the primary corticosteroids used to prevent and treat rejection of transplanted organs. Although an important part of immunosuppression, a goal of most transplantation programs, is to minimize, eliminate, or avoid corticosteroid use because of their numerous and significant side effects.[15]

Corticosteroids have multiple effects on most cells and tissues of the body, but it is their anti-inflammatory and, more importantly, their immunosuppressive properties that serve as the basis for their use in organ transplant recipients. These effects are exerted through specific intracellular glucocorticoid receptors. The corticosteroids bind with these receptors and interfere with RNA and DNA synthesis as well as transcription of specific genes. Cell function is altered, resulting in suppression or activation of gene transcription. Corticosteroids also affect RNA translation, protein synthesis, production and secretion of cytokines, and protein and cytokine receptor expression.

Even after a single dose, corticosteroids cause marked lymphocytopenia by redistribution of circulating lymphocytes to other lymphoid tissues, such as the bone marrow, rather than by cell lysis; they also transiently increase the number of circulating neutrophils. Corticosteroids inhibit IL-1 and IL-6 production from APC, a number of events associated with T-cell activation, and IL-2 and IFNY production. They interfere with the action of IL-2 and IL-2R on activated T cells, resulting in the inhibition of T helper 1 (T_{h1}) function. They can enhance Il-10 regulatory function and enhance T_{h2} cell function. Moderate- to high-dose corticosteroids also inhibit cytotoxic T-cell function by inhibiting cytokine production and lysis of T cells. They can inhibit early proliferation of B cells but have a minimal effect on activated B cells and immunoglobulin-secreting plasma cells. The corticosteroids affect most cells and substances associated with acute allograft rejection and inflammatory reactions. They inhibit accumulation of leukocytes at sites of inflammation; inhibit macrophage functions, including migration and phagocytosis; inhibit expression of class II MHC antigens induced by interferon-γ; block release of IL-1, IL-6, and TNF; inhibit the upregulation and expression of costimulatory molecules and neutrophil adhesion to endothelial cells; inhibit secretion of complement protein C3; inhibit phospholipase A_2 activity; and decrease production of prostaglandins.[16]

The plasma half-lives of prednisone and methylprednisolone are much shorter than their biologic half-lives. Prednisone is a prodrug that is rapidly converted to its active form, prednisolone. Bioavailability in transplant recipients is rapid and complete and similar to healthy subjects. In transplant recipients, plasma half-lives are approximately 2.5 to 4 hours for prednisolone and methylprednisolone. Prednisolone is metabolized extensively. Prednisolone and methylprednisolone are 70% to 90% protein bound. Clearance of the unbound fraction is reduced in renal and liver transplant recipients. These agents usually are given in fixed doses or dosing is based on body weight (mg/kg) with little regard for pharmacokinetic differences, despite the significant variability that exists.[17,18]

Calcineurin Inhibitors

Cyclosporine

The introduction of cyclosporine as an immunosuppressive agent has been the single most important factor in the current success of organ transplantation. Its use has increased patient and graft survival, reduced morbidity associated with rejection and infection, and extended the types and numbers of organ transplantations performed. Cyclosporine or tacrolimus are the primary agents used in almost all transplant recipients. In contrast to azathioprine and mycophenolate, cyclosporine has relatively nonmyelotoxic, immunosuppressive effects. It has been considered the prototype for agents such as tacrolimus and sirolimus, as well as some investigational immunosuppressive drugs.

Cyclosporine is an 11-amino acid undecapeptide metabolite extracted from a soil fungus, *Tolypocladium inflatum Gams.* The activity of cyclosporine is mediated through a reversible inhibition of T-cell function, particularly helper T cells. Its major effect is inhibiting the production of IL-2 and other cytokines, including interferon-γ. These actions result in an inhibition of the early events of T-cell activation, sensitization, and proliferation. Cyclosporine has little effect on activated mature cytotoxic T cells. Therefore, it has little usefulness in the treatment of acute rejection. Its site of action is within the cytoplasm of T cells after antigenic recognition and signaling occurs. Cyclosporine binds to an intracellular protein (immunophilin) called *cyclophilin.* Although binding to cyclophilin is required, it is not sufficient for immunosuppression. This cyclosporine–cyclophilin complex binds to a protein phosphatase, calcineurin. This is thought to prevent activation of nuclear factors involved in the gene transcription for IL-2 and other cytokines, including IFN.[19] Also, because of this inhibition, cyclosporine indirectly impairs the activity of other cells, macrophages, monocytes, and B cells in the immune response. Cyclosporine has no effect on hematopoietic cells or neutrophils. Cyclosporine is metabolized extensively in the liver to >25 metabolites. Two of these metabolites, AM1 (formerly M17) and AM9 (formerly M1), can elicit an immunosuppressive effect in vitro, but they have much lower activity than cyclosporine. The role of these metabolites in the development of toxicity with cyclosporine is unclear[22] (see Questions 15–17, 19–20).

Tacrolimus

Tacrolimus (formerly FK506) is isolated from a soil fungus, *Streptomyces tsukubaensis.* It is a macrolide with a different molecular structure than cyclosporine. Tacrolimus is as effective as cyclosporine in liver, kidney, kidney–pancreas or pancreas, heart, and lung transplantation recipients as the primary immunosuppressant in combination with corticosteroids or mycophenolate, azathioprine, sirolimus, and antibodies. It also is effective as rescue treatment in liver, kidney, kidney–pancreas or pancreas, heart, and lung transplant recipients experiencing acute or chronic rejection resulting from failure of standard immunosuppressive therapy. Tacrolimus has become the preferred CNI over cyclosporine in many transplant centers.[23,24]

The activity of tacrolimus is similar to that of cyclosporine, but the concentrations of tacrolimus needed to inhibit production of IL-2, which is its major effect, are 10 to 100 times lower than those of cyclosporine. Tacrolimus also inhibits production of other cytokines, including IL-3, IL-4, and interferon-γ, TNF, and granulocyte-macrophage colony-stimulating factor (GM-CSF). It has variable effects on B-cell response and also has anti-inflammatory effects. The action of tacrolimus on T cells is more difficult to reverse than cyclosporine. As with cyclosporine, tacrolimus binds to an intracellular, although different, protein: FK binding protein 12 (FKBP12). This protein, which interacts with calcineurin, inhibits gene transcription of cytokines and interferes with T-cell activation.[20] Further pharmacologic and pharmacokinetic descriptions of tacrolimus are presented in Questions 28–32.

Sirolimus

Sirolimus, formerly known as *rapamycin* (Rapamune), is an FDA-approved agent for prevention of acute rejection and for withdrawal of cyclosporine in kidney transplantation. It was isolated from soil samples in Rapa Nui (Easter Island) and is a macrolide, structurally related to tacrolimus. In multicenter clinical trials, sirolimus combined with cyclosporine and prednisone significantly reduced acute rejection episodes in kidney transplant recipients when compared with a combined regimen of cyclosporine, azathioprine, and prednisone. The rejection rate was decreased from approximately 30% to 40% to <20%. Positive results for sirolimus also have been observed in other transplantation populations; in situations in which it is used in combination with other agents, including antibodies, tacrolimus, and mycophenolate; and when it has been used for rescue therapy. Its major use appears to be primarily in calcineurin reduction or elimination protocols.[21]

Unlike tacrolimus and cyclosporine, which work earlier in the T-cell activation cycle and inhibit cytokine production, sirolimus is an inhibitor of late T-cell activation. It does not block cytokine production; rather, it inhibits signal transduction, which blocks the response of T cells and B cells to cytokines such as IL-2.

As with tacrolimus, sirolimus binds to intracellular proteins. Specifically, sirolimus binds to the same immunophilin bound by tacrolimus, *FK binding protein* (FKBP). This complex interferes with the action of certain enzymes or proteins. Both cyclosporine and tacrolimus inhibit calcineurin, whereas sirolimus influences a protein called the *mammalian target of rapamycin* (mTOR). Sirolimus also inhibits an enzyme called *P7056 protein kinase,* which is involved in microsomal protein synthesis. These effects result in cell-cycle arrest, blockage of messenger RNA (mRNA) production, and blockage of cell proliferation. Early in its development, in vitro studies indicated that tacrolimus and sirolimus were antagonistic. Clinical studies indicate that this is not true. Sirolimus and cyclosporine or tacrolimus appear to work synergistically. Sirolimus also inhibits proliferation of smooth muscle cells and may, although it is too early to tell, reduce the development of chronic rejection[21] (see Question 18).

Antithymocyte Globulins

Before monoclonal antibody preparations were developed to prevent and treat acute rejection, polyclonal antilymphocyte preparations, such as antilymphocyte globulin (ATG), were available. Products used today are administered IV and include equine (Atgam, lymphoglobulin) and rabbit (Thymoglobulin) globulin, which is considered the polyclonal antibody of choice.

The ATG preparations made in goats and sheep also have been synthesized for investigational study. However, the following discussion is limited to the products produced in horses (Atgam) and rabbits (Thymoglobulin). Regardless of the species from which they are produced, all ATG products have similar pharmacologic effects. Their potency and antibody specificity vary, however, from batch to batch and between products.[22] The production of polyclonal equine or rabbit antibody begins with the injection of homogenized human spleen or thymus preparations into the animals. This injection induces an immune response in the animals directed against human T lymphocytes; serum containing antibodies to T cells is collected from the animals and purified. Other antibodies to human cells are produced as well, however. These antibodies bind to all normal blood mononuclear cells in addition to T lymphocytes and B lymphocytes, resulting in depletion of lymphocytes, platelets, and leukocytes from the peripheral circulation. The mechanism of action of these agents is thought to be linked to lysis of peripheral lymphocytes, uptake of lymphocytes by the reticuloendothelial system, masking of lymphocyte receptors, apoptosis, and immunomodulation. These agents contain antibodies to a number of cell-surface markers on lymphocytes, including CD2, CD3, CD4, CD8, CD11a, CD25, CD44, CD45, HLA-DR, and HLA class I antigens. They also interfere with leukocyte adhesion and trafficking and also have effects against CD20+ B cells. ATG preparations can produce a rapid and profound depletion of circulating T cells, often within 24 hours of the initial dose. The duration of the effect can last several weeks after a course of therapy, particularly with Thymoglobulin. Antibodies can be produced to these products as well. This, however, does not appear to influence clinical outcomes.[23] The clinical use of Thymoglobulin is described further in Question 5.

Murine Monoclonal Antibody

Muromonab-CD3 (Orthoclone OKT3), the first therapeutic murine monoclonal antibody approved for use in humans, was developed to suppress T-cell–mediated rejection. It is used for induction therapy (prophylaxis) or to treat acute graft rejection.[24] With the introduction of Thymoglobulin, daclizumab, and basiliximab, the prophylactic use of OKT3 has significantly declined, although some centers still use it but in lower doses. With the introduction of Thymoglobulin for treatment of acute rejection, OKT3 is used if a patient is unresponsive.

Murine monoclonal antibodies are formed by immunizing a mouse with a specific antigen (in this case, human T lymphocytes). After the mouse produces B lymphocytes against the injected antigen, it is killed and the spleen is removed. All the lymphocytes derived from the spleen are suspended and mixed with mouse myeloma cells, a tumor cell line that can grow indefinitely in culture. The two cell types are mixed with polyethylene glycol (PEG), which allows the cells to fuse. This mixture of mouse spleen cells, myeloma cells, and hybridomas (fused spleen and myeloma cells) is grown in a medium that allows only hybridomas to grow. Hybridoma colonies that are producing the desired antibody are cloned, and the antibodies they produce are harvested from cell supernatants. Another method used to produce large amounts of monoclonal antibody is to inject the appropriate hybridoma into the peritoneum of a mouse. After 10 to 21 days, the ascitic fluid, which contains secreted antibodies, is harvested and purified to obtain the desired monoclonal antibody.

OKT3, an IV administered IgG_{2a} immunoglobulin, binds to the CD3 (cluster of differentiation 3) structure on CD3+ T lymphocytes located near the T-cell receptor complex. All mature T cells express CD3 and either the CD4 or CD8 surface antigen. Once OKT3 is bound to the CD3 region of T cells, it is thought to be opsonized and removed from the circulation by the reticuloendothelial system of the liver and the spleen. This removal occurs within minutes after IV administration. The first one to two doses, however, activate T cells thereby producing significant adverse effects known as the *cytokine release syndrome*. OKT3 also can modulate the antigen-recognition complex of T cells, which alters normal T-cell function. The third mechanism involves blocking killer T cells attached to the allograft. This occurs when high levels of OKT3 are achieved and the killer T cells are coated and rendered inactive. Once therapy is stopped, CD3+ cells return to measurable levels quickly, often within 24 hours.

$CD3^+$ cell counts of $<25/mm^3$ represent an appropriate response in most patients. Adequate response to OKT3 is delayed by up to 5 to 7 days after a second course, which is owing to a neutralizing antibody against OKT3.[24] Patients sometimes require two to three times the initial dose, or it may be contraindicated if anti-OKT3 antibody level is too high (see Questions 12–14).

Interleukin-2 Receptor Antagonists

Daclizumab and Basiliximab

Daclizumab (Zenapax) and basiliximab (Simulect) are two monoclonal antibodies approved for use in combination with other immunosuppressives to prevent acute cellular rejection in kidney transplantation. They are not considered treatment for acute rejection. Daclizumab is a humanized monoclonal antibody, which contains 90% human and 10% murine antibody sequences. Basiliximab is a chimeric antibody that contains both murine and human antibody sequences. In contrast to daclizumab, it contains higher amounts of murine antibody sequences.[25] These agents prevent episodes of acute rejection in kidney transplant recipients. Their use in combination with other agents is being studied in other transplant populations. Comparative studies between these agents or with other antibodies, such as Thymoglobulin, are being conducted. Advantages over these older agents include ease of administration, minimal side effects, low immunogenicity, no greater infections or malignancy rates, and fewer required doses. Both are well tolerated, although there are rare reports of anaphylaxis. These agents appear to be most effective in immunologically low-risk patients, whereas in high-risk patients, their use may be limited. These agents, as with other antibodies, are expensive. To date, the only perceived clinical difference between daclizumab and basiliximab is the dosing regimen. Daclizumab is given as 1 mg/kg on day 0 of the transplant and then every 2 weeks for four more doses. This regimen creates issues related to compliance, outpatient administration, and reimbursement. Basiliximab is given as a 20-mg dose on days 0 and 4 after transplantation. Several reports, however, have evaluated daclizumab regimens of one, two, or three doses given over the first few days after transplant.[25] Both daclizumab and basiliximab appear to have similar mechanisms. They bind to the α-subunit of the IL-2R, also known as *CD25* or the *TAC subunit*, which is expressed only on the surface of activated T cells; this subunit is critical to IL-2 activation of T cells in the acute rejection process. Daclizumab and basiliximab prevent the IL-2R from binding with IL-2, thereby blocking T-cell activation.[25]

Differences exist in the elimination half-life and duration of receptor saturation with these two agents, the significance of which remains to be determined. Daclizumab has a terminal half-life of 11 to 38 days, whereas that of basiliximab is 4 to 14 days. Daclizumab, using the approved five-dose regimen, saturates the IL-2R for about 120 days. Basiliximab, with the two-dose regimen, saturates the receptor for 36 days. Duration of IL-2 saturation was also found to be shorter in liver transplant recipients than that reported in kidney transplant recipients. The half-life and clearance of daclizumab and basiliximab have been shown to be shorter and faster, respectively, in liver transplant recipients. Total body clearance correlates positively with the volume of postoperative blood loss; basiliximab also is cleared through postoperative ascitic fluid.[26]

Alemtuzumab

Alemtuzumab (Campath-1H) is a humanized monoclonal antibody against CD52 proteins on the surface of T and B cells, natural killer cells, macrophages, and monocytes. It is approved for use in certain types of leukemias, but not in organ transplant. Because it causes a profound reduction or depletion in lymphocytes, especially T helper lymphocytes, a number of studies are evaluating its effect as induction therapy to prevent acute rejection after kidney transplant. Several studies are investigating its use in steroid avoidance or withdrawal regimens and calcineurin avoidance or withdrawal regimens. Short-term studies have indicated a role for this agent in these situations. Most protocols with this agent give a single 30 mg IV dose in the operating room. With this dose, significant neutropenia and lymphopenia can still occur, lasting for months to years in some patients. This single dose regimen has been successful in reducing the incidence of fungal and viral infections as compared with multiple dose regimens.[27]

Investigational Agents

A number of agents are in various stages of development. These include everolimus (SDZ-RAD), belatacept (LEA29Y), FTY720, deoxyspergualin, brequinar, mizoribine, leflunomide, FK-778, and AEB-071. These agents have more specific activity directed at T-cell and B-cell function and some interfere with costimulatory proteins. Everolimus is an analogue of sirolimus.[28] Belatacept is a CTL4-Ig, which blocks the costimulatory pathway of CD28 or CTL-A4: CD80/CD86 binding interactions. CTLA4-Ig binds to CD80/CD86 to a greater degree than CD28, resulting in inhibition of costimulation and T cell activation. Belatacept, which is given IV, once every few weeks in combination with other agents, is currently undergoing phase III trials as a replacement for CNI.[29] FTY720 interferes with lymphocyte migration from the lymph nodes. Leflunomide and its analogs, FK778, belong to a class of agents called malanitriloamides and target pyrimidine synthesis. Mizoribine and brequinar are inhibitors of DNA synthesis. Deoxyspergualin inhibits cell activation and maturation. In addition, a number of monoclonal antibodies and peptides have been developed and are undergoing investigation. The targets of these antibodies and peptides are antigen-binding sites, adhesion molecules, cytokines and enzymes such as tyrosine kinase.[31]

KIDNEY TRANSPLANTATION

Indications and Evaluation

1. G.P. is a 52-year-old, 72-kg black man with end-stage renal disease (ESRD) secondary to non–insulin-dependent diabetes mellitus, hypertension and hyperlipidemia. He has been undergoing hemodialysis three times a week for 4 years. Other medical problems include anemia, hypocalcemia, and hyperphosphatemia. G.P.'s medications include amlodipine 10 mg daily, ramipril 10 mg twice daily (BID), Lipitor 20 mg daily, Tums two tablets three times daily (TID) with meals, at bedtime, and in between meals, NPH insulin 30 U BID, regular insulin 8 U BID, and erythropoietin 8,000 U IV three times weekly. He has been on the kidney transplant waiting list for 2 years. He is called by the transplant coordinator and admitted for a possible deceased donor (formerly called cadaveric) kidney transplant. G.P. has the same blood type as the donor. His most recent PRA is 10%. Cross-match is negative, and HLA typing reveals a three-antigen match (A1, A2, B35) between donor and recipient. On admission to the hospital, his laboratory values are as follows: Na, 141 mEq/L (normal, 135–145); potassium (K), 4.7 mEq/L (normal, 3.4–4.6); Cl, 102 mEq/L (normal, 95–105); bicarbonate (HCO_3), 23 mEq/L (normal, 22–28); blood urea nitrogen (BUN), 44 mg/dL (normal, 8–18); serum creatinine (SrCr), 13.9 mg/dL (normal, 0.6–1.2); calcium (Ca), 7.8 mEq/L (normal, 8.8–10.3); phosphorus, 6.2 mg/dL (normal, 2.5–5.0); glucose, 225 mg/dL (normal, 65–110); WBC count, 8.4 cells/mm^3 (normal, 4,000–10,000); hemoglobin (Hgb), 10.8 g/dL (normal, 14–18); and hematocrit (Hct), 32% (normal, 39%–49%). His serology is negative for HIV, hepatitis B surface antigen, hepatitis C, and cytomegalovirus (CMV), and is positive for anti-HBS. What are the indications for and potential benefits of kidney transplantation in G.P.?

[SI units: Na, 141 mmol/L (normal, 135–145); K, 4.7 mmol/L (normal, 3.4–4.6); Cl, 102 mmol/L (normal, 95–105); Hco_3, 23 mmol/L (normal, 22–28); BUN, 15.7 mmol/L (normal, 3.0–6.5); SrCr, 1,228.8 μmol/L (normal, 50–110); Ca, 1.95 mmol/L (normal, 2.20–2.58); P, 2.0 mmol/L (normal, 0.77–1.45); glucose, 12.5 mmol/L (normal, 3.9–6.1); WBC count, 8.4 $\times$ 10^6 cells/L (normal, 4,000–10,000); Hgb, 108 g/L (normal, 115–155); Hct, 0.32 (0.39–0.49)]

All patients with ESRD are potential candidates for kidney transplantation unless contraindicated. The contraindications (absolute or relative) are determined by the individual transplant center. Absolute contraindications include current malignancy, active infection, active liver disease, HbsAg-positive, severe or symptomatic cardiac or pulmonary disease, specific renal diseases with an accelerated recurrence rate, substance abuse, and abnormal psychosocial and noncompliant behavior. Relative contraindications for the recipient of a kidney transplant include chronic liver disease, active infection, positive for hepatitis C, HIV-positive, morbid obesity, current positive cross-match, and age >70 years.[30] The relative contraindication for the elderly with ESRD is controversial because approximately 40% of the ESRD population is >65 years and an increasing number of these patients are undergoing kidney transplantation. Patients with ESRD need not wait until they are receiving dialysis before being considered for a kidney transplant because transplantation is associated with lower cost, better quality of life and longer survival than patients on dialysis awaiting transplantation. The primary diseases leading to ESRD and transplant are diabetes, glomerulonephritis, polycystic kidneys, and arterionephrosclerosis.

In G.P., diabetes and hypertension would be the most likely causes of his ESRD. For G.P., a renal transplant should return his renal function to near normal, improve his quality of life, and correct the complications of renal dysfunction such as anemia, hypocalcemia, and hyperphosphatemia, but not diabetes or hypertension or hyperlipidemia.

When evaluating a patient for any organ transplantation, the risk-to-benefit ratio must be considered. In general, kidney transplants are performed to improve the quality of life and avoid the complications and outcomes associated with dialysis and renal failure. It is also more cost effective than dialysis. In contrast, patients who are candidates for heart, lung, and liver transplantations will die if these vital organs fail. Therefore, the criteria established for organ transplantation must be evaluated carefully before it is offered to any patient.

Donor and Recipient Matching

2. What criteria are important in determining a good match between the donor and G.P.?

G.P. had a series of serologic tests to determine his genetic compatibility with the donor. He had a negative cross-match and low PRA of 10%, indicating that he is not already sensitized to this donor's antigens, which should result in a more favorable post-transplantation course. HLA matching also indicated a three-antigen match between G.P. and the donor. Matching of donor and recipient at the HLA-A, HLA-B, and HLA-DR loci is associated with better graft survival and longer half-lives for both living-related and deceased donor kidney transplants. Half-lives are longer with living donors (13–15 years) compared with deceased donors (8–20 years). For a group of recipients with a match similar to G.P., the 1-year and 3-year graft survival for a first deceased donor transplant is projected to be >90% and >80%, respectively. These positive factors may be offset, however, by his ethnicity. Patient and graft survival after kidney transplantation is reduced in the black population compared with others because of immunologic, medical, pharmacologic, pharmacokinetic, and socioeconomic reasons.[31] Along with black race, other risk factors associated with decreased survival include advanced donor age, recipient age <15 and >50 years, retransplantation, a high PRA (>20%–>50%), and delayed graft function. Recipients who fall into these categories are referred to as high-risk patients.[32]

Because of a limited number of donors, this pool has been expanded to include what are called expanded criteria donors (ECD). These are deceased donors (DD) who are either older, and have evidence of some pre-existing hypertension, higher serum creatinine, or death caused by cerebrovascular disease than the standard criteria DD. Survival appears to somewhat lower in recipients of organs from ECD. G.P.'s donor was a standard criteria DD donor.

Immunosuppressive Therapy

3. Before the transplant procedure, G.P. receives MMF 1 g orally (PO) and cefazolin 1 g IV. During surgery, just before reperfusion of his new kidney, he received methylprednisolone 500 mg IV and Thymoglobulin 100 mg IV. He is also given furosemide 100 mg IV after the kidney has been transplanted. Methylprednisolone 250 mg IV is to be given on the day after surgery. The methylprednisolone dose is to be decreased to 100 mg IV on the second postoperative day for one dose. Prednisone 60 mg (1 mg/kg/day) PO is to be given on the subsequent day for one dose and tapered by 0.3 mg/kg/day to 20 mg daily by day 7 after surgery. Tacrolimus nasogastric (NG) or orally (PO) 0.1 mg/kg/day or 3 mg Q 12 hr will be started within 12 hours after surgery if renal function improves. The dosage will be adjusted according to tacrolimus whole blood trough concentrations. MMF will be continued at 1g PO BID. He will also continue with antibody induction with Thymoglobulin 100 mg IV on days 1 and 3 after surgery. Why is G.P. being treated with this immunosuppressive regimen?

The major goal of immunosuppressive therapy is to prevent rejection and infection with minimal adverse side effects and to ensure long-term patient and graft survival. Overall acute rejection rates are <20% during the first year after kidney transplantation. Most of these episodes respond to acute antirejection therapy.

No consensus exists on the best immunosuppressive regimen, and the numerous dosing regimens in use primarily depend on the program and the specific organ to be transplanted. Although a number of studies have attempted to evaluate the superiority of various regimens, comparisons are influenced by variables such as differences in donor selection and condition, organ preservation and procurement, organ ischemic (cold and warm) time, recipient's pretransplant conditions, comorbid and high or low risk factors, surgical procedures and individual surgical techniques, postoperative management and monitoring, and length of follow-up. Another important consideration is that many of the newer agents show significant effects during the first year, but fail to show a significant impact on long-term effects such as chronic rejection and graft survival.[2] The choice of a particular regimen generally depends on the risk factors present at the time of transplantation. During this early time period, the number of agents and doses used are higher than later on after transplantation.

Most starting immunosuppressive drug regimens for the management of solid organ transplantations rely on three to four agents, although mono-or-dual therapy has been used, depending on organ type and risk factors. These combination regimens include a CNI (cyclosporine or tacrolimus) and MMF or sirolimus; or azathioprine and prednisone with or without a monoclonal antibody (alemtuzumab, basiliximab, daclizumab, OKT3); or polyclonal antibody (Atgam, Thymoglobulin). Several regimens are being studied that avoid the use of steroids and CNI; or use a short course in the early transplantation period, or are withdrawn sometime, usually several months, after transplantation in an attempt to avoid the long-term side effects of these agents.[33]

With DD kidney transplants, quadruple or triple therapy is used. The most commonly used regimen is one that contains an antibody with tacrolimus, MMF and prednisone. Cyclosporine or tacrolimus are the foundation of this type of regimen. Tacrolimus is used in >70% of new kidney transplant recipients.[20] In HLA-identical, living-related kidney transplants, conventional dual therapy (e.g., azathioprine or mycophenolate and prednisone) gives excellent results; however, acute rejection can still occur, and some programs may use dual therapy that contains either cyclosporine or tacrolimus. Combination therapy is used to take advantage of different mechanisms of action and to reduce drug toxicity by using sequential therapy and smaller doses of multiple agents rather than larger doses of any agent used alone. These multidrug combinations can lead, however, to increased drug costs, compliance issues, a higher incidence of infection and malignancy, and difficulty in assessing adverse effects.

In G.P., triple or quadruple therapy would be used. In many centers, an antibody such as Thymoglobulin, alemtuzumab, basiliximab, or daclizumab would be added to his current triple therapy, because G.P. is considered a high-risk recipient because he is black. Black recipients generally have a higher rate of acute rejection and graft loss than other ethnic groups after transplant.[34]

After the initial transplantation period, drug dosages are reduced over time and maintained at a stable dose for 6 months to 1 year. In G.P., tacrolimus, MMF, or the corticosteroid may be discontinued. Although the discontinuation of a drug may reduce adverse effects, it must be counterbalanced against the risk of acute rejection and graft loss. Monotherapy, generally with tacrolimus or cyclosporine, may be achieved in kidney, liver, and heart transplant recipients at some point after transplantation. Most patients, however, require lifetime immunosuppression.

4. What is induction therapy?

Induction therapy after transplantation refers to the use of an antibody, typically during the first week after transplant. Acute rejection can occur in the early transplant period and also delayed graft function (DGF). Both of these have a negative impact on graft survival. Antibodies, such as Thymoglobulin and OKT3, reduce the incidence of acute rejection and delayed graft function and have typically been used in immunologically high-risk patients. Their use in patients at low to moderate risk is increasing, however, often as a means of reducing or avoiding the use of CNI and steroids. The newer antibodies (e.g., basiliximab, daclizumab, and alemtuzumab) are playing a bigger role in these situations because they are easier to give and have a less severe adverse effect profile.[28] Recent data indicate that about 70% of all kidney transplants during 2004 to 2005 received induction therapy, with Thymoglobulin making up about 40%.[20]

Thymoglobulin and Antithymocyte Globulin (Atgam)

5. How would Thymoglobulin be administered and monitored in G.P.?

Dosing and Administration

Both Thymoglobulin and antithymocyte globulin are effective as induction therapy or as treatment of acute rejection. In general, Thymoglobulin appears to be more effective than antithymocyte globulin and has replaced Atgam as the polyclonal antibody of choice. Thymoglobulin, when used for induction, also has been reported to result in improved survival, fewer side effects, and less infection compared with OKT3. The dose of Thymoglobulin is 1.5 mg/kg/day, and the dose of antithymocyte globulin is 10 to 20 mg/kg/day. These drugs can be diluted in 0.9% sodium chloride for injection and administered over 4 to 6 hours. Both are usually infused into a high-flow central vein to reduce pain, erythema, and phlebitis at the injection site. Peripheral administration has been used successfully with Thymoglobulin by adding heparin and hydrocortisone to the IV solution.[25] Skin testing is recommended before horse-derived antithymocyte globulin use, but not rabbit-derived Thymoglobulin. Patients previously sensitized to horse serum are at risk for an anaphylactoid reaction, but the prevalence of anaphylaxis has diminished with improved purification of this product. Patients with a positive pretherapy skin test could undergo desensitization, but alternatives, such as Thymoglobulin and OKT3, are available.

Dose Regimen and Duration of Therapy

The first dose of Thymoglobulin is usually given intraoperatively rather than after transplant. Intraoperative administration of Thymoglobulin has been shown to reduce the incidence and severity of DGF as compared with postoperative adminstration.[34] Duration of therapy with Thymoglobulin and antithymocyte globulin ranges from 3 to 10 days for induction therapy. Protocols used to treat rejection commonly use a 7- to 14-day course of therapy.[20] In patients such as G.P., a three-dose regimen has been shown to be as effective as a daily regimen.[35]

Adverse Effects

A number of adverse effects have been related to the use of Thymoglobulin or antithymocyte globulin. Local phlebitis and pain usually can occur. Anaphylaxis is rare. Chills and fever, erythema, rash, hives, pruritus, headache, leukopenia, and thrombocytopenia are commonly encountered. Fever, chills, nausea, and vomiting may be caused by the release of cytokines, such as TNF and IL-6, from lysed lymphocytes. These symptoms can be minimized by premedication with acetaminophen and diphenhydramine before each dose. Methylprednisolone, up to 500 mg, is given 1 hour before Thymoglobulin for the first two doses to minimize infusion reactions. Serum sickness leading to acute glomerulonephritis, hypotension, and acute respiratory distress also has been associated with these agents. It may not be evident until the seventh day of therapy or within 2 weeks of discontinuation.[36] Opportunistic viral, (CMV and Epstein-Barr virus [EBV]), and fungal infections are the predominant delayed side effect. Susceptibility to malignancy, such as posttransplantation lymphoproliferative disease (PTLD) is also a concern (see Chapter 35, Questions 15–16). Because of the increased risk of CMV infection, patients are often given oral valganciclovir or IV ganciclovir during therapy, and then oral valganciclovir, which is continued up to several months after induction.

Monitoring

Vital signs should be monitored hourly during infusion, and WBC and platelet counts should be monitored daily. If the patient's WBC count drops to <3,000 cells/mm^3 or if the platelet count drops to <100,000 cells/mm^3, the dose of drug is decreased by 50% or held entirely until the counts return to desired levels. The decision to decrease or hold the dose is based on the status of the patient's rejection and the degree of thrombocytopenia and leukopenia.

Dosages also can be adjusted based on absolute lymphocyte counts or lymphocyte subsets as a way of maximizing efficacy and minimizing infectious complications. For example, the dose can be adjusted by using a target absolute T-lymphocyte count (CD2 or CD3) of <25 to 50 cells/mm^3. This latter approach results in a lower dose, less frequent dosing (e.g., every other day instead of daily), lower costs, and a lower rate of viral infection. Thymoglobulin produces a more profound and longer duration of effect on lymphocytes than antithymocyte globulin, but this does not result in a greater risk for infection and malignancy.[20]

6. Could daclizumab or basiliximab be used as an alternative to Thymoglobulin?

Daclizumab and basiliximab are agents approved for use as induction therapy in kidney transplantations. Although they are approved for use in kidney transplantations only, they are being used and studied in other organ transplant recipients. Studies with these agents have been in combination with cyclosporine or tacrolimus and steroids with or without an antimetabolite, such as azathioprine or MMF or sirolimus. These agents are well tolerated and have a better adverse event profile than Thymoglobulin or OKT3.[25] These agents have a limited role in high-risk populations, such as G.P. who is black, or patients with high PRA or long ischemic times, delayed graft function, patients who have received a previous transplant, and children. In these patients, induction with polyclonal antibodies is used in most centers. The large initial trials with these IL-2R antibodies included very few high-risk patients or excluded them altogether. More potent agents, such as Thymoglobulin, are still preferred in high-risk patients. A prospective study comparing Thymoglobulin with basiliximab in high-risk kidney transplants demonstrated that acute rejection rates were lower in patients receiving Thymoglobulin.[32] IL-2R antibodies can be used for low- to intermediate-risk patients and in patients where CNI minimization or steroid avoidance is implemented.[25]

Postoperative Course and Delayed Graft Function

7. G.P. is admitted to the transplant ward for initial post-transplantation management. His urine output during the next 3 hours has decreased from 300 to 40 mL/hour. He is receiving IV fluids at a rate equivalent to his urine output. He received 3 L of fluids in the operating room (OR). His blood pressure (BP)

is 140/83 mmHg, heart rate is 87 beats/minute, and temperature 36.9°C; he has no signs of dehydration. His BUN is 56 mg/dL (normal, 8–18), and his SrCr is 12.8 mg/dL (normal, 0.6–1.2). Another dose of furosemide 100 mg IV increased his urine output to 140 mL/hour, but his urine output returned to <40 mL/hour in a few hours. Fluids and IV furosemide were given again with similar results. Renal ultrasound indicates no urine leaks, fluid collections, or ureteral obstruction. A DPTA (diethylenetriamine penta-acidic acid) renal scan indicates good perfusion, but decreased accumulation and clearance. Over the next 2 days, G.P.'s BP is 150/93 mmHg, weight is 76 kg (4 kg higher than before the transplantation), urine output has fallen to <200 mL/day, and relevant laboratory values are as follows: BUN, 85 mg/dL; SrCr, 13.2 mg/dL; and K, 5.8 mEq/L (normal, 3.4–4.6). The decision is made to institute hemodialysis. What has happened to G.P.'s renal function? What is the most likely diagnosis?

[SI units: BUN, 20 mmol/L, 30.3 mmol/L (normal, 3.0–6.5); SrCr, 1,131.5 μmol/L, 1166.9 μmol/L (normal, 50–110); K, 5.8 mmol/L (normal, 3.4–4.6)]

After kidney transplantation, recipients require management and monitoring for fluid and electrolyte imbalance (potassium, magnesium, phosphorous and calcium), BP and blood glucose changes, surgical complications, gastrointestinal (GI) complications, infection, rejection, immunosuppressive dosing and toxicity, and, most important, kidney function. If all goes well, recipients should be discharged from the hospital within 3 to 5 days after transplantation. The initial renal function after kidney transplantation can reflect excellent, moderate, or slow graft function or DGF. In recipients with excellent function, a good diuresis begins immediately and continues; the serum creatinine rapidly declines to <2.5 mg/dL within the first few days after transplantation. Most living-related transplants and between 30% to 50% of DD transplants generally experience this excellent graft function pattern. Kidney transplant recipients with moderate or slow graft function usually experience a slower decline in serum creatinine, which stabilizes within the first week. Recipients with DGF usually experience anuria or oliguria, require dialysis in the early period, and take days to weeks to recover. DGF is most common in recipients of organs from deceased transplant donors, occurring in between 2% to 50% (average 25%) of cases.[37]

The diagnosis of DGF is based on clinical, laboratory, and diagnostic criteria that may vary among centers. DGF has been defined simply as the need for dialysis in the early transplantation period, whereas at others, the definition may be based on both a lack of improvement in the serum creatinine (e.g., it does not fall below 2.5 to 4 mg/dL or by 25%–30% from pretransplantation) and the presence of anuria or oliguria within the first 6 to 24 hours after other causes of acute tubular necrosis (ATN) are ruled out. Slow graft function (SGF) is another term that has been used to describe a lag in improvement and does not involve dialysis. DGF is influenced by conditions affecting the donor (age, condition of organ, prolonged ischemic time), intraoperative conditions (hypotension, fluid imbalance, ischemia or reperfusion injury), and recipient (prior transplantation, postoperative hypovolemia or hypotension, and nephrotoxic drugs).[37]

In G.P., poor urine output in the first hours after transplantation and subsequent oliguria, the exclusion of other causes of ATN, the results of the renal scan, the lack of improvement in BUN and serum creatinine, and the need for dialysis are indicative of DGF. DGF reduces kidney long-term graft survival, increases the risk of acute rejection, and influences a patient's early management by requiring dialysis, increasing the length of hospital stay, and increasing the costs of therapy. It also may make the assessment of acute rejection more difficult because the patient already has impaired renal function. In DGF, a renal biopsy is obtained if no improvement in serum creatinine is seen by day 7.[37]

8. What adjustments should be made in G.P.'s immunosuppressive regimen at this time?

The adverse renal effects of CNI can contribute to the onset of DGF as well as prolong its duration. Therefore, tacrolimus should be discontinued temporarily or its dose significantly reduced. Because of this effect, induction and sequential immunosuppressive protocols do not include CNI, or they use them only in low doses generally for the first week after a renal transplantation until renal function improves. These protocols include antibodies and provide more intense immunosuppression early after transplantation when the risk of acute rejection is highest. Thymoglobulin or OKT3 is used in patients with DGF because they have shortened the duration of DGF and the need for dialysis when compared with the CNI. These agents have an early positive impact on DGF but have failed to show a positive effect on long-term graft survival compared with standard therapies, such as CNI.[35] Another potential option would be to use one of the new IL-2R inhibitors, daclizumab or basiliximab, which have been shown to reduce acute rejection rates and extend the time to first rejection. They have been used primarily in low to moderate risk patients. Their use in high-risk patients (blacks, retransplantations, high PRA, prolonged ischemic time, DGF) is based primarily on single-center and retrospective studies with encouraging results, but their effectiveness in prospective studies in preventing acute rejection has not always been equal to other antibodies such as Thymoglobulin.[38] Another concern with use of the anti IL-2R agents is that a CNI may be required sooner than with Thymoglobulin because these agents do not provide as long a duration of protection from rejection.

In G.P., Thymoglobulin would be administered for between 5 to 10 days, depending on improvement in his SrCr and urine output, along with his current regimen of prednisone and mycophenolate. A typical dose would be 1.5 mg/kg/day or every other day, depending on his CD3+ level, and WBC and platelet counts. His tacrolimus could be held for a few days to a week and reintroduced at a lower dose of 0.025 mg/kg twice a day. Afterwards, a tacrolimus dosage of 0.05 mg/kg orally twice a day would be reasonable in G.P. with a goal of achieving whole blood trough concentrations of 8 to 12 ng/mL after transplant.

Rejection

9. G.P. was started on Thymoglobulin 1.5 mg/kg as a 6-hour IV infusion with further dosages to be adjusted to maintain CD3+ cell counts of <25/mm³ and lymphocyte counts of <20 cells/mm³ for a total of 7 days. He received this along with his prednisone

taper and MMF. He received three doses of Thymoglobulin, on days 1, 3, and 5 after transplant. Tacrolimus PO 3 mg BID was initiated on day 4 of Thymoglobulin therapy. G.P.'s urine output has increased gradually to ~1,600 mL/day 1 week after stopping Thymoglobulin. His weight has decreased to 73 kg, BP is 142/84 mmHg, heart rate is 82 beats/minute, temperature is 36.7°C, BUN is 23 mg/dL (normal, 8–18), SrCr is 2.3 mg/dL (normal, 0.6–1.2), and K is 4.6 mEq/L (normal, 3.4–4.6). He is on a regular diet and taking all oral medications. His current medications include MMF 500 mg BID, prednisone 10 mg daily, tacrolimus 5 mg BID, ranitidine 150 mg at bedtime, dioctyl sodium sulfosuccinate 100 mg BID, amlodipine 10 mg daily, metoprolol 50 mg PO BID, NPH insulin 28 U BID, regular insulin 10 U BID, valganciclovir 450 mg daily, and trimethoprim-sulfamethoxazole (TMP-SMX) DS, one tablet on Mondays, Wednesdays, and Fridays. Fifty days after stopping Thymoglobulin, G.P.'s weight increased to 74.6 kg, and his BP was 160/94 mmHg, heart rate was 98 beats/minute, temperature was 37.6°C, BUN was 30 mg/dL, SrCr was 3.4 mg/dL, K was 4.8 mEq/L, trough whole blood tacrolimus concentration was 5 ng/mL, and urine output decreased over the last 24 hours to 850 mL. He feels tired and has a decreased appetite, but his fluid intake has been adequate over the past day. What evidence is consistent with rejection in G.P.?

[SI units: BUN, 8.2 mmol/L, 10.7 mmol/L (normal, 3.0–6.5); SrCr, 212.2 μmol/L, 300.6 μmol/L (normal, 50–110); K, 4.6 mmol/L, 4.8 mmol/L (normal, 3.4–4.6)]

Although significant improvements in reduction in acute rejection and improved graft survival have occurred over the past decade, certain types of acute rejection and chronic rejection continue to be a major reason for graft loss in kidney transplants. Rejection episodes in all solid organ transplantations can be categorized as hyperacute, accelerated, acute, or chronic. Kidney biopsy is considered the gold standard for making the diagnosis of rejection after kidney transplant. Approved criteria are used to classify and grade the type of rejection.[39]

Hyperacute Rejection

Hyperacute rejection, which occurs within minutes to hours after transplantation of the allograft, is the result of preformed cytotoxic antibodies against donor-specific class I antigens. This type of rejection is rare because of ABO matching and improved HLA typing before transplant, but it remains associated with a poor prognosis. Clinically, the patient presents with anuria, hyperkalemia, hypertension, metabolic acidosis, pulmonary edema and, in some cases, disseminated intravascular coagulopathy (DIC). Diagnostic scan of the kidney would indicate no uptake. If other causes of anuria are excluded and this diagnosis is made, then the transplanted kidney must be removed.

Accelerated Rejection

Accelerated rejection usually occurs within a few days after organ transplantation. This is a result of prior sensitization to antigens that are similar to those of the donor and newly developed donor-specific antibodies. Accelerated rejections of transplanted kidneys occur primarily in recipients who have had prior transplantation, multiple pregnancies, or blood transfusions. These patients usually maintain good renal function for a few days before developing acute renal failure. Accelerated organ rejections generally are more resistant to pharmacologic therapy.

Acute Rejection

Acute rejection is the most common type of kidney rejection in transplant recipients and most episodes respond to therapy. Most episodes of acute rejection are T-cell mediated (cellular), although some can be B-cell (antibody or humoral) mediated, whereas others are a combination of both. Acute rejection of a transplanted kidney significantly reduces the half-life and survival of both living and DD transplants. The half-life refers to the time it takes for half of the grafts that survive the first year eventually to fail. Acute rejection can occur in the first week to months after kidney transplantation. The prophylactic use of antibody preparations may, however, delay the onset for several weeks, as illustrated by G.P.'s case. If acute rejection occurs, its onset is almost always within the first year, with most episodes occurring within the first 60 days after transplantation. Acute rejection can, however, also occur at any time after transplant and can be a result of patient nonadherence (also called noncompliance) to medications and monitoring. The clinical presentation of patients with acute rejection of a kidney ranges from an asymptomatic patient with mild renal dysfunction as indicated by an elevated serum creatinine, which is common, to patients presenting with a flulike illness and acute oliguric renal failure.[40]

G.P. presents with subjective complaints of malaise or tiredness and lack of appetite. Such nonspecific complaints occur often in patients with rejection and can be accompanied by myalgias as well as pain and tenderness at the graft site in some cases. Objectively, G.P.'s fever, increased weight, hypertension, decreased urine output, and increase in serum creatinine are consistent with acute kidney rejection. In addition, the tacrolimus concentration and mycophenolate doses are low, suggesting inadequate immunosuppressive coverage. Acute rejection of a transplanted kidney must be distinguished from CNI nephrotoxicity, and infections (e.g., pyelonephritis, CMV) also must be ruled out. Although the clinical evidence in G.P. probably represents an acute rejection, a kidney biopsy is the gold standard for establishing the diagnosis. Biopsy results usually are available within 6 to 8 hours. If there is acute rejection, the renal biopsy will show an interstitial infiltration of mononuclear cells with tubulitis or intimal arteritis in more severe cases. The severity of acute rejection would be classified and graded according to standardized pathologic criteria and can determine treatment. Less severe grades would receive high-dose steroids, whereas more severe grades would often receive Thymoglobulin or OKT3.[40]

Antibody-Mediated Rejection

Antibody-mediated (also called humoral) rejection can be either acute or chronic rejection mediated by antibodies. It differs histologically from acute cellular rejection in that there is no lymphocyte infiltration on biopsy. Presence of positive staining for the complement component C4d suggests antibody-mediated rejection. Humoral rejection can occur in hours to years after transplantation. Antibody-mediated rejection often is associated with hemodynamic compromise and is more resistant to drug therapy. In addition to standard therapy, such as steroids and Thymoglobulin, plasmapheresis, IVIG, and rituximab may be required to treat acute rejection episodes.[41]

Chronic Rejection

Chronic rejection is a major cause of long-term kidney graft loss after the first year. It can be either cellular or humorally mediated. It occurs slowly in most cases over several years. Because no specific treatment exists, therapy is supportive (e.g., dialysis in the case of a kidney transplantation). Ultimately, retransplantation is needed. Some data suggest that some patients may benefit from some of the newer agents, such as mycophenolate and sirolimus, which are considered non-nephrotoxic, but this requires further study. The diagnosis of chronic rejection is determined by clinical signs and biopsy findings indicative of obliterative fibrosis of hollow structures and vessels within the graft. The chronic rejection of a kidney must be distinguished from chronic CNI nephrotoxicity, chronic infection, and recurrence of the original kidney disease.[42]

Chronic Allograft Nephropathy

Chronic allograft nephropathy (CAN) is a term that has been used, generally, as a diagnosis of exclusion that indicates a slow deterioration of renal function over months to years after kidney transplant, with the exact cause unknown. Immunologic and nonimmunologic mechanisms play a role in CAN, a term that has been used to describe this overall process of graft deterioration. Another term, chronic renal allograft dysfunction (CRAD) is the functional result of CAN. It is a slow, insidious process that usually manifests as an increase in serum creatinine after about 1 year, although it can occur as early as 3 months after transplantation. The characteristic signs of chronic rejection are hypertension, proteinuria, and a progressive decline in renal function leading to renal failure. Immunologic factors that increase the likelihood of chronic rejection include a history of acute rejection, inadequate immunosuppression, noncompliance with immunosuppressive therapy, and previous infection, such as CMV. Nonimmunologic factors are donor related (age, hypertension, diabetes), increased ischemic times, recipient hypertension, hyperlipidemia, CNI nephrotoxicity, and elevated body mass index (BMI). CRAD is irreversible and unaffected by increased immunosuppressive therapy. Most recently, it has been recommended that the term CAN be eliminated from the pathologic diagnostic criteria for renal dysfunction because it is nonspecific and the end result of a number of different processes.[45]

Acute Rejection Treatment

10. A biopsy of G.P.'s transplanted kidney shows grade 1A, moderate acute rejection. G.P. is started on methylprednisolone 500 mg daily IV for three doses. His maintenance oral prednisone is discontinued, but his other medications are maintained. He will be placed on a high-dose oral prednisone tapering regimen after his IV doses. Why is methylprednisolone therapy of G.P.'s first acute episode of rejection appropriate?

High-dose or "pulse" IV methylprednisolone, IV OKT3, IV Thymoglobulin, IV ATG, or oral prednisone are several of the options used to treat acute rejection in all types of solid organ transplants. A high-dose corticosteroid (usually IV methylprednisolone) is considered first-line therapy because it works very quickly in decreasing lymphocyte responsiveness, is easy to administer, and reverses at least 75% of acute rejection episodes. Thymogloglobulin and OKT3 are usually reserved for steroid-resistant rejection or more severe grades of rejection. IVIG has also been used as an alternative for resistant rejection.[43] The ideal corticosteroid dosage, route, and regimen are unknown, and the number of corticosteroid protocols is as varied as the number of transplantation programs. IV methylprednisolone and oral prednisone are equally effective in reversing rejection, but oral corticosteroids are given for a longer period and have been associated with a higher incidence of adverse effects. Although as little as 50 mg of IV methylprednisolone has a similar lymphocyte suppressive effect as a 1-g IV dose of this drug, most programs use methylprednisolone 250 to 1,000 mg, most commonly 500 mg, IV every day for three doses and adjust the prerejection oral prednisone regimen accordingly. An example of an oral prednisone regimen is 100 to 200 mg/day tapered over 1 to 3 weeks to baseline maintenance dose.[44]

For G.P., IV methylprednisolone is appropriate because corticosteroids are considered first-line therapy for acute rejection of a transplanted kidney, and first rejection episodes (such as G.P.'s) are very responsive. In addition, G.P. has received a prophylactic course of Thymoglobulin recently. Thymoglobulin, ATG, or OKT3 therapy is associated with a higher risk of CMV infection and malignancy; it is more difficult to administer, requires more intensive monitoring, is more expensive, and usually is held in reserve for corticosteroid-resistant or more severe forms of rejection.

Nevertheless, high-dose corticosteroids are not without risk. They increase the risk of infection, and long-term therapy can induce ocular, bone, cardiovascular, and endocrine abnormalities. Although G.P. will be receiving high-dose IV methylprednisolone for only 3 days, because he is diabetic, he should be monitored for hyperglycemia and a change in his insulin requirements because corticosteroids can significantly alter glucose metabolism. Short-course methylprednisolone also can mask signs of infection (e.g., fever, changes in WBC counts, pain associated with inflammation) and delay the diagnosis. Insomnia, nervousness, euphoria, mood shifts, acute psychosis, and mania also can occur with short-term corticosteroid use. If this methylprednisolone regimen is effective in reversing the acute rejection of G.P.'s transplanted kidney, his serum creatinine concentration should decline within 2 to 5 days and his urine output should increase.

In addition, it would be appropriate to increase G.P.'s tacrolimus dosage to 7 mg twice a day because the concentration is low and a relationship exists between concentration and effect. Because small changes in tacrolimus dose can increase levels disproportionately, a trough whole blood concentration should be re-evaluated in 2 to 3 days. The mycophenolate dose could be increased to 1 g BID, because this dose in combination with a CNI has reduced acute rejection in black patients. If G.P. had been on cyclosporine, another option would be to change cyclosporine to tacrolimus, which has been shown to reduce future episodes of acute rejection.[45] Another important aspect for prevention of future rejection would be to assess G.P.'s adherence with, and understanding of, his medication regimen. Nonadherence is a cause of acute rejection and graft loss.[46]

11. After receiving three doses of IV methylprednisolone, G.P.s serum creatinine did not decrease and his urine output continued to be low. What is going on? Could this represent a steroid resistant acute rejection? If so, could muromonab (OKT3) be used if G.P.s acute rejection is steroid resistant?

OKT 3

Because of no improvement in his renal function, based on his serum creatinine and urine output, it appears that G.P. has steroid resistant rejection. Although most centers would generally treat steroid resistant rejection with Thymoglobulin, OKT3 is also an effective agent in this situation. OKT3 is a monoclonal antibody that binds to the CD3 receptor and effectively clears the body of T cells. It is indicated to prevent and treat rejection and is effective to treat severe rejection and steroid-resistant rejection. A typical regimen would be 5 mg IV daily for 5 to 10 days.

Cytokine Release Syndrome

12. One hour after receiving his first 5-mg IV dose of OKT3, G.P. began to experience chills, nausea, and severe muscle and joint aches. His temperature rose from 100.8°F to a maximum of 102.1°F, and his BP dropped to 100/50 mmHg. Which of these effects is consistent with OKT3 administration?

OKT3 produces many adverse effects, which occur with higher frequency after the first and second doses. G.P.'s adverse reaction after his first dose of OKT3 is consistent with this finding. This complex of symptoms is referred to as the *cytokine-release syndrome*. Flulike symptoms (e.g., fever, chills, myalgia, joint pains) are the earliest signal of this syndrome, but they can be accompanied by less common, but more specific, symptoms that reflect the involvement of various organ systems. For example, central nervous system (CNS) symptoms, such as seizures, headaches, photophobia, confusion, and hallucinations, have been reported, as have aseptic meningitis and encephalopathy. Acute reversible renal dysfunction, as evidenced by a rise in the serum creatinine concentration and a decrease in urine output over the first few days of therapy, also may occur. This renal dysfunction usually resolves with continued therapy. Intrarenal graft thrombosis has been reported after high doses (i.e., 10 mg) of OKT3. Patients with evidence of fluid overload on chest radiograph (or >3% over their base weight) should receive furosemide and some may require dialysis before initiating OKT3, because of the possible risk of rapid pulmonary edema and respiratory distress that are caused by cytokine-induced increases in capillary permeability. Anaphylaxis is rarely reported.[24]

A proposed cause is the release of cytokines, tumor necrosis factor-γ (TNF-γ), IL-2, and IFN-α by T cells after their initial binding with OKT3. OKT3 stimulation of cytokine production is another proposed explanation for the cause of these adverse effects. This effect is independent of cell lysis. The serum concentration of cytokines becomes acutely elevated within 1 to 4 hours after the first and second doses of OKT3, and these high concentrations correlate in time with the onset of the initial symptoms, which usually resolve in 4 to 6 hours. Furthermore, these cytokines have been associated with similar adverse effects in other patient populations.

Cardiovascular effects, including hypotension, hypertension, and tachycardia, can occur in heart transplant recipients and present as a biphasic response. The fever, hypertension, and tachycardia are followed by hypotension, hypoxemia, and decreased vascular resistance 5 to 7 hours later. The cardiopulmonary effects are secondary to a series of events involving a number of mediators, including TNF-α, leukotrienes, prostaglandins, thromboxane A_2, and arachidonic acid metabolites produced and released by endothelial cells, neutrophils, and muscle cells.[24]

Dosing Protocol

13. What special procedures should be followed in G.P. when using OKT3 therapy?

The high incidence of side effects associated with OKT3 therapy, especially after the first two doses, has prompted strict dosing protocols in most medical institutions. If G.P. had not had a chest radiograph within the last 24 hours, it would be ordered and reviewed before initiation of OKT3 therapy. If he had evidence of pulmonary edema, a dose of IV furosemide appropriate for the patient (commonly, 40 mg in an adult) or dialysis, if appropriate, would have been administered before the first OKT3 dose. G.P. should receive a dose of methylprednisolone 7 to 8 mg/kg (~500 mg) IV 60 minutes before the first dose of OKT3 and 4 mg/kg before the second dose to significantly reduce the amount of cytokine released after administration. Acetaminophen 650 mg orally or rectally (10 mg/kg in children) and diphenhydramine 50 mg orally or IV (1 mg/kg in children) also are administered before the first two doses of OKT3. Prophylactic IV ganciclovir (2.5 mg/kg/day) or oral valganciclovir (both adjusted for renal dysfunction) to prevent CMV infection also has been advocated.

Some transplant centers monitor peripheral T-lymphocyte populations, such as CD3+ T cells, during OKT3 therapy to determine dosing and effectiveness. The effectiveness of OKT3 can be evaluated by monitoring for the presence of CD3+ cells among T lymphocytes in the peripheral circulation. In some transplant centers, the number of soluble CD3+ cells is kept to <10 cells/mL, whereas others are willing to accept 20 to 50 CD3+ cells/mL. Anti-OKT3 titers, and CMV polymerase chain reaction (PCR) blood levels are monitored for at least 3 weeks after discontinuation of OKT3 therapy.

Antibodies to OKT3

14. Why would doses of G.P.'s immunosuppressive drugs need to be adjusted during OKT3 administration?

When OKT3 is administered, antibodies against OKT3 can be formed. These antibodies can be anti-idiotype, anti-isotype, or both, in most cases. Anti-isotype antibodies are formed against the murine proteins of OKT3, and anti-idiotype antibodies are formed against the specific CD3 region. In one study of renal transplant recipients, 60% had an anti-idiotype response and 44% had an anti-isotype response. Overall, an antibody response was detected in 75% of patients. A reduction in the dose of azathioprine, mycophenolate, and prednisone or a reduction in the dose of cyclosporine or tacrolimus while receiving OKT3 has lowered the titers of antibody against OKT3. Anti-idiotypic OKT3 antibodies have the potential to decrease the effectiveness of repeated courses of the drug. Multiple courses of treatment with OKT3 have been successful, however, particularly if antibody titers are low (<1:100).[24]

When treatment of G.P.'s acute rejection is initiated with OKT3, his tacrolimus dose should be reduced by 50% or temporarily held, his MMF should be held temporarily or decreased by 50%, and his prednisone dose should remain the same. On day 5 to 7 of his OKT3 treatment, his tacrolimus dose should be increased to the dose that he was taking before OKT3 therapy was initiated, and his MMF should be reinstituted or increased. He should be tested for an anti-OKT3 antibody titer 2 to 4 weeks after the end of OKT3 treatment, when the maximal anti-OKT3 antibody level is present, in the event that OKT3 would be required at a later time.

Cyclosporine

15. B.B. is a 27-year-old, 60-kg black man who received a deceased donor kidney transplant. Within 12 hours of the transplantation, his immunosuppression consisted of modified cyclosporine (Neoral) 300 mg PO BID, MMF 1.5 g PO BID, and prednisone. He was taking other medicines for hypertension and infection prophylaxis. Describe the pharmacokinetic characteristics of cyclosporine. Based on this information, is B.B.'s cyclosporine regimen appropriate?

Pharmacokinetics

Cyclosporine pharmacokinetic parameters (e.g., absorption, distribution, metabolism) exhibit significant intrapatient and interpatient variability, resulting in poor dose-response relationships. A number of factors are known to influence its pharmacokinetic behavior. These include age, transplant type, underlying disease, time after transplantation, GI metabolism and motility; biliary and liver function; metabolism, body weight, cholesterol, albumin, red blood cell mass; and drug interactions and formulation.[47] These factors can change cyclosporine's absorption, distribution, metabolism, and excretion and can influence therapeutic concentrations and, ultimately, outcomes.[48,49] For example, children, blacks, and patients with cystic fibrosis tend to have reduced absorption, increased clearance of cyclosporine, or both. Patients who are obese or who have decreased liver function will have reduced clearance. Oral absorption of cyclosporine, which has been characterized as slow, incomplete, and highly variable, is the parameter that is most significantly affected. Absorption can depend on the type of transplant, time after transplantation, presence of food and its composition, intestinal function (e.g., diarrhea, ileus), small bowel length, and presence or absence of external bile drainage.[50] The mean absorption of the original cyclosporine product (Sandimmune) in adults with relatively normal liver function after a liver transplantation is 27%, which is comparable to that observed in recipients of kidney (27%), heart (35%), and bone marrow (34%) transplants. Bioavailibility ranges from <5% to 90%.[51] In most transplant recipients, cyclosporine absorption increases over time.

Dosing

Because cyclosporine (Sandimmune) absorption is so poor and erratic, it is given IV for the first few days after transplantation, particularly after liver transplantation. Cyclosporine is given IV as a continuous infusion (2–3 mg/kg/day) or intermittently (2.5 mg/kg/day) over 2 to 6 hours two times a day. As the trough cyclosporine levels begin to rise, the IV dose is decreased gradually, while the oral dose is maintained or increased. This route may still be required in some patients with cystic fibrosis after lung transplantation.

B.B. was given modified cyclosporine (Neoral), a readily absorbed cyclosporine formulation in a solubilized microemulsified state. Neoral's bioavailability is better than that of Sandimmune, so less intrapatient and interpatient variability is seen in transplant recipients. Furthermore, Neoral absorption is much less dependent on bile and thus can be used in most liver transplant recipients early after transplant without the need for IV administration. However the doses used are initially higher (10–15 mg/kg/day) than those used after kidney and heart transplantation (5–10 mg/kg/day).[49]

Neoral and Sandimmune are not bioequivalent and, therefore, not interchangeable. Neoral produces a shorter time to C_{max} (T_{max}), higher maximum concentration (C_{max}), and higher area under the concentration-time curve (AUC) than Sandimmune. It has significantly less intrasubject and intersubject pharmacokinetic variability, and a better correlation exists between single doses and trough concentrations and AUC than seen with Sandimmune. The bioavailability of Neoral is approximately 20% higher than that of Sandimmune (absolute bioavailability is 10%–89%). When converting patients on Sandimmune to Neoral, a 1:1 dosage ratio is used unless patients are taking >10 mg/kg/day of Sandimmune. Trough concentrations are initially obtained within the first 4 to 7 days, and dosage adjustments are made accordingly. Most patients tolerate conversion well, although some develop concentrated-related headaches, tremors, or elevated serum creatinine levels that resolve with dose adjustment. In most patients, the Neoral dose is 10% to 20% lower than Sandimmune dose, but as much as a 50% difference can be seen in patients taking large doses (>10 mg/kg/day) of Sandimmune.[49]

The first generic cyclosporine, SangCya, is no longer available. SangCya was bioequivalent to Neoral but not Sandimmune. Three other capsule forms are now available, which are also AB-rated bioequivalent to Neoral (Gengraf from Abbott and modified cyclosporine from Eon and Sidmak). Neoral and Sandimmune are available as both capsule and liquid.

Cyclosporine is extensively distributed into red blood cells, about 60%, whereas in plasma it is highly bound to lipoproteins, about 90%. It is extensively metabolized by both the gut and liver P450 3A4 enzymes and transported by P-glycoprotein. The average half-life is about 15 to 20 hours.[47–49]

B.B. was started on Neoral 8 mg/kg/day BID. Because he is black, he may require even higher doses, because the absorption of cyclosporine has been reported to be reduced in this population.[50] His blood concentration will have to be monitored closely and adjusted if necessary. He should be watched closely for signs of rejection and toxicity.

Adverse Effects

16. What are some of the adverse effects associated with cyclosporine?

Cyclosporine can cause a number of adverse effects, of which acute or chronic nephrotoxicity is the most frequent and worrisome. Other major effects include hypertension, hyperlipidemia, tremors, headaches, seizures, paresthesias, hypomagnesemia, hypo- or hyperkalemia, hyperuricemia, hyperglycemia, gout, gingival hyperplasia, hirsutism, hemolytic-uremic syndrome, and hepatotoxicity. If these occur, they generally respond to a reduction in dose or discontinuation of cyclosporine.[49]

Therapeutic Drug Monitoring

17. B.B.'s cyclosporine levels are being measured by whole blood TDx® assay. How should cyclosporine levels be used to optimize his therapy?

Cyclosporine concentrations are monitored to prevent toxicity, optimize efficacy, and assess patient compliance to the prescribed regimen. Most institutions monitor trough cyclosporine levels. During the early postoperative period, cyclosporine levels should be measured daily, keeping in mind that these may not reflect steady-state concentrations, and that dosage changes should be made every few days. Once B.B. is home, cyclosporine monitoring can occur less frequently and eventually every 1 to 2 months. The target trough therapeutic concentration of cyclosporine during the first 2 months is 150 to 400 ng/mL with the monoclonal whole blood TDx assay. About 1 to 6 months after transplantation, the cyclosporine trough concentration target is lowered to 150 to 250 ng/mL. After 6 months, the targeted cyclosporine trough concentration is lowered even further to 50 to 150 ng/mL. These ranges may differ among institutions and also depend on the transplant type, time after transplantation, and other agents used. For example, lung and heart transplant recipients may require higher trough concentrations than kidney and liver transplant recipients. The range is reduced over time, given that less immunosuppression is required after transplantation and that the pharmacokinetics change over time.[47,48]

A number of assay methods are used to measure cyclosporine concentrations, and most institutions use the method that is most familiar to their transplant physicians. The type of cyclosporine assay used by a particular institution significantly influences interpretation of results because there are significant differences between methodologies. These issues have contributed to the debate on the value of monitoring cyclosporine concentrations. The pharmacologic effects of cyclosporine metabolites and whether the concentrations of these metabolites should be monitored individually, or in combination with cyclosporine, also need to be determined.[52]

Assays currently in use include high-performance liquid chromatography (HPLC), radioimmunoassay with polyclonal or monoclonal antibodies, enzyme immunoassay (EMIT)®, and fluorescence polarization immunoassay. Cyclosporine concentrations can be measured in either whole blood or plasma, but plasma cyclosporine levels can differ by as much as 50% if the plasma temperature is 21°C or 37°C; whole blood cyclosporine concentrations are recommended. The most commonly used assay is the whole blood monoclonal TDx.[52]

No assay appears to be superior in its ability to correlate cyclosporine trough levels with clinical events. Although many studies have attempted to correlate the clinical events of acute rejection or nephrotoxicity to trough concentrations of cyclosporine in recipients of solid organ transplants, results from these studies are conflicting. It may be that the ability to correlate a single blood level during the course of a day with a clinical event that takes place over a longer time period is influenced by too many other variables (e.g., other immunosuppressives, time since transplant, dosage regimen, route, transplant type, assay method, sample matrix, donor–recipient interaction). Nevertheless, most transplant programs, if not all, use cyclosporine concentrations to guide therapy decisions.

Because of the limitations of using a single cyclosporine level and the poor correlation between AUC and trough concentration, some programs use a more intensive sampling procedure (e.g., 6–10 samples collected over 12–24 hours) when cyclosporine concentrations are expected to be at steady state. The AUC and average steady-state concentrations are calculated and used to guide cyclosporine dosage adjustments. A more limited sampling strategy involving one to three samples (1–4 hours after a dose at steady state) collected over a dosing interval has also been advocated.[53–55] The more sophisticated pharmacokinetic monitoring programs have developed better correlations between the AUC and dose or AUC and rejection than correlations based on cyclosporine trough levels only. A number of studies have advocated the use of what is known as C2 monitoring of cyclosporine levels. This level is obtained 2 hours after the Neoral dose. In studies conducted in kidney and liver transplant recipients, a much better correlation was seen with AUC 0 to 4 hour, used as surrogate marker for AUC 0 to 12 hour for Neoral, compared with any other time point, including a C0 or trough levels. These studies indicate that C2 level is a more sensitive predictor of acute rejection and toxicity than C0 or trough values.[54] The limitation to this approach however, is that it requires training and re-education of staff and patients, potentially more personnel, modification of procedures, and a narrower window for timing of dose and sampling. Also, the concentrations ranges would be higher and different for kidney and liver transplant recipients with this approach.[55] Extrapolation to other populations, such as children, blacks, and patients with cystic fibrosis or diabetes will require further study.

As in all cases, pharmacokinetic data must be interpreted in conjunction with the patient's clinical condition. In addition, deference always must be given to trends established by multiple cyclosporine levels over that of a single level. Single levels may be erroneous because of variability in dose administration, incorrect sampling techniques (e.g., not being obtained at the correct time if drawn from an IV catheter in which IV cyclosporine had been infused), or assay error.

Sirolimus

18. B.B., developed GI intolerance to MMF and cannot take it anymore. A decision is made to use sirolimus instead. Describe the pharmacokinetic characteristics of sirolimus. What would be the appropriate regimen and monitoring parameters for this agent?

Pharmacokinetics

Pharmacokinetic data are derived primarily from kidney transplant recipients. Sirolimus, as with cyclosporine and tacrolimus, exhibits significant pharmacokinetic variability. It is rapidly absorbed after oral administration of the liquid with a median time to maximum concentration (T_{max}) of about 1 hour. Its average bioavailability is 15%; C_{max} and AUC are linear over a wide range of doses. Sirolimus is extensively distributed, with a mean apparent volume of distribution of 12 L/kg. It distributes primarily into red blood cells and is highly plasma protein bound, approximately 92%. It also binds to lipoproteins. Sirolimus is extensively metabolized in the gut and liver by CYP 3A4 isoenzymes, and it is a substrate for P-glycoprotein. Its drug interaction profile is very similar to that of cyclosporine and tacrolimus. Renal elimination accounts for only 2% of a dose. The terminal half-life generally ranges from 57 to 63 hours and the time to reach steady state occurs in 10 to 14 days. In children, it can be shorter.[56]

Dosing

Sirolimus can be used in the early transplantation period, although reports of impaired wound healing in kidney transplantations, hepatic artery thrombosis after liver transplantations, and bronchial anastamotic dehiscence in lung transplants during this time period have required reconsideration of its use in this capacity. In the case of liver or lung transplantations, its use is contraindicated in the early post-transplantation period. Sirolimus can be added later, as is the practice in many centers, as replacement for or minimization of cyclosporine, tacrolimus, steroids, or mycophenolate doses.[57] An initial loading dose is given followed by a once-daily maintenance dose. The starting maintenance dose range is 2 to 5 mg. The typical loading dose is 6 mg followed by 2 mg every day. In high-risk patients, such as blacks, a 15-mg loading dose and 5-mg daily dose is recommended along with cyclosporine. Other centers have used loading doses of 10 to 15 mg, followed by 5 to 10 mg/day for the first week with target levels of 10 to 15 ng/mL for the first month, and 5 to 10 ng/mL thereafter when used with tacrolimus.[58] Sirolimus is often given 4 hours after the morning dose of cyclosporine. If administered at the same time, sirolimus concentrations were, on average, 40% higher, than cyclosporine concentrations.[59]

Adverse Effects

As with other immunosuppressives, sirolimus is associated with a number of side effects, including oral ulcerations, diarrhea, arthralgias, epistaxis, rash, acne, leukopenia, thrombocytopenia, nausea and vomiting, lymphocele, hypokalemia, anemia, hypertension, and infection. The most concerning side effects are dose-related hypertriglyceridemia and hypercholesterolemia. This occurs within the first few weeks of therapy and is sufficiently significant to require intervention with lipid-lowering agents, although it will respond to dosage reduction to some degree.[57] Recently, there have been reports of sirolimus causing proteinuria in renal transplant recipients. The exact mechanism is unknown, but many transplant centers are now routinely monitoring for proteinuria in patients on sirolimus therapy.[60]

Therapeutic Drug Monitoring

Monitoring of blood concentrations plays an important role in the dosing of sirolimus. Trough concentrations are obtained and correlate well with sirolimus AUC. Because it has a longer half-life than the CNI, concentrations are obtained less frequently and only 5 to 7 days after a dose change. The target concentration range appears to be between 5 and 15 ng/mL; however, this continues to be refined with more experience. Early studies often achieved concentrations >15 ng/mL, especially if used without a CNI, which were associated with a higher degree of immunosuppression and adverse events.[61] Because sirolimus appears to work synergistically with the CNI, their target concentrations are reduced as well when these agents are used together. Target tacrolimus trough targets are 5 to 10 ng/mL, and the cyclosporine trough targets are 75 to 100 ng/mL.[62]

B.B. could be started on sirolimus at a loading dose of 6 mg, followed by 2 mg daily. Sirolimus blood trough concentration should be obtained 5 to 7 days after initiation. B.B.'s tacrolimus may need to be reduced if concentrations exceed 10 ng/mL. Monitoring parameters should include a fasting lipid panel, complete blood count (CBC), chemistries, and electrolytes.

CNI–Induced Nephrotoxicity

19. C.C. is a 60-year-old man who received a DD kidney transplant 3 years ago. His serum creatinine at 1 year after transplant was 1.8 mg/dL; at 2 years, it was 2.0 mg/dL; now it is 2.3 mg/dL. He says he feels fine. His BP is well controlled and urinalysis is negative for protein. A kidney biopsy conducted at this time indicates that he has no signs of acute or chronic rejection, but has evidence of CNI nephrotoxicity. His current regimen is cyclosporine 275 mg BID, MMF 500 mg BID, and prednisone 5 mg daily. Prednisone was reinstituted at 20 mg daily. His current cyclosporine blood concentration is 120 ng/mL (target 100–150 ng/mL). Why does C.C. have CNI nephrotoxicity?

With CNI nephrotoxicity, the rise in the serum creatinine concentration is more gradual and not as high as that seen with rejection. CNI concentrations may be elevated, although some patients may experience CNI nephrotoxicity even with levels below or within the targeted therapeutic range. Two forms of CNI nephrotoxicity have been identified: functional or acute renal dysfunction and chronic nephrotoxicity.[63]

Acute CNI nephrotoxicity is more likely to occur in the first months after transplantation in most patients receiving therapeutic doses because CNI doses and levels are highest and are being adjusted at this time, whereas chronic toxicity usually takes longer. Functional renal dysfunction, the most common form of renal dysfunction, is characterized by rapid reversal when the CNI dosage is held or reduced. This syndrome typically is not associated with histopathologic abnormalities, which suggests that it is related to severe vasoconstriction of the renal afferent arterioles. Repeated episodes of transient acute renal dysfunction can result in protracted acute renal dysfunction. Recovery of renal function after repeated episodes usually is not complete even when CNI is withdrawn. Protracted acute renal dysfunction can be associated with the development of thrombosis of glomerular arterioles or diffuse, interstitial fibrosis. Alternatively, cyclosporine may exacerbate intravascular thrombus formation or may serve as a stimulus to interstitial cell proliferation. Another syndrome is a chronic, usually irreversible, nephropathy, which often is associated with mild proteinuria and tubular dysfunction. Renal biopsies in allograft patients with chronic cyclosporine-related nephropathy showed tubulointerstitial abnormalities, sometimes with focal glomerular sclerosis.

Nephrotoxicity, one of the most common adverse effects associated with CNI, occurs to some degree in all patients. The pathophysiology of cyclosporine or tacrolimus-induced transient acute renal failure is not understood completely, but seems to be related to its effects on renal vessels. For example, CNI can induce glomerular hypoperfusion secondary to vasoconstriction of the afferent glomerular arteriole, thereby reducing glomerular filtration. One possible explanation for these effects is that cyclosporine alters the balance of prostacyclin and thromboxane A_2 in renal cortical tissue. Increased thromboxane A_2 results in renal vasoconstriction. Endothelin release from renal vascular cells stimulated by CNI also may contribute to this acute effect through its potent vasoconstrictive properties. CNI also can cause a reversible decrease in tubular function. The alterations in tubular function reduce magnesium reabsorption and decrease potassium and uric acid secretion. This may be a result of direct tubular toxicity and possibly the result of thromboxane A_2 stimulation of platelet activation and aggregation. A chronic nephropathy, usually seen after >6 months of therapy, can also occur and may become irreversible. In this situation, renal function progressively declines to a point that dialysis is required.[64]

Concern for chronic nephropathy has led to the development of cyclosporine or tacrolimus withdrawal or substitution protocols, using agents, such as mycophenolate or sirolimus, or protocols using low doses of cyclosporine or tacrolimus.[65] G.P.'s rise in serum creatinine and hypertension in conjunction with a high cyclosporine level suggests acute cyclosporine toxicity as the most likely cause of his findings. In this case, the total cyclosporine dose should be lowered by approximately 25% to 225 mg twice a day, and G.P. should be monitored closely for resolution of the symptoms or worsening if rejection results from lowering the dose. His elevated potassium, uric acid, and low magnesium should correct themselves with this dose reduction if it is acute CNI toxicity. In any case, magnesium should be replaced to maintain a level >1.5 mEq/L. If the nephrotoxicity is caused by cyclosporine, a decrease in the serum concentration of creatinine may be evident when the cyclosporine dose is reduced. If no such reduction occurs or if the serum concentration of creatinine continues to increase, then a renal biopsy is needed to rule out rejection, nephrotoxicity, or other causes.

CNI Avoidance, Withdrawal, or Minimization

20. Would it be appropriate to withdraw cyclosporine in C.C.? If attempted, how could this be accomplished?

Cyclosporine and tacrolimus are associated with a number of metabolic, cardiovascular, neurologic and cosmetic side effects but the most concerning is nephrotoxicity, which contributes to graft loss. The potential benefit of withdrawing cyclosporine would be to reduce toxicity, but this has to be weighed against the risk for rejection, graft loss, and toxicities of replacement agents.

IL-2R antibodies, sirolimus, and mycophenolate, which are not associated with nephrotoxicity, are being evaluated in protocols that attempt to avoid, minimize, or withdraw CNI. Alternative regimens that have included sirolimus, mycophenolate, and steroids; sirolimus and steroids; and daclizumab, mycophenolate, and steroids have been compared with cyclosporine-based regimens or historical data. Studies, which were usually done in low-risk populations, generally produced reduced serum creatinines and CNI-induced toxicities, but were associated with high rates of acute rejection (30%–50%). More recent trials in small numbers of patients that compared combinations of Thymoglobulin or basiliximab, sirolimus, mycophenolate, and steroids with either cyclosporine- or tacrolimus-containing regimens have shown equal effectiveness with acute rejection rates of <15%.[66]

In the case of cyclosporine withdrawal, a 10% to 20% increased risk of acute rejection appears to exist, but no change in graft survival. Several protocols are being developed that either withdraw the CNI or at least reduce the dose to a minimal level. Many are attempting to do this earlier after transplantation in the hope that the nephrotoxic effects can be reversed before significant chronic damage occurs. These approaches add mycophenolate, sirolimus, or both as the CNI is withdrawn or reduced in dose. Most protocols have been tested in small numbers of low-risk patients. A few larger studies have used a low-risk population.[67] In one of these, all patients received cyclosporine, sirolimus, and corticosteroids as their initial immunosuppressant regimen. In one arm, at 3 months after transplantation, cyclosporine was decreased and withdrawn over 6 to 8 weeks while sirolimus and steroids were maintained. In the other arm, cyclosporine, sirolimus, and corticosteroids were continued throughout the study period. Acute rejection rates were 9.8% in the CNI withdrawal group compared with 4.2% in the nonwithdrawal group. Renal function was better and BP lower, in the withdrawal group. In the withdrawal group, however, side effects associated with sirolimus, such as thrombocytopenia, hypokalemia, hyperlipidemia, and elevated liver function tests (LFT), were more frequent and many patients dropped out of the study. In a mycophenolate-based study, in which cyclosporine was withdrawn, improvements were seen in patients who did not develop acute rejection. Acute rejection episodes occurred in 10% in the withdrawal group with no graft loss and lower lipid profiles.[68] Usually, when sirolimus is added to the CNI regimen, the CNI dose is reduced by 50% initially and in some cases slowly withdrawn altogether over several weeks to months. Improvement in serum creatinine may be seen initially, which may be attributed to the diminution of the CNI vasoconstrictive effects.

This approach may not reverse the nephrotoxicity observed in C.C.'s biopsy, but it may slow the rate of deterioration of his renal function. Because C.C. is currently receiving mycophenolate, one approach would be to continue to reduce his cyclosporine, increase his mycophenolate and maintain steroids. Another approach would be to replace the mycophenolate with sirolimus, maintain steroids, and reduce or withdraw the cyclosporine. The best regimen for someone such as C.C. has not been established, since the long-term consequences of these changes are not known. If this approach is attempted, C.C. should be watched carefully for acute rejection, and side effects of these agents and infections should be closely monitored. In addition, BP control as well as control of hyperlipidemia and hyperglycemia could improve with reduction or withdrawal of cyclosporine and could also be important in minimizing renal injury.[52]

Steroid Avoidance or Withdrawal

21. D.T., a 60-year-old white woman, will receive a DD kidney transplant today because she has a negative cross-match to this donor and her previous PRA was <10%. She will be given one

dose of alemtuzumab 30 mg IV and 1 dose of methylprednisolone 500 mg IV intraoperatively. After transplant, she will be started on tacrolimus 0.025 mg/kg BID, adjusted to trough levels of 8 to 12 ng/mL for the first 3 months, along with MMF 750 mg BID. Methylprednisolone IV will be given as 250 mg IV on postoperative day (POD) 1, 125 mg IV on POD 2 and 3, and then discontinued. Is D.T. a good candidate for steroid avoidance or withdrawal?

Another important issue after kidney transplantation is the role of short- and long-term steroid use. Most transplant protocols incorporate steroid therapy, although an increasing number of protocols use steroids only in the early postoperative period.[20] The concept of either avoiding or discontinuing corticosteroids is appealing because they cause significant adverse effects such as diabetes, cataracts, infection, hypertension, hyperlipidemia, osteoporosis, and avascular necrosis, and have psychiatric, neurologic and cosmetic effects. Steroid withdrawal or avoidance, however, could increase the risk of acute rejection, compromise long-term graft function, and necessitate higher doses of the other immunosuppressives.[15]

Steroid avoidance is defined as either no steroid use or steroid use only for the first few days after transplant. Preliminary studies suggest no adverse impact on short-term graft survival exists and no need is seen for higher doses of other immunosuppressives when corticosteroids are not included in maintenance regimens. These protocols have included regimens such as alemtuzumab; daclizumab, basiliximab, or Thymoglobulin; mycophenolate or sirolimus; and cyclosporine or tacrolimus.[15,30,52,53]

Steroid withdrawal in the era of cyclosporine (Sandimmune)- and azathioprine-based regimens was associated with a high rate of acute rejection and late graft loss. With the introduction of newer agents, steroid avoidance or withdrawal has been viewed with renewed interest. Steroid withdrawal has been successful in at least 50% of kidney transplant recipients—resulting in reductions in BP and lipid levels. Some protocols have withdrawn corticosteroids within the first few days to weeks after the initial transplantation period, whereas others attempt to withdraw them 3 to 6 months or later after transplantation. The rate of success depends not only on the immunosuppressives used, but on the population (high risk vs. low risk) and timing of withdrawal. Regimens that appear most successful include an antibody with cyclosporine or tacrolimus, mycophenolate, or sirolimus. In terms of population, blacks, pediatric patients, patients who have retransplants, highly sensitized patients, and patients with a high serum creatinine (>2.5 mg/dL) those who have had a recent rejection episode are more difficult to withdraw from steroids. This is particularly true early (<3 months) after transplantation. Withdrawal in these cases is associated with a higher rate of rejection. Later withdrawal may be attempted, but the benefits in terms of side-effect profile may not be as great. Low-risk populations are candidates for steroid avoidance or early withdrawal. First-time transplantation, living-donor, well-matched transplantation, older age, and stable graft function without rejection are factors associated with a positive response to steroid withdrawal.[69]

D.T. would be considered a low-risk patient because of her low immunologic activity evidenced by a low PRA, her age, and ethnicity. Therefore a steroid avoidance protocol, such as the one indicated above, would be appropriate. As with other transplant recipients, she must be closely monitored for rejection and adverse effects.

BK Polyomavirus Infection

22. K.T., a 45-year-old white man, is now 16 months post-transplant. His post-transplantation course has been complicated by two rejection episodes. The first was severe and required Thymoglobulin therapy; the second was a mild rejection several weeks later that was adequately treated with three pulse-doses of 500 mg of IV methylprednisolone. His current immunosuppressant regimen consists of tacrolimus 8 mg PO BID, MMF 1 g PO BID, and prednisone 10 mg PO daily. In addition, he is receiving amlodipine 10 mg PO daily, benazepril 10 mg PO daily, pravastatin 40 mg PO at bedtime, and calcium with vitamin D 500 mg PO BID. Today, he is in the transplant clinic for a routine follow-up visit. He has no complaints and says he has been feeling "great," although he has noticed some blood in his urine over the past couple of weeks. Because of this, a urinalysis is ordered in addition to the standard laboratory values. The results are as follows: Na, 145 mEq/L (normal, 135–145); K, 4.2 mEq/L (normal, 3.4–4.6); Cl, 104 mEq/L (normal, 95–105); HCO_3, 26 mEq/L (normal, 22–28); BUN, 32 mg/dL (normal, 8–18); SrCr, 2.7 mg/dL (normal, 0.6–1.2); Ca, 10.1 mEq/L (normal, 8.8–10.3); phosphorus, 4.5 mg/dL (normal, 2.5–5.0); glucose, 110 mg/dL (normal, 65–110); amylase, 50 U/L (normal, 27–150); lipase, 32 U/L (normal, 10–50); WBC count, 7.7 cells/mm^3 (normal, 4,000–10,000); Hgb, 10.4 g/dL (normal, 14–18); and Hct, 31% (normal, 39%–49%); tacrolimus trough level of 9 ng/mL; urinalysis, color yellow (normal, clear–yellow); specific gravity, 1.013 (normal, 1.003–1.030); pH, 7.0 (normal, 5.0–7.0); protein 100 mg/dL (normal, negative–trace); glucose, negative (normal, negative); ketones, negative (normal, negative), bilirubin, negative (normal, negative), blood, moderate (normal, negative); nitrite, negative (normal, negative) leukocyte, negative (normal, negative); squamous epithelial cells, 3 cells/high power field (HPF) (normal, 0–5 cells/HPF); bacteria, negative (normal, negative). Urinalysis revealed "decoy" cells and plasma BKV PCR was $>10^4$. Because of the increasing serum creatinine, a percutaneous kidney biopsy is performed. The pathologist reviews the histology of the tissue sample and determines that it is consistent with BK virus nephritis. What is BK polyomavirus? How is it diagnosed and what are its clinical manifestations?

BK virus is a human polyomavirus, first isolated in 1971. Polyomaviruses are small, nonenveloped viruses with a closed, circular, double-stranded DNA sequence. Little is known about the transmission or about the primary infection of BK virus. It is believed that viremia during the initial exposure results in systemic seeding and subsequently into a latent infection. The kidney is the main site of BK virus latency in healthy people. More than 50% of the general population express BK virus antibodies by age 3. Immunosuppression after transplantation probably leads to the reactivation of the virus, but other factors, such as organ ischemia and coinfection with other pathogens, may contribute to reactivation. Reactivation inevitably leads to viruria or viral shedding into the urine. Asymptomatic viruria occurs in approximately 10% to 45% of renal transplant recipients.[70]

Diagnosis of BK virus nephritis is made by careful review of clinical, laboratory, and histologic findings. Patients are often asymptomatic, although hematuria has been noted in some patients. Clinically, BK virus nephritis mimics acute rejection very closely. Increases in serum creatinine often lead clinicians to perform a tissue biopsy. Tissue histology is very similar in cases of acute rejection and BK virus nephritis, with mononuclear infiltration as the predominant finding. The abundance of plasma cells, prominent tubular cell apoptosis, collecting duct destruction, and absence of endarteritis are features that may distinguish BK virus nephritis from acute cellular rejection. Although BK virus has been implicated in up to 5% of all cases of interstitial nephritis (of which 30% go on to graft failure), it is still unclear whether asymptomatic biopsy findings in the kidney transplant recipient is a prognostic indicator. Decoy cells in the urine and BKV-PCR in blood are used as screening tools. Blood or plasma BKV-PCR is a more sensitive and stable test and correlates better with renal dysfunction.[57]

Most cases of BK nephritis occur within the first 3 months after transplantation, although a number of cases have been reported as long as 2 years after transplantation. The major risk factor for the development of BK nephritis and subsequent graft dysfunction or loss is the degree of immunosuppression. In addition, accelerated graft loss has been demonstrated in patients who received antilymphocyte antibodies in the presence of BK virus nephritis misdiagnosed as an acute rejection episode. Because K.T. has received higher doses of immunosuppression recently to treat two acute rejection episodes, he is at higher risk for developing BK virus nephritis.

Treatment

23. **K.T. is told to stop taking MMF and to reduce his tacrolimus dose to 4 mg PO BID with target trough levels <6 ng/mL. Why was K.T.'s immunosuppressive regimen significantly reduced?**

Because BK virus reactivation and BK nephritis are strongly associated with the degree of immunosuppression, reduction in, or removal of, immunosuppressant agents is considered first-line therapy. Beneficial clinical responses have been demonstrated in some patients when the dose of CNI is reduced. Not all patients, however, respond to this maneuver. In addition, reduction in immunosuppression puts patients at higher risk for an acute rejection episode. Close clinical follow-up after reduction of immunosuppression is important to ensure adequate response and to make sure the patient does not develop an acute rejection episode. In K.T.'s case, an improvement of renal function can be expected, as seen by a reduction in serum creatinine over time. Also, monitoring viral loads both from the urine and serum have been shown to correlate with clinical disease.[57]

Antiviral Therapy

24. **Over the next 2 weeks, K.T.'s serum creatinine remains unchanged, and his serum and urine viral loads also remain approximately the same. Are there any additional treatment options for K.T.'s BK nephritis at this time?**

Cidofovir (Vistide), an antiviral agent indicated for the treatment of CMV retinitis, inhibits polyomavirus replication in vitro; however, to date, no well-conducted clinical trials have proved this agent to be effective in treating or preventing BK virus nephritis in the transplant population. In a small number of case reports and case-series, this agent was beneficial, but the appropriate dose and frequency are still undetermined. Most reports have used very small doses (0.25–1.0 mg/kg/dose) given IV either weekly or every other week; cidofovir was continued until renal dysfunction resolved and a decrease in the viral load occurred.

Cidofovir is associated with a high incidence of nephrotoxicity, especially at much higher doses; therefore, patients usually receive pre- and postdose hydration with 0.9% NaCl boluses. Close clinical monitoring of the patient is advised if this treatment option is used. Because the doses of cidofovir currently used are approximately 5% to 10% of the standard dose used to treat CMV (5 mg/kg/dose), use of probenecid as a premedication to prevent nephrotoxicity is not advocated. Other therapies that have been tried with or without success are IVIG and leflunomide in place of the discontinued antimetabolite, such as mycophenolate, and fluoroquinolones. Retransplantation has also been conducted with some success.[71]

New Onset Diabetes After Transplant (NODAT)

25. **J.F. is a 28-year-old black man who received a kidney transplant 6 weeks ago secondary to focal segmental glomerulosclerosis (FSGS), a glomerulonephridity of unknown etiology. His medical history is significant for hypertension and nephrotic syndrome. Before the transplant, he was taking lisinopril 20 mg PO daily, amlodipine 10 mg PO daily, and valsartan 160 mg PO daily. After the transplant, J.F. was started on tacrolimus, with his current dose being 12 mg PO BID, mycophenolate mofetil 1 gm PO BID, and a corticosteroid taper. He is currently receiving 20 mg PO BID of prednisone, and will be tapered down over the next 6 weeks to 10 mg PO daily. J.F.'s tacrolimus trough concentrations have been between 10 and 14 ng/L. Over the next 12 weeks, he will be maintained on a dose of tacrolimus to achieve trough concentrations between 8 and 12 ng/L. J.F. currently weighs 108 kg and is 6 feet tall. His BMI is 32 kg/m^2. After transplant, he has required a sliding-scale regular insulin regimen to maintain a blood glucose level between 120 and 180 mg/dL.**

What post-transplant complications are common and what is J.F. at risk of developing?

Post-transplantation diabetes mellitus (PTDM), or now more commonly referred to in the transplant literature as new onset diabetes after transplant (NODAT), is another common problem that appears to be on the increase in transplant recipients, similar to the increase in diabetes mellitus in the general population. Diabetes significantly affects morbidity and mortality in transplant recipients. It is often a pre-existing condition in renal transplant recipients and a cause of ESRD. In recipients of other organs, such as livers, diabetes is common as well, both as a pre-existing condition and as a post-transplantation complication. The definition of NODAT varies among studies. It has been based on symptoms and plasma glucose, oral glucose challenge results, or the need for insulin or oral antidiabetic drugs after transplantation.[72] Reported rates range from 3% to >40%, with most cases of NODAT occurring within the first year after transplantation. Risk factors, besides pre-transplantation diabetes, include advanced age, family history, CMV infection, certain HLA phenotypes, race (black or Hispanic), increased BMI, and infection with hepatitis C in the liver transplant population.[73]

One of the most critical factors in the development of NODAT is the immunosuppressive regimen. Cyclosporine, tacrolimus, sirolimus, and prednisone are all diabetogenic through a multitude of mechanisms. The CNI appear to have a direct toxic effect on the pancreatic beta cells leading to decreased insulin synthesis and secretion; this effect seems to be dose related and generally reversible.[74,75] Although still debated by a few clinicians, the literature now clearly suggests that tacrolimus is more likely to cause NODAT than cyclosporine.[74] Additionally, conversion from tacrolimus to cyclosporine has been useful in some patients with NODAT.[76] In evaluating these studies, other factors, such as CNI drug concentrations, steroid doses, black race, transplant type, and time lapsed following transplantation, must be considered.[77]

As with diabetes in the general population, a similar intensive approach in controlling blood glucose should be undertaken. Also, other conditions (e.g., hypertension and hyperlipidemia) should be managed aggressively. Another step includes reducing or withdrawing diabetes-inducing immunosuppression as much as possible without jeopardizing graft function or using agents that are nondiabetogenic, such as mycophenolate.[60,63] One important aspect of post-transplant diabetes management is to realize the differences in pharmacologic management is this patient population, as compared with patients who are not transplant recipients. Often, in the immediate post-transplant period, because of the rapidly changing organ function, and the dramatic tapering of corticosteroids, patient's antidiabetic medicines may need frequent adjustment. During this first 3 to 4 weeks post-transplant, insulin is the agent of choice owing to the ability to use sliding-scales and rapidly change dosing strategies. Once patients are stabilized on their immunosuppressant regimen, and their organ function has also stabilized, the use of oral agents can be introduced or restarted. Because of metformin's contraindications, it is usually not recommended for use in transplant recipients.[72]

J.F. is requiring insulin post-transplant. By some clinicians' definitions, he would be classified as having NODAT. Other definitions would wait to see if J.F. still required insulin after his immunosuppressant regimen was tapered to lower levels. In either regard, because J.F. is obese and is black, he is considered at high risk for the development of NODAT. At this point, J.F.'s diabetes should continue to be controlled on a sliding-scale insulin regimen. Once J.F.'s immunosuppression regimen is stable, he can be switched to oral antidiabetic agents if needed. J.F. should be counseled on diet and exercise to help control his blood glucose level. Other pharmacologic interventions that may help prevent long-term diabetes in J.F. is changing his tacrolimus to cyclosporine and reducing or withdrawing his prednisone. The risks and benefits of changing immunosuppressant regimens must always be weighed in patients such as J.F. For instance, changing his tacrolimus to cyclosporine may reduce his blood glucose level or prevent NODAT, but it also will put J.F. at higher risk of developing acute rejection. Additionally, reducing or removing J.F.'s steroids may also prevent NODAT, but will likely put J.F. at higher risk of acute rejection.

Post-Transplantation Osteoporosis

Rapid bone loss with the subsequent development of osteopenia or osteoporosis is another common post-transplantation disorder that must be evaluated, prevented, and treated. Osteoporosis, a silent disease, is characterized by low bone mass and microarchitectural deterioration of bone tissue, which increases bone fragility and eventually leads to fracture. Various epidemiologic and cross-sectional studies estimate that 7% to 11% of nondiabetic kidney transplant recipients, 45% of diabetic kidney transplant recipients, 18% to 50% of heart transplant recipients, and 24% to 65% of liver transplant recipients develop atraumatic fractures resulting from osteoporosis in the post-transplantation period.[78]

RISK FACTORS

Osteoporosis risk factors for transplant recipients, which are similar to those in the general population, include menopausal status, family history, smoking, alcohol use, lack of physical activity, poor nutritional status, and use of various medications, such as corticosteroids, phenytoin, thyroxine, heparin, warfarin, and loop diuretics.[78] Additional factors responsible for bone loss in organ transplant recipients depend on the underlying disease state and the particular organ system transplanted. For example, patients with ESRF commonly have at least some evidence of renal osteodystrophy, which includes hyperparathyroidism, osteomalacia, osteosclerosis, and adynamic or aplastic bone disease. Hypogonadism can also be present. Many renal transplant recipients have already been exposed to medications that can affect bone and mineral metabolism, such as corticosteroids, cyclosporine for immune complex disease, loop diuretics, or aluminum-containing phosphate binders.[79] Low bone mass and abnormal mineral metabolism are common in patients with several forms of chronic cholestatic liver disease, such as biliary cirrhosis. Therefore, liver transplant recipients are susceptible to this problem.[80]

Drugs used to prevent organ rejection predispose patients to osteoporosis, especially the corticosteroids.[81] Most transplant recipients, however, require steroids in combination with other immunosuppressive agents to prevent rejection. As noted, efforts are underway among transplant centers to develop corticosteroid-free or rapid-taper corticosteroid immunosuppressant regimens to help prevent post-transplant bone disease. Corticosteroids reduce net intestinal calcium absorption, increase urinary calcium excretion, increase parathyroid hormone, decrease production of skeletal growth factors, and decrease androgen and estrogen synthesis in the gonads and adrenal gland. They also decrease bone formation by osteoblasts and increase bone resorption.[81] The most dramatic reduction in bone loss after transplantation occurs within the first 3 to 6 months, when high doses of steroids are tapered to prednisone doses equivalent to 7.5 to 10 mg every day. Areas of the skeleton rich in trabecular or cancellous bone, such as the ribs, vertebrae, distal ends of long bones, and the cortical rim of the vertebral body, are most at risk for osteoporotic fracture because (a) a greater degree of bone remodeling or bone turnover occurs in these areas and (b) this is a target of corticosteroid activity.[78] Most studies suggest a minor effect from CNI on bone. Other currently used agents appear to have little or no effect.[79]

TREATMENT

Because rapid bone loss and fractures can occur during the first few months postoperatively, strategies to prevent bone loss and fractures should be initiated immediately after transplantation and if possible before transplantation. Most recommendations are based on the American College of Rheumatology's (ACR) guidelines for the prevention and treatment of corticosteroid-induced osteoporosis.[82] These recommendations focus on providing calcium (1,500 mg elemental calcium three times a day) and vitamin D (various dosing depending on kidney and liver functions) to patients who will be receiving continuous corticosteroid therapy. If patients are diagnosed with low bone mineral density (osteopenia) or even osteoporosis with bone mineral density scans using dual energy x-ray absorptionmetry (DXA) scans, calcium and vitamin D analogs are recommended in conjunction with either a bisphosphonate or calcitonin.[81]

Clinical trials have demonstrated that bisphosphonates and vitamin D analogs have had the best results in preventing and treating post-transplant bone disease. Because of their lack of size and short follow-up time, these studies have failed, however, to show a significant improvement in meaningful outcomes, including reduction in bone fracture rates, bone pain, or immobility owing to bone disease. Most studies show that these agents can minimize the loss of bone post-transplant, as demonstrated by stabilization of DXA scans.[83]

Although J.F. is young and likely does not have severe bone disease, a DXA scan should still be performed, and he should be given calcium and vitamin D because he is receiving steroids (unless he has a contraindication to this therapy, such as hypercalcemia). Based on the results of J.F.'s DXA scan, he may need to receive either a bisphosphonate or an activated vitamin D analog, such as calcitriol, and continue calcium supplementation. A repeat DXA scan should be performed in 1 to 2 years. J.F. should be carefully counseled on how to take his medicine correctly to minimize adverse effects and he should be monitored for hypo- or hypercalcemia.

LIVER TRANSPLANTATION

Indications

26. E.P., a 58-year-old, 78-kg man, with an 18-year history of chronic liver disease secondary to hepatitis C infection, arrives at the emergency room with a 2-day history of confusion, fever up to 102.2°F, and worsening jaundice, with scleral icterus. Because the patient has severe abdominal distention, a paracentesis is performed, and 7 L of fluid is drained from his peritoneal cavity. A diagnosis of spontaneous bacterial peritonitis is made.

E.P.'s clinical status over the next several days gradually worsens, and he is moved to the intensive care unit for closer monitoring and better supportive care. E.P. continues to be severely jaundiced, with worsening Liver Function Test (LFT). He becomes progressively more confused, and eventually comatose, requiring intubation. Within 3 days of admission into the intensive care unit (ICU), a suitable liver donor, matched for size and ABO blood group, is found, and E.P. receives an orthotopic liver transplant with a choledochocholedochostomy (duct-to-duct anastomosis). Cytomegalovines (CMV) serology for E.P. is negative, and the donor liver is CMV-positive.

After the transplantation, E.P. is started on fluid maintenance with 45% NS; nystatin suspension 5 mL four times daily (QID); tacrolimus 2 mg NG/PO BID; and high-dose methylprednisolone with a rapid taper: 50 mg IV Q 6 hours for four doses, 40 mg IV Q 6 hr for four doses, 30 mg IV Q 6 hours for four doses, 20 mg IV Q 6 hr for four doses, 20 mg IV Q 12 hours for two doses, then 20 mg IV daily; famotidine 20 mg IV Q 12 hr; and ganciclovir 150 mg IV daily. Ampicillin sulbactam 1.5 g IV Q 6 hr for 48 hours was begun just before transplantation. An order also is written to limit all pain medications and sedatives. E.P. returned from surgery with three abdominal Jackson-Pratt (J-P) drains, an nasogastric (NG) tube. Foley catheter, and Swan-Ganz central venous catheter. What was the indication for E.P. to receive a liver transplant?

E.P. was diagnosed with end-stage hepatic failure (cirrhosis) caused by chronic hepatitis C infection. The most common indication for liver transplantation in adults is cirrhosis from various causes. Each transplantation center varies with respect to the most common disease states that indicate transplantation, but nationwide, hepatitis C and alcohol-induced disease are the number one and two reasons for patients requiring liver transplantation. Indications for liver transplantation in adults include cholestatic liver disease (e.g., primary biliary cirrhosis and primary sclerosing cholangitis), hepatocellular liver disease (e.g., chronic viral hepatitis B or C, autoimmune, drug-induced, cryptogenic cirrhosis), vascular disease (e.g., Budd-Chiari), hepatic malignancy, inherited metabolic disorders, and fulminant hepatic failure (e.g., viral hepatitis, Wilson's disease, drug or toxin induced). Controversial indications include alcohol-induced disease and some types of hepatic malignancies. The concern with these indications is either recurrence of disease, as in the case of hepatic malignancies, or recidivism in the case of alcoholics.[84–86]

Contraindications to transplantation have decreased in numbers over the past few years. Current contraindications to liver transplantation include malignancy outside the liver, cholangiocarcinoma, active infection outside the biliary system, patients with alcoholic liver disease who continue to abuse alcohol, psychosocial instability and noncompliance, severe neurologic disease, and advanced cardiopulmonary disease. Patients with active infections are considered candidates after the infection has been eradicated.[86] HIV infection is not considered an absolute contraindication to transplantation.[87]

E.P. was within the age limitations for transplantation; he had severe progressive disease and was at risk for death if he had not received a liver transplant. Because he did not have any of the listed contraindications, a liver could be transplanted emergently. His anticipated survival after transplantation at 1 year is >80%; at 5 years it is >70%.[84]

Patient Monitoring

27. How should E.P. be monitored in the initial postoperative period?

A typical course is as follows. E.P. should be awake and alert within 12 to 24 hours after the operation, transferred from the ICU to a regular bed in 1 to 3 days, and discharged home within 7 to 14 days if he has a standard postoperative course with no severe complications. Because function of the transplanted liver is essential for the survival of the patient, extensive clinical, laboratory, and radiologic monitoring are necessary. E.P. has three J-P abdominal drains that must be monitored for output production. The serum concentrations of BUN, creatinine, LFT, albumin, potassium, sodium, magnesium, calcium, phosphate, and glucose should be monitored every 6 hours on the first postoperative day.[88] The surgical transplantation of a liver has been associated with coagulopathies and bleeding. Therefore, platelets, prothrombin time, fibrinogen, and factors V and VII also must be monitored and deficiencies rapidly corrected.[89]

Initial LFT results are highly variable; they can either increase for the first day or two after transplantation because of ischemic damage to the allograft, or they can decrease because of initial dilution by high-volume blood replacement. If the liver is functioning well, the LFT, bilirubin, and prothrombin time all should begin to trend toward normal within 4 to 5 days after the operation.

Magnesium, phosphate, and calcium levels may fall in the early postoperative period and should be monitored closely. Ionized calcium serum concentrations are monitored rather than total calcium because most patients have low serum albumin concentrations. Hypocalcemia can occur because these patients may receive large amounts of citrate through blood transfusions, which can lower serum calcium concentrations. Magnesium deficiency is common in patients with end-stage liver disease and may be exacerbated in the early post-transplantation period by tacrolimus or diuretics. Why patients develop hypophosphatemia is unclear, but increased demand for phosphate for incorporation into adenosine triphosphate is a possible explanation. Hypokalemia or hyperkalemia can occur, depending on renal function and fluid status. Electrolyte serum concentrations should be followed and electrolytes replaced if needed (see Chapter 11, Fluid and Electrolyte Disorders).

Hyperglycemia, which is a good indication of a properly functioning liver in this early period, may need to be controlled with a continuous IV infusion of insulin, initially, and then subcutaneous insulin dosed on the basis of periodic glucose measurements. In contrast, persistent hypoglycemia indicates a poorly functioning liver. Hypertension, which is multifactorial, also is seen during this time and usually is treated with calcium channel blockers, nitroglycerin, nitroprusside, or ß-blockers. Renal dysfunction and neurologic complications also can occur.[88,90] Neurologic complications, including those that are drug induced, include oversedation, acute psychosis, depression, tremor, headaches, peripheral neuropathy, cortical blindness, paresthesias, paresis, and seizures.[90]

Other complications that can occur within the first 3 days to 3 weeks include respiratory distress, intra-abdominal hemorrhage, biliary tract leaks and strictures, hepatic artery thrombosis, and primary graft nonfunction. Because infection is another early postoperative concern, E.P. should be monitored for bacterial, fungal, and viral infections.

Tacrolimus

Pharmacokinetics

28. Seven days after his liver transplantation, E.P.'s J-P abdominal drains, Foley catheter, and NG drain have been removed. Current medications include tacrolimus (Prograf) 2 mg PO Q 12 hours; prednisone 20 mg PO daily; nystatin suspension 500,000 U to swish and swallow QID; amlodipine 5 mg PO daily; TMP-SMX SS, one tablet every Monday, Wednesday, and Friday; and valganciclovir 900 mg PO daily. E.P.'s current laboratory values include the following: BUN, 27 mg/dL (normal, 8–18); SrCr, 0.9 mg/dL (normal, 0.6–1.2); AST, 170 U/L (normal, 0–35); ALT, 154 U/L (normal, 0–35); γ-glutamyl transferase (GGT), 320 U/L (normal, 0–30); total bilirubin, 3.4 mg/dL (normal, 0.1–1.0); and tacrolimus 9.4 ng/dL (whole blood by mass spectrometry). What important pharmacokinetic factors should be considered when using tacrolimus after transplantation?

[SI units: BUN, 9.6 mmol/L (normal, 3.0–6.5); SrCr, 79.6 μmol/L (normal, 50–110); AST, 170 U/L (normal, 0–35); ALT, 154 U/L (normal, 0–35); GGT, 320 U/L (normal, 0–30); total bilirubin, 58.14 μmol/L (normal, 2–18)]

Tacrolimus is a very lipophilic compound that is absorbed rapidly after oral administration in most patients. Peak blood concentrations are achieved in about 0.5 to 1 hour. Some patients have slower absorption or have a lag time of up to 2 hours in their absorption profiles. Oral bioavailability is usually poor, highly variable, and ranges from 4% to 89% (mean 25%). Protein binding is approximately 75% and is mainly to erythrocytes. Whole blood concentrations are significantly higher than serum concentrations for this reason. Tacrolimus has a large volume of distribution and accumulates in high concentrations in tissues, including the lungs, spleen, heart, kidney, brain, muscles, and liver. Tacrolimus is predominantly metabolized in the liver through the cytochrome P450 3A4 isoenzyme system and is primarily eliminated from the body as several inactive metabolites. Less than 1% of tacrolimus is eliminated as the parent compound in the urine, and renal dysfunction does not alter the pharmacokinetics of this agent. The elimination half-life ranges from 5.5 to 16.6 hours, with a mean of 8.7 hours, and plasma clearance averages 143 L/hour. Varying degrees of liver dysfunction, including cirrhosis and severe cholestasis, may have dramatic effects on the metabolism and excretion of tacrolimus. Pediatric patients appear to clear tacrolimus more rapidly and have a shorter half-life and larger volume of distribution compared with adults.[91] Black patients may require higher dosages.[92]

Dosing

29. How would you initiate the dosing of tacrolimus for E.P.?

Although tacrolimus can be administered as a continuous IV infusion through a central or peripheral infusion after transplantation (initial dose 0.025–0.05 mg/kg/day), it is preferable to give it via an NG tube or orally because adverse effects, such as headache, nausea, vomiting, neurotoxicity, and nephrotoxicity, occur more commonly with IV administration. If tacrolimus is given IV, patients should be converted as soon as possible to oral therapy (initial doses of 0.1–0.3 mg/kg/day in adults and 0.15–0.3 mg/kg/day in children divided into 12-hour intervals). Pediatric patients require two to three times the adult doses of tacrolimus.

In E.P., the initial starting dose was approximately 0.15 mg/kg/day given orally or through the NG tube every 12 hours. Oral tacrolimus should be administered on an empty stomach or taken consistently in relation to meals. Most institutions extemporaneously prepare an oral solution for NG tube administration because it is not commercially available.

30. How would you convert a patient from cyclosporine to tacrolimus?

Although E.P. was initiated on tacrolimus without prior exposure to cyclosporine, many patients are converted from cyclosporine to tacrolimus either because of a poor response (as evidenced by recurrent acute rejection episodes) or intolerance (as evidenced by persistent adverse drug reactions, most commonly gingival hyperplasia or unwanted hair growth). When switching from cyclosporine to tacrolimus, the cyclosporine should be discontinued 24 hours before initiating tacrolimus therapy or longer if cyclosporine concentrations are elevated. The concomitant administration of cyclosporine and tacrolimus has been accompanied by increases in the serum concentrations of creatinine and urea nitrogen, which decline after the discontinuation of cyclosporine. Thus, combination therapy with cyclosporine and tacrolimus is not recommended because of the additive or synergistic risk of nephrotoxicity.

Therapeutic Drug Monitoring

31. E.P.'s tacrolimus concentrations are being measured by whole blood IMx® immunoassay. Why is it important to monitor E.P.'s tacrolimus concentrations and how should his tacrolimus therapy be monitored?

Because of the large inter- and intrapatient variability, the narrow therapeutic index, and the large number of potential drug interactions associated with this agent, tacrolimus concentrations should be monitored in all patients receiving therapy. Concentrations are monitored to prevent toxicity, optimize efficacy, and assess patient compliance to the prescribed regimen. A relationship does appear to exist among concentration, efficacy, and toxicity.[93] The primary monitoring parameter used clinically is the trough concentration because, unlike cyclosporine, trough concentrations correlate well with overall total body exposure (AUC).[94] Because of accuracy in measuring the tacrolimus parent compound (without measuring inactive metabolites) and a rapid turnaround time (within hours), the microparticle enzyme immunassay (IMx®) assay method for tacrolimus that uses whole blood is the one most commonly used. The target range is 10 to 20 ng/mL for the first 3 months and 5 to 10 ng/mL thereafter, but this can vary with each transplantation center's protocols. More centers are now switching to using mass spectrometry to monitor all immunosuppressant concentrations. Mass spectrometry is a more reliable method of analysis that does not cross-react with metabolites.[95]

As in all cases, pharmacokinetic data must be interpreted in conjunction with the patient's clinical condition. In addition, deference always must be given to trends established by multiple tacrolimus concentrations over that of a single concentration.

Adverse Drug Reactions

32. What are the major adverse effects associated with tacrolimus and what clinical parameters should be monitored in E.P.?

Nephrotoxicity, which usually is the limiting adverse effect of tacrolimus, has been reported in >50% of patients in some studies.[96,97] This may have been related to the higher dosages used in earlier trials because dose reduction usually reverses the nephrotoxicity. The clinical presentation of tacrolimus-induced nephrotoxicity is similar to that of cyclosporine. Because IV administration of tacrolimus during the first week has been associated with acute renal failure in 20% of patients, very few centers use this route or rapidly convert to oral therapy. Presumably, liver recipients with poor graft function are unable to metabolize tacrolimus rapidly and are at a greater risk for acute renal failure.[96] In a multicenter study involving 529 patients, the efficacy and toxicity of tacrolimus was compared with cyclosporine in liver transplant recipients. Both agents increased serum creatinine and decreased glomerular filtration rate comparably.[97] Thus, E.P.'s renal function should be monitored closely.

Major neurologic toxicities (e.g., confusion, seizures, dysarthria, persistent coma) occur in approximately 10% of patients. Minor neurologic toxicities occur in approximately 20% to 60% of patients and include tremors, headache, and sleep disturbances.[97] Hypertension (40%) is another common finding in patients treated with tacrolimus. A greater number of tacrolimus-treated patients, however, are able to discontinue or limit their use of antihypertensives as compared with cyclosporine. Other adverse effects include diarrhea, nausea, vomiting and anorexia, hypomagnesemia, hyperkalemia, hemolytic anemia, hemolytic uremic syndrome, alopecia, increased susceptibility to infection and malignancy, and hyperglycemia. Hyperglycemia is reported to occur often with tacrolimus. This is most likely to be seen in patients with higher tacrolimus levels or higher steroid doses and in blacks. With reduction in tacrolimus and steroid doses, hyperglycemia appears to decrease. Hirsutism and gingival hyperplasia, in contrast to that which occurs with cyclosporine, are not complications of tacrolimus.

Rejection

33. E.P. was discharged from the hospital. He went to stay with his brother and was followed up with laboratory tests obtained three times a week. The following laboratory values were obtained 2 weeks later: AST, 36 U/L (normal, 0–35); ALT, 52 U/L (normal, 0–35); GGT, 65 U/L (normal, 0–30); and total/direct bilirubin, 1.0/0.3 mg/dL (normal, total 0.1–1.0, direct 0–0.3); and another week later: AST, 158 IU/L; ALT, 322 U/L; GGT, 321 U/L; and bilirubin, T/D 3.6/3.2 mg/dL.

E.P. was readmitted to the transplantation center because his LFT findings suggested liver dysfunction, and a percutaneous needle liver biopsy was obtained to determine the cause. On admission, he complained of tiredness, severe headaches, a mild tremor, and some pain over the area of the transplanted liver. E.P. also stated that he had not felt like eating for the last 2 to 3 days. The pathologist interpreted the liver biopsy as moderate rejection, and E.P. was given a 1-g IV bolus of methylprednisolone followed by rapidly tapered doses. This regimen used the following IV doses of methylprednisolone: 50 mg every 6 hours for four doses; 40 mg every 6 hours for four doses; 30 mg every 6 hours for four doses; 20 mg every 6 hours for four doses; 20 mg every 12 hours for two doses; then back to the pretapered oral prednisone dose. Three days into the recycle, E.P.'s liver enzyme values had not improved and Thymoglobulin therapy was initiated. Laboratory values after 10 days of Thymoglobulin IV 1.5 mg/kg/day were as follows: AST, 35 IU/L; ALT, 108 U/L; GGT, 169 U/L; and bilirubin, T/D 1.0/0.6 mg/dL. The 12-hour tacrolimus trough level at the end of the treatment course was 15.2 ng/mL by IMx immunoassay. E.P. was discharged and sent home with the following medications: tacrolimus 5 mg PO BID; prednisone 20 mg PO daily; clonidine 0.3 mg PO BID; felodipine 10 mg PO daily; furosemide 20 mg PO daily; co-trimoxazole one tablet daily Mondays, Wednesdays, and Fridays; and valganciclovir 900 mg PO daily. What subjective and objective evidence of liver rejection is present in E.P.?

[SI units: AST, 36 U/L, 158 U/L, 35 U/L (normal, 0–35); ALT, 52 U/L, 322 U/L, 108 U/L (normal, 0–35); GGT, 65 U/L, 321 U/L, 169 UL (normal,

0–30); bilirubin, 17.1/5.13 μmol/L, 61.56/54.72 μmol/L, 17.1/6.2 μmol/L (normal, 2–18)]

Rejection episodes in liver transplant recipients can be categorized as acute or chronic. Hyperacute rejection rarely occurs with liver transplantation. Treatment is supportive and retransplantation is needed.[98] Unlike other organs, however, the liver may function adequately, but survival is lower when the transplanted organ is incompatible.[99]

Acute Liver Rejection

Although acute liver rejection can occur at any time after the transplantation, it is most commonly experienced within the first week to 6 weeks in approximately 30% to 50% of patients treated with either cyclosporine or tacrolimus and prednisone.[98] Early data in patients treated with tacrolimus, mycophenolate, and prednisone indicate lower rejection rates up to 6 months after transplantation.[100,101] Late acute rejections often are a result of either a reduction in dose or a discontinuation of immunosuppressive agents. These rejection episodes, although common, rarely lead to graft loss.

E.P. presented with some of the common subjective complaints of patients experiencing rejection of their transplanted liver. Commonly, patients feel poorly and complain of anorexia, abdominal discomfort, and headache. Other symptoms, such as a low-grade fever, back pain, or respiratory distress, may occur. Objective evidence for rejection in E.P. included an abrupt rise in serum concentrations of transaminases and bilirubin and a liver biopsy that was interpreted as "moderate rejection" by the pathologist. These observations, in conjunction with the subjective signs, pointed to a diagnosis of rejection. Acute rejection is associated with mononuclear cell infiltration of the graft, edema, and parenchymal necrosis. Rejection should be diagnosed by biopsy using histologic criteria. Areas most commonly damaged are the bile ducts, veins, and arteries.[102]

Chronic Liver Rejection

Chronic liver rejection, also called *ductopenic rejection,* usually develops months to years after the transplant in about 5% of recipients. Characteristics of chronic liver rejection include occlusive arterial lesions, destruction of small intrahepatic bile ducts (often referred to as *vanishing bile duct syndrome*), intense cholestasis, accumulation of foamy macrophages within the portal sinusoids, and fibrosis, which can lead to the development of cirrhosis. Chronic rejection is irreversible and unaffected by increased immunosuppressive therapy. Retransplantation has been considered the only viable alternative. Some patients with ductopenic rejection unresponsive to cyclosporine-based therapy have responded to tacrolimus.[103]

Treatment of Rejection

34. Was the treatment of E.P.'s rejection of his transplanted liver appropriate?

E.P. was receiving maintenance immunosuppression with tacrolimus and prednisone. Double or triple therapy with tacrolimus or cyclosporine and prednisone commonly is used as chronic immunosuppressive therapy in liver transplant recipients. E.P.'s tacrolimus trough whole blood concentration was in the low normal therapeutic range (*Note:* normal values for therapeutic range vary with the institution). Although E.P.'s tacrolimus concentration appeared adequate, he was treated with a bolus dose of IV methylprednisolone because of clinical evidence that supported a diagnosis of graft rejection. This treatment decision was reasonable because high-dose corticosteroids can reverse acute rejection episodes of a transplanted liver.[98] The decision to monitor E.P.'s response to the initial bolus steroid dosage and the severity of rejection by biopsy also was appropriate before proceeding with further treatment. E.P. had experienced moderate rejection of his transplanted liver, and the subsequent initiation of another cycle of corticosteroids was reasonable because the mainstay for treatment of acute liver rejection is increased immunosuppression.

Adult liver transplant recipients usually are treated with 200 mg to 1,000 mg/day of IV methylprednisolone and tapered rapidly, as described for E.P. When patients fail to respond to recycle corticosteroid therapy, several options are available. E.P. was begun on Thymoglobulin therapy; other options include the use of OKT3 or potentially alemtuzumab. Most centers use Thymoglobulin as a second-line agent if there is no response to high-dose corticosteroids or it is used first-line if the rejection is severe. The typical dose is 1.5 mg/kg per day given as an infusion over 4 to 6 hours. Therapy is continued for 7 to 14 days. Treatment of corticosteroid-resistant rejection with Thymoglobulin is effective in about 70% to 80% of liver transplant recipients. Other adjustments in immunosuppression could include the addition of mycophenolate or possibly sirolimus.

Mycophenolate Mofetil

35. Following the rejection episode, E.P. is started on MMF. Describe MMF's pharmacokinetic characteristics and adverse effects. How will these characteristics affect the dosing and monitoring of MMF in this patient?

Mycophenolate mofetil is an alternative to azathioprine. In most transplantation centers, MMF has replaced azathioprine as the antiproliferative agent used in combination with antibodies, CNI, and prednisone. Several studies have shown significant reductions in acute rejection rates during the first year after liver transplant as compared with azathioprine. Results with longer follow-up, at 3 years, indicate no difference in survival, however.[91]

Pharmacokinetics

Mycophenolate mofetil is a prodrug for the active form, MPA. MMF is well absorbed (bioavailability 94%) and is rapidly hydrolyzed to MPA after absorption. The C_{max} for MPA occurs between 1 and 3 hours, and it is hepatically metabolized via glucuronidation to inactive MPAG, which is eliminated by the kidney and excreted into the bile. Once MPAG is excreted into bile, it undergoes enterohepatic recycling in the GI tract, where it is deconjugated to MPA, which is reabsorbed back into the systemic circulation. Because of this recycling, a second peak occurs 6 to 12 hours after dosing. MPA has an elimination half-life of 17 hours on average; the volume of distribution is 4 L/kg, and it is highly protein bound to albumin (98%). Protein binding correlates well with albumin and free MPA concentrations correlate with the immunosuppressive effect. Studies indicate that protein binding changes over time after transplantation, with the free fraction decreasing and total MPA concentrations increasing over time. Renal impairment, liver dysfunction, and elevated MPAG concentrations in transplant recipients can reduce protein binding. This may be a function of low albumin concentrations seen in these patients.[104]

Adverse Effects

The most commonly reported side effects for MMF are GI (anorexia, nausea, vomiting and diarrhea, gastritis), hematologic (leukopenia, thrombocytopenia, anemia), and infectious in nature. GI side effects are common, and all side effects are more common with higher dosages. If a patient complains, try giving the dose without other medications, giving smaller doses more frequently, or lowering the dosage and titrating upward as tolerated.[105] If the WBC count is <3,000 or absolute neutrophil count (ANC) is <1.3, the MMF dose should be reduced or discontinued.

Dosing

The usual starting dose in adults is 1 to 1.5 g twice daily. Some advocate the higher dosage in high-risk patients (e.g., patients receiving another transplant, patients with a high PRA, blacks). Excluding the early post-transplantation period, 1 g two times a day is the recommended regimen in patients with a glomerular filtration rate <25 mL/minute. In heart transplant recipients, the 1.5 g twice daily regimen is used. In children, 300 to 600 mg/M^2 two times a day or 23 mg/kg/day two times a day has been recommended.

Therapeutic Drug Monitoring

Monitoring MPA serum concentrations is controversial and not generally recommended at this time because of so much intrapatient and interpatient pharmacokinetic variability. Some studies, however, have shown a relation between effect and concentrations.[106]

Data in heart transplant recipients indicate that an MPA trough level of >2.5 mg/L is required for therapeutic effect. In kidney transplant recipients, AUC has been shown to correlate with acute rejection. Another approach is to measure free concentrations, but the primary limitation to using serum concentrations is the lack of a simple, commercially available assay. The preceding studies used an HPLC assay, but there are ongoing investigations with an EMIT immunoassay.[107]

Once started on MMF, the patient should be monitored for GI and hematologic side effects, as well as for any signs and symptoms of infection and rejection.

Drug Interactions With Immunosuppressives

36. C.C. is a 42-year-old woman who underwent a liver transplantation 5 days ago. She was noted to be febrile, with an elevated WBC. Cultures were obtained, and her J-P drainage grew *Candida albicans.* C.C. was started on fluconazole 400 mg daily. Her other medications included tacrolimus 3 mg BID, prednisone 20 mg daily, mycophenolate 500 mg BID, valganciclovir 450 mg daily, one-half TMP-SMX DS tablet daily, and esomeprazole 20 mg every night (QHS). The tacrolimus trough level is 11 ng/mL. What drugs interact with immunosuppressive agents? Will the initiation of fluconazole require any adjustments in current medication doses?

Because the immunosuppressants have complex and highly variable pharmacokinetic profiles with relatively narrow therapeutic indexes, drug–drug interactions represent a significant clinical problem. These drug interactions can be separated into two main categories: pharmacokinetic and pharmacodynamic. Pharmacokinetic drug interactions occur when one medication alters the absorption, distribution, metabolism, or elimination of the immunosuppressant agent.[108–110] Table 34-2 displays the most clinically relevant pharmacokinetic drug interactions that are likely to be encountered in transplant recipients and how to manage these interactions when they do occur. These include drugs that alter either the absorption or metabolism of the immunosuppressants. This table is not comprehensive.

Pharmacodynamic drug interactions with the immunosuppressant agents represent another significant problem in transplantation. These interactions occur when one medication either potentiates an adverse effect or alters the pharmacologic effects of the immunsuppressant agent.[108] An example of this would be the use of CNI (cyclosporine and tacrolimus) in combination with ACE inhibitors. Because both classes of agents can cause hyperkalemia and potentially can decrease renal function, toxicity may be more pronounced when these classes are given in combination.[111] Pharmacodynamic drug interactions are usually more difficult to identify and require a thorough knowledge of the pharmacologic effects of the agents being used. Often, little or no information in the literature on these types of interactions exists to guide the clinician in determining whether this drug interaction will occur. As a general rule, if an agent is known to cause a particular toxicity that is similar to a toxicity associated with the immunosuppressant agent, then there is a high likelihood that a pharmacodynamic interaction will occur. Another example is an interaction between metoclopramide and MMF. Both agents are known to cause diarrhea and a higher incidence or severity of diarrhea likely occurs when these agents are used together.[108] It is important to be alert for drugs with pharmacologic effects that may alter the efficacy of an immunosuppressant.[112] For example, a drug with immunosuppressant properties, such as cyclophosphamide, could lead to overimmunosuppression of the transplant recipient and a higher incidence or severity of opportunistic infections. Conversely, a drug with immunostimulant properties, such as the herbal medication echinacea, may reduce the efficacy of the immunsuppressant agent and increase the risk of rejection in the transplant recipient.[108,113] Although agents that have pharmacodynamic drug interactions with the immunosuppressants are not absolutely contraindicated, transplant recipients should be closely monitored for either increased risk of drug toxicity or decreased drug efficacy when these agents are used in combination with the immunosuppressants. When a transplant recipient adds any new medication—whether prescription, over-the-counter, or herbal—it should be thoroughly researched to determine whether there is a potential interaction with the immunosuppressant regimen.

In C.C., the addition of fluconazole will lead to a pharmacokinetic drug interaction and significantly increase (on average double) tacrolimus concentrations. This interaction is usually evident within 2 days, and a maximal effect is seen within a week of initiating fluconazole. Therefore, C.C.'s tacrolimus dose should be reduced by 50% when fluconazole is started. Tacrolimus blood levels should be monitored, as should signs and symptoms of toxicity and rejection. Fluconazole could also

Table 34-2 Immunosuppressant Drug Interactions

Immunosuppressant (IS)	Interacting Drugs	Mechanism	Consequence	Clinical Management	References
Calcineurin inhibitors (cyclosporine and tacrolimus) and sirolimus	Clarithromycin,[a] erythromycin,[a] telithromycin,[a] ketoconazole,[a] itraconazole,[a] fluconazole, voriconazole,[a] fluoxetine, fluvoxamine, citalopram, nefazodone,[a] diltiazem,[a] verapamil,[a] delaviridine,[a] ritonavir,[a] cimetidine,[a] grapefruit juice,[a] amiodarone, saquinavir, nelfinavir, indinavir, amprenavir, chloramphenicol[a]	Inhibit CYP450 3A4 isoenzyme in the liver and intestines.	Increase the concentration and total AUC of the IS.	Either prospectively decrease the IS dose or monitor trough concentrations more closely and adjust doses accordingly.	85, 86, 87, 246
Calcineurin inhibitors (cyclosporine and tacrolimus) and sirolimus	Carbamazepine,[a] dexamethasone, phenobarbital,[a] phenytoin,[a] St. John's Wort,[a] rifampin,[a] rifabutin,[a] efavirenz[a], nevirapine,[a] nafcillin, clindamycin	Induce CYP450 3A4 isoenzyme in the liver and intestines.	Decrease the concentration and total AUC of the IS.	Either prospectively increase the IS dose or monitor trough concentrations more closely and adjust doses accordingly.	86, 87, 245, 246, 247
Calcineurin inhibitors (cyclosporine and tacrolimus), sirolimus, mycophenolate mofetil, and mycophenolate sodium	Cholestyramine, colestipol, probucol, sevelamer, antacids (magnesium and aluminum containing),[b] iron containing products[b]	Bind to IS and prevent absorption.	Decrease the concentration and total AUC of the IS.	Avoid concomitant administration with IS and monitor trough concentrations.	86, 87, 248, 249, 250
Azathioprine	Allopurinol	Inhibits metabolism by inhibiting xanthine oxidase.	Increases the concentration and total AUC of azathioprine.	Avoid use together or prospectively reduce azathioprine dose to one-third or one-fourth normal dose and monitor for increased toxicity.	86, 251

AUC, area under the concentration-time curve.
[a] Indicates potent inhibitor or inducer.
[b] Only occurs with mycophenolate mofetil and mycophenolate sodium.

influence steroid metabolism, but specific recommendations are not available. In general, drug interactions can be managed and, in some cases, may require only separate administration times. In other cases, an alternative agent can be used within a pharmacologic class that does not interact with these agents.

Infection Prophylaxis

37. S.C. is a 20-year-old man who underwent liver transplantation for end-stage liver disease secondary to chronic hepatitis B. Besides his immunosuppressives, he received ampicillin sulbactam 1.5 g Q 8 hours for 24 hours perioperatively. After transplantation, he also was started on TMP-SMX one tablet Mondays, Wednesdays, and Fridays; nystatin 5 mL TID; lamivudine 100 mg daily; and valganciclovir 900 mg PO daily. Hepatitis B immunoglobulin (HBIG) 10,000 U was started intraoperatively and given every day for 8 days after transplantation. What is the rationale for all the aforementioned agents? Should other measures be considered to prevent infection?

Infection continues to be a major source of morbidity and mortality. Transplantation recipients have the same risk of infection from transplant surgery as any other immunocompromised patient having a surgical procedure. The percentage of transplantation recipients who develop infections has decreased since the advent of cyclosporine. Infection rates, however, remain high—50% in transplant recipients.[114]

Prophylactic antimicrobial therapy can decrease the risk of surgical infections in patients having transplantation surgery. As with other therapies in transplantation, prophylactic regimens and antibiotic therapies are highly institution dependent.[115] Kidney transplant recipients typically receive a first-generation cephalosporin, such as cefazolin, to cover uropathogens and staphylococci, both perioperatively and, in some cases, for 2 to 5 days postoperatively. Pancreas transplant recipients usually receive an antibiotic that covers both the skin flora and GI flora, such as ampicillin–sulbactam (Unasyn), because both are breached during the surgical procedure. In addition, because *Candida* is often within the GI flora and because postpancreas transplantation candidal infections occur frequently, prophylaxis with an antifungal such as fluconazole for 3 to 7 days is commonly used. Liver transplantations are associated with the highest rate of life-threatening bacterial infection. Ampicillin–sulbactam (Unasyn) commonly is used to cover staphylococci, enterococci, and *Enterobacteriaceae.* Heart transplant recipients routinely receive a first-generation cephalosporin, such as cefazolin, at anesthesia induction and for 48 hours postoperatively. Cefuroxime or vancomycin is an alternative for resistant organisms. For lung transplant candidates, common practice is to culture the patient's sputum

Table 34-3 Common Opportunistic Infections After Transplantation

Organisms	*Time of Onset After Transplantation*
CMV	1–6 months
HSV	2 weeks–2 months
EBV	2–6 months
VZV	2–6 months
Fungal	1–6 months
Mycobacterium	1–6 months
PCP	1–6 months
Listeria	1 month–indefinitely
Aspergillus	1–4 months
Nocardia	1–4 months
Toxoplasma	1–4 months
Cryptococcus	4 months–indefinitely

CMV, cytomegalovirus; EBV, Epstein-Barr virus; HSV, herpes simplex virus; PCP, *Pneumocystis carinii* pneumonia; VZV, varicella-zoster virus.

before transplantation, individualize the prophylactic regimen to reflect the resident flora, and include an antipseudomonal drug. Duration of therapy in these patients is individualized, based on the patient's postoperative recovery, but usually lasts 7 to 14 days.

Infections can occur at any time after transplantation, but there are predictable time patterns for certain kinds of infections.[114] The time of highest risk for infection in transplant recipients is during the first 6 months, because they are receiving the highest doses of immunosuppressive agents during this period. Another time of high risk is during and after treatment of acute rejection with high-dose immunosuppression. Patients can acquire new infections (*Pneumocystis carinii* pneumonia [PCP], CMV), reactivate old infections (e.g., CMV, BK virus), or develop recurrence of underlying disease (hepatitis B or C). Opportunistic infections are common during this time, as shown in Table 34-3. Because the infections shown in Table 34-3 occur at such a high rate, it is routine to provide specific prophylaxis for many of them. For example, nystatin suspension 500,000 U by "swish and swallow" (S&S) three to four times a day or fluconazole 100 mg every day are used to reduce fungal colonization of the GI tract; acyclovir, ganciclovir, valganciclovir, and immunoglobulins can be used for CMV and herpes virus infections; and TMP-SMX is used for *Pneumocystis* prophylaxis. For patients with sulfa allergies, alternatives, such as dapsone 50 to 100 mg PO daily or inhaled monthly doses of pentamidine 300 mg are used. These generally are given for the first 3 to 6 months after transplantation and, in some cases, up to 1 year or even for life.[116] In S.C., certainly a need exists for prophylaxis with TMP-SMX, valganciclovir, HBIG, and lamivudine or adefovir.

Hepatitis B

Another major concern for S.C. would be recurrence of hepatitis B in his new liver. Hepatitis B recurs and is associated with a poorer outcome.[117] Strategies that have been effective are the use of lamivudine, adefovir, entecavir, and telbivudine preoperatively and HBIG, with or without oral antiviral therapy, postoperatively.[118–121] S.C. was started on lamivudine and HBIG postoperatively because monotherapy with HBIG is associated with recurrence in 10% to 50% patients, whereas HBIG with lamivudine has been associated with development of resistance in 15% to 30% per year. In patients who develop a resistant form of hepatitis B to lamivudine, adefovir, entecavir, and telbivudine have been shown to be effective.[126] The combination of an antiviral with HBIG is currently preferred. After the first week of HBIG, S.C. will continue to receive 10,000 U IV as a 1- to 2-hour infusion weekly for 4 weeks, then 10,000 U monthly for the first 6 to 12 months after transplantation. During this time, anti-HBs titers are monitored and kept >500 U/L. Because HBIG is incredibly expensive to give in this regimen (up to $50,000 per patient per year), some transplantation centers now use lower titers (>100 U/L) and HBIG doses of 1,500 units intramuscularly (IM) every 3 to 4 weeks with lamivudine.[119]

Hepatitis C

Another virus that is a major cause for concern is hepatitis C. Hepatitis C is currently the most common reason for liver transplantation, and recurrence of hepatitis C viral replication after transplantation is universal.[122] Immunosuppression, especially overimmunosuppression, can have a significant detrimental effect on this disease after transplantation. Epidemiologic studies indicate that patient survival rates may be significantly lower at 5 years after transplant compared with patients who received liver transplants for nonhepatitis C causes.[123] Strategies to improve outcomes in hepatitis C-positive liver transplants include using antiviral therapies early post-transplant or waiting later until viral recurrence with pathologic changes on the transplanted liver can be documented. All strategies have varying degrees of efficacy, but the ideal regimen has not been elucidated.[124,125] In all cases, patients should be closely monitored for signs and symptoms of viral reactivation. If this does occur, a liver biopsy may be warranted to determine the severity of liver damage caused by the virus. In aggressive cases, the need for antiviral therapy and reduction in immunosuppression may be warranted.

Immunization

Another important element of S.C.'s care is the need for immunization. Although immunosuppression can blunt the response to some immunizations, the benefits outweigh the risks. At least 6 months after transplantation, he should receive a yearly flu vaccine. He also should receive the pneumococcal and hepatitis A vaccines if he has not yet done so. Live vaccines should be avoided.[126]

Treatment of infection in transplantation recipients should be based on principles established for other immunocompromised patients (see Chapter 68, Prevention and Treatment of Infections in Neutropenic Cancer Patients). One major difference between transplant recipients and other immunocompromised hosts is that the immunocompromised condition of transplant recipients is iatrogenic, secondary to their immunosuppression. Therefore, when a transplant recipient develops a life-threatening infection, the doses of immunosuppressants are usually decreased or, in some cases, discontinued. After the patient has recovered from the infection, immunosuppression can be restored to preinfection levels.

Cytomegalovirus

38. A.A., a 58-year-old, 76-kg man with end-stage liver disease caused by alcoholic cirrhosis, received an orthotopic liver transplant 16 weeks ago. He presents to the transplantation clinic with a 3-day history of generalized malaise, fatigue, nausea, vomiting, diarrhea, fever, and anorexia. At the time of transplantation, the liver he received was positive for CMV, but he had negative CMV serology. His postoperative immunosuppressant regimen included oral prednisone and tacrolimus 5 mg PO BID, with adjustments made to his dose to maintain a 12-hour trough concentration between 10 and 15 ng/mL. He was also given valganciclovir 450 mg PO daily for 3 months.

His postoperative course was complicated by an acute rejection episode on postoperative day 8, which was treated successfully with a pulse and taper of steroids. At that time, MMF 1 g PO BID was added to his immunosuppressant regimen. He was discharged from the hospital on postoperative day 12, with instructions to return to the transplant clinic in 4 days. Since then, he has done fairly well with no complaints until now, 4 months later. On admission to the hospital, a physical examination was remarkable for an oral temperature of 38.8°C, a BP of 112/79 mmHg, a heart rate of 104 beats/minute, a respiratory rate of 22 breaths/minute, and a mild tremor. All other findings on his examination were benign. Pertinent laboratory findings include the following: WBC count, 3,400 cells/mm^3 (normal, 4,000–10,000); platelet count, 34,000 cells/mm^3 (normal, 150,000–450,000); BUN, 29 mg/dL (normal, 5–22); SrCr, 1.4 mg/dL (normal, 0.6–1.1); total bilirubin, 2.2 mg/dL (normal, 0.0–1.2); AST, 62 U/L (normal, 14–38); ALT, 126 U/L (normal, 15–48); CMV PCR 184,000 copies/mL (normal <500 copies/mL); and 12-hour tacrolimus concentration, 18.3 ng/dL (normal, 5–15). His current medications include tacrolimus 6 mg PO BID; prednisone 10 mg PO daily; TMP-SMX 80 mg PO Mondays, Wednesdays, and Fridays; calcium carbonate 1.25 g PO TID; vitamin D 800 U PO daily; enteric-coated aspirin 325 mg PO daily; and nizatidine 150 mg PO BID. What is the most likely diagnosis for A.A.?

A major concern in A.A. at this time after transplantation is CMV infection, an infection that is commonly encountered within 1 to 6 months after both solid organ and bone marrow transplantation. It is a ubiquitous virus belonging to the herpes virus group. In healthy immunocompetent adults, infection with the virus is usually asymptomatic, whereas in immunocompromised patients, CMV can cause significant morbidity and mortality. CMV can potentiate the risk for developing both bacterial and fungal infections and induce chronic injury to the transplanted organ (arteriosclerosis in the heart, obliterative bronchiolitis in the lungs, vanishing bile duct syndrome in the liver, and chronic arteriopathy in the kidneys).[127]

Etiology

Cytomegalovirus infection in transplant recipients usually occurs when latent viruses from a seropositive donor organ are reactivated owing to immunosuppression. Transmission of CMV from a positive donor to a negative recipient leads to an 80% to 100% infection rate and a 40% to 50% disease rate; a positive donor to a positive recipient leads to a 40% to 60% reactivation rate and a 20% to 30% disease rate; and a negative donor to a negative recipient leads to a 0% to 5% infection rate. Transplant recipients at highest risk for developing the disease are (a) those who are or have serologically donor +/recipient − (D+/R−) at the time of transplant, (b) elderly, (c) those who received large amounts of perioperative blood transfusions, (d) those who received antilymphocyte antibodies, (e) those who received a retransplantation because of acute rejection, and (f) those who received larger amounts of immunosuppressive agents.[127] A.A. is at high risk because his CMV serology is D+/R−.

Diagnosis

Diagnosis of CMV is based on both clinical and laboratory findings. CMV may be detected by culturing body fluids, such as bronchoalveolar lavage, urine, blood, and tissue biopsies. CMV is contained within the host's leukocytes, which appear to have large intranuclear inclusion bodies. CMV PCR is now a readily available method for measuring viral loads in the patient's blood. Most transplant centers have the capability of performing this test at their site, with a turnaround time of hours. Documented viral shedding is not, however, diagnostic for active disease without clinical signs and symptoms.[127,128] A.A. certainly has laboratory criteria for the diagnosis of CMV infection: viral shedding, as indicated by the CMV PCR of 184,000 copies/mL, leukopenia, and thrombocytopenia.

Clinical Manifestations

In healthy immunocompetent adults, the CMV-infected patient is usually asymptomatic but may present with mild complaints of malaise, fever, and myalgias, as well as abnormal liver enzymes and lymphocytosis. More severe reactions are rare.[128] CMV may, however, be life threatening in the immunocompromised patient and is the most common opportunistic infection associated with solid organ transplantation. Evidence indicates that CMV infection is associated with graft rejection and that graft rejection in the setting of immunosuppression facilitates CMV infection. It often is unclear which comes first. The actual CMV course may be limited to fever and mononucleosis, or it may extend to organs presenting as pneumonia, hepatitis, gastroenteritis, colitis, disseminated infection, encephalopathy, or leukopenia.

A.A.'s clinical presentation meets the criteria for CMV disease: viremia with clinical signs and symptoms. At this time, it is unclear whether or not A.A. has any end-organ involvement. His liver enzyme concentrations are elevated and he is having numerous GI symptoms, which may be indicative of CMV hepatitis, CMV gastroenteritis, or CMV colitis, respectively. Alternatively, the increased total bilirubin and serum transaminases may be caused by acute rejection, and his GI problems may be a side effect he is experiencing from his medications (e.g., MMF). To fully differentiate among CMV hepatitis, CMV gastroenteritis, CMV colitis, acute rejection, and medication side effects, tissue biopsies should be obtained.

Treatment

39. What are the treatment options for A.A.'s diagnosed CMV disease? What doses should be used, and how should the effects of these drugs be monitored?

GANCICLOVIR

Before ganciclovir was available, CMV infection was "treated" by reducing the level of immunosuppression. This may be one of the explanations for an increased prevalence of rejection associated with CMV infections. Graft loss in kidney or pancreas recipients is undesirable; yet, it is not immediately life threatening. Reducing immunosuppression in liver, heart, or lung transplant recipients, however, could result in the patient's death owing to graft loss. Treatment has been attempted with acyclovir, adenine-arabinoside, and immune globulin, all of which have been largely unsuccessful. At present, ganciclovir is the first-line agent used for the treatment of CMV disease in solid organ transplant recipients, bone marrow transplant recipients, and patients with acquired immunodeficiency syndrome (AIDS). Although ganciclovir is highly efficacious in this regard, there is still a potential 20% relapse rate of CMV after ganciclovir therapy in liver transplant recipients.

Ganciclovir, a virustatic agent, is a nucleoside analog that is phosphorylated in infected cells to its active form and is then incorporated into replicating viral DNA. Although ganciclovir-resistant strains of CMV have been isolated, their occurrence is far more common in patients with HIV; currently, ganciclovir-resistant CMV in solid organ transplantation is not a large concern.[129] A.A. should receive ganciclovir IV; oral ganciclovir should not be used because its bioavailability is <10%. Because relapses of CMV disease after IV ganciclovir are still a concern, some suggest that patients should be placed on maintenance therapy with either oral ganciclovir, valganciclovir, or oral acyclovir after the IV course is completed.[129,130]

Dosing

The usual dose of ganciclovir in patients with normal renal function is 5 mg/kg/dose every 12 hours for 14 to 21 days. Dosage adjustment is necessary for patients with renal dysfunction: 2.5 mg/kg/dose every 12 hours for creatinine clearances 50 to 79 mL/minute; 2.5 mg/kg/dose every 24 hours for creatinine clearances 25 to 49 mL/minute; and 1.25 mg/kg/dose every 24 hours for creatinine clearances <25 mL/minute. Because A.A. has an estimated creatinine clearance of 60 mL/minute, he should receive 2.5 mg/kg/dose (190 mg) IV every 12 hours for 2 to 3 weeks, followed by either low-dose IV ganciclovir (2.5 mg/kg every day), valganciclovir, or oral ganciclovir for 2 to 4 weeks.

The most common adverse effect associated with ganciclovir therapy is neutropenia, which is seen in up to 27% of patients being treated with this drug.[129] Neutropenia is defined as an absolute neutrophil count of <500 to 1,000 cells/mm^3. The neutropenia usually resolves with a decrease in dosage or discontinuation of the drug, but colony-stimulating factors may help correct it.[131] Because CMV disease has a propensity to cause neutropenia as well, it is often difficult to distinguish the cause. If laboratory findings and clinical signs and symptoms of CMV disease are resolving and the patient remains neutropenic, the most likely cause is ganciclovir. Thrombocytopenia occurs in approximately 20% of ganciclovir recipients. Patients with initial platelet counts <100,000/mm^3 appear to be at greatest risk. Other adverse effects include CNS effects, fever, rash, and abnormal LFT findings.[129] A.A.'s WBC and platelet counts should be assessed every 3 to 4 days during therapy, and ganciclovir should be held if neutrophils fall to <500/mm^3 or platelets fall to <25,000/mm^3. To monitor either the regression or progression of A.A.'s CMV disease, a weekly CMV antigen test should be obtained.

IMMUNE GLOBULINS

The use of immunoglobulins to treat CMV disease in solid organ transplantation is controversial. Immunoglobulins provide passive immunization by potentiating an antibody-dependent, cell-mediated cytotoxic reaction. Basically, the immunoglobulins modify the immunologic response that damages host tissue. Some evidence suggests that immunoglobulins may have synergistic or additive effects with current antiviral drugs in the treatment of CMV disease.[132] Both unselective immunoglobulins and CMV hyperimmune globulin have been studied in combination with ganciclovir. CMV hyperimmune globulin is prepared from high-titer pooled sera that have a fourfold to eightfold enrichment of CMV titers compared with unscreened immunoglobulin.

Most of the literature involving combination therapy for CMV disease is in bone marrow transplant recipients. Initial response rates appear to favor the combination therapy in this group. In solid organ transplantation, the data are scarce. Most of the literature is in the form of case reports or small retrospective studies. It appears, however, that the combination of CMV immunoglobulin and ganciclovir may be more efficacious than ganciclovir alone in severe CMV disease (e.g., hepatitis, pneumonitis).[132] Although it is controversial, many clinicians would use combination therapy in patients with severe disease, as indicated by end-organ involvement, or in those who are refractory to monotherapy with ganciclovir.

Cytomegalovirus immunoglobulin may be given as 100 mg/kg/dose every other day for 14 days. This is the dose recommended for treatment of CMV when used in combination with ganciclovir. The most common adverse effects associated with the administration of immunoglobulins appear to be infusion related and include fever, chills, headache, myalgia, light-headedness, and nausea and vomiting.

FOSCARNET

Foscarnet is a virustatic pyrophosphate analog that inhibits DNA synthesis; however, unlike ganciclovir, no phosphorylation is required for activation. Because this drug has a high nephrotoxicity propensity and because most transplant recipients are already receiving drugs that are nephrotoxic, experience with the use of foscarnet in solid organ transplantation is limited. In most centers, foscarnet is a second- or third-line agent to be used only if intolerance or resistance develops with ganciclovir therapy.

The usual dosage of foscarnet is 60 mg/kg/dose every 8 hours for 14 to 21 days. The dosage should be adjusted downward in patients with renal dysfunction. The most serious adverse effect with foscarnet is nephrotoxicity, which occurs in up to 50% of patients and is probably induced by acute tubular necrosis. Therefore, prehydration is suggested to help minimize or avoid nephrotoxicity. GI effects, a decrease in hemoglobin and hematocrit, an increase in LFTs, and alteration of serum electrolyte concentrations are other side effects of foscarnet. All of these appear to be reversible on discontinuation of the drug. SrCr should be monitored daily during therapy.[128]

Prophylaxis

40. Is there any way to prevent CMV in high-risk patients, such as A.A.?

Because of its significant consequences, efforts should be made to prevent CMV disease in the transplantation population. One way to prevent primary CMV infections is to use seronegative donors and seronegative blood products, which should greatly reduce the risk. This solution is difficult if not impossible to implement because the availability of donor organs is insufficient. Therefore, CMV status is not considered in the donor-matching process. Many studies have tried to ascertain the easiest, most cost-effective regimen to prevent CMV disease. These studies have focused on the combined use of different agents as well as IV followed by oral therapies. Trials have also targeted high-risk patients.[129,132–138]

GANCICLOVIR

The use of both the IV and oral formulations of ganciclovir to prevent CMV disease has been studied in lung, heart, liver, kidney, and pancreas transplant recipients.[127] Very few relatively large trials have been conducted and most of the data in the solid organ transplantation population are from small uncontrolled trials. Another difficulty lies in that large discrepancies exist between the trials with regard to the terminology used to define prophylaxis and high-risk patients. Until the recent introduction of valganciclovir, ganciclovir has been the most widely used prophylactic agent.

Both oral and IV ganciclovir have been studied in lung transplant recipients to prevent CMV disease.[127,133] Although these studies had very small numbers of subjects, it does appear that both formulations can prevent CMV disease when used in the first 90 days after transplantation. The populations targeted in these trials were patients who were considered at risk for the development of CMV disease because of their serologic status or because antilymphocyte antibodies had been used as induction therapy. Long-term follow-up in these patients, however, revealed no difference in CMV disease rates when compared with placebo. This may indicate that, although ganciclovir therapy is effective in delaying CMV early in the post-transplantation period, it does not prevent the disease.

Studies using prophylactic IV ganciclovir in heart transplantation have found it to be both effective and ineffective as prophylaxis. Oral ganciclovir has been compared with other drug combinations and shown to be more effective.[134,135] Studies conducted in heart transplantation focused on patients at high risk for developing CMV disease. Most patients received antilymphocyte antibody induction therapy and were in the serologic high-risk groups as well (D+/R–, D+/R+, or D–/R+).[134,135]

The prophylactic use of ganciclovir in liver transplantation recipients has been evaluated as well. Trials have shown that oral ganciclovir, given for an average of 3 to 4 months after transplantation, significantly decreases the rates of CMV disease in this population. In addition, comparative trials have concluded that oral ganciclovir is more effective than oral acyclovir. Ganciclovir prophylaxis seems most effective when used in D+/R– patients.[136,137]

When ganciclovir prophylaxis, either oral or IV, is used in high-risk renal transplant recipients, it appears to reduce the incidence of CMV disease.[137,138] As in the liver transplantation population, ganciclovir is superior to oral acyclovir. In most studies, prophylaxis is continued for approximately 12 weeks after transplantation. As seen in A.A., CMV can, however, occur once prophylaxis is discontinued.

VALGANCICLOVIR

Valganciclovir was developed because oral ganciclovir has a very low bioavailability (<10%). Valganciclovir is the L-valyl ester of ganciclovir, which is a prodrug that is rapidly and completely converted into ganciclovir by hepatic and intestinal esterases once absorbed across the GI tract. The absolute bioavailability of valganciclovir is approximately 60%, so that a 900-mg single dose given with food has an AUC equivalent to a 5 mg/kg IV dose of ganciclovir. This is roughly twice the AUC achieved by 1,000 mg of ganciclovir given orally TID.[139] Valganciclovir is currently FDA approved for the treatment of HIV-associated CMV retinitis, and to prevent CMV disease in heart, lung, kidney, and pancreas transplantation.[140–141] Valganciclovir is not FDA approved for prevention of CMV disease in liver transplantation, although it is often utilized in such cases.[142] Several small studies have demonstrated that valganciclovir is effective in treating CMV infection preemptively and potentially preventing CMV disease.[143,144]

Similar to ganciclovir, valganciclovir is predominantly eliminated from the body through the kidney, and dosage adjustment is required in renal impairment. The incidence of adverse drug reactions is similar to IV ganciclovir and they include headache, neutropenia, nausea, diarrhea, and anemia. The incidence of neutropenia is significantly higher than oral ganciclovir, and dosage reduction or temporary withdrawal of the agent is recommended in patients with an ANC less than 1,000 cells/mm^3.[139,140,145]

ACYCLOVIR

Acyclovir is ineffective in the treatment of established CMV disease, but it does appear to have a beneficial preventive role. Since the introduction of oral ganciclovir, several trials have compared the prophylactic efficacy of high-dose acyclovir with oral ganciclovir.[137,138] As already noted, oral ganciclovir appears to be more effective in preventing CMV disease, especially in the D+/R– subgroup. Because of this, most consider oral acyclovir to be second-line therapy to IV or oral ganciclovir or valganciclovir as a CMV prophylactic agent.

CMV HYPERIMMUNE GLOBULIN

The role of CMV hyperimmune globulin in preventing CMV disease is controversial. Many studies have combined this agent with either oral acyclovir or ganciclovir, but because of its cost and IV route, its use as a prophylactic agent has decreased. In addition, in patients who are D+/R–, results have been mixed.[127,146]

VALACYCLOVIR

One recently published meta-analysis of 12 trials that included 1,574 patients evaluated valacyclovir as a prophylactic agent in transplant recipients.[147] Valacyclovir was found to be more effective than acyclovir in preventing herpes viruses, including CMV. Most transplantation centers, however, do not use valacyclovir for routine prophylaxis of CMV.

41. Should A.A. have received prophylactic therapy and, if so, which agent should be used?

A.A. has several risk factors that predispose him to developing CMV disease. At the time of transplantation, A.A. was CMV D+/R–, which means that he has about an 80% chance of developing CMV infection and a 40% chance of developing CMV disease. In addition, A.A. had an early acute rejection episode, which means he received higher doses of immunosuppression, also putting him at higher risk for developing CMV disease. Because of these risk factors, A.A. should have (and did) receive CMV prophylaxis for at least 3 months after transplantation. Immediately postoperatively, IV ganciclovir, at a dose of 5 mg/kg every day, should be used. Once A.A. is tolerating oral medications, he can be switched to oral valganciclovir at a dose of 900 mg daily with food. Because A.A. has renal insufficiency, his oral valganciclovir dose was adjusted to 450 mg daily.[145] As illustrated by A.A.'s case, a patient who has received prophylactic therapy does not preclude the development of CMV disease after the prophylaxis is withdrawn or, in rare instances, during prophylactic therapy. The incidence of CMV disease while receiving valganciclovir is significantly lower when compared to oral ganciclovir, probably because drug exposure is approximately two times higher.[140,141]

PRE-EMPTIVE THERAPY

Because of recent advances in the laboratory tests used to identify and quantify CMV; because prophylactic therapy is not always effective; and because it is often toxic and very expensive, pre-emptive therapy has been used in an attempt to prevent CMV disease. The technique involves withholding prophylactic therapy and monitoring laboratory tests to identify presymptomatic CMV viremia, usually by utilizing the CMV PCR. Once a patient develops viremia (CMV PCR viral load >2,000 copies/mL), he or she usually receives treatment with IV ganciclovir or oral valganciclovir. This strategy has been prospectively studied and is as effective as universal prophylaxis, with some potential cost advantages.[148]

REFERENCES

1. Port FK et al. Trends in organ donation and transplantation in the United States, 1996–2005. *Am J Transplant* 2007;7(Part2):131.
2. Tantaravahi JR et al. Why hasn't eliminating acute rejection improved graft survival. *Annu Rev Med* 2007;58:369.
3. Trivedi HL. Immunology of rejection and adaptation. *Transplant Proc* 2007;39:647.
4. Cecka JM et al. Histocompatibility testing, crossmatching, and allocation of kidney transplant. In: Danovitch DM, ed. *Handbook of Kidney Transplantation*. 4th ed. Lippincott Williams & Wilkins; 2004.
5. Jordan SC et al. Intravenous gammaglobulin (IVIG): a novel approach to improve transplant rates and outcomes in highly HLA-sensitized patients. *Am J Transplant* 2006;6:459.
6. Magee CC. Transplantation across previously incompatible immunological barriers. *Transpl Int* 2006;19:87.
7. Lennard L. The clinical pharmacology of 6-mercaptopurine. *Eur J Clin Pharmacol* 1992;43:329.
8. Chan GLC et al. Azathioprine metabolism pharmacokinetics of 6-mercaptopurine, 6-thiouric acid and 6-thioguanine nucleotides in renal transplant patients. *J Clin Pharmacol* 1990;30:358.
9. Kurzawski M et al. The impact of thiopurine s-methyltransferase polymorphism on azathioprine-induced myelotoxicity in renal transplant recipients. *Ther Drug Monit* 2005;27:435.
10. Romagnuolo J et al. Cholestatic hepatocellular injury with azathioprine: a case report and review of the mechanisms of hepatotoxicity. *Can J Gastroenterol* 1998;12:479.
11. Ciancio G et al. Review of major clinical trials with mycophenolate mofetil in renal transplantation. *Transplantation* 2005;80 (Suppl 2):s191.
12. Allison AC. Mechanisms of action of mycophenolate mofetil. *Lupus* 2005;14:s2.
13. Staatz C et al. Clinical pharmacokinetics and pharmacodynamics of mycophenolate in solid organ transplant recipients. *Clin Pharmacokinet* 2007;46:13.
14. Behrend M et al. Enteric-coated mycophenolate sodium: tolerability profile compared with mycophenolate mofetil. *Drugs* 2005;65:1037.
15. Bestard O et al. Corticosteroid-sparing strategies in renal transplantation. Are we still balancing rejection risk with improved tolerability? *Drugs* 2006;66:403.
16. Franchmont D. Overview of the action of glucocorticoids on the immune response. *Ann NY Acad Sci* 2004;1024:124.
17. Frey BM et al. Clinical pharmacokinetics of prednisone and prednisolone. *Clin Pharmacokinet* 1990;19:126.
18. Jeng S et al. Prednisone metabolism in recipients of kidney and liver transplants and in lung recipients receiving ketoconazole. *Transplantation* 2003;75:792.
19. Faulds D et al. Cyclosporin. A review of its pharmacodynamic and pharmacokinetic properties, and therapeutic use in immunoregulatory disorders. *Drugs* 1993;45:953.
20. Staatz CE et al. Clinical pharmacokinetics and pharmacodynamics of tacrolimus in solid organ transplantation. *Clin Pharmacokinet* 2004;43: 623.
21. Kuypers DR. Benefit-risk assessment of sirolimus in renal transplantation. *Drug Saf* 2005;28: 153.
22. Hardinger KL. Rabbit Antithymocyte globulin induction therapy in adult renal transplantation. *Pharmacotherapy* 2006;26:1771.
23. Zand MS. B-cell activity of polyclonal antithymocyte globulins. *Transplantation* 2006;82:1387.
24. ten Berge UM et al. Guidelines for the optimal use of muromonab CD3 in transplantation. *BioDrugs* 1999;11:277.
25. Vincenti F et al. Interleukin-2 receptor antagonist induction in modern immunosuppression regimens for renal transplant recipients. *Transpl Int* 2006;19:446.
26. Kovarik J et al. Disposition of and immunodynamics of basiliximab in liver allograft recipients. *Clin Pharmacol Ther* 1998;64:66.
27. Magliocca JF et al. The evolving role of alemtuzumab (campath-1H) for immunosuppressive therapy in organ transplantation. *Transpl Int* 2006;19:705.
28. Silva HT et al. Immunotherapy for de novo renal transplantation. What's in the pipeline? *Drugs* 2006;66:1665.
29. Vincenti F et al. Costimulation with belatacept in renal transplantation. *N Engl J Med* 2005;353:8.
30. Kasike BL et al. The evaluation of renal transplant candidates: clinical practice guidelines. *Am J Transplant* 2001;1:1.
31. Braun WE. The rocky road of limited immunosuppression for renal transplantation in African Americans. *Transplantation* 2007;83:267.
32. Brennan DC et al. Rabbit antithymocyte globulin versus basiliximab in renal transplantation. *N Engl J Med* 2006;355:1967.
33. Gaston RS. Current and evolving immunosuppressive regimens in kidney transplantation. *Am J Kid Dis* 2006;47(Suppl 2):1.
34. Goggins WC et al. A prospective randomized clinical trial of intraoperative versus postoperative Thymoglobulin in adult cadaveric renal transplant recipients. *Transplantation* 2003;76:798.
35. Peddi VR et al. Safety, efficacy and cost analysis of thymoglobulin induction therapy with intermittent dosing based on CD3+ lymphocyte counts in kidney and kidney-pancreas transplant recipients. *Transplantation* 2002;73:1514.
36. Lundquist AL et al. Serum sickness following rabbit antithymocyte-globulin induction in a liver transplant recipient: case report and literature review. *Liver Transplant* 2007;13:647.
37. Perico N et al. Delayed graft function in kidney transplantation. *Lancet* 2004;364:1814.
38. Sandrini S. Use of IL-2 receptor antagonists to reduce delayed graft function following renal transplantation: a review. *Clin Transplant* 2005;19:705.
39. Solez K et al. Banff of classification of renal pathology. Updates and future directions. *Am J Transplant* 2008;8:753.
40. Davis C. Transplant: immunology and treatment of rejection. *Am J Kid Dis* 2004;43:1116.
41. Colvin RB. Antibody mediated renal allograft rejection: diagnosis and pathogenesis. *J Am Soc Nephrol* 2007;18:1046.
42. Solez K et al. Banff meeting 05 report: differential diagnosis of chronic allograft injury and elimination of chronic allograft nephropathy (CAN). *Am J Transplant* 2007;7:518.
43. Casadei DH et al. A randomized and prospective study comparing treatment with high dose intravenous immunoglobulin with monoclonal antibodies for rescue of kidney grafts with steroid resistant rejection. *Transplantation* 2001;71:53.
44. Hricik DE et al. Trends in the use of glucocorticoids in renal transplantation. *Transplantation* 1994;57:979.
45. Cantarovich D et al. Switching from cysporine to tacrolimus. *Transplantation* 2005;79:72.
46. Butler JA et al. Frequency and impact of nonadherence to immunosuppressants after renal transplantation: a systematic review. *Transplantation* 2004;77:769.
47. Lindholm A et al. Influence of cyclosporine pharmacokinetics, trough concentrations, and AUC monitoring on outcome after kidney transplantation. *Clin Pharm Ther* 1993;54:205.
48. Kahan BD et al. Challenges in cyclosporine therapy: the role of therapeutic monitoring by area under the curve monitoring. *Ther Drug Monit* 1995;17:621.
49. Dunn CJ et al. Cyclosporin: an updated review of the pharmacokinetic properties, clinical efficacy and tolerability of a microemulsion-based formulation (neural) in organ transplantation. *Drugs* 2001;61:1957.
50. Min DL et al. Gender-dependent racial difference in disposition of cyclosporine among healthy African American and white volunteers. *Clin Pharmacol Ther* 2000;68:478.
51. Rossi SJ et al. Prevention and management of the adverse effects associated with immunosuppressive therapy. *Drug Saf* 1993;9:104.
52. Tsunoda SM et al. The use of therapeutic drug monitoring to optimize immunosuppressive therapy. *Clin Pharmacokinet* 1996;30:107.
53. Mahalati K et al. Neoral monitoring by simplified sparse sampling area under the concentration time curve: its relationship to acute rejection and cyclosporine nephrotoxicity early after kidney transplantation. *Transplantation* 1999;68:55.
54. Levy GA. C2 monitoring strategy for optimizing

cyclosporin immunosuppression from Neoral formulation. *BioDrugs* 2001;15:279.
55. Cole E et al. Recommendations for the implementation of Neoral C2 monitoring in clinical practice. *Transplantation* 2002;73:S19.
56. MacDonald A et al. Clinical pharmacokinetics and therapeutic monitoring of sirolimus. *Clin Ther* 2000;22(Suppl B);B101.
57. Ingle SR et al. Sirolimus: continuing the evolution of transplant immunosuppression. *Ann Pharmacother* 2000;34:1044.
58. El-Sabrout et al. Improved freedom from rejection after a loading dose of sirolimus. *Transplantation* 2003;75:86.
59. Kelly P. Review: metabolism of immunosuppressant drugs. *Cur Drug Metab* 2002;3:275.
60. Letavernier E et al. Proteinuria following a switch from calcineurin inhibitors to sirolimus. *Transplantation* 2005;80:1198.
61. Groth CG et al. Sirolimus (rapamycin)-based therapy in human renal transplantation: similar efficacy and different toxicity compared with cyclosporine. *Transplantation* 1999;67:1036.
62. MacDonald AS. Improving tolerability of immunosuppressive regimens. *Transplantation* 2001;72: S105.
63. Fellstrom B. Cyclosporine nephrotoxicity. *Transplant Proc* 2004;36(Suppl 2s):220s.
64. Campistol JM et al. Mechanisms of nephrotoxicity. *Transplantation* 2000;69:S5.
65. Yang H. Maintenance immunosuppression regimens: conversion, minimization, withdrawal, and avoidance. *Am J Kid Dis* 2006;47 (Suppl 2):1.
66. Wong W et al. Immunosuppressive strategies in kidney transplantation: which role for the calcineurin inhibitors? *Transplantation* 2005;80:289.
67. Land W et al. Toxicity sparing protocols using mycophenolate mofetil in renal transplantation. *Transplantation* 2005;80:s221.
68. Johnson RWG et al. Sirolimus allows early cyclosporine withdrawal in renal transplantation resulting in improved renal function and lower blood pressure. *Transplantation* 2001;72:777.
69. Woodle ES et al. Multivariate analysis of risk factors for acute rejection in early corticosteroid cessation regimens under modern immunosuppression. *American Journal of Transplantation* 2005;5: 2740.
70. Randhawa P et al. BK virus infection in transplant recipients: an overview and update. *American Journal of Transplantation* 2006;6:2000.
71. Trofe J et al. Polyomavirus-associated nephropathy: update of clinical management in kidney transplant patients. *Transpl Infect Dis* 2006;8:76.
72. Wilkinson A et al. Guidelines for the treatment and management of new-onset diabetes after transplantation. *Clin Transpl* 2005;19:291.
73. Vesco L et al. Diabetes mellitus after renal transplantation: characteristics, outcome, and risk factors. *Transplantation* 1996;61:1475.
74. Araki M et al. Posttransplant diabetes mellitus in kidney transplant recipients receiving calcineurin or mTOR inhibitor drugs. *Transplantation* 2006;81:335.
75. Johannes P et al. Evaluating mechanisms of posttransplant diabetes mellitus. *Nephrol Dial Transplant* 2004;19(Suppl 6):vi8.
76. Abouljoud MS et al. Neoral rescue therapy in transplant patients with intolerance to tacrolimus. *Clin Transplant* 2002;16:168.
77. Weir M. Impact of Immunosuppressive regimens on posttransplant diabetes mellitus. *Transplant Proc* 2001;33(Suppl 5A):23S.
78. Ebeling PR. Transplantation osteoporosis. *Current Osteoporosis Reports* 2007;5:29.
79. Heaf JG. Bone disease after renal transplantation. *Transplantation* 2003;75:315.
80. Hay JE. Osteoporosis in liver diseases and after liver transplantation. *J Hepatol* 2003;38:856.
81. Maalouf NM et al. Osteoporosis after solid organ transplantation. *J Clin Endocrinol Metab* 2005;90: 2456.
82. Hariharan S. Recommendations for outpatient monitoring of kidney transplant recipients. *Am J Kidney Dis* 2006;47:S22.
83. Palmer SC et al. Interventions for preventing bone disease in kidney transplant recipients: a systematic review of randomized controlled trials. *Am J Kidney Dis* 2005;45:638.
84. http://www.optn.org/organDatasource/about.asp?display=Liver;http://www.optn.org/organDatasource/about.asp?display=Liver Accessed June 11, 2007.
85. Tran TT et al. Advances in liver transplantation. New strategies and current care expand access, enhance survival. *Postgrad Med* 2004;115:73.
86. Neuberger J. Developments in liver transplantation. *Gut* 2004;53:759.
87. Roland ME et al. Review of solid-organ transplantation in HIV-infected patients. *Transplantation* 2003;75:425.
88. Keegan MT et al. Critical care issues in liver transplantation. *Int Anesthesiol Clin* 2006;44:1.
89. Porte RJ. Coagulation and fibrinolysis in orthotopic liver transplantation: current views and insights. *Semin Thromb Hemostat* 1993;19:191.
90. Wijdidicks EFM. Neurotoxicity of immunosuppressive drugs. *Liver Transpl* 2001;7:937.
91. Venkataramanan R et al. Clinical pharmacokinetics of tacrolimus. *Clin Pharmacokinet* 1995;29: 404.
92. Mancinelli LM et al. The pharmacokinetic and metabolic disposition of tacrolimus: a comparison across ethnic groups. *Clin Pharmacol Ther* 2001;69:24.
93. Kershner RP et al. Relationship of FK506 whole blood concentrations and efficacy and toxicity after liver and kidney transplantation. *Transplantation* 1996;62:920.
94. Holt DW et al. Clinical toxicology working group on immunosuppressive drug monitoring. *Ther Drug Monit* 2002;24:59.
95. Taylor PJ et al. Improved Therapeutic Drug Monitoring of Tacrolimus (FK506) by Tandem Mass Spectrometry. *Clin Chem* 1997;43:2189.
96. Porryko MK et al. Nephrotropic effects of primary immunosuppression with FK506 and cyclosporine regimens after liver transplantation. *Mayo Clin Proc* 1994;69:105.
97. Klintmahn GB. A comparison of tacrolimus (FK506) and cyclosporine for immunosuppression in liver transplantation. The U.S. Multicenter FK506 Liver Study Group. *N Engl J Med* 1994;331:1110.
98. Knechtle SJ et al. Rejection of the liver transplant. *Semin Gastrointest Dis* 1998;9:126.
99. Neumann, UP et al. Significance of a T-lymphocytotoxic crossmatch in liver and combined liver-kidney transplantation. *Transplantation* 2001;78:1163.
100. Fisher RA et al. A prospective randomized trial of mycophenolate mofetil with Neoral or tacrolimus after orthotopic liver transplantation. *Transplantation* 1998;66;1616.
101. Jani A et al. A prospective randomized trial of tacrolimus and prednisone versus tacrolimus, prednisone and mycophenolate mofetil in primary adult liver transplantation: a single center report. *Transplantation* 2001;72:1091.
102. Demetris AJ et al. Update of the International Banff Schema for Liver Allograft Rejection: working recommendations for the histopathologic staging and reporting of chronic rejection. An International Panel. *Hepatology* 2000;31:792.
103. Sher LS et al. Tacrolimus as rescue therapy in liver transplantation. *Transplantation* 1997;64:258.
104. Bullingham RE et al. Clinical pharmacokinetics of mycophenolate mofetil. *Clin Pharmacokinet* 1998;34:429.
105. Behrend M et al. Adverse gastrointestinal effects of mycophenolate mofetil. Aetiology, incidence, and management. *Drug Saf* 2001;24:645.
106. van Gelder T et al. Therapeutic drug monitoring of mycophenolate mofetil in transplantation. *Ther Drug Monit* 2006;28:145.
107. Cox VC et al. Mycophenolate mofetil for organ transplantation: does the evidence support the need for clinical pharmacokinetic monitoring. *Ther Drug Monit* 2003;25:137.
108. Neumayer HH et al. Protective effects of calcium antagonists in human renal transplantation. *Kidney Int Suppl* 1992;36:S87.
109. Anaizi N. Drug interactions involving immunosuppressive agents. *Graft* 2001;4:232.
110. Barone GW. Herbal supplements: a potential for drug interactions in transplant recipients. *Transplantation* 2001;71:239.
111. Dresser GK. Pharmacokinetic-pharmacodynamic consequences and clinical relevance of cytochrome P450 3A4 inhibition. *Clin Pharmacokinet* 2000;38:41.
112. Campana C et al. Clinically significant drug interactions with cyclosporine, An update. *Clin Pharmacokinet* 1996;30:141.
113. Ahmed AR. Cyclophosphamide (Cytoxan). *J Am Acad Dermatol* 1984;11:1115.
114. Fishman JA et al. Infection in organ transplant recipients. *N Engl J Med* 1998;338:1741.
115. ASHP therapeutic guidelines on antimicrobial prophylaxis in surgery. *Am J Health Syst Pharm* 1999;56:1839.
116. Gordon SM et al. Should prophylaxis for *Pneumocystis carinii* pneumonia in solid organ transplant recipients ever be discontinued? *Clin Infect Dis* 1999;28:240.
117. Samuel D et al. Liver transplantation in European patients with the hepatitis B surface antigen. *N Engl J Med* 1993;329:1842.
118. McGory RW et al. Improved outcome of orthotopic liver transplantation for a chronic hepatitis B cirrhosis with aggressive passive immunization. *Transplantation* 1996;61:1358.
119. Eisenbach C et al. Prevention of hepatitis B virus recurrence after liver transplantation. *Clin Transpl* 2006;20:111.
120. Hoofnagle JH et al. Management of hepatitis B: summary of a clinical research workshop. *Hepatology* 2007;45:1056.
121. Benhamou Y et al. Safety and efficacy of adefovir dipivoxil in patients co-infected with HIV-1 and lamivudine-resistant hepatitis B virus: an open-label pilot study. *Lancet* 2001;358:718.
122. Bloom RD et al. Emerging issues in hepatitis C virus-positive liver and kidney transplant recipients. *American Journal of Transplantation* 2006;6: 2232.
123. Forman LM et al. The association between hepatitis C infection and survival after orthotopic liver transplantation. *Gastroenterology* 2002;122:889.
124. Khalid SK et al. Management of hepatitis C in the setting of liver transplantation. *Clin Liver Dis* 2006;10:321.
125. Gane E. Treatment of recurrent hepatitis C. *Liver Transpl* 2002;8(10 Suppl 1):S28.
126. Munksgaard B. Guidelines for vaccination of solid organ transplant candidates and recipients. *American Journal of Transplantation* 2004;4(Suppl 10):160.
127. Biron KK. Antiviral drugs for cytomegalovirus diseases. *Antiviral Res* 2006;71:154.
128. Gerna G et al. Monitoring transplant patients for human cytomegalovirus: diagnostic update. *Herpes* 2006;1:3.
129. Noble S et al. Ganciclovir: an update of its use in the prevention of cytomegalovirus infection and disease in transplant recipients. *Drugs* 1998; 56:115.
130. Nankivell BJ. Maintenance therapy with oral ganciclovir after treatment of cytomegalovirus infection. *Clin Transplant* 1998;12:270.
131. Kutsogiannis DJ et al. Granulocyte macrophage colony-stimulating factor for the therapy of cytomegalovirus and ganciclovir-induced leukopenia in a renal transplant recipient. *Transplantation* 1992;53:930.
132. Snydman DR et al. A further analysis of the use of cytomegalovirus immune globulin in orthotopic liver transplant patients at risk for primary infection. *Transplant Proc* 1994;2(Suppl 1):23.
133. Avery RK. Special considerations regarding CMV

in lung transplantation. *Transplant Infect Dis* 1999;1(Suppl 1):13.
134. Rubin RH. Prevention and treatment of cytomegalovirus disease in heart transplant patients. *J Heart Lung Transplant* 2000;19:731.
135. Mullen GM et al. Effective oral ganciclovir prophylaxis against cytomegalovirus disease in heart transplant recipients. *Transplant Proc* 1998;30:4110.
136. Gane E et al. Randomized trial of efficacy and safety of oral ganciclovir in the prevention of cytomegalovirus disease in liver-transplant recipients. *Lancet* 1997;350:1729.
137. Turgeon N et al. Effect of oral acyclovir or ganciclovir therapy after preemptive intravenous ganciclovir therapy to prevent cytomegalovirus disease in cytomegalovirus seropositive renal and liver transplant recipients receiving antilymphocyte antibody therapy. *Transplantation* 1998;66:1780.
138. Flechner SM et al. A randomized prospective controlled trial of oral acyclovir versus oral ganciclovir for cytomegalovirus prophylaxis in high-risk kidney transplant recipients. *Transplantation* 1998;66:1682.
139. Brown F et al. Pharmacokinetics of valganciclovir and ganciclovir following multiple oral dosages of valganciclovir in HIV- and CMV-seropositive volunteers. *Clin Pharmacokinet* 1999;37:167.
140. Martin D et al. A controlled trial of valganciclovir as induction therapy for cytomegalovirus retinitis. *N Engl J Med* 2002;346:1119.
141. Pescovitz MD et al. Valganciclovir for prevention of CMV disease: 12 month follow up of a randomized trial of 364 transplant recipients. *American Journal of Transplantation* 2003;3:575.
142. Cvetkovi RS et al. Valganciclovir: a review of its use in the management of CMV infection and disease in immunocompromised patients. *Drugs* 2005;65:859.
143. Lopau K et al. Efficacy and safety of preemptive anti-CMV therapy with valganciclovir after kidney transplantation. *Clin Transpl* 2007;21:80.
144. Humar A et al. A prospective assessment of valganciclovir for the treatment of cytomegalovirus infection and disease in transplant recipients. *J Infect Dis* 2005;192:1154.
145. Product Information: Valcyte, valganciclovir. Roche Laboratories, Inc., Nutley, NJ; 4/2001.
146. Snydman DR et al. Cytomegalovirus immune globulin prophylaxis in liver transplantation. A randomized, double-blind, placebo-controlled trial. The Boston Center for Liver Transplantation. CMVIG Study Group. *Ann Intern Med* 1993;119:984.
147. Fiddian P et al. Valacyclovir provides optimum acyclovir exposure for prevention of cytomegalovirus and related outcomes after organ transplantation. *J Infect Dis* 2002;186(Suppl 1):S110.
148. Khoury JA et al. Prophylactic versus preemptive oral valganciclovir for the management of cytomegalovirus infection in adult renal transplant recipients. *American Journal of Transplantation* 2006;6:2134.

CHAPTER 35

Heart and Lung Transplantation

Tamara Claridge and Gilbert J. Burckart

INTRODUCTION

A general introduction to solid organ transplantation is provided in Chapter 34. This chapter addresses the indications for heart and lung transplantation, the appropriate use of immunosuppressive agents, and the management of postoperative and long-term complications. Although many of these issues are similar for all solid organ transplantations, unique issues exist for each organ.

HEART TRANSPLANTATION

Indications

1. M.S., a 60-year-old, 65-kg man (body mass index [BMI] 25 kg/m^2) with end-stage ischemic heart disease in stage D heart failure with functional class IV symptoms (according to New York Heart Association [NYHA]), is in the coronary intensive care unit, where he has been receiving continuous inotropic therapy for 1 month. He is on the heart transplant waiting list (status 1B). He had an acute myocardial infarction (MI) in 1995, coronary artery bypass graft in 1996 and 2003 along with several admissions for exacerbation of heart failure (HF) over the past year and an episode of sudden cardiac death 1 month ago. His most recent multiple gated acquisition (MUGA) scan to evaluate left ventricular function reveals a left ventricular ejection fraction (LVEF) of 14%, and echocardiography shows extensive anterior, septal, lateral, and apical akinesia, and severe mitral regurgitation. Right-sided heart catheterization shows mild pulmonary hypertension with a pulmonary vascular resistance of 2.8 Wood units. VO_2 (oxygen uptake via cardiopulmonary exercise testing) is 8 mL/kg/minute. Medical history also includes hypertension and hypercholesterolemia. He currently is being treated with dobutamine intravenous (IV) infusion, carvedilol 25 mg twice daily (BID), valsartan 80 mg daily, warfarin 2.5 mg daily, furosemide 80 mg BID, potassium chloride (KCl) 10 mEq BID, spironolactone 25 mg daily, digoxin 0.125 mg daily, and simvastatin 20 mg daily. His vital signs are as follows: blood pressure (BP), 122/82 mmHg; heart rate (HR), 70 beats/minute; respiratory rate (RR) 24 breaths/minute; and temperature, 36.6°C. His laboratory values are as follows: Na, 136 mEq/L (normal, 135–145); K, 4.3 mEq/L (normal, 3.4–4.6); Cl, 94 mEq/L (normal, 95–105); CO_2, 32 mEq/L (normal, 24–30); blood urea nitrogen (BUN), 23 mg/dL (normal, 8–18); serum creatinine (SrCr), 1.1 mg/dL (normal, 0.6–1.2); total bilirubin, 1.7 mg/dL (normal, 0.1–1.0); aspartate aminotransferase (AST), 40 U/L (normal, 0–35); alanine aminotransferase (ALT), 16 U/L (normal, 0–35); lactate dehydrogenase (LDH), 267 U/L (normal, 50–150); alkaline phosphatase, 100 U/L (normal, 30–120); 24-hour creatinine clearance (Cl_{Cr}), 60 mL/minute (normal, 75–125); cholesterol, 225 mg/dL (normal, <200); triglycerides, 99 mg/dL (normal, 1–249); high-density lipoprotein (HDL), 71 mg/dL (normal, 28–71); and low-density lipoprotein (LDL), 134 mg/dL (normal, <130). His other laboratory tests are negative for hepatitis B, human immunodeficiency virus (HIV), and Epstein-Barr virus (EBV), but positive for cytomegalovirus (CMV) and toxoplasmosis. What makes M.S. an appropriate candidate for heart transplantation?

[SI units: Na, 136 mmol/L (normal, 135–145); K, 4.3 mmol/L (3.4–4.6); Cl, 94 mmol/L (normal, 95–105); CO_2, 32 mmol/L (normal, 24–30); BUN, 8.2 mmol/L (normal, 3.0–6.5); SrCr, 97.2 μmol/L (normal, 50–110); total bilirubin, 29.1 μmol/L (normal, 2–18); AST 0.67 μkat/L (normal, 0–0.58); ALT, 0.27 μkat/L (normal, 0–0.58); LDH, 4.45 μkat/L (normal, 0.82–2.66); alkaline phosphatase, 1.67 μkat/L (normal, 0.5–2.0); Cl_{Cr}, 1.0 mL/sec (normal, 1.24–2.08); cholesterol, 5.82 mmol/L (normal, <5.20); triglycerides, 1.12 mmol/L (normal, 0.01–2.8); HDL, 1.83 mg/dL (normal, 0.72–1.83); LDL, 3.47 mmol/L (normal, 0.26–3.34)]

The success of heart transplantation has had a significant impact on the survival of patients with end-stage heart disease (ESHD). The 1- and 5-year survival rates are 85% to 90% and approximately 75%, respectively, with a graft half-life of 9.9 years. In contrast, the 1-year survival rate for patients with severe ESHD without transplant is 20% to 40%. Nonischemic cardiomyopathy and coronary artery disease account for 46%

and 42% of those having transplantation. Patients >50 years of age are the fastest-growing segment of the population having heart transplantation.[1,2]

The best candidates for heart transplantation are those who are least likely to survive without a transplant; that is, those with a low life expectancy and a high likelihood of a good quality of life after transplantation. The criteria for the selection of patients for heart transplantation varies from center to center, but general criteria for selection of appropriate candidates include NYHA functional class III or IV, having intolerable symptoms despite maximal medical and surgical management, lack of reversible factors, and a 1-year life expectancy of <50%. An ejection fraction of <20% alone is not an indication for transplantation. Secondary comorbid conditions also affect the selection of suitable patients for heart transplantation (e.g., irreversible renal, hepatic, or pulmonary disease; severe cerebrovascular or peripheral vascular disease; active infection; current malignancy; acute pulmonary embolus or pulmonary infarction; active gastrointestinal [GI] disease; insulin-dependent diabetes mellitus with end-organ damage; coexisting illness with poor prognosis; morbid obesity; severe osteoporosis; substance abuse; acute psychological disorder; noncompliance). One hemodynamic exclusion criterion specific for heart transplant is an elevated pulmonary vascular resistance >5 Wood units or a transpulmonary gradient >16 mmHg that does not reverse with treatment, indicating severe irreversible pulmonary hypertension. Patients with this characteristic are excluded as candidates for heart transplantation because they generally experience a poor outcome in the immediate post-transplantation period. These patients could be candidates for heart-lung transplant or, more commonly, the placement of a ventricular assist device as destination therapy, which also can be offered patients who do not qualify for heart transplant for other reasons.[3,4]

M.S. has considerable evidence of a progressively failing heart. His increasing number of admissions for HF exacerbations, an admission for sudden cardiac death, his need for chronic IV inotropic support, and his poor LVEF and VO_2 provide clear indications for heart transplantation. The status of his organ function and his negative infectious serology should clear the way for placement on the waiting list for transplantation. The placement of M.S. into the appropriate status category (1A, 1B, 2 or 7) for heart transplant is mainly dependent on his severity of illness including current medical management. Status is defined by United Network for Organ Sharing (UNOS) policy and bylaws. A 1A patient is considered to have the highest medically urgent need for a heart transplant. Qualifiers include continuous infusions of dobutamine at 7.5 mcg/kg/minute or higher, or milrinone at 0.5 mcg/kg/minute, or multiple inotropic infusions, all with a pulmonary artery catheter in place or continuous mechanical ventilation. Patients on mechanical assist devices automatically receive 30 days of 1A time once they are considered stable for listing and then they are downgraded to a 1B status. If they have a device complication, they may remain a 1A. Maintenance of 1A status requires recertification every 7 to 14 days, depending on the qualifier. The patient classified as a 1B has a mechanical assist device in place and has used up their 30 days of 1A status or is on continuous dobutamine or milrinone infusions at doses lower than those mentioned above. A status 2 patient does not meet the qualifiers for 1A or 1B, whereas the status 7 patient is considered temporarily inactive and unable to receive a heart transplant at this time.[5]

POSTOPERATIVE COURSE

2. M.S. receives oral (PO) mycophenolate 1 g, vancomycin 1 g IV, and cefepime 2 g IV before surgery. During reperfusion of his new heart, methylprednisolone 500 mg IV was given, and IV infusions of dopamine, nitroglycerin, dobutamine, and isoproterenol were started. A temporary pacemaker was placed in the new heart. M.S. is placed in the cardiac surgery ICU for post-transplantation care. The following medications were given IV: vancomycin 1 g every 12 hours, cefepime 1 g every 12 hours for 48 hours, pantoprazole 40 mg IV daily, methylprednisolone 125 mg every 8 hours × three doses and then a prednisone taper, mycophenolate 1g IV BID, thymoglobulin 1.5 g/kg IV × one subsequent dosing based on CD3 counts, tacrolimus 2 mg PO BID starting when SrCr was below 1.3 and ganciclovir 150 mg IV BID. He also is maintained on continuous IV infusions of nitroglycerin, dobutamine, and milrinone. Why would M.S. require vasopressor and inotropic therapy perioperatively and postoperatively?

Most heart transplant recipients recover rapidly from the transplantation procedure; they are extubated and taken off vasopressor or inotropic support within 24 to 48 hours. During the early postoperative period, however, the cardiac, respiratory, fluid, and electrolyte status of the patient must be monitored intensively. The transplanted heart is denervated such that contractility and sinus node function are temporarily impaired to varying degrees based on the condition of the donor heart, quality of preservation, ischemic time, surgical technique, myocardial depletion, and elevated pulmonary artery pressure. Soon after transplantation, both left and right ventricular dysfunction can present with elevated right and left heart filling pressures. For the first few days after transplantation, the heart depends on direct stimulation from exogenously administered catecholamines for inotropic and chronotropic support. At this time, the heart is especially sensitive to β-agonists, such as isoproterenol or dobutamine, because β-adrenergic receptors are upregulated.[6] Therefore, inotropic and chronotropic therapy should be guided by hemodynamic monitoring results (see Chapter 21, Shock). In addition, low-dose dopamine, diuretics, or both may be needed to maintain adequate fluid balance and urine output.

For recipients such as M.S., inotropic and chronotropic agents usually are started in the operating room when the new heart is being reperfused and cardiopulmonary bypass is being discontinued. The choice of agent or combination of agents is based on the aforementioned hemodynamic parameters. The patient is eventually weaned off these agents. Isoproterenol and epinephrine are the primary agents used to maintain a heart rate between 110 and 130 beats/minute to maximize cardiac output (CO). The inotropic effects of dobutamine or milrinone are used to increase CO, reduce left ventricular dysfunction, and reduce systemic vascular resistance. Dopamine, at low dosages, could improve renal blood flow. Nitroglycerin or nitroprusside reduces pulmonary arterial pressure and afterload. Temporary atrial pacing may be used to maintain the heart rate as well. If elevated pulmonary artery pressures are unresponsive to the above agents, leading to sustained right ventricular failure, sildenafil, inhaled nitric oxide, IV prostaglandin E_1, and norepinephrine may be required. If these interventions fail, insertion of a mechanical assistance device may be effective.[7,8]

Sinus Node Dysfunction

3. Two days later, M.S. is extubated and hemodynamically stable. Vasopressors are discontinued, and IV medications are switched to oral formulations. On day 9, his heart rate has decreased to 50 to 60 beats/minute. A continuous IV infusion of isoproterenol was restarted because M.S.'s temporary pacemaker had been removed 2 days earlier, resulting in a heart rate of 80 to 110 beats/minute. Theophylline extended release 150 mg BID is started and the dosage adjusted. Why is this appropriate therapy of M.S.'s bradycardia?

Sinus node dysfunction, which presents as nodal or sinus bradycardia and episodes of sinus arrest, is common in the early postoperative period. The donor sinus node serves as the heart's pacemaker, but because it is denervated, the transplanted heart cannot respond to cholinergic or vagal stimulation. Therefore, atropine, which commonly is used to treat bradycardia, is not effective. In most patients, the bradycardia is transient, and temporary use of isoproterenol or a pacemaker is needed. If resistance to vagal stimulation persists (as it does in ~5%–20% of patients), placement of a permanent pacemaker has been the traditional approach. The insertion of a permanent pacemaker may increase the risk of infection and interfere with the endomyocardial biopsy (EMB) procedure that is used to assess the status of rejection. Ultimately, up to 70% of patients with a permanent pacemaker return to normal sinus rhythm within 12 months.[9]

Theophylline has been associated with a restoration of normal vagal response, fewer days of temporary pacing and days of hospitalization, and a decreased need for a permanent pacemaker. It may antagonize the negative chronotropic and dromotropic effects of adenosine and increase catecholamine levels. The catecholamines stimulate the transplanted heart because of its increased sensitivity.[10]

Because M.S.'s temporary pacemaker was removed a few days earlier, the use of IV isoproterenol, followed by theophylline, is appropriate as long as he is hemodynamically stable. Although no specific dosing guidelines exist for this situation, oral theophylline extended release 150 mg every 12 hours or aminophylline IV infusion at 0.5 mg/kg/hour if the patient cannot take drugs orally are appropriate starting regimens. These regimens should be adjusted based on heart rate and achievement of therapeutic theophylline serum concentrations (10–15 mg/mL). A response should be evident within 4 days; if supraventricular tachyarrhythmias occur, the dosage of theophylline should be reduced and the drug may have to be discontinued. Terbutaline dosed three times daily PO is an alternative agent.

Cardiac Denervation

4. What is the effect of denervation on the physiology of the heart and what are the pharmacodynamic effects of cardiac medications after heart transplantation?

Although the transplanted heart usually functions very well, physiologic changes result in different responses to various stimuli when contrasted to the normal innervated heart. The transplanted heart has a higher resting heart rate than normal because of vagal tone loss. Therefore, as already noted, drugs that work via the parasympathetic pathway (e.g., atropine) will be ineffective. The transplanted heart also accelerates more slowly during exercise, usually taking several minutes to reach a maximal heart rate, which is still less than a normal innervated heart during exercise. Acute reflex changes in heart rate do not occur in response to increases or decreases in BP in the denervated transplanted heart, and the ability to feel anginal pain is lost. Therefore, the clinical response to antianginal medications is masked. CO and BP usually are normal in the nonrejecting heart.[6] Because the adrenergic system remains intact in the transplanted denervated heart, drugs such as isoproterenol, milrinone, epinephrine, norepinephrine, dopamine, phenylephrine, glucagon, and β-blockers still exert cardiac effects. The indirect chronotropic effect of digoxin on the sinus and atrioventricular nodes will not be manifested in the denervated heart, but the inotropic effect will be maintained. The usual increase in heart rate secondary to nifedipine-lowered BP usually is muted as well, and responses of the denervated heart to verapamil, diltiazem, quinidine, and disopyramide also may be altered.[9] Because the effect of nonprescription sympathomimetics on the transplanted heart has not been determined, these agents should be used cautiously.[11] Reinnervation has been reported in some patients.

Immunosuppression

5. What was the justification for using quadruple immunosuppressive therapy (i.e., thymoglobulin, tacrolimus, methylprednisolone, and mycophenolate) in M.S.? What is the appropriate therapeutic drug monitoring scheme for this regimen in M.S.?

After heart transplantation, immunosuppressive therapy with three or four drugs is administered aggressively during the early transplantation period when the risk of organ rejection is greatest. Calcineurin inhibitors (CNI) remain the mainstay of therapy, with tacrolimus being used a bit more frequently than cyclosporine; mycophenolate mofetil (MMF) 1 to 1.5 g BID is the antiproliferative agent of choice and corticosteroids are used as the third maintenance agent. Historically, regimens of azathioprine with prednisone or azathioprine, prednisone, and antithymocyte globulin were associated with survival rates of 50% and 60%, respectively. The addition of cyclosporine increased the rate of organ survival by 80% to 90%. Regimens containing oral tacrolimus (initial regimen of 0.05 mg/kg BID) are similar in efficacy to cyclosporine modified based regimens in regards to rejection episodes and graft survival, but with less hypertension and hyperlipidemia.[1,2,12,13] Long-term follow-up indicates that there may be less acute rejection, or acute rejection of lower severity, which may explain why more patients are receiving tacrolimus-based immunosuppressive therapy.[14,15] Because MMF is associated with lower rejection rates and improved survival, it has replaced azathioprine in heart transplantation at most U.S. centers.[16–18] Furthermore, data in patients converted from MMF to azathioprine late after transplant show a high rate of acute rejection.[19] Enteric-coated mycophenolate sodium 720 mg BID has been shown to be bioequivalent to MMF 1 g BID for mycophenolic acid in kidney transplant recipients and has a developing role in cardiac transplant recipients.[20]

The 20 times higher cost of MMF keeps azathioprine in use in the United States and extensively outside of North America. The active components of azathioprine are the 6-thioguanine nucleotides, which are metabolized by thiopurine methyltransferase (TPMT). The TPMT enzyme is polymorphically expressed, with heterozygous variants making up about 10% of the population and homozygous variants occurring in <1% of patients. If TPMT activity is decreased, 6-thioguanine nucleotides accumulate and exert their antiproliferative activity on white blood cells (WBC). Reports of excessive leukopenia in transplant recipients who are heterozygous for TPMT continue to appear in the literature.[21] Although the homozygous variant is rare, these patients would be at extreme risk of neutropenia and sepsis. The U.S. Food and Drug Administration (FDA)-approved information on azathioprine recommends TPMT genotyping before therapy.

The adverse effect profile of CNI, has led to an increased use of sirolimus (inhibitor of late T-cell function).[1] Sirolimus as a replacement for CNI in patients with renal failure showed mixed results.[22] When tacrolimus and sirolimus were used as initial therapy, an increase was seen in fungal infections, diabetes and nephrotoxicity.[23] Recently, tacrolimus or sirolimus or cyclosporine-modified, plus MMF and steroids were compared head to head. No difference was found in rejection at 6 months, whereas at 12 months an advantage was seen in the tacrolimus and sirolimus arms. When looking at other endpoints, however, sirolimus was associated with more fungal infections and wound healing issues. The authors concluded that the most advantageous initial maintenance regimen at this time includes tacrolimus, MMF, and a steroid.[24]

The use of antilymphocyte antibodies or antithymocyte globulin or IL-2 receptor (IL–2R) antagonists as induction therapy is increasing, with 50% of heart transplant recipients receiving one of the aforementioned agents, whereas OKT3 use continues to decline (<5%).[1] Induction therapy remains a controversial topic; some centers may choose induction therapy for every patient because it delays the onset of acute rejection. Others are more selective, using these agents only for patients who have pre- or postoperative renal insufficiency, which limits the early initiation of CNI, (as in M.S.'s case) or for sensitized patients (elevated panel reactive antibodies [PRA]) who are considered to have a higher risk of rejection.[25] Induction therapy also may allow for a more rapid discontinuation of maintenance corticosteroids.[26–28] IL-2R antagonists decrease the acute rejection rate when compared with placebo.[29–32] For basiliximab, patients receive two doses (perioperative and postoperative day 4), whereas daclizumab is labeled for five doses (1 mg/kg preoperative then every 2 weeks); however, two-dose therapy has been studied with no deleterious effects.[33,34] When IL-2R antagonists have been compared with antithymocyte globulins (also known as antilymphocyte antibodies) in head to head clinical trials, the results are mixed regarding acute rejection rates, and the long-term effects on chronic rejections rates and graft loss are not known.[35–37] The antithymocyte globulins are polyclonal immuneglobulins that contain antibodies that affect a variety of immune cell activities, including T-lymphocytes and B-lymphocytes, making them unable to generate a response to an immune stimulus. Thus, they can be used for both induction and rejection therapy. Their mechanism of action creates a profound immunosuppressed state that may lead to an increased rate of infection, adverse effect profile (cytokine release syndrome), and a higher risk of malignancy long term. Antithymocyte globulin rabbit (Thymoglobulin) is dosed at 1 to 1. 5 mg/kg/day, whereas antithymocyte globulin horse (ATGAM) is dosed at 10 to 15 mg/kg/day for 3 to 10 days. Studies have shown, however, that doses that are adjusted based on CD3 counts have a similar efficacy, with decreased total dose, length of stay, and lower costs. Overimmunosuppression may be avoided as well.[38,39] At U.S. transplant centers antithymocyte globulin rabbit has greater use. If muromonab-CD3 (OKT3), a murine monoclonal antibody to the CD3 receptor of the T-lymphocyte is used, the usual dose is 5 mg/kg IV daily for 7 days.

The corticosteroid could be discontinued within the first year depending on M.S.'s clinical course. Several reports have indicated that steroid withdrawal, generally begun >6 months after transplant, is possible in many patients who are considered low risk, such as whites with fewer and less severe acute rejection episodes.[40,41] A risk of late rejection always exists, and the impact of steroid discontinuation on long-term survival has not been thoroughly evaluated. Recent registry data indicate that ~75% of patients are still on prednisone therapy 12 months after transplant.[1] Corticosteroid withdrawal is particularly important in pediatric heart transplant recipients, because they decrease growth. Corticosteroids are substrates for the membrane transporter P-glycoprotein, which is very active in T cells. The genotype for higher P-glycoprotein pumping has been associated with the inability to wean pediatric heart transplant recipients off of corticosteroids 1 year after transplantation.[42]

Therapeutic drug monitoring for M.S. will include tacrolimus whole blood levels. The therapeutic range is 10 to 20 ng/mL early after transplant and 8 to 12 ng/mL once the patient is stabilized on the drug. The genotype of cytochrome P450 3A5 affects the dosage of tacrolimus required to achieve blood concentrations in heart and lung transplant recipients, with enzyme expressors requiring more drug to achieve the same levels as nonexpressors.[43,44] The availability of tacrolimus concentrations, however, negates the value of CYP3A5 genotyping in transplant recipients.[45] Although some centers measure mycophenolic acid plasma concentrations, most give an arbitrary MMF or mycophenolate sodium dosage and adjust doses as clinically indicated. Mycophenolic acid is very highly bound to albumin in plasma, so concentration measurement in the early postoperative period for heart or liver transplant recipients may be misleading until albumin concentrations stabilize.[46]

Transplant recipients older than 65 might experience lower rejection rates and higher rates of infections, malignancy, and toxicities. Although this requires further study, centers may target lower drug levels and doses of maintenance medications in this population.

Acute or Chronic Rejection

6. M.S. is discharged after 20 days in the hospital and returns for a routine clinic visit and scheduled EMB. Current medications include tacrolimus 3 mg PO BID; prednisone 20 mg daily; mycophenolate 1.5 g BID; valganciclovir 900 mg daily;

trimethoprim-sulfamethoxazole (TMP-SMX) double strength one tablet on Monday Wednesday, and Friday; diltiazem CD 180 mg daily; omeprazole 20 mg at bedtime; theophylline extended release 200 mg BID; pravastatin 40 mg daily; nystain swish four times daily (QID) and aspirin 81 mg daily. M.S.'s BP readings, which he monitors at home, range from 140–150/85–90 mmHg. Laboratory test results are as follows: Na, 134 mEq/L (normal, 135–147); K, 4.3 mEq/L (normal, 3.5–5.0); Cl, 103 mEq/L (normal, 95–105); CO_2, 26 mEq/L (normal, 22–28); BUN, 16 mg/dL (normal, 8–18); SrCr, 1.4 mg/dL (normal, 0.6–1.2); tacrolimus trough level 10 ng/mL; and theophylline level, 14 mg/mL. His vital signs are as follows: HR, 105 beats/minute; BP, 155/84 mmHg; and temperature, 36.8°C. Biopsy results indicate a mild grade 1R rejection of his transplanted heart. His tacrolimus dose is increased to 3 mg every morning and 4 mg every afternoon. A repeat EMB 1 week later now shows a grade 2R moderate rejection. What signs and symptoms indicate that M.S. is experiencing acute rejection of his transplanted heart?

[SI units: Na, 134 mmol/L (normal, 135–147); K, 4.3 mmol/L (normal, 3.5–5.0); Cl, 103 mmol/L (normal, 95–105); CO_2, 26 mmol/L (normal, 22–28); BUN, 5.7 mmol/L (3.0–6.5); creatinine, 173.3 μmol/L (normal, 50–110)]

Organ rejection can be classified as hyperacute, accelerated, acute, vascular, and chronic. (See Chapter 34 Question 9). Current data indicate that acute rejection rates are <30% after heart transplantation. Approximately 50% of these occurred within the first 6 weeks and 90% within the first 6 months, although rejection can occur at any time.[7] Acute rejection of a transplanted heart accounts for approximately 12% of deaths after transplantation.[1] Risk factors for acute rejection include younger recipient age, female gender (donor and recipient), donor heart ischemic time, number of human leukocyte antigen (HLA) mismatches, and retransplantation.

Most rejection episodes are asymptomatic. If clinical signs are present, however, they can include nonspecific signs of fatigue, malaise, and a low-grade temperature. In some cases, dyspnea and weight gain are seen. Heart transplant recipients do not experience cardiac chest pain because of denervation. When patients with a heart transplant present with significant hemodynamic cardiovascular symptoms, such as hypotension, increased jugular venous distention, S_3 sounds, and rales, it may indicate advanced severe rejection. Patients experiencing an acute rejection of a transplanted heart also may present with new-onset arrhythmias and congestive heart failure (CHF), although these usually occur late in the rejection process.[7] Therefore, acute rejection of a transplanted heart must be determined by an internal jugular transvenous EMB, the gold standard for diagnosis. A set of histologic criteria has been developed to standardize the severity of rejection. A grading scale of 0 to 3R is used to describe the degree of damage to cardiac tissue.[47]

Vascular or humoral rejection, which is an antibody-mediated process, also may occur.[48] This form of rejection is associated with a higher incidence of cardiac allograft vasculopathy and an increased mortality rate and is more difficult to treat. Because this rejection is antibody (B-lymphocyte) mediated, there have been several case reports of successful treatment using an anti-CD20 monoclonal antibody, rituximab.[49–51]

M.S. is asymptomatic, which is consistent with most patients who have biopsy-proved evidence of acute rejection but do not present with clinical symptoms. Although patients with mild, grade 1 rejection often are asymptomatic, 20% to 30% can go on to develop moderate, grade 2 to 3 rejection.[52] When rejection of a transplanted heart is detected, the EMB should be repeated within 1 week. A number of other noninvasive electrophysiologic, echocardiographic, immunologic, radioisotopic, and biochemical methods are being investigated for their value in detecting acute rejection of a transplanted heart.

A genomic test is being used to monitor heart transplant recipients for acute rejection, based on a study comparing a messenger RNA (mRNA) microarray of the peripheral blood to heart biopsy results.[53] Stable patients can now have a blood sample taken instead of having to undergo a heart biopsy. If the score of this test, called Allomap (XDx, Brisbane, California), suggests that the patient may be having acute rejection, then a heart biopsy is taken. This form of monitoring may be expanded in the future to include monitoring for renal dysfunction or adverse drug effects.

Chronic rejection of a transplanted heart is called *cardiac allograft vasculopathy* (CAV) and is sometimes referred to as *transplant coronary artery disease* (TCAD), *accelerated CAD,* or *graft arteriosclerosis.* It is a leading cause of death after the first year in many heart transplant recipients.[1] Despite immunosuppressive therapy, approximately 10% of patients experience chronic rejection of a heart transplant within the first year, and this increases to at least 50% within 8 years.[1] The clinical presentation is insidious, nonspecific, and similar to the clinical presentation associated with acute rejection. The first presenting signs may be CHF, arrhythmias, MI, or sudden death.[54] Therefore, patients must undergo routine coronary angiography or intravascular ultrasound, which is more sensitive, shortly after heart transplantation and every year subsequently. On angiography, chronic rejection of a transplanted heart diffusely affects both arteries and veins. The pathogenesis of this condition, which results in endothelial damage and a cascade of other related events, is unknown. However, a number of immunologic (acute rejection),[55,56] infectious (CMV), and nonimmunologic factors (graft ischemia, hyperlipidemia, hypertension, glucose intolerance, smoking, obesity), along with donor factors (age, male gender, hypertension [HTN], previous blood transfusion) are associated with its development.[54,57]

Pharmacologic therapy has been directed toward prevention of this condition. Antiplatelet agents, such as the aspirin used by M.S., are used routinely, but have not been shown to alter progression to CAV.[58] Diltiazem, which M.S. also is receiving for hypertension, inhibits progressive coronary obstruction as well.[59] Other maneuvers include diet modification and BP and lipid control.[60] Pravastatin and simvastatin initiated in the first days to weeks, decrease coronary artery disease and improve survival after transplantation, such that (HMG-CoA) reductase inhibitors are now considered as standard of care.[61–63] Sirolimus and everolimus (investigational in the United States) inhibit smooth muscle or fibroblastic cellular growth, which has been shown to delay the onset and slow the progression of CAV.[64–67] When these agents are added to therapy, the CNI dose is decreased or discontinued, or the MMF or azathioprine therapy is removed. Although the preceding pharmacologic interventions hold some promise, retransplantation is the only effective therapy for chronic rejection.

Treatment of Acute Rejection

7. What approach should be taken in the treatment of M.S.'s grade 1 acute cardiac rejection?

Rejection grade helps to form the basis for selecting pharmacologic management. Although the individual drugs usually are given at high doses over a short period, the doses, routes, and regimens vary from program to program. High-dose corticosteroids are the primary agents used to treat moderate to severe rejection, and IV methylprednisolone 1 g every day for 3 days is effective in 85% of the initial episodes of acute cardiac rejection.[68]

When M.S. was asymptomatic and had a grade 1R mild rejection, no treatment was indicated because many of these episodes resolve without intervention. An adjustment in maintenance immunosuppression is appropriate, and the increase in M.S.'s tacrolimus dose is reasonable, especially because his blood concentration was lower than desired. Nevertheless, some programs treat mild rejection because of the concern for progression to a more severe grade. As was done with M.S., a follow-up EMB, usually within 1 week of the initial diagnosis, should be performed. In M.S.'s case, the grade 1R (mild acute rejection) of his transplanted heart progressed to grade 2R. In this situation, high-dose methylprednisolone 500 to 1,000 mg IV or 10 mg/kg every day for 3 days would be given. Also, his maintenance prednisone regimen may be adjusted. Patients who were off of prednisone may have it reinstated. Alternatively, a high-dose prednisone regimen with a gradual dosage reduction could be instituted after the 3-day IV course of methylprednisolone was completed.[69] Oral prednisone 50 mg twice a day for 2 to 5 days and tapered over 7 to 14 days to the previous maintenance dose is another alternative because M.S. already is on prednisone, and hemodynamic compromise is not evident.[70]

After a course of high-dose methylprednisolone, M.S. should be monitored for any hemodynamic and functional changes that might indicate further progression of rejection, and the biopsy should be repeated. If M.S. develops severe rejection, he may receive another regimen of IV methylprednisolone, or therapy could be initiated with Thymoglobulin, ATG, or OKT3. When these antilymphocyte antibodies are used for patients unresponsive to corticosteroids, the treatment is known as *rescue therapy.* Thymoglobulin, ATG, and OKT3 are equally advantageous in this situation. A typical regimen is Thymoglobulin 1 to 1.5 mg/kg/day or ATG 10 mg/kg IV every day for 7 to 10 days and both could also be dosed using CD3 monitoring. OKT3, 5 mg IV every day for 7 to 10 days, can also be given.

In some patients, the acute rejection episode is refractory to high-dose corticosteroids, ATG, and OKT3. Treatment for refractory or recurrent rejection includes replacing cyclosporine with tacrolimus or azathioprine with mycophenolate.[71] Other therapies for this type of rejection include the addition of sirolimus,[72] methotrexate, or cyclophosphamide.

Hypertension

8. T.L., a 35-year-old woman, 15 months post heart transplant secondary to valvular cardiomyopathy, has noted an increase in the her home blood pressure readings. Her blood pressures have been ranging from 145–160/90–95 mmHg. T.L.'s current medication regimen includes tacrolimus 2 mg PO BID, sirolimus 2 mg daily, prednisone 2.5 mg daily, calcium and vitamin D 500 mg twice daily, famotidine 20 mg PO BID, atorvastatin 20 mg daily, aspirin 81 mg PO daily, and multivitamin PO daily. T.L. has no other comorbid conditions. In clinic, her BP is 150/85 mmHg, HR 90, BMI 23 kg/m^2, Na, 138 mEq/L (normal, 135–145); K, 4 mEq/L (normal, 3.4–4.6); Cl, 100 mEq/L (normal, 95–105); CO_2, 27 mEq/L (normal, 24–30); BUN, 30 mg/dL (normal, 8–18); SrCr, 1.3 mg/dL (normal, 0.6–1.2). What is the appropriate blood pressure regimen to institute in T.L.?

[SI units: Na, 136 mmol/L (normal, 135–145); K, 4.3 mmol/L (3.4–4.6); Cl, 94 mmol/L (normal, 95–105); CO_2, 32 mmol/L (normal, 24–30); BUN, 8.2 mmol/L (normal, 3.0–6.5); SrCr, 97.2 μmol/L (normal, 50–110)]

The prevalence of hypertension (HTN) increases following transplantation of all organs. Kidney and heart transplant recipients have a higher rate secondary to pre-existing HTN, which may have led to end-stage organ failure. Post-transplant HTN is a risk factor for the development of end-stage renal disease, cardiovascular morbidity and mortality, and decreased graft and patient survival.[73] Immunosuppressive medication is a confounding factor, because HTN is a side effect of many CNIs and corticosteroids. The target BP should be <140/90 mmHg, following published recommendations. Nonpharmacologic therapies (weight loss, low sodium diet, cessation of cigarette smoking) also play a role in treatment.

Selecting an appropriate antihypertensive must take into account the potential for significant drug interactions. Dihydropyridine calcium channel blockers (CCB), such as amlodipine (5 mg daily), have been considered first-line treatment. Amlodipine can ameliorate some of the CNI vasoconstrictive effects on the kidney allowing for both a reduction HTN and improvement in renal function with minimal effects on drug levels. Lower extremity edema and proteinuria can occur. In contrast, non-dihydropyridine CCBs (verapamil/diltiazem) have negative inotropic effects and can significantly elevate CNI levels as does nicardipine.

Angiotensin-converting enzymes inhibitors (ACEI) and angiotensin receptor blockers (ARB) may also be beneficial, especially when the patient also has diabetes, heart failure, proteinuria, or erythrocytosis.[74] They should be started cautiously because of their effects on renal perfusion, but they are not contraindicated. Studies in renal and cardiac transplant hypertensive populations show that CCB, ACEI, or ARB response rates are below 50% with monotherapy.[74–77] Thus, most transplant recipients, as with the general population, will require treatment with more than one antihypertensive agent. ACEIs and CCBs also decrease initimal thickening.[78,79]

β-blockers are important for patients with known coronary artery disease; however they can worsen post-transplant dyslipidemias, depression, and recognition of hypoglycemic symptoms; they also have negative chronotropic effects. Carvedilol may increase cyclosporine levels via P-glycoprotein inhibition.[80] Diuretic use is reasonable if there are signs of fluid overload; however, electrolytes and uric acid levels should be monitored. Difficult-to-treat HTN may require the use of vasodilators such as hydralazine or minoxidil.

In T.L., it is reasonable to start amlodipine 5 mg daily or a once-daily ACEI, while avoiding over aggressive titration which can lead to hypotension and compromised organ perfusion. Nonpharmacologic therapies should be strongly encouraged as well.

Hyperlipidemia

9. J.T., a 57-year-old black man, 22 months postorthotopic heart transplant, is seen in the clinic for follow-up of an abnormal lipid panel, HDL 40 mg/dL, LDL 170 mg/dL, triglycerides (TG) 300 mg/dL, and total cholesterol of 350 mg/dL. Other laboratory findings include an A1C of 8%, and an SrCr of 1.3 mg/dL. Current comorbid conditions include HTN, post-transplant diabetes, gout, and a BMI of 32 kg/m^2. His medications include cyclosporine-modified 150 mg PO BID, sirolimus 2 mg daily, prednisone 2.5 mg every other day, aspirin 81 mg daily, atorvastatin 10 mg daily, insulin glargine 15 U BID, correctional scale insulin aspart, calcium + D 500 mg BID, allopurinol 300 mg daily, amlodipine 10 mg daily, and quinapril 10 mg daily. How should his lipids be managed?

Cardiovascular disease after transplant is a major cause of morbidity and mortality. After heart transplant, use of HMG-CoA reductase inhibitors (statins) is a standard of care for most heart transplant centers as a way to decrease cardiac allograft vasculopathy.[81] Patients who develop concurrent hyperlipidemia, however, will need to have their therapy adjusted. The presence of confounding factors (e.g., concomitant diseases, medications, diet, and lack of physical exercise) can worsen the hyperlipidemia. J.T.'s risk factors for hyperlipidemia include male gender, ethnicity, obesity, and diabetes, along with the following medications: sirolimus, cyclosporine modified, and prednisone.

Several treatment options exist for hyperlipidemia including diet, physical activity, tight diabetes control, and lipid-lowering pharmacotherapy. A low-fat diet along with exercise may not be sufficient to control lipids in patients after transplant, and drug therapy is often needed. Drug therapy choices include fibric acid derivatives, niacin, bile-acid binders, statins, and cholesterol absorption inhibitors. Fibric acid derivatives, such as fenofibrates and gemfibrozil, primarily decrease TG levels rather than LDL. They also can affect the absorption of statins and increase their myotoxic effects when used concurrently with statins. Niacin can lower lipid levels; however, in J.T. it may worsen glucose control and precipitate a gout attack. Colestipol and cholestyramine, bile acid derivatives, have been reported to increase TG and may alter the absorption of cyclosporine. Ezetimibe, a cholesterol absorption inhibitor, reduces lipid levels as a single agent and in combination with statins.[82,83] Statins remain the mainstay of therapy for the treatment of dyslipidemias in transplant recipients with the following considerations. All statins—except pravastatin—are metabolized via CYP3A4 (minimal for fluvastatin) and may affect calcineurin inhibitor and sirolimus levels. The concurrent use of statins with CNIs and sirolimus may affect statin metabolism, leading to an increased risk of myotoxicity. Monitoring should be done for hepatotoxicity (liver function tests), myopathies (muscle cramps or pain, elevation in creatinine kinase). The use of statins in combination with other lipid-lowering agents may increase the occurrence of these side effects.

For J.T. the following may be considered: the cyclosporine modified can be changed to tacrolimus, although it is unclear whether its effects on dyslipidemia differ. Sirolimus is known to increase TG, especially when it is initiated. J.T.'s blood glucose levels should be more tightly controlled. His atorvastatin dose can be increased to at least 20 mg daily with close monitoring for side effects. Lastly, J.T.'s weight should be reduced with diet and exercise. If these measures do not result in significant changes, then the addition of ezetimibe therapy, 5 to 10 mg a day, could be considered.

LUNG TRANSPLANTATION

Postoperative Course

10. B.U., a 33-year-old, 54-kg man with a 12-year history of cystic fibrosis (CF), is admitted for bilateral lung transplantation. He had been doing reasonably well until 2 years ago. Since that time, he has been hospitalized five times for acute pulmonary exacerbations caused by *Pseudomonas aeruginosa.* In addition, he has been hospitalized twice in a 6-month period over the past year for hemoptysis secondary to pulmonary infarcts. He now requires continuous oxygen at 3 L/minute via nasal cannula for daily living. Other medical problems include diabetes mellitus, gastroesophageal reflux disease, pancreatic insufficiency, and sinusitis. His current medications are deoxyribonuclease (DNase) 2.5 mL BID, albuterol BID, 4 mL 7% sodium chloride BID, tobramycin 300 mg BID (with monthly holiday), all given via a nebulizer; ADEK vitamin one tablet BID, omeprazole 20 mg daily, insulin glargine 10 U BID, correctional scale insulin aspart, calcium supplement BID, and pancreatic enzymes with meals and snacks. While on 3 L/minute of oxygen, his oxygen saturation is 100%, forced expiratory volume in 1 second (FEV_1), 1.11 (22% predicted), forced vital capacity (FVC), 2.04 (34% predicted). His vital signs are as follows: temperature, 36.5°C; BP, 120/90 mmHg; RR, 20 breaths/minute; and HR, 96 beats/minute. His laboratory results are as follows: Na, 137 mEq/L (normal, 135–147); K, 4.2 mEq/L (normal, 3.5–5.0); Cl, 100 mEq/L (normal, 95–105); CO_2, 28 mEq/L (normal, 22–28); BUN, 24 mg/dL (normal, 8–18); SrCr, 1.2 mg/dL (normal, 0.6–1.2); glucose, 104 mg/dL (normal, 80–120); Ca, 9.0 mg/dL (normal, 8.8–10.3); protein, 8.3 g/dL (normal, 6.0–8.0); albumin 3.9 g/dL (normal, 4.0–6.0); bilirubin, 0.3 mg/dL (normal, 0.1–1.0); AST, 40 U/L (normal, 0–35); ALT, 46 U/L (normal, 0–35); WBC count, 8,000 (normal, 4,000–10,000); Hct, 30% (normal, 39%–49%); Hgb, 9.5 mg/dL (normal, 14.0–18.0); platelets, 340,000 (normal, 130,000–400,000); prothrombin time, 11.6 sec (normal, 9–12); and partial thromboplastin time, 26.4 seconds (normal, 22–37). He is CMV antibody negative.

In the operating room, B.U. was given preoperative mycophenolate mofetil 1,000 mg IV, tobramycin 350 mg IV, piperacillin/tazobactam 4.5 g IV with daclizumab 2 mg/kg IV and methylprednisolone 500 mg IV × 2 during the surgery. B.U. underwent a 12-hour surgery for double-lung transplantation. During the procedure, he received 8 L of fluids and dopamine to correct hypotension. He was admitted to the ICU on a ventilator, where he received tacrolimus 1 mg sublingual (SL) BID, mycophenolate 1 g BID IV, methylprednisolone 125 mg IV every 8 hours then transitioned to prednisone 20 mg daily by postoperative day (POD) 4, $D_5$1/2 normal saline at a rate to keep the vein open, insulin infusion, dopamine 3 mg/kg/minute IV, epidural and patient-controlled analgesia (PCA) morphine, tobramycin 350 mg

daily IV, piperacillin/tazobactam 4.5 g every 6 hours IV, pantoprazole 40 mg IV daily, ganciclovir 125 mg IV BID, CMV immune globulin × 1 on POD 1, cotrimoxazole daily, and albuterol nebulizer QID. The donor was CMV-positive. What complications can occur in B.U. during the early postoperative period?

[SI units: Na, 137 mmol/L (normal, 135–147); K, 4.2 mmol/L (normal, 3.4–4.6); Cl, 100 mmol/L (normal, 95–105); CO_2, 28 mmol/L (normal, 22–28); BUN, 8.6 mmol/L (normal, 3.0–6.5); SrCr, 106.1 (μmol/L (normal, 50–110); glucose, 5.8 mmol/L (normal, 3.9–6.1); Ca, 3.7 mmol/L (normal, 2.2–2.5); protein, 83 g/L (normal, 60–80); albumin, 39 g/L (normal, 40–60); bilirubin, 5.13 μmol/L (normal, 2–18); AST, 40 U/L (normal, 0–35); ALT, 46 U/L (normal, 0–35); WBC count, 4 × 10^9 cells/L (normal, 4,000–10,000); Hct, 0.3 (normal, 0.39–0.49); Hgb, 95 g/L (normal, 140–180); platelets, 340 × 10^8/L (normal, 130–400)]

Lung transplantation is a therapeutic option for end-stage pulmonary disease; >1,500 lungs worldwide are transplanted each year. The 1- and 5-year survival rates are approximately 78% and 49% with a median half-life of 5 years. Chronic obstructive pulmonary disease (COPD) and idiopathic pulmonary fibrosis (IPF) are the primary indications for a single-lung transplant (SLT). Cystic fibrosis and α_1-antitrypsin deficiency are the primary indications for bilateral lung transplant (BLT); however, the aforementioned diseases for SLT are also receiving more BLT.[2,8] Recently, the allocation of lungs has changed from time-on-the-list as priority (considering blood type, geographic location) to a lung allocation score (LAS) for recipients above the age of 12. The LAS score ranges from 0 to 100 (highest priority). Indications that a patient with CF should be evaluated for lung transplant include an FEV_1 below 30% or significant rapid decline and frequent antibiotic treated exacerbations. The use of oxygen, development of pulmonary hypertension, and increasing CO_2 indicate the need for listing.[84]

B.U.'s CF-associated pancreatic and GI problems will not be corrected by the double-lung transplantation. His pulmonary function should improve significantly, however, reaching normal levels within 3 to 12 months. After the transplant, B.U. should no longer require oxygen, achieve normal exercise capacity, and return to a good quality of life.

Patients such as B.U. usually leave the operating room under mechanical ventilation and should be extubated within 24 to 48 hours. In the early postoperative period, the transplanted lung(s) is susceptible to pulmonary edema, hemorrhage, dehiscence at the anastomotic sites, airway leaks, infection, and rejection. Hemorrhage, ischemic or reperfusion injury, and dehiscence have decreased as a result of improved donor preservation and surgical techniques. The most common serious complications are airway complications, reperfusion ischemic pulmonary edema, acute rejection, and infection. Significant incisional pain, which occurs in all patients, also can affect how quickly B.U. recovers. Altered GI function, such as gastroparesis, also is a typical problem in the initial period.

Immunosuppression

B.U. is on the most commonly used regimen for immunosuppression of lung transplants, which consists of tacrolimus, MMF, and steroids. Currently approximately 45% of lung transplant recipients receive induction therapy primarily with an anti-ILR2 antibody (daclizumab or basiliximab). Thymoglobulin and ATG are also used, with minimal use of OKT3.[8,85,86] The anti-IL2R antibodies reduce acute rejection compared with placebo, but when compared with antithymocyte globulin the data are mixed. These drugs have little impact on chronic rejection. A decreased risk of infection may be seen, but is variable in CMV mismatched patients.[87–90] Tacrolimus and cyclosporine have similar effects on graft survival, but tacrolimus is associated with fewer episodes of acute rejection and treated acute rejection and may slow the development of chronic rejection.[91,92] Early, low-dose prednisone (0.5 mg/kg/day tapered to 0.15 mg/kg/day) is used. B.U.'s tacrolimus regimen would be adjusted to maintain a whole blood concentration of 10 to 20 ng/mL (by monoclonal TDx).[93] Tacrolimus must be diluted before continuous IV administration. Because it is less stable in PVC containers and could leach out phthalates, it should be stored in glass or polyethylene containers and PVC tubing should not be used. To simplify administration when patients cannot take medications orally or have absorption problems (as in CF), some centers are giving tacrolimus sublingually. This route avoids the first-pass metabolism and has produced acceptable drug levels and rejection rates in small studies, but no prospective randomized trials have been conducted. Initial doses are 0.03 mg/kg/day.[94] MMF, instead of azathioprine, is used in approximately 50% of lung transplant recipients.[8,95] The role of sirolimus is increasing; however, use before 3 months postoperatively is avoided because it interferes with wound healing and can lead to weakened airway anastomosis.

Acute Rejection

11. At his 3 month visit, B.U. has his scheduled protocol biopsy. That afternoon, the transplant team is notified that he has an A1B2 rejection. What is the appropriate regimen to treat this rejection episode?

Rejection, both acute and chronic, occurs in all lung transplant recipients. Acute rejection is common in the early postoperative period, with up to 50% of patients having at least one treated episode within the first year.[8] Nevertheless, acute rejection can occur at any time.[96] The diagnosis of acute rejection is made using clinical and histologic criteria. Standardized criteria have been established for histologic grading of tissue from transbronchial biopsies (TBBX), which are scheduled routinely.[97] Clinical signs of acute rejection include fever, cough, dyspnea, rales, wheezes, infiltrates, and a decline in FEV_1. The FEV_1 and FVC are assessed daily by the patient using a hand-held spirometer. As little as a 10% decline in pulmonary function (i.e., FEV_1, FVC) can be significant in the absence of other causes of respiratory decline, particularly infection. Treatment for acute rejection can be initiated based on clinical signs only, although they are not always accurate. If clinical evidence of acute rejection is present, a TBBX is needed to firmly establish the diagnosis of rejection. The diagnosis of lung transplant rejection still can be established even in the face of a negative TBBX if other causes are ruled out.[97]

The primary treatment for acute rejection is methylprednisolone 500 to 1,000 mg/day IV or 10 to 15 mg/kg/day every day for 3 days. The dose of oral prednisone also can be increased to 1 mg/kg/day and then tapered down to the maintenance dose over 2 to 3 weeks. More than 90% of acute rejection episodes of transplanted lungs respond to corticosteroid therapy, with clinical response seen within 2 days in most patients.[98] OKT3, ATGAM, Thymoglobulin, tacrolimus, and experimental aerosolized cyclosporine have been used for refractory cases.[99–101]

Pharmacogenetic factors may play a role in resistance to treatment for acute rejection in lung transplant recipients. The homozygous and heterozygous ABCB1 genotypes that are associated with higher P-glycoprotein pumping had more persistent acute rejection that was resistant to drug therapy than the homozygous variant genotype.[102] The same association has been made between acute rejection in kidney transplant recipients and the ABCB1 high pumper genotype.

Chronic Rejection

12. B.U. is 36 months post transplant and is noticing a slight increase in shortness of breath when he exercises. His pulmonary function testing over the last two clinic visits has demonstrated a sustained change in his FEV_1. The FEV_1 has declined by 30% from his highest value post-transplant. The transplant team believes B.U. has chronic rejection. What is the appropriate management?

Chronic rejection is referred to as bronchiolitis obliterans (OB) or bronchiolitis obliterans syndrome (BOS). OB is a histologic finding of a fibroproliferative process in the small airways, which leads to progressive airway obstruction. The diagnosis of OB is based on clinical, physiologic, and histologic features.[103] Pulmonary function and exercise capacity progressively decline as a result of inflamed small airways and destruction of bronchioles. OB is found in 9% of patients at 1 year and in 45% at 5 years.[7] BOS represents the clinical description, defined as an otherwise unexplained and sustained fall in FEV_1 that is 20% or greater of the peak value after transplantation. This lung dysfunction is uncommon during the first 6 months after transplantation, but it can occur as early as 3 months after transplantation. The BOS staging system indicates that B.U. has BOS-2.[104] Once diagnosed with BOS or OB, patients may rapidly decline and experience early death. Alternatively, the decline in FEV_1 may stabilize or the patient may have alternating periods of decline and stabilization. Many proposed risk factors exist for the development of BOS or OB, including both immune and nonimmune factors.[105]

No evidence indicates superiority of one drug treatment over another for OB or BOS. The primary treatment of chronic rejection relies on short courses of high-dose corticosteroids, ATG, or OKT3 to stabilize and improve the patient's condition for a short time. Therapy generally stabilizes and slows down this process, but does not reverse it. Inhaled cyclosporine, antibodies, tacrolimus, mycophenolate, and methotrexate also have been used.[103] Only aerosolized cyclosporine has been shown to have an effect on lung transplant recipient survival in a placebo-controlled trial,[106] but the drug is not available for commercial use. Sirolimus has been used in a small number of patients with little effect, but with a significant number of side effects.[107] Azithromycin (250 mg PO every Monday, Wednesday, and Friday) may have an impact on the rate of progression of BOS and can be added to CNI therapy with minimal effect on CNI levels.[108–110] For B.U., a trial of short-course, high-dose IV methylprednisolone with the addition of azithromycin to his maintenance therapy may be considered.

Chronic rejection in lung transplant recipients has been associated with a genotype of the profibrotic cytokine, transforming growth factor-β.[111] A similar observation has been made for interferon-γ, but genotyping patients for these cytokines is not practical until chronic rejection in lung transplant recipients is better understood and treated.

Infection

13. B.U. has been talking to his fellow organ transplant recipients on the floor while awaiting discharge from his initial transplant episode, and he asks the transplant team why he is on more antimicrobials than some of the other patients? His regimen includes valganciclovir 900 mg daily, CMV immune globulin infusions until 16 weeks postoperative, TMP-SMX double strength (DS) every Monday, Wednesday, and Friday, clotrimazole troches 10 mg after meals and at bedtime, nebulized lipid complex amphotericin B 50 mg daily until discharge, and tobramycin nebulized 300 mg BID.

Risk

A patient's overall infection risk depends on their net state of immunosuppression, the environment, and the surgical procedure. The first few months after transplant can be considered the period of highest risk. There is a temporal pattern to the infection type and how infections present in transplant recipients. Infection is the leading cause of death in the first 60 days after lung transplantation and contributes significantly to the number of deaths thereafter. There are several reasons for this problem. These patients may be colonized with organisms along the upper airways and sinuses; the donor lung may contain organisms at the time of transplantation; and the transplanted organ may have ischemic damage. After lung transplantation, patients lack a cough reflex because of denervation. Consequently, pulmonary secretions that accumulate can serve as a medium for bacterial growth. Furthermore, the transplanted lung's mucociliary clearance may be impaired; alveolar macrophages may not function properly; and patients are immunocompromised. Most infections present as bacterial sepsis or pneumonia, primarily associated with *Pseudomonas aeruginosa, Enterobacter,* other gram-negative organisms, and staphylococci. In patients with CF, *Candida* and *Aspergillus* infections also are common. Patients with CF still have a CF airway above their anastomosis site and should continue their pretransplant nebulized antibiotic regimen to prevent colonization of the new lungs. Besides bacterial infections, viral and fungal infections are a concern. Most transplant centers adopt universal prophylaxis protocols in the early transplant period. At least 50% of lung transplant recipients develop infections despite prophylaxis. The most common infections for which patients receive prolonged prophylaxis are CMV (see Chapter 34 Kidney and Liver Transplant) *pneumocystis jiroveci* pneumonia, thrush, and other fungal infections.

Pneumocystis jiroveci (PJP)

Pneumocystis jiroveci (formerly called *Pneumocystis carinii*), an opportunistic pathogen, can cause pneumonia in immunocompromised patients. The incidence of PJP is highest in thoracic organ recipients. The first 6 months after transplant is the period of highest risk for nonlung transplant recipients. Prophylaxis is very effective; life-long treatment is used for lung transplant recipients or others deemed to have an increased risk.[112] TMP-SMX given as a daily single strength or double strength tablet is the agent of choice; three times a week prophylaxis has also been used.[113] Nebulized pentamidine 300 mg every month, dapsone 100 mg daily, and atovaquone 1,500 mg daily are alternatives for patients intolerant or allergic to TMP-SMX.[114,115] For documented infection, the primary agent is TMP-SMX (20 mg/kg/day of TMP); however, the above alternatives may be used with pentamidine given IV instead of nebulized at 2 to 4 mg/kg/day.

FUNGAL INFECTIONS

The use of fungal prophylaxis is based on a patient's presumed risk, considering type of transplant, center patterns, colonization, or previous infection status, and the patient's overall state of immunosuppression.[116] Prophylaxis to prevent the occurrence of thrush may include nystatin or clotrimazole troches or oral triazoles that can cover other fungal organisms, including nonalbicans *Candida*, and *Aspergillus*. The timeline for fungal infections ranges from *Candida* in the early postoperative period along with some *Aspergillus*, then opportunistic infections for the next 6 months. After 6 months, infections are caused by other fungal organisms, including cryptococcus, zygomycetes, and endemic mycoses along with the previous mentioned organisms.[117] Drug interactions between the triazole antifungal agents, CNI, and sirolimus create challenges for prophylaxis. Triazole antifungals, such as fluconazole, itraconazole, voriconazole and posaconazole, are inhibitors of CYP3A4, resulting in supertherapeutic immunosuppressive levels. Because voriconazole use with sirolimus has resulted in a ninefold elevation of sirolimus levels, the FDA label contraindicates the use of the combination. Transplant recipients may still receive this drug combination, especially if the patient is infected with *Aspergillus*, but close monitoring of sirolimus levels is obviously required. Echinocandins are not used for long-term prophylaxis because no orally bioavailable product exists. These agents are used because they have fewer effects on immunosuppressive drug levels, especially micafungin and anidulafungin. Commonly, these agents may be used in combination with triazole antifungals in the treatment of invasive *Aspergillus* infections.[118] Intravenous amphotericin B in the conventional or lipid-based formulations would be used to treat fungal infections, but not for prophylaxis. Nebulized amphotericin B (or lipid based formulations) has been used, however, for prophylaxis in lung transplant populations because it allows for delivery of the antifungal agent to an area of high risk lung tissue without the systemic complications associated with IV therapy. Nebulized lipid complex amphotericin B was better tolerated in one lung transplant population than the conventional product.[119] Zygomycosis infections remain a challenge to treat; however, posaconazole with its spectrum of activity may have a role, keeping in mind that this agent requires administration with high fat meals for best absorption.

Cyclosporine Bioavailability

14. M.R. a 30-year-old woman status post bilateral lung transplant 5 years ago for interstitial pulmonary fibrosis (IPF) has called the transplant clinic because the cyclosporine she picked up from her local pharmacy does not look like the capsules she has received in the past. She reads the label to the pharmacist as Apotex cyclosporine 100 mg capsules. Reviewing the chart, M.R.'s cyclosporine is listed as GenGraf (generic Neoral) 125 mg BID. M.R. is asked to come to the clinic to clarify her medications.

Cyclosporine was initially introduced as a non-microemulsified product branded as Sandimmune, which demonstrated great interpatient variability in absorption and drug levels. Neoral, a microemulsion of cyclosporine, improved the absorption characteristics resulting in more predictable cyclosporine concentrations in lung transplant recipients. In general, the time to C_{max} (T_{max}) for Neoral is shorter, the maximum concentration (C_{max}) is higher, and the AUC is greater.[120] The two branded agents are not interchangeable; however, they both are available as generics. M.R. has received the generic for Sandimmune instead of her usual generic of GenGraf, the generic for Neoral, and is at risk for subtherapeutic cyclosporine levels. To rectify the situation, M.R. needs to have her local pharmacy dispense GenGraf instead. To minimize this inappropriate interchange, the clinician should specifically indicate the cyclosporine type on prescriptions.

SECONDARY MALIGNANCY

POST-TRANSPLANTATION LYMPHOPROLIFERATIVE DISORDER

Risk Factors

15. A.L., a 17-year-old, 42-kg girl with CF, had a double-lung transplant 1 year ago. She now presents with low-grade fever, malaise, pain, redness and swelling at her Port-A-Cath site, and a 1-week history of decreased appetite. She has experienced four episodes of rejection that were treated with 1 to 2 g of methylprednisolone each time. She also received ATG, azathioprine, prednisone, and cyclosporine after transplantation and has been on the latter three agents chronically along with ketoconazole, TMP-SMX, lactulose, and pancreatic enzymes. She has just finished the last of two courses of IV ganciclovir (6 weeks) for CMV infection. The donor was CMV-positive and she is CMV-positive. Her EBV IgG-VCA (viral capsid antigen) titer is now elevated, although at the time of transplantation it was negative (<1:40). On physical examination, she was noted to have mediastinal adenopathy. She denies chills, sweats, nausea, vomiting, or diarrhea. A chest computed tomography (CT) scan revealed a mediastinal mass. Vital signs and all laboratory tests are within normal limits. Her cyclosporine level is 221 ng/mL. Seven days after admission, a biopsy of this mass shows a thoracic lymphoproliferative lesion identified as a thoracic immunoblastic lymphoma adherent to the right side of the heart. Ten days later, she developed tachy/brady syndrome and a pacemaker was implanted. Given the location of her lymphoma and symptoms, surgery and radiation therapy are not viable options, and chemotherapy is started the next day. What clinical signs and risk factors in A.L. are associated with lymphoma?

A.L. has developed a post-transplantation lymphoproliferative disorder (PTLD), one of many types of malignancies that have been reported after solid organ transplantation. The exact etiology of this condition is unclear and probably multifactorial. The presentation of PTLD varies significantly. Patients can present asymptomatically, with mild mononucleosis-like symptoms or with multiorgan failure. A.L. presents with fever, lymphadenopathy, malaise, and lack of appetite. Although these symptoms are consistent with PTLD, they also are consistent with infection and episodes of rejection. Because PTLD can involve various organ systems, patients can present with organ-specific symptoms (e.g., acute abdominal pain, perforation, obstruction, bleeding if a tumor is in the GI tract). Depending on its location, a tumor can impinge on the function of other organs as seen in A.L.[121]

Besides immunosuppression, two factors that have been strongly associated with PTLD are the presence of EBV and the age of the patient. Children have a higher incidence of PTLD.[122] A.L. seroconverted from a negative to a positive EBV titer, indicating that she had been exposed to this virus at the time of transplantation or afterward. EBV also can be transmitted from the donor lung and blood products. Also, EBV-positive recipients at the time of transplantation can experience reactivation of this virus as a result of immunosuppression.

A.L. received a significant amount of immunosuppression. This could lead to an inability to suppress an active viral infection by cytotoxic T cells and result in uncontrolled B-cell proliferation and polyclonal and monoclonal expansion. In addition to this T-cell defect, an imbalance or alteration in cytokine production in response to EBV, which infects B lymphocytes, may contribute to the exaggerated B-cell expansion and transformation; most are classified as non-Hodgkin lymphomas primarily of B-cell origin. Small percentages are of T-cell origin, however, and are harder to treat.[123]

The incidence and detection of PTLD has increased. Newer, more potent agents used in different combinations, increased numbers of transplantation procedures, and closer monitoring certainly contributes to this phenomenon. When cyclosporine-based regimens were compared with azathioprine-based or cyclophosphamide-based regimens, lymphomas made up 26% and 11% of all cancers, respectively. The lymphomas occurred, on average, within 15 months in the cyclosporine group versus 48 months in the azathioprine group. One-third of these malignancies occurred in the first 4 months in the cyclosporine group compared with only 11% in the latter group.[123]

The incidence of PTLD increases with ATG, Thymoglobulin, and OKT3 therapy and appears to be related to a cumulative dose and multiple courses. PTLD is not caused by any single agent but probably reflects the intensity of immunosuppression with multiple agents. Chronic antigenic stimulation by foreign antigens, repeated infections, genetic predisposition, and indirect or direct damage to DNA are other variables that might affect the development of PTLD.[123] A.L. had two recent CMV infections, which also could have contributed to this process.

As a percentage of all malignancies, PTLD occurs more commonly in thoracic than in renal transplant recipients and is even more common in children.[122] Lymphomas develop in about 1% of renal transplantations, 2% of liver transplantations, 2% to 10% of heart transplantations, and 5% to 9% of lung transplantations. These tumors often appear early and progress rapidly. The overall prevalence of malignancies in the transplantation population averages about 6%, and the risk of cancer increases with time after a transplantation. Major organ transplant recipients are 100 times more likely to have cancer than the general population.[124] Furthermore, the most common types of cancer observed in transplant recipients (e.g., lymphomas, cancer of the skin and lips) are uncommon in the general population. The development of skin and lip cancers in the transplant population has been attributed partially to exposure to sunlight and sensitization of skin to sunlight by an azathioprine metabolite, methylnitrothioimidazole.[125]

TREATMENT AND OUTCOMES

16. What are the therapeutic maneuvers and outcomes that would be expected in A.L.?

Treatment of a PTLD depends on timing, presentation, symptoms, extent of involvement, histologic type, and transplant type. Early experiences with PTLD indicated that reduction or discontinuation of immunosuppression led to regression of the cancer. Therefore, the first step in treating PTLD is to consider the discontinuation of all immunosuppressives. This course of action is not feasible for A.L., however, because her transplanted lungs are essential for her life. The discontinuation of immunosuppressive therapy also is not an option for heart and liver transplants, but immunosuppressive drugs can be discontinued in kidney transplant recipients because dialysis is available. A.L. will need chemotherapy for her cancer. Therefore, her azathioprine probably should be discontinued to minimize the potential for severe bone marrow toxicity. If her cyclosporine levels were high, a reduction in dose could be attempted, but her cyclosporine concentration of 221 ng/mL is in the lower range for this type of transplantation, and prednisone is reduced to the lowest dose possible. If her immunosuppressive drug therapy is diminished, she should be monitored closely for rejection of her transplanted lungs.

Antiviral therapy with IV acyclovir or ganciclovir has been used to inhibit EBV replication in an effort to treat PTLD. Response is variable and may depend on the type and extent of PTLD. A.L. already has received ganciclovir for 6 weeks during which time she presented with PTLD. Surgery, radiation therapy, and chemotherapy are used to treat PTLD depending on the situation. Interferon and immune globulin have been effective in a few cases that appeared unresponsive to other therapies. Monoclonal or immunoblastic, disseminated, rapidly progressive PTLD responds poorly to traditional therapy and has a mortality rate as high as 70%.[126] Rituximab (an anti–B-cell, anti-Cd20 antibody) is considered first-line therapy for CD20-postive B-cell PTLD along with reduction or withdrawal of immunosuppression if possible. Patients usually get 375 mg/m^2 weekly for 4 weeks; some groups have used prolonged therapy.[127–129] Patients may have relapse or disease progression that may respond to chemotherapy regimens such as cyclophosphamide, adriamycin, vincristine, prednisone or dexamethasone (CHOP), CHOP plus rituximab (CHOP-R), cyclophosphamide, doxorubicin, etopside, prednisone, cytarbine and bleomycin (PROMACE-cytaBOM).[130,131] Transplant recipients have a higher risk of myelotoxic side effects, depending on their maintenance immunosuppression.[132] A.L.'s prognosis is poor given the type and extent of her PTLD, which would have been more responsive to therapy if it had been diagnosed early before it had metastasized. Polyclonal PTLD responds well to reduction or discontinuation of immunosuppression and high-dose acyclovir or ganciclovir therapy for several weeks to months. The roles of prophylactic antivirals, immunoglobulins, and EBV polymerase chain reaction (PCR) monitoring in the prevention of PTLD are currently under study.[133,134]

REFERENCES

1. Taylor DO et al. Registry of the international society of heart and lung transplantation: twenty-fourth official adult heart transplantation report-2007. *J Heart Lung Transplant* 2007;26:769.
2. Garrity ER et al. Heart and lung transplantation in the United States, 1996–2005. *Am J Transplant* 2007;7(Part 2):1390.
3. Mehra MR et al. Listing criteria for heart transplantation: international society for heart and lung transplantation guidelines for the care of cardiac transplant candidates—2006. *J Heart Lung Transplant* 2006;25:1024.
4. Cimato TR et al. Recipient selection in cardiac transplantation: contraindications and risk factors for mortality. *J Heart Lung Transplant* 2002;21:1161.
5. United Network of Organ Sharing. "Policy 3.7 Organ Distribution: Allocation of Thoracic Organs." December 2007. United Network of Organ Sharing Home Page. http://www.unos.org/PoliciesandBylaws2/policies/pdfs/policy_9.pdf. Accessed July 2007.
6. Young JB et al. 24th Bethesda conference: Cardiac Transplantation Task Force 4: Function of the heart transplant recipient. *J Am Coll Cardiol* 1993;22:31.
7. Kobashigawa JA. Postoperative management following heart transplantation. *Transplant Proc* 1999;31:2038.
8. Trulock EP et al. Registry of the international society of heart and lung transplantation: twenty-fourth official adult lung and heart-lung transplantation report—2007. *J Heart Lung Transplant* 2007;26:782.
9. Cotts WG et al. Function of the transplanted heart. *Am J Med Sci* 1997;314:164.
10. Redmond JM et al. Use of theophylline for treatment of prolonged sinus node dysfunction in human orthotopic heart transplantation. *J Heart Lung Transplant* 1993;12:133.
11. Lake KD et al. Over the counter medications in cardiac transplant recipients: guidelines for use. *Ann Pharmacother* 1992;26:1566.
12. Taylor DO et al. A randomized, multicenter comparison of tacrolimus and cyclosporine immunosuppressive regimens in cardiac transplantation: decreased hyperlipidemia and hypertension with tacrolimus. *J Heart Lung Transplant* 1999;18:336.
13. White M et al. Conversion from cyclosporine microemulsion to tacrolimus-based immunoprophylaxis improves cholesterol profile in heart transplant recipients with treated but persistent dyslipidemia: the Canadian Multicentre Randomized Trial of Tacrolimus vs. Cyclosporine Microemulsion. *J Heart Lung Transplant* 2005;24:798.
14. Kobashigawa JA et al. Five-year results of a randomized, single-center study of tacrolimus vs. microemulsion cyclosporine in heart transplant patients. *J Heart Lung Transpl* 2006;25:434.
15. Grimm M et al. Superior prevention of acute rejection by tacrolimus vs. cyclosporine in heart transplant recipients—a large European trial. *Am J Transpl* 2006;6:1387.
16. Kobashigawa J et al. A randomized active: controlled trial of mycophenolate mofetil in heart transplant recipients. Mycophenolate mofetil investigators. *Transplantation* 1998;66:507.
17. Hosenpud JD et al. Mycophenolate mofetil compared to azathioprine improves survival in patients surviving the initial cardiac transplant hospitalization: an analysis of the joint ISHLT/UNOS Thoracic Registry. *J Heart Lung Transplant* 2000;19:72.
18. Eisen HJ et al. Three-year results of a randomized, double-blind, controlled trial of mycophenolate mofetil versus azathioprine in cardiac transplant recipients. *J Heart Lung Transplant* 2005;24:517.
19. Taylor DO et al. Increased incidence of allograft rejection in stable heart transplant recipients after late conversion from mycophenolate to azathioprine. *Clin Transplant* 1999;13:296.
20. Kobashigawa JA et al. Similar efficacy and safety of enteric-coated mycophenolate sodium (EC-MPS, Myfortic) compared with mycophenolate mofetil (MMF) in de novo heart transplant recipients: results of a 12-month, single-blind, randomized, parallel-group multicenter study. *J Heart Lung Transplant* 2006;25:935.
21. Kurzawski A et al. The impact of thiopurine s-methyltransferase polymorphism on azathioprine-induced myelotoxicity in renal transplant recipients. *Ther Drug Monit* 2005;27:435.
22. Groetzner J et al. Mycophenolate mofetil and sirolimus as calcineurin inhibitor-free immunosuppression for late cardiac-transplant recipients with chronic renal failure. *Transplantation* 2004;77:568.
23. Zucker MJ et al. De novo immunosuppression with sirolimus and tacrolimus in heart transplant recipients compared with cyclosporine and mycophenolate mofetil: a one-year follow-up analysis. *Transplant Proc* 2005;37:2231.
24. Kobashigawa JA et al. Tacrolimus with mycophenolate mofetil (MMF) or sirolimus vs. cyclosporine with MMF in cardiac transplant patients: 1-year report. *Am J Transplant* 2006;6:1377.
25. Uber PA et al. Induction therapy in heart transplantation: is there a role? *J Heart Lung Transplant* 2007;26:205.
26. Wilde MI et al. Muromonab CD3: a reappraisal of its pharmacology and use as prophylaxis of solid organ rejection. *Drugs* 1996;51:865.
27. Copeland JG et al. Rabbit antithymocyte globulin: a 10-year experience in cardiac transplantation. *J Thorac Cardiovasc Surg* 1990;99:852.
28. Scnetzler B et al. A prospective randomized controlled study on the efficacy and tolerance of two antilymphocytic globulins in the prevention of rejection in first heart transplant recipients. *Transpl Int* 2002;15:317.
29. Hershberger RE et al. Daclizumab to prevent rejection after cardiac transplantation. *N Engl J Med* 2005;352:2705.
30. Rosenberg PB et al. Induction therapy with basiliximab allows delayed initiation of cyclosporine and preserves renal function after cardiac transplantation. *J Heart Lung Transplant* 2005;24:1327.
31. Kobashigawa J et al. Daclizumab is associated with decreased rejection and no mortality in cardiac transplant patients receiving MMF, cyclosporine and corticosteroids. *Transplant Proc* 2005;37:1333.
32. Beniaminovitz A et al. Prevention of rejection in cardiac transplantation by blockade of the interleukin-2 receptor with a monoclonal antibody. *N Engl J Med* 2000;342:613.
33. Ortiz V et al. Induction therapy with daclizumab in heart transplantation- how many doses. *Transplant Proc* 2006;38:2541.
34. Cantarovich JD et al. Early experience with two-dose daclizumab in the prevention of acute rejection in cardiac transplantation. *Clin Transplant* 2004;18:493.
35. Carrier M et al. Basiliximab and rabbit antithymocyte globulin for prophylaxis of acute rejection after heart transplantation: a non-inferiority trial. *J Heart Lung Transplant* 2007;26:258.
36. Flaman F et al. Basiliximab versus rabbit antithymocyte globulin for induction therapy in patients after heart transplantation. *J Heart Lung Transplant* 2006;25:1358.
37. Carlsen J et al. Induction therapy after cardiac transplantation: a comparison of anti-thymocyte globulin and daclizumab in the prevention of acute rejection. *J Heart Lung Transplant* 2005;24:296.
38. Uber WE et al. CD3 monitoring and thymoglobulin therapy in cardiac transplantation: clinical outcomes and pharmacoeconomic implications. *Transplant Proc* 2004;36:3245.
39. Krasinskas AM et al. CD3 monitoring of antithymocyte globulin therapy in thoracic organ transplantation. *Transplantation.* 2002;73:1339.
40. Fekel TO et al. Survival and incidence of acute rejection in heart transplant recipients undergoing successful withdrawal from steroid therapy. *J Heart Lung Transplant* 2002;21:530.
41. Opelz G et al. Long-term prospective study of steroid withdrawal in kidney and heart transplant recipients. *Am J Transplant* 2005;5:720.
42. Zheng B et al. The MDR1 polymorphisms at exons 21 and 26 predict steroid weaning in pediatric heart transplant patients. *Hum Immunol* 2002;63:765.
43. Zeng HX et al. Tacrolimus dosing in pediatric heart transplant patients is related to CYP3A5 and MDR1 gene polymorphisms. *Am J Transplant* 2003;3:477.
44. Zeng HX et al. Tacrolimus dosing in adult lung transplant patients is related to cytochrome P450 3A5 gene polymorphism. *J Clin Pharmacol* 2004;44:135.
45. Burckart GJ. Looking beneath the surface of CYP3A5 polymorphism. *Pediatr Transplant* 2007;11:239.
46. Psupati J et al. Intraindividual and interindividual variations in the pharmacokinetics of mycophenolic acid in liver transplant patients. *J Clin Pharmacol* 2005;45:34.
47. Stewart SS et al. Revision of the 1990 working formulation for the standardization of nomenclature in the diagnosis of heart rejection. *J Heart Lung Transplant* 2005;24:1710.
48. Reed EF et al. Acute antibody-mediated rejection of cardiac transplants. *J Heart Lung Transplant* 2006;25:153.
49. Aranda JM et al. Anti-CD20 monoclonal antibody (rituximab) therapy for acute cardiac humoral rejection: a case report. *Transplantation* 2002;73:907.
50. Garrett HE et al. Treatment of humoral rejection with rituximab. *Ann Thorac Surg* 2002;74:1240.
51. Baran DA et al. Refractory humoral cardiac allograft rejection successfully treated with a single dose of rituximab. *Transplant Proc* 2004;36:3164.
52. Yeogh TJ et al. Clinical significance of mild rejection of the cardiac allograft. *Circulation* 1992;86(Suppl 2):II267.
53. Deng MC et al. Noninvasive discrimination of rejection in cardiac allograft recipients using gene expression profiling. *Am J Transplant* 2006;6:150.
54. Weis M. Cardiac Allograft vasculopathy: prevention and treatment options. *Transplant Proc* 2002;34:1847.
55. Yamani MH et al. Does acute cellular rejection correlate with cardiac allograft vasculopathy? *J Heart Lung Transplant* 2004;23:272.
56. Stoica SC et al. The cumulative effect of acute rejection on development f cardiac allograft vasculopathy. *J Heart Lung Transplant* 2006;25:420.
57. Caforio et al. Immune and nonimmune predictors of cardiac allograft vasculopathy onset and severity: multivariate risk factor analysis and role of immunosuppression. *Am J Transplant* 2004;4:962.
58. de Lorgenil M et al. Low-dose aspirin and accelerated coronary disease in heart transplant recipients. *J Heart Lung Transplant* 1990;9:339.
59. Schroeder JS et al. A preliminary study of diltiazem in the prevention of coronary artery disease in heart-transplant recipients. *N Engl J Med* 1993;328:164.
60. Mehra MR. Contemporary concepts in prevention and treatment of cardiac allograft vasculopathy. *Am J Transplant* 2006;6:1248.
61. Wenke K et al. Simvastatin reduces graft vessel disease and mortality after heart transplantation: a four-year randomized trial. *Circulation* 1997;96:1398.
62. Kobashigawa JA et al. Effect of pravastatin on outcomes after cardiac transplantation. *N Engl J Med* 1995;333:621.
63. Wenke K et al. Simvastatin initiated early after heart transplantation: 8-year prospective experience. *Circulation* 2003:07:93.
64. Eisen HJ et al. Everolimus for the prevention of allograft rejection and vasculopathy in cardiac-transplant recipients. *N Engl J Med* 2003;349:847.
65. Ruygrok PN et al. Angiographic regression of cardiac allograft vasculopathy after introducing sirolimus immunosuppression. *J Heart Lung Transplant* 2003;22:1276.

66. Keogh A et al. Sirolimus in de novo heart transplant recipients reduces acute rejection and prevents coronary artery disease at 2 years: a randomized clinical trial. *Circulation* 2004;110:2694.
67. Mancini D et al. Use of rapamycin slows progression of cardiac transplantation vasculopathy. *Circulation* 2003:108:48.
68. Miller LW. Treatment of cardiac allograft rejection with intravenous corticosteroids. *J Heart Transplant* 1990;9(3 Pt 2):283.
69. Kobashigawa JA et al. Is intravenous glucocorticoid therapy better than an oral regimen for asymptomatic cardiac rejection: a randomized trial. *J Am Coll Cardiol* 1993;21:1142.
70. Lonquist JL et al. Reevaluation of steroid tapering after steroid pulse therapy for heart rejection. *J Heart Lung Transplant* 1992;11:913.
71. Kirklin JK et al. Treatment of recurrent heart rejection with mycophenolate mofetil: initial clinical experience. *J Heart Lung Transplant* 1994;13:444.
72. Miller L et al. Treatment of acute cardiac allograft rejection with rapamycin: a multicenter dose ranging study. *J Heart Lung Transplant* 1997;16:44.
73. Kunst H et al. Hypertension as a marker for later development of end-stage renal failure after lung and heart-lung transplantation: a cohort study. *J Heart Lung Transplant* 2004;23:1182.
74. Brozena SC et al. Effectiveness and safety of diltiazem or lisinopril in treatment of hypertension after heart transplantation: results of a prospective, randomized multicenter trial. *J Am Coll Cardiol* 1996;27:1707.
75. Formica RN et al. A randomized trial comparing losartan with amlodipine as initial therapy for hypertension in the early post-transplant period. *Nephrol Dial Transplant* 2006;21:1389.
76. Midtvedt K et al. Efficacy of nifedipine or lisinopril in the treatment of hypertension after renal transplantation: a double-blind randomized comparative trial. *Clin Transplant* 2001;15:426.
77. Opie LH et al. Antihypertensive effects of angiotensin converting enzyme inhibition by lisinopril in post-transplant patients. *Am J Hypertens* 2005;15:911.
78. Mehra MR et al. An intravascular ultrasound study of the influence of angiotensin-converting enzyme inhibitors and calcium entry blockers on the development of cardiac allograft vasculopathy. *Am J Cardiol* 1995;75:853.
79. Erinc K et al. The effect of combined angtiotensin-converting enzyme inhibition and calcium antagonism on allograft coronary vasculopathy validated by intravascular ultrasound. *J Heart Lung Transplant* 2005;24:1033.
80. Bader FM et al. The effect of B-blocker use on cyclosporine level in cardiac transplant recipients. *J Heart Lung Transplant* 2005;24:2144.
81. de Denus S et al. Dyslipidemias and HMG-CoA reductase inhibitor prescription in heart transplant recipients. *Ann Pharmacother* 2004;38:1136.
82. Patel AR et al. Treatment of hypercholesterolemia with ezetimibe in cardiac transplant recipients. *J Heart Lung Transplant* 2007;26:281.
83. Buchanan C et al. A retrospective analysis of ezetimibe treatment in renal transplant recipients. *Am J Transplant* 2006;6:770.
84. Orens JB et al. International guidelines for the selection of lung transplant candidates: 2006 update—a consensus report from the pulmonary scientific council of the international society of heart and lung transplantation. *J Heart Lung Transplant* 2006;25:745.
85. Palmer SM et al. Rabbit antithymocyte globulin decreases acute rejection after lung transplantation: results of a randomized prospective study. *Chest* 1999;116:127.
86. Brock MV et al. Induction therapy in lung transplantation: a prospective, controlled clinical trial comparing OKT3, anti-thymocyte globulin, and daclizumab. *J Heart Lung Transplant* 2001;20:1282.
87. Borro JM et al. Comparative study of basiliximab treatment in lung transplantation. *Transplant Proc* 2005;37:3996.
88. Burton CM et al. The incidence of acute cellular rejection after lung transplantation: a comparative study of anti-thymocyte globulin and daclizumab. *J Heart Lung Transplant* 2006;25:638.
89. Mullen JC et al. A randomized, controlled trial of daclizumab vs anti-thymocyte globulin induction for lung transplantation. *J Heart Lung Transplant* 2007;26:504.
90. Lischke R et al. Induction therapy in lung transplantation: initial single-center experience comparing daclizumab and antithymocyte globulin. *Transplant Proc* 2007;39:205.
91. Treede H et al. Tacrolimus versus cyclosporine after lung transplantation: a prospective, open, randomized two-center trial comparing two different immunosuppressive protocols. *J Heart Lung Transplant* 2001;20:511.
92. Bhorade SM et al. Comparison of three tacrolimus-based immunosuppressive regimens in lung transplantation. *Am J Transplant* 2003;3:1570.
93. Garrity ER et al. Suggested guidelines for the use of tacrolimus in lung transplant recipients. *J Heart Lung Transplant* 1999;18:175.
94. Reams BD et al. Sublingual tacrolimus for immunosuppression in lung transplantation a potentially important therapeutic option in cystic fibrosis. *Am J Respir Med* 2002;1:91.
95. Palmer SM et al. Results of a randomized, prospective, multicenter trial of mycophenolate versus azathioprine in the prevention of acute lung allograft rejection. *Transplant* 2001;71:1772.
96. Knoop C et al. Acute and chronic rejection after lung transplantation. *Semin Respir Crit Care Med* 2006;27:521.
97. Yousem SA et al. Revision of the 1990 working formulation for the standardization of nomenclature in the diagnosis of heart and lung rejection: lung rejection study group. *J Heart Transplant* 1996; 15:1.
98. Trulock EP. Management of lung transplant rejection. *Chest* 1993;103:1566.
99. Shenib H et al. Efficacy of OKT_3 therapy for acute rejection in isolated lung transplantations. *J Heart Lung Transplant* 1994;13:514.
100. Iacono AT et al. Dose-related reversal of acute lung rejection by aerosolized cyclosporine. *Am J Respir Crit Care Med* 1997;155:1690.
101. Vitulo P et al. Efficacy of tacrolimus rescue therapy in refractory acute rejection after lung transplantation. *J Heart Lung Transplant* 2002:21:435.
102. Zeng HX et al. The impact of pharmacogenomic factors on acute rejection in adult lung transplant patients. *Transpl Immunol* 2005;14:37.
103. Estenne M et al. Bronchiolitis obliterans after human lung transplantation. *Am J Respir Crit Care Med* 2002;166:440.
104. Estenne M et al. Bronchiolitis obliterans syndrome 2001: an update of the diagnostic criteria. *J Heart Lung Transplant* 2002;21:297.
105. Chan A et al. Bronchiolitis obliterans: an update. *Curr Opin Pulm Med* 2004;10:133.
106. Iacono AT et al. A randomized trial of inhaled cyclosporine in lung-transplant recipients. *N Engl J Med* 2006;354:141.
107. Cahill BC et al. Early experience with sirolimus in lung transplant recipients with chronic allograft rejection. *J Heart Lung Transplant* 2003;22:169.
108. Yates B et al. Azithromycin reverses airflow obstruction in established bronchiolitis obliterans syndrome. *Am J Respir Crit Care Med* 2005;172:772.
109. Verleden GM et al. Azithromycin reduces airway neutrophilia and interleukin-8 in patients with bronchiolitis obliterans syndrome. *Am J Respir Crit Care Med* 2006;174:566.
110. Shitrit D et al. Long-term azithromycin use for treatment of bronchiolitis obliterans syndrome in lung transplant recipients. *J Heart Lung Transplant* 2005;24:1440.
111. Burckart GJ et al. Pharmacogenomics and lung transplantation: clinical implications. *Pharmacogenomics J* 2006;6:301.
112. Gordon SM et al. Should prophylaxis for pneumocystis carinii pneumonia in solid organ transplant recipients ever be discontinued? *Clin Infect Dis* 1999;28:240.
113. American Society of Transplant Surgeons and the American Society of Transplantation. *Pneumocystis jiroveci* (formerly pneumocystis carinii). *Am J Transplant* 2004;4(Suppl 10):135.
114. Nathan SD et al. Utility of inhaled pentamidine prophylaxis in lung transplant recipients. *Chest* 1994;105:417.
115. Meyres B et al. Pneumocystis carinii pneumonia prophylaxis with atovaquone in trimethoprim-sulfmethoxazole-intolerant orthotopic liver transplant patients: a preliminary study. *Liver Transpl* 2001;7:750.
116. Kubak BM. Fungal infections in lung transplantation. *Transplant Infect Dis* 2002;4 (Suppl 3):24.
117. Anonomyous. Fungal Infections. *Am J Transplant* 2004;(Suppl)10:110.
118. Singh N et al. Combination of voriconazole and caspofungin as primary therapy for invasive aspergillosis in solid organ transplant recipients: a prospective, multicenter, observational study. *Transplantation* 2006;81:320.
119. Palmer SM et al. Safety of aerosolized amphotericin B lipid complex in lung transplant recipients. *Transplantation* 2001;72:545.
120. Kesten S et al. Pharmacokinetic profile and variability of cyclosporine versus Neoral in patients with cystic fibrosis after lung transplantation. *Pharmacotherapy* 1998;18:847.
121. Dror Y et al. Lymphoproliferative disorders after organ transplantation in children. *Transplantation* 1999;67:990.
122. Penn I. De novo malignancy in pediatric organ transplantation. *Pediatr Transplant* 1998;2:56.
123. Penn I. Post-transplant malignancy. The role of immunosuppression. *Drug Saf* 2000;23:101.
124. Penn I. The problem of cancer in organ transplant recipients. *Transplantation Science* 1994;4:423.
125. Euvrard S et al. Skin cancer after organ transplantation. *N Engl J Med* 2003;348:1681.
126. Swinnen LJ. Treatment of organ transplant-related lymphoma. *Hematol Oncol Clin North Am* 1997;11:963.
127. Blaes AH et al. Rituximab therapy is effective for posttransplant lymphoproliferative disorders after solid organ transplantation. *Cancer* 2005;104:1661.
128. Jain AB et al. Rituximab (chimeric anti-CD20 antibody) for posttransplant lymphoproliferative disorder after solid organ transplantation in adults: long-term experience from a single center. *Transplantation* 2005;80:1692.
129. Svoboda J et al. Management of patients with post-transplant lymphoproliferative disorder: the role of rituximab. *Transplant Int* 2006;19:259.
130. Buell JF et al. Chemotherapy for posttransplant lymphoproliferative disorder: the Israel Penn transplant tumor registry experience. *Transplant Proc* 2005;37:956.
131. Trappe R et al. Salvage chemotherapy for refractory and relapsed posttransplant lymphoproliferative disorders (PTLD) after treatment with single-agent rituximab. *Transplantation* 2007;83:912.
132. Verschuuren EA et al. Treatment of posttransplant lymphoproliferative disease with rituximab: the remission, the relapse, and the complication. *Transplant* 2002;73:100.
133. McDiarmid SV et al. Prevention and preemptive therapy of posttransplant lymphoproliferative disease in pediatric liver recipients. *Transplantation* 1998;66:1604.
134. Green M et al. Serial measurement of Epstein-Barr viral load in peripheral blood in pediatric liver transplant recipients during treatment for posttransplant lymphoproliferative disease. *Transplantation* 1998;66:1641.

SECTION EIGHT

NUTRITION ISSUES

Marcus Ferrone

SECTION EDITOR

CHAPTER 36

Adult Enteral Nutrition

Carol J. Rollins and Yvonne Huckleberry

Enteral nutrition refers to nutrition provided via the gastrointestinal (GI) tract. However, as the term is commonly used, enteral nutrition (EN) is synonymous with delivery of nutrients into the GI tract by tube (e.g., nasogastric or jejunostomy feeding). Tube feeding allows continued use of the GI tract when one or more steps in the normal process of obtaining nutrients from oral intake is disrupted. Chewing or swallowing may be completely disrupted but some digestive and absorptive function must remain for tube feeding to be a viable option.

Patient Selection

Patients generally are considered at risk of nutrient depletion and associated increased morbidity and mortality when intake is inadequate to meet nutritional requirements for 5 to 7 days or when weight loss exceeds 10% of pre-illness weight within a 6-month period.[1,2] For adequately nourished patients, specialized nutrition support is generally not warranted when support will only be needed for fewer than 10 days.[3] Nutrition screening is used to identify patients who may be at nutritional risk. Parameters, such as weight, height, diagnosis, recent weight loss, and serum albumin, are evaluated. Nutrition assessment expands screening by including other data (hemoglobin [Hgb], hematocrit [Hct], creatinine, cholesterol, nitrogen balance, total iron-binding capacity [TIBC], prealbumin [transthyretin]), calculation of energy requirements, dietary history, and medical history. Completion of nutrition assessment helps identify potential candidates for EN. (See Chapter 37, Adult Parenteral Nutrition, for further information on nutrition assessment.)

Routes of nutrition intervention may include modified oral diet including oral supplements, EN by tube, or parenteral nutrition (PN). Tube feeding is considered the route of choice in patients with a functional GI tract whose oral nutrient intake is insufficient to meet estimated needs.[1,3]

Table 36-1 lists functional anatomic units of the GI tract along with major steps occurring in preparing nutrients for

Table 36-1 Functional Units of the GI Tract

Functional Unit	Major Steps	Conditions/Diseases
Mouth and oropharynx	Chew and lubricate food; swallow	Amyotrophic lateral sclerosis, muscular dystrophy, severe RA, CVA, end-stage Parkinson's disease, paralysis, coma, anorexia due to other disease: cardiac or cancer cachexia, renal failure and uremia, liver failure, neurologic disease
Esophagus	Transport food to the stomach	Esophageal disease: ulcer, cancer, obstruction, fistula, esophagectomy, CVA
Stomach	Hold food for mixing and grinding; add acid and enzymes; release chyme to small bowel; osmoregulation	Severe gastritis or ulceration, gastroparesis, gastric outlet obstruction, gastric cancer, severe gastroesophageal reflux
Duodenum	Osmoregulation; neutralize stomach acid	Severe duodenal ulcer, duodenal fistula, cancer: gastric, pancreatic
Small bowel: jejunum and ileum	Digestion; absorption	Enterocutaneous fistula, severe enteric infection, malnutrition, malabsorption, Crohn's disease, celiac disease, ileus and dysmotility syndrome
Pancreas	Secretion of digestive enzymes	Pancreatitis, pancreatic cancer, pancreatic injury, pancreatic fistula
Colon	Absorb fluid; ferment soluble fiber and unabsorbed carbohydrate; absorb water	Ulcerative colitis, Crohn's disease, colon cancer, colocutaneous fistula, colovaginal fistula, diverticulitis, colitis of any etiology, colon surgery

CVA, cerebrovascular accident; GI, gastrointestinal; RA, rheumatoid arthritis.

absorption and it provides examples of conditions potentially impairing each region. EN may be appropriate for patients with the disorders listed, depending on the extent to which normal intake, transport, digestion, and absorption of nutrients is impaired. Clinical circumstances, not specific diagnoses, should be the determining factor for initiating tube feeding. EN should be used with caution in patients with severe necrotizing or hemorrhagic pancreatitis, distal high-output enterocutaneous fistulae, hypotension with significant inotropic support, GI ischemia, and partial bowel obstruction.[1,3] Contraindications to EN generally include diffuse peritonitis, complete bowel obstruction, paralytic ileus, intractable vomiting or diarrhea, severe malabsorption, severe GI bleed, inability to access the GI tract, and when aggressive intervention is not warranted or desired. Frequent reassessment is recommended because patients may become candidates for EN as the condition improves or resolves. With advances in GI access and formula composition over the past decade, many patients once requiring PN are now treated successfully with EN.

Route of Tube Feeding

The route for EN is determined by the anticipated duration of tube feeding, disrupted region or process in the GI tract, and the risk of aspiration. Figure 36-1 illustrates the two basic types of tube placement—nasal versus ostomy—and the sites available for formula delivery (i.e., gastric, duodenal, or jejunal). The name of the feeding route usually includes both the type of tube placement and the site of formula delivery. For example, *nasogastric* (NG) indicates nasal placement with gastric delivery of formula, whereas *gastrostomy* indicates ostomy placement with gastric delivery of formula.

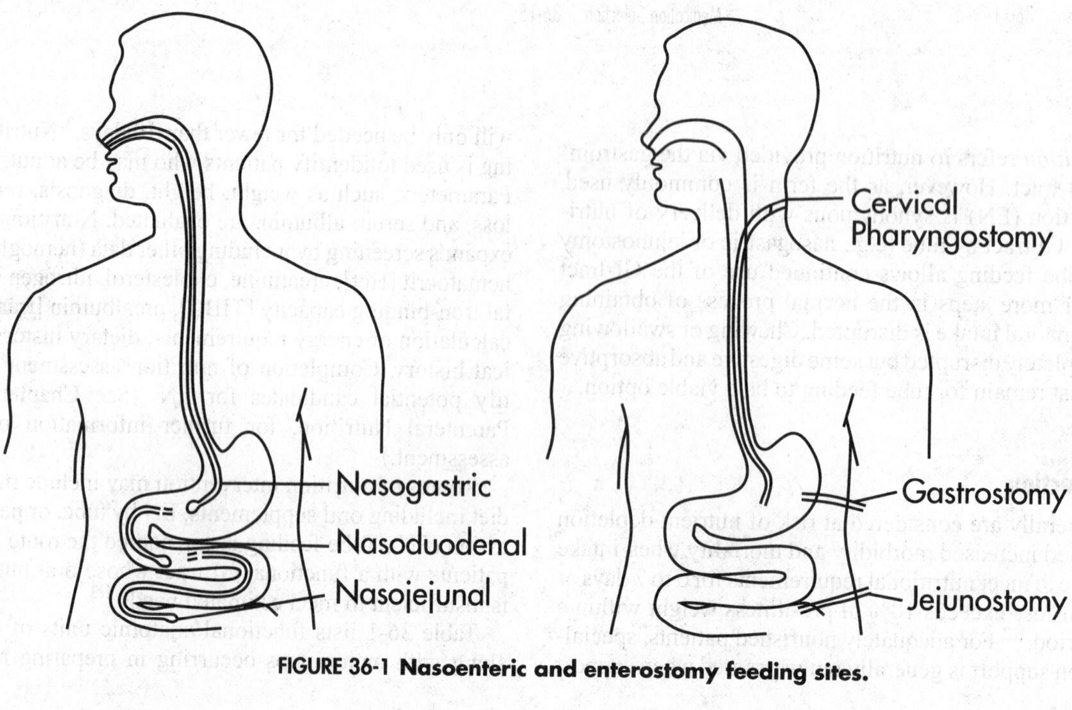

FIGURE 36-1 Nasoenteric and enterostomy feeding sites.

Tube Placement

NASAL

Nasal tube placement is preferred for short-term use in patients expected to resume oral feeding and without obstruction of nasal, pharyngeal, or esophageal passages. Clinically evident injury from nasal intubation is very low, but patients may suffer mucosal trauma in the nasopharynx.[4–6] Perforation of the hypopharynx, esophagus, or stomach is a rare complication.[7,8] Pharyngitis, sinusitis, otitis media, and incompetence of the lower esophageal sphincter are associated with nasal tubes, especially large-bore tubes. The incidence of inadvertent pulmonary placement of small-bore feeding tubes is 4% or less.[4] Radiographic confirmation of tube placement is mandatory to rule out pleural perforation and pulmonary intubation in unconscious patients and remains the standard to ensure correct tube placement in all patients. Tube displacement is a potential complication occurring in 25% to 41% of cases.[4]

FEEDING OSTOMIES

Feeding ostomies (tube enterostomies) generally are reserved for long-term EN, interpreted as anywhere from 4 weeks to 6 months, depending on clinical circumstances and the type of tube enterostomy placed. Nasal tubes are seldom tolerated for more than 6 weeks in alert patients. Access for enterostomies can be achieved through open surgery, laparoscopy, or percutaneously. Most surgical enterostomies require general anesthesia for placement.[4]

Percutaneous access is usually performed under local anesthesia or conscious sedation by endoscope (percutaneous endoscopic gastrostomy [PEG] or jejunostomy [PEJ]) or by radiography (PRG or PRJ), including fluoroscopy, ultrasound, or computed tomography (CT).[4,9,10] The major advantage of radiographic compared with endoscopic placement is reduced contamination of the puncture site by oral pharyngeal microorganisms, which are implicated in the 5.4% to 30% incidence of site infections.[7] Most patients requiring long-term EN receive a PEG, with 216,000 procedures reported annually.[11] Endoscopic placement is contraindicated when obstruction prevents passage of the endoscope but radiographic placement may be possible in such cases. Relative contraindications to percutaneous feeding tube placement include inability to see the endoscopic light through the abdominal wall (e.g., morbid obesity, massive ascites), peritoneal dialysis, coagulopathy, gastric varices, portal hypertension, hepatomegaly, and neoplastic or infiltrative disease of the gastric or jejunal wall.[4,5,7,9,10,12] Prior total or subtotal gastrectomy prevents percutaneous gastrostomy placement, but percutaneous jejunostomy may be possible. Major advantages of percutaneous access are shorter procedure time and lower cost, because morbidity and mortality appear to be similar to surgical feeding tube access.[5,12] Major complications, such as aspiration, peritonitis, hemorrhage, gastrocutaneous fistula formation, necrotizing fasciitis, gastric perforation, and migration of the tube through the gastric wall, are generally low but have been reported in up to 2.5% of patients.[4,13]

SITE OF DELIVERY

The preferred site for formula delivery is the stomach because this is the most physiologically normal feeding site. Stimulation of normal digestive processes and hormonal responses associated with eating occur with gastric feeding. The stomach serves as a reservoir, typically allowing tolerance of bolus, and intermittent or continuous feeding. Gastric feeding, either by NG tube or gastrostomy, requires adequate gastric motility to prevent accumulation of formula in the stomach. Patients with gastric outlet obstruction, gastroparesis, gastric distention, or gastroesophageal reflux are poor candidates for gastric feeding.

Transpyloric feeding into the duodenum or jejunum may be appropriate when gastric dysfunction or disease is present, when risk of aspiration is high, or for early postoperative feeding when gastric emptying may be impaired. In healthy volunteers, negligible reflux to the stomach occurs with dye infused into the fourth portion of the duodenum or proximal jejunum (beyond the ligament of Treitz), suggesting insignificant risk of aspiration with feeding tube placement in these positions.[14] Nevertheless, despite widespread use of postpyloric feeding tube placement, evidence of reduced aspiration remains controversial.[15] Tube migration from the duodenum into the stomach and equal risk of aspiration between postpyloric and intragastric tube placement has been observed.[16] Critically ill patients are at risk for aspiration and ventilator-associated pneumonia, with a 25% to 40% incidence of aspiration in patients with long-term nasoenteric feeding.[17,18] Tube placement beyond the ligament of Treitz may be best for patients at risk of tube migration and aspiration; however, rigorous randomized trials comparing feeding sites are lacking. Poor differentiation between aspiration of oral secretions and aspiration of feedings may result in erroneously high rates for aspiration of postpyloric feedings.

FORMULA SELECTION

Polymeric Formulas

Enteral formula selection is based on nutrient requirements, fluid restrictions, and the extent of impaired digestion and absorption. Many enteral formulas are available but few are typically necessary on the formulary to meet patient needs. Categorizing formulas as listed in Table 36-2 simplifies the formula selection process.

Polymeric formulas are most common. Use of whole (i.e., intact) proteins in these formulas requires that patients have full digestive capability for proteins. Carbohydrate and fat sources also require full digestive function. Osmolality is decreased and palatability increased with use of relatively intact nutrients. Administration of approximately 1.5 to 2 L of most polymeric formulas provides 100% of Dietary Reference Intakes (DRI) for vitamins and minerals; thus, these formulas sometimes are called "complete" formulas. Polymeric formulas tend to be the least expensive, although prices can vary considerably based on specific nutrient content (e.g., omega-3 [Ω-3FA] fatty acids, fiber). Table 36-3 provides a relative cost summary for enteral formulas.

Nutrient Source

Enteral products are typically *lactose-free* and these formulas are the standard for tube-fed patients owing to presumed lactose intolerance in many hospitalized patients.[19,20] Reduced disaccharidase production during fasting, malnutrition, and various GI tract diseases contribute to lactose intolerance in hospitalized patients.[21] In addition, most ethnic groups, except northern Europeans, have reduced lactase production in adulthood,

Table 36-2 Generic Groups and Subgroups of Enteral Formulas

Polymeric Formulas
Nutrient Source
Blenderized
Lactose free
Fiber Content
Fiber-free
Low fiber (1–9 g/1,000 kcal)
Moderate fiber (9.1–13.9 g/1,000 kcal)
High fiber (14 g or higher/1,000 kcal)
Caloric Density
Standard density (1–1.2 kcal/mL)
Moderate density (1.5 kcal/mL)
Calorically dense (1.8–2 kcal/mL)
Protein or Nitrogen Content
Low nitrogen (6%–9% of kcal)
Standard nitrogen (11%–15% of kcal)
High nitrogen (16%–25% of kcal)
Oligomeric Formulas
Elemental
Peptide based
Specialized Formulas
Renal Failure
Essential amino acid enriched
Low protein and electrolytes
Hepatic Failure (High BCAA, Low AAA)
Stress or Critically Ill
Branched-chain amino acid enriched
High nitrogen plus conditionally essential nutrients
Immune modulating
Pulmonary Disease
Traditional, high fat content
Immune modulating
Glucose Control
Modular Components
Carbohydrate
Protein
Fats

BCAA, branched-chain amino acids; AAA, aromatic amino acids.

leading to lactose intolerance. Lactose can cause bloating, flatulence, abdominal cramps, and watery diarrhea in patients with permanent or transient lactose intolerance. Milk protein concentrate does not contain lactose. Lactose-free formulas leave little residue in the colon and their viscosity is low unless fiber is added.

Table 36-3 Relative Cost of Enteral Formulas[a]

Type of Formula	*Relative Cost (dollars)*
Polymeric Formulas	
Lactose free, standard caloric density, standard nitrogen content plus	
Fiber free for oral supplement or tube feeding[b]	1
Low to moderate fiber (1–8 g/1,000 kcal)	1.5
Moderate to high fiber (>8 g/1,000 kcal)	1.7
Lactose free, standard nitrogen content, fiber-free plus	
Standard caloric density (1–1.2 kcal/mL)[b]	1
Moderate density (1.5 kcal/mL)	1.3
Calorically dense (1.8–2 kcal/mL)	1.3
Lactose free, standard caloric density, fiber-free plus	
Low nitrogen (6%–10% of kcal as protein); low electrolyte	3
Standard nitrogen (11%–15% of kcal as protein)[b]	1
High nitrogen (16%–25% of kcal as protein)	1.3
Oligomeric Formulas	
Elemental (free amino acids)	16.8
Peptide-based	
High protein	14.4
Very high protein	18.2
Specialized Formulas	
Renal failure	
Essential amino acid enriched	19
Low protein and electrolytes	3
Hepatic failure (high BCAA, low AAA)[c]	25
Stress or critically ill	
Branched-chain enriched	22
High nitrogen plus conditionally essential nutrients	2.5
Immune modulating	19.5
Pulmonary disease (standard; not immune modulating)	2.1
Glucose control	4.6

[a]Based on average cost per 1,000 calories for equivalent formulas on contract from 2005–2007.
[b]Index product; given a relative value of 1.
[c]BCAA, branched-chain amino acids; AAA, aromatic amino acids.

Fiber Content

Fiber content provides a second criterion for subdividing polymeric formulas. Fiber has potential physiologic benefits, including increased fecal bulk, decreased transit time in patients susceptible to constipation, increased transit time in patients with diarrhea, reduction of serum cholesterol, and improved glycemic control in patients with diabetes. Recommended fiber intake for healthy Americans is 21 to 25 g for women and 30 to 38 g for men, with the lower end of these amounts for people 51 years of age or older.[22,23] Adequate intake is determined by calorie intake and fiber intake observed to protect against coronary artery disease (14 g/1,000 calories). Optimal fiber intake for ill persons has not been determined. *Fiber-supplemented formulas* vary considerably in fiber content. There is no standardized terminology for low-, moderate-, and high-fiber content. Fiber intake to protect against coronary artery disease is typically considered a high-fiber diet; thus, fiber at 14 g or higher per 1,000 calories is considered high fiber. Diets providing 9 g fiber or less per 1,000 calories generally requires excessive calories to meet recommended fiber intake and are

Table 36-4 Fiber Amount and Sources for Selected Enteral Formulas

Formula Name	Total Dietary Fiber (g/L)	Kcal to Provide 25–38 g Dietary Fiber Daily	Insoluble Fiber	Soluble Fiber	FOS
Ensure with fiber	12	2,083–3,167	x	x	x
Glucerna	14.4	1,736–2,639	x		
Glucerna Select	21.1	1,185–1,800	x	x	x
Jevity 1 Cal	14.4	1,736–2,639	x		
Jevity 1.5 Cal	22	1,705–2,590	x	x	x
Nutren 1.0 with fiber	14	1,786–2,714	x		
Nutren Glytrol	15.2	1,645–2,500	x	x	
Nutren Probalance	10	3,000–4,560	x	x	
Nutren Replete with fiber	14	1,786–2,714	x	x	
Peptamen AF	5.2	4,808–7,307		x	

FOS, fructo-oligosaccharides.

considered low-fiber diets. EN formulas with 9 g or less per 1,000 calories are considered low-fiber formulas, and fiber content above 9 g but below 14 g per 1,000 calories is classified as moderate fiber content.

Fiber is added to enteral formulas primarily to reduce the rapid intestinal transit associated with fiber-free formulas.[24] Insoluble fiber is associated with changes in fecal bulk and transit time, whereas soluble fiber tends to be responsible for effects on cholesterol and glycemic control. Enteral formulas may contain one or both types of fiber, as indicated in Table 36-4. Soluble fibers, such as pectin, psyllium, and certain gums, tend to form gels and are seldom used as a single fiber source.

The most common fiber source for enteral formulas is soy polysaccharide, or soy fiber. Benefits associated with both soluble and insoluble fibers have been noted with soy fiber despite its primarily insoluble fiber content.[25] Although soy polysaccharide demonstrates beneficial effects in healthy subjects and patients non-critically ill, studies do not provide clear evidence of improved bowel function in critically ill patients.[26] Given the current data, stable patients on long term EN appear most likely to benefit from fiber-supplemented formulas. Some patients on short-term EN without GI pathology who experience altered stool consistency may benefit from fiber supplementation. The effect of fiber on patients with bowel pathology is less clear, however, and it may be detrimental in the hypotensive patient with subclinical ischemia.[27]

Addition of fiber to enteral formulas creates some potential problems. Fiber tends to increase formula viscosity, which may necessitate a pump for administration through feeding tubes. GI symptoms from fiber can include increased gas production and abdominal discomfort.[24,28] Gradual introduction of fiber may help reduce these symptoms. Bezoar formation also has been reported in a patient receiving fiber-containing tube feedings and medications that suppressed GI motility.[26] Caution is advised for the use of fiber-containing formulas in patients with poor GI motility, underlying GI dysfunction, or those who are critically ill.[24,27,28] Inadequate fluid intake may also contribute to the risk of bezoar formation and intestinal blockage with fiber.

Fructo-oligosaccharides (FOS) are naturally occurring sugars that are added to some enteral formulas (Table 36-4). Glycosidic linkages between fructose units and glucose in the FOS are not split by GI enzymes but can be fermented to short-chain fatty acids by *Bifidobacterium* in the colon.[26,29] Soluble fibers also are fermented to short-chain fatty acids by colon bacteria; they stimulate colonic blood flow, enhance fluid and electrolyte absorption, and provide a trophic effect in the colon. This may account for the association between soluble fibers and beneficial effects on colonocytes (e.g., regulation of cell growth and adhesion, including inhibition of neoplastic cell growth). Improvement in constipation has been noted with FOS administration; however, intake of >45 g/day may cause diarrhea.[30] Use of FOS in enteral formulas has increased over the past several years as FOS appear to offer the benefits of soluble fiber without the same physicochemical limitations.

Caloric Density

Caloric density is another method of subdividing polymeric enteral formulas. The standard caloric density is 1 to 1.2 kcal/mL. Moderate density formulas contain approximately 1.5 kcal/mL, and calorically dense formulas contain 2 kcal/mL. Increased caloric density increases formula osmolality. Gastric emptying can be reduced when osmolality exceeds 800 mOsm/kg and this may result in feeding intolerance.[31] GI intolerance (e.g., nausea, flatulence, abdominal discomfort) also can occur if the capacity of intestinal enzymes is overwhelmed by infusion of a calorically dense formula. The risk of dehydration increases with increasing caloric density; however, standard caloric density formulas can result in fluid overload in patients with congestive heart failure, renal failure, or other fluid-sensitive conditions.

Protein Content

The fourth method of subdividing polymeric formulas is by protein content, either as a percentage of calories from protein or as the nonprotein calorie:nitrogen ratio (NPC:N). Grams of protein times 4 equals protein calories, and grams of protein divided by 6.25 equals grams of nitrogen, assuming protein is 16% nitrogen. Protein needs increase disproportionately to caloric needs during injury and critical illness. High-nitrogen enteral formulas, designed to supply this increased protein requirement provide approximately 16% to 25% of calories from protein. The NPC:N ratios in these formulas range from 75:1 to 130:1. Standard protein content is 11% to 15% of calories, with NPC:N approximately 140:1 to 200:1. Low-nitrogen formulas with 6% to 9% of calories from protein and a ratio >250:1 are available for patients requiring protein restriction.

Oligomeric Formulas

Oligomeric formulas, also called *predigested, monomeric* or *chemically defined formulas,* require minimal digestive function and produce little residue in the colon. Pancreatic enzyme activity is required for digestion of oligosaccharides and fats. Brush-border disaccharidase activity also is required. Minimal digestion is required, however, for the hydrolyzed protein and medium-chain triglyceride (MCT) components. These formulas can be used for patients with pancreatic insufficiency, reduced mucosal absorption, or reduced hydrolytic capability. Patients most likely to benefit from oligomeric formulas are those with severe pancreatic insufficiency or short bowel syndrome.[1] Although the Canadian Clinical Practice Guidelines for Nutrition Support in Mechanically Ventilated, Critically Ill Adult Patients (CCPG) noted patients with these and other GI complications may benefit from oligomeric formulas, insufficient data were available to make recommendations regarding use of such formulas.[32] Pancreatic enzyme supplementation with polymeric formulas may be tried before oligomeric formulas for some patients with pancreatic insufficiency (e.g., cystic fibrosis).

Two subgroups of oligomeric formulas can be differentiated based on the protein source. True "elemental" formulas contain free amino acids, whereas "peptide-based" formulas contain oligopeptides plus dipeptides, tripeptides, and free amino acids from hydrolysis of protein. Amino acids require no digestion, but the sodium-dependent active transport mechanism appears to be somewhat slow and inefficient with only about one-third of dietary protein absorbed as free amino acids; the remaining two-thirds are absorbed as di- and tripeptides.[30,31,33,34] Specific carriers for di- and tripeptides absorption located in small bowel mucosa do not compete with the free amino acid transport system. Peptides longer than three amino acids require further hydrolysis within the lumen of the small bowel before they are absorbed. Most peptide-based formulas contain a significant portion of peptides that require hydrolysis before absorption.

Some data suggest enteral diets high in peptides stimulate protein synthesis and tissue recovery better than free amino acids; however, the clinical relevance is unclear.[35] No well-designed, randomized, controlled trials have clearly delineated clinical differences in elemental (free amino acid) versus peptide-based formulas. Elemental formulas generally have the lowest fat content (10% f.a.a. (see Table 36-5)). Peptide formulas typically contain one-fourth to one-third of calories from fat, but provide 20% to 70% of the fat as MCT to minimize the risk of malabsorption. Crucial, Optimental, Peptamen products, and Perative are examples of formulas containing peptides.

Oligomeric formulas are typically hypertonic owing to their partially digested nature, although peptide-containing formulas tend to be only slightly hypertonic. Osmotic diarrhea can occur because of the hyperosmolality; however, the CCPG meta-analysis found no difference in diarrhea occurrence between patients receiving intact protein and those receiving peptide-rich formulas.[32] Taste and cost are disadvantages of oligomeric formulas. Flavoring packets are available and newer formulas may be better accepted, but patients commonly complain of a bitter taste when these formulas are taken orally. In general, patients do not tolerate adequate oral consumption of an oligomeric formula to meet daily requirements. As shown in Table 36-3, oligomeric formulas tend to cost several times more than polymeric formulas.

Specialized Formulas

Specialized formulas are designed for specific disease states or conditions, but their use and clinical benefits are controversial. Formulas generally have a good theoretic basis for use, yet lack conclusive clinical evidence of improved efficacy compared with standard formulas. Well-designed studies showing a difference in outcome between specialized and standard enteral formulas providing equal nitrogen and equal calories are difficult to find. Given the high cost of most specialized formulas, it often is difficult to justify their use without evidence of improved clinical efficacy compared with standard formulas.

Renal Failure

Specialty enteral formulas designed for patients with renal failure have enriched essential amino acid content. Theoretically, recycling of urea nitrogen for nonessential amino acid synthesis reduces the accumulation of blood urea nitrogen (BUN).[19,35,36] Clinically significant recycling of nitrogen and incorporation into nonessential amino acids does not appear to occur, however. Essential amino acid formulas may be appropriate for patients with chronic renal failure with glomerular filtration rates <25 mL/minute/1.73 m^2 who are receiving very-low-protein diets and for whom dialysis is not an option.[1,35] Use should be limited to no more than 2 to 3 weeks, because hyperammonemia and metabolic encephalopathy have been associated with longer use. These formulas are not appropriate for patients in acute renal failure or for those receiving dialysis. The NPC:N is generally >300:1 in these formulas. Appropriate vitamin and mineral supplements must be provided with essential amino acid formulas because the formulas themselves are incomplete. Renalcal contains higher-than-normal essential amino acids in combination with nonessential amino acids.

Polymeric enteral formulas designed for renal failure or renal insufficiency are now the standard for patients with impaired renal function. A systematic review, however, found data were insufficient to complete a meta-analysis comparing outcomes with renal versus standard enteral formulas in patients on chronic dialysis.[37] These formulas are not enriched with essential amino acids and use a lower NPC:N ratio (e.g., 140:1 or 160:1) than essential amino acid-enriched formulas. Lower-than-normal concentrations of potassium, phosphorus, and magnesium, as well as higher caloric concentrations (1.8–2 kcal/mL) are used in these formulas to minimize fluid and electrolyte problems. Polymeric enteral formulas meet 100% of the DRI with <2,000 mL/day. Examples of intact protein renal formulas include Suplena, Nepro, and Nutren Renal.

Hepatic Failure

Hepatic failure formulas contain 45% to 50% of protein as branched-chain amino acids (BCAA), compared with 15% to 20% in standard formulas, and lower-than-normal concentrations of aromatic amino acids (AAA), especially phenylalanine. Theoretically, increasing BCAA and decreasing AAA improves hepatic encephalopathy by reducing inhibitory and false neurotransmitter formation.[19,35,36] Prospective, randomized, controlled trials comparing BCAA-enriched formulas with comparable enteral formulas containing standard protein sources are limited. Most studies have not shown a clear advantage for hepatic failure formulas, especially with respect to mortality, and most patients with liver disease tolerate formulas with standard protein sources.[1,19,35] NutriHep is a ready-to-use high BCAA formula containing appropriate vitamin content for patients with end-stage liver disease. Hepatic-Aid II is a powder that must be mixed with water; supplementation of vitamins, minerals, and electrolytes is necessary because it contains negligible amounts of these nutrients.

Stress or Critically Ill

Specialized *stress formulas* designed for critically ill, hypercatabolic patients generally contain a NPC:N ratio of <100:1 (i.e., high nitrogen content) and >35% of protein content as BCAA, without reduced AAA concentrations. Thus, stress and hepatic failure formulas are not therapeutically interchangeable. The theory behind stress formulas is as follows: BCAA are used preferentially for energy production in skeletal muscle of critically ill patients and exogenous BCAA reduces skeletal muscle breakdown and improves protein synthesis.[19,35,36] Studies evaluating the effectiveness of BCAA in stressed patients have primarily involved parenteral BCAA, although results for both parenteral and enteral administration are conflicting and controversial, with no significant improvement in clinical outcome, including morbidity and mortality. Objective criteria for defining critical illness and determining entry into studies may contribute to the inconclusive and controversial results when these studies are viewed as a group.

Enteral formulas having a NPC:N ratio of ≤125:1, but without BCAA supplementation, are commonly marketed as stress or critical care formulas. Several of these formulas, as listed in Table 36-5, also contain arginine, glutamine, or nucleic acid supplementation, a modified fat component, or both. Such formulas are often referred to as "immune-modulating" formulas based on their proposed beneficial modulation of biologic responses to stress. Study formulas frequently contain varying portions of potentially immune modifying components making it difficult to determine the effect of any given component. In addition, effects of immunonutrition in critically ill patients are difficult to isolate from other effects of critical illness and studies are not conclusive for the role of these formulas in most cases. Properties of each of the main immunonutrition substrates are discussed below.

Arginine. The postulated role of arginine in critical illness is related to protein synthesis, cellular growth, and lymphocyte blastogenesis. Arginine is a nonessential amino acid synthesized by the urea cycle during detoxification of ammonia and it is normally available in sufficient quantities for growth and tissue repair. Endogenous synthesis may, however, become inadequate during metabolic stress, making it conditionally essential. Studies in healthy and elderly volunteers have shown beneficial effects from arginine supplementation on T-lymphocyte response and collagen deposition in artificial wounds used as markers of wound healing.[38–40] In burn patients, reduced wound infections, hospital length of stay (LOS), and mortality have been demonstrated with supplemental arginine.[41] Arginine supplementation at two to seven times normal dietary intake (~5.4 g/day in the United States) was suggested as safe for nonseptic burn patients in a review, but further study was considered necessary in septic patients.[40,42] Few studies with surgery and critically ill patients have used arginine alone and results with arginine plus other immune modulating components, most commonly Ω-3FA, nucleotides, glutamine, and antioxidants, are controversial. A recent meta-analysis found no difference in clinical outcomes (e.g., infectious complications, ventilator days, LOS) and mortality for critically ill patients receiving immunonutrition versus standard EN.[43] This meta-analysis was heavily weighted by the results of a large multicenter trial that showed no difference in the outcome parameters of 597 critically ill patients randomized to isonitrogenous high protein, isocaloric formulas, and study formula that contained 9 g/L arginine, 13 g/L glutamine, high Ω-3FA, antioxidants, and low-fiber content.[44] Several earlier meta-analyses and systematic reviews indicated improved clinical outcomes but no difference in mortality with combined immune-modulating components.[19,40,42,45] Inclusion of multiple prospective, double-blind, randomized controlled studies in patients with upper GI cancers undergoing major surgery likely contributed to these results.[40] One meta-analysis suggested high arginine (>12 g/day) was associated with potential enhanced immune function and reduced infections in patients having elective surgery, yet advised of potential harm in some subpopulations of critically ill patients, particularly septic patients.[45]

Arginine produces some of its versatile physiologic effects through a nitric oxide (NO) dependent pathway. The synthesis of NO, a potent vasodilating agent, requires arginine as a substrate. Although NO production increases during sepsis (thereby creating a negative arginine balance), the exact role of this effector molecule remains controversial. Many believe that excess NO is part of an adaptive response directed toward limiting infection, ischemia, coagulation, inflammation, and tissue injury.[42] One study indicates that a population of septic patients, mostly with pneumonia, receiving a high–arginine-containing, immune-enhancing formula (>12 g/L) had significant decreases in the incidence of bacteremia and decreased mortality.[45,46] On the other hand, a number of other studies and subgroup analysis of higher quality studies reveal that arginine supplementation in the critically ill patient population may be detrimental owing to an enhanced systemic inflammatory response and hemodynamic instability.[45,47–49]

Bertolini et al.[49] reported about a 31% higher mortality with an immune-modulating EN formula (supplemented with arginine, glutamine, nucleic acids, and Ω-3FA) compared with PN in septic patients. Patients with pneumonia receiving arginine, Ω-3FA, and antioxidant-supplemented feeding also may be at increased risk for death.[50] High plasma arginine concentrations in critically ill patients with hepatic failure have been reported and the conclusion was that supplemental arginine could be harmful in this patient population.[51] Use of arginine-containing, immune-enhancing diets is not recommended by CCPG because higher-quality studies indicated no effect on mortality with these formulas and increased mortality was reported for septic patients in some studies.[32] No randomized studies were available for arginine alone in critically ill patients. A consensus statement published by another group also

Table 36-5 Selected High-Protein Enteral Formulas With Altered Protein or Fat Sources[a]

Formula[b,c]	kcal/mL (mOsm/kg)	Free Water (%)	Protein g/L (% kcal)	NPC:N Ratio	Protein Source	ARG g/L[d]	GLN g/L[d]	Fat g/L (% kcal)	Fat Sources	Fat kcal as MCT (%)	Ratio of n-6 to n-3 FA[d]	Fiber g/L[d]
Crucial[c]	1.5 (490)	77	94 (25)	67:1	Hydrolyzed casein; L-arginine	15	–	67.6 (39)	MCT oil; fish oil (<2%); Soybean oil; lecithin	50	1.5:1	–
f.a.a[c]	1.0 (850)	85	50 (20)	100:1	Crystalline amino acids	–	–	11.2 (10)	Soybean oil; MCT	25	–	–
Jevity 1 Cal[b]	1.06 (300)	83.5	44 (16.7)	125:1	Sodium and calcium caseinates; soy protein isolates	–	–	35 (29)	Canola oil; corn oil; MCT oil; lecithin	19	–	14.4
Jevity 1.2 Cal[b]	1.2 (450)	80.7	55.5 (18.5)	110:1	Sodium and calcium caseinates; soy protein isolates	–	–	39.3 (29)	Canola oil; corn oil; MCT oil; lecithin	19	–	18 (8 g FOS)
Optimental[b]	1.0 (540)	83.2	51 (20.5)	97:1	Soy protein hydrolysate; partially hydrolyzed sodium caseinate; L-arginine	5.5	–	28.4 (25)	Structured lipid (interesterified sardine oil [EPA, DHA] and MCT); canola oil, soy oil	NA	–	5 FOS
Osmolite 1 Cal[b]	1.06 (300)	84	44 (16.7)	125:1	Sodium and calcium caseinates; soy protein isolates	–	–	34.7 (29)	Canola oil; corn oil; MCT oil; lecithin	20	–	–
Osmolite 1.2 Cal[b]	1.2 (360)	82	55.5 (18.5)	110:1	Sodium and calcium caseinate	–	–	39 (29)	High-oleic safflower oil; canola oil; MCT oil; lecithin	20	–	–
Osmolite 1.5[b]	1.5 (525)	76	62.7 (16.7)	125:1	Sodium and calcium caseinates; soy protein isolates	–	–	49 (29)	High-oleic safflower oil; canola oil; MCT oil; lecithin	20	–	–
Oxepa[b]	1.5 (535)	78.5	62.5 (16.7)	125:1	Sodium and calcium caseinates	–	–	93.8 (55)	Canola oil; MCT oil; sardine oil; borage oil	25	–	–
Peptamen VHP[c]	1.0 (270–380)	84	62.4 (25)	75:1	Hydrolyzed whey protein	–	–	39 (33)	MCT oil; soybean oil (<2%); lecithin	70	7.4:1	–
Peptamen AF[c]	1.2 (390)	81	75.6 (21)	76:1	Hydrolyzed whey protein	–	–	54.8 (39)	MCT oil; soybean oil (<2%); fish oil (<2%); lecithin	50	1.8:1	5.2 (FOS and other fibers)
Perative[b]	1.3 (460)	79	66.6 (20.5)	97:1	Partially hydrolyzed sodium caseinate; whey protein hydrolysate; L-arginine	6.5	–	37.4 (25)	Canola oil; MCT oil; corn oil	40	–	6.5 FOS
Pivot 1.5 Cal[b]	1.5 (595)	75.9	93.8 (25)	75:1	Partially hydrolyzed sodium caseinate; whey protein hydrolysate	13	6.5	50.8 (30)	Structured lipid (interesterified sardine oil [EPA, DHA] and MCT); soy oil; canola oil	20	–	7.5 FOS
Nutren ProBalance[c]	1.2 (350–450)	81	54 (18)	114:1	Calcium-potassium caseinate	–	–	40.8 (30)	Canola oil; MCT oil (<2%); corn oil (<2%); lecithin	20	3.6:1	10
Nutren Replete[c]	1.0 (300–350)	84	62.4 (25)	75:1	Calcium-potassium caseinate	–	–	34 (30)	Canola oil; MCT oil (<2%); lecithin	25	2.3:1	–
Nutren Replete with fiber[c]	1.0 (310–390)	84	62.5 (25)	75:1	Calcium-potassium caseinate	–	–	34 (30)	Canola oil; MCT oil (<2%); lecithin	25	2.3:1	14

[a]Changes periodically occur in nutrient sources and content; use this table as a general reference only and not for specific patient care issues.
[b]Abbott (Ross) product.
[c]Nestle product.
[d]None or unknown indicated by "-".
ARG, arginine; DHA, docosahexenoic acid; EPA, eicosapentenoic acid; FOS, fructo-oligosaccharides; GLN, glutamine; HN, high nitrogen; MCT, medium-chain triglycerides; NPC:N, nonprotein calorie to nitrogen; n-3FA, Ω-3 fatty acids; n-6FA, Ω-6 fatty acids; VHP, very high protein; VHN, very high nitrogen.

recommends against use of arginine-enriched formulas in critically ill patients.[52] Clearly, the role of arginine-supplemented EN remains controversial. Additional studies with well-defined patient populations are necessary to determine appropriate arginine doses, the effects of arginine alone versus combinations of immune-modulating components (arginine, glutamine, nucleic acids, Ω-3FA), and to identify which patient populations would benefit from this amino acid.

Nucleic acids or *nucleotides*. Purines and pyrimidines, including RNA and DNA, comprise the nucleotides. Evidence for including nucleotides in the diet comes primarily from animal studies that suggest a need for preformed pyrimidines to develop and activate T cells in the immune system.[53] Diets lacking nucleotides may be immunosuppressive; however, little data are available on the role of nucleotides in EN formulas. Nucleotide use in EN formulas has only been in conjunction with other immune-modulating components and studies are needed to clarify their effects.

Glutamine. The proposed role of glutamine in critical illness is enhanced neutrophil function and maintenance of intestinal barrier function, thereby preventing translocation of bacteria and endotoxins from the GI tract into systemic circulation and reducing bacteremia.[54–56] Glutamine potentially reduces the inflammatory response, lowers the risk of insulin resistance, and maintains acid-base balance. Glutamine is a nonessential amino acid synthesized in sufficient quantities for its roles in transamination, as an intermediate in numerous metabolic pathways, such as gluconeogenesis and renal ammoniagenesis, as a fuel source for rapidly dividing lymphocytes and enterocytes, and in the synthesis of glutathione. Endogenous synthesis may become inadequate during metabolic stress, however, making glutamine conditionally essential. Large, abrupt drops in plasma and muscular glutamine concentrations, which appear to correlate with increased mortality, have been reported in patients who are critically ill or septic.[55,57] Although this observation does not necessarily indicate depletion, it is used as a hypothesis for the supplementation of glutamine in certain patient populations. Although a number of benefits have been attributed to the provision of glutamine, study results are often conflicting. Decreased methotrexate-induced enterocolitis, improved rates of GI tract recovery after radiation therapy, and a reduction in the severity or duration of mucositis have all been reported following glutamine administration.[58,59] Although glutamine supplementation has been associated with improvements in the indicators for protein catabolic rate and immune function in critically ill patients, improvements in nitrogen balance and visceral protein status are rarely noted. The reports of less pneumonia, bacteremia, and septic events in critically ill patients receiving glutamine supplementation do not translate into reduced mortality.[60] Glutamine supplementation may however be linked to a decrease in complications and mortality rates when parenteral, high-dose glutamine is utilized. Data from a meta-analysis confirm the previous hypothesis of many investigators that the beneficial effect of glutamine in the critically ill may be very dependent on dose and route of administration.[54]

Protein-bound glutamine is present in all enteral formulas. Free glutamine is unstable in ready-to-use formulas, however, and it is generally administered separately from the formula. Glutamate is stable in water and functions in many roles attributed to glutamine. Additional research is needed to determine whether physiologic effects are equivalent for glutamate, protein-bound glutamine, and free glutamine. Until such questions are answered, supplementation of free glutamine separately from the formula is likely to continue despite its uncertain role in many patient populations and suggestions that it is not necessary.[61] The currently recommended maximal dose of glutamine is 0.57 g/kg/day, although lower doses are used in most studies and >0.2 g/kg/day was adequate to see benefit in one meta-analysis.[38,62] Doses of enteral glutamine used in studies reviewed for the CCPG varied from 0.16 to 0.5 g/kg/day, and the committee decided a reasonable dose would be 0.3 g/kg/day.[32,63] Although available data do not indicate a harmful effect of glutamine, there are theoretic concerns associated with providing a large quantity of one amino acid that shares transport systems with other amino acids in the body and that has a role in ammoniagenesis. Glutamine supplementation should be avoided in patients with total bilirubin >10 mg/dL or creatinine clearance <30 mL/minute because ammonia excretion could be impared.[64] Monitoring for potential complications with glutamine supplementation is advised given these theoretic concerns.

Alteration in the fat component of enteral formulas. Stress or critical care and immune-modulating formulas contain different sources of fat to alter the type of fatty acids provided. Fat sources commonly include MCT, along with predominantly canola oil, high oleic oils, or fish oils as long-chain fatty acids. Usual polyunsaturated vegetable oils (i.e., corn, soy, and safflower oils) are avoided or provided in relatively small quantities to limit omega-6 fatty acids (Ω-6FA), which are precursors to arachidonic acid and therefore to dienoic or "2" series prostaglandins, prostacyclins, and thromboxanes, and to "4" series leukotrienes. These compounds, taken as a whole, are potent inflammatory, vasoconstrictive, and platelet-aggregating agents.[65,66] The source of Ω-6FA may, however, also influence the type of prostaglandins produced.[67] Dietary α-linoleic acid is converted to γ-linoleic acid (GLA), then to dihomo-GLA, and subsequently to arachidonic acid. As a dietary supplement, GLA is converted to dihomo-GLA, which effectively competes with arachidonic acid in the pathways for prostaglandin synthesis rather than being elongated to arachidonic acid. The resulting "1" series prostaglandins have lower proinflammatory effects, similar to "3" series prostaglandins. Small amounts of Ω-6FA are required in the diet to prevent deficiency of linoleic acid an essential fatty acid not provided by MCT and fish oils.

Fish oils, including menhaden oil, provide fatty acids primarily from the Ω-3 family, with the very long-chain fatty acids eicosapentenoic acid (EPA) and docosahexenoic acid (DHA) predominating. The proposed role of Ω-3FA in critical illness is to reduce infectious complications and death in selected patient populations. The Ω-3FA are precursors to the "3" series prostaglandins, prostacyclins, and thromboxanes, and "5" series leukotrienes. In total, these compounds are less inflammatory and more vasodilatory than compounds from Ω-6FA.[65,66,68] This may be beneficial in critically ill patients, but few data are available evaluating effects of only fat modification. Combinations of immune-modulating components may produce different effects than single nutrients. For example, in vitro data demonstrate an interaction between prostaglandins and arginine metabolism. Greater arginase induction and lower nitrate levels exist with "1" and "2" series compared to "3" series prostaglandins.[69]

Improved clinical outcomes for postsurgical and critically ill patients have been associated with EN containing Ω-3FA, usually in conjunction with other immune-modulating components, although the effects remain controversial.[19,40,42,45,68] Studies suggest a minimum of 5 to 7 days of supplementation with immune-modulating components, including Ω-3FA, is necessary to see beneficial effects on postoperative outcomes.[70–72] Incorporation of Ω-3FA into cell membranes has been demonstrated in humans with supplementation for 5 days.[73] Decreased wound infections and reduced mortality have been demonstrated in burn patients with low-fat diets containing 50% of fat as fish oil.[41] Other studies, however, have shown no benefit in this population.[65] Fat modification to provide high Ω-3FA content also has been studied in acute respiratory distress syndrome (ARDS) and acute lung injury, as discussed under pulmonary formulas.

Further research is needed to elucidate effects of Ω-3FA alone and to determine their safety and efficacy in various disease states. Effects of Ω-3FA on antioxidant levels, especially vitamin E, and the need for supplementation require study. Appropriate quantities of Ω-3FA and the most beneficial ratios of Ω-6FA to Ω-3FA also must be determined before routine supplementation with Ω-3FA can be recommended beyond modifying the diet to include foods rich in Ω-3FA (i.e., fish, such as salmon). Current ratios of Ω-6FA to Ω-3FA in diets range from about 4:1 in Japan to 16:1 in the United States, although a specific intake amount resulting in adverse effects has not been determined for either Ω-6FA or Ω-3FA.[61,64] No data exist to guide the use in various illnesses.

Canola oil and high-oleic oils are other fat sources used in EN. These oils are common in standard formulas, as well as those used for stress and critical illness. Canola oil contains approximately two-thirds monounsaturated fatty acids, compared with less than half this amount in polyunsaturated vegetable oils. High-oleic safflower and sunflower oils also have a high monounsaturated fatty acid content. Monounsaturated fatty acids have been popularized by reports of low cardiovascular disease in populations using olive oil, but further research is needed to determine the role of these fatty acids in ill patients. The combination of canola oil and high-oleic oil does increase the content of linolenic acid.

Enteral formulas often contain MCT to improve fat absorption. Absorption of MCT is relatively independent of pancreatic enzymes and bile salts; thus, they can be absorbed in patients experiencing malabsorption of the long-chain triglycerides. Rapid, carnitine-independent metabolism occurs with MCT, whereas long-chain triglycerides require carnitine for metabolism. Therefore, use of long-chain triglycerides is compromised when carnitine deficiency occurs, but MCT metabolism is unaffected. Formulas containing a relatively large percentage of fat calories as MCT are frequently marketed for critically ill patients with malabsorption. Examples of formulas with higher percentages of fat calories as MCT include Nutren 1.5 and Crucial with 50% to 65%, Nutren 2.0, NutriHep, and Peptamen products with 65% to 80%, and Portagen with over 85% of fat calories as MCT.

Carnitine. An important compound in normal nutrition, carnitine is required for transport of long-chain triglycerides into the mitochondria for metabolism and export of acyl-coenzyme A (CoA) compounds out of the mitochondria. Formulas marketed for critical care may contain higher amounts than standard formulas, but most formulas contain an adequate quantity of carnitine to prevent deficiency.

Taurine. A sulfur-containing amino acid, taurine protects cell membranes by attenuating toxic substances and acting as an osmoregulator.[74] Taurine may improve fat absorption in patients with malabsorption through effects on bile acid production and micelle formation. Taurine also is essential for normal neuronal and retinal development in infants and children; thus, pediatric formulas include taurine as an essential nutrient.[74] Dietary taurine is adequate for adults, except possibly those with catabolic illness such as cancer, chemotherapy, radiation, burns, and operative injury. Taurine is typically added to formulas marketed for stress and critical illness because these populations may be at risk of inadequate intake.

The results of clinical trials examining the effects of immune-modulating enteral formulations on mortality, hospital LOS, intensive care unit (ICU) days, incidence of nosocomial infection, duration of mechanical ventilation, and GI complications are conflicting.[32,41–50,52,54–56,61–63,68,70–77] Differences in study design, patient population, enteral formulation (immune-modulating components and doses), time to EN commencement, and volume of formula received, make it difficult to compare study results reliably. Meta-analyses of major studies reveal particular subsets of patients who may benefit from certain immune-modulating components whereas other subgroups may exhibit increased mortality. Patients with sepsis, pneumonia, and possibly other infections appear potentially to be at risk of harm. Arginine has been identified as the component most likely responsible for poor outcomes, but no studies with arginine as a single supplemental ingredient are available. Formulas generally include some combination of arginine, glutamine, Ω-3FA, and antioxidants, making it difficult to identify the effects of any single component clearly. Elective surgical patients, especially upper GI surgery, appear to be most likely to benefit from immunonutrition, with significant reductions in infectious complications and lower hospital LOS without mortality effect. Further research is needed to examine this controversial area of nutrition. A need exists to define which patients will benefit from immunonutrition, and the optimal components, doses, and timing of immune modulators for different patient subgroups. Until such information is available, the immune-modulating formulas must be used with caution and careful evaluation of each patient. Guidelines, consensus statements, and recommendations have been developed to help the clinician provide evidence-based nutrition therapy; however, many barriers to implementation exist.[1,28,32,52,63,72,75,78]

Pulmonary Disease

The percentage of calories from fat is relatively high (40%–55%) in formulas marketed for patients with pulmonary disease. The premise for higher fat content is that fat oxidation produces less carbon dioxide (CO_2) than carbohydrate oxidation, thereby reducing the work load of the lungs. Fats, particularly long-chain triglycerides, have a lower respiratory quotient (RQ) than carbohydrates, meaning less CO_2 is produced per volume of oxygen consumed during fat metabolism. Early studies comparing isocaloric, high-fat, low-carbohydrate diets with higher carbohydrate diets showed improved respiratory parameters in ambulatory patients with chronic obstructive pulmonary disease (COPD) as well as reduced time on the ventilator and decreased arterial CO_2 concentrations in mechanically ventilated patients.[19,35,36,77] Calories at 1.7 to 2.25 times measured energy expenditure in these studies were excessive by current standards and excess calories contribute to higher CO_2 production.[79] Preventing overfeeding is as important for control of CO_2 as high-fat, low-carbohydrate diets.[19,20] In addition, improved respiratory parameters with a high-fat EN product are unlikely to be seen in patients without excess CO_2 production or retention. A more recent study in 60 malnourished, underweight patients with COPD does suggest respiratory status in this population is more likely to benefit from a high-fat, low-carbohydrate (28% of calories) formula compared with a high-carbohydrate (60%–70% of calories) formula.[80] Although the percent of calories from fat (55%) in the high-fat formula was similar to traditional pulmonary formulas, fat distribution was considerably different with 20% of fat as MCT and a predominance of monounsaturated fat. During a period of overfeeding for weight gain, pulmonary formulas may be reasonable; however, they are not warranted for routine use.

An immune-modulating pulmonary (IMP) formula has been studied in patients with ARDS and acute pulmonary injury.[81] Two high-fat formulas, the IMP formula containing fish oil, borage oil, and antioxidants (vitamins C and E, beta-carotene) and a typical pulmonary formula with high Ω-6FA content were compared. The IMP formula was associated with fewer days of supplemental oxygen, fewer days of mechanical ventilation, decreased ICU days, and fewer new organ failures. However, the choice of control formula in this study has been questioned since there is some evidence of harmful effects from administration of Ω-6FA-rich fats in critically ill patients.[32] Mortality was not improved. This was the only study meeting inclusion criteria for the CCPG using fish oils in critically ill adults.[32] Due to the potential need for higher antioxidant intake with Ω-3FA and because of inability to separate effects of the combined components in the IMP formula, the CCPG recommendation is to consider using IMP formulas containing a combination of fish oils, borage oils, and antioxidants in patients with ARDS. Another study not available for CCPG evaluation used the same IMP formula and found lower alveolar membrane permeability and reduced leukotriene B4 and total neutrophils in bronchoalveolar lavage (BAL) fluid of patients with ARDS.[82] As for all immune-modulating formulas, the cost of the IMP formula is relatively high (Table 36-3).

Delayed gastric emptying is associated with high-fat diets, and must be considered when evaluating possible benefits and adverse effects of high-fat EN. Abdominal distention, increased gastric residuals, nausea, and vomiting can result from delayed gastric emptying. Delivery of a high-fat load, especially long-chain triglycerides, into the small bowel may overwhelm pancreatic lipase activity in some patients, leading to fat malabsorption. Formulas typically classified as pulmonary formulas include Nutren Pulmonary and Pulmocare. Oxepa is an IMP formula.

Glucose Control

Formulas for hyperglycemic patients, known as diabetic formulas, have caloric distributions of 31% to 40% carbohydrate, 42% to 49% fat, and 16% to 20% protein. The fat content is higher than recommended for healthy persons with diabetes, but high monounsaturated fat sources predominate.[83–85] The source and type of carbohydrates in diabetic formulas varies, with a predominance of more complex carbohydrates (i.e., oligosaccharides, cornstarch, fiber) and insulin-independent sugars (i.e., fructose) despite total carbohydrate content probably being more important than carbohydrate type.[19,85] For tube feeding the American Diabetes Association suggests either a standard formula with 50% carbohydrate or a formula containing 33% to 40% carbohydrate.[86] Practice guidelines for nutrition support suggest no changes in macronutrients compared with the standard diet recommendations for diabetes, including 45% to 65% of calories from carbohydrate.[1] Fiber sources associated with improved glycemic control, mainly soluble fibers but also soy polysaccharide, are included in these formulas to help minimize postprandial hyperglycemia.[24] Fiber content ranges from 14 to 21 g/L and formulas are 1 kcal/mL; thus, the recommended fiber intake of 25 to 38 g daily generally can be achieved with <2,000 kcal/day.[22,23]

Results of studies with diabetic formulas have been mixed. Early studies showing improvement in glucose response were conducted in healthy volunteers, whereas patients with type 2 diabetes in a long-term care facility showed no improvement compared with a standard EN formula.[19,28,87] Studies showing reductions in blood glucose frequently fail to achieve tight control (i.e., 80–110 mg/dL) and lack improvement in clinical outcomes, including infectious complications, hospital LOS, and mortality.[88,89] Current evidence is insufficient to support routine use of diabetic formulas; thus, starting with a standard formula in conjunction with insulin use and changing to a diabetes formula if insulin causes difficulties with glucose control has been suggested.[28,53,87,90,91] Problems with delayed gastric emptying or fat malabsorption must be weighed against possible benefits of improved glucose control with diabetic formulas. Clearly, treatment goals for EN in patients with diabetes mellitus should include individualization of macronutrient composition, avoidance of excess calories, and maintenance of euglycemia.[1] Formulas marketed for glucose control include Glucerna, Glucerna Select and Nutren Glytrol.

Modular Components

Modular components are individual nutrient substrates designed for addition to oral diets or enteral formulas. Glucose polymers are used to supplement calories as carbohydrate. They do not increase osmolality or alter food or formula flavor. Powdered carbohydrate modules contain 20 to 30 kcal/tablespoon, whereas liquids contain 2 kcal/mL. Protein modules are powders containing 3 to 5 g protein/tablespoon. Most protein modules are intact protein. Arginine and glutamine are available as individual packets to allow supplementation as a single amino acid. Modular components typically are mixed with water and administered through the feeding tube rather than being mixed directly into the formula.

TUBE-FEEDING ADMINISTRATION REGIMEN

The feeding route, formula selected, and anticipated duration of feeding influence the administration regimen. Patient location (e.g., hospital, nursing facility, home) and cost also are considered when developing the regimen, including delivery schedule, formula strength or concentration for initiating and advancing feedings, and the administration method (i.e., syringe, gravity drip, pump). Limited scientific data exist regarding EN administration regimens; thus, expert opinion plays an important role and different regimens can be used in various settings, all of which appear to meet the needs of the patients and personnel. Practice guidelines or protocols for initiation and advancement of EN have been suggested to minimize variations in quality of care and facilitate optimal delivery of nutrients and appropriate monitoring.[92] The CCPG found insufficient data to recommend the use of feeding protocols in critically ill patients.[32] With or without a protocol, the administration regimen should be adjusted as necessary for feeding intolerance.

Four basic schedules for formula delivery are available to provide the daily volume of formula: continuous infusion, cyclic infusion, intermittent infusion, and bolus delivery of formula. *Continuous infusion* provides formula at a continuous rate over 24 hours/day. In contrast, *cyclic infusion* provides formula at a continuous rate for <24 hours daily. *Intermittent infusion* provides formula in a specified number of feedings daily. Each of three to eight daily feedings is administered over 20 to 60 minutes via gravity drip or infusion pump. *Bolus delivery* is similar to intermittent infusion except that each feeding is administered via a syringe or by gravity over a few minutes up to 20 minutes.

Continuous Infusion

Continuous infusion can be used with any route of feeding. Intragastric continuous infusion is most commonly used for hospitalized patients, although small bowel feeding may be more appropriate in certain settings (e.g., ICU).[32] Risks of gastric distention and aspiration may decrease with continuous infusion compared with intermittent gastric infusion.[18,93,94] In addition, continuous infusion may be better tolerated as judged by stool frequency and time to attain full nutrition support, especially in the elderly and in metabolically unstable patients.[77,92,95,96] Insufficient evidence exists to include a recommendation for continuous infusion versus other administration methods for critically ill patients in the CCPG.[32] Feeding into the duodenum or jejunum is best initiated with continuous infusion because rapid infusion of large formula volumes into the small bowel can result in symptoms consistent with a dumping syndrome, including sweating, lightheadedness, abdominal distention, cramping, hyperperistalsis, and watery diarrhea. With time, the jejunum may adapt to larger volumes over a shorter time allowing cyclic or longer intermittent infusions.

Cyclic Feeding

Cyclic feeding most commonly is used for patients who need supplemental nutrition because of an inability to consume adequate oral nutrients, during transition to an oral diet, and for long-term home EN patients. Infusions are typically given at night over 8 to 12 hours to minimize interference with oral intake during the day and normal activities such as work or school, although cycles can be as long as 20 hours. Formula volume and osmolality can limit tolerance to cyclic feedings, especially jejunal feedings, and transition from continuous to cyclic infusion may require several days to weeks depending on the cycle length and patient tolerance.

Intermittent or Bolus Feedings

The stomach's reservoir capacity allows administration of relatively large-volumes on an *intermittent* or *bolus schedule.* This is more physiologic than continuous feeding and more convenient for patients in nursing facilities and ambulatory patients at home on EN. Patients are typically started on continuous infusion feedings, then transitioned to intermittent infusions, and eventually to the shorter administration time of bolus feedings. Patients may need feedings over at least 15 minutes to avoid bloating, cramping, nausea, and diarrhea. A rate of <60 mL/minute is suggested to minimize symptoms of GI intolerance with bolus feedings.[97,98] In small studies, healthy volunteers tolerated bolus feedings of up to 750 mL at 60 mL/minute, but intolerance developed at the next higher rate of 85 mL/minute.[97]

Initiation of Feedings

The rate and strength, or concentration, of formula used for initiating EN primarily depends on the site of feeding and condition of the patient's GI tract. Diluted formula and a low infusion rate were standard "starter regimens" for intragastric tube feedings in the past and still are used in some institutions based on concern for GI intolerance during the first few days of feeding when full-strength formula or a large volume of formula is administered, because adaptation to osmolality and volume has not occurred. Controlled studies do not support this theory.[95–99] Dilution delays delivery of adequate nutrients without significantly affecting the incidence of GI intolerance. Hypertonic formulas are diluted rapidly in the GI tract, reaching isotonicity before or shortly beyond the ligament of Treitz.[98] Rapid infusion of formula may, however, increase the incidence of nausea, cramping, and abdominal discomfort.

For intermittent feeding, rates of 200 to 300 mL over 20 to 60 minutes every 4 to 6 hours are generally tolerated; bolus feedings are better tolerated when the rate is <60 mL/minute.[97,99] Volumes up to 750 mL every 4 to 6 hours may be tolerated.[92,98] Although studies have demonstrated tolerance with initiation of feedings at goal rate, starting slower is appropriate for most patients. Various recommendations for continuous infusion intragastric feedings include starting at 50 mL/hour for 6 to 10 hours then advancing to the goal rate in 20 to 25 mL/hour increments every 6 to 8 hours; starting at 20 to 50 mL/hour and advancing by 20 to 25 mL every 4 to 6 hours; or starting at 10 to 40 mL/hour, advancing in increments of 10 to 20 mL/hour every 8 to 12 hours.[92,95–98,100] For critically ill patients, those with abnormal GI function, patients without use of the GI tract for a prolonged time, those at risk of refeeding syndrome, and when calorically dense or high-osmolality formulas are used, the slower start and advancement may be preferable although it is not an "evidence-based" practice.[92,97,101,102] Feedings into the small bowel are initiated at 10 to 40 mL/hour, with rate increases of 10 to 25 mL/hour every 8 to 12 hours until goal rate is reached.[77,96,97] Isotonic formulas can start at 30 to 40 mL/hour; hypertonic formulas may require a slower rate. A general rule for EN is to change one parameter at a time; thus, the formula and rate or concentration should not be changed concurrently.

MONITORING ENTERAL FEEDING

Appropriate monitoring of patients receiving EN via tube is essential to recognize and prevent complications. Complications can be divided into three groups: mechanical, GI, and metabolic (Table 36-6).

Mechanical Complications

Mechanical complications often can be avoided with good nursing technique and careful observation of feeding tolerance. Frequent assessment of tube placement by auscultation, location of markings on the tube, and withdrawal of gastric contents is important to prevent pulmonary aspiration of the formula. Tube placement should be evaluated every 4 to 6 hours with continuous feeding, or before each intermittent or bolus feeding.[97,99,103,104] Withdrawal of gastric contents through the feeding tube using a syringe allows both confirmation of tube placement and evaluation of volume in the stomach (gastric residual volume [GRV]).

Gastric residual volume varies based on the volume and timing of previous feeds, especially for intermittent or bolus feeds, feeding tube characteristics, and patient position and activity.[97,99] Gastrostomy tubes may yield less volume than NG tubes because of their more anterior position in the stomach. Soft, small-bore feeding tubes may collapse when GRV is checked, preventing accurate measurement. GRV is not usually checked through tubes placed in the postpyloric region because of (a) problems with tube collapse and (b) the small bowel does not serve as a reservoir for residuals. If the patient has an NG tube in addition to a small bowel feeding tube, GRV can be checked through the NG tube to assess whether the formula is "backing-up" or refluxing into the stomach. Previously, methylene blue or blue food coloring was added to the formula to evaluate reflux; however, reports of mortality associated with this practice have resulted in its abandonment.[18,105–107] The use of glucose oxidase test strips to detect the presence of enteral formula in tracheobronchial secretions lacks sensitivity and specificity, and the results have not been shown to correlate with aspiration.[92,97]

Promotility agents (e.g., metoclopramide, erythromycin) should be considered in the systematic management of a high GRV.[18,32,108,109] These agents may improve feeding tolerance and formula delivery and the risk of aspiration may be decreased. Postpyloric tube placement generally is recommended when the GRV is persistently high or for patients who have experienced aspiration. Elevating the head of the bed to 30 to 45 degrees, with 45 degrees preferred in critically ill patients, during and after feedings also is recommended to reduce the risk of aspiration.[32,104]

Gastrointestinal Complications

Gastrointestinal complications are frequently associated with tube feeding. Diarrhea occurs in 2% to 70% of patients, depending on the definition used, and is one of the most difficult problems for nurses, patients, and caregivers to address.[97–99,110] Predisposing illnesses, including diabetes mellitus, GI infections, pancreatic insufficiency, and malabsorption syndromes, are more likely to cause diarrhea in patients receiving EN than the formula itself.[77,92,97,111] Formula-related GI infections occur owing to contamination of an opened can or package. Sources of contamination include the water used for reconstitution or dilution, transfer to the delivery bag, formula kept in the delivery bag for a prolonged period, and poorly cleaned feeding bags or administration sets. Closed enteral feeding systems using ready-to-hang bags of formula decrease contamination by reducing manipulation of the bag and formula. Concurrent drug therapy is another major contributor to diarrhea in tube-fed patients, potentially accounting for 61% of diarrhea cases.[97]

Metabolic Complications

Metabolic complications of EN include hyperglycemia, electrolyte abnormalities, and fluid imbalance. Although rigorous evaluation of monitoring frequency is lacking, regular biochemical determinations similar to those used for PN are recommended to identify metabolic abnormalities and to correct before severe abnormalities occur. Baseline values for serum glucose, creatinine, BUN, and electrolytes should be available to guide selection of the enteral formula. Fingerstick glucose measurements every 6 hours or an insulin protocol are recommended before EN starts in diabetic or hyperglycemic patients or if hyperglycemia is anticipated. After EN is initiated, serum glucose, sodium (Na), potassium (K), chloride (Cl), and bicarbonate should be determined daily until they are stable in hospitalized patients, usually 4 to 5 days. Monitoring frequency is decreased to once or twice weekly when results are stable, but typically continue daily or every other day in critically ill patients. Patients discharged to home or a nursing facility before reaching their tube feeding goal should have serum glucose and electrolytes determined two to three times during the first week of therapy, then weekly for 2 to 3 weeks in stable patients after the EN is at goal rate. Serum creatinine (SrCr) and BUN are determined daily for a few days in critically ill patients, then by the same schedule as electrolytes. These laboratory values may be needed only two to three times in the first week, then weekly in relatively stable hospitalized patients.

Monitoring schedules for SrCr, BUN, calcium, phosphorus, and magnesium for patients in a nursing facility or at home are the same as for electrolytes. For hospitalized patients, calcium, phosphorus, and magnesium are determined two to three times during the first week, then once weekly if the patient is stable. Nutrition monitoring also is recommended, including serum albumin and prealbumin or transferrin weekly while the patient is hospitalized. For patients receiving long-term EN, the frequency of laboratory monitoring gradually is decreased. Laboratory monitoring should be done once or twice yearly in stable patients without significant medical problems. Patients who have medical problems that can affect nutrient, electrolyte, or trace element requirements or tolerances should be monitored as appropriate to the medical condition.

Weight and fluid status are important parameters to monitor throughout EN therapy. For hospitalized patients, weight is primarily a reflection of fluid status, whereas in long-term patients it is an important parameter for adequacy of caloric intake. Consistent increases or decreases from the required

Table 36-6 Complications of Tube Feeding

Complication	Cause/Contributing Factor	Treatment/Prevention
Mechanical Complications		
Aspiration	Deflated tracheostomy cuff	Inflate tracheostomy cuff before feeding; keep inflated 1 hr after feeding; consider small-bore feeding tube placed past the ligament of Treitz
	Displaced feeding tube	Reinsert tube, check placement; consider hand restraints or feeding tube bridle
	Reduced gastric emptying	Check residuals every 4–6 hrs for gastric tube; raise head of bed 30–45 degrees; use lower fat formula; use prokinetic medication; use small bowel feeding tube
	Lack of gag reflex; coma	Place feeding tube into jejunum; keep head of bed elevated to 45 degrees; provide continuous feeding
Nasal or pharyngeal irritation or necrosis; esophageal erosion; otitis media	Large-bore, polyvinyl chloride tube for long periods of time	Reposition tube daily, change tape; use smaller-bore tube; position tube to avoid pressure on tissues; moisten mouth and nose several times daily
Tube obstruction	Poorly crushed medications	Crush medications thoroughly, dissolve in water; use liquid medications whenever possible; check compatibility of medication with tube and formula
	Inadequate flushing after medications or thick formula	Flush tube with 50–150 mL water after medications or thick formula and every 4–6 hr with 20 mL minimum
	Poorly dissolved or mixed formula	Use blender to mix powdered formula (check manufacturer's mixing guidelines); use ready-to-use formula
	Formula mixed with low pH substance	Avoid checking gastric residuals when safe to do so; use larger-diameter tubes when checking residuals; avoid administering acidic medications through small-diameter tubes; consider a nonacidic therapeutic alternative; flush with a minimum of 30 mL water before and immediately after medication administration
Metabolic Complications		
Hyperglycemia, glycosuria (can lead to dehydration, coma, or death)	Stress response; diabetes mellitus	Monitor fingerstick glucose every 6 hr, use sliding scale insulin plus appropriate routine insulin (e.g., insulin drip in critically ill)
	High-carbohydrate formula	Change formula
	Drug therapy (steroids)	Monitor intake and output accurately
Excess CO_2 production (high RQ)	High percentage of carbohydrate calories or excess calories from any source	Reduce total calories to avoid overfeeding; consider formula with higher fat calories
Hyponatremia	Dilutional (fluid excess, SIADH); inadequate sodium intake; excess GI losses	Use full-strength formula or change to 1.5–2 kcal/mL formula; add salt to tube feeding (1 tsp = 2 g Na = 90 mEq); use diuretics if appropriate; replace GI losses
Hypernatremia	Inadequate free water intake	Use 1 kcal/mL formula; monitor intake and output accurately; temperature and weight daily; increase flush volume
	Excess water losses (diabetes insipidus; osmotic diuresis from hyperglycemia; fever)	Correct hyperglycemia and the cause of fever or diabetes insipidus
Hypokalemia	Medications (diuretics, antipseudomonal penicillins, amphotericin B)	Monitor serum potassium; give PO or IV potassium replacement PRN
	Intracellular or extracellular shifts (insulin therapy, acidosis)	Correct underlying problem
	Excess GI losses (NG suction, small bowel fistula, diarrhea)	Routinely provide potassium in replacement fluid
Hyperkalemia	Potassium-sparing medications (triamterene, amiloride, spironolactone, ACE inhibitors); potassium-containing medications (penicillin G potassium)	Monitor serum potassium; change to medications without potassium-sparing effect or without potassium salts
	Renal failure	Monitor renal function; change to formula with lower potassium content
Hypercoagulability	Warfarin antagonism due to formula	Use lower vitamin K formula; hold formula 1–2 hr before and after warfarin dose; monitor coagulation status

ACE, angiotensin-converting enzyme; GI, gastrointestinal; ICU, intensive care unit; IV, intravenous; NG, nasogastric; PO, oral; PRN, as needed/ RQ, respiratory quotient; SIADH, syndrome of inappropriate antidiuretic hormone secretion.

enteral formula volume can have significant effects on weight. For example, a weight loss of 12.5 pounds over a year can be expected if the daily intake of a 1-kcal/mL formula is 120 mL less than required.

Fluid status must be monitored closely with EN therapy, especially in patients with unusual losses, an inability to recognize thirst, or voluntarily adjust their oral fluid intake. Enteral formula contains solutes, as well as water. Only free water in the formula contributes toward meeting fluid requirements. Standard caloric density formulas are approximately 80% to 85% free water and 65% to 80% is typical for calorically dense formulas. Manufacturers generally list the free water content of formulas in product labeling.

Water used to irrigate, or flush, the feeding tube can contribute a significant volume of fluid daily. Protocols for flushing feeding tubes have not been well studied, but it generally is agreed that the tube should be flushed before and after each intermittent administration of formula or medication and after each GRV evaluation. Tube patency is maintained by flushing the tube every 4 to 6 hours for continuous feedings.[97,99,103,104] Each flush is generally 20 to 60 mL of water. For patients with signs of fluid overload, a flush volume of 20 to 30 mL can be used and the number of flushes should be kept to a minimum. Patients requiring more daily fluid may benefit from increased flush volume, number of flushes, or both.

MEDICATIONS AND ENTERAL NUTRITION BY TUBE

Patients receiving EN often receive medications through the same tube. Feeding tube occlusion, adverse effects caused by changes in pharmaceutical dosage forms, and alteration of medication pharmacokinetics and pharmacodynamics are among the potential problems. Interactions related to pharmacologic or physiologic effects of medications or enteral nutrients also may occur. For this reason, oral medication administration should be considered unless a strict "nothing by mouth" status is required.

The incidence of feeding tube occlusion is 1.6% to 66%.[7,103,112] Pump malfunction, lack of periodic tube flushing, formula characteristics, and tube characteristics are non–medication-related factors affecting tube occlusion. Important tube characteristics include the inner diameter (bore size), tube material, and the arrangement and number of delivery holes (ports) at the distal end. The most important formula characteristic appears to be the protein source. In vitro studies suggest formulas with intact protein, particularly caseinates or soy, coagulate and clump when exposed to an acidic pH, whereas formulas with hydrolyzed protein do not.[31,113]

Medication-related factors influencing feeding tube occlusion include the administration method, dosage form, pH, and viscosity. Medications admixed with formula have the greatest potential for occluding tubes owing to alteration of the texture, viscosity, or physical form of the medication or formula. Therefore, medications rarely should be admixed directly with formula. Stopping the enteral formula infusion, flushing the tube with a minimum of 10 to 20 mL water before and after medication administration and a minimum of 5 mL between each medication, limit the contact between medications and formula within the tube lumen and decrease the risk of occlusion.[97,104,113]

Restoring Feeding Tube Patency

When a feeding tube occludes, it must be replaced unless patency can be restored. Frequent tube replacement disrupts nutrient delivery and increases patient discomfort as well as the cost of care.

The initial treatment for tube occlusion is to flush the tube with warm water using a large syringe, at least 20 mL but preferably 50 mL, to avoid generation of excessive pressure that could rupture the tube. When a specific cause for occlusion can be identified (e.g., a specific medication) and physiochemical characteristics of the responsible product are known (e.g., solubility, pH), it may be possible to select a more appropriate flush preparation than water. In most cases, however, use of an acidic or basic flush preparation could worsen the occlusion. Acidic liquids (e.g., cranberry juice, diet soda, regular soda) may perpetuate or extend the occlusion, especially when coagulated proteins are the cause.[36,103,113,114] When water fails to restore patency, activated pancreatic enzymes prepared with one crushed Viokase tablet and one sodium bicarbonate tablet (324 mg) dissolved in 5 mL of warm water just before instillation may be useful.[97,113] Alternatively, a commercial product containing multiple enzymes, buffers, and antibacterial agents in a powder form (Clog Zapper, Corpak Medical Systems, Wheeling, IL) can be used.

Medication Selection

Solid dosage forms are the greatest challenge to administer by feeding tube. Whenever possible, liquid dosage forms should be selected, but these are not without problems. Liquids, especially those with a high viscosity, should be diluted before administration to avoid coating the tube interior. Pharmaceutical syrups with a pH of 4 or less must be used with caution because immediate clumping and tackiness of formulas mixed with the syrups have been reported.[113,114]

For medications not available in liquid form, a therapeutically equivalent medication in a liquid form can be considered. Extemporaneous preparation of a liquid also may be considered but can increase cost significantly. Simple compressed tablets can be crushed, then dissolved or suspended in 10 to 30 mL of water before administration through the tube. Medications in a soft gelatin capsule are best delivered by dissolving the capsule in warm water. Undissolved gelatin should not be administered, because this may occlude the tube. Powder in hard gelatin capsules can be poured into water and mixed thoroughly before administration. Failure to dissolve any of these dosage forms thoroughly in water before administration through the tube can result in occlusion. Omeprazole, potassium chloride, phenytoin, multivitamins, lansoprazole, protein supplements, sucralfate, pentoxifylline, zinc salts, calcium salts, and iron salts were identified by nurses as the products most frequently contributing to feeding tube occlusion.[110,112]

Crushing a medication and mixing the powder in water results in an altered pharmaceutical dosage form, and this may affect its efficacy or patient tolerance. The safety and efficacy of simple compressed tablets are not affected by crushing and dissolving in water immediately before use. Crushing a sustained release product, however, destroys slow release mechanisms, resulting in the immediate release of several hours worth of the medication at one time. An exaggerated therapeutic response may be seen initially, followed by a loss of response part way through the dosing interval. Therefore, sustained-release or long-acting dosage forms should not be crushed.[115] Instead, an immediate-release dosage form can be used with appropriate adjustment of dose and dosing interval, or an alternate administration routes (e.g., morphine suppositories rather than slow-release tablets).

Enteric-coated tablets are designed to release medication in the small bowel because the medication is either acid labile or irritates the stomach. Protection for the medication or stomach is lost when enteric-coated tablets are crushed and delivered via feeding tube into the stomach, resulting in decreased efficacy of the medication or increased gastric irritation. When an irritating medication must be given by tube into the stomach, diluting the medication in at least 60 mL of water is recommended.[113] Administering buccal or sublingual dosage forms via feeding tube may result in altered absorption or destruction of the medication by stomach acid. Therefore, therapeutically equivalent medications (e.g., isosorbide dinitrate rather than sublingual nitroglycerin) or an alternate route of administration (e.g., nitroglycerin ointment or transdermal system rather than sublingual nitroglycerin) should be used.

Pharmacokinetic parameters can be altered when medications are administered by feeding tube. The medication delivery site can affect bioavailability, although few studies address this issue. Medications taken orally are delivered to the stomach, where dissolution occurs for most dosage forms and hydrolysis of some medications may occur. Delivery into the small bowel may alter these processes, thereby affecting bioavailability. For instance, recovery of digoxin from intrajejunal dosing is higher than with oral administration, primarily because of reduced intragastric hydrolysis.[31,113] Bioavailability of medications also can be affected by the presence of enteral formula in the GI tract. Medications affected by the presence of food are expected to be affected in a similar manner by the presence of formula. For example, administration of tetracycline with formula present is expected to reduce tetracycline bioavailability because of interactions with divalent cations. A similar interaction is expected between ciprofloxacin and enteral formula, although some evidence suggests a mechanism other than binding with divalent cations is responsible for reduced ciprofloxacin concentrations with enteral feeding.[31]

Phenytoin is particularly troublesome to manage in patients receiving EN, with reduced phenytoin concentrations reported in numerous case reports and small studies. Methods suggested for management include using a meat-based formula, administering phenytoin capsules rather than the suspension, and stopping formula delivery for 1 to 2 hours before and after the phenytoin dose.[113,116] Holding formula administration before and after phenytoin dosing is usually recommended. None of these methods, however, clearly prevents low phenytoin concentrations; thus, monitoring of serum concentrations is important whenever EN is started or altered. Large-scale, controlled trials are needed to determine the most appropriate method for managing the phenytoin–EN interaction.

Reversal of warfarin anticoagulation by the vitamin K included in enteral formulas is an important pharmacologic interaction.[31] The vitamin K content of most enteral formulas today is unlikely to interfere with anticoagulation, but should be evaluated if adequate anticoagulation is difficult to achieve. In addition, binding of warfarin to a component of enteral formulas, likely protein, has been proposed to explain warfarin resistance with formulas containing low vitamin K content.[31] Stopping formula administration for an hour before and after warfarin administration appears to prevent this type of interaction.

Diarrhea is a potential problem related to physiologic effects of hypertonic medications. Diluting hypertonic medications (e.g., potassium chloride) with 30 to 60 mL of water before administration is suggested. Dividing the medication dose and separating doses by about 2 hours also decrease GI effects of hypertonic medications. In addition, selection of brands and dosage forms with minimal sorbitol can reduce the risk of diarrhea. Cumulative sorbitol doses >5 g can cause bloating and flatulence, whereas larger doses may act as a cathartic.[113]

PATIENT ASSESSMENT

Evaluation of Nutrition Status

1. J.K., an 81-year-old man, was hospitalized 6 days ago after collapsing at the golf course. Physical examination on admission revealed left-sided paralysis and overall muscle weakness. He was confused and disoriented, and his mucous membranes were dry. J.K. was diagnosed with mild dehydration and was thought to have had a cerebrovascular accident (CVA). His condition has changed little since admission. J.K. is estimated to be 5 ft 9 in tall; his admission weight by bed scale was 132 lb (60 kg). His maintenance IV is 5% dextrose/0.45% sodium chloride with KCl 20 mEq/L at 100 mL/hour. Laboratory evaluation today shows a serum albumin of 3.1 g/dL, down from 3.8 on admission. Other biochemical data are within normal limits: glucose, 89 mg/dL (normal, 70–110); creatinine, 0.8 mg/dL (normal, 0.6–1.2); Na, 140 mEq/L (normal, 135–145); K, 4.4 mEq/L (normal, 3.5–5.5); and Cl, 104 mEq/L (normal, 95–105). Assess J.K.'s nutrition status. Identify factors placing him nutritionally at risk. Is nutrition support indicated at this time?

J.K. has mild malnutrition based on his weight for height and serum albumin concentration. Low serum albumin in the elderly is a risk factor for malnutrition, sarcopenia, and mortality.[117,118] He is at risk for developing more severe malnutrition during hospitalization, and possibly death. Serum albumin at the time of admission was falsely elevated because of dehydration; therefore, today's albumin should be used to evaluate his visceral protein status. Mild visceral protein depletion may have resulted from metabolic stress associated with his CVA. Weight loss to 85% of ideal body weight (IBW, 70.7 kg) most likely is owing to chronic deficiency in total energy intake but may also be associated with significant loss of lean mass, especially in older men.[119]

At 85% of IBW, J.K. should appear underweight. If not, the estimated height may be wrong. The weight of 60 kg was obtained at admission and is expected to be falsely low (by a few kilograms at most) because of J.K.'s dehydration. Records of clinic visits and hospitalizations may provide information on chronic or recent illnesses that may be contributing to his weight loss.

Socioeconomic factors contributing to nutrition risk also should be considered.[120] Low income is associated with food insecurity and inadequate nutrition. Social conditions also may influence nutrition. A nursing note states, per his friend, that they were playing golf like they usually do two to three times weekly since J.K.'s wife died a few months ago. He says J.K. spends too much time alone staring out his window at the golf course rather than getting out to play. This indicates J.K. lives alone but also suggests he is probably not low income.

J.K. most likely has been without oral intake since admission because he is unable to feed himself; he is expected to have difficulty chewing and swallowing as a result of the CVA. The low amount of dextrose in his maintenance IV is inadequate to minimize protein breakdown for gluconeogenesis. Patients with inadequate intake for 5 to 7 days or those who are not expected to have adequate intake for 5 to 7 days are considered candidates for specialized nutrition support.[1] Malnourished patients should be considered for nutrition support sooner. Because J.K. has mild malnutrition and is not likely to take adequate nutrients by mouth within the next few days, specialized nutrition support is indicated.

Estimation of Nutrition Requirements

2. What are J.K.'s requirements for calories, protein, and fluid? Does he have any special nutrient requirements?

Because J.K. is below IBW for height, his actual weight should be used to estimate energy and protein requirements. It would be best to use a weight after J.K. was rehydrated. His chart indicates a weight of 62 kg the past 3 days, which will be used for calculations. Use of IBW to estimate requirements for malnourished patients may result in fluid and electrolyte imbalance. Once the patient is stabilized on nutrition support, calories can be increased, if necessary, to achieve weight gain.

J.K.'s level of metabolic stress is relatively low. He has no surgical wounds, no fractures or skeletal trauma, no burns, and no major infections. Therefore, caloric requirements are only slightly higher than basal needs. Although the term *calorie* is used interchangeably with kilocalorie (kcal) in nutrition literature, the large "Calorie" or kilocalorie technically is correct and energy requirements generally are listed as kcal/day or kcal/kg body weight when specific numbers are given for a patient. Requirements can be estimated using predictive equations such as Harris-Benedict or one of the many other equations.[2,36] Indirect calorimetry (metabolic cart measurements) is an expensive procedure and probably is unnecessary in a mildly stressed patient. Metabolic cart measurements determine energy (or "metabolic") requirements from oxygen consumption and carbon dioxide production. They account for individual variations in energy expenditure not adequately accounted for by predictive equations or by the kcal/kg method of determining energy requirements, especially in highly complex patients. An estimation of 20 to 25 kcal/kg actual weight also can be used based on J.K.'s low level of metabolic stress but higher caloric intake may be needed for weight gain after he is stable. Protein requirements for healthy elderly people are estimated to be to be 1 g/kg/day, which is slightly higher than the DRI of 0.8 g/kg/day.[120]

Mild visceral protein depletion and metabolic stress are expected to increase J.K.'s protein needs to at least 1 to 1.2 g/kg actual weight per day. Renal function appears adequate for J.K. to tolerate up to 1.2 g/kg/day without developing azotemia. SrCr, however, may provide a poor estimate of renal function in underweight patients owing to below-normal muscle mass. Daily fluid requirements for geriatric patients can be estimated at 30 to 35 mL/kg, with a minimum of 1,500 mL daily, plus replacement of excess losses from hyperthermia, vomiting, or diarrhea.[1,120] Baseline requirements of 1,500 mL for the first 20 kg plus 20 mL per each additional kilogram of body weight also can be used to estimate fluid requirements. Based on caloric intake, fluid requirements can be estimated as 1 mL/kcal ingested.[1] J.K. does not appear to have any excess fluid losses at this time; therefore, calculation of baseline fluid requirements should provide adequate fluids.

J.K.'s estimated daily requirements are approximately 1,240 to 1,550 total calories, 62 to 74 g protein, and 1,860 to 2,168 mL of fluid. These are estimated requirements that should be adjusted based on frequent reassessment of J.K.'s response to therapy and changes in his clinical situation. Additional calories and protein may be needed for repletion of weight and protein status.

J.K.'s apparently suboptimal nutrition before hospitalization increases his risk for vitamin deficiencies. Vitamins of particular concern are antioxidants (i.e., vitamin C and beta carotene) and those that influence plasma concentrations of homocysteine (i.e., vitamin B_{12}, folic acid, and pyridoxine). Vitamins A and D also are of concern since free-living, generally healthy elderly have deficient intake of these vitamins.[120] No medical, medication, or dietary histories are available to determine nutritional risks associated with specific conditions. Factors that predispose patients to vitamin deficiencies include weight loss of >5% of usual body weight in 1 month or >10% of usual body weight in 6 months, prolonged periods of dietary restriction, high levels of physiologic stress as occurs with trauma and large areas of burn, significant alterations in biochemical tests such as serum glucose and albumin, abnormal or protracted body fluid losses, administration of medications that alter vitamin absorption or metabolism, and diagnoses associated with alteration in vitamin absorption or requirements. J.K.'s age, along with his acute illness and mild mixed protein-calorie malnutrition, increase his risk of vitamin deficiencies, and it is likely that he has at least some subclinical deficiencies. J.K. should receive 100% up to 200% of the DRI for vitamins and minerals daily. A daily multivitamin preparation providing 100% of the DRI should be considered in addition to an oral diet or EN. If actual deficiencies are identified, J.K. will require higher, therapeutic doses of the specific vitamins that are deficient.

Enteral Nutrition Route

3. The health care team decides to initiate specialized nutrition support via tube feeding. What route for tube feeding is most appropriate for J.K.?

It is likely J.K. has problems with chewing and swallowing, in addition to difficulty getting food to his mouth. Otherwise, J.K.'s GI tract is expected to be functional. Nothing indicates that J.K. has risks associated with aspiration. Some patients have a poor gag reflex after a CVA, but J.K. has no reported coughing or choking. The duration of tube feeding is uncertain because J.K. may improve with time. An NG tube is the least invasive feeding route at this time. Measures to prevent J.K. from pulling the feeding tube may be necessary.

Enteral Formula Selection

4. What type of enteral formula is most appropriate for J.K.?

J.K. has full digestive capability; therefore, a polymeric formula is most appropriate. Standard caloric density (1–1.2 kcal/mL) should be used because J.K. has no fluid restriction and no evidence of fluid overload. A high-nitrogen formula will provide protein at the upper end of the estimated requirement (1.2 g/kg/day), whereas a standard nitrogen formula will provide between 0.8 and 1 g/kg/day. A high-nitrogen formula may replete J.K.'s visceral protein status sooner but it may not provide adequate calories for weight gain. The decision to use a high- versus standard-nitrogen formula depends on the exact nutrient composition of available formulas.

Fiber can be included in the formula if desired. The benefits of fiber for short-term feeding are not clearly defined, so a fiber-free formula is an equally appropriate selection at this time. If a fiber-containing formula is selected initially, the formula should contain a low to moderate fiber content or be started at a low rate and advanced slowly to minimize gas and abdominal distention.

Fluid Provision

5. How much fluid is necessary to meet J.K.'s estimated daily fluid requirements?

The free water content of EN must be calculated to determine the volume of additional fluid that must be provided to J.K. Formulas with 1 to 1.2 kcal/mL generally contain 80% to 85% free water. Assuming a goal volume of 1,440 mL/day (six cans) of a 1 kcal/mL, 0.044 g protein/mL formula, approximately 1,150 to 1,225 mL of free water is provided daily. Using 30 mL/kg/day as J.K.'s fluid requirement, he will need 1,860 mL daily. Therefore, the volume of fluid needed in addition to the enteral formula is 635 to 710 mL/day, which can be provided with medications and tube irrigation (flushes). The feeding tube should be irrigated with a minimum of 20 mL of fluid every 4 to 6 hours, as well as before and after administration of each medication through the tube.[97,99,103,104] Using five flushes daily with 125 mL of water each will provide 625 mL of fluid.

Selection of a 2 kcal/mL, 0.075 g protein/mL formula for J.K. would require approximately 720 mL (three cans) of formula daily to meet his caloric and protein requirements. Formulas with 2 kcal/mL contain approximately 65% to 80% free water, meaning J.K. would receive about 470 to 575 mL of free water from the formula and still need an additional 1,285 to 1,390 mL of fluid daily. Large flushes of water would be necessary. Diluting the formula to half-strength is not recommended because this increases the risk of error and contamination. Thus, a 1 kcal/mL formula is more appropriate for J.K. than a 2 kcal/mL product.

Enteral Nutrition Administration

6. Recommend a plan for initiating and advancing J.K.'s tube feeding.

J.K. receives gastric feeds; therefore, continuous infusion, intermittent infusion, or bolus feedings can be used. Continuous infusion most commonly is used for hospitalized patients despite no clearly established difference in tolerance compared with intermittent infusion.

Full-strength formula should be used to initiate feedings. J.K. is assumed to have full digestive capacity and is being fed into the stomach; therefore, diluting the formula is not expected to improve tolerance to either an isotonic or hypertonic formula. Dilution or starting the feedings at a very low rate also is likely to delay reaching J.K.'s nutrition goals. The standard of practice in most institutions for patients without GI disease who are not critically ill is to start continuous infusion polymeric feedings at 40 to 50 mL/hour and advance by 20 to 25 mL/hour every 4 to 8 hour, as tolerated, until the goal rate is achieved.

The goal volume of enteral nutrition for J.K. is 1,440 mL/day of a 1 kcal/mL formula, or 60 mL/hour continuous infusion. The infusion can be started at 40 mL/hour for 4 to 6 hours, then increased to 60 mL/hour. If J.K. experiences diarrhea, abdominal distention, or a large GRV, the feeding may be held at the initial rate for 24 hours, then increased only 10 to 15 mL/hour every 12 to 24 hour as tolerated. If the formula is not advanced to goal rate within 24 hours of initiating feedings, extra care must be taken to ensure he receives an adequate fluid intake.

Continuous infusion enteral feeding can be administered by gravity drip or by enteral pump. With gravity drip, the infusion rate must be adjusted frequently to maintain a consistent flow rate and the formula flow must be checked regularly to ensure that the flow has not stopped because of kinked administration tubing or an empty delivery container. Gravity infusion has no alarms to alert nurses to these problems. Enteral pumps provide a consistent flow rate and alarms to alert nurses if there are problems with the infusion, but they are more expensive than gravity drip. Pumps often are used for hospitalized patients to help maintain delivery of the prescribed volume of enteral formula. Either gravity drip or an enteral pump could be used for J.K., depending on the hospital's protocol for enteral feeding. To prevent inadvertent IV infusion of enteral formula when an enteral pump is used, the connector at the distal (patient) end of the delivery set should not be compatible with IV devices.[83]

Monitoring Enteral Nutrition Support

7. Recommend a plan for monitoring J.K.'s response to enteral nutrition, including clinical and biochemical parameters.

Monitoring patients on enteral nutrition is necessary to prevent complications and to assess appropriateness of therapy. Clinical parameters to monitor include tube placement, GRV, GI symptoms, respiratory status, vital signs, and weight. Tube placement should be evaluated every 4 to 6 hours, by auscultation, location of markings on the tube, and GRV. A tube displaced into the esophagus or pharynx could result in pulmonary aspiration of the formula.

High GRV has been assumed to increase the risk of esophageal reflux and pulmonary aspiration. No consensus exists, however, on the frequency for GRV assessment or the volume at which feedings should be held. GRV is typically checked every 4 to 8 hours, although this practice has been questioned because it may contribute to feeding tube occlusion.[103] The incidence of tube occlusion was reduced from 66% to 7.6% when one institution eliminated GRV evaluation in their EN protocol.[7] Few data are available from prospective, randomized, controlled trials to define an appropriate GRV at which to hold EN, or even to demonstrate a correlation between GRV and gastroesophageal reflux or aspiration.[18,98,104,108,111] Endogenous secretions from saliva and gastric fluids are about 4,500 mL/day in normal adults receiving food.[98] This represents about 185 mL/hour crossing the pyloric sphincter and food or formula increases the volume. Continuing EN with a GRV <500 mL has been recommended, along with careful bedside assessment and a systematic approach to managing a GRV of 200 to 500 mL.[18,108] Other authors suggest acceptance of GRV up to 250 or 300 mL.[32,98] Nonetheless, many institutions hold feedings if the GRV is >200 mL, which may compromise nutrient delivery. In general, a GRV of 200 to 500 mL should prompt clinical assessment of EN tolerance and feedings should continue unless volumes are persistently high, a trend of a rising GRV is evident, or other evidence of feeding intolerance is present. Setting the residual volume too low can result in inadequate nutrition because feedings are stopped frequently. Residuals should be checked every 4 to 8 hours as long as no residual is above the volume for holding feeding. If the feeding is held because of a high GRV, hourly evaluation of the GRV is recommended until the volume is <200 to 250 mL and the feeding is restarted. The fluid withdrawn for GRV assessment should be infused through the tube back into the stomach to avoid electrolyte imbalances.

Assessment of GI symptoms is important for determining EN tolerance. Abdominal distention and bloating should be evaluated at least every 8 hours while J.K. is hospitalized. Small-bore feeding tubes may collapse during withdrawal of the gastric residual, resulting in a falsely low residual volume. Abdominal distention may be an indication of accumulating formula. Gas formation secondary to lactose intolerance or rapid increases in fiber intake, and poor gastric emptying secondary to a high-fat formula, medications, recent surgery, critical illness, or an underlying disease such as diabetes are among the conditions associated with distention. When considerable distention is present, the formula should be held temporarily, and the patient evaluated further to rule out a contraindication to EN. Gastric outlet obstruction, complete or partial small bowel obstruction, or severe ileus preclude restarting EN until the condition resolves. If no contraindication to EN is found, feeding can be restarted, preferably with the feeding tube placed into the small bowel, a formula with lower fat or fiber content, or medications to promote gastric emptying (e.g., metoclopramide or erythromycin). Feeding should be restarted at a rate of 25 to 40 mL/hour, and J.K. should be observed closely for signs of feeding intolerance. The head of the bed should be elevated 30 to 45 degrees during feeding.[32,104]

Nausea, vomiting, abdominal cramping, diarrhea, and constipation are other GI symptoms monitored as indicators of EN tolerance. Vomiting creates the most immediate concern because tube displacement and pulmonary aspiration can occur. Nausea and vomiting commonly occur with a high GRV, severe gastric distention, poor gastric emptying during gastric feeding, GI tract obstruction, or poor GI motility. Lactose intolerance and bolus feeding into the jejunum can lead to diarrhea and abdominal cramping, as well as nausea and vomiting. Initiation of EN with a hypertonic formula, a rapid rate of infusion or a large volume, and use of formula at refrigerator temperature are other factors often cited as causing GI symptoms. Although controlled studies have not supported these factors as significant contributors to GI intolerance, subjective evidence suggests they are important. Constipation is most likely to occur with long-term tube feeding in nonambulatory patients. Inadequate fluid intake and lack of fiber may be factors associated with constipation.

Respiratory status should be evaluated every 8 hours in hospitalized patients, to help recognize pulmonary aspiration and pulmonary edema. A stethoscope should be used for assessment at least two times per week, but simple observation of the patient's breathing pattern is adequate at other times unless altered respirations are noted. Coughing or respiratory distress may be indications of aspiration or other developing respiratory problems. Vital signs also may provide clues to aspiration or other problems, such as dehydration, fluid overload, or infection.

Weight and fluid input and output should be monitored daily in hospitalized patients. Day-to-day changes in weight reflect fluid status. Increasing weight for 3 or 4 consecutive days may be an indication fluid intake needs to be reduced, whereas decreasing weight may indicate a need for increased fluid. Generally, total fluid can be adjusted by the number of times the feeding tube is flushed daily and the volume of each flush. Caloric density of the formula can be changed when altering the number or volume of flushes is not adequate for fluid control. For patients with a stable fluid status, the week-to-week weight change can be used as an indicator of appropriate caloric intake. An upward trend in weight (e.g., ≥3 consecutive weeks with an increase) may indicate a need for fewer calories unless weight gain is a goal. A downward trend may indicate a need to increase caloric intake, unless weight loss is desired.

Regular monitoring of biochemical parameters is important for identifying metabolic abnormalities before they become critical problems. Serum glucose, sodium, potassium, chloride, and bicarbonate should be determined daily in J.K. for 4 to 5 days after feeding starts. Monitoring can then be decreased to once or twice weekly if J.K. has no evidence of tube feeding intolerance or metabolic abnormalities. Fingerstick glucose measurements should be ordered every 6 hours after tube feeding starts; then, based on the results, a decision can be made whether fingersticks are needed routinely. Because J.K. has a normal serum glucose (89 mg/dL) while receiving 5% dextrose in his IV fluid and is not highly stressed, hyperglycemia is not a major concern with EN.

During the first week of EN, SrCr, BUN, calcium, phosphorus, and magnesium should be monitored a minimum of three times. Daily monitoring of SrCr and BUN for a few days may even be considered in J.K. because of his recent dehydration. Daily phosphorus and magnesium also may be considered for a few days in J.K. because of his low body weight. Chronic malnutrition can lead to intracellular depletion of potassium, phosphorus, and magnesium, while serum concentrations are maintained. When specialized nutrition support begins, refeeding syndrome may develop as these electrolytes move from the extracellular space into the cells, causing a decrease in serum concentrations over the first few days of feeding.[101,102] Failure to monitor the patient and replace electrolytes as necessary can result in serious electrolyte abnormalities. If SrCr, BUN, phosphorus, and magnesium are stable after the first 4 or 5 days, the frequency of monitoring could be reduced to once or twice weekly.

Biochemical parameters used to assess response to protein provision should be monitored. For example, prealbumin (i.e., transthyretin) and transferrin are short-term indicators of visceral protein response to nutrition support and can be monitored every 3 to 4 days (transthyretin) or weekly (transferrin). Because of J.K.'s age, transferrin would not be an appropriate parameter to use, because transferrin levels are significantly reduced in the elderly as a result of increased tissue iron stores.[120] Albumin is a long-term indicator that requires 2 to 3 weeks to reflect a response to nutrition therapy; however, it may be included on a weekly monitoring schedule to allow adjustment of serum calcium for hypoalbuminemia. Nitrogen balance can be used as an alternative to prealbumin, but it requires an accurate 12- to 24-hour urine collection to be useful.

Electrolyte Abnormalities

8. J.K. has been receiving EN for 4 days. Feeding was started at 40 mL/hour for 8 hours, then increased to 60 mL/hour (goal rate). The IV fluids were stopped when the tube feeding reached the goal rate. Laboratory evaluation today shows the following: K, 2.9 mEq/L (decreased from 3.5 mEq/L yesterday, 3.9 mEq/L the previous day, and 4.6 mEq/L when tube feeding started); Cl, 95 mEq/L (normal, 95–105); calcium, 7.9 mg/dL (normal, 9–11); Mg, 2.4 mEq/L (normal, 2.5–3.5), decreased from 3.5 mEq/L 2 days ago; phosphorus, 3.5 mg/dL (normal, 3.5–4.5), decreased from 4.4 mg/dL 2 days ago; and albumin, 2.6 g/dL. Micro-K (8 mEq KCl/capsule) has been ordered as six capsules via feeding tube and calcium carbonate (260 mg elemental calcium/tablet) as two tablets twice daily (BID) via feeding tube. Is the electrolyte replacement appropriate as ordered? What changes, if any, should be considered?

Calcium carbonate, a simple compressed tablet, can be crushed, suspended in 10 to 30 mL of water, and administered through the feeding tube. Calcium salts, however, have been identified by nurses as among the products most frequently contributing to feeding tube occlusion.[110] Risk of tube occlusion from an inadequately crushed tablet may be decreased by use of calcium carbonate suspension (500 mg Ca/5 mL), if available. Administration of either crushed and suspended tablets or commercial suspension requires flushing the tube with at least 10 to 20 mL of water before and after medication administration.[97,104,113] Diluting the suspension 1:1 with water and flushing with 75 to 100 mL may be advisable because suspensions may otherwise coat the tube. The appropriateness of calcium supplementation should be questioned, however, because J.K.'s serum calcium concentration is within normal limits after correction for his low serum albumin concentration. Administering any medication via the feeding tube may occlude the tube. The oral route should be used for medications whenever appropriate. Many patients receiving EN are allowed some oral intake, and oral medications are frequently acceptable. J.K.'s risk for aspiration may be too high at this time to allow oral medications, however. Alternative dosage forms for electrolytes are limited to IV forms so the easiest and most cost effective route is via feeding tube if J.K. cannot take oral medications.

Potassium is below normal today and has been decreasing since tube feeding began. Potassium supplementation should have been considered yesterday, rather than waiting until hypokalemia developed because a definite trend downward in serum potassium was evident. The selected potassium supplement is inappropriate for administration by tube because Micro-K is a slow-release product. Crushing slow-release products destroys the slow-release mechanism. Potassium chloride powder for solution (three packets with 15 mEq KCl/packet) or liquid (10% KCl 35 mL, 15% KCl 25 mL, or 20% KCl 15–20 mL) should be ordered rather than the slow-release product. Dividing the potassium dose into two or three smaller doses and diluting each dose with 60 mL of water is recommended. Giving 45 to 50 mEq of potassium as a single dose may cause nausea, vomiting, abdominal discomfort, or diarrhea. These symptoms might be mistaken as intolerance to EN, resulting in the tube feeding being stopped temporarily. The larger fluid volume for administration also may help reduce the gastric irritation associated with potassium doses.

Consideration also should be given to changes occurring in other electrolytes. J.K. appears to be developing mild refeeding syndrome.[101,102] Magnesium and phosphorus are slightly below the normal range and have decreased significantly over the past 2 days. Supplements should be started today so that smaller daily quantities can be used before electrolytes are critically low. This may decrease the risk of diarrhea and GI upset caused by the administration of magnesium or phosphate. Magnesium supplementation could be accomplished with a magnesium oxide tablet (400 or 500 mg) administered two to four times daily. These are simple compressed tablets that can be crushed and suspended for administration via feeding tube. An alternative would be magnesium hydroxide suspension 5 mL two to four times daily. Magnesium doses are distributed through the day to avoid the cathartic action.

Phosphate supplementation could be accomplished by changing part of the potassium ordered to Neutra-Phos-K, which provides 8.1 mmol of phosphate and 14.2 mEq of potassium per 250 mg capsule. Contents of each capsule are designed to be dissolved in 75 mL of water for administration, so dissolution is not a concern. One Neutra-Phos-K twice a day plus KCl liquid to provide 20 mEq potassium is the same potassium dose as is ordered currently. The liquid KCl should be given at least 2 hours before or after the Neutra-Phos-K to minimize GI effects. The feeding tube must be flushed adequately before and after each dose of electrolyte replacement. The flush volume should be a minimum of 10 to 20 mL, although 75 to 100 mL following the magnesium dose may be better to ensure the electrolyte preparation is out of the tube. Intermittent tube flushes can be accomplished with medication administration to limit the total fluid intake to the estimated requirement of 1,860 to 2,168 mL, or 635 to 710 mL in addition to that provided by a 1 kcal/mL formula.

With the current electrolyte abnormalities, it is important to monitor potassium, magnesium, and phosphorus for the next several days. The extent of electrolyte depletion in the body is difficult to evaluate, but 1 day of electrolyte replacement is not expected to replete intracellular stores. It is difficult to provide large quantities of potassium, phosphate, and magnesium via feeding tube secondary to the GI intolerance they cause.

Therefore, IV electrolyte replacement may be necessary if intracellular depletion is extensive.

Transfer to a Nursing Facility

9. J.K. has received EN for 10 days. During this time he removed his feeding tube twice despite mittens to hinder his ability to grab the tube. Feedings were off for approximately 5 to 8 hours each time the tube was removed. J.K.'s electrolyte abnormalities have been corrected with 3 days of electrolyte replacement. He has tolerated his tube feeding without metabolic abnormalities or electrolyte replacement for the past 2 days. J.K. remains confused and disoriented. The prognosis for improvement in J.K.'s ability to feed himself is poor. Plans are made to discharge J.K. in 1 to 2 days to a nursing facility. What changes in the care plan would be appropriate relative to nutrition support goals?

J.K. should be evaluated for gastrostomy placement because he is expected to need EN for a prolonged period. Gastrostomy placement also should solve the problem of repeated tube displacement, although this alone is not an appropriate reason to place a gastrostomy. Placement of a percutaneous gastrostomy can be accomplished with local anesthesia, which may be advantageous given J.K.'s age and lack of another reason for general anesthesia. Percutaneous gastrostomy placement is less expensive and typically requires less time to perform than surgical gastrostomies, but the incidence of major complications remains essentially the same at up to 2.5%.[4,9,12]

If fiber-free formula was selected initially, fiber-containing formula should be considered. Fiber may prevent GI tract changes associated with prolonged use of fiber-free formulas.[24] Constipation is frequently a problem in elderly and bedridden patients. Increased stool weight and frequency has been demonstrated in patients with constipation receiving fiber-containing formula versus fiber-free formula. Starting with a low to moderate fiber content may minimize gas and abdominal distention. To approach the recommended fiber intake of 30 g/day, however, a high-fiber formula is necessary.[22,23] Fiber content can be gradually increased by providing half the daily formula volume as a fiber-free formula and half as a formula containing 15 g fiber/1,000 kcal for a few days, then changing completely to the fiber-containing formula. With 1,440 mL daily, the fiber provided will be slightly below recommended amounts; however, it would be reasonable to assess stooling pattern before adding another fiber source to J.K.'s regimen. Fiber can be problematic for tube occlusion.[24,110] The fiber-free and fiber-containing formulas should not be mixed directly without prior in vitro observation of compatibility. Although the likelihood of incompatibility is low, mixing different formulas together could result in gelling or separation of formula components.

J.K. should transition to an intermittent schedule before discharge. Many nursing facilities do not routinely use enteral pumps because of increased cost. Without a pump, delivery of the prescribed volume of formula at a consistent rate may not be reliable. Transitioning from 60 mL/hour continuous infusion to intermittent delivery of formula can be accomplished by various methods. An overlapping regimen of gradually decreasing the continuous infusion rate and increasing the intermittent volume appears to be economic and efficient.[92] For J.K., change the continuous rate to 40 mL/hour and add four intermittent feedings of 120 mL over 60 minutes every 6 hours initially. If tolerated, decrease continuous infusion to 20 mL/hour and increase intermittent feeding to 240 mL. Finally, stop continuous feeding and increase intermittent feedings to 360 mL, or add a fifth feeding to keep the intermittent volume at 285 to 300 mL. Other methods stop the continuous feedings and progressively infuse larger intermittent volumes, starting with the equivalent volume of 2 to 4 hours of continuous infusion, over shorter time periods, starting with 2- to 3-hour infusions and ending with 20- to 60-minute infusions, with fewer daily infusions. Start with 180 mL over 2 hours for J.K, allowing an hour between each of eight feedings, then decrease infusion time to 60 minutes with 2 hours between feedings. If tolerated, the volume increases to 240 mL over 60 minutes every 4 hours, then to 360 mL every 6 hours. The time between feedings can be decreased further to allow feedings during typical meal hours and the infusion time for each feeding can be decreased down to 20 minutes, if tolerated. Ideally, the transition will be completed before he is discharged to the nursing facility.

The discharge EN prescription should state clearly the desired caloric density, protein content, fiber content per 1,000 kcal and formula volume, or the daily calories, protein, fiber, and fluid to be provided. The brand name may be included, but the nursing facility may not have the same brand of formula. Any special considerations for the feeding schedule also should be communicated (e.g., J.K. does not tolerate feeding after 9 PM; raise the head of the bed to 45 degrees for 3 hours after the last daily feeding to avoid regurgitation).

Twice-weekly monitoring of glucose, creatinine, and electrolytes should be recommended during the first week after discharge. Careful monitoring of fluid status and tolerance to the intermittent delivery schedule also is recommended. J.K. will have been on the new schedule for only a short time before discharge, so a full evaluation of tolerance to the new regimen will not have been completed.

Transfer to Home on Enteral Nutrition

10. J.K.'s overall status has improved during 3 weeks at the nursing facility, and he is now ready for discharge. J.K. has made no progress toward an oral diet; dysphagia and aspiration continue to be severe on "per swallow" studies. He is not to take solids or liquids by mouth at this time, and swallow studies are not to be repeated for 6 months. Intermittent tube feedings with a total of 1,680 mL (seven cans) daily of a 1 kcal/mL, 0.044 g protein/mL, 15 g fiber/1,000 kcal polymeric formula are to continue. His weight has increased 2 kg since hospital discharge. J.K. still needs assistance with some activities of daily living; thus, he will be staying with his sister. She is concerned about insurance coverage for the EN therapy and states J.K. has a Medicare Part D prescription plan. Will Medicare cover EN?

Strict guidelines exist for home EN coverage, Medicare Part B (not Part D) will cover 80% of the cost if criteria are met.[121–123] EN must be medically necessary to "maintain weight and strength commensurate with overall health status" and there must be a functional disability of the GI tract (e.g., dysphagia, swallowing disorder) that is expected to be "permanent."[124] The formula must be delivered by feeding tube (i.e., not oral supplements) and must provide most of the patient's nutritional requirements (i.e., not supplemental

Table 36-7 Medicare Categories for Enteral Formulas

Category	*Description*	*Examples (Partial Listing)*
Category I	Semisynthetic intact protein or protein isolates	Ensure fiber w/FOS, Jevity 1 Cal, Monogen, Osmolite 1 Cal, Osmolite 1.2 Cal *Disease-specific formulas:* Glytrol
Category II	Intact protein or protein isolates; calorically dense	Ensure Plus, Ensure Plus HN, Jevity 1.5 Cal, Nutren 1.5, Nutren 2.0
Category III[a]	Hydrolyzed protein or amino acids	Optimental, Peptamen 1.5, Peptamen AF Documentation that *may* provide justification for use: dumping syndrome, uncontrolled diarrhea, evidence of malabsorption on appropriate semisynthetic formulas (e.g., isotonic, low long-chain fat content, lactose free) that resolves with an oligomeric formula or documentation of the disease process causing malabsorption
Category IV[a]	Defined formula for special metabolic need (i.e., disease-specific formulas)	Advera, Alitraq, Glucena, Glucerna Select, Modulen, NutriHep, NutriRenal, Peptamen, Peptamen VHP, Pulmocare, Renalcal, Replete Documentation that *may* provide justification for use: evidence of inability to meet nutritional goals with category I or II products without compromising patient safety and documentation of the specific diagnosis for which a formula is intended
Category V[a]	Modular components for protein, fat, and carbohydrate	*Protein:* Complete amino acid mix, Propac, Propass, Protifar *Carbohydrate:* Moducal, Polycal, Polycose *Fat:* MCT oil Documentation that *may* provide justification for use: inability to meet specific nutrient requirements (i.e., protein, carbohydrate, or fat) with a commercially available formula

[a]Failure to provide adequate documentation of medical necessity for the specific formula will likely result in denial of claim or payment at the lower category I rate for Medicare Part B insurance coverage.
MCT, medium-chain triglyceride.

nutrition). Approval is on an individual basis, requires a physician's written order, and sufficient documentation must be available to support the need for EN. Calories above or below 20 to 35 kcal/kg/day require additional documentation and 90 days or more meets the test of permanence. J.K.'s therapy falls within these guidelines. In addition, the formula J.K. receives is in a category that does not require him to meet additional eligibility criteria related to the formula itself. Additional documentation would be needed to justify a pump if J.K. was receiving EN via pump.

Enteral formulas are divided into five categories for reimbursement purposes by Medicare Part B (Table 36-7). Formula manufacturers typically list the Medicare category on the product label. Medicare intermediaries may also list formula categories.[125] Most polymeric formulas containing intact (whole) protein and 1 to 1.2 kcal/mL are in category I. These products have the lowest reimbursement rate and do not require documentation of medical necessity for the specific formula itself but still require documentation of the need for EN. Clear documentation of medical need for formulas in specific categories (e.g., category III and IV) is required for their higher reimbursement rates. Appropriate forms available from the Centers for Medicare and Medicaid (CMS) must be completed for Medicare reimbursement of any EN therapy.[126]

Evaluation of Nutrition Status

11. R.L., a 29-year-old woman, was admitted to the hospital 52 days ago following a motor vehicle crash. She sustained multiple rib fractures, pelvic fracture, cardiac contusion, and liver laceration. She required endotracheal intubation shortly after admission and a tracheostomy was placed 2 weeks later when prolonged intubation was expected owing to ARDS. She developed an enterocutaneous fistula about a month after admission and more recently a large perihepatic abscess was noted on a CT scan. During her hospitalization, R.L. has had several exploratory laparotomies and has been treated for multiple infections, including pneumonia, sepsis, and wound infection. She has been treated for *Clostridium difficile* diarrhea but has not had diarrhea since therapy was completed 3 weeks ago. Lysis of adhesions, closure of an enterocutaneous fistula, and placement of a feeding jejunostomy tube (J tube) were done during the last laparotomy 8 days ago.

After admission, EN was considered but ruled out based on high-dose inotropic support and abdominal distension. PN was started on hospital day 3. R.L.'s current PN regimen contains 250 g dextrose, 96 g amino acid, and 50 g fat, with a rate of 85 mL/hour. EN is to start today. R.L. is 5 ft tall and weighs 88 kg. Her weight before surgery 8 days ago was 79 kg and admission weight was 75 kg. The electronic medical record shows her weight at 64.4 kg in a clinic note 3 weeks prior to the accident. Laboratory evaluation today shows the following: Na, 133 mEq/L (normal, 135–145); Cl, 98 mEq/L (normal, 95–105); glucose, 128 mg/dL (normal, 70–110); BUN, 35 mg/dL (normal, 8–20); creatinine, 0.8 mg/dL (normal, 0.6–1.2); triglycerides, 145 mg/dL (normal, <160); C-reactive protein (CRP), 8 mg/dL (normal <0.8); albumin, 2.6 g/dL (normal, 4–6); and the prealbumin, 7 mg/dL (normal, 10–40). One week ago the CRP was 17 mg/dL and prealbumin was 15 mg/dL. A urine collection ending last night shows a volume of 2,500 mL/24-hour collection and a urine urea nitrogen (UUN) of 560 mg/dL. R.L. has been afebrile the past week, but remains on broad-spectrum antibiotics. Assess R.L.'s nutrition status and identify factors that place her at risk nutritionally.

R.L. is obviously at risk owing to her injuries, multiple surgeries, multiple complications, and duration of hospitalization. Currently, she appears to be malnourished based on low visceral protein concentrations. Her weight has increased because of fluid retention. Large urinary nitrogen losses indicate she is highly catabolic. This also is evident from the low serum prealbumin concentration despite a daily intake of 2.1 g protein/kg of IBW. Nutrition status should have been maintained with PN, but visceral protein status has declined during the past week.

R.L. has an increased risk of nutrient deficiencies because of her critical illness, long-term hospitalization, antibiotic therapy, highly catabolic condition, and complications, including a fistula.[1,63,100,127–129] Vitamin and trace element supplementation in PN formulations generally is adequate, but highly catabolic, critically ill patients may have increased requirements for micronutrients with antioxidant properties, including vitamins C and E plus copper, selenium, zinc, and manganese.[1,128] Niacin, thiamine, calcium, and vitamin D are other problematic micronutrients in the critically ill.[128,129] Increased GI losses of zinc occur in patients with diarrhea and GI tract fistulas, both of which were problems for R.L. before the latest laparotomy. It is assumed excess losses of vitamins and trace elements have been managed appropriately in the PN formulation. Thus, R.L. should not have overt deficiencies. Measurement of most vitamin and trace element serum concentrations is difficult in the clinical setting in metabolically unstable patients, and interpretation of values may be equally difficult. Therefore, objective measures of marginal vitamin deficiencies rarely are available. Clinical impressions must be relied on. R.L. should receive 100% to 200% of the DRI for all vitamins and minerals.

Estimation of Nutrition Requirements

12. What are R.L.'s requirements for calories, protein, and fluid?

R.L.'s current weight is significantly above her IBW of 45.5 kg. Some of the "extra" weight most likely is water. The admission weight may not be reliable, because R.L. likely received fluid resuscitation before she was weighed. Her clinic weight is most reliable as an indicator of nutrition status. The appropriate weight, actual or adjusted, for energy calculations in obese patients remains controversial.[130–132] R.L.'s clinic weight should be used as the "dosing" weight if no adjustment is done or to calculate an adjusted weight for dosing. Using an adjusted weight may reduce the risk of overfeeding. An adjustment of 40% of weight over IBW is based on aminoglycoside pharmacokinetics and is commonly used by pharmacists.[131] Using this adjustment, the weight for calculations is 55 kg.

Calories and protein provided by the PN give an indication of R.L.'s requirements. A decline in CRP, especially <10 to 15 mg/dL, should result in a rise of 0.5 to 1 mg/dL/day in prealbumin.[133] Because prealbumin has declined despite a large protein intake and decreasing CRP, the nitrogen (N) balance should be calculated. (N balance = daily N intake from all sources minus N output that includes daily UUN and obligatory losses.) Intake of nitrogen is calculated from grams of protein (g protein/6.25 = g N). The UUN for nitrogen balance is based on total urine urea loss per 24 hours and must be calculated as follows:

$$560\ \text{mg N}/100\ \text{mL urine} \times 2{,}500\ \text{mL urine}/24\ \text{hours} = 14{,}000\ \text{mg N/day} \qquad \textbf{36-1}$$

Obligatory losses generally are estimated as 2 to 4 g/day of nitrogen. Thus, the nitrogen balance for R.L. is calculated as follows:

$$\text{N balance} = \frac{96\ \text{g protein from PN}}{6.25} - (14\ \text{g N from UUN} + 3\ \text{g}) \qquad \textbf{36-2}$$

where N is nitrogen, PN is parenteral nutrition, and UUN is urine urea nitrogen.

R.L. is negative approximately 1.6 g N or 10 g of protein (1.6 g N × 6.25). In addition, because R.L. has wounds to heal, a positive nitrogen balance of approximately 3 to 5 g of nitrogen is desirable. Therefore, R.L. needs another 4.6 to 6.6 g N/day or 29 to 41 g protein/day more than the 96 g protein currently provided by PN. Optimal conditions for wound healing may actually require N balance results of 5 to 10 g positive when using insensible losses but not wound exudate.[127] In addition, urea accounts for only about 80% of total urine N (TUN).[34] Use of TUN is more reliable than UUN, when available, or an estimate of TUN can be made by adding 20% of UUN losses along with the 2 to 4 g obligatory losses. Thus, the calculated N balance for R.L. may under estimate her protein requirement. Maintaining positive nitrogen balance may not be feasible in such highly catabolic patients and some question if protein >1.5 g/kg/day promotes positive N balance or lean tissue accretion.[129] So long as R.L. does not demonstrate adverse effects, such as azotemia or hyperammonemia, from the high protein intake it is reasonable to aim for a positive N balance.

R.L. currently receives 1,734 kcal daily (31.5 kcal/kg/day); 1,350 as nonprotein calories (NPC). With R.L.'s highly catabolic state, maintaining the current NPC:N ratio of approximately 90:1 or down to 75:1 is advisable as long as R.L. can tolerate the extra protein. Estimating caloric requirements in patients such as R.L. is subject to greater error than in patients with low metabolic stress, but the most appropriate method to determine energy requirements is unclear.[134] Use of indirect calorimetry is considered the gold standard, although data were insufficient for the CCPG to recommend this method versus predictive equations in critically ill adults.[32] In a study of patients in a surgical ICU, use of indirect calorimetry was no better than Harris-Benedict calculations multiplied by 1.5 or 30 kcal/kg adjusted body weight for determining energy requirements.[135] Other studies indicate unbiased and precise results in critically ill patients using adjusted body weight with Harris-Benedict equations multiplied by 1.2, or 1.6.[136,137] Predictive equations, including Swinamer, Ireton-Jones, and Penn State, have also been developed for critically ill patients and produce varying results in different studies.[36,134,136–138] It is reasonable to consider indirect calorimetry for R.L. If a metabolic cart is not available, the total caloric intake from the PN formulation plus calories from another 30 g of protein can be calculated as a guideline for R.L.'s caloric requirement:

$$1{,}734\ \text{kcal from PN} + (30\ \text{g of protein for positive balance} \times 4\ \text{kcal/g}) = 1{,}854\ \text{total kcal} \qquad \textbf{36-3}$$

Fluid requirements for younger patients (i.e., those <65 years) can be estimated at 35 to 40 mL/kg/day plus replacement of excess losses from hyperthermia, vomiting, diarrhea, fistulae, or wound drainage. Based on this method, R.L.'s fluid requirements are 1,925 to 2,200 mL/day. Estimated fluid needs also may be based on 1 mL/kcal ingested or on 1,500 mL plus 20 mL/kg over 20 kg.[1] R.L. should receive a minimum of 1 mL/kcal owing to her high-protein intake but she is likely to need at least 35 to 40 mL/kg/day.

Enteral Nutrition Therapy (Tube Feeding)

13. Enteral feeding is to start today via the J tube. What type of formula is most appropriate for R.L.?

R.L.'s hospitalization has been unusually long and complicated. She may have impaired absorptive function because of her prolonged period without GI tract stimulation. Some practice-based publications suggest consideration of an oligomeric formula for patients whose GI tract has not been used for >7 days.[1,127,133] The CCPG recommend initiation of EN with a polymeric formula.[32] Only four studies comparing oligomeric with polymeric formulas in critically ill patients were found for the CCPG, and none met the criteria for the highest level of study. Available data did not indicate a clinically important benefit for oligomeric formulas. Given the limited data and conflicting suggestions for formula selection, implementing the CCPG can be difficult.[78] Formula selection may instead be determined by physician preference and the calorie, protein, and fat content of formulas on the formulary. To obtain the necessary NPC:N ratio, a high or very high protein formula is needed, or a modular protein component must be added to the EN regimen.

One very high nitrogen polymeric formula and one oligomeric formula are available on formulary. The very high nitrogen formula has a caloric distribution of 25% protein (NPC:N = 75:1), 45% carbohydrate, and 30% fat with a 25:75 MCT:long-chain triglyceride ratio. This formula provides 1,000 kcal and 62.5 g protein/L. The hydrolyzed protein formula has a caloric distribution of 20% protein (NPC:N = 115:1), 65% carbohydrate, and 15% fat with a 50:50 MCT:long-chain triglyceride ratio. This formula provides 1,000 kcal and 50 g protein/L.

The oligomeric formula is selected based on current practice in the ICU. The osmolality is 460 mOsm/kg and the free water content is 830 mL/L (83%). The goal volume is 1,920 mL (80 mL/hour) to provide 1,920 kcal, 96 g protein, and 1,594 mL fluid. The remaining fluid requirement will be met by flushing the tube three to four times daily and by IV medications. The enteral formula provides slightly more calories than the estimated requirements (Eq. 36-3), but it is acceptable at 34.9 kcal/kg/day. The formula does not meet R.L.'s protein requirement based on nitrogen balance. At some point, the formula should be changed to a higher protein formula or 30 g of a modular protein component must be added. This is a significant amount of protein; thus, it would be preferable to transition R.L. to a very high nitrogen formula. The primary concern with the formulary product listed earlier will be whether R.L. can tolerate the more complex nutrients and higher fat content.

Additional Nutrients

14. Overall, R.L. appears to be improving despite the perihepatic abscess. She no longer requires inotropic support and ventilatory parameters have improved, although she continues to require mechanical ventilation. Should additional nutrients, such as those associated with immune modulation, be considered for R.L.?

Based on the CCPG, EN with fish oils, borage oils, and antioxidants should be considered for patients with ARDS, which R.L. was diagnosed with early in her hospitalization.[32] Protein content of the pulmonary formula matching CCPG recommendations is 16.7% of calories (~42 g/1,000 kcal) and would require an exceptionally large dose of supplemental protein to meet R.L.'s requirement. This would increase the risk of tube occlusion, as well as the risk of inadequate protein provision. Soon after R.L.'s diagnosis of ARDS, the immune-modulating pulmonary formula might have received higher consideration but with her improving ventilatory status it is not warranted.

The CCPG does not recommend formulas supplemented with arginine and other selected nutrients for use in critically ill patients by owing to a potentially higher mortality rate associated with their use, especially in septic patients.[32,48] Although R.L. does not appear septic at this time, no impetus exists to use an arginine-supplemented formula.

Glutamine should be considered based on the CCPG recommendation.[32] One moderate quality study in trauma patients reported a significant reduction in infectious complications, leading CCPG to include consideration of enteral glutamine for trauma patients. It is questionable whether glutamine will provide any benefit to R.L. because she is improving overall; however, she does have a recently diagnosed intra-abdominal (perihepatic) abscess. No data indicate harm from enteral glutamine; therefore, it is reasonable to add 0.3 g/kg/day of glutamine to the EN regimen.[63] Glutamine powder, available in individual packets, is mixed with water and administered via the feeding tube.

Enteral Nutrition Administration

15. Recommend a plan for initiating and advancing R.L.'s tube feeding.

Enteral nutrition should be initiated slowly because R.L. has not used her GI tract for a prolonged period and may have both impaired absorption and digestion.[92,97] Initiation at 10 to 40 mL/hour is typical in patients such as R.L., with rate increases of 10 to 25 mL/hour every 8 to 12 hours until the goal rate is reached.[77,96,97] EN in R.L. is probably best started at 10 to 20 mL/hour for 8 to 12 hours and increased in 10- to 15-mL/hour increments every 8 to 12 hours until 80 mL/hour (goal rate) is reached, assuming tolerance with each step. An enteral infusion pump should be used to maintain consistent flow. Small-bore feeding tubes can occlude if the flow is disrupted and surgery may be required to replace the J tube if the tract has not matured adequately for nonsurgical tube replacement.

Protein in the PN formula may remain at the current level, or be increased to provide protein for a 3- to 5-g positive nitrogen balance because transition to EN is expected to be slow. The selected enteral formula is hypertonic; nonetheless, full-strength formula should be started and the formula diluted only if full strength formula causes abdominal distention, diarrhea, or other signs of intolerance. A transition plan from the PN to EN must also be developed. Typically, the PN rate is gradually decreased as tolerance to EN is established. The sum of enteral and parenteral calories and protein should be monitored closely to avoid complications of overfeeding while ensuring adequate nutrition provision. For R.L., maintaining adequate protein intake is critical; thus, cumulative protein intake (i.e., protein from PN plus EN) should be kept at 125 g/day or higher.

Tube Feeding Intolerance

16. R.L. develops diarrhea approximately 18 hours after EN is increased to 80 mL/hour. The PN formulation is at 20 mL/hour. What is the likely cause of the diarrhea? Should the EN be stopped and the PN formulation increased to goal rate again?

Diarrhea affects 15% to 30% of patients in the ICU.[129] In patients receiving EN, diarrhea is multifactorial. Factors associated with diarrhea, but not related to EN, include medications, partial small bowel obstruction or fecal impaction, bile salt malabsorption, intestinal atrophy, hypoalbuminemia, infections such as *C. difficile,* and underlying conditions affecting the GI tract.[97,99,104,111,113,114,129] Tube feeding-related causes of diarrhea include high fat content, lactose content, and bacterial contamination. Formula temperature, caloric density, osmolality, formula strength, lack of fiber content, and method of delivery also have been associated with diarrhea, although a cause-and-effect relationship is not clear.

R.L.'s diarrhea may be related to increasing the formula volume. The jejunum adapts slowly to changes in volume or concentration, and formula volume was increased <24 hours before diarrhea started. Changing back to the previous volume or slightly less should decrease stool output within 24 hours if the volume change was responsible. If R.L. does not respond to decreasing formula volume, the formula may be held for 24 hours to assess whether diarrhea decreases or stops. Diarrhea related directly to EN usually is an osmotic diarrhea that stops within 24 hours of stopping the formula.[104] The PN rate should be increased to 85 mL/hour (goal rate) if EN is stopped for more than 2 days or so. A more objective approach than stopping the formula is to measure stool osmolality. Enteral formula-induced diarrhea is associated with a large osmotic gap, whereas secretory diarrhea (e.g., infectious diarrhea) is associated with a low or negative osmotic gap.[104]

Evaluate other potential causes of diarrhea before stopping R.L.'s EN. The current formula is lactose free and low in long-chain triglyceride content. As a ready-to-use formula, bacterial contamination from mixing technique is not of concern. Cleanliness during formula transfer to the delivery bag, the period of time formula is in the bag, and methods of cleaning the delivery bag may contribute to bacterial contamination of formula. Closed enteral systems (i.e., ready-to-hang formula-filled containers) virtually eliminate transfer-related contamination when proper technique is used. Any addition (e.g., medication, carbohydrate, fat or protein module, MCT oil) to the prefilled container before hanging can contaminate the system as well, and guidelines (e.g., hang-time, set changes) for an open enteral system should be followed.

Medications are a major contributor to diarrhea in tube-fed patients.[97] Study results implicating antibiotic therapy in diarrhea have been questioned because of failure to report stool frequency and consistency as well as lack of a clear definition of diarrhea.[139] Treatment of antibiotic-associated diarrhea can include administration of *Lactobacillus acidophilus* preparations via the feeding tube to restore normal GI flora, administering antidiarrheal agents, changing antibiotics, or stopping therapy when appropriate to do so. Infectious causes of diarrhea require appropriate antibiotic therapy. Antidiarrheal agents decreasing motility should not be used when *C. difficile* is present, but adsorbents such as Kaolin may be beneficial.

R.L. currently receives antibiotics and has for some time. *C. difficile* may have relapsed after her previous treatment. Stool specimens should be sent for culture and *C. difficile* toxin. Evaluation of R.L.'s medications may reveal medications associated with diarrhea (e.g., sorbitol-containing products, antacids, oral magnesium, potassium chloride, phosphate supplements, H_2-receptor antagonists) for which therapeutic alternatives or different routes of administration could be considered.[97] High osmolality liquid medications should be diluted before administration to reduce GI side effects.[113,114]

Malnutrition and hypoalbuminemia are associated with diarrhea in the ICU and might contribute to R.L.'s diarrhea given her low serum albumin and prolonged PN course without GI tract stimulation.[129] Diarrhea would be expected within 24 to 48 hours of starting feedings if this were the primary cause. Malabsorption should be limited in R.L. by use of an oligomeric formula containing only 15% of calories from fat and 50% of fat calories from MCT. Continued use of the GI tract is encouraged when malabsorption and hypoalbuminemia are the primary causes of diarrhea.

R.L.'s GI tract should continue to be used to the extent possible. EN appears to be better than PN for maintaining the GI tract barrier and host immunologic function.[1,41,63,72,75,127,133,140] Based on 13 moderate to high level studies, the CCPG strongly recommend use of EN over PN in critically ill patients.[32] The risk of sepsis increases without enteral stimulation of the GI tract. Whether this occurs through bacterial translocation, an unproved process in humans in which enteric bacteria or endotoxin cross the GI mucosa into mesenteric lymph nodes and portal circulation or through another mechanism is unclear. In addition, the GI tract serves an immune function, especially with respect to IgA secretion. Respiratory tract infections, such as pneumonia, may increase without proper stimulation of the GI tract, owing to less-effective protection from IgA. Compared with PN, EN attenuates catabolism in highly stressed patients, although initiation of feedings soon after the stressing event may be required to obtain this response. Before a decision is made to stop R.L.'s EN, possible benefits of improved fluid and electrolyte balance by stopping EN should be weighed against the potential benefits of reduced infections from continued use of the GI tract.

Medication Administration via Feeding Tube

17. It is determined that R.L. has *C. difficile* in her stool again. The tube feeding is at 30 mL/hour and the PN formulation is at 55 mL/hour. Kaolin has been ordered for administration via tube feeding. Is this an appropriate order?

It generally is better to administer medication separate from the enteral formula, because interactions are more likely to occur if the medication is admixed with the formula. Interactions can lead to feeding tube occlusion, loss of nutrients, or loss of medication. Addition of kaolin directly into the enteral formula could result in nutrient losses because adsorption by kaolin is not selective and may include nutrients as well as bacteria, toxins, noxious materials, and drugs.[141] Administration via a small inner-diameter jejunostomy also is likely to occlude the tube. To the extent possible, medications should be given by a route other than the feeding tube because of the risk of tube occlusion. Occlusion of the feeding tube would be more detrimental to the overall plan of transitioning R.L. to tube feedings than stopping the tube feeding for 2 or 3 days until treatment of *C. difficile* resolves the diarrhea. PN should be increased to goal rate if EN is stopped owing to severe diarrhea. Stopping the tube feeding is not expected to resolve R.L.'s infectious diarrhea, however, and kaolin should not be administered through the jejunostomy tube even if tube feeding is stopped. Other methods of controlling diarrhea should be investigated.

REFERENCES

1. ASPEN Board of Directors and the Clinical Guidelines Task Force. Guidelines for the use of parenteral and enteral nutrition in adult and pediatric patients. *JPEN* 2002;26(Suppl 1):1SA.
2. Russell MK et al. Nutrition screening and assessment. In: Gottschlich MM et al., eds. *The ASPEN Nutrition Support Core Curriculum: A Case-Based Approach—The Adult Patient.* Silver Spring: American Society for Parenteral and Enteral Nutrition; 2007:163.
3. Marian M et al. Overview of enteral nutrition. In: Gottschlich MM et al., eds. *The ASPEN. Nutrition Support Core Curriculum: A Case-Based Approach—The Adult Patient.* Silver Spring: American Society for Parenteral and Enteral Nutrition; 2007:187.
4. Bankhead RR et al. Enteral access devices. In: Gottschlich MM et al., eds. *The ASPEN. Nutrition Support Core Curriculum: A Case-Based Approach—The Adult Patient.* Silver Spring: American Society for Parenteral and Enteral Nutrition; 2007:233.
5. Kirby DF et al. Enteral access and infusion equipment. In: Merritt R et al., eds. *The ASPEN. Nutrition Support Practice Manual.* 2nd ed. Silver Spring: American Society for Parenteral and Enteral Nutrition; 2005:54.
6. Cresci G. Enteral access. In: Charney P et al. eds. *ADA Pocket Guide to Enteral Nutrition.* Chicago: American Dietetic Association; 2006:26.
7. Baskin WN. Acute complications associated with bedside placement of feeding tubes. *Nutrition in Clinical Practice* 2006;21:40.
8. Vanek V. Ins and outs of enteral access, Part I: short-term enteral access. *Nutrition in Clinical Practice* 2002;17:272.
9. Vanek V. Ins and outs of enteral access, Part 2: Long term access—esophagostomy and gastrostomy. *Nutrition in Clinical Practice* 2003;18:50.
10. Vanek V. Ins and outs of enteral access, Part 3: Long-term access—jejunostomy. *Nutrition in Clinical Practice* 2003;18:201.
11. Lynch CR et al. Prevention and management of complications of percutaneous endoscopic gastrostomy (PEG) tubes. *Pract Gastroenterol* 2004;28:66.
12. Bankhead RR et al. Gastrostomy tube placement outcomes: comparison of surgical, endoscopic, and laparoscopic methods. *Nutrition in Clinical Practice* 2005;20:1.
13. Bankhead R et al. Access to the gastrointestinal tract. In: Rolandelli RH et al., eds. *Clinical Nutrition. Enteral and Tube Feeding.* 4th ed. Philadelphia: Elsevier Saunders; 2005:202.
14. Gutske RF et al. Gastric reflux during perfusion of the proximal small bowel. *Gastroenterology* 1970;59:890.
15. McClave SA et al. Complications of enteral access. *Gastrointest Endosc* 2003;58:739.
16. Heyland DK et al. Optimizing the benefits and minimizing the risks of enteral nutrition in the critically ill: role of small bowel feeding. *JPEN* 2002;26:S51.
17. Heyland DK et al. Aspiration and the risk of ventilator-associated pneumonia. *Nutrition in Clinical Practice* 2004;19:597.
18. McClave SA et al. North American summit on aspiration in the critically ill patient: consensus statement. *JPEN* 2002;26(Suppl):S80
19. Lefton J et al. Enteral formulations. In: Gottschlich MM et al., eds. *The ASPEN. Nutrition Support Core Curriculum: A Case-Based Approach—The Adult Patient.* Silver Spring: American Society for Parenteral and Enteral Nutrition; 2007:209.
20. Marian M et al. Enteral formulations. In: Merritt R et al., eds. *The ASPEN. Nutrition Support Practice Manual.* 2nd ed. Silver Spring: American Society for Parenteral and Enteral Nutrition; 2005:63.
21. Sheehy TW et al. Disaccharidase activity in normal and diseased small bowel. *Lancet* 1965;2(7401):1.
22. Food and Nutrition Board, Institute of Medicine, National Academy of Sciences. Dietary reference intakes for individuals, macronutrients. Dietary Reference Intakes for Energy, Carbohydrates, Fiber, Fat, Protein and Amino Acids, 2002. Available at www.iom.edu/object.file/Master/21/372/0.pdf. Accessed April 22, 2007.
23. Food and Nutrition Board, Institute of Medicine, Dietary, functional, and total fiber. Dietary Reference Intakes for Energy, Carbohydrates, Fiber, Fat, Protein and Amino Acids (Macronutrients). Washington, DC: National Academy of Sciences, 2002. Available at www.nap.edu/openbook.php?isbn=0309085373/html/285-333.html. Accessed April 22, 2007.
24. Slavin J. Dietary fiber. In: Matarese LE et al., eds. *Contemporary Nutrition Support Practice: A Clinical Guide.* 2nd ed. Philadelphia: WB Saunders; 2003:173.
25. Campbell SM. An anthology of advances in enteral tube feeding formulations. *Nutrition in Clinical Practice* 2006;21:411.
26. Bliss DZ et al. Fiber. In: Gottschlich MM et al., eds. *The ASPEN. Nutrition Support Core Curriculum: A Case-Based Approach—The Adult Patient.* Silver Spring: American Society for Parenteral and Enteral Nutrition; 2007:88.
27. McClave SA et al. Feeding the hypotensive patient: does enteral feeding precipitate or protect against ischemic bowel? *Nutrition in Clinical Practice* 2003;18:279.
28. Malone A. Enteral formula selection. In: Charney P et al., eds. *ADA Pocket Guide to Enteral Nutrition.* Chicago: American Dietetic Association; 2006:63.
29. Bengmark S et al. Prebiotics and synbiotics in clinical medicine. *Nutrition in Clinical Practice* 2005;20:244.
30. Speigel JE et al. Safety and benefits of fructooligosaccharides as food ingredients. *Food Technology* 1994;48:85.
31. Rollins CJ. Drug-nutrient interactions in enteral nutrition. In: Boullata JI et al., eds. *Handbook of Drug Nutrient Interactions.* Totowa: Humana Press; 2004:515.
32. Heyland DK et al. Canadian clinical practice guidelines for nutrition support in mechanically ventilated, critically ill adult patients. *JPEN* 2003;27:355.
33. Matthews DE. Protein and amino acids. In: Shils ME et al., eds. *Modern Nutrition in Health and Disease.* 10th ed. Baltimore: Lippincott Williams & Wilkins; 2006:23.
34. Young LS et al. Protein. In: Gottschlich MM et al., eds. *The ASPEN. Nutrition Support Core Curriculum: A Case-Based Approach—The Adult Patient.* Silver Spring: American Society for Parenteral and Enteral Nutrition; 2007:71.
35. Matarese LE. Rationale and efficacy of specialized enteral and parenteral formulas. In: Matarese LE et al., eds. *Contemporary Nutrition Support Practice: A Clinical Guide.* 2nd ed. Philadelphia: WB Saunders; 2003:263.
36. Rollins CJ. Basics of enteral and parenteral nutrition. In: Wolinsky I et al., eds. *Nutrition in Pharmacy Practice.* Washington, DC: American Pharmaceutical Association; 2002:213.
37. Stratton RJ et al. Multinutrient oral supplements and tube feeding in maintenance dialysis: a systematic review and meta-analysis. *Am J Kidney Dis* 2005;46:387.
38. Stechmiller JK et al. Wound healing. In: Gottschlich MM et al., eds. *The ASPEN. Nutrition Support Core Curriculum: A Case-Based Approach—The Adult Patient.* Silver Spring: American Society for Parenteral and Enteral Nutrition; 2007:405.
39. Thompson C et al. Nutrients and wound healing: still searching for the magic bullet. *Nutrition in Clinical Practice* 2005;20:331.
40. Basu HN et al. Arginine: a clinical perspective. *Nutrition in Clinical Practice* 2002;17:218.
41. Mayes T et al. Burns and wound healing. In: Matarese LE et al., eds. *Contemporary Nutrition Support Practice: A Clinical Guide.* 2nd ed. Philadelphia: WB Saunders; 2003:595.
42. Zaloga GP et al. Arginine: mediator or modulator of sepsis. *Nutrition in Clinical Practice* 2004;19:201.
43. Heyland D et al. Immunonutrition in the critically ill: from old approaches to new paradigms. *Intensive Care Med* 2005;31:501.
44. Kieft H et al. Clinical outcome on immunonutrition in a heterogenous intensive care population. *Intensive Care Med* 2005;31:524.
45. Heyland DK et al. Should immunonutrition become routine in critically ill patients? A systemic review of the evidence. *JAMA* 2001;286:944.
46. Galban C et al. An immune-enhancing enteral diet reduces mortality rate and episodes of bacteremia in septic intensive care unit patients. *Crit Care Med* 2000;28:643.
47. Suchner U et al. Immune-modulating actions of arginine in the critically ill. *Br J Nutr* 2002; 87(Suppl 1):S121.
48. Heyland DK et al. Does immunonutrition in septic patients do more harm than good? *Intensive Care Med* 2003;29:669.
49. Bertolini G et al. Early enteral immunonutrition in patients with severe sepsis; results of an interim analysis of a randomized multicenter clinical trial. *Intensive Care Med* 2003;29:834.
50. Dent DL et al. Immunonutrition may increase mortality in critically ill patients with pneumonia: results of a randomized trial. *Crit Care Med* 2003;30:A17.
51. Jijveldt RJ et al. High plasma arginine concentrations in critically ill patients suffering from hepatic failure. *Eur J Clin Nutr* 2004;58:587.

52. MacFie J. European round table: the use of immunonutrients in the critically ill. *Clin Nutr* 2004;23:1426.
53. Charney P et al. Enteral formulations. In: Rolandelli RH et al., eds. *Clinical Nutrition: Enteral and Tube Feeding.* 4th ed. Philadelphia: Elsevier Saunders; 2005:216.
54. Wischmeyer PE. Clinical applications of L-glutamine: past, present, and future. *Nutrition in Clinical Practice* 2003;18:377.
55. Coeffier M et al. The role of glutamine in intensive care unit patients: mechanisms of action and clinical outcomes. *Nutr Rev* 2005;63:65.
56. Grimble RF. Immunonutrition. *Curr Opin Gastroenterol* 2005;21:216.
57. Alpers DH. Glutamine: do the data support the cause for glutamine supplementation in humans? *Gastroenterology* 2006;130:S106.
58. Savarese DM et al. Prevention of chemotherapy and radiation toxicity with glutamine. *Cancer Treat Rev* 2003;29(6):501.
59. Anderson PM et al. Oral glutamine reduces the duration and severity of stomatitis after cytotoxic cancer chemotherapy. *Cancer* 1998;83:1433.
60. Moore FA. Effects of innune-enhanncing diets on infectious morbidity and multiple organ failure. *JPEN* 2001;25:S36.
61. Buchman A. Clinical controversies. The role of glutamine: counterpoint. *Nutrition in Clinical Practice* 2003;18:391.
62. Novak F et al. Glutamine supplementation in serious illness: a systematic review of the evidence. *Crit Care Med* 2002;30:2022.
63. Heyland DK. Critical care nutrition. Available at hhp://www.criticalcarenutrition.com. Accessed May 2, 2007.
64. Sacks GS. Clinical controversies. The role of glutamine. *Nutrition in Clinical Practice* 2003;18:386.
65. Hise ME et al. In: Gottschlich MM et al., eds. *The ASPEN. Nutrition Support Core Curriculum: A Case-Based Approach—The Adult Patient.* Silver Spring: American Society for Parenteral and Enteral Nutrition; 2007:48.
66. Kelley MJ. Lipids. In: Matarese LE et al., eds. *Contemporary Nutrition Support Practice: A Clinical Guide.* 2nd ed. Philadelphia: WB Saunders; 2003:112.
67. Lee S et al. Current clinical applications of W-6 and W-3 fatty acids. *Nutrition in Clinical Practice* 2006;21:323.
68. Calder PC. n-3 fatty acids, inflammation, and immunity—relevance to postsurgical and critically ill patients. *Lipids* 2004;39:1147.
69. Bansal V et al. Interactions between fatty acids and arginine metabolism: implications for the design of immune-enhancing diets. *JPEN* 2005;29:S75.
70. Braga M et al. Nutritional approach in malnourished surgical patients: a prospective randomized study. *Arch Surg* 2002;137:174.
71. Gianotti L et al. A randomized controlled trial of preoperative oral supplementation with a specialized diet in patients with gastrointestinal cancer. *Gastroenterology* 2002;122:1763.
72. Cresci G. Targeting the use of specialized nutritional formulas in surgery and critical care. *JPEN* 2005;29:S92.
73. Senkal M et al. Preoperative oral supplementation with long-chain W-3 fatty acids beneficially alters phospholipid fatty acid patterns in liver, gut mucosa, and tumor tissue. *JPEN* 2005;29:236.
74. Chessman KH. Infant nutrition and special nutritional needs of children. In: Berardi RR et al., eds. *Handbook of Nonprescription Drugs. An Interactive Approach to Self-Care.* 15th ed. Washington, DC: American Pharmacists Association; 2006:521.
75. Kudsk KA et al. Consensus recommendations from the U.S. Summit on immune-enhancing enteral therapy. *JPEN* 2001;25(Suppl):S61.
76. Hall JC et al. A clinical trial evaluating enteral glutamine in critically ill patients. *Am J Clin Nutr* 2002;75(Suppl):415S.
77. DeChicco RS et al. Determining the nutrition support regimen. In: Matarese LE et al., eds. *Contemporary Nutrition Support Practice: A Clinical Guide.* 2nd ed. Philadelphia: WB Saunders; 2003:181.
78. Jones NF et al. Implementation of the Canadian Clinical Practice Guidelines for Nutrition Support: a multiple case study of barriers and enablers. *Nutrition in Clinical Practice* 2007;22:449.
79. Malone AM. The use of specialized enteral formulas in pulmonary disease. *Nutrition in Clinical Practice* 2004;19:557.
80. Cai B et al. Effect of supplementing a high-fat, low-carbohydrate enteral formula in COPD patients. *Nutrition* 2003;19:229.
81. Gadek JE et al. Effect of enteral feeding with eicosapentaenoic acid, gamma-linolenic acid, and antioxidants in patients with acute respiratory distress syndrome. *Crit Care Med* 1999;27:1409.
82. Pacht ER et al. Enteral nutrition with eicosapentaenoic acid, gamma-linolenic acid, and antioxidants reduces alveolar inflammatory mediators and protein influx in patients with acute respiratory distress syndrome. *Crit Care Med* 2003;31: 491.
83. Sheard NF et al. Dietary carbohydrate (amount and type) in the management of diabetes. *Diabetes Care* 2004;29:2266.
84. Franz MJ. 2002 diabetes nutrition recommendations: grading the evidence. *Diabetes Education* 2002;28:756.
85. American Diabetes Association. Nutrition principles and recommendations in diabetes. *Diabetes Care* 2004;27(Suppl):S36.
86. American Diabetes Association. Diabetes nutrition recommendations for health care institutions. *Diabetes Care* 2004;27:555.
87. Malone A. Enteral formula selection: a review of selected product categories. *Practical Gastroenterology* 2005;24:44.
88. Leon-Sans M et al. Glycemic and lipid control in hospitalized type 2 diabetic patients: evaluation of 2 enteral nutrition formulas (low carbohydrate-high monounsaturated fat vs high carbohydrate). *JPEN* 2005;29:21.
89. Mesejo A et al. Comparison of a high-protein disease-specific enteral formula with a high-protein enteral formula in hyperglycemic critically ill patients. *Clin Nutr* 2003;22:295.
90. Charney P et al. Management of blood glucose and diabetes in the critically ill patient receiving enteral feeding. *Nutrition in Clinical Practice* 2004;19:129.
91. Russell MK et al. Is there a role for specialized enteral nutrition in the intensive care unit? *Nutrition in Clinical Practice* 2002;17:156.
92. Thompson C. Initiation, advancement, and transition of enteral feedings. In: Charney P et al., eds. *ADA Pocket Guide to Enteral Nutrition.* Chicago: American Dietetic Association; 2006:123.
93. Scolapio JS. Methods for decreasing risk of aspiration pneumonia in critically patients. *JPEN* 2002;26(6):S58.
94. Methany NA. Risk factors for aspiration. *JPEN* 2002;26(Suppl 6):S26.
95. Stroud M et al. Guidelines for enteral feeding in adult hospital patients. *Gut* 2003;52(Suppl 7):vii1.
96. Clohessy S et al. Administration of enteral nutrition: initiation, progression, and transition. In: Rolandelli RH et al., eds. *Clinical Nutrition. Enteral and Tube Feeding.* 4th ed. Philadelphia: Elsevier Saunders; 2005:243.
97. Lord L et al. Enteral nutrition implementation and management. In: Merritt RJ et al., eds. *The ASPEN. Nutrition Support Practice Manual.* 2nd ed. Silver Spring: American Society for Parenteral and Enteral Nutrition; 2005:76.
98. Parrish CR. Enteral feeding: the art and the science. *Nutrition in Clinical Practice* 2003;18:76.
99. Malone AM et al. Complications of enteral nutrition. In: Gottschlich MM et al., eds. *The ASPEN. Nutrition Support Core Curriculum: A Case-Based Approach—The Adult Patient.* Silver Spring: American Society for Parenteral and Enteral Nutrition; 2007:246.
100. Biffl WL et al. Nutrition support of the trauma patient. *Nutrition* 2002;18:960.
101. McCray S et al. Much ado about refeeding. *Practical Gastroenterology* 2005;24:26. Available at http://www.healthsystem.virginia.edu/internet/digestive-health/nutritionarticles/McCrayAricle.pdf. Accessed April 21, 2007.
102. Kraft MD et al. Review of the refeeding syndrome. *Nutrition in Clinical Practice* 2005;20:625.
103. Lord LM. Restoring and maintaining patency of enteral feeding tubes. *Nutrition in Clinical Practice* 2003;18:422.
104. Russell MK. Monitoring complications of enteral feedings. In: Charney P et al., eds. *ADA Pocket Guide to Enteral Nutrition.* Chicago: American Dietetic Association; 2006:155.
105. Maloney JP et al. Detection of aspiration in enterally fed patients: a requiem for bedside monitors of aspiration. *JPEN* 2002;26:S34.
106. U.S. Food and Drug Administration. FDA Public Health Advisory: Report of blue discoloration and death in patients receiving enteral tube feedings tinted with dye, FD&C Blue No. 1. September 29, 2003. Available at: http://www.cfan.fda.gov/~dms/col-ltr2.html. Accessed May 3, 2007.
107. Maloney JP et al. Food dye use in enteral feedings: a review and a call for a moratorium. *Nutrition in Clinical Practice* 2002;17:168.
108. McClave SA et al. Clinical use of gastric residual volumes as a monitor for patients on enteral tube feeding. *JPEN* 2002;26:S43.
109. Booth C et al. Gastrointestinal promotility drugs in the critical care setting: a systematic review of the evidence. *Crit Care Med* 2002;30:1429.
110. Seifert CF et al. Drug administration through enteral feeding catheters [Letter]. *Am J Health Syst Pharm* 2002;59:378.
111. Beyer P. Complications of enteral nutrition. In: Matarese LE et al., eds. *Contemporary Nutrition Support Practice: A Clinical Guide.* 2nd ed. Philadelphia: WB Saunders; 2003:315.
112. Seifert CF et al. A nationwide survey of long-term care facilities to determine the characteristics of medication administration through enteral feeding catheters. *Nutrition in Clinical Practice* 2005;20:354.
113. Rollins CJ. General pharmacologic issues. In: Matarese LE et al., eds. *Contemporary Nutrition Support Practice. A Clinical Guide.* Philadelphia. 2nd ed. WB Saunders; 2003:303.
114. Nyffeler MS et al. Drug-nutrient interactions. In: Gottschlich MM et al., eds. *The ASPEN. Nutrition Support Core Curriculum: A Case-Based Approach—The Adult Patient.* Silver Spring: American Society for Parenteral and Enteral Nutrition; 2007:118.
115. Mitchell JF et al. Oral dosage forms that should not be crushed. *July 2007 Chart: Hospital Pharmacy,* St. Louis: Wolters-Kluwer Health; 2007.
116. Au Yeung SC et al. Phenytoin and enteral feedings: does evidence support an interaction? *Ann Pharmacother* 2000;34:896.
117. Kagansky N et al. Poor nutritional habits are predictors of poor outcome in very old hospitalized patients. *Am J Clin Nutr* 2005;82:784.
118. Visser M et al. Lower serum albumin concentration and change in muscle mass: the Health, Aging and Body Composition Study. *Am J Clin Nutr* 2005;82:531.
119. Newman AB et al. Weight change and the conservation of lean mass in old age: the Health, Aging and Body Composition Study. *Am J Clin Nutr* 2005;82:872.
120. Chernoff R. Normal aging, nutrition assessment, and clinical practice. *Nutrition in Clinical Practice* 2003;18:12.
121. Pattinson A et al. Home enteral nutrition. In: Merritt R et al., ed. *The ASPEN. Nutrition Support Practice Manual.* 2nd ed. Silver Spring: American Society for Parenteral and Enteral Nutrition; 2005: 193.
122. DeLegge MH et al. Home care. In: Gottschlich MM et al., eds. *The ASPEN. Nutrition Support Core*

Curriculum: A Case-Based Approach—The Adult Patient. Silver Spring: American Society for Parenteral and Enteral Nutrition; 2007:725.

123. Rollins CJ. Nutrition therapies: parenteral nutrition, enteral nutrition, and hydration. In: Monk-Tutor MR, ed. *NHIA Home Infusion Pharmacy Certificate Program.* Alexandria: National Home Infusion Association; 2004.
124. Department of Health and Human Services. Health Care Financing Administration. Medicare Coverage Issues Manual-Transmittal 133. December 7, 2000. Page 7, 65-10.2. Available at www.cms.hhs.gov/transmittals/downloads/R133CIM.pdf. Accessed May 22, 2007.
125. Palmetto GBA-SADMERC. Enteral nutrition product classification list. Available at www2.palmettogba.com/classifications/enteral%20nutrition.pdf. Accessed May 25, 2007.
126. Department of Health and Human Services. Centers for Medicare and Medicaid Services. DME Information Form. CMS-10126-Enteral and Parenteral Nutrition. Available at http://www.cms.hhs.gov/medicare. Accessed May 12, 2007.
127. Cresci G et al. Trauma, surgery, and burns. In: Gottschlich MM et al., eds. *The ASPEN. Nutrition Support Core Curriculum: A Case-Based Approach—The Adult Patient.* Silver Spring: American Society for Parenteral and Enteral Nutrition; 2007:455.
128. Berger MM. Antioxidant micronutrients in major trauma and burns: evidence and practice. *Nutrition in Clinical Practice* 2006;21:438.
129. Hollander JM et al. Nutrition support and chronic critical illness syndrome. *Nutrition in Clinical Practice* 2006;21:587.
130. Krenitsky J. Adjusted body weight, Pro: evidence to support the use of adjusted body weight in calculating calorie requirements. *Nutrition in Clinical Practice* 2005;20:468.
131. Ireton-Jones C. Adjusted body weight, Con: why adjust body weight in energy-expenditure calculations. *Nutrition in Clinical Practice* 2005;20:474.
132. Dickerson RN et al. Hypocaloric enteral tube feeding in critically ill obese patients. *Nutrition* 2002;18:241.
133. Kozar RA et al. Trauma. In: Merritt R et al., ed. *The ASPEN. Nutrition Support Practice Manual,* 2nd ed. Silver Spring: American Society for Parenteral and Enteral Nutrition; 2005:271.
134. Ireton-Jones C. Clinical dilemma: which energy expenditure equation to use? *JPEN* 2004;28:282.
135. Davis KA et al. Nutritional gain versus financial gain: the role of metabolic carts in the surgical ICU. *J Trauma* 2006;61:1436.
136. MacDonald A et al. Comparison of formulaic equations to determine energy expenditure in the critically ill. *Nutrition* 2003;19:233.
137. Alexander E et al. Retrospective evaluation of commonly used equations to predict energy expenditure in mechanically ventilated, critically ill patients. *Pharmacotherapy* 2004;24:1659.
138. Frankenfield D et al. Validation of two approaches to predicting resting metabolic rate in critically ill patients. *JPEN* 2004;28:259.
139. Haddad RY et al. Enteral nutrition and enteral tube feeding: review of the evidence. *Clin Geriatr Med* 2002;18:87.
140. Braunschweig CL et al. Enteral compared with parenteral nutrition: a meta-analysis. *Am J Clin Nutr* 2001;74:534.
141. Walker PC. Diarrhea. In: Berardi RR et al., eds. *Handbook of Nonprescription Drugs: An Interactive Approach to Self-Care.* 15th ed. Washington, DC: American Pharmacists Association; 2006:327.

CHAPTER 37

Adult Parenteral Nutrition

Jane M. Gervasio and Jennifer L. Ash

Since the mid-1600s, efforts have been made to provide nutrients intravenously. Peripheral veins were cannulated and various feeding solutions, including salt water, cow's milk, and glucose, were administered. Unfortunately, peripheral venous access necessitated the administration of large volumes (up to 5 L/day) of solutions with low nutrient content to provide sufficient calories to a patient. This method of feeding often resulted in thrombophlebitis or fluid overload.

It was not until the 1960s that Dudrick et al. introduced the technique of placing an intravenous (IV) catheter into the superior vena cava, a large vessel with rapid blood flow. Hemodilution of fluids administered into this vessel allowed delivery of small volumes of solutions with high concentrations of nutrients.[1]

Since then, many advances in the techniques for IV cannulation and formulation of IV nutrient solutions have been made. Today, the IV provision of complex mixtures of nutrients, known as parenteral nutrition, is an integral part of the medical management of patients, both hospitalized and at home, who cannot eat or ingest nutrients by the gastrointestinal (GI) tract.

MALNUTRITION

Adequate nutrition is important to maintain optimal health. Malnutrition occurs when there is any disorder of nutrition status, including disorders resulting from a deficiency of nutrient intake, impaired nutrient metabolism, or overnutrition. Clinically, a more useful definition of malnutrition is the state induced by alterations in dietary intake, which results in subcellular, cellular, and/or organ function changes that expose the individual to increased risks of morbidity and mortality and can be reversed by adequate nutritional support.[2]

The incidence of malnutrition among hospitalized patients has been reported to be as high as 55%.[3,4] In the hospitalized patient, acute malnutrition occurs when nutrient intake is inadequate in the face of injury or stress (e.g., trauma, infection, major surgery), and nutrient stores are rapidly depleted. Acute stress or injury increases energy needs to repair tissues. When this energy is not provided exogenously, the body turns to endogenous sources of energy by breaking down skeletal muscle to release amino acids for the production of glucose. This iatrogenic malnutrition can occur rapidly even in individuals who were well nourished prior to the stress. Once the illness or injury improves and normal nutrient intake is resumed, this acute malnutrition usually resolves.

In contrast, starvation or semistarvation states, without stress or injury, allow humans to adapt slowly to inadequate nutrient intake. This adaptation results in the use of endogenous fat stores for energy and a slow loss of muscle proteins. Nevertheless, energy and protein stores are not unlimited, and with total starvation, death occurs in normal-weight individuals in about 60 to 70 days.[5,6] Patients with a history of chronic malnutrition who are faced with stress or injury are at the greatest risk of developing malnutrition.

Protein-calorie malnutrition, the most common type of nutrition deficiency in hospitalized patients, is manifested by depletion of both tissue energy stores and body proteins. Malnourished patients are at a higher risk of developing complications during therapy. These nutrition-associated complications, as a result of organ wasting and functional impairment, can include weakness, decreased wound healing, altered hepatic metabolism of drugs, increased respiratory failure, decreased cardiac contractility, and infections such as pneumonia and abscesses. These complications increase the length of hospital stay and costs of care.[7–9]

SPECIALIZED NUTRITION SUPPORT

Patients with inadequate intake for 7 to 14 days or those with an unintentional weight loss of 10% of their preillness weight are considered malnourished or at risk of developing malnutrition. Nutritional intervention should be considered for these patients.[10,11] Patients who cannot meet their nutritional needs by consuming enough food by mouth should be considered for some type of specialized nutrition support. *Specialized nutrition support* is the provision of specially formulated and/or delivered parenteral or enteral nutrients to maintain or restore nutrition status.[12] For those who cannot eat by mouth but who have a functional GI tract, a method of enteral nutrition or tube feeding should be the first line of consideration (see Chapter 36).

When possible, the GI tract should be used for providing nutrients. Nutrients administered enterally may be more beneficial and less expensive than those provided by the parenteral route.[13] Stimulation of the intestine with enteral nutrients maintains the mucosal barrier structure and function and has been associated with decreased infectious morbidity in critically ill patients compared with those receiving nutrients parenterally.[14–18] For these reasons, parenteral nutrition (formerly referred to as total parenteral nutrition) is reserved for patients whose GI tracts are not functional or cannot be accessed and patients whose GI tracts do not absorb enough nutrients to maintain adequate nutrition status.[10]

PATIENT ASSESSMENT

An assessment of the nutritional status of a patient incorporates the analysis of body composition and evaluation of physiological function. Proper patient assessment should include the examination of multiple factors and should not rely on any one parameter. This evaluation is important in order to determine the presence and severity of malnutrition or the risk of developing malnutrition. The need for specialized nutrition support, as well as whether the goal of therapy is to maintain current nutrition status or to replete fat and lean body mass, is also determined following a complete patient assessment.

Table 37-1 Components of a Nutrition History

Medical history
Chronic illnesses
Surgical history
Psychosocial history
Socioeconomic status
History of gastrointestinal problems (nausea, vomiting, or diarrhea)
Diet history, including weight loss or weight gain diets
Food preferences and intolerances
Medications
Weight history
Increase or decrease
Intentional or unintentional
Time period for weight change
Functional capacity

Nutrition History

A nutrition history is critical in assessing nutrition status. Information can be obtained by interviewing the patient or the patient's family and reviewing the medical record to identify factors that may contribute to malnutrition or increase the risk of developing malnutrition.

Multiple factors can contribute to the development of malnutrition, including the patient's underlying disease states, past medical history, and financial and social environment. Medications can adversely affect nutrition status by decreasing the synthesis of nutrients, minimizing food intake through alteration of appetite and taste, changing the absorption or metabolism of nutrients, or increasing nutrient requirements. A nutrition history should also include evaluation of body weight. The components of a nutrition history are summarized in Table 37-1.

Weight History

Weight and weight history are important in evaluating nutrition status. Weight loss is a sign of negative energy and negative protein balance and is associated with poor outcome in hospitalized patients.[3,19] An unintentional weight loss of more than 10% is considered significant for malnutrition.[12]

A patient's current weight often is compared with a standard for ideal body weight (IBW). Percentage of IBW is determined as shown in Equation 37-1:

$$\%\,\text{IBW} = \frac{\text{Current weight}}{\text{IBW}}(100) \quad (37\text{-}1)$$

This method of assessing weight has its shortcomings because the patient's weight is compared with a population standard rather than using the individual patient as the reference point. For example, a patient who is significantly overweight and has lost large amounts of weight may still be more than 100% of IBW and therefore not considered at risk for developing malnutrition. A more patient-specific method of evaluating weight is to compare current weight with the patient's usual weight. This can be determined using Equation 37-2:

$$\%\ \text{Usual body weight} = \frac{\text{Current weight}}{\text{Usual body weight}}(100) \quad \textbf{(37-2)}$$

Using this method, the obese patient who has lost weight may be determined to be less than 90% of usual weight (weight loss of more than 10%) and therefore nutritionally at risk. It is also important to assess over what time period the change has occurred. Involuntary weight loss is considered severe if loss exceeds 5% of usual weight within 1 month, or 10% of usual weight within 6 months. The pattern of weight loss must be evaluated to determine whether the loss is continuing or stabilized. Continuing weight loss is a more serious concern than if the weight loss has stabilized. Weight gain after a significant weight loss is a positive sign.

Physical Examination

A physical examination may reveal signs of nutrition deficiencies that require further evaluation. General evidence of muscle and fat wasting (commonly noticed in the temporal area), loss of subcutaneous fat and muscle in the shoulders, and loss of subcutaneous fat in the interosseous and palmar areas of the hands are readily identifiable. Other physical parameters that may be less obvious are hair for color and sparseness; skin for turgor, pigmentation, and dermatitis; mouth for glossitis, gingivitis, cheilosis, and color of the tongue; nails for friability and lines; and the abdomen for ascites or enlarged liver.

Anthropometrics

Physical examination may include anthropometrics that measure subcutaneous fat and skeletal muscle mass. Assessment of fat stores provides information about fat loss or gain and assumes fat is gained or lost proportionally over the entire body. Approximately 50% of body fat is in the subcutaneous compartment. Triceps skinfold and subscapular skinfold thickness measurements are examples of methods used to assess subcutaneous fat and therefore estimate total body fat.

The values obtained are compared with reference standards. Somatic protein mass or skeletal muscle mass can be estimated by measuring mid-arm circumference and then calculating arm muscle circumference. These values are also compared with standards, and the amount of muscle mass is estimated.

When used for the long-term study of large, nutritionally stable populations, anthropometric measurements accurately reflect total body fat and skeletal muscle mass. However, anthropometric measurements of hospitalized patients are of little value. During acute illness and stress, changes in subcutaneous fat may not be proportional to changes in weight, and peripheral edema can result in inflated values for skinfold thickness and mid-arm circumference.[3,19]

Biochemical Assessment

Biochemical assessment of nutrition status includes measuring concentrations of serum proteins. The visceral proteins most commonly used to assess nutrition status are albumin, prealbumin, transferrin, and retinol-binding protein. These proteins are synthesized by the liver and reflect its synthetic capability. Serum concentrations decrease with hepatic insufficiency or when intake of substrates is inadequate for synthesis of these proteins. During stress or injury, inflammatory cytokines are released and substrates are shunted away from the synthesis of these proteins to synthesize other proteins such as C-reactive protein, haptoglobin, fibrinogen, and others; these are the acute phase proteins.[20] Serum concentrations of proteins are altered by acute stress or inflammatory states and chronic starvation.[19,20]

Albumin is the classic visceral protein used to evaluate nutrition status and is a prognostic indicator. Serum concentrations of <3 g/dL correlate with poor outcome and increased length of stay of hospitalized patients.[21] Albumin serves as a carrier protein for fatty acids, hormones, minerals, and drugs, and is necessary for maintaining oncotic pressure. Albumin has a large body pool of 3 to 5 g/kg, and 30% to 40% is localized to the intravascular space. The normal hepatic rate of albumin synthesis is 150 to 250 mg/kg/day. Because albumin has a half-life of 18 to 21 days, a decrease in serum albumin concentrations is generally not observed until after several weeks of inadequate nitrogen intake. Serum albumin concentrations decrease rapidly in response to stress (which causes albumin to shift from the intravascular to the extravascular space), burns, nephrotic syndrome, protein-losing enteropathy, overhydration, and decreased synthesis with liver disease.[19,21]

Transferrin is responsible for the transport of iron. It has a half-life of 8 to 10 days and therefore is more sensitive than albumin to acute changes in nutrition status. Normal serum concentrations for transferrin are 250 to 300 mg/dL.

Even more sensitive to changes in energy and protein intake is prealbumin (transthyretin), which has a small body pool (10 mg/kg) and a half-life of 2 to 3 days. Prealbumin transports both retinol and retinol-binding protein. Normal serum prealbumin concentrations are 15 to 40 mg/dL.

Retinol-binding protein has the shortest half-life, 12 hours; normal serum concentrations are 2.5 to 7.5 mg/dL. However, because serum concentrations of retinol-binding protein change rapidly in response to alterations in nutrient intake, monitoring it has limited use in clinical practice. The visceral proteins commonly used for nutrition assessment are summarized in Table 37-2.

Other proteins, such as fibronectin and somatomedin-C (insulinlike growth factor-1), are also used as markers of nutrition status. Fibronectin is a glycoprotein found in blood, lymph, and many cell surfaces. Somatomedin-C is important in regulating growth. Both fibronectin and somatomedin-C have half-lives of <1 day and respond to fasting and refeeding. Urinary measurement of 3-methylhistidine, a byproduct of muscle metabolism that is excreted unchanged, has been used to estimate skeletal muscle mass. Although these markers have potential use in nutrition assessment, they are used primarily as research tools and are not readily available for routine clinical use.[19]

Table 37-2 Visceral Proteins for Nutrition Assessment

Visceral Protein	*Half-Life (Days)*	*Normal Serum Concentration*
Albumin	18–21	3.5–5 g/dL
Transferrin	8–10	250–300 mg/dL
Transthyretin (prealbumin)	2–3	15–40 mg/dL
Retinol-binding protein	0.5	2.5–7.5 mg/dL

The interpretation of serum protein concentrations in hospitalized patients may be difficult because factors more important than hepatic synthesis rate alter serum concentrations. These factors may include renal, hepatic, or cardiac dysfunction; hydration status; and metabolic stress. Visceral proteins, as with any nutrition assessment parameter, must be used in conjunction with other parameters and comprehensive consideration of the patient's clinical status.

Nutrition assessment based on determinations of body composition using anthropometrics and biochemical parameters has many limitations. Newer techniques (e.g., bioelectrical impedance, dexa-energy x-ray absorptiometry, isotope dilution, neutron activation) are increasingly being used to determine body composition. Other parameters such as hand grip and forearm dynamometry may be used to assess skeletal muscle function, which relates changes in body composition to body function.[3,19]

Another nutrition assessment method, subjective global assessment (SGA), combines objective parameters and physiologic function. This method is based on a history of weight change, dietary intake, presence of significant GI symptoms, functional capacity, and physical examination to assess the loss of subcutaneous fat and muscle and edema. Using the SGA system, patients are rated as well nourished, moderately malnourished, or severely malnourished. This subjective assessment is easy to use and useful in diagnosing malnutrition.[22]

Classification of Malnutrition

Protein-calorie malnutrition is divided classically into three categories: marasmus, kwashiorkor, and a mixed protein-calorie. Marasmus, which means a "dying away state," is seen in individuals who have a chronic deficiency primarily in the intake of energy (calories) over a prolonged period (i.e., partial starvation). Physical examination reveals severe cachexia through loss of both fat and muscle mass; however, visceral protein (e.g., albumin, prealbumin) production is preserved. Patients with anorexia or suffering from chronic wasting diseases such as cancer are likely to present with marasmus malnutrition.

Kwashiorkor malnutrition results from a diet adequate in calories but limited in protein or in patients extremely catabolic from their medical complication (sepsis) or injury (trauma, thermally injured). Insulin is produced to metabolize the carbohydrates; it also prevents lipolysis and promotes the movement of amino acids into muscle. To meet protein needs, protein is mobilized from internal organs and circulating visceral proteins such as albumin. Thus, an individual with kwashiorkor malnutrition has adequate fat and muscle mass but depleted serum proteins.

Hospitalized patients commonly exhibit components of both marasmus and kwashiorkor malnutrition and are classified as having mixed protein-calorie malnutrition. This often occurs when an injury or stress compounds chronic starvation or semistarvation, resulting in wasting of fat and muscle mass, as well as depletion of serum proteins.

Estimation of Energy Expenditure

An important aspect of patient evaluation is estimating energy expenditure. A common approach used to determine energy requirements (and simplest method) is based on body weight in kilograms. The energy requirements are standardized and are determined by the metabolic condition of the patient (Table 37-3).

Table 37-3 Estimation of Energy Expenditure

Basal Energy Expenditure (BEE)	
Harris-Benedict Equations	
BEE_{men} (kcal/day) = 66.47 + 13.75 W + 5.0 H − 6.76 A	
BEE_{women} (kcal/day) = 655.10 + 9.56 W + 1.85 H − 4.68 A	
or	
20–25 kcal/kg/day	
Energy Requirements	
Hospitalized patient, mild stress	20–25 kcal/kg/day
Moderate stress, malnourished	25–30 kcal/kg/day
Severe stress, critically ill	30–35 kcal/kg/day

A, age in years; H, height in cm; W, weight in kg.

Many predictive equations for estimating expenditure have been described in the literature.[23,24] The traditional method of assessing energy expenditure is the basal energy expenditure (BEE), the amount of energy (kilocalories [kcal]) needed to support basic metabolic functions in a state of complete rest, shortly after awakening, and after a 12-hour fast. BEE is most commonly calculated using the Harris-Benedict equations. Alternatively, BEE can be estimated at 20 to 25 kcal/kg/day.

Basal metabolic rate (BMR) is the energy expended in the postabsorptive state (2 hours after a meal) and is approximately 10% greater than BEE. Determination of BEE or BMR does not include additional energy needed for stress or activity. The Harris-Benedict equations can be modified to include stress and physical activity factors, or these variables can be estimated at 20 to 35 kcal/kg/day for moderate to severe stress (Table 37-3).

Energy expenditure can be determined more accurately by indirect calorimetry, which uses a machine ("metabolic cart") to measure the patient's breathing or respiratory gas exchange. The machine measures oxygen (O_2) consumption and carbon dioxide (CO_2) production when standard testing conditions are maintained. The amount of O_2 consumed and CO_2 produced for carbohydrate, fat, and protein is constant and known. Through a series of equations, the energy expenditure, including stress, for that point in time is calculated and then extrapolated for 24 hours.[17,25] This is the measured energy expenditure (MEE). Because the measurement is usually conducted while the patient is at rest, activity is not included in MEE.

Indirect calorimetry is available to many clinicians and is considered the gold standard for energy expenditure determination. It is especially valuable in the energy assessment of critically ill or obese patients.

Estimation of Protein Goals

Estimation of protein needs must also be included in nutrition assessment. Protein needs are calculated based on body weight, degree of stress, and disease state. The recommended dietary allowance for the United States is 0.8 g of protein per kilogram per day. Well-nourished, hospitalized patients with minimal stress need 1 to 1.2 g of protein per kilogram per

Table 37-4 Estimation of Protein Requirements

U.S. recommended dietary allowance	0.8 g/kg/day
Hospitalized patient, minor stress	1–1.2 g/kg/day
Moderate stress	1.2–1.5 g/kg/day
Severe stress	1.5–2 g/kg/day

day to maintain lean body mass. The requirement for protein intake may be as high as 2 g/kg/day for a patient in a hypermetabolic, hypercatabolic state secondary to trauma or burns. In addition, patients with renal or hepatic dysfunction may require decreased protein intake as a result of altered metabolism. Guidelines for protein needs are summarized in Table 37-4.

VENOUS ACCESS SITES

When parenteral nutrition is necessary, the type of venous access must be selected. Parenteral nutrient formulations may be administered via peripheral veins or central veins, depending on the anticipated duration of parenteral nutrition therapy, nutrient requirements, and availability of venous access.[10]

Peripheral

Peripheral administration may be considered when parenteral nutrition is expected to be necessary for more than 10 days and when the patient has fairly low energy and protein needs due to minimal stress. Candidates for peripheral parenteral nutrition must have good peripheral venous access and must be able to tolerate large volumes of fluids.[26]

Parenteral nutrient formulations for administration via peripheral veins have traditionally contained relatively low concentrations of dextrose (5%–10%) and amino acids (3%–5%), providing <1 kcal/mL. Therefore, several liters may be needed daily to meet energy and protein needs. Although dilute with nutrients, the osmolarity of these formulations is 600 to 900 mOsm/L. These hypertonic formulations are irritating to peripheral veins and can cause thrombophlebitis. This necessitates frequent site rotations (at least every 48–72 hours), which may quickly exhaust venous access sites. Caloric density can be increased with only a modest increase in osmolarity by administering IV lipids concurrently or by adding them to the dextrose and amino acid mixtures. Lipids may also protect the vein against irritation through dilution and a buffering effect.[27,28]

Central

Administration of parenteral nutrient formulations through a central vein is preferred for patients whose GI tracts are nonfunctional or should be at rest for more than 7 days, who have limited peripheral venous access, or who have energy and protein needs that cannot be met with peripheral nutrient formulations.[10,26,29]

Traditionally, the central venous catheter is percutaneously inserted in the subclavian vein and threaded through the vein so the tip rests in the upper portion of the superior vena cava (SVC) just above the right atrium. A newer catheter technique involves the use of a peripherally inserted central catheter (PICC) that is inserted in the antecubital vein and advanced until the end of the catheter reaches the upper SVC.[29,30] The internal and external jugular veins may also be used to thread a catheter into the SVC. However, maintaining a sterile dressing on these sites is more difficult than with the subclavian approach or PICC. The SVC is an area of rapid blood flow, which quickly dilutes concentrated parenteral nutrient formulations, thereby minimizing phlebitis or thrombosis. Some patients are not candidates for placement of catheters in the SVC and require a femoral vein insertion with the tip of the catheter in the inferior vena cava. There may be a greater risk for infection with catheters placed using this technique.[29]

Central venous catheters can have single or multiple lumens. Multilumen catheters permit the administration of several therapies through the same IV site. Unlike peripheral venous sites, the central venous access site does not require frequent rotation. In fact, some patients requiring parenteral nutrition for months to years may have permanently placed central venous catheters.[31] Parenteral nutrient formulations designed for administration through central veins can contain relatively high concentrations of dextrose (20%–35%), amino acids (5%–10%), and lipids providing a caloric density of >1 kcal/mL in a solution with an osmolarity of >2,000 mOsm/L.

COMPONENTS OF PARENTERAL NUTRIENT FORMULATIONS

Parenteral nutrient formulations are very complex mixtures containing carbohydrate, protein, lipid, water, electrolytes, vitamins, and trace minerals. These admixtures must be prepared under aseptic conditions as described by the American Society of Health-System Pharmacists and U.S. Pharmacopeia standards.[32,33] Although parenteral feeding is an important adjuvant therapy for patients with many disease states, errors have occurred in managing this complex therapy, resulting in patient harm and death. Guidelines for safe practices have been developed for the situations in which inconsistent practices have the potential to cause harm. Pharmaceutical problem areas that are addressed in the Safe Practices for Parenteral Nutrition Formulations are compounding, formulas, labeling, stability, and filtering of parenteral nutrient formulations.[34] These practice guidelines have become standards of practice for parenteral nutrition therapy.

The three macronutrients used in parenteral nutrient formulations, carbohydrate, fat, and protein are available from various manufacturers. Water, as sterile water for injection, is also used to dilute the macronutrients to achieve the prescribed final concentrations of dextrose, amino acids, and lipids, as well as the final volume of the parenteral nutrient formulation.

Carbohydrate

Dextrose in water is the most common carbohydrate for IV use. It is available commercially in concentrations ranging from 2.5% to 70%. These dextrose solutions are mixed with other components of the parenteral nutrient formulation and diluted to various final concentrations. From these concentrations of dextrose, all parenteral nutrient formulations can be compounded. IV dextrose is monohydrated and provides 3.4 kcal/g, in comparison with dietary carbohydrate, which has a caloric density of 4 kcal/g.

Glycerol, a sugar alcohol with a caloric density of 4.3 kcal/g, is also available (as a 3% mixture with 3% amino acids) for administration as a peripheral parenteral nutrient formulation.

Unfortunately, because of the dilute formula necessary for peripheral administration, large volume of formula may be necessary to meet the patient's caloric requirements, limiting the usefulness of the formulation. Other carbohydrates such as fructose, sorbitol, and invert sugar have been used investigationally in parenteral nutrient formulations but are associated with adverse effects and are not available commercially.

Lipid

Lipid for IV use is supplied as emulsions of either soybean oil or a 50:50 physical mixture of soybean and safflower oils that provide long-chain fatty acids (>16 carbon length). The soybean oil emulsion is available in three concentrations: 10%, 20%, and 30%. The soybean/safflower oil emulsion is available as 10% and 20%. The 10% and 20% IV lipid emulsions may be administered concurrently (IV piggyback) with dextrose/amino acid solutions or admixed with dextrose and amino acids. The 30% IV lipid emulsion should not be used for IV piggyback administration. It is used exclusively for compounding formulations that combine dextrose, amino acids, and lipid in the same container.

Although lipid has a caloric density of 9 kcal/g, the caloric density of the IV lipid emulsions is increased to approximately 10 kcal/g by the addition of glycerol, which is added to adjust the osmolarity. Egg phospholipids are also added as emulsifiers. The phospholipids are derived from egg yolks; therefore, IV lipids are contraindicated in patients with severe egg allergies, especially egg yolk allergies. Phospholipids also contribute approximately 15 mmol/L of phosphorus.

Medium-chain triglycerides (MCTs) are used investigationally. MCTs are 6 to 12 carbons in length and provide 8.3 kcal/g. Physical mixtures of soybean oil and MCTs are being evaluated for potential use in the United States and are already commercially available in other countries.[35]

Research investigating the use of lipid formulations enhanced with omega-3 fatty acids is also being performed, with results showing improved patient outcomes (decreased length of hospital stay, decreased infections).[36] However, similar to the MCT mixtures, commercially available products are not available in the United States at this time.

Amino Acids

Protein for parenteral administration is available as synthetic amino acids and serves as the source of nitrogen. Nitrogen is the building block of cell structure and is used to produce enzymes, peptide hormones, and serum proteins. Amino acid concentrations of 3.5% to 20% are available commercially and vary slightly from one product to another in the specific amounts of each amino acid, electrolyte content, and pH. Generally, amino acid products are characterized as "standard" mixtures, which provide a balanced mix of essential, nonessential, and semiessential amino acids, or "specialty" mixtures, which are modified for specific disease states. For example, the specialty amino acid mixture for use in patients with hepatic failure contains increased amounts of the branched-chain amino acids and decreased amounts of the aromatic amino acids. Protein formulations designed for critically ill patients are supplemented with branched-chain amino acids but have normal amounts of the other amino acids. Amino acid products for patients experiencing renal failure have increased amounts of the essential amino acids or provide only essential amino acids.[37] Amino acid products designed to meet the special needs of neonates also are available (see Chapter 97).

Table 37-5 Caloric Density of Intravenous Nutrients

Nutrient	kcal/g	kcal/mL
Amino acids	4	
Amino acids 5%		0.2
Amino acids 10%		0.4
Dextrose	3.4	
Dextrose 10%		0.34
Dextrose 50%		1.7
Dextrose 70%		2.38
Fat	10	
Fat emulsion 10%		1.1
Fat emulsion 20%		2
Fat emulsion 30%		3
Glycerol	4.3	
Glycerol 3%		0.129
Medium-chain triglycerides	8.3	

Protein or amino acids have a caloric density of 4 kcal/g. Protein calories have not always been included in the calculation of energy needs for patients receiving parenteral nutrient formulations. Ideally, protein is used to stimulate protein synthesis and tissue repair and is not oxidized for energy; however, the human body cannot compartmentalize energy metabolism this way. Today, the conventional wisdom is to include the protein calories in these total calorie calculations. Table 37-5 summarizes available nutrients and their caloric density.

Micronutrients

Micronutrients are the electrolytes, vitamins, and trace minerals needed for metabolism. These nutrients are available from various manufacturers as either single entities or in combinations. For example, the trace element zinc is available commercially as a single trace element product or as a combination product with the other trace elements: copper, chromium, manganese, and selenium. It is important to be aware of the specific products available in each institution to avoid providing inadequate or excessive amounts of various micronutrients.

PARENTERAL NUTRITION

Patient Assessment: Woman in No Acute Stress

1. S.D., a 39-year-old cachectic woman, is admitted to the hospital with shortness of breath and pleuritic chest pain. She has a history of moderate scleroderma (fibrosis of the skin, blood vessels, and visceral organs) diagnosed 3 years ago. She presents to the hospital with an increasing weight loss over the past 3 months accompanied with regurgitation, vomiting, and poor appetite. Approximately 3 months ago, S.D. weighed 130 lb. Her weight on admission is 98 lb; height is 64 in. Past medical history is also significant for hypertension. Physical examination reveals a thin woman with wasting of subcutaneous fat in the temporal area and squared-appearing shoulders. Attempts at enteral nutrition with

tube feeds have resulted in sustained gastric residual volumes of >400 mL.

Admission laboratory values are sodium (Na), 135 mEq/L (normal, 135–145); potassium (K), 4.0 mEq/L (normal, 3.5–5.0); chloride (Cl), 100 mEq/L (normal, 100–110); bicarbonate (HCO_3^-), 25 mEq/L (normal, 24–30); blood urea nitrogen (BUN), 4 mg/dL (normal, 8–20); creatinine, 0.6 mg/dL (normal, 0.8–1.2); glucose 87 mg/dL, (normal, 85–110); calcium (Ca), 8.2 mg/dL (normal, 8.5–10); magnesium (Mg), 2.0 mg/dL (normal, 1.6–2.2); phosphorus (P), 3.0 mg/dL (normal, 2.5–4.5); total protein, 6.0 g/dL (normal, 6.8–8.3); albumin, 3.5 g/dL (normal, 3.5–5.0); and prealbumin, 15 mg/dL (normal, 15–40). Her white blood cell (WBC) count is 6,800/mm^3 (normal, 4,000–12,000).

Based on history and physical findings, S.D.'s working diagnosis includes aspiration pneumonia and advanced scleroderma with cutaneous, joint, and GI involvement. Assess her nutrition status.

[SI units: Na, 135 mmol/L (normal, 135–145); K, 4.0 mmol/L (normal, 3.5–5.0); Cl, 100 mmol/L (normal, 100–110); HCO_3^-, 25 mmol/L (normal, 24–30); BUN, 1.43 mmol/L (normal, 3–6.4); creatinine, 53 μmol/L (normal, 50–110); glucose, 4.83 mmol/L (normal, 4.7–6.1); Ca, 2.04 mmol/L (normal, 2.3–2.7); Mg, 10 mmol/L (normal, 8–11); P 0.97 mmol/L (normal, 0.81–1.45); albumin, 35 g/L (normal, 35–50); WBC count, 6.8 $\times$ 10^9/L (normal, 4–12)]

Assessment of nutrition status requires evaluation of multiple factors. S.D.'s nutrition history indicates that she is unable to eat because of the gastroparesis, and the scleroderma diagnosis raises the question of nutrient malabsorption. Most striking about S.D.'s history is her weight loss of 30 lb in 3 months, or about 2.5 lb/week. S.D. is now 75% of her usual weight (Eq. 37-2). Another way of analyzing this is that she has lost 25% of her original weight, which is a severe weight loss. S.D.'s physical findings of cachectic appearance, temporal wasting, and loss of subcutaneous fat and muscle in her shoulders are significant. No anthropometric measurements are available. S.D.'s visceral proteins are also in low-normal ranges, indicating both short-term (prealbumin) and longer-term (albumin) malnutrition.

Consideration of these factors leads one to conclude that S.D. is severely malnourished. Her cachectic appearance with loss of subcutaneous fat and muscle, but normal visceral proteins, would be best classified as marasmus malnutrition. If S.D. were to be faced with stress or injury (e.g., major surgery, infection) necessitating use of visceral proteins for energy production, she would likely exhibit characteristics of both marasmus and kwashiorkor, or mixed protein-calorie malnutrition in which fat, muscle, and visceral proteins are all depleted.

2. Why is S.D. a candidate for parenteral nutrition therapy?

S.D. is admitted to the hospital for tests to evaluate her scleroderma, weight loss, and aspiration pneumonia. Many of the expected diagnostic tests will require that S.D. remain NPO. The subjective and objective evidence points to a nonfunctioning GI tract. If the diagnosis of advanced GI scleroderma is accurate, S.D. may require long-term parenteral nutrition therapy. In addition, attempts at enteral nutrition were unsuccessful with continued increased gastric residual volumes indicating decreased GI motility. With her malnourished state, continued inadequate nutrition in the hospital will result in further deterioration of her nutrition status. Parenteral nutrition should be implemented.

Goals of Therapy

CALORIE AND PROTEIN GOALS

3. Calculate calorie and protein goals for S.D.

S.D.'s initial calorie goals are to meet her current energy expenditure needed for basal metabolism and activity of ambulating. S.D. would fall into the category of "moderate stress, malnourished" requiring 25 to 30 kcal/kg/day (Table 37-3). For this calculation, S.D.'s actual weight of 98 lb (44.5 kg) should be used because her metabolism and current energy expenditure reect this decrease in body mass. Using usual weight or ideal body weight in patients who have severe weight loss may result in overfeeding. For S.D., her caloric goal should be 1,112 to 1,335 kcal/day.

Protein goals are estimated based on weight, degree of stress, and disease state. Because S.D. has not had surgery and her stress is minimal, her protein goal should be based on the desire to maintain her current protein status. Using the guidelines provided in Table 37-4, S.D.'s protein dose is 1.2 to 1.5 g/kg/day, or 53.4 to 66.7 g/day. As with energy expenditure, calculations of protein needs are only estimates; the patient's clinical course should be monitored, and the protein dose adjusted accordingly. The protein source for parenteral nutrition is synthetic amino acids. Generally, 1 g of protein is equivalent to 1 g of amino acids. S.D. will need 53.4 to 66.7 g/day of amino acids. If S.D. requires parenteral nutrition following a surgery, her energy or calorie goals should be reassessed to include a stress factor.

ACCESS

4. S.D. has a peripheral IV, and her peripheral access appears to be adequate. Is she a candidate for using a peripheral parenteral nutrition formulation?

With good peripheral access, S.D. meets one of the criteria for peripheral parenteral nutrition. Furthermore, she should be able to tolerate the volume of a peripheral parenteral nutrition formulation necessary to meet her goals. A common complication (up to 70%) of peripheral parenteral nutrition is phlebitis, which occurs within 72 hours.[27,38] Phlebitis is usually attributed to the acidic pH or hyperosmolarity of the nutrient formulation. The osmolarity of typical peripheral parenteral feedings ranges from 600 to 900 mOsm/L. Osmolarity of a dextrose/amino acid formulation can be approximated quickly by multiplying the % dextrose concentration by 50 and the % amino acid concentration by 100. Alternatively, the osmolarity can be estimated by multiplying the number of grams of dextrose by 5 and the number of grams of amino acids by 10, then dividing by the total volume in liters. Approximately 150 mOsm/L should be added for contribution of electrolytes, vitamins, and trace elements. Although the concurrent administration of fat emulsions (up to 60% of nonprotein calories) decreases osmolarity, buffers the pH, and improves peripheral vein tolerance, it does not eliminate the risk of thrombophlebitis.[39]

Because parenteral nutrition is anticipated to be a long-term therapy for S.D., it would be most appropriate to obtain central venous access. Central access allows for longer-term access, more concentrated solutions, and has no osmolarity restrictions.

FORMULATION DESIGN

Macronutrients and Micronutrients

5. Design a parenteral nutrient base formulation for S.D. based on the caloric and protein goals determined previously.

S.D.'s caloric goal was determined to be approximately 1,300 kcal/day and 60 g protein/day. Giving 60 g of protein per day would provide 240 kcal/day (1 g protein = 4 kcal). Subtracting these protein calories from total desired calories results in the amount of nonprotein calories (to be provided by carbohydrates and fat) needed. For S.D., this would be 1,300 total calories – 240 protein calories = 1,060 nonprotein calories needed. Typically, dextrose should account for 60% to 70% of nonprotein calories, and lipids would account for the remaining 30% to 40% of nonprotein calories. Providing S.D. with 742 kcal of dextrose (approximately 218 g of dextrose; 1 g dextrose = 3.4 kcal) would supply 70% of nonprotein calories as dextrose. The remaining 30% of nonprotein calories would be provided by lipids at 318 kcal (31.8 g of lipids; 1 g of IV lipids = 10 kcal).

As with any medical therapy, the parenteral nutrition formula should be adjusted based on patient response and tolerance. If S.D. had complications of hyperglycemia, the dextrose component could be reduced with a subsequent increase in the lipid proportion of nonprotein calories. If hypertriglyceridemia resulted, the lipid component may be reduced with a subsequent increase in dextrose.

S.D.'s nutrient formulation should also contain standard amounts of electrolytes, as well as a daily dose of IV multivitamins and trace elements.

6. The pharmacy has the following stock solutions available for compounding the parenteral nutrition formula: dextrose 70%, amino acids 10%, and IV lipids 20%. How much of each stock solution is needed to compound the parenteral nutrition formula determined previously?

For dextrose, a 70% stock solution provides 70 g of dextrose/100 mL. To obtain 218 g of dextrose, 311 mL of the stock solution are needed:

$$\text{mL} = \frac{218 \text{ g dextrose} \times 100 \text{ mL}}{70 \text{ g dextrose}} = 311.4 \text{ mL} \qquad \text{(37-A)}$$

Similarly, the volume necessary to provide 60 g of amino acids is 600 mL. IV lipids at 20% provide 20 kcal/mL or 20 g/100 mL. Using this stock solution, 159 mL would provide 31.8 g of lipids. The total volume of the compounded solution would be 1,070 mL/day.

Fluids

7. The institution uses a total nutrient admixture (TNA) system, and S.D.'s parenteral nutrient formulation is provided in 1,070 mL/day. Will this meet S.D.'s maintenance fluid requirements?

Maintenance fluid needs can be estimated using several methods. The simplest method uses 30 to 35 mL/kg/day as the basis. Another method is to provide 1,500 mL for the first 20 kg body weight plus an additional 20 mL/kg for actual weight beyond the initial 20 kg. Both methods provide estimates of fluid needs for basic maintenance, and additional fluid must be provided for increased losses such as vomiting, nasogastric (NG) tube output, diarrhea, or large open wounds. S.D.'s fluid needs are estimated as follows:

$$\begin{aligned} \text{mL/day} &= 1{,}500 \text{ mL} + [(20 \text{ mL/kg})(44.5 \text{ kg} - 20 \text{ kg})] \\ &= 1{,}500 \text{ mL} + (20 \text{ mL/kg})(24.5 \text{ kg}) \\ &= 1{,}500 \text{ mL} + 490 \text{ mL} \\ &= 1{,}990 \text{ mL} \end{aligned} \qquad \text{(37-B)}$$

The peripheral parenteral nutrient formulation will not meet S.D.'s needs of 1,990 mL/day. The parenteral nutrition formula may be supplemented with sterile water to make the final formula 1,990 mL. Another option would be to provide the additional fluids via a separate IV line. It is important to not supply fluids in excess. The extra fluid intake may put patients at risk for becoming fluid overloaded, manifesting as hypervolemic, hypotonic hyponatremia. Therefore, S.D. should be monitored for signs of fluid overload, including peripheral edema, shortness of breath, daily intake exceeding daily output, hyponatremia, and rapidly increasing weight.

Monitoring and Management of Complications

8. What metabolic complication is a potential concern due to S.D.'s malnutrition?

Refeeding syndrome is the term used to define the severe hypophosphatemia and associated metabolic complications that occur when malnourished patients receive a concentrated source of calories via parenteral or enteral nutrition. This phenomenon was first reported when the Holocaust victims and prisoners of war in World War II were rescued and given normal food and liquid intake. Complications coinciding with refeeding these individuals included hypertension, cardiac insufficiency, seizures, coma, and death. These complications were reported later in the 1970s and 1980s, with the introduction of parenteral nutrition in chronically ill, essentially starved hospitalized patients.

Metabolic complications from refeeding are associated primarily with severe hypophosphatemia, but hypokalemia, hypomagnesemia, vitamin deficiencies, fluid intolerance, and glucose alterations may occur. In the starved, depleted individual, there is a loss of lean body mass, water, and minerals. Individuals may preserve some intracellular electrolytes, including phosphorus. When these individuals are given a concentrated source of calories, the carbohydrates are converted to glucose. Glucose, in turn, results in the secretion of insulin. The release of insulin enhances the uptake of glucose, water, phosphorus, and other intracellular electrolytes. The combination of phosphorus depletion and intracellular uptake causes severe hypophosphatemia.

To minimize the risk of refeeding syndrome in S.D., all electrolyte abnormalities must be corrected before any nutrition is initiated. Because S.D.'s electrolytes are within normal range, no adjustments are necessary. Nutrition should then be implemented slowly and vitamins administered routinely. Electrolytes, including phosphorus, potassium, magnesium, and glucose, should be monitored at least daily over the first week. Although electrolyte and mineral abnormalities may not be avoided, careful recognition of and close monitoring for refeeding syndrome will prevent serious complications.[40,41]

9. **Members of the medical team are anxious to have S.D. gain weight and are concerned by her malnourished appearance. Therefore, there is a desire to increase the calories provided to S.D. What potential complications could result from overfeeding S.D.?**

Overfeeding should be avoided in all patients, especially those with respiratory concerns (i.e., mechanically ventilated, chronic obstructive airway disease). Overfeeding with carbohydrates is particularly detrimental because of the amount of CO_2 produced relative to the amount of O_2 consumed. This results in CO_2 retention that may lead to acid–base disturbances. Complete oxidation of carbohydrate is demonstrated at dextrose infusions of 4 to 5 mg/kg/minute. Infusions exceeding this rate increase CO_2 production and may cause respiratory distress. In designing a parenteral nutrient formulation for S.D., it is important to provide a moderate calorie dose and to limit her dextrose dose to <4 mg/kg/minute.[42,43] S.D.'s current parenteral nutrition formulation provides 3.4 mg/kg/minute of dextrose.

For adults, the daily lipid intake should not exceed 2.5 g/kg/day. However, current literature supports a maximum of 1 g/kg/day. S.D.'s formulation provides approximately 32 g of lipid daily, or 0.72 g/kg/day. It is also important to monitor serum triglyceride levels to assess tolerance to this dose of IV lipid. If the blood sample is obtained while the triglycerides are infusing, as with the TNA formulation, a serum triglyceride concentration of 400 mg/dL, although elevated, is acceptable.[44] Hypertriglyceridemia can sometimes be noted quickly by gross observation of the blood sample.

Patient Assessment: Man in Moderate Stress

10. **D.C., a 38-year-old man with a 12-year history of Crohn's disease, is admitted to the hospital after being evaluated in the clinic for a complaint of increasing abdominal pain, nausea, and vomiting for 9 days, and no stool output for 5 days. Questioning reveals that over the past week he has been drinking only liquids secondary to nausea and vomiting, and his weight has decreased 10 lb during that time. D.C.'s medical history is significant for frequent exacerbations of his Crohn's disease during the past 2 years. His surgical history includes an exploratory laparotomy 6 months ago for resection of 10 cm of ileum. Family and social histories are noncontributory. His current medications include mesalamine 1,000 mg orally (PO) four times a day (QID) and prednisone 10 mg PO every day. Review of systems is positive for severe abdominal pain. On physical examination, D.C. appears thin, and his abdomen is distended. Vital signs are notable for a temperature of 38.3°C, heart rate of 98 beats/minute, and a blood pressure (BP) of 108/71 mmHg. He is 6 feet tall and weighs 60.5 kg. His medical record indicates that 1 month ago he weighed 64 kg, and 6 months ago, his weight was 70 kg. Abdominal radiographs are consistent with a small bowel obstruction.**

Admission laboratory values are Na, 131 mEq/L (normal, 135–145); K, 3.2 mEq/L (normal, 3.5–5.0); Cl, 98 mEq/L (normal, 100–110); HCO_3^-, 28 mEq/L (normal, 24–30); BUN, 19 mg/dL (normal, 8–20); creatinine, 0.9 mg/dL (normal, 0.8–1.2); glucose, 105 mg/dL (normal, 85–110); albumin, 3.2 g/dL (normal, 3.5–5.0); WBC count, 10,900/mm^3 (normal, 4,000–12,000); hematocrit (Hct), 46% (normal, 34%–50%); alanine aminotransferase (ALT), 29 U/L (normal, 20–70); aspartate aminotransferase (AST), 25 U/L (normal, 20–55); alkaline phosphatase, 45 U/L (normal, 40–125); and total bilirubin, 0.5 mg/dL (normal, 0–1.2).

D.C. is admitted with a diagnosis of a small bowel obstruction secondary to a stricture or narrowed area in his small intestine. The plan is to manage him with IV fluids, bowel rest, decompression, and possible surgery. Why is D.C. a candidate for parenteral nutrition?

[SI units: Na, 131 mmol/L (normal, 135–145); K, 3.2 mmol/L (normal, 3.5–5.0); Cl, 96 mmol/L (normal, 100–110); HCO_3^-, 28 mmol/L (normal, 24–30); BUN, 6.78 mmol/L (normal, 3–6.4); creatinine, 54 μmol/L (normal, 50–110); glucose, 6.5 mmol/L (normal, 4.7–6.1); albumin, 32 g/L (normal, 35–50); WBC count, 10.9 × 10^9/L (normal, 4–12); Hct, 0.46 (normal, 0.34–0.50); ALT, 0.334 μkat/L (normal, 0.03–0.4); AST, 0.25 μkat/L (normal, 0.1–0.28); alkaline phosphatase, 0.75 μkat/L (normal, 0.48–1.5); total bilirubin, 8.5 μmol/L (normal, 0–20)]

Parenteral nutrition should be considered when the patient's nutrient intake has been inadequate for 7 days or longer and the GI tract is not functioning. D.C. has eaten little in the past week, and his 5% decrease in weight is of concern. Furthermore, his weight has decreased by more than 10% over the past 6 months, which is considered a severe weight loss. D.C. is not expected to resume oral intake because his small bowel obstruction is being managed conservatively with bowel rest and decompression.

Assessment of weight loss should include evaluation of hydration status, especially because D.C.'s vomiting and minimal oral intake for the past week place him at risk of dehydration. Loss of lean body mass is probably less than that reflected by the decrease in weight. Although D.C. may be dehydrated, he also may have significant loss of muscle resulting from his chronic intake of prednisone, which stimulates gluconeogenesis and muscle breakdown for amino acids. In addition, D.C.'s admission serum albumin concentration is low at 3.2 g/dL. His hydration status should be considered when evaluating this visceral protein, since D.C.'s serum albumin concentration will probably decrease further after he is rehydrated.

One factor contributing to his low serum albumin is the loss of proteins from the GI tract (protein-losing enteropathy) during exacerbations of his Crohn's disease. Continued inadequate nutrient intake increases his risk of malnutrition. Some type of specialized nutrition support should be initiated, and because D.C.'s GI tract is not functioning, parenteral nutrition is indicated.

11. **What type of malnutrition does D.C. have?**

At this point, D.C. exhibits some loss of fat and muscle, as well as depletion of visceral proteins. He has components of both marasmus and kwashiorkor malnutrition; therefore, he would be considered to have mixed protein-calorie malnutrition.

Calorie and Protein Goals

12. **After hydration with IV fluids, D.C.'s weight is 62.5 kg. Parenteral nutrition therapy was delayed because, within 24 hours after admission, D.C. developed severe abdominal pain and distention and required surgery. An exploratory laparotomy was performed, and 25 cm of ileum was resected to remove the area of bowel with severe disease and a stricture that was causing the obstruction. A small abscess near his colon was also drained. His postoperative medications include hydrocortisone 100 mg IV Q 8 hr and piperacillin-tazobactam 4.5 g IV Q 6 hr. Bowel sounds**

are absent. He has a right subclavian triple-lumen central venous catheter and a nasogastric (NG) tube output of 1,800 mL/day. His urine output is 1,400 mL/day. Parenteral nutrition is to begin on postoperative day 1. Calculate energy and protein goals for D.C.

Using the Harris-Benedict equation for men, his current weight of 62.5 kg, height of 182.9 cm, and age of 38 years, D.C.'s BEE is 1,583 kcal/day (Table 37-3). To estimate his total energy expenditure, the BEE should be modified with an activity factor for being confined to bed of 1.2 and a stress factor of 1.2 for surgery. These modifications result in an estimated energy expenditure of 40% greater than his BEE, or 2,216 kcal/day. Using the simpler method for moderate stress (27 kcal/kg/day) results in an estimated energy expenditure of 1,875 kcal/day. Therefore, an energy goal of 2,000 kcal/day is reasonable. In a similar manner, his protein goal (Table 37-4) for moderate stress is 75 to 94 g/day of protein (1.2–1.5 g/kg/day).

Formulation Design

13. Design a single daily bag, TNA parenteral nutrient formulation for D.C. that provides 2,200 kcal and 90 g of amino acids with a nonprotein calorie distribution of 75% carbohydrate and 25% lipid. The macronutrients available on the formulary for compounding the parenteral nutrient formulations are 70% dextrose, 30% lipid emulsion, and 10% amino acids.

1. Amino acids calculation

$$\text{Calories from amino acids (protein)} = 90\text{ g} \times 4.0\text{ kcal/g} = 360\text{ kcal}$$

$$\text{mL of 10\% amino acids} = \frac{90\text{ g}}{0.1\text{ g/mL}} = 900\text{ mL} \quad \text{(37-C)}$$

2. Dextrose calculation

$$\text{Calories from dextrose} = (2{,}200 - 360)(0.75) = 1{,}380\text{ kcal}$$

$$\text{g of dextrose} = \frac{1{,}380\text{ kcal}}{3.4\text{ kcal/g}} = 406\text{ g} \quad \text{(37-D)}$$

$$\text{mL of 70\% dextrose} = \frac{406\text{ g}}{0.7\text{ g/mL}} = 580\text{ mL}$$

3. Lipid emulsion calculation

$$\text{Calories from lipid} = (2{,}200 - 360)(0.25)\text{ or }(1{,}840 - 1{,}380) = 460\text{ kcal}$$

$$\text{mL 30\% lipid emulsion} = \frac{460\text{ kcal}}{3.0\text{ kcal/mL}} = 153\text{ mL} \quad \text{(37-E)}$$

4. Calculation of final volume

$$\begin{array}{r} 900\text{ mL amino acids 10\%} \\ 580\text{ mL dextrose 70\%} \\ 153\text{ mL lipid emulsion 30\%} \\ \hline 1{,}633\text{ mL total volume} \end{array} \quad \text{(37-F)}$$

Other additives such as electrolytes, vitamins, and trace elements are included in the parenteral nutrient formulation and slightly increase the final volume to 1,800 mL/day. The infusion rate for this formulation can be calculated as follows:

$$\text{Hourly infusion rate (mL/hr)} = \frac{1{,}800\text{ mL/day}}{24\text{ hr/day}} = 75\text{ mL/hr} \quad \text{(37-G)}$$

D.C.'s parenteral nutrient formulation of 1,800 mL/day will not meet his maintenance fluid needs of 2,350 mL/day (see question 7). He will require extra fluid to meet the remainder of his basic fluid needs plus additional fluid to replace the fluid loss from his NG tube. These additional fluids should be provided through another IV.

Monitoring and Management of Complications

METABOLIC COMPLICATIONS: ESSENTIAL FATTY ACID DEFICIENCY

14. What consequences are associated with providing only dextrose and amino acids to meet D.C.'s nutrient needs?

A small amount of lipid is necessary to prevent essential fatty acid deficiency (EFAD). The essential fatty acids, linoleic and alpha-linolenic, are those that cannot be synthesized by humans. Of these, linoleic acid appears to be the only one required by adults. The continuous infusion of hypertonic dextrose from the parenteral nutrition is associated with high circulating concentrations of insulin. Because insulin promotes lipogenesis rather than lipolysis, linoleic acid cannot be released from adipose tissue.[45]

Clinical symptoms of EFAD are dry, thickened, scaly skin, hair loss, poor wound healing, and thrombocytopenia, which may be observed after a few weeks to months of lipid-free parenteral feedings.[46] Biochemical evidence of EFAD, determined by a triene:tetraene ratio of >0.4, may be seen after 1 week of lipidfree parenteral feedings and is characterized by a decrease in the serum concentrations of linoleic and arachidonic acids and an increase in the concentration of 5,8,11-eicosatrienoic acid.[45] The requirement for essential fatty acids is 1% to 4% of total caloric intake and can usually be met by the administration of 500 mL of a 10% lipid emulsion twice weekly or 500 mL of a 20% lipid emulsion once a week to patients receiving a dextrose/amino acid parenteral nutrient formulation.[10,45] The lipid emulsions should be infused at a rate of <0.11 g/kg/hour to prevent adverse effects, which include impaired hepatic, pulmonary, immune, and platelet function.[35]

METABOLIC CONSEQUENCES OF EXCESSIVE DEXTROSE ADMINISTRATION

15. What are the benefits of using a mixed-fuel system, combining dextrose and fat to meet energy needs?

Providing a portion of nonprotein calories as fat may reduce the metabolic consequences of excessive dextrose administration. The maximum rate of dextrose metabolism in humans is 5 to 7 mg/kg/minute, or approximately 7 g/kg/day. In doses of

>7 g/kg/day, dextrose is used inefficiently and is converted to fat.[46] The conversion to fat may be associated with respiratory compromise and hepatic dysfunction.[47–49] Hyperglycemia, another complication of excessive dextrose infusion, is associated with electrolyte and acid–base disturbances, osmotic diuresis, increased risk of infections (especially *Candida albicans*), and altered phagocyte and complement function. Furthermore, using a mixed-fuel system allows the administration of a small amount of IV lipid daily and avoids the need for larger boluses of lipid twice weekly to prevent EFAD. Rapid administration of IV lipids has been associated with alterations in the reticuloendothelial system that are not observed with continuous administration of small doses.[50] Typically, a mixed-fuel system provides 15% to 30% of nonprotein calories as fat, 70% to 85% as carbohydrate.

Total Nutrient Admixtures

16. What are the advantages to combining the dextrose, fat, and amino acids in one container?

The system of providing one container per day offers the advantage of convenience to pharmacy staff, nursing personnel, and the patient. The pharmacy department usually prepares TNA only once per day and therefore requires fewer supplies and inventory; waste of unused feeding formulations is minimized as well. Nursing time to administer TNAs is decreased because only one bag is hung per day, minimizing venous catheter interruptions and avoiding the need to manipulate a secondary infusion of lipid emulsions, as well as additional IV tubing and an infusion pump.[51]

Although there are many practical benefits to using TNA parenteral feeding formulations, this system is not without concerns. These formulations must be mixed in plastic containers constructed with ethylvinylacetate. Containers with diethylhexylphthalate (DEHP) should be avoided because this toxic material may by extracted by the lipid and may harm patients. The addition of lipid to the traditional mixture of dextrose and amino acids converts this solution to a complex emulsion formulation with physiologic differences that alter the stability of the product.[52] These differences must be considered in the compounding of TNA parenteral feeding formulations.

STABILITY

17. How stable are the TNA parenteral feeding formulations?

IV lipid emulsions alone gradually deteriorate over time because of increased formation of free fatty acids and a resultant decrease in pH. When lipids are mixed with dextrose and amino acids, this process is accelerated. IV lipid products commercially available in the United States use an anionic egg yolk phosphatide emulsifier, which stabilizes the lipid droplets of the dispersed phase with the aqueous external phase and maintains the integrity of the dispersion. Because the emulsifier is anionic, the addition of any substance with cationic properties can neutralize the negative charge of the emulsifier and alter the emulsion's stability. When the emulsion becomes unstable or breaks down, the fat particles begin to aggregate and the particle size increases.

Destabilization of the emulsion occurs in steps that begin with creaming and end with the coalescence of the lipid particles, or "cracking" of the emulsion. A decrease in pH and the addition of divalent cations (Mg^{2+}, Ca^{2+}) increase fat particle size. Although dextrose decreases the pH, the addition of amino acids provides an adequate buffer for this variable. The amount of divalent cations added to TNAs should be limited to minimize the risk of emulsion instability. Trivalent cations such as iron should never be added to a TNA parenteral nutrient formulation. Nutrient formulations containing lipid must be assessed visually for signs of phase separation, in which the instability of the emulsion is manifested by "oiling out," indicated by a continuous layer of oil or individual fat droplets. Fat emulsion particles have an average size of 0.5 μm. A destabilized emulsion is not visibly apparent until the lipid particles are 40 to 50 μm. Fat particles as small as 5 μm may occlude pulmonary capillaries.[51,52] Therefore, the use of a 1.2-μm filter is recommended to protect against the infusion of enlarged lipid particles.[34,51]

Using dual-chamber bags may extend the shelf life of TNAs because they allow the lipid to be physically separated from the dextrose, amino acids, and other additives until it is time to administer the feeding. The use of dual-chamber bags has the greatest advantage for the home care setting, where up to a week's supply of parenteral feedings are prepared at one time.[51]

After preparation, TNAs should be refrigerated (4°C) to preserve stability. Once the bag is removed from the refrigerator, it may be warmed to room temperature and the contents mixed well before administration. Mixing is best accomplished by gently inverting the container up and down to ensure top-to-bottom transfer of the fluid. Vigorous shaking should be avoided because it introduces air, which can destabilize the emulsion.[51,52]

MICROBIAL GROWTH

18. How does the microbial growth in TNAs compare with that of dextrose/amino acid formulations?

Dextrose/amino acid parenteral nutrient formulations are not conducive to growth of most organisms because of their high osmolarity (>2,000 mOsm/L) and acidic pH. Lipid emulsions alone, however, are isotonic and have a physiologic pH, providing an optimal growth medium. Combining these three substrates in a TNA provides a formulation with a microbial growth potential that is intermediate between these two.[51,52] The number of central venous catheter violations or manipulations correlates strongly with the incidence of catheter-related infections. From an infection control perspective, the use of a single daily bag TNA system limits the number of manipulations of the central venous catheter to one per day, thereby minimizing touch contamination. The Centers for Disease Control and Prevention guidelines allow TNA or dextrose/amino acid formulations to hang for up to 24 hours. However, because of concerns about the potential of lipid emulsions to support microbial growth, the hang time for lipids when administered alone is 12 hours.[51]

MICRONUTRIENTS

Electrolytes

19. D.C.'s current laboratory values are Na, 137 mEq/L; K, 4.5 mEq/L; Cl, 102 mEq/L; HCO_3^-, 26 mEq/L; BUN, 9 mg/dL; creatinine, 0.8 mg/dL; glucose, 148 mg/dL; Ca, 8.9 mg/dL (normal, 8.5–10.0); Mg, 1.9 mg/dL (normal, 1.6–2.2); P, 2.8 mg/dL (normal,

Table 37-6 Guidelines for Daily Electrolyte Requirements

Electrolyte	*Amount*
Sodium	80–100 mEq
Potassium	60–80 mEq
Chloride	50–100 mEq[a]
Acetate	50–100 mEq[a]
Magnesium	8–20 mEq
Calcium	10–15 mEq
Phosphorus (phosphate)	20–40 mmol

[a] As needed to maintain acid–base balance.

2.4–4.5); and albumin, 3.0 mg/dL. Which electrolytes should be included in D.C.'s parenteral nutrient formulation?

[SI units: Na, 137 mmol/L; K, 4.5 mmol/L; Cl, 102 mmol/L; HCO_3^-, 26 mmol/L; BUN, 3.2 mmol/L; creatinine, 48 μmol/L; glucose, 8.2 mmol/L; Ca, 2.22 mmol/L; Mg, 9.5 mmol/L; P, 0.9 mmol/L; albumin, 30 g/L]

Electrolytes added are sodium, potassium, chloride, acetate (which is metabolized to bicarbonate), magnesium, calcium, and phosphate. Electrolytes should be added to the parenteral nutrient formulation based on the individual patient's needs. However, patients without significant fluid and electrolyte losses, hepatic or renal dysfunction, or acid–base disturbances do well with maintenance doses of electrolytes. Electrolytes may be added individually or as commercially available combination products of maintenance doses, but the electrolyte content of the amino acid solution should be considered. General guidelines for electrolyte requirements for parenteral feedings are included in Table 37-6.

Vitamins and Trace Elements

20. What doses of multiple vitamins and trace elements should D.C. receive in his parenteral nutrient formulation?

Vitamins and trace elements are essential for normal metabolism and should be included in a patient's daily parenteral nutrition regimen. Guidelines for the 13 essential vitamins have been established by the Nutrition Advisory Group of the American Medical Association[53] (Table 37-7).

Guidelines for daily doses of the trace elements zinc, copper, chromium, and manganese have also been developed.[54] In addition to these trace elements, many practitioners provide selenium on a daily basis. Recommended doses of the trace elements are listed in Table 37-8. As with vitamins, trace elements are available as single entities or combination products. Molybdenum and iodine are also available commercially.

21. D.C.'s daily parenteral nutrient formulation of 1,800 mL provides 2,200 calories (75% nonprotein calories as carbohydrate, 25% as fat) and 90 g of amino acids with the following additives per daily volume: NaCl, 75 mEq; K acetate, 70 mEq; phosphate as Na, 27 mmol; $MgSO_4$, 16 mEq; calcium gluconate, 10 mEq; and standard doses of adult multivitamins and multiple trace elements providing copper, chromium, manganese, selenium, and zinc. The infusion is initiated at a rate of 40 mL/hour. Why is this slow infusion rate selected?

Standard practice for administering parenteral nutrient formulations containing hypertonic dextrose is to begin at a slow infusion rate of <250 g during the first 24 hours for most patients and <150 g for patients with known diabetes mellitus or hyperglycemia. The infusion is increased slowly over the next 24 to 48 hours to the goal infusion rate. This initial period allows the clinician to assess the patient's ability to tolerate the nutrient formulation components and to avoid metabolic complications, primarily hyperglycemia.[45] If D.C.'s serum glucose level remains <150 mg/dL, the parenteral nutrient formulation infusion rate can be increased to his goal rate of 75 mL/hour.

Table 37-7 Recommended Adult Daily Doses of Parenteral Vitamins

Vitamins	*Dose*
Fat-Soluble Vitamins	
A	3,300 IU (990 retinol equivalents)
D	200 IU (5 mg cholecalciferol)
E	10 IU (6.7 mg/dL-α-tocopherol)
K	150 mcg
Water-Soluble Vitamins	
Thiamine (B_1)	6 mg
Riboflavin (B_2)	3.6 mg
Niacin (B_3)	40 mg
Pyridoxine (B_6)	6 mg
Cyanocobalamin (B_{12})	5 mcg
Folic acid	600 mg
Pantothenic acid	15 mg
Biotin	60 mcg
Ascorbic acid (C)	200 mg

Monitoring and Management of Complications

METABOLIC COMPLICATIONS

Parenteral nutrition therapy may be associated with multiple metabolic complications. The most common abnormalities are hypokalemia, hypomagnesemia, hypophosphatemia, and hyperglycemia. The plan for parenteral nutrition therapy should include routine monitoring of these serum chemistries to identify complications early and institute methods to manage or prevent complications.

22. Over the next 24 hours, D.C.'s infusion rate is increased to the goal rate of 75 mL/hour. A comparison of his intake and output reveals an overall negative fluid balance because a high volume of gastric fluid is being removed via the NG tube. Laboratory values at this time are Na, 138 mEq/L; K, 3.1 mEq/L; Cl, 91 mEq/L; HCO_3^-, 33 mEq/L; BUN, 28 mg/dL; creatinine, 0.9 mg/dL; glucose, 279 mg/dL; Ca, 7.8 mg/dL; Mg, 1.4 mg/dL; P, 1.8 mg/dL;

Table 37-8 Recommended Daily Adult Doses of Parenteral Trace Elements

Trace Element	*Dose*
Zinc	2.5–5 mg
Copper	0.3–0.5 mg
Chromium	10–15 mcg
Manganese	60–100 mcg
Selenium	20–60 mcg

and albumin, 2.8 g/dL. Arterial blood gas (ABG) results are pH, 7.46 (normal, 7.37–7.44); PO_2, 98 (normal, 85–100); PCO_2, 47 (normal, 35–45); and HCO_3^-, 31 (normal, 24–30). What factors contribute to these metabolic abnormalities?

[SI units: Na, 130 mmol/L; K, 3.1 mmol/L; Cl, 91 mmol/L; HCO_3^-, 33 mmol/L; BUN, 8.96 mmol/L; creatinine, 75 μmol/L; glucose, 15.5 mmol/L; Ca, 1.92 mmol/L; Mg, 0.8 mmol/L; P, 0.58 mmol/L; albumin, 28 g/L]

Hypokalemia

Hypokalemia, a common metabolic abnormality associated with the initiation of parenteral nutrition, usually occurs within 24 to 48 hours. Potassium moves, along with dextrose, from the extracellular to the intracellular space. Furthermore, building lean body mass (i.e., anabolism) requires approximately 3 mEq of potassium per gram of nitrogen provided by the amino acids. Administering dextrose promotes repletion of glycogen stores, which also requires potassium.[41,45,55]

D.C.'s decreased serum potassium concentration is compounded by metabolic alkalosis caused by his loss of gastric secretions through the NG tube and the administration of hydrocortisone. With this type of metabolic alkalosis, the renal excretion of potassium is increased. Additional potassium should be administered and can be provided in D.C.'s parenteral feeding or through another IV.

Hypomagnesemia

Magnesium, like potassium, is primarily an intracellular cation and is considered an anabolic electrolyte. It is common to observe decreases in magnesium serum concentrations during the administration of parenteral nutrient formulations. Synthesis of lean tissue requires 0.5 mEq magnesium per gram of nitrogen.[41,45,55] Additional magnesium can be added to the parenteral nutrient formulation. However, when a TNA formulation is used, the amount of magnesium must stay within the guidelines for the cation content to maintain the stability of the lipid emulsion.

Hypophosphatemia

Hypophosphatemia occurs when phosphorus moves into the cells for the synthesis of adenosine triphosphate (ATP), an important energy carrier. Phosphorus is depleted quickly with the administration of hypertonic dextrose, especially in malnourished patients (see question 8 for discussion of refeeding syndrome). The phosphorus is used for ATP synthesis, primarily in the liver and skeletal muscle. Alkalosis also decreases phosphate stores by stimulating the phosphorylation of carbohydrates. As a component of 2,3-diphosphoglycerate (2,3-DPG), found in red blood cells (RBCs), phosphorus is necessary for the disassociation of oxygen from hemoglobin.[55]

Clinical signs and symptoms of hypophosphatemia usually occur when serum concentrations fall below 1.0 mg/dL; they include lethargy, muscle weakness, impaired WBC function, glucose intolerance, rhabdomyolysis, seizures, hemolytic anemia, reduced diaphragmatic contractility, and death. Moderate to severe, complicated hypophosphatemia can be managed by administering up to 0.625 mmol/kg of phosphate IV.[41,55–57] Although D.C.'s serum phosphorus is not <1.0 mg/dL, it is low (1.8 mg/dL), and he should receive 15 to 30 mmol phosphate in the parenteral nutrient formulation per day. Additional supplements may be necessary to replete his phosphorus stores.[56]

Metabolic Alkalosis

D.C. has evidence of a metabolic alkalosis based on his ABG results, hypochloremia, and elevated bicarbonate level. The continued loss of fluid and HCl from the NG tube is the most probable cause of his metabolic alkalosis. Management of this type of metabolic alkalosis is to replace the fluid and chloride through another IV. Because acetate is converted to bicarbonate and can further contribute to the alkalosis, the acetate salts in the parenteral nutrient formulation can be changed to chloride salts.[55] Nevertheless, the parenteral nutrient formulation is not the primary vehicle for adjusting and supplementing electrolytes and fluids. Instead, the fluid and electrolyte balance should be adjusted with maintenance IV fluid and electrolyte supplements.

Hyperglycemia

Hyperglycemia is a common metabolic complication of parenteral nutrition therapy, especially in stressed patients. Stress alone increases gluconeogenesis, and the administration of hypertonic dextrose compounds the potential for hyperglycemia.[58] D.C. is at particular risk for hyperglycemia because he is recovering from surgery and is receiving steroids, which increase gluconeogenesis.

Persistent hyperglycemia leads to glucosuria and an osmotic diuresis, resulting in dehydration and concomitant electrolyte abnormalities. It also compromises the immune response by causing abnormalities in chemotaxis and phagocytosis and by impairing complement function. Hyperglycemia is associated with an increased risk of infections, especially *C. albicans*. In extreme cases, hyperglycemia progresses to hyperosmolar, nonketotic acidosis and coma, a condition associated with 40% mortality.

Hyperglycemia can be minimized by limiting the dextrose infusion rate to <4 mg/kg/minute.[59] (D.C.'s parenteral nutrient formulation provides 4 mg/kg/minute.) Other measures that will minimize the risk of hyperglycemia include gradually increasing the parenteral nutrient formulation infusion rate, frequently monitoring capillary blood glucose concentrations, and advancing therapy only when the serum glucose is consistently <150 mg/dL for stable patients and <120 mg/dL for critically ill patients. Insulin therapy should be considered if serum glucose concentrations exceed these parameters and can be administered subcutaneously according to a sliding scale, IV by continuous infusion, or by adding insulin to the parenteral nutrient formulation.[60,61] Only regular insulin can be added to a parenteral nutrient formulation. A reasonable strategy for adding insulin to the parenteral nutrient formulation is to begin with 0.1 U of regular insulin per gram of dextrose. This dosage is adjusted depending on serum glucose concentrations.[60] Clinical evidence suggests that treatment of hyperglycemia and maintenance of euglycemia may reduce morbidity and mortality, length of stay, and hospital costs.[61–65]

Formulation Design

Compatibility

23. In response to these serum chemistries, the electrolytes in D.C.'s parenteral nutrient formulation are changed to the following per liter: NaCl, 160 mEq; KCl, 140 mEq; phosphate as K, 60 mmol; $MgSO_4$, 54 mEq; and calcium gluconate, 30 mEq. How

do the doses of calcium and phosphate compare to maintenance doses? What calcium and phosphate incompatibilities should be anticipated? Will the calcium and magnesium content alter the lipid stability?

The dose of calcium ordered for D.C. is more than three times the usual maintenance dose (Table 37-7). This amount of calcium is not necessary because the observed hypocalcemia merely reflects D.C.'s low serum albumin concentration; therefore, less calcium is bound to albumin. D.C. probably does not have true hypocalcemia because his free (or ionized) calcium, which is critical for physiological function, has not changed. If available, obtaining an ionized calcium concentration is advised. However, some laboratories do not have this test available. In this situation, a "corrected" calcium formulation may be used. For every 1-g/dL decrease in serum albumin concentration, there will be about a 0.8-mg/dL reduction in the serum calcium concentration.[66] For D.C., a serum calcium of 7.8 mg/dL will correct to a serum concentration of 8.8 mg/dL ([4.0–2.8 g/dL albumin][0.8] + 7.8 mg/dL calcium).

The amount of phosphate prescribed for D.C. at this time exceeds the usual recommended dose of 15 to 30 mmol/day (Table 37-6). Although D.C. has a low serum phosphorus concentration and needs additional phosphate, increasing the dosage in the parenteral nutrient formulation to 60 mmol/day may be incompatible with the calcium content, resulting in calcium phosphate precipitation. Administering a parenteral nutrient formulation containing calcium phosphate crystals may occlude blood flow, especially in the lungs, and has been associated with adverse events, such as respiratory distress and death.[34,67]

It is important to consider the factors that affect calcium phosphate solubility and to take measures that ensure the solubility limits are not exceeded when preparing parenteral nutrient formulations. The *in vitro* precipitation of calcium phosphate depends on multiple factors, including the calcium salt, concentrations of calcium and phosphate, amino acid concentration, temperature, pH of the formulation, and infusion time. Using calcium gluconate rather than the chloride salt can enhance calcium phosphate solubility. In solution at equimolar concentrations, calcium chloride dissociates more than calcium gluconate, thereby increasing the yield of free calcium available for binding with phosphate.

The amounts of calcium and phosphorus in the formulation are critical. Multiple investigators have varied the calcium and phosphate concentrations in parenteral nutrient formulations and have developed precipitation curves to assist practitioners in determining the amounts of calcium and phosphate that can be added safely to nutrient formulations. These guidelines help predict the points at which calcium phosphate precipitation is likely to occur. However, extrapolating these data to parenteral nutrient formulations different from those described is difficult because these mixtures are extremely complex, and numerous variables affect the interrelationship between calcium and phosphate.

The solubility of calcium and phosphate must be determined based on the volume of the formulation at the time the calcium and phosphate are mixed together, not the final volume. For example, if the electrolytes including calcium and phosphate are added to 1,000 mL of a dextrose/amino acid mixture and then 300 mL of IV fat is added, the calcium phosphate solubility is based on the 1,000 mL, not the final 1,300 mL volume. In addition, some amino acid products contain phosphate ions, and these should be considered when determining calcium phosphate solubility.[34]

Last, calcium and phosphate should not be added to the parenteral nutrient formulation in close sequence. It is recommended to add phosphate first and calcium last, thereby taking advantage of the maximum parenteral volume. Also, during preparation, the parenteral nutrient formulation should be agitated periodically and inspected for precipitates.[68] Other guidelines for improving the solubility of calcium are a final amino acid concentration of >2.5% and a pH <6. Temperature is a critical variable, and an increase in the ambient temperature can facilitate the precipitation of calcium phosphate. Formulations should be infused within 24 hours after compounding if stored at room temperature; if refrigerated, they should be infused within 24 hours after rewarming. Furthermore, slow infusions may decrease solubility. Increasing temperature and slow infusions may result in precipitation in the IV catheter, even if precipitation has not occurred in the infusion container.[34]

The amount of divalent cations, calcium (20 mEq) and magnesium (30 mEq), exceeds the general guidelines for maximum amounts that can be added safely to a TNA without disrupting the stability of the lipid emulsion. A limit of 20 divalent cations per liter is a general guideline. The amount prescribed for D.C.'s regimen is excessive because it provides 50 divalent cations in 1.8 L (28 divalent cations/L) and may result in a potentially unstable admixture.

Last, a 1.2-μm air-eliminating filter should be used when infusing TNA parenteral nutrient formulations, and a 0.22-μm air-eliminating filter should be used for non–lipid-containing admixtures.[34]

Medication Additives

24. In addition to his parenteral nutrient formulation, D.C. is receiving ranitidine 50 mg IV Q 8 hr and hydrocortisone 100 mg IV Q 8 hr, and now he needs insulin. Can these medications be mixed with his parenteral nutrient formulation to simplify his medication regimen?

Patients receiving parenteral nutrition therapy often require concomitant drug therapy. Most patients have adequate venous access or have multiple-lumen central venous catheters, so that mixing medications with the parenteral nutrient formulation is not an issue. However, for some patients with limited venous access, directly added medications or piggybacking medications via a secondary infusion must be considered.

The stability of medications when mixed with parenteral nutrient formulations is a complex issue. Some medications may be added directly to the parenteral nutrient formulation, whereas others should be administered via a secondary infusion set (piggybacked). Many medications have been studied for physical compatibility, but few have been evaluated for pharmacologic activity. Furthermore, the study conditions vary, and different nutrient formulations have been used; therefore, interpretation and application of data from a particular scientific study to a specific nutrient formulation may be difficult. This area of knowledge is growing rapidly, and current information regarding compatibility and stability is available in standard references such as Trissel's *Handbook of Injectable Drugs*.[69]

Although insulin, antibiotics, chemotherapeutic agents, H_2-receptor antagonists, and heparin have been considered for addition to parenteral nutrient formulations in some specific circumstances, the routine addition of medications to parenteral nutrient formulations is discouraged. The addition of insulin to parenteral nutrient formulations may be an option, as described in question 23.

MONITORING PARAMETERS

25. Design a plan to monitor the adequacy of D.C.'s specialized nutrition support and to identify and prevent adverse complications.

Routine evaluation of patients receiving nutrition support should include an assessment of nutrition and the metabolic effects of therapy. Goals for nutrition therapy are estimates of a patient's needs; therefore, the adequacy of therapy to meet these needs must be evaluated. Daily monitoring parameters must include vital signs, body weight, temperature, serum chemistries, hematologic indices, nutrition intake, and fluid intake and output.

The adequacy of nutrition therapy should be assessed weekly. This may include measuring serum concentrations of visceral proteins (Table 37-2). Because prealbumin has a half-life of only 2 to 3 days, serum concentrations of this protein should increase with adequate nutrition and improving clinical status. Albumin, with a much longer half-life, may not change for several weeks to months despite provision of adequate nutrients. In addition, it is reasonable to perform indirect calorimetry to reassess energy expenditure.

Another method to assess the adequacy of protein intake is to evaluate nitrogen balance. This test is designed to estimate the amount of nitrogen retained by comparing the amount of nitrogen administered to the amount of nitrogen excreted (amount "in" vs. amount "out"). The nitrogen "in" is provided by the amino acid component of the parenteral nutrient formulation and other sources from tube feeding or an oral diet. Each commercially available amino acid formulation has a slightly different amount of nitrogen per gram of amino acids, and the manufacturer's product information should be consulted to obtain this value. An average value is 6.2 g of nitrogen per gram of amino acids.

Most of the nitrogen is excreted as byproducts of protein breakdown for energy. This nitrogen is excreted in the urine as urea nitrogen, which increases with increasing stress. To determine this value, urine must be collected for 24 hours and the amount of urea nitrogen (UUN) measured. Some laboratories have the capability of measuring total urine nitrogen, which measures all nitrogen entities in the urine. In addition, some nitrogen lost via skin, respiration, and stool is not measurable but is estimated to be 2 to 4 g/day.

$$\begin{aligned}\text{Nitrogen balance} &= \text{Nitrogen in} - \text{Nitrogen out}\\ &= \frac{\text{AA(g)}}{6.2} - (\text{UUN(g)} + 3\text{ g}) \qquad (37\text{-}3)\\ &= \text{g}\end{aligned}$$

Achieving a positive nitrogen balance is difficult, if not impossible, in critically ill patients; therefore, the calculation may result in a negative number or zero. For convalescing patients, a nitrogen balance of plus 2 to 4 g is acceptable. A negative nitrogen balance prompts a re-evaluation of the amount of protein and energy a patient is receiving. For patients with a negative nitrogen balance, it may be helpful to increase intake of both calories and protein.

Table 37-9 Routine Monitoring Parameters for Parenteral Nutrition

Before Initiating Therapy
Body weight
Serum electrolytes (Na, K, Cl, HCO_3^-, BUN, creatinine)
Glucose
Ca, Mg, P
Albumin, transthyretin
Triglycerides
Complete blood count
Liver-associated tests (AST, ALT, alkaline phosphatase, bilirubin)
INR, Prothrombin time
Daily
Body weight
Vital signs (pulse, respirations, temperature)
Fluid intake
Nutritional intake
Output (urine, other losses)
Serum electrolytes (Na, K, Cl, HCO_3^-, BUN, creatinine)
Glucose
Two or Three Times a Week
CBC
Ca, Mg, P
Weekly
Albumin, transthyretin
Liver-associated tests (AST, ALT, alkaline phosphatase, bilirubin)
INR, prothrombin time
Nitrogen balance

ALT, alanine aminotransferase; AST, aspartate aminotransferase; BUN, blood urea nitrogen; Ca, calcium; CBC, complete blood count; Cl, chloride; HCO_3^-, bicarbonate; INR, international normalized ratio; K, potassium; Mg, magnesium; Na, sodium; P, phosphorus.

As with all tests, assessment should include monitoring several parameters, including the patient's clinical status. Most important is the identification of trends that may alert one to impending complications. A suggested schedule for monitoring is provided in Table 37-9.

Home Therapy

Enterocutaneous Fistulas

26. S.A. is a 24-year-old female hospitalized following an abdominal trauma injury. Her hospital course includes abdominal surgery to repair a small bowel perforation. On hospital day 10, she presents with a fever and green, purulent fluid draining from a small hole in her previous abdominal incision site. She is diagnosed with an enterocutaneous fistula, which is a communication between her intestine and the skin. The fluid loss from S.A.'s fistula is about 1,300 mL/day. Management will include nothing by mouth (NPO) and parenteral nutrition for 4 to 6 weeks in anticipation that the fistula will heal and further surgery can be avoided. The physician would like to begin parenteral nutrition therapy in the hospital with the plan to discharge S.A. home in a few days. S.A. is 5 feet 4 inch and weighs 54 kg.

Parenteral nutrition therapy in the home has allowed patients such as S.A. to be discharged after a much-shortened hospital stay. Candidates for home therapy must be physically and medically stable, have a strong support network in the home setting to assist with care, and have an appropriate home environment; they must be educated regarding the prescribed therapy.[70]

The first step in designing a parenteral nutrition regimen is to estimate energy and protein needs. S.A. is 10 days post injury, and her estimated requirements would be 25 to 30 kcal/kg/day or 1,550 to 1,620 kcal/day. Protein goals must include adequate nitrogen (protein) for wound healing and replacement for losses from the enterocutaneous fistula. A goal of 1.5 to 1.8 g/kg/day (81–97 g) is reasonable.

To simplify her nutrition and fluid regimen, all of S.A.'s fluids, including parenteral nutrients, electrolytes, vitamins, trace minerals, and water, should be provided in one container per day. S.A.'s home parenteral nutrient formulation can be provided in 3,000 mL/day to meet maintenance requirements (30–35 mL/kg/day) and to replace losses from her enterocutaneous fistula (1,300 mL/day). Nutrients provided include 95 g amino acids (390 kcal); 217 g dextrose (750 kcal); 38 g lipid (375 kcal); and electrolytes, vitamins, and minerals to maintain normal serum chemistries. Initially, daily intake and output must be monitored; therapy should be adjusted based on this information and S.A.'s clinical status.

Adjustments in fluids and electrolytes may be needed. The fluids secreted by the GI tract are rich in electrolytes, including sodium, potassium, chloride, and bicarbonate. Measurement of the electrolyte content of the fistula fluid will determine those that must be replaced, and in what quantities. Both fluid and electrolytes should be replaced to prevent dehydration and electrolyte and acid–base imbalances.

In addition to losses of fluids and electrolytes, the trace element zinc is lost in fluid from the small intestine. Approximately 12 mg of zinc is lost in each liter of small bowel fluid, and this should be replaced to prevent zinc deficiency. Furthermore, zinc may play a role in wound healing.[70] Management of enterocutaneous fistulas may include octreotide 50 to 100 mg given subcutaneously two or three times daily or added to the parenteral nutrient formulation to decrease fistula output.[71]

A home infusion pharmacy will be responsible for preparing S.A.'s parenteral nutrient formulations. Typically, nutrient formulations for 7 days are prepared and delivered to the patient's home. These formulations must be refrigerated until administration; however, formulations should be warmed to room temperature and visually inspected for particulate matter before being administered. Because some additives such as multivitamins are not stable for long periods, the patient or caregiver must add these to the parenteral nutrient formulation just before administration.

Patients and caregivers preparing for home parenteral nutrition therapy must be taught how to manage home therapy. This includes assessment of fluid status, care of a central venous catheter, infection, and the technical aspects of administering parenteral feeding formulations.[72]

Preparation for home parenteral nutrition will include placement of a central venous access device. Various devices are available for long-term therapy.[29,31] However, because the duration of S.A.'s therapy is expected to be 4 to 6 weeks, she may be a good candidate for a PICC.

Cyclic Therapy

27. What other measures can be used to simplify S.A.'s parenteral feeding regimen and encourage ambulation?

After S.A.'s daily nutrient and fluid needs are consolidated and she is stable on that regimen, her parenteral nutrient regimen can be cycled. *Cycling* means infusing the parenteral nutrient formulation over <24 hours so there is some time free from therapy. Cycling is usually done gradually and depends on the patient's ability to tolerate the changes in fluid and dextrose intake. Initially, the infusion period is decreased by 2 to 6 hours, and the infusion rate is increased to compensate for the shorter infusion period. For example, a 24-hour infusion at 100 mL/hour would be changed to a 20-hour infusion at 120 mL/hour. This gradual adjustment is more likely to ensure that all nutrients are infused and well tolerated. With each incremental decrease in time, the infusion rate should be increased.

Vital signs, fluid intake and output, and serum electrolytes and glucose concentrations should be monitored during this period. The serum glucose concentration should be evaluated 30 minutes after the infusion is completed to be sure that hypoglycemia does not occur as the result of the rapid cessation of the nutrient formulation. If hypoglycemia occurs, the infusion rate can be tapered at the end of the infusion because a gradual decrease in glucose intake should minimize the potential for hypoglycemia. Furthermore, the infusion can be gradually increased to minimize sudden hyperglycemia at the beginning of the infusion. Infusion management devices used at home can automatically make these adjustments in the infusion rate. Eventually, the nutrient formulation can be infused over 10 to 12 hours during the night, leaving S.A. free from her infusion bag during the day.

METABOLIC COMPLICATIONS: ELEVATED LIVER-ASSOCIATED ENZYMES

28. After receiving home parenteral nutrition for 3 weeks, S.A.'s liver function tests are found to be elevated. Current values are bilirubin, 0.8 mg/dL (normal, 0–1.2); AST, 70 U/L (normal, 19–25); ALT, 90 U/L (normal, 19–72); and alkaline phosphatase, 100 U/L (normal, 38–126). Could her parenteral nutrition be contributing to these abnormalities?

Elevations in liver function tests are common in adults receiving long-term parenteral nutrition therapy and may be noted as early as 2 to 3 weeks after beginning therapy. The abnormalities are usually mild and transient and do not progress to significant liver dysfunction in adults. The predominant type of hepatobiliary dysfunction is steatosis, whereas other patients develop cholestasis or cholelithiasis. Liver-associated enzyme elevations usually resolve when parenteral nutrition therapy is discontinued. Rarely does this dysfunction proceed to hepatic failure.[73,74]

Although parenteral nutrition-associated liver abnormalities were first noted more than 30 years ago, a cause-and-effect relationship has been difficult to establish because patients have many confounding factors that can also cause liver dysfunction, including medications, inflammatory bowel disease, and sepsis. Other contributing factors are overfeeding with parenteral nutrient formulations containing high amounts of carbohydrate, amino acid deficiencies, excess fat, EFAD, carnitine deficiency, choline deficiency, toxic effects of the amino acid degradation products, bacterial overgrowth in the small intestine, and lack of stimulation of the GI tract.[73,74] Other than avoiding overfeeding with carbohydrate and lipid, there are few options to prevent or manage parenteral nutrition–associated liver abnormalities. Potential treatments include metronidazole and supplements of ursodeoxycholic acid, choline, and carnitine. Patients with progressive liver disease may be candidates for liver and small bowel transplantation.[74]

The elevations in S.A.'s liver enzymes should be monitored weekly for continued increases. Because she may not need lifelong parenteral nutrition therapy, the mild elevations are likely to resolve.

USE OF PARENTERAL NUTRITION IN SPECIAL DISEASE STATES

Hepatic Failure

29. V.G. is a 42-year-old woman with a 15-year history of alcohol abuse, cirrhosis, ascites, and esophageal varices who was admitted to the hospital 5 days ago with an upper GI bleed after a weekend drinking binge. She was supported initially with IV fluids, packed RBCs, and fresh frozen plasma. Endoscopic examination showed bleeding esophageal varices, which were banded. V.G.'s hospital course is now complicated by primary bacterial peritonitis causing a paralytic ileus. On physical examination, V.G. is cachectic, with a large protuberant abdomen and ascites; bowel sounds are absent. She is alert, oriented, and without evidence of encephalopathy. V.G. has a central venous catheter. The plan is to begin parenteral nutrition because she has not eaten in 8 days and is not expected to eat for several more days when her peritonitis resolves. Is V.G. a candidate for a specialty amino acid product specifically designed for use in hepatic failure?

Aromatic Amino Acids and Branched-Chain Amino Acids

Patients with chronic hepatic failure, especially those with alcohol-induced disease, are malnourished and prone to complications such as GI bleeding and infection. The metabolism of glucose, fat, and protein is altered in liver disease. Amino acid metabolism is particularly affected because blood is shunted around the liver.

In patients with hepatic insufficiency, adequate protein must be provided to support regeneration of the liver and other vital functions such as the immune system. However, administration of protein may result in hepatic encephalopathy, a severe complication of hepatic failure. Encephalopathy is characterized by progressive depression and impaired neurologic function. The pathogenesis of encephalopathy is controversial, although several theories have been proposed. It is probably caused by the inability of the diseased liver to remove neurotoxins, which accumulate in the brain, resulting in abnormal neurotransmitters. Substances implicated as neurotoxins include ammonia, benzodiazepines, and aromatic amino acids.

Cirrhosis and chronic hepatic failure are associated with significant protein breakdown. The branched-chain amino acids (BCAAs) (e.g., leucine, isoleucine, valine) are used in the muscle as an energy source rather than being released into the circulation. Although the BCAAs are used for energy, the aromatic amino acids (AAAs; phenylalanine, tyrosine, and free tryptophan) are released, increasing circulating concentrations of these amino acids. This results in increased plasma concentrations of the AAAs and methionine and subnormal concentrations of the BCAAs. Both AAAs and BCAAs share a common pathway across the blood–brain barrier and compete for entry into the cerebrospinal fluid (CSF). The "false neurotransmitter" theory proposes that because the concentration of AAAs is greater, more are transported across the blood–brain barrier, where they accumulate and form "false neurotransmitters" such as octopamine and serotonin, an inhibitory neurotransmitter. These compete with normal neurotransmitters for binding sites and impair normal neurotransmission and brain activity.[75]

Based on these theories, an amino acid mixture was designed to provide adequate protein for anabolism while also treating hepatic encephalopathy. To normalize the amino acid profile in the brain, specially designed products with increased amounts of BCAAs and decreased amounts of both AAAs and methionine are available (Table 37-10). Controversy exists with regard to the ability of this special amino acid mixture to improve encephalopathy by altering the amino acid profile of the CSF.[75–77] Generally, this amino acid mixture is reserved for patients with significant hepatic encephalopathy.

Because V.G. is alert, oriented, and without signs of encephalopathy, use of this product is not warranted at this time. Furthermore, protein restriction is not necessary. She should receive 1 to 1.2 g/kg/day of a standard amino acid product, and she should be monitored for signs of encephalopathy. Should she develop hepatic encephalopathy while receiving the standard amino acids, temporary protein restriction of 0.6 to 0.8 g/kg/day is reasonable while the etiology of the encephalopathy is determined and treated. The use of the increased BCAA–decreased AAA mixture may be appropriate for patients with chronic encephalopathy who are unresponsive to pharmacotherapy.[10]

30. What other amino acid mixtures are enriched with BCAAs?

BCAAs have metabolic properties that are considered beneficial during physiological stress (multiple trauma, sepsis, and major surgery). BCAAs can be used as an alternative energy source by the heart, brain, and skeletal muscle. These BCAAs can increase protein synthesis in muscle and liver, decrease excessive proteolysis in muscle, and normalize abnormal plasma amino acid profiles. These unique properties led to the design of commercially available amino acid mixtures that provide about 45% of the amino acids as BCAAs. In comparison, most standard amino acid mixtures contain 19% to 25% BCAAs.

Multiple trials have evaluated the effects of BCAA-enriched amino acid formulations in critically ill patients. Although most evidence suggests that these formulations may improve nitrogen retention, they do not appear to improve clinical outcome.[78,79] It is important to appreciate the differences between the amino acid composition of the mixtures for hepatic failure and those designed for stress. They are not therapeutically equivalent, and one should not be substituted for the other.

Renal Failure

31. O.M. is a 75-year-old man with a long history of hypertension, coronary artery disease, and peripheral vascular disease. Four days ago, he was admitted to the hospital complaining of

Table 37-10 Amino Acid Product Comparison

Description	Product Name	Supplier	Available Concentrations (%)
Standard Formulations			
Contain essential[a] and nonessential[b] amino acids, some available with electrolytes[c]	Aminosyn, Aminosyn II	Abbott	3.5,[c] 5, 7,[c] 8.5,[c] 10,[c] 15
	FreAmine III	B. Braun	3, 8.5, 10
	Novamine	Baxter	15
	ProSol	Baxter	20
	Travasol	Baxter	3.5,[c] 5.5,[c] 8.5,[c] 10
Hepatic Failure Formulations			
Contain essential and nonessential amino acids with a proportion of branched-chain amino acids (leucine, isoleucine, valine)	HepatAmine	B. Braun	8
	HepAtasol	Baxter	8
Renal Failure Formulations			
Contain primarily essential amino acids; RenAmin also contains a complement of nonessential amino acids	Aminess	Baxter	5.2
	Aminosyn-RF	Abbott	5.2
	NephrAmine	B. Braun	5.4
	RenAmin	Baxter	6.5
Stress Formulations			
Contain percentages of leucine, isoleucine, and valine, as well as all essential and nonessential amino acids	Aminosyn HBC	Abbott	7
	FreAmine HBC	B. Braun	6.9
Supplements			
Contain only branched-chain amino acids (isoleucine, leucine, valine); must be used with a general formulation	BranchAmin	Baxter	4

[a]Essential amino acids: isoleucine, leucine, lysine, methionine, phenylalanine, thionine, tryptophan, valine, histidine.
[b]Nonessential amino acids: cysteine, arginine, alanine, proline, glycine, glutamine, aspartate serine, tyrosine.
[c]These concentrations are available with or without electrolytes.
Adapted from references 42 and 43.

severe abdominal pain and was diagnosed with a ruptured abdominal aortic aneurysm, which was repaired surgically. Hypotension and hemodynamic instability requiring pressors, respiratory distress necessitating endotracheal intubation and mechanical ventilation, and renal failure with oliguria have complicated his postoperative course. Furthermore, there is concern that O.M. has an ischemic bowel, which precludes using his GI tract for enteral feeding. Serum chemistries are Na, 130 mEq/L; K, 5.2 mEq/L; Cl, 99 mEq/L; HCO_3^-, 15 mEq/L; BUN, 79 mg/dL; creatinine, 4.0 mg/dL; glucose, 143 mg/dL; Ca, 7.9 mg/dL; Mg, 2.4 mg/dL; P, 5.8 mg/dL; and albumin, 2.7 g/dL. The decision is made to initiate parenteral nutrition therapy via a central venous catheter. In view of O.M.'s acute renal failure, what adjustments should be made in the amount and type of protein (amino acid) provided in the parenteral feeding formulation?

[SI units: Na, 130 mmol/L; K, 5.2 mmol/L; Cl, 99 mmol/L; HCO_3^-, 15 mmol/L; BUN, 28 mmol/L; creatinine, 240 μmol/L; glucose, 9.6 mmol/L; Ca, 1.96 mmol/L; Mg, 12 mmol/L; P, 1.9 mmol/L; albumin, 27 g/L]

The protein dose in acute renal failure should be reduced to 0.6 to 1 g/kg/day because the kidneys have a limited ability to excrete nitrogenous byproducts of protein metabolism.[80] The use of essential amino acids (EAAs) orally has been demonstrated to improve uremic symptoms. Based on this experience, parenteral amino acid mixtures containing only EAAs were investigated. These studies compared parenteral feedings containing dextrose and EAAs to the administration of only dextrose; there was an improved rate of recovery in the group that received the EAA and dextrose. Subsequent studies comparing parenteral nutrient formulations containing a standard mix of both EAAs and nonessential amino acids to EAAs alone have not demonstrated any difference in urea appearance or nitrogen balance.[80,81] The use of EAAs alone in parenteral nutrient formulations for patients with acute renal failure offers no clinical advantage over formulations providing a balanced mixture of EAAs and nonessential amino acids.

32. What other adjustments should be made in formulating a parenteral nutrient formulation for O.M.?

O.M.'s nutrient needs should be provided in the least amount of fluid possible. This can be accomplished by using the most concentrated macronutrients of 70% dextrose, 20% amino acids, and 30% lipid. Using these substrates, a patient's entire needs can often be provided in <1,200 mL/day. Electrolytes should also be adjusted. Initially, patients with acute renal failure may not require potassium, magnesium, and phosphorus because they cannot excrete them. However, once parenteral feedings begin and an anabolic state occurs, these patients commonly experience decreases in the serum concentrations of these minerals and will require small daily doses to maintain normal serum concentrations.

Renal Replacement Therapies

33. O.M.'s renal failure progresses, and he requires renal replacement therapy. Because of his hemodynamic instability,

continuous venovenous hemodialysis (CVVHD) is initiated. How should his nutrition therapy be altered?

Continuous renal replacement therapies (CRRTs), including CVVHD, continuous arteriovenous hemodialysis, continuous venovenous hemofiltration, continuous venovenous hemodiafiltration, and slow continuous ultrafiltration delivery provide a means to remove large volumes of water, nitrogenous byproducts, and electrolytes. Consequently, the delivery of unlimited quantities of fluids, nutrients, and electrolytes is possible. Several factors must be considered in the nutritional management of a patient requiring these therapies. First, a dialysate solution of 1.5% to 2.5% dextrose may be used. If so, some dextrose is absorbed during the process and contributes to the caloric intake. A solution with a 1.5% dextrose concentration at a rate of 1 L/hour delivers approximately 5.8 g of glucose per hour. Increasing the dextrose concentration of the dialysate solution to 2.5% increases the glucose delivery to 11.5 g/hour. The amount of glucose absorbed (550–700 kcal/day) must be considered when designing the amount of calories that will be provided in the parenteral nutrient formulation.[80–85]

The second nutritional consideration is the loss of amino acids across the dialysis filter, which can range from 20 to 28 g of nitrogen per day. Sufficient amino acids should be provided to compensate for this daily loss of 120 to 175 g of amino acids (approximately 6.25 g of amino acids per gram of nitrogen).[80,82,84,85] Protein requirements for patients on CRRT may be as high as 2.5 g/kg/day to promote positive nitrogen balance.[86]

Last, the rapid loss of electrolytes must be considered. Patients may experience dramatic decreases in potassium, magnesium, and phosphorus once CRRT is initiated. This requires frequent monitoring and replacement of these electrolytes, usually as IV supplements rather than as additions to the parenteral feeding formulation.

34. **After several days of CVVHD, O.M. is changed to intermittent (three times a week) hemodialysis. What alterations in his parenteral nutrition are necessary?**

Hemodialysis also allows the passage of amino acids through a semipermeable membrane. The loss is approximately 1 g of amino acids for each hour of hemodialysis with a glucosefree dialysate. This loss is reduced by 50% when a glucose-containing dialysate solution is used. These losses should be considered when determining the dosage of protein that will be provided by the parenteral nutrient formulation. The recommended protein dosage for patients requiring hemodialysis is 1.2 to 1.3 g/kg/day,[80,84,85] but dosages up to 1.8 g/kg/day have been reported.[80,87] In addition, hemodialysis can increase energy expenditure by increasing oxygen consumption and gluconeogenesis; therefore, energy goals should range between 25 to 35 kcal/kg/day.[80] Patients requiring chronic hemodialysis may require protein doses of 1.2 to 1.4 g/kg/day to maintain a positive nitrogen balance and prevent protein malnutrition. Patients requiring peritoneal dialysis have higher losses of protein through the peritoneal cavity and may need 1.2 to 1.5 g/kg/day of protein. In contrast to patients on hemodialysis, those on peritoneal dialysis require fewer calories provided by parenteral feedings because 600 to 800 cal/day may be absorbed through the peritoneal membrane from the glucose-containing dialysate.[80,84,85]

Diabetes, Obesity, and Short Bowel Syndrome

35. **F.L., a 51-year-old man with a history of diabetes mellitus, is hospitalized after receiving a gunshot wound to the abdomen. His injuries included a lacerated spleen, requiring a splenectomy, and several tears in his small and large intestine, necessitating resection of these areas. A feeding jejunostomy tube is placed at the time of surgery, and enteral tube feedings are begun on postoperative day 2. Five days later, F.L. is noted to have a temperature of 39.6°C; a WBC count of 18,900/mm^3; and a distended, tender abdomen. He requires surgery for a small bowel perforation at the site of the feeding jejunostomy and peritonitis. The jejunostomy tube is removed, but F.L. is not expected to have return of bowel function for 7 to 10 days. Parenteral nutrition is to be initiated. F.L. is 5 feet 8 inches tall, and his usual weight is 215 lb. What adjustments should be made in determining F.L.'s energy goals?**

First, F.L. is considered obese, and an adjusted body weight should be calculated and used in nutrition calculations. Obesity is defined as weight exceeding 120% of IBW or a body mass index (BMI) of >27 kg/m^2. F.L. weighs 215 lb, or 98 kg, which is 142% of his IBW of 69 kg –10%. BMI is determined as shown by Equation 37-4.

$$\begin{aligned} BMI &= \frac{\text{Weight (kg)}}{\text{Height (m)}^2} \\ &= \frac{98 \text{ kg}}{(1.73 \text{ m})^2} \\ &= 32.7 \text{ kg/m}^2 \end{aligned} \qquad (37\text{-}4)$$

Obese patients should have their weight adjusted because adipose tissue is not metabolically active. However, about one-fourth of the adipose tissue is composed of some supporting tissue that is metabolically active. Adjusted weight for obesity is calculated using Equation 37-5.[88]

$$\begin{aligned} \text{Adjusted weight} &= (0.25)(\text{Actual Weight} - \text{IBW}) + \text{IBW} \\ &= (0.25)(98 - 69) + 69 \\ &= 76 \text{ kg} \end{aligned} \qquad (37\text{-}5)$$

Using an adjusted weight will decrease the risk of overfeeding, which can further increase adipose tissue and complicate glucose management, especially in a patient with a history of diabetes mellitus. Another approach is to use the Ireton-Jones predictive equation that includes a factor for obesity. Using indirect calorimetry to obtain an MEE may more accurately assess energy expenditure and avoid overfeeding.

36. **What special considerations should be addressed in designing a parenteral nutrient regimen for F.L.?**

Patients without a history of diabetes mellitus may develop hyperglycemia under conditions of stress. Even greater derangements in glucose metabolism may be observed in patients with diabetes mellitus during a critical illness. Dextrose should be limited to 150 g during the first 24 hours of therapy, and the amount of dextrose should not be increased until serum glucose concentrations are consistently <150 mg/dL. It can be anticipated that F.L. will need supplemental insulin when his parenteral nutrient regimen is infused. Insulin may be added to the parenteral nutrient formulation. Initial insulin therapy of 0.1 U of regular insulin per gram of dextrose is a good starting point and should be adjusted to achieve serum glucose levels between 80 to 120 mg/dL. Alternatively, a separate insulin infusion may be used. Frequent capillary glucose monitoring is required in these patients, and it may be necessary to provide additional subcutaneous insulin.[62,63,89] (See question 22 for additional discussion on management of hyperglycemia.)

37. F.L. has a prolonged hospital course complicated by multiple intra-abdominal abscesses, poor wound healing, and necrotic bowel, requiring removal of all but 55 cm of his small intestine but leaving his colon intact. F.L. is given a diagnosis of short bowel syndrome (SBS). What issues should be addressed in the nutrition and metabolic management of this patient?

SBS is characterized by maldigestion, malabsorption, dehydration, and both macronutrient and micronutrient abnormalities. Severe malnutrition will develop without adequate nutrition support. To maintain adequate nutrition status, F.L. will require parenteral nutrition until his remaining intestine begins to adapt. This adaptive period may take several weeks to months to years. Adaptation is enhanced by stimulation of the enterocytes with nutrients, which is best provided by small, frequent oral meals or tube feeding.[10,90,91]

First, F.L. should be continued on parenteral nutrition support, including therapy at home, to meet his nutrient and fluid requirements. After extensive small bowel resection, F.L. may experience severe diarrhea. This increase in GI losses may lead to dehydration and electrolyte abnormalities, including hyponatremia, hypokalemia, hypomagnesemia, hypocalcemia, and metabolic acidosis.[91] F.L.'s fluid status must be monitored and evaluated daily for clinical signs of dehydration or fluid overload.

Medication therapy plays an important role in managing fluid and electrolyte imbalances secondary to excessive GI fluid losses. H_2-receptor antagonists are useful in decreasing gastric secretion, thereby reducing fluid and electrolyte losses and enhancing absorption. Antimotility agents should be used to decrease diarrhea. Octreotide also may have a role in decreasing diarrhea in patients with SBS. Patients with extensive small bowel resections and an intact colon, such as F.L., may develop diarrhea as a result of bile salt depletion.[10,90,91]

Patients with SBS are at risk for developing vitamin deficiencies, especially folate and B_{12}. These patients should receive supplemental B_{12} and IV parenteral or oral liquid multivitamin supplements. GI losses of trace minerals, particularly zinc and selenium, are increased in SBS, and these minerals should be supplemented.[90,91]

Pancreatitis, Respiratory Failure

38. K.R., a 59-year-old woman, is admitted to the hospital complaining of increasing abdominal pain and vomiting. She is diagnosed with pancreatitis. This is her third admission for acute pancreatitis during the past year. Her past medical history is significant for ethanol abuse and chronic obstructive airway disease. An NG tube is inserted, and she is to be NPO. IV fluids are begun for hydration. Over the next 5 days, K.R.'s abdominal pain subsides, her pancreatitis resolves, and she is started on an oral diet. Two days after beginning an oral diet, K.R. complains of severe abdominal pain and is vomiting. She is febrile, her WBC count has increased to 21,000/mm^3, and she is hypotensive, requiring large volumes of IV fluids. Furthermore, she develops respiratory distress and requires endotracheal intubation and mechanical ventilation. Her most recent ABG is notable for pH, 7.36 (normal, 7.37–7.44); PCO_2, 51 mmHg (normal, 35–45); PO_2, 88 mmHg (normal, 85–100); and HCO_3^-, 28 mEq/L (normal, 24–30). This clinical presentation is consistent with severe pancreatic necrosis. A small-bore nasojejunal feeding tube is placed and enteral nutrition therapy is begun. However, K.R. develops severe abdominal pain and distention and bowel sounds are absent, so the enteral feeding is discontinued. The decision is made to begin parenteral nutrition because K.R. is not expected to have a functional GI tract in the near future and her nutrient intake has been inadequate during her hospitalization. What special considerations should be addressed in designing a parenteral feeding formulation for K.R.? Is the use of fat contraindicated in patients with pancreatitis?

Several observations have caused concern over the use of IV lipid emulsions in patients with pancreatitis. The oral ingestion of fats may stimulate pancreatic exocrine function and should be restricted in patients with pancreatitis. Although hyperlipidemia has been well described in patients with alcohol-induced pancreatitis, it is unlikely that it is primarily responsible for initiating the pancreatitis. Hypertriglyceridemia associated with acute pancreatitis is most often seen in patients with hereditary or acquired defects in lipid metabolism. Furthermore, pancreatitis alone may be associated with hypertriglyceridemia.[92]

Several investigators have evaluated the effects of parenteral nutrient formulations containing fat emulsions in patients with acute pancreatitis and have found no stimulation of pancreatic exocrine function. Furthermore, IV lipids did not result in abdominal pain or relapse in patients with a history of pancreatitis. Available data suggest that IV lipid emulsions are a safe and efficacious form of calories for patients with pancreatitis.[92]

Monitoring serum triglyceride concentrations should be part of routine management for patients with pancreatitis and those receiving parenteral nutrient formulations containing lipids. Serum triglyceride concentrations should be maintained at <400 mg/dL with a continuous infusion of lipids and <250 mg/dL when checked 4 hours after the infusion for patients receiving intermittent lipid infusions.[10,44,92] If serum concentrations exceed these parameters, consideration must be given to decreasing or eliminating the IV lipid from the parenteral nutrient regimen.

39. K.R. is recovering from her pancreatitis, and the small-bore nasojejunal enteral feeding tube is reinserted. Tube feeding is considered because she cannot eat by mouth secondary to the endotracheal tube and mechanical ventilation. How should she be transitioned from parenteral to enteral feedings?

Tube feedings can begin with a full-strength isotonic enteral feeding formulation at a slow infusion rate (25 mL/hour). Concurrently, the parenteral nutrient formulation should be decreased to avoid fluid overload and to keep the calorie and protein intake constant. It can be anticipated that K.R. can transition from parenteral to enteral feedings in 24 to 48 hours (see Chapter 36).

REFERENCES

1. Dudrick SJ et al. Long-term parenteral nutrition with growth, development and positive nitrogen balance. *Surgery* 1968;64:134.
2. Grant JP. Nutritional assessment in clinical practice. *Nutr Clin Pract* 1986;1:3.
3. Shopbell JM, et al. Nutrition screening and assessment. In: Gottschlich MM, ed. *The Science and Practice of Nutrition Support*. Dubuque, IA: Kendall/Hunt; 2001:107.
4. McWhirter JP, Pennington CR. Incidence and recognition of malnutrition in the hospital. *Br Med J* 1994;308:945.
5. Leiter LA, Marliss EB. Survival during fasting may depend on fat as well as protein stores. *JAMA* 1982;248:2306.
6. Keys A et al. *The Biology of Human Starvation*. Minneapolis: University of Minnesota Press; 1950.
7. Robinson G et al. Impact of nutritional status on DRG length of stay. *JPEN J Parenter Enteral Nutr* 1987;11:49.
8. Reilly JJ et al. Economic impact of malnutrition: a model system for hospitalized patients. *JPEN J Parenter Enteral Nutr* 1988;12:371.
9. Detsky AS et al. Is this patient malnourished? *JAMA* 1994;271:54.
10. A.S.P.E.N. Board of Directors and the Clinical Guidelines Task Force. Guidelines for the use of parenteral and enteral nutrition in adult and pediatric patients. *JPEN J Parenter Enteral Nutr* 2002;26(Suppl):18SA.
11. A.S.P.E.N. Board of Directors and Task Force on Standards for Specialized Nutrition Support for Hospitalized Adult Patients. Standards for specialized nutrition support: adult hospitalized patients. *Nutr Clin Pract* 2002;17:384.
12. A.S.P.E.N. Board of Directors. Definitions of terms used in A.S.P.E.N. guidelines and standards. *Nutr Clin Pract* 1995;10:1.
13. Lipman TO. Grains or veins: is enteral nutrition really better than parenteral nutrition? A look at the evidence. *JPEN J Parenter Enteral Nutr* 1998;22:167.
14. Braunschweig CL et al. Enteral compared with parenteral nutrition: a meta-analysis. *Am J Clin Nutr* 2001;74:534.
15. Beier-Holgersen R. Influence of postoperative enteral nutrition on postsurgical infections. *Gut* 1996;39:833.
16. Hernandez G et al. Gut mucosal atrophy after a short enteral fasting period in critically ill patients. *J Crit Care* 1999;14:73.
17. Kudsk KA et al. Enteral versus parenteral feeding. *Ann Surg* 1992;215:503.
18. Moore FA et al. Early enteral feeding, compared with parenteral, reduces septic complications: the results of a meta-analysis. *Ann Surg* 1992;216:172.
19. Charney P. Nutrition assessment in the 1990's: where are we now? *Nutr Clin Pract* 1995;10:131.
20. Gabay C, Kushner I. Acute-phase proteins and other systemic responses to inflammation. *N Engl J Med* 1999;340:448.
21. Vanek VW. The use of serum albumin as a prognostic or nutritional marker and the pros and cons of IV albumin therapy. *Nutr Clin Pract* 1998;13:110.
22. Detsky AS et al. What is subjective global assessment of nutritional status? *JPEN J Parenter Enteral Nutr* 1987;11:8.
23. Garrel DR et al. Should we still use the Harris and Benedict equations? *Nutr Clin Pract* 1996;11:99.
24. Frakenfield D. Energy and macrosubstrate requirements. In: Gottschlich MM, ed. *The Science and Practice of Nutrition Support*. Dubuque, IA: Kendall/Hunt; 2001:31.
25. McClave SA, Snider HL. Use of indirect calorimetry in clinical nutrition. *Nutr Clin Pract* 1992;7:207.
26. Krzywda EA et al. Parenteral access devices. In: Gottschlich MM, ed. *The Science and Practice of Nutrition Support*. Dubuque, IA: Kendall/Hunt; 2001:225.
27. Payne-James J, Kwahaja HT. First choice for total parenteral nutrition: the peripheral route. *JPEN J Parenter Enteral Nutr* 1993;17:468.
28. Kane KF et al. High osmolality feedings do not increase the incidence of thrombophlebitis during peripheral IV nutrition. *JPEN J Parenter Enteral Nutr* 1996;20:194.
29. Vanek VW. The ins and outs of venous access: part 1. *Nutr Clin Pract* 2002;17:85.
30. Alhimyary A et al. Safety and efficacy of total parenteral nutrition delivered via a peripherally inserted central venous catheter. *Nutr Clin Pract* 1996; 11:199.
31. Vanek VW. The ins and outs of venous access: part 2. *Nutr Clin Pract* 2002;17:142.
32. ASHP Technical Assistance Bulletin on quality assurance for pharmacy-prepared sterile products. *Am J Hosp Pharm* 1993;50:2386.
33. Total parenteral nutrition/total nutrient admixture. *USP DI Update*. United States Pharmacopeial Convention, Inc.; Rockville, MD; 1996:66.
34. Task Force for the Revision of Safe Practices for Parenteral Nutrition. Safe practices for parenteral nutrition. *JPEN J Parenter Enteral Nutr* 2004;28:S39.
35. Driscoll EF. Intravenous lipid emulsions: 2001. *Nutr Clin Pract* 2001;16:215.
36. Heller AR et al. Omega-3 fatty acids improve the diagnosis-related clinical outcome. *Crit Care Med* 2006;34:972.
37. Kearns LR et al. Update on parenteral amino acids. *Nutr Clin Pract* 2001;16:219.
38. Bayer-Berger M et al. Incidence of phlebitis in peripheral parenteral nutrition: effect of the different nutrient solutions. *Clin Nutr* 1989;8:81.
39. Daly JM et al. Peripheral vein infusion of dextrose/amino acid solutions—20% fat emulsion. *JPEN J Parenter Enteral Nutr* 1985;9:296.
40. Solomon SM, Kirby DK. The refeeding syndrome: a review. *J Parenter Enteral Nutr* 1990;14:90.
41. Brooks MJ, Melnik G. The refeeding syndrome: an approach to understanding its complications and preventing its occurrence. *Pharmacotherapy* 1995;15:713.
42. Mowatt-Larssen, Brown RO. Specialized nutritional support in respiratory disease. *Clin Pharm* 1993;12:276.
43. Talpers SS et al. Nutritionally associated increased carbon dioxide production. *Chest* 1992;102:551.
44. Sacks GS. Is IV lipid emulsion safe in patients with hypertriglyceridemia? Adult patients. *Nutr Clin Pract* 1997;12:120.
45. Matarese LE. Metabolic complications of parenteral nutrition therapy. In: Gottschlich MM, ed. *The Science and Practice of Nutrition Support*. Dubuque, IA: Kendall/Hunt; 2001:269.
46. Driscoll DF. Clinical issues regarding the use of total nutrient admixtures. *DICP* 1990;24:296.
47. Wolfe RR. Glucose metabolism in burn injury: a review. *J Burn Care Rehab* 1985;6:408.
48. Delafoss BY et al. Respiratory changes induced by parenteral nutrition in postoperative patients undergoing inspiratory pressure support ventilation. *Anesthesiology* 1986;66:393.
49. Quigley EMM et al. Hepatobiliary complications of total parenteral nutrition. *Gastroenterology* 1993;286:301.
50. Seidner DL et al. Effects of long-chain triglyceride emulsions on reticuloendothelial system function in humans. *JPEN J Parenter Enteral Nutr* 1989;13:614.
51. Barber JR et al. Parenteral feeding formulations. In: Gottschlich MM, ed. *The Science and Practice of Nutrition Support*. Dubuque, IA: Kendall/Hunt; 2001:251.
52. Driscoll DF. Total nutrient admixtures: theory and practice. *Nutr Clin Pract* 1995;10:114.
53. *Federal Register*, April 20, 2000 (Volume 65, Number 77).
54. Task Force for the Revision of Safe Practices for Parenteral Nutrition. Safe practices for parenteral nutrition. *JPEN J Parenter Enteral Nutr* 2004;28:S54.
55. Baumgartner TG. Enteral and parenteral electrolyte therapeutics. *Nutr Clin Pract* 2001;16;226.
56. Brown KA et al. A new graduated dosing regimen for phosphorus replacement in patients receiving nutrition support. *JPEN J Parenter Enteral Nutr* 2006;30:209.
57. Rosen GH et al. Intravenous phosphate repletion regimen for critically ill patients with moderate hypophosphatemia. *Crit Care Med* 1995;23:1204.
58. Mizock BA. Alterations in carbohydrate metabolism during stress: a review of the literature. *Am J Med* 1995;98:75.
59. Rosemarin DK et al. Hyperglycemia associated with high, continuous infusion rates of total parenteral nutrition. *Nutr Clin Pract* 1996;11:151.
60. McMahon MM. Management of hyperglycemia in hospitalized patients receiving parenteral nutrition. *Nutr Clin Pract* 1997;12:35.
61. Van den Berghe G et al. Intensive insulin therapy in the critically ill patients. *N Engl J Med* 2001;345:1359.
62. Van den Berghe G et al. Outcome benefit of intensive insulin therapy in the critically ill: insulin dose versus glycemic control. *Crit Care Med* 2003;31:359.
63. Montori VM et al. Hyperglycemia in acutely ill patients. *JAMA* 2002;288:2167.
64. Furnary AP et al. Continuous intravenous insulin infusion reduced the incidence of deep sternal would infection in diabetic patients after cardiac surgical procedures. *Ann Thorac Surg* 1999;67:352.
65. Zerr KJ et al. Glucose control lowers the risk of wound infection in diabetics after open heart operations. *Ann Thorac Surg* 1997;63:356.
66. Rose BD. *Clinical Physiology of Acid–Base and Electrolyte Disorders*. 4th ed. New York: McGraw-Hill; 1994:891.
67. Knowles JB et al. Pulmonary deposition of calcium phosphate crystals as a complication of home parenteral nutrition. *JPEN J Parenter Enteral Nutr* 1989;13:209.
68. McKinnon BT. FDA safety alert: hazards of precipitation associated with parenteral nutrition. *Nutr Clin Pract* 1996;11:59.
69. Trissel LA. *Handbook of Injectable Drugs*. 14th ed. Bethesda, MD: American Society of Hospital Pharmacists; 2006.
70. Malone AM. Supplemental zinc in wound healing: is it beneficial? *Nutr Clin Pract* 2000;15:253.
71. Seidner DL et al. Can octreotide be added to parenteral nutrition solutions? Point-counterpoint. *Nutr Clin Pract* 1998;13:84.
72. Hammond KA et al. Transitioning to home and other alternative sites. In: Gottschlich MM, ed. *The Science and Practice of Nutrition Support*. Dubuque, IA: Kendall/Hunt; 2001:701.
73. Quigley EMM et al. Hepatobiliary complications of total parenteral nutrition. *Gastroenterology* 1993;104;286.
74. Buchman A. total parenteral nutrition–associated liver disease. *JPEN J Parenter Enteral Nutr* 2002;26:S43.
75. Teran FC, McCullough AF. Nutrition in liver diseases. In: Gottschlich MM, ed. *The Science and Practice of Nutrition Support*. Dubuque, IA: Kendall/Hunt; 2001:537.
76. Marchesini G et al. Nutritional treatment with branched-chain amino acids in advanced liver cirrhosis. *J Gastroenterol* 2000;35:S1.
77. Fabbri A et al. Overview of randomized clinical trials of oral branched-chain amino acid treatment in chronic hepatic encephalopathy. *JPEN J Parenter Enteral Nutr* 1996;20:159.
78. Skeie B et al. Branch-chain amino acids: their metabolism and clinical utility. *Crit Care Med* 1990;18:549.
79. Oki JC, Cuddy PG. Branched-chain amino acid support of stressed patients. *DICP* 1989;23:399.
80. Wolk R et al. Renal disease. In: Gottschlich MM, ed. *The A.S.P.E.N. Nutrition Support Core Curriculum: A Case-Based Approach—The Adult Patient*. Silver Spring, MD: American Society for Parenteral and Enteral Nutrition; 2007:585.
81. Oldrizzi L et al. Nutrition and the kidney: how to manage patients with renal failure. *Nutr Clin Pract* 1994;9:3.

82. Bellomo R et al. Continuous arteriovenous hemodiafiltration in the critically ill: influence on major nutrient balances. *Intensive Care Med* 1991;17:399.
83. Frankenfield DC et al. Glucose dynamics during continuous hemodiafiltration and total parenteral nutrition. *Intensive Care Med* 1995;21:1016.
84. Charney P, Charney D. Nutrition support in acute renal failure. In: Shikora SA et al, eds. *Nutritional Considerations in the Intensive Care Unit*. Dubuque, IA: Kendall/Hunt; 2002:209.
85. Charney P, Charney D. Nutrition support in renal failure. *Nutr Clin Pract* 2002;17:226.
86. Wooley JA et al. Metabolic and nutritional aspects of acute renal failure in critically ill patients requiring continuous renal replacement therapy. *Nutr Clin Pract* 2005;20:176.
87. National Kidney Foundation. K/DOQI clinical practice guidelines for nutrition in chronic renal failure. *Am J Kidney Dis* 2000;35:S1.
88. Choban PS et al. Nutrition support of obese hospitalized patients. *Nutr Clin Pract* 1997;12:149.
89. McMahon M, Rizza RA. Nutritional support in hospitalized patients with diabetes mellitus. *Mayo Clin Proc* 1996;71:587.
90. Bernard DKH, Shaw MJ. Principles of nutrition therapy for short-bowel syndrome. *Nutr Clin Pract* 1993;8:153.
91. Kelly DG, Nehra V. Gastrointestinal disease. In: Gottschlich MM, ed. *The Science and Practice of Nutrition Support*. Dubuque, IA: Kendall/Hunt; 2001:517.
92. Seidner DL, Fuhrman MP. Nutrition support in pancreatitis. In: Gottschlich MM, ed. *The Science and Practice of Nutrition Support*. Dubuque, IA: Kendall/Hunt; 2001:553.

DERMATOLOGIC DISORDERS

Wayne Kradjan
SECTION EDITOR

CHAPTER 38

Dermatotherapy and Drug-Induced Skin Disorders

Richard N. Herrier

ANATOMY AND PHYSIOLOGY OF THE SKIN

The skin is the largest organ in the body and constitutes, on average, 17% of a person's body weight. The skin's thickness ranges from 3 to 5 mm. Figure 38-1 shows a cross-section of the anatomy of human skin. The major function of the skin is to protect underlying structures from trauma, temperature variations, harmful penetrations, moisture, humidity, radiation, and invasion of micro-organisms. There are three layers of skin: the epidermis, the dermis, and subcutaneous tissue.[1–6]

Epidermis

The epidermis consists of four distinct layers: stratum corneum, stratum lucidum, stratum spinosum, and stratum germinativum. The major function of the epidermis is to serve as a barrier. This layer keeps chemicals and other substances from penetrating into the body and prevents the loss of water from the skin and underlying tissues. The maturation of keratinocytes from the stratum germinativum to the stratum corneum is critical for this barrier function. As keratinocytes

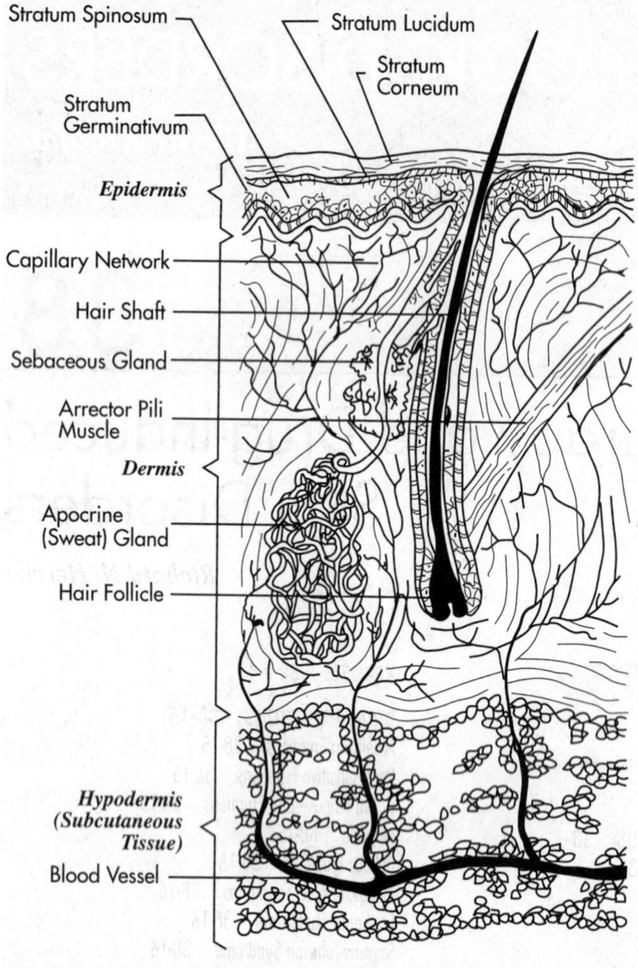

FIGURE 38-1 Cross-section of the anatomy of human skin.

migrate to the skin surface, they change from living cells to dead, thick-walled, nonnucleated cells containing keratin, a hard fibrous protein. It normally takes 26 to 28 days for a keratinocyte to divide, differentiate, move up to the stratum corneum, and be sloughed off.

The *stratum corneum,* which is composed of the dead cells, provides the greatest resistance to the percutaneous absorption of chemicals and drugs. It behaves as a semipermeable membrane through which drugs are absorbed by passive diffusion. Factors that can affect drug absorption are hydration of the skin and damage to the stratum corneum. In general, the greater the damage to the stratum corneum, the greater is the absorption of topically applied drugs. Skin diseases affecting only the epidermis heal without scarring.[1–6]

Dermis

The dermis, which ranges in thickness from 1 to 4 mm, is composed of collagen fibers, elastic fibers, and an extrafibrillar gel of mucopolysaccharides called *glycosaminoglycans* (formally called *ground substances*). The major function of the dermis is to protect the body from mechanical injury and to support the dermal appendages (i.e., apocrine and eccrine sweat glands, sebaceous glands, hair follicles) and the epidermis. It also provides capillary, lymphatic, and nerve supply to the skin and its appendages. The capillary network plays a major role in temperature regulation and provides nutrition to the epidermis. The nerves transmit sensations of touch and pain. Finally, the dermis contains large amounts of water, thus serving as a water storage organ. All but the most superficial injuries to the dermis generally result in scarring as the wound heals.[1–6]

Drugs passing through the epidermis penetrate directly into the dermis and may be absorbed into the general circulation through the capillary network. Generally, only small amounts of topically applied drugs enter the dermis via the sweat glands or the pilosebaceous units.

Subcutaneous Layer

The subcutaneous layer supports the dermis and epidermis, and serves as a fat storage area. This layer helps regulate temperature, provide nutritional support, and cushion the outer skin layers.[1–6]

INFLAMMATORY LESIONS

One of the dermatologic axioms regarding therapy is particularly useful in selecting dosage forms. “If it’s wet, dry it; if it’s dry, wet it.” Paradoxically, wet dressings are most useful in drying acute, inflamed lesions, because they draw out fluid as they evaporate. Ointment types bases are most useful for chronic, lichenified, scaling lesions. The choice of vehicle for chronic lesions is often based on what the patient has found to work best or is willing to use. Frequently, patients with chronic dermatologic conditions use multiple types of vehicles concomitantly (e.g., cream bases [which are drying]) during the day, as they are cosmetically acceptable, and ointment bases at night (greasy, but better emollients).

Acute Lesions

Acute inflammatory lesions are characterized by vesiculation, erythema, swelling, warmth, pruritus, oozing, and/or weeping. Generally, the more severe the dermatitis, the milder is the initial topical therapy. For instance, cool water in the form of an aqueous vehicle, preferably a wet dressing, soak, or bath, is more effective as the initial therapeutic agent than a potent topical corticosteroid applied to a warm, erythematous, weeping dermatitis. The specific approach depends on the part(s) of the body involved.

Subacute and Chronic Lesions

Subacute lesions are characterized by decreasing vesiculation and oozing, and are often covered with crusts. They still require cleaning and drying with aqueous preparations, but for a shorter duration than with acute lesions. Chronic inflammatory lesions are characterized by erythema, scaling, lichenification, dryness, and pruritus. There are no absolute rules for treating chronic lesions. If the lesion is dry, an oleaginous or occlusive base should be used, perhaps with a keratolytic agent.

DERMATOLOGIC DRUG DELIVERY SYSTEMS

A range of dermatologic formulations are available: solutions, suspensions or shake lotions, powders, lotions, emulsions, gels, creams, ointments, and aerosols. Each dermatologic delivery vehicle has specific characteristics and uses based on the type, relative acuteness, and location of the lesion.

Solutions

Solutions provide evaporative cooling, vasoconstriction, and resultant mild antipruritic effects. They soothe and cool inflamed skin, dry oozing lesions, soften crusts, aid in cleaning wounds, and assist in the drainage of purulent wounds. Aqueous solutions are most useful for acutely inflamed, oozing lesions; erosions; and ulcers. In most instances, solutions should be the sole therapy until the oozing or weeping subsides. If other topical medications are applied to oozing or weeping lesions, they will be washed away and will not provide the desired effect. The most commonly used solutions are normal (0.9%) saline and aluminum acetate 5% solution (Burow's solution) diluted 1:10 to 1:40. Solutions are often applied as wet dressings.

The most important component of a solution is water. Although active or inert substances may be added to solutions, the cleansing, drying and cooling effect of water provides the major therapeutic benefit. Some of the products (e.g., Burow's solution) also have *astringent* properties that alter the skin surface and interstitial spaces to cause contraction and wrinkling. Water penetration is reduced to minimize edema, inflammation, and exudation. Table 38-1 lists the most commonly used solutions. Boric acid should not be used as a topical agent because it can be absorbed through the skin, causing systemic toxicity.[7]

Depending on the affected area and its size, a patient may soak the affected area directly in the solution for 15 to 30 minutes three to six times per day. If larger areas are involved or if the affected area cannot be easily soaked (e.g., a shoulder), a clean towel or cloth soaked in the solution (lightly wrung out) is directly applied to the lesion(s) as a wet dressing. The soaked cloth should be left in place for 5 to 10 minutes, then resoaked in the solution and reapplied. The patient may repeat this procedure for 15 to 30 minutes three times daily. Solutions applied with a cloth should have the cloth material wrapped around the lesions several times, if possible. If large areas are involved, the patient may draw a bath, add appropriate amounts of medications, and soak for 15 to 30 minutes three to six times per day. It is impractical to prepare a Burow's solution bath at the 1:10 to 1:40 concentration. Again, the concentration of the Burow's solution is probably insignificant because the major effect of the solution is produced by the water. In general, no more than one-third of the body should be soaked in this manner at any time. One should be aware that evaporation can concentrate solutions, potentially making them too irritating to use. Small volumes of a 1:40 concentration of Burow's solution left standing open at room temperature after 30 to 60 minutes may yield a 1:10 solution. This problem is not as significant with larger volumes or if the solution is stored in a closed container. For this reason, wet dressings should always be freshly prepared (i.e., within 24 hours), kept in closed containers, and never reused. Wet dressings are most comfortable if they are slightly cool or warm, depending on the patient's preference. When drying the affected area after a wet dressing has been used, care must be taken not to irritate the inflamed skin by rubbing it with a towel. The proper technique for drying the skin is to pat the area gently with a soft, clean towel.[7]

Baths

In addition to wet dressings and soaks, topical solutions can be applied to large areas of the body through bathing. In using this type of treatment, the bath should be about half full. Soothing and antipruritic colloidal bath additives may be used to treat widespread eruptions such as lichen planus, pityriasis rosea, urticaria, and other weeping or crusting dermatoses. Colloidal oatmeal (1 cup of oatmeal [Aveeno] mixed with 2 cups of cold tap water and poured into 6 inches of a lukewarm bath) produces a pleasing and soothing bath. Alternatively, a starch bath using 2 cups of hydrolyzed starch (Linit) or cornstarch mixed with 4 cups of tap water and added to a bath may

Table 38-1 Solutions for Wet Dressings or Drying Weeping Lesions

Agent[a]	*Strength*	*Preparation (H_2O)*	*Germicidal Activity*	*Astringent Activity*	*Comments*
Normal saline	0.9% NaCl	1 tsp NaCl per pint H_2O	None	None	Inexpensive; easy to prepare
Aluminum acetate (Burow's solution) (Domeboro packets/tablets)	5%	Dilute to 1:10–1:40 (0.5%–0.125%) One packet/tablet to a pint of water yields a 1:40 solution; two packets/tablets yields a 1:20 solution	Mild	+	
Potassium permanganate	65- and 330-mg tablets	Dilute to 1:4,000–1:16,000; 65-mg tablet to 250–1,000 mL; 330-mg tablet to 1,500–5,000 mL	Moderate	None	Stains skin, clothing
Silver nitrate	0.1%–0.5%	1 tsp of 50% stock solution to 1,000 mL will yield a 0.25% solution	Good	+	Stains; can cause pain
Acetic acid[b]	1%	Dilute 1 pint of standard 5% household vinegar with 5 parts H_2O	Good	+	Unpleasant odor; can be irritating

[a] Although many substances are added to wet dressings, the cleansing and drying effect of the water is the major benefit.
[b] Used primarily for *Pseudomonas aeruginosa* infections.
Adapted from reference 7.

be used. A mixture of equal parts baking soda and starch may also be used. Epsom salt baths, made by dissolving 3 cups of magnesium sulfate in 6 inches of lukewarm water in a tub, are useful in treating pyodermas, furuncles, and necrotic acne (especially when the back, shoulders, and buttocks are affected). Water-soluble coal tar preparations applied via a bath for the treatment of psoriasis may be the most acceptable way to apply this medication. Ointments or creams containing coal tar are malodorous and have a tendency to stain materials on contact.

A variety of bath oils are available: Alpha-Keri, Domol, Lubriderm, and Nutraderm. Adding bath oil directly to the bath is not recommended because it makes the tub slippery and potentially dangerous. The concentration of the oil in the water becomes almost insignificant anyway (5–10 mL in 20–40 gal). Five to 10 mL of bath oil may be applied directly to wet skin on leaving a bath and patted dry with a towel for a more significant effect. This is most useful in preventing and treating mild cases of xerosis (dry skin). With moderate to severe cases of xerosis, additional topical oleaginous products are generally required to improve the condition. Patients may make their own bath oil by adding 2 oz of olive oil or Nivea oil to a cup of milk and applying it following a bath.[7]

Powders

Powders are drying and cooling; they absorb moisture and create more surface area for evaporation. They are used mainly in intertriginous areas (e.g., groin, under the breasts or in skin folds) to decrease friction, which can cause mechanical irritation. They also are useful in the treatment of chafing, tinea pedis (athlete's foot), tinea cruris (jock itch), and diaper dermatitis (diaper rash). Occasionally, powders are applied on top of ointments to protect clothing from the ointment. The liberal use of powders on bedridden patients helps prevent pressure ulcers (bed sores).

Powders can be applied with a cotton puff or shaker. Care should be taken to minimize breathing the powder because this can lead to respiratory tract irritation, particularly in infants. Powders that contain starch or cellulose should be washed off before reapplication, as continued buildup can produce mechanical irritation. Corn starch–containing powders should not be used for intertrigo (inflammation of body folds—thighs, armpits, under breasts or enlarged abdomen; aggravated by heat, moisture, and maceration) because starch can serve as a substrate for *Candida albicans*. Powders should not be applied to oozing lesions because they tend to cake into hard granules, making them difficult and painful to remove and promoting maceration. Concerns regarding the association of routine cosmetic talc use and ovarian cancer and granulomatous lung changes are without convincing evidence.[8] The most commonly used powders are talc and the antifungal, nystatin.

Lotions

Lotions are suspensions or solutions of powder in a water vehicle. They are usually cooling and drying, but may provide some lubrication, depending on the formulation. Lotions are used to treat superficial dermatoses, especially if there is slight oozing. They are useful if large or intertriginous (see previous definition) areas are affected, and they are especially advantageous in the treatment of conditions characterized by significant inflammation and tenderness. In these situations, creams or ointments may cause pain on application. Sunburn, acute contact dermatitis, and poison ivy/oak are examples of conditions in which this principle may apply. Generally, lotions are applied three or four times daily, with each fresh application placed over previous application, unless there is significant oozing present, which could promote caking of dried solid ingredients. If this is the case, the area should be cleansed before repeat application. Because many lotions are suspensions, it is advisable to shake the lotion well before application. Generally, 6 oz of lotion covers the entire body of an average adult.[7]

Emulsions

Emulsions are solid or liquid and can be divided into two classes: *oil-in-water* and *water-in-oil* emulsions. Cream preparations are generally oil-in-water emulsions, whereas ointment preparations are water-in-oil emulsions. As the amount of oil increases, the viscosity of the emulsion will also increase.

The indications for liquid oil-in-water emulsions are similar to those for lotions, except that this dosage form provides greater occlusion and is more useful in conditions where dry skin predominates. Liquid water-in-oil emulsions have similar indications to ointments, except they can be applied more easily than ointments. Water-in-oil emulsions are most useful in conditions where dry skin predominates; application to hairy or intertriginous areas should be avoided. As with lotions, 6 oz of a liquid emulsion will cover all exposed skin on an average adult.[7]

Table 38-2 lists some commercially available oil-in-water and water-in-oil emulsion bases.

Gels

Gels are a form of ointment (semisolid emulsion) that contain propylene glycol and carboxypolymethylene. They are clear, nongreasy, nonstaining, nonocclusive, and quick drying. They are thixotropic (i.e., become thinner with rubbing and may sting on application). Gels are most useful when applied to hairy areas or other areas such as the face or scalp, where it is considered cosmetically unacceptable to have the residue of a vehicle remain on the skin. Because of their ingredients, gels tend to be more drying.

Table 38-2 Commercially Available Emulsion Bases

Oil-in-Water	Water-in-Oil
Acid mantle cream	Aquaphor
Aquaphilic	Eucerin
Cetaphil	Lubriderm
Dermabase	Nivea Cream
Dermovan	Nutraderm
Hydrophilic ointment USP	Polysorb
Keri Lotion	Vanicream
Lanaphilic	Velvachol
Unibase	

Adapted from reference 7, with permission.

Table 38-3 Amount of Topical Medication Needed for Various Dosage Regimens

Area Treated	Single Application (g)	BID for 1 week (g)	BID for 1 month (g)
Hands, head, face, anogenital area	2	28	120
On arm, anterior or posterior trunk	3	42	180
One leg	4	56	240
Entire body	30–60	420–840 kg (14–28 oz)	1.8–3.6 kg (60–120 oz)

Adapted from reference 7.

Table 38-4 Appropriate Dermatologic Vehicle Selection Across the Range of Dermatologic Lesions

Range of Lesions	Range of Vehicles
Acute inflammation: Oozing, weeping, vesication, edema, pruritus	Aqueous vehicles and water, and then powders solutions, lotions, sprays, and aerosols
↓	↓
Subacute inflammation: Crusting, less oozing, pruritus	Creams, gels
↓	↓
Chronic inflammation : Lichenification, dryness, erythema, pruritus, scaling	Ointments

Creams

Creams are the most commonly used vehicle in dermatology. Most are oil-in-water emulsions and are intended to be rubbed in well until they vanish (vanishing creams). Because creams do not provide much occlusiveness, they are most often recommended for subacute lesions and occasionally for chronic lesions without significant lichenification. The most common mistake made by patients when applying creams is that they use too much and/or do not rub them in fully. Generally, if the cream can be seen on the skin after application, the patient has made one or both of these application mistakes. Ultimately, they are wasting the preparation or are not getting the full therapeutic benefits. One gram of cream should cover 100 cm^2 of surface area. Table 38-3 lists the approximate amount of cream required for application to various parts of the body.[7]

Ointments

Ointments are made of inert bases such as petrolatum or may consist of droplets of water suspended in a continuous phase of oleaginous material (water-in-oil emulsions). Ointments are most useful on chronic lesions, relieving dryness, brittleness, and protecting fissures due to their occlusive properties. They should not be used on acutely inflamed lesions. Ointments should not be applied to intertriginous or hairy areas because they tend to trap heat and promote maceration. Ointments are greasy and may be cosmetically unacceptable.

Aerosols

Aerosols are the most expensive and inefficient way to apply dermatologic medications. Their only advantage over other dosage forms is that they do not require direct mechanical contact with the skin and may be useful if application causes intolerable pain for the patient. If an aerosol is used, it should be shaken well before use, and the patient should be cautioned not to spray the product around the face where it could get into the eyes or nose, or could be inhaled. Generally, aerosols should be sprayed from approximately 6 inches above the skin in bursts of 1 to 3 seconds. Aerosols are also useful for application to hairy areas if a special application nozzle is used. Aerosols have a drying effect and should not be used for a long period of time.

Other Delivery Systems

The addition of solvents, such as dimethyl sulfoxide, may enhance dermal absorption, allowing the delivery of many drugs directly through the skin. Skin patch delivery systems have also been designed to deliver drugs directly through the skin. Examples include scopolamine, nitroglycerin, clonidine, nicotine, opioids, and various hormones. These dermatologic drug delivery systems, or similar ones, offer great potential for the sustained delivery of pharmaceuticals over extended periods of time.

Selection of a Delivery System

Dermatologic vehicles should be matched to the type of lesion for which they will be used. Acute lesions require aqueous vehicles until the lesions become dry. Subacute lesions also benefit from aqueous vehicles, but for shorter periods of time before switching to creams or gels. Chronic lesions usually require ointments because of their dry, lichenified characteristics. Although there are exceptions, these principles are depicted on Table 38-4.

ASSESSING THE DERMATOLOGIC PATIENT

1. C.B., a 23-year-old, 66-kg woman, complains of a rash. What types of questions should C.B. be asked to help determine the appropriate diagnosis and treatment?

The diagnosis of dermatologic conditions can be simplified by considering six primary factors: morphology (what the lesions look like, pattern of the lesions); location or distribution of the lesions on the body; symptoms, both local and systemic; history of the present condition as well as related conditions; age of the patient; and patient gender. These six factors are discussed in the following sections, along with their significant qualifying characteristics.

Morphology

Table 38-5 provides a listing of common dermatologic lesions, their respective definitions, and some well-known clinical examples. Lesions may also be classified as either primary or secondary. Primary lesions are lesions as they first appear on the skin, whereas secondary lesions develop from primary lesions. A papule (primary lesion) might progress to a pustule (secondary lesion). A pustule may also be a primary lesion if it

Table 38-5 Dermatologic Lesions, Definitions, and Clinical Examples

Name	Definition	Examples
Primary Lesions		
Macule	Nonpalpable, flat, change in color, <1 cm	Freckles, flat moles
Patch	Nonpalpable, flat, change in color, >1 cm	Vitiligo, cafe au lait spots, chloasma
Papule	Palpable, solid mass, may have change in color, <1 cm	Verrucae, noninflammatory acne (comedone), raised nevus
Nodule	Palpable, solid mass, most often below the plane of the skin, 1–2 cm	Erythema nodosum, severe acne
Tumor	Palpable, solid mass, >2 cm, most often above and below the plane of the skin	Neoplasms
Plaque	Flat, elevated, superficial papule with surface area greater than height, >1 cm	Psoriasis, seborrheic keratosis
Wheal	Superficial area of cutaneous edema, fluid not confined to cavity	Urticaria (hives), insect bite
Vesicle	Palpable, fluid-filled cavity, <1 cm, filled with serous fluid (blister)	Herpes simples, herpes zoster, contact dermatitis
Bulla	Palpable, fluid-filled cavity, >1 cm, filled with serous fluid (blister)	Pemphigus vulgaris, second-degree burn
Pustule	Similar to vesicle, but filled with purulent fluid	Acne, impetigo, folliculitis
Special Primary Lesions		
Comedone	Plugged opening of sebaceous gland	Acne, blackhead, whitehead
Cyst	Palpable lesion filled with semiliquid material or fluid	Sebaceous cyst
Abscess	Accumulation of purulent material in dermis or subcutaneous layers of skin; purulent material not visible on surface of skin	
Furuncle	Inflammatory nodule involving a hair follicle, following an episode of folliculitis	Small boil
Carbuncle	A coalescence of several furuncles	Large boil
Secondary Lesions		
Erosion	Loss of part or all the epidermis	
Ulcer	Loss of epidermis and dermis	Ecthyma
		Stasis ulcer
Fissure	Linear crack from epidermis into dermis	Tinea pedis
Excoriation	Self-induced linear, traumatized area caused by intense scratching	Atopic dermatitis, extreme pruritus
Atrophy	Thinning of skin with loss of dermal tissue	Striae
Crusts	Dried residue of pus, serum, or blood from a wound, pustule, or vesicle	Impetigo, scabs
Lichenification	Thickening of epidermis, accentuated skin markings, usually induced by scratching or chronic inflammation	Atopic dermatitis, allergic contact dermatitis

originally developed as a pustule. The ability to recognize and describe specific lesions is critical to a successful diagnosis and communication regarding response to therapy.

In addition, many lesions present in a particular distribution or pattern. Poison ivy lesions are commonly distributed linearly. Herpetic lesions are so typical that the term herpetiform is used for lesions due to other conditions that have a herpes-like distribution. The specific size of the lesion is also important in assessing a patient's condition. Dermatologic terms related to lesion distribution or pattern are shown in Table 38-6. The lesion's consistency (firm vs. soft), borders, and color are also important diagnostic considerations.

Location

"Location, location, location" is another axiom of dermatology. Simply put, certain lesions or conditions almost always occur in certain body locations. Table 38-7 provides a list of anatomic sites with common dermatoses occurring in those locations. For example, diseases of the sebaceous glands (e.g., acne, seborrheic dermatitis, rosacea) occur only in sites with high concentrations of sebaceous glands, such as the scalp, head, neck, chest, and umbilicus. Atopic dermatitis shows a predilection for the flexor surfaces of the body (i.e., antecubital and popliteal fossae).

Symptoms

Most skin conditions have only localized symptoms with the most common symptom being pruritus. Occasionally, localized burning or pain is the predominant symptom.

History

Although a diagnosis may often be made from morphology, location, and symptoms, the patient history provides useful diagnostic and therapeutic information. Similar to the historical information obtained for any acute medical problem, the following questions should always be asked:

1. When and how did the problem start?
2. How has it progressed or changed since its onset? How have the lesions changed in size, color, appearance, or severity?
3. What is the patient's past and current medical history? What other symptoms might indicate that this is a dermatologic manifestation of a systemic disease?
4. What are the patient's symptoms?
5. What kind of allergies does the patient have?
6. What makes the condition worse or better?
7. What events or happenings have occurred with the onset or worsening of the condition (e.g., increased stress, exposure to new products, recent travel, changes in climate)?

Table 38-6 Descriptive Dermatologic Terms

Term	*Characteristics*	*Examples*
Annular	Ring shaped	Tinea
Arcuate	Shaped like an arc	Syphilis
Circinate	Circular	Tinea
Confluent	Lesions run together	Psoriasis, tinea
Discrete	Lesions remain separate	Psoriasis, tinea
Eczematous	General term for vesiculation, crusting, and lichenification	Contact dermatitis, atopic dermatitis
Geographic	Shaped like islands or continents; maplike	Generalized psoriasis
Grouped	Lesions clustered together	Herpes
Herpetiform	Appears like herpes simplex	Herpes simplex
Intertrigo	Irritant dermatitis in skin folds	Diaper dermatitis
Iris	Looks like a bull's eye, lesion within a lesion, target lesion	Erythema multiforme
Keratotic	Horny thickening	Psoriasis, corn, callus
Linear	Shaped in lines	Poison ivy
Multiform	More than one type or shape of lesion	Erythema multiforme
Papulosquamous	Papules with desquamation	Psoriasis
Serpiginous	Snakelike lesions	Cutaneous larva migrans
Zosteriform	Appears like herpes zoster	Herpes zoster

8. What have you used to treat the condition, and how have the treatments worked?
9. How did the patient use any previous therapy, and for how long did they use it?

Age

Many conditions occur predominantly in certain age groups, such as acne in neonates and those ages 11 to 20 years, seborrheic dermatitis in neonates and those ages 11 to 12 years, rosacea in those older than 30 years, and atopic dermatitis primarily in children younger than 6 years. In fact, atopic dermatitis begins and ends prior to age 6 years in 95% of patients. It is equally important to realize that many conditions, such as primary irritant and allergic contact dermatitis, occur independent of age. In addition, the skin of children and patients older than 65 years is more penetrable, thus more responsive and more susceptible to adverse effects from therapy with topical agents. Topical therapeutic agent potency and delivery systems must be carefully evaluated before usage.

Table 38-7 Common Skin Diseases by Body Location

Location	*Skin Diseases*
Scalp	Seborrheic dermatitis, dandruff
Face	Acne, rosacea, seborrheic dermatitis, perioral dermatitis, impetigo, herpes simplex
Ears	Seborrheic dermatitis
Chest/abdomen	Tinea versicolor, tinea corporis, pityriasis rosea, acne, herpes zoster
Back	Tinea versicolor, tinea corporis, pityriasis rosea
Genital area	Tinea cruris, scabies, pediculosis, condyloma acuminate (venereal warts)
Extremities	Atopic dermatitis
Hands	Tinea manuum, scabies, primary irritant contact dermatitis, warts
Feet	Tinea pedis, contact dermatitis, onychomycosis
Generalized or localized	Primary irritant or contact dermatitis, photodermatitis

Gender

Although most dermatologic conditions occur in both genders, sometimes frequency and severity are gender dependent. Rosacea occurs more frequently in females, but is often more serious in males.

TOPICAL CORTICOSTEROIDS

General Principles of Therapy

Table 38-8 lists the most common topical corticosteroid preparations by their degree of potency. The following principles are used to guide the choice of agent and application technique.

- Topical corticosteroids should be applied twice daily. Increasing the application from twice daily to four times daily does not produce superior responses and is more expensive.[9]
- Preparations should be rubbed in thoroughly and, when possible, applied while the skin is moist (e.g., after bathing).[7] Hydration of the skin increases percutaneous absorption and the resultant therapeutic effect of topical steroids.
- Appropriate-strength preparations should be used to control the condition. For maintenance, most dermatologic conditions requiring topical corticosteroids can be managed with medium- or low-strength corticosteroid preparations (i.e., 1% hydrocortisone or a low-strength fluorinated corticosteroid such as triamcinolone acetonide 0.025%).[9,10]
- Occluded areas and certain, thin-skinned areas of the body, such as the face and flexures, are more prone to the development of side effects.[9,11] If corticosteroids must be used on the face or flexures, hydrocortisone or other nonfluorinated topical steroids should be used to reduce the probability of side effects.
- Children, elderly patients, and patients with liver failure are at risk for systemic corticosteroid toxicities. In addition, patients who use the highest-potency preparations for longer than 2 weeks are susceptible to percutaneous absorption and systemic toxicity.[9–11]

Table 38-8 Topical Corticosteroid Preparations

Corticosteroid	*Brand Name(s)*	*Vehicle*
1 (Most Potent)		
Betamethasone dipropionate	Diprolene 0.05%	Ointment, optimized vehicle
Clobetasol propionate	Temovate 0.05%	Cream, ointment, optimized vehicle
Diflorasone diacetate	Psorcon 0.05%	Ointment
Halobetasol propionate	Ultravate 0.05%	Cream, ointment
2		
Amcinonide	Cyclocort 0.1%	Cream, lotion, ointment
Betamethasone dipropionate	Diprolene AF 0.05%	Cream
Betamethasone dipropionate	Diprosone 0.05%	Ointment
Desoximetasone	Topicort 0.25%	Cream, ointment
Desoximetasone	Topicort 0.05%	Gel
Diflorasone diacetate	Florone, Maxiflor 0.05%	Ointment
Fluocinonide	Lidex 0.05%	Cream, ointment, gel
Halcinonide	Halog 0.1%	Cream
Mometasone furoate[a]	Elocon 0.1%	Ointment
Triamcinolone acetonide	Kenalog 0.5%	Cream, ointment
3		
Amcinonide	Cyclocort 0.1%	Cream, lotion
Betamethasone	Benisone, Uticort 0.025%	Gel
Betamethasone benzoate	Topicort LP 0.05%	Cream (emollient)
Betamethasone dipropionate	Diprosone 0.05%	Cream
Betamethasone valerate	Valisone 0.1%	Ointment
Diflorasone diacetate	Florone, Maxiflor 0.05%	Cream
Fluocinonide	Cutivate 0.005%	Ointment
Fluticasone propionate	Lidex E 0.05%	Cream
Halcinonide	Halog 0.1%	Ointment
Triamcinolone acetate	Aristocort A 0.1%	Ointment
Triamcinolone acetate	Aristocort HP 0.5%	Cream
4		
Betamethasone benzoate	Benisone, Uticort 0.025%	Ointment
Betamethasone valerate	Valisone 0.1%	Lotion
Desoximetasone	Topicort-LP 0.05%	Cream
Fluocinolone acetonide	Synalar-HP 0.2%	Cream
Fluocinolone acetonide	Synalar 0.025%	Ointment
Flurandrenolide	Cordran 0.05%	Ointment
Halcinonide	Halog 0.25%	Cream
Hydrocortisone valerate[a]	Westcort 0.2%	Ointment
Mometasone furoate[a]	Elocon 0.1%	Cream
Triamcinolone acetonide	Aristocort, Kenalog 0.1%	Ointment
5		
Betamethasone benzoate	Benisone, Uticort 0.025%	Cream
Betamethasone dipropionate	Diprosone 0.02%	Lotion
Betamethasone valerate	Valisone 0.1%	Cream
Clocortolone	Cloderm 0.1%	Cream
Fluocinolone acetonide	Synalar 0.025%	Cream
Flurandrenolide	Cordran 0.05%	Cream
Fluticasone propionate	Cutivate 0.05%	Cream
Hydrocortisone buryrate[a]	Locoid 0.1%	Cream
Hydrocortisone valerate[a]	Westcort 0.2%	Cream
Prednicarbate	Dermatop 0.1%	Cream
Triamcinolone acetonide	Aristocort 0.25%	Cream
6		
Alclometasone dipropionate	Aclovate 0.05%	Ointment
Betamethasone valerate	Valisone 0.1%	Lotion
Desonide[a]	Tridesilon 0.05%	Cream
Fluocinolone acetonide	Synalar 0.01%	Solution
Triamcinolone acetonide	Kenalog 0.1%	Cream, lotion
7 (Least Potent)		
Hydrocortisone[a]	Generic 0.5, 1.0, 2.5%	Cream, ointment
Dexamethasone	Decadron 0.1%	Cream

[a] Nonfluorinated corticosteroid.

- With chronic conditions such as atopic eczema, it is best to discontinue therapy gradually. This reduces the potential for rebound flares of topical lesions.[7]

Indications

A topical corticosteroid is often the drug of choice for inflammatory and pruritic eruptions. In addition, topical corticosteroids are useful with hyperplastic and infiltrative disorders. The following conditions generally respond well to topical corticosteroids: primary irritant and allergic contact dermatitis, alopecia areata, atopic eczema, discoid lupus erythematosus, granuloma annulare, hypertrophic scars and keloids, lichen planus, lichen simplex, lichen striatus, various nail disorders, pretibial myxedema, psoriasis, sarcoidosis, and seborrheic dermatitis.

Contraindications

The following conditions (predominantly infectious etiologies) are worsened by topical corticosteroids: acne vulgaris, ulcers, scabies, warts, molluscum contagiosum, fungal infections, and balanitis. However, during the acute phase, topical corticosteroids are sometimes combined with other active ingredients (e.g., antifungal agents) for a few days if marked inflammation is present.

Side Effects

Although relatively infrequent, both localized (i.e., at the application site) and systemic side effects (from percutaneous absorption) can be caused by topical corticosteroids. The risks for adverse reactions are influenced by the potency of preparation used, frequency of application, duration of use, anatomical site of application, and individual patient factors. Any of the previously discussed factors that increase potency, such as inflammation and occlusion, increase the chances of side effects.[9]

Epidermal and dermal atrophy (thinning of the skin), telangiectasia, localized fine hair growth, bruising, hypopigmentation, and striae can result from repeated application of topical corticosteroids.[11] Epidermal changes consisting of a reduction in cell size may begin within several days of therapy and are generally reversible after therapy is stopped.[9] Exposed areas are most vulnerable to epidermal atrophy.

Dermal atrophy generally takes several weeks to occur and is usually reversible, depending on how long the patient has used the corticosteroid and on individual host factors such as skin age. Inguinal, genital, and perianal areas are most vulnerable to dermal atrophy. Most cases of dermal atrophy are reversible within 2 months after stopping the corticosteroid.[11]

Telangiectasia, which occurs most often on the face, neck, groin, and upper chest, may not be reversible after stopping corticosteroid therapy. Striae, which occur most commonly in the groin, axillary, and inner thigh areas, are usually permanent.[11] Fine hair growth may be particularly bothersome to female patients using corticosteroid preparations on the face. This problem is generally reversible after stopping therapy. Hypopigmentation, predominantly a problem of dark-skinned patients, is generally reversible after therapy is discontinued.[11]

Prolonged (several weeks or months) of application of high-potency steroids to large areas of the body, especially if occlusion is used, can lead to systemic absorption and subsequent adrenal suppression. Rarely, typical cushingoid features are observed.

Atopic Dermatitis

2. **P.K., a 17-year-old boy, presents to a dermatology clinic with 30% of his body covered with a pruritic, eczematous rash. There is extensive involvement of popliteal and cubital fossae bilaterally. There is evidence of excoriation with cosmetic disfigurement in the antecubital fossae, around the neck, and on his forehead.**

Family History: P.K.'s mother and aunt have asthma. One sister (L.K.), age 15, has seasonal allergic rhinitis and atopic eczema. His father and younger brother, age 11, appear to have no atopic manifestations.

Past Medical History: A rash was first noted 1 month after birth. The scalp, face, and neck were the only areas affected, and the rash continued with varying degrees of severity until age 2 years, when it spontaneously resolved. A similar rash reappeared at age 12, was diagnosed as atopic eczema, and has not disappeared since that time. P.K. developed seasonal allergic rhinitis at age 6 years and has had occasional attacks of asthma (last attack, age 15). He has had a difficult time trying to follow provided nondrug recommendations for eczema. He has used over-the-counter topical hydrocortisone cream to cool down flare-ups over the years. He reports a variable course; clearing in the summer and during periods of little stress, and worsening during the winter and periods of stress.

Physical Examination: P.K. is a well-nourished, well-developed, adolescent male with no abnormal physical findings other than marked allergic shiners, pale boggy nasal mucosa, and Dennie's lines noted near the eyes, plus extensive skin lesions. Oozing, crusted, erythematous, eczematous, lichenified, maculopapular, and fine vesicular eruptions are on his face, neck, flexor aspects of both arms and legs, hands, and chest. There is some evidence of secondary bacterial infection in both cubital fossae and on portions of the left leg. Identify the presenting history, symptoms, and signs characteristic of eczema.

Atopic dermatitis, a form of eczema, can be acute or subacute, but is more commonly a chronic pruritic inflammation of the epidermis and dermis. Roughly two-thirds of the patients have a personal or family history of allergic rhinitis, eczema, or asthma. Atopic dermatitis in infants may be a prelude to the development of other atopic disorders later in life (i.e., allergic rhinitis or asthma). Presence of these disorders many times is the key to differential diagnosis. About 80% of patients with atopic dermatitis have a type I (IgE-mediated) hypersensitivity reaction occurring as a result of the release of vasoactive substances from both mast cells and basophils that have been sensitized by the interaction of the antigen with IgE. An allergy workup is rarely helpful in determining the allergen. The disorder affects 0.5% to 1.0% of the general population, although its prevalence in children is 5% to 10%. In infants and young children, the dermatitis often occurs on the scalp, face, and extensor surfaces. In older children and adults, it tends to localize to the flexural areas, especially the cubital and popliteal fossae and the neck. In addition, the rash may affect the hands and feet, sometimes in the absence of eczema elsewhere. Most patients become afflicted between infancy and age 12, with 60% being affected by the first year; another 30% are seen for the first time by age 5, with the final 10% developing atopic dermatitis between 6 and 20 years of age.

Pruritus is the hallmark of atopic dermatitis. The constant scratching leads to a vicious cycle of itch-scratch-rash-itch, with the rash consisting primarily of lichenification of the skin. Atopic dermatitis has been described as "the itch that rashes, rather than the rash that itches." In other words, the itching precedes the rash. Wool, detergents, soaps, a change in room temperature, and mental and/or physical stress precipitate itching. Patients tend to have dry skin (xerosis). This is due to a reduced water-binding capacity and a higher transdermal water loss. Xerosis is worsened during periods of low humidity, such as winter in northern latitudes.

P.K.'s family and medical history are classic for atopic dermatitis. His family history is significant for asthma, allergic rhinitis, and atopic dermatitis. He had his initial outbreak at age 1 month and then developed seasonal allergic rhinitis and asthma. His skin examination reveals findings of both acute and chronic atopic eczema, with typical lesion location and description.

3. What are the relevant biopharmaceutic considerations for selecting a topical corticosteroid for P.K.?

Topical corticosteroids are classified into potency categories (Table 38-8). The relative potency assigned to a topical corticosteroid is determined by the ability of the preparation to penetrate the skin after release from the vehicle, the intrinsic activity of the corticosteroid at the receptor, and the rate of clearance from the receptor. Activity of corticosteroids may be enhanced by the use of a more occlusive vehicle, the addition of penetration-enhancing substances (i.e., urea, salicylic acid, propylene glycol), and modifications of the steroid molecule. Hydrocortisone was the initial local corticosteroid discovered, and since then, the molecule has been modified in several ways. The addition of a fluorine atom protects the steroid ring from metabolic conversion, resulting in more potent activity. The introduction of an acetonide bond and/or lipophilic ester groups increases skin penetration. Many newer topical corticosteroids have incorporated one or more of these molecular changes, resulting in increased-potency agents and a growing armamentarium of agents.

It is believed that topical corticosteroids penetrate into the stratum corneum by passive diffusion, which varies considerably, depending on the part of the body to which the preparation is applied. When a standard hydrocortisone preparation was applied to various parts of the body, absorption was found to be 0.14% on the plantar surface of the foot, 1% on the forearm, 4% on the scalp, 7% on the forehead, 13% on the cheeks, and 36% on the scrotum. Because penetration is high in the groin, axillae, and face, lower-potency nonfluorinated topical preparations such as hydrocortisone 0.5% to 1% should be used on these areas.[9,10] In areas where penetration is poor, owing to thickening of the stratum corneum, such as the elbows, knees, palms, or soles, higher-strength preparations should be used.[9]

For P.K., a 1% hydrocortisone cream should be used on his face and other areas of high penetrability to reduce the possibility of complications.[9] A high-potency cream (intermediate- or higher-potency classification from Table 38-8) should be used initially on acutely inflamed areas or where high penetration is not a problem. This will "cool down" these lesions quickly.

If equal amounts of a corticosteroid are incorporated into ointments, gels, creams, and lotion bases, the gel and ointment preparations are generally more active than creams and lotions.[9,10] However, with the increased use of optimized vehicles, that rule is not as true as in the past. The addition of certain substances enhances penetration and potency. Using these principles, pharmaceutical manufacturers have increasingly developed optimized vehicles that maximize diffusion of individual corticosteroids into the stratum corneum. Therefore, for new products, the only reliable way to ascertain potency is to consult the manufacturer's literature for its Stoughton classification. Increasing the concentration of a corticosteroid in a preparation also increases its potency, but not in a linear fashion. Because P.K. has a fine vesicular eruption, a cream should be used initially, to facilitate drying. However, patients often express a preference (e.g., cream or gel), and this should be considered.

Occlusion

4. It has been some time since P.K.'s atopic eczema has been aggressively treated. He has many acute, inflamed lesions. Should occlusive therapy be used? What complications could develop from occlusion? How would you describe the use of occlusion to P.K.?

As discussed previously (see Dermatologic Delivery Systems section), occlusion traps heat and promotes maceration. This same mechanism increases the hydration of the skin and resultant absorption of corticosteroid preparations, thus producing a heightened therapeutic effect. As a general rule, occlusion enhances the potency of corticosteroids by a factor of 10. Occlusion can be accomplished by selecting an ointment-based corticosteroid, applying a nonmedicated ointment base over another corticosteroid preparation (gel, cream, lotion, or aerosol), or by enveloping the medicated area with plastic (e.g., plastic wrap, gloves, or plastic suit [space suit]).[5,7,9,11] Several hours of occlusion are all that is necessary to increase potency; thus, relatively short periods of occlusion are clinically useful. Occlusion can be uncomfortable, and can lead to sweat retention and an increased risk of bacterial and candidal infections. To reduce these problems and the chances of systemic side effects, occlusion should not be maintained for more than 12 hours in a 24-hour period. Occlusion should not be used for acute lesions, which already have increased absorptive capability and need the vasoconstrictive effects of cooling first. Occlusion is best used for chronic lesions that are thick and scaly, where drug absorption is impaired. Most patients with atopic dermatitis do not tolerate occlusion because their itch threshold is low, and heat, sweat retention, and maceration increase pruritus. The long-term benefit of occlusion in a patient with atopic dermatitis is reduced by the increased pruritus, which may lead to noncompliance. When using occlusion in patients with eczema, care should be taken not to occlude unaffected skin (because of the low itch threshold). For other chronic dermatologic conditions (e.g., psoriasis) that are not associated with severe pruritus, occlusion could be used for prolonged periods if necessary. Increasing the hydration of the skin (after a shower or bath) also increases the effects of medications immediately applied after the bath or shower, which would be an appropriate recommendation for P.K.

Product Selection

Pharmacokinetic Considerations

5. P.K. received a prescription for halcinonide (Halog) 0.1% cream, 80 g, to be applied at bedtime, with five refills. Comment on the appropriateness of this prescription based on pertinent biopharmaceutic considerations.

Corticosteroids tend to penetrate human skin very slowly, leading to a reservoir effect. With low-potency preparations, this reservoir effect persists for several days, and with the most potent preparations under occlusion, the effects may persist for up to 14 days.[9,10] The clinical implication of this reservoir effect on chronic conditions is a cumulative effect with repeated application of topical corticosteroids. As a result, the number of applications per day can be reduced, and less potent preparations can be used after the acute inflammatory process has been brought under control. Results from P.K.'s treatment regimen might be improved by providing more frequent (twice-daily) application or a more potent preparation for twice-daily administration to control inflamed lesions. Once control is achieved, a less-potent preparation could be used for maintenance and the number of applications may be reduced. Due to the reservoir effect, control can be maintained in many cases with intermittent regimens such as once daily, every other day, or every third day use of topical corticosteroids. In addition, intermittent regimens can involve alternating corticosteroids and agents such as pimecrolimus.

Side Effects

Acne

6. After several months of continuous corticosteroid therapy in a maintenance format, P.K. presents with four pustules and two closed comedones on his forehead and multiple pustules on both cheeks. What problems from the use of topical corticosteroid therapy on the face does this represent?

The face is particularly vulnerable to corticosteroid side effects because of enhanced penetration.[11] Acne, acne rosacea, and perioral dermatitis can develop after several weeks to months of application. Corticosteroid-induced conditions can generally be distinguished from naturally occurring disorders. Corticosteroid-induced acne lesions are uniformly at the same level of development throughout the affected area and are present only in areas treated with the corticosteroid. Generally, steroid acne, acne rosacea, and perioral dermatitis resolve after discontinuing the drug. Application of corticosteroid preparations (particularly the potent preparations) to areas around the eye can lead to increased intraocular pressure, glaucoma, cataracts, increased risk of ocular mycotic infections, and exacerbation of pre-existing herpes simplex infections.[11] Hydrocortisone or nonfluorinated topical corticosteroids are often the agents of choice for facial lesions.

P.K.'s acneiform lesions may get worse after the application of topical corticosteroids. He should be instructed to apply the corticosteroid preparation only to the atopic eczema and to avoid areas where acne exists. If the atopic eczema and acne lesions are in the same area and his acne gets worse after using the topical corticosteroid, P.K. must make a decision as to which of these two dermatologic conditions bothers him more and treat the condition that is most disturbing. Some improvement in corticosteroid-exacerbated acne may be achieved by decreasing the strength of the topical product applied to the face and reducing the frequency of application. An alternative to this approach, if P.K.'s acne is severe, would be to continue topical corticosteroid therapy, but treat the acne systemically.[5,6] (See Chapter 39 for a more extensive discussion.)

Idiosyncratic/Allergic Reactions

7. P.K.'s sister, L.K., who also has atopic eczema, started using a new topical corticosteroid preparation (halcinonide) 10 days ago. She has been complaining of a burning sensation lasting for 1 hour after every application of this product. She stopped using the product 2 days ago because of this. Is it possible that she has developed an allergy to a corticosteroid-containing medication?

Cortisol is endogenously secreted by the adrenal gland and is essential to life. As a result, allergic reactions to topical corticosteroid preparations are rare. When allergic symptoms do occur, they are generally not due to the corticosteroid, but to the preservatives (e.g., paraben) or other ingredients in the formulation or the base (e.g., lanolin). Allergic sensitization can occur within 2 weeks of therapy, but may be difficult to diagnose because the corticosteroid can modify the allergic reaction.[12] One should suspect an allergic reaction if lesions change appearance after starting therapy, if healing does not occur within the expected period of time, or if the condition improves and then abruptly gets worse. Most case reports of allergic reactions (dryness, itching, burning, or irritation) to topical corticosteroids are nonspecific and have been in patients with atopic eczema.[12] Atopic individuals are more likely to react to the vehicle base than the active corticosteroid ingredient.

Because of the time course of the burning sensation in L.K. (starting the first day and lasting only 1 hour), it is doubtful that she is actually allergic to this product. However, atopic eczema patients often have "sensitive" skin that reacts idiosyncratically to a variety of topical preparations.[12] To remedy this situation, L.K. should be given another topical corticosteroid preparation with a different formulation (base and preservatives). If the reaction continues with a new product, an allergy workup may be necessary and patch testing could be considered.

Adrenal Axis Suppression/Risk of Infection

8. P.K. recently sustained a knee injury and corrective surgery is being considered. Should he receive a systemic corticosteroid during the perioperative period as a precaution against adrenal insufficiency? Should he wear a Medic-Alert tag while using long-term topical corticosteroids? Is he at risk for developing an infection after surgery?

Systemic adrenal axis suppression from topically applied corticosteroids appears to be more of a theoretic risk than a clinical entity in adults, except when the highest-potency preparations are used[13] or other risk factors are present (Table 38-9). Although suppression has been reported with use of mild to moderately potent agents, these cases can be attributed to excessive use or to application of corticosteroids over large areas of the body for prolonged periods under

Table 38-9 Risk Factors for Systemic Side Effects From Topical Corticosteroids

Duration of application
Prolonged application (>3–4 wk)
Potency of corticosteroid
Weak or moderately strong, 100 g/wk without occlusion
Very potent, >45 g/wk without occlusion
Application location
Thin stratum corneum results in easier penetration (eyelids, forehead, cheeks, armpits, groin, and genitals)
Age of patient
Very young children and elderly people have very thin epidermis
Manner of application
Occlusion
Presence of penetration-enhancing substances
Propylene glycol
Salicylic acid
Urea
Condition of the skin
General factors
Compromised liver function

occlusion. If suppression does occur, it reverses within 2 to 4 weeks after application is stopped. Patients using more than 45 g/week of a high-potency corticosteroid are at risk for adrenal axis suppression.[13] Therefore, the use of preparations such as clobetasol (Temovate) should be limited to no more than 45 g/week for 2 weeks or less. In addition, these preparations should not be used under occlusion and should be reserved for dermatoses that are unresponsive to less potent preparations.

Because young children absorb corticosteroids to a greater extent, they have a greater risk of developing adrenal axis suppression and other systemic side effects.[13] To reduce this risk, hydrocortisone topical preparations should be used in children, and their use should be limited to short periods of time. Patients whose corticosteroid clearance is impaired (e.g., liver failure) should also use hydrocortisone and be monitored closely for signs of systemic toxicity.[11]

The risk of developing an Addisonian crisis during surgery or at other times of stress secondary to adrenal suppression from topical steroids is extremely low. Patients who have used potent topical corticosteroids over large areas of their bodies (>30%) or those who have used occlusion are at greater risk (see previous discussion) and are often given systemic hydrocortisone prophylactically before surgery. Because P.K. is not likely to require such supplementation, a MedicAlert tag is unnecessary.

Infection secondary to topically administered corticosteroids is also a theoretic risk, but is uncommon. Although anecdotal reports of secondary bacterial infections appear in the literature, there is scant evidence to suggest that they occur with any frequency. Topical corticosteroids do not alter normal skin flora.[14]

Topical Antibiotics with Corticosteroids

9. P.K.'s atopic eczema presentation is complicated with areas of erythematous, honey-colored, crusted lesions on his forehead, arm, and leg. Can a corticosteroid and an antibiotic preparation be used together? What are the risks associated with topical antibiotics?

It is determined that P.K. has impetigo superimposed on his atopic dermatitis. Because impetigo can be treated with topical antibiotics such as mupirocin, combination therapy with a corticosteroid-antibiotic preparation appears to be a logical choice. The corticosteroid suppresses the clinical signs of infection and helps re-establish the normal skin barrier function. This, in combination with an appropriate antibiotic, allows the skin's normal defense mechanisms to ward off the infection. However, because staphylococci toxins act as superantigens, eliciting the production of IgE, thus worsening the atopic dermatitis, almost all clinicians treat impetiginized atopic dermatitis with oral antibiotics such as penicillin, dicloxacillin, erythromycin, or cephalexin, in combination with topical corticosteroids for the eczema.[15–17] Oral antibiotics reduce the bacterial counts faster and have a lower incidence of recurrent impetigo compared with topical agents. In areas where community methicillin-resistant *Staphylococcus aureus* rates are high, other more effective antibiotic therapy might be indicated.

Otitis externa, certain intertriginous eruptions, and possibly seborrheic dermatitis may respond favorably to combination antibiotic-corticosteroid preparations. Table 38-10 describes the spectrum of activity of common topical antibiotics. Although mupirocin may be an appropriate alternative for topical dermatologic infections, the current over-the-counter topical antibiotics (bacitracin, neomycin, and polymyxin) are ineffective for most dermatologic infections and are indicated only for the prophylaxis of skin infections. Mupirocin resistance occurs with overuse.[18]

P.K. would most likely benefit from a treatment course of an oral antibiotic plus a topical corticosteroid preparation.

Table 38-10 Spectrum of Activity of Antibiotics Available for Topical Use

Bacitracin
Effective against all anaerobic cocci, most strains of streptococci, staphylococci, and pneumococci. Not effective against most gram-negative organisms.
Gentamicin
Effective against most gram-negative organisms (similar to neomycin), including *Pseudomonas* and many strains of *Staphylococcus aureus*.
Mupirocin
Very effective against *S. aureus* and does not interfere with wound healing. Currently, the only topical antibiotic that has been proved to be more effective than the vehicle based on U.S. Food and Drug Administration guidelines.
Gramicidin
Effective against most gram-positive organisms. Not effective against most gram-negative organisms.
Neomycin
Effective against most gram-negative organisms (except *Pseudomonas*) and some gram-positive organisms. Group A streptococci are resistant.
Polymyxin B
Effective against most gram-negative organisms (including *Pseudomonas*). Most strains of *Proteus, Serratia,* and gram-positive organisms are resistant.

Table 38-11 Systemic Diseases Associated With Pruritus

Brain abscesses	Iron-deficiency anemia
Carcinoid syndrome	Multiple myeloma
Carcinoma of the breast, lung, or stomach	Multiple sclerosis
Central nervous system infarct	Mycosis fungoides
Diabetes mellitus	Obstructive biliary disease
Gout	Polycythemia vera
Hodgkin disease and other lymphomas	Pregnancy (first trimester)
Hypertension	Thyroid disease (both hyper- and hypothyroidism)
	Uremia

Side Effects

There have been many reports of contact dermatitis caused by topical antimicrobials, particularly neomycin.[19] Neomycin sensitivity has been reported in 4% of the general population by patch testing and in 40% of patients with a history of allergic contact dermatitis or a history of recurrent use of topical antibiotics.[19,20] The corticosteroid contained in many neomycin preparations does not prevent these allergic reactions, although it may decrease the severity of the reaction.

Pruritus

10. As stated in Question 2, one of P.K.'s complaints is pruritus. What could you recommend for relief of pruritus?

Pruritus (itching) is the most common cutaneous symptom. It has many different causes and has been associated with a variety of systemic diseases, several of which are listed in Table 38-11.[5,7,21] In the absence of a cutaneous manifestation, a careful history and physical examination should be performed to rule out one of the systemic causes of pruritus. In addition, a chest radiograph, stool examination for occult blood, complete blood count with differential, thyroid panel, blood urea nitrogen, creatinine, liver function panel, glucose, and urinalysis may be necessary to help screen for the aforementioned systemic diseases.[21]

Scratching, which can damage or fatigue receptor nerve endings, is the most common method of relieving pruritus. One would, therefore, expect topically applied local anesthetics or antihistamines to be effective in dulling the sensation. However, this approach is often disappointing, probably because the intact epidermis poorly absorbs the salt forms of these drugs. Also, low concentrations are used in many over-the-counter preparations. If adequate concentrations of local anesthetics are used (benzocaine 20% or lidocaine 3%–4%), pruritus or pain may be reduced for up to 45 minutes. These agents are most useful for relieving pruritus or pain for short periods of time (e.g., when trying to go to sleep at night).[21] A drawback to the use of benzocaine and topical antihistamine preparations are their propensity to induce allergic contact dermatitis.[22–24]

P.K. could also try cold water or ice cubes, which effectively relieve pruritus via vasoconstriction, as do products containing aluminum acetate (Burow's solution), tannic acid, or calamine. A cool bath may be useful for the relief of pruritus from dermatologic lesions if they are widespread.

Moisturizing mixtures such as Keri Lotion, Lubriderm, or, simply, mineral or baby oil are useful in the treatment of pruritus caused by dry skin. This problem is often encountered in the elderly and others during the winter months. Bathing should be restricted to avoid washing away normal body oils, the drying effect of water, the irritant effect of alkaline soaps, and the trauma of toweling.[7]

Topical corticosteroid applications can be very effective. They reduce inflammation and are often contained in a cream base, which helps soothe the affected area.

Systemic antihistamines are effective antipruritics, although their major beneficial effect may be due to sedation. The newer, nonsedating antihistamines are notably ineffective at relieving itch, with the exception of cetirizine.[25] There is disagreement over which antihistamine or antiserotonin agents are most effective for treatment of pruritus.[21,25,26] Many practitioners consider hydroxyzine to be the antihistamine of choice; doses of 10 to 25 mg three to four times a day are commonly used. Other practitioners favor cyproheptadine. There is little evidence that antihistamines are effective in treating non–histamine-mediated pruritus, except that their inherent sedative effect may be somewhat beneficial in all pruritic conditions. Doxepin, a tricyclic antidepressant with potent H_1-blocking properties, is valuable as a second-line antihistamine topically or systemically if others fail.[27] Because P.K.'s pruritus is worse at night as is typical with atopic dermatitis, the use of any of the four H_1-blockers mentioned at bedtime would be appropriate.[28]

Nondrug Recommendations for Atopic Dermatitis

11. In addition to prescriptions for topical corticosteroids (triamcinolone acetonide cream 0.1%/augmented betamethasone dipropionate 0.05%) for flare-ups, a systemic antibiotic (erythromycin 250 mg QID × 10 days), and an oral antihistamine (hydroxyzine 25 mg, 1–2 tablets HS as needed), what nondrug interventions should be suggested for P.K.?

The general goals of therapy for atopic dermatitis are to decrease pruritus, suppress inflammation, lubricate the skin, and reduce anxiety. The nondrug recommendations shown in Table 38-12 are useful adjuncts and mainstays between disease flares, for patients such as P.K. with eczema or any other irritant dermatitis. Often careful attention to nonpharmacologic measures can reduce the incidence of disease flare. Because

Table 38-12 Nondrug Recommendations for Patients With Atopic Eczema or Other Irritant Dermatitis

- Clothing should be soft and light. Cotton or corduroy is preferred. Wools and coarse, heavy synthetics should be avoided.
- Heat should be avoided because it often makes eczema worse. The environment should be well ventilated, cool, and low in humidity (30%–50%). Rapid changes in ambient temperature should be avoided.
- Bathing should be kept to a minimum (no longer than 5 minutes), and the patient should use a nonirritating soap (e.g., Basis soap). A colloid bath or the use of appropriate amounts of bath oil may be useful.
- The skin should be kept moist with frequent applications of emollients (e.g., Keri, Lubriderm, Nivea, Aquaphor, Eucerin, or petrolatum).
- Primary irritants such as paints, cleansers, solvents, and chemical sprays should be avoided.

even nonlesional skin in patients with atopic dermatitis has reduced moisture, the use of emollients should include all skin surfaces.

P.K. should be warned to avoid people with active herpes simplex infections because severe disseminated infections can occur. Similarly, based on the anthrax bioterrorism attack in October 2001, debate has emerged on the advisability of reinitiating routine vaccination against smallpox. Vaccinia virus was the live poxvirus used throughout the world as the vaccine against smallpox. Because of the increased risk for eczema vaccinatum, vaccinia vaccine should not be administered to persons with eczema of any degree, those with a past history of eczema, household contacts who have active eczema, or household contacts who have a history of eczema.[26,29]

Tachyphylaxis/Specialized Corticosteroid Dosage Forms/Antihistamines

12. P.K. responded well to the previous treatment plan and now requests a refill of his topical corticosteroid prescriptions. The bacterial superinfected areas have cleared. He continues to have problems with his fingers. He has applied betamethasone dipropionate to his hands five to six times daily for the past 3 weeks without any noticeable improvement. Triamcinolone cream resolved the rash on other areas of his body. Other than occasional sedation early on from the hydroxyzine and when he uses it intermittently, he has not had any other adverse effects. As P.K. continues to follow other nondrug recommendations, he inquires if anything else could be done for his hands. Assess P.K.'s use and response to the corticosteroids.

P.K. is overusing the potent topical corticosteroid and may have developed tachyphylaxis. Tachyphylaxis can occur within 1 week of therapy, but generally takes several weeks to a month to occur.[30] To treat this problem, P.K. should stop applying the betamethasone preparation for 4 to 7 days and then restart therapy in a more appropriate manner (i.e., twice daily). Limited courses of treatment separated by short periods of rest may be more effective than continuous treatment. However, clinicians commonly misdiagnose tachyphylaxis. Failure of topical corticosteroids to clear difficult atopic dermatitis after an initial improvement may give the false impression of tachyphylaxis when the actual problem is a primary failure of the treatment.[31] This could be caused by either inappropriate application technique by the patient or the choice of a product with inadequate potency.

Flurandrenolide 4 mg/cm^2 tape (Cordran) may be useful after P.K. stops his other corticosteroids for 4 to 7 days. Although this product is expensive, it is effective for small areas because the tape serves as a protectant and provides occlusion. It is a good choice for use on the hands, particularly the fingers, where P.K. is having problems, because other vehicles are often quite messy when applied to the hands. When using Cordran tape, the general principles previously outlined for occlusion should be followed.

Topical tacrolimus (Protopic) is an effective alternative to topical corticosteroids and is safe for use in children.[32,33] In addition to its inhibitory effect on cytokine production, topical tacrolimus has been shown to cause alterations in epidermal antigen-presenting dendritic cells that may result in decreased immunologic response to antigens. Transient burning, erythema, and pruritus are the most common adverse effects. Pimecrolimus cream (Elidel) 1% is an immunomodulatory agent with properties similar to those of cyclosporine and tacrolimus, but it does not appear to affect the systemic immune response and might, therefore, be better tolerated for long-term therapy.[34] Neither pimecrolimus nor tacrolimus causes skin atrophy, making them attractive alternatives for patients with lesions on the face and neck. Recently, issues regarding the long-term safety of these products has led the U.S. Food and Drug Administration to place a temporary black box warning in the manufacturer's literature regarding a potential increased cancer risk.

XEROSIS

13. C.R., a 64-year-old woman, requests something for dry skin on her arms and back. She has had this problem for a number of years. It is generally not a problem in the summer, with most symptoms troubling her in the winter. She has no other medical conditions and only takes an occasional aspirin for "arthritis." How would you advise C.R. to manage this condition?

C.R.'s complaints represent a common problem of the elderly, xerosis (dry skin). The seasonal cycle described is frequently called "winter itch." Most cases of dry skin are caused by dehydration of the stratum corneum.[35] Table 38-13 gives general recommendations for the treatment of dry skin.

Table 38-13 General Recommendations for Treatment of Dry Skin

1. Use room humidifiers.
2. Keep room temperature as low as comfortable to prevent sweating and water loss from the skin.
3. Keep bathing to a minimum (every 1–2 days) with warm, but not hot, water. After bathing, the patient should immediately apply an emollient (Table 38-2). When the skin is soaked for 5 to 10 minutes, the stratum corneum can absorb as much as six times its weight in water. Application of an emollient immediately after bathing will trap the water in the skin and reduce dryness.
4. Eliminate exposure to solvents, drying chemicals, harsh soaps, and cleaners. These substances remove oils from the skin and reduce its barrier function. As the barrier function is lost, water loss from the skin is increased up to 75 times higher than normal. Exposure to cold, dry winds will also enhance water loss.
5. Apply emollients (Table 38-2) three to six times a day, especially after bathing to help retain moisture in the skin from bathing.
6. The selection of emollients depends on the atmospheric moisture content of the region. In dry parts of the western United States where humidity is very low, water-in-oil emollients such as Lubriderm, Eucerin, or Nivea are preferred because the high oil content prevents the loss of moisture from the skin. In those areas, a general rule is to avoid products where glycerin is one of the top four ingredients on the label because glycerin is hygroscopic and in low humidity will pull moisture out of the dermis leading to drier, cracked skin. In areas with higher humidity such as the eastern United States, glycerin in both types of emollients pulls moisture from the atmosphere into the skin. Regardless of region, if application of an emollient appears to be ineffective, switching to a product with less glycerin and more oil may resolve the dryness.
7. If scaling is a problem, a keratolytic (Lac-Hydrin, AmLactin) or a higher-strength, urea-containing preparation (20%) may be useful.
8. If inflammation is present, a mild to moderately potent topical corticosteroid may be useful (Table 38-8). An ointment vehicle is more effective than others.

However, before recommending therapy, the following differential should be considered: ichthyosis vulgaris (familial history usually present), atopic eczema, psoriasis, contact dermatitis, and hypothyroidism. Usually, simple questioning can rule out these conditions.

DRUG ERUPTIONS

Clinically recognizable adverse drug reactions are manifested on the skin more often than any other organ or organ system.[36,37] An estimated 1% to 5% of hospitalized patients develop a drug eruption.[37] Outpatient statistics are more difficult to obtain, but are probably within the same range. There is no correlation between age, diagnosis, or severity of illness and the likelihood of developing a drug eruption. Women appear to be twice as likely as men to develop a drug eruption.

The most common type of eruption encountered in clinical practice, and probably the one most often overlooked, is the exanthematic (bursting out) eruption. This type of reaction comprises both morbilliform (measles-like) and scarlatiniform (scarlet fever–like) eruptions. Stevens-Johnson syndrome (SJS), toxic epidermal necrolysis, drug hypersensitivity syndrome, vasculitis, serum sickness, coagulant-induced skin necrosis, and angioedema are the most important severe reactions and require immediate attention and management. Many of the common dermatologic reactions that can be induced by drugs have other causes as well, so a complete workup must include other nondrug etiologies. Viral, fungal, and bacterial infections, as well as certain systemic diseases and foods, have been identified as causes for common reactions such as urticaria, erythema multiforme, and erythema nodosum. The diagnosis of drug eruptions is best made by identifying the type of lesions observed and associating the lesions with specific drug therapy. The most important diagnostic criterion is an accurate assessment of the skin lesions. With this critical information, the clinician can then refer to a drug information source to associate any current or past drug therapy with the specific lesions observed.

Acneiform Eruptions

Acneiform eruptions appear very much like common acne. They may be distinguished from acne by their sudden occurrence, the absence of comedones, uniform appearance (i.e., all at the same stage of development), and the fact that they may occur on any part of the body. Cysts and scarring are rarely associated with drug-induced acne. Eruptions can also occur during any period of the patient's life; thus, drug-induced acne should be suspected when the lesions appear in persons outside the typical age bracket for acne. Drugs implicated include adrenocorticotropic hormone, anabolic steroids, azathioprine, danazol, glucocorticoids, halogens (iodides, bromides), isoniazid, lithium, and oral contraceptives. For patients with acne vulgaris, these drugs may worsen existing lesions (see Chapter 40).

Photosensitive Eruptions

Photosensitivity eruptions require the presence of both a drug (or chemical) and a light source of appropriate wavelength. These eruptions are divided into two subtypes: phototoxic and photoallergic. *Phototoxic* reactions, the most common drug-induced photodermatosis, manifest themselves as an exaggerated sunburn or increased sensitivity to sunburn. The ultraviolet A (UVA) light source alters the drug to a toxic form, resulting in tissue damage independent of any allergic response and occurs in everyone who gets high enough skin levels of the offending drug. This eruption can occur on first exposure to a drug, is dose related, usually has no cross-sensitivity, and will continue as long as the skin concentration of the drug exceeds the threshold level for the reaction to occur. *Photoallergic* reactions, which are very uncommon, may appear as a variety of lesions, including urticaria, bullae, and sunburn. UVA light alters the drug so it becomes an antigen or acts as a hapten. Photoallergic eruptions require previous contact with the offending drug, are not dose related, exhibit cross-sensitivity with chemically related compounds, and are secondary to the use of topical agents. Unfortunately, outside light through a window and fluorescent lighting permits passage of or can emit UVA light. In addition, until recently, there were inadequate topical preparations that provide protection against UVA light. Avobenzone, while covering much of the UVA spectrum, is photolabile, losing 60% of its effectiveness in <1 hour. New products containing ecamsule appear to offer an advance in protection against UVA rays. In some instances, a drug may produce both photoallergic and phototoxic reactions. Most phototoxic and photoallergic reactions occur fairly soon after exposure to light. Implicated drugs are numerous, including, among others, antibiotics (tetracyclines, fluoroquinolones), antidepressants (tricyclics), antihypertensives (hydrochlorothiazide, β-blockers), hypoglycemics (sulfonylureas), nonsteroidal anti-inflammatory drugs, sunscreens (PABA), oral contraceptives, and antipsychotics (phenothiazine) (see Chapter 42).

Lichen Planus–Like Eruptions

Lichen planus–like lesions appear as flat-topped papules that have a distinctive sheen. Pruritus is usually quite pronounced. Any part of the body can be affected (most commonly the arms and legs), including mucous membranes. The lesions are sometimes confused with fixed eruptions, but can easily be differentiated histologically. Implicated drugs include angiotensin-converting enzyme inhibitors, antimalarials, phenothiazine derivatives, thiazide diuretics, and sulfonylurea hypoglycemic agents among others.

Alopecia

Alopecia (hair loss) is not a true drug eruption, but hair may occasionally be lost when other drug reactions such as exfoliative dermatitis and erythema multiforme occur. Hair loss can be caused by a direct toxic action of a drug (e.g., a cancer chemotherapeutic agent) or from interference with the normal growth phases of hair (e.g., warfarin).

Bullous Eruptions

Bullous (blister-like) lesions can occur in combination with other drug eruptions, such as erythema multiforme and toxic epidermal necrolysis or by themselves. The lesions may be round or irregular and contain a clear, serous fluid. The fluid-filled sacs may be tense or flaccid and can occur on both mucous membranes and skin. These lesions are similar to those associated with pemphigus and pemphigoid reactions. Lesions

Table 38-14 Frequent Contact Sensitizers

Substance	Found In
Ammonia	Soaps, chemicals, hair dyes
Balsam of Peru	Cosmetics
Benzyl alcohol	Medications, cosmetics
"Caine" anesthetics	Medications (e.g., over-the-counter benzocaine products)
Carba	Rubber
Chromium	Jewelry
Epoxy resin	Glue
Ethylenediamine	Stabilizer in topical products (e.g., aminophylline)
Formaldehyde	Shoes, clothing, soaps, insulations
Mercaptobenzothiazol	Rubber
Naphthyl	Rubber
Neomycin	Topical medications (e.g., Neosporin)
Nickel sulfate	Jewelry, fasteners
Paraben	Preservative in many topical products
Paraphenylenediamine	Hair dyes, leather
Potassium dichromate	Shoes, leather
Thiomersal	Preservatives, contact lens products
Thiram	Rubber products
Turpentine	Paint products
Wool alcohols	Lanolin-containing products, clothes

usually resolve after discontinuation of the drug, but occasionally become chronic. Implicated drugs include amiodarone, barbiturates, coumarin, gold, penicillins, and sulfonamides.

Allergic Contact Dermatitis

Topical administration of a sensitizing agent produces localized lesions limited to areas of contact with the topical product. Neomycin, benzocaine, and diphenhydramine are well-known topical sensitizers (Table 38-14). Systemic administration of a drug to a patient previously sensitized to the drug by topical application can provoke widespread eczematous dermatitis. Implicated systemically or topically administered drugs that reactivate allergic contact dermatitis include procaine/benzocaine, radiographic contrast media/iodine, and streptomycin and gentamicin/neomycin among others.

Erythema Multiforme

As the name implies, erythema multiforme (EM) eruptions take on a varied spectrum of morphologic forms, ranging from the mildest with tiny maculovesicular lesions to more severe forms such as SJS and toxic epidermal necrolysis syndrome (TENS) with extensive bullous lesions and routine involvement of mucous membranes. Although all forms have been reported to have oral lesions, they are much more severe in SJS and TENS, where genital, nasal, and ocular mucosas are also involved. Target lesions are usually present in all forms of the disorder, which characteristically are erythematous, iris-shaped papules and vesiculobullous lesions typically involving the extremities (especially the palms and soles) in EM and the torso in SJS/TENS. The lesions take on the appearance of a circular target with a bulls-eye in the middle, thus the term target lesion. However, questions have recently been raised about the shared pathological nature of these forms of erythema multiforme.[38] EM in its mildest forms, EM minor and EM major, is more common in children and young adults, and is self-limited in nature with only transient hypo- or hyperpigmentation as complications. Sometimes malaise, a low-grade fever, and itching or burning may accompany this type of eruption. Etiologic factors associated with EM include drugs, mycoplasma and herpes infections, radiation therapy, foods, and sometimes neoplasms. Allopurinol, barbiturates, phenothiazine, and sulfonamides are the drugs most often implicated in EM eruptions.

Stevens-Johnson Syndrome

SJS is probably the most common type of severe drug eruption. The syndrome is usually a moderate mucocutaneous and systemic reaction. Blisters and atypical target lesions involve less than 10% of body surface area, with some epidermal detachment, which can cause scarring in some cases. With more extensive involvement, clinical findings are almost indistinguishable from toxic epidermal necrolysis. The skin can become hemorrhagic, and pneumonia and joint pains may occur. Serious ocular involvement is common and can culminate in partial or complete blindness. Besides drugs, this syndrome has been associated with infections, pregnancy, foods, deep radiographic therapy, and neoplasms. Mortality is estimated to be in the range of 5% to 18%. The duration of the syndrome is usually 4 to 6 weeks. The long-acting sulfonamides are most often implicated. Allopurinol, carbamazepine, fluoroquinolones, hydantoin, phenylbutazone, and piroxicam are also possible causative agents.

Toxic Epidermal Necrolysis Syndrome

Epidermal necrolysis, a severe, life-threatening mucocutaneous and systemic reaction, may be preceded by a prodrome characterized by malaise, lethargy, fever, and occasionally throat or mucous membrane soreness. Epidermal changes follow and consist of erythema and massive bullae formations that easily rupture and peel, giving the skin a scalded appearance. Hairy parts of the body are usually not affected, but mucous membrane involvement is common. Blisters cover >30% of body surface area, with extensive epidermal detachment that can result in scarring. Approximately 30% of patients with toxic epidermal necrolysis succumb, often within 8 days after bullae appear. The usual cause of death is infection complicated by massive fluid and electrolyte loss, similar to patients with extensive burns. Although the skin takes on a grave appearance, healing occurs within 2 weeks in approximately 70% of patients, with some potential for scarring. In addition to drugs, certain bacterial infections and foods are believed to cause this type of eruption. Most causes of toxic epidermal necrolysis in children are due to infection (e.g., *Staphylococcus aureus*). There appears to be a higher incidence of this type of drug eruption in HIV-positive patients. Drugs most frequently implicated include allopurinol, aminopenicillins, carbamazepine, hydantoin, phenylbutazone, piroxicam, and sulfa drugs.

Erythema Nodosum

Erythema nodosum eruptions appear as red, indurated, inflammatory nodules on the shins and knees. In addition to the unusual distribution, the lesions are tender when palpated. Occasionally, these lesions are accompanied by mild constitutional symptoms, but there is usually no mucous membrane involvement. Etiologic factors associated with the development of erythema nodosum include drugs, female gender, rheumatic fever, sarcoidosis, leprosy, certain bacterial infections (e.g., tuberculosis), and systemic fungal infections such as coccidioidomycosis. Usually, the lesions heal slowly over several weeks after the offending agent is removed. Oral contraceptives are the most frequently implicated drug with this type of eruption. Other implicated drugs include sulfonamides and analgesics.

Drug Hypersensitivity Syndrome

This severe systemic reaction is also known as anticonvulsant hypersensitivity syndrome and as drug reaction with eosinophilia and systemic symptoms (DRESS). Symptoms begin with a high fever followed by widespread maculopapular-pustular rash on the trunk, arms, and legs that may lead to exfoliative dermatitis with large areas of skin sloughing. Hair and nails are sometimes lost. Eosinophilia occurs in >50% of cases, 30% have abnormal lymphocytosis, and 20% have lymphadenopathy. Internal organ damage appears late in the syndrome with elevations of liver function and/or renal function laboratory values. These may be accompanied by other general systemic symptoms such as headache and malaise. Secondary bacterial infections can occur. Approximately 10% of patients die, many due to infection. If exfoliative dermatitis occurs, it can take weeks or months to resolve, even after withdrawal of the offending agent. The most commonly implicated drugs are sulfonamides, antimalarials, anticonvulsants, and penicillin. Although rarely reported in the literature, its broad range of symptoms, confusing nomenclature, and symptom overlap with other drug-related adverse effects may lead to underdiagnosis and reporting.

Fixed Drug Eruptions

Fixed drug eruptions, unlike the previously mentioned reactions, are caused exclusively by drugs. The lesions are erythematous and sharply bordered, and have a tendency to be darker than the surrounding, unaffected skin. Eruptions can be eczematous, urticarial, vesicular, bullous, or nodular. Lesions appear 30 minutes to 8 hours after readministration in sensitized individuals. Because these lesions have a marked propensity to recur at the same location with each drug exposure, the word *fixed* is applied. The face and genitalia are common sites for this type of drug eruption. Although the eruptions heal after withdrawal of the causative drug, there is usually a marked hyperpigmentation of the area that may take months to resolve. The mechanism by which fixed drug eruptions occur has not been elucidated, but is believed to be allergic in nature. It can be described figuratively as islands of hypersensitivity; one area of the skin having the ability to evoke an allergic response and other areas lacking this ability. Commonly implicated drugs include antimicrobial agents (tetracycline, sulfonamides, metronidazole, nystatin), anti-inflammatory drugs (salicylates, nonsteroidal anti-inflammatory drugs), barbiturates, oral contraceptives, and phenolphthalein-containing laxatives.

Maculopapular Eruptions

Maculopapular eruptions are subdivided into two groups: scarlatiniform and morbilliform. Most drug eruptions fall within one of these two groups. *Scarlatiniform* eruptions are erythematous and usually involve extensive areas of the body. They are differentiated from streptococcal-induced scarlet fever by the lack of other diagnostic signs and laboratory studies. *Morbilliform* eruptions usually begin as discrete, reddish-brown maculae that may coalesce to form a diffuse rash. These eruptions are differentiated from measles by the lack of fever and other typical clinical signs. In either type of maculopapular eruption, pruritus may or may not be present. Generally, this type of eruption appears within 1 week after the causative drug (with penicillins, 2 or more weeks) has been started and completely clears within 7 to 14 days after stopping it. Morbilliform eruptions commonly are caused by ampicillin, amoxicillin, and allopurinol.

Purpura

Purpuric lesions are characterized as hemorrhages into the skin. They are purplish and sharply bordered, and have a tendency to become brownish as they get older. These lesions may or may not be associated with thrombocytopenia. Etiologic factors other than drugs that are associated with purpura are vitamin C deficiency, snake bites, and infections. The mechanism by which these lesions are produced is not known, but they have a tendency to recur with re-exposure to the causative agent. Sometimes purpura may develop concurrent with other types of eruptions, such as erythema multiforme.

Urticaria

Urticarial eruptions are immediate hypersensitivity reactions (IgE mediated) and usually appear as sharply circumscribed (raised), edematous, and erythematous lesions (wheals) with an abrupt onset. In most cases, the lesions disappear within a few hours, rarely last longer than 24 hours, and are associated with an intense itching, stinging, or prickling sensation. Commonly called *hives,* urticarial eruptions are frequently associated with certain drugs, foods, psychic upsets, and serum sickness. Rarely, parasites or neoplasms can precipitate hives. The most frequently implicated drugs with this type of reaction are aspirin, penicillin, and blood products. Patients who develop urticaria due to a drug are at increased risk of anaphylaxis if re-exposed to the same medication in the future.

Angioneurotic Edema

Angioneurotic edema (also called angioedema) is a more severe form of urticaria in which giant hives penetrate more deeply into surrounding tissues. Lips, mouth, tongue, and eyelids are common locations. Extensive involvement of the tongue, throat, or larynx can be fatal. Angiotensin converting enzyme inhibitors (ACEIs) are the most common drug cause of angioedema. Patients taking ACEIs should be warned to look out for any unusual swelling in the facial/oral area and, if present, should go immediately to the nearest emergency room for treatment. Although it usually occurs within the first several months of treatment, cases have been reported up to as long as 3 years after initiation of ACEI therapy (see Chapter 18, Heart Failure).

14. D.Z., a 42-year-old man with a chronic seizure disorder and long-standing anxiety was recently given a prescription for penicillin V 250 mg QID for a group A, α-hemolytic streptococcal-positive pharyngitis. Chronic medications include carbamazepine 200 mg TID and clonazepam 2 mg BID. One week later, D.Z. presents with urticarial lesions on his chest and arms. Is this a typical time of onset for a drug-induced dermatologic reaction? How should the drug eruption in D.Z. be managed?

Although most drug eruptions occur within 1 to 2 weeks after starting therapy, it may take 3 to 4 weeks after an initial exposure to a medication for the reaction to occur. Repeated exposure to the same offending agent can reduce the time of onset of the reaction to a few days or even within hours of ingestion. Because D.Z. has been taking clonazepam and carbamazepine chronically and penicillin for only 8 days, the temporal relationship would logically lead to the conclusion that penicillin is a highly probable cause. However, before labeling penicillin as the cause of his drug eruption, a thorough history to rule out other common causes should be done.

For D.Z., a different antibiotic should be substituted for penicillin (to complete the 10-day course of therapy). The lesion should begin to clear in 24 hours (if the penicillin is the cause of the urticaria). If the urticaria does not begin to clear in a few days, another cause should be investigated.

Treatment is primarily supportive, and use of an oral antihistamine (e.g., diphenhydramine 25–50 mg BID-QID) for several days would be recommended. If the reaction is severe, a 1- to 2-week course of prednisone 40 to 60 mg/day will control most symptoms within 48 hours.

ALLERGIC CONTACT DERMATITIS: POISON IVY/OAK/SUMAC

Poison ivy (*Rhus*) dermatitis is the major cause of allergic contact dermatitis in the United States, exceeding all other causes combined. It is estimated that 50% to 95% of the population is sensitive to the plant to some degree. The severity of the condition varies from mild discomfort to an extremely painful, debilitating condition. *Rhus* dermatitis is caused by sensitization to an allergic substance in the leaves, stems, and roots of poison ivy, poison oak, and poison sumac plants. All three plants contain the same sensitizing oleoresin, urushiol oil, which contains pentadecacatechol, the actual sensitizing agent. Therefore, the dermatitis caused by the three different plants is identical.

Direct contact with the plant is unnecessary for the rash to occur. Highly sensitive persons may develop severe dermatitis merely from exposure to *Rhus* oleoresin carried by pollen or by smoke from burning leaves. The oleoresin may remain active for months on clothing, shoes, tools, and sporting equipment. Once the toxic substance comes in contact with the skin, it can be spread by the hands to other areas of the body (e.g., genitals or eyes) or to people who may come into close contact with the exposed person. Although washing with soap and water will not prevent the dermatitis, even if it is done within 15 minutes of exposure, it will prevent spread of the oleoresin to other parts of the body.

Rhus dermatitis can be contracted throughout the year, even in winter, by contact with the roots of the plant. The virulence of the leaf sap varies little during the foliage period. The incidence of poison ivy is higher during the spring because the leaves are tender and bruise easily, and people spend more time outdoors. Sensitive individuals should be instructed to avoid contact with the offending plant. If contact is inevitable, every effort should be made to shield exposed areas of the skin with appropriate clothing, and bentoquatam (Ivy Block), a topical organoclay compound, should be considered. A 5% lotion applied to the skin 15 minutes before exposure and reapplied every 4 hours has reduced or prevented contact dermatitis induced by experimental challenge with urushiol in sensitive individuals. Cost may limit its routine use.

Exposed individuals should bathe or shower as soon as they come in from outdoors and should wash their clothes. A nonprescription topical cleanser called Tecnu Extreme claims to remove urushiol oil embedded in the skin through the action of microfine scrubbing beads and surfactants, thus possibly preventing the rash or limiting spread. It also contains the homeopathic agent Grindelia as an antipruritic. It is formulated as a thick, creamy gel that is applied to exposed areas of the skin, followed by vigorous scrubbing, and rinsed off after application.

After an initial incubation period of 5 to 21 days, a patient would be expected to react to the oleoresin in 12 to 48 hours after re-exposure. A mild exposure to these plants in a sensitized person results in a typical erythematous, vesicular, linear, and sometimes, oozing rash after 2 to 3 days; complete clearing occurs in 1 to 3 weeks. If a large area is exposed, lesions appear within 6 to 12 hours and may appear blistered and eroded; in some cases, ulcers may appear. Healing occurs more slowly, often requiring 2 to 3 weeks for complete resolution. The following factors contribute to the development of poison ivy/oak/sumac: the concentration of the oleoresin to which the skin is exposed, area of exposure (i.e., the thickness of the stratum corneum), duration of exposure, site of exposure, genetic factors, and immune tolerance. It is important to determine the areas of the body that are affected. If the eyes, genital areas, mouth, respiratory tract, or >15% of the body is affected, the patient should receive a course of systemic corticosteroids.

Because different sites of the body differ in their sensitivity to the oleoresin and because patients spread the *Rhus* oleoresin to different parts of their bodies over a period of time, lesions often erupt over a period of several days. A common misconception many people have is that the fluid from the *Rhus*-induced vesicles will spread the disease to unaffected areas. A more likely explanation is the presence of residual resin underneath poorly washed fingernails, soiled clothes (including gloves used in yard work), and pet fur.

Treatment

15. K.P., a 27-year-old woman, has recently returned from an outing in the woods. She now has vesicular eruptions that appear in a linear pattern on one arm and hand. She believes that she has had a poison oak reaction and requests therapy. What should be recommended at this point? What should be recommended if the condition becomes more severe?

Weeping lesions should be treated with aqueous vehicles (e.g., Burow's solution or saline) as outlined in the beginning of this chapter. Lesions that are not wet or weeping should be treated with calamine lotion applied two to four times daily. The zinc oxide in calamine lotion may act as a mild astringent, although some people find this preparation to be unacceptable because of its pink color, which can stain clothes. Alternatively, a topical corticosteroid appropriate for the body part affected could be used. If K.P.'s poison oak reaction becomes more severe, additional treatment with prednisone 1 mg/kg/day for at least 2 or 3 weeks will be required; such therapy should be withdrawn slowly (over 1–2 weeks) to prevent recurrence of the lesions.

Systemic Therapy

16. Z.T., a 19-year-old man, has just returned from a fishing trip and now has an erythematous, linear, dry eruption on his leg and arm, and a generalized eruption on his hands and face. He has been in areas that have dense poison ivy growth, and he may have burned some in the campfire. Z.T. has washed himself and his clothes thoroughly. How should he be treated?

The fact that Z.T.'s facial rash is not linear (as one would expect if he had just contacted the plant) suggests that he may have contacted the smoke of a burning poison ivy plant. This can be quite serious because the oleoresin can be carried in smoke and, if inhaled, can cause severe respiratory problems. Z.T. should be observed for signs of respiratory difficulties and should be treated with a course of systemic corticosteroids.

Relapse

17. Z.T.'s physician prescribed prednisone for his rash. He was instructed to take 80 mg/day for 14 days and to decrease the dose by 5 mg/day each day thereafter. Calamine lotion (TID to affected areas) also was prescribed. After 12 days, Z.T. complains that the lesions seem to be getting worse. The lesions had cleared after 8 days of treatment, and he began rapidly tapering the prednisone at that time. Why is he experiencing a relapse?

Two weeks is the absolute minimum course of treatment when systemic corticosteroids are used for severe cases of poison ivy/oak/sumac. The oleoresin remains fixed in the skin, and if the systemic corticosteroid is withdrawn too soon, the lesions return. This is probably the most common reason for treatment failure with systemic corticosteroids.

Allergic Contact Dermatitis

18. Z.T.'s corticosteroid therapy was reinstated. After 3 weeks, most of the lesions had disappeared, and the prednisone therapy was discontinued. However, Z.T. continued to complain of a rash on his hands. Further questioning revealed that he was continuing to apply an over-the-counter topical calamine lotion containing diphenhydramine. What is a potential drug-related cause of this persistent rash?

Topical application of diphenhydramine and other antihistamines may cause allergic contact dermatitis.[24] Z.T. should stop using this product to see if his rash clears. A list of common contact sensitizers is found in Table 38-14.

The treatment for sensitivity reactions is basically the same as that outlined for poison ivy/oak/sumac.

REFERENCES

1. Hall JC. Sauer's Manual of Skin Diseases. 9th ed. Philadelphia: Lippincott Williams & Wilkins; 2006.
2. Hood AF et al. Primer of Dermatopathology. 3rd ed. Philadelphia: Lippincott Williams & Wilkins; 2002.
3. Odom RB. Andrew's Diseases of the Skin. 10th ed. Philadelphia: WB Saunders; 2005.
4. Champion RH et al. Rook's Textbook of Dermatology. 7th ed. Oxford, England: Blackwell Scientific; 2004.
5. Freedberg IM et al. Fitzpatrick's Dermatology in General Medicine. 6th ed. New York: McGraw-Hill; 2003.
6. Habif TP et al. Clinical Dermatology: A Color Guide to Diagnosis and Therapy. 3rd ed. St. Louis, MO: Mosby; 1967.
7. Arndt KA et al. Manual of Dermatologic Therapies. 6th ed. Philadelphia: Lippincott Williams & Wilkins; 2002.
8. Wehner AP. Biological effects of cosmetic talc. Food Chem Toxicol 1994;32:1173.
9. Lee NP et al. Topical corticosteroids: back to basics. *West J Med* 1999;171:351.
10. Giannotti B et al. Topical corticosteroids. Which drug and when? *Drugs* 1992;44:65.
11. Fisher D. Adverse effects of topical corticosteroid use. *West J Med* 1995;162:123.
12. Butani L. Corticosteroid-induced hypersensitivity reactions. *Ann Allergy Asthma Immunol* 2002;89: 439.
13. Levin C et al. Topical corticosteroid-induced adrenocortical insufficiency: clinical implications. *Am J Clin Dermatol* 2002;3:141.
14. Chan HL et al. Effect of topical corticosteroid on microbial flora of human skin. *J Am Acad Dermatol* 1982;7:346.
15. George A et al. A systematic review and meta-analysis of treatments for impetigo. *Br J Gen Pract* 2003;53:480.
16. Guay DR. Treatment of bacterial skin and skin structure infections. *Expert Opin Pharmacother* 2003;4:1259.
17. Brown J et al. Impetigo: an update. *Int J Dermatol* 2003;42:251.
18. Walker ES et al. Mupirocin-resistant, methicillin-resistant *Staphylococcus aureus:* does mupirocin remain effective? *Infect Control Hosp Epidemiol* 2003;24:342.
19. Kimura M et al. Contact sensitivity induced by neomycin with cross-sensitivity to other aminoglycoside antibiotics. *Contact Dermatitis* 1998;39:148.
20. Yung MW et al. Delayed hypersensitivity reaction to topical aminoglycosides in patients undergoing middle ear surgery. *Clin Otolaryngol* 2002;27:365.
21. Charlesworth EN et al. Pruritic dermatoses: overview of etiology and therapy. *Am J Med* 2002;113(Suppl 9A):25S.
22. Prystowsky SD et al. Allergic contact hypersensitivity to nickel, neomycin, ethylenediamine, and benzocaine: relationships between age, sex, history of exposure, and reactivity to standard patch tests and use tests in a general population. *Arch Dermatol* 1979;115:959.
23. Marks JG, DeLeo VA. Evaluation and treatment of patients with contact dermatitis. In: Marks JG, DeLeo VA, eds. Contact and Occupational Dermatology. 2nd ed. St. Louis, MO: Mosby; 1997:14.
24. Heine A. Diphenhydramine: a forgotten allergen? *Contact Dermatitis* 1996;35:311.
25. Dimson S, Nanayakkara C. Related articles. Do oral antihistamines stop the itch of atopic dermatitis? *Arch Dis Child* 2003;88:832.
26. Herman SM et al. Antihistamines in the treatment of atopic dermatitis. *J Cutan Med Surg* 2003; epub ahead of print.
27. Gupta MA et al. The use of antidepressant drugs in dermatology. *J Eur Acad Dermatol Venereol* 2001;15:512.
28. Akdis CA et al. Diagnosis and treatment of atopic dermatitis in children and adults: European Academy of Allergology and Clinical Immunology/American Academy of Allergy, Asthma and Immunology/PRACTALL Consensus Report. *J Allergy Clin Immunol* 2006;118:152
29. Wharton M et al. Advisory Committee on Immunization Practices: Healthcare Infection Control Practices Advisory Committee. Recommendations for using smallpox vaccine in a pre-event vaccination program. Supplemental recommendations of the Advisory Committee on Immunization Practices (ACIP) and the Healthcare Infection Control Practices Advisory Committee (HICPAC). *MMWR Recomm Rep* 2003;52(RR-7):1.
30. Senter TP. Topical fluocinonide and tachyphylaxis. *Arch Dermatol* 1983;119:363.
31. Miller JJ et al. Failure to demonstrate therapeutic tachyphylaxis to topically applied steroids in patients with psoriasis. *J Am Acad Dermatol* 1999;41: 546.
32. Kapp A et al. Atopic dermatitis management with tacrolimus ointment (Protopic). *J Dermatol Treat* 2003;14(Suppl 1):5.
33. Patel RR et al. The safety and efficacy of tacrolimus therapy in patients younger than 2 years with atopic dermatitis. *Arch Dermatol* 2003;139:1184.
34. Weinberg JM et al. Atopic dermatitis: a new treatment paradigm using pimecrolimus. *J Drugs Dermatol* 2003;2:131.
35. Norman RA. Xerosis and pruritus in the elderly: recognition and management. *Dermatol Ther* 2003;16:254.
36. Fiszenson-Albala F et al. A 6-month prospective survey of cutaneous drug reactions in a hospital setting. *Br J Dermatol* 2003;149:1018.
37. Cutaneous drug reaction case reports: from the world literature. *Am J Clin Dermatol* 2003;4:727.
38. Williams MP, Conklin RJ. Erythema multiforme: a review and contrast from Stevens-Johnson syndrome/topic epidermal necrolysis. *Dent Clin N Am* 2005;49:67.

CHAPTER 39

Acne

Ellen E. Rhinard

Definition, Clinical Signs, and Symptoms

The term *acne* usually refers to acne vulgaris, a common disease in which the pilosebaceous units of the skin become plugged and distended (see Fig. 38-1 in Chapter 38). It differs from rosacea (formerly called *acne rosacea*), which causes facial erythema, telangiectasia, and papules, and occurs later in life. *Acne cosmetica* and *acne mechanica* are terms describing aggravation of the condition by cosmetics or by mechanical irritation such as that from helmet straps.

Acne lesions generally appear on the face, but the chest, back, or upper arms may also be affected. Comedones, plugged follicular openings, are noninflammatory lesions that may be closed ("whiteheads") or open ("blackheads"). The dark pigmentation in open comedones is caused by oxidation of sebaceous material or melanin rather than by dirt, a common misperception.[1] Inflammatory lesions are typically erythematous and can include pustules (raised, superficial, pus-filled lesions), papules (raised, solid lesions up to several millimeters in diameter), and nodules (like papules but larger and deeper in the skin); in severe cases (acne conglobata), multiple lesions coalesce into abscesses with draining sinus tracts.[2] Although no single severity scale has emerged as standard, clinicians must use some acne grading scale consistently to evaluate treatment options and clinical response. Often, clinicians describe acne as mild (few lesions, little or no inflammation), moderate (many lesions, significant inflammation), or severe (numerous lesions, extreme inflammation and/or nodules, significant scarring).[3] The Combined Acne Severity Classification is one recommended codification system (Table 39-1).[4] Lesion counts per se are not practical for clinicians, but are used by researchers.

Acne can cause psychological distress, low self-esteem, and social withdrawal, affecting quality of life as much as more physically disabling diseases such as asthma and diabetes.[5] Considerable psychological morbidity can result from even mild to moderate acne.[6] Questionnaires have been developed to identify the psychosocial impact of acne.[7] The major long-term complication of acne is scarring, usually "ice pick" pitting with significant disfigurement. Scarring can be exacerbated by tissue excoriation caused by picking at or squeezing the lesions. Early initiation of effective therapy is critical to prevent scarring.[8]

Acne occurs in people of all ages, but acne vulgaris primarily afflicts teenagers and young adults. Acne is also associated with systemic diseases such as SAPHO (synovitis, acne, pustulosis, hyperostosis, osteitis) and Apert syndromes.[9,10] The differential diagnosis of acneiform eruptions includes acne vulgaris; rosacea; folliculitis caused by gram-negative bacteria, *Pityrosporum*, or mechanical irritation; drug-induced acne such as that caused by topical or systemic corticosteroids, or by anabolic steroids, including those abused by athletes; and perioral dermatitis.[11–14] Detailed discussions of severe acne variants, such as acne conglobata and acne fulminans, are beyond the scope of this chapter.[11,15]

Incidence and Prevalence

Acne vulgaris affects more than 50 million people in the United States[16] and about 90% of all adolescents.[17] Studies suggest that it is primarily an inherited disorder with environmental factors playing a secondary role.[8] Although no gender preference exists, females typically develop acne at a younger age and have milder cases than males.[15] Acne can occur in children as young as 8 years; however, it is most prevalent in adolescents between 14 and 19 years of age.[18] Although most cases resolve by the time patients reach their mid-20s, acne persists into later life in

Table 39-1 Combined Acne Severity Classification

Acne Severity Grade	Description[a]
Mild	<20 comedones; or <15 papules; or <30 lesions total; no nodules
Moderate	20–100 comedones; or 15–50 inflammatory lesions; or 30–125 lesions total; nodules may be present
Severe	>5 nodules; or >100 comedones; or >50 inflammatory lesions; or >125 lesions total

[a]Stage acne in the most severe applicable grade.
Adapted from reference 4.

7% to 17% of patients, more often in women than men.[15] Acne may be slightly less common in patients with darker skin, but some believe research in prevalence is confounded by poorer access to health care among patients of color; most studies find that acne is the top dermatologic complaint in patients of all skin tones.[19] Severe nodular acne is more common in light-skinned patients, but dark-skinned patients show more inflammation at the histologic level than in light-skinned patients with similar clinical lesion severity. Dark-skinned individuals are also more likely to contend with postinflammatory hyperpigmentation (PIH) and keloid scar formation in the wake of acne lesions.[19,20] Females treated with antiepileptic drugs such as phenytoin or phenobarbital experience acne more commonly than age-matched controls (80% vs. 30%).[21]

Etiology and Risk Factors

The development of acne is related to increased sebum production, abnormal keratinization within the pilosebaceous canal (hypercornification), bacterial colonization, and immune-mediated inflammation. Multiple exogenous and endogenous factors can affect the development of acne vulgaris. Diet (with rare individual exceptions), cleanliness, and sexual activity do not contribute to the severity of acne or the frequency of its exacerbations, but some evidence does support the popular belief that psychological stress may promote exacerbations in predisposed patients.[1] Premenstrual exacerbations of acne are common.[15] Oil-based cosmetics, pomades, and moisturizers may also encourage the development of acne.[22] Hot and humid conditions that stimulate sweating often worsen acne.[1]

Studies of sunlight exposure have found contradictory results; ultraviolet light may make sebum more comedogenic, but some of the visible wavelengths may reduce the follicular bacterial population.[1,23] Occupational or environmental exposure to halogenated compounds, ultraviolet light, animal fats, dioxin, or petroleum derivatives may cause "chloracne" or other acneiform lesions.[24,25] It is important to identify drug-induced acne (see Chapter 38) because treatment success likely depends on drug therapy modification. Mechanical skin irritation caused by headbands, hats, chin straps, backpacks, or shoulder pads may also induce acne mechanica.[3]

Pathogenesis

The key pathophysiologic change leading to acne occurs when keratinocytes in the follicular epithelial lining proliferate and undergo changes in cellular differentiation. Keratinization increases and the cells adhere more to each other, interfering with normal desquamation. Cellular debris and sebum accumulate to plug sebaceous follicles and form clinically undetectable microcomedones.[2] If the superficial portion of the follicular opening dilates from the pressure of the impaction, an open comedo forms. Such lesions rarely become inflamed because as pressure builds from further sebum production and cellular accumulation, follicular contents can escape to the skin surface.[22] If the follicular opening remains narrow and a closed comedo forms, increased pressure ruptures the follicular wall and infiltration of foreign matter into the dermis incites an inflammatory response. The depth and extent of this occurrence determine whether a pustule, papule, or nodule results.[11]

Androgen-enhanced sebocyte activity and bacterial colonization mediate lesion development. Testosterone, of testicular origin in males or ovarian and adrenal origin in females, is metabolized in the skin by 5-α-reductase to dihydrotestosterone (DHT), which in turn stimulates sebum biosynthesis.[2] Increased sebum production dilutes the availability of linoleic acid and increases the production of interleukin-1-α, triggering hypercornification and thus comedogenesis.[2,22] Increased sebum production also creates a lipid-rich, microaerophilic environment favorable to the growth of *Propionibacterium acnes*. This gram-positive rod releases proteases, hyaluronidases, lipases, and chemotactic factors that attract neutrophils, T cells, and macrophages.[26] Even after being engulfed by macrophages, this organism can persist intracellularly.[27] Hydrolytic enzymes released by macrophages may contribute to weakening the follicular wall, hastening rupture and the resulting progression of comedo to inflammatory lesion.[22] Inflammatory mediators traverse the follicular wall into the dermis and initiate the inflammatory process even prior to wall rupture.[15] Interleukins and tumor necrosis factor-α released by macrophages and lymphocytes complement activation by *P. acnes*, and antibody- and cell-mediated immunologic mechanisms activated by *P. acnes* all participate in the inflammatory response.[2] Finally, a genetic predisposition may exist in which patients with acne have enhanced cytochrome P450 1A1 activity, which reduces levels of protective endogenous retinoids.[28]

Therapy

No known cure exists for acne, but treatment can reduce its severity and minimize complications of scarring. In most cases, especially in severe forms, treatment is more an "art" than a science and must be individualized, depending on the particular clinical presentation of the patient. The goals of treatment are to relieve discomfort, improve skin appearance, prevent scarring, and minimize the psychosocial impact of the condition.

Treatment is largely preventive because little can be done for existing lesions. Slow improvement over weeks to months is the rule for all treatments. Patients can generally expect 20%, 60%, and 80% resolution of lesions within 2, 6, and 8 months, respectively, after effective therapy is begun (slower resolution with hormonal therapies, faster resolution with oral isotretinoin).[15] Therefore, treatment regimens should not be modified more often than every 6 to 8 weeks. Patients should be counseled on the basic pathophysiology of acne, proper drug administration or application technique, delay in onset of therapeutic effect, potential adverse effects, and steps to take if adverse effects

Table 39-2 Pertinent Historical Components To Be Obtained From a Patient With Acne

- Duration, including onset and peak severity
- Location and distribution
- Seasonal variation
- For female patients, relation to menstrual periods, pregnancy status, scalp hair thinning, contraceptive method (if used)
- Present and past treatments, topical and systemic, prescription and over the counter
- Family history, including severity
- Other skin disorders or medical problems
- Medications and drug allergies
- Occupational exposure to chemicals or oils
- Skin care routine; use of cosmetics, moisturizers, hairstyling products (pomades)
- Areas of skin friction or irritation

occur. Clinical practice guidelines are available.[4,29,30] Therapy is tailored to patient-specific data (Table 39-2).

Nondrug Therapy

Nondrug therapy plays a minimal role in the management of acne. In general, patient education regarding nondrug therapy boils down to "first, do no harm." Twice-daily washing with warm water and a mild facial cleanser is sufficient; acne is not a disorder of poor hygiene, and aggressive skin washing and abrasive cleansers needlessly traumatize the skin.[15] Manipulation (e.g., squeezing, picking) of acne lesions should be strongly discouraged because it can lead to scarring. Drugs known to cause acne, oil-based cosmetics, and other known precipitants should also obviously be avoided. However, oil-free, noncomedogenic moisturizers formulated for facial skin can improve the penetration and tolerability of many topical acne drugs by improving the skin's hydration, especially in patients with sensitive skin. Many such moisturizers also contain sunscreen, which is recommended for use with many of the available acne therapies.[16]

Dermatologists may use physical modalities to treat acne, especially as adjuncts to medication in severe cases. Options include surgical comedo extraction, dermabrasion, cryotherapy, and experimental light and laser therapies.[11,31,32] No prospective, controlled trials comparing medical and physical measures for managing severe acne exist. Acne scarring is treated with dermabrasion, laser therapy, chemical peels, and recollagenation, but systematic randomized trials are needed to fully assess safety and comparative efficacy.[11,33,34]

Drug Therapy

Although many drugs either alone or in combination may ultimately be used in acne treatment, all therapies are based on treating one or more of the primary pathogenic factors.[35,36] Effective drugs work by (a) normalizing follicular keratinization (e.g., retinoids, benzoyl peroxide, azelaic acid); (b) decreasing sebum production (e.g., isotretinoin, hormonal therapies); (c) suppressing *P. acnes* (e.g., antibiotics, benzoyl peroxide, azelaic acid, systemic isotretinoin); and (d) reducing inflammation (e.g., antibiotics, retinoids).

Topical therapy is generally preferable for mild to moderate acne. Common choices include a retinoid for mild comedonal acne or benzoyl peroxide for mild inflammatory acne, initially augmented in moderate acne with a course of topical antibiotics. Treatments are applied to the entire acne-prone area, not just to existing lesions, because the mechanisms of action more effectively prevent than resolve lesions. With topical therapy, choice of vehicle is as important to treatment success as choice of drug. Gels and solutions are highly drying and suitable for oily skin, whereas less drying creams and moderately drying lotions are preferred in dry and/or sensitive skin; ointments are generally too comedogenic to be useful in acne. Comedolytic therapies such as retinoids and benzoyl peroxide are often initiated at low concentrations and application frequencies using a vehicle appropriate to the patient's skin type, and titrated up in strength, frequency, and drying effect as tolerated to achieve desired outcomes.

Moderate to severe acne often requires combination therapy using agents with different mechanisms of action, such as topical benzoyl peroxide and/or a topical retinoid plus a systemic antibiotic. Hormonal therapies (e.g., oral contraceptives) are an option in female patients who are not pregnant and not planning to become pregnant. Severe acne requires oral isotretinoin. Because oral isotretinoin addresses every known pathophysiologic mechanism of acne, combining it with other medications is unnecessary.

RETINOIDS

Vitamin A and its analogs have been used to treat acne for more than 50 years.[37,38] Retinoids normalize keratinization by decreasing horny cell cohesiveness and stimulating epidermal cell turnover. These actions combine to unplug follicles and prevent microcomedo formation.[39] Retinoids also reduce inflammation by inhibiting the production of inflammatory mediators.[40] Topical retinoids have no antibacterial properties, but systemic (oral) isotretinoin indirectly reduces *P. acnes* colonization by reducing the production of sebum, which *P. acnes* requires for survival.[2] Systemic isotretinoin therefore exhibits all four of the mechanisms of action outlined previously, making it uniquely effective monotherapy.

As the most potent comedolytic agents, topical retinoids are preferred therapy in mild acne cases with mostly noninflammatory lesions.[41] They may also be used in combination with antibiotics and/or other therapies to manage moderate to severe acne. They are usually applied once daily at bedtime. Common side effects include skin irritation, peeling, erythema, and dryness; patients should be advised to use sunscreen because the newly exfoliated skin is prone to burn. Patients should also be warned that acne may initially worsen before improvement is noted,[42] although this rarely occurs if topical antibiotics are also being used.[43] Tretinoin (Retin-A®), also called all-*trans*-retinoic acid, is the naturally occurring form of vitamin A acid and is available for topical application as a cream (0.025%, 0.05%, 0.1%) and gel (0.01%, 0.025%). Newer dosage forms are less irritating (and more expensive): delayed-release cream and gel (0.025%; Avita®) and microsphere gel (0.04%, 0.1%; Retin-A® Micro). Another topical retinoid, adapalene (Differin®), is available as a 0.1% cream and gel. It binds to different receptors than tretinoin[44] and has more anti-inflammatory activity.[40] Adapalene is at least as effective as tretinoin and may cause less skin irritation than other topical retinoids.[45] Irritation from topical tretinoin can darken skin if used too aggressively in dark-skinned patients, but adapalene may reduce hyperpigmentation in such patients.[40] The newest agent in the class, tazarotene (Tazorac®), is available in cream and gel formulations (0.05% and 0.1%). It may not only be the most effective, but also the least well tolerated, of the topical retinoids.[42] Among the topical retinoids, only the older dosage forms of tretinoin are available generically. Topical isotretinoin is not yet available in the United States. Because benzoyl peroxide inactivates tretinoin, combination therapy with these two agents should be avoided. However, benzoyl peroxide can be used in combination with either adapalene or tazarotene to provide potential additive benefit.[46]

Isotretinoin (Accutane®, Amnesteem™, Claravis™, Sotret®), a synthetic 13-*cis*-isomer of tretinoin, has greater pharmacologic activity than tretinoin. It is administered orally as 10-, 20-, 30-, and 40-mg capsules and is the only effective agent for severe nodular acne. Essentially all patients will respond to systemic isotretinoin; in most cases, one or two 5-month-long courses of therapy induce a remission lasting for several months or even years after the drug is stopped. Use of oral isotretinoin is perhaps more cost effective than use of long-term oral antibiotics in patients with severe acne, due to its superior efficacy and the long-term cost savings realized by a shorter total duration of therapy.[47] The common adverse effects of systemic isotretinoin, invariably including drying of skin and mucous membranes, can usually be managed without having to stop the drug. However, the risk of serious adverse effects from oral isotretinoin, the high cost of the drug, and its potential for overuse necessitate strict guidelines for its rational use (Table 39-3).[29,48] Table 39-4 summarizes common and significant adverse effects of isotretinoin. Patients should also be warned that acne may worsen initially because flares occur in about half of patients.[49]

Retinoids, even for topical use, must be avoided during pregnancy because the drug class is notoriously teratogenic.

Table 39-3 Guidelines for Isotretinoin Use in Acne

Patient Selection	
	Severe nodular acne
	Moderate acne, but resistant to combination conventional therapies or inducing significant scarring
	Unusually severe acne variants (conglobata, fulminans)
Dosage and Duration of Therapy	
	0.5–1 mg/kg/day in two divided doses with food; use lower initial dose to minimize flaring
	Usual course about 20 weeks (best results if cumulative dose reaches 120–150 mg/kg)
	Use higher dosage in young patients, males, those with severe acne, patients with acne involving the trunk (up to 2 mg/kg/day)
	Consider pretreatment or concomitant oral corticosteroids for severely inflamed acne
Relapse Rate	
	Repeat courses required in 10%–20% of patients, often younger patients or patients who received lower doses
	Allow 2–3 months between courses
	Very rarely, patients may require three to five courses

Adapted from references 11, 29, and 58.

A strict risk management program called iPLEDGE regulates the prescription and distribution of isotretinoin in the United States.[50] The program requires all patients, prescribers, pharmacies, and even drug wholesalers involved in distribution and use of the drug to register with a national database. Proper patient monitoring and education, including negative pregnancy tests in female patients of child-bearing potential, must be documented in the database each month before initial or refill medication can be dispensed to a patient. Female patients of child-bearing potential must use two forms of contraception for at least a month before, all during, and for at least a month following isotretinoin therapy. All isotretinoin patients, male and female, must refrain from donating blood during or for a month after therapy to ensure no isotretinoin-contaminated blood products are unknowingly administered to a pregnant woman.

BENZOYL PEROXIDE

Topical benzoyl peroxide primarily works as an antibacterial agent, but also has comedolytic properties. Lipophilic, it penetrates to the site of *P. acnes* growth and releases oxygen free radicals that damage bacterial cell walls.[51] Because resistance cannot develop to this bactericidal mechanism, benzoyl peroxide is often paired with oral antibiotics to prevent the development of antibiotic resistance. The irritant effects of benzoyl peroxide also cause vasodilation and increase blood flow, which may hasten resolution of inflammatory lesions. Benzoyl peroxide improves both inflammatory and noninflammatory lesions; it is similar to topical retinoids in improving comedonal acne and preferred for inflammatory acne.[52,53]

Benzoyl peroxide is available over the counter (OTC) and by prescription in a variety of dosage forms (cleansers, lotions, creams, and gels) and concentrations (2.5%–10%). It is usually applied to the affected area once or twice daily. Cleansers allow little contact time compared to other dosage forms, but they can enhance adherence to therapy when patients must apply medication to the trunk because the cleanser can be conveniently applied and left on for a few minutes in the shower. Patients should be instructed to use sunscreen while using benzoyl peroxide because the skin is more prone to burn. Patients must also be advised that benzoyl peroxide can bleach or discolor towels, pillowcases, rugs, or other fabrics on which it is wiped or spilled.

Benzoyl peroxide has been associated with tumors in mice, but long-term use has not been associated with skin cancer.[54] The World Health Organization International Agency for Research on Cancer concluded that there is inadequate evidence to determine the human carcinogenicity risk with benzoyl peroxide.[55]

AZELAIC ACID

Azelaic acid 20% cream (Azelex®) carries an indication for acne vulgaris, while the 15% gel (Finacea®) formulation is indicated for rosacea. This dicarboxylic acid normalizes keratinization and also reduces inflammation by suppressing *P. acnes*.[56,57] *P. acnes* resistance has not been reported.[41]

Azelaic acid causes less skin irritation than other topical therapies (except for antibiotics), but may not be as effective.[2,29,58] In addition to being less irritating than other comedolytic therapies, azelaic acid inhibits tyrosinase and thereby melanin production, giving it a useful niche in treating

Table 39-4 Adverse Effects of Systemic Retinoids

Body System	Adverse Effect	Management
Common, Pharmacologic		
Reproductive	Teratogenicity (birth defects, premature birth, neonatal death)	Avoid pregnancy; patients should not donate blood during therapy
Skin	Dryness, peeling, pruritus, photosensitivity	Use moisturizers, sunscreens, protective clothing; avoid skin waxing, dermabrasion, and other dermatologic procedures during and 6 months following therapy
Hair, nails	Hair dryness, hair thinning, nail fragility	None; discontinue drug if severe
Mucous membranes	Cheilitis, dry mouth, dry nose, nosebleeds, dry eyes, blepharoconjunctivitis	Use lip balms, sugarless gum/candy, saline nasal spray, artificial tears or ophthalmic ointment; avoid contact lenses; lower dosage if severe or bothersome
Metabolic	Elevated triglycerides, cholesterol; lowered HDL (rare reports of pancreatitis)	Reduce/eliminate alcohol; consume low-fat diet; consider dosage reduction or drug discontinuation
Uncommon, Toxic		
CNS	Pseudotumor cerebri, hearing loss, tinnitus	Discontinue drug if patient develops severe headache, nausea, vomiting, papilledema, visual changes (suggest pseudotumor cerebri) or hearing changes
Bones	Pain	Monitor at each visit
	Bone mineral density loss (osteopenia), premature epiphyseal closure, hyperostosis	Routine monitoring is not recommended for usual durations of therapy
Muscle, ligaments	Pain, calcifications	Monitor; more likely in physically active patients; discontinue if severe
Eyes	Impaired night vision, corneal opacities	Patients should use caution when driving
Liver	Elevated transaminases; hepatitis	Monitor if transaminase elevation is mild; avoid in patients with previous liver dysfunction; discontinue drug if hepatitis occurs
Hematologic	Anemia, neutropenia, thrombocytopenia	Monitor CBC
Psychiatric	Depression, suicide	Monitor for depressed mood and suicidal thoughts

CBC, complete blood count; CNS, central nervous system; HDL, high-density lipoprotein.
Adapted from reference 49.

patients of color with postinflammatory hyperpigmentation.[59] A small amount of azelaic acid cream is applied twice daily. Patients should protect their skin with sunscreen. Due to its cost and possibly lower efficacy, it is usually reserved for patients who cannot tolerate benzoyl peroxide or topical retinoids.

MISCELLANEOUS TOPICAL AGENTS

Salicylic acid, sulfur, and resorcinol have been used for many years in acne, but are not well studied. Topical salicylic acid, a concentration-dependent keratolytic, is more effective than placebo, but less effective than topical benzoyl peroxide or tretinoin.[29] It may be useful in patients with mild acne who cannot tolerate other comedolytics and may augment the effectiveness of other agents when used in combination. It is available in nonprescription creams, lotions, and gels in strengths ranging from 0.5% to 2%. Chronic use over large body surfaces should be avoided because of the risk of percutaneous absorption that could cause systemic salicylate toxicity.[46] Sulfur preparations have mild comedolytic properties, but can produce skin discoloration and odor, and may be comedogenic with continued use.[60] Anecdotally, however, sulfur products succeed for some patients who have failed first-line therapies. They are available in strengths of 2% to 10%, in a variety of vehicles, often in nonprescription combination products. Resorcinol alone is ineffective,[15] but is combined in a 2% concentration with sulfur preparations to enhance the keratolytic effect. It can cause dark scaling on some patients.[60] Topical nicotinamide, a form of vitamin B_3, appears as effective as 1% clindamycin gel monotherapy in treating inflammatory acne.[15]

ANTIBIOTICS

Acne is not an "infectious" disease per se and is certainly not contagious. Rather, *P. acnes* helps transform comedones into inflammatory pustules or papules. Antibiotics do not resolve existing lesions, but they can prevent future lesions by decreasing *P. acnes* colonization. Antibiotic courses used in acne are months long, unlike the short courses used in most infectious diseases. One reason for this may be that *P. acnes* colonies encase themselves within a polysaccharide biofilm that shields them from antibiotics.[26] Another is that antibiotics can exert anti-inflammatory effects independent of their antibacterial activity. Tetracyclines and macrolides can reduce neutrophil chemotaxis and inhibit cytokines, even at subminimal inhibitory concentrations.[61,62] As a result, clinical efficacy does not correlate perfectly to reductions in bacterial load; unlike in standard antibiotic treatment, successful antibiotic courses do not necessarily eradicate *P. acnes*.[63] Just 20 mg orally twice daily of doxycycline, far lower than usual doses, was shown to reduce acne lesion counts despite causing no changes in the numbers or resistance patterns of bacteria on the skin surface.[64] However, the efficacy of this regimen has not been compared to that of traditional regimens.

Topical Antibiotics

Topically applied antibiotics avoid systemic exposure and achieve high follicular concentrations. They can augment topical retinoids when initiating therapy in mild to moderate acne cases involving inflammatory lesions, or they can be added to patients failing benzoyl peroxide monotherapy.[65] Topical antibiotic monotherapies are more effective than placebo, but they are not superior to benzoyl peroxide monotherapy.[46,66] Topical antibiotic and benzoyl peroxide combinations outperform either ingredient alone.[46,65]

Clindamycin and erythromycin are most commonly used. Clindamycin (e.g., Cleocin T®) is available as a 1% gel, lotion, solution, and foam; 1% gel in combination with 5% benzoyl peroxide (BenzaClin®, Duac™); and 1.2% gel in combination with 0.025% tretinoin (Ziana™). Erythromycin (e.g., Erygel®) is available as 2% solution, gel, ointment, and pledgets, and as 3% gel in combination with 5% benzoyl peroxide (Benzamycin®). Sodium sulfacetamide is not as well studied, but offers an option in patients who have failed first-line agents.[3] It is available at 10% strength, often with 5% sulfur, in a variety of vehicles.

Topical antibiotics are usually applied once or twice a day for 2 to 3 months. Although rare reports of systemic side effects exist, topical effects such as stinging and tingling are the most common adverse effects, and even these occur more rarely with topical antibiotics than with other topical therapies.

Oral Antibiotics

Oral antibiotics should be paired with topical retinoids and/or benzoyl peroxide in patients with moderate to severe acne, especially if lesions are in widespread or difficult-to-reach areas. Oral antibiotics can also replace topical antibiotics when other topical combination regimens fail.

Tetracycline and doxycycline are effective.[67] Minocycline is sometimes tried if other antibiotics fail, but is significantly more expensive and not clearly better in efficacy, even in resistant acne.[68] It is also associated with a higher rate of serious adverse effects than other tetracycline antibiotics (Table 39-5). Tetracyclines cannot be prescribed in children due to potential impairment of bone growth and discoloration of forming teeth. Pregnant women must avoid tetracyclines due to similar effects on the fetus. Trimethoprim-sulfamethoxazole is effective, but has a less favorable side effect profile than tetracyclines.[11] Erythromycin is associated with higher rates of resistance, but can be useful in patients who cannot use the drugs previously mentioned, such as pregnant women. Azithromycin has also been studied.[69,70] Clindamycin is not used systemically to treat acne due to the risk of pseudomembranous colitis.

Oral antibiotics are initiated with twice daily dosing for 6 to 8 weeks; if a good clinical response is noted, dose frequency may be reduced to once daily for maintenance (Table 39-6). To minimize the emergence of bacterial resistance, the patient should attempt to discontinue antibiotic therapy after achieving treatment success for a few months.

Table 39-5 Potentially Serious Adverse Effects Associated With Minocycline

- Lupuslike syndrome
- Necrotizing vasculitis of uterine cervix
- Hepatotoxicity
- Eosinophilic pneumonitis
- Polyarteritis nodosa
- Arthralgia, arthritis, or other autoimmune phenomena
- Intracranial hypertension or pseudotumor cerebri
- Discoloration or hyperpigmentation of the skin or gums
- Hypersensitivity (e.g., fever, rash, neutropenia, eosinophilia)

Adapted from references 68 and 95.

Table 39-6 Frequently Used Oral Antibiotics

Drug	Initial Dose	Maintenance Dose
Doxycycline	100 mg PO BID	100 mg PO daily
Tetracycline	500 mg PO BID	250–500 mg PO daily
Minocycline	50–100 mg PO BID	50–100 mg PO daily
Erythromycin	250–500 mg PO BID	250–500 mg PO daily
Trimethoprim/ sulfamethoxazole	160/800 mg PO BID	160 mg/800 mg PO daily

Adapted from reference 77.

Antibiotic Resistance

Resistance of *P. acnes* to antibiotics frequently used for acne is increasing and correlates to prescribing patterns. Erythromycin resistance is highest; clindamycin resistance follows similar patterns, and cross-resistance between these two agents is high.[71] More than half of European patients harbor resistant bacteria.[72] At one British site, resistance rates almost doubled over a span of 6 years.[71] Resistance to tetracyclines is less common and is increasing at a slower rate than resistance to other antibiotics. Nonetheless, up to 20% of European patients and nearly one-third of patients in the United States are colonized with tetracycline-resistant strains (reflecting higher historical use of tetracyclines to treat acne in the United States than in Europe).[63,71] One reason tetracycline resistance may lag behind erythromycin and clindamycin resistance is that, in environments free of tetracycline, tetracycline-resistant bacteria do not grow as well as susceptible bacteria. Because the genetic material that allows survival in tetracycline-containing environments is a liability in normal environments, selection pressure reduces resistance levels once tetracycline use is discontinued. However, erythromycin/clindamycin-resistant bacteria grow about as well as susceptible strains in antibiotic-free environments, so resistance to these antibiotics fades less quickly after antibiotic use stops.[71] Tetracycline resistance is often accompanied by erythromycin and clindamycin resistance.[63]

The increasing rates of antibiotic resistance have had limited impact on prescribing patterns because resistance is not consistently linked to treatment failure in prescribers' everyday clinical experience, and research on the significance of resistance has been conflicting and sparse. However, notwithstanding the extra-antimicrobial mechanisms of action of antibiotics, bacterial resistance to erythromycin and tetracyclines has appeared to cause higher rates of treatment failure in the few trials that have specifically examined this issue.[73–75] Increasing bacterial resistance is also postulated to explain why recent clinical trials of erythromycin obtain far lower efficacy rates than trials from earlier decades.[76] Although acne treatment failure may not be clearly linked to antibiotic resistance, it is also not the only possible consequence. Acne patients are likelier to carry not only resistant *P. acnes*, but also resistant strains of more clinically significant pathogens such as *Streptococci* and *Staphylococci*.[63,65] As a result, guidelines increasingly emphasize that antibiotics should be reserved for acne of at least moderate severity; should be used for courses of no more than 3 to 6 months' duration; and should not be used as monotherapy, but rather should be teamed with drugs exerting additional mechanisms of action. Furthermore, combinations of two antibiotics should be avoided.[29,30,63,65,66,77] Many prescribers habitually extend patients' antibiotic therapy almost indefinitely to prevent relapse, but studies show that topical retinoids can be as effective as antibiotics for maintenance therapy after successful courses of antibiotics.[78]

HORMONAL THERAPIES

Hormonal therapies with antiandrogenic effects, such as androgen receptor antagonists and combination oral contraceptives, are the only treatments besides oral isotretinoin to attack acne by reducing sebum production. Hormonal therapies may be helpful in patients with normal serum androgen levels, as well as in patients with elevated serum androgen levels, because hypersensitivity to androgens sometimes occurs at the follicular level despite normal circulating androgen levels.[79] Well-conducted comparative studies are needed to clarify the place of these therapies relative to other treatments suitable for moderate to severe acne, such as antibiotics, but they are good options for women with acne who are not pregnant and not planning to get pregnant.[80] However, their systemic effects limit the use of hormonal therapies to female patients, and because of their "upstream" mechanism of action, response to hormonal therapies can be delayed 3 to 6 months.[58]

Androgen Receptor Antagonists

Cyproterone (Androcur®), an antiandrogen with orphan drug status in the United States, and the antiandrogenic progestins chlormadinone and dienogest are each available abroad in combination with ethinyl estradiol in contraceptive products that have been shown to improve acne.[81] More accessible to U.S. patients, spironolactone (Aldactone®) is an androgen receptor antagonist and inhibits 5-α-reductase.[82] Doses of 50 to 200 mg/day have been used successfully in acne due to its antiandrogenic effects,[83] although higher-quality data are needed.[84] Flutamide (Eulexin®), an antiandrogen licensed for metastatic prostate cancer, is effective but potentially hepatotoxic.[82] Antiandrogens are avoided in males because gynecomastia is likely to develop. Female patients not taking concomitant estrogens often develop menstrual irregularities when taking these drugs. Patients must use contraception because antiandrogen exposure impairs the sexual development of male fetuses.[83]

Combination Oral Contraceptives

Estrogen, usually administered as ethinyl estradiol in a cycled combination oral contraceptive (OC), improves acne in females by reducing ovarian androgen production and by increasing sex hormone binding globulin concentrations in the serum, thereby lowering free testosterone levels.[79] The manufacturers of Ortho Tri-Cyclen® (ethinyl estradiol, norgestimate), Estrostep® Fe (ethinyl estradiol, norethindrone acetate), and Yaz® (ethinyl estradiol, drospirenone) specifically sought and obtained U.S. Food and Drug Administration approvals for acne indications, but acne improvement may be seen with any combination OC relative to baseline. Studies of ethinyl estradiol in combination with levonorgestrel, desogestrel, or gestodene (not available in the United States) demonstrate efficacy in acne for those products as well.[80] Comparative trials have not yet clearly established clinically significant superiority of one product over another.[79,80,85] In individual patients, products containing progestins with androgenic effects (e.g., norgestrel, levonorgestrel) may override the effect of ethinyl estradiol and worsen acne. Conversely, patients already on a combined OC may improve when switched to a formulation with a less androgenic progestin.[81] Other estrogen-containing contraceptives (transdermal patches, vaginal rings) may have similar beneficial effects to OCs, but studies have not been conducted.

CORTICOSTEROIDS

Although corticosteroids sometimes cause acne, under some circumstances they can be used to treat severe acne. To avoid potentially severe flaring when oral isotretinoin is begun, patients may pretreat 1 to 2 weeks with prednisone 40 to 60 mg/day and continue concomitant prednisone for the first 2 weeks of isotretinoin therapy.[11] Corticosteroids are used concomitantly with isotretinoin when treating acne fulminans to decrease the inflammatory response.[15] In acne patients with diagnosed adrenal hyperplasia, prednisone 5 to 10 mg/day may be given in the evening to suppress diurnal corticotropin release and thus adrenal hypersecretion of endogenous steroids.[86] Intralesional triamcinolone injections markedly improve severe nodules, but repeated or careless use of the technique can lead to atrophic scarring.[4] Topical application of corticosteroids is not effective.

CLINICAL ASSESSMENT

1. L.Y., a fair-skinned, 15-year-old, Caucasian girl presents to her physician complaining of worsening "zits." Several of her classmates are taking antibiotics for acne, and she wants to move up from nonprescription treatments to "strong medicine." The problem began when she was 13 and has progressively worsened. At first, lesions occasionally appeared on her chin and forehead; now she consistently has four to eight lesions, which have spread to her cheeks and nose. She uses a nonprescription 10% benzoyl peroxide gel as needed on lesions when her acne "gets really bad," but it is too drying for everyday use. She tried a "medicated" soap in the past, but stopped because it caused excessively dry skin. She has no other medical problems and takes no chronic prescription medications. She has had normal menstrual periods since menarche at age 12. Both her older brothers have acne,

one mild and one severe. L.Y. denies alcohol, tobacco, or illicit drug use. She has a boyfriend but denies sexual intercourse. After school, she works part time at a fast food restaurant, plays varsity tennis, and practices violin. She wears a sweatband around her head while playing tennis and uses a hair styling gel.

Examination reveals three pustules and two closed comedones on her forehead, three papules on her cheeks and chin (which are covered with makeup), two well-healing areas on her nose, and no open comedones or nodules. Her skin is only slightly oily. Her chest, back, and arms are clear. She has no facial hair, and her voice is normal in pitch. What are the key components in the clinical assessment of L.Y.'s acne?

The clinical assessment of L.Y.'s acne should include evaluating each of the following factors:

- Type, number, and distribution of lesions. This patient has relatively few lesions that are mostly inflammatory (pustules) and located on the face.
- Contributing factors such as family history of acne (noted in brothers), work-related exposures (oils from fast food restaurant), systemic or topical medications, cosmetic or hair care products (makeup and hair gel), or mechanical pressure on the skin (sweatband and violin chin rest).
- Hormonal influences that indicate androgen excess or atypical menstrual cycles. This patient has no signs of virilization (normal voice and lack of facial hair), and her menstrual periods are normal.
- A detailed medical history. This patient is healthy and does not have epilepsy, liver disease, alcohol abuse, or dyslipidemia.
- Effectiveness of current or past treatments. This patient's response to two therapies was suboptimal, but because she used them erratically, effectiveness is difficult to assess.
- Psychosocial impact of acne on her quality of life. This appears to be very important to her based on her plea for effective therapy.

2. What subjective and objective data support a diagnosis of acne vulgaris?

This patient's age (teenager) puts her in the highest prevalence category. The facial distribution of lesions, while sparing most other areas, further supports acne, as does a positive family history. The fact that her condition has waxed and waned but progressively worsened is consistent with acne. Her condition also worsened because of mechanical irritation caused by sweatband use and violin playing. The lesion type and severity rule out more severe variants such as gram-negative folliculitis or acne fulminans.

MILD ACNE

Benzoyl Peroxide

3. Evaluate L.Y.'s current acne medication regimen.

L.Y.'s current antiacne regimen is suboptimal, which explains her progressively worsening course. Benzoyl peroxide is excellent for mild to moderate inflammatory acne, but 2.5% and 5% concentrations are less irritating than 10% concentrations and equally effective overall.[87] The product is failing to control L.Y.'s acne because she applies it infrequently to existing lesions only. Routine use over the entire susceptible area is required for long-term acne control.

4. Why should other treatment options be avoided at this time?

Topical retinoids are more expensive and may not be as effective for inflammatory lesions as benzoyl peroxide. Azelaic acid is more expensive and should be reserved for patients who cannot tolerate other comedolytic topical therapies. A course of topical antibiotics may be added if appropriate benzoyl peroxide therapy is ineffective. Oral antibiotics should not be added because her acne is mild and distributed in a small area. Although oral isotretinoin would be very effective, it is not warranted at this time because of high cost, significant bothersome adverse effects, need for close monitoring, and potential teratogenicity. Combination oral contraceptives would have been a reasonable choice if L.Y. were sexually active or had menstrual abnormalities.

Skin Irritation

5. How can L.Y. reduce the risk of developing skin irritation and dryness while using benzoyl peroxide?

Topical application of benzoyl peroxide may cause transient warmth or stinging, significant drying, or skin irritation. Mild skin redness or drying is acceptable and indicates proper dosage and optimal therapeutic response. Factors that worsen skin irritation include increased benzoyl peroxide concentration and contact time, gels or lipophilic vehicles, thin and sensitive skin, low environmental humidity, use of irritating adjunctive therapies, and increased application frequency.[88] Initiating regular benzoyl peroxide use in a less drying vehicle (cream) and at lower strength (2.5%) would minimize the risk of intolerable skin irritation while still achieving the desired therapeutic effect. L.Y. could apply the product every other day for the first week or two, and then advance to daily application as tolerated. The cream should be applied at bedtime, ideally half an hour after washing the face with a mild cleanser, and washed off in the morning (or after several hours, if excessive skin dryness or peeling occurs). In a few weeks, she may be able to tolerate a second daily application half an hour after washing the face in the morning. L.Y. should be reminded of the product's potential to bleach fabrics.

To minimize skin irritation, L.Y. should also discontinue use of medicated cleansers. Oilfree moisturizer increases skin hydration and comfort, and can perform double duty if it also contains sunscreen. Patients using benzoyl peroxide should use a sunscreen every day that blocks ultraviolet (UV) light in both A and B wavelengths and that provides a sun protection factor (SPF) of at least 15. (See Chapter 41 for a more detailed discussion of sunscreens.) If L.Y. is applying benzoyl peroxide in the morning, she should apply it before applying the moisturizer with sunscreen.

Topical Antibiotics

6. How should L.Y.'s benzoyl peroxide therapy be modified if the desired effect is not achieved?

If L.Y. notices no improvement after 6 to 8 weeks of consistent twice-daily use and feels like the product is not having any effect on her skin, she should switch to gel and/or increase the strength of her benzoyl peroxide. Titration should continue to the point of mild, tolerable skin irritation. Alternatively, if she experiences inadequate improvement despite 6 to 8 weeks of benzoyl peroxide therapy strong enough to cause mild redness and drying, she should be given a course of topical antibiotics, applying the antibiotic in the morning while benzoyl peroxide is applied at bedtime. Combination products are convenient but often expensive; a recent community-based trial found no advantage, in efficacy or in preventing antibiotic resistance, to using Benzamycin® (3% erythromycin, 5% benzoyl peroxide gel) twice daily over 2% erythromycin gel in the morning and benzoyl peroxide 5% gel in the evening.[75] If a 2- to 3-month antibiotic course is successful, L.Y. should continue maintenance therapy with just benzoyl peroxide.

Adverse Effects to Topical Medications

7. R.P., a fair-skinned, 17-year-old Hispanic male, has been using a benzoyl peroxide 5% gel (Benzac®-W) for 2 months. Since he began using this treatment, his acne has slightly improved. The treatment caused some peeling at first, but soon only barely noticeable redness and dryness. About 1 week ago, he began noticing significant redness and itching in the areas where he had applied the gel. He denies any changes in sun exposure or skin care routine. He stopped using the medication until last night, when the irritation had almost resolved. Last night, he attempted to resume benzoyl peroxide therapy. Within 10 minutes after applying a small amount of gel, his skin became reddened, and began to burn and itch. He immediately washed the area well with cool, soapy water, but the skin irritation prevented him from getting a good night's sleep. The area is better this morning, but remains red and itchy. Currently, his acne consists of several noninflammatory and about 10 inflammatory lesions located primarily in the T-zone (forehead and nose). Is this a typical adverse reaction to benzoyl peroxide?

No. Because sun exposure or dryness from a change in skin cleanser did not appear to provoke the skin reaction, it is unlikely due to benzoyl peroxide's direct irritating effects. The intense itching and burning following rechallenge is more consistent with an allergic-type contact dermatitis, which occurs in up to 2.5% of patients.[46] Those who develop such contact dermatitis should discontinue benzoyl peroxide use.

8. R.P.'s treatment with benzoyl peroxide was discontinued. What alternative therapy is indicated at this time?

After the allergic reaction has resolved, R.P. should resume comedolytic therapy with a more tolerable formulation of tretinoin, or with adapalene or azelaic acid. Because benzoyl peroxide monotherapy was not achieving optimal results, therapy can be intensified by adding a course of topical clindamycin. Erythromycin is more associated with the development of resistance than clindamycin, and benzoyl peroxide cannot be used concomitantly to prevent resistance. The entire face, not just the lesions, should be treated for optimal results. An oral antibiotic is not indicated at this time because only a small area is affected.

MODERATE ACNE

9. R.P. moved away to go to college and returns for follow-up care after 2 months. He has been applying Ziana® gel (1.2% clindamycin and 0.025% tretinoin) regularly. Nevertheless, his inflammatory lesions have increased in number and have spread to his chest and back. He has one painful nodule on his cheek and another on his back. R.P. is embarrassed by the appearance of his skin, especially on his trunk, which is exposed when he wears his basketball jersey while playing on the school team. How would you assess his acne now? Why might his acne be worsening?

R.P.'s acne is now moderate in severity, as defined by the extensive distribution of lesions. For unknown reasons, perhaps hormonal changes that are increasing keratinization of the pilosebaceous unit, the acne has clearly progressed. The hot and humid conditions associated with playing basketball and potentially colonization with clindamycin-resistant *P. acnes,* or the stress of college, may also be contributing to his acne flare.

Systemic Antibiotics

10. Suggest modifications to R.P.'s treatment regimen to help him achieve better control of his acne. Provide a rationale for your choice.

Because R.P.'s lesions are primarily inflammatory in nature, antibiotics remain a good choice. However, the area affected is more widespread, so oral antibiotics should now be used in addition to a topical retinoid. Topical clindamycin should be discontinued, a retinoid-only topical product initiated (perhaps adapalene, or the higher concentration of tretinoin available as microsphere gel, if the patient can afford it), and doxycycline initiated at 100 mg PO BID with food. Doxycycline may cause gastrointestinal effects such as heartburn, nausea, and diarrhea, and dermatologic effects, such as rash and photosensitivity. Patients should be advised to take the drug with a full glass of water to avoid esophageal erosions from prolonged esophageal contact, and to wear protective clothing and use UV-A/UV-B sunscreen with an SPF of at least 15 on a daily basis. Because tetracycline may cause less photosensitivity, it may be an alternative to doxycycline if the patient spends a lot of time outdoors (although a sunscreen should still be used).[77] However, tetracycline must be taken at least 1 hour before or 2 hours after eating because food, particularly dairy, impairs its absorption.

If gram-negative folliculitis is suspected, oral trimethoprim/sulfamethoxazole should be considered. However, this is probably not the case in this patient. Rather than continued gradual deterioration, gram-negative folliculitis usually presents as worsening of acne in long-term antibiotic patients whose control had improved. Gram-negative organisms overgrow in the anterior nares and cause pustules on the central and lower face, often in the nasolabial folds. With their usual history of multiple antibiotic courses, gram-negative folliculitis patients often require isotretinoin therapy.[58]

11. How should R.P.'s doxycycline regimen be monitored and the dosage adjusted?

If tolerated, doxycycline should be continued for 6 to 8 weeks, at which point changes can be made if there is no improvement.[75,77] If therapy is effective at that point, the frequency can be lowered from BID to daily to minimize the risk of adverse effects (the same could be done for any of the other frequently used antibiotics; Table 39-6).[77] Routine laboratory monitoring is not necessary for most young, healthy patients receiving long-term oral tetracyclines or erythromycin because the incidence of serious adverse effects is low.[89] Antibiotics should be discontinued after the acne has been controlled for about 2 months in order to limit antibiotic exposure; courses are generally 3 to 6 months long. Longer courses are associated with little additional clinical improvement, but with the development of antibiotic resistance.[65] Topical retinoid therapy should continue during doxycycline therapy and then after the antibiotic course to maintain treatment benefit. If R.P. relapses again in the future after successful use of an oral antibiotic, another course of the same antibiotic should be used.[77]

Retinoids in Postinflammatory Hyperpigmentation

12. J.H., a 23-year-old African American woman with medium brown skin tone, has had acne vulgaris for the past 10 years. During this time, she has tried several medications. Benzoyl peroxide was somewhat helpful, but even low concentrations caused excessive irritation. She also tried extended courses of topical erythromycin and clindamycin, with little clinical improvement. Oral tetracycline was moderately effective, but caused her to get frequent yeast infections. A year ago, she began using Yaz® for contraception and has noticed improvement in her acne as well. However, she still has about 20 open and closed comedones on her forehead, cheeks, and chin. She has 2 papules on her nose and 1 papule along the jawline. J.H.'s biggest concern about her skin is that lesions "take forever to clear completely." She shows you 8 hyperpigmented macules on her cheeks and forehead at the sites of lesions that healed over the past 6 months. Recommend a new treatment strategy for J.H.

Because J.H.'s acne is mostly comedonal, a topical retinoid would likely be an effective addition to the hormonal therapy provided by her contraceptive. However, given her history of sensitive skin and propensity toward postinflammatory hyperpigmentation (PIH), it is important that therapy not be so irritating as to prompt severe inflammation. Adapalene would be a good option because it has less irritation potential than tretinoin and can reduce PIH as well. Cream is a less irritating vehicle than gel. She should apply the cream to her entire face every night. Some acne might appear worsened within the first 1 to 2 weeks because preclinical lesions may become visible. Sun exposure significantly intensifies skin irritation, so all patients regardless of skin color (and especially those prone to PIH) should be instructed to apply sunscreen to sun-exposed areas when using comedolytic therapies.[90] It is also important to ask J.H. about her skin care regimen and use of hair products to identify the use of any counterproductive cleansing strategies or comedogenic hair pomades.

Like many patients with PIH, J.H. is more distressed by the splotchy aftermath of her acne than by the acne itself.[20] She should be assured that the adapalene cream will likely aid the resolution of her current hyperpigmentation in addition to interrupting the comedogenic process behind future lesions. If the hyperpigmentation shows no signs of improvement when J.H. returns for follow-up in 6 weeks, once- or twice-daily application of nonprescription skin-lightening hydroquinone 2% cream can be added to speed resolution.[19] Hydroquinone is applied only to the areas of hyperpigmentation and only until they fade, typically 1 to 3 months. If it is being applied at the same time of day as acne medication, it should be applied following the acne medication.

SEVERE ACNE

Isotretinoin

Dose

13. Four years ago, K.S., an olive-skinned, 24-year-old, Hispanic woman, was diagnosed with moderate noninflammatory and inflammatory acne that was primarily located on her face and back. She tried topical benzoyl peroxide and systemic erythromycin with limited success. Two years ago, she was diagnosed with polycystic ovary syndrome and began taking Ortho Tri-Cyclen®, after which her acne improved but remained inadequately treated. Five months ago, she also began taking minocycline 100 mg PO BID. After a few months, she experienced significant improvement, but she has not been able to reduce her dosage to 100 mg daily because of predictable flare-ups. In fact, her acne has worsened over the past 2 months, and she now has at least a dozen nodules widely distributed among multiple papules and pustules on her face and back.

K.S. is 5′6″ and weighs 180 lb (81.8 kg). She has no other health problems. She does not smoke, but she occasionally drinks three to four alcoholic beverages on weekends. She is sexually active with one partner, her husband. A month ago, a comprehensive metabolic panel, thyroid-stimulating hormone level, complete blood count with platelets, and lipid panel were normal. Suggest a therapeutic plan for K.S.'s acne.

K.S. has severe acne based on the large number of lesions, wide distribution on multiple body sites, and presence of multiple inflammatory lesions, including nodules. The most effective medication for K.S. will be oral isotretinoin at an initial dose of 20 mg twice daily (approximately 0.5 mg/kg). The dosage should be increased to 40 mg twice daily (1 mg/kg) as tolerated after 1 month. A single treatment course is most effective if a cumulative dose of approximately 120 mg/kg, which should take almost 5 months to complete, is attained. Higher dosages are associated with an increased risk of adverse effects. K.S. should stop taking minocycline when isotretinoin therapy begins because isotretinoin is effective monotherapy, and coadministration of isotretinoin and tetracyclines increases the risk of intracranial hypertension.[77] Her acne should significantly improve within the first month of therapy and gradually resolve by the third or fourth month. A second course of therapy is usually not necessary.

Teratogenicity

14. What should K.S. be told about avoiding pregnancy while taking isotretinoin?

Because of isotretinoin's teratogenic effects (e.g., severe birth defects, premature birth, neonatal death), the iPLEDGE program emphasizes repeated patient education regarding contraception.[91] The program requires that all female patients of child-bearing potential use two forms of contraception, of which at least one must be a "primary" method, for a month before, all during, and for a month after therapy. K.S. is already using an approved primary method with Ortho Tri-Cyclen®; approved primary methods include bilateral tubal ligation, partner's vasectomy, some intrauterine devices, or hormonal methods (other than progestin-only minipills). However, she must also begin using a backup method, such as condoms. The program requires that all female patients of child-bearing potential must have two negative pregnancy tests before beginning isotretinoin therapy, one at the time of screening and then another, from an appropriately certified laboratory, after a month on their chosen contraception regimen. The program also requires a negative pregnancy test before each monthly refill is prescribed, immediately after therapy, and a month following therapy. K.S. and her prescriber will both have to verify with the program on a monthly basis that she has been counseled again regarding contraception. K.S. must also be reminded to avoid donating blood during therapy and for a month following therapy because blood products created from her donation could potentially be used in pregnant patients.

Laboratory Monitoring Parameters

15. In addition to the pregnancy testing discussed, which baseline and periodic laboratory monitoring parameters should be followed in this patient?

Before beginning isotretinoin therapy, baseline values for the following laboratories should be obtained for all patients, male and female: a fractionated lipid panel; a liver function panel, including both serum transaminases and bilirubin; and a complete blood count, including platelets.[11,29]

If a particular patient's other medical history suggests potential risk, providers might order baseline serum glucose levels, erythrocyte sedimentation rate, and creatine phosphokinase.[92] For accurate triglyceride results, the blood sample should be collected at least 36 hours after alcohol consumption and 10 hours after eating food. The laboratory results measured a month ago will suffice for K.S. because they likely would not be significantly different now.

A fractionated lipid panel should be redrawn 4 weeks and 8 weeks into isotretinoin therapy to document the effect of the drug.[11] About 20% of patients develop significant triglyceride elevations.[49] Triglyceride levels >400 mg/dL should be treated with diet and reduced alcohol intake; monthly monitoring should continue throughout isotretinoin therapy. In the unusual event that triglyceride levels exceed 800 mg/dL, isotretinoin should be discontinued, or continued at a reduced dosage with concomitant gemfibrozil therapy to reduce the risk of pancreatitis.[11] If pancreatitis develops, isotretinoin must be discontinued. High-density lipoprotein concentrations may decrease slightly, and total cholesterol concentrations may increase during isotretinoin therapy; however, the clinical significance is unknown. These lipid abnormalities usually resolve within several weeks of completion of therapy.[49]

Liver function tests and blood counts only need to be redrawn during therapy if symptoms suggestive of hepatitis or blood dyscrasias appear,[11] although some guidelines suggest periodic monitoring.[29] Mild elevations in serum transaminases may simply be monitored if they occur. However, isotretinoin dosage reduction or drug discontinuation should be considered in asymptomatic patients with persistent enzyme elevations greater than twice the upper limit of normal. Clinical hepatitis occurs rarely, but requires drug discontinuation if suspected.

Adverse effects on bone such as hyperostosis, premature epiphyseal closure, and reduced bone mineral density have not been observed when isotretinoin is used at the doses and durations typical in acne treatment, so monitoring for this toxicity is not required unless a patient is undergoing multiple isotretinoin courses or has pertinent medical history.[29,48]

Adverse Effects

16. How should K.S. be counseled with regard to adverse effects of isotretinoin?

Severe photosensitivity can occur in any patient taking isotretinoin; K.S. should be advised to wear protective clothing and to use UV-A and UV-B blocking, high-SPF sunscreen daily, even if she does not anticipate sun exposure. She should also be cautioned about limiting alcohol consumption, which can enhance isotretinoin-induced hypertriglyceridemia and hepatotoxicity. She should expect significant skin and mucous membrane dryness, which is reported by virtually all patients taking isotretinoin. Another possible adverse effect is muscle or joint pain, especially if she exercises more than usual. She should avoid waxing, dermabrasion, and other skin procedures during and for 6 months after therapy because her skin would be likelier than usual to scar. She should drive with caution, paying attention to any potential vision changes, particularly at night. Bone growth is not impaired when isotretinoin is used in recommended dosages. Refer to Table 39-4 for a list of other noteworthy potential adverse effects caused by isotretinoin.

17. The package insert for isotretinoin warns against possible drug-induced depression. How significant is this risk?

Isotretinoin product labeling includes a warning that isotretinoin may cause depression, including suicide attempts, psychosis, and violent behavior. Case reports suggest that isotretinoin causes psychiatric symptoms in some patients. However, severe acne is itself associated with depression, and prospective trials and literature reviews have not established a causal relationship between isotretinoin and depressive symptoms.[93] Although the absolute risk is low, drug-induced depression is a possible idiosyncratic reaction to isotretinoin in individual patients. In any case, all patients with severe acne, whether receiving isotretinoin or not, should be monitored for the development or worsening of depression.[29]

18. After 3 weeks of therapy, K.S. complains of dry eyes, dry skin, and cracks with bleeding at the corners of her mouth. How might these bothersome mucocutaneous side effects be managed?

K.S. should use artificial tears to relieve the discomfort of her dry eyes; if she is still uncomfortable after several days, she can also apply lubricating ophthalmic ointment at bedtime. Dry skin may be treated with frequent application of moisturizer, particularly after bathing (see Chapter 38). Frequent application of a lip balm or emollient, ideally one containing sunscreen, is recommended to treat cheilitis. If the symptoms become intolerable, a small reduction in the isotretinoin dose (e.g., reduction of 10–20 mg/day) usually decreases the intensity of skin and mucous membrane reactions. Drug discontinuation is rarely necessary.[49]

ACKNOWLEDGEMENT

The author wishes to thank Terry L. Seaton. This is an update of his chapter in the last edition.

REFERENCES

1. Goodman G. Acne: natural history, facts, and myths. *Aus Fam Physician* 2006;35:613.
2. Gollnick H. Current concepts of the pathogenesis of acne: implications for drug treatment. *Drugs* 2003;63:1579.
3. Feldman S et al. Diagnosis and treatment of acne. *Am Fam Physician* 2004;69:2123.
4. Institute for Clinical Systems Improvement. ICSI Health Care Guideline: Acne Management. 3rd ed. Bloomington, MN: ICSI; May 2006. Available at: http://www.icsi.org/guidelines_and_more/guidelines_order_sets_protocols/other_health_care_conditions/acne/acne_management_of_2.html.
5. Mallon E et al. The quality of life in acne: a comparison with general medical conditions using generic questionnaires. *Br J Dermatol* 1999;140:672.
6. Gupta MA, Gupta AK. Psychiatric and psychological co-morbidity in patients with dermatologic disorders: epidemiology and management. *Am J Clin Dermatol* 2003;4:833.
7. Dreno B. Assessing quality of life in patients with acne vulgaris: implications for treatment. *Am J Clin Dermatol* 2006;7:99.
8. Goulden V. Guidelines for the management of acne vulgaris in adolescents. *Pediatr Drugs* 2003;5:301.
9. Cuerda E et al. Acne in Apert's syndrome: treatment with isotretinoin. *J Dermatolog Treat* 2003;14:43.
10. Olivieri I et al. Pharmacological management of SAPHO syndrome. *Expert Opin Investig Drugs* 2006;15:1229.
11. Thiboutot DM, Strauss JS. Diseases of the sebaceous glands. In: Freedberg IM et al., eds. *Fitzpatrick's Dermatology in General Medicine.* 6th ed., Vol. I. New York: McGraw-Hill; 2003:672.
12. Cheung MJ et al. Acneiform facial eruptions: a problem for young women. *Can Fam Physician* 2005;51:527.
13. Munroe M, Crutchfield C. Steroid acne. *Dermatol Nurs* 2003;15:365.
14. Walker SL, Parry EJ. Acne induced by 'Sus' and 'Deca.' *Clin Exp Dermatol* 2006;31:297.
15. Simpson NB, Cunliffe WJ. Disorders of the sebaceous glands. In: Burns T et al., eds. *Rook's Textbook of Dermatology.* 7th ed., Vol. 3. Malden, MA: Blackwell Science; 2004:43.1.
16. Roebuck HL. Acne: intervene early. *Nurs Prac* 2006;31:24.
17. White GM. Recent findings in the epidemiologic evidence, classification, and subtypes of acne vulgaris. *J Am Acad Dermatol* 1998;39(Suppl 2):S34.
18. Lucky AW. A review of infantile and pediatric acne. *Dermatology* 1998;196:95.
19. Callender VD. Acne in ethnic skin: special considerations for therapy. *Dermatol Ther* 2004;17:184.
20. Taylor SC. Enhancing the care and treatment of skin of color, part 1: the broad scope of pigmentary disorders. *Cutis* 2005;76:249.
21. Swart E, Lochner JD. Skin conditions in epileptics. *Clin Exp Dermatol* 1992;17:169.
22. Kerkemeyer K. Acne vulgaris. *Plastic Surg Nursing* 2005;25:31.
23. Magin P et al. A systematic review of the evidence for 'myths and misconceptions' in acne management: diet, face-washing, and sunlight. *Fam Pract* 2005;22:62.
24. Marks JG et al. Contact & Occupational Dermatology. 3rd ed. St. Louis, MO: Mosby; 2002:306.
25. Yamamoto O, Tokura Y. Photocontact dermatitis and chloracne: two major occupational and environmental skin diseases induced by different actions of halogenated chemicals. *J Dermatol Sci* 2003;32:85.
26. Burkhart CN, Burkhart CG. Microbiology's principle of biofilms as a major factor in the pathogenesis of acne vulgaris. *Int J Dermatol* 2003;42:925.
27. Perry AL, Lambert PA. Under the microscope: propionibacterium acnes. *Lett Appl Microbiol* 2006;42:185.
28. Paraskevaidis A et al. Polymorphisms in the human cytochrome P-450 1A1 gene (CYP1A1) as a factor for developing acne. *Dermatology* 1998;196:171.
29. Strauss JS et al. Guidelines of care for acne vulgaris management. *J Am Acad Dermatol* 2007;56:651.
30. Gollnick H et al. Management of acne: a report from a Global Alliance to Improve Outcomes in Acne. *J Am Acad Dermatol* 2003;49:S1.
31. Ortiz A et al. A review of lasers and light sources in the treatment of acne vulgaris. *J Cosmet Laser Ther* 2005;7:69.
32. Ross EV. Optical treatments for acne. *Dermatol Ther* 2005;18:253.
33. Jordan RE et al. Laser resurfacing for facial acne scars (Cochrane Review). In: *The Cochrane Library*, Issue 1, 2007. Oxford, UK: Update Software.
34. Goodman G. Post-acne scarring: a review. *J Cosmet Laser Ther* 2003;5:77.
35. Oberemok SS, Shalita AR. Acne vulgaris, I: pathogenesis and diagnosis. *Cutis* 2002;70:101.
36. Liao DC. Management of acne. *J Fam Pract* 2003;52:43.
37. Straumfjord JV. Vitamin A: its effects in acne vulgaris. *Northwest Med* 1949;42:219.
38. Shalita A. The integral role of topical and oral retinoids in the early treatment of acne. *J Eur Acad Derm Venereol* 2001;15(Suppl 3):43.
39. Lavker RM et al. An ultrastructural study of the effects of topical tretinoin on microcomedones. *Clin Ther* 1992;14:773.
40. Chivot M. Retinoid therapy for acne: a comparative review. *Am J Clin Dermatol* 2005;6:13.
41. Haider A, Shaw JC. Treatment of acne vulgaris. *JAMA* 2004;292:726.
42. Rolewski S. Clinical review: topical retinoids. *Dermatol Nurs* 2003;15:447.
43. Guenther LC. Optimizing treatment with topical tazarotene. *Am J Clin Dermatol* 2003;4:197.
44. Shroot B. Pharmacodynamics and pharmacokinetics of topical adapalene. *J Am Acad Dermatol* 1998;39(Part 3):S17.
45. Waugh J et al. Adapalene: a review of its use in the treatment of acne vulgaris. *Drugs* 2004;64:1465.
46. Akhavan A, Bershad S. Topical acne drugs: review of clinical properties, systemic exposure, and safety. *Am J Clin Dermatol* 2003;4:473.
47. Honein MA, Paulozzi LJ. Cost-effectiveness of oral isotretinoin. *Dermatology* 1999;198:404.
48. Goldsmith LA et al. American Academy of Dermatology Consensus Conference on the safe and optimal use of isotretinoin: summary and recommendations. *J Am Acad Dermatol* 2004;50:900.
49. Kaymak Y, Ilter N. The results and side effects of systemic isotretinoin treatment in 100 patients with acne vulgaris. *Dermatol Nurs* 2006;18:576.
50. U.S. Food and Drug Administration. Isotretinoin (marketed as Accutane) capsule information. Rockville, MD: Author; October 26, 2007. Available at: http://www.fda.gov/cder/drug/infopage/accutane/default.htm.
51. Taylor GA, Shalita AR. Benzoyl peroxide-based combination therapies for acne vulgaris: a comparative review. *Am J Clin Dermatol* 2004;5:261.
52. Hughes BR et al. A double-blind evaluation of topical isotretinoin 0.05%, benzoyl peroxide gel 5% and placebo in patients with acne. *Clin Exp Dermatol* 1992;17:165.
53. do Nascimento LV et al. Single-blind and comparative clinical study of the efficacy and safety of benzoyl peroxide 4% gel (BID) and adapalene 0.1% gel (QD) in the treatment of acne vulgaris for 11 weeks. *J Dermatolog Treat* 2003;14:166.
54. Kraus AL et al. Benzoyl peroxide: an integrated human safety assessment for carcinogenicity. *Reg Toxicol Pharmacol* 1995;21:87.
55. International Agency for Research on Cancer (IARC). Benzoyl peroxide. IARC Monogr Eval Carcinog Risks Hum 1999;71(Part 2):345–358. Available at: http://www.inchem.org/documents/iarc/vol71/007-benzoylperox.html.
56. Nguyen QH, Bui TP. Azelaic acid: pharmacokinetic and pharmacodynamic properties and its therapeutic role in hyperpigmentary disorders and acne. *Int J Dermatol* 1995;34:75.
57. Hjorth N, Graupe K. Azelaic acid for the treatment of acne: a clinical comparison with oral tetracycline. *Acta Derm Venereol Suppl (Stockh)* 1989;143:45.
58. James WD. Clinical practice: acne. *N Engl J Med* 2005;352:1463.
59. Halder RM et al. Acne in ethnic skin. *Dermatol Clin* 2003;21:609.
60. Foster KT, Coffey CW. Acne. In: Berardi RR et al., eds. *Handbook of Nonprescription Drugs.* 15th ed. Washington, DC: American Pharmacists Association; 2006:810.
61. Sapadin AN, Fleischmajer R. Tetracyclines: nonantibiotic properties and their clinical implications. *J Am Acad Dermatol* 2006;54:258.
62. Voils SA et al. Use of macrolides and tetracyclines for chronic inflammatory diseases. *Ann Pharmacother* 2005;39:86.
63. Eady EA et al. Is antibiotic resistance in cutaneous propionibacteria clinically relevant? Implications of resistance for acne patients and prescribers. *Am J Clin Dermatol* 2003;4:813.
64. Skidmore R et al. Effects of subantimicrobial-dose doxycycline in the treatment of moderate acne. *Arch Dermatol* 2003;139:459.
65. Dreno B. Topical antibacterial therapy for acne vulgaris. *Drugs* 2004;64:2389.
66. Tan HH. Topical antibacterial treatments for acne vulgaris: comparative review and guide to selection. *Am J Clin Dermatol* 2004;5:79.
67. Purdy S, de Berker D. Acne: clinical review. *BMJ* 2006;333:949.
68. Garner SE et al. Minocycline for acne vulgaris: efficacy and safety (Cochrane Review). In: The Cochrane Library, Issue 1, 2007. Oxford, UK: Update Software.
69. Kus S et al. Comparison of efficacy of azithromycin vs. doxycycline in the treatment of acne vulgaris. *Clin Exp Dermatol* 2005;30:215.
70. Fernandez-Obregon AC. Azithromycin for the treatment of acne. *Int J Dermatol* 2000;39:45.
71. Coates P et al. Prevalence of antibiotic-resistant propionibacteria on the skin of acne patients: 10-year surveillance data and snapshot distribution study. *Br J Dermatol* 2002;146:840.
72. Ross JI et al. Antibiotic-resistant acne: lessons from Europe. *Br J Dermatol* 2003;148:467.
73. Leyden JJ et al. Propionibacterium acnes resistance to antibiotics in acne patients. *J Am Acad Dermatol* 1983;8:41.
74. Eady EA et al. Erythromycin resistant propionibacteria in antibiotic treated acne patients: association with therapeutic failure. *Br J Dermatol* 1989;121:51.
75. Ozolins M et al. Comparison of five antimicrobial

regimens for treatment of mild to moderate inflammatory facial acne vulgaris in the community: randomised controlled trial. *Lancet* 2004;364:2188.
76. Simonart T, Dramaix M. Treatment of acne with topical antibiotics: lessons from clinical studies. *Br J Dermatol* 2005;153:395.
77. Tan HH. Antibacterial therapy for acne: a guide to selection and use of systemic agents. *Am J Clin Dermatol* 2003;4:307.
78. Zane LT. Acne maintenance therapy: expanding the role of topical retinoids? *Arch Dermatol* 2006; 142:638.
79. Van Vloten W, Sigurdsson V. Selecting an oral contraceptive agent for the treatment of acne in women. *Am J Clin Dermatol* 2004;5:435.
80. Arowoloju AO et al. Combined oral contraceptive pills for treatment of acne (Cochrane Review). In: *The Cochrane Library,* Issue 1, 2007. Oxford, UK: Update Software.
81. Raudrant D, Rabe T. Progestogens with antiandrogenic properties. *Drugs* 2003;63:463.
82. Williams C, Layton AM. Persistent acne in women: implications for the patient and for therapy. *Am J Clin Dermatol* 2006;7:281.
83. Yemisci A et al. Effects and side-effects of spironolactone therapy in women with acne. *J Eur Acad Dermatol Venereol* 2005;19:163.
84. Farquhar C et al. Spironolactone versus placebo or in combination with steroids for hirsutism and/or acne (Cochrane Review). In: *the Cochrane Library*, Issue 1, 2007. Oxford, UK: Update Software.
85. Thorneycroft IH et al. Superiority of a combined contraceptive containing drospirenone to a triphasic preparation containing norgestimate in acne treatment. *Cutis* 2004;74:123.
86. Shaw JC. Acne: effect of hormones on pathogenesis and management. *Am J Clin Dermatol* 2002;3:571.
87. Swanson JK. Antibiotic resistance of propionibacterium acnes in acne vulgaris. *Dermatol Nurs* 2003;15:359.
88. Ives TJ. Benzoyl peroxide. *Am Pharm* 1992;33:S32.
89. Webster GF. Topical tretinoin in acne therapy. *J Am Acad Dermatol* 1998;39(Pt 3):S38.
90. iPLEDGE: Committed to Pregnancy Prevention website. Available at: https://www.ipledgeprogram.com/.
91. Isotretinoin. In: Lacy CF et al. *Drug information handbook.* 14th ed. Hudson, OH: Lexi-Comp; 2006:874.
92. Chia CY et al. Isotretinoin therapy and mood changes in adolescents with moderate to severe acne: a cohort study. *Arch Dermatol* 2005;141:557.
93. Lehman HP, Robinson KA. Management of Acne, Volume 1: Evidence Report and Appendixes. Evidence Report/Technology Assessment, Number 17. AHRQ Publication No. 01-E019, September 2001. Rockville, MD: Agency for Healthcare Research and Quality. Available at: http://www.ncbi.nlm.nih.gov/books/bv.fcgi?rid=hstat1.section.24941.
94. Gruber F et al. Azithromycin compared with minocycline in the treatment of acne comedonica and papulo-pustulosa. *J Chemother* 1998;10: 469.
95. Smith K, Leyden JJ. Safety of doxycycline and minocycline: a systematic review. *Clin Ther* 2005; 27:1329.

CHAPTER 40

Psoriasis

Timothy J. Ives and Kathryn L. Kiser

Epidemiology

Psoriasis, a chronic, proliferative skin disease is one of the most common immune-mediated disorders occurring in 1.5% to 3% of the population worldwide, with northern Europeans and Scandinavians affected most.[1,2] It is characterized by well-delineated, thickened erythematous epidermis or dermal plaques covered with a distinctive silvery scale. Of patients, 75% present with symptoms of psoriasis before the age of 46 years.[2] A family history of psoriasis is found in nearly half of patients. At least nine chromosomal loci have been identified that increase psoriasis susceptibility.[3,4] The primary genetic determinant is PSORS1, a region of the major histocompatability complex on chromosome 6p2, which accounts for 35% to 50% of the heritability of the disease.[2,3] Environmental triggers also play a major role in disease expression.

Pathogenesis

Innate and adaptive immunity are both involved in the initiation and maintenance of psoriatic plaques. Indeed, because the epidermis is the body's main barrier to environmental insult, epidermal hyperplasia forms a key component of the innate immune response. Natural killer cells and natural killer T cells are part of the cutaneous inflammation in psoriasis.[5]

As CD4+ and CD8+ T-lymphocytic cells constitute most of the leukocyte infiltrate found in plaques early in the development of lesions, current evidence supports an autoimmune mechanism for psoriasis. Cytokines such as interferon-α_2 or interleukin 2 are also found in psoriatic plaques.[6] T cells in the cutaneous infiltrate are positive for cutaneous lymphocyte-associated antigen (CLA), a marker for skin-homing leucocytes. Pathogenesis also involves vascular and inflammatory changes, which precede epidermal changes.[7] The alterations in the dermal vasculature also appear to be a result of angiogenesis, the development of new blood vessels, similar to a number of other disease processes, including tumor growth. Many commonly used therapeutic agents for psoriasis have antiangiogenic activity.[1]

The epidermal changes of psoriasis are based on the time required for affected epidermal cells to travel to the surface and be cast off, which is markedly reduced (3–4 days, vs. 26–28 days in normal cells).[8] This sixfold to ninefold transit time decrease does not allow the normal events of cell maturation and keratinization to take place and is reflected clinically as diffuse scaling. T cells contribute to this keratinocyte hyperproliferation through the secretion of various growth factors.[9,10] Memory T lymphocytes marked with CLA, to remember the anatomic site where they first encountered antigen, migrate to the (epi)dermis by a number of immunologic and inflammatory triggering mechanisms released from keratinocytes after minor trauma. On entry into the skin, these T cells complex with epidermal self-antigens presented by major histocompatibility complex molecules that confer the risk of psoriasis. The subsequent release of T-cell cytokines results in further inflammation, the recruitment of additional marked (i.e., with CLA) T cells, and ultimately the development of psoriatic lesions in susceptible persons.[9,10]

Signs and Symptoms

Most psoriatic lesions are asymptomatic, but not always. Pruritus, for example, is noted in 50% of patients, and it can be severe.[11] The primary psoriatic lesion is a relapsing eruption of scaling papules that rapidly coalesce or enlarge to form circumscribed, erythematous, scaly, plaques. The scale is adherent and silvery white, and may reveal bleeding points when removed (*Auspitz sign*). Scales can become extremely dense on the scalp or macerated and dispersed in intertriginous areas. (Web sites, such as www.dermnet.com or www.psoriasiscafe.org/psoriasis-pictures, provide representative pictures of psoriatic lesions.)

Lesions of active psoriasis can develop at the site of epidermal trauma (*Koebner phenomenon*). Scratch marks, sunburn, or surgical wounds may heal, leaving psoriatic lesions in their place. The elbows, knees, scalp, gluteal cleft, fingernails, and toenails are favored areas of involvement. Extensor surfaces are affected more than the flexor surfaces, but the disease usually spares the palms, soles, and face. Nail beds may show punctate pitting, profuse collections of keratotic material, yellow-brown subungual discoloration ("oil spot"), or onycholysis (nail plate separation) in approximately 50% of patients.[12] Psoriatic arthritis is a seronegative inflammatory arthritis that occurs in approximately 25% of all patients with psoriasis, with combined features of both rheumatoid arthritis and the seronegative spondyloarthropathies.[2,11]

Most patients (90%) have chronic localized disease (plaque-type or *psoriasis vulgaris*), but there are several other presentations. The most severe form of the disease is *erythrodermic psoriasis,* which describes a condition of acute inflammatory erythema and scales involving >90% of body surface area. *Pustular psoriasis* is generally localized to palms and soles, but there is also a generalized version. Both generalized *pustular psoriasis* and *erythrodermic psoriasis* can be accompanied by systemic symptoms (hyperthermia, tachycardia, edema, dehydration, shortness of breath) and can have life-threatening consequences (hypovolemia, electrolyte imbalance, septicemia) if not promptly treated.[13] Lesions of *Guttate psoriasis* are small, fine, erythematous scales, usually found on the trunk, arms, or legs, classically following β-hemolytic streptococcal pharyngitis. *Flexural* or *inverse psoriasis* is shiny, red, and typically lacks scales and looks more like intertrigo.[2] Interestingly, psoriatic skin is rarely secondarily infected, because of the overexpression of endogenous peptides (cathelicidins and beta-defensins).[14]

Systemic disorders that can have a causative association with psoriasis include type 2 diabetes mellitus, Crohn's disease, metabolic syndrome, depression, and cardiovascular disease.[2,15,16] This increased risk is thought to be caused by the presence of endothelial activation, proinflammatory cytokines and hyperlipidemia.[2,13,15] In a prospective cohort study, the relative risk of myocardial infarction was significantly increased with a greater risk in younger patients with more severe disease.[15]

Prognosis

Similar to those with diabetes, cancer, and heart disease, patients with psoriasis experience a decreased quality of life related to social, psychological, and physical functioning.[16,17] It is important to emphasize that psoriasis is a treatable disease, but with no known cure. Optimism and encouragement are justified and make it easier for patients to conscientiously apply sometimes awkward and messy topical treatments or take medications that have significant adverse effects. The goal of therapy should be to achieve complete clearing of psoriatic lesions, particularly during emotionally critical times, such as the commencement of school, puberty, and the summer months.

The Self-Administered Psoriasis Area and Severity Index (SAPASI) is a validated, structured instrument that can be used for patient assessment of psoriasis severity and response to therapy. It closely correlates with the standard clinician assessment instrument, Psoriasis Area and Severity Index (PASI), which includes quantification of the percentage of body involvement and severity of lesions.[18] PASI 75 (a $\geq$75% decrease in PASI score) at 3 months from baseline has become the most prominent marker to assess systemic agent efficacy.[19]

The National Psoriasis Foundation recently released a clinical consensus statement on the classification of severity of disease. Rather than using a mild, moderate, or severe classification system, the statement recommends two categories for patients, those who are candidates for localized (i.e., topical) therapy, and those who are candidates for systemic or phototherapy (e.g., methotrexate or immunomodulators). The National Psoriasis Foundation (http://www.psoriasis.org) is a good resource for both patients and providers for information on treatment options as well as psychosocial support.[20,21]

TOPICAL PHARMACOTHERAPY

Many topical and systemic therapeutic agents are available, varying from simple topical emollients to systemic, highly potent immunosuppressant drugs for more recalcitrant conditions. Treatment modalities are chosen on the basis of disease severity, patient preference (including cost and convenience), and response. Patients with mild disease can generally be treated with topical therapy (Table 40-1). Patients with psoriasis covering >20% of the body need more specialized systemic treatment programs (Table 40-2).

Topical Corticosteroids

Topical corticosteroids, the most widely prescribed treatment for psoriasis, are effective in the treatment of psoriasis because of their anti-inflammatory, antimitotic, immunosuppressant, and antipruritic properties.[22,23] These properties are explained by a reduction in phospholipase A_2, DNA synthesis, and epidermal mitotic activity, as well as their vasoconstrictive actions. They provide prompt relief, and patients find them convenient and acceptable, but some are expensive. Tachyphylaxis occurs, and long-term use after skin has returned to a normalized state leads to typical corticosteroid adverse effects (atrophy, telangiectasia, and striae). Thin-skinned areas (facial and intertriginous) are particularly susceptible. Psoriasis is generally a relatively corticosteroid-resistant disease; therefore, the more potent corticosteroids are frequently necessary, often with occlusion, for best results. (See Table 38-8 in Chapter 38, Dermatotherapy and Drug Induced Skin Disorders, for a listing of topical corticosteroids by potency.) Less potent agents are more appropriate in intertriginous areas, on the face, and for maintenance. Potent corticosteroids clear psoriasis in 25% of patients in 3 to 4 weeks, with 75% clearing in 50% of treated patients.[24]

Intermittent dosing or "pulse therapy" seems to yield the best long-term results and minimizes tachyphylaxis and adverse effects. An additional drawback of chronic corticosteroid

Table 40-1 Topical Agents for the Treatment of Psoriasis (Mild to Moderate; <20% Body Involvement)

Treatment Modality	*Advantages*	*Disadvantages*
Emollients	Basic adjunct for all treatments; safe, inexpensive, reduces scaling, itching, and related discomfort	Provide minimal relief alone
Keratolytics (salicylic acid, urea, α-hydroxy acids [i.e., glycolic and lactic acids])	Reduce hyperkeratosis; enable other topical modalities to better penetrate; inexpensive	Provide minimal relief individually; nonspecific; salicylism (tinnitus, nausea, vomiting) with salicylic acid if applied extensively
Topical corticosteroids	Rapid response; control inflammation and itching; best for intertriginous areas and face; convenient, not messy; mainstay topical treatment modality for psoriasis	Temporary relief; less effective with continued use (tachyphylaxis occurs); withdrawal can produce flares; atrophy, telangiectasia, and striae with continued use after skin returns to normalized state; expensive; adrenal suppression possible
Coal tar	Particularly effective for "flaky" scalp lesions; new preparations "pleasant"; efficacy enhanced in combination with UVB (i.e., Goeckerman regimen)	Effective only for mild psoriasis or scalp psoriasis; inconvenient—difficult to apply; stains clothing and bedding, not skin; strong smelling; folliculitis and contact allergy (bronchospasm in atopic patient with asthma after inhalation of vapor); carcinogenic in animals
Anthralin	Effective for widespread, refractory plaques; produces long remissions; short, concentrated programs preferred; enhanced efficacy in combination with UVB (i.e., Ingram regimen)	Purple-brown staining (skin, clothing, and bath fixtures); irritating to normal skin and flexures; careful application required (inpatient?); can precipitate generalized psoriasis
Calcipotriene (Dovonex)	As effective as topical corticosteroids, although slower onset, without long-term corticosteroid adverse effects; convenient, well tolerated	Slow onset; expensive; potential effects on bone metabolism (hypercalcemia); irritant dermatitis on face and intertriginous areas; contraindicated during pregnancy
Tazarotene (Tazorac)	Extended response; convenient (applied daily, in gel formulation); maintenance therapy; effective on scalp and face; used in combination with topical corticosteroids	Slow onset; local irritation and pruritus; teratogenic (adequate contraception is required)
Ultraviolet B (UVB)	Effective as maintenance therapy; eliminates problems of topical steroids	Expensive (insurance reimburses); office-based therapy; sunburn (exacerbates psoriasis); photoaging; skin cancer

Table 40-2 Agents for the Treatment of Severe Psoriasis (>20% Body Involvement)

Treatment Modality	*Advantages*	*Disadvantages*
UVA and psoralen (PUVA)	80% efficacy; "suntan" cosmetically desirable	Time-consuming; expensive, office-based therapy (restrictive); sunburn (exacerbates psoriasis); photoaging; both nonmelanoma skin cancer and melanoma; contraindicated during pregnancy and lactation
Acitretin (Soriatane)	Not as effective as other systemic agents; efficacy enhanced if given with PUVA or UVB (i.e., RePUVA or ReUVB); less hepatotoxic than methotrexate	Teratogenic (contraception required); contraindicated with liver or renal dysfunction, drug or alcohol abuse, hypertriglyceridemia, hypervitaminosis A
Methotrexate	Effective for both skin lesions and arthritis as well as psoriatic nail disease	Hepatotoxicity (periodic liver biopsy?); bone marrow toxicity; folic acid protects against stomatitis (not against hepatic or pulmonary toxicity); drug interactions; contraindicated during pregnancy and lactation, drug or alcohol abuse; caution during acute infections
Cyclosporine	Toxicities and short-lived remissions; used in patients with extensive disease—not responsive to other agents; however, given changing pathophysiology and increasing experience at lower dosages, increasing role in rotational therapy to induce remissions	Renal impairment; suppressive therapy (relapse occurs when discontinued); increased risk of skin cancer, lymphomas, and solid tumors; phototoxic; contraindicated during pregnancy and lactation, and with hypertension, hyperuricemia, hyperkalemia, acute infections
Immunomodulators (alefacept, efalizumab, etanercept, infliximab)	Specific, targeted therapy; effective for moderate to severe both skin lesions and arthritis; maintains remission	Expensive; parenteral (often office-based) therapy; long-term safety unknown; increased risk of serious infections

PUVA, psoralens plus ultraviolet A light; RePUVA, retinoid-PUVA; UVA, ultraviolet A; UVB, ultraviolet B.

therapy is an associated acute flare-up of psoriasis when corticosteroid therapy is terminated.[25] Continuous application for >3 to 4 weeks should be discouraged in patients with psoriasis, and systemic corticosteroids have no place in therapy.[24,26] Topical corticosteroids occasionally can cause a reversible suppression of the hypothalamic-pituitary-adrenal (HPA) axis, as indicated by a decrease in the morning plasma cortisol level.[26] For anything more extensive than mild disease, topical corticosteroids are best used in an adjunctive role. During a flare, corticosteroids help reduce inflammation, redness, and irritation and prepare the involved area for initiation of other potentially irritating, but more appropriate, maintenance topical treatments (e.g., coal tar, anthralin, calcipotriene, or tazarotene).

Coal Tar

Crude coal tar is a complex mixture of thousands of hydrocarbon compounds.[27] It is a time-honored modality for treating psoriasis. It affects psoriasis by enzyme inhibition and antimitotic action (antiproliferative and anti-inflammatory).[27] The efficacy of the combination of tar and ultraviolet B (UVB) light (i.e., Goeckerman regimen) led to its increased popularity beginning in the 1920s. Tar preparations of 2% to 10% are processed as creams, ointments, lotions, gels, oils, shampoos, and coal tar solution (liquor carbonis detergens). Newer purified preparations, using refined coal tar, are less messy and more cosmetically acceptable, but perhaps not as effective.[27] Tar may be helpful for patients with mild to moderate disease, and tar shampoos are useful for psoriasis of the scalp. The potential severity of adverse drug effects from topical tar products is less than that from anthralin, and much less than that from topical corticosteroids. Because tar, in every form, is messy, stains the skin, and has an odor, it has been relegated to second-line therapy for most patients, despite its moderate price.[28]

Tar preparations generally are used once or twice daily, and bedtime application (as a shampoo or cream overnight) is particularly useful in psoriasis of the scalp and overcomes some of the negative cosmetic bias. Patients should be warned about the staining properties of tar on clothing and bedding. Other adverse effects include photosensitivity, acneiform eruptions, folliculitis, and irritation dermatitis. Care should be taken to avoid use of tar on the face, flexures, and genitalia and with inflammatory psoriasis because of tar's irritant properties.

The polyaromatic hydrocarbons contained in coal tar may be metabolized to active carcinogens by epidermal microsomal enzymes. The incidence of hyperkeratotic lesions, including squamous-cell carcinomas, is increased after prolonged industrial exposure to tar; however, extensive reviews of patients who have used tar preparations in psoriasis have not revealed an increased risk of carcinoma.[29]

Anthralin

Anthralin (dithranol in the United Kingdom) is a hydroxyanthrone derivative that inhibits DNA synthesis, mitotic activity, and a variety of enzymes crucial to reducing cell proliferation.[24] It is effective for treatment of widespread, discrete psoriatic plaques. It is applied as a stiff paste (anthralin in Lassar's paste) overnight and used in conjunction with coal tar baths and UVB light (i.e., Ingram regimen). Most cases of chronic plaque psoriasis clear in 3 weeks. The primary disadvantages of anthralin are its irritant and staining properties to skin and clothing. Anthralin also can precipitate generalized psoriasis if applied to unstable psoriasis (i.e., plaque transformation to pustular form).

The standard anthralin regimen involves liberal application of gradually increasing concentrations (0.1%–0.2% up to no more than 3%–5%) for 8 to 12 hours (often overnight), depending on degree of irritation and clinical response. To minimize brownish to purplish staining (of hair, skin, clothing, furniture, and bedding), plastic gloves should be used, as well as old bed linens and clothing for sleep. Contact with the face, eyes, mucous membranes, and nonpsoriatic skin should be avoided because of irritant properties. Application of petrolatum ointment around the psoriatic lesion prevents perilesional irritation. Removal of the anthralin application is facilitated with a bath (often containing coal tar) or mineral oil in the morning. A corticosteroid cream may be used during the day.

Alternative, shorter contact (10–60 minutes twice daily) regimens (e.g., short-contact anthralin therapy [SCAT]) have been developed to minimize application time and staining. These SCAT regimens are most appropriate for the outpatient setting.[24,30] Higher concentrations of anthralin are used in the shorter-contact regimens and irritation is more of a problem. Both methods are used daily for clearing of psoriasis, then once or twice weekly for maintenance therapy, which is instituted after a response is seen at 2 to 3 weeks. Short-course regimens clear 32% of lesions and produce >75% improvement in 50% of patients after 5 weeks. These regimens are comparable in effectiveness to the Ingram regimen and topical corticosteroids are associated with fewer adverse drug events.[24,30]

Calcipotriene (Dovonex)

Calcipotriene (calcipotriol in Europe), a topical vitamin D_3 analog that suppresses keratinocyte proliferation and that has anti-inflammatory effects,[31] can be applied twice daily as a cream, ointment, or solution. Although systemic absorption is slight and the vitamin D effects of calcipotriene on calcium and bone metabolism are about 100 to 200 times less that that of 1,25-dihydroxyvitamin D_3, serum calcium levels and urinary calcium excretion should be monitored to prevent serious effects on calcium and bone metabolism. Other adverse effects of calcipotriene include lesional and perilesional irritation, burning, stinging, pruritus, erythema, and scaling, especially in facial and intertriginous areas.[22] About 30% of patients using calcipotriene develop skin irritation.[32]

Most patients see improvement, although not clearing, of psoriatic plaques at 2 weeks when treated with calcipotriene, often in combination with potent topical corticosteroids. A maximal response is usually seen at 6 to 8 weeks. Of treated patients, 57% experience >75% clearance of psoriatic plaques, which is comparable to that achieved with corticosteroids, albeit slower in onset and associated with more dermal irritation.[24,32] Tachyphylaxis has not been a problem.[33] A formulation of calcipotriene and betamethasone (Taclonex) is available.

Tazarotene (Tazorac)

Tazarotene is a topical synthetic retinoid that is rapidly converted to its biologically active metabolite, tazarotenic acid.[34] By interacting with the predominant retinoid receptors on the skin surface regulating gene transcription, retinoic acids normalize abnormal keratinocyte differentiation, reduce hyperproliferation, and decrease inflammation associated with psoriasis.[34] Treatment success rates compare favorably with corticosteroids (52% clearing of all lesions; 70% clearing of trunk and limb lesions). The antipsoriatic effects of tazarotene are sustained for a longer period after treatment compared with corticosteroids.[24,35] Because local skin irritation and pruritus are common adverse effects of tazarotene use, combination therapy with corticosteroids not only provides additive antipsoriatic effects, but also reduces retinoid-induced irritation.[36] Oral retinoids are known *teratogens*, and tazarotene is not recommended for use during pregnancy. Women should be warned of potential risk and the need to use adequate contraception while using these preparations.[34,35]

PHOTOTHERAPY

Ultraviolet B

Ultraviolet B light (sunburn spectrum, 290–320 nm) induces pyrimidine dimers, inhibits DNA synthesis, and depletes intraepidermal T cells found in psoriatic epidermis (i.e., UVB has antiproliferative and local immunologic effects).[22] UVB light, unlike ultraviolet A (UVA) light, is effective without additional sensitizers (i.e., psoralens). UVB therapy is generally considered pleasant to use and relatively nontoxic. Typically, 60% of patients with chronic plaque psoriasis experience clearing, and an additional 34% achieve a 75% clearance with UVB treatment for 7 to 8 weeks.[24] Heat and humidity from sunlight provide additional positive effects. Narrow-band UVB (NBUVB) phototherapy, 311 nm, has been found to be more effective than broad-band UVB (BBUVB)[19]; however, it is not as effective as psoralens plus ultraviolet A light (PUVA) therapy in terms of clearing psoriatic lesions.[37] The greater efficacy of PUVA, however, may be offset by the short-term adverse effects of psoralens (e.g., nausea, headaches), the greater incidence of phototoxic reactions (erythema), the inconvenience of wearing photoprotective eyewear after treatments, and the extra cost. Although not currently proved, it is hypothesized that NBUVB will produce less long-term photodamage and fewer skin cancers than PUVA.

Ultraviolet B treatments are administered three times weekly. The use of pretreatment emollients (e.g., petrolatum, mineral or "baby" oil, Eucerin) applied before UVB exposure, long thought to improve results, actually inhibits the penetration of UVB and should not be used.[38] After the skin clears, therapy is discontinued gradually over 2 to 4 months to prolong remissions. The risks of UVB radiation and sunlight are similar: sunburn, photoaging, and skin cancer.

Regimens combining UVB with anthralin (Ingram regimen) or tar (Goeckerman regimen) have been used for years, theoretically, taking advantage of the photosensitizing properties of tar and anthralin. The Goeckerman regimen involves daily application of coal tar for at least 4 hours along with exposure to UVB light. The Ingram regimen combines daily application of anthralin plus tar baths with exposure to UVB light.[24] Both the Goeckerman and Ingram regimens can clear widespread psoriasis in 3 to 4 weeks, induce remissions that last for weeks to months, and may reduce the long-term adverse effects of UVB exposure.[24]

A recent development in UVB therapy involves use of a high-energy, 308-nm excimer laser. Laser treatment allows exposure of only involved skin, thus higher doses of UVB can be administered during a given treatment. After only 10 twice-weekly treatments, 84% and 50% of patients achieved 75% or better and 90% or better clearing of plaques, respectively. Adverse drug effects include erythema and blistering, but are generally well tolerated.[39]

Photochemotherapy

Photochemotherapy combines psoralens with UVA light in the 320 to 400 nm spectrum. The psoralens (methoxsalen, 8-methoxypsoralen, and trioxsalen) are a group of photoactive compounds that on absorption of UV light, are both antiproliferative and immunomodulatory. When photoactivated by UVA, psoralens form monofunctional adducts and cross-links with pyrimidine bases. PUVA also inhibits cytokine release and depletes both epidermal and dermal T cells. As measured by extent of T-cell depletion and decreases in delayed hypersensitivity, PUVA has greater immunomodulatory effects in the skin than UVB. Use of PUVA for scalp or nail involvement is limited, however, because of lower exposure.[22,40] Remissions are longer in duration than with UVB. Psoralens are not active without UVA.

Photochemotherapy is used to control severe, recalcitrant, disabling plaque psoriasis. After 10 to 20 treatments over 4 to 8 weeks, >80% of patients experience clearing of symptoms, which can be maintained with periodic (twice monthly) treatments.[24] UVA penetrates the skin more deeply than UVB and may have marked effects on the dermis. The use of PUVA requires careful consideration and adherence to strict photoprotective measures. Patients unwilling to adhere to PUVA-related precautions may prefer UVB treatment because it is much less restrictive.

The peak range for UVA light's therapeutic action is between 320 and 335 nm. 8-Methoxypsoralen (8-MOP) is the most widely used agent, taken at an oral dosage of 0.6 to 0.8 mg/kg of body weight rounded to the nearest 10 mg, 1.25 to 1.5 hours before exposure to UVA light.[37] The initial dose is selected based on the patient's skin type (i.e., ease of sunburn and inherent skin color). Other options for combination therapy with UVA include calcipotriol-PUVA (D-PUVA) and retinoid-PUVA (RePUVA). Both of these modalities have shown to have greater efficacy as compared to PUVA alone.[19]

Acute adverse phototoxic effects, such as erythema and blistering, are dose related and, therefore, controllable. Other acute adverse drug effects include nausea, lethargy, headaches, pruritus, and hyperpigmentation. Topical steroid therapy should be continued until the psoriasis is brought under control. If topical steroids are discontinued at the start of PUVA, an exacerbation of psoriasis usually occurs. Patients should wear protective clothing (with long sleeves and high necklines), use sunscreens that filter out both UVA and UVB, and wear sunglasses that block UVA after PUVA (see Chapter 41, Photosensitivity and Burns). Because methoxsalen has a short half-life and 80% is eliminated within 6 to 8 hours, physical barriers are most important during the 8 hours immediately following PUVA therapy.

Of greater concern are the potential long-term adverse effects: mutagenicity, carcinogenicity, and cataract formation. Squamous cell carcinoma has been associated with cumulative PUVA treatments (11-fold increase in patients who receive >260 treatments compared with patients who received <160 treatments).[24] Male patients have an increased risk of developing genital squamous cell carcinoma.[24] More controversial is the relationship of exposure to PUVA and the risk of malignant melanoma. At present, there appears to be a dose-dependent increase in the risk of melanoma associated with high-dose exposure to PUVA. The risk is first manifested ≥15 years after initial exposure to PUVA.[41–43] Long-term maintenance and high cumulative dosages should be avoided. Shielding the face and genitalia during treatment and performing annual examinations to detect skin cancer at an early stage may lessen the risk of long-term adverse effects of photochemotherapy.

Topical psoralens are extremely photosensitizing, hence difficult to administer. Application of methoxsalen 0.1% followed by small UVA doses (i.e., ≤ 20% of the level of usual doses for oral PUVA) has been used, however, to treat localized areas and to prevent adverse gastrointestinal effects.[24]

SYSTEMIC PHARMACOTHERAPY

Acitretin (Soriatane)

Second-generation systemic retinoids are effective for treatment of recalcitrant psoriatic disease. Antipsoriatic effects stem from the drug's ability to modulate epidermal differentiation and immunologic function in addition to an anti-inflammatory action.[44] This latter effect may alleviate the arthritis that accompanies psoriasis.[22,44] Acitretin is the principal metabolite of etretinate. It is less lipophilic, has a considerably shorter half-life (50 hours vs. 120 days),[44] and has a favorable adverse drug effect profile; however, patients taking any retinoid product should still be monitored closely.

Systemic retinoids are not as effective in psoriasis as are other systemic agents. Acitretin 50 mg/day completely cleared psoriatic plaques in 11% of patients and provided >75% clearance in 40% of patients treated for 8 to 12 weeks.[24] When the combination RePUVA or ReUVB phototherapy (about 50% of usual phototherapy dose) was used, however, the oral retinoids were highly effective, resulting in superior clinical efficacy. Acitretin 30 to 35 mg/day with UVB cleared psoriatic plaques in 55% of patients and provided >75% improvement in an additional 20% of patients treated for 6 to 8 weeks.[24,45] Acitretin is indicated for patients who have received extensive radiation with PUVA, pretreatment for PUVA (1–3 weeks) to accelerate the response rate, for patients who fail to respond to UVB with anthralin or tar, or for patients who are not candidates for methotrexate. Most patients require maintenance or intermittent therapy to prevent relapses.[46]

Numerous other adverse effects are associated with acitretin use, including hypervitaminosis A syndrome (i.e., dry skin, skin thinning and fragility, chapped lips, dry nasal mucosa, skin peeling, alopecia, and nail dystrophy), retinoid rash, extraspinal tendon and ligament calcification and bone changes in children, hyperlipidemia with elevated levels of serum triglycerides and cholesterol, and liver enzyme alteration and hepatitis.[47]

Many patients find the adverse effects of the retinoids intolerable and discontinue treatment. Topical corticosteroids can reduce some of the cutaneous retinoid adverse effects. With continued therapy, retinoids accumulate in adipose tissue and the liver and may be detectable in serum for >2 years after discontinuation of therapy. Appropriately, pregnancy should be avoided after treatment with acitretin for 3 years, because of its teratogenicity.[47]

Immunosuppressive Agents

Methotrexate

Methotrexate (MTX), a folic acid analog, inhibits dihydrofolate reductase needed for synthesis of several amino acids, pyrimidines, purines, and subsequently DNA, RNA, and protein synthesis. MTX therapy greatly suppresses rapidly proliferating cells, such as those in psoriatic skin. Antipsoriatic mechanisms of MTX action include inhibition of keratinocyte differentiation and immunomodulation by destruction of lymphoid cells.[22,24]

Unlike other cytotoxic drugs, MTX produces antipsoriatic effects at dosages that are much lower than those used in cancer chemotherapy. Methotrexate in 10- to 25-mg weekly doses cleared psoriatic plaques in 50% of patients treated for 3 to 4 weeks and resulted in >75% improvement in an additional 40% of patients. Prolonged remissions are expected with continued therapy.[24] MTX is relatively safe and well tolerated, but the long-term concerns for hepatotoxicity (fibrosis and cirrhosis) and the need for periodic liver biopsies can discourage many patients and physicians from using it.[48] Alcohol and methotrexate are a particularly potent hepatotoxic combination. Patients with psoriasis receiving MTX have a 2.5- to 5-fold higher incidence of advanced liver changes than patients with rheumatoid arthritis receiving comparable regimens.[49] Methotrexate hepatotoxicity may be related to both cumulative doses and constant blood levels. Daily administration has been replaced by weekly dosage schedules for this reason. Liver chemistry tests (i.e., serum alanine aminotransferase [ALT], serum aspartate aminotransferase [AST], serum albumin, bilirubin) can be within normal limits, even in the presence of methotrexate-induced liver disease.[48,49] Therefore, consensus guidelines call for a liver biopsy in all patients with psoriasis at baseline and then at intervals of approximately 1- to 1.5-g cumulative MTX dose. Liver chemistry, including AST, ALT, bilirubin, and albumin, should be monitored every 3 months.[50] A high degree of vigilance is necessary in methotrexate-treated psoriatic patients.

Bone marrow depression, nausea, diarrhea, and stomatitis are other adverse effects associated with MTX. Pneumonitis can occur early in the course of treatment, particularly when MTX is given at higher dosages similar to those used in cancer chemotherapy regimens. Folic acid, 1 mg daily, may prevent some of these adverse events, but not hepatitis or pulmonary toxicities. Teratogenesis and miscarriage have occurred, and MTX may cause reversible oligospermia. A number of clinically significant drug interactions may enhance the toxicity of methotrexate. Drug interactions are most likely to be clinically relevant problems in patients with decreased renal function.[50]

Relative contraindications to treatment with MTX include decreased renal function, significant abnormalities in liver function (i.e., fibrosis, cirrhosis, hepatitis), pregnancy or breastfeeding, anemia, leukopenia, thrombocytopenia, active peptic ulcer disease or infectious disease (tuberculosis, pyelonephritis), alcohol abuse, and patient unreliability.[50]

Conception must be avoided during MTX therapy and for at least 3 months after cessation of MTX in men or one full ovulatory cycle in women.[50] Monthly monitoring of complete blood count with differential should be performed as well as renal function tests (specifically serum creatinine) every 3 months.

Hydroxyurea, thioguanine, and azothioprine are additional antineoplastic agents that have antipsoriatic activity. Their effects are not as potent as methotrexate, but they cause less hepatotoxicity with continuous use.[51,52] Dose-dependent myelosuppression is a bigger concern with these agents compared with MTX.[24,52]

Cyclosporine

The positive dermatologic effects of cyclosporine, an immunosuppressive agent, highlight the importance of immune alterations in the pathogenesis of psoriasis. The toxicity and the short duration of remissions induced by the immunosuppressant agents cyclosporine and tacrolimus limit their usefulness, however. Cyclosporine is generally reserved for patients with extensive psoriasis who have not responded adequately to topical agents, UVB, PUVA, and other systemic agents.

In psoriasis, cyclosporine most likely acts via its effect on lymphocytes. Cyclosporine inhibits calcineurin, which is necessary for production of interleukin (IL)-2. IL-2 amplifies helper T cells and cytotoxic lymphocytes. Decreased IL-2 production leads to a decline in activated CD4 and CD8 cells in the epidermis. Cyclosporine also inhibits tumor necrosis factor-α (TNF-α) and interferon-α_2, both of which are involved in the chemotaxis of inflammatory cells; it inhibits release of cytokines and the growth of keratinocytes.[53]

Cyclosporine is used at lower dosages for the treatment of psoriasis than for prevention of organ transplant rejection. In general, 3 to 5 mg/kg of cyclosporine is recommended for the treatment of psoriasis. Rapid improvement of plaque psoriasis is expected, with 30% of patients experiencing clearing of psoriatic plaques and 50% achieving >75% clearing of lesions within 10 weeks at 2 to 3 mg/kg/day. Increasing the dosage to 5 mg/kg/day cleared psoriatic lesions in 97% of those treated for 10 weeks.[24] Most people relapse 2 to 4 months after the discontinuation of cyclosporine therapy.[24] Cyclosporine showed comparable efficacy to methotrexate in patients with psoriasis with average doses of 4.5 mg/kg/day and 20.6 mg/wk, respectively.[54]

Drug-induced renal impairment is common with cyclosporine use, but usually reversible. Hypertension, secondary to vasoconstrictive effects on the smooth muscle of renal blood vessels or drug-induced arteriolar hyalinosis, is dose dependent and insidious in onset. Blood pressure and serum concentrations of creatinine should be monitored closely in patients receiving cyclosporine.[55] Hypokalemia, hypomagnesemia, hyperuricemia, gingival hyperplasia, hypercholesterolemia, hypertriglyceridemia, adverse gastrointestinal effects, hypertrichosis, fatigue, myalgia, and arthralgia also have been attributed to cyclosporine therapy.[56] The risk of skin cancer, lymphomas, and solid tumors also can increase.[57,58] Patients should be cautioned about excessive sun exposure and should not receive concurrent UVB or PUVA treatment during cyclosporine therapy.[56] Both systemic tacrolimus and mycophenolate mofetil are also reported to be highly effective and well tolerated in the treatment of severe recalcitrant psoriasis. More clinical experience with these agents is needed.[59,60]

Immunomodulatory Drugs

Advances in biotechnology immunomodulatory therapy, specifically the use of anticytokines, are becoming important treatment alternatives for moderate to severe plaque and arthritis type psoriasis that is resistant to other systemic therapies. These agents are thought to work owing to the immune-mediated and elevated levels of TNF found in psoriasis. These biotechnology agents are expensive, estimated to cost $13,000 to $20,000/year.

Alefacept and Efalizumab

The agents, alefacept and efalizumab, act as immunosuppressants mainly by inhibiting activation of T lymphocytes in plaques. The mechanism is by binding to CD2 on memory effector T lymphocytes (alefacept) or binding to a subunit of leukocyte function antigen-1 (LFA-1). They are U.S. Food and Drug Administration (FDA) approved for the treatment of plaque psoriasis. Administered subcutaneously or intramuscularly on a weekly regimen, benefit includes approximately 25% obtaining PASI 75 after 12 weeks of alefacept and 30% obtaining PASI 75 after 12 weeks of efalizumab compared with placebo. Some patients have sustained clinical response even after cessation of therapy.[61,62] Alfacept is also effective in combination with NBUVB phototherapy.[63] Because of immunosuppression, these agents are contraindicated in pregnancy or in patients already immunocompromised because of malignancy, infection, or medications. Monitoring includes complete blood counts monthly for the first 9 months and liver function tests every 3 months for the first 3 months.[64]

Infliximab, Etanercept, and Adalimumab

The TNF-α inhibitors, infliximab, etanercept, and adalimumab, are FDA approved for the treatment of both plaque and arthritic psoriasis, except for adalimumab, which is only approved for arthritic psoriasis. Their mechanism of action is through blocking the interaction of TNF-α with cell-surface TNF receptors. Dosing is either subcutaneous injection (etanercept and adalimumab) or intravenous infusion (infliximab) on a weekly or every other weekly schedule for initiation. These agents have been proved to produce rapid, well-tolerated, beneficial responses compared with placebo, with infliximab showing the greatest benefit. Benefit is seen anywhere from 2 weeks to 12 weeks with ≥80% of patients obtaining PASI 75 after 10 weeks of infliximab, ≥50% obtaining PASI 75 after 12 weeks of entanercept, and ≥50% obtaining PASI 75 after 48 weeks of adalimumab treatment.[65–67] Contraindications to therapy include active infection, including tuberculosis, and New York Heart Association (NYHA) III-IV heart failure. All three are a pregnancy category B. However, during pregnancy, they should be used only if clearly necessary.[64,66] An association of increased rate of lymphoma has been seen in patients with psoriasis and treatment with TNF-α inhibitor.[68]

ALTERNATIVE THERAPY

Balneology (bathing in the sea) and spa therapy are not accepted as mainline dermatologic treatment modalities for psoriasis; however, these approaches are used throughout the world. The antipsoriatic properties of the Dead Sea area may be attributed to its unique climatic characteristics and natural resources. Mechanisms may involve mechanical, thermal, and chemical effects.[69] Favorable results of climatotherapy have been reported from specialized treatment centers along the Dead Sea, the German North Sea coast, and the Mediterranean Sea.[69] Climatotherapy is the combination of bathing in the sea (thalassotherapy or balneotherapy) and exposure to sunlight (heliotherapy). A major aspect of climatotherapy, in addition to daily sunbathing, is bathing in salt (sea) water. Relaxation, rest, and simple topical remedies (e.g., petrolatum) are also important. When rigorously studied, little difference is found in therapeutic outcomes of bathing in salt water or tap water, or the application of various topical ointments (e.g., 2% salicylic acid in white petrolatum, Eucerin, or mineral oil) when used in the current UVB phototherapy protocols.[70] Psychological factors (especially relaxation), however, may contribute substantially to the favorable results of natural heliobaleotheapy. If UV phototherapy is administered via artificial UV sources on an outpatient basis, the psychological effect will certainly be much less than when the patient receives this treatment far from home, when cares and social problems are left behind.[70]

Traditional Chinese medicine provides an alternative method of therapy that emphasizes the importance of using many herbs that are combined in different formulations for each patient. This has become popular among some segments of the population. Both topical and systemic use of herbs has been administered to treat psoriasis, as well as a combination of herbal medications with UVA. For example, *Radix angelicae dahuricae*, combined with UVA, was not significantly different from 8-MOP and UVA.[71]

Amphiregulin is an autocrine growth factor that is overexpressed in psoriatic lesions. Keratinocytes produce protein-bound and free heparin sulfate, which function physiologically as an amphiregulin antagonist. Because glucosamine promotes keratinocyte synthesis of heparin sulfate, it may provide a therapeutic benefit in psoriasis. Clinical trials evaluating the efficacy of amphiregulin are unavailable.[72]

MILD TO MODERATE (<20% BODY) PSORIASIS

Classic Presentation

1. M.M., a 35-year-old man, presents with worsening psoriasis. Approximately 1 year before presentation, he was given triamcinolone 0.025% cream to apply to several thick, well-defined erythematous plaques on his elbows and knees that were covered with silvery scales. He recently returned from a trip to the Dominican Republic, where he noted gradual worsening of redness and scaling, despite adherence to a twice-daily triamcinolone regimen. He is emotionally distraught because of this "flare-up," which disrupted his vacation. On examination, besides erythematous, scale-covered plaques on his elbows and knees, several scattered, circumscribed, erythematous, scaly plaques are noted on the flexural surfaces of both arms and legs. A dense scale was evident on his scalp (forehead). These and other areas, demonstrating typical psoriatic involvement, including the gluteal fold and fingernails, now total approximately 20% of his body area. His medical history is noncontributory. His only medication besides the topical corticosteroid product is a recently completed course of chloroquine for malaria prophylaxis during recent travel. Characterize the classic psoriatic lesions demonstrated by M.M.

The classic plaques of psoriasis appear symmetrically on the extensor surfaces of the elbows and knees as distinctive, chronic, erythematous plaques covered with silvery scales, as typified by M.M.'s presentation. Patients can present a broad clinical spectrum, ranging from only scalp involvement to scattered plaques on the trunk and extremities to, in the most serious cases, a generalized erythroderma accompanied by a rheumatoid factor-negative symmetric arthritis. In addition, the finding of very small pits in the nail plates of the hands and feet ("oil spots"), the presence of gluteal "pinking" (erythema and slight scaling of the intergluteal cleft), and the occurrence of lesions conforming to specific sites of skin trauma (Koebner phenomenon) help characterize psoriatic plaques from seborrheic dermatitis and eczema. Most psoriatic lesions are asymptomatic, but pruritus is noted in 50% of patients.

2. What part does emotional support play in the total management of M.M.'s psoriasis?

Psoriasis is often more emotionally or psychologically disturbing than is recognized, and it may cause a reluctance of the patient to participate in sports, which may expose their skin. Although exposure to sunlight helps most patients with psoriasis, there is an unwillingness to sunbathe if the lesions can be seen. Furthermore, if the psoriatic lesions become pruritic and are scratched, there can be further deterioration at the site. Many patients alter their lifestyles or use nontraditional medicine (perhaps irrationally) in desperation.

Emotional support should begin with explanation of the psoriatic condition. M.M. needs to be reassured that many other people have the same affliction, that the disorder is not contagious or fatal, and that it can be controlled although, as yet, no cure exists. The National Psoriasis Foundation website (http://www.psoriasis.org) contains much useful information for patients afflicted with psoriasis.[20] Patients usually are comforted in the knowledge that a wide range of treatments are available. Clinical optimism and psychological encouragement and support are justified and make it easier for the patient to conscientiously apply sometimes awkward and messy topical treatments or to take toxic medications.

3. What are the potential causes of M.M.'s psoriatic exacerbation? List other factors that can precipitate or aggravate psoriasis.

A thorough medical history may reveal a cause for exacerbations of psoriatic lesions. Most patients report that hot weather, sunlight, and humidity help clear psoriasis, whereas cold weather has an adverse effect on its course. Anxiety or psychological stress is believed to contribute adversely. Viral or bacterial infections, especially streptococcal pharyngitis may precipitate the onset or flare-up of psoriasis. Trauma to the uninvolved skin can cause a lesion to appear at the site of injury (Koebner phenomenon). Cuts, burns, abrasions, injections, and other trauma can elicit this reaction. Any drug that causes a skin eruption to develop can exacerbate psoriasis via this response.

Drug-Induced Psoriasis

A number of drugs have been reported to exacerbate preexisting psoriasis, induce psoriatic lesions on apparently

Table 40-3 Drugs Reported to Induce Psoriasis

Anesthetics	Procaine
Antimicrobials	Amoxicillin, ampicillin, imiquimod, penicillin, sulfonamides, vancomycin, terbinafine, tetracycline
Anti-inflammatory drugs	Corticosteroids (following withdrawal), NSAID (indomethacin, salicylates)
Antimalarials	Chloroquine, hydroxychloroquine
Cardiovascular drugs	Acetazolamide, amiodarone, angiotensin-converting enzyme inhibitors (captopril, enalapril), β-blockers (atenolol, propranolol, timolol [topical]), calcium channel blockers (dihydropyridines, diltiazem, verapamil), clonidine, digoxin, gemfibrozil, quinidine
H_2-antagonists	Cimetidine, ranitidine
Hormones	Oxandrolone, progesterone
Opioid analgesics	Morphine
Psychotropics	Lithium carbonate, valproic acid, fluoxetine
Miscellaneous	Potassium iodide, mercury

NSAID, nonsteroidal anti-inflammatory drugs.
Adapted from Dika E et al. Drug-induced psoriasis: an evidence-based overview and the introduction of psoriatic drug eruption probability score. *Cutan Ocul Toxicol* 2006;25:1, with permission.

normal skin in patients with psoriasis, or precipitate psoriasis in persons with or without a family history of psoriasis (Table 40-3).[73] Antimalarial agents, such as chloroquine (taken by M.M.), may have an adverse effect on the course of psoriasis and can cause exfoliative erythroderma.[74] Hydroxychloroquine, however, has not shared this association (except for one recent case report) and usually induces a beneficial response in 75% of patients with psoriatic arthritis.[74] It is preferred over chloroquine in patients with psoriasis who need prophylactic treatment for malaria when both are effective against the particular plasmodium species in the area (see Chapter 74, Parasitic Infections).[74]

Lithium also can precipitate psoriasis and contribute to resistance to treatment through its effects on cell kinetics (increase in circulating neutrophils, accelerated neutrophil turnover, increased epidermal cell proliferation).[73] Psoriasis is not a general contraindication, however, to lithium therapy. More intensive psoriasis treatment can be used if these reactions occur and lithium must be continued.[73]

β-Blockers and some nonsteroidal anti-inflammatory drugs (NSAIDs) also can precipitate a psoriasiform state.[73] As both lithium and propranolol inhibit cyclic adenosine monophosphate (cAMP), cyclic nucleosides may play a role in the onset and clinical course of psoriasis. Chemotactic substances, including 12-HETE and leukotrienes, may accumulate in the epidermis of some patients taking indomethacin, thereby precipitating psoriasis. When compared with other NSAIDs, indomethacin may selectively inhibit cyclooxygenase more than lipoxygenase pathways of arachidonic acid metabolism. As a result, indomethacin may have a more significant adverse psoriatic effect than other NSAIDs that have been reported to ameliorate psoriasis.[73]

Flare-ups of pustular psoriasis also can be precipitated by withdrawal from systemic corticosteroids or withdrawal from high-potency topical corticosteroids that are applied under occlusion to large areas.[22] Systemic corticosteroids are not routinely used to treat psoriasis because of this problem, and because fatalities have been associated with systemic corticosteroid use and withdrawal.

Chloroquine prophylaxis, a Caribbean sunburn, and triamcinolone tachyphylaxis probably all contributed to the exacerbation of M.M.'s psoriasis.[22,74]

Topical Corticosteroids

4. Are additional potent topical corticosteroids appropriate for treatment of M.M.'s psoriasis? Outline the place of steroids in the pharmacotherapy of psoriasis.

For isolated hyperkeratotic plaques, potent topical corticosteroids are the most widely used initial treatment for psoriasis. They give fast relief, especially in reducing inflammation and in controlling itching. Patients find them convenient and acceptable, however, their relief is temporary because they become less effective with continued use (tachyphylaxis).[26] In addition, psoriasis is a relatively steroid-resistant disease that responds only to potent or superpotent agents.[26] Long-term use of potent agents also leads to predictable adverse effects (i.e., atrophy, telangiectasia, and striae). For these reasons, topical corticosteroids are best used in an adjunctive role unless used to treat mild disease for short periods. Continuous application of topical corticosteroids for >3 weeks, particularly after skin normalization, should be discouraged. An interval of several weeks between successive courses of therapy is recommended. High-potency corticosteroids produce better clinical results than low-potency corticosteroids, but the potential for adverse drug effects is greater. Potent topical steroids can suppress the HPA axis as a result of cutaneous absorption, especially when large areas of the body are involved.[26]

A short course of a potent topical corticosteroid is appropriate for this "flare-up" of erythematous plaque psoriasis in M.M. With plastic occlusion (e.g., plastic food wrap on top of the steroid-treated area), topical corticosteroids help reduce inflammation, redness, and irritation before initiation of more appropriate chronic topical treatments, such as calcipotriene, coal tar, or anthralin with UVB, all of which are potentially irritating. Topical corticosteroids also may continue to be useful on the face and flexures, where the alternative topical agents are poorly tolerated. Potent fluorinated corticosteroid preparations should be used cautiously and only for short periods on the face and flexures, if at all. Scalp psoriasis can be treated with steroid preparations in gels, lotions, or aerosol sprays, but a coal tar shampoo lathered into the scalp for 5 to 10 minutes, then rinsed out, generally is more effective for scaling and pruritus.

The response to once- or twice-daily corticosteroid application is as effective or better than that observed with more frequent regimens (due to a steroid reservoir effect) and is much less expensive. Patients should apply steroids after a bath, at bedtime with occlusion, and possibly again during the day without occlusion. As the lesions subside, occlusion should be decreased or omitted, emollient use should increase, and steroid potency should decrease. After lesions have flattened, steroids can be continued intermittently (e.g., 1–2 weeks on, 1–2 weeks off; or on alternate days [e.g., days 1, 3, 5, 7]).

Alternative Topical Treatments

5. Assuming that a short course of a potent topical corticosteroid is effective in reducing the acute flare-up, what alternative topical therapeutic regimens are available for patients such as M.M. who have localized disease (involving <20% of the body)?

Four effective alternative topical therapies are available for patients with localized, mild to moderate psoriasis. Older, well-known agents are crude coal tar and anthralin, with more recent additions of calcipotriene and tazarotene. Although anthralin has irritating properties and both coal tar and anthralin generally stain clothing and skin, and are somewhat inconvenient to apply, their efficacy is well established, and may be an option to consider for initial management. Tachyphylaxis does not occur with chronic use of any of these alternative agents. Once corticosteroids have flattened acute psoriatic lesions and diminished erythema significantly, daily application of one of these alternative agents can be used until the lesions are totally clear.

Ointment vehicles are favored for patients with psoriasis because ointments help moisturize the plaques (in contrast to creams, which dry the plaques further). Moisturizers or emollients alone are often helpful for psoriasis.

Coal tar, although effective, is of low potency when compared with anthralin. Topical tar products (e.g., Tegrin, T/Gel), or 1% to 5% crude coal tar ointment (messy, but more effective), are commonly applied to lesions at night, even during the initial corticosteroid phase. Short-contact tar therapy, unlike anthralin, generally is ineffective. A number of tar shampoos (e.g., T/Gel, Zetar) and bath additives (Balnetar Therapeutic Tar Bath) are available. The combination of coal tar with salicylic acid, in concentrations from 2% to 6%, (e.g., Coco-Scalp) is useful in reducing scaling. Both tar (Goeckerman regimen) and anthralin (Ingram regimen) can be used in combination with UVB, with results superior to UVB monotherapy. These two regimens are reported to clear plaques in 75% of patients treated for 6 weeks for chronic plaque psoriasis (vs. 56% with UVB alone). The total number of treatments and the total UVB dose required for clearing are less in the combination groups.[24]

Once the inflammation and erythema have lessened with corticosteroid use or when a twice-daily, high-potency corticosteroid regimen along with bedtime application of tar is ineffective, calcipotriene ointment applied twice daily or tazarotene gel applied once daily is effective in treating flare-ups and maintaining remission.

Calcipotriene may be the topical maintenance treatment of choice in patients with generalized mild to moderate psoriasis. The drug is usually effective, relatively easy to apply, odorless, and nonstaining (cream, ointment, or scalp solution). It is generally considered to be about as effective as moderate- to high-potency topical corticosteroid products. It has a slower onset of action than corticosteroids, and about 10% of patients develop irritation. This irritation precludes use on the face or in intertriginous areas. Sequential or simultaneous use of topical corticosteroids and vitamin D derivatives may provide synergy and reduce irritation. Tachyphylaxis does not occur. Patient use must be monitored to ensure that a 100-g/week limit is not exceeded; exceeding this limit results in negative effects on calcium and bone metabolism. When used concurrently with topical salicylic acid, calcipotriene will be chemically inactivated.

Similar to calcipotriene, tazarotene works slowly and can be irritating. It is formulated as a gel, which many patients find more cosmetically appealing than an ointment. It is also effective in a once-daily regimen, which might help to improve compliance. The ointment should be used in combination with a high-potency topical corticosteroid to increase efficacy and to reduce irritation. Because of a potential for retinoids to be teratogenic, tazarotene should not be used in women who are pregnant or who are contemplating becoming pregnant.

Topical anthralin, generally reserved for resistant cases, clears lesions in some patients within 2 to 3 weeks. Although overnight regimens are available, short-contact therapy, which is more appealing, starts with 0.1% anthralin applied for 20 to 30 minutes and then washed off. Irritation should be checked for at least 48 hours. According to tolerance, potency can be increased (up to 1%) and the contact time shortened, or for resistant plaques, increased. This regimen is used daily for clearing, then once or twice weekly for maintenance therapy.

Phototherapy also is an option. If available locally, UV light can be used as an outpatient modality; it produces comparatively long-lasting remissions, is pleasant to use, and is relatively nontoxic. Different protocols require exposure daily or multiple times per week for varied lengths of time, depending on patient variables. The optimal effect of UVB on psoriasis is a dose that produces minimal erythema at 24 hours. The usual time to induce clearing of psoriasis is approximately 4 to 6 weeks.

In summary, the first step in the treatment of mild localized disease is to start with a high-potency corticosteroid ointment twice daily along with tar ointment at night. If this is ineffective, either calcipotriene ointment can be added twice daily, or tazarotene gel can be used once a day for 8 weeks. Once control is achieved, patients may use calcipotriene or tazarotene without topical corticosteroids; these products do not cause corticosteroid atrophy and they do not have the potential for systemic adverse effects associated with topical corticosteroids. Topical anthralin, with or without UVB, can be used for resistant cases.

SEVERE (>20% BODY) PSORIASIS

Psoralens and Ultraviolet A Light

6. G.L., a 35-year-old man with a several-year history of psoriasis (generally fairly localized) presents with diffuse, erythematous plaquelike lesions now extending over 80% of his body surface area. The areas have become inflamed, and application of his maintenance topical medication (anthralin) causes pain and irritation. He expresses frustration with the messiness of the current topical regimen. He has reinstituted topical steroids, which helped the redness and itching but are too expensive to use long term. He is free of cardiovascular, renal, or hepatic disease and takes no systemic medications. He is self-employed as a business consultant. Which "systemic" therapy would be most appropriate for G.L. at this point?

Systemic therapies for psoriasis include PUVA; the systemic retinoid, acitretin; methotrexate; and cyclosporine. Newer biologics, including the TNF inhibitors infliximab, etanercept, and adalimumab and the immunosuppressants alefacept and efalizumab, have also been used for skin lesions. These agents prevent the activation and reduce the number of memory T lymphocytes.

Although PUVA and methotrexate are used most often, cyclosporine and the newer immunomodulatory agents are being used increasingly as more experience is gained with them for treatment of severe psoriasis.[22,68] The choice of agents depends on patient and drug characteristics. Because patients with psoriasis generally have the disease for the rest of their lives, the goal of treatment is not just safe and effective resolution of disease at a specific point in time, but also safe and effective maintenance therapy for long periods. Anecdotal experience suggests that long-term maintenance therapy for psoriasis can generally be achieved even with weaning or discontinuation of UVB, PUVA, and methotrexate. From a histologic perspective, these drugs have been shown to induce remittive cellular changes. In contrast, partial to full doses of acetretin or cyclosporine are necessary to maintain the therapeutic effects of these two drugs, because they induce suppressive rather than remittive histopathologic changes. For example, relapse will occur in most patients in a predictable manner 2 to 4 months after cyclosporine is discontinued.[75]

Rotational Therapy

No form of therapy used in psoriasis today is without toxicity. Rotational therapy involves the use of alternating monotherapies, which allows the patient to experience extended intervals off a particular treatment. When used in long-term maintenance, rotational therapy limits adverse effects associated with either long-term use of one specific agent or the additive or synergistic interactions when multiple therapies are used concurrently. As discussed, the relative risk of skin cancer associated with PUVA increases after 160 treatments. If a patient in remission is rotated off PUVA to another treatment after 100 exposures, the skin has time to recuperate from the light therapy, and PUVA can eventually be reinstated presumably with lesser risk. Rotational therapy assumes that the patient can tolerate three to four alternative treatments with unrelated toxicity profiles.[75] By rotating each treatment after 12 to 18 months of cumulative use, the potential for long-term toxicity associated with any single treatment is minimized. With this theoretic rationale, cyclosporine could be used for a limit of possibly 3 to 6 months, thus inducing a remission. The patient could then be rotated to another treatment (e.g., methotrexate or PUVA) for maintenance.

Psoralens and UVA irradiation become noticeably effective in 80% to 90% of patients in 6 to 8 weeks.[24] The regimen is time-consuming because UV radiation treatments must be administered at least three times a week. Adverse long-term effects (premature photoaging, dyskaryotic or precancerous dermal changes, skin cancer [including melanoma], immunologic changes, and cataracts) can be minimized with appropriate patient selection and monitoring. More immediate adverse effects (e.g., itching, nausea, headache, lethargy, erythematous phototoxic reactions with overexposure, skin pain, and hyperpigmentation) are common. Male patients have increased risk of developing genital squamous-cell cancer (the groin should be shielded during therapy), wrinkling, lentigines (brown macule resembling a freckle), irregular pigmentation, and cataracts (if protective eye wear is not used). Generally, 8-MOP is administered (0.6–0.8 mg/kg of body weight), followed by UVA (dose selected based on skin type, ease of sunburn, and inherent skin color) about 75 to 90 minutes later when psoralen blood levels peak. PUVA-induced erythema generally appears later than with UVB therapy, reaching a peak by 48 hours. Consequently, treatment should not be administered more frequently than every second day. The time to produce clearing of psoriatic plaques with PUVA takes longer than with UVB therapy (average 10 weeks compared with ≤3 weeks for UVB).[40] PUVA treatment must be decreased slowly once plaques have been cleared (frequency of treatment is reduced over 2–3 months) to prevent recurrence of psoriatic plaques. In contrast, UVB therapy can be ceased abruptly. Taking time off from work three times weekly for photochemotherapy can be disruptive to some patients' work or school schedules.

Psoralens and UVA should be avoided in patients with a history of skin cancer, in children, during pregnancy, in patients who are immunosuppressed, and in those who have light-colored skin that burns rather than tans. Absolute contraindications to treatment with PUVA include a history of photosensitivity diseases (i.e., lupus erythematosus, porphyria), idiosyncratic or allergic reactions to psoralens, arsenic intake, exposure to ionizing radiation, skin cancer (relative contraindication), pregnancy, and lactation. Techniques to minimize cumulative dosage of radiation and reduce the risk of long-term adverse effects of photochemotherapy include use of sunscreen, protective clothing, and sunglasses; and use of combination therapy (RePUVA). Other photosensitizing drugs (e.g., fluoroquinolones, phenothiazines, sulfonamides, sulfonylureas, tetracyclines, thiazides) should be avoided in patients receiving PUVA.

In summary, PUVA is effective in 80% to 90% of patients, and G.L.'s severe, extensive, plaque psoriasis should be expected to respond accordingly. The systemic drugs (e.g., methotrexate, cyclosporine) may be preferred if G.L. had systemic symptoms (e.g., psoriatic arthritis). Although thrice-weekly PUVA treatments can be disruptive to work schedules, G.L. is self-employed and presumably has some flexibility in his working hours. Rotational therapy could be considered at a later time depending on G.L.'s response and tolerance of PUVA.

Psoriatic Arthritis

7. R.T. is a 38-year-old male aerospace machinist with psoriasis and increasing joint complaints. He describes a flare-up over the last month involving predominantly the middle finger of the right hand. He also has arthralgias of the shoulders, knees, and the rest of his hands. Concomitantly, his skin disease has once again become active, despite nightly betamethasone dipropionate (Diprolene) administration. He has a history of chronic depression and alcoholism, although he is currently sober and not being treated with antidepressant medications. Physical examination reveals a significant amount of tenderness of the right third metacarpophalangeal joint, without a great deal of active synovitis. He also has a moderate effusion of his right knee, but the rest of the joint examination is otherwise benign. Active psoriatic lesions are noted on his feet, knees, and elbows, and he has characteristic psoriatic nail changes. An erythrocyte sedimentation

rate is mildly elevated. Which systemic therapy would be most appropriate for both R.T.'s skin and joint complaints?

Psoriatic arthritis is a distinct form of inflammatory arthritis that is usually seronegative for rheumatoid factor. In various reports, 6% to 42% of patients with psoriasis experience arthritis, and the prevalence is increased among patients with severe cutaneous disease.[76] Nail involvement occurs in >80% of patients with psoriatic arthritis, as compared with 30% of patients with only cutaneous psoriasis.[76] Five clinical subsets of psoriatic arthritis have been identified: distal interphalangeal arthritis (classic, 5%–10%, often accompanied by nail changes), arthritis mutilans (5%, starts in early age, accompanied by osteolysis with severe deformities of fingers and toes), symmetric polyarthritis (rheumatoidlike, <25% incidence, milder course), asymmetric oligoarthritis (most prevalent, 70%, proximal and distal interphalangeal joints, metacarpophalangeal joints, knee and hip), and spondylitis (5%–40%, often asymptomatic).

The presentation of R.T. is representative of asymmetric oligoarthritis. Treatment of this form of psoriatic arthritis consists of an NSAID, local corticosteroid injections, and immunosuppressive agents, including TNF inhibitors. NSAIDs suppress symptoms, but do not induce remissions and can exacerbate cutaneous symptoms.[73] Systemic corticosteroids are avoided because they destabilize psoriasis (transformation to pustular forms), induce resistance to other effective therapies, and re-exacerbate the skin disease during withdrawal.[26,77] PUVA and acitretin have negligible antiarthritic efficacy.

Methotrexate

Methotrexate has traditionally been the drug claimed to produce benefit in both the cutaneous and the articular manifestations of psoriatic arthritis.[76] Despite its widespread use in psoriatic arthritis, data on its effectiveness are sparse. In a meta-analysis of the published randomized trials of second-line drugs for psoriatic arthritis, only sulfasalazine (no activity against skin disease) and methotrexate were proved to be effective.[77] Cyclosporine was not considered because no controlled study met the inclusion criteria for this particular meta-analysis. Another study compared low-dose methotrexate (up to 15 mg/week) with cyclosporine. Both were found to be effective, but methotrexate was better tolerated (28% vs. 41% withdrawal rate).[78] After a sufficient trial of an NSAID, initiation of methotrexate therapy is a reasonable second-line agent for R.T.'s arthralgias in his shoulders, knees, and hands and his active skin disease.

Therapy with methotrexate usually is initiated with a 2.5-mg test dose. If no idiosyncratic reaction occurs, doses are gradually increased to a maintenance dose of 10 to 25 mg/week. Methotrexate is best given in a single weekly oral dose or in three 2.5- to 7.5-mg doses at 12-hour intervals during a 24-hour period (e.g., 8 AM, 8 PM, and again at 8 AM). Folic acid 1 mg daily should be prescribed concomitantly to protect against common adverse effects, such as stomatitis. Folate does not protect against hepatic or pulmonary toxicity, and monitoring for these complications is necessary during therapy. Regular blood counts, urinalysis, and renal and liver function tests should be evaluated. An aspiration needle biopsy of the liver should be performed at or near the initiation of treatment.[50] More practically, if no risk factors for hepatotoxicity exist, the liver biopsy can be postponed for 2 to 4 months until the drug's efficacy and lack of toxicity have been established for the patient and long-term therapy is about to be initiated. Delaying the biopsy for this period does not pose a risk because it is rare for life-threatening liver disease to develop with the first 1.0 to 1.5 g of methotrexate.[49,50]

Hepatotoxicity, however, may not be apparent on routine laboratory evaluation. When liver chemistry tests are obtained, there should be at least a 1-week interval after the last methotrexate dose because liver chemistry values are often elevated 1 to 2 days after methotrexate therapy. If a significant abnormality in liver chemistry is noted, methotrexate therapy should be withheld for 1 to 2 weeks and the battery of liver chemistry tests repeated. Liver chemistry values should return to normal in 1 to 2 weeks. If significantly abnormal liver chemistry values persist for 2 to 3 months, a liver biopsy should be considered. Liver biopsy is recommended when the cumulative dosage level reaches 1.5 g and after each subsequent 1.5-g increase in the cumulative dose. Risk factors for hepatotoxicity include daily methotrexate administration, heavy alcohol intake, diabetes, obesity, intravenous drug abuse, previous exposure to hepatotoxic drugs, and pretreatment of liver dysfunction. Liver function abnormalities may improve after cessation of MTX therapy for 6 months.

8. During a follow-up visit to his family doctor several months later, R.T. had several somatic complaints that led to a diagnosis of recurrent depression. Subsequent history reveals that he also has resumed use of alcohol. He tends to drink four to five beers a night on weekends or when he is feeling low, although he does admit that his level of alcohol use is sometimes higher. His skin disease is relatively well controlled, but joint complaints have persisted. What additional options now exist for R.T.?

Methotrexate should be discontinued because the risks probably now exceed the benefits, particularly because rheumatic complaints have not been controlled and alcohol consumption has resumed. RT should be referred for physical and occupational therapy, encouraged to exercise, and (if needed) referred for orthotics. An NSAID can be given symptomatically. Sulfasalazine and hydroxychloroquine might be beneficial for joint symptoms alone, and cutaneous manifestations may be controlled with topical agents. Alternative second-line agents include immunomodulatory agents, cyclosporine, anticytokines, TNF inhibitors, infliximab, and etanercept.

Immunomodulatory Agents

Oral cyclosporine is given in divided daily doses in the range of 2.5 to 5 mg/kg, lower than for organ transplantation. Improvement is generally observed within 4 weeks. In one study, pain, number of painful and swollen joints, and duration of morning stiffness all decreased by 30% to 50%, along with 52% improvement in skin scores and serum C-reactive protein.[79] Another open-label study of 99 patients randomized to cyclosporine, sulfasalazine, or placebo reported beneficial effects from cyclosporine compared with placebo, but not sulfasalazine over 6 months, in terms of pain and tender, swollen joints counts.[80] Hypertension (13.9%), declining renal function (27.8%), and a variety of neurologic complaints (19.4%) were common in the cyclosporine-treated group. Skin disease also abated more in the cyclosporine group. Close monitoring is required because these toxicities often limit the long-term use of cyclosporine.

Both methotrexate and cyclosporine reduce inflammatory joint activity in the short term, but it remains to be seen whether they actually modify the long-term disease process. It is clear that better therapies for psoriatic arthritis are necessary.

Tumor necrosis factor-α is a potent cytokine involved in inflammation and joint damage. Inhibition of this cytokine reduces direct actions as well as the action of other proinflammatory cytokines. Etanercept is a TNF-α receptor blocker. In a 3-month, double-blind, placebo-controlled study of 60 patients with psoriatic arthritis, an etanercept response was observed in 73% of patients (vs. 13% with placebo) and skin condition improved in 50% (vs. 0% with placebo).[81] Infliximab is a human/mouse chimeric anti–TNF-α antibody. Patients given infliximab intravenously 10 mg/kg at 0, 2, and 6 weeks, reported 91% clinical response (vs. 18%, placebo) at 10 weeks and 82% (vs. 18%, placebo) had at least 75% improvement in PASI. The median time to response was 4 weeks. No serious adverse events occurred during this short trial.[65] In two other 1-year, open-label trials, infliximab at 5 mg/kg every 4 to 8 weeks produced significant reduction in both psoriatic skin lesions and joint symptoms, which was maintained with continued 5 mg/kg doses every 14 weeks.[82,83]

For patients such as R.T., whose disease cannot be treated successfully or safely with methotrexate, proceed with an anti–TNF-α agent. If available, etanercept (25–50 mg subcutaneously twice weekly) is preferred for convenience. Screening for tuberculosis before beginning therapy with anti-TNF agents is prudent, and those with evidence of prior tuberculous chest infection or with a positive skin test for tuberculosis should be offered prophylactic antitubercular therapy. If further studies confirm long-term effectiveness and safety of the anti-TNF treatments, these may become the preferred treatments for patients with moderate to severe disease.

REFERENCES

1. Bowcock AM et al. Getting under the skin: the immunogenetics of psoriasis. *Nature* 2005;5:699.
2. Griffiths CEM, Barker JNWN. Pathogenesis and clinical features of psoriasis. *Lancet* 2007;370:263.
3. Capon F et al. An update on the genetics of psoriasis. *Dermatol Clin* 2004;22:339.
4. Dika E et al. Environmental factors and psoriasis. *Curr Probl Dermatol* 2007;35:118.
5. Landgren E et al. Psoriasis in Swedish conscripts: time trend and association with T-helper 2-mediated disorders. *Br J Dermatol* 2006;154:332.
6. Gaspari AA. Innate and adaptive immunity and the pathophysiology of psoriasis. *J Am Acad Dermatol* 2006;54(S2):S67.
7. Robert C et al. Inflammatory skin diseases, T cells, and immune surveillance. *N Engl J Med* 1999;341: 1817.
8. Galosi A et al. Abnormal epidermal cell proliferation on the elbow in psoriatic and normal skin. *Arch Dermatol Res* 1980;267:105.
9. Leonardi CL et al. Etanercept as monotherapy in patients with psoriasis. *N Engl J Med* 2003;349:2014.
10. Reich K et al. Infliximab induction and maintenance therapy for moderate-to-severe psoriasis: a phase III, multicentre, double-blind trial. *Lancet* 2005;366: 1367.
11. Gladman DD et al. Psoriatic arthritis: epidemiology, clinical features, course, and outcome. *Ann Rheum Dis* 2005;64:14.
12. Jiaravuthisan MM et al. Psoriasis of the nail: anatomy, pathology, clinical presentation, and a review of the literature on therapy. *J Am Acad Dermatol* 2007;57:1.
13. Bonifati C et al. Recognition and treatment of psoriasis. Special considerations in elderly patients. *Drugs Aging* 1998;12:1.
14. Ong PY et al. Endogenous antimicrobial peptides and skin infections in atopic dermatitis. *N Engl J Med* 2002;347:1151.
15. Gelfand JM et al. Risk of myocardial infarction in patients with psoriasis. *JAMA* 2006;293:1735.
16. Smith CH et al. Psoriasis and its management. *BMJ* 2006;333:380.
17. Jobling R. A patient's journey. Psoriasis. *BMJ* 2007; 334:953.
18. Feldman SR et al. The self-administered psoriasis area and severity index is valid and reliable. *J Invest Dermatol* 1996;106:183.
19. Leon A et al. An attempt to formulate an evidence-based strategy in the management of moderate to severe psoriasis: a review of the efficacy and safety of biologics and prebiologic options. *Expert Opin Pharmacother* 2007;8:617.
20. http://www.psoriasis.org, The National Psoriasis Foundation. Accessed October 2007.
21. Pariser DM et al. National Psoriasis Foundation clinical consensus on disease severity. *Arch Dermatol* 2007;143:239.
22. Menter A et al. Current and future management of psoriasis. *Lancet* 2007;370:272.
23. Mason J et al. Topical preparations for the treatment of psoriasis: a systemic review. *Br J Dermatol* 2002;146:351.
24. Tristani-Firouzi P et al. Efficacy and safety of treatment modalities for psoriasis. *Cutis* 1998;61:11.
25. Gottleib AB. Therapeutic options in the treatment of psoriasis and atopic dermatitis. *J Am Acad Dermatol* 2005;53(Suppl 1):S3.
26. Katz HI. Topical corticosteroids. *Dermatol Clin* 1995;13:805.
27. Roelofzen JH et al. Coal tar in dermatology. *J Dermatolog Treat* 2007;12:1.
28. Thami GP et al. Coal tar: past, present and future. *Clin Exp Dermatol* 2002;27:99.
29. Zackheim HS. Should coal tar products carry cancer warnings? *Cutis* 2004;73:333.
30. Harris DR. Old wine in new bottles: the revival of anthralin. *Cutis* 1998;62:201.
31. Pearce DJ et al. Trends in on and off-label calcipotriene use. *Journal of Dermatological Treatment* 2006;17:308.
32. Kragballe K et al. Calcipotriol cream with or without concurrent topical corticosteroid in psoriasis: tolerability and efficacy. *Br J Dermatol* 1998;139:649.
33. Bleiker TO et al. Long-term outcome of severe chronic psoriasis following treatment with high dose topical calcipotriol. *Br J Dermatol* 1998;139:285.
34. Marks R. Pharmacokinetics and safety review of tazarotene. *J Am Acad Dermatol* 1998;39:S134.
35. Dando TM et al. Topical tazarotene: a review of its use in the treatment of plaque psoriasis. *Am J Clin Dermatol* 2005;6:255.
36. Rigopoulos D et al. Treatment of psoriatic nails with tazarotene cream 0.1% vs. clobetasol propionate 0.05% cream: a double-blind study. *Acta Derm Venereol* 2007;87:167.
37. Markham T et al. Narrowband UV-B phototherapy vs. oral 9-methoxypsoralen psoralen-UV-A for the treatment of chronic plaque psoriasis. *Arch Dermatol* 2003;139:325.
38. Diffey BL et al. The challenge of follow-up in narrowband ultraviolet B phototherapy. *Br J Dermatol* 2007;157:344.
39. Feldman SR et al. Efficacy of the 308-nm excimer laser for treatment of psoriasis: results of a multicenter study. *J Am Acad Dermatol* 2002;46:900.
40. Stern RS. Psoralen and ultraviolet A light therapy for psoriasis. *N Engl J Med* 2007;357:682.
41. Stern RS. Malignant melanoma in patients treated for psoriasis with PUVA. *Photodermatol Photoimmunol Photomed* 1999;15:37.
42. Lindelof B. Risk of melanoma with psoralen/ultraviolet: a therapy for psoriasis. *Drug Saf* 1999;20:289.
43. Stern RS. The risk of melanoma in association with long-term exposure to PUVA. *J Am Acad Dermatol* 2001;44:755.
44. Saurat JH. Retinoids and psoriasis: novel issues in retinoid pharmacology and implications for psoriasis treatment. *J Am Acad Dermatol* 1999;41:S2.
45. Lebwohl M. Acitretin in combination with UVB or PUVA. *J Am Acad Dermatol* 1999;41:S22.
46. Roenigk HH et al. Effects of acitretin on the liver. *J Am Acad Dermatol* 1999;41:584.
47. Ling MR. Acitretin: optimal dosing strategies. *J Am Acad Dermatol* 1999;41:S13.
48. Ahern MJ et al. Methotrexate hepatotoxicity: what is the evidence? *Inflamm Res* 1998;47:148.
49. Whiting-O'Keege QE et al. Methotrexate and histologic hepatic abnormalities: a meta-analysis. *Am J Med* 1991;90:711.
50. Roenigk HH et al. Methotrexate in psoriasis: consensus conference. *J Am Acad Dermatol* 1998;38: 478.
51. Smith CH. Use of hydroxyurea in psoriasis. *Clin Exp Dermatol* 1999;24:2.
52. Jackson CG. Immunomodulating drugs in the management of psoriatic arthritis. *Am J Clin Dermatol* 2001;2:367.
53. Wong RL et al. The mechanisms of action of cyclosporin A in the treatment of psoriasis. *Immunol Today* 1993;14:69.
54. Heydendael VMR et al. Methotrexate versus cyclosporine in moderate to severe chronic plaque psoriasis. *N Engl J Med* 2003;349:658.
55. Powles AV et al. Renal function after 10 years' treatment with cyclosporin for psoriasis. *Br J Dermatol* 1998;138:443.
56. Lebwohl M et al. Cyclosporine consensus conference: with emphasis on the treatment of psoriasis. *J Am Acad Dermatol* 1998;39:464.
57. Paquet P et al. Breast and lung cancers in two cyclosporin-A-treated psoriatic women. *Dermatology* 1998;196:450.
58. Paul C et al. Risk of malignancy associated with cyclosporin use in psoriasis. *Dermatology* 1999;198: 320.
59. Ruzicka T et al. Tacrolimus. The drug for the turn of the millennium? *Arch Dermatol* 1999;135:574.

60. Nousari HC et al. Mycophenolate mofetil in autoimmune and inflammatory skin disorders. *J Am Acad Dermatol* 1999;40:265.
61. Dubertret L et al. Clinical experience acquired with the efalizumbab (CLEAR) trial in patients with moderate to severe plaque psoriasis: results from a phase II international randomized, placebo-controlled trial. *Br J Dermatol* 2006;155:170.
62. Lebwohl M et al. An international, randomized, double-blind placebo-controlled phase III trial of intramuscular alefacept in patients with chronic plaque psoriasis. *Arch Dermatol* 2003;139:719.
63. Legat FJ et al. Narrowband UV-B phototherapy, alefacept, and clearance of psoriasis. *Arch Dermatol* 2007;143:1016.
64. Nast A et al. German evidence-based guidelines for the treatment of psoriasis vularis (short version). *Arch Dermatol Res* 2007;299:111.
65. Chaudhari U et al. Efficacy and safety of infliximab monotherapy for plaque-type psoriasis: a randomised trial. *Lancet* 2001;357:1842.
66. Gladman DD et al. Adalimumab for long-term treatment of psoriatic arthritis. *Arthritis Rheum* 2007;56:476.
67. Tyring S et al. Long-term safety and efficacy of 50 mg of etanercept twice weekly in patients with psoriasis. *Arch Dermatol* 2007;143:719.
68. Rott S et al. Recent developments in the use of biologics in psoriasis and autoimmune disorders. *BMJ* 2005;330:716.
69. Halevy S et al. Different modalities of spa therapy for skin diseases at the Dead Sea area. *Arch Dermatol* 1998;134:1416.
70. Boer J. The influence of mineral water solutions in phototherapy. *Clin Dermatol* 1996;14:665.
71. Koo J et al. Traditional Chinese medicine for the treatment of dermatologic disorders. *Arch Dermatol* 1998;134:1388.
72. McCarty MF. Glucosamine for psoriasis? *Med Hypotheses* 1997;48:437.
73. Dika E et al. Drug-induced psoriasis: an evidence-based overview and the introduction of psoriatic drug eruption probability score. *Cutan Ocul Toxicol* 2006;25:1.
74. Vine JE et al. Pustular psoriasis induced by hydroxychloroquine: a case report and review of the literature. *J Dermatol* 1996;23:357.
75. Koo J. Systemic sequential therapy of psoriasis: a new paradigm for improved therapeutic results. *J Am Acad Dermatol* 1999;41:S25.
76. Gladman DD et al. Psoriatic arthritis: epidemiology, clinical features, course, and outcome. *Ann Rheum Dis* 2005;64:14.
77. Salvarani C et al. Psoriatic arthritis. *Curr Opin Rheum* 1998;10:299.
78. Spadaro A et al. Comparison of cyclosporin A and methotrexate in the treatment of psoriatic arthritis: a one-year prospective study. *Clin Exp Rheumatol* 1995;13:589.
79. Mahrle G et al. Anti-inflammatory efficacy of low-dose cyclosporin A in psoriatic arthritis. A prospective multicentre study. *Br J Dermatol* 1996;135:752.
80. Salvarani C et al. A comparison of cyclosporine, sulfasalazine, and symptomatic therapy in the treatment of psoriatic arthritis. *J Rheumatol* 2001;28:2274.
81. Mease PJ et al. Etanercept in the treatment of psoriatic arthritis and psoriasis: a randomised trial. *Lancet* 2000;356:385.
82. Ogilvie AL. Treatment of psoriatic arthritis with antitumor necrosis factor-α antibody clears skin lesions of psoriasis resistant to treatment with methotrexate. *Br J Dermatol* 2001;144:587.
83. Van den Bosch F et al. Effects of a loading dose regimen of three infusions of chimeric monoclonal antibody to tumour necrosis factor-α (infliximab) in spondyloarthropathy: an open pilot study. *Ann Rheum Dis* 2000;59:428.

CHAPTER 41

Photosensitivity, Photoaging, and Burns

Timothy J. Ives

PHOTOSENSITIVITY

Effects of Ultraviolet Radiation

Changing lifestyles have considerably increased human exposure to sunlight: more outdoor recreational activities, more emphasis on tanning, longer life spans, and seasonal population shifts to the Sunbelt. Public attitudes toward tanning and sun exposure have not changed although epidemiologic evidence clearly implicates sunlight as a causative factor in many skin diseases. Squamous cell carcinoma (SCC) and basal cell carcinoma (BCC), which together account for more than half of all malignancies in the United States, are linked closely to exposure to ultraviolet radiation (UVR).[1] Malignant melanoma, the incidence of which has increased >100% in the last decade, most likely is linked to UVR exposure.[2] Sunburn, photoaging, immunologic changes in the skin, cataracts, photodermatoses, phototoxicity, and photoallergy are other commonly encountered photosensitivity reactions. The appropriate use of sunscreens or other photoprotective behaviors can help mitigate the incidence of the adverse effects of UVR.

Ultraviolet Radiation Spectrum

Ultraviolet radiation, the primary inducer of photosensitivity reactions in humans, is divided into ranges according to the effects of the four primary wavelengths: UVA1 (340–400 nm), UVA2 (320–340 nm), UVB (290–320 nm), and UVC (200 to 290 nm) (Fig. 41-1). UVA, with a wavelength of 320 to 400 nm, is closest in wavelength to visible light.[3] Unlike UVB rays,

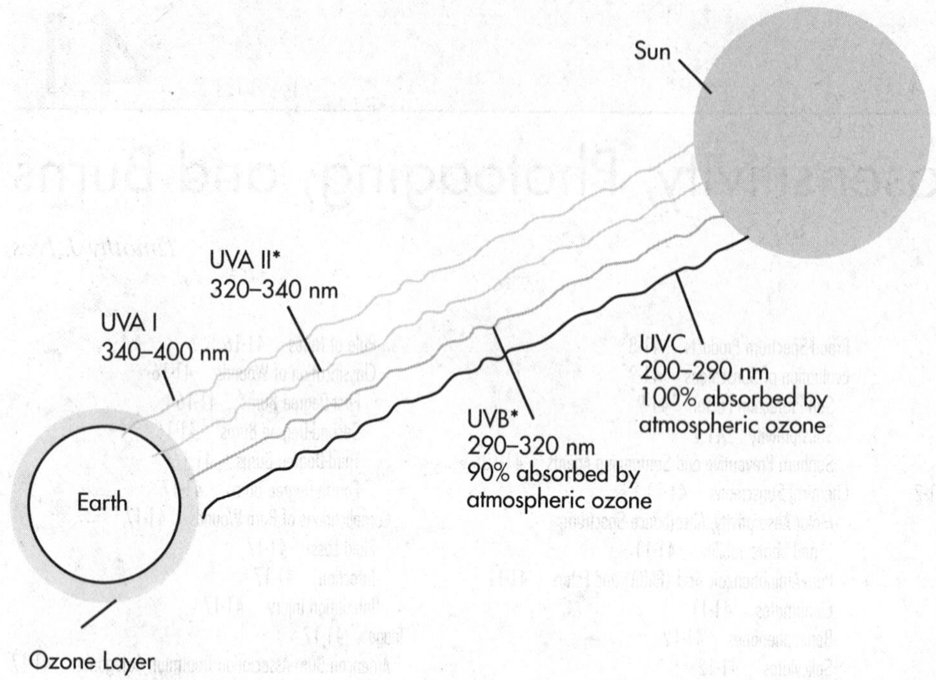

FIGURE 41-1 Ultraviolet radiation (UVR) spectrum. *Erythro-genic and melanogenic bands of UVR.

UVA radiation levels have small fluctuations during the day, and are present from sunrise to sunset every day, all year round, even in the winter and on cloudy days. It is considerably less likely than a comparable dose of UVB to cause a similar degree of erythema.[4,5] Unlike UVB, however, UVA penetrates to the dermal layer and may cause harmful effects not caused by UVB.[3] About 10 to 100 times more UVA reaches the earth's surface than UVB. Consequently, UVA may contribute up to 15% of the erythemal response at midday.[3,6] UVB is the most erythemogenic and melanogenic of the three UVR bands.[3,7] Up to 90% of UVB is blocked by the earth's stratospheric ozone layer, and it is absorbed completely by the epidermal layer of the skin.[8,9] The only known beneficial effect of UVR in humans is exposure to small amounts of UVB, most commonly through sunlight, which converts 7-dehydrocholesterol to cholecalciferol (vitamin D_3). Vitamin D enhances calcium homeostasis and has direct and indirect effects on cells involved with bone remodeling. As a result, vitamin D can decrease the risk of rickets in childhood and fractures and osteomalacia in adults.[10]

The UVC wavelengths are absorbed completely by the earth's stratospheric ozone layer. Artificial sources of UVC have been used in the sterilization and preservation of food and in minimizing bacterial growth in laboratories and hospital operating rooms by germicidal lamps, which can cause erythema or cataracts if mishandled.[3,7]

Environmental Effects on UVR

OZONE AND CHLOROFLUOROCARBONS

The amount of UVR that reaches the earth's surface is influenced by many factors. Concern has been focused on the implications of depletion of the ozone layer.[6,9,11] In the decade after it was first detected in 1983, ozone levels above the Antarctic had fallen to 50% of normal.[11] In the early 1990s, worldwide estimates from the Environmental Protection Agency (EPA) predicted an additional 40% depletion of ozone by the year 2075 if controls on chlorofluorocarbons (CFC) were not enacted. The EPA also concluded that for every 1% decrease in ozone, UVB radiation reaching the earth's surface would increase by 2% per year, possibly resulting in a 1% to 3% increase per year in nonmelanoma skin cancer.[12] In addition, UVB radiation can alter the immune system. As demonstrated by the worldwide meteorologic phenomena known as *El Nino* and *La Nina,* an impaired immune system can increase the incidence of certain cancers, including skin cancers.[9] These losses in the ozone layer are thought to be caused by man-made pollutants (e.g., nitrous oxides from jet airliners in stratospheric aviation and CFC as propellants and refrigerants). The effect of the ban on the commercial use of CFC by many of the industrialized nations has begun to be seen, as evidenced by a slow decline in these ozone-depleting compounds. Because ozone depletion takes place approximately a decade after CFC expression in the stratosphere, this recovery may take place later than expected.[13] Because UVA is only slightly filtered by the ozone layer, any decrease in the ozone layer would result in a disproportionate increase in UVB reaching the earth.

TIME OF DAY, CLOUD COVER, AND SURFACE REFLECTION

The time of day influences the amount of UVR reaching the earth's surface; 20% to 30% of the total daily UVR is received from 11 AM to 1 PM, with 75% between 9 AM and 3 PM. Cloud cover can decrease UV intensity by 10% to 80% and decreases infrared radiation to an even greater extent. This greater attenuation of infrared radiation by cloud cover can lead to an increased risk of UVR overexposure because less infrared radiation will be absorbed by the body and transformed into heat, resulting in less warning of overexposure to UVR. Reflection of UVR by substances (e.g., sand, water, snow) also may be important. For example, sand reflects about 25% of incident UVB radiation; therefore, sitting under an umbrella at the beach may not offer adequate protection. In general, whenever someone's shadow is shorter than his or her height, care should be taken; the shorter the shadow, the more likely a sunburn will occur. Fresh snow can reflect 50% to 95% of incident sunlight. Water reflects approximately 5% of erythemal UVR, whereas 75% of the radiation is transmitted through 2 m of water, offering swimmers little protection.[3] Seasonal changes, geographic latitude, and altitude also influence the amount of UVR reaching the earth's surface.

UV INDEX

The UV Index, offered by the EPA, the National Weather Service, and the Centers for Disease Control and Prevention, is a public health education service that is available in 58 U.S. cities.[14] This Index, with a scale from 1 (minimal exposure) to 10 (very high exposure), forecasts the probable intensity of skin-damaging UVR expected to reach the surface during the noon hour when the sun is highest in the sky. Theoretically, the UV Index can range from 0 (e.g., during the night) to 15 or 16 (in the tropics at high elevations under clear skies). The higher the UV Index, the greater the dose received of skin- and eye-damaging UVR, and the less time it takes before skin damage occurs.

The amount of UVR exposure needed to damage an individual's skin is affected by the elevation of the sun in the sky, the amount of ozone in the stratosphere, and the amount of clouds present. Clear skies transmit 100% of UVR to the earth's surface, with scattered clouds 89%, broken clouds 73%, and overcast clouds 32%. The darker an individual's skin tone, the longer (or the more UVR) it takes to cause erythema.

Erythema, Sunburn, and Tanning

ERYTHEMA AND OXYGEN-FREE RADICALS

Excessive exposure of the epidermal and dermal layers of the skin to UVR can result in an inflammatory erythematous reaction. Excess UVA and UVB causes the release of vasodilatory mediators (e.g., histamine, prostaglandins, cytokines), resulting in increased blood flow, erythema, tissue exudates, swelling, increased sensation of warmth, and a characteristic sunburn.[3,7] Severe UVR exposure, primarily UVB, can cause blister formation, desquamation, fever, chills, weakness, and shock. Erythema caused by UVB begins within 3 to 5 hours after exposure, is maximal after 12 to 24 hours, and usually resolves over the ensuing 3 days.[7] In contrast, erythema caused by UVA begins immediately, plateaus between 6 and 12 hours, and remains for 24 hours. UVA-induced changes in the dermis are characterized by greater damage to the vasculature and dense cellular infiltrates that penetrate to deeper levels of the skin.[7] The dermis also may be damaged when endogenous components of the skin absorb UVR energy and subsequently interact with oxygen to form tissue-damaging oxygen-free radicals.[9]

HISTOLOGY OF SUNBURN

The skin undergoes adaptive changes in response to UVR exposure. When keratinocytes in the epidermis are damaged and lose their typical organization, both the epidermis and the stratum corneum thicken[6] and attempt to serve as a barrier to UVR, particularly to UVB. The skin's normal protective immune response, however, is altered with exposure to UVR. Metalloproteinase proteins, proteolytic enzymes that are induced with low-dose UVR exposure, cause degradation of collagen and elastin in the dermal matrix.[15] Langerhans' cells (i.e., antigen-presenting cells in the skin) are decreased in number and function even after small doses of UVB.[15] These cells abnormally activate suppressor T-lymphocytes and lose their ability to activate normal effector pathways of the immune system.[16]

IMMEDIATE PIGMENT DARKENING AND DELAYED TANNING

Tanning is an adaptive mechanism of the skin to UVR. Tanning occurs by two different mechanisms: immediate pigment darkening (Meirowsky phenomenon) and delayed tanning. The primary cell involved in tanning is the melanocyte, which produces the radiation-absorbing protein, melanin.[3,6] Immediate pigment darkening begins during the actual exposure to UVA and certain bands of visible light,[3,6] and the oxidation of existing melanin in the epidermis transiently turns the skin grayish brown. The degree of immediate pigment darkening depends on the duration and intensity of exposure, the extent of previous tanning (or amount of pre-existing melanin), and the skin type of the individual.[3] Immediate pigment darkening is not protective against UVB erythema.[6]

Delayed tanning occurs 48 to 72 hours after exposure to either UVA or UVB. It is most intense 7 to 10 days after UV exposure and can last for weeks to months.[3] Delayed tanning is the result of increased production of melanin, an increase in the size and dendricity of the melanocyte, and the rate of transfer of melanosomes (particulate bodies of melanin) to keratinocytes.[3,6] The keratinocyte, now pigmented with melanosomes, migrates to the epidermis, producing the characteristic suntan. Delayed tanning caused by UVA is less protective against sunburn than delayed tanning caused by UVB, as epidermal thickening is not induced by UVA.[3]

SKIN TYPES

1. L.M., a 26-year-old woman, and G.M., her 28-year-old husband, have planned a 2-week cruise to the Caribbean and are inquiring about sunscreens for the trip. L.M. has fair complexion with blonde hair and blue eyes, and G.M. has a light brown complexion with brown hair and brown eyes. On first exposure to the sun with about an hour of intense midday sunlight, L.M. almost always develops a deep red, painful sunburn, with only minimal subsequent tanning. She freckles easily when exposed to sunlight and remembers being severely sunburned on several occasions as a child. When G.M. is first exposed to the sun in the summer, he usually develops mild erythema, followed by moderate tanning. He cannot recall being severely sunburned as a child, but does recall becoming moderately tanned each summer as a child and adolescent. L.M. is employed as a receptionist for an accounting firm, and G.M. works outdoors for a construction company. Both spend considerable amounts of time participating in outdoor activities. What data in this history would influence your recommendation of a sunscreen product for G.M. and L.M.?

One of the most important pieces of information to include in the patient history is the patient's skin type.[17] Patients can be classified into six sun-reactive skin types based on their response to initial sun exposure, skin color, tendency to sunburn, ability to tan, and personal history of sunburn (Table 41-1). This skin typing system has been used by the U.S. Food and Drug Administration (FDA) since 1978 in its guidelines for sunscreen agents. L.M.'s fair complexion, propensity to

Table 41-1 Suggested SPF for Various Skin Types

Complexion	Skin Type	Skin Characteristics	Suggested Product SPF
Very fair	I	Always burns easily; never tans	20–30
Fair	II	Always burns easily; tans minimally	15–20
Light	III	Burns moderately; tans gradually	10–15
Medium	IV	Burns minimally; always tans well	8–10
Dark	V	Rarely burns; tans profusely	8
Very dark	VI	Never burns; deeply pigmented	8

SPF, sun protection factor.

sunburn, and minimal tanning classify her as skin type II. G.M.'s light brown complexion, minimal sunburn reaction, and moderate tanning classify him as skin type IV. Hair and eye colors also provide an indication to skin reactiveness to sunlight. People who have blonde, red, or light brown hair or blue or green eyes tend to have greater skin reactivity to sunlight than people with darker-colored hair or eyes. A history of severe sunburn also can be associated with skin reactivity to sunlight, although self-reported patient histories of sunburn or tanning may not be consistently reliable, and personal interviews may be a more reliable indicator. L.M.'s propensity to freckle and her history of severe sunburns as a child may give an indication as to her skin's sun reactiveness. Other important information to consider in the patient history includes a medication history, history of sun-reactive dermatoses, history of allergies (particularly contact hypersensitivities to cosmetics or other topical agents), and the intended activities during sunscreen use.

Photocarcinogenesis

RISK FACTORS

2. What subjective and objective evidence do L.M. and G.M. exhibit that places them at risk for the long-term adverse effects of UVR? What are the risk factors for these long-term adverse effects of UVR?

The long-term effects of UVR include photocarcinogenesis and premature aging of the skin (photoaging). The associated risks for development of these long-term effects are directly related to the congenital pigmentation of an individual (which includes skin type and hair and eye color) and intensity, duration, and frequency of exposure to UVR. With a type II skin type, L.M. is at high risk for carcinogenesis and photoaging, whereas G.M., with skin type IV, may be at a lower risk. Excessive sun exposure, especially during childhood, increases the risk of nonmelanoma and melanoma skin cancers. During the first 18 years of life, the average child receives three times the dose of UVB of the average adult; consequently, most sun exposure occurs during childhood.[18,19] A history of frequent sunburn or intermittent high-intensity exposures to UVR may be associated with the occurrence of malignant melanoma, whereas large cumulative doses of UVR over a lifetime may contribute to the incidence of nonmelanoma skin cancers. L.M.'s history of several severe sunburns as a child may more than double her risk of cutaneous malignant melanoma (CMM).[18,19] Cumulative doses of UVR received unintentionally from working outdoors (as in G.M.) or from participating in outdoor recreational activities also can contribute significantly to the risk of photocarcinogenesis and photoaging.[4] A large number of moles, congenital moles >1.5 cm wide, and abnormal moles also appear to be a risk factor for malignant melanoma.[20] Risk for skin cancer is increased among first-degree relatives of patients with skin cancer,[21] because frequent sunburns, suboptimal sunscreen use, and high rates of tanning bed use are common among the children with a personal or family history of skin cancer.[22]

SQUAMOUS CELL AND BASAL CELL CARCINOMA

The association of skin cancer in humans to UVR exposure is based primarily on clinical and epidemiologic evidence. Nonmelanoma skin cancers, such as SCC and BCC, occur most commonly on areas that are maximally exposed to sunlight (e.g., the face, neck, arms, back of the forearms, and hands).[3] The prevalence of nonmelanoma skin cancers is inversely related to geographic distance from the equator and to the melanin content of the skin, with SCC more strongly linked than BCC to UVR.[3,20] Persons of skin types most sensitive to sunlight, as well as persons working outdoors, have higher incidences of nonmelanoma skin cancers.[3] A family history of SCC and BCC increases the risk at least twofold, depending on the histology, number of lesions, and degree of invasiveness.[23] Albinism, a genetic disease characterized by partial or total absence of pigment in the skin, hair, and eyes, is associated with increased and premature development of skin cancers.[3]

CUTANEOUS MALIGNANT MELANOMA

The development of CMM also may be linked to UVR exposure, specifically exposures that induce sunburn. A history of five or more severe sunburns during adolescence more than doubles the risk of CMM.[20] CMM, as does nonmelanoma skin cancers, demonstrates an inverse relationship to geographic distance from the equator and melanin content of the skin.[3] Unlike nonmelanoma skin cancers, however, CMM does not demonstrate a clear relationship to the cumulative dose of UVR, and it occurs on areas of the body exposed to the sun intermittently (e.g., on the back in men and the lower legs in women). In addition, it occurs most commonly in the middle-aged and individuals who work indoors, as well as those whose sun exposure is limited to weekends and vacations.[20] A family history of melanoma increases the risk of melanoma two- to eightfold.[24]

MECHANISMS OF CARCINOGENESIS

Mechanisms of carcinogenesis may include damage to DNA and alterations in immunologic status. Epidermal and dermal DNA can absorb UVR, which can contribute to abnormal formation of pyrimidine dimers. Normally, these pyrimidine dimers are excised and repaired; however, if left uncorrected, these DNA lesions can lead to interruption of transcription, with possible mutagenesis and malignancy.[25]

TANNING BOOTHS

3. B.P., a 32-year-old woman, is preparing for a business trip to Cancun. She is seeking advice about the use of a tanning bed to stimulate melanin for the prevention of sunburn while on her trip. B.P. has skin type III and light brown hair and green eyes. She recently heard, however, that a tan produced by artificial sunlight may not protect against sunburn and may even cause skin cancer. What advice will you offer her? What precautions would you recommend if she decides to visit a tanning salon?

Most tanning beds, booths, or salons use an artificial light source that emits about 95% UVA with minimal (i.e., 1% to 5%) UVB.[26,27] Although UVA is much less likely to produce photoaging and photocarcinogenic changes of the skin than UVB, high doses of UVA received during a tanning session, as well as increasing cumulative UVA doses over time, and increased exposure to sunlight in general, raise great concern over the long-term effects of UVA.[28] UVA causes many of the same effects on the skin as UVB, including immunologic, degenerative, and neoplastic changes, as well as damage to DNA and the formation of reactive oxygen species.[29] UVA also contributes to cataract formation and the activation of herpetic lesions.[30] In addition, UVA may augment the photocarcinogenic effect of UVB,[2] and growing evidence indicates the relationship between indoor tanning and melanoma.[31] This issue is compounded by a recent study that suggests that excessive UV exposure may have a behavioral component.[32]

With a skin type III, B.P. may be able gradually to achieve a moderate tan with minimal burning, thus providing some protection from UVR because of increased melanization of the skin. This UVA-induced tan, however, may not be as protective as a tan achieved under normal sunlight conditions because UVA does not thicken the stratum corneum.[33] An artificially produced tan plus subsequent sun exposure has not been found to provide any net reduction in long-term damage to the skin when compared with the same amount of tan obtained by sunbathing alone.[33] For these reasons, B.P. should not use the tanning booth to obtain a protective tan, and she should use appropriate photoprotective measures during her trip.

If B.P. decides to artificially tan despite your recommendation, she should undertake some precautions. Because she has skin type III, her UVR exposure should be limited to 30 to 50 half-hour sessions a year and she should keep a record of total joules of exposure that she has received over time.[3] To minimize cataract development, B.P. always should wear protective eye wear that absorbs all UVA, UVB, and visible light up to 500 nm; simply closing her eyes or wearing regular sunglasses provides no protective effect against eye damage.

Photoaging

NORMAL AGING AND HISTOLOGY OF PHOTODAMAGED SKIN

Photoaging, or premature aging of the skin, involves skin changes that differ from those associated with normal chronologic aging.[34,35] Normal aging of the skin involves fine wrinkling of the skin, atrophy of the dermis, and a decrease in the amount of subcutaneous adipose tissue, all of which lead to a state of hypocellularity of the skin.[34] Photoaging involves a chronic inflammatory state induced by long-term exposure to sunlight, leading to a hypermetabolic state of the skin.[33] Photodamaged skin is characterized histologically by an accumulation of excessive quantities of thickened, degenerated elastic connective tissue fibers (elastosis).[34] Type I collagen predominates in normal skin, but in photodamaged skin, type III collagen increases about fourfold and the mature matrix of type I collagen slightly decreases.[29] These degenerative changes in connective tissue may be caused by hyperactive fibroblasts or by enzymatic degradation via cellular infiltrates in inflamed skin.[3] The elastic connective tissue then replaces the collagen in upper parts of the dermis.[33] The ground substance, composed of proteoglycans and glycosaminoglycans, also is increased considerably in photoaged skin.[3] Capillaries in the dermis become dilated and tortuous, resulting in telangiectasias, ecchymosis, and purpura.[35] The epidermis thickens, and epidermal cells become hyperplastic and possibly neoplastic. Actinic keratosis, a premalignant lesion found mostly in the older population, is a risk factor for the development of BCC, because a low percentage of these lesions transform into SCC.[35,36] Large cumulative doses of UVA, UVB, and possibly infrared radiation over the course of a lifetime are strongly implicated as the cause of these changes in photoaged skin.[3]

Photodamaged skin is characterized as being wrinkled, yellowed, and sagging. Mildly affected skin becomes irregularly pigmented, rough, and dry, with mild wrinkles. Moderately affected skin becomes deeply wrinkled, sagging, thickened, and leathery, with vascular lesions.[35] Largely irreversible, severely affected skin can become deeply furrowed, permanently (and irregularly) pigmented, and may manifest premalignant and malignant lesions.[35] Areas of the body most commonly affected are the face, back of the neck, back of the arms and hands, the V-line of the neck of women, and balding areas of the head of men.

TOPICAL RETINOIDS

4. P.B. is a 38-year-old woman who has enjoyed many outdoor activities over the years. She lives in a moderate climate, with hot, sunny summers and cold winters. She feels that she appears older than other women her age because of wrinkling and color changes of her skin. Her facial color is somewhat yellowish in appearance and the fine wrinkles at the corners of her eyes and mouth have become more obvious. She has noticed the formation of small brown spots mottling parts of her face, hands, and forearms. P.B. has skin type III; a clear complexion; and skin that is sensitive to soaps, heavy cosmetics, and perfumes. Would P.B. be an appropriate candidate for therapy with a topical retinoid product (e.g., tretinoin)?

Tretinoin (transretinoic acid) is available as a cream (0.025%, 0.05%, and 0.1%), gel (0.01%, 0.025%, 0.04% [in microspheres], 0.1% [in microspheres]), or liquid (0.05%). Tazarotene, another retinoic acid, is available as a 0.05% or 0.1% cream. Adapalene is available as a 0.1% cream, and a 0.1% or 0.3% gel. These agents are effective in partially reversing some of the clinical and histologic changes of photoaging by lessening fine wrinkles, mottled pigmentation, and the tactile roughness associated with photoaged skin.[37–40] Adverse drug events include erythema, peeling, burning, and stinging. These adverse effects, as well as the clinical and histologic improvements, are thought to be dose dependent. Mild to moderate reactions decrease gradually after the second week of therapy. Additional benefits of retinoid therapy include the formation of new dermal collagen and vessels, reduction in the number and melanization of freckles, resorption of degenerated connective tissue fibers, and treatment of premalignant and malignant skin lesions.[41] In one of the initial trials, all subjects treated (100%) demonstrated global improvement in the signs of photoaging, with 53% showing moderate changes and the remainder having at least slight improvement. Of the clinical parameters assessed, the most impressive improvements were found with facial skin sallowness, with respondents developing a healthy, rosy glow.[38]

Patient Selection

Topical retinoid therapy is most effective for patients 50 to 70 years of age with moderate to severe photoaging and for prophylactic use in patients undergoing the initial changes of photoaging.[37] Recently, P.B. has noticed some of the skin changes consistent with early photoaging and would be a good candidate for prophylactic therapy with topical tretinoin. Treatment may improve her sallow skin color; lessen the mottling on her face, forearms, and fine wrinkles at the corners of her eyes and mouth; as well as prevent worsening of the photoaging process that she is experiencing.

Patient Counseling

5. P.B.'s physician asks if tretinoin 0.05% cream would be a good starting dose. What do you recommend? What patient counseling should P.B. be given?

Because both the beneficial and adverse effects of topical retinoid therapy are dose dependent, the underlying goal is to provide the maximal benefit by using the highest concentration that causes minimal skin irritation. Considering P.B.'s skin sensitivity to soaps, cosmetics, and perfumes, her skin is likely to be irritated easily by tretinoin; therefore, it would be best to initiate therapy with the lowest strength (e.g., tretinoin 0.025% cream). An alternative retinoid is tazarotene 0.1% cream. These agents are usually applied every night at bedtime, but in some instances, they are applied initially on an every-other-night basis until the skin accommodates to the irritant effects. The likelihood of irritation depends on the type of vehicle, more than on the concentration of the agent.[41] The cream formulation causes the least skin irritation and would be preferred for initiating therapy for P.B. Tretinoin is also available as a gel with an alcohol base, with a tendency to be drying and irritating. It is preferred for patients with persistent acne or for those with focal actinic lesions. The vehicle in the gel formulation of tretinoin can evaporate, resulting in the potentiation of its effects. Younger patients often prefer the gel because it leaves no residue and is compatible with most cosmetics. The solution and gel may be better tolerated in older patients with oily, thick, pigmented skin.

Before applying the cream to her face at bedtime, P.B. should wash her face gently, using her fingertips and mild soap, then patting her skin dry with a towel. If gentle washing with her fingers does not remove the dry, peeling skin, a washcloth can be used gently on the face. The treated stratum corneum is fragile, and erosions could occur if P.B. is not careful when washing. After waiting about 15 minutes, she should apply a pea-sized amount of cream to her forehead and spread the cream evenly over her entire face. Care should be exercised while applying the cream to the areas adjacent to the eyes and mouth because tretinoin can cause irritation and burning of mucous membranes.

Skin irritation can be expected to start in the first 3 to 5 days of therapy and, hopefully, will subside in 1 to 3 months. If P.B. experiences excessive irritation, she can reinitiate the regimen on a slower timeline by applying the cream on an every-other-night or every-third-night basis for the first 2 weeks to reduce skin irritation, or she can also apply a topical corticosteroid product such as hydrocortisone 1% cream. As she begins to tolerate the therapy, her frequency of applications and strength of cream should be titrated to cause mild scaling with only occasional mild erythema. A thicker film of cream can be applied to photodamaged areas. After 9 to 12 months of therapy, she can begin maintenance therapy, which consists of application two or three nights a week indefinitely.

Because these agents can dry the skin, P.B. should be counseled to use moisturizers during the day to help decrease the dryness and irritation of the skin. Nighttime application of moisturizers should be discouraged when topical tretinoin is being used because the moisturizers can cause a pH incompatibility with the cream and possibly dilute the concentration of tretinoin. With a thinning of the stratum corneum, P.B.'s skin may be more susceptible to the effects of UVR. For this reason, as well as to prevent further actinic damage, P.B. should begin prophylactic daytime application of a sunscreen. Considering her skin type (III) and early photoaging changes, a sunscreen with a sun protective factor (SPF) of at least 30 would be appropriate. P.B. should be counseled not to become discouraged by any apparent lack of response; her skin damage is mild, her response to therapy will be gradual, and part of the goal of therapy is to prevent further damage. Her wrinkles may actually appear to worsen early in therapy owing to an initial buildup of the stratum corneum. P.B. should avoid facial saunas and irritating soaps and cosmetics.

Phototoxicity and Photoallergy

PATIENT HISTORY

6. D.L., a 16-year-old, blond-haired, blue-eyed teenager with skin type II, presents with a severe sunburn. He states that he started a new summer job 2 days ago with typical sun exposure. He is surprised at the severity of this sunburn, which is worse than normal for the same amount of sun exposure. What nonprescription remedies might you recommend for D.L. at this time?

Treatment recommendations for D.L.'s sunburn are inappropriate without first obtaining additional data (e.g., a history and brief visual examination of the condition). Information that may be important in the history of the condition include the temporal relationship between sun exposure and onset of symptoms; the nature and duration of symptoms; recent ingestion or topical application of medications; possible exposure to photosensitizers, chemical irritants, or plants that can cause allergic contact dermatitis (e.g., poison ivy); and the potential for arthropod bites. Information that may be important from the physical examination includes the distribution and morphology of the reaction, as well as areas of the body spared of the reaction.

A drug-induced photosensitivity reaction most commonly appears as a sunburn of greater severity than would normally be expected or as a rash in areas exposed to the sun or tanning apparatus. With an increased emphasis on health that includes exercise and physical activity outdoors, the incidence of these reactions is common, with a greater frequency during both the summer and winter. Further, with an increase in the use of complementary or alternative medications, many people are unaware that some of these products (e.g., St. John's Wort) can also cause photosensitivity reactions. Chemicals with photosensitization potential are found in medications, cosmetics, shampoos, moisturizing lotions, hair dyes or tints, soaps, and other topically applied medications and agents.

Drug-induced photosensitivity reactions can be subdivided into phototoxic and photoallergic reactions. The same medication or agent may produce both phototoxic and photoallergic reactions, and it may at times be difficult to differentiate clinically between the two types of reactions.

PHOTOSENSITIZERS AND SYMPTOMS OF PHOTOTOXICITY

7. On further questioning, you discover that D.L. first experienced painful erythema of the extensor surface of his hands and forearms, the anterior aspect of his neck, and parts of his face within hours of starting his new job at an outdoor garden and greenhouse. Besides painful erythema, the symptoms also included an immediate prickling and burning sensation. The symptoms continued to worsen until the following morning, about 24 hours after initial exposure to the sun. D.L. does not recall orally ingesting or topically applying any medication or other preparation to his skin, nor does he recall exposure to any chemical irritants, or poison ivy or oak. The morphology of the skin lesions is that of an exaggerated sunburn. The skin lesions are patchy in distribution with greater density on his forearms and hands than on his neck and face. The posterior aspect of his neck and covered areas of his body were spared completely. What are some possible causes of his exaggerated sunburn reaction?

The most likely explanation for D.L.'s exaggerated sunburn reaction is *phototoxicity,* secondary to contact with psoralen-like chemicals from the plants at his job at the outdoor garden and greenhouse. Phototoxicity is an immediate or delayed inflammatory reaction that occurs when a compound with photosensitizing ability absorbs a sufficient concentration of UVR in or on the skin, and when the skin is exposed simultaneously to a specific wavelength of light.[42] This spectrum of offending UVR occurs from the UVB to the UVA range. These compounds include many drugs (see Table 38-8 in Chapter 38, Dermatotherapy and Drug Induced Skin Disorders) and naturally occurring psoralen-like (furocoumarin) compounds that are found in many plants (e.g., limes, parsley, celery, figs).[43] When the photosensitizing compound is deposited on the skin surface, the photosensitizer absorbs the radiologic energy and transfers the energy to surrounding molecules, which then become destructive to the surrounding tissue.[3,42]

The most common type of drug-induced photosensitivity reaction is phototoxicity, in which the offending agent is thought to act as a chromophore, absorbing UVR. When the chromophore reaches a sufficient concentration in or on the skin and when the skin is exposed to the appropriate wavelength of UVR, energy is emitted, which damages the adjacent tissue to cause a phototoxic reaction. The wavelength of radiation necessary to produce such a reaction depends on the absorption spectrum of the offending agent.

Phototoxic photosensitivity reactions are dose dependent and occur in almost any person who takes or applies an adequate amount of the offending agent. The dose necessary to produce such a reaction varies from person to person and depends on such factors as complexion, hair and eye color, usual ability to tan, and type and amount of UVR exposure. Phototoxic photosensitivity reactions are not immunologically mediated or true allergic reactions; they can occur on first exposure to the agent, and generally show no cross-sensitivity to chemically related agents.

A phototoxic reaction usually has a rapid onset, often within several hours after UVR exposure and presents as an exaggerated or intensified sunburn with erythema, pain, and prickling or burning. Blistering, desquamation, and hyperpigmentation can occur in severe cases.[42] Symptoms generally peak 24 to 48 hours after the initial exposure and are usually limited to the areas of UVR-exposed skin. Because phototoxicity reactions do not involve the immune system, prior exposure to the photosensitizer is unnecessary for this reaction to occur.

Presumably, D.L. came into contact with psoralen-containing plants and simultaneous exposure to sunlight. With an unusual distribution of lesions on his hands, forearms, neck, and face, the lack of lesions on areas not contacted by the plants or sunlight, the temporal relationship between the exposure and onset of symptoms place phototoxicity higher in the differential diagnosis.

PHOTOSENSITIZERS AND SYMPTOMS OF PHOTOALLERGY

Photoallergy is another possible cause of D.L.'s symptoms. Although much less common than phototoxicity, photoallergy requires prior or prolonged exposure to the photosensitizing compound. Photoallergy results from a similar mechanism to phototoxicity, except that the immune system is involved. Most commonly, it is caused by polycyclic photosensitizers that react with UVA to form antigenic macromolecules, evoking a delayed hypersensitivity response. Clinically, photoallergy differs from phototoxicity in that it produces an intensely pruritic, eczematous form of dermatitis.[42] The rash is preceded by pruritus and may subside within an hour. In 5% to 10% of cases, persistent hypersensitivity to light occurs, even after the offending chemical has been eliminated.[42]

In photoallergic photosensitivity reactions, the suspected medication or chemical agent is altered in the presence of UVR to become antigenic or to become a hapten (i.e., an incomplete antigen), which can combine with a tissue antigen. These antigen-antibody or immune-mediated processes differentiate photoallergic from phototoxic reactions. Photoallergic reactions do not occur on first exposure to the medication, but as with other allergic reactions, they require prior or prolonged exposure (sensitization period) to the offending agent.[42] Once sensitization has occurred, subsequent exposure to even small amounts of the offending product will produce a photoallergic reaction.

Photoallergic reactions are not dose related, and eruptions can also be caused by chemically related agents owing to a cross-sensitivity or cross-allergenicity. As a type of delayed hypersensitivity reaction, time is required to develop an immune response and the onset of a photoallergic reaction is often delayed for 1 to 3 days. These reactions can present as macular, bullous, or purpuric lesions. Acute urticaria can occur within minutes after UVR exposure. Recovery is slower than from a phototoxic reaction, and it can persist after the offending product has been removed. These reactions may present with erythema and possible edema secondary to the inflammation, but are most commonly found to be eczematous, characterized by erythema; pruritus (possible severe); and papules, vesicles, or both, with weeping, oozing, and crusting. Scaling, lichenification, and pigmentation may occur later.

In a small percentage of cases, hypersensitivity to UVR can persist after the suspected agent is discontinued. Photoallergic reactions primarily occur on the skin at sites that are exposed to UVR, but may extend to nonexposed areas. These reactions are more common in adults, usually caused by topical medications or chemicals, but also can be seen with the use of systemic medications.

D.L. is unlikely to have a photoallergic reaction because of the lack of a delayed temporal relationship between the onset of symptoms and combined exposure to plant furocoumarins and sunlight. Unlike phototoxicity reactions, photoallergic reactions can spread to areas that have not been exposed to sunlight; however, D.L.'s lesions were limited to areas of skin exposed to sunlight.

MANAGEMENT

8. What recommendations should you give D.L. for management of his photosensitivity?

General recommendations for the management of phototoxicity and photoallergy reactions are focused on the removal of exposure to the potential photosensitizer and reduced exposure to the sun. Patients should be counseled not to take any medications, orally or topically, without first consulting with their health care provider to minimize exposure to other photosensitizers. D.L. should try wearing long-sleeved shirts, pants, and gloves when working to limit exposure to plant photosensitizers. He also may try applying a broad-spectrum sunscreen to protect his skin from UVB and UVA radiation. If these measures do not prevent further photosensitivity reactions, D.L. should consider a different type of employment. His presenting symptoms should be managed in a manner similar to that for an exaggerated sunburn.

Photoprotection

Broad-Spectrum Products

Sunscreens are used to prevent sunburn and reduce the incidence of premature aging and carcinogenesis.[36,44,45] The original formulations were developed to protect against the effects of UVB radiation because the potential adverse effects of UVA were not yet recognized. Because UVA plays a significant role in many of the adverse effects associated with UVR exposure, broad-spectrum sunscreen products with absorption spectra in the UVA range have become commercially available, in combination with UVB absorbers. These broad-spectrum products provide additional benefit for patients with photosensitivity reactions caused by wavelengths not covered by single-ingredient sunscreens.

Numerous public health information programs have targeted sun protection for younger children. These programs are used to counter the fact that starting in the years of early adolescence, use of sun protective measures continually decrease, with the nadir by the high school to college-level years of early adulthood.[46] Sunscreens should be considered as only one component of an overall program to reduce UV exposure and protect against long-term photodamage.[47–49] The American Cancer Society has adopted the "*Slip, Slop, Slap*" slogan from an Australian public health skin cancer prevention campaign, and recommends that anyone going out into the sun should slip on a shirt, slop on sunscreen, and slap on a hat. Since the Australian campaign was introduced in 1981, the overall incidence of skin cancer in Australia has decreased. This program was extended in later years to encourage the use of sunglasses (i.e., slip on a shirt, slop on the sunscreen, slap on a hat, and wrap on some sun glasses: "*Slip, Slop, Slap, Wrap*").

For health care providers and their patients, the tenets of this program can be recalled with the acronym C-H-E-S-S:

C Clothing that is sun protective (i.e., tightly woven and in dark colors)
H Hats with wide brims all around
E Eyeglasses that block both UVA and UVB light
S Sunscreen with an SPF of at least 15 that is applied appropriately
S Shade, especially between 10 AM and 4 PM

Table 41-2 lists the available sunscreen chemicals that have been judged to be both safe and effective.

Table 41-2 Sunscreens and UVR Absorbance

Sunscreen	*Absorbance*
Anthranilates	
Meradimate (menthyl anthranilate)	260–380
Benzophenones	
Dioxybenzone	250–390
Oxybenzone (benzophenone-3)	270–350
Sulisobenzone (Eusolex 4360)	260–375
Cinnamates	
Cinoxate (diethanolamine p-methoxycinnamate)	280–310
Octocrylene	250–360
Octinoxate (octyl methoxycinnamate, Parsol MCX)	290–320
Dibenzoylmethanes	
Avobenzone (butyl methoxydibenzoylmethane, Parsol 1789)	320–400
Aminobenzoic Acid and Ester Derivatives	
Lisadimate (Glyceryl PABA)	264–315
Para-aminobenzoic acid (PABA)	260–313
Padimate O (octyl dimethyl PABA)	290–315
Roxadimate	280–330
Salicylates	
Homosalate	295–315
Octisalate (octyl salicylate)	280–320
Triethanolamine salicylate	260–320
Trolamine salicylate	260–320
Camphor Derivatives	
Benzoate-4 methylbenzylidene camphor	290–300
Ecamsule (terephthalylidene dicamphor sulfonic acid; Mexoryl)	290–400
Others	
Ensulizole (phenylbenzimidazole sulfonic acid)	290–340
Physical Sunscreens	
Red petrolatum	290–365
Titanium dioxide	290–700
Zinc oxide	290–700

UVR, ultraviolet radiation.

Evaluation of Sunscreens

SUN PROTECTION FACTOR

The effectiveness of a sunscreen formulation is based on its SPF and its substantivity.[50] SPF is a measure of how much solar energy (UV radiation) is required to produce sunburn on protected skin (i.e., in the presence of sunscreen) relative to the amount of solar energy required to produce sunburn on unprotected skin. As the SPF value increases, sunburn protection increases. It is defined as the ratio of the minimal dose of UVR required to produce an erythemal response in sunscreen-protected skin compared with unprotected skin.[36] SPF are based on tests of volunteers with skin types I through III, using either natural sunlight or a solar simulator that generates both UVB and UVA.[36,50] Because the SPF can be influenced by the composition, chemical properties, emollient properties, and pH of the vehicle, sunscreen formulations must be evaluated on an individual basis.[50] SPF also is influenced by the amount applied to the skin, the time of initial application before UVR exposure, the frequency of application, and environmental factors, such as photodegradation during UVR exposure; therefore, the SPF achieved during actual use can be significantly less than indicated on the label.[51–55] Consumers have been shown to routinely apply only one fourth to one-half thickness of the layer of sunscreen used to determine the SPF prior to marketing.[56]

A popular misconception is that SPF relates to time of solar exposure. For example, many people believe that if they normally get sunburn in 1 hour, then an SPF 15 sunscreen allows them to stay in the sun for 15 hours (i.e., 15 times longer) without getting sunburn. This is untrue because SPF is not directly related to time of solar exposure, but to the amount of solar exposure. Although solar energy amount is related to solar exposure time, other factors have an impact on the amount of solar energy. For example, the intensity of the solar energy has an impact on the amount. Generally, it takes less time to be exposed to the same amount of solar energy at midday compared with early morning or late evening because the sun is more intense at midday relative to the other times. The following exposures may result in the same amount of solar energy: 1 hour at 9:00 AM versus 15 minutes at 1:00 PM. Solar intensity is also related to geographic location, with greater solar intensity occurring at lower latitudes. Also, as clouds absorb solar energy, solar intensity is generally greater on clear days than on cloudy days.

In 1978, the FDA Over-the-Counter (OTC) Review Panel on sunscreens reclassified sunscreens from cosmetics to drugs intended to protect the structure and function of the human integument against actinic damage. In 1999, the FDA finalized its regulations for OTC sunscreens. Manufacturers of cosmetic tanning preparations that do not contain a sunscreen were required to include a warning statement (see the following discussion) on their products. These regulations list the active ingredients that can be used in sunscreens, labeling and testing requirements, and also provide for uniform, streamlined labeling for all OTC products intended for use as sunscreens to assist consumers in making decisions on sun protection. These regulations include the following:

- Similar labeling requirements for all OTC products intended for use as sunscreens (including sunscreen–cosmetic combinations, such as makeup products carrying sun protection claims) to provide good, useful information to consumers.
- Uniform, streamlined labeling for all sunscreens. Accommodations in labeling must be made for sunscreens that are labeled for use only on specific small areas of the face (e.g., lips, nose, ears, or around eyes).
- A list of 16 allowed sunscreen active ingredients, with zinc oxide and avobenzone being the two most recent additions.
- Both required and optional label claims, warnings, and directions.
- Required SPF testing for all agents.
- A new SPF category of "30" plus (or "30%") for SPF values above 30.
- Simplification of the previously proposed five product sun protection categories down to three:
  - *Minimum* (corresponding to the current SPF of 2 to 12)
  - *Moderate* (corresponding to an SPF of 12 to 30)
  - *High* (corresponding to an SPF of 30 or greater)
- A "Sun Alert" statement that reflects the important role that sunscreens play in a total program to reduce the harmful effects of the sun (i.e., "Sun alert: Limiting sun exposure, wearing protective clothing, and using sunscreens may reduce the risks of skin aging, skin cancer, and other harmful effects of the sun").
- Cessation of unsupported, absolute, or misleading and confusing terms such as *sun block, waterproof, all-day protection, deep tanning,* and *visible and/or infrared light protection.*

In addition to the aforementioned changes, cosmetic regulations require tanning preparations that do not contain a sunscreen ingredient to display the following warning: "Warning—this product does not contain a sunscreen and does not protect against sunburn. Repeated exposure of unprotected skin while tanning may increase the risk of skin aging, skin cancer, and other harmful effects to the skin even if you do not burn."

In 2006, the FDA introduced final regulations on sunscreen labeling. The term *sunscreen* was redefined[12]: "A product with active ingredients to affect the structure or function of the body by absorbing, reflecting, or scattering the harmful, burning rays of the sun, thereby altering the normal physiological response to solar radiation". These ingredients also help to prevent diseases such as sunburn and may reduce the chance of premature skin aging, skin cancer, and other harmful effects due to the sun when used in conjunction with limiting sun exposure and wearing protective clothing. Sunscreen ingredients may also be used in some products for nontherapeutic, nonphysiologic uses (e.g., as a color additive or to protect the color of the product). Further, for sunscreen products that retain SPF after 40 minutes of activity in the water, sweating, or perspiring, the term *water resistant* is used. For products that retain SPF activity after 80 minutes, the term *very water resistant* is allowed. Further, the following phases may be used for sunscreen products: *reapply as needed or after towel drying, swimming, or sweating* (or *perspiring*).

SUBSTANTIVITY

Substantivity is a measure of the sunscreen formulation's effectiveness. The substantivity of a sunscreen formulation is its ability to be adsorbed by, or adhere to, the skin while swimming

Table 41-3 Examples of Commercially Available Sunscreen Products

Name (Active Ingredients)	Formulation	SPF
Anthelios SX (avobenzone, ecamsule, octocrylene)	Cream	15
Banana Boat Baby Sunblock (octinoxate, octisalate, homosalate, titanium dioxide)	Lotion	50
Banana Boat Sport Sun Gear Sunblock (avobenzone, homosalate, octocrylene, oxybenzone, octisalate)	Lotion	50
Banana Boat Quik Blok Kids (octinoxate, homosalate, octisalate, oxybenzone, avobenzone)	Lotion	25+
Banana Boat Sport Sunblock (octinoxate, octisalate, oxybenzone, octocrylene)	Lotion	50
Blistex Ultra Protection (homosalate, meradimate, octinoxate, octisalate, oxybenzone)	Lip balm	30
Blue Lizard Australian Suncream (octinoxate, octocrylene, oxybenzone, zinc oxide)	Lotion	30+
Bullfrog Superblock (octocrylene, octinoxate, oxybenzone)	Lotion	45
Bullfrog For Kids (octocrylene, octinoxate, oxybenzone, octisalate, titanium dioxide, meradimate)	Gel	36
Bullfrog Extreme Sport (octocrylene, octinoxate, octisalate, oxybenzone)	Lotion	30
Bullfrog Sunblock (octinoxate, oxybenzone, octisalate, octocrylene)	Gel	36
ChapStick (padimate O)	Lip balm	15
ChapStick Ultra (octocrylene, octinoxate, oxybenzone, octisalate)	Lip balm	30
ChapStick Sunblock (oxybenzone, padimate O)	Lip balm, or ointment	15
Coppertone BUG & SUN for Adults (with DEET; octocrylene, octinoxate, oxybenzone)	Lotion	30
Coppertone KIDS Quick Cover Sunblock (avobenzone, octocrylene, octisalate, oxybenzone, homosalate)	Lotion/Spray	50
Coppertone Sport (octinoxate, oxybenzone, octisalate)	Lotion	15/30/50
Coppertone Ultra Sheer Faces (avobenzone, homosalate, octisalate, octocrylene, oxybenzone)	Lotion	30
DuraScreen (octinoxate, octisalate, oxybenzone, ensulizole, titanium dioxide)	Lotion/Stick	15, 30
Eau Thermale Avene (titanium dioxide, zinc oxide)	Cream	25, 50
Hawaiian Tropic Ozone (octocrylene, oxybenzone, avobenzone)	Lotion	70
Hawaiian Tropic Kids (avobenzone, octocrylene, oxybenzone)	Lotion	60+
Hawaiian Tropic 45 Plus Sunblock (octinoxate, octisalate, titanium dioxide)	Lotion	45
Neutrogena MoistureShine Lip Soother (octinoxate, oxybenzone)	Lip balm	20
Neutrogena Healthy Defense Oil-Free Sunblock (avobenzone, homosalate, octinoxate, octisalate)	Lotion/Spray/ Stick	30, 45
Neutrogena Age Shield Sunblock (avobenzone, homosalate, octocrylene, octisalate, oxybenzone)	Lotion	30, 45
Neutrogena Ultra Sheer Dry-Touch Sunblock (octinoxate, octocrylene, homosalate, octisalate, oxybenzone, avobenzone)	Lotion	30, 45 55, 70
Off! Skintastic with Sunscreen (with DEET; octinoxate, octocrylene, oxybenzone)	Lotion	30

SPF, sun protective factor.

or perspiring. In the past, labeling of a product as "waterproof" or "water-resistant" indicated that the SPF of the product was maintained after 80 minutes of moderate activity or 40 minutes while swimming, respectively. Because testing is performed indoors under close to ideal conditions (e.g., lower humidity), the effects of the actual environment where it is used and the evaporation of the vehicle may reduce considerably the overall effectiveness of the sunscreen. The substantivity of a product largely depends on the vehicle, as well as the active ingredient (Table 41-3).[57] The affinity of a sunscreen to the keratinaceous layer of the stratum corneum is directly related to the keratin or vehicle partition coefficient. The saturation of the active agent in keratin depends on the drug's lipophilicity, whereas its substantivity is independent of its lipophilicity. Sunscreen compounds with a high solubility in the product's vehicle penetrate the skin most easily. Classically, vehicles such as water-in-oil emulsions or ointments tend to have a higher degree of substantivity. Some of the newer products have improved substantivity with the addition of a polymer, such as polyacrylamide, to the formulation.

SUNBURN PREVENTIVE AND SUNTANNING AGENTS

Sunburn preventive agents are those active ingredients that absorb >95% of UVB radiation, and have the potential to prevent sunburn. Suntanning agents are those with active ingredients that absorb 85% to 95% of UVB radiation, thereby allowing suntanning without significant sunburn in the average individual. Chemical sunscreens include both of the aforementioned designations. Opaque sunblocks, or physical sunscreens, are those active ingredients that reflect or scatter all UVA, UVB, and visible light, thereby preventing or minimizing sunburn and suntanning.[58] Limiting UV exposure by starting sunscreen use during childhood can reduce the lifetime risk of nonmelanoma skin cancers by up to 78%[59]; however, some investigators have suggested that sunscreen use, through increased UV exposure, may actually cause melanoma, perhaps because its use allows for a longer exposure to the sun.[60,61] Also, sunscreen use appears to be associated with the occurrence of nevi (pigmented "moles"), which is a strong predictor of melanoma development[25,62]; however, epidemiologic analyses have refuted this proposed association.[63,64]

Of note, *sunless tanner*, a commercial term, denotes a product that provides a tanned appearance without exposure to the sun or other sources of UVR. One commonly used ingredient in these products is dihydroxyacetone (DHA), a color additive that darkens the skin to orange-brown by reacting with amino acids in the stratum corneum. The term *bronzer* is used to describe a variety of products intended to achieve a temporary tanned appearance. For example, among the products that are marketed as bronzers are tinted moisturizers and brush-on powders. These produce a temporary effect, similar to other types of makeup, and wash off over time. Some products are marketed with other ingredients in addition to DHA to provide a tanned appearance. Neither sunless tanners nor bronzers provide any protective activity to UV exposure by themselves.[65] Effective May 22, 2000, the FDA required that all suntanning preparations that do not contain sunscreen ingredients are required to carry the following warning statement on the label: "Warning—This product does not contain a sunscreen and does not protect against sunburn. Repeated exposure of unprotected skin while tanning may increase the risk of skin aging, skin cancer, and other harmful effects to the skin even if you do not burn."

Tanning pills are promoted for tinting the skin by ingesting massive doses of color additives, usually canthaxanthin. At large doses, canthaxanthin is deposited in various organs, including skin, imparting an orange-bronze color. This color varies from individual to individual. This colorization is not the result of an increase in the skin's supply of melanin. Although canthaxanthin is approved by FDA for use as a color additive in foods, where it is used in small amounts, its use in these so-called tanning pills is not approved. Reported adverse events include drug-induced retinopathy, nausea, gastrointestinal cramping, diarrhea, pruritus, and urticaria. None of the above noted unapproved agents should be recommended for use.

Chemical Sunscreens

Chemical sunscreens are compounds capable of absorbing UVR, thereby protecting the skin structures from the adverse effects of the selective wavelengths absorbed.[36] After application to the skin, these aromatic compounds convert the high UVR energy into harmless longer-wave radiation, which may or may not be perceived as warmth.[36] Chemical sunscreens usually are nonopaque because they do not absorb the wavelengths of visible light.

MOLAR ABSORPTIVITY, ABSORBANCE SPECTRUM, AND PHOTOSTABILITY

The molar absorptivity and absorption spectrum determines the effectiveness of an individual chemical sunscreen agent, mostly by its chemical structure. *Molar absorptivity* is a measure of the amount of UVR absorbed by a particular sunscreen, and it depends on the concentration of the sunscreen in the product and the amount applied to the skin. Sunscreens with an absorbance spectrum in the UVB range with a maximal absorption between 310 and 320 nm, are the most effective at preventing a sunburn.[50] Chemical sunscreens with absorption spectra in the UVB range are para-aminobenzoic acid (PABA) and its esters, cinnamates, and the salicylates. Sunscreens with absorption spectra that extend into the UVA range are the anthranilates (e.g., meradimate), dibenzoylmethanes (e.g., azobenzene), and benzophenones (e.g., oxybenzone). *Photostability* means the ability to stabilize under sunlight. The process of photostability is a key factor in sunscreen protection efficacy. High photostability means the sunscreen will maintain a higher UVA protective barrier longer, and not degrade as quickly as other UVA filters when exposed to the sun.

Seventeen chemical ingredients that act as sunscreens are currently approved in the United States (with their FDA-allowable maximal concentration in sunscreen products listed in parentheses):

- P-aminobenzoic acid (PABA; up to 15%)
- Avobenzone (3%)
- Cinoxate (3%)
- Dioxybenzone (3%)
- Ecamsule (3%)
- Ensulizole (4%)
- Homosalate (15%)
- Meradimate (5%)
- Octocrylene (10%)
- Octinoxate (7.5%)
- Octisalate (5%)
- Oxybenzone (6%)
- Padimate O (8%)
- Sulisobenzone (10%)
- Titanium dioxide (25%)
- Trolamine salicylate (12%)
- Zinc oxide (25%)

PARA-AMINOBENZOIC ACID (PABA) AND ESTERS

Commonly used in the past, PABA absorbs UVR in the UVB range from 260 to 313 nm, with maximal absorbance around 290 nm; its molar absorptivity is considered to be high.[50] PABA readily penetrates and binds to the stratum corneum and, after several days of application, may remain in the skin and provide protection even after swimming, perspiration, and bathing.[50] It is commonly formulated as an alcoholic mixture, which can cause stinging, dryness, or tightness, particularly when applied to the face. Its major disadvantage is the potential to cause contact or photocontact dermatitis. Responsible for more sensitivity reactions than any other sunscreen,[53] PABA can also cause cross-sensitivity reactions with benzocaine, thiazides, sulfonamides, paraphenylenediamine (a common ingredient in hair dyes), and other PABA derivatives. It can cause discoloration of clothes as well. The use of PABA in commercial sunscreens has decreased to the point where many of the newer sunscreens are promoted as being PABA-free.

The PABA esters include octyldimethyl PABA (Padimate O) and glyceryl PABA. These esters are incorporated easily into formulations, demonstrate good substantivity, and do not discolor clothing. Their absorption spectra are similar to that of PABA (Table 41-2). With a maximal absorbance of 311 nm, Padimate O has the lowest likelihood of any PABA ester to cause cross-sensitivity reactions or contact and photocontact dermatitis.[66] Glyceryl PABA can cause contact dermatitis and cross-sensitivities, both of which may be caused by benzocaine impurities in the commercial products.[67]

CINNAMATES

Cinnamates have UVB-absorbing qualities. Octinoxate (octyl methoxycinnamate, Parsol MCX), which has high molar absorptivity and a maximal absorbance of 305 nm, is the most commonly used cinnamate.[68] Cinnamates are related chemically to balsam of Peru, balsam of Tolu, coca leaves, cinnamic acid, cinnamic aldehyde, cinnamic oil, ingredients that are used in perfumes, topical medications, cosmetics, and flavorings.[67] These agents do not bind well to the stratum corneum, leading to poor substantivity. Cinnamate-based sunscreens tend to be comedogenic because the vehicle may contain other occlusive ingredients that are added to improve the substantivity. Cinnamates, which absorb only UVB radiation, are often used in combination with benzophenones, appear to be nonstaining, and rarely cause contact dermatitis.[68]

BENZOPHENONES

Benzophenones, such as oxybenzone and dioxybenzone, are UVB-absorbing sunscreens that have absorbance spectra extending into the UVA range.[69] Benzophenones are also found in shampoos, soaps, hair sprays and dyes, paints, varnishes, and lacquers. The maximal absorbance for each is about 290 nm, but both are limited because of poor substantivity and sensitization.[69] Photocontact dermatitis with oxybenzone and contact dermatitis with dioxybenzone occur commonly, with the latter usually occurring as a contact urticaria.

SALICYLATES

Salicylates are weak UVB absorbers often found in PABA-free products. Topical salicylates are considered among the safest sunscreens, even though they are used in high concentrations.[70] Salicylates have low molar absorptivities, are incorporated easily into formulations, and are used to boost the SPF of combination products. Sensitization to the salicylates is rare[70]; however, it has been reported with the use of octyl salicylate.[71]

ANTHRANILATES

Anthranilates, such as meradimate (menthylanthranilate), are weak UVB-absorbing sunscreens with an absorbance spectrum extending into the UVA range. As with the salicylates, they have low molar absorptivity, with a maximal absorbance of approximately 336 nm.[50] Meradimate has a low risk of sensitization and a desirable absorbance spectrum, especially when it is used in combination with other sunscreens to give broad-spectrum protection.[70]

DIBENZOYLMETHANES

As a prototype of the dibenzoylmethanes class, avobenzone (butyl methoxydibenzoylmethane, Parsol 1789) has high molar absorptivity and absorption spectra exclusively in the UVA range, with maximal absorbance at approximately 360 nm.[72] It is commonly formulated with UVB sunscreens to broaden UVR coverage. Even though protection is provided throughout the UVA and UVB ranges in these combination products, it is unknown whether sufficient protection is available for patients who are highly UVA sensitive. Avobenzone loses approximately 35% of its absorbance capacity about 15 minutes after UVR exposure, because of the photoinstability of the compound.[2] When UVA and UVB inorganic protective filters were first introduced using cosmetically acceptable concentrations, they provided minimal protection against UVA rays. Avobenzone was approved for use in 1992; however, it was discovered that when used by itself, avobenzone degrades when exposed to the sun, thereby reducing its UVA protection efficacy. One molecule of avobenzone can absorb UVA radiation only once, making it inactive from that time forward as opposed to zinc oxide or titanium dioxide that can reflect UVA radiation over and over again with minimal decay. All of the avobenzone applied to the skin is virtually rendered inactive after 5 hours of UVA exposure.

In 2006, the FDA approved the combination of 2% ecamsule/2% avobenzone/10% octocrylene cream (*Anthelios SX*, L'Oreal USA) for the prevention of sunburn and protection from UVA and UVB rays. This OTC product is only available in the United States as a moisturizing cream with a SPF rating of 15, although it is available in Europe up to SPF 50. The actions of the individual components of this combination are as follows: (*a*) octocrylene, to protect against UVB rays, (*b*) avobenzone protects against long UVA rays and is stabilized by octocrylene, and (*c*) ecamsule (Mexoryl), a camphor derivative, protects against short UVA rays. This combination provides continuous protection across most of the UV spectrum (290–400 nm range), with ecamsule providing protection within the short UVA range (320–340 nm), filling the gap between octocrylene and avobenzone capabilities (210–290 nm, and 340–400 nm, respectively). The photostability of the ecamsule and octocrylene–avobenzone combination provides residual protection at 1 and 5 hours (1 hour, 100% UVB protection and 97% UVA protection; 5 hours, 90% UVB protection and 80% UVA protection, respectively). Adverse events associated with its use are infrequent and include acne, dermatitis, dry skin, eczema, erythema, pruritus, skin discomfort, and sunburn.

There are two additional formulations of ecamsule. Mexoryl SX is a water-soluble form suitable for daytime sunscreens, including sunscreen-containing moisturizers and facial foundations. Mexoryl XL, an oil-soluble formulation, is suitable for water-resistant sunscreen formulations, including those worn on the beach and during vigorous physical exercise.

The other extended spectrum agent on the market in the United States at present is Helioplex, a combination of avobenzone, oxybenzone, and a photostabilizing solvent, Hallbrite TQ. Neutrogena uses it in products such as UltraSheer Dry-Touch Sunblock SPF 30/45/55/70, Age Shield Sunblock SPF 30/45, Fresh Cooling Body Mist Sunblock SPF 30/45, and Moisture Rich Sunless Tanner SPF 20.

ANTIOXIDANTS

Antioxidants have received increased attention for use as photoprotective agents, particularly because of the observation that vitamin C levels in the skin can be severely depleted after UVR exposure.[73] Vitamins C and E, either taken orally or applied topically (incorporated into a commercially available sunscreen product), may provide additive protection against both UVA- and UVB-induced photodamage.[73,74] Topically applied antioxidants do not have adequate diffusion into the epidermal layer, however, and are susceptible to chemical instability.[75]

PHYSICAL SUNSCREENS

Physical sunscreens are opaque formulations made of particulate insoluble compounds, incorporated into a vehicle. The skin is shielded from sunlight by reflection and scattering of both UV and visible radiation; both size of the particles and thickness of the film determine the degree of protection.[76] The most effective and commonly used physical sunscreens are titanium dioxide and zinc oxide, which reflect and scatter UVR as well as reflect and scatter.[76,77] Other physical sunscreens include magnesium oxide, red veterinarian petrolatum, iron oxides, kaolin, ichthammol, and talc.

These compounds are used in conjunction with chemical sunscreens to formulate products of higher SPF and as single-ingredient sunblocks. When used alone, they are usually placed in an ointment base designed specifically for vulnerable parts of the body, such as the nose, cheeks, lips, ears, and shoulders.[58]

Physical sunscreens are important in individuals who are unusually sensitive to UVA and visible light, such as those with vitiligo, a skin condition with amelanotic lesions (white patches) surrounded by areas of normally pigmented skin. Appropriately colored formulations can be used to camouflage and protect these vulnerable amelanotic lesions.[58] Physical sunscreen agents are preferred for persons who need absolute UVR and visible light protection (e.g., young children; persons with skin types I through IV who receive constant exposure; and persons with drug photosensitivity reactions, xeroderma pigmentosa, lupus erythematosis, and other photosensitive skin reactions).[58]

Physical sunscreens are not widely accepted because they are visible to others, messy, and occlusive when applied to the skin. They have a higher substantivity, but may melt in the heat of the sun, limiting their protection to a few hours. Physical sunscreen products tend to be so occlusive that they may cause or worsen acne or obstruct sweat glands.[58] Neutrogena Sensitive Skin Sunblock Lotion SPF 30 (titanium dioxide 9.1%) is an example of a physical sunscreen with cosmetically appealing properties (e.g., ease of application).

Product Selection

9. R.J. and her husband J.J. are parents of two children: P.J., a 6-month-old girl, and L.J., an 18-month-old boy. They are spending a week in August vacationing on the Outer Banks of North Carolina, with plans for time at the beach, bicycling, and sailing. R.J. is 25 years of age, has type V skin, brown hair and brown eyes, and has no history of photosensitivity reactions or medication allergies. She has a history of contact dermatitis on her scalp and around her hairline on several occasions after dying her hair and using certain shampoos. J.J. is 27 years of age and has skin type II with blonde hair and blue eyes. As a teenager, he suffered from frequent sinus infections and often was treated with trimethoprim-sulfamethoxazole (TMP-SMX [Septra/Bactrim]) because of an allergy to penicillin. He remembers developing a severe sunburn after minimal exposure to the sun while taking the sulfa-containing antibiotic. He recently has been started on hydrochlorothiazide (HCTZ), 12.5 mg PO QD, for hypertension. What considerations are important in recommending sunscreens for R.J. and J.J.? Recommend an appropriate sunscreen for each member of the family with appropriate directions for application while on vacation.

CROSS-SENSITIVITY

The first consideration for recommending an appropriate sunscreen for R.J. and J.J. is their skin type. R.J. has skin type V, suggesting that a sunscreen with an SPF of at least 8 would provide adequate protection for her (Table 41-1). J.J. has skin type II, suggesting that a sunscreen with an SPF of 30 would be required to provide adequate protection for him. Furthermore, the history of contact dermatitis and photosensitivity reaction exhibited by R.J. and J.J., respectively, is important when recommending use of a sunscreen.[78] The contact dermatitis that R.J. experienced from hair dyes and shampoos may have been caused by para-phenylenediamine, an ingredient of hair dyes,[65] or a benzophenone, which sometimes is included in products such as hair dyes and shampoos.[69] Because a cross-reactivity between para-phenylenediamine and PABA or its derivatives is possible, a sunscreen for R.J. that does not contain PABA or a benzophenone should be recommended. A wide-spectrum PABA-free sunscreen that does not contain a benzophenone may be ideal for R.J. because cinnamates and anthranilates rarely cause contact dermatoses.

Because both contain sulfa moieties, the photosensitivity reaction that J.J. experienced while taking TMP-SMX may indicate that he might be susceptible to a cross-sensitivity reaction with PABA or its derivatives. This reaction to TMP-SMX also indicates that J.J. may be susceptible to a photosensitivity reaction with HCTZ. If a photosensitivity reaction is likely, it is advisable to recommend an SPF of 30. Because drug-induced photosensitivity reactions are caused by UVA, a PABA-free, broad-spectrum sunscreen that absorbs UVA as well as UVB would be necessary to provide J.J. with adequate protection. Broad-spectrum chemical sunscreens commonly contain a benzophenone and a cinnamate. A broad-spectrum sunscreen containing both of these chemical classes (e.g., Shade Sunblock Lotion, with octyl methoxycinnamate, oxybenzone, homosalate, and octyl salicylate; [Table 41-3]) would be an acceptable broad-spectrum product. Alternatively, because Padimate O is the least likely of the PABA ester derivatives to cause photocontact dermatitis,[65] a broad-spectrum combination product that contains Padimate O could be recommended for J.J. If the photosensitivity reaction is caused by visible light, it would also be necessary to recommend a physical sunscreen to block all sunlight or complete avoidance of the sun.[54] With all of these issues considered, it may be preferable to recommend an alternative antihypertensive medication for J.J. that would not place him at risk for a photosensitivity reaction.

APPLICATION

Because R.J. and J.J. are planning to be active on the beach, sunscreens that are water-resistant or waterproof are recommended (Table 41-3). Before complete application of the sunscreen to the body, because of the risk of cross-sensitivity reactions, patients can perform a patch test by applying small quantity of the sunscreen to the inner aspect of the forearm and covering with a small bandage overnight. Most persons apply 20% to 60% of the required amount of sunscreen needed to achieve the SPF of their product.[52,56] Because of this, a method has been developed to determine an approximate volume of sunscreen product needed for adequate protection.[79] One study of sunscreen application techniques at the beach demonstrated inadequate application at all body sites.[80] The worst protected areas were the ears and top of the feet, and the back was poorly protected if sunscreen was self-applied.

Dosing for sunscreen can be calculated using the formula for body surface area and subsequently subtracting the area covered by clothing that provides effective UV protection. The dose used in FDA sunscreen testing is 2 mg/cm^2. Considering only the face, this translates to about one fourth to one-third of a teaspoon for the average adult face. For protection in the beach environment, for example, an average-size adult should apply and rub in 2 to 2.5 ounces evenly to all exposed skin surfaces at least 30 to 45 minutes before exposure.[79] Patients should be reminded to apply sunscreen on those often forgotten areas, such as the hands, cheeks, neck, ears, and dorsum of the feet. It is best to reapply the sunscreen every 1 to 2 hours or after sweating, swimming, or toweling off.

10. How long might J.J. expect to be protected with the sunscreen properly applied? Do products with an SPF >15 provide any additional benefit?

If J.J. (skin type II) normally burns after 30 minutes of exposure to the sun, a sunscreen with an SPF of 15 to 30 may provide up to 7.5 hours (0.5 hours 15 [SPF 15]) of photoprotection from UVB. However, a high SPF product may provide only partial protection against UVA, with little or no protection from infrared radiation.[50] Because of this, sun exposure should be limited to 90 to 120 minutes for each outing after appropriate sunscreen application. Further, environmental factors, such as elevated atmospheric humidity, and inadequate application techniques may reduce photoprotection by as much as half.

Sunscreen formulations with SPF as high as 50 can be made using combinations of chemical and physical sunscreen agents (e.g., Hawaiian Tropic Baby Faces Sunblock Lotion, with octinoxate, octocrylene, oxybenzone, octisalate, and titanium dioxide; [Table 41-3]).[3] Individuals who are extremely sensitive to the sun may benefit from formulations with higher SPF, but the average fair-skinned person gains adequate protection for sunbathing or for average daily exposure from a product with an SPF of 30.[52]

Photoprotection for Children

11. What photoprotective measures should be provided for P.J. and L.J.? What nonsunscreen protection is appropriate for use with children?

AGE-RELATED RECOMMENDATIONS AND OTHER PROTECTIVE BEHAVIOR

Sun protection during childhood is very important, considering that most of a person's lifetime of sun exposure occurs in childhood and that the harmful effects of UVR are cumulative.[62] The FDA has recommended that sunscreen agents not be used for children younger than 6 months of age because of the possible chemical absorption through the skin and lowered ability of children of this age to metabolize the absorbed drug.[81] P.J. needs to be kept out of direct sunlight and, when outside, must be protected with proper clothing and shading.[82–85] The FDA has recommended that children <2 years of age be treated with an SPF >4 because of inadequate UVR protection with lower SPF products for most individuals.[81]

L.J. should be protected with a PABA-free sunscreen with an SPF of at least 15. Regular use of a sunscreen with an SPF of at least 15 for the first 18 years of life can reduce the lifetime incidence of nonmelanoma skin cancers by about three-fourths.[85] If L.J. is in the sun during 6 hours of maximal exposure (i.e., 10 AM–4 PM), or otherwise for an extended period, he should wear protective clothing, covering as much of his body as possible.[84] Tightly woven clothing, long sleeves, and pants protect the skin from almost all UVR, whereas loosely woven clothing or wet T-shirts can allow up to 30% of UVR to pass through to the skin. Although not complete, water is thought to reduce UVR scattering, thus decreasing its transmission. An average-weight cotton T-shirt provides only an SPF of 7 or 8.[84] The transmission of UVR through a fabric is measured using a spectrophotometer or spectroradiometer. The ultraviolet protection factor (UPF), rather than SPF, has been recommended as a measure of the sun-protective properties of fabrics.[86,87] It is calculated using a formula based on UV transmission through the fabric and the erythema response for human skin. For example, if a fabric has a UPF of 20, then only one-twentieth of the UVR at the surface of the fabric actually passes through it. Table 41-4 compares the UPF with the amount of effective UVR transmitted and absorbed.

Table 41-4 Relative Ultraviolet Protection Factor (UPF) by Ultraviolet Ray (UVR) Transmission and Absorption

UVR Transmitted (%)	UVR Absorbed(%)	UPF	Protection Category
10	90.0	10	Moderate protection
5	95.0	20	High protection
3.3	96.7	30	Very high protection
2.5	97.5	40	Extremely high protection
<2.0	>98.0	50	Maximal protection

No woven fabric provides complete coverage because the holes between the threads permit UVR transmission. A baseball cap shields little more than the upper central forehead. Broad-rimmed hats can protect the ears, neck, nose, and cheeks, but may provide inadequate protection against SCC of the head or neck.[88] The use of an ultraviolet-absorbing ingredient for fabric softeners (e.g., Tinosorb-FD, Ciba) are promoted to reduce transmission of excessive UVA and UVB radiation through fabrics to the skin, through absorption of UV radiation without impairing whiteness. This chemical absorbance process has a high affinity for cotton fibers at various washing temperatures. Available as a laundry additive (e.g., detergent or fabric softener), it works by binding to laundered fibers, and through accumulation, it increases the UV protection through repeated wash and rinse cycles.[89,90]

PRODUCT SELECTION

Two types of sunscreens are appropriate for use in children. A lotion is preferred for total body application versus an alcoholic lotion or gel because alcoholic preparations can cause stinging, burning, and irritation of the skin and eyes. Physical sunscreens (e.g., zinc oxide) are available in bright colors and are recommended for selected body areas, such as the nose, cheeks, and shoulders. PABA and its derivatives are considered potentially harmful to a child's tender skin. For adolescents with acne vulgaris, the use of an oil-free, noncomedogenic sunscreen formulation (e.g., Neutrogena Healthy Defense Oil-Free Sunblock) and a lip balm that contains a sunscreen of at least SPF 15 (e.g., ChapStick or Blistex Regular (SPF 15), Blistex Ultra (SPF 30) or ChapStick Ultra (SPF 30) would be appropriate.

Photoeffects on the Eye

12. Why should R.J. and J.J. be concerned about the effect of prolonged sunlight on their eyes? Recommend appropriate protective eyewear for them while they are on vacation.

CATARACT FORMATION

Age-related opacification of the ocular lens, or senescent cataracts, has been attributed to a lifetime of exposure to sunlight. The incidence of cataracts increases steadily after age 50, reaching nearly 50% in individuals over the age of 75.[30] UVB is absorbed by the cornea and lens, which slowly results in protein oxidation and precipitation within the lens. UVA penetrates the ocular lens and can cause cumulative damage to deeper structures of the eye. Decreased transmittance and increased scattering of light by the opacified lens eventually result in blurred vision, rings or halos around lights, changes in color perception, and blindness.[91] In advanced cases, the only treatment is surgical removal of the cataract.

High exposure of the eye to UVR (which can range from a few seconds of exposure to arc welding, a few minutes of exposure to a UVC-emitting germicidal lamp, commercial tanning, or UVR reflection by snow or sand) can cause conjunctivitis or photokeratitis, a painful inflammation of the cornea. Photokeratitis usually begins 30 minutes to 24 hours after the exposure and time to onset depends on the intensity of the exposure.[92] Conjunctivitis commonly accompanies photokeratitis and is characterized by the sensation of a foreign body or grit in the eyes. Varying degrees of photophobia, lacrimation, and blepharospasm also may accompany photokeratitis.[92] Because the corneal epithelium has a great regenerative capacity, photokeratitis tends to be transient, with regression in 24 to 48 hours. Treatment consists of cool, wet compresses and mild anti-inflammatory analgesics, such as ibuprofen, aspirin, or naproxen sodium.

PROTECTIVE EYEWEAR

R.J. and J.J. should wear sunglasses when outdoors to decrease their lifelong exposure to solar radiation and while at the beach to prevent high exposure of UVR and possible photokeratitis or conjunctivitis. Many manufacturers of sunglasses label their products according to three categories: cosmetic, general purpose, and special purpose. Cosmetic sunglasses block at least 70% of UVB, at least 20% of UVA, and <60% of visible light and are appropriate for casual wear when high exposure to UVR is unlikely. General-purpose sunglasses block at least 95% of UVB, at least 60% of UVA, 60% to 92% of visible light, and are appropriate for most activities in sunny environments.[93] Special-purpose sunglasses block at least 99% of UVB, at least 60% of UVA, and at least 97% of visible light and are appropriate for very bright environments, such as ski slopes or tropical beaches.[93] Special- or general-purpose sunglasses are appropriate recommendations for R.J. and J.J. to wear while on vacation.

TREATMENT OF SUNBURN

13. G.B., a 31-year-old man with skin type IV, returned a few hours ago from an afternoon of activity in the sun. His shoulders, back, neck, and arms are bright red and are beginning to feel hot, stretched, and painful. G.B. has been otherwise healthy, has no significant medical history, and has no known allergies to medications. What treatment recommendations would you give G.B. for his sunburn?

Sunburn is a self-limiting condition, and treatment is usually symptomatic. Suggested treatments that G.B. can try for his first-degree burn are oral (e.g., ibuprofen, aspirin) or topical (e.g., camphor, menthol) analgesics, topical anti-inflammatory agents (e.g., hydrocortisone cream or aloe vera gel), cooling compresses (tap water, saline, or aluminum acetate solution [Burow's solution]) applied to the skin, or cool protectant baths (e.g., colloidal oatmeal). Nonsteroidal anti-inflammatory drugs (NSAID), such as aspirin or ibuprofen, may be preferred over acetaminophen because of blockade of the inflammatory prostaglandin-mediated sunburn process.[94] Topical NSAID use, commonly seen as a cream formulation of indomethacin, possesses anti-inflammatory activity, especially if applied before UVR exposure, which may prove impractical for many individuals.

Treatment beyond self-management is unnecessary unless the sunburn is extensive with constitutional symptoms (i.e., severe first- or second-degree burns), involves second-degree burns on the eyes or genitalia, or becomes infected. In such cases, referral of the patient to his/her continuity provider is indicated as a short course (i.e., up to 3 days) of an oral corticosteroid may need to be given (e.g., 1 mg/kg of prednisone or equivalent, given once daily).

Topical anesthetics, such as benzocaine or lidocaine, provide only transient analgesia for up to 15 to 45 minutes. These agents should not be used in large quantities or applied more than three or four times a day. In addition, they should not be used on raw, blistered, or abraded skin. Benzocaine has minimal systemic toxicities, but is associated with contact sensitization.[95] In contrast, lidocaine is associated with a low incidence of contact sensitization, but has the potential to cause significant systemic toxicity (e.g., cardiovascular) if adequate serum drug concentrations are reached as a result of cutaneous absorption.[96]

If G.B. desires to try one of these agents, application or administration is recommended when the pain is particularly bothersome, such as at bedtime. Topical 1% hydrocortisone, when applied to mild to moderate sunburn, may provide some additional benefit. If G.B. experiences fever, chills, nausea, vomiting, and prostration, he should be referred to his health care provider. These symptoms generally respond to oral prednisone 20 mg/day for 3 days. Antihistamines may help control pruritus associated with sunburn, as well as aid with sleep, if taken at bedtime.

MINOR BURNS

Burn injuries rank second only to motor vehicle accidents as the leading cause of death in children between 1 and 4 years of age and rank third after motor vehicle accidents and drowning as the leading cause of injury and death in persons between 0 and 19 years of age.[97] Of the 2 million Americans treated for burns yearly, >80,000 require hospitalization; burns cause an overall yearly mortality of approximately 6,500.[98,99] Complications such as fluid and electrolyte imbalances, metabolic derangements, respiratory failure, sepsis, scarring, and functional impairment are the primary causes of hospitalization for these cases. Most burns, however, are minor and can be managed in an ambulatory environment, provided the burned patient is evaluated carefully, the severity of the burn is assessed accurately, and proper and continuous follow-up care is ensured. Most partial thickness burns in this country are managed by practitioners in hospital and community settings who do not treat burns on a regular basis.[100]

Epidemiology

Burn injuries range from relatively minor, superficial injuries to severe, extensive skin loss resulting from contact with hot solids and liquids, steam, chemical agents, electricity, or other physical agents, such as UVR or infrared radiation. House fires, commonly caused by cigarettes or malfunctioning heating or electrical equipment, are responsible for 84% of fire- and burn-related deaths.[97] The peak incidence of burn injuries occurs in up to 10% of preschool-aged children, who are often scalded by or immersed into hot liquids, frequently as a result of child abuse and neglect that crosses all socioeconomic classes.[98,101–103] School-aged children and adolescents often are injured when experimenting with matches or gasoline or in association with cars, motorcycles, fireworks, or flammables.[97] Teenagers and adults between 17 and 30 years of age most commonly are involved in accidents with flammable liquids, but the mortality associated with clothing ignition continues to decrease as a result of the use of flame-retardant forms of fabric in clothing. Categories of individuals who have a higher reported incidence of burn injuries are the very young, elderly, males, blacks, economically disadvantaged, individuals who have ingested alcohol, handicapped children, and children with previous history of burn.[99]

With the development of multidisciplinary burn centers and a better understanding of the pathophysiology of the burn wound, survival of patients with second- and third-degree burns has improved by five to six times over the last three decades.[104] An increased national focus on burn treatment and prevention, societal changes such as an overall decrease in tobacco use, decreased alcohol abuse, changes in home cooking practices, and reduced industrial employment have contributed to the lower national burn incidence.[99] The techniques of improved burn wound management that have contributed to this decline include topical antimicrobial therapy, early excision or enzymatic débridement of devitalized tissue, and skin grafting or substitutes.[105–107]

Zones of Injury

The skin functions as a protective barrier of the underlying organ systems from trauma, temperature variations, harmful penetrations, moisture, humidity, radiation, and invasion by microorganisms (see Fig. 38-1 in Chapter 38.) It also is involved with carbohydrate, protein, fat, and vitamin D metabolism; it produces secretions that lubricate the skin, is involved with the immune response, and provides the body with the sense of touch.

Burn wounds caused by thermal injury can be described by varying zones of injury.[106,107] The most peripheral area of injury is the *zone of hyperemia.* The tissue in this area is characterized by inflammatory changes with minimal tissue damage. The *zone of stasis* is the next area of injury, extending inward from the zone of hyperemia. This area involves ischemic, damaged tissue, with blood vessels only partially thrombosed. The damaged endothelial linings of blood vessels within this zone of injury may trigger further thrombosis, resulting in further ischemia, cell death, and deepening of the burn wound. This process of further injury can occur 24 to 48 hours after the initial injury. Drying of the burn wound or infection can cause deepening of the burn wound by preventing re-establishment of circulation to injured tissue. The central-most area, or the *zone of coagulation,* is characterized by thrombotic vessels and necrotic tissue. This area absorbs the most thermal energy, resulting in the greatest tissue damage. Minor burns may involve only the most peripheral zones of injury, whereas severe burns encompass all three zones of injury.

Extent of Injury

RULE OF NINES

Burn severity is proportional to the percent of body surface area (BSA) involvement and wound depth. The percent of BSA for adults can be estimated by using the "rule of nines," in which each arm constitutes 9% of the BSA, the head 9%, each leg 18%, the front and back of the torso 18% each, and the genitalia 1%. For children <10 years of age, the percent BSA must be adjusted because their bodies have different proportions. The Lund and Browder chart has been used for this purpose.[108] At birth, the infant's head constitutes about 19% of the BSA. For each additional year of age, the head decreases by about 1% and the BSA of the legs increases by about 1% of the patient's total body surface area (TBSA), so a quick estimation of the percent BSA of a burn can be made.[101]

CLASSIFICATION OF WOUNDS

Burn wounds also are classified according to the depth of tissue damage. Determining the depth of the burn wound can be difficult during the first 24 to 48 hours because of the presence of edema and continued tissue ischemia and infection, both of which can cause deepening of the wound. In addition, the depth of destruction can vary within the same burn, and skin surface characteristics may not match underlying tissue damage, making assessment of the burn wound difficult.[106]

First-Degree Burns

First-degree burns result from injury to the superficial cells of the epidermis. A common example is a mild sunburn. The burned skin does not form blisters, but it does become erythematous and mildly painful. This partial-thickness burn heals within 3 to 4 days without scarring.

Second-Degree Burns

Second-degree burns may be superficial or deep, depending on the depth of dermal involvement. Superficial second-degree burns involve the epidermis and the upper layer of the dermis. The burn surface often is erythematous, blistered, weeping, painful, and very sensitive to stimuli. The erythema blanches with pressure, and the hair follicles, sweat, and sebaceous glands are spared. Superficial second-degree burns heal spontaneously within 3 weeks with little, if any, scarring. Deep second-degree burns involve the deeper elements of the dermis and may be difficult to distinguish from third-degree burns. The burn surface is pale, feels indurated or boggy, and does not blanch with pressure. This wound is less painful than more superficial wounds; some areas may be insensitive to stimuli. Healing occurs slowly over about 35 days with eschar formation and possible severe scarring and permanent loss of hair follicles and sweat and sebaceous glands.

Third-Degree Burns

Third-degree burns entail complete destruction of the full thickness of the skin, including all skin elements. The wound may appear pearly white, gray, or brown and is dry and inelastic. Pain is sensed only when deep pressure is applied. If the wound is small, healing over several months can occur by epithelial migration from the margins of the injury, with scar and contracture formation. Third-degree burns are repaired most often by excision and grafting of the wound to prevent contractures of the skin.[109]

Fourth-Degree Burns

Fourth-degree burns are similar to third-degree burns except that devitalized tissue extends into the subcutaneous tissue, fascia, and bone. These burns are blackened in appearance; they are dry and generally painless (because of destruction of nerve endings) and are at great risk for infection.

Complications of Burn Wounds

FLUID LOSS

In severe burns, release of vasoactive mediators and capillary injury cause sequestration of large amounts of body fluid, plasma, and electrolytes in extravascular compartments, resulting in edema both locally and throughout the entire body. This redistribution of fluid is compounded by the loss of large amounts of fluid, electrolytes, and protein into the open wound. The cumulative effect is a marked decrease in blood volume, a fall in cardiac output, and decreased tissue and organ perfusion. During the first 24 to 48 hours after a severe burn injury, adequate fluid must be given to replace fluid lost from the vascular space to prevent shock and, possibly, multiple organ failure, and death.[109]

INFECTION

The most important threat to survival of the fully resuscitated patient is infection, with burn wound sepsis and pneumonia being the leading causes of death.[109] The local mechanical defenses of the skin and respiratory tract often are damaged in burn victims, making these common foci for fatal infections. Loss of circulation to the burn wound margins disallows proper functioning of cellular and humoral defense mechanisms, which increases susceptibility to infection. Devitalized tissue and tissue exudates provide an ideal environment for the proliferation of bacteria. Colonization of gram-positive bacteria occurs if topical antimicrobial therapy is not initiated promptly, and gram-negative bacteria may predominate by the fifth day after injury.[109] Systemic antibiotics are of limited benefit in full-thickness burns and are used only to treat infections documented by wound biopsy, which reveal $>10^5$ bacteria/g of burn tissue.[109] Topical antimicrobials, local wound care, and strict infection control practices are the mainstays of controlling burn wound infections. Devitalized tissue initiates and perpetuates a sepsislike state in the absence of an identifiable focus of infection.[109] For this reason, as well as for infection control, early excision of devitalized tissue and closure of the burn wound by skin grafting or substitutes have been adopted by many burn centers.

INHALATION INJURY

Burn injuries complicated by inhalation injury are associated with greatly increased mortality rates. Injury to the tracheobronchial mucosa is caused by inhalation of smoke or flames and may result in bronchospasm, ulceration of the mucous membranes, damage to cell membranes, edema, and impairment of bacterial ciliary clearance. Even patients with minor burns can have inhalation injury and require hospital admission. The early symptoms of pulmonary injury (hoarseness, dyspnea, tachypnea, and wheezing) may not be evident for 24 to 48 hours, so patients with suspected inhalation injury (i.e., facial burns or entrapment in a closed space) must be examined carefully. Singed nasal hair, soot-coated tongue or oropharynx, and upper airway edema are indications of inhalation injury. The diagnosis is established by bronchoscopy, and management may include endotracheal intubation and mechanical ventilation. Maintenance of the patient's fluid status is essential. Corticosteroids do not influence survival rates and should not be routinely administered to patients with inhalation injury. They can also increase morbidity and mortality associated with burns and inhalation injury by increasing the risk of infection.[109] The use of exogenous surfactant in the treatment of inhalation burns in patients with adult respiratory distress syndrome (ARDS) improves the survival of these high-risk patients.[110]

Triage

14. **S.T., a 17-year-old, nonobese boy, has just burned the calf of his right leg on the muffler of his motorcycle. Immediately after being burned, S.T. was able to rinse his leg with cool water from a garden hose. The burn on his leg is about twice the size of the palm of his hand and appears erythematous and weeping. He sustained no other injury, but now he is in considerable pain. S.T. has no significant medical history. Should S.T. be referred to a health care provider or can he safely self-treat his burn? What patient information is necessary to consider in making this decision?**

Before recommending treatment for a patient with a minor burn, it is important to accurately assess the patient to determine whether he or she can self-treat safely or whether referral or hospitalization is necessary. The location and severity of the burn, the patient's age and state of health, and the cause of the burn injury all must be considered.

American Burn Association Treatment Categories

Three treatment categories for burn injuries are recommended by the American Burn Association: major burn injuries; moderate, uncomplicated burn injuries; and minor burn injuries.[111]

- *Major burn injuries* are second-degree burns with >25% BSA involvement in adults (20% in children); all third-degree burns with 10% BSA involvement; all burns involving the hands, face, eyes, ears, feet, and perineum that may result in functional or cosmetic impairment; high-voltage electrical injury; and burns complicated by inhalation injury, major trauma, or poor-risk patients (elderly patients and those with debilitating disease).
- *Moderate, uncomplicated burns* are second-degree burns with 15% to 25% BSA involvement in adults (10%–20% in children); third-degree burns with 2% to 10% BSA involvement; and burns not involving risk to areas of specialized function, such as the eyes, ears, face, hands, feet, or perineum.
- *Minor burn injuries* include second-degree burns with <15% BSA involvement in adults (10% in children), third-degree burns with <2% BSA, and burns not involving functional or cosmetic risk to areas of specialized function.

Patients with minor burn injuries may be treated on an outpatient basis if no other trauma is present; if circumferential burns of the neck, trunk, arms, or legs are not present; and if the patient is able to comply with therapy. After initial evaluation by a health care provider, patients may self-treat a second- or third-degree burn only if <1% BSA is involved.

Major or moderate, uncomplicated burns necessitate hospital admission, and surgical referral is recommended for patients of all ages who have deep second- or third-degree burns covering 3% of the TBSA.

Both the American Burn Association and the American College of Surgeons recommend transfer to a burn center for all acutely burned patients who meet any of the following criteria[111]:

- Partial-thickness burns ≥20% TBSA in patients aged 10 to 50 years
- Partial-thickness burns ≥10% TBSA in children aged 10 or adults aged 50 years
- Full-thickness burns ≥5% TBSA in patients of any age
- Patients with partial- or full-thickness burns of the hands, feet, face, eyes, ears, perineum, or major joints
- Patients with high-voltage electrical injuries, including lightning injuries
- Patients with significant burns from caustic chemicals
- Patients with burns complicated by multiple trauma in which the burn injury poses the greatest risk of morbidity or mortality (in such cases, if the trauma poses the greater immediate risk, the patient may be treated initially in a trauma center until stable before being transferred to a burn center)
- Patients with burns who suffer an inhalation injury
- Patients with significant ongoing medical disorders that could complicate management, prolong recovery, or affect mortality
- Patients who were taken to hospitals without qualified personnel or equipment for the care of children
- Burn injury in patients who will require special social, emotional, or long-term rehabilitative support, including cases involving suspected child abuse or substance abuse

Age-Related Recommendations

Children <2 years of age and elderly patients with a burn injury should be referred for evaluation because these patients may not tolerate any trauma associated with the burn. In addition to medical issues, children with burns that result from suspected child abuse should be hospitalized for legal, psychosocial, and protective reasons. Burns in varying stages of healing, demarcated patterns of burns (e.g., stocking or glove distribution), or more than two burn sites may be clues in identifying an abused child.[103]

Disease-Related Recommendations

Burn patients with any other medical condition, such as diabetes mellitus, cardiovascular disease, immunodeficiency disorders (e.g., human immunodeficiency virus [HIV]-associated disease, patients receiving cancer chemotherapy), renal disease, obesity, or alcoholism, may be more susceptible to complications from the burn and may have compromised wound healing.

Etiology

The etiology of a burn should always be considered because this may provide some insight into the burn presentation and its management. Electrical burns can appear to be superficial because external injury may occur at only the entrance and exit sites of the current. These burns, however, can cause extensive damage to underlying nerve and muscle tissue that is not initially evident. Except for very minor electrical burns, these patients should be referred for further evaluation. S.T. has sustained a superficial second-degree burn over about 2% of his BSA. Even though the burn wound on his leg was caused by thermal injury and is relatively minor, S.T. should be referred for further evaluation and treatment.

Treatment

15. How should S.T.'s burn be treated? What treatment alternatives may be used for S.T.? What immunization should S.T. be questioned about?

Goals of Treatment and Immediate Care

Treatment goals for first- and second-degree burns are to relieve the pain associated with the burn; to prevent desiccation and deepening of the wound, and infection; and to provide a protective environment for healing. Immediate care of the wound should be application of cold, wet compresses or immersion in cool water. S.T. may have prevented extension of the burn to deeper layers of tissue and alleviated some of his pain from the burn by immediately irrigating the wound with cool water. Next, the area should be cleansed with a mild hypoallergenic soap (e.g., Basis, Purpose) and water. A sterile, nonadherent, fine-mesh gauze dressing that is impregnated with hydrophilic petrolatum (Xeroflo, Adaptic) should be placed over the wound. This type of dressing prevents the gauze from adhering to the wound and allows the burn exudate to flow freely through the dressing, thus preventing maceration.

A second layer of absorbent gauze should be placed over the petrolatum gauze and a supportive layer of rolled gauze can be used to keep the dressing in place. The outer layer must not be too constricting, and the dressing should be replaced every 48 hours after recleansing the area and inspecting for signs of infection. If S.T.'s wound continues to weep, it may be beneficial to soak his wound or apply a towel saturated with water, normal saline, or Burow's solution (diluted 1:20 or 1:40) for 15 to 30 minutes at least four times daily (see Chapter 38). The use of butter, grease, or similar home remedies should be avoided in the treatment of burns because these measures tend to retain the thermal energy sustained in the burn and may increase the area of thermal injury. Because burn patients are susceptible to secondary tetanus infections, S.T. should receive a tetanus toxoid booster if he has not been immunized within the previous 10 years.

Skin Substitutes/Synthetic Dressings

Advances in the development of skin substitutes are being used to achieve the elusive goal of finding a skin replacement to mimic completely the interaction and functions of dermis and epidermis. Although this goal has yet to be achieved, a growing number of synthetic and biologic products are available that can serve important roles in caring for burn patients.[112] Some of the current modalities are as follows:

HUMAN CADAVER SKIN

Fresh human cadaver skin (allograft) is considered the *sine qua non* for temporary closure of burn wounds. It adheres well to a healthy wound bed, resulting in reduced contamination and reduced protein, heat, and water loss. Cost, rejection, and disease transmission (e.g., hepatitis) are the most commonly perceived disadvantages of human cadaver skin, thus, appropriate cadaveric screening is essential.

EPIDERMAL SUBSTITUTE: CULTURED EPITHELIAL ALLOGRAFTS

The technique of culturing autologous human epidermal cells grown from a single full-thickness skin biopsy into confluent keratinizing sheets suitable for grafting has been available for over two decades and is especially useful for patients with large wounds.[113] A lack of mechanical stability of cultured epithelium, causing an imperfect cover, remains a major concern; therefore, the development of a dermal substitute (or a vascularized remnant of allogenic dermis) in combination with cultured epithelial allografts to increase mechanical stability and decrease wound contracture, or a laboratory-derived autologous composite continues to receive scientific investigation.[114]

ANIMAL SUBSTITUTE: PIG SKIN

Pig skin (xenograft) has gained acceptance as a temporary dressing alternative to allograft because of its lower cost and greater availability. At 0°C, frozen pig skin has a storage life of 6 to 18 months from the date of manufacture. As with an allograft, it has the desirable properties of being able to adhere initially to a clean wound; to cover nerve endings to decrease pain; to function as an autograft test graft; and to diminish heat, protein, and electrolyte loss. A premeshed, de-epithelialized, shelf-stored form is available (EZ-Derm, Brennen Medical), which is thought to be more resistant to bacterial degradation.

DERMAL SUBSTITUTES: ALLODERMAL GRAFTS

Unlike the epidermis, the dermis can be rendered acellular and still perform its basic protective and supportive functions. With removal of the dermal cells, the antigenic elements are also eliminated; therefore, an alloplastic transplantation can occur without rejection. The principle of allodermal grafting is that an ultrathin (0.01 cm) meshed autograft laid on top of the allodermis provides skin quality that is comparable to that obtained from thick partial-thickness skin grafts. AlloDerm (LifeCell) is a shelf-stored, freeze-dried, acellular human cadaveric dermal matrix. Integra (Integra Life Sciences) is used in life-threatening burns. The inner layer of this material is a 2-mm thick combination of collagen fibers isolated from bovine tissue and the glycosaminoglycan chondroitin-6-sulfate that has a 70 to 200 μm pore size to facilitate host fibrovascular ingrowth. The outer layer is a 0.009-inch polysiloxane polymer with vapor transmission characteristics that simulate normal epithelium.[87]

SEMISYNTHETIC/SYNTHETIC DRESSINGS

Biobrane (Bertek) is a bilaminar, semisynthetic, temporary skin substitute made of silicone bonded to nylon mesh. Its adherence is facilitated by collagen peptides bonded to the nylon underlayer. This substitute has been shown to be as effective as frozen human allograft for the temporary coverage of freshly excised full-thickness burn wounds before autografting.[113] Duoderm (ConvaTec) (Bristol-Myers Squibb) is a hydrocolloid dressing, whereas OpSite (Smith & Nephew) and Tegaderm (3M) are elastomeric polyurethane films. Comfeel (Coloplast) is a semipermeable polyurethane film coated with a flexible, cross-linked adhesive mass containing sodium carboxy-methylcellulose (NaCMC) as the principal absorbent and gel-forming agent. This product is permeable to water vapor but impermeable to exudates and microorganisms. In the presence of an exudate, NaCMC absorbs fluids and swells to form a cohesive gel that does not disintegrate or leave residues in the wound bed.

Alternatives in treating S.T.'s second-degree burn include the use of synthetic dressings and topical antimicrobial agents. Synthetic dressings serve as skin substitutes that are applied to fresh, clean, and moist burns. They are trimmed to about the size of the burn and left in place until the burn is healed or the dressing separates from the wound spontaneously. The synthetic dressings keep the wound warm and moist, require absorbent dressings that must be changed daily, and are indicated for superficial second-degree burns. The chief advantage over gauze dressings is that synthetic dressings prevent mechanical injury from daily cleansing and dressing changes.[115]

TISSUE-ENGINEERED BIOLOGICAL DRESSINGS

Tissue-engineered biological dressings, although relatively new, have promise in the treatment of burns, chronic ulcers, surgical wounds, and other desquamating dermatologic conditions.[116,117] Although expensive, repeated applications of skin cells, whether these be keratinocytes or fibroblasts, autologous (the patients own) or allogeneic (from human donors), can all offer some benefit to chronic nonhealing wounds in prompting them to restart healing. In this setting, cultured cells assist the body's own wound repair mechanisms. Products include Dermagraft, Apligraf, and Epicel (cultured epidermal autograft). As an example, Apligraf is a bilayer approximating the structure of normal skin. The product is applied in a polyethylene bag containing a 10% CO_2:air ratio and agarose nutrient medium and must be stored at 20°C to 23°C until use. The first intended indication for Apligraf was full-thickness burns. In a multicenter trial, the use of meshed Apligraf in conjunction with meshed autograft resulted in better scores on the Vancouver Scar Assessment Scale than the use of meshed autograft alone. In most patients, Apligraf-treated burns were judged to have healed better than those treated with meshed autograft alone. Investigators rated Apligraf-treated sites superior to control in 58% of patients, equivalent in 16%, and worse in 16%.[118] The principle of using an appropriate biologically active matrix is now well established for accelerating wound healing and achieving skin reconstruction. Cellular components migrate to the wound from preexisting cell populations in adjacent tissue. Increasing evidence suggests that both circulating marrow-derived stem cells and preexisting organ-specific stem cells can contribute to tissue regeneration.[116] Although important issues concerning wound pretreatment, choice of matrix support for cell growth, and the use of allogenic cells remain to be fully resolved, tissue-engineered approaches to wound repair still offer significant therapeutic possibilities. Such benefits may include the following:

- Reduced donor site morbidity in burn wounds
- Increased potential for healing of recalcitrant lesions
- Reduced rates of lesion recurrence (as a result of improved dermal quality)
- Reduced wound contracture and scarring

- More rapid closure (epithelialization) of large acute excisional wounds
- Delivery of exogenous growth factors (autologous, allogenic, or genetically engineered)
- Reduced overall treatment costs and hospital stay.

Topical Antimicrobial Agents

SILVER SULFADIAZINE

Silver sulfadiazine (Silvadene) is the usual agent of choice because it has broad-spectrum gram-positive and gram-negative antibacterial activity, provides reasonable eschar penetration, and is easy and painless to apply and wash off. The cream is a 1% suspension of silver sulfadiazine in a water-miscible base. As a consequence of poor water solubility, the active agent shows only limited diffusion into the eschar. Silver sulfadiazine cream is most effective when applied to burn wounds immediately after thermal injury to prevent bacterial colonization of the burn wound surface as a prelude to intraeschar proliferation. This agent has the advantages of being painless when applied to the wound and being free from acid-base and electrolyte disturbances. The limitations of silver sulfadiazine cream include neutropenia,[119] which usually reverses when application is discontinued; hypersensitivity, which is rare; and ineffectiveness against certain strains of *Pseudomonas* organisms and virtually all strains of *Enterobacter cloacae.* A evidence-based review of use of silver sulfadiazine in burns suggested that whereas there is evidence of antibacterial activity, no direct evidence is seen of improved healing or reduced infection over normal dressings.[120] This agent should not be applied around the eyes or mouth in patients with hypersensitivity to sulfonamides or in pregnant or breastfeeding women.

MAFENIDE ACETATE

Mafenide acetate (Sulfamylon) is an 11.1% cream formulation of mafenide acetate in a water-dispersible base, or a 5% powder for topical solution. As a water-soluble agent, mafenide diffuses freely to establish an effective antibacterial concentration throughout the eschar and at the interface of viable-nonviable tissue, where bacteria characteristically proliferate before invasion. Because of this characteristic, mafenide is the best agent for use if the patient to be treated has heavily contaminated burn wounds, if treatment is delayed for several days after the burn occurred, or if a dense bacterial population already exists on and within the eschar. Adverse effects include hypersensitivity reactions in 7% of patients (usually responsive to antihistamines), pain or discomfort of 20 to 30 minutes duration when applied to partial-thickness burns (seldom a cause for discontinuation), and inhibition of carbonic anhydrase. The inhibition of carbonic anhydrase can produce both an early bicarbonate diuresis and an accentuation of postburn hyperventilation. The resulting overall reduction of serum bicarbonate levels renders such patients liable to a rapid shift from an alkalotic to an acidotic state. If acidosis should develop during use of mafenide, the frequency of application should be reduced to once daily, or it should be omitted for 24 to 48 hours, with buffering used as necessary, and with efforts made to improve pulmonary function.

Either topical silver sulfadiazine or mafenide should be applied in a one-eighth inch thick layer to the entire burn wound with a sterile gloved hand immediately after initial débridement and wound care. Twelve hours later, to ensure continuous topical treatment, a one-eighth inch coat of cream should be reapplied to those areas of the burn wound from which it has been abraded by clothing. The topical cream should be cleansed gently once each day from all of the burn wound and the wound inspected. Daily débridement should be carried out to a point of bleeding or pain without the use of general anesthesia. After débridement, the wound should be covered again by the topical cream.

SILVER NITRATE

If topical antimicrobial creams are unavailable, multilayered occlusive gauze dressings, saturated with a 0.5% solution of silver nitrate, can be used. These soaks are changed two or three times each day and moistened every 2 hours. Evaporation should be avoided to prevent raising the silver nitrate concentration to cytotoxic levels within the soaks. Transeschar losses of sodium, potassium, chloride, and calcium should be anticipated and appropriately replaced. Similar to therapy with silver sulfadiazine cream, silver nitrate soak therapy is best for bacterial control in burn patients who are received immediately after injury before significant microbial proliferation has occurred. Silver nitrate is immediately precipitated on contact with proteinaceous material; it does not penetrate the eschar and, consequently, is ineffective in the treatment of established burn wound infection. For these reasons, it is not routinely recommended.

In S.T.'s case, *silver sulfadiazine cream* could be chosen to treat his burn on an outpatient basis if an assessment determines that he is at particular risk for infection. The cream would be applied in a thin layer over the wound and covered with absorbent gauze and wrapped with rolled gauze. The dressing must be changed twice daily to maintain an application of cream that is biologically active. Topical bacitracin and the combination of polymyxin B and bacitracin are transparent formulations that also can be used but, because of limited efficacy, may be desirable for use only on small, second-degree burns on the face.

Oral Analgesics and Topical Protectants

S.T.'s burn pain can be treated with oral OTC analgesics, aspirin, acetaminophen, or ibuprofen. If these analgesics do not provide adequate relief, oxycodone or acetaminophen (or equivalent) may be of additional benefit. Topical protectants, such as allantoin, calamine, white petrolatum, or zinc oxide, are safe and effective in treating first-degree and minor second-degree burns. These agents protect the burn from mechanical irritation caused by friction and rubbing and prevent drying of the stratum corneum.

Postwound Care

Postwound care is an essential part of total burns management to ensure adequate follow-up subsequent to wound healing, including psychological support. Good burns care that helps to alleviate physical discomfort, pain and scarring, and that promotes good wound healing will also provide psychological benefits for the patient. Healed wounds should be moisturized on a regular basis. Pruritus can be a major problem after burn injury. To reduce itching, moisturizers can be applied, and oral antihistamines may be necessary.[121] Protection from the sun will help to prevent further thermal damage or pigmentation changes to the affected area. Patients in this population should avoid the sun following a burn injury whenever possible, and use of a sunscreen with SPF of at least 25 is recommended.[122] If surface changes occur (e.g. skin becomes hypertrophic, or blisters or new wounds appear), the patient should be advised to return for evaluation.

REFERENCES

1. Green A et al. Daily sunscreen application and beta carotene supplementation in prevention of basal-cell and squamous-cell carcinomas of the skin: a randomised controlled trial. *Lancet* 1999;354:723.
2. Beddingfield FC 3rd. The melanoma epidemic: res ipsa loquitur. *Oncologist* 2003;8:459.
3. Council on Scientific Affairs. Harmful effects of ultraviolet radiation. *JAMA* 1989;262:380.
4. Ferrini RL et al. American College of Preventive Medicine Practice Policy Statement: skin protection from ultraviolet light exposure. *Am J Prev Med* 1998;14:83.
5. Leffell DJ et al. Sunlight and skin cancer. *Sci Am* 1996;275:52.
6. National Institutes of Health Consensus Development Panel. National Institutes of Health summary of the consensus development conference on sunlight, ultraviolet radiation, and the skin. *J Am Acad Dermatol* 1991;24:608.
7. Diffey BL. What is light? *Photodermatol Photoimmunol Photomed* 2002;18:68.
8. McMichael AJ et al. Climate change and health: implications for research, monitoring and policy. *BMJ* 1997;315:870.
9. World Meteorological Organization, Scientific Assessment of Ozone Depletion: 1998, WMO Global Ozone Research and Monitoring Project Report No. 44, Geneva; 1998.
10. Wolpowitz D et al. The vitamin D questions: how much do you need and how should you get it? *J Am Acad Dermatol* 2006;54:301.
11. Thrush B. Causes of ozone depletion. *Nature* 1988;332:784.
12. Salawitch RJ. A greenhouse warming connection. *Nature* 1998;392:551.
13. Shindell DT et al. Increased polar stratospheric ozone losses and delayed eventual recovery owing to increasing greenhouse-gas concentrations. *Nature* 1998;392:589.
14. Coldiron BM. The UV Index: a weather report for skin. *Clin Dermatol* 1998;16:441.
15. Fisher GJ et al. Molecular basis of sun-induced premature skin aging and retinoid antagonism. *Nature* 1996;379:335.
16. Fourtanier A et al. Protection of skin biological targets by different types of sunscreens. *Photodermatol Photoimmunol Photomed* 2006;22:22.
17. Fitzpatrick TB. The validity and practicality of sun-reactive skin types I through VI. *Arch Dermatol* 1988;124:869.
18. Gallagher RP et al. Broad-spectrum sunscreen use and the development of new nevi in white children: a randomized controlled trial. *JAMA* 2000;283:2955.
19. Buller DB et al. Skin cancer prevention for children: a critical review. *Health Educ Behav* 1999;26:317.
20. Bentham G et al. Incidence of malignant melanoma of the skin in Norway, 1955–1989: associations with solar ultraviolet radiation, income and holidays abroad. *Int J Epidemiol* 1996;25:1132.
21. Geller AC et al. Skin cancer prevention and detection practices among siblings of patients with melanoma. *J Am Acad Dermatol* 2003;49:631.
22. Geller AC et al. Sun protection practices among offspring of women with personal or family history of skin cancer. *Pediatrics* 2006;117:688.
23. Hemminski K et al. Familial invasive and in situ squamous cell carcinoma of the skin. *Br J Cancer* 2003;88:1375.
24. Ford D et al. Risk of cutaneous melanoma associated with a family history of the disease. The International Melanoma analysis group (IMAGE). *Int J Cancer* 1995;62:377.
25. Wolf P et al. Phenotypic markers, sunlight-related factors and sunscreen use in patients with cutaneous melanoma: an Austrian case-control study. *Melanoma Res* 1998;8:370.
26. Gerber B et al. Ultraviolet emission spectra of sunbeds. *Photochem Photobiol* 2002;76:664.
27. Culley CA et al. Compliance with federal and state legislation by indoor tanning facilities in San Diego. *J Am Acad Dermatol* 2001;44:53.
28. Levine JA et al. The indoor UV tanning industry: a review of skin cancer risk, health benefit claims, and regulation. *J Am Acad Dermatol.* 2005;53:1038.
29. Fisher GJ et al. Mechanisms of photoaging and chronological skin aging. *Arch Dermatol* 2002;138:1462.
30. West SK et al. Sunlight exposure and risk of lens opacities in a population-based study. The Salisbury Eye Evaluation Project. *JAMA* 1998;280:714.
31. Abdulla FR et al. Tanning and skin cancer. *Pediatr Dermatol* 2005;22:501.
32. Warthan MM et al. UV light tanning as a type of substance-related disorder. *Arch Dermatol* 2005;141:963.
33. Fisher GJ et al. Pathophysiology of premature skin aging induced by ultraviolet light. *N Engl J Med* 1997;337:1419.
34. Uitto J. Understanding premature skin aging [Editorial]. *N Engl J Med* 1997;337:1463.
35. Gilchrest BA. A review of skin aging and its medical therapy. *Br J Dermatol* 1996;135:867.
36. Naylor MF et al. The case for sunscreens. A review of their use in preventing actinic damage and neoplasia. *Arch Dermatol* 1997;133:1146.
37. Kang S et al. Photoaging and topical tretinoin: therapy, pathogenesis, and prevention. *Arch Dermatol* 1997;133:1280.
38. Kang S et al. Photoaging therapy with topical tretinoin: an evidence-based analysis. *J Am Acad Dermatol* 1998;39:S55.
39. Kang S et al. Tazarotene cream for the treatment of facial photodamage. *Arch Dermatol* 2001;137:1597.
40. Phillips TJ et al. Efficacy of 0.1% tazarotene cream for the treatment of photodamage. *Arch Dermatol* 2002;138:1486.
41. Kligman AM. Guidelines for the use of topical tretinoin (Retin A) for photoaged skin. *J Am Acad Dermatol* 1989;21:650.
42. Gonzalez E et al. Drug photosensitivity, idiopathic photodermatoses and sunscreens. *J Am Acad Dermatol* 1996;35:871.
43. Gonzalez E et al. Bilateral comparison of generalized lichen planus treated with psoralens and ultraviolet A. *J Am Acad Dermatol* 1984;10:958.
44. Darlington S et al. A randomized controlled trial to assess sunscreen application and beta carotene supplementation in the prevention of solar keratoses. *Arch Dermatol* 2003;139:451.
45. Hawk JLM. Cutaneous photoprotection [Editorial]. *Arch Dermatol* 2003;139:527.
46. Coogan PF et al. Sun protection practices in adolescents: a school-based survey of almost 25,000 Connecticut schoolchildren. *J Am Acad Dermatol* 2001;44:512.
47. Adam JE. Living a "shady life": sun-protective behaviour for Canadians. *CMA J* 1999;160:1471.
48. Diffey B. Sunscreen isn't enough. *J Photochem Photobiol B* 2001;64:105.
49. Rigel AS. Hat-wearing patterns in persons attending baseball games. *J Am Acad Dermatol* 2006;54:918.
50. Gasparro FP et al. A review of sunscreen safety and efficacy. *Photochem Photobiol* 1998;68:243.
51. Diffey BL. When should sunscreen be reapplied? *J Am Acad Dermatol* 2001;45:882.
52. Autier P et al. European Organization for Research and Treatment of Cancer Melanoma Co-operative Group. Quantity of sunscreen used by European students. *Br J Dermatol* 2001;144:288.
53. Teichmann A et al. Investigation of the homogeneity of the distribution of sunscreen formulations on the human skin: characterization and comparison of two different methods. *J Biomed Opt* 2006;11:064005.
54. Robinson JK et al. Sun protection by families at the beach. *Arch Pediatr Adolesc Med* 1998;152:466.
55. Wright MW et al. Mechanisms of sunscreen failure. *J Am Acad Dermatol* 2001;44:781.
56. Faurschou A et al. The relation between sun protection factor and amount of sunscreen applied in vivo. *Br J Dermatol* 2007;156:716.
57. Hagedorn-Leweke U et al. Accumulation of sunscreens and other compounds in keratinous substrates. *Eur J Pharm Biopharm* 1998;46:215.
58. Patel NP et al. Properties of topical sunscreen formulations: a review. *J Dermatol Surg Oncol* 1992;18:316.
59. Stern RS et al. Risk reduction for nonmelanoma skin cancer with childhood sunscreen use. *Arch Dermatol* 1986;122:537.
60. Weinstock MA. Do sunscreens increase or decrease melanoma risk: an epidemiologic evaluation. *J Investig Dermatol Symp Proc* 1999;4:97.
61. Westerdahl J et al. Sunscreen use and malignant melanoma. *Int J Cancer* 2000;87:145.
62. Autier P et al. Sunscreen use, wearing clothes, and the number of nevi in 6- or 7-year-old European children. *J Natl Cancer Inst* 1998;90:1873.
63. Bastuji-Garin S et al. Cutaneous malignant melanoma, sun exposure, and sunscreen use: epidemiological evidence. *Br J Dermatol* 2002; 146(Suppl. 61):24.
64. Dennis LK et al. Sunscreen use and the risk of melanoma: a quantitative review. *Ann Intern Med* 2003;139:966.
65. Faurschou A et al. Sunprotection effect of dihydroxyacetone. *Arch Dermatol* 2004;140:886.
66. Schauder S et al. Contact and photocontact sensitivity to sunscreens. Review of a 15-year experience and of the literature. *Contact Dermatitis* 1997;37:221.
67. Dromgoole SH et al. Sunscreening agent intolerance: contact and photocontact sensitization and contact urticaria. *J Am Acad Dermatol* 1990;22:1068.
68. Fisher AA. Sunscreen dermatitis. Part II: The cinnamates. *Cutis* 1992;50:253.
69. Fisher AA. Sunscreen dermatitis. Part III: The benzophenones. *Cutis* 1992;50:331.
70. Fisher AA. Sunscreen dermatitis. Part IV: The salicylates, the anthranilates, and physical agents. *Cutis* 1992;50:397.
71. Singh M et al. Octyl salicylate: a new contact sensitivity. *Contact Dermatitis* 2007;56:48.
72. Gange RW et al. Efficacy of a sunscreen containing butyl methoxydibenzoylmethane against ultraviolet A radiation in photosensitized subjects. *J Am Acad Dermatol* 1986;15:494.
73. Humbert P. Topical vitamin C in the treatment of photoaged skin. *Eur J Dermatol* 2001;11:172.

74. Eberlein-Konig B et al. Protective effect against sunburn of combined systemic ascorbic acid (vitamin C) and d-alpha-tocopherol (vitamin E). *J Am Acad Dermatol* 1998;38:45.
75. Kullavanijaya P et al. Photoprotection. *J Am Acad Dermatol* 2005;52:937.
76. Kollias N. The absorption properties of "physical" sunscreens. *Arch Dermatol* 1999;135:209.
77. Tan MH et al. A pilot study on the percutaneous absorption of microfine titanium for sunscreens. *Australas J Dermatol* 1996;37:185.
78. Scheuer E et al. Sunscreen allergy: a review of epidemiology, clinical characteristics, and responsible allergens. *Dermatitis* 2006;17;3–11.
79. Schneider J. The teaspoon rule of applying sunscreen. *Arch Dermatol* 2002;138:838.
80. Lademann J et al. Sunscreen application at the beach. *Journal of Cosmetic Dermatology* 2004; 3:62.
81. Notice of proposed rule-making on sunscreen drug products for over-the-counter use: tentative final monograph. *Fed Regist* 1993;58:282.
82. Buller DB et al. Sun protection policies and environmental features in US elementary schools. *Arch Dermatol* 2002;138:771.
83. Emmons KM et al. Preventing excess sun exposure: it is time for a national policy. *J Natl Cancer Inst* 1999;91:1269.
84. Adam JE. Sun protective clothing. *J Cutan Med Surg* 1998;3:1.
85. Committee on Environmental Health. American Academy of Pediatrics. Ultraviolet light: a hazard to children. *Pediatrics* 1999;104:328.
86. Gambichler T et al. Protection against ultraviolet radiation by commercial summer clothing: need for standardised testing and labelling. *BioMed Central Dermatol* 2001;1:6.
87. Stanford DG et al. Sun protection by a summer-weight garment: the effect of washing and wearing. *Med J Aust* 1995;162:422.
88. Gambichler T et al. Role of clothes in sun protection. *Recent Results Cancer Res* 2002;160:15.
89. Wang SQ et al. Reduction of ultraviolet transmission through cotton T-shirt fabrics with low ultraviolet protection by various laundering methods and dyeing: clinical implications. *J Am Acad Dermatol* 2001;44:767.
90. Edlich RF et al. Revolutionary advances in sun-protective clothing-an essential step in eliminating skin cancer in our world. *J Long Term Eff Med Implants* 2004;14:95.
91. de Gruijl FR et al. Health effects from stratospheric ozone depletion and interactions with climate change. *Photochem Photobiol Sci* 2003;2:16.
92. Longstreth J et al. Health risks. *J Photochem Photobiol* 1998;46:20.
93. Sliney DH. Photoprotection of the eye UV radiation and sunglasses. *J Photochem Photobiol* 2001;64:166.
94. Hughes GS et al. Synergistic effects of oral nonsteroidal drugs and topical corticosteroids in the therapy of sunburn in humans. *Dermatology* 1992;184:54.
95. Sidhu SK et al. A 10-year retrospective study on benzocaine allergy in the United Kingdom. *Am J Contact Dermat* 1999;10:57.
96. Cuesta-Herranz J et al. Allergic reaction caused by local anesthetic agents belonging to the amide group. *J Allergy Clin Immunol* 1997;99:427.
97. McLoughlin E et al. The causes, cost, and prevention of childhood burn injuries. *Am J Dis Child* 1990;144:607.
98. Ryan CM et al. Objective estimates of the probability of death from burn injuries. *N Engl J Med* 1998;338:362.
99. Brigham PA et al. Burn incidence and medical care use in the United States: estimate, trends, and data sources. *J Burn Care Rehabil* 1996;17:95.
100. Alsbjrn B et al. Guidelines for the management of partial-thickness burns in a general hospital or community setting. Recommendations of a European working party. *Burns* 2007;33:155.
101. Morrow SE et al. Etiology and outcome of pediatric burns. *J Pediatr Surg* 1996;31:329.
102. Hultman CS et al. Return to jeopardy: the fate of pediatric burn patients who are victims of abuse and neglect. *J Burn Care Rehabil* 1998;19:367.
103. Stratman E et al. Scald abuse. *Arch Dermatol* 2002;138:318.
104. Demling RH. The advantage of the burn team approach. *J Burn Care Rehabil* 1995;16:569.
105. Sheridan RL et al. Skin substitutes in burns. *Burns* 1999;25:97.
106. Dziewulski P. Burn wound healing: James Ellsworth Laing memorial essay for 1991. *Burns* 1992;18:466.
107. Sheridan RL. Burns. *Crit Care Med* 2002;30:S500.
108. Miller SF et al. Burn size estimate reliability: a study. *J Burn Care Rehabil* 1991;12:546.
109. Monafo WW. Initial management of burns. *N Engl J Med* 1996;335:1581.
110. Pallua N et al. Intrabronchial surfactant application in cases of inhalation injury: first results from patients with severe burns and ARDS burns. *Burns* 1998;24:197.
111. American Burn Association. Hospital and prehospital resources for optimal care of patients with burn injury: guidelines for development and operation of burn centers. *J Burn Care Rehabil* 1990;11: 98.
112. Hopper RA et al. Use of skin substitutes in adult Canadian burn centres. *Canadian Journal of Plastic Surgery* 1997;5:112.
113. Purdue GF et al. Biosynthetic skin substitute versus frozen human cadaver allograft for temporary coverage of excised burn wounds. *J Trauma* 1987; 27:155.
114. Takahashi Y et al. Wound management of allgeneic cultural dermal substitutes (CDS). *Burns* 2007;3S:S131.
115. Poulsen TD et al. Polyurethane film (Opsite) vs. impregnated gauze (Jelonet) in the treatment of outpatient burns: a prospective, randomized study. *Burns* 1991;17:59.
116. Ehrenreich M et al. Update on tissue-engineered biological dressings. *Tissue Eng* 2006;12:2407.
117. MacNeil S. Progress and opportunities for tissue-engineered skin. *Nature* 2007;445:874.
118. Waymack P et al. The effect of a tissue engineered bilayered living skin analog, over meshed split-thickness autografts on the healing of excised burn wounds. The Apligraf Burn Study Group. *Burns* 2000;26:609.
119. Caffee F et al. Leukopenia and silver sulfadiazine. *J Trauma* 1982;22:586.
120. Hussain S et al. Best evidence topic report. Silver sulphadiazine cream in burns. *Emerg Med J* 2006;23:929.
121. Willebrand M et al. Pruritis, personality traits and coping in long-term follow-up of burn-injured patients. *Acta Derm Venereol* 2004;84:375.
122. DeChalain TM et al. Burn area color changes after superficial burns in childhood: can they be predicted? *J Burn Care Rehabil* 1998;19(1 Pt 1):39.

ARTHRITIC DISORDERS

CHAPTER 42

Gout and Hyperuricemia

KarenBeth H. Bohan and Tricia M. Russell

Gout is a disease that most commonly manifests as recurrent episodes of acute joint pain and inflammation secondary to the deposition of monosodium urate (MSU) crystals in the synovial fluid and lining. MSU deposition in the urinary tract can cause urolithiasis and urinary obstruction.[1] Patients with gout cycle between flares of acute joint pain and inflammation and intercritical gout (i.e., periods of quiescence with no symptoms of the disease). In addition, they can also develop chronic tophaceous gout and hyperuricemia. (Tophi are hard nodules of MSU crystals that have deposited in soft tissues and are most commonly found in the toes, fingers, and elbows.) Although gout is often associated with hyperuricemia, elevated serum uric acid (SUA) is not a prerequisite for this painful condition.[2] Hence, *gout* should be considered as a clinical diagnosis and *hyperuricemia* as a biochemical one. These two terms are not synonymous and are not interchangeable.

PATHOPHYSIOLOGY

Uric Acid Disposition

Uric acid serves no biological function; it is merely the end product of purine metabolism. Unlike animals, humans lack the enzyme uricase, which degrades uric acid into more soluble products for excretion. As a consequence, uric acid is not metabolized in humans and primarily is excreted renally, although up to one third of the daily uric acid produced can be eliminated through the gastrointestinal (GI) tract.[3,4] Increased SUA concentrations, therefore, can result from an increase in production or a decrease in renal excretion of uric acid, or a combination of these two mechanisms.

Overproduction

Overproduction of uric acid, accounting for about 10% of gout cases,[3] can result from excessive *de novo* purine synthesis, which is associated primarily with rare genetic enzyme mutation defects; neoplastic diseases (e.g., multiple myeloma, leukemias, lymphomas, Hodgkin disease); and myeloproliferative disorders (e.g., myeloid metaplasia, polycythemia vera). Aggressive cytotoxic chemotherapy can cause tumor lysis syndrome and increased uric acid production from increased nucleoprotein turnover. Overproduction of uric acid can also be the result of excessive intake of dietary purines from meat, seafood, dried peas and beans, certain vegetables (e.g., mushrooms, spinach, asparagus), beer, and other alcoholic beverages.[5,6] Many patients attempt to avoid intake of these foods; however, dietary restrictions are seldom of much benefit (with the exception of avoiding excessive alcohol, yeast, or liver supplements), and patients should feel comfortable in eating "modest" quantities of meats, seafood, and vegetables.

Underexcretion

A defect in the renal clearance of uric acid is the main cause of hyperuricemia and gout in about 90% of patients. Uric acid is filtered in the renal glomerulus and is almost completely (98%–100%) reabsorbed in the proximal tubule. Uric acid is then secreted distal to the proximal tubular reabsorption site, and most is reabsorbed again.[2,3] In normal patients, homeostasis between reabsorption and secretion of urate is maintained. However, many factors (e.g., renal impairment, certain drugs, alcohol excess, metabolic syndrome, hypertension [HTN], cardiovascular disease [CVD]) can cause this balance to fail, resulting in excess serum concentrations of uric acid and tissue deposition.[4,7]

ACUTE GOUT

Epidemiology

The risk of gouty arthritis is approximately the same for both men and women at any given SUA concentration; however, many more men are hyperuricemic. For example, men are six times more likely than women to have SUA concentrations >7 mg/dL. Overall, gout occurs as often in postmenopausal elderly women as in men.[8]

Classically, gout presents during middle age; in one study, the average age at the time of the first attack was 48 years.[9] The onset of gout is uncommon in prepubertal children, premenopausal women, and men younger than 30 years of age. The appearance of gout in these populations should alert the clinician to the possibility of a renal parenchymal disease, which decreases urate clearance, or to a genetic enzymatic defect that is associated with increased *de novo* purine production.

Clinical Features

1. E.J., a 52-year-old male school bus driver, reports to the emergency department of his local hospital with the primary complaint of extreme pain in his right elbow. He admits to playing several tennis matches yesterday followed by a few beers with friends. He awoke in the early hours of the morning with a sore and stiff elbow, which he self-medicated with acetaminophen before trying to get back to sleep. When his pain escalated, he sought medical attention. Pertinent medical history includes the recent diagnoses of HTN, hyperlipidemia, impaired fasting glucose, and obesity. E.J. has not had regular medical care since graduating from high school, and only recently started seeing a primary care physician at the urging of his wife after his father died of an ischemic stroke. At that visit 1 month ago, E.J. was prescribed hydrochlorothiazide 12.5 mg once daily, which is his only medication. He was also encouraged to go on a diet and to increase his exercise. He states that he has no drug or food allergies and is tolerating the antihypertensive well. On physical examination, the right elbow is exquisitely tender and erythematous, and his vital signs are all within normal limits. The elbow is warm to the touch and has moderate swelling. What information in this case leads you to a consideration of gout as an explanation for E.J.'s elbow pain?

First, E.J.'s symptoms of severe, acute pain and an obviously inflamed joint are consistent with the usual presentation of gout. Next, epidemiologically, E.J.'s gender and age are consistent with the epidemiological data that are commonly associated with gout.

Pain

The pain of gout rapidly reaches its maximum within 6 to 12 hours of onset and is usually accompanied by erythema.[10] It is often so severe that patients cannot even tolerate a sheet lying on top of the affected area. E.J.'s symptoms are consistent with this description.

Number and Type of Joints

Acute gout attacks affect a single joint 85% to 90% of the time, and most often affect a joint of the lower extremity.[3] The first metatarsophalangeal joint (the great toe) is the most common joint affected and the term, *podagra,* specifically refers to gout in this joint. In a study of dietary intake and the occurrence of gout in North American men, 88% of those reporting gout episodes experienced podagra.[6] An explanation for the predilection of the great toe to acute gouty arthritic attacks is based on the premise of a transient local increase in the concentration of monosodium urate in this joint, as well as lower body temperature in the extremities.[11] Because urate diffuses more slowly than water across a synovial membrane, resorption of synovial effusion from traumatic joints when the patient is in a recumbent position increases the urate concentration within a joint.[12,13] Synovial effusions are also increased in the great toe during the day because of degenerative changes in that joint: the first metatarsophalangeal joint is the most common and often the only joint affected in degenerative joint disease of the foot. This tendency for degenerative changes in the big toe appears less often in non-European and non–North American populations as compared to Western societies and perhaps can be attributed to differences in traditional footwear, climate, and other variables associated with gout.[14]

Although initial gout attacks are primarily monoarticular, as many as 39% of the patients in one study experienced polyarticular involvement as their first manifestation of gout.[15] Generally, recurrent attacks are of longer duration than first attacks, more likely to be polyarticular, and more smoldering in onset.[16] Gout presenting initially in an elbow joint is much less common than podagra, but it certainly can occur[3] and does not rule out gout as a diagnosis for E.J.'s pain.

Nocturnal Occurrence

Acute gouty arthritis commonly begins at night. Thomas Sydenham's 18th-century classic description of an acute gouty attack begins, "The victim goes to bed and sleeps in good health. About two o'clock in the morning he is awakened by a severe pain in the great toe; more rarely in the heel, ankle, or instep."[11] According to the Simkin hypothesis,[11] small amounts of effusion fluid gravitationally enter into degenerative joints of the feet (or other joints) during the day, when most people are busily walking around, and are reabsorbed during the night when the lower extremities are elevated. Thus, the onset of pain in E.J. during the night is typical of gout.

Physical Stress

Gouty attacks also seem to be more common during episodes of increased physical exercise. Long walks, hikes, golf games, or tight new shoes have historically been associated with the subsequent onset of podagra.[11] Thus, this acute episode of elbow pain experienced by E.J. after a tennis match is compatible with the association of gout with increased physical exercise.

Risk Factors

2. What findings in the previous case put E.J. at risk for gout?

The recent diagnoses of HTN, dyslipidemia, impaired fasting glucose, and obesity in E.J. are disorders that have all been associated with gout and hyperuricemia.[7]

Metabolic Syndrome

E.J.'s recent diagnoses fulfill the criteria for *metabolic syndrome,* and it is well-known that this set of diseases increases the risk for CVD. Interestingly, hyperuricemia is often present in patients who have these diseases as well, so does that mean hyperuricemia is a risk factor for CVD? Although this relationship is strong, causality is controversial. Even though the Framingham study group found that the presence of gout was a risk for CVD in men, it is likely that this is just a marker for CVD rather than a trigger.[18] In other studies, hyperuricemia was noted to be an independent risk factor for CVD and unlikely to be a cause of CVD.[19] Impaired glucose utilization, often called "insulin resistance syndrome," also has a relationship with hyperuricemia. This may be mediated via reduced renal excretion of sodium and urate in hyperinsulinemia, although the complete mechanism has not been fully elucidated.[20] Because of these close linkages, patients who present with gout and/or hyperuricemia should be monitored closely for the development of CVD and diabetes, even if currently well.

Renal Dysfunction

Uric acid excretion is decreased in patients with renal dysfunction due to decreased glomerular filtration, and as a consequence, hyperuricemia is a common finding. The hyperuricemia does not need to be treated unless patients manifest gouty arthritis.[21] E.J.'s workup for his sore elbow and possible gout should include a metabolic panel for blood urea nitrogen (BUN), serum creatinine (SCr), and electrolytes to clarify the status of his renal function.

Ethanol Consumption

Overindulgence of alcohol has been linked to acute gout attacks. In one case-control study, the weekly intake of alcohol was more than doubled in patients with gout compared to matched controls without gout.[22] Ethanol-induced gout/hyperuricemia has been attributed to reduced renal urate excretion when acute alcohol intake causes lactic acidosis, degradation of the purines in beer and other alcoholic beverages increases uric acid production, and possible lead exposure from moonshine whiskey or port wine.[20] E.J.'s intake of a "few beers" after playing in a rigorous tennis tournament, when combined with possible dehydration from vigorous exercise and lactic acidemia from muscle energy expenditure, place the diagnosis of an acute gout attack near the top of the list of possible causes for his elbow pain and inflammation.

Lead Exposure

Chronic lead exposure is associated with renal dysfunction. Patients with renal dysfunction and concurrent gout have higher lead levels than gouty patients with normal renal function.[23] Unexpectedly, the serum concentrations of lead in healthy subjects with no known lead exposure were noted to be higher (albeit within normal limits) in those with gout than those without gout.[24] Lead exposure, however, is not a likely risk factor for gout for E.J.

Diagnosis

3. What objective data would be of value in assisting in the diagnosis of E.J.'s elbow pain and inflammation?

Laboratory Tests

Because uric acid primarily is excreted renally and renal impairment is a risk factor for gout, the serum concentrations of E.J.'s BUN and SCr should be measured along with a serum uric acid concentration, especially in light of his history of HTN, hydrochlorothiazide therapy, hyperlipidemia, and impaired glucose tolerance. A subsequent urinalysis could also be evaluated for proteinuria and glucose if his laboratory blood tests demonstrate that further workup might be warranted. Although infection, in particular, *septic arthritis*, could also present as sudden onset of joint pain and inflammation, it is not likely in this case. An elevated systemic white blood cell (WBC) count would be consistent with infection or gout. If joint infection is of genuine concern, synovial fluid aspiration could differentiate between infection and gout.

Radiography

Radiographic findings during the early phase of gout are nonspecific and generally characterized by asymmetric soft tissue swelling overlying the involved joint. When gout has been long standing, bony changes can be noticed on x-ray, along with calcium deposition and increased density in the areas of soft tissue swelling.[25] An x-ray of E.J.'s elbow should be obtained if other *musculoskeletal disorders* (e.g., bone fracture) are likely; however, the history and physical examination of E.J. do not provide adequate support for an x-ray at this juncture.

Joint Fluid Aspiration

A definitive diagnosis of gout only can be established by finding MSU crystals in the aspirated synovial fluid of the affected joint. The absence, however, of MSU crystals in the synovial fluid does not rule out the diagnosis of gout. In one study, when synovial fluid was aspirated from the knees of 50 patients with asymptomatic, nontophaceous gout (synovial fluid monosodium urate crystals had been previously documented in the knees or other joints of these patients), urate crystals were only found in 58% of these asymptomatic patients.[26] Urate crystals, however, can be found on repeated search of other involved joints,[27] or even of the same joint a few hours later.[28,29] If synovial fluid is aspirated from an inflamed joint, it should also be analyzed for bacteria and a WBC count obtained. In gouty arthritis, the WBC count is likely to range from 5,000 to 50,000/L.[2] In septic arthritis, the WBC count of the synovial fluid is usually >50,000/L, and a Gram stain of the synovial fluid is often positive for bacteria.[30] In clinical practice, primary care providers generally do not aspirate an inflamed joint to diagnose gout (see Criteria for Diagnosis section).

Pseudogout

Deposition of microcrystals (i.e., calcium pyrophosphate, calcium oxalate, calcium hydroxyapatite) into joints can cause acute or chronic arthritis in a manner similar to that caused by monosodium urate deposition.[31] The role of these microcrystals in causing acute synovitis has been greater than previously expected because improved crystallographic technology (e.g., electron microscopy, x-ray diffraction) can differentiate these diagnoses from that of acute gout. Crystal-induced diseases tend to occur in older patients because prior joint disease, especially osteoarthritis (which is generally a disease of the elderly), predisposes them to crystal deposition and acute episodes of joint inflammation. The elderly are also more prone to microcrystal-induced arthritis because these crystals generally accumulate over a long period, and must attain a sufficient concentration and size before they precipitate into the synovial fluid and cause inflammation.[32]

Criteria for Diagnosis

According to the American College of Rheumatology (ACR), only 6 of the 12 criteria listed in Table 42-1 (derived from a 1977 report)[33] need to be present to confirm a diagnosis of gout when synovial fluid has not been aspirated from an inflamed joint. Routine synovial fluid aspirates are not obtained by most practitioners due to the technical expertise required for obtaining and analyzing the specimen, as well as the pain to the patient, during the procedure. Newer evidence-based guidelines for the diagnosis (Table 42-2) and management (Table 42-3) of gout have been developed by the European League Against Rheumatism (EULAR) using the Delphi method of expert consensus to determine standard of care.[10,34] The experts' consensus of the strength of a recommendation is listed as a percentage of concurrence in the right-hand columns of Tables 42–2 and 42–3.

Table 42-1 Criteria for Diagnosis of Gout (at least six criteria are needed for diagnosis unless MSU crystals are present in joint fluid aspirate)

1. More than one acute attack of arthritis
2. Attack of monoarticular arthritis
3. Joint inflammation maximal within 1 day
4. Negative synovial joint fluid culture
5. Erythema over involved joint(s)
6. Podagra (first metatarsophalangeal joint)
7. Unilateral podagra
8. Unilateral attack involving tarsal joint
9. Tophi
10. Hyperuricemia
11. Asymmetric swelling within a joint on radiograph
12. Subcortical cysts without erosions on radiograph

Adapted from reference 3.

Table 42-2 EULAR Propositions for Diagnosis of Gout

Recommendation	*SOR (%)*
1. In acute attacks, the rapid development of acute pain, swelling, and tenderness that reaches peak intensity within 6–12 hours, especially with overlying erythema, highly suggest crystal inflammation (although not specific for gout).	88
2. For typical presentations of gout (e.g., recurrent podagra with hyperuricemia), a clinical diagnosis alone is reasonably accurate, but not definitive without crystal confirmation.	95
3. Demonstration of MSU crystals in synovial fluid or a tophus permits a definitive diagnosis of gout.	96
4. A routine search for MSU crystals is recommended in all synovial fluid samples obtained from undiagnosed joints.	90
5. Identification of MSU crystals from asymptomatic joints may allow for definite diagnosis in intercritical gout.	84
6. Gout and sepsis can coexist. When septic arthritis is suspected, synovial fluid should be Gram stained and cultured for bacteria even if MSU crystals are identified.	93
7. Serum uric acid concentrations, although the most important risk factor for gout, do not confirm or exclude gout. Many with hyperuricemia do not develop gout, and serum uric acid concentrations during acute attacks can be normal.	95
8. Renal uric acid excretion should be assessed in selected gout patients, especially those with a family history of young-onset gout, onset of gout at younger than 25 years, or those with renal calculi.	72
9. Although radiographs can be useful for differential diagnosis and can show typical features of chronic gout, they are not useful in confirming the diagnosis of early or acute gout.	86
10. Risk factors for gout and comorbidity should be assessed, including features of the metabolic syndrome (obesity, hyperglycemia, hyperlipidemia, hypertension).	93

SOR, strength of recommendation.
Adapted from reference 10.

4. Laboratory tests were ordered for E.J., and the results are SUA of 7.5 mg/dL, BUN of 10 mg/dL, SCr of 1 mg/dL, and a WBC count of 10.2×10^3/mm^3. An x-ray of his elbow shows soft tissue swelling with no evidence of tophi. Does E.J. have gout?

E.J.'s objective and clinical presentation fulfills five of the ACR criteria (i.e., 2, 3, 5, 10, 11) in Table 42-1; however, at least 6 of the 12 criteria must be met to achieve a diagnosis of gout. According to the EULAR propositions (Table 42-2), criteria 1 and 7 are met and consistent with, but not diagnostic

Table 42-3 EULAR Propositions for Gout Management

Propositions	SOR (%)
1. Optimal treatment of gout requires nonpharmacologic and pharmacologic modalities tailored to specific risk factors (SUA levels, prior attacks); clinical phase of gout; and general risk factors (age, comorbidity, drug interactions)	96
2. Patient education and lifestyle modifications (e.g., weight loss if obese, reduced beer and other alcohol consumption) are important.	95
3. Associated comorbidity and risk factors (e.g., hyperlipidemia, HTN, hyperglycemia, obesity, smoking) should be addressed.	91
4. Oral NSAIDs or colchicine are first-line agents for systemic treatment of acute gout. In the absence of contraindications, an NSAID is a convenient and well accepted treatment.	94
5. High doses of colchicine cause side effects and low doses (e.g., 0.5 mg TID) can be sufficient.	83
6. Intra-articular aspiration and injection of a long-acting steroid is an effective and safe treatment for an acute attack.	80
7. Urate lowering therapy is indicated in patients with recurrent acute attacks, arthropathy, tophi, or radiographic changes of gout.	97
8. The therapeutic goal of urate lowering (i.e., SUA less than the saturation point for MSU of 6 mg/dL) is to promote crystal dissolution and prevent crystal formation.	91
9. Allopurinol, an appropriate long-term urate-lowering agent, should be initiated at 100 mg/day and increased by 100 mg every 2–4 weeks, if required. The dose must be adjusted in patients with renal impairment. If toxicity occurs, options include other xanthine oxidase inhibitors, a uricosuric agent, or allopurinol desensitization (in mild rash).	91
10. Uricosuric agents (e.g., probenecid, sulfinpyrazone) can be alternatives to allopurinol in patients with normal renal function, but relatively contraindicated in patients with urolithiasis. Benzbromarone can be used in patients with moderate renal insufficiency, but carries a small risk of hepatotoxicity.	87
11. Prophylaxis against acute attacks during the first months of urate lowering therapy can be achieved by colchicine (0.5–1 mg/day) and/or NSAID (with gastroprotection, if indicated).	90
12. When gout is associated with diuretic therapy, discontinue the diuretic if possible.	88

SOR, strength of recommendation.
Adapted from reference 34.

of, gout. An important difference between the EULAR guidelines and those of the ACR is the emphasis on synovial fluid examination. Item 2 indicates that only "typical" gout presentations such as podagra can be accurately diagnosed without examination of the synovial fluid, and E.J.'s elbow involvement is an atypical presentation. An aspiration of synovial fluid from the inflamed elbow joint fluid would help diagnose gout and rule out infection, although both gout and infection could coexist. Although E.J. is reluctant to undergo this procedure, he relents, and his aspirate is positive for 25,000 WBC/L and for MSU crystals. E.J. now can be considered as having acute gout.

Treatment of Acute Gout

Goals of Therapy

5. What is the primary goal in the treatment of this acute gout attack in E.J.?

The primary goal in the treatment of an acute attack of gout is to relieve pain and inflammation. The immediate goal of therapy should not be aimed at decreasing the SUA concentration with hypouricemic agents such as allopurinol (Zyloprim) or probenecid (Benemid). Patients most likely have been hyperuricemic for several months or years, and it is not necessary to treat the hyperuricemia immediately. Furthermore, a decrease in the serum urate concentration at this time might mobilize urate stores and precipitate yet another acute gouty attack.

Drug Therapy Overview

6. What are the pharmacotherapeutic options for the treatment of E.J.'s acute pain?

Acute gouty arthritis can be effectively treated in most instances by a nonsteroidal anti-inflammatory drug (NSAID), colchicine, or corticosteroids.

NONSTEROIDAL ANTI-INFLAMMATORY DRUGS

Indomethacin (Indocin), naproxen (Naprosyn), and sulindac (Clinoril) are U.S. Food and Drug Administration (FDA)-approved for the treatment of pain associated with acute gout attacks,[35–37] but other nonselective NSAIDs are also effective, including ibuprofen (Motrin),[38] fenoprofen (Nalfon),[39] piroxicam (Feldene),[40,41] fluribiprofen (Ansaid),[42] ketoprofen (Orudis),[43] tolmetin (Tolectin),[44] and meclofenamate (Meclomen).[45] GI bleeding and/or ulceration and inhibition of platelet aggregation are two of the most common serious adverse effects of these nonselective NSAIDs, and both adverse effects compound the risk of bleeding when given concomitantly with anticoagulants (e.g., warfarin). The NSAIDs, which are selective cyclo-oxygenase-2 (COX-2) inhibitors, do not inhibit platelets at normal doses; however, the efficacy of celecoxib (Celebrex), the only COX-2 inhibitor currently available in the United States, has not been evaluated for the treatment of gout. Etoricoxib, a COX-2 inhibitor available outside the United States, has been approved for the treatment of acute gouty arthritis in New Zealand.[46,47] Among the nonselective NSAIDs, ibuprofen is the least likely to cause GI adverse effects and is perhaps the safest nonselective NSAID for use in patients at risk for GI bleeding. Piroxicam and indomethacin are among the worst offenders.[48]

The potential adverse cardiovascular effects of NSAIDs are of concern. In 2005, the FDA issued an advisory requiring all manufacturers of over-the-counter and prescription NSAIDs to alert patients and health care professionals to increased cardiovascular risks (e.g., myocardial infarction, stroke) from selective and nonselective COX-2 inhibitors.[49] NSAIDs can also aggravate HTN, cause renal failure by inhibiting vasodilatory renal prostaglandins, inhibit diuretic-induced increases in renal sodium excretion[50–53], and decrease the hypotensive effect of diuretics and other antihypertensive drugs (e.g., beta-blockers).[54,55] Although hypertensive patients are not likely to experience problems when using NSAIDs for only a few days, three isolated cases of hyperkalemia and renal insufficiency have occurred after indomethacin treatment of gouty arthritis.[56] Patients with CVD and renal insufficiency can be treated for a short duration with nonselective NSAIDs, albeit with much caution. The nonselective NSAIDs are safe for patients with stable, controlled HTN when given for only a few days and with closer monitoring of blood pressure.

CORTICOSTEROIDS

Corticosteroids, effective in the management of an acute gouty attack, are usually considered second-line therapy because of the potential for serious adverse effects and adrenal suppression when used long term and because of the potential for rebound pain when abruptly discontinued.[2,57] If the acute gout episode involves only one or two joints, intra-articular corticosteroid administration could minimize adverse effects. When corticosteroid oral doses equivalent to 30 to 60 mg of prednisone/day are used, doses are tapered over 2 to 3 weeks to minimize the potential for rebound.[2] Corticosteroids are especially useful for elderly patients or those with renal or CVD who cannot tolerate NSAIDs.[2,34,57] Corticosteroid adverse effects (e.g., osteoporosis, myopathy, peptic ulcer disease, central nervous system effects, HTN, predisposition to infections) are not likely with the short courses of treatment for gout attacks. Glucose intolerance, however, can occur with short-term therapy.

COLCHICINE

At one time, colchicine was the agent of choice for the treatment of an acute attack of gout. This drug not only provided symptomatic relief to more than 95% of patients when administered early in the course of an attack of gout, but it also provided diagnostic confirmation because of its relative specificity for relieving only the symptoms of acute gout. Colchicine's mechanism of action is quite unique because it is an inhibitor of microtubule polymerization, which results in inhibition of inflammatory mediators such as cytokines and chemokines.[58] It is only indicated for the treatment of gout.[59] For the fully developed acute attack, the traditional dose of colchicine has been one or two 0.5- to 0.6-mg tablets initially (only 0.6-mg tablets are available in the United States today), followed by 0.5 to 0.6 mg hourly or every other hour, until joint pain was relieved or GI effects (i.e., diarrhea, nausea, vomiting) intervened. A colchicine 0.5-mg (or 0.6-mg) TID regimen until symptoms resolve has been successful in treating patients who do not respond to, or cannot use, NSAIDs or corticosteroids.[34,60] The dose of colchicine must not exceed 6 mg/gout episode because of significant adverse effects and a narrow therapeutic index.

INTRAVENOUS COLCHICINE

Colchicine is available for intravenous (IV) injection for patients who cannot tolerate oral colchicine, but IV colchicine for *acute gout* is no longer recommended because of a potential for bone marrow suppression, myocardial injury, muscle paralysis, acute organ failure, and fatalities.[57] The usual initial colchicine IV dose of 2 mg is instilled slowly over 2 to 5 minutes directly into a large vein that has normal saline infusing. It must not be administered subcutaneously or intramuscularly because it can cause extensive tissue necrosis, and caution must be undertaken with IV infusions to prevent extravasation into surrounding tissue. An IV dose of 0.5 mg can be repeated every 6 hours until relief of pain, but no more than 4 mg per 24 hours or 4 mg per acute episode of gout.

OPIATE ANALGESICS

When an occasional patient requires more pain control, a dose or two of a narcotic analgesic can be a reasonable adjunct to blunt the pain of acute gouty arthritis while awaiting the apparent benefits of NSAIDs or corticosteroids. Most patients, however, generally experience benefits from NSAIDs and corticosteroids soon after a dose of either of these anti-inflammatory drugs.

Choice of Agent

7. What therapeutic intervention would be most appropriate for E.J. at this time?

An NSAID is first-line therapy for the acute treatment of gout, and although E.J. does have HTN and metabolic syndrome, his renal function is normal. Assuming his blood pressure is adequately controlled, a short course of ibuprofen 800 mg now and Q 8 hr for 3 days is appropriate. The ibuprofen should be prescribed on a scheduled basis rather than "as needed" to reduce inflammation and prevent breakthrough pain. The dose of 2,400 mg/day does not exceed the maximum recommended dose of 3,200 mg/day.

8. If E.J. were 72-years-old instead of 52 and/or his BP was 160/96 mm Hg, what therapeutic option would be appropriate?

These patient-specific parameters are relative contraindications or precautions for the use of NSAIDs for the treatment of acute gout so alternative treatments should be considered. Because E.J.'s pain is monoarticular (his elbow), an intra-articular dose of corticosteroid could be administered, but the possibility of bone necrosis from intra-articular corticosteroids would probably result in the choice of oral prednisone, which could be administered and tapered over 10 to 21 days. As an alternative, oral colchicine could be considered. IV colchicine should not be considered, and if E.J. were unable to tolerate oral therapies, then parenteral or intra-articular corticosteroids should be administered.

Management Guidelines

Gout is one of few rheumatologic diseases that can be treated successfully and even cured in many patients.[61] However, despite the availability of adequate pharmacologic interventions, a survey of rheumatologists and internists in the United States found that drug therapy is often not used based on scientific evidence for both acute and chronic gout.[62] Furthermore, in a survey of Chinese physicians, most agreed that synovial fluid aspiration from a joint in a search for crystals should be performed for a definitive diagnosis, but such joint aspiration was rarely undertaken. A comparable survey of physicians in the United States might reach similar conclusions. Also, oral colchicine was considered first-line therapy by 77% of physicians in China, which is contrary to current management guidelines.[63] In consideration of these issues, the EULAR gout task force developed recommendations for the management of gout (Table 42-3) and the percentage consensus for a given recommendation.[34]

Nonpharmacologic Interventions

ICE

The benefit of ice application to the affected joint in acute gouty arthritis should not be overlooked. In a small randomized study, the application of ice to an affected joint significantly reduced the pain of a gouty attack when used in conjunction with oral steroids or colchicine.[64]

ALCOHOL CONSUMPTION

Excessive alcohol intake has been known to be a risk factor for acute gout episodes since the time of Hippocrates[5]; however, lead was also a contributory factor when it was used as a flavoring agent for wine in early Roman times. Beer was also believed to be more problematic for gout than other alcoholic beverages because of its high purine content; however, current thinking is that the quantity of alcohol consumed in the 24 hours prior to an acute attack is more important than the type of beverage consumed.[65] Moderation in alcohol consumption should be advocated.

DIET MODIFICATION

Diet has a twofold effect on the epidemiology of gout. First, obese patients are at a greater risk of developing elevated SUA levels, and gout might, in part, be related to insulin resistance of obesity.[5] Weight reduction via a caloric- and carbohydrate-restricted diet has been associated with decreased SUA and frequency of gout attacks.[66] Furthermore, in a prospective, longitudinal study of male health professionals, weight gain was strongly associated with an increased risk of gout, and weight loss was associated with a decreased risk.[67]

Second, much of the uric acid produced daily comes from metabolism of food. The excessive dietary intake of purine-rich foods, without a concomitant increase in urinary excretion, can lead to elevated serum urate concentrations.[5,6] However, the type of protein and purine-rich foods that are detrimental, and the true impact of these foods on the incidence of increased SUA and gout episodes, are controversial issues.[68,69] Using the NHANES-III survey (Third National Health and Nutrition Examination Survey) data, diets rich in dairy protein were noted to be helpful in preventing elevated SUA levels, while diets high in meat and seafood were detrimental.[68] Interestingly, in that survey, the type of protein was more important than the total protein intake. The more yogurt or milk servings consumed per day, the lower the SUA.

Delay of Hypouricemic Therapy

9. Why should (or should not) allopurinol be prescribed for E.J. before he leaves the emergency department?

Hypouricemic therapy should be initiated only when patients with gout have frequent acute attacks, urate tophi, or evidence of urate nephropathy (e.g., uric acid stones or renal damage). If these indications are absent, hypouricemic drug therapy should await the natural course of events because nothing is lost by waiting. The acute attack can be treated when it appears and usually resolves within days. Long-term hypouricemic medications should not be started for E.J. at this time because criteria for therapy (see EULAR proposition 7 in Table 42-3) are not met, and initiation of urate-lowering therapy during an acute episode can mobilize urate from tissues and compound the problem. E.J. should not be treated with hypouricemic drugs at this time.

HYPERURICEMIA

Chronic Gout

10. E.J. has experienced about four to five acute gouty arthritis attacks, which were treated successfully with ibuprofen over the past year. His HTN, metabolic syndrome, and obese condition have all improved. On a routine clinic visit, his SUA is 7.5 mg/dL, and his renal function and CBC are normal. Would it be appropriate to initiate hypouricemic therapy at this time?

Drug therapy to lower SUA is warranted for patients who have recurrent gout attacks, arthropathy, tophi, or radiographic changes related to gout (Table 42-3).[34] Because E.J. has experienced several episodes of acute gout, hypouricemic therapy consideration is appropriate. The decision to begin hypouricemic therapy, however, should be preceded by a consideration of whether *drug-induced hyperuricemia* could be a mitigating factor.

Drug-Induced Hyperuricemia

A patient's complete medication list should be reviewed to rule out drug-induced hyperuricemia (Table 42-4) before adding a medication to decrease SUA. Perhaps the only treatment needed would be to discontinue the offending agent. Until recently, the mechanisms by which many drugs induce hyperuricemia were unknown. A urate transporter, URAT-1, is now believed to be the primary protein responsible for reabsorption of urate into the systemic circulation from the lumen of the proximal tubule of the nephron.[70] URAT-1 also appears to be the site at which some drugs (e.g., losartan, probenecid) inhibit urate reabsorption, and where other drugs (e.g., pyrazinamide, nicotinic acid) stimulate urate reabsorption and, thereby, increase SUA.[2] As the role of URAT-1 and other transporters are better understood, new drug therapies may be discovered.

DIURETICS

The association of hyperuricemia and diuretics is well known, and the mechanism, although not fully elucidated, is likely secondary to diuretic-induced sodium and water excretion, which in turn increases reabsorption of uric acid in the proximal tubule.[71] The importance of diuretic-induced hyperuricemia, however, is now somewhat more controversial. When variables in addition to diuretic use were controlled in a study of patients with HTN, heart failure, and myocardial infarction, the risk of gout was increased in the hypertensive patients more than the risk of gout in patients on diuretics.[72] In a case cross-over survey, however, thiazides and loop diuretic use in the 48 hours before an acute gout attack had increased their risk for this attack.[73] Although diuretics increase SUA concentrations, the antioxidant properties of uric acid could be beneficial and perhaps sufficient to account for their favorable outcomes in the ALLHAT study.[74] Because diuretics are associated with hyperuricemia in both hypertensive and nonhypertensive patients, and because hyperuricemia has an association with acute gout

Table 42-4 Drugs Associated With Hyperuricemia

Drug	*Mechanism*	*Comments*
Certain antiretrovirals[121–125]	Catabolic effect; NRTIs may increase urate through mitochondrial toxicity	NRTIs: Uric acid blood increases of 0.5–5 mg/dL have occurred in patients receiving >9.6 mg/kg/day of didanosine. Stavudine also was associated with increased uric acid. PIs: Have been associated with elevated uric acid. Ritonavir and ritonavir boosting have been associated with gout.
Cyclosporine[126,127]	Decreased urate renal clearance, either via a tubular mechanism or decrease in GFR	Cyclosporine-induced hyperuricemia may cause gout in patients with risk factors (renal dysfunction, concurrent diuretics, and male gender).
Cytotoxic chemotherapy[85]	Rapid cell lysis	Occurs primarily with lymphomas and leukemias. Uric acid nephropathy, acute renal failure, and nephrolithiasis can result.
Diuretics[128–132]	Secondary to volume contraction and increased uric acid reabsorption in the proximal tubules for all diuretics; thiazides may also competitively inhibit proximal tubular secretion	Dose- and duration-dependent elevations in uric acid
Ethambutol[133]	Decreased urate renal clearance	Hyperuricemia and gout have been demonstrated. A majority of patients were receiving 20 mg/kg/day orally.
Ethanol[65,134]	Increased uric acid production due to adenine nucleotide turnover, lead-tainted moonshine and/or high purine content in some alcoholic beverages, such as beer	Associated with increased uric acid and acute gout. Even a light-to-moderate amount triggers recurrent gout attacks within 24 hours.
Filgrastim[135]	Increased WBC production	Transient effect, seen more often with higher doses (30–60 mg/kg/day).
Isotretinoin[136]	Hypervitaminosis A	Hyperuricemia and rare gout cases have been reported.
Levodopa[137]	Inhibition of urate excretion	Patients taking therapeutic doses have experienced hyperuricemia and gout. Secondarily, interference with colorimetric assay of uric acid may contribute a false-positive increment.
Niacin[138,139]	Decreases excretion of urate	Hyperuricemia and gout have occurred.
Pancreatic enzymes: pancreatin and pancrelipase[140]	Ingestion of pancreatic enzyme products having high purine content.	Hyperuricemia, hyperuricosuria, and uric acid crystalluria have occurred with high dosages.
Pyrazinamide[141,142]	Inhibition of renal tubular urate secretion	Hyperuricemia is more common with daily than with intermittent administration. Gouty attacks have occurred in those with a history of gout. Asymptomatic hyperuricemia was the only manifestation seen in one trial of pediatric patients.
Ribavirin and interferon[143]	Mechanism unclear; commonly associated with hemolysis	Nephrolithiasis developed in a patient with diabetes and hypertension. Hyperuricemia noted in 24% of those receiving ribavirin with interferon.
Aspirin (low dose)[87]	Inhibition of proximal tubular secretion of urate	Doses <1 g/day cause hyperuricemia.
Tacrolimus[144,145]	Reduced urate excretion	Associated with hyperuricemia and cases of gout; however, two prior case reports demonstrated resolution of polyarticular gout after switching cyclosporine to tacrolimus.
Teriparatide[146]	Mechanism unknown	Elevated uric acid levels, mainly with higher doses and with moderate renal impairment, but no association with increased gout, arthralgia or nephrolithiasis.
Theophylline[147,148]	Interference with uric acid assay	False-positive elevation with automated Bittner adapted method. Interference does not appear to occur with phosphotungstate assay method.

NRTI, nucleoside reverse transcriptase inhibitors; PI, protease inhibitors; GFR, glomerular filtration rate; WBC, white blood cell.

attacks, most clinicians would discontinue the diuretic, irrespective of possible ancillary benefits from hyperuricemia if alternatives to the diuretics are available and appropriate for a particular patient.[34] The hyperuricemic effect of diuretics is dose related.[75]

Goal of Hypouricemic Therapy

The general goals for lowering serum concentrations of uric acid are the elimination of acute gout attacks and the mobilization of urate crystals from soft tissue. The SUA concentration in a patient who has clinical gout should be decreased to

<6 mg/dL, which is below the saturation point for monosodium urate (NB: a 1 mg/dL change in SUA is equivalent to about 60 μmol/L SI units).[34]

Uric Acid Urine Quantification

Urinary uric acid excretion can be determined by measuring a 24-hour collection of urine to ascertain whether the patient overproduces or underexcretes uric acid. In theory, an "overproducer" should be treated with a drug that inhibits production of uric acid (e.g., xanthine oxidase inhibitors), and an "underexcretor" should be treated with a drug that increases excretion of uric acid. Because both groups of patients usually respond to xanthine oxidase inhibitors, drugs such as allopurinol have become the first-line agents for the treatment of hyperuricemia. Alternatively, urinary uric acid overproducers can be identified by use of uric acid:creatinine (or creatinine clearance [Cl_{Cr}]) ratios based on spot-midmorning serum and urine samples.[76,77]

Drug Therapy of Hyperuricemia

XANTHINE OXIDASE INHIBITORS

Allopurinol

Allopurinol (Xyloprim), the only available xanthine oxidase inhibitor in the United States, inhibits the production of uric acid and thereby decreases SUA concentrations. As first-line therapy of hyperuricemia, allopurinol should be initiated at a 100 mg once daily dose and the dose increased by 100 mg/day increments every 2 to 4 weeks until the SUA is at the desired goal of <6 mg/dL (Table 42-3). The ability of allopurinol to lower SUA is dose related: the higher the dose of allopurinol, the greater the decrease in uric acid serum concentration. An allopurinol dose of 200 to 300 mg/day is usually needed to normalize hyperuricemia in patients with mild disease and larger doses of 400 to 600 mg/day are needed for those with more severe disease.[78] Allopurinol doses should be adjusted for patients with renal dysfunction to minimize the potential for toxicity; however, patients with decreased doses might not achieve adequate uric acid suppression if SUA concentrations are not appropriately monitored.[79] Allopurinol doses for patients with renal insufficiency should be based on recommended guidelines for varying degrees of renal insufficiency, adjusted according to periodic evaluations of SUA concentrations, and appreciated for the increased association of adverse events, including hypersensitivity reactions, in patients with renal dysfunction.

Febuxostat

Febuxostat, a nonpurine xanthine oxidase inhibitor, is currently in Phase III trials and awaiting FDA approval for use in the management of hyperuricemia. Febuxostat is more selective than allopurinol for xanthine oxidase and does not inhibit other enzymes involved in purine and pyrimidine metabolism. In a double-blind, randomized, 52-week multicenter trial, oral febuxostat (80 or 120 mg/day) was significantly more effective than allopurinol (300 mg/day) in decreasing SUA concentrations from >8 mg/dL to an end point of <6 mg/dL.[80] It is not known if allopurinol would have been more effective if titrated further. Adverse effects were similar across all treatment groups and consisted primarily of mild to moderate diarrhea, headaches, abnormal liver function tests, and joint- or muscle-related nonspecific symptoms. During the first 8 weeks of febuxostat treatment, naproxen or colchicine was provided concurrently as prophylaxis against flares of acute gout attacks. Nevertheless, more patients in the higher-dose febuxostat treatment arm discontinued therapy because of the greater prevalence of gout flares and adverse events. The role of febuxostat for the management of hyperuricemia needs further study.[81]

RASBURICASE

Uricase, an enzyme endogenous in many animal species other than humans, converts uric acid to allantoin, which is much more soluble than uric acid and, therefore, more readily excreted into urine. Rasburicase (Elitek), a recombinant urate oxidase enzyme, similarly enhances the solubilized uric acid metabolic product into the urine. It is now approved for the management of hyperuricemia in children who are susceptible to hyperuricemia resulting from chemotherapy and tumor lysis. Rasburicase is especially useful in children with leukemia, lymphoma, or solid tumor malignancies about to undergo cytotoxic therapy. In a multicenter, randomized trial of 52 children with leukemia or lymphoma, IV rasburicase (0.2 mg/kg once daily), during initial chemotherapy, decreased serum urate concentrations more effectively and with a quicker onset of action than oral allopurinol (median doses of 300 mg/day).[82] The rasburicase dose (0.15 or 0.20 mg/kg) should be infused over a 30-minute period once daily for 5 days for a single course of treatment, and about 4 to 24 hours before the initiation of chemotherapy.[83] Rasburicase should be reserved for patients who cannot undertake allopurinol therapy and who are at high risk for tumor lysis syndrome (see Chapter 90). Although it is not currently approved by the FDA for use in adults, rasburicase has been shown to be safe and effective for the prophylaxis or treatment of hyperuricemia in adults with leukemia or lymphoma.[84,85] This drug is significantly more costly than allopurinol.

Rasburicase is contraindicated (a black box warning in the labeling) for patients with glucose-6-phosphate dehydrogenase deficiency, or a known history of hypersensitivity, anaphylactic, or hemolytic reactions. It also has been associated with fever, neutropenia, respiratory distress, sepsis, and mucositis. This drug can interfere with uric acid assays when a blood sample is left in room temperature and has been associated with spuriously low uric acid serum concentrations in laboratory reports.

URICOSURIC AGENTS

The uricosuric agents, probenecid (Benemid) and sulfinpyrazone (Anturane), are alternatives to allopurinol for patients who are unable to tolerate allopurinol (Table 42-3).[34] These uricosurics should not be administered to patients with impaired renal function or urolithiasis.

Probenecid

Probenecid is well absorbed orally, and plasma concentrations peak within 2 to 4 hours. Its biological half-life is 6 to 12 hours, and its active metabolites extend the duration of action. The usual initial dose of probenecid (250 mg twice daily for the first week of therapy) can be increased to 500 mg twice a day. If necessary, the dose can be increased further to 2 g/day. Uricosuric therapy should begin with small doses because the excretion of large amounts of uric acid increases the risk of urate stone formation in the kidney. High fluid intake to maintain urine flow of at least 2 L/day also minimizes renal stone formation. This gradual approach to the initiation of hypouricemic therapy also decreases the likelihood of precipitating an acute attack of gout.

Drug Interactions. Probenecid inhibits secretion of penicillins into the renal tubule, and thereby prolongs the serum half-life of penicillin and increases penicillin serum concentrations. Probenecid can also compete with salicylates for renal tubular transport, but its interactions with salicylates involve several mechanisms.[86] Two 300-mg tablets of aspirin every 6 hours can completely antagonize the uricosuric effects of 2 g of probenecid. Doses of salicylate that do not produce serum salicylate levels of >5 mg/dL do not significantly affect probenecid uricosuria.[55] Therefore, low-dose aspirin for cardioprotection is unlikely to interfere with probenecid therapy. Interestingly, high-dose aspirin (e.g., >1 g) has uricosuric activity of its own.[87] Acetaminophen (Tylenol) and NSAIDs do not interfere with probenecid, and are reliable alternatives for antipyresis and mild analgesia in patients taking uricosuric agents.

Sulfinpyrazone and Benzbromarone

Sulfinpyrazone (Anturane), another effective uricosuric agent, inhibits the tubular secretion of uric acid at low doses and inhibits the tubular reabsorption of uric acid at usual therapeutic doses. As with probenecid, therapy should be initiated slowly and the dose increased gradually. Benzbromarone, another uricosuric agent, is not available in the United States because of its association with hepatotoxicity.

ASCORBIC ACID

Vitamin C has a hypouricemic effect that is believed to be mediated by competition with urate for renal tubular reabsorption.[88] In a study of 184 healthy, nonsmoking adults, ascorbic acid 500 mg daily for 2 months significantly decreased SUA concentrations.[89] Overall, ascorbic acid reduced the SUA concentration a mean of 0.5 mg/dL (range, 0.3–0.7), but the decrease in subjects with baseline SUA levels of >7 mg/dL was a mean of 1.5 mg/dL. This would have brought those patients' SUA below goal, if they required treatment for their hyperuricemia. Further investigation into the potential benefits of vitamin C in the treatment of hyperuricemia either alone or as adjunct therapy is needed.

Choice of Agent

11. E.J.'s hydrochlorothiazide was discontinued about 4 weeks ago, but his SUA only has decreased from 7.5 to 7.2 mg/dL. As a result, allopurinol is to be initiated. What dose of allopurinol should be prescribed for E.J., and what parameters should be monitored for efficacy and toxicity?

Allopurinol 100 mg daily should be started, and a SUA should be obtained no earlier than 2 weeks after the initiation of therapy. If urate-lowering therapy is successful, treatment should continue for a long period of time before attempting a trial to discontinue the allopurinol. An acute attack of gout is not a catastrophic event and perhaps the future discontinuation of allopurinol is a worthwhile risk to undertake in an effort to minimize potential future difficulties when any drug is taken over a lifetime.

ONSET OF EFFECTS

SUA levels usually begin to fall within 1 to 2 days after initiation of allopurinol therapy; maximal uric acid suppression in response to a given dosage usually requires 7 to 10 days.[78,90] Clinically observable improvement takes longer. After approximately 6 months, one should observe a gradual decrease in the size of established urate tophi, as well as the absence of new tophaceous deposits if these were present. A baseline SUA should be obtained, and then 2 to 4 weeks after onset of therapy, and after every dose change until SUA is maintained at goal (<6 mg/dL).

ONCE-DAILY DOSING

Allopurinol has a half-life of <2 hours, but its active metabolite, oxypurinol, has a serum half-life of 13 to 18 hours; therefore, once-daily dosing is effective. In renal impairment, oxypurinol accumulates and dosage adjustments should be considered.[91,92]

ADVERSE EFFECTS

Allopurinol generally is well tolerated, with few significant adverse effects. Occasionally, GI intolerance, bone marrow suppression, renal or hepatic toxicities, and mild skin rash are reported. Hyperuricemic patients receiving allopurinol might be more susceptible to "ampicillin rash"[93] and to interactions with other drugs (Table 42-5). Allopurinol's interaction with azathioprine is well documented and is of major clinical significance; however, in one survey of 24 transplant patients taking both drugs, the dose of azathioprine was decreased in only 14 of 24 patients.[94] This survey exposes one weakness in our understanding of how best to adjust azathioprine dosages despite the widely acknowledged need for dosage adjustment.[14]

Whether allopurinol causes cataracts is controversial. In one study, allopurinol use for longer than 2 years was associated with the formation of cataracts.[95] This adverse reaction has been attributed to above-average exposure to sunlight that enhances the photobinding of allopurinol in the lens, resulting in cataracts.[95] This report disputes the finding of the Boston Collaborative Drug Surveillance Program that any association between allopurinol and cataracts was coincidental.[96] In addition, a subsequent study found no evidence to confirm a higher risk of cataract formation in allopurinol users than in nonusers.[97]

HYPERSENSITIVITY REACTIONS

Of the adverse drug reactions sometimes encountered with allopurinol, hypersensitivity-type reactions have been the most notorious. These generally present as mildly erythematous, dusky red purpuric, or scaly maculopapular skin eruptions. When allopurinol is discontinued promptly, these hypersensitivity reactions should subside without sequelae. However, the continued administration of allopurinol to hypersensitive individuals has resulted in progression of these symptoms and several fatalities.[98–107] The cutaneous reactions often progressed to include necrosis of the skin and mucous membranes, exfoliative dermatitis, Stevens-Johnson syndrome, or toxic epidermal necrolysis. Hepatomegaly, jaundice, hepatic necrosis, and renal impairment often accompanied these reactions.[108] The hepatic and renal changes were usually reversible when the drug was discontinued, and these organ failures were not correlated with any one cutaneous reaction pattern. Patients with renal insufficiency, those receiving thiazide diuretics, and

Table 42-5 Allopurinol Drug Interactions

Major Documentation

Azathioprine (Imuran). Metabolized to 6-mercaptopurine (6-MP) and then to inactive metabolites by xanthine oxidase. Allopurinol inhibition of xanthine oxidase ↑ the serum concentration of 6-MP and the risk of bone marrow depression. When azathioprine (or 6-MP) is used concurrently with allopurinol, use extreme caution, and the azathioprine dose should be ↓ to one fourth of the recommended dose.
Mercaptopurine (Purinethol). See Azathioprine.

Moderate Documentation

ACE Inhibitors. Specifically, captopril and enalapril can predispose patients to severe allopurinol hypersensitivity reactions (e.g., Stevens-Johnson syndrome). Concurrent renal impairment can be an important variable.
Anticoagulants. Occasionally, patients on oral anticoagulants and allopurinol develop enhanced anticoagulant effects; however, this interaction is unpredictable and primarily based on isolated case reports.
Cyclophosphamide. Allopurinol may ↑ cyclophosphamide-induced bone marrow depression based on epidemiologic data.

Anecdotal Documentation

Ampicillin. Concomitant allopurinol might increase ampicillin rash based on epidemiologic data.
Antacids. Aluminum hydroxide inhibited the GI absorption of allopurinol in three patients on hemodialysis; however, the interaction can be avoided by the administration of allopurinol ≥3 hours before or 6 hours after aluminum hydroxide.
Chlorpropamide. Allopurinol or its metabolites might compete with chlorpropamide for renal tubular secretion and can result in an ↑ chlorpropamide effect.
Cyclosporine. Allopurinol may ↑ cyclosporine concentrations and toxicity based on case reports.
Phenytoin. Allopurinol seemed to inhibit the metabolism of phenytoin in one patient.
Probenecid. Allopurinol can inhibit the metabolism of probenecid, and probenecid can enhance the renal elimination of the active oxypurinol.
Theophylline. Allopurinol in high doses can ↑ mean theophylline AUC by approximately 27% and half-life by 25%; clearance can be ↓ approximately 21%. An active metabolite (1-methylxanthine) also can accumulate.[149,150]
Vidarabine. An active metabolite of vidarabine is metabolized by xanthine oxidase, and accumulation of this metabolite can ↑ neurotoxicity.

ACE, angiotensin-converting enzyme; GI, gastrointestinal; AUC, area under the concentration–time curve.
Adapted from reference 55.

those with chronic alcoholism or severe liver disease have been the most commonly afflicted with this syndrome.

The toxic syndrome generally appeared within the first 5 weeks of therapy; however, it has appeared as part of a delayed hypersensitivity reaction as late as 25 months after the initiation of therapy.[107] The mechanism by which this toxicity syndrome occurs is unknown. The cutaneous reaction and renal failure have been consistent with a diffuse systemic vasculitis, and the nonfatal cases did not improve until large steroid doses were instituted, despite the discontinuation of allopurinol. Biopsy specimens from patients provide support for the premise that vasculitis results from an immune hypersensitivity reaction to allopurinol.[98,101,104,108] Although no specific mechanism or causative agent producing this toxicity has been identified, the accumulation of allopurinol or a metabolite is postulated to be a primary factor, especially because 80% of patients with this syndrome had significantly impaired renal function before the initiation of allopurinol.[109] In one particular incident, allopurinol serum concentrations were 50 times normal values.[107] Therefore, dose adjustments of allopurinol should be considered in renal impairment, but especially in patients who develop acute renal failure or have worsening renal function over time. Patients who have been titrated on allopurinol to goal SUA level, have stable but reduced renal function, and are tolerating the drug do not necessarily need a dosage decrease.

Patients who have recovered from an allopurinol hypersensitivity syndrome should avoid the future use of this drug because most will probably experience a similar reaction on re-exposure. However, a few hypersensitive individuals may tolerate low dosages (50–100 mg/day). If there is no reaction after a few days, the allopurinol dosage can be increased gradually. Nevertheless, severe toxic reactions have been produced by doses of allopurinol as low as 1 mg. Some hypersensitive patients have been desensitized with daily doses as small as 0.05 mg that were increased gradually over a period of 30 days. Although the cautious reintroduction of allopurinol through graded oral doses can be attempted in patients with cutaneous rash who have failed other options,[110] the risk of serious hypersensitivity is significant, and an alternative agent would be appropriate.

PROPHYLAXIS AGAINST ACUTE GOUT

Symptoms of acute gout might be slightly exacerbated during the first 6 weeks of allopurinol or uricosuric therapy because of uric acid mobilization from tissues. Concurrent administration of an NSAID or low-dose daily colchicine (0.5–1 mg daily) should be prescribed for the first few months of urate-lowering therapy to prevent acute gout attacks (see proposition 11 in Table 42-3).[34] If a uricosuric drug is preferred, a combination product (i.e., ColBenemid) is available that contains both colchicine and probenecid. If this is used, the ColBenemid should be replaced with the single drug entity (i.e., probenecid) after a few months because the colchicine component of this fixed-combination product is only needed short term.

Comorbid Conditions

Dyslipidemia

12. L.M. is a 57-year-old man who presents to his family physician for a regular checkup. He is currently controlled on allopurinol 300 mg/day for the management of hyperuricemia. For his dyslipidemia, L.M. takes simvastatin (Zocor) 40 mg/day. Although his low-density lipoprotein (LDL) is at goal of <130 mg/dL, he requires further lowering of his non–high-density lipoprotein (non-HDL) cholesterol (goal of <160 mg/dL). What would be the best option to consider in this patient?

In addition to therapeutic lifestyle changes, fibrates (i.e., gemfibrozil, fenofibrate) or niacin are effective in lowering total cholesterol, LDL, and triglycerides. These drugs can also increase the beneficial HDL. A fibrate or niacin can also be used in combination with this patient's current simvastatin. However, with a history of gout and hyperuricemia, a fibrate would be preferred over niacin because niacin can induce hyperuricemia (Table 42-4). Specifically, fenofibrate has been shown to decrease uric acid serum concentrations and could be beneficial in this dyslipidemic patient with a history of gout; however, the selection of a medication to manage dyslipidemia or other comorbid conditions also involves other clinical variables that might be equally applicable.[34,111,112] Fenofibrate modestly increases renal urate excretion.[88]

Hypertension

13. Because one of the first-line agents for the treatment of HTN, thiazide diuretics, is known to increase SUA, what other antihypertensives might be particularly beneficial for hyperuricemic patients?

Both amlodipine and losartan have positive effects on SUA levels. Amlodipine, a calcium channel blocker, decreased serum urate levels by increasing glomerular filtration rate in a study of renal transplant patients taking cyclosporine.[113] Losartan (Cozaar), an angiotensin II receptor blocker (ARB), appears to increase renal excretion of uric acid by interacting with the URAT-1 protein in the proximal tubule of the nephron.[2] When used with diuretics, it appears to alleviate the hyperuricemic effect of the diuretic.[88] This does not seem to be a class effect of ARB's because, in one study, patients on losartan achieved significantly lower SUA concentrations than an irbesartan-treated group.[114] Some advocate losartan for patients with hyperuricemia.[34] Because both fenofibrate and losartan have hypouricemic effects and often patients with hyperuricemia have HTN and dyslipidemia as comorbid conditions, the use of these two drugs in combination is of potential benefit under appropriate circumstances. In one study of five healthy male patients, concurrent daily losartan 100 mg and fenofibrate 300 mg decreased SUA concentrations by a mean of about 1 mg/dL (53.6 mol/L SI units) compared to the decrease during treatment alone with these drugs.[111] If further studies show promise, some patients with hyperuricemia might be managed better by selecting drugs to manage comorbid conditions rather than requiring the use of the more traditional hypouricemic agents.

Asymptomatic Hyperuricemia

14. T.M., a 50-year-old man, is seen by his physician for a routine evaluation. His physical examination is unremarkable, and his laboratory evaluations are all within normal limits except for a SUA concentration of 9.5 mg/dL, which is noted on a basic metabolic panel. Should this hyperuricemia be treated?

Individuals with high SUA levels are more likely to develop acute gouty arthritis than normouricemic individuals, and the magnitude of the risk increases with increasing degrees of hyperuricemia. Nevertheless, it would be excessive to treat all hyperuricemic individuals with uric acid–lowering medications for a lifetime solely to prevent acute attacks of gouty arthritis. A large percentage of hyperuricemic patients may never experience an acute attack of gout.[115] If an attack should occur, it can be treated easily within 48 to 72 hours, and after the acute episode has subsided, uric acid–lowering medications can then be considered.

The key issue in the treatment of hyperuricemia concerns the effect of uric acid on renal function. Renal disease was commonly associated with gout, and renal failure was believed to be the eventual cause of death in as many as 25% of gouty patients. Thus, treatment of asymptomatic hyperuricemia is justifiable if renal disease is prevented. However, this renal damage was noted to occur in a setting that included HTN, diabetes, renal vascular disease, glomerulonephritis, pyelonephritis, renal calculi, or some other cause of primary nephropathy independent of gout.[116] In fact, the coexistence of gout and renal insufficiency without HTN is so rare that its presence should raise the suspicion of chronic lead toxicity.[23,117] Therefore, the consensus now seems to be that hyperuricemia by itself has no deleterious effect on renal function.[118,119] Considering the financial costs, risks of adverse drug reactions, and practical considerations such as patient compliance, drug treatment of asymptomatic hyperuricemia is difficult to justify.[115]

The relationship of hyperuricemia to HTN in individuals who have not experienced gout was studied prospectively in 124 hyperuricemic subjects. None of these patients had evidence of gout, HTN, or cardiovascular, renal, or other diseases. After 10 years, 22.5% of these individuals with "asymptomatic hyperuricemia" had developed HTN, and 5.4% had developed atherosclerotic heart disease. The incidences of HTN and atherosclerotic heart disease in the control group were 2.1% and 0.5%, respectively.[120] Atherosclerosis and HTN apparently were more serious problems in this population than renal disease. Although hyperuricemia may represent an important risk factor for the development of CVD,[18] the evidence is not sufficiently compelling to justify the treatment of asymptomatic hyperuricemia at this time.

REFERENCES

1. Terkeltaub R et al. Recent developments in our understanding of the renal basis of hyperuricemia and the development of novel antihyperuricemic therapeutics. Arthritis Res Ther 2006;8(Suppl): S4.
2. Teng GG et al. Pathophysiology, clinical presentation and treatment of gout. Drugs 2006;66:1547.
3. Wortmann RL, Kelley WN. Gout and hyperuricemia. In: Harris ED Jr. et al., eds. Kelley's Textbook of Rheumatology. 7th ed. Philadelphia: Elsevier Science; 2005:1981.
4. Lee SJ, Terkeltaub RA. New developments in clinically relevant mechanisms and treatment of hyperuricemia. Curr Rheum Rep 2006;8:224.
5. Fam AG. Gout, diet, and the insulin resistance syndrome. J Rheum 2002;29:1350.
6. Choi HK et al. Purine-rich foods, dairy and protein intake, and the risk of gout in men. N Engl J Med 2004;350:1093.
7. Saag KG, Choi H. Epidemiology, risk factors, and lifestyle modifications for gout. Arthritis Res Ther 2006;8(Suppl):S2.
8. Agudelo CA, Wise CM. Crystal-associated arthritis in the elderly. Rheum Dis Clin North Am 2000;26:527.
9. Hall AP et al. Epidemiology of gout and hyperuricemia: a long-term population study. Am J Med 1967;42:27.
10. Zhang W et al. EULAR evidence based recommendations for gout. Part 1: diagnosis. Report of a task force of the standing committee for international clinical studies including therapeutics (ESCISIT). Ann Rheum Dis 2006;65:1301.
11. Simkin PA. The pathogenesis of podagra. Ann Intern Med 1977;86:230.
12. Simkin PA, Pizzorno JE. Trans-synovial exchange of small molecules in normal human subjects. J Appl Physiol 1974;36:581.
13. Simkin PA. Synovial permeability in rheumatoid arthritis. Arthritis Rheum 1979;22:689.
14. Simkin PA. Gout and hyperuricemia. Curr Opin Rheum 1997;9:268.
15. Hadler NM et al. Acute polyarticular gout. Am J Med 1974;56:715.

16. Hermann G, Bloch C. Gout. In: Taveras JM, ed. Radiology: Diagnosis, Imaging, Intervention. Philadelphia: JB Lippincott; 1994:1.
17. Saag KG, Choi H. Epidemiology, risk factors, and lifestyle modifications for gout. Arthritis Res Ther 2006;8(Suppl.1):S2.
18. Abbott RD et al. Gout and coronary heart disease: the Framingham study. J Clin Epidemiol 1988;41:237.
19. Baker JF et al. Serum uric acid and cardiovascular disease: recent developments, and where do they leave us? Am J Med 2005;118:816.
20. Fam AG. Gout, diet, and the insulin resistance syndrome. J Rheum 2002;29:1350.
21. Brady HR et al. Acute renal failure. In: Brenner BM et al., eds. Brenner and Rector's The Kidney. 7th ed. Philadelphia: Saunders; 2007:1261.
22. Sharpe CR. A case-control study of alcohol consumption and drinking behaviour in patients with acute gout. Can Med Assoc J 1984;131:563.
23. Batuman V et al. The role of lead in gout nephropathy. N Engl J Med 1981;304:520.
24. Lin JL et al. Environmental lead exposure and urate excretion in the general population. Am J Med 2002;113:563.
25. Cardenosa G, Deluca SA. Radiographic features of gout. Am Fam Physician 1990;4:539.
26. Bomalaski JS et al. Monosodium urate crystals in the knee joints of patients with asymptomatic nontophaceous gout. Arthritis Rheum 1986;29:1480.
27. Abeles M, Urman JD. Acute gouty arthritis: the diagnostic importance of aspirating more than one involved joint. JAMA 1977;238:2526.
28. Schumacher HR et al. Acute gouty arthritis without urate crystals identified on initial examination of synovial fluid: report on nine patients. Arthritis Rheum 1975;18:603.
29. Romanoff NR et al. Gout without crystals on initial synovial fluid analysis. Postgrad Med J 1978;54:95.
30. Ho G Jr. et al. Infection and arthritis. In: Harris: Kelley's Textbook of Rheumatology. 7th ed. Philadelphia: Elsevier Saunders; 2005:1622.
31. Reginato AJ. Gout and other crystal arthropathies. In: Braunwald E et al., eds. Harrison's Principles of Internal Medicine. 15th ed. New York: McGraw-Hill; 2001:1994.
32. Finch W. Acute crystal-induced arthritis: gout and a whole lot more. Postgrad Med 1989;85:273.
33. Wallace SL et al. Preliminary criteria for the classification of the acute arthritis of primary gout. Arthritis Rheum 1977;20:895.
34. Zhang W et al. EULAR evidence based recommendations for gout. Part II: Management. Report of a task force of the EULAR standing committee for international clinical studies including therapeutics (ESCISIT). Ann Rheum Dis 2006;65:1312.
35. Roche Laboratories, Inc. Naprosyn package insert. Nutley, NJ: 2007.
36. Merck and Company, Inc. Indocin package insert. Whitehouse Station, NJ: March 2007.
37. Watson Laboratories, Inc. Sulindac package insert. Corona, CA: February 2006.
38. Franck WA, Brown MM. Ibuprofen in acute polyarticular gout. Arthritis Rheum 1976;19:269.
39. Wanasukapunt S et al. Effect of fenoprofen calcium on acute gouty arthritis. Arthritis Rheum 1976;19:933.
40. Widmark PH. Piroxicam: its safety and efficacy in the treatment of acute gout. Am J Med 1982; 72:63.
41. Bluestone RH. Safety and efficacy of piroxicam in the treatment of gout. Am J Med 1982;72:66.
42. Lomen PL et al. Flurbiprofen in the treatment of acute gout: a comparison with indomethacin. Am J Med 1986;80(Suppl 3A):134.
43. Tamisier JN. Ketoprofen. Clin Rheum Dis 1979;5: 381.
44. Petera P et al. Treatment of acute gout attacks with tolmetin. Wien Med Wochenschr 1982;132:43.
45. Eberl R, Dunky A. Meclofenamate sodium in the treatment of acute gout: results of a double-blind study. Arzneimittelforschung 1983;33:641.
46. Schumacher HR et al. Randomised double blind trial of etoricoxib and indomethacin in treatment of acute gouty arthritis. Br Med J 2002;324:1488.
47. Merck Sharp and Dohme (NZ), Ltd. Arcoxia (etoricoxib) package insert. Auckland, New Zealand: May 2007.
48. Henry D et al. Variability in the risk of major gastrointestinal complications from non-aspirin nonsteroidal anti-inflammatory drugs. Gastroenterology 1993;105:1078.
49. U.S. Food and Drug Administration, Center for Drug Evaluation and Research. COX-2 Selective (includes Bextra, Celebrex, and Vioxx) and Non-Selective Non-Steroidal Anti-Inflammatory Drugs (NSAIDs). July 18, 2005. Available at: http://www.fda.gov/cder/drug/infopage/COX2/default.htm. Accessed December 13, 2007.
50. Patak RV et al. Antagonism of the effects of furosemide by indomethacin in normal and hypertensive man. Prostaglandins 1975;10:649.
51. Frolich JC et al. Suppression of plasma renin activity by indomethacin in man. Circ Res 1976;39:447.
52. Smith DE et al. Attenuation of furosemide's diuretic effect by indomethacin: pharmacokinetic evaluation. J Pharmacokinet Biopharm 1979;7:265.
53. Brater DC. Analysis of the effect of indomethacin on the response to furosemide in man: effect of dose of furosemide. J Pharmacol Exp Ther 1979;210:386.
54. Durao V et al. Modification of antihypertensive effect of beta-adrenoceptor-blocking agents by inhibition of endogenous prostaglandin synthesis. Lancet 1977;2:1005.
55. Hansten PD, Horn JR. Drug Interactions & Updates Quarterly. St. Louis, MO: Facts and Comparisons; 2007.
56. Findling JW et al. Indomethacin-induced hyperkalemia in three patients with gouty arthritis. JAMA 1980;244:1127.
57. Cronstein BN, Terkeltaub R. The inflammatory process of gout and its treatment. Arthritis Res Ther 2006;8(Suppl 1):S3.
58. Niel E, Scherrmann JM. Colchicine today. Joint Bone Spine 2006;73:672.
59. Bedford Laboratories. Intravenous colchicine package insert. Bedford, OH: April 1999.
60. Morris I et al. Colchicine in acute gout. BMJ 2003;327:1275.
61. Wortmann RL. The management of gout: it should be crystal clear. J Rheumatology 2006;33:1921.
62. Schlesinger N et al. A survey of current evaluation and treatment of gout. J Rheumatology 2006;33: 10.
63. Fang W et al. The management of gout at an academic healthcare center in Beijing: a physician survey. J Rheumatology 2006;33:2041.
64. Schlesinger N et al. Local ice therapy during bouts of acute gouty arthritis. J Rheumatology 2002;29:331.
65. Zhang Y et al. Alcohol consumption as a trigger of recurrent gout attacks. Am J Med 2006; 119: 800.e13.
66. Dessein PH et al. Beneficial effects of weight loss associated with moderate calorie/carbohydrate restriction, and increased proportional intake of protein and unsaturated fat on serum urate and lipoprotein levels in gout: a pilot study. Ann Rheum Dis 2000;59:539.
67. Choi HK et al. Obesity, weight change, hypertension, diuretic use, and risk of gout in men. Arch Int Med 2005;165:742.
68. Choi HK et al. Intake of purine-rich foods, protein, and dairy products and relationship to serum levels of uric acid. Arthritis Rheum 2005;52:283.
69. Johnson RJ, Rideout BA. Uric acid and diet-insights into the epidemic of cardiovascular disease. N Engl J Med 2004;350:1071.
70. Terkeltaub R et al. Recent developments in our understanding of the renal basis of hyperuricemia and the development of novel antihyperuricemic therapeutics. Arthritis Res Therapy 2006;8(Suppl 1):S4.
71. Pascual E, Perdiguero M. Gout, diuretics and the kidney. Ann Rheum Dis 2006;65:981.
72. Janssens HJ et al. Gout, not induced by diuretics? A case-control study from primary care. Ann Rheum Dis 2006;65:1080.
73. Hunter DJ et al. Recent diuretic use and the risk of recurrent gout attacks: the online case-crossover gout study. J Rheumatology 2006;33:1341.
74. Reyes AJ, Leary WP. The ALLHAT and the cardioprotection conferred by diuretics in hypertensive patients: a connection with uric acid? Cardiovasc Drugs Ther 2002;16:485.
75. Sica DA. The argument against. J Clin Hypertension 2005;7:117.
76. Simkin PA et al. Uric acid excretion: quantitative assessment from spot, midmorning serum and urine samples. Ann Intern Med 1979;91:44.
77. Wortmann RL, Fox IH. Limited value of uric acid to creatinine ratios in estimating uric acid excretion. Ann Intern Med 1980;93:822.
78. Rundles RW et al. Allopurinol in the treatment of gout. Ann Intern Med 1966;64:229.
79. Dalbeth N et al. Dose adjustment of allopurinol according to creatinine clearance does not provide adequate control of hyperuricemia in patients with gout. J Rheumatology 2006;33:1646.
80. Becker MA et al. Febuxostat compared with allopurinol in patients with hyperuricemia and gout. N Engl J Med 2005;353:2450.
81. Bruce SP. Febuxostat: a selective xanthine oxidase inhibitor for the treatment of hyperuricemia and gout. Ann Pharmacother 2006;40:2187.
82. Goldman SC et al. A randomized comparison between rasburicase and allopurinol in children with lymphoma or leukemia at high risk for tumor lysis. Blood 2001;97:2998.
83. Sanofi-Synthelabo, Inc. Elitek package insert. New York: January 2007.
84. Pui CH et al. Recombinant urate oxidase for the prophylaxis or treatment of hyperuricemia in patients with leukemia or lymphoma. J Clin Oncol 2001;19:697.
85. Sood AR et al. Clarifying the role of rasburicase in tumor lysis syndrome. Pharmacotherapy 2007;27:111.
86. Yu TF et al. Mutual suppression of the uricosuric effects of sulfinpyrazone and salicylate: a study in interactions between drugs. J Clin Invest 1963;42: 1330.
87. Reyes AJ. Cardiovascular drugs and serum uric acid. Cardio Drugs Ther 2003;17:397.
88. Daskalopoulou SS et al. Effect on serum uric acid levels of drugs prescribed for indications other than treating hyperuricaemia. Curr Pharm Design 2005;11:4161.
89. Huang HY et al. The effects of vitamin C supplementation on serum concentrations of uric acid. Arthritis Rheum 2005;52:1843.
90. Yu TF, Gutman AB. Effect of allopurinol [4-hydroxypyrazolo-(3,4-d)pyrimidine] on serum and urinary uric acid in primary and secondary gout. Am J Med 1964;37:885.
91. Elion GB et al. Renal clearance of oxypurinol, the chief metabolite of allopurinol. Am J Med 1968;45:69.
92. Rodnan GP et al. Allopurinol and gouty hyperuricemia: efficacy of a single daily dose. JAMA 1975;231:1143.
93. Boston Collaborative Drug Surveillance Program. Excess of ampicillin rashes associated with allopurinol or hyperuricemia. N Engl J Med 1972;286:505.
94. Cummins D et al. Myelosuppression associated with azathioprine-allopurinol interaction after heart and lung transplantation. Transplantation 1996;61:1661.
95. Fraunfelder FT, Lerman S. Allopurinol and cataracts [letter]. Am J Ophthalmol 1985;99:215.
96. Jick H, Brandt DE. Allopurinol and cataracts. Am J Ophthalmol 1984;98:355.
97. Clair WK et al. Allopurinol use and the risk of cataract formation. Br J Ophthalmol 1989;73: 173.
98. Kantor GL. Toxic epidermal necrolysis, azotemia, and death after allopurinol therapy. JAMA 1970;212:478.

99. Mills RM. Severe hypersensitivity reactions associated with allopurinol. JAMA 1971;216:799.
100. Young JL Jr. et al. Severe allopurinol hypersensitivity. Association with thiazides and prior renal compromise. Arch Intern Med 1974;134:553.
101. Boyer TD et al. Allopurinol-hypersensitivity vasculitis and liver damage. West J Med 1977;126:143.
102. Al-Kawas FH et al. Allopurinol hepatotoxicity: report of two cases and review of the literature. Ann Intern Med 1981;95:588.
103. Lang PG Jr. Severe hypersensitivity reactions to allopurinol. South Med J 1979;72:1361.
104. Hande KR et al. Severe allopurinol toxicity. Description and guidelines for prevention in patients with renal insufficiency. Am J Med 1984;76:47.
105. Singer JZ, Wallace SL. The allopurinol hypersensitivity syndrome: unnecessary morbidity and mortality. Arthritis Rheum 1986;29:82.
106. Rundles RW. Metabolic effects of allopurinol and alloxanthine. Ann Rheum Dis 1966;25:615.
107. Tam S, Carroll W. Allopurinol hepatotoxicity. Am J Med 1989;86:357.
108. Jarzobski J et al. Vasculitis with allopurinol therapy. Am Heart J 1970;79:116.
109. Arellano F, Sacristán JA. Allopurinol hypersensitivity syndrome: a review. Ann Pharmacother 1993;27:337.
110. Fam AG. Difficult gout and new approaches for control of hyperuricemia in the allopurinol-allergic patient. Curr Rheumatol Rep 2001;3:29.
111. Ka T et al. Effects of a fenofibrate/losartan combination on the plasma concentration and urinary excretion of purine bases. Int J Clin Pharm Ther 2006;44:22.
112. Feher MD et al. Fenofibrate enhances urate reduction in men treated with allopurinol for hyperuricemia and gout. Rheumatology 2003;42:321.
113. Chanard J et al. Amlodipine reduces cyclosporine-induced hyperuricaemia in hypertensive renal transplant recipients. Nephrol Dial Transplant 2003;18:2147.
114. Dang A et al. Effects of losartan and irbesartan on serum uric acid in hypertensive patients with hyperuricaemia in Chinese population. J Hum Hypertension 2006;20:45.
115. Liang MH, Fries JF. Asymptomatic hyperuricemia: the case for conservative management. Ann Intern Med 1978;88:666.
116. Berger L, Yu TF. Renal function in gout. IV. An analysis of 524 gouty subjects including long-term follow-up studies. Am J Med 1975;59:605.
117. Reif MC et al. Chronic gouty nephropathy: a vanishing syndrome? [editorial]. N Engl J Med 1981;304:535.
118. Yu TF et al. Renal function in gout. V. Factors influencing the renal hemodynamics. Am J Med 1979;67:766.
119. Yu TF, Berger L. Impaired renal function in gout: its association with hypertensive vascular disease and intrinsic renal disease. Am J Med 1982;72:95.
120. Fessel WJ et al. Correlates and consequences of asymptomatic hyperuricemia. Arch Intern Med 1973;132:44.
121. Yarchoan R et al. Long-term toxicity/activity profile of 2-,3-dideoxyinosine in AIDS or AIDS-related complex. Lancet 1990;336:526.
122. Cooley TP et al. Once-daily administration of 2-,3-dideoxyinosine (ddI) in patients with acquired immunodeficiency syndrome or AIDS-related complex: results of phase I trial. N Engl J Med 1990;322:1340.
123. Creighton S et al. Is ritonavir boosting associated with gout? Int J STD AIDS 2005;16:362.
124. Walker UA et al. High serum urate in HIV-infected persons: the choice of the antiretroviral drug matters [letter]. AIDS 2006;20:1556.
125. Bagnis CI et al. Changing electrolyte and acido-basic profile in HIV-infected patients in the HAART era. Nephron Physiology 2006;103:131.
126. Laine J, Holmberg C. Mechanisms of hyperuricemia in cyclosporine-treated renal transplanted children. Nephron 1996;74:318.
127. Zurcher RM et al. Hyperuricaemia in cyclosporine-treated patients: GFR-related effect. Nephrol Dial Transplant 1996;11:153.
128. Hopkinson N, Doherty M. In patients with chronic cardiac failure who have diuretic induced gout, are certain diuretics less prone at causing problems? Br J Rheum 1991;30:225.
129. Waller PC, Ramsay LE. Predicting acute gout in diuretic-treated hypertensive patients. J Human Hyperten 1989;3:457.
130. Friedel HA, Buckley MMT. Torsemide: a review of pharmacological properties and therapeutic potential. Drugs 1991;41:81.
131. Achimastos A et al. The effects of the addition of micronised fenofibrate on uric acid metabolism in patients receiving indapamide. Cur Med Res Opin 2002;18:59.
132. Curry CL et al. Clinical studies of a new, low-dose formulation of metolazone for the treatment of hypertension. Clin Ther 1986;9:47.
133. Khanna BK et al. Ethambutol-induced hyperuricaemia. Tubercle 1984;65:195.
134. Nishimura T et al. Influence of daily drinking habits on ethanol-induced hyperuricemia. Metabolism 1994;43:745.
135. Morstyn G et al. Effect of granulocyte colony stimulating factor on neutropenia induced by cytotoxic chemotherapy. Lancet 1988;1:667.
136. Mawson AR. Hypervitaminosis A toxicity and gout. Lancet 1984;1:1181.
137. Bierer DW, Quebbemann AJ. Effect of L-dopa on renal handling of uric acid. J Pharmacol Exp Ther 1982;223:55.
138. Keith MP, Gilliland WR. Updates in the management of gout. Am J Med 2007;120:221.
139. Knodel LC, Talbert RL. Adverse effects of hypolipidaemic drugs. Med Toxicol 1987;2:10.
140. Stapleton FB et al. Hyperuricosuria due to high-dose pancreatic extract therapy in cystic fibrosis. N Engl J Med 1976;295:246.
141. Sanchez-Albisua I et al. Tolerance of pyrazinamide in short-course chemotherapy for pulmonary tuberculosis in children. Pediatr Infect Dis J 1997;16:760.
142. Solangi GA et al. Pyrazinamide induced hyperuricemia in patients taking anti-tuberculous therapy. J Coll Physicians Surg Pak 2004;14:136.
143. Fontana RJ. Uric acid nephrolithiasis associated with interferon and ribavirin treatment of hepatitis C. Dig Dis Sci 2001;46:920.
144. Pilmore HL et al. Tacrolimus for treatment of gout in renal transplantation: two case reports and review of the literature. Transplantation 2001;72:1703.
145. Gerster JC et al. Gout in liver transplant patients receiving tacrolimus. Ann Rheum Dis 2004;63:894.
146. Miller PD et al. Teriparatide in postmenopausal women with osteoporosis and mild or moderate renal impairment. Osteoporos Int 2007;18:59.
147. Yamamoto T et al. Theophylline-induced increase in plasma uric acid-purine catabolism increased by theophylline. Int J Clin Pharmacol Ther Toxicol 1991;29:257.
148. Shimizu T et al. Effect of theophylline on serum uric acid levels in children with asthma. J Asthma 1994;31:387.
149. Manfredi RL, Vesell ES. Inhibition of theophylline metabolism by long-term allopurinol administration. Clin Pharmacol Ther 1981;29:224.
150. Grygiel JJ et al. Effects of allopurinol on theophylline metabolism and clearance. Clin Pharmacol Ther 1979;26:660.

CHAPTER 43

Rheumatic Disorders

Steven W. Chen

Epidemiology

The term *arthritis* refers to more than 100 diseases causing pain, swelling, and damage to joints and connective tissue.[1] The prevalence of arthritis is on the rise: 46.4 million Americans, or 21.6% of U.S. adults have been diagnosed with arthritis, an increase from the 2002 estimate of 42.7 million.[2] Arthritis is the most common chronic condition in persons older than 15 years of age, individuals who are overweight or inactive, and those without a high school education. The prevalence rate is higher in women (25.4%) than men (17.6%), and in the elderly (50.0% of those ≥65 years of age versus 29.3% of those between 45 and 64 years of age). A major objective from *Healthy People 2010* is to reduce the proportion of arthritis sufferers who have a limited ability to work due to their disease (about 33% of American adults fall into this category, with prevalence rates exceeding 50% in some states).[3] As more Americans work beyond 65 years of age, along with increasing arthritis prevalence with increasing age, this disease will become a growing source of economic and quality of life burden in the United States.

Table 43-1 Criteria for Diagnosis of RA

Morning stiffness in and around joints lasting ≥1 hr before maximal involvement[a]
Soft tissue swelling (arthritis) of ≥3 joint areas observed by a physician[a]
Swelling (arthritis) of the proximal interphalangeal, metacarpophalangeal, or wrist joints[a]
Symmetric arthritis[a]
Subcutaneous nodules
Positive test for RF
Radiographic erosions or periarticular osteopenia in hand or wrist joints

[a]Criteria 1 to 4 must be present for ≥6 weeks; ≥4 criteria must be present.
RA, rheumatoid arthritis; RF, rheumatoid factor.
Adapted from reference 4.

Table 43-2 Criteria for Complete Clinical Remission in RA

A minimum of five of the following requirements must be fulfilled for at least 2 consecutive months in a patient with RA[a]:

1. Morning stiffness not >15 minutes
2. No fatigue
3. No joint pain
4. No joint tenderness or pain on motion
5. No soft tissue swelling in joints or tendon sheaths
6. ESR (Westergren's) <30 mm/hour (females) or 20 mm/hr (males)

[a] Exclusions: Manifestations of active vasculitis, pericarditis, pleuritis, myositis, or unexplained recent weight loss or fever secondary to RA prohibit designation of complete clinical remission.
ESR, erythrocyte sedimentation rate; RA, rheumatoid arthritis.
Adapted from reference 11.

Rheumatoid arthritis (RA) is a chronic systemic inflammatory disorder characterized by potentially deforming polyarthritis and a wide spectrum of extra-articular manifestations. The diagnosis of RA primarily is based on clinical criteria (Table 43-1) because no single chemical or laboratory finding is specific for this disease.[4] The prevalence of RA is estimated to be 1% worldwide.[5] In the United States, RA afflicts approximately 1.3 million individuals, occurring nearly twice as often in women as men.[6] The onset of RA typically occurs between the third and fourth decades of life, and prevalence increases with advancing age up to the seventh decade.[1,5] The average age of RA prevalence has increased from 63.3 years in 1965 to 66.8 years in 1995. RA-related morbidity, mortality, and disability are expected to increase substantially in future years as large numbers of the boomer population age.[6]

The cause of RA seems to be an interplay among multiple factors (e.g., genetic susceptibility, environmental influences, the effects of advancing age on somatic changes in the musculoskeletal and immune systems).[5] Support for the concept of genetically controlled susceptibility comes from studies demonstrating an association between RA and class II gene products of the major histocompatibility complex (MHC). Although epidemiologic associations have not been clearly established, cigarette smoking might increase the production of rheumatoid factor (RF), which often precedes the clinical presentation of RA.[7] In a case-control study of 2,625 men and women (1,095 with RA and 1,530 healthy adults), a history of smoking increased risk for RA in men, but not in women.[8] A possible explanation for this gender-dependent difference is that female hormones might interfere with smoking-induced RF production and subsequent RA development.

The course of RA is variable and can be categorized as *polycyclic*, *monocyclic*, or *progressive*.[9] The *polycyclic* course occurs in approximately 70% of patients, who initially experience mild intermittent symptoms that resolve over the course of several weeks to months. The patient can be symptom free for several weeks to months and then experience symptoms that can be more severe than those experienced initially. *Monocyclic* patients (~20% of patients) experience a rather sudden onset of symptoms followed by a prolonged clinical remission of disease activity. *Progressive* patients (~10% of patients) experience progressive uninterrupted disease that usually evolves over the course of a few months, but the rate of disease progression in this group can be rapid or slow. Patients within this group can be divided further into a subgroup that responds to "aggressive" therapy and a subgroup that does not. Patients with more aggressive disease (multiple joint involvement, positive RF) have a >70% probability of developing damage or erosions to joints within 2 years of disease onset.[10]

The rate of RA disease remission was low before the increased use of medications capable of halting or slowing disease progression. The application of standardized criteria for remission (Table 43-2)[11] to rheumatology clinic patients reported a remission rate of about 1%.[12] In another clinic, 18% of patients were in remission at some time over 2.5 years (including >10% of patients not receiving disease-modifying drugs).[13] Remissions, however, were temporary with fewer than 4% experiencing a remission lasting up to 2 years and only 1.2% experiencing a remission lasting up to 3 years. Some clinical trials using disease-modifying drugs early in the course of RA reported remission rates of 16% to 31% at 2 years with monotherapy and up to 37% at more than 6 years with combination drug therapy.[14–17] In a more recent evaluation of a large dataset of RA patients, however, the use of anti-tumor necrosis factor (TNF) medications was associated with a remission rate (i.e., no disease activity) of only 7% and a minimum disease activity rate of just over 20%.[18] This significant difference in treatment response rates could be due to less standardization of patients in a general RA population versus clinical trials.

In several studies, survival rates of RA patients were not different compared with the general population during the first 10 years of the disease.[19,20] However, in analyses of more recent data, patients with RA had a lower life expectancy (median age at death was 4 years less than non-RA populations), and life expectancy was less with more severe disease.[21] The excess mortality has been attributed primarily to accelerated cardiovascular disease, which in turn might be due to RA-induced vascular inflammation, hyperhomocysteinemia, dyslipidema, or elevations in TNF-α.[22] RA is associated with a two- to threefold increased rate of myocardial infarction (MI), as well as lower MI survival. About one-third to one-half of RA patient deaths is due to cardiovascular disease. In comparison, only about one-fourth to one-fifth of deaths among adults without

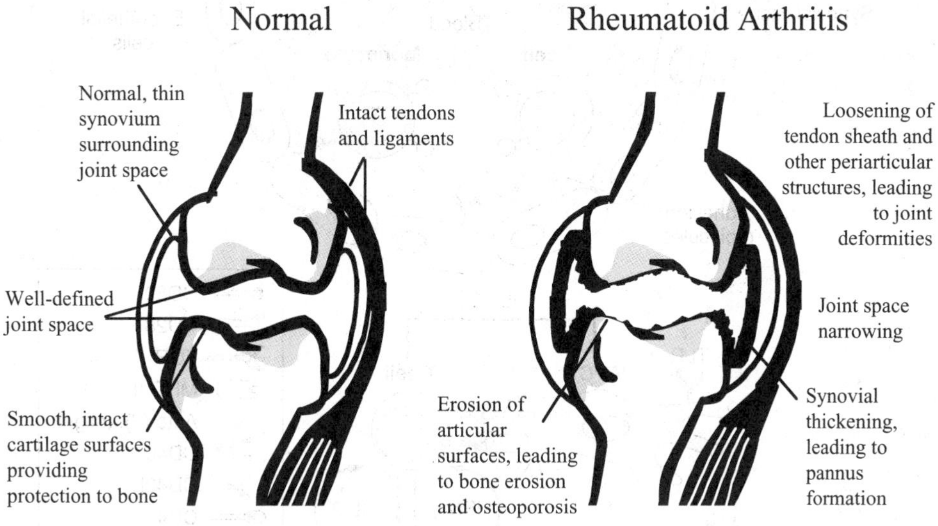

FIGURE 43-1 Overview of joint changes in RA.

RA have been attributed to cardiovascular disease. Guidelines for reducing cardiovascular disease risk in RA patients recommend the following: (a) consideration of RA as a potential independent risk factor for cardiovascular disease; (b) correction of modifiable cardiovascular risk factors (e.g., hypertension, dyslipidemia, diabetes mellitus); (c) treatment with the lowest possible dose of glucocorticoid to reduce the risk of glucocorticoid-associated cardiovascular events; (d) consideration of the use of methotrexate (MTX) therapy owing to its association with reduced cardiovascular mortality in RA patients; (e) inclusion of active RA into the consideration of cardiovascular risk factors when determining low-density lipoprotein cholesterol targeting; and (f) consideration of daily low-dose aspirin therapy for prevention of cardiovascular events with appropriate caution when other nonsteroidal anti-inflammatory drugs (NSAIDs) are being used because of possible increased risk of serious gastrointestinal (GI) toxicity.[23,24]

Pathophysiology

RA-induced joint destruction begins with inflammation of the synovial lining.[25] This normally thin membrane, which surrounds the joint space, proliferates and becomes transformed into the synovial pannus. The pannus, a highly erosive enzyme-laden inflammatory exudate, invades articular cartilage (leading to narrowing of joint spaces), erodes bone (resulting in osteoporosis), and destroys periarticular structures (ligaments, tendons) resulting in joint deformities (Fig. 43-1).

Familiarity with the basic cellular processes involved in tissue destruction and sustained inflammation in rheumatoid synovium is essential to understanding pharmacologic therapies for RA.[25–27] Under normal circumstances, the body can distinguish between self (i.e., proteins found within the body) and non-self (i.e., foreign substances such as bacteria and viruses). On occasion, immune cells (T or B lymphocytes) can react to a self-protein while developing in the thymus or bone marrow. These developing cells are usually killed or inactivated; however, a self-targeted immune cell can escape destruction and become activated years later to initiate an autoimmune response. Some believe the activation is initiated by bacteria (possibly streptococcus) or a virus containing a protein with an amino acid sequence similar to tissue protein. When this activation source (i.e., the self-targeted immune cell) reaches the joint, complex cell-to-cell interactions take place leading to the pathology associated with RA.

The initiating interaction for an autoimmune response takes place between antigen-presenting cells (APC), which display complexes of class II MHC molecules, and CD4-lineage T-cell lymphocytes (Fig. 43-2). In addition, B cells (previously thought to have little to do with the inflammatory response) can become activated, which leads to antibody formation (including RF and anticyclic citrullinated peptide), proinflammatory cytokine production, and accumulation of polymorphonuclear leukocytes that release cytotoxins and other substances destructive to the synovium and joint structures. B cells also act as APCs, leading to T-cell activation and acceleration of the inflammatory process.[27] T-cell activation requires two signals: (a) an antigen-specific signal occurring when an MHC class II antigen molecule on an APC binds to a T-cell receptor; and (b) binding of CD39 on the T-cell to either CD80 or CD86 on the APC. T-cell activation leads to activation of macrophages and secretion of cytotoxins and cytokines. Cytotoxins can directly destroy cells and tissues. Cytokines are polypeptides that serve as important mediators of inflammation. Proinflammatory cytokines such as interleukin (IL)-1 and TNF-α stimulate both synovial fibroblasts and chondrocytes in neighboring articular cartilage to secrete enzymes that lead to tissue destruction by degrading proteoglycans and collagen. In healthy individuals, the inflammatory process is regulated by balancing the ratios of proinflammatory cytokines (e.g., IL-1, IL-6, TNF-α) with anti-inflammatory cytokines—for example, IL-1 receptor antagonist (IL-1Ra), IL-4, IL-10, and IL-11. In the synovium of RA patients, however, this balance is heavily weighted toward

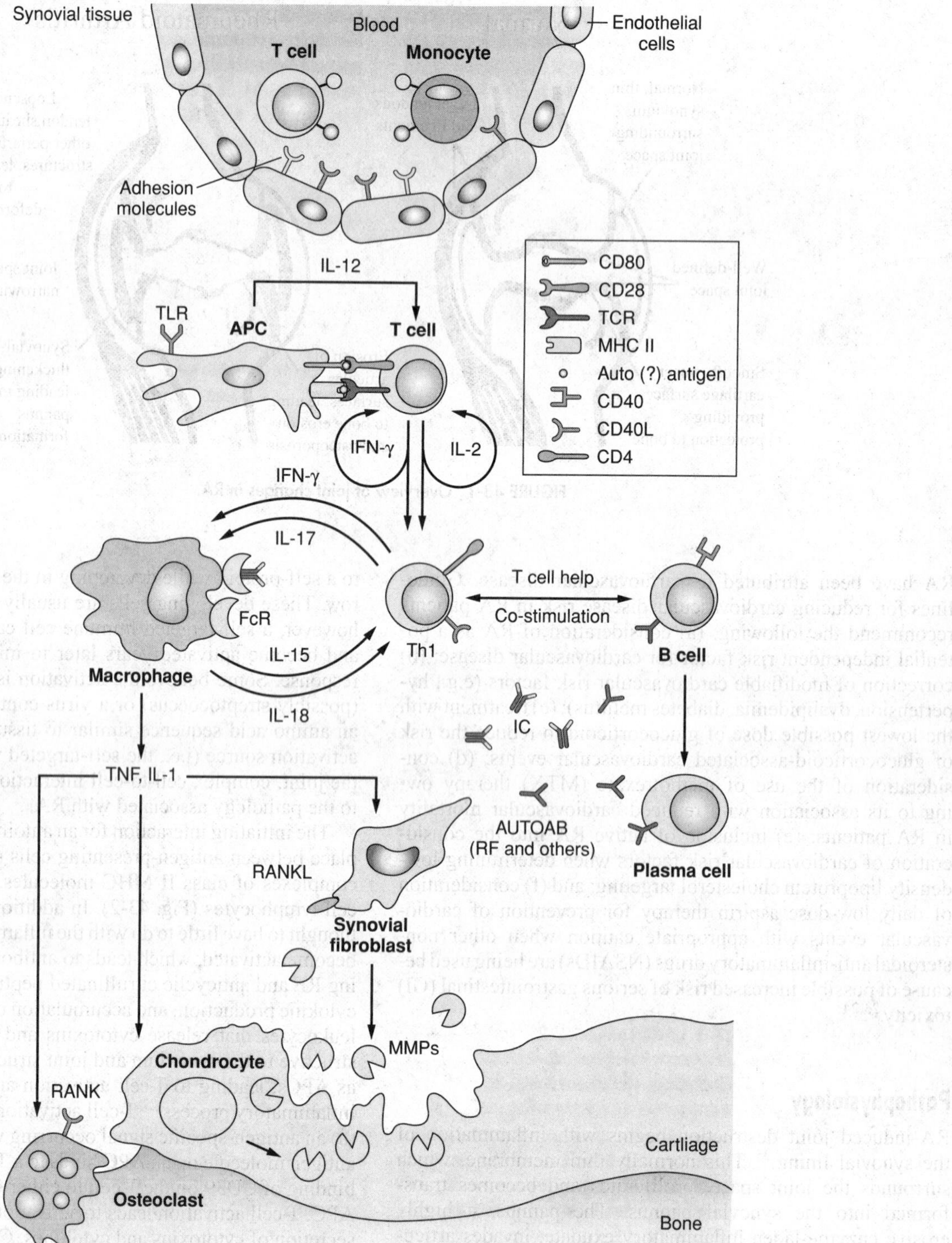

FIGURE 43-2 Schematic representation of events occurring in RA T cells invading the synovial membrane are primarily CD4^{+} memory cells, which produce interleukin-2 (IL-2) and interferon- (IFN-γ) to a similar extent as antigen-triggered T cells, and which are either already preactivated or become (further) activated by APCs in conjunction with arthritogenic (auto)antigen(s) and appropriate MHC class II molecules, costimulation (mainly through CD80/81 and CD28) and certain cytokines (IL-1, IL-15, IL-18). Through cell-cell contact (e.g., through CD11- and CD69-mediation) and through different cytokines, such as IFN-γ, tumor necrosis factor-α (TNF-α) and IL-17, these T cells activate monocytes, macrophages, and synovial fibroblasts. The latter then overproduce proinflammatory cytokines, mainly TNF-α, IL-1, and IL-6, which seem to constitute the pivotal event leading to chronic inflammation. Through complex signal transduction cascades, these cytokines activate a variety of genes characteristic of inflammatory responses, including genes coding for various cytokines and matrix metalloproteinases (MMPs) involved in tissue degradation. TNF-α and IL-1 also induce RANK expression on macrophages which, when interfering with RANKL on stromal cells or T cells, differentiate into osteoclasts that resorb and destroy bone. In addition, chondrocytes also become activated, leading to the release of MMPs. Initial events might also involve activation of APCs through Toll-like receptors (TLRs) before T-cell engagement. RANK, receptor activator of nuclear factor-κB; RANKL, RANK ligand; RF, rheumatoid factor; TCR, T-cell receptor. (Reprinted with permission from reference 314.)

the proinflammatory cytokines, which results in sustained inflammation and tissue destruction.[28]

Treatment

The treatment of RA involves a combination of interventions, which include rest, exercise (physical therapy), emotional support, occupational therapy, and drugs.[10] Specific treatment should be individualized based on joint function, degree of disease activity, patient age, gender, occupation, family responsibilities, drug costs, and results of previous therapy. The ultimate goal of RA treatment is disease remission; however, in light of the fact that complete and sustained remission is uncommon, minimizing disease activity (i.e., providing pain relief, maintaining activities of daily living, maximizing quality of life, slowing of joint damage) is also a goal.

An old standard for treatment of RA, known as the "pyramid approach," was based on the assumption that RA is a slowly progressing, benign disease that is not life threatening (Fig. 43-3).[29] Based on the pyramid approach, the initial treatment for any RA patient was a basic program of rest, exercise, and education along with NSAID therapy. If trials of several NSAIDs proved to be ineffective, treatment with disease-modifying antirheumatic drugs (DMARDs) was initiated with the relatively least toxic agent. As disease progressed, the patient "ascended" up the pyramid to receive more toxic DMARDs, with the "peak" of the pyramid consisting of experimental drugs and procedures. The problems with the pyramid approach are as follows: RA is not a benign condition for most patients; NSAIDs are associated with significant toxicities; DMARDs are not as toxic as once believed; and, perhaps most important, the pyramid approach has not made an impact on functional, clinical, or radiographic evidence of disease progression.[10] Although symptoms of RA can be controlled in most patients by conservative management, the disease progresses in most patients, and more aggressive therapy often is needed. Unfortunately, primary care clinicians who adopt the pyramid approach to RA management might delay consultation with rheumatologists and delay the use of important DMARDs.

Current treatment guidelines still support the use of NSAIDs to provide rapid anti-inflammatory and analgesic effects.[10] However, because NSAIDs do not prevent or slow joint destruction, DMARD therapy should be initiated within the first 3 months of RA diagnosis. Traditional DMARDs (e.g., hydroxychloroquine [HCQ], sulfasalazine [SSZ], MTX, leflunomide [LEF], gold, azathioprine [AZA], or D-penicillamine [DPEN]) have the potential to slow disease progression; however, DPEN is seldom utilized because of a very slow onset of action and numerous toxicities.[30] These agents, alone or in combination, should be considered as initial therapy for most RA patients. The newest class of DMARDs, biological agents (also referred to as anticytokines, biologicals, biological modifiers, or biological response modifiers), include etanercept (Enbrel), infliximab (Remicade), anakinra (Kineret), adalimumab (Humira), abatacept (Orencia), and rituximab (Rituxan). These agents target the physiological proinflammatory and joint-damaging effects of TNF-α, IL-1, T-cell activation, or B cells.

MTX is the initial treatment of choice for most RA patients because of its efficacy and safety profile.[10,30,31] TNF-α biologicals are recommended for patients who fail to achieve an adequate response either with MTX alone or MTX in combination with other traditional DMARDs, or for patients intolerant to MTX. The TNF-α biologicals, however, can worsen heart failure in patients with preexisting heart failure, and possibly increase their risk of death.[32,33] The newer biologicals, abatacept and rituximab, are effective in patients who have an inadequate response to TNF-α biologicals and seem to be free of cardiovascular adverse effects. Abatacept and rituximab, however, are expensive, are associated with serious side effects, and the long-term effects of these agents have yet to be

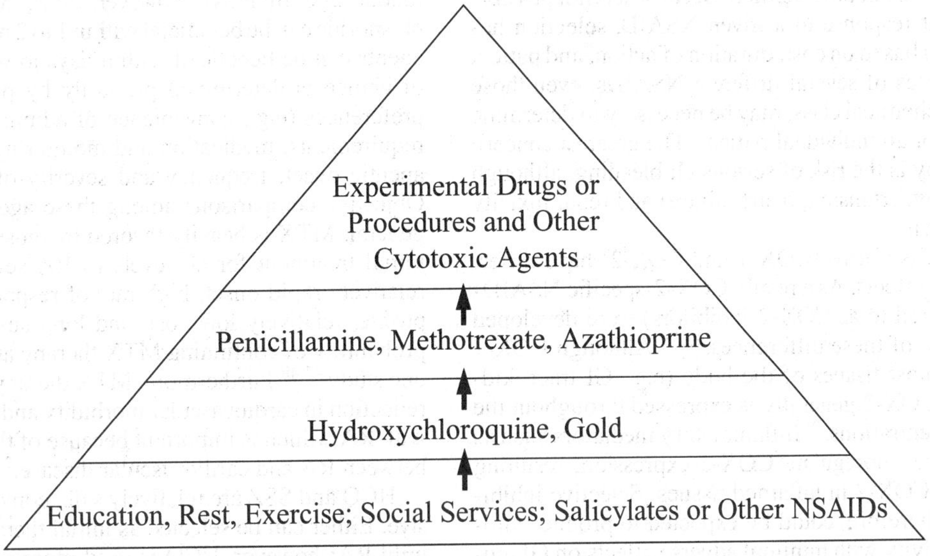

FIGURE 43-3 Traditional pyramid approach for treatment of RA. ↑ indicates worsening disease.

determined. As a result, abatacept and rituximab warrant cautious and judicious use. The glucocorticoids also are potent anti-inflammatory agents that seem to slow the progression of joint damage in RA; however, these generally are reserved for brief periods of active disease (low-dose oral therapy), or for isolated joints experiencing disease flares (local intra-articular injection), because of serious adverse effects associated with long-term systemic use. Alkylating cytotoxic drugs, although effective, are also toxic and are normally reserved for severe disease uncontrolled by other drug therapies.

Nonsteroidal Anti-Inflammatory Drugs

Aspirin, an acetylated salicylate, is inexpensive, has a long history of established efficacy, and continues to be the standard by which the effectiveness of all other NSAIDs is measured. However, aspirin (particularly nonenteric coated) is associated with a higher incidence of GI bleeding than other NSAIDs and is no longer commonly used for the treatment of RA.[34] Many other NSAIDs are available, including nonacetylated salicylates and nonsalicylate NSAIDs.

Although NSAIDs differ in chemical structure, they generally have similar pharmacologic properties (e.g., antipyresis, analgesia, anti-inflammatory activity, inhibition of prostaglandin synthesis), mechanisms of action (i.e., inhibition of cyclo-oxygenase [COX]; activity), harmful side effects largely attributable to COX inhibition (e.g., GI intolerance, nephrotoxicity, risk of bleeding), and pharmacokinetic properties (e.g., highly protein bound and extensively metabolized to inactive metabolites that are excreted renally).[34] The nonacetylated salicylates, however, have virtually no effect on COX and their mechanism of action remains unknown. The lack of COX activity and smaller early studies initially suggested that nonacetylated salicylates are less GI toxic than nonselective NSAIDs; however, in more recent comparisons both the GI and renal toxicities of nonacetylated salicylates are no different than nonselective NSAIDs.[35,36] (Note: For simplicity and clarity, the term *NSAID* is used henceforth to describe NSAIDs other than acetylated [i.e., aspirin] and nonacetylated [e.g., diflunisal, salsalate] salicylates.)

Although NSAIDs are more similar to, than different from, aspirin, they often are better tolerated. Because it is not possible to predict patient response to a given NSAID, selection has traditionally been based on cost, duration of action, and patient preference. Courses of several different NSAIDs, even those within the same chemical class, may be necessary to determine the best choice for an individual patient. The greatest concern of NSAID therapy is the risk of serious GI bleeding, although cardiovascular (hypertension, heart failure) and renal toxicity are also of concern.

The two COX isoforms (COX-1 and COX-2) have different physiological effects. As a result, COX-2-specific NSAIDs (commonly referred to as COX-2 inhibitors) were developed to take advantage of these differences.[37,38] Although COX-1 is expressed in most tissues of the body (e.g., GI tract, kidneys, platelets), COX-2 generally is expressed throughout the body in low concentrations.[39] Inflammatory mediators such as cytokines, however, upregulate COX-2 expression, resulting in high levels of COX-2 in inflamed tissues. Selective inhibition of COX-2, therefore, could be expected to produce anti-inflammatory activity with minimal adverse effects on GI mucosa (leading to less GI bleeding) and on cells (e.g., platelets). However, after several years of blockbuster sales of COX-2 inhibitors such as celecoxib (Celebrex), rofecoxib (Vioxx), and valdecoxib (Bextra), only celecoxib remains available in the United States. Rofecoxib and valdecoxib were withdrawn from the market because of a two- to four-fold increased risk of cardiovascular events (e.g., MI, stroke) when compared with placebo-treated patients.[39,40]

The potential risk of thrombosis and subsequent cardiovascular events associated with COX-2-specific inhibition was a recognized concern well before the first COX-2 inhibitor was marketed in the United States.[41,42] COX-1 and COX-2 balance a multitude of physiological processes, including hemostasis and vascular tone.[43,44] Thromboxane, a promoter of platelet activation and vasoconstriction, is produced primarily in platelets via the COX-1 enzyme. Prostacyclin, an inhibitor of platelet aggregation and a vasodilator, is produced in the vascular endothelium by COX-1 and COX-2 enzymes. Based on these facts alone, COX-2-specific inhibition has the potential to suppress prostacyclin while leaving thromboxane production unattenuated; the net clinical effect is a prothrombotic state. Celecoxib remains on the market because usual doses (up to 400 mg/day) have not been associated with an increased rate of cardiovascular events. One possible explanation for this difference in cardiovascular risk between the COX-2 inhibitors is that celecoxib is four to five times less selective for COX-2 than rofecoxib or valdecoxib.[45]

Traditional Disease-Modifying Antirheumatic Drugs

DMARD therapy should be considered for all RA patients and initiation of therapy should not be delayed beyond 3 months of RA diagnosis for the majority of patients.[10] Corticosteroid therapy (i.e., injections into isolated joints or low oral doses for multiple joint involvement) and NSAIDs can be used to control symptoms of pain and swelling initially and intermittently as needed. Although DMARDs have the potential to cause serious toxicity, they can substantially reduce joint inflammation, reduce or prevent joint damage, maintain joint function and integrity, and ultimately reduce health care costs and allow patients to remain productive.[10]

The onset of action of most traditional DMARDs is slow (about 3–6 months); however, SSZ, MTX, LEF, and cyclosporine can be beneficial within 1 to 2 months and biological agents can be beneficial within days to weeks.[30,31] The agent of choice is determined primarily by physician and patient preferences (e.g., convenience of administration, monitoring requirements, medication and monitoring costs, time to therapeutic onset, frequency and severity of adverse reactions). Objective comparisons among these agents are limited.[46] In general, MTX is heavily favored by most rheumatologists for initial treatment for all levels of RA severity because of its relatively rapid onset, high rate of response, mild side effect profile, relatively low cost, and long sustained efficacy. The probability of continuing MTX therapy at 5 years was 62% in one study.[47,48] Furthermore, MTX therapy is associated with a reduction in cardiovascular morbidity and mortality in patients with RA, which is important because of the strong association between RA and cardiovascular disease.[22,24]

HCQ and SSZ are relatively safe, convenient, and inexpensive. Either can be selected as initial therapy for patients with mild RA; however, HCQ is used more often than SSZ, even though it is less potent.[49–51] LEF is an attractive option for treatment of severe RA because its onset of effect can occur as soon as 4 weeks and its overall efficacy (including retarding of radiographic progression) is similar to MTX.[52–54]

Injectable gold is effective, but can be inconvenient and causes numerous intolerable adverse effects. Interestingly, a follow-up study of patients with early RA who discontinued injectable gold after about 1 year of treatment because of side effects, noted that these patients experienced sustained disease improvement (i.e., remission) for several years thereafter.[55] The rate of clinical remission among these patients was similar to that of patients who *continued* gold or MTX therapy over a 6-year period. The oral form of gold, auranofin (AUR) is rarely used because of poor GI tolerance, slow onset of action (up to 6 months), and low efficacy.

In a meta-analysis, parenteral gold, MTX, SSZ, and penicillamine were the most effective of the traditional DMARD therapies.[56] In comparison, HCQ was relatively less effective and AUR was the least effective. Parenteral gold seemed to be most toxic, whereas AUR and antimalarials were best tolerated. LEF was not evaluated in this study. Although AZA is effective, it usually is reserved for patients with severe disease who do not respond to safer alternatives because of potential myelosuppression and hepatotoxicity. DPEN is one of the slowest acting DMARDs (e.g., doses should be adjusted only once every 3 months). DPEN is seldom used because it has a relatively low response rate and is associated with rare, but serious, autoimmune diseases (e.g., systemic lupus erythematous, myasthenia gravis, Goodpasture syndrome). Cyclosporine is reserved for severe, refractory RA because of potential toxicity (renal insufficiency and hypertension) and cost. Although cyclosporine has been associated with an increased risk of malignancy in organ transplant patients, this adverse effect does not seem to be significant in the treatment of RA patients.[57]

Biological Agents

Since the late 1990s, the earliest biological agents targeted proinflammatory cytokines such as TNF-α, IL-1 (specifically IL-1α and IL-1β), and IL-6, which seem to be key inflammatory mediators in RA.[58] These cytokines are abundant in rheumatoid synovial tissues and fluid. Most cytokines can independently induce expression of the others, and IL-1 is capable of upregulating its own expression.[59] Excessive macrophage-produced cytokines (e.g., TNF-α, IL-1, IL-6, IL-8) correlate closely with RA disease activity and severity. Most importantly, RA improves when the physiological action of TNF-α and/or several different ILs are suppressed.

TNF-α is a proinflammatory cytokine produced by activated macrophages and T cells in RA-affected joints. TNF-α also plays a role in keeping infections localized by increasing platelet activation and adhesion, resulting in local blood vessel occlusion and containment of infection. This action of TNF-α is responsible for its tumor necrosis properties, thus leading to the name.

TNF-α exerts its physiological effects by binding to two different cell-surface receptors known as p55 (i.e., 55kD) and p75 (i.e., 75kD) on inflammatory cells.[59] These receptors, with portions extending from within the cell cytoplasm to the cell exterior, are capable of binding TNF to the domains extending above the cell surface. Soluble forms of these receptors can be found in the serum and synovial fluid and seem to play a role in regulating TNF-α.

Two approaches have targeted the action of TNF-α: (a) the use of soluble TNF receptors with high TNF binding affinity (e.g., etanercept); and (b) antibodies against TNF-α (e.g., infliximab, adalimumab).[58] Etanercept (Enbrel) is a recombinant TNF-receptor Fc fusion protein with the extracellular portion of two p75 receptors fused to the Fc portion of human immunoglobulin (Ig)-G1.[60] Infliximab (Remicade) is a chimeric IgG antibody directed against TNF-α; adalimumab is a genetically engineered human IgG1 monoclonal antibody. All three TNF-α inhibitors (Enbrel, Remicade, and Humira) render TNF biologically unavailable and are highly effective in reducing RA disease activity. It is not clear whether one agent is superior to the other. Anti-infliximab antibodies can develop with the long-term use of infliximab, but these can be prevented by concomitant immunosuppression with MTX.

In healthy individuals, IL-1 overexpression is prevented by naturally occurring IL-1Ra.[59,61] Consequently, inadequate production of IL-1Ra, relative to IL-1, is hypothesized to be an important contributor to active RA. In addition to proinflammatory properties, IL-1 augments cartilage damage and inhibits bone formation. Although TNF-α seems to be key in RA inflammation regulation and symptomatology, IL-1 may be largely responsible for bony erosion and periarticular osteoporosis. In animal studies, the combination IL-1Ra with anti-TNF-α has synergistic benefits.[62] Nevertheless, this combination is not recommended for use in humans because of a high risk of neutropenia and subsequent severe infections.[63]

TNF-α and IL-1 serve important physiological functions (e.g., protection against infections).[10,59] The incidence of serious infections in patients receiving biological agents was not increased during clinical trials; however, hospitalizations and deaths secondary to sepsis, tuberculosis, atypical mycobacterial infections, fungal infections, and opportunistic infections have developed in patients treated with biological agents.[10,63] Although these infections occurred primarily among patients with significant risk factors for infection (e.g., poorly controlled diabetes, concurrent corticosteroid or DMARD therapy), biological agents should not be given to patients with active infection, history of recurring infections, or medical conditions predisposing them to infection.

Increased serum levels of TNF-α seem to be associated with worsening of heart failure through mechanisms that are not entirely clear.[22] Some proposed mechanisms contributing to the onset or worsening of heart failure include accelerated left ventricular remodeling, cardiac contractile abnormalities that result in negative inotropic effects, and increased aptosis of myocytes and endothelial cells. However, despite the association between TNF-α and worsening of heart failure, clinical trials with anti-TNF therapy (which have included etanercept and infliximab) have not reduced mortality and heart failure-related hospitalizations. Furthermore, significantly more deaths have occurred in infliximab-treated patients with moderate to severe heart failure than in placebo-treated patients.[64] As a result, anti-TNF therapy is not recommended for RA patients with moderate to severe (New York Heart Association [NYHA] class III and IV) heart failure. Anti-TNF therapy can be used with caution in patients with mild (NYHA class I and II) heart failure, but patients should be closely monitored for cardiac decompensation.[31]

The newest biological agents target T cells and B cells.[31] Abatacept (Orencia), a fusion protein of cytotoxic T-lymphocyte-associated antigen attached to IgG1, inhibits T-cell activation by preventing the binding of CD80 and CD86 ligands on the surface of APCs to the CD28 receptor on the T-cell. Rituximab (Rituxan) has been available since 1997 for the treatment of B-cell lymphoma.[65] Rituximab, a chimeric (mouse-human) monoclonal antibody, binds to the CD20 antigen on the surface of pre-B cells and mature B cells, resulting in the depletion of B cells from peripheral blood, lymph nodes, and bone marrow. Stem cells, pro-B cells, and antibody-producing plasma cells do not express CD20 and, therefore, are not affected by rituximab. Owing to its chimeric composition, rituximab must be administered with MTX to reduce the risk of human antichimeric antibody (HACA) formation.[66] Inhibition of T-cell activation and depletion of proinflammatory B cells result in significant reductions in RA-related inflammation and joint destruction.

Safety data reflecting up to 5 years of abatacept therapy indicate that abatacept is generally safe, but associated with significant adverse effects.[67] All infections (54% vs. 48%) and serious infections (3.0% vs. 1.9%) occurred at a slightly higher rate among abatacept-treated versus placebo-treated patients, respectively.[68] When combined with anti-TNF therapy, these infection rates are significantly higher. The most common serious infections associated with abatacept included pneumonia, cellulitis, urinary tract infection, bronchitis, diverticulitis, and acute pyelonephritis. Thus far, the overall risk of malignancy seems to be no different than with placebo; however, several cases of malignancy have been reported with abatacept when combined with anti-TNF therapy. Abatacept-treated patients with chronic obstructive pulmonary disease experienced significantly more pulmonary and serious adverse effects than placebo-treated patients in one study.[68] Rituximab has a good safety profile overall, but it has several black box warnings regarding serious and potentially fatal adverse effects (e.g., fatal cardiorespiratory infusion reactions that most commonly occur within 24 hours of the first infusion, tumor lysis syndrome, severe mucocutaneous reactions, progressive multifocal leukoencephalopathy).[69] Mild infusion reactions (e.g., fever, chills, urticaria, headache, rhinitis, bronchospasm, angioedema, hypotension) occur in about 40% of RA patients treated with rituximab, especially upon administration of the first dose. These infusion reactions can be minimized by administration of methylprednisolone 100 mg IV 30 minutes before infusion of rituximab. Rituximab is also associated with a slightly increased risk of serious infection (e.g., septic arthritis, pneumonia) when compared with placebo (3% vs. 1%, respectively), including reactivation of hepatitis B and tuberculosis infections.[69]

Corticosteroids

Corticosteroids administered orally at low dosages (i.e., the equivalent of 10 mg of daily prednisone or less) or through local injections are effective in relieving symptoms of active RA.[10] Oral corticosteroids seem to slow the rate of disease progression, particularly when used for less than 1 year.[70] Long-term use of corticosteroids, however, is associated with many serious adverse effects (e.g., osteoporosis, weight gain, diabetes, cataract formation, adrenal suppression, hypertension, infections, impaired wound healing).[71] As a result, oral corticosteroid dosing should be limited to daily doses of 7.5 to 10 mg of prednisone (or equivalent) and should be administered for as short a time as possible. Oral corticosteroids are particularly useful when patients are waiting the onset of DMARD action or during brief flares of active RA involving multiple joints. Local corticosteroid injections are useful when flares involve only a few joints. Frequent corticosteroid injections over an extended period have the potential to accelerate bone and cartilage deterioration; therefore, the same joint should not be injected more than once every 3 months.[71]

Alkylating Cytotoxic Agents

Cyclophosphamide and chlorambucil are effective in the treatment of severe progressive cases of RA, but they also carry the risk of potentially serious toxicity (e.g., malignancy, infections).[29] Thus, use of these drugs usually is limited to patients with progressive RA unresponsive to more conservative management or, in some cases, potentially life-threatening complications of RA (e.g., rheumatoid vasculitis).[30]

Other Therapies

Minocycline seems to be a useful adjunctive agent in the treatment of RA, and its successful use supports a speculation that RA might have an infectious etiology. A double-blind, placebo-controlled trial, involving 46 patients with recent-onset RA, evaluated the benefit of the addition of minocycline 100 mg twice daily to conventional therapy with NSAIDs, DMARDs, and corticosteroids.[72] At 4-year follow-up, eight minocycline-treated patients without DMARD or steroid therapy were in remission compared with one patient in the placebo group ($p = 0.02$). Perhaps even more impressive are the results of a randomized trial comparing minocycline 100 mg BID to HCQ 200 mg/day in patients with early onset RA.[73] At 2 years, significantly more minocycline-treated patients experienced relief of RA signs and symptoms, required less prednisone, and were more likely to be completely tapered off prednisone.

Apheresis with the Prosorba column is an effective therapeutic option for patients with severe RA refractory to several DMARDs.[74] The Prosorba column, a medical device, contains highly purified staphylococcal protein A bound to a silica matrix that has a high affinity for IgG and complexes of IgG and IgM, including RF and circulating immune complexes. A plasmapheresis machine is used to withdraw blood from the patient, separate blood cells from plasma, pass the plasma through the Prosorba column to remove selected immunoglobulins and immune complexes, and recombine the plasma with the blood cells for return to the patient. Removal of these immunoglobulins and immune complexes results in immunomodulation and improvement in RA symptoms. In a randomized, double-blind, sham-controlled trial, the effect of weekly apheresis with the Prosorba column in patients with severe RA (i.e., average disease duration, 15.5 years; average number of failed DMARDs per patient, 4.2; average number of tender and swollen joints, 36.6 and 24.2, respectively) on improvement of symptoms was evaluated. According to American College of Rheumatology (ACR) criteria for response, 32% of the Prosorba-treated and 11.4% of the sham-treated patients improved ($p < 0.019$) at

19- or 20-week follow-up. The trial was stopped early by the data safety monitoring board because of overwhelming benefit with the Prosorba column. No differences in harmful adverse effects were found; both treatment groups experienced short-term joint pain flares and swelling after treatment, which were thought to be caused by the plasmapheresis procedure. However, because of the difficulty and expense of weekly treatments, combined with a limited duration of response, this treatment should be reserved for patients with RA refractory to multiple DMARDs.[10]

Cyclosporine is an effective treatment option, either alone or in combination with MTX.[10] Cyclosporine therapy, however, is complicated by the potential for serious side effects (particularly dose-related renal toxicity and hypertension), the inconvenience of necessary drug level monitoring, drug interactions, and high cost. As a result, consideration of cyclosporine is limited to patients with refractory RA.

Thalidomide also is a TNF-α inhibitor that is effective in treatment-resistant RA.[75] Although thalidomide is associated with serious adverse effects (e.g., teratogenesis, peripheral neuropathy), strict treatment guideline adherence and diligent monitoring make thalidomide a treatment consideration for selected cases of refractory RA.

Two **new classes of NSAIDs** in development may provide GI protection without COX-2 specificity.[76] *Nitric oxide NSAIDs*, also known as COX-inhibiting-nitric oxide donors, consist of standard NSAIDs linked to a nitric oxide moiety. By donating nitric oxide to the gastric mucosa, nitric oxide NSAIDs produce the same the same gastroprotective effect as prostaglandins.[77] The second class of new NSAIDs broadens the pharmacologic effects of currently available NSAIDs by inhibiting both enzymatic pathways of arachidonic acid metabolism (i.e., both COX and 5-lipoxygenase). Although COX inhibition is clearly associated with GI toxicity, inhibition of both enzymatic pathways of arachidonic acid metabolism has been GI-sparing in animal and initial human safety studies.[78] Interestingly, both of these new NSAID classes seem to provide extended anti-inflammatory activity and, as a result, may have disease-modifying properties.[77]

Vaccine therapy has been evaluated for RA prevention. In a double-blind, placebo-controlled phase II study of a T-cell receptor peptide vaccine in 99 patients with active RA, doses of 90 or 300 mcg were administered at baseline and at 4, 8, and 20 weeks. At 20-week follow-up, significantly more patients receiving the 90-mcg vaccine dose experienced improvement in RA signs and symptoms.[79] Although both vaccine dosage groups did not improve significantly when compared with placebo, a trend toward improvement was noted and no patients withdrew because of treatment-related adverse effects.

Clinical Use of Disease-Modifying Antirheumatic Drugs

Traditional DMARDs (e.g., gold, penicillamine, antimalarials, AZA, SSZ, MTX) are effective in attenuating clinical and laboratory manifestations of RA.[56] For example, a meta-analysis of the four published placebo-controlled trials that used strict research methodologies supports parenteral gold as an effective intervention.[80] Using a strict definition of improvement, 27% of patients treated with gold achieved 50% reduction in active joint count compared with 11% of placebo-treated patients within 6 months.[81] Nevertheless, long-term, positive therapeutic outcomes have not been realized for these drugs. With the exception of MTX, sustained treatment with any of these therapies is uncommon. Fewer than 20% of individuals, who were treated initially with parenteral gold, penicillamine, or antimalarials continued with their initial therapy for up to 5 years.[82] Many discontinue therapy because of the loss of responsiveness and still more discontinue because of toxicity. Over a 20-year period, traditional DMARDs may improve function during the first 10 years, but joint function declines considerably during the following 10 years, resulting in severe disability.

In a prospective study of 245 patients with recently diagnosed RA, long-term treatment with traditional DMARDs (i.e., HCQ, SSZ, gold, penicillamine) was evaluated by survival analysis.[83] When indexed for side effects, 40% of gold, 12% of HCQ, 19% of SSZ, and 13% of penicillamine regimens were discontinued at 2 years. When this study was indexed for lack of efficacy, 61% of HCQ, 46% of SSZ, 43% of gold, and 43% of penicillamine regimens were discontinued by 2 years. These studies reveal the limited effectiveness of most traditional DMARDs in RA and provide important insight on the inability of relatively short-term efficacy studies to fully characterize therapeutic outcomes achievable for chronic diseases.

In another prospective trial, DMARD therapy (injectable gold, SSZ, HCQ, DPEN, AUR, MTX, AZA) was initiated early in patients with early onset RA. In this study, one or more DMARD was used continuously for an average of 6.2 years (range, 18-111 months). Throughout the study, if efficacy seemed to be inadequate or if adverse effects occurred, another DMARD was substituted. For example, MTX use continued to rise throughout the study until 37% of patients were taking MTX by the end of the study. The use of all of the other DMARDs either fell dramatically (particularly injectable gold) or remained constant at a low level of use.[84] This approach achieved a remission rate that increased with time to 32% at final follow-up. In this trial, the beneficial effects of active and continual traditional DMARD therapy persisted for at least 6 years and yielded better long-term outcomes than those achieved in previous trials. Nevertheless, this approach is far from adequate for all patients as because RA progressed in 25% of the study patients.

MTX remains efficacious significantly longer than other traditional DMARDs.[85] In one study, about 400 patients with RA were successfully treated with continuous MTX monotherapy for an average of 42 months, and some patients continued MTX as long as 60 months. In another study, only half of 600 patients with RA were able to continue therapy with any DMARD (except MTX) beyond 9 to 24 months.[86] In contrast, 62% of patients receiving MTX were able to continue with MTX therapy after 5 years of treatment. Nevertheless, MTX monotherapy seldom results in complete disease remission; only one-third of patients are able to maintain improvement by 50% after 2 to 4 years of treatment.[87]

In a comprehensive review of the literature, the Agency for Healthcare Research and Quality compared the efficacy and adverse effects of various traditional and biological DMARDs, including monotherapies and combination therapies.[46] The efficacy of traditional DMARDs (MTX, SSZ, LEF) was deemed similar. Although MTX is the preferred first-line DMARD, SSZ or LEF seem to be reasonable options for patients who are unable to tolerate MTX. All of the anti-TNF biologicals (etanercept, infliximab, adalimumab) seem to have similar efficacy. Although the IL-1Ra, anakinra, might be less efficacious than anti-TNF therapies; this preliminary assessment was based only on adjusted indirect comparisons.

In comparative trials of monotherapies of *traditional* DMARDs and *biological* DMARDs, adalimumab and etanercept monotherapies were equal in efficacy to MTX monotherapy; however, the biological DMARDs performed significantly better than MTX based on radiographic outcomes.[46] Although this seems to be an important difference, the relationship between radiographic differences in clinical trails and long-term disease progression has not been clearly established. Both etanercept and adalimumab improved functionally capacity more than MTX.

The tight control of RA, utilizing dose escalation and several different combinations of DMARDs, is key to achieving remission, or at least a satisfactory response, to DMARD therapy.[88] In addition, the combination of various biological DMARDs with MTX is more efficacious than either biological DMARD or MTX therapy alone, and not associated with greater prevalence of adverse effects. Biological DMARDs, however, are still relatively new, and insufficient time has passed to clearly establish long-term safety (especially for abatacept and rituximab). The biological DMARDs have not been compared with DMARDs other than MTX.

The combination of MTX, SSZ, and HCQ is more effective than any one or two of these therapies for up to 2 years. This triple combination has not been compared with biological DMARDs. Combinations of two biological DMARDs do not show additional benefit over biological DMARD monotherapy and serious adverse effects (e.g., cellulitis, pneumonia, herpes zoster, pneumonitis, pyelonephritis) are increased significantly by combining two biological DMARDs.[89] Corticosteroid therapy combined with traditional DMARDs significantly improves functional capacity and radiographic outcomes when compared with traditional DMARD monotherapy, thereby reemphasizing the ability of corticosteroid therapy to modify disease. Corticosteroid therapy, however, should be limited to intermittent periods of use to manage disease flares or exacerbations because of significant adverse effects associated with long-term therapy.

Inadequate studies are available to resoundingly conclude which combination of DMARDs is most effective. The BeSt study, the only randomized controlled trial comparing different DMARD treatment strategies, found that two different treatment approaches (MTX + SSZ + high-dose tapering prednisone [60 mg tapered down to 7.5 mg/day over 7 weeks] or MTX + infliximab) resulted in less radiographic progression of RA than either sequential DMARD therapy (MTX to SSZ to LEF) or step-up combination DMARD therapy (starting with MTX, adding SSZ then HCQ then prednisone 7.5 mg/day if disease remains active) at 1- and 2-year follow-up.[8] However, all treatment groups experienced a similar improvement in functional capacity, as measured by Health Assessment Questionnaire (HAQ) scores, and disease activity, as measured by Disease Activity Score (DAS).

Biological agents (alone or in combination with MTX) seem to more rapidly improve signs and symptoms and slow disease progression (based on radiographic evidence) of RA than traditional DMARDs. These drugs should be considered for RA patients with moderate to severe disease, as well as for patients who fail to respond to an adequate trial of MTX.[30,46,58] Nevertheless, the long-term efficacy and safety of biological DMARDs is unknown because these drugs are relatively new and clinical studies have been of limited duration. The routes of administration, dosing frequencies, and propensity for infusion reactions of biological agents are listed in Table 43-3.

Quantifying Response to Drug Therapy

RA drug therapy, historically, has been evaluated subjectively by evaluating patient self-reported changes in disease activity. The subjectiveness of patient self-reporting of RA activity is being replaced increasingly by more objective and comprehensive measures of disease control (e.g., laboratory test results, radiographic changes). This shift has been prompted by the fact that better disease remission rates (e.g., after 6–12 months of therapy) have been reported in DMARD clinical trials than from observational studies.[90,91] The use of validated clinical assessment tools should yield a more accurate assessment of disease activity and improve the likelihood of attaining disease remission through modifications of drug therapy.[92,93]

Table 43-3 Dosing and Administration of Biological Disease-Modifying Antirheumatic Drugs

Biological DMARD	Route of Administration	Dosing Interval	Any Infusion Reaction Reported?	Fatal Infusion Reactions Reported?	Can Be Self-Administered?
Abatacept (Orencia)	IV	Every 2 weeks ×3 doses, then every 4 weeks	Yes	No	No
Adalimumab (Humira)	SC	Every 1–2 weeks	No	No	No
Anakinra (Kineret)	SC	Daily	No	No	No
Etanercept (Enbrel)	SC	1–2 times per week	No	No	No
Infliximab (Remicade)	IV	Every 8 weeks	Yes	Yes	No
Rituximab (Rituxan)	IV	Variable (usually every 24 weeks)	Yes	Yes	Yes

IV, intravenous; SC, subcutaneous.

Successful integration of objective clinical measurements into a standard of practice requires that the measurement tools used are validated, can be quickly administered, and are simple to use. Until recently, most large RA treatment trials utilized ACR standards to quantify response to therapy such as ACR-20, which refers to a 20% reduction in tender and swollen joint counts and 20% improvement in at least three of the following: patient's assessment of pain, patient's global assessment, physician's global assessment, patient's assessment of disability, and acute phase reactant measures (i.e., erythrocyte sedimentation rate [ESR] or C-reactive protein [CRP]). ACR-50 and ACR-70 are other common thresholds used to evaluate response to therapy, and attempts are being made to improve ACR-20 standards for clinical trials.[94] ACR evaluation reflects a minimum 6-week period of evaluation and, consequently, is of limited use in clinical practice because clinicians modify therapy based on an evaluation at a particular moment in time. The DAS 28 or 44 (corresponding to a 28 or 44 joint count) is a relatively newer tool used in more recent clinical trials to evaluate response to RA drug therapy.[95] However, the DAS is also not practical for clinical use because a very complex mathematical calculation is required.[96]

New tools for measurement of RA disease activity that are more suited for clinical use have been developed. The *Clinical Disease Activity Index* (CDAI) and the *Simplified Disease Activity Index* (SDAI) are very similar in that they are determined through a simple sum of swollen joint count, tender joint count, and patient global disease activity and evaluator global disease activity (both measured by a visual analog scale [VAS]).[97] The difference between the two is that the SDAI includes CRP in the summation, whereas the CDAI does not. The *Global Arthritis Scale* (GAS) utilizes a summation of tender joint count, modified Health Assessment Questionnaire, and patient self-assessment of pain and function levels. The *Routine Assessment of Patient Index Data* (RAPID) measurement tool includes assessments of pain and function levels along with patient global assessment of disease activity.[98–100] More recently, the *Easy Rheumatoid Activity Measure* (ERAM),[96–99] a summation of patient and clinician global disease activity using a VAS with swollen joint counts from 28 joints, demonstrated a high level of correlation with DAS28, SDAI, and CDAI.[99] An important additional finding is that the ERAM required only an average of 2.67 minutes to complete. All of these tools have distinctly defined threshold scores corresponding to high disease activity, low moderate disease activity, low disease activity, and remission. For example, remission scores for DAS, CDAI, SDAI, and GAS are $\leq$2.6, $\leq$2.8, $\leq$3.3, and $\leq$3, respectively.

Although no single tool has been adopted as a standard of practice, RA disease activity measurement tools are becoming simpler to use in clinical settings and provide a more objective and comprehensive assessment of disease status. These tools, however, should not be solely relied upon for making RA treatment decisions because radiographic changes also should be considered when making RA treatment decisions. Radiographic changes, considered the gold standard for evaluating arthritis-related joint damage, occur in more than one-half of patients categorized as in remission based on DAS score.[101]

EARLY AND PROGRESSIVE RHEUMATOID ARTHRITIS

See Questions 1 to 16 for the role of nondrug and NSAID therapy, Questions 17 to 38 for traditional DMARDs, and Questions 39 to 47 for biological agents and corticosteroid therapy.

Signs and Symptoms

1. T.W., a previously healthy 42-year-old, 60-kg woman, has been suffering from morning stiffness that persists for several hours, anorexia, fatigue, and generalized muscle and joint pain over the past 4 months. In addition, she reports that her eyes seem red most of the time and are unusually dry. Her symptoms have been much worse during the past month and a half, and she has limited her physical activities. She also can no longer wear her wedding ring because of swelling of her hand.

Physical examination reveals bilaterally symmetrical swelling, tenderness, and warmth of the metacarpophalangeal (MCP) and proximal interphalangeal (PIP) joints of the hands and the metatarsophalangeal (MTP) joints of the feet. A subcutaneous nodule is evident on the extensor surface of the left forearm. Pertinent laboratory findings include the following: ESR by the Westergren method, 52 mm/hour (normal for women, <20 mm/hour if <50 years old, <30 if >50 years old; men, <15 mm/hour if <50 years old, <20 if >50 years old); hemoglobin (Hgb), 10.6 g/dL (normal, 12–16 g/dL); hematocrit (Hct), 33% (normal, 36%–47%); platelets, 480,000/mm^3 (normal, 140,000–400,000/mm^3); albumin, 3.8 g/dL (normal, 4.3–5.6 g/dL); serum uric acid, 3.0 μg/dL (normal, 2–8 mg/dL); serum iron, 40 μg/dL (normal, 60–180 mg/dL); total iron-binding capacity, 275 mg/dL (normal, 200–400 mg/dL); positive anti-cyclic citrullinated peptide (anti-CCP) at 82 U (normal, <20 U; weak positive, 20–39 U; moderate positive, 40–59 U; strong positive, >60 U) and positive RF performed by latex fixation method in a dilution of 1:320. Tests for antinuclear antibodies (ANA) and tuberculin sensitivity are negative. Radiographic films of the hands and feet show soft tissue swelling, narrowing of joint spaces, and marginal erosions of the second and third MCP and PIP joints bilaterally with no evidence of tophi or calcification. Other routine laboratory data and physical findings are normal. What signs and symptoms of RA are manifested by T.W.?

[SI units: Hgb, 6.6 mmol/L (normal, 7.4–9.9); albumin, 38 g/L (normal, 35–50); uric acid, 178.4 mol/L (normal, 202–416); iron, 7.2 μmol/L (normal, 9–26.9); total iron-binding capacity, 49.2 mol/L (normal, 45–73)]

The presentation of RA at onset can vary, but characteristically 50% to 70% of cases have a rather insidious onset of disease over weeks to months.[9] Early nonspecific symptoms such as fatigue, malaise, diffuse musculoskeletal pain, and morning stiffness may precede more specific symptoms. *Fatigue* and *morning stiffness* are prominent features of RA in T.W. About half of patients with RA initially experience fatigue that later in the disease serves as a useful index of disease activity. Patients usually experience prolonged morning stiffness upon awakening. This stiffness usually lasts 30 to 60 minutes, but can be present all day with decreasing intensity after arising. Duration of morning stiffness also can be a useful index of disease activity.

Over time, nonspecific *musculoskeletal pain* localizes to the joints bilaterally. Bilaterally symmetrical joint swelling and

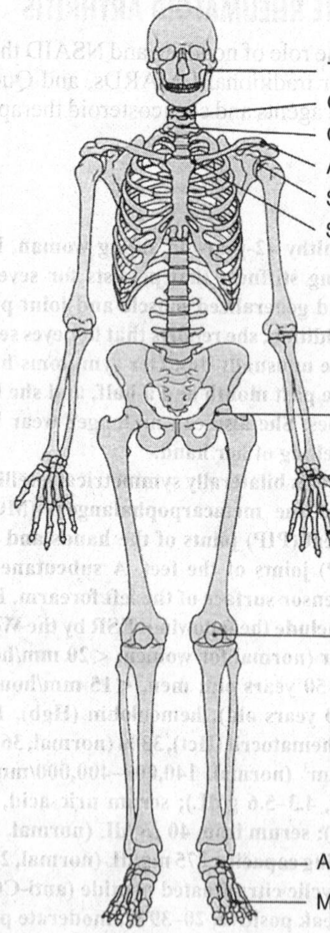

FIGURE 43-4 Frequency of involvement of different joint sites in established RA.

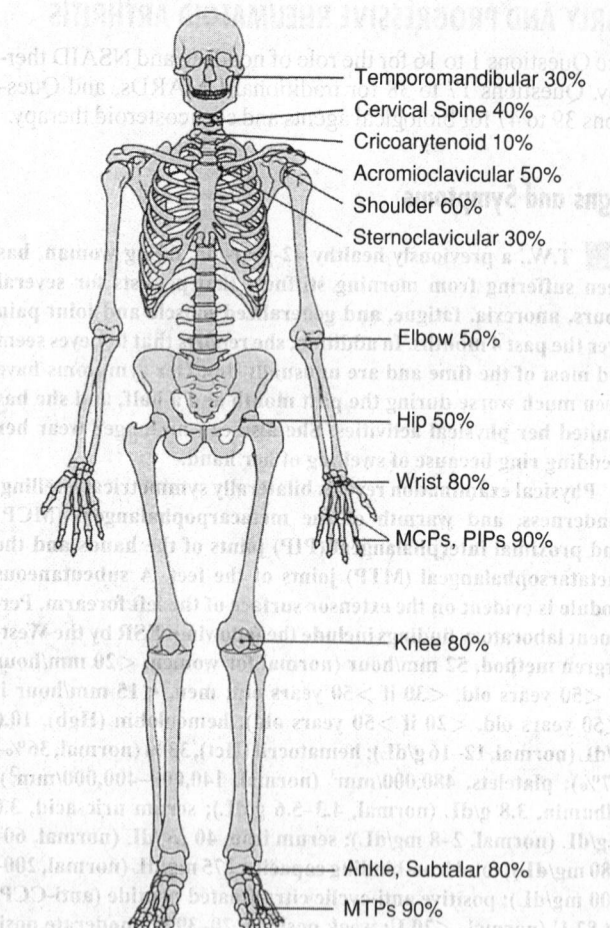

pain, involving the MCP and PIP joints of the hands and MTP joints of the feet, as illustrated by T.W., are characteristic of RA. The peripheral joints of the hands, wrists, and feet usually are involved first. Although MCP and PIP joints of the hands often are affected, the distal interphalangeal (DIP) joints usually are spared. Ultimately, any or all of the diarthrodial joints (elbows, knees, shoulders, ankles, hips, temporomandibular joints, sternoclavicular joints, glenohumeral joints) can be involved Fig. 43-4). *Joint involvement* is characterized by soft tissue swelling and warmth, decreased range of motion (ROM), and sometimes muscle atrophy around affected joints. Progressive disease is characterized by irreversible joint deformities such as ulnar deviation of the fingers (Fig. 43-5), boutonniere deformities (hyperextension of the DIP joint and flexion of the PIP joint), or swan neck deformities (hyperextension of the PIP joint and flexion of the DIP joint; Fig. 43-6). Similar irreversible deformities also can involve the feet.

RA is a systemic disease, which is reflected by the extra-articular manifestations that can accompany joint involvement. *Subcutaneous nodules* are found in up to 35% of individuals with RA.[9] As in the case of T.W., these nodules usually develop along extensor surfaces (e.g., olecranon process, proximal ulna), but occasionally are found in the hands, sacral areas, eyes, lungs, heart, soles of the feet and along the Achilles tendon. Patients who develop rheumatoid nodules almost always are RF positive.

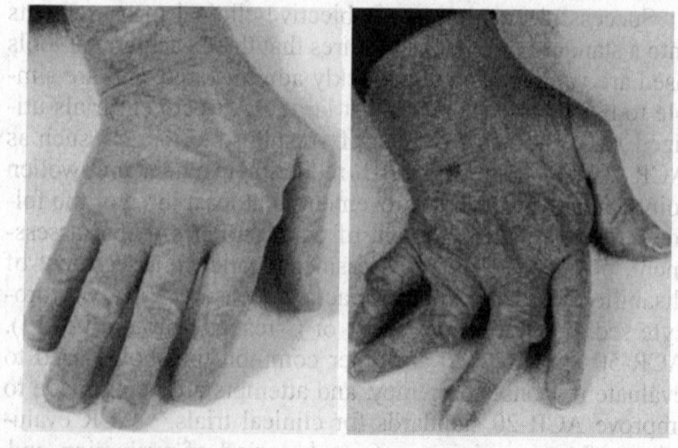

FIGURE 43-5 Ulnar deviation and MCP synovitis (*left*). This may progress to more marked lateral deviation with subluxation of the extensor tendons (right finger; *right*).

Organ system involvement may be extensive. *Pleuropulmonary manifestations* (e.g., pleuritis, development of pulmonary nodules, interstitial fibrosis, pneumonitis, and rarely arteritis of the pulmonary vasculature) also can accompany the articular involvement of RA.[9] *Cardiac involvement* can present as pericarditis or myocarditis. In addition, rheumatoid nodules can produce conduction defects or valve defects.

Some extra-articular manifestations occur as syndromes. *Sjogren syndrome* includes dry eyes (keratoconjunctivitis sicca), dry mouth (xerostomia), and connective tissue disease.[102] T.W.'s eye complaints may be an extra-articular manifestation of her RA. *Felty syndrome* is characterized by chronic arthritis, splenomegaly, and neutropenia; thrombocytopenia, anemia, and lymphadenopathy also may be present.[25]

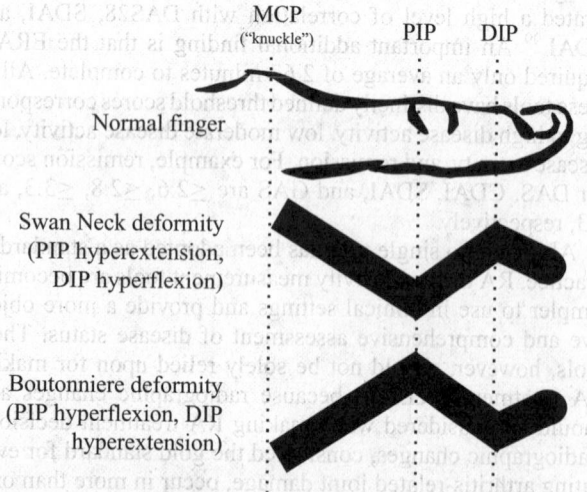

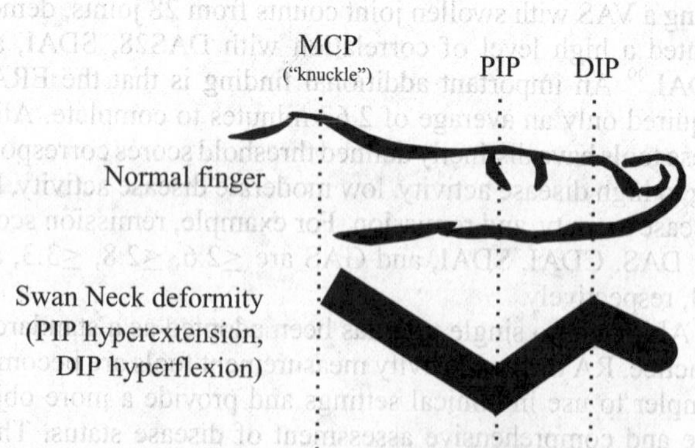

FIGURE 43-6 Characteristic finger deformities in RA. DIP, distal interphalangeal joint; MCP, metacarpophalangeal joint; PIP, proximal interphalangeal joint.

Vasculitis, another extra-articular manifestation of RA, can involve any organ system and can vary in seriousness from mild to potentially life-threatening (see Chapter 44).

2. What abnormal laboratory values in T.W. could be used to monitor the efficacy of drug therapy or disease progression?

The laboratory findings in RA are characteristic of a chronic systemic inflammatory disease. No test is specific for RA. T.W.'s elevated ESR is a nonspecific indication of inflammation. Alternatively, CRP plasma concentrations can be tested instead of ESR.[103] Levels of CRP, a plasma protein of the acute-phase response, correlate with RA disease activity better than ESR; however, CRP is also not disease specific. T.W.'s hematologic findings are consistent with a mild anemia of chronic inflammation. Although her serum iron concentration is decreased, her normal iron-binding capacity makes a diagnosis of iron-deficiency anemia unlikely. Her anemia probably results from a failure of iron release from the reticuloendothelial tissues and would not be expected to respond to iron therapy. The mild thrombocytosis is additional evidence of a systemic inflammatory response. The laboratory manifestations of inflammation should improve with effective drug therapy and, along with many of the clinical features of RA, are useful parameters for monitoring disease activity and response to therapy (Table 43-4).

T.W.s serum albumin concentration is low (3.8 g/dL). The low serum albumin concentration in RA patients can result in higher free drug serum concentrations because of decreased protein binding of drugs (e.g., salicylates).[104]

RF, an autoantibody (usually IgM or IgG) that reacts with the Fc portion of antigenic IgG to form an immune complex in vitro, is in the serum of approximately 75% of patients with RA.[105] RF is not in the serum of all patients with RA. It also can be present in 3% to 5% of healthy individuals and in patients with diseases other than RA, including almost any condition associated either with immune complex formation or with hypergammaglobulinemia (e.g., chronic infections, lymphoproliferative and hepatic diseases, systemic forms of autoimmunity). Therefore, RF does not establish the diagnosis of RA. An RF titer of at least 1:160 is considered a positive test.[106] Patients with RA typically have titers of at least 1:320. Although RF titers do not parallel disease activity, high titers (>1:512) early in the disease course are associated with more severe and progressive disease. In T.W., the test for ANA ruled out systemic lupus erythematosus. The ANA, however, can be positive in 10% to 70% patients with RA.

Although RF lacks specificity for RA, the presence of RF remains one of the ACR criteria for establishing the diagnosis of RA.[10] Citrullin, a nonstandard amino acid, also is established as a key component of RA antigenicity. Citrullinated proteins and anti-CCP antibodies are abundant in inflamed RA synovium. Anti-CCP antibodies can be detected in 50% to 60% of early RA patients, and the specificity of anti-CCP is very high at 95% to 98%[107] In a study of 136 patients with a broad range of RA disease duration (3 months–30 years), the sensitivity of anti-CCP for the diagnosis of RA was 63% and the specificity was 89%, versus 85% and 65%, respectively, for RF. Another study found a sensitivity of 55% and a specificity of 97% for RA when both anti-CCP and RF were positive in the early cases of arthritis. Anti-CCP was detectable 1.5 to 9 years before the onset of RA (thereby suggesting a possible pathogenic role for these antibodies for RA).[108] A positive anti-CCP also correlates with an increase likelihood of a more erosive course of RA than either a negative anti-CCP or a positive RF.[108] In summary, a positive anti-CCP antibody test is highly specific for RA, predictive of the development of RA, and is a marker of an erosive disease course. Studies are currently ongoing attempting to define the optimal manner in which to incorporate anti-CCP into RA therapy management.

Table 43-4 Parameters Used to Assess Disease Activity and Drug Response in RA

- Duration and intensity of morning stiffness
- Number of painful or tender joints
- Number of swollen joints; severity of joint swelling
- Range of joint motion
- Time to onset of fatigue
- ESR or CRP
- Anti-CCP
- Radiographic changes: osteopenia, joint space narrowing, bony erosions
- Hgb/Hct
- Subcutaneous nodules, pleuritis, pneumonitis, myocarditis, vasculitis
- AIMS
- HAQ
- Validated clinical assessment tools: See general treatment section Quantifying Response to Drug Therapy

AIMS, arthritis impact measure scale; anti-CCP, anti-cyclic citrullinated peptide; CRP, C-reactive protein; ESR, erythrocyte sedimentation rate; HAQ, health assessment questionnaire; Hct, hematocrit; Hgb, hemoglobin; RA, rheumatoid arthritis.

Treatment

Nondrug Treatment

3. What nondrug therapy should be included in the management of T.W.'s RA?

Treatment objectives in RA are reduction of joint pain and inflammation, preservation of joint function, and prevention of deformity. This is best achieved by instructing patients on proper regular exercise, joint protection and energy conservation, in combination with effective symptom-relieving and disease-modifying drug therapy.[10,109,110] Insufficient literature evidence is available to support the use of spa therapy and thermotherapies such as ultrasound, electrotherapies (e.g., transcutaneous nerve stimulation, electrostimulation of muscles), and laser therapy. Heat treatments in general should be avoided during periods of active joint inflammation, because heat can further exacerbate pain and swelling. Overall, physical and occupational therapy can provide valuable assistance to patients with compromised activities of daily living, and thereby, maximize the potential for self-sufficiency.

EXERCISE

Passive exercise (e.g., ROM exercises) should be prescribed for T.W. until the acute inflammation subsides. Passive exercise minimizes muscle atrophy and flexion contractures and maintains joint function without increasing inflammation or radiographic progression of disease.[109] A properly defined exercise program should be developed with specific exercises on a scheduled basis that are not harmful to inflamed joints. Examples of ideal exercises include cycling (stationary if outdoor movement is considered unsafe), water exercises (e.g., swimming, water aerobics), and walking (assuming weight-bearing joints can tolerate the patient's bodyweight).

JOINT PROTECTION AND ENERGY CONSERVATION

Systemic and articular rest (achieved by splinting the affected joints) can reduce inflammation significantly.[109,110] Restful and adequate sleep are important for general health and particularly important in a chronic, fatigue-inducing disease such as RA. Prolonged rest, however, can induce rapid losses in strength and endurance. Therefore, RA patients experiencing acute inflammation, such as T.W., should rest often, but daytime rest periods should be limited to 30 to 60 minutes. Splinting of joints is typically prescribed throughout the day and night during periods of active inflammation, then only at night for several weeks after cessation of inflammation.

Some orthoses, which are medical devices secured to any part of a patients body designed to support, immobilize, align, correct or prevent deformity, or improve functioning, can reduce pain and inflammation and/or improve joint function in targeted joints for RA patients.[109] For example, wrist and finger/thumb splints can reduce wrist and hand pain while improving grip strength; however, these can worsen dexterity. Finger splints for patients with swan neck deformities have been shown to improve hand function and finer stability. Special shoes and sole inserts also can reduce pain and disability.

EMOTIONAL SUPPORT

Emotional support should be provided to all patients such as T.W. A patient's reaction to RA can be affected by age, personality, and the environment at work and at home. As with all chronic debilitating diseases, the potential loss of independence, loss of self-esteem, altered interpersonal relationships with friends and family, and potential loss of employment can result in a two- to threefold increase in depression.[111] Depending on each patient's needs, the expertise of different health care disciplines (e.g., physical therapists, social workers, health educators, psychiatrists, clinical psychologists, podiatrists, vocational rehabilitation therapists, pharmacists) should be consulted. For example, pharmacists in capitated outpatient clinical practices can monitor RA drug therapy for therapeutic and adverse effects under collaborative practice agreements with other practitioners and can counsel patients on proper medication use and clarify expectations.[112]

Drug Treatment (Fig. 43-7)

NONSTEROIDAL ANTI-INFLAMMATORY DRUGS AND ASPIRIN

4. T.W. will be treated with a DMARD and concurrent NSAID therapy initially to rapidly control inflammation and swelling. What should be the role of NSAIDs for T.W.?

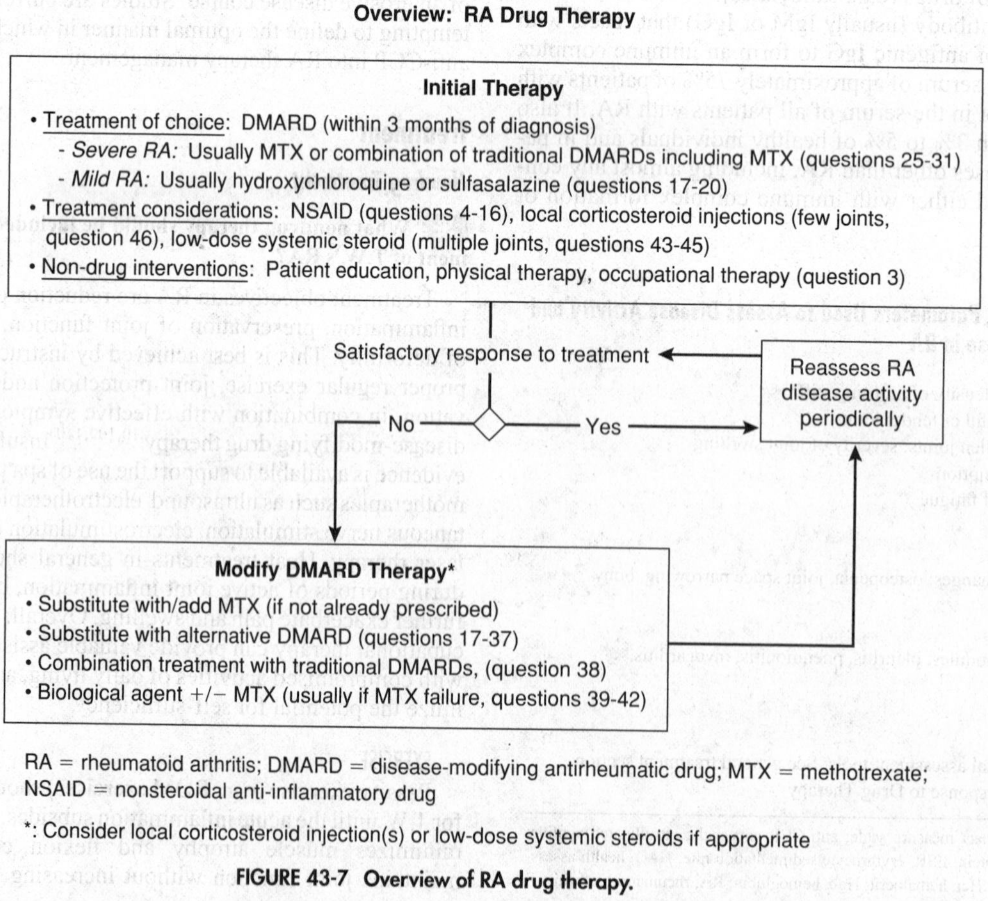
Overview: RA Drug Therapy
Initial Therapy
• Treatment of choice: DMARD (within 3 months of diagnosis)
- Severe RA: Usually MTX or combination of traditional DMARDs including MTX (questions 25-31)
- Mild RA: Usually hydroxychloroquine or sulfasalazine (questions 17-20)
• Treatment considerations: NSAID (questions 4-16), local corticosteroid injections (few joints, question 46), low-dose systemic steroid (multiple joints, questions 43-45)
• Non-drug interventions: Patient education, physical therapy, occupational therapy (question 3)
Satisfactory response to treatment
No
Yes
Reassess RA disease activity periodically
Modify DMARD Therapy*
• Substitute with/add MTX (if not already prescribed)
• Substitute with alternative DMARD (questions 17-37)
• Combination treatment with traditional DMARDs, (question 38)
• Biological agent +/− MTX (usually if MTX failure, questions 39-42)
RA = rheumatoid arthritis; DMARD = disease-modifying antirheumatic drug; MTX = methotrexate; NSAID = nonsteroidal anti-inflammatory drug
*: Consider local corticosteroid injection(s) or low-dose systemic steroids if appropriate

FIGURE 43-7 **Overview of RA drug therapy.**

T.W.s clinical presentation clearly warrants DMARD therapy (see Question 17 and section on Clinical Use of Disease-Modifying Agents). The purpose of NSAID therapy, which has no disease-modifying activity, is to provide rapid pain relief and reduction of joint inflammation.

At one time, aspirin was the first line of treatment for RA patients who were able to tolerate it; however, aspirin currently seldom is the NSAID of choice because of well-documented GI toxicity and the availability of safer and more convenient NSAIDs.[10,113]

Aspirin is low cost, and serum salicylate levels correlate well with both efficacy and toxicity.[34] Anti-inflammatory effects of aspirin can be achieved with dosages sufficient to provide serum salicylate concentrations of 15 to 30 mg/dL.[34] A reasonable initial aspirin dose is 45 mg/kg/day divided into 4- or 6-hour intervals; however, the anti-inflammatory dose of aspirin varies widely because of interindividual variations in metabolism.

After intestinal absorption, aspirin is hydrolyzed rapidly to salicylate (or salicylic acid), which subsequently is metabolized via multiple pathways. Metabolism to salicyluric acid and salicyl phenolic glucuronide is capacity limited.[34] The serum salicylate half-life after a single 650-mg dose of aspirin is 3.5 to 4.5 hours, but large daily doses of aspirin (e.g., 4.5 g/day) result in a serum salicylate half-life of 15 to 20 hours. The pharmacokinetics of salicylate are complex and affected by both first-order and Michaelis-Menten elimination processes. When utilizing anti-inflammatory doses of aspirin, 5 to 7 days of therapy are needed before steady-state serum concentrations of salicylate are attained.

5. A.L., a patient with RA, had her aspirin dosage increased to 975 mg QID approximately 1 week ago. She now complains of, "... ringing in my ears all the time!" What is the most probable cause of this symptom?

Aspirin-induced tinnitus (i.e., a ringing or high-pitched buzzing sensation in the head) is noticeable to most patients with normal hearing when serum levels are 10 to 30 mg/dL; however, in some patients tinnitus might not be encountered until serum levels exceed 25 mg/dL.[34] Serum salicylate concentrations usually are within the therapeutic range when tinnitus is apparent. Tinnitus, therefore, can be used to titrate patients to therapeutic doses of aspirin; however, patients with preexisting hearing loss might not experience tinnitus despite potentially toxic concentrations.[114]

Alternative Formulations

6. P.D., a man with an alleged aspirin allergy, avoids aspirin because it has upset his stomach in the past. However, he can take large doses of an enteric-coated aspirin (Ecotrin) without experiencing GI intolerance. What are appropriate alternatives for patients who cannot tolerate therapeutic doses of aspirin?

Patients who complain of GI side effects commonly use aspirin formulations that contain buffering agents (e.g., Alka-Seltzer, Ascriptin, Bufferin). The antacid content in Alka-Seltzer is insufficient to reduce acute GI microbleeding and symptoms, and contributes more than a gram of sodium for each 650 mg of aspirin. Ascriptin and Bufferin contain too little antacid to appreciably reduce GI microbleeding,[115] but occasionally are better tolerated than regular aspirin.

Enteric-coated aspirin is associated with fewer GI complaints than uncoated aspirin.[115] Although enteric coating increases the likelihood of incomplete absorption, Measurin was absorbed reliably in one study involving small numbers of patients,[116] and other newer enteric-coated aspirin preparations can be absorbed reliably as well. Enteric-coated aspirin can be a useful alternative to regular aspirin for some patients.

Sustained-release (SR) aspirin (e.g., ZORprin, Measurin) is intended to provide more stable salicylate concentrations with less frequent administration. Twice-daily dosing of Measurin produces average serum salicylate concentrations comparable to equal doses of aspirin administered four times daily.[117] However, the elimination half-life of regular aspirin in anti-inflammatory doses already is sufficiently long to support relatively stable serum salicylate concentrations with twice-daily dosing.[118,119] The relative advantage of SR aspirin compared with regular or enteric-coated aspirin remains unclear. Nevertheless, some patients tolerate these SR aspirin dosage forms better than regular aspirin.

In summary, various aspirin dosage forms are available. Enteric-coated preparations, despite their expense and potential for incomplete absorption, are alternatives for patients with a history of gastroduodenal ulcers. Alternatively, some newer NSAIDs are equally effective and associated with less GI toxicity (see Question 11).

Aspirin and Nonsteroidal Anti-Inflammatory Drug Allergy

7. Aspirin was ordered for the relief of pain in C.S., who was hospitalized for evaluation and treatment of his RA. An allergy to aspirin is noted in C.S.'s medical chart. Why might another NSAID, also be contraindicated for this patient?

C.S. should be asked to describe his reaction to aspirin to determine whether his symptoms are consistent with a hypersensitivity reaction. Many patients who claim to be allergic to aspirin merely experience GI distress. In these patients, aspirin is not contraindicated and can be tolerated if administered with food or as an enteric-coated preparation.

Aspirin intolerance (hypersensitivity), especially in association with asthma, is cause for serious concern. Challenge with aspirin in these patients can precipitate an acute, life-threatening, bronchospastic reaction.[120] About 10% of asthmatics have a history of aspirin-induced bronchospasm, more often women than men and rarely in children.[121] A somewhat smaller number of patients with recurrent rhinitis also experience this problem.[122] The frequency of aspirin intolerance in patients with nasal polyps can be as high as 22%, and 70% of these patients have asthma.[123] All these patients also can experience a high degree of cross-reactivity to indomethacin (Indocin), naproxen (Naprosyn), ibuprofen (Motrin), fenoprofen (Nalfon), mefenamic acid (Ponstel), sodium benzoate (a widely used preservative), and tartrazine dye (FD&C Yellow No. 5), which is used in foods and some drugs. These substances are structurally dissimilar, but most are inhibitors of prostaglandin synthesis. Therefore, this reaction could be the result of an abnormal response to a common pharmacologic effect. Weak prostaglandin synthesis inhibitors (e.g., sodium and choline salicylate), have been administered to such aspirin-intolerant patients without untoward reactions.

COX-2 inhibitors also have been used safely in aspirin-sensitive asthmatics.[124,125] In theory, these agents might be safer because they allow COX-1 to continue producing prostaglandin E_2. Prostaglandin E_2 is an important mediator of multiple physiological processes, including reduction of leukotriene synthesis, suppression of the release of inflammatory mediators from mast cells, and prevention of aspirin-induced bronchoconstriction.

Some patients with chronic urticaria, as well as patients with rhinitis and aspirin allergy might be at increased risk to develop urticaria or angioedema on exposure to aspirin.[123] The pathogenic mechanism for this urticarial form of aspirin intolerance is unknown.

Prolongation of Bleeding Time

8. A.C. is scheduled to have an impacted wisdom tooth removed. She states that she is taking an aspirinlike product for arthritis. Why would the specific NSAID she is taking affect this dental procedure?

Aspirin, nonacetylated salicylates, nonaspirin NSAIDs, and COX-2 inhibitors have different effects on platelet function. Aspirin alters hemostasis most significantly and should be discontinued before surgery.[34] Low doses of aspirin irreversibly impair platelet aggregation throughout the life of the platelet by irreversible binding to COX and, thereby, prolong bleeding time for several days because new platelets must be released into the circulation before the bleeding time normalizes. Salicylates also can enhance blood fibrinolytic activity, and very large salicylate doses can induce a hypoprothrombinemia that is reversible by vitamin K. Salicylate-induced hypoprothrombinemia usually is not clinically significant, but it can be the cause of bleeding when associated with severe liver dysfunction or malnutrition.[126] Bleeding times normalize within 3 to 6 days after discontinuation of aspirin. Therefore, aspirin should be discontinued about 7 days before surgery.

Nonaspirin NSAIDs also can prolong bleeding times by inhibiting platelet aggregation, but these drugs bind reversibly to COX resulting in reversible platelet inhibition.[34] Therefore, nonaspirin NSAIDs should be discontinued about 5 half-lives before surgical procedures. Generally, the impairment of platelet aggregations is reversed within 2 days after the discontinuation of nonaspirin NSAIDs. Nonacetylated salicylates have minimal effects on COX and platelet function, and are of little concern in presurgical patients.[34] Likewise, COX-2 inhibitors are not expected to alter platelet function because COX-2 is not found in platelets.[127]

Use in Pregnancy

9. K.H., a 28-year-old pregnant woman with RA, is concerned about the possible effects of NSAIDs on her baby. What are the risks to the fetus with uninterrupted consumption of NSAIDs? What are maternal- and lactation-related effects of these medications?

Although NSAIDs, including aspirin, are not teratogenic, they must be used cautiously in women who are pregnant and who plan to breast-feed infants.[128] Fetal effects of NSAIDs include possible premature ductus arteriosus closure, increased cutaneous and intracranial bleeding, transient renal impairment, and a reduction in urine output. High doses of aspirin (>3 g/day) and NSAIDs can inhibit uterine contraction, resulting in prolonged labor. NSAIDs also can increase peripartum blood loss and anemia. Aspirin and nonaspirin NSAIDs should be used sparingly at lowest effective doses during in pregnancy and discontinued at least 6 to 8 weeks before delivery to minimize adverse fetal and maternal effects.

Aspirin generally should be avoided for women who plan to nurse their baby because salicylate serum concentrations in breastfed neonates raise concerns about the potential for metabolic acidosis, bleeding, and Reye syndrome. According to the American Academy of Pediatrics, the nonaspirin NSAIDs (e.g., ibuprofen, naproxen) generally are compatible with breastfeeding.[129]

NONASPIRIN NONSTEROIDAL ANTI-INFLAMMATORY DRUGS

Choice of Agent

10. NSAIDs and DMARD therapy are to be initiated for T.W. (Questions 1–4). What is the NSAID of choice for T.W.?

In general, there is no "NSAID of choice" for treatment of RA.[10,34] There is no significant difference among the NSAIDs in efficacy, and it is difficult to predict a given patient's response to a particular NSAID. The selection of an NSAID is based primarily on patient preference, convenience, cost, and safety.[8] A 1- to 2-week trial of any NSAID (Table 43-5) at a moderate to high dose on a scheduled basis (i.e., not "as needed") is the best method of determining anti-inflammatory efficacy. The analgesic and antipyretic effects are relatively prompt in onset. Although aspirin is effective, the nonaspirin NSAIDs usually are preferred.[113] Nonacetylated salicylates, derivatives of salicylic acid, are weak inhibitors of COX in vitro, but have risks of GI and renal toxicity similar to nonselective NSAIDs.[130–132]

The nonsalicylate NSAIDs (e.g., ibuprofen) have important differentiating properties.[34] For example, indomethacin penetrates the blood-brain barrier better than any other NSAID, achieving levels in the cerebrospinal fluid of up to 50% of serum levels. As a result, the incidence of central nervous system side effects of indomethacin often precludes the use of optimal anti-inflammatory doses, particularly in the elderly.[133] Loose stools or diarrhea can be dose limiting for some patients receiving meclofenamate. Piroxicam, a longer acting NSAID, has been associated with a higher frequency of peptic ulcer disease and GI bleeding[113] and, therefore, should be avoided. Several NSAIDs, including celecoxib and high doses of either ibuprofen or diclofenac, seem to increase the risk of MI, whereas naproxen seems to have the best cardiovascular safety.[134]

The relative GI safety of partially COX-2-selective NSAIDs (e.g., nabumetone, etodolac, meloxicam) versus nonselective NSAIDs is unclear. The only remaining COX-2-specific inhibitor that is available in the United States, celecoxib, has no effect on COX-1 and the GI protective effect of celecoxib is questionable owing to a major protocol violation in the largest GI safety study involving celecoxib[135] (see Question 11).

A low-cost NSAID with a good safety profile (e.g., ibuprofen) is a good choice for T.W. because she is relatively young and does not have any concomitant illnesses. If convenience of administration is a more important consideration, a longer acting NSAID (e.g., naproxen) would be preferable. If the first chosen NSAID is ineffective or not well tolerated, other NSAIDs can be tried to identify the optimal one for this patient.

Adverse Effects

11. Naproxen 500 mg BID with meals has been prescribed for T.W. If T.W. were to develop dyspepsia during therapy, should she

Table 43-5 Nonsteroidal Anti-inflammatory Drugs (NSAIDs)

NSAID Generic Name (Brand Name)	Product Availability	Usual Dosing Interval	Maximum Daily Dose (mg)	Cost/30-Day Supply ($)[a]
Salicylates (acetylated and nonacetylated)[b]				
Aspirin, enteric-coated[c]	*Tablets:* 325 mg; 325, 500, 800, 975 mg SR	QID	6,000	12.00
Salsalate (Disalcid)[c]	*Tablets:* 500, 750 mg	BID-TID	4,800	18.00
Diflunisal (Dolobid)[c]	*Tablets:* 250, 500 mg	BID	1,500	35.00
Magnesium choline salicylate (Trilisate)[c]	*Tablets:* 500, 750, 1,000 mg *Liquid:* 500 mg/5 mL	QD-TID	4,800	30.00
Propionic acid derivatives				
Fenoprofen (Nalfon)[c]	*Capsules:* 200, 300 mg *Tablets:* 600 mg	TID-QID	3,200	22.50
Flurbiprofen (Ansaid)[c]	*Tablets:* 50, 100 mg	BID-QID	300	26.50
Ibuprofen (Motrin)[c]	*Tablets:* 200, 400, 600, 800 mg *Suspension:* 100 mg/5 mL	TID-QID	3,200	13.80
Ketoprofen (Orudis, Orudis ER)[c]	*Capsules:* 25, 50, 75 mg	TID-QID ER: QD	300 ER: 200	17.50 ER: 67.50
Naproxen (Naprosyn)[c]	*Tablets:* 250, 375, 500 mg; 375, 500 mg SR *Suspension:* 125 mg/5 mL	BID	1,500	37.80
Naproxen sodium (Anaprox)[c]	*Tablets:* 275, 550 mg	BID	1,375	39.60
Oxaproxin (Daypro)[c]	*Tablet or capsule:* 600 mg	QD	1,800	34.80
Acetic acid derivatives				
Diclofenac (Voltaren, Voltaren XR)[c]	*Tablets:* 25, 50, 75 mg; 100 mg XR	BID-TID XR: QD	200 XR: 100 mg	54.60 XR: 68.40
Etodolac (Lodine, Lodine XL)[c]	*Capsules:* 200, 300 mg *Tablets:* 400, 500 mg; 400, 500, 600 mg XL	BID-TID XL: QD	1,200 XL: 1,000	69.00 40.50
Indomethacin (Indocin, Indocin SR)[c]	*Capsules:* 25, 50 mg; 75 mg SR *Suppository:* 50 mg *Suspension:* 25 mg/5 mL	TID-QID SR: QD-BID	200 SR: 150	55.00 SR: 65.00
Ketorolac (Toradol)[c]	*Tablet:* 10 mg	QID	40	1015.00
Nabumetone (Relafen)	*Tablet:* 500, 750 mg	QD	2,000	84.00
Sulindac (Clinoril)[c]	*Tablets:* 150, 200 mg	BID	400	54.00
Tolmetin (Tolectin)[c]	*Tablets:* 200, 600 mg *Capsules:* 400 mg	TID-QID	1,800	46.20
Anthranilic acids				
Meclofenamate sodium (Meclomen)[c]	*Capsules:* 50, 100 mg	TID-QID	400	91.00
Oxicam derivatives				
Piroxicam (Feldene)[c]	*Capsule:* 10, 20 mg	QD	20	75.00
Meloxicam (Mobic)[c]	*Tablets:* 7.5, 15 mg	QD	15	5.40
COX-2 inhibitors				
Celecoxib (Celebrex)	*Capsules:* 50, 100, 200, 400 mg	BID	400	111

[a] From reference 30. Average cost to patient based on usual dose for RA; price is for generic version if available (see footnote c).
[b] Highly variable half-life; anti-inflammatory doses associated with salicyclate serum concentrations from 15 to 30 mg/dL.
[c] Generic version available.
BID, twice a day; ER, extended release; QD, daily; QID, four times a day; SR, sustained release; TID, three times a day.

be given misoprostol (or other antiulcer therapy) for prophylaxis against GI complications of NSAID therapy or would a COX-2 selective NSAID be preferable? What is the correlation between dyspepsia and gastroduodenal mucosal injury?

About 5% and 15% of patients with RA discontinue NSAID therapy because of dyspepsia,[37] and about 1.3% of patients taking NSAIDs for RA experience a serious GI complication.[136] As expected, the rate is somewhat lower for patients using NSAIDs for osteoarthritis (OA; 0.7%) because these patients generally use analgesics only on an as-needed basis. Serious NSAID-induced GI complications account for about 103,000 hospitalizations annually in the United States and for approximately 16,500 NSAID-related deaths each year.[37] Although these figures warrant concern, most patients who experience NSAID-induced gastropathy suffer only superficial and self-limiting injury. Nevertheless, prevention of NSAID-induced

GI bleeding should be an important focus, particularly in high-risk patients.

NSAID-induced gastroduodenal mucosal damage primarily results from inhibition of COX-1 in the mucosal lining.[37] This inhibition of COX-1 decreases bicarbonate secretion, mucosal blood flow, formation of protective mucus, proliferation of gastric epithelium, and the ability of the mucosa to resist injury. NSAID-induced direct topical injury to the mucosa can occur, but direct injury plays a smaller role than COX-1 inhibition. NSAID-induced gastropathy can be managed by: (a) treatment of NSAID-related dyspepsia, (b) prevention of NSAID-associated gastroduodenal ulcers, and (c) management of NSAID-related gastroduodenal ulcers.

Dyspepsia can be managed by ingesting the NSAID with meals or a large glass of water; however, these measures usually are ineffective in preventing GI ulcers. In addition, dyspepsia correlates poorly with endoscopically confirmed mucosal injury.[37] Histamine-2 (H_2)-receptor antagonists (e.g., ranitidine, famotidine) significantly reduce dyspepsia among NSAID users; however, NSAID users with RA who take a H_2-receptor antagonist might have a higher risk of developing serious GI complications compared with those who did not take these medications (odds ratio, 2.14; 95% confidence interval, 1.06–4.32).[137] The suppression of dyspepsia can give a false sense of security to the patient and physician, leading to higher doses of NSAIDs and increased risk of major gastropathy. Therefore, H_2-receptor antagonists are not recommended for routine use in asymptomatic patients receiving NSAIDs. Proton pump inhibitors (PPIs; e.g., lansoprazole 30 mg/day or omeprazole 20 mg/day) relieve dyspepsia better than H_2-receptor antagonists and prevent the development of NSAID-induced gastroduodenal ulcers.[37,138,139] PPIs are safe and effective for the treatment of NSAID-induced dyspepsia and should be considered if symptoms develop in T.W.

Routine concomitant antiulcer prophylactic therapy is not warranted for all patients taking NSAIDs.[10,34] The most effective means of preventing NSAID-related gastroduodenal ulcers is obviously to avoid their use. If NSAIDs must be used, the patient's risk for GI ulcer development must be assessed to determine the need for ulcer prevention measures.[37] Established risk factors for NSAID-induced GI bleeding include advancing age (>60 years of age), a history of ulcers, use of ulcer-promoting medications (corticosteroids, high-dose NSAIDs, concurrent use of more than one NSAID or aspirin at any dose, anticoagulants), and daily alcohol consumption.[140] *Helicobacter pylori* infection may also increase the risk of NSAID-induced GI bleeding; however, *H. pylori* eradication has a minimal impact on preventing NSAID-related gastroduodenal injury.[141] Patients requiring NSAID therapy who are at high risk for GI bleeding should receive concomitant ulcer prevention therapy. Misoprostol (200 mcg three or four times daily), a prostaglandin E_1 analog, and a PPI are effective in preventing NSAID-induced gastroduodenal mucosal injury.[141] PPI cotherapy is more commonly prescribed because of the convenience of once-daily dosing and better tolerability. Dose-related GI upset, particularly diarrhea and abdominal pain, is a frequent cause of misoprostol intolerance. No evidence is available to support the use of H_2-receptor antagonists, sucralfate, and antacids in preventing NSAID-related GI injury.

Active NSAID-induced gastroduodenal ulcers are best treated by discontinuing the NSAID and initiating either a H_2-receptor antagonist (e.g., cimetidine 800 mg, ranitidine 150 mg, nizatidine 150 mg, famotidine 40 mg) or a PPI (same dosing as for ulcer prevention). In general, a PPI is preferred because of rapid healing rates and shorter duration of treatment (4–8 weeks). If discontinuation of the NSAID is not feasible, ulcer healing can still be accomplished with a PPI but requires a longer duration of therapy (8–12 weeks).[37] Patients who test positive for *H. Pylori* should undergo *H. Pylori* eradication therapy. Misoprostol, and antacids are ineffective treatments for NSAID-induced ulcers.

The development of NSAIDs highly selective for COX-2 introduced the potential to reduce inflammation without the worrisome adverse effects of nonselective NSAIDs, particularly gastropathy (see general treatment section and Table 43-6). COX-2-selective inhibitors (e.g., celecoxib, rofecoxib, valdecoxib) do not interfere with COX-1 at therapeutic plasma concentrations in humans.[142–145] Although COX-2 inhibitors are associated with significantly less endoscopically confirmed gastroduodenal ulcers when compared with nonselective NSAIDs, their effect on clinically significant gastropathy is unclear.[146] The incidence of clinically significant gastropathy was evaluated in two large clinical trials involving celecoxib (Celecoxib Long-Term Safety Study [CLASS]) and rofecoxib (Vioxx Gastrointestinal Outcomes Research [VIGOR]).[135,147] The CLASS trial compared celecoxib to ibuprofen (800 mg TID) and diclofenac (75 mg BID), and the VIGOR trial compared rofecoxib to naproxen (500 mg BID). Up to 325 mg/day of aspirin use was allowed in CLASS (taken by 21% of patients). The primary endpoint for CLASS at 6 months of treatment was complicated ulcers and the secondary endpoint for CLASS included both symptomatic and complicated ulcers.

In the CLASS study, only the secondary endpoint proved to significantly favor celecoxib over ibuprofen and diclofenac. The conclusions of CLASS are controversial. The published CLASS data consisted of roughly half of the treatment

Table 43-6 Comparison of Cyclo-oxygenase (COX)-1 and COX-2 Isoforms[282]

COX Isoform	*COX-1*	*COX-2*
Expression: continuous or induced?	Primarily continuous, although some evidence of induction	Primarily induced, but present continuously in several organs
Common organs/tissues	Nearly all organs, including stomach, kidneys, platelets, vasculature	Induced at sites of inflammation and neoplasms Continuously active in kidneys, small intestine, pancreas, brain, ovaries, uterus
Primary role	Housekeeping/maintenance May be important when induced in response to inflammation	Inflammation, repair, neoplasia May be important in housekeeping/maintenance of organs which continuously express COX-2

duration specified in the original study design.[146] The study design for CLASS consisted of two separate long-term comparisons with diclofenac (12 months) and ibuprofen (16 months). The reporting of only 6 months of data seems to seriously violate the study protocol. Complete results, available through the U.S. Food and Drug Administration (FDA)'s website, indicates that the twofold reduction in combined symptomatic and complicated ulcers associated with celecoxib is only significant when compared with ibuprofen; no gastropathy advantage was identified when compared with diclofenac.[148] In fact, when an alternate definition of ulcer-related complications is applied to the CLASS trial (which was preplanned by the FDA), a nonsignificant trend in favor of diclofenac was found.[146] Consequently, the FDA has not approved of product labeling that suggest GI-sparing advantages associated with celecoxib. Although the results from VIGOR led to FDA approval of labeling to reflect reduction in serious GI complications,[149] rofecoxib has since been withdrawn from the market because of increased risk of cardiovascular events (see discussion in general treatment section).

Without risk factors other than NSAID use, T.W. does not need concurrent ulcer prophylaxis medication at this time.

Use in Renal Disease

12. T.Z., a 68-year-old man with heart failure previously managed with furosemide 40 mg/day, digoxin 0.125 mg/day, metoprolol 50 mg BID, and lisinopril 40 mg/day, returns for a prescription refill of ibuprofen 600 mg TID, which he takes for his RA. He has noted increased leg swelling over the past 2 weeks associated with a weight gain of several pounds, increasing shortness of breath (SOB), and easy fatigability. Why might these signs and symptoms be associated with ibuprofen?

Mild fluid retention occurs in approximately 5% of NSAID users, and NSAID-induced kidney disease occurs in <1% of patients.[150] NSAID therapy should be monitored carefully in patients with heart failure, liver disease with associated ascites, compromised renal function, or when diuretics are administered concomitantly. In these situations, renal function highly depends on local production of prostaglandin E_2 within the kidney to offset the vasoconstrictor effects of high concentrations of angiotensin, vasopressin, and catecholamines.[151] Inhibition of COX by NSAIDs within the kidney reduces prostaglandin concentrations and unopposed vasoconstriction. Consequently, urine output declines, serum blood urea nitrogen and serum creatinine levels rise, and fluid is retained. This potential complication is associated with all of the currently marketed NSAIDs.[152] In addition, ibuprofen is among several NSAIDS (e.g., celecoxib, high doses of diclofenac) that are associated with an increased risk of MI, which is a concern for T.Z. owing to his risk for cardiac events.[134]

T.Z. should be informed that his leg swelling, weight gain, SOB, and fatigability might be caused by ibuprofen.

13. How should this drug-related problem be managed in T.Z.?

If T.Z.s symptoms have been objectively attributed to some degree of renal dysfunction, his ibuprofen (Motrin) should be discontinued, NSAID therapy should not be restarted until renal function normalizes, and alternative approaches for management of his RA should be considered. In several studies, sulindac (Clinoril) had been associated with less adverse effects on the kidney than other NSAIDS.[153–156] The reason(s) for this are unclear, but one explanation is that the active sulfide metabolite undergoes renal metabolism and, therefore, might not achieve tissue concentrations within the kidney sufficient to reduce prostaglandin production.[157] Unfortunately, patients do not seem to benefit from sulindac as much as from other NSAIDs. Nabumetone (Relafen), an NSAID with moderate COX-2 selectivity, has less of an effect on glomerular filtration than sulindac or ibuprofen.[158] The nonacetylated salicylates have minimal prostaglandin-inhibiting activity and could be alternatives for T.Z., although they too have been associated with renal toxicity. The COX-2 inhibitor, celecoxib, also has been associated with renal adverse effects such as edema (2.1%), new hypertension (0.8%), and exacerbation of preexisting hypertension (0.6%).[159] The incidence for these particular adverse events is similar to those associated with nonselective NSAIDs. Although celecoxib was associated with a slightly lower risk of death and heart failure exacerbation when compared with traditional NSAIDs,[160] it is not a reasonable initial option for T.Z. because celecoxib also is associated with an increased risk of MI.

NSAIDs should be used at lowest effective doses for minimal periods of time for T.Z. High-dose ibuprofen and celecoxib should be avoided owing to potential MI risk. Although acetaminophen is not an anti-inflammatory, it can provide analgesic relief. Intra-articular corticosteroid injections can be useful if inflamed joints are limited in number, or a short course of oral corticosteroids can provide rapid control of inflammation while reducing the need for longer courses of anti-inflammatory therapy. If T.Z. is not being treated with a DMARD, it should be seriously considered because all patients with RA are candidates for DMARDs, which could obviate T.Z.'s need for an NSAID. If an NSAID or short course of systemic corticosteroid is selected, close monitoring of renal function and fluid retention status is warranted.

14. What other renal syndromes are associated with NSAID therapy?

In addition to acute renal failure, NSAIDs can induce various adverse renal effects (e.g., nephrotic syndrome, interstitial nephritis, hyponatremia, abnormalities of water metabolism, hyperkalemia).[161] The nephrotic syndrome, unlike NSAID-induced acute renal failure, can appear anytime (i.e., from days to years) after starting therapy; and can resolve as quickly as 1 month, or as long as 1 year, after discontinuation of the NSAID. Hematuria, pyuria, and proteinuria without prior renal disease differentiates nephrotic syndrome from other NSAID-induced renal problems. Histologically, NSAID-induced nephrotic syndrome is characterized by interstitial lymphocytic infiltrates, vacuolar degeneration of proximal and distal tubules, and fusion of epithelial foot processes of glomeruli.

Prostaglandin-mediated inhibition of active chloride transport, regulation of medullary blood flow within the kidney, and antagonism of antidiuretic hormone can be suppressed by NSAIDs. As a result, urine is maximally concentrated, free water clearance is limited, and water retention that is disproportionate to sodium retention can occur. The resulting hyponatremia can be severe and could be potentiated by thiazide diuretics.[162]

Local prostaglandin synthesis also can stimulate renin production within the kidney. NSAID therapy can critically attenuate this regulatory mechanism in some situations, resulting in reduced aldosterone-mediated potassium excretion and hyperkalemia.

Although the mechanism is poorly understood, some NSAIDs have been associated with sustained mean arterial pressure increases of 5 to 6 mm Hg,[163] presumably the result of COX-2 inhibition and sodium/water retention. However, in several studies, only patients taking antihypertensive medications experienced NSAID-induced mean arterial pressure elevations, whereas those who controlled their hypertension without medications were unaffected by NSAID therapy. It seems, therefore, that NSAIDs can interfere with the action of antihypertensive drug therapy by a mechanism that has yet to be identified.

Laboratory Test Monitoring for Nonsteroidal Anti-Inflammatory Drug Therapy

15. When should routine renal or liver function be tested during NSAID therapy?

Patients at high risk for NSAID-induced renal disease (see Questions 12–14) should have their serum creatinine checked weekly for several weeks after initiation of therapy because renal insufficiency more commonly occurs early in the course of therapy.[162] NSAID-induced nephrotic syndrome and allergic interstitial nephritis occur, on average, about 6.6 months and 15 days after NSAID initiation, respectively.

In most cases, liver function testing (LFT) is unnecessary.[162] Although NSAIDs can elevate liver enzymes, severe hepatotoxicity is rare. Abnormal LFTs without clinical symptoms have no impact on patient outcome and have not been associated with severe hepatotoxicity. However, patients who seem to be at greater risk for hepatotoxicity are those with established or suspected intrinsic liver disease and those receiving diclofenac. These patients should have liver function tested no later than 8 weeks after initiation of therapy because liver toxicity manifests early in therapy if at all.

Patient Instructions

16. What instructions should be provided to a RA patient receiving a NSAID prescription?

Patients should be informed that NSAID therapy is being prescribed to provide relief of pain and inflammation associated with RA, but does not slow or stop the progression of the disease. It should be explained that the latter only can be accomplished by DMARD therapy. Patients should also understand that moderate to high daily doses of NSAIDs are required for anti-inflammatory activity, as opposed to analgesic and antipyretic effects which can be achieved with single and low doses.

Patients should be instructed to keep the NSAID container tightly closed and to avoid storing NSAIDs, particularly aspirin, in moist environments (e.g., bathrooms). Aspirin is hydrolyzed to salicylic acid and acetic acid with moisture. Prescription NSAIDs and aspirin come in childproof safety containers, but many arthritic patients have difficulty with these safety closures because of diminished grip strength and hand deformities. If an NSAID is dispensed in a conventional closure container, it is necessary to explain the hazards of accidental ingestion by children and, as required by law in most states, obtain a signed release form.

Patients should be taught to recognize the signs and symptoms of GI bleeding (e.g., nausea, vomiting, anorexia, gastric pain), GI bleeding as manifested by melena (described to the patient as "dark, tarry stool"), or emesis of coagulated blood (described to the patient as, "coughing or vomiting up what seems to be coffee grounds"). It should be emphasized that GI bleeding can occur without gastric pain. The patient should be instructed to contact their health care provider immediately for further instructions if any of these signs or symptoms occur.

TRADITIONAL DISEASE-MODIFYING ANTIRHEUMATIC DRUGS

17. Which traditional DMARD therapies are most appropriate for T.W.?

Every newly diagnosed RA patient is a candidate for DMARD therapy, which should be started within 3 months of diagnosis.[10] For most patients, MTX is the initial DMARD of choice because of high rate of clinical response for all levels of RA severity and radiographic evidence of slowing joint erosion, which is most rapid during the first several years of active disease[164,165] (Fig. 43-8). Although most DMARDs are associated with potentially serious adverse effects, these generally are reversible and seldom lead to serious complications if the patient has been monitored appropriately.

Most patients with active RA are treated with at least one DMARD and with an NSAID.[10] In addition, low-dose oral corticosteroids are often prescribed on an "as needed" basis for brief periods of severe disease activity or while awaiting the onset of DMARD action. During periods of disease remission, NSAID therapy can be discontinued; however, attempts to discontinue traditional DMARDs have resulted in disease reactivation or "rebound flare" and resumption of the discontinued traditional DMARD is not always successful in reestablishing control. Therefore, successful traditional DMARD therapy should be continued indefinitely. Safety and efficacy data, which reflect several years of DMARD therapy combined with biological agents, have been excellent, and the combination is now commonly prescribed for patients who fail MTX monotherapy (see Questions 39 and 43). The selection of DMARDs (see General Treatment section) and their use in combination seems more effective than DMARD monotherapy (see Question 38).

Antimalarials

Dosing

18. Although T.W.'s presentation could warrant a more potent DMARD, treatment was initiated with HCQ. What dosages would be appropriate, and when should clinical improvement be expected?

Although the manufacturer's literature recommends an initial HCQ adult dose of 400 to 600 mg/day (310–465 mg of base), dosages for HCQ generally range from 2 to 6.5 mg/kg/day.[29] If the patient responds well, the maintenance dose can be reduced by 50% and the medication continued at a dose of 200 to 400 mg/day (155–310 mg of base). About two-thirds of patients who tolerate HCQ respond favorably. Benefits usually are apparent within 2 to 4 months of therapy, but can vary between 1 and 6 months.[10] About 37% of patients discontinued HCQ within a year and 54% within 2 years primarily owing to lack of efficacy.[166]

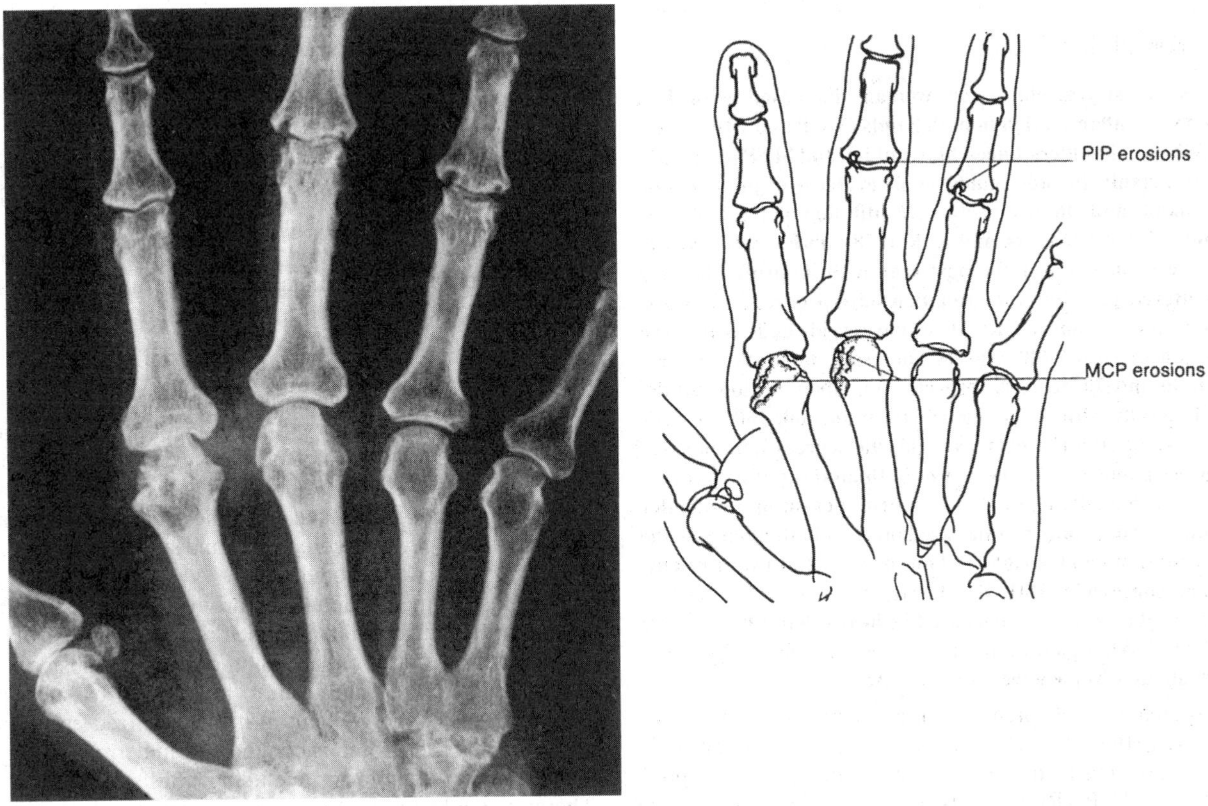

FIGURE 43-8 Radiograph of the hand in RA showing both active erosions at the metacarpophalangeal joints (MCPs) and old well-demarcated erosions at the proximal interphalangeal joints (PIPs).

Risk of Retinopathy

19. How great is the risk of retinopathy from antimalarials when used for the treatment of RA? What monitoring parameters are appropriate?

HCQ seems to be the least toxic of all DMARDs. The most serious toxicity, retinal damage and subsequent visual impairment, is rare.[162] Risk of retinopathy seems to correlate with cumulative dose (>800 g) and age (>70 years). The increased risk of retinopathy in the elderly seems to be related to the increased prevalence of macular disease in this age group. HCQ doses exceeding 6.0 to 6.5 mg/kg are associated with increased risk of retinal damage, particularly in patients with renal or hepatic dysfunction.

Patients should be instructed to stop therapy immediately and undergo an ophthalmologic evaluation if experiencing symptoms of antimalarial-associated retinopathy (e.g., difficulty seeing faces or entire words, glare intolerance, poor night vision, loss of peripheral vision).[162] The fully developed lesion of antimalarial retinopathy is seen on ophthalmoscopy as a pigmentary disturbance with a characteristic "bull's eye" appearance in the macular region. The 4-amino-quinolines bind to melanin, and as a result, concentrate in the uveal tract and retinal pigment epithelium. The retinopathy can be progressive even after discontinuation of the drug.

Baseline eye examination is not required in patients younger than 40 with no family history of eye disease. The first ophthalmologic examination is recommended after 6 months of HCQ therapy, followed by an examination with central field testing every 6 to 12 months. More frequent testing is recommended for patients with renal dysfunction or patients who have received HCQ therapy for >10 years. Benign corneal deposits of antimalarial drug may occur during therapy. Although this adverse effect may be symptomatic, it is harmless, reversible when the antimalarial drug is discontinued, and not related to the more serious and less common retinopathy.[167]

Sulfasalazine

20. If SSZ were chosen as initial therapy for T.W., when should therapeutic effects become apparent and what adverse effects might be anticipated?

The onset of SSZ effect is generally more rapid than HCQ and can become apparent within a month[10]; however, a clinical response might be delayed for 4 months, and doses should be adjusted only after this period has elapsed.

Compared with other DMARDs, adverse effects associated with SSZ are relatively mild, consisting of nausea, abdominal discomfort, heartburn, dizziness, headaches, skin rashes, and, rarely, hematologic effects such as leukopenia (1%–3%) or thrombocytopenia (rare).[168] A complete blood count (CBC) is recommended every 2 to 4 weeks for the first 3 months of therapy, then every 3 months thereafter. Leukopenia more commonly manifests within the first 6 months of therapy. To minimize GI-related adverse effects, SSZ is initiated at 500 mg/day or 1 g/day and the dosage is increased at weekly intervals by 500 mg until 1,000 mg two or three times daily is reached.

Gold

Preparations and Adverse Reactions

21. S.S., a 41-year-old Asian woman diagnosed with RA, presents with inflammation in both hands (MCP and PIP joints), wrists, elbows, shoulders, knees, hips, ankles, and MTP joints. Objective test results include radiographic evidence of joint erosion in both hands and elbows, positive RF (dilution of 1:1,280), positive anti-CCP at 102 units, and ESR of 78 mm/hour. Her symptoms were managed over the past year with ibuprofen 800 mg TID; however, pain and inflammation have progressively worsened over several months. ROM testing reveals deficits in wrist flexion and extension (20 degrees bilaterally for both motions; normal, 90 and 70 degrees, respectively), elbow flexion (90 degrees bilaterally with flexion contracture; normal, 160 degrees), shoulder abduction (70 degrees right, 90 degrees left; normal, 180 degrees), and plantar flexion of both ankles (20 degrees bilaterally; normal, 45 degrees). Three firm, pea-sized, nontender moveable subcutaneous nodules are found on both elbows at the ulnar border, two on the right and one on the left. In your discussion about considering DMARD therapy, S.S. states that she does not want gold therapy "... because I've heard that it has terrible side effects." What gold preparations are available, and is S.S.'s concern about adverse effects warranted?

Two parenteral gold preparations are available: gold sodium thiomalate (Myochrysine), an aqueous solution, and aurothioglucose (Solganal), an oil suspension. Although an oral gold formulation, AUR (Ridaura), is also available, it is slow in onset (4–6 months) and is less efficacious.[10] The parenteral formulations, containing approximately 50% gold by weight expressed as milligrams of complex, are equally effective.[29] Aurothioglucose must be shaken thoroughly before withdrawal from its vial and a large-bore needle is necessary to draw up this viscous suspension. Lumps at the intramuscular injection site sometimes can be troublesome to the patient.

Toxicities with both injectable gold preparations are numerous and largely responsible for their high rate of discontinuation. In a 6-year prospective trial, nearly half of patients receiving gold sodium thiomalate discontinued therapy, with 95% of those discontinuing because of toxicity.[55] The toxicity profiles of the parenteral gold preparations differ. A vasomotor reaction (also termed *nitritoid reaction*), which manifests as nausea, weakness, flushing, tachycardia, and/or syncope, can occur in up to 5% of patients receiving gold sodium thiomalate. These reactions generally are mild, are transient, and often can be alleviated by having the patient lie down.

Gold-induced myocardial ischemia or infarction is rare and possibly related to the vehicle or preservative in the thiomalate preparation because it has not been reported with aurothioglucose.[169] Patients with concomitant cardiovascular disease or patients who experience a nitritoid reaction after an injection of gold sodium thiomalate can be treated with aurothioglucose, although treatment with MTX, biological agents, or other alternatives should be considered.

Nonvasomotor reactions, consisting of transient stiffness, arthralgias, and myalgias, developed in 15% of patients after initiation of gold sodium thiomalate therapy,[170] and substituting aurothioglucose for the thiomalate formulation decreased severity of this adverse reaction in 40% of the patients.

Skin eruptions, stomatitis, and albuminuria are more common in patients who receive the aqueous gold sodium thiomalate preparation than in patients who received the oil suspension of aurothioglucose.[171] Aurothioglucose also is more commonly associated with renal toxicity than gold sodium thiomalate, although the overall incidence is rare.[172] Membranous nephropathy (most common), nephrotic syndrome, and interstitial nephritis have been reported. Hematuria and proteinuria may be early indicators of membranous nephropathy; however, proteinuria can occur transiently in up to 50% of patients receiving aurothioglucose. Patients who develop proteinuria should undergo a renal evaluation and a urinalysis. Gold therapy should be discontinued if protein excretion is >500 mg/24 hr.

Parenteral gold preparations have been associated with sudden occurrence of idiosyncratic thrombocytopenia (1%–3%) or aplastic anemia (<1%).[172] Screening for urine protein and a CBC should be performed before each weekly injection for the first 20 to 22 weeks, then before every other injection. In addition, patients should be asked about the occurrence of pruritus, skin eruptions, purpura, sore throat, and stomatitis before each dose of gold is administered.

Pruritus, erythema, or a fine morbilliform rash on the neck or extremities can develop after the first few injections of gold. These cutaneous reactions are common, usually subside within several days, and do not seem to be affected by subsequent injections. Although a highly pruritic localized eruption resembling pityriasis rosea is common, gold dermatitis may assume many different forms, including exfoliative dermatitis.[29] Therapy should be discontinued if a pruritic dermatitis develops. Mild dermal reactions may be managed with topical corticosteroids.[172]

If discontinued, gold can be reintroduced in a reduced dosage after resolution of rashes (see Question 23). Gold treatments should be discontinued if white blood cells (WBCs) decline to <3,500 cells/mm^3, if platelets fall to <100,000 cells/mm^3, or if the Hgb concentration falls rapidly.[162] Although eosinophilia may be associated with toxic reactions, it is not a reliable predictor of gold toxicity and is not an indication to discontinue gold therapy.[173]

Thrombocytopenia can be life threatening and sometimes is difficult to treat because of the long half-life of gold.[172] Most cases respond to cessation of gold therapy, but platelet or red cell transfusions might be needed for severe cases. Antibiotics should be administered to patients with fever and an absolute neutropenia count of <1,000/mm^3.[172]

Other unusual but potentially serious complications of gold therapy include colitis, pneumonitis, and cholestatic hepatitis.[174–177] Corneal chrysiasis also can occur but does not lead to ocular complications.[178]

AUR capsules, containing 3 mg of gold, are 25% bioavailable.[179] The recommended AUR daily dose of 6 mg can be given either as single or divided doses. AUR is better tolerated than parenteral gold formulations, but is significantly less effective.[10] Like parenteral chrysotherapy, benefit can occur as early as 6 to 8 weeks after starting AUR, but objective benefits might not be apparent for several months. Overall, AUR has a slower onset of action when compared with gold sodium thiomalate.[180] AUR must be monitored in a manner similar to parenteral therapy. Proteinuria and bone marrow suppression occur with AUR, but the incidence is low.[181] The incidence of rashes necessitating AUR withdrawal is lower than with parenteral gold therapy, but loose stools and diarrhea are encountered more commonly (47%).

S.S.'s concerns have merit. Although gold is an effective DMARD and can induce complete RA remission, none of the gold formulations are ideal. Gold sodium thiomalate is easier to administer, but is associated with more frequent side effects compared with aurothioglucose. Aurothioglucose carries a low but serious risk of nephrotoxicity. Both parenteral forms of gold are commonly discontinued because of side effects. AUR is the best tolerated gold preparation, but the least effective and is associated with significant diarrhea.

Dosing

22. How is parenteral gold administered? Is serum drug monitoring of value in gold therapy?

The standard treatment schedule for parenteral gold consists of an initial intramuscular test dose of 10 mg followed by a 25 mg IM dose 1 week later. The third and subsequent weekly intramuscular injections of 25 to 50 mg should be continued until the cumulative dose reaches 1 g, toxicity occurs, or major benefit is derived.[29,172] If a satisfactory response is achieved, maintenance doses of 25 to 50 mg every other week are recommended. If the disease remains stable, doses can be administered every third and subsequently every fourth week for an indefinite period.[172]

Attempts to correlate serum gold concentrations with clinical outcomes generally have been unsuccessful.[182,183] Furthermore, toxicity has not been correlated with serum gold concentrations.[182]

23. After 10 weeks of treatment with aurothioglucose (total, 435 mg), L.T. developed pruritus and a rash on her abdomen. Gold was withheld and she was given a prescription for triamcinolone cream. Should L.T's gold therapy be discontinued?

Dermatologic reactions to gold occur in 15% to 30% of patients.[172] Because of fears of subsequent exfoliative dermatitis and the belief that dermatologic reactions recur upon rechallenge, there is a natural reluctance to continue gold treatment after the appearance of dermatitis or stomatitis. However, in one series of patients, gold treatments were reinstituted successfully in 28 of 30 patients in whom dermatologic reactions developed.[184] One of these patients who presented initially with severe exfoliative dermatitis was treated successfully with gold several years later. Gold therapy was reinstituted in these patients as follows. After waiting at least 6 weeks after the lesions had healed completely, a 1-mg test dose of gold was administered intramuscularly. Subsequent doses were increased to 2 mg, then to 5 mg, and then to 10 mg at 2- to 4-week intervals. Thereafter, 5-mg increments were added until a dose of 50 mg/week was attained. Dermatologic reactions did not develop in any of these patients subsequently. Gold therapy, therefore, need not be abandoned in L.T.

Auranofin

24. J.M., a patient receiving gold sodium thiomalate for 1 year and responding well to a maintenance regimen of 50 mg IM Q 4 wk asks about switching to AUR. Will switching to AUR from parenteral gold maintain J.M.'s RA under good control? Can patients who have discontinued parenteral therapy because of adverse side effects be treated with AUR?

Some patients originally treated with parenteral therapy can be switched to AUR and remain well controlled.[185,186] This experience is not universal, however, and it is not possible to predict which patients can be switched successfully to oral therapy.

When parenteral gold is injected weekly, the relative cost of parenteral gold therapy (including office visits and monitoring) is more than the costs associated with daily AUR therapy. When gold injections are given every 2 to 3 weeks, the cost of parenteral and oral therapy is similar, depending on local laboratory and medical costs. When injections are given monthly, the cost of parenteral therapy usually is less than for oral therapy. Because this patient is well controlled, little is to be gained by switching from parenteral therapy to AUR, either from an economic or therapeutic standpoint.

Data are limited on the use of AUR in patients who experienced side effects from parenteral gold. Because rashes usually are mild and proteinuria is reversible if the patient is properly monitored, a trial of AUR in patients withdrawn from parenteral gold for these reasons may be justified.[187] It is inadvisable, however, to initiate AUR in patients who were withdrawn from parenteral gold because of bone marrow suppression.

Methotrexate

25. S.S. (from Question 21) will be treated with MTX. Why is MTX a good selection for her?

S.S. has many indicators of severe disease (e.g., young age of onset, multiple joint involvement, extra-articular manifestations [i.e., subcutaneous nodules], radiographic evidence of erosions, elevated ESR, and positive RF with a high titer of 1:1,280 [positive RF is generally a titer ≤1:20 and titers correlate with disease severity]). The disease prognosis for S.S. is clearly poor, and a relatively potent DMARD should be initiated to maximize the preservation of joint function as much as possible because the patient is young and likely to have many years of life ahead of her. MTX is currently the initial DMARD of choice among most rheumatologists, particularly for patients with severe disease.[10] MTX has a rapid onset (usually 1–2 months before a "plateau" of effectiveness), a high efficacy rate, and the most predictable benefit of any DMARD.[10] In one study, the probability of continuing MTX therapy for at least 5 years was 62%.[48] In contrast, the use of other traditional DMARDs only results in about half of the patients being able to continue therapy beyond 9 to 24 months.[85] MTX is good choice for treating S.S.'s very active RA.

Dosing

26. How should MTX be administered when it is used in the treatment of RA?

MTX generally is administered orally at an initial dose of 7.5 mg once a week. Liquid MTX is a less expensive and equally efficacious alternative to the more-commonly administered tablet formulation.[30] The MTX commonly is administered as a single weekly dose, or it can be divided into 2.5 mg every 12 hours for a total of three doses (i.e., "pulse dosing"). Pulse dosing of the weekly MTX is as effective as single weekly dosing and may be associated with less hepatotoxicity.[188] If the patients RA shows no objective response in 6 weeks (i.e., the time at which the plateau of therapeutic effectiveness occurs), the dose is increased to 15 mg/week (or 5 mg every 12 hours for three doses) for at least 12 additional weeks.[189] If no response is seen at this time, the dose can be (a) increased to the maximum of 25 mg/wk, (a) the dose can be administered as a subcutaneous or intramuscular injection to address bioavailability concerns, (c) the same dose can be continued for a longer period of time, or (d) MTX can be discontinued.[10,30,190] When subcutaneous MTX was compared with oral MTX in a 6-month randomized controlled trial of 384 MTX-naive patients with active RA,[191] 78% of patients treated with subcutaneous MTX achieved an ACR-20 response, and only 70% of those treated with oral MTX achieved a similar response. At week 16 of this study, patients treated with oral MTX, who failed to attain an ACR-20 response, were switched to subcutaneous MTX; patients treated with subcutaneous MTX patients, who failed to attain an ACR-20 response, were given a larger MTX dose (20 mg) subcutaneously. The patients who were converted from oral dosing to subcutaneous dosing and the patients who were given a larger subcutaneous dose had a 30% and 23% ACR response rate at week 24, respectively. As a result, subcutaneous MTX seems to be more effective than oral MTX and not associated with a higher incidence of adverse effects.

In a 6-month clinical trial, RA patients with a short disease duration (i.e., <3 years), who achieve disease remission with weekly MTX therapy, remained in remission when the same MTX dose was administered every other week (i.e., monthly dose reduced by 50%).[192] It is unknown, however, whether every-other-week dosing of MTX prevents joint destruction as effectively as weekly dosing.

Adverse Effects

27. What subjective and objective data should be evaluated for evidence of MTX adverse effects in RA patients treated with MTX?

Nausea and other GI distress, malaise, dizziness, mucositis, and mild alopecia are commonly encountered adverse effects associated with low-dose MTX therapy.[162] More serious, but less common, adverse effects include myelosuppression, pneumonitis, and hepatic fibrosis and cirrhosis.[162] A CBC, LFTs, and a serum creatinine concentration should be evaluated at baseline, monthly for the first 6 months of therapy, and then every 4 to 8 weeks during MTX therapy. Renal dysfunction can result in accumulation of MTX and higher risk of myelosuppression. Hypersensitivity pneumonitis, occurring in 1% to 2% of patients, has no known risk factors for development, although it may be more common in patients with a history of lung disease.[30] In addition, hypersensitivity pneumonitis can occur at any time during therapy and at any MTX dosage. A baseline chest radiograph is recommended within the year before MTX initiation. If the patient is found to have preexisting lung disease, MTX treatment should be reconsidered because further pulmonary damage could be devastating to the patient. Patient also should be monitored carefully for cough, dyspnea on exertion, and SOB at each clinic visit.

MTX-induced liver disease is rare, but increased age, long duration of therapy, obesity, diabetes mellitus, ethanol consumption, and a history of hepatitis B or C increase the risk of hepatotoxicity.[162] MTX should be prescribed with great caution, if at all, in patients with preexisting liver disease. The serum concentrations of liver enzymes commonly are modestly increased after administration for 1 to 2 days. MTX, however, should be withheld if liver enzymes increase to three times the baseline value or if the liver enzyme serum concentrations remain elevated for sustained periods during therapy.[193] The ability of LFT monitoring to predict risk for serious hepatotoxicity is unclear. In one study of psoriatic patients receiving MTX, liver enzyme elevations did not predict risk of serious hepatotoxicity; however, serum concentrations of liver enzymes were evaluated only on the day of biopsy rather than at regular intervals throughout therapy.[194] Patients taking MTX should avoid alcohol and be instructed to report symptoms of jaundice or dark urine to their primary care provider. Routine liver biopsies to monitor for MTX-induced hepatotoxicity are unnecessary (see Question 28).

28. Should a baseline liver biopsy be performed before starting MTX?

At one time, routine liver biopsies were recommended for RA patients receiving MTX because cirrhosis developed in up to 26% of psoriasitic patients.[195] In RA patients, however, serial liver biopsies are neither recommended nor cost effective. Nevertheless, the liver should be biopsied before treatment in patients with suspected liver disease and in patients with persistent LFT abnormalities during, or after discontinuation of, MTX therapy (Table 43-7).[196]

29. When should folate (or folinic acid) be administered to reduce the risk of MTX-related toxicity?

In early studies, folate supplementation effectively prevented, or managed, GI disturbances, mucositis (mouth or

Table 43-7 Proposed Criteria for Liver Biopsies During MTX Therapy

Baseline liver biopsy if patient has:
1. History of significant regular ethanol consumption, arbitrarily defined as 3 drinks/day
2. History of hepatitis, jaundice, or liver disease
Liver biopsy during therapy if:
1. Six of 12 monthly determinations of AST are elevated into the abnormal range
2. Baseline normal serum albumin falls to 3.3 g/dL
3. Three to 5 of 12 monthly elevations of AST are in the abnormal range for 3 consecutive years
Liver biopsy results:
Biopsy showing Roenigk class I, II, or IIIA (minimal fibrosis) would be grouped as a "benign" hepatic outcome and a repeat biopsy would be performed only if serum albumin falls to |Ld3.3 g/dL. Roenigk Class IIIB (significant hepatic fibrosis) or IV (cirrhosis) would be cause to permanently discontinue MTX

AST, aspartate aminotransferase; MTX, methotrexate.
Adapted from reference 196.

GI ulcerations), and possibly alopecia attributable to MTX therapy.[197–201] In larger randomized controlled trials, folic acid or folinic acid (leucovorin) was only able to decrease the incidence of alanine aminotransferase (ALT) elevation.[202,203] When folic acid (1 mg/day), folinic acid (2.5 mg/week), or placebo was added to MTX therapy (7.5 mg/week, titrated up to 25 mg/week) to more than 400 RA patients, hepatotoxicity developed in 26% in the placebo group, but in only 4% of patients in the folic acid and folinic acid groups ($p < 0.001$ for treatment groups versus placebo). Because hepatotoxicity is one of most common reasons for MTX discontinuation, the benefit of folate supplementation is clearly important.

A slightly higher dose of MTX might be needed in folate users to produce clinical benefits similar to that achieved by patients without folate supplementation, perhaps because MTX is a folate antagonist.[204] Clinically, however, there does not seem to be a significant attenuation of MTX efficacy associated with concomitant folate supplementation and, very importantly, folate supplementation reduces the incidence of MTX discontinuation secondary to ALT elevation.

Although either folic acid or folinic acid is effective, folic acid 1 mg/day or 7 mg once a week is preferred over folinic acid because of cost and ease of administration.[162]

30. S.S. is treated with MTX 7.5 mg and with folic acid 7 mg orally once a week. Nine weeks later, she returns to the clinic with subjective and objective improvement in morning stiffness, fatigability, and joint tenderness and swelling. However, she has noted increased SOB and dyspnea over the past week. Why might these symptoms be related to MTX?

Pneumonitis, a rare complication of MTX therapy, is characterized by a nonproductive cough, malaise, and fever, progressing to severe dyspnea.[205] Recognition of this unusual reaction is important to ensure that MTX is discontinued before the pneumonitis progresses to respiratory failure (see Question 27). After discontinuation of MTX, pulmonary function improves. Corticosteroids can accelerate improvement in pulmonary symptoms associated with pneumonitis. S.S.'s dyspnea and SOB might be related to MTX. If appropriate tests rule out other causes for her pulmonary complaints, MTX-induced pulmonary toxicity should be considered and MTX treatment discontinued.

31. What major MTX food and drug interactions need to be considered by patients and providers?

NSAIDs increase MTX serum concentrations and increase the risk of toxicity.[30] MTX doses should be adjusted cautiously in patients taking NSAIDs concurrently. Trimethoprim can increase the risk of MTX-induced bone marrow suppression. The concurrent use of MTX and LEF has been associated with major liver damage, including fatalities; as a result, this combination should be avoided. When 39 MTX-treated RA patients consumed low doses of caffeine (<120 mg/day), morning stiffness and joint pain were improved by more than 30% compared with high caffeine consumption (>180 mg/day).[206] Caffeine may interfere with the anti-inflammatory effects of MTX. Because MTX is protein bound and renally excreted, other drugs (e.g., salicylates, etretinate, probenecid, penicillin, ciprofloxacin) also might interact with MTX.

Leflunomide

Place in Therapy

32. B.W., a 36-year-old woman, has severe, progressive RA and is not responding sufficiently to MTX therapy. Would LEF be a reasonable consideration for her?

LEF (Arava), an oral traditional DMARD, seems to be similar in efficacy to MTX with regards to ACR-20, radiographic response, and work productivity.[46] The onset of benefit (as early as 4 weeks) and the percentage of patients who discontinue LEF therapy because of either lack of efficacy or toxicity are similar for LEF, MTX, and SSZ.[30,207–211] Nevertheless, postmarketing surveillance of LEF has noted more than 130 severe liver-related adverse events, including 12 liver-related fatalities.[212] In one clinical evaluation, more than 75% of patients ($n = 369$) who received etanercept or infliximab continued with therapy after 20 months compared with only 22% of LEF-treated patients.[213] Although the incidence of hepatotoxicity was not specifically reported, adverse effects were the primary reason for LEF discontinuation during the first 6 months of treatment.

LEF is as safe and effective as MTX or SSZ in and can be combined with MTX therapy (see Question 38); however, postmarketing reports are a reminder that diligent patient monitoring is crucial. It is not known whether the addition of other DMARDs to MTX therapy is a better therapeutic option than substituting LEF for MTX (see Question 38).

Dosing

33. How would you initiate LEF in B.W.? How would you monitor B.W. for adverse effects?

The active metabolite of LEF, A771726 or M1, is responsible for virtually all the pharmacologic activity of LEF.[214] The serum half-life of the M1 metabolite is approximately 2 weeks. As a result, LEF should be initiated with a loading dose of 100 mg once daily for 3 days to reduce time to steady state, followed by 20 mg once daily. If this dose is not tolerated, the dose should be reduced to 10 mg once daily.

Monitoring for Adverse Effects

Diarrhea (20%–30%), rash (10%), alopecia (10%–17%), and reversible liver enzyme elevations more than three times the upper limit of normal (ULN; 2%–4%) are common adverse effects of LEF.[211,214] Routine laboratory testing includes a baseline ALT followed by monthly ALT testing for several months. When it is evident that ALT results are stable and within normal limits, testing can be performed less often according to the clinician's judgment. Because of the risk of liver toxicity and the need for activation by the liver to the M1 active metabolite, LEF is not recommended in patients with preexisting liver disease, including hepatitis B or C.

Potential hepatotoxicity is the greatest concern with LEF. The rate of LEF-induced liver enzyme elevation is not significantly different than MTX. Guidelines for managing potential hepatotoxicity include dosage reduction from 20 to 10 mg/day if ALT increases more than twofold the ULN.[214] If ALT elevations remain steady between two to three times the ULN and treatment continuation is desired, a liver biopsy is recommended. If ALT elevations are persistently more than three times the ULN despite dosage reduction and cholestyramine administration to enhance elimination (see Question 34), then the drug should be discontinued and another course of cholestyramine elimination therapy should be given.

Enhancement of Elimination With Cholestyramine

34. After 2 months of therapy, B.W. does not respond to LEF and the treatment discontinued, especially because she is beginning to consider starting a family. What precautions must be taken when discontinuing LEF?

LEF (pregnancy category X) has not been tested in pregnant women, but greatly increases the risk of fetal death or teratogenicity in animals receiving as little as 1% of human equivalent doses.[214] After discontinuation of therapy, however, up to 2 years may need to elapse before plasma M1 metabolite levels of LEF are undetectable. As a result, cholestyramine is recommended for all women who discontinue LEF and who are hoping to become pregnant. After stopping the medication, cholestyramine 8 g TID is administered for 11 days (which need not be consecutive). Plasma levels of the M1 metabolite are reduced by 40% to 65% in 24 to 48 hours and should become nondetectable (<0.02 mg/L) at the end of therapy. The patients blood should be tested at least 14 days apart to verify the absence of the metabolite. If plasma M1 levels remain >0.02 mg/L, more cholestyramine should be administered. Cholestyramine also can be used to enhance elimination of LEF in patients who experience hepatotoxicity or who overdose with this drug. Activated charcoal also can reduce plasma M1 levels by 50% after 48 hours, and can be an effective alternative to cholestyramine when LEF overdosages need to be managed.

Azathioprine

Indications and Adverse Effects

35. In considering options for B.W., AZA is mentioned. B.W. knows someone who is using AZA for prevention of kidney transplant rejection and thinks AZA is a highly toxic drug. How can adverse effects to AZA be minimized?

AZA is FDA approved for transplant rejection prophylaxis and for treatment of severe RA. The starting dose of AZA for RA is 1 mg/kg/day in single or divided doses.[10] If the patient does not respond, the dose can be increased by 0.5 mg/kg/day after 6 to 8 weeks; and subsequently increased by the same magnitude every 4 weeks if needed until a maximum dose of 2.5 mg/kg/day is reached.

The most common adverse effect of AZA is GI intolerance and about 10% of patients discontinue therapy because of this problem.[162] Myelosuppression can occur, but is reversible upon discontinuation of therapy. Patients with renal insufficiency are at increased risk for myelosuppression and doses should be adjusted accordingly for renal insufficiency. Allopurinol decreases metabolism and elimination of AZA via inhibition of xanthine oxidase, thereby increasing the risk of toxicity of AZA because of increased serum concentrations. If concomitant allopurinol therapy cannot be avoided, the dose of AZA must be reduced by 75%. Monitoring for AZA adverse effects should include a baseline CBC, renal function, and LFTs. When AZA doses are increased, a CBC should be monitored every 1 to 2 weeks; thereafter, a CBC should be monitored every 1 to 3 months. Although serious adverse effects have limited the use of AZA for RA; diligent laboratory and clinical monitoring can minimize risk to patients.

Penicillamine

Considerations for Use

36. When would you consider penicillamine therapy for B.W.? How is penicillamine dosed and monitored?

Penicillamine is rarely used for the treatment of progressive RA because of a lengthy dose titration schedule and serious toxicities (e.g., myelosuppression, autoimmune diseases).[10,30]

Dosing

A "go low, go slow" approach is recommended for penicillamine dosing.[172] The initial dose usually is 250 mg/day, and the dose is increased to 500 mg/day after 4 to 8 weeks. If therapeutic benefits are not observed after an additional 4 to 8 weeks, the dosage is increased to 750 mg/day, then occasionally to 1,000 mg. Up to 6 months of therapy may be necessary before therapeutic benefits become apparent.

Adverse Effects

Rash, stomatitis, and dysgeusia are the most common adverse effects associated with penicillamine.[162] Myelosuppression (particularly thrombocytopenia), proteinuria, renal toxicity, and autoimmune syndromes (e.g., systemic lupus erythematosus, myasthenia gravis, polymyositis, Goodpasture syndrome) have been reported but are rare. Gradual increases in DPEN doses of 125 to 250 mg every 3 months seem to reduce the risk of thrombocytopenia. Laboratory monitoring includes a baseline renal function test. A renal function test, CBC, and urine protein assay should be obtained at baseline. In addition, the latter two tests should be monitored every 2 weeks until dosing is stabilized, then every 1 to 3 months thereafter.

Although B.W. has failed to respond to MTX and LEF, DMARDs other than penicillamine have a more rapid onset of action, greater efficacy, and less toxicity, and are therefore preferable.

37. A patient with RA, M.M., is allergic to penicillin. Could he receive penicillamine for RA treatment?

Metabolites of penicillin, rather than penicillin itself, are responsible for allergic reactions. The penicilloyl group is the major haptenic determinant in penicillin allergy, but other metabolites (e.g., penicillinate, penicillate, penicillamine) also can cause allergy. Penicillamine be prescribed with caution to penicillin-allergic patients because in vitro studies note cross-sensitivity to penicillamine in 44% to 65% of penicillin-allergic patients.[215] However, none of these patients received an oral penicillamine challenge. When 40 patients with histories of penicillin allergy, confirmed by positive skin tests in 80%, were given penicillamine 250 mg orally in another study, none experienced an immediate or delayed reaction.[216] Three RA patients, who had positive penicillin skin test reactions, subsequently received penicillamine without experiencing hypersensitivity reactions during therapy. Penicillamine, therefore, need not be withheld in patients with a history of penicillin allergy. The potential for cross-reactivity, although real, seems to be small.

Traditional Disease-Modifying Antirheumatic Drug Combination Therapy

38. What evidence supports the early and safe use of DMARDs in combination?

Because most RA patients develop joint erosions within the first 2 years of disease, the initiation of disease-modifying agents early in the course of therapy, and using them in combination, have been associated with improved patient outcomes. The rationale for combination therapy is based on the premise that a combination of drugs might improve outcomes because of different pharmacological mechanisms of action or different sites of actions. A combination of drugs also may allow the use of lower doses of individual drugs, thereby reducing the risk of toxicity while maintaining or possibly increasing efficacy. The early use of combinations of potent disease-modifying agents also can expose the patient to increased risks of drug adverse effects.

A multitude of possible study designs (e.g., different DMARD combinations, variable doses, varying durations of therapy, number of patients enrolled) make it difficult to draw valid comparative conclusions from various clinical trials.[31] Studies, most applicable to clinical practice, should compare the efficacy of MTX against a combination of drugs that incorporate MTX in the regimen because MTX is the single most effective traditional DMARD. Nevertheless, MTX alone, improves only one-third of patients by 50% after 2 to 4 years.[87]

The triple combination of MTX, HCQ, and SSZ seems to be a very effective treatment approach for RA.[217–219] In one study, this triple combination resulted in a 2-year disease remission rate of 37% versus 21% in patients treated with SSZ or MTX monotherapy with no significant differences in adverse effects.[217] Another trial compared the triple drug regimen with MTX alone and with the combination of HCQ and SSZ.[218] At 2-year follow-up, 77% of the triple-drug-treated patients responded significantly as compared with 33% of the patients treated with MTX monotherapy ($p < 0.001$) and 40% of the patients treated with SSZ plus HCQ ($p = 0.003$). Toxicity did not differ between the treatment groups. A follow-up abstract of the same study reported that triple-drug therapy remained efficacious and safe in 36 of 58 patients (62%) after 5 years.[219]

In a randomized controlled trial of 263 MTX-treated patients with active persistent RA, the addition of LEF resulted in significant clinical improvement without an increase in adverse event and treatment discontinuation rates.[220] However, anecdotal reports of serious liver disease, including fatalities, have prompted some to conclude that the combination of MTX with LEF is unsafe.[30]

Aggressive DMARD therapy has been implemented through many historic approaches, including the "step-down," "sawtooth," and "graduated step-up" strategies.[221–223] Although each strategy differs in specifics, they share the concepts of starting DMARD therapy earlier and a willingness to combine DMARDs to achieve improved short-term as well as long-term outcomes. After an initial response to a DMARD, disease progression accelerates (even on therapy), according to one hypothesis used to reconcile the apparent paradox of short-term improvement with failure to alter long-term outcomes in RA.[221] Under this premise, DMARD treatment makes disease progression to disability irregular, like the tooth of a saw. The initiation of DMARDs as soon as possible, before joints are substantially damaged by the disease, therefore, should improve outcomes while keeping overall drug toxicity near traditional levels. In this sawtooth strategy, one or multiple DMARDs are used continually, throughout the entire disease course, while monitoring for evidence of disease progression. A ceiling is set in terms of progression, which triggers treatment changes. DMARD therapy is changed serially, alone or in combination, at each decision point. Analgesics and NSAIDs are used only as adjunctive therapy for symptomatic relief as required. The longest prospective study of the sawtooth strategy for DMARD therapy was conducted among 135 patients over 15 years.[224] A total of 606 monotherapy or combination DMARD therapies were initiated. Five hundred twenty-eight (87.1%) of these therapies were discontinued after a median time of 10 months, with most discontinuing because of inefficacy (51.1%) rather than adverse effects (28.2%). Thus, the main factor limiting the sawtooth strategy was the loss of efficacy as opposed to harmful adverse effects.

The "step-down" more aggressive approach initiates treatment with prednisone 10 mg/day for 1 month.[222] If active RA is still evident, multiple DMARDs are added all at once to induce disease remission as quickly as possible. One DMARD at a time is then tapered and discontinued, eventually leaving a single agent as monotherapy.

The slightly more conservative "graduated step" approach matches disease severity and activity to "appropriate" initial and long-term therapy.[223] This strategy increases objectivity of therapeutic decision making throughout the course of disease treatment and exposes only those patients with sufficiently active disease to the risks of combination DMARD therapy. Patients are reevaluated at 3-month intervals and disease activity is categorized as mild, moderate, or severe based on a quantified scoring system utilizing measures of pain, tender and swollen joint count, and ESR or CRP. Scores reflecting severe RA or poor disease control are indicators for treatment escalation. Subsequent treatment changes may require consideration of additional information beyond disease activity criteria (e.g., time of onset of afternoon fatigue, change in grip strength, change in Hgb concentration, onset or worsening of extra-articular disease manifestations).

As described in the Quantifying Response to Drug Therapy section, clinical assessment tools (DAS, CDAI, SDAI, GAS, RAPID, ERAM) integrate measures of RA activity (e.g., swollen joint count, tender joint count, pain, questionnaire-derived patient- and clinician-evaluated global disease activity) into a simple summary score.[96–99] These scores can be used to categorize disease severity and modify DMARD or biological agent therapy accordingly. The BeSt Study utilized the DAS-44 (44 joints) to compare four different treatment approaches for patients with early onset RA (<2 years). Three of these treatments included exclusively traditional DMARDs.[88] Group 1 patients initially received MTX monotherapy, with dose escalation and sequential addition of SSZ and LEF if DAS-44 was >2.4. Group 2 patients also began therapy with MTX, followed by additions of SSZ, HCQ, and then prednisone if DAS-44 was >2.4. In contrast, Group 3 patients started with a prednisone taper (60 mg/day tapered down to 7.5 mg/day after 7 weeks), MTX, and SSZ. Group 4 started with infliximab and MTX. DAS-44 was evaluated every 3 months. After 1 year of treatment, all groups had similar remission rates (defined by DAS-44 <1.6), average DAS-44 scores, and adverse events. The BeSt Study demonstrated that an aggressive,

DAS-based titration regimen, utilizing a variety of traditional-based DMARDs, is a successful method of using combination DMARD therapy for early RA.

In summary, with very few exceptions every RA patient should receive DMARD therapy within the first 3 months of diagnosis, either as monotherapy or as combination therapy. Loss of efficacy and intolerable adverse effects seem to be the first and second most common reasons for DMARD discontinuation, respectively. Various combinations of traditional DMARDs, when titrated aggressively, have proven to be very effective in RA management. Nevertheless, the availability and greater efficacy of biological agents in slowing joint erosions have provided additional important therapeutic alternatives to traditional DMARDs.

BIOLOGICAL AGENTS

Etanercept

Place in Therapy

39. B.W., the patient with severe RA in Question 32, begins etanercept after both MTX and LEF therapy failed. Why is etanercept a reasonable therapeutic option?

Etanercept (Enbrel) is the first biological response modifier to be approved by the FDA for reducing the signs and symptoms of moderate to severe active RA, either alone or in combination with MTX.[32] Etanercept also is approved for use in juvenile RA and psoriatic arthritis. Etanercept is a soluble TNF receptor that competitively binds two TNF molecules, rendering both inactive. Etanercept consists of two extracellular portions of the TNF receptor; and TNF primarily exists as a trimer in the human body. The dimeric structure of etanercept is believed to have a higher binding affinity for the trimeric TNF than the naturally occurring monomeric receptor.

In a randomized, placebo-controlled trial of 234 patients with active RA, significantly more patients met ACR-20 criteria after 6 months of treatment with etanercept 10 mg (51% of patients) and 25 mg (59% of patients) than placebo-treated patients (11%).[225] The etanercept was administered subcutaneously twice weekly for 26 weeks. The definition of ACR-20 criteria is described in the Quantifying Response to Therapy section. All patients who were enrolled in this study had experienced an inadequate response to at least one of several DMARDs. Most patients (about 90%) had tried MTX at one time or another, followed by HCQ (about 68%), injectable gold and SSZ (about 50% each), AZA (about 30%), DPEN (about 20%) and gold (about 25%). Furthermore, 24% and 40% of the patients taking etanercept 10 mg and 25 mg, respectively, met ACR-50 response criteria compared with 5% of the placebo group ($p < 0.001$ for both doses compared with placebo, no significant difference between doses). Significant ACR-20, ACR-50, and ACR-70 responses to either etanercept dose were seen after only 2 weeks of therapy.

Another randomized, placebo-controlled trial evaluated the use of combination MTX and etanercept therapy in 89 patients with active RA refractory to at least 6 months of MTX therapy.[226] A dose of 25 mg etanercept or placebo was given subcutaneously twice weekly, and a stable dose of MTX (between 15 and 25 mg/week) was provided to all patients. At 24 weeks of follow-up, an ACR-20 response was found in 71% of the MTX plus etanercept group and 27% of the MTX plus placebo group ($p < 0.001$). Similarly, 39% of the MTX plus etanercept group met ACR-50 response criteria compared with 3% of the MTX plus placebo group ($p < 0.001$). Etanercept was also associated with significantly greater improvement in ESR or CRP test results. The addition of etanercept to MTX provided greater clinical efficacy when compared with MTX monotherapy.

In the Early Rheumatoid Arthritis trial of 632 moderate to severe early RA patients, etanercept (25 mg twice a week) was associated with significantly greater improvement in clinical and radiologic measures within the first 6 months of therapy than MTX.[227] No significant therapeutic differences were found between etanercept and MTX at 12-month follow-up; however, at the conclusion of the 24-month trial, significantly less radiographic progression of disease was found among the etanercept patients. The Sharp score, which quantifies a composite of joint space narrowing and erosions, served as the basis for the radiographic evaluation. Etanercept provides rapid and significant improvement in subjective and objective measures of RA, either alone or in combination with MTX. In other studies, etanercept has demonstrated long-term safety and efficacy.[228,229] Although cost is a significant consideration, etanercept is a reasonable choice for B.W.

Dosing and Monitoring

40. How would you initiate etanercept therapy and monitor B.W. for therapeutic and adverse effects?

The FDA-approved dose of etanercept for the treatment of active RA is 25 mg subcutaneously twice weekly.[32] The medication may be self-injected by the patient after proper training. Etanercept must be reconstituted using only the diluent supplied; the contents should be swirled, not shaken, to avoid excessive foaming. Injection sites (e.g., thigh, abdomen, upper arm) should be rotated. Clinical response usually appears within 1 to 2 weeks of treatment, and nearly all patients respond within 3 months. In fact, patients who fail to respond to DMARD or biological agent therapy within 3 months should receive consideration for an alternative treatment. When pooled data from early RA trials, which evaluated MTX, anti-TNF, and the combination of MTX with anti-TNF, a significant response at 3 months correlated with response 1 year after start of therapy based on SDAI, CDAI, and DAS28 scores.[230]

Injection site reactions (37% vs. 10% with placebo), upper respiratory infections (29% vs. 10% with placebo), and the development of autoantibodies are encountered with etanercept treatments. Injection site reactions generally are mild to moderate in severity and usually occurred within the first month of treatment with decreased frequency over time. Upper respiratory infections (e.g., sinusitis) occur at a rate of 0.82 events per patient-year in patients treated with etanercept versus 0.68 events per patient-year in the placebo group. Autoantibodies that developed during etanercept treatment included ANA (11% vs. 5% in placebo group) and new positive anti-double-stranded DNA antibodies (15% vs. 4% in placebo group). No patients developed clinical signs of autoimmune disease, and the long-term effect of etanercept on the development of autoimmune disease is unknown. Patients with severe heart failure (e.g., NYHA class III or IV) may be at increased risk for heart failure exacerbation and mortality when taking any anti-TNF agent.[31] Although not a contraindication, caution is advised if etanercept is prescribed for patients with heart failure. Although an increased incidence of lymphoma has been observed among RA patients receiving any of the available anti-TNF agents, causation has not been established because both RA and MTX are associated with an increased rate of lymphoma.[32] Other adverse effects, in order of decreasing frequency, include headache, rhinitis, dizziness, pharyngitis, cough, asthenia, abdominal pain, and rash.

The greatest concern with etanercept therapy is the risk of immunosuppression and subsequent serious infections, including sepsis. TNF is a key mediator of inflammation and plays a major role immune system regulation. Approximately 6 months after FDA approval of etanercept, 30 patients receiving etanercept developed serious infections.[231] Although the number of reports was not more than what was expected from clinical trials, six of these patients died within 2 to 16 weeks of starting therapy. Postmarketing reports of other infections such as tuberculosis (a black box warning for all anti-TNF agents), mycobacterial infections, and fungal infections further reinforces the strong recommendation against the initiation of etanercept therapy in patients with sepsis or any chronic or localized active infection.[10,30] *Mycobacterium tuberculosis* skin testing and a baseline chest radiograph should be undertaken before initiation of anti-TNF therapy. Therapy should be postponed for patients identified as having latent tuberculosis until appropriate antituberculosis therapy has been completed. Clinicians also must be cautious when prescribing etanercept to patients with a history of recurring infection or with underlying illnesses that predispose them to infection (e.g., diabetes).

B.W. should receive a tuberculosis skin test, undergo a chest radiograph, and be warned of the potential adverse effects of etanercept, particularly the risk of immunosuppression and subsequent infection. Any sign of infection must be reported immediately to her health care provider.

Infliximab and Adalimumab

Dosing and Place in Therapy

41. After 3 weeks of etanercept therapy, B.W. seems to respond well. However, she dislikes the subcutaneous administration of etanercept twice weekly and wants another medication that can be administered on a much more convenient basis. How do the other TNF-inhibitors differ from etanercept, and is B.W. a candidate for one of these alternatives?

Two anti-TNF monoclonal antibodies are FDA approved for the treatment of RA. The first, infliximab (Remicade), is a chimeric (mouse/human) IgG antibody directed against TNF that is approved for the treatment of Crohn disease and for the treatment of RA in patients who have not responded adequately to MTX.[33] The usual dose of infliximab is 3 mg/kg intravenously at 0, 2, and 6 weeks, then every 8 weeks thereafter; thus, the convenience of infrequent dosing is tempered by the need for supervised intravenous administration. Infliximab should be given with MTX therapy to prevent the formation of antibodies to infliximab.

In a randomized, placebo-controlled trial of 101 patients with active RA who responded suboptimally to MTX therapy, 60% of patients receiving 3 or 10 mg/kg of infliximab with or without MTX (7.5 mg/week) responded to treatment after 26 weeks.[232] A control group received intravenous placebo with MTX 7.5 mg weekly. Response to treatment was defined as a 20% Paulus response (i.e., 20% reduction in at least four of the following six criteria: [a] number of swollen joints; [b] number of tender joints; [c] duration of morning stiffness; [d] reduction in ESR; [e] a two-grade improvement in the patient's global assessment of disease severity; and [f] a two-grade improvement in the physician's global assessment of disease severity). Patients, who received a 1-mg/kg dose of infliximab, without MTX, did not respond. Although a significant number of patients receiving 1 mg/kg infliximab with MTX met the 20% Paulus response criteria after 16 weeks of treatment, this response was no longer significant at week 26.

Serious infections have occurred in patients treated with infliximab. In one case, bacterial endophthalmitis resulted in enucleation (complete removal) of the affected eye. In another case, a patient died within 24 hours of emergency admission for staphylococcal septic shock. The development of antibodies to infliximab (human antichimeric antibodies [HACA]) occurred at a rate of 53%, 21%, and 7% of patients receiving the 1-, 3-, and 10-mg/kg doses of infliximab alone, respectively. These rates were lower when MTX was given concurrently (15%, 7%, and 0%, respectively). High doses of infliximab or concurrent use of MTX apparently minimize HACA formation.

In a randomized, double-blind, multicenter, placebo-controlled trial (ATTRACT) of 428 active RA patients who failed to respond adequately to at least 12.5 mg/week of MTX, infliximab 3 or 10 mg/kg or placebo was administered every 4 or 8 weeks along with MTX therapy. This study was unblinded after 1 year because of radiographic evidence of disease modification in patients receiving infliximab. Analysis of radiographic results after 2 years demonstrated that infliximab significantly protected against joint erosion.[233,234]

The second anti-TNF monoclonal antibody, adalimumab (Humira), is a genetically engineered, fully humanized IgG1 monoclonal antibody, as opposed to the chimeric infliximab. Adalimumab, generally is self-administered subcutaneously by the patient as a 40-mg injection every other week, whether as monotherapy or in combination with traditional DMARDs (e.g., MTX).[235] When administered weekly, or every other week, monotherapy with adalimumab 40 mg significantly improved ACR-20 response rates in a randomized controlled trial of 283 RA patients refractory to traditional DMARDs.[236] Patients receiving 40 mg/week had a higher response rate than patients who received the drug every other week. When adalimumab 40 mg every other week was added to the treatment regimen of RA patients receiving stable MTX doses, significantly more adalimumab-treated patients (67%) achieved an ACR-20 response than those receiving only MTX after 24 weeks.[237] In radiographic data reflecting 1 or 2 years of treatment, adalimumab slowed the progression of joint damage.[238] Data are available supporting the efficacy and safety of adalimumab for up to 7 years.[239]

Adverse Effects of Anti-Tumor Necrosis Factor Antibodies

Infliximab and adalimumab have treatment risks and side effect profiles very similar to etanercept (e.g., injection site pain, local reactions, upper respiratory tract infections, nausea, flulike symptoms, rash).[238] Serious adverse effects (e.g., serious infections, increased incidence of lymphoma) are similar as well. As with all anti-TNF agents, a tuberculosis skin test result and chest radiograph must be obtained before initiating treatment. The development of antibodies against infliximab occurs frequently with monotherapy owing to the chimeric nature of the medication, and concurrent use with MTX decreases the formation of these HACA antibodies (see Question 41). Although adalimumab is a fully humanized product, approximately 5% of RA patients develop antibodies against it at least once during therapy when used as a single agent.[236] This reaction is attenuated with weekly dosing of adalimumab or concurrent use of MTX.

Patients who switch from one anti-TNF agent to another owing to loss of efficacy of the initial agent are able to attain a good response from the second.[240–242] About 40% to 60% of patients in clinical studies were able to maintain good ACR-20 scores following the switch, and many patients respond even better to the second drug.[243]

B.W. seems to be a reasonable candidate for either infliximab or adalimumab therapy. Her interest in a biological agent with less frequent dosing is understandable. Although clinical trials have not compared the biological agents, key differentiating variables between these drugs need to be considered. No evidence suggests that there are any significant efficacy differences between etanercept, infliximab, and adalimumab. Although infliximab is ultimately administered every 2 months, it must be administered intravenously and in combination with MTX (or possibly at a higher dose) to minimize HACA formation. Adalimumabs ease of administration (self-injected subcutaneous injection) and infrequent dosing interval compares favorably with etanercept (twice weekly injections) and anakinra (daily injections), but it is administered more frequently than infliximab (Table 43-3). At FDA-approved doses, all biological agents (etanercept, infliximab, adalimumab, anakinra) are priced similarly (~$1,300–$1,500 per month retail based on 2007 prices from www.drugstore.com). Additional therapeutic benefit might be achieved from weekly dosing of adalimumab. If adalimumab is administered weekly, the cost of adalimumab therapy will be considerably more than the other biological agents.

Anakinra

42. B.W. would prefer to avoid anakinra [Kineret] because it requires daily subcutaneous injection dosing. Apart from this inconvenience, what are its therapeutic advantages over the anti-TNF agents?

Anakinra is currently the only available IL-1Ra that is almost identical in composition to human IL-1Ra (see biological agents in the general treatment section). The recommended dose of anakinra is 100 mg daily by self-administered subcutaneous injection.[244] Anakinra significantly, but modestly, improves signs and symptoms and radiographic evidence of joint erosion in RA patients.[30,245] In a study of 472 patients with serious active RA, three different doses of anakinra monotherapy (30, 75, and 150 mg/day) were compared with placebo.[246] At 24-week follow-up, 34% of patients receiving anakinra 75 mg demonstrated an ACR-20 response; however, 27% of placebo patients achieved the same response. Although modest, this difference is statistically significant. Although the higher dose of 150 mg produced improvement in 43% of patients, this dose exceeds the manufacturer's recommended dose. The combination of anakinra and MTX seems to be more effective than anakinra monotherapy. A 24-week randomized controlled trial compared five different doses of anakinra (0.04, 0.1, 0.4, 1.0, and 2.0 mg/kg/day) to placebo among 419 RA patients receiving at least 3 months of fixed MTX doses.[247] Significantly more patients receiving the higher daily doses of anakinra (1.0 and 2.0 mg/kg) experienced the ACR-20 response (42% and 35%, respectively) versus placebo (23%) at 24-week follow-up. Local injection site reactions were frequently encountered.[30] Although neutropenia and severe infections are more common with anakinra than placebo, there have been no reports of patients experiencing tuberculosis reactivation. Combining anakinra with an anti-TNF agent seems to be logical based on their different mechanisms of action; however, the combination is not recommended because of a significantly increased incidence of serious infections and leukopenia.[248] Unlike anti-TNF agents, anakinra is not associated with decompensation of heart failure.[248]

Although the anti-TNF agents have not been compared directly, anakinra seems to be relatively less effective. In addition, the advantage of being able to self-administer anakinra is offset by the need for daily injections. Anakinra is a therapeutic alternative for RA patients in whom traditional DMARD treatment fails; however, it seems to offer no advantages and some real and potential disadvantages when compared with the anti-TNF agents.

43. S.K., a 71-year-old woman, was diagnosed with RA approximately 15 years ago. Her initial drug therapy included MTX, followed by the addition of SSQ and HCQ, which seemed to keep her RA in near-remission until 2002. She began etanercept along with MTX (without SSZ and HCQ) with good results until 2005. In response to declining disease control, infliximab was substituted for MTX with excellent results. Then last month, she experienced a flare in RA activity. At that time, her CRP was 5.1 mg/dL, ESR was 90 mm/hour, and anti-CCP was positive at 112 units. She also experienced morning stiffness lasting several hours, and multiple joints with swelling ($n = 26$) and tenderness ($n = 38$). What are reasonable treatment options for S.K. at this stage of her disease?

Most patients who lose responsiveness to an initial trial of anti-TNF therapy (i.e., etanercept, infliximab, or adalimumab) can often be successfully treated with an alternative anti-TNF agent (see Question 41). However, no evidence supports switching to a third anti-TNF agent if two of the three fail. The newest biological agents, abatacept (inhibitor of T-cell activation) and rituximab (selective depletor of $CD20^+$ B cells) are have great potential to fill this void; both have demonstrated excellent efficacy in patients with inadequate response to traditional DMARD (e.g., MTX) as well as anti-TNF therapy (see discussion in general treatment: Biological Agents).[68,69]

Abatacept

The Abatacept in Inadequate Responders to Methotrexate study compared abatacept 10 mg/kg plus MTX versus placebo plus MTX.[249] At 12-month follow-up, significantly more patients in the abatacept group than the placebo group attained an ACR-20 response (73.1% vs. 39.7%, respectively, $p < 0.001$) and better quality of life survey scores. Fewer patients experienced a change in joint erosion score (0.0 vs. 0.26, respectively, $p = 0.029$).

The Abatacept Trial in Treatment of Anti-TNF Inadequate Responders study evaluated patients on background DMARD therapy (about 80% were using MTX) who did not achieve an adequate treatment response (despite sufficient doses given for ≥3 months) to etanercept, infliximab, or both.[250] Patients were randomized to receive abatacept or placebo along with a fixed dose of background DMARD therapy. At 6-month follow-up, ACR response rates were dramatically better in the abatacept-treated patients. The ACR 20 response was 50.4% and 19.5%, ACR-50 was 20.3% and 3.8%, and ACR-70 was 10.2% and 1.5% in the abatacept and placebo treatment groups, respectively. More patients receiving abatacept were able to achieve a significant improvement in physical functioning (measured by HAQ). Efficacy and safety date reflecting 5 years of abatacept therapy indicate that abatacept maintains ACR-20, ACR-50, and ACR-70 scores over this time period, with no change in safety profile.[67]

The side effects of greatest concern include infections (significantly more common when combined with anti-TNF therapy) such as pneumonia, cellulitis, urinary tract infection, bronchitis, diverticulitis, and acute pyelonephritis (see general treatment section: Biological Agents).[68] A few case reports of malignancy have been associated with abatacept, and chronic obstructive pulmonary disease patients are noted to suffer from more respiratory-related and non-respiratory-related adverse effects than chronic obstructive pulmonary disease patients treated with placebo.[68]

Rituximab

In a placebo-controlled trial of 161 RA patients who responded inadequately to MTX therapy (≥10 mg/week), subjects were randomized to one of four treatment groups: MTX >10 mg per week; rituximab 1,000 mg IV given on days 1 and 15; rituximab plus cyclophosphamide 750 mg IV given on days 3 and 17; or rituximab plus MTX.[251] At 24-week follow-up, ACR-50 response was significantly higher among treatment groups receiving rituximab (33%, 41%, and 43% in the rituximab only, rituximab plus cyclophosphamide, and rituximab plus MTX groups, respectively) versus the MTX only group (13%). At week 48, however, significantly more patients in the rituximab plus MTX group (35%) maintained an ACR-50 response than patients in the rituximab plus cyclophosphamide group (27%). Although cyclophosphamide is reserved for severe cases of RA (usually involving rheumatoid vasculitis), the combination of rituximab plus cyclophosphamide does not seem to be as effective as rituximab plus MTX.

The Dose-Ranging Assessment: International Clinical Evaluation of Rituximab in Rheumatoid Arthritis trial evaluated 465 patients with RA with an inadequate response to DMARD therapy.[252] Nearly one-third of participants previously had tried a biological agent. Patients were randomized to receive either placebo, rituximab 500 mg, or rituximab 1,000 mg on days 1 and 15. Furthermore, each of the three study groups were further randomized to receive either no premedication, IV premedication with methylprednisolone, or IV premedication plus oral premedication with prednisone for a total of 9 treatment groups. All subjects received MTX at a dose of 10 to 25 mg/week. At 24-week follow-up, significantly more subjects receiving either dose of rituximab achieved an ACR-20 response (55% and 54% for the 500 mg and 1,000 mg groups, respectively) than placebo group subjects (28%). These findings were consistent with DAS-28 scores. Premedication with IV methylprednisolone reduced the frequency and intensity of first infusion adverse drug reactions, and the addition of prednisone was not additionally beneficial. Overall, rituximab was well tolerated, with no difference in types and severity of infections compared with placebo-treated patients.

The REFLEX (Randomized Evaluation of Long-Term Efficacy of Rituximab in RA) trial evaluated the use of rituximab (two IV infusions 2 weeks apart, 1,000 mg/infusion) plus MTX versus placebo plus MTX in 499 patients with active, long-standing RA who responded inadequately to one or more anti-TNF medications.[253] At 24-week follow-up, significantly more patients in the rituximab group demonstrated an ACR-20 response than the placebo group (51% vs. 18%, respectively). Peripheral $CD20^+$ B cells were depleted among rituximab-treated patients at about 4 to 5 months after treatment. Average IgG, IgM, and IgA levels remained consistent and within normal ranges. The incidence of all side effects was similar in the two treatment groups (85% of rituximab patients, 88% of placebo patients), as were side effects identified as being related to any of the study drugs, including placebo (39% and 47%, respectively). Infusion reactions were common during or soon after the first dose among rituximab-treated patients (23% vs. 18% of placebo patients). Interestingly, more placebo-treated patients experienced an infusion reaction during or soon after the second infusion (11% vs. 8% of rituximab patients). The rate of infections was slightly higher among rituximab patients (41%) than placebo patients (38%). Similarly, the rate of serious infections was higher among rituximab (5.2 per 100 patient-years) than placebo-treat patients (3.7 per 100 patient-years). No cases of tuberculosis or opportunistic infections were reported. In a 56-week follow-up report of the REFLEX trial, rituximab significantly inhibited radiographic progression of joint damage.[254] These findings support the efficacy of rituximab for RA patients refractory to anti-TNF therapy, a very challenging population.

Dosing for Abatacept and Rituximab

Abatacept is supplied as a lyophilized powder in preservative-free, single-use vials containing 250 mg of abatacept. Abatacept must be reconstituted with 10 mL of sterile water for injection, using only the silicone-free syringe provided, along with an 18- to 21-gauge needle. Reconstitution using a siliconized syringe can result in the development of translucent particles in the medication solution; solutions prepared using siliconized syringes must be discarded. Abatacept dosing is based on body weight (500 mg for patients <60 kg, 750 mg for patients 60-100 kg, and 1,000 mg for patients >100 kg) and should be infused intravenously over 30 minutes. The abatacept dose should be repeated at 2 and 4 weeks after the first dose, then every 4 weeks thereafter. Abatacept can be given as monotherapy or in combination with DMARDs other than anti-TNF agents.[68]

Rituximab, provided in 100- and 500-mg single-use vials at a concentration of 10 mg/mL, is administered as two 1,000-mg IV infusions separated by 2 weeks. Rituximab must be diluted to a final concentration of 1 to 4 mg/mL with either 0.9% sodium chloride or 5% dextrose in water. To reduce the incidence and severity of infusion-related adverse effects, premedication with IV methylprednisolone 100 mg, or its equivalent, 30 minutes before each infusion is strongly recommended; other premedications (e.g., acetaminophen, antihistamine) may also be beneficial. Antihypertensive medications should be discontinued 12 hours before rituximab administration to avoid transient hypotension, which has been reported during rituximab infusions. Rituximab must be given with MTX for maximum efficacy based on clinical trials and to help reduce the risk of developing HACA, which occurs in approximately 9% of patients receiving rituximab.[69]

The first IV infusion of rituximab solution should be administered at a rate of 50 mg/hour. In the absence of infusion reactions, the infusion rate can be increased in 50-mg/hour increments every 30 minutes to a maximum rate of 400 mg/hour. In the event of an infusion reaction, the infusion should be halted or slowed until symptoms improve, at which time the infusion can continue at one-half the previous rate. In patients who tolerated the first infusion well, subsequent infusions of rituximab can be administered at a higher rate (100 mg/hour) and increased by 100 mg/hour increments every 30 minutes to a maximum rate of 400 mg/hour. Patients poorly tolerant to the first infusion should receive subsequent rituximab infusions at 50 mg/hour.[69]

The results of several large trials support the therapeutic value of either abatacept or rituximab for S.K. Efficacy has been demonstrated in patients with inadequate response to DMARDs, including anti-TNF agents. Both abatacept and rituximab are generally well-tolerated and have not been associated with cardiovascular events or worsening of heart failure, unlike the anti-TNF agents. However, some serious adverse effects have been associated with abatacept and rituximab that warrant consideration and diligent monitoring. Rituximab has several black box warnings (see general treatment section entitled Biological Agents) for serious and potentially fatal adverse effects (e.g., fatal cardiorespiratory infusion reactions, tumor lysis syndrome, severe mucocutaneous reactions, and progressive multifocal leukoencephalopathy).[69] Experience with both abatacept and rituximab is limited; therefore, the full range of adverse effects from these agents has not been fully manifested. In summary, abatacept and rituximab are potent treatment options with novel mechanisms of action and proven efficacy at improving RA symptoms and slowing joint erosion. However, based on a combination of current research findings, lack of long-term safety data, and cost, abatacept and rituximab should not be used before a trial with anti-TNF agents, except for patients with relative contraindications to anti-TNF agents (e.g., multiple sclerosis, moderate to severe heart failure).

Corticosteroids

Indications

44. W.M., a 57-year-old man, has progressive RA that has not been responsive to SSZ. He is having difficulty working a full day and is seeking an alternative medication. After a discussion of therapeutic options, W.M. declines MTX therapy and asks to start HCQ. Would it be appropriate to initiate corticosteroids concurrently?

Despite the potential for serious adverse effects with long-term therapy, the judicious use of low-dose corticosteroids represents an important component of treatment during the course of unremitting disease. In addition, low-dose corticosteroids may have disease-modifying properties, particularly in the first year or two of treatment.[10,30] Considering that W.M.'s RA is sufficiently active to compromise his ability to earn an income, MTX is a much better DMARD selection. Regardless, concurrent initiation of a DMARD and an intermediate-acting corticosteroid (e.g., prednisone in a daily or divided dose of 5–10 mg) is justified.[10] In large cohort studies, prednisone doses >7.5 mg/day have been associated with a greater than twofold increase risk of cardiovascular events (MI, stroke, heart failure), as well as the risk of developing hypertension with long-term use (≥6–12 months).[255,256] Therefore, the lowest effective corticosteroid dose is preferred for the shortest duration of time possible. The onset of action of corticosteroids is relatively rapid and their immediate benefits will allow W.M. to maintain his current employment and continue taking care of home responsibilities. The corticosteroid dose can be decreased gradually and eventually discontinued as W.M. begins to respond to HCQ therapy. An important goal of low-dose corticosteroid treatment is to provide bridge therapy until the DMARD therapy becomes effective, in hopes of then being able to taper and discontinue the corticosteroid.[29]

Dosing

45. Why are corticosteroids administered occasionally in divided daily doses rather than as single daily doses or on an every-other-day regimen when used to treat RA?

Administering intermediate- or short-acting corticosteroids as a single daily dose each morning most closely mimics the early morning physiological secretion of cortisol, and, thereby, minimizes hypothalamic-pituitary-adrenal axis suppression. Administering corticosteroids on alternate mornings further reduces the risk of hypothalamic-pituitary-adrenal axis suppression by allowing the adrenal glands to respond to hypothalamic and pituitary mediators during the "off" day.[257] Once-a-day and alternate-day steroid therapies are most advantageous when used to prevent reactivation of some diseases (e.g., asthma, ulcerative colitis, chronic active hepatitis, sarcoidosis).[258] In contrast, when corticosteroids are used to provide symptomatic relief in RA during periods of active, ongoing inflammation, switching patients to single daily doses or every-other-day regimens frequently results in increased symptoms during the latter part of each day and during the "off" day. The anti-inflammatory effect of prednisone or prednisolone is attenuated after 12 hours, and is either diminished or absent after 24 hours. As a result, daily prednisone doses may need to be divided in half and administered twice daily to ensure 24-hour anti-inflammatory activity. Although a larger single daily dose may provide comparable therapeutic benefits, dividing the daily dose of prednisone is preferable because larger doses are associated with more frequent and severe adverse effects.

Osteoporosis

46. What therapeutic interventions can prevent steroid-induced osteoporosis?

Chronic corticosteroid therapy induces osteoporosis by inhibiting bone formation and enhancing bone resorption. Steroids impair bone formation by inhibiting the production of bone-forming osteoblasts and enhance bone resorption by reducing GI calcium absorption and increasing the renal excretion of calcium.[258] In addition, corticosteroids reduce the secretion of luteinizing hormone from the pituitary, resulting in a reduction in estrogen production in women and testosterone production in men.[259] This leads to deficiencies in circulating levels of anabolic hormones (e.g., estradiol, estrone, androstenedione, progesterone), which contribute to the development of osteoporosis. Trabecular bone of the spine and ribs seems to be affected primarily by corticosteroid therapy, with most rapid skeletal wasting occurring during the first 6 months.[259]

Before starting long-term (i.e., 6 months) corticosteroid therapy at a dose of 7.5 mg of daily prednisone or equivalent, bone mineral density should be evaluated.[258,259] Anteroposterior measurement of the lumbar spine or hip by dual-energy x-ray absorptiometry is the preferred procedure. Follow-up measurements can be repeated up to every 6 months to monitor for corticosteroid-related bone loss, or annually for patients already receiving bone loss prevention treatment. A complete history should be obtained to identify potentially modifiable osteoporosis risk factors (e.g., smoking, alcohol consumption, other drugs that can induce osteoporosis, calcium and vitamin D intake, indicators of hormone deficiency such as menopause in women and infertility or impotence in men, lack of participation in weight-bearing exercises). Height and weight should be measured. Lifestyle changes should be encouraged to modify those risk factors that do not require drug therapy. Physical therapy referral is recommended.

All patients on corticosteroid therapy should receive calcium (1,000 mg/day) and vitamin D (800 IU/day) or an activated form of vitamin D (e.g., alfacalcidiol or calcitriol) to maintain calcium balance. Supplementation with calcium and an activated form of vitamin D is needed to prevent bone loss in patients receiving medium- to high-dose corticosteroid therapy (e.g., prednisone $\geq$5 mg/day).[258,259]

Bisphosphonates effectively prevent and treat corticosteroid-induced bone loss.[258] In radiographic studies, bisphosphonates effectively reduced vertebral fractures in postmenopausal women with corticosteroid-induced osteoporosis. Bisphosphonate therapy is recommended for men and postmenopausal women receiving >5 mg/day of prednisone, or its equivalent, to prevent bone loss. In addition, bisphosphonates are recommended for men and postmenopausal women receiving long-term corticosteroids with a bone mineral density T-score below normal at either the lumbar spine or hip. Bisphosphonates should be considered for premenopausal women receiving corticosteroids, even though data in this population are limited. However, premenopausal women receiving bisphosphonates must be counseled about contraception because bisphosphonates are classified as FDA pregnancy risk category C. Bisphosphonates adversely affect fetal skeletal development in animals, and reduce serum calcium. Although data are limited, hypogonadal patients receiving long-term corticosteroid treatment should be offered hormone replacement therapy. Thiazide diuretics reduce urinary calcium excretion and maintain bone mineral content.[260] A thiazide diuretic is recommended if hypercalciuria is present.

Intra-Articular Corticosteroids

47. Do intra-articular corticosteroid injections provide any benefit in RA?

Intra-articular corticosteroid injections are safe and effective for patients with RA and are often underutilized. This strategy is most sensible when flaring occurs in one or a few joints.[10] Systemic side effects are minimal when compared with oral corticosteroid therapy. Although onset of action is virtually immediate, effects are often short lived; however, a corticosteroid injection alone can be sufficient to relieve a temporary RA flare. If the decision is made to reinject a given joint, the injection site should be rotated and administration frequency should be no more than every 3 months.

JUVENILE IDIOPATHIC ARTHRITIS

In the United States, all chronic arthritis of childhood is identified as juvenile idiopathic arthritis (JIA), formerly known as juvenile rheumatoid arthritis.[261] JIA affects all races and afflicts approximately 294,000 children in the United States.[262]

By definition, JIA usually begins before the age of 16 and must present with objective signs of joint inflammation (e.g., swelling, pain, limited ROM, warmth, erythema) for at least 6 weeks in at least one joint or at least two of the following: tenderness, pain with movement, joint warmth, or limited motion.[263] In addition, other conditions causing arthritis such as infectious arthritis and malignancy must be excluded.[261] The onset of disease is rare before 6 months of age, and the peak age of onset ranges from 1 to 3 years. However, new cases are seen throughout childhood.

Signs and Symptoms

As with adult RA, JIA begins with synovial inflammation.[261,263] Morning stiffness and joint pain probably occur in JIA as frequently as in RA; however, children should be observed carefully for symptoms because they often cannot articulate complaints. The morning stiffness and joint pain may manifest as increased irritability, guarding of involved joints, or refusal to walk. Fatigue and low-grade fever, anorexia, weight loss, and failure to grow are other manifestations. JIA can be divided into several subsets based on characteristic signs and symptoms during the first 4 to 6 months of disease. Currently, patients are categorized according to one of six distinct subsets of symptoms: (a) polyarticular, (b) pauciarticular or oligoarthritic, (c) systemic arthritis, (d) enthesitis related, (e) psoriatic, and (f) other.[263]

Patterns of Onset

JIA is classified under the subgroup "polyarticular" when the disease involves five or more joints with few or no systemic manifestations of disease.[261,263] Two types of polyarticular JIA exist: seronegative (i.e., RF negative affecting 20%–25% of all JIA patients) and seropositive (i.e., RF positive affecting 5%–10% of all JIA patients) disease. Both affect girls more often than boys, with seronegative arthritis more common in children younger than 5 years and seropositive arthritis more common in children older than 8 years. Although the onset of disease can be acute, it more commonly is insidious. Generally, the large, fast-growing joints (e.g., knees, wrists, elbows, ankles) are affected, but the small joints of the hands and feet also may be involved. Although the joints at onset usually are symmetrically involved, asymmetric patterns also can occur. Temporomandibular joint involvement is relatively common and may lead to limitation of bite and micrognathia. Systemic manifestations of disease in children with polyarticular disease are rare and include low-grade fever, slight hepatosplenomegaly, lymphadenopathy, pericarditis, and chronic uveitis. Subcutaneous nodules are seen most typically in children with "polyarthritis onset" JIA. When present, nodules are associated with positive RF in >75% of patients. Approximately 30% to 35% of JIA presents as polyarticular.

Oligoarthritic JIA, formerly known as pauciarticular juvenile rheumatoid arthritis, accounts for approximately 40% to 60% of children with JIA, which usually involves four or fewer joints and occasionally up to as many as nine joints.[261] Joint involvement in these children most commonly involves large joints in an asymmetric distribution. The two major subgroups of pauciarticular arthritis: *early childhood onset* (more common, usually affecting girls between the ages of 1 and 5 years of age); and *late childhood onset* (less common, usually affecting boys after 8 years of age).

Approximately 20% to 30% of children with early onset oligoarthritic JIA develop iridocyclitis (inflammation of the iris and ciliary body, also known as uveitis) within the first 10 years of the disease (see Question 53). ANA testing is positive in approximately 60% of these patients. Joints commonly affected include the knees (56%), ankles (20%), hands—especially PIP joints (10%)—feet 6%, and wrists (4%).[264] When only one joint is involved, the knee is the most common joint affected. Hip and sacroiliac joint involvements are rare. On the other hand, children with late-onset pauciarticular JIA do not test positive for ANA, have no extra-articular manifestation of the disease, and often have hip involvement in addition to other lower-limb joints (e.g., knees, ankle, feet). Arguably, this late-onset subgroup may be grouped with the spondyloarthropathies well-known in adult patients (e.g., ankylosing spondylitis).

A smaller percentage (10%–20%) of children experience severe systemic involvement associated with or preceding the onset of arthritis.[261] The hallmarks of the "systemic-onset" category of JIA, which can afflict children at any age, are a high spiking fever and a rheumatoid rash. Once or twice daily, the body temperature can increase to 103°F or higher. The temperature increase may be accompanied by a rash consisting of small, discrete erythematous morbilliform macules, which commonly appear on the trunk and proximal extremities. The lesions tend to be migratory and of short duration in any one location. Other manifestations of "systemic-onset" JIA are hepatosplenomegaly, lymphadenopathy, and pericarditis; these occur in about two-thirds of patients.

Enthesitis-related JIA is manifested as inflammation of the enthesis (the site of attachment of tendon to bone) along with arthritis.[261] Children with enthesitis-related JIA commonly have two of the following: inflammatory spinal pain, sacroiliac joint tenderness, HLA B27 positivity, a family history of enthesitis-related JIA, acute anterior uveitis, and onset of polyarthritis or oligoarthritis in a boy >8 years of age. These children commonly develop a spondyloarthropathy (e.g., reactive arthritis, juvenile ankylosing spondylitis), and inflammatory bowel disease-associated arthritis. The relative proportion of JIA patients with enthesitis-related JIA is unknown.

Psoriatic JIA accounts for approximately 5% of all JIA and is diagnosed if chronic arthritis and definite psoriasis is evident.[261] Children may also be diagnosed with psoriatic JIA if any two of the following are present: dactylitis (finger or toe inflammation), onycholysis or nail pitting, or family history of psoriasis. The arthritis may develop peripherally only or both peripherally and axially; children with axial arthritis and psoriasis are HLA B27 positive. Joint destruction in children with psoriatic JIA can be chronic and destructive, requiring DMARD or biological therapy similar to patients with polyarthritic JIA.

In contrast with adult RA, in which joint destruction is common within the first year of the disease, 70% to 90% of children with JIA experience no long-term disability. However, complete remission is uncommon, occurring in approximately one-third of all JIA patients over a 10-year period.[265] Preservation of joint function is least favorable in children with seropositive polyarticular JIA (severe arthritis in >50%). Children with pauciarticular JIA experience the least joint disease, and those with early-onset pauciarticular JIA experience the worst uveitis. Children with systemic-onset are most prone to develop life-threatening or fatal complications with approximately 25% developing severe arthritis.

Diagnosis of Systemic Juvenile Idiopathic Arthritis

47. J.R., a 4-year-old girl, is hospitalized for high fever and arthritis. Several weeks before admission, J.R. developed a daily fever ranging from 103°F to 106°F. One week before admission, her knees became painful and swollen. J.R. is listless and irritable during her physical examination. The rectal temperature is 102.4°F. She refuses to walk. The right hip is tender and the right wrist and both knees are warm, red, and swollen. Minimal generalized lymphadenopathy and splenomegaly are present. The Westergren ESR is 82 mm/hour, the WBC count 37,000 cells/mm^3 with a mild left shift, and Hct 33%. Cultures of the throat, urine, stool, and blood are negative. An intermediate-strength purified protein derivative, antistreptolysin-O titer, ANA titer, and RF titer all are normal. Radiographs of the chest and involved joints all are normal. An electrocardiogram reveals only tachycardia. After hospitalization and withholding aspirin, an evanescent rash becomes apparent in conjunction with fever spikes. What signs and symptoms of JIA does J.R. manifest?

The signs and symptoms (i.e., the spiking fever episodes, evanescent rash, arthritis, lymphadenopathy, splenomegaly) that J.R. experienced are characteristic of systemic-onset JIA. These children also may have a normocytic, hypochromic anemia, elevated ESR, thrombocytosis, and leukocytosis. Leukocytosis is common and a WBC count of 30,000 to 50,000 cells/mm^3 is seen occasionally. A positive RF titer is uncommon in JIA and is present in only 5% to 10% of all cases.[261] The ANA titer more often is positive and is most prevalent in young girls and children with early-onset pauciarticular arthritis and uveitis.

Treatment

The goal of JIA treatment is to minimize the destructive effects of inflammation, control pain, preserve or restore ROM, and promote development and growth, to facilitate an acceptable quality of life.

Nonsteroidal Anti-Inflammatory Drugs

SELECTION AND DOSING

48. What is the initial drug therapy for treatment of JIA?

NSAID therapy is the treatment of choice for treating the joint manifestations as well as the febrile episodes in systemic-onset JIA.[261,263] Up to two-thirds of JIA patients achieve good disease control with NSAID therapy.[266] In most cases, at least two different NSAIDs should be tried before ruling out this group of medications. Failure to respond to an NSAID in a particular chemical class does not rule out the efficacy of others in the same class. As with adults, it is not possible to predict a patient's response to any one NSAID.

The most commonly prescribed NSAID for JIA is naproxen, used in over 50% of patients.[261] Naproxen is dosed at 10 to 15 mg/kg/day (maximum, 750 mg) in two daily divided doses, and is advantageous in school-age children because of the convenient dosing interval and availability in liquid or tablet formulations.[34] Oxaprozin can be administered once daily as a 600-mg dose if weight is between 22 and 31 kg, 900 mg if weight is between 32 and 54 kg, and 1,200 mg if weight is >55 kg. Although not FDA approved, nabumetone is also frequently used for JIA because of convenient once daily dosing. Ibuprofen doses should not exceed 40 to 50 mg/kg/day and, like naproxen, is available in liquid (suspension) form. Tolmetin usually is dosed at 20 mg/kg/day in three to four divided doses. The usual Tolmetin maintenance doses are between 15 and 30 mg/kg/day in three to four divided doses, with a maximum daily dose of 1,800 mg. Aspirin is seldom used because of its association with Reye syndrome (see Question 49). Aspirin is initiated in divided doses totaling 60 to 80 mg/kg/day.[34] The dosage should be increased slowly to 130 mg/kg/day to achieve anti-inflammatory serum salicylate concentrations ranging from 20 to 30 mg/dL.

REYE SYNDROME

49. Should aspirin be discontinued in a JIA patient who experiences chickenpox because of the potential for causing Reye syndrome?

Unrelated to the mild, reversible, dose-related transaminitis, Reye syndrome occurs in association with the use of aspirin as an antipyretic in children during the prodromal phase of viral illnesses such as influenza and chickenpox. Reye syndrome is characterized by fatty vacuolization of the liver producing hepatic injury, vomiting, hypoglycemia, and progressive encephalopathy. The suggestion that aspirin might be a factor in the development of Reye syndrome first was proposed in the early 1960s.[267] Subsequently, retrospective case-controlled studies revealed a statistically significant difference in the prevalence of salicylate use in patients with Reye syndrome compared with controls.[268–270] Virtually all cases of Reye syndrome were exposed to salicylates during an antecedent illness. In the control population, salicylate use varied from approximately 40% to 70%. Based on these findings, the Committee of Infectious Diseases of the American Academy of Pediatrics issued a statement that aspirin should not be given to febrile children who are at risk for Reye syndrome by virtue of possible infection with either influenza virus or chickenpox.[271]

The risk of Reye syndrome in children receiving salicylate therapy for JIA is unknown. However, in a retrospective study, 6 of 176 patients with biopsy-confirmed Reye syndrome were treated with salicylates for connective tissue disease.[272] Three of these children experienced a preceding upper respiratory tract infection; the other three experienced no apparent prodromal illness. Therefore, patients with JIA also should avoid salicylate ingestion during febrile illnesses that represent possible infection with either influenza or chickenpox.

DISEASE-MODIFYING ANTIRHEUMATIC DRUG THERAPY

50. When should DMARDs be used in JIA?

The heterogeneity of JIA is an important consideration in approaching treatment. Fortunately, most children with JIA improve significantly with NSAID treatment, particularly those with pauciarticular disease. Only a small number of these patients are considered for DMARD therapy, usually because of the evolution of their condition into the polyarticular type. Patients with polyarticular, RF-positive disease and patients with early-onset polyarthritis in association with systemic-onset disease both have poor prognosis in terms of ultimate joint function and should receive early consideration for DMARD therapy. Children with polyarticular-onset, RF-negative disease generally have a better prognosis than patients with polyarticular involvement. One may wait considerably longer before introducing a DMARD for these patients.

Most DMARDs used for adult RA are not effective for JIA,[261] and DPEN is no more effective than placebo. MTX is clearly the DMARD of choice for polyarthritic JIA.[273] The recommended dose of MTX for JIA treatment is 5 to 15 mg/m^2 (0.15–0.5 mg/kg) orally or subcutaneously each week. Pediatric patients are often prescribed the injectable form of MTX for oral consumption via a suspension. Food reduces the bioavailability of MTX, so MTX should be administered on an empty stomach. However, in general, oral MTX dosesk >12 mg/m^2 are poorly absorbed; as a result, higher doses of MTX are usually given parenterally (subcutaneous or intramuscular). JIA patients with oligoarthritis seem to respond best to MTX, while systemic arthritis patients experience little to no benefit. Depending on the definition of response to therapy, 33% to 100% of JIA patients respond to dosages of MTX between 7.1 and 30 mg/m^2 (0.15 and 1 mg/kg) per week. MTX at a dose of 10 to 15 mg/m^2 seems to require an average of 13 months of treatment until remission is achieved in most JIA patients. Radiologic evidence of improvement or slowing of joint damage has been demonstrated in JIA patients who responded to MTX therapy over a 2-year period.[274]

The prognosis of JIA-related joint damage is much better than that associated with adult RA; therefore, discontinuation of MTX should be attempted when disease remission is apparent. The optimal length of time between achievement of disease remission and MTX discontinuation remains to be defined; however, it probably should not be discontinued sooner than 1 year after disease remission, with slower withdrawal in patients at high risk for relapse.[275,276] In one trial involving all types of JIA subgroups, MTX discontinuation was attempted approximately 6 to 8 months after disease control was achieved.[277] After 11 months, 50% of patients relapsed; patients younger than 4.5 years old at the time of diagnosis seemed to be at higher risk of relapse. However, all patients who relapsed responded to MTX retreatment at prediscontinuation doses. In another study, patients with pauciarticular JIA who progressed to polyarticular disease were at greatest risk for relapse.[276]

Children tolerate MTX therapy well and generally experience few serious or troublesome adverse effects (e.g., transient liver enzyme elevations, nausea, vomiting, oral ulcerations).[275] These adverse effects are reduced with daily folic acid therapy

(1 mg) or weekly folinic acid (the day after MTX dosing). Liver biopsy studies of patients with JIA receiving cumulative MTX doses up to 5,300 mg for up to 6 years have all been normal with the exception of a single case report in 1990. Liver toxicity monitoring in JIA, therefore, is the same as the guidelines recommend for MTX therapy in adult RA, including biopsy recommendations (see Questions 27 and 28).The combination of MTX and other DMARDs has not been fully evaluated.

If MTX is not tolerated or is ineffective, SSZ is often the next DMARD selected.[261,263] SSZ (30–50 mg/kg/per day in two divided doses with a maximum of 2 g/day) is effective for pauciarticular and polyarticular JIA, but numerous adverse effects (e.g., liver enzyme elevations, leukopenia, hypoimmunoglobulinemia, hematomas, diarrhea, anorexia) lead to discontinuation of therapy in about 30% of patients.[278] HCQ may be considered if SSZ fails, but efficacy data from well-designed randomized controlled trials are not available.[261,263]

Biological Agents

51. What biological agents are effective in JIA?

Etanercept (Enbrel), the only FDA-approved biological agent for the treatment of JIA, is indicated for patients 4 years of age and older whose conditions have failed to respond to one or more DMARDs.[32] The recommended dose is 0.4 mg/kg (maximum, 25 mg) subcutaneously twice weekly. Etanercept monotherapy at this dose would be expected to yield about a 76% response rate (i.e., a minimum 30% improvement in at least three of six and ≥30% worsening in no more than one of six JIA core set criteria, including physician and patient global assessment, active joint count, limitation of motion, functional assessment, and ESR). The safety of etanercept in children is comparable to adults with the exception of significantly more abdominal pain (17% of JIA patients vs. 5% of adult patients with RA) and vomiting (14.5% of patients with JIA vs. <3% of adult patients with RA). JIA patients should be current on immunizations before initiation of etanercept therapy because the effect of etanercept on vaccine response is unknown. Safety and efficacy data reflecting up to 8 years of treatment support the long-term use of etanercept for JIA.[279]

Other biological agents, including infliximab, adalimumab, anakinra, and abatacept, are not FDA approved for JIA but have been studied.[273,280–282] Trials involving these agents are primarily short term and relatively small in number of participants, but available data suggest that all of these treatments may be safe and effective for JIA with no evidence of significant risk for serious adverse reactions.

In summary, NSAID therapy is normally the first medication administered for JIA. If response to NSAID therapy is inadequate, two of the three most common forms of JIA (oligoarthritis, polyarthritis) have a high response rate to MTX. Patients with systemic arthritis unresponsive to NSAID therapy or patients with oligoarthritis or polyarthritis who have a suboptimal response to MTX should receive a trial of etanercept. The use of other anti-TNF agents, anakinra, and abatacept is promising.[273]

Intra-Articular Corticosteroid Therapy

52. What is the evidence to support the use of intra-articular corticosteroid therapy in JIA?

Intra-articular corticosteroid therapy seems to be highly efficacious in JIA. Full disease remission of injected joints lasting longer than 6 months can be expected in 84% of patients with JIA, and 60% of patients could be expected to be able to discontinue all oral medications, with even greater success in patients with pauciarticular JIA (75%).[283] In one study, after an average of 30 months of follow-up, long-term negative effects of corticosteroid therapy (e.g., joint stability, osteonecrosis, soft tissue atrophy) were not encountered. As a result, intra-articular corticosteroid therapy seems to be a safe and effective option for JIA, particularly in pauciarticular disease limited to a few troublesome joints.[261]

Uveitis

53. J.R. is scheduled to be seen by an ophthalmologist every 6 months to screen for uveitis. How should her uveitis be managed?

Uveitis associated with JIA is a nongranulomatous inflammation involving the iris and ciliary body. This type of uveitis, sometimes is referred to as iridocyclitis, can occur in 2% to 4% of patients with JIA.[284] The posterior uveal tract, or choroid, rarely is affected.[261] Chronic uveitis can progress, leading to cataracts, glaucoma, and blindness; however, careful screening and early detection are effective at preventing these conditions. Uveitis is most common in ANA-positive oligoarthritis JIA and usually occurs within 4 to 7 years of JIA diagnosis. Fewer than 1% of patients with systemic JIA develop uveitis.

Uveitis rarely presents with symptoms, and even if symptoms occur, children may have difficulty recognizing them. If symptoms of uveitis (e.g., ocular pain, decreased vision, headaches, red eye, unequal pupils) occur, urgent eye examination is warranted.

Prevention of uveitis relies on compliance with regularly scheduled slit-lamp examinations performed by an ophthalmologist.[284] Direct ophthalmoscopy cannot detect uveitis. All JIA patients must have a baseline slit-lamp examination within 1 month of diagnosis. The highest-risk JIA patients for uveitis (e.g., ANA-positive oligoarthritis or polyarthritis, ≤6 years of age at JIA onset and ≤4 years JIA duration) require slit-lamp examination every 3 months. At the opposite extreme, low-risk oligoarthritis or polyarthritis patients (i.e., >7 years JIA duration, >6 years of age at JIA onset and >4 years JID duration, ≤6 years of age at JIA onset and >4 years JIA duration who are ANA negative, >6 years of age at JIA onset and ANA negative) and systemic JIA patients require slit-lamp examination once a year.

If detected early, the prognosis for uveitis is very good. The initial drug of choice is a topical corticosteroid (e.g., dexamethasone, prednisolone), which usually reduces ocular inflammation rapidly. More severe and chronic uveitis may require a 1- to 3-day course of intravenous methylprednisolone (30 mg/kg once daily, maximum 1 g/dose). Uveitis that responds poorly to corticosteroids should be treated with systemic NSAIDs, followed by serial trials of by MTX and anti-TNF agents if responses are inadequate.[261]

OSTEOARTHRITIS

OA, also referred to as degenerative joint disease, is the most common form of arthritis in the United States. Approximately 27 million Americans have clinical OA.[286] OA is the single most common cause of rheumatic symptoms, and no other disease is responsible for more loss of time from work. Patients with OA are more dependent on others in climbing stairs and walking than any other disease, and OA is second only to heart disease as the most common disability leading to the receipt of Social Security benefits.

The prevalence of OA rises dramatically with age, increasing from two- to tenfold from age 30 to age 65, respectively. Although men are affected more commonly in early adulthood, men and women are generally affected equally. At age 65, OA is twice as prevalent in women, and women are more likely to have proximal and DIP joint involvement presenting with Bouchard's nodes or Heberden's nodes. Although only 30% of patients are symptomatic, >90% of all individuals older than 40 years of age have radiographic evidence of joint damage in weight-bearing joints consistent with OA.[287]

Risk factors for the development of OA include advancing age, obesity, quadriceps muscle weakness,[288] joint overuse/injury from vocational or sports activities, genetic susceptibility,[289] and developmental abnormalities.[287] Obesity increases OA risk because of excess weight placed on weight-bearing joints (e.g., hips, knee). However, metabolic factors other than excess weight may also play a role in the development of OA in obese individuals. Excess adipose tissue can produce abnormal levels of hormones or growth factors that can affect cartilage or underlying bone, predisposing individuals to OA.[290] A weight loss of 5 kg is associated with a 50% reduction in the odds of developing symptomatic knee OA.

Quadriceps muscle weakness is strongly predictive of both radiographic and symptomatic OA of the knee. The risk of knee damage associated with quadriceps weakness is more pronounced in relation to body weight. Vocational or athletic activities also can contribute to OA as the result of repetitive joint use or trauma subjected to the joints. This is consistent with the traditional "wear and tear" concept used to explain the etiology of OA. However, OA is much more complicated than simply a disease of wearing-down of joints. Under normal conditions, chondrocytes in articular cartilage, which undergo active cell division, balance matrix degradation and repair. Biomechanical stress placed on the joint is believed to stimulate cytokine-mediated release of enzymes (e.g., matrix metalloproteinase, plasmin, cathepsins) that degrade the proteoglycan and collagen components of cartilage, possibly predisposing affected joints to the development of OA.[287]

Signs and Symptoms

The clinical presentation of OA is variable and depends on the particular joints involved. Unlike RA, which is characterized by synovial proliferation within multiple joints and systemic disease, the symptoms of OA are limited to the joints in which progressive degeneration of cartilage with secondary reactive bone changes (i.e., osteophyte formation) occurs. Occasionally, secondary synovial inflammation can contribute to symptoms. The primary symptom is a deep aching pain localized to the affected joint(s). The joints most commonly involved are the DIP (known as Heberden's nodes), PIP (known as Bouchard's nodes), first carpometacarpal, knees, hips, cervical and lumbar spine, and the first MTP joints. Shoulder, elbow, and rarely the MCP joints also can become involved. In addition to joint pain, common OA symptoms include morning stiffness and stiffness after rest during the day lasting less than 20 to 30 minutes, limited to involved joints. Joint motion may be limited secondary to loss of integrity of the joint surfaces, development of osteophytes, intra-articular loose bodies, and protective muscle spasm. Crepitus, a palpable grating or crackling due to roughened articular surfaces, may be associated with both passive and active motion of involved joints.[287]

54. G.R., a 190-lb, 60-year-old school teacher, developed painful, tender swelling in the right knee approximately 1 year ago. Since then, she has experienced intermittent pain in the right knee and hip. She now has moderate morning stiffness in the hip and knee and some joint stiffness after inactivity. Her pain is increased significantly by ambulation. Examination of her joints revealed Heberden's nodes in both hands, limitation of flexion of the right hip to 45 degrees, patellar crepitus, and mild tenderness at the joint margin of the right knee. Laboratory studies were all normal, including negative RF. What signs and symptoms of OA are present in G.R.?

Symptoms of OA usually are referable to the particular joint or joints involved. Common complaints include joint pain (particularly with motion) and stiffness after periods of rest for weight-bearing joints with aching during periods of inclement weather. Crepitation upon joint motion, limitation of motion, and changes in the shape of the joint may be detected on physical examination. The joint(s) may be tender to palpation, but signs of inflammation are relatively uncommon with the exception of effusion, which may be noted after trauma or vigorous use of the involved joint. The Heberden's nodes observed in G.R.'s hands are bony protuberances (osteophytes) at the margins on the dorsal surfaces of the DIP joints. These nodes are more common in women, have a genetic predisposition, and often are associated with a more severe disease course involving multiple joints. OA of the hip is usually rapidly progressive, possibly due to constant weight-bearing, eventually leading to limitation of ROM. Knee OA is observed frequently in older women, particularly when obesity and weak quadriceps muscles are contributing factors, and is associated with crepitus, loss of ROM, and flexion deformities. Other common manifestations of OA that are not present in G.R. include vertebral column involvement and Bouchard's nodes (i.e., osteophytes on PIP joints).

Results of laboratory studies are usually normal unless an underlying disease coexists. ESR may be elevated in patients with generalized OA characterized by involvement of three or more joint groups with evidence of local inflammation (e.g., soft tissue swelling, redness, warmth). RF is usually negative; however, as discussed previously, approximately 3 to 5% of non-RA individuals test positive for RF. Synovial fluid analysis may reveal mild inflammation-induced increase in volume, decreased viscosity, mild pleocytosis, and a slight increase in synovial fluid protein.[287]

Treatment

Nonpharmacologic and First-Line Therapy

55. How should G.R. be treated?

Because of the degenerative nature of OA, nonpharmacologic interventions aimed at preserving joint function and ROM while maintaining muscle strength are essential. Medications are used to reduce symptoms and have no impact on the disease course. G.R. has significant pain in both the hip and knees. She should understand the pathology of OA and taught appropriate self-management techniques. Examples of effective nonpharmacologic measures include exercises that avoid stress on joints while strengthening periarticular muscles (e.g., aerobic aquatic exercises, stationary bicycle), avoidance of excessive loading of the hip or knee joints by using assistive devices (e.g., canes, walkers, orthopedic shoe), weight reduction for obese individuals, education on principles of joint protection, and thermal modalities.[291]

If possible, G.R. should be referred to a physical therapist, who can help to develop an exercise program appropriate for OA patients. Occupational therapists can provide valuable techniques and assistance devices to help with activities of daily living.

OA treatment goals are to relieve pain, maintain or improve joint function, minimize disability, enhance quality of life and functional independence, minimize risks of therapy, and educate patients and their families. Because the cause and much of the pathophysiology pertaining to OA remain unexplained, drug therapy is empiric and directed toward providing symptomatic relief. Drugs have not been proven to prevent, delay the progression of, or reverse the pathologic changes of OA in humans.

In a comprehensive review of 351 OA clinical trials, acetaminophen was only effective for the treatment of mild pain, whereas NSAIDs were more effective for moderate to severe OA pain.[134] Furthermore, acetaminophen should be considered the treatment of choice for mild pain because of a lower risk of GI complications compared with NSAIDs. (See Nonsteroidal Anti-inflammatory Drugs section). In a 4-week study of patients with symptomatic OA of the knee,[292] acetaminophen, up to 4 g/day, was comparable to an analgesic regimen of ibuprofen (1.2 g/day) and an anti-inflammatory regimen (2.4 g/day). In a multicenter, randomized, double-blind, 2-year comparison of naproxen 750 mg/day with acetaminophen 2.6 g/day, no significant differences were noted between the treatments, knee flexion and walking time in the were improved in the naproxen group.[293]

NSAIDs should be prescribed for OA patients with moderate to severe pain; however, the risk of serious adverse effects, particularly GI bleeding, must be considered. Risk factors (e.g., older age, history of prior GI bleeding, concurrent use of antiplatelets or anticoagulants) may warrant the use of PPIs or misoprostol concurrently with NSAID therapy. As in the case of RA, all NSAIDs are equally efficacious for OA; patient response to a given NSAID is not predictable.[134] Therefore, a trial of several different NSAIDs, even those within the same chemical class, may be required before satisfactory analgesic effects are achieved.

Alternatives to Simple Analgesics

56. G.R. starts a regimen of acetaminophen 1 g QID PRN and returns to the clinic 4 weeks later. She states that most joint-related symptomatically and general functioning have improved; however, she claims that the pain and stiffness in her right knee is more bothersome now than 1 month ago. What is the best treatment option for G.R. at this visit?

If joint symptoms persist despite an adequate trial with acetaminophen, several options may be considered. Locally applied medications offer the advantage of minimizing the potential for systemic adverse effects associated with oral medications. Although not FDA approved, topical NSAIDs (diclofenac, ibuprofen) have been as effective as oral NSAIDs, particularly in patients with OA of the knee.[134] Evidence supporting the use of capsaicin cream is not as strong as topical NSAIDs, but is better than placebo in providing pain relief. Capsaicin cream, derived from vanillyl alkaloids found in hot peppers and related plants, induces analgesic effects by depleting local sensory nerve endings of substance P. Topical salicylates are not effective for relief of OA symptoms. Intra-articular corticosteroid injections are very effective for the treatment of pain and inflammation in isolated joints (see Corticosteroids section). A poor response to local treatment warrants consideration of NSAID use.

Nonsteroidal Anti-Inflammatory Drugs and Cyclo-Oxygenase-2 Inhibitors

57. What is the role of the NSAIDs and/or COX-2 inhibitors in managing G.R.'s OA?

Because G.R. is overweight and has experienced OA symptoms for more than 1 year, her condition is most likely more than a mild form of OA. The treatment of choice for moderate to severe OA is NSAID therapy.[134] NSAIDs or COX-2 inhibitors are also preferred for patients who have not responded adequately to maximum doses of acetaminophen and patients with joint effusions. Some patients may benefit from a combination acetaminophen plus an NSAID.[294,295] This combination would allow for lower doses of NSAIDs when used with acetaminophen. In one study, acetaminophen 4 g/day in combination with naproxen 500 mg/day was as effective as 1,000 to 1,500 mg/day of naproxen alone in patients with OA of the hip.[295] Patients with inflammatory OA (clinically defined as having detectable effusion in their joints) may respond better to NSAIDs.[296]

Although NSAIDS are effective for controlling pain and inflammation associated with OA, the risk of GI-related complications, including ulceration, hemorrhage, and death, must be considered.[134,136] (See complete discussion regarding adverse effects of NSAIDs and COX-2 inhibitors in Question 11.) NSAID use is associated with a 2.5- to 5.5-fold increased risk of GI-related hospitalization and 16,500 deaths per year among arthritis patients. Risk factors for GI complications, include NSAID dose, concurrent prednisone use, history of GI bleeding, and old age, may warrant the concurrent use of gastroprotective agents such as misoprostol or PPIs. NSAIDs are also associated with other serious adverse effects including renal dysfunction, elevated blood pressure, fluid retention, and heart failure exacerbation. In one study, NSAID use was associated with approximately 19% of hospital admissions for heart failure.[297] The burden of illness from NSAID-related heart failure may exceed the burden associated with gastropathy.

COX-2 inhibitors are similar to nonselective NSAIDs with regard to virtually all adverse effects, including sodium retention and reductions in glomerular filtration rate.[298] The published results of a large trial suggesting that the only remaining COX-2 inhibitor available in the United States, celecoxib, is associated with fewer serious GI complications when compared to nonselective NSAIDs are questionable (see Question 11). Therefore, until more reliable data are available, the safest course of action is to consider celecoxib as having the same side effect profile as nonselective NSAIDs.

The synthetic opioid tramadol is an alternative to the nonselective NSAIDs or COX-2 inhibitors for patients who have contraindications to the COX inhibitors. Tramadol relieves moderate to severe pain and is comparable to ibuprofen for the treatment of OA of the hip and knee, and may be used as adjunctive therapy to NSAIDs.[292] Because tramadol is a synthetic opioid, nausea, constipation, and drowsiness are common side effects. Although the abuse potential for tramadol is very low, the FDA MedWatch adverse effect surveillance program has received 766 reports of abuse and 482 cases of withdrawal associated with tramadol between 1995 and 2004.[299,300] Therefore, tramadol seems to be safest for the short-term treatment of acute pain. If tramadol is used for chronic pain, closes monitoring for abuse or addiction is warranted.

Corticosteroids

Systemic corticosteroids are not commonly prescribed for patients with OA because inflammation is not a primary component of OA pathophysiology. Intra-articular injection of a corticosteroid can be of value when isolated joints with effusions are painful and swollen. The aspiration of effusion fluid followed by an injection of a corticosteroid such as triamcinolone hexacetonide (up to 40 mg) can be effective for reducing pain and increasing muscle strength. The injections can be used as monotherapy or as adjunctive therapy along with an analgesic or NSAID. Symptomatic improvement from intra-articular corticosteroids may last only a few days, but also may persist for a month or longer. The initial relief of pain may permit more effective physical therapy and appropriate balance of rest and exercise, thus attenuating the need for repeated injections.[291] On the other hand, symptomatic improvement may lead to overuse of the joint and potentially accelerate the degenerative process. The safe frequency of repeated corticosteroid injections into the same joint is unclear. In one study, repeated weekly joint injections for up to 9 weeks in animals resulted in histologic evidence of cartilage degeneration and depressed collagen and proteoglycan synthesis.[301] In RA patients, corticosteroid injections up to 10 times per joint per year over a 10-year period were not associated with cartilage loss.[302] In one randomized, placebo-controlled trial, corticosteroid injections as often as every 3 months did not worsen joint space loss over a period of 2 years.[303]

The intra-articular injection of crystalline steroid suspension can precipitate a flare of synovitis, which usually is temporary and can be relieved with cold compresses and analgesics. Other potential, but rare, complications of intra-articular injections include osteonecrosis, tendon rupture, microcrystalline corticosteroid deposition in the synovial fluid, and joint capsule calcification.[304] Thus, frequent injections into the same joint, particularly weight-bearing joints, should be avoided. Although the mechanism of benefit of intra-articular corticosteroids in OA is still unclear, patient response is very high, as demonstrated by the fact that a corticosteroid injection is given in one of every six patient care encounters with a rheumatologist.[305] Although not evaluated in clinical trials, it is common practice to mix a small about of 1% or 2% lidocaine with corticosteroid to provide temporary analgesia upon injection.

Viscosupplements

Viscosupplements, classified by the FDA as a "medical devices," are used as substitutes for the natural hyaluronic acid in the joint fluid that breaks down in patients with OA. Two viscosupplements are currently available in the United States, hyaluronan (sodium hyaluronate) and hylan. Hyaluronan, polysaccharide molecules that occur naturally in synovial fluid, help to create a viscous environment, cushion joints, and maintain normal function. The viscosupplements (derived compound from rooster combs) act as lubricants and shock absorbers in weight-bearing joints, possibly protecting cartilage from damage.[306,307]

The hyaluronans are usually administered when analgesics and other measures fail for knee OA. The affected knee is first aspirated and hyaluronan is administered intra-articularly into the knee as a series of three to five injections on a weekly basis. In some clinical trials, the hyaluronans provide pain relief comparable to NSAIDs for 6 months or longer after a course of treatment, longer than the duration of relief achievable by intra-articular corticosteroids. Nevertheless, in a systematic review and meta-analysis, intra-articular hyaluronic acid provided no clinical benefits for knee OA.[308]

Hyaluronan is generally well-tolerated, with the most common adverse event being mild to moderate pain, inflammation, and effusion at the injection site.[309,310] Patients allergic to avian proteins and products, including eggs and feathers, should avoid all hyaluronans with the exception of ferring (Euflexxa), the only bioengineered formulation.

Corticosteroids or hyaluronans administered intra-articularly may provide temporary relief of pain and, if present, inflammation. Corticosteroids seem to offer a higher response rate at a much lower cost (medication cost <\$2 per injection, 2007 pricing, www.drugstore.com), although hyaluronans may provide a longer duration of effect. Both have the advantage of avoiding systemic adverse effects of oral medications, and may provide the support necessary to allow for the therapeutic success of other key interventions (e.g., weight loss, exercise and muscle strengthening, knee replacement).

Glucosamine and Chondroitin

Glucosamine, used for many years in the United States for arthritis in dogs and horses, was hypothesized to halt or reverse OA. Endogenous glucosamine, an amino-monosaccharide synthesized from glucose, is integral to the biosynthesis of proteoglycans and the glycosaminoglycans, which are building blocks of cartilage. Chondroitin sulfate reportedly provides substrate for the formation of a healthy joint matrix and blocks enzymes responsible for breaking down old cartilage. These products are often sold as combination products for the treatment of OA, but there is no evidence that the combination produces better results than glucosamine sulfate alone.[311] Almost all of the clinical trials of glucosamine and chondroitin have produced weak conclusions because of small sample size or other deficiencies in study design.[312]

As a result of the widespread promotion and use of glucosamine with or without chondroitin for OA and the lack of strong clinical trial evidence, the National Institutes of

Health sponsored a large study to end all speculation. The Glucosamine/chondroitin Arthritis Intervention Trial evaluated 1,583 patients randomized to receive either placebo, celecoxib, glucosamine, chondroitin, or glucosamine with chondroitin.[313] The study required investigators to manufacture their own pharmaceutical-grade glucosamine hydrochloride and chondroitin because of the inability to identify a manufacturer of a product with acceptable lot-to-lot consistency (glucosamine and chondroitin are natural products unregulated by the FDA). At 24-week follow-up, glucosamine and chondroitin, either alone or in combination, were found to be no different than placebo at achieving the primary endpoint of a 20% reduction in knee pain from baseline. On the other hand, significantly more patients treated with celecoxib achieved the primary endpoint when compared with placebo ($p = 0.008$). A preplanned subgroup analysis of 354 patients with baseline moderate to severe pain revealed a significantly higher response rate with combination glucosamine and chondroitin versus placebo (79.2% vs. 54.3%, respectively, $p = 0.002$). In general, successful treatment of more severe pain is easier to achieve than treatment of mild pain, for which there is little room for improvement. Rates of adverse events and treatment withdrawals were low and similar between all study groups. Celecoxib-treated patients had a higher incidence of blood pressure elevation, and chondroitin-treated patients had the highest incidence of nonspecific musculoskeletal and connective tissue events.

The combination of glucosamine and chondroitin is well-tolerated and may only be beneficial for moderate to severe OA. However, clinicians and patients should keep in mind that these are natural products unregulated by the FDA and, as a result, consistency in potency, safety, purity, and efficacy cannot be assured.

ACKNOWLEDGMENTS

The author acknowledges Mircea Florea, MD, for his guidance and mentoring in the evaluation and management of arthritic disorders, and William Gong, PharmD for his contributions to the earlier editions of this chapter.

REFERENCES

1. Arthritis Foundation. Disease Center: Rheumatoid Arthritis. Available at: http://www.arthritis.org/disease-center.php?disease_id=31, Accessed September 2007.
2. Prevalence of doctor-diagnosed arthritis and arthritis-attributable activity limitation—United States, 2003–2005. *MMWR* 2006;55:1089.
3. State-specific prevalence of arthritis-attributable work limitation—United States, 2003. *MMWR* 2007;56:1045.
4. Arnett FC et al. The American Rheumatism Association 1987 revised criteria for the classification of rheumatoid arthritis. *Arthritis Rheum* 1988;31:315.
5. Felson DT. Epidemiology of the rheumatic diseases. In: Koopman WJ ed. *Arthritis and Allied Conditions [Online]*, 15th ed. Baltimore: Lippincott Williams & Wilkins; 2005.
6. Helmick CG et al. Estimates of the prevalence of arthritis and other rheumatic conditions in the United States, Part I. *Arthritis Rheum* 2008;58:15.
7. Tuomi T et al. Smoking, lung function, and rheumatoid factors. *Ann Rheum Dis* 1990;49:753.
8. Krishnan E et al. Smoking-gender interaction and risk for rheumatoid arthritis. *Arthritis Res Ther* 2003;5:R158.
9. O'Dell JR. Rheumatoid arthritis: the clinical picture. In: Koopman WJ ed. *Arthritis and Allied Conditions [Online]*, 15th ed. Baltimore, MD: Lippincott Williams & Wilkins; 2005.
10. American College of Rheumatology Subcommittee on Rheumatoid Arthritis Guidelines. Guidelines for the management of rheumatoid arthritis. *Arthritis Rheum* 2002;46:328.
11. Pinals RS et al. Preliminary criteria for clinical remission in rheumatoid arthritis. *Arthritis Rheum* 1981;24:1308.
12. Alarcon GS et al. Evaluation of the American Rheumatism Association preliminary criteria for remission in rheumatoid arthritis: a prospective study. *J Rheumatol* 1987;14:93.
13. Wolfe F, Hawley DJ. Remission in rheumatoid arthritis. *J Rheumatol* 1985;12:245.
14. Mottonen T et al. Comparison of combination therapy with single-drug therapy in early rheumatoid arthritis: a randomised trial. *Lancet* 1999;353:1568.
15. Mottonten T et al. Outcome in patients with early rheumatoid arthritis treated according to the "saw-tooth" strategy. *Arthritis Rheum* 1996;39:996.
16. van Jaarsveld CFM et al. Aggressive treatment in early rheumatoid arthritis: a randomized controlled trial. *Ann Rheum Dis* 2000;59:468.
17. The North American Rheumatoid Arthritis Disease Management Study Group. A population-based assessment of disease activity, quality of life and cost of care in early rheumatoid arthritis. *Arthritis Rheum* 1998;41:S127.
18. Wolfe F et al. Minimal disease activity, remission, and the long-term outcomes of rheumatoid arthritis. *Arthritis Rheum* 2007;57:935.
19. Lindqvist E, Eberhardt K. Mortality in rheumatoid arthritis patients with disease onset in the 1980s. *Ann Rheum Dis* 1999;58:11.
20. Kroot EJA et al. No increased mortality in patients with rheumatoid arthritis: up to 10 years of follow up from disease onset. *Ann Rheum Dis* 2000;59:954.
21. Gerli R et al. Precocious atherosclerosis in rheumatoid arthritis: role of traditional and disease-related cardiovascular risk factors. *Ann N Y Acad Sci* 2007;1108:372.
22. Sarzi-Puttini P et al. TNF-alpha, rheumatoid arthritis, and heart failure: a rheumatological dilemma. *Autoimmun Rev* 2005;4:153.
23. Wei L et al. Taking glucocorticoids by prescription is associated with subsequent cardiovascular disease. *Ann Intern Med* 2004;141:764.
24. Pham T et al. Cardiovascular risk and rheumatoid arthritis: clinical practice guidelines based on published evidence and expert opinion. *Joint Bone Spine* 2006;73:379.
25. Hale LP. Pathology of rheumatoid arthritis and associated disorders. In: Koopman WJ ed. *Arthritis and Allied Conditions [Online]*, 15th ed. Baltimore, MD: Lippincott Williams & Wilkins; 2005.
26. Arend W. The pathophysiology and treatment of rheumatoid arthritis. *Arthritis Rheum* 1997;40:595.
27. Carter RH. B cells in health and disease. *Mayo Clin Proc* 2006;81:377.
28. Feldmann M et al. Rheumatoid arthritis. *Cell* 1996;85:307.
29. Zvaifler NJ, Corr M. The evaluation and treatment of rheumatoid arthritis. In: Koopman WJ ed. *Arthritis and Allied Conditions [Online]*, 15th ed. Baltimore, MD: Lippincott Williams & Wilkins; 2005.
30. Abramowicz M. Drugs for rheumatoid arthritis. *Treat Guidel Med Lett* 2005;3:83.
31. Furst DE et al. Updated consensus statement on biologic agents for the treatment of rheumatoid arthritis and other rheumatic diseases. *Ann Rheum Dis* 2002;61(Suppl ii):ii2.
32. Etanercept (Enbrel) package insert. Thousand Oaks, CA: Immunex; 2006.
33. Infliximab (Remicade) package insert. Malvern, PA: Centocor; 2007.
34. Sundy J. Nonsteroidal anti-inflammatory drugs. In: Koopman WJ ed. *Arthritis and Allied Conditions [Online]*, 15th ed. Baltimore, MD: Lippincott Williams & Wilkins; 2005.
35. Mann J, Evans T. Gastrointestinal-related complications in a long-term care population taking NSAIDs versus COX-2 inhibitor therapy. *Consultant Pharmacist* 2004;19:602.
36. Greene JM, Winickff RN. Cost-conscious prescribing of nonsteroidal anti-inflammatory drugs for adults with arthritis. *Arch Intern Med* 1992;152:1995.
37. Wolfe MM et al. Medical progress: gastrointestinal toxicity of nonsteroidal anti-inflammatory drugs. *N Engl J Med* 1999;340:1888.
38. Cryer C, Feldman M. Cyclooxygenase-1 and cyclooxygenase-2 selectivity of widely used nonsteroidal anti-inflammatory drugs. *Am J Med* 1998;104:413.
39. Bresalier RS et al; Adenomatous Polyp Prevention on Vioxx (APPROVe) Trial Investigators. Cardiovascular Events Associated with Rofecoxib in a Colorectal Adenoma Chemoprevention Trial. *N Engl J Med* 2005;352:1092.
40. Nussmeier NA et al. Complications of the COX-2 Inhibitors Parecoxib and Valdecoxib after Cardiac Surgery. *N Engl J Med* 2005;352:1080.
41. Schafer AI. Effects of nonsteroidal antiinflammatory drugs on platelet function and systemic hemostasis. *J Clin Pharmacol* 1995;35:209.
42. FitzGerald GA, Patrono C. The coxibs, selective inhibitors of cyclooxygenase-2. *N Engl J Med* 2001;345:433.
43. Buttar NS, Wang KK. The aspirin of the new millennium: cyclooxygenase-2 inhibitors. *Mayo Clin Proc* 2000;75:1027.
44. Halter F et al. Cyclooxygenase 2-implications on maintenance of gastric mucosal integrity and ulcer healing: controversial issues and perspectives. *Gut* 2001;49:443.
45. Abramowicz M. Valdecoxib (Bextra)- a new COX-2 inhibitor. *Med Letter* 2002;44:39.
46. Donahue KE et al. Comparative effectiveness of drug therapy for rheumatoid arthritis and psoriatic

arthritis in adults. Comparative effectiveness review no. 11. Rockville, MD: Agency for Healthcare Research and Quality. November 2007. Available at: www.effectivehealthcare.ahrq.gov/reports/final.cfm.
47. Felson DT et al. Use of short-term efficacy/toxicity trade-offs to select second-line drugs in rheumatoid arthritis. *Arthritis Rheum* 1992;35:1117.
48. Buchbinder R et al. Methotrexate therapy in rheumatoid arthritis: a life table review of 587 patients treated in community practice. *J Rheumatol* 1993;20:639.
49. Nowlin NS et al. DMARDs in the nineties: the UW experience. *Arthritis Rheum* 1998;41:S153.
50. Suarez-Almazor ME. Practice patterns in the management of rheumatoid arthritis: increased use of combination therapy. *Arthritis Rheum* 1998; 41:S153.
51. Wang BWE et al. Frequency of two-DMARD combinations in the treatment of rheumatoid arthritis. *Arthritis Rheum* 1998;41:S59.
52. Smolen JS et al. Efficacy and safety of leflunomide compared with placebo and sulphasalazine in active rheumatoid arthritis: a double-blind, randomised, multicentre trial. *Lancet* 1999;353:259.
53. Leflunomide (Arava) [package insert]. Bridgewater, NJ: Sanofi-Aventis Pharmaceuticals; 2007.
54. Cohen S et al. Two-year, blinded, randomized, controlled trial of active rheumatoid arthritis with leflunomide compared with methotrexate. *Arthritis Rheum* 2001;44:1984.
55. Sander O et al. Prospective six year follow-up of patients withdrawn from a randomised study comparing parenteral gold salt and methotrexate. *Ann Rheum Dis* 1999;58:281.
56. Felson DT et al. The comparative efficacy and toxicity of second-line drugs in rheumatoid arthritis. *Arthritis Rheum* 1990;33:1449.
57. Van den Borne B et al. No increased risk of malignancies and mortality in cyclosporin A-treated patients with rheumatoid arthritis. *Arthritis Rheum* 1998;41:1930.
58. O'Dell JR. Anticytokine therapy—a new era in the treatment of rheumatoid arthritis? *N Engl J Med* 1999;340:310.
59. Jenkins JK et al. Biologic modifier therapy for the treatment of rheumatoid arthritis. *Am J Med Sci* 2002;323:197.
60. Moreland LW et al. Etanercept therapy in rheumatoid arthritis: a randomized, controlled trial. *Ann Intern Med* 1999;130:478.
61. Louie SG et al. Biologic response modifiers in the management of rheumatoid arthritis. *Am J Health System Pharm* 2003;60:346.
62. Bendele AM et al. Combination benefit of treatment with the cytokine inhibitors interleukin-1 receptor antagonist and PGEylated soluble tumor necrosis factor receptor type I in animal models of rheumatoid arthritis. *Arthritis Rheum* 2000;43:2648.
63. Ault A. Rheumatoid arthritis drug linked to infections. *Lancet* 1999;353:1770.
64. Packer M et al. Randomized placebo-controlled dose-ranging trial of infliximab, a monoclonal antibody to tumor necrosis factor-a, in moderate to severe heart failure. Paper presented at Annual Meeting of the Heart Failure Society of America; September 25, 2002; Boca Raton, FL.
65. Abramowicz M. Rituximab for non-Hodgkins lymphoma. *Med Lett Drugs Ther* 1998;40:65.
66. Van Vollenhoven RF et al. Safety of rituximab in rheumatoid arthritis: results of a pooled analysis (Poster no. FR10151). Presented at the 2006 annual meeting of the European League Against Rheumatism; Amsterdam, The Netherlands; June 21–24, 2006.
67. Westhovens R et al. Maintained efficacy and safety of abatacept in rheumatoid arthritis patients receiving background methotrexate through 5 years of treatment. Program and abstracts of the American College of Rheumatology 2007 Annual Scientific Meeting; November 6–11, 2007; Boston, Massachusetts. Abstract 950.
68. Abatacept (Orencia) package insert. Princeton, NJ: Bristol-Myers Squibb; 2008.
69. Rituximab (Rituxan) package insert. South San Francisco, CA: Biogen Idec and Amgen; 2008.
70. Conn DL. Resolved: low-dose prednisone is indicated as standard treatment in patients with rheumatoid arthritis. *Arthritis Rheum* 2001;45:462.
71. Saag KG. Resolved: low-dose glucocorticoids are neither safe nor effective for the long-term treatment of rheumatoid arthritis. *Arthritis Rheum* 2001;45:468.
72. O'Dell JR et al. Treatment of early seropositive rheumatoid arthritis with minocycline: four-year follow-up of a double-blind, placebo-controlled trial. *Arthritis Rheum* 1999;42:1691.
73. O'Dell JR et al. Treatment of early seropositive rheumatoid arthritis: a two-year, double-blind comparison of minocycline and hydroxychloroquine. *Arthritis Rheum* 2001;44:2235.
74. Felson DT et al. The Prosorba column for treatment of refractory rheumatoid arthritis. *Arthritis Rheum* 1999;42:2153.
75. Ossandon A et al. Thalidomide: focus on its employment in rheumatologic diseases. *Clin Exp Rheumatol* 2002;20:709.
76. Skelly MM, Hawkey CF. Potential alternatives to COX 2 inhibitors. *BMJ* 2002;324:1289.
77. Hawkey C et al. Gastrointestinal safety of AZD 3582: a new chemical entity with a novel multipathway mechanism of action [Abstract 446]. *Gastroenterology* 2002;122:a446.
78. Palmer RH et al. Licofelone (ML 3000) an inhibitor of COX-1, COX-2, and 5-LO is associated with less gastric damage than naproxen and is similar to placebo in man [Abstract 445]. *Gastroenterology* 2002;122:a445.
79. Moreland LW. T-cell receptor peptide vaccination in rheumatoid arthritis: a placebo-controlled trial using a combination of V-beta3, V-beta14, and V-beta14 peptides. *Arthritis Rheum* 1998;41:1919.
80. Clark P et al. Meta-analysis of injectable gold in rheumatoid arthritis. *J Rheumatol* 1989;16:442.
81. Ward JR et al. Comparison of auranofin, gold sodium thiomalate, and placebo in the treatment of rheumatoid arthritis. *Arthritis Rheum* 1983; 26:1303.
82. Scott DL et al. Long-term outcome of treating rheumatoid arthritis: results after 20 years. *Lancet* 1987:1108.
83. Thompson PW et al. Practical results of treatment with disease-modifying antirheumatoid drugs. *Br J Rheumatol* 1985;24:167.
84. Mottonen T et al. Outcome in patients with early rheumatoid arthritis treated according to the "saw-tooth" strategy. *Arthritis Rheum* 1996;39:996.
85. Ortendahl M et al. Influence of time on methotrexate in rheumatoid arthritis. *Arthritis Rheum* 1998;41:S156.
86. Morand EF et al. Life table analysis of 879 treatment episodes with slow acting antirheumatic drugs in community rheumatology practice. *J Rheum* 1992;19:704.
87. Cannella AC, O'Dell, JR. Is there still a role for traditional disease-modifying antirheumatic drugs (DMARDs) in rheumatoid arthritis? *Curr Opin Rheumatol* 2003;15:185.
88. Goekoop-Ruiterman YP et al. Clinical and radiographic outcomes of four different treatment strategies in patients with early rheumatoid arthritis (the BeSt study): a randomized, controlled trial. *Arthritis Rheum* 2005;52:3381.
89. Genovese MC et al. Combination therapy with etanercept and anakinra in the treatment of patients with rheumatoid arthritis who have been treated unsuccessfully with methotrexate. *Arthritis Rheum* 2004;50:1412.
90. Weisman MH et al. Analysis at 2 years of an inception cohort of early rheumatoid arthritis: the Study of North American Patients Diagnosed with New-Onset Rheumatoid Arthritis (SONORA) study. *Ann Rheum Dis* 2004;63(Suppl):70.
91. Wallace DJ et al. Etanercept or infliximab in combination with methotrexate in the treatment of rheumatoid arthritis: results from the Rheumatoid Arthritis DMARD Intervention and Utilization Study (RADIUS) registry. *Arthritis Rheum* 2005;52:S721.
92. van der Bijl AE et al. Persistent good clinical response after tapering and discontinuation of initial infliximab therapy in patients with early rheumatoid arthritis: 3-year results from the Behandel Strategieen (BeSt) trial. Presented at the European League Against Rheumatism Annual Meeting; June 21–24, 2006; Amsterdam, The Netherlands. Abstract OP0180.
93. Grigor C, Capell H, Stirling A et al. Effect of a treatment strategy of tight control for rheumatoid arthritis (the TICORA study): a single-blind randomised controlled trial. *Lancet* 2004;364:263.
94. Felson D et al. A proposed revision to the ACR20: the hybrid measure of American College of Rheumatology response. *Arthritis Rheum* 2007;57:193.
95. Smolen J et al. Improved Clinical and Simplified Disease Activity Index (CDAI, SDAI) scores with rituximab in patients with rheumatoid arthritis (RA) and an inadequate response to TNF inhibitors. Program and abstracts of the American College of Rheumatology (ACR) 71st Annual Meeting; November 6–11, 2007; Boston, Massachusetts. [Abstract #272]
96. DAS-Score.nl. Home of the DAS in Rheumatoid Arthritis, Dept of Rheumatology, University Medical Centre- the Netherlands. Available at: http://www.das-score.nl/www.das-score.nl/index.html. Accessed December 2007.
97. Aletaha D, Smolen J. The Simplified Disease Activity Index (SDAI) and the Clinical Disease Activity Index (CDAI): a review of their usefulness and validity in rheumatoid arthritis. *Clin Exp Rheumatol* 2005;23(Suppl 39):100.
98. Cush JJ. Global Arthritis Score: a rapid practice tool for rheumatoid arthritis (RA) assessment. Presented at the American College of Rheumatology 2005 Annual Scientific Meeting; November 12–17, 2005; San Diego, CA. Abstract 1854.
99. Fleischmann RM et al. A new composite measure for assessing RA activity in clinical practice. Program and abstracts of the American College of Rheumatology (ACR) 71st Annual Meeting; November 6–11, 2007; Boston, Massachusetts. [Abstract #173]
100. Yazici Y. Monitoring response to treatment in rheumatoid arthritis: which tool is best suited for routine real world care? *Bull NYU Hosp Joint Dis* 2007;65(Suppl 1):25.
101. Cohen G et al. Radiological damage in patients with rheumatoid arthritis on sustained remission. *Ann Rheum Dis* 2007;66:358.
102. Jonsson R et al. Sjogren's syndrome. In: Koopman WJ ed. *Arthritis and Allied Conditions* [*Online*], 15th ed. Baltimore, MD: Lippincott Williams & Wilkins; 2005.
103. Chatham WW, Blackburn WD Jr. Laboratory findings in rheumatoid arthritis. In: Koopman WJ ed. *Arthritis and Allied Conditions* [*Online*], 15th ed. Baltimore, MD: Lippincott Williams & Wilkins; 2005.
104. Dromgoole SH et al. Rational approaches to the use of salicylates in the treatment of rheumatoid arthritis. *Semin Arthritis Rheum* 1981;11:257.
105. Bridges SL Jr, Davidson A. Rheumatoid factor. In: Koopman WJ ed. *Arthritis and Allied Conditions* [*Online*], 15th ed. Baltimore, MD: Lippincott Williams & Wilkins; 2005.
106. Schwinghammer TL. Rheumatic diseases. In: Traub SL ed. *Basic Skills in Interpreting Laboratory Data,* 3rd ed. Bethesda, MD: American Society of Health-Systems Pharmacists; 2004:563.
107. Kavanaugh A et al. The Use of Anti-cyclic Citrullinated Peptide (anti-CCP) Antibodies in RA. ACR Hotline, available at: http://www.rheumatology.org/publications/hotline/1003anticcp.asp. Accessed December 2007.
108. Sharif S et al. Comparative study of anti-CCP and RF for the diagnosis of rheumatoid arthritis. *APLAR Journal of Rheumatology* 2007;10:121.

109. Vliet Vlieland TPM. Non-drug care for RA- Is there an evidence-based practice approaching? *Rheumatology* 2007;46:1397.
110. Shih VC, Chang RW. Rehabilitation for persons with arthritis and rheumatic disorders. In: Koopman WJ ed. *Arthritis and Allied Conditions* [*Online*], 15th ed. Baltimore, MD: Lippincott Williams & Wilkins; 2005.
111. Rogers MP et al. Psychological care of adults with rheumatoid arthritis. *Ann Intern Med* 1982;96: 344.
112. Dickens C et al. Depression in rheumatoid arthritis: a systematic review of the literature with meta-analysis. *Psychosom Med* 2002;64:52.
113. Roth SH. NSAID gastropathy: a new understanding. *Arch Intern Med* 1996;156:1623.
114. Anderson RJ et al. Unrecognized adult salicylate intoxication. *Ann Intern Med* 1976;85:745.
115. Lanza FL et al. Endoscopic evaluation of the effects of aspirin, buffered aspirin, and enteric-coated aspirin on the gastric and duodenal mucosa. *N Engl J Med* 1980;303:136.
116. Orozco-Alcala JJ, Baum J. Regular and enteric coated aspirin: a reevaluation. *Arthritis Rheum* 1979;22:1034.
117. Karahalios WJ et al. Comparative bioavailability of sustained-release and uncoated aspirin tablets. *Am J Hosp Pharm* 1981;38:1754.
118. Cassell S et al. Steady-state serum salicylate levels in hospitalized patients with rheumatoid arthritis. *Arthritis Rheum* 1979;22:384.
119. Mann CC, Boyer JT. Once-daily treatment of rheumatoid arthritis with choline magnesium trisalicylate. *Clin Ther* 1984;6:170.
120. Szczeklik A. Aspirin-induced asthma. In: Vane JR, Botting RM eds. *Aspirin and Other Salicylates.* London: Chapman & Hall Medical; 1993:548.
121. Szczeklik A, Stevenson DD. Aspirin-induced asthma: advances in pathogenesis and management. *J Allergy Clin Immunol* 1999;104:5.
122. Slepian IK et al. Aspirin-sensitive asthma. *Chest* 1985;87:386.
123. Settipane GA. Aspirin and allergic diseases: a review. *Am J Med* 1983;74:102.
124. Woessner KM et al. The safety of celecoxib in patients with aspirin-sensitive asthma. *Arthritis Rheum* 2002;46:2201.
125. Martin-Garcia C et al. Safety of a cyclooxygenase-2 inhibitor in patients with aspirin-sensitive asthma. *Chest* 2002;121:1812.
126. Goldsweig HG et al. Bleeding, salicylates, and prolonged prothrombin time: three case reports and a review of the literature. *J Rheumatol* 1976;3:37.
127. May N et al. Selective COX-2 inhibitors: a review of their therapeutic potential and safety in dentistry. *Oral Surg Oral Med Oral Pathol Oral Rediol Endod* 2001;92:399.
128. Janssen NM, Genta MS. The effects of immunosuppressive and anti-inflammatory medications on fertility, pregnancy, and lactation. *Arch Intern Med* 2000;160:610.
129. Committee on Drugs. The transfer of drugs and other chemicals into human milk (American Academy of Pediatrics). *Pediatrics* 2001;108:776.
130. Morris HG et al. Effects of salsalate (nonacetylated salicylate) and aspirin on serum prostaglandins in humans. *Ther Drug Monit* 1985;7:435.
131. Cryer B et al. Comparison of salsalate and aspirin on mucosal injury and gastroduodenal mucosal prostaglandins. *Gastroenterology* 1990;6:1616.
132. Mann J, Evans T. Gastrointestinal-related complications in a long-term care population taking NSAIDs versus COX-2 inhibitor therapy. *Consult Pharm* 2004;19:602.
133. Brooks PM, Day RO. Nonsteroidal anti-inflammatory drugs—differences and similarities. *N Engl J Med* 1991;324:1716.
134. Chou R et al. Comparative effectiveness and safety of analgesics for osteoarthritis. Comparative effectiveness review No. 4. Rockville, MD: Agency for Healthcare Research and Quality. Available at: www.effectivehealthcare.ahrq.gov/reports/final.cfm. Accessed September 2006.
135. Silverstein FE et al. Gastrointestinal toxicity with celecoxib vs. nonsteroidal anti-inflammatory drugs for osteoarthritis and rheumatoid arthritis: the CLASS study: A randomized controlled trial. Celecoxib Long-term Arthritis Safety Study. *JAMA* 2000;284:1247.
136. Sing G, Triadafilopoulus G. Epidemiology of NSAID-induced GI complications. *J Rheumatol* 1999;26:(Suppl 26):18.
137. Singh G et al. Gastrointestinal tract complications of nonsteroidal anti-inflammatory drug treatment in rheumatoid arthritis: a prospective observational cohort study. *Arch Intern Med* 1996;156:1530.
138. Ad Hoc Committee on Practice Parameters of the American College of Gastroenterology. A guideline for the treatment and prevention of NSAID-induced ulcers. *Am J Gastroenterol* 1998;93:2037.
139. Graham DY et al. Ulcer prevention in long-term users of nonsteroidal anti-inflammatory drugs. *Arch Intern Med* 2002;162:169.
140. Rostom et al. Prevention of NSAID-induced gastroduodenal ulcers. [update of Cochrane Database Syst Rev. 2000;(4):CD002296; PMID: 11034748]. *Cochrane Database of Systematic Reviews* 2002; 4:CD002296.
141. Barkin J. The relation between *Helicobacter pylori* and nonsteroidal anti-inflammatory drugs. *Am J Med* 1998;105:22S.
142. Celecoxib (Celebrex) package insert. New York: Pfizer; August 2002.
143. Rofecoxib (Vioxx) package insert. Whitehouse Station, NJ: Merck; April 2003.
144. Valdecoxib (Bextra) package insert. New York: Pfizer; October 2002.
145. Hawkey CJ. Cox-2 inhibitors. *Lancet* 1999;353: 307.
146. Juni P et al. Are selective Cox-2 inhibitors superior to traditional non steroidal anti-inflammatory drugs? *BMJ* 2002;321;1287.
147. Bombardier C et al. VIGOR Study Group. Comparison of upper gastrointestinal toxicity of rofecoxib and naproxen in patients with rheumatoid arthritis. VIGOR Study Group. *N Engl J Med* 2000;343:1520,
148. Witter J. Medical Officer Review. Available at: http://www.fda.gov/ohrms/dockets/ac/01/briefing/3677b1_03_med.pdf. Accessed June 2003.
149. FDA Talk Paper. FDA approves new indication and label changes for the arthritis drug, Vioxx. 2002, Available at: http://www.fda.gov/bbs/topics/ANSWERS/2002/ANS01145.htm. Accessed June 2003.
150. Dunn MJ et al. Nonsteroidal anti-inflammatory drugs and renal function. *J Clin Pharmacol* 1988; 28:524.
151. Patrono C, Dunn MJ. The clinical significance of inhibition of renal prostaglandin synthesis. *Kidney Int* 1987;32:1.
152. Rossat J et al. Renal effects of selective cyclooxygenase-2 inhibition in normotensive salt-depleted subjects. *Clin Pharmacol Ther* 1999; 66:76.
153. Ciabottoni G et al. Effects of sulindac and ibuprofen in patients with chronic glomerular disease. *N Engl J Med* 1984;310:279.
154. Swainson CP, Griffiths P. Acute and chronic effects of sulindac on renal function in chronic renal disease. *Clin Pharmacol Ther* 1985;37:298.
155. Berg KJ, Talseth T. Acute renal effects of sulindac and indomethacin in chronic renal failure. *Clin Pharmacol Ther* 1985;37:447.
156. Sedor JR et al. Effects of sulindac and indomethacin on renal prostaglandin synthesis. *Clin Pharmacol Ther* 1984;36:85.
157. Miller MJS et al. Renal metabolism of sulindac: functional hypothesis. *J Clin Pharmacol Exp Ther* 1984;231:449.
158. Cook ME et al. Comparative effects of nabumetone, sulindac, and ibuprofen on renal function. *J Rheumatol* 1997;24:1137.
159. FitzGerald GA, Patrono C. Drug therapy: the coxibs, selective inhibitors of cyclooxygenase-2. *N Engl J Med* 2001;345:433.
160. Hudson M et al. Differences in outcomes of patients with congestive heart failure prescribed celecoxib, rofecoxib, or non-steroidal anti-inflammatory drugs: population based study. *BMJ* 2005;330:1370.
161. Clive DM, Stoff JS. Renal syndromes associated with nonsteroidal anti-inflammatory drugs. *N Engl J Med* 1984;310:563.
162. American College of Rheumatology Ad Hoc Committee on Clinical Guidelines. Guidelines for monitoring drug therapy in rheumatoid arthritis. *Arthritis Rheum* 1996;39:723.
163. Johnson AG et al. NSAIDs and increased blood pressure: what is the clinical significance? *Drug Safety* 1997;17:277.
164. Weinblatt ME. Rheumatoid arthritis: treat now, not later. *Ann Intern Med* 1996;124:773.
165. Schattner A. Treatment considerations in early rheumatoid arthritis. *J Intern Med* 1997;241: 445.
166. Morand EF et al. Continuation of long term treatment with hydroxychloroquine in systemic lupus erythematous and rheumatoid arthritis. *Ann Rheum Dis* 1992;51:1318.
167. Bernstein HN. Ophthalmologic considerations and testing in patients receiving long-term antimalarial therapy. *Am J Med* 1983;75:25.
168. Farr M et al. Side effects profile of 200 patients with inflammatory arthritides treated with sulphasalazine. *Drugs* 1986;32:49.
169. Gottlieb NL, Brown HEJ. Acute myocardial infarction following gold sodium thiomalate induced vasomotor (nitritoid) reaction. *Arthritis Rheum* 1977;20:1026.
170. Halla JT et al. Postinjection nonvasomotor reactions during chrysotherapy: constitutional and rheumatic symptoms following injection of gold salts. *Arthritis Rheum* 1977;20:1188.
171. Lawrence JS. Comparative toxicity of gold preparations in treatment of rheumatoid arthritis. *Ann Rheum Dis* 1976;35:171.
172. Chatham WW. Traditional disease-modifying antirheumatic drugs: gold compounds d-penicillamine sulfasalazine and antimalarials. In: Koopman WJ ed. *Arthritis and Allied Conditions* [*Online*], 15th ed. Baltimore, MD: Lippincott Williams & Wilkins; 2005.
173. Edelman J et al. Prevalence of eosinophilia during gold therapy for rheumatoid arthritis. *J Rheumatol* 1983;10:121.
174. Podell TE et al. Pulmonary toxicity with gold therapy. *Arthritis Rheum* 1980;23:347.
175. Smith W, Ball GV. Lung injury due to gold treatment. *Arthritis Rheum* 1980;23:351.
176. Stein HB, Urowitz MB. Gold-induced enterocolitis: case report and literature review. *J Rheumatol* 1976;3:21.
177. Favreau M et al. Hepatic toxicity associated with gold therapy. *Ann Intern Med* 1977;87:717.
178. Gottlieb NL, Major JC. Ocular chrysiasis correlated with gold concentrations in the crystalline lens during chrysotherapy. *Arthritis Rheum* 1978;21: 704.
179. Gottlieb NL. Comparative pharmacokinetics of parenteral and oral gold compounds. *J Rheumatol* 1982;9(Suppl 8):99.
180. Ward JR et al. Comparison of auranofin, gold sodium thiomalate and placebo in the treatment of active rheumatoid arthritis: response by treatment duration. In: Capell HA et al eds. *Auranofin: Proceedings of a Smith Kline & French International Symposium.* Amsterdam: Excerpta Medica; 1982:115.
181. Morris RW et al. Worldwide clinical experience with auranofin. *Clin Rheumatol* 1984;3(Suppl 1):105.
182. Gottlieb NL. Serum gold levels. *Arthritis Rheum* 1975;18:626.
183. Dahl SL et al. Lack of correlation between gold concentrations and clinical response in patients with definite or classical rheumatoid arthritis receiving auranofin or gold sodium thiomalate. *Arthritis Rheum* 1985;28:1211.

184. Klinefelter HF. Reinstitution of gold therapy in rheumatoid arthritis after mucocutaneous reactions. *J Rheumatol* 1975;2:21.
185. Hull RG et al. A double-blind study comparing sodium aurothiomalate and auranofin in patients with rheumatoid arthritis previously stabilized on sodium aurothiomalate. *Int J Clin Pharmacol Res* 1984;4:395.
186. Wenger ME et al. Therapy of rheumatoid arthritis. Transferring treatment from injectable gold to auranofin. In: Capell HA et al eds. *Auranofin: Proceedings of a Smith Kline & French International Symposium.* Amsterdam: Excerpta Medica; 1982:201.
187. Tosi S et al. Injectable gold dermatitis and proteinuria: retreatment with auranofin. *Int J Clin Pharmacol Res* 1985;5:265.
188. Dahl MG et al. Methotrexate hepatotoxicity in psoriasis comparison of different dose regimens. *Br Med J* 1972;1:654.
189. Williams HJ et al. Comparison of low-dose oral pulse methotrexate and placebo in the treatment of rheumatoid arthritis. *Arthritis Rheum* 1985;28:721.
190. Kremer HM. Rational use of new and existing disease-modifying agents in rheumatoid arthritis. *Ann Intern Med* 2001;134:695.
191. Braun, et al. Comparison of the clinical efficacy and safety of subcutaneous versus oral administration of methotrexate in patients with active rheumatoid arthritis. *Arthritis Rheum* 2008;58:73.
192. Magdalena L et al. Comparison of two dosing schedules for administering oral low-dose methotrexate (weekly versus every-other-week) in patients with rheumatoid arthritis. *Arthritis Rheum* 1999;42:2160.
193. Health and Public Policy Committee AC of P. Methotrexate in rheumatoid arthritis. *Ann Intern Med* 1987;107:418.
194. Tobias H, Auerbach R. Hepatotoxicity of long-term methotrexate therapy for psoriasis. *Arch Intern Med* 1973;132:391.
195. Zachariae H et al. Methotrexate induced liver cirrhosis: studies including serial liver biopsies during continued treatment. *Br J Dermatol* 1980;102:407.
196. Kremer JM. Liver biopsies in patients with rheumatoid arthritis receiving methotrexate: where are we going? *J Rheumatol* 1992;19:189.
197. Tishler M et al. The effects of leucovorin (folinic acid) on methotrexate therapy in rheumatoid arthritis. *J Rheumatol* 1988;31:906.
198. Buckley LM et al. Administration of folinic acid after low dose methotrexate in patients with RA. *J Rheumatol* 1990;17:1158.
199. Shiroky JB et al. Low dose methotrexate with leucovorin (folinic acid) rescue in the management of rheumatoid arthritis. Results of a multicenter randomized, double-blind, placebo-controlled trial. *Arthritis Rheum* 1993;36:795.
200. Weinblatt ME et al. Low dose leucovorin does not interfere with the efficacy of methotrexate in rheumatoid arthritis: an 8 week randomized placebo controlled trial. *J Rheumatol* 1993;20:950.
201. Morgan SL et al. The effect of folic acid supplementation on the toxicity of low-dose methotrexate in patients with rheumatoid arthritis. *Arthritis Rheum* 1990;33:9.
202. Stewart KA et al. Folate supplementation in methotrexate-treated rheumatoid arthritis patients. *Semin Arthritis Rheum* 1991;20:332.
203. van Ede AE et al. Effect of folic or folinic acid supplementation on the toxicity and efficacy of methotrexate in rheumatoid arthritis: a fort-eight-week, multicenter, randomized, double-blind, placebo-controlled study. *Arthritis Rheum* 2001;44:1515.
204. Hoekstra M et al. Factors associated with toxicity, final dose, and efficacy of methotrexate in patients with rheumatoid arthritis. *Ann Rheum Dis* 2003;62:423.
205. Carson CW et al. Pulmonary disease during the treatment of rheumatoid arthritis with low dose pulse methotrexate. *Semin Arthritis Rheum* 1987;16:186.
206. Nesher G et al. Effect of caffeine consumption on efficacy of methotrexate in rheumatoid arthritis. *Arthritis Rheum* 2003;48:571.
207. Furst D et al. Onset of effect and duration of response to leflunomide treatment of active rheumatoid arthritis compared to placebo or methotrexate. *Arthritis Rheum* 1998;41:S155.
208. Weaver A et al. Treatment of active rheumatoid arthritis with leflunomide compared to placebo or methotrexate. *Arthritis Rheum* 1998;41:S131.
209. Scott DL et al. Treatment of active rheumatoid arthritis with leflunomide: two year follow-up of a double blind, placebo controlled trial versus sulfasalazine. *Ann Rheum Dis* 2001;60:913.
210. Sharp JT et al. Treatment with leflunomide slows radiographic progression of rheumatoid arthritis. *Arthritis Rheum* 2000;43:495.
211. Osiri M et al. Leflunomide for the treatment of rheumatoid arthritis: a systematic review and meta-analysis. *J Rheumatol* 2003;30:1182.
212. Barbehenn E et al. Petition to the FDA to ban the rheumatoid arthritis drug leflunomide (ARAVA) (HRG publication #1614) Public Citizen. March 28, 2002. http://www.citizen.org/documents/1614.pdf". Accessed June 2003.
213. Geborek P et al. Etanercept, infliximab, and leflunomide in established rheumatoid arthritis: clinical experience using a structured follow up programme in southern Sweden. *Ann Rheum Dis* 2002;61:793.
214. Leflunomide (Arava) package insert. Bridgewater, NJ: Sanofi-Aventis Pharmaceuticals; 2007.
215. Assem ESK, Vickers MR. Immunological response to penicillamine in penicillin-allergic patients and in normal subjects. *Postgrad Med J* 1974;50(Suppl 2):65.
216. Bell C, Graziano F. The safety of administration of penicillamine to penicillin-sensitive individuals. *Arthritis Rheum* 1983;26:801.
217. O'Dell J et al. Treatment of rheumatoid arthritis with methotrexate alone, sulfasalazine and hydroxychloroquine, or a combination of all three medications. *N Engl J Med* 1996;1287.
218. Mottonen T et al. Comparison of combination therapy with single-drug therapy in early rheumatoid arthritis: a randomised trial. *Lancet* 1999;353:1568.
219. O'Dell, et al. Combination DMAARD therapy with methotrexate-sulfasalazine-hydroxychloroquine in rheumatoid arthritis: continued efficacy with minimal toxicity at 5 years. *Arthritis Rheum* 1998;41:S132.
220. Kremer JM et al. Concomitant leflunomide therapy in patients with active rheumatoid arthritis despite stable doses of methotrexate. *Ann Intern Med* 2002;137:726.
221. Fries JF. Reevaluating the therapeutic approach to rheumatoid arthritis: the "sawtooth" strategy. *J Rheumatol* 1990;17(Suppl 22):12.
222. Wilske KR, Healey LA. Challenging the therapeutic pyramid: a new look at treatment strategies for rheumatoid arthritis. *J Rheumatol* 1990;17(Suppl 25):4.
223. Wilke WS, Clough JD. Therapy for rheumatoid arthritis: combinations of disease-modifying drugs and new paradigms of treatment. *Semin Arthritis Rheum* 1991;21(Suppl 1):21.
224. Sooka T, Hannonen P. Utility of disease modifying antirheumatic drugs in "sawtooth" strategy. A prospective study of early rheumatoid arthritis patients up to 15 years. *Ann Rheum Dis* 1999;58:61.
225. Moreland, et al. Etanercept therapy in rheumatoid arthritis: a randomized, controlled trial. *Ann Intern Med* 1999;130:478.
226. Weinblatt M et al. A trial of etanercept, a recombinant tumor necrosis factor receptor: Fc fusion protein, in patients with rheumatoid arthritis receiving methotrexate. *N Engl J Med* 1999;253.
227. Bathon JM et al. A comparison of etanercept and methotrexate in patients with early rheumatoid arthritis. *N Engl J Med* 2000;343:1586.
228. Koike, et al. Safety outcomes from a large Japanese post-marketing surveillance for etanercept. Program and abstracts of the American College of Rheumatology 2007 Annual Scientific Meeting; November 6–11, 2007; Boston, Massachusetts. Abstract #344.
229. Van der Heijde D et al. Efficacy of etanercept in early versus long-term rheumatoid arthritis: posthoc analysis of 3-year TEMPO data. Program and abstracts of the American College of Rheumatology 2007 Annual Scientific Meeting; November 6–11, 2007; Boston, Massachusetts. Abstract #265.
230. Aletaha D et al. Disease activity early in the course of treatment predicts response to therapy after one year in rheumatoid arthritis patients. *Arthritis Rheum* 2007;56:3226.
231. Ault A. Rheumatoid arthritis drug linked to infections. *Lancet* 1999;353:1770.
232. Ravinder MN et al. Therapeutic efficacy of multiple intravenous infusions of anti-tumor necrosis factor (alpha) monoclonal antibody combined with low-dose weekly methotrexate in rheumatoid arthritis. *Arthritis Rheum* 1998;41:1552.
233. Lipsky P et al. Long-term control of signs and symptoms of rheumatoid arthritis with chimeric monoclonal anti-TNF (alpha) antibody (infliximab) in patients with active disease on methotrexate. *Arthritis Rheum* 1998;41:S364.
234. St Clair EW. Infliximab treatment for rheumatic disease: clinical and radiological efficacy. *Ann Rheum Dis* 2002;61(Suppl iii):ii67.
235. Humira (adalimumab) package insert. North Chicago, IL: Abbott Laboratories; January 2003.
236. van de Putte LB et al. Efficacy and safety of adalimumab (D2E7), the first fully human anti-TNF monoclonal antibody, in patients with rheumatoid arthritis who failed previous DMARD therapy: 6-month results from a phase 3 study. Program #467. Abstract presented at: The European Congress of Rheumatology; June 12–15, 3003; Stockholm, Sweden.
237. Weinblatt ME et al. Adalimumab, a fully human anti-tumor necrosis factor-alpha monoclonal antibody, for the treatment of rheumatoid arthritis in patients taking concomitant methotrexate: the ARMADA Trial. *Arthritis Rheum* 2003;48:35.
238. Abramowicz M ed. Adalimumab (Humira) for rheumatoid arthritis. *Met Lett* 2003;45:25.
239. Weinblatt ME et al. Change over time in the safety, efficacy, and remission profiles of patients with rheumatoid arthritis receiving adalimumab for up to 7 years. Program and abstracts of the American College of Rheumatology 2007 Annual Scientific Meeting; November 6–11, 2007; Boston, Massachusetts. Abstract 294.
240. Sidiropoulos P et al. Comparable response rates between first and second anti-TNF alpha therapies in rheumatoid arthritis patients under treatment with anti-TNF agents. Program and abstracts of the American College of Rheumatology 2007 Annual Scientific Meeting; November 6–11, 2007; Boston, Massachusetts. Abstract 295.
241. Blom M et al. Effectiveness of switch to a second anti-TNFalpha in primary nonresponders, secondary nonresponders and failure due to adverse events. Program and abstracts of the American College of Rheumatology 2007 Annual Scientific Meeting; November 6–11, 2007; Boston, Massachusetts. Abstract 299.
242. Burmester G et al. Effectiveness and safety of adalimumab (HUMIRA) after failure of etanercept or infliximab treatment in patients with rheumatoid arthritis, psoriatic arthritis, or ankylosing spondylitis. Program and abstracts of the American College of Rheumatology 2007 Annual Scientific Meeting; November 6–11, 2007; Boston, Massachusetts. Abstract 945.
243. Hyrich KL et al. Effect of switching to a second anti-TNF therapy on haq response in rheumatoid arthritis patients with lack of response to their first anti-TNF therapy: results from the BSR biologics register (BSRBR). Program and abstracts of EULAR 2007; June 13–16, 2007; Barcelona, Spain. Abstract THU0157.
244. Abramowicz M ed. Anakinra (Kineret) for rheumatoid arthritis. *Med Lett* 2002;44:18.

245. Bresnihan B. Effects of anakinra on clinical and radiological outcomes in rheumatoid arthritis. *Ann Rheum Dis* 2002;61(Suppl ii):ii74.
246. Bresnihan B et al. Treatment of rheumatoid arthritis with recombinant human IL-1 receptor antagonist. *Arthritis Rheum* 1998;41:2196.
247. Cohen S et al. Treatment of rheumatoid arthritis with anakinra, a recombinant human interleukin-1 receptor antagonist, in combination with methotrexate: results of a twenty-four-week, multicenter, randomized, double-blind, placebo-controlled trial. *Arthritis Rheum* 2002;46:574.
248. Anakinra (Kineret) package insert. Thousand Oaks, CA: Amgen; 2006.
249. Kremer, et al. Effects of abatacept in patients with methotrexate-resistant active rheumatoid arthritis. *Ann Intern Med* 2006;144:865876.
250. Genovese M et al. Abatacept (CTLA4Ig) in patients with rheumatoid arthritis and an inadequate response to tumor necrosis factor-a inhibitors. *N Engl J Med* 2005;353:1114.
251. Edwards JC et al. Efficacy of B-cell-targeted therapy with rituximab in patients with rheumatoid arthritis. *N Engl J Med* 2004;350:2572.
252. Emery P et al. The efficacy and safety of rituximab in patients with active rheumatoid arthritis despite methotrexate treatment: results a phase IIB randomized, double-blind, placebo-controlled, dose-ranging trial. *Arthritis Rheum* 2006;54:1390.
253. Cohen SB et al. Rituximab for rheumatoid arthritis refractory to anti-tumor necrosis factor therapy: Results of a multicenter, randomized, double-blind, placebo-controlled, phase III trial evaluating primary efficacy and safety at twenty-four weeks. *Arthritis Rheum* 2006;54:2793.
254. Cohen S et al. Consistent Inhibition of Structural Damage Progression by Rituximab in Medically Important Subgroups of Patients with an Inadequate Response to TNF Inhibitors: Week 56 REFLEX Results. Program and abstracts of the American College of Rheumatology 2007 Annual Scientific Meeting; November 6–11, 2007; Boston, Massachusetts. Abstract 267.
255. Panoulas VF et al. Long-term exposure to medium-dose glucocorticoid therapy associates with hypertension in patients with rheumatoid arthritis. *Rheumatology* 2008;47:72.
256. Wei L et al. Taking glucocorticoids by prescription is associated with subsequent cardiovascular disease. *Ann Intern Med* 2004;141:764.
257. Myles AB et al. Single daily dose of corticosteroid treatment. *Ann Rheum Dis* 1976;35:73.
258. Tassiulas I et al. Corticosteroids. In: Koopman WJ ed. *Arthritis and Allied Conditions* [*Online*], 15th ed. Baltimore, MD: Lippincott Williams & Wilkins; 2005.
259. American College of Rheumatology Task Force on Osteoporosis Guidelines. Recommendations for the prevention and treatment of glucocorticoid-induced osteoporosis: 2001 update. *Arthritis Rheum* 2001;441496.
260. Wasnich RD et al. Thiazide effect on mineral content of bone. *N Engl J Med* 1983;309:344.
261. Warren RW et al. Juvenile idiopathic arthritis (juvenile rheumatoid arthritis). In: Koopman WJ ed. *Arthritis and Allied Conditions*[*Online*], 15th ed. Baltimore, MD: Lippincott Williams & Wilkins; 2005.
262. Helmick CG et al. Estimates of the prevalence of arthritis and other rheumatic conditions in the United States, Part I. *Arthritis Rheum* 2008;58:15.
263. Goldmuntz EA, White PH. Juvenile idiopathic arthritis: a review for the pediatrician. *Pedatr Rev* 2006; 27:e24.
264. Sharma S, Sherry DD. Joint distribution at presentation in children with pauciarticular arthritis. *J Pediatr* 1999;134:642.
265. Fantini F et al. Remission in juvenile chronic arthritis: a cohort study of 683 consecutive cases with a mean 10 year followup. *J Rheumatol* 2003;30:579.
266. Levinson JE et al. Comparison of tolmetin sodium and aspirin in the treatment of juvenile rheumatoid arthritis. *J Pediatr* 1977;91:799.
267. Mortimer EA et al. Varicella with hypoglycemia possibly due to salicylates. *Am J Dis Child* 1962; 103:583.
268. Starko KM et al. Reye's syndrome and salicylate use. *Pediatrics* 1980;66:859.
269. Waldman RJ et al. Aspirin as a risk factor in Reye's syndrome. *JAMA* 1982;247:3089.
270. Halpin TJ et al. Reye's syndrome and medication use. *JAMA* 1982;248:687.
271. Committee on Infectious Diseases AA of P. Aspirin and Reye syndrome. *Pediatrics* 1982;69:810.
272. Rennebohm RM et al. Reye syndrome in children receiving salicylate therapy for connective tissue disease. *J Pediatr* 1985;107:877.
273. Hashkes PJ, Laxer RM. Medical treatment of juvenile idiopathic arthritis. *JAMA* 2005;294:1671.
274. Ravelli A et al. Radiologic progression in patients with juvenile chronic arthritis treated with methotrexate. *J Pediatr* 1998;133:262.
275. Wallace CA. The use of methotrexate in childhood rheumatic diseases. *Arthritis Rheum* 1998;41:381.
276. Cassidy JT. Outcomes research in the therapeutic use of methotrexate in children with chronic peripheral arthritis. *J Pediatr* 1998;133:179.
277. Gottlieb BS et al. Discontinuation of methotrexate treatment in juvenile rheumatoid arthritis. *Pediatrics* 1997;100:994.
278. Van Rossum MAJ et al. Salazine in the treatment of juvenile chronic arthritis: a randomized, double-blind, placebo-controlled, multicenter study. *Arthritis Rheum* 1998;41:808.
279. Lovell DJ et al. Long-term safety and efficacy of etanercept in children with polyarticular-course juvenile rheumatoid arthritis. *Arthritis Rheum* 2006;54:1987.
280. Giannini EH et al. Efficacy of abatacept in different sub-populations of juvenile idiopathic arthritis (JIA): results of a randomized withdrawal study. Program and abstracts of the American College of Rheumatology 2007 Annual Scientific Meeting; November 6–11, 2007; Boston, Massachusetts. Abstract 679.
281. Lovell DJ et al. Abatacept treatment of juvenile idiopathic arthritis (JIA): safety report. Program and abstracts of the American College of Rheumatology 2007 Annual Scientific Meeting; November 6–11, 2007; Boston, Massachusetts Abstract 680.
282. Lovell DJ et al. Adalimumab is safe and effective during long-term treatment of patients with juvenile rheumatoid arthritis: results from a 2-year study. Program and abstracts of the American College of Rheumatology 2007 Annual Scientific Meeting; November 6–11, 2007; Boston, Massachusetts. Abstract 681.
283. Padeh S, Passwell JH. Intra-articular corticosteroid injection in the management of children with chronic arthritis. *Arthritis Rheum* 1998;41:1210.
284. Cassidy J et al. Ophthalmologic examinations in children with juvenile rheumatoid arthritis. *Pediatrics* 2006;117:1843.
285. Weiss AH et al. Methotrexate for resistant chronic uveitis in children with juvenile rheumatoid arthritis. *J Pediatr* 1998;133:266.
286. Lawrence RC et al. Estimates of the prevalence of arthritis and other rheumatic conditions in the united states. *Arthritis Rheum* 2008;58:26.
287. Hooper MM et al. Clinical and laboratory findings in osteoarthritis. In: Koopman WJ ed. *Arthritis and Allied Conditions* [*Online*], 15th ed. Baltimore, MD: Lippincott Williams & Wilkins; 2005.
288. Slemenda C et al. Quadriceps weakness and osteoarthritis of the knee. *Ann Intern Med* 1997;127:97.
289. Holderbaum D et al. Genetics and osteoarthritis: exposing the iceberg. *Arthritis Rheum* 1999;43:397.
290. Freidich MJ. Steps toward understanding, alleviating osteoarthritis will help aging population. *JAMA* 1999;11:1023.
291. Recommendations for the medical management of osteoarthritis of the hip and knee: 2000 update. American College of Rheumatology Subcommittee on Osteoarthritis Guidelines. *Arthritis Rheum* 2000;43:1905.
292. Bradley JD et al. Comparison of an anti-inflammatory dose of ibuprofen, an analgesic dose of ibuprofen, and acetaminophen in the treatment of patients with osteoarthritis of the knee. *N Engl J Med* 1991;325:87.
293. Williams HJ et al. Comparison of naproxen and acetaminophen in a two-year study of treatment of osteoarthritis of the knee. *Arthritis Rheum* 1993;36:1196.
294. Schnitzer TJ. Update of ACR guidelines for osteoarthritis: role of the coxibs [discussion S31]. *J Pain Sympt Manage* 2002;23:S24.
295. Seideman P et al. Naproxen and paracetamol compared with naproxen only in coxarthrosis: increased effect of the combination in 18 patients. *Acta Orthop Scand* 1993;64:285.
296. Schumacher HR et al. Effect of a nonsteroidal anti-inflammatory drug on synovial fluid in osteoarthritis. *J Rheumatol* 1996;23:1774.
297. Page J, Henry D. Consumption of NSAIDs and the development of congestive heart failure in elderly patients: an underrecognized public health problem. *Arch Intern Med* 2000;160:777.
298. Brater DC. Renal effects of cyclooxygyenase-2-selective inhibitors. *J Pain Sympt Manage* 2002;23:S15.
299. Brinker A et al. Abuse, dependence, or withdrawal associated with tramadol. *Am J Psychiatry* 2002;159:881.
300. Adverse Event Reporting System. Freedom of Information Report. Rockville, MD: Office of Drug Safety, U.S. Food and Drug Administration: Search November 1997 to September 2004.
301. Behrens F et al. Metabolic recovery of articular cartilage after intra-articular injections of glucocorticoids. *J Bone Joint Surg* 1976;58:1157.
302. Gray RC et al. Corticosteroid treatment in rheumatic disorders. *Semin Arthritis Rheum* 1981; 10:231.
303. Abramowicz M. Intra-Articular Injections for osteoarthritis of the Knee. *Med Lett Drug Ther* 2006; 48:25.
304. Gray RG et al. Local corticosteroid injection treatment in rheumatic disorders. *Semin Arthritis Rheum* 1981;10:231.
305. Creamer P. Intra-articular corticosteroid injections in osteoarthritis: do they work and if so, how? *Ann Rheum Dis* 1997;56:634.
306. Abramowicz M. Intra-articular injections for osteoarthritis of the knee. *Med Lett* 2006;1231: 25.
307. Altman RD. Status of hyaluronan supplementation therapy in osteoarthritis. *Curr Rheumatol Rep* 2003;5:7.
308. Arrich J et al. Intra-articular hyaluronic acid for the treatment of osteoarthritis of the knee: systematic review and meta-analysis. *CMAJ* 2005;172:1039.
309. Altman RD, Moskowitz R. Intraarticular sodium hyaluronate (Hyalgan) in the treatment of patients with osteoarthritis of the knee: a randomized clinical trial. *Hyalgan Study Group J Rheumatol* 1998;25:2203.
310. Altman RD. Intra-articular sodium hyaluronate in osteoarthritis of the knee. *Semin Arthritis Rheum* 2000;30:11.
311. Kelly GS. The role of glucosamine sulfate and chondroitin sulfates in the treatment of degenerative joint disease. *Alt Med Rev* 1998;3:27.
312. da Camara CC, Dowless GV. Glucosamine sulfate for osteoarthritis. *Ann Pharmacother* 1998;32:580.
313. Clegg DO et al. Glucosamine, Chondroitin Sulfate, and the Two in Combination for Painful Knee Osteoarthritis. *N Engl J Med* 2006;354:795.
314. Smolen JS, Steiner G. Therapeutic strategies for rheumatoid arthritis. *Nat Rev Drug Discovery* 2003:2.

CHAPTER 44

Connective Tissue Disorders: The Clinical Use of Corticosteroids

William C. Gong

Despite new knowledge in the immunology and the pathogenesis of the different connective tissue diseases (CTDs), their etiology and classification remains elusive.[1] Different textbooks approach the connective tissues disease in varied fashions. Some textbooks group systemic lupus erythematosus (SLE), progressive systemic sclerosis, inflammatory muscle disease, Sjögren's syndrome, and the systemic vasculitides together loosely. Other textbooks put them in separate sections.[2] The diagnosis of the different CTDs is a matter of clinical judgment as patients present with constellations of symptoms, physical findings, and laboratory features that permit their recognition. Patients may present with findings consistent with more than one CTD. There is also overlap CTD representing the presence of two defined CTDs. Examples of this include SLE/RA or what is known as lupus and myositis/scleroderma resulting in sclerodermatomyositis or scleromyositis. Complicating matters, there is also the mixed connective tissue disease (MCTD), which includes examples, such as myositis/scleroderma/RA/SLE first described in 1972.[1]

Sustained inflammation is the hallmark of CTDs. The inflammatory effector mechanisms can engage mast cells, platelets, neutrophils, endothelial cells, mononuclear phagocytes, and lymphocytes as well as trigger the complement, kinin, and coagulation cascades. The diversity of the potential mechanisms activated during inflammation can lead to a broad spectrum of clinical manifestations. Environmental factors can also serve as stimuli to the particular mechanism activated. For example, biologic agents such as group A β-hemolytic streptococci can lead to rheumatic fever or *Borrelia burgdorferi* leading to Lyme disease, drugs such as hydralazine and procainamide can lead to drug-induced lupus, and vinyl chloride can lead to progressive systemic sclerosis.[2]

GENERAL SIGNS AND SYMPTOMS

Many patients can have arthralgias and arthritis as part of the inflammatory disease associated with their CTD, such as those patients with SLE. Inflammatory disease is suggested by morning stiffness of >1 hour (a similar problem occurs with sitting or resting), swelling, fever, weakness, and systemic fatigue. In some patients, activities of daily living and function may be excellent despite pain and deformity; in others, because of psychologic and systemic disease, there may be poor function with minimum articular involvement. Other psychosocial aspects of their life, including sexuality, may be affected by many of the inflammatory disorders.

Dermatologic changes are often associated with a particular rheumatic disease. Examples include alopecia with SLE, onycholysis, and keratoderma blenorrhagica with Reiter's syndrome, buccal or genital ulcers with SLE or Reiter's syndrome, Raynaud's phenomenon with SLE or systemic sclerosis, calcinosis and rash over the knuckles (Gottron's papule) with dermatomyositis, and sun sensitivity malar rash with SLE. The presence of nodules, tophi, telangiectasia, or vasculitic changes also may be detected, helping the clinician differentiate which inflammatory disease is present and what management is necessary.

The CTDs are commonly associated with musculoskeletal changes. Joints may display warmth, redness and effusion, synovial thickening, deformities, decreased range of motion, pain on motion, tenderness on palpation, and decreased function. Often, a patient's hand and arm function, as well as gait, may be altered. In addition to the signs and symptoms used to differentiate various rheumatic diseases, laboratory evaluation of patients with rheumatic complaints can often define the extent of disease or detect other organ systems that may be involved.

NONPHARMACOLOGIC AND PHARMACOLOGIC TREATMENT

The aim of present therapy is to provide pain relief, decrease joint inflammation, and more importantly, maintain or restore joint function and prevent bone and cartilage destruction. The current approach to treatment is to interrupt the complex inflammatory process. The general treatment program consists of patient education, balance between rest and exercise, physical and occupational therapy, adequate nutrition, local heat, use of supportive or rehabilitative devices, and orthopedic surgery. Depending on the disorder being treated, various drugs may be used, including the salicylate class of drugs, nonsteroidal anti-inflammatory drugs (NSAIDs), disease-modifying antirheumatic drugs (DMARDs), and corticosteroids. All drugs other than corticosteroids have been reviewed extensively in other chapters.

These agents and especially the corticosteroids used in the treatment of CTDs and systemic rheumatic disorders may have systemic toxicity as well. A good understanding of corticosteroids and their effects can help the clinician monitor the patient appropriately and order laboratory studies, such as renal or liver function tests, complete blood counts (CBCs), muscle enzyme levels, or urinalysis. More sophisticated tests may be necessary to differentiate hypothalamic-pituitary-adrenal (HPA) axis abnormalities from effects of chronic corticosteroid therapy.[3] Functional evaluation and health status outcome measurements are ultimately the most important measurement tools in evaluating treatment. Psychologic function typically is assessed in terms of affective domains, such as depression and anxiety, whereas social function usually is measured in terms of social interactions and social support.

SELECTED CONNECTIVE TISSUE DISEASES

CTDs and rheumatic diseases encompass a wide range of disorders that are inflammatory in nature and related to the immune system. The following are some of the conditions that are encountered in clinical practice, which necessitates the use of corticosteroids as part of their therapy.

LUPUS ERYTHEMATOSUS: SYSTEMIC AND DISCOID

SLE is the most diverse of the autoimmune diseases as it is a multisystem CTD caused by several autoantibodies and immune complexes.[4] Disease manifestations depend on the tissues targeted and often have musculoskeletal involvement. It generally involves one organ system at the onset, but can affect other organ systems subsequently displaying a broad range of clinical manifestations.[5] SLE is a dynamic disease in a sense that many patients have fluctuations or flare-ups that necessitate the use of steroids and other potent immunosuppressive agents. Discoid lupus erythematosus is a form of lupus erythematosus in which cutaneous lesions appear on the face and elsewhere. These are atrophic plaques with erythema, hyperkeratosis, follicular plugging, and telangiectasia. These are chronic cutaneous lesions and have few if any systemic manifestations. The lesions are usually sharply demarcated and can be round; therefore, the term *discoid* (or disclike) is used.[6]

Epidemiology

SLE generally affects women of childbearing age; this population accounts for >90% of all cases. However, SLE can affect people of all ages and gender, including children, men, and the elderly. SLE can begin at any age but occurs most frequently in women between16 and 45 years of age. It is more common in African Americans than in whites, and the mean age for diagnosis of African American females is younger than that of white females. Its prevalence ranges from 17 to 50 per 100,000 in American European white females as compared with 60 to 280 per 100,000 in African American females.[4,7] Asian and Hispanic patients are also susceptible with the prevalence in Chinese patients being similar to that seen in whites. There are currently no published data on the incidence in Hispanic Americans.[7,8] Genetic epidemiology of SLE has generated strong evidence of hereditary predisposition to this disorder.[7]

Clinical Presentation

SLE is the prototype autoimmune disease as it can affect almost any organ system, and most patients have multiorgan involvement. Clinical signs of SLE are presented in Table 44-1.[9]

Table 44-1 Signs of SLE

Organ System	*Sign*
Cutaneous	Malar rash, discoid rash, mouth/nasal sores, Raynaud phenomenon, cutaneous vasculitis, alopecia
Musculoskeletal	Polyarthritis, especially of the small joints of hands and wrists, myositis
Renal	Proteinuria, hematuria, red blood cell casts, nephrotic syndrome, elevated creatinine
Cardiopulmonary	Pericarditis, pleurisy, pleural effusions, pneumonitis, pulmonary emboli, pulmonary hypertension, myocardial infarction
Hematologic	Anemia, leucopenia, thrombocytopenia, elevated sedimentation rate, lupus anticoagulant, anticardiolipin
Neurologic	Seizure, psychosis, stroke, encephalopathy, transverse myelitis, mononeuritis multiplex, peripheral neuropathy
Gastrointestinal	Esophageal dysmotility, intestinal vasculitis, protein-losing enteropathy
Constitutional	Fever, weight loss, lymphadenopathy

The most common organ systems affected include cutaneous, musculoskeletal, and renal systems. The most common sign of SLE is cutaneous involvement occurring in about 90% of the patients. Rashes are photosensitive in about 70% of the patients, and maculopapular rashes are usually indicative of disease flare-ups. The malar rash or butterfly rash is reported in 20% to 60% of the SLE patients. The rash is often precipitated by exposure to sunlight.[10] Discoid lesions occur primarily in the face, but also occur in the ears and on forearms. Most patients with SLE experience fatigue and suffer from some form of arthralgias and myalgias, which mimic rheumatoid arthritis with symmetrical involvements of the joints. However, unlike rheumatoid arthritis, the affected joints of lupus arthritis are rarely erosive. Renal involvement, occurring in about 50% of the whites and 75% of the African Americans with SLE, is manifested by proteinuria, hematuria, and red blood cell casts. The more severe cases of renal involvement can lead to renal failure if not controlled early. Hematologic manifestations of lupus are frequent and can be life-threatening. Anemia generally is consistent with anemia of chronic disease and iron-deficiency anemia. Leukopenia is common, but rarely severe (i.e., <2,000 cells/mm^3). Mild chronic thrombocytopenia is common, but can be sudden and life-threatening. Lupus patients can also present with neurologic and gastrointestinal signs as presented in Table 44-1. Vague constitutional signs of SLE (e.g., fatigue, malaise, fever, anorexia, nausea, weight loss) occur in 95% of patients during the course of their disease. Because of its multisystem organ involvement, the diagnosis of SLE may be difficult. The American College of Rheumatology has published criteria for the classification of patients having SLE. The Diagnostic and Therapeutic Criteria originally published in 1982 and updated in 1997 lists 11 characteristic signs, symptoms, and laboratory values most often associated with a positive diagnosis of SLE (Table 44-2). The presence of four or more of these criteria, either serially or simultaneously, during any period of observation, confers >97% sensitivity and 98% specificity for the diagnosis of lupus.[11–13]

Prognosis

Although disability of varying degrees is common in patients with SLE, most will live nearly normal lives. Survival rates are 90% to 95% at 2 years, 82% to 90% at 5 years, 71% to 80% at 10 years, and 63% to 75% at 20 years.[5] The prognosis is poor in patients with high serum creatinine levels (>1.4 mg/dL), hypertension, nephrotic syndrome, anemia, hypoalbuminemia, and hypocomplementemia at the time of diagnosis. Another 50% of the patients who go into remission remain in remission for decades. The leading causes of death are generally from complications of renal failure or infections.[5]

Treatment

Because there is no cure for SLE, therapy generally involves (a) controlling the acute symptoms of SLE and (b) providing maintenance therapy to prevent exacerbations and to keep clinical manifestations of SLE at acceptable levels. Approximately 25% of patients with SLE have mild symptoms without any life-threatening situations. These patients are normally treated for their symptoms of arthritis, arthralgias, myalgias, fever, and mild serositis with NSAIDs and salicylates. More potent agents and immunosuppressives are used for more active disease. Corticosteroids are used for the more severe life-threatening and severely disabling manifestations unresponsive to immunosuppressive agents.[5]

DRUG-INDUCED LUPUS

The first case of drug-induced lupus was reported in 1945 in a patient receiving sulfadiazine.[14] Since then, approximately 75 drugs have been identified that induce a lupus-like syndrome or exacerbate pre-existing SLE. Classes of drugs that have been linked to the lupus-like syndrome include antihypertensives, antimicrobials, anti-inflammatory agents, anticonvulsants, immunosuppressive agents, recombinant cytokines, psychotropic agents, and antithyroid and hormonal drugs. Drug-induced LE occurs in at least two forms. One is characterized by serositis and the finding of a positive antihistone antibody. This form has been associated with procainamide, hydralazine, minocycline, and isoniazid. The second form involves positive anti-Ro (SS-A) antibody findings[15] and is most prominently linked to hydrochlorothiazide and calcium channel blockers.[16] The most common drugs causing drug-induced LE are procainamide and hydralazine followed by chlorpromazine, isoniazid,

Table 44-2 1997 Revised Criteria for Classification of SLE

Criteria	*Explanation*[a]
Malar rash	Fixed erythema, flat or raised
Discoid rash	Erythematosus raised patches with adherent keratotic scaling and follicular plugging; atrophic scarring may occur in older lesions
Photosensitivity	Skin rash resulting from an unusual reaction to sunlight by patient history or observed by physician
Oral ulcers	Painless oral or nasopharyngeal ulcers observed by physician
Arthritis	Nonerosive arthritis involving two or more peripheral joints; characterized by tenderness, swelling, or effusion
Serositis	Evidence of pleuritis or pericarditis documented by ECG or rub heard by physician or evidence of pericardial effusion
Renal disorder	As manifested by persistent proteinuria (>0.5 g/day or >3+) or cellular casts
Neurologic disorder	Seizures or psychosis occurring without any other explanation
Hematologic disorder	Leukopenia (<4,000/mm^3), or hemolytic anemia, or lymphopenia (<1,500/mm^3), or thrombocytopenia (<100,000/mm^3)
Immunologic disorder	Anti-double stranded DNA antibody, or anti-Sm antibody, or anti-phospholipid
Antinuclear antibody	An abnormal ANA titer in the absence of drugs known to be associated with drug-induced lupus

[a]The diagnosis of SLE is made when a patient has 4 or more of the 11 criteria at any time during the course of the disease with 98% specificity and 97% sensitivity.

methyldopa, penicillamine, quinidine, and sulfasalazine. The most commonly reported drug associated with drug-induced lupus is procainamide, which has resulted in the syndrome in approximately one third of patients who have taken it over a 1-year period. The drug-induced lupus-like syndrome onset can occur as soon as 1 month of therapy or as late as 12 years from the initiation of procainamide. Hydralazine follows procainamide, with a prevalence of drug-induced lupus-like syndrome being reported between 2% and 21%, with the wide range reflecting differences in duration of treatment, dosage, and acetylator phenotype. Drug-induced lupus from hydralazine appears to be associated with daily dosage >200 mg or a cumulative dose of 100 g. Drug-induced cutaneous lupus erythematosus occurs in 15,000 to 20,000 people yearly in the United States and is often unrecognized.[17–19] New cases of drug-induced LE continue to occur with newer drugs such as terbinafine and celecoxib.[15,20] In particular for celecoxib, this may be another precaution to keep mind since the COX-2 inhibitors are being widely used in the treatment of rheumatic diseases. Patients who develop drug-induced lupus have symptoms (e.g., arthralgias, myalgias, fever) similar to those of patients with idiopathic SLE; however, renal disease is rare.[14,21] Fever, rash, anemia, and cardiac problems occur slightly less frequently than with spontaneous lupus. Although the lupus erythematosus (LE) cell and antinuclear antibody (ANA) titer can be positive, antibodies to native or double-stranded DNA are not found. Drug-induced lupus typically improves rapidly after discontinuation of the drug and usually does not require specific therapy. However, in some situations (e.g., symptoms present for a long time or patients are significantly symptomatic), a short course of low- to moderate-dose prednisone is beneficial.

SYSTEMIC SCLEROSIS (SCLERODERMA)

Systemic sclerosis, also called scleroderma (*skleros,* meaning hard; *derma,* meaning skin), is a multisystem disorder of connective tissues characterized by inflammation, fibrosis, and degenerative changes in the blood vessels, skin, synovium, skeletal muscle, and some internal organ systems (e.g., gastrointestinal tract, lung, heart, kidney). Systemic sclerosis is an acquired, noncontagious, rare disorder that affects all races worldwide. The incidence in the United States is 19 to 20 per million per year with a prevalence of 19 to 75 cases per 100,000.[22] Overall, females are affected three times as often as males, and the female-to-male ratio is increased during the childbearing years when the ratios of women to men may reach 7:1 to 12:1. Onset of systemic sclerosis generally begins in people between 30 and 50 years of age. It is rare in childhood and after age 80. Environmental factors including occupational silica and organic solvent exposure have been implicated in predisposing or precipitating systemic sclerosis. It is a disease of unknown etiology, but most investigators believe the key players are endothelial cells, activated immune cells, and fibroblasts. It is hypothesized that the process is initiated by an immune attack on the endothelium resulting in endothelial cell activation and/or injury. This is followed by activation of the fibroblasts resulting in subendothelial connective tissue proliferation, narrowing of the vascular lumen, and Raynaud's phenomenon. T cells are then selectively activated and populate the affected areas such as the dermis and lung. These cells produce cytokines that simulate resident fibroblast to produce excessive amounts of procollagen, which is then converted extracellularly to mature collagen. Later and when the inflammatory process subsides, the fibroblasts revert back to normal.

Systemic sclerosis is divided into two major classes: diffuse cutaneous and limited cutaneous disease, which are distinguished from one another based on the degree and extent of skin involvement. The term *overlap syndrome* is used when features common in one or more of the other CTDs are also present. In most cases of limited cutaneous systemic sclerosis, the initial complaint is Raynaud's phenomenon. Patients with diffuse cutaneous systemic sclerosis most often have generalized swelling of the hands, skin thickening, or arthritis as the first manifestation. The diffuse cutaneous systemic sclerosis patients will present with fatigue or lack of energy, musculoskeletal complaints, and sclerosis of the skin and certain organs. The degree and the rate of organ involvement vary among patients. The skin is taut, firm, and edematous and is firmly bound to subcutaneous tissue; it feels tough and leathery, may itch, and later becomes hyperpigmented. The dermatologic manifestations usually precede the development of signs of visceral involvement. The combination of *C*alcinosis with *R*aynaud's phenomenon, esophageal dysfunction, *S*clerodactyly, and *T*elangiectasias normally found in limited cutaneous systemic sclerosis is called the *CREST syndrome.* Patients with limited cutaneous systemic sclerosis may have Raynaud's phenomenon for years before other signs of disease become evident. They are less likely than those with diffuse cutaneous systemic sclerosis to develop severe lung, heart, or kidney disease, although all these diseases can occur. In contrast to limited cutaneous systemic sclerosis, diffuse cutaneous systemic sclerosis develops only with a short interval between the onset of Raynaud's phenomenon and significant organ involvement.

The overall course of systemic sclerosis is highly variable and unpredictable. However, after a remission occurs, relapse is uncommon. The diffuse form of the disease generally has a worse prognosis with a 10-year survival rate of 40% to 60%, compared with a >70% 10-year survival rate in those with limited cutaneous systemic sclerosis. The prognosis is worse in white males and African American females. There is no specific therapy for systemic sclerosis. Supportive therapy is indicated for the organ systems affected. Because multisystem organs are involved, treatment is directed toward alleviating the affected organ systems. Because of potential toxicities, including precipitating acute renal failure, corticosteroids are not generally used and are typically restricted to patients with inflammatory myopathy or symptomatic serositis not adequately controlled with NSAIDs. D-Penicillamine significantly improves diffuse cutaneous systemic sclerosis symptoms in patients with skin thickening, reduces subsequent renal involvement, and increases survival. Vasodilators, such as the calcium channel blocker, nifedipine, and the angiotensin converting enzyme receptor blocking agent, losartan, have proved useful in alleviating Raynaud's phenomenon. Angiotensin-converting enzyme (ACE) inhibitors are the drugs of choice to manage renal complications and hypertension associated with systemic sclerosis. Metoclopramide, erythromycin, nifedipine, proton pump inhibitors, and H_2 blockers can alleviate specific gastrointestinal symptoms.[23]

POLYMYALGIA RHEUMATICA AND TEMPORAL ARTERITIS (GIANT CELL ARTERITIS)

Polymyalgia rheumatica (PMR) and temporal arteritis or giant cell arteritis (GCA) are clinical syndromes that usually affect the elderly population, and both can occur in the same patient. The incidence of PMR and GCA increases in patients after the age of 50 and peaks in those 70 to 80 years of age.[24] The occurrence of PMR is two to five times more likely than GCA. Up to 15% of patients with PMR can have GCA, and PMR is found in 40% to 60% of patients with GCA.[25] The incidence of PMR increases with age and has been estimated to be as high as 400 cases per 100,000 in individuals older than 65 years of age.[26–28] Women are affected twice as much as men.[24] PMR generally affects whites and is uncommon in African Americans, Hispanics, Asians, and Native Americans.[25] A viral cause has been suspected but not confirmed in PMR and GCA, because the prevalence of antibodies against parainfluenza virus type 1 is increased in patients with PMR and GCA.[29]

Patients with PMR generally present with malaise, weight loss, night sweats, and occasional fever. There is intense pain and stiffness in the neck, shoulder, and buttocks, and the patient may have difficulty arising from bed in the morning. The most useful supporting evidence in support of a clinical diagnosis of PMR is the ESR. It is usually in excess of 50 mm/hour and may exceed 100 mm/hour.[25] The C-reactive protein has been found to be a more sensitive indicator of disease activity than the ESR.[24,30] Also, levels of interleukin-6 appear to be a sensitive indicator of active disease, but most clinical laboratories do not yet have the means to measure these levels.[28] As with other CTDs, the diagnosis if PMR is made based on clinical presentation despite well-recognized laboratory abnormalities. No pathognomonic laboratory test exists. Nonspecific clinical features and the frequent absence of physical signs make diagnosis difficult.

GCA is a connective tissue disorder that involves the inflammation of the medium and large arteries and almost always occurs in whites. It is more common in women and rare in African Americans. GCA rarely affects patients younger than 50 year of age, and the incidence increases with age. It is closely associated with PMR and affects many arteries throughout the body, producing symptoms and signs that mimic other medical and surgical conditions. Carotid artery involvement lends itself to the name *temporal arteritis* when the temporal arteries are distended, are tender, and pulsate early in the disease. These arteries can become occluded and lead to visual disturbances and blindness from ischemic optic neuritis. The symmetric and proximal muscle pain and stiffness of PMR are often associated with GCA.

Corticosteroids are essential for the treatment of PMR and GCA because they rapidly relieve symptoms and reduce the incidence of blindness associated with GCA. The therapeutic goal in PMR is to alleviate stiffness and constitutional features. The corticosteroids are the drugs of choice and the NSAIDs are used when PMR symptoms are mild.[25] For patients with PMR, the current recommendation is to start with prednisone 15 to 20 mg/day. Most patients respond significantly within 24 hours, but it may take up to 48 to 72 hours to achieve a good response in a few patients. The results are dramatic. If patients do not obtain relief of symptoms after a few days, another diagnosis should be considered.[24] If the patient's symptoms are not reduced by the initial dose, prednisone can be increased by an additional 10 mg/day for control. After the symptoms are controlled, the dosage of prednisone can be decreased by 2.5 mg Q 2 weeks for as long as the symptoms remain improved until 10 mg/day is reached. Afterwards, the prednisone is titrated at 1-mg decrements Q 4 weeks while following the clinical response and the ESR.[25] Although patients respond quickly to the corticosteroids, treatment is often required for several years. Duration of treatment may be related to the severity of the disease as measured by the ESR. High pretreatment ESRs indicate more severe disease, and these patients require longer duration of therapy.[28] Typically, corticosteroid treatment is required for 6 to 24 months. For patients with mild PMR disease, the NSAIDs can effectively manage their symptoms.

For patients with GCA, corticosteroid treatment must be initiated immediately as soon the diagnosis is made because GCA can lead to severe visual loss and potential blindness.[24] Treatment for GCA is more aggressive than PMR and usually begins with prednisone 40 to 60 mg as a single or a divided dose. Initial pulsed intravenous does of methylprednisolone (1,000 mg/day for 3 days) may be given to patients with recent or impending visual loss. Corticosteroids may prevent, but usually do not reverse, visual loss.[24,25] After the clinical symptoms and laboratory findings of inflammation have subsided for about 1 month, decreases in the prednisone dose should be initiated. Sometimes, it may take several months at doses of 15 to 25 mg/day before prednisone may be decreased. Prednisone dosages should be decreased gradually in 1- to 2-week intervals by a maximum of 10% of the total daily dose. Excessively rapid tapering of the prednisone dose may result in relapses and recurrence of symptoms.[24] The decrease in the dosage of prednisone should be based on the patient's clinical status rather than on laboratory results.[27] Treatment of GCA should be continued for 1 to 2 years to minimize the potential for relapse.[25] If the patients do not achieve clinical remission or do not respond to low doses of the corticosteroids, immunosuppressive agents, such as azathioprine, should be considered. Monitoring ESR or the C-reactive protein value is the most useful in determining disease activity.[24] Another study suggested that measurement of interleukin-6 levels after 4 weeks of therapy was helpful.[28] PMR and GCA are among the most rewarding diseases for a clinician to diagnose and treat because the unpleasant symptoms and serious consequences of these two disorders can be relieved rapidly and prevented by corticosteroids.[25]

REITER'S SYNDROME

Reiter's syndrome is a form of reactive arthritis defined as peripheral arthritis often accompanied by one or more extra-articular manifestations that appear shortly after certain infections of the genitourinary or gastrointestinal tracts. Reactive arthritis typically begins acutely 2 to 4 weeks after venereal infections or bouts of gastroenteritis.[31] Some evidence also suggests that respiratory infection with *Chlamydia pneumoniae* may also trigger the disease.[32] Most of the cases affect young men, with the ratio of male to female patients of 9:1. The classic triad of Reiter's syndrome is arthritis, urethritis, and conjunctivitis. Urethritis usually appears first in this syndrome, which occurs mainly in young men.[33] Mild dysuria and a mucopurulent urethral discharge are the most typical symptoms in men. Women may have dysuria, vaginal discharge, and purulent cervicitis and/or vaginitis. Reiter's syndrome has its peak onset during the third decade of life, but has been reported in children and octogenarians.[34]

There is no specific therapy for Reiter's syndrome. Interventions should include joint protection and relief of pain, suppression of inflammation, and when appropriate, eradication of infection. The arthritis is treated symptomatically with NSAIDs. Systemic corticosteroids are relatively ineffective in the routine management of patients with seronegative spondyloarthropathies such as Reiter's syndrome.[34] Aggressive and unremitting Reiter's syndrome may benefit from immunosuppressive drugs.

POLYMYOSITIS AND DERMATOMYOSITIS

Polymyositis and dermatomyositis are autoimmune diseases of unknown etiology. Polymyositis is predominately a disease of adults. Dermatomyositis affects both children and adults, and more women than men. Polymyositis includes inflammation of a number of voluntary skeletal muscles simultaneously. The onset is insidious, and patients initially complain of muscle weakness of the trunk, shoulders, hip girdles, upper arms, thighs, neck, and pharynx. These patients usually report increasing difficulties in everyday tasks requiring the use of proximal muscles such as getting up from a chair, climbing stairs, stepping onto a curb, lifting objects and combing hair. Polymyositis spares the skin; however, dermatomyositis is a progressive polymyositis condition that is associated with a skin rash. The rash accompanies or more often precedes the muscle weakness of polymyositis. The rash is erythematous, scaly, and eczematous and generally affects the eyelids, bridge of the nose, cheeks, forehead, chest, elbows, knees, and knuckles and around nail beds. One-third of these cases are associated with various connective tissue disorders such as rheumatoid arthritis, SLE, and progressive sclerosis; one-tenth are associated with a malignancy. Edema, inflammation, and degeneration of muscles characterize both polymyositis and dermatomyositis.[35]

The goal of therapy is to improve muscle weakness, thereby improving the activities of daily living. Supportive therapy such as bed rest, physiotherapy, warm baths, and moist heat applications to the affected areas can improve muscle stiffness. If mouth lesions are present, irrigation of these lesions with warm saline solution is helpful. Oral prednisone (e.g., 1–2 mg/kg/day) is the initial treatment of choice and should be initiated as soon as possible. After the symptoms are brought under control in approximately 3 to 4 weeks, the dosage of the steroid is tapered slowly over a period of 10 weeks to 1 mg/kg every other day. Afterward, the dose is further decreased to the lowest possible dose to control symptoms and to avoid adverse effects of the corticosteroids as long-term steroid usage can cause steroid myopathy. This can further confuse the issue of whether the muscle weakness is due to increased disease activity or to adverse effects of steroid therapy. Generally, there should be objective increase in muscle strength and activities of daily living by the end of the third month of therapy. Approximately 75% of these patients may require immunosuppressive therapy if their conditions do not respond to prednisone after 3 months.[35]

CLINICAL USE OF CORTICOSTEROIDS

Corticosteroids play an important role in the treatment of a wide variety of disease states. In physiologic doses, they are used to replace deficiencies of this endogenous hormone. In pharmacologic doses, they are used to treat and, more often, provide supportive therapy for a variety of diseases. In the past 40 years, much has been learned about the corticosteroids; however, the exact mechanism by which corticosteroids exert their anti-inflammatory and immunosuppressive effects remains unclear. Corticosteroids may be used for the treatment of many rheumatologic disorders, including ankylosing spondylitis, bursitis, tenosynovitis, acute gouty arthritis, RA, osteoarthritis, dermatomyositis, PMR, acute rheumatic carditis, SLE, mixed CTD, polymyositis, and vasculitis.

Predictable Pharmacologic Effects Relative to the Corticosteroids

1. J.L., a 62-year-old man with a 1-year history of scleroderma, is being treated with prednisone 60 mg/day and azathioprine 50 mg/day. At a recent clinic visit, his vital signs and laboratory test results were as follows: weight, 292 lb; blood pressure (BP), 180/102 mmHg; pulse, 62 beats/minute and regular; and fasting plasma glucose (FPG), 196 mg/dL. J.L. complains of occasional headaches, a "swollen face," a modest weight gain, and increases in urinary frequency. Based on J.L.'s presentation, are any of his symptoms related to his drug therapy?
[SI unit: FPG, 10.9 mmol/L]

His "swollen face" could represent a cushingoid feature resulting from long-term corticosteroid use. Hypercortisolism alters normal body fat distribution, resulting in moon facies, buffalo hump, truncal obesity, and other localized fatty deposits. J.L.'s complaint of headaches could be related to his increased BP (180/102 mmHg) in part to fluid retention resulting from his corticosteroid use, even though hypertension usually is asymptomatic (see Chapter 14, Essential Hypertension). Although corticosteroids with the greatest mineralocorticoid activity are more likely to produce fluid retention and increase BP, even those without mineralocorticoid action (Table 44-3) can increase BP. Hypertension can also be induced by high-dose glucocorticoids due to the permissive effects of the glucocorticoids on the action of vasoactive substances (angiotensin II, catecholamines) on the vessel wall and myocardium that results in increased systemic vascular resistance and increased cardiac contractility.[36] A history of high BP and advanced age can predispose individuals to corticosteroid-induced increases in BP. Whether hypertension is related to the dose or duration of corticosteroid therapy is unknown; it rarely occurs in patients receiving alternate-day therapy. The hypertension usually resolves after discontinuation of the steroid. In J.L., however, the hypertension also can be attributed to other possible etiologies (e.g., scleroderma). J.L. also has urinary frequency and elevated fasting plasma glucose that could be attributed to using

Table 44-3 Comparison of Corticosteroid Preparations

Compound	*Equiv. Potency (mg)*	*Anti-Inflammatory Potency*	*Na-Retaining Potency (Mineralocorticoid Activity)*	*Plasma $t_{1/2}$(min)*	*BIOLOGIC $t_{1/2}$ (hr)*
Short Acting					
Cortisone	25	0.8	2+	30	8–12
Hydrocortisone (Cortisol)	20	1	2+	80–118	8–12
Prednisone	5	4	1+	60	18–36
Prednisolone	5	4	1+	115–212	18–36
Methylprednisolone	4	5	0	78–188	18–36
Triamcinolone	4	5	0	200	12–36
Long Acting					
Dexamethasone	0.75	20–30	0	110–210	36–54
Betamethasone	0.6	20–30	0	300+	36–54

high doses of glucocorticoids. The increases in glucose are mainly mediated through decreased peripheral utilization of glucose and induction of gluconeogenesis in the liver. In patients whose glucose levels remain elevated and the continued use of the glucocorticosteroid is warranted, antihyperglycemic agents may be started.

The equivalent potency, sodium-retaining potency, plasma half-life, and biologic half-life of several synthetic analogs of cortisol are listed in Table 44-3. The corticosteroids are used primarily for their anti-inflammatory, immunosuppressive, or antiallergic activity. Cortisone and hydrocortisone have the highest sodium-retaining potency and, therefore, are seldom prescribed for long-term anti-inflammatory therapy. They are useful when sodium and water retention properties are desirable (e.g., adrenal insufficiency after surgery for Cushing's syndrome). All corticosteroids are 21-carbon steroid molecules. The chemical structures of the corticosteroids have been modified, resulting in large differences in duration of action, anti-inflammatory potency, and mineralocorticoid activity.[37] The body synthesizes cortisol by converting cholesterol to pregnenolone, which in turn is converted to progesterone and ultimately to cortisol, the major corticosteroid in humans.[38]

Active Corticosteroid Compounds

2. M.H. is a 43-year-old woman with RA awaiting a liver transplant. Her total bilirubin is 3.1 mg/dL, aspartate aminotransferase (AST) is 93 U/L, and alanine aminotransferase (ALT) is 65 U/L. She has been well maintained on prednisone for her arthritis until recently, when her arthritis failed to respond despite escalating doses of prednisone. Why has prednisone seemed to have stopped being effective? What factors need to be considered when selecting an alternative corticosteroid for M.H.?

[SI units: bilirubin, 53.01 μmol/L; AST, 93 U/L; ALT, 65 U/L]

Although orally administered corticosteroids are well absorbed, exogenously administered corticosteroids, which are 11-keto compounds, are devoid of corticosteroid activity until converted in vivo into active 11 β-hydroxyl compounds.[39] Cortisone and prednisone must be converted to the active compounds, cortisol and prednisolone, respectively, in the liver.[39] M.H. has very little hepatic capacity and, theoretically, might not have been converting the prednisone to its active prednisolone metabolite. To circumvent this possibility, M.H. should be given prednisolone or perhaps a different corticosteroid (e.g., methylprednisolone). Although this explanation is logical given this patient's end stage liver disease, dosage adjustments for hepatically metabolized drugs in the setting of liver disease are difficult to predict because hepatic metabolism is complex and involves numerous oxidative and conjugative pathways that are variably affected in hepatic disease. M.H.'s ability to adhere to her medication regimen because of encephalopathic changes and other potential variables also should be considered as explanations for her decreased responsiveness to prednisone.

Approximately 95% of cortisol is bound to α-globulin transcortin or cortisol-binding globulin (CBG), and the remaining 5% is bound to albumin after this carrier is saturated.[40] However, the bond between cortisol and albumin is weak, and about 25% of the steroid disassociates from albumin and is free to circulate in the plasma. Although the dosing of corticosteroids is not a very precise science, it is important to consider adjusting dosages for patients who have decreased serum albumin concentrations. In these patients, a greater amount of free hormone will result in increased pharmacologic effects. Because albumin is synthesized by the liver, M.H. is likely to have decreased serum albumin concentrations and could be more susceptible to the pharmacologic effects of corticosteroids when given an active corticosteroid moiety.

When selecting an alternative corticosteroid to replace M.H.'s prednisone, the clinician should not base the dosing interval of the replacement corticosteroid strictly on the plasma half-lives shown in Table 44-3. Corticosteroids have biologic half-lives that are 2 to 36 times longer than their plasma half-lives. In addition, the onset of biologic effects lags behind peak plasma levels. Practitioners must always be mindful that the serum or plasma half-life of a drug might not be synonymous with the biologic half-life. For example, prednisone with a plasma half-life of only about 1 hour can be dosed on alternate days for some disorders.

Clinical Presentation of SLE

3. H.R., a 33-year-old African American woman with recently diagnosed lupus erythematosus, has experienced a recent weight loss of 15 lb (down to 130 lb), joint pain, fatigue, and a worsening of

Table 44-4 Systemic Lupus Erythematosus Disease Activity and Use of Corticosteroids

Indication	*Corticosteroid Regimen*
Cutaneous manifestations	Topical or intralesional corticosteroids
Minor disease activity	Prednisone (or equivalent) at a dosage of <0.5 mg/kg in a single or divided daily dose (5–30 mg prednisone daily)
Major disease activity	Oral: Prednisone (or equivalent) at a dosage of 1–2 mg/kg in a single or divided daily dose
	IV bolus: Methylprednisolone (1 g or 15 mg/kg) over 30 minutes; dose often repeated for 3 consecutive days for life-threatening situations

her facial rash. She has a temperature of 105°F, serum creatinine (SrCr) of 2.8 mg/dL, Westergren ESR of 50 mm/hour, ANA titer of 1:320, and positive anti-dsDNA and anti-Sm tests. Urinalysis (UA) reveals 3% proteinuria and a modest amount of casts. What subjective and objective data are consistent with SLE, and would therapy be likely to reflect resolution of these signs and symptoms?

[SI unit: SrCr, 247.52 μmol/L]

According to some of the objective data (fever, increased Westergren ESR, proteinuria, weight loss, high ANA titer, increased SrCr, positive anti-dsDNA and anti-Sm tests) and subjective data (fatigue, joint pain, worsening facial rash), H.R. is experiencing a flare of her SLE (major disease activity shown on Table 44-4). Three major patterns of SLE exist. The classic pattern, one of exacerbations, or "flares" of disease activities, now is called the "relapsing remitting pattern."[18] Newly diagnosed lupus continue to evolve more than 5 years after initial diagnosis and flares of lupus occur with a median time of 12 months, even in patients with longstanding disease and treatment.[41] This disease tends to wax and wane, and the aggressiveness of therapy should be adjusted to accommodate these changes.

Role of Corticosteroids in SLE

4. Why might corticosteroids be indicated for H.R.?

The general management of SLE stresses patient education through which patients need to understand their disease processes. H.R. is definitely experiencing a flare of her SLE and needs aggressive therapy to control her symptoms. Normally, she would be maintained with NSAIDs (including the COX-2 inhibitors) for her joint pains and possibly an immunosuppressive agent such as hydroxychloroquine since she was recently diagnosed.[42] H.R.'s fever, joint pain, fatigue, and worsening facial rash all reflect an inflammatory response to her SLE. These subjective symptoms along with the objective measurements of her disease activity (e.g., increased ESR, ANA, SrCr) are mediated by leukotrienes, prostaglandins, lymphocytes, and the other inflammatory responses described earlier. Therefore, corticosteroids are indicated for the treatment of H.R.

Selection of Appropriate Corticosteroid Therapy

5. What would be a reasonable corticosteroid dosage for H.R.?

Because of the great variety of clinical applications and the wide variety of corticosteroid compounds and dosages, the selection of the most appropriate dosage of a corticosteroid is as much an art as it is a science. Generally, higher dosages and shorter dosing intervals of the corticosteroid translate into an increased anti-inflammatory effect and increased side effects.[36] Therefore, the need to modify disease activity must be balanced against the need to minimize toxicities.

There are multiple dosage forms and uses of corticosteroids in SLE, including topical preparations for inflammatory rashes, intralesional injections for discoid lupus, low-dose oral therapy for mild active disease, and high-dose oral or bolus intravenous infusions for acute, severe manifestations. These indications and the corresponding dose of corticosteroid are listed in Table 44-4.[42]

A review of H.R.'s subjective and objective data suggests that her disease activity probably represents a major flare-up of her SLE. Uncontrolled disease activity can be both debilitating and life-threatening and thus demands rapid an effective intervention. Therefore, a short course of a high-dose corticosteroid regimen probably would be a reasonable treatment for this episode of SLE in H.R.

A short course of steroids or even a single treatment with a high-dose corticosteroid typically can result in prompt and complete resolution of most manifestations of lupus SLE. Pulse therapy with methylprednisolone 1,000 mg intravenously daily for 1 to 3 days has proven effective for SLE, vasculitis, and RA.[36] High-dose steroid pulses must be considered on an individualized basis because adverse effects can be more likely with this dosing regimen. Normally, the pulse methyl prednisone therapy of 1,000 mg/day for 3 days is not given more frequently than at monthly intervals because high doses of glucocorticoids are invariably toxic.[36] Alternatively, the use of mini pulses of oral prednisone (100–200 mg/day) for several days also may help in disease control. In some situations, the addition of a potent immunosuppressive agent such as cyclophosphamide in combination with the corticosteroid pulse therapy may be necessary to bring the patient under control.[43] In any case, depending on how high the dose of glucocorticoid initiated, tapering of the glucocorticoid should be initiated within one to two weeks following initiation of therapy.[36] Table 44-5 provides a summary of different steroid regimens that may be used for severe and active SLE.[44] Assuming that H.R. had been taking a higher dose of oral prednisone, the rationale for IV pulse therapy seems applicable to H.R.

6. After finishing her bolus "pulse" therapy of methylprednisolone (1 g/day IV for 3 days), H.R.'s lupus has responded well. Her joint pain is decreased, and her temperature decreased to normal. The current laboratory test results are as follows: Westergren ESR, 22 mm/hour; SrCr, 2.5 mg/dL; ANA titer, 1:80; and positive anti-dsDNA. H.R. wishes to go home to finish her recovery. What dosage of oral corticosteroid would be reasonable to prescribe for H.R. at her discharge from the hospital?

Along with adjustments of the other medications that she may be taking (e.g., NSAIDs or other immunosuppressive agents), H.R. needs to have her IV doses of methylprednisolone converted to an oral formulation (Table 44-6) and consideration given to reducing the steroid dosage. Because the steroid dosage H.R. received is considered massive supraphysiologic,

Table 44-5 Usual Regimens of Systemic Corticosteroid Therapy in Severe, Active SLE

Preparations	*Dose*	*Rationale*	*Toxicities*
Regimen 1: Daily oral short-acting (prednisone, prednisolone, methylprednisolone)	1–2 mg/kg/day; begin in divided doses	Controls disease activity rapidly	High–infections, sleeplessness, mood swings, hyperglycemia, psychosis, hypertension, weight gain, hypokalemia, fragile skin, bruising, osteoporosis, osteonecrosis, irregular menses, muscle cramps, acne, hirsutism, cataracts
Regimen 2: Intravenous methylprednisolone	500–1,000 mg/day for 3–5 days; then, 1–1.5 mg/kg/day of oral corticosteroids	Controls disease activity rapidly, may achieve results more rapidly than daily oral therapy; some nonresponders to oral regimen respond to the intravenous regimen	High–same as above except more rapid taper of daily maintenance steroid dose may be possible, leading to lower cumulative doses
Regimen 3: Combination of either regimen 1 or 2 with cytotoxic or immunosuppressive agent			

the corticosteroid effects on lymphocyte function can be expected to be prolonged. Therefore, the residual benefits from the supraphysiologic doses of methylprednisolone will be additive to the effect of the oral steroid that will be prescribed for her upon departure from the hospital. Because of this fact, H.R. does not require an oral corticosteroid dose that is equivalent to the IV dose, and a lower oral daily dose can be prescribed, because she responded well to her IV doses. In some patients with presumably modest disease activity, alternate-day dosing of corticosteroids may be adequate to maintain disease suppression as there are less adverse effects associated with alternate-day dosing.[36,41] However, more study is needed to better determine the role of alternate-day dosing of corticosteroids, because there is less efficacy in patients renal nephritis taking alternate-day therapy as compared to those taking daily glucocorticoids.[36,41]

In the United States, prednisone is the most commonly prescribed corticosteroid for oral use in the treatment of CTDs. Prednisone is rapidly and substantially absorbed following oral administration, has an intermediate duration of action (12–36 hours), is available in many dosage forms and strengths, and is relatively inexpensive. The recommended dosage of prednisone for most CTDs is 1 mg/kg/day in three to four divided doses. Administration of corticosteroids in daily divided doses given two to four times per day provides a more rapid onset and a greater degree of anti-inflammatory effect. Considering the severity of H.R.'s lupus flare-up, this dosing appears appropriate. The dosing of oral corticosteroids is a balancing act to minimize toxicity while preventing flare-up of disease activity.[36] For H.R., who weighs approximately 59 kg, a maintenance regimen of prednisone 20 mg three times a day (for a total of 60 mg/day) or an equivalent dose of another corticosteroid should be prescribed. H.R. also might need an immunosuppressive agent, such as azathioprine or cyclophosphamide, because of her increased SrCr and possibility of lupus nephritis. These latter drugs would not be initiated in H.R. because she seems to be responding to her methylprednisolone without adverse sequelae thus far. The addition of immunosuppressive agents may have a "steroid-sparing" effect and could allow for steroid dosage reduction.[36]

Table 44-6 Routes of Administration of Various Corticosteroids

Corticosteroid	*Route of Administration*
Betamethasone	PO, IM, intra-articular, intrasynovial, intradermal, soft-tissue injection
Cortisone	PO, IM
Dexamethasone	PO, IM, IV, intra-articular, intradermal, soft-tissue injection
Hydrocortisone	IM, IV, PO
Methylprednisolone	PO, IM, IV
Prednisolone	PO, IM, IV, intra-articular, intradermal, soft-tissue injection
Prednisone	PO
Triamcinolone	PO, IM, intra-articular, intrasynovial, intradermal, soft-tissue injection

IM, intramuscularly; IV, intravenously; PO, oral.

Once-daily Dosing

7. H.R. was discharged from the hospital taking ibuprofen 600 mg QID with food and prednisone 20 mg TID. After 3 weeks, her flare-up has subsided, and her symptoms are now back at her previous baseline. Why should a change in her medication be considered?

Once the patient's lupus flare-up is under control and has responded to steroids, the divided daily doses of a steroid can be consolidated into a single daily dose, usually administered in the morning. Endogenous cortisol levels are normally highest at about 7 to 8 AM and decline to their lowest at midnight. Thus, a once-a-day morning corticosteroid dose coincides in time with high endogenous plasma cortisol. Because this is the time that the patient's tissues would normally be exposed to the highest levels of endogenous cortisol, suppression of the HPA axis is minimized somewhat. If the divided dose regimen has been used for <2 weeks, the dose can be combined into a single daily dose immediately; however, if the divided dose regimen has been used for >2 weeks, the dose should be converted over a 2-week period to a single daily dose because patients who have taken glucocorticoids for more than 2 weeks are candidates for more HPA suppression and their dose needs to be tapered more slowly.[45] Because H.R. received her dosage for 3 weeks, the daily dose should be converted to 60 mg each morning over a 2-week period.

Hypothalamic-Pituitary-Adrenocortical Axis Suppression

8. R.S., a 48-year-old, 135-lb, 5 feet 5 inch man, has recently been diagnosed with polyarteritis. After a recent hospitalization, R.S. was discharged home taking 15 mg prednisone QID. He has been adhering to this regimen for approximately 1 month, and his symptoms are well controlled. R.S. now is scheduled for major surgery. His laboratory test evaluation revealed the following: SrCr, 1.4 mg/dL; blood urea nitrogen (BUN), 17 mg/dL; white blood cell (WBC) count, 11,200 cells/mm^3; and Westergren ESR, 29 mm/hour. Why should R.S.'s corticosteroid regimen be adjusted?

[SI units: SrCr, 123.76 μmol/L; BUN, 6.07 mmol/L urea; WBC, 11.2×10^3 ESR, 29 mm/hour]

The HPA axis regulates the amount of circulating cortisol.[36,45] Corticotropin-releasing factor, a hormone secreted by the hypothalamus, stimulates the release of adrenocorticotropin (ACTH) from the anterior pituitary. ACTH, in turn, stimulates the adrenal cortex to secrete cortisol.[45] As serum cortisol levels rise, a negative-feedback mechanism inhibits corticotropin-releasing factor and ACTH secretion, resulting in decreased secretion of cortisol (Fig. 44-1). Under normal conditions, about 10 to 30 mg/day of cortisol is secreted by the adrenal cortex in accordance with the circadian cycle of an individual.[39,40] Under stress and illnesses the amount of cortisol increases to up to 10-fold or 250 to 300 mg/day for patients undergoing surgery or prolonged major stress.[39,40]

Corticosteroid doses can be classified as physiologic (i.e., replacement) or pharmacologic (i.e., supraphysiologic). A physiologic dose of a corticosteroid is equal to the amount of corticosteroid usually secreted by the adrenal cortex each day and is equal to about 5 mg/day of prednisone. A dosage of prednisone of 0.1 to 0.25 mg/kg/day is a low supraphysiologic dosage; 0.5 mg/kg/day of prednisone is a supraphysiologic dose; 1 to 3 mg/kg/day is a high-supraphysiologic dose; and 15 to 30 mg/kg/day is a massive supraphysiologic dose.

Shortly after cortisone and ACTH were accepted into clinical practice, adrenocortical insufficiency and subsequent adrenal atrophy were noted in patients who received doses of exogenous corticosteroids that exceeded the normal amount needed for hormone replacement. When corticosteroids are discontinued abruptly in the patients who had been treated with supraphysiologic doses of corticosteroids for a prolonged period, the HPA axis cannot respond to situations in which there is a need for increased cortisol (e.g., illness, stress, surgery).[45] The minimum dose, dose interval, and therapy duration required to suppress the HPA axis are difficult to assess. The best predictor of HPA axis suppression is the patient's current corticosteroid dosage and duration of the corticosteroid therapy. There is a strong correlation between prednisone maintenance doses >5 mg/day and a subnormal ACTH-stimulation test result.[3] Following long-term therapy, this suppression can last up to 1 year. The duration of adrenal suppression following a short course of corticosteroid therapy is unknown. Even though there is HPA axis suppression in short-term treatment of 1 week or less, clinically evident adrenal insufficiency is probably extremely rare and the suppression lasts only for a few days.[3] Because R.S. is receiving prednisone 1 mg/kg/day, he is receiving a massive supraphysiologic dose that is capable of suppressing endogenous cortisol secretion. Surgery is a stressful event and supplemental doses of a corticosteroid with mineralocorticoid effects probably are warranted for R.S., because he most likely has some degree of HPA axis suppression. Although corticosteroids can decrease wound healing, this is a minor consideration relative to HPA axis suppression.

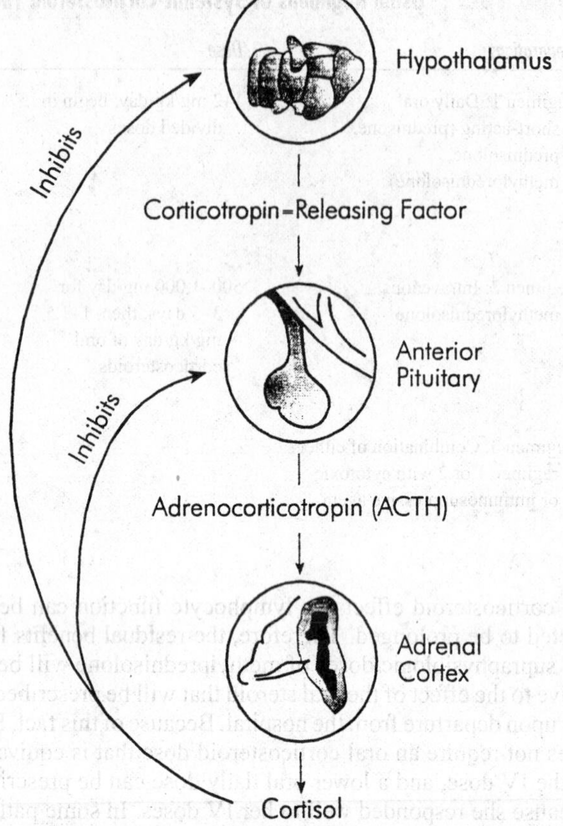

FIGURE 44-1 Hypothalamic-pituitary-adrenocortical axis regulation.

Adrenal Function Testing

9. How can the degree of adrenal suppression in R.S. be assessed?

The clinician has two options when HPA axis suppression is suspected. The first option is to treat the suspected patient as though adrenocortical insufficiency is present. The second is to try to quantify the adrenocortical reserves of the pituitary and hypothalamus. In today's environment of cost containment, the former approach usually is taken. There are currently five well-established stimulatory tests of HPA axis function. The most commonly used test to diagnose adrenal insufficiency is the short 250-μg ACTH (cosyntropin) stimulation test. This test directly assesses adrenal gland responsiveness to exogenous ACTH. The test measures baseline cortisol plasma concentrations both before the rapid injection of a highly supraphysiologic dose of a synthetic ACTH analog and the cortisol level 30 to 60 minutes after injection. Patients with normal adrenal gland function should be able to generate a poststimulation cortisol concentration of 20 mcg/ dL. Plasma cortisol concentrations of <495 nmol/L (18 mcg/dL) suggest adrenal insufficiency.[40] The remaining four tests—insulin-induced hypoglycemia, overnight metyrapone, CRH stimulation, and low-dose (1 mcg) ACTH stimulation—are more sensitive than the 250-g ACTH stimulation test, because they depend on a completely intact HPA axis for a normal result.[3] With the exception of the low-dose (1 mcg) ACTH stimulation, these tests tend to be labor intensive and expensive. The low-dose ACTH stimulation not only measures adrenal gland responsiveness, but may be able to detect subtle degrees of adrenal atrophy caused by central adrenal insufficiency.[46,47]

Dosing During Stressful Events

10. R.S. has a cosyntropin test performed, and it demonstrates an increase of 80 mmol/L to a level of 190 mmol/L. In the consideration of this laboratory report, what dosages of corticosteroid should be ordered to prevent an addisonian crisis during R.S.'s surgery?

A normal response includes an increase in plasma cortisol of >170 mmol/L (6 mcg/dL) from baseline to a level >495 nmol/L (18 mcg/dL).[40] R.S. apparently has adrenal insufficiency and needs cortisol supplementation during periods of stress. Depending on the amount of stress and how prolonged the stress, recommendations for corticosteroid replacement regimen for patients with suppressed HPA axis has been somewhat arbitrary (e.g., hydrocortisone 100 mg Q 6–8 hr).[45] Newer recommendations propose that the amount and duration of corticosteroid coverage should be determined by (a) the preoperative dose of corticosteroid taken by the patient, (b) the preoperative duration of the corticosteroid administration, and (c) the nature and anticipated duration of surgery.[48] Because the adrenal gland can secrete as much as 300 mg/day during acute stress, 150 mg of hydrocortisone every 6 hours is a reasonable regimen for R.S. on the day of his surgery.

Leukocytosis

11. R.S. was doing fine until 3 days after surgery when his temperature spiked to 103°F. R.S. has been back on his original prednisone dosage. Urine, blood, and sputum cultures were ordered as well as a STAT CBC, drawn at 4 PM. His CBC revealed an increase in WBCs with a differential showing an increase in segmented neutrophils (granulocytes 16,000/mm^3 from 11,000 at baseline) along with decreases in both total lymphocyte and monocyte count from baseline. No "left shift" was noted. What could be causing these results?

At first, it would be reasonable to assume there may be an infectious process present. The effects of prednisone on peripheral or circulating WBC counts are well documented and predictable (e.g., granulocytosis along with lymphopenia and monocytopenia). T-cell lymphocytes are decreased more than B-cell lymphocytes. The occurrence of a "left shift" (e.g., an increase in immature leukocytes, such as bands) is variable, and only slight if present. The increase in granulocytes (PMNs) and decrease in lymphocytes and monocytes is most significant 4 to 6 hours after a prednisone dose; these values return to normal in 24 hours. The decrease in monocyte accumulation at tissue sites of inflammation may persist for several days.

Prednisone increases granulocytes by an average of 4,000/mm^3 with a range of 1,700 to 7,500/mm^3. The increase in granulocytes results primarily from release of cells from bone marrow and secondarily from the shift of cells from the marginal or noncirculating cell pool to the circulating or peripheral pool.[49] The temporal relationship of WBC changes in patients taking multiple doses of corticosteroids is less predictable because of the constant flux in steroid effect.

The results from R.S.'s most recent CBC should be compared with his baseline CBC. The temporal relationship to his prednisone dose also should be determined. Because a STAT CBC, at the time of a temperature spike, was obtained only 7 hours after his prednisone dose was administered, the CBC changes (leukocytosis, monocytopenia, and lymphocytopenia) are difficult to interpret. Another CBC, 24 hours after his dose, was ordered to differentiate the cause of his CBC abnormalities. This CBC was normal, indicating that the abnormalities on the first CBC were probably steroid induced.

Alternate-day Therapy

12. One month later, R.S. states he feels much better. He has recovered from his surgery, and his polyarteritis is now asymptomatic; his WBC count, BUN, SrCr, and Westergren ESR are returning toward the normal range. Why should R.S.'s prednisone dosage be adjusted at this time?

Once a stable clinical response is attained with a single daily dose of a corticosteroid, R.S.'s corticosteroid dosage should be decreased to the lowest effective dosage and, if possible, to taper the steroid to an alternate-day regimen.[3,45] If used appropriately, alternate-day corticosteroid therapy can help minimize HPA axis suppression and undesirable side effects, while allowing effective treatment of the disease process. A corticosteroid with a short or intermediate duration of action should be chosen for alternate-day therapy to minimize accumulation from subsequent doses that would negate the benefits of every-other-day dosing. If the dosing interval is substantially longer than the biologic half-life (e.g., giving prednisone every 48 hours), nearly normal hypophyseal-pituitary-adrenal function can be maintained. This can minimize the risks of daily therapy. Although alternate-day steroid dosing can be used to maintain disease suppression in chronic therapy, control of the active disease process usually necessitates more intensive dosage schedules.

Conversion to Alternate-day Therapy

13. How would you convert R.S.'s current 60 mg/day dosage to alternate-day therapy?

Before converting a patient to alternate-day therapy, the minimum effective daily dosage must be determined.

Generally, the optimum every-other-day dose is 2.5 to 3 times the minimal daily dose.[45,50] The dose on the "off" day should be tapered gradually by the equivalent of 2.5 to 5 mg of prednisone or its equivalent per week until the patient is taking the steroid every other day. Tapering of the alternate-day dosage can continue until the minimum dosage sufficient to control the underlying disorder is achieved. For R.S., one approach would be to decrease the dosage of prednisone by 5 mg/week until the minimum daily dose is reached that controls his polyarteritis. For illustrative purposes, assume this dosage is 30 mg/day. The 30-mg dose is multiplied by 2.5, so R.S. would take 75 mg on one day, alternating with 30 mg of prednisone the next. The 30-mg dose would then be tapered each week by 5 mg/week until discontinued. R.S. would then be taking 75 mg of prednisone every other day. Should R.S. be asymptomatic at this dosage, a taper of the 75 mg could then be attempted. Tapering should be 2.5 mg/week until the lowest possible dosage that will control his disease is achieved.

Discontinuation of Therapy

14. R.S. has now received prednisone 60 mg QOD for 5 months, and his polyarteritis is well controlled. What would be a reasonable dosing schedule for implementing the gradual discontinuation of R.S.'s corticosteroid?

Many methods of tapering steroid dosages have been tried.[3] Some suggest decreasing the corticosteroid dosage by the equivalent of 2.5 to 5 mg of prednisone every 3 to 7 days until the physiologic dose is reached. Another recommends the daily dose of prednisone (or its equivalent) can be decreased by 5% to 10% per week until a dose of 0.25 to 0.5 mg/kg/day is reached and more slowly thereafter, aiming for either a complete withdrawal or, if not possible, for a low dose of corticosteroid.[36] Others suggest decreasing the dosage by 2.5 mg of prednisone (or the equivalent of another corticosteroid) every 1 to 2 weeks if on daily therapy or by 5 mg of prednisone every 1 to 2 weeks if on alternate-day therapy, until it can be discontinued. Some clinicians follow this procedure until a physiologic dose is reached and, at that time, will convert the patient to hydrocortisone 20 mg/day. After 2 to 4 weeks, this dosage can be decreased by 2.5 mg every week until 10 mg/day is achieved. At this time, the patient should have a plasma cortisol concentration measured. If this is normal, the hydrocortisone can be discontinued.[45,50] During the tapering process, disease flare-up is a definite possibility; therefore, the patient must be monitored closely. Also, if the patient is stressed during this period, exogenous corticosteroid supplementation may be necessary. Abrupt withdrawal of steroids following long-term, high-dose therapy should be avoided because this may produce a steroid withdrawal syndrome manifested by the presence of nausea, vomiting, anorexia, headache, joint pain, fever, lethargy, myalgia, hypotension, and weight loss. These symptoms are thought to occur as a consequence of rapidly falling serum corticosteroid concentrations rather than the presence of low concentrations.

R.S.'s prednisone dosage of 60 mg every other day can now be decreased by 5 mg at 1- to 2-week intervals until he is receiving 5 mg on alternate days. R.S. can then be converted to hydrocortisone 20 mg/day for 2 to 4 weeks. Weekly reductions of the hydrocortisone by 2.5 mg could be undertaken until the daily dose of 10 mg is reached. At this point, R.S.'s morning dose should be held and a cortisol level taken.

If the serum cortisol concentration is normal (>10 mcg/dL), the hydrocortisone can be discontinued. This is but one of the many possible approaches.[45,51] All approaches to discontinuing corticosteroids must be modified based on factors such as dose, duration of therapy, disease status, patient condition, and existence of adverse effects.

Adverse Effects

In addition to suppression of the HPA axis, corticosteroid therapy produces inevitable side effects.[36,39,45] A compilation of documented complications and adverse effects associated with various organ systems is listed in Table 44-7.[52]

Osteoporosis

15. D.L., a 28-year-old, 5 feet 4 inch, 105-lb woman, is diagnosed with SLE. After an acute episode of lupus nephritis, D.L. has been maintained on high-dose prednisone, currently at a level of 15 mg/day. Her lupus seems well controlled, but she comes in today with complaints of back pain. A physical examination reveals no apparent joint involvement typical of a lupus flare-up. What are possible explanations for her back pain, and what additional data are needed to assist in the differential diagnosis?

Table 44-7 Adverse Effects of Corticosteroid Therapy

Organ System	*Complication*
Immunologic	Increased susceptibility to infections, decreased inflammatory responses, suppressed delayed hypersensitivity, neutrophilia, lymphocytopenia
Musculoskeletal	Osteoporosis, fractures, osteonecrosis, myopathy
Gastrointestinal	Peptic ulcers and gastrointestinal bleeds associated with NSAID use, pancreatitis
Cardiovascular	Hypertension, fluid retention accelerated atherosclerosis
Dermatologic	Acne, hirsutism, purple striae, skin fragility, ecchymoses
Neuropsychiatric	Altered mood, emotional lability, euphoria, insomnia, depression, psychosis, pseudotumor cerebri
Ophthalmologic	Cataracts, glaucoma
Endocrine-metabolic	Glucose intolerance, weight gain, fat redistribution (Cushing's syndrome), negative nitrogen balance, growth suppression, muscle wasting, impaired wound healing, fluid retention, hypokalemia, impotence, irregular menses, HPA suppression, acute renal insufficiency

HPA, hypothalamic-pituitary-adrenal; NSAID, nonsteroidal anti-inflammatory drug.

A good medical history combined with a physical examination and laboratory tests should be obtained to determine whether D.L. is having arthralgias due to SLE or other etiologies. It also is important to note that osteoporosis and osteonecrosis are common adverse effects of corticosteroid therapy, and that 30% to 50% of patients treated with chronic corticosteroids develop osteoporosis. During the first 3 to 6 months of corticosteroid therapy, there is a rapid bone loss of up to 12%, which slows down to 2% to 5% annually.[36] Prednisone dosages of >10 mg/day result in a 10% to 12% annual reduction in the bone mineral content of the lumbar spine.[53,54] Dosages as low as prednisolone 7.5 mg/day appear to be the threshold dose for the development of osteoporosis.[54] Bone loss leading to fractures at sites such as the spine, hip, and ribs are well-recognized complications of corticosteroid therapy. Osteoporosis in postmenopausal women with RA is more evident at the hip than the spine, and the most important determinants of bone loss are disability and cumulative corticosteroid dose.[55]

The mechanism of corticosteroid-induced osteoporosis is uncertain, but it appears to be different from that of postmenopausal osteoporosis. Corticosteroid-induced osteoporosis is attributable, in part, to decreased osteoblast activity, decreased matrix synthesis, and decreased active life span of osteoblasts. In general, bone formation is decreased and bone resorption may be increased as well.[53] The degree of bone loss correlates to the dose of the corticosteroid and the duration of treatment; however, the absolute amount and duration of corticosteroid therapy have not been determined. When large corticosteroid doses are used, vertebral bone loss can be rapid, and compression fractures can occur within weeks to months after initiation of therapy.[53] D.L. has multiple risk factors for osteoporosis (young, female, and small stature); therefore, her bone mineral density (BMD) should be evaluated and a vertebral radiograph should be taken to look for a compression fracture. D.L.'s bone mineral density test results will determine whether she is a candidate for either primary or secondary prevention and treatment. Primary prevention with prophylactic calcium and calcitriol, with or without calcitonin, should be initiated for any patient with multiple risk factors who possibly will be maintained on the equivalent of prednisone 7.5 mg/day or more of corticosteroids.[53] Primary prevention is indicated for D.L. if her bone density is not decreased. Because D.L. has been taking prednisone 15 mg/day for an extended time, she most likely would require secondary prevention and treatment. Secondary prevention and treatment are indicated when bone density is low, regardless of whether fractures are present.[53] Primary and secondary interventions include the bisphosphonates, calcitriol (for primary prevention only), vitamin D and calcium, calcitonin, fluoride, and selective estrogen receptor modulators (e.g., raloxifene) for postmenopausal women (also see Chapter 48, The Transition Through Menopause). The statins may have promise as they have been preliminarily studied to have bone anabolic activity, block osteoporosis and osteonecrosis, resulting in lower rates of fractures in human studies.[56–58] For D.L., a bisphosphonate such as cyclical etidronate would be a good choice especially at the initiation of corticosteroid when bone loss is the worse. Although there is some concern with prolonged use of these agents in young individuals, due to their long retention in bones, this should not discourage their use when they are clearly indicated in young SLE patients. The bisphosphonates should not be used in pregnancy or moderate-severe renal failure, and their discontinuation should be considered when the corticosteroids doses have been substantially tapered with stabilization of BMD.[36] If she is not able to tolerate etidronate or if safety is a concern, calcitriol may be used, although it requires regular serum calcium monitoring at 4 weeks, 3 and 6 months, and 6-month intervals afterwards.[53] The pathogenesis of osteonecrosis is not well-known. Symptoms of osteonecrosis usually take a few months to a few years to develop after exposure to corticosteroids.[59,60] The risk increases with both the dose and duration of corticosteroid therapy. Corticosteroid therapies of short-term high doses, adrenal insufficiency replacement dose, and intraarticular injections have all been implicated.[36]

Gastrointestinal

16. C.W., a 66-year-old, 5 feet 6 inch, 68-kg woman, is newly diagnosed with PMR. She is an occasional drinker and smoker (1–2 packs/week). She started prednisone 15 mg/day and naproxen 500 mg Q 12 hr PRN 1 week ago and has shown dramatic improvement in the muscle pain of her shoulder and pelvic girdle. She comes in today to begin a taper of her prednisone and comments she's been having some "stomach" problems. What may be the cause of her stomach problems, and how may it be addressed?

Whether corticosteroids lead to peptic ulcer disease is controversial despite early observations of a probable correlation.[45,61,62] The prevalence of peptic ulcer disease is increased with the combined use of NSAIDs and corticosteroids.[63] Corticosteroids and NSAIDs commonly are prescribed concomitantly because many patients with connective tissue disorders have symptoms, such as arthralgias, inflammation, and pain. Corticosteroids can induce tissue atrophy and probably enhance the ulcerogenic potential of other drugs. The risk also depends on the underlying disease and the dose and duration of the steroid therapy. Several risk factors can contribute to C.W.'s stomach problems. First, she probably has been taking her prescribed naproxen, a nonspecific cyclooxygenase inhibitor (COX) for her chronic aches and pains until her diagnosis of PMR. The nonspecific COX inhibitors (see Chapter 43, Rheumatic Disorders) have been used significantly in the United States and are well documented to precipitate gastrointestinal complications. C.W. is also at increased risk for gastrointestinal complications because of her gender, advanced age, and her smoking and drinking history. At this time, she should have her naproxen switched to a COX-2 inhibitor (e.g., celecoxib, rofecoxib), which, theoretically, should be expected to decrease the potential for developing serious gastrointestinal complications, despite the paucity of substantive documentation. Because prednisone probably will be needed for an extended period by C.W., prophylactic therapy against ulceration may be reasonable.

Hyperglycemia

17. G.P., a 58-year-old man, has a medical history of dermatomyositis, type 2 diabetes mellitus (5 years), hypercholesterolemia, and obesity. G.P.'s current medications are prednisone 80 mg/day (started 2 months ago), lovastatin 20 mg Q HS, and glyburide 5 mg Q am. He came into clinic this morning with the following physical findings: weight, 285 lb; BP, 140/90 mmHg; pulse, 50 beats/minute and regular; and FPG, 189 mg/dL. G.P.'s diabetes

has been controlled for 3 years. What are likely explanations for his hyperglycemia?

[SI unit: FPG, 10.5 mmol/L]

Hyperglycemia in G.P. can be attributed to corticosteroid stimulation of gluconeogenesis or impairment of peripheral glucose utilization[36]; however, other etiologies (e.g., missed glyburide dose) also should be considered. Corticosteroids can promote pancreatic glucagon secretion with resultant glycogenolysis and formation of sugar from breakdown of amino acids and lactate produced during glycogenolysis. This process is not generally ketosis producing. Corticosteroids also decrease peripheral glucose utilization by decreasing glucose cell entry and cell membrane insulin receptors. The effects of the corticosteroids on carbohydrate metabolism in susceptible patient are dose related.[36] Increases in blood glucose are usually mild and dosages of prednisone as low as 15 mg/day can cause this effect. Alternate-day therapy has been proposed to minimize, but does not prevent, this adverse effect and in fact produces alternate-day hyperglycemia. Hyperglycemia peaks 2 to 4 hours after administration of the corticosteroid and can last from 12 to 24 hours, depending on the size of the dose.

G.P.'s diabetes has been well controlled in the past; therefore, immediate medication changes are not warranted. He should self-monitor his blood glucose (SMBG) on a regular basis and report the results on the next clinic visit. Corticosteroid-induced hyperglycemia can occur in nondiabetic patients as well. Blood sugars in many nondiabetic patients will return to normal as the patient adjusts to the excess glucose concentration. G.P.'s diabetes should be managed aggressively because he is overweight and at increased risk for cardiovascular complications with hypercholesterolemia. If his fasting blood glucose remains above the American Diabetes Association (ADA) guidelines on subsequent clinic visits, his glucose control may necessitate modifications in his medication management (e.g., increasing the glyburide dosage).

Ecchymosis

18. Several weeks after discharge, R.D. began noticing large purple blotches on her arms that did not blanch upon application of local pressure. Also, these "bruises" did not seem to disappear very rapidly. Why is this dermatologic effect probably prednisone induced?

Ecchymosis, easy bruisability, is a common side effect of prolonged corticosteroid use; it occurs most often in the elderly and is associated with continued use of supraphysiological corticosteroid doses.[39] Steroids destroy the collagen support of small blood vessels, resulting in leakage of blood into surrounding tissue. The anti-inflammatory effects of steroids reduce the normal resorption of blood leakage into tissue, making the "bruise" last longer. A reduction in the dosage of prednisone or the use of an alternate-day prednisone dosing regimen should lessen the purpura.[64] Unfortunately, patients such as R.D. often are already receiving the lowest dosage of corticosteroid that is compatible with keeping the clinical condition under control.

REFERENCES

1. Alarcon GS. Unclassified or undifferentiated connective tissue disease. In: Koopman WJ et al., eds. *Clinical Primer of Rheumatology*. Philadelphia: Lippincott Williams & Wilkins; 2003:213.
2. Kimberly RP. Connective-tissue diseases. In: Klippel JH et al., eds. *Primer of the Rheumatic Diseases*. 12th ed. Atlanta: Arthritis Foundation; 2001:325.
3. Krasner AS. Glucocorticoid-induced adrenal insufficiency. *JAMA* 1999;282:671.
4. Karpouzas FA et al. Systemic lupus erythematosus. In: Smolen JS et al., eds. *Targeted Therapies in Rheumatology*. London: Taylor & Francis Group PLC; 2003:563.
5. Hahn BH. Systemic lupus erythematosus. In: Braunwald E et al., eds. *Harrison's Principles of Internal Medicine*. 15th ed. New York: McGraw-Hill; 2001: 1922.
6. Callen JP. Lupus erythematosus. In: Callen JP et al., eds. *Dermatological Signs of Internal Disease*. 3rd ed. Philadelphia: WB Saunders; 2003:1.
7. Rus V et al. The epidemiology of systemic lupus erythematosus. In: Wallace DJ et al., eds. *Dubois's Lupus Erythematosus*. 6th ed. Philadelphia: Lippincott Williams & Wilkins; 2002:65.
8. McCarty DJ et al. Incidence of systemic lupus erythematosus. Race and gender differences. *Arthritis Rheum* 1995;38:1260.
9. Petri M. Systemic lupus erythematosus. In: Koopman WJ et al., eds. *Clinical Primer of Rheumatology*. Philadelphia: Lippincott Williams & Wilkins; 2003:164.
10. Sontheimer RD et al. Cutaneous manifestations of lupus erythematosus. In: Wallace DJ et al., eds. *Dubois' Lupus Erythematosus*. 6th ed. Philadelphia: Lippincott Williams & Wilkins; 2002:575.
11. Tan EM et al. The 1982 revised criteria for the classification of systemic lupus erythematosus. *Arthritis Rheum* 1982;25:1271.
12. Hochberg MC. Updating the American College of Rheumatology revised criteria for the classification of systemic lupus erythematosus. *Arthritis Rheum* 1997;40:1725.
13. Guidelines for referral and management of systemic lupus erythematosus in adults. American College of Rheumatology Ad Hoc Committee on Systemic Lupus Erythematosus Guidelines. *Arthritis Rheum* 1999;42:1785.
14. Morelock SY et al. Drugs and the pleura. *Chest* 1999;116:212.
15. Callen JP et al. Subacute cutaneous lupus erythematosus induced or exacerbated by terbinafine: a report of 5 cases. *Arch Dermatol* 2001;137:1196.
16. Crowson AN et al. Subacute cutaneous lupus erythematosus arising in the setting of calcium channel blocker therapy. *Hum Pathol* 1997;28:67.
17. Callen JP. Drug-induced cutaneous lupus erythematosus, a distinct syndrome that is frequently unrecognized. *J Am Acad Dermatol* 2001;45: 315.
18. Petri MA. Systemic lupus erythematosus: clinical aspects. In: Koopman WJ, ed. *Arthritis and Allied Conditions: A Textbook of Rheumatology*. 14th ed. Philadelphia: Lippincott William & Wilkins; 2001:1455.
19. Rubin RL. Drug-induced lupus. In: Wallace DJ et al., eds. *Dubois' Lupus Erythematosus*. 6th ed. Philadelphia: Lippincott Williams & Wilkins; 2002: 885.
20. Poza-Guedes P et al. Celecoxib-induced lupus-like syndrome. *Rheumatology (Oxford)* 2003;42:916.
21. Yung RL et al. Drug-induced lupus. *Rheum Dis Clin North Am* 1994;20:61.
22. Medsger TA Jr. Systemic sclerosis and Raynaud syndrome. In: Koopman WJ et al., eds. *Clinical Primer of Rheumatology*. Philadelphia: Lippincott Williams & Wilkins; 2003:171.
23. Legerton CW et al. Systemic sclerosis (scleroderma). Clinical management of its major complications. *Rheum Dis Clin North Am* 1995;21:203.
24. Salvarani C et al. Polymyalgia rheumatica and giant-cell arteritis. *N Engl J Med* 2002;347:261.
25. Kumar R. Polymyalgia rheumatica and temporal arteritis. In: Koopman WJ et al., eds. *Clinical Primer of Rheumatology*. Philadelphia: Lippincott William & Wilkins; 2003:207.
26. Kyle V et al. Polymyalgia rheumatica/giant cell arteritis in a Cambridge general practice. *Br Med J (Clin Res Ed)* 1985;291:385.
27. Swannell AJ. Polymyalgia rheumatica and temporal arteritis: diagnosis and management. *BMJ* 1997;314:1329.
28. Weyand CM et al. Corticosteroid requirements in polymyalgia rheumatica. *Arch Intern Med* 1999;159: 577.
29. Duhaut P et al. Giant cell arteritis, polymyalgia rheumatica, and viral hypotheses: a multicenter, prospective case-control study. Groupe de Recherche sur l'Arterite a Cellules Geantes. *J Rheumatol* 1999;26:361.
30. Evans JM et al. Polymyalgia rheumatica and giant cell arteritis. *Rheum Dis Clin North Am* 2000;26:493.
31. Amor B. Reiter's syndrome: diagnosis and clinical features. *Rheum Dis Clin North Am* 1998;24:677.
32. Hannu T et al. Chlamydia pneumoniae as a triggering infection in reactive arthritis. *Rheumatology (Oxford)* 1999;38:411.
33. Arnett FC. Seronegative spondyloarthropathies B. Reactive arthritis and enteropathy arthritis. In: Klippel JH et al., eds. *Primer on Rheumatic Diseases*. 12th ed. Atlanta: Arthritis Foundation; 2001:245.
34. Boulware DW et al. The seronegative spondyloarthropathies. In: Koopman WJ et al., eds. *Clinical Primer of Rheumatology*. Philadelphia: Lippincott Williams & Wilkins; 2003:127.

35. Dalakas MC. Polymyositis, dermatomyositis, and inclusion body myositis. In: Braunwald E et al., eds. *Harrison's Principles of Internal Medicine*. 15th ed. New York: McGraw-Hill; 2001:2524.
36. Kirou KA et al. Systemic glucocorticoid therapy in systemic lupus erythematosus. In: Wallace DJ et al., eds. *Dubois' Lupus Erythematosus*. 6th ed. Philadelphia: Lippincott Williams & Wilkins; 2002:1173.
37. Fullerton DS. Steroids and therapeutically related compounds. In: Delgado JN et al., eds. *Wilson and Gisvold's Textbook of Organic Medicinal and Pharmaceutical Chemistry*. 10th ed. Philadelphia: Lippincott-Raven; 1998:727.
38. Kehrl JH et al. The clinical use of glucocorticoids. *Ann Allergy* 1983;50:2.
39. Schimmer BP et al. Adrenocorticotropic hormone; adrenocortical steroids and their synthetic analogs; inhibitors of the synthesis and actions of adrenocortical hormones. In: Hardman JG et al., eds. *Goodman and Gilman's The Pharmacological Basis of Therapeutics*. 10th ed. New York: McGraw-Hill; 2001:1649.
40. Williams GH et al. Disorders of the adrenal cortex. In: Braunwald E et al., eds. *Harrison's Principle of Internal Medicine*. 15th ed. New York: McGraw-Hill; 2001:2084.
41. Petri M. Systemic lupus erythematosus (including pregnancy and antiphospholipid antibody syndrome). In: Weisman MH et al., eds. *Treatment of Rheumatic Diseases*. Philadelphia: WB Saunders; 2001:274.
42. Manzi S. Systemic lupus erythematosus. C. treatment. In: Klippel JH, ed. *Primer on the Rheumatic Diseases*. 12th ed. Atlanta: Arthritis Foundation; 2001:346.
43. Illei GG et al. Combination therapy with pulse cyclophosphamide plus pulse methylprednisolone improves long-term renal outcome without adding toxicity in patients with lupus nephritis. *Ann Intern Med* 2001;135:248.
44. Hahn BH. Management of systemic lupus erythematosus. In: Ruddy S et al., eds. *Kelley's Textbook of Rheumatology*. 6th ed. Philadelphia: WB Saunders; 2001:1125.
45. Baxter JD. Advances in glucocorticoid therapy. *Adv Intern Med* 2000;45:317.
46. Dickstein G et al. One microgram is the lowest ACTH dose to cause a maximal cortisol response: there is no diurnal variation of cortisol response to submaximal ACTH stimulation. *Eur J Endocrinol* 1997;137:172.
47. Abdu TA et al. Comparison of the low dose short synacthen test (1 microg), the conventional dose short synacthen test (250 microg), and the insulin tolerance test for assessment of the hypothalamo-pituitary-adrenal axis in patients with pituitary disease. *J Clin Endocrinol Metab* 1999;84:838.
48. Salem M et al. Perioperative glucocorticoid coverage: a reassessment 42 years after emergence of a problem. *Ann Surg* 1994;219:416.
49. Bishop CR et al. Leukokinetic studies. 13. A nonsteady-state kinetic evaluation of the mechanism of cortisone-induced granulocytosis. *J Clin Invest* 1968;47:249.
50. Walton J et al. Alternate-day vs. shorter-interval steroid administration. *Arch Intern Med* 1970;126:601.
51. Kountz DS et al. Safely withdrawing patients from chronic glucocorticoid therapy. *Am Fam Physician* 1997;55:521.
52. Stein MC et al. Glucocorticoids. In: Ruddy S et al., eds. *Kelley's Textbook of Rheumatology*. 6th ed. Philadelphia: WB Saunders; 2001:823.
53. Eastell R et al. A UK Consensus Group on management of glucocorticoid-induced osteoporosis: an update. *J Intern Med* 1998;244:271.
54. Eastell R. Management of corticosteroid-induced osteoporosis. UK Consensus Group Meeting on Osteoporosis. *J Intern Med* 1995;237:439.
55. Hall GM et al. The effect of rheumatoid arthritis and steroid therapy on bone density in postmenopausal women. *Arthritis Rheum* 1993;36:1510.
56. Wang PS et al. HMG-CoA reductase inhibitors and the risk of hip fractures in elderly patients. *JAMA* 2000;283:3211.
57. Meier CR et al. HMG-CoA reductase inhibitors and the risk of fractures. *JAMA* 2000;283:3205.
58. Schlienger R et al. HMG-CoA reductase inhibitors in osteoporosis: do they reduce the risk of fracture. *Drugs Aging* 2003;20:321.
59. Mankin HJ. Nontraumatic necrosis of bone (osteonecrosis). *N Engl J Med* 1992;326:1473.
60. Simkin PA et al. Osteonecrosis: pathogenesis and practicalities. *Hosp Pract (Off Ed)* 1994;29:73.
61. Keenan GF. Management of complications of glucocorticoid therapy. *Clin Chest Med* 1997;18:507.
62. Conn HO et al. Corticosteroids and peptic ulcer: meta-analysis of adverse events during steroid therapy. *J Intern Med* 1994;236:619.
63. Piper JM et al. Corticosteroid use and peptic ulcer disease: role of nonsteroidal anti-inflammatory drugs. *Ann Intern Med* 1991;114:735.
64. Yanovski JA et al. Glucocorticoid action and the clinical features of Cushing's syndrome. *Endocrinol Metab Clin North Am* 1994;23:487.

WOMEN'S HEALTH

CHAPTER 45

Contraception

Jennifer L. Hardman

The term "contraception" is defined as the intentional prevention of pregnancy. Contraceptives are therefore pharmaceuticals or devices that prevent pregnancy. The goal of contraception "therapy" is to prevent unintended pregnancy without causing adverse effects and to preserve fertility, when desired. Medically, pregnancy is defined by the U.S. Food and Drug Administration (FDA) and the National Institutes of Health (NIH) as being synonymous with implantation. An unintended pregnancy (also referred to as unplanned pregnancy) is a pregnancy that was unplanned or unwanted at the time of conception and includes pregnancies occurring in women who were using contraceptives during the month the pregnancy occurred.

In the United States, nearly half of all the pregnancies each year (~3 million) are unintended.[1] The rate of unintended pregnancy in the United States is higher than that of other developed countries with comparable medical resources.[2,3] Unintended pregnancy is common in the United States and affects women of all ages and socioeconomic groups. Although a significant number (47%) of unintended pregnancies occur in the 7% of women at risk for pregnancy who do not use a method of contraception, most unintended pregnancies (53%) occur in the 94% of women at risk for pregnancy who were using a contraceptive method during the month they became pregnant.[4] Unintended pregnancy rates are highest among women <18 years of age and decline with age until age 40. More than one-half of unintended pregnancies in the United States are terminated by elective abortion.[5] An unintended pregnancy has significant negative consequences to both the woman and to society. The consequences to a woman from an unintended pregnancy are obvious. The consequences to society are public health issues. An unintended pregnancy results in a lost opportunity to prepare for pregnancy in ways that reduce fetal and maternal morbidity and mortality, including folic acid supplementation, management of preexisting conditions, and changes in lifestyle, such as avoidance of alcohol or tobacco.

Contraception choices have medical, personal and public health considerations. The personal aspects include issues related to sexuality, religious, or cultural beliefs. Medical conditions that affect contraceptive selection or the risks associated with pregnancy also must be considered. Public health issues include relative risk from contraceptive use, medical complications of childbearing, and abortion rates. The safety and efficacy of contraceptive options have improved significantly; however, misconceptions regarding contraception are common. A 1993 Gallup poll found that 65% of women believe oral contraceptives are at least as risky as pregnancy.[6] The risk of death from pregnancy is more than five times the risk of death from oral contraceptive use in nonsmoking women. In the same Gallup survey, 58% of respondents could not name one noncontraceptive benefit from using oral contraceptives. The survey also found that 29% of women believed oral contraceptives cause cancer and 31% believed the failure rate to be at least 10%; both of these are incorrect. As members of the health care team, the pharmacist can play a critical role in helping women and their partners choose and use from the available methods as safely and effectively as possible.

Is it estimated that nearly 20% of adolescents have had sex before the age of 15. About 15% of 14-year-old girls who have had sex report having been pregnant.[7] Contraceptive policies in the United States and worldwide will help determine how quickly the population will grow and can help reduce the number of unwanted pregnancies.

MENSTRUAL CYCLE PHYSIOLOGY

Biological feedback mechanisms involving the hypothalamus, anterior pituitary gland, ovaries, and endometrial lining of the uterus control the average 28-day menstrual cycle.[8,9] The hypothalamus synthesizes gonadotropin-releasing hormone (GnRH) and secretes the hormone in a pulselike manner with varying frequencies throughout the menstrual cycle. GnRH stimulates the anterior pituitary to produce and release follicle-stimulating hormone (FSH) and luteinizing hormone (LH). FSH and LH act on the ovaries to produce estrogen and progesterone. Estrogen in turn acts on the hypothalamus and anterior pituitary, in a negative feedback manner, to stop FSH and LH secretion (Fig. 45-1).

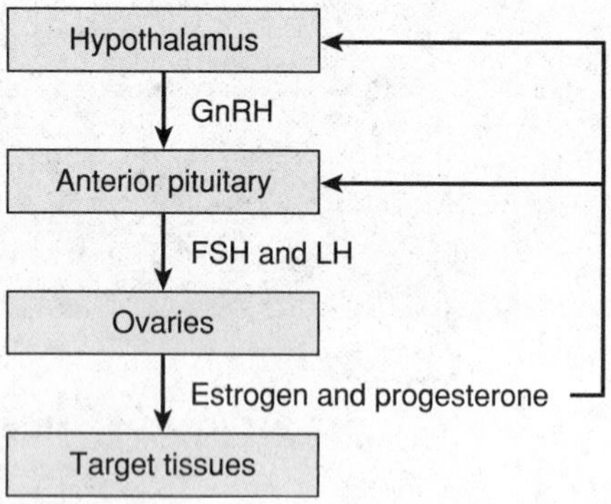

FIGURE 45-1 Menstrual cycle physiology. GnRH, gonadotropin-releasing hormone; FSH, follicle-stimulating hormone; LH, luteinizing hormone.

The menstrual cycle is divided into three phases: the follicular phase, ovulation, and the luteal phase (Fig. 45-2).[8,9] By convention, the day bleeding begins is referred to as the first day (or day 1) of the menstrual cycle. Menstrual bleeding usually occurs between days 1 to 5 of the cycle. The follicular phase begins at the onset of menstruation (menstrual phase) and lasts approximately 10 to 14 days (Fig. 45-2). Also at the beginning of the follicular phase, several follicles begin to develop within the ovary. In the second half of the follicular phase, most of the developing follicles atrophy except for one "dominant" follicle that will develop further and produce increasing amounts of estrogen. Elevated estradiol levels cause a surge of both LH and FSH. This LH surge is responsible for final-stage growth and maturation of the follicle, ovulation, and the formation of the corpus luteum. Ovulation usually occurs 14 days before the last day of the cycle. After ovulation, the dominant follicle develops further and produces estrogen and progesterone in increasing amounts. In 90% of women, the luteal phase lasts 13 to 15 days and is the least variable part of the human reproductive cycle. During this progesterone-dominant phase, the corpus luteum produces both progesterone and estrogen. Progesterone prepares the endometrium for implantation of a fertilized ovum. If implantation does not occur, corpus luteum regression causes a decrease in the levels of estrogen and progesterone. When these hormone levels decrease, the endometrium cannot be maintained and is sloughed off (menstrual phase). Using the average 28-day cycle as an example, day 28 is the last day of the cycle and is the day before bleeding begins again for the next menstrual cycle.

COMPARISON OF CONTRACEPTIVE METHOD EFFECTIVENESS

The effectiveness of any contraceptive method depends on its mechanism of action, availability (e.g., if a prescription is required, cost), adherence, and acceptability (e.g., side effects, ease of use, religious and social beliefs). Any or all of these reasons can account for the discrepancy between the lowest observed failure rate (so called "perfect use") and the actual failure rate in typical users observed in clinical practice. Table 45-1 compares the first-year failure rates of various contraceptive methods.[9]

HORMONAL CONTRACEPTION PHARMACOLOGY

Estrogens prevent the development of the dominant follicle by suppressing FSH secretion. Estrogens also stabilize the

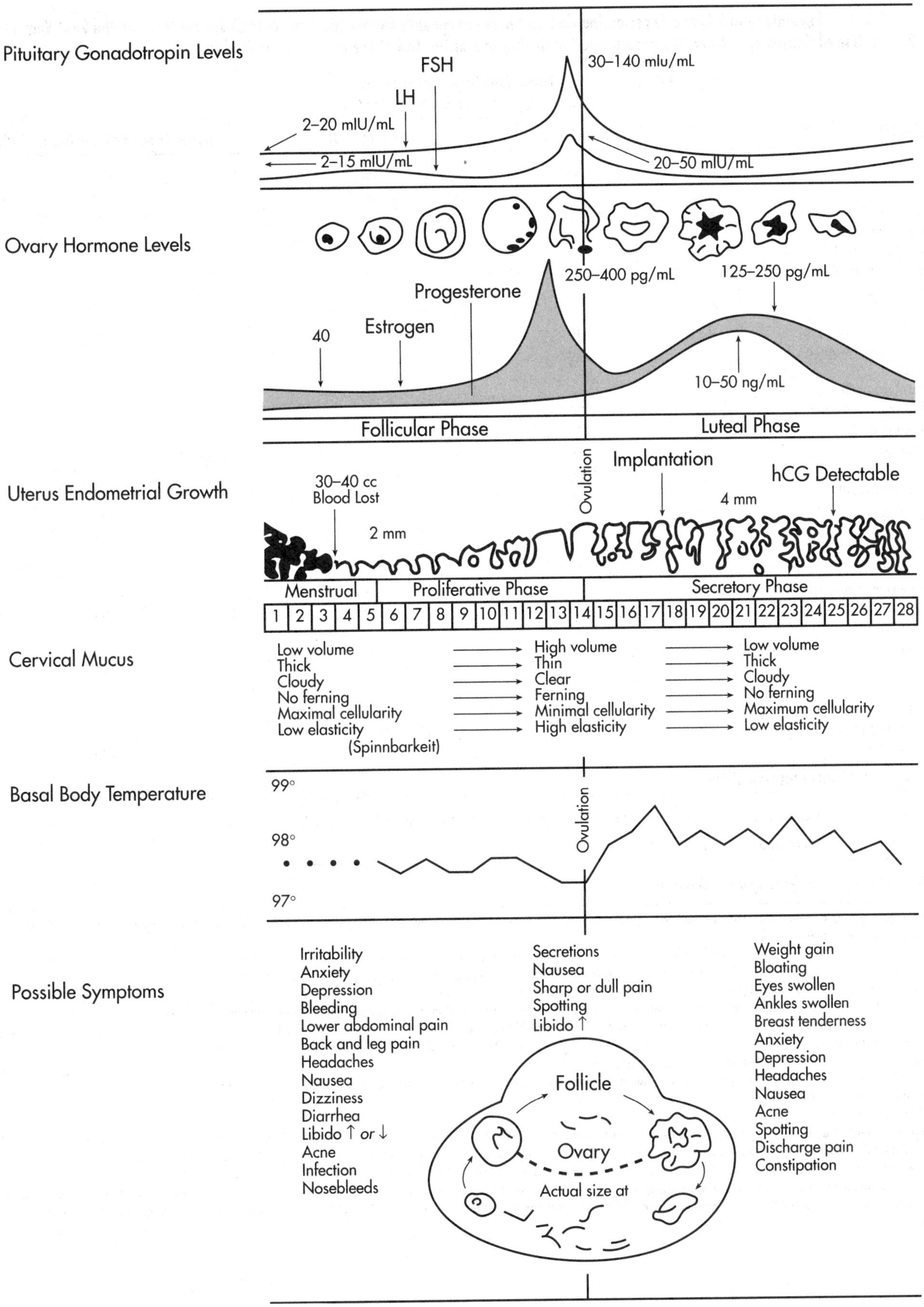

FIGURE 45-2 The menstrual cycle. FSH, follicle-stimulating hormone; hCG, human chorionic gonadotropin; LH, luteinizing hormone. (Adapted from Hatcher RA et al. *Contraceptive Technology*. 18th ed. New York: Ardent Media; 2004, with permission.)

Table 45-1 Percentage of Women Experiencing an Unintended Pregnancy During the First Year of Typical Use and the First Year of Perfect Use of Contraception and the Percentage Continuing Use at the End of the First Year: United States

	Women Experiencing an Unintended Pregnancy Within the First Year of Use (%)		
Method (1)	*Typical Use[a] (2)*	*Perfect Use[b] (3)*	*Women Continuing Use at One Year[c] (%) (4)*
Chance[d]	85	85	
Spermicides[e]	26	6	40
Periodic abstinence	25		63
Calendar		9	
Ovulation method		3	
Symptothermal[f]		2	
Postovulation		1	
Cap[g]			
Parous women	40	26	42
Nulliparous women	20	9	56
Sponge			
Parous women	40	20	42
Nulliparous women	20	9	56
Diaphragm[g]	20	6	56
Withdrawal	19	4	
Condom[h]			
Female (Reality)	21	5	56
Male	14	3	61
Pill	5		71
Progestin only		0.5	
Combined		0.1	
Intrauterine contraceptive device (IUD)			
Copper T 380A	0.8	0.6	78
LNg 20	0.1	0.1	81
Depo-Provera	0.3	0.3	70
Patch		1	
Ring		1–2	
Norplant and Norplant-2	0.05	0.05	88
Female sterilization	0.5	0.5	100
Male sterilization	0.15	0.10	100

Emergency Contraceptive Pills

Treatment initiated within 72 hr after unprotected intercourse reduces the risk of pregnancy by at least 75%.[i]

Lactational Amenorrhea Method (LAM)

LAM is a highly effective, *temporary* method of contraception.[j]

[a] Among *typical* couples who initiate use of a method (not necessarily for the first time), the percentage who experience an accidental pregnancy during the first year if they do not stop use for any other reason.

[b] Among couples who initiate use of a method (not necessarily for the first time) and who use it *perfectly* (both consistently and correctly), the percentage who experience an accidental pregnancy during the first year if they do not stop use for any other reason. For patch and ring, the percentage comes from the package insert.

[c] Among couples attempting to avoid pregnancy, the percentage who continue to use a method for 1 year.

[d] The percentages becoming pregnant in columns (2) and (3) are based on data from populations where contraception is not used and from women who cease using contraception to become pregnant. Among such populations, about 89% become pregnant within 1 year. This estimate was lowered slightly (to 85%) to represent the percentages who would become pregnant within 1 year among women now relying on reversible methods of contraception if they abandoned contraception altogether.

[e] Foams, creams, gels, vaginal suppositories, and vaginal film.

[f] Cervical mucus (ovulation) method supplemented by calendar in the preovulatory and basal body temperature in the postovulatory phases.

[g] With spermicidal cream or jelly.

[h] Without spermicides.

[i] The treatment schedule is one dose within 72 hours after unprotected intercourse, and a second dose 12 hours after the first dose. The U.S. Food and Drug Administration has declared the following brands of oral contraceptives to be safe and effective for emergency contraception: Ovral (1 dose is 2 white pills); Alesse (1 dose is 5 pink pills); Nordette or Levlen (1 dose is 4 light-orange pills); Lo/Ovral (1 dose is 4 white pills); Triphasil or Tri-Levlen (1 dose is 4 yellow pills).

[j] However, to maintain effective protection against pregnancy, another method of contraception must be used as soon as menstruation resumes, the frequency or duration of breastfeeding is reduced, bottle feeds are introduced, or the baby reaches 6 months of age. Adapted from Hatcher RA et al. *Contraceptive Technology*. 18th ed. New York: Ardent 2004.

Table 45-2 Commercially Available Brand-Name and Generic Oral Contraceptive and Progesterone-Only Pills

Brand Name	Generic Name	Progestin Type and Dose	EE Dose (mcg)	Progestin Activity	Estrogen Activity	Androgen Activity
Monophasic COC						
Alesse	Aviane	Levonorgestrel 0.1 mg	20	L	L	L
Demulen 1/35	Zovia 1/35	Ethynodiol diacetate 1 mg	35	H	L	L
Desogen	Apri	Desogestrel 0.15 mg	30	H	I	L
Levlen	Levora, Portia	Levonorgestrel 0.15 mg	30	I	L	I
Levlite	Lessina	Levonorgestrel 0.1 mg	20	L	L	L
Lo-Ovral	Cryselle, Low-Ogestrel	Norgestrel 0.3 mg	30	I	L	I
Loestrin 1.5/30[a]	Microgestin Fe 1.5/30	Norethindrone acetate 1.5 mg	30	H	L	H
Loestrin 1/20[a]	Microgestin Fe 1/20	Norethindrone acetate 1 mg	20	H	L	I
Mircette[b]	Kariva	Desogestrel 0.15 mg	20	H	L	L
Modicon	Brevicon, Nortel 0.5/35 Necon 0.5/35	Norethindrone 0.5 mg	35	L	H	L
Nordette	Levora, Portia	Levonorgestrel 0.15 mg	30	I	L	I
Ortho Cyclen	Sprintec, MonoNessa	Norgestimate 0.25 mg	35	L	I	L
Ortho-Cept	Apri	Desogestrel 0.15 mg	30	H	I	L
Ortho-Novum 1/35	Norinyl 1+ 35, Nortrel 1/35, Necon 1/35, Genora 1/35	Norethindrone 1 mg	35	I	H	I
Ovcon-35		Norethindrone 0.4 mg	35	L	H	L
Yasmin		Drosperinone 3 mg	30	No data	I	None
Biphasic COC						
Ortho-Novum 10/11	Necon 10/11, Jenest	Norethindrone 0.5, 1 mg	35	I	H	L
Triphasic COC						
Cyclessa		Desogestrel 0.1, 0.125 0.15 mg	25	H	L	L
Estrostep[a]		Norethindrone acetate 1 mg	20, 30, 35	H	L	I
Ortho Tri-Cyclen	Tri-Sprintec	Norgestimate 0.18, 0.215, 0.25 mg	35	L	I	L
Ortho Tri-Cyclen Lo		Norgestimate 0.18, 0.215, 0.25 mg	25	L	L	L
Ortho-Novum 7/7/7	Necon 7/7/7, Nortrel 7/7/7	Norethindrone 0.5, 0.75, 1 mg	35	I	H	L
Tri-Norinyl		Norethindrone 0.5, 1, 0.5 mg	35	L	H	L
Tri-Levlen	Enpresse, Trivora	Levonorgestrel 0.05, 0.075, 0.125 mg	30, 40, 30	L	I	L
Triphasil	Enpresse, Trivora	Levonorgestrel 0.05, 0.075, 0.125 mg	30, 40, 30	L	I	L
Progesterone-Only Pills						
Micronor	Errin	Norethinedrone 0.35 mg	None			
Nor-QD	Nora-BE, Camila	Norethinedrone 0.35 mg	None			
Ovrette		Norgestrel 0.075 mg	None			

[a] Also available with iron tablets instead of placebo tablets during the usual placebo week.
[b] as 2 days of placebo followed by 5 days of EE 10 mg during the usual placebo week.
COC, combined oral contraceptive; EE, ethinyl estradiol; H, high; I, intermediate; L, low.

endometrial lining to minimize the breakthrough bleeding seen with oral contraceptive (OC) use.[9,10]

Progestins have multiple mechanisms of action providing contraception. Progestins may prevent ovulation by suppressing LH secretion. In addition, progestins may impede the transport of sperm through the cervical canal by thickening cervical mucus. Progestins also may inhibit implantation by causing alterations or transformation of the endometrial lining or alter the transport of sperm or ovum within the fallopian s tubes.[9]

COMBINATION ORAL CONTRACEPTIVE PILLS (COC)

Manipulating the normal physiologic feedback mechanisms of the menstrual cycle using estrogen and progestin has proved to be an effective method of contraception. COC containing estrogen and a progestin and are the most commonly used reversible method of contraception in the United States. In 1960, the U.S. Food and Drug Administration (FDA) released the first COC, Enovid 10.[3,9] Enovid 10 (containing 150 mcg mestranol and 9.85 mg norethynodrel) contained much higher doses of estrogen and progestin than are in today's pills. The side effects caused by the early high dose COC prompted a search for lower dose, better tolerated products. Table 45-2 lists many of the available brand-name and generic COCs.

Currently available COCs are very effective in preventing pregnancy. The failure rate ranges from 0.1 to 5 pregnancies per 100 women-years (Table 45-1).[9] Virtually all of the COCs

Table 45-3 Estrogenic, Progestogenic, and Androgenic Effects of Oral Contraceptive Pills

Estrogenic Effects	*Progestogenic Effects*	*Androgenic Effects*
• Nausea • Increased breast size (ductal and fatty tissue) • Cyclic weight gain owing to fluid retention • Leukorrhea • Cervical eversion or ectopy • Hypertension • Rise in cholesterol concentration in gallbladder bile • Growth of leiomyomata • Telangiectasia • Hepatocellular adenomas or hepatocellular cancer (rare) • Cerebrovascular accidents (rare) • Thromboembolic complications including pulmonary emboli (rare) • Stimulation of breast neoplasia (exceedingly rare) (Most pills with >50 mcg of ethinyl estradiol do not produce troublesome estrogen-mediated side effects or complications.)	Both the estrogenic and the progestational components of oral contraceptives may contribute to the development of the following adverse effects: • Breast tenderness • Headaches • Hypertension • Myocardial infarction (rare)	All low-dose combined pills suppress a woman's production of testosterone, which has a beneficial effect on acne, oily skin, and hirsutism. The progestin component may have androgenic as well as progestational effects: • Increased appetite and weight gain • Depression, fatigue, tiredness • Decreased libido and/or enjoyment of intercourse • Acne, oily skin • Increased breast tenderness or breast size • Increased low-density lipoprotein (LDL) cholesterol levels • Decreased high-density lipoprotein (HDL) cholesterol levels • Decreased carbohydrate tolerance; increased insulin resistance • Pruritus

Adapted with permission from Hatcher RA et al. *Contraceptive Technology*. 18th ed. NY: Ardent Media; 2004:419, Table 19-4.

available in the United States contain the synthetic estrogen ethinyl estradiol (EE). Mestranol is another estrogen that has been used. Mestranol is inactive (prodrug) and is converted in the body to EE. Mestranol 50 mcg has approximately the same activity as EE 35 mcg.[3,9] COCs contain one of the following synthetic progestins: ethynodiol diacetate, desogestrel, drospirinone, levonorgestrel, norethindrone, norethindrone acetate, norgestimate, or norgestrel. Norgestrel is a mixture of dextronorgestrel and levonorgestrel. Dextronorgestrel appears to be progestationally inert compared with levonorgestrel.[3,10] These progestins differ significantly in their progestational potency and also in the extent of their metabolism to estrogenic substances. Progestins have both estrogenic and antiestrogenic effects. Because the progestins have a chemical structure similar to that of 19-nortestosterone, they have varying degrees of androgenic activity (Table 45-3).[10] The androgenic effects are largely mitigated by the estrogen-induced increase in sex-hormone binding globulin (SHBG), which binds progestins. Minor structural changes in all of the progestins may lead to significant changes in their progestational, estrogenic, antiestrogenic, and androgenic activities in tissue culture. The clinical significance of these differences may vary widely in effect from woman to woman (Table 45-2).

Different terminology is used to describe the classes of pills that have been approved over the years. The COCs most commonly used today are also called "low-dose" COCs. They contain <35 mcg/day of EE. In the literature, COCs have been referred to by "generations," as well.[8,11] First-generation COCs contain >50 mcg/day of EE and are not currently in use. Second-generation COCs contain 30 to 35 mcg of EE with one of the following progestins levonorgestrel, norgestimate, norethindrone, norethindrone acetate, or ethynodiol diacetate. Third-generation COCs contain desogestrel and 20 to 30 mcg EE. There are also references to generations related to the progestin used. First-generation progestins include norethindrone and its derivatives. Second-generation progestins include levonorgestrel and norgestrel, and third-generation progestins include desogestrel, norgestimate, and gestodene (gestodene is not available in the United States).[3,10]

Contraindications to Oral Contraceptive Use

1. M.F., a healthy 32-year-old woman, wants to know if she is a good candidate for COC. She smokes a pack of cigarettes per day. What contraindications to COC therapy must be considered? Is she a good candidate for COC?

To determine if any contraindications or precautions exist, the clinician should first obtain baseline health information from M.F.[10] (Table 45-4). M.F. should be encouraged to stop smoking. She does not currently have any contraindications to COC use, but she should be informed that COCs may no longer be prescribed for her in a few years if she continues to smoke (see Question 8). Because she does not have any medical problems, she is an acceptable candidate for a COC.

Choice

2. M.F. has decided to start COC. Which COC should be selected for her?

All COCs are considered to be equally effective. For most women, the selection of any product containing 35 mcg or less of EE is preferred. Few studies have compared one product with another. For some women, formulary restrictions may also need to be considered. The information in Figure 45-3 may be used to select an initial COC or to change pill formulations

Table 45-4 Medical Eligibility Criteria for Contraceptive Use

Condition	OC	CIC	POP	DMPA	Norplant	Cu-IUD	LNG-IUD
	Contraceptive Method						
				I = Initiation, C = Continuation			
Personal Characteristics and Reproductive History							
Smoking							
a) Age <35	2	2	1	1	1	1	1
b) Age >35							
(i) <15 cigarettes/day	3	2	1	1	1	1	1
(ii) >15 cigarettes/day	4	3	1	1	1	1	1
Obesity >30 kg/m122 body mass index (BMI)	2	2	1	2	2	1	2
Cardiovascular Disease							
Multiple Risk Factors for Arterial Cardio-vascular Disease (e.g., older age, smoking, diabetes and hypertension)	3/4	3/4	2	3	2	1	2
Hypertension							
a) History of hypertension where blood pressure *cannot* be evaluated (including hypertension during pregnancy)	3	3	2	2	2	1	2
b) Adequately controlled hypertension, where blood pressure *can* be evaluated	3	3	1	2	1	1	1
c) Elevated blood pressure levels (properly taken measurements)							
(i) Systolic 140–159 or diastolic 90–99	3	3	1	2	1	1	1
(ii) Systolic >160 or diastolic >100	4	4	2	3	2	1	2
d) Vascular disease	4	4	2	3	2	1	2
History of High Blood Pressure During Pregnancy (where current blood pressure is measurable and normal) Deep Venous Thrombosis (DVT) or Pulmonary Embolism (PE)	2	2	1	1	1	1	1
a) History of DVT/PE	4	4	2	2	2	1	2
b) Current DVT/PE	4	4	3	3	3	1	3
c) Family history (first-degree relatives)	2	2	1	1	1	1	1
d) Major surgery							
(i) With prolonged immobilization	4	4	2	2	2	1	2
(ii) Without prolonged immobilization	2	2	1	1	1	1	1
e) Minor surgery without immobilization	1	1	1	1	1	1	1
Superficial Venous Thrombosis							
a) Varicose veins	1	1	1	1	1	1	1
b) Superficial thrombophlebitis	2	2	1	1	1	1	1
Stroke (history of cerebrovascular accident)			I C		I C		
	4	4	2 3	3	2 3	1	2
Known Hyperlipidemias (screening is NOT necessary for safe use of contraceptive methods)	4	4	2	2	2	1	2
Neurologic Conditions							
Headaches	I C	I C	I C	I C	I C		I C
a) Nonmigrainous (mild or severe)	1 2	1 2	1 1	1 1	1 1	1	1 1
b) Migraine							
(i) Without focal neurologic symptoms							
Age <35	2 3	2 3	1 2	2 2	2 2	1	2 2
Age >35	3 4	3 4	1 2	2 2	2 2	1	2 2
(ii) With focal neurologic symptoms (at any age)	4 4	4 4	2 3	2 3	2 3	1	2 3
Epilepsy	1	1	1	1	1	1	1

(continued)

Table 45-4 Medical Eligibility Criteria for Contraceptive Use *(Continued)*

Condition	*OC*	*CIC*	*POP*	*DMPA*	*Norplant*	*Cu-IUD*	*LNG-IUD*
	Contraceptive Method						
Reproductive Tract Infections and Disorders							
Unexplained Vaginal Bleeding (suspicious for serious condition)						I C	I C
Before evaluation	2	2	2	3	3	4 2	4 2
Endometriosis	1	1	1	1	1	2	1
Benign Ovarian Tumors (including cysts)	1	1	1	1	1	1	1
Cervical Intraepithelial Neoplasia (CIN)	2	2	1	2	2	1	2
Cervical Cancer (awaiting treatment)						I C	I C
	2	2	1	2	2	4 2	4 2
Breast Disease							
a) Undiagnosed mass	2	2	2	2	2	1	2
b) Benign breast disease	1	1	1	1	1	1	1
c) Family history of cancer	1	1	1	1	1	1	1
d) Cancer							
(i) Current	4	4	4	4	4	1	4
(ii) Past and no evidence of current disease for 5 years	3	3	3	3	3	1	3
Endometrial Cancer						I C	I C
	1	1	1	1	1	4 2	4 2
Ovarian Cancer						I C	I C
	1	1	1	1	1	3 2	3 2
Uterine Fibroids							
a) Without distortion of the uterine cavity	1	1	1	1	1	1	1
b) With distortion of the uterine cavity	1	1	1	1	1	4	4
Pelvic Inflammatory Disease (PID)							
a) Past PID (assuming no current risk factors of STD)						I C	I C
(i) With subsequent pregnancy	1	1	1	1	1	1 1	1 1
(ii) Without subsequent pregnancy	1	1	1	1	1	2 2	2 2
b) PID-current or within the last 3 months	1	1	1	1	1	4 2	4 2
HIV or AIDS							
High Risk of HIV	1	1	1	1	1	2	2
HIV-Positive	1	1	1	1	1	2	2
AIDS	1	1	1	1	1	3/2	3/2
Endocrine Conditions							
Diabetes							
a) History of gestational disease	1	1	1	1	1	1	1
b) Nonvascular disease							
(i) Noninsulin dependent	2	2	2	2	2	1	2
(ii) Insulin dependent	2	2	2	2	2	1	2
c) Nephropathy, retinopathy, or neuropathy	3/4	3/4	2	3	2	1	2
d) Other vascular disease or diabetes of >20 years' duration	3/4	3/4	2	3	2	1	2
Gastrointestinal Conditions							
Gallbladder Disease							
a) Symptomatic							
(i) Treated by cholecystectomy	2	2	2	2	2	1	2
(ii) Medically treated	3	2	2	2	2	1	2
(iii) Current	3	2	2	2	2	1	2
b) Asymptomatic	2	2	2	2	2	1	2

Table 45-4 Medical Eligibility Criteria for Contraceptive Use *(Continued)*

	Contraceptive Method						
Condition	*OC*	*CIC*	*POP*	*DMPA*	*Norplant*	*Cu-IUD*	*LNG-IUD*
Viral Hepatitis							
a) Active	4	3/4	3	3	3	1	3
b) Carrier	1	1	1	1	1	1	1
Cirrhosis							
a) Mild (compensated)	3	2	2	2	2	1	2
b) Severe (decompensated)	4	3	3	3	3	1	3
Liver Tumors							
a) Benign (adenoma)	4	3	3	3	3	1	3
b) Malignant (hepatoma)	4	3/4	3	3	3	1	3
Anemias							
Sickle Cell Disease	2	2	1	1	1	2	1
Iron Deficiency Anemia	1	1	1	1	1	2	1

1, a condition for which there is no restriction for the use of the contraceptive method;
2, a condition where the advantages of using the method generally outweigh the theoretical or proven risks;
3, a condition where the theoretical or proven risks usually outweigh the advantages of using the method;
4, a condition which represents an unacceptable health risk if the contraceptive method is used.
AIDS, acquired immunodeficiency syndrome; CIC, combined injectable contraceptive; Cu-IUD, copper intrauterine device; DMPA, depot medroxyprogesterone acetate; HIV, human immunodeficiency virus; LNG-IUD, levonorgestrel intrauterine device; OC, oral contraceptive; POP, progestin-only pills; STD, sexually transmitted diseases.
Adapted from reference 10, with permission.

if side effects become intolerable.[10] Any pill containing 20 to 35 mcg EE can be used for M.F. because she is a healthy woman without medical complications. Her blood pressure and weight should be obtained before starting the pills A body weight >70.5 kg has been associated in some studies with increased COC failure, therefore a product with a higher dose of EE (e.g., 35 mcg) may be a better choice if she weighs more than 70.5 kg.[12]

21-Day versus 28-Day Cycle

Most 28-day COC pill packs contain 21 days of active pills (pills that contain estrogen and progestin) followed by 7 days of placebo or iron tablets. The 21-day pill packs contain only the active pills. Many clinicians prefer the use of 28-day cycle COC to minimize confusion and to promote adherence. With a 28-day pack, users take one tablet daily regardless of whether it is in the active or placebo phase of the cycle. After taking the last tablet of a 28-day pack, a new pack should started the next day. When continuous ovarian suppression is used for extended cycles or to treat estrogen-dependent disorders, such as endometriosis, the 21-day cycle packs may preferred. Many products are only available in 28-day cycle packs. If M.F. will not be taking a COC continuously, a 28-day pack is recommended.

Multiphasic Oral Contraceptives

3. Should M.F. start a monophasic or triphasic COC? What are the advantages and disadvantages of the triphasic products relative to other regimens?

Because of metabolic and physiologic effects related to the progestin component of monophasic COCs, the biphasic and triphasic products were formulated to contain a lower total monthly dose of progestin than the monophasic products (with the exception of Mircette). These products attempt to lower doses of progestin and provide adequate endometrial support while also providing adequate contraception.[11]

The multiphasic products contain varying amounts of progestin and estrogen during each of the active phases. Currently, Necon 10/11, Ortho-Novum 10/11, and Jenest 28 are the only biphasic COCs marketed in the United States, and they are rarely used. Mircette can be classified as either a monophasic or biphasic OC. Mircette provides a novel regimen containing 21 days of 0.15 mg desogestrel plus 20 mcg EE (fixed doses as with a monophasic product), then only 2 days of placebo, and finally followed by 5 days of 10 mcg EE alone. The woman does not need to take missed 10 mcg EE doses or use a backup method if those tablets are missed. The 5 days of 10 mcg EE alone help minimize breakthrough bleeding with this product and may be useful for women who have estrogen deficiency symptoms, such as headaches, during the hormone-free week.

The triphasic COCs (e.g., Ortho-Novum 7/7/7, Tri-Levlen, Triphasil, Ortho Tri-Cyclen) appear to support the endometrium more consistently than the biphasic COCs.[13] No studies, however, show superior efficacy of one triphasic over another or over monophasic COCs. The reduced progestin content may be desirable for women who experience progestin-related side effects caused by too much progestin or for women who have cardiovascular disease or metabolic abnormalities.[9,14] Women with side effects related to progestin deficiency (e.g., late-cycle bleeding) who desire extended cycles or who have conditions necessitating progestin dominance (e.g., benign breast disease) may do better with a monophasic formulation.

One drawback associated with triphasic COC use is the confusion caused by the different-colored tablets in each of the three different phases, making the missed-dose instructions more complicated. Monophasic formulations are preferred for women who will be taking pills continuously (i.e., skipping the placebo pills). M.F. may be started on either a monophasic or triphasic product.

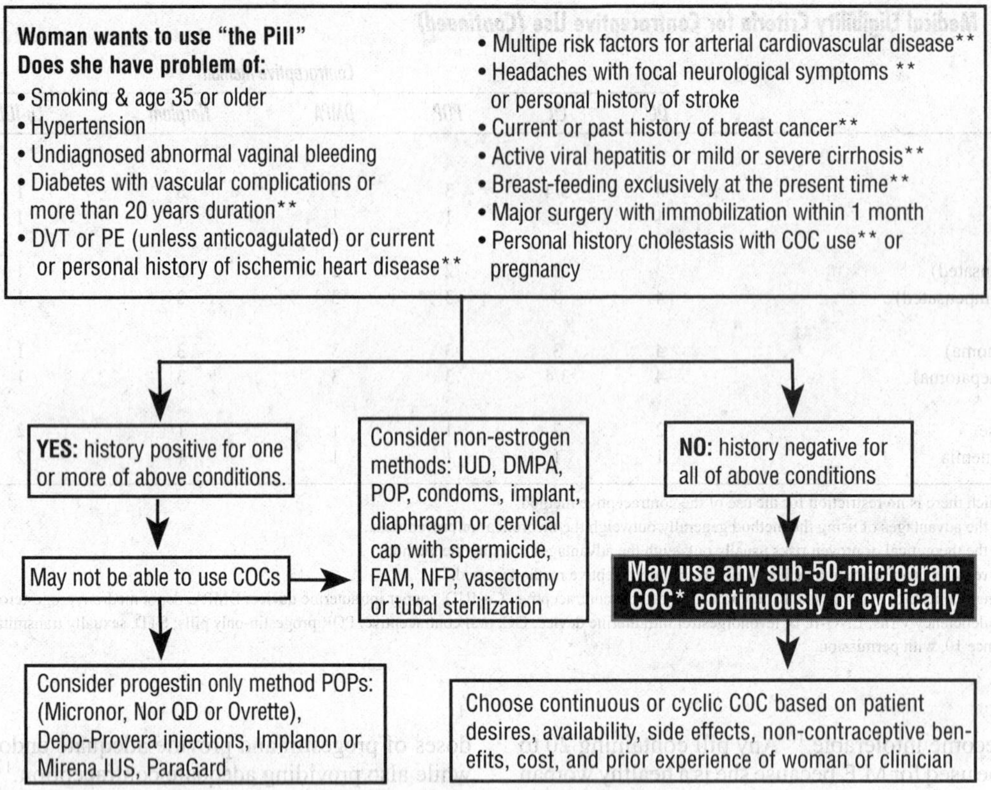

Woman wants to use "the Pill"
Does she have problem of:
• Smoking & age 35 or older
• Hypertension
• Undiagnosed abnormal vaginal bleeding
• Diabetes with vascular complications or more than 20 years duration**
• DVT or PE (unless anticoagulated) or current or personal history of ischemic heart disease**
• Multipe risk factors for arterial cardiovascular disease**
• Headaches with focal neurological symptoms ** or personal history of stroke
• Current or past history of breast cancer**
• Active viral hepatitis or mild or severe cirrhosis**
• Breast-feeding exclusively at the present time**
• Major surgery with immobilization within 1 month
• Personal history cholestasis with COC use** or pregnancy
YES: history positive for one or more of above conditions.
May not be able to use COCs
Consider non-estrogen methods: IUD, DMPA, POP, condoms, implant, diaphragm or cervical cap with spermicide, FAM, NFP, vasectomy or tubal sterilization
Consider progestin only method POPs: (Micronor, Nor QD or Ovrette), Depo-Provera injections, Implanon or Mirena IUS, ParaGard
NO: history negative for all of above conditions
May use any sub-50-microgram COC* continuously or cyclically
Choose continuous or cyclic COC based on patient desires, availability, side effects, non-contraceptive benefits, cost, and prior experience of woman or clinician

- The World Health Organization and the Food and Drug administration both recommend using the **lowest dose pill** that is effective. All combined pills with less that 50 μg of estrogen are considered "low –dose" and are effective and safe
- There are no studies demonstrating a decreased risk for deep vein thrombosis (DVT) in women on 20-μg pills. Data on higher dose pills have demonstrated that the less the estrogen dose, the lower the risk for DVT
- All COC's lower free testosterone. Class labeling in Canada for all combined pills states that use of pills may improve acne
- To minimize discontinuation due to spotting and breakthrough bleeding, warn women in advance, reassure that spotting and breakthrough bleeding become better over time.
- The package insert for women on Yasmin and Yaz states *[Berlex-2001]*: "Yasmin is different from other birth control pills because it contains the progestin drospirenone. Drospirenone may increase potassium. Therefore, you should not take Yasmin if you have kidney, liver or adrenal disease, because this could cause serious heart and health problems. Other drugs may also increase potassium. If you are currently on daily, long term treatment for a chronic condition with any of the medications below, you should consult your healthcare provider about whether Yasmin is right for you, and during the first month that you take Yasmin, you should have a blood test to check your potassium level: NSAIDs (ibuprofen [Motrin®, Advil®], naproxen [Naprosyn®, Aleve®, and others] when taken long-term and daily for treatment of arthritis or other problems]; potassium-sparing diuretics (spironolactone and others); potassium supplementation; ACE inhibitors (Capoten®, Vasotec®, Zestrik® and others); Angiotensin-II receptor antagonists (Cozaar®, Diovan®, Avapro®and others); heparin"

**These are conditions that receive a WHO:3 or a WHO:4

FIGURE 45-3 Choosing a pill.

Reprinted with permission from Zieman M, Hatcher RA, Managing Contraception 2007–2009 (fig 26–2).

Patient Instructions

4. **M.F. has heard that she can skip periods by skipping the placebos. What can you tell her about this? What instructions should be given to M.F. about her COC?**

When to Start Oral Contraceptives

M.F. should start the first cycle of pills according to the manufacturer's package instructions or according to one of the following recommendations:[9,10]

1. Day 1 Start: Take the first tablet in the pack on the first day of menses. This offers the advantage of more rapid contraceptive effects.
2. Sunday Start: Take the first tablet in the pack on the first Sunday after the beginning of menstruation. If menses begins on Sunday, start that day. Back-up contraception must be used for at least the first 7 days. The advantage is that bleeding usually does not occur on weekends.
3. Quick Start: This is a newer method for initiating COC.[15] In Quick Start, the woman takes her first COC tablet at any

point in her cycle. She also uses back-up contraception for at least 7 days. This method can minimize confusion about when to start the first pack and can increase rates of method continuation. The quick start method provides contraceptive protection sooner and, therefore, would likely lower the risk of unintended pregnancy.

Any woman who is a candidate for COCs can use them continuously (i.e. skipping the placebo tablets and taking no break between pill packs). Any product may be used continuously, however monophasic pills usually are selected. Any duration of continuous pill use is acceptable, but many providers recommend taking the active pills from 3 to 4 pill packs and then stopping for 2-7 days. Alternatively, providers may prescribe products that are specifically packaged for continuous use (Seasonale and generics, Seasonique, Lybrel). Continuous pill use usually results in more breakthrough bleeding or spotting (see question 8) than usual pill use, so women should be informed about this. If M.F. is willing to tolerate more irregular bleeding during the first 6-12 months of continuous COC use, then she can use them continuously.

When to Use a Back-Up Method of Contraception

Some clinicians recommend that women use an alternative method of contraception (back-up) for the entire first cycle. Using a back-up method for one full cycle is recommended because many new users of COCs do not complete the first cycle of pills. Most pill package inserts state that a back-up method of contraception (e.g., condoms) is not necessary if women use the Day 1 start method.[9,16] When using the Sunday start or Quick start methods, back-up contraception should be used for the first week (7 days) of the cycle. A back-up method is also recommended when doses are missed, as described in the following section. M.F. has decided to use the Sunday start method, so she will need to use a back-up method (e.g., condoms, diaphragm) for the first week of the cycle.

Proper Pill Taking

M.F. should take the COC tablets at exactly the same time each day. If she experiences nausea, she may find that the nausea is reduced if she takes her pill at bedtime or with food. The best time for pills to be taken depends on her schedule. The optimal time for M.F. is the time when she will have the fewest problems remembering to take her pill. Missed pills are common in COC users; estimates as high as 40% of users miss one pill in each cycle, therefore reviewing the instructions for missed pills is an important part of medication counseling.

If M.F. forgets to take one pill, she should take the missed pill as soon as she remembers and refer to the instructions in the package insert for further information.[9,10,16] Most manufacturers recommend that if one pill is missed, the woman should take two pills when she remembers (e.g., if she forgets to take her one pill on Monday, she should take two pills on Tuesday when she remembers). Then, she should take the remaining pills in the pack as usual. A back-up method of contraception usually is not considered necessary. If she misses two tablets in a row in weeks 1 or 2 of her pack, she should take two pills on the day she remembers and two the following day (e.g., if she forgets her pill on Monday and Tuesday, she should take two pills on Wednesday and two on Thursday). Then, she should take the remaining pills as usual. She should use an alternative method of contraception for 7 days of taking active pills.

If a woman misses two tablets in a row in the third week (for Day 1 starters), she can either discard the rest of the pack and start a new pack on that same day or continue taking one pill daily until her usual stop day (skipping the placebos) and start a new pack. For Sunday starters, she can continue taking one pill every day until Sunday and start a new pack on Sunday without taking the placebos. She must use an alternative method of contraception for 7 days after missing the pills. She may not have her menstrual period this month.

If a woman misses three or more pills in a row anytime during the period taking the active pills she will likely experience bleeding or spotting. At the time she remembers, she can discard the rest of her pack and start a new pack that same day; or Sunday starters should keep taking one pill every day until Sunday, then start a new pack on Sunday. After missing three pills, she should use an alternative method of contraception for 7 days of taking active pills. She may not have a menstrual period this month. She may also want to consider emergency contraception if she has been sexually active (see Question 44).

Drug Interactions

Antibacterials

5. G.H. is a 26-year-old woman whose last menstrual period (LMP) was 7 weeks ago. She has a history of regular menstrual cycles both before and during the use of COC. Six weeks ago, she developed an *Escherichia coli* urinary tract infection and was treated with oral (PO) sulfamethoxazole trimethoprim (TMP-SMX) BID × 3 days for 7 days. This coincided with the first seven tablets of her cycle. She has been taking Ortho-Novum 1/35 for 3 years and tetracycline 250 mg PO every day (QD) for acne. What is the clinical significance of the potential drug interactions in G.H.?

Ethinyl estradiol is conjugated in the liver, excreted in the bile, hydrolyzed by intestinal bacteria, and reabsorbed as active drug.[17] Certain broad-spectrum antibiotics, by reducing the population of intestinal bacteria, may interrupt the enterohepatic circulation of the estrogen, resulting in a decreased concentration of circulating estrogen. The existence of similar antibiotic interactions with contraceptive progestins is unlikely. Although this mechanism for the drug interaction is not well established, various antibiotics have been reported to decrease COC efficacy, resulting in unintended pregnancy or abnormal bleeding patterns. The antibiotics rifampin and griseofulvin are known to cause contraceptive failure, but NOT by this mechanism. These agents reduce contraceptive efficacy by increasing the metabolism of estrogen.

Theoretically, any broad-spectrum antimicrobial with significant effects on intestinal bacterial flora could affect COC efficacy by interfering with the enterohepatic recycling of exogenous estrogen. Numerous reports of changes in bleeding patterns and contraceptive failure have been documented.[17] About 30 case reports of contraceptive failure with concomitant COC and antibiotic use have been published. The antibiotics in the case reports include rifampin, ampicillin, penicillin G, tetracycline, and minocycline.[17a] In addition, surveys of women in clinics have revealed about 20 other cases of

OC failure. A major limitation of survey data is that it relies on patients' memories, which are often unreliable. The Committee on the Safety of Medicines in the United Kingdom received 63 reports of unplanned pregnancies between 1968 and 1984 in women on antibiotics and COC. Penicillins, tetracyclines, sulfamethoxazole-trimethoprim, metronidazole, cephalosporins, and erythromycin were among the antibiotics used. Finally, more than 200 reports of COC failure have been documented in women seeking family planning services.

The probability of a clinically significant drug interaction between COC and antimicrobials depends on several factors: the hormonal content of the COC relative to the woman's requirements, the dosage and duration of use of the interacting drug, variation in the response to bacterial flora alteration, and her inherent fertility.[17,18,19] The number and complexity of these variables make prediction of outcome in a specific woman exceedingly difficult. Even if a drug produces a several-fold increase in unwanted pregnancies in women taking COC, the likelihood of pregnancy in a given woman is still low because COC are so effective. Long-term, low-dose tetracycline use for G.H.'s acne therapy (tetracycline 250 mg daily) is unlikely to interfere with her COC efficacy, but no good data exist to support this supposition. Topical antibiotics often can control acne, do not interfere with COC, and can be recommended as alternatives to oral tetracycline.[17]

A practical approach to managing coadministration of COC and antibiotics is to educate women about the potential for increased risk of pregnancy and to recommend a back-up method of contraception until menses occurs. In addition, the clinician should discuss what is described in the literature about these interactions (Table 45-5). Whether TMP-SMX inhibits COC efficacy is not certain; however, clinical data are consistent with the premise that it occasionally impairs COC efficacy. In this case, G.H. should take a pregnancy test.

Liver Enzyme Induction

6. S.R., a 22-year-old woman, is taking phenytoin (Dilantin) 300 mg PO QD and phenobarbital 60 mg PO twice daily (BID). Her serum concentrations of these drugs have been consistently in the therapeutic range for at least 2 years, and she has not experienced seizures for 18 months. Is S.R. a good candidate for COC?

Ethinyl estradiol is a substrate of cytochrome P450 3A4 (CYP3A4); therefore, medications that induce CYP3A4 may decrease COCs efficacy. With the older high-dose COCs, efficacy was not decreased significantly by many drug–drug interactions because of their high hormone content. The estrogen and progestin doses in newer COC are much lower. The case reports of menstrual irregularities (e.g., spotting, breakthrough bleeding [BTB]) and unintended pregnancies attributable to drug interactions have been increasing with lower dose formulation (Table 45-5).

Carbamazepine, phenytoin, phenobarbital, and primidone are CYP3A4 inducers known to cause increased metabolism of COCs. Another inducer of CYP3A4 is St. John's wort.[20] The newer anticonvulsants topiramate and oxcarbazepine have also been shown to lower serum levels of estrogen.

Although drug interactions that reduce the efficacy of contraceptives are of the greatest concern, COCs also can affect

Table 45-5 Oral Contraceptive Drug Interactions

Interacting Drug	*Net Effect*
Drugs that increase or may increase the metabolism of OCs	
	Spotting, breakthrough bleeding, or pregnancy
Aprepitant	
Bexarotene	
Bosentan	
Carbamazepine	
Darunavir	
Felbamate	
Fosphenytoin/Phenytoin	
Griseofulvin	
Modafanil	
Mycophenolate mofetil	
Nevirapine	
Oxcarbazepine	
Phenobarbital	
Pioglitazone	
Primidone	
Rifabutin	
Rifampin	
Ritonavir	
Secobarbital	
St John's Wort	
Topiramate	
Miscellaneous drug interactions with OCs	
Amprenavir/ fosamprenavir	Decrease concentrations of amprenavir; increase or decrease concentrations of EE or progestin
Atanazir	Increase in EE concentrations
Atorvastatin	30% increase in norethindrone concentration; 20% increase in EE concentration
Benzodiazepines	Reduced metabolism of benzodiazepines
Corticosteroids	Reduced metabolism of corticosteroids
Cyclosporine	Doubling of cyclosporine level
Fluconazole	Increase or decrease in EE and levonorgestrel levels
Fosphenytoin/ Phenytoin	Increase or decrease in phenytoin concentration
Ginseng	Additive estrogenic effects
Lamotrigine	Increase or decrease in lamotrigine concentration
Nelfnavir	Increase or decrease in EE and progestin concentrations
Paclitaxel	Reduced metabolism of paclitaxel
Red Clover	May increase or decrease OC effects
Rosuvastatin	Increase in EE and norgestrel concentrations
Selegiline	Increase in selegiline concentration
Succinylcholine	Inhibits plasma cholinesterase activity
Tacrine	Increase in tacrine concentrations
Tacrolimus	Increase in tacrolimus concentrations
Theophylline	33% reduction in theophylline clearance
Tizanidine	50% reduction in tizanidine clearance
Tricyclic antidepressants	Decreased antidepressant effects yet can cause TCA toxicity
Valdecoxib	Increase in EE and norethindrone concentrations
Voriconazole	Increase in EE, norethindrone and valdecoxib concentrations
Warfarin	Increase of decrease in anticoagulation
Zolmitriptan	Increase in adverse effects

AUC, area under the time-concentration curve; EE, ethinyl estradiol; OC, oral contraceptives.

DRUGDEX® System (electronic version). Klasco RK (ed) Thomson Healthcare, Greenwood Village, Colorado, USA. Available at: http://csi.micromedex.com. Accessed June 1, 2007.

the activity of other drugs. COCs have been reported to increase or decrease serum levels of lamotrigine and can affect seizure control. COCs may increase the activity of some benzodiazepines. One report claims that COCs might increase serum phenytoin concentrations substantially.[22]

Unlike many drug classes that are carefully dosed to maintain a therapeutic range of monitored blood levels, contraceptive estrogen and progestin blood levels are obtained only in clinical drug studies. Therefore, users are managed by monitoring side effects and by changes in menstrual patterns. It is no wonder, therefore, that the drug interaction literature is less than satisfactory and management of the interactions is largely empiric. Although some prescribers suggest using a 50-mcg EE formulation in women taking enzyme-inducing drugs, most others would recommend that S.R. use a contraceptive method other than a COC. An alternative recommendation is to use a second method of contraception for 3 months of the combined therapies and monitor bleeding patterns. If no intracycle bleeding occurs, the secondary method can be discontinued.[9]

Oral Contraceptive Risks and Adverse Effects

Some women may not be candidates for a COC because of the risks and adverse effects associated with use. Other women may experience minor side effects with COC that may be managed by changing to a formulation with a different type or dose of estrogen or progestin.

Breakthrough Bleeding, Spotting, and Amenorrhea

7. V.S. comes to the family planning clinic after taking Ovcon-35 for 2 months. She had been started on Ovcon-35 to help with her acne. Her only complaint is spotting at various times during her past two menstrual cycles. What action should be taken to correct V.S.'s bleeding pattern?

Bleeding during active pills days of the cycle (intermenstrual bleeding) that requires the use of a pad or tampon is designated *breakthrough bleeding* (BTB), whereas a lesser amount of intermenstrual bleeding that does not require protection is called *spotting*. Spotting and BTB are the most frequent reasons cited by women for the discontinuation of COCs.[21]

Most clinicians will continue with the same formulation for at least 3 months if irregular bleeding is the only complaint because BTB or spotting usually resolves without intervention.[21,22] Early-cycle intermenstrual bleeding, which usually starts before the 14th day of the menstrual cycle (or never ceases completely after menses), may be caused by insufficient estrogen. Late-cycle intermenstrual bleeding, which occurs after day 14, may caused by insufficient progestational support of the endometrium. The most common cause of BTB or spotting, especially in long-term users of COCs, is missed pills or irregular pill taking. Before making formulation adjustments, adherence should be assessed. Other possible causes of BTB or spotting include drug interactions (see Questions 5 and 6) or infection.

The balance between estrogen and progestin components in COCs determines endometrial activity and, therefore, the likelihood of intermenstrual bleeding problems. It is helpful to envision the estrogen component as the basic building block or "brick" of the endometrium and the progestational component providing the mortar that holds the bricks together. In addition, the estrogenic activity of the progestational component increases the number of bricks, whereas its antiestrogenic activity decreases their numbers. If bricks or mortar are insufficient or if they are present in the wrong proportions, the wall will crumble and bleeding will ensue (Table 45-2).

If V.S.'s intermenstrual bleeding continues to occur late in her cycle after 3 months of consistent use, a formulation with the same estrogen dose and more progestin should be prescribed. Desogen or Ortho-Cept would be a good choice because progestational activity would be increased and estrogenic activity would be maintained with minimal androgenic liability (Table 45-2). If V.S. develops intermenstrual bleeding early in the cycle after several months of use, she should be changed to a pill with a higher ratio of estrogen to progesterone or should try Mircette, which provides a low dose of estrogen during the placebo week.

Some women experience amenorrhea while taking COC. If this occurs, pregnancy should first be ruled out. If she is not pregnant and amenorrhea is acceptable to her, then the formulation need not be changed. If she prefers a monthly menstrual period, then a product with more estrogen or less progestin or a triphasic formulation can be tried.

Cardiovascular Disease

8. M.F. (from Questions 1–4) and her fiancé, who is with her in the health care provider's office, have been reading in the lay press about the cardiovascular risks of estrogen. What are her potential risks for cardiovascular disease from taking COC?

In women who do not smoke or use a COC, the risk of death from cardiovascular disease is 0.59 per 100,000 women <35 years of age and 3.18 per 100,000 women >35 years of age.[23] This risk is increased by 0.06 and 3.03 for COC users <35 years or >35 years, respectively. For COC users who smoke, the risk is increased by 1.73 and 19.4 for women <35 or >35, respectively.

Both the Royal College of General Practitioners and the Oxford Family Planning Association OC studies showed that women <35 years taking the new low-dose COC did not have a significantly increased mortality risk from cardiovascular disease, regardless of smoking status.[23–25] The increase in mortality reported from COC is significant only for smokers >35 years of age.

Several studies have reported the effects of COC on serum lipoprotein concentrations because of the association between lipoproteins and atherosclerotic cardiovascular disease.[26–28] High serum concentrations of total cholesterol (TC), triglycerides (TG), low-density lipoprotein (LDL) cholesterol, and very-low-density lipoprotein (VLDL) cholesterol are associated with the risk of developing atherosclerotic circulatory diseases, whereas high-density lipoprotein (HDL) cholesterol has an inverse relationship. Apolipoprotein levels also affect atherosclerotic risk (e.g., Lp(a) elevations increase risk).[29]

Estrogen tends to increase serum concentrations of HDL. Progestins, depending on the dose and potency, may decrease HDL concentrations.[27,28] Progestins can modify the composition of total HDL by changing the relative amounts of HDL_2

and HDL_3.[30,31] HDL_2 is protective against cardiovascular disease, unlike HDL_3.[32] Decreases in HDL are associated with increasing age, weight, and cigarette smoking. Increased triglyceride serum concentrations are related to the estrogen content of the COC as well as to the antiestrogenic effect of the progestin component.

Studies evaluating the effect of COC on lipids have reported similar results.[27–29] One study found an increase in HDL from baseline with a low-androgenic progestin compared with a high-androgenic progestin.[27] Another study compared COC with phasic EE and levonorgestrel or desogestrel.[26] After six cycles, significant increases in HDL_3 and apolipoproteins (apo A-I, apo A-II, and apo B) were seen in both groups. HDL_2 also increased significantly in the desogestrel group but decreased in the levonorgestrel group. After nine cycles, levels of TG and VLDL in both groups and HDL in the desogestrel group were significantly increased from baseline. HDL did not change significantly in the levonorgestrel group after six cycles. In another study, a reduction in the COC doses of EE and levonorgestrel by one-third improved levels of LDL, TG, Lp(a), and HDL.[28]

Lipid serum concentrations also are altered in adolescent (ages 12–17 years) users. These adolescents had significantly higher TC levels compared with nonusers, although the type of COC used was not specified.[33]

Women taking COCs containing levonorgestrel may be more likely to have a myocardial infarction (MI) than users of COCs containing desogestrel or gestodene.[34] When confounding factors for cardiovascular disease were accounted for, women taking levonorgestrel-containing COC were 2.5 times more likely to have an MI than nonusers. Another study found the opposite effect of the two types of COC, but the results were not significant.[35] Heavy smoking, especially in women >35 years of age, increases the risk of MI.

M.F. and her fiancé should understand that the risk of a cardiovascular adverse effect may be increased with COC use, but the risk is still very low regardless of which COC is used. Cigarette smoking is a much more significant risk factor for MI, causing a reported 8 to 13 times increase in risk.

Cervical Dysplasia and Cervical Cancer

9. J.M., a 24 year-old woman, has an older sister who had cervical dysplasia that progressed to carcinoma in situ. Her sister never took OC. What can you tell J.M. about the risks of cervical dysplasia and cancer associated with COCs?

An estimated 11,070 new cases of, and 3,870 deaths from, cervical cancer will occur in the United States in 2008.[36] The human papilloma virus (HPV) infection is the most common cause of cervical cancer. Women at highest risk for cervical cancer are positive for certain subtypes of HPV, are immunosuppressed, or are smokers.[9] Sexual behaviors that increase the risk of HPV infection and with cervical cancer include beginning sexual activity at a young age, having multiple male sexual partners, or having a male sexual partner who has had multiple partners. Women at low risk for cervical cancer have two or fewer partners, use condoms, and do not smoke.[5]

Pooled data from eight case-control studies on cervical cancer risk for COC users who are positive for HPV indicate they are more likely to develop cervical cancer.[37] Women who had ever used a COC and those who had used a COC for >5 years were 1.5 and 3.4 times, respectively, more likely to develop cervical cancer. This is consistent with older studies that suggest that COC users have an increased risk of developing or dying of cervical cancer; however, COCs are not thought to cause cervical cancer. In contrast, a large cohort study conducted in England found no significant increase in deaths caused by cervical cancer in women who had ever used OC.[38]

Epidemiologic comparisons of the prevalence of cervical cancer in COC users versus nonusers often are difficult to interpret because factors other than the hormone use need to be considered. Women using COCs are less likely to have partners using condoms and are more likely to have regular medical examinations (e.g., Pap smears), resulting in early detection and treatment of precancerous lesions.[39] Health care providers may wish to perform Pap smears every 6 months in women who have used a COC for >5 years who are at a higher risk because of multiple partners or a history of sexually transmitted diseases (STD).[8] J.M. should be counseled about avoiding risk factors for cervical cancer and should be encouraged to have a Pap smear annually. Women between 9 and 26 years of age, such as J.M., are candidates for the HPV vaccine. The vaccine, given as a series of three injections, provides substantial (but not complete) protection from cervical cancer. Use of the vaccine in older women or in men is not currently approved but is being studied.

Headache

10. G.R., a 32-year-old woman, comes to the clinic complaining of headaches, which predominantly occur during the 7-day placebo phase of her 28-day cycle of Nordette. The throbbing headaches are preceded by blurred vision, nausea, and vomiting. Aspirin and acetaminophen, which normally relieve her other headaches, are ineffective. Lying down in a dark room provides some relief. Her family history is pertinent because her mother and maternal grandmother have migraine headaches. Are these headaches a relative contraindication for the continued use of a COC?

Headache is a common complaint in women, including those taking a COC. Headaches can occur while taking the active pills (estrogen related) or during the placebo week, owing to the withdrawal of estrogen.[21] Women with migraines may find that their headaches either lessen or worsen when COCs are initiated.

Mild headaches may abate over time or if the woman is changed to a pill with less estrogen or progestin. Headaches that occur during the placebo week can be managed by trying Mircette or taking a COC continuously (i.e., skipping placebo pills). Women with severe headaches should discontinue COC use and should be evaluated by their health care provider.

Ischemic stroke is more likely to occur in COC users with a history of classic migraines (migraines with aura), especially if they are smokers.[40] Women with classic migraines should use COCs with caution or not at all, particularly if they smoke, are >35 years of age, or have other significant medical problems. Clinical experience indicates that women having increasing migraine attacks with COCs are not likely to have relief from them when the formulation is changed to one with a different hormone balance. Women with menstrual migraine (migraine associated with menses) may have fewer headaches while taking a COC and may prefer continuous use.

G.R.'s symptoms are typical of classic migraine headache and, because she also has a family history of migraine headaches, she may need to discontinue her COC and use another method of contraception. Subsequent to a thorough medical evaluation of her headaches, she should be monitored carefully if COCs are continued.

Hypertension

11. A.M., an obese 26-year-old woman, experienced hypertension during all of her pregnancies. She restarted Lo-Ovral after her last pregnancy. She continues to smoke a half-pack of cigarettes per day. Her blood pressure (BP) before starting the COC was 126/76 mmHg. Today, her BP is 146/96 mmHg. What is the mechanism of COC-induced hypertension? Can she continue taking Lo-Ovral considering her history of hypertension during pregnancy?

The underlying mechanisms for COC-induced hypertension may be sodium and water retention and increased renin activity.[41,42] Hypertension secondary to COC use may develop slowly over 3 to 36 months and may not decline for 3 to 6 months after discontinuing their use.[43]

Women taking older and more potent oral contraceptives (e.g., 50 mcg EE) have been reported to have a two to three times higher incidence of hypertension (BP >140/90 mmHg) than nonusers.[42–44] Small studies have found systolic BP to increase by 7 to 8 mmHg and diastolic BP to increase by 6 mmHg in normotensive or mildly hypertensive women.[43] Population-based, case-control studies have shown differing results on whether women with hypertension who use COC are more likely to have an MI than nonusers. A small study of adolescent women showed similar systolic and diastolic BP in users versus nonusers.[33]

For A.M., it is reasonable to consider using a 20-mcg EE formulation such as Alesse/Apri/Levlite or one with less progestin and estrogen such as Ortho TriCyclen Lo. The effect of this change in medication on her BP should be monitored to determine whether continued use is indicated.

Liver Effect

12. T.A.'s physician is concerned about the possibility of hepatic tumors. What is the risk of hepatomas in patients using COC?

The incidence of benign liver tumors for women using low-dose COC is very low, 3.3 per 100,000 users per year compared with 0.1 per 100,000 users per year in nonusers or short-term users.[45] The incidence increases after 4 years of use. Although the tumors generally are benign, death can result from intrahepatic or extrahepatic tumor rupture and hemorrhagic shock.[46,47] Because animal studies suggest that both estrogen and progestin can accelerate abnormal liver cell proliferation, the lowest effective tolerable COC dose should be used.[45,48] A significant increase in death from liver disease or cancer was not seen in one large cohort study.[37]

Cholestatic jaundice also has been associated with COC use.[49] T.A. can monitor for signs or symptoms of cholestatic jaundice, because this disorder usually presents as malaise, nausea, anorexia, and pruritus; these usually appear 4 weeks after the initiation of COC use. Discontinuation results in complete clinical remission within a month.

Thromboembolic Events

13. B.C., a 21-year-old woman, is interested in starting COC. After taking a complete history, the provider learns that her sister and mother have both had a deep vein thrombosis (DVT). Do COC contribute to the development of a DVT or pulmonary embolism (PE)? If so, which women are at the highest risk? Should B.C. start COC?

OCs contribute to thromboembolic events by several mechanisms. Estrogens increase coagulability and thereby increase the possibility of clot formation. Although they have been shown to significantly increase some clotting factors, other studies have shown no changes or decreases in prothrombotic factors.[27,30] Long-term OC use is associated with an increased platelet count and increased platelet aggregation similar to that seen late in pregnancy; this is generally thought to be caused by the estrogen component. More recent data showing increased thrombosis rates in users of third-generation progestins [desogestrel and gestodene (not available in the U.S.)] suggest that progestin may also has a role in thromboembolism risk.[4]

The baseline risk of venous thrombosis is low, at 4-8 for every 100,000 women per year.[50,51] The best studies looking at thromboembolism in OC users found that most users have a three- to six-fold increased risk of developing superficial or deep venous thrombosis or PE. Therefore, the risk is still quite low, at approximately 10 to 30 per 100,000 women per year; less than the risk during pregnancy of 60 per 100,000 women per year. Patients requiring emergency major surgery while on OCs are more prone to thromboembolism than nonusers. The risk of venous thrombosis does not seem to be associated with duration of OC use, past OC use, mild obesity, or cigarette smoking. A greater risk is associated with EE doses >35 meg.

Women with a mutation in clotting factor V (also called factor V Leiden) or a deficiency in protein C, protein S, or antithrombin are more likely to develop a venous thrombosis with OC use than women without a hereditary prothrombotic defect.[51] Women with blood types other than O may also be more susceptible to clotting due to higher levels of factor VIII.

Whether third-generation progestins (desogestrel, gestodene) are associated with a higher risk of venous thromboembolism (VTE) relative to other progestins is controversial.[50,51] It was believed that the risk of thrombosis with third-generation progestins would be lower than other progestins since they have more beneficial effects on HDL. However, most studies that compared the risk of thrombosis with third-generation progestins to second-generation progestins found that desogestrel and gestodene are associated with a greater VTE risk. Although the risk may be increased, the overall rate of thrombosis is still low. All patients using OCs should be counseled about the VTE warning signs (ACHES; Table 45-6).

The minimal risk of thrombosis associated with OCs in the general population does not justify the cost of routine screening for deficiencies in the coagulation system; however, when a patient has a family history of thrombosis, measurement of antithrombin III, protein C, activated protein C resistance ratio, protein S, anticardiolipin antibodies, prothrombin G mutation, and homocysteine levels should be considered.[51]

Table 45-6 Pill Early Danger Signs (ACHES)

Signals	*Possible Problem*
Abdominal pain (severe)	Gallbladder disease, hepatic adenoma, blood clot, pancreatitis
Chest pain (severe), shortness of breath, or coughing up blood	Blood clot in lungs or myocardial infarction
Headaches (severe)	Stroke, hypertension, or migraine headache
Eye problems: blurred vision, flashing lights, or blindness	Stroke, hypertension, or temporary vascular problem
Severe leg pain (calf or thigh)	Blood clot in legs

B.C. should be evaluated for hereditary prothrombotic defects. If any exist, she should avoid OC use. If none exist, she may still wish to consider a method without estrogen but should be educated on the signs and symptoms of thrombosis if she decides to start OCs.

Benefits of Oral Contraceptives

Acne

14. D.S., a 20-year-old woman, has had severe acne since menarche at age 13. She is currently taking no medications but wants to begin COC. What effect, if any, would oral contraceptives have on her acne? Which formulation would you recommend for D.S.?

Depending on the woman, COC use may cause acne to appear, disappear, or significantly improve.[12,16] Most women will have improvement in acne with any COC used, only a few formulations are FDA approved for this indication. Progestins with higher androgenic activity may be more likely to increase acne because they stimulate sebaceous glands to produce more sebum. Higher doses of estrogen may decrease acne by suppressing the activity of sebaceous glands, decreasing the production of androgens, and increasing the synthesis of SHBG. SHBG binds androgens and thereby diminishes the effects.[52] The triphasics are modestly estrogen-dominant contraceptives, lower in progestin potency, and may significantly reduce the overall incidence of acne. Both desogestrel- and norgestimate-containing COCs are less androgenic, thereby increasing SHBG levels and decreasing acne.[53]

D.S.'s acne should improve with COC use. Products to consider starting with are OrthoTriCyclen, Estrostep, and Ovcon 35.

Benign Breast Disease

15. A young woman has a family history of fibrocystic breast disease. What influence do COC have on fibrocystic breast disease?

A 50% to 75% reduction in the risk of fibroadenomas, chronic cystic breast disease, and breast biopsies appears to exist in COC users.[15] Protection seems directly related to length of use. Because the progestin component may be primarily responsible for this protection, progestin-dominant COCs that contain a less estrogenic progestin, such as levonorgestrel, are preferred.[9,14,54] The progestin-only minipill could be of use here, except that progestin-only pills are less effective contraceptives than a COC. In addition, it does not provide the same level of endometrial stability (leading to more BTB and spotting) or other benefits of a COC such as decreased dysmenorrhea, iron deficiency anemia, acne, and hirsutism (more irregular bleeding).

Dysmenorrhea and Premenstrual Syndrome

16. C.P. has a history of premenstrual syndrome (PMS) and worsened menstrual cramping with a copper intrauterine device (IUD). What effect on PMS and dysmenorrhea might she expect from a COC?

Dysmenorrhea, or painful menstruation, may be of unknown etiology; it may be caused by endometriosis or uterine fibroids. Complaints of menstrual pain may be decreased by >60% after starting COCs.[10] A formulation with decreased estrogenic and increased progestational activity may be the best at relieving dysmenorrhea.

Premenstrual tension has been reported to be reduced 29% in COC users, and other premenstrual symptoms seem to be relieved as well.[55,56] Nevertheless, the effect of COCs on PMS symptoms is inconsistent and unpredictable, probably because PMS symptoms are neither consistent nor predictable. There may be augmentation of depression and mood swings by the progestational component. Although the probability of this effect is low with a low-dose product, C.P. should be monitored for changes in her PMS symptoms. (See Chapter 47, Disorders Related to the Menstrual Cycle, for further discussion of dysmenorrhea and PMS.)

Endometrial Cancer

17. C.P. is hesitant to take a COC because her grandmother, who had been receiving estrogen replacement therapy for 5 years, died of endometrial cancer in 1970. What is the relationship between COC use and endometrial cancer?

Clinical data suggest that cyclic COCs contain sufficient progestin to prevent endometrial hyperplasia and to reduce the risk of endometrial cancer by about 50% to 70%.[39] The protection is directly related to duration of use and may persist for many years after discontinuation. A meta-analysis of 11 studies showed a 56%, 67%, and 72% reduction in endometrial cancer risk after 4, 8, and 12 years of COC use, respectively.[57]

C.P. should be reassured that COC use will not cause endometrial cancer and will likely reduce her chances of developing this disease. She may want to find out more about her grandmother's cancer, because it may have been caused by treating her menopausal symptoms with estrogen alone rather than with estrogen plus a progestin.

Menorrhagia (Heavy Menstrual Bleeding)

18. M.V. has iron deficiency anemia attributed to heavy menses secondary to her previous use of a copper IUD. What will be the effect of COC use on her iron deficiency anemia?

The total amount of menstrual flow in established COC users is decreased by up to 40%,[58–60] which may caused by the progressive thinning of the endometrium induced by use or a lack of irregular bleeding. Bleeding may be decreased the most by COCs that have a high ratio of progestin to estrogen, because endometrial thinning is maximized.[8] Another option would be to have her take a COC continuously so she has fewer bleeding episodes.

Ovarian Cancer and Functional Ovarian Cysts

19. C.P. (from Questions 16 and 17) is concerned also about ovarian cysts and cancer. Can COC cause ovarian problems?

The risk of developing functional ovarian cysts is decreased, pre-existing cysts are more rapidly resolved, and surgery rates for ovarian masses are reduced in women taking COCs.[60–62] This is likely owing to reducing ovulation, suppressing androgen production, or increasing progesterone levels.

Each year of COC use decreases the relative risk of developing ovarian cancer by 7% to 9%.[60] The risk reduction continues to be seen in women using a COC for >15 years and persists after discontinuation.

C.P. should be reassured that COC use will decrease, not increase, her likelihood of developing ovarian cancer.

Pelvic Inflammatory Disease and Ectopic Pregnancy

20. M.A., a 20-year-old woman who has several sexual partners, arrives at the emergency department with a temperature of 38.2°C (normal, 37°C) and lower abdominal cramping. Examination is compatible with the diagnosis of pelvic inflammatory disease (PID), based on her cervical motion tenderness, abdominal pain, and adnexal (ovary and fallopian tube) tenderness. Can COC be used for M.A.?

Many clinicians prefer to prescribe COCs with condoms for STD protection to young women with multiple sexual partners because PID has been found to be less prevalent with this combination of contraceptive methods.[8,63] In one study, COC users were half as likely to develop PID as nonusers.[64] Although early studies failed to distinguish between gonococcal and nongonococcal PID, the PID protective effects of COCs may depend on the organism. A Swedish study found that COCs protect against both gonococcal and chlamydial PID.[65] In contrast, one report suggested that COCs may promote chlamydial PID; and another concluded that COC users were neither more nor less likely to develop PID.[66,67] A 1990 case-control study showed protection against symptomatic PID in women infected with chlamydia but not in those infected with gonococcus.[68]

Despite the contradictory data, it is logical that the thickening of cervical mucus caused by COCs may prevent bacteria from ascending into the uterus and fallopian tubes, thereby minimizing hospitalizations as well as deaths stemming from PID. The risk of ectopic pregnancy is greater for women who already have had PID, and COC use has been shown to prevent hospitalizations and deaths stemming from ectopic pregnancies.[69,70]

In view of these data, a COC may be initiated for M.A. if no contraindications are present. Patients and clinicians should be alert for the symptoms of cervicitis or salpingitis in women who are at high risk for STDs.

Other Issues with Oral Contraceptives

Breast Cancer

21. The medical history and physical examination of S.M. are negative for breast disease, except for a history of breast cancer in her maternal grandmother. How will COC use affect her risk of breast cancer?

Studies on the use of COCs and breast cancer have yielded conflicting results. Some studies have suggested an increased risk of breast cancer in young, nulliparous women using COC with high progestin activity.[71,72] In addition, the Royal College of General Practitioners' Oral Contraceptive Study in 1981 reported a significant increase in risk for breast cancer in women 30 to 34 years of age who use COCs.[73] Another study found an increased risk of breast cancer in women with a first-degree family history of breast cancer who had ever used a COC.[74]

In contrast, other studies found no association between current or former use and breast cancer.[37,75] In addition, both the Oxford/Family Planning Association Contraceptive Study in 1977 and the Walnut Creek Contraceptive Drug Study in 1981 found no association between breast cancer and COC use in any age group.[76–78] The Centers for Disease Control Cancer and Steroid Hormone Study in 1983 reported a relative risk of 0.9 for COC users compared with never-users, despite other risk factors for breast cancer, such as early menarche, later age at first birth and menopause, family history of breast cancer, or benign breast disease.[79] The ongoing Nurses' Health Study identified 3,383 cases of breast cancer from 1976 to 1992 among 1.6 million person-years of COC use and found that long-term past COC use (10 years), either overall or before a first full-term pregnancy, does not appreciably increase breast cancer risk in women >40 years of age.[80]

Users of COCs tend to have a greater awareness of breast cancer, examine their breasts more frequently, and are examined by clinicians more often than nonusers. Thus, early detection of breast abnormalities can preclude the progression of these abnormalities into cancerous lesions.[81] A COC would not be expected to increase the risk of breast cancer in S.M. She should be instructed to perform monthly self-breast examinations and to return annually for a physical examination by her health care provider.

Depression

22. K.G. is a 24-year-old woman with persistent mild depression. Taking into account her depression, would a formulation with high or low estrogen or progestin balance be preferred for her?

Usually women notice improved mood or premenstrual symptoms when taking a COC.[16] COC-related depression has been attributed to progestin or estrogen excess, however. Some COC users experience deterioration in mood during the pill-free period. Other causes of depression, such as hypothyroidism or vitamin B_6 deficiency, also should be considered. If depression worsens or is severe, the COC may be discontinued.

On further questioning, K.G. states that she noticed only a minor change in mood, denies suicidal or homicidal ideations, and desires to continue taking a COC. She can be changed from Nordette to a formulation with less estrogenic activity (e.g., Lo-Estrin 1/20), less progestational activity (e.g., Ovcon 25), or both (e.g. Alesse/Levlite/Apri) (Table 45-2). If she reports that her depression is worse during the hormone-free week, then changing her to continuous-use may be helpful.

Diabetes

23. R.D., a 33-year-old woman, experienced glucose intolerance during pregnancy that resolved after delivery. She has a father and sister with diabetes. Would a COC be appropriate for R.D.?

Generally, low-dose COCs do not alter glucose tolerance.[26,27] Results of one controlled, randomized, prospective study showed no adverse effect on carbohydrate or lipid metabolism in women with a history of gestational diabetes after 6 to 13 months of low-dose COC use.[81] Both the users and nonusers showed a significant and similar deterioration in glucose tolerance with an overall prevalence of 14% impaired glucose tolerance and 17% diabetes mellitus. The authors concluded that low-dose COC could be prescribed safely and that serum lipids and glucose tolerance should be monitored closely, regardless of contraceptive choice.

Women with a history of gestational diabetes and those with a strong family history of diabetes in parents or siblings are at greater risk for COC-induced glucose intolerance.[13,16,46] COCs have complex effects on carbohydrate metabolism. Progestins decrease and estrogens increase the number of insulin receptors on the cell membrane. Progestins also may alter insulin receptor affinity. The different progestins have different propensities to induce glucose intolerance. Norgestrel appears to have the greatest insulin-antagonizing activity. Ethynodiol diacetate, norethindrone, norethindrone acetate, desogestrel, and norgestimate have significantly less effect. In general, carbohydrate metabolism is not affected to an important degree in most diabetic women using low-dose COC.

For R.D., Levlen (Levora/Nordette) would be poor choices because they are known to cause glucose intolerance in women with previous history of gestational diabetes.[82] Interestingly, the triphasic levonorgestrel product TriLevlen, Trivora, containing 39% less progestin than the monophasic product, did not alter glucose tolerance, and Alesse (Levlite/Apri), which contains 33% less EE, also should not alter glucose tolerance. Lowering the estrogen content without changing progestin content also has improved glucose tolerance and increased insulin secretion.[83,84]

For women without diabetes, COC use may protect against developing diabetes. One large prospective, observational study found that both white and black COC users had lower fasting glucose levels and lower odds of diabetes.[85]

R.D. can be started on a COC. If she smokes or has other medical problems such as hypertension, nephropathy, retinopathy, or other vascular diseases, however, a COC probably should be avoided. It seems prudent to put R.D. on a low dose of estrogen and progesterone and to monitor for any changes in glucose control.

Gallbladder Disease

24. L.S., a 26-year-old woman, arrives at the emergency department with acute epigastric pain accompanied by nausea, vomiting, and diarrhea. She has been taking a COC for 1 year. She is diagnosed as having gallstones. What is the association between gallbladder disease and COC use? What would be an appropriate contraceptive for L.S.?

The incidence of cholelithiasis has been reported to increase with COC use. Estrogens and progestins may contribute to bile stasis and cholelithiasis by reducing cholesterol clearance and altering bile acid composition.[14,86] The incidence of gallbladder disease has been reported to increase during the first year of use but then to decline steadily to a rate lower than that of controls.[87] In another large study, long-term users experienced slightly lower rates of gallbladder disease than nonusers.[88] Finally, another study found that women who had ever used COCs were not more likely to have symptomatic gallstones, but current and long-term users were. An analysis of 482 women with benign gallbladder disease from the Oxford Family Planning Association Contraception Study concluded that it is unlikely that COCs cause gallbladder disease.[89]

The newer COCs with lower progestin and estrogen concentrations should have little effect, if any, on gallstone formation in health patients. Women who are obese, young, or long-term users may be the most likely to develop gallstones.

In L.S., it is not known whether COC use contributed to her development of gallstones. A history of or the current presence of gallstones is not a contraindication to COC use, so L.S. may continue to use a COC if desired.

Use During Pregnancy and Breastfeeding

25. P.S., a 25-year-old woman, was started on Triphasil 2 months ago because of a history of abnormal menstrual periods. Unknowingly, she was pregnant at that time and continued taking her COC for two complete cycles. What can you tell P.S. about the possible effects of COC use on her unborn child?

The fact that COCs are classified as pregnancy category X (contraindicated, fetal risks clearly outweigh maternal benefit) is very misleading.[90] Although an association between COC use during pregnancy with cardiac or limb anomalies has been reported, other contraceptive studies have not noted a teratogenic effect. Simpson[91] summarized all available data on contraceptive steroid exposure during pregnancy and concluded that COC use did not substantially increase the risk of anomalies over that expected in other uneventful pregnancies.

Clearly, a COC should not be started in a woman known to be pregnant. P.S. should be reassured, however, that the risks to her fetus from the use of a low-dose COC during the first trimester should be minimal.

P.S. may resume COC use after she has her baby even if she is breastfeeding, although it may be preferable for her to use a progesterone-only method.[9,90] For women without contraindications, the American Academy of Pediatrics considers COC use to be compatible with breastfeeding.[92] COCs have been reported to decrease milk quantity and quality, however, especially if used early in the postpartum period before milk is well established (see Question 27).[90] Therefore, many providers suggest avoiding or delaying the use of a COC in women who are exclusively breastfeeding. If a postpartum woman would like to start COC, she should wait to begin them until at least 3 to 4 weeks postpartum or use progestin-only formulations. By waiting 3 to 4 weeks, the increased risk of thrombosis that occurs during pregnancy should be reduced to baseline and initiation of a COC is appropriate.

CONTRACEPTIVE PATCH AND RING

26. K.H. is a 16-year-old who started taking a COC 3 months ago. She is very concerned about getting pregnant because she has trouble remembering to take her pill each day. She likes all the noncontraceptive benefits but is wondering if there are dosage forms other than pills. What do you tell her?

Contraceptive Patch

Contraceptive patch users experience about 1 pregnancy per 100 women-years of use (Table 45-1). The contraceptive patch (Ortho Evra) contains 6 mg norelgestromin and 750 mcg EE and delivers transdermally, 150 mcg of norelgestromin (a metabolite of norgestimate) and 20 mcg EE daily into the bloodstream.[93] The product is a thin, beige 20-cm^2 square patch with rounded corners. The patch uses a 4-week cycle similar to that of pills. A new patch is applied once weekly for 3 consecutive weeks, followed by 1 week with no patch. Then this cycle is repeated. Menses should begin during the patch-free week.

The contraceptive patch may be worn on the buttock, abdomen, upper torso, or upper outer arm.[93] K.H. should not apply the patch to the same exact spot but rather rotate within or between sites. The patch should not be applied to the breasts. When applying the patch, K.H. should select the application site and be sure it is clean and dry. She should press firmly on the patch for 10 seconds and trace her finger around the edge of the patch to be sure it sticks properly. The patch should stay attached during usual activities, including exercising, swimming, and bathing. If the patch falls off for <24 hours, she should reapply it to the same spot or apply a new patch as soon as possible, keeping her patch-change day will stay the same. No back-up contraception is needed. If the patch is off for >24 hours, she should start a new apply a new patch and begin a new 4-week cycle, she will have a new patch-change day, and she should use back-up contraception for 1 week.

The patch may be started using the Sunday start, Day 1 start, or Quick Start method, and the recommendations for back-up contraception are the same as described earlier with COC.[93] If K.H. forgets to start the first patch of a cycle, she should apply it as soon as she remembers. This day will become her new patch-change day, and she should use back-up contraception for 1 week. If she forgets to change the patch for 1 or 2 days during week 2 or at the end of week 1 or 2, she should apply a new patch as soon as she remembers. This becomes her new patch-change day. No back-up contraception is needed. If she leaves the patch on for >9 days at the end of week 3, she should remove the patch when she remembers and apply the new patch "on schedule" even if that is only 1 or 2 days later. No back-up contraception is needed. If she forgets to remove the patch for >2 days at the end of week 1 or 2, she should apply a new patch as soon as she remembers. This becomes her new patch change day. No back-up contraception is needed. If she forgets for >2 days, she should start a new cycle as soon as she remembers. She will need to use back-up contraception for 1 week and will have a new patch-change day.

Because the patch contains similar hormones to those in COCs, the risks and benefits are thought to be similar. The package insert lists the same contraindications and precautions with the use of the patch as for a COC (Table 45-4).[93] Because the delivery system and serum levels are different, future studies may find, however, that differences exist in certain risks or benefits between the products. One difference with the patch is that efficacy is reduced in users weighing >90 kg. Therefore, providers may choose to recommend another method for heavier women. The most common side effects reported with the patch are breast tenderness, headache, application site reaction, and nausea.

Contraceptive Ring

The contraceptive ring (NuvaRing) delivers 120 mcg etonogestrel (an active metabolite of desogestrel) and 15 mcg EE through the vaginal mucosa.[94] The ring is flexible, transparent, and has a diameter of just over 2 inches. The ring is inserted vaginally and kept in place for 3 weeks in a row. After 3 weeks, the ring is removed and a new ring is inserted 1 week later. The NuvaRing must be refrigerated in the pharmacy before dispensing. On dispensing, the pharmacist should apply the label provided in the packaging indicating a 4-month expiration date when the ring is stored at room temperature. The "used" ring should be discarded in the foil package provided by the manufacturer to avoid environmental hormone exposure in trash. The failure rate for the contraceptive ring is 1 or 2 pregnancies per 100 woman-years.

The ring may be placed anywhere in the vagina, so K.H. does not need to worry about its exact position.[94] To insert the ring, she should compress it so the opposite sides of the ring are touching, and gently insert it into the vagina. If she feels discomfort with the ring, it has probably not been inserted far enough into the vagina. Most women do not feel the ring once it is in place. To remove the ring, K.H. should grasp the ring between two fingers or hook one finger inside the ring and pull it out. Menses will usually begin within 3 days following removal of the ring. If the ring slips out, it should be rinsed with cool water and reinserted. If the ring is out for <3 hours, back-up contraception is not needed. If the ring is out for >3 hours, back-up contraception should be used for 1 week. If the ring has been left in the vagina for 3 to 4 weeks (late removal of the ring), she should remove the ring when she remembers, wait 1 week, then reinsert a new ring. If the ring has been in place for >4 weeks, she should remove it, confirm that she is not pregnant, reinsert a new one right away, and use back-up contraception for 1 week.

The initial contraceptive ring should be inserted anytime during the first 5 days of the menstrual cycle.[94] Back-up contraception should be used for the first week of use. When changing from other hormonal methods to the ring, the woman should insert the ring within 7 days of the last active pill or at the end of the patch-free week. No back-up contraception is needed.

As with the patch, the ring has the same contraindications and precautions as COCs (Table 45-4).[94] The most common side effects with the ring are vaginal infections, irritation, and discharge, headache, weight gain, and nausea.

PROGESTERONE-ONLY PILL (MINIPILL)

27. P.K., a 39-year-old woman, plans to breastfeed her infant and to begin some type of contraception following her discharge from the hospital. Her previous experience with condoms and concurrent spermicidal foams or gels resulted in itching and burning, and a copper IUD caused severe cramping and bleeding. She has a strong family history of cardiac disease and smokes two packs of cigarettes a day. What are the advantages of the minipill as a contraceptive method for P.K.?

Advantages

The minipill is devoid of some of the nuisance side effects (Table 45-4) caused by estrogen (e.g., headaches, chloasma).[9] More importantly, estrogen-mediated hypertension and clotting factor changes will be avoided in this smoker, who has a strong family history of cardiovascular disease. Confusion with pill taking is minimized because there is no placebo week and all 28 tablets in each pack are the same. Therefore, the missed-dose directions are the same whenever any pill is missed: take two pills as soon as possible and use back-up contraception for 48 hours. The minipill is less effective for preventing pregnancy than a COC. Minipills have noncontraceptive benefits, including decreased dysmenorrhea and bleeding. They also may protect against PID and endometrial cancer.

Theoretically, progestin use in the early postpartum period may decrease milk production, because milk production is triggered by the decline in progesterone that occurs after delivery. No data, however, have consistently shown this to be a problem in postpartum women.[90] Once breastfeeding has been established, progestins have not been shown to interfere with the quantity or quality of milk produced by a nursing mother. Thus, a progestin-only contraceptive may be preferred for a woman who plans to breastfeed her infant.

Disadvantages

28. What disadvantages of the minipill should you discuss with P.K.?

The minipills, with a failure rate of 0.5% to 5%, are less effective than COC (Table 45-1).[9] Because minipills must be taken on a more regular schedule than a COC, minipills are not often used except in women who are breastfeeding or who have contraindications to estrogen (see instructions below). Most women using progestin-only pills have fewer bleeding days because there is no withdrawal bleeding induced by pill-free days. Some women on minipills will continue to ovulate and experience regular cyclic bleeding whereas others will have little or no bleeding for extended periods. The contraceptive actions of progestins include alteration of cervical mucus, endometrial changes, and tubal transport changes and, therefore, most users do not experience contraceptive failure despite continuing to ovulate. Some women using minipills will consistently have ovulatory cycles whereas others will shift back and forth between ovulatory and anovulatory cycles. Women who consistently have regular menses on the minipill are potentially at higher risk of pregnancy and may be advised to either use a back-up method of contraception or change to a different method.

Bleeding changes, including decreased duration and amount volume of menstrual flow, spotting, or amenorrhea commonly occur while taking the minipill.[9] Because of this, some women may be concerned that they may be pregnant. Women who are exclusively breastfeeding usually will have amenorrhea. The high incidence of irregular menses associated with the minipill may mask underlying pathology. Other side effects reported with minipills include headaches, breast tenderness, mood changes, and nausea.

Minipills should be avoided if when there is a personal history of breast cancer or undiagnosed vaginal bleeding. Caution should be exercised when using minipills in women with hepatic disease, certain cardiovascular conditions, a current DVT or PE, or complicated diabetes (Table 45-4).[10]

Patient Instructions

29. What instructions should P.K. receive regarding the use of a minipill?

P.K. should begin taking the minipill when she is discharged from the hospital or after her first postpartum visit (3–6 weeks postpartum). If she were not postpartum, she would begin her first pack on the first day of her menses.[16] Waiting for 4 to 6 weeks postpartum often is recommended to minimize complaints of irregular bleeding and to confirm that milk flow is established. Back-up contraception is not needed with a Day 1 start or when started within 4 weeks of delivery in a women who is breastfeeding. When back-up contraception is needed, it should be used for 48 hours. She can begin immediately postpartum or wait 3 weeks to start.

P.K. should be instructed to take the pill at the exact same time each day. If she is >3 hours late taking a pill, she should take the pill as soon as she remembers and should use back-up contraception for 48 hours. This is quite different from the directions for a COC, so this point should be stressed during consultation.

LONG-ACTING INJECTIONS: DEPO-PROVERA AND LUNELLE

Depo-Provera

30. A.K., a 35-year-old woman who is breastfeeding, returns to the gynecology clinic for her second injection of depot medroxyprogesterone acetate (Depo-Provera; DMPA). She is a smoker with a history of thromboembolism. She was given her first injection 3 months ago, immediately postpartum. She is experiencing frequent BTB and has gained 2 pounds since her injection. Is this to be expected? What are the benefits and risks of DMPA? How are the side effects to be managed?

Depo-Provera is most often given as a 150-mg deep intramuscular injection in the deltoid or gluteus maximus every 11 to 13 weeks.[9] Since its development in the early 1960s, DMPA has been approved for use in >90 countries and has been used by >30 million women worldwide.[95] The FDA approved DMPA in 1992. DMPA inhibits ovulation, thickens the cervical mucus, and suppresses endometrial growth, making it a very effective contraceptive. A newer lower-dose 104-mg formulation for subcutaneous injection also is available. The 104-mg formulation also is given every 11 to 13 weeks and has been reported to have fewer side effects, including weight gain.

Advantages

Depo-Provera is a good contraceptive choice for A.K. because she is at risk for estrogenic side effects. She is 35 years old, smokes, and has a history of thromboembolism. Among its benefits are a low failure rate of 0.3% (Table 45-1), ease of use, lack of estrogenic side effects, decreased dysmenorrhea, reduced monthly blood loss, and a reduced risk of endometrial cancer and PID.[9,96] Other noncontraceptive benefits may include decreasing pain and frequency of sickle cell crises, reduction in seizure frequency in epileptic patients, and a possible reduction in ovarian cancer.[9,97] Furthermore, contraceptive efficacy is not reduced by the concurrent use of anticonvulsants as is seen with COC.

Disadvantages

The package insert states women with breast cancer should not use DMPA.[98] DMPA should be used with caution in women with undiagnosed vaginal bleeding, certain cardiovascular diseases or multiple risk factors for cerebrovascular disease, or a current DVT or PE (Table 45-4). Some experts disagree with the Depo-Provera package insert, which lists a history of prior thromboembolism as a contraindication, because clotting factors have not been shown to be clinically affected by DMPA.[99] Some clinicians also begin DMPA immediately postpartum rather than waiting 6 weeks postpartum, as directed by the package insert. Women starting DMPA earlier are more likely to report frequent episodes of bleeding or spotting, however.[99,100]

Estrogen production declines in women using DMPA, so A.K. should be told that DMPA may decrease bone mineral density (BMD).[101] Numerous studies have found that women receiving DMPA injection have lower BMD compared with nonusers. Other studies have found that DMPA does not affect BMD. Although there have been reports of stress fractures in DMPA users, no studies to date have documented an increased rate of hip or vertebral fractures in DMPA users.[102,103] Also, BMD has been shown to recover after discontinuation of the injections.[101] Product labeling advises limiting use to 2 years unless advantages outweigh the potential risk of reduced BMD.[98]

A.K. can be reassured that, although DMPA frequently causes irregular bleeding or spotting during the first few months of use or more, the irregular bleeding diminishes with continued use. Bleeding is caused by insufficient estrogen to maintain the endometrium. After 1 and 2 years of use, 55% and 68% of women experience amenorrhea, respectively. Amenorrhea leads to discontinuation of DMPA in 13% of patients women.[95] Women beginning Depo-Provera should be informed that during the first year of use, they might have menstrual changes. If unusually heavy or continuous bleeding occurs, A.K. should be evaluated. She should be counseled and reassured that her irregular bleeding probably will resolve in the next few months. If the bleeding is bothersome to her, a 4- to 21-day course of oral estrogen (e.g., conjugated estrogen 0.625–2.5 mg/day) or a COC with 20 mcg EE can be added to minimize or eliminate the bleeding.[18] The bleeding may, however, recur after discontinuation of the estrogen. Low-dose estrogen may be continued if bleeding recurs. The mean weight gain after 1 year of therapy with DMPA was about 5 pounds in two-thirds of users. Users typically gain a total of about 8 pounds over 2 years, nearly 14 pounds over 4 years, and 16.5 pounds over 6 years. Other side effects include mood changes, hair loss, and headaches.

Following a 150-mg DMPA injection, return to fertility is delayed by approximately 10 months after the last injection in half of users.[98] The remaining users took longer to become pregnant, with nearly all users becoming pregnant by 18 months.

Lunelle

31. A.K. is concerned about the menstrual changes with DMPA but likes the idea of an injectable method of contraception. Are there any other options for her?

Although currently not available in the United States, another injectable contraceptive, Lunelle, contains medroxyprogesterone 25 mg and estradiol cypionate 5 mg; it is administered intramuscularly every 28 to 33 days.[104] With this injection, women may experience spotting initially but should have regular menses about 2 to 3 weeks after each injection. The first injection should be given within 5 days of menstrual bleeding, and no back-up contraception is needed. Unlike DMPA, ovulation resumes more rapidly, within 2 to 3 months of discontinuing Lunelle. The most common side effects of Lunelle are irregular menses, weight gain (an average of 4 pounds in the first year), fluid retention, breast symptoms, nausea, headache, and mood changes.[104]

Lunelle was available in vials and prefilled syringes until manufacturing problems caused the product production to be discontinued. Lunelle is no longer marketed for business reasons in the United States. Lunelle has not been available since October 2002. Pfizer medical information (the product owner) does not know if it will ever become available again. At this time, A.K. will have to select an alternate method or continue DMPA.

SUBDERMAL IMPLANTS

32. A.K. returns to the gynecology clinic on the first day of her flow after missing three consecutive DMPA injections because she cannot remember to come in for her shots and does not like the weight gain and prolonged intermenstrual irregular bleeding that occurred over 6 months. A friend of hers has used Norplant in the past, and she would like to try it. What information should be given to her about this product?

The Norplant System brand of subdermal levonorgestrel implants, is not currently available in the United States. Norplant, approved by the FDA in 1990, is a device consisting of six Silastic capsules 2.4 mm wide and 34 mm long that are implanted under the skin in the upper arm.[9] Norplant contains a total of 216 mg of levonorgestrel that is released at a constant rate of only 20 to 30 mcg/day over 5 years, after which time they are replaced.

Certain lot numbers of Norplant were recalled in 2000 however because of efficacy concerns, and users were encouraged to use back-up contraception. Further research found that the recalled lots did not have reduced efficacy, so back-up contraception is no longer required for the affected women. Wyeth does not plan to reintroduce the system.

A new implant, Implanon, a single rod containing 68 mg of etonogestrel (active metabolite of desogestrel) was approved in the United States in 2006 but has not yet been marketed (release is expected in 2008). Implanon provides highly effective, reversible contraception for 3 years. Etonogestrel side effects are similar to those seen with other progestin-only methods, including irregular bleeding, weight gain, and a potential for drug interactions with 3A4 inducers.

INTRAUTERINE DEVICES AND INTRAUTERINE SYSTEMS

Background and Mechanism of Action

33. R.P., a 23-year-old woman with hydrocephalus, is brought to the gynecology clinic by her mother, S.P., to determine the best method of contraception for her mentally impaired daughter. R.P. has never given birth or been pregnant. She is in a monogamous relationship with a mentally impaired partner. According to S.P., R.P. wishes to put off pregnancy for many years, and any method of

contraception that necessitates compliance is virtually impossible for the couple. DMPA has been considered but has not been used because of the possibility of menstrual irregularities that would upset R.P. and may not be a good long-term method owing to bone density concerns. R.P. and her mother have never heard of intrauterine devices or intrauterine systems (IUS) before. Counsel her on what is available and how they work.

The IUD and IUS available to women today are safe and effective long-term methods of contraception. The devices are not as popular in the United States (only 1%–2% of women are users) as compared with other areas of the world (15%–18% of married women of reproductive age are users).[105,106] In the 1960s and 1970s several IUD were available to women in the United States including Lippes Loop, Safe-T-Coil, Copper-7, Tatum T, and Progestasert. The Dalkon Shield IUD introduced in the United States in 1971 and removed from the market in 1974 is responsible for much of the negative "press" related to IUD and IUS. The Dalkon Shield was removed from the market owing to increased susceptibility to PID, with subsequent tubal scarring and infertility reported in users. Although the higher incidence of PID was not seen with the other types of IUD, the negative publicity hurt the use of all IUD. By 1976, the only IUD still available in the United States was the Progestasert, which was discontinued in 2001. Currently, two devices are available in the United States, the ParaGard IUD introduced in 1988 and the Mirena IUS introduced in 2000. Although the safety issues raised by the Dalkon Shield have been reassessed and resolved, the myths and misinformation associated with IUD and IUS have continued.

The ParaGard IUD, also known as the Copper-T IUD, has a polyethylene body that is wrapped with copper wire. Once inserted, the ParaGard may be left in place for 10 years.[9,107] The Mirena IUS also has a polyethylene body, with a levonorgestrel reservoir in the vertical stem of the T.[108] Mirena is effective for 5 years. The failure rate of ParaGard is 0.6 to 0.8 pregnancies per 100 woman-years compared with 0.1 for Mirena (Table 45-1). IUD and IUS are inserted by a health care provider in the office. The procedure usually takes only a few minutes and does not require sedation. Many providers will recommend that patients take a dose of an NSAID before the insertion visit. The devices are frequently inserted during or within 5 days of menses to eliminate the possibility of pregnancy at the time of insertion; however, the devices can be inserted at any time in the cycle.

The mechanisms of action for ParaGard include prevention of fertilization and implantation and by interfering with sperm transport, viability, or number. A secondary mechanism, interfering with implantation may explain the effectiveness of ParaGard for emergency contraception. Mirena contains a progestin and works by thickening the cervical mucus, preventing sperm from entering the uterus, altering the endometrial lining, preventing ovulation, and altering sperm activity.[108] A secondary mechanism of action for Mirena, interfering with implantation has also been proposed. The myth that IUD and IUS are abortifacient is widespread and inaccurate.

Advantages

34. R.P.'s mother thinks that an IUD or IUS is a good option for her daughter, but R.P. is not sure. What are the advantages of IUD or IUS that R.P. should be aware of?

Both the Mirena and ParaGard are both safe, highly effective, reversible, long-term methods that do not require regular action by the user. The ParaGard IUD is a good option for women who want a highly effective nonhormonal contraceptive method; however, increased menstrual bleeding and cramping are seen more often with ParaGard than with Mirena. The Mirena IUS is a good option for women who want a long-lasting method and also are good candidates for progestins. Mirena can be left in place for 5 years, is rapidly reversible and has the added advantages of reducing menstrual bleeding and cramping. Mirena is used worldwide to manage heavy bleeding and dysmennorrhea. User satisfaction with IUD or IUS is higher than for all other methods of contraception. Reasons for low use of IUD or IUS in the United States include lack of awareness of the method (only 50% of women are aware), those aware are uncertain about safety (71%) or efficacy (58%), and lack of trained health care providers to insert them.[105]

Although the initial cost of inserting an IUD or IUS is higher than the initial cost of pills or injections (around $500 for the device and insertion costs), there are no monthly recurring costs to R.P. as there would be with the other methods. Therefore, women who use an IUD or IUS for >1 year have an overall lower monthly overall cost than women who use COC or the contraceptive ring or patch.

Disadvantages

Insertion of an IUD or IUS requires an office visit for the minor procedure. IUD or IUS are contraindicated in women with certain anatomic abnormalities of the uterus that might interfere with insertion, unexplained vaginal bleeding, cervical cancer, and those with active untreated PID or genital infections (Table 45-4).[18,109] The device may be safely used in women with human immunodeficiency virus (HIV) infection (World Health Organization [WHO] Category 2).[110–112] The Mirena IUS should not be used in women with active breast cancer and should be used with caution in women with a current DVT or PE or a history of breast cancer. Breast cancer is hormonally sensitive, and the disease may be worsened by the use of levonorgestrel. Although the serum levels of levonorgestrel are low with the Mirena IUS, the manufacturer currently does not recommend that women with active or past breast cancer use the device.

It has been widely believed that IUD users are more likely to develop PID than nonusers. Users of IUD or IUD have similar rates of PID infection as nonusers. Long-term use, defined as beyond 21 days, is not associated with increased risk. The transient increase in risk of PID from IUD or IUD use occurs shortly after insertion (in the first 21 days) and is usually related to a pre-existing untreated STD at the time of insertion.[109,111] To reduce the risk of PID associated with the device insertion, screening for gonorrhea and chlamydia before insertion is recommended. Women who are positive for either STD should consider an alternative form of contraception until treatment is completed. In addition, IUD and IUS have previously been reserved for women in monogamous relationships or who have strict use of condoms because of concerns about STD and PID; however, current product labeling no longer contains these restrictions (product labeling updated 2006). IUD and IUS have also previously not been recommended for women who have not delivered a child; this is also no longer the case. They can be safely and appropriately used in nulliparous women.

Table 45-7 Intrauterine Device or Intrauterine System (IUD/IUS) Early Danger Signs (PAINS)

Period late (pregnancy) or abnormal spotting or intermenstrual bleeding
Abdominal pain or pain with intercourse
Infection exposure (e.g., gonorrhea) or abnormal vaginal discharge
Not feeling well, fever, chills
String missing, shorter, or longer

The IUD and IUS devices are almost as effective as sterilization for preventing pregnancy. In the unlikely event that an IUD or IUS user becomes pregnant, there is a higher risk that the pregnancy may be ectopic. This, however, is more a reflection of the effectiveness of the method and not because the devices cause ectopic pregnancy (i.e., the ratio of ectopic to uterine pregnancies is higher in IUD or IUS users than nonusers).[107,108] If a woman using an IUD or IUS becomes pregnant, the device should be removed because her risk for spontaneous abortion, sepsis, or premature delivery are increased if the device is left in place.

Continuation rates for IUD and IUS users are high. Approximately 10% to 15% of IUD are removed because of excessive uterine bleeding, spotting, or pain.[107,108] Another 2% to 6% of women spontaneously expel their IUD within the first year. Rarely, and IUD or IUS may become embedded in the endometrium or partially or totally perforate the uterine wall. R.P. should be instructed to look for the warning signs of a possible complication with IUD or IUS use (Table 45-7).

DIAPHRAGM

Mechanism of Action

35. R.C., a 25-year-old woman who is breastfeeding her 6-week-old infant, will consider only a barrier method of contraception. How do diaphragms prevent pregnancy?

The diaphragm is a soft, latex device with a metal spring reinforcing the rim.[9,18] The device is inserted vaginally and placed over the cervical to mechanically block access of sperm to the cervix. It is held in place by the spring tension of the rim, vaginal muscle tone, and the pubic bone. Because the diaphragm does not fit sufficiently tightly to be a complete barrier to sperm, spermicidal gel must be placed in the dome before use.[9]

The first-year failure rate with diaphragms is 6 to 20 pregnancies per 100 woman-years (Table 45-1).[9] R.C. should be counseled that diaphragms are less effective than other available methods and may increase her risk of UTI. Because breastfeeding offers some protection against pregnancy, breastfeeding women may be the best candidates for the diaphragm. Women allergic to latex or spermicide should not use the method.

Types

36. What types of diaphragms are available?

Diaphragms must be properly fitted to be effective. Currently available devices are made of latex, available in a range of sizes (50–95 mm in diameter) and types of circular rim construction.[9,18] The coil spring rim diaphragm folds flat and may be used with a diaphragm introducer. These diaphragms are indicated for women with average vaginal muscle tone and for those who can tolerate the sturdy rim and firm spring strength. The rim of the arcing spring rim diaphragm arcs when folded. Most women, even those with lax vaginal muscle tone, can tolerate the firm spring strength of the arcing spring rim diaphragm. The flat spring rim diaphragm is good for women with firm vaginal muscle tone, because the rim is less firm than the other styles. The wide-seal rim diaphragm (available as an arcing spring or coil spring) has a flexible flange designed to hold spermicide in place and to create a better seal between the diaphragm and vaginal wall.

R.C. would likely be able to tolerate any of the diaphragms. Perhaps she will find that one type is more comfortable than the others when she is fitted and the best fit can be selected during the office visit. The importance of using the diaphragm with spermicide during every act of intercourse should be stressed during counseling.

Fitting

37. How is a diaphragm size selected?

The goal of fitting a diaphragm is to select the largest rim size that is comfortable for the woman.[9,18] A diaphragm that is too small may become dislodged during intercourse because vaginal depth increases during sexual arousal. Conversely, a diaphragm that is too large may cause vaginal pressure, abdominal pain or cramping, vaginal ulceration, or recurrent urinary tract infections.

Patient Instructions

38. What instructions should be provided to R.C. concerning the use of a diaphragm?

The diaphragm should not remain in the vagina for longer than 24 hours.[9] Toxic shock syndrome (TSS) has been associated with diaphragm use and women should be alert to its symptoms, which include fever, diarrhea, vomiting, muscle aches, and a sunburnlike rash. Allergic reactions to the latex or spermicides also have been reported.

Before insertion, R.C. should inspect the diaphragm for holes or puckering. R.C. should be counseled that the diaphragm should always be inserted before intercourse if contraception is to be maximized. It can be inserted as much as 6 hours before intercourse if necessary. The diaphragm should not be removed for at least 6 hours after intercourse. One teaspoon of spermicidal gel should be placed into the dome (on the side adjacent to the cervix) and along the rim of the diaphragm before insertion. If intercourse is repeated, a new application of spermicide should be inserted vaginally without removal of the diaphragm.

When the diaphragm is removed, it should be washed with mild soap and water, rinsed and dried, and stored in its plastic container. Talcum or perfumed powders should not be used on the diaphragm because these may damage the diaphragm or cause irritation of the vagina or cervix. Oil-based products also may decompose the diaphragm and should not be used. Contraceptive gel, however, may be used if vaginal lubrication is needed. If R.C. gains or loses 10 to 20 pounds, has a pregnancy, or has abdominal or pelvic surgery, the fit of her diaphragm should be checked.

CERVICAL CAP

39. R.C. is also interested in the cervical cap. What is it, how well does it work, and what information should be provided to cervical cap users?

The cervical cap is a small, flexible, cuplike device made of latex and designed to fit closely around the base of the cervix; it is available in 22-, 25-, 28-, and 31-mm internal rim diameter sizes.[9,18] The cervical cap is less effective in women who have delivered a child, with pregnancy rates of 26 to 40 pregnancies per 100 woman-years in nulliparous women and 9 to 20 pregnancies per 100 woman-years in parous women. Women generally prefer other methods of contraception to cervical caps. In one study, 50% of women discontinued using cervical caps after 6 months, and 50% were pregnant after 2 years of use.[113]

To use the cervical cap, R.C. should fill the cap about one-third full with spermicidal gel, insert it vaginally, and place it over the cervix.[9,18] Suction holds it in place. It should be left in place at least 8 hours after intercourse but no longer than 48 hours, according to the manufacturer. Most experts recommend removal after 24 hours because of problems with vaginal odor at 36 to 48 hours and the theoretic risk of TSS.

As with the diaphragm, patient users should check the cap for holes before using. Also, R.C. should avoid using oil-based lubricants or medications when using the cervical cap.

CONDOMS

40. J.D. is a 45-year-old unmarried woman who has sex infrequently. She would like a method to protect against pregnancy as well as STD. How effective are condoms in preventing pregnancy? What types of condoms are available?

Condoms are an effective method of contraception when used properly. The failure rate with condoms is 3 to 12 pregnancies per 100 woman-years of use (Table 45-1).[9,16] The female condom is slightly less effective, with 5 to 21 pregnancies per 100 woman-years. Many different brands of condoms are available in the United States. The brands differ in size, shape, color, material, and the presence or absence of lubricants or spermicide. Most practitioners recommend lubricated condoms with reservoir ends to collect the ejaculate and to prevent breakage. Spermicides may increase the risk of HIV transmission.

The most commonly used male condom is made of latex.[9,10] Male condoms made of polyurethane and lambskin, which are also available, are recommended for men or women when one partner is allergic to latex. Polyurethane condoms, however, are more expensive and harder to find than latex condoms and natural or lambskin condoms do not offer the same protection against STD. Female condoms are made of polyurethane.

41. What are the advantages and disadvantages of condoms? How are they used?

Because the pre-ejaculatory secretions may contain sperm, the male condom should be applied before vaginal contact.[9,10] Female condoms should also be inserted before sexual contact; they may be inserted up to 8 hours before intercourse. Condoms should be used by their expiration date and should not be reused. They should be stored in a cool, dry place, not somewhere they will be exposed to prolonged periods of heat or light.

The chief noncontraceptive benefit of condoms is the prevention of STD (including gonorrhea, chlamydia, and HIV), and they can be used for vaginal, anal, or oral sex.[9,18] Condoms are also readily available without a prescription and do not cause systemic side effects like the hormonal methods. Latex male condoms are inexpensive. Some complain, however, that condoms reduce sensitivity and spontaneity. Female condoms are more costly (about $3 each), can be noisy, and can be difficult to insert.[18] Condoms may also break; this is less likely with the female condom. Oil-based products can degrade latex and should be avoided when using male, latex condoms. Oil-based lubricants can be used with female condoms or male polyurethane or lambskin condoms.

When using a male condom, the man or his partner holds the tip of the condom and unrolls it down to the base of the erect penis.[9,18] The female condom consists of a smaller circular ring at one end (which secures the device around the cervix like a diaphragm) and a larger ring at the other end. The inner ring should be compressed and inserted vaginally as far as it will go, and the larger ring remains outside of the vagina, protecting the external genitalia.

VAGINAL SPERMICIDES

42. J.D. would like to use a spermicide along with condoms. What options does she have, and how effective are spermicides when used alone?

Vaginal spermicides currently are available without a prescription as gels (jellies), suppositories, foams, and films.[8,18,114] Most of these products use a nonionic surfactant, nonoxynol-9, as the spermicide; the balance use octoxynol-9. The in vitro spermicidal potencies of the various preparations are highest with foam, followed by cream, jelly, and gel, respectively. When used in combination with a male condom, spermicides provide effective contraception.

43. What dosage form should J.D. use? How should she be instructed to use a vaginal spermicide? What side effects can be anticipated?

Table 45-8 compares the different spermicidal products.[9,18,114] The different characteristics of the products can help guide J.D. when selecting a dosage form. Regardless of the dosage form, a new dose of spermicide should be applied before each act of intercourse.

Spermicides can cause genital irritation and, in some patients, lead to ulceration. For this reason, spermicides have been shown to increase the transmission of STD, including HIV, gonorrhea, and chlamydia.

EMERGENCY CONTRACEPTION

Emergency Contraceptive Pills

44. B.P., a 24-year-old woman, has just returned home from a vacation in Europe. Her luggage containing her COC was stolen

Table 45-8 Comparison of Vaginal Spermicides

Formulation	Brand Name Examples	How to Use	Onset of Action	Duration of Action
Gel	Conceptrol, Gynol II	Fill applicator, insert applicator vaginally as far as it will comfortably go, press plunger of applicator to deposit spermicide near the cervix.	Immediate	1 hr
Film	VCF	Fold film in half, fold over finger, use finger to insert as far as it will comfortably go.	15 min	3 hr
Foam	Delfen, Koromex, VCF	Shake foam canister, fill applicator, insert applicator vaginally as far as it will comfortably go, press plunger of applicator to deposit spermicide near the cervix.	Immediate	1 hr
Suppository	Conceptrol, Encare	Unwrap, use finger to insert as far as it will comfortably go.	15 min	1 hr

2 weeks ago, and she had unprotected midcycle intercourse 24 hours ago. What can be done to prevent an unwanted pregnancy at this time?

Emergency contraception (also known EC), sometimes referred to as the morning-after pill, is a method of contraception that can be used after intercourse to prevent pregnancy.[115] Indications for EC are failure to use a contraceptive during intercourse (e.g., forgot, were assaulted) or method failure (e.g., broken condom or missed oral contraceptives). Emergency contraceptive pills (ECP) reduce the risk of pregnancy by 75% to 89% when taken up to 120 hours after unprotected intercourse. The mechanism of action for EC has been widely debated. A 2006 article discussing the mechanism of action concluded the primary mechanism of actions is delayed or inhibited ovulation. EC may also interfere with fertilization (most likely owing to altered tubular transport of the sperm or ovum). Alternations to the endometrial lining that may affect implantation have not been reported from the use of levonorgestrel only EC; however, the possibility can not be excluded.[116]

Although ECP use is on the rise, many women are not aware that it is available. In a 1998 survey, 686 of 1,000 women aged 18 to 44 had ever heard of emergency contraception. Of those aware of EC, only 5% had learned about it from a health care professional, 44% identified the source as a television news program, and another 16% read about it in a magazine. Approximately 12% of obstetricians and gynecologists interviewed in the same survey feared women would use ECP for routine contraception.[117] A more recent survey from 2004 found similar results. In the more recent survey, many of the women indicated awareness of EC, were not aware that is was available in the United States, confused it with Mifiprex (RU-486), or did not know that EC is taken after unprotected intercourse.[118]

Available Emergency Contraceptive Pills

PROGESTIN ONLY EMERGENCY CONTRACEPTIVE PILLS

Plan B is a progestin-only ECP approved for nonprescription sale by pharmacies and clinics to consumers (men and women) age 18 and older and by prescription to women 17 years and under. The Plan B pack consists of two white levonorgestrel 0.75-mg tablets and detailed instructions for use.[119–121] One tablet is to be taken as soon as possible and the second is taken 12 hours later. An alternative dosing regimen that is not currently FDA approved is to take both tablets (1.5 mg levonorgestrel) at once. The single-dose regimen (1.5 mg) is available in Canada and Europe and may be more effective than the two doses 12 hours apart.[118] Progestin-only EC is the regimen of choice because it is more effective and has significantly fewer side effects than estrogen and progestin ECPs.[118]

The risk of pregnancy is reduced by 89% when Plan B is taken within 72 hours after a single act of intercourse. If taken within the first 24 hours after intercourse, levonorgestrel may reduce the risk of pregnancy by 95%. Although the reduction in pregnancy is greatest when used within 24 hours after unprotected intercourse, use as long as 120 hours after has been shown to be effective.[119] The progesterone-only pill, Ovrette, may also be used for emergency contraception. This product is rarely used, however, because the woman would need to take 20 pills per dose to get the proper amount of progestin.

ESTROGEN AND PROGESTIN EMERGENCY CONTRACEPTIVE PILLS

An alternative to the progestin-only EC regimen is the Yuzpe regimen. An FDA-approved product (Preven) was released in 1999 utilizing the Yuzpe regimen but Preven is no longer being marketed in the United States. The Yuzpe regimen of emergency contraception utilizes commercially available COC to deliver 0.5 mg levonorgestrel and 100 mcg EE per dose.[9,122] Women should take two doses 12 hours apart. Table 45-9 shows

Table 45-9 Oral Contraceptive Pills That May Be Used As Emergency Contraception

Brand	Tablets per Dose (N)	Color
Alesse	5	Pink
Aviane	5	Orange
Cryselle	4	White
Enpresse	4	Orange
Lessina	5	Pink
Levlen	4	Light-orange
Levlite	5	Pink
Levora	4	White
Lo-Ovral	4	White
Low-Ogestrel	4	White
Nordette	4	Light-orange
Ogestrel	2	White
Ovral	2	White
Ovrette	20	Yellow
Plan B	1	White
Portia	4	Pink
Preven	2	Blue
Tri-Levlen	4	Yellow
Triphasil	4	Yellow
Trivora	4	Pink

which COC may be used and how many tablets need to be taken per dose.[121–123] It is very important to counsel women about which pills to take, because the tablet color and number differ depending on the brand chosen. This coupled with an increase in side effects makes this method less desirable than levonorgestrel-only regimens (discussed above). As with progestin-only regimens, the reduction in pregnancy is greatest when used within 24 hours after unprotected intercourse; however, the use after as long as 120 hours has been shown to be more effective than estrogen and progestin ECP.[119,122] The Yuzpe regimen reduces the risk of pregnancy by 89% after a single act of intercourse when taken within 72 hours.

Patient Instructions

The ECP are most effective when taken as soon as possible after intercourse; therefore, treatment should not be delayed.[115,119,122] In the FDA-approved regimens, the first dose is to be taken within 72 hours after intercourse; however, ECP have been shown to be effective when the first dose is taken within 5 days of unprotected sex.[118,120] The most common side effects with ECP are nausea and vomiting; however, most women do not experience side effects from the progestin-only regimen. Gastrointestinal adverse effects are more likely with the estrogen and progestin ECP than with the progestin-only ECP. B.P. should be instructed that if she vomits within 1 hour of taking either dose of medication, the dose should be repeated. When a Yuzpe regimen is used, an antiemetic (e.g., prochlorperazine or meclizine) can be given 30 to 60 minutes before each dose of ECP to prevent nausea or vomiting.[115]

B.P.'s menses may come early or late, but she should take a pregnancy test if her menses do not come within 3 weeks of taking ECP.

Women under age 18 may call the Emergency Contraception Hotline (1-888-NOT-2-Late or 1-888-668-2528) to find a provider near them who will prescribe ECP. Women may also find information about ECP at the Emergency Contraception website website (http://www.not-2-late.com). As of January 2008, pharmacists can prescribe EC under collaborative protocol agreements in nine states.[118]

IUD for Emergency Contraception

The copper IUD is also an effective method of emergency contraception when inserted within 5 days of unprotected sex.[124] Because some women are not good candidates for IUD (see discussion above) and because IUD must be inserted by a health care provider, they are not used as regularly for emergency contraception in the United States. The biggest advantage of using of an IUD for emergency contraception is that it provides ongoing contraception and the Paragard is significantly more effective in preventing pregnancy than oral regimens (1 failure in 10,000 insertions vs. 1:100 for pills).

MEDICAL ABORTION

45. G.H. was given a pack of OCs last month, but could not remember how to start them. She has just discovered that she is 4 weeks pregnant. She is 23 yo and single and is considering terminating the pregnancy. What options are there for medical abortion?

It is estimated that about one half of pregnancies are unintended, so it is important for these women to hav safe options. G.H. should be counseled extensively about her options including keeping the baby, adoption, and medical or surgical abortion. Compared with surgical abortion, medical abortion does not require a surgical procedure so it is less likely to cause infection and is less costly.[51] Also some women feel more in control when choosing this option. However, some patients may not prefer medical abortion because it usually takes more medical visits and follow-up, has a slightly lower success rate (94–97%; failures will need a surgical procedure), and involves more bleeding and cramping which usually lasts for 2 weeks.

There are many variations in how medical abortions are carried out, but the general treatment remains the same.[51] G.H. would first have baseline labs done including blood type and hemoglobin. She would be given mifepristone that same day to stop development of the pregnancy. In the U.S., mifepristone, and antiprogestin, is more commonly used. Then misoprostol is given to induce uterine contractions and expel the pregnancy.

Typically, if using mifepristone, G.H. would be given 200 mg orally on day 1 then misoprostol orally or vaginally on day 2 or 3.[51] Misoprostol is FDA approved for oral use. It may be given as 400 or 600 mcg orally, given sublingually or given as early as 6–8 hours after mifepristone.[123–125] Vaginal use of misoprostol is not approved and it's use is under review.

REFERENCES

1. Henshaw S. Unintended Pregnancy in the United States. *Family Planning Perspectives* 1998;30.
2. Hansten PD et al. Inhibition of oral contraceptive efficacy. *Drug Interactions Newsletter* 1985;5:7.
3. Speroff L et al. *A Clinical Guide to Contraception*. 32nd ed. Baltimore: Lippincott Williams & Wilkins; 2001.
4. Jones RK et al. Contraceptive use among U.S. women having abortions in 2000–2001. *Perspect Sex Reprod Health* 2002;34:294.
5. Jones RK et al. Patterns in the socioeconomic characteristics of women obtaining abortions in 2000–2001. *Perspect Sex Reprod Health* 2002;34:226.
6. Peipert JF et al. Oral contraceptive risk assessment: a survey of 247 educated women. *Obstet Gynecol* 1993;82:112.
7. National Campaign to Reduce Teen Pregnancy. 14 and Younger: The Sexual Behavior of Young Adolescents. Washington, DC; 2003.
8. Speroff L et al., eds. *Clinical Gynecologic Endocrinology and Infertility*. 6th ed. Philadelphia: Lippincott Williams & Wilkins; 1999.
9. Hatcher RA et al. *Contraceptive Technology*. 18th ed. New York: Ardent Media; 2004.
10. Dickey RP. *Managing Contraceptive Pill Patients*. 12th ed. Dallas: Essential Medical Information Systems; 2004.
11. Upton GW. The phasic approach to oral contraception: the triphasic concept and its clinical application. *Int J Fertil* 1983;28:121.
12. Holt VL et al. Body weight and risk of oral contraceptive failure. *Obstet Gynecol* 2002;99:820.
13. Briggs MH. Choosing contraceptive steroids and doses. *J Reprod Med* 1983;28(Suppl 1):57.
14. Goldzieher JW et al. Comparative studies of the ethinyl estrogens used in oral contraception. II: Antiovulatory potency. *Am J Obstet Gynecol* 1975;122:619.
15. Westhoff C et al. Initiation of oral contraceptives using quickstart vs. compared with a conventional start: a randomized controlled clinical trial. *Obstet Gynecol* 2007;109:1270.
16. Drug Facts and Comparisons. 57th ed. St Louis: Facts and Comparisons; 2002.
17. Dickinson BD et al. Drug interactions between oral contraceptives and antibiotics. *Obstet Gynecol* 2001;98:853.

17a. Back DJ et al. Evaluation of Committee on Safety of Medicines yellow card reports on oral contraceptive drug interactions with anticonvulsants and antibiotics. *Br J Clin Pharmacol* 1988;25:527.

18. Family and Reproductive Health Programme. Improving Access to Quality Care in Family Planning. Medical Eligibility Criteria for Contraceptive Use. 3rd ed. Geneva: World Health Organization; 2004.
19. Hansten PD et al. Inhibition of oral contraceptive efficacy. *Drug Interactions Newsletter* 1985;5:7.
20. Roby CA et al. St John's wort: effect of CYP3A4 activity. *Clin Pharmacol Ther* 2000;67:451.
21. Vandenbroucke JP et al. Oral contraceptives and the risk of venous thrombosis. *N Engl J Med* 2001;344:1527.
21a. Rosenberg MJ et al. Oral contraceptive discontinuation: a prospective evaluation of frequency and reasons. *Am J Obstet Gynecol* 1998;179:577.
22. DeLeacy EA et al. Effects of subjects' sex, and intake of tobacco, alcohol, and oral contraceptives on plasma phenytoin levels. *Br J. Clin Pharmacol* 1979;8:33.
23. Schwingl PJ et al. Estimates of the risk of cardiovascular death attributable to low-dose oral contraceptives in the United States. *Am J Obstet Gynecol* 1999;180:241.
24. Royal College of General Practitioners' Oral Contraceptive Study. Incidence of arterial disease among oral contraceptive users. *J R Coll Gen Prac* 1983;33:75.
25. Vessey MP et al. Mortality in oral contraceptive users. *Lancet* 1981;1:549.
26. Vessey MP et al. Mortality among oral contraceptive users: 20-year follow-up of women in a cohort study. *BMJ* 1989;299:1487.
27. Knopp RH et al. Comparison of the lipoprotein, carbohydrate, and hemostatic effects of phasic oral contraceptives containing desogestrel or levonorgestrel. *Contraception* 2001;63:1.
28. Merki-Feld GS et al. Long-term effects of combined oral contraceptives on markers of endothelial function and lipids in healthy premenopausal women. *Contraception* 2002;65:231.
29. Miller NE et al. Relation of angiographically defined coronary artery disease to plasma lipoprotein subfractions and apolipoprotein. *BMJ* 1981;282:1741.
30. Endrikat J et al. An open-label, comparative study of the effects of a dose-reduced oral contraceptive containing 20 mcg ethinyl estradiol and 100 mcg levonorgestrel on hemostatic, lipids, and carbohydrate metabolism variables. *Contraception* 2002;65:215.
31. Tikkanen MJ et al. High-density lipoprotein-2 and hepatic lipase: reciprocal changes produced by estrogen and norgestrel. *J Clin Endocrinol Metab* 1982;54:1113.
32. Tikkanen MH et al. Reduction of plasma high-density lipoprotein-2 cholesterol and increase of post-heparin plasma hepatic lipase activity during progestin treatment. *Clin Chim Acta* 1981;115:63.
33. Paulus D et al. Oral contraception and cardiovascular risk factors during adolescence. *Contraception* 2000;62:113.
34. Tanis BC et al. Oral contraceptives and the risk of myocardial infarction. *N Engl J Med* 2001;345: 1787.
35. Dunn N et al. Oral contraceptives and myocardial infarction: results of the MICA case-control study. *BMJ* 1999;318:1579.
36. American Cancer Society. Cancer Facts and Figures 2008. Atlanta: American Cancer Society; 2008.
37. Moreno V et al. Effect of oral contraceptives on risk of cervical cancer in women with human papillomavirus infection: the IARC multicentric case-control study. *Lancet* 2002;359:1085.
38. Beral et al. Mortality associated with oral contraceptive use: 25-year follow-up of cohort of 46,000 women from Royal College of General Practitioners' oral contraception study. *BMJ* 1999;318:96.
39. Irwin KL et al. Oral contraceptives and cervical cancer risk in Costa Rica. Detection bias or causal association? *JAMA* 1988;259:59.
40. Seibert C et al. Prescribing oral contraceptives for women older than 35 years of age. *Ann Intern Med* 2003;138:54.
41. Tapla HR et al. Effect of oral contraceptive therapy on the renin angiotensin system in normotensive and hypertensive women. *Obstet Gynecol* 1973;41:643.
42. Fisch TR et al. Oral contraceptives and blood pressure. *JAMA* 1977;237:2499.
43. Ramcharan S et al. The occurrence and course of hypertensive disease in users and nonusers of oral contraceptive drugs. In: Ramcharan S, ed. *The Walnut Creek Contraceptive Drug Study: A Prospective Study of the Side Effects of Oral Contraceptives.* Vol 2. Washington, DC: Government Printing Office; 1976:1. DHEW publication no. (NIH) 74-562.
44. Fisch TR et al. Oral contraceptives, pregnancy and blood pressure. In: Ramcharan S, ed. *The Walnut Creek Contraceptive Drug Study: A Prospective Study of the Side Effects of Oral Contraceptives.* Vol 1. Washington, DC: Government Printing Office; 1974:105. DHEW publication no. (NIH) 74-562.
45. American College of Obstetrics and Gynecology. The use of hormonal contraception in women with coexisting medical conditions. *ACOG Practice Bulletin Number* 8; July 2000.
46. Rooks JB et al. Epidemiology of hepatocellular adenoma: the role of oral contraceptive use. *JAMA* 1979;242:644.
47. Bein NN et al. Recurrent massive hemorrhage from benign hepatic tumors secondary to oral contraceptives. *Br J Surg* 1977;64:433.
48. Klatskin G. Hepatic tumors: possible relationship to use of oral contraceptives. *Gastroenterology* 1977;73:386.
49. Desser-Wiest L. Promotion of liver tumors by steroid hormones. *J Toxicol Environ Health* 1979;5: 203.
50. Gomes MPV et al. Risk of venous thromboembolic disease associated with hormonal contraceptives and hormone replacement therapy: a clinical review. *Arch Int Med* 2004;164:1964.
51. Hatcher RA et al. *A Pocket Guide to Managing Contraception.* Tiger, GA: Bridging the Gap Foundation; 2005.
52. Cunliffe WJ. Acne, hormones and treatment. *BMJ* 1982;285:912.
53. Speroff L et al. Evaluation of a new generation of oral contraceptives. *Obstet Gynecol* 1993;81:1034.
54. Brinton LA et al. Risk factors for benign breast disease. *Am J Epidemiol* 1981;113:203.
55. Royal College of General Practitioners. Oral Contraceptives and Health: An Interim Report From the Oral Contraception Study of the Royal College of General Practitioners. Pitman, NY: Royal College of General Practitioners; 1974.
56. Speroff L. PMS: looking for new answers to an old problem. *Contemporary Obstetrics and Gynecology* 1983;21:102.
57. Darney PD. Evaluating the pill's long-term effects. *Contemporary Obstetrics and Gynecology* 1982;20:57.
58. Barber HRK. The pill: noncontraceptive benefits. *Female Patient* 1982;7:12.
59. Halbert DR. Noncontraceptive uses of the pill. *Clin Obstet Gynecol* 1981;24:987.
60. Schlesselman JJ. Risk of endometrial cancer in relation to use of combined oral contraceptives. A practioner's guide to meta-analysis. *Hum Reprod* 1997;12:1851.
61. Siskind V et al. Beyond ovulation: oral contraceptives and epithelial ovarian cancer. *Epidemiology* 2000;11:106.
62. Susannel G et al. Declining ovarian cancer rates in U.S. women in relation to parity and oral contraceptive use. *Epidemiology* 2000;11:102.
63. Sherris JD et al. Infertility and sexually transmitted disease: a public health challenge. *Popul Rep L* 1983;11:113.
64. Rubin GL et al. Oral contraceptives and pelvic inflammatory disease. *Am J Obstet Gynecol* 1982;140:630.
65. Wolner-Hanssen P et al. Laparoscopic findings and contraceptive use in women with signs and symptoms suggestive of acute salpingitis. *Obstet Gynecol* 1985;66:233.
66. Washington AE et al. Oral contraceptives, chlamydia trachomatous infection, and pelvic inflammatory disease. *JAMA* 1985;253:2246.
67. Cramer DW et al. Tubal infertility and the intrauterine device. *N Engl J Med* 1985;312:941.
68. Wolner-Hanssen P et al. Decreased risk of symptomatic chlamydial pelvic inflammatory disease associated with oral contraceptive use. *JAMA* 1990;263:54.
69. Ory HW. The noncontraceptive health benefits from oral contraceptive use. *Family Planning Perspective* 1982;14:182.
70. Rubin GL et al. Ectopic pregnancy in the United States, 1970–1978. *JAMA* 1983;249:1725.
71. McPherson K et al. Oral contraception and breast cancer [Letter]. *Lancet* 1983;2:144.
72. Pike MC et al. Breast cancer in young women and use of oral contraceptives: possible modifying effect of formulation and age of use. *Lancet* 1983;2:926.
73. Royal College of General Practitioners' Oral Contraception Study. Breast cancer and oral contraceptives: findings in Royal College of General Practitioners' Study. *BMJ* 1981;282:2088.
74. Grabrick DM et al. Risk of breast cancer with oral contraceptive use in women with a family history of breast cancer. *JAMA* 2000;284:1791.
75. Marchbanks PA et al. Oral contraceptives and the risk of breast cancer. *N Engl J Med* 2002;346: 2025.
76. Ramcharan S et al. General summary of findings: general conclusions; implications. In: Ramcharan S et al., eds. *The Walnut Creek Contraceptive Drug Study: A Prospective Study of the Side Effects of Oral Contraceptives.* Vol 3. *An interim report: a comparison of disease occurrence leading to hospitalization or death in users and nonusers of oral contraceptives.* Bethesda, MD: Center for Population Research; 1981:1.
77. Vessey MP et al. Mortality among women participating in the Oxford/Family Planning Association Contraceptive Study. *BMJ* 1977;282:731.
78. Vessey MP et al. Breast cancer and oral contraceptives: findings in Oxford/Family Planning Association Contraceptive Study. *BMJ* 1981;282:2093.
79. The Centers for Disease Control Cancer and Steroid Hormone Study. Oral contraceptive use and the risk of breast cancer. *JAMA* 1983;249:1591.
80. Matthews PN et al. Breast cancer in women who have taken contraceptive steroids. *BMJ* 1981;282: 774.
81. Kjos SL et al. Effect of low-dose oral contraceptives on carbohydrate and lipid metabolism in women with recent gestational diabetes: results of a controlled, randomized, prospective study. *Am J Obstet Gynecol* 1990;163:1822.
82. Skouby SO. Low-dosage oral contraception in women with previous gestational diabetes. *Obstet Gynecol* 1982;59:325.
83. Skouby SO et al. Triphasic oral contraception: metabolic effects in normal women and those with previous gestational diabetes. *Am J Obstet Gynecol* 1985;153:495.
84. Briggs MH et al. Randomized prospective studies on metabolic effects of oral contraceptives. *Acta Obstet Gynecol Scand* 1982;105(Suppl):25.
85. Kim C et al. Oral contraceptive use and association with glucose, insulin, and diabetes in young adult women; the CARDIA Study. *Diabetes Care* 2002;25:1027.
86. Grodstein, et al. A prospective study of symptomatic gallstones in women: relation with oral contraceptives and other risk factors. *Obstet Gynecol* 1994;84:207.
87. Royal College of General Practitioners' Oral Contraception Study. Oral contraceptives and gallbladder disease. *Lancet* 1982;2:957.
88. Ramcharan S et al. *The Walnut Creek Contraceptive Drug Study: A Prospective Study of the Side Effects of Oral Contraceptives.* Vol 3. *An interim report: a comparison of disease occurrence leading to hospitalization or death in users and nonusers of oral contraceptives.* Bethesda, MD: Center for

Population Research; 1981; NIH publication no. 81564:349.

89. Vessey M, Painter R. Oral contraceptive use and benign gallbladder disease; revisited. *Contraception* 1994;50:167.
90. Briggs GG et al., eds. *A Reference Guide to Fetal and Neonatal Risk. Drugs in Pregnancy and Lactation*. 6th ed. Philadelphia: Lippincott Williams & Wilkins; 2001.
91. Simpson JL. Relationship between congenital anomalies and contraception. *Adv Contracept* 1985; 1:3.
92. Committee on Drugs, American Academy of Pediatrics. The transfer of drugs and other chemicals into human milk. *Pediatrics* 1994;93:137.
93. Ortho Evra package insert. Raritan, NJ: Ortho-McNeil Pharmaceuticals; 2001.
94. NuvaRing package insert. West Orange, NJ: Organon; 2001.
95. Kaunitz AM. Injectable contraception. *Clin Obstet Gynecol* 1989;32:356.
96. WHO Collaborative Study of Neoplasia and Steroid Contraceptives. Depot medroxyprogesterone acetate (DMPA) and risk of endometrial cancer. *Int J Cancer* 1991;49:186.
97. de Abood M et al. Effect of Depo-Provera or Microgynon on the painful crises of sickle cell anemia patients. *Contraception* 1997;56:313.
98. Depo-Provera package insert. Kalamazoo, MI: Pharmacia & Upjohn; 2002.
99. Kaunitz AM et al. Injectable contraception with depot medroxyprogesterone acetate. *Current Status Drugs* 1993;45:857.
100. Archer B et al. Depot medroxyprogesterone. Management of side effects commonly associated with its contraceptive use. *J Nurse Midwif* 1997;42:104.
101. Cundy T et al. Recovery of bone density in women who stop using medroxyprogesterone acetate. *BMJ* 1994;308:247.
102. Lappe JM et al. The impact of lifestyle factors on stress fracture in female Army recruits. *Osteoporosis Int* 2001;12:35.
103. Cromer B. Recent clinical issues related to the use of depot medroxyprogesterone acetate (Depo-Provera). *Curr Opin Obstet Gynecol* 1999;11:467.
104. Lunelle package insert. Kalamazoo, MI: Pharmacia & Upjohn; 2001.
105. Stanwood NL et al. Young pregnant women's knowledge of modern intrauterine devices. *Obstet Gynecol* 2006;108:1417.
106. Stanwood NL et al. Obstetrician-gynecologists and the intrauterine device: a survey of attitudes and practice. *Obstet Gynecol* 2002;99:275.
107. ParaGard package insert. Raritan, NJ: Ortho-McNeil Pharmaceuticals; 2002.
108. Mirena package insert. Montville, NJ: Berlex Laboratories; 2000.
109. Lee NC et al. The intrauterine device and pelvic inflammatory disease revisited: new results from the Women's Health Study. *Obstet Gynecol* 1988;72:1.
110. Morrison CS et al. Is the intrauterine device appropriate contraception for HIV-infected women? *Br J Obstet Gynaecol*. 2001;108:784.
111. World Health Organization. Medical Eligibility Criteria for Contraceptive Use. 3rd ed. Geneva: WHO; 2004.
112. Richardson B et al. Effect of intrauterine device use on cervical shedding of HIV-1 DNA. *AIDS* 1999; 13:2091.
113. Smith GG et al. The use of cervical caps at the University of California, Berkeley: a survey. *Contraception* 1984;30:115.
114. Berardi RR et al., eds. *Handbook of Nonprescription Drugs*. 13th ed. Washington, DC: American Pharmaceutical Association; 2002.
115. Wellbery C. Emergency contraception. *Archives of Family Medicine* 2000;9:642.
116. Davidoff F et al. Plan B and the politics of doubt. *JAMA*; 2006:296.
117. Demott K. Ob Gyns not discussing "morning-after pill." *Obstet Gynecol News* 1998;33:14.
118. The Emergency Contraception Website. http://ec.princeton.edu/. Accessed March 31, 2008.
119. Rodrigues I et al. Effectiveness of emergency contraceptive pills between 72 and 120 hours after unprotected sexual intercourse. *Am J Obstet Gynecol* 2001;184:531.
120. Foster DG et al. Pharmacy Access to Emergency Contraception in California. *Perspect Sex Reprod Health* 2006;38.
121. American Pharmaceutical Association. Emergency contraception: the pharmacist's role. Washington, DC: American Pharmaceutical Association; 2000.
122. Task Force on Postovulatory Methods of Fertility Regulation. Randomised controlled trial of levonorgestrel versus the Yuzpe regimen of combined oral contraceptives for emergency contraception. *Lancet* 1998;352:428.
123. Gemzell-Danielsson K et al. Studies on uterine contractility following mifepristone and various routes of misoprostol. *Contraception* 2006;74:31.
124. Tang OS, Ho PC. The pharmacokinetics and different regimens of misoprostol in early first trimester medical abortion. *Contraception* 2006;74:26.
125. Schaff E. Evidence for shortening the time interval of prostaglandin after mifepristone for medical abortion. *Contraception* 2006;74:42.

CHAPTER 46

Obstetric Drug Therapy

Kimey D. Ung and Jennifer McNulty

PREGNANCY

More than 4 million live births were registered in the United States in 2004, with an estimated 83.9% of women beginning prenatal care in the first trimester.[1] Although much improved, prenatal care is still not accessible to all women. The timing and quality of prenatal care can influence an infant's health and survival. Early comprehensive care can promote healthier pregnancies through early detection of risk factors, disease state management, and encouragement of healthy behaviors. Appropriate preconception counseling and treatment of women with pre-existing high-risk medical conditions, such as diabetes, hypertension and epilepsy, can greatly improve pregnancy outcomes. Essential preconception and early prenatal care, critical for normal fetal organogenesis, may not be sought because 40% of pregnancies in an American woman's lifetime are unplanned.[2] In 2004, the mortality rate (from birth through the first year of life) for infants of mothers beginning prenatal care after the first trimester, or not at all, was 37% higher (8.35 per 1,000 live births) than the rate for infants whose mothers' prenatal care began in the first trimester (6.11 per 1,000 births).[1]

The goal of prenatal care, to promote a safe and successful pregnancy and the delivery of a healthy infant, can be achieved through education and by monitoring the health of the mother and fetus. The first prenatal visit should occur no later than the second missed menstrual period, generally 8 weeks after missed menses.[2]

Placental Physiology

Conception begins with the fertilization of an ovum. The time after conception is the conceptional or developmental age. The gestational age or menstrual age, is the time from the start of the last menstrual period (LMP) and generally exceeds the developmental age by 2 weeks.[3] The fertilized ovum, or zygote, undergoes mitotic divisions that lead to the formation of the blastocyst, a hollow fluid-filled sphere.[4] The outer cell mass of the blastocyst differentiates into trophoblasts, whereas the internal cell mass gives rise to the embryo. About 5 to 6 days after fertilization, the blastocyst adheres to the endometrial epithelium, where it undergoes implantation between postconception day 7 to 12.[3] The outer cell mass, or trophoblasts, invades the endometrium, and the blastocyst becomes completely buried within the endometrium. Once trophoblastic invasion of the endometrium occurs, the endometrium is transformed into the decidua, the functional layer of the pregnant endometrium, and is referred to by this term throughout pregnancy.[5]

The trophoblast secretes human chorionic gonadotropin (hCG), which maintains the corpus luteum so that menstruation is prevented and pregnancy can continue.[6] (See Chapter 45, Contraception, for a detailed discussion of the menstrual cycle.) As more of the decidua is invaded, the walls of the decidual capillaries are eroded, thereby leaking maternal blood into spaces called lacunae.[4] This initial contact with the maternal blood allows hCG to enter the maternal circulation by day 11 of gestation when it can be measured to aid in the diagnosis of pregnancy.[6] The trophoblasts are the only cells of the conceptus that are in direct contact with maternal tissue or blood; embryonic cells never come in contact with maternal tissues.[4]

As the embryo within the blastocyst grows, the thickness of the decidua decreases. The part of the decidua directly below the site of implantation becomes the *decidua basalis*, and the part that lies over the growing blastocyte, which separates it from the rest of the uterine cavity, is the *decidua capsularis*; this part of the decidua contacts the chorion leave, the extraembryonic, avascular, fetal membrane. The rest of the uterus is lined by the decidua parietalis. By 14 to 16 weeks, the gestational sac is sufficient large to fill the entire uterine cavity, at which time the decidua capsularis has lost its blood supply and fuses with the decidua parietalis (which is sometimes referred to as the *decidua vera*).[5]

The vessels (spiral arteries) supplying blood to the decidua parietalis retain their endothelium and smooth muscle wall and therefore continue to respond to vasoactive agents.[5] By contrast, the spiral arteries supplying the decidua basalis undergo trophoblastic invasion whereby they are transformed into wide-bore uteroplacental vessels that empty directly into the intervillous space in fountainlike spurts.[3,4] This process creates a low-resistance arteriolar circuit that allows maximal placental blood flow necessary for the growing fetus.[7] Unlike the rest of the maternal and fetal vasculature, the resistance within these uteroplacental vessels does not change in response to vasoactive agents. The resistance is fixed and therefore directly dependent on maternal perfusion pressure.[6] If the maternal perfusion pressure decreases, blood flow to the placenta decreases. Likewise, placental blood flow is increased when the maternal perfusion pressure is increased. Incomplete trophoblastic invasion of the spiral arteries in the myometrium results in decreased placental perfusion and ischemia. This is believed to be a factor in the pathogenesis of pre-eclampsia.[7]

The placenta has both fetal and maternal components. The placenta is made up of the amnion, chorion, chorionic villi and intervillous spaces, decidual plate, and the myometrium.[3] The fetal surface of the placenta is covered by the amnion beneath which the fetal chorionic vessels cross. Figure 46-1 describes the structure of the placenta and its maternal–fetal circulation. Maternal–fetal circulation to the intervillous space is not fully established until the second trimester.[3] Maternal uteroplacental arteries perfuse the intervillous spaces, and as the maternal blood flows around the villi, exchanges (oxygen and nutrients) occur with fetal blood contained within capillaries found inside these villi.[3] Although the placenta serves as a strong barrier between the fetal and maternal circulations, a few cells are able to cross between the two circulations.[3] Except for pathologic conditions, fetal blood and maternal blood do not make contact. Placental blood flow reaches the fetus through a single umbilical vein. At the juncture of the placenta and umbilicus, the umbilical vein and arteries repeatedly branch and traverse the fetal surface of the placenta (between the amnion and the chorionic plate) forming capillary networks that terminate within the villi. These vessels are termed the *chorionic veins and arteries*. Fetal blood flow reaches the placenta through two umbilical arteries; carbon dioxide and waste products diffuse into the intervillous spaces and are carried away by the maternal decidual veins.[3] A description of fetal circulation can be found in Chapter 94, Neonatal Therapy.

The placenta has many functions in pregnancy.[3] In addition to respiratory functions, the placenta also has excretory functions, similar to those of the postnatal kidney (e.g., maintaining water and pH balance). The placenta also has resorptive functions similar to those of the gastrointestinal (GI) tract.[3] The placenta and the fetus regulate the course of pregnancy. This fetoplacental unit functions as the endocrine portion of the fetal–maternal communication system, producing several hormones responsible for regulating and maintaining pregnancy (e.g., hCG, estrogens, progesterone, placental lactogen).[6] The placenta also produces many other hormones, enzymes, proteins, and releasing factors.[6]

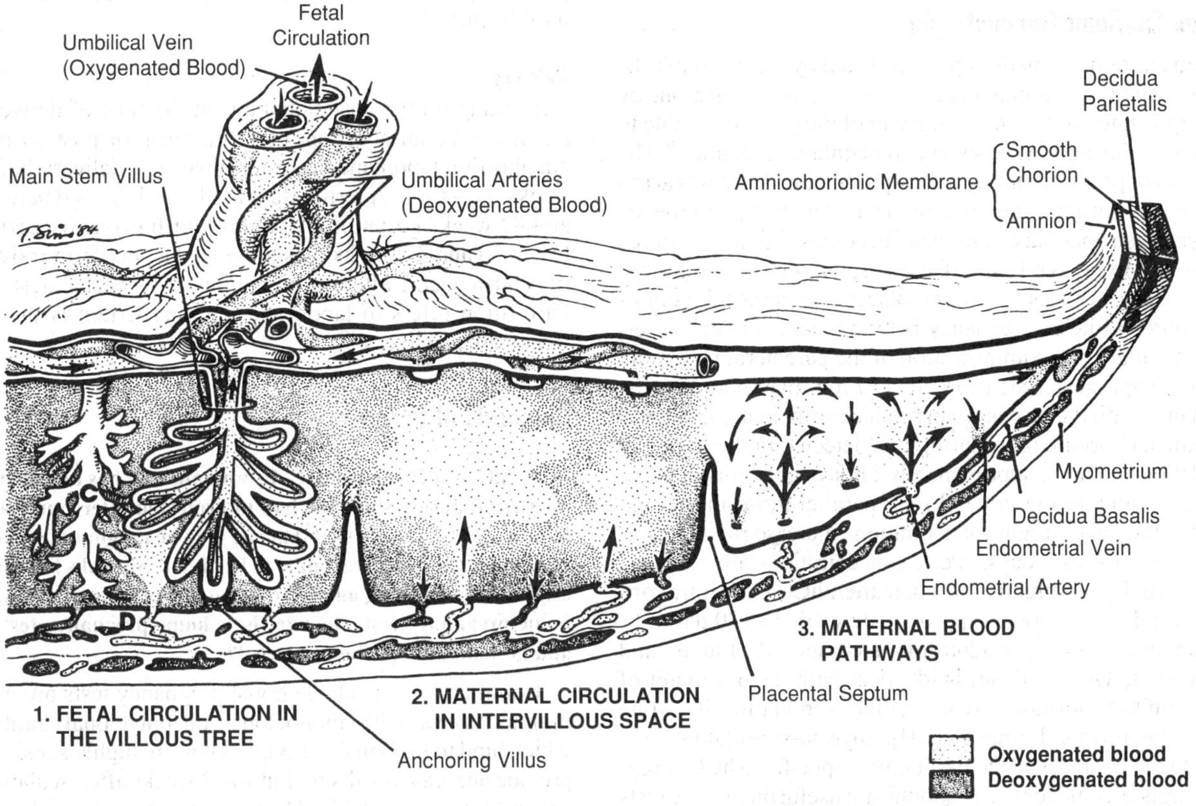

FIGURE 46-1 Term placenta. 1. The relation of the villous chorion (*C*) to the decidua basalis (*D*) and fetal placental circulation. 2. The maternal placenta circulation. Maternal blood flows into the intervillous spaces in the funnel-shaped spurts, and exchanges occur with the fetal blood as the maternal blood flows around the villi. 3. The inflowing arterial blood pushes venous blood into the endometrial veins, which are scattered over the entire surface of the decidua basalis. Note also that the umbilical arteries carry deoxygenated fetal blood to the placenta and that the umbilical vein carries oxygenated blood to the fetus. From reference 42, with permission.

Fetal Membranes

The fetal membranes are made up of an innermost membrane, the amnion, and an outer membrane, the chorion. These make up the "water bag." The amnion at term gestation is a tough but pliable membrane whose integrity is vital for the continuation and progression of pregnancy.[4] The fluid-filled space between the amnion and the embryo is the amniotic cavity. The membranes surround the developing fetus and function to contain the amniotic fluid and assist in its formation. This fluid provides a mechanically buffered, stable environment in which the fetus develops. The amniotic fluid has both maternal and fetal sources and is the paracrine arm of the fetal–maternal communication unit. The maternal source is plasma filtrate and, as pregnancy advances, the fetal contribution is from urine and lung fluids. The volume of amniotic fluid increases from 50 mL at 12 weeks' gestation to a maximum of 1,000 mL at 36 weeks, and declines at term.[8] The composition of the amniotic fluid includes water, fetal cells, hormones, lecithin, sphingomyelin, electrolytes, creatinine, and urea.[8] Amniotic fluid can be obtained by amniocentesis and tested for the presence of some of these substances to aid in fetal assessment. For example, the lecithin-to-sphingomyelin ratio is used as a marker of fetal lung maturity when preterm delivery is being contemplated for obstetric reasons (e.g., severe pre-eclampsia).[8]

Human Chorionic Gonadotropin

Human chorionic gonadotropin, produced by the trophoblasts, is responsible for maintaining the synthesis of progesterone by the corpus luteum within the ovary until the placenta is able to synthesize the amount necessary to maintain pregnancy.[9] The synthesis of progesterone by the corpus luteum decreases at approximately 6 weeks' gestation (menstrual age). After 8 weeks, the syncytiotrophoblast (placenta) becomes the major source for progesterone synthesis. If the corpus luteum is removed or its function ceases before the placenta becomes the dominant source of hCG, pregnancy is terminated.[9] In such cases, intramuscular (IM) administration of the parenteral progestin, 17-hydroxyprogesterone caproate 150 mg, may maintain the pregnancy until the placenta can produce sufficient quantities.[9]

Human chorionic gonadotropin is detected in the maternal circulation and urine approximately 11 days after conception.[6] Concentrations in the urine closely parallel those in the maternal blood. hCG serum concentrations increase rapidly, doubling every 1.4 to 2 days.[9] Peak concentrations are achieved at 60 to 70 days of pregnancy. Thereafter, hCG concentrations decline and reach a low at approximately 100 to 130 days.

Human chorionic gonadotropin is composed of an α- and a β-subunit. The α-subunit is identical with the α-subunit of other pituitary hormones (e.g., follicle-stimulating hormone [FSH], luteinizing hormone [LH], thyroid-stimulating hormone [TSH]); however, the β-subunit is specific to hCG. Pregnancy tests specific for this β-subunit are useful diagnostic tests for confirming pregnancy.[9]

Definitions

Parity and Gravida

Parity and *gravida* are terms used to describe a pregnant woman. Parity is the number of deliveries after 20 weeks' gestation. A delivery before the completion of 20 weeks' gestation is considered an abortion and can be either elective or spontaneous. Parity is independent of the number of fetuses delivered (live or stillborn, single fetus, or twins) or the method of delivery. *Gravida* refers to the number of pregnancies a woman has had regardless of the outcome. For example, a woman who is currently pregnant and has previously delivered one set of twins and had two spontaneous abortions is described as a gravida 4 para 1 (G_4P_1).[10]

Trimesters of Pregnancy

The average pregnancy is approximately 280 days or 40 weeks when calculated from the first day of the LMP. Pregnancy is typically divided into three trimesters, approximately 13 to 14 weeks each.[10] The time between the end of the 22nd week of gestation and the end of the 28th day after birth is considered the perinatal period.[2]

Pregnancy also can be divided into time periods, based on development, and refers to the conceptional age. The developmental or conceptional age is the time after fertilization and is about 2 weeks less than the gestational age.[3]

The first 2 weeks after fertilization is the pre-embryonic period. The embryonic period is from the second week of conception through the eighth week. Organogenesis occurs from the fourth through the seventh developmental week. The fetal period begins after the eighth conceptional week and continues until birth.[3]

Delivery

Depending on the gestational age at the time of delivery, the result can be an abortion, preterm, term, or post-term birth. An abortion (spontaneous or terminal) is a delivery before 20 weeks' gestation. A term infant is a fetus delivered between 37 and 42 weeks gestation. A preterm birth is one occurring between 20 and 37 weeks' gestation, and a post-term (postmaturity) birth occurs after the beginning of 43 weeks' gestation.[10] Parturition refers to labor, and the puerperium is the 6 to 8 weeks after delivery.[10]

Diagnosis of Pregnancy

1. S.C. is a 29-year-old, G_1P_1 woman, who has not started her menstrual period since she had unprotected intercourse about a month ago. She is worried that she may be pregnant. S.C. cannot remember the exact start date of her LMP. She asks her pharmacist for help selecting an over-the-counter commercially available home pregnancy test. How do these home pregnancy tests work and how should S.C. be counseled?

Commercially available home pregnancy tests are enzyme immunoassays with monoclonal or polyclonal antibodies, which bind to hCG in the urine.[11] They are highly sensitive and provide accurate results within 1 to 2 weeks after ovulation.[9,11] Several kits are available. The tests can be performed privately and quickly, and are easily interpreted. The results are obtained rapidly—within 1 and 5 minutes—and are highly accurate when performed at the start of the first missed menstrual period. Although home pregnancy tests are reportedly 98% to 100% accurate when used correctly, consumer studies have documented accuracy rates as low as 50% to 75% if product directions are not precisely followed.[11] Many home pregnancy tests include a second test, which should be repeated at a specified time after the first negative test result.

S.C. should purchase a product containing two tests and follow the instructions carefully. If the first test result is negative, S.C should repeat the test in 1 week if she has not started menstruating. False–negative results occur when testing is done before the first day of a missed period or if the urine is not at room temperature.[11] False–negative results can also occur with an ectopic (outside the uterus) pregnancy or ovarian cysts and in women receiving menotropins or chorionic gonadotropin.[11] If the test is positive, S.C. should be counseled on the possible fetal effects of any medications or herbal products she may be taking and advised to see her physician as soon as possible.

A positive urine or blood test result for hCG is still considered a probable diagnosis of pregnancy. The diagnosis of pregnancy is positively made with the identification of fetal heart sounds, perception of active fetal movements by an examiner, or visualization of embryo or fetus by sonography.[9]

Date of Confinement (Due Date)

2. What is S.C.'s "due date?"

The assessment of gestational age is important to determine the expected date of confinement (EDC), schedule a cesarean section, or determine when it is safe to end a pregnancy prematurely. Gestational age can be determined by several methods, including the date of the LMP, pelvic examination, uterine size, and measurement of fetal parameters by ultrasound. The onset date of the LMP is most commonly used to estimate the gestational age of the fetus.

Because the day of conception rarely is known, it is more practical to measure the duration of pregnancy from the first day of the LMP. The EDC is generally determined by adding 7 days to the first day of the LMP, counting back 3 months, and adding 1 year (Nagele rule).[12] This method assumes that ovulation occurs on day 14 of a 28-day menstrual cycle. The problems with this method are that many pregnant women do not know the date of their LMP, and it is inaccurate in women with irregular or prolonged menstrual cycles. S.C.'s first day of her LMP was estimated to be 6 weeks ago on August 6. It is now September 17; therefore, her EDC or "due date" is May 13. Although this may not be an accurate date, a more exact date will be estimated using first trimester sonography.

Pregnancy-Induced Pharmacokinetic Changes

Important physiologic changes occur in almost all maternal organs during pregnancy to support the growth and development of the fetus. These physiologic changes affect the cardiovascular, respiratory, and GI systems;, plasma volume, renal function, and hepatic enzymes, which can alter the absorption, distribution, metabolism, and elimination of drugs.[13] Alterations in the pharmacokinetics of drugs are influenced by mainly by two factors: (*a*) maternal physiologic changes and (*b*) the effects of the placental–fetal compartment.[14]

Absorption

Pregnancy-induced changes affecting drug absorption are (*a*) a decrease in intestinal motility, owing to smooth muscle relaxation by progesterone, resulting in a 30% to 50% increase of gastric and intestinal emptying time; (*b*) 40% decrease in gastric acidity, which increases gastric pH; and (*c*) altered bioavailability or absorption attributable to increased incidence of nausea and vomiting. Bioavailability may be increased for acid-labile drugs and decreased for drugs that require acid medium for stability. A prolonged gastric and intestinal emptying time may decrease the maximum concentration (C_{max}) of a drug and the time to reach C_{max}, whereas the increased intestinal transit time may increase the area under the curve (AUC) and bioavailability of a drug. In contrast, pregnancy-induced vomiting may decrease amount of drug ingested; it is therefore better to schedule medications during the evening when the incidence of nausea and vomiting is lower or to use the rectal route for drug administration. In summary, the effect of pregnancy on drug absorption is variable and depends greatly on the physicochemical properties of the drug.[14] Increased blood flow to maternal skin, which helps dissipate fetal heat production, may also increase the absorption of a topically (transdermal) administered medication.[13]

Distribution

Changes in protein binding and increased plasma volume can theoretically increase the apparent volume of distribution of drugs during pregnancy. Plasma volume increases by 6 to 8 weeks' gestation and continues to expand to 40% to 50% above pregnancy volumes by 32 to 34 weeks' gestation.[13,14] Plasma volume expands even more with multiple gestations. The total body water (TBW) increases by 8 L; 40% of this increase can be attributable to the mother and 60% to the fetal–placental unit. This increase in TBW necessitates larger loading doses of water-soluble drugs (e.g., aminoglycosides) because of the increase in volume of distribution (Vd). A decrease in the peak serum concentration (C_{max}) would be expected.

Plasma albumin concentrations decrease during pregnancy, mostly because of dilution by the increased plasma volume.[13,14] Albumin concentrations may be decreased because of decreased synthesis or increased catabolism.[13] In addition, increased concentrations of steroid and placental hormones may decrease protein-binding sites for drugs.[15] These changes in protein binding generally result in decreased protein binding, increased free fraction (f_u) of drugs, and increased clearance of drugs when clearance is dependent on f_u (e.g., valproic acid, carbamazepine).[16] When both f_u and intrinsic clearance are increased as is the case with increased cytochrome P450 enzyme activity, both the total and free concentrations are decreased (e.g., phenytoin, phenobarbital).[16] Total protein and α_1-acid glycoprotein concentrations remain fairly unchanged.

Metabolism

Protein binding, activity of hepatic enzymes, and liver blood flow determine the hepatic clearance of drugs. Increases in estrogen and progesterone during pregnancy affect the hepatic metabolism by stimulating or decreasing different hepatic enzymes of the cytochrome P-450 system.[17] CYP3A4 and CYP2D6 activities are increased during pregnancy, which results in the increased metabolism of certain drugs such as phenytoin.[14,17] On the other hand, CYP1A2, xanthine oxidase, and *N*-acetyltransferase activity are decreased, resulting in reduced hepatic elimination of drugs such theophylline and caffeine.[15,16,18] The clearance of caffeine can be decreased by 70%.[18] Hepatic blood flow, as a percentage of the cardiac output, is decreased; however, the rate (L/min) remains unchanged.[13] The activity of nonhepatic enzymes (e.g., plasma cholinesterase) is also decreased.[16] The extent of effect on drug therapy of these hepatic physiologic changes during pregnancy is difficult to quantify.

Elimination

The glomerular filtration rate (GFR) begins to rise in the first half of the first trimester and increases by 50% by the beginning of the second trimester.[15] Renal blood flow also increases by 25% to 50% early during gestation. As a result, renal drug excretion (e.g., β-lactams, digoxin, enoxaparin) can increase.[14,18] This increase in GFR necessitates dosage adjustments up to 20% to 65% for renally excreted drugs throughout pregnancy to maintain therapeutic concentrations.[17] The increased cardiac output and regional blood flow (e.g., renal blood flow), primarily are caused by increased stroke volume and increased heart rate, which can increase drug distribution and drug excretion.

During pregnancy, the serum creatinine concentration is lower because of the increased GFR, resulting in normal serum creatinine values of 0.3 to 0.7 mg/dL in the first and second trimesters.[19] A normal value for serum creatinine in nonpregnant adults is 0.6 to 1.2 mg/dL.[19] Similar changes occur with serum urea nitrogen and uric acid concentrations. These differences have important implications when assessing renal function in a pregnant patient. A serum creatinine indicative of normal renal function in a nonpregnant woman may be indicative of renal insufficiency in a woman who is pregnant in her third trimester.

Placental–Fetal Compartment Effect

Maternal and fetal drug concentrations are dependent on the amount of drug that crosses the placenta, the extent of metabolism by the placenta, and fetal distribution and elimination of drug (Fig. 46-2).[14] Diffusion across the placenta is the main mechanism of drug transfer giving nonionized lipophilic substances easy passage and making less lipid soluble ionized substances more difficult to cross.[14] Highly protein bounded or large molecular weight drugs (e.g., heparin and insulin) do not cross the placenta. Both the immature fetal liver and placenta can metabolize drugs. Fetal drug accumulation can be problematic secondary to limited metabolic enzymatic activity along with the concern that approximately half of blood flow from the umbilical vein bypasses the fetal liver and goes to the cardiac and cerebral circulations.[14] Another mechanism that can also lead to prolonged effects of drugs in the fetal compartment is ion trapping. This phenomenon occurs because the fetal plasma pH is more acidic than the maternal plasma, causing weak bases (e.g., usually nonionized and lipophilic substances) to diffuse across the placental barrier and become ionized in the more acidic fetal blood. The net effect is movement of drugs from the maternal to fetal compartment.[14] This equilibrium between the maternal–fetal compartment becomes important when therapeutic fetal drug concentrations are desired (e.g., digoxin therapy for intrauterine fetal arrhythmias). Drugs are eliminated by the fetus primarily through diffusion back to the maternal compartment. As the fetal kidney matures, metabolites of drugs are excreted into the amniotic fluid.[14]

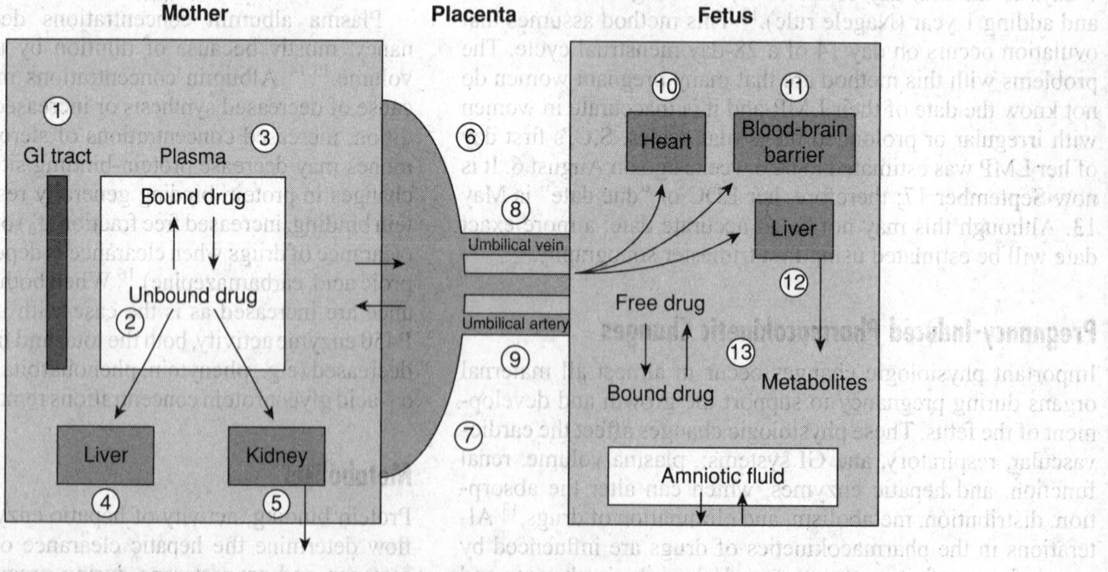

FIGURE 46-2 Drug disposition in the maternal–placental fetal system. The factors affecting the pharmacokinetcs and drug effects on mother and fetus are (1) altered maternal absorption; (2) increased maternal unbound drug fraction; (3) increased maternal plasma volume; (4) altered hepatic clearance; (5) increased maternal renal blood flow and glomerular filtration rate; (6) placental transfer; (7) possible placental metabolism; (8) placental blood flow; (9) maternal-fetal blood pH; (10) preferential fetal circulation to the heart and brain; (11) undeveloped fetal blood–brain barrier; (12) immature fetal liver enzyme activity; and (13) increased fetal unbound drug fraction. GI, gastrointestinal. From reference 292, with permission.

VITAMINS AND MINERALS

3. What vitamin and mineral supplementation would you recommend for S.C. and when should she begin taking these products?

A balanced diet that provides S.C. with multiple B vitamins, oil-soluble vitamins (A, E, D, and K), folic acid, and minerals (iron, calcium, phosphorus, magnesium, iodine, zinc) should be encouraged. S.C should be started on a prenatal multivitamin if she has not yet started taking one. Prenatal vitamins should be taken months before conception to ensure that proper nutritional requirements are met during critical periods of organogenesis and fetal growth.

Iron Requirements

Iron requirements increase during pregnancy because of maternal blood volume expansion, fetal needs, placenta and cord needs, and blood loss at time of delivery.[20] Maternal iron deficiency can cause anemia during infancy, spontaneous abortion, premature delivery, and delivery of a low-birth-weight infant.[20]

A woman needs about 18 to 21 mg of iron/day during pregnancy; the body compensates by increasing iron absorption from the GI tract by about 15% to 50%.[20] The average diet of women in the United States does not meet these requirements because only about 6 mg of iron are absorbed from 1,000 kcal of food. In addition, some women may already have inadequate body stores of iron before pregnancy. For these reasons, the Food and Nutrition Board of the National Research Council recommends a daily elemental iron supplementation of 30 mg during the second and third trimesters of pregnancy.[21] Prenatal vitamins usually contain 30 to 60 mg of elemental iron. Women with iron deficiency anemia should be given 60 to 120 mg of elemental iron daily. Iron deficiency anemia during pregnancy generally is associated with a hemoglobin and hematocrit <11% and <33%, respectively, during the first and third trimesters or below 10.5% and 32%, respectively, during the second trimester. Anemic women are more likely to suffer adverse effects from blood loss during delivery, hemorrhage secondary to other causes, or infections after delivery.[22]

S.C.'s hemoglobin and hematocrit should be assessed now and again at 26 to 28 weeks' gestation. If her hemoglobin and hematocrit are normal, she will not need more iron than what is already available in a prenatal vitamin.

Folate Requirements

Folic acid is essential in the synthesis of DNA and RNA. Pregnant women who take 0.4 to 0.8 mg of folic acid daily during the first trimester of pregnancy are significantly less likely to have a child with neural tube defects (NTD), such as spina bifida and anencephaly.[23,24] NTD can lead to stillbirth, neonatal death, or serious disabilities. Approximately 4,000 pregnancies in the United States are affected by NTD each year.[25]

Neural tube defects can develop within the first month of pregnancy at a time when many women are unaware of their pregnancy. More than half of pregnancies in the United States are unplanned.[24,25] In 1992, the US Public Health Service recommended that all women with child-bearing potential should consume 0.4 mg/day of folic acid to reduce the risk of an NTD-affected pregnancy.[24] If this practice were implemented in the United States, the incidence of NTD could possibly be reduced by 50%.

It may be difficult to meet the recommended daily allowance (RDA) for folic acid because foods contain only a small amount of this vitamin; overcooking and high fiber diets also can reduce the amount of available folic acid from food.[20] Most prenatal vitamins contain 0.8 to 1 mg of folic acid.

Folic acid supplementation is especially important in women with a history of infants born with NTD. Women who have had an NTD-affected pregnancy should receive genetic counseling because they have a 2% to 3% risk of having another such outcome. Women with previous NTD-affected pregnancies, who plan another pregnancy, should take 4 mg/day of folic acid at least 1 month before conception and through the first 3 months of pregnancy.[26]

Women who require 4 mg/day of folic acid should be prescribed folic acid tablets as an addition to combination prenatal multivitamins (which contain folic acid), rather than just increasing the number of multivitamin tablets. When several fixed-combination multivitamin tablets are taken daily, the mother could be exposed to a potentially teratogenic dose of vitamin A. High doses of folic acid do not prevent NTD better than 0.4 mg/day in women without a previous history of NTD-affected pregnancies and may complicate the diagnosis of a B_{12} deficiency.[24]

S.C. should be counseled about the risks for NTD. She should receive adequate folic acid during the remainder of her pregnancy from a daily prenatal vitamin.

Calcium Requirements

Calcium is needed during pregnancy for adequate mineralization of the fetal skeleton and teeth, especially during the third trimester when teeth are formed and skeletal growth is greatest.[20] The RDA for calcium during pregnancy is 1,200 mg/day.[20] Large maternal stores can provide calcium if dietary intake is inadequate; however, depleting maternal stores may put S.C. at risk for osteoporosis later in life. Foods rich in calcium (e.g., milk, cheese, yogurt, legumes, nuts, dried fruits) or calcium supplements can be used to meet the calcium RDA.[15]

COMMON COMPLAINTS OF PREGNANCY

Nausea and Vomiting

4. Now S.C. is 10 weeks pregnant, and the nausea and vomiting has worsened. How long is her nausea and vomiting likely to last?

Nausea and vomiting during pregnancy (NVP) is a common condition occurring in approximately 50% to 80% of pregnancies, during weeks 5 to 12 of gestation.[27] For most women, NVP is a self-limiting condition that resolves after the first trimester with no long-term detrimental effect on the fetus.[28] The effects of NVP can have an impact on a woman's daily activities, work productivity, and quality of life. Studies estimate $130 million per year is spent on the hospitalization for severe NVP.[28] The cause of NVP is unknown, but is most likely multifactorial including hormonal, psychological, and neurologic factors.[28,29] Changes in hormonal levels of estrogen, progesterone, and hCG have been implicated as a possible cause of NVP.[28,29] Mild to moderate NVP has been associated with lower rates of miscarriage, preterm delivery, and stillbirth.[30]

Severe NVP can persists in less than 1% of pregnancies leading to a condition called *hyperemesis gravidarum*, which can lead to detrimental effects on the mother and fetus.[29,30] Weight loss of >5% of prepregnancy weight, ketonuria, and electrolyte abnormalities are associated with this condition. Treatment of hyperemesis gravidarum often requires hospitalization for parental fluid administration, electrolyte replacement, vitamin supplementation, and antiemetic therapy.[28] Metabolic acidosis, ketosis, hypovolemia, electrolyte disturbances, and weight loss may ensue if patients are not treated.[28] Reductions in lower esophageal pressure, gastric peristalsis, and gastric emptying may worsen nausea and vomiting.

S.C. may be evaluated for other causes of nausea and vomiting if her symptoms persist (e.g., gastroenteritis, cholecystitis, pancreatitis, hepatitis, peptic ulcer disease, pyelonephritis, and fatty liver of pregnancy).[28]

Nonpharmacologic Management

5. How should S.C.'s NVP be managed?

Most mild forms of NVP can be managed with psychological support, and lifestyle and dietary changes.[28,29] Eating smaller frequent meals consisting of a low-fat, bland, and dry diet (e.g., bananas, crackers, rice, toast), avoiding spicy and highly aromatic foods, and eliminating pills with iron may alleviate some of the symptoms.[28] Meals high in protein were more likely to alleviate NVP than carbohydrate or fatty meals.[29] Rest and avoidance of sensory stimuli that contribute to the effects of NVP can also be helpful.[28]

Pharmacologic Management

6. S.C. does not respond to nonpharmacologic treatment of her nausea and vomiting. What antiemetic would be appropriate for her?

Antiemetics are indicated for the treatment of moderate to severe nausea and vomiting that fails to respond to nonpharmacologic interventions or when the nausea or vomiting threatens the mother's metabolic or nutritional status (e.g., hyperemesis gravidarum). Traditionally, medications for NVP have been avoided during the first trimester because of fear of the possible teratogenic effects. Most antiemetic therapies (e.g., antihistamines, multivitamins, phenothiazines) are classified in pregnancy category B or C as listed in Table 46-1. The goal of antiemetic therapy is to choose an effective medication to improve a woman's quality of life by maintaining her nutrition and hydration needs, while ensuring fetal safety.

Doxylamine with pyridoxine (vitamin B_6) can be considered first-line therapy for the treatment of NVP.[29] This combination, formerly known as Bendectin, was commercially available from 1958 to 1983 and withdrawn from the market owing to claims of teratogenicity.[29] Subsequently, a meta-analysis including 17,427 first-trimester exposures failed to find an association between the medication and an increased risk of malformations.[31] Several randomized, controlled trials have demonstrated its effectiveness in reducing NVP.[28] Because of its safety and efficacy profile, doxylamine and pyridoxine are still considered a first-line therapy and are available separately as over-the-counter products.[28,29]

Other antihistamine H_1 receptor blockers (e.g., diphenhydramine, hydroxyzine, meclizine) have been studied for NVP.[27–29] The safety of antihistamines was supported in a meta-analysis including >200,000 first-trimester exposures,

Table 46-1 Medications Used for Nausea and Vomiting during Pregnancy

Drug	Dose	Pregnancy Category
Pyridoxine	10–25 mg PO three to four times daily	A
Doxylamine	12.5–25 mg PO three to four times daily	B
Diphenydramine	25–50 mg PO, IV, IM every 4–6 hrs	B
Droperidol	0.5–2 mg IV or IM every 3–4 hrs	C
Meclizine	25 mg PO every 4–6 hrs	B
Hydroxyzine	25–50 mg PO every 6–8 hrs	C
Promethazine	12.5–25 mg PO, PR every 6 hrs	C
Prochlorperazine	5–10 mg PO every 6–8 hrs	C
Metoclopramide	5–10 mg PO, IM, IV every 8 hrs	B
Ondansetron	4–8 mg PO, IV every 8 hrs	B

IM, intramuscular; IV, intravenous; PO, oral.
Category A: Controlled studies in women fail to demonstrate risk to the fetus.
Category B: Either animal studies have not demonstrated a risk and no controlled studies have been done in women, or animal studies have shown a risk that has not been confirmed in humans.
Category C: Either studies in animals have shown an adverse effect on the fetus and no controlled studies have been done in women, or no studies in women or animals are available.
Category D: There is evidence of fetal harm, but the benefit of the medication may outweigh the risk.
Category X: There is evidence of fetal harm, and no benefit of the medication outweighs the risk.
From reference 33, with permission

which did not find an increase in teratogenic risk.[32] Phenothiazines are generally considered safe for both the mother and fetus if used occasionally in low doses.[33] Although there are some isolated reports of congenital malformations *in utero* with its use, most evidence examining the use of phenothiazines, such as prochlorperazine and promethazine, in NVP has not shown an increase in malformations.[27,28] Trimethobenzamide has also been used in pregnancy to treat nausea and vomiting without observation of adverse effects in the fetus.[33]

Metoclopramide can control vomiting and gastric reflux associated with pregnancy. Despite the limited safety data on metoclopramide, it is the antiemetic of choice in many European countries.[27,29] Data supporting the use of ondansetron, a 5 hydroxytryptamine (5-HT_3) antagonist, during pregnancy is limited including only a small randomized trial and a few case reports with no malformations reported with first trimester use.[27] More studies are needed to confirm the safety and establish its efficacy in NVP. Limited experience with droperidol use in hyperemesis gravidarum has been documented in a small controlled trial.[27] Human and animal data suggest droperidol carries a low risk of major anomalies to the fetus.[33] Corticosteroids may improve the symptoms of NVP. Corticosteroid use during the first trimester is associated, however, with a small but significant risk of fetal oral clefts.[27]

Alternative therapies (e.g., vitamin B_6, ginger root, acupuncture, acupressure) have improved NVP in small number of patients.[28] Intravenous (IV)fluids, total parenteral nutrition, and enteral nutrition may be needed in hyperemesis gravidarum.[29] S.C. may be started doxylamine and pyridoxine because of its safety and efficacy profile. Drug selection for S.C. mostly depends on the tolerability of adverse effects.

Reflux Esophagitis

7. S.C. is now 30 weeks pregnant and no longer complains of nausea or vomiting. However, now she has heartburn that worsens when she lies down. What causes reflux esophagitis in pregnancy and how should S.C. manage this problem?

Reflux esophagitis or heartburn is a normal occurrence in pregnancy affecting approximately two-thirds of women.[34] The enlarging uterus increases intra-abdominal pressure, and estrogen and progesterone relax the esophageal sphincter.[34] These two factors cause the reflux of stomach acid into the lower esophagus, producing symptoms of substernal burning worsened by eating, lying down, or bending over. Lifestyle and dietary modifications, such as eating smaller meals, avoiding late meals close to bedtime, and elevation of the head of the bed, should be tried first.[34] Avoidance of salicylates, caffeine, alcohol, and nicotine are encouraged to reduce the symptoms of reflux and fetal exposure to these harmful substances.[34]

If these modifications are not successful, S.C. should try a calcium carbonate antacid. Animal studies have not shown antacids to cause teratogenic effects, and human data are limited.[33] Sodium bicarbonate can cause metabolic alkalosis and fluid overload and should be avoided.[34] Despite evidence of fetal toxicity with aluminum, available data suggest that usual doses of aluminum-containing medications are not harmful to the fetus of a pregnant woman with normal renal function.[33,34] Sucralfate, which contains aluminum, appears to be safe in pregnancy. The American College of Gastroenterology has classified sucralfate as a medication with benefits that outweigh the risks when used in pregnant women.[33]

H_2-receptor antagonists can be used when necessary because most studies in animals and humans have not found fetal harm with cimetidine, ranitidine, famotidine, or nizatidine.[33,34] Proton pump inhibitors should be reserved for complicated reflux disease.[34] Animal data with lansoprazole have been reassuring, but few human data are available.[33] The proton pump inhibitors should be avoided during the first trimester, but preferably during any part of gestation because birth defects have been reported in animal pregnancies in which omeprazole was used.[33,34]

PREVENTION OF RH D ALLOIMMUNIZATION

Maternal–Fetal Rh Incompatibility

8. G.G., a 34-year-old primigravida, had her ABO blood group and Rh status determined during her initial prenatal visit. She is was found to be type O, Rh-negative. Her husband is type O, Rh-positive. What are the risks associated with Rh incompatibility that could affect G.G.'s unborn?

Blood group incompatibility between a pregnant woman and her fetus can result in alloimmunization of the mother and hemolytic anemia in the fetus. When a woman is exposed during pregnancy, labor, or delivery to a fetal erythrocyte antigen (i.e., AB, Rh-complex) that is not found on her own erythrocytes, she forms antibodies against that antigen. This is referred to as *alloimmunization*. Antibodies of the IgG class cross the placenta and can interact with the fetal erythrocyte antigens, resulting in their destruction and leading to hemolytic disease of the fetus and newborn (HDN). Most serious cases of HDN are caused by Rh alloimmunization involving the D antigen. The other four alleles of the Rh gene complex code for the antigens C, c, E, and e. They are also serious, but less common, causes of alloimmunization.[35]

An Rh D-negative mother becomes immunized after exposure to fetal erythrocytes that carry the D antigen. The likelihood of having an Rh D-positive offspring is determined by whether an Rh D-positive father is homozygous or heterozygous for the D antigen. If the father is homozygous for the D antigen, all of his offspring will be D positive (Rh-positive). If he is heterozygous for the D antigen, then there is a 50% chance that his offspring will be Rh-positive.

Pregnant women can produce detectable IgG antibodies to Rh antigens within 6 weeks to 6 months.[36] These antibodies can cross the placenta during subsequent pregnancies and destroy fetal Rh D-positive red blood cells (RBC). Of Rh D-negative women, 175% will become alloimmunized during a term pregnancy, with most cases occurring at the time of delivery.[37] Approximately 1% to 2% of women will, however, become sensitized from antepartum fetomaternal hemorrhage, generally in the third trimester.[38] As little as 0.1 mL of blood can immunize a human. A concomitant ABO incompatibility between an Rh D-positive fetus and the Rh D-negative mother decreases the chance of alloimmunization.[37] This is because the ABO-incompatible RBC are rapidly hemolyzed and sequestered in the liver, wherein a lower potential for antibody production exists.

The severity of Rh-associated HDN or erythroblastosis fetalis depends on the concentration of maternal antibodies. The placental transfer of large amounts of antibody can cause substantial erythrocyte destruction. This initially results in anemia and hyperbilirubinemia with compensatory extramedullary erythropoiesis (e.g., liver, spleen). In severe hemolytic diseases, the fetus might develop hepatosplenomegaly, portal hypertension, edema, ascites, and hepatic and cardiac failure. The clinical presentation of profound anemia, anasarca, hepatosplenomegaly, cardiac failure, and circulatory collapse is termed *hydrops fetalis*.

The severity of Rh-associated HDN generally worsens with each pregnancy in the alloimmunized mother if her fetus is Rh positive. Thus, it is important to discuss the consequences of alloimmunization with any woman who is known to be alloimmunized and wishes to have more children in the future.

Rh_o(D) Immunoglobulin

9. What interventions should be undertaken to prevent G.G. from becoming alloimmunized?

Antepartum Prophylaxis

G.G. should have antibody screens at the beginning of each pregnancy, and postpartum. Although the American Association of Blood Banks recommends that an antepartum screen should also be obtained at 28 weeks, the cost-effectiveness of such screening has not been studied and it is estimated that sensitization before 28 weeks occurs at a rate of <0.18%. Therefore, the American College of Obstetrics and Gynecology (ACOG) has suggested that the decision to obtain a third-trimester antibody screen should be dictated by individual circumstances.[39] As pregnancy progresses, both the incidence and the degree of fetomaternal hemorrhage increase. Administrating Rh_o(D) immune globulin to G.G. before or shortly after exposure to fetal Rh D-positive erythrocytes will prevent her from becoming alloimmunized. Giving Rh_o(D) immune globulin at 28 weeks' gestation has been shown to decrease the antepartum sensitization rate from approximately 2% to 0.1%.[38] One mechanism by which Rh_o(D) immune globulin might prevent sensitization is by suppression of the primary immune response to the D antigen.[36] The anti-D immune globulin binds the D antigen, and this complex is filtered by the spleen and lymph nodes whereby it inhibits D antigen-specific B cells from proliferating.

Postpartum Prophylaxis

A second dose of Rh_o(D) immune globulin should be repeated within 72 hours of delivery. A larger dose is needed if a large transplacental bleed occurs at the time of delivery (0.4% of cases). Therefore, all Rh_o(D)-negative women who deliver an Rh_o(D)-positive newborn should be tested to detect fetal RBC in maternal blood (e.g., Kleihauer-Betke test) to calculate the correct dose of Rh_o(D) immune globulin. If a woman at risk for sensitization has not been given Rho_o(D) immune globulin within 72 hours, she should still be treated as soon as possible as it has been demonstrated that protection can be seen in some individuals up to 13 days after exposure to Rh positive red cells.[40]

Adverse Effects Rh(D) Immune Globulin

The plasma from which immune globulin is obtained is tested for viral infections and the manufacturing process used to produce Rh_o(D) immune globulin inactivates viruses such as human immunodeficiency virus (HIV), hepatitis B virus (HBV), and hepatitis C virus (HCV).[36,39] Adverse reactions associated with the use of anti-D immune globulin are rare. Pain and swelling at the injection site and rash are the most common adverse reactions.[36] Hypersensitivity reactions such as anaphylaxis, although rare, can occur owing to a small amount of IgA in the product.

Prophylaxis for First- and Second-Trimester Events and Procedures

10. G.G. will undergo amniocentesis at 16 weeks' gestation. Will she need a dose of Rh_o(D) at that time?

Rh_o(D) immune globulin should be given after all clinical events (e.g., spontaneous abortion) or procedures (e.g., abortion, amniocentesis, fetal blood sampling, or chorionic villus sampling) in which fetomaternal hemorrhage is a risk in an Rh-incompatible pregnancy. Although little evidence supports the need for prophylaxis in the early first trimester, adverse effects are rare and potential benefits are thought by most experts to outweigh the risks.[41] Although a 50-mcg dose is available for first trimester use (e.g., chorionic villus sampling or abortion), many hospitals do not stock this dose and so a 300-mcg standard dose is often given.

Length of Protection

11. G.G. had an amniocentesis at 16 weeks for which she received Rh_o(D) IGIM 300 mcg IM. Will she need another dose at 28 weeks' gestation? How long will this dose protect G.G. against alloimmunization?

G.G. will still need a dose of 300 mcg repeated at 28 weeks' gestation and within 72 hours postpartum if her infant is Rh_o(D)-positive. The half-life of Rh_o(D) immune globulin is approximately 24 to 25 days.[39] Without a large fetomaternal hemorrhage, a standard dose of 300 mcg will protect against alloimmunization for up to 12 weeks. If $>$12 weeks have lapsed between receipt of anti-D immune globulin and delivery, many practitioners recommend administering another antepartum dose.[36,39]

Failure of Immunoprophylaxis

12. What are the most common reasons for Rh D alloimmunization during pregnancy?

The most common reasons for Rh D alloimmunization are (*a*) failure to give a dose of anti-D immune globulin at 28 weeks' gestation; (*b*) failure to give Rh_o(D) immune globulin in a timely manner postpartum to women who have delivered an Rh_o(D)-positive or untyped fetus; and (*c*) failure to recognize clinical procedures and situations that increase maternal risk for alloimmunization (i.e., amniocentesis, abortions).[35]

Thus, G.G. should be told that with proper prophylaxis with anti-D immune globulin, there is little chance for her to become alloimmunized. She need not worry about her present pregnancy or future pregnancies.

DIABETES MELLITUS

Diabetes mellitus is the most common maternal medical complication during pregnancy. Diabetes during pregnancy can be detected before or during pregnancy and can be separated in two groups: (*a*) *pregestational diabetes,* which includes women who have been diagnosed before pregnancy with either insulin-dependent or insulin-independent diabetes mellitus or (*b*) *gestational diabetes mellitus* (GDM) defined as carbohydrate intolerance first detected during pregnancy.[42]

More prevalent than pregestational diabetes, GDM accounts for $>$90% of diabetes cases during pregnancy and affects approximately 4.4% of live births each year.[43,44] More than half of women with GDM will go on to develop type 2 diabetes later in life.[43] Some believe that GDM is a diagnosis of type 2 diabetes that has been discovered during pregnancy.[42]

Pregestational diabetes accounts for the remaining 10% of cases. In the United States, $>$8 million women have pregestational diabetes affecting about 1% of live births each year.[43] Most women with pregestational diabetes have type 2 diabetes characterized by peripheral insulin resistance and relative insulin deficiency. The incidence of type 2 pregestational diabetes has been rapidly rising in the past decade, most likely because of the increasing prevalence of obesity.[42,43] In contrast to type 2 diabetes, type 1 diabetes is characterized by complete insulin deficiency resulting from autoimmune destruction of pancreatic β-cells. Less than 0.5% of all pregnancies in the United States are complicated by type 1 diabetes.[45]

Fluctuating glucose levels during the first trimester may be the first signs of pregnancy for women with pregestational diabetes owing to increased insulin resistance and reduced sensitivity to insulin action. Placental hormones (e.g., human

Table 46-2 Modified White's Classification of Diabetes During Pregnancy

Class Gestational Diabetes Mellitus	Criteria
A_1	Diagnosed during pregnancy Controlled by diet and exercise
A_2	Diagnosed during pregnancy Requires use of medication therapy (i.e., insulin) along with diet and exercise
Pregestational Diabetes Mellitus	
B	Age of onset ≥20 yrs Duration of disease <10 yrs Absence of vascular disease
C	Onset of age between 10 and 19 yrs Duration of disease between 10 and 20 yrs Absence of vascular disease
D	Onset of age <age 10 yrs Duration of disease ≥20 yrs Background retinopathy observed Hypertension
F	Nephropathy (>500 mg/day proteinuria)
H	Arteriosclerotic heart disease
R	Proliferative retinopathy or vitreous hemorrhage
T	After renal transplantation

From references 42 and 46 with permission.

placental lactogen, progesterone, prolactin, placental growth hormone, and cortisol) are thought to be responsible for the increase in insulin resistance during pregnancy.[43] The ACOG classifies diabetes in pregnancy according to the White Classification, modified to include gestational diabetes according to glycemic control.[42] The White Classification relies on age at onset, duration of diabetes, and presence of vascular complications for patient classification (Table 46-2).[42,46]

Pre-existing Diabetes Mellitus

Fetal and Infant Risks

13. K.H., a 27-year-old, 60-kg, woman known to have type 1 diabetes since age 12, has married recently and wishes to have children. She has been conscientious in her diabetes care and self-monitors her blood glucose concentrations with a glucometer. Over the past month, her fasting blood glucose (FBG) concentrations have ranged from 90 to 140 mg/dL. Today, her FBG and HbA_{1c} laboratory results are 134 mg/dL (normal, 70–110) and 7.8% (normal, 4.5–6.5), respectively. Her blood pressure (BP) is 145/94 mm Hg, renal function is normal, serum creatinine is 0.8 mg/dL (normal, 0.6–1.2), and no proteinuria. K.H. reports tingling and pain in her toes. Her current human insulin regimen consists of a combination of 16 U of isophane insulin (NPH) and 8 U of regular insulin 30 minutes before breakfast, and 8 U of NPH and 4 U of regular 30 minutes before supper. How will diabetes affect the health of a child she would like to conceive?

Perinatal mortality for infants of diabetic mothers has declined dramatically with strict maternal metabolic control, improved fetal surveillance, and neonatal intensive care.[47] Fetal and neonatal mortality rates are approximately 2% to 4%, and the risk of spontaneous abortion in well-controlled type 1 diabetics is equal to that of women without diabetes.[48] The incidence of stillbirth is greatest after 36 weeks' gestation in women with poor glycemic control, fetal macrosomia (see below), maternal vascular disease, ketoacidosis, or preeclampsia.[42]

The leading cause of perinatal mortality is major congenital anomalies that occur in 6% to 12% of infants born to mothers with diabetes. The major malformations observed are usually neural tube defects and other anomalies involving the cardiac, renal, and GI systems, and rarely caudal regression syndrome.[43] Many of these congenital anomalies occur before the seventh week of gestation, a time when organogenesis is occurring.[49] The risk of giving birth to an infant with a major congenital anomaly correlates with the degree of glycemic control during the time just before and the 2 months after conception.[42,47] A direct correlation exists between higher glycosylated hemoglobin levels and increased frequency of anomalies. Women with higher HbA_{1c} values during this time have a significantly higher incidence of infants with anomalies compared with women with HbA_{1c} closer to the normal range.[48] The risk of fetal anomalies increases dramatically to 20% to 25% when HbA_{1c} levels are near 10%.[43] HbA_{1c} levels >12% are associated with the same risk of anomalies as infants exposed to known teratogens such as thalidomide, isotretinoin, or alcohol during organogenesis.[33,50] HbA_{1c} values up to 1% above normal, however, are associated with rates of spontaneous abortions and congenital malformations similar to those of nondiabetic pregnancies.[47]

Macrosomia, defined as birthweight >4 kg, occurs in 20% to 25% of pregnancies complicated by diabetes. It is thought to be caused in part by fetal hyperglycemia and hyperinsulinemia.[42] Fetal hyperglycemia occurs when glucose crosses the placenta and subsequently stimulates fetal pancreatic β-cells to release excessive insulin. Hyperinsulinemia can promote excessive fetal growth in adipose tissue causing disproportional fat concentration around the shoulders and chest, doubling the risks of trauma (e.g., shoulder dystocia) during vaginal delivery.[43]

Infants of diabetic mothers (IDM) also are at increased risk for prolonged hypoglycemia after delivery, respiratory distress syndrome (RDS), hypocalcemia, polycythemia, and hyperbilirubinemia during the neonatal period.[43]

K.H. should be informed that tight glucose control, especially early in the first trimester, will maximize her chance of having a healthy baby. She should be educated before pregnancy about the healthy practices she can institute now to improve a successful pregnancy outcome.

Maternal Risks

14. K.H. wants to know what health risks she might incur from becoming pregnant and what measures could minimize these risks.

A prepregnancy assessment, including a history and physical examination, is necessary to determine the risks or contraindications to pregnancy for K.H. She should be evaluated for ischemic heart disease, neuropathies, or retinopathy, and her renal status must be assessed.[47] Pregnancy can exacerbate the vascular complications of diabetes. For instance, diabetic retinopathy can worsen if strict glycemic control is implemented quickly in pregnant women with proliferative retinopathy; progression to end-stage renal disease can occur in women with mild to moderate renal insufficiency (e.g., serum creatinine >1.5 mg/dL or proteinuria >3 g/24 hours; myocardial infarction may occur with preexisting symptomatic ischemic heart disease secondary to the hemodynamic changes that occur during pregnancy).[43] The presence of gastroparesis should be noted, because it will make controlling her glucose more difficult.[47]

Controlling K.H.'s diabetes before she becomes pregnant may benefit her hypertension and neuropathies and will minimize maternal and fetal problems. Good metabolic control of her diabetes can minimize progression of her diabetes.[47]

Preconception Management

15. What prepregnancy interventions relative to her general health and diabetes should K.H. undertake before she attempts to become pregnant?

K.H. should be started on prenatal vitamins containing at least 400 mcg of folic acid, and re-educated about diet and glycemic control of her diabetes. Her insulin therapy should be titrated to reduce her preprandial (capillary whole blood) glucose to 70 to 100 mg/dL and her 2-hour postprandial glucose to below 140 mg/dL.[47] Good glycemic control (HbA_{1c} levels up to >1% above normal) should be achieved months before conception to minimize risks of major congenital anomalies.[50] K.H.'s current regimen may not achieve euglycemia (see Chapter 50, Diabetes Mellitus).

Her BP of 145/94 mm Hg is high and should be decreased to a diastolic BP of about 80 mm Hg to minimize risks for preeclampsia or exacerbation of her disorder. Many women with pregestational diabetes are likely on an angiotension converting enzyme inhibitor (ACEI) or angiotension receptor blocker for hypertension treatment. K.H. should consider other antihypertensives (e.g., methyldopa or calcium channel blockers) because recent studies have observed increased rates of congenital cardiac malformation associated with the use of ACEI in the first trimester.[51]

Treatment

16. After lowering her BP to 125/80 mm Hg with a calcium channel blocker and HbA_{1c} to 7.3% K.H. discontinues her oral contraceptive and returns to clinic 5 months later and is noted to be about 4 weeks pregnant. How should her diabetes be managed at this time?

GOALS OF THERAPY

The overall goals of treatment of K.H.'s diabetes are to reduce the maternal and fetal morbidity and mortality associated with diabetes. Treatment of diabetes (Chapter 50, Diabetes Mellitus), should include dietary management, appropriate maternal weight gain, insulin therapy to normalize glycemic control, and exercise.

DIETARY MANAGEMENT

The goals of dietary management for diabetes during pregnancy are directed at ensuring fetal growth and development, appropriate maternal weight gain, and normalizing maternal glucose concentrations. Patients often benefit from individualized diets developed by a dietitian.[47,49] Neonatal macrosomia has been associated with high postprandial glucose levels; therefore, a reduction in postprandial hyperglycemia is an important goal.[52]

INSULIN THERAPY

Insulin is the hypoglycemic of choice during pregnancy because it does not cross the placenta and has an established safety record for both mother and fetus.[33,43] The goal with insulin therapy is to imitate the glucose levels of a healthy pregnant woman.

Insulin requirements may vary, depending on the trimester. The first trimester is characterized by unstable diabetes, followed by a stable period.[42] During the first trimester, glucose and gluconeogenic substances in the blood are taken up by the fetus, which can lead to a decrease in maternal insulin requirements and increased episodes of hypoglycemia. On average, insulin dosages range from 0.7 to 0.8 U/kg/day in the first trimester.[43] If K.H. experiences nausea and vomiting during this time, glycemic control may be unstable and should be monitored closely. At about 24 weeks' gestation, insulin requirements begin to increase to 0.8 to 1 U/kg/day and insulin doses may need to be adjusted every 5 to 10 days.[43] These needs continue to increase during the third trimester to 0.9 to 1.2 U/kg/day, which may be twice as much as the prepregnancy dose, in part, because of the placental hormones (i.e., lactogen, prolactin, estrogen, and progesterone), which antagonize the action of insulin.[42,43] Weight-based dosing may not accurately assess the insulin requirements in all pregnant women, especially in the obese population. Insulin regimens must be individualized for each patient, taking into consideration their educational level, compliance, and schedule constraints. Dosage adjustments must take into account the level of activity, meal plan, and other factors (e.g., steroid use, stress, infections) that may affect glucose control. Some women may be admitted into the hospital in the first trimester to (*a*) rapidly gain glucose control, (*b*) accurately assess their insulin requirements, and (*c*) institute an individualized insulin regimen under careful monitoring of blood sugars.[42]

An insulin regimen with three to four daily injections is most successful at maintaining adequate glucose control. Biosynthetic human insulin (e.g., regular and NPH insulin) is the usual treatment of choice in pregestational diabetes mellitus because of its chemical, biological, and immunological equivalency to pancreatic human insulin. These insulins have the most established safety profile during pregnancy, but they require more stringent timing of meals during the day.

Recent additions of rapid and long-acting insulin analogs (e.g., lispro, aspart, glargine) have sparked interest in their use during pregnancy. Insulin analogs are genetically engineered by recombinant DNA technology and usually differ by a few amino acids from human insulin.[52] Concerns about insulin analog use during pregnancy include teratogenicity, placental drug transfer, and antibody formation.[52] The use of insulin lispro (Humalog) during pregnancy is supported by several studies that found minimal passage to the placenta, an absence of antibody formation, and no adverse maternal or fetal effects noted.[53] Although the rapid onset of insulin lispro can increase adherence and patient satisfaction, it also may increase the incidence of hypoglycemia.[43] Insulin aspart (Novolog), another rapid-acting insulin analog, has not been studied as extensively as lispro and remains a pregnancy category C drug, meaning that the risk cannot be excluded.[52] Insulin glargine (Lantus), the first long-acting insulin analog developed, allows for once daily dosing and produces a peakless basal level of insulin. Only several case reports have examined the safety and efficacy of insulin glargine during pregnancy, making it a pregnancy category C drug.[52]

ORAL HYPOGLYCEMICS

Oral hypoglycemics are used commonly to treat type 2 diabetes in nonpregnant women. With more than half of pregnancies being unplanned, many discover their pregnancy status while taking these medications. A switch to insulin therapy is recommended before conception,if possible, or at the time the pregnancy is confirmed because many patients have inadequate control with oral hypoglycemic agents.[43] Control of blood glucose levels during the preconception period and early first trimester is of utmost importance to decrease the risk of congential malformations.[43,50] If insulin is not started before conception, women should be counseled to stay on oral hypoglycemics to adequately control blood glucose until insulin therapy can be implemented. Often, patients will discontinue oral hypoglycemics from fear of taking any medication in pregnancy, resulting in hyperglycemia during the critical period of organogenesis.

The ACOG recommends that the use of oral hypoglycemics for the treatment of type 2 diabetes during pregnancy be individualized until more safety and efficacy data become available.[43] There is limited experience with oral hypoglycemic use in type 2 diabetes during pregnancy. Metformin, a biguanide, has been used during pregnancy for hyperinsulinemic insulin resistance or in the treatment of infertility in women with polycystic ovarian syndrome (PCOS).[43,52,54] (See Chapter 47, Treatment of Menstrual and Menstrual-Related Disorders.) Metformin was shown to cross the human placenta; it was detected in cord serum levels and can potentially affect the fetal cellular function and development of the embryo.[52] Studies are underway to determine the safety and efficacy of metformin in pregnancy. Until these studies can establish the role of metformin in pregnancy, women taking metformin should be switched to insulin therapy unless specific circumstances (e.g., high insulin requirements during second or third trimester) warrant its use.[52,54]

BLOOD GLUCOSE AND HBA_{1C} MONITORING

K.H. should measure her glucose at fasting, before and after meals, at bedtime, if she feels symptomatic, and occasionally at 3:00 AM to rule out nocturnal hypoglycemia (i.e., about five to seven times daily). The goal of therapy is to maintain fasting glucose levels <95 mg/dL, premeal values of <100 mg/dL, 1-hour postprandial levels of 140 mg/dL, and 2-hour postprandial levels <120 mg/dL.[43] Adjusting therapy based on postprandial glucose levels (as opposed to preprandial levels) can lower HbA_{1c} levels and decrease the risk of macrosomia and neonatal hypoglycemia.[49] HbA1c levels can be drawn at each trimester to reveal the glycemic control over the previous 3 months.[43]

Gestational Diabetes Mellitus

Diagnostic Criteria

17. J.B. is a 22-year-old, Asian woman in the 26th week of her first pregnancy. She is 5 feet 2 inches, 75 kg (prepregnancy weight), and her BMI is 30. At her regular prenatal visit, her obstetrician recommends an oral glucose-screening test for GDM. Although her mother has diabetes, J.B. has had no glucosuria during pregnancy. Why is J.B. at risk for GDM?

Gestational diabetes mellitus is defined as carbohydrate intolerance that develops or is recognized during pregnancy regardless of severity, necessity for treatment, time of onset, or persistence after pregnancy.[55,56] GDM occurs in about 7% (range, 1%–14%), and the prevalence varies with the population and methods of detection.[55] Complications noted in the offspring of affected women include macrosomia, hypocalcemia, hypoglycemia, polycythemia, and jaundice.[55] Women with GDM are more likely to develop pregnancy-induced hypertensive disorders or require a cesarean delivery. They also are at risk for type 2 diabetes later, and their children have an increased risk for obesity and diabetes later in life.[55]

Risk factors for GDM include age >25 years, obesity (BMI ≥25), family history of diabetes, previous delivery of an infant >4 kg, a history of a stillbirth, a history of glucose intolerance, or current glycosuria.[55,56] Blacks, Hispanic, Asian, and Native-American women also are at increased risk for GDM.[55,56] Some practitioners screen all pregnant women for GDM, whereas others do not screen low-risk women. Those considered at low risk must meet all of the following criteria: age <25 years, BMI ≤25, member of a low-risk ethnic group, no history of abnormal glucose tolerance, no known diabetes in a first-degree relative, and no history of poor obstetric outcome.[55]

The most common method of initial screening for GDM is the 50-g, 1-hour glucose challenge administered at 24 to 28 weeks gestation.[57] Women are instructed to drink a pure 50-g load of glucose and have their venous blood drawn. If the results are >140 mg/dL, a 100-g, 3-hour oral glucose tolerance test (OGTT)will be conducted.[57] If the results of the initial screen >200 mg/dL, most clinical practices may skip the 3-hour OGTT and obtain a fasting blood sugar level to diagnose GDM. Plasma glucose results from the 3-hour OGTT are used to diagnose GDM using either criterion. High-risk women should undergo OGTT early in pregnancy, and the test should be repeated in women who do not initially meet the diagnostic criteria for GDM.[55]

J.B. is at risk for GDM because she is Asian, obese, and has a family history of diabetes. Because she is at risk for GDM, J.B. should undergo OGTT. The diagnosis of GDM is important to the mother and the fetus because of the increased risks related to fetal hypersinsulinemia and macrosomia.[42,58] GDM does not have the same negative effect on pregnancy outcomes as pregestational diabetes.[42]

Treatment

18. J.B. is screened with a 1-hour OGTT, resulting in 160 mg/dL. A 3-hour OGTT is then recommended. The results of a 3-hour test show a fasting plasma glucose of 115 mg/dL, a 1-hour of 185 mg/dL, a 2-hour of 175 mg/dL, and a 3-hour of 150 mg/dL. These results confirm that J.B. has GDM. How should she be managed?

Most women with gestational diabetes can control their glucose with dietary modifications and regular exercise; however, insulin therapy should be initiated if dietary management fails to maintain fasting plasma blood glucose concentrations ≤95 mg/dL, a 1-hour postprandial plasma concentration <140 mg/dL, or 2-hour postprandial plasma glucose concentrations <120 mg/dL.[57] Treatment of GDM with insulin therapy is implemented similarly to the treatment for pregestational diabetes. An optimal insulin regimen for GDM has not been determined. The insulin regimen must be tailored specifically to the needs of the woman to successfully achieve target blood glucose levels. More recently, the role of oral hypoglycemics for the treatment of GDM has come into question. Traditionally, oral hypoglycemics have not been used during pregnancy because early animal studies implicated some agents as teratogens.[52] The studies failed to show whether the primary teratogen was the drug itself or the effect of hyperglycemia and altered maternal metabolism.[52] Glyburide, a second-generation sulfonyurea, has been used in several studies as an alternate treatment modality in women with GDM who have relatively mild hyperglycemia.[59] A gestational age of >30 weeks, fasting blood glucose levels,110 mg/dL, and 1-hour postprandials <140 mg/dL are parameters that have been shown in one study to predict glyburide success in women with GDM who have failed diet therapy.[60] In a randomized trial, glyburide therapy was compared with an intensive insulin protocol in women between 11 and 33 weeks of gestation with GDM who failed to achieve target blood glucose goals with diet alone.[59] Equivalent glycemic control was achieved with treatment of glyburide or insulin therapy. In addition, both groups had similar pregnancy outcomes, including rates for cesarean delivery, preeclampsia, macrosomia, and neonatal hypoglycemia. Analysis of the cord serum of the infant did not detect any glyburide.[59] More randomized trials are needed to further determine and to better understand the role of oral hypoglycemics in pregnancy.

J.B. requires more extensive education than patients with type 1 diabetes who know about the disease before becoming pregnant. She needs to be educated about diabetes, the signs and symptoms of hyper- and hypoglycemia, and the use of a glucometer. If insulin is started, she will also need to learn about injection technique, and how to mix and store insulin. She is most likely not a good candidate for glyburide therapy because she is <30 weeks' gestation and has a fasting blood sugar level >110 mg/dL.[60]

Risk of Developing Diabetes Mellitus

19. Why is J.B. at risk for developing diabetes mellitus after delivery?

Glucose tolerance normalizes after delivery for most women. Women with GDM, however, have a 17% to 63% chance of developing nongestational diabetes within 5 to 16 years.[56] The highest risk is in women who are obese, diagnosed before 24 weeks' gestation, or women who had marked hyperglycemia during or soon after pregnancy.[46] The risk of developing GDM in a future pregnancy is estimated to be 50% to 70%.

J.B. should try to minimize the potential for development of insulin resistance by exercising and maintaining a normal weight. She should also have her glucose checked with a 2-hour OGTT at her postpartum appointment 6 weeks after delivery and then at least every 3 years.[55] In addition, J.B. should be instructed about the importance of using an effective birth control method to prevent unplanned pregnancies. She also needs to schedule regular appointments with her primary care physician.

HYPERTENSION AND PRE-ECLAMPSIA

Classification and Definitions

Hypertensive disease occurs in 5% to 10% of all pregnancies and is a major cause of maternal and perinatal morbidity and mortality.[61] From 15% to 24% of maternal deaths in developed countries are attributed to hypertensive disorders in pregnancy.[62,63] *Hypertension in pregnancy* is defined as a systolic BP ≥140 mm Hg or a diastolic BP ≥90 mm Hg on two separate occasions at least 6 hours apart.

Women with pregnancy-associated hypertension can be grouped into the following categories: chronic hypertension, pre-eclampsia–eclampsia, pre-eclampsia superimposed on chronic hypertension, and gestational hypertension.[61] After delivery, *gestational hypertension* is ultimately delineated as either (*a*) transient hypertension of pregnancy if pre-eclampsia is absent during delivery and BP normalizes by 12 weeks postpartum or (*b*) chronic hypertension if BP remains elevated.[61]

Chronic hypertension is defined as hypertension diagnosed before conception or before the 20th week of gestation, or hypertension persisting beyond 12 weeks postpartum.[61] Hypertension noted after the 20th week of gestation might be difficult to classify, particularly if a woman has had inadequate prenatal care without appropriate BP monitoring.

Pre-eclampsia is a pregnancy-specific condition usually occurring after 20 weeks' gestation and consisting of hypertension with proteinuria.[61] The signs and symptoms of pre-eclampsia can affect multiple organ systems (e.g., kidney, liver, hematologic, CNS); they are often unpredictable and can be mistaken for other disorders. Because edema is so common in normal pregnancy and is not specific, it is no longer used as a criterion for the diagnosis of pre-eclampsia. Pre-eclampsia is a consequence of progressive placental and maternal endothelial cell dysfunction, increased platelet aggregation, and loss of arterial vasoregulation.[7] A variant of pre-eclampsia is HELLP syndrome, which consists of hemolysis (H), elevated liver enzymes (EL), and low platelet count (LP). HELLP can be also be life-threatening despite sometimes minimal proteinuria and increase in BP.[64]

When women with pre-eclampsia develop seizures, the term "*eclampsia*" is applied. Women with pre-eclampsia may unpredictably progress rapidly from mild to severe pre-eclampsia and to eclampsia within days or even hours. Eclampsia is a potentially preventable complication of pre-eclampsia (see Questions 30 to 34). About 20% of women who develop eclampsia have a diastolic BP <90 mm Hg or no proteinuria.[65]

The term "*gestational hypertension*" is used when BP is increased during pregnancy or is increased in the first 24 hours postpartum in a woman without signs or symptoms of pre-eclampsia and without pre-existing hypertension.[61] Women with gestational hypertension are at high risk of recurrence during subsequent pregnancies.

Chronic Hypertension

Clinical Presentation

20. T.D., a 37-year-old G_1P_0, obese black woman was diagnosed with stage 1 hypertension several months before her pregnancy (BP 135 to 145 mm Hg systolic and 90 to 95 mm Hg diastolic pressure). She had no cardiovascular risk factors (i.e., smoking,

diabetes mellitus, dyslipidemias) and was prescribed a trial of lifestyle modification (i.e., weight loss and exercise). When she initiated prenatal care at 16 weeks' gestation, her BP ranged from 130 to 135 mm Hg systolic pressure and 82 to 85 mm Hg diastolic pressure. Her BP today at 28 weeks is 142/90 mm Hg. Her serum chemistry values are creatinine (Cr) 0.6 mg/dL (normal, 0.5–0.6); and uric acid (UA) 4 mg/dL (normal, 2.5–5.9). A random urinalysis did not demonstrate proteinuria. Ultrasound confirms an adequately growing fetus at 28 weeks' gestation. What is the likelihood T.D. has pre-eclampsia?

Women with chronic hypertension commonly have a normal BP during the first half of pregnancy because of the normal physiologic decline of BP during the second trimester.[66] Blood pressure usually returns to the prepregnancy level by the third trimester. T.D.'s diastolic pressure decreased from the prepregnancy levels of 90 to 95 mm Hg to 86 to 90 mm Hg during the second trimester. It is normal for T.D.'s BP to increase during the third trimester. These changes in BP make it difficult to differentiate chronic hypertension from pre-eclampsia during the second half of pregnancy in women with late prenatal care or inadequate BP monitoring. It is also difficult to diagnose pre-eclampsia superimposed on existing hypertension using BP measurements alone. A sharp increase in T.D.'s pressure of >30 mm Hg systolic or >15 mm Hg diastolic could be consistent with pre-eclampsia. Without co-existing proteinuria (≥0.3 g/24-hour or ≥1+ in a random urine) or evidence of renal dysfunction, a diagnosis of pre-eclampsia would be a reach.[61] T.D. has no proteinuria, and a normal serum creatinine and serum uric acid. It is unlikely that T.D. has pre-eclampsia at this time.

Risk Factors for Pre-eclampsia

21. What risk factors does T.D. have for developing pre-eclampsia?

Pre-eclampsia occurs most commonly during the first pregnancy (two-thirds of cases). Obesity and increasing maternal age are risk factors.[67] Chronic diseases that increase the risk for pre-eclampsia include diabetes mellitus or insulin resistance, and renal disease. Pregnancy-associated risk factors include multifetal gestations, urinary tract infection, certain fetal chromosomal anomalies, and hydatiform moles. A family history of a sister or mother with pre-eclampsia significantly increases the risk of developing pre-eclampsia. Women with previous pre-eclampsia are at high risk for recurrence in subsequent pregnancies, particularly if it developed before 30 weeks' gestation.[67,68] In addition to her age and obesity, chronic hypertension is the most significant aspect of T.D.'s medical history, which confers a 25% risk of developing superimposed pre-eclampsia.[69]

MONITORING

22. What subjective and objective data should be monitored in T.D. for the development of pre-eclampsia?

T.D. should have her BP monitored frequently. If protein is detected in a random urinalysis, then a 24-hour urine collection for protein and creatinine can be repeated to determine accurately the degree of proteinuria and severity of disease.[61] Periodic ultrasounds should be obtained to assess fetal growth because intrauterine growth retardation (IUGR) is common in pregnant women with chronic hypertension. T.D. should be taught to recognize and immediately report all signs and symptoms of pre-eclampsia, such as nondependent edema, headaches, and visual disturbances. The latter two are signs of severe pre-eclampsia and may indicate impending eclampsia. Upper abdominal pain also can be a sign of severe pre-eclampsia, indicating hepatic subcapsular hemorrhage.[67] Because T.D. has chronic hypertension, worsening of hypertension alone may not be a reliable sign of superimposed pre-eclampsia. Proteinuria is the best indicator of superimposed pre-eclampsia in a pregnant woman with chronic hypertension and no renal disease.[65]

ANTIHYPERTENSIVE DRUG THERAPY

23. Why should (or should not) T.D.'s chronic hypertension be treated with antihypertensive drugs to prevent pre-eclampsia?

The goal of antihypertensive therapy for women with chronic hypertension during pregnancy is to minimize the risks to the mother of an elevated BP without compromising placental perfusion.[61] The value of treating pregnant women with chronic antihypertension drugs remains an area of ongoing debate. A sustained diastolic BP of >100 mm Hg may cause maternal vascular damage, especially if the diastolic pressure is >105 to 110 mm Hg.[67] Morbidity is unlikely with a diastolic BP of <100 mm Hg. Therefore, many clinicians recommend treatment with antihypertensive drugs to lower diastolic pressures of >100 to 110 mm Hg.[61] Treatment of a diastolic BP of <100 mm Hg should be reserved for women with chronic hypertension and target organ damage (e.g., left ventricular hypertrophy) or underlying renal disease because antihypertensive drugs can decrease placental blood flow, which might increase fetal growth restriction.[70,71] Treatment of mild to moderate hypertension is associated with a decrease in the risk of developing severe hypertension by approximately 50%, but the overall risk of developing pre-eclampsia is unchanged.[72] Moreover, women treated with antihypertensives were more likely to develop adverse drug effects compared with those who received placebo or were untreated. Antihypertensive therapy, however, is required to reduce the risk of cardiovascular morbidity such as heart or renal failure, and acute risk of stroke in pregnant women with severe hypertension (diastolic >110 mm Hg).

T.D. has normal renal function and her BP is <100 mm Hg; she does not need antihypertensive drug treatment at this time. If T.D. had been on drug therapy before conception, some experts would have her continue during the pregnancy.[61,65,70] In such cases, however, the doses of the antihypertensive agents often need to be lowered or discontinued altogether to prevent hypotension because the maternal BP naturally decreases during the second trimester. The only antihypertensive drugs absolutely contraindicated during pregnancy are ACEI and angiotensin II-receptor blockers because of the association with fetal and newborn morbidity and mortality.[70] Atenolol use also should be avoided because of the reported association with a high incidence of IUGR.[70]

Perinatal outcomes in women with untreated chronic hypertension who do not progress to pre-eclampsia are similar to those of the general obstetric population.[65] Although chronic hypertension is a major risk factor for pre-eclampsia, treating T.D.'s uncomplicated mild chronic hypertension is unlikely to prevent the development of pre-eclampsia.

METHYLDOPA

Methyldopa (Aldomet) is a centrally-acting α-agonist that decreases sympathetic outflow to decrease BP. It is the antihypertensive most commonly used for chronic treatment of hypertension in pregnancy in the United States. The usual starting dose of 750 to 1,000 mg/day, to be administered in three to four daily divided doses, can be increased to 2 or 3 g/day if needed. Higher doses may be needed to control BP in pregnancy.[73]

Methyldopa, classified as category B for fetal risk, has the longest and best safety record of all antihypertensive agents during pregnancy. Despite its common use, few adverse effects have been reported in neonates exposed to methyldopa *in utero*. In addition, no congenital anomalies are associated with methyldopa.[33]

Dizziness and sedation, accompanied by a loss of energy, are among the most common adverse effects reported by pregnant women.[73] Generally, these adverse effects occur early in therapy and tend to subside, but may recur with an increased dosage. Problems with postural hypotension usually do not occur in pregnant females.[73] Patients should be monitored for methyldopa-induced liver damage.[65] Other drugs used to treat hypertension in pregnancy include labetalol and calcium channel blockers. A review of drug therapies for the treatment of chronic hypertension in pregnancy is listed in Table 46-3.

Mild Pre-eclampsia

Etiology and Pathogenesis

The causes of pre-eclampsia currently remain unknown. Although the pathogenesis begins early in pregnancy, the disease is not clinically evident until the latter half of the pregnancy and persists until the fetus is delivered.[7,74] Incomplete physiologic placental vascular bed changes and endothelial cell dysfunction are integral to the pathogenesis of pre-eclampsia (see Placental Physiology).

PLACENTAL ISCHEMIA

Early in a normal pregnancy, the trophoblastic migration and invasion of the uterine spiral arteries result in physiologic changes within the placental vascular bed that facilitate maximal intervillous blood flow. The physiologic changes within these spiral arteries are responsible for creating a fixed low-resistance arteriolar circuit, which increases blood supply to the growing fetus. In pre-eclampsia, these physiologic changes do not occur completely, resulting in decreased perfusion and consequently, placental ischemia.[7,74,75]

ENDOTHELIAL DAMAGE

An intact vascular endothelium assists in preserving the integrity of vasculature, mediating immune and inflammatory responses, preventing intravascular coagulation, and modulating the contractility of the underlying smooth muscle cell.[75]

In normal pregnancy, prostacyclin is increased 8 to 10 times, creating an increased ratio of prostacyclin to thromboxane A_2.[74] The biologic dominance of prostacyclin along with nitric oxide plays an important role in maintaining vasodilation throughout pregnancy. Prostacyclin may be responsible for vascular refractoriness to angiotensin II in normal pregnancy. In pre-eclampsia, the ratio of prostacyclin to thromboxane A_2 is reversed. Thromboxane A_2 is biologically

Table 46-3 Drugs For Treatment of Chronic Hypertension In Pregnancy

Drug	Dose	Comments
Methyldopa	750–1000 mg/day start, increase up to 2–3 g/day, divided in three to four doses	Longest safety record in pregnancy. Considered a first-line drug.[66] Dizziness, sedation, and lack of energy are common symptoms, which tend to resolve. Can cause liver toxicity. Low breast milk concentrations so considered safe in breast-feeding.
Labetolol	200–400 mg/day start, increase to up to 2,400 mg/day, divided in two or sometimes three doses	Combined α- and β-receptor antagonist properties. Considered a first-line drug.[66] Increasingly preferred to methyldopa owing to fewer side effects. Neonatal effects could include bradycardia and hypotension. Low concentration in breast milk and generally considered safe in breast-feeding.[235]
Other β-Blockers	Various	Atenolol in particular associated with decreased placental weight and IUGR.[287,288] IUGR thought to be related to β-blocker–induced increased vascular resistance in mother and fetus. Atenolol, acebutolol, metoprolol, nadolol, and sotalol can have high milk-to-plasma ratios and accumulate in breast milk, creating potential risk for neonatal-blockade.[289,290] Propanolol found in only small amounts in breast milk and generally considered safe, but infants should be monitored for hypotension, bradycardia, and blood glucose changes.
Nifedipine, long acting	30 mg/day start, increase to up to 120 mg/day, single dose	Limited pregnancy data on nifedipine or other calcium channel blockers such as verapamil, iltiazem, and amlodipine. Concentrations of nifedipine in breast milk are low and considered compatible with breast-feeding.[235,291]
Diuretics	Various	Not first-line agents, although probably safe.[61] Concern regarding potential interference with normal blood volume expansion in pregnancy. Avoid if pre-eclampsia or IUGR already present. Concentration low in breast milk, but may decrease milk production.
ACEI or ARB	Contraindicated	Contraindicated in pregnancy in all trimesters. Fetal renal failure when used after first trimester, resulting in oligohydramnios, limb contractures, pulmonary hypoplasia, skull hypoplasia, and irreversible neonatal renal failure.[33] Increased risk major birth defects with first trimester ACEI exposure.[51] Minimal amounts of captopril and enalapril in breast milk and both considered compatible with breast feeding.[235] Minimal amounts of benezepril in breast milk. Limited or no data on other ACEI or ARB.

* ACEI, angiotensin-converting enzyme inhibitor. ARB, angiotensin II receptor blocker. IUGR, intrauterine growth restriction.

dominant during pre-eclampsia, leading to increased vascular sensitivity to angiotensin II and norepinephrine.[74] The increased release of thromboxane A_2 is believed to be caused by endothelial cell dysfunction. The end result is vasospasm, which further increases endothelial cell dysfunction, and increases BP.[7,74] Reduced activity of nitric oxide synthase and decreased nitric oxide-dependent or nitric oxide-independent endothelium-derived relaxing factor are believed to increase the vasoconstrive potential of pressors such as angiotensin II.[61]

Endothelial cell dysfunction in pregnancy is thought to be caused by oxidative stress. Intermittent hypoxic and reperfusion injury that occurs as a consequence of decreased placental perfusion may increase oxidative stress.[74,75] Endothelial damage eventually leads to the disruption of the vascular lining, which causes leaking capillary membranes, allowing fluid to leak into the interstitium.[75] In severe pre-eclampsia, this results in hypovolemia, hemoconcentration, and consequently an increase in hematocrit. The loss of plasma volume, vasospasm, and microthrombi decrease perfusion of the kidney, CNS, liver, and other organs. The loss of intravascular proteins in the urine secondary to renal damage, and through damaged epithelia, decreases plasma oncotic pressure and leads to a rapid onset of nondependent edema. The imbalance of endogenous procoagulants and anticoagulants produces platelet consumption and results in thrombocytopenia and coagulation defects.[75]

Clinical Presentation

24. T.D. returns to her obstetrician 3 weeks later at 31 weeks' gestation complaining of mild hand and leg edema. She has 1+ proteinuria by dipstick and her BP is 155/102 mm Hg. An ultrasound demonstrates fetal growth restriction. Laboratory results are serum Cr 0.9 mg/dL (normal, 0.5–0.7); UA 6.0 mg/dL (normal, 2.5–5.9); aspartate aminotransferase (AST) 25 U/L (normal, 0–35); alanine aminotransferase (ALT) 16 U/L (normal, 0–35); platelets 230,000/mm^3 (normal, 203,000–353,000. What signs and laboratory evidence are consistent with pre-eclampsia in T.D.? Does she have mild or severe pre-eclampsia?

T.D.'s diastolic BP is now higher than it was before her pregnancy and has increased by 12 mm Hg in the last 3 weeks. Although an increase in BP by itself is not diagnostic of pre-eclampsia, the new finding of proteinuria confirms the diagnosis. Other evidence for pre-eclampsia includes the elevated serum uric acid concentration, which is a sensitive marker for pre-eclampsia, and elevated creatinine.[67] T.D. denies headaches, visual disturbances, and abdominal pain, which are symptoms of severe pre-eclampsia. The transaminases and platelet count are normal; therefore she does not have HELLP syndrome at this time. T.D.'s clinical presentation is consistent with mild pre-eclampsia; however, a 24-hour urine collection should be obtained to measure protein excretion, quantify the urine output, and further rule out severe pre-eclampsia.

Treatment

GENERAL PRINCIPLES

25. T.D. is admitted to the hospital. The 24-hour urine protein is 500 mg/24 hours. Although fetal growth is restricted, all other fetal testing is reassuring. After 24 hours, her BP decreased to 140/95. Her platelet counts remained stable and >200/mm^3 and transaminases were normal. No other signs and symptoms of pre-eclampsia were noted. How should T.D.'s mild pre-eclampsia be managed?

The delivery of the fetus is the only cure for pre-eclampsia and would be the best treatment option for T.D. if she were >weeks' gestation.[7] T.D. has mild disease, however, and is not close to term. Her delivery should be postponed because premature delivery increases neonatal morbidity and mortality. T.D.'s fetus is somewhat growth restricted, which is common in women with chronic hypertension, with or without superimposed pre-eclampsia. If T.D.'s fetus is severely growth restricted or if subsequent fetal biophysical testing is abnormal, premature delivery would be indicated.[61] Because neither of these is evident in the present circumstances, T.D. should carry her fetus under very close medical supervision. It has been suggested that continued hospitalization is appropriate for women with preterm onset of mild pre-eclampsia, such as T.D.[61] This would allow for rapid intervention in case of rapid progression of disease or associated complications. Probably a role exists for outpatient monitoring of some select women with very frequent maternal and fetal monitoring, and rehospitalization for worsening disease.[61]

T.D. is also a candidate for administration of glucocorticoids for fetal lung maturation (see also Question 55). Bedrest in the lateral decubitus position is usually suggested and may help reduce BP and promote diuresis by decreasing vasoconstriction and improving renal and uteroplacental perfusion. T.D. should have her BP measured regularly each day. Her urine should be checked daily for protein. Liver transaminases, platelets, and creatinine should be measured periodically and whenever her clinical status changes. She also should be assessed for symptoms of severe pre-eclampsia (e.g., headaches, visual disturbances, epigastric or right upper quadrant pain). Fetal surveillance is indicated.[61] One approach is to perform a modified biophysical profile twice a week and whenever maternal clinical status changes, and an ultrasound for fetal growth every 3 to 4 weeks.

Severe Pre-eclampsia

Clinical Presentation

26. T.D.'s BP for about 2 weeks ranged from 140 to 150 mm Hg systolic and 90 to 100 mm Hg diastolic with bedrest. Her proteinuria remained stable at 1+ to 2+ by dipstick. During the past 2 days T.D.'s BP started to increase again, and today her BP is 160/112 mm Hg and her urine dipstick is 3+. She complains of headaches, dizziness, and visual disturbances and has significant edema in her face, hands, legs, and ankles. T.D. is transferred to the Labor and Delivery Unit for delivery. Pertinent laboratory results are Cr 1.3 mg/dL (normal, 0.5–0.6); UA 6.7 mg/dL (normal, 2.5–5.9); AST 30 U/L (normal, 0–35); ALT 16 U/L (normal, 0–35); total bilirubin 1 mg/dL (normal, 0.1–1); platelets, 95,000/mm^3 (normal, 203,000–353,000); hematocrit 38% (normal, 32.7%–36%), hemoglobin 13 g/dL (normal, 10.9–13.5); random urine protein 4+. Estimated fetal weight by ultrasound is 1,700 g, which is between the 10th and 25th percentile for a gestational age of 34 weeks. What signs, symptoms, and laboratory evidence of severe pre-eclampsia supports this diagnosis in T.D.?

T.D. has developed severe pre-eclampsia.[64] Her systolic and diastolic BP are above 160 and 112 mm Hg, respectively. She has >3+ protein in a random urine sample and her serum creatinine is >1.2 mg/dL. She complains of headaches and visual disturbances. T.D. is also thrombocytopenic as her platelet count is 95,000/mm^3. Although her liver transaminases are currently normal, she may be developing HELLP syndrome, a variant of severe pre-eclampsia associated with a high incidence of maternal and perinatal morbidity and mortality. Therefore, her laboratory values should continue to be monitored even as delivery is being planned.

Complications

27. To what complications of severe pre-eclampsia would T.D. be exposed?

T.D. is at risk for cerebral hemorrhage, cerebral edema, encephalopathy, coagulopathies, pulmonary edema, liver failure, renal failure, and eclamptic seizures.[7,65] Severe pre-eclampsia is not only dangerous to T.D., but also to her fetus because uteroplacental perfusion is compromised. T.D. requires drug treatments to both lower her BP and prevent eclampsia.

Acute Treatment of Severe Hypertension

HYDRALAZINE

28. How should T.D.'s severe hypertension be treated?

The goal of antihypertensive therapy in T.D. is to prevent cerebral complications (e.g., encephalopathy, hemorrhage).[65] Although it is important to reduce the maternal BP, it must be accomplished gradually while the fetus is *in utero* because a sudden large drop in maternal BP could result in the reduction of uteroplacental perfusion.[67] Because of the potential for fetal bradycardia during or after acute treatment of maternal hypertension, continuous fetal heart rate monitoring should be considered.

Hydralazine, a direct arterial smooth muscle dilator, has been the drug of choice for the acute treatment of severe hypertension in pregnancy.[65,73] This drug induces a baroreceptor-mediated tachycardia and increases cardiac output, which increases uterine blood flow as the BP is lowered.[67] Hydralazine 5 mg IV over 1 to 2 minutes should be administered to T.D. and repeated in doses of 5 to 10 mg every 20 to 30 minutes to a cumulative dose of 20 mg.[7,65]

T.D. should have repeated measurements of her BP at 15-minute intervals. Because intervillous blood flow depends on maternal perfusion pressure, the goal is to decrease the diastolic pressure to not less than 90 mm Hg.[7,65] Lowering the maternal BP excessively may decrease uteroplacental perfusion and compromise the fetus. The onset of antihypertensive effect for hydralazine ranges from 10 to 20 minutes and duration of action ranges from 3 to 6 hours after an IV dose.[67] Therefore, doses of hydralazine should not be repeated more frequently than every 20 to 30 minutes to prevent drug accumulation.[73] T.D. should also be monitored for nausea, vomiting, tachycardia, flushing, headache, and tremors. Some of these hydralazine-induced adverse effects mimic symptoms associated with severe pre-eclampsia and imminent eclampsia, making it difficult for a clinician to differentiate between drug-associated and disease-related problems.[73] Fetal hydralazine serum concentrations are reportedly the same as or higher than maternal serum concentrations, but drug-associated fetal abnormalities have not been reported.[33]

ALTERNATIVE ANTIHYPERTENSIVE DRUGS

29. After receiving two doses of IV hydralazine (total dose 15 mg), T.D.'s BP decreased to 150/100 mm Hg. What other antihypertensive drugs could have been used to treat her severe hypertension?

Labetalol

Labetalol (Trandate) is the second most commonly used drug to treat severe hypertension during pregnancy. It should be administered IV in increasing doses of 20, 40, and 80 mg every 10 minutes to a cumulative dose of 300 mg or until the diastolic pressure is <100 mm Hg.[76] The onset of action is within 5 minutes, and its effect peaks in 10 to 20 minutes with a duration of action ranging from 45 minutes to 6 hours.

Intravenous labetalol is as effective as intravenous hydralazine in lowering BP in patients with hypertension during pregnancy, but has fewer reported adverse effects.[73,77] In a meta-analysis of β-blocker trials for the treatment of hypertension in pregnancy, labetalol was associated with less maternal hypotension, fewer cesarean deliveries, and no increase in perinatal mortality.[77] Labetalol also does not appear to decrease uteroplacental blood flow even with a decrease in maternal BP.[73] Labetalol reduces cerebral perfusion pressure, which occurs in up to 43% of women with severe pre-eclampsia, without negatively affecting cerebral blood flow.[78] Decreased cerebral perfusion pressure may prevent progression to eclampsia. It, however, should be avoided in women with asthma and heart failure.[61] Labetalol has also been associated with higher rates of neonatal bradycardia and hypotension than hydralazine, but not higher rates of neonatal intensive care admission.[79,80]

Nifedipine

Nifedipine (Procardia, Adalat) has been used in doses of 10 mg for acute treatment of severe hypertension during pregnancy because it can be given orally.[73] Nifedipine is effective in decreasing BP without reducing uteroplacental blood flow or decreasing fetal heart rate. Short-acting nifedipine capsules are no longer recommended for the treatment of acute hypertensive urgency, however, because of the risk of stroke or myocardial infarction, and it was never US Food and Drug Administration (FDA) approved for this indication. Immediate-release nifedipine continues to be used to treat hypertension in pregnancy, however, because this unique patient population may not be at high risk for ischemic events secondary to atherosclerotic disease.[70] Calcium gluconate or calcium chloride should be available for IV administration in the event of sudden hypotension. Caution should be used when giving nifedipine to women concomitantly treated with magnesium sulfate because these drugs have synergistic effects, causing hypotension and neuromuscular blockade.[81]

Several studies comparing oral nifedipine with IV labetalol in hypertensive emergencies of pregnancy have found them to be equally effective in lowering BP.[82,83] Nifedipine lowers BP to <160 mm Hg systolic and <100 mm Hg diastolic earlier than labetalol,[82] but it increases cardiac index[83] (see Chapter 20, Hypertensive Emergencies).

Eclampsia

Magnesium Sulfate Prophylaxis

30. T.D. was given magnesium sulfate 4 g IV for 30 minutes and then started on a continuous IV infusion of 2 g/hour. Labor was induced, and T.D. subsequently delivered vaginally. Why was T.D.'s drug therapy appropriate?

Magnesium sulfate was given to T.D. to prevent eclamptic seizures during labor.[61] Although termination of the pregnancy is the definitive treatment for severe pre-eclampsia, the intrapartum and immediate postpartum periods are also the periods of greatest risk for eclampsia.[67] Although the incidence of eclampsia is extremely low, maternal morbidity and mortality are high.[84] In the United States, it has been usual practice to treat all pre-eclamptic women with magnesium sulfate during labor and for 12 to 24 hours postpartum.[61,65] In the United Kingdom, it is common to reserve magnesium sulfate therapy for severe pre-eclampsia.[85] The evidence for magnesium sulfate prevention of the progression of disease in mildly pre-eclamptic women has been largely anecdotal. In a large international study of more than 10,000 women, magnesium sulfate clearly decreased the risk of eclampsia in pre-eclamptic women by 58% compared with placebo.[85] An observational study of nearly 2,500 women with mild pre-eclampsia (BP of 140/90 and 1+ protein) found an incidence of eclampsia of about 1%, without the use of seizure prophylaxis.[86]

In a prospective, randomized study, magnesium sulfate was superior to phenytoin for the prevention of eclampsia in hypertensive pregnant women.[84] In addition, magnesium sulfate was more effective than nimodipine for seizure prophylaxis in severely pre-eclamptic women.[87]

A regimen of magnesium sulfate 4 to 6 g IV as a loading dose followed by a continuous infusion of 2 g/hour is the most commonly used regimen in the United States.[88] Continuous infusion of 1 g/hour has been associated with treatment failures.[89] Intravenous loading doses of 6 g followed by continuous infusions of 2 g/hour maintain therapeutically effective magnesium serum concentrations between 4 to 8 mg/dL.[89] Using a loading dose of 4 g consistently resulted in subtherapeutic serum levels (<4 mg/dL), prompting a protocol change to a 6-g load in one study.[86] A magnesium sulfate 50% solution can be used to administer 10 g IM in two divided doses into the upper outer quadrant of each buttock followed by 5 g IM every 4 hours, although this protocol is not commonly used.[88] Because magnesium is excreted by the kidneys and will accumulate in cases of renal dysfunction, the continuous infusion rate must be lowered with oliguria or an elevated serum creatinine.

Because of the potential for infusion errors and significant patient morbidity and even mortality with accidental overdoses of magnesium sulfate, the Institute of Medicine has identified magnesium sulfate as a high-risk medication.[90] All infusions of magnesium sulfate must be given through a controlled pump designed to protect against free flow. If such an infusion pump is not available, the IM route of administration should be used. Dispensing premixed IV bags from central pharmacy with a standardized concentration of magnesium sulfate and limiting the total grams of magnesium sulfate in each dispensed IV bag also can help guard against inadvertent overdose. Dispensing the loading dose in a separate small bag (e.g., 4 g in 100 mL) from the maintenance bag (e.g., 20 g in 200 mL) also may be helpful.[91]

31. What is the proposed mechanism of action of magnesium sulfate in the prevention and treatment of eclamptic seizures?

The precise mechanism of anticonvulsant action of magnesium for the prevention and treatment of eclamptic seizures is unknown. The anticonvulsant activity may be partly mediated through blockade of an excitatory amino acid receptor, *N*-methyl-d-aspartate (NMDA).[81] Seizures are thought to be caused by decreased cerebral blood flow because of vasospasm. Magnesium sulfate is a potent cerebral vasodilator and increases the synthesis of prostacyclin, an endothelial vasodilator. It also causes a dose-dependent decrease in systemic vascular resistance, which may explain its transient hypotensive effect. Magnesium may also protect against oxidative injury to endothelial cells.[81]

Monitoring Magnesium Sulfate Therapy

32. What subjective and objective data should be monitored during treatment of T.D. with magnesium?

Deep tendon reflexes (patellar reflex), respiratory rate, and urine output should be monitored periodically during treatment with magnesium sulfate.[84] The loss of patellar reflexes, the first sign of magnesium toxicity, generally occurs at serum concentrations of 8 to 12 mg/dL. The respiratory rate should be monitored hourly and should be >12 breaths/minute. Respiratory arrest can occur with serum concentrations of >13 mg/dL. Urine output should be carefully monitored and should be at least 100 mL every 4 hours (or 25 mL/hour).[84] Magnesium serum concentrations are not routinely measured unless renal dysfunction is evident with oliguria or elevated serum creatinine, because magnesium is almost entirely excreted by the kidney.[81,84] Hypocalcemia and hypocalcemic tetany also can occur secondary to hypermagnesemia and can be reversed by calcium gluconate 1 g (10 mL of a 10% solution) slow IV push over 3 minutes.[7] Neuromuscular depression can occur in infants whose mothers received magnesium sulfate.[33] Parenteral magnesium sulfate is safe and rarely causes maternal or neonatal toxicity when administered properly but requires built-in system safeguards to avoid unintended dosing errors.[91]

Treatment

33. What is appropriate drug therapy for eclampsia?

Diazepam, phenytoin, and magnesium sulfate have all been used to treat eclampsia. The use of magnesium sulfate to treat these seizures results in less maternal morbidity and mortality and less neonatal morbidity.[84,92] Generally, higher serum concentrations of magnesium sulfate are needed to treat than to prevent eclamptic seizures. The same therapeutic range guides both prophylaxis and treatment, however.[88] Seizures unresponsive to magnesium sulfate treatment should prompt an evaluation for other cerebrovascular events (e.g., cerebral hemorrhage or infarction).[88]

34. How long should magnesium sulfate be continued in T.D.?

Depending on the severity of pre-eclampsia, magnesium sulfate therapy usually is continued for 24 hours after delivery.[93] Attempts are being made to identify patient-specific criteria that can be used to determine the optimal duration of therapy. Women with severe pre-eclampsia or pre-eclampsia superimposed on chronic hypertension are at greater risk for disease exacerbation when magnesium sulfate is discontinued too soon.

INDUCTION OF LABOR

Mechanisms of Term Labor

In pregnancy, many hormones and peptides, including progesterone, prostacyclin, relaxin, nitric oxide, and parathyroid hormone-related peptide inhibit uterine smooth muscle contractility. Labor at term occurs because the myometrium is released from its quiescent state.[94] For example, as progesterone concentrations decrease near term gestation, estrogen may stimulate uterine contractility.

Uterine activity is divided into four phases: quiescence (phase 0), activation (phase 1), stimulation (phase 2), and involution (phase 3). Each of these phases is stimulated or inhibited by several factors.[94] During activation, uterotropins, such as estrogen, and possibly others stimulate a complex series of uterine changes (e.g., increased myometrial prostaglandin and oxytocin receptors and myometrial gap junctions), which are important for the coordination of contractions. These changes help prime the myometrium and cervix for stimulation by the uterotonins oxytocin and prostaglandins E_2 and $F_{2\alpha}$. The cervix softens, shortens, and dilates, a process referred to as *cervical ripening*. Uterine stimulation is responsible for the change in myometrial activity from irregular to regular contractions. During phase 3, involution of the uterus occurs after delivery and is mediated mostly by oxytocin.[94]

The exact stimulus of the biochemical scheme leading to labor in humans is unknown. The fetus may help facilitate this process by affecting placental steroid production through mechanical distention of the uterus and by activating the fetal hypothalamic-pituitary-adrenal axis. Ultimately, these lead to increased production of oxytocin and prostaglandins by the fetoplacental unit.

Labor is divided into three stages.[95] Weak, irregular, rhythmic contractions (Braxton-Hicks contractions or "false labor") may happen for weeks before the onset of true labor. The first stage begins with the start of regular uterine contractions and ends with complete cervical dilation. Stage 1 is divided further into the latent phase, active phase, and deceleration phase. During the latent phase, the cervix effaces (thins) but dilates minimally. The contractions become progressively stronger and longer, better coordinated, and more frequent. The duration of the latent phase is the most varied and unpredictable of all aspects of labor and can continue intermittently for days. During the active phase, contractions are strong and regular, occurring every 2 to 3 minutes. The cervix dilates from 3 to 4 cm to full dilation, usually 10 cm. The second stage starts with complete cervical dilation and ends with the delivery of the fetus. The third stage of labor is the time between the delivery of the fetus and the delivery of the placenta.[95]

Indications, Contraindications, and Requirements

35. J.T., a 28-year-old primigravida, is admitted to the labor and delivery suite for labor induction. She is at 42 weeks' gestation by dates and ultrasound and has a normal obstetric examination. Cervical examination reveals an unfavorable cervix for labor induction; Bishop score is 4. What are the indications and contraindications for labor induction in J.T.?

The induction of labor involves the artificial stimulation of uterine contractions that lead to labor and delivery.[96] Induction of labor is indicated when the continuation of pregnancy jeopardizes maternal or fetal health (e.g., pre-eclampsia, chorioamnionitis [infection of the fetal membranes}, fetal demise, IUGR, $Rh_o(D)$ alloimmunization, maternal medical problems, post-term pregnancy).[96] Post-term pregnancy ($\geq$42 weeks' gestation), as in J.T.'s case, is the most common indication and most commonly encountered problem leading to induction of labor.[96,97] Contraindications to labor induction are similar to those for spontaneous labor and vaginal delivery and include, but are not limited to, active genital herpes infection, placenta previa (abnormally implanted placenta), prior classic uterine incision, transverse fetal lie, and prolapsed umbilical cord. If uterine activity is appropriately monitored, induced labor yields similar maternal and perinatal outcomes as those with spontaneous labor.[96]

A complete assessment of both mother and fetus should be performed before inducing labor.[96–98] Previous labor complications or cesarean deliveries in the mother should be considered. Fetal maturity must be assessed accurately before the induction of labor to avoid the inadvertent delivery of a preterm fetus.[96,98] Every attempt should be made to ensure fetal lung maturation before inducing labor when termination of pregnancy is necessary before 34 weeks' gestation, and antenatal corticosteroids should be administered.[99]

The degree of cervical ripeness and readiness for induction of labor should be assessed because the success of labor induction depends on the degree of cervical ripeness.[96,100] The state of the cervix is assessed using a pelvic scoring method. The Bishop method assigns a score based on the station of the fetal head relative to the maternal spine and the extent of cervical dilation, effacement, consistency, and position.[98,100] Bishop scores of >8 are associated with a 100% induction rate and short labor.[96,100] Bishop scores $\leq$4, as is documented in J.T., are associated with a high likelihood of failed inductions and cesarean deliveries. Women with Bishop scores $\leq$2 who undergo cervical ripening before induction of labor still, however, have high incidence of failure and cesarean deliveries.[100]

Cervical ripening can be accomplished by the administration of prostaglandins (E_2 and E_1) or low-dose oxytocin. Alternatively, cervical dilators or separation of the chorioamniotic membranes from the internal surface of the uterus can ripen the cervix.[96,98,100] Osmotic or hygroscopic dilators (e.g., Dilapan, Lamicel) work by absorbing cervical mucus and gradually swelling, thereby dilating the cervical canal.[98,100] The hygroscopic dilators require less monitoring of the mother when compared with the administration of prostaglandins; however, they do not appear to decrease the incidence of cesarean deliveries.[98,100] Labor induction is accomplished most commonly by amniotomy (artificial rupture of the fetal membranes) and oxytocin administration.[96,98]

Although labor induction is medically indicated in J.T. to decrease the risk of an adverse fetal outcome with continuing a post-term pregnancy, her cervix is unfavorable for induction.

Cervical Ripening

Prostaglandin E_2 (Dinoprostone)

36. When should dinoprostone be used to induce labor?

Prostaglandins (e.g., dinoprostone) induce cervical ripening and enhance myometrial sensitivity to oxytocin by promoting the breakdown of collagen and increasing the submucosal hyaluronic acid and water content.[96,98,100] A Bishop score of ≤4 is a definite indication for cervical ripening. Although not universally accepted, intermediate Bishop scores of 5 to 7 indicate a need for cervical ripening.[101] Patients with intermediate Bishop scores undergoing cervical ripening with prostaglandins are more likely to achieve labor without oxytocin.[96] Dinoprostone is the drug used most commonly for cervical ripening.[98] Up to half of the women treated with dinoprostone experience labor and deliver within 24 hours, some without oxytocin.[102–104] Dinoprostone cervical gel (Prepidil Gel) contains dinoprostone 0.5 mg/3 g (2.5 mL gel) and is administered endocervically. Dinoprostone vaginal insert (Cervidil) contains dinoprostone 10 mg and is inserted vaginally.[105] Prepidil Gel must be refrigerated and Cervidil vaginal inserts must remain frozen until administration. Women with unfavorable cervices, such as J.T., should undergo a trial of cervical ripening with dinoprostone before labor induction. Post-term women with unfavorable cervices who receive dinoprostone have shorter durations of labor, require lower doses of oxytocin, and may have a decreased incidence of cesarean deliveries.[100,102–104]

37. Which dinoprostone dosage form should be used in J.T.?

Both dinoprostone products are effective for cervical ripening, leading to successful induction of labor.[100,102–104] The two dinoprostone formulations differ in dosing and application.[105,106]

DINOPROSTONE GEL (PREPIDIL)

Prepidil 0.5 mg should be administered endocervically at room temperature in or near the labor and delivery suite.[96,106] After administration, the patient should remain in a recumbent position for at least 30 minutes to minimize leakage from the cervix.[96,106] Fetal heart rate and uterine activity should be monitored before administration and continuously for at least 2 hours after administration. The cervix should be reassessed and the dose repeated every 6 hours if needed or until a maximal cumulative dose of 1.5 mg (three doses) has been administered in 24 hours.[106] Most women need more than one application, and at least 50% need three doses.[107] The average wholesale price for one dose of Prepidil Gel has been about $172/0.5-mg dose.[108]

Once the cervix has ripened but the patient is not in active labor, oxytocin may be started if at least 6 hours have elapsed from the time the last dinoprostone dose was administered.[105,109] Waiting at least 6 to 12 hours may decrease the incidence of uterine hyperstimulation, which is defined as uterine contractions occurring more frequently than every 2 minutes or lasting longer than 90 seconds, with or without fetal heart rate changes.[110]

DINOPROSTONE VAGINAL INSERT (CERVIDIL)

The dinoprostone 10-mg vaginal insert, Cervidil, slowly releases dinoprostone 0.3 mg/hour over a 12-hour period.[105] The insert is contained within a knitted pouch attached to a long tape. This is a major advantage because it can be removed quickly at the beginning of active labor or in the event of uterine hyperstimulation.[105,109] The use of this vaginal insert requires continuous monitoring of fetal heart rate and uterine activity for as long as the insert is in place and for at least 15 minutes after its removal because of possible uterine hyperstimulation anytime during its administration.[103,109] The dinoprostone vaginal insert allows for a shorter dosing interval for oxytocin, which can be infused as soon as 30 minutes after the removal of the dinoprostone vaginal insert.[105] The total cost of using Cervidil may be considerably less than Prepidil.

EFFICACY OF DINOPROSTONE GEL VERSUS VAGINAL INSERT

The number of prospective, randomized trials comparing the efficacy of dinoprostone endocervical gel and the controlled-release vaginal insert for preinduction cervical ripening are limited.[107,111] In one study, women treated with the vaginal insert experienced shorter cervical ripening and delivery times, decreased need for oxytocin, and decreased lengths of hospital stay.[107] A second prospective, randomized comparison of the two products showed no difference in the number of women delivering within 24 hours, time to delivery, or cesarean deliveries.[111] Women treated with the vaginal insert achieved a greater change in Bishop score and active labor, negating the need for oxytocin.

ADVERSE EFFECTS

The most serious side effect associated with dinoprostone administration is uterine hyperstimulation with or without abnormal fetal heart rate tracings. The incidence of uterine hyperstimulation associated with the use of dinoprostone intravaginal insert is about 5%; the rate of occurrence for dinoprostone endocervical gel is about 1%.[96,109] Uterine hyperstimulation occurs more frequently if the Bishop score is >4 before administration of dinoprostone and can occur up to 9.5 hours after placement of the intravaginal insert.[96,97] Most episodes of uterine hyperstimulation with the use of the vaginal insert occur during active labor and resolve within a few minutes after removal of the insert.[103] Uterine contraction abnormalities may be avoided if the insert is promptly removed at the onset of labor.[112]

Both dinoprostone formulations are associated with fever, nausea, vomiting, and diarrhea; and neither are associated with adverse neonatal outcomes.[96,105,106] Therefore, either formulation of dinoprostone is appropriate for cervical ripening in J.T. Cervidil may be more cost effective.

Misoprostol (Cytotec)

38. What advantages does misoprostol have over dinoprostone when used for cervical ripening?

Misoprostol (Cytotec) is a prostaglandin E_1 analog approved for use in the prevention of nonsteroidal anti-inflammatory drug (NSAID)-induced peptic ulcer disease. It also has been used for cervical ripening and the induction of labor in women despite the lack of approval by the FDA for these latter indications.[112,113] In two large meta-analyses, misoprostol was more effective for cervical ripening and labor induction than either placebo or treatment with dinoprostone.[112,113] Failure to deliver within 24 hours and the need for supplemental oxytocin were both higher in women treated with dinoprostone compared with women treated with misoprostol. Women treated with misoprostol experienced labor more often during cervical ripening and had a reduced rate of cesarean deliveries, a shorter delivery time, and a greater incidence of vaginal delivery within 24 hours, but a higher incidence of uterine contraction abnormalities.[112–114] In other comparisons, intravaginal misoprostol resulted in shorter times to delivery than either dinoprostone vaginal insert or dinoprostone endocervical gel.[115,116] Again, uterine hyperstimulation without fetal heart rate abnormalities was most common with misoprostol use. Maternal and neonatal outcomes were similar in both groups. The need for oxytocin is decreased significantly in women treated with misoprostol compared with women treated with dinoprostone.[117]

Misoprostol has been given both orally and intravaginally, but intravaginal doses of 25 mcg every 4 hours are more effective than oral doses of 50 mcg every 4 hours for cervical ripening and labor induction.[118] Misoprostol 25 mcg (one-fourth of a 100-mcg tablet) is inserted into the posterior vaginal fornix and repeated as needed every 3 to 6 hours.[114,117] Higher doses of 50 mcg are associated with increased uterine contractile abnormalities.[112,117] Continuous fetal heart rate and uterine monitoring is recommended throughout the administration of misoprostol.[116]

Misoprostol should not be used in women with previous uterine scars because of the risk for uterine rupture.[114,115] Misoprostol appears to be an effective, and much less costly method of cervical ripening, but the incidence of uterine hyperstimulation appears to be increased relative to dinoprostone, especially with higher doses. Although misoprostol is a known teratogen in the first trimester of pregnancy, there are no reports of teratogenic effects with exposure beyond the first trimester.[114] Misoprostol's low cost and ease of administration are advantages over dinoprostone; however, its lack of FDA approval for cervical ripening and induction of labor is a disadvantage.

Oxytocin (Pitocin)

Mechanism of Action

39. Twelve hours after administration of dinoprostone vaginal insert, J.T.'s cervix has responded and her Bishop score is now 9, but she has not developed a consistent pattern of uterine contractions. What drug therapy should be initiated at this point?

Synthetic oxytocin should be administered to J.T. to stimulate uterine contractions for accomplishing delivery. Oxytocin increases the frequency, force, and duration of uterine contractions.[119] The uterine response to oxytocin increases throughout pregnancy beginning at approximately 20 weeks' gestation and increases considerably at 30 weeks' gestation.[119] Oxytocin is indicated for both the induction and augmentation of labor. A prolonged latent phase or dystocia (difficult labor) caused by uterine hypocontractility in the active phase of labor is indication for augmentation with oxytocin.[120]

Dosing and Administration

40. How should oxytocin be administered to J.T.?

Oxytocin should be administered by continuous IV infusion using a controlled infusion device. The goal of oxytocin administration is to induce uterine contractions that dilate the cervix and aid in the descent of the fetus while avoiding uterine hyperstimulation and fetal distress.[121] There are two opposing views about oxytocin administration for the induction or augmentation of labor. One view is that oxytocin infusions should mimic physiologic doses in the range of 2 to 6 mU/minute with the goal being vaginal delivery with as little as possible uterine hyperstimulation and fetal distress.[115] The other view is that oxytocin should be used in pharmacologic doses to cause strong uterine contractions with the goals being shortened labor, timely correction of dysfunctional labor, decreased cesarean deliveries, and reduced maternal morbidity.[111,120]

Oxytocin plasma concentrations increase linearly with increasing doses and steady-state is reached within 20 to 40 minutes. Oxytocin serum concentrations correlate poorly with uterine activity, however.[122] Factors that may affect response to oxytocin include parity, gestational age, and cervical dilation.[120,122]

Despite many randomized, controlled trials and much experience with oxytocin, the optimal starting doses, dosage increments, dosing intervals, and maximal doses are different in the various protocols (Table 46-4).[110,119,121] Starting doses range from 0.5 to 0.6 mU/minute and dose increment intervals range from 15 to 60 minutes.[96,110,121] Waiting for 30 to 40 minutes between each dosage rate increase allows time to assess the response at steady-state. Most low-dose protocols usually start oxytocin at 1 to 2 mU/minute and increase the rate of infusion by 1 to 2 mU/minute every 30 to 40 minutes.[121,123] High-dose protocols start oxytocin at 3 to 6 mU/minute with incremental increases of 3 to 6 mU/minute every 20 to 40 minutes. The maximal dose of oxytocin for augmentation of delivery and for induction of labor are 20 mU/minute and 40 mU/minute, respectively.[121] The American College of Obstetricians and Gynecologists recommends a low-dose oxytocin protocol starting at 0.5 to 2 mU/minute and increasing by 1 to 2 mU/minute every 30 to 60 minutes, using a cervical dilation rate of 1 cm/hour as a gauge of adequate progression of active labor.[96]

Table 46-4 Oxytocin Regimens for Induction and Augmentation of Labor

Regimen	*Starting Dose*	*Incremental Increase*	*Dosage Interval*	*Maximum Dose*	*Reference*
Low-dose	1 mU/min	1 mU/min up to 8 U/min then 2 mU/min	20 min	20 mU/min	131
High-dose	6 mU/min	6 mU/min[a]	20 or 40 min	42 mU/min	130
	4 mU/min	4 mU/min	15 min	Until adequate contractility reached	132

[a]Uterine hyperstimulation: reduce incremental increase to 3 mU/min; recurrent hyperstimulation: reduce to 1 mU/min.

Oxytocin protocols using higher doses or shorter dose adjustment intervals (15–20 minutes) for augmentation of labor generally result in fewer cesarean deliveries for labor dystocia.[123–125] The incidence of uterine hyperstimulation during labor induction is higher with high-dose protocols (initial dose of 6 mU/minute with incremental increases of 6 mU/minute), however, when compared with shorter dosing adjustment intervals of 20 minutes or with longer dose adjustment intervals of 40 minutes.[123] Women undergoing labor induction with high-dose oxytocin have a higher incidence of uterine stimulation and cesarean deliveries for fetal distress, but a reduced incidence of failed inductions and neonatal sepsis compared with women treated with low-dose oxytocin.[124] In general, lower maximal doses are needed for augmentation of labor than for induction of labor.[121,124]

J.T. should be started on an infusion of oxytocin 10 or 20 U diluted in 1,000 mL of an isotonic solution (concentration = 10 and 20 mU/mL, respectively) at 1 mU/minute. She should have continuous uterine and fetal heart rate monitoring throughout the infusion to detect abnormal uterine contraction patterns or fetal heart rate patterns. The goal is to establish a pattern of three to five uterine contractions of 60 to 90 seconds duration per 10-minute period.[110] The oxytocin infusion should be increased by 1 to 2 mU/minute every 30 to 40 minutes as needed for inadequate progression of labor (cervical dilation rate of <1cm/hour).[96] Fluid intake and urine output should be assessed hourly.

Adverse Effects

41. What are the adverse effects and complications of oxytocin for which J.T. should be monitored?

Uterine hyperstimulation with fetal heart rate deceleration is the most common adverse effect of oxytocin.[119,120] Uterine hyperstimulation, usually associated with excessive maternal dosing or increased myometrial sensitivity to oxytocin, may result in uterine rupture, vaginal and cervical lacerations, precipitous delivery, abruptio placentae, emergency cesarean delivery for fetal distress, and postpartum hemorrhage secondary to uterine atony. In general, neonatal outcomes associated with oxytocin use do not differ from those achieved by spontaneous labor.[110] Although oxytocin has only weak antidiuretic properties, water intoxication resulting in seizures, coma, and death have been reported.[96] Intravenous bolus administration may cause paradoxical relaxation of vascular smooth muscle leading to hypotension and tachycardia.[119]

POSTPARTUM HEMORRHAGE

Prevention

42. What are other uses for oxytocin during delivery other than induction or augmentation of labor?

Oxytocin is administered routinely following the delivery of the placenta to promote uterine contraction and vasoconstriction.[119,126] Uterine contraction leading to vasoconstriction is important for hemostasis.[126] Uterine atony, the condition in which the uterus fails to contract after delivery of the placenta, is the most common cause of postpartum hemorrhage.[119,126,127] Risks for uterine atony include induction with oxytocin, prolonged labor, overdistended uterus, and previous postpartum hemorrhage.[126–128] Oxytocin 10 to 20 U IM or diluted in 0.5 to 1 L of parenteral fluid and given as an IV infusion of 200 mU/minute until the uterus is firmly contracted reduces the risk for postpartum hemorrhage secondary to uterine atony.[119,129] Oxytocin should never be administered undiluted as a bolus dose because it can cause severe hypotension and cardiac dysrhythmias.[129]

Misoprostol

Misoprostol 400 to 600 mcg can be administered orally in the third stage of labor to prevent postpartum hemorrhage.[130,131] In a comparison of 600 mcg oral misoprostol with parenteral Oxytocin for prevention of postpartum hemorrhage, Oxytocin was, however, marginally but statistically more effective and had fewer side effects.[132] Misoprostol also can be administered rectally. The vaginal route is not preferred in the setting of bleeding. Rectal administration is associated with a lower incidence of fever and shivering, which is common with orally administered misoprostol during the third stage of labor.[130] The rectal route of administration also is associated with lower maximal serum concentrations and lower time to maximal concentrations than when the drug is administered orally.

Treatment

43. Within a few hours of delivering her fetus, J.T. has visible vaginal bleeding. She has a distended uterus and the hemorrhage is attributed to uterine atony. Uterine massage and infusion of oxytocin do not control the bleeding. What other pharmacologic options are available to treat her?

Ergot Alkaloids

If the postpartum hemorrhaging does not respond to oxytocin administration, ergonovine maleate (Ergotrate) and its semisynthetic derivative, methylergonovine maleate (Methergine) can be used because of their potent uterotonic effects. Iintramuscular administration is associated with less frequent adverse effects (nausea, vomiting, hypertension, headache, chest pain, dizziness, tinnitus, diaphoresis) than the intravenous route.[127,133] Ergot alkaloids should be avoided in hypertensive and eclamptic patients because of the potential for arrhythmias, seizures, cerebrovascular accidents, and rarely myocardial infarction. The dose of both drugs is 0.2 mg administered IM every 2 hours as needed. This may be followed by 0.2 to 0.4 mg administered orally two to four times daily for 2 to 7 days to promote involution of the uterus.[133]

15-Methyl Prostaglandin F_2 (Carboprost Tromethamine)

Bleeding caused by uterine atony that is unresponsive to oxytocin can be treated with 15-methyl prostaglandin $F_{2\alpha}$-tromethamine, also known as carboprost tromethamine (Hemabate).[126,128] Carboprost tromethamine, as with naturally occurring prostaglandins, stimulates uterine contraction and decreases postpartum hemorrhage; it is more potent and has a longer duration of effect than its parent compound, prostaglandin $F_{2\alpha}$.

Carboprost tromethamine is approved for IM use, but also has been also administered through direct myometrial injection[126,127] and intrauterine irrigation.[126] Intramyometrial administration has been associated with severe hypotension and pulmonary edema.[134] An initial dose of 0.25 mg IM is given followed by 0.25 mg every 15 to 90 minutes.[127,135] The dose may be increased to 0.5 mg if a patient does not respond adequately to several 0.25-mg IM doses. The total cumulative dose should not exceed 2 mg.[135] Carboprost tromethamine is effective in treating 60% to 85% of women with uterine atony who have failed standard treatment.[127] Improvement in bleeding typically occurs after one to two injections.

The most common adverse effects of carboprost tromethamine are gastrointestinal, including nausea, vomiting, and diarrhea. Flushing and fever also occur frequently. Many of the adverse effects are related to the contractile effect of this drug on smooth muscle.[135] Hypertension, although rare, typically occurs in women with pre-existing hypertension or preeclampsia. The potent vasoconstricting and bronchoconstricting properties of carboprost can cause uterine rupture, as well as pulmonary and cardiac problems. Carboprost is contraindicated in women with active pulmonary, cardiac, renal, or hepatic disease as well as in women with acute pelvic inflammatory disease.[127,128,135]

Misoprostol

Several case series and small randomized trials have reported that misoprostol might be useful in the treatment of postpartum hemorrhage caused by uterine atony. The available data are very limited, however, and large randomized trials are needed to clarify the efficacy of misoprostol compared with standard therapies, as well as the optimal dose and route of administration.[136]

PRETERM LABOR

Preterm delivery occurred in 12.7% of births in the United States in 2004, representing a 20% increase since 1990.[137] Approximately 55% of singleton preterm births follow spontaneous preterm labor and approximately 8% follow preterm premature rupture of the chorioamniotic membranes.[138] Premature birth is the leading cause of neonatal mortality (infant death <1 month of age), resulting in approximately 70% of deaths. Furthermore, prematurity is the second leading cause of infant mortality under the age of 1 year, and has resulted in 36% of such deaths in 2004.[1]

Etiology

Spontaneous preterm labor is a heterogeneous syndrome and several known pathways can lead to preterm birth. These pathways include excessive uterine distension, decidual hemorrhage, activation of the maternal and fetal hypothalamic pituitary system, and intrauterine infection leading to inflammation. These pathways ultimately lead to a final common response with production of uterine and cervical proteases and uterotonins, which result in progressive cervical ripening and dilation; weakening of the chorioamniotic membranes, which leads to rupture; and uterine contractions. Ultimately, delivery of the infant occurs. Infection triggers an inflammatory response that results in the release of cytokines, prostaglandins, and proteases, which stimulate uterine activity, induce cervix softening and dilation, and weaken the chorioamniotic membranes.[139] Variations in maternal and fetal genes coding for cytokines have been implicated in the apparent genetic predisposition to preterm birth found in some families and racial groups.[140] Thrombin is another uterotonic that has been implicated in causing preterm labor associated with vaginal bleeding caused by placental abruption.[141] Studies have shown a relationship between increasing maternal corticotropin-releasing hormone (CRH) and delivery timing.[142] Maternal and fetal stress can activate the hypothalamic pituitary system and result in the rapid increase of maternal CRH before premature birth. Infection can also activate the fetal hypothalamic pituitary system, increasing CRH, cortisol, and ultimately, prostaglandins.[139,141] Despite some progress in recent years, much remains unknown about the etiology of preterm birth, and little is known about how preterm birth can be prevented.

Clinical Presentation and Evaluation

44. B.B., a 17-year-old white girl, G_2P_1, 29 weeks' gestation, is admitted to the obstetrical unit with complaints of backache, cramps, and uterine contractions. She has no symptoms of preterm premature rupture of the membranes (PPROM). She had a previous preterm birth at 32 weeks' gestation. Cervicovaginal secretions are positive for fetal fibronectin. A pelvic examination reveals that her cervix is 2 cm dilated and 80% effaced, which is increased from 1 cm at her prenatal visit last week. Cervical cultures for *Chlamydia trachomatis* and *Neisseria gonorrhoeae* from her previous visit are negative. Vaginal wet preparations are also negative for bacterial vaginosis and *Trichomonas vaginalis*. Vital signs, urinalysis, and CBC with differential are normal. Uterine contractions and fetal heart tones are being monitored. Ultrasound reveals a fetus of 30 weeks' size with an estimated weight of 1,200 g. What signs, symptoms and laboratory evidence support a diagnosis of preterm labor?

B.B. has backache and uterine contractions, which are symptoms of preterm labor. Most women with preterm contractions are not in labor, however, which results in frequent overdiagnosis.[141] In addition, contractions during preterm labor are frequently not painful, are not detected by the woman and, thus, are not a sensitive marker for preterm labor. Fibronectin, a protein that serves as an adhesive between the fetal membranes and decidua, normally disappears from the cervical secretions after the first half of pregnancy, reappearing only at term as labor approaches.[141] A negative fibronectin test can exclude imminent preterm delivery in a woman at risk for preterm delivery, between 24 to 34 weeks' gestation with intact amniotic membranes, and with cervical dilatation of <3 cm.[143] Because of fibronectin's high negative predictive value of >95% for delivery in the next 1 to 2 weeks, it can be used to avoid overdiagnosis of preterm labor. Although fibronectin testing will yield false–positive results in the presence of blood, vaginal bleeding itself is independently associated with preterm birth. B.B. has the criteria necessary to establish a firm diagnosis of preterm labor. Not only is her fibronectin test positive, but she has persistent contractions with a documented change in cervix dilatation.

Risk Factors

45. What risk factors does B.B. have for spontaneous preterm labor?

B.B. has several risk factors for preterm delivery. The strongest predictor of preterm birth is prior preterm birth. She has a fourfold increased risk of preterm delivery because of one previous preterm delivery.[141] If this pregnancy also ends prematurely, her risk for a third preterm birth in her next pregnancy will be sixfold higher than that in the normal population. Her young age may also be a risk factor. A maternal age <18 or >35 years is associated with spontaneous preterm birth, although it is difficult to separate age from the confounding factors associated with age.[141] Black race is an independent risk factor for both preterm labor and lower neonatal birthweight. Other risk factors include low maternal weight before pregnancy, smoking, second or third trimester bleeding, multiple gestation, and uterine anomalies.[94,141] Studies of cervix length by transvaginal ultrasound imaging have demonstrated that shorter lengths are associated with greater risk for preterm delivery; however, the positive predictive value varies widely.[141,143] Maternal infections, such as untreated urinary tract infections and pneumonia, are associated with preterm delivery. In addition, genital organisms such as *Gardnerella vaginalis*, *Chlamydia trachomatis*, *Neisseria gonorrhoeae*, *Ureaplasma urealyticum*, and *Trichomonas vaginalis*, are also associated with preterm births.[139] Although it is important to identify women at risk for spontaneous preterm delivery, only half of all preterm deliveries occur in women with known risk factors.[141]

Tocolysis

Goals of Therapy

46. What are the goals of tocolysis?

Treatment of spontaneous preterm labor primarily has been directed at slowing or stopping contractions which are the obvious, although likely late, sign of impending preterm birth. It has been presumed that if successful, this should prevent or delay preterm birth. Few placebo controlled trials have been conducted of agents used to diminish contractions (tocolytics), and most data suggest delay of delivery by at most 1 to 2 days. This might be because of the heterogeneous causes of spontaneous preterm birth, and because tocolytic agents may not arrest the underlying process that led to contractions. Most studies have been unable to demonstrate a clear benefit of tocolysis on neonatal morbidity and mortality. Instead they have evaluated surrogate endpoints, such as pregnancy prolongation or number of preterm births prior to various cutoff points.[144] The value of prolonging pregnancy will vary by gestational age, and might be substantial if time is gained to administer glucocorticoids to improve fetal lung maturation and decrease the risk of intraventricular hemorrhage (see section on Antenatal Glucocorticoid Administration). All women at risk for preterm birth within 7 days and between 24 to 34 weeks should be considered for glucocorticoid therapy.[145,146] Delay of delivery can also allow transport to a facility best equipped to care for both mother and premature newborn.

Numerous factors affect the decision to treat preterm labor with a tocolytic agent. Fetal factors precluding tocolysis include non-reassuring fetal monitoring, significant IUGR, and lethal congenital anomalies. Maternal factors include evidence of chorioamnionitis, other significant maternal infections or illness, pre-eclampsia, and advanced labor.[141] Tocolysis is less likely to be effective in women with cervical dilation of >3 cm and is usually unsuccessful if the patient is in advanced labor (cervical dilation >5 cm).[141] Because the etiology of preterm labor is multifactorial, B.B. should be evaluated thoroughly and periodically for potential causes of preterm labor and treated appropriately when diagnosed. For example, urinary tract infections are associated with preterm labor and they should be diagnosed and treated if present.[141] Additionally, some would also perform amniocentesis to exclude subclinical chorioamnionitis as a cause of preterm labor before initiating or continuing tocolysis, and to evaluate lung maturity at later gestational ages.[145] B.B. has no evidence of overt infection or other complications and has no contraindications to tocolysis. Prolonging gestation, even for a few days, would be beneficial because B.B. is only 29 weeks' gestation.

Magnesium Sulfate

47. Magnesium sulfate 6 g IV loading dose for 30 minutes followed by 2 g/hour continuous IV infusion through a controlled infusion pump has been ordered. How effective is magnesium sulfate for tocolysis?

Magnesium sulfate is the most frequently used parenteral tocolytic agent in the United States and is also prescribed for the prevention and treatment of eclampsia. Magnesium sulfate relaxes uterine smooth muscle at maternal serum levels of 5 to 8 mg/dL.[141] The mechanism by which it exerts this effect is not understood completely, but involves inhibition of myosin light-chain kinase activity by competition with intracellular calcium, reducing myometrial contractility.[144]

Despite its widespread use, the evidence for magnesium's efficacy in prolonging gestation is inadequate. In two published randomized, placebo-controlled trials, no benefit in mean prolongation of pregnancy or mean neonatal birthweight was demonstrated. In meta-analyses of both placebo-controlled trials of magnesium for tocolysis compared with other active drugs, no prolongation of pregnancy was seen with magnesium.[147,148] Several small randomized, controlled studies have directly compared magnesium with parenteral β-adrenergic agonists, mostly ritodrine.[148] Three of the four showed no differences in birth outcomes. One of the four suggested prolonged pregnancy with magnesium added to ritodrine compared with ritodrine alone. Studies on the efficacy of β-adrenergic agonists (mostly ritodrine) versus placebo have been mixed but on balance suggest delay of delivery for 48 hours, but not for 7 days. Therefore, because most trials comparing magnesium with β-adrenergic agonists did not show differences, it has been presumed that magnesium is equally effective. Magnesium is better tolerated than the β-adrenergic agonists, with fewer maternal side effects.[148] Magnesium is contraindicated in patients with myasthenia gravis, and renal failure.

MONITORING FOR EFFICACY AND TOXICITY

49. How should magnesium sulfate therapy in B.B. be monitored for efficacy and safety?

The hourly rate of magnesium administration for B.B. may be increased until she has one or fewer contractions per 10 minutes or a maximum of 4 g/hour is attained. B.B.'s deep tendon reflexes, respiratory rate, and urine output should be monitored regularly. Close monitoring of fluid balance is important because fluid overload has been associated with pulmonary edema and the drug is renally excreted.[149]

Magnesium serum concentrations are commonly evaluated every 6 to 12 hours in an effort to minimize adverse effects.[150] The patellar reflex disappears with magnesium serum concentrations between 9 and 10 mg/dL, and as long as deep tendon reflexes are present, many practitioners will not measure concentrations. To prevent inadvertent overdoses, a controlled infusion device should always be used to deliver magnesium as a continuous infusion. Hypocalcemia and tetany can occur with hypermagnesemia. Neuromuscular blockade and respiratory arrest develop with magnesium serum concentrations of 15 to 17 mg/dL, and cardiac arrest develops with greater concentrations. The toxic effects of magnesium can be rapidly reversed with 1 g of parenteral calcium gluconate, which should be readily available where patients are receiving magnesium infusion.[151]

The most common side effects of magnesium loading doses are transient hypotension, flushing, a sense of warmth, headache, dizziness, lethargy, nystagmus, and dry mouth.[141,149] Other adverse effects reported with magnesium are hypothermia, paralytic ileus, and pulmonary edema, which may occur in 1% to 2% of patients treated with magnesium sulfate.[149] Pulmonary edema occurs less frequently with magnesium sulfate than with parenteral β-sympathomimetics and is more commonly encountered with prolonged infusions, multifetal pregnancy, and the use of multiple tocolytics.[149,151] Treatment consists of discontinuing magnesium sulfate and administration of the diuretic furosemide.

Fetal magnesium serum concentrations are similar to maternal concentrations.[149] The most common neonatal adverse effects are hypotonia and sleepiness. Hypotonia may continue for 3 or 4 days in the neonate because of decreased renal elimination of magnesium. Rarely, assisted mechanical ventilation for neuromuscular depression may be needed.[149] A possible role for magnesium sulfate in the prevention of cerebral palsy is an area of ongoing investigation.[152]

β-Adrenergic Agonists

EFFICACY

50. Could B.B. have been treated with a β-adrenergic agonist?

β-Adrenergic agonists are not the first-line choice for preterm labor because of high costs and the significant potential for maternal adverse effects described below.[141,148] Both ritodrine, the only medication approved by the FDA for the treatment of preterm labor, and terbutaline, bind to β_2-adrenergic receptors in uterine smooth muscle and ultimately inhibit smooth muscle cell contractility. Results of randomized, controlled trials of ritodrine have been mixed; however, a meta-analysis which included 1,320 women treated with β-agonists demonstrated fewer births at 48 hours but no change in number of births at 7 days. No benefit on neonatal morbidity or mortality was seen; however, the studies are limited by sample size.[153,154] The continued use of β-agonists can result in the development of tachyphylaxis to its effects on the myometrium and may in part explain treatment failures with these drugs.[141,153]

Terbutaline is available for IV, subcutaneously (SC), and oral administration. One SC dose of terbutaline is often administered to women with mild contractions and cervical dilation <2 cm. Intravenous β-sympathomimetics are used in cases with more severe and frequent contractions and cervical dilation >2 cm.

MATERNAL AND FETAL ADVERSE EFFECTS

51. What adverse effects are associated with terbutaline?

β-Adrenergic agonists are not selective for myometrial β_2-adrenergic receptors at pharmacologic doses, and this accounts for their high incidence of adverse effects.[151] Maternal adverse effects such as pulmonary edema, palpitations, tachycardia, myocardial ischemia, hyperglycemia, hypokalemia, and hepatoxicity result in discontinuation of therapy in up to 10% of patients.[141] Pulmonary edema can occur and, if not recognized promptly, can lead to adult RDS and death.[141,151] β-Sympathomimetics should not be used in women with underlying cardiac disease or arrhythmias, hypertension, diabetes mellitus, severe anemia, or thyrotoxicosis.[141]

The most commonly reported fetal or neonatal adverse effects associated with β-agonist therapy include tachycardia, hypotension, hypoglycemia, and hypocalcemia.[151] Maternal hyperglycemia causing fetal hyperglycemia and hyperinsulinemia can lead to neonatal hypoglycemia if not properly monitored postnatally. Fetal tachycardia rarely leads to fetal myocardial ischemia or hypertrophy.[151] The use of β-sympathomimetic drugs was reported to be associated with an increased risk of neonatal intraventricular hemorrhage in some early studies but not in others.[141,148]

Other Tocolytic Drugs

52. What other drugs are commonly used for tocolysis?

INDOMETHACIN

Prostaglandins $F_{2\alpha}$ and especially E_2 are important regulators of myometrial contractility and cervical ripening.[94] Prostaglandin synthetase inhibitors, such as indomethacin, decrease prostaglandin production and thereby decrease contractions and inhibit cervical change. As with other tocolytics, these drugs have not been adequately studied in multiple randomized controlled trials. A review of available randomized trials of indomethacin (Indocin) compared with placebo found significant reductions in women delivering at <37 weeks, an increase in gestational age at delivery, and a trend toward fewer deliveries at 48 hours and 7 days.[155] In three of eight trials comparing cyclo-oxygenase (COX) inhibitors with other tocolytics, a reduction in both delivery before 37 weeks and in maternal drug reactions, was noted. Also, seen in these studies was a trend toward a reduction in delivery within 48 hours.[155] Indomethacin is well tolerated, and GI upset can be mitigated by antacids when it occurs. The available studies are inadequately powered to evaluate neonatal outcomes.[156]

Although well tolerated by the mother, concerns exist about the fetal and neonatal effects of prostaglandin synthetase inhibition. Indomethacin crosses the placenta rapidly, and fetal levels rapidly approach maternal levels.[151,156] Because indomethacin can decrease fetal urine output leading to oligohydramnios, the amniotic fluid index (AFI) should be followed and indomethacin discontinued if it falls below 5 cm. Oligohydramnios generally resolves within 48 to 72 hours of the discontinuation of indomethacin. The ductus arteriosus—a fetal vessel important in maintaining fetal circulation—constricts in 25% to 50% of fetuses exposed to indomethacin *in utero* and generally is reversible.[141] Permanent closure of the ductus arteriosus, however, has led to intrauterine demise. The risk for neonatal adverse effects is increased with drug exposure of >48 hours, as well as use after 32 weeks when premature closure of the ductus occurs more frequently.[141] An increased risk for maternal postpartum hemorrhage has also been reported with indomethacin use but did not reach significance in a meta-analysis.[155] Indomethacin should not be used in the presence of oligohydramnios or suspected fetal renal or cardiac anomaly (see Chapter 94, Neonatal Therapy).

More serious fetal and neonatal effects have been reported in some retrospective and observational studies, including neonatal necrotizing enterocolitis, intraventricular hemorrhage, and renal failure.[156–158] It is difficult, however, to discern whether these complications are causally related to indomethacin or to the use of the drug in cases of refractory preterm labor caused by subclinical intra-amniotic infection.[156,159] The randomized trials have limited power to assess these serious neonatal complications. An analysis of the risks and benefits of indomethacin suggested its continued use as second-line treatment for preterm labor between 24 to 32 weeks in women with contraindications to other tocolytics.[156] Typical dosing regimens include a loading dose of 50 to 100 mg either rectally or orally followed by maintenance doses of 25 to 50 mg orally every 4 to 8 (most commonly given every 6 hours) hours for 24 to 48 hours.[157]

COX-2 INHIBITORS

Only amniotic cyclooxygenase-2 (COX-2), and not COX-1, activity is increased during labor, and tocolysis with COX-2 specific inhibitors might result in fewer adverse effects than with indomethacin or other nonspecific COX inhibitors.[160] In a randomized, double-blind, placebo-controlled trial, celecoxib was comparable to indomethacin in efficacy and did not negatively affect ductal patency when used to treat preterm labor.[160] Both drugs decreased AFI; however, fluid reaccumulation was prolonged when indomethacin was discontinued, an effect not observed with the discontinuation of celecoxib. Another small double-blinded trial demonstrated a similar reversible decrease in AFI and ductus arteriosus flow from COX-2 inhibition with sulindac or nimesulide, compared with COX-1 inhibition with indomethacin.[161] More studies with larger number of subjects are needed to determine the safety and efficacy of COX-2 enzyme inhibitors relative to indomethacin.

CALCIUM CHANNEL BLOCKERS

The calcium channel blockers nifedipine and nicardipine inhibit preterm contractions by decreasing calcium influx into uterine smooth muscle and inhibiting myometrial contractions. No placebo-controlled trials have been performed with nifedipine, the most commonly used calcium channel blocker. Meta-analysis of 12 randomized trials including a total of 1,029 women evaluated the effectiveness of calcium channel blockers compared with other tocolytics, mostly betamimetics.[162] Calcium channel blockers were found to be superior in reducing preterm births within 7 days and before 34 weeks. In addition, fewer maternal side effects were seen. A more recent study of 192 women comparing nifedipine with magnesium sulfate for preterm labor found no differences in delivery in 48 hours, gestational age at delivery, or deliveries before 32 or 37 weeks.[163] Maternal side effects were significantly fewer in patients receiving calcium channel blockers compared with other tocolytics.[162,163] Maternal side effects can include tachycardia, headache, flushing, dizziness, nausea, and hypotension in the hypovolemic patient.[151] Nifedipine does not adversely affect uteroplacental blood flow or fetal circulation. Concurrent use with magnesium should be avoided because the combination may potentiate neuromuscular blockade.[81,151] Nifedipine appears to be an attractive alternative for short-term tocolysis. The starting dose is usually 10 mg orally with repeated doses of 10 mg every 15 to 20 minutes for persistent contractions up to a maximum of 40 mg in the first hour.[164,165] Depending on the tocolytic effect, nifedipine is then maintained at 10 to 20 mg orally every 4 to 6 hours.[164] The appropriate duration of treatment has not been established, but typically it is continued through the 34th week of gestation.[164,162]

DURATION OF TOCOLYSIS

ACUTE THERAPY

53. B.B. has been maintained on magnesium sulfate continuous IV infusion for approximately 48 hours. The dose was increased to 3 g/hour shortly after the start of the infusion. B.B. has had no contractions for the past 24 hours. How long does she need to be treated? Should she be "weaned" off magnesium sulfate?

B.B.'s contractions have completely stopped for 24 hours. Some protocols maintain magnesium sulfate for 12 to 24 hours after successful tocolysis, or for the time it takes to complete the course of corticosteroids. After successful acute tocolysis is achieved, the magnesium infusion sometimes is discontinued gradually.[164] The weaning of magnesium sulfate is likely unnecessary, however, and simple discontinuation of the magnesium infusion is an easier and less costly option.[150]

CHRONIC MAINTENANCE THERAPY

54. Should B.B. be started on chronic maintenance tocolytic therapy?

Maintenance tocolysis has been used to prevent recurrence of preterm labor and prolong gestation in women in whom preterm labor was terminated successfully with parenteral tocolytics.[166] The use of continuous SC low-dose terbutaline infusion through a portable pump has been used widely in outpatient tocolysis and in conjunction with home uterine activity programs.[166,167] Although continuous SC low-dose terbutaline is associated with fewer cardiopulmonary adverse effects compared with IV β-adrenergic therapy, the FDA issued a "Dear Colleague" letter in 1997 alerting practitioners about the lack of effectiveness and potential danger of continuous SC terbutaline for the treatment and prevention of preterm labor.[166] After additional review, the FDA reaffirmed this position in 2000. A subsequent review reached similar conclusions.[168] Other tocolytics, including β-adrenergic agents and oral calcium channel blockers have been evaluated for maintenance therapy. Results of meta-analysis of trials comparing placebo or no treatment with betamimetics for maintenance therapy after acute preterm labor, which included more than 900 women, showed no benefit in delay of delivery, births at <34 or 37 weeks, or neonatal complications.[169] Moreover, increases in maternal adverse effects occurred, primarily tachycardia, hypotension, and palpitations. Inadequate data exist to support the use of calcium channel blockers as maintenance therapy and the single randomized, controlled trial was relatively small.[145,170–172] B.B. should not be started on chronic maintenance tocolysis.

Antenatal Glucocorticoid Administration

55. While receiving the loading dose of magnesium sulfate, B.B. was given betamethasone 12 mg IM with a second dose in 24 hours. Why was betamethasone given?

B.B. was given betamethasone to facilitate fetal lung maturation by increasing production of fetal lung surfactant, thereby reducing the incidence and severity of RDS.[99] Antenatal corticosteroid administration (betamethasone and dexamethasone) also decreases the incidence of intraventricular hemorrhage, necrotizing enterocolitis, and neonatal death.[99] The greatest reduction in RDS occurs when delivery can be delayed 24 hours up to 7 days after starting treatment. Repeat weekly corticosteroid courses are discouraged because of the association with decreased birthweight and head circumference, hypothalamic-pituitary-adrenal axis suppression, deleterious effects on cerebral myelination and lung growth, and neonatal death (particularly in neonates born to mothers who received three or more courses).[146,173]

The National Institutes of Health (NIH) Consensus Panel and the ACOG recommend antenatal betamethasone or dexamethasone for all women in preterm labor between 24 to 34 weeks' gestation.[99] Betamethasone, however, might be the preferred agent because fewer IM injections are needed and because in meta-analysis it was associated with a greater reduction in RDS compared with dexamethasone.[173] That conclusion, however, is not based on direct comparison of betamethasone with dexamethasone and should be interpreted with caution. One study, although limited by its retrospective nature, also suggested an advantage of betamethasone over dexamethasone in the reduction of periventricular leukomalacia, a finding associated with later risks for cerebral palsy.[174] In cases of PPROM, the NIH Consensus recommends that corticosteroids may be given up to 32 weeks' gestation in the absence of chorioamnionitis.[99] Recent meta-analysis supports the efficacy of corticosteroids in the reduction of neonatal death, RDS, duration of ventilator use, and intraventricular hemorrhage in infants born after ruptured membranes.[173] Women >32 weeks' gestation can be considered for amniotic fluid testing for the presence of phosphatidylglycerol or lecithin-to-sphingomyelin (L:S) ratio (>2) because these are indicators of fetal lung maturation.[175] Corticosteroids are not recommended for use in pregnant women who are >34 weeks' gestation unless there is an indication of fetal lung immaturity (see Chapter 94, Neonatal Therapy).

Antibiotic Therapy

56. What is the role of antibiotic therapy in the prevention or management of preterm labor? Is B.B. a candidate for a trial of antibiotics?

Antibiotics are given during preterm labor to treat bacterial vaginosis, occult or documented intra-amniotic infections in PPROM, and prophylactically against neonatal group B *Streptococcus* (GBS) infection.

Bacterial Vaginosis

All pregnant women should be screened and treated for sexually transmitted diseases and bacteriuria. In addition, some, but not all studies have demonstrated that screening and treating asymptomatic women for bacterial vaginosis (BV) who are at high risk for preterm delivery may reduce the risk of preterm birth.[144,176] A polymicrobial overgrowth of mostly anaerobic bacteria, BV is one of the most common genital infections in pregnancy and it is associated with an increased risk of preterm delivery.[177] Treatment of women with BV who had a prior preterm delivery with oral metronidazole (Flagyl) in combination with erythromycin decreased the risk of recurrent preterm delivery in one randomized clinical trial.[178] The use of vaginal antibiotics, antibiotic regimens not including metronidazole, or the treatment of BV in women without a history of preterm birth does not appear, however, to decrease the risk of preterm birth.[139,179] In addition, a meta-analysis including 622 women with prior preterm birth, found no reduction in the risk of preterm birth before 37 weeks after treatment of BV with antibiotics.[179] B.B. does not have BV; therefore, treatment with metronidazole is unnecessary (also see GBS resistance to erythromycin in Chapter 96, Pediatric Infections Diseases).

Preterm Premature Rupture of Membranes

Increasing evidence associates preterm labor with intra-amniotic infections.[139,180] Of preterm births, 20% to 40% may be caused by an infectious-inflammatory process.[181] Intrauterine infection is associated with approximately 80% of early preterm deliveries.[139] Most of the bacteria found in amniotic fluid and the placenta are believed to have ascended from the vagina.[180] It has been suggested that the microbes responsible for preterm birth are already present in the endometrium before conception, causing a chronic, subclinical infection weeks to months before eventually causing PPROM or labor.[139,141]

Antibiotic therapy during preterm labor is indicated in select cases. When PPROM has occurred, spontaneous labor and delivery occurs on average within 7 days, although longer intervals from PROM to delivery occur with earlier gestational ages.[177] Additionally, the use of antibiotics has been shown to prolong the period between PPROM and delivery (the latency period), and decrease neonatal morbidity.[177] In the largest and best designed trial of antibiotic treatment of PPROM, women between 24 to 32 weeks' gestation treated with ampicillin and erythromycin had both prolonged pregnancies and lower rates of chorioamnionitis.[182] Their newborns experienced decreased mortality, as well as decreased morbidity including RDS, and necrotizing enterocolitis. These effects were not owing to tocolytics or corticosteroids because these were exclusionary factors. These results were confirmed by the results of a large meta-analysis including >6,000 women, although information on the best choice of antibiotics was less clear.[183] Therefore, women with PPROM benefit from antibiotic therapy with a broad-spectrum regimen and IV ampicillin plus erythromycin for 48 hours followed by 5 days of oral amoxicillin plus erythromycin for a total of 7 days treatment is a reasonable choice.[182]

Antibiotics should also be given to women if delivery is anticipated resulting either from preterm labor with intact

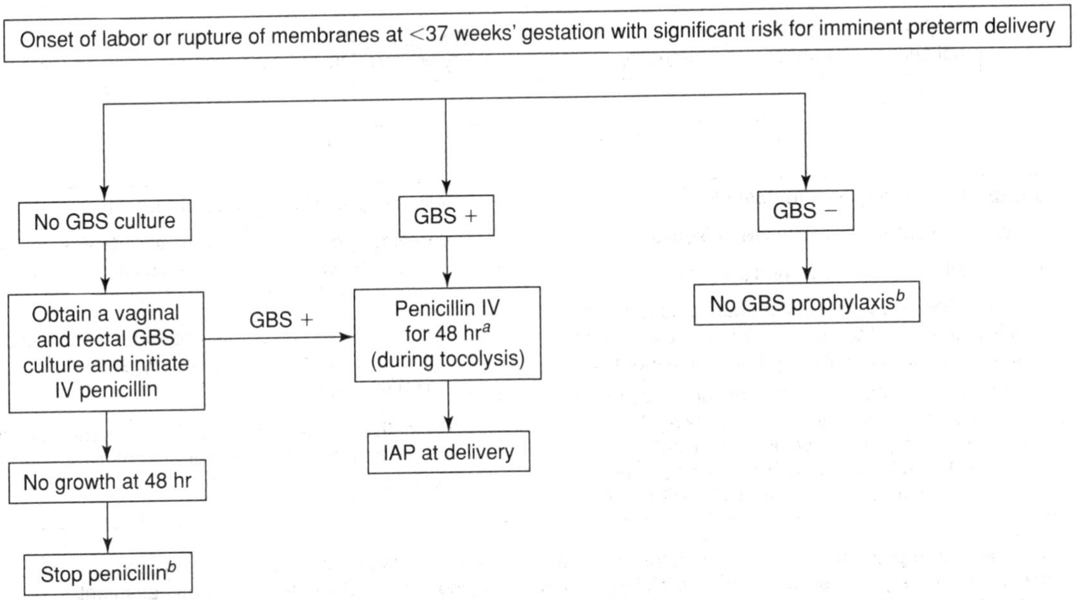
Onset of labor or rupture of membranes at <37 weeks' gestation with significant risk for imminent preterm delivery
No GBS culture
GBS +
GBS −
Obtain a vaginal and rectal GBS culture and initiate IV penicillin
GBS +
Penicillin IV for 48 hr[a] (during tocolysis)
No GBS prophylaxis[b]
IAP at delivery
No growth at 48 hr
Stop penicillin[b]

[a] Penicillin should be continued for a total of at least 48 hours, unless delivery occurs sooner. At the physician's discretion, antibiotic prophylaxis may be continued beyond 48 hours in a GBS culture positive woman if delivery has not yet occurred. For women who are GBS culture positive, antibiotic prophylaxis should be reinitiated when labor likely to proceed to delivery occurs or recurs.

[b] If delivery has not occurred within 4 weeks, a vaginal and rectal GBS screening culture should be repeated and the patient should be managed as described, based on the result of the repeat culture.

GBS, group B streptococcus; IAP, intrapartum antibiotic prophylaxis.

Reprinted from Centers for Disease Control and Prevention. Prevention of perinatal Group B streptococcal disease. Revised guidelines. MMWR 2002;51(No. RR-11):8.)

FIGURE 46-3 Sample algorithm for group B streptococcus (GBS) prophylaxis for women with threatened preterm delivery. This algorithm is not an exclusive course of management. Variations that incorporate individual circumstances or institutional preferences may be appropriate.

membranes or after preterm PPROM, to prevent group B streptococcal infection in the newborn. Other broad-spectrum antibiotic therapy to prevent preterm delivery should not be given routinely to women in preterm labor with intact membranes. Antibiotics have not been proved to prevent premature births in the setting of acute preterm labor.[145,181]

Because B.B. does not have PPROM or signs of chorioamnionitis (temperature ≥100.4°F or 38°C), she should not be treated with broad-spectrum antibiotics. She should receive penicillin G, however, to prevent perinatal group B streptococcus infection (Fig. 46-3).

Group B Streptococcus Intrapartum Prophylaxis

Ten to 30% are colonized with GBS in the vagina or rectum, and 1% to 2% of neonates born to colonized women develop early-onset invasive GBS disease. One-fourth of all cases of neonatal GBS infections occur in preterm newborns. B.B.'s fetus, therefore, is at risk for invasive GBS or *Streptococcus agalactiae* infection from vertical transmission (mother to infant) of bacteria during labor or delivery.[184] The mortality rate for GBS is reported to be between 5% and 20%. During pregnancy, GBS infection causes maternal urinary tract infection, amnionitis, endometriosis, and wound infection.[184] Antibiotics given to the mother during preterm labor and delivery prevent neonatal GBS disease. In the past decade, the routine administration of intrapartum antibiotic prophylaxis to certain subsets of pregnant women has led to a 70% reduction in the overall incidence of GBS disease (see Chapter 94, Neonatal Therapy). The decision to treat women with intrapartum antibiotics has been based on either a positive vaginal GBS culture or one or more of the following risk factors without culture screening: (a) previous infant with invasive GBS disease; (b) GBS bacteriuria during current pregnancy; (c) preterm labor of <37 weeks' gestation; (d) PROM ≥18 hours; and (e) intrapartum temperature ≥38°C (100.4°F).[184] This treatment algorithm prevents an estimated 85% of all early-onset GBS disease (Fig. 46-4). A multistate, retrospective cohort study identified the culture-screening process as being 50% more effective than the risk-based process.[185] Consequently, the Centers for Disease Control and Prevention (CDC) and ACOG no longer recommend the risk-based approach, except in situations for which no culture results are available before delivery.[186]

Vaginal and rectal GBS cultures should be obtained from B.B., and she should be given a loading dose of penicillin G injection 5 MU, followed by 2.5 MU IV every 4 hours until delivery, while awaiting success of tocolysis and culture results. CDC guidelines recommend that the benchmark for optimal prophylaxis should be antibiotics given at least 4 or more hours before delivery. Penicillin G is preferred over ampicillin because it has a narrower spectrum of antimicrobial activity. If B.B. had a history of anaphylaxis to penicillin, sensitivities to clindamycin and erythromycin should be requested at the time

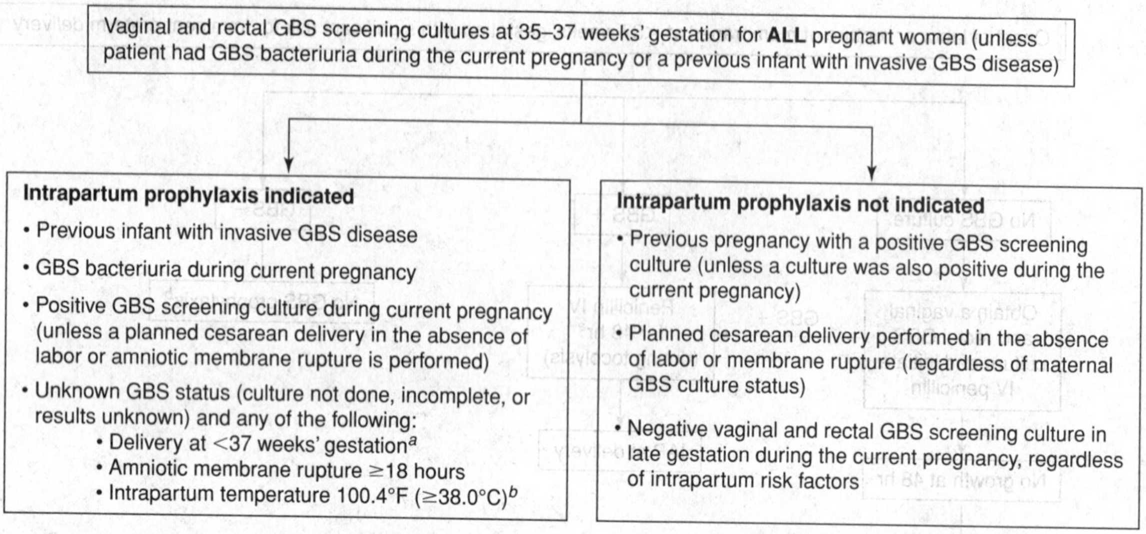
Vaginal and rectal GBS screening cultures at 35–37 weeks' gestation for ALL pregnant women (unless patient had GBS bacteriuria during the current pregnancy or a previous infant with invasive GBS disease)
Intrapartum prophylaxis indicated
• Previous infant with invasive GBS disease
• GBS bacteriuria during current pregnancy
• Positive GBS screening culture during current pregnancy (unless a planned cesarean delivery in the absence of labor or amniotic membrane rupture is performed)
• Unknown GBS status (culture not done, incomplete, or results unknown) and any of the following:
• Delivery at <37 weeks' gestation[a]
• Amniotic membrane rupture ≥18 hours
• Intrapartum temperature 100.4°F (≥38.0°C)[b]
Intrapartum prophylaxis not indicated
• Previous pregnancy with a positive GBS screening culture (unless a culture was also positive during the current pregnancy)
• Planned cesarean delivery performed in the absence of labor or membrane rupture (regardless of maternal GBS culture status)
• Negative vaginal and rectal GBS screening culture in late gestation during the current pregnancy, regardless of intrapartum risk factors

[a] If onset of labor or rupture of amniotic membranes occurs at <37 weeks' gestation and there is a significant risk for preterm delivery (as assessed by the clinician), a suggested algorithm for GBS prophylaxis management is provided (Figure 46-2).
[b] If amnionitis is suspected, broad-spectrum antibiotic therapy that includes an agent known to be active against GBS should replace GBS prophylaxis.
Reprinted from Centers for Disease Control and Prevention. Prevention of perinatal Group B streptococcal disease. Revised guidelines. MMWR 2002;51(No.RR-11):8.

FIGURE 46-4 Indications for intrapartum antibiotic prophylaxis to prevent perinatal group B streptococcus (GBS) disease under a universal prenatal screening strategy based on combined vaginal and rectal cultures collected at 35–37 weeks' gestation from all pregnant women.

of culture in the event GBS is found, because of increasing resistance to these drugs. Antibiotic regimens for intrapartum antimicrobial prophylaxis are listed in Table 46-5.

57. B.B.'s culture results are negative for GBS growth. She is still at high risk for imminent delivery. Should penicillin G administration be discontinued?

Penicillin should be discontinued at this time. Vaginal and rectal cultures need not be repeated if B.B. delivers within the next 4 weeks. If tocolysis is successful and delivery is delayed for more than 4 weeks, obtaining cultures and starting penicillin G pre-emptively should be repeated at that time. Intrapartum prophylaxis is effective only if antibiotics can be given immediately before and during delivery.

Table 46-5 Recommended Regimens for Intrapartum Antimicrobial Prophylaxis for Perinatal GBS Disease Prevention[a]

Recommended: Penicilin G, 5 million units IV initial dose, then 2.5 million units IV every 4 hours until delivery	
Alternative: Ampicillin, 2 g IV initial dose, then 1 g IV every 4 hours until delivery If penicillin allergic[b]	
Patients not at high risk for anaphylaxis:	Cefazolin, 2 g IV initial dose, then 1 g IV every 8 hours until delivery
Patients at high risk for anaphylaxis[c]*:*	
GBS-susceptible to clindamycin and erythromycin[d]:	Clindamycin, 900 mg IV every 8 hours until delivery or Erythromycin, 500 mg IV every 6 hours until delivery
GBS-resistant to clindamycin or erythromycin or susceptibility unknown:	Vancomycin,[e] 1 g IV every 12 hours until delivery

[a] Broader-spectrum agents, including an agent active against GBS, may be necessary for treatment of chorioamnionitis.
[b] History of penicillin allergy should be assessed to determine whether a high risk for anaphylaxis is present. Penicillin-allergic patients at high risk for anaphylaxis are those who have experienced immediate hypersensitivity to penicillin including a history of penicillin-related anaphylaxis; other high-risk patients are those with asthma or other diseases that would make anaphylaxis more dangerous or difficult to treat, such as persons being treated with beta-adrenergic-blocking agents.
[c] If laboratory facilities are adequate, clindamycin and erythromycin susceptibility testing should be performed on prenatal GBS isolates from penicillin-allergic women at high risk for anaphylaxis.
[d] Resistance to erythromycin is often but not always associated with clindamycin resistance. If a strain is resistant to erythromycin but appears susceptible to clindamycin, it may still have inducible resistance to clindamycin.
[e] Cefazolin is preferred over vancomycin for women with a history of penicillin allergy other than immediate hypersensitivity reactions, and pharmacologic data suggest it achieves effective intra-amniotic concentrations. Vancomycin should be reserved for penicillin-allergic women at high risk for anaphylaxis.
GBS, group B streptococcus.
(Reprinted from Centers for Disease Control and Prevention. Prevention of Perinatal Group B Streptococcal Disease. Revised guidelines. MMWR 2002;51 (No. RR-11):10.)

TERATOGENICITY

Medication Use During Pregnancy

Drug use during pregnancy presents a great challenge to clinicians because of the potential adverse effect on the embryo, fetus, and newborn. The limited availability of scientific data from randomized trials complicates the decision to prescribe and recommend medications for pregnant women, even when they are medically necessary. Most drugs are not labeled by the manufacturer for use during pregnancy because of the medical and legal implications. The potential benefits of medication therapy must be weighed against the possible risks to the fetus. Currently, only a few therapeutic agents of the thousands of drug therapies are adequately studied and considered relatively low risk on the development of the embryo and fetus. Knowledge of the teratogenic potential of these agents can be used to prevent or limit fetal exposure during the course of a pregnancy.

Many women have the general perception that use of any medication during a pregnancy can harm the developing fetus. This thought may lead to consideration of terminating wanted pregnancies or withholding necessary drug therapy during the course of the pregnancy. A thorough assessment, including knowledge of the teratogenic potential of the drug, the critical period of exposure, and magnitude of risk must be compared with the background risk. The basic principles of teratogenicty can help to assess the risk of exposure and interpretation of limited studies during pregnancy.

Rates of Drug Consumption During Pregnancy

Pregnancy is a symptom-producing condition. As a result, many drugs regularly are consumed during gestation, including some that are potential teratogens. The critical period to avoid or limit drug therapy exposure is during organogenesis (5–10 weeks after the last menstrual period or 20–55 days after conception) when most vital organs in the embryo are developing.[187] During these early weeks of pregnancy, the embryo is the most susceptible to medication exposure when many women are not yet aware of the pregnancy.

Earlier epidemiologic studies attempting to identify patterns of drug exposure during pregnancy have estimated that women consumed on average five to nine medications. A more recent epidemiologic collaborative study, conducted under the auspices of the World Health Organization (WHO) Drug Utilization Research Group, assessed the pattern of drug use in pregnancy in 22 countries.[188] This survey of 14,778 women estimated that approximately 14% did not take any medications during pregnancy. In the group that did consume drugs, the average number of drugs taken was 2.9. Vitamin and iron supplements were those most commonly used, followed by anti-infectives, and analgesics, antipyretics, and anti-inflammatory agents.[188] The proportion of women who consumed medications and the pattern of drug use varied by geographic distribution.

Proven Human Teratogens

The term *teratogen* is used to denote an agent that has the potential under certain exposure conditions to produce abnormal development in the fetus.[187] The extent to which a drug will affect the development of the fetus depends on the physical and chemical properties of the drug as well as the dose, duration, route, and timing of exposure; and genetic composition and biological susceptibility of the mother and fetus.[189] Numerous drugs have been associated with congenital anomalies, but only in a few cases has a consensus been reached that a specific agent is teratogenic. Table 46-6 lists those agents generally considered or suspected to be proven human teratogens. Not all these teratogens will cause development toxicity with every exposure, however. Table 46-7 lists some medications that can be used selectively during pregnancy when indicated.

The largest concern with medication use during pregnancy is the risk of congential malformations. Congenital malformations are defined as "structural abnormalities of prenatal origin that are present at birth and that seriously interfere with viability or physical well-being."[190] Congenital anomalies or birth defects are the leading cause of infant mortality in the United States, accounting for 20% of all infant deaths.[191] The economic impact of anomalies from the 18 most clinically significant structural birth defects is approximately \$8 billion annually.[192] This estimate does not include minor anomalies or the psychological and emotional impact to the child and family. Some drug-induced defects relate to changes in functions or conditions that are not structural abnormalities (e.g., mental retardation, CNS depression, deafness, tumors, or biochemical changes). The broader term *congential anomalies* include the four major manifestations of abnormal fetal development which include growth alterations, functional deficits, structural malformations, and fetal death.[187]

Prevalence of Congenital Malformations

The background incidence of birth defects in the general population must be taken into consideration when interpreting the risk of drug-induced teratogenicity. The prevalence of major congenital malformations discovered at or shortly after birth in the general population is approximately 3%.[193] This number has been derived from large epidemiologic studies completed over the past several decades and depends on how terms are defined (e.g., major versus minor congenital malformations), the thoroughness with which the infant is examined, and how long the exposed person is followed after birth.[187] Although the collection of data on the occurrence of malformations would seem to be straightforward, it is in fact a complicated task subject to numerous errors and biases. Some studies examined only "significant anomalies," others "major malformations," whereas still others reported only "live births" or "single births" or "birth weights >500 g." Stillbirths and spontaneous abortions, both often associated with congenital malformations, often were excluded from epidemiologic data. Neurodevelopmental delays and growth retardation also are potential long-term effects that will not be diagnosed in the immediate postpartum period. The prevalence of congential anomalies is likely >3% if minor anomalies and long-term adverse effects are considered.

Despite the significant impact of drug-induced birth defects, it is difficult and unethical to conduct randomized, controlled trials to assess the risk of fetal exposure to drugs in humans. Much of the data available are derived from epidemiologic

Table 46-6 Drugs With Suspected or Proven Teratogenic Effects in Humans[a]

Alcohol	Growth restriction, mental retardation, midfacial hypoplasia, renal and cardiac defects
Aminopterin, methotrexate	Central nervous system (CNS) and limb malformations
Angiotensin converting enzyme (ACE) inhibitors and angiotensin receptor blockers (ARB)	Renal failure in the fetus and neonates, decreased skull ossification, renal tubular dysgenesis
Antithyroid drugs	Fetal and neonatal goiter and hypothyroidism, aplasia cutis (with methimazole)
β-Blockers (without intrinsic sympathomimetic activity)	Intrauterine growth restriction
Carbamazepine	Neural tube defects, minor craniofacial defects, fingernail hypoplasia
Cigarette smoking	Oral clefts
Cocaine	Bowel atresias, heart, limbs, face, and genitourinary tract malformations; microcephaly, cerebral infarctions, growth restriction
Corticosteroids	Oral clefts
Cyclophosaphamide	CNS malformations, secondary cancer
Danazol and testosterone	Masculinization of female fetus
Diethylstilbestrol	Vaginal carcinoma and other genitourinary defects
Lithium	Ebstein anomaly
Misoprostol	Moebius sequence and spontaneous abortions
Nonsteroidal anti-inflammatory drugs	Constriction of the ductus arteriosus, oral clefts, cardiac defects, and possible spontaneous abortion
Paramethadione and trimethadione	Facial and CNS defects
Phenytoin	Fetal hydantoin syndrome, growth retardation, CNS deficits
Streptomycin and kanamycin	Hearing loss, eighth cranial damage (no ototoxicity reported with gentamicin use)
Systemic retinoids (isotretinoin and etretinate)	CNS, craniofacial, cardiovascular, and other defects
Tetracycline	Anomalies of teeth
Thalidomide	Limb shortening defects, internal organ defects
Trimethoprim	CNS deficits, possible cardiac defects and oral clefts
Vaccines (live)	Live attenuated vaccines can potentially cause fetal infection
Valproic acid	Neural tube defects
Vitamin A (high dose)	Deficiency and excess can cause teratogenicity. High dose (>25,000 IU/day): craniofacial and CNS anomalies, facial palsy and clefts, cardiac defects, limb reductions, gastrointestinal (GI) atresias, and urinary tract defects
Warfarin	Dandy Walker syndrome, skeletal and CNS defects

[a]Teratogenic effects include the four major manifestations of abnormal fetal development which include growth alterations, functional deficits, structural malformations, and fetal death.

[b]Only drugs that are teratogenic when used at clinically recommended doses are listed.

From references, 33 and 210, with permission.

studies, anecdotal experiences in humans, and animal studies. Because birth defects are species specific and influenced by many factors including genetic predisposition, the data must be carefully interpreted and the results not over generalized.

Although once thought to be rare occurrences, the tragedy with thalidomide in the early 1960s highlights the detrimental effects of fetal exposure to drugs. With >7,000 cases, observed defects included various forms of limb defects, including phocomelia, as well as other major organ abnormalities.[187] The embryotoxic effects were unexpected because no teratogenicity was observed in different animal species, and only mild adverse effects were reported in human adults. Other examples of iatrogenic major birth defects include diethylstilbestrol (DES), which causes vaginal adenocarcinoma in female offspring (detected only in later years of life), and valproic acid, which causes neural tube defects.[33] Classifying thalidomide as a teratogen means that it has the potential to cause developmental toxicity under specific conditions. For example, a single 50-mg dose of thalidomide increases the risk for a major structural malformation if given on the 26th day after conception, and confers minimal risk if taken in the 10th week after conception. Furthermore, a 1-mg dose of thalidomide taken at anytime during pregnancy has no observable effects on the fetus.[194]

Causes of Malformations

Classification

Causes of congenital malformations are generally classified into one of five categories: (*a*) monogenic origin; (*b*) chromosomal abnormalities; (*c*) multifactorial inheritance; (*d*) environmental factors; and (*e*) unknown.[193,195] Single gene and chromosomal-related defects account for approximately 25% of all congenital malformations in live-born infants (monogenetic, 7.5%–20%; chromosomal, 5%–6%).[190,195] *Multifactorial inheritance* refers to defects that are polygenic in origin; it has an environmental component. One surveillance program estimated that this interaction between genetic and environmental factors causes 23% of defects.[193] Congenital dislocation of the hip is an example of a defect in this category: the depth of the acetabular socket and joint laxity are genetically determined, and a frank breech malposition is one of the environmental factors.[196] In most cases, however, the environmental factors in multifactorial inheritance are unknown.

Environmental factors account for approximately 10% of malformations.[195] These include maternal conditions, mechanical effects, chemicals and drugs, and certain infectious agents. Maternal diseases associated with malformations include diabetes, phenylketonuria, virilizing tumors, and

Table 46-7 Medications Which Can Be Used Selectively During Pregnancy When Indicated, According to Condition

Condition	Drugs of Choice	Alternative Drugs	Comments
Acne	Topical: erythromycin, clindamycin, benzoyl peroxide	Systemic: erythromycin, topical tretinoin (vitamin A acid)	Isotretinoin is contraindicated
Allergic rhinitis	Topical: glucocorticoids, cromolyn, decongestants, xylometazoline, oxymetazoline, naphazoline Systemic: diphenhydramine, dimenhydrinate		
Constipation	Docusate sodium, glycerin, Milk of Magnesia, Metamucil, sorbitol, lactulose	Bisacodyl	Enema use should be avoided
Cough	Diphenhydramine, phenergan, dextromethorphan, guaifenesin		
Depression	Tricyclic antidepressants, bupropion, selective serotonin reuptake inhibitors (SSRI) but avoid paroxetine, serotonin-norepinephrine reuptake inhibitors (SNRI)		Exposure to paroxetine during the first trimester has been associated with an increased risk for cardiac malformations. Persistent pulmonary hypertension and neonatal withdrawal syndrome may occur in infants with maternal SSRI, SNRI use.
Diabetes	Insulin (human)	Insulin analogs (lispro, aspart, glargine), glyburide	Limited experience with metformin, studies mostly in polycystic ovarian syndrome patients. The role of other hypoglycemics not evaluated yet.
Headache (tension)	Acetaminophen	Aspirin and nonsteroidal anti-inflammatory drugs (NSAID), benzodiazepines	Aspirin and NSAID should be avoided in third trimester owing to concerns of oligohydramnios and premature closure of the ductus arteriosus, which can lead to pulmonary hypertension in the newborn. Small risk of malformations and spontaneous abortions with NSAID use in first trimester.
Migraine	Acetaminophen, codeine, dimenhydrinate	β-adrenergic receptor antagonists, tricyclic antidepressants (used for prophylaxis)	Limited experience with ergotamine has not revealed evidence of teratogenicity, but there is concern about potent vasoconstriction and uterine contraction.
Hyperthyroidism	Propylthiouracil	Methimazole, β-adrenergic receptor antagonists (for symptomatic relief)	Surgery may be required; radioactive iodine should be avoided (especially after 10 weeks gestation). Small risk of aplasia cutis with methimazole use.
Infections	Penicillins, cephalosporins, clindamycin, erthryomycin, nitrofuratoin	Gentamicin, vancomycin	Theoretic risk of hyperbilirubinemia in newborn with sulfamethoxazole in third trimester. Possible risk of hemolytic anemia in newborn with nitrofuratoin if taken close to term.
Mania (and bipolar affective disorders)	Lithium, chlorpromazine, haloperidol	For depressive episodes, tricycle antidepressants drugs, SSRI (avoid paroxetine), valproic acid	If lithium is used in first trimester, fetal echocardiogram is recommended because of small risk of cardiac anomalies; valproic acid may be given after the first trimester.
Nausea and vomiting	Doxylamine with pyridoxine (Vitamin B_6)	Chlorpromazine, metoclopramide, diphenhydramine, dimenhydrinate, meclizine, ondansetron	
Peptic ulcer disease	Antacids, magnesium hydroxide, aluminum hydroxide, calcium carbonate, ranitidine	Sucralfate, bismuth subsalicylate	Proton pump inhibitors (PPI) should be reserved for severe reflux. Omeprazole is only PPI with a pregnancy category D listing.
Pruritis	Topical: aluminum acetate, zinc oxide, calamine, glucocorticoids Systemic: hydroxyzine, diphenhydramine	Topical: local anesthetics	Small risk of oral clefts in first trimester if oral corticosteroids are used.
Smoking cessation	Nicotine lozenges, gums	Nicotine patches	Avoid during first trimester if possible, wear patches 16 hours during day to reduce nicotine exposure. Off during night.
Thrombophlebitis, deep vein thrombosis	Heparin, low-molecular weight heparins, antifibrinolytic, streptokinase		Streptokinase is associated with risk of bleeding; warfarin should be avoided

Adapted from reference 210, with permission.
Modified and updated data taken from reference 33, with permission.

maternal hyperthermia. About 9% (range, 6.6%–13.0%) of infants of diabetic mothers develop major congenital defects, primarily consisting of cardiovascular, neural tube, and skeletal malformations.[197] Mechanical effects, such as intrauterine compression and abnormal cord constriction, may result in fetal deformations.[195,197]

Probably the best known of the teratogenic viruses is rubella, which can cause a fetal rubella syndrome consisting of cataracts, heart disease, and deafness.[198] *In utero* exposure to rubella in the first trimester can cause defects in up to 85% of fetuses. Cytomegalovirus (CMV) infection occurs in 0.5% to 1.5% of newborns in the United States, resulting in deafness and mental retardation in 5% to 10% of these infants.[190] Characteristics of cytomegalic inclusion disease, the syndrome produced by CMV, include IUGR, microcephaly, and at times chorioretinitis, seizures, blindness, and optic atrophy.[199] Herpes simplex 1 and 2 and varicella may be associated with malformations.[195] The data on varicella are controversial.[198]

The protozoan generally accepted as a teratogen is *Toxoplasma gondii*.[190] Most infants infected with *T. gondii* show no symptoms and develop normally. When toxicity does occur, the anomalies may consist of hepatosplenomegaly, icterus, maculopapular rash, chorioretinitis, cerebral calcifications, and hydrocephalus or microcephalous.[199] *Treponema pallidum* (syphilis) can cross the placenta and cause congenital syphilis as well as other defects, such as hydrocephaly, chorioretinitis, and optic atrophy.[195,198] *In utero* exposure to syphilis after the fourth month of pregnancy is associated with higher risk.

The final category, defects of unknown cause, comprises the greatest percentage of congenital malformations, accounting for about 60% to 65% of the total.[193]

Basic Principles of Teratogenicity

Several critical factors are to be considered in evaluating the effects of drug exposure in human pregnancies. Because every pregnancy has the risk of an abnormal outcome regardless of drug exposure, the objective of evaluating data on drug exposure during pregnancy is to ascertain if a particular drug increases the risk of developmental toxicity in the fetus beyond the background rate. The following basic principles of teratogenicity should be applied when assessing the potential for teratogenicity of drugs.

Critical Stage of Exposure

After fertilization, the development of the embryo and fetus is divided into three main stages: pre-embryonic period, embryonic period, and fetal period.[195,200] In the first 2 weeks after fertilization or the pre-embryonic period (0–14 days), little is known about the effects of drugs on human development. Exposure to a teratogenic agent during this period usually produces an "all or none" effect on the ovum[201]: the ovum either dies from exposure to a lethal dose of a teratogenic drug, or it regenerates completely after exposure to a sublethal dose. Some animal studies have suggested, however, that exposure to some drugs during the preimplantation stage can halt growth and development before implantation.[202] Although the damage can be repaired, intrauterine growth may be retarded in the offspring.

During the embryonic period (14–56 days after fertilization), when organogenesis occurs, the embryo is most susceptible to the effects of teratogens or other chemicals.[200] Exposure during this sensitive period may produce major morphologic changes. These stages of development differ significantly from other species, and knowledge of these stages is essential for the interpretation of the relationship between congenital malformations and drugs. For example, if a specific drug exposure occurs after the time of organ development, then a structural defect in that organ is less likely to be caused by that specific drug.

The fetal period (57 days to term) includes most of the stages of histogenesis and functional maturation, although the latter continues for some time after birth.[195,200] Minor structural changes are still possible during histogenesis, but anomalies are more likely to involve growth and functional aspects such as mental development and reproduction.

Dose-Response Curve

All teratogens follow a toxicologic dose-response curve.[187] All teratogens have a threshold dose below which adverse effects will not occur. The threshold dose is the dosage in which the incidence of structural malformations, rate of fetal death, growth restriction, and functional deficits does not exceed the background rate in the general population.[187] Conversely, developmental toxicity may occur when the fetus is exposed to doses above the maximum or threshold dose. There may be an increase in the severity and incidence of malformations when the fetus is exposed to increasingly higher dosages. For example, the risk for major congenital malformations, including NTD and minor anomalies, are increased statistically in patients taking valproic acid dosages >1,000 mg/day during the first trimester.[203]

Extrapolation From Animal Studies

In the absence of human trials, data derived from animal studies is used to assess the level of risk of developmental toxicity in humans. Most newly marketed drugs often have to rely on preclinical data to develop an estimation of teratogenic risk based on animal studies until human data becomes available. The dose used in experimental animal data is expressed as multiples of the human dose using plasma or serum AUC or dose per unit based on body surface area (BSA).[33] The drug appears to have a low risk for teratogenicity if the toxic dose in animals (based on AUC or mg/m^2 comparison) is greater than 10 times the anticipated human dose.[204] Risk assessment using animal data is more complicated than just considering the dosage alone. Other major factors, including the effects of metabolism and active metabolites, species differentiation, route of administration, and type of defects, must be considered.[187]

Genetic Variability

The most potent teratogenic agent will not produce malformations with every exposure.[187] The teratogenic potential of some drugs is influenced by the genotype of both the mother and fetus. Although the effects of known teratogens can be predictable in the general population, the possibility of individual assessment is difficult. The same dose of a teratogenic agent exposed at the same gestational window will produce variable outcomes in different people. Genetic variability can confer differences in cell sensitivities, placental transport, drug metabolism, enzyme composition, and receptor binding, which may affect how much active drug will reach fetal tissues.[205]

One study showed an increased susceptibility to the teratogentic effect of phenytoin most likely caused by elevated levels of oxidative metabolites (epoxides). These epoxides are normally eliminated from the systemic circulation by enzymes called microsomal epoxide hydrolase. Women who are homozygous for the recessive allele produce low levels of epoxide hydrolase, which may expose the fetus to higher levels of epoxides. These fetuses may be at a higher risk for fetal hydantoin syndrome.[206]

Specific Grouping of Defects

Most human teratogens generally produce specific defects or grouping of defects.[187] These congential malformations occur after exposure during a critical period of embryonic development. One theory suggests that a teratogenic agent can possibly be identified by grouping individual malformations by understanding their embryologic tissue of origin.[187] For instance, isotretinoin interferes with the neural crest cell migration and leads to malformations of the ear, heart, and neural tube.[33] Thalidomide causes limb, spine, and CNS defects.[33] The rate of malformations in these teratogens must be compared with the background incidence in the general population.

Placental Transfer of Drugs

At one time, the placenta was thought to present a barrier to the passage of drugs and noxious chemicals to the fetus. It is now known, however, that most medications cross the placenta to the fetus and, in general, what the mother consumes also is consumed by the fetus. Although the placenta acts as a biologic membrane, it initially is composed of four layers effectively separating two distinct individuals.[207] These layers are (*a*) the endothelial lining of fetal vessels, (*b*) the connective tissue in the core of the villus, (*c*) the cytotrophoblastic layer, and (*d*) the covering syncytium. During gestation, the placenta's surface area increases while its thickness decreases from approximately 25 microns during the first trimester to 2 to 6 microns at term. Both processes tend to favor the transfer of chemicals to the fetus.

Drugs, nutrients, and other substances cross the placenta by five mechanisms: (*a*) simple diffusion (e.g., most drugs), (*b*) facilitated diffusion (e.g., glucose), (*c*) active transport (e.g., some vitamins, amino acids), (*d*) pinocytosis (e.g., immune antibodies), and (*e*) breaks between cells (e.g., erythrocytes).[200,207] The latter two mechanisms are of no practical importance in the transfer of drugs.

Several factors influence the rate of drug transfer across the placenta, including molecular weight (MW), lipid solubility, ionization, protein binding, uterine and umbilical blood flow, and maternal diseases.[200] Drugs with molecular weights <600 cross easily, whereas those $>1,000$ (e.g., heparin) cross with difficulty or not at all. Because most drugs have molecular weights <600, it is safe to assume that most drugs reaching the mother's circulatory system also will reach the fetus. As with other biologic membranes, lipid-soluble substances are transferred rapidly, with the rate of entry primarily governed by the lipid solubility of the nonionized molecule. Conversely, those molecules that are ionized at physiologic pH (e.g., the cholinergic quaternary amines) cross slowly, whereas weak acids and bases with pKa values between 4.3 and 8.5 are transferred rapidly to the fetus. The penetration of highly protein-bound drugs also is inhibited; only the free, unbound drugs cross the placenta.

Uterine blood flow, a major factor in determining the rate of drug transfer, increases throughout gestation. Several variables can affect uterine blood flow and the rate of drug transfer, including maternal blood pressure, cord compression, and drug therapy. Maternal hypotension reduces uterine blood flow and the rate at which substances are delivered to the membrane. Cord compression reduces the blood flow on the fetal side of the membrane. The use of drugs with α-adrenergic property (e.g., epinephrine) may constrict uterine vessels and thereby reduce blood flow.[208] Maternal diseases, such as pregnancy-induced hypertension, erythroblastosis, and diabetes, change the permeability of the placenta and may reduce or increase transfer.[200]

Food and Drug Administration Risk Factors

In 1979, the FDA introduced a system of rating pregnancy risks associated with pharmacologic agents. This system categorizes all drugs approved after 1983 into one of five pregnancy risk categories (see Table 46-1). It establishes the level of risks to the fetus based on available animal and human data and recommends the degree of caution that should be undertaken with each drug. The risk factors assigned are sometimes difficult to interpret because they may be ambiguous, outdated, and do not provide information regarding the full range of potential developmental toxicity (i.e., structural defects, growth restriction, functional deficits, and fetal death).[204] Level of risks also have been described and categorized by teratology specialists, and they may or may not concur with manufacturers' ratings.[208,209] The FDA is currently working on revising the pregnancy labeling and category system to include narrative text to provide more clinical management advice that includes consideration of both animal and human data[204] Table 46-6. lists some drugs that are considered contraindicated during pregnancy. These lists are not all-inclusive, and a review of specialty resources on drug use in pregnancy is recommended.[199,208,209] Teratogen information programs also are available in the United States and Canada to respond to questions concerning the risks of drug exposure during pregnancy. These programs are usually affiliated with medical or university settings.[210,211] Because the potential for fetal risks cannot be entirely disregarded for many drugs, the need to medicate during pregnancy should be evaluated carefully.

LACTATION

Lactation is controlled primarily by prolactin (PRL), but the entire process is under the intricate control of several hormones. Breast tissue maturation during pregnancy is influenced by many factors, including estrogen, progesterone, PRL, insulin, growth hormone, cortisol, thyroxine, and human placental lactogen.[212] PRL concentrations gradually increase during pregnancy, but high estrogen and progesterone concentrations inhibit milk secretion by blocking PRL's effect on the breast epithelium.[212,213] It is the dramatic decrease in progesterone that triggers lactogenesis or milk secretion for the first 3 days following delivery. Infant suckling at the breast is necessary to maintain an adequate milk supply beyond postpartum day 3 or 4. Nipple stimulation transmits sensory impulses to the hypothalamus to initiate PRL release from the anterior pituitary and oxytocin from the posterior pituitary. Prolactin stimulates the production and secretion of breast milk and oxytocin stimulates the contraction of the myoepithelial cells in the breast alveoli and ducts so that milk can be ejected from the breast (milk letdown). Oxytocin also can be secreted through other sensory pathways, which is why women can release milk on hearing, smelling, or even thinking about their infants. Prolactin, however, is released only in response to nipple stimulation.

Prolactin synthesis and release depend on the inhibition of hypothalamic prolactin inhibitory factor (PIF) secretion. Prolactin secretion is regulated primarily by dopamine-releasing neurons. Activating the dopamine receptors on the prolactin-secreting cells of the anterior pituitary inhibits the release of prolactin. PIF is believed to be closely associated with dopamine.[212,213]

Although prolactin controls the volume of milk produced, once lactation is established, milk production is regulated by infant demand. Lactation eventually ceases if milk is not removed from the breast. Absence of suckling stops milk letdown and restores the normal production of PIF. Decreased blood flow to the breast reduces oxytocin delivery to the myoepithelium. Consequently, milk secretion stops within a few days.[212,213]

Stimulation

Nonpharmacologic Measures

58. C.C., a 22-year-old woman, vaginally delivered her first child, a healthy term infant. C.C. plans to breast-feed and was educated about breast-feeding during obstetric visits and prenatal classes. After giving birth, C.C. tried to breast-feed in the delivery room with great difficulty. Afterward, she became extremely apprehensive and continued to have trouble breast-feeding. What can be done to encourage C.C. and help her with lactation?

The most effective stimulus for lactation is suckling. Many women nurse in the delivery room after uncomplicated vaginal deliveries because nursing increases maternal–infant bonding and helps establish good milk production. If a mother does not nurse immediately after delivery, she should be encouraged to do so as soon as she is physically able. C.C. did try to nurse after delivery, but experienced problems that may have been related to her emotional or physical state, or to the physical state of her infant. The nursing staff should encourage and support C.C. emotionally to help her relax, be comfortable, and relieve her anxiety about breast-feeding. Health care personnel also should emphasize appropriate feeding techniques and proper positioning for breast-feeding. Allowing C.C.'s infant to sleep in her room, rather than the nursery, may help C.C. develop a breast-feeding routine.

Most new mothers who have difficulty breast-feeding initially respond to the emotional and educational support of a good obstetric nursing staff. Few require pharmaceutical intervention.

Enhancement of Milk Production

59. C.C. was successful in establishing breast-feeding. Despite good technique and adequate nutrition, she, however, had trouble maintaining adequate milk production after about 2 to 3 weeks and was forced to supplement her infant with formula. How can C.C.'s milk production be enhanced?

Although not an FDA-approved indication, metoclopramide is used to stimulate lactation in women with decreased or inadequate milk production.[33,214–218] Metoclopramide, a dopamine-antagonist, increases PRL secretion. This is particularly useful in women whose infants do not breast-feed effectively (e.g., preterm infants).[214] Metoclopramide 10 mg orally three times daily for 1 to 2 weeks is effective in restoring milk production.[33,214–217] Improvement in lactation occurs within 2 to 5 days of starting therapy and persists after discontinuing metoclopramide.

The estimated total daily dose of metoclopramide ingested by the nursing infant of a woman on 30 mg/day is 1 to 45 mcg/kg/day.[33] This is below the maximal recommended infant daily dose of 0.5 mg/kg/day. Maternal doses of 30 mg/day do not alter PRL, thyroid-stimulating hormone, or free thyroxin serum concentrations in breast-fed infants.[218] The only adverse effect reported in nursing infants has been intestinal gas.[33,216] The short-term use of metoclopramide for re-establishing lactation appears to be both safe and effective, even in preterm infants.[33,214,217] The American Academy of Pediatrics (AAP), however, considers metoclopramide use in breast-feeding women to be of concern because of the potential for adverse CNS effects in infants.[33]

Suppression

60. After delivery, J.G., a 26-year-old G_2P_2, informs her obstetrician that she does not wish to breast-feed. What methods are available to suppress lactation?

Suppression of lactation is indicated for women who do not want to breast-feed, women who have delivered a stillborn infant, and those who have had an abortion. Both drugs and nonpharmacologic methods have been used. In 1988, the FDA, however, recommended against drug-induced suppression of lactation.[219] The only drug therapy that the FDA recommends in women who are not breast-feeding are analgesics for the relief of breast pain. Bromocriptine (Parlodel) was approved for the postpartum suppression of lactation; however, the FDA rescinded its approval for that indication because of cardiovascular complications (e.g., stroke, myocardial infarction) associated with its use.[213]

If breast stimulation is avoided (with or without the use of a breast binder), breast milk production will continue, leading to engorgement and distention of breast alveoli. This leads to the termination of lactation after several days. Approximately 40% of women using this method experience breast discomfort and pain; 30% experience milk leakage from their nipples.[219,220] Ice packs may be applied to the breasts for comfort and a mild analgesic used if necessary.

DRUG EXCRETION IN HUMAN MILK

Breast milk is recognized as the optimal source of nutrition for infants, with documented benefits not only to infants but also to mothers, families, and societies.[221] Evidence indicates that breast-feeding decreases the incidence or severity of many infectious processes (e.g., otitis media, respiratory infections, urinary tract infections) in infants. In children and adults who were breast-fed, the risk of developing certain medical illnesses also may decrease (e.g., obesity, inflammatory bowel disease, celiac disease, childhood leukemia).[222] Breast-feeding may also positively influence cognitive and intellectual development in children and young adults.[223] Numerous benefits to the mother also have been identified, such as decreased postpartum blood loss, more rapid uterine involution, earlier return to prepregnancy weight, and decreased risks of breast cancer, ovarian cancer, and osteoporosis.[221]

The AAP recommends that mothers breast-feed for ≥12 months. Recognition of the importance of breast-feeding is highlighted in *Healthy People 2010,* a national health promotion and disease prevention program that helps the nation address public health issues by establishing objectives and goals. In the United States, breast-feeding during the early postpartum period increased from 54% in 1988 to 73.8% in 2004.[224] The percentage of women who are still breast-feeding at 6 months decreases to 41.5%. Although encouraging, these figures are still below the *Healthy People 2010* targets of 75% for early postpartum and 50% at 6 months.

The perception that nursing should be discontinued while the mother is medicated persists, although only a finite number of drugs are absolutely contraindicated during lactation. This misconception is likely a result of the uncertainty surrounding the effects of exposure of many drugs in nursing infants because of the inherent difficulties in accessing risks in controlled environments (e.g., clinical trials). Unlike the use of drugs during pregnancy, when the effects of fetal exposure are difficult to predict, drug excretion in breast milk can be approximated to a certain extent. Actual measurements of drug concentrations in milk and clinical observations in breast-fed infants have been published for selected drugs. An understanding of the basic physiochemical principles of drug excretion in breast milk and the factors that affect this process allows for better prediction of the risk of drug exposure to the nursing infant.

Pharmacokinetics

Different pharmacokinetic models of drug excretion in milk have been described.[225–227] A two-compartment open model presents the maternal fluids as one compartment and breast milk as the other. After ingestion, the drug gets absorbed into the maternal compartment, with a proportion of drug passing into breast milk and the remaining portion distributed in and eliminated from the maternal system. Drugs reaching breast milk will ultimately leave this compartment either by diffusing back into maternal fluids or through milk production and nursing.[226,227] A more popular model describes drug excretion in milk using a three-compartment model that incorporates the pharmacokinetics of the mother, mammary tissues, and infant.[225,226] The overall risk to the infant depends on the amount of drug bioavailable to the mother, the amount reaching breast milk, and the actual amount of drug ingested and bioavailable to the nursing infant.

Transfer of Drugs From Plasma to Milk

Transfer of drugs from maternal plasma to milk is generally through passive diffusion.[228] Low-molecular-weight, water-soluble substances diffuse through small, water-filled pores, whereas lipid-soluble compounds pass through lipid membranes.[229] Many factors affect the excretion of drugs in breast milk, and they should be carefully assessed before making a recommendation. The extent of drug passage into breast milk is often expressed quantitatively as the milk-to-plasma (M:P) ratio. This ratio should not be used as the sole determinant of whether a drug is safe for use during breast-feeding (see Estimating Infant Exposure).

Table 46-8 Factors Affecting the Fate of Drugs in Milk and the Nursing Infant

Maternal Parameters	• Drug dosage and duration of therapy • Route and frequency of administration • Metabolism • Renal clearance • Blood flow to the breasts • Milk pH • Milk composition
Drug Parameters	• Oral bioavailability (to mother and infant) • Molecular weight • pKa • Lipid solubility • Protein binding
Infant Parameters	• Age of the infant • Feeding pattern • Amount of breast milk consumed • Drug absorption, distribution, metabolism, elimination

From references 225, 228, 230, and 231, with permission.

Several parameters affect drug excretion into breast milk (Table 46-8). The pKa of a drug partially determines how much drug can reach the milk, because only the nonionized portion of free drug is transferred. Human milk, with an average pH of 7.1, is slightly more acidic than plasma. In general, drugs that are weak acids (e.g., penicillin) tend to have a higher concentration in plasma than milk (M:P <1). Conversely, the concentration of weak bases (e.g., erythromycin) in milk is more likely to be higher or to reach an equilibrium with that measured in plasma (M:P ≥1).[225,227] Once in the milk, the proportion of ionized weak base rises in the relatively acidic solution, and thus drug "trapping" occurs. Drug reabsorption has been found for some agents, and the prevention of passage back into the plasma by "trapping" may be clinically important. Lipid solubility also is determined to a large extent by the degree of ionization because drugs with relatively high lipid solubility exist in the nonionized form. Diffusion through lipid membranes is probably the most important pathway for drug transfer. Although pH, pKa, and lipid solubility are important elements, other factors may significantly modify predictions based solely on these chemical characteristics. Two of these other factors are protein binding and molecular weight.[228–230] Drugs with high molecular weights such as insulin (MW >6,000) are less likely to transfer into breast milk, whereas those with molecular weights <300 transfer more readily.[231] Highly protein-bound drugs such as glyburide (99% protein bound) are less likely to be transferred into breast milk, although infants should still be monitored for signs of hypoglycemia.

Drug transfer also is influenced by the yield of milk, which is related to blood flow and prolactin secretion.[225] Lactation is associated with a high blood flow to the breasts, but little is known about this flow during or between feedings. The milk yield (volume) differs slightly depending on the duration of lactation and the time of day. A diurnal pattern has been observed, with highest yields at 6 AM and lowest yields at 6 PM or 10 PM. The mean composition of mature human milk is approximately 87% aqueous solution, 3.5% lipids, 8% carbohydrate (83% of which is lactose), 0.9% protein, and 0.2% nitrogen.[232] The proportions of these components may vary widely from woman to woman and even within the same woman. For example, hind milk contains four- to fivefold the fat content of foremilk, whereas colostrum contains little fat. Fat content also has exhibited a diurnal variation.

After a drug reaches the milk, it equilibrates between the aqueous and lipid phases. The nature of this equilibration can modify how much drug actually reaches the infant. Infant feeding patterns differ significantly from one baby to another. The time spent suckling at each breast and the volume of milk taken in also determine the amount of drug ingested, especially if the drug has partitioned into one phase more so than the other. Once the infant ingests the drug via breast milk, the pharmacologic and adverse effects on the infant will be determined by the extent of oral bioavailability, distribution, metabolism, and rate of elimination. These pharmacokinetic parameters differ, depending on the infant's age and whether he or she was born prematurely or at term.

Estimating Infant Exposure

Understanding the transfer of drugs into breast milk is important because the primary objective is to minimize infant exposure to these substances. The actual amount an infant will ingest is difficult to determine owing to varying maternal, drug, and infant parameters. Available data generally are from single or small numbers of case reports or pharmacokinetic studies involving few mother–infant pairs. An M:P ratio is sometimes used alone as the basis for a recommendation, but this should be avoided because its accuracy can be affected by many factors. The time of sampling after maternal ingestion (peak versus steady-state), dose, length of therapy, route of administration, and milk composition are a few of the variables that can influence the M:P ratio.[225,227,230] Sampling during maternal peak drug concentration attempts to approximate the highest amount of drug that can reach the infant. This assumption is inherently flawed because peak drug concentration in the mother does not necessarily equate with peak drug concentration in milk at that same point in time.[226,230] The amount of drug an infant actually receives also depends on the volume of milk ingested. Even if a drug has a high M:P ratio, the actual amount received by the infant could be low if only a small volume of milk was consumed. Therefore, an M:P ratio describes the likelihood of drug excretion into breast milk, but it does not indicate the level of infant exposure. In general, drugs with lower M:P ratios (<1) are preferred over those with higher M:P ratios (>1) during breast-feeding, but other parameters such as maternal condition and therapeutic efficacy should be considered.

Infant exposure to a drug via ingestion of breast milk can be estimated for some drugs. The M:P ratio is used to estimate the drug concentration in milk (Equation 46-1) and the dose the infant may ingest (Equation 46-2).[211,226,230] The variables required to calculate Equation 46-1 can be located in the published literature, but only for some drugs. The actual volume of milk ingested by the infant is difficult to estimate, but the average consumption is approximately 150 mL/kg/day.[230] The estimated infant dose can then be used to calculate a "relative infant dose" (RID) (Equation 46-3), which is expressed as a percentage of the maternal dose.[233] A RID $<10\%$ is generally interpreted as an acceptable level. This must be interpreted with caution, however, taking into account other variables, such as the age and health of the infant and the safety profile of the drug. It is also important to note that these are estimated values, often based on data collected from one or only a few individuals. Applying these equations using measurements specific to a woman and her infant is not clinically practical, however. Compared with the M:P ratio, experts believe that the RID is a better estimate of infant exposure.

$$\text{Drug concentration in milk} = \text{Maternal plasma drug concentration} \times \text{M/P} \quad \textbf{(46-1)}$$

$$\text{Infant dose (mg/kg/day)} = \text{Drug concentration in milk} \times \text{Milk volume (mL/Kg/day)} \quad \textbf{(46-2)}$$

$$\text{RID (\%)} = (\text{Infant dose [mg/kg/day]})/(\text{Maternal dose [mg/kg/day]}) \times 100 \quad \textbf{(46-3)}$$

Reducing Risk of Exposure

If pharmacologic treatment is medically necessary for a nursing mother, every attempt should be made to minimize infant exposure to the drug. Methods of reducing risks have been proposed.[226,227,234] Table 46-9 summarizes critical factors that should be considered. Except for drugs that are contraindicated during lactation, the decision to continue or discontinue nursing while receiving medication is ultimately the mother's.

Table 46-9 Reducing Risk of Infant Exposure to Drugs in Breast Milk[226, 227, 233, 234]

A drug should be used only if medically necessary and treatment cannot be delayed until the infant is ready to be weaned.
Drug Selection
Consider whether the drug can be safely given directly to the infant.
Select a drug that passes poorly into breast milk with the lowest predicted M:P ratio, and a RID $<10\%$.
Avoid long-acting formulations (e.g., sustained-release).
Consider possible routes of administration that can reduce drug excretion into milk.
Determine length of therapy and if possible avoid long-term use.
Feeding Pattern
Avoid nursing during times of peak drug concentration.
If possible, plan breast-feeding before administration of the next dose.
Other Considerations
Always observe the infant for unusual signs (e.g., sedation, irritability, rash, decreased appetite, failure to thrive).
Discontinue breast-feeding during the course of therapy if the risks to the fetus outweigh the benefits of nursing.
Provide adequate patient education to increase understanding of risk factors.

RID, relative infant dose; M:P, milk to plasma ratio.

Table 46-10 Drugs Considered Contraindicated During Lactation[a]

Drug or Drug Class	*Effects on Nursing Infants*
Amphetamine[b]	Accumulate in breast milk and may cause irritability and poor sleep patterns[208,235]
Antineoplastics	Potential for immune suppression; cytotoxic effects on drugs on dividing cells in infants unknown[235]
Cocaine[b]	Excreted in milk; contraindicated because of central nervous system (CNS) stimulation and intoxication[208,235]
Ergotamine	Potential for suppressing lactation; vomiting, diarrhea, and convulsions have been reported.[208] Considered contraindicated by some clinicians. American Academy of Pediatrics (AAP) recommends using with caution[235]
Heroin[b]	Possible addiction if sufficient amounts ingested[208,235]
Immunosuppressants	Potential for immune suppression[235]
Lithium	Milk and serum concentrations average 40% of maternal serum levels. Potential for toxicity exists.[208,231] Considered contraindicated by some clinicians. AAP recommends using with caution.[235]
Lysergic acid diethylamide (LSD)[b]	Probably excreted in milk[208]
Marijuana[b]	Excreted in milk[208,235]
Misoprostol	Excretion in milk has not been studied but contraindicated because of potential for severe diarrhea in infant[208]
Phencyclidine[b]	Potent hallucinogenic properties[208,235]
Phenindione	Massive scrotal hematoma and wound oozing after herniotomy in one infant; contraindicated[208,235]
Requiring Temporary Cessation of Breast-Feeding	
Metronidazole (after single-dose therapy)	Diarrhea and secondary lactose intolerance in one infant; mutagenic and carcinogenic in some species; AAP recommends halting breast-feeding for 12–24 hrs to allow clearance of drug from the milk if single-dose therapy administered.[231,235]
Radiopharmaceuticals	Halt breast-feeding temporarily to allow clearance of radioactivity from milk. Suggested times for individual agents are[235]: Copper-64 (^{64}Cu) 50 hrs; Gallium-67 (^{67}Ga) 2 wks; Indium-111 (^{111}In) 20 hrs; Iodine-123 (^{123}I) 36 hrs; Iodine-125 (^{125}I) 12 days; Iodine-131 (^{131}I) 2–14 days; Radioactive Sodium 96 hrs; Technetium-99m (^{99m}Tc) 15 hrs–3 days; ($^{99m}TcO_4$) (^{99m}Tc macroaggregates) 15 hrs–3 days.

[a] This list is not all-inclusive. Selected drugs are listed by drug class and not by individual names.
[b] All drugs of abuse are contraindicated during lactation.

Therefore, patient education is an integral component in this decision-making process. The mother should be informed of the potential risks, or lack thereof, associated with a drug. She also should be made aware that certain risks may be minimized by altering feeding pattern and drug administration time and by carefully monitoring the infant for early signs of adverse effects.

Resources for Drugs and Lactation

Comprehensive sources reviewing drug use in lactation are available to assist clinicians in weighing the potential risks versus benefits of mothers using medications while breast-feeding. Table 46-10 lists some medications that are contraindicated during lactation. The AAP Committee on Drugs reviews periodically the transfer of drugs and other chemicals into human milk and publishes their findings.[235] The Committee identifies drugs that should be avoided during breast-feeding, drugs that should be used with caution, drugs whose effects on infants are unknown but of concern, and those considered usually compatible with breast-feeding. This rigorous review is an ongoing process, and new guidelines are published every few years; therefore, the reader should locate the latest AAP recommendations available. In addition to the AAP guidelines, several other references also offer comprehensive information and recommendations on drug use in lactation.[208,230]

Most drugs are excreted into breast milk to some extent, the reader is referred to specialty sources for an in-depth review of the drug in question. The best sources for information regarding drugs in lactation are (a) *Drugs in Pregnancy and Lactation* by Briggs, Freeman, and Yaffe[33] and (b) TOXNET, an online lactation database (LactMed) sponsored by the NIH, assessible at http://toxnet.nlm.nih.gov and click on LactMed. These two databases are peer-reviewed and referenced sources. Categories assigned to these drugs may change as new data become available for specific drugs.

THERAPEUTIC DILEMMAS IN PREGNANT AND LACTATING WOMEN

Anticoagulation

Warfarin

FETAL WARFARIN SYNDROME

61. H.P. is a 25-year-old woman with a 5-week intrauterine pregnancy. She recently was diagnosed with a distal deep vein thrombosis (DVT) in her lower left extremity. She has a significant history of having multiple DVTs in her prior pregnancies and her thrombophilia workup was negative. Currently, she is taking warfarin 5 mg/day and just found out that she is pregnant. Does warfarin present a therapeutic problem to the fetus? If so, what changes should be made?

Warfarin (Coumadin) crosses the placenta and is generally considered contraindicated in pregnancy except under specific circumstances.[236] Use of warfarin in the first trimester has been associated with a characteristic pattern of defects collectively known as the fetal warfarin syndrome (FWS).[237] The susceptible period seems to be between weeks 6 and 12 of gestation.[237,238] Nasal hypoplasia and a depressed nasal bridge are common to all known cases of FWS. The nares and air passages may be constricted to such a degree that respiratory distress results. As seen roentgenographically, stippling in uncalcified epiphyseal regions occurs in most newborns with FWS but may not be evident after the first year of life.[237] The axial skeleton, proximal femurs, and calcanei are the sites primarily involved in FWS, and this pattern of distribution distinguishes it from other syndromes and genetic disorders.[237] Less common features are reduced birthweight, eye and ear defects, hypoplasia of extremities, development retardation, congenital heart disease, laryngeal calcification, and death.[209,239]

The exact incidence of warfarin-induced anomalies is unknown, but it is estimated to range from 17% to 37%.[208,240] The rate of FWS reported is approximately 3% to 10%.[208,209] Therefore, the use of warfarin in H.P. is controversial. Discontinuation of warfarin should be considered, especially during the critical period between weeks 6 and 12 of gestation.

Warfarin exposure after this critical period may increase the risk of CNS anomalies in the fetus. These anomalies appear to be a result of abnormal growth arising from an earlier fetal hemorrhage and subsequent scarring.[232] Two distinct patterns of CNS damage may occur: (a) dorsal midline dysplasia, characterized by agenesis of the corpus callosum, Dandy-Walker malformation, midline cerebellar atrophy, and encephaloceles in some; and (b) ventral midline dysplasia, characterized by optic atrophy.[232,234] The effects of CNS defects include mental retardation (ranging from mild to severe), blindness, hydrocephalus, deafness, spasticity, seizures, scoliosis, growth failure, and death. Fetal complications from warfarin may be dose dependent, as demonstrated in two retrospective studies.[240a,240b] Cotrufo et al.[240b] observed that daily warfarin doses >5 mg were associated with more pregnancy complications, including adverse fetal outcomes.

Heparin and more recently low-molecular-weight heparin (LMWH) are the preferred anticoagulants in pregnancy for most indications, including prevention and treatment of DVT.[238] The efficacy of heparin and LMWH in pregnant women with prosthetic heart valves is less clear, although they have a better safety profile for the fetus. If heparin or LMWH is used in H.P., close monitoring for thromboembolic complications is required.[241]

Heparin

62. Heparin therapy (10,000 U SC every 8 hours) is initiated, and warfarin is discontinued. What are the fetal and maternal risks of using heparin in H.P.?

Heparin is a large molecule (MW 12,000) and does not cross the placenta. According to the Seventh American College of Chest Physicians (ACCP) Consensus Conference, heparin is one of the preferred anticoagulants during pregnancy for most thromboembolic conditions because of its efficacy and more favorable safety profile compared with warfarin.[238] Although earlier cases reported that the rate of fetal complications associated with heparin use may be as high as those reported with warfarin (22% versus 27%, respectively),[237] subsequent evaluations demonstrated that the rate of adverse fetal outcome with heparin therapy is comparable to that reported in the normal population.[209,240] The high incidence of fetal abnormalities reported earlier can be attributed to the use of heparin in pregnancies with comorbid conditions known to increase risks.

Nevertheless, the use of heparin during pregnancy may pose several risks to the mother. The risk of bleeding from heparin during pregnancy is approximately 2%.[238] Heparin-induced thrombocytopenia (HIT) is a well-recognized complication and may require discontinuation of therapy if it is an immune-mediated response. The frequency of HIT during pregnancy is unknown but has been estimated at 3% in non-pregnant patients.[238]

Prolonged administration of heparin (>1 month) increases the risk of developing osteoporosis. Although the occurrence of symptomatic fractures is uncommon (2%–3%), the development of osteopenia may occur in up to one third of pregnant women on chronic heparin therapy.[242–246] This reduction in bone mineral density (BMD) may be reversible after discontinuation of heparin.[243,245] Heparin-induced osteoporosis may be associated with higher doses of heparin and longer duration of use. In a prospective, cohort study of 184 cases by Dahlman,[244] the incidence of osteoporosis was higher in women who received a mean dose of 25,000 units/24 hours versus a mean dose of 16,500 units/24 hours. The average duration of treatment was 25 weeks (range, 7–27 weeks). A definitive dose–response relationship cannot be confirmed, however, because reductions in BMD have been reported with lower dosages and shorter duration of heparin use. The mechanism behind this effect is thought to be heparin inhibition of the renal activation of calcifediol (25-hydroxyvitamin D_3, a major transport form of vitamin D) to calcitriol, one of the active forms of vitamin D_3. Several recent studies have suggested that LMWH may pose a lower risk of osteoporosis than unfractionated heparin (UFH).

63. H.P. presents again at 20 weeks' gestation complaining of mild muscle pain and tingling in the lower left extremity. Laboratory workup confirmed an activated partial thromboplastin time (aPTT) of 1.5 times control despite an adjusted heparin dosage of 15,000 units SC every 8 hours several weeks ago. H.P. is now in her second trimester. What subjective and objective evidence does H.P. exhibit that indicates a need to change anticoagulant therapy?

H.P. is at increased risk for thromboembolic complications because her aPTT is not within the therapeutic range and her heparin dosage is not currently adequate to maintain anticoagulation. Higher doses are generally required because of increases in plasma volume, renal clearance, heparin-binding proteins, and decreased bioavailability of heparin because of degradation by the placenta.[247] To minimize H.P.'s risk of developing thrombotic complications and osteoporosis, an adjusted-dose regimen with SC heparin every 8 hours is warranted. The lowest effective heparin dose to achieve a mid-interval aPTT at least two times control should be maintained.[238]

H.P.'s symptoms are consistent with thromboembolism. Her low aPTT level despite a high dosage of heparin suggests an increased requirement for heparin. Because H.P. already is on high-dose heparin, prolonged administration will significantly increase her risk of osteoporosis. Of special concern is her apparent resistance to heparin therapy. An alternative anticoagulant should be considered to minimize her risk for further thrombotic complications.

Low-Molecular-Weight Heparin

64. Is LMWH an alternative for H.P.?

As with heparin, LMWH does not cross the placenta to the fetus. LMWH offers a better bioavailability profile, more convenient dosing, and it may be associated with less thrombocytopenia, bleeding, and osteoporosis than UFH.[238] It is often preferred in most patients because it requires less monitoring of laboratory values than UFH. A starting dosage of 1 mg/kg given SC every 12 hours should be used. Regular antifactor Xa levels drawn 3 to 4 hours after a dose at steady-state to achieve a level of 0.5 to 1.2 U/mL is recommended.[238] As H.P.'s pregnancy progresses and her weight increases, the volume of distribution for LMWH also will change. Adjustments to the dosage of LMWH can be made through weight-based changes or in response to antifactor Xa levels drawn. Preliminary data suggest LMWH does not increase the risk of adverse birth outcomes.[248,249] Although it is an effective alternative to heparin in general, its role in preventing thromboembolic complications in pregnant women with prosthetic heart valves has not been determined.

Heparin and LMWH in the Third Trimester Near Delivery

65. H.P. is now at 38 weeks' gestation and has a scheduled cesarean section in 1 week. She currently is on enoxaparin 100 mg SC every 12 hours. What advice should be given to help her manage her anticoagulation just before surgery?

To minimize bleeding complications during delivery, the Seventh ACCP Conference on Antithrombotic and Thrombolytic Therapy suggests that heparin and LMWH be discontinued 24 hours before elective induction of labor or cesarean section.[238] If spontaneous labor occurs before her scheduled cesarean section, neuroaxial anesthesia can become complicated if H.P. is anticoagulated. If the aPTT or antifactor Xa is markedly prolonged near delivery, protamine sulfate may be required to decrease the risk of bleeding.

Graduated compression stockings should be used during and after H.P.'s cesarean section because some data have suggested that some patients (i.e., prior venous thromboembolism, thrombophilia, age >35 years, obesity, prolonged bedrest) are at high risk for thromboembolic complications.[238] Anticoagulation with heparin should be reinitiated after surgery once H.P. is hemodynamically stable and the risk of bleeding is low. H.P is at an increased risk for venous thrombosis during both pregnancy and the postpartum period.

Breast-Feeding

66. After vaginal delivery, H.P. is restarted on low-dose heparin and then changed to warfarin on day 5. H.P. also is breast-feeding. Does either of these drugs present a risk to the nursing infant?

Heparin does not cross into breast milk (see Drug Excretion in Human Milk) because of its high molecular weight (~12,000). Therefore, the risk from this anticoagulant is minimal. Warfarin is a weakly acidic drug (pKa 5.05) that is highly ionized at physiologic pH (>99%) in maternal serum.[229] It also is highly protein bound (97%).[239] These pharmacokinetic parameters make warfarin unlikely to transfer into breast milk. Case reports in lactating mothers confirm that warfarin was not detected in breast milk or infant plasma, or that very low amounts were detected in breast milk.[208] The AAP lists warfarin under the category of "usually compatible with breast-feeding."[235] As a precaution, the mother should observe the infant for bruising or other signs of hemorrhage, although the apparent risk is low.

Antiepileptic Drugs

Phenytoin

67. L.F. is a 30-year-old woman with epilepsy who is planning to start a family. Her generalized tonic–clonic seizures have been well controlled with oral phenytoin 100 mg four times daily (QID), and L.F. has had no seizures for the past 3 years. She is otherwise healthy and is not taking any medication besides phenytoin. Should L.F. become pregnant, what are the risks of phenytoin to the fetus?

Approximately 90% of women with epilepsy who receive antiepileptic drugs (AED) have uneventful pregnancies. A few women have an increased risk for fetal abnormalities, with both major and minor malformations reported. Controversy exists over whether maternal epilepsy increases the rate of malformations; however, newer studies suggest this increased incidence is most likely caused by AED therapy.[250–252] The risk of fetal abnormalities is lowest with monotherapy and is generally considered to be two- to threefold higher than in the general population.[253] In a prospective study by Holmes et al.[252] conducted between 1986 and 1993, congenital malformations occurred more frequently in infants exposed to one AED compared with controls (20.6% versus 8.5%; odds ratio [OR] 2.8; 95% confidence interval [CI] 1.1–9.7). The rate was even higher for infants exposed to two or more AED compared with control (28% versus 8.5%; OR 4.2; 95% CI 1.1–5.1). Abnormalities most commonly observed with the use of AED are major congenital malformations (e.g., cardiac malformations, cleft lip or palate), microcephaly, hypoplasia of the midface and fingers, and growth retardation.[252,254,255] Preliminary data also proposed that children exposed to AED *in utero* may be more likely to have developmental delay, childhood medical problems, and behavior disorders.[256] More studies are needed to confirm these initial findings.

FETAL HYDANTOIN SYNDROME

Phenytoin (Dilantin) can cause a recognizable pattern of malformations collectively known as the *fetal hydantoin syndrome* (FHS). It is now recognized that this syndrome is not restricted to phenytoin use and can be linked to other AED. Infants of mothers who were treated with AED have a 10% to 30% chance of developing some aspects of FHS, but the full-blown syndrome is less common.[257–259]

Common features identified with FHS are varying degrees of craniofacial malformations, including lip and palatal changes; limb anomalies, such as hypoplasia of nails and distal phalanges; congenital heart disease; and mental and physical growth retardation.[208,257,258].

PROPOSED MECHANISMS OF TERATOGENICITY

A study published in 1990 demonstrated a relationship between levels of activity of the enzyme epoxide hydrolase and the risk of FHS.[257] Toxic oxidative metabolites of phenytoin normally are removed by epoxide hydrolase, which appears to be regulated by a single gene with two allelic forms. The level of enzyme activity was measured using amniocytes obtained through amniocentesis. Fetuses of women with low activity of this enzyme appear to be at an increased risk from phenytoin. If further studies confirm these findings, this would be an example of an interaction between the mother's genetic predisposition and the environment (in this case, a drug). Two other AED, phenobarbital and carbamazepine, also are metabolized via this route.

A second proposed mechanism is altered folate concentration by AED. Phenytoin, carbamazepine, and barbiturates have been shown to decrease serum folate concentration. Valproic acid also decreases this by interfering with folate metabolism. Decreased folate concentration is correlated with an increased risk of developing NTD.[251,260,261]

CARCINOGENIC POTENTIAL

Phenytoin may be a human transplacental carcinogen: several tumors have been observed in children exposed to this drug during gestation.[208] The reported tumors are neuroblastoma (five cases), ganglioneuroblastoma (one case), melanotic neuroectodermal tumor (one case), extrarenal Wilms tumor (one case), mesenchymoma (one case), lymphangioma (one case), and ependymoblastoma (one case). Exposed children must be evaluated closely for several years because tumors may take that long to appear.

HEMORRHAGIC DISEASE OF THE NEWBORN

The use of phenytoin and other AED during the third trimester increases the risk of HDN.[208] Both early HDN (onset, 0–24 hours) and classic HDN (onset, 2–5 days) may occur in gestationally exposed infants. The hemorrhage is often life-threatening, with intracranial bleeding common. It is thought to result from phenytoin induction of fetal liver microsomal enzymes that further deplete the already low reserves of fetal vitamin K. Suppression of the vitamin K-dependent clotting factors, II, VII, IX, and X, results from the hypovitaminosis. Phenytoin-induced thrombocytopenia also may play a role in the bleeding. Vitamin K_1 (phytonadione) 1 mg should be given IM to the neonate at birth for prophylaxis against HDN.[250,258]

Teratogenicity of Nonhydantoin Antiepileptic Drugs

68. Do other AED offer an advantage over phenytoin in pregnancy?

For patients with generalized tonic–clonic seizures, the drugs that offer the most effective therapy are phenytoin, carbamazepine (Tegretol), and valproic acid (Depakene). Primidone (Mysoline), phenobarbital, and clonazepam (Klonopin) may be effective as alternative or adjunctive agents, whereas ethosuximide (Zarontin) and trimethadione (Tridione) are not indicated. Whether these AED offer any advantage over phenytoin depends on many variables, including fetal risks to drug exposure and the likelihood of maintaining seizure control if phenytoin were discontinued or another AED initiated.

CARBAMAZEPINE

Carbamazepine, an AED structurally related to the tricyclic antidepressants, has been used frequently in pregnancy. It was once thought to be the AED of choice because earlier reviews failed to demonstrate a relationship with congenital malformations.[262,263] Evidence since has linked carbamazepine to fetal abnormalities.[208,209] Numerous case reports and epidemiologic studies have been published involving carbamazepine-induced anomalies. Earlier reports described a pattern of malformations similar to FHS.[264] It has been postulated that carbamazepine and phenytoin may cause a similar pattern of fetal abnormalities because both are metabolized through the arene oxide pathway to produce an oxidative intermediate that is embryotoxic.[264,265] Matalon et al.[266] conducted a meta-analysis of 1,255 *in utero* exposures to carbamazepine that confirmed a 2.89 times increased risk of major congenital anomalies in exposed children compared with healthy controls. No significant difference in congenital anomalies was observed in untreated epileptic women compared with controls. Anomalies reported with carbamazepine include cardiac defects, urinary tract defects, craniofacial defects, cleft palate, fingernail hypoplasia, and low birthweight.[264,266,267] In addition, exposure to carbamazepine *in utero* carries a 0.5% to 1% risk of developing NTD, including spina bifida.[261,268] If possible, carbamazepine should be avoided in women with family histories of NTDs.[250]

VALPROIC ACID

In utero exposure to valproic acid is associated with a broad range of major and minor congenital anomalies often referred to as *fetal valproate syndrome* (FVS).[209,269] Abnormalities may involve craniofacial defects, organ malformations, and growth and developmental defects. In a review of 70 cases of valproic acid exposure, some of the more common features were small or broad nose (57%), small or abnormal ears (46%), long or flat philtrum (43%), and hypertelorism (27%).[269] Use of valproic acid during pregnancy is associated with a 1% to 2% risk of NTD, ranging from spina bifida to meningomyelocele.[208] Other major adverse fetal effects observed with this drug include craniofacial, cardiac, digital, skeletal and limb, urogenital, skin and muscle, and miscellaneous anomalies.[208] A small observational study of nine infants from mothers who received valproic acid during pregnancy suggests that valproic acid may cause immediate and long-term (evaluated at 6 years of age) neurologic dysfunction in some children.[270] If valproic acid must be used during pregnancy, the total dose should be divided over three or four administrations per day to avoid high plasma concentrations, because NTD may be dose dependent.[250,258,271] Dosages >1,000 mg/day may be associated with an increased risk of congenital anomalies.[269] As with carbamazepine, valproic acid should be avoided in women with a family history of NTD.[250] High serum concentration of the free fraction of valproic acid during labor and at birth may be responsible for a fetal or newborn toxicity consisting of fetal distress and low Apgar scores.[272] Because of the high incidence of teratogenicity, valproic acid does not offer any advantage over phenytoin in L.F.

PHENOBARBITAL

Phenobarbital often is used in combination with phenytoin, although it is used much less frequently as a single agent for the treatment of the type of seizures that L.F. has. Although a recognizable pattern of malformations, such as FHS, does not occur in epileptic women treated only with phenobarbital, some of the minor anomalies composing FHS are observed.[208] In three cases, women treated during the first trimester with only primidone, a structural analog of phenobarbital, bore infants with malformations similar to those with FHS. Another pharmacologically related AED is mephobarbital (Mebaral), which is partially demethylated by the liver to phenobarbital. The teratogenic potential of mephobarbital is unknown because information about its use during pregnancy is limited.[208]

All of these agents may induce maternal folic acid deficiency, a situation similar to that observed with phenytoin. Low folate concentration is linked to NTD. Hemorrhagic disease of the newborn has been reported after phenobarbital or primidone exposure and should be expected after mephobarbital use as well. The mechanism of this effect and its treatment are the same as that described for phenytoin.

In addition, barbiturate withdrawal has been observed in newborns exposed to phenobarbital during gestation. The average onset of symptoms was 6 days (range, 3–14 days) after birth, and withdrawal has been reported with daily doses as low as 64 mg.[208] Neonates should be monitored for withdrawal symptoms for 2 to 6 weeks because phenobarbital has a long elimination half-life (100 hours).[251] Recent data also suggest that infants exposed to phenobarbital *in utero* may experience some decline in cognitive performance.[258] Use of phenobarbital could be considered for L.F.; however, carbamazepine, valproic acid, and phenytoin are the preferred AED for tonic–clonic seizures.

ALTERNATIVE ANTIEPILEPTIC DRUGS

Experience with clonazepam as an AED is limited in human pregnancy. One infant exposed *in utero* and delivered prematurely at 36 weeks' gestation developed apnea, cyanosis, lethargy, and hypotonia at 6 hours of age.[273] Although congenital malformations were not evident, the toxic symptoms persisted for several days. Clonazepam usually is given in combination with other AED; hence, an increased rate of malformations caused by the agent would be difficult to detect. Thus, too little information is available to recommend this drug.

NEWER ANTIEPILEPTIC DRUGS

69. Several AED have been approved in the past few years. Have they been associated with teratogenicity, and do they offer any advantage over phenytoin for L.F.?

Most of the newer AED are approved as adjunctive therapy for partial seizures; currently, they are not first-line therapy for generalized tonic–clonic seizures. Their safety in women with epilepsy during pregnancy is yet to be determined because little information is available to assess their teratogenic potential.

Of the newer AED, preliminary pregnancy outcomes are available for lamotrigine (Lamictal). The manufacturer of lamotrigine, GlaxoSmithKline, initiated the International Lamotrigine Pregnancy Registry in 1992 to monitor the occurrence of major structural birth defects associated with *in utero* exposure to lamotrigine. As of September 30, 2001, birth outcomes for 389 pregnancies were prospectively collected and analyzed.[274] Of these, 168 infants were exposed to lamotrigine monotherapy. Three cases (1.8%) of major birth defects (esophageal malformation, cleft soft palate, right clubfoot) were observed. The occurrence of birth defects was higher in women on polytherapy, especially those who received lamotrigine and valproic acid (5 of 50; 10%). In comparison, the rate of major birth defects for infants exposed to lamotrigine polytherapy without valproic acid was 4.3% (5 of 116). Lamotrigine is rated pregnancy risk category C and has been found to cross the placenta in one case report.[275]

Other new AED available include felbamate (Felbatol), gabapentin (Neurontin), levetiracetam (Keppra), oxcarbazepine (Trileptal), tiagabine (Gabitril), topiramate (Topamax), and zonisamide (Zonegran). The teratogenic risk of these new agents has not been determined. They are rated pregnancy risk category C, and malformations have been reported in animals exposed to these agents.[276] The use of felbamate in any epileptic patient is limited because of the risk of aplastic anemia and acute liver failure. Until more data become available, these new AED do not appear to offer any advantage for L.F.

Reducing Fetal Risks

70. If L.F. chooses to become pregnant, what steps should her physician implement to lessen the risks of AED toxicity to her fetus?

Preconception planning with patient education is an extremely important component in epileptic women desiring to bear a child. Achieving good seizure control before conception is imperative. Although no clear consensus on the AED of choice during pregnancy has been reached, discontinuation of the agent should be considered in women who have been free of seizures for at least 2 to 5 years.[258] The dose should be tapered over 1 to 3 months. In patients for whom withdrawal is not an option, monotherapy is preferred, and the lowest effective dose of the appropriate AED should be used.[250,253,258] Because L.F. has had no seizure activity for the past 3 years, her phenytoin should be gradually discontinued before conception. If discontinuation is not an option, a careful reduction of her dose may be possible.

Close monitoring of phenytoin plasma concentrations is required during pregnancy to ensure maintenance of therapeutic levels and to help prevent seizures, which may increase the risk of fetal malformations. Consideration also should be given to changing L.F.'s drug therapy to another AED effective for tonic–clonic seizures. Any change to her regimen should be initiated and seizure control achieved before conception is attempted.

SUPPLEMENTAL FOLIC ACID

Folic acid deficiency increases the risk of NTD, such as spina bifida and anencephaly. The Medical Research Council (MRC) vitamin study evaluated the protective effects of folic acid in 1,817 pregnant women carrying fetuses at high risk for NTD.[277] High-dose folic acid (4 mg once daily), given from the date of randomization until 12 weeks of pregnancy, reduced the risk of NTD by 72%. Women with epilepsy were excluded from this study because of concerns that elevated folate concentrations might interfere with AED therapy. It is now recommended that all women of childbearing age take 0.4 mg folic acid as a daily supplement. Women at high risk of having a child with NTD should consult with their health care provider and consider supplementing with 4 mg folic acid daily from at least 1 month before conception through the first 3 months of pregnancy.[258,271] Because AED can significantly decrease folate concentrations, supplementation with folic acid 4 mg daily in epileptic women may be warranted to decrease the risk of NTD.

L.F. is at risk of having a child with NTD because of phenytoin therapy. The addition of folic acid 4 mg daily to her drug regimen should be considered, especially before conception and during the first 3 months of pregnancy.

Phenytoin in Breast Milk

71. If L.F. decides to breast-feed her newborn, would the use of phenytoin be expected to cause any problems?

Phenytoin is readily bioavailable after oral administration, but its high protein binding (95%) hinders its passage into breast milk.[239] The estimated M:P ratio of 0.13:0.45 is low.[230] Because an infant may receive about 5% of the maternal dose,[227] the AAP considers maternal use of phenytoin compatible with breast-feeding.[235] L.F. should be counseled on ways to reduce the risk of exposure (Table 46-9).

Isotretinoin

72. P.J., a 19-year-old woman with severe, recalcitrant nodular acne, has been treated with isotretinoin. After several months of therapy, P.J. suspects she is pregnant. What is the risk to P.J.'s fetus from isotretinoin exposure in early pregnancy?

Isotretinoin (Accutane), an isomer of vitamin A, was introduced in 1982 as a treatment for severe, recalcitrant nodular acne. The drug is rated pregnancy risk category X and is a known human teratogen.[276] Serious fetal abnormalities, including spontaneous abortion, can occur with any amounts, even for a short duration of use after conception. A recognized pattern of embryopathy is reported with isotretinoin,[209,276] which includes defects of the skull, ear (e.g., microtia or anotia), eye (e.g., microphthalmia), face, CNS, thymus, and cardiovascular system. Other adverse outcomes reported include cleft palate, rare limb defects, and low IQ scores.

To prevent unintended pregnancies in women, such as P.J., on isotretinoin, the manufacturer of Accutane established a more stringent prescribing program known as the System to Manage Accutane-Related Teratogenicity (SMART).[276] Both the physician and patient are required to follow the steps of this program before isotretinoin is prescribed and dispensed. In general, routine pregnancy avoidance counseling, regular pregnancy testing, and use of two forms of effective contraception are required. Pregnancy should be avoided for at least 1 month after stopping therapy. The health care provider should refer to the package insert and contact the manufacturer for details.

Isotretinoin must be discontinued immediately for P.J. She has a significant chance of spontaneously aborting her fetus. Should her pregnancy continue to term, the likelihood of delivering an infant with a major congenital malformation is high. Her health care provider must discuss these risks with P.J. and closely monitor her for adverse fetal outcomes. After this pregnancy, whether P.J. remains a candidate for isotretinoin must be carefully reassessed.

Tretinoin

73. If P.J. had been treated with topical retinoic acid (tretinoin), another vitamin A derivative used for acne vulgaris, would this have placed her fetus at risk?

Tretinoin, as with other retinoids, is a potent teratogen when taken systemically. Topical use, however, is associated with minimal risk because, at most, only about one-third of a topical dose is absorbed.[208] Assuming a 1-g/day application of a 0.1% preparation, this would amount to about one-seventh of the vitamin A activity received from a typical prenatal vitamin supplement. P.J.'s fetus would not have been at risk from this degree of exposure.

Antidepressants

Selective Serotonin Receptor Inhibitors (SSRI) Use in First Trimester

74. B.C. has been diagnosed with major depressive disorder since 3 years ago when she was started on oral fluoxetine 10 mg daily. She has recently had some sleep disturbances, decreased libido, and fatigue. Her dosage was increased to 20 mg daily a few months ago. Today, B.C. learns that she is pregnant at 6 weeks' gestation. The pregnancy was unplanned. B.C has recently heard in the news that paroxetine can affect the development of a baby's heart. Because she is on fluoxetine, she is worried that it may have the same effects. What effects do SSRI have on the developing fetus during the first trimester?

Clinical depression can affect up to 20% of pregnant women.[278] Depression during pregnancy can have adverse effects on the fetus and the mother if untreated. Pharmacotherapy is often needed in many cases. A recent study in 2006 showed an increase in relapse of major depression up to 68% in patients who discontinued their antidepressant medications during pregnancy compared with 26% of those who maintained treatment.[279] Possible effects of antidepressants on pregnancy outcome have not yet been established. Antidepressants used during pregnancy have been associated with preterm delivery, low birthweight, growth impairment, neonatal toxicity, and physical and behavioral teratogenicity.[278]

Selective serotonin receptor inhibitors (e.g., fluoxetine, fluvoxamine, paroxetine, sertraline, escitalopram, and citalopram) are the most common antidepressants used in pregnancy. Although all the SSRI share a similar mechanism of action, their chemical structures differ.[33] These differences may also confer differences on pregnancy outcomes but further studies are needed to define the effects.

Recent studies have suggested that paroxetine may be associated with a small but significant increase in congenital malformations. Two epidemiologic studies found that paroxetine use during the first trimester increased the risk for congenital malformations 1.8 times and increased the risk for cardiac defects 1.5 to 2.0 times.[280] Doses of paroxetine above 25 mg/day were more likely associated with major malformations and cardiac defects.[281] In December 2005, the FDA changed the pregnancy category for paroxetine from C to D and advised that it should be avoided if possible in the first trimester of pregnancy.[282] Two case control studies published in 2007 found that the absolute risk of any birth defects from paroxetine and other SSRI is small.[283,284] The absolute risk for right ventricular outflow tract obstruction defects and all congenital heart defects would probably not exceed 1% and 2% respectively.[285]

Because B.C. has a history of major depressive disorder that has been well controlled on fluoxetine, she should continue on her antidepressant because she may be at high risk for relapse of a major depressive episode if she discontinues treatment. Fluoxetine, the most studied SSRI in pregnancy, was not associated with an increased risk of cardiac anomalies.[278,283,284] The risk of fetal harm must be weighed against the possible risk of untreated depression. The decision to continue or start antidepressants during pregnancy must be made on a case-by-case basis that involves a thorough discussion examining the risks.

Effect of SSRI in Third Trimester and in the Neonate

75. What are some risks to the fetus associated with SSRI use in third trimester and in the neonate after delivery?

Exposure to SSRI's use after 20 weeks' gestation was associated with persistent pulmonary hypertension in the newborn (PPHN). A case control study in 2006 found the absolute risk to be about 1%.[286] Developmental toxicities are also associated with SSRI use during pregnancy, including spontaneous abortions, low birth-weight, premature delivery, poor neonatal adaptation syndrome, and possible long-term neurocognitive effects.[278]

ACKNOWLEDGMENT

The author acknowledges Gerald G. Briggs, B.Pharm., for his contributions to this chapter in earlier editions.

REFERENCES

1. Mathews TJ et al. Infant mortality statistics from the 2004 period linked birth/infant death data set. *National vital statistics reports*, vol 52 no. 15. Hyattsville, MD: National Center for Health Statistics; 2007.
2. Cunningham FG et al, eds. Obstetrics in broad perspective. In: *Williams Obstetrics.* New York: McGraw-Hill; 2001: 3.
3. Cunningham FG et al., eds. The placenta and fetal membranes. In: *Williams Obstetrics.* New York: McGraw-Hill; 2001: 95.
4. Craven C, Ward K. Embryo, fetus, and placenta: normal and abnormal. In: Scott JR et al., eds. *Danforth's Obstetrics and Gynecology.* Philadelphia: Lippincott Williams & Wilkins; 1999: 29.
5. Cunningham FG et al., eds. The endometrium and decidua: menstruation and pregnancy. In: *Williams Obstetrics.* New York: McGraw-Hill; 2001: 69.
6. Buster JE et al. Endocrinology and diagnosis of pregnancy. In: Gabbe SG et al., eds. *Obstetrics: Normal and Problem Pregnancies.* New York: Churchill Livingstone; 1996: 31.
7. Lockwood CJ et al. Preeclampsia and hypertensive disorders. In: Cohen WR, ed. *Cherry and Merkatz's Complications of Pregnancy.* Philadelphia: Lippincott Williams & Wilkins; 2000: 207.
8. Cunningham FG et al., eds. Fetal growth and development. In: *Williams Obstetrics.* New York: McGraw-Hill; 2001: 129
9. Cunningham FG et al., eds. Pregnancy: overview, organization, and diagnosis. In: *Williams Obstetrics.* New York: McGraw-Hill; 2001: 15.
10. Farrington PF et al. Normal labor, delivery, and puerperium. In: Scott JR et al., eds. *Danforth's Obstetrics and Gynecology.* Philadelphia: Lippincott Williams & Wilkins; 1999: 91.
11. Rosenthal WM et al. Home testing and monitoring devices. In: Young LL, ed. *Handbook of Nonprescription Drugs.* Washington: American Pharmaceutical Association; 2002: 1017.
12. Cunningham FG et al., eds. Prenatal care. In: *Williams Obstetrics.* New York: McGraw-Hill; 2001: 221.
13. Frederiksen MC. Physiologic changes in pregnancy and their effect on drug disposition. *Semin Perinatol* 2001;25:120.
14. Loebstein R et al. Clinical relevance of therapeutic drug monitoring during pregnancy. *Ther Drug Monit* 2002;24:15.
15. Little BB. Pharmacokinetics during pregnancy: evidence-based maternal dose formulation. *Obstet Gynecol* 199;93:858.
16. McAuley JW et al. Treatment of epilepsy in women of reproductive age. Pharmacokinetic considerations. *Clin Pharmacokinet* 2002;41:559.
17. Anderson G. Pregnancy-induced changes in pharmacokinetics: a mechanistic-based approach. *Clin Pharmacokinet* 2005;44:989.
18. Harris RZ et al. Gender effects in pharmacokinetics and pharmacodynamics. *Drugs* 1995;50:222.
19. Bowers D et al. Clinical laboratory referent values. In: Cohen WR, ed. *Cherry and Merkatz's Complications of Pregnancy.* Philadelphia: Lippincott Williams & Wilkins; 2000: 873.
20. Worthington-Roberts BS. Nutrition. In: Cohen WR, ed. *Cherry and Merkatz's Complications of Pregnancy.* 5th ed. Philadelphia: Lippincott Williams & Wilkins; 2000: 17.
21. National Research Council. Trace elements. In: *Recommended Dietary Allowances.* Washington, DC: National Academy Press; 1989: 195.
22. Cunningham FG et al., eds. Hematological disorders. Prenatal care. In: *Williams Obstetrics.* New York: McGraw-Hill; 2001: 1307.
23. Czeizel AE et al. Prevention of the first occurrence of neural-tube defects by periconceptional vitamin supplementation. *N Engl J Med* 1992;327: 1832.
24. Centers for Disease Control and Prevention. Recommendations for the use of folic acid to reduce the number of cases of spina bifida and other neural tube defects. *Morbid Mortal Wkly Rep* 1992; 41:RR-14.
25. Centers for Disease Control and Prevention. Neural tube defect surveillance and folic acid intervention—Texas-Mexico border, 1993–1998. *Morbid Mortal Wkly Rep* 2000;49:1.
26. Centers for Disease Control and Prevention. Use of folic acid for prevention of spina bifida and other neural tube defects—1983–1991. *Morbid Mortal Wkly Rep* 1991;40:513.
27. Magee LA et al. Evidence-based view of safety and effectiveness of pharmacologic therapy for nausea and vomiting of pregnancy. *Am J Obstet Gynecol* 2002;186:s256.
28. Badell ML et al. Treatment options for nausea and vomiting during pregnancy. *Pharmacotherapy* 2006;26(9):1273.
29. ACOG Practice Bulletin. Nausea and vomiting of Pregnancy. *Obstet Gynecol* 2004;52:803.
30. Nelson-Piercy C. Treatment of nausea and vomiting in pregnancy: when should it be treated and what can be safely taken? *Drug Saf* 1998;19:155.
31. McKeigue PM et al. Bendetin and birth defects: a meta-analysis of the epidemiologic studies. *Teratology* 1994;50:27.
32. Seto A et al. Pregnancy outcome following first trimester exposure to antihistamines: meta-analysis. *Am J Perinatol* 1997;14:119.
33. Briggs GG et al., eds. *Drugs in Pregnancy and Lactation.* 7th ed. Philadelphia: Lippincott William & Williams; 2005.
34. Richter JE. The management of heartburn in pregnancy. *Aliment Pharmacol Ther* 2005;22:749.
35. Anonymous. ACOG practice bulletin. Management of alloimmunization during pregnancy. *Obstet Gynecol* 2006;108:457.
36. Moise KJ. Hemolytic disease of the fetus and newborn. In: Creasy RK et al., eds. *Maternal-Fetal Medicine: Principles and Practice.* Philadelphia: WB Saunders; 2004: 537.
37. Ascari WQ et al. Incidence of maternal Rh immunization by ABO compatible and incompatible pregnancies. *BMJ* 1969;1:399.
38. Bowman JM et al. Rh isoimmunization during pregnancy: antenatal prophylaxis. *Can Med Assoc J* 1978;118;623.
39. Anonymous. ACOG practice bulletin. Prevention of Rh D alloimmunization. *Int J Gynecol Obstet* 1999;66:63.
40. Samson D et al. Effect on primary Rh immunization of delayed administration of anti-Rh. *Immunology* 1975;28:349.
41. Jabara S. Is Rh immune globulin needed in early first-trimester abortion? A review. *Am J Obstet Gynecol* 2003;188:623.
42. Cunningham FG et al., eds. Diabetes. In: *Williams Obstetrics.* New York: McGraw-Hill; 2005: 1359.
43. Pregestational diabetes mellitus. ACOG Practice Bulletin No. 60. American College of Obstetricians and Gynecologists. *Obstet Gynecol* 2005;105:675.
44. Martin JA et al. Expanded health data from the new birth certificate, 2004. *National vital statistics reports*; vol 55 no 12. Hyattsville, MD: National Center for Health Statistics; 2007.
45. Garner P. Type I diabetes mellitus and pregnancy. *Lancet* 1995;346:157.
46. White P. Classification of obstetric diabetes. *Am J Obstet Gynecol* 1978;130:228.
47. American Diabetes Association. Preconceptional care of women with diabetes. *Diabetes Care* 2003;26:S91.
48. Diabetes Control and Complications Trial Research Group. Obstetrics: pregnancy outcomes in the diabetes control and complications trial. *Am J Obstet Gynecol* 1996;174:1343.
49. Homko CJ et al. Ambulatory care of the pregnant woman with diabetes. *Clin Obstet Gynecol* 1998;41:584.
50. Greene MF et al. First-trimester hemoglobin A, and risk for major malformation and spontaneous abortion in diabetic pregnancy. *Teratology* 1989;39:225.
51. Cooper WO et al. Major congential malformations after first-trimester exposure to ACE inhibitors. *N Engl J Med* 2006;354:2443.
52. Homko CJ et al. Insulins and oral hypoglycemic agents in pregnancy. *J Matern Fetal Neonat Med* 2006;19(11):679.
53. Jovanovic L et al. Metabolic and immunologic effects of insulin lispro in gestational diabetes. *Diabetes Care* 1999;22:1422.
54. Brown FM et al. Metformin in pregnancy: its time has not yet come [Letter]. *Diabetes Care* 2006;29:485.
55. American Diabetes Association. Gestational diabetes mellitus. *Diabetes Care* 2003;26:S103.
56. Kjos SL et al. Gestational diabetes mellitus. *N Engl J Med* 1999;341:1749.
57. Gestational Diabetes. ACOG Practice Bulletin No. 30. American College of Obstetricians and Gynecologists. *Obstet Gynecol* 2001;98:525.

58. Brody SC et al. Screening for gestational diabetes: A summary of the evidence for the U.S. Preventive Services Task Force. *Obstet Gynecol* 2003;101:380.
59. Langer O et al. A comparison of glyburide and insulin in women with gestational diabetes mellitus. *N Engl J Med* 2000;343:1134.
60. Chmait R et al. Prospective observational study to establish predictors of glyburide success in women with gestational diabetes mellitus. *J Perinatol* 2004;24:617.
61. National High Blood Pressure Education Program Working Group report on high blood pressure in pregnancy. Report of the national High Blood Pressure Education Program Working Group on high blood pressure in pregnancy. *Am J Obstet Gynecol* 2000;183(Suppl):S1.
62. Wildman K et al. Maternal mortality as an indicator of obstetric care in Europe. *BJOG* 2004;111:164.
63. Chang J et al. Pregnancy-related mortality surveillance—United States, 1991–1999. *MMWR CDC Surveill Summ* 2003;52:1.
64. Anonymous. ACOG practice bulletin. Diagnosis and management of preeclampsia and eclampsia. *Obstet Gynecol* 2002;99:159.
65. Sibai BM. Treatment of hypertension in pregnant women. *N Engl J Med* 1996;335:257.
66. Anonymous. ACOG practice bulletin. Chronic hypertension in pregnancy. *Obstet Gynecol* 2001;98:177.
67. Roberts JM. Pregnancy-related hypertension. In: Creasy RK et al., eds. *Maternal-Fetal Medicine.* Philadelphia: WB Saunders; 2004: 859.
68. Sibai B et al. Pre-eclampsia. *Lancet* 2005;365:785.
69. Caritis S et al. Low-dose aspirin to prevent preeclampsia in women at high risk. *N Engl J Med* 1998;338:701.
70. Chobian AV et al. The Seventh Report of the Joint National Committee on Prevention, Detection, Evaluation, and Treatment of High Blood Pressure. *Hypertension* 2003;42:1206.
71. von Dadelszen P et al. Fall in mean arterial pressure and fetal growth restriction in pregnancy hypertension: a meta-analysis. *Lancet* 2000;355:87.
72. Abalos AE. Antihypertensive drug therapy for mild to moderate hypertension during pregnancy. *Cochrane Database Syst Rev* 2003;1:1.
73. Kyle PM et al. Comparative risk-benefit assessment of drugs used in the management of hypertension in pregnancy. *Drug Saf* 1992;7:222.
74. Dekker GA et al. Etiology and pathogenesis of preeclampsia: current concepts. *Am J Obstet Gynecol* 1998;179:1359.
75. Patrick T et al. Current concepts in preeclampsia. *MCN Am J Matern Child Nurs* 1999;24;193.
76. Mabie WC. Management of acute severe hypertension and encephalopathy. *Clin Obstet Gynecol* 1999;42:519.
77. Magee LA et al. Risks and benefits of β-receptor blockers for pregnancy hypertension: overview of the randomized trials. *Eur J Obstet Gynecol Reprod Biol* 2000;8:15.
78. Belfort MA et al. Labetalol decreases cerebral perfusion pressure without negatively affecting cerebral blood flow in hypertensive gravidas. *Hypertens Pregnancy* 2002;21:185.
79. Magee LA et al. Hydralazine for treatment of severe hypertension in pregnancy: meta-analysis. *BMJ* 2003;327:955.
80. Vigil-De Gracia P et al. Severe hypertension in pregnancy: hydralazine or labetalol a randomized clinical trial. *Eur J Obstet Gynecol Repro Biol* 2006;128:157.
81. Idama TO et al. Magnesium sulphate: a review of clinical pharmacology applied to obstetrics. *Br J Obstet Gynaecol* 1998;105:260.
82. Vermillion ST et al. A randomized, double-blind trial of oral nifedipine and intravenous labetalol in hypertensive emergencies of pregnancy. *Am J Obstet Gynecol* 1999;181:858.
83. Scardo JA et al. A randomized, double-blind, hemodynamic evaluation of nifedipine and labetalol in preeclamptic hypertensive emergencies. *Am J Obstet Gynecol* 1999;181:862.
84. Lucas MJ et al. A comparison of magnesium sulfate with phenytoin for the prevention of eclampsia. *N Engl J Med* 1995;333:201.
85. Magpie Trial Collaborative Group. Do women with pre-eclampsia, and their babies, benefit from magnesium sulphate? The Magpie Trial: a randomized placebo-controlled trial. *Lancet* 2002;359:1877.
86. Alexander JM et al. Selective magnesium sulfate prophylaxis for the prevention of eclampsia in women with gestational hypertension. *Obstet Gynecol* 2006;108:826.
87. Belfort MA et al. A comparison of magnesium sulfate and nimodipine for the prevention of eclampsia. *N Engl J Med* 2003;348:304.
88. Witlin AG. Prevention and treatment of eclamptic convulsions. *Clin Obstet Gynecol* 1999;42: 507.
89. Sibai BM et al. Reassessment of intravenous $MgSO_4$ therapy in preeclampsia-eclampsia. *Obstet Gynecol* 1981;57:199.
90. Kohn, LT et al. *To err is human: building a safer health system.* Washington, DC: Institute of Medicine and the National Academy Press; 1999.
91. Simpson KR et al. Obstetrical accidents involving intravenous magnesium sulfate. *MCN Am J Matern Child Nurs* 2004;29:161.
92. The Eclampsia Trial Collaborative Group. Which anticonvulsant for women with eclampsia? Evidence from the collaborative eclampsia trial. *Lancet* 1995;345:1455.
93. Isler CM et al. Postpartum seizure prophylaxis: using maternal clinical paramenters to guide therapy. *Obstet Gynecol* 2003;101:66.
94. Norwitz ER et al. The control of labor. *N Engl J Med* 1999;341:660.
95. Farrington PF et al. Normal labor, delivery, and puerperium. In: *Danforth's Obstetrics and Gynecology.* Philadelphia: Lippincott Williams & Wilkins; 1999: 91.
96. Anonymous. ACOG technical bulletin. Induction of labor. *Int J Gynecol Obstet* 1996;53:65.
97. Anonymous. ACOG practice patterns. Management of postterm pregnancy. *Int J Gynecol Obstet* 1997;60:86.
98. Laube DW. Induction of labor. *Clin Obstet Gynecol* 1997;40:485.
99. NIH Consensus Development Panel on the Effect of Corticosteroids for fetal Maturation on Perinatal Outcomes. Effect of corticosteroids for fetal maturation on perinatal outcomes. *JAMA* 1995;273: 413.
100. Riskin-Mashiah S et al. Cervical ripening. *Obstet Gynecol Clin North Am* 1999;26:243.
101. Xenakis EMJ et al. Induction of labor in the nineties: conquering the unfavorable cervix. *Obstet Gynecol* 1997;90:235.
102. Rayburn WF. Prostaglandin E_2 gel for cervical ripening and induction of labor: a critical analysis. *Am J Obstet Gynecol* 1989;160:529.
103. Witter FR et al. A randomized trial of prostaglandin E_2 in a controlled-release vaginal pessary for cervical ripening at term. *Am J Obstet Gynecol* 1992;166:830.
104. Rayburn WF et al. An intravaginal controlled-release prostaglandin E_2 pessary for cervical ripening and initiation of labor at term. *Obstet Gynecol* 1992;79:374.
105. Cervidil package insert. St. Louis, MO: Forrest Pharmaceuticals, Inc; 1997.
106. Prepidil Gel package insert. Kalamazoo, MI: Pharmacia & Upjohn Company; 1999.
107. Chyu JK et al. Prostaglandin E_2 for cervical ripening: a randomized comparison of Cervidil versus Prepidil. *Am J Obstet Gynecol* 1997;177;606.
108. Cohen HE, ed. *Drug Topics Red Book.* Montvale, NJ: Thomson Medical Economics Company; 2002.
109. Anonymous. ACOG committee opinion. Monitoring during induction of labor with dinoprostone. *Int J Gynecol Obstet* 1999;64:200.
110. Shyken JM et al. The use of oxytocin. *Clin Perinatol* 1995;22:907
111. Ottinger WS et al. A randomized clinical trial of prostaglandin E_2 intracervical gel and slow release vaginal pessary for preinduction cervical ripening. *Am J Obstet Gynecol* 1998;179:349.
112. Sanchez-Ramos L et al. Misoprostol for cervical ripening and labor induction: a meta-analysis. *Obstet Gynecol* 1997;89:633.
113. Hofmeyr GJ et al. Vaginal misoprostol for cervical ripening and induction of labour. *Cochrane Database Syst Rev* 2003;3:1.
114. Wing DA, A benefit-risk assessment of misoprostol for cervical ripening and labour induction. *Drug Saf* 2002;25:665.
115. Blanchette HA et al. Comparison of the safety and efficacy of intravaginal misoprostol (prostaglandin E_1) with those of dinoprostone (prostaglandin E_2) for cervical ripening and induction of labor in a community hospital. *Am J Obstet Gynecol* 1999;180:1551.
116. Sanchez-Ramos L et al. Labor induction with prostaglandin E_1 misoprostol compared with dinoprostone vaginal insert: a randomized trial. *Obstet Gynecol* 1998;91:401.
117. Wing DA et al. A comparison of orally administered misoprostol with vaginally administered misoprostol for cervical ripening and labor induction. *Am J Obstet Gynecol* 1999;180:1155.
118. Wing DA. Labor induction with misoprostol. *Am J Obstet Gynecol* 1999;181:339.
119. Dudley DJ. Complications of labor. In: Scott JR et al., eds. *Danforth's Obstetrics and Gynecology.* Philadelphia: Lippincott Williams & Wilkins; 1999: 437.
120. Anonymous. ACOG technical bulletin. Dystocia and the augmentation of labor. *Int J Gynecol* 1996;53:73.
121. Dudley DJ. Oxytocin: use and abuse, science and art. *Clin Obstet Gynecol* 1997;40:516.
122. Perry RL et al. The pharmacokinetics of oxytocin as they apply to labor induction. *Am J Obstet Gynecol* 1996;174:1590.
123. Satin AJ et al. High-dose oxytocin: 20-versus 40-minute dosage interval. *Obstet Gynecol* 1994;83:234.
124. Satin AJ et al. High- versus low-dose oxytocin for labor stimulation. *Obstet Gynecol* 1992;80:111.
125. Xenakis EMJ et al. Low-dose versus high-dose oxytocin augmentation of labor—a randomized trial. *Am J Obstet Gynecol* 1995;173:1874.
126. Ripley DL. Uterine emergencies. atony, inversion, and rupture. *Obstet Gynecol Clin North Am* 1999;26:419.
127. Cohen WR. Postpartum hemorrhage and hemorrhagic shock. In: Cohen WR, ed. *Cherry and Merkatz's Complications of Pregnancy.* Philadelphia: Lippincott Williams & Wilkins; 2000: 803.
128. Alamia V et al. Peripartum hemorrhage. *Obstet Gynecol Clin North Am* 1999;26:385.
129. Cunningham FG et al., eds. *Conduct of normal labor and delivery. In Williams Obstetrics.* New York: McGraw-Hill; 2001: 309.
130. Khan RU et al. Pharmacokinetics and adverse-effect profile of rectally administered misoprostol in the third stage of labor. *Obstet Gynecol* 2003;101:968.
131. Caliskan E et al. Oral misoprostol for the third stage of labor: a randomized controlled trial. *Obstet Gynecol* 2003;101:921.
132. Gulmezoglu, AM et al. WHO multicentre randomized trial of misoprostol in the management of the third stage of labour. *Lancet* 2001;358:689.
133. Ergonovine maleate/Methylergonovine maleate. In: McEvoy G, ed. *AHFS Drug Information.* Bethesda, MD: American Society of Health-System Pharmacists: 2003: 3098.
134. O'Brien WF. The role of prostaglandins in labor and delivery. *Clin Perinatol* 1995;22:973.
135. Pharmacia & Upjohn Company. Hemabate package insert. Kalamazoo, MI: Pharmacia & Upjohn Company; 1999.
136. Blum J et al. Treatment of postpartum

hemorrhage with misoprostol. *Int J Gynaecol Obstet* 2007;99:S202.
137. Hamilton BE et al. Births: preliminary data for 2005. National Vital Statistics Reports; Vol 55 no. 11. Hyattsville, MD: National Center for Health Statistics; 2007.
138. Ananth C et al. Trends in preterm birth and perinatal mortality among singletons: United States, 1989 through 2000. *Obstet Gynecol* 2005;105:1084.
139. Goldenberg RL et al. Intrauterine infection and preterm delivery. *N Engl J Med* 2000;342:1500.
140. Esplin MS. Preterm birth: a review of genetic factors and future directions for genetic study. *Obstet Gynecol Surv* 2006;61:800.
141. Iams JD et al. Preterm labor and delivery. In: Creasy RK et al., eds. *Maternal-Fetal Medicine.* Philadelphia: WB Saunders; 2004: 623.
142. Smith R. Parturition. *N Engl J Med* 2007;356:271.
143. Anonymous. ACOG practice bulletin. Assessment of risk factors for preterm birth. *Obstet Gynecol* 2001;98:709.
144. Simhan HN et al. Prevention of preterm delivery. *N Engl J Med* 2007;357:477.
145. Anonymous. ACOG practice bulletin. Management of preterm labor. *Obstet Gynecol* 2003;101:1039.
146. Anonymous. ACOG committee opinion. Antenatal corticosteroid therapy for fetal maturation. *Obstet Gynecol* 2002: 99:871.
147. Crowther CA et al. Magnesium sulphate for preventing preterm birth in threatened preterm labour. *Cochrane Database Syst Rev* 2002;4:CD001060.
148. Berkman ND et al. Tocolytic treatment for the management of preterm labor: a review of the evidence. *Am J Obstet Gynecol* 2003;188:1648.
149. Lewis DF. Magnesium sulfate: the first-line tocolytic. *Obstet Gynecol Clin North Am* 2005;32: 485.
150. Lewis DF et al. Successful magnesium sulfate tocolysis: is "weaning" the drug necessary? *Am J Obstet Gynecol* 1997;177:742.
151. Goldenberg RL. The management of preterm labor. *Obstet Gynecol* 2002;100:1020.
152. Crowther CA et al. Effect of magnesium sulfate given for neuroprotection before preterm birth: a randomized controlled trial. *JAMA* 2003;290:2669.
153. The Canadian Preterm Labor Investigators Group. Treatment of preterm labor with the beta-adrenergic agonist ritodrine. *N Engl J Med* 1992; 327:308.
154. Anotayanonth S. et al. Betamimetics for inhibiting preterm labour. *Cochrane Database Syst Rev* 2004;4:CD004352.
155. King J et al. Cyclo-oxygenase (COX) inhibitors for treating preterm labour. *Cochrane Database Syst Rev* 2005;2:CD001992.
156. Macones GA. The controversy surrounding indomethacin for tocolysis. *Am J Obstet Gynecol* 2001;184:264.
157. Iannucci TA et al. Effect of dual tocolysis on the incidence of severe intraventricular hemorrhage among extremely low-birth-weight infants. *Am J Obstet Gynecol* 1996;175:1043.
158. Norton ME et al. Neonatal complications after the administration of indomethacin for preterm labor. *N Engl J Med* 1995;329:1602.
159. Loe SM et al. Assessing the neonatal safety of indomethacin tocolysis. A systematic review with meta-analysis. *Obstet Gynecol* 2005;106:173.
160. Stika CS et al. A prospective randomized safety trial of celecoxib for treatment of preterm labor. *Am J Obstet Gynecol* 2002;187:653.
161. Sawdy RJ. A double-blind randomized study of fetal side effects during and after the short-term maternal administration of indomethacin, sulindac, and nimesulide for the treatment of preterm labor. *Am J Obstet Gynecol* 2003;188:1046.
162. King JF et al. Calcium channel blockers for inhibiting preterm labour. *Cochrane Database Syst Rev* 2003;1:CD002255.
163. Lyell D et al. Magnesium sulfate compared with nifedipine for acute tocolysis of preterm labor. A randomized controlled trial. *Obstet Gynecol* 2007;110:61.
164. Glock JL et al. Efficacy and safety of nifedipine versus magnesium in the management of preterm labor: a randomized study. *Am J Obstet Gynecol* 1993;169:960.
165. Papatsonis DNM et al. Nifedipine and ritodrine in the management of preterm labor: a randomized multicenter trial. *Obstet Gynecol* 1997;90:230.
166. Guinn DA et al. Terbutaline pump maintenance therapy for prevention of preterm delivery: a double-blind trial. *Am J Obstet Gynecol* 1998;179:874.
167. Perry KG Jr et al. Incidence of adverse cardiopulmonary effects with low-dose continuous terbutaline infusion. *Am J Obstet Gynecol* 1995; 173:1273.
168. Nanda K et al. Terbutaline pump maintenance therapy after threatened preterm labor for preventing preterm birth. *Cochrane Database Syst Rev* 2002;4:CD003933.
169. Dodd JM et al. Oral betamimetics for maintenance therapy after threatened preterm labour. *Cochrane Database Syst Rev* 2006;1:CD003927.
170. Carr DB et al. Maintenance oral nifedipine for preterm labor: a randomized clinical trial. *Am J Obstet Gynecol* 1999;181:822.
171. Gaunekar NN et al. Maintenance therapy with calcium channel blockers for preventing preterm birth after threatened preterm labour. *Cochrane Database System Rev* 2005;3:CD004071.
172. Thornton JG. Maintenance tocolysis. *BJOG* 2005;112:118.
173. Roberts D et al. Antenatal corticosteroids for accelerating fetal lung maturation for women at risk of preterm birth. *Cochrane Database Syst Rev* 2006;3:CD004454.
174. Baud O et al. Antenatal glucocorticoid treatment and cystic periventricular leukomalacia in very premature infants. *N Engl J Med* 1999;341:1190.
175. Chen B et al. Antenatal corticosteroids in preterm premature rupture of membranes. *Clin Obstet Gynecol* 1998;41:832.
176. Anonymous. ACOG practice bulletin. Assessment of risk factors for preterm birth. *Obstet Gynecol* 2001: 98:709.
177. Goldenberg RL et al. Medical progress: prevention of premature birth. *N Engl J Med* 1998;339:313.
178. Hauth JC et al. Reduced incidence of preterm delivery with metronidazole and erythromycin in women with bacterial vaginosis. *N Engl Med* 1995;333;1732.
179. McDonald HM et al. Antibiotics for treating bacterial vaginosis in pregnancy. *Cochrane Database Syst Rev* 2007;1:CD000262.
180. Carey JC et al. Metronidazole to prevent preterm delivery in pregnant women with asymptomatic bacterial vaginosis. *N Engl J Med* 2000;342:534.
181. Gibbs RS et al. Use of antibiotics to prevent preterm birth. *Am J Obstet Gynecol* 1997;177:375.
182. Mercer BM et al. Antibiotic therapy for reduction of infant morbidity after preterm premature rupture of the membranes. *JAMA* 1997;278:989.
183. Kenyon S. Antibiotics for preterm rupture of membranes. *Cochrane Database Syst Rev* 2003;2:CD001058.
184. Centers for Disease Control and Prevention. Prevention of perinatal group B streptococcal disease: a public health perspective. *Morbid Mortal Wkly Rep* 1996;45(No. RR-7):1.
185. Schrag SJ et al. A population-based comparison of strategies to prevent early onset group B streptococcal disease in neonates. *N Engl J Med* 2002;347:233.
186. Schrag S. Prevention of perinatal group B streptococcal disease. Revised guideline from CDC. *MMWR Recomm Rep* 2002;51:1.
187. Schardein JL. *Chemically Induced Birth Defects.* 3rd ed. New York: Marcel Dekker: 2000.
188. Collaborative Group on Drug Use in Pregnancy. Medication during pregnancy: an intercontinental cooperative study. *Int J Gynecol Obstet* 1992;39:185.
189. American College of Obstetricians and Gynecologists. Teratology. ACOG Educational Bulletin 236. Washington, DC: ACOG; 1997.
190. Kalter H et al. Congenital malformations. Etiologic factors and their role in prevention. Part I. *N Engl J Med* 1983;308:424.
191. Mathews TJ et al. Infant mortality statistics from the 1999 period linked birth/infant death data set. *National Vital Statistics Reports*, Vol. 50, no. 4. Hyattsville, MD: National Center for Health Statistics; 2002.
192. Economic costs of birth defects and cerebral palsy—United States, 1992. *MMWR* 1995;44:694.
193. National Research Council. *Scientific Frontiers in Developmental Toxicology and Risk Assessment.* Washington, DC: National Academy Press; 2000.
194. Brent RL et al. Clinical and basic science lessons from the thalidomide tragedy: what have we learned about the causes of limb defects? *Teratology* 1998;38:241–251.
195. O'Rahilly R et al., eds. *Human Embryology & Teratology*. 3rd ed. New York: Wily-Liss; 2001.
196. Carter CO. Genetics of common single malformations. *Br Med Bull* 1976;32:21.
197. Beckman DA et al. Mechanism of known environmental teratogens: drugs and chemicals. *Clin Perinatol* 1986;13:649.
198. Seaver LH et al. Teratology in pediatric practice. *Pediatr Clin North Am* 1992;39:111.
199. Shepard TH. *Catalog of Teratogenic Agents.* 10th ed. Baltimore: Johns Hopkins University Press; 2001.
200. Polin RA et al., eds. *Fetal and Neonatal Physiology*. 2nd ed. Philadelphia: WB Saunders; 1998.
201. Shepard TH. Teratogenicity of therapeutic agents. *Curr Prob Pediatr* 1979;10:1.
202. Fabro S et al. Chemical exposure of embryos during the preimplantation stages of pregnancy: mortality rate and intrauterine development. *Am J Obstet Gynecol* 1984;148:929.
203. Koren G et al. Major malformations with valproic acid. *Can Fam Physician* 2006;52:441.
204. Scialli AR et al. *Birth Defects Res (Part A)* 2004;70:7–12.
205. Polifka JE et al. Clinical teratology: identifying teratogenic risks in humans. *Clin Genet* 1999;56:409–420.
206. Buehler BA et al. Prenatal prediction of risk of the fetal hydantoin syndrome. *N Engl J Med* 1990;322:1567–1572.
207. Nishimura H et al. *Clinical Aspects of the Teratogenicity of Drugs.* New York: American Elsevier; 1976.
208. Briggs GG et al. Drugs in Pregnancy and Lactation. A Reference Guide to Fetal and Neonatal Risk, 7th ed. Philadelphia: Lippincott Williams & Wilkins; 2005.
209. Heitland G et al., eds. *REPRORISK System.* MICROMEDEX, Greenwood Village, CO: Pharmacia & Upjohn Company. (Edition expires 6/2003).
210. Koren G et al. Drugs in pregnancy. *N Engl J Med* 1998;338:1128.
211. Koren G ed. *Maternal-Fetal Toxicology: A Clinician's Guide.* New York: Marcel Dekker; 1990.
212. Lawrence RA. Anatomy of the human breast. In: *Breastfeeding: A Guide for the Medical Profession*. 4th ed. St. Louis: Mosby-Year Book; 1994:37.
213. Neville MC et al. Effects of drugs on milk secretion and composition. In: Bennett PN, ed. *Drugs and Human Lactation*. 2nd ed. New York: Elsevier Science; 1996: 15.
214. Ehrenkranz RA et al. Metoclopramide effect on faltering milk production by mothers of premature infants. *Pediatrics* 1986;78:614.
215. Gupta AP et al. Metoclopramide as a lactagogue. *Clin Pediatr* 1985;24:269.
216. Kauppila A et al. A dose response relation between improved lactation and metoclopramide. *Lancet* 1981;1:1175.

217. Toppare MF et al. Metoclopramide for breast milk production. *Nutr Res* 1994;14:1019.
218. Kauppila A et al. Metoclopramide and breast feeding: efficacy and anterior pituitary responses of the mother and the child. *Eur J Obstet Gynecol Reprod Biol* 1985;19:19.
219. Spitz A. Treatment for lactation suppression: little progress in one hundred years. *Am J Obstet Gynecol* 1998;179:1485.
220. Lawrence RA. Breastfeeding and medical disease. *Med Clin North Am* 1989;73:583.
221. American Academy of Pediatrics. Breastfeeding and the use of human milk. *Pediatrics* 1997; 100:1035.
222. Zembo CT. Breastfeeding. *Obstet Gynecol Clin North Am* 2002;29:51.
223. Mortensen EL et al. The association between duration of breastfeeding and adult intelligence. *JAMA* 2002;287:2365.
224. National Center for Health Statistics. *Healthy People 2010 Final Review.* Hyattsville, MD: Public Health Service; 2004.
225. Wilson JT, ed. *Drugs in Breast Milk.* Sydney: ADIS Press; 1981.
226. Anderson PO. Drug use during breastfeeding. *Clin Pharm* 1991;10:594.
227. Lawrence RA et al. Drugs in breast milk. In: *Breastfeeding: A Guide for the Medical Profession.* St. Louis: Mosby; 1999: 351.
228. Dillon AE et al. Drug therapy in the nursing mother. *Obstet Gynecol Clin North Am* 1997; 24:675.
229. Breitzka RL et al. Principles of drug transfer into breast milk and drug disposition in the nursing infant. *J Hum Lact* 1997;12:1155.
230. Bennett PN et al., eds. *Drugs and Human Lactation.* 2nd ed. New York: Elsevier; 1996.
231. Hale TW et al. *Drug Therapy and Breastfeeding: From Theory to Clinical Practice.* Boca Raton, FL: Parthenon Publishing Group; 2002.
232. Picciano MF. Nutrient composition of human milk. *Pediatr Clin North Am* 2001;48:53.
233. Begg EJ et al. Studying drugs in human milk: time to unify the approach. *J Hum Lact* 2002;18: 323.
234. Howard CR et al. Drugs and breastfeeding. *Clin Perinatol* 1999;26:447.
235. Committee on Drugs. American Academy of Pediatrics. The transfer of drugs and other chemicals into human milk. *Pediatrics* 2001;108:776.
236. ACOG practice bulletin: thromboembolism in pregnancy. *Int J Gynecol Obstet* 2001;75:203.
237. Hall JG et al. Maternal and fetal sequelae of anticoagulation during pregnancy. *Am J Med* 1980;68:122.
238. Bates SM et al. Use of antithrombotic agents during pregnancy: The Seventh ACCP Conference on Antithrombotic and Thrombolytic Therapy. *Chest* 2004;126;627.
239. McEvoy GK, ed. *AHFS Drug Information 2003.* Bethesda, MD: American Society of Health-System Pharmacists; 2003.
240. Ginsberg JS et al. Risks to the fetus of anticoagulant therapy during pregnancy. *Thromb Haemost* 1989;61:197.
240a. Vitale N et al. Dose-dependent fetal complications of warfarin in pregnant women with mechanical heart valves. *J Am Coll Cardiol* 1999;33:1637.
240b. Cotrufo M et al. Risk of warfarin during pregnancy with mechanical valve prostheses. *Obstet Gynecol* 2002;99:35.
241. Stein PD et al. Antithrombotic therapy in patients with mechanical and biological prosthetic heart valves. *Chest* 2001;119:220s.
242. Barbour LA et al. A prospective study of heparin-induced osteoporosis in pregnancy using bone densitometry. *Am J Obstet Gynecol* 1994;170: 862.
243. Dahlman TC et al. Osteopenia in pregnancy during long-term heparin treatment: a radiologic study post partum. *Br J Obstet Gynaecol* 1990;97:221.
244. Dahlman TC. Osteoporotic fractures and the recurrence of thromboembolism during pregnancy and the puerperium in 184 women undergoing thromboprophylaxis with heparin. *Am J Obstet Gynecol* 1993;168:1265.
245. Dahlman TC et al. Bone mineral density during long-term prophylaxis with heparin in pregnancy. *Am J Obstet Gynecol* 1994;170:1315.
246. Douketis JD et al. The effects of long-term heparin therapy during pregnancy on bone density. *Thromb Haemost* 1996;75:254.
247. Barbour LA. Current concepts of anticoagulant therapy in pregnancy. *Obstet Gynecol Clin North Am* 1997;24:499.
248. Sorensen HT et al. Birth outcomes in pregnant women treated with low-molecular-weight heparin. *Acta Obstet Gynecol Scand* 2000;79:655.
249. Rowen JA et al. Enoxaparin treatment in women with mechanical heart valves during pregnancy. *Am J Obstet Gynecol* 2001;185:633.
250. Delgado-Escueta AV et al. Consensus guidelines: preconception counseling, management, and care of the pregnant woman with epilepsy. *Neurology* 1992;42(Suppl 5):149.
251. Nulman I et al. Treatment of epilepsy in pregnancy. *Drugs* 1999;57:535.
252. Holmes LB et al. The teratogenicity of anticonvulsant drugs. *N Engl J Med* 2001;344:1132.
253. Eller DP et al. Maternal and fetal implications of anticonvulsive therapy during pregnancy. *Obstet Gynecol Clin North Am* 1997;24:523.
254. Arpino C et al. Teratogenic effects of antiepileptic drugs: use of an international database on malformations and drug exposure (MADRE). *Epilepsia* 2000;41:1436.
255. Fonager K et al. Birth outcomes in women exposed to anticonvulsant drugs. *Acta Neurol Scand* 2000;101:289.
256. Dean JCS et al. Long-term health and neurodevelopment in children exposed to antiepileptic drugs before birth. *J Med Genet* 2002;39:251.
257. Buehler BA. Prenatal prediction of risk of the fetal hydantoin syndrome. *N Engl J Med* 1990;322:1567.
258. ACOG educational bulletin: seizure disorders in pregnancy. *Int J Gynecol Obstet* 1997;56:279.
259. Punnonen R et al. Oestrogen-like effect of ginseng. *BMJ* 1980;281:1110.
260. Dansky LV et al. Mechanisms of teratogenesis: folic acid and antiepileptic therapy. *Neurology* 1992;42(Suppl 5):32.
261. Morrell MJ. Guidelines for the care of women with epilepsy. *Neurology* 1998;51(Suppl 4):S21.
262. Nakane Y et al. Multi-institutional study on the teratogenicity and fetal toxicity to antiepileptic drugs: a report of a collaborative study group in Japan. *Epilepsia* 1980;21:633.
263. Paulson GW et al. Teratogenic effects of anticonvulsants. *Arch Neurol* 1981;38:140.
264. Jones KL et al. Pattern of malformations in the children of women treated with carbamazepine during pregnancy. *N Engl J Med* 1989;320:1661.
265. Chang SI et al. Pharmacotherapeutic issues for women of childbearing age with epilepsy. *Ann Pharmacother* 1998;32:794.
266. Matalon S et al. The teratogenic effect of carbamazepine: a meta-analysis of 1255 exposures. *Reprod Toxicol* 2002;16:9.
267. Diav-Citrin O et al. Is carbamazepine teratogenic? A prospective controlled study of 210 pregnancies. *Neurology* 2001;57:321.
268. Rosa FW. Spina bifida in infants of women treated with carbamazepine during pregnancy. *N Engl J Med* 1991;324:674.
269. Kozma C. Valproic acid embryopathy: report of two siblings with further expansion of the phenotypic abnormalities and a review of the literature. *Am J Med Gene A* 2001;98:168.
270. Koch S et al. Antiepileptic drug treatment in pregnancy: drug side effects in the neonate and neurological outcome. *Acta Paediatr* 1996;85:739.
271. Recommendations for the use of folic acid to reduce the number of cases of spina bifida and other neural tube defects. *MMWR* 1992;41(RR14):1.
272. Jager-Roman E et al. Fetal growth, major malformations, and minor anomalies in infants born to women receiving valproic acid. *J Pediatr* 1986;108:997.
273. Fisher JB et al. Neonatal apnea associated with maternal clonazepam therapy: a case report. *Obstet Gynecol* 1985;66(Suppl):34S.
274. Tennis P et al. Preliminary results on pregnancy outcomes in women using lamotrigine. *Epilepsia* 2002;43:1161.
275. Tomson T et al. Lamotrigine in pregnancy and lactation: a case report. *Epilepsia* 1997;38:1039.
276. *Physicians' Desk Reference*. 57th ed. Montvale, NJ: Thomson; 2003.
277. MRC Vitamin Study Research Group. Prevention of neural tube defects: results of the Medical Research Council Vitamin Study. *Lancet* 1991;338:131.
278. Way CM. Safety of Newer Antidepressants in Pregnancy. *Pharmacotherapy* 2007;27:546.
279. Cohen LS et al. Relapse of major depression during pregnancy in women who maintain or discontinue antidepressant treatment. *JAMA* 2006;295:499.
280. Kallen B et al. Antidepressant drugs during pregnancy and infant congenital heart defect. *Reprod Toxicol* 2006;21:221.
281. Berard A et al. First trimester exposure to paroxetine and risk of cardiac malformations in infants: the importance of dosage. *Birth Defects Res B Dev Reprod Toxicol* 2007;80:18.
282. FDA Public Health Advisory. Paroxetine. December 8, 2005. Available at http://www.fda.gov/cder/drug/advisory/paroxetine200512.htm. Accessed June 30, 2007.
283. Alwan S et al., for the National Birth Defects Prevention Study. Use of selective serotonin-reuptake inhibitors in pregnancy and the risk of birth defects. *N Engl J Med* 2007;356:2684.
284. Louik C et al. First-trimester use of selective serotonin reuptake inhibitors and the risk of birth defects. *N Engl J Med* 2007;356:2675.
285. Greene MF. Teratogenicity of SSRIs: serious concern or much ado about little? *N Engl J Med* 2007;356:2732.
286. Chambers CD et al. Selective serotonin-reuptake inhibitors and risk of persistent pulmonary hypertension in the newborn. *N Engl J Med* 2006;354 :579.
287. Butters L et al. Atenolol in essential hypertension during pregnancy. *BMJ* 1990;301:587.
288. Lydakis C et al. Atenolol and fetal growth in pregnancies complicated by hypertension. *Am J Hypertens* 1999;12:541.
289. Ito S. Drug therapy for breast-feeding women. *N Engl J Med* 2000;343:118.
290. Shannon ME et al. Beta blockers and lactation: an update. *J Hum Lact* 2000;16:240.
291. Shannon ME et al. Calcium channel antagonists and lactation: an update. *J Hum Lact* 2000;16:60.
292. Loebstein R et al. Pharmacokinetic changes during pregnancy and their clinical relevance. *Clin Pharmacokinet* 1997;33:328.

CHAPTER 47

Disorders Related to the Menstrual Cycle

Laura B. Hansen and Karen Gunning

POLYCYSTIC OVARY SYNDROME

Polycystic ovary syndrome (PCOS) affects approximately 6% to 8%, or 1 of 15 women of reproductive age, making it the leading cause of anovulatory infertility and the most common endocrine abnormality for this age group.[1] This syndrome, or constellation of symptoms, was first described in 1935 by Stein and Leventhal when they reported infertility and amenorrhea in seven women with enlarged cystic ovaries.[2] Excessive male-patterned hair growth and obesity were added later to the description of this syndrome.[3] PCOS also has been referred to as Stein-Leventhal syndrome, polycystic ovary, polycystic ovarian disease, hyperandrogenic chronic anovulatory syndrome, and functional ovarian hyperandrogenism. The name "polycystic ovary syndrome" has been most widely accepted because it best describes the heterogeneous nature of this disorder.

Diagnostic Criteria

The diagnosis of PCOS is complicated by variations among women of the presenting signs and symptoms and because diagnostic criteria have changed over time. Precise and uniform criteria for diagnosis have not been firmly established. Three major diagnostic criteria for PCOS have been proposed by different organizations (Table 47-1).

The initial diagnostic criteria were developed in 1990 during an expert conference sponsored by the National Institutes of Health (NIH) and National Institute of Child Health and Human Development (NICHD). The panel concluded that the major criteria for PCOS should include (in order of importance): (a) hyperandrogenism (clinical signs of hyperandrogenism such as hirsutism) or hyperandrogenemia (biochemical signs of hyperandrogenism such as elevated testosterone

Table 47-1 Criteria for Defining Polycystic Ovary Syndrome (PCOS)

	Proposed Definitions		
Clinical Criteria	*NIH 1990 (all marked with ×)*	*ESHRE/ASRM (Rotterdam) 2003 (2 of first 3 criteria and last)*	*AES 2006 (first criterion, 1 of criteria 2 or 3, and last)*
1. Hyperandrogenism or hyperandrogenemia	×	×	×
2. Oligo-ovulation or anovulation	×	×	×
3. Polycystic ovaries (by ultrasound)	—	×	×
4. Exclusion of related disorders	×	×	×

AES, Androgen Excess Society; ESHRE/ASRM, European Society for Human Reproduction and Embryology/ American Society for Reproductive Medicine; NIH, National Institutes of Health.
Adapted from references, 4–6.

levels), (b) oligo-ovulation (infrequent or irregular ovulation with fewer than nine menses per year), and (c) exclusion of other known disorders such as hyperprolactinemia, thyroid abnormalities, and congenital adrenal hyperplasia.[4] The second set of criteria was proposed at an expert conference in Rotterdam sponsored by the European Society for Human Reproduction and Embryology (ESHRE) and the American Society for Reproductive Medicine (ASRM) in 2003.[5] They concluded that the presence of two of the following three features, after exclusion of related disorders, confirmed diagnosis of PCOS: (a) oligo-ovulation or anovulation, (b) clinical or biochemical signs of hyperandrogenism, or (c) polycystic ovaries. The third set of criteria was developed by a task force of the Androgen Excess Society (AES) in 2006.[6] They concluded hyperandrogenism, hyperandrogenemia (highest priority), or both and ovarian dysfunction, as evidenced by oligo-ovulation, polycystic ovaries, or both must be present after exclusion of other androgen excess or related disorders. Strengths and weaknesses exist in each of the criteria proposed, but it is clear that the definition of and diagnostic criteria for PCOS will continue to evolve as new information is released.

Clinical Characteristics

Common clinical signs of PCOS include hirsutism, acne, and alopecia. Hirsutism, the most common of these characteristics, occurs in 60% to 70% of women with PCOS.[6] It is defined as an excess of thickly pigmented body hair in a male pattern distribution and commonly found on the upper lip, lower abdomen, and around the nipples. Women seeking treatment for hirsuitism may be evaluated for PCOS. Acne affects 15% to 25% of women with PCOS, but this prevalence may not be different than in the general population. Alopecia occurs in approximately 5% of women with PCOS and presents as scalp hair loss in the crown and vertex areas.[7]

Ovulatory dysfunction in PCOS is typically described as oligo-ovulation or anovulation, presenting clinically as a woman with irregular menstrual cycles. Overall, 60% to 85% of women with PCOS and oligo-ovulation have menstrual dysfunction, usually oligomenorrhea or amenorrhea.[1] The menstrual disturbances usually begin in the peripubertal years. An increased luteinizing hormone (LH) to follicle-stimulating hormone (FSH) ratio >2 or 3 may provide evidence for irregular ovulation. This occurs in 20% to 60% of women with PCOS.[1]

Obesity occurs in approximately 30% to 60% of women with PCOS.[1] Central or abdominal obesity is the typical pattern. Central obesity is a risk factor for the development of diabetes and heart disease and, when present in a woman with PCOS, worsens the clinical features (e.g., anovulation, hyperandrogenism, insulin resistance) of the syndrome.[8] Therefore, lifestyle modification with appropriate diet and exercise is a cornerstone of therapy for many women with PCOS.

Pathophysiology

The pathophysiology of PCOS is complex. The primary defect in PCOS is unknown, but at least three potential mechanisms, acting alone or synergistically, appear to create the characteristic clinical presentation. These mechanisms include inappropriate gonadotropin secretion, excessive androgen production, and insulin resistance with hyperinsulinemia. Figure 47-1 displays the closely integrated relationship between these mechanisms in the development of PCOS.

A genetic basis for PCOS has been postulated, but its mode of transmission is unclear.[9] Theories include an autosomal-dominant model and a polygenic model with genetic–environmental interactions. The complex presentation and various mechanisms make it impossible to target just one gene locus; in fact, >50 candidate genes have been proposed. A familial pattern to the development of PCOS may exist, because the incidence is higher in women with relatives with the disorder.

Gonadotropin Secretion

In normal menstrual cycles, ovulation occurs when the hypothalamus produces gonadotropin-releasing hormone (GnRH), a neurohormone that regulates the release of FSH and LH from the anterior pituitary in a pulsatile fashion every 60 to 90 minutes. FSH is important to stimulate growth of ovarian follicles and LH is critical for ovulation and sex steroid production. Typically, FSH concentrations rise during the follicular phase, stimulating the growth and development of a small group of follicles until a dominant follicle emerges late in the follicular phase. Estrogen levels rise during this time, generating the LH surge and resulting in ovulation. During the luteal phase that follows, progesterone is synthesized and secreted, which is necessary for implantation of an embryo should pregnancy occur. If pregnancy does not occur, progesterone concentrations decrease and menstruation occurs.

In PCOS, there is an increased frequency of GnRH stimulation, leading to an increase in LH pulse frequency and amplitude, while FSH secretion remains normal. The development

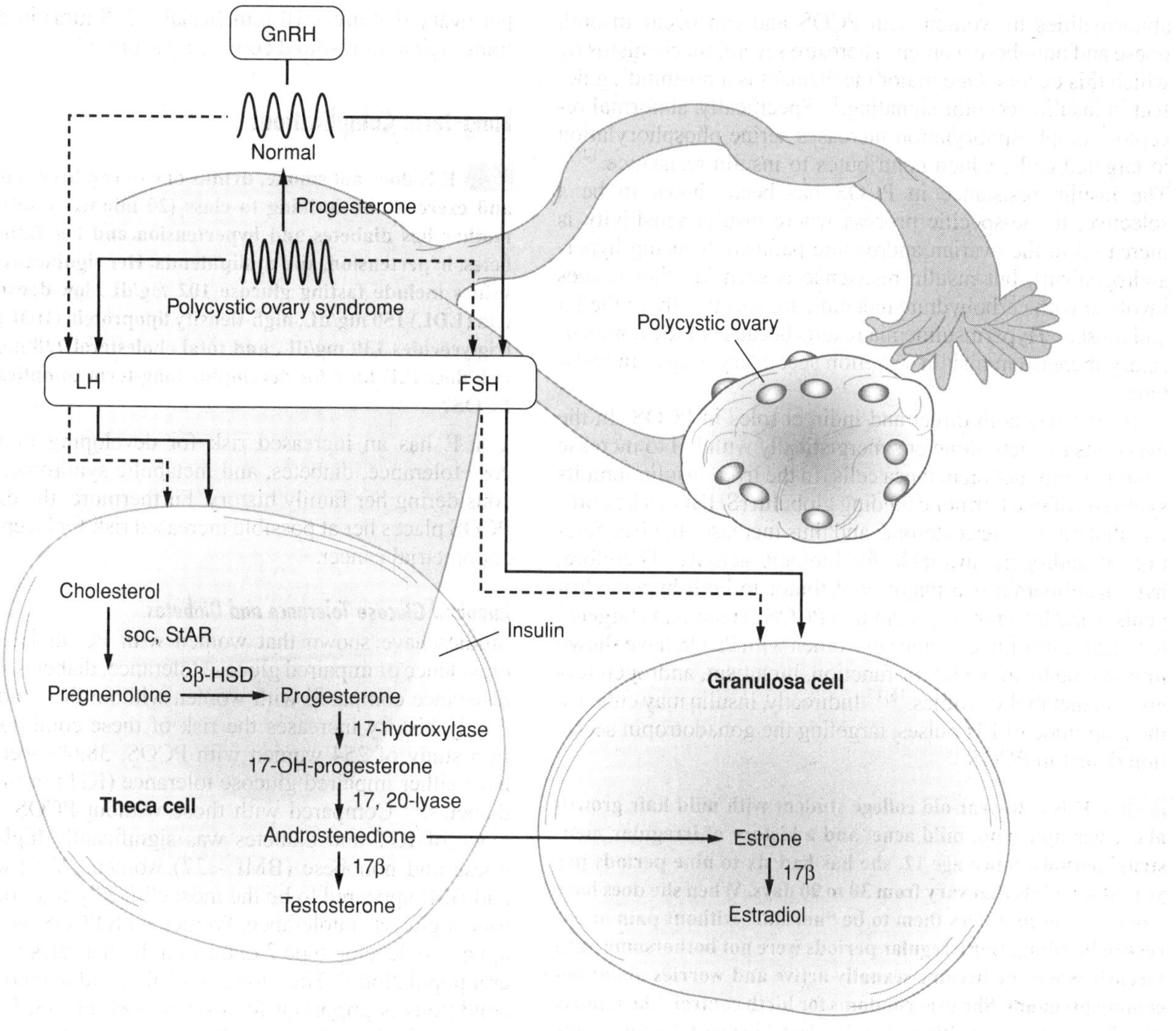

FIGURE 47-1 Relationship of gonadotropin secretion, androgen production, and insulin in polycystic ovary syndrome (PCOS). From reference 10, with permission.

of a dominant follicle does not occur because LH secretion occurs too early in the menstrual cycle. Therefore, a woman is left with several immature follicles and usually will not ovulate. It is not clear whether the abnormal pulse frequency of GnRH is an intrinsic problem in the GnRH pulse generator or a result of relatively low progesterone concentrations from infrequent ovulation.[10] A woman with this abnormality does not enter the luteal phase of her menstrual cycle, leaving estrogen unopposed. Unopposed estrogen leads to endometrial hyperplasia and increases the risk for endometrial cancer. Increased LH stimulation also leads to increased steroidogenesis in the ovary, leading to excess androgen production.

Excess Androgen Production

Androgen production occurs in the theca cell of the ovary to facilitate follicular growth and estradiol synthesis in the granulosa cell. In women with PCOS, hypersecretion of LH and insulin increase the production of androgens, causing abnormal sex steroid synthesis, hyperandrogenism, and hyperandrogenemia. The dysregulation in steroid synthesis and metabolism is believed to result primarily from a dysfunction of the cytochrome P450c17 enzyme in the ovaries, an enzyme with 17-hydroxylase and 17,20-lyase activities that are required to form androstenedione.[10,11] Androstenedione is then converted to testosterone or is aromatized by the aromatase enzyme to form estrone. Theca cells in women with PCOS are more efficient at the conversion to testosterone than normal theca cells.[12] Also, a similar steroid pathway occurs in the adrenal cortex and, when hyperandrogenism or hyperinsulinemic states exist, androgen production is exacerbated.

Elevated androgen levels are seen in approximately 60% to 80% of women with PCOS, mostly as increased free testosterone concentrations.[6] Assays for testosterone tend, however, to be highly variable and inaccurate, so measurement of androgen concentrations should be used only as an adjuvant test and never as the sole criterion for diagnosis. Clinical assessment is the primary tool for assessment of excess androgen.

Insulin

Women with PCOS experience an increased risk of insulin resistance with compensatory hyperinsulinemia.[1] Insulin resistance is associated with reproductive and metabolic abnormalities in women with PCOS and can occur in both obese and nonobese women. There are several mechanisms by which this occurs. One major mechanism is a postbinding defect in insulin-receptor signaling.[13] Specifically, abnormal receptor autophosphorylation increases serine phosphorylation in targeted cells, which contributes to insulin resistance.[14,15] The insulin resistance in PCOS has been shown to be a selective, tissue-specific process where insulin sensitivity is increased in the ovarian androgenic pathway (causing hyperandrogenism), but insulin resistence is seen in other tissues involved with carbohydrate metabolism, specifically in the fat and muscle. Hyperinsulinemia results because of the compensatory increase in insulin secretion secondary to insulin resistance.

Insulin has both direct and indirect roles in PCOS. In the ovary, insulin acts alone or synergistically with LH to increase androgen production in theca cells. In the liver, insulin inhibits synthesis of sex-hormone binding globulin (SHBG), a key protein that binds to testosterone, and thus increases the free fraction of androgens available for biologic activity. Therefore, hyperinsulinemia is a major contributor to both hyperandrogenism and hyperandrogenemia in PCOS. Treatments targeted to improve insulin resistance in women with PCOS have shown improvements in ovulatory function, hirsutism, androgen levels, and metabolic profiles.[16,17] Indirectly, insulin may enhance the amplitude of LH pulses, targeting the gonadotropin secretion defect in PCOS.[18]

1. E.F. is a 20-year-old college student with mild hair growth above her upper lip, mild acne, and a history of irregular menstrual periods. Since age 12, she has had six to nine periods per year at intervals that vary from 30 to 90 days. When she does have a period, she considers them to be "normal" without pain or excessive bleeding. Her irregular periods were not bothersome until recently when she became sexually active and worries about becoming pregnant. She uses condoms for birth control. She reports no other medical conditions. E.F. is 5 feet 7 inches tall and weighs 180 pounds (body mass index [BMI] 28.2). Her vital signs today are BP 118/84 mmHg, heart rate (HR) 70 beats/minute, temperature 98.6°F, respiratory rate (RR) 18. Her physical examination is normal, with the exception of noted excessive facial hair and mild acne. She takes a multivitamin daily and acetaminophen as needed for headaches. She has no known medication allergies. What signs and symptoms does E.F. have that are consistent with PCOS?

E.F. exhibits several signs and symptoms that would indicate the presence of PCOS. According to the criteria of all organizations, her history of abnormal menstrual periods (oligomenorrhea) and clinical signs of hyperandrogenism, including hirsutism and acne, would indicate PCOS. E.F. is overweight, which is common in women with PCOS but is not considered a criterion for diagnosis. Before a diagnosis of PCOS is made, laboratory testing to exclude other related causes of her symptoms would have to be performed. Studies may include prolactin, thyroid-stimulating hormone, testosterone, and 17-hydroxyprogesterone concentrations to rule out hyperprolactinemia, hypothyroidism, virilizing tumor, and congenital adrenal hyperplasia, respectively. PCOS is primarily diagnosed by clinical assessment; therefore, these tests assist only in confirming or excluding a diagnosis. To determine the presence of polycystic ovaries, defined as more than eight follicles per ovary that are <10 mm (usually 2–8 mm) in diameter, a transvaginal ultrasound could be performed.

Long-term Complications

2. E.F. does not smoke, drinks one to two beers on weekends, and exercises by walking to class (20 minutes total) daily. Her mother has diabetes and hypertension and her father has diabetes, hypertension, and dyslipidemia. Her significant laboratory values include fasting glucose 102 mg/dL, low-density lipoprotein (LDL) 150 mg/dL, high-density lipoprotein (HDL) 52 mg/dL, triglycerides 130 mg/dL, and total cholesterol 228 mg/dL. What risk does E.F. have for developing long-term complications from PCOS?

E.F. has an increased risk for developing impaired glucose tolerance, diabetes, and metabolic syndrome, especially considering her family history. Furthermore, the diagnosis of PCOS places her at possible increased risk for sleep apnea and endometrial cancer.

Impaired Glucose Tolerance and Diabetes

Studies have shown that women with PCOS have a higher prevalence of impaired glucose tolerance, diabetes, and insulin resistance compared with women without the syndrome.[19] A family history increases the risk of these conditions further. In a study of 254 women with PCOS, 38.6% were found to have either impaired glucose tolerance (IGT) or undiagnosed diabetes.[20] Compared with those without PCOS, the prevalence of IGT and diabetes was significantly higher in both obese and nonobese (BMI <27) women. Waist-to-hip ratio and BMI appeared to be the most clinically important predictors of glucose intolerance. Women with PCOS who have IGT appear to develop type 2 diabetes at higher rates than the general population.[19] Therefore, screening and diagnosis of these conditions is important for women with PCOS. E.F.'s mildly elevated fasting glucose and obesity suggest that she may be at increased risk for impaired glucose tolerance.

Glucose tolerance should be assessed in all women with PCOS using a fasting and 2-hour oral (75 g) glucose tolerance test.[19] Routine screening for diabetes with an oral glucose tolerance test should be performed for all women with PCOS by the age of 30 years.[21] The American Diabetes Association or World Health Organization criteria should be used for the appropriate diagnosis of IGT or diabetes. Insulin concentrations are typically not obtained in clinical settings because they are inaccurate.

Metabolic Syndrome and Cardiovascular Risk

Approximately one-third to one-half of women with PCOS have a metabolic syndrome using the National Cholesterol Education Panel-Adult Treatment Panel III (NCEP-ATP III) criteria (Table 47-2).[22–25] The incidence of a metabolic syndrome in women with PCOS is significantly higher than the rate for the general U.S. population (45% vs. 6% ages 20–29 years, 53% vs. 14% ages 30–39 years) and independent of body weight.[22] It is believed that insulin resistance is the primary contributing factor to metabolic syndrome in women with PCOS.[26] Insulin resistance in the metabolic syndrome has been associated with a twofold increased risk of cardiovascular disease and a fivefold increased risk of type 2 diabetes.[27] Low

Table 47-2 NCEP ATP III Criteria for Metabolic Syndrome[22]

Three or more of the following:
Central obesity: >40 inches in males, >35 inches in females (may need to adjust lower when individuals or ethnic groups are prone to insulin resistance)
Elevated triglycerides: ≥150 mg/dL or on drug treatment for this lipid abnormality
Reduced high-density lipoprotein cholesterol (HDL-C): <45 mg/dL in males, <50 mg/dL in females, or on drug treatment for this lipid abnormality
Hypertension: systolic blood pressure ≥135 mmHg or diastolic blood pressure ≥85 mmHg, or on drug treatment for hypertension
Elevated fasting plasma glucose: ≥100 mg/dL

NCEP ATP, National Cholesterol Education Program Adult Treatment Panel.

HDL cholesterol (HDL-C) is seen most frequently in women with PCOS (68%), followed by increased BMI and waist circumference (67%), high blood pressure (45%), hypertriglyceridemia (35%), and elevated fasting glucose (4%).[23] Another group found that elevated fasting insulin concentrations, obesity, and a family history of diabetes conferred higher risk of having the metabolic syndrome in women with PCOS.[25]

Compared with women without PCOS, women with PCOS are reported to have a higher prevalence of cardiovascular risk factors, including hypertension, dyslipidemia, and surrogate markers for early atherosclerosis (e.g., increased C-reactive protein concentrations).[26] With increasing age, and especially as women with PCOS become postmenopausal, the risk of hypertension increases. Postmenopausal women with PCOS have a twofold increased risk of hypertension compared with age-matched controls.[28] Dyslipidemia in women with PCOS typically presents as decreased HDL-C (which is a strong predictor of cardiovascular disease in women), elevated triglycerides, elevated LDL cholesterol (LDL-C), and higher LDL-to-HDL ratios.[29] Women with PCOS are noted to have more atherogenic, small dense LDL-C compared with controls and this substantially increases cardiovascular risk.[30] Women with PCOS may have other surrogate markers for early atherosclerosis and cardiovascular disease, impaired endothelial dysfunction, and other markers of cardiovascular risk such as coronary artery calcifications and increased carotid intima-media thickness.[26] Although cardiovascular risk exists, women with PCOS do not appear to have markedly higher rates of mortality from cardiovascular disease.

Obstructive Sleep Apnea

Obstructive sleep apnea is cessation of breathing that occurs during sleep. It can disrupt sleep and cause daytime fatigue. Patients may not be aware that they are having the symptoms of sleep apnea, which include snoring and a gasping or snorting when breathing resumes. Studies indicate that the prevalence of obstructive sleep apnea in the PCOS is higher than expected and cannot be explained by obesity alone.[31–33] Insulin resistance appears to be a strong predictor of sleep apnea—more so than age, BMI, or the circulating testosterone concentration.[31]

Endometrial Hyperplasia and Cancer

Chronic anovulation in women with PCOS results in an endometrium that is exposed to the prolonged effects of estrogen unopposed by progesterone. Therefore, PCOS is a risk factor for endometrial hyperplasia. It is unknown if this translates into an increased risk for endometrial cancer because it is a rare occurrence in young women (4% of all cases occur in women <40 years of age).[34] It is considered prudent management to induce artificial withdrawal bleeding by administering a course of progestin at least every 3 months to prevent endometrial hyperplasia in women with PCOS who experience either amenorrhea or oligomenorrhea. Alternatively, ultrasound scans can also be used to measure endometrial thickness and morphology every 6 to 12 months.

Treatment Goals

3. E.F. worries about becoming pregnant when she does not have regular periods. She also has mild hair growth above her upper lip which is somewhat bothersome. Given these concerns, what are the treatment goals for E.F.?

The primary goals for E.F. are to prevent pregnancy and address her hirsutism. Additionally, treatment goals in E.F. would include maintaining a normal endometrium, blocking the actions of androgens at target tissues, reducing insulin resistance and hyperinsulinemia, reducing weight, and preventing long-term complications. Other goals of treatment in patients with PCOS may include correcting anovulation or oligo-ovulation and improve fertility.

Therapy goals should encompass both long- and short-term objectives because response to nonpharmacologic and pharmacologic therapy is slow, often requiring 3 to 9 months. Addressing long-term goals can minimize the risk for future complications and specifying short-term goals can improve motivation and adherence to therapy.

Nonpharmacologic Treatment

4. E.F. has indicated that she would like to lose weight. What nonpharmacologic method(s) would be most effective?

Weight reduction programs designed for a modest weight loss (5%–10%) with the incorporation of fitness are effective in reducing metabolic disease and improving ovulatory potential. Diet modification and exercise are the most efficient, cost-effective, and safe ways to produce weight loss and improve the endocrine and metabolic parameters of PCOS. Weight reduction should be considered first-line therapy in all overweight or obese women with PCOS.

Impact of Weight Loss in PCOS

A minimum 5% weight loss has consistently demonstrated restoration of regular menstrual cycling and ovulation in overweight and obese women with PCOS.[8,35,36] When lifestyle modification is implemented, free testosterone concentrations decrease, but clinical outcomes of acne and hirsutism are not often reported.[8] Obesity in PCOS is associated with a higher risk of developing endometrial cancer, but very limited evidence exists to determine the impact of weight loss on the incidence of endometrial cancer.[8] Studies of weight loss in women without PCOS indicate a 25% to 50% reduced risk of endometrial cancer, so it is logical that addressing weight reduction may lower that risk as well.[37,38] The Diabetes Prevention Program trial demonstrated a 53% prevalence of metabolic syndrome; the incidence of this was reduced 41% in the lifestyle modification group.[39,40] This was significantly better than treatment with metformin. Studies specifically evaluating cardiovascular improvements with weight loss in women with PCOS are limited, but improvements in dyslipidemia and insulin sensitivity have been noted.

Diet Composition

No single diet has been proven to be ideal for women with PCOS. A diet low in saturated fat and high in fiber from mostly low-glycemic-index-carbohydrate foods may, however, be suitable and is recommended.[8,41] Glycemic index is a classification of carbohydrates based on the blood glucose response over 2 hours. Low-glycemic index foods include bran cereals, mixed grain breads, broccoli, peppers, lentils, and soy. High-glycemic index foods, or those that should be minimized, include white rice and bread, potatoes, chips, and foods containing simple sugars (e.g., juice). It has been shown that in women with PCOS, oral glucose intake causes larger fluctuations in plasma glucose, increased hyperinsulinemia, and stimulated adrenal steroid secretion; protein was found to be a preferred nutrient over glucose.[42] The composition of a diet should be individualized to promote adherence and achieve specific goals.

Exercise

Exercise is a key component in the attainment and maintenance of weight loss. Exercise with muscle strengthening improves insulin sensitivity.[8] The American Heart Association recommends 1 hour daily of physical activity for weight reduction and 30 minutes daily for all adults. The American Diabetes Association recommends at least 150 minutes per week of moderate to vigorous activity spread over at least 3 days for individuals with IGT and 1 hour daily of exercise for long-term weight loss.

Pharmacologic Treatment

5. E.F. would like to improve her menstrual irregularity, and be sure that she will not get pregnant. If possible, she would also like to minimize her hirsutism and acne. What pharmacologic treatment options would be appropriate to recommend for E.F.?

Several different pharmacologic options could be recommended to E.F (Table 47-3). A combined oral contraceptive (COC) will address her concerns about irregular menstruation, hyperandrogenism, and pregnancy prevention. An insulin sensitizer would improve her menstrual irregularity and possibly reduce her hirsutism and acne, but it does not address her desire to prevent pregnancy. An antiandrogen, such as spironolactone, would address only hyperandrogenism and other agents would have to be used concurrently to address pregnancy prevention and the other hormonal and metabolic alterations in PCOS.

Combined Oral Contraceptives

Estrogen-progestin combination therapy with a COC is the treatment of choice for women seeking regularity in menstrual cycles and relief from hyperandrogenic symptoms. The estrogen component suppresses LH, resulting in a reduction of androgen production, and increases hepatic production of

Table 47-3 Selected Treatment Options for PCOS

Drug Class (example)	Purpose of Therapy	Mechanism of Action	Effective Dose	Side Effects	Pregnancy Category
Combined oral contraceptive (estrogen and progestin)	Menstrual cyclicity, hirsutism, acne	Suppresses LH (and FSH) and thus ovarian androgen production; increases sex hormone-binding globulin, which decreases free testosterone	One tablet orally daily for 21 (or 24) days, then 7-day (or 4-day) pill-free interval	Breast tenderness, breakthrough bleeding, mood swings, libido changes	X
Progestins (medroxyprogesterone)	Menstrual cyclicity	Creates withdrawal bleeding by transforming proliferative endometrium into secretory endometrium	5–10 mg orally daily for 10–14 days every 1–2 months	Breakthrough bleeding, spotting, mood swings	X
Biguanide (metformin)	Menstrual cyclicity, ovulation induction, hirsutism, acne, insulin lowering	Decreases hepatic glucose production, secondarily reducing insulin levels; may have direct effects on steroidogenesis	500 mg orally 3 times daily (up to 2,550 mg/day)	Gastrointestinal problems, diarrhea, abdominal pain	B
Thiazolidinediones (pioglitazone or rosiglitazone)	Menstrual cyclicity, ovulation induction, hirsutism, acne, insulin lowering	Improve insulin sensitivity at target-tissue level (muscle, adipocyte); may have direct effects on steroidogenesis	Pioglitazone: 45 mg orally daily Rosiglitazone: 4 mg orally twice daily	Edema, headache, fatigue, weight gain	C
Antiandrogen (spironolactone)	Hirsutism, acne	Inhibit androgens from binding to androgen receptor	50–100 mg orally twice daily	Hyperkalemia, polymenorrhea, headache, fatigue	C
Antiestrogen (clomiphene citrate)	Ovulation induction	Increases GnRH secretion, which Induces rise in FSH and LH	50 mg orally daily for 5 days; may increase to 100 mg	Vasomotor symptoms, gastrointestinal problems	X

FSH, follicle-stimulating hormone; GnRH, gonadotropin-releasing hormone; LH, luteinizing hormone.

sex-hormone–binding globulin (SHBG), thereby reducing free testosterone. The progestins in various COCs possess variable androgenic effects, so the choice of the COC is important. The potential effects of COCs on insulin resistance, glucose tolerance, and lipids have been debated and should be considered when choosing a progestin component.[43,44] Caution should be used in those who have insulin resistance, a high propensity to develop type 2 diabetes, or abnormal lipid profiles.

6. What oral contraceptive agent should be initiated in E.F.?

Combined oral contraceptive therapy in PCOS should be initiated with a formulation that contains a low- or very-low dose of estrogen (≤35 mcg ethinyl estradiol) and a progestin with low androgenic or antiandrogen properties. Most COCs manufactured today have low- or very-low estrogen doses. Desogestrel and norgestimate are progestins with low androgen potential and drospirenone is an antiandrogen. A COC containing ethinyl estradiol and drospirenone would prevent pregnancy, improve menstrual cycle regularity, and reduce E.F.'s signs of hyperandrogenism (hirsutism and acne). If E.F. desired monthly cycles, she could take the typical 21/7 regimen (21 days active pill, 7 days inactive pill) or a 24/4 regimen (24 days active pill, 4 days inactive pill). Although not specifically evaluated in women with PCOS, a monophasic regimen may also be prescribed using extended cycles of 84 or even 365 days. Extended regimens reduce the number of cycles per year while providing contraception. Regardless of the COC selected, one of the long-term benefits is that her risk for endometrial cancer would be reduced by 50%, even up to two decades after discontinuation.[45–47]

7. What other therapy options may be beneficial for E.F. if a COC was not tolerated?

Insulin Sensitizers

A reduction in insulin levels by using insulin sensitizers can ameliorate the sequelae of hyperinsulinemia and hyperandrogenemia. Currently available insulin sensitizers include metformin, rosiglitazone, and pioglitazone. More efficacy data are available regarding the use of metformin compared with the thiazolidinediones. Metformin is statistically significantly better in women with PCOS for ovulation induction when compared with rosiglitazone.[48] For these reasons, metformin tends to be the preferred insulin sensitizer for women with PCOS.

METFORMIN

Metformin inhibits hepatic glucose output, providing lower insulin concentrations and reducing androgen production in the ovary. Metformin also appears to influence ovarian steroidogenesis directly.[49] Most studies demonstrate that metformin improves menstrual cycle regulation, ovulation, and fertility in both obese and lean patients with PCOS.[50] Metformin has been used in ovulation induction protocols and has been shown to be very effective when used alone or with clomiphene citrate for inducing ovulation.[51,52] Data also indicate that insulin and free testosterone concentrations may be decreased 20% to 50% with metformin when used in women with PCOS.[53,54] Although few studies have been published on other clinical outcomes in PCOS, results suggest that metformin will produce reductions in hirsutism, acne, and BMI (especially in obese patients).[50]

The most commonly used and most effective dose of metformin in PCOS is 500 mg three times daily (TID). It should be titrated slowly to this effective dose; doses up to 2,000 mg daily or 2,550 mg daily may be necessary for individual circumstances. The gastrointestinal (GI) side effects of diarrhea, nausea, vomiting, and abdominal bloating are usually transient and dose related, and do not require discontinuation of the drug. Serum creatinine should be evaluated at least annually in women using metformin because it is contraindicated in women who have a serum creatinine >1.4 mg/dL.

THIAZOLIDINEDIONES

Rosiglitazone and pioglitazone have been evaluated in women with PCOS, but studies have been small in number. These agents improve insulin action in the liver, skeletal muscle, and adipose tissue. They also are reported to directly affect ovarian steroid synthesis.[55] Rosiglitazone and pioglitazone are extremely effective at reducing insulin and androgen concentrations and have modest effects on hirsutism.[10] Rosiglitazone has demonstrated significantly better ovulation rates in women with PCOS compared with placebo, but it is less effective than metformin.[48] Other abstracts have indicated rosiglitazone may be beneficial for menstrual regularity, hyperandrogenism, and insulin sensitivity. Pioglitazone has proved to be as effective as metformin in small studies of women with PCOS and may be especially beneficial when used in combination with metformin for clinical and biochemical improvements.[56,57]

Recommended doses for rosiglitazone and pioglitazone are the same as those used for the treatment of type 2 diabetes. Adverse effects include edema, headache, fatigue, and potential liver enzyme elevations. Liver enzymes should be measured before initiation of treatment and periodically thereafter. It should be noted that rosiglitazone also appears to have a negative effect on the lipid profile, an unwanted outcome considering the potential long-term consequences of PCOS.

Agents for Hirsutism

Antiandrogenic agents are beneficial therapeutic options for hirsutism and acne. They often are used alone or combination with COC for moderate to severe hirsutism or acne. Although frequently used, antiandrogens are not approved for the treatment of female hirsutism or acne in the United States. Spironolactone is commonly prescribed to women for hirsutism, but drospirenone is an antiandrogen found in COC and it has also been evaluated in the long-term treatment of hirsutism.[58] Finasteride has been used for female hirsutism, but its lack of specificity for type I 5α-reductase in the pilosebaceous unit and toxicity may make this a suboptimal treatment choice. Flutamide is effective for hirsuitism, but it is not used because of hepatoxicity. Cyproterone acetate is used in Europe but is not available in the United States. Eflornithine hydrochloride has been approved for topical use in treating facial hirsutism, but has not been evaluated in women with PCOS.

SPIRONOLACTONE

Spironolactone acts by competitively inhibiting dihydrotestosterone (DHT) from interacting with its androgen receptor. This causes a decrease in activity of ovarian-produced testosterone. Spironolactone reduces hair growth by 40% to 88%; however, it takes 6 to 9 months for improvement.[59] Spironolactone may be associated with possible teratogenicity (feminization of the male fetus), so it is prudent to advise women to avoid pregnancy for at least 4 months after the discontinuation of spironolactone. It is recommended that spironolactone be used with a COC to avoid teratogenicity, as well as the side effect of polymenorrhea (more frequent menses) when used as monotherapy. Spironolactone in combination with a COC would also improve hormonal and metabolic manifestations of PCOS as well. The usual effective spironolactone dose is 50 to 100 mg twice daily (BID) for 6 to 12 months. Serum potassium and renal function should be monitored because this aldosterone antagonist can cause hyperkalemia. Furthermore, spironolactone should not be used with a COC containing drospirenone because of a potential risk for hyperkalemia.

FINASTERIDE

Finasteride is a type II 5α-reductase inhibitor, which decreases the conversion of testosterone to DHT. It provides an approximate 30% reduction from baseline for hirsutism. Compared with spironolactone, finasteride is as or less effective in women with hirsutism.[60] The dose of 5 mg to 7.5 mg daily typically takes 6 months for clinical improvement. It is critical to avoid pregnancy while taking this drug owing to the potential teratogenic effect of abnormal genitalia in the male fetus. Finasteride should not be touched or handled by women who are or may be pregnant. This danger limits the usefulness of finasteride in women with PCOS because most are of childbearing age or desire pregnancy.

8. E.F. successfully used oral contraceptives for 10 years. After getting married 3 years ago, E.F. and her husband decided to have children. She lost 30 pounds with diet and exercise when she got married and has been able to maintain that weight loss. They have been trying to get pregnant for the last 18 months. The reason for infertility has been identified as oligo-ovulation associated with PCOS. What treatments for ovulation induction should be used and why?

Anovulation or oligo-ovulation in women with PCOS is usually first treated with diet, exercise, and weight reduction. Weight loss improves pregnancy rates and reduces miscarriage rates in women with PCOS.[61] E.F. has been successful at losing weight and now must consider agents for ovulation induction. Clomiphene citrate is the pharmacologic agent of choice in women with PCOS. Ovulation induction and conception occur in about 50% to 80% and 35% to 40% of women with PCOS, respectively, using clomiphene citrate. Although side effects (e.g., bloating, nausea, vomiting, and multiple gestation) can occur, the benefit of this therapy outweighs the risk for E.F.

Agents for Ovulation Induction

CLOMIPHENE CITRATE

Clomiphene citrate induces ovulation via an antiestrogenic effect on the hypothalamus. GnRH secretion is increased, which increases LH and FSH production. The increase in FSH concentrations causes appropriate follicle development and estrogen secretion, which produces a positive feedback on the hypothalamic-pituitary system to create a LH surge for ovulation.

The usual initial dose of clomiphene citrate is 50 mg orally daily for 5 days, started on day 5 after a spontaneous or progestin-induced menses. The clinician must determine if ovulation occurs with each cycle through laboratory testing, ultrasound monitoring, or both. If ovulation does not occur, the dose can be increased by 50 mg daily up to 150 mg daily; however, doses >100 mg daily for 5 days are not recommended by the manufacturers.[62] A repeat cycle can be administered as early as 30 days after the previous cycle as long as pregnancy has not occurred. If conception does not occur, women can use clomiphene for three to four cycles before considering another regimen. Long-term cyclic therapy is not recommended beyond a total of six cycles because of potential ovarian cancer risk. Most women respond to clomiphene citrate within three to four ovulatory cycles, but 5% to 10% have demonstrated clomiphene resistance and need to consider other options.[61,62] For women who are clomiphene citrate resistant, dexamethasone can be used in conjunction with clomiphene or an aromatase inhibitor can be used (e.g., letrozole, anastrozole) as an alternative for infertility in PCOS.[63–66]

In the 1990s, it was suggested that the combination of clomiphene citrate plus metformin produced higher ovulation rates than either agent alone.[67] The most clinically relevant outcome for infertility, live birth, however, had not been fully investigated.[52] Investigators recently performed a randomized, controlled study to determine the live-birth rates in 626 women with PCOS taking metformin, clomiphene citrate, or both.[68] The live-birth rate was 22.5% in the clomiphene citrate group, 7.2% in the metformin group, and 26.8% in the combination group ($p < 0.001$ for metformin versus clomiphene citrate and combination therapy). They concluded that clomiphene citrate was superior to metformin in achieving live-birth rates, although multiple births occurred in 6% (3/50) of live births.

OTHER AGENTS

Although clomiphene citrate is the pharmacologic agent of choice in women with PCOS for infertility, it can only be used for a limited number of cycles and resistance can occur. If clomiphene citrate alone is no longer an option, other regimens, including metformin (alone or in combination with clomiphene citrate), dexamethasone (in combination with clomiphene citrate), aromatase inhibitors, ovarian drilling or controlled ovarian stimulation with gonadotropins can be recommended.[69] Based on the evidence available, it would be reasonable to start with combination clomiphene citrate and metformin.[62] If that is not successful, dexamethasone 0.25 mg at bedtime can be used in combination with clomiphene citrate. Aromatase inhibitors and ovarian drilling are the next alternatives, followed by administration of gonadotropins or in vitro fertilization. Gonadotropins are effective, but are generally reserved as one of the last options because of ovarian hyperstimulation syndrome. Egg retrieval and in vitro fertilization may be used in conjunction with gonadotropins to increase pregnancy rate and minimize the likelihood of multiple pregnancies by limiting the number of transferred embryos.[62]

Treatment Decisions in PCOS

9. E.F. and her husband are overwhelmed by the number of options available to treat her PCOS. What is the best approach in evaluating E.F. and making appropriate recommendations?

Woman with PCOS exhibit unique clinical features and have individual concerns that should be addressed when making treatment recommendations. Assessment should include gathering relevant medical information, such as menstrual history, signs and symptoms of hyperandrogenism, time course of symptoms, weight history, previous agents tried, and family history. If PCOS is suspected, laboratory assessments should be performed to rule out any other related disorders. Once a diagnosis has been made, a recommendation about treatment must consider the patient's priorities and motivation.

In any obese patient, weight loss is a first step to improve many of the clinical and biochemical endocrine and metabolic abnormalities in PCOS. If contraception is desired, COCs will improve menstrual cycles and hyperandrogenism. If contraception is not needed, metformin will address menstrual cycle regulation, hyperandrogenism, and insulin resistance. COCs also will address menstrual cycle regulation, hyperandrogenism, and insulin resistance. Other agents, such as thiazolidinediones, can be used if metformin or COCs are contraindicated or have caused serious side effects. If pregnancy is desired, clomiphene citrate is the first-line pharmacologic option for ovulation induction. Other alternatives, including metformin, dexamethasone, aromatase inhibitors, gonadotropins, ovarian drilling, and in vitro fertilization, can be used if clomiphene citrate alone is not effective.

Appropriate follow-up for women such as E.F. may include quality-of-life measures, laboratory monitoring when necessary, and medication adherence monitoring. Providers should be educators, facilitators, and empathetic listeners to help women with PCOS become informed and actively engaged in their therapy plan.

DYSMENORRHEA

Dysmenorrhea, or painful cramping that occurs with the onset and first days of menstruation, can be categorized as either primary, without underlying uterine pathology, or secondary, owing to underlying uterine pathology. Secondary dysmenorrhea can result from uterine conditions, including endometriosis, uterine polyps, or fibroids; complications of intrauterine contraceptive device (IUD) use; or pelvic inflammatory disease.

Up to 93% of adolescents report some pain with menstruation, and up to 15% experience pain that is sufficiently severe and disabling to interfere with activities of daily life.[70] Dysmenorrhea is the single largest cause of lost productivity and school absence among adolescent girls. It most commonly begins within 1 to 2 years after the onset of menses.[71] The prevalence of primary dysmenorrhea decreases with age.[72]

Clinical Characteristics

10. A.B., a 17-year-old girl, presents at the pharmacy with complaints of severe cramping pain associated with her menstrual cycles. The pain predictably begins with the onset of menses and has been occurring for the past 5 years, but is now limiting A.B.'s ability to play sports in high school. A.B. states that she experienced her first menstrual period at age 11. The pain usually is "like a fist, clenching and relaxing," and it starts in the pelvic area, and radiates to her lower back. She reports no headache, but usually has diarrhea and some nausea, without vomiting. Her symptoms are most severe during the first 12 to 24 hours of her menses, then subside over the next few days. She usually takes two acetaminophen 325-mg tablets when her pain begins and then one tablet every 4 to 6 hours, as needed, with little relief. She has taken no other medications for her symptoms, has no known allergies to medications, and is not taking any other medications. She has no other medical problems. Her physical examination was within normal limits. What clinical manifestations in A.B. are consistent with primary dysmenorrhea?

No specific diagnostic criteria exist for primary dysmenorrhea. Typically, the diagnosis is one of exclusion, and is based on response to known effective therapy. Thus, if patients do not respond to therapy, an investigation of pelvic pathology and secondary dysmenorrheal should occur.[73] A.B.'s symptoms that are typical of primary dysmenorrhea include cramping pain in the suprapubic area, which may radiate into the back and thighs, nausea, and diarrhea. Some women also experience vomiting, fatigue, headache, lightheadedness, flushing, loss of appetite, irritability, nervousness, and insomnia.[72] Symptom severity seems to correlate with women who have early menarche (onset of menses), and those with increased duration and quantity of menstrual flow.[74] Risk factors for dysmenorrhea include age <20 years, depression or anxiety, nulliparity, menorrhagia, and smoking.[75]

Primary dysmenorrhea occurs only with ovulatory cycles, which typically begin after the first year following menarche. Dysmenorrhea occurring several years after menarche is most likely secondary dysmenorrhea, and should be investigated as such. Because A.B.'s pain began within 1 year of menarche and her physical examination is normal, a trial of an effective therapy can be initiated without further investigation into secondary causes of dysmenorrhea. The typical pattern of dysmenorrhea is to have pain beginning up to 12 hours before menses, increasing in severity for up to 24 hours, and continuing with reduced intensity for 24 to 72 hours.[72] A.B.'s description of pain, as a cramping–relaxing cycle, is typical for dysmenorrhea. Likely, her symptoms will decrease with age, after the onset of sexually activity, as well as after childbirth.[74]

Pathophysiology

11. What underlying pathophysiology explains A.B.'s symptoms?

In the normal menstrual cycle, prostaglandins are released by the endometrium in the late luteal phase inducing contraction of the uterine smooth muscle and subsequent sloughing of the endometrium, leading to menstrual flow and the beginning of the follicular phase of the next cycle. Women with primary dysmenorrhea appear to have increased prostaglandin secretion, inducing more intense uterine contractions, leading to decreased uterine blood flow and uterine hypoxia, which results in the cramping and pain that are the hallmarks of dysmenorrhea.[73] The decreasing levels of progesterone in the late luteal phase trigger the release of arachidonic acid from cell membranes, ultimately resulting in the production of prostaglandins and leukotrienes.[73]

The importance of prostaglandin secretion in the pathology of primary dysmenorrhea is confirmed by studies of the exogenous administration of prostaglandin $F_2\alpha$ ($PGF_2\alpha$), and PGE_2, each of which produce pain and uterine contractions similar to those observed in women with primary dysmenorrhea.[76] These prostaglandins, with potent platelet disaggregation and vasodilatory properties, also induce nausea, vomiting, and diarrhea. Thus, A.B.'s pain, nausea, and diarrhea may caused by elevated prostaglandin levels. This also explains the rationale for the effectiveness of the two main treatments for primary dysmenorrhea: nonsteroidal anti-inflammatory drugs (NSAID), which inhibit prostaglandin synthesis, and combined oral contraceptives, which minimize the progesterone increase typically seen in the luteal phase.

Nearly 85% to 90% of women initially thought to have primary dysmenorrhea respond to NSAID with or without oral contraceptive therapy. The remaining women deserve further investigation into potential causes of secondary dysmenorrhea.[77]

Treatment

Nonpharmacologic Treatment

12. What nonpharmacologic therapies may be effective for the treatment of A.B.'s symptoms of primary dysmenorrhea?

A.B. should be educated about the causes of primary dysmenorrhea, its associated symptoms, and the rationale behind nonpharmacologic and pharmacologic treatment options. Nonpharmacologic therapies that may have benefit in the relief of A.B.'s symptoms include aerobic exercise, heat therapy, tobacco use cessation, omega-3 polyunsaturated fatty acids, and transcutaneous electrical nerve stimulation (TENS).

Exercise, particularly aerobic exercise, has been correlated with decreased menstrual symptoms in observational studies, and is, in all patients, associated with positive general health benefits.[78] The benefit may be owing to improved pelvic blood flow and decreased ischemia, or increased release of β-endorphins. Application of local heat to the lower abdomen has been studied in two clinical trials, one comparing a heated wrap patch with ibuprofen 400 mg, the other comparing it with acetaminophen 1,000 mg.[79,80] Heat plus ibuprofen demonstrated a reduction in the time to pain relief compared with an unheated patch plus ibuprofen; and heat provided better relief than acetaminophen. With few adverse effects, heat, in the form of a heating pad or heated patch or wrap device, represents a reasonable suggestion for women with dysmenorrhea.

Women should be advised and assisted in efforts to stop tobacco use. Although no direct evidence links smoking cessation with improvement in dysmenorrhea, an association exists with increased risk and severity of dysmenorrhea in women who smoke.[74] Increased intake of omega-3 polyunsaturated fatty acids, a low-fat vegetarian diet, or both may decrease the intensity and duration of symptoms.[81–83]

Transcutaneous electrical nerve stimulation has been evaluated in seven small trials, and when high frequency stimulation was utilized, it was more effective than placebo in achieving pain relief.[84] Acupuncture may also be effective, although few trials, utilizing heterogeneous techniques and study designs have been conducted, which makes interpretation difficult.[84] In extreme cases, surgical interruption of pelvic nerve pathways has been utilized as a last resort, with continued pain control up to 12 months in clinical trials.[85]

A.B.'s therapy should be based on her specific symptoms, response to previous therapy, and any adverse effects of therapy. The regimen of acetaminophen that A.B. is currently using is not providing relief owing to its lack of effect on prostaglandin activity. Discussion of the nonpharmacologic therapies, particularly heat, exercise, and smoking cessation, provide low risk, potentially beneficial and low-cost suggestions for pain relief, in addition to drug therapy.

Pharmacologic Therapy

Pharmacologic therapy for primary dysmenorrhea is focused on reducing prostaglandin activity. Anti-inflammatory drugs act by directly inhibiting prostaglandin synthesis. Hormonal contraceptives reduce the amount of endometrial proliferation and, as a result, decrease the amount of prostaglandins secreted. By inhibiting ovulation, hormonal contraceptives eliminate the cyclic changes in progesterone that induce prostaglandin release. Both NSAID and hormonal contraceptives provide relief from the symptoms of primary dysmenorrhea for most women.

Choice of therapy depends on the need for contraception, concomitant medical conditions, and patient preference. Treatment efficacy can be monitored by evaluating pain relief, improved functionality, reduced absenteeism, and relief of other symptoms (e.g., diarrhea, nausea) associated with dysmenorrhea. Nonsteroidal agents should be tried for two to three cycles before switching to other agents. Hormonal contraceptives may require 3 or more months to provide maximal relief of symptoms. The goals of therapy, namely reduction in pain and associated symptoms, as well as improvement in functionality, should be explained to the patient, and reviewed at each contact.

ANTI-INFLAMMATORY DRUGS

Mechanism of Action

Prostaglandins, leukotrienes, thromboxanes, and prostacyclin are synthesized via the arachidonic acid pathway. Free, unesterified fatty acids, such as arachidonic acid (derived from phospholipids, cholesterol, and triglycerides), are prostaglandin precursors. Arachidonic acid may be synthesized from phospholipids found in cell membranes of the menstruating uterus through hydrolysis by the lysosomal enzyme, phospholipase A_2. It is then metabolized by one of two enzyme systems. Lipoxygenase converts arachidonic acid to 5-hydroperoxyeicosatetraenoic acid, which is converted to leukotrienes. Cyclooxygenase metabolizes arachidonic acid to unstable cyclic endoperoxides (PGG_2 and PGH_2), which are then converted to prostacyclin (PGI_2), thromboxane A_2, and the prostaglandins PGF_2 and PGE_2 by the action of prostacyclin synthetase, thromboxane synthetase, or isomerase reductase, respectively.[86] Cyclooxygenase I (COX-1) is responsible for the synthesis of prostaglandins involved in normal physiologic processes. Cyclooxygenase 2 (COX-2) is an inducible enzyme that produces prostaglandins involved in an inflammatory response.(See Chapter 43, Rheumatic Disorders, for additional information). In addition to the inhibition of prostaglandin synthesis, NSAIDs relieve pain through their analgesic effects.

Choice of Agent

13. A.B.'s family physician decides to initiate naproxen sodium 550 mg orally at the beginning of menses, followed by 275 mg every 8 hours thereafter for the 2 to 3 days she experiences dysmenorrhea. What criteria should be used to select an NSAID for primary dysmenorrhea? Explain to A.B why she should take it according to the regimen above.

Table 47-4 NSAID and Dosing Regimens for Primary Dysmenorrhea

Groups	Drugs	Dosages	Dosing Regimen (Maximum Daily Dose)	Approved for Primary Dysmenorrhea
Salicylic acids	Aspirin	325, 500, 650, 975 mg	500–600 mg PO Q 4–6 hr	No
Indole acetic acids	Diclofenac	50 mg (as potassium)	50 mg PO TID; some patients may need a first dose of 100 mg followed by 50 mg TID; (150 mg/day, may give 200 mg on first day)	Yes
Propionic acids	Ibuprofen	300–800 mg doses	400 mg PO Q 4–6 hr[a] (3.2 g/day)	Yes
	Ketoprofen	12.5, 25, 50, 75 mg	25–50 mg Q 6–8 hr[b] (300 mg/day)	Yes
	Naproxen	250, 375, 500 mg	500 mg PO first dose; 250 mg PO Q 6–8 hr (1,250 mg/day)	Yes
	Naproxen sodium	220, 275 mg	550 mg PO first dose; 275 mg PO Q 6–8 hr (1,375 mg/day)[c]	Yes
Fenamates	Meclofenamate sodium	50, 100 mg	100 mg TID for up to 6 days (300 mg/day)	No
	Mefenamic acid	250 mg	500 mg PO first dose; 250 mg PO Q 6 hr for 2–3 days (1 g/day; may give 1.25 g on first day)	Yes
COX-2 selective agents	Celecoxib	100, 200, 400 mg	400 mg PO first dose; 200 mg BID	Yes

[a]Dosing recommended for dysmenorrhea when using the prescription product is higher than the over-the-counter (OTC) dosing of 200 mg Q 4–6 hr; may wish to start with the OTC dosing when an OTC product is used.
[b]Dosing recommended for dysmenorrhea when using the prescription product is higher than the OTC dosing of 12.5 Q 6–8 hr; may wish to start with the OTC dosing when an OTC product is used.
[c]Dosing recommended for dysmenorrhea when using the prescription product is higher than the OTC dosing of 220 mg Q 8–12 hr; may wish to start with the OTC dosing when an OTC product is used.
NSAID, nonsteroidal anti-inflammatory drug.
BID, twice daily; PO, orally; TID, three times daily.
From references 72, 73, 87, 93.

The NSAIDs are effective for treatment of dysmenorrhea (Table 47-4). Initial selection of therapy should be based on effectiveness, incidence of adverse effects, cost, patient history of previous benefit, and availability. Naproxen (as the sodium salt), ibuprofen, and ketoprofen are approved without a prescription for the treatment of primary dysmenorrhea. In a Cochrane review, 63 trials of NSAIDs for treatment of primary dysmenorrhea were reviewed to assess for any differences in efficacy or safety among the different NSAIDs.[87] When compared with placebo, NSAIDs were significantly more effective (odds ratio [OR] 7.91, 95% confidence interval [CI] 5.65–11.09). In limited head-to-head trials comparing NSAIDs, no significant differences in efficacy were seen, with the exception of aspirin being slightly less effective than other NSAIDs when directly compared. Adverse effects seen in these trials were generally mild GI (nausea, upset stomach) and neurologic (sleepiness, dizziness, headache) complaints. When directly compared with each other, no NSAID was found to be better tolerated than another. Naproxen and ketoprofen offer the advantage of less frequent dosing compared with ibuprofen.

A.B.'s physician suggested taking a loading dose of the naproxen sodium (550 mg). A randomized trial demonstrated increased relief from dysmenorrhea symptoms in adolescents treated with an NSAID regimen that started with a loading dose, versus those who utilized a flat dosing regimen.[88] Loading doses generally are twice the regular dose. Although all NSAIDs that have been studied for the treatment of dysmenorrhea appear to be equally effective at reducing pain, there may be theoretic advantages to those that achieve peak serum concentrations 30 to 60 minutes after administration (ibuprofen, naproxen sodium, and meclofenamate). Some claim that meclofenamate is more beneficial for the treatment of dysmenorrhea because of its ability to block both the cyclooxygenase and the lipoxygenase pathway in the formation of prostaglandins, but this pharmacologic difference does not appear to confer a clinically significant advantage.[72] If A.B. experienced adverse effects with the higher loading dose, an alternative strategy is to initiate dosing 24 hours before menses is expected to start, based on the calendar if the patient has predictable cycles, or based on the start of premenstrual syndrome-type symptoms. This prophylactic dosing may be helpful especially for patients who have severe dysmenorrhea with absenteeism and decreased work or school productivity.[73,87] A.B.'s provider also has suggested she take the regimen on a scheduled basis, versus "as needed". Although no specific evidence supports this practice for dysmenorrhea, avoiding as needed ("PRN") dosing may provide consistent serum levels to maintain reduced prostaglandin levels. As the duration of therapy is typically limited to 2 or 3 days, risk of adverse effects tends to be outweighed by the potential benefit of loading doses, prophylactic dosing, and scheduled versus PRN therapy.

Although the COX-2 selective inhibitor, celecoxib, is approved for the treatment of primary dysmenorrhea, it has not been directly compared with conventional NSAID for effectiveness for pain control. The U.S. Food and Drug Administration (FDA) approved dosing of celecoxib at a 400-mg loading dose, followed by 200 mg that same day if needed, then 200 mg twice daily thereafter. Increased cost, lack of increased benefit, and limited data regarding differences in GI safety make celecoxib a second-line therapy for primary dysmenorrhea.

Adverse Effects

14. What adverse effects might A.B. experience from her NSAID?

All NSAIDs have a similar adverse effect profile. Nausea, vomiting, indigestion, anorexia, diarrhea, constipation, abdominal pain, melena, and bloating are common GI complaints. Central nervous system (CNS) adverse effects include headache, vertigo, dizziness, visual disturbances, depression, drowsiness, irritability, excitation, insomnia, fatigue, tremors, and confusion. In addition, adverse effects also may involve cardiovascular, hepatic, renal, or hematologic systems (see Chapter 43, Rheumatic Disorders).

Careful attention should be given to previous trials of NSAID for dysmenorrhea and other conditions, because women may respond favorably to one NSAID over another. If a 2- or 3-month trial of one NSAID is unsuccessful, another agent from a different class may be tried. Because dysmenorrhea is most prevalent in younger women, who tend to be healthy, the risk of adverse events may be lower than would be expected in an older population.

Contraindications

15. What medical history information is important to avoid serious adverse effects?

A.B should be questioned about medication allergies, any prior history of ulceration, or GI bleeding, and history of cardiovascular and renal disease elicited before prescribing therapy. A thorough medication history, including over-the-counter (OTC) agents and dietary supplements should be conducted. Particular attention should be paid to any potential therapeutic duplications (i.e., prescription and OTC NSAIDs), drug–drug (e.g., warfarin), and drug–disease (hypertension) interactions.

Women who are allergic to aspirin or have a history of allergic reaction to any NSAID should not use NSAIDs or celecoxib. Celecoxib should also be avoided in women who are allergic to sulfa drugs. A.B. has not had a previous allergic reaction to NSAID or aspirin; she is not taking any medications that may interact and does not have any history of medical problems that would prevent her from a trial of NSAID therapy.

HORMONAL CONTRACEPTION

Oral Contraceptives

16. After 6 months of treatment, A.B. has some relief of her pain, nausea, and diarrhea with the naproxen sodium, and has not missed a soccer game in 5 months. She is asking about other treatment options for further pain relief. When would the use of an oral contraceptive be an appropriate choice for A.B.?

Oral contraceptives (OC) suppress ovulation, decrease menstrual fluid volume, and subsequently decrease prostaglandin production and uterine cramping.[70,72] OCs alone, or in combination with an NSAID, are appropriate as first-line treatment in women without a need for contraception. OC relieve dysmenorrhea symptoms in 50% to 80% of women within 3 to 6 months after beginning hormone therapy.[89] A study of healthy adolescent women with primary dysmenorrhea evaluated the effects of a 20-mcg ethinyl estradiol/100-mcg levonorgestrel oral contraceptive pill as compared with placebo over a 3-month period.[90] With OC use, women reported decreased severity of pain, and used less pain medication. A Cochrane review of oral contraceptives and primary dysmenorrheal failed to demonstrate a significant difference between various OC formulations.[89] Selection of an OC should be based on factors presented in Chapter 45, Contraception. Although many providers prescribe extended cycles of oral contraceptives to treat primary dysmenorrhea, no evidence suggests that this practice is more effective than the customary 21/7, and a to change from traditional dosing to continuous dosing may be considered if symptoms occur during the placebo week.[77,91]

Adverse effects and contraindication associated with OC use must be considered. Although serious complications from OC use are uncommon in young, healthy women, breakthrough bleeding and spotting, nausea, and breast tenderness may occur, especially early in treatment. A.B. may choose to add an OC to her naproxen sodium, with potentially improved pain relief compared with either agent alone. If pain does not respond to either course of therapy, investigation via laparoscopy for causes of secondary dysmenorrhea may be necessary.

Other Hormonal Contraceptive Agents

Other hormonal contraceptive agents that suppress ovulation have also been used in the treatment of primary dysmenorrhea, although none have undergone rigorous trials for this indication.[77] The levonorgestrel intrauterine system (IUS) is associated with amenorrhea and decreased dysmenorrhea over time, unlike the copper IUD, which may result in increased pain, cramping, and blood loss. Three years after insertion, fewer women with a levonorgestrel IUS reported menstrual pain (60% baseline, 29% after 3 years), with 47% of women with amenorrhea.[92] In women with primary dysmenorrhea at low risk of sexually transmitted infections, and desiring long term contraception, the levonorgestrel IUS would be an option.

Medroxyprogesterone depot injection is another hormonal contraceptive agent that has been used to treat primary dysmenorrhea. Nearly two-thirds of adolescents reported fewer symptoms of dysmenorrhea with injections every 3 months.[72] Negative effects of medroxyprogesterone injections on bone density should be weighed with potential benefit when considering this option.

OTHER AGENTS

18. What are other agents that can be recommended for the treatment of A.B.'s primary dysmenorrhea?

Although NSAID and hormonal contraceptives have the most evidence supporting their use for the treatment of primary dysmenorrhea, a variety of other agents have been evaluated. In adolescents, 91% reported using OTC medications to treat primary dysmenorrhea, usually without consultation from a health care professional.[71] This lack of professional advice resulted, however, in nearly 70% of women using <50% of the maximal dose of medication on day 1 of pain. Only 66% of patients choose to use ibuprofen, whereas 44% selected acetaminophen, 30% selected acetaminophen–pyrilamine combinations, and 10% acetaminophen, magnesium salicylate, pamabrom combination products. Acetaminophen does not suppress prostaglandin synthesis and is of limited efficacy in the treatment of dysmenorrhea, when compared with NSAID or hormonal contraception.[93] Narcotic analgesics do not have a role in the treatment of primary dysmenorrhea.

Leukotriene receptor antagonists have also been studied in the treatment of primary dysmenorrhea, because the leukotriene pathway to prostaglandin formation is relatively unaffected by NSAID. Although the pharmacology is promising, small trials in patients with primary dysmenorrhea with the leukotriene receptor antagonist montelukast have not demonstrated significant pain reduction.[94]

Transdermal nitroglycerin ointment and transdermal patches provide rapid relief of dysmenorrhea in up to 90% of patients, but use is limited by adverse effects, including headache in up to 25% of patients.[95] Nitroglycerin serves to increase nitric oxide concentrations, which results in uterine relaxation. Guaifenesin 2,400 mg daily has been evaluated in a small trial, with a nonsignificant trend toward benefit, potentially owing to thinning effects on cervical secretions.[96]

Vitamin B_1 100 mg daily, magnesium, vitamin B_6, and omega-3 fatty acids have all shown some benefit in pain relief compared with placebo, with Vitamin B_1 and magnesium showing the most promise.[83] Other dietary supplements, including fennel, vitamin E, neptune krill oil, and toki-shakuyaju-san, have been evaluated in small trials and need further study.[77]

ENDOMETRIOSIS

Endometriosis is defined as the presence of functional endometrial tissue occurring outside the uterine cavity. It is the most common cause of secondary dysmenorrhea in young women, and can result in chronic pelvic pain, infertility, and dyspareunia.[72] The ovaries are commonly the site of endometriosis, which can also be found in the pelvic peritoneum, cervix, vagina, vulva, rectosigmoid colon, and appendix. Less common sites of implantation of endometrial tissue include the umbilicus, scar tissue resulting from surgery, kidneys, lungs, and even arms and legs.[97] Endometriosis is present in up to 45% of women with infertility. Overall, it is difficult to determine the prevalence of endometriosis, because many women do not experience symptoms or seek treatment, and formal diagnostic criteria currently require visual identification of endometrial tissue during surgery. In women who have laparotomies for any reason, endometriosis is identified in 5% to 15%. This increases to 33% in women with chronic pelvic pain.[97] In contrast to primary dysmenorrhea, endometriosis usually occurs in women who have been menstruating for some time; it can provoke pain that is not limited to the time of the menses, but can occur anytime throughout the cycle. Endometriosis is rarely seen in women near the menarche, after menopause, or in amenorrheic women. Given the many women with endometriosis; the expense of diagnosis and treatment; and the infertility associated with it, endometriosis represents a significant area of cost in the health care system.[98]

Diagnostic Criteria

Diagnosis of endometriosis is difficult, with a delay in diagnosis in the range of 8 to 12 years from initial symptom presentation.[99] Endometriosis, interstitial cystitis, irritable bowel syndrome, and pelvic adhesions represent the four most common causes of chronic pelvic pain (defined as pain not associated with the menses, severe in nature, resulting in functional disability, and lasting at least 6 months).[100] The delay in diagnosis is the unfortunate consequence of the lack of diagnostic laboratory markers, and its similarities to these other conditions. The physical examination is often normal, although the most common physical finding is a fixed retroverted uterus, with scarring and tenderness. A definitive diagnosis is only possible with visualization of endometriosis on laparoscopy, although this is not considered as absolutely necessary today as it has been in the past.[101] Although no diagnostic criteria currently exist, endometriosis can be staged at the time of laparoscopy according to the Revised American Fertility Society Classification of Endometriosis.[102] The stages are minimal (stage I), mild (stage II), moderate (stage III), and severe (stage IV) as determined by an accumulated point total, with points based on the location of the endometrial lesions, the size of the lesions, the presence and extent of the adhesions, and the degree of obliteration of the posterior cul-de-sac. The classification system is designed to document the location and extent of endometriosis and does not predict infertility, aid in treatment selection or outcomes, or predict recurrence of disease. Making diagnosis and prognosis more difficult is that the reported severity of pelvic pain and level of functional disability do not seem to be correlated to the stage of endometriosis.[97]

Clinical Characteristics

19. N.H. is a 32-year-old mechanical engineer who has been married for 6 years, and is currently using the vaginal contraceptive ring to prevent pregnancy. She and her spouse have been contemplating the timing of a pregnancy, but have not yet attempted to become pregnant. She presents to her gynecologist to discuss preconceptual planning, and reports that she has been having severe lower abdominal cramps, associated with her menses, occurring on day 1 and lasting until day 4 or 5. This has been occurring for the past 4 years after many years of pain-free cycles, and has recently been increasing in severity. The pain is slightly relieved by ibuprofen 400 mg TID, and over the past 6 months she has had to work from home at least 1 to 2 days per month owing to pain that has been increasing in frequency. On further questioning, she also reports mild to moderate pain that occurs randomly in her cycle, associated with low back pain, constipation with painful defecation, and pain with intercourse. Her menstrual history reveals menarche at age 10 with regular cycles every 26 to 27 days and heavy menses for 6 to 7 days. She reports discussing her symptoms with her mother, who described similar symptoms during her childbearing years.

Her physical examination is normal, with the exception of tenderness on palpation of the posterior fornix, and a fixed retroverted uterus. A pregnancy test, and tests for gonorrhea and chlamydia are negative, and a pap smear is within normal limits. What subjective and objective data in N.H.'s presentation is compatible with a diagnosis of endometriosis?

A woman presenting with endometriosis may have signs and symptoms that are difficult, initially, to distinguish from primary dysmenorrhea [103] (Table 47-5) N.H.'s symptoms of lower abdominal cramps accompanying her menses are often mistaken for primary dysmenorrhea when other history details are not evaluated in total. N.H.'s age and her nulliparity are consistent with the characteristics of women with endometriosis. Although endometriosis has been diagnosed in women of all ages, it most commonly occurs in women in their late 20s and early 30s who have delayed pregnancy or who have infrequent pregnancies.

Table 47-5 Primary Versus Secondary Dysmenorrhea

Characteristic	*Primary Dysmenorrhea*	*Secondary Dysmenorrhea*
Onset	Around menarche	Any age (while menstruating)
Timing in menstrual cycle	Worse day 1, lasts 24–48 hr	Increases in severity, may last days
Change over time	Stable, predictable	Increasing pain with increasing age
Symptoms	Low back pain, premenstrual syndrome (PMS), nausea, bloating	Low back pain, dyspareunia, diarrhea or constipation, dysuria, infertility
Signs	Normal pelvic examination	Fixed retroverted uterus, tenderness, but may be completely normal

Adapted from reference 103, with permission.

N.H.'s menstrual pattern of short cycle length with prolonged flow is characteristic of women with endometriosis. Risk factors for endometriosis are related to exposure to estrogen (i.e., early menarche and late menopause), and shorter menstrual cycle length (<28 days) with longer duration of menstrual flow (≥6 days), as well as having a mother or sister with endometriosis, as may be true with N.H.'s mother.[104] Potential, but not yet confirmed, risk factors that have been identified include genetic factors, higher social class, exposure to dioxins, and intake of caffeine and alcohol. Increased BMI and cigarette smoking appear to reduce the risk for endometriosis.[105,106]

N.H.'s chief complaints center on her progressive pelvic pain occurring throughout the cycle, with worsening during menses, constipation, and pain with intercourse (dyspareunia). Women who report pain during intercourse may have a fixed, retroverted uterus (as N.H. does) or endometriosis located in the posterior fornix of the vagina or along the uterosacral ligaments.[97] This pain may persist for several hours after intercourse. Other symptoms such as the constipation and painful defecation N.H. is experiencing, are associated with endometriosis and may (but not always) depend on the organs affected by the location of the endometrial tissue[107,108] (Table 47-6). Depression also is a common symptom in patients with endometriosis, particularly those with chronic pelvic pain, and may express as sadness, somatic complaints, inability to work, or carry on activities of normal living.[109]

Although it is unclear yet whether infertility will be a problem in N.H., endometriosis occurs in up to 45% of women with infertility.[97] The cause of endometriosis-associated infertility is not clear, but is probably caused by a combination of factors, which may include physical distortion of the pelvic architecture, inflammatory factors (including prostanoids, cytokines, and growth factors that may interfere with normal reproductive processes), impaired folliculogenesis, or defects in fertilization or implantation.[110,111] Treatment for endometriosis, in inducing a "pseudo-menopause," results in impaired fertility while actively being treated.

N.H.'s limited physical findings are not uncommon in women with endometriosis; physical findings, other than visualization of endometrial tissue during exploratory surgery, may not be present, and outward physical findings may have no correlation with the stage of endometriosis determined with surgery. Many symptoms and physical findings of endometriosis can be associated with other gynecologic conditions or diseases (particularly irritable bowel disease as mentioned) and, if the patient is not responsive to empiric therapy, laparoscopy is indicated to confirm the diagnosis. N.H.'s negative pregnancy, chlamydia, and gonorrhea tests, as well as her normal pap smear are reassuring. Other laboratory tests that have been evaluated to diagnose endometriosis have not been sufficiently sensitive or specific in clinical trials to be routinely used. Tests, such as CA-125 are not sufficiently specific as a single test to diagnose endometriosis, but may have potential in combination with others as markers of disease severity and of treatment efficacy, and their utility is currently being investigated.[112]

Table 47-6 Location of Endometriosis and Associated Symptoms

Sites	*Symptoms*
Most Common	
Pelvic	
Cervix	Abnormal uterine bleeding
Ovaries	Dysmenorrhea
Peritoneum	Dyspareunia
Rectovaginal septum	Infertility
Uterosacral ligaments	Pelvic pain
Intestinal	
Abdominal scars	Intestinal obstruction
Sigmoid colon	Midabdominal pain
Small intestines	Nausea
	Painful defecation
	Rectal bleeding
Urinary Tract	
Bladder	Cyclic flank pain
Ureter	Hematuria
	Hydronephrosis
	Hydroureter
Least Common	
Miscellaneous	
Breasts	Hemoptysis
Diaphragm	Sciatica
Extremities	Subarachnoid bleeding
Gallbladder	
Pleura	
Sciatic notch	
Spleen	
Stomach	
Subarachnoid space	

From references 107, 108, with permission.

Pathophysiology

Although the first description of endometriosis was made in the 1860s, the precise etiology of endometriosis remains a mystery. Several theories exist regarding the origins of endometriosis, and the exact etiology is probably a complex interplay between physical and individual patient-specific immunologic factors.[97]

The most commonly cited theory is that of retrograde menstruation, or the flow of menstrual fluid, endometrial cells, and other debris backward through the fallopian tubes resulting in implantation in the peritoneal cavity. Once endometrial cells reach the peritoneum, stimulated angiogenesis (potentially by estrogen, among other factors) appears to be a determinant of the development and growth of lesions.[113,114] Also at this point, the lesion stimulates an immune response, triggering the activation of macrophages, as well as cytokine and growth factor release. Peritoneal lesions may contribute to more distant disease by spread via hematogenous or lymphatic routes, or even by movement owing to iatrogenic causes, such as cesarean sections and other forms of gynecologic surgery. Outflow obstruction of the genital tract may also contribute to retrograde menstruation and endometriosis, particularly in adolescents with primary amenorrhea. Investigation and removal of obstruction(s) may impede the course of the disease in those patients.[97,105,114] Although the retrograde menstruation theory makes scientific sense, it has been discovered that retrograde menstruation occurs in nearly all menstruating women (90%), and not all women have endometriosis. This suggests that an additional factor, such as genetic susceptibility or altered immunity, must be present for the pathogenesis of endometriosis in certain patients.

Another theory for the etiology of endometriosis is the coelomic metaplasia theory. This theory rests on the belief that the coelomic epithelium, the fetal originator tissue for the reproductive tract, retains its ability to differentiate into multiple cell types.[97,105,115] The trigger for differentiation is thought to be, in part, estrogen or environmental factors. This theory would explain the presence of endometriosis in prepubertal girls, in women born without a uterus, and in the rare cases of endometriosis seen in men. Genetics also play a role in the development of endometriosis. There is a six times higher rate of endometriosis in first degree relatives in women with severe endometriosis when compared with those who do not have endometriosis; they also have more severe disease and disease that appears earlier in life.[97,115] More than 15 different gene and gene product abnormalities have been documented in women with endometriosis. Environmental factors, as discussed, are intriguing in their role as potential causative factors, but are not definitive.[106,115]

Once endometrial tissue becomes implanted, hormones are necessary for their continued growth. As with intrauterine endometrium, the implants of endometriosis possess estrogen, progesterone, and androgen receptors. The endometrial implants may, however, respond differently to hormonal stimulation than normal endometrium. In general, estrogens stimulate the implants, whereas androgens or lack of estrogen results in implant atrophy. Because of their complex hormonal effects, progestins have variable effects on the implants.[102,116] (See Chapter 46 Obstetric Drug Therapy for the effects of estrogens and progestins on the endometrium.) In addition, lesions also show high levels of estrogen biosynthesis, owing to abnormally increased aromatase activity, with a concomitant decrease in the inactivation of estrogen, resulting in high intralesional estrogen concentrations.[115,117] The responsiveness of endometrial implants to ovarian hormones plays a role in the pathology of endometriosis. Withdrawal of estrogen and progesterone causes the endometrial implants to bleed, leading to an inflammatory response in the adjacent tissues. Repetitive cycles of bleeding and inflammation lead to the development of scar tissue and adhesions between adjacent peritoneal tissues. On laparoscopy, these areas of involvement appear as multiple hemorrhagic foci composed of endometrial epithelium, stroma, and glands. Ovarian endometriosis usually involves the formation of endometriomas, blood-filled cysts ("chocolate cysts") ranging in size from microscopic to 10 cm. Nodules may form on uterosacral ligaments. Fibrosis usually is present with the endometrial implants, and extensive adhesions may form between pelvic structures.[118]

Treatment

20. Given the potential mechanisms behind the pathophysiology of endometriosis, what therapeutic approaches are available for the treatment of endometriosis in N.H.?

Therapy for endometriosis should be individualized, and consider N.H.'s desire for future fertility, severity of symptoms, extent of disease, and potential for infertility. This should be done with the knowledge that a high likelihood exists of recurrence and a lack of good prognostic indicators for future severity. The goals of treatment are to relieve symptoms and, if desired, to preserve or improve fertility. Options currently available to treat endometriosis include definitive and conservative surgery, hormonal therapy with estrogen–progestin combinations or progestins alone, danazol, aromatase inhibitors, or the GnRH agonists, and expectant management. Pharmacologic treatment of endometriosis is based on manipulation of this hormonal response: danazol, GnRH agonists, progestins, aromatase inhibitors, and estrogen–progestin combination all cause endometrial tissue atrophy. No treatment has been shown to provide 100% protection against recurrence when discontinued; even surgical removal of the uterus and ovaries is associated with recurrence rates of up to 10%.[114]

Pain Management: Nonpharmacologic Therapy

"DEFINITIVE" SURGERY

Definitive surgery, referring to total abdominal hysterectomy, bilateral salpingo-oophorectomy, and removal of all visible endometriosis, theoretically should eliminate the risk of recurrence of the disease. These procedures are not an option for the many women with endometriosis who desire pregnancy in the future. It is invasive surgery, reserved for those patients whose pain is unresponsive to other therapies or to conservative surgery. Furthermore, removal of all endometriosis is difficult, and recurring pain is not uncommon. Sinaii et al.[119] surveyed patients with endometriosis regarding treatments and benefits, and found that, of the 1,160 women surveyed, 12% had had definitive surgery, with 40% reporting the surgery was successful, 33% reporting partial benefit, 5.6% reporting no benefit, and 6% of patients actually reported increased pain and symptoms after surgery.

CONSERVATIVE SURGERY

In contrast to definitive surgery, conservative surgery (involving ablation and removal of implants, and lysis of adhesions) preserves fertility, and is commonly conducted during the initial diagnostic laparoscopy. In the Sinaii et al. survey,[119] 70% of patients had undergone laparoscopy with removal of lesions, with 30% considering the procedure a success, 50% reporting partial benefit, 15% with no difference in symptoms, and 10% who reported increased symptoms. On average, women reported having three surgical procedures.[119] Drug treatment is used after conservative surgery, as it is not possible to remove all lesions, many of which are difficult to visualize. Clinical trials utilizing GnRH agonists for up to 6 months after conservative surgery have provided mixed results, and danazol and medroxyprogesterone trials have shown similar results.[120] Oral contraceptives and progestin intrauterine devices have not been evaluated for prevention of recurrence after surgery.

Pain Management: Pharmacologic Therapy

NSAID

Nonsteroidal anti-inflammatory agents, particularly those available as OTC products, are often the first medications that women try for relief of pain from endometriosis, often before they are officially diagnosed. Although typically not thought of as "disease modifying agents," NSAIDs may have a role beyond pain control because of the presence of increased cyclooxygenase (both I and II) expression in endometriosis lesions.[117] Although evidence at this point is predominantly in animal models, a potential exists for non–pain-related benefits with NSAIDs in endometriosis. NSAIDs may provide some relief of mild symptoms, particularly in women with endometriosis who have pain associated with the menses (see Dysmenorrhea section), and are an appropriate first choice for women with mild symptoms who desire conception. They should not be the only therapy offered to patients with confirmed endometriosis.[121] Pharmacists should be aware of and consider the potential for endometriosis in patients with noncyclic pain, including pain that does not respond to an appropriate trial of an NSAID. N.H. has been taking ibuprofen with some relief; a higher dose or trial of another NSAID is an appropriate strategy at this time. Additional treatment should be considered once her response to therapy with a different NSAID has been evaluated.

ORAL CONTRACEPTIVES

For women who do not receive pain relief from a trial of an NSAID, a reasonable next step for those women desiring contraception is the use of oral contraceptives because they are considerably better tolerated over the long term versus other hormonal options. They may be used alone or in combination with NSAIDs. OCs improve symptoms of endometriosis by inhibiting ovulation, decreasing hormone levels, reducing menstrual flow, potentially to the point of amenorrhea. These mechanisms contribute to atrophy of endometrial implants. When used, the most appropriate regimen is continuous OC dosing, so that there is not a "placebo week" that allows for growth of endometrial implants. In a trial of patients who did not respond to cyclic OCs, use of continuous dosing resulted in significant pain reduction.[122] A recent Cochrane review found that the benefits of OCs (≤35 mcg of ethinyl estradiol) are similar those seen with the GnRH agonist implants (goserelin).[123]

Investigators in Japan also evaluated women with dysmenorrhea and endometriosis in a placebo-controlled trial with a low-dose OC. Over the course of three cycles, patients reported that contraceptive use decreased disability caused by pain, and reduced the number of days when analgesics were required, with minimal side effects.[124] It is important to note that these benefits were seen although the drug was administered in a cyclic fashion.

PROGESTINS

Similarly to oral contraceptives, progestins reduce symptoms of endometriosis by inhibiting ovulation, reducing hormone levels, and inducing endometrial atrophy. They may be particularly useful if estrogen use is contraindicated. Regimens used include oral medroxyprogesterone in high doses (30–100 mg daily), depot medroxyprogesterone in the usual doses (150 mg intramuscularly [IM] every 3 months or 104 mg subcutaneously [SC] every 3 months). More recent studies have evaluated the use of the levonorgestrel IUS as a means of providing consistent progestin dosing. The IUS has the advantage of providing longer term contraception. When compared with leuprolide depot, the levonorgestrel IUS provided similar benefits in reducing pelvic pain, with a decreased potential for hypoestrogenic effects, and an increased potential for early breakthrough bleeding, followed by eventual amenorrhea.[125] Progestins, although as effective as GnRH agonists in the treatment of pain, have increased side effects when compared with OCs, primarily weight gain, initial breakthrough bleeding followed by amenorrhea, and decreased bone density with prolonged use, placing them after OCs in choice of therapy.[126]

GONADOTROPIN-RELEASING HORMONE AGONISTS

Gonadotropin-releasing hormone agonists induce a pseudomenopausal state, resulting in relief of endometriosis symptoms. Because the GnRH agonists have a longer half-life than endogenous GnRH, their binding to GnRH receptors in the pituitary results in downregulation of the hypothalamic-pituitary-ovarian axis, decreasing release of FSH and LH, leading to low estrogen levels and amenorrhea.[127] GnRH agonists are available in a variety of dosage forms, outlined in Table 47-7. When compared in clinical trials, GnRH agonists have efficacy that is similar to oral contraceptives, progestins, and danazol, but their increased cost, and adverse effect profile (including menopausal-type symptoms and decreased bone density) make them second-line agents, after OCs, and progestins (see Questions 25–27).[128]

AROMATASE INHIBITORS

The most recently studied therapy for endometriosis, aromatase inhibitors (AIs), were originally developed for use in patients with breast cancer. Aromatase, the enzyme responsible for the synthesis of estrogens, is required for the conversion of androstenedione and testosterone to estrone and estradiol.[129] Although aromatase inhibitors, OCs, progestins, and GnRH agonists all decrease serum levels of estrogen, only AIs decrease secretion and production of estrogen by endometrial tissue itself. Anastrozole and letrozole are type II aromatase inhibitors, binding reversibly to the enzyme to produce a beneficial effect on endometriosis symptoms.[129] Although the end result of GnRH agonists and AIs is similar, the adverse effects of the AIs are decreased, with fewer hot flashes, and primarily

Table 47-7 GnRH Agonists

GnRH Agonist (Brand Name)	Strength	Dosage Form	Dosage Regimen
Nafarelin (Synarel)	2 mg/mL delivers 200 mcg/spray	Intranasal	200–400 mcg BID
Leuprolide (Lupron)	3.75, 7.5, 11.25 mg	IM depot	3.75 mg/month
Goserelin (Zoladex)	3.6 mg	SC implant	3.6 mg/month
Histrelin[a] (Supprelin)	120 mcg/0.6 mL 300 mcg/0.6 mL 600 mcg/0.6 mL	SC injection	100 mcg/day

[a]Not U.S. Food and Drug Administration (FDA) approved for treatment of endometriosis.
BID, twice daily; GnRH, gonadotropin-releasing hormone; IM, intramuscular; SC, subcutaneous.

mild headache, nausea, and diarrhea. Although few long term trials have been conducted, decreased bone density is suspected with the use of AIs and add-back therapy is appropriate.

Aromatase inhibitors have been studied alone and in combination with oral contraceptives, progestins and GnRH agonists. All studies, although small, have demonstrated reduction in pain and reduced lesion size. The largest study to date utilized a combination of anastrozole with GnRH agonists compared with GnRH agonists alone in patients after surgery.[130] Although effective at controlling pain, the combination resulted in significantly more bone loss than either regimen alone at 6 months, but no difference was seen at the 2-year follow-up.[130] Further research is needed to determine the role of AIs in the treatment of endometriosis, because currently they do not have an FDA indication for the treatment of endometriosis. Their use should be reserved at this time for those patients with severe endometriosis who have failed other therapies.

DANAZOL

Danazol, an androgenic drug derived from 17-ethinyl testosterone, also induces a pseudomenopausal state by increasing androgen levels and decreasing estrogen levels. It inhibits the enzymes involved in ovarian steroidogenesis and increases the metabolic clearance of estradiol. By creating a hypoestrogenic, hypoprogestogenic state, danazol causes anovulation, amenorrhea, and atrophy of endometrial implants. Although effective at decreasing pelvic pain, danazol is poorly tolerated because of its significant side effects, which include weight gain, voice changes, edema, acne, hot flashes, vaginal dryness, hirsutism, liver disease, and increased cholesterol; these occur in up to 85% of treated patients.[114] Because of safety concerns, use should be limited to 6 months at a time, and should only be initiated in women after all other therapy options have failed.[128]

Clinical Application

21. N.H.'s pain is uncontrolled after trials of three different NSAID and she would like relief so she would be able to function at work and home. Although she is interested in having children in the future, she is not interested in conception in the next few years. What is the treatment of choice for N.H.?

Clinical trials in endometriosis have not singled out one treatment as the treatment of choice for all women, with most investigations demonstrating equivalence of the studied therapies. An NSAID and combined hormonal contraception (e.g., N.H.'s contraceptive vaginal ring) are the drugs of choice for initial management, owing to their safety profile, and in this case, the contraceptive agent's dual utility in preventing conception. As a next step, progestins, GnRH agonists, and AI are options. Because of adverse effects and poor tolerability, danazol should be reserved as an agent of last choice. If N.H. were uninterested in having children in the future, surgical sterilization would be an option. Conservative surgery, including removal of endometriomas and adhesions, and ablation of visible lesions is not curative, but may provide pain relief in 50% to 95% of patients at 1 year.[127] A combination of conservative surgery, followed by postoperative progestin, GnRH agonists, or danazol has been shown to prolong the duration of pain relief and decrease recurrence after surgery.[127] Oral contraceptives have not been studied as a postsurgery treatment option.

22. N.H. is 5 feet 7 inches and weighs 145 pounds. She smokes one-half pack of cigarettes per day, and does not drink alcohol. She plays recreation league basketball and softball, but does not have a regular exercise regimen. She usually eats five servings of fruits or vegetables per day, but does not like to drink milk. She has been told she has inherited her father's high cholesterol, and is concerned because he had a cardiac stent placed at age 40. She has not had a problem in the past tolerating a variety of contraceptive products, but does have some problems with daily medication adherence, and would like to avoid needles if possible. How does this information assist in the selection of therapy for her endometriosis?

N.H. is a smoker, with poor calcium intake, and some cardiovascular risk factors (family history, "high cholesterol"), who would rather avoid injectable medication and has trouble with daily medication taking. Danazol, with its ability to increase cardiovascular risk factors, and extensive side effects, is not a good option. Although some GnRH analoges are available as nasal sprays or injectable implants, the significant risk of decreased bone density, and menopausal-like adverse effects place it as a second-line option. Progestins, particularly the long-acting progestins, either in the form of the medroxyproesterone acetate 3-month depot injection, or the levonorgestrel IUS make these appropriate first-line options for N.H., although the risk of diminished bone density remains an issue.

23. N.H. elects to start the levonorgestrel IUS, but her insurance company will not pay for it to be used in the treatment of endometriosis because of its lack of FDA indication. She decides to start depot medroxyprogesterone acetate. What information

can you provide her regarding use, and the benefits and risks of treatment?

Depot medroxyprogesterone acetate (DMPA) is available in two dosage forms: 150 mg to be given IM every 3 months, and a 104-mg formulation given SC every 3 months. Product choice may be based on insurance coverage, or preference of the patient to self-administer (in this case, the SC product may be more patient friendly). Because N.H. does not want to use needles, either choice, administered by her provider's office, or pharmacy if law allows, would be an appropriate option. Although the DMPA does provide the contraception N.H. desires, she should be informed that it may take longer than usual (up to 1 year) to become pregnant after its use. More than 80% of patients treated with progestins will experience partial or complete pain relief.[131] Although devoid of the menopausal-like adverse effects of other medications used to treat endometriosis, DMPA is associated with weight gain, which may be significant in some patients; bloating, and irregular periods or bleeding for several months, with most users eventually experiencing amenorrhea. To reduce bone density loss, which is significant but less than with GnRH agonists, N.H. should be advised to increase her calcium and vitamin D intake by diet or supplementation, counseled to stopping smoking, and start a regular weight-bearing exercise regimen.[132] She should be monitored for pain relief, weight gain, amenorrhea or bleeding changes, and adherence to the quarterly injections. When N.H. desires conception, significant planning is required, and she may require a different therapy for her endometriosis as she regains fertility.

Gonadotropin-Releasing Hormone Agonists

DOSING

24. M.F., a 24-year-old single woman with a history of moderate to severe endometriosis, has been treated with some benefit with an NSAID, oral contraceptives, and the levonorgestrel IUS. She has no desire for conception, and is looking for pain relief. She has also had two conservative laparoscopic surgical procedures, each of which was successful, with pain relief lasting 6 months to 1 year. She recently had her "last ever" surgical procedure, and is looking to extend the improvement she has seen previously after surgery. She does not mind injections, but has had trouble with adherence in the past. Her physician has prescribed leuprolide 11.25 mg IM every 3 months. Why did she select this product, and how long should M.F. continue the medication?

Leuprolide, nafarelin, and goserelin are GnRH analogs (agonists) typically used for the treatment of endometriosis (Table 47-7). Although GnRH analogs have not been shown to produce better results than the therapies M.F. has already used, they may provide her with pain relief. Choice of GnRH agonist is driven by patient choice of administration method (nasal BID with nafarelin, monthly SC implant with goserelin, or IM injection either once monthly or once every 3 months with leuprolide). In M.F's case, the once every 3 months dosing with leuprolide would be most desirable for her, eliminating the need for daily administration. Efficacy is similar for all the GnRH agonists. Before use of these agents, pregnancy, undiagnosed vaginal bleeding, and breastfeeding should be ruled out. Because M.F. does not desire conception, and use of the GnRH agonists is contraindicated in pregnancy, she should be counseled regarding choices of nonhormonal contraceptive agents.

Onset of response to GnRH therapy depends on the phase in the menstrual cycle during which the agent is initiated. Administration beginning in the luteal phase causes decreased estrogen levels within 2 to 3 weeks, and amenorrhea within 4 to 5 weeks versus the 6 to 8 weeks if started in the follicular phase.[97]

Usual therapy duration is 6 months, although a small recently published pilot study suggested long-term treatment (up to 10 years) with add-back therapy (see Question 25) is without major adverse effects, with continued efficacy.[133] Therapy beyond 3 to 6 months requires the use of add-back therapy to reduce the risk of hypoestrogenic complications. Monitoring for efficacy includes monitoring for amenorrhea, decreases in pain and dyspareunia, and quality of life. After discontinuation of GnRH agonists, menses and ovarian function return to normal in 6 to 12 weeks, whereas benefits may be maintained for another 6 to 12 months.[97]

ADVERSE EFFECTS

Adverse effects should be discussed in detail with M.F. because they differ significantly from the other therapies she has tried. Adverse effects are related to the induction of the pseudomenopausal state (Table 47-8). Nearly all patients experience hot flushes; vaginal dryness and insomnia also are common. GnRH agonists do not affect SHBG or testosterone levels, so the androgenic side effects of danazol, including changes in lipid profiles, are not experienced with these agents.[97] Significant bone loss can occur, necessitating preemptive actions to decrease loss (see Question 26).

Hypoestrogenic Effects

25. M.F has read a significant amount about the use of GnRH agonists for endometriosis. She is confused by the use of estrogen and progestin with GnRH agonists. Explain to M.F. what is meant by "add-back" therapy.

Add-back therapy is the addition of a progestin or estrogen plus progestin to GnRH agonist therapy to decrease the hypoestrogenic adverse effects related to their use, while maintaining the therapeutic benefit of the GnRH agonist. This therapy is based on the concept of an "estrogen threshold hypothesis," formulated by Barbieri,[118] which states that there is a critical amount of estrogen that exacerbates endometriosis, and below that level, the presence of estrogen serves to decrease adverse effects, but does not have an adverse effect on the disease itself. Add-back therapy can be initiated at the beginning of GnRH agonist therapy to try to reduce the occurrence of all hypoestrogenic adverse effects (the most common regimen), or wait until 3 to 6 months into therapy, to assess patient-specific adverse effects.

Estrogen-containing OCs contain a dose of estrogen that is above the "threshold," and they should not be used for add-back therapy. Doses of estrogen equivalent to 0.625 mg of conjugated equine estrogen have been studied in combination with either medroxyprogesterone 2.5 mg daily, or norethindrone 5 mg daily. This dose of norethindrone alone, or a dose of 20 mg of medroxyprogesterone alone, has also demonstrated benefit.[114] To prevent bone loss, a regimen of a progestin plus a bisphosphonate has been studied with positive results. No

Table 47-8 Adverse Reactions With Danazol and the GnRH Agonists[170]

	Danazol (%)	Nafarelin (%)	Leuprolide (%)	Goserelin (%)
Antiestrogenic Effects				
Hot flushes	67–69	90	84	96
Vaginal dryness or vaginitis	7–43	19	28	75
Abnormal vaginal bleeding[a]	+	+	28	+
Breast atrophy	16–42	10	6	33
Decreased libido	7–44	22	11	61
Androgenic Effects				
Weight gain	23–28	8	13	3
Voice alteration	8	NR	<5	3
Hirsutism	6–7	2	<5	15
Acne	20–42	13	10	55
Central Nervous System Effects				
Sleep disturbances	4	8	<5	11
Headaches	21–63	19	32	75
Depression or emotional lability	18–60	9–15	22	54–56
Other				
Peripheral edema	34	8	7	21
Nausea	14	NR	13	8
Seborrhea	17–52	8	10	26
Nasal irritation	NR	10	NR	NR
Injection site reactions	NR	NR	<5	6
Joint pain	+	<1	8	=

[a] Amenorrhea is expected consequence of these medications.
+, reported but percentages not given; NR, not reported.

studies have demonstrated superior efficacy or safety of one regimen over another.

Bone Demineralization

26. How significant is the bone loss associated with Gn-RH agonists?

Reduction in bone density is a significant concern with Gn-RH agonists, even at 3 months after the onset of therapy, and is particularly concerning because these agents are being used in young women, many of whom have not reached their peak bone mass. Studies have demonstrated a loss of 3.2% in lumbar spine bone mineral density (BMD) after 6 months, and a 6.3% decrease after 12 months of GnRH agonist treatment.[128] It has also been reported that endometriosis itself is also a risk factor for decreased bone density, although a long-term study did not find any associated between endometriosis and fracture risk over a 20-year follow-up period.[134] Interestingly, this same study did not find any association between fracture risk and Gn-RH agonist therapy, although a significant number of women in the study did take add-back therapy.

Monitoring for decreases in bone density should be accomplished via dual-energy x-ray absorptiometry (DXA) scan every 24 months if GnRH therapy is continued. Women such as M.F. should also be counseled regarding adequate calcium and vitamin D intake, smoking cessation, and a regimen of weight-bearing exercise.

Management of Endometriosis-Related Infertility

27. K.L. is a 34-year-old woman with a history of stage II endometriosis. She currently is using a levonorgestrel IUS for both contraception and control of her pain, with positive results. She also takes ibuprofen on a regular basis. She and her spouse would like to have a child. About 6 years ago, they attempted to conceive without success after 24 months. K.L is concerned that she will now have even more difficulty becoming pregnant, given her advanced age. What are the recommendations for improving infertility associated with endometriosis?

Of women presenting to the health care system with infertility, 30% to 45% have endometriosis, and 30% to 50% of women with endometriosis are infertile.[135] Proposed mechanisms contributing to infertility include adhesions that impair oocyte transport, changes in the peritoneum not compatible with fertility, changes in hormonal function, endocrine or ovulation dysfunction, and disorders of implantation. No evidence suggests that hormonal therapy, including therapy with GnRH agonists, improves conception rates for women with stage I/II endometriosis, similar to K.L's. On the other hand, surgical ablation or resection of visible endometriosis implants is beneficial in improving pregnancy rates in women with stage I/II endometriosis.

For K.L., removal of her IUS, followed by laparoscopic ablation or resection of visible implants may improve her ability to conceive, barring other factors influencing fertility (e.g.,

PCOS, male factor infertility, tubal patency). For patients with more advanced disease, or in those patients >35 years of age, a more aggressive treatment regimen is appropriate. Options include the use of agents to induce superovulation (clomiphene), and the use of in vitro fertilization techniques with embryo transfer (IVF-ET). In women with endometriosis, the success of IVF-ET is decreased by as much as 20% when compared with women without endometriosis.[97] For women contemplating IVF-ET, three prospective clinical trials have demonstrated a potential benefit in women with stage II–IV endometriosis who were treated for 3 to 6 months or more with Gn-RH agonists before IVF-ET. The treated subjects had significantly higher pregnancy rates compared with women who did not use Gn-RH agonists before IVF-ET.[136]

For women who have not yet demonstrated an inability to conceive, a "wait and see" approach, with use of NSAID for pain, emotional support, and reassurance for 6 to 12 months is appropriate in women <35 years of age.

Table 47-9 ACOG Diagnostic Criteria for PMS

Affective Symptoms	*Somatic Symptoms*
Depression	Breast tenderness
Angry outbursts	Abdominal bloating
Irritability	Headache
Anxiety	Swelling of extremities
Confusion	
Social withdrawal	

ACOG, American College of Obstetricians and Gynecologists; PMS, premenstrual syndrome.
1. Diagnosis made if at least one affective and one somatic symptom is reported in the three prior menstrual cycles during the 5 days before the onset of menses.
2. The symptoms must resolve within 4 days of onset of menses and do not recur until after day 12 of the cycle.
3. The symptoms must be present in at least two cycles during prospective recording.
4. The symptoms must adversely affect social or work related activities.
From reference 139, with permission.

PREMENSTRUAL SYNDROME AND PREMENSTRUAL DYSPHORIC DISORDER

Premenstrual symptoms occur in up to 90% of reproductive-age women.[137] Approximately 20% to 40% of these women have more bothersome symptoms of premenstrual syndrome (PMS) and it is estimated that 3% to 8% meet the criteria for premenstrual dysphoric disorder (PMDD), a more severe variant of PMS.[137] More than 200 premenstrual symptoms have been described as occurring during the days before menstruation, including positive symptoms, such as increased energy, libido, and ability to relax, as well as negative symptoms including abdominal distention, fatigue, headaches, and crying spells.[138] It is not until the symptoms have a decidedly negative influence on the physical, psychological, or social function of a woman that PMS exists. In essence, the symptoms must induce a reduction or loss of life quality to be considered PMS or PMDD.[138]

Diagnosis

No specific physical findings or laboratory tests can be used to make a diagnosis of PMS. The American College of Obstetricians and Gynecologists (ACOG) published a Practice Bulletin in 2000 that defined diagnostic criteria using cyclical patterns of symptoms in women.[139] PMS can be diagnosed if at least one of the affective and one of the somatic symptoms listed in Table 47-9 is reported 5 days before the onset of menses in the three previous cycles. The symptoms must be prospectively recorded in at least two cycles and must cease within 4 days of onset of menses and not recur until after day 12 of the menstrual cycle. A key factor that separates PMS from "normal" premenstrual symptoms is that work or social activities are adversely affected in PMS. Other diagnoses that may explain premenstrual symptoms should be excluded, including psychological, thyroid, and gynecologic disorders.[140]

The American Psychiatric Association has developed criteria for PMDD (Table 47-10).[141] The criteria for PMDD focus on the mood and mental health symptoms, leading to a higher level of dysfunction compared with PMS. Criteria for PMS and PMDD, however, share three essential characteristics: (a) symptoms must occur in the luteal phase and resolve within a few days of menstruation; (b) symptoms are documented over at least two menstrual cycles and are not better explained by other physical or psychological conditions; and (c) symptoms are sufficiently severe to disrupt normal activities.[140]

The symptoms of PMS and PMDD experienced by women can vary widely. Risk factors for PMS include advancing age (>30 years) and genetic factors.[140] Symptoms, however, can begin in adolescents around age 14, or 2 years postmenarche,

Table 47-10 Diagnostic Criteria for Premenstrual Dysphoric Disorder

- In most menstrual cycles during the past year, at least five of the symptoms below (including one core symptom) were present for most of the time 1 week before menses (luteal phase), began to remit within a few days after the onset of menses, and were absent the week after menses (follicular phase).
  - Core symptoms
    - Markedly depressed mood, feelings of hopelessness or self-deprecating thoughts
    - Persistent and marked anger or irritability or increased interpersonal conflicts
    - Marked anxiety, tension
    - Marked affective lability (i.e., feeling suddenly sad or tearful)
  - Other symptoms
    - Decreased interest in usual activities (e.g., friends, hobbies)
    - Subjective sense of difficulty in concentrating
    - Lethargy, easy fatigability, or marked lack of energy
    - Marked change in appetite, overeating, or specific food cravings
    - Hypersomnia or insomnia
    - A subjective sense of being overwhelmed or out of control
    - Other physical symptoms (e.g., breast tenderness, bloating, weight gain, headache, joint or muscle pain)
- The symptoms seriously interfere with work or school, usual activities, or relationships with others.
- Symptoms are not merely an exacerbation of another disorder, such as major depression, panic disorder, dysthymia, or a personality disorder (although it may be superimposed on any of these disorders).
- Three major criteria above are confirmed by prospective daily self-ratings for at least two consecutive symptomatic cycles.

Adapted from reference 141, with permission.

and persist until menopause.[142] Some studies suggest that women with mothers reporting PMS are more likely to develop PMS than those with unaffected mothers (70% vs. 37%, respectively).[143,144] One article found that traumatic events, such as physical threat, childhood sexual abuse, and severe accidents, increased the risk of developing PMDD.[145]

Pathophysiology

The wide range of symptoms exhibited in patients with PMS or PMDD can be explained by multiple possible mechanisms, probably a result of interactions between sex steroids and central neurotransmitters.[146] Alterations in neurotransmitters, primarily reductions in serotonin, triggered by normal hormonal fluctuations of the menstrual cycle appear to be the most probable factors for the development of PMS or PMDD. Other neurotransmitters, including endorphins and γ-aminobutyric acid (GABA), have also been implicated.[147,148] The levels of estrogen, progesterone, and testosterone are normal in women with PMS, but they may be more vulnerable to normal fluctuations.[148] These potential mechanisms provide a rationale basis for the symptoms that appear in PMS and PMDD, but also support the therapeutic benefits of treatments that increase serotonin or GABA levels. Many treatments have limited and variable efficacy, which reinforces the argument that PMS or PMDD is a result of multiple factors. Furthermore, placebo responses in trials can be as high as 50% to 80%, which points to an important psychosomatic component and the consideration that PMS or PMDD has relevant biological, psychological, and social factors.[138]

29. C.P., a 27-year-old woman, visits her family physician complaining of significant mood changes that occur the week before her menstrual cycle. She experiences increased irritability and anxiety as well as breast tenderness and abdominal bloating. These symptoms usually subside the first or second day after her menses begin. For 2 to 3 weeks after her menstrual period, C.P. is her "normal, usual self" until the symptoms begin again just before her next menstruation. She has had these symptoms every month for the past several years. She states that she is very uncomfortable when these symptoms occur. Although she is able to work most of the time, she typically avoids going out with her friends when she has these symptoms. Her menstrual cycles are regular, occurring every 28 to 30 days with a light flow lasting 3 to 4 days.

Pelvic, cardiovascular, and neurologic examinations are normal and all laboratory assessments are within normal limits. Her serum pregnancy test was negative. She has no history of an affective disorder. Her physician makes a preliminary diagnosis of PMS. What symptoms does C.P. have that are consistent with this diagnosis?

C.P. has symptoms that meet the ACOG criteria for PMS. Her affective symptoms include irritability and anxiety and somatic symptoms include breast tenderness and abdominal bloating. These symptoms occur during the luteal phase of the menstrual cycle, resolve within 4 days of menses, and do not recur until after day 12 of her cycle. C.P.'s symptoms appear to be affecting her social activities. She states that these symptoms have been present for years and that they occur every month, although she has not prospectively recorded this information. C.P. does not meet the criteria for PMDD because her symptoms are not severe or markedly impairing her ability to participate in daily activities.

Treatment: PMS

28. C.P. asks about nonprescription therapy. What options are available and what is the evidence for use of these products?

Nonprescription options that have been studied and have demonstrated at least minimal benefit include calcium, magnesium, pyridoxine, chaste tree or chasteberry, and some mind–body approaches. NSAIDs and acetaminophen may be beneficial for the physical symptoms of PMS, but diuretics found in various OTC products (e.g., ammonium chloride, caffeine, pamabrom) have limited data and unproved efficacy. Given the high placebo response rate in PMS, only agents with clinically proved efficacy should be used.

Calcium

Increased estrogen during the middle of a normal menstrual cycle decreases calcium. In women with PMS, intact parathyroid hormone (PTH) increases in response to this change compared with no PTH change in women without PMS.[149] Therefore, women with PMS have midcycle elevations of intact PTH with transient, secondary hyperparathyroidism. This explains why calcium has demonstrated some benefit in women with PMS.

Three calcium trials have shown efficacy of PMS symptoms. A randomized, double-blind cross-over trial of 33 women receiving 1,000 mg elemental calcium daily or placebo for 3 months reported a significant overall 50% reduction in PMS symptoms for women taking calcium compared with placebo.[150] In a double-blind study of 10 women assigned to dietary calcium intake, 1,336 mg daily was found to benefit mood, behavior, pain, and water retention symptoms significantly during the menstrual cycle.[151] Perhaps the most convincing evidence comes from a prospective, multicenter, randomized, double-blind, placebo-controlled, parallel-group trial conduced in 466 women with PMS.[152] Elemental calcium 1,200 mg daily (given as 600 mg BID) for three menstrual cycles significantly decreased negative affect, water retention, food cravings, and pain compared with placebo. Overall, the calcium-treated group had a 48% reduction in symptoms compared with a 30% reduction in the placebo group. Because calcium is well tolerated and may provide other benefits (e.g., osteoporosis prevention) calcium supplementation should be recommended to women with symptoms of PMS if inadequate through diet or other supplementation.

Magnesium

Low levels of red cell magnesium have been correlated with women experiencing PMS, therefore magnesium supplementation has been evaluated for PMS symptoms.[153] A Cochrane Library analysis of three small trials comparing magnesium and placebo in women with dysmenorrhea concluded that magnesium was more effective for pain associated with PMS and the need for additional medication was less for those taking magnesium.[154] Magnesium doses that have been studied for PMS vary from 200 to 360 mg daily. Trials have reported improvements in fluid retention and negative affect, but findings have not been consistent.[155] The conflicting results may be caused by differences in the dosing regimens of the magnesium

Table 47-11 Menstrual Cycle Daily Diary Chart

Month 1

Grading Severity of Symptoms:
1 = Mild; general awareness of discomfort but does not interfere with daily activities
2 = Moderate symptoms present; interferes with activities but not disabling
3 = Severe; symptoms disabling, unable to meet daily social, family, or work obligations

Day of month	1	2	3	4	5	6	7	8	9	10
Day of cycle	18	19	20	21	22	23	24	25	26	27
Menses										
Breast tenderness and pain				1	1	1	1	1	1	1
Sadness or depression				1	2	3	3	3	3	3
Fatigue				3	3	3	3	3	3	3
Irritability					2	2	3	3	3	3
Inability to concentrate							2	2	3	3
Daily weight	130	130	130	130	130	130	130	130	130	130
Basal body temperature	98.0	98.2	98.0	98.2	98.0	98.0	98.2	97.8	98.0	97.8

Month 2

Day of month	1	2	3	4	5	6	7	8	9	10
Day of cycle	21	22	23	24	25	26	27	28	1	2
Menses									*	*
Breast tenderness and pain				1	1	1	1	1	1	
Sadness/depression		1	2	3	3	3	3	3	2	2
Fatigue		2	2	3	3	3	3	3	2	1
Irritability	1	2	2	2	3	3	3	3	3	2
Inability to concentrate			1	1	2	2	3	3		
Daily weight	128	128	128	128	128	128	128	129	129	129
Basal body temperature	98.0	98.2	98.4	98.0	98.2	97.8	98.0	97.4		

and differing levels of magnesium stores in the study subjects. Available data support the use of magnesium in PMS, but more research is needed.

Pyridoxine (Vitamin B_6)

Vitamin B_6 has been noted to have positive effects on neurotransmitters, such as serotonin.[156] The most comprehensive information for this nutrient comes from a systematic review of nine trials representing 940 patients with PMS.[157] The overall assessment of the review was that women with PMS are likely to benefit from vitamin B_6 supplementation at a dose of 50 to 100 mg daily. An analysis of four of the trials, which specifically examined depressive symptoms, showed that pyridoxine was more effective than placebo in reducing depressive symptoms (OR 1.69; 95% CI 1.39–2.06). Although the conclusions of this review were positive, the authors felt there was insufficient evidence of high quality to recommend vitamin B_6 for PMS. Because neuropathy has been reported with pyridoxine dosages as low as 100 mg/day, patients should be advised to monitor for symptoms and to discontinue therapy and seek medical attention if they occur.

Chastetree or Chasteberry

The mechanism of action of chasteberry (*Vitex agnus-castus*) relative to PMS is unclear, but several trials have reported its beneficial effects. In a study of 1,542 women with PMS taking chasteberry extract, 33% of subjects reported total relief of symptoms whereas an additional 57% reported partial relief after 4 months.[158] Of patients, 2% complained of adverse events including nausea, allergy, diarrhea, weight gain, heartburn, hypermenorrhea, and gastric complaints. A randomized, double-blind, placebo-controlled trial of 170 women taking chasteberry extract 20 mg daily for three menstrual cycles showed a treatment response rate of 52% compared with 24% for placebo ($p < 0.001$).[159] Individual symptoms of irritability, mood alteration, anger, headache, and breast fullness were reduced. Bloating was not significantly altered compared with placebo. The incidence of side effects was low, but long-term safety is unknown. In general, data indicate that chasteberry may be effective for PMS.

Mind–Body Approaches

Evidence regarding mind–body approaches for PMS is somewhat limited. Because these modalities are risk free and they are generally accepted as components of a healthy lifestyle, they are favored in the treatment of PMS. Mind–body approaches that have demonstrated benefit in PMS include relaxation response, cognitive-behavioral therapy, yoga, aerobic exercise, and light therapy.[160]

NSAIDs and Diuretics

Nonsteroidal anti-inflammatory drugs have been used to relieve the physical symptoms (e.g., headache, joint pain) of PMS, but do not improve the mood symptoms.[140] Regimens have included taking naproxen or mefenamic acid during the luteal phase and stopping therapy after menses begin. Diuretics

Each Day:
1. List the major symptoms (mood, physical, emotional, behavioral) that you experience during your menstrual cycle
2. Grade the severity of the symptom
3. Record daily weight
4. Record basal body temperature
5. Check the days of the cycle when menstrual flow occurs

11	12	13	14	15	16	17	18	19	20	21	22	23	24	25	26	27	28	29	30	31
28	1	2	3	4	5	6	7	8	9	10	11	12	13	14	15	16	17	18	19	20
	*	*	*	*																
1																				
3	2	1																		
3	2	1																		
3																				
3																				
130	131	131	131	130	130	130	130	130	130	129	129	129	128	128	129	128	128	128	128	128
97.6					97.8	97.8	97.6	97.8	97.6	97.8	97.8	97.6	97.4	98.4	98.0	98.4	98.6	98.0	98.2	98.0

11	12	13	14	15	16	17	18	19	20	21	22	23	24	25	26	27	28	29	30
3	4	5	6	7	8	9	10	11	12	13	14	15	16	17	18	19	20	21	22
*	*																		
1																			
2	1																		
128	128	128	128	128	128	128	128	128	128	128	128	128	128	128	129	128	128	128	128
		97.6	97.6	97.8	97.8	97.6	97.8	97.6	97.6	97.6	97.2	97.2	97.0	98.4	98.6	98.0	98.2	98.2	98.0

commonly found in OTC products, such as ammonium chloride, caffeine, and pamabrom, are not effective. Spironolactone 100 mg daily given on days 15 through 28 may have some positive effects on somatic (e.g., breast tenderness, bloating) and affective symptoms, but data are not conclusive.[140]

30. **C.P. has been taking a multivitamin daily with adequate amounts of calcium, magnesium, and vitamin B_6 for PMS relief. She also has been taking naproxen sodium 220 mg BID without significant reduction of her symptoms. Her physician requests that she keep a daily dairy for two consecutive cycles to document her symptoms. What information should be included in this tool?**

C.P. should keep a daily diary for two consecutive menstrual cycles to demonstrate a temporal relationship between her symptoms during the luteal phase and to document the severity of these symptoms (Table 47-11). In addition, she should indicate the presence of menstrual flow, weight, and daily basal body temperature readings to help determine when ovulation occurs. The diary establishes a baseline for each patient and documents the most troublesome symptoms. Once therapy is selected for these symptoms, the diary can aid in assessing patient response.

Treatment: PMDD

31. **C.P. returns to clinic with the diary presented in Table 47-11. The physician determines that C.P. actually has PMDD. What evidence supports this diagnosis and what should be recommended for treatment?**

C.P. meets the criteria for PMDD as evidenced by her symptoms during the 1 week before her menstrual cycle (luteal phase). Specifically, she has at least five symptoms required for the diagnosis of PMDD: sadness or depression (core symptom), fatigue, irritability, inability to concentrate, breast tenderness, and bloating. She rated several of those symptoms as severe, which indicates the symptoms are disabling and she is unable to meet her daily obligations. There is no reason to suspect any other disorder based on her history. PMDD seems to be the most likely diagnosis for C.P.

Therapy options at this time include lifestyle modifications, psychosocial interventions, and pharmacologic therapy. Psychotropic drugs targeted to her most severe symptoms may include selective serotonin reuptake inhibitors (SSRI), serotonergic tricyclic antidepressants, and anxiolytics. An oral contraceptive has also been approved for PMDD and could be considered.

Selective Serotonin Reuptake Inhibitors

Serotonin is critical in the pathogenesis of PMDD and for that reason, SSRIs have become the treatment of choice for PMDD and severe PMS (Table 47-12).[161] SSRIs have demonstrated efficacy in reducing irritability, depressed mood, dysphoria, psychosocial function, and the physical symptoms of PMDD, including bloating, breast tenderness, and appetite changes.

Table 47-12 Psychotropic Drugs for the Management of PMDD and Severe PMS

Drug (Brand Name)	Daily Dosing Regimen (mg)	Intermittent Dosing Regimen (mg)[a]
SSRI		
Citalopram (Celexa)	5–20	10–30
Escitalopram (Lexapro)	10–20	10–20
Fluoxetine (Prozac)	20–60	20 or 90 weekly
Fluvoxamine (Luvox)	50–150	NS
Paroxetine (Paxil)	10–30	NS
Paroxetine controlled release (Paxil CR)	12.5–25	12.5–25
Sertraline (Zoloft)	50–150	100
Other Serotonergic Antidepressants		
Nefazodone (Serzone)	200–600	NS
Venlafaxine (Effexor)	50	NS
Anxiolytics		
Alprazolam (Xanax)	NS	1–2[b]
Buspirone (BuSpar)	NS	25–60

[a]Day 14 until onset of menses.
[b]Dose to be tapered over 2 days after onset of menses to prevent withdrawal symptoms.
NS, not studied; PMS, premenstrual syndrome; SSRI, selective serotonin reuptake inhibitors.

Fluoxetine, sertraline, and paroxetine controlled release each have an approved indication for PMDD.

The onset of effect of SSRI in women with PMDD or severe PMS is much more rapid than when these agents are used for treatment of major depression or anxiety disorders.[161] Women may experience symptom relief or resolution within the first menstrual cycle versus the 4 to 8 weeks for other psychological disorders. Several different dosing strategies have been studied, including continuous dosing (once daily), intermittent dosing (last 2 weeks of menstrual cycle), and semi-intermittent dosing (continuous administration throughout the cycle with increased doses during luteal phase). Continuous dosing would be reasonable for women with concurrent mood or anxiety disorders or those who may have difficulty remembering the timing of the intermittent dosing. Intermittent dosing should be considered for patients with: regular menstrual cycles who are able to adhere to the regimen, an absence of symptoms during the follicular phase, concerns about long-term affects (e.g., sexual dysfunction), and few side effects at treatment initiation. Studies evaluating these dosing strategies have reported conflicting results regarding the most effective method; treatment should be individualized based on patient history, willingness to adhere to therapy, and drug response.

In a meta-analysis of 15 randomized, placebo-controlled trials including 904 women, SSRI treatment demonstrated a significant reduction in overall PMS symptoms (OR 6.91; 95% CI 3.9–12.2).[162] SSRIs were effective in treating both physical and behavioral symptoms of PMS. No detectable difference was found in PMS symptoms when comparing continuous or intermittent dosing. SSRIs are generally well tolerated; however, in this analysis, the discontinuation rate in women taking SSRI was 2.5 times higher than in those taking placebo.[162] Common side effects reported with SSRI use were insomnia, fatigue, decreased libido, nausea, and dry mouth.

Other Psychotropic Agents

Non-SSRI antidepressants that affect serotonin are also beneficial in treating PMS (Table 47-12). Venlafaxine, dosed daily, is significantly better than placebo at relieving psychological and physical symptoms of PMS.[163] Alprazolam is a short-acting benzodiazepine that has been assessed for the treatment of PMS in several studies with differing results.[164] With conflicting data and concerns about dependence, alprazolam should be reserved for women who are unresponsive to other PMS treatments. Luteal-phase dosing may limit the risk of drug dependence of this benzodiazepine, but the dose should be tapered over several days to minimize mild withdrawal symptoms. Buspirone, a partial 5 hydoxytryptamine (5HT) receptor agonist, demonstrated significant reduction in irritability when given daily, but does not seem to affect the physical symptoms of PMS.[165]

Combination Oral Contraceptives

32. C.P. is considering a COC. What agent(s) would be appropriate and how might this affect her PMS?

A low-dose COC formulation containing 20 mcg ethinyl estradiol and 3 mg drospirenone (an antimineralocorticoid spironolactone analog) with a 4-day hormone-free interval is approved for the treatment of emotional and physical symptoms of PMDD.[166] Studies using this agent have shown efficacy for reduced mood, physical, and behavioral symptoms of PMDD, including a 48% improved response with this agent compared with a 36% response using placebo ($p = 0.015$).[167] Side effects occurring in at least 10% of women treated with this medication included intermenstrual bleeding, headache, nausea, breast pain, and upper respiratory infection. For women desiring contraception, this particular agent is approved and has data supporting its use in PMDD. The effects of other contraceptive agents for PMDD symptoms are currently under investigation.

Other Agents

33. What other therapeutic modalities are available to treat symptoms of PMS and what evidence exists to support their use?

Treatment with Gn-RH agonists has been used for the physical and psychological symptoms of PMS.[168] These agents are not typically used for long periods of time, however, because of vasomotor symptoms and the potential for negative long-term effects on bone. They also have to be administered by injection or nasal spray which may affect adherence. This treatment is reserved for women with very severe PMDD who do not respond to other treatments.

Danazol has been investigated for the treatment of PMS with moderate results. Danazol 200 mg BID provides greater symptom relief than placebo for symptoms of severe PMS; however, luteal phase treatment does not appear effective for PMS symptoms.[169] Potential side effects are also a concern with this agent and, therefore, its use in women should be limited to those who have failed other therapies.

34. The physician working with you recognizes your strong knowledge base in PMS and PMDD through your recommendations for C.P. He requests a brief "take home" summary of the treatment strategy for PMS and PMDD. How would you respond?

If mild to moderate symptoms of PMS exist, supportive therapy can be recommended with healthy nutrition, aerobic exercise, calcium supplements, and possibly magnesium, vitamin B_6 and chasteberry. If physical symptoms are also present, NSAIDs could be initiated. When mood symptoms predominate and are markedly impairing functionality, an SSRI should be started in either a continuous or intermittent manner. An anxiolytic could be tried for symptoms not relieved by the SSRI. If no response is seen with these agents, a GnRH agonist could be initiated, but should be done in consultation with a gynecologist.

REFERENCES

1. Trivax B et al. Diagnosis of polycystic ovary syndrome. *Clin Obstet Gynecol* 2007;50:168.
2. Stein IF et al. Amenorrhea associated with bilateral polycystic ovaries. *Am J Obstet Gynecol* 1935;29:181.
3. Stein IF. Bilateral polycystic ovaries. *Am J Obstet Gynecol* 1945;50:385.
4. Zawadski JK et al. Diagnostic criteria for polycystic ovary syndrome: towards a rational approach. In: Dunaif A et al., eds. *Polycystic Ovary Syndrome.* Boston: Blackwell Scientific Publications; 1992:377.
5. The Rotterdam ESHRE/ASRM-Sponsored PCOS consensus workshop group. Revised 2003 consensus on diagnostic criteria and long-term health risks related to polycystic ovary syndrome. *Fertil Steril* 2004;81:19.
6. Azziz R et al. Position statement: criteria for defining polycystic ovary syndrome as a predominantly hyperandrogenic syndrome: an Androgen Excess Society guideline. *J Clin Endocrinol Metab* 2006;91:4237.
7. Azziz R et al. Androgen excess in women: experience with over 1,000 consecutive patients. *J Clin Endocrinol Metab* 2004;89:453.
8. Hoeger KM. Obesity and lifestyle management in polycystic ovary syndrome. *Clin Obstet Gynecol* 2007;50:277.
9. Menke MN et al. Genetics of polycystic ovary syndrome. *Clin Obstet Gynecol* 2007;50:188.
10. Ehrmann DA. Polycystic ovary syndrome. *N Engl J Med* 2005;352:1223.
11. Ehrmann DA et al. Polycystic ovary syndrome as a form of functional ovarian hyperandrogenism due to dysregulation of androgen secretion. *Endocr Rev* 1995;16:322.
12. Nelson VL et al. The biochemical basis for increased testosterone production in theca cells propagated from patients with polycystic ovary syndrome. *J Clin Endocrinol Metab* 2001;86:5925.
13. Dunaif A. Insulin resistance in women with polycystic ovary syndrome. *Fertil Steril* 2006;86(Suppl 1):S13.
14. Dunaif A et al. Excessive insulin receptor serine phosphorylation in cultured fibroblasts and in skeletal muscle: a potential for insulin resistance in the polycystic ovary syndrome. *J Clin Invest* 1995;96:801.
15. Corbould A et al. Insulin resistance in the skeletal muscle of women with PCOS involves intrinsic and acquired defects in insulin signaling. *Am J Physiol Endocrinol Metab* 2005;288:E1047.
16. Baillargeon JP et al. Insulin sensitizers for polycystic ovary syndrome. *Clin Obstet Gynecol* 2003;46:325.
17. Meyer C et al. Effects of medical therapy on insulin resistance and the cardiovascular system in polycystic ovary syndrome. *Diabetes Care* 2007;30:471.
18. Tsilchorozidou T et al. The pathophysiology of the polycystic ovary syndrome. *Clin Endocrinol* 2004;60:1.
19. Lorenz LB, Wild RA. Evaluation and management of diabetes and cardiovascular risks for today's clinician. *Clin Obstet Gynecol* 2007;50:226.
20. Legro RS et al. Prevalence and predictors of risk for type 2 diabetes mellitus and impaired glucose tolerance in polycystic ovary syndrome: a prospective, controlled study in 254 affected women. *J Clin Endocrinol Metab* 1999;84:165.
21. American Association of Clinical Endocrinologists. American Association of Clinical Endocrinologists position statement on metabolic and cardiovascular consequences of polycystic ovary syndrome. *Endocr Pract* 2005;11:126.
22. Expert Panel on Detection, Evaluation, and Treatment of High Blood Cholesterol in Adults (Adult Treatment Panel III). Executive summary of the third report of the National Cholesterol Education Program (NCEP). *JAMA* 2001;285:2486.
23. Apridonidze T et al. Prevalence and characteristics of the metabolic syndrome in women with polycystic ovary syndrome. *J Clin Endocrinol Metab* 2005;90:1929.
24. Glueck CJ et al. Incidence and treatment of metabolic syndrome in newly referred women with confirmed polycystic ovarian syndrome. *Metabolism* 2003;52:908.
25. Ehrmann DA et al. Prevalence and predictors of the metabolic syndrome in women with polycystic ovary syndrome. *J Clin Endocrinol Metab* 2006;91:48.
26. Essah PA. The metabolic syndrome in polycystic ovary syndrome. *Clin Obstet Gynecol* 2007;50:205.
27. Grundy SM et al. Diagnosis and management of the metabolic syndrome. An American Heart Association/National Heart, Lung, and Blood Institute scientific statement. *Circulation* 2005;112:2735.
28. Dahlgren E et al. Women with polycystic ovary syndrome wedge resected in 1956 to 1965: a long-term follow-up focusing on natural history and circulating hormones. *Fertil Steril* 1992;57:505.
29. Talbott E et al. Coronary heart disease risk factors in women with polycystic ovary syndrome. *Arterioscler Thromb Vasc Biol* 1995;15:821.
30. Pirwany IR et al. Lipids and lipoprotein subfractions in women with PCOS: relationship to metabolic and endocrine parameters. *Clin Endocrinol* 2001;54:447.
31. Vgontzas AN et al. Polycystic ovary syndrome is associated with obstructive sleep apnea and daytime sleepiness: role of insulin resistance. *J Clin Endocrinol Metab* 2001;86:517.
32. Fogel RB et al. Increased prevalence of obstructive sleep apnea syndrome in obese women with polycystic ovary syndrome. *J Clin Endocrinol Metab* 2001;86:1175.
33. Gopal M et al. The role of obesity in the increased prevalence of obstructive sleep apnea syndrome in patients with polycystic ovary syndrome. *Sleep Med* 2002;3:401.
34. Balen A. Polycystic ovary syndrome and cancer. *Human Reprod Update* 2001;7:522.
35. Huber-Buchholz MM et al. Restoration of reproductive potential by lifestyle modification in obese polycystic ovary syndrome: role of insulin sensitivity and luteinizing hormone. *J Clin Endocrinol Metab* 1999;84:1470.
36. Moran LJ et al. Dietary composition in restoring reproductive and metabolic physiology in overweight women with polycystic ovary syndrome. *J Clin Endocrinol Metab* 2003;88:812.
37. Trentham-Dietz A et al. Weight change and risk of endometrial cancer. *Int J Epidemiol* 2006;35:151.
38. Schouten LJ et al. Anthropometry, physical activity, and endometrial cancer risk: results from the Netherlands Cohort Study. *J Natl Cancer Inst* 2004;96:1635.
39. Knowler WC et al. Reduction in the incidence of type 2 diabetes with lifestyle intervention or metformin. *N Engl J Med.* 2002;346:393.
40. Orchard TJ et al. The effect of metformin and intensive lifestyle modification on the metabolic syndrome: the Diabetes Prevention Program randomized trial. *Ann Intern Med* 2005;142:611.
41. Marsh K et al. The optimal diet for women with polycystic ovary syndrome? *Br J Nutr* 2005;94:154.
42. Kasim-Karakas SE et al. Relation of nutrients and hormones in polycystic ovary syndrome. *Am J Clin Nutr* 2007;85:688.
43. Diamanti-Kandarakis E et al. A modern medical quandary: polycystic ovary syndrome, insulin resistance, and oral contraceptive pills. *J Clin Endocrinol Metab* 2003;88:1927.
44. Cibula D et al. Insulin sensitivity in non-obese women with polycystic ovary syndrome during treatment with oral contraceptives containing low androgenic progestin. *Human Reprod* 2002;17:76.
45. Pike MC et al. Estrogen-progestin replacement therapy and endometrial cancer. *J Natl Cancer Inst* 1997;89:1110.
46. Weiderpass E et al. Use of oral contraceptives and endometrial cancer risk. *Cancer Causes Control* 1999;10:277.
47. Vessey MP et al. Endometrial and ovarian cancer and oral contraceptives-findings in a large cohort study. *Br J Cancer* 1995;71:1340.
48. Baillargeon JP et al. Effects of metformin and rosiglitazone, alone and in combination, in nonobese women with polycystic ovary syndrome and normal indices of insulin sensitivity. *Fertil Steril* 2004;82:893.
49. Mansfield R et al. Metformin has direct effects on human ovarian steroidogenesis. *Fertil Steril* 2003;79:956.
50. Harborne L et al. Descriptive review of the evidence for the use of metformin in polycystic ovary syndrome. *Lancet* 2003;361:1894.
51. Nestler JE et al. Effects of metformin on spontaneous and clomiphene-induced ovulation in the polycystic ovary syndrome. *N Engl J Med* 1998;338:1876.
52. Palomba S et al. Prospective parallel randomized, double-blind, double-dummy controlled clinical trial comparing clomiphene citrate and metformin as the first-line treatment for ovulation induction in nonobese anovulatory women with polycystic ovary syndrome. *J Clin Endocrinol Metab* 2005;90:4068.
53. Lord JM et al. Metformin in polycystic ovary syndrome: systematic review and analysis. *BMJ* 2003;327:951.
54. Morin-Papunen LC et al. Metformin therapy improves the menstrual pattern with minimal endocrine and metabolic effects in women with polycystic ovary syndrome. *Fertil Steril* 1998;69:691.

55. Mitwally MF et al. Troglitazone: a possible modulator of ovarian steroidogenesis. *J Soc Gynecol Investig* 2002;9:163.
56. Glueck CJ et al. Pioglitazone and metformin in obese women with polycystic ovary syndrome not optimally responsive to metformin. *Human Reprod* 2003;18:1618.
57. Ortega-Gonzalez C et al. Responses of serum androgen and insulin resistance to metformin and pioglitazone in obese, insulin-resistant women with polycystic ovary syndrome. *J Clin Endocrinol Metab* 2005;90:1360.
58. Bautukan C et al. Efficacy of a new oral contraceptive containing drospirenone and ethinyl estradiol in the long-term treatment of hirsutism. *Fertil Steril* 2006;85:436.
59. Ganie MA et al. Comparison of efficacy of spironolactone with metformin in the management of polycystic ovary syndrome: an open label study. *J Clin Endocrinol Metab* 2004;89:2756.
60. Moghetti P et al. Comparison of spironolactone, flutamide, and finasteride efficacy in the treatment of hirsutism: a randomized, double blind, placebo-controlled trial. *J Clin Endocrinol Metab* 2000;85:89.
61. Palomba S et al. Is ovulation induction still a therapeutic problem in patients with polycystic ovary syndrome? *J Endocrinol Invest* 2004;27:796.
62. Guzick DS. Ovulation induction management of PCOS. *Clin Obstet Gynecol* 2007;50:255.
63. Elnashar A et al. Clomiphene citrate and dexamethasone in the treatment of clomiphene-resistant PCOS: a prospective placebo-controlled study. *Hum Reprod* 2006;21:1805.
64. Holzer H et al. A new era in ovulation induction. *Fertil Steril* 2006;85:277.
65. Mitwally MF et al. Aromatase inhibition: a novel method of ovulation induction in women with polycystic ovarian syndrome. *Reprod Technol* 2000;10:244.
66. Al-Omari WR et al. Comparison of two aromatase inhibitors in women with clomiphene-resistant polycystic ovary syndrome. *Int J Gynaecol Obstet* 2004;85:289.
67. Nestler JE et al. Effects of metformin on spontaneous and clomiphene-induced ovulation in the polycystic ovary syndrome. *N Engl J Med* 1998; 338:1876.
68. Legro RS et al. Clomiphene, metformin, or both for infertility in the polycystic ovary syndrome. *N Engl J Med* 2007;356:551.
69. Palomba S et al. Ovulation induction in women with polycystic ovary syndrome. *Fertil Steril* 2006;86:S26.
70. Davis AR et al. Primary dysmenorrhea in adolescent girls and treatment with oral contraceptives. *J Pediatr Adolesc Gynecol* 2001;14:3.
71. O'Connell K et al. Self-treatment patterns among adolescent girls with dysmenorrhea. *J Pediatr Adolesc Gynecol* 2006;19:285.
72. Harel Z. Dysmenorrhea in adolescents and young adults: etiology and management. *J Pediatr Adolesc Gynecol* 2006;19:363.
73. Dawood MY. Primary dysmenorrhea. Advances in pathogenesis and management. *Obstet Gynecol* 2006;108:428.
74. Latthe P et al. Factors predisposing women to chronic pelvic pain: systematic review. *BMJ* 2006;332:749.
75. French L. Dysmenorrhea. *Am Fam Physician* 2005;71:285.
76. Harlow SD et al. Epidemiology of menstruation and its relevance to women's health. *Epidemiol Rev* 1995;17:265.
77. Society of Obstetrics Gynecology Canada (SOGC). Primary Dysmenorrhea Consensus Guideline. *JOGC* 2005;169:1119.
78. Golomb LM et al. Primary dysmenorrhea and physical activity. *Med Sci Sports Exerc* 1998;30: 906.
79. Akin M et al. Continuous low-level topical heat wrap therapy as compared to acetaminophen for primary dysmenorrhea. *J Reprod Med* 2004;49:739.
80. Akin MD et al. Continuous low level topical heat in the treatment of dysmenorrhea. *Obstet Gynecol* 2001;97:343.
81. Harel Z et al. Supplementation with omega-3 polyunsaturated fatty acids in the management of dysmenorrhea in adolescents. *Am J Obstet Gynecol* 1996;174:1335.
82. Barnard ND et al. Diet and sex hormone binding globulin, dysmenorrhea, and premenstrual symptoms. *Obstet Gynecol* 2000;95:245.
83. Proctor ML et al. Herbal and dietary therapies for primary and secondary dysmenorrhea. *Cochrane Database Syst Rev* 2003;1.
84. Procter ML et al. Transcutaneous electrical nerve stimulation and acupuncture for primary dysmenorrhea (Cochrane Review). *Cochrane Database Syst Rev* 2002:CD002123.
85. Latthe PM et al. Surgical interruption of pelvic nerve pathways in dysmenorrhea: a systematic review of effectiveness. *Acta Obstet Gynecol* 2007;86:4.
86. Smyth EM et al. Lipid derived autacoids: eicosanoids and platelet activating factor. In: Brunton L et al., eds. *Goodman & Gillman's Pharmacological Basis of Therapeutics*. 11th ed. New York: McGraw-Hill; 2006:653.
87. Marjoribanks J et al. Nonsteroidal anti-inflammatory drugs for primary dysmenorrhoea. *Cochrane Database Syst Rev* 2003;4:CD001751.
88. DuRant RH et al. Factors influencing adolescents' responses to regimens of naproxen for dysmenorrhea. *Am J Dis Child* 1985;139:489.
89. Proctor ML et al. Combined oral contraceptive pill (OCP) as treatment for primary dysmenorrhea. *Cochrane Database Syst Rev* 2001;2:CD002120.
90. Davis AR et al. Oral contraceptives for dysmenorrhea in adolescent girls: a randomized trial. *Obstet Gynecol* 2005;106:97.
91. Gerschultz KL et al. Extended cycling of combined hormonal contraceptives in adolescents: physician views and prescribing practices. *J Adolesc Health* 2007;40:151.
92. Baldaszti E et al. Acceptability of the long term contraceptive levonorgestrel releasing intrauterine system: a three year follow up study. *Contraception* 2003;67:87.
93. Zhang WY et al. Efficacy of minor analgesics in primary dysmenorrhoea: a systematic review. *Br J Obstet Gynaecol* 1998;105:780.
94. Harel Z et al. The use of the leukotriene receptor antagonist montelukast in the management of dysmenorrhea in adolescents. *J Pediatr Adolesc Gynecol* 2004;17:183.
95. Ghazizadeh S et al. Local application of glyceril trinitrate ointment for primary dysmenorrhea. *Int J Gynecol Obstet* 2002;79:43.
96. Marsden J et al. Guaifenesin as a treatment for primary dysmenorrhea. *J Am Board Fam Pract* 2004;17:240.
97. Lobo R. Endometriosis: etiology, pathology, diagnosis and management. In: Katz V et al., eds. *Comprehensive Gynecology*. 5th ed. Philadelphia: Mosby Elsevier; 2007.
98. Gao X et al. Economic burden of endometriosis. *Fertil Steril* 2006;86:1561.
99. Kennedy S. Should a diagnosis of endometriosis be sought in all symptomatic women? *Fertil Steril* 2006;86:1312.
100. Boardman R et al. Below the belt: approach to chronic pelvic pain. *Can Fam Physician* 2006;52:1557.
101. Jackson B et al. Managing the misplaced: approach to endometriosis. *Can Fam Physician* 2006;52:1422.
102. American Fertility Society. Revised American Fertility Society for Reproductive Medicine classification of endometriosis: 1996. *Fertil Steril* 1997;67:817.
103. Reddish S. Dysmenorrhea. *Aust Fam Physician* 2006;35:844.
104. Mousey AL et al. Diagnosis and management of endometriosis. *Am Fam Physician* 2006;74:594.
105. Farquhar C. Endometriosis. *BMJ* 2007;334:249.
106. Missmer SA et al. Incidence of laparoscopically confirmed endometriosis by demographic, anthropometric, and lifestyle factors. *Am J Epidemiol* 2004;160:784.
107. Fauconnier A et al. Endometriosis and pelvic pain: epidemiological evidence of the relationship and implications. *Hum Reprod Update* 2005;11:595.
108. Fauconnier A et al. Relation between pain symptoms and the anatomic location of deep infiltrating endometriosis. *Fertil Steril* 2002;78:719.
109. Lorencatto C et al. Depression in women with endometriosis with and without chronic pelvic pain. *Acta Obstet Gynecol Scand* 2006;85:88.
110. Mahutte NG et al. New advances in the understanding of endometriosis related infertility. *J Reprod Immunol* 2002;55:78.
111. Cahill DJ. What is the optimal medical management of infertility and minor endometriosis? *Hum Reprod* 2002;17:1135.
112. Seeber B et al. Panel of markers can accurately predict endometriosis in a subset of patients. *Fertil Steril* 2008;89:1073.
113. Ferrero S et al. Antiangiogenic therapies in endometriosis. *Br J Pharmacol* 2006;149:133.
114. Winkel CA. Evaluation and management of women with endometriosis. *Obstet Gynecol* 2003;102:397.
115. Giudice LC et al. Endometriosis. *Lancet* 2004;364: 1789.
116. Lin SY et al. Reproducibility of the revised American Fertility Society classification of endometriosis using laparoscopy or laparoscopy. *Int J Gynaecol Obstet* 1998;60:265.
117. Ferrero S et al. Future perspectives in the medical treatment of endometriosis. *Obstet Gyn Survey* 2005;60:817–826.
118. Barbieri RL. Endometriosis and the estrogen threshold theory: relation to surgical and medical treatment. *J Reprod Med* 1998;43:287.
119. Sinaii N et al. Treatment utilization for endometriosis symptoms: a cross-sectional survey study of lifetime experience. *Fertil Steril* 2007;87:1277. Epub 2007 Feb 12.
120. Practice Committee of the American Society for Reproductive Medicine. *Treatment of pelvic pain associated with endometriosis*. 2006;86(Suppl 4):S18.
121. Allen C et al. Non-steroidal anti-inflammatory drugs for pain in women with endometriosis. *Cochrane Database Syst Rev* 2005;4:CD004753. DOI: 10.1002/14651858.CD004753.pub2.
122. Verellini P et al. Continuous use of an oral contraceptive for endometriosis associated recurrent dysmenorrhea that does not respond to a cyclic pill regimen. *Fertil Steril* 2003;80:560.
123. Davis L et al. Modern combined oral contraceptives for pain associated with endometriosis. *Cochrane Database Syst Rev* 2007;3:CD001019. DOI: 10.1002/14651858.CD001019.pub2.
124. Harada T et al. Low-dose oral contraceptive pill for dysmenorrhea associated with endometriosis: a placebo controlled double-blind, randomized trial. *Fertil Steril* 2007; Dec 26. Epub ahead of print.
125. Petta C et al. Randomized clinical trial of a levonorgestrel-releasing intrauterine system and a depot GnRH analogue for the treatment of chronic pelvic pain in women with endometriosis. *Hum Reprod* 2005;20:1993.
126. Schlaff W et al. Subcutaneous injection of depot medroxyprogesterone acetate compared with leuprolide acetate in the treatment of endometriosis-associated pain. *Fertil Steril* 2006;85:314.
127. The practice committee of the American Society for Reproductive Medicine. Treatment of pelvic pain associated with endometriosis. *Fertil Steril* 2006;86(Suppl 4):S18.
128. Crosignani P et al. Advances in the management of endometriosis: an update for clinicians. *Hum Reprod Update* 2006;12:179.
129. Attar E et al. Aromatase inhibitors: the next generation of therapy for endometriosis. *Fertil Steril* 2006;85:1307.
130. Soysal S et al. The effects of post-surgical administration of goserelin plus anastrozole compared with

goserelin alone in patients with severe endometriosis: a prospective randomized trial. *Hum Reprod* 2004;19:160.
131. Nasir L et al. Management of pelvic pain from dysmenorrhea or endometriosis. *J Am Board Fam Pract* 2004;17:S43.
132. Crosignanai PG et al. Subcutaneous depot medroxyprogesterone acetate versus leuprolide acetate in the treatment of endometriosis associated pain. *Hum Reprod* 2006;21:248.
133. Bedaiwy M et al. Treatment with leuprolide acetate and hormonal add-back for up to 10 years in stage IV endometriosis patients with chronic pelvic pain. *Fertil Steril* 2006;86:220.
134. Melton LJ et al. Long term fracture risk among women with proven endometriosis. *Fertil Steril* 2006;86:1576.
135. The practice committee of the American Society for Reproductive Medicine. Endometriosis and infertility. *Fertil Steril* 2006;86(Suppl 4):S156.
136. Tavmergen E et al. Long term use of gonadotropin releasing hormone analogues before IVF in women with endometriosis. *Curr Opin Obstet Gynecol* 2007;19:284.
137. Winer SA et al. Premenstrual disorders: prevalence, etiology and impact. *J Reprod Med* 2006;51:339.
138. Campagne DM et al. The premenstrual syndrome revisited. *Eur J Obstet Gynaecol Reprod Biol* 2007;130:4.
139. American College of Obstetricians and Gynecologists. ACOG practice bulletin: premenstrual syndrome. Washington, DC: ACOG, April 2000:15.
140. Braverman PK. Premenstrual syndrome and premenstrual dysphoric disorder. *J Pediatr Adolesc Gynecol* 2007;20:3.
141. American Psychiatric Association. Diagnostic and Statistical Manual of Mental Disorders. 4th ed. DSM-IV-Text Revision. DSM-IV-TR, Washington, DC: American Psychiatric Association; 2000.
142. Mishell DR. Premenstrual disorders: epidemiology and disease burden. *Am J Manag Care* 2005;11:S473.
143. Dalton K et al. Incidence of premenstrual syndrome in twins. *BMJ* 1987;295:1027.
144. Van der Akker OB et al. Genetic and environmental variation in 2 British twin samples. *Acta Genet Med Gemellol* 1987;36:541.
145. Perkonigg A et al. Risk factors for premenstrual dysphoric disorder in a community sample of young women: the role of traumatic events and posttraumatic stress disorder. *J Clin Psychiatry* 2004;65:1314.
146. Mortola JF. Premenstrual syndrome-pathophysiologic considerations. *N Engl J Med* 1998;338:256.
147. Halbreich U et al. Low plasma GABA during the late luteal phase of women with premenstrual dysphoric disorder. *Am J Psychiatry* 1996;153:718.
148. Steiner M et al. Premenstrual dysphoric disorder and the serotonin system: pathophysiology and treatment. *J Clin Psychiatry* 2000;61(Suppl 12):17.
149. Thys-Jacobs S et al. Calcium-regulating hormones across the menstrual cycle: evidence of a secondary hyperthyroidism in women with PMS. *J Clin Endocrinol Metab* 1995;80:2227.
150. Thys-Jacobs S et al. Calcium supplementation in premenstrual syndrome. *J Gen Intern Med* 1989;4:183.
151. Penland JG et al. Dietary calcium and manganese effects on menstrual cycle symptoms. *Am J Obstet Gynecol* 1993;168:1417.
152. Thys-Jacobs S et al. Calcium carbonate and the premenstrual syndrome: effects on premenstrual and menstrual symptoms. *Am J Obstet Gynecol* 1998;179:444.
153. Rosenstein DL et al. Magnesium measures across the menstrual cycle in premenstrual syndrome. *Biol Psychiatry* 1994;35:557.
154. Proctor ML et al. Herbal dietary therapies for primary and secondary dysmenorrhea (Cochrane Review). *The Cochrane Library*, Issue 2, 2002.
155. Stevinson C et al. Complementary/alternative therapies for premenstrual syndrome: a systematic review of randomized trials. *Am J Obstet Gynecol* 2001;185:227.
156. Ebadi M et al. Pyridoxal phosphate and neurotransmitters in the brain. In: Tryiates G, ed. *Vit B6: Metabolism and the Role in Growth*. Westport: Food and Nutrition Press; 1980:223.
157. Wyatt KM et al. Efficacy of vitamin B-6 in the treatment of premenstrual syndrome: systematic review. *BMJ* 1999;318:1375.
158. Dittmar G et al. Premenstrual syndrome: treatment with a phytopharmaceutical. *TW Gynakol* 1992;5:60.
159. Schellenberg R. Treatment for the premenstrual syndrome with agnus castus fruit extract: prospective, randomized, placebo controlled study. *BMJ* 2001;332:134.
160. Girman A et al. An integrative medicine approach to premenstrual syndrome. *Am J Obstet Gynecol* 2003;188:S56.
161. Steiner M et al. Expert guidelines for the treatment of severe PMS, PMDD, and comorbidities: the role of SSRIs. *J Womens Health (Larchmt)* 2006;15:57.
162. Dimmock PW et al. Efficacy of selective serotonin-reuptake inhibitors in premenstrual syndrome: a systematic review. *Lancet* 2000;356:1131.
163. Freeman EW et al. Venlafaxine in the treatment of premenstrual dysphoric disorder. *Obstet Gynecol* 2001;98:737.
164. Kroll R et al. Treatment of premenstrual disorders. *J Reprod Med* 2006;51:359.
165. Landen M et al. Compounds with affinity for serotonergic receptors in the treatment of premenstrual dysphoria: a comparison of buspirone, nefazodone and placebo. *Psychopharmacology* 2001;155:292.
166. Brown C et al. A new monophonic oral contraceptive containing drospirenone: effect on premenstrual symptoms. *J Reprod Med* 2002;47:14.
167. Yonkers KA et al. Efficacy of a new low-dose oral contraceptive with drospirenone in premenstrual dysphoric disorder. *Obstet Gynecol* 2005;106:492.
168. Sundstrom I et al. Treatment of premenstrual syndrome with gonadotropin-releasing hormone agonist in a low dose regimen. *Acta Obstet Gynaecol Scand* 1999;78:891.
169. O'Brien PMS et al. Randomized controlled trial of the management of premenstrual syndrome and premenstrual mastalgia using luteal phase-only danazol. *Am J Obstet Gynecol* 1999;180:18.
170. Donnez J. Today's treatments: medical, surgical and in partnership. *Int J Gynaecol Obstet* 1999;64:S5.

CHAPTER 48

The Transition Through Menopause

Louise Parent-Stevens

THE TRANSITION THROUGH MENOPAUSE

The perimenopause, or climacteric, is the phase in the female aging process between the reproductive and nonreproductive years and is characterized by waning ovarian function and irregular menstrual cycles. Menopause is the last spontaneous episode of physiologic uterine bleeding confirmed by 12 months of amenorrhea and typically occurs 4 to 5 years after the beginning of the perimenopause. The postmenopausal state is characterized by significantly decreased hormone levels that may contribute to an increased risk of disease.

Although female life expectancy has increased significantly over the past century, the average age of women at menopause has remained relatively constant at 51 years.[1] Thus, women today may spend one-third of their lives with reduced ovarian hormone concentrations. Age at menopause appears to be genetically determined and is not influenced by race, physical characteristics, age at menarche, age at last pregnancy, socioeconomic status, or oral contraceptive use. Cigarette smoking decreases age of menopause by 1 to 2 years.[1] As the U.S. population ages, the number of women at risk for postmenopausal related issues will increase. Recent census data estimates that there are 47 million women age 50 years and older in the United States.[2]

Pathophysiology

The perimenopause results from an age-related decline in the number and competence of ovarian follicles. Loss of negative feedback due to decreased inhibin production by the failing ovary triggers increased production of FSH. Despite this increase in FSH levels, the rate of follicular maturation declines and anovulatory cycles predominate during this phase. However, ovulation can still occur and contraception should be used if pregnancy is not desired. After all ovarian follicles have been depleted, menopause ensues. This corresponds with a 10- to 20-fold increase in FSH levels and a threefold increase in LH levels which peak 1 to 3 years after menopause.[1] Postmenopausally, estrogen production decreases to approximately 10% of premenopausal production because the ovary is no longer making estrogen. Estrogen levels after menopause are derived from peripheral conversion of the androgen, androstenedione. The aromatase enzyme responsible for this conversion is predominantly found in fat, liver, and skin and increases with age and body weight, resulting in higher estrogen levels with women with greater body fat.[1,3] The primary estrogen no longer is estradiol, but the less potent agent, estrone.[1,3] Estrogen concentrations do not vary in a cyclic fashion as they do in women who are in their reproductive years (Table 48-1). Progesterone levels after menopause are generally undetectable in the absence of corpus luteum formation by the failed ovary.[4] Androgen production by the postmenopausal ovary increases, but overall postmenopausal androgen levels are decreased by 25% to 50% resulting from decreased conversion of androstenedione to testosterone.[1,4] The androgen:estrogen ratio increases markedly after menopause due to the greater drop in estrogen levels, which may result in mild symptoms of androgenism, such as hirsutism.[1]

Clinical Presentation

Although menopause is a natural consequence of aging, the concurrent decrease in estrogen production can result in clinical symptoms, such as hot flushes and vaginal atrophy. Postmenopausal osteoporosis may also result from estrogen deficiency (see Chapter 102: Osteoporosis). In addition to their presence in the sex organs, the two estrogen receptors (ERα and ERβ) are found in many tissues throughout the body, including the brain, bladder, lung, bone, and skin.[5,6] The

Table 48-1 Plasma Levels of Hormones in Pre- and Postmenopausal Women[10]

	Premenopausal	*Postmenopausal*
Estradiol	50–350 pg/mL	5–25 pg/mL
Estrone	30–110 pg/mL	20–70 pg/mL
Progesterone:		0.17 ng/mL
follicular	0.2–0.7 ng/mL	
luteal	3–21 ng/mL	
Testosterone	0.3 ng/mL	0.25 ng/mL
Androstenedione	1.5 ng/mL	0.6 ng/mL

impact of estrogen deficiency and replacement therapy on these organs is not yet fully elucidated.

Hot Flushes

Signs and Symptoms

1. D.R., a 51-year-old woman, has been having sudden feelings of warmth over her chest accompanied by a patchy flushing of her skin and increased sweating for the past month, especially after drinking coffee or wine or if she is upset. She now visits her physician because she has been waking up shivering from a perspiration-drenched gown nightly for the past week. D.R. does not take any medications. She has not had a menstrual period for at least 6 months; her physical examination was normal for a 51-year-old woman. What is the assessment based on the data provided for D.R.?

It appears that D.R. is experiencing hot flushes, a vasomotor symptom experienced by 50% to 85% of all women during the menopause transition.[1,7] The onset of vasomotor symptoms may precede the last menstrual period, but the prevalence is highest during the 2 years after menopause and declines over time.[1] Symptoms persist for longer than 1 year in 80% and longer than 5 years in 25% of women.[1,8] Women with surgically induced menopause, including bilateral oophorectomy, are more likely to experience moderate to severe hot flushes compared to women with natural menopause.[9] Symptoms include a feeling of warmth in the chest, neck, and facial areas that may be accompanied by visible red flushing. An average hot flush is approximately 4 minutes in duration.[8] The flushes are characteristically episodic rather than continuous, but may be as frequent as hourly in women with severe symptoms.[10] An increased environmental temperature, the ingestion of hot liquids or alcohol, and mental stress also may provoke hot flushes.

Other symptoms associated with the perimenopause may include irritability, inability to concentrate, forgetfulness, headaches, dizziness, joint stiffness, and fatigue.[10,11] Nocturnal hot flushes may lead to insomnia and sleep deprivation. Mood changes, including depression, are not uniformly associated with menopause, but are reported more frequently in women during the perimenopausal period.[12]

2. What are the underlying causes of the hot flushes associated with the perimenopause?

The exact trigger for hot flushes is unknown, but they are clearly associated with the declining estrogen concentrations that occur during menopause. Estrogen therapy (ET) is more effective than placebo in reducing hot flushes, and withdrawal of ET results in resumption of hot flushes. It is postulated that the drop in estrogen production leads to a decrease in 5-HT levels and an increase in the levels of norepinephrine and its metabolite, MHPG. This in turn alters thermoregulatory sensitivity and lowers temperature set point, triggering an autonomic reaction directed at cooling the body.[1,7,8]

Treatment

First-line treatment for hot flushes includes avoidance of known triggers (e.g., hot beverages, alcohol, warm environments), regular exercise, biofeedback, and relaxation techniques.[8] If the patient continues to experience bothersome symptoms, drug therapy should be considered. It is important to note that there is a high placebo response in clinical trials evaluating interventions for hot flushes.

ESTROGEN WITH OR WITHOUT A PROGESTIN

3. D.R. has tried lifestyle modifications for management of her hot flushes without much relief. Her physician is recommending hormone therapy but she expresses concern about its risks. How should D.R. be counseled about the risks and benefits of hormone therapy?

Hormone therapy has received a great deal of attention through the widely-publicized results of the Women's Health Initiative (WHI). The WHI prospectively studied estrogen and progestin therapy (EPT) versus placebo in 16,608 postmenopausal women and estrogen therapy (ET) versus placebo in 10,739 postmenopausal women without a uterus. Other large cohort studies, including the Million Women Study and the Nurses Health Study, have also contributed important information to the understanding of postmenopausal hormone therapy. Prior to selecting a treatment option, women should be counselled about the possible risks and benefits of ET/EPT (Table 48-2). Absolute and relative contraindications to the use of postmenopausal hormones are listed in Table 48-3.

Vasomotor Symptoms

Numerous clinical trials have established the efficacy of estrogen in reducing the frequency and severity of hot flushes compared to placebo. Oral and transdermal estrogen are equally efficacious and the addition of a progestin does not appear to alter this benefit. Some studies report a dose-response

Table 48-2 Risks and Benefits of ET/EPT (change in event frequency per 10,000 women years of exposure)[29,34,42]

	ET	*EPT*
Osteoporotic Hip Fracture	−6[a]	−5
Colorectal Cancer	NS[b]	−6
Breast Cancer	NS	+8[c]
Myocardial infarction	NS	+7
Thromboembolism (DVT/PE)	+7	+18
Stroke	+12	+8

[a]Negative sign indicates that hormone therapy provides protective effect.
[b]NS: no significant change in risk.
[c]positive sign indicates an increased risk with hormone therapy.

Table 48-3 Contraindications to ET[10,94]

Absolute Contraindications
Active thromboembolic disease or history thereof (e.g., DVT, PE, stroke, MI)
Undiagnosed abnormal genital bleeding
Known, suspected or history of estrogen dependent neoplasia (e.g., breast cancer, endometrial cancer)
Impaired liver function
Known or suspected pregnancy
Relative Contraindications (diseases that may be (exacerbated by estrogens/progestins)
Gallbladder Disease
Hypertriglyceridemia
Asthma
Migraine headache
Epilepsy
Systemic lupus erythematosus
Porphyria

relationship.[13] In women with hot flushes, EPT has been shown to improve quality of life and depressive symptoms.[14] Combination hormonal contraceptives are effective in reducing vasomotor symptoms and preventing pregnancy in women during perimenopause.

Osteoporosis

There are strong clinical data on the efficacy of estrogen, with or without a progestin, in preventing the bone loss associated with menopause. Estrogen has also been shown to decrease the risk of osteoporotic hip and vertebral fractures by approximately 25%.[15] Multiple oral and transdermal estrogen products are FDA-approved for the prevention of osteoporosis (Table 48-4); however, based on its risks and the availability of effective alternate treatments, ET/EPT should not be used solely for the prevention of osteoporosis. In women using systemic estrogen for menopausal symptoms, bone density will be maintained. After estrogen is discontinued, bone loss will resume so alternate protective therapies should be considered in women at risk (see Chapter 102: Osteoporosis).[15]

Endometrial Cancer

Stimulation of the endometrium by exogenous estrogen causes endometrial proliferation leading to endometrial hyperplasia rates of 8 to 62% after 1 to 3 years of use.[16] Continuous exposure to unopposed estrogen can lead to the development of endometrial cancer. Use of ET alone in a woman with a uterus increases the risk of endometrial cancer by twofold to 10-fold, with higher estrogen dose and duration associated with greater risk. The elevated risk persists for at least 5 years after discontinuation of ET.[17] Addition of a progestin can significantly attenuate or eliminate the increased risk of endometrial cancer, with combined-continuous regimens possibly offering greater endometrial protection than intermittent regimens[16–18] (see Question 3).

Breast Cancer

Randomized and observational studies support a 20% increased risk of breast cancer with EPT use, beginning 5 years after initiation, increasing with continued use and returning to baseline approximately 5 years after EPT is stopped.[19,20] Risk appears to be similar between oral and transdermal estrogen but a dose-response relationship has not been established. The effect of ET on breast cancer is less clear. Some studies, including the estrogen only arm of the WHI, found no increased risk of breast cancer after 7 years of treatment, whereas others reported an increased risk, particularly with long-term use.[21–23]

Ovarian Cancer

Several studies have documented an increased risk of ovarian cancer with postmenopausal hormone use.[24–28] The risk increases with increasing duration of use and occurs with both ET and EPT. Limited data suggest that the type and route of therapy do not influence risk. It is unclear if long-term past use confers an increased risk of ovarian cancer.

Thromboembolic Disease

Current ET use increases the risk for venous thromboembolic disease, including DVT and pulmonary embolism, up to twofold.[29,30] The greatest risk, up to 3.5-fold, is within the first year of treatment. Women who are older or have a higher BMI are at elevated risk.[31] Concurrent use of estrogen and progestin may incur a greater risk than use of unopposed estrogen but transdermal estrogen may significantly decrease the risk compared to oral estrogen.[32,33]

Some, but not all, studies have documented an increased risk for stroke with ET/EPT use.[23] In the WHI, ET and EPT increased the risk of ischemic, but not hemorrhagic, stroke by approximately 40%.[34,35] The Women's Estrogen for Stroke Trial (WEST) found that use of estrogen soon after a stroke or transient ischemic attack was associated with adverse outcomes compared to placebo.[36]

Cardiovascular Disease

Cardiovascular disease is the leading cause of death among women, accounting for more deaths than all cancer types.[37] Some, but not all, studies report a non-age-related increase in coronary heart disease (CHD) in postmenopausal women.[10] Estrogens have beneficial effects on lipids and endothelial function, suggesting a pharmacologic basis for a heart-protective effect.[38] However, the cardiovascular effects of ET remain controversial despite numerous studies addressing this issue. Case-control and cohort studies, such as the Nurses' Health Study (NHS), found that, compared with never users, postmenopausal women who used ET or EPT had a lower risk of CHD-related death.[39] However, the HERS trial, a prospective study of EPT in postmenopausal women with pre-existing heart disease, showed an increased risk of CHD during the first year of the study and no overall benefit on CHD after 4.1 years of follow-up.[40] The ERA Trial, which compared the effects of ET and placebo on the angiographic progression of pre-existing CHD, showed no benefit of ET.[41] In the WHI, which was specifically designed to answer questions about ET/EPT and primary prevention of cardiovascular disease, increased cardiovascular events in the EPT group led to early termination of that arm of the study. The estrogen-only arm was also stopped early due to an increased risk of stroke without evidence of cardiovascular protection.[29,42] A major criticism of the WHI was that the average age of the study participants, 63 years, did not reflect the typical age at which symptomatic menopausal women were most likely to use ET/EPT. Further analysis of the WHI data found a trend towards reduced CHD risk and lower total mortality in women aged 50 to 59 years

Table 48-4 Agents Used in ET/EPT Therapy

Drug (Brand Name)	Initial Daily Dosage
Estrogens	
Conjugated equine estrogens (CEE)[a] (Premarin)	0.3 mg
Synthetic conjugated estrogens (Cenestin, Enjuvia)	0.3 mg
Estropipate[a] (piperazine estrone sulfate) (Ogen, Ortho-Est)	0.625 mg
Micronized estradiol[a] (Estrace, Gynodiol)	0.5 mg
Estradiol transdermal system[a] (various brand name products)	0.014–0.025 mg/24-hr patch applied weekly or twice weekly
Esterified estrogen[a] (Estratab, Menest)	0.3 mg
Estradiol acetate tablet (Femtrace)	0.45 mg
Estradiol acetate vaginal ring (Femring)	0.05 mg/24-hr ring inserted vaginally every 90 days
Estradiol topical emulsion/gel (Elestrin, Estrogel, Estrasorb)	1 packet daily
Progestins	
Medroxyprogesterone acetate (Provera and generic products)	5 mg for cyclic regimens/2.5 mg for continuous regimens
Norethindrone acetate (various brand name products)	2.5 mg for cyclic regimens/0.5 mg for continuous regimens
Progesterone (Prometrium)	200 mg for cyclic regimens/100 mg for continuous regimens
Progesterone vaginal gel (Prochieve, Crinone)	1 full applicator of 4% gel every other day
Levonorgestrel-releasing IUD (Mirena)	20 mcg/day
Estrogen and Progestin Combinations	
Prempro[a]	0.3 mg CEE and 1.5 mg MPA
Premphase[a]	0.625 mg CEE for 28 days with 5 mg MPA for last 14 days
CombiPatch	0.05 mg estradiol with either 0.14 or 0.25 mg norethindrone
Femhrt[a]	2.5 mcg EE[b] and 0.1 mg norethindrone acetate
Activella[a]	0.5 mg estradiol and 0.5 mg norethindrone acetate
Prefest[a]	1 mg estradiol and 0.09 mg norgestimate
Climara Pro[a]	0.045 mg estradiol/0.015 mg levonorgestrel/24 hr patch once weekly
Estrogen and Androgen Combinations[c]	
Esterified estradiol and Methyltestosterone (Estratest, Covaryx)	0.625 mg esterfied estrogens and 1.25 mg MT
Vaginal Estrogens (localized effect only)	
Conjugated Equine Estrogen cream (Premarin)	Initial: 1 gm cream (0.625 mg CEE) daily Maintenance: 1 gm cream once/twice weekly
Estradiol cream (Estrace)	Initial: 2–4 gm cream (0.2–0.4 mg estradiol) daily Maintenance: 1 gm cream (0.1 mg estradiol) twice weekly
Estradiol ring (Estring)	2 mg ring (0.0075 mg/day) every 90 days
Estradiol hemihydrate tablets (Vagifem)	1 tablet (0.025 mg) daily for 2 wk, then one tablet twice weekly

[a] Approved by the FDA for prevention of osteoporosis.
[b] EE: ethinyl estradiol.
[c] Requires addition of progestin in women with uterus.

who began therapy within 10 years of menopause.[43] The WHI-Coronary Artery Calcium Study, a WHI substudy, also found a lower calcified plaque burden in 50- to 59-year-old women who took ET as compared to placebo, suggestive of a protective effect of estrogen on CHD when used early after the onset of menopause.[44] The NHS analyzed CHD risk based on age at initial hormone use and found a 65% to 72% reduction in risk for women who began use within 10 years of menopause compared with no change in CHD risk for women who initiated first use more than 10 years after menopause.[45]

Although there are still unanswered questions regarding the cardiovascular effects of ET/EPT, it appears to be safer than previously thought when used for symptom control soon after menopause. However, there is no clear indication that ET/EPT should be used for the prevention of CHD in asymptomatic women.[46]

Gallbladder Disease

Estrogen, with or without progestin, increases the risk of gallbladder disease by approximately 60%.[47] In the WHI and HERS studies, use of ET/EPT was associated with a significant increase in the risk for gallbladder surgery.[47,48]

Other Risks and Benefits

Oral estrogen therapy has beneficial effects on lipids, increasing HDL while decreasing total cholesterol, LDL and lipoprotein(a). However, it can also significantly increase triglyceride levels.[49,50] Transdermal estrogen has similar but less pronounced effects on cholesterol levels.[50] Addition of a progestin attenuates the beneficial changes of ET on HDL but may also ameliorate ET's triglyceride-elevating effects. Of the commonly used progestins, micronized progesterone appears to have the least deleterious effect on the lipid profile.[17]

Observational studies have suggested that postmenopausal hormone use reduced the risk colorectal cancer during the time of use.[51] In the WHI study, EPT was associated with a significantly decreased risk of colorectal cancer; however, this decreased risk was not seen with use of ET alone.[29,52]

The effects of postmenopausal hormone therapy on cognitive function are unclear. While observational trials indicated that ET/EPT protects against mental decline, the WHI Memory Study (WHIMS), a substudy of the WHI, found that, in women aged 65 years or older at time of hormone initiation, ET and EPT increased the risk of dementia and mild cognitive impairment.[53–56] Other studies suggest that when therapy is begun in recently postmenopausal women, ET/EPT may provide a protective effect on mental status.[57,58] More data are needed on the effects of various regimens and time of use before a definitive answer about the effects of ET/EPT on cognitive function can be made.

The WHI study found a decreased incidence of new-onset diabetes mellitus in both the ET and EPT treatment groups and the HERS trial documented a similar reduction in risk.[23] Additional data are needed before hormone therapy can be recommended for the prevention of diabetes.

Dosing Regimens

4. What is an appropriate regimen of estrogen for the management of D.R.'s hot flushes?

There are a number of estrogen and estrogen/progestin products currently available for the management of vasomotor symptoms (Table 48-4). Conjugated equine estrogens (CEE) have traditionally been the products most frequently used in the United States; however, use of alternate agents, including oral and transdermal estradiol, is increasing. Oral and transdermal estrogen appear to be equally efficacious in treating hot flushes.[13] Transdermal estrogen is associated with a decreased risk for TED and hypertension but has less of a beneficial effect on the lipid profile compared to oral estrogen. The effect of transdermal estrogen on cardiovascular and gallbladder disease has not been well studied. Current recommendations are to initiate estrogen at a low dose (e.g., 0.3 mg of CEE or 0.025 mg of transdermal estradiol) with titration as needed for symptom control.

In women with an intact uterus, such as D.R., a progestin must also be added to the regimen to minimize the risk of endometrial cancer.[23] Currently, there is no indication for adding a progestin to ET in women without a uterus. Oral progestins used in the United States to antagonize the endometrial effects of estrogen are listed in Table 48-4. For medroxyprogesterone acetate (MPA), the most commonly used EPT progestin, 5 mg/day for at least 12 days/month is needed to prevent endometrial hyperplasia when used in cyclic regimens (Table 48-5). For continuous regimens, 2.5 mg/day may be adequate. Oral micronized progesterone 100 to 300 mg/day for 12 days/month or the progestin-releasing IUD also appear to protect against endometrial hyperplasia from ET.[17]

EPT may result in resumption of uterine withdrawal bleeding. The pattern and frequency of bleeding is dependent on the EPT regimen used (Table 48-5). For women using cyclic

Table 48-5 ET/EPT Regimens and Expected Vaginal Bleeding Patterns

Estrogen/Progestin Dosing	*Hormone Free Interval*	*Typical Bleeding Pattern*
Combined Regimens (EPT) for Patient with intact uterus		
CYCLIC REGIMEN		
Estrogen (PO or TD) : days 1–25 of each month	3–6 days	Withdrawal bleeding 1–2 days after progestin dosing ended[a]
Progestin: days 10–25 or 14–25 of each month		80% experience regular bleeding
CYCLIC COMBINED		
Estrogen (PO or TD) and Progestin: days 1–25 of each month	3–6 days	Withdrawal bleeding 1–2 days after progestin dosing ended[a]
		Lower incidence than cyclic regimen
CONTINUOUS CYCLIC		
Estrogen (PO or TD): daily	none	Withdrawal bleeding 1–2 days after progestin dosing ended[a]
Progestin: 10–14 days every month		80% experience regular bleeding
LONG-CYCLE CYCLIC		
Estrogen (PO or TD): daily	none	Withdrawal bleeding 1–2 days after progestin dosing ended[a]
Progestin: 14 days every third month		~70% experience regular bleeding
CONTINUOUS COMBINED		
Estrogen (PO or TD) and Progestin: daily	none	40% have irregular bleeding for first 6–12 months[b]
		75%–89% become amenorrheic within 12 months
CONTINUOUS PULSED		
Estrogen PO × 3 days then	none	~70% experience spotting early during treatment
Estrogen + Progestin PO × 3 days		80% are amenorrheic at the end of 12 months[b]
Repeat continuously		
Estrogen only Regimens (ET) for Patients without uterus		
CONTINUOUS REGIMEN		
Estrogen (PO or TD): daily	none	none

[a]Bleeding earlier than 11 days after beginning progestin suggests need for endometrial evaluation.
[b]Bleeding after 6 months of therapy requires endometrial evaluation.

regimens, studies suggest that the use of progestin every 3 months rather than monthly is protective of the endometrium and may improve patient acceptance.[59] Patient preference regarding bleeding patterns should be considered when selecting an EPT regimen.

There is increasing consumer interest in "natural" ("bioidentical") hormone therapy as a safer alternative to conventional estrogen products. "Natural hormone therapy" is extemporaneously compounded and does not carry the standardized FDA-approved warnings. However, there is no good clinical evidence to support claims of greater safety with these products.[60,61]

Because hot flushes are self-limiting, discontinuation of ET/EPT should be attempted every 6 to 12 months. Abrupt discontinuation of ET/EPT may trigger recurrence of hot flushes; therefore, tapering is recommended. However, there are no specific guidelines; a taper regimen should be developed for each patient individually.[62]

Adverse Effects

5. How should D.R. be counselled about possible side effects of ET/EPT?

In addition to being counselled about the serious risks of ET/EPT, D.R. should be advised regarding "nuisance" side effects from hormone therapy. These most commonly include resumption of vaginal bleeding (see Question 3) and breast tenderness.[13] Nausea, weight gain, edema, headache, PMS-like symptoms, and increased vaginal discharge have also been reported. Skin irritation may occur with the use of transdermal products. Frequently, these side effects diminish with time or may respond to a change in dosage or product. Although ET/EPT has not been shown to consistently induce or worsen hypertension, patients should be monitored for increases in blood pressure.[63]

6. D.R. has decided that she does not wish to take EPT for her hot flushes. What alternate therapy would be appropriate to try?

PROGESTINS

Progestins, given alone, appear to be similar to ET in relieving the symptoms of hot flushes. Regimens that have been shown to be effective include megestrol acetate, 40 mg/day PO, and medroxyprogesterone acetate, 10 mg/day PO or 150 mg IM Q 3 months or 500 mg IM on days 1, 14, and 28.[64,65] Adverse effects of progestins include vaginal bleeding, fluid retention, increased appetite, breast tenderness, acne, hirsutism, headaches, mood swings, fatigue, and depression. In the absence of ET, progestins do not appear to increase the risk of thromboembolic disease.[17] Progestins are a reasonable alternative for women who cannot take estrogen but need highly effective therapy for hot flushes.

ANDROGENS

Androgens do not relieve vasomotor symptoms in postmenopausal women. However, some clinical trials have shown that testosterone therapy in postmenopausal women can improve sexual function and may also improve energy levels and sense of wellbeing.[66,67] Only methyltestosterone, in combination with estrogen, is FDA-approved for the management of menopausal symptoms (Table 48-4). Currently available gels and patches deliver an inappropriately high dose of androgen for women; however, use of smaller quantities of gel may provide adequate therapy (e.g., 5 mg of testosterone) while minimizing the risk of undesired side effects, such as acne, hirsutism, and masculinization. Products specifically designed for use in women are under development. A short-term trial of androgen therapy can be given to women taking ET/EPT who experience low libido. If improvement is not seen after several months of testosterone, it should be discontinued.

NONHORMONAL AGENTS

Nonhormonal agents are modestly effective in reducing hot flush frequency and severity. These agents include some serotonergic antidepressants, antiseizure, and antihypertensive drugs. Table 48-6 lists the agents and doses which have been

Table 48-6 Nonhormonal Agents for the Management of Vasomotor Symptoms[71-73]

Drug	Daily Dose Used in Clinical Trials	Placebo Controlled Trial?	Adverse Reactions Reported
Serotonergic Antidepressants			
Citalopram (Celexa)	20 mg	Yes	Dry mouth, ↓ libido, rash/hives, insomnia, somnolence, bladder spasm, palpitations, arthralgias
Fluoxetine (Prozac)	20–30 mg	Yes	Nausea, dry mouth,
Mirtazapine (Remeron)	15–30 mg	No	↑ appetite, dry mouth
Paroxetine (Paxil)	10–25 mg	Yes	Headache, nausea, insomnia, drowsiness
Sertraline (Zoloft)	50 mg	Yes	Nausea, fatigue/malaise, diarrhea, anxiety/nervousness
Venlafaxine (Effexor)	37.5–150 mgXR	Yes	Dry mouth, ↓ appetite, nausea, constipation
Antiseizure Agents			
Gabapentin (Neurontin)	900 mg	Yes	Somnolence, fatigue, dizziness, rash, palpitations, peripheral edema
Antihypertensive Agents			
Clonidine	PO: 0.05–0.15 mg TD: 0.1 mg/24 hr	Yes	Headache, dry mouth, drowsiness, skin reaction/itching (patch)

shown to be effective along with adverse effects most commonly seen.[68–70,71–73]

PHYTOESTROGENS

Phytoestrogens, including isoflavones and lignans, are plant-based substances that exert mild estrogenic effects. Epidemiologic studies have found an association between higher dietary soy intake and fewer menopausal symptoms.[74] However, the results of clinical trials of isoflavones, including soy and red clover extracts, are mixed. Several meta-analyses concluded that phytoestrogens have minor, if any, benefits[70,74,75] on menopausal symptoms. This apparent lack of benefit may be related to the source and dose of isoflavones being evaluated. In general, isoflavones are well tolerated. The most commonly reported side effect is gastrointestinal intolerance. A 5-year study documented an increased risk of endometrial hyperplasia with phytoestrogen use.[76] Due to their estrogenic effects, phytoestrogens should be avoided or used cautiously in women with a history of estrogen-dependent disease.

BLACK COHOSH

Black cohosh (*cimicifuga racemosa*) is one of the most popular herbs for the management of menopausal symptoms. It does not appear to have estrogenic effects, but may exert a serotonergic effect.[77] Clinical studies of black cohosh for hot flushes have shown mixed results.[78–81] Several trials have suggested that black cohosh may have a beneficial effect on mood symptoms associated with menopause.[77] The typical dose of black cohosh is 20 mg BID.[82] It is generally well tolerated, but use beyond 6 months has not been evaluated. The most common adverse effects are gastrointestinal in nature. For women who do not wish to use hormonal agents, black cohosh would be a reasonable alternate treatment.

OTHER THERAPY

Studies on the use of wild yam extract, DHEA, ginseng, evening primrose oil, and dong quai do not support a beneficial effect of these agents in the management of hot flushes.[82–84]

Genitourinary Atrophy

Signs and Symptoms

7. R.J., a 60-year-old woman who has remarried recently, complains of pain associated with intercourse. She also complains of vaginal dryness and pain during intercourse. Upon physical examination, she is noted to have sparse, gray pubic hair. Her labia minora have a pale, dry appearance, whereas the labia majora appear flattened. Her vagina is small with a pale, dry epithelium. How would you assess R.J.'s problem?

R.J. appears to be experiencing symptoms associated with genitourinary atrophy. Estrogen is the dominant hormone of vaginal physiology. With the postmenopausal loss of estrogen production, the vagina decreases in size and loses its rugal pattern: its mucosa becomes pale, thin, and dry and vaginal blood flow decreases. A decrease in lactobacillus production of lactic acid leads to an increase in vaginal pH to 5.0 or greater (compared to a premenopausal pH of 3.5–4.5).[85,86] These changes make the vagina more susceptible to infection from bacterial colonization and localized trauma secondary to intercourse. Unlike hot flushes, vaginal atrophy does not abate with time since menopause.

Symptoms of atrophic vaginitis include dryness, itching, pain and dyspareunia. About 10% to 40% of postmenopausal women experience symptoms, however, only 25% of those affected seek medical attention.[85] Postmenopausal women who engage in regular coital activity have less atrophic vaginal changes compared with those of similar age and estrogen levels who do not have regular intercourse. Also, postmenopausal women who have breaks in their sexual intercourse patterns, such as that experienced by R.J. between the death of her first husband and remarriage, tend to experience dyspareunia (painful coitus) with the resumption of intercourse.

Treatment

VAGINALLY ADMINISTERED ESTROGENS

8. What would be an appropriate regimen for R.J. to decrease her vaginal symptoms?

Estrogen therapy reverses vaginal epithelial thinning, decreases the vaginal pH and improves the symptoms of vaginal atrophy. If hot flushes are also present, oral or transdermal estrogen may be used. For treatment of vaginal symptoms alone, low-dose vaginal administration is the preferred route of administration.[85,87] Absorption of estrogen through the vaginal mucosa is efficient and can produce estrogen levels adequate to relieve systemic symptoms such as hot flushes (e.g. 50–100 mcg/day estradiol acetate vaginal ring.) Limited data suggest that low-dose vaginal administration of estrogen does not significantly alter serum estradiol levels.[87] Low-dose vaginal estrogen is available in several dosage formulations (see Table 48-4). The various products appear to be equivalent in restoring vaginal cytology and pH and relieving symptoms of vaginal dryness, pruritus, and dyspareunia; product selection should be based on patient preference.[85] Vaginal creams and tablets are initiated with once daily dosing; after symptoms have resolved, the patient should be switched to maintenance dosing of once or twice weekly administration. The low-dose vaginal ring releases a constant dose of estrogen over 90 days.

The most common adverse effects of vaginal estrogens are vaginal irritation and bleeding and breast tenderness. Studies of limited duration suggest that the risk of endometrial hyperplasia from low-dose vaginal estrogen is small and the addition of a progestin is generally considered unnecessary.[85,87] Women at high risk for endometrial cancer, using higher than usual doses of vaginal estrogen, or experiencing vaginal bleeding during intravaginal ET should be evaluated for endometrial hyperplasia.[85]

OTHER TREATMENT

If a woman with vaginal atrophy is unwilling or unable to use estrogen, a vaginal bioadhesive (Replens) has been shown to significantly improve vaginal pH and atrophy symptoms, although to a lesser degree than vaginal ET.[88] Nonhormonal treatments, such as SSRIs and orally consumed herbal treatments (e.g., black cohosh, isoflavones), do not appear to improve vaginal atrophy symptoms.[86]

Urinary Incontinence

9. Would ET/EPT be an appropriate choice of therapy if R.J. were experiencing urinary incontinence?

Estrogen has multiple effects on the urinary tract, including maintaining urethral pressure and collagen synthesis and controlling micturition. While the incidence of incontinence and urinary tract infections (UTI) increase with age, it is not clear that loss of estrogen production contributes to these problems.[89] Despite their theoretic benefits on the urinary tract, multiple studies have failed to show a benefit of ET/EPT on the symptoms of urinary incontinence.[90] In the WHI and NHS studies, ET and EPT increased the risk of developing urinary incontinence and worsened symptoms in women with pre-existing urinary incontinence.[91,92] For women with recurrent UTI, 3 of 5 controlled trials showed a benefit of oral or vaginal estrogen in decreasing the frequency of infections.[93] Estrogens should not be used for management of urinary incontinence but could be given a trial in women with recurrent UTIs.

ACKNOWLEDGMENT

I would like to thank Dr. Rosalie Sagraves, Professor, University of Illinois at Chicago College of Pharmacy, Dr. Jennifer Hardman, Clinical Assistant Professor, University of Illinois at Chicago College of Pharmacy, and Dr. Nancy Letassy, Clinical Associate Professor, College of Pharmacy, University of Oklahoma Health Sciences Center, for their outstanding work on previous editions of this chapter.

REFERENCES

1. Speroff L. The perimenopause: definitions, demography, and physiology. *Obstet Gynecol Clin N Am* 2002;29:397.
2. U.S. Census Bureau. *Statistical abstract of the United States: 2007.* 126th ed. Washington, DC: U.S. Government Printing Office; 2006.
3. Grow DR. Metabolism of endogenous and exogenous reproductive hormones. *Obstet Gynecol Clin N Am* 2002;29:425.
4. Burger HG et al. Hormonal changes in the menopause transition. *Recent Prog Horm Res* 2002;57:257.
5. Hall G, Phillips TJ. Estrogen and skin: the effects of estrogen, menopause, and hormone replacement therapy on the skin. *J Am Acad Dermatol* 2005;53:555.
6. Nilsson S, Gustafsson JA. Biological role of estrogen and estrogen receptors. *Crit Rev Biochem Mol Biol* 2002;37:1.
7. Pinkerton JV, Zion AS. Vasomotor symptoms in menopause: where we've been and where we're going. *J Womens Health* 2002;15:135.
8. Stearns V et al. Hot flushes. *Lancet* 2002;360:1851.
9. Gallicchio L et al. Type of menopause, patterns of hormone therapy use, and hot flashes. *Fertil Steril* 2006;85:1432.
10. Nathan L, Judd HL. Menopause & postmenopause. In: DeCherney AH et al., eds. *Current Diagnosis and Treatment: Obstetrics & Gynecology.* 10th ed. Columbus: McGraw-Hill Companies; 2007: 1018.
11. Avis NE et al. A universal menopausal syndrome? *Am J Med* 2005;118:37S.
12. Schmidt PJ. Mood, depression, and reproductive hormones in the menopausal transition. *Am J Med* 2005;118:54S.
13. Nelson HD. Commonly used types of postmenopausal estrogen for treatment of hot flashes: scientific review. *JAMA* 2004;291:1610.
14. Hlatky MA et al. Quality-of-life and depressive symptoms in postmenopausal women after receiving hormone therapy. *JAMA* 2002;287:591.
15. North American Menopause Society. Management of osteoporosis in postmenopausal women: 2006 position statement of the North American Menopause Society. *Menopause* 2006;13:340.
16. Yeh IT. Postmenopausal hormone replacement therapy: endometrial and breast effects. *Adv Anat Pathol* 2007;14:17.
17. North American Menopause Society. Role of progestogen in hormone therapy for postmenopausal women; position statement of The North American Menopause Society. *Menopause* 2003;10:113.
18. Million Women Study Collaborators. Endometrial cancer and hormone-replacement therapy in the Million Women Study. *Lancet* 2005;365:1543.
19. Collins JA et al. Breast cancer risk with postmenopausal hormonal treatment. *Hum Reprod Update* 2005;11:545.
20. Li CI et al. Relationship between long durations and different regimens of hormone therapy and risk of breast cancer. *JAMA* 2003;289:3254.
21. Beral V et al. Breast cancer and hormone-replacement therapy in the Million Women Study. *Lancet* 2003;263:419.
22. Chelbowski RT et al. Influence of estrogen plus progestin on breast cancer and mammography in healthy postmenopausal women. *JAMA* 2003;289:3243.
23. North American Menopause Society. Estrogen and progestogen use in peri- and postmenopausal women: March 2007 position statement of the North American Menopause Society. *Menopause* 2007;14:168.
24. Million Women Study Collaborators. Ovarian cancer and hormone replacement therapy in the million women study. *Lancet* 2007;369:1703.
25. Anderson GL et al. Effects of estrogen plus progestin on gynecologic cancers and associated diagnostic procedures: the women's health initiative randomized trial. *JAMA* 2003;290:1739.
26. Danforth KN et al. A prospective study of postmenopausal hormone use and ovarian cancer risk. *Br J Cancer* 2007;96:151.
27. Lacey JV et al. Menopausal hormone therapy and ovarian cancer risk in the National Institutes of Health–AARP diet and health study cohort. *J Natl Cancer Inst* 2006;98:1397.
28. Lacey JV et al. Menopausal hormone replacement therapy and risk of ovarian cancer. *JAMA* 2002;288:334.
29. Women's Health Initiative Steering Committee. Effects of conjugated equine estrogen in postmenopausal women with hysterectomy: the Women's Health Initiative randomized controlled trial. *JAMA* 2004;291:1701.
30. Miller J et al. Postmenopausal estrogen replacement and risk for venous thromboembolism: a systematic review and meta-analysis for the U.S. Preventive Services Task Force. *Ann Intern Med* 2002;136:680.
31. Gompel A et al. The EMAS 2006/2007 update on clinical recommendations on postmenopausal hormone therapy. *Maturitas* 2007;56:227.
32. Canonico M et al. Hormone therapy and venous thromboembolism among postmenopausal women: impact of the route of estrogen administration and progestogens: the ESTHER study. *Circulation* 2007; 115:840.
33. Scarabin PY et al. Differential association of oral and transdermal oestrogen-replacement therapy with venous thromboembolism risk. *Lancet* 2003;362:428.
34. Wassertheil-Smoller S et al. Effect of estrogen plus progestin on stroke in postmenopausal women: the Women's Health Initiative: a randomized trial. *JAMA* 2003;289:2673.
35. Hendrix SL et al. Effects of conjugated equine estrogen on stroke in the Women's Health Initiative. *Circulation* 2006;113:2425.
36. Hurn PD, Brass LM. Estrogen and Stroke: a balanced analysis. *Stroke* 2003;34:338.
37. Wingo PA et al. How does breast cancer mortality compare with that of other cancers and selected cardiovascular diseases at different ages in U.S. women? *J Womens Health Gend Based Med* 2000;9:999.
38. Mendelsohn ME, Karas HR. The protective effects of estrogen on the cardiovascular system. *N Engl J Med* 1999;340:1801.
39. Grodstein F et al. A prospective, observational study of postmenopausal hormone therapy and primary prevention of cardiovascular disease. *Ann Intern Med* 2000;133:933.
40. Hulley S et al. Randomized trial of estrogen plus progestin for secondary prevention of coronary heart disease in postmenopausal women. *JAMA* 1998;280:605.
41. Herrington DM et al. Effects of estrogen replacement on the progression of coronary-artery disease. *N Engl J Med* 2000;343:522.
42. Writing Group for the Women's Health Initiative Investigators. Risks and benefits of estrogen plus progestin in healthy postmenopausal women: principle results from the Women's Health Initiative randomized controlled trial. *JAMA* 2002;288:321.
43. Rossouw JE et al. Postmenopausal hormone therapy and risk of cardiovascular disease by age and years since menopause. *JAMA* 2007;297:1465.
44. Manson JE et al. Estrogen therapy and coronary-artery calcification. *N Engl J Med* 2007;356:2591.
45. Grodstein F et al. Hormone therapy and coronary heart disease: the role of time since menopause and age at hormone initiation. *J Womens Health* 2006;15:35.
46. Mendelsohn ME, Karas RH. HRT and the young at heart. *N Engl J Med* 2007;356:2639.
47. Cirillo DJ et al. Effect of estrogen therapy on gallbladder disease. *JAMA* 2005;293:330.
48. Simon JA et al. Effect of estrogen plus progestin on risk for biliary tract surgery in postmenopausal women with coronary artery disease. *Ann Intern Med* 2001;135:493.
49. Dias AR et al. Effects of conjugated equine estrogens or raloxifene on lipid profile, coagulation and fibrinolysis factors in postmenopausal women. *Climacteric* 2005;8:63.
50. Hemelaar M et al. Oral, more than transdermal, estrogen therapy improves lipids and lipoprotein(a) in postmenopausal women: a randomized, placebo-controlled study. *Menopause* 2003;10:550.
51. Grodstein F et al. Postmenopausal hormone therapy

and the risk of colorectal cancer: a review and meta-analysis. *Am J Med* 1999;106:574.
52. Chelbowski RT et al. Estrogen plus progestin and colorectal cancer in postmenopausal women. *N Engl J Med* 2004;350:991.
53. Espeland MA et al. Conjugated equine estrogens and global cognitive function in postmenopausal women: women's health initiative memory study. *JAMA* 2004;291:2959.
54. Rapp SR et al. Effect of estrogen plus progestin on global cognitive function in postmenopausal women. The Women's Health Initiative Memory Study: a randomized controlled trial. *JAMA* 2003;289:2663.
55. Shumaker SA et al. Estrogen plus progestin and the incidence of dementia and mild cognitive impairment in postmenopausal women: the Women's Health Initiative Memory Study: a randomized controlled trial. *JAMA* 2003;289:2651.
56. Shumaker SA et al. Conjugated equine estrogens and incidence of probable dementia and mild cognitive impairment in postmenopausal women. *JAMA* 2004;291:2947.
57. MacLennan AH et al. Hormone therapy, timing of initiation, and cognition in women aged older than 60 years: the REMEMBER pilot study. *Menopause* 2006;13:28.
58. Maki PM. A systematic review of clinical trials of hormone therapy on cognitive function: effects of age at initiation and progestin use. *Ann N Y Acad Sci* 2005;1052:182.
59. Odmark IS et al. Endometrial safety and bleeding pattern during a five-year treatment with long-cycle hormone therapy. *Menopause* 2005;12:699.
60. Boothby LA et al. Bioidentical hormone therapy: a review. *Menopause* 2004;11:356.
61. ACOG Committee on Gynecologic Practice. Compounded bioidentical hormones. *Obstet Gynecol* 2005;106:1139.
62. Grady D, Sawaya GF. Discontinuation of postmenopausal hormone therapy. *Am J Med* 2005;118:163S.
63. Mueck AO, Seeger H. Effect of hormone therapy on BP in normotensive and hypertensive postmenopausal women. *Maturitas* 2004;49:189.
64. Prior JC et al. Medroxyprogesterone and conjugated oestrogen are equivalent for hot flushes: a 1-year randomized double-blind trial following premenopausal ovariectomy. *Clinical Science* 2007;112:517.
65. Bertelli G et al. Intramuscular depot medroxyprogesterone versus oral megestrol for the control of postmenopausal hot flashes in breast cancer patients: a randomized study. *Ann Oncol* 2002;13:883.
66. Liu JH. Therapeutic effects of progestins, androgens, and tibolone for menopausal symptoms. *Am J Med* 2005;118:88S.
67. North American Menopause Society. The role of testosterone therapy in postmenopausal women: position statement of the North American Menopause Society. *Menopause* 2005;12:497.
68. Gordon PR et al. Sertraline to treat hot flashes: a randomized controlled, double-blind, crossover trial in a general population. *Menopause* 2006;13:568.
69. Kimmick GG et al. Randomized, double-blind, placebo-controlled, crossover study of sertraline (Zoloft) for the treatment of hot flashes in women with early stage breast cancer taking tamoxifen. *Breast J* 2006;12:114.
70. Nelson HD et al. Nonhormonal therapies for menopausal hot flashes: systematic review and meta-analysis. *JAMA* 2006;295:2057.
71. Kalay AE et al. Efficacy of citalopram on climacteric symptoms. *Menopause* 2007;14:223.
72. Perez DG et al. Pilot evaluation of mirtazapine for the treatment of hot flashes. *J Support Oncol* 2004;2:50.
73. Barton DL et al. Pilot evaluation of citalopram for the relief of hot flashes. *J Support Oncol* 2003;1:47.
74. Krebs EE et al. Phytoestrogens for treatment of menopausal symptoms: a systematic review. *Obstet Gynecol* 2004;104:824.
75. Howes LG et al. Isoflavone therapy for menopausal flushes: a systematic review and meta-analysis. *Maturitas* 2006;55:203.
76. Unfer V et al. Endometrial effects of long-term treatment with phytoestrogens: a randomized, double-blind, placebo-controlled study. *Fertil Steril* 2004;82:145.
77. Geller SE, Studee L. Botanical and dietary supplements for mood and anxiety in menopause. *Menopause* 2007;14:1.
78. Osmers R et al. Efficacy and safety of isopropanolic black cohosh extract for climacteric symptoms. *Obstet Gynecol* 2005;105:1074.
79. Frei-Kleiner S et al. Cimicifuga racemosa dried ethanolic extract in menopausal disorders: a double-blind placebo-controlled clinical trial. *Maturitas* 2005;51:397.
80. Pockaj BA et al. Phase III double-blind, randomized, placebo-controlled crossover trial of black cohosh in the management of hot flashes: NCCTG Trial N01CC. *J Clin Oncol* 22006;24:2836.
81. Newton KM et al. Treatment of vasomotor symptoms of menopause with black cohosh, multibotanicals, soy, hormone therapy, or placebo. *Ann Intern Med* 2006;145:869.
82. McKee J, Warber SL. Integrative therapies for menopause. *South Med J* 2005;98:319.
83. Komesaroff PA et al. Effects of wild yam extract on menopausal symptoms, lipids and sex hormones in healthy menopausal women. *Climacteric* 2001;4:144.
84. Speroff L. Alternative therapies for postmenopausal women. *Int J Fertil* 2005;50:101.
85. North American Menopause Society. The role of local vaginal estrogen for treatment of vaginal atrophy in postmenopausal women: 2007 position statement of the North American Menopause Society. *Menopause* 2007;14:357.
86. Van Voorhis BJ. Genitourinary symptoms in the menopause transition. *Am J Med* 2005;118:47S.
87. Crandall C. Vaginal estrogen preparations: a review of safety and efficacy for vaginal atrophy. *J Womens Health* 2002;11:857.
88. Bygdeman M, Swahn ML. Replens versus dienoestrol cream in the symptomatic treatment of vaginal atrophy in postmenopausal women. *Maturitas* 1996;23:259.
89. Robinson D, Cardozo LD. The role of estrogens in female lower urinary tract dysfunction. *Urology* 2003;62:45.
90. Waetjen LE, Dwyer PL. Estrogen therapy and urinary incontinence: what is the evidence and what do we tell our patients? *Int Urogynecol J* 2006;17:541.
91. Hendrix SL et al. Effects of estrogen with and without progestin on urinary incontinence. *JAMA* 2005;293:935.
92. Grodstein F et al. Postmenopausal hormone therapy and risk of developing urinary incontinence. *Obstet Gynecol* 2004;103:254.
93. Hextall A. Oestrogens and lower urinary tract function. *Maturitas* 2000;36:83.
94. Mitchell JL et al. Postmenopausal hormone therapy: a concise guide to therapeutic uses, formulations, risks, and alternatives. *Prim Care Clin Office Pract* 2003;30:671.

SECTION TWELVE

ENDOCRINE DISORDERS

Mary Anne Koda-Kimble

SECTION EDITOR

CHAPTER 49

Thyroid Disorders

Betty J. Dong

OVERVIEW

Thyroid disease is common, affecting approximately 5% to 15% of the general population. Females are three to four times more likely than males to develop any type of thyroid disease. The typical thyroid disorders emphasized in this chapter are hypothyroidism, hyperthyroidism, and nodular disease. Thyroid cancer is discussed briefly. The reader is referred to standard medical textbooks for more detailed medical and diagnostic information.

Triiodothyronine (T_3) and thyroxine (T_4) are the two biologically active thyroid hormones produced by the thyroid gland in response to hormones released by the pituitary and hypothalamus. The hypothalamic thyrotropin-releasing hormone (TRH) stimulates release of thyrotropin (i.e., thyroid-stimulating hormone [TSH]) from the pituitary in response to low circulating levels of thyroid hormone. TSH in turn promotes hormone synthesis and release by increasing thyroid activity. When sufficient synthesis has occurred, high circulating thyroid hormone levels block further production by inhibiting TSH release. The intrapituitary deiodination of T_4 to T_3 also plays a critical role in the inhibition of TSH secretion. As the serum concentrations of thyroid hormone decrease, the hypothalamic-pituitary centers again become responsive by releasing TRH and TSH.

T_3 is four times more potent than T_4, but its serum concentration is lower. T_4 is the major circulating hormone secreted by the thyroid. In contrast, about 80% of the total daily T_3 production results from the peripheral conversion of T_4 to T_3 through deiodination of T_4. T_4 has intrinsic biological activity and does not function solely as a prohormone. Approximately 35% to 40% of secreted T_4 is converted peripherally to T_3; another 45% of secreted T_4 undergoes peripheral conversion to inactive reverse T_3 (rT_3). Certain drugs and diseases can modify the conversion rate of T_4 to T_3 and decrease the serum T_3 levels (Table 49-1; see question 2).

T_3 and T_4 exist in the circulation in free (active) and protein-bound (inactive) forms. About 99.97% of circulating T_4 is bound: 70% to thyroxine-binding globulin (TBG), 15% to thyroxine-binding prealbumin (TBPA), and the rest to albumin. Only 0.03% exists as the free form. This affinity for plasma proteins accounts for T_4's slow metabolic degradation and long half-life ($t_{1/2}$) of 7 days. In contrast, T_3 is considerably less strongly bound to plasma proteins (99.7%); about 0.3% exists as free hormone. The lower protein-binding affinity of T_3 accounts for its threefold greater metabolic potency and its shorter half-life of 1.5 days.

Hypothyroidism is a clinical syndrome that results from a deficiency of thyroid hormone. The prevalence of hypothyroidism is 1.4% to 2% in females and 0.1% to 0.2% in males. The incidence increases in persons older than 60 years to 6% of women and 2.5% of men. Hypothyroidism can be caused by either primary (thyroid gland) or secondary (hypothalamic-pituitary) malfunction. Primary hypothyroidism is more common than secondary causes.

Table 49-1 Factors That Can Significantly Alter Thyroid Function Tests in Euthyroid Patients

↑ TBG Binding Capacity	*Drugs/Situations*
↑ TT_4	Estrogens,[27,28] tamoxifen,[30] raloxifene[29]
↑ TT_3	Oral contraceptives[7]
Normal TSH	Heroin[26]
Normal FT_4I, FT_4	Methadone maintenance[26]
Normal FT_3I, FT_3	Genetic ↑ in TBG
	Clofibrate
	Active hepatitis[1]
↓ TBG Binding Capacity/Displacement T_4 From Binding Sites	
↓ TT_4	Androgens[7]
↓ TT_3	Salicylates,[7,18,19] disalcid,[19] salsalate[19]
Normal TSH	High-dose furosemide
Normal FT_4I, FT_4	↓ TBG synthesis-cirrhosis/hepatic failure
Normal FT_3I, FT_3	Nephrotic syndrome[1,7]
	Danazol[1,7]
	Glucocorticoids[1,7]
↓ Peripheral $T_4 \rightarrow T_3$ Conversion	
↓ TT_3	PTU
Normal TT_4	Propranolol[174]
Normal FT_4I, FT_4	Glucocorticoids[3,7]
Normal TSH	
↓ Pituitary and Peripheral $T_4 \rightarrow T_3$	
↓ TT_3	Iodinated contrast media (e.g., ipodate)[161–165]
↑ TT_4	Amiodarone[31–33]
↑ TSH (transient)	Euthyroid sick syndrome[8–10]
↑ FT_4I	
↑ T_4 Clearance by Enzyme Induction/↑ Fecal Loss[a]	
↓ TT_4	Phenytoin[20,21]
↓ FT_4I	Phenobarbital[20]
Normal or ↓ FT_4	Carbamazepine[20–25]
Normal or ↓ TT_3	Cholestyramine, colestipol[98]
Normal or ↑ TSH	Rifampin[20]
	Bexarotene[92]
↓ TSH Secretion	
	Dopamine[1,7] dobutamine[34]
	Levodopa[7] cabergoline[35]
	Glucocorticoids[3,7]
	Bromocriptine[3,7]
	Octreotide[2]
	Metformin[36]
	Bexarotene[188]
↑ TSH Secretion	
	Metoclopramide[1,3,7]
	Domperidone[1,3,7]

[a] Can also cause hypothyroidism in patients receiving levothyroxine therapy.

FT_3, free triiodothyronine; FT_4, free thyroxine; FT_3I, free triiodothyronine index; FT_4I, free thyroxine index; PTU, propylthiouracil; T_3, triiodothyronine; T_4, thyroxine; TBG, thyroxine-binding globulin; TSH, thyroid-stimulating hormone; TT_3, total triiodothyronine; TT_4, total thyroxine.

Hashimoto's thyroiditis, an autoimmune disorder, is the most common cause of primary hypothyroidism and appears to have a strong genetic predisposition. The pathogenesis of Hashimoto's thyroiditis results from an impaired immune surveillance, causing dysfunction of normal "suppressor" T lymphocytes and excessive production of thyroid antibodies by plasma cells (differentiated B lymphocytes). The destruction of thyroid cells by circulating thyroid antibodies produces an underlying defect or block in the intrathyroidal, organo-binding of iodide. As a result, inactive hormones or insufficient amounts of active hormones are synthesized, and this eventually produces hypothyroidism. However, the clinical presentation of Hashimoto's thyroiditis can be variable, depending on the time of diagnosis. Although the typical presentation is hypothyroidism and goiter (thyroid gland enlargement), patients can present with hypothyroidism and no goiter, with euthyroidism and goiter, or rarely (<5%) with hyperthyroidism (Hashi-toxicosis).

Hashimoto's thyroiditis might be related to Graves' disease, a common cause of hyperthyroidism. Both diseases share similar clinical features: positive antibody titers, goiter with lymphocytic infiltration of the gland, familial tendency, and predilection for women. Both diseases can coexist in the same gland. Thyrotoxicosis can precede the onset of Hashimoto's hypothyroidism, and the end result of Graves' hyperthyroidism is often hypothyroidism. These common clinical features suggest that Graves' disease and Hashimoto's thyroiditis might be the same disease manifesting in different ways.

Other common causes of hypothyroidism are presented in Table 49-2 and include iatrogenic destruction of the gland after radioiodine therapy or surgery and hypothyroidism secondary to nontoxic multinodular goiter. Drug-induced hypothyroidism (e.g., iodides, amiodarone, lithium, interferon-α) occurs in susceptible persons (i.e., Hashimoto's thyroiditis) with a preexisting thyroid abnormality.

The typical symptoms of hypothyroidism include weight gain, fatigue, sluggishness, cold intolerance, constipation, heavy menstrual periods, and muscle aches. A goiter might or might not be present. Patients with end-stage hypothyroidism, or myxedema coma, can also present with hypothermia, confusion, stupor or coma, carbon dioxide retention, hypoglycemia, hyponatremia, and ileus. Symptoms of "slowing down" would be expected because thyroid hormone is essential for the function and maintenance of all body systems and metabolic processes. In general, the more severe the degree of hypothyroidism, the greater the number of clinical findings. The exception is the older patient with hypothyroidism, who often presents with minimal or atypical symptoms (e.g., weight loss, deafness, tinnitus, carpal tunnel syndrome). Patients with mild and subclinical hypothyroidism might also have few or no symptoms. Laboratory findings that are diagnostic for overt hypothyroidism include elevated TSH and low free thyroxine (FT_4) levels; those for subclinical or early hypothyroidism are elevated TSH and normal FT_4 levels. The common clinical symptoms, physical findings, and laboratory abnormalities of overt hypothyroidism are summarized in Table 49-3.

Table 49-2 Causes of Hypothyroidism

Nongoitrous (No Gland Enlargement)

Primary Hypothyroidism (Dysfunction of the Gland)
- Idiopathic atrophy
- Iatrogenic destruction of thyroid
- Surgery
- Radioactive iodine therapy
- X-ray therapy
- Postinflammatory thyroiditis
- Cretinism (congenital hypothyroidism)

Secondary Hypothyroidism
- Deficiency of TSH due to pituitary dysfunction
- Deficiency of TRH due to hypothalamic dysfunction

Goitrous Hypothyroidism (Enlargement of Thyroid Gland)
- Dyshormonogenesis: defect in hormone synthesis, transport, or action
- Hashimoto's thyroiditis
- Congenital cretinism: maternally induced
- Iodide deficiency
- Natural goitrogens: rutabagas, turnips, cabbage

Drug-Induced
- Aminoglutethimide[7]
- Amiodarone[31–33]
- Bexarotene[92,188]
- Ethionamide[237]
- Iodides and iodide-containing preparations[143]
- Rifampin[91]
- Sunitinib[238,239]
- Interleukin[240,241]
- Interferon-α[226–229]
- Lithium[219–221]
- Thiocyanates, phenylbutazone, sulfonylureas[7]

TRH, thyrotropin-releasing hormone; TSH, thyroid-stimulating hormone.

Levothyroxine (L-thyroxine) is the preferred thyroid replacement preparation. Several brand name and less costly generic preparations are available, and they are interchangeable in most patients. The signs and symptoms of

Table 49-3 Clinical and Laboratory Findings of Primary Hypothyroidism

Symptoms	*Physical Findings*	*Laboratory*
General: weakness, tiredness, lethargy, fatigue	Thin brittle nails	↓ TT_4
Cold intolerance	Thinning of skin	↓ FT_4I
Headache	Pallor	↓ FT_4
Loss of taste/smell	Puffiness of face, eyelids	↓ TT_3
Deafness	Yellowing of skin	↓ FT_3I
Hoarseness	Thinning of outer eyebrows	↑ TSH
No sweating	Thickening of tongue	Positive antibodies (in Hashimoto's)
Modest weight gain	Peripheral edema	↑ Cholesterol
Muscle cramps, aches, pains	Pleural/peritoneal/pericardial effusions	↑ CPK
Dyspnea	↓ DTRs	↓ Na
Slow speech	"Myxedema heart"	↑ LDH
Constipation	Bradycardia (↓ HR)	↑ AST
Menorrhagia	Hypertension	↓ Hct/Hgb
Galactorrhea	Goiter (primary hypothyroidism)	

AST, aspartate aminotransferase; CPK, creatinine phosphokinase; DTRs, deep tendon reflexes; Hct, hematocrit; Hgb, hemoglobin; HR, heart rate; LDH, lactate dehydrogenase; Na, sodium; FT_3I, free triiodothyronine index; FT_4I, free thyroxine index; FT_4, free thyroxine; TSH, thyroid-stimulating hormone; TT_3, total triiodothyronine; TT_4, total thyroxine.

Table 49-4 Treatment of Hypothyroidism

Patient Type/Complications	*Dose (L-thyroxine)*	*Comment*
Uncomplicated adult	1.6–1.7 mcg/kg/day; 100–125 mcg/day average replacement dose; usual increment 25 mcg q6–8wk	*Onset of action:* 2–3 wk; *max effect:* 4–6 wk. Reversal of skin and hair changes may take several months. An FT_4 or FT_4I and TSH should be checked 6–8 wk after initiation of therapy because T_4 has a half-life of 7 days and three to four half-lives are needed to achieve steady state. Levels obtained before steady state can be very misleading. Because 80% is bioavailable, adjust IV doses downward. Small changes can be made by varying dose schedule (e.g., 150 mcg daily except Sunday).
Elderly	≤1.6 mcg/kg/day (50–100 mcg/day)	Initiate T_4 cautiously. Elderly may require less than younger patients. Sensitive to small dose changes. A few patients older than 60 yr require ≤50 mcg/day.
Cardiovascular disease (angina, CAD)	Start with 12.5–25 mcg/day. ↑ by 12.5–25 mcg/day q2–6wk as tolerated	These patients are very sensitive to cardiovascular effects of T_4. Even subtherapeutic doses can precipitate severe angina, MI, or death. Replace thyroid deficit slowly, cautiously, and sometimes even suboptimally.
Long-standing hypothyroidism (>1 yr)	Dose slowly. Start with 25 mcg/day. ↑ by 25 mcg/day q4–6wk as tolerated	Sensitive to cardiovascular effects of T_4. Steady state may be delayed because of ↓ clearance of T_4.[a] Correct replacement dose is a compromise between prevention of myxedema and avoidance of cardiac toxicity.
Pregnant	Most will require 45% ↑ in dose to ensure euthyroidism	Evaluate TSH, TT_4, and FT_4I. *Goal:* normal TSH and TT_4/FT_4I in upper normal range to prevent fetal hypothyroidism.
Pediatric (0–3 mo)	10–15 mcg/kg/day	Hypothyroid infants can exhibit skin mottling, lethargy, hoarseness, poor feeding, delayed development, constipation, large tongue, neonatal jaundice, piglike facies, choking, respiratory difficulties, and delayed skeletal maturation (epiphyseal dysgenesis). The serum T_4 should be increased rapidly to minimize impaired cognitive function. In the healthy term infant, 37.5–50 mcg/day of T_4 is appropriate. Dose decreases with age (Table 49-9).

[a] In severely myxedematous patients, steady state may require ≥6 months. In patients who are clinically euthyroid but have ↑ TT_4 and FTI, use TT_3 and TSH as guide to dose adjustments.

CAD, coronary artery disease; FT_4, free thyroxine; FT_4I, free thyroxine index; IV, intravenous; MI, myocardial infarction; q, every; QD, every day; T_4, thyroxine; TSH, thyroid-stimulating hormone; TT_4, total thyroxine.

hypothyroidism can be reversed easily in most patients by the administration of L-thyroxine on an empty stomach at average oral replacement dosages of 1.6 to 1.7 mcg/kg/day. Exceptions include older patients, patients with severe and long-standing hypothyroidism, and patients with cardiac disease, in whom administration of full replacement doses might cause cardiac toxicity (Table 49-4). In such patients, minute T_4 doses should be started initially and the dosage titrated upward as tolerated; complete reversal of hypothyroidism might not be indicated or possible. In myxedema coma, intravenous (IV) therapy with large initial doses of L-thyroxine (e.g., 400 mcg) is necessary to increase the active free hormone level by saturating the empty thyroid-binding sites and to prevent the 60% to 70% mortality rate. In subclinical hypothyroidism, it is controversial whether T_4 replacement therapy is beneficial. There is no justification for treating patients with hypothyroid symptoms and normal laboratory findings with T_4.

The goal of therapy is to reverse the signs and symptoms of hypothyroidism and normalize the TSH and FT_4 levels. Some improvement of hypothyroid symptoms is often evident within 2 to 3 weeks of starting T_4 therapy. Overreplacement of L-thyroxine (manifested by below-normal or suppressed serum concentrations of TSH) is associated with osteoporosis and cardiac changes. The optimal T_4 replacement dosage must be administered for ~6 to 8 weeks before steady-state levels are reached. Evaluation of thyroid function tests before this time is misleading. Once a euthyroid state is attained, laboratory tests can be monitored every 3 to 6 months for the first year and then yearly thereafter. Medications that interfere with T_4 absorption (e.g., iron, aluminum-containing products, some calcium preparations, cholesterol resin and phosphate binders, raloxifene) should not be coadministered with T_4.

Hyperthyroidism or thyrotoxicosis is the hypermetabolic syndrome that occurs when the production of thyroid hormone is excessive. Hyperthyroidism affects about 2% of females and about 0.1% of males. The prevalence of hyperthyroidism in older patients varies between 0.5% and 2.3% but accounts for 10% to 15% of all thyrotoxic patients, depending on the population studied.

Graves' disease is the most common cause of hyperthyroidism. Toxic autonomous nodular goiters, both multi- and uninodular, account for a large proportion of the remaining

Table 49-5 Causes of Hyperthyroidism

Graves' disease (toxic diffuse goiter); may be caused by polymorphisms in the TSH receptor[4]
Toxic uninodular goiter (Plummer's disease)
Toxic multinodular goiter
Nodular goiter with hyperthyroidism caused by exogenous iodine (Jod-Basedow)
Exogenous thyroid excess through self-administration (factitious hyperthyroidism)
Tumors (thyroid adenoma, follicular carcinoma, thyrotropin-secreting tumor of the pituitary, and hydatidiform mole with secretion of a thyroid-stimulating substance)
Drug induced (iodides,[142] amiodarone,[31–33] interleukin,[7,240] interferon-α,[226,229] lithium[223,224])

Table 49-6 Clinical and Laboratory Findings of Hyperthyroidism

Symptoms

Heat intolerance
Weight loss common, or weight gain caused by ↑ appetite
Palpitations
Pedal edema
Diarrhea/frequent bowel movements
Amenorrhea/light menses
Tremor
Weakness, fatigue
Nervousness, irritability, insomnia

Physical Findings

Thinning of hair (fine)
Proptosis, lid lag, lid retraction, stare, chemosis, conjunctivitis, periorbital edema, loss of extraocular movements
Diffusely enlarged goiter, bruits, thrills
Wide pulse pressure
Pretibial myxedema
Plummer's nails[a]
Flushed, moist skin
Palmar erythema
Brisk DTRs

Laboratory Findings

↑ TT_4
↑ TT_3
↑ FT_4I/FT_4
↑ FT_3I/FT_3
Suppressed TSH
⊕ TRAb
⊕ ATgA
⊕ TPO
RAIU >50%
↓ Cholesterol
↑ Alkaline phosphatase
↑ Calcium
↑ AST

[a]The fingernail separates from its matrix, but only one or two nails are generally affected.

AST, aspartate aminotransferase; ATgA, antihydroglobulin antibody; DTRs, deep tendon reflexes; FT_3, free triiodothyronine; FT_4, free thyroxine; FT_3I, free triiodothyronine index; FT_4I, free thyroxine index; RAIU, radioactive iodine uptake; TPO, thyroperoxidase antibody; TRAb, thyroid-receptor antibodies; TSH, thyroid-stimulating hormone; TT_3, total triiodothyronine; TT_4, total thyroxine.

causes. Other causes of hyperthyroidism, including iatrogenic ones, are outlined in Table 49-5. Graves' disease is an autoimmune disorder characterized by one or more of the following features: hyperthyroidism, diffuse goiter, ophthalmopathy (exophthalmos), dermopathy (pretibial myxedema), and acropachy (thickening of fingers or toes). The production of excessive quantities of thyroid hormone is attributed to a circulating IgG or thyroid receptor antibody (TRAb), which has a TSH-like ability to stimulate hormone synthesis. The abnormal production of TRAb by plasma cells (differentiated B lymphocytes) results from a deficiency of suppressor T-cell lymphocytes. The peak incidence of Graves' disease occurs in the third or fourth decade of life, the duration of the disease is unknown, and its clinical course is characterized by remission and relapse.

The classic symptoms of hyperthyroidism, summarized in Table 49-6, mimic a hypermetabolic state and include nervousness, heat intolerance, palpitations, weight loss despite increased appetite, insomnia, proximal muscle weakness, frequent bowel movements, amenorrhea, and emotional lability. Hyperthyroid symptoms can be present for 3 to 12 months before the diagnosis is made. The typical symptoms are often absent in the older patient, producing a masked or "apathetic" picture. Because the clinical presentation of hyperthyroidism in the older patient is atypical, occult hyperthyroidism always must be considered, especially in patients with new or worsening cardiac findings (e.g., atrial fibrillation). Untreated hyperthyroidism can progress to thyroid storm, a life-threatening form of hyperthyroidism characterized by "exaggerated" symptoms of thyrotoxicosis and the acute onset of high fever (sine qua non). The diagnosis of hyperthyroidism is confirmed by high serum concentrations of FT_4 and/or an undetectable TSH level. Positive thyroid antibodies confirm an autoimmune origin for the hyperthyroidism (e.g., Graves' disease).

The primary treatment options for hyperthyroidism are antithyroid drugs (thioamides), radioiodine, and surgery. All three modalities are effective, and the treatment of choice is influenced by the etiology of the hyperthyroidism, the size of the goiter, the presence of ophthalmopathy, comorbid conditions (e.g., angina), likelihood of pregnancy, patient age, patient preference, and physician bias. Older patients and those with coexisting cardiac disease, ophthalmopathy, and hyperthyroidism secondary to a toxic multinodular goiter are treated best with radioactive iodine (RAI). Surgery is preferable if obstructive symptoms are present or concomitant malignancy is suspected. Pregnant patients can be managed with thioamides or surgery in the second trimester; RAI is absolutely contraindicated.

The thioamides are used as primary therapy for hyperthyroidism and as adjunctive short-term therapy to produce euthyroidism before surgery or RAI. The thioamides (e.g., methimazole [Tapazole], propylthiouracil [PTU]) primarily prevent hormone synthesis but do not affect existing stores of thyroid hormone. Therefore, hyperthyroid symptoms will continue for 4 to 6 weeks after beginning thioamide therapy, and initial treatment with β-blockers or iodides is often required for symptomatic relief. The onset of action of PTU is more rapid than methimazole because PTU has an additional mechanism of action, which is to inhibit the peripheral conversion of T_4 to T_3. Therefore, PTU is the thioamide of choice for thyroid storm. PTU is also preferred during pregnancy because congenital defects have been reported with methimazole. Although both drugs are secreted in breast milk, no adverse effects have been reported in the exposed infants. Otherwise, methimazole is preferred over PTU to enhance adherence; it can be administered once daily, whereas PTU must be given two or three times daily. The duration of treatment is empiric, and thioamides typically are prescribed for 12 to 18 months in hopes of long-term spontaneous remission once the drug is discontinued. Although thioamides maintain euthyroidism, they do not change the natural course of the disease, and the likelihood of spontaneous remission, once treatment is discontinued, is about 50%. The expectation that the combination of thioamide and T_4 therapy might increase the likelihood of remission has been disappointing. The major adverse effects from thioamides include skin rash, gastrointestinal (GI) complaints, agranulocytosis, and hepatitis. Cross-sensitivity between the thioamides is not complete, and the alternative drug can be used if rash or GI complaints do not resolve. This is not true for agranulocytosis, and the alternative agent is not recommended.

Nodular goiters, both multi- and uninodular, are common thyroid problems. The estimated prevalence is 4% to 5% of the adult population. The origin of thyroid nodules is unknown, although TSH stimulation, iodine deficiency, goitrogens (e.g., iodides, lithium, amiodarone), and radiation exposure are contributory. The nodular goiter is usually found on routine physical examination in asymptomatic and euthyroid patients. However, patients can present with hyperthyroidism caused by autonomous functioning "hot" nodules, overt hypothyroidism, or obstructive symptoms of dysphagia and respiratory difficulty. Thyroid function tests, including TSH and FT_4 levels, and antibodies should be obtained. Additional information can be obtained from radioactive iodine uptake (RAIU), ultrasound, fine-needle aspiration (FNA), or magnetic resonance imaging.

Treatment options include surgery, RAI, or thyroid replacement therapy if necessary to correct the hypothyroidism. All goitrogens should be removed if possible. L-thyroxine suppression therapy is no longer recommended since the dangers from supraphysiologic dosages of T_4 (e.g., osteoporosis and the potential for cardiac arrhythmias) exceed the benefits of therapy.

Malignancy must be considered if there is recent growth in a "cold" single or dominant nodule, a firm nodule clinically suspicious for cancer on a physical examination, a history of thyroid irradiation, or a strong family history of medullary thyroid carcinoma. A FNA of the thyroid nodule can document an underlying malignancy. The risk of malignancy in a toxic multinodular goiter is small, and definitive treatment with RAI is usually required to manage any hyperthyroid symptoms. Surgery is indicated if malignancy is highly suspected or if any obstructive or respiratory symptoms are present.

Following a total thyroidectomy for thyroid cancer, RAI ablation is usually given to remove any remaining thyroid tissue. This dosage is higher than the dosage required for treatment of Graves' disease. A yearly evaluation for detection of recurrence of some thyroid cancers requires the patient to be off T_4 for 4 to 6 weeks so that a repeat radioactive uptake and scan can be completed. An elevated TSH level is also necessary to allow thyroglobulin levels, a tumor marker, to rise if any malignant tissue is present. Recurrence of the thyroid cancer is likely if there are positive findings on the scan or an elevation in thyroglobulin levels. The administration of recombinant human TSH (Thyrogen) may improve quality of life because comparable elevations in TSH occur without stopping L-thyroxine therapy, reducing the duration of hypothyroidism.

THYROID FUNCTION TESTS

The principal laboratory tests recommended in the initial evaluation of thyroid disorders are the TSH and the FT_4 levels.[1–3] Positive thyroid antibodies indicate an autoimmune thyroid etiology. Adjuncts to the previous tests include the total T_3 (TT_3), free T_3 (FT_3) or FT_3 index (FT_3I), RAIU and scan, TRAb, ultrasound, and FNA biopsy (Table 49-7).

Measurements of Free and Total Serum Hormone Levels

Free Thyroxine, Free Thyroxine Index, Free Triiodothyronine, and Free Triiodothyronine Index

The FT_4 and FT_3 are the most reliable tests for the evaluation of hormone concentrations, especially when thyroid hormone binding abnormalities exist. The FT_3 is most useful in hyperthyroidism but can be normal or low in hypothyroidism. If a direct measure of the free hormone levels are not available, the estimated free hormone indices (FT_4I, FT_3I) can provide comparable information. However, these indices do not correct for changes observed in patients with "euthyroid sick" nonthyroidal illnesses whose TBG binding affinity is altered. In these circumstances, the FT_4 and FT_3 are preferable.

Total Thyroxine and Total Triiodothyronine

The total thyroxine (TT_4) and total triiodothyronine (TT_3) measure both free and bound (total) serum T_4 and T_3. Because the bound fraction is the major fraction measured, situations that change the hormone's affinity for TBG or the TBG level will influence the results. For example, falsely elevated levels of TT_4 and TT_3 are common in the euthyroid pregnant woman (see question 4). In addition, the TT_3 is often low in older patients and in many acute and chronic nonthyroidal illnesses because the peripheral conversion of T_4 to T_3 is decreased (see questions 2 and 3). Therefore, careful interpretation of these tests is necessary in situations that alter thyroid hormone binding, TBG levels, or T_4 to T_3 conversion (Table 49-1). The TT_3 is particularly helpful in detecting early relapse of Graves' disease and in confirming the diagnosis of hyperthyroidism despite normal TT_4 levels. The TT_3 is not a good indicator of hypothyroidism because TT_3 can be normal. Measurement of only the total hormone levels is less reliable than either the free or estimated free hormone levels when alterations in thyroid-binding globulin or nonthyroidal illnesses exist.

Tests of the Hypothalamic-Pituitary-Thyroid Axis

Thyroid-Stimulating Hormone

The serum TSH or thyrotropin is the most sensitive test to evaluate thyroid function.[1–3] TSH, secreted by the pituitary, is elevated in early or subclinical hypothyroidism (when thyroid hormone levels appear normal) and when thyroid hormone replacement therapy is inadequate. TSH can be abnormal even if the FT_4 remains within the normal range because the TSH is specific for each person's physiological set point. Polymorphisms in the TSH receptor contribute to this interindividual variability.[4] Consequently, low normal free hormone levels can stimulate the pituitary to synthesize increased amounts of TSH. This test cannot be used to differentiate between primary hypothyroidism (thyroid failure), which is characterized by elevated TSH levels and secondary (pituitary or hypothalamus failure) hypothyroidism. In the latter instance, TSH levels may be low or normal. However, the TSH assay can quantitate the upper and lower limits of normal so that a suppressed TSH level is highly suggestive of hyperthyroidism or exogenous thyroid overreplacement. Of note, TSH is not entirely specific for thyroid disease because abnormal levels are observed in euthyroid patients with nonthyroidal illnesses and in patients receiving drugs that can interfere with TSH secretion. TSH secretion is increased at bedtime and is affected by lack of sleep and exercise.[5] TSH secretion is suppressed physiologically by dopamine, which antagonizes the stimulatory effects of TRH. Therefore, both dopaminergic agonists and antagonists can alter TSH secretion (see Question 5). Whether the upper

Table 49-7 Common Thyroid Function Tests

Tests	Measures	Normals[a]	Assay Interference	Comments
Measurement of Circulating Hormone Levels				
FT_4	Direct measurement of free thyroxine	0.7–1.9 ng/dL (9–24 pmol/L)	No interference by alterations in TBG	Most accurate determination of FT_4 levels; might be higher than normal in patients on thyroxine replacement
FT_4I	Calculated free thyroxine index	*T_4 uptake method*: 6.5–12.5 *$TT_4 \times RT_3U$ method*: 1.3–4.2	Euthyroid sick syndrome (see question 2)	Estimates direct FT_4 measurement; compensates for alterations in TBG
TT_4	Total free and bound T_4	5–12 mcg/dL (64–154 mmol/L)	Alterations in TBG (Table 49-1)	Specific and sensitive test if no alterations in TBG
TT_3	Total free and bound T_3	70–132 ng/dL (1.1–2 nmol/L)	Alterations in TBG levels; T_4 to T_3 (Table 49-1). Euthyroid sick syndrome (see question 2)	Useful in detecting early, relapsing, and T_3 toxicosis. Not useful in evaluation of hypothyroidism
FT_3	Direct measurement of free T_3	0.2–0.42 ng/dL (3.5–6.5 pmol/L)	No interference by alterations in TBG	Most accurate determination of FT_4 levels; might be lower than normal in patients on thyroxine replacement
FT_3I	Calculated free T_3 index	17.5–46	Euthyroid sick syndrome (see question 2)	Estimates direct FT_3 measurement; compensates for alterations in TBG
Tests of Thyroid Gland Function				
RAIU	Gland's use of iodine after trace dose of either ^{123}I or ^{131}I	5%–35%	False decrease with excess iodide intake; false elevation with iodide deficiency	Useful in hyperthyroidism to determine RAI dose in Graves'; does not provide information regarding hormone synthesis
Scan	Gland size, shape, and tissue activity after ^{123}I or ^{99m}Tc	—	^{154}I scan blocked by antithyroid/thyroid medications	Useful in nodular disease to detect "cold" or "hot" areas
Test of Hypothalamic-Pituitary-Thyroid Axis				
TSH	Pituitary TSH level	0.5–5 μU/mL	Dopamine, glucocorticoids, metoclopramide, thyroid hormone, amiodarone, metformin (Table 49-1)	Most sensitive index for hyperthyroidism, hypothyroidism, and replacement therapy
Tests of Autoimmunity				
ATgA	Antibodies to thyroglobulin	<1 IU/mL	Nonthyroidal autoimmune disorders	Present in autoimmune thyroid disease; undetectable during remission
TPO	Thyroperoxidase antibodies	<1 IU/mL	Nonthyroidal autoimmune disorders	More sensitive of the two antibodies; titers detectable even after remission
TRAb	Thyroid receptor stimulating antibody	<125%	—	Confirms Graves' disease; detects risk of neonatal Graves'
Miscellaneous				
Thyroglobulin	Colloid protein of normal thyroid gland	<56 ng/mL	Goiters; inflammatory thyroid disease	Marker for recurrent thyroid cancer or metastases in thyroidectomized patients

[a] At University of California laboratories.

ATgA, antibodies to thyroglobulin; FT_3, free triiodothyronine; FT_4, free thyroxine; FT_3I, free triiodothyronine index; FT_4I, free thyroxine index; RAI, radioactive iodine; RAIU, radioactive iodine uptake; T_3, triiodothyronine; T_4, thyroxine; TBG, thyroxine-binding globulin; TPO, thyroperoxidase antibodies; TRAb, thyroid-receptor antibodies; TSH, thyroid-stimulating hormone; TT_3, total triiodothyronine; TT_4, total thyroxine.

limits of normal for TSH should be lowered to 2.5 μU/mL is controversial.[4,5]

Tests of Gland Function

Radioactive Iodine Uptake

RAIU, a measure of iodine utilization by the gland, is an indirect measure of hormone synthesis. It is elevated in hyperthyroidism and in early hypothyroidism when the failing gland is trying to increase hormone synthesis. A low or undetectable RAIU occurs in hypothyroidism, thyrotoxicosis factitia, and subacute thyroiditis. Typically, RAIU is used to calculate the dose of RAI therapy for treatment of Graves' disease and to determine the activity of one or several nodules in a gland. The RAIU is not necessary to diagnose classic Graves' disease or hypothyroidism.

A tracer dose of ^{131}I is administered, and the radioactivity of the gland is measured at 5 and 24 hours after ingestion. It is necessary to measure both the 5- and 24-hour RAIU so that patients with rapid turnover of iodine will not be missed. In some hyperthyroid patients, the 5-hour uptake is elevated, but the 24-hour uptake can fall to normal or subnormal levels.

The normal range of the RAIU (Table 49-7) is affected by any condition that alters iodine intake. Iodine depletion caused by rigorous diuretic therapy or an iodine-deficient diet increases uptake because of replenishment of depleted total iodide pools. Conversely, dilution of ^{131}I with exogenous iodide sources (e.g., contrast dyes) decreases RAIU.

Imaging Studies

THYROID SCAN

A scan of the gland is performed simultaneously with the RAIU or after ingestion of technetium (^{99m}Tc) pertechnetate. The scan provides information concerning gland size and shape, and identifies hypermetabolic ("hot") and hypometabolic ("cold") areas. The possibility of carcinoma must be considered if cold areas are present. A scan should be considered in the patient with nodular thyroid disease.

Thyroid Ultrasound

A thyroid ultrasound can provide information about gland size and number of clinically palpable or nonpalpable nodules or cysts in the thyroid gland.

Tests of Autoimmunity

Thyroperoxidase and Antithyroglobulin Antibodies

Thyroperoxidase (TPO) and antithyroglobulin (ATgA) antibodies to the thyroid gland indicate an autoimmune process, although the nature of the problem is undetermined.[1,3] About 60% to 70% of patients with Graves' disease and 95% of patients with Hashimoto's thyroiditis have positive antibodies to both thyroid antigens. Positive antibodies alone do not indicate thyroid disease because 5% to 10% of asymptomatic patients, as well as patients with other nonthyroidal autoimmune disorders, have positive antibodies.

Clinically, the TPO is more specific than ATgA in assessing disease activity. Although both antibodies are elevated during acute flares of the disease, lower titers of TPO remain positive during quiescent periods of the disease, while ATgA levels revert to negative.

Thyroid Receptor Antibodies

TRAbs are IgG immunoglobulins that are present in virtually all patients with Graves' disease.[1,3] Like TSH, these immunoglobulins can stimulate the thyroid gland to produce thyroid hormones. High titers of TRAb are useful in diagnosing otherwise asymptomatic Graves' disease (i.e., ophthalmopathy), in predicting the risk of relapse of Graves' disease after discontinuing medication, and in predicting the risk of neonatal hyperthyroidism in utero through transplacental passage of TRAb from the pregnant mother. Otherwise, TRAb measurement is expensive and offers no additional information in the patient with a typical Graves' disease presentation.

Clinical Application and Interpretation

Euthyroidism and Nonthyroidal Illness Syndrome

1. R.K., an obese 42-year-old woman, is admitted to the hospital because of increasing fatigue, sluggishness, shortness of breath (SOB), and pitting edema of the legs during the past 3 weeks. Bilateral pleural effusions found on her chest radiograph indicate a worsening of her congestive heart failure (CHF). Her other medical problems include cirrhosis of the liver, diabetes, and chronic bronchitis, for which she takes glipizide 10 mg every day (QD) and Lugol's solution three times a day (TID).

Pertinent physical findings include a palpable but normal-size thyroid, bibasilar rales, cardiomegaly, hepatomegaly, 4 + pitting edema, and normal deep tendon reflexes (DTRs). A diagnosis of worsening CHF secondary to hypothyroidism is suspected based on the following laboratory findings: cholesterol, 385 mg/dL (normal, <200); RAIU at 24 hours, 13% (normal, 5%–35%); scan, normal-size gland with homogenous uptake; TT_4, 1.4 mcg/dL (normal, 5–12); TT_3, 22 ng/dL (normal, 70–132); TSH, 4 μunits/mL (normal, 0.5–4.7); FT_4I, 3.5 (normal, 6.5–12.5); TPO, 30 IU/mL (normal, <1); and ATgA, 3 IU/mL (normal, <1). Evaluate and explain R.K.'s thyroid status based on her clinical and laboratory findings.

[SI units: cholesterol, 9.96 mmol/L (normal, <5.2); TT_4, 18 nmol/L (normal, 64–154); FT_4I, 45 (normal, 84–161); TT_3, 0.3 nmol/L (normal, 1.1–2); TSH, 4 mIU/L (normal, 0.5–4.7)]

Although low-output failure can be a presenting sign of hypothyroidism, the normal TSH definitely indicates that R.K. is euthyroid, despite the confusing results of her other thyroid function tests. The depressed RAIU is consistent with her history of iodide ingestion and dilution of the ^{131}I. The low TT_4, TT_3, and FT_4I may be explained by her cirrhosis and nonthyroidal illness syndrome (see question 2). The negative thyroid antibodies, the normal scan, and normal DTRs further substantiate the diagnosis of euthyroidism. In hypothyroidism, a lower rate of cholesterol degradation can produce an elevated serum cholesterol level. However, because many extrathyroidal factors influence the serum concentration of cholesterol, this test is an imprecise reflection of thyroid status. In this case, the elevated cholesterol level is not related to hypothyroidism.

2. Assess the results and explain the significance of R.K.'s TT_4, FT_4I, and TT_3 values.

R.K.'s thyroid function test results are consistent with nonthyroidal illness syndrome. Abnormal thyroid function tests are commonly found in euthyroid patients with various serious systemic diseases, including starvation, infections, sepsis, acute psychiatric disorders, HIV infection, myocardial infarction (MI), bone marrow transplantation, and severe chronic cardiac, pulmonary, renal, hepatic, and neoplastic diseases.[1,3,7–14] This "euthyroid sick" syndrome occurs in 37% to 70% of chronically ill or hospitalized patients and must be recognized. In general, the sicker the patient, the greater the degree of abnormal thyroid function findings, even though the patient has no thyroid disease.

The extent of laboratory changes varies with the severity of the illness. Typical changes include a low TT_3 (e.g., 15–20 ng/dL), a high rT_3, a normal or low TT_4 and FT_4I, and a suppressed (uncommon), normal or borderline-high compensatory TSH as patients recover from illness. In more serious illness, the TT_4 and FT_4I are often low. Free hormone levels (e.g., FT_4, FT_3) are often normal or low, which might be related to variations in the assays used. However, these inconsistent findings fuel the controversy over whether thyroid hormone therapy is beneficial or detrimental. These findings are believed to be explained by alterations in the peripheral conversion of T_4 to T_3 and by complex changes in the hypothalamic-pituitary-thyroid relationships. The low serum T_3 levels and high inactive rT_3 levels are caused by decreased activity of 5′-deiodinase, an enzyme that is necessary for the peripheral conversion of T_4 to T_3. Impaired protein synthesis of thyroid-binding prealbumin and an increase in the proportion of a lower-binding-capacity form of TBG might account for the lower bound hormone levels, but the concomitant increase in the free hormone concentrations would maintain a euthyroid state. Furthermore, circulating substances that inhibit the binding of T_4 and T_3 to the serum-binding proteins might also be present.

Less common changes include a modestly elevated TT_4 and FT_4I in patients with acute viral hepatitis, psychiatric disorders, renal failure, and advanced HIV infection. The TT_3 is usually normal but can be low in critically ill patients. Modest elevations in hormonal binding affinity and increased synthesis of TBG explain these findings.

Several studies have shown a strong inverse correlation between mortality and total serum T_4, T_3, and rT_3 levels.[10–12] Of 86 hospitalized, intensive care patients, 84% of those with a serum T_4 of <3 mcg/dL died, whereas 85% of those with a serum T_4 of >5 mcg/dL survived. In 331 patients with acute MI, rT_3 levels >0.41 nmol/L were significantly associated with a greater risk of death at 1 year. During recovery, TSH levels increase and hormone levels start to normalize. Therefore, a favorable outcome is associated with reversal of the hormone indices.

Thyroid experts are divided about whether patients with euthyroid sick syndrome should be treated, and few randomized studies are available to guide therapeutic decisions.[8,9–17] The few available studies found no survival benefits or favorable clinical outcomes following hormone therapy, although cardiac hemodynamics improved. The benefits of hormone replacement are unproven, and might be detrimental. In one trial, the mortality of patients with acute renal failure treated with T_4 was 43% versus 13% in the control group.[14] Opponents argue that T_4 therapy, by inhibiting TSH, may interfere with normal thyroid recovery, whereas proponents argue that there is no clear evidence that therapy is toxic.

In summary, T_4 and T_3 measurements are of limited value in the diagnosis of thyroid dysfunction in patients with significant nonthyroidal illness. A normal or near-normal TSH is necessary to establish euthyroidism in sick patients with nonthyroidal illness. The available data are not supportive of starting thyroid hormone treatment now. The abnormal laboratory findings should reverse when R.K.'s nonthyroid illness is corrected. To confirm euthyroidism, the slightly elevated TSH should be repeated once R.K.'s medical condition improves.

Drug Interference With Thyroid Function Tests

3. J.R., a 45-year-old man, complains of fatigue, dry skin, and constipation. His other medical problems include alcoholism for 10 years, cirrhosis, grand mal seizures treated with phenytoin (Dilantin) 300 mg/day and phenobarbital 90 mg at night, and rheumatoid arthritis for which he takes aspirin 325 mg, 20 tablets/day.

The results of his thyroid function tests are TT_4, 4.2 mcg/dL (normal, 5–12); FT_4, 0.6 ng/dL (normal, 0.7–1.9); and TSH, 2.5 μunits/mL (normal, 0.5–4.7). How should these laboratory findings be interpreted? What factors are responsible for the observed changes?

[SI units: TT_4, 54 nmol/L (normal, 64–154); FT_4, 8 pmol/L (normal, 9–24); TSH, 2.5 mIU/L (normal, 0.5–4.7)]

Despite complaints that could be consistent with hypothyroidism (e.g., fatigue, dry skin, constipation) and findings of low serum hormone values, J.R. is euthyroid, as evidenced by the normal TSH level. Secondary hypothyroidism is unlikely at this age without a history of central nervous system (CNS) trauma or tumor. Some nonthyroidal factors could account for J.R.'s low TT_4 and FT_4 values.[7] Anti-inflammatory doses of salicylates >2 g/day and salicylate derivatives (i.e., Disalcid, salsalate) can displace T_4 from both TBG and TBPA, causing these abnormal findings.[7,18,19] Elevation in free T_4 levels and suppression of TSH below normal occur transiently (i.e., no longer than first 3 weeks of administration) but normalize with chronic administration. Cirrhosis, stress, severe infections, and hereditary factors can also decrease TBG and TBPA synthesis to produce similar TT_4 findings. A medication history for drugs such as androgens or glucocorticoids that can lower TBG levels, and therefore TT_4 levels, should be elicited (Table 49-1).[7]

Enzyme inducers, such as rifampin and anticonvulsants, (phenytoin [Dilantin], phenobarbital, valproic acid [Depakene], carbamazepine [Tegretol]), can alter serum thyroid hormone levels.[7,20–25] A 40% to 60% reduction in total T_4 serum concentrations results from an increase in the metabolism (nondeiodination) of T_4 and from hormone displacement in patients receiving chronic anticonvulsant therapy. Serum T_3 levels are normal or slightly decreased. In addition, therapeutic levels of phenytoin and carbamazepine interfere with the FT_4 assay, causing a 20% to 40% lower FT_4 than would be expected in euthyroid persons.[21] TSH levels remain normal and patients are euthyroid; however, those who previously required T_4 therapy may need a dosage increment to maintain euthyroidism.[24,25] Valproic acid is reported to have similar but less potent effects on thyroid function.[20,22] Phenobarbital can increase T_4 uptake by the liver and increase the fecal excretion of T_4. Serum binding of thyroid hormones is unaffected by phenobarbital.

In summary, J.R. is taking several drugs that can further compromise the already low serum T_4 levels resulting from his liver disease. FT_4 remains subnormal in euthyroid persons receiving phenytoin, but normal TSH confirms euthyroidism.

4. S.T., a 23-year-old, sexually active woman whose only medication is birth control pills comes to the clinic complaining of extreme nervousness, diaphoresis, and scanty menstrual periods. Although she appears healthy, the possibility of hyperthyroidism is considered on the basis of the following laboratory values: TT_4, 16 mcg/dL (normal, 5–12); FT_4, 1.2 ng/dL (normal, 0.7–1.9); and TSH, 1.2 μunits/mL (normal, 0.5–4.7). Based on this information, what would be a reasonable assessment of S.T.'s thyroid status?

[SI units: TT_4, 206 nmol/L (normal, 64–154); FT_4, 16 pmol/L (normal, 9–24); TSH, 1.2 mIU/L (normal, 0.5–4.7)]

The normal FT_4, TSH, and calculated FT_4I confirm that S.T. is not hyperthyroid. The elevated TT_4 is consistent with increased TBG levels observed in patients with acute hepatitis; in pregnancy; and in persons taking estrogen, oral contraceptives, tamoxifen, raloxifene, heroin, or methadone.[7,26–30] Because TBG and therefore bound T_4 levels are increased by estrogens in S.T., total serum T_4 measurements are falsely elevated. In patients requiring L-thyroxine, the use of estrogens can increase requirements of hormone replacement because the increased pituitary secretion of TSH cannot increase thyroid production needed to offset the increased binding of T_4.[27] Thyroid function tests should return to normal within 4 weeks after oral contraceptives are discontinued. Progesterone-only oral contraceptives do not affect protein binding and therefore do not alter thyroid function tests.

5. J.P., a 55-year-old woman, complains of 3 months of progressive tremors, dizziness, and ataxia. Two months ago, she had a silent MI complicated by malignant ventricular ectopy that was responsive only to amiodarone (Cordarone) therapy. Her other medical problems include Parkinsonism, insulin-dependent diabetes, and diabetic gastroparesis. Her current medications include amiodarone, insulin, metformin, metoclopramide (Reglan), bromocriptine (Parlodel), and levodopa/carbidopa (Sinemet). Physical examination of the thyroid was unremarkable. Thyroid function tests show TT_4, 14.5 mcg/dL (normal, 5–12); FT_4, 2.3 ng/dL (normal, 0.7–1.9); TSH, 3.8 μunits/mL (normal, 0.5–4.7); TT_3, 40 ng/dL (normal, 70–132); and TPO antibodies, 40 IU/L (normal, <1). How should J.P.'s laboratory values be interpreted?

[SI units: TT_4, 187 nmol/L (normal, 64–154); FT_4, 30 pmol/L (normal, 9–24); TSH, 3.8 mIU/L (normal, 0.5–4.7); TT_3, 0.63 nmol/L (normal, 1.1–2)]

Although the symptoms of tremors, dizziness, and weight loss are suggestive of hyperthyroidism, the low TT_3, negative antibodies, normal TSH, and normal thyroid examination make this diagnosis unlikely. Side effects of amiodarone could be responsible for J.P.'s symptoms. Her drug therapy could also explain her laboratory findings.

Amiodarone produces complex changes in thyroid function tests that are confusing if not properly interpreted.[31–33] Because amiodarone inhibits both the peripheral and pituitary conversion of T_4 to T_3, FT_4 levels are elevated above normal, and TT_3 levels are subnormal in euthyroid patients. Transient elevations in TSH levels occur (usually <20 μU/mL) during the first few weeks of therapy but return to normal in approximately 3 months. If TSH levels do not normalize, then amiodarone-induced thyroid disease should be considered. Amiodarone can cause either hypothyroidism or hyperthyroidism in susceptible patients (see question 54).

The other drugs J.P. is taking—bromocriptine, levodopa, metformin, and metoclopramide—also add to the diagnostic confusion. Although these drugs do not affect the actual circulating hormone levels, they affect the dopaminergic system that controls both TSH and TRH secretion.[2,3,7] Infusions of dopamine and dobutamine can decrease both TSH secretion and the TSH response to TRH in euthyroid and hypothyroid patients.[2,3,7,34] Therefore, dopamine agonists such as bromocriptine, cabergoline, and levodopa can blunt the normal TSH response.[2,7,35] In addition, metformin suppresses TSH levels by as yet an unknown mechanism of action.[36] Conversely, dopamine antagonists such as metoclopramide or domperidone can elevate TSH levels.[2,7] Fortunately, the alterations in TSH caused by these agents are usually not substantial enough to completely obscure the true thyroid abnormality.

HYPOTHYROIDISM

Clinical Presentation

6. M.W., a 70-kg, 23-year-old voice student, thinks that her neck has become "fatter" over the past 3 to 4 months. She has gained 10 kg, feels mentally sluggish, tires easily, and finds that she can no longer hit high notes. Physical examination reveals puffy facies, yellowish skin, delayed DTRs, and a firm, enlarged thyroid gland. Laboratory data include FT_4, 0.6 ng/dL (normal, 0.7–1.9); TSH, 60 μunits/mL (normal, 0.5–4.7); and TPO antibodies, 136 IU/L (normal, <1). Assess M.W.'s thyroid status based on her clinical and laboratory findings.

[SI units: FT_4, 8 pmol/L (normal, 9–24); TSH, 60 mIU/L (normal, 0.5–4.7)]

M.W. presents with many of the clinical features of hypothyroidism as presented in Table 49-3. These include weight gain, mental sluggishness, easy fatigability, lowering of the voice pitch, puffy facies, yellowish tint of the skin, delayed DTRs, and enlarged thyroid.[37] The diagnosis of hypothyroidism is confirmed by her laboratory findings of a low FT_4, an elevated TSH value, and positive TPO antibodies.

A firm goiter, thyroid antibodies, and clinical symptoms of hypothyroidism strongly suggest Hashimoto's thyroiditis. She has no history of prior antithyroid drug use, surgery, or RAI treatment, which are common causes of iatrogenic hypothyroidism. She is also not taking any goitrogens or drugs known to cause hypothyroidism (Table 49-2).

Table 49-8 Thyroid Preparations

Drug/Dosage Forms	Composition	Dosage Equivalent	Comments
Thyroid USP (Armour) *Tab:* 0.25, 0.5, 1, 1.5, 2, 3, 4, and 5 gr	Desiccated hog, beef, or sheep thyroid gland Standardized iodine content	1 gr[a] —	Unpredictable T_4:T_3 ratio; supraphysiologic elevations in T_3 levels might produce toxic symptoms; Armour brand preferred
L-thyroxine (Levoxyl, Levothroid, Synthroid, Unithroid, various)	Synthetic T_4	60 mcg[a]	Stable, predictable potency; well absorbed; more potent than desiccated thyroid. When changing from >2 gr desiccated thyroid to L-T_4, a lower dosage of L-T_4 might be needed to avoid toxicity. Weight should be considered in dosing (1.6–1.7 mcg/kg/day). L-T_4 absorption can be impaired by iron, aluminum-containing products (e.g., antacids, sucralfate), Kayexalate, calcium preparations, proton pump inhibitors, cholesterol resin and phosphate binders, raloxifene, soy, bran, fiber enriched foods. L-T_4 metabolism increased by anticonvulsants, rifampin, imatinib, bexarotene, and pregnancy
Tab: 0.025, 0.050, 0.075, 0.088, 0.112, 0.125, 0.137, 0.15, 0.175, 0.2, and 0.3 mg	—	—	
Inj: 200 and 500 mcg	—	—	
l-Triiodothyronine (Cytomel)	Synthetic T_3	25–37.5 mcg	Complete absorption; requires multiple daily dosing; toxicity similar to all T_3-containing products; see desiccated thyroid comments
Tab: 5, 25, and 50 mcg	—	—	
Inj: 10 mcg/mL (Triostat)	—	—	
Liotrix (Thyrolar)	60 mcg T_4:15 mcg T_3	Thyrolar-1	No need for liotrix because T_4 is converted to T_3 peripherally; expensive, stable, and predictable content
Tab: 0.25, 0.5, 1, 2, and 3 gr	50 mcg T_4:12.5 mcg T_3	—	

[a] 60 mg (1 gr) of desiccated thyroid = 60 mcg of T_4.[42]
gr, grain; Inj, injection; L-T_4, levothyroxine; T_3, triiodothyronine; T_4, thyroxine; Tab, tablet; USP, United States Pharmacopeia.

Treatment With Thyroid Hormones

Thyroid Hormone Products

7. What thyroid preparation should be used to treat M.W.'s hypothyroidism? Are differences, advantages, or disadvantages significant among the various generic and brand name formulations of thyroid hormones?

The principal goals of thyroid hormone therapy are to attain and maintain a euthyroid state. Thyroid preparations (Table 49-8) are synthetic (L-thyroxine [various], L-triiodothyronine [Cytomel], liotrix [Thyrolar]) or natural (desiccated thyroid). The latter come from animal tissues.

DESICCATED THYROID

Desiccated thyroid (U.S. Pharmacopeia [USP]) is derived from pork thyroid glands, although beef and sheep also are used. Today, starting patients on desiccated thyroid is not justified. The USP requires only that desiccated thyroid contain 0.17% to 0.23% organic iodine by weight. These requirements do not seem stringent enough because potency may vary with changes in the proportion of the two active hormones (T_3 and T_4) or with changes in the amount of organic iodine present.[38,39] This variable potency seems to be particularly true of generic formulations compared with the biologically standardized Armour brand of desiccated thyroid. Inactive desiccated thyroid preparations that contain negligible amounts of T_3 and T_4 or even iodinated casein instead of active hormone have been identified in various brands sold in retail pharmacies and in over-the-counter products found in health food stores.[39–41] Likewise, preparations with greater-than-expected activity caused by an abnormally high T_3 content have resulted in thyrotoxicosis.

Allergic reactions to the animal protein are another concern. In addition, desiccated thyroid suffers from two problems inherent to all T_3-containing preparations. Because T_3 is absorbed more rapidly than T_4, supraphysiological elevations in plasma T_3 levels occur after oral ingestion, which can produce mild thyrotoxic symptoms in some patients. FT_4 levels are low during T_3 administration and, if misinterpreted, can result in the erroneous administration of more hormone. These problems with T_3 are easily missed unless T_3 levels are routinely monitored. Because significant amounts of T_4 are converted to T_3 peripherally, oral administration of T_3 offers no advantage and is not usually needed. (See Triiodothyronine section.)

Loss of tablet potency can occur from prolonged storage of desiccated thyroid preparations, but this instability is not as important as once believed. Because the only apparent advantage of desiccated thyroid is its low cost, it should not be considered the drug of choice for replacement therapy. Patients maintained on desiccated thyroid should be encouraged to change to L-thyroxine (T_4). Although 60 mg (1 gr) of desiccated thyroid is theoretically equal in potency to 75 to 100 mcg of T_4,[42] this equivalency may not hold true if the desiccated thyroid preparation is less active than its labeled content. The patient's weight also should be considered when switching therapy (see Question 8).

The synthetic thyroid preparations differ from one another in their relative potency, onset of action, and biological half-life.

LEVOTHYROXINE OR L-THYROXINE

L-thyroxine is the thyroid replacement of choice.[43] Its advantages include stability, uniform potency, relatively low cost, and lack of allergenic foreign protein content. The long half-life of 7 days permits once-a-day dosing and, if necessary, the creation of special convenience schedules, such as the omission of medication on weekends. The mean absorption of a commonly used branded preparation is 81%.[44] Spuriously low absorption values noted in earlier studies resulted from an overestimation of L-thyroxine tablet content. Absorption is optimal on an empty stomach, at least 60 minutes before or 2 hours after meals or at bedtime.[45] Several medications can also impair L-thyroxine absorption (see Question 15).

Concerns about generic and branded L-thyroxine tablet stability and potency, bioavailability, and product interchangeability existed because L-thyroxine preparations were grandfathered in by the 1938 Food, Drug, and Cosmetic Act. To address these concerns, the U.S. Food and Drug Administration (FDA) required that all manufacturers of L-thyroxine products submit a New Drug Application (NDA) by August 2001 or cease production by 2003 if the NDA was not filed.[46] Several FDA-approved brand (e.g., Levoxyl, Levothroid, Synthroid, Unithroid) and generic (e.g., Genpharm, Mylan Pharmaceuticals, Sandoz, Vintage) formulations approved under the NDA received AB or BX ratings, indicating interchangeability for some generic and brand preparations (e.g., Synthroid, Sandoz, Mylan). Raising concerns about the methodology the FDA used to determine bioequivalence, the American Thyroid Association, The Endocrine Society, and the American Association of Clinical Endocrinologists issued joint position statements expressing their displeasure with the FDA's conclusions of interchangeability.[47] Abbot Laboratories, the manufacturer of Synthroid, and others also disagreed with the FDA's findings.[48] Although this issue remains controversial, the preponderance of the evidence supports the FDA ratings and suggests that these preparations are likely to be interchangeable in the majority of patients.[49–52]

TRIIODOTHYRONINE

T_3 (Cytomel) is not recommended for routine thyroid hormone replacement because of the problems identified earlier with T_3 administration (see Desiccated Thyroid section).[43] Numerous randomized studies now conclude that replacement with combination T_4 and small dosages of T_3 offer no advantage to T_4 alone, despite an initial study showing improved cognitive performance and mood changes.[53,54] Its use in coronary bypass surgery is controversial.

Although T_3 is well absorbed, it has a relatively short half-life (1.5 days), necessitating multiple daily dosing to ensure a uniform response. Other disadvantages include higher expense and a greater potential for cardiotoxicity. Its primary use is for patients who require short-term hormone replacement therapy and those in whom T_4 conversion to T_3 might be impaired. Proponents favoring thyroid treatment of the "euthyroid sick" syndrome identify T_3 as the hormone replacement of choice. T_3 therapy should be monitored using the TSH and TT_3 or FT_3 levels.

LIOTRIX

Liotrix (Thyrolar) is a combination of synthetic T_4 and T_3 in a physiological ratio of 4:1. This preparation is subject to the same disadvantages common to all T_3-containing preparations. It is also stable and potent, but it is more expensive than other thyroid preparations. Because oral administration of T_3 is not needed and there is no advantage of adding T_3 to T_4 therapy, this expensive preparation is not recommended.[53,54] Patients should be changed to an equivalent dosage of L-thyroxine.

Thyroxine

DOSAGE

8. What would you recommend as appropriate starting and maintenance dosages of T_4 for M.W.?

The maintenance dosage for M.W. can be estimated from her weight. Average replacement doses of 1.6 to 1.7 mcg/kg/day (e.g., 100–125 mcg) are sufficient in most patients to normalize the TSH.[37,43] L-thyroxine dosages that suppress TSH levels to below normal or undetectable levels (subclinical hyperthyroidism) should be avoided to prevent osteoporosis and cardiac toxicity.[43,55–59] Excessive L-thyroxine can cause tachycardia, atrial arrhythmias, impaired ventricular relaxation, reduced exercise performance, and increased risk of cardiac mortality.[55] These considerations are especially important in older patients, who might require less T_4 than their younger counterparts and who are particularly sensitive to minute changes in T_4 doses (see Question 11). As patients age, the dosage should be evaluated yearly and decreased if necessary to maintain a normal TSH level.

How rapidly T_4 replacement can proceed depends on the likelihood of invoking cardiac toxicity in susceptible patients. Minute doses of T_4 (e.g., <75 mcg) can increase heart rate, stroke volume, oxygen consumption, and cardiac workload before euthyroidism occurs. One double-blind study compared the clinical outcome between starting full replacement doses versus gradual 25-mcg incremental doses in relatively young hypothyroid subjects with asymptomatic cardiac disease and concluded that those receiving full doses normalized thyroid function tests more rapidly (4 weeks) and without any toxicity.[60] Although this strategy may improve symptoms more quickly, further confirmation is needed to eliminate concerns about potential cardiac toxicity. Because M.W. has no identifiable risk factors (see Question 21) for cardiotoxicity that require careful dosage titration (e.g., old age, cardiac disease, long duration of hypothyroidism), she can be started on an estimated full replacement dose of 125 mcg daily of L-thyroxine (70 kg × 1.7 mcg/kg/day = 120 mcg). An alternative conservative approach would be to start with 100 or 112 mcg/day, check the FT_4 or FT_4I and TSH tests after 6 to 8 weeks of therapy, and if the TSH is still elevated without any symptoms of toxicity, increase the dosage to 125 mcg/day. The appropriate replacement dose will produce a TSH of 1 to 2 μunits/mL, normalize FT_4 or FT_4 I levels, and reverse clinical symptoms of hypothyroidism. Generally, dosing adjustments should not exceed monthly increments of 12.5 to 25 mcg/day.

MONITORING THERAPY

9. Ten days after starting L-thyroxine therapy, M.W. continues to complain of tiredness, fatigue, and difficulty singing despite excellent adherence. Thyroid function tests show a TT_4 of 4 mcg/dL (normal, 5–12), an FT_4 of 0.5 ng/dL (normal, 0.7–1.9), and a TSH of 40 μunits/mL (normal, 0.5–4.7). What therapeutic

options are available? How should M.W.'s thyroid function tests be interpreted?

[SI units: TT_4, 52 nmol/L (normal, 64–154); FT_4, 6 pmol/L (normal, 9–24); TSH, 40 mIU/L (normal, 0.5–4.7)]

Clinical improvement in the signs and symptoms of hypothyroidism and normalization of laboratory parameters are appropriate therapeutic end points. If the replacement dose is sufficient, some correction of her symptoms should occur after 2 to 3 weeks, but maximal effects will not be evident for 4 to 6 weeks. Typically, improvement of anemia and hair and skin changes is delayed and requires several months of treatment before resolution.[36,42]

In patients with severe myxedema, a transiently elevated T_4 level might occur at 6 weeks because the metabolic clearance of T_4 is decreased by the hypometabolic state associated with hypothyroidism.

FT_4 or FT_4I and TSH should be checked about 6 to 8 weeks after the initiation of therapy because T_4 has a half-life of 7 days, and three to four half-lives are needed to reach steady-state levels. Levels obtained before this time (as in M.W.) may be misleading and should be interpreted cautiously. No change in her L-thyroxine dosage should be attempted at this time.

10. Eight weeks later, on a routine follow-up visit, M.W. still feels tired and not back to her normal self. She denies any symptoms of hyperthyroidism. Her thyroid function tests show a TT_4 of 14 mcg/dL (normal, 5–12), a TT_3 of 50 ng/dL (normal, 70–132), FT_4 of 1.9 ng/dL (normal, 0.7–1.9), and a TSH of 3.5 μunits/mL (normal, 0.5–4.7). How should M.W.'s thyroid function tests be interpreted? What changes, if any, should be recommended in her therapeutic regimen?

[SI units: TT_4, 180 nmol/L (normal, 64–154); FT_4, 24 pmol/L (normal, 9–24); TT_3, 0.7 nmol/L (normal, 1.1–2); TSH, 3.5 mIU/L (normal, 0.5–4.7)]

Patients treated with L-thyroxine may develop an elevated TT_4 concentration and FT_4 without overt clinical signs of hyperthyroidism.[61,62] Despite these elevated levels, patients are euthyroid, as evidenced by a normal TSH. Because T_3 is not being released from the nonfunctioning thyroid gland, a higher concentration of T_4 is necessary to increase the amount of T_3 obtained from peripheral conversion. Woeber reported that the mean FT_4 was significantly higher (16 pmol/L) and the mean FT_3 lower (4 pmol/L) in patients receiving L-thyroxine than in those with thyroid disease not on L-thyroxine (FT_4, 14 pmol/L; FT_3, 4.2 pmol/L).[61] As expected, patients receiving L-thyroxine who had an elevated TT_4, an elevated TT_3, and an elevated T_3:T_4 ratio also had symptoms of hyperthyroidism. Thus, the TSH appears to be the best indicator of euthyroidism in patients treated with L-thyroxine.

Another possibility is that the elevated thyroid levels may only be an artifact of the laboratory collection time. Before any changes in her dosing regimen are made, M.W. should be asked about the time she takes the drug and its relationship to the time of her blood draw. Random sampling of FT_4 and TSH levels can be significantly different when compared with trough levels.[63,64] In one study, the FT_4 level was 12% higher and the TSH level 19% lower when obtained from random samples compared with trough samples.[64] Transient elevations in FT_4 levels were detected for 9 hours after ingestion of the oral L-thyroxine.

The symptoms of fatigue that M.W., is experiencing is likely not due to her hypothyroidism. Patients may continue to have symptoms of hypothyroidism despite normalization of the TSH value. Although some have suggested that the goal TSH be titrated to 1 to 2 μunits/mL for replacement therapy, this is controversial. One study found that changes in T_4 dosing to achieve TSH concentrations of 2 to 4.8 μunits/mL, 0.3 to 1.9 μunits/mL, or <0.3 μunits/mL in hypothyroid patients did not result in improvements in well-being, psychological, or hypothyroid symptoms, or quality of life.[65]

In conclusion, if an elevated TT_4 and FT_4 are noted without any symptoms of thyrotoxicosis (as in M.W.), the dosage should not be decreased; rather, a trough TT_4, TT_3, and TSH should be obtained to evaluate excessive dosing. The repeat values should be in the normal range with the correct dosing. An excessively suppressed TSH confirms a dosage that is too high. In M.W., the lack of hyperthyroid symptoms suggests euthyroidism, and no changes in her therapeutic regimen should be attempted until the trough levels are available. Evaluation for other causes of fatigue should be explored.

Triiodothyronine

11. C.B., a 65-year-old woman, complains of fatigue and vague muscle aches and pains, which she attributes to insufficient thyroid medication. On physical examination, the thyroid gland is palpable but not enlarged, and DTRs are 2 plus and brisk. Her dose of T_3 (Cytomel) was increased from 25 mcg TID to 50 mcg TID about 2 weeks ago based on the results of a recent FT_4 of 0.5 ng/dL (normal, 0.7–1.9). She denies taking any other medications. Is C.B.'s thyroid hormone replacement appropriate?

[SI units: FT_4, 6 pmol/L (normal, 9–24)]

As noted previously, Cytomel is not the drug of choice for thyroid replacement. The use of L-thyroxine would simplify her dosing regimen and facilitate monitoring.

The low FT_4 did not justify increasing C.B.'s dose of Cytomel. Because she is receiving T_3, the FT_4, which is a measure of free T_4, will always be low and will never reach normal levels. In fact, her vague complaints may be related to hyperthyroidism because she is receiving the equivalent of 0.2 to 0.3 mg of L-thyroxine daily. TSH and FT_3 levels are most useful in monitoring patients receiving T_3 therapy. A TSH level should be obtained to evaluate her thyroid function. A suppressed TSH and an elevated FT_3 would indicate hyperthyroidism. It is important to remember that in an older patient, hyperthyroidism might not always produce symptoms because of an "apathetic" sympathetic system.

L-thyroxine should be initiated cautiously in older patients to avoid exacerbating any pre-existing arteriosclerotic heart disease that might be masked by the hypothyroidism (see Questions 20 and 21). In general, older patients require smaller replacement dosages (approximately $\leq$1.6 mcg/kg/day of T_4) than their younger counterparts.[66–68] Dosages of <50 mcg/day of T_4 are common in patients older than 60 years. However, this lower T_4 dosage is not universal for all older subjects.[68] The reason that older patients need lower dosages is unclear, but it has been suggested that the lower requirements result from an age-related decrease in T_4 degradation rates. Because dosage requirements change with age, patients should be reassessed annually to determine whether the original dosage prescribed is still appropriate.

In C.B., who had been on T_3 without any evidence of cardiac toxicity, a less cautious approach in changing to T_4 can be attempted. An empiric L-thyroxine dosage of 68 mcg/day (40 kg × 1.6 mcg/kg/day) is an approximate dosing end point for C.B. The Cytomel should be discontinued and T_4 initiated in a dosage of 50 mcg/day; this dosage can be adjusted as needed based on C.B.'s symptoms and thyroid function tests. After T_3 therapy is discontinued, its effects will disappear over 3 to 5 days. In contrast, T_4 levels rise slowly over 4 to 5 days, so no overlap in T_3 administration is necessary to prevent hypothyroidism.

PARENTERAL DOSING

12. G.F., a 70-year-old man with long-standing hypothyroidism, has been receiving L-thyroxine 0.2 mg/day. Currently, he is in the hospital with a stroke and paralysis that prohibits him from swallowing oral medications. His last thyroid function tests were normal. What is a reasonable method of administering thyroid hormone to G.F.?

Because L-thyroxine has a half-life of 7 days, administration can be delayed for up to 1 week, assuming G.F. can resume oral intake at that time. However, if parenteral administration is required, L-thyroxine is available as an intramuscular (IM) or IV injection. The IV route is preferred because IM absorption may be slow and unpredictable, particularly if the circulation is compromised. Because the oral absorption of T_4 is approximately 80%,[44] parenteral doses should be decreased. Once IV L-thyroxine replacement is successful, maintenance with a once-weekly IM injection is successful if oral ingestion is not feasible.[69]

IN PREGNANCY

13. P.K. is a 35-year-old woman with Hashimoto's thyroiditis who is 6 weeks pregnant. Laboratory test results showed TT_4, 5 mcg/dL (normal, 5–12) and FT_4, 0.7 ng/dL (normal, 0.7–1.9). She takes her medications in the morning, which include L-thyroxine 0.1 mg/day and a prenatal vitamin enriched with iron and calcium. What dosing adjustments are required because of P.K.'s pregnancy?

[SI units: TT_4, 64 nmol/L (normal, 64–154); FT_4, 9 pmol/L (normal, 9–24)]

Inadequately treated or undiagnosed maternal hypothyroidism can be detrimental to the mother and the developing fetus.[70–74] Miscarriage, spontaneous abortion, hypertension, pre-eclampsia, and higher rates of cesarean sections and stillbirths have been reported with maternal hypothyroidism. Congenital defects, congenital hypothyroidism (see Question 14), abnormal fetal development, and impaired cognitive development in the newborn have been attributed to maternal hypothyroidism. The IQ scores of children born to mothers with undiagnosed hypothyroidism during pregnancy averaged 7 points lower than children born to euthyroid mothers.[71] A delay in both mental and motor development was observed in children ages 1 to 2 years old who were born to mothers with hypothyroxinemia but normal TSH levels during the first trimester of pregnancy.[74] Because thyroid hormone does not cross the placenta in significant amounts, the effect of maternal hypothyroidism on the fetus (if it occurs) must be indirect. The risk of congenital hypothyroidism is small if maternal antibodies from Hashimoto's thyroiditis cross the fetal circulation. The infant's cord blood should be assayed at birth to ensure that TSH is normal and that the child is euthyroid.

The majority of women with primary hypothyroidism will require a 30% to 50% increase in the prepregnancy T_4 dosage to maintain euthyroidism during the first trimester of pregnancy.[75,76] The only evidence of increased T_4 demands is an elevated TSH level (e.g., subclinical hypothyroidism) that occurs between weeks 5 (but can be as early as 3) and 16 of gestation. Often, no clinical symptoms of hypothyroidism are evident, and the FT_4 and the index are normal. Because of the adverse consequences associated with maternal hypothyroidism, some have advocated universal TSH screening of all pregnant women[77] as well as empirically increasing the prepregnancy T_4 dosage by 30% (extra two pills/week) as soon as pregnancy is confirmed.[76]

Some authors have challenged the dogma that pregnancy per se increases T_4 demands. Rather, they propose that these increments were recommended before it was recognized that coadministration of iron- and calcium-containing prenatal vitamins reduced T_4 absorption (see question 15) and that these drug interactions may be primarily responsible for these increased needs. When prenatal vitamins with iron and calcium were separated by 4 hours from T_4 administration, only 31% of women required an increase in T_4 dose.[78] Nevertheless, women should be followed closely during pregnancy and the FT_4 and TSH levels evaluated monthly during the first trimester. If necessary, the T_4 dosage should be adjusted to maintain a normal TSH and an FT_4 or FT_4I in the upper limits of normal. Because TBG is elevated, the TT_4 should be kept above the normal range; it is not the best indicator of adequate replacement.

P.K.'s low TT_4 and FT_4 are concerning. The TT_4 should be much higher because of pregnancy-associated increases in TBG. The TSH level should be obtained, and the daily dosage of T_4 should be increased to 125 mcg after eliminating the possibility of patient nonadherence and drug interactions. Ingestion of the prenatal vitamins with iron and calcium should be separated by at least 4 hours from T_4. PK could also be instructed to take the T_4 at night for better absorption.[45] The TSH should be repeated in 6 weeks, and the dosage should be adjusted as needed to keep the TSH in the normal range. After delivery, the dosage should be reduced to prepregnancy levels and the FT_4 and TSH rechecked to ensure euthyroidism.

Congenital Hypothyroidism

14. P.K. delivered a healthy baby, T.K., at term without difficulty. T.K.'s postpartum screening serum T_4 level was 5 mcg/dL (normal, 5–12), and TSH was 35 μunits/mL (normal, 0.5–4.7). At home, T.K. became lethargic, had a weak cry, sucked poorly, and failed to thrive. Assess the situation (including a treatment plan and prognosis). How is mental development affected?

[SI units: T_4, 64 nmol/L (normal, 64–154); TSH, 15 mIU/L (normal, 0.5–4.7)]

T.K.'s symptoms are suggestive of congenital hypothyroidism, although in most infants the clinical signs and symptoms are so subtle and nonspecific that they are easily missed until the child is several months old. The early clinical findings include prolonged jaundice, skin mottling (cutis marmorata), lethargy, poor feeding, constipation, hypothermia, hoarse cry, large fontanels, distended abdomen, hypotonia, slow reflexes, and piglike facies. Respiratory difficulties, delayed skeletal maturation, and choking (but not palpable goiter) may be present. These infants are also at risk for additional congenital defects or complications.[79] Mass neonatal screening programs have been successful in detecting congenital hypothyroidism within the first few weeks of life before clinical manifestations are apparent and before irreversible changes occur.

The postpartum low serum T_4 concentration and elevated TSH level (>20 μunits/mL) in T.K. are of concern and should be verified. Transient hypothyroidism can result from intrauterine exposure to thioamides or excess iodides, or from transplacental passage of TRAb from the mother. Thyroid function tests often normalize without treatment in 3 to 6 months as the TRAb is cleared by the infant.[79] The diagnosis of hypothyroidism should be confirmed by a low serum T_4, a low FT_4, and an elevated TSH concentration during the next few weeks. Serum T_3 concentrations are often in the normal range and are not helpful. Normal serum T_4 concentrations are higher in the first few weeks of life and gradually return to normal by 2 to 4 months of life. The FT_4I may also be elevated. Because of these confusing changes, thyroid serum levels should be compared with the normal range for the approximate postnatal age.

Thyroid hormones play a critical role in normal growth and development, particularly of the CNS, during the first 3 years of life. If untreated, dwarfism and irreversible mental retardation occur. T.K.'s normal mental (IQ) and physical development will be determined by the age at which treatment is started, the initial dosage of T_4, the serum T_4 level attained during therapy, the adequacy with which treatment is maintained, and the cause and severity of the initial deficiency.[80–86]

Sodium L-thyroxine is the preparation of choice for replacement. T_4 tablets can be crushed and mixed with breast milk or formula; suspensions are not stable and should not be used. T_3 also can be used, but this form is less desirable because its short half-life causes a greater fluctuation in plasma levels (Table 49-8). The initial replacement dose of T_4 should raise the serum T_4 as rapidly as possible to minimize the consequences of hypothyroidism on cognitive function. A delay in starting therapy of even a few days has resulted in a poorer IQ outcome.[81,82,86] A minimum T_4 dosage of 10 to 15 mcg/kg/day is recommended to raise the serum T_4 to >10 mcg/dL (129 nmol/L) by 7 days.[80] However, some suggest that higher than previously recommended dosages of 12 to 17 mcg/kg/day might be more effective, but concern about negative neurologic outcomes exists.[79,81,82] In the full-term healthy infant, full initial replacement T_4 doses are appropriate unless the infant has underlying heart disease or is extremely sensitive to the effects of thyroid hormones. In these infants, reduced doses of T_4 (approximately 25%–33% of the recommended dose) can be started and increased gradually by similar increments until the therapeutic dose is achieved. The recommended replacement dose decreases with age and is shown in Tables 49-4 and 49-9.

Mental development and attainment of normal growth are not severely impaired if adequate T_4 treatment is initiated before 3 months of age to achieve a serum T_4 level >10 mcg/dL (129 nmol/L).[79–82,84] Nevertheless, children with the most severe congenital hypothyroidism (i.e., athyreosis) scored 8 IQ points lower than their siblings.[83] Young adults 20 years after congenital hypothyroidism showed impaired motor and intellectual outcomes after suboptimal T_4 (<7.8 mcg/kg/day) therapy compared to sibling controls.[84] However, those receiving optimal therapy still had some deficits in memory, attention, and behavior versus the siblings.[87] Newborns detected by screening programs who start therapy within the first 4 to 6 weeks of life have mean IQs of 100 to 109, similar to the control populations. The mean IQ drops if treatment is delayed until 6 weeks and 3 months (mean IQ, 95), or until 3 and 6 months (mean IQ, 75). When treatment is not started until 6 months to 1 year of age, normal mental development is impaired despite subsequent treatment (mean IQ, 55). Higher IQs also were found in children who received dosages of T_4 >10 mcg/kg/day compared to lower dosages and achieved a mean serum T_4 level >14 mcg/dL (181 nmol/L) in the first month of therapy.[81,82,86,88] Neurologic deficits are also more likely to occur in infants whose thyroid replacement is delayed or inadequate (as evidenced by a serum T_4 <8 mcg/dL [103 nmol/L] within 30 days of therapy and delayed suppression [18–24 months] of the TSH into the normal range). Additional risk factors for a low IQ and poor motor and speech skills despite adequate therapy include clinical signs of hypothyroidism during fetal life, more marked chemical hypothyroidism at birth (T_4 <2 mcg/dL), thyroid aplasia, and retarded bone age.[79,80,82]

The goal of therapy is a T_4 in the upper normal range (e.g., 10–18 mcg/dL [129–232 nmol/L]) and/or an FT_4 of 2 to 5 ng/dL (27–64 pmol/L) during the first 2 weeks of therapy, and then a lower target thereafter: a T_4 of 10 to 16 mcg/dL (129–206 nmol/L) and/or an FT_4 of 1.6 to 2.2 ng/dL [20–30 pmol/L]). IQs are improved if TSH levels are normalized within the first month of therapy, but no later than 3 months.[81,82,86,88] Thyroid function tests should be routinely monitored 2 to 4 weeks after starting therapy, then every 1 to 2 months during the first year of life and every 2 to 3 months during the next 2 years of life. Although TSH suppression is the most reliable index of adequate replacement in older children, normalization of the TSH should not be used as the sole monitoring parameter in infants because the TSH may lag behind correction of the T_4 and/or FT_4 levels. Overtreatment should be avoided to prevent brain dysfunction, acceleration of bone age, and premature craniosynostosis. Normal growth and development should also be a treatment goal. Other clinical end points include an improvement in activity level, skin color, temperature, facial appearance, and reversal of other symptoms and signs of hypothyroidism. The child will require lifelong replacement therapy.

Table 49-9 T_4 Recommended Replacement Dose

Age	***Daily mcg/kg T_4***
3–6 mo	10–15
6–12 mo	5–7
1–10 yr	3–6
>10 yr	2–4

T_4, thyroxine.

Unresponsiveness to Levothyroxine and Drug–Drug Interactions

15. R.T., a 45-year-old woman, complains of weight gain, heavy menses, sluggishness, and cold intolerance. Her present medical problems include Hashimoto's thyroiditis, treated with L-thyroxine 150 mcg daily; hypercholesterolemia treated with

cholestyramine (Questran) 4 g QID; anemia, treated with $FeSO_4$ 325 mg twice a day (BID); menorrhagia treated with conjugated estrogens 1.25 mg QD; and a history of peptic ulcer disease, treated with antacids and sucralfate 1 g BID. She was recently started on calcium carbonate 1 g BID and raloxifene (Evista) 60 mg QD to protect her bones. Her laboratory data include a cholesterol serum concentration of 280 mg/dL (normal, <200), a TSH of 21 μunits/mL (normal, 0.5–4.7), an FT_4 of 0.6 ng/dL (normal, 0.7–1.9), and positive ATgA and TPO antibodies. R.T. admits that she has increased her L-thyroxine dose because she feels better on the higher dose. Why is R.T. apparently unresponsive to thyroid therapy?

[SI units: cholesterol, 7.2 nmol/L (normal, <5.2); FT_4, 8 pmol/L (normal, 9–24); TSH, 21 mIU/L (normal, 0.5–4.7)]

R.T.'s complaints and laboratory values confirm inadequate treatment of hypothyroidism despite thyroid therapy. Possible causes of therapeutic failure include nonadherence, error in diagnosis, poor absorption, subpotent medication, rapid metabolism, and tissue resistance.[43,89,90] Thyroid resistance is rare, and nonadherence, error in diagnosis, and rapid metabolism do not appear to be reasonable explanations in R.T. An increase in L-thyroxine requirements can result from concomitant anticonvulsants (see Question 3), rifampin,[91] bexarotene,[92] and imatinib therapy by increasing the metabolism of L-thyroxine. In hypothyroid patients receiving T_4, imatinib increased TSH levels 384%, necessitating a 10% to 47% increase in the L-thyroxine dosage.[93]

The most likely explanations are poor bioavailability and/or a subpotent preparation. The timing of T_4 administration with her meals should be ascertained because its bioavailability is improved when it is taken on an empty stomach and at night.[43,45,94] Simultaneous coadministration of T_4 with soy proteins or high-fiber diets (e.g., oat bran, soybean) should also be avoided because T_4's absorption can be impaired.[95,96] R.T.'s history does not include surgical bowel resection or GI disorders (e.g., steatorrhea, malabsorption) or cholesterol resin binders that can interfere with the enterohepatic circulation of orally administered thyroid and lead to excessive fecal loss.[90] Evidence for incomplete absorption of the hormone can be obtained by comparing R.T.'s response to oral and parenteral T_4.[89]

L-thyroxine bioavailability can also be compromised by the numerous medications that R.T. is taking. Estrogen therapy can increase T_4 requirements by increasing TBG to increase T_4 binding.[27] Cholestyramine, colestipol, iron sulfate, antacids, sucralfate, calcium preparations, particularly the carbonate salt, and raloxifene can impair thyroid absorption if these medications are administered at the same time.[43,97–104] Cholesterol-lowering agents (e.g., lovastatin) and phosphate binders are also reported to interfere with thyroid absorption.[100,105] R.T. should be questioned about the time she takes her thyroid medication. She should be instructed to take it on an empty stomach or at night,[45] and at least 12 hours apart from the raloxifene and 4 hours apart from the iron, calcium, and cholestyramine.[97–104] Aluminum-containing products (i.e., antacids, sucralfate) should be discontinued because separating the concurrent administration of T_4 and her aluminum-containing preparations does not consistently correct this interaction.[101,102] R.T. should be changed to an aluminum- and calcium free antacid (e.g., Riopan) and, if necessary, an H_2-receptor antagonist. Proton pump inhibitors (e.g., omeprazole) should be avoided because decreased acid secretion may reduce T_4 absorption, although data are conflicting.[106,107] After R.T. has been instructed on the proper times of administration for her medications, the therapeutic response and thyroid function tests should be reevaluated in 6 to 8 weeks before any changes are made.

16. Could R.T.'s hypothyroidism be responsible for her hypercholesterolemia?

Type IIa hypercholesterolemia is the most common lipid abnormality observed in patients with primary hypothyroidism.[108] Although the rate of cholesterol synthesis is normal in hypothyroid patients, the rate of cholesterol clearance is decreased. Similarly, slow removal of triglycerides may result in hyperlipidemia. Hypercholesterolemia is frequently observed before the appearance of clinical hypothyroidism. Treatment with T_4 alone should lower the cholesterol levels if no other causes are contributing.

Myxedema Coma

Clinical Presentation

17. R.B., a 65-year-old, agitated woman arrived at the emergency department complaining of chest pain unrelieved by nitroglycerin (NTG). Her medical problems include alcoholic cardiomyopathy, angina, and hypothyroidism. Although she has been advised repeatedly to take her T_4 regularly, she continues to take it sporadically. An FT_4I drawn 4 months ago was 1 (normal, 6.5–12.5). Haloperidol (Haldol) 2 mg IM and morphine sulfate 10 mg IM were given for the agitation. After the injection, the nurse noticed mental depression, lethargy, and shallow breathing. R.B.'s oral temperature was 34.5°C, and she exhibited chills and shakes. What is your assessment of R.B.'s subjective and objective data?

[SI units: FT_4I, 13 (normal, 84–161)]

R.B. has several symptoms consistent with myxedema coma.[109] Myxedema coma is the end stage of long-standing, uncorrected hypothyroidism. The classic features are hypothermia, delayed DTRs, and an altered sensorium that ranges from stupor to coma. Other predominant features include hypoxia, carbon dioxide retention, severe hypoglycemia, hyponatremia, and paranoid psychosis. Typical physical findings (Table 49-3) include a puffy face and eyelids, a yellowish discoloration of the skin, and loss of the lateral eyebrows. Pleural and pericardial effusions and cardiomegaly may be present. Because myxedema coma frequently occurs in older women, it is often difficult to distinguish the signs and symptoms from dementia or other disease states, as illustrated by R.B. Precipitating factors include cold weather or hypothermia, stress (e.g., surgery, infection, trauma), coexisting disease states such as MI, diabetes, hypoglycemia, or fluid and electrolyte abnormalities (especially hyponatremia), and medications such as sedatives, narcotic analgesics, antidepressants, and other respiratory depressants and diuretics.

Haloperidol and morphine might be responsible for what appears to be impending myxedema coma in R.B. In severely myxedematous patients, respiratory depressants (anesthetics, narcotic analgesics, phenothiazines, sedative-hypnotics) alone or in combination with the hypothermic effects of the phenothiazines can aggravate the pre-existing hypothermia and carbon dioxide retention to precipitate myxedema coma.[109,110] Tranquilizers such as haloperidol should not be given; small doses of less depressive sedative-hypnotics such as the benzodiazepines should be used only when necessary. Myxedematous patients are also inherently sensitive to the respiratory depressant effects of narcotic analgesics, especially morphine. A dose as small as 10 mg may induce coma in a hypothyroid patient or cause death in a patient who is already comatose. If morphine is required, the dose should be decreased to one-third to one-half the usual analgesic dose, and the respiratory rate should be monitored closely.

Treatment

18. What would be a reasonable therapeutic plan for the management of R.B.'s myxedema coma?

Emergency treatment, usually in the intensive care unit, of myxedema coma is directed toward thyroid replacement, maintenance of vital functions, and elimination of precipitating factors. Despite immediate and aggressive therapy with large replacement doses of thyroid, mortality rates of 60% to 70% are common.[109]

Whether T_4 or T_3 is the drug of choice in myxedema coma is controversial because no comparative trials have been conducted. Although T_3 is potentially more cardiotoxic, it has been recommended because its more rapid onset might reverse coma faster, and the peripheral conversion from T_4 to the biologically active T_3 might be inhibited in severe systemic disease.[110,111–114] T_4 alone, T_3 alone, and a combination of the two have all been used successfully to treat myxedema coma. However, L-thyroxine is generally regarded as the hormone of choice because of greater clinical experience with T_4 than with T_3. Also, mortality has occurred despite the higher T_3 levels achieved after T_3 administration.[114] T_3 might be considered after failure of T_4 or if concomitant systemic illness (e.g., heart failure) is likely to impair conversion of T_4 to T_3. Supraphysiological elevations in T_3 levels occur only after oral administration but are not seen after IV T_3 infusion. Factors associated with a higher mortality 1 month after therapy include older age, cardiac complications, and T_4 replacement $\geq$500 mcg/day or T_3 replacement $>$75 mcg/day.[110,114]

L-thyroxine 400 to 500 mcg should be given IV initially in patients $<$55 years of age without cardiac disease to saturate the TBG and raise the serum T_4 level to 6 to 7 mcg/dL.[109,115] This initial dose can be adjusted based on the patient's weight and other restrictive factors (e.g., age, cardiac disease). The initial T_4 dosage for R.B. should be reduced to 300 mcg/day to avoid worsening her angina. If the proper dosage is given, consciousness, restoration of vital signs, and decreased TSH levels should occur within 24 hours. If T_3 is preferred, the usual dose is 10 to 20 mcg IV, followed by 10 mcg every 4 hours for the first 24 hours, and then 10 mcg every 6 hours for a few days until oral therapy can be started.[109]

Maintenance doses should be titrated to the patient's clinical response. Because myxedema can impair oral absorption, the IV route is preferred to ensure adequate drug concentrations. Oral administration is permitted once GI function returns to normal. The smallest dosage (without untoward effects) administered should be 50 to 100 mcg/day of T_4 or 10 to 15 mcg of T_3 every 12 hours.[109,115]

Supportive measures include assisted ventilation, glucose for hypoglycemia, restriction of fluids for hyponatremia, and the use of blood or plasma expanders to prevent circulatory collapse and to maintain blood pressure. The use of blankets to treat R.B.'s hypothermia is not advised because vasodilation will occur and further compromise the cardiovascular components of shock. Although steroids have not been shown to be clearly beneficial in primary myxedema, they may be lifesaving in patients with hypopituitarism masquerading as myxedema coma. Because it is difficult to distinguish between primary and secondary myxedema, hydrocortisone 50 to 100 mg every 6 hours should be given empirically.[109]

Appropriate measures should be taken to relieve R.B.'s chest pain while ruling out the possibility of an MI. The use of a narcotic antagonist such as naloxone may be beneficial in this instance because it can reverse the effects of the morphine. Naloxone can also arouse comatose patients intoxicated with alcohol.

Hypothyroidism With Congestive Heart Failure

Clinical Presentation

19. E.B., a 45-year-old woman, is admitted with complaints of substernal pressure and chest pain, SOB, dyspnea on exertion, and orthopnea. Other subjective and objective data suggest CHF complicated by MI. Significant past medical history reveals exertional angina and Graves' disease, which was treated with RAI ablation 10 years ago. Symptoms have not recurred. Physical examination reveals cardiomegaly, diastolic hypertension, obesity, facial edema and puffiness, delayed DTRs, and nonpitting pretibial edema. Pertinent laboratory findings include FT_4, 0.2 ng/dL (normal, 0.7–1.9); TSH, 100 μunits/mL (normal, 0.5–4.7); creatinine kinase, 300 units/L (normal, 32–267); aspartate aminotransferase (AST), 80 units/L (normal, 7–26); lactate dehydrogenase (LDH), 250 units/L (normal, 80–230); and troponin, 0.3 ng/mL (normal, 0.3–1.5). A chest radiograph reveals cardiomegaly and pericardial effusions, and an electrocardiogram (ECG) shows bradycardia and flattened T waves with ST depression. Diuretics, nitrates, angiotensin II inhibitor, and digitalis are instituted. E.B.'s symptoms improve, but her cardiac abnormalities are not reversed. Why do these clinical findings suggest hypothyroidism?

[SI units: FT_4, 5 pmol/L (normal, 9–24); TSH, 100 mIU/L (normal, 0.5–4.7); creatinine kinase, 300 units/L (normal, 32–267); AST, 80 units/L (normal, 7–26); LDH, 250 units/L (normal, 80–230); troponin, 0.3 g/L (normal, 0.3–1.5)]

E.B.'s abnormal thyroid function tests, symptoms, physical findings, and history of RAI therapy are consistent with severe hypothyroidism. "Myxedema heart" can be confused with low-output CHF because the symptoms are similar: cardiomegaly, dyspnea, edema, pericardial effusions, and abnormal ECG.[55,109] Therefore, hypothyroidism should be excluded in all patients with new or worsening symptoms of cardiovascular disease (e.g., angina, arrhythmia). Although hypothyroidism alone rarely causes CHF, it can worsen an underlying cardiac condition. Rarely, ventricular arrhythmia, including torsades de pointes, can occur from a prolonged QT interval.

Although E.B.'s enzyme elevations (i.e., AST, CK, LDH) are suggestive of an MI, they all may be moderately or significantly increased from chronic skeletal or cardiac muscle damage or from decreased enzyme clearance secondary to hypothyroidism. The enzymes can be fractionated to determine their origin. The normal troponin level eliminates the possibility of an MI.

Treatment

20. What might be the effect of hypothyroidism on the cardiac treatment and status of E.B.?

If E.B.'s cardiac abnormalities are caused by hypothyroidism rather than organic disease, adequate doses of T_4 will restore the heart size, normalize the diastolic blood pressure, reverse the ECG findings, and normalize the serum enzyme elevations within 2 to 4 weeks. However, improvement in myocardial function begins only at dosages of 50 to 75 mcg/day of T_4, which may be tolerated poorly by cardiac patients.

The relationship between the altered lipid metabolism of hypothyroidism and increased risk of atherosclerosis is controversial and poorly documented.[108] Interestingly, angina pectoris and MI are rather uncommon among hypothyroid patients. Theoretically, the hypometabolic state associated with hypothyroidism may protect the ischemic myocardium by reducing metabolic demands. However, hypothyroidism actually aggravates subendocardial ischemia during an acute MI by decreasing erythrocyte production of 2,3-diphosphoglycerate, which shifts the oxyhemoglobin dissociation curve to the left. This effect further diminishes oxygen delivery to already ischemic tissues. Angina or premature beats can develop or worsen with the institution of T_4 therapy,[116–118] so doses should be titrated carefully (see Question 21). Without organic disease, digitalis is ineffective and may even be harmful. Hypothyroid patients show an increased sensitivity to digitalis, and digitalis toxicity is possible unless the maintenance dose is decreased (see Question 26).[119,120] Nitrates may precipitate hypotension and/or syncope in hypothyroid patients because these patients have a low circulating blood volume and their response to vasodilation can be exaggerated. Furthermore, if β-blockers are required, the cardioselective β-blockers are preferred. The noncardioselective β-blockers have produced coronary spasm by exacerbating the compensatory increase in norepinephrine levels and α-adrenergic tone found in hypothyroidism.

21. How aggressively should thyroid hormone therapy be initiated in a patient like E.B. who has angina? What is the hormone replacement of choice in patients with cardiac disease?

Patients with long-standing hypothyroidism, arteriosclerotic cardiac disease, or advanced age tend to be extremely sensitive to the cardiac effects of thyroid hormone. Initiation of normal or even subtherapeutic doses in these patients might produce severe angina, MI, supra- and ventricular premature beats, cardiac failure, or sudden death. These effects underscore the need to replace thyroid cautiously, and sometimes suboptimally, to avoid cardiac toxicity.[116–118,121]

The angina and cardiac status should be controlled before initiating T_4 therapy. In the patient with poorly controlled angina, cardiac catheterization is warranted to assess the coronary artery status before starting hormone therapy. Coronary bypass has been performed safely with minimal complications in the hypothyroid patient to control the angina and may allow institution of full replacement doses without cardiotoxicity.[122]

For E.B., 12.5 to 25 mcg of T_4 should be initiated cautiously and increased as tolerated by similar increments of T_4 every 4 to 6 weeks until a therapeutic dosage is reached. The rapidity with which the increments can proceed is determined by how well each increased dose is tolerated. If cardiac toxicity occurs, therapy should be stopped immediately. Once symptoms resolve, therapy can be restarted using smaller dosage increments and longer intervals between dosage adjustments. If cardiac symptoms recur, further T_4 therapy should be stopped pending cardiac evaluation. In some patients with severe cardiac sensitivity, complete euthyroidism might never be achieved. In these patients, the correct replacement dosage is a compromise between prevention of myxedema and avoidance of cardiac toxicity.[118] E.B.'s clinical status and ECG should be monitored closely during the titration period. T_4 should be discontinued or decreased at the first sign of cardiac deterioration. It is not necessary to monitor thyroid function tests (e.g., TSH or FT_4) during the titration period because the results will remain low until adequate replacement is achieved. Thyroid function tests should be obtained once maximally tolerated or estimated euthyroid dosages are achieved.

Some suggest that T_3 (Cytomel) is the agent of choice in patients with cardiac abnormalities. The onset of action of T_3 is 1 to 3 days compared with 3 to 5 days for T_4. After therapy is withdrawn, the effects of T_3 dissipate in 3 to 5 days, while a period of 7 to 10 days is needed for T_4. Thus, if toxicity occurs, the effects of T_3 will disappear rapidly on cessation of therapy, a theoretical advantage in the cardiac patient. Nevertheless, T_3 is not recommended because its greater potency requires finer and more difficult dosage titration to ensure smooth and uniform blood levels. Furthermore, the high serum T_3 levels that occur after oral administration might cause more cardiac toxicity, especially angina.

Subclinical Hypothyroidism

22. M.P., a healthy 53-year-old woman, comes in for her regular checkup. She denies any symptoms of hypothyroidism and feels well. She has no other medical problems, takes no medications, and has no known allergies. Her physical examination is within normal limits. Routine screening laboratory tests are normal except for an FT_4 of 1.2 ng/dL (normal, 0.7–1.9) and a TSH of 8 μunits/mL (normal, 0.5–4.7). Does M.P. require thyroid treatment, based on her clinical presentation and laboratory findings?

[SI units: FT_4, 16 pmol/L (normal, 9–24); TSH, 8 mIU/L (normal, 0.5–4.7)]

M.P.'s free thyroid levels are normal, but her TSH level is elevated, indicating subclinical hypothyroidism (SH). The prevalence of SH ranges from 4% to 10% and increases to 26% in the elderly population, particularly women.[57,58] It is unclear whether SH represents the early stages of thyroid failure. The estimated risk of developing overt hypothyroidism after 10 years in untreated patients by Kaplan-Meier curves was 0% for a TSH level of 4 to 6 mIU/L, 42.8% for a TSH level of 6 to 12 mIU/L, and 76.9% for a TSH level >12 mIU/L. This risk increased in patients with positive thyroid antibodies.[123] Because the most common clinical scenarios involve asymptomatic patients with TSH levels <10 mIU/L, negative thyroid antibodies, and no history of prior thyroid disease, routine thyroid screening has been recommended, particularly in elderly women.[58]

Mild symptoms of hypothyroidism, including psychiatric and cognitive abnormalities, are found in approximately 30% of patients with SH, but the average TSH level usually exceeds 11 mIU/L. Cardiac dysfunction, including impaired left ventricular diastolic function at rest, systolic dysfunction with exercise, atherosclerosis, CHF, and MI has been reported.[55,58,124–126] Data showing an increased risk of coronary heart disease (CHD) is conflicting and is influenced by the severity of SH, study design, and length of follow-up. A meta-analysis noted a 1.6 times increased risk of CHD,[127] a cross-sectional analysis noted an odds ratio of 2.2 only in those with TSH levels of ≥10 mIU/L, whereas the 20-year longitudinal analysis found a significant risk (hazard ratio of 1.7) regardless of the degree of TSH elevation.[128] However, a large prospective cohort study found no significant association with atherosclerotic disease or cardiac mortality but observed an increase in all-cause mortality at 10 years of follow-up.[189] Other atypical and nonspecific signs and symptoms reflecting dysfunction of any part of the body may occur, primarily in the elderly. Failure to thrive, mental confusion, weight loss with poor appetite, incontinence, depression, inability to walk, carpal tunnel syndrome, deafness, ileus, anemia, hypercholesterolemia, and hyponatremia have been reported.[57,58,124–126]

Treatment of subclinical hypothyroidism with T_4 is controversial because study results are conflicting. Potential benefits of treatment include (a) preventing progression to hypothyroidism, (b) improving the lipid profile and reducing cardiac risks, and (c) reversing symptoms of hypothyroidism. Patients with higher TSH levels (e.g., >10 mIU/L), a history of previously diagnosed thyroid disease, elevated lipid levels, or evidence of positive thyroid antibodies gained the most benefit from L-thyroxine therapy.[55,123,126,129] L-thyroxine significantly reduced total cholesterol by 0.2 to 0.4 mmol/L (7.9–15.8 mg/dL) and low-density cholesterol concentrations by 0.33 mmol/L (10 mg/dL); serum HDL and triglyceride concentrations remain unchanged.[58,125,126,129] Improvement of elevated intraocular pressures, memory, mood, somatic complaints, and diastolic dysfunction has also been reported after T_4 replacement.[123,125,126,129] However, in patients with mild TSH elevations (e.g., <10 mIU/L), well-designed studies showed no improvement in clinical symptoms of hypothyroidism with T_4 supplementation.[57,58,125,126]

Treatment of older patients requires an assessment of the risks versus benefits of therapy. Thyroid therapy carries the risk of unmasking underlying cardiac disease in older patients. Nevertheless, thyroid replacement appears reasonable in asymptomatic patients with TSH levels >10 mIU/L and especially those with symptoms of mild hypothyroidism, dyslipidemia, laboratory abnormalities, or end-organ alterations.[57,58,123–126,129] Patients with asymptomatic subclinical hypothyroidism and a TSH level <10 mIU/L do not warrant immediate therapy, but close follow-up is warranted.

Because M.P. is asymptomatic and has a TSH level <10 mIU/L, it is reasonable to delay therapy and recheck the TSH in a few months.

Hypopituitarism and T_4 Replacement With a Normal Thyroid-Stimulating Hormone Level

23. J.P. is a 65-year-old woman who complains of fatigue, cold intolerance, dry skin, and weight gain for the past several months. Her thyroid examination and DTRs are within normal limits. A TSH level was 2.5 μunits/mL (normal, 0.5–4.7). She denies taking any other medications. J.P. is started empirically on a 3-month trial of L-thyroxine. How should the TSH level be interpreted? Is T_4 therapy indicated, based on her presenting findings?

[SI units: TSH, 2.5 mIU/L (normal, 0.5–4.7)]

Despite complaints that could be consistent with hypothyroidism (e.g., fatigue, cold intolerance, dry skin, weight gain), the normal TSH level indicates that J.P. is euthyroid. However, because a diagnosis of hypopituitarism (i.e., TSH level could be normal or low) cannot be ruled out, an FT_4 level should be obtained; a low level would increase the likelihood of hypopituitarism. Some argue that hypopituitarism is underdiagnosed and would advocate adding FT_4 to the primary screening tests.[130]

If the FT_4 level is normal, indicating euthyroidism, then hypopituitarism is unlikely and L-thyroxine therapy is not indicated. A randomized, double-blind, placebo-controlled crossover trial found that T_4 supplementation in patients with hypothyroid symptoms and normal thyroid function tests was not more effective than placebo in improving cognitive function or psychological well-being despite changes in the TSH and FT_4 levels.[131,132]

In J.P., the T_4 should be discontinued because there is no evidence of its efficacy in euthyroid individuals.

HYPERTHYROIDISM

Clinical Presentation

24. S.K., a 48-year-old woman, is admitted to the hospital for a possible MI. Her complaints include chest pain that is unrelieved by NTG, increasing SOB with exercise, nervousness, palpitations, muscle weakness, weight loss despite an increased appetite, and epistaxis; she also bruises easily. She has a history of deep venous thrombosis treated with warfarin (Coumadin) 5 mg/day; her last prothrombin time (PT) was 18 seconds (normal, 10.5–12.1), and an international normalized ratio (INR) was 1.8 (normal, 1; therapeutic, 2–3). She has angina, treated with NTG 0.4 mg, and CHF, treated with digoxin (Lanoxin) 0.25 mg/day.

Physical examination reveals a thin, flushed, hyperkinetic, nervous woman. Blood pressure (BP) is 180/90 mmHg; pulse is 130 beats/minute, irregularly irregular; respiratory rate is 30 breaths/min; and temperature is 37.5°C. Other pertinent findings include a lid lag with stare, proptosis with tearing, decreased visual acuity, a diffusely enlarged thyroid gland without nodules, a bruit in the left lobe of the thyroid, positive jugular venous distention (JVD), bibasilar rales, warm moist skin with multiple bruises, new-onset atrial fibrillation (AF), slight diarrhea, hepatomegaly, acropachy, 2+ pitting edema, a fine tremor, proximal muscle weakness, and irregular scant menses.

Laboratory data include FT_4, 2.9 ng/dL (normal, 0.7–1.9); TSH, <0.5 μunits/mL (normal, 0.5–4.7); RAIU at 24 hours, 80% (normal, 5%–35%); PT, 40 seconds (normal, 10.5–12.1); INR,

4.8 (normal, 1; therapeutic, 2–3); TPO, 200 IU/mL (normal, <1); alkaline phosphatase, 200 units/L (normal, 41–133); total bilirubin, 1.1 mg/dL (normal, 0.1–1.2); AST, 60 units/L (normal, 7–26); and alanine aminotransferase (ALT), 55 units/L (normal, 3–23). A scan shows a diffusely enlarged gland, three to four times normal size. What subjective and objective data are suggestive of hyperthyroidism in S.K.?

S.K. presents with many of the clinical and laboratory features[133] associated with an increased metabolic state resulting from excessive T_4 (Table 49-6). Her ocular symptoms are consistent with Graves' disease and include lid lag (lid falls behind the movement of the eye and a narrow white rim of sclera becomes visible between the upper lid and cornea, producing a "staring" appearance), ophthalmopathy (protrusion of the eyeball), and decreased visual acuity. The thyroid bruit, palpitations, exertional dyspnea, worsening CHF (JVD, bibasilar rales, edema, hepatomegaly), diarrhea, irregular scant menses, nervousness, tremor, muscle weakness, weight loss despite increased appetite, increased perspiration, and flushing of the skin are consistent with a hypermetabolic state. Although sinus tachycardia is the most common arrhythmia in hyperthyroidism, new-onset AF is the presenting symptom in 5% to 20% of patients with hyperthyroidism, particularly in those older than 70 years.[134] Together with S.K.'s symptoms, a diagnosis of Graves' disease is confirmed by an elevated FT_4 level, an undetectable TSH level, an increased RAIU, positive TPO antibodies, and a diffusely enlarged goiter. Her cardiac status and other medical problems are aggravated by the hyperthyroidism. (Table 49-5 lists the causes of hyperthyroidism.)

Hypoprothrombinemia

25. What factors contribute to S.K.'s hypoprothrombinemia? What effect could this have on her subsequent drug treatment?

The hypoprothrombinemia and bleeding observed in S.K. are most likely related to an exaggerated response to warfarin. This may be related to a decrease in the hepatic metabolism of warfarin (secondary to hepatic congestion), but it is more likely that S.K.'s findings are due to the combined effects of hyperthyroidism and warfarin on vitamin K–dependent clotting factors.

Warfarin Metabolism

Warfarin metabolism and the metabolism of vitamin K–dependent clotting factors can be altered by thyroid status. Net circulating levels of vitamin K–dependent clotting factors are generally not altered in hyperthyroid patients because both the synthesis and catabolism of these clotting factors are increased. However, an enhanced anticoagulant response occurs when the warfarin-induced decrease in clotting factor synthesis is combined with the hyperthyroidism-induced increase in clotting factor catabolism.[33,135] This may explain S.K.'s elevated prothrombin time, bruising, and history of epistaxis.

The opposite occurs in hypothyroidism, in which a decrease in both the metabolism and synthesis of clotting factors occurs. In hypothyroid patients, the response to oral anticoagulants is delayed because the clotting factors are eliminated more slowly.[33,135] Therefore, hyperthyroid patients need less warfarin, whereas hypothyroid patients require more warfarin to achieve the same hypoprothrombinemic response. The anticoagulant response to warfarin should be monitored carefully in patients with thyroid abnormalities, and the dosage adjusted as the thyroid status changes.

Thioamide Effects

Because S.K.'s hyperthyroidism will most likely be treated with a thioamide, caution must be exercised. Treatment of hyperthyroid patients with thioamides, especially PTU, has been associated with hypoprothrombinemia, thrombocytopenia, and bleeding, albeit rarely.[136] These drugs can depress the bone marrow and the synthesis of clotting factors II, VII, III, IX, X, and XIII; vitamin K and prothrombin times may remain depressed for up to 2 months after discontinuation of therapy. These effects may be caused by a subclinical hepatic alteration in synthesis or hepatotoxicity (see question 38).[137–139] Symptoms occur 2 weeks to 18 months after starting therapy. The bleeding is responsive to vitamin K or blood transfusions. (Also see questions 31 and 32 for further discussion of treatment with thioamides.)

Response to Digoxin

26. After treatment with RAI, S.K.'s daily dose of digoxin was increased to 0.5 mg because of persistent AF and rapid ventricular response. Six weeks later, she returns with complaints of nausea and vomiting. The gland remains palpable but is decreased considerably in size. The ECG shows ST depression, atrioventricular (AV) block, and occasional bigeminy. Assess these subjective and objective data.

S.K.'s nausea and vomiting, together with the ECG changes of AV block and bigeminy, strongly suggest digitalis toxicity. Although a high dosage of digoxin is appropriate while a patient is thyrotoxic, continuation of this same dose as the hyperthyroidism resolves increases the likelihood of digitalis toxicity.[119,120]

27. Why was such a large dose of digoxin required initially? What other options can be used to control the ventricular rate?

The AF of hyperthyroidism is often resistant to digitalis. When euthyroid patients with AF were given digitalis before and after exogenous T_3 administration, the daily dose of digoxin required to maintain a ventricular rate of 70 was increased from 0.2 to 0.8 mg after T_3 administration.[140] Higher dosages of digoxin without side effects might be tolerated better by the hyperthyroid patient.[119,120,140] Nevertheless, the goal of digoxin therapy should be a higher target heart rate (i.e., 100 beats/minute) than that achieved with digoxin in the euthyroid patient with AF to minimize cardiac toxicity. If additional rate control is required, β-blockers or calcium channel blockers (e.g., diltiazem or verapamil) can be added. Unless contraindicated by severe bronchospasm, β-blockers rather than calcium channel blockers are preferred because they are more effective in controlling the ventricular rate and are less likely to cause hypotension.

This apparent resistance to digitalis is attributed to intrinsic changes in myocardial function, to an increased volume of distribution for digoxin, and to an increased glomerular filtration of the glycoside.[119,120,140] Conversely, hypothyroid patients are inordinately sensitive to the effects of digitalis and require smaller doses to achieve a therapeutic response. Regardless of the mechanism, one should be aware that higher-than-normal doses might be required in patients with thyrotoxicosis and that the initial dosage should be reduced as the hyperthyroid state resolves.

Cardioversion

28. If the AF persists, when should cardioversion be attempted in S.K.? Is other treatment indicated?

Because S.K. received RAI 6 weeks ago, her thyroid function tests should be rechecked to determine her present thyroid status. Cardioversion, either medical or electrical, should not be attempted if she is still toxic because the success rate is low. AF spontaneously reverted to normal sinus rhythm (NSR) in 56% to 62% of patients within the first 3 to 4 months after control of the hyperthyroidism.[134] Spontaneous conversion is highly unlikely if the duration of the hyperthyroidism-induced AF exceeds 13 months or if the AF persists after 4 months of euthyroidism.[134] Older patients with or without underlying heart disorders (except CHF) are also less likely to spontaneously convert to NSR. Patients who meet these criteria are candidates for cardioversion at about the third or fourth month after achieving euthyroidism. Age and the duration of thyrotoxicosis are important determinants of successful cardioversion. Ninety percent of patients achieved NSR after cardioversion; of these, 57% and 48% maintained NSR at 10 and 14 years, respectively, of follow-up.[134]

S.K. should be maintained on warfarin because of a high prevalence of systemic embolization in thyrotoxic patients with AF. Anticoagulation should be started when the AF is first diagnosed and continued until S.K. is euthyroid and in NSR. This is especially true for younger patients at low risk of bleeding with Coumadin. The risks versus benefits of anticoagulation should be weighed before therapy (see Chapter 16). Because an increased sensitivity to warfarin is observed, close monitoring is warranted (see Question 25).

Thyrotoxicosis: Clinical Presentation

29. C.R., a 27-year-old woman, has a 3-month history of intermittent heat intolerance, sweats, tremor, and severe muscle weakness, which has limited her ability to climb stairs. Her weight has increased because of increased appetite. She is also bothered by the pounding of her heart and some minor difficulty in swallowing. There is a family history of thyroid disease, but she denies taking any thyroid medications or any history of radiation to her neck. C.R. previously received iodide drops with symptomatic improvement, but her disease recurred despite its continued administration. Her other medical problems include diabetes, which is controlled with diet, and osteoarthritis, which is treated with aspirin 2.5 g/day. She has a history of noncompliance with her clinic visits.

Pertinent physical findings include a BP of 180/90 mmHg, a pulse of 110 beats/minute, hyperreflexia, lid lag, and a diffusely enlarged thyroid gland that is about four times normal (about 100 g). Laboratory data include TT_4, 6 mcg/dL (normal, 5–12); FT_4, 2 ng/dL (normal, 0.7–1.9); TSH, <0.01 μunits/mL (normal, 0.5–4.7); TPO, 350 IU/mL (normal, <1); and blood glucose, 350 mg/dL (normal, 60–115). Assess these subjective and objective data.

[SI units: TT_4, 77 nmol/L (normal, 64–154); FT_4, 28 pmol/L (normal, 9–24); TSH, <0.01 mIU/L (normal, 0.5–4.7); blood glucose, 19.4 mmol/L (normal, 3.3–6.4)]

C.R.'s clinical findings verify an autoimmune hyperthyroid state. However, the serum FT_4 is elevated only slightly and is disproportionately low relative to the severity of her symptoms, the undetectable TSH level, and her other laboratory findings. The low normal TT_4 could be explained by displacement of T_4 from TBG by aspirin (see Question 3). The possibility of a variant type of hyperthyroidism known as T_3 toxicosis should be considered. The clinical features include signs and symptoms of thyrotoxicosis, normal or borderline high FT_4, an undetectable TSH level, and elevated T_3 levels. The latter occurs through preferential secretion and peripheral conversion of T_4 to T_3. A T_3 level should be obtained to establish the diagnosis.

Asymptomatic elevations of T_3 levels often precede elevation of T_4 levels and the development of overt hyperthyroidism. T_3 toxicosis probably represents an early stage of classic T_4 toxicosis and is useful for early diagnosis or as an early indicator of relapse after discontinuation of thioamide therapy.

Iodides

30. Why were the iodide drops initially effective in improving C.R.'s symptoms and later ineffective? When are iodides indicated? What is their mechanism of action?

Iodides have several effects: They inhibit thyroid hormone release, they block iodotyrosine and iodothyronine synthesis by blocking organification, and they decrease the vascularity of the thyroid gland.[141] However, large doses may accentuate hyperthyroidism because they provide a significant increase in available substrate for hormone synthesis (see question 54).[141,142]

The inhibitory effect of exogenous iodides on the intrathyroidal organification of iodides is known as the Wolff-Chaikoff effect. This is an inherent autoregulatory function of the normal gland to prevent excessive hormone synthesis in the event of a large iodide load. The Wolff-Chaikoff effect occurs when intrathyroidal concentrations of iodides reach a critical level, and this is not overcome by TSH stimulation. However, as illustrated by C.R., the gland can "escape" from this block even with continued iodide use. The gland escapes by decreasing iodide transport or by leaking iodide. Both mechanisms decrease the critical intrathyroidal iodide level, thereby decreasing the block to organification. This effect is illustrated in C.R. Therefore, iodides should not be used as primary therapy for Graves' disease.

Conversely, some patients are responsive to iodide therapy, including (a) patients who already have high intrathyroidal iodine stores (i.e., "hot" nodules, Graves' disease); (b) patients with underlying defects in organic binding mechanisms (i.e., Hashimoto's); (c) patients who develop drug-induced thyroid disorders (see questions 52–55); and (d) patients with Graves' disease made euthyroid with RAI or surgery and who are receiving no thyroid replacement.

These patients are so sensitive that small doses of iodide can elicit the Wolff-Chaikoff effect, resulting in either amelioration of hyperthyroid symptoms or precipitation of hypothyroidism.[141–143] For this reason, patients with recurrent hyperthyroidism after surgery or RAI can often be managed with iodides alone.

The most important pharmacologic effect of iodides is their ability to promptly inhibit thyroid hormone release when dosages of 6 mg/day are given.[141,143] The mechanism is unknown, but it is not related to the Wolff-Chaikoff effect, which may take several weeks to manifest. Unlike the Wolff-Chaikoff effect, this effect can be overcome partially by an increase in TSH secretion. Thus, the normal gland can escape in 7 to 14 days because inhibition of thyroid hormone release stimulates a reflex increase in TSH secretion. Because patients with hyperthyroidism experience an improvement in symptoms within 2 to 7 days of initiation of therapy, inhibition of hormone release must be the predominant mechanism of action for the iodides. This rapid onset is the reason iodides are used in the treatment of thyroid storm and as an ameliorative measure while awaiting the onset of the therapeutic effects of thioamides or RAI.

Large doses of iodides are also used 2 weeks before thyroid surgery to increase the firmness of the thyroid gland by decreasing its size, vascularity, and friability. Iodides facilitate a smoother, less complicated surgery and reduce the risk of postoperative complications by inducing a euthyroid state.[141]

Stable iodine can be administered orally either as an unpleasant-tasting Lugol's solution (5% iodine and 10% potassium iodide), containing 8 mg/drop of iodide, or as the more palatable saturated solution of potassium iodide (SSKI), containing 50 mg/drop of iodide. The minimum effective daily dose is 6 mg,[141] although larger doses (e.g., 5–10 drops QID of SSKI) are often administered.

The advantages of iodide therapy are that it is simple, inexpensive, and relatively nontoxic and involves no glandular destruction. Disadvantages include "escape," accentuation of thyrotoxicosis, allergic reactions, relapse after discontinuation of treatment, and subsequent interference with RAI if used before therapy.

Treatment Modalities

31. What are the advantages and disadvantages of the different treatment modalities available for C.R.?

The three major treatment modalities for Graves'-related hyperthyroidism are the thioamides, RAI, and surgery (Table 49-10).[133] In most cases, any of these three modalities can be used, and there is controversy as to which is the most effective therapy. Often the final decision is empiric, depending on the physician's available resources and the patient's desires. A review of treatment guidelines published by the major endocrine organizations found that RAI is the most common treatment, while surgery is the least common.[144] Patients who are older and those with cardiac disease, concomitant ophthalmopathy, and hyperthyroidism caused by a toxic multinodular goiter are treated best with RAI. Surgery is the preferred therapy for pregnant women who are drug intolerant, when obstructive symptoms are present, or if malignancy is suspected.

Thioamides

The thioamides are the preferred treatment for children, pregnant women, and young adults with uncomplicated Graves' disease.[133,145,146] This is the only treatment that leaves the thyroid gland intact and does not carry the added risk of permanent hypothyroidism often associated with RAI or surgery.

Because the thyrotoxicosis of Graves' disease might be self-limiting, thioamides are used to control the symptoms until spontaneous remission occurs. Thioamides should also be given before treatment with RAI or surgery to deplete the gland of stored thyroid hormone, which prevents subsequent thyroid storm. Although hyperthyroidism from toxic nodules will also respond to thioamides, more definitive therapy (surgery or RAI) is needed because these conditions do not undergo spontaneous remission.

Disadvantages of thioamide therapy include the numerous tablets required, patient adherence, possible drug toxicity, the long duration of treatment, and the low remission rates after discontinuation of therapy (see Question 42).

The use of thioamides in C.R. has several potential drawbacks. Her relatively large gland and severe disease make the prognosis for spontaneous remission somewhat less favorable. A delay in the onset of thioamide's effect may be expected if intraglandular stores of thyroid have been increased by her prior iodide therapy. Furthermore, her nonadherence and difficulty swallowing may necessitate another means of treatment. Thioamides may also be prepared for administration by the rectal routes.[147–149]

Surgery

Surgery is considered the treatment of choice[133,150–152] when (a) malignancy is suspected; (b) esophageal obstruction, evidenced by difficulty swallowing, is present; (c) respiratory difficulties are present; (d) contraindications to the use of thioamides (e.g., allergy) or RAI (e.g., pregnancy) exist; (e) a large goiter that regresses poorly on RAI or thioamide therapy is present; or (f) it is the patient's preference. Some argue that surgery is underused in the treatment of Graves' disease.[150] In a prospective, randomized trial comparing the three treatment modalities, surgery produced euthyroidism more quickly and was associated with a lower relapse rate than either RAI or thioamides.[151] A meta-analysis of 35 studies encompassing 7,241 patients with Graves' disease found that thyroidectomy was successful in 92% of patients with a low recurrence (7.2%) of hyperthyroidism.[153] If C.R.'s minor difficulty in swallowing persists because of poor regression of goiter size with drug therapy, then surgery is a reasonable alternative. If surgery is contemplated, C.R. must be brought to surgery in a euthyroid state to prevent rapid postoperative rises in T_4 levels and subsequent thyroid storm (see Question 50). A total or near-total rather than a subtotal thyroidectomy is the procedure of choice when performed by an experienced surgeon.[150,152,153] Although subtotal thyroidectomy theoretically avoids the predictable risk of hypothyroidism from total thyroidectomy; the likelihood of recurrent hyperthyroidism increases in proportion to the amount of residual thyroid tissue remaining.[150,151] Recurrent thyrotoxicosis following a subtotal thyroidectomy should be treated with RAI because the incidence of surgical complications increases with a second surgery.

Surgical complication rates are low when the procedure is performed by a competent surgeon and when the patient is adequately prepared for surgery. The disadvantages of surgery are expense, hospitalization, hypothyroidism, the small risk of postoperative complications, and the patient's fear of surgery (see Question 40).[150,151,153]

Table 49-10 Treatment for Hyperthyroidism

Modality	Drug/Dosage	Mechanism of Action	Toxicity	Indication
Primary Treatment				
Thioamides				
PTU 50 mg tablet; rectal formulation can be made[147,148]	100–200 mg PO q6–8h (*max:* 1,200 mg/d) for 6–8 wk or until euthyroid; then maintenance of 50–150 mg QD PO × 12–18 mo	Blocks organification of hormone synthesis, blocks peripheral conversion of T_4 to T_3 (PTU only)	Skin rashes, GI symptoms, arthralgias, ↑ transaminases, hepatitis, agranulocytosis	DOC in thyroid storm, pregnancy, and breast-feeding
Methimazole (Tapazole) 5-, 10-mg tablet; rectal suppositories can be made[149]	Methimazole 30–40 mg PO QD or in two divided doses (*max:* 60 mg/d) for 6–8 wk or until euthyroid, then maintenance of 5–10 mg/d PO × 12–18 mo	Similar to PTU except does not block conversion of T_4 to T_3	Similar to PTU; cholestatic jaundice, reports of aplasia cutis	Thioamide DOC (see PTU) because QD dosing and better compliance
Surgery	Preoperative preparation with iodides, thioamides, or β-blockers before surgery; see specific operative agent	Near total thyroidectomy	Hypothyroidism, cosmetic scarring, hypoparathyroidism, risks of surgery, and anesthesia, vocal cord damage	Obstruction, choking, malignancy, pregnancy in second trimester, contraindication to RAI or thioamides
RAI	^{131}I radioactive isotope; 80–100 μCi/g thyroid tissue. Average dose, ≈10 mCi; pretreatment with corticosteroids indicated in patients with ophthalmopathy	Destruction of the gland	Hypothyroidism; worsening of ophthalmopathy; fear of radiation-induced leukemia; genetic damage; malignancy; rarely, radiation sickness	Adults, older patients who are poor surgical risks or have cardiac disease; patients with a history of prior thyroid surgery; contraindications to thioamide usage; increasingly used in kids
Adjuncts to Primary Usage				
Iodides				
Lugol's solution 8 mg/drop (5% iodine, 10% potassium iodide; saturated [SSKI] 50 mg/drop)	5–10 drops TID PO for 10–14 days before surgery; minimum effective dose 6 mg/day	↓ vascularity of gland and ↑ firmness; blocks release of thyroid hormone	Hypersensitivity reactions, skin rashes, mucous membrane ulcers, anaphylaxis, metallic taste, rhinorrhea, parotid and submaxillary swelling; fetal goiters and death	Preoperative preparation before surgery; thyroid storm, provides symptomatic relief of symptoms. *Do not use before RAI or chronically during pregnancy*
β-Blockers				
Propranolol or equivalent β-blocker. *Avoid* those with ISA	Propranolol 10–40 mg PO q6h or PRN to control HR <100 beats/min; IV 0.5–1 mg slowly	Blocks effects of thyroid hormone peripherally, no effect on underlying disease; blocks T_4 to T_3 conversion	Related to β-blockade; bradycardia, CHF, blocks hyperglycemic response to hypoglycemia, bronchospasm, CNS symptoms at high doses; fetal bradycardia	Symptomatic relief while awaiting onset of thioamides, RAI; preoperative preparation for surgery; thyroid storm
Calcium channel blockers				
	Diltiazem 120 mg TID–QID PO or verapamil 80–120 mg TID–QID PO PRN to control HR <100 beats/min	Blocks effects of thyroid hormone peripherally, no effect on underlying disease	Bradycardia, peripheral edema, CHF, headache, flushing, hypotension, dizziness	Alternative for symptomatic relief of hyperthyroid symptoms in patients who cannot tolerate β-blockers
Corticosteroids				
	Prednisone or equivalent corticosteroids 50–140 mg/day PO in divided doses; IV hydrocortisone 50–100 mg q6h or equivalent for thyroid storm	↓ TRAb, suppression of inflammatory process; blocks T_4 to T_3 conversion	Complications of steroid therapy	Ophthalmopathy, thyroid storm (use IV steroid), pretibial myxedema, pretreatment before RAI therapy in patients with ophthalmopathy

CHF, congestive heart failure; CNS, central nervous system; DOC, drug of choice; GI, gastrointestinal; HR, heart rate; ISA, intrinsic sympathomimetic activity; IV, intravenous; mCi, millicurie; PO, orally (by mouth); PRN, as needed; PTU, propylthiouracil; q, every; QD, every day; QID, four times a day; RAI, radioactive iodine; SSKI, saturated solution of potassium iodide; T_3, triiodothyronine; T_4, thyroxine; TID, three times a day; TRAb, thyroid receptor antibody; μCi, microcurie.[57–59]

Radioactive Iodine

RAI, the most common treatment modality in the United States, is the preferred treatment for (a) debilitated, cardiac, or older patients who are poor surgical candidates; (b) patients who fail to respond to drug therapy or who experience adverse drug reactions; and (c) patients who develop recurrent hyperthyroidism after surgery.[133,144,151]

Pregnancy is an absolute contraindication to RAI therapy. Previously, the use of RAI was restricted to adults older than an arbitrary age of 20 to 35 years because it was feared that RAI could result in genetic damage or neoplasia. However, its use in adolescents is increasing after more than 50 years of clinical experience with RAI showing that it is safe and effective.[154–156] There is no reported evidence of genetic damage after ^{131}I ingestion, and the dose of radiation to the gonads is <3 rads, which is comparable to other radiographic diagnostic tests (e.g., barium enemas).[157] The incidence of leukemia or malignancy is no higher in recipients of ^{131}I than in thyrotoxic patients treated with drugs or surgery.[154,158] In a retrospective review of 98 adolescents followed for 36 years after receiving ^{131}I, no cancers of the thyroid or leukemia were reported.[156] One interesting finding is that patients receiving RAI should be warned that they can set off radiation detectors at airport screening terminals for up to 12 weeks after RAI and that they should carry documentation of their treatment.[159,160]

RAI is painless, effective, economical, and quick, but unsubstantiated fears about radiation and malignancy, as well as the high incidence of hypothyroidism, may deter its use. RAI could be used safely in this nonpregnant young patient. However, C.R.'s prior use of iodides will dilute the ^{131}I pool. Thus, it will be impossible to achieve therapeutic thyroid concentrations of RAI for as long as 3 to 6 months.

Iodinated Contrast Media

The unavailability in the United States of radiographic iodinated contrast agents (e.g., ipodate, iopanoic acid, sodium tyropanoate) effective in the short-term management of hyperthyroidism may increase the use of less well-studied agents.[161] Iodinated contrast media act by inhibiting the 5-monodeiodinase enzyme responsible for the pituitary and peripheral conversion of T_4 to T_3 and also inhibit thyroid hormone secretion. Each gram of the iodinated contrast agents contains 600 to 650 mg iodine. The onset of their therapeutic effect is more rapid than that of the thioamides. After administration of ipodate 0.5 to 1 g/day, a rapid decline in T_3 concentrations by 58% and T_4 levels by 20% occurred within 24 hours; the agent was more effective than 600 mg of PTU, which decreases T_3 levels by only 23%.[162] Significant clinical improvement and maximal reductions of hormone levels were evident within 3 to 7 days. Ipodate and other contrast media are useful adjuncts to thioamides in the early treatment of severe hyperthyroidism and with RAI therapy.[163] However, long-term use is not reasonable because the antithyroid effects are transient. Serum T_3 levels can return to baseline or hyperthyroid levels within 1 month despite continued administration; subsequent response to thioamides might also be impaired.[161,162] When used as sole therapy, loss of efficacy occurs after 2 to 12 weeks.[161,162,164,165]

Treatment With Thioamides

Propylthiouracil Versus Methimazole

32. C.R. is started on PTU 200 mg q8h after baseline FT_4I and TSH levels have been obtained. Three weeks later, she angrily complains that her symptoms are worse and that the medication is not working; however, she reluctantly admits missing doses because of difficulty swallowing, nausea, vomiting, diarrhea, fatigue, a cough, and a sore throat. What are the advantages of using either PTU or methimazole in the treatment of hyperthyroidism?

Both thioamides are effective in treating hyperthyroidism. The antithyroid effectiveness of the thioamides primarily depends on their ability to block the organification of iodines, thereby inhibiting thyroid hormone synthesis.[145,146] Thyroid autoantibody synthesis may also be suppressed. In most hyperthyroid situations, methimazole should be considered the drug of choice rather than PTU because patient adherence and ease of administration are improved.

DOSING AND ADMINISTRATION

Methimazole is effective when administered initially as a single dose compared with the multiple-dose regimen required with PTU to achieve a euthyroid state.[145,146] Although a single-dose regimen of PTU has been tried acutely, it is most effective when given in divided doses (see Question 41). Compared to PTU, methimazole is also less expensive, requires daily ingestion of fewer numbers of tablets, and is not associated with a bitter tablet taste. However, PTU is preferred over methimazole in thyroid storm because, unlike methimazole, it also blocks the peripheral conversion of T_4 to T_3.[166] Within 24 to 48 hours after PTU administration, a 25% to 40% reduction in peripheral T_3 production is seen, which contributes to PTU's therapeutic effectiveness. A significantly greater fall in T_3 concentration and the T_3:T_4 ratio can be demonstrated in hyperthyroid patients treated acutely with PTU and iodine than with methimazole and iodides. Last, PTU is preferred over methimazole in breast-feeding and pregnant patients (see Question 44).

33. Why was the thioamide therapy ineffective in C.R.? Was the dose of PTU appropriate?

The inadequate response in C.R. suggests poor adherence to the thioamide dosing regimen or a delayed response caused by prior iodide loading of the gland.

The onset of action of the thioamides is slow because they block the synthesis rather than the release of thyroid hormone. Therefore, hormone secretion will continue until the glandular stores of hormone are depleted. If adequate doses were given, some improvement of clinical symptoms should be noted after 2 or 3 weeks.[146]

The dosage of PTU is appropriate. Thioamide dosing consists of two phases: initial therapy to achieve euthyroidism, and maintenance therapy to achieve remission. Initially, high blocking dosages of PTU (400–800 mg/day, depending on the severity of the toxicosis) should be given in three or four divided doses, as in C.R.[133,145,146] Rarely, dosages of 1,200 mg/day of PTU or its equivalent may be required in patients with severe disease or storm.[166] Equipotent doses of methimazole (which is 10 times more potent than PTU on a mg-per-mg basis) can also be used. However, it is usually unnecessary to use >40 mg/day of methimazole to restore a euthyroid state.[133,145,146]

Toxicity is also less common (see questions 38 and 39). True resistance to thioamides is rare; thus, most cases of unresponsiveness are caused by poor patient adherence, as in C.R.

C.R.'s adherence is also hindered by the frequency of PTU administration. The serum half-life of PTU is short (1.5 hours), but it is the intrathyroidal drug concentrations that should determine the dosing intervals because they are most clearly related to the drug's antithyroid effects[146] (see question 41). PTU must be dosed every 6 to 8 hours initially, or as frequently as every 4 hours in cases of severe hyperthyroidism and thyroid storm. In contrast, methimazole has a serum half-life of 6 to 8 hours, remains in the thyroid for 20 hours, and has a duration of activity of up to 40 hours.[146,167]

If C.R. is taking her PTU as directed, then an increase in the PTU dosage to 200 mg every 6 hours is reasonable. However, poor adherence is often difficult to ascertain and is more likely when multiple daily doses are required. The best option for C.R. is to change to 30 to 40 mg of methimazole, given once daily to improve adherence, or divided into two doses to decrease GI distress. After methimazole is given for 4 to 6 weeks to achieve euthyroidism, the daily dosage can be reduced gradually by 25% to 30% monthly to a dosage that maintains euthyroidism, usually 5 to 10 mg/day of methimazole or 50 to 150 mg/day of PTU. If C.R. remains hyperthyroid despite adequate doses of thioamides, then the most likely reason is nonadherence.

MONITORING THERAPY

34. What additional objective baseline data should be obtained to monitor both the efficacy and toxicity of thioamides?

Before thioamides are administered, a baseline FT_4 and TSH should be obtained. A baseline white blood cell (WBC) count with differential can also help differentiate the leukopenia associated with hyperthyroidism from drug-induced leukopenia and/or agranulocytosis (see Question 39). Baseline liver function tests can assist in the evaluation of thioamide-induced hepatotoxicity (see Question 38). A repeat FT_4 and TSH should be obtained after 4 to 6 weeks on therapy and 4 to 6 weeks after any change in the dosing regimen. Once the patient is euthyroid on maintenance dosages, thyroid function tests can be obtained every 3 to 6 months.

DURATION OF THERAPY

35. How long should C.R. be continued on thioamide treatment?

Traditionally, thioamide therapy is continued for 1 to 2 years despite the lack of data regarding the optimal treatment period.[133,145,146] The goal of treatment is to control the symptoms of Graves' disease until spontaneous remission occurs. Graves' disease remits spontaneously in about 25% to 30% of patients.[168] Because it is unknown when or if remission will occur, it is understandable why the optimal duration of therapy is unclear. Short-term therapy (i.e., <6 months) has been advocated to save time and money and improve adherence because earlier studies suggested remission rates comparable to a longer course of therapy. However, short-term therapy is not recommended because longer follow-ups of patients receiving short-term therapy have noted remission rates comparable to those observed with spontaneous remission.[145,146]

Most data support a 12- to 18-month course of treatment to achieve remission rates of approximately 60%.[145,146,169,170] Two prospective randomized trials found that extending treatment from 6 to 18 months was beneficial but that 42 months of therapy was not significantly better than 18 months.[169,170] However, one retrospective study of patients treated for >12 months observed remission rates of only 17.5%.[171] These conflicting results underscore the fact that determining the optimal treatment period is confounded by the large variability that exists with regard to spontaneous remission. Nevertheless, treatment periods of 1 to 2 years are justifiable in adherent patients. Therapy can be reinstituted if hyperthyroidism reappears shortly after therapy is discontinued. Thioamides can also be continued indefinitely if there are no side effects and treatment with either RAI or surgery is not desired. In C.R., this goal might not be achievable, given her history of nonadherence.

Precautions

36. Can thioamide therapy affect any of C.R.'s pre-existing medical conditions?

Thyrotoxicosis can activate or intensify diabetes, primarily by increasing the basal hepatic glucose production and the metabolism of insulin.[172] Therefore, effective therapy with thioamides may restore control of C.R.'s diabetes.

C.R.'s arthritis should not be affected by the PTU, although both PTU and methimazole are associated with the development of lupus erythematosus (LE), lupuslike syndromes, and vasculitis.[146,173] These adverse drug reactions are rare; the incidence is <0.1%. Lupuslike syndromes include skin ulcers, splenomegaly, migratory polyarthritis, pleuritis and pericarditis, periarteritis, and renal abnormalities. Serologic abnormalities may also occur with these connective tissue disorders and include hyperglobulinemia, positive LE preparations, and positive antinuclear antibodies. Recovery occurs with adequate steroid therapy and withdrawal of the thioamides. Because cross-reaction between methimazole and PTU is likely to occur, patients exhibiting these reactions should be treated with surgery or RAI. C.R.'s treatment should be monitored with this lupuslike adverse effect in mind, but the occurrence of this syndrome is so uncommon that a troublefree course of therapy can be anticipated.

Adjunctive Therapy

37. What adjunctive therapy might help alleviate some of C.R.'s symptoms while awaiting the onset of thioamide's effects?

Iodides (see question 30), β-adrenergic blocking agents without intrinsic sympathomimetic activity, or calcium channel blockers can be used acutely to ameliorate some of C.R.'s symptoms.[174,175] Because iodides were previously ineffective in C.R., a β-blocker should be tried.

β-adrenergic blocking agents rapidly decrease the nervousness, palpitations, fatigue, weight loss, diaphoresis, heat intolerance, and tremor associated with thyrotoxicosis, probably because many of the signs and symptoms mimic sympathetic overactivity.[133,174] An increase in the number of β-adrenergic receptors rather than an elevation in catecholamine levels is probably responsible for this overactivity. Because the underlying disease process and thyroid hormone levels are not affected significantly by β-blockers, patients generally remain mildly symptomatic and fail to gain weight. For this reason, they should not be used as the sole treatment for thyrotoxicosis.

All β-blockers without intrinsic sympathetic activity (e.g., atenolol, metoprolol, propranolol) are effective in alleviating the hyperthyroid symptoms, but propranolol (Inderal) is the only β-blocker that inhibits peripheral conversion of T_4 to T_3.[174] Thyroid function tests are generally not affected except for a mild decrease in the T_3 level.

In summary, β-blockers are (a) effective adjuncts in the management of thyroid storm, (b) useful to prepare patients for surgery, and (c) useful in the short-term management of thyrotoxicosis during pregnancy.[150,166,174] Surprisingly, propranolol also improves many of the neuromuscular manifestations of hyperthyroidism, including thyrotoxic periodic paralysis.

Diltiazem or verapamil are effective alternatives when β-blockers are contraindicated.[175] Diltiazem 120 mg TID or QID can be tried. The dihydropyridine calcium channel blockers are unlikely to be effective.

Because of C.R.'s history of diabetes, the effects of β-adrenergic blocking drugs in patients with diabetes must be considered (see Chapter 50). If β-blockers are instituted, a cardioselective β-blocker would be a better choice. The appropriate dosage should be based on clinical and objective improvement of hyperthyroid symptoms, such as a reduction in heart rate. Metoprolol 25 to 50 mg BID can be started initially and the dosage titrated to maintain the heart rate at <90 beats/minute. Otherwise, diltiazem, verapamil, or a retrial of iodides is warranted.

Adverse Effects

38. A pruritic area over the pretibial aspects of both legs, as well as several maculopapular erythematous patches and abdominal tenderness, were noticed during C.R.'s physical examination. Do these reactions require the discontinuation of her PTU?

THIOAMIDE RASH

Although C.R. may be experiencing a drug rash from PTU, pretibial myxedema or the dermopathy of Graves' disease may also be possibilities because of the location of the pruritic area. About 4% of patients with Graves' disease who exhibit infiltrative exophthalmos also have dermatologic changes. The skin is thickened, erythematous, and nonpitting because of mucopolysaccharide infiltration and accentuation of hair follicles. Pruritus or pain may be present. Treatment includes topical corticosteroids, control of the Graves' disease, and reassurance.

Both PTU and methimazole can produce a maculopapular pruritic rash in 5% to 6% of treated patients.[146] The rash can occur at any time but is more common early in therapy. If the rash is mild, drug therapy can be continued while the patient's symptoms are treated with an antihistamine and a topical steroid; such rashes generally subside spontaneously. Alternatively, another thioamide can be substituted because cross-sensitivity to this side effect is uncommon. If the rash is urticarial or is associated with other systemic manifestations of a drug reaction (e.g., fever, arthralgias), thioamides should be stopped and nondrug treatment considered.

HEPATITIS

C.R.'s symptoms of nausea, vomiting, diarrhea, fatigue, and abdominal tenderness require further evaluation. Her symptoms could be consistent with mild GI side effects from her PTU therapy or with impending thyroid storm from nonadherence (see Question 50). Taking the PTU after meals or changing to methimazole could improve medication tolerability and adherence. However, the possibility of drug-induced hepatitis should be considered. Typically, PTU-induced hepatotoxicity is hepatocellular in nature, but cholestasis, hepatic necrosis, and fulminant hepatic failures have been reported.[137,138,146] Transient elevations in transaminases occur in approximately 30% of asymptomatic patients within the first 2 months of PTU therapy and may not require drug discontinuation.[137] The liver enzymes usually normalize within 3 months of reducing the PTU to maintenance dosages despite drug continuation. However, PTU should be stopped immediately in patients with clinical symptoms of hepatitis to ensure complete recovery. The mechanism of PTU-induced hepatotoxicity appears to be autoimmune because circulating autoantibodies and in vitro peripheral lymphocyte sensitization to PTU have been detected.[138] Overt hepatitis typically occurs during the first 2 months of PTU therapy and is not dose related. In contrast, methimazole typically produces a cholestatic jaundice picture and might be more common in older patients and in those receiving higher dosages (i.e., >40 mg/day).[139] In patients with thioamide-induced hepatitis, changing to the alternative thioamide is not recommended because fatalities have been reported on rechallenge. In such patients, either radioactive therapy or surgery should be used.

The thyroid function tests, transaminases, and bilirubin should be checked in C.R. and the PTU stopped until these results are available. Routine monitoring of liver function tests is not recommended because patients can be asymptomatic. However, routine monitoring might be indicated in patients with a history of liver disease and risk factors for hepatitis (e.g., alcohol use). All patients receiving thioamides should be questioned closely during the first 2 months of therapy for symptoms of hepatitis, and hepatic function tests should be obtained if appropriate.

AGRANULOCYTOSIS

39. Assess C.R.'s complaints of sore throat and cough.

C.R.'s complaints should not be dismissed casually because they might indicate PTU-induced agranulocytosis. Agranulocytosis (<500/mm^3 of neutrophils) is the most severe adverse hematologic reaction associated with the thioamides and should be considered strongly in C.R.[146,176] In contrast, drug-induced leukopenia is usually transient, is not associated with impending agranulocytosis, and is not an indication to discontinue thioamide therapy. An accurate history should be obtained from C.R. The clinician should be particularly alert for a temperature of 101°F for 2 or more days, malaise, or other flulike findings that appeared temporally with her sore throat. If subjective or objective data are consistent with agranulocytosis, the PTU should be discontinued immediately until the results of a repeat WBC count with a differential are obtained. Traditionally, routine serial determinations of WBC counts are not recommended for monitoring the development of agranulocytosis because the onset is so abrupt. Instead, patients should be instructed to immediately report rash, fever, sore throat, or any flulike symptoms. However, one study suggested that weekly monitoring of the WBC count with a differential during the first 3 months of antithyroid therapy might identify asymptomatic patients with agranulocytosis before infection occurs.[176]

The prevalence of agranulocytosis is about 0.5% but ranges from 0.5% to 6%.[146,176] The risk factors for agranulocytosis are unknown. There is no predilection for either gender, and the reaction may be idiosyncratic or dose related. Some reports suggest that patients older than 40 years or those taking high dosages of methimazole (e.g., >40 mg/day) might be more susceptible than those on any dosage of PTU. Although controversial, patients receiving low dosages of methimazole (e.g., <40 mg/day) might be at less risk than those receiving high or conventional dosages of PTU.[146,176]

Agranulocytosis typically develops within the first 3 months of treatment, although it can occur at any time and as late as 12 months after starting thioamide therapy.[146] A delayed reaction is more common with methimazole therapy than with PTU. In 55 patients who developed agranulocytosis while taking thioamides, the duration of PTU therapy (17.7 ± 9.7 days) was significantly shorter than for methimazole therapy (36.9 ± 14.5 days).[176] The mechanism of thioamide-induced agranulocytosis is unknown. Both allergic- (idiosyncratic) and toxic-type (dose-related) reactions have been suggested. An autoimmune reaction with circulating antineutrophil antibodies and lymphocyte sensitization to antithyroid drugs has been demonstrated.[177] Death usually results from overwhelming infection.

If agranulocytosis is diagnosed, the drug should be discontinued, the patient monitored for signs of infection, and antibiotics instituted if necessary. Granulocyte colony-stimulating factors may shorten the recovery period.[146,178] If the patient recovers, granulocytes begin to reappear in the periphery within a few days to 3 weeks; a normal granulocyte count occurs shortly thereafter.[176,178]

Although some cases of granulocytopenia have resolved with substitution or continuation of thioamides, the risks of drug rechallenge clearly outweigh the benefits, and other treatments should be instituted. Changing to an alternative thioamide should also be avoided because of possible cross-sensitivity between these agents.[146]

In summary, all patients receiving thioamide therapy should be well educated regarding the signs and symptoms of agranulocytosis. If these symptoms develop, they should be advised to contact their physician or pharmacist. If they cannot reach their own physician, patients should inform the emergency physician that they are taking thioamides, and a WBC count with differential should be obtained. Routine monitoring of a WBC and differential is not recommended until further studies justify that it is indicated and cost effective.

Preoperative Preparation

40. C.R.'s PTU is discontinued because she developed agranulocytosis and hepatitis, and surgery is scheduled when her granulocyte level returns to normal. What thyroid preparation is needed for C.R. before thyroidectomy? What postoperative complications are associated with thyroidectomy?

C.R. should be in a euthyroid state at the time of surgery to avoid precipitation of thyroid storm and morbidity. Generally, iodides (see Question 30), thioamides, or propranolol can be used.[141,166,174] The combination of iodides and propranolol is more effective than either used alone. Propranolol used alone has been associated with thyroid crisis postoperatively and may be less effective than iodides in decreasing gland friability and vascularity.[174]

Because C.R. received only 1 week of thioamide therapy, it is likely that her gland still contains large stores of hormone; therefore, pretreatment is necessary.

In addition to the risks of anesthesia and surgery, postoperative complications include hypoparathyroidism, adhesions, laryngeal nerve damage, bleeding, infection, and poor wound healing. However, the surgery can be uneventful if it is performed by experienced surgeons.[150–153,179] Complications are also higher if a total rather than a subtotal thyroidectomy is performed, but there is a lower risk of recurrent hyperthyroidism. Development of hypothyroidism, especially subclinical hypothyroidism, is greatest during the first year after surgery, with an insidious rise in incidence over the next 10 years. The incidence of permanent hypothyroidism varies from 6% to 75% and is related inversely to the amount of remnant tissue left behind.[150–153,179] Thyroid function tests should be monitored annually after surgery.

Single Daily Dosing

41. J.R., a 23-year-old man newly diagnosed with Graves' disease, remains hyperthyroid after 6 weeks of PTU 200 mg q8h. He admits he has trouble remembering to take it three times a day and desires a more simplified regimen. Could J.R. be placed on a single daily dose of PTU?

A single daily dose of PTU should not be used as initial therapy because euthyroidism is achieved in only 39% to 68% of hyperthyroid patients using this approach.[146,180] However, once euthyroidism occurs, single daily doses of PTU are effective. In contrast, several clinical studies have documented that a single daily dose of methimazole is as effective as multiple daily doses in >90% of treated patients.[145,146] Although a lower dosage of methimazole (e.g., 10–15 mg QD) can produce euthyroidism with fewer side effects, higher initial dosages of 20 to 40 mg/day are recommended to increase the likelihood of euthyroidism in 6 weeks.[133,145,146]

Methimazole is the preferred agent for once-a-day dosing because of its longer intrathyroidal duration of action (40 hours).[146,167] However, as previously noted, PTU is preferable in thyroid storm because it acts more rapidly. Despite its short plasma half-life of 4 to 6 hours, a single 30-mg dose of methimazole has a duration of action of 40 hours.[167] The duration of action of PTU is unknown, but it is shorter than methimazole. Apparently, the duration of action of the antithyroid agents correlates best with the size of the dose and the intrathyroidal concentration of the drug.

J.R. should be changed to 20 to 40 mg of methimazole given once daily. Thyroid function tests should be obtained after 4 to 6 weeks and the dosage reduced as necessary to maintain euthyroidism. An effective single daily dose regimen of methimazole should increase patient acceptance and adherence.

Remission Rates With Thioamides

42. B.D., a 30-year-old woman, has been maintained on PTU 100 mg QD for >2 years. Her PTU has been discontinued twice in the past, and each time her hyperthyroidism recurred. She refuses either surgery or RAI therapy. Although she is clinically

euthyroid on the PTU, her gland is larger than normal and has never decreased with therapy. Recent laboratory tests showed an FT_4 of 1 ng/dL (normal, 0.7–1.9) and a TSH level of 6.5 μunits/mL (normal, 0.5–4.7). What is responsible for the enlarging gland? What subjective or objective data in B.D. would influence her remission rate and justify a longer course of thioamide therapy? Would the addition of T_4 be helpful?

[SI units: FT_4, 14 pmol/L (normal, 9–24); TSH, 6.5 mIU/L (normal, 0.5–4.7)]

The high TSH level suggests that TSH stimulation caused by excessive suppression of hormone synthesis by PTU is contributing to the enlarging thyroid gland. The easiest solution to this problem is to decrease the maintenance dose of PTU to 50 mg daily to normalize the TSH value and minimize gland stimulation.

Long-term remission rates achieved with the thioamides are disappointing. Remission rates within 6 years after discontinuing therapy average 50% (range, 14%–75%),[145,146,169–171] although relapse rates are as high as 80%. The rate of permanent remission is usually <25% if the follow-up period is long enough.[145,146,181] Why some patients remain in remission while others relapse once thioamides are discontinued is unclear, although patients who remain euthyroid for >10 to 15 years after discontinuing therapy probably do so because of disease progression to Hashimoto's thyroiditis rather than as a direct result of treatment.[168] In other words, the natural course of Graves' hyperthyroidism might be eventual hypothyroidism regardless of the treatment modality used. Several factors have a limited role in predicting relapse and remission and have been used to guide therapy.

A longer duration of thioamide treatment (see Question 35) improved the remission rate by changing the basic underlying abnormality of Graves' disease.[145,169–171] Numerous studies show that titers of antithyroid receptor (TRAb) and antimicrosomal antibodies fall during therapy with the thioamides but are unchanged during therapy with placebo or β-blockers.[145,146,170,182] Patients with low or undetectable TRAb titers at the end of 12 to 24 months of thioamide therapy had a 45% chance of remission compared to a <10% chance of remission for those with higher TRAb titers within 1 to 5 years after completing therapy.[181–184] The best response was obtained in those with smaller goiters, those with less severe disease, and nonsmokers. A higher dosage of thioamides does not appear to improve the remission rate but causes a higher incidence of toxicity, including agranulocytosis, arthralgias, dermatitis, gastritis, and hepatotoxicity.[145,169,181]

Some clinical features might be predictive of a higher rate of remission and may help clinicians identify patients who deserve a longer trial of drug treatment before changing to RAI or surgery. These clinical features include smaller goiter, mild symptoms of short duration, a reduction in goiter size during treatment, nonsmokers, absence of ophthalmopathy, and undetectable or low TRAb levels.[146,181,182] Smokers should be advised to discontinue smoking to increase the chance of remission.[185]

In a preliminary study, the addition of L-thyroxine to maintenance doses of thioamides given for 1 year, followed by an additional year of L-thyroxine alone, significantly reduced the risk of relapse after thioamides were discontinued.[184] Those receiving the T_4-methimazole combination experienced significant reductions in TSH receptor antibody titers compared to those receiving methimazole alone. At 3 years, the combination-treated patients had a lower rate of recurrence (1.7%) than those receiving methimazole alone (recurrence rate, 34.7%) after all therapy was discontinued. Unfortunately, several prospective studies evaluating the addition of T_4 to thioamides have not validated these initial favorable results.[181,183,186,187] Support for this therapeutic approach has waned, and the addition of T_4 to existing thioamide therapy is not recommended.

B.D.'s large goiter reduces her chance of remission with longer therapy. Although thioamide therapy can be continued indefinitely if well tolerated, surgery or RAI therapy should seriously be considered for B.D., who already has received PTU for >2 years. Alternative therapy is especially crucial if she plans to become pregnant within the next few years (see Question 44).

Subclinical Hyperthyroidism

43. J.C. is a 68-year-old male who is found to have a TSH level of 0.25 μunits/mL (normal, 0.5–4.7) with normal FT_4 and FT_3 hormone levels on routine blood tests. He is otherwise healthy and denies any symptoms of thyroid dysfunction. On physical exam, his thyroid gland is normal. He denies any family history of thyroid disease and is taking no medications. How should these tests be interpreted? How should J.C. be managed?

[SI units: TSH, 0.25 mIU/L (normal, 0.5–4.7)]

J.C.'s laboratory values of a suppressed TSH value with normal free thyroid hormone levels are consistent with subclinical hyperthyroidism (SHyper). Other causes of a suppressed TSH value that are unlikely in J.C. include medication suppression (e.g., metformin, bexarotene) of the TSH level (Table 49-1), pituitary hypothyroidism, and euthyroid sick syndrome (see Question 2).[36,188] A suppressed TSH may also be a normal finding in healthy elderly patients.

The dangers of SHyper are similar to those of overt hyperthyroidism, and include cardiac findings (e.g., atrial and ventricular premature beats, atrial fibrillation [AF], left ventricular hypertrophy), loss of bone mineral density in postmenopausal women, and if present, subtle symptoms of hyperthyroidism. In elderly patients, hyperthyroid symptoms, even if overtly hyperthyroid, may not be apparent or "apathetic" due to impaired responsiveness of the sympathetic nervous system. A significant relationship between atrial fibrillation and degree of SHyper is clear, whereas an association with increased atherosclerotic heart disease or mortality is weak.[189] The relative risk of AF in SHyper may be as high as 5.2 and increased by older age, male gender, higher FT_4 levels, and degree of TSH suppression. In two cohorts followed for 10 to 13 years, the relative risk of atrial fibrillation ranged from 1.6 to 3.1, depending on the degree of TSH suppression.[189,190]

The management of subclinical hyperthyroidism is controversial, especially in asymptomatic patients, because data evaluating treatment outcomes are limited.[57–59] An expert panel concluded that treatment of subclinical hyperthyroidism should be considered in "elderly" patients and in those with cardiac disease and osteoporosis with TSH levels <0.1 μunits/mL.[57,58] For patients with TSH levels of 0.1 to

0.45 μunits/mL, the evidence was insufficient to recommend therapy. A recent review recommends RAI or thioamide therapy only if the TSH level is <0.1 μunits/mL in postmenopausal women, those older than 60 years, patients with a history of heart disease, osteoporosis, or hyperthyroid symptoms.[59] For patients with TSH levels of 0.1 to 0.4 μunits/mL, antithyroid therapy can be considered if they are in the aforementioned groups; otherwise, therapy is not recommended.

In J.C., his thyroid function tests should be repeated. An RAI update and scan should be obtained to detect any hyperactive areas or nodules that might be responsible for the suppressed TSH. Because J.C. is generally healthy, treatment can be considered if there are concerns about cardiac disease or bone loss; otherwise, no therapy is also reasonable based on the available evidence. Close monitoring of thyroid function tests is recommended every 6 months to a year. If hyperthyroid symptoms or changes in cardiac or bone function occur, then RAI therapy is recommended.

In Pregnancy

44. N.N., a 32-year-old woman who is 3 months pregnant, is referred for management of her Graves' disease. What are the therapeutic ramifications of managing thyrotoxicosis during pregnancy?

Hyperthyroidism develops in 0.02% to 1.4% of pregnant women and often precedes conception.[191] Symptoms of thyrotoxicosis are typically ameliorated during the second and third trimesters and exacerbated early in the postpartum period. Treatment is crucial to prevent damage to the fetus and to maintain the pregnancy. RAI, chronic iodide therapy, and iodine-containing compounds are contraindicated during pregnancy because they will cross the placenta to produce fetal goiter and athyreosis.[191–193] As little as 12 mg/day of iodide has produced neonatal goiter and death. The long-term use of propranolol should also be avoided because it is associated with fetal respiratory depression, a small placenta, intrauterine growth retardation, impaired response to anoxia, and postnatal bradycardia and hypoglycemia.[191,192] However, if rapid control of hyperthyroidism is required, short-term use (<1 week) of propranolol or the iodides is safe.[191–193]

Either surgery or thioamide is the treatment of choice for hyperthyroidism in the pregnant patient. Surgery is safe during the second trimester with adequate preoperative preparation. During both other trimesters, thioamides are preferred because surgery can precipitate spontaneous abortion. PTU is preferable, although both thioamides are equally efficacious,[194] demonstrate similar placental crossing properties,[195] and produce similar thyroid hormone concentrations in fetal umbilical cord blood samples.[196] Of concern, methimazole has been associated with anecdotal reports of congenital scalp defects (e.g., aplasia cutis) and an embryopathy syndrome (esophageal and choanal atresia).[197–200] However, the risks of reversible aplasia cutis were not greater in women receiving methimazole (e.g., 2.7%) compared to PTU (e.g., 3%) or hyperthyroid controls (e.g., 6%).[194,197,198] Therefore, methimazole can be considered in pregnancy if there is intolerance or nonadherence to PTU.[191,192,194] (See Chapter 47.) Methimazole may be preferred by some because its longer half-life allows once-daily dosing.

Fetal hypothyroidism and goiter can develop when large doses of either thioamide are administered to the mother, even if the mother is still hyperthyroid.[191,192] Therefore, to avoid goiter and suppression of the fetal thyroid gland, which begins to function at about 12 to 14 weeks of gestation, any thioamide should be prescribed in the lowest effective doses that will maintain the mother's T_4 level in the upper ranges of normal. Control of maternal hyperthyroidism increases the risk of fetal hypothyroidism. Initiate therapy with PTU (e.g., maximum of 450 mg/day in three divided doses) or methimazole (e.g., maximum of 20–30 mg given once daily) until control is achieved, and then taper the dosage to 50–150 mg/day of PTU or 5–15 mg/day of methimazole for the remainder of the pregnancy. Some patients can discontinue thioamides in the second half of pregnancy.[191] Such modest doses of thioamides provide satisfactory control of maternal hyperthyroidism and should not cause clinically evident thyroid dysfunction in the neonate. Patients requiring more than the maximum recommended thioamide dosages for control may need to consider the possibility of surgery in the second trimester.

Nevertheless, a small but significant reduction in neonatal serum T_4 occurs even when small (100–200 mg) doses of PTU are administered during pregnancy to mothers with Graves' disease.[191,192,199] It is unclear whether this mild, transient reduction in serum T_4 causes long-term impairment of mental development or is otherwise detrimental to the newborn. To date, no significant differences in intellectual development have been noted between children exposed to PTU or methimazole in utero and their unexposed siblings.[201–203] However, children exposed in utero to >300 mg/day of PTU had lower IQs.[201,202]

Although transient fetal or neonatal hypothyroidism does not appear to be a major threat to the baby, it is advisable to maintain the mother in a mildly hyperthyroid state.[191,192] Mild maternal hyperthyroidism seems to be well tolerated, but maternal hypothyroidism is poorly tolerated by both the mother and the fetus (see Question 13). T_4 levels should be maintained in the upper ranges of normal because normal thyroid function tests are suggestive of hypothyroidism during pregnancy (high TBG and TBPA levels). A normal TSH level should not be the goal of therapy but should remain suppressed because control of maternal hyperthyroidism increases the risk of fetal hypothyroidism.

It is not rational to add thyroid hormone to the mother's regimen to prevent fetal goiter or hypothyroidism because thyroid hormones do not reach the fetal circulation. Thyroid supplementation only complicates the treatment of maternal hyperthyroidism by increasing thioamide requirements, which can further compromise fetal thyroid hormone production.[191] If the mother has not been thyrotoxic throughout pregnancy, a normal infant can be expected. All pregnant patients with a history of or active Graves' disease should be screened during pregnancy for TRAb to assess the risk of neonatal hyperthyroidism.[191] Last, both thioamides can be safely used in the lactating mother if the maximal dose of PTU does not exceed 200 mg/day (up to 750 mg/day in one report)[204] and 10 to 20 mg daily for methimazole.[205] Propranolol and iodides are secreted in breast milk and should be avoided. (See Chapter 47.)

Treatment With Radioactive Iodine

Pretreatment

45. B.J., a 35-year-old woman, has newly diagnosed Graves' disease complicated by CHF and angina. After a few days of treatment with PTU 200 mg TID and Lugol's solution, 5 drops/day, B.J. received RAI therapy. Six months later, she is still symptomatic. Evaluate the influence of B.J.'s pretreatment therapy on the efficacy of her RAI therapy.

Patients with severe hyperthyroidism, patients with hyperthyroidism and cardiac disease, and those who are debilitated or older should receive antithyroid treatment before RAI therapy. The goal of pretreatment is to deplete stored thyroid hormone. This minimizes post-RAI hyperthyroidism (which occurs during the first 10 days after ^{131}I administration) and thyroid storm, which is caused by leakage of hormones from the damaged thyroid gland.[146,166,206] Other patients with hyperthyroidism can be treated safely with RAI without pretherapy.

Lugol's solution or other iodides should not be given before RAI because iodides decrease the effectiveness of this therapy by decreasing the gland's uptake of RAI. This effect of iodides persists for several weeks. Iodides can be used for 1 to 7 days after RAI treatment if they are needed to rapidly control symptoms of hyperthyroidism.

The thioamides can be used before RAI therapy to achieve a euthyroid state, but pretreatment with thioamides may lower the cure rate and increase the need for subsequent doses of RAI.[146,207–211] A meta-analysis of 14 trials found that use of thioamides (PTU, methimazole, carbimazole) before and after RAI was associated with an increased risk of treatment failure (relative risk of 1.28; 95% CI, 1.07–1.52) and a 32% reduced risk of hypothyroidism regardless of the thioamide used.[211] Purportedly, higher RAI failure rates occur with PTU than with methimazole due to the presence of the radioprotective sulfhydryl group in PTU.[207–210] To facilitate optimal uptake and retention of ^{131}I by the gland, PTU should be stopped at least 7 days before and methimazole at least 4 days before RAI administration.[207,208,210] If necessary, thioamides can be restarted after RAI administration without impairing its efficacy. β-Adrenergic blocking agents can be used before, during, and after RAI therapy without interfering with its uptake.

B.J. remains symptomatic because pretreatment with the PTU and iodides decreased the effectiveness of RAI therapy. Propranolol should be given to B.J. before RAI therapy to ameliorate symptoms of hyperthyroidism because she has received only a short course of thioamide. Iodides might be preferable to propranolol following RAI therapy if B.J.'s CHF worsens. For subsequent RAI doses, pretreatment with methimazole may be preferable to PTU because it can be stopped a few days prior to RAI therapy, thereby causing a shorter duration of hyperthyroidism.

Onset of Effects

46. B.J. still is symptomatic 2 weeks after a second dose of RAI. When can she expect to experience the therapeutic effects of RAI therapy?

Although some benefits from RAI therapy are evident within 1 month, a period of 8 to 12 weeks is generally required for maximal effects.[133,206] Euthyroidism or, more commonly, hypothyroidism occurs in approximately 80% to 90% of patients treated with a single nonablative dose of RAI; the remaining 10% to 20% become euthyroid or hypothyroid after two or more doses. This slow onset is a disadvantage, but symptomatic control can be obtained quickly by administration of a β-adrenergic blocking agent, or iodides starting 1 to 14 days after the ^{131}I dose. Iodides are less preferable if a second dose of RAI is necessary. Thioamides can also be given, although their therapeutic effects are delayed for 3 to 4 weeks.

At least 3 months should elapse before a second radioactive dose of iodide is administered, and most recommend waiting 6 months before repeating ^{131}I administration, unless the patient remains severely thyrotoxic. It is inadvisable to give a second dose before the major effects of the first dose have become apparent. Although the use of iodides before RAI in B.J. may have decreased the amount of ^{131}I retained by her thyroid, it still is advisable to wait at least 3 months before a second dose is given.

Iatrogenic Hypothyroidism

47. S.D., a 54-year-old woman, returns to the thyroid clinic after being lost to follow-up for 6 months. She initially received RAI 3 years ago but required a repeat dose of RAI 1 year ago for recurrence of hyperthyroidism. She currently has no other medical problems and is not taking any medications. She is a mildly obese, puffy-faced woman wearing several layers of clothing. She complains of fatigue and lack of energy. Her reflexes are delayed, and her skin is cool and dry. What is a likely explanation for her symptoms?

S.D.'s clinical presentation and history are compatible with hypothyroidism secondary to RAI therapy. An FT_4 and a TSH level would confirm this diagnosis. Iatrogenic hypothyroidism is the major complication of ^{131}I therapy, although transient hypothyroidism may be seen in the first 3 to 6 weeks after RAI therapy.[133] The incidence of iatrogenic myxedema is often reported as 7% to 8%, but it increases at a constant rate of 2.5% per year. The reported prevalence of this complication ranges from 26% to 70% after 1 to 14 years.[206]

The best predictor of eventual hypothyroidism is the dose of ^{131}I administered. Prevention of iatrogenic hypothyroidism is directed toward calculation of a dose that will produce neither recurrent hyperthyroidism nor hypothyroidism. Unfortunately, when lower doses of ^{131}I were used to avoid hypothyroidism, the cure rate was reduced but the incidence of hypothyroidism was unaffected. Thus, the appearance of iatrogenic hypothyroidism may be inevitable with time. However, hypothyroidism is managed easily and is an acceptable therapeutic end point. Because hypothyroidism after RAI therapy is latent and often insidious, patients should be informed of this and monitored closely at monthly intervals for subsequent hypothyroidism. Awareness of a transient hypothyroidism soon after RAI therapy should minimize the institution of unnecessary hormone replacement.

Ophthalmopathy

Clinical Presentation

48. H.R., a 50-year-old man, first developed "large eyes with stare," weakness, diaphoresis, and thyroid enlargement when he was diagnosed with Graves' disease. RAI therapy caused some worsening of his eye symptoms. Although he is clinically

euthyroid, physical examination reveals severe bilateral conjunctival edema and injection, proptosis of the right eye, incomplete lid closure, and decreased visual acuity. He complains of photophobia, tearing, and extreme irritation, which is worse after smoking cigarettes. His other medical problems include diabetes treated with metformin and pioglitazone. What is the association of H.R.'s ocular changes with Graves' disease?

H.R. presents with symptoms consistent with the infiltrative ophthalmopathy of Graves' disease.[212,213] The eye signs of Graves' disease are the most striking abnormality of this disorder. Rarely, ophthalmopathy can occur without any evidence of hyperthyroidism. Fortunately, severe ophthalmopathy occurs in only 3% to 5% of patients, while 25% to 50% have some eye findings. Eye disease is more severe in older patients and in men than women. Smokers often have higher levels of TRAb and more severe ophthalmopathy.[185,213,214]

It is unknown why the eye and its muscles are attacked in Graves' disease. Histologic examination reveals lymphocytic infiltration, increased mucopolysaccharides, fat (due to increased adipogenesis and glycosaminoglycans), and water in all retrobulbar tissue. Ocular symptoms include edema, chemosis, excessive lacrimation, photophobia, corneal protrusion (proptosis), scarring, ulceration, extraocular muscle paralysis with loss of eye movements, and blindness from retinal and optic nerve damage.

The eye involvement can occur at any time and is usually bilateral. The ocular symptoms usually subside or remain stable once the patient is euthyroid; however, some cases will progress during the euthyroid period or following RAI treatment of the hyperthyroidism (see Question 49). Pioglitazone may also increase eye protrusion by 1 to 2 mm by stimulating adipogenesis and increasing retrobulbar fat production.[215]

Management of Eye Symptoms

49. Was previous treatment of H.R.'s hyperthyroidism appropriate? How should his current ocular symptoms be managed?

The optimal treatment of hyperthyroidism and its effect on the course of ophthalmopathy remain controversial.[212,213,216] Thioamides might improve eye symptoms through an immunosuppressive mechanism of action and control of the hyperthyroidism or exert a neutral effect.[212] Many clinicians believe that gland ablation with RAI or surgical removal is preferable because it removes the antigen source and prevents progression of the ophthalmopathy.[150,212] However, several studies have confirmed development or worsening of eye symptoms immediately after RAI therapy.[214,216] One randomized study demonstrated that the concomitant use of 0.4 to 0.5 mg/kg of prednisone begun 2 to 3 days post-RAI and continued for a total of 3 months after RAI therapy in those with any degree of ocular involvement was well tolerated and prevented further deterioration of eye symptoms.[214,216] Regardless of the treatment used, control of the hyperthyroidism often improves most eye findings, except for proptosis.

In H.R., prednisone 40 to 60 mg/day should have been started after his RAI treatment and continued for 2 to 3 months until the eye symptoms improved. Because the pathophysiology of the ophthalmopathy is unclear, treatment is limited to symptomatic and empiric measures once the patient is euthyroid.[212,213] H.R. should also be encouraged to stop smoking to prevent progression of the ophthalmopathy.[185] His pioglitazone should be discontinued as well because thiazolidinediones can increase eye protrusion by 1 to 2 mm via adipogenesis stimulation to increase retrobulbar fat.[215]

Periorbital edema and chemosis are worse in the morning after being in the horizontal position; elevating the head of the bed, treatment with diuretics, and restricting salt intake may be helpful. Protective glasses can relieve photophobia and external irritation. Topical corticosteroid drops are effective in decreasing local irritation, but they should be used cautiously because they increase the risk of infection. Ocular irritants such as smoke and dust should be avoided. Bothersome symptoms (e.g., dry eye, redness, tearing) caused by eyelid retraction can be ameliorated with artificial tears and lubricants.[212] Incomplete lid closure predisposes the patient to corneal scarring and ulceration, so lubricant eyedrops should be applied several times daily and at night to keep the bulbs moist. Taping the eyelids shut at night helps prevent drying and scarring. Lateral surgical closure of the lids (tarsorrhaphy) may be required to improve lid closure.

When the ophthalmopathy is severe and progressive, an aggressive approach is necessary. Systemic corticosteroids can produce either dramatic or marginal results in the emergency treatment of progressive exophthalmos associated with decreasing visual acuity. Prednisone at dosages of 35 to 80 mg/day is often effective, although dosages as high as 100 to 140 mg/day may be necessary.[212,213] Pain, irritation, tearing, and other subjective complaints often respond within 24 hours of administration. Therapy for about 3 months is necessary to improve eye muscle and optic nerve function disturbances. Initial large doses should be tapered rapidly once the desired response is obtained to minimize adverse effects. Subconjunctival and retrobulbar injections of steroids are not as effective.

X-ray therapy to the orbit also relieves congestive and inflammatory symptoms.[212] The combination of orbital irradiation and systemic steroids may be required to achieve maximal benefits. Plasmapheresis and immunosuppressive agents, such as cyclophosphamide, azathioprine, cyclosporine, and methotrexate, have also been used with limited success in combination with steroids.[212]

When the previous measures and thyroid ablation fail to arrest the progression of visual loss and exophthalmos, then surgical orbital decompression should be considered.

Thyroid Storm

Clinical Presentation

50. H.L., a 48-year-old woman, is admitted to the hospital with a 3-week history of fatigue, weakness, dyspnea on exertion, SOB, palpitations, and inability to keep food and liquids down. One year before admission, she began noticing a preference for cold weather and an increase in nervousness and emotional lability. After her husband died a few days ago, she experienced increased nausea and vomiting, irritability, insomnia, tremor, and a 104°F fever, which she attributed to an upper respiratory tract infection. She denies taking any current medications. Her laboratory data obtained on admission included an FT_4 of 4.65 ng/dL (normal, 0.7–1.9) and an undetectable TSH level. Assess H.L.'s subjective and objective data.

[SI unit: FT_4, 60 pmol/L (normal, 9–24)]

The presentation is consistent with thyroid storm, a life-threatening medical emergency that might have been precipitated by the stress associated with the death of her husband. The clinical manifestations of thyroid storm[166] include the acute onset of high fever (sine qua non), tachycardia, and tachypnea, and involvement of the following organ systems: cardiovascular (tachycardia, pulmonary edema, hypertension, shock), CNS (tremor, emotional lability, confusion, psychosis, apathy, stupor, coma), and GI (diarrhea, abdominal pain, nausea and vomiting, liver enlargement, jaundice, nonspecific elevations of bilirubin and PT). Hyperglycemia was a clinical finding in 12 of 18 episodes.

Thyroid storm develops in about 2% to 8% of hyperthyroid patients. The pathogenesis of thyroid storm is not well understood, but the condition can be described as an "exaggerated" or decompensated form of thyrotoxicosis. The term *decompensated* implies failure of body systems to adequately resist the effects of thyrotoxicosis. It is not attributed solely to the release of massive quantities of hormones, which can occur after surgery or RAI therapy. Catecholamines also play an important role; the increased quantities of thyroid hormone in conjunction with increased sympathetic and adrenal output contribute to many of the manifestations of thyroid storm. Although thyroid hormones exert an independent effect, many of the symptoms of hyperthyroidism are ameliorated by catecholamine-blocking agents such as β-blockers and calcium channel blockers (e.g., diltiazem, verapamil).

Treatment

51. What treatment plan (including route of administration) should be initiated promptly in H.L.?

Accurate, continuous, and immediate treatment can decrease the mortality of thyroid storm significantly. Mortality rates as low as 7% and survival rates as high as 50% are reported. Treatment of thyroid storm should be directed against four major areas discussed in the following sections.[166]

DECREASE IN SYNTHESIS AND RELEASE OF HORMONES

High dosages of thioamides, preferably PTU 800 to 1,200 mg/day or methimazole 60 to 100 mg/day, should be given orally in four divided doses. If H.L. cannot take oral doses, a rectal formulation of PTU (better bioavailability with enema than suppository) or methimazole, which is as effective as the oral route, can be administered.[147–149] No commercial parenteral preparation is available for either drug, limiting their use by the IV route. PTU is the thioamide of choice because it acts more rapidly than methimazole by blocking the peripheral conversion of T_4 to T_3, a dominant source of the hormone.

Iodides, which rapidly block further release of intraglandular stores of T_4, should be given at least 1 hour after thioamide administration. Given in this way, the substrate for hormone synthesis is not increased, and the therapeutic effect of thioamide is not blocked. The addition of iodides (e.g., Lugol's solution 15 to 30 drops/day orally in divided doses) to the thioamides often ameliorates symptoms within 1 day.

Cholestyramine 4 g orally (PO) QID may assist in lowering hormone levels rapidly but should be administered apart from other agents to prevent inhibiting their absorption.[217] Other effective modalities include plasmapheresis, charcoal hemoperfusion, and plasma exchange.

REVERSAL OF THE PERIPHERAL EFFECTS OF HORMONES AND CATECHOLAMINES

β-adrenergic blocking drugs are the preferred agents to decrease the tachycardia, agitation, tremulousness, and other symptoms of excessive adrenergic stimulation seen in thyroid storm. Propranolol is the β-blocker of choice because its clinical efficacy in storm is well documented and because it inhibits the peripheral conversion of T_4 to T_3.[166,174] If rapid effects are necessary, propranolol 1 mg by slow IV push can be given every 5 minutes to lower the heart rate to 90 to 110 beats/minute. A 5- to 10-mg/hour IV infusion can be given to maintain the desired heart rate. IV esmolol 50 to 100 mcg/kg/minute can also be given. If perfusion is maintained, oral β-blockers (e.g., propranolol, 40 mg every 6 hours; atenolol, 50–100 mg BID; metoprolol, 50–100 mg daily; nadolol, 40–80 mg daily), titrated to response, can also be given.

SUPPORTIVE TREATMENT OF VITAL FUNCTIONS

This may include sedation, oxygen, IV glucose, vitamins, treatment of infections with antibiotics, digitalization to maintain the cardiac status, rehydration, and treatment of hyperpyrexia with cooling blankets, sponge baths, and the judicious use of antipyretics. Because hypoadrenalism is often suspected, hydrocortisone 100 to 200 mg should empirically be given IV every 6 hours. Because pharmacologic doses of steroids acutely depress serum T_3 levels, a beneficial effect in storm, their routine use is recommended.

ELIMINATION OF PRECIPITATING CAUSES OF STORM

Factors associated with the induction of thyroid storm include infection (most common), trauma, inadequate preparation before thyroidectomy, surgical operations, stress, diabetic acidosis, pregnancy, emboli, discontinuation or withdrawal of antithyroid medications, drug therapy, and RAI therapy.[166]

DRUG-INDUCED THYROID DISEASE

Lithium and Antidepressants

52. D.A., a 56-year-old man, complains of sluggishness, cold intolerance, fatigue, and a "rundown" feeling, which doctors attribute to the depressive phase of his bipolar affective illness. He previously had been well controlled with sertraline (Zoloft) 100 mg/day, but lithium carbonate (Eskalith) 900 mg/day was added 4 months ago because of unreasonable mirthfulness and uncontrollable gift-buying tendencies. Physical examination reveals a puffy face and a large goiter. What is a reasonable assessment of these subjective and objective data?

Thyroid function tests (i.e., TSH, FT_4) should be obtained to evaluate the possibility of lithium- and possibly sertraline-induced hypothyroidism and goiter.[218–221] If appropriate, T_4 should be initiated. Although the incidence of goiter and hypothyroidism in the manic-depressive population is unknown, the incidence of baseline elevated TSH might be higher than in the general population; one study reported an incidence of 15%.[221]

The antithyroid effects of lithium were noted first in manic-depressive patients. The exact mechanism of lithium's antithyroid effect on the gland is unclear, although it is highly concentrated by the gland. Similar to the iodides, chronic lithium therapy inhibits the release of thyroid hormone from the gland.

The fall in serum T_4 and T_3 hormone levels leads to a compensatory and transient increase in serum TSH levels until a new steady state is achieved.[219–221]

The incidence of subclinical hypothyroidism (i.e., increased TSH level) occurs in approximately 19% of patients on chronic lithium therapy.[221] Typically, the serum thyroid hormone levels decrease and the TSH levels increase during the first few months of treatment, returning to pretreatment levels after 1 year. In one study, TSH levels increased within 10 days after starting therapy. Normalization of the TSH level is less likely to occur in patients with pre-existing positive thyroid antibodies before lithium therapy. Induction of thyroid antibodies and increases in baseline antibody titers also occur after chronic lithium therapy. Because abnormal thyroid function tests can be transient, a longer period of observation is justified before starting thyroid hormone therapy in patients with subclinical hypothyroidism.

Lithium-induced goiter, with or without hypothyroidism, appears in a small percentage of the population after 5 months to 2 years of therapy.[219–221] Overt hypothyroidism develops most often during the first 2 years of treatment in women with a history of positive antibodies before lithium therapy. A direct goitrogenic effect of lithium might explain the occurrence of euthyroid goiter. The goiters respond to discontinuation of lithium or to suppression with thyroid hormone despite continuation of lithium therapy. Surgical removal of the goiter is required if there are local obstructive symptoms. In D.A.'s case, sertraline could be exerting an additive or synergistic antithyroid effect with lithium because antithyroid effects have also been associated with this drug.[218]

Most patients with lithium-induced thyroid abnormalities are women older than 50 years, have a prior history of compromised thyroid function (e.g., Hashimoto's thyroiditis), positive thyroid antibodies before lithium therapy, or a strong family history of thyroid disease.[219–221] Therefore, baseline thyroid function tests (i.e., FT_4, TSH), antibodies, and thyroid ultrasound should be obtained before starting lithium therapy, and levels should be checked annually thereafter or more frequently if clinically indicated. Patients should also be questioned about a positive history or family history for thyroid disease and the concurrent use of other, potentially goitrogenic medications (e.g., tricyclic antidepressants, iodides, iodinated expectorants).

53. A.B., a 66-year-old, otherwise healthy man, is admitted for evaluation of new-onset AF. His only other medical problem is a history of bipolar affective disorder treated with lithium for 1 year. However, A.B. discontinued the lithium 1 month before hospitalization without the knowledge of his physician. His laboratory studies are within normal limits except for a TT_3 of 380 ng/dL (normal, 70–132 ng/dL). What is the potential cause of A.B.'s AF?

[SI unit: TT_3, 6 nmol/L (normal, 1.1–2)]

AF may be the only manifestation of thyrotoxicosis in older patients.[190,222] Thyrotoxicosis is reported following lithium withdrawal, and A.B.'s AF most likely is the result of excessive thyroid hormone activity. Lithium's antithyroid action is substantial and is comparable to that of the thioamides; T_4 levels decline by 20% to 35%. Therefore, A.B.'s underlying hyperthyroidism has probably been unmasked by his discontinuation of the lithium. Rarely, lithium-induced thyrotoxicosis occurs.[219,223,224]

Although lithium is not considered the standard of care for hyperthyroidism, it is recommended as an adjunct to RAI therapy in patients allergic to conventional treatment modalities because it does not interfere with ^{131}I uptake. Furthermore, lithium can increase ^{131}I retention by decreasing its rate of elimination from the gland. The increased thyroidal half-life of ^{131}I by lithium is beneficial in localizing the dose of radiation to the gland and producing faster control of the hyperthyroidism.[224]

Because clinical experience with lithium in the treatment of thyrotoxicosis is limited and because it has such a narrow therapeutic index, its use should be restricted to situations when rapid suppression of thyroid hormone secretion is needed, and when thioamides and iodides are contraindicated.

Iodides and Amiodarone

54. C.Y., a 54-year-old man with chronic obstructive pulmonary disease (COPD), presents with a 6-month history of weakness, fatigue, tremor, heat intolerance, palpitations, and cardiac tachyarrhythmias, previously controlled for the last 2 years on amiodarone 400 mg/day. Physical examination reveals a 50-g multinodular gland, which C.Y. says has "been there forever." He denies any family history of thyroid disease or ingestion of any thyroid medication. He recently started to use an iodinated expectorant for his COPD. His current complaints began after an intravenous pyelogram (IVP). What might be responsible for C.Y.'s hyperthyroid symptoms?

The iodine load from the IVP, the iodinated expectorant, or the amiodarone could be responsible for C.Y.'s hyperthyroid symptoms.[31–33,141,142] Iodide-induced hyperthyroidism, known as the Jod-Basedow phenomenon, was first described in the 1800s when patients residing in iodide-deficient areas became toxic when given adequate iodide supplementation. Other reports have appeared since then. Both T_3 toxicosis and classic T_4 toxicosis have occurred following iodide ingestion or injection of roentgenographic contrast media.

Although it is presumed that both iodide deficiency and a multinodular goiter, as in C.Y., are required to invoke the Jod-Basedow phenomenon, iodide-induced disease has been reported in patients residing in iodide-sufficient areas, as well as in euthyroid patients with normal glands and no apparent risk factors (e.g., family history).[141,142]

Amiodarone can cause hypo- or hyperthyroidism in susceptible patients because of its high iodine content.[31–33,141–143] Twelve milligrams (37%) of free iodine is released per 400-mg dose of amiodarone. Patients with multinodular goiters who lose the ability to turn off organification of iodide with increasing iodide loads (Wolff-Chaikoff effect) are most likely to develop iodide-induced thyrotoxicosis. Conversely, patients with positive antibodies or with underlying Hashimoto's thyroiditis who cannot escape from the Wolff-Chaikoff block are most likely to develop hypothyroidism.

Amiodarone-induced hypothyroidism may occur at any time during therapy and does not appear to be related to the cumulative dose. A normal FT_4 and a persistently elevated TSH (see Question 5) are consistent with amiodarone-induced hypothyroidism, which occurs in 6% to 10% of long-term users. The hypothyroidism responds readily to T_4 therapy, and the amiodarone can often be continued.[31,32]

In contrast, the development of amiodarone-induced thyrotoxicosis occurs early and suddenly during therapy, so that routine monitoring of thyroid function tests is often not useful. Elevated hormone levels, an undetectable TSH level, and clinical symptoms consistent with hyperthyroidism are the best indicators of amiodarone-induced thyrotoxicosis, which occurs in 1% to 5% of long-term users. Worsening of tachyarrhythmias may be the first clinical clue to amiodarone-induced thyrotoxicosis.

Amiodarone-induced hyperthyroidism can be classified as either type I or type II.[30,31,33] Type I occurs in patients with underlying risk factors for thyroid disease (e.g., multinodular goiter) and is related to the iodine load. The formation of large amounts of preformed hormone from the massive iodine load produces a protracted course of hyperthyroidism, which is challenging to manage. Type II amiodarone-induced hyperthyroidism results from a direct destructive type of thyroiditis, causing excessive release of thyroid hormone into the systemic circulation. This occurs most often in patients with normal thyroid glands. Unique laboratory findings include a low RAIU and elevated interleukin-6 levels.

The management of amiodarone-induced thyrotoxicosis is complicated because it is not always possible to identify the type of hyperthyroidism. Stopping amiodarone alone does not immediately improve the hyperthyroidism because of the drug's long half-life (22–55 days) and its sequestration in fat. RAI ablation is never appropriate because the high iodine load from amiodarone will suppress therapeutic uptake of the ^{131}I. The combination of methimazole and potassium perchlorate is the treatment of choice for type I hyperthyroidism.[31–33,141,142] The addition of corticosteroids to block T_4 to T_3 conversion is less effective because of the already potent inhibitory effects of amiodarone on T_4 to T_3 conversion. However, in patients with type II hyperthyroidism, β-blockers, corticosteroids, and iodinated contrast media if available, rather than the aforementioned agents, are the most appropriate choices.[31,32,142,225] A total thyroidectomy can be effective by rapidly controlling the thyrotoxicosis, permitting continued therapy with amiodarone if necessary. Despite underlying cardiac disease in these patients, uneventful surgery and a low complication rate were observed if patients were treated before surgery with a short course of an oral cholecystographic agent.[225]

Large doses of iodides should be avoided in patients with nontoxic multinodular goiters who are predisposed to thyrotoxicosis (see Questions 5 and 30).

Interferon-α

55. P.R., a 56-year-old woman, complains of hoarseness, fatigue, "slow movement," and forgetfulness. She is troubled by these new symptoms, which have worsened during the past few weeks. Her medical history includes persistent hepatitis C, which is responding to the combination of pegylated interferon-α injections and ribavirin. She notes that her mother had a history of Graves' disease treated with RAI ablation. Her medications include pegylated interferon and an over-the-counter dietary supplement, Cellasene, to reduce cellulite. On examination, facial edema, coarse skin, an enlarged thyroid gland without nodules, and delayed DTRs are noted. Thyroid function tests, including thyroid antibodies, are pending. What might be responsible for her new complaints?

The medications that P.R. is taking could be responsible for her complaints and physical findings, which are consistent with hypothyroidism. A detailed history of any other dietary and herbal supplements, especially those containing thyroid or iodine (e.g., kelp tablets), should be obtained. Cellasene, a dietary supplement promoted to reduce cellulite, contains a significant amount of iodine (e.g., 310 mcg of iodine per capsule) and could cause thyroid illness in susceptible patients (see Questions 30 and 54).

Another possible cause for hypothyroidism could be the pegylated interferon-α injections that she has been receiving for the hepatitis C infection.[226–228] The prevalence of thyroid abnormalities observed with interferon-α ranges from 15% to 46%. Development de novo or aggravation of pre-existing antithyroid antibodies is the most common abnormal finding. The presence of pre-existing antithyroid antibodies (seropositivity) before interferon-α therapy or its persistence at the end of therapy is a significant risk factor for the development of overt thyroid dysfunction. Other predisposing risk factors include female gender, older patients, and Asian ethnicity.[227] The incidence of thyroid dysfunction was 46% in a seropositive group compared to 5.4% in the seronegative group.[227] Likewise, in a group of 114 patients with no pre-existing thyroid disease, those who were seropositive at the end of therapy had the highest risk of developing subclinical hypothyroidism 6.2 years later (odds ratio of 38.7).[228]

Hypothyroidism, from Hashimoto's thyroiditis or a nonautoimmune basis, is more common (40%–50% of patients) than hyperthyroidism (10%–30%). There are two types of hyperthyroidism, an autoimmune Graves'-like disorder with positive antibodies, and a hyperthyroid thyroiditis, similar to the type II amiodarone hyperthyroidism (see question 54). This is due to a direct toxic effect of interferon on the gland. Approximately 20% of patients with a thyroiditis will first have transient symptoms of hyperthyroidism followed by hypothyroidism (biphasic thyroiditis).[229]

In patients with positive thyroid antibodies, reversal of thyroid dysfunction is less likely. However, thyroid dysfunction appears to be transient in most patients without positive antibodies, and treatment is not always necessary. L-thyroxine is required only if hypothyroid symptoms are bothersome; otherwise, therapy can be withheld because symptoms often resolve spontaneously within 2 to 3 months after stopping therapy. If T_4 is begun, it should be stopped after 6 months to re-evaluate the need for continued thyroid replacement. Similarly, transient hyperthyroid laboratory indices do not require therapy with β-blockers unless the patient is symptomatic or laboratory values are dangerously elevated. Rarely, thyroid dysfunction is permanent, but it may take up to 17 months after stopping therapy for findings to resolve.

P.R. should be advised to stop taking the Cellasene and to avoid other iodide-containing herbal or dietary supplements. Once the laboratory values confirm hypothyroidism, T_4 should be started concurrently with the interferon-α because of the severity of her symptoms. Once interferon therapy is completed, L-thyroxine should be tapered off to evaluate the need for continued replacement. The presence of thyroid antibodies may increase the risk of permanent hypothyroidism.

Iodide Prophylaxis for Radiation Emergencies

56. J.M. is a healthy, 43-year-old Russian woman who lives near a nuclear reactor with her two young children. She has relatives living in Chernobyl who were exposed to the 1986 radiation fallout and developed various thyroid abnormalities, including cancer. J.M. would like to protect herself and her children. What prophylaxis and benefits, if any, might be indicated for J.M. in case of a nuclear accident?

The most accurate data for irradiation-induced thyroid abnormalities come from the 1986 Chernobyl incident, where massive amounts of RAI was released into the environment, contaminating air, food, and water supplies. Significant increases in thyroid cancer were found, primarily in children, who received ≥5 cGy ^{131}I exposures.[230]

The thyroid can be protected against radiation-induced thyroid cancer if potassium iodide (KI) is taken immediately before, coincident with, or possibly 3 to 4 hours after the radiation exposure.[231] Administration of KI 130 mg in adults and 65 mg in school-age children lasts approximately 24 hours and should be continued until the risk of exposure is over. Adolescents close to 70 kg should receive the full 130-mg dose; neonates should receive 16 mg. Repeat dosing is not recommended in pregnant women, neonates, or during lactation unless there is ongoing contamination because the risks of repeated KI administration (e.g., neonatal and fetal hypothyroidism) outweigh their protective benefits. In the aforementioned conditions, when repeated doses of KI are not advisable, and in those intolerant to KI, protective measures (e.g., sheltering, evacuation, control of the food supply) should be implemented. Hypothyroidism can be managed with T_4 supplementation. If repeat dosing is necessary during continued contamination, close monitoring for toxicity is recommended. Short-term administration of KI is safer in children than in adults.

Adverse effects include sialadenitis, GI disturbances, rash, and other allergic reactions, which are increased in patients with dermatitis herpetiformis and hypocomplementemic vasculitides. Hyperthyroidism, goiter, and hypothyroidism can occur, especially in adults with underlying thyroid disorders (see Question 54).

NODULES

"Hot" Nodule

57. N.S., a 20-year-old woman, noticed a "lump" in the right side of her neck. There is no history of irradiation and no family history of thyroid disease. She has no local symptoms and no symptoms suggestive of hypo- or hyperthyroidism. The right lobe of the thyroid is occupied by a 3 × 3-cm firm, immovable nodule; the left lobe is barely palpable. All thyroid function tests are within normal limits. A scan shows a large "hot" nodule occupying the right lobe and a nonexistent left lobe. How should N.S.'s single "hot" nodule, or Plummer's disease, be managed?

Hot nodule is a term used to describe a "hyperfunctioning" or iodine-concentrating area of the thyroid as shown on scan; it appears as an area of greater density than the rest of the gland. The hyperfunctioning autonomous nodule typically suppresses activity in the remainder of the gland, but it need not produce clinical or chemical evidence of hyperthyroidism and may remain unchanged for years. Some nodules may develop into toxic goiters, causing overt symptoms of toxicosis. Most hot nodules are benign; malignancies are rarely reported.[232]

Treatment of the hot nodule depends on the existing clinical situation. If it is suppressing the other lobe of the thyroid, is not causing toxic symptoms, and is the only source of thyroid production, the patient should be left alone and monitored closely for signs of toxicity. A toxic hot nodule is best treated surgically or with RAI ablation. Because hot nodules do not spontaneously resolve, antithyroid drugs are not the treatment of choice. Because the normal thyroid tissue is suppressed, RAI is concentrated only by the hot nodule, sparing the suppressed tissue. After treatment, the suppressed tissue should begin functioning again.

"Cold" Nodule

58. P.L., a 29-year-old woman, is found to have a left thyroid nodule on routine physical examination. She has no history of neck irradiation, no family history of thyroid disease, and no symptoms suggestive of hypo- or hyperthyroidism. A firm, nontender 1-cm nodule occupies the left lobe of the gland. Thyroid function tests are within normal limits. The scan shows a "cold" nodule and the ultrasound reveals a solid mass, ruling out the possibility of a cyst. The results of the fine-needle aspiration (FNA) are pending. Antibodies are negative. What is the significance of a cold nodule, and how should it be managed?

A cold nodule is a "hypofunctioning" area of the thyroid that fails to collect radioiodine. It is depicted on the scan as a lighter or less dense area. The differential diagnosis includes Hashimoto's thyroiditis, benign adenomas, cysts, and malignant tumors. The absence of thyroid antibodies and identification of a solid mass on ultrasound rules out the possibility of a cyst or Hashimoto's thyroiditis. Most cold nodules turn out to be benign adenomas rather than cancers. The FNA can help distinguish a benign from a malignant nodule. However, a benign biopsy in a suspicious nodule or in a patient with risk factors for malignancy does not eliminate the possibility of malignancy. In these patients, surgery is recommended. The incidence of malignancy in a cold nodule varies between 10% and 20%.[232] A history of irradiation increases the likelihood of cancer in a nodule, and surgery is recommended in these instances. The nature of the nodule is important. Fixation of the nodule to the strap muscles or the trachea, a hard bulging mass, any pain or tenderness, or voice hoarseness can indicate malignancy.

If the nodule is benign, then close follow-up every 6 to 18 months is recommended to detect any growth. If the nodule increases in size, a repeat FNA is recommended to rule out any malignancy. Although T_4-suppressive therapy can be considered, only about 10% to 20% of nodules shrink with therapy.[233,234] Furthermore, L-thyroxine may not actually shrink the nodule itself, but rather the surrounding thyroid tissue, making the nodule appear smaller. Spontaneous resolution of the nodule can also occur. The dangers of excessive L-thyroxine therapy (e.g., osteoporosis, cardiac arrhythmias) exceed the benefits of benign nodule suppression.[56,190] Therefore, watchful waiting, with no therapy, is recommended.

Multinodular Goiter

59. G.D., a 35-year-old woman, is referred for a "goiter" discovered on routine physical examination. She denies any symptoms of hyper- or hypothyroidism or any history of irradiation. Her grandmother had hypothyroidism and a goiter. A large "lumpy, bumpy" gland is present, but she has no problems with breathing or swallowing. The FNA shows a benign lesion. The assessment is a nontoxic multinodular goiter. How should this be managed?

Nontoxic multinodular goiter is a common finding, occurring in about 5% of the population.[232] In low-risk patients, long-standing asymptomatic nodules that have not exhibited recent growth are likely to be benign and can be followed or excised surgically for cosmetic reasons. If the patient develops symptoms (swallowing or respiratory difficulty), surgery is the treatment of choice. Observation with close follow-up is the preferred treatment option for most benign multinodular goiters.

T_4 suppression therapy to decrease TSH stimulation and further gland enlargement can be considered if the patient has no cardiac contraindications. Whether T_4 suppression is effective is controversial; studies have noted both reductions in nodular growth and no changes.[232–234] Some gland shrinkage should be noted 3 to 6 months following the initiation of T_4 0.1 to 0.2 mg/day to suppress the TSH to subnormal levels. If so, maintenance therapy can be continued. However, the dangers of long-term thyroid suppression therapy (e.g., osteoporosis, cardiac toxicity) outweigh any potential benefits.[55–59] Patients should be carefully monitored for the development of hyperthyroidism. Most multinodular goiters contain autonomously functioning nodules that are independent of TSH control and could produce excessive thyroid hormone secretion spontaneously.[232] Toxic multinodular goiters are optimally treated with RAI therapy.[206] If the nodules grow while the patient is receiving T_4 therapy, rebiopsy or surgery should be considered. Nodular responsiveness to T_4 does not rule out malignancy.

Thyrotropin-α and Thyroid Suppression Therapy for Thyroid Cancer

60. J.R., a 28-year-old man, had a total thyroidectomy last year for papillary cancer followed by RAI therapy. He is clinically euthyroid on 200 mcg L-thyroxine daily with a TSH level of <0.2 μunits/mL (normal, 0.5–4.7). He is hesitant to discontinue his L-thyroxine so that an RAIU scan and thyroglobulin testing can be done to evaluate for tumor recurrence. His doctor is concerned about his suppressed TSH level and is also worried about taking J.R. off his L-thyroxine because the patient says he "feels incapacitated" while carrying out these tests. What can you tell his physician about the TSH level and the need to stop L-thyroxine during these tests?

[SI units: TSH, 0.2 mIU/L (normal, 0.5–4.7)]

In patients with thyroid cancers, total thyroidectomy, followed by RAI and L-thyroxine therapy to suppress the TSH to subnormal levels, were associated with improved overall survival.[235] The actual degree of thyroid suppression required is unclear but will depend on the severity of the thyroid cancer. An expert task force recommends a TSH level <0.1 μunits/mL to 0.5 μunits/mL for the majority of patients.[232] A low normal TSH of 0.3 to 2 μunits/mL can be considered for disease free patients.

Annually, it is important to assess recurrence of the malignancy by determining whether any residual cancerous or normal thyroid tissue remains. This is done by raising endogenous TSH levels. A rise in thyroglobulin concentrations and/or positive RAIU scan is an indication for additional RAI therapy. If no thyroid tissue is detected, patients are considered free of cancer and an evaluation is repeated in 1 year. Before recombinant human TSH or thyrotropin alfa (Thyrogen) was available, it was necessary to allow recovery of endogenous TSH secretion by discontinuing T_4 for 4 to 6 weeks. The development of hypothyroidism during this withdrawal period is often distressing. Now, thyrotropin-α is indicated as an adjunctive tool for the follow-up assessment of patients with thyroid cancer.[236]

Thyrotropin-α is intended to improve the quality of life in these patients by allowing these procedures to be undertaken without stopping the T_4. Clinical trials show that thyrotropin is comparable to the traditional method of T_4 withdrawal to detect distant metastases but that thyroid withdrawal is still superior in identifying recurrent thyroid cancers. Thyrotropin-α failed to detect localized tumor recurrence in 7% of patients compared to 100% detection after hormone withdrawal but detected 100% of patients with metastatic disease.[232,236]

Thyrotropin-α is generally well tolerated. Nausea, headaches, and asthenia are the most common adverse effects noted. Recombinant human TSH is available as a 0.9-mg vial and is administered once daily for 2 days IM. Thyrotropin costs approximately $1,118 per two-vial kit and is covered under most health plans. Improved quality of life, avoidance of hypothyroidism, and increased patient productivity may offset the direct costs of thyrotropin. However, concerns exist about the efficacy of thyrotropin-α to detect tumor recurrence compared with the current standard of practice, which is withdrawal of T_4 therapy. Further studies are needed to identify its role in care.

J.R. should be maintained on his current L-thyroxine suppression dosage because his TSH level is appropriately suppressed without hyperthyroidism.

REFERENCES

1. Demers LM, Spencer CA. Laboratory Medicine Practice Guidelines. Laboratory support for the diagnosis and monitoring of thyroid disease. *Thyroid* 2003;13:19.
2. Ross DS. Serum thyroid-stimulating hormone measurement for assessment of thyroid function and disease. *Endocrinol Metab Clin North Am* 2001;30:245.
3. Surks MI et al. ATA guidelines for use of laboratory tests in thyroid disorders. *JAMA* 1990;263:1529.
4. Peeters RP et al. Genetic variation in the thyroid hormone pathway genes; polymorphisms in the TSH receptor and the iodothyronine deiodinases. *Eur J Endocrinol* 2006;155:655.
5. Surks MI et al. The thyrotropin reference range should remain unchanged. *J Clin Endocrinol Metab* 2005;90:5489.

6. Wartofsky L, Dickey RA. The evidence for a narrower thyrotropin reference range is compelling. *J Clin Endocrinol Metab* 2005;90:5483.
7. Surks MI, Sievert R. Drugs and thyroid function. *N Engl J Med* 1995;333:1688.
8. DeGroot LJ. Non-thyroidal illness syndrome is a manifestation of hypothalamic-pituitary dysfunction, and in view of current evidence, should be treated with appropriate replacement therapies. *Crit Care Clin* 2006;22:57.
9. Fliers E et al. The hypothalamic-pituitary-thyroid axis in critical illness. *Best Pract Res Clin Endocrinol Metab* 2001;15:453.
10. Plikat K, et al Frequency and outcome of patients with nonthyroidal illness syndrome in a medical intensive care unit. *Metabolism* 2007;56:239.
11. Slag MF et al. Hypothyroxinemia in critically ill patients as a predictor of high mortality. *JAMA* 1981;245:43.
12. Friberg L et al. Association between increased levels of reverse triiodothyronine and mortality after acute myocardial infarction. *Am J Med* 2001; 111:699.
13. Stathatos N, Wartofsky L. The euthyroid sick syndrome: is there a physiologic rationale for thyroid hormone treatment? *J Endocrinol Invest* 2003; 26:1174.
14. Acker CG et al. Thyroid hormone in the treatment of post-transplant acute tubular necrosis (ATN). *Am J Transplant* 2002;2:57.
15. Brent GA, Hershman JM. Thyroxine therapy in patients with severe nonthyroidal illnesses and lower serum thyroxine concentration. *J Clin Endocrinol Metab* 1986;63:1.
16. Becker RA et al. Hypermetabolic low triiodothyronine syndrome of burn injury. *Crit Care Med* 1982;10:870.
17. Wyne KL. The role of thyroid hormone therapy in acutely ill cardiac patients. *Crit Care* 2005;9:333.
18. Wang R et al. Salsalate administration: a potential pharmacological model of the sick euthyroid syndrome. *J Clin Endocrinol Metab* 1998;83:3095.
19. McDonnell RJ. Abnormal thyroid function test results in patients taking salsalate. *JAMA* 1992; 267:1242.
20. Curran PG, Degroot LJ. The effect of hepatic enzyme-inducing drugs on thyroid hormones and the thyroid gland. *Endocrinol Rev* 1991;12:135.
21. Surks MI, DeFesi CR. Normal serum free thyroid hormone concentrations in patients treated with phenytoin or carbamazepine: a paradox resolved. *JAMA* 1996;275:1495.
22. Isojarvi JIT et al. Thyroid function in men taking carbamazepine, oxcarbazepine, or valproate for epilepsy. *Epilepsia* 2001;42:930.
23. Tiihonen M et al. Thyroid status of patients receiving long-term anticonvulsant therapy assessed by peripheral parameters: a placebo-controlled thyroxine therapy trial. *Epilepsia* 1995;36:1118.
24. Blackshear JL et al. Thyroxine replacement requirements in hypothyroid patients receiving phenytoin. *Ann Intern Med* 1983;99:341.
25. DeLuca F et al. Changes in thyroid function tests induced by 2 month carbamazepine treatment in L-thyroxine-substituted hypothyroid children. *Eur J Paediatr* 1986;145:77.
26. English TN et al. Abnormalities in thyroid function associated with chronic therapy with methadone. *Clin Chem* 1988;34:2202.
27. Arafah BM. Increased need for thyroxine in women with hypothyroidism during estrogen therapy. *N Engl J Med* 2001;344:1743.
28. Marqusee E et al. The effect of droloxifene and estrogen on thyroid function in postmenopausal women. *J Clin Endocrinol Metab* 2000;85:4407.
29. Hsu SHJ et al. Effect of long-term use of raloxifene, a selective estrogen receptor modulatory on thyroid function test profiles. *Clin Chem* 2001;10:1865.
30. Kostoglour-Athanassiou I et al. Thyroid function in postmenopausal women with breast cancer on tamoxifen. *Eur J Gynaecol Oncol* 1998;19:150.
31. Basaria S, Cooper DS. Amiodarone and the thyroid. *Am J Med* 2005;118:706.
32. Martino E et al. The effects of amiodarone on the thyroid. *Endocr Rev* 2001;22:240.
33. Kurnik D et al. Complex drug–drug–disease interactions between amiodarone, warfarin, and the thyroid gland. *Medicine* 2004;83:107.
34. Lee E et al. Effect of acute high-dose dobutamine administration on serum thyrotropin (TSH). *Clin Endocrinol* 1999;50:486.
35. Keogh MA, Wittert GA. Effect of cabergoline on thyroid function in hyperprolactinaemia [letter]. *Clin Endocrinol* 2002;57:699.
36. Vigersky RA et al. Thyrotropin suppression by metformin. *J Clin Endocrinol Metab* 2006;91:225.
37. Roberts CGP, Ladenson PW. Hypothyroidism. *Lancet* 2004;363:793.
38. Rees-Jones RW, Larsen PR. Triiodothyronine and thyroxine content of desiccated thyroid tablets. *Metabolism* 1977;26:1213.
39. Rees-Jones RW et al. Hormonal content of thyroid replacement preparations. *JAMA* 1980;243:549.
40. Csako GA et al. Therapeutic potential of two over-the-counter thyroid hormone preparations. *Drug Intell Clin Pharm* 1990;24:26.
41. Sawin CT, London MH. "Natural" desiccated thyroid, a health food thyroid preparation. *Arch Intern Med* 1989;149:2117.
42. Sawin CT et al. A comparison of thyroxine and desiccated thyroid in patients with primary hypothyroidism. *Metabolism* 1978;27:1518.
43. Wiersinga WM. Thyroid hormone replacement therapy. *Horm Res* 2001;56(Suppl 1):74.
44. Fish LH et al. Replacement dose, metabolism, and bioavailability of levothyroxine in the treatment of hypothyroidism. *N Engl J Med* 1987;316:764.
45. Bolk N et al. The effect of thyroxine is greater when taken at bedtime. *Clin Endocrinol (Oxf)* 2007; 66:43.
46. Hennessey JV. Levothyroxine a new drug? Since when? How could that be? *Thyroid* 2003;13:279.
47. AACE, TES, and ATA joint position statement on the use and interchangeability of thyroxine products. *Thyroid* 2004;14:486.
48. Blakesley VA. Current methodology to assess bioequivalence of levothyroxine sodium products is inadequate. *AAPS J* 2005;7:E42.
49. Toft A. Which thyroxine? *Thyroid* 2005;15:124.
50. Gibaldi M. Bioequivalence of thyroid preparations: the final word? *AAPS J* 2005;7:E59.
51. Bolton S. Bioequivalence studies for levothyroxine. *AAPS J* 2005;7:E47.
52. Klein I, Danzi S. Evaluation of the therapeutic efficacy of different levothyroxine preparations in the treatment of human thyroid disease. *Thyroid* 2003;13:1127.
53. Escobar-Morreale HF et al. Review: treatment of hypothyroidism with combinations of levothyroxine plus liothyronine. *J Clin Endocrinol Metab* 2005;90:4946.
54. Grozinsky-Glasberg S et al. Combined thyroxine and triiodothyronine therapy is not more effective than thyroxine alone in patients with hypothyroidism. *J Clin Endocrinol Metab* 2006;91:2592.
55. Fazio S et al. Effects of thyroid hormone on the cardiovascular system. *Recent Prog Horm Res* 2004;59:31.
56. Murphy E, Williams GR. The thyroid and the skeleton. *Clin Endocrinol* 2004;61:285.
57. Surks MI et al. Subclinical thyroid disease: scientific review and guidelines for diagnosis and management. *JAMA* 2004;291:228.
58. Col NF et al. Subclinical thyroid disease: clinical applications. *JAMA* 2004;291:239.
59. Cooper DS. Approach to the patient with subclinical hyperthyroidism. *J Clin Endocrinol Metab* 2007;92:3.
60. Annemieke R et al. The starting dose of levothyroxine in primary hypothyroidism treatment: a prospective, randomized, double-blind trial. *Arch Intern Med* 2005;165:1714.
61. Woeber KA. Levothyroxine therapy and serum free thyroxine and free triiodothyronine concentrations. *J Endocrinol Invest* 2002;25:106.
62. Grund FM, Niewoehner CB. Hyperthyroxinemia in patients receiving thyroid replacement therapy. *Arch Intern Med* 1989;149:921.
63. Dong BJ et al. Bioequivalence of generic and brand-name levothyroxine products in the treatment of hypothyroidism. *JAMA* 1997;277:1205.
64. Ain KB et al. Thyroid hormone levels affected by time of blood sampling in thyroxine-treated patients. *Thyroid* 1993;3:81.
65. Walsh JP et al. Small changes in thyroxine dose do not alter well-being or symptoms in patients with hypothyroidism. *J Clin Endocrinol Metab* 2006;91:2624.
66. Sawin CT et al. Aging and the thyroid: decreased requirements for thyroid hormone in older hypothyroid patients. *Am J Med* 1983;75:206.
67. Davis FB et al. Estimation of a physiologic replacement dose of levothyroxine in elderly patients with hypothyroidism. *Arch Intern Med* 1984;144:1752.
68. Kabadi UM. Variability of L-thyroxine replacement dose in elderly patients with primary hypothyroidism. *J Fam Pract* 1987;24:473.
69. Grebe SKG et al. Treatment of hypothyroidism with once-weekly thyroxine. *J Clin Endocrinol Metab* 1997;82:870.
70. Casey BM et al. Subclinical hypothyroidism and pregnancy outcomes. *Obstet Gynecol* 2005;105: 239.
71. Haddow JE et al. Maternal thyroid deficiency during pregnancy and subsequent neuropsychological development of the child. *N Engl J Med* 1999; 341:549.
72. Allan WC et al. Maternal thyroid deficiency and pregnancy complications: implications for population screening. *J Med Screen* 2000;7:127.
73. Kooistra L et al. Neonatal effects of maternal hypothyroxinemia during early pregnancy. *Pediatrics* 2006;117:161.
74. Pop VJ et al. Maternal hypothyroxinemia during early pregnancy and subsequent child development: a 3-year follow-up study. *Clin Endocrinol* 2003;59:282.
75. Mandel SJ et al. Increased need for thyroxine during pregnancy in women with primary hypothyroidism. *N Engl J Med* 1990;323:91.
76. Alexander EK et al. Timing and magnitude of increases in levothyroxine requirements during pregnancy in women with hypothyroidism. *N Engl J Med* 2004;351:241.
77. Vaidya B et al. Detection of thyroid dysfunction in early pregnancy: universal screening or targeted high-risk case finding? *J Clin Endocrinol Metab* 2007;92:203.
78. Chopra IJ, Baber K. Treatment of primary hypothyroidism during pregnancy: is there an increase in thyroxine dose requirement in pregnancy? *Metabolism* 2003;52:122.
79. LaFranchi S. Congenital hypothyroidism: etiologies, diagnosis, and management. *Thyroid* 1999;9: 735.
80. Rovet JF. In search of the optimal therapy for congenital hypothyroidism. *J Pediatr* 2004;144:698.
81. Salerno M et al. Effect of different starting doses of levothyroxine on growth and intellectual outcome at four years of age in congenital hypothyroidism. *Thyroid* 2002;12:45.
82. Bongers-Schokking JJ et al. Influence of timing and dose of thyroid hormone replacement on mental, psychomotor, and behavioral development in children with congenital hypothyroidism. *J Pediatr* 2005;147:768.
83. Rovet JF. Children with congenital hypothyroidism and their siblings: do they really differ? *Pediatrics* 2005;115:e52
84. Oerbeck B et al. Congenital hypothyroidism: influence of disease severity and L-thyroxine treatment on intellectual, motor, and school-associated outcomes in young adults. *Pediatrics* 2003;112:923.
85. Simoneau-Roy J et al. Cognition and behavior at school entry in children with congenital hypothyroidism treated early with high-dose levothyroxine. *J Pediatr* 2004;144:747.
86. Heyerdahl S, Oerbeck B. Congenital hypothyroidism: developmental outcome in relation to

levothyroxine treatment variables. *Thyroid* 2003; 13:1029.
87. Oerbeck B et al. Congenital hypothyroidism: no adverse effects of high dose thyroxine treatment on adult memory, attention, and behavior. *Arch Dis Child* 2005;90:132.
88. Selva KA et al. Initial treatment dose of L-thyroxine in congenital hypothyroidism. *J Pediatr* 2002;141:786.
89. Ain KB et al. Pseudomalabsorption of levothyroxine. *JAMA* 1991;266:2118.
90. Sherman SI, Malecha SE. Absorption and malabsorption of levothyroxine. *Am J Ther* 1995;2:814.
91. Takasu N et al. Rifampin-induced hypothyroidism. *J Endocrinol Invest* 2006;29:645.
92. Smit JW et al. Bexarotene induced hypothyroidism: bexarotene stimulates the peripheral metabolism of thyroid hormones. *J Clin Endocrinol Metab* 2007;92:2496.
93. deGroot JWB et al. Imatinib induces hypothyroidism in patients receiving levothyroxine. *Clin Pharmacol Ther* 2005;78:433.
94. Benvenga S et al. Delayed intestinal absorption of levothyroxine. *Thyroid* 1995;5:249.
95. Liel Y et al. Evidence for a clinically important adverse effect of fiber-enriched diet on the bioavailability of levothyroxine in adult hypothyroid patients. *J Clin Endocrinol Metab* 1996;80:857.
96. Bell DS, Ovalle F. Use of soy protein supplement and resultant need for increased dose of levothyroxine. *Endocr Pract* 2001;7:193.
97. Siraj ES et al. Raloxifene causing malabsorption of levothyroxine. *Arch Intern Med* 2003;163:1367.
98. Harmon SM, Seifert CF. Levothyroxine-cholestyramine interaction reemphasized [letter]. *Ann Intern Med* 1991;115:658.
99. Campbell NRC et al. Ferrous sulfate reduces thyroxine efficacy in patients with hypothyroidism. *Ann Intern Med* 1992;117:1010.
100. Demke DM. Drug interaction between thyroxine and lovastatin [letter]. *N Engl J Med* 1989; 321:1341.
101. Sperber AD, Liel Y. Evidence for interference with the intestinal absorption of levothyroxine sodium by aluminum hydroxide. *Arch Intern Med* 1992; 152:183.
102. Havrankova J, Lahaie R. Levothyroxine binding by sucralfate [letter]. *Ann Intern Med* 1992;117: 445.
103. Singh N et al. Effect of calcium carbonate on the absorption of levothyroxine. *JAMA* 2000;283:2822.
104. Singh N et al. The acute effect of calcium carbonate on the intestinal absorption of levothyroxine. *Thyroid* 2001;11:967.
105. Diskin CJ et al. Effect of phosphate binders upon TSH and L-thyroxine dose in patients on thyroid replacement. *Int Urol Nephrol* 2007;39:599.
106. Centanni M et al. Thyroxine absorption is decreased in patients with *Helicobacter pylori*-related gastritis and atrophic gastritis and by omeprazole therapy. *N Engl J Med* 2006;354:1787.
107. Dietrich JW et al. Absorption kinetics of levothyroxine is not altered by proton-pump inhibitor therapy. *Horm Metab Res* 2006;38:57.
108. Duntas LH. Thyroid disease and lipids. *Thyroid* 2002;12:287.
109. Wartoksky L. Myxedema coma. *Endocrinol Metab Clin North Am* 2006;35:687.
110. Yamamoto T et al. Factors associated with mortality of myxedema coma: report of eight cases and literature survey. *Thyroid* 1999;9:1167.
111. MacKerrow SD et al. Myxedema-associated cardiogenic shock treated with intravenous triiodothyronine. *Ann Intern Med* 1992;117:1014.
112. Pereira VG et al. Management of myxedema coma: report on three successfully treated cases with nasogastric or intravenous administration of triiodothyronine. *J Endocrinol Invest* 1982;5:331.
113. Ladenson PW et al. Rapid pituitary and peripheral tissue responses to intravenous L-triiodothyronine in hypothyroidism. *J Clin Endocrinol Metab* 1983;56:1252.
114. Hylander B, Rosenqvist U. Treatment of myxedema coma: factors associated with fatal outcome. *Acta Endocrinol (Copenh)* 1985;108:65.
115. Ariot S et al. Myxoedema coma: response of thyroid hormones with oral and intravenous high-dose L-thyroxine treatment. *Intensive Care Med* 1991;17:16.
116. Kohno A, Hara Y. Severe myocardial ischemia following hormone replacement in two cases of hypothyroidism with normal coronary arteriogram. *Endocrinol J* 2001;48:565.
117. Fadeyev VV et al. Levothyroxine replacement therapy in patients with subclinical hypothyroidism and coronary artery disease. *Endocr Pract* 2006;12:5.
118. Levine D. Compromise therapy in the patient with angina pectoris and hypothyroidism. *Am J Med* 1980;69:411.
119. Lawrence JR et al. Digoxin kinetics in patients with thyroid dysfunction. *Clin Pharmacol Ther* 1977;22:7.
120. Doherty JE et al. Digoxin metabolism in hypo- and hyperthyroidism. *Ann Intern Med* 1966;64:489.
121. Myerowitz PD. Diagnosis and management of the hypothyroid patient with chest pain. *J Thorac Cardiovasc Surg* 1983;86:57.
122. Becker C. Hypothyroidism and atherosclerotic heart disease: pathogenesis, medical management and the role of coronary artery bypass surgery. *Endocrinol Rev* 1985;6:432.
123. Staub HG et al. Prospective study of the spontaneous course of subclinical hypothyroidism: prognostic value of thyrotropin, thyroid reserve, and thyroid antibodies. *J Clin Endocrinol Metab* 2002;87: 3221.
124. McDermott MT, Ridgway EC. Subclinical hypothyroidism is mild thyroid failure and should be treated. *J Clin Endocrinol Metab* 2001;86:4585.
125. Kong WM et al. A 6-month randomized trial of thyroxine treatment in women with mild subclinical hypothyroidism. *Am J Med* 2002;112:348.
126. Meier C et al. TSH-controlled L-thyroxine therapy reduces cholesterol levels and clinical symptoms in subclinical hypothyroidism: a double blind placebo-controlled trial (Basel Thyroid Study). *J Clin Endocrinol Metab* 2001;86:4860.
127. Rodondi N et al. The risk of coronary heart disease is increased in subclinical hypothyroidism. *Am J Med* 2006;119:541.
128. Walsh JP et al. Subclinical thyroid dysfunction as a risk factor for cardiovascular disease. *Arch Intern Med* 2005;165:2467.
129. Danese MD et al. Effect of thyroxine therapy on serum lipoproteins in patients with mild thyroid failure: a quantitative review of the literature. *J Clin Endocrinol Metab* 2000;85:2993.
130. Wardle CA et al. Pitfalls in the use of thyrotropin concentration as a first-line thyroid function test. *Lancet* 2001;357:1013.
131. Pollock MA et al. Thyroxine treatment in patients with symptoms of hypothyroidism but thyroid function tests within the reference range: randomised double-blind placebo-controlled crossover trial. *Br Med J* 2001;323:891.
132. Weetman AP. Thyroxine treatment in biochemically euthyroid but clinically hypothyroid individuals. *Clin Endocrinol* 2002;57:25.
133. Cooper DS. Hyperthyroidism. *Lancet* 2003;362: 459.
134. Shimizu T et al. Hyperthyroidism and the management of atrial fibrillation. *Thyroid* 2002;12:489.
135. Loeliger EA et al. The biological disappearance rate of prothrombin factors VII, IX, X from plasma in hypo-, hyper-, and during fever. *Thromb Diath Haemorrh* 1964;10:267.
136. Lipsky JJ, Gallego MO. Mechanism of thioamide antithyroid drug-associated hypoprothrombinemia. *Drug Metab Drug Interact* 1988;6:317.
137. Liaw Y et al. Hepatic injury during propylthiouracil therapy in patients with hyperthyroidism: a cohort study. *Ann Intern Med* 1993;118:424.
138. Williams KV et al. Fifty years of experience with propylthiouracil-associated hepatotoxicity: what have we learned? *J Clin Endocrinol Metab* 1997;82:1727.
139. Woeber KA. Methimazole-induced hepatotoxicity. *Endocr Pract* 2002;8:222.
140. Frye RL, Braunwald E. Studies on digitalis III: the influence of triiodothyronine on digitalis requirement. *Circulation* 1961;23:376.
141. Burman KD, Wartoksky L. Iodine effects on the thyroid gland: biochemical and clinical. *Rev Endocrinol Metab Disord* 2000;1:19.
142. Roti E, Uberti ED. Iodine excess and hyperthyroidism. *Thyroid* 2001;11:493.
143. Markou K et al. Iodine-induced hypothyroidism. *Thyroid* 2001;11:501.
144. Arbelle JE, Porath A. Practice guidelines for the detection and management of thyroid dysfunction: a comparative review of the recommendations. *Clin Endocrinol* 1999;51:11.
145. Abraham P et al. Antithyroid drug regimen for treating Graves' hyperthyroidism [review]. *Cochrane Database Syst Rev* 2005;Apr 18:CD003420.
146. Cooper DS. Antithyroid drugs. *N Engl J Med* 2005;352:905.
147. Jongjaroenprasert W et al. Rectal administration of propylthiouracil in hyperthyroid patients: comparison of suspension enema and suppository form. *Thyroid* 2002;12:627.
148. Yeung SCJ et al. Rectal administration of iodide and propylthiouracil in the treatment of thyroid storm. *Thyroid* 1995;5:403.
149. Nabil N et al. Methimazole: an alternative route of administration. *J Clin Endocrinol Metab* 1982; 54:180.
150. Alsanea O, Clark OH. Treatment of Graves' disease: the advantages of surgery. *Endocrinol Metab Clin North Am* 2000;29:321.
151. Torring O et al. Graves' hyperthyroidism: treatment with antithyroid drugs, surgery, or radioiodine: a prospective, randomized study. *J Clin Endocrinol Metab* 1996;81:2986.
152. Boostrom S, Richards ML. Total thyroidectomy is the preferred treatment for patients with Graves' disease and a thyroid nodule. *Otolaryngol Head Neck Surg* 2007;136:278.
153. Palit TK et al. The efficacy of thyroidectomy for Graves' disease: a meta-analysis. *J Surg Res* 2000;90:161.
154. Ron E et al. Cancer mortality following treatment for adult hyperthyroidism: Cooperative Thyrotoxicosis Therapy Follow-up Study Group. *JAMA* 1998;280:347.
155. Rivkees SA. The management of hyperthyroidism in children with emphasis on the use of radioactive iodine. *Pediatr Endocrinol Rev* 2003;1(Suppl 2):212.
156. Read CH et al. A 36-year retrospective analysis of the efficacy and safety of radioactive iodine in treating young Graves' patients. *J Clin Endocrinol Metab* 2004;89:4229.
157. Robertson J, Gorman CA. Gonadal radiation dose and its genetic significance in radioiodine therapy of hyperthyroidism. *J Nucl Med* 1976;17:826.
158. Holm LE. Thyroid cancer after exposure to radioactive ^{131}I. *Acta Oncol* 2006;45:1037.
159. Zuckier L et al. *Sensitivity of personal Homeland Security radiation detectors to medical radionuclides and implications for counseling of nuclear medicine patients*. Paper presented at RSNA '04, 90th Scientific Assembly and annual meeting of the RSNA; Chicago, IL; November 30.
160. Gangopadhyay KK et al. Patients treated with radioiodine can trigger airport radiation sensors for many weeks. *BMJ* 2006;333:293.
161. Fontanilla JC et al. The use of oral radiographic contrast agents in the management of hyperthyroidism. *Thyroid* 2001;22:561.
162. Wu SY et al. Comparison of sodium ipodate (Oragrafin) and propylthiouracil in early treatment of hyperthyroidism. *J Clin Endocrinol Metab* 1982;54:630.
163. Bal CS et al. Effect of iopanoic acid on radioiodine therapy of hyperthyroidism: long-term outcome of a randomized controlled trial. *J Clin Endocrinol Metab* 2005;90:6536.
164. Roti E et al. Sodium ipodate and methimazole in the

long-term treatment of hyperthyroid Graves' disease. *Metabolism* 1993;42:403.
165. Martino E et al. Therapy of Graves' disease with sodium ipodate is associated with a high recurrence rate of hyperthyroidism. *J Endocrinol Invest* 1991;14:847.
166. Nayak B, Burman K. Thyrotoxicosis and thyroid storm. *Endocrinol Metab Clin North Am* 2006;35:663.
167. Cooper DS et al. Methimazole pharmacology in man: studies using a newly developed radioimmunoassay for methimazole. *J Clin Endocrinol Metab* 1984;58:473.
168. McIver B, Morris JC. The pathogenesis of Graves' disease. *Endocrinol Metab Clin North Am* 1998;27:73.
169. Allannic H et al. Antithyroid drugs and Graves' disease: a prospective randomized evaluation of the efficacy of treatment duration. *J Clin Endocrinol Metab* 1990;70:675.
170. Maugendre D et al. Antithyroid drugs and Graves' disease: prospective randomized assessment of long-term treatment. *Clin Endocrinol* 1999;50:127.
171. Bolanos F et al. Remission of Graves' hyperthyroidism treated with methimazole. *Rev Invest Clin* 2002;54:307.
172. Nijs HG et al. Increased insulin action and clearance in hyperthyroid newly diagnosed IDDM patient: restoration to normal with antithyroid treatment. *Diabetes Care* 1989;12:319.
173. Aloush V et al. Propylthiouracil-induced autoimmune syndromes: two distinct clinical presentations with different course and management. *Semin Arthritis Rheum* 2006;36:4.
174. Geffner DL, Hershman JM. Beta-adrenergic blockade for the treatment of hyperthyroidism. *Am J Med* 1992;93:61.
175. Milner MR et al. Double-blind crossover trial of diltiazem versus propranolol in the management of thyrotoxic symptoms. *Pharmacotherapy* 1990;10:100.
176. Tajiri J et al. Antithyroid drug-induced agranulocytosis: the usefulness of routine white blood cell count monitoring. *Arch Intern Med* 1990;150:621.
177. Wall JR et al. In vitro immunosensitivity to propylthiouracil, methimazole, and carbimazole in patients with Graves' disease: a possible cause of antithyroid drug-induced agranulocytosis. *J Clin Endocrinol Metab* 1984;58:868.
178. Jakucs J, Pocsay G. Successful treatment of methimazole-induced severe aplastic anemia with recombinant human granulocyte colony-stimulating factor and high-dosage steroids. *J Endocrinol Invest* 2006;29:74.
179. Gaujoux, S et al. Extensive thyroidectomy in Graves' disease. *J Am Coll Surg* 2006;202:868.
180. He CT et al. Comparison of single daily dose of methimazole and propylthiouracil in the treatment of Graves' hyperthyroidism. *Clin Endocrinol* 2004;60:671.
181. Orgiazzi J, Madec AM. Reduction of the risk of relapse after withdrawal of medical therapy for Graves' disease. *Thyroid* 2002;12:849.
182. Vitti P et al. Clinical features of patients with Graves' disease undergoing remission after antithyroid drug treatment. *Thyroid* 1997;3:369.
183. Glinoer D et al. Effects of L-thyroxine administration, TSH-receptor antibodies and smoking on the risk of recurrence in Graves' hyperthyroidism treated with antithyroid drugs: a double-blind prospective randomized study. *Eur J Endocrinol* 2001;144:475.
184. Hashizume K et al. Administration of thyroxine in treated Graves' disease: effects on the level of antibodies to thyroid-stimulating hormone receptors and on the risk of recurrence of hyperthyroidism. *N Engl J Med* 1991;324:947.
185. Vestergaard P. Smoking and thyroid disorders—a meta-analysis. *Eur J Endocrinol* 2002;146:153.
186. Hoermann R et al. Relapse of Graves' disease after successful outcome of antithyroid drug therapy: results of a prospective randomized study on the use of levothyroxine. *Thyroid* 2002;12:1119.
187. McIver B et al. Lack of effect of thyroxine in patients with Graves' hyperthyroidism who are treated with an antithyroid drug. *N Engl J Med* 1996;334:220.
188. Golden WM et al. The retinoid receptor agonist bexarotene inhibits thyrotropin secretion in normal subjects. *J Clin Endocrinol Metab* 2007;92:124.
189. Cappola AR et al. Thyroid status, cardiovascular risk, and mortality in older adults. *JAMA* 2006;295:1033.
190. Sawin CT et al. Low serum thyrotropin concentrations as a risk factor for atrial fibrillation in older patients. *N Engl J Med* 1994;331:1249.
191. Mestman JH. Hyperthyroidism in pregnancy. *Best Pract Res Clin Endocrinol Metab* 2004;18:267.
192. Atkins P et al. Drug therapy for hyperthyroidism in pregnancy: safety issues for mother and fetus. *Drug Safety* 2000;23:229.
193. ACOG Practice Bulletin. Thyroid disease in pregnancy. *Obstet Gynecol* 2002;100:387.
194. Wing DA et al. A comparison of propylthiouracil versus methimazole in the treatment of hyperthyroidism in pregnancy. *Am J Obstet Gynecol* 1994;170:90.
195. Mortimer RH et al. Methimazole and propylthiouracil equally cross the perfused human term placental lobule. *J Clin Endocrinol Metab* 1997;82:3099.
196. Momotani N et al. Effects of propylthiouracil and methimazole on fetal thyroid status in mothers with Graves' hyperthyroidism. *J Clin Endocrinol Metab* 1997;82:3633.
197. Momotani N et al. Maternal hyperthyroidism and congenital malformation in the offspring. *Clin Endocrinol* 1984;20:695.
198. Van Dijke CP et al. Methimazole, carbimazole, and congenital skin defects [letter]. *Ann Intern Med* 1987;106:60.
199. Momotani N et al. Antithyroid drug therapy for Graves' disease during pregnancy: optimal regimen for fetal thyroid status. *N Engl J Med* 1986;315:24.
200. Wolf D et al. Antenatal carbimazole and choanal atresia: a new embryopathy. *Arch Otolaryngol Head Neck Surg* 2006;132:1009.
201. Eisenstein Z et al. Intellectual capacity of subjects exposed to methimazole or propylthiouracil in utero. *Eur J Pediatr* 1992;151:558.
202. Burrow GN et al. Intellectual development in children whose mothers received propylthiouracil during pregnancy. *Yale J Biol Med* 1978;51:151.
203. Messer MP et al. Antithyroid drug and Graves' disease in pregnancy: long-term effects on somatic growth, intellectual development and thyroid function of the offspring. *Acta Endocrinol* 1990;123:311.
204. Momotani N et al. Thyroid function in wholly breast-feeding infants whose mothers take high doses of propylthiouracil. *Clin Endocrinol* 2000; 53:177.
205. Azizi F et al. Thyroid function and intellectual development of infants nursed by mothers taking methimazole. *J Clin Endocrinol Metab* 2000;85:3233.
206. Iagaru A, McDougall IR. Treatment of thyrotoxicosis. *J Nucl Med* 2007;48:379.
207. Andrade V et al. The effect of methimazole pretreatment on the efficacy of radioactive iodine therapy in Graves' hyperthyroidism: one-year follow-up of a prospective randomized study. *J Clin Endocrinol Metab* 2001;86:3488.
208. Imseis RE et al. Pretreatment with propylthiouracil but not methimazole reduces the therapeutic efficacy of iodine-131 in hyperthyroidism. *J Clin Endocrinol Metab* 1998;83:685.
209. Tuttle RM et al. Treatment with propylthiouracil before radioactive iodine therapy is associated with a higher treatment failure rate than therapy with radioactive iodine alone in Graves' disease. *Thyroid* 1995;5:243.
210. Braga M et al. The effect of methimazole on cure rates after radioiodine treatment for Graves' hyperthyroidism: a randomized clinical trial. *Thyroid* 2002;12:135.
211. Walter MA et al. Effects of antithyroid drugs on radioiodine treatment: systemic review and meta-analysis of randomised controlled trials. *BMJ* 2007;334:514
212. Bartalena L et al. Management of Graves' ophthalmopathy: reality and perspectives. *Endocrinol Rev* 2000;21:168.
213. Wiersinga WM. Management of Graves' ophthalmopathy. *Nat Clin Pract Endocrinol Metab* 2007;3:396.
214. Bartalena L et al. Relation between therapy for hyperthyroidism and the course of Graves' ophthalmopathy. *N Engl J Med* 1998;338:73.
215. Dorkhan M et al. Treatment with a thiazolidinedione increases eye protrusion in a subgroup of patients with type 2 diabetes. *Clin Endocrinol (Oxf)* 2006;65:35.
216. Marcocci C et al. Relationship between Graves' ophthalmopathy and type of treatment of Graves' hyperthyroidism. *Thyroid* 1992;2:171.
217. Tsai WC et al. The effect of combination therapy with propylthiouracil and cholestyramine in the treatment of Graves' hyperthyroidism. *Clin Endocrinol* 2005;62:521.
218. McCowen KC et al. Elevated serum thyrotropin in thyroxine treated patients with hypothyroidism given sertraline [letter]. *N Engl J Med* 1997; 337:1010.
219. Bocchetta A, Loviselli A. Lithium treatment and thyroid abnormalities. *Clin Pract Epidemol Ment Health* 2006;2:23.
220. Bocchetta A et al. Ten-year follow-up of thyroid function in lithium patients. *J Clin Psychopharmacol* 2001;21:594.
221. Kleiner J et al. Lithium-induced subclinical hypothyroidism: review of the literature and guidelines for treatment. *J Clin Psychiatr* 1999;60: 249.
222. Gammage MD et al. Association between serum free thyroxine concentration and atrial fibrillation. *Arch Intern Med* 2007;167:928.
223. Barclay ML et al. Lithium associated thyrotoxicosis: a report of 14 cases, with statistical analysis of incidence. *Clin Endocrinol* 1994;40:759.
224. Dang AH, Hershman JM. Lithium-associated thyroiditis. *Endocrinol Pract* 2002;8:232.
225. Bogazzi F et al. Preparation with iopanoic acid rapidly controls thyrotoxicosis in patients with amiodarone-induced thyrotoxicosis before thyroidectomy. *Surgery* 2002;132:1114.
226. Mandac JC et al. The clinical and physiological spectrum of interferon alpha induced thyroiditis: toward a new classification. *Hepatology* 2006;43:661.
227. Dalgard O et al. Thyroid dysfunction during treatment of chronic hepatitis C with interferon alpha: no association with either interferon dosage or efficacy of therapy. *J Intern Med* 2002;251:400.
228. Carella C et al. Long-term outcome of interferon-induced thyroid autoimmunity and prognostic influence of thyroid autoantibody pattern at the end of treatment. *J Clin Endocrinol Metab* 2001;86:1925.
229. Wong V et al. Thyrotoxicosis induced by alpha-interferon therapy in chronic viral hepatitis. *Clin Endocrinol* 2002;56:793.
230. Becker DV et al. Childhood thyroid cancer following the Chernobyl accident: a status report. *Endocrinol Metab Clin North Am* 1996;25:197.
231. U.S. Department of Health and Human Services, Food and Drug Administration, Center for Drug Evaluation and Research. *Guidance document: Potassium iodide as a thyroid blocking agent in radiation emergencies*. December 2001. Available at: http://www.fda.gov/cder/guidance/4825fnl.htm. Accessed July 16, 2007.
232. The ATA Guidelines Taskforce. Management guidelines for patients with thyroid nodules and differentiated thyroid cancer. *Thyroid* 2006;16:109.
233. Wemeau JL et al. Effects of thyroid-stimulating hormone suppression with levothyroxine in reducing the volume of solitary thyroid nodules and improving extranodular nonpalpable changes: a randomized, double-blind, placebo-controlled trial by the French Thyroid Research Group. *J Clin Endocrinol Metab* 2002;87:4928.

234. Castro MR et al. Effectiveness of thyroid hormone suppressive therapy in benign solitary thyroid nodules: a meta-analysis. *J Clin Endocrinol Metab* 2002;87:4154.
235. Jonklaas J et al. Outcomes of patients with differentiated thyroid carcinoma following initial therapy. *Thyroid* 2006;16:1229.
236. Basaria M et al. The use of recombinant thyrotropin in the follow-up of patients with differentiated thyroid cancer. *Am J Med* 2002;112:721.
237. McDonnell ME, Braverman LE, Bernardo J. Hypothyroidism due to ethionamide. *N Engl J Med* 2005;352:2757.
238. Rini BI et al. Hypothyroidism in patients with metastatic renal cell carcinoma treated with sunitinib. *J Natl Cancer Inst* 2007;99:81.
239. Desai J et al. Hypothyroidism after sunitinib treatment for patients with gastrointestinal stromal tumors. *Ann Intern Med* 2006;145:660.
240. Krouse RS et al. Thyroid dysfunction in 281 patients with metastatic melanoma or renal carcinoma treated with interleukin-2 alone. *J Immunother Emphasis Tumor Immunol* 1995;18:272.
241. Weijl NI et al. Hypothyroidism during immunotherapy with interleukin-2 is associated with antithyroid antibodies and response to treatment. *J Clin Oncol* 1993;11:1376.
242. Bogazzi F et al. Treatment with lithium prevents serum thyroid hormone increase after thioamide withdrawal and radioiodine therapy in patients with Graves' disease. *J Clin Endocrinol Metab* 2002;87:4490.
243. Auer J et al. Subclinical hyperthyroidism as a risk factor for atrial fibrillation. *Am Heart J* 2001;142:838.

CHAPTER 50

Diabetes Mellitus

Lisa A. Kroon, Mitra Assemi, and Betsy A. Carlisle

An estimated 20.8 million people, or 7.0% of the United States population, currently has diabetes.[1] Of these, 6.2 million or about one-third were undiagnosed. In 2005 alone, over 1.5 million new cases in adults were diagnosed. Globally, the prevalence of diabetes for all ages is estimated to be 2.8% in 2000 and projected to increase to 4.4% by 2030.[2] The Centers for Disease Control and Prevention predicts the national incidence of diabetes will rise by 37.5% by the year 2025. The incidence of type 2 diabetes is now epidemic, with alarming increases in prevalence in both adults and children. The dramatic increase in type 2 diabetes is related to obesity and decreased physical activity levels. Additional factors include genetic predisposition, increased insulin resistance, and progressive β-cell failure. Clinical studies have affirmed that type 2 diabetes can be delayed or prevented in high-risk populations and that good glycemic control and other interventions can slow its devastating complications. Therefore, broad implementation of guidelines and goals established by the American Diabetes Association (ADA) and others, as well as progress in processes of care, which could help to eliminate health disparities, need to be national priorities.[3]

Definition, Classification, and Epidemiology

Diabetes is a chronic condition caused by a relative or an absolute lack of insulin. Its hallmark clinical characteristics are symptomatic glucose intolerance resulting in hyperglycemia and alterations in lipid and protein metabolism. Over the long term, these metabolic abnormalities contribute to the development of complications such as retinopathy, nephropathy, and neuropathy.

Genetically, etiologically, and clinically, diabetes is a heterogeneous group of disorders. Nevertheless, most cases of diabetes mellitus can be assigned to type 1 or type 2 diabetes (Table 50-1). The term gestational diabetes mellitus (GDM) is used to describe glucose intolerance that has its onset during pregnancy. Glucose intolerance that cannot be ascribed to causes consistent with these three classifications include specific genetic defects in β-cell function or insulin action; diseases of the exocrine pancreas; endocrinopathies; drug or chemical-induced; infections; and other genetic syndromes.[4] Subclinical glucose intolerance or "prediabetes" is identified as impaired fasting glucose (IFG) and/or impaired glucose tolerance (IGT).

Approximately 5% to 10% of the diagnosed diabetic population has type 1 diabetes, which usually results from autoimmune destruction of the pancreatic β-cells.[4] At clinical presentation, these patients have little or no pancreatic reserve, have a tendency to develop ketoacidosis, and require exogenous insulin to sustain life. The incidence of autoimmune-mediated type 1 diabetes peaks during childhood and adolescence, but can occur at any age. A minority of patients diagnosed with type 1 diabetes, mostly of African or Asian ancestry, have no evidence of autoimmunity; the etiology is, therefore, unknown. In these individuals, the rate of pancreatic destruction seems to occur more slowly, leading to a later onset and less acute presentation.

Most people with diabetes have type 2 diabetes, a heterogeneous disorder that is characterized by obesity, β-cell dysfunction, resistance to insulin action, and increased hepatic glucose production. Both the incidence and prevalence of diabetes increase dramatically with age. For example, the prevalence of self-reported diagnosed diabetes is 1.7% among persons 20 to 39 years of age and 15.8% among persons over 65 years of age.[5] One study estimates that the prevalence of diabetes in persons over 65 years of age increased 62% from 2003 to 2004.[6] The prevalence of type 2 diabetes also differs among ethnic populations. Relative to Caucasians, the prevalence of diagnosed

Table 50-1 Type 1 and Type 2 Diabetes

Characteristics	*Type 1*	*Type 2*
Other names	Previously, type I; insulin-dependent diabetes mellitus (IDDM); juvenile-onset diabetes mellitus	Previously, type II; non–insulin-dependent diabetes mellitus (NIDDM); adult-onset diabetes mellitus
Percentage of diabetic population	5–10%	90%
Age at onset	Usually <30 yr; peaks at 12–14 yr; rare before 6 mo; some adults develop type 1 during the fifth decade	Usually >40 yr, but increasing prevalence among obese children
Pancreatic function	Usually none, although some residual C-peptide can sometimes be detected at diagnosis, especially in adults	Insulin present in low, "normal," or high amounts
Pathogenesis	Associated with certain HLA types; presence of islet cell antibodies suggests autoimmune process	Defect in insulin secretion; tissue resistance to insulin; ↑ hepatic glucose output
Family history	Generally not strong	Strong
Obesity	Uncommon unless "overinsulinized" with exogenous insulin	Common (60–90%)
History of ketoacidosis	Often present	Rare, except in circumstances of unusual stress (e.g., infection)
Clinical presentation	Moderate to severe symptoms that generally progress relatively rapidly (days to weeks): polyuria, polydipsia, fatigue, weight loss, ketoacidosis	Mild polyuria, fatigue; often diagnosed on routine physical or dental examination
Treatment	Insulin MNT Physical activity Amylin mimetic (pramlintide)	MNT Physical activity Antidiabetic agents (biguanides, nonsulfonylurea insulin secretagogues, sulfonylureas, thiazolidinediones, α-glucosidase inhibitors, incretin mimetics/analogs, DPP-4 inhibitors) Insulin Amylin mimetic (pramlintide)

MNT, medical nutrition therapy; HLA, human leukocyte antigen; DPP-4, dipeptidyl peptidase-4.

and undiagnosed diabetes is higher in African Americans (1.8 times), Hispanics/Latinos (1.7 times), American Indians and Alaskan Natives (2.2 times), and Asian Americans and Pacific Islanders (>2.0 times).[1] Growth in the aging population as well as greater racial and ethnic diversity in the USA are causing predicted increases in the prevalence of diagnosed diabetes from 5.6% to 12% by 2050.[7]

Diabetes is a serious condition that places people at risk for greater morbidity and mortality relative to the nondiabetic population. Diabetes is the sixth leading cause of death in the United States, although deaths attributed to diabetes and its complications are likely to be underreported.[1] Compared with the general population, the mortality rate for people with diabetes is about twice that for people without diabetes. In addition, disparities in morbidity and mortality attributed to acute and chronic complications associated with diabetes have been documented in certain groups, such as underrepresented minorities and the uninsured.[8]

Medical management of persons with diabetes is costly. In 2007, the total cost of diabetes in the United States was estimated to be $174 billion, with 1 out of 5 health care dollars being spent on people with diabetes.[9] The average health care expenditures for people with diabetes were approximately 2.3 times higher than those for individuals without diabetes. The majority (56%) of all health care expenditures attributed to diabetes are used by persons age 65 years and older. Hospital inpatient costs, nursing facility resources, home care, physician visits, and medications (not just insulin and oral agents) made up the majority of these expenditures. Because many expenditures are related to treatment of long-term complications, considerable effort has been directed toward early diagnosis and metabolic control of patients with diabetes.

Carbohydrate Metabolism[10]

An understanding of the signs and symptoms associated with diabetes is based on a knowledge of glucose metabolism and the metabolic effects of insulin in nondiabetic and diabetic subjects during the fed (postprandial) and fasting (postabsorptive) states.[10] Homeostatic mechanisms maintain plasma glucose concentrations between 55 and 140 mg/dL (3.1–7.8 mmol/L). A minimum concentration of 40 to 60 mg/dL (2.2–3.3 mmol/L) is required to provide adequate fuel for the central nervous system, which uses glucose as its primary energy source and is independent of insulin for glucose utilization. When blood glucose concentrations exceed the reabsorptive capacity of the kidneys (~180 mg/dL), glucose spills into the urine, resulting in a loss of calories and water. Muscle and fat, which use glucose as a major source of energy, require insulin for glucose uptake. If glucose is unavailable, these tissues are able to use other substrates such as amino acids and fatty acids for fuel.

Postprandial Glucose Metabolism in the Nondiabetic Individual

After food is ingested, blood glucose concentrations rise and stimulate insulin release. Insulin is the key to efficient glucose utilization. It promotes the uptake of glucose, fatty acids, and amino acids and their conversion to storage forms in most tissues. Insulin also inhibits hepatic glucose production by suppressing glucagon and its effects. In muscle, insulin promotes the uptake of glucose and its storage as glycogen. It also stimulates the uptake of amino acids and their conversion to protein. In adipose tissue, glucose is converted to free fatty acids and stored as triglycerides. Insulin also prevents a breakdown of these triglycerides to free fatty acids, a form that may be transported to other tissues for utilization. The liver does not require insulin for glucose transport, but insulin facilitates the conversion of glucose to glycogen and free fatty acids. The latter are esterified to triglycerides, which are transported by very-low-density lipoproteins (VLDLs) to adipose and muscle tissue.

Fasting Glucose Metabolism in the Nondiabetic Individual

As blood glucose concentrations drop toward normal during the fasting state, insulin release is inhibited. Simultaneously, a number of counter-regulatory hormones that oppose the effect of insulin and promote an increase in blood sugar are released (e.g., glucagon, epinephrine, growth hormone, glucocorticoids). As a result, several processes maintain a minimum blood glucose concentration for the central nervous system. Glycogen in the liver is broken down into glucose (glycogenolysis). Amino acids are transported from muscle to liver, where they are converted to glucose through gluconeogenesis. Uptake of glucose by insulin-dependent tissues is diminished to conserve glucose for the brain. Finally, triglycerides are broken down into free fatty acids, which are used as alternative fuel sources.

Type 1 Diabetes

Pathogenesis[11]

The loss of insulin secretion in type 1 diabetes mellitus results from autoimmune destruction of the insulin-producing β-cells in the pancreas, which is thought to be triggered by environmental factors, such as viruses or toxins, in genetically susceptible individuals.[11] This form of diabetes is associated closely with histocompatibility antigens (human leukocyte antigen [HLA]-DR3 or HLA-DR4) and the presence of circulating insulin antibodies, including insulin antibody, glutamic acid decarboxylase antibody, islet cell antibody (ICA), and islet cell antibody 512 (a tryosine phosphatase antibody). The capacity of normal pancreatic β-cells to secrete insulin far exceeds the normal amounts needed to control carbohydrate, fat, and protein metabolism. As a result, the clinical onset of type 1 diabetes is preceded by an extensive asymptomatic period during which β-cells are destroyed (Fig. 50-1). β-Cell destruction may occur rapidly, but is more likely to take place over a period of weeks, months, or even years. The earliest detectable abnormality in insulin secretion is a progressive reduction of immediate or *first-phase* plasma insulin response. However, this initial impairment has few detrimental effects on overall glucose homeostasis, and plasma glucose concentrations remain normal. Most affected individuals have circulating antibodies to islet cells or to their own insulin at this stage of the disease. These represent markers of an ongoing autoimmune process that culminates in type 1 diabetes. Fasting hyperglycemia occurs when the β-cell mass is reduced by 80% to 90%. Initially, only postprandial hyperglycemia occurs, but as insulin secretion becomes further compromised, progressive fasting hyperglycemia is seen.

On presentation, approximately 65% to 85% of patients have circulating antibodies directed against islet cells and 20%

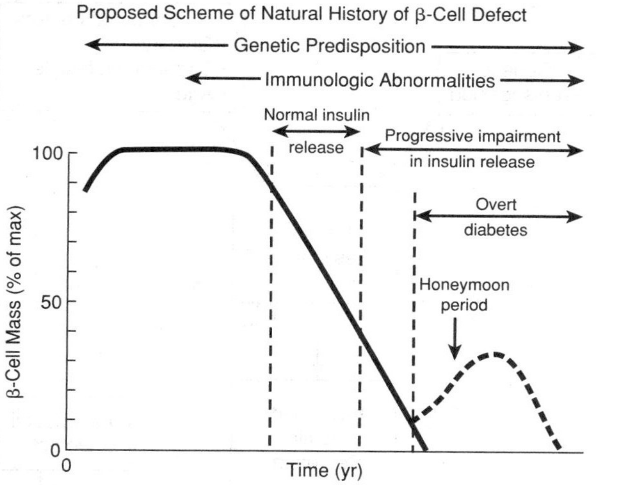

Timing of trigger in relation to immunologic abnormalities is unknown. Note that overt diabetes is not apparent until insulin secretory reserves are <10–20% of normal.

FIGURE 50-1 Pathogenesis of type 1 diabetes. In an individual with a genetic predisposition, an event (such as a virus or toxin) triggers autoimmune destruction of the pancreatic β-cells, probably over a period of several years. When the number of β-cells diminishes to approximately 250,000, the pancreas is unable to secrete sufficient insulin and intolerance to glucose ensues. At this point, a stressful event, such as a viral infection, can produce acute symptoms of hyperglycemia and ketoacidosis. Once the acute event has passed, the pancreas temporarily recovers, leading to a remission (honeymoon period). Continued destruction of the β-cell ultimately leads to an insulin-dependent state.

to 60% of patients have measurable antibodies directed against insulin. Within 8 to 10 years of clinical presentation, β-cell loss is complete and insulin deficiency is absolute.

Clinical Presentation

Although the onset of type 1 diabetes seems to be abrupt, evidence now exists for an extended *preclinical period* that can precede obvious symptoms by several years. As insulin secretion becomes compromised, progressive fasting hyperglycemia occurs. When plasma glucose concentrations exceed the normal renal threshold of approximately 180 mg/dL (10 mmol/L), glucosuria results in an osmotic diuresis, producing the classic symptoms of polyuria with compensatory polydipsia. If symptoms are untreated, weight loss occurs as glucose calories are lost in the urine and body fat and protein stores are broken down owing to increased rates of lipolysis and proteolysis. Muscle begins to metabolize its own glycogen stores and fatty acids for fuel, and the liver begins to metabolize free fatty acids that are released in response to epinephrine and low insulin concentrations. An absolute lack of insulin may cause excessive mobilization of free fatty acids to the liver, where they are metabolized to ketones. This can result in ketonemia, ketonuria, and, ultimately, ketoacidosis. Patients present with complaints of fatigue, significant weight loss, polyuria, and polydipsia. A significant elevation in glycosylated hemoglobin confirms weeks or months of preceding hyperglycemia.

Because glucose provides an excellent medium for microorganisms, patients may present also with recurrent respiratory, vaginal, and other infections. Patients also may experience blurred vision secondary to osmotically induced changes in the lens of the eye. Treatment with insulin is essential to prevent severe dehydration, ketoacidosis, and death.

Honeymoon Period

Within days or weeks after the initial diagnosis, many patients with type 1 diabetes experience an apparent remission, which is reflected by decreased blood glucose concentrations and markedly decreased insulin requirements. This is called the *honeymoon period* because it may last for only a few weeks to months. Once hyperglycemia, metabolic acidosis, and ketosis resolve, endogenous insulin secretion recovers temporarily (Fig. 50-1). Although the honeymoon period may last for up to a year, increasing exogenous insulin requirements are inevitable and should be anticipated. During this time, patients should be maintained on insulin even if the dose is very low, because interrupted treatment is associated with a greater incidence of resistance and allergy to insulin (see Question 26).

Type 2 Diabetes

Pathogenesis

Type 2 diabetes is characterized by impaired insulin secretion and resistance to insulin action. In the presence of insulin resistance, glucose utilization by tissues is impaired, hepatic glucose production is increased, and excess glucose accumulates in the circulation. This hyperglycemia stimulates the pancreas to produce more insulin in an attempt to overcome insulin resistance. The simultaneous elevation of both glucose and insulin levels is strongly suggestive of insulin resistance. Genetic predisposition may play a role in the development of type 2 diabetes. People with type 2 diabetes have a stronger family history of diabetes than those with type 1. There is no association with HLA types, however, and circulating ICAs are absent.[4,12] People with type 2 diabetes also exhibit varying degrees of tissue resistance to insulin, impaired insulin secretion, and increased basal hepatic glucose production. Finally, environmental factors such as obesity and a sedentary lifestyle also contribute to the development of insulin resistance.

Despite being the most common form of diabetes, the exact pathogenesis of type 2 is the least understood. Basal insulin levels are typically normal or elevated at diagnosis. First- or early-phase insulin release in response to glucose often is reduced and pulsatile insulin secretion is absent, resulting in postprandial hyperglycemia. The effects of other insulinotropic substances such as incretin hormones, which contribute to meal-stimulated insulin release, are also altered.[13] Over time, β-cells lose their ability to respond to elevated glucose concentrations, leading to increasing loss of glucose control. In patients with severe hyperglycemia, the amount of insulin secreted in response to glucose is diminished and insulin resistance is worsened (glucose toxicity).

Most individuals with type 2 exhibit decreased tissue responsiveness to insulin.[12] Overeating and/or hyperglycemia may contribute to hyperinsulinemia, which over time may lead to a decrease in or downregulation of the number of insulin receptors on the surface of target tissues and organs. Evidence suggests that decreased peripheral glucose uptake and utilization in muscle is the primary site of insulin resistance and results in prolonged postprandial hyperglycemia. Resistance may be secondary to decreased numbers of insulin receptors on the cell surface, decreased affinity of receptors for insulin, or defects in insulin signaling and action that follows receptor binding. Defects in insulin signaling and action are referred to as *postreceptor* or *postbinding* defects and are likely to be the primary sites of insulin resistance.

Patients with type 2 diabetes also exhibit increased hepatic glucose production (glycogenolysis and gluconeogenesis) reflected by an elevated fasting plasma or blood glucose concentration.[12] As noted, hepatic glucose production is the primary source of glucose in the fasting state. In patients with type 2 diabetes, altered hepatic glucose production may also contribute to or cause postprandial hyperglycemia. Glucagon, produced by the α-cells in the pancreatic islets and secreted in response to low blood glucose, stimulates hepatic glucose production.[14] Its production is inhibited by insulin. Glucagon response to carbohydrate ingestion is altered in patients with type 2 diabetes who have a defective or absent early insulin response secondary to β-cell dysfunction or failure. For patients with type 2 diabetes, untreated fasting and postprandial hyperglycemia caused by decreased glucose uptake and increased hepatic glucose production, hyperinsulinemia and insulin resistance, lead to a vicious cycle that inflicts ongoing damage to tissues and organs.

Patients with type 2 diabetes are often subclassified based on weight. Obese individuals account for over 80% of patients with type 2 diabetes.[12] Patients with type 2 diabetes who are not obese often have increased body fat distributed primarily in the abdominal area. Nonobese individuals account for about 10% of the type 2 population. Typically, they develop a mild form of diabetes during childhood, adolescence, or as young adults (usually before age 25), and their insulin levels are low in response to a glucose challenge. Included in this group are patients who have maturity-onset diabetes of the young (MODY).[4,12] MODY is associated with a strong family history that suggests an autosomal-dominant transmission. The underlying defect is heterogeneous and to date, abnormalities at 6 different loci on different chromosomes have been discovered. More common defects include those for hepatic transcription factors and glucokinase (the "glucose sensor" in β-cells). Patients with MODY may present with moderate to severe symptoms with or without ketosis. Unlike type 1 diabetes, however, the disease generally is mild and controlled easily with diet, oral agents, or low doses of insulin (<40 units).

Type 2 diabetes is associated with a variety of disorders, including hyperlipidemia, hypertension, and atherosclerosis (Fig. 50-2). Dr Gerald Reaven, who referred to this association as syndrome X, insulin resistance syndrome, or metabolic syndrome, proposed that either the insulin resistance itself, or the compensatory hyperinsulinemia resulting from insulin resistance, may be the fundamental underlying pathophysiological process responsible for the frequent occurrence of these conditions in the same patient.[15] The concept of a single defect explaining this cluster of disorders, however, remains the subject of considerable debate and research activity. Metabolic syndrome is common in the United States, with an estimated prevalence of more than 20% in adults older than 20 years and more than 40% among adults 60 to 69 years of age.[16] Because it is highly correlated with cardiovascular events, the National Cholesterol Education Program has suggested criteria for the diagnosis and treatment of metabolic syndrome to prevent cardiovascular events and diabetes.[17] Not all individuals with the metabolic syndrome progress to IGT or diabetes, but those who do may be genetically predisposed to β-cell dysfunction.

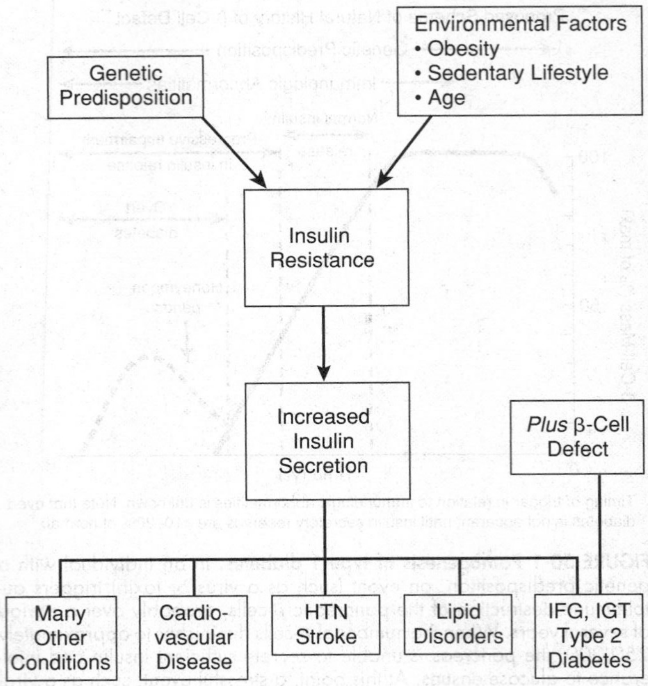

FIGURE 50-2 Metabolic syndrome (insulin resistance syndrome, syndrome X). Genetic and environmental factors (visceral obesity, sedentary lifestyle, aging) predispose some individuals to insulin resistance. To overcome the resistance, the pancreas secretes more insulin, leading to hyperinsulinemia. People with insulin resistance and hyperinsulinemia commonly develop a cluster of medical problems and biochemical abnormalities: cardiovascular disease, hypertension, dyslipidemia, hyperuricemia, and type 2 diabetes mellitus. Only those individuals who are further genetically predisposed to β-cell failure go on to develop IGT and diabetes mellitus. Many people with type 2 diabetes already have evidence of cardiovascular disease at the time of diabetes diagnosis. The cause-and-effect relationships between insulin resistance and/or hyperinsulinemia and these clinical conditions has not been clarified. See text for expanded discussion. DM, diabetes mellitus; HTN, hypertension; IFG, impaired fasting glucose; IGT, impaired glucose tolerance.

Clinical Presentation

Type 2 diabetes is typically diagnosed incidentally during a routine physical examination or when the patient seeks attention for another complaint. This is because symptoms are so mild and their onset so gradual that they can easily be "explained away." When giving a history of their illness, people with type 2 diabetes acknowledge fatigue, polyuria, and polydipsia. Because these patients have sufficient insulin concentrations to prevent lipolysis, there is usually no history of ketosis except in situations of unusual stress (e.g., infections, trauma). Weight loss is therefore uncommon because relatively high endogenous insulin levels promote lipogenesis. Macrovascular disease is also often evident at diagnosis. Microvascular complications at diagnosis suggest the presence of undiagnosed or subclinical diabetes for 7 to 10 years. Because type 2 diabetes patients retain some pancreatic reserve at the time of diagnosis, they generally can be treated with medical

Table 50-2 Normal and Diabetic Plasma[a] Glucose Levels in mg/dL (mmol/L) and Normal and Diabetic Plasma Glucose Levels for the Oral Glucose Tolerance Test[4,19]

	Fasting	½, 1, 1½ hr	2 hr
Normal	<100 (5.6)	<200 (11.1)	<140 (7.8)
Impaired glucose tolerance	<126 (7.0)	≥200 (11.1)	140–200 (7.8–11.1)
Impaired fasting glucose	100–125 (5.6–6.9)		
Diabetes (nonpregnant adult)	≥126 (7.0)	≥200 (11.1)	≥200 (11.1)

[a]Equivalent *venous whole blood* glucose concentrations are approximately 12%–15% lower. *Arterial* samples are higher than venous samples postprandially because glucose has not yet been removed from peripheral tissues. *Capillary whole blood* samples contain a mixture of arterial and venous blood. Fasting levels are equivalent to whole blood venous samples. One hour after a 100-g glucose load, capillary samples may be 30–40 mg/dL higher than venous samples.

nutrition therapy (MNT), physical activity, and oral antidiabetic medications for several years. Nevertheless, many eventually require insulin for control of their symptoms.

Gestational Diabetes Mellitus

GDM affects about 7% of all pregnancies and is defined as "any carbohydrate intolerance with onset or first recognition during pregnancy."[4,18] The onset of diabetes during pregnancy and its duration affect the prognosis for a good obstetric and perinatal outcome (see Chapter 46).

Diagnosis

Diagnostic Criteria

The normal fasting plasma glucose (FPG) values and those for diabetes mellitus, along with the glucose values for the oral glucose tolerance test (OGTT) are listed in Table 50-2.[4,19] The Expert Committee of the ADA has established the diagnostic criteria for diabetes for nonpregnant individuals of any age. For these individuals, a diagnosis of diabetes can be made when one of the following is present[4]:

1. Classic signs and symptoms of diabetes (polyuria, polydipsia, ketonuria, and unexplained weight loss) combined with a random plasma glucose ≥200 mg/dL (11.1 mmol/L).
2. A FPG ≥126 mg/dL (7.0 mmol/L). *Fasting* means no caloric intake for at least 8 hours.
3. After a standard oral glucose challenge (75 g glucose for an adult or 1.75 g/kg for a child), the venous plasma glucose concentration is ≥200 mg/dL (11.0 mmol/L) at 2 hours and >200 mg/dL (11.0 mmol/L) at least one other time during the test (0.5, 1, 1.5 hours); this is the OGTT.

The diagnosis must be confirmed on a subsequent day by any one of these conditions in the absence of unequivocal hyperglycemia with acute metabolic complications.

At times, it may be difficult to classify patients as having type 1 or type 2 diabetes mellitus. Type 1 is more likely when a patient is younger than 30 years of age, lean, has an elevated FPG and signs and symptoms of diabetes. The presence of moderate ketonuria with hyperglycemia in an otherwise unstressed patient also strongly supports a diagnosis of type 1 diabetes. Absence of ketonuria, however, is not of diagnostic value. The presence of antibodies to islet cell components may also indicate the need for eventual insulin therapy.[11] Relatively lean older adults believed to have type 2 diabetes because they are initially responsive to oral agents or low doses of insulin may be subsequently diagnosed with type 1 diabetes. In addition, clinicians are beginning to observe more cases of type 2 diabetes in obese children and adolescents.[20]

Individuals with FPG values or OGTT values that are intermediate between normal and those considered diagnostic of diabetes are considered to have "prediabetes" or IFG or IGT. These individuals are not given the diagnosis of diabetes because of broad social, psychological, and economic implications. The categories of FPG values are as follows:

1. A normal FPG is <100 mg/dL (5.6 mmol/L).
2. An FPG of 100 to 125 mg/dL (5.6–6.9 mmol/L) is IFG.
3. An FPG ≥126 mg/dL (7.0 mmol/L) indicates a *provisional* diagnosis of diabetes that must be confirmed, as described.

The corresponding categories when the OGTT is used for diagnosis are as follows:

1. A 2-hour postload glucose (2-hPG) <140 mg/dL (7.8 mmol/L) indicates normal glucose tolerance.
2. A 2-hPG ≥140 mg/dL (7.8 mmol/L) and <200 mg/dL (11.1 mmol/L) indicates IGT.
3. A 2-hPG ≥200 mg/dL (11.1 mmol/L) indicates a *provisional* diagnosis of diabetes, which must be confirmed by a second test.

Many factors can impair glucose tolerance or increase plasma glucose. These must be excluded before a definitive diagnosis is made. For example, an individual who has not fasted for a minimum of 8 hours may have an elevated FPG, and one who has fasted too long (>16 hours) or has ingested insufficient carbohydrates before testing may have an IGT. Patients who are tested for glucose tolerance during, or soon after, an acute illness (e.g., a myocardial infarction [MI]) may be misdiagnosed because of the presence of high concentrations of counter-regulatory hormones that increase glucose concentrations. Glucose tolerance often returns to normal in these individuals. Pregnancy, many forms of stress, and lack of physical activity can similarly affect glucose tolerance. Many drugs may alter glucose tolerance due to their effects on insulin release and tissue response to insulin, and their direct cytotoxic effects on the pancreas. Drugs and other chemicals also may falsely elevate the plasma glucose concentrations through interference with specific analytic methods.

Screening for Type 2 Diabetes

The ADA advises against routine screening for type 2 diabetes outside of the health care setting because of the low likelihood

Table 50-3 Risk Factors for Type 2 Diabetes Mellitus[22]

Adults	*Children*[a]
Overweight (≥25 kg/m^2)	Overweight (BMI >85th percentile for age and sex; or weight >120% of ideal for height)
Family history of diabetes (first-degree relative)	Family history of diabetes (first- or second-degree relative)
Physical inactivity	Ethnic predisposition[b]
Ethnic predisposition[b]	
Previous IFG or IGT	
History of PCOS, GDM, or macrosomia	Maternal history of diabetes (including GDM)
Clinical conditions associated with insulin resistance (e.g., severe obesity and acanthosis nigricans)	Signs of insulin resistance (e.g., acanthosis nigricans)
Hypertension (≥140/90 mmHg or on antihypertensive therapy)	Conditions associated with insulin resistance (e.g., hypertension, dyslipidemia, or PCOS)
Dyslipidemia	
HDL-C <35 mg/dL (0.90 mmol/L)	
Triglyceride >250 mg/dL (2.82 mmol/L)	
Cardiovascular disease	

[a]Children = <18 years of age.
[b]Ethnic predisposition = individuals of African American, Hispanic or Latino, Native American, Asian, or Pacific Islander descent.
IFG, impaired fasting glucose; IGT, impaired glucose tolerance; PCOS, polycystic ovarian syndrome; GDM, gestational diabetes mellitus.

of follow-up care and testing in the case of both negative and positive results.[21] The FPG is the preferred over the OGTT as a screening test based on cost and convenience. Adults should be screened starting at age 45.[22] Repeat testing should take place every 3 years. Adults may be tested at a younger age and more frequently if they are overweight (body mass index [BMI] ≥25 kg/m^2) and have one or more of the risk factors listed in Table 50-3. Asymptomatic children who are age 10 or who experience the onset of puberty before age 10 should be screened every 2 years for type 2 diabetes if they are overweight (BMI >85th percentile for age and sex; weight for height >85th percentile; or weight >120% of ideal for height) and have two or more of the risk factors listed in Table 50-3.

Long-Term Complications and Their Relation to Glucose Control

The long-term sequelae of diabetes account for most of the morbidity and mortality in the diabetic population. Complications are typically designated as microvascular or macrovascular in nature. Glucose toxicity seems to contribute most to the development and progression of microvascular complications (retinopathy, nephropathy, and neuropathy).[23] Diabetes is the leading cause of new cases of adult blindness and kidney failure in the United States.[1] About 70% of people with diabetes also have some manifestation of peripheral and/or autonomic neuropathy. Severe peripheral neuropathy coupled with abnormalities in immune function likely contribute to the high rate of lower extremity amputations among patients with diabetes.[1,24] Finally, poor glucose control promotes development of dental and oral complications and increases the risk of complications during pregnancy for both mother and fetus.[25,26]

Diabetes mellitus itself is also one of many risk factors for macrovascular disease (peripheral vascular disease, cardiovascular disease [CVD], stroke). These risk factors tend to cluster in people prone to type 2 diabetes. Epidemiologic studies also show, however, a general relationship between degree of glucose control and risk for cardiovascular events.[27] In addition, patients with diabetes demonstrate rheological changes, such as platelet hypersensitivity to platelet aggregants and elevated thromboxane production, which may contribute to peripheral and cardiovascular complicataions.[28] Thus, the primary goal for both type 1 and type 2 diabetic individuals is to bring glucose concentrations as close to normal values as is safely possible.

Results of the Diabetes Complications and Control Trial (DCCT) definitively established that intensive treatment of type 1 diabetes can prevent or slow the onset of long-term microvascular complications.[29] In this landmark study, intensive treatment reduced the risk of clinically meaningful retinopathy, nephropathy, and neuropathy by approximately 60%. The Epidemiology of Diabetes Interventions and Complications (EDIC) study has followed DCCT cohorts. Patients originally assigned to the intensive treatment group, have enjoyed a persistently lower incidence of microvascular complications even though their glucose control has since been equivalent to the conventional group.[30,31] The EDIC study has also shown a significant reduction in cardiovascular complications among patients previously assigned to the intensive therapy DCCT arm.[32] See Table 50-4 for the glycemic goals of intensive insulin therapy (referred to by these authors as physiological or basal-bolus therapy).

The United Kingdom Prospective Diabetes Study (UKPDS) was the first to report the effect of tight blood glucose control on the microvascular and cardiovascular complications associated with type 2 diabetes.[33] Epidemiologic analysis of the data from this landmark study demonstrated a continuous relationship between glycemia and the risks of microvascular complications. For every percentage point reduction in hemoglobin A_{1C} (HbA_{1c}), there was a 35% reduction in the risk of complications. Whether intensive therapy designed to attain sustained normoglycemia decreased the risk of macrovascular disease was less clear. Although a 21% reduction in the risk of combined fatal and nonfatal MI and sudden death was seen, this combined outcome failed to reach statistical significance ($p = .52$).

Other studies support the use of a more comprehensive approach to preventing microvascular and macrovascular complications in patients with type 2 diabetes. In a UKPDS group substudy, tight blood pressure control (<130/85 mmHg) reduced the risk of stroke by 44% ($p = .013$) and microvascular endpoints by 37% ($p = .0092$).[33] The Steno group found that multifactorial intensive treatment of patients with type 2 diabetes and microalbuminura for a mean of 7.8 years reduced the risk of microvascular complications and cardiovascular events by 50% compared with conventional treatment. Their interventions included lifestyle education and aggressive use of drugs to lower HbA_{1c}, and blood pressure (BP), and achieve a normal lipid profile.[34] See Table 50-5 for the metabolic goals for adults with diabetes.

Table 50-4 Goals of Physiological (Basal-Bolus) Insulin Therapy[a]

Monitoring Parameter	Adults (mg/dL)	School Age (6–12 years) (mg/dL)	Adolescents and Young Adults (13–29 years) (mg/dL)	Pregnancy (mg/dL)
Fasting plasma glucose	70–130	90–180	90–130	60–90
2 hr postprandial plasma glucose	<180	Not routinely recommended	Not routinely recommended	≤120
2–4 am plasma glucose	>70	100–180	90–150	>60
HbA_{1c}[b]	<7.0%[c]	<8.0%	<7.5%[d]	5–6%
Urine ketones[e]	Absent to rare	Absent to rare	Absent to rare	Rare

[a]Modified and extrapolated from references 22, 29, and 344. See Questions 4 and 22 for discussion. Physiological insulin therapy is a complete therapeutic program of diabetes management and requires a team approach.
[b]HbA_{1c}, glycosolated hemoglobin. Normal values vary; normalize to laboratory.
[c]Acceptable values should be individualized to levels that are attainable without creating undue risk for hypoglycemia. These results are similar to the results achieved in the DCCT trial. ADA recommends HbA_{1c} goal within 1% or upper limit of normal and consideration for <6% as an individual goal. These values may be inappropriate for patients with hypoglycemic unawareness, counter-regulatory insufficiency, angina pectoris, or other complicating features (Table 50-12).
[d]A lower goal (<7%) is reasonable if can be achieved without creating excessive risk for hypoglycemia.
[e]Does not apply to type 2 diabetes patients.

Early in 2008, researchers announced that the glucose-lowering arm of the Action to Control Cardiovascular Risk in Diabetes (ACCORD) trial was stopped prematurely because of a higher rate of mortality in the intensive treatment arm. The ACCORD study is a National Heart, Lung and Blood Institute study of approximately 10,000 patients with type 2 diabetes with known heart disease or two cardiovascular risk factors. Patients had an average duration of diabetes of 10 years, average age of 62 years, and baseline HbA_{1c} of 8.2%. In the glycemic control portion of the trial, researchers were testing whether intensive glucose control (goal HbA_{1c} <6%) reduced the rate of cardiovascular events compared with less intensive glucose control (goal HbA_{1c} 7.0%–7.9%). At the time the trial was stopped, the median HbA_{1c} in the intensive and standard treatment groups were 6.4% and 7.5%, respectively. The intensive arm had an excess of three deaths per 1,000 participants per year compared with the standard group over an average of 4 years on treatment (257 vs. 203 deaths). The higher mortality rate could not be attributed to a specific drug therapy or hypoglycemia.[35] Approximately 1 week later, preliminary results from a very similar study, the ADVANCE trial, were released demonstrating no increases in mortality risk in intensively treated patients with type 2 diabetes. ADVANCE, an international study, enrolled over 11,000 patients with type 2 diabetes, (about one-third with known CVD) average age of 66 years, and average duration of diabetes of 10 years. The intensive-therapy group's HbA_{1c} goal was 6.5% or below. The same as the intensive arm in ACCORD. The actual average HbA_{1c} achieved was 6.4%. In the face of these new data, the ADA continues to recommend an HbA_{1c} goal of less than 7% for most people with diabetes. The ADA recommends that patients with type 2 diabetes and CVD or multiple risk factors for CVD discuss their treatment goals with their providers.[36]

Table 50-5 American Diabetes Association Goals for Adults With Diabetes Mellitus[22,58]

Glycemic goals	
• HbA_{1C}	<7.0% (normal, 4–6%)[a]
• Preprandial plasma glucose	70–130 mg/dL (3.9–7.2 mmol/L)[b]
• Postprandial plasma glucose	<180 mg/dL (<10.0 mmol/L)[c]
Blood pressure	<130/80 mmHg
Lipids	
• Low-density lipoproteins	<100 mg/dL (<2.6 mmol/L)[d]
• Triglycerides	<150 mg/dL (<1.7 mmol/L)
• High-density lipoproteins	
– Men	>40 mg/dL (>1.0 mmol/L)
– Women	>50 mg/dL (>1.3 mmol/L)

Goals must be individualized to the patient. See Questions 4, 45, 73, 76, and 77 for broader discussion.
[a]More stringent goals (i.e., <6%) can be considered for select individuals. American Association of Clinical Endocrinologists/American College of Endocrinology recommends HbA_{1C} goal ≤6.5%.
[b]American Association of Clinical Endocrinologists recommends a fasting blood glucose goal of <110 mg/dL (6.1 mmol/L).
[c]American Association of Clinical Endocrinologists/American College of Endocrinology recommends goal <140 mg/L (7.8 mmol/L).
[d]More stringent goals (i.e., <70 mg/dL [1.8 mmol/L]) may be considered for individuals with overt cardiovascular disease.

Prevention of Type 1 and Type 2 Diabetes Mellitus

Because the clinical symptoms of type 1 diabetes mellitus are the overt expression of an insidious pathogenic process that begins years earlier, investigators are focusing attention on strategies that alter the natural history of the disease (Fig. 50-1). First-degree relatives of individuals with type 1 diabetes mellitus have an increased risk for developing the diabetes and can be identified by the presence of immune markers that may herald the disease by many years.[11] This has led to attempts at immune intervention at the prediabetes stage with such drugs as nicotinamide and low doses of insulin, but neither was found to delay or prevent diabetes.[37–39] In contrast, treatment of newly diagnosed diabetes with agents that modify cytotoxic T cells may slow pancreatic destruction and progression of diabetes.[40]

In addition to the 20.8 million people with diabetes in the United States, an estimated additional 41 million Americans have prediabetes (IGT or IFG).[1] The annual risk of progression to type 2 diabetes mellitus in persons with IGT is 1% to 5%.[41] Persons at risk for IGT and who are eligible for further screening include those who are overweight and/or lead a sedentary lifestyle, have a family history of diabetes, are a member of a high-risk ethnic population (e.g., African American, Hispanic/Latino, Native American, Asian American,

Pacific Islander), have a history of gestational diabetes or who have delivered a baby weighing more than 9 lb, and have with a medical history of a high blood glucose test without a diagnosis of diabetes.[42]

The Diabetes Prevention Program Research Group studied a diverse group of individuals at high risk for developing diabetes to determine if lifestyle interventions or metformin (850 mg PO BID) would prevent or delay the onset of type 2 diabetes.[43] Results of the study found that relative to the placebo group, the incidence of diabetes was reduced by 58% and 31% in the intensive lifestyle and metformin groups, respectively. A repeat OGTT was performed in the metformin group who had not developed diabetes 1 to 2 weeks after the drug had been discontinued to determine whether the drug simply masked diabetes through its antihyperglycemic effects. The incidence of diabetes was still reduced by 25% relative to the placebo group.[44] Other studies have confirmed the value of lifestyle intervention and other drugs (acarbose, troglitazone, orlistat, and rosiglitazone) in the prevention of type 2 diabetes.[42,45] Lifelong medication therapy, however, is not without its own risks and complications. Current recommendations regarding the treatment for individuals with IFG, IGT, or both include lifestyle modification (5%–10% weight loss and 30 minutes of moderately intense physical activity per day).[22] For patients at very high risk of diabetes (age <60, BMI $\geq$35 kg/m^2, combined IFG and IGT, and at least one risk factor), the addition of metformin may be considered. Until further evidence becomes available to support their use in the delay or prevention of complications of diabetes and/or cost effectiveness has been established, the use of other pharmacologic agents to prevent the development of type 2 diabetes is not recommended.[46]

1. R.P. is a 43-year-old woman visiting the drop-in clinic to obtain a routine physical examination for her new job. Her past medical history is significant for GDM. She was told during her two pregnancies (last child born 3 years ago) that she had "borderline diabetes," which resolved each time after giving birth. Her family history is significant for type 2 diabetes (mother, maternal grandmother, older first cousin), hypertension, and CVD. She appears black and when asked identifies herself as African American. She denies tobacco or alcohol use. She states she tries to walk 15 minutes twice a week. Physical examination is significant for moderate central obesity (5 feet 4 inches; 160 lbs; BMI, 30.2 kg/m^2) and BP 145/85 mmHg. R.P. denies any symptoms of polyphagia, polyuria, or lethargy. Upon checking her electronic medical record, she has documented hypertension and an FPG value of 119 mg/dL, measured 2 months prior. What features of R.P.'s history and examination are consistent with an increased risk of developing type 2 diabetes?

The features of R.P.'s history that are consistent with an increased risk of developing type 2 diabetes include her age, ethnicity, weight, family history of diabetes, history of GDM, and a documented IFG. In addition, type 2 diabetes is also often associated with other disorders such as hypertension. The fact that R.P. has hypertension that is not well controlled and has a family history of hypertension and CVD may indicate that she is predisposed to insulin resistance, further putting her at risk for developing type 2 diabetes.

2. The physician orders another FPG for R.P., which comes back at 122 mg/dL. How should R.P. be managed at this time?

R.P. should be educated about her risk for developing type 2 diabetes. Working with her physician and/or other health care providers, R.P. should be encouraged and educated on how to institute lifestyle modifications (MNT, physical activity) that will help her to lose weight, improve her cardiovascular health, and decrease her risk for developing type 2 diabetes. A weight loss goal of 5% to 10% should be recommended and she should increase her level of moderate physical activity to at least 150 minutes/week. Her hypertension should be managed. At this time, the use of pharmacologic agents (i.e., metformin) to prevent the development of type 2 diabetes is not recommended.

Treatment

There are three major components to the treatment of diabetes: diet, drugs (insulin and oral hypoglycemic agents, and other antihyperglycemic agents), and exercise. Each of these components interacts with the others to the extent that no assessment and modification of one can be made without knowledge of the other two. Target blood glucose values for pregnant diabetics are very strict.

Medical Nutrition Therapy[47]

PRINCIPLES

MNT plays a crucial role in the therapy of all individuals with diabetes. Unfortunately, patient acceptance and adherence to diet and meal planning is often poor, but revised evidence-based recommendations that are more flexible than previous approaches offer new opportunities to increase the effectiveness of nutrition therapy.

Nutrition therapy is designed to help patients achieve appropriate metabolic and physiological goals (e.g., glucose, lipids, BP, proteinuria, weight), select healthy foods, and to take into consideration personal and cultural preferences. Appropriate levels and types of physical activity to achieve a healthier status are incorporated into the nutrition plan.

NUTRITION THERAPY AND TYPE 1 DIABETES MELLITUS

For patients with type 1 diabetes taking fixed doses of insulin, a meal plan is designed to provide adequate carbohydrates timed to match the peak action of exogenously administered mealtime insulin. Regularly scheduled meals and snacks should contain consistent carbohydrate amounts, which are required to prevent hypoglycemic reactions. Fortunately, newer insulins and insulin regimens provide much more flexibility in the amount and timing of food intake. Patients who are taught to "count carbohydrates" can inject rapid- or short-acting insulin doses designed to match their anticipated intake. Integration of food intake, physical activity, and insulin dose is critical and discussed extensively in the cases that follow.

NUTRITION THERAPY AND TYPE 2 DIABETES MELLITUS

For patients with type 2 diabetes, meal plans emphasize normalizing plasma glucose and lipid levels as well as maintaining a normal BP to prevent or mitigate cardiovascular morbidity. Although weight loss reduces insulin resistance and improves glycemic control, traditional dietary strategies incorporating hypocaloric diets have not been effective in achieving long-term weight loss. A sustainable weight loss of 5% to 7% can be achieved within structured programs that emphasize lifestyle changes, physical activity, and food intake that modestly reduces caloric and fat intake. For weight loss, the ADA recently updated their recommendation on types of diets to include either low-carbohydrate (new recommendation in 2008) or low-fat, calorie-restricted diets for up to 1 year.[47]

SPECIFIC NUTRITION COMPONENTS

MNT is an integral and critical component of diabetes care. For a more extensive discussion of the principles underlying nutrition therapy, the reader is directed to other sources.[47,48] A few key principles are briefly noted below because they are common sources of misunderstanding.

Carbohydrates and Artificial Sweeteners

Carbohydrates include sugar, starch, and fiber and they are liberally incorporated into the diet of a person with diabetes. In fact, the amount of dietary carbohydrate is the main determinant of insulin demand and is commonly used to determine the premeal insulin dose. Furthermore, patients using fixed doses of insulin or antihyperglycemic medications (e.g., sulfonylureas) must eat meals containing consistent amounts of carbohydrate to avoid hypoglycemia. Avoiding "sugar" or *sucrose* does not prevent "sugar diabetes." Because isocaloric amounts of sucrose and starch produce the same degree glycemia, sucrose can be substituted for a portion of the total carbohydrate intake and should be incorporated into an otherwise healthful diet.

Whole grains, fruits, and vegetables high in *fiber* are recommended for people with diabetes, as they are for the general population. There is no evidence that larger amounts produce a differential metabolic benefit with regard to plasma glucose and lipid levels. *Non-nutritive sweeteners* (saccharin, aspartame, neotame, acesulfame potassium, sucralose) and sugar alcohols have been rigorously tested by the FDA for safety in people with diabetes and are safe at approved daily intakes. Fructose and the reduced calorie sweeteners called *sugar alcohols* produce lower postprandial glucose responses than sucrose, glucose, and starch. When sugar alcohols (e.g., sorbitol, mannitol, lactitol, xylitol, and maltitol) are consumed, it is recommended to subtract half of their grams from the total carbohydrate amount, because their effect on blood glucose is less. Patients should be advised that when these sweeteners are used in foods labeled "dietetic" or "sugar free," they still add to the carbohydrate content and provide substantial calories (2 cal/g). Furthermore, excessive intake of sorbitol-sweetened foods (e.g., 30–50 g/day) can induce an osmotic diarrhea, and excessive amounts of fructose can increase total and LDL cholesterol.

Counting Carbohydrates

When patients are taught to estimate the grams of carbohydrate in a meal they are given the following guideline: One carbohydrate serving = 1 starch or 1 fruit or 1 milk = 15 g carbohydrate. Patients vary with regard to their insulin: carbohydrate ratio throughout time and throughout the day; however, a typical starting point is 1 unit/15 g carbohydrate. Examples of one carbohydrate serving include 1 slice bread, 1/4 bagel, 1/2 English muffin or hamburger bun, 3/4 c dry cereal, 1/2 c cooked cereal, 1/2 c legumes, 1/3 c *cooked* pasta or rice, 1/4 large baked potato, 4 c popcorn, 1 small fruit, 1/2 c fruit juice, 1 c milk, 1/2 c ice cream, and 2 small cookies.

Fat

CVD is a major cause of morbidity and mortality in patients with diabetes. Therefore, a reduced fat diet (<30% of the total calories) with <7% of calories from saturated fats is recommended. The intake of *trans* fat should be minimized. The recommended cholesterol intake is <200 mg/day for patients with diabetes. Two servings per week of fish to provide *n*-3 polyunsaturated fatty acids and omega-3 fatty acids is advised.

Protein

Data are insufficient to support special dietary protein recommendations for persons with diabetes if kidney function is normal. Generally, 15% to 20% of the daily caloric intake comes from animal and vegetable protein sources in the U.S. diet. This amount may be liberalized in pregnant and lactating women or in elderly people. With the onset of nephropathy, a lower protein intake of 0.8 to 1.0 g/kg/day is considered sufficiently restrictive. For patients in later stages of nephropathy, reduction of protein intake to 0.8 g/kg/day is recommended. High protein diets are not recommended as a long-term method for weight loss, because the effects on kidney function are not known.

Sodium

The ADA recommends a reduced sodium intake of <2,300 mg/day in normotensive and hypertensive individuals. For patients with diabetes and symptomatic heart failure, sodium should be further restricted to <2,000 mg/day to help reduce symptoms. For all other patients, the ADA has no particular restrictions on sodium intake, but recommends individualizing amounts based on the patient's sensitivity to salt and concurrent conditions such as hypertension or nephropathy.

Alcohol

The ADA's recommendation for alcohol is consistent with general recommendations of no more than two alcoholic drinks per day for men or one drink per day for women. A drink is equivalent to 12 oz beer, 5 oz wine, or 1.5 oz distilled spirits (each contains about 15 g carbohydrate). Nevertheless, its caloric contribution must be considered (1 alcoholic beverage = 2 fat exchanges), and it should always be taken with food to minimize its hypoglycemic effect. In patients with diabetes, light to moderate alcohol intake (one to two drinks per day) is associated with a decreased risk of CVD. A note of caution: Evening consumption of alcohol in type 1 diabetes may increase the risk of nocturnal and fasting hypoglycemia.

Exercise

Exercise is a key factor in the treatment of diabetes, particularly in type 2 diabetes, because obesity and inactivity contribute to the development of glucose intolerance in genetically predisposed individuals. Regular exercise reduces cholesterol levels, lowers BP, augments weight reduction diets, reduces the dose requirements or need for insulin or antihyperglycemic agents, enhances insulin sensitivity, and improves psychological well-being by reducing stress. Exercise increases glucose utilization, which is provided initially from the breakdown of muscle glycogen and, subsequently, from hepatic glycogenolysis and gluconeogenesis. These effects are mediated through norepinephrine, epinephrine, growth hormone, cortisol, and glucagon, along with the suppression of insulin secretion. In insulin-dependent diabetic patients, hyperglycemia, normoglycemia, or hypoglycemia can occur secondary to exercise depending on the degree of control, recent administration of insulin, and food intake. Exercise in patients taking insulin must be tempered by increased food intake, potential delay in insulin administration, decreased doses of insulin, or a combination of these actions to minimize hypoglycemia (see Question 29).

In the type 2 diabetic population, plasma glucose concentrations usually decrease in response to exercise; symptomatic hypoglycemia is uncommon. Because diabetic individuals are predisposed to CVD, attention has been focused on the metabolic response of a patient with diabetes to exercise. In general, moderate, regular exercise is highly recommended for individuals with type 2 diabetes treated with diet and/or antidiabetic agents and encouraged in individuals taking insulin if special precautions are taken.

The ADA's recommendation is for people with diabetes to perform at least 150 min/week of moderate-intensity aerobic physical activity (50%–70% of maximal heart rate). Resistance exercise has been shown to improve insulin sensitivity. Therefore, in the absence of any contraindications, patients with type 2 diabetes are encouraged to perform resistance training three times per week. Patients with conditions that may preclude certain types of physical activity (e.g., coronary artery disease, uncontrolled hypertension, severe autonomic neuropathy, severe peripheral neuropathy or history of foot lesions, and advanced retinopathy) that may preclude certain types of physical activity should be carefully evaluated before starting an exercise regimen.

Pharmacologic Treatment

Insulin, along with diet, is crucial to the survival of individuals with type 1 diabetes and plays a major role in the therapy of people with type 2 diabetes when their symptoms cannot be controlled with diet or non-insulin antidiabetic agents. Insulin also is used for patients with type 2 diabetes during periods of intercurrent illness or stress (e.g., surgery, pregnancy). The use of antidiabetic agents is reserved for the treatment of patients with type 2 diabetes whose symptoms cannot be controlled with diet and exercise alone (however, metformin is an exception to this). The clinical use of these agents and the complications associated with their use are discussed later in this chapter.

Pancreas and Islet Cell Transplants

Pancreas transplantation, by either whole pancreas or pancreatic islet cells, is the only available treatment for type 1 diabetes mellitus that induces an insulin-independent, normoglycemic state. Benefits can include improvement in quality of life, retinopathy, and nephropathy.[49,50] Whole organ pancreas transplantation continues to be widely used in uremic diabetic patients because it can be performed at the same time as kidney transplantation (simultaneous kidney and pancreas transplant [SPK]) or after (pancreas after kidney transplant [PAK]). SPK graft survival rates are 86% and 71% at years 1 and 5, respectively. For PAK, survival rates are slightly lower, at 78% and 57% at years 1 and 5, respectively.[51] Another option is for pancreas transplantation alone; survival rates are similar to PAK. The pancreatic graft is usually placed peritoneally, with duct management by enteric drainage or less commonly by bladder drainage. However, pancreatic transplantation alone in a patient with diabetes mellitus remains controversial because the disadvantages of exogenous insulin therapy are replaced with risks of the transplantation procedure itself and the complications of immunosuppressive medications.[52] The International Pancreas Transplant Registry tracks whole organ pancreas transplantation. As of December 2004, 23,043 pancreas transplants were reported to the International Pancreas Transplant Registry, with 17,127 performed in the United States. SPK accounted for the majority of pancreas transplants.

Islet cell transplants (infusions) have received increased attention with the success of the "Edmonton Protocol," which used a steroid-free immunosuppression regimen as well as other techniques. All patients achieved insulin independence after 1 year in contrast with a previous success rate of 8%.[53] At 5 years, approximately 80% of patients had C-peptide present, but only 10% maintained insulin independence with a median duration of insulin independence of 15 months.[54] Since then, an international trial of the Edmonton Protocol, organized by the Immune Tolerance Network, was published demonstrating proof of concept that the protocol could be replicated.[55] At 1 year, 44% of patients were insulin independent with adequate glycemic control, and 31% of these remained insulin independent at 2 years. Twenty-eight percent had complete graft loss at 1 year. Although islet cell transplantation does not achieve sustained insulin independence, it can improve quality of life, mainly from reduced hypoglycemia.[55,56] Currently, islet cell transplantation is considered for patients with type 1 diabetes with severe, recurrent hypoglycemia and hypoglycemic unawareness. Most protocols use sirolimus and tacrolimus for maintenance immunosuppression and a monoclonal anti-CD25 antibody for induction immunosuppression at the first islet infusion.[57] The Collaborative Islet Transplant Registry reported 319 recipients of islet infusion procedures from 1999 to 2005 in North America. Many issues remain regarding islet cell transplantation, including availability of islet cell transplant material, islet cell preparation, types of immunosuppression, and assessment of long-term outcomes.

Overall Goals of Therapy

The overall goal of diabetes management is to prevent acute and chronic complications. Periodic assessments of HbA_{1c} coupled with regular measurement of fasting, preprandial, and postprandial glucose levels should be utilized to assess therapy. The following overall goals of therapy are agreed upon by most endocrinologists:

1. Strive for glycemic control achieved in DCCT and UKPDS. The landmark randomized, prospective trials of various interventional therapies in patients with both types 1 and 2 diabetes have clearly demonstrated that reductions in hyperglycemia significantly decreases microvascular complications. In general, these trials demonstrated an overall reduction in microvascular complications by 30% to 35% with a 1% absolute reduction in HbA_{1c}. In both the UKPDS and the DCCT, a trend toward a significant reduction in macrovascular complications was observed. Target blood glucose goals may need to be adjusted for patients with frequent, severe hypoglycemia or hypoglycemia unawareness (see questions 35 and 38), or CVD. In addition, established renal insufficiency, proliferative retinopathy, severe neuropathy, and other advanced complications are not likely to be improved by tight glucose control. See Table 50-5 for the ADA glycemic goals. The American Association

of Clinical Endocrinologists and the American College of Endocrinology established glycemic goals as well (Table 50-5).[58] These authors elected to discuss ADA guidelines throughout this chapter.

2. Try to keep patients free of symptoms associated with hyperglycemia (polyuria, polydipsia, weight loss, fatigue, recurrent infection, ketoacidosis) or hypoglycemia (hunger, anxiety, palpitations, sweatiness).
3. Maintain normal growth and development in children. Intensive therapy is not recommended for children younger than 7 years of age and should be used cautiously in children ages 7 to 13 years old (see Questions 22 and 23).
4. Eliminate or minimize all other cardiovascular risk factors (obesity, hypertension, tobacco use, hyperlipidemia; see Table 50-5 for BP and lipid goals).
5. Try to integrate the patient into the health care team through intensive education. The patient's knowledge and understanding of this disease can favorably influence its outcomes (see Table 50-16).

Methods of Monitoring Glycemic Control

In addition to monitoring signs and symptoms associated with hyperglycemia, hypoglycemia, and the long-term complications of diabetes, an ongoing assessment of metabolic control is an integral component of diabetes management. Ideally, self-monitored blood glucose (SMBG) results combined with laboratory measures of acute and chronic glycemia can be used to evaluate and adjust therapy. Several chemical measurements may be used by the patient and clinician to assess glycemic control directly or indirectly.[59] SMBG and HbA_{1c} levels continue to be the two primary methods used to access glycemic control. Recently, continuous glucose monitoring (CGM) of interstitial fluid has become available for people with diabetes. CGM is discussed somewhat briefly here, because this method still is currently recommended for consideration, along with SMBG, for patients with type 1 diabetes only, especially those with hypoglycemic unawareness.[22]

Urine Ketone Testing

Urine ketone testing is recommended for patients with gestational and type 1 diabetes. Urine ketones should be evaluated when glucose concentrations consistently exceed 300 mg/dL (16.7 mmol/L) or during acute illness.[59] Persistently high glucose concentrations of this magnitude signal insulin deficiency that can, in turn, lead to lipolysis and ketoacidosis. A positive test may indicate impending or established ketoacidosis and demands a more extensive diagnostic workup. Testing also is recommended during pregnancy and if the patient has symptoms of ketoacidosis. Although there are generally no ketones in the urine, they may be present in people who are on extremely low caloric diets and in the first morning sample of women who are pregnant. Also, see discussions of sick day management and ketoacidosis in other sections of this chapter (Questions 30 and 39 through 43).

Plasma Glucose

FPG concentrations (normal FPG, 3.9–5.6 mmol/dL or 70–100 mg/dL) are commonly used to assess glycemic control in the fasting state because this is when glucose concentrations are most reproducible. FPG concentrations generally reflect glucose derived from hepatic glucose production because this is the primary source of glucose in the postabsorptive state. The FPG is the most frequent test performed by patients when self-monitoring. Postprandial glucose concentrations (1–2 hours after the start of the meal) also are used to assess glycemic control when fasting glucose concentrations are within normal limits or when there is a need to assess the effects of food or drugs (e.g., rapid-acting insulins, α-glucosidase inhibitors) on meal-related glycemia. In nondiabetic individuals, glucose concentrations generally return to below 140 mg/dL (7.8 mmol/L) within 2 hours after a meal. One- to 2-hour postprandial concentrations primarily reflect the efficiency of insulin-mediated glucose uptake by peripheral tissue.

Because any glucose concentration can be affected by various factors (e.g., meals, medications, stress), measurement at a single point in time cannot be used to assess a patient's overall control. Most laboratories measure plasma glucose concentrations rather than whole blood because these values are not subject to changes in the hematocrit. The majority of glucose monitors report plasma-referenced glucose concentrations. Whole blood glucose concentrations are approximately 10% to 15% lower than plasma glucose concentrations because glucose is not distributed into red blood cells. To convert plasma glucose concentrations (mg/dL) to whole blood glucose values (and vice versa), the following equation can be used:

- Whole blood glucose (mg/dL) = plasma glucose (mg/dL) ÷ 1.12
- To convert a glucose concentration in mg/dL to mmol/L, a factor of 18 is used:

$$\text{Plasma glucose (mmol/L)} = \text{plasma glucose (mg/dL)} \div 18$$

Self-Monitored Blood Glucose

SMBG has made euglycemia, both preprandially and postprandially, an achievable goal (80–140 mg/dL). Patients and their health care providers can use SMBG to assess directly the effects of drug dose changes, meals, exercise, and illness on daily blood glucose concentrations. With improved technology, decreasing costs, and increased coverage by health plans, SMBG is the day-to-day monitoring test of choice for all patients with diabetes. However, SMBG remains expensive for patients without health insurance, is invasive, and is technique dependent. Furthermore, to achieve maximum benefit from SMBG, both the clinician and patient must be motivated and willing to spend the time required to interpret the data and modify therapy to improve glycemic control. Based on the results of the DCCT and UKPDS, most persons with diabetes should attempt to achieve and maintain blood glucose levels as close to normal as is safely possible. This goal can realistically be achieved only by using SMBG. The frequency and timing of performing SMBG should be dictated by the individual's needs and goals. Selection and use of SMBG testing materials are discussed in questions 11 and 12. Patients in whom blood glucose self-monitoring is particularly valuable include the following:

- *Patients with type 1 diabetes*: Frequent blood glucose measurements help the patient to correlate meals, exercise, and insulin dose with blood glucose concentrations. This instant feedback gives the patient an increased sense of control and motivation, leading to improved glucose control.

- *Pregnant patients*: Infant morbidity and mortality are associated with the mother's overall glucose control. Using SMBG, the mother with diabetes who achieves normoglycemia before conception and throughout pregnancy, improves her chances of delivering a live, healthy infant.
- *Patients having difficulty recognizing hypoglycemia*: Over time, many patients with diabetes develop a sluggish counterregulatory response to hypoglycemia whereby hypoglycemic symptoms are blunted or even absent. This is often referred to as *hypoglycemic unawareness*. Routine SMBG to detect asymptomatic hypoglycemia is essential in these individuals (see question 38). In addition, acute anxiety attacks or signs and symptoms associated with a rapidly falling blood glucose concentration may mimic a true hypoglycemic reaction. This can be evaluated easily by measuring a fingerstick blood glucose concentration.
- *Patients who are using physiological (e.g., basal-bolus) insulin therapy*: Individuals who are on multiple daily doses of insulin or those using an insulin pump should use SMBG to evaluate the effectiveness of their insulin regimens and meal plans and to check for hypoglycemic or hyperglycemic reactions (see Question 12). Knowledge of preprandial, postprandial, bedtime, and nocturnal (e.g., 2 AM) blood glucose concentrations is essential in determining basal and preprandial insulin requirements.

Continuous Glucose Monitoring

CGM has become available in recent years and provides real time information on glucose concentrations. Commercially available CGM monitors currently measure SC interstitial glucose levels. The four main CGM systems in the United States are DexCom STS 3- and 7-day systems, MiniMed Paradigm REAL-Time system (communicates with the Paradigm 522 and 722 insulin pumps), MiniMed Guardian REAL-Time system, and the Abbott FreeStyle Navigator. The CGM systems use electrochemical sensors that are inserted into the skin. Sensor probe length varies from 5 to 16 mm. Depending on the system, the sensors are good for 3 to 7 days. The sensors transmit a signal to a transmitter (wired or wireless), and then to a receiver for display. The system transmits glucose information to the receiver; receivers then display the glucose reading every 1 minute (Navigator) or 5 minutes (DexCom and MiniMed systems). The sensors require a warmup or initialization period and have very specific calibration requirements (e.g., at 2 and 6 hours, then every 12 hours for the life of the sensor with the MiniMed systems). Calibration is performed by using a blood glucose monitor. Interstitial glucose concentrations are displayed on the receiver every 1 or 5 minutes depending on the system. Interstitial glucose levels lag behind plasma or blood glucose levels by 8 to 18 minutes, depending on the glucose rate of change.[60] Therefore, if a person's glucose is low, or trending downward, SMBG is required. An issue with CGM is severe skins reactions to the adhesive for either the sensor or transmitter. CGM systems have alarms that can go off at certain high and low glucose thresholds. The ability to detect hypoglycemia during the night with these alarms has been a very attractive reason for using CGM. Another key feature is the ability to follow trends and rates of change in blood glucose levels. Small, short-term studies have demonstrated modest improvements in HbA_{1c} (0.3%–0.6% reductions) in adults and children with type 1 diabetes.[61–64] CGM does not replace SMBG, but provides a new tool for patients to actively manage their diabetes. A noninvasive, watchlike device called the GlucoWatch G2 Biographer (Animas Corporation, West Chester, PA) used to be available, but the manufacturer ceased selling this in 2007. This device used iontophoresis to obtain glucose samples through intact skin via interstitial fluid.

Glycosylated Hemoglobin

The glycosylated hemoglobin, or HbA_{1c}, has become the gold standard for measuring chronic glycemia and is the clinical marker for predicting long-term complications, particularly microvascular complications. HbA_{1c} is most commonly measured because it comprises the majority of glycosylated hemoglobin and is the least affected by recent fluctuations in blood glucose. HbA_{1c} measures the percentage of hemoglobin A that has been irreversibly glycosylated at the *N*-terminal amino group of the β-chain; the plasma glucose level and the life span of a red blood cell (RBC; ~120 days) determine its value. Thus, HbA_{1c} is an indicator of glycemic control over the preceding 2 to 3 months. In patients without diabetes, HbA_{1c} comprises approximately 4% to 6% of the total hemoglobin. Values may be three times this level in patients with diabetes.

The current HbA_{1c} assay actually measures several different molecules of hemoglobin A (HbA_{1c}, HbA_{1a}, HbA_{1b}, HbA_0), not just HbA_{1c}. Each laboratory establishes its own normal values for the HbA_{1c} test (most are referenced to the normal range of 4%–6%). The International Federation of Clinical Chemistry has developed a new reference method that only measures glycated HbA_{1c} (with a new unit of mmol HbA_{1c} per mol total hemoglobin).[65] The downside of this method is that the HbA_{1c} values are 1.3% to 2.0% lower than the current values, which would cause great confusion among practitioners. Another movement is to report estimated average glucose (units mg/dL or mmol/L), which is calculated using HbA_{1c} measurements and correlating them to actual glucose measurements (using 7-point blood glucose profiles with SMBG and CGM) over a 3-month period.[66] The International HbA_{1c}-derived Average Glucose trial will provide new correlations of HbA_{1c} with estimated average glucose and is due to be published in 2008. The current correlation between HbA_{1c} and mean plasma glucoses that is reported is based on DCCT values (see below).[22,67] In these data, a 1% change in the glycosylated hemoglobin represents a 35-mg/dL change in the mean plasma glucose concentration.

	Mean Plasma Glucose Levels	
HbA_{1c} (%)	(mg/dL)	mmol/L
6	135	7.5
7	170	9.5
8	205	11.5
9	240	13.5
10	275	15.5
11	310	17.5
12	345	19.5

Alterations in RBC survival such as hemoglobinopathies, anemias, acute or chronic blood loss, and uremia may affect HbA_{1c} values, resulting in inaccurate indications of glycemic control. Antioxidants such as vitamins C and E also may interfere with the glycosylation process[68,69] (Table 50-6).

Table 50-6 Factors Affecting HbA_{1c}

Cause	*Effect on HbA_{1c}*
Alterations in RBC Survival	
Hemoglobinopathies	Decreased
Anemias	
Hemolytic	Decreased
Iron deficiency	Decreased[a]
Blood loss	Decreased
Assay Interference	
Uremia	Increased or no change[b,c]
Hemodialysis	No change[b]
Antioxidants	Decreased[d]

[a] For patients receiving iron replacement therapy. Normal levels would be expected in untreated patients.
[b] Interference seen in assays using high-pressure liquid chromatography and electroendosmosis. Affinity chromatography seems unaffected.
[c] Carbamylated hemoglobin equaling 0.063% of total hemoglobin is formed for every 1 mmol/L of serum urea.
[d] Reported with vitamins C (1 g/day) and E (1,200 mg/day). Possible mechanism is competitive inhibition of hemoglobin glycosylation.
HbA_{1c}, glycosylated hemoglobin; RBC, red blood cell.

HbA_{1c} can be measured without any special patient preparation (e.g., fasting) and generally is not subject to acute changes in insulin dosing, exercise, or diet. Normalization can indicate whether euglycemia has been achieved. However, HbA_{1c} does not replace the day-to-day monitoring of blood glucose concentrations, which is essential for evaluating acute changes in blood glucose concentrations. These values are needed to adjust the meal plan or medication doses.

CLINICAL USE

Currently, the HbA_{1c} value is used as an adjunct to assessing overall glycemic control in patients with diabetes. Often, it is used to verify clinical impressions related to glucose control and patient adherence. Some also have suggested the use of HbA_{1c} values for diabetes screening and diagnosis; however, until the test is standardized and more studies are completed, it cannot be recommended for these purposes. HbA_{1c} should be measured quarterly in patients who do not meet treatment goals, and at least semiannually in stable patients who are meeting treatment goals.

Glycated Serum Protein, Glycated Serum Albumin, and Fructosamine

Assays for glycated serum proteins reflect the extent of glycosylation of a variety of serum proteins, including glycated serum albumin.[59] The fructosamine assay is one of the most widely used methods to measure glycated proteins (normal, 2–2.8 mmol/L). Because the half-life of albumin is approximately 14 to 20 days, fructosamine provides an indication of glycemic control over a shorter time frame (1–2 weeks) than does the HbA_{1c}. The ADA does not consider measurement of fructosamine equivalent to that of HbA_{1c}, although it correlates well with this value. Fructosamine levels may be useful as an adjunct to HbA_{1c} in determining whether a patient is improving or worsening in the short term (e.g., a patient on insulin therapy undergoing multiple dosage adjustments; for women with type 2 diabetes during pregnancy or gestational diabetes) or in patients with conditions such as hemolytic anemia in whom the HbA_{1c} test is inaccurate (Table 50-6). However, the exact role of glycated serum protein in monitoring glycemic control requires further study.

INSULIN

Insulin is a hormone secreted from the pancreatic β-cell in response to glucose and other stimulants (e.g., amino acids, free fatty acids, gastric hormones, parasympathetic stimulation, β-adrenergic stimulation).[70,71] The hormone is made up of two polypeptide chains (a 21-amino acid α chain and a 30-amino acid β chain), which are connected by two disulfide bonds (Fig. 50-3). Proinsulin, the precursor of insulin, is a single-chain, 86-amino acid polypeptide. In the storage granule of the β-cell, the connecting or C-peptide is cleaved from proinsulin to produce equimolar amounts of insulin and C-peptide. Thus, measurable C-peptide levels indicate the presence of endogenously produced insulin and functioning β-cells. Insulin is crucial to the survival of individuals with type 1 diabetes, whose β-cells have been destroyed. It also plays a major role in the therapy of individuals with type 2 diabetes when their symptoms cannot be controlled with diet and exercise alone or a combination of antidiabetic agents. Insulin also is used in patients with type 2 diabetes during pregnancy or periods of intercurrent illness or stress (e.g., surgery).

Commercially available insulin products differ in their immunogenicity, physical and chemical properties, pharmacokinetics, and pharmacodynamics.

Immunogenicity

Modern manufacturing processes have virtually eliminated contaminants from current products, and most people now use human insulin. Consequently, immunologically mediated sequelae, such as lipodystrophy, hypersensitivity, and insulin resistance caused by "blocking" antibodies, are rare.

Regular insulin is a solution that can be administered by any parenteral route: intravenously, intramuscularly, or subcutaneously. Insulin lispro, insulin aspart, and insulin glulisine are rapid-acting analogs. These insulins are also clear solutions approved by the U.S. Food and Drug Administration (FDA) for SC use. Insulin glargine and insulin detemir, two long-acting insulins are also clear solutions, but neither should be administered IV. Insulin glargine is designed to precipitate at physiological pH and insulin detemir binds to plasma albumin. NPH insulin, an intermediate insulin, is a suspension in which regular insulin has been complexed with protamine to extend its action. Two previously available insulins, Lente and Ultralente, were removed from the market in 2005. NPH insulin must be mixed well before administration and should never be administered IV. All insulin products have a neutral pH, except for insulin glargine, which has a pH of 4.0.

Pharmacokinetics: Absorption, Distribution, and Elimination

After SC injection, insulin is absorbed directly into the bloodstream, bypassing the lymphatic system. The rate-limiting step of insulin activity after SC administration is absorption of

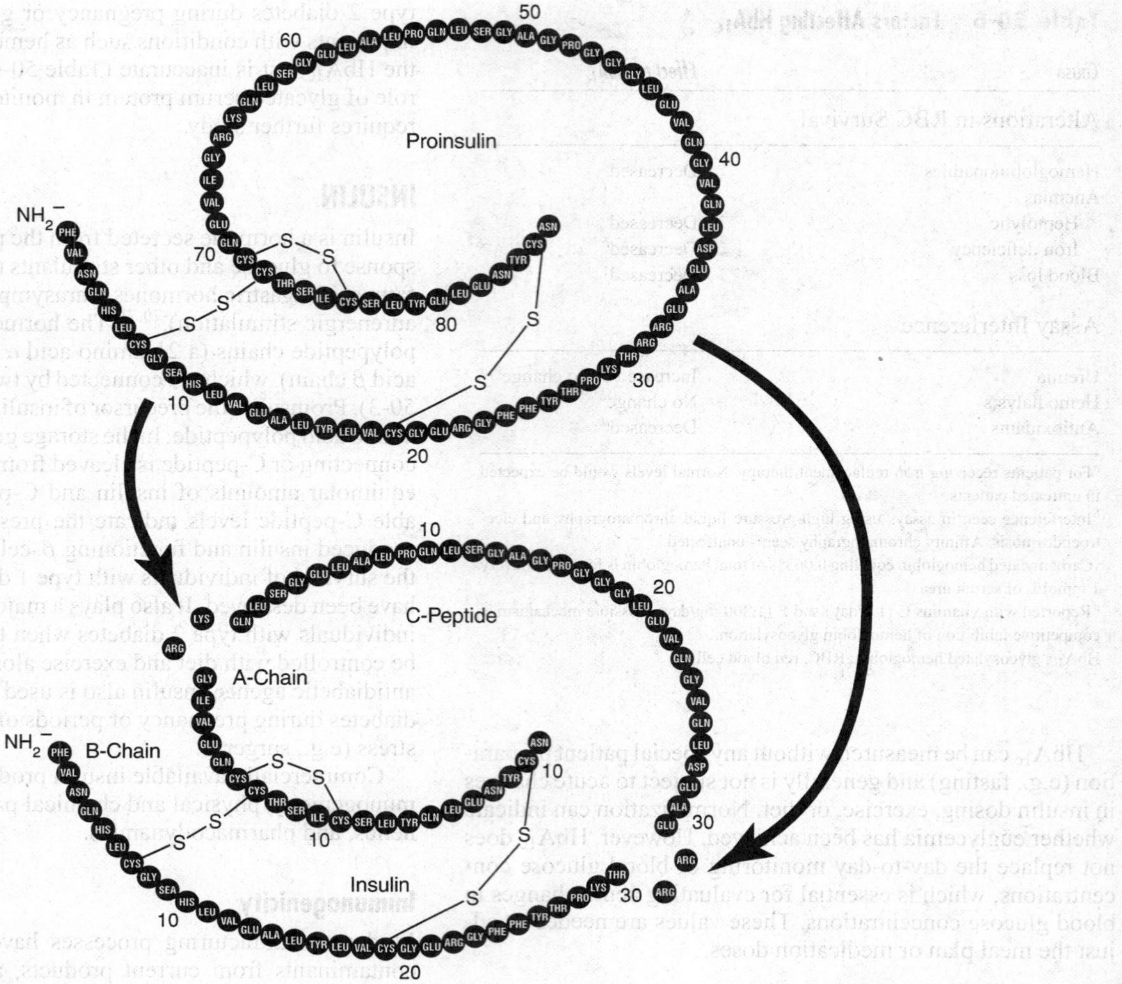

FIGURE 50-3 Proinsulin. Insulin is secreted from the pancreas as proinsulin. The connecting or C-peptide is cleaved to release the active insulin molecule. Thus, C-peptide levels are measured in study conditions to confirm the presence of a working pancreas. Insulin is a 51-amino acid protein made up of an A chain and a B chain connected by two disulfide bonds. (Reproduced with permission from reference 341.)

insulin from the injection site, which depends on the type of insulin administered, as well as a multitude of other factors. Although SC absorption generally follows a simple exponential course, it is highly irregular. Coefficients of variation for the time until 50% of the insulin dose is absorbed are approximately 25% within an individual and up to 50% among patients for all insulins studied.[72] A primary cause of this variation is attributed to changes in blood flow around the injection site.

Exogenous insulin is degraded at both renal and extrarenal (liver and muscle) sites. Degradation also takes place at the cellular level after internalization of the insulin-receptor complex. Approximately 30% to 80% of insulin is cleared from the systemic circulation by the kidneys, which have a larger role in clearing exogenously administered insulin. Endogenous insulin is secreted directly into the portal circulation and is primarily cleared by the liver in nondiabetic individuals (60%).[70] Insulin is filtered by glomerular capillaries, but more than 99% is reabsorbed by the proximal tubules. The insulin is then degraded in glomerular capillary cells and postglomerular peritubular cells.[73] See Question 31 for changes in insulin requirement in renal dysfunction.

When insulin is given IV, the half-life for three compartments are 2.3 to 2.4 minutes, 14 minutes, and 133 minutes. Insulin action most closely corresponds to last compartment.[72] Therefore, it is unnecessary to adjust the dose more frequently than Q 2 hr.

Pharmacodynamics

Clinically, the most important differences between insulin products relate to their onset, peak, and duration of action (not the actual insulin levels, which is pharmacokinetics). Current insulin products can be categorized as rapid acting, short acting, intermediate acting, and long acting. Products available in the United States are listed in Table 50-7, and the onset of action, peak effect, and durations of action of each insulin category are listed in Table 50-8. However, these data are derived primarily from studies in normal, healthy volunteers in the fasting state or in well-controlled patients with diabetes

Table 50-7 Insulins Available in the United States

Type/Duration of Action	Brand Name	Manufacturer
Rapid Acting		
Insulin lispro	Humalog	Lilly
Insulin aspart	NovoLog	Novo Nordisk
Insulin glulisine	Apidra	Sanofi-Aventis
Short Acting		
Regular	Humulin R	Lilly
	Novolin R	Novo Nordisk
Intermediate Acting		
NPH (isophane insulin suspension)	Humulin N	Lilly
	Novolin N	Novo Nordisk
Long Acting		
Insulin glargine	Lantus	Sanofi-Aventis
Insulin detemir	Levemir	Novo Nordisk
Combination Insulins		
NPH/regular mixture (70%/30%)	Humulin 70/30	Lilly
	Novolin 70/30	Novo Nordisk
NPH/regular mixture (50%/50%)	Humulin 50/50	Lilly
Insulin aspart protamine/insulin aspart mixture (70%/30%)	Novolog Mix 70/30	Novo Nordisk
Insulin NPL/insulin lispro mixture (75%/25%)	Humalog Mix 75/25	Lilly
Insulin NPL/insulin lispro mixture (50%/50%)	Humalog Mix 50/50	Lilly

stabilized in a metabolic ward. In actuality, intersubject and intrasubject variations in response to insulin can be substantial because an individual pattern of response to insulin can be affected by numerous factors (e.g., the formation of insulin hexamers, the presence of insulin-binding antibodies, dose, exercise, site of injection, massage of the injection site, ambient temperature, and interactions between insulins that have been

Table 50-8 Insulin Pharmacodynamics[a,110,254]

Insulin	Onset (hr)	Peak (hr)	Duration (hr)	Appearance
Rapid acting (insulin lispro, aspart and glulisine)	5–25 min	30–90 min	<5	Clear
Regular	0.5–1	2–3	5–8	Clear
NPH	2–4	4–12	12–18	Cloudy
Insulin glargine	1.5	No pronounced peak	20–24	Clear[b]
Insulin detemir	3–8	Relatively flat	5.7–23.2	Clear[b]

[a] The onset, peak, and duration of insulin activity may vary considerably from times listed in this table. See text and Table 50-12.
[b] Should not be mixed with other insulins or administered IV. Some patients require twice-daily dosing.

Table 50-9 Components of Physiological Insulin Therapy

- Multicomponent insulin regimen of basal plus preprandial insulin doses
- Balance of carbohydrate intake, exercise, and insulin dosage
- Daily, multiple self-monitoring of blood glucose levels
- Patient self-adjustment of carbohydrate intake and insulin dosage with use of correction/supplemental rapid- or short-acting insulin according to a predetermined plan
- Individualized target blood glucose and HbA_{1c} levels
- Frequent contact between patient and diabetes team
- Intensive patient education
- Psychological support
- Regular objective assessment (as measured by HbA_{1c})

HbA_{1c}, glycosylated hemoglobin.
Modified from reference 100.

mixed together; Table 50-10 and Question 16).[72,74] Nevertheless, knowledge of when one might expect the various insulins to exert their effects is absolutely essential to the rational adjustment of insulin dosages.

Rapid-Acting Insulin

INSULIN LISPRO

Insulin lispro [Lys(B28),Pro(B29)]-human insulin (Humalog, Eli Lilly, Indianapolis, IN) was the first available rapid-acting insulin analog and received FDA approval in 1996. The natural amino acid sequence of the insulin β-chain at positions 28 (proline) and 29 (lysine) is inverted to form lispro. This change results in an insulin molecule that more loosely self-associates into hexamers than does regular insulin. Consequently, the active monomeric form is more readily available, resulting in an onset of activity (15 minutes), peak action (60–90 minutes), and duration (3–4 hours) that more closely simulates physiological insulin secretion relative to meals. Because it can be injected shortly before eating (0–15 minutes), lispro, and all rapid-acting insulins, provide patients greater flexibility in lifestyle. These insulins lower 2-hour postprandial blood glucose levels, and decrease the risk for late postprandial and nocturnal hypoglycemia compared with regular insulin formulations.[75] Patients who use an insulin pump most often use a rapid-acting insulin instead of regular insulin. One randomized, two-way, cross-over, open-label study compared lispro with regular insulin administered for 3 months by continuous SC insulin infusion.[76] Lispro resulted in HbA_{1c} values that were significantly lower than those produced by regular insulin (7.41% vs. 7.65%). There were no differences in adverse events. Because lispro has a shorter duration of action than regular insulin, hyperglycemia and ketosis may occur more rapidly if insulin delivery is inadvertently interrupted. Insulin lispro is approved for use in pediatric patients, age 3 and older.[77] It is pregnancy category B.

INSULIN ASPART

Insulin aspart (NovoLog, Novo Nordisk, West Princeton, NJ) is a rapid-acting insulin analog that differs from human insulin by substitution of aspartic acid at B28. Insulin aspart is approved for use in pediatric patients, age 6 and older.[78] It is pregnancy category B. Insulin aspart controls postprandial glucose excursions similar to insulin lispro.

Table 50-10 Factors Altering Onset and Duration of Insulin Action

Factor	Comments
Route of administration	Onset of action more rapid and duration of action shorter for IV>IM>SC[137]
	Intrapulmonary insulin has more rapid onset and shorter duration than SC insulin, resembling IV pharmacokinetics[72]
Factors altering clearance	
Renal function	Renal failure lowers insulin clearance; may prolong and intensify action of exogenous and endogenous insulin
Insulin antibodies	IgG antibodies bind insulin as it is absorbed and release it slowly, thereby delaying and/or prolonging its effect[339]
Thyroid function	Hyperthyroidism increases clearance, but also increases insulin action, making control difficult; patients stabilize as they become euthyroid
Factors altering SC absorption	Factors that raise SC blood flow ↑ absorption rates of regular insulin; effect on intermediate- and long-acting insulins minimal
Site of injection	Rate of absorption fastest from the abdomen, intermediate from the arm, and slowest from the thigh; less variation observed in type 2 patients; less variation observed with lispro insulin
	Site — *Half-life absorption (min)*
	Abdomen — 87 ± 12
	Arm — 141 ± 23
	Hip — 153 ± 28
	Thigh — 164 ± 15
Exercise of injected area	Strenuous exercise of an injected area within 1 hr of injection can increase absorption rate; rate of absorption of regular insulin is increased, but little effect on intermediate-acting insulin[72,134]
Ambient temperature	Heat (e.g., hot weather, hot bath, sauna) increases absorption rate; cold has opposite effect[70,72]
Local massage	Massaging injected area for 30 min substantially increases absorption rate of regular insulin as well as longer acting insulins
Smoking	Controversial; vasoconstriction may down decrease absorption rate[72]
Jet injectors	Insulin absorption more rapid, probably secondary to increases surface area for absorption
Lipohypertrophy	Insulin absorption is delayed from lipohypertrophic sites
Insulin preparation	More soluble forms of insulin are absorbed more rapidly and have shorter durations of action (see Table 50-8 and text); human insulin may have shorter action than animal insulin
Insulin mixtures	The short-acting properties of raid-acting insulins may be blunted if mixed with NPH insulin (see Question 17)
Insulin concentration	More dilute solutions (e.g., U-40, U-10) are absorbed more rapidly than more concentrated forms (U-100, U-500)[70]
Insulin dose	Lower doses are absorbed more rapidly and have a shorter duration of action than larger doses

IgG, immunoglobulin G; IM, intramuscular; IV, intravenous; SC, subcutaneous.

INSULIN GLULISINE

Insulin glulisine (Apidra, Sanofi-Aventis, Bridgewater, NJ) is a rapid-acting insulin analog that differs from human insulin by substitution of lysine for asparagine at position B3 and glutamic acid for lysine at position B23. Insulin glulisine is currently not FDA approved for use in pediatric patients.[79] It is pregnancy category C. Insulin glulisine lowers postprandial glucose excursions similar to insulin lispro and insulin aspart.

Short-Acting Insulin

Regular insulin has an onset of action of 30 to 60 minutes, a peak effect at 2 to 4 hours, and a duration of action of 5 to 7 hours. The broad range in peak effect and duration reflects the many variables that affect insulin action (Table 50-8). The 30- to 60-minute onset of action requires proper timing of premeal regular insulin, which is difficult for most patients. Use of regular insulin in patients with type 1 diabetes is much less common with the advent of the rapid-acting insulins.

Previously, an inhaled human insulin powder (Exubera, Pfizer, New York, NY) was available. In October 2007, Pfizer announced that it would no longer make this insulin owing to its infrequent use. In March 2008, Lilly announced that it was cancelling the trials of its inhaled insulin, AIR, which it was developing with Alkermes, Inc. Similarly, Novo Nordisk in January 2008 announced it would discontinue studies of its insulin inhaler AERx.

Intermediate-Acting Insulin

NPH

NPH (neutral protamine hagedorn or isophane) is an intermediate-acting insulin. Its onset of action is approximately 2 hours (range, 1–3), peak effects occur at approximately 6 to 14 hours, and the duration of action of NPH is approximately 16 to 24 hours. Again, it must be emphasized that this pattern of response is at best a generalization. Patients may have a variable pattern of response to NPH insulin over time, and those on higher doses are likely to have a later peak and a longer duration of action. Up to 80% of these day-to-day fluctuations in blood glucose responses can be accounted for by variation in the absorption of this intermediate-acting insulin.[72]

Long-Acting Insulin

INSULIN GLARGINE

Insulin glargine (Lantus, Sanofi-Aventis) was approved by the FDA in April 2000 and is pregnancy category C. It is approved for once a day SC administration for the treatment of adult and pediatric patients (age ≥6) with type 1 diabetes or adult patients with type 2 diabetes who require basal (long-acting) insulin for the control of hyperglycemia. It can be administered anytime during the day, but it is important to take it at the same time each day. It is usually administered at bedtime (this was the original approved administration time) or, second most commonly, in the morning.

Insulin glargine is an insulin analog in which asparagine in position A21 is substituted with glycine and two arginines are added to the C-terminus of the β-chain. This change in the amino acid sequence causes a shift in the isoelectric point from pH 5.4 to 6.7, making it more soluble at an acidic pH.[80] Once injected, insulin glargine (which is a clear solution with a pH of 4.0) precipitates at physiological pH forming a depot that releases insulin slowly over 24 hours. This results in delayed absorption and a less pronounced peak compared with NPH insulin.[81] Zinc is added to further prolong the duration of insulin glargine. In clinical trials of patients with types 1 and 2 diabetes, once-daily injections of insulin glargine were as effective as NPH in lowering HbA_{1c} values with less nocturnal hypoglycemia.[82] Insulin glargine is associated with more injection site pain compared with NPH (6.1% vs. 0.3% in one study and 2.7% vs. 0.7% in another), which is likely due to its acidity.[83,84] Some patients report that they "feel" the insulin glargine injection more than other insulins.

INSULIN DETEMIR

Insulin detemir (Levemir, Novo Nordisk), was approved in June 2005 and joins insulin glargine as the second basal insulin marketed in the United States. It is pregnancy category C. Unlike other insulin analogs, in which the amino acid sequence is modified, for insulin detemir, a fatty acid moiety is added to the last amino acid on the end of the β-chain. Insulin detemir is a neutral, soluble insulin preparation in which the B30 threonine has been removed and the B29 lysine residue has been covalently bound to a 14-carbon fatty acid. The result is an insulin that is more slowly absorbed in the SC tissue because the fatty acid moiety binds to albumin, creating a long-acting insulin.[85] Insulin determir's kinetics and dynamics are dose dependent.[86] When used in type 1 diabetes, two injections daily are usually required to provide adequate basal coverage. Insulin detemir demonstrates less intrasubject variability than NPH or insulin glargine.[87] The clinical significance and impact of this observation is unclear.

Premixed Insulin

Products that contain premixed NPH and regular insulin in a fixed ratio of 70:30 are available from Lilly as Humulin 70/30 and Novo Nordisk as Novolin 70/30. Lilly also makes a premixed formulation in a 50:50 ratio (Humulin 50/50). Additional premixed formulations are available wherein both insulin lispro and insulin aspart have been co-crystallized with protamine to create an intermediate-acting insulin similar to NPH. Humalog Mix 75/25 and Humalog Mix 50/50 (Lilly) are products with lispro protamine and insulin lispro in a fixed ratio of 75:25 and 50:50, respectively. Novolog Mix 70/30 (Novo Nordisk) is aspart protamine and insulin aspart in a fixed ratio of 70:30. These premixed insulins are available for patients who have difficulty measuring and mixing insulins and are dosed twice daily. These insulins are compatible when mixed together and retain their individual pharmacodynamic profiles (see Question 16).

TREATMENT OF TYPE 1 DIABETES: CLINICAL USE OF INSULIN

Clinical Presentation of Type 1 Diabetes

3. A.H., a slender, 18-year-old woman who was recently discharged from the hospital for severe dehydration and mild ketoacidosis is referred to the Diabetes Clinic from the University Student Health Service (no records available). A fasting and a random plasma glucose ordered subsequently were 190 mg/dL (normal, 70–100) and 250 mg/dL (normal, 140 to <200). Approximately 4 weeks before she was hospitalized, A.H. had moved across the country to attend college—her first time away from home. In retrospect, she remembers that she had symptoms of polydipsia, nocturia (six times a night), fatigue, and a 12-lb weight loss over this period, which she attributed to the anxiety associated with her move away from home and adjustment to her new environment. Her medical history is remarkable for recurrent upper respiratory infections and three cases of vaginal moniliasis over the past 6 months. Her family history is negative for diabetes, and she takes no medications.

Physical examination is within normal limits. She weighs 50 kg and is 5 feet 4 inches tall. Laboratory results are as follows: FPG, 280 mg/dL (normal, <100); HbA_{1c}, 14% (normal, 4%–6%); and trace urine ketones as measured by Keto-Diastix (normal, negative). On the basis of her history and laboratory findings, the presumptive diagnosis is type 1 diabetes. Which findings are consistent with this diagnosis in A.H.?

[SI units: FPG, 15.5 mmol/L (normal, <5.6); HbA_{1c}, 0.14 (normal, 0.04–0.06)]

A.H. meets several of the diagnostic criteria for diabetes. She has classic symptoms of the disease (polyuria, polydipsia, weight loss, glucosuria, fatigue, recurrent infections), a random plasma glucose above 200 mg/dL, and an FPG of 126 mg/dL or higher on at least two occasions[4] (Tables 50-1 and 50-2). The elevated HbA_{1c} also is consistent with diabetes mellitus. Features of A.H.'s history that are consistent with type 1 diabetes, in particular, include the relatively acute onset of symptoms in association with a major life event (moving away from home), ketones in the urine, negative family history, and a relatively young age at onset.

Treatment Goals

4. A.H. will be started on insulin therapy on this visit. What are the goals of therapy? Will normoglycemia prevent the development or progression of long-term complications?

The goal of diabetes management is the prevention of acute and chronic complications. As discussed in the introduction to this chapter, the results of the DCCT and DCCT-EDIC convincingly demonstrated that lowering blood glucose concentrations through intensive insulin therapy in persons with type 1 diabetes slows or prevents the development of microvascular complications.[29,30] The ADA recommends an HbA_{1c} goal of less than 7% for patients in general and an individual goal as close to normal as possible (<6%) without significant hypoglycemia.

It is important to understand that physiological or basal-bolus insulin therapy involves a *complete* program of diabetes management that includes a balanced meal plan, exercise, frequent SMBG, and insulin adjustments based on these factors (Tables 50-4 and 50-9). Because the patient is the key member of the team, A.H. must be highly motivated and able to learn about the complex metabolic interplay between insulin and lifestyle.

In summary, A.H. is a patient newly diagnosed with type 1 diabetes who has not yet developed any signs or symptoms of long-term complications. Therefore, she is an ideal candidate for basal-bolus insulin therapy and, if she is willing and motivated, normoglycemia with rare hypoglycemic reactions is a reasonable long-term goal. This goal should be achieved gradually over several months with insulin therapy, diet, education, and strong clinical support. A desirable goal is an HbA_{1c} value as close to the normal range as possible with rare hypoglycemic reactions.

Basal-Bolus (Physiological) Insulin Therapy

5. What methods of insulin administration are available to achieve optimal glucose control?

A physiological insulin regimen is designed to mimic normal insulin secretion as closely as possible.[88] Problems with insulin delivery include factors that affect the SC absorption of insulin (Table 50-10). Before the development of the rapid-acting insulin analogs and basal insulins, previous insulins lacked pharmacodynamic profiles that allowed one to closely simulate the basal-bolus model (see text that follows). Clinicians now have more tools to mimic the pancreatic release of the hormone. In the nondiabetic individual, the pancreas secretes boluses of insulin in response to snacks and meals. Between meals and throughout the night, the pancreas secretes small amounts of insulin that are sufficient to suppress lipolysis and hepatic glucose output (basal insulin). Two methods have been used to achieve a similar pattern of insulin release: (a) insulin pump therapy (previously referred to as "continuous subcutaneous infusion of insulin") and (b) basal-bolus insulin regimens consisting of once to twice daily doses of basal insulin coupled with pre-meal doses of rapid or short-acting insulin (see Question 6).

Insulin Pump Therapy

The use of an insulin pump is currently the most precise way to mimic normal insulin secretion. This consists of a battery-operated pump and a computer that can program the pump to deliver predetermined amounts of regular insulin, insulin lispro, insulin aspart, or insulin glulisine from a reservoir to a subcutaneously inserted catheter or needle (e.g., MiniMed Paradigm 722, Northridge, CA; Animas 2020).[89,90] These systems are portable and designed to deliver various basal amounts of insulin over 24 hours as well as meal-related boluses. A bolus of regular insulin can be released by the patient 30 minutes before food ingestion. Most patients using an insulin pump, however, prefer to use the rapid-acting insulin analogs in their pump. For meal coverage, the rapid-acting insulin can be given 0 to 15 minutes before eating. The delivery of the bolus can be adjusted depending on the type of food eaten (e.g., piece of cake versus slice of pizza). Caveat: If SC delivery is discontinued, check for rise in glucose and urine ketones after 2 or 3 hours. Because there is no SC pool, effects dissipate quickly.

The preferred meal planning approach for patients using an insulin pump is carbohydrate counting. The "insulin to carbohydrate ratio" or how much carbohydrate is covered by 1 unit of insulin must be determined. One method is to use the "500 Rule." The number 500 (or 450 for regular insulin) is divided by the total daily dose of insulin the patient is using to determine the insulin to carbohydrate ratio (see Question 13). Insulin pumps are capable of delivering many basal insulin rates. The basal insulin infusion rate may be adjusted depending on the situation. Many patients find it advantageous to decrease the basal rate during the middle of the night when nocturnal hypoglycemia is most likely to occur. The basal rate also may be increased before awakening to avoid hyperglycemia secondary to the "dawn phenomenon"—adjustments that are not possible using subcutaneous basal insulin injections. Features of the current pump models include "bolus wizard," which calculates accurate boluses based on preset carbohydrate-to-insulin ratios and correction factors, carbohydrate counts for selected foods, and an "insulin-on-board" feature, which avoids stacking of insulin doses by indicating how much insulin from a previously administered dose is still available. Most insurance plans provide coverage for insulin pumps for patients with type 1 and some patients with type 2 diabetes. Factors to consider when choosing a pump include safety features, durability, ability of the manufacturer to provide service, availability of training, clinically desirable features, and cosmetic attractiveness for the user.[89,91]

MULTIPLE DAILY INJECTIONS

6. How can insulin injections be administered to A.H. in a way that mimics the physiological release of insulin from the pancreas?

Endocrinologists have developed a variety of insulin regimens that are intended to mimic the release of insulin from the pancreas.[92] Examples of these are displayed in and illustrated in Figure 50-4. A total daily dose of insulin is estimated empirically (e.g., 0.5 unit/kg/day) or according to guidelines listed in Table 50-11. The total daily dose of insulin then is split into several doses. In general, the basal dose comprises approximately 50% of the total daily dose.

A regimen much less commonly used in patients with type 1 diabetes involves injecting a mixture of intermediate-acting and regular or rapid-acting insulin twice daily, before breakfast and before dinner (Fig. 50-4A). The morning dose of regular/rapid-acting insulin is intended to take care of the breakfast meal; the morning dose of NPH takes care of the noon meal and provides basal insulin throughout the day; the evening dose of regular/rapid-acting insulin takes care of the evening meal; and the evening dose of NPH provides basal insulin levels during the night and takes care of any evening snack that is ingested. Because NPH is an intermediate-acting insulin and has a peak effect, it does not provide true basal insulin coverage. Also, when NPH is injected in the morning, the patient must eat lunch on time because of this peak effect, otherwise they will experience hypoglycemia. Also, when NPH is taken with mealtime insulin before dinner, the patient is at risk for nocturnal hypoglycemia from the peak effect of the evening dose of NPH. The advantage of using a rapid-acting insulin (e.g., insulin lispro, insulin aspart, or insulin glulisine) instead of regular insulin in this regimen is to facilitate the patient being able to take their insulin doses immediately before

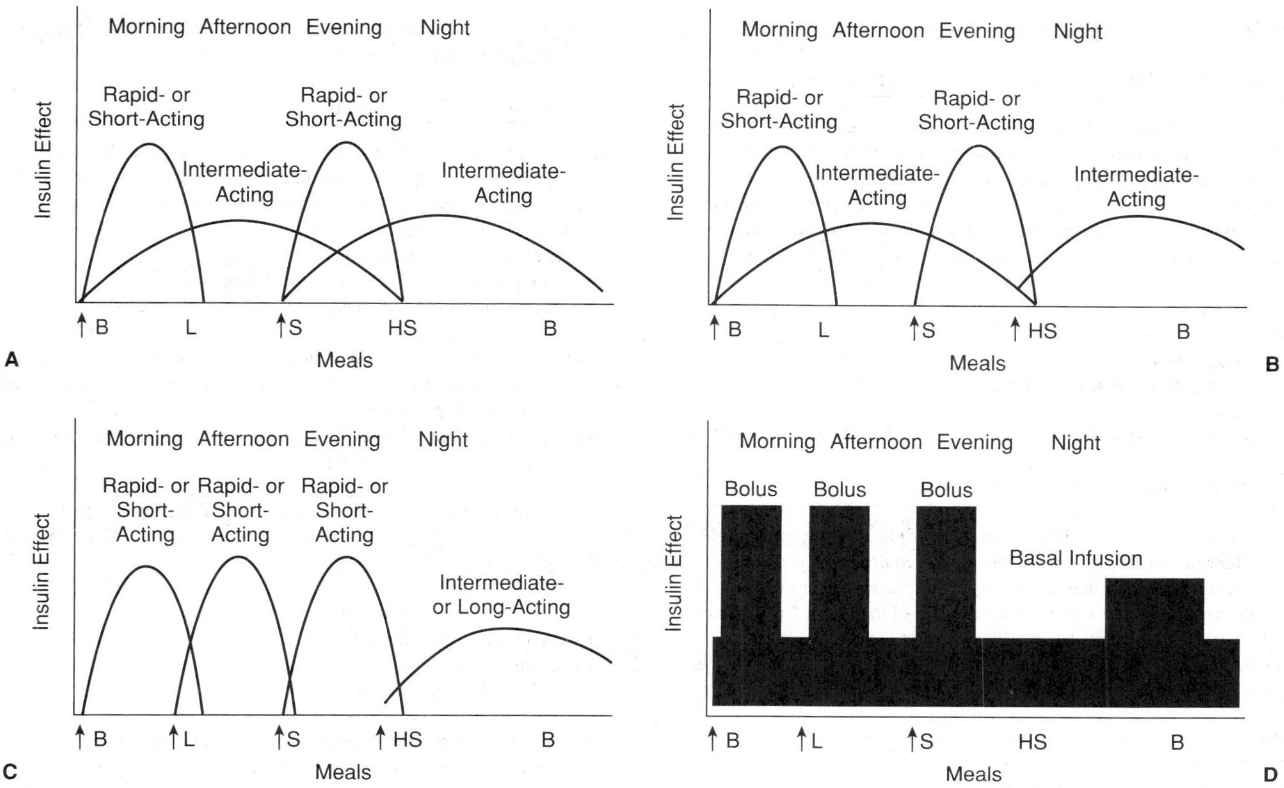

FIGURE 50-4 Theoretical insulin effect provided by various insulin regimens. A: Two daily injections of rapid-acting (insulin aspart, glulisine, or lispro) or short-acting (regular) and intermediate-acting insulin (NPH). **B:** Morning injection of rapid or short-acting insulin and an intermediate-acting insulin, a presupper injection of rapid or short-acting insulin, and a bedtime injection of intermediate-acting insulin. Suggested for patients with early morning hypoglycemia followed by rebound hyperglycemia or for patients with early morning hyperglycemia (rebound phenomenon). **C:** Preprandial injections of rapid or short-acting insulin and long-acting (e.g., insulin glargine or detemir) or intermediate-acting insulin (NPH) at bedtime. **D:** Continuous subcutaneous insulin infusion. B, breakfast; HS, bedtime snack; L, lunch; S, supper. *Arrows,* time of insulin injection (<15 minutes before meals for rapid-acting insulin and ~30 minutes before meals for short-acting insulin). (Adapted from reference 342.)

a meal. However, the peak effect of the NPH component in this combined dose still presents the same problems. Caveat: When patients are switched to a rapid-acting insulin from regular insulin in this type of regimen, the doses of NPH may have to be increased to minimize preprandial hyperglycemia. This type of insulin regimen does not mimic physiological insulin release.

Figure 50-4B depicts a variation of this method. It is the same except that the evening dose of NPH is given as a third injection at bedtime. This shifts the time of peak effect from approximately 2 to 3 AM to approximately 7 AM. By administering NPH at bedtime, nocturnal hypoglycemia is reduced and peak insulin activity occurs when the patient is more likely to be awake and ingesting food. This method may be useful for patients in whom nocturnal hypoglycemia and fasting hyperglycemia are particularly troublesome; however, this regimen also does not mimic physiological insulin release.

The regimen that most closely mimics physiological insulin release besides the use of an insulin pump, is the use of a once-daily basal insulin such as insulin glargine or insulin detemir to provide basal insulin levels throughout the day, along with doses of regular, insulin lispro, insulin aspart or insulin glulisine before meals (Fig. 50-4C depicts the long-acting insulin given at bedtime, but it can be given alternatively in the morning). When smaller doses are used, twice-daily insulin detemir and possibly insulin glargine will be required for 24-hour coverage.[93–95] This method theoretically provides insulin similar to the insulin pump works: constant basal levels plus small boluses for meals and snacks. In doing so, it offers some of the same advantages of the pump in that it permits some degree of flexibility in the patient's lifestyle. For example, if a patient with diabetes chooses to skip a meal, he or she omits a premeal bolus; if the patient chooses to eat a larger meal than usual, he or she increases the premeal bolus. Similar dose adjustments can be made to accommodate snacks, exercise patterns, and acute illnesses. Caveat: Insulin glargine and insulin detemir must be injected separately; that is, they may not be mixed in same syringe with other insulins.

7. Should A.H. use an insulin pump or multiple insulin injections?

Indications for basal-bolus insulin therapy are listed in Table 50-12. Patients with type 1 diabetes should be placed on a basal-bolus insulin regimen. A.H. is an ideal candidate to strive for an HbA_{1c} <6%. She is newly diagnosed, has not yet

Table 50-11 Empiric Insulin Doses

Estimating Total Daily Insulin Requirements

These are initial doses only; they must be refined using SMBG results. Patients may be particularly resistant to insulin if their blood glucose concentrations are high (glucose toxicity); once glucose concentrations begin to drop, insulin requirements often decrease precipitously. The weight used is actual body weight. Insulin dose requirements can change dramatically over time depending on circumstances (e.g., a growth spurt, modest weight gain or loss, illness).

Type 1 diabetes	
Initial dose	0. 3–0.5 unit/kg
Honeymoon phase	0. 2–0.5 unit/kg
With ketosis, during illness, during growth	1. 0–1.5 units/kg
Type 2 diabetes	
With insulin resistance	0. 7–1.5 units/kg

Estimating Basal Insulin Requirements

These are empiric doses only and should be adjusted using appropriate SMBG results (fasting or premeal). Basal requirements vary throughout the day, often increasing during the early morning hours. Basal requirements are approximately 50% of total daily insulin needs. The basal requirement also is influenced by the presence of endogenous insulin, the degree of insulin resistance, and body weight. The basal insulin dose is approximately 50% of total daily dose.

Estimating Premeal Insulin Requirements

The "500 rule" estimates the number of grams of carbohydrate that will be covered by 1 unit of rapid-acting insulin. The rule is modified to the "450 rule" if using regular insulin.

500/total daily dose of insulin (TDD) = number of grams covered

Example: For a patient using 50 U/day, 500/50 = 10. Therefore, 10 g carbohydrate would be covered by 1 unit of insulin lispro, glulisine, or aspart. This equation works very well for type 1 patients in estimating their premeal insulin requirements. Because patients with type 2 diabetes have insulin resistance, the rule may underestimate their insulin requirements.

Determining the "Correction Factor"

Supplemental doses of rapid-acting insulin are administered to acutely lower glucose concentrations that exceed the target glucose concentration. These doses must be individualized for each patient and again are based on the degree of sensitivity to insulin action. For example, if the premeal or bedtime blood glucose target is 140 mg/dL and the patient's value is 190 mg/dL, additional units of insulin might be added to the premeal dose or an additional supplemental bedtime dose of rapid-acting insulin might be given. The correction factor determines how far the blood glucose drops per unit of insulin given and is known as the "1700 rule." For regular insulin, the rule is modified to the "1500 rule." The equation is as follows:

1700/TDD = point drop in blood glucose per unit of insulin

Example: If a patient uses 28 U/day of insulin, their correction factor (or insulin sensitivity) would be 1700/28 = 60 mg/dL. Therefore, the patient can expect a 60 mg/dL drop for every unit of rapid acting insulin administered. Patients with a higher sensitivity factor have lower insulin requirements. Individuals with a lower sensitivity factor (higher insulin requirements) typically achieve a smaller reduction in blood glucose per unit of insulin.

SMBG, self-monitored blood glucose; TDD, total daily dose.
Adapted from references 88, 92, and 102.

Table 50-12 Basal-Bolus (Physiological) Insulin Therapy: Indications and Precautions

Patient Selection Criteria

Type 1, otherwise healthy patients (>7 years of age) who are highly motivated and compliant individuals. Must be willing to test blood glucose concentrations multiple times daily and inject 4 doses of insulin daily, on average
Women with diabetes who plan to conceive
Pregnant patients with diabetes (pre-existing)
Patients poorly controlled on conventional therapy (includes type 2 patients)
Technical ability to test blood glucose concentrations
Intellectual ability to interpret blood glucose concentrations and adjust insulin doses appropriately
Access to trained and skilled medical staff to direct treatment program and provide close supervision

Avoid or Use Cautiously in Patients Who Are Predisposed to Severe Hypoglycemic Reactions or in Whom Such Reactions Could be Fatal

Patients with counter-regulatory insufficiency
β-Adrenergic blocker therapy
Autonomic insufficiency
Adrenal or pituitary insufficiency
Patients with coronary or cerebral vascular disease
(*Note*: Counter-regulatory hormones released in response to hypoglycemia may have adverse effects in these individuals)
Unreliable, noncompliant individuals, including those who abuse alcohol or drugs and those with psychiatric disorders

developed the long-term complications of diabetes, and should derive the benefits of normoglycemia. Assuming A.H. will be able to comply with basal-bolus insulin therapy, individualized target blood glucose levels that strive for the best level of glucose control possible without placing her at undue risk for hypoglycemia should be prescribed. She must be willing to test her blood glucose concentrations four or more times daily and inject herself four times daily or learn about the use and care of an insulin pump. She also must be willing to keep detailed blood glucose and food records and participate in an extensive education program that enables her to adjust her insulin doses based on blood glucose concentrations, physical activity, and the carbohydrate content of her snacks and meals.

Transition to an insulin pump is facilitated by patients being able to attain these skills using multiple daily SC insulin injections before insulin pump initiation. The ADA recommends that the use of insulin pumps be limited to highly motivated individuals under the guidance of a health care team trained and knowledgeable in their use. Pumps offer the patient the ability to use multiple basal rates over the 24-hour period and assist with the calculation of bolus and correction insulin doses. Most studies have shown that pump therapy provides equivalent and sometimes better glycemic control than does intensive management with multiple injections.[89,96]

Insulin pumps are particularly useful in patients with frequent, unpredictable hypoglycemia or marked dawn phenomena (see Question 20). Others have described the methods by which insulin doses are established and altered in patients using the insulin pump.[88,91] Because A.H. has just been diagnosed, she should be initiated on a basal-bolus SC insulin therapy. Once she has acquired these skills, she may be considered for pump therapy.

Clinical Use of Insulin

Initiating Insulin Therapy

8. How should multiple-dose insulin therapy be initiated in A.H.?

A conservative total daily dose of insulin is estimated empirically or according to guidelines similar to those listed in Table 50-12 in newly diagnosed patients. For a basal-bolus insulin regimen, insulin glargine (Lantus) or insulin detemir (Levemir) is used as the basal insulin with bolus doses of a rapid- or short-acting insulin (insulin lispro, insulin aspart, insulin glulisine or regular) given at meal time. However, the cost of insulin glargine and insulin detemir, their availability on formularies, and their incompatibility with other insulins in the same syringe may force some clinicians and patients to use NPH insulin.

During the initial visit, A.H. needs to learn how to inject her insulin (see question 10), how to test her blood glucose (Table 50-13), how and when to test her urine for ketones, and how to recognize and treat hypoglycemia (Table 50-14). She also needs to understand the importance of meal planning and the relationship between carbohydrate intake and insulin action (Table 50-15). It is very important not to overwhelm A.H. with information on the first visit. One should be particularly sensitive to the psychological impact of this diagnosis on A.H., address her major concerns, and provide only the information that is absolutely essential before the next visit. Between visits, she should be assessed and provided information on an as-needed basis by phone. Table 50-16 lists important areas of patient education.

A reasonable first approach for A.H. is to provide a total daily dose of insulin of 24 units (~0.5 unit/kg). Because 50% of the daily dose should be given as basal insulin with the remainder given as rapid-acting insulin divided into three doses, A.H. would take the following: 12 units of insulin glargine (Lantus) once daily (morning or bedtime) with 4 units of insulin aspart (Novolog) given with each meal. An alternative regimen using NPH would be 8 units of NPH in the morning with 8 units of Novolog, 4 units of Novolog with dinner, and

Table 50-13 Self-Monitored Blood Glucose Testing: Areas of Patient Education

When and how often to test

Technique

How and when to calibrate the glucose monitor.

Review all "buttons" and their purposes. Identify battery case. Review cleaning procedures, if applicable.

Preparation

1. Calibrate monitor/set code for batch of test strips, if required.
2. Insert test strip to turn machine on (some meters require user to turn machine on).
3. Prepare all materials: tissue, strip, lancet.
4. Remember to close the lid of the strip container immediately. Strips exposed to air and moisture deteriorate rapidly.
5. Wash hands with warm water. *Dry thoroughly.* A wet finger causes blood to spread rather than form a drop. Milk the finger from the base to ensure an adequate flow of blood.
6. Lance the tip of the finger. Avoid the pads of the finger where nerve endings are concentrated.
7. Hold the finger *below* the heart with the lanced area pointing toward the floor.
8. Once a sufficient amount of blood is available, *quickly* apply blood to designated area of the test strip. Depending on the strip type, the blood sample is placed in an area on the surface of the strip or it is applied to the side of the strip where it is taken up by capillary action.

Record results in a log book and bring to all clinician visits. Include relevant information regarding diet or exercise.

How to use results to achieve normoglycemia

Table 50-14 Hypoglycemia

Definition

Blood glucose concentration <60 mg/dL: Patient may or may not be symptomatic. Blood glucose <40 mg/dL: Patient is generally symptomatic. Blood glucose <20 mg/dL can be associated with seizures and coma.

Signs and Symptoms

Blurred vision, sweaty palms, generalized sweating, tremulousness, hunger, confusion, anxiety, circumoral tingling, and numbness. Patients vary with regard to their symptoms. Behavior can be confused with inebriation. Patients become combative and use poor judgment.

Nocturnal hypoglycemia: nightmares, restless sleep, profuse sweating, morning headache, morning "hangover." In one study, 80% of patients with nocturnal hypoglycemia had no symptoms.

Clinical Considerations

Irregular eating patterns
↑ Physical exercise
Gastroparesis (delayed gastric emptying)
Defective counter-regulatory responses
Excessive dose of sulfonylurea
Alcohol ingestion
Drugs

Treatment

Ingest 10–20 g rapidly absorbed carbohydrate. Repeat in 15–20 min if glucose concentration remains <60 mg/dL or if patient is symptomatic. Follow with complex carbohydrate/protein snack if meal time is not imminent.

The following are examples of food sources that provide 15 g of carbohydrate:

Orange, grapefruit, or apple juice; regular, nondiet soda	1/2 cup
Fat-free milk	1 cup
Grape juice, cranberry juice cocktail	1/3 cup
Sugar	1 T or 3 cubes
Lifesavers	5–6 pieces
Glucose tablets	3–4 tablets

If patient is unconscious the following measures should be initiated:

Glucagon 1 mg SC, IM, or IV (mean response time, 6.5 min)
Glucose 25 g IV (dextrose 50%, 50 mL; mean response time, 4 min)

IM, intramuscular; IV, intravenous; SC, subcutaneous.

Table 50-15 Interpreting Self-Monitored Blood Glucose Concentrations[a]

Test Time	Target Insulin Dose	Target Meal/Snack
Prebreakfast (fasting)	Predinner/bedtime intermediate- or basal insulin	Bedtime snack
Prelunch	Prebreakfast regular or rapid-acting insulin	Breakfast/midmorning snack
Predinner	Prebreakfast intermediate-acting insulin and/or prelunch regular or rapid-acting insulin	Lunch/midafternoon snack
Bedtime	Predinner regular or rapid-acting insulin	Dinner
2-hour postprandial	Premeal regular or rapid-acting insulin	Preceding meal or snack
3 AM or later	Predinner intermediate-acting insulin or basal insulin if given in am	Dinner/bedtime snack

[a] Considerations: (a) Assumes a normal meal pattern. For patients who travel, have odd working or sleeping hours, or irregular meal patterns, these rules may not apply. (b) Assumes administration of regular insulin 30–60 min before meals or rapid-acting insulin 0–15 min before meals and a normal pattern of insulin response (see for factors that can alter insulin absorption and response). (c) If prebreakfast concentrations are high, rule out reactive hyperglycemia (Somogyi reaction or posthypoglycemic hyperglycemia). Consider contribution of dawn phenomenon as well. Whenever blood glucose concentrations are high, consider reactive hyperglycemia (excessive insulin doses). (d) Consider accuracy of reported test results: (i) Do they correlate with HbA_{1c} and patient's signs and symptoms? (ii) What is the patient's compliance? Could results be fabricated? (iii) Is patient's technique appropriate? Check timing, adequate blood sample, machine, strips, and calibration (Table 50-13). (iv) Are insulin kinetics altered? (v) Meals: Consider content, quality, and regularity.

4 units of NPH at bedtime. Caveat: As A.H.'s glucose concentration returns to normal, glucose toxicity will recede and she may require less insulin.

Selecting an Insulin Syringe

9. What kind of insulin syringe should be prescribed for A.H.?

Delivery of insulin with a syringe is still the most common method of insulin administration in the United States. Insulin syringes are plastic, disposable syringes with needles that are very fine (28–31 gauge), sharp, and well lubricated to ease insertion. Needles and syringes have been improved so that insulin injections are relatively painless if proper technique is used. Less pain is associated with the smaller, 30- or 31-gauge needles. The "dead space" (air space at the hub of the needle) has been virtually eliminated so that mixing and measuring problems previously associated with its presence are no longer a concern. The lengths of needles are 5/16 inch, 3/8 inch, or 1/2 inch. The shortest needle can be used for children or patients with little SC fat.[90] A longer needle length (1/2 inch) may be required in patients with excess abdominal fat; use of a short needle (e.g., 3/16 inch) may result in insulin leakage.

Manufacturers produce 1-, 0.5-, and 0.3-mL syringes for U-100 insulin. For patients such as A.H., using fewer than <30 units of insulin per injection, the 0.3-mL syringe is preferred for ease of reading the dose markings on the syringe. This allows the patient to measure insulin more easily. Insulin syringes are available in 1-U increments or 0.5-U increments (BD Ultra-Fine Short Needle Syringe and Precision Sure Dose, 3/10 mL only).[90] One-half-unit increments are useful for pediatric patients and for patients who are carbohydrate counting, because meal time insulin doses can be rounded to the 0.5 unit.

A 0.3-mL U-100 insulin syringe with a 5/16 inch (8 mm), 30- or 31-gauge needle should be prescribed for A.H. Needle length can be adjusted depending on patient comfort. Cost and patient preference will govern the brand selected. Subjectively, patients can "feel" the difference between different brands, or they may prefer the "ease of bubble removal," physical characteristics, or packaging of one syringe over another.

Insulin pen and dosing devices (e.g., Innolet) are also available for injecting insulin. Pen devices are gaining in popularity because they make insulin administration much easier, especially for patients who need to take their insulin doses away from home. They also can increase dosing accuracy. These devices are useful in patients with visual or dexterity problems in whom use of a vial and syringe method is difficult. Pens eliminate the need to withdraw insulin, and the insulin dose is dialed up on the device. Pen devices are available to dose insulin in 2-U, 1-U (most), and 0.5-U increments (NovoPen Junior and HumaPen Luxura HD). Pen needles are available in 29, 30, and 31 gauge and 3/16 inch (5 mm), 1/4 inch (6 mm) 5/16 inch (8 mm), or 1/2 inch (12.7 mm) lengths.[90,97]

Table 50-16 Areas of Patient Education

Diabetes: Pathogenesis and the complications
Hyperglycemia: Signs and symptoms
Ketoacidosis: Signs and symptoms (Table 50-23)
Hypoglycemia: Signs, symptoms, and appropriate treatment (Table 50-14)
Exercise: Effect on blood glucose concentrations and insulin dose (Table 50-21)
Diet: See text. Emphasis placed on carbohydrate counting because the carbohydrate is responsible for 90% of the rise in blood glucose after a meal.
Insulins:
- Injection technique
- Types of insulin
- Onset and peak actions
- Storage
- Stability (look for crystallization and precipitation with NPH insulin)

Therapeutic goals: HbA_{1c}, fasting, preprandial and postprandial blood glucose levels, cholesterol, triglycerides, blood pressure
SMBG testing: Table 50-15
Interpretation of SMBG testing results
Foot care: Inspect feet daily; wear well-fitted shoes; avoid self-care of ingrown toenails, corns, or athlete's foot; see a podiatrist
Sick day management: Table 50-22
Cardiovascular risk factors: Tobacco use, high blood pressure, obesity, elevated cholesterol
Importance of annual ophthalmologic examinations; tests for microalbuminuria; keeping up-to-date with immunizations

Measuring and Injecting Insulin

10. How should A.H. be instructed to administer her insulin injections?

INJECTION

A.H. should prepare an area for injection. Alcohol swabs may be used to clean the rubber stopper of the insulin vial (or pen device). To inject the insulin subcutaneously, A.H. should be instructed to firmly pinch up the area to be injected (this creates a firm surface for the injection) and to quickly insert the needle perpendicularly (90-degree angle) into the center of this area. The syringe should be held toward the middle or back of the barrel, like a pencil. Anxious patients have a tendency to "choke" the hub of the syringe, and this prevents proper needle insertion. A 45-degree angle of injection may be used for infants and very thin individuals who have little SC fat, especially in the thigh area. The skin pinch should be released and the insulin injected.[97] Gentle pressure should be applied at the site of injection for 5 to 8 seconds to prevent back leakage of the insulin as the needle is removed. The site should not be massaged, because this may accelerate the absorption and onset of action of insulin (Table 50-10). When using an insulin pen or other delivery, the needle should be embedded within the skin for about 5 to 10 seconds after depressing the dosing knob to ensure full delivery of the insulin dose.

Patients who are anxious about self-injection can be helped by applying an ice cube to the site before injection or by using an injection aid. However, injection aids are generally unnecessary once the patient realizes that injections are relatively pain free with proper technique.

ROTATING INJECTION SITES

The primary sites used for injecting insulin are the lateral thigh, abdomen (avoid 2-inch radius around the navel) and upper arm. Previously, patients were advised to rotate injection sites between the arms, thighs, abdomen, and buttocks (Fig. 50-5). The ADA recommends that insulin injections be rotated within the same anatomic region to decrease chances of variability in insulin absorption.[97] Many practitioners recommend insulin injections into the abdominal area because absorption from this site is least affected by exercise and the most predictable. Alternatively, A.H. can be instructed to rotate her morning injection within one region (e.g., the abdomen) and her evening injection in another anatomic region. This minimizes the variables that can alter her response to insulin.

Rotating injection sites also was recommended at one time to avoid the lipodystrophic effect of insulin (lipohypertrophy and lipoatrophy); however, because insulin has been purified, these complications are less common and the importance of rotation is less critical. Nevertheless, repetitive use of the same site of injection may still result in lipohypertrophy and it does toughen the skin, making needle penetration more difficult. Furthermore, insulin absorption from lipohypertrophic sites can be slowed.[97]

AGITATION

A.H. does not need to agitate Lantus or Novolog because these are clear insulins. For NPH insulin, which is a suspension, the vial and must be agitated before insulin is withdrawn. A new, unused vial of NPH insulin may require vigorous agitation to loosen the sediment, which may have become packed down with storage. The vial should be rolled between the palms of the hands to minimize foaming. Agitation is only required for insulin suspensions (e.g., insulin 70/30 or other insulin mixtures).

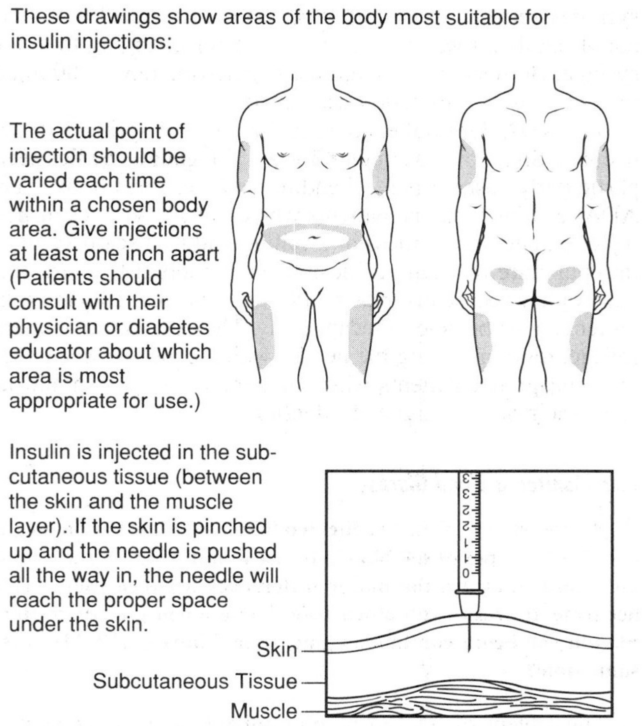
These drawings show areas of the body most suitable for insulin injections:
The actual point of injection should be varied each time within a chosen body area. Give injections at least one inch apart (Patients should consult with their physician or diabetes educator about which area is most appropriate for use.)
Insulin is injected in the subcutaneous tissue (between the skin and the muscle layer). If the skin is pinched up and the needle is pushed all the way in, the needle will reach the proper space under the skin.
Skin
Subcutaneous Tissue
Muscle

FIGURE 50-5 Selecting insulin injection sites. (Used with permission from reference 343.)

MEASUREMENT

First, A.H. should make sure her hands and the injection site are clean (it is not necessary to use alcohol to clean the site). She should withdraw the plunger to the level of insulin she intends to inject (e.g., 12 units for her Lantus dose); then she should insert the needle into the vial and inject the air to prevent creation of a vacuum within the vial. The vial then should be inverted with the syringe inserted, and 12 units of insulin glargine should be withdrawn. The bevel of the needle should be well below the surface of the insulin to avoid withdrawing air or bubbles into the syringe. Lantus must not be mixed in the same syringe with her insulin aspart, and it should be injected into a different site if it is injected at the same time as her Novolog dose.

The barrel of the syringe should be held at eye level to check for air bubbles and to allow accurate placement of the plunger tip at the 12-U mark. If bubbles are present, they should be removed by tapping the syringe gently to coax the bubbles to the top of the barrel, where they can be injected back into the insulin vial. To remove air bubbles in an insulin pen, prime the needle with 2 units of insulin before each use (repeat until insulin drop appears at tip of pen needle). Also, remove the needle from the pen device in between uses to prevent air bubbles from accumulating.

REUSING INSULIN SYRINGES AND NEEDLES

Those who work with patients with diabetes know that they are extremely resourceful in cutting their health care costs. A frequently encountered practice is the reuse of disposable syringes. In a survey of 254 adult insulin users, 45% reused their syringes for an average of 4 days, 16% refrigerated their syringes between uses, and 35% wiped their needles with alcohol. Dullness was the major reason for changing to a new syringe. Borders et al.[98] examined approximately 2,800 injection sites, and no infection was noted.

The ADA does not encourage the reuse of syringes or pen needles. Some of the smaller 30- and 31-gauge needles seem particularly susceptible to bending and can form hooks. The ADA recommends that patients who do reuse syringes inspect injection sites for redness or swelling and to discard syringes into puncture-resistant, disposable containers if they are dull, bent, or have come in contact with surfaces other than the skin. Patients must be able to recap safely. They do not recommend refrigeration or wiping the needle with alcohol between uses, only recapping. Patients who reuse their syringes should inspect their skin for signs of infection.[97]

Self-Monitored Blood Glucose

11. How should A.H. be educated to self-monitor her blood glucose? What types of self blood glucose monitoring tests are available, and what are the major differences between them? How accurate are results obtained from home blood glucose testing? Should she begin continuous glucose monitoring (CGM) at the same time?

The advent of SMBG revolutionized the management of diabetes mellitus by providing a simple and portable method for periodic and repeated measurement of blood glucose in the ambulatory care setting. The ADA recommends that most individuals with diabetes should attempt to attain and achieve normoglycemia as safely as possible. For patients with type 1 diabetes, this can be achieved by using SMBG; therefore, all treatment programs should include the routine use of daily glucose monitoring. SMBG is also important in (a) pregnancy complicated by diabetes, (b) patients with unstable diabetes, (c) patients with a propensity to severe ketosis or hypoglycemia, (d) patients prone to hypoglycemia who may not experience the usual warning symptoms, and (e) patients on insulin pumps. SMBG has been widely accepted by both patients and clinicians. Because blood glucose testing materials constitute a multimillion dollar business, the market has been flooded with a multitude of monitors, and the technology in this area is changing rapidly. New monitors with advanced features are introduced yearly.[90]

All monitors use test strips and are self-timing, requiring no patient action after the blood is placed on the strip. Several factors should be taken into account when evaluating a monitor and its appropriateness for an individual. The primary considerations are ease of use, accuracy relative to a reference standard, reliability, insurance coverage, and cost.[90,99] Convenience factors include coding requirements (some new monitors do not require coding for test strips), meter size, volume of blood required for testing, site to obtain sample (e.g., finger versus alternate site such as forearm), capacity of the meter to store blood glucose values (memory) and data management, required testing time, size of readout, general availability of strips, ability to turn off audible signals, and availability of technical support. Some devices are less reliable for use in anemic patients (e.g., renal transplant patients), and all function most reliably within certain temperature ranges (usually 60–95°F) and humidity (generally <90%) conditions. Strips are sensitive to light, moisture, and temperature extremes and must be stored and handled with care.

Periodically, patients should compare the results they get on their monitor with the laboratory blood glucose test for accuracy. The majority of monitors are calibrated to plasma levels (i.e., plasma referenced). Only a few monitors report whole blood glucose; in these monitors, capillary values measured are likely to be 10% to 15% lower than values measured by the laboratory.

Patient education regarding coding procedures, testing procedures, the importance of recording results, and test times are critical. Ultimately, A.H. should be taught how to use blood glucose values to adjust her insulin dose, dietary intake, and exercise pattern (Table 50-17).

Used properly, available monitors provide accurate, precise results that can be used by patients to manage their diabetes. However, several factors can affect the accuracy of monitor results—most commonly, equipment malfunction and human error. Problems with a monitor can be detected by performing a quality-control test once weekly and with each new vial of strips; human error can be minimized with adequate training. If at any time patients think their monitor is not working properly, they can call the 1-800 support service number on the back of the monitor for immediate assistance. Table 50-18 lists factors that can affect results of SMBG test results. Anytime SMBG values are inconsistent with the patient's symptoms or HbA_{1c} values, sources of error should be evaluated. A.H.'s technique should be reviewed periodically, because clinical decisions are based on the patient's blood glucose testing record.

Because A.H. is just starting insulin therapy and SMBG, it would be reasonable to hold off on considering CGM until she becomes comfortable with these skills. Then, she and her practitioner could assess whether CGM would be useful.

Testing Frequency

12. How often should A.H. test her blood glucose concentrations?

Although the exact frequency and timing of blood glucose tests should be dictated by individualized patient goals, most patients with type 1 diabetes using basal-bolus insulin regimens should perform SMBG at least three times daily or more according to the ADA.[22] Glucose monitoring should also be performed more frequently whenever therapy is modified. Because A.H. is being initiated on insulin therapy with the goal of normoglycemia, she should self-monitor her blood glucose a minimum of three times per day. Most practitioners recommend at least premeal and bedtime blood glucose testing (at least four times daily).

The objective of ongoing, frequent blood glucose testing is to determine whether normoglycemia is being achieved and to assess the action of specific insulin doses as well as the impact of meals, food, illness, or exercise on blood glucose levels. Ideally, patients should test their blood glucose concentration before meals, 90 to 120 minutes after meals to assess postprandial glycemic control and to determine their "insulin to carbohydrate ratio," at bedtime, and occasionally, at 2 or 3 AM (i.e., eight times daily). However, most patients are unable to adhere to such a rigorous regimen. At the minimum, to determine her daily insulin requirements, A.H. should test her blood glucose concentrations four times daily: before each

Table 50-17 Guidelines for Dosing Insulin

Basic Insulin Dose

First, adjust the basic insulin dose (i.e., the dose that the patient will be instructed to take daily). This assumes that diet and physical activity are stable. Set a reasonable goal initially. This may mean the upper limits of the acceptable concentrations may be high initially (e.g., <200 mg/dL). Move toward a more ideal goal slowly.

Only adjust insulin doses if a *pattern* of response is observed under stable diet and exercise circumstances. That is, the same response to insulin is observed for ≥3 days. It is important to verify the stability of diet and exercise. Consider adjusting these variables as well.

Unless all levels are >200 mg/dL, try to adjust one component of insulin therapy at a time.

Start with the insulin component affecting the fasting blood glucose concentration. This glucose level often is the most difficult to control and often affects all other glucose concentrations measured throughout the day.

Adjust the basic insulin dose by 1–2 units at a time. The amount prescribed is based on the individual patient's response to insulin. This can be determined by looking at the patient's total daily dose using the "500 rule" (see the following, and Table 50-11).

Supplementary Insulin Doses

Once the basic dose of insulin has been established, supplemental doses of rapid- or short-acting insulin can be prescribed to correct *preprandial* hyperglycemia. For example, if the goal is 140 mg/dL, and the glucose value is 190 mg/dL, administer one additional unit. Supplemental doses also can be used when the patient is ill (Table 50-22).

Algorithms for correction doses are based on the patient's sensitivity to insulin using the "1500 or 1700 rule" (Table 50-11).

If premeal glucose concentrations are <60–70 mg/dL, the dose of lispro, aspart, glulisine, or regular insulin administered before the meal is ↓ by 1–2 U; insulin administration is delayed until just before the meal; the meal should include an extra 15 g of glucose if the value is <50 mg/dL.

If supplemental doses before a given meal are required for ≥3 days, the basic insulin dose should be adjusted appropriately. For example, if a patient taking lispro before meals requires an extra 2 units before lunch for ≥3 days, 2 units should be added to the prebreakfast dose.

Anticipatory Insulin Doses

The basic insulin dose is increased or decreased based on the anticipated effects of diet or physical activity.

Increase lispro/aspart/glulisine or regular insulin by 1 unit for each additional 15 g of carbohydrate ingested (e.g., holiday meal) or decrease the usual dose by 1–2 units if the meal is smaller than usual (Table 50-11).

See Table 50-21 for recommended insulin adjustments for exercise.

meal and at bedtime. She also should set her alarm for 3 AM two or three times per week and test her blood glucose. Blood glucose concentrations measured premeals allow patients and clinicians to determine if the rapid-acting insulin dose is appropriate for the amount of carbohydrate consumed; FPG levels are used to determine if the basal insulin dose is adequate; and the 2 to 3 AM blood glucose level is used to identify nocturnal hypoglycemia. For example, the blood glucose measured before dinner reflects the action of A.H.'s prelunch Novolog dose on food she has eaten for lunch, as well as hepatic glucose production between meals. Increasingly, patients who use

Table 50-18 Factors That Can Alter Self-Monitored Blood Glucose Test Results: Troubleshooting

Glucose monitor not coded for batch of test strips[a]
An inadequate amount of blood applied to test strip[b]
Dirty glucose monitor[a]
Low battery[a]
Test performed outside of temperature and humidity operating conditions[a]
Low[c] or high[b] hematocrit
Dehydration[b]
Hyperosmolar, nonketotic state[b]
Lipemia[a]
High levels of ascorbic acid or salicylates (rare)[b]

[a] Effect unpredictable.
[b] Values tend to be lower.
[c] Values tend to be higher.

carbohydrate counting with rapid-acting insulins are being advised to test 2-hour postprandial levels on initiating therapy to enhance proper dosage adjustment (Table 50-15).

The importance of frequent blood glucose testing cannot be overemphasized. When blood glucose is tested less frequently than four times daily, glucose control deteriorates to baseline levels. This is because complete profiles are no longer available, and it is impossible to adjust insulin doses based on random blood glucose concentrations.[100] If patients refuse to test four times daily, they should be encouraged to test four times daily on representative days of the week or to test at different times of the day each day so that a weekly profile can be developed. A.H. also should be encouraged to test her blood glucose concentration any time she is feeling unusual, if she is experiencing hypoglycemic symptoms, or to evaluate the effect of unusual circumstances on her blood glucose concentration (e.g., increased physical exercise, a large holiday meal, final examinations, a family crisis).

Using Blood Glucose Test Results to Evaluate Insulin Doses

13. A.H. was instructed to inject herself with 12 units of Lantus each morning and give 4 units of Novolog with each meal. She was asked to test her blood glucose four times daily (before meals and at bedtime), to record her results and other unusual events or symptoms during the day, and to bring her records to the clinic. A.H. was also instructed to keep a food diary and record the number of carbohydrates she ingested at each meal. The initial goal of therapy is to achieve preprandial blood glucose concentrations of <180 mg/dL and to eliminate symptoms of hyperglycemia. One week later, trends in her blood glucose concentrations were as follows.

Time	*Glucose Concentration (mg/dL)*	*mmol/L*
7 AM	160–200	8.8–11.1
Noon	220–260	2.2–14.4
5 PM	130–180	7.2–10.0
11 PM	140–180	7.8–10.0

Occasional 3 AM tests averaged 160 mg/dL and A.H.'s urine is negative for ketones. She eats approximately four carbohydrate servings for breakfast (60 g) and two to four carbohydrate servings for lunch and dinner (30–45 g). Subjectively, A.H. feels a bit better, and her weight has stabilized, but she still urinates two to three

times nightly. How would you interpret these results, and how should A.H.'s insulin doses be altered?

Health care providers should use the data obtained from self-monitoring to (a) set glycemic goals, (b) develop recommendations for pharmacologic therapy, (c) evaluate the effectiveness of pharmacologic therapy, (d) instruct patients to interpret and respond to blood glucose patterns, (f) evaluate the impact of dietary factors on glycemic control, (g) modify therapy during acute/intercurrent illness or whenever patients receive medications known to affect glycemic control, (h) modify the management plan in response to a change in activity levels, and (i) identify hypoglycemic unawareness.[59]

Before using A.H.'s blood glucose results to adjust her insulin dose, it is important to observe and reassess her testing technique. One also should determine whether there were any unusual circumstances in her life, diet changes, or exercise patterns over the past week that might have affected her response to insulin. Once these have been ruled out as confounding factors, one can begin making gross adjustments in A.H.'s insulin dose, realizing that fine-tuning will be impossible until a consistent diet and exercise pattern have been instituted.

Several principles must be kept in mind whenever blood glucose tests are used to adjust a patient's basic insulin dose (Table 50-19). Because many factors can alter a patient's response to insulin, it is important to use blood glucose concentration *trends* measured over a minimum of 3 days to adjust the basic insulin dose (i.e., the dose the patient will use every day). The only exception to this rule is the use of supplemental insulin doses to correct exceptionally high glucose concentrations after A.H. has acquired sophisticated insulin adjustment skills (see Questions 18 and 19). SMBG results should be evaluated in conjunction with other parameters such as HbA_{1c} and periodic laboratory blood glucose measurements.

The daily dose of Lantus is inadequately controlling A.H.'s fasting blood glucose and should be increased to by 2 to 4 U. Although published algorithms would recommend to increase her dose to 16 units each morning, a more conservative approach would be to increase it to 14 units (or bedtime, whichever she will be able to do consistently) and further titrate as needed.[101] She is achieving some response from her lunchtime dose of Novolog, but there is room for improvement in her meal insulin coverage overall. The blood glucose concentration of 160 mg/dL at 3 AM indicates that rebound hyperglycemia is an unlikely cause of her high fasting levels (see Questions 15 and 20). As an initial step toward control, A.H.'s daily dose of Lantus could be increased in an attempt to control her fasting hyperglycemia. However, this approach does not address A.H.'s elevated prelunch values. Her intake of carbohydrates also varies from meal to meal. Thus, a more appropriate method would be to calculate the insulin-to-carbohydrate ratio for A.H. and allow her to determine her premeal Novolog dose based on the amounts of carbohydrates she will ingest at each meals. A typical starting point for the insulin-to-carbohydrate ratio is 1 unit to every 15 g carbohydrate. To calculate her insulin-to-carbohydrate, the "500 rule" is used: Divide the number 500 by her total daily dose of insulin (14 units Lantus plus 12 units of Novolog for meal coverage = 26 units):

$$500/26 = 19 \text{ g of carbohydrate covered by 1 unit of insulin}$$

Because most single servings of carbohydrate contain 15 g, A.H. decides to start with a ratio of 1 unit for every 15 g or single serving of carbohydrates she consumes at each meal. If A.H. were using regular insulin for meal coverage, she could use the "450 rule": 450/total daily insulin dose = grams of carbohydrate covered by 1 unit of insulin.

To evaluate the accuracy of her insulin:carbohydrate ratio, A.H. will need to check her blood glucose values 2 hours after each meal (postprandial blood glucose checks) to assess the appropriateness of her meal insulin calculation. She agrees to test her blood glucose level eight times per day and return in 2 weeks.

Table 50-19 Factors That Can Alter Blood Glucose Control

Diet	Insufficient calories (e.g., alcoholism, eating disorders, anorexia, nausea, and vomiting) Overeating (e.g., during the holidays) Irregularly spaced, skipped or delayed meals Dietary content (e.g., fiber, carbohydrate content)
Physical Activity	See Table 50-21 and Question 29
Stress	Infection Surgery/trauma Psychological
Drugs	Certain medications can increase or decrease blood glucose levels. It is important to assess for potential effects on the blood glucose when starting new medications.
Hormonal Changes	Menstruation: Glucose concentrations may increase premenstrually and return to normal postmenses. Pregnancy Puberty: hyperglycemia probably related to high growth hormone levels
Gastroparesis	Delays gastric emptying time. Peak insulin action and meal-related glucose excursions may become mismatched.
Altered Insulin Pharmacokinetics	See Table 50-10
Insulin Injection Technique	Measuring Timing Technique
Inactive Insulin	Outdated insulin Improperly stored insulin (heat or cold) Crystallized insulin

14. A.H. is getting more comfortable with carbohydrate counting and adjusting her insulin doses accordingly. A review of her

food diary reveals that for the most part, she is able to determine the appropriate serving sizes for 15 g of carbohydrate. She admits to difficulty determining carbohydrate amounts when eating out. As a result, A.H. notices that her preprandial blood glucose concentrations exceed her goal of 80 to 120 mg/dL on occasion. Sometimes they are as high as 200 mg/dL. Evaluate A.H.'s blood glucose trends. How should occasional preprandial glucose concentrations that exceed the desired goal of 80 to 120 mg/dL be managed?

Once the basal insulin dose and insulin-to-carbohydrate insulin dose have been established, one can begin to teach A.H. how to use a correction factor to adjust her dose of insulin when preprandial blood glucose concentrations fall above or below the range of blood glucose concentrations that have been established as her goal of therapy (70–130 mg/dL per the ADA or roughly 80–120 mg/dL; Table 50-17).

A correction insulin dose is used to compensate for unusually high blood glucose concentrations (high sugar correction). To reemphasize, this assumes there are no unusual changes in the patient's overall diet or exercise patterns. Many clinicians favor rapid-acting insulin over regular insulin because its action is brief and patients do not have to worry about residual effects 3 to 4 hours after its injection. This is particularly valuable when correctional doses of insulin are needed at bedtime.

The patient's sensitivity to insulin, as reflected by his or her total daily dose on a unit per kilogram basis is a major determinant of any algorithm developed. Previously, it was advised that 1 to 2 units of supplemental insulin should be given for each 30 to 50 mg/dL elevation above the target level. However, this relationship was observed to apply only to a person of average size on average doses of insulin (i.e., the 70-kg patient on 50 U/day of insulin). A very small person on 10 U/day or a very obese individual with type 2 diabetes on 100 U/day has different responses to a given dose of insulin. An alternative method of estimating the drop in a person's blood glucose per unit of regular insulin is the "1500 rule."[88] The 1500 rule was developed by Paul Davidson, MD, in Atlanta, Georgia, during the 1990s. The derived value is referred to as the "sensitivity factor": The rule was modified to the "1800 rule" for use with rapid-acting insulin (insulin lispro, aspart, or glulisine). Because these insulins tend to drop the blood glucose level faster and farther, so 1500 turns out to be too aggressive. Others (e.g., Bruce Bode, John Walsh) have recommended other numerators such as 1600, 1700, 2000, and 2200.[102] For this case, the "1700 rule" will be used. The calculation for A.H. would be as follows:

$$1700/24 = 70 \text{ mg/dL}$$

Thus, 1 unit of regular insulin for A.H. will drop her blood glucose level by about 70 mg/dL. The 1500 rule and the 1700 rule have proved to be a valuable way to initiate an algorithm for supplemental insulin. People with a lower sensitivity factor (higher insulin requirements) typically achieve a smaller reduction in blood glucose per unit of insulin compared to those with a higher sensitivity factor (lower insulin requirement). Thus, an algorithm of 1 unit of regular insulin for every 70 mg/dL excursion above her goal of 120 mg/dL is a reasonable place to begin. If this dose of insulin is insufficient, one can increase the dose of insulin or decrease the blood glucose excursion required per unit of insulin dose. Correctional insulin doses also are used for sick day management (see Question 30). The following is an example of an algorithm for A.H.:

Glucose Concentrations (mg/dL)	*Insulin Aspart*
<80	1 unit less
80–120	Usual dose
120–190	1 unit extra
191–260	2 units extra
261–330[a]	3 units extra
331–400[a]	4 units extra

[a] Check urine ketones. If urine ketones are positive and blood glucose concentrations remain >300 mg/dL for ≥12 hours, call the physician for directions.

Evaluating Fasting Hyperglycemia

15. A.H. returns after 1 month. She is currently using 14 units of Lantus each morning, 1 unit of Novolog for each 15 g of carbohydrate ingested at meal time and a correction factor of 1 unit of Novolog for every 70 mg/dL above 120 mg/dL. Her SMBG results are as follows:

Time	*Glucose Concentration mg/dL*	*mmol/L*
7 AM	140–180	7.8–10.0
Noon	120–150	6.7–8.3
5 PM	90–130	5.0–7.2
11 PM	90–120	5.0–6.7
3 AM	60–90	3.3–5.0

Overall, A.H. feels her diabetes is in good control. Her energy level has returned to normal and her nocturia has diminished, but she occasionally gets up one or two times nightly to urinate. A.H. has also noticed that nightmares or "sweats" sometimes awaken her. When this occurs, she generally has something to eat because she is "famished." She is able to get back to sleep, but wakes up the next morning with a "splitting headache" and a "hungover" feeling. A.H.'s weight remains the same, and she has begun to develop some consistency in her dietary patterns with the help of a dietitian. She has been consistently correcting her prelunch and predinner insulin doses by adding or subtracting 2 units from her premeal insulin doses based on her carbohydrate counts. The HbA_{1c} from her last visit is 7.3%. Evaluate A.H.'s blood glucose values. What are possible causes of A.H.'s fasting hyperglycemia?

When evaluating morning hyperglycemia, several causes must be considered:

- An insufficient basal dose of insulin. If the basal dose is insufficient, hepatic glucose output during the fasting state will be excessive, thereby producing hyperglycemia.
- Reactive hyperglycemia in response to a nocturnal hypoglycemic episode (Somogyi effect or rebound hyperglycemia).
- An excessive bedtime snack.
- The dawn phenomenon (see Question 20).
- Somogyi effect or rebound hyperglycemia

The presence of normoglycemia at bedtime, low blood glucose concentrations at 3 AM, and symptoms of nocturnal hypoglycemia (nightmares, sweating, hunger, morning headache) in A.H. are consistent with a rebound hyperglycemic reaction in the morning (i.e., posthypoglycemic hyperglycemia; Somogyi effect).[103] Theoretically, this effect occurs after any episode of severe hypoglycemia and is secondary to an excessive increase in glucose production by the liver that is activated by insulin counter-regulatory hormones such as cortisol, glucagon, epinephrine, and growth hormone. The waning effects of the basal insulin dose can also be a cause of fasting hyperglycemia because insulin is needed to suppress hepatic glucose output during the fasting state; however, this is not likely in A.H.'s.[93] Asymptomatic nocturnal hypoglycemia can occur in 33% of patients taking evening doses of insulin and may account for morning hyperglycemia in more than 10% of patients. Another potential consequence of nocturnal hypoglycemia is prolonged insulin resistance (perhaps a consequence of glucose toxicity), as signified by high postbreakfast glucose concentrations. By correcting the nocturnal hypoglycemia, normalization of A.H.'s fasting hyperglycemia also may be achieved. Thus, a decrease in the daily dose of Lantus by 2 units is warranted. A.H. should continue to monitor her blood glucose concentrations at 3 AM.

Caveat: If A.H. were using NPH BID to supply her basal insulin, one option would be to shift the evening injection of NPH from predinner to bedtime. This preferred method effectively shifts the peak action of NPH to the early morning, when she is awake, and decreases the risk of nocturnal hypoglycemia.[92,104] This peak action also corresponds to the dawn phenomenon (see Question 20) and the breakfast meal.

Another option if a patient is using NPH and experiencing nocturnal hypoglycemia is to change from NPH to either insulin glargine (Lantus) or insulin detemir (Levemir) because these insulins are associated with less nocturnal hypoglycemia.[105,106] In this case, the daily dose of NPH should be decreased by 20% to determine the Lantus dose. When switching from NPH to Levemir, a one-to-one dose conversion may be used, although higher doses of Levemir may be required. In one cross-over study of type 1 diabetes patients, the average Levemir basal dose was approximately double that of the NPH basal dose.[107]

Mixing Insulins

16. If A.H. were to use NPH as basal insulin, how should she be instructed to measure and withdraw this insulin mixture?

The procedure used to mix and withdraw NPH and mealtime insulin (regular or rapid-acting insulin) is basically the same as that described in Question 8. The major difference is that an adequate volume of air must be injected into the NPH vial before the regular or insulin aspart is measured and withdrawn. Also, the mealtime clear insulin is measured and withdrawn into the insulin syringe *first* to avoid contamination of the vial of regular, aspart, lispro, or glulisine insulin with NPH. For example, contamination with NPH ultimately alters the NPH:regular insulin ratio that is administered. When patients withdraw NPH insulin first, the vial of regular insulin eventually becomes cloudy. In contrast, contamination of the NPH insulin with regular insulin probably is insignificant because the protamine contained in NPH can bind the regular insulin (see Question 17). The procedure A.H. should use to mix her insulins is described in the following section, using her morning dose as an example.

- After dispersing the NPH insulin suspension, inject 14 units of air into the NPH vial and withdraw the needle.
- Inject 7 units of air into the insulin aspart or regular insulin vial, and withdraw the 7 units of insulin as described in Question 10.

Table 50-20 Compatibility of Insulin Mixtures

Mixture	*Proportion*	*Comments*
Regular + NPH	Any proportion	The pharmacodynamic profiles of regular and NPH insulin are unchanged when premixed and stored in vials or syringes for up to 3 months.
Regular + normal saline	Any proportion	Use within 2–3 hours of preparation.
Regular + insulin diluting solution	Any proportion	Stable indefinitely.
Rapid-acting + NPH	Any proportion	The absorption rate and peak action of the rapid-acting insulins are blunted; total bioavailability is unaltered. Rapid-acting insulin and NPH should be mixed just before use (within 15 minutes).
Insulin glargine and detemir	Do not mix with other insulins	Pharmacodynamics could be modified.

- Insert the needle into the NPH vial, and pull the plunger down to the 21-U mark (14 units of NPH plus 7 units of mealtime insulin).

Stability of Mixed Insulins

17. Will mixing NPH with a rapid-acting or regular insulin blunt the rapid action of the mealtime insulins? How stable are other insulin mixtures (Table 50-20)?

Regular insulin and all of the rapid-acting insulin analogs (aspart, lispro, and glulisine) may be mixed with NPH. In general, it is recommended to mix the insulins just before administration.

REGULAR PLUS NPH

The onset and duration of action of regular and NPH insulin administered as a mixture are similar to those observed when the two insulins are administered by separate injections. The pharmacodynamic profiles of these insulins are retained in premixed preparations stored in vials or syringes for 3 months (Table 50-20).[97,108] This is true even though protamine in NPH binds regular insulin in vitro.

RAPID-ACTING INSULIN PLUS NPH

Insulin aspart, glulsine, and lispro are compatible with human NPH insulin manufactured by NovoNordisk (Novolin N), and Eli Lilly and Company (Humulin N). However, relative to aspart, glulisine, and lispro alone, the absorption rate is slowed and the peak concentrations are blunted. The total bioavailability is unaltered. The manufacturers recommend mixing the two insulins just before administration, which should be scheduled 15 minutes before meals. The compatibility of insulin aspart, glulisine, and lispro with other brands of human NPH insulin or animal source NPH is unknown.[77–79,97]

RAPID-ACTING INSULIN PLUS INSULIN GLARGINE

The long-acting insulin glargine (Lantus) must not be mixed with any other insulins. If Lantus is mixed or diluted with other insulins, its pH will be increased, which will affect its absorption kinetics. The onset of action and duration of effect may be altered unpredictably.[93] However, small studies with pediatric patients have demonstrated that insulin glargine when mixed with a rapid-acting analog is effective for glycemic control.[109]

INSULIN GLARGINE

Insulin glargine is a long-acting analog that is soluble at pH 4.0; it is designed to precipitate when injected into the neutral pH of subcutaneous tissue. Because all other insulin products have a pH of 7.0, it should not be mixed in the same syringe with other insulins.[93]

INSULIN DETEMIR

Insulin detemir should not be mixed or diluted with any other insulin.[110]

Midmorning Hyperglycemia

18. Evaluate A.H.'s noon blood glucose concentration of 120 to 150 mg/dL.

Midmorning hyperglycemia frequently represents the maximum glucose excursion in patients with diabetes and often is the most difficult to manage. The following are possible explanations for midmorning hyperglycemia:

- An insufficient dose of Novolog insulin before breakfast. For A.H., this means that her insulin-to-carbohydrate ratio needs to be adjusted.
- Poor synchrony between meal intake and insulin action. This could be caused by administration of rapid-acting insulin too long before or after the meal (e.g., ≥30 minutes). If regular insulin is used, this could be caused by administering regular insulin just before or after meals.
- Delayed onset of Novolog insulin owing to binding with insulin-blocking antibodies.[339] Because A.H. is a newly diagnosed patient with diabetes, it is unlikely that she has developed significant concentrations of insulin-blocking antibodies.
- An insufficient dose of evening Lantus insulin to suppress hepatic glucose production (glycogenolysis and gluconeogenesis) during the fasting state or the dawn phenomenon (see Question 20).
- Excessive carbohydrate ingestion at breakfast.
- Increased peripheral resistance to insulin action caused by high fasting glucose levels (glucose toxicity).

When evaluating midmorning hyperglycemia, it is important to remember that the FPG concentration can contribute up to 50% of this plasma glucose excursion. Therefore, a key to the control of midmorning hyperglycemia may be to normalize the fasting glucose concentration.

Since insulin glargine has been decreased to correct the morning reactive hyperglycemia, this should be the approach used for A.H.

If control of her fasting hyperglycemia does not correct the midmorning hyperglycemia, the following interventions may be considered:

- Increase the dose of Novolog before breakfast. Her insulin-to-carbohydrate ratio should be changed to 1 unit of Novolog for every 12 g of carbohydrate for each meal.
- If regular insulin were used, inject the morning dose of regular insulin 45 to 60 minutes before breakfast in an attempt to match peak insulin concentrations with postmeal glucose excursions. If this maneuver is used, the patient should be warned of possible hypoglycemia before breakfast.
- Alter the carbohydrate content of the meals. This may include decreasing the amount of carbohydrate in the breakfast meal, changing the type of carbohydrate ingested, or adding fiber to that meal to minimize glucose excursions.

Preprandial Hypoglycemia: Use of Rapid-Acting Insulin

19. A.H. is now taking Lantus 12 units each night and using an insulin-to-carbohydrate ratio of 1:15 (1 unit of Novolog for every 15 g of carbohydrate) for each meal. She is continuing with the same high sugar premeal correction of 1 unit of Novolog for every 70 mg/dL over her premeal blood glucose target of 120 mg/dL. Two weeks later, she brings in her blood glucose concentration records.

Time	*Glucose Concentration (mg/dL)*	*mmol/L*
7 AM	110–120	6.1–6.7
Noon	90–110	5.0–6.1
5 PM	60–110	3.3–6.1
11 PM	80–110	4.4–6.1
3 AM	80–110	4. 4–6.1

A.H. feels that she is now "back to normal." She has no signs or symptoms of hyperglycemia, and her weight has remained stable. Occasionally, she becomes hypoglycemic before dinner, but this most often occurs when her dinner is delayed because of a hectic work schedule. Evaluate A.H.'s blood glucose trends. What could be the cause of her predinner hypoglycemia and how could she be managed?

A.H.'s blood glucose concentrations indicate that her basic insulin regimen is generally adequate to achieve the overall goal of preprandial blood glucose concentrations of less than 120 mg/dL. Note that correction of A.H.'s FPG concentration ultimately corrected her midmorning hyperglycemia. In fact, if one were to evaluate A.H.'s blood glucose concentrations from the previous visit, it is evident that the prebreakfast dose of Novolog was working well. This domino effect on blood glucose concentrations emphasizes the importance of correcting one blood glucose concentration at a time.

The hypoglycemia A.H. is experiencing before dinner could be caused by insufficient carbohydrate intake at lunch, increased activity during the day, or an excessive dose of Novolog insulin (insulin-to-carbohydrate ratio too high). Thus, the problem could be resolved by augmenting A.H.'s lunch meal, adjusting the lunch insulin-to-carbohydrate ratio to 1 unit of Novolog for every 18 (or 20) g carbohydrate, or adding a midafternoon snack.

Dawn Phenomenon

20. R.D., a 37-year-old man, has had type 1 diabetes since age 14. Over the past 2 years, he has been very well controlled on the following insulin regimen: 20 units Lantus each morning with 3 to 4 units insulin lispro depending on carbohydrate intake before

meals. On this regimen, his blood glucose concentrations for the past 2 weeks have been as follows.

Time	*Glucose Concentration (mg/dL)*	*mmol/L*
7 AM	140–170	7. 8–9.4
Noon	100–120	5. 5–6.7
5 PM	100–130	5. 5–7.2
11 PM	115–140	6. 4–7.8
3 AM	100–120	5. 5–6.7

What are the likely causes of R.D.'s fasting hyperglycemia?

As discussed in question 15, fasting hyperglycemia may be the result of insufficient doses of insulin in the evening, a decline in the effect of insulin over time, and, possibly, reactive hyperglycemia. In R.D.'s case, the dawn phenomenon also must be considered.[111] The *dawn phenomenon* is a rise in the blood glucose concentration that occurs between 4 and 8 AM after a physiological nadir in the blood glucose concentration that occurs between midnight and 3 AM. This 30 to 40 mg/dL increase in the morning blood glucose concentration cannot be attributed to increases in counter-regulatory hormones secondary to an antecedent hypoglycemic event, but it may be secondary to rising growth hormone levels. This phenomenon is inconsistently observed in individuals with types 1 and 2 diabetes as well as nondiabetic individuals; furthermore, it is inconsistently present from one day to the next.[112]

R.D.'s normal 3 AM blood glucose concentration indicates that posthypoglycemic hyperglycemia is an unlikely cause of his fasting hyperglycemia. Thus, the modest increase in his blood glucose concentration between 3 and 8 AM may be attributed to the waning effects of insulin or the dawn phenomenon. In both cases, an increase in R.D.'s daily dose of insulin glargine would be indicated. Another option would be to switch R.D. to an insulin pump. He has demonstrated a desire and ability for intensive management with multiple daily injections, frequent blood glucose monitoring, record-keeping skills, the ability to make appropriate insulin dose adjustments, and accurate carbohydrate counting. The advantage to using a pump is the ability to program an increase in the basal infusion rate at approximately midnight. Because it takes 3 to 4 hours to observe a biologic response following a change in the infusion rate, the response would occur at approximately 3 to 4 AM, when the dawn phenomenon begins.[113]

Type 1 Diabetes in Children

Diagnosis and Clinical Presentation

21. J.C., a 7-year-old, 30-kg (95th percentile), 50 inches tall (90th percentile) girl, was brought to the emergency department (ED) by her parents because of nausea, vomiting, and a persistent "stomach ache" secondary to the flu. For the past week, J.C. had flu-like symptoms, resulting in a 6-lb weight loss. Initial laboratory values revealed a blood glucose of 600 mg/dL, serum pH of 6.8 with bicarbonate level of 13 mEq/L, plasma ketone level of 5.2 mmol/L, and positive ketonuria. J.C. was diagnosed with diabetic ketoacidosis (DKA) secondary to new-onset type 1 diabetes. In retrospect and on further questioning, J.C.'s parents realized that she probably had symptoms as early as 4 weeks before her hospitalization. While on a driving vacation, she drank large quantities of juice and had to stop hourly to urinate. She began experiencing enuresis, which her parents attributed to her increased fluid intake. What signs and symptoms are consistent with the diagnosis of type 1 diabetes in a child?

The diagnosis of type 1 diabetes in children is generally straightforward. Presenting symptoms include a several-week history of polyuria, polydipsia, polyphagia, and weight loss, with hyperglycemia, glucosuria, ketonemia, and ketonuria. J.C.'s presentation is typical for a child newly diagnosed with diabetes who is brought in for medical attention because of severe symptoms related to the flu. An acute viral illness can trigger autoimmune destruction of the pancreas and abdominal pain, which may masquerade as gastroenteritis. Abdominal pain is a common presenting symptom of diabetic ketoacidosis (DKA).[114] J.C.'s weight loss probably represents fluid and caloric loss secondary to uncontrolled diabetes as well as decreased caloric intake from the flu. The symptoms of polyuria are less obvious in an infant and are frequently missed until metabolic derangement has occurred. Unlike J.C., infants frequently present with severe dehydration and metabolic acidosis despite a negative history of diarrhea or significant vomiting.

Goals of Therapy

22. What are the goals of therapy for J.C.? Do the results of the DCCT apply to children such as J.C.? Are there age-specific goals?

The goals of therapy for children such as J.C. and adolescents with diabetes mellitus are as follows: (a) achieve normal growth and development, (b) obtain optimal glycemic control, (c) facilitate positive psychosocial adjustment to diabetes, and (d) prevent acute and chronic complications. Attainment of these goals requires a tremendous amount of support and education for the parents and can be best provided by a multidisciplinary team of professionals, including a physician, nurse educator, pharmacist, dietitian, and psychosocial expert.

Growth serves as an important clinical indication of overall general health and well-being in children with diabetes. Height and weight should be measured at each visit and plotted on standard growth grids. If, at the time of diagnosis, a child has fallen behind in height or weight, prompt and appropriate treatment should quickly return the child to the appropriate percentile and pattern of growth. An obese child should be encouraged to achieve a more appropriate percentile of weight gradually, over a period of several months.

Although recommendations for glycemic control are based on data from studies in adult patients with diabetes, achieving the same near normalization of blood glucose levels in children and adolescents is recommended. However, special consideration must be given to the unique risks and consequences of hypoglycemia in young children. A cohort of adolescents included in the DCCT was analyzed separately. The intensive group achieved an HbA_{1c} about 1% higher than the current ADA recommendations for patients in general.[115] Similar to the adults in the DCCT, adolescents had sustained benefits from intensive management with little further progression to proliferative retinopathy 4 years after the DCCT was terminated.[116] Thus, J.C.'s pediatrician must strive for the best glucose control that she, her family circumstances, and currently available treatment regimens will permit.

The risk of hypoglycemia and potential neuropsychological impairment is of the greatest concern for children younger than 6 years. This is because the young child may be unable to mount an adequate adrenergic response to hypoglycemia and be unable to effectively communicate symptoms of hypoglycemia. In addition, food intake and physical activity are unpredictable in this age group. To minimize the risk of hypo- and hyperglycemia, an HbA_{1c} value between 7.5% and 8.5% is recommended.[117]

The management of diabetes in children 6 to 12 years of age, such as J.C., is particularly challenging because many children require insulin with lunch or at other times when they are away from home. Administration of insulin at school demands flexibility and close communications between the parents, the health care team and school personnel. An HbA_{1c} goal of 8% or lower is recommended (Table 50-4).[22,117]

The greatest amount of evidence-based data exist for adolescents with diabetes (13–19 years). As mentioned, teenagers included in the DCCT achieved a mean HbA_{1c} level of 8.06% in an era before the availability of rapid-acting or basal insulins. An HbA_{1c} goal of <7.5% is recommended in this age group.[117]

Insulin Therapy

23. How should J.C. be started on insulin? Is the use of an insulin pump appropriate in children such as J.C.?

Generally, rapid-acting insulin analogs, short-acting insulin, intermediate-acting insulin, and basal insulin analogs are used in children. Insulin requirements are generally based on body weight, age, and pubertal status. Newly diagnosed children with type 1 diabetes usually require an initial total daily dose of approximately 0.5 to 1.0 unit/kg. The small insulin requirements of infants and toddlers may be delivered by using diluted insulin to measure doses less than 1 U. Diluents are available for specific types of insulin from the insulin manufacturers. Insulin syringes and pens that deliver insulin in 0.5-U increments are also very useful. Most children are treated with two or three doses of rapid-acting or short-acting insulin combined with intermediate-acting insulin. Multiple daily insulin injection regimens combined with carbohydrate counting are attractive regimens for middle and high school students. Basal/bolus insulin regimens have demonstrated lower fasting blood glucose levels with less nocturnal hypoglycemia versus regimens using NPH in children and adolescents.[118] However, many families are reluctant to commit to six to seven insulin injections per day. Children who have lunch at a consistent time and are willing to eat a consistent amount of carbohydrate at lunch do well with a breakfast dose of NPH given to provide meal coverage for lunch and a bedtime dose of a basal insulin such as Lantus or Levemir. Many patients find rapid-acting insulins more convenient because they can be injected 0 to 15 minutes before a meal so that little preplanning is involved. Because children often have erratic eating habits, an advantage of rapid-acting insulins over regular insulin is that they can also be injected immediately after a meal. J.C. should be started on a total daily dose of 14 units given as 4 units of NPH plus 3 units of Novolog at breakfast, 3 units of Novolog with dinner, and 4 units of Lantus at bedtime (three injections per day).[117,119]

When J.C. gets older and can self-administer her injections, a basal-bolus regimen can be initiated. Also, the use of an insulin pump can be considered. The use of insulin pumps in the pediatric population is increasing rapidly.[120,121] Young children (not just adolescents) are now recommended for consideration of insulin pump therapy.[122] Adult support both at home and school is critical for successful pump use until the child is able to manage his or her diabetes independently.

Injection Sites

24. Are the recommended sites of injection different for children? Does the age of the child play a factor?

Although many studies exist in adults investigating the rate of SC insulin absorption depending on the site and depth of injection, it is not clear whether these results are applicable to children. For infants with abundant SC tissue, injection sites are usually plentiful. For some toddlers who have lost their "baby fat," locating an appropriate site for injection can be difficult. Injecting insulin into the abdomen of children with minimal SC abdominal fat or in very young children may not be advisable. Rotation of injection sites between arms, thighs, and the upper-outer quadrant of the buttock or hip area, as well as the abdominal area in older children, is recommended. To achieve consistent absorption, insulin injections can be patterned; for example, using the arms for the morning injection and the thighs for the evening injection. Unfortunately, many children and teens consistently inject their insulin into a single area for convenience, accessibility, and comfort. This results in the development of fatty deposits and scar tissue secondary to insulin action at the local tissue level. Insulin absorption from these hypertrophied areas is generally poor and may make glycemic control quite variable. Insulin pen devices are very helpful for use in children because they are less intimidating. Also, spring-loaded injection devices may be helpful in reducing the child's fear of needles and easing access to difficult-to-reach injection sites such as the back of the arms or buttocks.

Blood Glucose Monitoring

25. How often should J.C. monitor her blood glucose?

The eventual goal for children with diabetes is self-management, with insulin dosing decisions based on interpretation of blood glucose results. Self-management skills and basal-bolus insulin regimens rely on frequent SMBG. For children with type 1 diabetes, four or more blood glucose tests per day are generally necessary. Most of the newer meters allow alternative site testing (arm or thigh), which decreases the discomfort of fingersticks. For infants, the earlobes and heel provide alternative blood sources to fingersticks. Enthusiasm for frequent blood glucose testing tends to wane with duration of diabetes. However, families who are instructed on managing diabetes on the basis of test results are better motivated to persevere with SMBG. CGM may also hold promise for improved assessment of metabolic control in pediatric patients. J.C. should test her blood glucose before each meal and at bedtime, at a minimum. The results will construct a useful profile of her daily fluctuations. Additional tests should be performed whenever J.C. experiences hypoglycemia or ketonuria or when she becomes acutely ill.

Honeymoon Period

26. Over the next 2 months, J.C.'s insulin requirements decreased to a total daily dose of 10 units (~0.3 unit/kg). Has her diabetes gone into remission?

Approximately 20% to 30% of individuals with type 1 diabetes go into a remission phase (honeymoon period) within days to weeks of their diagnosis.[123] During this time, which can last for weeks to months, C-peptide can be measured, indicating a return of pancreatic function; insulin requirements may diminish partially or completely. As illustrated by J.C., this presents clinically as markedly decreased insulin requirements to maintain normoglycemia. Although it is tempting to discontinue insulin, diabetes invariably recurs. To minimize the possibility of inducing insulin allergy secondary to intermittent insulin exposure and to avoid engendering a sense of false hope in J.C. that her disease has been cured, many clinicians continue insulin even if the doses are minuscule. J.C. should be followed closely for rising blood glucose concentrations.

Hypoglycemia

27. J.C.'s parents contacted the clinic to report that J.C. is having nightmares and is awakening in the middle of the night complaining of a headache and stomach pain. However, these symptoms resolve by noon the following day. Her current insulin regimen is NPH 3 units with Novolog 2 units before breakfast, 2 units of Novolog with dinner and 3 units of Lantus at bedtime. Could J.C. be experiencing nocturnal hypoglycemia? How do the symptoms of hypoglycemia differ in a child compared with an adult? How can the risk of hypoglycemia be minimized for J.C.?

J.C.'s parents are appropriately worried. Hypoglycemia is a serious and often life-threatening complication of diabetes management in children, and the risk of hypoglycemia increases with attempts to maintain meticulous control of blood glucose levels. Common causes of hypoglycemia include changes in meal amounts, late or skipped meals or snacks, exercise or unusual activity, and administration of excessive insulin. Because very young children may not be able to identify or express symptoms of hypoglycemia, caretakers must observe the child closely and identify symptoms or behaviors associated with a falling blood glucose. Symptoms of hypoglycemia may include crankiness, sudden crying, restless sleep, or nightmares as seen in J.C.

Hypoglycemia is more frequent in children with lower HbA_{1c} values, a prior history of severe hypoglycemia, larger insulin doses, and younger children.[124] Additional risk factors for hypoglycemia include a longer duration of diabetes and male gender. Nocturnal hypoglycemia is reported in 14% to 47% of children with type 1 diabetes and is thought to be due to impaired counter-regulatory response to hypoglycemia during sleep.[125] Bedtime blood glucose levels are poor predictors of nocturnal hypoglycemia. J.C.'s parents should be instructed to test her blood glucose at 2 AM closely over the next few nights, and then continue to check at least twice weekly. In children, Lantus can exhibit a small peak effect during the initial 3 to 5 hours after administration, increasing the risk for nocturnal hypoglycemia.[117] The Lantus dose should be moved to dinner time. If this does not correct the nocturnal hypoglycemia, then the dose should be reduced. Use of Lantus as basal insulin is associated with less nocturnal hypoglycemia (and asymptomatic nocturnal hypoglycemia) compared with NPH insulin in children and adolescents.[126,127] A bedtime snack may also be needed. Treatment of hypoglycemia is addressed in Question 37.

Using Insulin in Special Situations

Insulin Stability: Factors Altering Control

28. T.M., a 31-year-old farmer, has had type 1 diabetes for 20 years. He has been relatively well controlled on his current regimen of premeal Humalog and twice daily NPH human insulin for some time. During the winter and spring seasons, his blood glucose concentrations have ranged from 90 to 140 mg/dL, and the HbA_{1c} measured at his last clinic visit 3 months ago was 7.5%. It is now August. For the past 2 months, T.M. has noticed that his diabetes is not under good control. His blood glucose concentrations vary widely from concentrations as low as 60 mg/dL (3.3 mmol/L) to as high as 240 mg/dL (13.3 mmol/L). He has no explanation for this. On inspection, his vial of insulin lispro is cloudy and a white precipitate is clinging to the NPH vial, giving it a frosted appearance. Both vials are approximately one-third full. What factors may be contributing to T.M.'s poor glycemic control?

[SI units: blood glucose concentrations, 5.0–7.8 mmol/L; HbA_{1c}, 0.085 (normal, 0.04–0.06)]

Many factors may be contributing to T.M.'s poor control. These are discussed in the subsequent sections. Physical changes in insulin are addressed here.

PHYSICAL CHANGES

Both of T.M.'s insulin vials have changed in appearance. T.M. should be instructed not to use his insulin lispro if it is discolored; has become cloudy or thickened; or contains small, threadlike or other solid particles. As discussed in Question 17, the cloudiness may be caused by contamination of insulin lispro with NPH. If T.M. reuses his syringes, this also may be caused by the silicone oil that is used to coat needles of disposable syringes.[128] The silicone oil can denature the insulin, reducing its pharmacologic effect.

FLOCCULATION

NPH can sometimes flocculate or crystallize onto the insulin bottle.[129] This results in a significant loss of potency, with insulin concentrations in the remaining suspensions varying from 6 to 64 U/mL (labeled 100 U/mL). This phenomenon can occur precipitously, generally after 3 to 6 weeks of use. Incorporation of additional zinc into these preparations during the manufacturing process has minimized this problem. Nevertheless, all patients should be warned to inspect their vials carefully before each injection and to discard or exchange them if they have crystallized (Fig. 50-6).

TEMPERATURE

Insulin is a fragile molecule that can be damaged by temperature extremes. All commercially available insulins are stable for at least 28 days (e.g., ~1 month) at room temperature (68–75°F), and the ADA recommends avoiding temperature extremes (<36°F or >86°F).[97] In practice, most patients store vials currently in use at room temperature because injection of cold insulin is uncomfortable. All unopened, extra vials or pen devices should be stored in the refrigerator. The *United States Pharmacopeia* recommends that patients discard vials that have not been completely used in 1 month if they have been kept at room temperature.

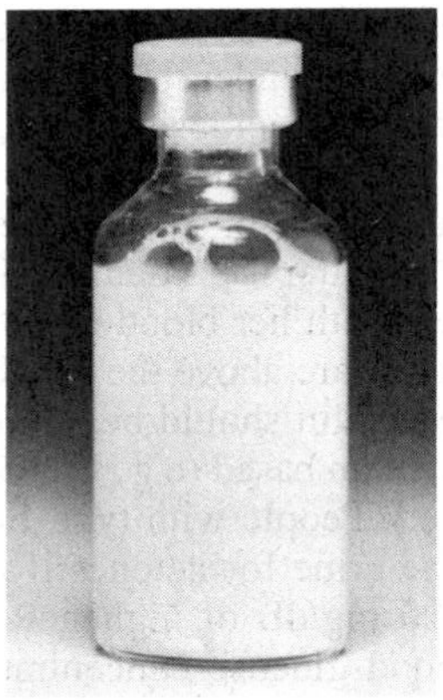

FIGURE 50-6 Insulin vial with crystallized insulin. (Used with permission from reference 341.)

The stability of insulin at temperatures of 75°F to 100°F is unknown, but all insulins lose significant potency within 1 to 2 months at 100°F. T.M. lives in an area where temperatures frequently exceed 100°F during the summer months. Therefore, it is important that he not store his insulin in an automobile or in the sun, where it may be subject to deterioration. An insulated container or cooling packet (such as the FRIO Wallet) is recommended for T.M. It also is of interest that many wholesale drug distributors and some mail-order pharmacies do not take special packaging precautions when delivering insulins to pharmacies or homes during the summer months. Thus, inadvertent exposure to high temperatures during these months may alter the potency and actions of insulins. Freezing apparently does not affect the potency of insulin, but may cause aggregation of the precipitate. This could alter the absorption kinetics of the preparation.[130]

OTHER FACTORS ALTERING RESPONSE TO INSULIN

Many other factors may be altering T.M.'s response to insulin. The heat in the summer months may increase circulation to the injected site, thus speeding the onset and shortening the duration of action of his insulin. Exercise of the injected limb may affect insulin action similarly. During the summer months, farmers typically are more physically active and, as a consequence, require less insulin than usual. Other factors that can alter insulin action are listed in Tables 50-10 and 50-19.

When patients like T.M. observe that their insulin seems to work less well even when the product is well within the expiration date and there are no obvious physical changes, we recommend that they inject insulin from a fresh vial to assess whether insulin from the original vial has deteriorated. If the response remains the same, they should work with a clinician to identify other reasons for their decreased responsiveness to insulin.

Exercise and Insulin Requirements

29. J.S. is a 17-year-old, nonobese, patient with type 1 diabetes who was diagnosed at age 12. He currently is moderately well controlled on a single daily dose of Lantus 18 units at bedtime with 4 to 6 units of insulin aspart with meals (depending on carbohydrate intake). His HbA_{1c} is 7.8%, and his blood glucose levels before meals range from 150 to 190 mg/dL (8.3–10.5 mmol/L). Fasting blood glucose concentrations in the clinic range from 130 to 170 mg/dL (7.2–9.4 mmol/L). He has rare hypoglycemic reactions that are associated with skipped meals, and he generally is compliant with his prescribed meal plan. J.S. would like to begin a jogging program. What effect is jogging likely to have on his diabetic control? What precautions, if any, should he take?

[SI unit: HbA_{1c}, 0.10]

Exercise has varying effects on plasma glucose levels in patients, such as J.S., who are taking insulin. In the resting state, muscle derives approximately 10% of its metabolic requirement from glucose. In contrast, almost all of the muscle's metabolic requirements are derived from glucose during moderate to heavy exercise. Muscle glycogen stores are depleted quite rapidly, after which glucose is derived from the peripheral circulation. To meet the increased glucose demands, hepatic glycogenolysis and gluconeogenesis increase. This is mediated primarily through suppression of insulin secretion and increased secretion of counter-regulatory hormones such as glucagon. Low, permissive levels of insulin are required for glucose utilization by the muscle. In nondiabetic individuals, hepatic glucose output and peripheral utilization are balanced such that euglycemia is maintained during exercise.[131,132]

In a patient like J.S., exercise may cause hyperglycemia or hypoglycemia if he does not take proper precautions. If he is insulin deficient when he commences exercise, hepatic glucose output will be increased, but peripheral utilization will be decreased and hyperglycemia will ensue. Thus, patients like J.S. with type 1 diabetes should not exercise if their blood glucose concentrations exceed 250 mg/dL and they have ketosis or if levels exceed 300 mg/dL (with or without ketosis), because these levels usually indicate insulin deficiency.[132]

Conversely, excess insulin enhances peripheral utilization of glucose by muscle and suppresses hepatic glucose output. Both can contribute to hypoglycemia. Hypoglycemia is more likely to occur in patients whose blood glucose concentrations are normal or low just before exercise. Thus, if J.S.'s blood glucose concentration is normal or low (<100 mg/dL) before he begins exercise, he should eat a carbohydrate snack (10–20 g) and have additional carbohydrates readily available during and after exercise.[132] He should delay his dose of insulin lispro until after exercising and adjust the amount according to his postexercise blood glucose level.

It is less well appreciated that peripheral glucose utilization remains high after exercise has been discontinued. This is thought to be related to the replenishment of glycogen stores in the liver and muscle. Thus, if appropriate adjustments are not made in diet and insulin dose after exercise, hypoglycemia can occur 10 to 12 hours thereafter.[133]

For patients who inject insulin into their thighs, jogging may enhance insulin absorption. The absorption of regular insulin is increased when it is administered just before exercise (within 5 minutes), but it does not appear to be affected if injected 30 to 40 minutes before exercise. Absorption of the intermediate-acting or long-acting insulins is less likely to be augmented by exercise.[134] Some have suggested that insulin be injected at a site that is not exercised, for example, the abdomen, to minimize this effect. J.S. should inject his insulin in the abdomen.

In summary, J.S. should be encouraged to begin an exercise program. He should test his blood glucose concentrations before, during, and after exercise and adjust his insulin doses

Table 50-21 Exercise in Patients With Diabetes

1. Test blood glucose concentrations before, during, and after exercise.
2. For moderate exercise (e.g., bicycling or jogging for 30–45 min), ↓ the preceding dose of regular rapid-acting insulin by 30%–50%. If glucose concentration is normal or low before exercise, supplement the diet with a snack containing 10–15 g of carbohydrate.
3. To avoid ↑ absorption of regular insulin by exercise, inject into the abdomen or exercise 30–60 min after injection. Avoid exercise when rapid-acting insulin is peaking.
4. Individuals with low glycogen stores may be predisposed to the hypoglycemic effects of exercise. Examples include alcoholics, fasted individuals, or patients on extremely hypocaloric (<800 calories), low-carbohydrate (<10 g/day) diets.
5. Patients taking insulin are more susceptible to hypoglycemia than those taking sulfonylureas. Patients with type 2 diabetes mellitus treated with diet are unlikely to develop hypoglycemia.
6. Watch for postexercise hypoglycemia. Individuals who have been exercising during the day (e.g., skiing) should ↑ their carbohydrate intake and test their blood glucose concentration during the night to detect nocturnal hypoglycemia. Hypoglycemia can occur 8–15 hr after exercise.
7. If the glucose concentration is >240–300 mg/dL, the patient should not exercise. This indicates severe insulin deficiency. These patients are predisposed to hyperglycemia secondary to exercise.
8. Patients with severe proliferative retinopathy or retinal hemorrhage should avoid jarring exercise or exercise that involves moving the head below the waist.

and food intake accordingly. In general, exercise should be avoided at times corresponding to peak insulin action, because high levels can suppress counter-regulatory hormones that stimulate hepatic glucose production (Table 50-21). Regular exercise may increase tissue sensitivity to insulin and eventually lower J.S.'s insulin requirements. Vigorous exercise is contraindicated in patients with retinal or vitreous hemorrhages because retinal detachment may occur.

In overweight or obese individuals with type 2 diabetes mellitus who are treated with diet, exercise is unlikely to cause hypoglycemia. An extremely low-calorie diet (<800 calories) that also is low in carbohydrates may decrease an individual's exercise endurance because muscle glycogen stores are not maintained.[131] Patients with type 2 diabetes who are treated with insulin secretagogues or insulin may become hypoglycemic if insulin levels are high enough to increase peripheral utilization of glucose and suppress hepatic glucose output. Thus, patients with type 2 diabetes who are normoglycemic before exercise also should consider increasing their carbohydrate intake.[135] Because patients with type 2 diabetes do not have an absolute lack of insulin, they are less likely to become hyperglycemic in response to exercise.

Sick Day Management

30. R.D., a 32-year-old woman with type 1 diabetes, has been well controlled on basal-bolus regimen (four injections daily) for the past 6 months. However, 2 days ago, she began to develop signs and symptoms consistent with the flu. This has made her anorexic and nauseated and now she has begun to vomit; consequently, her food intake has been minimal. Because R.D. is not eating at this time, should she discontinue her insulin?

Insulin requirements always increase in the presence of an infection or acute illness, even if food intake is diminished. Patients with type 1 diabetes, such as R.D., commonly decrease or eliminate insulin doses under these circumstances, and it is in just this setting that ketoacidosis occurs.

Therefore, R.D. should be instructed to maintain her usual dose of insulin and test her blood glucose and urine ketones every 3 to 4 hours; the latter is particularly important if she has become nonadherent with her blood glucose testing. If blood glucose concentrations are above the usual range, extra doses of her rapid-acting insulin should be administered according to a prescribed algorithm based (e.g., 1 U/50 mg/dL above her blood glucose target). People with type 1 diabetes should be instructed to test the urine for ketones if their blood glucose concentration is 300 mg/dL of higher. R.D. should call her physician if her blood glucose concentration remains above 240 mg/dL after three corrective insulin doses; if she has moderate to large amounts of ketones in her urine, if she has been vomiting or having diarrhea for longer than 6 hours; or if she begins to develop signs and symptoms related to ketoacidosis (polyuria, polydipsia, dehydration, ketonuria, and a fruity breath; (see Question 39). R.D. also should attempt to maintain her fluid, mineral, and carbohydrate intake with easily digested food and fluids (Table 50-22).[136]

Insulin Requirements in Renal Failure

31. M.B., a 32-year-old woman, has had type 1 diabetes for 15 years. Over the past 2 years, a gradual deterioration of her renal function—as reflected by increased proteinuria, serum creatinine (SrCr), and blood urea nitrogen (BUN) values—has been observed. What are the anticipated effects of decreased renal function on M.B.'s insulin requirements?

The effects of renal failure on insulin requirements are complex and, under various circumstances, insulin requirements may increase or decrease. The kidney is the most important site of extrahepatic insulin metabolism and excretion. Renal clearance of insulin is 190 to 270 mL/minute, approximately two-thirds of hepatic clearance (320–400 mL/minute). In nondiabetic individuals, the liver extracts approximately 40% to 50% of insulin secreted endogenously before it reaches the peripheral circulation.[70,137] Because exogenous insulin is

Table 50-22 Sick Day Management

1. Continue taking your basic dose of insulin *even* if you are not eating well or have nausea or vomiting.
2. Test your blood glucose more frequently: every 3–4 hr.
3. If indicated, give yourself extra doses (high sugar correction) of lispro, aspart, glulisine, or regular insulin: for example, 1–2 units for every 30–50 mg/dL over an agreed-upon target glucose concentration (e.g., 150 mg/dL). Correction doses must be individualized based on the patient's sensitivity to insulin (Table 50-11).
4. Begin testing your urine for ketones if you have type 1 diabetes. If you have type 2 diabetes, begin testing especially when glucose readings exceed 300 mg/dL.
5. Try to drink plenty of fluid (1/2 cup/hr for adults) and maintain your caloric intake (50 g carbohydrate Q 4 hr). Foods such as gelatin, noncarbonated soft drinks, crackers, soup, and soda may be used.
6. Call a physician if your blood glucose concentration remains >300 mg/dL; or your urine ketones remain high after two or three supplemental doses of insulin; or your blood glucose level remains >240 mg/dL for more than 24 hours.

delivered directly to the periphery, the kidneys play a more important role in its elimination. Insulin is filtered by the glomerulus and reabsorbed in the proximal tubules, where it is destroyed enzymatically. The kidney also clears insulin from the peritubular circulation.[73,138] At that site, insulin can enhance the reabsorption of sodium, which may account for the edema occasionally observed after the initiation of insulin therapy in some individuals.

Diminished renal function can be accompanied by decreased clearance of endogenous and exogenous insulin, resulting in increased plasma concentrations of insulin. Therefore, M.B.'s insulin requirements may diminish as her renal disease progresses. Patients with moderate degrees of renal failure (glomerular filtration rate [GFR] >22.5 mL/minute) remove 39% of insulin from arterial plasma, similar to normal subjects. In contrast, patients with severe renal insufficiency (GFR <6 mL/minute) have a marked reduction in insulin removal from arterial plasma (9%).[139] Decreased insulin clearance in conjunction with the anorexia, nausea, and decreased food intake associated with uremia can lead to hypoglycemia in such individuals. In some patients with diabetes, particularly those with residual endogenous insulin secretion (type 2), glucose tolerance may normalize as renal function diminishes, eliminating the need for insulin.

In contrast, severe uremia is associated with glucose intolerance. This seems to be related to tissue resistance to insulin secondary to an unknown factor that can be removed by dialysis. Other factors that may alter blood glucose control in patients with renal failure include dialysis against glucose-containing dialysates and high-dose glucocorticoids in patients who have undergone renal transplantation.

As M.B.'s renal function worsens, a reduction in her insulin requirements should be anticipated. During this time, M.B. should monitor her blood glucose concentrations closely and adjust her insulin according to an algorithm.

Traveling With Diabetes

32. J.R. is a 42-year-old woman with type 1 diabetes mellitus who has just taken a position that requires extensive overseas air travel. She is concerned about potential problems she may encounter managing her diabetes under these circumstances. What are some basic travel tips J.R. should consider?

J.R.'s predeparture preparations depend on the duration and destination of her trip. The following sections discuss basic considerations for people with diabetes when traveling. Before a trip, she should obtain a letter from her health care provider indicating her diagnosis (type 1 diabetes), therapy, and the supplies she requires (e.g., syringes). She should also obtain a prescription for her insulins and syringes (or other delivery devices) in case of an emergency.

SUPPLIES

When going through airport security, J.R. should alert the security officer that she has diabetes and is carrying her supplies with her. All diabetes medications, supplies, and equipment are allowed through the checkpoint once they have been screened.

J.R. should carry a plentiful backup supply of insulin, syringes, blood-testing supplies (including an extra battery for her meter), and glucose tablets. She should double her anticipated insulin needs in case of loss, destruction, or unavailability of comparable products in foreign countries. For example, only U-40 and U-80 insulin are available in some parts of the world. J.R.'s insulin supply should be insulated (e.g., using a FRIO Wallet) and separated in various bags she will carry with her. Most sources advise against placing insulin in checked luggage, because its effectiveness might be altered by x-ray scanning or by freezing that could occur in the unpressurized baggage compartment. J.R. should take with her a brief medical history and a prescription for insulin for emergency situations.

IDENTIFICATION

J.R. should carry some identification that alerts medical personnel or others to her diagnosis in emergency situations. This can take the form of a wallet card or a medical alert bracelet. In certain situations, she could consider informing key individuals that she has diabetes (e.g., airline personnel, hotel managers, tour guides, traveling companions). She should review her insurance policy carefully so that she knows how to obtain care out of the country and bring along her policy and claim forms. Finally, she should provide friends or relatives with a detailed itinerary so that medical care can be summoned promptly if difficulties are encountered.

FOOT CARE

J.R. should wear comfortable shoes and not go barefoot. She should avoid wearing new shoes to prevent formation of blisters. She should check her feet daily, looking for blisters, cuts, and sores and seek medical care if she sees any signs of infection or inflammation.

MEAL PLANNING

J.R. should try to maintain some regularity in her diet (time and amounts). When it is the custom to take the evening meal later than is usual in the United States, a late afternoon or early evening snack should be planned. When flying, she can request a low-carbohydrate/low-fat meal. She should inject her rapid-acting insulin only when her meal has been served to her (or sees the food coming down the aisle) to prevent hypoglycemia. To avoid unforeseen events (e.g., travel delays), J.R. should carry sufficient food and snacks with her on the plane. Anticipating the likely composition of her diet in a foreign country also will help her to design a diet that maintains her pattern of carbohydrate and caloric intake.

INSULIN DOSES

J.R. needs to adjust her basal insulin doses when she flies across several time zones to account for time lost or gained.[48] When traveling east, the insulin dose should be decreased proportionately for the time lost and a shorter day. Conversely, when traveling west, the basal insulin dose should be increased for the time gained and a longer day. The principle is to provide the same amount of basal insulin per hour. For example, if J.R. is using 10 units of Lantus insulin and is traveling from New York to London (a 5-hour difference), her dose would be reduced to 8 units. This is because she is receiving about 0.4 unit/hour and she will be losing 5 hours as she crosses the time zones ($0.4 \times 5 = 2$ units). When she arrives in London and changes her watch, she may resume her Lantus 10 units at the usual time of administration. When drawing up her insulin dose while on an airplane, J.R. should inject only half as much air into the vial (if at all); because the cabin pressure is lower than ground pressure, less pressure is needed inside the vial to balance the insulin she withdraws.

JET LAG

Because jet lag may be indistinguishable from symptoms of hypoglycemia or hyperglycemia, J.R. should test her blood glucose concentrations more frequently to better assess her symptoms.

Perioperative Management

33. A.G., a 55-year-old, 60-kg woman with a 35-year history of type 1 diabetes, was admitted to the critical care unit for an abdominal hysterectomy. Before admission, she was well controlled on 24 units insulin glargine at bedtime and premeal doses of insulin aspart. How should A.G.'s diabetes be managed while in the critical care unit?

The hospital management of a patient with diabetes is complex because so many variables can influence insulin requirements. Accordingly, common practice has been to aim for blood glucose concentrations in the range of 150 to 200 mg/dL. Over the past decade, much literature has been published looking at the management of hyperglycemia in critically ill hospitalized patients and the effects of hyperglycemia on mortality and morbidity. The initial Diabetes and Insulin Glucose Infusion in Acute Myocardial Infarction study compared intensive insulin therapy (insulin glucose infusion for ≥24 hours followed by SC insulin four times daily for ≥3 months) in patients with diabetes after acute MI with standard insulin therapy. Intensive insulin therapy improved long-term survival at 1 year and continued for 3.5 years, with an absolute risk reduction in mortality of 11%.[140] Three more recent studies—Diabetes and Insulin Glucose Infusion in Acute Myocardial Infarction-2, CREATE-ECLA, and HI-5—did not show significant reductions in mortality in post-MI patients using intensive insulin-glucose infusions.[141–143] In a study of surgical patients in the intensive care unit (ICU) with hyperglycemia (some with diabetes), in which liberal glucose control (blood glucose concentrations of 180–200 mg/dL) was compared with tight control (blood glucose concentrations of 80–110 mg/dL), tight control decreased overall in-hospital mortality and systemic infection.[144] The same researcher performed a subsequent, similarly designed study in medical ICU patients and demonstrated reduced morbidity, but not mortality, in the intensively treated group. Interestingly, patients who were treated for 3 or more days with intensive insulin infusion therapy did have a significant reduction in in-hospital mortality, suggesting that the initial length of intensive insulin therapy (via infusion) in these patients may be an important factor.[145] The incidence of severe hypoglycemia (blood glucose level <40 mg/dL) was 18.7%, which was much higher than the 5.1% observed in the surgical ICU population.[146] Overall, studies suggest insulin therapy in critically ill patients has a beneficial effect on short-term morality in different hospital units.[147] Implementation of insulin infusion protocols using tight blood glucose targets (e.g., 80–110 mg/dL) should be carefully implemented, but with careful tracking for hypoglycemia.[148] For patients on general medical-surgical units, blood glucose targets below 180 to 200 mg/dL are reasonable.[22]

For perioperative insulin needs, A.G. should receive her usual basal insulin dose (Lantus 24 units) on the night before surgery. If the basal insulin is normally administered in the morning, the usual dose can still be give for patients with type 1 diabetes; for those with type 2 diabetes, 50% to 100% of the basal insulin is administered the morning of surgery. Correction doses of rapid-acting insulin can be administered the morning of surgery if the blood glucose is above 180 mg/dL.[149] If a current HbA_{1c} is not available, it should be measured to assess the patient's glycemic control before admission.

Most insulin infusion protocols include the use of intravenous regular insulin and maintenance IV fluids; D5W, D5W 1/2 NS, or D10W (for fluid restriction or renal failure).[149] The adjustment algorithms are used by nursing to change the rate of infusion depending on the blood glucose level. Most often, the insulin infusion is prepared in a solution of 1 U/1 mL normal saline (e.g., 100 units of regular insulin in 100 mL normal saline). A dedicated IV line is used for the insulin infusion to avoid iatrogenic hypoglycemia. The insulin infusion is connected to the maintenance IV containing dextrose (can be Y-connected). Because insulin binds to plastic, the insulin solution should be flushed (e.g., with 20 mL) through the IV tubing before the line is connected to the patient. An IV dextrose infusion is maintained while a patient is on an insulin infusion. Most patients need 5 to 10 g of glucose per hour (or D5W or D5W-1/2 normal saline at 100–200 mL/hour). Additional maintenance fluids (and electrolytes) can be administered via a different port or line. Some protocols include an initial bolus dose of insulin. The initial insulin infusion rate is primarily based on current blood glucose level and BMI; other factors such as body weight, current daily insulin requirements, and renal function should be taken into consideration. A rate of 1 unit/hour is a typical initial rate (can range from 0.5 unit/hour to ≥2 units/hour). Adjustments in the insulin infusion rate are determined by fingerstick blood glucose levels every 30 to 60 minutes hour until the blood glucose is stable and close to target. Then the frequency of blood glucose testing may be reduced to every 2 to 3 hours. Algorithms should consider both the current and previous blood glucose level, the rate of change of the blood glucose level, and the current infusion rate.[22]

Insulin infusion should be started at least 2 to 3 hours before the surgery to titrate to the desired level of glucose control. Examples of protocols are available on the Institute for Healthcare Improvement's website (available at http://www.ihi.org/IHI/Topics/PatientSafety/MedicationSystems/Tools/) and many are published in the medical literature.[150,151]

Thus, A.G.'s usual SC insulin regimen should be discontinued, and she should be initiated on an insulin infusion that is adjusted according to an algorithm. Throughout the perioperative period, she should receive a minimum of 100 g glucose daily to prevent starvation ketosis.

Alternative Routes of Administration

34. W.C. is a 22-year-old male college student with type 1 diabetes, who is currently injecting multiple doses of insulin lispro throughout the day and insulin glargine at bedtime; however, he finds the traditional insulin injection process using vials and syringes time consuming and cumbersome. He would like to find an easier, more convenient, and more discreet way to inject his insulin while at school. What insulin delivery devices are

available for W.C.? What alternative routes of insulin delivery may be available for W.C. in the future?

PEN DEVICES AND PREFILLED SYRINGES

Pen devices and prefilled syringes eliminate the need to carry syringes and insulin vials separately. Insulin pens are available as prefilled pens, which are disposable, or reusable pens (referred to as durable pen devices). Prefilled pens contain a built-in, single-use insulin cartridge designed to deliver 300 units of insulin. Novolog and Humalog and their insulin mixtures (Novolog Mix 70/30, Humalog Mix 75/25, and Humalog Mix 50/50) are available in prefilled pens. Lilly has the KwikPen (1-U increments; 60-U maximum dose), which is easier to dial than their original prefilled pens that are still available (1-U increments; 60-U maximum dose). NovoNordisk has the Flexpen (1-U increments; 60-U maximum dose). Lantus insulin is available in a prefilled pen called SoloStar (1-U increments; 80-U maximum dose). Prefilled pens are helpful for patients who have difficulty handling the cartridges in reusable pens or for patients with busy schedules who prefer not to have to change cartridges.

Most durable pens use 3.0-mL cartridges, each holding 300 units. A 1.5-mL cartridge is available for some insulins, but these are used infrequently. A patient inserts an insulin cartridge into the pen's delivery chamber. This may allow greater flexibility for some patients, such as the ability to change the type of insulin injected without needing to purchase another pen if the insulin prescription changes. NovoNordisk makes the NovoPen Junior (0.5-unit increments; 35-units maximum dose) and the NovoPen 3 (1-unit increments; 70-units maximum dose). Lilly makes the HumaPen Luxura HD (0.5-unit increments; 30-units maximum dose) and the HumaPen Memoir (1-unit increments; 60-units maximum dose), which records and displays the last 16 insulin doses given. Sanofi-Aventis insulins (Lantus, Apidra) use the OptiClik pen device (1-unit increments; 80-units maximum dose), which unfortunately is only distributed to physicians (not to pharmacies). Patients are advised to use a new disposable needle for each injection. Pen needles are available in 29- to 31-guage and needle lengths of 3/16 inch (5 mm), 1/4 inch (6 mm), 5/16 inch (8 mm), and 1/2 inch (12.7 mm).

The pens are particularly useful for patients with (a) regimens consisting of multiple daily doses of rapid- or short-acting insulin before meals and snacks (such as W.C.), (b) a fear of needles, (c) impaired hand dexterity, (d) hectic work/lifestyle, or (e) for training alternate individuals who administer insulin (e.g., school nurses, siblings).

INSULIN PUMPS

Insulin pumps were discussed in Question 5 and have been reviewed elsewhere.[152]

INHALED INSULIN

Developing alternative routes for insulin delivery to avoid injections has been under investigation for several decades. Alternative routes evaluated include gastrointestinal (GI), intranasal, buccal, transdermal, and intrapulmonary. Inhalation of insulin via the lungs is ideal in that the insulin protein passes into the small alveoli, which has enormous surface area, high blood flow, and a thin membrane. Exubera, inhaled human (rDNA origin) and made by Pfizer received FDA approval in January 2006, but is no longer available. Pfizer decided to cease manufacturing due to its lack of use. Other inhaled insulin products may be approved in the future.

Adverse Effects of Insulin

Hypoglycemia

35. G.O., a 42-year-old, slightly overweight (5 feet 11 inches, 180 lbs) man, has had a history of type 1 diabetes mellitus for 17 years. G.O.'s medical care was sporadic until 1 year ago when he referred himself to a diabetes clinic because he was beginning to develop pain and numbness in his feet. At that time, he was poorly controlled on a single daily dose of 45 units Humulin 70/30. He had not been testing his blood glucose concentrations, and his HbA_{1c} was 13%.

On physical examination, G.O. was found to have an elevated BP (160/94 mmHg), background retinopathy, and decreased pedal pulses bilaterally. He had decreased sensation to vibration and monofilament testing in both feet. G.O. also complained of impotence and "shooting pains" in both legs. A spot collection for microalbuminuria was 450 mg of albumin/g creatinine (normal, 30–299 mg/g creatinine).

G.O. was transitioned to a basal-bolus insulin regimen. His physician gave him a premeal blood glucose target of 70 to 130 mg/dL.[22] Over the last several months, he has been treated with the following regimen: 14 to 18 units insulin glulisine before breakfast; 14 to 18 units insulin glulisine before lunch; 16 to 18 units insulin glulisine before dinner; and 40 units insulin glargine at bedtime. If his blood glucose level is high after lunch, he takes additional glulisine (~2 hours after eating). If his blood glucose is high at bedtime (e.g., >150 mg/dL), he takes additional insulin glulisine (7–10 units) because his doctor told him his blood glucose level needed to be lowered significantly. Blood glucose concentrations have been as follows.

Time	*Glucose Concentration (mg/dL)*
7 AM	60–320
Noon	140–280
5 PM	40–300

Over the past year, G.O.'s HbA_{1c} has decreased to 7.1%. Currently, he has approximately five hypoglycemic episodes per week, primarily in the late afternoon and evenings. These are characterized by intense hunger, sweating, palpitations, and (according to his wife) a short temper. He has found that he can avoid nocturnal hypoglycemia (night sweats, nightmares, and headaches) by eating a large bedtime snack. Over the past 3 months, he has gained 15 lb. Are G.O.'s signs and symptoms consistent with mild, moderate, or severe hypoglycemia? What are the causes?

[SI units: blood glucose 7 AM, 5.5–8.3 mmol/L; 12 PM, 15.5 mmol/L; 5 PM, 2.2–15.5 mmol/L; HbA_{1c}, 0.72]

G.O.'s case illustrates one of the major hazards of aggressive blood glucose targets and intensive insulin therapy: hypoglycemia. Hypoglycemia is a fact of life for patients with type 1 diabetes, virtually all of whom experience a hypoglycemic episode at one time or another. An estimated 4% of deaths related to type 1 diabetes are caused by hypoglycemia.[29,153,154]

Hypoglycemia is a blood glucose concentration below 60 mg/dL (<2.7 mmol/L), and its occurrence is potentially fatal if not promptly recognized and treated. However, the exact level at which a patient experiences symptoms is difficult to define. Clinical hypoglycemia is associated with typical autonomic (neurogenic) and neuroglycopenic symptoms relieved by the administration of a quickly absorbed carbohydrate.

PATHOPHYSIOLOGY

Normal brain function depends on glucose, the exclusive fuel for cerebral metabolism. Because the brain is unable to synthesize or store glucose, it must be provided with a constant exogenous quantity via the brain's blood supply. As blood glucose concentrations fall, a series of physiological responses occur to restore glucose levels. These responses create symptoms warning a patient to take corrective action by consuming carbohydrates. If these counter-regulatory responses fail to alert the patient and blood glucose concentrations fall below a critical level, cognitive function becomes impaired and confusion and coma may ensue.

In people without diabetes, the peripheral responses to hypoglycemia are so efficient that clinically important hypoglycemia probably never occurs. As glucose levels fall between 50 and 60 mg/dL (2.7–3.3 mmol/L), a series of neuroendocrine events occur, raising the plasma glucose concentration back toward normal by increasing hepatic glucose output. The major hormone responsible for producing acute recovery from insulin-induced hypoglycemia is glucagon; however, epinephrine alone also can produce near-normal recovery. Rising levels of adrenergic and cholinergic hormones generate warning symptoms of hypoglycemia. When hypoglycemia is prolonged, growth hormone and cortisone play a greater role in producing recovery.

Patients with type 1 diabetes who maintain insulin depots throughout the day are predisposed to severe hypoglycemic reactions because deficiencies in the normal feedback system occur over time. Glucagon secretion becomes deficient within the first 2 to 5 years after diagnosis, and by 10 years or longer, epinephrine secretion may become impaired. The latter defect leads to asymptomatic hypoglycemia or hypoglycemic unawareness (see Question 38).

Certain circumstances predispose patients with type 1 diabetes to severe hypoglycemia. These include (a) a defective counter-regulatory hormonal response to hypoglycemia (see Question 38), which may be further diminished with frequent hypoglycemia, (b) medications such as β-blockers that diminish early warning signs of impending hypoglycemia, (c) intensive insulin therapy that can alter secretion of counter-regulatory hormones, (d) skipped meals or inadequate carbohydrate intake relative to the insulin dose, (e) physical activity, and (e) excessive alcohol intake (Table 50-14).

SYMPTOMS

The signs and symptoms associated with hypoglycemia vary in intensity according to the presence of cognitive deficits and the patient's ability to self-treat the reaction. They vary substantially from one patient to another. Symptoms are conventionally divided into two categories: neurogenic (or autonomic) and neuroglycopenic.[153]

Autonomic symptoms include sweating, intense hunger, palpitations, tremor, tingling, and anxiety. Epinephrine is thought to mediate many of the neurogenic responses to hypoglycemia.

Neuroglycopenic symptoms resulting from neuronal fuel deprivation (glucose) include difficulty concentrating; lethargy; confusion; agitation; weakness; and possibly, slurred speech, dizziness, and fainting. Profound behavioral changes, seizures, and coma are more severe manifestations of neuroglycopenia. Prolonged, severe neuroglycopenia ultimately results in death. Symptoms of mild, moderate, severe, and nocturnal hypoglycemia are as follows:

- *Mild hypoglycemia*: Symptoms include tremor, palpitations, sweating, and intense hunger. Diminished cerebral function is not present and patients are capable of self-treating mild reactions.
- *Moderate hypoglycemia*: Moderate hypoglycemic reactions include neuroglycopenic as well as autonomic symptoms: headache, mood changes, irritability, decreased attention, and drowsiness. Patients may require assistance in treating themselves because of the presence of impaired judgment or weakness. Symptoms are more severe, usually last longer, and often require a second dose of a simple carbohydrate.
- *Severe hypoglycemia*: Symptoms of severe hypoglycemia include unresponsiveness, unconsciousness, or convulsions. These reactions require assistance from another individual for appropriate treatment. Approximately 10% of patients treated with insulin develop at least one severe, disabling episode of hypoglycemia per year that requires emergency treatment with parenteral glucagon or IV glucose.[153]
- *Nocturnal hypoglycemia*: Tingling of the lips and tongue are common complaints of patients who develop nocturnal hypoglycemia. These patients also may complain of headache and difficulty arising in the morning, nightmares, or nocturnal diaphoresis.[153] Family members should be conscious of any unusual sounds or activity while the patient is sleeping.

G.O. has mild to moderate hypoglycemic reactions, which he is able to self-treat. These are likely due to overinsulinization and insulin "stacking" with his rapid-acting insulin.

Overinsulinization

36. Evaluate G.O.'s overall control. What signs and symptoms in G.O. are consistent with overinsulinization and insulin "stacking"? How should he be managed?

The following is a list of signs and symptoms of overinsulinization in G.O.:

- A total daily insulin dose of more than 1.0 unit/kg. This dose is unusually high for a patient with type 1 diabetes, who should not be resistant to the action of insulin.
- Weight gain over the past several months. This is secondary to the anabolic effects of insulin as well as G.O.'s increased carbohydrate intake to match his high insulin doses or treatment of hypoglycemia.
- Frequent hypoglycemic reactions.
- High glycemic variability (i.e., blood glucose concentrations that fluctuate wildly between hypoglycemia and hyperglycemia). In G.O.'s case, high blood glucose concentrations may represent reactive hyperglycemia or overtreatment of hypoglycemic episodes. His low blood glucose level may represent excessive rapid-acting insulin at bedtime and insulin "stacking" of his rapid-acting insulin after lunch. At lunchtime, he is administering a high sugar correction dose

of insulin glulisine too soon; his mealtime glulisine is still likely at a peak action and working to lower his prandial blood glucose. By administering additional glulisine soon after the meal, the two insulin doses are adding up, or "stacking," causing hypoglycemia.

- Near-normal HbA_{1c} levels indicate mean blood glucose concentrations that must be within the normal range even though the patient has recorded numerous high blood glucose concentrations. Patients treated with intensive insulin therapy in the DCCT experienced hypoglycemic episodes three times more often than patients treated with standard insulin therapy.[29] HbA_{1c} levels were approximately 7.2%.

G.O. should be managed by discontinuing his high sugar corrections at bedtime and after lunch. He should SMBG premeal, 1 to 2 hours after meals, and at bedtime to obtain a better picture of his glucose patterns and insulin requirements. He should avoid the large bedtime snack. He should also begin testing his blood glucose at 2 or 3 AM to assess if he is still experiencing nocturnal hypoglycemia after stopping the bedtime insulin glulisine. It will be important that he record the actual dose he administers before each meal and bring the record to clinic so that his insulin doses can be fine tuned. Next, if he is capable, an algorithm for adjusting his preprandial insulin glulisine doses should be provided to minimize hypoglycemic and hyperglycemic reactions (see Question 14), eventually he can transition to counting carbohydrates (see Question 13).

Treatment of Hypoglycemia

37. How should G.O.'s hypoglycemic episodes be managed?

As G.O. illustrates, many patients with diabetes are frightened of hypoglycemia and have a tendency to overtreat their reactions with, for example, large quantities of juice or several candy bars. This should be discouraged because overcorrection together with glucose generated by counter-regulatory hormones ultimately results in hyperglycemia.

The key to successful management of hypoglycemia is recognition and prevention. Because early warning symptoms of hypoglycemia vary from person to person, it is important that G.O. study and learn to recognize his earliest warning symptoms and treat early. Patients generally can recall prodromal symptoms after recovery from a severe hypoglycemic reaction if they have not developed hypoglycemic unawareness (see Question 38). As a caveat, these authors occasionally have seen patients who "feel" hypoglycemic after their blood glucose concentrations have been normalized from very high levels with intensive insulin therapy. We encourage patients to test their blood glucose level any time they "feel unusual" to verify a low blood glucose concentration before treatment. G.O. should treat his symptoms only if he is truly hypoglycemic.

A second component of prevention is determining its cause and taking preventive or corrective action. This entails assessment of his diet (did he skip or delay a meal or change its content?), exercise pattern, time of insulin administration, insulin dose, and accuracy of dose administered. If hypoglycemic reactions consistently occur at a certain time of day, he should determine whether this corresponds with a mealtime dose of his rapid-acting insulin and reduce that insulin dose by 1 to 2 U. If his FBG is running low, his Lantus insulin dose can be reduced.

If a reaction occurs, G.O. should be instructed to treat it as follows (Table 50-14).

MILD HYPOGLYCEMIA

Most hypoglycemic reactions are managed readily with the equivalent of 10 to 20 g of glucose (see Table 50-14 for examples of carbohydrate sources containing 15 g of glucose). If the blood concentration remains low after 15 minutes, the patient should ingest another 10 to 20 g of carbohydrate. This quick-acting source of glucose should be followed by a small complex carbohydrate or protein snack (e.g., milk, peanut butter sandwich) to provide a continual source of glucose if a meal is not scheduled within the next 1 to 2 hours. An easy rule of thumb that can be used by patients is "15-15-15": 15 g of glucose followed by a second 15 g if the patient is still symptomatic after 15 minutes.

Glucose tablets are available and have the added benefit of being premeasured to prevent overtreatment of hypoglycemia. Glucose gels or small tubes of cake frosting are useful for children or patients who become uncooperative and combative when hypoglycemic.

MODERATE TO SEVERE HYPOGLYCEMIA

Glucagon can be injected by the SC or intramuscular (IM) route into the deltoid or anterior thigh region. Glucagon is used when a patient is unable to self-treat their hypoglycemia. The dose of glucagon recommended to treat moderate or severe hypoglycemia for a child younger than 5 years of age is 0.25 to 0.5 mg; for children 5 to 10 years of age, 0.5 to 1 mg; and for patients older than 10 years, 1 mg. Parents, spouses, or other close contacts should be taught how to mix, draw up, and administer glucagon during emergency situations. Kits with prefilled syringes containing 1 mg glucagon are available. Patients who are given glucagon should be positioned so that their face is turned toward the floor to prevent aspiration in the event of vomiting. As soon as the patient awakens (10–25 minutes), he or she should be fed.

Intravenous Glucose

If glucagon is unavailable, the patient should be taken to the hospital's emergency department, where he or she can be treated with IV glucose (~10–25 g administered as 20–50 mL of 50% dextrose over 1–3 minutes) in preference to glucagon. Following the bolus injection of glucose, IV glucose (5–10 g/hour) should be continued until the patient has gained consciousness and is able to eat.

Hypoglycemic Unawareness

38. M.M., a 35-year-old, 75-kg, unemployed man, has had type 1 diabetes since the age of 3. As a consequence of the diabetes, he has developed proliferative retinopathy and progressive diabetic nephropathy (current SrCr, 3.0 mg/dL). M.M. has an erratic lifestyle. Because he does not work, he often stays out late at night and sleeps late into the morning. His insulin is injected whenever he awakens, and his meals are irregularly spaced. Each time he comes to the clinic, he brings with him a complete log of glucose concentrations that range from 80 to 140 mg/dL. He has two to three severe hypoglycemic reactions a month that require emergency treatment with IV glucose. On several occasions, his blood

glucose concentration has been 30 mg/dL and he states he may feel a little weak, but otherwise feels "not too bad." M.M.'s last HbA_{1c} was 10%. He says that he adheres to the following insulin regimen: 18 units NPH/11 units regular insulin before breakfast, 10 units regular insulin before lunch and dinner, and 14 units NPH at bedtime.

At this visit, M.M. comes with his girlfriend. He has a large gash on his nose that occurred 3 days ago when he lost consciousness at approximately 1:30 PM while pushing his stalled car. He was unable to eat lunch at the usual hour because he had problems with his car. Assess M.M.'s hypoglycemic reactions and blood glucose control. Should his current insulin regimen be continued? How should he be managed?

[SI units: SrCr, 265 μmol/L; blood glucose, 4.4–7.8 mmol/L; HbA_{1c}, 0.10]

M.M. illustrates a patient with type 1 diabetes who has defective glucose counter-regulation and, as a result, is unable to counteract a hypoglycemic reaction effectively. He also is an example of a patient who should not have aggressive blood glucose targets because he does not feel the symptoms of a low blood sugar and has already developed end-stage organ damage (proliferative retinopathy and nephropathy). Neither are likely to be reversed with improved glycemic control. In fact, proliferative retinopathy may actually worsen with intensive insulin therapy initially.[29] In the DCCT study, severe hypoglycemic reactions were three times more common among patients treated with intensive insulin therapy, and nocturnal hypoglycemia accounted for 41% of the total hypoglycemic episodes.[29] In patients with defective counter-regulation, the risk of severe hypoglycemia may be 25 times higher than in patients with adequate counter-regulatory mechanisms treated with intensive insulin therapy.[153] M.M. is at great risk for death secondary to hypoglycemia.

M.M.'s lifestyle is erratic, he eats irregularly, and his reported blood glucose concentrations (80–140 mg/dL) do not correspond to his elevated HbA_{1c} value. This may indicate that M.M.'s technique is incorrect or that he simply fills in the log with fictitious numbers before he comes to the clinic. Irregular entries in different colored inks and blood stains usually indicate authentic records.

As noted, the primary hormones that are secreted in response to a low blood glucose concentration are glucagon and epinephrine. In patients who have had type 1 diabetes for longer than 2 to 5 years, a deficiency in glucagon secretion is a relatively consistent finding, and these patients must rely on epinephrine to reverse low blood glucose concentrations. Unfortunately, approximately 40% of patients with long-standing type 1 diabetes (8–15 years) have defective epinephrine secretion as well, and this may be related to the development of autonomic neuropathy. Patients whose diabetes is tightly controlled also have reduced counter-regulatory hormone responses to hypoglycemia. As illustrated by M.M., patients with defective epinephrine secretory responses also lose the warning signs and symptoms of hypoglycemia. These patients are said to have "hypoglycemia unawareness" because they have no awareness of blood glucose concentrations below 50 mg/dL. In these individuals, loss of consciousness, seizures, or irrational behavior may be the first objective signs of exceedingly low blood glucose concentrations. The glycemic threshold for symptoms also is lowered in patients on intensive insulin therapy whose glucose concentrations have been lowered to normal or near-normal levels.[153] Consequently, their hypoglycemic reactions may go unnoticed and untreated until they lose consciousness. M.M. should be managed as follows.

- Because his waking, sleeping, and eating patterns are highly irregular, M.M. should be treated with an insulin regimen that addresses his lifestyle. For example, he could be instructed to give himself a rapid-acting insulin just before he actually intends to eat. A dose of insulin glargine or detemir could be given before his first meal to supply a basal level of insulin between meals.
- Because M.M. has no warning symptoms for hypoglycemia, the importance of regular blood glucose testing should be emphasized. When blood glucose testing was reviewed with M.M., it was discovered that his eyesight was so poor that he was unable to distinguish between the right and wrong side of the glucose test strip. Furthermore, because he had lost his depth of field, he was unable to apply the drop of blood into the test strip. To address this situation, M.M.'s girlfriend was taught how to perform blood glucose testing. Also, a glucose monitor that requires a very small blood sample and beeps with an adequate blood sample (e.g., Abbott Freestyle Freedom) was provided to him.
- M.M.'s girlfriend also was taught how to recognize and treat symptoms of hypoglycemia. Often, patients ignore early warning symptoms and progress to a point that they lose the judgment needed to treat the condition. If M.M. has not yet become combative, a quick-acting carbohydrate source should be offered. If he has lost consciousness, glucagon should be injected.

All of these maneuvers diminished the frequency of M.M.'s severe hypoglycemic reactions. On the whole, his blood glucose concentrations were maintained below 180 mg/dL, and he remained relatively free of hyperglycemic symptoms. M.M.'s HbA_{1c} using this insulin regimen was 8.0%.

DIABETIC KETOACIDOSIS

39. J.L., a 25-year-old, 60-kg woman with an 8-year history of type 1 diabetes, is moderately well controlled on 24 units insulin glargine plus premeal doses of insulin lispro. Her family brings her to the emergency department, where she complains of abdominal tenderness, nausea, and vomiting. According to her family, J.L. was well until 2 days ago when she awoke with nausea, vomiting, diarrhea, and chills. Because she was unable to eat, she omitted her usual morning dose of insulin. Her GI symptoms progressed, and she was brought to the emergency department when she became lethargic.

Physical examination reveals an ill-appearing woman who is lethargic but responsive. Her temperature is 37°C. Skin turgor is poor, mucous membranes are dry, and her eyeballs are shrunken and soft. J.L.'s lungs are clear, but respirations are deep and her breath has a fruity odor. Cardiac examination is within normal limits.

In the supine position, J.L.'s pulse rate is 115 beats/minute (normal, 60–100) and her BP is 105/60 mmHg. In the upright position, her pulse increased to 140 beats/minute, and her BP dropped to 85/40 mmHg. There is mild, diffuse tenderness over her abdomen.

Laboratory results on admission disclosed the following: blood glucose, 750 mg/dL; sodium (Na), 148 mEq/L (normal, 135–147); potassium (K), 5.4 mEq/L (normal, 3.5–5.0); chlorine (Cl),

106 mEq/L (normal, 95–105); HCO_3, 6 mEq/L (normal, 22–28); SrCr, 2.0 mg/dL (normal, 0.6–1.2); hemoglobin, 14.7 g/dL (normal, 11.5–15.5); hematocrit, 49% (normal, 33%–43%); white blood cell (WBC) count, 15,000/mm^3 (normal, 3,200–9,800) with 3% bands (normal, 3%–5%), 70% polymorphonuclear neutrophils (normal, 54%–62%), and 27% lymphocytes (normal, 25%–33%); serum ketones were moderate at 1:10 dilution (normal, negative). The urinalysis showed 2% glucose (normal, 0); moderate ketones (normal, 0); pH, 5.5 (normal, 4.6–8); and a specific gravity of 1.029 (normal, 1.020–1.025); there were no WBCs, RBCs, bacteria, or casts. Arterial blood gas results were as follows: pH, 7.05 (normal, 7.36–7.44); Pco_2, 20 mmHg (normal, 35–45); Po_2, 120 mmHg (normal, 90–100). What supports the diagnosis of DKA in J.L.?

[SI units: blood glucose, 41.6 mmol/L; Na, 148 mmol/L; K, 5.4 mmol/L; Cl, 106 mmol/L; HCO_3, 6 mmol/L; SrCr, 176.8 μmol/L; hemoglobin, 147 g/L; hematocrit, 0.49; WBC count, 15 × 10^8/L with 0.03 bands; polymorphonuclear neutrophils, 0.70; lymphocytes, 0.27; Pco_2, 2.6 kPa; Po_2, 16.0 kPa]

The fact that J.L. has type 1 diabetes puts her at risk for developing ketoacidosis. An absolute or relative insulin deficiency promotes lipolysis and metabolism of free fatty acids to β-hydroxybutyrate, acetoacetic acid, and acetone in the liver. Excess glucagon enhances gluconeogenesis and impairs peripheral ketone utilization. Stress can contribute to the development of DKA by stimulating release of insulin counterregulatory hormones such as glucagon, catecholamines, glucocorticoids, and growth hormone. Common stress factors include infection, pregnancy, pancreatitis, trauma, hyperthyroidism, and acute MI.

J.L. presented with symptoms of nausea, vomiting, diarrhea, and chills, and these are suggestive of an acute viral gastroenteritis. Patients such as J.L. commonly discontinue their insulin in this setting, which further predisposes them to the development of DKA (see Question 30). Table 50-23 lists patient education points with regard to DKA.

As illustrated by J.L., patients with DKA present with moderate to high serum glucose concentrations secondary to decreased peripheral utilization and increased hepatic production (Table 50-24). This increases serum osmolality, which initially shifts fluid from the intracellular to the extracellular space. When glucose concentrations exceed the renal threshold, osmotic diuresis ensues and water, sodium, potassium, and other electrolytes are depleted. J.L. also has lost fluid and electrolytes from vomiting and diarrhea. Eventually, as losses exceed input, the patient becomes dehydrated (dry mucous membranes; dry skin; soft, shrunken eyeballs; increased hematocrit) and intravascular volume becomes depleted (orthostatic BP and pulse changes).

Evidence of excessive ketone production in J.L. includes ketonuria, ketonemia, and the characteristic fruity odor of acetone on the breath. Elevated levels of these organic acids increase the anion gap and decrease the pH and carbonate levels. The respiratory rate is increased to compensate for the metabolic acidosis leading to hypercapnia.[114,155]

Treatment

40. How should J.L. be treated?

Treatment of patients with DKA is aimed at expansion of intravascular and extravascular volume, restoration of renal perfusions, correction of dehydration, fluid and electrolyte losses, and hyperosmolarity (hyperglycemia; Table 50-25).

Fluids

Rapid correction of fluid loss is most crucial. The usual fluid deficit approximates 6 to 10 L or 10% of body weight in most patients with DKA. In the absence of cardiac compromise, hypernatremia or significant renal dysfunction, isotonic saline (0.9% NaCl) should be used.[114]

Table 50-23 Diabetic Ketoacidosis: Patient Education

Definition: DKA occurs when the body has insufficient insulin.

Questions to Ask

1. Has insulin use been discontinued or a dose skipped for any reason?
2. If an insulin pump is being used, is the tubing clogged or twisted? Has the catheter become dislodged?
3. Has the insulin being used lost its activity? Is the bottle of rapid-acting/regular or basal insulin cloudy? Does the bottle of NPH look frosty?
4. Have insulin requirements increased owing to illness or other forms of stress (infection, pregnancy, pancreatitis, trauma, hyperthyroidism, or MI)?

What to Look For

1. Signs and symptoms of hyperglycemia: thirst, excessive urination, fatigue, blurred vision, consistently elevated blood glucose concentrations (>300 mg/dL)
2. Signs of acidosis: fruity breath odor, deep and difficult breathing
3. Signs of dehydration: dry mouth; warm, dry skin; fatigue
4. Others: stomach pain, nausea, vomiting, loss of appetite

What to Do

1. Review "Sick Day Management" (Table 50-22)
2. Test blood glucose ≥4 times daily
3. Test urine for ketones when blood glucose concentration is >300 mg/dL
4. Drink plenty of fluids (water, clear soups)
5. Continue taking insulin dose
6. Contact physician immediately

Table 50-24 Common Laboratory Abnormalities in Diabetic Ketoacidosis

Glucose	>250 mg/dL
Serum osmolarity	Variable, can be >320 mOsm/kg in presence of coma
Sodium	Low, normal, or high[a]
Potassium	Normal or high
Ketones	Present in urine and blood
pH	Mild: 7.25–7.30 Moderate: 7.00–7.24 Severe: <7.00
Bicarbonate	Mild: 15–18 Moderate: 10 to <15 Severe: <10
WBC count	15,000–40,000 cells/mm even without evidence of infection

[a] Total body sodium is always low.
DKA, diabetic ketoacidosis; WBC, white blood cell.

Table 50-25 Management of Diabetic Ketoacidosis[114]

Fluid Administration
Start IV fluids using normal saline (0.9% NaCl) unless patient has cardiac compromise.
Rate is 15–20 mL/kg body weight or 1–1.5 L during first hour
Then, if corrected sodium is normal or elevated, use 0.45% NS at a rate of 4–14 mL/kg/hr (250–500 mL/hr). Use 0.9% NS if corrected sodium is low.
Once serum glucose reaches 200 mg/dL, change to 5% dextrose with 0.45% NaCl at 150–250 mL/hr.
Insulin
Continuous IV infusion of regular insulin is preferred. Use IM route only if infusion is not available.
Bolus dose: 0.1 unit/kg IV
Maintenance dose: 0.1 unit/kg/hr IV
If blood glucose level has not decreased by 50–75 mg/dL after 1 hr, double infusion rate.
Once blood glucose reaches 200 mg/dL, reduce infusion rate to 0.05–0.1 unit/kg/hr and change fluid to 5% dextrose with 0.45% NaCl (do not stop insulin infusion).
When SC insulin can be initiated, administer dose 1–2 hr before discontinuing IV infusion.
For uncomplicated DKA, SC rapid-acting insulin can be considered. A bolus dose of 0.2 unit/kg followed by 0.1 unit/kg every hour *or* an initial dose of 0.3 unit/kg followed by 0.2 unit/kg Q 2 hr until the blood glucose reaches <250 mg/dL; then the SC insulin dose is decreased by half (to either 0.05 or 0.1 unit/kg every 1–2 hr).
Potassium
Establish adequate renal function (urine output ~50 mL/hr). If K is <3.3 mEq/L, hold insulin and give 20–40 mEq/hr until K >3.3 mEq/L. If K is >5.5mEq/L, do not give K and check serum K Q 2 hr. If K is >3.3 but <5.3 mEq/L, give 20–30 mEq in each liter IV fluid to maintain K between 4–5 mEq/L.
Phosphate
Initiate if level <1 mg/dL, or in patients with cardiac dysfunction, anemia, or respiratory depression. Use potassium phosphate salt, 20–30 mEq added to replacement fluid. Rarely needed.
Bicarbonate
Replacement is controversial and may be dangerous.
For adults with pH <6.9, 100 mmol sodium bicarbonate may be added to 400 mL sterile water with 20 mEq KCl; infuse over 2 hr (200 mL/hr). For adults with pH of 6. 9–7.0, 50 mmol sodium bicarbonate diluted in 200 mL sterile water with 10 mEq KCL; infuse over 1 hr (200 mL/hr). No bicarbonate is necessary if pH >7.0.

NS, normal saline.

J.L. has evidence of significant dehydration and intravascular volume depletion. A rough calculation indicates that approximately 6 to 7 L will be needed (10% of body weight). It is recommended that fluids be replaced at the rate of 15 to 20 mL/kg/hour during the first hour (~1 to 1.5 L in the average adult). The subsequent choice for fluid replacement depends on the patient's state of hydration, serum electrolyte levels, and urinary output. If the corrected sodium is normal or elevated, 0.45% NaCl infused at a rate of 4 to 14 mL/kg/hour is appropriate. If the corrected serum sodium is low, 0.9% NaCl is preferred.[114] When serum glucose concentrations approach 200, solutions should be changed to 5% glucose in half-normal saline. Glucose is added to prevent hypoglycemia and the cerebral edema that can occur if the osmolality is reduced too rapidly. The use of dextrose also allows for continued insulin administration that is required to resolve the ketoacidosis (see Question 41). These recommendations for fluid replacement must be adjusted in the elderly or those with compromised renal or myocardial function. In these patients, fluid administration must be titrated against the central venous pressure.[114,155]

Sodium

Total body sodium usually is depleted by 7 to 10 mEq/kg of body weight in patients with DKA. In assessing serum sodium in these patients, it is important to remember that falsely low values (i.e., pseudohyponatremia) may be the result of hyperglycemia and hypertriglyceridemia. A corrected sodium value can be estimated by adding 1.6 mEq/L to the observed sodium value for every 100 mg/dL glucose >100 mg/dL. Sodium is replaced adequately with normal saline.[114]

Potassium

Potassium balance is altered markedly in patients with DKA because of combined urinary and GI losses. Invariably, total potassium is depleted; however, the serum potassium concentration may be high, normal, or low, depending on the degree of acidosis and volume contraction. Usual potassium deficits in this situation average 3 to 5 mEq/kg of body weight, although they may be as high as 10 mEq/kg.[114,155]

Thus, J.L. needs approximately 200 to 350 mEq of potassium to replenish her body stores, assuming her normal weight is 70 kg. To prevent hypokalemia, potassium replacement should be started after her serum potassium concentrations decreases to <5.3 mEq/L (assuming an adequate urine output of 50 mL/hour). Generally IV solutions containing 20 to 30 mEq/L are sufficient to maintain the serum potassium between 4 and 5 mEq/L. However, in cases with low serum potassium (<3.3 mEq/L) at presentation, potassium replacement should be initiated with fluid therapy, and insulin therapy delayed until the potassium level is >3.3 mEq/L to avoid cardiac arrest, arrhythmias, and respiratory muscle weakness. In these cases, initial IV solutions should contain KCl 20 to 30 mEq/L.

Phosphate

Routine use of phosphate in the treatment of DKA has resulted in no clinical benefit to patients.[114] Phosphate is lost as the result of increased tissue catabolism, impaired cellular uptake, and enhanced renal excretion. Like other electrolytes, serum levels initially may seem normal, even though body stores are depleted. Overzealous replacement can result in severe hypocalcemia. Hypophosphatemia can cause cardiac and skeletal muscle weakness and respiratory depression. To avoid this, phosphate can be carefully replaced in patients with cardiac dysfunction, anemia, respiratory depression, and those with phosphate concentrations below 1.0 mg/dL. Potassium phosphate can be added to the replacement fluids in the amount of 20 to 30 mEq/L.

Insulin

41. What is an appropriate insulin dose and route of administration for J.L.?

Unless the episode of DKA is mild (pH 7.25–7.30) and uncomplicated, regular insulin by continuous infusion is the treatment of choice. Once hypokalemia (K^+ <3.3 mEq/L) is excluded, an IV bolus of regular insulin at 0.1 unit/kg followed by a continuous infusion at a dose of 0.1 unit/kg/hour should be administered. This should decrease the plasma glucose at a rate of 50 to 75 mg/dL/hour. If this does not occur in the first hour, then the rate may be doubled every hour until a steady glucose decline is achieved. Once the plasma glucose reaches 200 mg/dL, the insulin infusion can be decreased to 0.05 to 0.1 unit/kg/hour. At this point, dextrose should be added to the IV fluids (i.e., fluids changed to D_5W with 0.45% NaCl). Thereafter, the rate of insulin administration or the concentration of dextrose is adjusted to maintain the glucose value at around 200 mg/dL until the acidosis is resolved.[114] Thus, for J.L., an IV bolus dose of 6 units followed by an infusion rate of 6 units/hour is appropriate.

For uncomplicated DKA, SC rapid-acting insulin has been studied with no differences in patient outcomes. The advantage is that patients can be treated in a non-ICU setting, thus reducing hospital costs. The dosing for rapid-acting insulin is included in Table 50-25.

Sodium Bicarbonate

42. J.L. was treated with fluids, electrolytes, and insulin as discussed in previous questions. Laboratory and clinical data 4 hours after therapy are as follows: pH, 7.1; blood glucose, 400 mg/dL; K, 3.8 mEq/L; SrCr, 3.1 mg/dL; and serum ketones strongly positive at a 1:40 dilution. Her BP was 120/70 mmHg with no orthostatic changes. Urine output over the last 3 hours has been 500 mL. Because serum ketones have increased, should J.L. receive more insulin? Should she receive bicarbonate therapy?

[SI units: blood glucose, 22 mmol/L; K, 3.8 mmol/L; SrCr, 274 μmol/L]

The assumption that ketosis is worse in J.L. is incorrect. In DKA, low levels of insulin and elevated glucagon levels promote the metabolism of free fatty acids in the liver to acetoacetate and β-hydroxybutyrate. The standard nitroprusside reaction test for ketones measures only acetoacetate, even though β-hydroxybutyrate is the more important ketone. The conversion of acetoacetic acid to β-hydroxybutyrate is coupled closely with the NADH:NAD ratio. If this ratio is high (as in the presence of alcohol) so much β-hydroxybutyrate may be formed that acetoacetate is virtually undetectable; thus, the absence of ketones in the serum does not rule out ketoacidosis.

Conversely, treatment with insulin begins to suppress lipolysis and fatty acid oxidation; NAD is regenerated shifting the reaction back in favor of acetoacetate.[114,155] Thus, even though there seems to be higher concentrations of ketones in the serum, J.L.'s declining blood glucose concentration, improved bicarbonate concentrations, and improved acid–base and cardiovascular responses indicate that she is responding appropriately. Therefore, no change in the insulin dose is indicated. It is important to emphasize that the glucose concentrations normalize before ketones (4–6 hours vs. 6–12 hours) because the latter are metabolized more slowly. For this reason, it is important to continue insulin to maintain suppression of lipolysis until plasma and urine ketones have cleared.

The use of bicarbonate in patients with DKA has been controversial.[114] Most investigators discourage its routine use, reserving it for patients with severe acidemia (pH <7.0) or those in clinical shock. Coma is correlated most closely with blood glucose concentrations (>700 mg/dL) and hyperosmolality (calculated osmolality >340 mOsm/kg).[114] In a randomized, prospective study, bicarbonate did not affect recovery in patients with severe DKA (arterial pH, 6.9–7.14).[156] Thus, even though J.L.'s acidosis seemed severe on admission (pH, 7.05; bicarbonate, 6 mEq/L; Kussmaul respirations), bicarbonate was not administered. It is apparent that with fluid and insulin therapy alone, her acidosis is beginning to improve.

43. What is the expected course of DKA in J.L.?

After 3 L of fluid and a constant insulin infusion of 6 units/hour for 3 hours, J.L.'s glucose concentration had dropped to 400 mg/dL and she had no orthostatic BP changes, reflecting recovery from her volume-depleted status. Potassium (40 mEq/L) was added to her fluids, which were administered at a reduced rate of 300 mL/hour.

Three hours later, the glucose concentration had dropped to 350 mg/dL and her pH had increased to 7.21. The serum potassium remained low-normal at 3.4 mEq/L, and serum sodium increased to 151 mEq/L. In view of these changes, the IV infusion fluid was changed to half-normal saline with 5% dextrose to which 40 mEq/L of potassium was added. The rate was slowed to 250 mL/hour, and the insulin infusion was continued at 6 units/hour.

Four hours later (10 hours after admission), the blood glucose was 205 mg/dL and the serum potassium was 3.5 mEq/dL. The IV fluids were changed to 5% dextrose with 40 mEq/L of KCl, administered at a rate of 250 mL/hour, and the regular insulin infusion was decreased from 6 to 3 units/hour. J.L. continued to improve over the next 12 hours, and she began taking full oral liquids by the second hospital day. At that time, her IV infusion rate was decreased to 200 mL/hour, but her insulin infusion was continued.

Approximately 24 hours after admission, J.L.'s blood glucose concentration was 175 mg/dL, potassium was 4.6 mEq/L, and sodium was 144 mEq/L. There were no ketones in the plasma. The urine contained 1% glucose and moderate amounts of ketones. IV fluids were discontinued and a rapid-acting insulin was administered subcutaneously 1 hour before the insulin infusion was discontinued. J.L. continued to receive rapid-acting insulin subcutaneously every 4 hours according to a sliding scale (see Question 14). Thirty-six hours after admission, J.L. was given her usual dose of insulin glargine and insulin lispro and was sent home for follow-up in the clinic.

TREATMENT OF TYPE 2 DIABETES: ANTIDIABETIC AGENTS

Type 2 diabetes must be managed in the context of the metabolic syndrome. At the time of diagnosis, many people with type 2 diabetes already have evidence of macrovascular and microvascular disease. Every effort to lower glucose concentrations toward normal values, control BP, and lower cholesterol is important to delay the onset or slow the progression of these complications, improve the overall quality of the patient's life, and save the health care system millions of dollars in hospitalization costs to treat these complications. MNT, physical activity, and other lifestyle changes are cornerstones in treating of people with type 2 diabetes. Unfortunately, these measures alone are usually not successful in achieving control for the majority of patients, and drug therapy is eventually

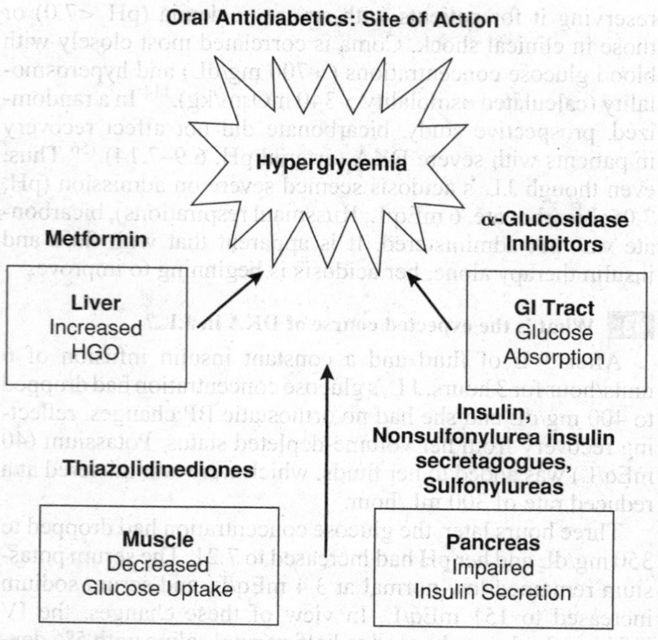

FIGURE 50-7 Sources of hyperglycemia in type 2 diabetes and site of action of oral antidiabetic agents. GI, gastrointestinal; HGO, hepatic glucose output.

required. Because these patients also often require a number of medications to treat related conditions (e.g., hypertension, hypercholesterolemia, and depression) and may also be medicating themselves with over-the-counter drugs, herbal products, and/or nutritional supplements, the aim of therapy for type 2 diabetes should be the simplest and safest regimen that provides the best glycemic control possible.

Figure 50-7 depicts the sources of hyperglycemia in people with type 2 diabetes and the primary site of action for each class of agents. Table 50-26 and Table 50-27 summarize the comparative pharmacology, pharmacokinetics, and dosing of the non-insulin antidiabetic drugs. The clinical use of these agents in specific situations is illustrated in cases presented later in this chapter.

Biguanides

Metformin (Glucophage) belongs to the biguanide class of oral antidiabetic agents. It has been available in the United States since 1995 and became generically available in 2002. The clinical pharmacology of metformin has been extensively reviewed.[157]

Mechanism of Action[157]

The biguanides are described more accurately as antihyperglycemic agents. Although they lower blood glucose concentrations in people with type 2 diabetes, they do not cause hypoglycemia in nondiabetic individuals. The precise mechanisms by which metformin lowers blood glucose concentrations remain to be elucidated. Evidence suggests metformin lowers FPG concentrations by decreasing hepatic gluconeogenesis and increasing insulin-stimulated glucose uptake by skeletal muscle and adipose tissue. Metformin also lowers plasma free fatty acid levels and subsequent oxidation. This observation may explain its ability to reduce hepatic glucose production and increase insulin-mediated glucose disposal in the muscle. Metformin also slightly lowers total cholesterol (5%–10%) and triglycerides (10%–20%) and may maintain or improve high-density lipoprotein (HDL) cholesterol levels.[158] The observed effects on lipid metabolism as well as others on clotting factors, platelet function, and vascular function have generated interest in the potential favorable effects of metformin on CVD and outcomes. Unlike the sulfonylureas, thiazolidinediones (TZDs), and insulin, weight loss rather than weight gain is more likely to occur with metformin therapy (mean weight loss of 1.2 kg compared with 1.7 kg increase).[159]

Pharmacokinetics

Approximately 50% to 60% of metformin is absorbed from the small intestine. It is eliminated entirely by the kidney unchanged and has a plasma half-life of 6.2 hours and a whole blood half-life of 17.6 hours. It is not bound to plasma proteins.[158,160]

Adverse Effects

GASTROINTESTINAL EFFECTS

Transient side effects include diarrhea and other GI disturbances such as nausea, abdominal discomfort, metallic taste, and anorexia.[158] Relative to placebo, diarrhea is the most common GI complaint (53.2% metformin vs 11.7% placebo-treated patients). Symptoms can be minimized by taking metformin with food and slowly titrating the dose. To enhance adherence to therapy, patients should be informed of the possibility of GI side effects that will likely subside with time and instructed to discuss any suspected side effects with their provider before discontinuing therapy (see Question 47).

LACTIC ACIDOSIS

Much of the perceived risk of lactic acidosis secondary to metformin use is based on historical data for phenformin, a biguanide that was withdrawn from the market in 1977.[161] The risk of lactic acidosis secondary to metformin is 10 to 20 times lower than with phenformin.[157] Unlike phenformin, metformin is not metabolized, does not inhibit peripheral glucose oxidation, and does not enhance peripheral lactate production.[162] However, it may decrease conversion of lactate to glucose (decreased gluconeogenesis) and increase lactate production in the gut and liver.[157] Metformin has rarely been associated with lactic acidosis. The few patients in whom this event has been reported had renal, liver, or cardiorespiratory contraindications to the use of biguanides. Patients should be warned to bring the following symptoms of lactic acidosis to the attention of their physician: weakness, malaise, myalgias, abdominal distress, and heavy, labored breathing (see Question 62).

Contraindications and Precautions

Patients with renal impairment, hepatic disease, congestive heart failure (CHF) requiring pharmacologic treatment or other states predisposing them to hypoxia, acute or chronic metabolic

Table 50-26 Comparative Pharmacology of Antidiabetic Agents

Agent Generic Name Brand Name Mechanism	*FDA Indications*	*Efficacy*	*Adverse Effects*	*Comments*
Insulin Replaces or augments endogenous insulin	Monotherapy; combined with any oral agent	↓ HbA_{1c} ∞ ↓FPG ∞ ↓ PPG ∞ ↓ TG	Hypoglycemia, weight gain, lipodystrophy, local skin reactions.	Offers flexible dosing to match lifestyle and glucose concentrations. Rapid onset. Safe in pregnancy, renal failure, and liver dysfunction. Drug of choice when patients do not respond to other antidiabetic agents.
Insulin-Augmenting Agents				
Nonsulfonylurea secretagogues (Glinides) Repaglinide (Prandin) Nateglinide (Starlix) Stimulate insulin secretion.	Monotherapy; combined with metformin or TZD	↓ HbA_{1c} 1.7% ↓ FPG 61 mg/dL ↓ PPG 48 mg/dL	Hypoglycemia, weight gain.	Take only with meals. If a meal is skipped, skip a dose. Flexible dosing with lifestyle. Safe in renal and liver failure. Rapid onset.
Sulfonylureas Various; see Table 50-27. Stimulate insulin secretion. May decrease hepatic glucose output and enhance peripheral glucose utilization.	Monotherapy; combined with metformin; combined with insulin (glimepiride)	↓ HbA_{1c} 1. 5–1.7% FPG 50–70 mg/dL ↓ PPG 92 mg/dL	Hypoglycemia, especially long-acting agents; weight gain (5–10 lb). Rash, hepatotoxicity, alcohol intolerance, and hyponatremia are rare.	Very effective agents, Some can be dosed once daily. Rapid onset of effect (1 wk).
Incretin-Based Therapies				
Glucagon-like peptide -1 receptor agonists/Incretin Mimetic Exenatide (Byetta) Stimulates insulin secretion, delays gastric emptying, reduces postprandial glucagon levels, improved satiety	Combined with metformin, SFU or TZD, combined with metformin + SFU; combined with metformin + TZD	↓ HbA_{1c} 0.8%–0.9% ↓ FPG 10 mg/dL ↓ PPG 71 mg/dL	GI: nausea, vomiting, diarrhea. Hypoglycemia (with SFUs); weight loss; reports of acute pancreatitis	Take within 60 min before morning and evening meals or before two main meals of the day (≥6 hr apart). Do not use in patients with gastroparesis or severe GI disease. Administered by SC injection; pen device in use does not need to be refrigerated.
DPP-4 Inhibitors Sitagliptin (Januvia) Stimulates insulin secretion and reduces postprandial glucagon levels	Monotherapy; combined with metformin, SFU or TZD	↓ HbA_{1c} 0.7%–0.8% ↓ FPG 12–17 mg/dL ↓ PPG 49–62 mg	Headache, nasopharyngitis, hypoglycemia (with SFU), rash (rare)	Dosed once daily. Taken with or without food. No weight gain or nausea. Need to dose adjust in renal dysfunction. Reduce dose of SFU when combined.
Amylin Receptor Agonists				
Amylin mimetic Pramlintide (Symlin) Stimulates insulin secretion, delays gastric emptying, reduces postprandial glucagon levels, improved satiety	Type 1: Adjunct to mealtime insulin Type 2: Adjunct to mealtime insulin; ± SFU and/or metformin	T1: ↓ HbA_{1C} 0.33% T2: ↓ HbA_{1c} 0.40%	GI: nausea, decreased appetite. Headache; hypoglycemia; weight loss (mild)	Take only immediately before meals; administered by SC injection. Do not use in patients with gastroparesis.
Insulin Sensitizers				
Biguanides Metformin (Glucophage) ↓ Hepatic glucose output; ↑ Peripheral glucose uptake	Monotherapy; combined with SFU and/or TZD; or with insulin	↓ HbA_{1c} 1.5%–1.7% ↓ FPG 50–70 mg/dL ↓ PPG 83 mg/dL	GI: nausea, cramping, diarrhea. Lactic acidosis (rare).	Titrate dose slowly to minimize GI effects. No hypoglycemia or weight gain; weight loss possible. Mild reduction in cholesterol. Do not use in patients with renal or hepatic dysfunction or CHF requiring treatment.

(continued)

Table 50-26 Comparative Pharmacology of Antidiabetic Agents (*continued*)

Agent Generic Name Brand Name Mechanism	*FDA Indications*	*Efficacy*	*Adverse Effects*	*Comments*
Thiazolidinediones Rosiglitazone (Avandia) Pioglitazone (Actos) Enhance insulin action in periphery; increase glucose utilization by muscle and fat tissue; decrease hepatic glucose output	Monotherapy; combined with SFU, TZD or insulin; combined with SFU + TZD	Monotherapy: ↓ HbA_{1c} 0.8%–1.5% Combination: ↓ HbA_{1c} 0.6%–1.2%	Mild anemia; fluid retention and edema, weight gain, macular edema, fractures (in women)	Can cause or exacerbate CHF; do not use in patients with symptomatic heart failure or class III or IV CHF. Rosiglitazone may increase risk of MI. Increased risk of distal fractures in older women. Slight reduction in TG with pioglitazone; slight increase in LDL-C with rosiglitazone. LFTs must be measured at baseline and periodically thereafter. Slow onset (2–4 wk).
Delayers of Carbohydrate Absorption				
α-Glucosidase inhibitors Acarbose (Precose) Miglitol (Glyset) Slow absorption of complex carbohydrates.	Monotherapy; combined with SFUs	↓ HbA_{1c} 0.5%–1.0% ↓ FPG 20–30 mg/dL ↓ PPG 25–50 mg/dL	GI: flatulence, diarrhea. Elevations in LFTs seen in doses >50 mg TID of acarbose.	LFTs should be monitored every 3 months during the first year of therapy and periodically thereafter. Because miglitol is not metabolized, monitoring of LFTs is not required. Titrate dose slowly to minimize GI effects. No hypoglycemia or weight gain. If used in combination with hypoglycemic agents, advise patients to treat hypoglycemia with glucose tablets because absorption is not inhibited as with sucrose.

CHF, congestive heart failure; FPG, fasting plasma glucose; GI, gastrointestinal; HbA_{1c}, hemoglobin A_{1C}; LDL-C, low-density lipoprotein cholesterol; LFTs, liver function tests; MI, myocardial infarction; PPG, postprandial glucose; SC, subcutaneously; SFU, sulfonylureas; TG, triglycerides; TZD, thiazolidinediones.

acidosis, or a history of lactic acidosis should be excluded from therapy. Metformin can accumulate in patients whose renal function is impaired, thereby increasing their risk for lactic acidosis. Its use is not recommended in patients with decreased GFRs (<60 mL/minute) or elevated creatinine levels (≥1.4 mg/dL for females or ≥1.5 mg/dL for males). Because even a temporary reduction in renal function could cause lactic acidosis in patients taking metformin, the manufacturer recommends withholding it after some radiologic procedures (see Drug Interactions). Other predisposing factors for lactic acidosis include the following: excessive alcohol ingestion, dehydration, surgery, CHF, hepatic failure, shock, or sepsis. Because aging is associated with reduced renal function, metformin should be titrated to the minimum effective dose and renal function should be monitored regularly. A creatinine clearance (ClCr) to ensure adequate renal function should be measured in patients over the age of 80 years, because these patients are more susceptible to developing lactic acidosis.[158]

Drug Interactions

- Alcohol potentiates the effect of metformin on lactate metabolism. Patients should be warned against excessive alcohol intake while taking metformin.
- Cimetidine increases peak metformin plasma concentrations by 60%; use of an alternative H2 blocker or a reduction in metformin dose is recommended.
- Parenteral contrast studies (e.g., pyelography or angiography) that use iodinated materials can result in acute renal failure and metformin-induced lactic acidosis. For patients requiring such a study, metformin should be withheld at the time of, or before, and for 48 hours after the procedure. Metformin should be reinstituted only after renal function has been reevaluated and determined to be normal.

Efficacy

As monotherapy, metformin can be expected to reduce the HbA_{1c} by 1.5% to 1.7% and the FPG by 50 to 70 mg/dL. In patients who have developed secondary failure to sulfonylureas, the addition of metformin can be expected to produce a similar or slightly greater improvement in the FPG and HbA_{1c}.[157] Research suggests that certain genetic variations may impact patient response to metformin therapy. Patients exhibiting reduced function polymorphisms of organic cation transporter 1, which is involved in the hepatic uptake of metformin, may be less responsive to metformin therapy.[163]

Table 50-27 Antidiabetic Pharmacokinetic Data

Drug (Brand Name) Available Tablet Strengths (mg)	Typical Dosing Regimen (mg)	Usual Minimum and Maximum Total Daily Dose/How Divided	Mean Half-Life	Approximate Duration of Activity	Bioavailability Metabolism, and Excretion	Comments
α-Glucosidase inhibitors						
Acarbose (Precose) 25, 50, 100 mg	25–100 mg with first bite of each meal. Begin with 25 mg; ↑ by 25 mg/meal every 4–8 weeks.	Minimum: 25 mg TID; Maximum dose is 50 mg TID if ≤60 kg; 100 mg TID if >60 kg.	2.8 hr	Affects absorption of complex carbohydrates in a single meal	F = 0.5%–1.7%; extensively metabolized by GI amylases to inactive products; 50% excreted unchanged in the feces	Titrate doses slowly to avoid GI effects
Miglitol (Glyset) 25, 50, 100 mg	25–100 mg with first bite of each meal. Begin with 25 mg; ↑ by 25 mg/meal every 4–8 weeks.	Minimum: 25 mg TID Maximum: 100 mg TID	2 hr	Affects absorption of complex carbohydrates in a single meal	Dose of 25 mg is completely absorbed; dose of 100 mg 50–70% absorbed; elimination by renal excretion as unchanged drug	
Biguanides						
Metformin (Glucophage) 500, 850, 1000 mg; 500 mg/mL liquid	Begin with 500 mg QD or /BID; ↑ by 500 mg QD every 1–2 weeks.	0.5–2.5 g BID or TID	Plasma, 6.2 hr Whole blood, 17.6 hr	6–12 hr	F = 50%–60%; excreted unchanged in urine	Take with food. Avoid in patients with renal dysfunction or those who could be predisposed to lactic acidosis (e.g., alcoholism, CHF, severe respiratory disorders, liver failure)
Metformin extended-release (Glucophage XR) 500, 750, 1000 mg	500–1,000 mg/QD with evening meal; ↑ by 500 mg every 1–2 weeks.	1,500–2,000 mg QD	As for metformin, but active drug is released slowly	24 hr	As for metformin	As for metformin
Nonsulfonylurea Insulin Secretagogues (Glinides)						
Repaglinide (Prandin) 0.5, 1, 2 mg	If HbA_{1c} is <8% or if this is first drug, begin with 0.5 mg with each meal. For others, begin with 1–2 mg/meal.	0.5–4 mg with each meal (16 mg/day)/TID–QID	1 hr	C_{max} is at 1 hr; duration is approximately 2–3 hr	F = 56%; 92% metabolized to inactive products by the liver; 8% excreted as metabolites unchanged in the urine	Take only with meals. Skip dose if meal is skipped. Maximum dose per meal is 4 mg.
Nateglinide (Starlix) 60, 120 mg	120 mg TID 1–30 min before meals; 60 mg TID for patients with near-normal HbA_{1c} at initiation.	60 or 120 mg TID	1.5 hr	Onset, 20 min; peak, 1 hr; duration, 2–4 hr	F = 73%; metabolized to inactive products (predominantly) that are excreted in the urine (83%) and feces (10%)	Skip dose if meal is skipped.
First-Generation Sulfonylureas						
Acetohexamide (Dymelor) 250, 500 mg	250 or 500 mg/QD; ↑ by 250 mg daily every 1–2 weeks.	0. 25–1.5 g QD or BID	5 hr (active metabolite)	12–18 hr	Activity of metabolite greater then parent drug. Metabolite excreted, in part, by kidney	Caution in elderly and patients with renal disease, Significant uricosuric effects
Chlorpropamide (Diabinese) 100, 250 mg	100 or 250 mg/QD; ↑ by 100 or 250 mg every 1–2 weeks.	0.1–0.5 g QD	≥35 hr	24–72 hr	Inactive and weakly active metabolites; 20% excreted unchanged; varies widely	Caution in elderly and patients with renal impairment. Highest frequency of side effects relative to other sulfonylureas

(continued)

Table 50-27 Antidiabetic Pharmacokinetic Data (*Continued*)

Drug (Brand Name) Available Tablet Strengths (mg)	Typical Dosing Regimen (mg)	Usual Minimum and Maximum Total Daily Dose/How Divided	Mean Half-Life	Approximate Duration of Activity	Bioavailability Metabolism, and Excretion	Comments
First-Generation Sulfonylureas (*continued*)						
Tolazamide (Tolinase) 100, 250, 500 mg	100–250 mg/QD; ↑ by 100 or 250 mg every 1–2 weeks.	0.2–1 g QD or BID	7 hr (4–25)	12–24 hr	Some metabolites with moderate activity excreted via kidney	Active metabolites may accumulate in renal failure
Tolbutamide (Orinase) 250, 500 mg	250 mg/BID before meals; ↑ by 250 mg daily every 1–2 weeks	0.5–3 g BID or TID	7 hr	6–12 hr	Metabolized to compounds with negligible activity	No special precautions. Shortest-acting sulfonylurea
Second-Generation Sulfonylureas						
Glimepiride (Amaryl) 1, 2, 4 mg	1–2 mg/QD initially; usual maintenance dose is 1–4 mg.	1–8 mg QD	9 hr	24 hr	F = 100% completely metabolized by liver. Principal metabolite is slightly active (30% of parent compound). Excreted by the urine (60%) and feces (40%)	Probably safe in patients with renal failure, but low initial doses recommended for older patients and those with renal insufficiency. Incidence of hypoglycemia may be lower than other long-acting sulfonylureas
Glipizide (Glucotrol) 5, 10 mg	2.5 mg/QD in elderly, 5 mg QD in others; ↑ by 2.5 or 5 mg every 1–2 weeks.	2.5–40 mg QD or BID[a]	2–4 hr	12–24 hr	Metabolized to inactive compounds	No special precautions daily dose >15 mg should be divided. Dose 30 min before meals
Glipizide extended–release (Glucotrol XL) 5 mg	5 mg/QD; ↑ by 5 mg every 1–2 weeks.	5–20 mg QD	4–13 hr	24 hr	Same as glipizide	Use with caution in patients with preexisting GI narrowing owing to possible obstruction
Glyburide (Diabeta, Micronase) 1.25, 2.5, 5 mg	1.25 mg/QD in elderly, 2.5 mg QD in others; ↑ by 1.25 or 2.5 mg every 1–2 weeks.	1.25–20 mg QD or BID	4–13 hr	12–24 hr	Metabolized to inactive/weakly inactive compounds; 50% excreted in urine and 50% in feces	Caution in elderly patients with renal failure and others predisposed to hypoglycemia. Daily doses >10 mg should be divided
Micronized Glyburide (Glynase presTab) 1.5, 3 mg	1.5 mg/QD; ↑ by 1.5 mg every 1–2 weeks.	1.0–12 mg QD	4 hr	24 hr	Metabolized to inactive/weakly inactive compounds; 50% excreted in urine and 50% in feces	Daily doses >6 mg should be divided. ↑ bioavailability relative to original formulation. Resulted in reduced dose
Thiazolidinediones						
Rosiglitazone (Avandia) 2, 4, 8 mg	4 mg QD; ↑ to 8 mg QD (or 4 mg BID)	4–8 mg daily in single or divided doses	3–4 hr	Onset and duration poorly correlated with half-life because of mechanism of action. Onset at 3 weeks; max at ≥4 weeks. Offset likely to be similar	F = 99%; extensively metabolized in liver into inactive metabolites; excreted 2/3 in urine and 1/3 in feces	Food has no effect on absorption. BID dosing may have greater HbA_{1c} lowering effect. No dose adjustments required in renal failure. Avoid in patients with liver disease and heart failure.
Pioglitazone (Actos) 15, 30, 45 mg	15–30 mg QD; ↑ to 45 mg QD. If used with insulin, ↓ insulin dose by 10%–25% once FPG <120 mg/dL.	15–45 mg QD	3–7 hr (16–24 hr for all metabolites)	Same as previous	Extensively metabolized in liver; 15%–30% excreted in urine, remainder eliminated in the feces	Food delays absorption but is not clinically significant. No dose adjustments required in renal disease. Avoid in patients with liver disease and heart failure.

GLP-1 receptor agonists/incretin mimetics						
Exenatide (Byetta)	5 mcg SC BID; ↑ to 10 mcg SC BID after 1 month	5–10 mcg BID	2.4 hr	C_{max} is at 2.1 hr; duration 10 hr	Glomerular filtration	Take within 60 min before morning and evening meal. Nausea usually subsides over time
DPP-4 Inhibitors						
Sitagliptin (Januvia)	100 mg QD CrCl ≥30 to <50 mL/min: 50 mg QD CrCl <30 mL/min: 25 mg QD	100 mg QD	12.4 hr	24 hr	F = 87%; ~79% excreted unchanged in urine.	Requires dose adjustment in renal insufficiency.
Amylin Mimetics						
Pramlintide (Symlin)	Type 1 DM: 15 mcg SC before major meals; ↑by 15-mcg increments after minimum of 3 days Type 2 DM: 60 mcg SC before major meals; ↑ to 120 mcg after 3–7 days	Type 1: 15–60 mcg before major meals Type 2: 60 or 120 mcg before major meals	48 min	C_{max} is 20 minutes	F = 30%–40%; metabolized by kidneys	Reduce mealtime insulin dose by 50%. Titrate dose if no significant nausea.
Combination Products						
Glipizide/metformin (Metaglip) 2.5/250 mg, 2.5/500 mg, 5/500 mg	*Initial therapy:* 2.5/250 mg QD *2nd-line therapy:* 2.5–5/500 mg BID; ↑ every 2 weeks	5/1,000–20/2,000 mg in two divided doses	See metformin and glyburide	See metformin and glyburide	See metformin and glyburide	See Glucovance
Glyburide/Metformin (Glucovance) 1.25/500, 2.5/500 mg 5.0/500 mg	2.5/500 mg QD or BID; ↑ by 2.5/500 mg every 1–2 weeks.	7.5/1,500–10/2,000 mg in 2–3 divided doses with meals	See metformin and glyburide	See metformin and glyburide	See metformin and glyburide	Effect should be similar to the two agents given in combination. Minimum dose of 1,500 mg metformin is needed for effect. No need to exceed 10 mg glyburide
Rosiglitazone/metformin (Avandamet) 1/500 mg, 2/500 mg, 4/500 mg	2/500 mg BID	4/1,000–8/2,000 mg in two divided doses with meals	See metformin and rosiglitazone	See rosiglitazone	See metformin and rosiglitazone	Dose titration schedule is dependent on which drug is being adjusted.
Pioglitazone/metformin (ActoPlus Met) 15/500 mg, 15/850 mg	15/500 mg or 15/850 mg QD or BID	30/1,000–45/2,550 mg in two divided doses with meals	See pioglitazone and metformin	See pioglitazone and metformin	See pioglitazone and metformin	Dose titration schedule is dependent on which drug is being adjusted.
Pioglitazone/glimepiride (Duetact) 30/2 mg, 30/4 mg	30/2 mg or 30/2 mg QD	30/2–30/4 mg QD	See pioglitazone and glimepiride	See pioglitazone and glimepiride	See pioglitazone and glimepiride	Dosed once daily with first main meal.
Rosiglitazone/Glimepiride (Avanadryl) 4/1 mg, 4/2 mg, 4/4 mg, 8/2 mg, 8/4 mg	4/1 mg or 4/2 mg QD	4/1–8/4 mg QD	See rosiglitazone and glimepiride	See rosiglitazone and glimepiride	See rosiglitazone and glimepiride	Dose titration schedule is dependent on which drug is being adjusted.
Sitagliptin/Metformin (Janumet) 50/500 mg, 50/1000 mg	50/500 mg BID	100/1,000–100/2,000 mg in two divided doses with meals	See sitagliptin and metformin	See sitagliptin and metformin	See sitagliptin and metformin	Starting dose depends on current regimen. Metformin dose is titrated.

BID, twice a day; CHF, congestive heart failure; CrCl, creatinine clearance; DM, diabetes mellitus; DPP-4, dipeptidyl peptidase-4; FPG, fasting plasma glucose; GI, gastrointestinal; HbA_{1c}, hemoglobin A_{1c}; QD, daily; SC, subcutaneously; TID, three times a day.

Dosage and Clinical Use

Metformin is the first line of therapy for type 2 diabetes.[22] It is usually initiated as monotherapy in combination with lifestyle interventions (e.g., MNT, physical activity) upon diagnosis. To minimize GI side effects, metformin should be initiated at 500 mg once or twice daily, to be taken with food, followed by weekly or biweekly increases in increments of 500 mg daily. Metformin is dosed two to three times daily (500–1,000 mg/dose; maximum dose, 2,550 mg/day or 850 mg PO TID), unless an extended-release preparation is prescribed. Clinicians should obtain a SrCr and hepatic function tests at baseline and then annually. Metformin should not be used in patients older than 80 years unless a ClCr demonstrates normal renal function. Patients are candidates for treatment if the ClCr is above 60 mL/minute. For patients unable to achieve goals of therapy with metformin alone within 3 to 6 months of initiating therapy, addition of insulin or another agent should be considered (also see Questions 54–58).

Nonsulfonylurea Insulin Secretagogues (Glinides)

Repaglinide (Prandin) and nateglinide (Starlix) are nonsulfonylurea insulin secretagogues (i.e., they stimulate insulin secretion).[70,164,165] They belong to a class of agents referred to as meglitinides and amino acid derivatives, respectively. Repaglinide was approved by the FDA in December 1997 and nateglinide was approved in December 2000 (Table 50-26).

Mechanism of Action

These agents close the adenosine triphosphate (ATP)-sensitive potassium channels in the β-cell, which leads to cell membrane depolarization, an influx of Ca^{2+}, and secretion of insulin.[164,165] Unlike the sulfonylureas, they have a rapid onset and shorter duration of action, so they are given with meals to enhance postprandial glucose utilization.

Pharmacokinetics

Repaglinide has a bioavailability of 56% and is rapidly absorbed and excreted.[164] Its C_{max} occurs at approximately 1 hour and its half-life is 1 hour. Repaglinide is highly (>98%) protein bound (volume of distribution [Vd], 31 L). It is completely metabolized (CYP 3A4) by the liver to inactive products, with 90% excreted in the feces and 8% excreted in urine. Nateglinide has a bioavailability of 73%.[165] It is rapidly absorbed with a C_{max} occurring within 1 hour after dosing and a half-life of 1.5 hours. Nateglinide is metabolized (CYP2C9, 70%; CYP3A4, 30%) to less potent compounds, which are 75% excreted in the urine and 10% in the feces. Sixteen percent is excreted unchanged in the urine. It is highly (98%) protein bound, primarily to albumin, and, to a lesser extent, to α_1-acid glycoprotein.

Adverse Effects

Mild hypoglycemia may occur, particularly if patients delay or forget to eat after the dose.[164,165] A weight gain of 0.9 to 3 kg compared with baseline has been observed. Rare side effects include elevated hepatic enzymes and hypersensitivity reactions. There has been at least one case report of repaglinide-induced hepatic toxicity.[166]

Contraindications and Precautions

Because a functioning pancreas is required, these agents should not be used in people with type 1 diabetes. They should be used with caution in patients with liver dysfunction.[164,165] Repaglinide clearance is reduced in patients with severe renal insufficiency, but may still be used safely at a reduced dose. Nateglinide's clearance is not affected in patients with moderate to severe renal insufficiency.

Drug Interactions

Clinically relevant drug interactions include those that occur when these drugs are taken in combination with other glucose-lowering agents or drugs known to induce or inhibit their metabolism.[167] Therefore, blood glucose levels should be closely monitored when either drug is taken in combination with other agents known to lower blood glucose or affect their metabolism. Repaglinide is metabolized by CYP2C8 and 3A4.[164] Studies have shown that repaglinide has no pharmacokinetic effects on digoxin or warfarin. Cimetidine does not affect its absorption or efficacy. Gemfibrozil should be avoided in combination with repaglinide owing to the risk of hypoglycemia. The combination of gemfibrozil and itraconazole synergistically inhibits repaglinide metabolism and should be avoided. Nateglinide is metabolized largely by CYP2C9 (70%) and to a lesser extent by 3A4 (30%).[165] When evaluated in clinical studies, there were no clinically relevant interactions with nateglinide and glyburide, metformin, digoxin, diclofenac, or warfarin. Concomitant use of either repaglinide or nateglinide with rifampin may lower their efficacy.[167]

Efficacy

The efficacy of repaglinide is comparable to metformin and the sulfonylureas.[168] When used as monotherapy, the mean decrease in FPG, postprandial glucose, and the HbA_{1c} values were 61 mg/dL, 104 mg/dL, and 1.7%, respectively, compared with placebo (−31.0 mg/dL, −47.6 mg/dL, and −0.6% compared with baseline). Newly diagnosed patients who have never been treated with oral agents and those whose HbA_{1c} is below 8% respond more profoundly than poorly controlled individuals already on treatment. Nateglinide as monotherapy results in a mean decrease in FPG and HbA_{1c} of 13.6 mg/dL and 0.7%, respectively, compared with placebo (−4.5 mg/dL and −0.5% compared with baseline). In comparison with metformin monotherapy, both drugs produce a similar or slightly smaller reduction in HbA_{1c}. When either drug is used in combination with metformin, a clinically significant additional reduction in HbA_{1c} is observed over metformin alone.

Dosage and Clinical Use

Repaglinide and nateglinide are approved to treat people with type 2 diabetes as monotherapy or in combination with metformin. Repaglinide is also approved for use with TZDs. Because they have the same mechanism of action as the sulfonylureas, combining these agents does not produce any additional benefit. The agents are usually added to therapy for patients with high postprandial glucose values. When repaglinide is used as the initial treatment in patients who are "naive" to oral antidiabetic therapy or in patients with HbA_{1c} values below 8%, the recommended starting dose is 0.5 mg with each meal. When used in patients who have failed sulfonylureas or in those with HbA_{1c} values above 8%, the initial dose is 1 to 2 mg with each meal. Doses can be titrated weekly at a rate of 1 mg/meal to a maximum of 4 mg/dose or 16 mg/day. The recommended starting dose of nateglinide is 120 mg TID 0 to 30 minutes before meals. For patients close to their HbA_{1c} goal, a dose of 60 mg TID may be used. Doses should be omitted if a meal is skipped and added if an extra meal is ingested (repaglinide only). Repaglinide should be initiated at a 0.5-mg dose in patients with severe renal dysfunction and should be titrated cautiously in patients with liver dysfunction.

Sulfonylureas

Until metformin and other antidiabetics became available in the United States, sulfonylureas were the first-line pharmacologic treatment for people with type 2 diabetes who had failed diet and exercise therapy. Six different sulfonylureas are available in the United States. The three first-generation sulfonylureas (chlorpropamide [Diabinese], tolazamide [Tolinase], and tolbutamide [Orinase]) are considered equally effective despite differences in their pharmacokinetic properties and adverse effect profiles (see the following discussion and Table 50-25).

Glipizide (Glucotrol) and glyburide (DiaBeta, Glynase, Micronase), two second-generation sulfonylureas, were first introduced into the United States in May 1984. Glimepiride (Amaryl) was approved for use in 1995. Despite being approximately 100 times more potent than the first-generation sulfonylureas on a milligram-for-milligram basis, these agents are not more clinically effective. They have a relatively favorable side effect profile and have a duration of activity that allows for once or twice daily dosing.

Mechanism of Action

PANCREATIC EFFECTS

Sulfonylureas stimulate the release of insulin from pancreatic β-cells and enhance β-cell sensitivity to glucose. A specific sulfonylurea receptor closely linked to the ATP-sensitive potassium ion channel exists on the β-cell. Sulfonylureas are believed to inhibit this potassium ion channel, thus blocking the efflux of potassium and lowering the membrane potential to cause depolarization. The voltage-dependent calcium channels then open, increasing intracellular calcium concentration. The increased intracellular concentration of calcium ultimately stimulates insulin secretion.[70] Insulin levels tend to return to baseline values after a few months of continued sulfonylurea use.

EXTRAPANCREATIC EFFECTS

Sulfonylureas can normalize hepatic glucose production and partially reverse insulin resistance in the peripheral tissues of people with type 2 diabetes. Whether these "extrapancreatic" effects of the sulfonylureas are direct effects or secondary to improved insulin release and lower glucose concentrations remains to be established.[169] In any case, tissues become more responsive to lower concentrations of endogenous insulin in type 2 patients treated with sulfonylureas.[170]

Pharmacokinetics

The duration of hypoglycemic activity is related to the half-life of these compounds only in very general terms and may correlate poorly in some cases.[170] All sulfonylureas are highly protein bound (90%–100%), mainly to albumin. Binding characteristics, however, vary among individual sulfonylureas. Food does not impair the extent of drug absorption, but may delay the time to peak levels of some agents. The relationship between sulfonylurea doses and their blood glucose-lowering effect remains unclear. Studies of glyburide and glipizide suggest that these agents may operate within a narrow range of plasma concentrations that may be achieved with low (10 mg/day) doses.[171–173] The maximum recommended daily doses of 40 mg for glipizide and 20 mg for glyburide may therefore not be more effective. Furthermore, insulin may be indicated for patients no longer responding to 10 mg or higher doses of glyburide or glipizide.

Chlorpropramide has the longest serum half-life and duration of hypoglycemic activity and a variable rate of renal excretion.

Glipizide is an intermediate-acting second-generation agent with a half-life of 2 to 4 hours, but a duration of action of 12 to 24 hours.[70] Patients receiving <20 mg/day may require only once daily dosing. Food delays its rate of absorption, but not its bioavailability. Patients may therefore take it with or without food. Glipizide is extensively metabolized by the liver to inactive products that are eliminated primarily by the kidney.[170,174] A sustained-release formulation of glipizide (Glucotrol XL) also is available.

Glyburide (or glibenclamide) is a longer acting second-generation agent similar to glipizide. The half-life is approximately 1.5 to 4 hours after single-dose studies and up to 13.7 hours when chronically administered.[175] Nevertheless, as with glipizide, the duration of action can last for up to 24 hours in many patients, allowing for once daily dosing with small to intermediate doses (<15 mg). Food does not delay the rate or extent of absorption. Glyburide is metabolized completely by the liver to active metabolites, half of which are excreted in the urine and the remainder eliminated via the biliary tract.[176] The micronized tablets (e.g., Glynase Prestabs) are not bioequivalent to the conventionally formulated tablets.[70] Thus, patients switched between the conventional form and the micronized product must be retitrated.

Glimepiride is a long-acting second-generation sulfonylurea. Its half-life is 9 hours and its duration of action is 24 hours, allowing for once-daily dosing.[177] The absorption of glimepiride is unaffected by food, and its peak effect on plasma glucose concentrations is observed 2 to 3 hours after each dose. Glimepiride is completely metabolized by the liver, and its principal metabolite has 30% of the activity of the parent drug. Metabolites are excreted in feces and urine.

Adverse Effects

The primary side effects of the sulfonylureas are hypoglycemia (particularly for those that are long acting) and weight gain (see questions 63 and 71).[178] Other adverse effects attributed to the sulfonylureas generally are so infrequent and mild that fewer than 2% of patients discontinue these agents because of them. In general, the type, incidence, and severity of reported side effects are similar for all the sulfonylureas. An important exception is chlorpropamide, which has several unique adverse effects (see following discussion). Adverse reactions to the sulfonylureas include GI symptoms (nausea, fullness, bloating that can be relieved if taken with meals), rare blood dyscrasias, allergic dermatologic reactions, hepatotoxicity, and hypothyroidism (also see Questions 63–65).

A disulfiram (Antabuse-like) reaction occurs when patients take certain oral sulfonylurea drugs and drink ethanol. It is most frequently associated with chlorpropamide, occurring in approximately one-third of all patients receiving it. The flushing reaction is rare with other sulfonylureas.

SYNDROME OF INAPPROPRIATE ANTIDIURETIC HORMONE SECRETION

Chlorpropamide, and to a much lesser extent, tolbutamide, may enhance the release of antidiuretic hormone centrally, enhance the effect of antidiuretic hormone on the kidney, and override the inhibitory effects of waterloading on antidiuretic hormone release, resulting in syndrome of inappropriate antidiuretic hormone secretion.[170,178] This antidiuretic effect has been used clinically to treat diabetes insipidus. In the UKPDS study, the increase in BP seen in patients on chlorpropamide was likely due to water retention.[33] In contrast to chlorpropamide and tolbutamide, glipizide, glyburide, tolazamide, and acetohexamide have a mild diuretic effect.

Contraindications and Precautions

Contraindications to the use of sulfonylureas include the following[178]:

1. Type 1 diabetes
2. Pregnancy or breast-feeding, because these agents (except glyburide) can cross the placental barrier and can be excreted into breast milk
3. Documented hypersensitivity to sulfonylureas
4. Severe hepatic or renal dysfunction
5. Severe, acute intercurrent illness (e.g., infection, MI), surgery, or other stress that can unduly affect blood glucose control

Drug Interactions

Drug interactions with sulfonylureas have a pharmacodynamic or pharmacokinetic basis. Pharmacodynamic interactions are discussed later in this chapter in sections addressing drug-induced hypoglycemia and hyperglycemia. Most of the reported pharmacokinetic drug interactions with the sulfonylureas involve chlorpropamide and tolbutamide. Because most of the clinically significant interactions occur with drugs that alter liver metabolism or urinary excretion, possible interactions with all of the sulfonylureas must be anticipated, even though the outcomes may be quite different. Second-generation sulfonylureas (glipizide, glyburide, and glimepiride) are dosed in milligram rather than gram quantities and are thus less likely to interact with other drugs on a pharmacokinetic basis. Glipizide and glyburide also differ from the first-generation agents in that they are highly bound to albumin at nonionic rather than ionic sites.[170,174] On this basis, these agents are unlikely to interact with other highly protein-bound drugs, such as phenylbutazone, salicylates, or certain sulfonamide antibiotics that have been reported to enhance the effects of the first-generation sulfonylureas. These highly protein-bound drugs, however, seem to interact with the sulfonylureas by altering their hepatic metabolism as well. Therefore, glipizide and glyburide should be used cautiously with drugs reported to interact with first-generation sulfonylureas.

Efficacy

Like metformin, the sulfonylureas decrease the HbA_{1c} by 1.5% to 1.7% and the FPG by 50% to 70%. In patients who have developed secondary failure to maximum doses of metformin, the addition of sulfonylureas produces similar improvements in the HbA_{1c} and FPG, unless the disease has progressed and the pancreas is no longer able to respond appropriately. Whether sulfonylureas actually contribute to β-cell dysfunction and decline remains to be clearly determined.[179]

Dosage and Clinical Use

The sulfonylureas are very effective, relatively safe, relatively inexpensive, and easy to titrate. Sulfonylureas are usually added on to therapy in patients unable to achieve blood glucose goals on metformin monotherapy. Sulfonylureas may also be considered as monotherapy or first-line agents in patients with contraindications to metformin therapy. The doses of the sulfonylureas are displayed in Table 50-27. As a general rule, one should begin with low doses and titrate upward every 1 to 2 weeks until the desired goal is achieved. Exceeding maximum doses is not likely to produce improvement, but may put the patient at risk for adverse effects (see Questions 53, 70, and 71).

Thiazolidinediones

Rosiglitazone (Avandia, GlaxoSmithKline) and pioglitazone (Actos, Takeda Pharmaceuticals) were approved in 1999 and are the two available TZDs in the United States.

Mechanism of Action

The TZDs are often referred to as insulin sensitizers. The precise molecular actions of these agents remain to be clarified. TZDs bind to and activate a nuclear receptor (peroxisome proliferator-activated receptor-γ [PPAR-γ]), which is expressed in many insulin-sensitive tissues, including adipose, skeletal muscle, and liver tissue.[70] PPAR-γ regulates transcription of genes that influence glucose and lipid metabolism. For example, PPAR-γ stimulation increases the transcription of GLUT-4, a glucose transporter that stimulates glucose uptake.[180] Reduced expression of GLUT-4 may contribute to the development of insulin resistance.

TZDs either directly or indirectly sensitize adipose tissue to insulin action.[70,169,180] The effects may include stimulating apoptosis of large adipocytes, increasing the number of small adipose cells, and promoting fatty acid uptake and storage in adipose tissue. The subsequent reduction in free circulating fatty acids may spare other insulin sensitive tissues (e.g., liver, skeletal muscle, β-cells) from the effects of lipotoxicity. TZDs also lower expression of tumor necrosis factor-α, a cytokine produced by adipose tissue that may contribute to insulin resistance and fatty acid release.[169,180] In fact, TZD interaction with adipocytes may be their primary mechanism of action in sensitizing other tissues to insulin action.

Other observed effects of TZDs that may prove to be beneficial in patients with type 2 diabetes and metabolic syndrome include favorable effects on lipids, reduction of inflammatory mediators, inhibition of vascular smooth muscle cell proliferation, improved endothelial function, and enhanced fibrinolysis.[169,180]

In summary, the TZDs clinically decrease insulin resistance in muscle and liver, which enhances glucose utilization and decreases hepatic glucose output. Alleviation of insulin resistance also reduces insulin, glucose, and free fatty acid levels and has positive effects on lipid levels.

Pharmacokinetics

Rosiglitazone is completely absorbed, with peak plasma concentrations reached in approximately 1 hour.[181] Pioglitazone has a bioavailability of 83%, with peak plasma concentrations reached within 2 hours.[182,183] Food does not alter absorption of either drug. Both TZDs are extensively (>99%) protein bound, primarily to albumin. The plasma elimination half-life of rosiglitazone is 3 to 7 hours. Pioglitazone has a serum half-life of 3 to 7 hours, and its metabolites have a serum half-life of 16 to 24 hours. Rosiglitazone is extensively metabolized in the liver by CYP 2C8 and to a much lesser extent by 2C9. Its conjugated metabolites are considerably less potent than the parent drug and are excreted two-thirds in urine and one-third in feces. Pioglitazone is hepatically metabolized, mainly by CYP 2C8 and 3A4, into two active metabolites. Approximately 15% to 30% of the dose is recovered in the urine as metabolites, with the remainder excreted into the bile either as unchanged drug or as metabolites.

Because the action of the TZDs relies on gene transcription and protein production, the onset and duration of action are unrelated to the plasma half-life.[70] The onset of their effect occurs in 1 to 2 weeks, although maximum effects are not usually seen before 8 to 12 weeks. No dose adjustment is necessary in patients with renal impairment or failure.

Adverse Effects

HEPATOTOXICITY

Troglitazone, the first TZD to be approved by the FDA in 1997, was associated with idiosyncratic hepatotoxicity leading to hepatic failure and death in some patients, which became apparent during postmarketing surveillance. During clinical trials, fewer than 2% of troglitazone-treated patients experienced asymptomatic, reversible elevations in liver transaminase (alanine transaminase [ALT]) levels that were greater than three times the normal values.[184] In contrast, the elevations in liver transaminase levels observed during preapproval clinical trials for pioglitazone and rosiglitazone (0.26% and 0.2%, respectively) were similar to placebo (0.25% and 0.2%).[181,182] Liver failure has been very rarely reported with either rosiglitazone or pioglitazone, although causality in most cases remains uncertain.[185–187] For both drugs, monitoring of liver function tests (LFTs) is recommended at baseline, and then periodically thereafter (see Contraindications and Precautions).

HEMATOLOGIC EFFECTS

TZD therapy may result in small decreases in hemoglobin and hematocrit and, infrequently, anemia.[169,180] Transient decreases in neutrophil counts occurred infrequently within the first 4 to 8 weeks of TZD therapy. These effects may be due to dilutional effects (see below).

WEIGHT GAIN

Dose-related weight gain (2–3 kg for every 1% decrease in HbA_{1c}) has been seen with rosiglitazone and pioglitazone.[180] The cause of weight gain is likely due to fluid retention and/or fat accumulation. The weight gain seems to be associated with an increase in peripheral adipose tissue along with a reduction in visceral adiposity.[169,180]

VASCULAR AND CARDIOVASCULAR EFFECTS

Increases in plasma volume and peripheral edema (4%–6%), possibly caused by an increased endothelial cell permeability, have been reported with the TZDs.[180] The incidence of peripheral edema is greatly increased when TZDs are used in combination with insulin.

Although no CHF was observed in original clinical trials with either drug, patients with New York Heart Association (NYHA) class III and IV cardiac status were not included. In 2007, the FDA added black box warnings to rosiglitazone and pioglitazone based on association of their use with an increased risk of developing or exacerbating CHF in patients with type 2 diabetes. Recent meta-analyses and retrospective studies have suggested that TZD use may be associated with an increased risk of MI and mortality.[188,189–193] Whether or not TZDs actually increase rates of MI and morbidity and mortality owing to cardiovascular causes remains to be clearly determined. Some prospective studies are currently underway.

Based on these effects and observations, TZDs are contraindicated for use in patients with NYHA class III or IV CHF. In addition, they should be avoided in patients with symptomatic CHF, such as those requiring nitrate therapy. TZDs should be used with caution in patients with preexisting edema, which may increase the risk of developing new-onset CHF or exacerbating preexisting CHF.

OTHER EFFECTS

Hypersensitivity reactions including rash, pruritus, urticaria, angioedema, anaphylactic reaction, and Stevens-Johnson syndrome have been rarely reported with rosiglitazone.[181] Macular edema has been rarely reported with TZDs.[181,182,194] Patients experiencing changes or worsening in vision should be referred to an ophthalmologist for follow-up. In some cases, macular edema improved or resolved after discontinuation of TZD therapy. An increased risk of distal limb bone fractures (e.g., forearm, hand, wrist, foot, and ankle) and bone loss have been observed women receiving TZDs.[181,182,191,195] Potential for fractures in older female patients should be carefully considered before using a TZD.

Contraindications and Precautions

- *Type 1 diabetes:* Because insulin is required for their action, TZDs should not be used in people with type 1 diabetes.
- *Patients with type 2 diabetes using insulin:* TZDs should be used with caution due to the increased risk of developing edema.
- *Preexisting hepatic disease:* Pioglitazone and rosiglitazone should not be used in patients whose ALT is more than 2.5 times normal. TZDs should be discontinued if the ALT is

more than 3 times normal, if serum bilirubin levels begin to rise or if the patient complains of any symptoms that could be attributed to hepatitis (e.g., fatigue, nausea, vomiting, abdominal pain, and dark urine).

- *Symptomatic or severe (NYHA classes III and IV) CHF:* See previous discussion.
- *Premenopausal anovulatory women:* TZDs may cause resumption of ovulation and menstruation in women with polycystic ovarian syndrome, placing these patients at risk for an unwanted pregnancy.
- *History of hypersensitivity to TZDs.*
- *Drugs metabolized by CYP 3A4:* See the Drug Interactions section for further details.

Drug Interactions

Coadministration of a TZD with other antidiabetic medications or insulin does not alter the pharmacokinetics of either drug, but may increase the patient's risk for hypoglycemia. Pioglitazone induces CYP 3A4 and may, therefore, decrease effectiveness of other drugs metabolized by this enzyme, such as estrogens, cyclosporine, tacrolimus, and 3-hydroxy-3-methylglutaryl-coenzyme A (HMG-CoA) reductase inhibitors.[182] Patients taking oral contraceptives or estrogen replacement therapy should be informed of the possible risk of decreased effectiveness of estrogen therapy. Rosiglitazone does not seem to inhibit any of the major CYP enzymes.[181] Rifampin decreases the area under the plasma concentration–time curve (AUC) for both rosiglitazone and pioglitazone, although the clinical significance of this interaction is unknown.[196] Gemfibrozil significantly increases the AUC of both drugs. For patients receiving both a TZD and gemfibrozil, a dose reduction of the TZD may be warranted.

Efficacy

The effects of TZDs on HbA_{1C} and FPG are intermediate between that of acarbose and the sulfonylureas or metformin.[169,180] When combined with other antidiabetic agents in a poorly controlled type 2 patient, one can expect to see an augmented effect on the HbA_{1c} (0.9%–1.3% decrease with a sulfonylurea, 0.8%–1.2% decrease with metformin, and 0.6%–1.0% decrease with insulin).[181,182] When added to the therapy of a type 2 patient taking insulin, rosiglitazone and pioglitazone can enhance glycemic control while decreasing insulin requirements. Individuals who are minimally responsive or unresponsive to TZD therapy may include those who are not obese and have lower levels of endogenous insulin.

Other potential benefits of the TZDs are their favorable, but variable, effects on lipids.[180–182] Pioglitazone and to a lesser extent rosiglitazone may decrease triglycerides. Both drugs may increase HDL levels by 10%. Their effects on LDL levels are less clear. Rosiglitazone has been observed to increase LDL cholesterol by 8% to 16%, whereas pioglitazone may not affect LDL. Increases in LDL may be due to a shift from smaller, dense particles to larger, more buoyant ones, which are less susceptible to oxidation.[169] As noted, TZD therapy has been associated with weight gain and this may be substantial when used in combination with sulfonylureas or insulin.

Dosage and Clinical Use

TZDs are usually indicated in patients who are unable to take or have failed metformin or sulfonylurea monotherapy or who have not responded to combination therapy with other oral antidiabetic agents. A greater glucose-lowering effect has been observed when rosiglitazone is given as two divided doses rather than as a single daily dose. For monotherapy, a typical dose is 4 mg once daily or 2 mg twice daily with or without food. If the response is inadequate, the dosage can be increased to 8 mg once daily or 4 mg twice daily. For combination therapy with a sulfonylurea, metformin, or insulin, rosiglitazone can be initiated at 4 mg once daily and titrated to a maximum daily dose of 8 mg.

For monotherapy or combination therapy with a sulfonylurea, metformin, or insulin, the starting dose for pioglitazone is 15 or 30 mg once daily with or without food. The dose can be titrated up to a maximum of 45 mg/day.

Glucosidase Inhibitors

Acarbose (Precose) and miglitol (Glyset) are the two available oral agents in the α-glucosidase inhibitor class of antidiabetic agents.

Mechanism of Action

The α-glucosidase inhibitors reversibly inhibit glucosidases present in the brush-border of the mucosa of the small intestine.[70] These enzymes break down complex polysaccharides and disaccharides into glucose and other absorbable monosaccharides. Enzyme inhibition delays carbohydrate digestion and subsequent glucose absorption. Postprandial blood glucose concentrations are therefore lowered when these agents are taken with a meal containing complex carbohydrates.

Pharmacokinetics

Acarbose is minimally absorbed from the GI tract, with an oral bioavailability of parent drug of <2.0%.[197] It is extensively metabolized by GI amylases to inactive metabolites. The elimination half-life for acarbose is 2.8 hours, although there may be a longer terminal half-life. Unlike acarbose, miglitol is absorbed.[198] Absorption is saturable at higher doses (>25 mg). The drug is primarily distributed in extracellular fluids and is not metabolized. After a 25-mg dose, 95% of the drug is excreted unchanged by the kidneys within 24 hours.

Adverse Effects

GASTROINTESTINAL EFFECTS

Flatulence, diarrhea, and abdominal pain are the most frequently reported adverse effects of α-glucosidase inhibitors.[199] In placebo-controlled trials of acarbose, these complaints were experienced by 74%, 31%, and 19% of subjects, respectively. GI side effects are due to fermentation of unabsorbed carbohydrate in the small intestine and can be minimized by slowly titrating the dose of either agent. GI discomfort usually improves with continued therapy as induction of the α-glucosidase enzymes occurs in the distal jejunum and terminal ileum.

ELEVATED LIVER FUNCTION TESTS

In studies using doses of acarbose 300 mg/day or more, a transient increase in serum hepatic transaminases was reported.[197] The manufacturer recommends monitoring hepatic transaminases every 3 months for the first year of therapy and periodically thereafter. If an elevation of serum transaminases occurs, the dose should be decreased or discontinued if elevations persist. Because miglitol is not metabolized, it does not seem to affect hepatic function.

Contraindications and Precautions[197,198]

GASTROINTESTINAL CONDITIONS

Because of their profound GI effects (flatulence, diarrhea), acarbose and miglitol are contraindicated in patients with malabsorption, inflammatory bowel disease, or other marked disorders of digestion or absorption, or intestinal obstruction.

RENAL IMPAIRMENT

Acarbose has not been studied in patients with severe renal impairment (SrCr >2.0 mg/dL) and should not be used in these patients.[197]

Drug Interactions

Patients who use acarbose or miglitol in combination with other antidiabetic agents may develop hypoglycemia. These reactions should be treated with dextrose because acarbose may limit the availability of the disaccharide, sucrose (table sugar). Because acarbose and miglitol delay carbohydrate passage through the bowel, they could influence the absorption kinetics of concomitantly administered drugs. Conversely, because their own absorption may be diminished by digestive enzyme preparations and charcoal, they should not be taken concomitantly with these agents.[197,198] Acarbose and miglitol do not affect the absorption of glyburide in individuals with diabetes. The bioavailability of digoxin can be reduced and may require dose adjustment. Miglitol decreases the bioavailability of ranitidine and propranolol by 60% and 40%, respectively.[198]

Efficacy

By delaying the absorption of glucose following ingestion of complex carbohydrates and disaccharides, the α-glucosidase inhibitors can lower postprandial plasma glucose concentrations in patients with type 2 diabetes by 25 to 50 mg/dL.[199] FPG concentrations remain unchanged or are slightly lowered (20–30 mg/dL), but this effect may be related to decreased glucose toxicity, which improves insulin secretion and action. Mean HbA_{1c} values decline by 0.5% to 1%. Acarbose and miglitol have no effect on weight or lipid profiles.

Dosage and Clinical Use

Because of their more limited effects on HbA_{1c} and side effect profile, α-glucosidase inhibitors are usually used as add-on therapy in patients who have failed monotherapy or combination therapy with other oral antidiabetic agents. The recommended initial dose of either drug is up to 25 mg three times daily, taken at the start of each meal.[197,198] The dosage can be gradually increased (e.g., 25 mg/meal) every 4 to 8 weeks to a maximum of 50 mg three times daily for individuals weighing 60 kg or less, or 100 mg three times daily for individuals weighing more than 60 kg. A maximum response is observed at 6 months.

Incretin-Based Therapies

The most recent advances in therapy for type 2 diabetes have revolved around the discovery and exploration of the effects of incretins. Incretins are insulinotropic hormones secreted from specialized neuroendocrine cells in the small intestinal mucosa in response to carbohydrate ingestion and absorption.[13] The two hormones accounting for most incretin effects are glucose-dependent insulinotropic polypeptide (GIP) and glucagonlike peptide-1 (GLP-1). GIP and GLP-1 stimulate pancreatic β-cells in a glucose-dependent manner, contributing to the early phase insulin response. GLP-1 also inhibits pancreatic α-cells, thus reducing glucagon secretion and hepatic glucose production. Incretin action is efficient, but short lived. As they enter the blood vessels, incretins undergo rapid metabolism via proteolytic cleavage by dipeptidyl peptidase-4 (DPP-4) to inactive metabolites. Thus, only small amounts are needed to exert their effects on glucose metabolism.

Glucagonlike Peptide-1 Receptor Agonists (GLP-1 Mimetics/Analogs)

At the time of writing, exenatide (Byetta) is the only available GLP-1 mimetic in the United States. A long-acting release formulation of exenatide is currently under development.[200] Another agent, liraglutide (NN2211, Novo-Nordisk), is currently in phase III clinical trials.[201]

Mechanism of Action

GLP-1 mimetics and analogs that have stability in the presence of DPP-4 have been developed, resulting in a longer duration of action than endogenous GLP-1. Exenatide is a synthetic form of exendin-4, a peptide originally discovered from the saliva of the Gila monster.[200] Exendin-4 shares 50% of its amino acid sequence with GLP-1, demonstrating similar affinity for receptor sites but a strong resistance to DPP-4. Liraglutide is a GLP-1 analog with partial resistance to DPP-4. Both agents augment early or first-phase insulin response in response to elevated glucose concentrations, moderate glucagon secretion, and decrease hepatic glucose production without impairing the normal glucagon response to hypoglycemia. In addition, both agents slow gastric emptying, thereby reducing the rate at which glucose is absorbed. They suppress appetite, which may contribute to the prevention of weight gain and the weight loss (1.5–5 kg) observed in patients.

Pharmacokinetics

After subcutaneous (SC) injection, exenatide reaches median peak plasma concentrations in 2.1 hours, with a Vd of 28.3 L and a circulating half-life of 60 to 90 minutes.[200,202] The injection site (abdomen, thigh, or arm) does not significantly alter its kinetics. Exenatide is eliminated predominantly by glomerular filtration with subsequent proteolytic degradation. The mean terminal half-life is 2.4 hours, substantially longer than endogenous GLP-1, thus allowing for twice daily dosing. Its metabolism and elimination are dose independent; exenatide concentrations are measurable for up to 10 hours after injection. Liraglutide is highly protein bound (>98%), with a half-life of about 10 to 14 hours, allowing for once-daily dosing.[200]

Adverse Effects

GI side effects are common and dose dependent; 40% of patients report mild to moderate nausea and 15% report vomiting and/or diarrhea.[200,202] These side effects may be lessened by starting patients on low doses, ensuring correct timing and administration of the drug, and titrating the dose slowly. Other reported side effects have included decreased appetite and injection site reactions. Hypoglycemic risk can be increased in patients who are also taking a hypoglycemic oral agent (e.g., sulfonylurea) or insulin.

Exenatide use has been rarely related to hypersensitivity reactions, acute pancreatitis, and reversible renal impairment or failure requiring hemodialysis. Patients should be educated about symptoms of acute pancreatitis, including severe abdominal pain accompanied by vomiting, and instructed to report to their practitioner immediately. Patients in whom acute pancreatitis is confirmed with no other probable cause should not be rechallenged with exenatide.

About 40% to 50% of patients taking exenatide develop antibodies with weak binding affinities and low titers. In some patients, high antibody titers may result in treatment failure. Patients who demonstrate adherence to therapy, yet experience no change or worsening in glycemic control, should discontinue therapy and be switched to alternative agents.

Contraindications and Precautions

Exenatide is contraindicated in patients with known hypersensitivity.[201,202] Exenatide is not recommend for use in patients with severe GI disease, severe renal impairment (CrCl <30 mL/minute), end-stage renal failure, or those requiring hemodialysis.[202]

Drug Interactions

Exenatide may increase the risk for hypoglycemia when used with other hypoglycemic agents such as nonsulfonylurea secretagogues, sulfonylureas, and insulin.[202] Because of its mechanism of action, exenatide may reduce the rate and extent of absorption of orally administered drugs. Exenatide should therefore be used with caution in patients taking medications that require rapid GI absorption and are dose dependent on threshold concentrations for efficacy, such as antibiotics and oral contraceptives. In these cases, patients may be instructed to take the affected medications at least 1 hour before exenatide injection. There have been case reports of an increased International Normalized Ratio, sometimes associated with bleeding, in patients taking exenatide and warfarin. Patients should be closely monitored, with dose adjustments to warfarin therapy made as needed.

Efficacy

In clinical trials, maximum doses of exenatide combined with a sulfonylurea, metformin, a TZD, or sulfonylurea plus metformin therapy over 30 weeks reduced fasting blood glucose by 8 to 20 mg/dL, 2-hour postprandial blood glucose by 60 to 70 mg/dL, and HbA_{1c} by 0.8% to 1.0%.[200,202] Exenatide use over 80 weeks has been reported to reduce body weight by 4 to 5 kg. Clinical trials conducted to date with liraglutide monotherapy demonstrate decreases in fasting blood glucose of 30 to 60 mg/dL, HbA_{1c} of 0.6% to 1.75%, and weight of 2 to 3 kg.[200,201,203]

Dosage and Clinical Use

GLP-1 mimetics and analogs are indicated as add-on agents in patients with type 2 diabetes who have been unable to reach target goals on monotherapy or combination therapy with other oral agents and/or insulin. In addition, these agents may be helpful in patients with type 2 diabetes who are obese and struggling with weight loss. The starting dose of exenatide is 5 mcg injected SC into the abdomen, thigh, or arm twice daily within 60 minutes before morning and evening meals. Patients who experience severe GI side effects may try injecting just before meals initially and then move to 30 to 60 minutes before meals. If a patient tolerates the 5 mcg dose, then it can be titrated after 1 month of therapy to the maximum dose of 10 mcg SC twice daily. At the time of this writing, the dosing for liraglutide remains to be determined.

Dipeptidyl Peptidase-4 Inhibitors

At the time of writing, sitagliptin (Januvia) is the only available DPP-4 inhibitor in the United States. Vildagliptin (Galvus, Novartis), is expected to be approved sometime in 2009.[204] Saxagliptin (BMS-477118, Bristol-Myers Squibb) and denagliptin (GW823093, GlaxoSmithKline) are in phase III clinical trials.

Mechanism of Action

The DDP-4 inhibitors inhibit the degradation of GIP and GLP-1 upon entering the GI vasculature, thus increasing the effects of these endogenous incretins on first-phase insulin secretion and glucagon inhibition.[200] Both sitagliptin and vildagliptin reduce DPP-4 activity by 80%, with some inhibition maintained for up to 24 hours after an oral dose.

Pharmacokinetics

Sitagliptin is rapidly absorbed, with an absolute bioavailability of 87%.[205] Absorption is unaffected by food. Peak plasma concentrations occur in 1 to 4 hours, with a dose-proportional increase in plasma AUC, a Vd of 198 L, and terminal half-life of 12.4 hours. Only 38% of sitagliptin is plasma protein bound. Seventy-nine percent of the parent drug is excreted unchanged in the urine, primarily by active renal tubular secretion and may involve p-glycoprotein and human organic anion transporter-3. Metabolism by CYP3A4, and to a much lesser extent, CYP2C8, plays a minimal role in the excretion of metabolites in the feces.

Vildagliptin is rapidly absorbed, with an absolute bioavailability of 85%.[206,207] Food does not affect its absorption.[208] Absorption may take place at two sites and median time to peak plasma concentrations occurs 1 hour after oral administration.[206,207] Body weight may impact the Vd. Plasma AUC increases in a dose-proportional manner and the terminal half-life ranges from 1.32 to 2.43 hours. Renal clearance accounts for 21% of elimination, and may be greater in men than women.

Adverse Effects

Because these agents differ significantly in chemical structure from one another, some adverse events may be unique to the individual agent and may not be indicative of a class-wide effect.[200] The most commonly reported side effects with sitagliptin and vildagliptin in clinical trials include increased risk of infection [nasopharyngitis (3.5%–7.9% and 5.8%–9.3%, respectively), upper respiratory tract infection

(4.0%–8.0% and 5.3%–8.6%, respectively), sinusitis (1.4%–3.4% and 0.3%–4.1%, respectively), urinary tract infection (2.1%–4.6% and 1.5%–8.3%, respectively)] and headache (2.9%–4.5% and 5.0%–8.0%, respectively).[209] Vildagliptin has also been associated with cough (4.8%–7.4%) and other mild effects including dizziness, dyspepsia, nausea, constipation, and diarrhea.[210] Case reports of severe hypersensitivity reactions, including anaphylaxis, angioedema, and exfoliative skin reactions—including Stevens-Johnson syndrome—occurring after the first dose to as long as 3 months of therapy have been reported with sitagliptin.[205] Some authors have mentioned patients experiencing increased BP as well as musculoskeletal and connective tissue disorders in clinical trials with vildagliptin.[204,210] Because DPP-4 is expressed on many cell types, including lymphocytes, additional clinical experience and postmarketing studies are needed to clearly establish the long-term safety of these agents.

Contraindications and Precautions

Sitagliptin is contraindicated in patients with a history of serious hypersensitivity reaction to the drug.[205] It should be used with caution in combination with antidiabetic agents that cause hypoglycemia such as nonsulfonylurea secretagogues, sulfonylureas, and insulin. In such situations, patients should be instructed to closely monitor their blood glucose and if warranted, have the dose of their nonsulfonylurea secretagogue, sulfonylurea, and/or insulin adjusted. The dose of sitagliptin should be reduced in patients with moderate (CrCL 30–50 mL/minute) to severe (CrCl <30 mL/minute) renal insufficiency and in those with end-stage renal disease (ESRD) requiring hemodialysis or peritoneal dialysis.

Drug Interactions

Sitagliptin is not significantly protein bound.[205] It also does not inhibit CYP isoenzymes or induce CYP3A4; therefore, it is not expected to interact with other drugs that are metabolized by these pathways. Despite a lack of documented pharmacokinetic interactions from pharmacokinetic studies and clinical trials, because sitagliptin is a substrate for p-glycoprotein, patients taking digoxin should be monitored for any signs or symptoms of digoxin toxicity.[204] Limited information is available regarding drug interactions with vildagliptin. One pharmacokinetic study reports no interactions with digoxin in healthy volunteers.[211]

Efficacy

In clinical trials versus placebo, sitagliptin and vildagliptin lower fasting glucose by 15 to 30 mg/dL and HbA_{1c} by 0.62% to 0.85%.[200,209] In addition, clinical trials with sitagliptin demonstrate reductions in 2-hour postprandial glucose by 63 to 71 mg/dL.[205] Clinical trials of vildagliptin have reported statistically significant decreases in 4-hour postprandial glucose (-34.2 ± 9 mg/dL; $p < .0001$).[209,210] Unlike the GLP-1 mimetics and analogs, sitagliptin and vildagliptin do not seem to significantly affect body weight, appetite, or satiety.[200,209,210] As is the case for the GLP-1 mimetics/analogs, further studies are needed to more clearly determine the DDP-4 inhibitor effects on long-term preservation of β-cell function.

Dosage and Clinical Use

DDP-4 inhibitors seem to be useful as add-on therapy in combination with sulfonylureas, biguanides, TZDs, and insulin for patients who have been unsuccessful in reaching target goals. Sitagliptin may be initiated at 100 mg taken once daily with or without food.[205] Renal function should be assessed before initiation with sitagliptin therapy and periodically thereafter. In patients with moderate renal insufficiency (CrCl 30–50 mg/dL), the dose should be reduced to 50 mg once daily. In patients with severe renal insufficiency (CrCl <30 mg/dL) or those in end-stage renal failure requiring dialysis, the sitagliptin dose should be reduced to 25 mg once daily. Sitagliptin may be administered without regard to the timing of hemodialysis. For patients taking sitagliptin in combination with other antidiabetic agents that may cause hypoglycemia, the dose of the other agent (e.g., sulfonylurea) may need to be reduced.

Amylin Receptor Agonists (Amylinomimetics)

Amylin, or islet amyloid polypeptide, is a hormone found in the β-cells where it is co-manufactured, stored, and released with insulin in response to food intake.[212] Its actions seem to be centrally mediated and include slowing gastric emptying, suppressing glucagon secretion, and modulating the regulation of appetite. Amylin is absent in patients with type 1 diabetes. In patients with type 2 diabetes, its concentrations are altered to mirror those of insulin at different points in the progression of the disease. Pramlintide (Symlin) is currently the only approved amylin mimetic available in the United States for the adjunctive treatment of both types 1 and 2 diabetes.

Mechanism of Action

Pramlintide is a synthetic amylin analog, differing from the endogenous human substance by three amino acids.[213] These modifications render pramlintide equipotent, but with an increased solubility and decreased aggregability compared with endogenous amylin.

Pharmacokinetics

The absolute bioavailability of subcutaneously injected pramlintide is 30% to 40%.[213] Injection into the abdomen and thigh allow for more predictable absorption and distribution than injection into the arm. Body mass does not affect absorption or bioavailability. Approximately 40% of the drug is unbound in plasma. The half-life is about 48 minutes. Pramlintide is metabolized by the kidneys to an active metabolite with a half-life similar to the parent drug. It does not seem to accumulate with repeat dosing.

Adverse Effects

GI symptoms—including mild to moderate nausea (up to 95%), vomiting (8%–11%), anorexia (9%–17%), and abdominal pain (8%)—are the most frequently reported adverse reactions associated with therapy.[213] GI symptoms are usually transient, subsiding after 4 to 8 weeks of treatment and/or with dose reduction and slow dose escalation. Other reported adverse events from clinical trials include headache, dizziness, fatigue, coughing, pharyngitis, injection site reactions, and allergic reactions. There is a substantial increased risk of severe insulin-induced hypoglycemia within 3 hours of injection (see

Contraindication and Precautions section). There have been no reports of antibody formation to date.

Contraindications and Precautions

Pramlintide is contraindicated in patients with a known hypersensitivity to the drug or any of its components (e.g., metacresol), patients with hypoglycemic unawareness, and those with diagnosed gastroparesis. Severe hypoglycemia can occur when used in combination with insulin or another hypoglycemic agent (e.g., sulfonylurea) due to delayed gastric emptying, which slows carbohydrate absorption. Patients with type 1 diabetes seem to be at greatest risk. The package insert contains a black box warning for individuals while driving, those who operate heavy machinery, and those who engage in other high-risk activities in which serious injuries could result during a hypoglycemic episode. Patients should be closely monitored and have their insulin or oral hypoglycemic agent dose reduced upon initiation of therapy (see Dosage section).

Drug Interactions

As noted, severe hypoglycemia can occur in patients who are concurrently taking an oral hypoglycemic agent (e.g., sulfonylurea) or insulin (see Dosage section).[213] There have been no other reported drug interactions to date with pramlintide. Patients concurrently taking anticholinergics or agents that slow gastric absorption should be closely monitored for worsening GI symptoms.[212] Patients taking any medications that depend on rapid absorption for efficacy (e.g., antibiotics, oral contraceptives, pain medications) should be instructed to take those medications at least 1 hour before or 2 hours after pramlintide injection.

Efficacy

In clinical studies of patients with type 2 diabetes with doses up to 120 mcg/day for 52 weeks, pramlintide combined with oral hypoglycemic agents and/or insulin decreased HbA_{1c} significantly by 0.3% to 0.6% and weight by 0.5 to 4 kg.[212] Studies suggest that patients with significant obesity (BMI >35 kg/m^2) demonstrate the greatest weight reduction when treated with pramlintide versus placebo.

Clinical studies of patients with type 1 diabetes taking insulin in combination with pramlintide or placebo over 29 to 52 weeks demonstrate significant HbA_{1c} reductions of 0.3% to 0.5% and weight loss of 0.3 to 1.8 kg.[212] In three studies, patients were able to reduce their total daily insulin dose by 3% to 12%.

Dosage and Clinical Use

In clinical practice, pramlintide is considered an add-on agent primarily for patients with type 1 diabetes who have failed to achieve target blood glucose goals on insulin therapy alone. Its practical use is more limited to obese patients with type 2 diabetes who have failed to achieve target blood glucose levels with a regimen that includes a sulfonylurea or insulin. Pramlintide should not be considered for patients who have poor adherence to regular SMBG, medication therapy, and/or maintaining regularly scheduled visits with their health care providers.

Pramlintide is available in a vial and pen device (SymlinPen pen injector).[213] It cannot be mixed with any type of insulin. In addition, complex calculations are required to prepare a dose from a multidose vial and insulin syringes. This can impact proper dosage administration and adherence for even highly health literate patients. The pen device is therefore a more practical option when considering pramlintide therapy. Both vials and pens in use may be stored at room temperature (86°F or 30°C) for up to 30 days. Storing pramlintide at room temperature may minimize injection site reactions.

For patients with type 1 diabetes, the initial dose is 15 mcg and for patients with type 2 diabetes the initial dose is 60 mcg. Pramlintide is injected SC into the abdomen or thigh immediately before every major meal. A major meal is one that contains 30 g or more of carbohydrate or 250 kcals or more. If a meal is skipped, the pramlintide dose should be skipped and resumed before the next major meal. Injection sites should be rotated within the same anatomical area at every dose and sites used to inject insulin should be avoided.

When initiating pramlintide therapy, the dose of sulfonylureas, nonsulfonylurea secretagogues and premeal insulins must be reduced. It is recommended to reduce premeal insulin doses by at least 50%. Patients should be closely monitored and instructed to intensively monitor and record blood glucose (fasting, pre-, and postprandial) levels until control has stabilized. Any hypoglycemic episodes should be recorded and reported to the provider. Doses of hypoglycemic oral agents and insulin should then be titrated to optimal blood glucose control.

Pramlintide is titrated based upon achieving optimal glucose control with minimal side effects (e.g., nausea). For patients experiencing moderate to severe nausea, the dose may be reduced. If nausea does not subside, pramlintide therapy should be discontinued and the medication regimen adjusted accordingly. The dose may be increased when no clinically significant nausea has occurred for 3 to 7 days. For patients with type 1 diabetes, doses may be increased in 15-mcg increments up to a maximum meal dose of 60 mcg. For patients with type 2 diabetes, the dose may be increased to 120 mcg before every major meal. Pramlintide should be discontinued in patients who experience recurrent unexplained severe hypoglycemic episodes requiring medical attention.

TREATMENT OF PATIENTS WITH TYPE 2 DIABETES

Clinical Presentation

44. L.H. is a 45-year-old, moderately overweight, Mexican-American woman with central obesity (height, 5 feet 5 inches; weight, 160 lbs; BMI 26.6 kg/m^2). She was referred to the diabetes clinic when her gynecologist, who had been treating her for recurrent monilial infections, noted glucosuria on routine urinalysis. Subsequently, on two separate occasions she was found to have an FPG of 150 mg/dL and 167 mg/dL. L.H. denies any symptoms of polyphagia or polyuria, although lately she has been more thirsty than usual. She does complain of lethargy and often takes afternoon naps.

L.H.'s other medical problems include hypertension, which is well controlled on lisinopril 20 mg/day, and recurrent monilial

infections, which are treated with fluconazole. She has given birth to four children (birth weights, 7, 8.5, 10, and 11 lb) and was told during her last pregnancy that she had "borderline diabetes." She currently works as a loan officer in a local bank and spends her weekends "catching up on her sleep" and reading. L.H. has been smoking one pack of cigarettes per day for 20 years and drinks an occasional glass of wine. She drinks at least two regular sodas daily and has "large" glass of orange juice every morning. Her family history is significant for a sister, aunt, and grandmother with type 2 diabetes; all have "weight problems." L.H.'s mother is alive and well at age 77; her father died of a heart attack at age 47.

Laboratory assessment reveals an FPG of 147 mg/dL (normal, 70–100); fasting plasma triglycerides of 400 mg/dL (normal, <150 mg/dL); and an HbA_{1c} of 9.2% (normal, 4%–6%). All other values (including the complete blood count, electrolytes, LFTs, and renal function tests) are within normal limits. L.H. is given the diagnosis of type 2 diabetes. What features in L.H.'s history and physical examination are consistent with this diagnosis?

[SI units: plasma glucose, 8.3, 9.3, and 8.1 mmol/L; plasma triglycerides, 6.77 mmol/L; HbA_{1c}, 0.09 (normal, 0.04–0.07)]

The features of L.H.'s history that are consistent with type 2 diabetes include an FPG concentration of 126 mg/dL or higher on more than one occasion, an elevated HbA_{1c}, high BMI with central obesity, age greater than 40, family history of diabetes, and Mexican American descent. L.H. also has delivered large babies, which suggests that she may have had undiagnosed gestational diabetes, a condition that places women at high risk for subsequently developing type 2 diabetes. Diagnosis on routine examination and mild signs and symptoms of hyperglycemia (including increased thirst and lethargy), recurrent monilial infections, hypertriglyceridemia, and indications of CVD (hypertension) also are typical in patients with type 2 diabetes (see Type 2 Diabetes and Table 50-1).

Treatment Goals

45. What should the goals of therapy be for L.H. and other patients with type 2 diabetes? Which biochemical indices should be monitored?

The beginning of this chapter discussed general goals of therapy for all people with diabetes, which include eliminating acute symptoms of hyperglycemia, avoiding hypoglycemia, reducing cardiovascular risk factors, and preventing or slowing the progression of both microvascular and macrovascular diabetic complications. The ADA recommends that otherwise healthy patients with type 2 diabetes strive to achieve the same biochemical goals as those recommended for people with type 1 diabetes[22,214] (Table 50-4 and Table 50-5).

The UKPDS was the longest and largest study of patients with type 2 diabetes. It conclusively demonstrated that improved blood glucose control reduces the risk of developing retinopathy, nephropathy, and, potentially, neuropathy.[33] A 25% overall reduction in microvascular complication rate was observed among those patients receiving intensive therapy versus conventional therapy. An additional finding of the UKPDS was that aggressive control of BP also significantly reduced strokes, diabetes-related deaths, heart failure, microvascular complications, and vision loss.[215,216]

When determining treatment goals for L.H. and others with type 2 diabetes, the same individual characteristics should be considered as for type 1 diabetes, such as the patient's capacity to understand and carry out the treatment regimen, the patient's risk for severe hypoglycemia, and other patient-specific factors that may increase the risk or decrease the benefit of intensive treatment (e.g., advanced age, ESRD, advanced cardiovascular or cerebrovascular disease, or other coexisting diseases that may shorten life expectancy). Emphasis should be placed on assessment of all cardiovascular risk factors, including hypertension, tobacco use, dyslipidemia, and family history.

Macrovascular disease is the primary cause of death in this population, and its underlying pathogenesis may or may not be related to hyperglycemia per se. This is a subject of great complexity and controversy. Although the prevalence of cardiovascular morbidity and mortality correlates with HbA_{1c} levels in observational and epidemiologic studies, no prospective, randomized, controlled trials have established a relationship between macrovascular disease and the degree of glycemic control.[27] Whether intensive insulin therapy is appropriate for people with type 2 diabetes also has been questioned. Some have worried that hyperinsulinemia associated with intensive insulin therapy or the sulfonylureas actually could accelerate atherosclerosis or increase the risk of cardiovascular events. However, the UKPDS showed no increase in cardiovascular events or mortality in patients assigned to sulfonylurea or insulin therapy, despite their fasting plasma insulin levels being higher than those of the conventionally treated patients.[33] There is also concern that the counter-regulatory hormones released in response to hypoglycemia could endanger those with existing CVD. These views are summarized and analyzed by Colwell[217,218] and others,[219] who suggest taking a more aggressive stance toward glycemic control, while attending to the reduction of all risk factors for CVD (e.g., hypertension, dyslipidemia, platelet hyper-reactivity, microalbuminuria).

Glycemic goals for patients with type 2 diabetes must be individualized. Given the conflicting preliminary data from the ACCORD and ADVANCE trials, patients with type 2 diabetes and CVD or multiple CVD risk factors should be carefully assessed before determining their metabolic goals (See Long-term Complications and Their Relation to Glucose Control).[35,36] For example, less aggressive HbA_{1c} goals should be considered for patients with advanced age or significant cerebrovascular or coronary artery disease because of the serious consequences related to hypoglycemia. However, many treatment options available today are associated with a very low risk of hypoglycemia.

Because L.H. is relatively young and has no symptoms of microvascular disease or neuropathy, every effort should be made to normalize her glucose concentrations to prevent these complications. Furthermore, a lipid panel should be ordered and steps taken to achieve normal LDL cholesterol, HDL cholesterol, and triglyceride levels. Often, triglyceride levels improve as blood glucose concentrations decline and the metabolic response to insulin improves.

(Management of dyslipidemia is addressed more fully later in this chapter.)

Biochemical indices that should be followed to monitor L.H.'s response to therapy include fasting, postprandial, and preprandial blood glucose concentrations, HbA_{1c} values, fasting triglyceride levels, as well as LDL and HDL cholesterol concentrations. Initial metabolic goals for L.H. should be an HbA_{1c} value of <7%, an FPG of <130 mg/dL, postprandial glucose concentrations below 180 mg/dL, LDL-cholesterol below 100 mg/dL, and triglycerides below 150 mg/dL.

Treatment: A Stepped-Care Approach

Lifestyle Interventions and Initial Therapy With Metformin (Step 1)

46. How should L.H. be managed initially?

Initial therapy of type 2 diabetes is aimed at lifestyle changes that will minimize insulin resistance and risk for CVD. In L.H.'s case and in the case of other overweight (BMI 25.0–29.9) or obese (BMI ≥30.0) type 2 individuals, this includes a lower calorie, low-fat, low-cholesterol diet; regular exercise; smoking cessation (see Chapter 85) and aggressive management of dyslipidemia and hypertension. Because obesity is associated with increased tissue resistance to endogenous insulin, L.H. should be strongly encouraged to decrease her caloric intake and lose weight. When signs and symptoms are mild, diet and exercise alone can correct glucose intolerance. SMBG monitoring should be encouraged and education that addresses the serious nature of diabetes mellitus and its long-term consequences also should begin. This is discussed in the previous sections, Medical Nutrition Therapy and Exercise, under Treatment (Table 50-16).

INITIAL PHARMACOLOGIC THERAPY WITH METFORMIN

In 2006, the ADA and the European Association for the Study of Diabetes published a consensus algorithm for the initiation and adjustment of therapy in type 2 diabetes.[220] The major change to the typical approach for glycemic control in type 2 diabetes was the recommendation to begin metformin along with lifestyle intervention as part of the initial therapy. The reasoning behind this recommendation is that patients with type 2 diabetes often fail to achieve the aggressive glycemic goals with lifestyle intervention alone leading to prolonged elevations in HbA_{1c} (Fig. 50-8).

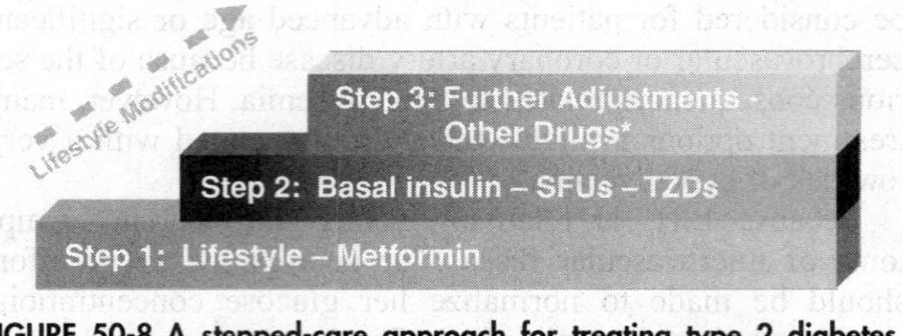

FIGURE 50-8 A stepped-care approach for treating type 2 diabetes. Treatment plans should be individualized. Lifestyle interventions (diet, exercise, weight loss, tobacco cessation, lipid and blood pressure management) are reinforced at every visit. *α-Glucosidase inhibitors, glinides, exenatide, dipeptidyl peptidase-4 inhibitors, glinides, pramlintide. SFUs, sulfonylureas; TZDs, thiazolidinediones.

Although the UKPDS demonstrated that the sulfonylureas, metformin, and insulin reduce glucose with equal effectiveness (TZDs were not studied), metformin is favored as a first-choice agent for overweight, type 2 diabetic patients by many endocrinologists as long as there are no contraindications to its use. This is because metformin lowers blood glucose by decreasing hepatic glucose output and insulin resistance (indirectly) without causing weight gain or hypoglycemia. Metformin also has beneficial effects on plasma lipid concentrations as well.[33,221] One must always keep in mind that the primary goal is to normalize glucose concentrations, because hyperglycemia has been most closely correlated to the development of long-term complications. Thus, agents that may cause weight gain (e.g., sulfonylureas) are still very effective.

A drawback to metformin is that it requires multiple daily dosing and its dose also must be titrated to minimize GI effects. After the dose is established, it is possible to use a long-acting product that can be dosed once daily. Renal function tests should be evaluated before the drug is initiated. L.H. does not have any contraindications (renal or hepatic dysfunction, cardiorespiratory disease, binge alcohol use) to the use of metformin that could predispose her to its most significant side effect, lactic acidosis (see Question 62). Because L.H. exhibits the typical features of insulin resistance syndrome, has no contraindications for its use, and her HbA_{1c} is about 2% above her goal of <7%, she should be started on metformin. L.H. should take metformin 500 mg twice daily with food. If her HbA_{1c} was much closer to 7%, it would be reasonable to try lifestyle intervention alone before instituting pharmacologic therapy. However, most patients with type 2 diabetes require at least one medication to achieve the glycemic goals set forth by the ADA.

TITRATING METFORMIN DOSES

47. L.H. is started on metformin 500 mg BID with food and instructed to increase her dosage to 500 mg Q AM and 1,000 mg Q PM after 1 week. Three days after starting metformin, she phones the clinic complaining of nausea and diarrhea. She admits to taking her doses on an empty stomach. How should L.H.'s symptoms be addressed?

GI disturbances such as diarrhea, bloating, anorexia, abdominal discomfort, nausea, and metallic taste often dissipate with time and can be minimized by initiating metformin in a single, 500- or 850-mg dose at breakfast or with the patient's largest meal of the day. Consistently taking metformin with food significantly minimizes the GI side effects. The dosage should be slowly increased (e.g., 500 mg/day every 2 weeks) until the appropriate clinical effect is achieved or the patient is taking the maximum dose (1,000 mg twice daily or 850 mg three times a day). Therefore, L.H.'s metformin dose should be reduced to 500 mg daily with her largest meal, and she should be titrated more slowly over a period of several weeks to 500 mg three times a day or higher as tolerated. Metformin is typically dosed two to three times daily (the long-acting formulation is dosed once daily with dinner). If she continues to experience GI symptoms, an alternative approach is to use the extended-release formulation; small studies have demonstrated improved tolerability with the extended-release tablets over the immediate release dosage form.[222] A drawback to these tablets is their very large size.

MONITORING METFORMIN THERAPY

48. How should metformin therapy be monitored in N.H.?

As is standard with other agents, L.H. should be encouraged to perform SMBG (see Question 49) and have an HbA_{1c} test performed quarterly until she achieves consistent values of <7%. Additional evidence of metformin's therapeutic benefits may include an improved lipid profile and some weight loss. Initially, it is important to follow GI problems and, although lactic acidosis is unlikely, L.H. should be warned to bring to the attention of her physician any sudden symptoms of shortness of breath, weakness, and malaise. A baseline SrCr, LFTs, and complete blood count should be obtained for L.H. and repeated yearly.

Self-Monitoring Blood Glucose in Type 2 Diabetes

49. L.H. is interested in learning how to perform blood glucose testing. What are the advantages and disadvantages of SMBG tests? When and how often should L.H. be instructed to test her blood glucose concentrations?

SMBG is an important self-management tool for patients such as L.H. to assess the efficacy of therapy and guide adjustments in nutrition, exercise, and medications. Performing SMBG also helps patients to monitor for and prevent hypoglycemia. Disadvantages include cost of testing, inadequate understanding by both health care providers and patients regarding the benefits and proper use of SMBG results, patient psychological and physical discomfort associated with obtaining a blood sample, and the inconvenience of testing. However, with the current advances in meter technology and proper patient education, most of these potential barriers can be overcome.

The ADA recommends SMBG for all patients taking insulin, but its stance with regard to patients with type 2 diabetes treated with diet or diet plus antidiabetic agents (other than insulin) is less clear. A meta-analysis of SMBG effects in patients with type 2 diabetes who are not taking insulin concluded the overall effect on HbA_{1c} was a 0.4% reduction; however, these studies often included multiple interventions such as education, diet, and medication adjustments. [223] The ADA does suggest that the "optimal frequency and timing of SMBG for patients with type 2 diabetes on noninsulin therapy is not known but should be sufficient to facilitate reaching glucose goals."[22] We often recommend SMBG for motivated type 2 patients who are learning to adjust their carbohydrate intake and portion sizes and want to measure how well medications and lifestyle changes are working to improve their glucose control. Initially, we may suggest testing four times daily before meals and at bedtime for 1 week so that the patient can observe his or her glucose profiles. Later, once the desired HbA_{1c} has been achieved, we recommend a minimum of testing blood glucose twice daily, but at various times to evaluate fasting glucose concentrations, 2-hour postmeal concentrations, and preprandial concentrations. A study of type 2 patients treated with diet with or without oral agents, but not insulin, observed that 2-hour postlunch values (<150 mg/dL) and predinner values (<125 mg/dL) most closely correlated with HbA_{1c} values of less than 7%.[224] As emphasized by the ADA, intensive patient education regarding testing technique and interpretation are vital to the cost-effective use of this monitoring tool. The patient must be able to assess his or her glucose profile and institute lifestyle changes that can have a favorable effect.

50. L.H. was quite motivated to improve her glucose control because her grandmother "lost a leg" to diabetes and her aunt is undergoing dialysis because "her kidneys have failed." She is taking metformin 1,000 mg PO BID and tolerating it reasonably well (she occasionally gets some stomach discomfort, but states she is fine with it). She is proud that she remembers to take the metformin everyday as instructed. She met with a dietitian who suggested an 1,800-calorie diet and 45-minute walks three times weekly. After 3 months, L.H. had lost 6 pounds. L.H. stopped drinking regular sodas and juices, but eats either breads or two large tortillas at each meal. She admits to eating only small amounts of "greens" and vegetables. She has not been able to implement her walks three times weekly; more often she only walks once a week. Although her FPG fell to 130 mg/dL (normal, 70–100), more than 50% of her postprandial blood glucose levels were often above 180 mg/dL (normal, <140). Her HbA_{1c} is 7.4% (normal, 4%–6%), and fasting triglyceride levels are now 260 mg/dL (normal, <150). How should her therapy be adjusted? What factors should be considered when deciding on the next steps for pharmacologic therapy?

L.H.'s HbA_{1c} has improved by 1.8%. However, she has not fully instituted lifestyle interventions. Although she has cut out juices and regular sodas, she can improve her diet and lower her postprandial blood glucose (to <180 mg/dL) by eating lower carbohydrate meals and increasing her vegetable intake. She also can increase her physical activity to at least three times weekly. Although the HbA_{1c} is not below 7%, a reasonable approach would be to continue metformin at 1,000 mg PO BID and reinforce lifestyle changes at this point before modifying her pharmacocologic therapy.

Type 2 diabetes is a progressive condition, which is highly likely to require drug therapy. In the UKPDS, only 16% and 19% of the subjects achieved a FPG below 108 and HbA_{1c} below 7%, respectively, after 3 years of dietary therapy.[225] By 9 years, only 9% were able to maintain their glycemic goals using diet therapy alone. For patients who elect to start with lifestyle changes, we recommend monotherapy followed by combination therapy with two antidiabetic agents if therapeutic goals are not met. For patients who start with metformin at the time of diagnosis, as in the case of L.H., the next step would be to add a second antidiabetic agent.[220,226] Selecting an antidiabetic agent to treat type 2 diabetes has become more complex as new agents with unique mechanisms of action have been introduced into the market. As with all therapeutic decisions, clinicians should also blend their knowledge of the drug (e.g., its efficacy, safety, side effects, dosing methods, and cost) with the unique characteristics of the patient (e.g., level of glycemic control, organ function, other concurrent diseases and medications, ability to adhere to complex medication regimens, health care coverage) when making a choice of drug products.[227] The current HbA_{1c} level and

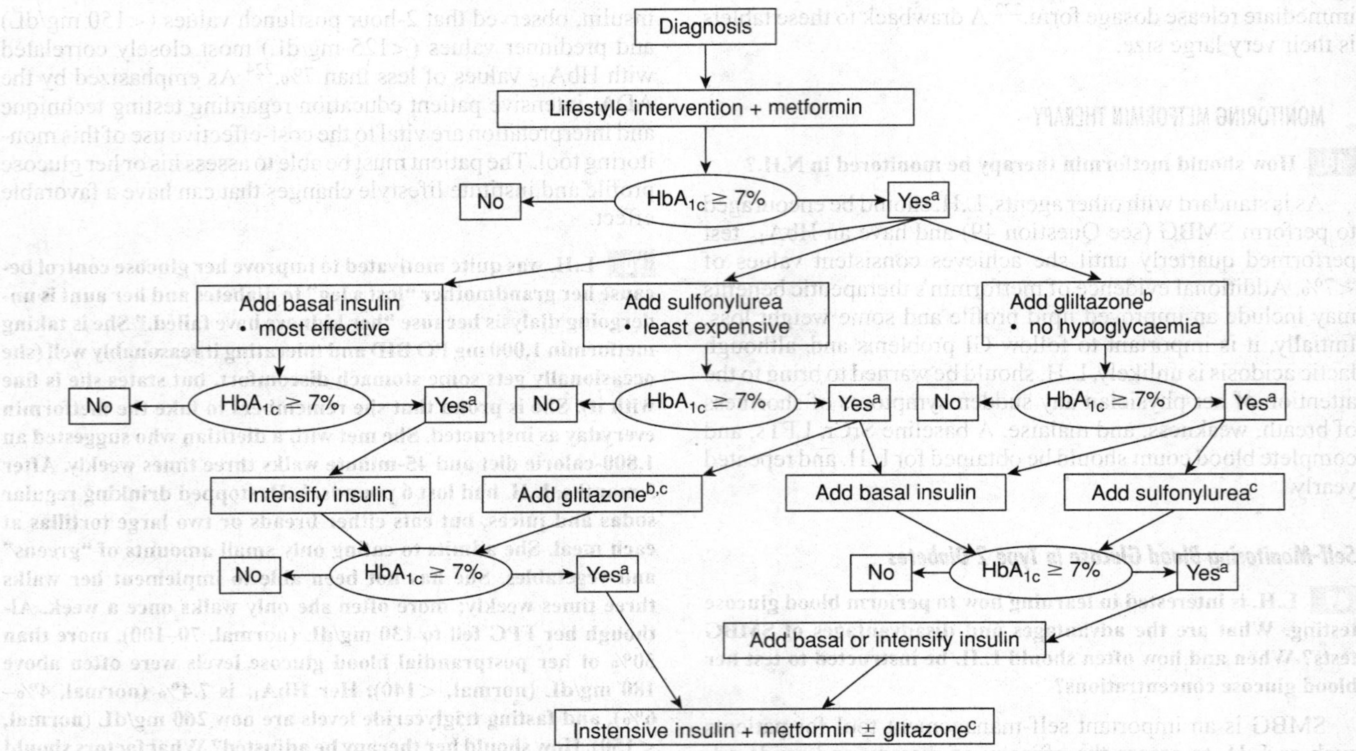

FIGURE 50-9 Suggested treatment algorithm for type 2 diabetes. [a]Check HbA_{1c} every 3 months until it is below 7%, and then at least every 6 months. [b]Associated with an increased risk of fluid retention, heart failure, and fractures. Rosiglitazone, but probably not pioglitazone, may be associated with an increased risk of MI. [c]Although three oral agents can be used, initiation and intensification of insulin therapy may be preferred based on effectiveness and lower costs. (Used with permission from reference 226.)

reduction required to reach the HbA_{1c} goal is also an important consideration. Practitioners should attempt to avoid unnecessarily complex therapy that may confuse the patient, increase drug costs, and complicate the clinician's ability to assess each medication's contribution to the overall therapeutic outcome (Fig. 50-8). The algorithm proposed by Nathan et al., and endorsed by the ADA, recommends consideration of initiating insulin therapy (most often basal insulin) if the HbA_{1c} is above 8.5%. However, in clinical practice, most would continue to select noninsulin combination therapy until the HbA_{1c} reaches a higher level, closer to 10% (Fig. 50-9). To use the algorithm, practitioners need to take into account the patient's underlying pathogenesis. The pathogenic features are deduced from the patient's body weight. If the patient is obese, it is presumed there is an element of insulin resistance and increased hepatic glucose output. If the patient is lean, he or she is presumed to be insulin deficient. Antidiabetic therapy is chosen to target the pathogenic problem(s).

Table 50-26 compares and contrasts the efficacy, advantages, and disadvantages of antidiabetic agents used to treat type 2 diabetic patients and can be used in conjunction with the basic algorithm to select drugs for a specific patient. Table 50-28 summarizes treatment of type 2 diabetes under special circumstances.

If patients fail therapy with two oral agents, one could move to triple therapy (noninsulin) or add insulin. To avoid injections, many patients and caregivers opt for triple combination therapy (using oral agents with different mechanisms of action), but this is less well studied.[228–231,232] One study compared triple oral therapy with insulin 70/30 mix plus metformin in patients with type 2 diabetes poorly controlled on two oral agents.[233] Both treatments were about equally effective in lowering HbA_{1c} and FPG values (1.77% and 55 mg/dL; and 1.96% and 65 mg/dL, respectively). However, 10.2% of patients in the triple-therapy group were switched to the insulin plus metformin therapy because of an inadequate response, but these patients had higher HbA_{1c} levels (average 10.6%) at baseline. The cost of triple therapy (drug cost plus LFT monitoring for the TZDs) was higher. Other combination options exist now with the availability of exenatide (which is injected), the DPP-4 inhibitors, and pramlintide (although this is very infrequently used).

The combined use of insulin plus oral therapy was once considered a bridge to insulin monotherapy. However, a substudy of the UKPDS demonstrated that the early addition of insulin to patients with inadequate responses to oral sulfonylureas (FPG >108) improved glycemic control over insulin therapy alone over an average follow-up period of 6 years. Patients on combined therapy with insulin suffered 50% more episodes of major hypoglycemia, but weight gain was comparable.[234] If this fails, the patient is treated with insulin monotherapy. Insulin is being considered earlier in therapy now for patients with type 2 diabetes to achieve glycemic goals. For patients who are gaining weight because they require large insulin doses, metformin can be added to achieve control with lower doses in insulin. Although TZDs have been shown to allow for lower

Table 50-28 Treating Type 2 Diabetes Under Special Circumstances

Circumstance	*Avoid*	*Consider*
Patients with decreased renal function	Acarbose[a] Long-acting SFUs (e.g., glyburide) Metformin	Glipizide Glimepiride Insulin Glinides (Repaglinide/nateglinide) Sitagliptin Thiazolidinediones
Patients with impaired liver function	Acarbose[a] Metformin Thiazolidinediones ? SFUs (severe liver dysfunction)	Insulin Repaglinide[b] Exenatide Sitagliptin Miglitol
Patients who are obese or gaining excessive weight	Insulin[c] Sulfonylureas Repaglinide ? Thiazolidinediones[d]	Acarbose Miglitol Metformin
Patients with preexisting edema	Thiazolidinediones	SFUs Glinides Exenatide Sitagliptin
Patients with heart failure	Thiazolidinediones Metformin	SFUs Glinides Exenatide Sitagliptin Insulin
Patients experiencing hypoglycemia due to irregular eating patterns	Insulin Long-acting SFUs	Acarbose Metformin Repaglinide/nateglinide Thiazolidinediones Exenatide Sitaglipin

[a]This is a labeled recommendation. Although very little acarbose is absorbed into the systemic circulation, the small amount available relies on the kidneys for elimination. This accumulation and doses ≥300 mg/day rarely have been associated with elevated liver enzymes. Plasma concentrations of miglitol in renally impaired volunteers were proportionally increased relative to the degree of renal dysfunction.
[b]The manufacturer recommends more cautious dose titration in these cases.
[c]This recommendation presumes that the patient can be controlled on other antidiabetic agents. Often by the time insulin is required in type 2 diabetes, pancreatic function may have deteriorated considerably.
[d]Rosiglitazone and pioglitazone are associated with mild to moderate weight gain owing to fluid retention and fat accumulation. However, because of their mechanism of action, they are effective in improving glycemic control in insulin-resistant patients who are often overweight or obese.
SFUs, sulfonylureas.

insulin doses, their use is associated with weight gain and more edema when combined with insulin.

Clinical Use of Antidiabetic Agents

Selecting an Oral Agent

51. Which other antidiabetic agents could be considered for L.H. as monotherapy?

Although the treatment algorithm recommends the use of metformin as step 1 therapy, other antidiabetic agents are approved for use as monotherapy as well.

L.H. is a typical overweight type 2 patient with early evidence of CVD (hypertension), but with no evidence of microvascular complications. Her liver, renal, and GI functions are normal. Patients like L.H. with moderate to severe type 2 diabetes have varying degrees of β-cell dysfunction and tissue resistance to insulin. In these individuals, pulsatile insulin secretion and first-phase insulin release are absent, and the pancreas is "blind" or unresponsive to high glucose concentrations (glucotoxicity). Because target tissues are less responsive to insulin, hepatic glucose output typically is increased and patients may require higher concentrations of insulin to achieve the same degree of peripheral glucose utilization observed in people without diabetes mellitus. At this stage, technically all classes of oral antidiabetic agents and insulin are likely to work equally well, although metformin is still considered the preferred agent. Insulin causes more weight gain and hypoglycemia than the other antidiabetic agents and is usually reserved for combination therapy unless the initial HbA_{1c} at diagnosis is very elevated (>10%) or ketonuria is present.[220]

Often, *acarbose* is eliminated from consideration because slow titration is required to minimize GI effects; anecdotally, however, people of Mexican American origin, such as L.H., seem less susceptible to flatulence and diarrhea. Also, because acarbose has less dramatic effects on the FPG (20–30 mg/dL decrease) and HbA_{1c} (0.5%–1.0% decrease) than the other agents, biochemical goals are less likely to be achieved in patients whose HbA_{1c} is 8.5% or higher.

Rosiglitazone or *pioglitazone* also can be used as monotherapy and, like metformin, neither is likely to cause hypoglycemia, but weight gain and edema are likely. Their effects on FPG and HbA_{1c} are intermediate between those of acarbose and metformin or the sulfonylureas, so that it is likely that the goals established for L.H. could be achieved with either agent as monotherapy.[220] On the positive side, the TZDs have been shown to have better "glycemic durability" compared with metformin and the SFUs. In a double-blind, randomized, controlled trial of 4,360 patients with type 2 diabetes, time to monotherapy failure, defined as FPG above 180 mg/dL was assessed for rosiglitazone, metformin, and glyburide (A Diabetes Outcome Progression Trial [ADOPT]).[235] Patients were treated for a median of 4 years. The Kaplan-Meier analysis showed that the cumulative incidence of failure at 5 years was 15% for rosiglitazone, 21% for metformin, and 34% for glyburide ($p < .0001$). The suggested explanation for the favorable rosiglitazone results was that it slowed the rate of β-cell function decline. On the negative side, several meta-analyses have called into question the safety of rosiglitazone.[189,190,236,237] Given the recent data suggesting a 30% to 40% relative increase in risk of MI, many practitioners are using rosiglitazone more cautiously. Other analyses, however, have not continued an increased risk of MI for either rosiglitazone or pioglitazone, which may even have a protective effect.[192,238,239] Both rosiglitazone and pioglitazone are associated with an approximate twofold increased risk of heart failure.[238–240] In the long-term ADOPT trial, rosiglitazone was associated with a mean weight gain of 4.8 kg, whereas weight decreased by 2.9 kg in the metformin group; glyburide-treated patients had a mean weight gain of 1.6 kg during the first year, and then remained stable.[235] Given these adverse effects, most practitioners reserve TZDs for combination therapy.

Sitagliptin, which is approved for monotherapy, is generally reserved for add-on (combination) therapy. However, it can be used as monotherapy for patients in whom the use of other oral agents is precluded (such as renal dysfunction for metformin or severe heart failure for the TZDs).

Finally, one should not forget that until the newer agents became available, sulfonylureas were used quite successfully to treat obese patients with type 2 diabetes. These agents are relatively trouble free with regard to side effects (weight gain and occasional hypoglycemia), and many can be dosed once daily. They are very effective and many are now available in generic form, making them quite affordable when cost is a primary consideration (Table 50-27).

Several new products that combine two oral agents into one medication are available. Although these products are approved as first-line therapy, thus skipping the monotherapy step, we recommend that they be reserved for use in patients whose medication regimens must be simplified to enhance adherence.

Based on this discussion, we favor the use of metformin as initial therapy in L.H.

Thiazolidinediones

52. N.H. is a 46-year-old, obese (BMI 33 kg/m^2) man with a history of type 2 diabetes, hypertension, recurrent deep venous thrombosis, and hyperlipidemia. He presents with complaints of fatigue and nocturia. N.H. has smoked 2 packs of cigarettes/day for 15 years and has a strong family history of coronary heart disease (CHD). At diagnosis 3 months ago, he had a random plasma glucose >200 mg/dL on two occasions (248 and 207 mg/dL); a FPG of 150 mg/dL (normal, <126 mg/dL), and an HbA$_{1c}$ of 8.5% (normal, 4%–6%) confirming the diagnosis of type 2 diabetes. Tests of liver and renal function are within normal limits. Current medications include enalapril and lovastatin. N.H. started metformin but stopped taking it because of GI symptoms (loose stools); he refuses to try this medication again. After a 1-month trial of diet and exercise, his glucose concentrations remain above 200 mg/dL. What is a reasonable next monotherapy option for N.H.?

Unfortunately, N.H. did not tolerate metformin. Although this is less common if patients take metformin with food and the dose titrated slowly, some do not overcome the GI adverse effects. N.H. is refusing to even consider a retrial. With a BMI of 33 kg/m^2, hypertension, and dyslipidemia, N.H. has many components of the metabolic syndrome and insulin resistance (see Pathogenesis). We would not select sulfonylureas or insulin as a next choice of drug of choice for N.H. because they do not exert a favorable effect on plasma lipids and generally are associated with weight gain. We acknowledge that some sulfonylureas remain the least expensive oral antidiabetic agents, and this may be an important factor in the initial selection of therapy for some patients. Although sulfonylureas or insulin decrease blood glucose concentrations in patients like N.H., they do so by increasing insulin concentrations. Patients such as N.H. are likely to have β-cell dysfunction, as evidenced by poor first-phase insulin release; however, in the early stages of type 2 diabetes, they also are likely to exhibit high insulin concentrations, which suggests resistance of peripheral tissues to insulin action. This can be overcome by increasing insulin levels, but hyperinsulinemia promotes fuel storage and often is accompanied by hunger, occasional hypoglycemia, and weight gain. Interestingly, research suggests that the sulfonylureas may close ATP-sensitive potassium channels in cardiac tissue, similar to their action at the β-cell. In the heart, this effect could limit circulation to an ischemic area.[198,217]

In light of N.H.'s HbA$_{1c}$ value (8.5%), acarbose as monotherapy is not likely to attain near-normal plasma glucose concentrations. Rosiglitazone or pioglitazone improve peripheral target tissue responses to insulin and lipid profiles. N.H. is taking several other medications, and the convenience of a single-daily-dose therapy may be beneficial to him. In addition to the increased risk of MI demonstrated with rosiglitazone (see Question 52), edema, weight gain, and heart failure are adverse effects associated with TZDs; rosiglitazone and pioglitazone have also been shown to increase the risk of bone fractures. However, this risk has only been seen in older women.[235,241] It is thought to be due to reduced osteoblast differentiation as a result of increased adipogenesis in the bone marrow.[242] TZDs should be used cautiously in older women and patients on chronic steroids.

For N.H., whose liver function is normal, pioglitazone 15 to 30 mg/day is the next reasonable option. He should be started on pioglitazone 15 to 30 mg/day. Liver function tests (ALT) should be performed at baseline (done already), and then periodically thereafter according to the manufacturer.[182] Many practitioners check the LFTs every 3 to 6 months during the first year of therapy and then every 6 to 12 months thereafter.

Clinical Note: N.H. was successful in reducing his HbA$_{1c}$ to 7.1% through a combination of lifestyle modifications and pioglitazone. He was able to lose 10 pounds with walking and reduction in fatty food, despite being on a TZD, which can cause weight gain secondary to fluid retention and fat accumulation. The modest weight loss and improved glucose concentrations likely reduced his insulin resistance, thereby improving tissue responsiveness to his endogenous insulin. N.H. enrolled in a smoking cessation program, but has been unable to quit smoking completely (see Chapter 85).

Sulfonylureas

53. K.M. is a 64-year-old Asian woman with a BMI of 22 kg/m^2 who was diagnosed with type 2 diabetes. Her HbA$_{1c}$ is 9.0%. Because she is thin, with no evidence of abdominal obesity, the diabetes interdisciplinary team agrees that she is likely insulinopenic and should be treated with a sulfonylurea. Which agents could be used? How should they be dosed?

A minority of patients who are diagnosed with type 2 diabetes are thin, with little to no abdominal obesity. In this type of patient, the major cause of hyperglycemia is likely insulin deficiency, or a β-cell defect. A sulfonylurea would be a reasonable first choice of therapy because it increases insulin secretion. Patients likely to respond most favorably to oral sulfonylureas include those who are older than 40 years of age, have been diagnosed within the last 5 years, are within 110% to 160% of ideal body weight, and have an FPG of more than 200 mg/dL. If patients have been treated with insulin, those whose requirements are <40 units/day (indicating endogenous pancreatic reserve) are most likely to respond.[170] N.H. fulfills these criteria and does not have any contraindications to sulfonylurea use (see Antidiabetic Agents). Approximately two-thirds to three-fourths of the patients who meet all of the previously specified criteria will achieve satisfactory control initially. The remainder (16%–36%) fail to respond to a 1-month trial of maximum therapeutic doses and are considered primary failures.[170]

There is little evidence that any particular oral sulfonylurea is more effective than another in properly selected patients with type 2 diabetes. However, as discussed, there are differences in duration of action and side effects that should be considered in the selection of these agents. (see Table 50-26 and Table 50-27 and the section on Antidiabetic Agents.)

The first-generation agents (chlorpropamide, acetohexamide, tolbutamide, and tolazamide) are less potent than the second-generation agents on a milligram for milligram basis. Because they are now rarely used, they will not be addressed.

Glimepiride, glipizide, and glyburide are second-generation agents. Glipizide is metabolized to inactive products and has an intermediate duration of action. Many patients can be controlled on single daily doses, but twice-daily doses are recommended for patients who require more than 15 mg. Because glyburide has a longer duration of action, it is associated more frequently with severe, prolonged hypoglycemia than is glipizide. For this reason, it should be used cautiously in frail, elderly individuals or in those who, for any reason, are predisposed to hypoglycemia (see Questions 65 and 70). Glimepiride can be dosed once daily and may be associated with a slightly lower incidence of hypoglycemia than glyburide.

For K.M., glimepiride, glipizide, or glyburide would be the agents of choice because they are reasonably safe, can be dosed once daily, and are relatively inexpensive. She should be initiated on low dosages (e.g., 1–2 mg glimepiride, 5 mg glipizide, or 1.25–2.5 mg glyburide) once daily. Every 1 to 2 weeks, the dosage can be increased until the therapeutic goals are achieved or maximum doses of these agents have been reached (Table 50-27). The manufacturers of glipizide and glyburide recommend twice-daily dosing of these agents once a specified dose has been exceeded; whether this actually is necessary has not been documented. Many clinicians recommend taking these agents 30 minutes before meals so that the onset of action more closely matches food absorption[170]; this may be less important in patients taking these agents chronically, particularly for the intermediate-acting and longer acting agents.[243,244] If GI intolerance occurs, these agents should be taken with food.

Because K.M. is starting a medication that can cause hypoglycemia, it is important that she be counseled not to skip meals and taught SMBG. She should be educated about symptoms of hypoglycemia and how to treat them (see Self-Monitored Blood Glucose in Type 2 Diabetes and Table 50-13 and Table 50-14).

Clinical Note: K.M. was successfully treated with diet, exercise, and relatively low doses of glyburide (5 mg/day). Within 4 months, her HbA_{1c} dropped to 6.9% and her SMBG results ranged from 120 to 160 mg/dL.

Failure of Antidiabetic Monotherapy

Pathogenesis

FAILURE OF ORAL MONOTHERAPY

54. Q.R. is a 68-year-old, 5 feet 1 inch, 155-lb (BMI 29.3 kg/m²) woman with an 8-year history of type 2 diabetes who has been treated with diet, exercise, and metformin. According to clinic records, she was well controlled initially (HbA_{1c} 6.7%–7.2%) for the first 5 years. When her glycemic control worsened (FPG, 130–160 mg/dL; HbA_{1c}, 7.5%–8.5%), her metformin dose was increased over time, from an initial dose of 500 mg PO BID to her current dose of 850 mg PO TID. Recent chart notes indicate that Q.R.'s chief complaints have included loss of appetite and fatigue. She has lost 15 lb over the past year, and her current HbA_{1c} is 8.6%. Other medical problems include hypertension managed with hydrochlorothiazide 25 mg daily and mild peripheral neuropathy managed with naproxen 500 mg twice daily. Her estimated GFR is 70 mL/minute.

At this clinic visit, Q.R., who is well known to you, seems particularly listless and flat in her affect. Her blood glucose records, which are typically meticulous, are incomplete. Blood glucose values consistently exceed 200 mg/dL and range from 202 to 340 mg/dL. While taking her history, you discover that her husband passed away last year and that one of her adult children has recently been diagnosed with a terminal illness. What factors may be contributing to Q.R.'s poor glucose control?

Several factors may be contributing to Q.R.'s deteriorating blood glucose control and apparent lack of responsiveness to maximum dose of metformin over the past year (as evidenced by her elevated blood glucose and HbA_{1c}, listlessness, and weight loss). When SFUs were used exclusively for oral monotherapy (before other oral agents were available), this loss of glycemic control, called *secondary failure,* was fairly common, occurring at a rate of approximately 5% to 10% per year in patients who initially were well controlled on these agents.[170] Monotherapy failure is characterized by progressively poor glucose control that occurs after a 1-month to a several-year period of good response. The cause of failure may be related to progressive pancreatic failure; poor compliance with diet, exercise, or medications; and exogenous diabetogenic factors such as obesity, illness, or drugs that induce hyperglycemia.

The UKPDS confirmed that monotherapy failure represents a natural progression of type 2 diabetes. The investigators found failure occurred at the same rate regardless of the initial treatment selected: glyburide, chlorpropamide, metformin, or ultralente insulin. In all the monotherapy treatment groups, patients required additional therapies over the study duration.[225] At 3 years, fewer than 55% of patients randomized to single pharmacologic therapy could maintain an HbA_{1c} below 7%, and by 9 years this dropped to about 25% of patients. In the ADOPT study, patients were able to maintain HbA_{1c} levels below 7% using monotherapy for 60, 45, and 33 months with rosiglitazone, metformin, and glyburide, respectively.[235] The reason for glycemic deterioration is likely due to the natural progression of type 2 diabetes in which β-cell function declines with increased duration of disease. Also, when the blood glucose becomes very elevated (FPG >250–300 mg/dL; preprandial glucose concentrations ≥200 mg/dL), the pancreas's ability to secrete insulin is diminished and postreceptor (postbinding) defects in insulin activity become more important. Postreceptor defects are characterized by a reduced responsiveness of tissues to any level of insulin. If glucose concentrations can be normalized, postreceptor defects and pancreatic responsiveness to glucose can be improved. This may be related to the hypothesis that high glucose concentrations in and of themselves may be toxic to the β-cells and peripheral tissues (glucotoxicity).[245]

Q.R.'s deteriorating control on maximum doses of metformin after 5 years of reasonable response is consistent with the natural progression of type 2 diabetes. However, the stress and depression arising out of her life situation have no doubt contributed to her poor control. The latter may have led to a change in her usual compliance with diet, exercise, and medications and should resolve with time and appropriate management. Although hyperglycemia has been attributed to hydrochlorothiazide, the dose prescribed for Q.R. has few adverse metabolic effects.

Managing Monotherapy Failure

55. How should Q.R. be managed? Should she be switched to another antidiabetic agent?

Q.R. is exhibiting symptoms of depression (e.g., listlessness and flat affect). Her depression likely started after her husband's death. Every effort must be made to address Q.R.'s depression because it is unlikely that she will be able to effectively implement more aggressive treatment of her diabetes until her situation is improved. Resources that may be used include her family, a therapist, and a social worker.

Treatment of monotherapy failure includes identifying and correcting any diabetogenic factors and altering her drug therapy. When failure to any oral agent occurs, one should always add another agent rather than switch to another. This is supported by a study that evaluated the effect of metformin alone in a population of patients who had failed oral sulfonylureas and the effect of metformin plus the sulfonylureas. Substitution of metformin for glyburide did not produce any significant change in glycemic control, but the addition of metformin to glyburide therapy substantially improved glucose concentrations.[246] Many combinations of antidiabetic agents can be used. The key is that they should have different mechanisms of action. For example, it is not reasonable to combine a sulfonylurea with a "glinide" (i.e., repaglinide and nateglinide) because they are both insulin secretagogues. It makes more sense to maintain the current agent and add another rather than to change to two new medications. Options for Q.R. include adding one of the following to metformin: insulin secretagogue (sulfonylurea or glinide), acarbose, TZD, sitagliptin, or exenatide.

Table 50-26 summarizes the FDA-approved combination therapy indications. One also could introduce insulin therapy at this time. According to Nathan's algorithm (Fig. 50-9), basal insulin therapy could certainly be initiated. However, because Q.R.'s HbA_{1c} should be effectively lowered with an additional oral agent, we recommend using two noninsulin antidiabetic agents to avoid an unreasonably complicated intervention.

In summary, patients such as Q.R. who are unresponsive to the maximum dose metformin are unlikely to respond to monotherapy with another agent. They should therefore be initiated on combination therapy.

Combination Antidiabetic Therapy (Step 2)

56. As anticipated, Q.R. refuses to consider insulin therapy at this time. Which combination of antidiabetic agents is preferred?

When agents from different antidiabetic classes are combined, their effects are essentially additive. With the availability of many antidiabetic agents, there is no one best combination therapy. As discussed, the choice of therapy should take into account the patient's organ function, amount of HbA_{1c} lowering required to reach an individual's goal, possible adverse effects of a particular drug or drug combination, cost, and patient preference.

Acarbose has been used successfully in combination with both sulfonylureas and metformin, lowering the HbA_{1c} by approximately 1%. However, an agent that can be titrated more quickly than acarbose, does not have significant GI side effects (especially when used with metformin), and one that is more likely to have a profound effect on blood glucose concentrations should be used in Q.R. The TZDs are approved for use in combination with sulfonylureas and metformin. Pioglitazone 30 mg added to metformin monotherapy reduced the FPG by a mean of 38 mg/dL and the HbA_{1c} by 0.8%.[182] Rosiglitazone 4 mg/day added to metformin reduced HbA_{1c} and FPG by 1.0% and 40 mg/dL, respectively, compared with metformin alone.[181,247]

Metformin also has been used successfully in combination with the sulfonylureas. The combination lowers fasting glucose concentrations by approximately 80 mg/dL and HbA_{1c} values by 2% when metformin is given in full dose (2,500 mg/day in three divided doses).[246] In the later stages of the UKPDS, 537 obese and nonobese patients who failed sulfonylurea monotherapy were randomly assigned to continue sulfonylurea monotherapy or to have metformin added. Interestingly, an intention-to-treat analysis of this substudy showed that those patients assigned to the combined metformin–sulfonylurea therapy had a 96% increase in diabetes-related deaths ($p < .039$) and a 60% increase in all-cause deaths ($p < .041$) compared with the sulfonylurea monotherapy group.[221] However, these detrimental effects have been questioned because there was no placebo control and the treatments could not be masked. The ADA currently does not recommend any change in the current guidelines, which include the use of metformin and sulfonylureas in combination. They will await a new, appropriately designed, randomized, placebo-controlled trial that can affirm an adverse interaction between these two drugs.

The addition of sitagliptin to metformin results in a 0.7% HbA_{1c} reduction compared with baseline[248] and the addition of exenatide to metformin results in a 0.8% HbA_{1c} reduction.[249] A disadvantage to exenatide is that it requires an injection; its advantage is that it may result in weight loss.

Although Q.R. has recently lost weight, she remains overweight. Thus, metformin should be maintained and a second agent added. Q.R. would like to remain on oral medications if possible. Sitagliptin may result in slightly less HbA_{1c} lowering compared with adding a sulfonylurea. Therefore, she is started on glimepiride 2 mg PO daily.

Combination Antidiabetic Therapy (Step 3)

57. Q.R. is titrated to glimepiride 4 mg/day and continued on metformin 850 mg PO TID. This improved her FPG and HbA_{1c} modestly for approximately 12 months (FPG, 120–150 mg/dL; currently HbA_{1c}, 7.6%). She remains resistant to starting insulin, despite a 10-minute conversation discussing the rationale for its

use. She has heard about a new diabetes medication called Byetta, and would like to try it because it can cause weight loss.

When a combination of oral agents fails, practitioners often add a third agent before considering insulin. Although this is tempting, depending on a patient's current level of glycemic control, this practice only delays insulin therapy, which is likely to be required to achieve HbA_{1c} goals. However, because Q.R. is close to an HbA_{1c} level of <7%, it is reasonable to try a third, noninsulin antidiabetic agent. Although glimepiride 8 mg/day is the maximum dose, there is little difference in clinical efficacy compared to 4 mg/day. Therefore, increasing glimepiride to 8 mg/day is not likely to achieve her glycemic goals.[250]

Exenatide (Byetta) is approved for use in patients taking metformin, sulfonylurea. or a TZD alone, or a combination of metformin plus a TZD or metformin plus a sulfonylurea. When added to patients on a sulfonylurea and metformin, exenatide at 10 mcg BID resulted in a 0.8% HbA_{1c} reduction compared with baseline.[251] Thus for Q.R., the addition of exenatide could result in an HbA_{1c} of <7%. The use of exenatide with a sulfonylurea is associated with an increased risk of mild to moderate hypoglycemia (28% when used with sulfonylurea and metformin and 36% when use with sulfonylurea alone).[249,251] Most practitioners reduce the dose of the sulfonylurea upon initiation of exenatide and then make adjustments based on the patient's response to exenatide.

Q.R. should be started on exenatide 5 mcg subcutaneously BID, taken within 60 minutes of the two main meals of the day and at least 6 hours apart. She should be counseled about nausea, which is the most frequent side effect; 44% of patients will develop nausea, but there is only 3% dropout rate in the clinical trials. The glimepiride should be reduced to 2 (or 3) mg/day. After 1 month, if she is tolerating exenatide, the dose should be increased to 10 mcg subcutaneously BID. Her HbA_{1c} should be monitored within 3 months of using the 10-mcg dose. An advantage of exenatide (over sitagliptin) is the potential for weight loss. In a 30-week blinded study of exenatide added onto sulfonylurea and metformin, patients on the 10-mcg dose had an average weight loss of 1.6 kg.[251] In the three open-label, noncontrolled extension trials with exenatide, at 3 years exenatide progressively reduced (−5.3 kg) and sustained weight loss at 3 years.[252]

A small proportion of patients will form anti-exenatide antibodies. At high titers, these antibodies could result in failure to achieve adequate improvement in glycemic control. If there is worsening glycemic control or failure to achieve targeted glycemic control while on exenatide, the formation of blocking antibodies should be considered as a reason. A long-acting release formulation of exenatide that is dosed once weekly should be available shortly.[253]

Combination Antidiabetic (Step 3) With Insulin Therapy

58. If Q.R. was willing to start insulin, why would it be reasonable to use insulin in combination with oral agents? How should it be combined with oral agents? Is this combination more effective than insulin alone?

Most patients with type 2 diabetes eventually require insulin. The combined use of insulin with a variety of oral agents has been extensively evaluated, but the studies differ in their design. In some studies, single doses of an intermediate- or long-acting insulin or once or twice daily doses of premixed insulin are added to a single or combination of oral antidiabetic agents in poorly-controlled patients. The primary outcomes that have been evaluated include measures of glycemic control (e.g., HbA_{1c}, FPG) and the extent to which insulin doses have been decreased. Dewitt and Hirsch published a comprehensive review of these studies and readers are referred to this excellent article for this evidence.[254] The combined use of insulin and oral agents can be considered at both steps 2 and 3 in the ADA algorithm (Fig. 50-8 and Fig. 50-9).

The traditional approach to adding insulin therapy to an oral agent (i.e., a sulfonylurea) was called BIDS therapy (bedtime insulin, daytime sulfonylurea). Now, with the many available noninsulin antidiabetic options, bedtime basal insulin (using NPH, glargine, or detemir) can be added to single or combination (usually only two) oral agent therapy. Combining a sulfonylurea with insulin can lower the insulin requirements by 25% to 50%, which results in less weight gain. Similarly, use of metformin with insulin has decreased mean insulin requirements by 25%.[255] Although metformin is an antihyperglycemic agent, one must be alert for increased susceptibility to hypoglycemia when it is used in combination with insulin. Studies seem to confirm potential advantages of metformin over sulfonylureas when used in combination with insulin. These include its favorable effects on the lipid profile, insulin concentrations, and lack of weight gain. The risk for hypoglycemia may also be lower with metformin than with combined use of sulfonylureas.[221,256,257] Use of a TZD with insulin is effective in reducing insulin doses and HbA_{1c}.[258] However, the disadvantage with this combination is weight gain and significant edema (~15%).

In Q.R.'s case, it makes the most sense to add a single dose of basal insulin to metformin and glimepiride. Advantages attributed to adding insulin to an oral agent as the "next step" after failure, as opposed to using insulin alone, include the following[254,259,260].

- Lower insulin dosages can be used, and this minimizes weight gain and hypoglycemia.
- Simpler, single-dose insulin regimens are possible (vs. monotherapy with insulin).
- Lowering the fasting glucose concentrations improves glucose control throughout the day because glucose excursions related to meals are layered over lower values. Furthermore, lower glucose values improve β-cell responsiveness to glucose and enhance tissue responsiveness to insulin action.
- Use of the insulin sensitizers may enhance the effect of exogenous insulin while minimizing weight gain and hyperinsulinemia. They also may have beneficial effects on lipid profiles and other cardiovascular defects.

However, lowering glucose concentrations is the first priority, not attempting to use lower insulin doses. Q.R. should be started on 10 units or 0.2 unit/kg of NPH, insulin glargine, or insulin detemir at bedtime. This dose is based on empiric use of insulin in a variety of studies (0.1–0.35 unit/kg)[220,261] and a conservative estimate for basal insulin of approximately 0.5 unit/hour (Q.R. weighs 155 pounds, or 70.5 kg). The dose also takes into account the possibility that Q.R. is secreting some basal insulin of her own and will have some residual stimulation of insulin secretion by glipizide. The basal dose should be titrated upward based on the FPG for 3 consecutive days. A common titration method used is the "treat-to-target" schedule:[262,263]

FPG (mmol/L)	Adjustment of Basal Insulin Dose (U)
≥180 (≥9.90)	8
160–180 (8.80–9.90)	6
140–159 (7.70–8.75)	4
120–139 (6.60–7.65)	2
100–119 (5.50–6.55)	1
80–99 (4.40–5.45)	Maintain dose
60–79 (3.30–4.35)	−2
<60 (<3.30)	−4 or more

Alternatively, the basal insulin dose can be increased by 2 units every 3 days until the FPG is in a target range (70–130 mg/dL).[220] If the FPG is above 180 mg/dL, larger increments can be used (e.g., by 4 units every 3 days). If hypoglycemia occurs or the FPG is less than 70 mg/dL, the dose should be reduced by at least 4 units, or by 10% if the dose is more than 60 units. If there is no improvement in glycemic control after 3 months, Q.R. should be converted to multiple daily insulin injections (see Question 59 and 60).

An alternative for Q.R. is to discontinue all oral agents and begin insulin monotherapy using methods similar to those described for type 1 patients. This option also is rational based on the observation that patients like Q.R. are likely to require insulin therapy because of progressive β-cell failure. Furthermore, insulin monotherapy may be less expensive and easier to assess than combination oral agents plus insulin therapy. Nevertheless, many clinicians use single doses of basal insulin in combination with oral agents as a bridge to eventual insulin monotherapy, especially for those patients unwilling to adhere to multiple daily insulin injections.

Insulin Monotherapy in Patients With Type 2 Diabetes

Insulin Regimens

59. Q.R.'s insulin glargine dose was eventually titrated to 25 units at bedtime. In combination with glimepiride 4 mg/day and metformin 850 mg TID, her fasting glucose levels fell to the 120s and 130s on most occasions; her HbA_{1c} dropped to 7.5%. However, after 1 year, she began to note a gradual rise in glucose concentrations throughout the day. This resulted in a further increase in her bedtime insulin glargine to 40 units (0.57 unit/kg). Currently, her morning glucose concentrations are 120 to 140 mg/dL, and glucose concentrations measured before or after meals range between 170 and 200 mg/dL. A recent HbA_{1c} value was 8.8%. For the past 6 months or so, Q.R. has noted increasing fatigue, bouts of blurred vision, and recurrence of her monilial infections. How should she be managed now?

The next step in managing Q.R.'s diabetes is to institute prandial insulin therapy, which is needed as indicated by her daytime hyperglycemia. Like type 1 patients, those with long-standing type 2 disease may require regular insulin, insulin aspart, glulisine, or lispro before meals to minimize postprandial excursions. Insulin lispro has been shown to decrease postprandial glucose concentrations to a greater extent than regular insulin (30% lower at 1 hour and 53% lower at 2 hours) and was associated with a lower rate of hypoglycemia, particularly between midnight and 6 AM (36%). However, HbA_{1c} levels were not significantly different after 6 months.[264] A similar response with insulin aspart and glulisine would be expected.

Because Q.R. is on insulin glargine, the most appropriate next step is to add prandial insulin using a rapid-acting insulin. This requires four injections daily. She needs to be able to handle and be adherent to multiple daily injections. Initiation of basal-bolus insulin regimens are discussed in detail in the type 1 insulin therapy section (see Question 6). Patients with type 2 diabetes may require large insulin total daily doses (>1 units/kg) to reach HbA_{1c} targets below 7%. Because she is taking prandial insulin, glimepiride should be discontinued. Although not technically insulin monotherapy, metformin is often continued to assist in reducing insulin resistance and minimizing weight gain with insulin.

Premixed Insulins

60. Q.R. has difficulty adhering to a basal-bolus insulin regimen. She is currently taking insulin glargine 38 units at nighttime and 7 units of insulin aspart before each meal. What options are available for Q.R.?

Because people with type 2 diabetes retain some pancreatic function, it often is possible to achieve an acceptable level of control with twice-daily doses of intermediate-acting insulin in combination with rapid or short-acting insulins, which are available as premixed insulins. These are referred to as split-mixed insulin regimens. Although convenient, they do limit flexibility in dosing, and thus HbA_{1c} lowering ability without increasing hypoglycemia risk. In the United States, fixed mixtures of NPH and regular insulin in a 70:30 ratio and a 50:50 ratio are available (Table 50-7). Commercial combinations of the rapid-acting insulins plus an intermediate-acting insulin also are available as Humalog Mix 75/25 (a mixture of insulin lispro plus NPL- neutral protamine lispro), Humalog Mix 50/50 (a mixture of insulin lispro plus NPL), and Novolog Mix 70/30 (a mixture of insulin aspart plus aspart protamine suspension). These fixed mixtures are available in prefilled syringes, which can add to their flexibility and convenience for administration.

Q.R. is currently receiving a total daily dose of insulin of 59 U, or 0.84 unit/kg/day. To convert her to a premixed insulin, one could begin with a conservative total daily dose of 0.5 to 0.6 unit/kg/day, split two-thirds in the morning and one-third in the evening. However, many type 2 patients do better splitting the dose 50/50. When starting an insulin-naive type 2 patient on premixed insulin, doses of 5 to 6 units twice daily (administered before breakfast and dinner) are often used, with the doses being titrated prebreakfast (to adjust the dinner dose) and predinner (to adjust the breakfast dose).[262,265]

If the premixed insulin does not achieve adequate glycemic control, an option is to mix the short- or rapid-acting insulin with NPH in the same syringe. By doing this, each insulin dose can be individually adjusted. A disadvantage to this is the chance for patients to make errors in measuring and mixing insulin, especially the elderly. Alternatively, a prandial dose of insulin (a third injection) can be added at lunch; the breakfast dose of premixed insulin should be decreased as well.[254] Q.R. should be instructed to inject the regular/NPH insulin mixture 30 minutes before breakfast and dinner. If she were to use a premixed insulin with either insulin aspart or lispro, she would need to inject the insulin immediately before eating (within 15 minutes of eating).

Q.R. should be started on a rapid-acting premixed insulin twice daily, administered within 15 minutes of eating (for

NPH/R mixture, this would be 30 minutes). A dose of 20 units subcutaneously BID represents a conservative starting dose.

Use of Antidiabetic Agents in Special Situations

Cardiovascular Effects

61. J.A., a 47-year-old man was diagnosed with type 2 diabetes when he developed "very high blood sugars in the 300s" while being treated for a foot infection. He states he has had "borderline diabetes" for longer than 10 years. Other medical problems include hypertension and class III CHF, which is currently well controlled on benazepril (10 mg/day), furosemide (40 mg/day), and digoxin (0.25 mg/day). For the past 3 months, he has adhered to a low-fat diet and exercise program and has managed to lose 10 pounds (J.A. is currently 5 feet 9 inches tall and weighs 190 lbs; BMI, 28.1 kg/m^2). FPG concentrations measured over the past 2 months were 160 mg/dL and 145 mg/dL. Liver and renal function tests are within normal limits. How will J.A.'s cardiovascular history affect the choice of oral agents? The package insert for all sulfonylureas includes a special warning on increased risk of cardiovascular mortality. What is the basis of this warning? Are sulfonylureas contraindicated in patients such as J.A. with a history of CVD?

Because J.A. has class III CHF and is under treatment, the use of metformin is not recommended. This is because when metformin-associated cases of lactic acidosis were analyzed, virtually all patients had concurrent conditions that predisposed them to this potentially fatal condition. One of these was clinically significant CHF, a condition that could decrease circulation to the periphery, thereby predisposing the patient to anaerobic metabolism (see Question 62).[266,267] Although TZDs should not be used in patients with NYHA class III or IV heart failure, practitioners often avoid their use altogether in patients with heart failure because of a concern for CHF exacerbation.

Sulfonylureas are not contraindicated in individuals with a history of CVD. However, the FDA required all manufacturers of sulfonylureas to include in their package inserts a special "black box" warning prescribers of an increased risk for cardiovascular mortality. This was based on an unexpected finding of the University Group Diabetes Program study in 1970. This was a cooperative, prospective study to evaluate the effectiveness of antidiabetic therapy in preventing vascular and other late complications of diabetes in mild type 2 diabetic patients. Unexpectedly, twice as many cardiovascular deaths occurred in the tolbutamide-treated group than in the placebo- and insulin-treated groups.[268]

After publication of the University Group Diabetes Program results, a great controversy regarding the study's validity and clinical implications appeared in both the professional and lay press; these are summarized elsewhere.[269] Strong evidence that normalization of glucose concentrations may in fact delay long-term complications has diminished any concerns for cardiovascular adverse effects associated with the sulfonylureas. In fact, the UKPDS found no increase in the rates of MI or diabetes-related deaths when participants treated intensively with a sulfonylurea were compared with those treated conventionally.[33]

Thus, current evidence indicates that the benefits of sulfonylureas far outweigh their risks in type 2 diabetic patients with CVD. On this basis, their use is not contraindicated.

Lactic Acidosis

62. M.R. is a 76-year-old, 5 feet 11 inch, 150-lb man (BMI, 20.9 kg/m^2) with type 2 diabetes who was hospitalized when his son found him in a "near-unconscious state." According to his son, M.R.'s diabetes had been adequately managed with glipizide 10 mg BID and acarbose 100 mg TID with each meal until approximately 2 months ago, when M.R. was hospitalized for pneumonia. Because M.R. lived alone and adamantly refused to take "shots," he was discharged on metformin, which was to be added to his other medications. A review of the hospital records revealed a SrCr of 1.4 mg/dL and several random blood glucose concentrations above 190 mg/dL. He also has a history of chronic obstructive pulmonary disease (COPD). His current dose of metformin is 850 mg TID with meals.

On physical examination, the patient was oriented, but appeared acutely ill. Temperature, pulse, and BP were within normal limits. The respiratory rate was 32 breaths/minute. Significant laboratory values included the following: Na, 140 mEq/L(normal, 135–145); K, 6.2 mEq/L (normal, 3.5–5); Cl, 103 mEq/L (normal, 95–105); HCO_3, 5 mEq/L (normal, 22–28); arterial pH, 6.8 (normal, 7.36–7.42); SrCr 3.2 mg/dL (normal, 0.7–1.4); blood glucose, 130 mg/dL (normal, 70–140); serum acetones, negative; serum lactate, 12.3 mmol/L (normal, 0.7–2.0); and serum pyruvate, 0.49 mmol/L (normal, 0.05–0.08).

A diagnosis of lactic acidosis was made. What signs and symptoms are consistent with this diagnosis? What is the relation between metformin and lactic acidosis, and what are the predisposing factors?

The most notorious side effect associated with metformin—although extremely rare—is lactic acidosis. Lactic acidosis is a metabolic acidosis characterized by a significant reduction in the arterial pH and an accumulation of serum lactate, a product of anaerobic metabolism. It is a condition that is highly lethal (50% mortality) and resistant to therapy. Lactic acidosis occurs when there is an increased production of or decreased utilization of lactate. Decreased utilization of lactate occurs when tissues are unable to oxidize lactate to pyruvate (these two substances are normally present in the serum in a ratio of 10:1). Metformin might predispose a patient to lactic acidosis by augmenting anaerobic metabolism or by decreasing the kidney's ability to handle an acid load. Other factors that might contribute to lactic acidosis include severe cardiac or pulmonary disease (anoxia, increased lactate production), septic shock, renal dysfunction (retention of metformin and lactate), and excessive alcohol intake (increased lactate production and decreased utilization).

Signs and symptoms generally are acute in onset and commonly include nausea, vomiting, diarrhea, and hyperventilation. Hypovolemia, hypotension, confusion, and coma also may occur; death is usually secondary to cardiovascular collapse.

As illustrated by M.R., typical laboratory findings include a low serum bicarbonate and PCO_2, a low arterial pH, an elevated potassium, a normal or low serum chloride, elevated lactate and pyruvate levels, an increased L:P ratio, and an anion gap of 30 mEq/L or higher.

Treatment is empiric and includes correction of any underlying cause of anoxia and elimination of factors predisposing to lactic acidosis, large doses of sodium bicarbonate with frequent arterial pH determinations, hemodialysis, and glucose plus insulin infusion. The latter are administered in an attempt to improve the metabolic utilization of lactate and pyruvate.[270,271]

Although metformin rarely is associated with lactic acidosis, the manufacturer and the FDA have taken extreme measures to prevent its improper use because another biguanide, phenformin, which induced this life-threatening condition was removed from the market in 1977.[259] The estimated rate of phenformin-induced lactic acidosis was 0.25 to 4 cases per 1,000 users versus 5 to 9 cases per 100,000 users for metformin.[266,272,273] A group of clinicians from the FDA summarized 47 confirmed cases of metformin-related lactic acidosis (lactate levels ≥5 mmol/L) that had been reported to the FDA between May 1995 and June 1996.[273] Unfortunately, the condition continues to be resistant to treatment; the mortality rate was 43%. Importantly, 43 of the 47 cases (91%) had concurrent conditions that predisposed them to lactic acidosis. These included cardiac disease (64%), decreased renal function (28%), and chronic pulmonary disease (6%). Several patients (17%) were over the age of 80 years and may have had decreased renal function despite normal SrCr concentrations. Interestingly, 38% of the patients had CHF, and those who died were more likely to be under treatment with digoxin and furosemide. The mean daily dose of metformin was well within the therapeutic range and was not higher in the group that succumbed (1,259 ± 648 mg in the group that died and 1,349 ± 598 mg in the group that survived).

As a consequence of this analysis, the manufacturer has changed its labeling to warn against the use of metformin in individuals who are being treated for CHF. Furthermore, metformin should not be initiated in patients over 80 years old unless a GFR or ClCr evaluation confirms normal renal function. The drug should not be used when patients are septic.[158]

Unfortunately, studies assessing the appropriate use of metformin (according to the manufacturer's recommendations) reveal that metformin is frequently used in patients in whom it is contraindicated.[274–277] A retrospective cohort study of 1,847 patients found that 24.5% of patients who received metformin had conditions for which it was contraindicated (21.0% had CHF and were receiving loop diuretics, and 4.8% had renal impairment).[274] Medicare patients hospitalized with the primary diagnosis of heart failure and concomitant diabetes were assessed for metformin and TZD use, both of which are contraindicated in this situation.[277] Between 1998 and 1999, 7.1% and 7.2% of patients were treated with metformin and a TZD, respectively, at discharge; these numbers increased between 2000 and 2001 to 11.2% and 16.1%. In patients with renal dysfunction (SrCr ≥1.5 mg/dL), metformin was used in 9.3% and 15.2% of patients in 1998 through 1999 and 2000 through 2001, respectively. See question 61 for discussion of TZDs and heart failure. Clinicians need to carefully assess patients for contraindications before initiating antidiabetic agents.

M.R.'s pulmonary disease may have caused an anoxic state, which predisposed him to lactic acidosis. Furthermore, even though his SrCr was below 1.5 mg/dL, this value may not have reflected normal renal function in this elderly gentleman.[278] Finally, dehydration caused by extensive vomiting and diarrhea has caused prerenal failure, which is likely contributing to the acidosis.

Clinical Note: M.R. recovered after aggressive treatment with fluids and sodium bicarbonate. Metformin was discontinued and he was managed with insulin.

Hypoglycemia

63. C.A., a 68-year-old woman who has had a 20-year history of type 2 diabetes and a 5-year history of mild renal failure (SrCr, 1.5 mg/dL; BUN, 30 mg/dL), is admitted to the hospital in a coma. According to her daughter, C.A.'s diabetes has been well controlled over the past several months with glyburide 10 mg BID. She took her last dose approximately 5 hours before admission. Three days before admission C.A. developed anorexia, nausea, and vomiting in association with the flu and became progressively lethargic. Laboratory results on admission are as follows: plasma glucose, 20 mg/dL (normal, 70–140); SrCr, 3.0 mg/dL (normal, 0.6–1.2); and BUN, 80 mg/dL (normal, 7–20). What is C.A.'s diagnosis? Were there any predisposing factors?

[SI units: SrCr, 132.6 and 265.2 μmol/L; BUN, 10.7 and 28.6 mmol/L; plasma glucose, 1.1 mmol/L]

C.A. has developed a case of severe hypoglycemia secondary to glyburide. Hypoglycemia is the most common (incidence, 2.4 per 100 patients per year) and potentially severe (4%–7% mortality) adverse effect of the sulfonylureas. The incidence and severity of this effect increase with the duration of action and potency of the agents. Thus, the incidence of severe, prolonged hypoglycemia secondary to chlorpropamide and glyburide is approximately two times higher than that for glipizide and approximately five times higher than that for tolbutamide.[170,279] The sulfonylureas account for almost all cases of drug-induced hypoglycemia in individuals older than age 60.

Most sulfonylurea-induced hypoglycemia occurs in patients who are predisposed to hypoglycemia in some way, and C.A. is no exception. She is an elderly woman with renal impairment who was on relatively high doses of an agent, a portion of which is excreted unchanged in the urine. Even in the face of decreased carbohydrate intake (anorexia and vomiting), she continued to take her usual dose of glyburide. Even though the stress of illness most often raises glucose levels, the decreased intake and vomiting probably led to dehydration and further compromised her renal function.

Because glyburide and chlorpropamide have a long duration of action, hypoglycemia induced by these agents may last for several hours, or days in the case of chlorpropamide. Therefore, patients such as C.A. must be hospitalized and treated with continuous glucose infusions until oral intake resumes. Otherwise, severe hypoglycemia may recur.

Renal Dysfunction

64. Glyburide was withheld and C.A.'s kidney function stabilized with fluid replacement (estimated GFR, 37 mL/min/1.73 m^2). Because she lives alone, has impaired eyesight secondary to cataracts, and has severe arthritis, insulin treatment is impractical. Oral agents are to be continued. Which agents should be avoided? Which agents could be used?

Once C.A.'s plasma glucose concentrations and renal function have stabilized, reinstitution of antidiabetic therapy must be considered. Sulfonylurea compounds that are metabolized to active products that depend on the kidney for elimination (e.g., acetohexamide, chlorpropamide glyburide, and tolazamide) should be avoided in the elderly and in patients with decreased renal function. Sulfonylureas that are completely metabolized to inactive or weakly active products may be used (i.e., glipizide, glimeperide, or tolbutamide). Although glyburide is unlikely to accumulate in patients with a ClCr above 30 mL/min, it should not be used in C.A. because it caused a severe hypoglycemic reaction. Furthermore, even patients who are not taking sulfonylureas are more likely to experience hypoglycemic reactions if they have renal insufficiency; therefore, any oral hypoglycemic agent should be initiated at a low dose and titrated slowly (Table 50-28). C.A. should be instructed to eat regularly, because skipped meals may result in recurrent hypoglycemia.[174,280]

Metformin is contraindicated in C.A. because her renal function is abnormal (see Question 62). Decreased renal function can result in accumulation of metformin, which can, in turn, predispose her to lactic acidosis.

The TZDs are primarily metabolized by the liver and are not contraindicated in patients with mild renal failure. The use of rosiglitazone or pioglitazone, beginning with low doses, could be considered as can acarbose, which is poorly absorbed from the GI tract. Sitagliptin can be used, but the dose is reduced in renal dysfunction. Exenatide can be used in patients with ClCr above 30 mL/minute and the dose does not need to be adjusted. None of these agents cause hypoglycemia when used as monotherapy.

Hepatic Dysfunction

65. B.R., a 60-year-old man with cirrhosis of the liver, is found to have type 2 diabetes. Glipizide 10 mg/day is initiated. How will B.R.'s liver function affect the disposition of glipizide and his response to this agent?

Because hepatic metabolism is the primary route of elimination for most sulfonylureas, including glipizide, patients with hepatic disease should be expected to have an exaggerated response to those drugs metabolized to less active products.

Tolbutamide, a first-generation sulfonylurea, has been studied most extensively with respect to liver disease. In a double-blind, placebo-controlled trial of 50 cirrhotic patients, hypoglycemia was a complication in 20% of the tolbutamide-treated group.[281] Tolbutamide's elimination half-life in subjects with cirrhosis has been reported to be increased or unaltered in different studies.[282] A complicating factor is that alcohol can induce hepatic enzymes, markedly increasing tolbutamide metabolism in alcoholic patients with cirrhosis.

Liver disease can be a separate predisposing factor for severe, prolonged hypoglycemia because glycogenolysis and gluconeogenesis are impaired; thus, sulfonylureas are relatively contraindicated for cirrhotic patients. If they are used, shorter acting agents are preferred and small initial doses should be used. For B.R., glipizide could be initiated at a dose no greater than 2.5 mg/day and increased if needed by 2.5-mg increments at no less than weekly intervals. Other options are low doses of repaglinide (0.5 mg) or nateglinide (60 mg) with meals.

Diabetes in the Elderly

Clinical Presentation

66. J.M. is a frail, 82-year-old, unresponsive man, who is brought to the emergency department. According to J.M.'s family, he has become increasingly confused, dizzy, and lethargic, with a recent weight loss of 10 lb. J.M. lives by himself and has been generally healthy with the exception of mild to moderate COPD and arthritis. Fasting serum chemistry reveals the following: Na, 128 mEq/L (normal, 135–145); glucose, 798 mg/dL (normal, 70–140); and serum osmolality, 374 mOsm/L (normal, 280–295 mOsm/kg H_2O). His serum is negative for ketones. On physical examination, J.M. has poor skin turgor, dry mucous membranes, and is responsive only to deep pain. His BP is 90/60 mmHg with a pulse of 96 beats/minute. He has rales at the left lower base of his lung, and a chest radiograph confirms pneumonia. Despite aggressive fluid replacement, J.M.'s blood glucose remains consistently above 250 mg/dL and his HbA_{1c} is 11% (normal, ≤6%). J.M. presents with very high glucose concentrations, but has no history of diabetes mellitus. What special factors contribute to a late and atypical presentation of diabetes in the elderly?

[SI units: Na, 128 mmol/L (normal, 135–145); glucose, 44.3 and >13.9 mmol/L (normal, 3.9–6.1); serum osmolality, 374 mmol/kg; HbA_{1c}, 0.11]

Diabetes in the elderly commonly is underdiagnosed and undertreated because it often presents atypically.[283–285] Classic symptoms associated with diabetes mellitus may be masked by other illnesses, may be entirely absent, or may be explained away by the normal aging process. For example, polyuria is minimized by higher renal thresholds for glucose or may be confounded by urinary incontinence or "prostate problems." Thirst is commonly blunted in elderly persons, increasing their risk of dehydration and electrolyte imbalance. Hunger can be altered by medications or depression. Fatigue often is discounted as "part of getting old," and weight loss, although sometimes profound, may be so gradual that it goes unnoticed for months to years. (See Table 50-29 for a comparison of presenting symptoms for diabetes mellitus in elderly patients compared with younger patients.)

Hyperosmolar Hyperglycemic State

67. J.M. is diagnosed with hyperosmolar hyperglycemic state (HHS). Why are the elderly predisposed to this condition and what signs and symptoms are consistent with this diagnosis?

HHS is a condition characterized by extremely elevated plasma glucose concentrations (>600 mg/mL) and high serum osmolality (>320 mOsm/L) without ketoacidosis. Because patients with type 2 diabetes have some residual insulin production, they are usually protected against excessive lipolysis and ketone production. Measurements of serum ketones and blood pH differentiate this condition from DKA (see Question 39). The condition occurs when urinary fluid and electrolyte losses

Table 50-29 Presentation of Diabetes Mellitus in Elderly Patients Compared With Younger Patients

Metabolic Abnormality	Symptoms in Young Patients	Symptoms in Elderly Patients
Serum osmolality	Polydipsia	Dehydration, confusion, delirium
Glycosuria	Polyuria	Incontinence
Catabolic state owing to insulin deficiency	Polyphagia	Weight loss, anorexia

secondary to glucosuria are inadequately replaced by oral fluid intake.[114,286]

HHS primarily occurs in the elderly because several factors predispose this population to hypodipsia. These include an inability to recognize thirst,[287] an inability to ask for fluids (e.g., dementia, sedation, intubation), and an inability to get fluids on demand (e.g., physical disabilities or restraints). Infections or other acute illnesses (e.g., MI, GI bleeding, pancreatitis) that exacerbate diabetes can interact with the hyperosmolar diuresis and hypodipsia to produce severe dehydration and hyperglycemia. Drugs that increase plasma glucose concentrations (e.g., glucocorticoids), increase diuresis, or decrease mentation also can contribute to this unfortunate situation.

J.M. presents with several symptoms of HHS dehydration, including osmolality greater than 320 mOsm, plasma glucose greater than 600 mg/dL, decreased skin turgor, hypotension, and the absence of serum ketones. His pneumonia was probably the precipitating factor. The mortality rate for this disorder is 3% in patients younger than 50 years of age; it increases to 30% for those older than 50.[288] Treatment involves rapid IV hydration. Fluid replacement is provided in the same manner as with DKA. See Question 40 and Table 50-25 for details.[114] Insulin infusion is given simultaneously. The initiation and rate adjustments are the same as with DKA, except that the plasma glucose cutoff to reduce the insulin infusion rate is 300 mg/dL (not 200 mg/dL as with DKA; see Question 41 and Table 50-25 for details). Rehydration and insulin administration corrected J.M.'s metabolic imbalance, allowing his diabetes control to be addressed.

Goals of Therapy

68. What are the goals of therapy for J.M.?

It is widely recognized that strict glycemic control is associated with an increased incidence of hypoglycemia.[29] In the elderly patient with age-related autonomic dysfunction, hypoglycemia may present without the usual premonitory symptoms and can result in severe adverse effects such as angina, seizures, stroke, or MI. Therefore, the general tendency when treating elderly diabetic patients is to aim for slightly more liberal outcome objectives.

The basic principles of management are to set less aggressive glycemic goals. Thus, a fasting blood glucose target of 100 and 140 mg/dL with postprandial glucose values below 180 mg/dL and an HbA_{1c} goal of 8%, while avoiding hypoglycemia, is appropriate in this frail patient.[289]

Diet and Exercise

69. How should diet and exercise recommendations be modified for elderly diabetic patients such as J.M.?

NUTRITION

Because most elderly patients have type 2 diabetes, nutrition and exercise programs are the initial steps in therapy. In 2001, the prevalence of obesity in the United States was 20.9%.[290] Elderly persons between the ages of 60 and 69 had a 25.3% prevalence of obesity and people at 70 and older had a prevalence of 17.1%. Older people with diabetes, especially those in a long-term care facility, have a tendency to be underweight rather than overweight.[47] Therefore, caution should be used when considering a weight loss diet, because this could cause malnutrition or dehydration. For obese individuals, a modest weight loss of 5% to 10% may be indicated. However, an involuntary weight gain or loss of more than 10 pounds or 10% of body weight in <6 months should be carefully assessed.[47]

Several factors can adversely affect proper nutrition in the elderly. They include an impaired ability to shop for and prepare food, limited finances, an age-related decline in taste perceptions, and coexisting illnesses. Ill-fitting dentures, difficulty in chewing and swallowing, and lack of companionship during meals also can contribute to malnutrition as well.

High-fiber diets may lower blood glucose and improve plasma lipids. However, high-fiber diets in frail, elderly patients, particularly those who are bedridden, should be used cautiously because they can be constipating and result in fecal impaction. Ambulatory patients, on the other hand, generally benefit from increased dietary fiber. Because many elderly patients are malnourished, a daily multivitamin preparation containing the recommended daily allowance of each vitamin should be prescribed.[47]

EXERCISE

Exercise in the elderly provides all the benefits derived by younger individuals. It increases well-being and glucose stability, and may decrease a propensity to fall. Exercise also improves BP, the lipid profile, hypercoagulability, and bone density. Physical activity is necessary to minimize any lean body mass loss that can occur with caloric restriction. For patients with arthritis, aquatic exercise may be substituted. Before such an exercise program is initiated, careful evaluation is mandatory to avoid myocardial ischemia or the acceleration of retinopathy.[132]

Selecting an Antidiabetic Agent in the Elderly

70. Why is it important to institute drug therapy to treat J.M.'s diabetes? What considerations should be made in selecting an initial treatment regimen?

As in all patients with diabetes mellitus, poor glycemic control increases the risk of long-term complications. Although it is tempting to minimize the importance of glycemic control because these complications take so long to develop, patients such as J.M. may have had unrecognized hyperglycemia for many years before clinical diagnosis. Thus, many have already begun to develop complications. Furthermore, as life expectancy increases one can expect that these individuals will live long enough to experience morbidity related to diabetes if they are not treated. Therefore, pharmacologic treatment should be strongly considered in J.M. and most elderly patients whether or not they are symptomatic.[291]

The general approach to treating an elderly patient with type 2 diabetes is basically the same as described in questions 46, 50, and 51. The initial choice of an antidiabetic agent should be based on the severity of hyperglycemia. Other considerations include body weight, coexisting diseases, and cost of the agent. Patients with IFG (FPG >100, but <126 mg/dL) should be treated with diet and exercise tailored to their individual capabilities. For patients with diabetes (FPG ≥126 mg/dL or 2-hour postprandial blood glucose >200 mg/dL), acarbose, a short-acting insulin secretagogue (e.g., nateglinide or repaglinide), a TZD, and sitagliptin are all appropriate options. Sulfonylurea-induced hypoglycemia is a concern in these patients. However, if inability to adhere to the multiple-daily regimen is problematic, a short-acting sulfonylurea is an appropriate alternative agent. In J.M.'s case, metformin should probably be avoided because he has COPD. Also, he is older than age 80 and requires an assessment of his GFR. Use of ClCr often overestimates renal function in elderly individuals owing to their reduced muscle mass. There is a strong relationship between the pharmacokinetics of metformin and both kidney function and age. In healthy elderly patients, renal clearance of metformin was 35% to 40% lower than respective values for healthy young individuals.[160] Finally, the favorable effect metformin has on weight is irrelevant in J.M. Thus, although the efficacy of metformin is comparable to that of sulfonylureas, it is not the agent of first choice for elderly patients such as J.M.[289]

Patients with an FPG above 300 mg/dL and no overt stress should be considered insulin deficient and started on insulin therapy.

Selecting a Sulfonylurea

71. Because his FPG concentrations remain 200 to 250 mg/dL (normal, 70–100), the decision is made to start J.M. on a sulfonylurea. What factors should be considered in selecting a sulfonylurea for J.M.?

There are several age-associated problems with the use of oral hypoglycemic agents. Hepatic blood flow and oxidative metabolism are decreased with aging, resulting in prolonged half-lives of hepatically metabolized drugs. Serum albumin is reduced in the elderly, and this affects the highly protein-bound first-generation sulfonylureas, resulting in increased serum levels of free drug.[292] Response to hypoglycemic counter-regulatory hormones is diminished in the elderly, predisposing them to prolonged hypoglycemia. The decreased renal function and mass that occurs with aging decreases the clearance and increases the half-lives of oral agents excreted renally, specifically acetohexamide, chlorpropamide, and glyburide. Chlorpropamide should not be used in the elderly population owing to its long half-life (≥35 hours) and high incidence of hypoglycemia and hyponatremia.[292] Of the second-generation agents, glipizide is preferred over glyburide in frail, elderly patients like J.M. This is because its duration of action is shorter than that of glyburide and it is metabolized to inactive products. Consequently, it is 50% less likely to cause severe and prolonged hypoglycemia in the elderly population.[293] This is a concern because several factors predispose the elderly to drug-induced hypoglycemia. These include anorexia, irregular or inadequate food intake, and other factors affecting nutrition (see Question 69). Tolbutamide (which is converted to inactive metabolites), glimepiride (which has been studied in renal insufficiency), and repaglinide[294] and nateglinide (which are very short-acting) are also appropriate options.

Maturity-Onset Diabetes of the Young

72. B.L. is a 34-year-old, slender (5 feet 6 inches, 120 lbs, BMI 19.4 kg/m^2) woman who developed diabetes at the age of 23. Until recently, her diabetes was very well controlled (HbA$_{1c}$, 6%–7%) on glipizide 5 mg/day. Approximately 3 months ago, her physician discontinued glipizide and began treating her with very low doses of insulin (7 units of 70/30 insulin twice daily) when she announced her intention to become pregnant. However, she is experiencing frequent hypoglycemic reactions and would like to switch back to glipizide. B.L. has no other medical problems, and her physical examination is within normal limits. B.L.'s mother (onset at age 32) and younger sister (onset at age 25) also have diabetes and are well controlled on oral agents. Assess B.L.'s diabetes. How should she be managed?

It is quite likely that B.L. has a relatively rare form of diabetes often referred to as *maturity-onset diabetes of the young* (MODY).[295] Typically, the patient is normal weight, has a strong family history of diabetes, and is diagnosed during his or her young adult years.[296] Unlike obese patients with type 2 diabetes, tissue sensitivity to insulin action is normal, but insulin secretion in response to glucose is defective. Consequently, patients such as B.L. respond to oral sulfonylureas and low doses of insulin. The physician's decision to treat B.L. with insulin is rational because she intends to conceive and oral sulfonylureas cross the placental barrier; however, it seems as though her dose and regimen will have to be adjusted.

Complications

Note to the reader: A thorough discussion addressing the clinical presentation of the complications of diabetes is beyond the scope of this chapter. Thus, the following cases and responses are presented to provide an introduction to some of the most common complications and a general approach to their treatment. Also see Chapters 12, 13, and 31.

Hypertension

73. L.S. is a 46-year-old, obese man with an 8-year history of type 2 diabetes. His current problems include a BP of 155/103 mmHg (documented on two occasions), blurry vision, and sexual impotence, which he now admits has troubled him for the last few years. Physical examination reveals decreased pedal pulses bilaterally, loss of sensation to monofilament testing, and evidence of an amputated toe on the right foot. His laboratory values are as follows: FPG, 170 mg/dL (normal, 70–100); HbA$_{1c}$, 7.8% (normal, 4%–6%); fasting cholesterol, 240 mg/dL (normal, <200); and triglycerides, 160 mg/dL (normal, <150). L.S. has normal electrolyte values and microalbuminuria (180 mg/g creatinine). His only medication is metformin 500 mg PO BID. Describe the pathogenesis of hypertension in patients such as L.S. Why is it so important to treat his hypertension?

[SI units: FPG, 9.4 mmol/L; fasting cholesterol, 13.3 mmol/L; triglycerides, 8.9 mmol/L]

More than 70% of adults with diabetes have a BP greater than 130/80 mmHg or use medication to treat diagnosed hypertension.[1] Patients with type 1 diabetes are usually normotensive in the absence of nephropathy. Hypertension in type 1 diabetes is usually of renal parenchymal origin and occurs 1 to 2 years after the onset of nephropathy as indicated by microalbuminuria (see Question 75).[297] The relationship between type 2 diabetes and hypertension is more complex and not as closely correlated to nephropathy. In type 2 diabetes, hypertension is often part of the metabolic syndrome of insulin resistance and may be present for years before diabetes is actually detectable.

Patients with diabetes and hypertension have an increased risk for developing microvascular complications such as retinopathy and nephropathy. They are also at a twofold increased risk of developing CVD.[297] A 5 mmHg reduction in mean diastolic BP can produce a 37% reduction in microvascular complications, and a 10 mmHg reduction in mean systolic BP reduces the risk of MI by 11% and death related to diabetes by 15%.[215,216,297] Aggressive management is therefore essential for patients with both diabetes and hypertension, such as L.S. Treatment includes weight management, exercise, sodium restriction, smoking cessation, and antihypertensive therapy. Many patients require two or three medications to achieve the target BP goal of $<130/80$ mmHg.[22]

74. What must be considered in selecting an antihypertensive agent for L.S.?

Numerous studies have documented the effectiveness of angiotensin-converting enzyme inhibitors (ACEIs) and angiotensin-receptor blockers (ARBs) in delaying the development and progression of nephropathy. All patients with diabetes and hypertension should be treated with a regimen that includes either an ACEI or ARB.[297] If one class is not tolerated, patients should be switched to the other. For patients failing to reach target BP goals on an ACEI or ARB alone, a diuretic should be added. Second-line add-on agents include β-blockers and calcium channel blockers. Other classes of agents are considered for use as add-on therapy after patients have failed combination therapy with the five classes listed. The management of hypertension in people with diabetes is discussed further in Chapter 13.

Nephropathy

75. What is the significance of the presence of albumin in L.S.'s urine? How should it be managed?

Diabetic nephropathy, characterized by nephrotic syndrome and azotemia, accounts for 35% of all patients with ESRD. It is a major cause of death in patients with type 1 diabetes and is an increasing source of morbidity in type 2 diabetic individuals.[298] Thickening of the glomerular capillary basement membranes is the hallmark of diabetic nephropathy.[299] Diffuse deposition of basement membrane–like material expands the mesangium. This process narrows the capillary lumina, impedes blood flow, and thereby reduces the filtering surface area in the glomerulus. Hyperglycemia causes intraglomerular hypertension and renal hyperfiltration. Hyperfiltration is followed by microalbuminuria with minimal glomerulosclerosis, which still is potentially reversible. If left untreated, overt proteinuria (macroalbuminuria) occurs and the patient usually progresses to nephrotic syndrome. Progression of diabetic renal disease can be accelerated in the presence of hypertension, proteinuria, and diabetic retinopathy. Lipid abnormalities also may contribute to the progression of glomerulosclerosis. Management includes early detection through screening for microalbuminuria; tight glucose control; ACEIs and ARBs for patients with microalbuminuria (to slow progression); aggressive management of hypertension, which can accelerate deterioration of renal function; aggressive management of dyslipidemia; and smoking cessation. A thorough discussion on the management of diabetic nephropathy and ESRD is discussed in Chapter 31.

SCREENING FOR AND CONFIRMATION OF MICROALBUMINURIA

The preferred method of screening for microalbuminuria is measurement of the albumin-to-creatinine ratio in a random spot collection (preferably the first-void or morning sample). Microalbuminuria is defined as a urinary albumin excretion 30 mcg or more albumin/mg creatinine (or mg albumin/g creatinine) during a spot collection.[298] Because of day-to-day variability in albumin excretion, two of three urine samples collected in a 3- to 6-month period need to abnormal before a designation is made. Annual screening should be performed in patients with type 1 diabetes with duration of at least 5 years and in patients with type 2 diabetes from the time of diagnosis. More frequent screening is indicated if hypertension, any increase in SrCr, and/or retinopathy develop. Urine albumin concentrations can be falsely elevated by exercise within 24 hours, fever, infection, uncontrolled diabetes, uncontrolled hypertension, and CHF. Screening should therefore be delayed if a patient has one of these conditions.

Based on established criteria, L.S. has microalbuminuria (180 mg albumin/g creatinine). Management includes tight blood glucose control, lowering the BP, and correction of his dyslipidemia with medications. An ACEI or ARB to treat the microalbuminuria (L.S. should already be receiving one of these agents to treat his hypertension as noted). After initiation of therapy, continued monitoring of the microalbuminuria is recommended to assess the response to therapy and progression of disease.[22] Serum potassium and creatinine levels should be followed as well. A thorough discussion on the management of diabetic nephropathy and ESRD is discussed in Chapter 31.

Cardiovascular Disease

76. L.S. is treated with lisinopril 20 mg/day, which controls his BP and improves his microalbuminuria. His dose of metformin is titrated to 1,000 mg twice daily. Recent laboratory values include an FPG of 130 mg/dL (normal, 70–100), HbA_{1c} of 6.0% (normal, 4%–6%), a triglyceride level of 170 mg/dL (normal, <150 mg/dL), total cholesterol of 204 mg/dL (normal, <200 mg/dL), LDL cholesterol 135 mg/dL (normal depends), and HDL cholesterol of 35 mg/dL (normal, >40 mg/dL). How does the risk of heart disease for patients such as L.S. compare with persons without diabetes? What is the pathogenesis of CHD in persons with diabetes?

[SI units: FPG, 7.2 mmol/L; HbA_{1c}, 0.07; triglycerides, 2.77 mmol/L; total cholesterol, 11.3 mmol/L; HDL, 0.91 mmol/L]

CHD is the leading cause of premature death in the type 2 population and accounts for 50% of the deaths in people with diabetes. Renal complications of type 1 diabetes were previously the principal causes of death; however, with the advent of dialysis and renal transplantation, cardiovascular complications have become the principal cause of morbidity and mortality. Relative to nondiabetic individuals, those with diabetes are two to three times more likely to develop CHD, and their risk of death after an MI also is two to three times higher than their nondiabetic counterparts. Women with diabetes, regardless of their age or menopausal status, have equal risk for CHD to that of nondiabetic men. These sobering figures point to the importance of minimizing or eliminating all other preventable risk factors for CVD in patients with diabetes (i.e., tobacco use, hypertension, hypercholesterolemia, obesity) through the prescription of exercise, diet, and appropriate medications.[300]

PATHOGENESIS

The pathogenesis of CVD in people with diabetes is complex. The metabolic syndrome with its attendant cardiovascular risk factors, dyslipidemia, inflammation, and hemostatic abnormalities are only some of the mechanisms under study.[17,301]

The most common lipid abnormality in type 2 diabetes is hypertriglyceridemia (>150 mg/dL) with low levels of HDL cholesterol (<40 mg/dL in men or <50 mg/dL in women), similar to the lipid profile seen in L.S.[302] Poor control of type 1 diabetes also is associated with elevated LDL cholesterol levels as well as hypertriglyceridemia.[303] All of these lipid abnormalities contribute to the risk for CVD.

In patients with diabetes, clinical trials (primarily with statins) have demonstrated primary and secondary CHD prevention. Although the evidence for the reduction in "hard" CVD outcomes (e.g., CHD death and nonfatal MI) is stronger in diabetic patients who have a high baseline CVD risk (i.e., known CVD and/or very high LDL-C levels), the overall benefits of statins in patients with diabetes at moderate or high risk for CVD is convincing.[22] Readers are referred to the ADA Standards of Medical Care for more detailed information on the CVD clinical trials in patients with diabetes.

Dyslipidemia

77. Should L.S. be treated with drug therapy for his dyslipidemia?

Adults with diabetes should be screened annually for serum lipoprotein levels, including triglycerides, total cholesterol, LDL cholesterol, and HDL cholesterol. A total cholesterol level of less than 200 mg/dL, triglyceride level <150 mg/dL, and LDL cholesterol levels maintained at 100 mg/dL or lower are acceptable. In almost all instances, a statin should be used in patients with diabetes. The ADA now recommends statin therapy in patients over the age of 40 who have one or more other CVD risk factors regardless of baseline LDL levels.[22] For those patients with diabetes and overt CVD, a statin is overwhelmingly indicated.

Diet and exercise are cornerstones in the management of dyslipidemia in patients such as L.S. Weight loss is associated with improvements in insulin sensitivity and glucose control, as well as a reduction in triglycerides, total cholesterol, and LDL cholesterol. Physical activity enhances weight loss and increases HDL cholesterol levels. Thus, L.S.'s diet and exercise habits should be reassessed and instruction in both reinforced as appropriate. Blood glucose concentrations should be optimally controlled with diet, exercise, and oral agents or insulin when indicated. However, the attainment of diabetes control in patients with type 2 diabetes does not necessarily correct lipid abnormalities, as seen in L.S. Because insulin resistance may be the underlying cause of elevated lipids in these patients, efforts should be devoted to reversing insulin resistance as well. Because L.S.'s FPG and HbA_{1c} values indicate that he has achieved diabetes control, a lipid-lowering agent (i.e., a statin) is warranted.

STATIN THERAPY

Simvastatin, pravastatin, lovastatin, fluvastatin, atorvastatin, and rosuvastatin inhibit HMG-CoA reductase, a key regulatory enzyme for cholesterol biosynthesis. As a result, hepatic cholesterol synthesis declines, surface LDL particle receptors increase, and LDL cholesterol clearance increases. The statins' lipid effects are dose dependent. Rosuvastatin and higher doses of atorvastatin and simvastatin can have a substantial effect on triglycerides, which is helpful in patients with elevations in both LDL cholesterol and triglycerides. They raise HDL cholesterol slightly.

OTHER LIPID-LOWERING MEDICATIONS

Bile acid sequestrants primarily lower total and LDL cholesterol levels with little effect on HDL cholesterol. These agents can elevate triglyceride levels and may be problematic as monotherapy for patients such as L.S. with mild to moderate hypertriglyceridemia. Low doses of bile acid sequestrants may be useful as adjunctive therapy when combined with a fibric acid derivative or an HMG-CoA reductase inhibitor. Of note, colesevelam (Welchol) received FDA approval in January 2008 to be used as adjunctive therapy (added on to metformin, sulfonylurea, or insulin) to improve glycemic control in type 2 diabetes.

Gemfibrozil and fenofibrate are the fibric acid derivatives currently available in the United States. These drugs activate lipoprotein lipase, which reduces triglycerides and increases HDL cholesterol. They exert a variable but generally modest LDL cholesterol-lowering effect. Gemfibrozil or fenofibrate may be useful in patients like L.S. whose dyslipidemia is predominantly characterized by hypertriglyceridemia. Gemfibrozil should not be used in combination with repaglinide or the TZDs because it increases their effects and potential for toxicity.

Niacin effectively lowers LDL cholesterol. However, it has a dose-dependent effect in increasing plasma glucose. Although precise mechanisms by which this occurs are unknown, it may be due to accentuation of insulin resistance. Therefore, niacin's use as first-line therapy for dyslipidemia in people with diabetes is not recommended.[302] Although two studies have demonstrated a minimal glycemic effect (increases in blood glucose by 9 mg/dL and HbA_{1c} 0.3%), practitioners still reserve its use as third-line therapy when combination therapy is indicated.[304,305]

Because L.S.'s LDL cholesterol is 135 mg/dL and his goal is less than 100 mg/dL (<70 mg/dL if he had overt CVD), he should be started on a statin. The choice of statin is primarily based on formulary coverage; however, potential for drug–drug interactions with each agent should be assessed before starting (see Chapter 12, and reviews on this subject).[302]

Retinopathy

78. L.S. is referred to the ophthalmologist for his persistent complaints of vision problems despite improvement in his glycemic control. He is diagnosed with mild background retinopathy. Should L.S. be concerned?

Ocular disorders related to diabetes are the leading cause of new cases of legal blindness in Americans. Patients with diabetes may experience blurred vision associated with poor glycemic control, but retinopathy, senile-type cataracts, and glaucoma are the complications that threaten sight. Diabetic retinopathy appears as early as 3 years after diagnosis and is evident in 90% of type 1 diabetic individuals after 15 years. Comparable figures for patients with type 2 diabetes treated with insulin and type 2 patients treated with diet and oral agents are 80% and 55%, respectively. Proliferative retinopathy is less prevalent, but nevertheless is present in 30% of people with type 1 diabetes and in 10% to 15% of insulin-treated patients with type 2 diabetes who have had diabetes for 15 years or longer.[8,41,306,307]

Patients with type 1 diabetes should have a dilated retinal examination within 3 to 5 years of diagnosis; evaluation is not necessary before 10 years of age. Patients with type 2 diabetes should have a comprehensive eye examination soon after diagnosis. The ADA recommends annual comprehensive eye examinations.[22,307] Less frequent eye examinations (every 2–3 years) can be considered in patients with normal examinations based on the advice of an ophthalmologist.[307]

Current theories addressing the possible causes of this complication have been thoroughly reviewed.[306] Microvascular disease characterized by thickening of the capillary membrane may be the underlying lesion for two forms of retinopathy. The first and most common presentation is a nonproliferative retinopathy, which is characterized by microaneurysms that may progress to hard, yellow exudates, signifying chronic leakage, retinal edema, and punctate hemorrhage. This form of retinopathy may be associated with loss of central vision, but generally is associated with excellent visual prognosis. Focal laser photocoagulation of the retina in patients with nonproliferative diabetic retinopathy and macular edema decreases the likelihood of visual loss by 50%.

A second, less common presentation is proliferative retinopathy. This form is characterized by neovascularization (presumably owing to retinal hypoxia) and occurs in approximately 45% of people with type 1 diabetes and in 15% of people with type 2 diabetes who have had the disease for 15 years. Neovascularization ultimately leads to fibrosis, vitreous hemorrhage, and retinal detachment. Photocoagulation therapy may arrest progression and decrease loss of vision associated with neovascularization.[306] Because hypertension, smoking, uremia, and hyperglycemia may lead to more rapid progression of the retinopathy, every effort should be made to eliminate these risk factors for L.S.

Autonomic Neuropathy: Gastroparesis

79. H.D. is a 36-year-old man with a 20-year history of type 1 diabetes. He is in poor glycemic control (HbA_{1c}, 12%) and complains of frequent, severe hypoglycemic reactions that do not make sense. According to H.D., "I have insulin reactions right after I eat, but later on, my glucose concentrations are sky high." H.D. presents to the diabetes clinic with a 2-month history of nausea, postprandial fullness, and occasional vomiting, all of which are unrelieved by antacids. H.D. also has peripheral neuropathy involving both his hands and feet and manifestations of autonomic neuropathy (impotence and orthostatic hypotension). An upper GI series was ordered to rule out peptic ulcer disease and reflux esophagitis, but the preliminary diagnosis was diabetic gastroparesis. What is the cause of diabetic gastroparesis? How should H.D. be treated?

Autonomic neuropathy may present as gastroparesis with feelings of fullness and nausea, urinary retention, impotence in men (manifested as retrograde ejaculation or an inability to attain an erection), postural hypotension, tachycardia, and diarrhea with incontinence of stool.[308] The presence of autonomic insufficiency may have profound effects on the patient's response to vasodilating drugs and ability to counteract hypoglycemia.[309]

Impaired diabetic control with "unexplained" hypoglycemia may result from the disrupted delivery of food to the intestine; that is, glucose delivery does not correspond with prandial insulin action. Many patients with diabetic gastroparesis, like H.D., have had diabetes for many years and also have evidence of peripheral and autonomic neuropathies.

Conventional antiemetic therapy is usually not helpful in the treatment of gastroparesis. Prokinetic agents, such as metoclopramide, are considered first-line therapy. Metoclopramide increases gut motility through indirect cholinergic stimulation of the gut muscle. However, symptomatic improvement does not always correlate with improved gastric emptying, which implies that the effectiveness of metoclopramide also is due to its centrally mediated antiemetic activity. A usual starting dose of metoclopramide is 10 mg orally four times daily, 30 minutes before meals and at bedtime. Although treatment may not eliminate all symptoms, it should minimize most of the patient's complaints. If oral therapy is ineffective for H.D., metoclopramide may be effective in extemporaneously compounded suppository form. Other pharmacotherapeutic interventions include domperidone (not available in the United States), cisapride (withdrawn from the U.S. market), erythromycin, and cholinergic agonists.[310] They are reviewed by Vinik et al.[309] A key component to treating H.D.'s gastroparesis is improving his glycemic control.

Peripheral Neuropathy

80. Six months after institution of metoclopramide 10 mg QID and several insulin adjustments, H.D.'s GI symptoms have been alleviated, and his diabetes is now reasonably well controlled as evidenced by elimination of hypoglycemic episodes and a recent HbA_{1c} of 7.5% (normal, 4%–6%). However, H.D. has been complaining of increasing bilateral foot and leg pain, which he describes as a burning or aching sensation. An examination of his feet reveals cool extremities with absent pulses and loss of monofilament sensation. Outline appropriate steps that can be taken to alleviate H.D.'s peripheral neuropathy.

Diabetic neuropathy may be a consequence of metabolic disturbances in the neurons, microangiopathy affecting the capillary supply to neurons, or an autoimmune process. It affects 60% to 70% of the diabetic population and has a broad spectrum of presentation. Clinically, it most commonly presents as a diffuse symmetric sensorimotor syndrome, as carpal tunnel syndrome, or as autonomic neuropathy. Symptomatic diabetic peripheral neuropathy (DPN) occurs in 25% of patients with diabetes. It is characterized by paresthesia and pain in the lower extremities that may be mild or severe and unrelenting; decreased sensation to monofilament testing; decreased ankle and knee jerks; and decreased nerve conduction velocity. The decreased sensation associated with peripheral neuropathy contributes to the progression of foot injuries and infections that may go unnoticed by the patient until they are severe.[311,312] The management of diabetic neuropathies has been reviewed.[311]

SIMPLE ANALGESICS

Painful neuropathy may respond to simple analgesics (e.g., acetaminophen) or nonsteroidal anti-inflammatory drugs. The analgesic selected should be based on the patient's history of responsiveness to these agents as well as their duration of action and side effect profiles. Side effects include GI upset and bleeding, and renal and hepatic toxicity.

TRICYCLIC ANTIDEPRESSANTS

For painful neuropathy that becomes incapacitating and is unrelieved by simple analgesics, tricyclic antidepressants (TCAs) can be effective and are the most thoroughly studied. TCAs relieve pain by inhibiting reuptake of serotonin and norepinephrine; by a quinidine-like local analgesic effect; or by other, as yet unexplained, mechanisms. Amitriptyline and imipramine are the most commonly prescribed TCAs because of their favorable effects on DPN. Low to moderate (25–150 mg) daily doses have been used, but usually 75 to 100 mg are required for adequate pain relief. The onset of analgesia is evident in 1 to 4 weeks. To minimize side effects, attempts should be made to use antidepressants alone and at bedtime.

81. **Amitriptyline (Elavil) 25 mg at bedtime was begun in H.D. with the dose titrated to 100 mg at bedtime over 1 month. H.D. experienced moderate relief of pain, and both his psychological and somatic complaints of depression lessened dramatically. However, H.D. also experienced intolerable constipation, dry mouth, and urinary hesitancy. Attempts to taper the dose of amitriptyline while maintaining pain relief were unsuccessful. What other drugs are effective for treating DPN?**

Most of the adverse effects of psychotropic drug therapy (sedation, anticholinergic effects, extrapyramidal reactions, cardiovascular effects) are dose related, except for tardive dyskinesia. Patients with autonomic neuropathy and the elderly are at increased risk for complications. Because desipramine and nortriptyline are less likely to cause sedation, anticholinergic side effects, and orthostatic hypotension, we recommend their preferential use over amitriptyline.

ANTICONVULSANTS

Carbamazepine

For cases of extremely painful DPN resistant to simple analgesics and TCAs, carbamazepine can be tried. Doses have varied from 100 to 400 mg three times daily.[22] Dizziness and drowsiness are common, but often transient, and GI disturbances or dermatologic reactions are observed in 5% to 10% of patients. Carbamazepine is now rarely used because of its side effects. Phenytoin (Dilantin) generally is not of value in the treatment of diabetic neuropathy because toxicity (such as nystagmus, ataxia, and sedation) often develops before a therapeutic effect is seen. Furthermore, phenytoin potentially decreases insulin secretion in type 2 patients.

Gabapentin and Pregabalin

Gabapentin and pregabalin's exact mechanism of action in treating neuropathic pain is not known, but it may be through its modulation of calcium channels.[313] A randomized, double-blind, placebo-controlled, 8-week trial evaluated the use of gabapentin in 165 patients with painful diabetic neuropathy.[314] Gabapentin was titrated from 900 mg daily (divided TID) in the first week up to 3,600 mg/day (divided TID) to assess its efficacy and tolerability. Gabapentin significantly improved pain compared with placebo. Although gabapentin was associated with more dizziness and somnolence, only 2 of the 84 patients treated with gabapentin withdrew because of side effects. Backonja and Glanzman[313] reviewed data from five clinical trials of gabapentin and recommends a starting dose of 900 mg/day (300 mg on the first day, 600 mg on the second day, and 900 mg/day on the third day taken in three divided doses); the dose should be titrated to 1,800 to 3,600 mg/day for effective relief of neuropathic pain. An advantage of gabapentin is its lack of significant drug interactions. It needs to be dose adjusted in renal impairment.

Pregabalin is FDA approved for the treatment of painful diabetic neuropathy. It has better bioavailability compared with gapapentin (at higher doses). Doses studied range from 150, 300, and 600 mg per day (divided TID or BID), with 600 mg/day having the greatest effect.[315] The starting dose is 50 mg PO TID. The most common side effects are dizziness, somnolence, and edema.

Other Anticonvulsants

Lamotrigine and topiramate have been found to be effective in the treatment of painful diabetic neuropathy.[181,316,317] Lamotrigine can be started at 25 to 50 mg/day and titrated by 50-mg increments to 400 mg/day; patients should be closely monitored for rash. Topiramate can be started at 25 mg/day and increased in 25-mg increments to 400 mg/day (taken in two to three divided doses).

In January 2008, the FDA released information about an increased risk for suicidal thoughts and behaviors (suicidality) in patients taking antiepileptics. They advise that patients be closely monitored and counseled about these risks.

OTHER AGENTS

Another analgesic, tramadol, which binds to μ-opioid receptors and weakly inhibits norepinephrine and serotonin uptake, has been shown to be effective in DPN.[318,319] Patients can be started on 50 mg/day and titrated in 50-mg increments to 400 mg/day. In one clinical trial, an average dose of 210 mg of tramadol was found to be significantly more effective than placebo in treating painful diabetic neuropathy.[318]

Duloxetine is a selective serotonin norepinephrine reuptake inhibitor that is FDA approved for painful diabetic neuropathy. A recent analysis looked at the number needed to treat at doses of 60 mg/day or BID; the number needed to treat was only 5.2 and 4.9, respectively.[320] Duloxetine should be administered at 60 mg once or twice daily.[321]

The antiarrhythmics, mexiletine and lidocaine, can be beneficial in the treatment of resistant neuropathy.[322] However, because of inconsistent therapeutic benefits and an increased risk of side effects, these agents are reserved for cases that cannot be treated successfully with other, less toxic agents. The use of clonidine (Catapres) also has been studied for the treatment of DPN because peripheral vasodilation may decrease neuronal ischemia. Transdermal clonidine has also been shown to relieve painful diabetic neuropathy in a subpopulation of patients.

Topical application of 0.075% capsaicin (Zostrix), the active ingredient in hot peppers, is used to treat postherpetic neuralgia and has been recommended for diabetic neuropathy. This nonprescription preparation enhances the release and prevents the reaccumulation of substance P in nerve terminals of type C nociceptive fibers. In this way, it impedes the conduction and transmission of peripheral pain impulses. Because capsaicin acts to deplete substance P from nerve fiber terminals, initial high levels are released from the fibers, resulting in a burning and stinging sensation. H.D. should be advised that benefit from capsaicin may not occur for several weeks. Patients should use gloves or an applicator to apply capsaicin and avoid contact with the eyes or mucous membranes. Capsaicin may be useful in diabetic patients intolerant of oral medications.[311]

The treatment of DPN continues to center on providing symptomatic relief. Gabapentin, pregabalin, duloxetine, or TCAs provide the most effective analgesia. A variety of other medications may provide relief in refractory patients.

82. Can anything be done for H.D.'s peripheral vascular disease?

Peripheral vascular disease or peripheral arterial disease (PAD) presents as diminished or absent foot pulses (35%), intermittent claudication (24%–35%), skin ulcers, gangrene, or amputation. People with diabetes are two to ten times more likely to develop symptoms of PAD than those without diabetes, and half of all nontraumatic amputations in the United States are performed in patients with diabetes. In one study that followed type 2 patients for 7 years, 5.5% had an amputation. The prevalence of this condition increases with age, duration of diabetes, and the presence of risk factors such as hypertension or smoking.[311,323]

Signs and symptoms of PAD include leg pain, which is relieved by rest; cold feet; nocturnal leg pain, which is relieved by dangling the feet over the bed or walking; absent pulses; loss of hair on the foot and toes; and gangrene. Treatment of this condition includes elimination and treatment of risk factors such as smoking, dyslipidemia, hypertension, and hyperglycemia; antiplatelet therapy; exercise, the mainstay of therapy; and revascularization surgery.[323] H.D. should be thoroughly educated regarding proper foot care and have frequent foot examinations.[324,325]

83. Should L.S. be started on aspirin therapy?

L.S. has several cardiovascular risk factors (microalbuminuria, dyslipidemia, hypertension, obesity, and age) and should be started on aspirin therapy as primary prevention. The ADA recommends aspirin therapy as secondary prevention in patients with a history of CVD (e.g., MI, vascular bypass procedure, peripheral vascular disease, stroke or transient ischemic attack, claudication, and/or angina).[22,28] Primary prevention is indicated in diabetic individuals over 40 years of age or in those who have additional risk factors (a family history of CVD, smoking, hypertension, albuminuria, dyslipidemia). L.S. should take an enteric-coated aspirin, 81 mg/day.

DRUG-INDUCED ALTERATIONS IN GLUCOSE HOMEOSTASIS

Persons with diabetes are likely to take more drugs over their lifetime than any other group of patients. Patients with type 2 diabetes present with a constellation of chronic conditions, including hypertension, dyslipidemia, and CVD, all of which are amenable to drug therapy. Drugs to manage depression, intermittent infections, obesity, and neurologic and ophthalmologic conditions also are commonly prescribed. Because we know that the actions of drugs are complex, and that for every desired effect there are several other unwanted effects, each time a drug is added to the regimen of someone with diabetes, it is important to assess the patient's situation to determine whether a potential exists for a drug–drug or drug–disease interaction or if the benefit of the newly prescribed drug is likely to outweigh its risks. With the availability of online drug information databases to assist in assessment of drug–drug and drug–disease interactions, a detailed listing of drugs that can exacerbate hyperglycemia and hypoglycemia is not provided. Below, a few case examples are illustrated. The subject has been reviewed by others.[326] Some medications that can have significant hyperglycemic effects include atypical antipsychotics, protease inhibitors, corticosteroids, immunosuppressants (e.g., tacrolimus, cyclosporine), niacin (higher doses), and pentamidine (can also cause hypoglycemia). Patients should be monitored closely for a medication's possible effect on the blood glucose levels.

Drug-Induced Hyperglycemia

Corticosteroids

84. A.L., a 37-year-old obese woman with systemic lupus erythematosus, has been taking 60 mg/day of prednisone for 6 months. During this period, her weight has increased by 30 lb and she has developed glycosuria (no ketones). She was referred to the diabetes clinic, where her FPG was found to be 160 mg/dL. Physical examination shows a 5 feet 2 inch, 150-lb, depressed woman with truncal obesity and an acneiform rash. Her mother and one sister have type 2 diabetes. How do corticosteroids contribute to diabetes mellitus? How should A.L. be treated?

The term *steroid diabetes* was first used to describe the hyperglycemia and glycosuria seen in patients with Cushing syndrome. Now, it is associated more commonly with exogenously administered glucocorticoids and has been a side effect of parenteral, oral, and even topical therapy.[327] Corticosteroids are one of the most common drug groups that unmask latent diabetes or aggravate preexisting disease, and they may produce hyperglycemia and overt diabetes in individuals who are not otherwise predisposed.

Corticosteroids increase hepatic gluconeogenesis and decrease tissue responsiveness to insulin. Although steroid-induced diabetes generally is mild and rarely associated with ketonemia, a wide spectrum of severity may be encountered—from asymptomatic, abnormal glucose tolerance tests to difficult-to-control, insulin-requiring disease. The onset of glucose tolerance can occur within hours to days or after months to years of chronic therapy. The effect generally is considered dose dependent and usually is reversible upon discontinuation of the drug; reversal may take several months.[328,329]

A.L. exhibits many symptoms that can be attributed to supraphysiological doses of corticosteroids: truncal obesity, depression, acneiform rash, and diabetes. Mildly elevated glucose levels in obese individuals, as in A.L.'s case, sometimes can be controlled by diet, but may require treatment with antidiabetic medications. A person with diabetes before glucocorticoid use, whose condition is aggravated by use of a glucocorticoid, should modify treatment appropriately to restore glycemic control. It is important to anticipate the need to modify insulin or other antidiabetic therapy as corticosteroid doses are increased or decreased.

Sympathomimetics

85. R.C., a 41-year-old man with type 1 diabetes, is well controlled on a basal-bolus insulin regimen and has been taking pseudoephedrine 30 mg QID for 7 days and Robitussin DM 10 mL QID (which contains 2.92 g/5 mL sugar) for a cold. Recently, glucose concentrations have been higher than usual. Can pseudoephedrine or the cough preparation be the cause of his poor glycemic control? Discuss the use of sympathomimetics and cough preparations in patients with diabetes.

Over-the-counter drug products, such as decongestants and diet aids, which contain sympathomimetics, carry warning labels that caution against their use in patients with diabetes. Standard sugar- and ethanol-containing cough preparations also carry such warning labels. However, clinically significant drug-induced glucose intolerance probably is very infrequent. It is well established that parenterally administered epinephrine increases blood glucose concentrations secondary to increased glycogenolysis and gluconeogenesis. Other sympathomimetics generally do not have as potent an effect on blood glucose as epinephrine, and their use usually does not pose a practical problem in diabetic patients. Nevertheless, therapeutic to high oral doses of phenylephrine caused hyperglycemia and acetonuria in three nondiabetic children.[330,331] Furthermore, the effects of sympathomimetics on BP must be considered in many patients with diabetes. Therefore, we recommend antihistamines or occasional use of nasal sprays for severe congestion.

In summary, pseudoephedrine or the cough preparation may be aggravating R.C.'s diabetic control, although at these low to normal therapeutic doses, it is quite unlikely. The stress related to R.C.'s underlying cold is more likely to be impairing his glucose tolerance than these low doses of sympathomimetic agents or the small amounts of sugar contained in the cough syrup.

Drug-Induced Hypoglycemia

Ethanol

86. C.F., a 22-year-old woman with newly diagnosed type 1 diabetes, enjoys a glass or two of wine with her evening meal. What effect does alcohol have on a patient with diabetes, particularly one using insulin? Is alcohol contraindicated in C.F. or any person with diabetes?

Clinicians often are reluctant to permit the use of alcoholic beverages in patients with diabetes. However, barring contraindications that are similar in the nondiabetic and diabetic alike (e.g., alcoholism, hypertriglyceridemia, gastritis, pancreatitis, pregnancy), a person with diabetes can safely enjoy a moderate alcohol intake as long as certain precautions are taken. For an in-depth discussion, the reader is referred to two comprehensive reviews of alcohol and diabetes, parts of which are summarized in the following list.[332,333]

- Drink in moderation. The ADA defines this as a daily intake of one drink for adult women and two drinks for adult men (5 oz wine, 12 oz beer, 1.5 oz distilled liquor). The patient should be aware of his or her own sensitivity to the intoxicating effects of ethanol and adjust consumption downward, if needed. This is particularly important for insulin-dependent patients. When having a drink, be sure to have it with a meal.
- Avoid drinks that contain large amounts of sugar, such as liqueurs, sweet wines, and sugar-containing mixes. Instead, consider dry wines, light beers, and distilled spirits. Not only does the simple sugar content add an additional source of glucose and calories to the diet, but ethanol ingested with simple sugar-containing mixers enhances reactive hyperglycemia.
- Remember to count the calories in alcohol (calories = [0.8] × [proof] × [oz]); substitute 1 oz of alcohol for two fat exchanges.
- Be aware that the symptoms of alcohol intoxication and hypoglycemia are similar. If hypoglycemia is mistaken for intoxication by others, appropriate and potentially life-saving treatment can be delayed.
- Be aware of alcohol–sulfonylurea drug interactions, specifically the alcohol-induced enzyme induction of tolbutamide metabolism and the chlorpropamide–alcohol flush reaction.

REFERENCES

1. Centers for Disease Control and Prevention. National diabetes fact sheet: general information and national estimates on diabetes in the United States, 2005. Atlanta, GA: U.S. Department of Health and Human Services, Centers for Disease Control and Prevention; 2005.
2. Wild S et al. Global prevalence of diabetes: Estimates for the year 2000 and projections for 2030. *Diabetes Care* 2004;27:1047.
3. Saaddine JB et al. Improvements in diabetes processes of care and intermediate outcomes: United States, 1998–2002. *Ann Intern Med* 2006;144:465.
4. American Diabetes Association. Diagnosis and classification of diabetes mellitus. *Diabetes Care* 2008;31(Suppl 1):S55.
5. Cowie CC et al. Prevalence of diabetes and impaired fasting glucose in adults in the U.S. *Diabetes Care* 2006;29:1263.
6. Sloan FA et al. The growing burden of diabetes mellitus in the U.S. elderly population. *Arch Intern Med* 2008;168:192.
7. Narayan KMV et al. Impact of recent increase in incidence on future diabetes burden. *Diabetes Care* 2006;26:2114.
8. Agency for Healthcare Research and Quality (AHRQ). 2006 National Healthcare Disparities Report. Rockville, MD: USDHHS, AHRQ; December 2006. AHRQ Pub No. 07-0012.
9. American Diabetes Association. Economic costs of diabetes in the U.S. in 2007. *Diabetes Care* 2008;31:1.
10. Shulman GI et al. Integrated fuel metabolism. In: Porte D Jr et al., eds. *Ellenberg's and Rifkin's Diabetes Mellitus*. 6th ed. Stamford, CT: Appleton & Lange; 2003:1.
11. Naik RG et al. The pathophysiology and genetics of type 1 (insulin-dependent) diabetes. In: Porte D Jr et al., eds. *Ellenberg's and Rifkin's Diabetes Mellitus,* 6th ed. Stamford, CT: Appleton & Lange; 2003: 301.
12. Kahn S, Porte D Jr. The pathophysiology and genetics of type 2 diabetes mellitus. In: Porte D Jr et al., eds. *Ellenberg's and Rifkin's Diabetes Mellitus*. 6th ed. Stamford, CT: Appleton & Lange; 2003: 331.
13. D'Alessio D. Incretins: glucose-dependent insulinotropic polypeptide and glucagon-like peptide 1. In: Porte D Jr et al., eds. *Ellenberg and Rifkin's Diabetes Mellitus*. 6th ed. Stamford, CT: Appleton & Lange; 2003:85.
14. Amatruda JM, Livingston JN. Glucagon. In: Porte D Jr et al., eds. *Ellenberg's and Rifkin's Diabetes Mellitus*. 6th ed. Stamford, CT: Appleton & Lange; 2003:97.
15. Reaven GM. Pathophysiology of insulin resistance in human disease. *Physiol Rev* 1995;75:473.
16. Ford ES et al. Prevalence of the metabolic syndrome among U.S. adults: findings from the third National Health and Nutrition Examination Survey. *JAMA* 2002;287:356.
17. Executive Summary of The Third Report of The National Cholesterol Education Program (NCEP) Expert Panel on Detection, Evaluation, and

Treatment of High Blood Cholesterol In Adults (Adult Treatment Panel III). *JAMA* 2001;285:2486.
18. American Diabetes Association (ADA) Position Statement. Gestational Diabetes Mellitus. *Diabetes Care* 2004;27(Suppl 1):S88.
19. American Diabetes Association. The Expert Committee on the Diagnosis and Classification of Diabetes Mellitus: follow-up report on the diagnosis of diabetes. *Diabetes Care* 2003;26:3160.
20. Hannon TS et al. Childhood obesity and type 2 diabetes mellitus. *Pediatrics* 2006;116:473.
21. American Diabetes Association. Position Statement. Screening for type 2 diabetes. *Diabetes Care* 2004;27(Suppl 1):S11.
22. American Diabetes Association. Standards of medical care in diabetes—2008. *Diabetes Care* 2008;31(Suppl 1):S12.
23. Skyler JS. Relationship of glycemic control to diabetic complications. In: Porte D Jr et al., eds. *Ellenberg and Rifkin's Diabetes Mellitus*. 6th ed. Stamford, CT: Appleton & Lange; 2003:909.
24. Currie BP, Casey JI. Host defense and infections in diabetes mellitus. In: Porte D Jr et al., eds. *Ellenberg and Rifkin's Diabetes Mellitus*. 6th ed. Stamford, CT: Appleton & Lange; 2003:601.
25. Ship JA. Diabetes and oral health. *J Am Dent Assoc* 2003;134(Suppl):43S.
26. American Diabetes Association. Preconception care of women with diabetes. *Diabetes Care* 2004;27(Suppl):S76.
27. Stratton IM et al. Association of glycaemia with macrovascular and microvascular complications of type 2 diabetes (UKPDS 35): prospective observational study. *Br Med J* 2000;321:405.
28. American Diabetes Association. Aspirin therapy in diabetes. *Diabetes Care.* 2004;27(Suppl 1):S72.
29. The effect of intensive treatment of diabetes on the development and progression of long-term complications in insulin-dependent diabetes mellitus. The Diabetes Control and Complications Trial Research Group. *N Engl J Med* 1993;329:977.
30. DCCT-EDIC. Retinopathy and nephropathy in patients with type 1 diabetes four years after a trial of intensive therapy. The Diabetes Control and Complications Trial/Epidemiology of Diabetes Interventions and Complications Research Group. *N Engl J Med* 2000;342:381.
31. Martin CL et al. Neuropathy among the diabetes control and complications trial cohort 8 years after trial completion. *Diabetes Care* 2006;29:340.
32. Nathan DM et al. Intensive diabetes treatment and cardiovascular disease in patients with type 1 diabetes. *N Engl J Med* 2005;353:2643.
33. Intensive blood-glucose control with sulphonylureas or insulin compared with conventional treatment and risk of complications in patients with type 2 diabetes (UKPDS 33). UK Prospective Diabetes Study (UKPDS) Group. *Lancet* 1998;352:837.
34. Gaede PH et al. [The Steno-2 study. Intensive multifactorial intervention reduces the occurrence of cardiovascular disease in patients with type 2 diabetes]. Ugeskr Laeger 2003;165:2658.
35. National Heart, Lung, and Blood Institute. ACCORD telebriefing prepared remarks. Available at: http://www.nhlbi.nih.gov/health/prof/heart/other/accord/remarks.pdf. Accessed February 6, 2008.
36. American Diabetes Association. Statement from the American Diabetes Association in related to the ACCORD trial announcement. Available at: http://www.diabetes.org/for-media/pr-ada-statement-related-to-accord-trail-announcement-020608.jsp. Accessed February 6, 2008.
37. Schatz DA, Bingley PJ. Update on major trials for the prevention of type 1 diabetes mellitus: the American Diabetes Prevention Trial (DPT-1) and the European Nicotinamide Diabetes Intervention Trial (ENDIT). *J Pediatr Endocrinol Metab* 2001; 14(Suppl 1):619.
38. Diabetes Prevention Trial–Type 1 Diabetes Study Group. Effects of insulin in relatives of patients with type 1 diabetes mellitus. *N Engl J Med* 2002;346:1685.
39. Gale EA. Intervening before the onset of Type 1 diabetes: baseline data from the European Nicotinamide Diabetes Intervention Trial (ENDIT). *Diabetologia* 2003;46:339.
40. Herold KC et al. Anti-CD3 monoclonal antibody in new-onset type 1 diabetes mellitus. *N Engl J Med* 2002;346:1692.
41. Harris MI et al. Prevalence of diabetes, impaired fasting glucose, and impaired glucose tolerance in U.S. adults. The Third National Health and Nutrition Examination Survey, 1988–1994. *Diabetes Care* 1998;21:518.
42. ADA and NIDDK. Prevention or delay of type 2 diabetes. *Diabetes Care* 2004;27(Suppl 1):S47.
43. Knowler WC et al. Reduction in the incidence of type 2 diabetes with lifestyle intervention or metformin. *N Engl J Med* 2002;346:393.
44. The Diabetes Prevention Program Research Group. Effects of withdrawal from metformin on the development of diabetes in the diabetes prevention program. *Diabetes Care* 2003;26:977.
45. DREAM (Diabetes REduction Assessment with ramipril and rosiglitazone Medication) Trial Investigators, Gerstein HC et al. Effect of rosiglitazone on the frequency of diabetes in patients with impaired glucose tolerance or impaired fasting glucose: a randomised controlled trial. *Lancet* 2006;368:1096.
46. Nathan DM et al. Impaired fasting glucose and impaired glucose tolerance: implications for care. *Diabetes Care* 2007;30:753.
47. American Diabetes Association. Nutrition recommendations and interventions for diabetes—2008. *Diabetes Care* 2008;31(Suppl 1):S61.
48. Franz MJ. Medical nutrition therapy. In: Franz MJ, ed. *Diabetes Management Therapies*. 4th ed. Chicago: American Association of Diabetes Educators; 2001:3.
49. Giannarelli R et al. Effects of pancreas-kidney transplantation on diabetic retinopathy. *Transpl Int* 2005;18:619.
50. Fioretto P et al. Remodelling of renal interstitial and tubular lesions in pancreas transplant patients. *Kidney Int* 2006;69:907.
51. Pavlakis M, Khwaja K. Pancreas and islet cell transplantation in diabetes. *Curr Opin Endocrinol Diabetes Obes* 2007;14:146.
52. Robertson RP et al. Pancreas transplantation for patients with type 1 diabetes. *Diabetes Care* 2004;27(Suppl 1):S105.
53. Shapiro AM et al. Islet transplantation in seven patients with type 1 diabetes mellitus using a glucocorticoid-free immunosuppressive regimen. *N Engl J Med* 2000;343:230.
54. Ryan EA et al. Five-year follow-up after clinical islet transplantation. *Diabetes* 2005;54:2060.
55. Shapiro AM et al. International trial of the Edmonton protocol for islet transplantation. *N Engl J Med* 2006;355:1318.
56. Gross CR, Zehrer CL. Health-related quality of life outcomes of pancreas transplant recipients. *Clin Transplant* 1992;6:165.
57. Meloche RM. Transplantation for the treatment of type 1 diabetes. *World J Gastroenterol* 2007;13:6347.
58. AACE Diabetes Mellitus Clinical Practice Guidelines Task Force. American Association of Clinical Endocrinologists medical guidelines for clinical practice for the management of diabetes mellitus. *Endocr Pract* 2007;13(Suppl 1):1.
59. Goldstein DE et al. American Diabetes Association Position Statement. Tests of glycemia in diabetes. *Diabetes Care* 2004;27(Suppl 1):S91.
60. Buckingham B et al. Real-time continuous glucose monitoring. *Curr Opin Endocrinol Diabetes Obes* 2007;14:288.
61. Diabetes Research in Children Network (DirecNet) Study Group, Buckinham B et al. Continuous glucose monitoring in children with type 1 diabetes. *J Pediatr* 2007;151:388.
62. Bailey TS et al. Reduction in hemoglobin A1C with real-time continuous glucose monitoring: results from a 12-week observational study. *Diabetes Technol Ther* 2007;9:203.
63. Garg SK et al. Continuous home monitoring of glucose: improved glycemic control with real-life use of continuous glucose sensors in adult subjects with type 1 diabetes. *Diabetes Care* 2007;30:3023.
64. Weinzimer S et al. Freestyle navigator continuous glucose monitoring system use in children with type 1 diabetes using glargine-based multiple daily dose regimens. *Diabetes Care* 2007;31:525.
65. Gorus F et al. How should HbA1c measurements be reported? *Diabetologia* 2006;49:7.
66. Nathan DM, Turgeon H, Regan S. Relationship between glycated haemoglobin levels and mean glucose levels over time. *Diabetologia* 2007;50:2239.
67. Rohlfing CL et al. Defining the relationship between plasma glucose and HbA(1c): analysis of glucose profiles and HbA(1c) in the Diabetes Control and Complications Trial. *Diabetes Care* 2002;25:275.
68. Ceriello A et al. Vitamin E reduction of protein glycosylation in diabetes. New prospect for prevention of diabetic complications? *Diabetes Care* 1991;14:68.
69. Davie SJ et al. Effect of vitamin C on glycosylation of proteins. *Diabetes* 1992;41:167.
70. Nolte MS, Karam, JH. Pancreatic hormones and antidiabetic drugs. In: Katzung B, ed. *Basic and Clinical Pharmacology*, 10th ed. New York: Lange Medical Books/McGraw Hill; 2007:693.
71. DeFelippes M et al. Insulin chemistry and pharmacokinetics. In: Porte DS et al., eds. *Ellenberg and Rifkin's Diabetes Mellitus*. 6th ed. New York: McGraw-Hill; 2003:481.
72. Binder C, Brange J. Insulin chemistry and pharmacokinetics. In: Porte D et al., eds. *Ellenberg's and Rifkin's Diabetes Mellitus*. 5th ed. Stamford, CT: Appleton & Lange; 1997:689.
73. Rabkin R et al. The renal metabolism of insulin. *Diabetologia* 1984;27:351.
74. Burge MR, Schade DS. Insulins. *Endocrinol Metab Clin North Am* 1997;26:575.
75. Holleman F et al. Reduced frequency of severe hypoglycemia and coma in well-controlled IDDM patients treated with insulin lispro. The Benelux-UK Insulin Lispro Study Group. *Diabetes Care* 1997;20:1827.
76. Raskin P et al. A comparison of insulin lispro and buffered regular human insulin administered via continuous subcutaneous insulin infusion pump. *J Diabetes Complications* 2001;15:295.
77. Eli Lilly and Company. Humalog Package Insert. September 2007.
78. Novo Nordisk Inc. Novolog Package Insert. January 2007.
79. Sanofi-Aventis U.S. LLC. Apidra Package Insert. April 2007.
80. Bolli GB, Owens DR. Insulin glargine. *Lancet* 2000;356:443.
81. Lepore M et al. Pharmacokinetics and pharmacodynamics of subcutaneous injection of long-acting human insulin analog glargine, NPH insulin, and ultralente human insulin and continuous subcutaneous infusion of insulin lispro. *Diabetes* 2000;49:2142.
82. Dunn CJ et al. Insulin glargine: an updated review of its use in the management of diabetes mellitus. *Drugs* 2003;63:1743.
83. Raskin P et al. A 16-week comparison of the novel insulin analog insulin glargine (HOE 901) and NPH human insulin used with insulin lispro in patients with type 1 diabetes. *Diabetes Care* 2000;23:1666.
84. Sanofi-Aventis U.S. LLC. Lantus Package Insert. March 2007.
85. Kurtzhals P. Pharmacology of insulin detemir. *Endocrinol Metab Clin North Am* 2007;36(Suppl 1):14.
86. Plank J et al. A double-blind, randomized dose-response study investigating the pharmacodynamic and pharmacokinetic properties of the long-acting insulin analog detemir. *Diabetes Care* 2005;28:1107.
87. Heise T et al. Lower within-subject variability of insulin detemir in comparison to NPH insulin and insulin glargine in people with type 1 diabetes. *Diabetes* 2004;53:1614.

88. Walsh J, Roberts R. *Pumping Insulin*. 3rd ed. San Diego, CA: Torrey Pine Press; 2000.
89. ADA. American Diabetes Association Position Statement. Continuous subcutaneous insulin infusion. *Diabetes Care* 2004;27(Suppl 1):S110.
90. ADA. Resource Guide. Diabetes Forecast 2008; January.
91. Pickup J, Keen H. Continuous subcutaneous insulin infusion at 25 years: evidence base for the expanding use of insulin pump therapy in type 1 diabetes. *Diabetes Care* 2002;25:593.
92. Hirsch IB. Implementation of intensive insulin therapy for IDDM. *Diabetes Review* 1995;3:288.
93. Ashwell SG et al. Twice-daily compared with once-daily insulin glargine in people with type 1 diabetes using meal-time insulin aspart. *Diabet Med* 2006;23:879.
94. Bott S et al. Insulin detemir under steady-state conditions: no accumulation and constant metabolic effect over time with twice daily administration in subjects with type 1 diabetes. *Diabet Med* 2660;23:522.
95. Porcellati F et al. Comparison of pharmacokinetic and dynamics of the long-acting insulin analogs glargine and determir at steady state in type 1 diabetes: a double-blind, randomized, crossover study. *Diabetes Care* 2007;30:2447.
96. Lenhard MJ, Reeves GD. Continuous subcutaneous insulin infusion: a comprehensive review of insulin pump therapy. *Arch Intern Med* 2001;161:2293.
97. American Diabetes Association. Position Statement. Insulin administration. *Diabetes Care* 2004; 27(Suppl 1):S106.
98. Borders LM et al. Traditional insulin-use practices and the incidence of bacterial contamination and infection. *Diabetes Care* 1984;7:121.
99. Anon. Bringing medicine home: self-test kits monitor your health. Consumer Reports 1996, October.
100. Skyler JS. Tactics for type I diabetes. *Endocrinol Metab Clin North Am* 1997;26:647.
101. Gomis R et al. ATLANTUS Study Group. Improving metabolic control in sub-optimally controlled subjects with type 1 diabetes: comparison of two treatment algorithms using insulin glargine. *Diabetes Res Clin Pract* 2007;77:84.
102. Walsh J et al. Using Insulin. San Diego, CA: Torrey Pine Press; 2003:342.
103. Perriello G et al. The effect of asymptomatic nocturnal hypoglycemia on glycemic control in diabetes mellitus. *N Engl J Med* 1988;319:1233.
104. Fanelli CG et al. Administration of neutral protamine hagedorn insulin at bedtime versus with dinner in type 1 diabetes mellitus to avoid nocturnal hypoglycemia and improve control. *A randomized, controlled trial. Ann Intern Med* 2002;136:504.
105. Ratner RE et al. Less hypoglycemia with insulin glargine in intensive insulin therapy for type 1 diabetes. U.S. Study Group of Insulin Glargine in Type 1 Diabetes. *Diabetes Care* 2000;23:639.
106. De Leeuw I et al. Insulin detemir used in basal-bolus therapy in people with type 1 diabetes is associated with a lower risk of nocturnal hypoglycemia and less weight gain over 12 months in comparison to NPH insulin. *Diabetes Obes Metab* 2005;7:73.
107. Hermansen K et al. Comparison of the soluble basal insulin analog insulin detemir with NPH insulin. *Diabetes Care* 2001;24:296.
108. Peters AL, Davidson MB. Effect of storage on action of NPH and regular insulin mixtures. *Diabetes Care* 1987;10:799.
109. Hassan K et al. A randomized, controlled trial comparing twice-a-day insulin glargine mixed with rapid-acting insulin analogs versus standard neutral protamine hagedorn (NPH) therapy in newly diagnosed type 1 diabetes. *Pediatrics* 2008;121:e466.
110. Novo Nordisk Inc. Levemir Package Insert. June 2005.
111. Campbell PJ et al. Pathogenesis of the dawn phenomenon in patients with insulin-dependent diabetes mellitus. Accelerated glucose production and impaired glucose utilization due to nocturnal surges in growth hormone secretion. *N Engl J Med* 1985;312:1473.
112. Bolli GB, Gerich JE. The "dawn phenomenon"—a common occurrence in both non-insulin-dependent and insulin-dependent diabetes mellitus. *N Engl J Med* 1984;310:746.
113. Zinman B et al. Insulin lispro in CSII: results of a double-blind crossover study. *Diabetes* 1997;46:440.
114. Kitabachi AE et al. Hyperglycemic crisis in adult patients with diabetes. A consensus statement from the American Diabetes Association. *Diabetes Care* 2006;29:2739.
115. Diabetes Control and Complications Trial Research Group. Effect of intensive diabetes treatment on the development and progression of long-term complications in insulin-dependent diabetes mellitus. Diabetes Control and Complications Trial. *J Pediatr* 1994;125:177.
116. White NH et al. Beneficial effects of intensive therapy of diabetes during adolescence: outcomes after the conclusion of the Diabetes Control and Complications Trial (DCCT) *J Pediatr* 2001;139: 804.
117. Silverstein J et al. Care of children and adolescents with type 1 diabetes. *Diabetes Care* 2005;28: 186.
118. Murphy NP et al. Randomized cross-over trial of insulin glargine plus lispro or NPH insulin plus regular human insulin in adolescents with type 1 diabetes on intensive insulin regimens. *Diabetes Care* 2003;26:799.
119. Chase HP et al. Reduced hypoglycemic episodes and improved glycemic control in children with type 1 diabetes using insulin glargine and neutral protamine hagedorn insulin. *J Pediatr* 2003;143:737.
120. Ahern JA et al. Insulin pump therapy in pediatrics; a therapeutic alternative to safely lower HbA1c levels across all age groups. *Pediatr Diabetes* 2002;3:10.
121. Bode BW et al. Diabetes management in the new millennium using insulin pump therapy. *Diabetes Metab Res Rev* 2002;18(Suppl 1):S14.
122. Moshe P et al. Use of insulin pump therapy in the pediatric age-group. Consensus statement from the European Society for Paediatric Endocrinology, the Lawson Wilkins Pediatric Endocrine Society, and the International Society for Pediatric and Adolescent Diabetes, endorsed by the American Diabetes Association and the European Association for the Study of Diabetes. *Diabetes Care* 2007;30: 1653.
123. Agner T et al. Remission in IDDM: prospective study of basal C-peptide and insulin dose in 268 consecutive patients. *Diabetes Care* 1987;10:164.
124. Davis EA et al. Impact of improved glycaemic control on rates of hypoglycaemia in insulin dependent diabetes mellitus. *Arch Dis Child* 1998;78:111.
125. Jones TW et al. Decreased epinephrine responses to hypoglycemia during sleep. *N Engl J Med* 1998; 338:1657.
126. Deiss D et al. Treatment with insulin glargine reduces asymptomatic hypoglycemia detected by continuous subcutaneous glucose monitoring in children and adolescents with type 1 diabetes. *Pediatr Diabetes* 2007;8:157.
127. Murphy NP et al. Randomized cross-over trial of insulin glargine plus lispro or NPH insulin plus regular human insulin in adolescents with type 1 diabetes on intensive insulin regimens. *Diabetes Care* 2003;26:799.
128. Bernstein RK. Clouding and deactivation of clear (regular) human insulin: association with silicone oil from disposable syringes? *Diabetes Care* 1987;10:786.
129. Benson EA et al. Flocculated humulin N insulin. *N Engl J Med* 1987;316:1026.
130. Storvick WO, Henry HJ. Effect of storage temperature on stability of commercial insulin preparations. *Diabetes* 1968;17:499.
131. Qing Shi Z et al. Metabolic implications of exercise and physical fitness in physiology and diabetes. In: Porte D Jr, Sherwin R, eds. *Ellenberg's and Rifkin's Diabetes Mellitus*. 5th ed. Stamford, CT: Appleton & Lange; 1997:653.
132. American Diabetes Association. Physical activity/exercise and diabetes mellitus. *Diabetes Care* 2004;27(Suppl 1):S58.
133. MacDonald MJ. Postexercise late-onset hypoglycemia in insulin-dependent diabetic patients. *Diabetes Care* 1987;10:584.
134. Koivisto VA, Felig P. Effects of leg exercise on insulin absorption in diabetic patients. *N Engl J Med* 1978;298:79.
135. Kemmer FW et al. Mechanism of exercise-induced hypoglycemia during sulfonylurea treatment. *Diabetes* 1987;36:1178.
136. American Diabetes Association. When you're sick. Available at: http://www.diabetes.org/type-1-diabetes/sick.jsp. Accessed March 16, 2008.
137. Turnheim K. Basic aspects of insulin pharmacokinetics. In: Brunetti P, Waldhausl W, eds. *Advanced Models for the Therapy of Insulin-Dependent Diabetes*. New York: Raven Press; 1987:91.
138. Rubenstein AH, Spitz I. Role of the kidney in insulin metabolism and excretion. *Diabetes* 1968;17:161.
139. Rabkin R et al. Effect of renal disease on renal uptake and excretion of insulin in man. *N Engl J Med* 1970;282:182.
140. Malmberg K. Prospective randomised study of intensive insulin treatment on long term survival after acute myocardial infarction in patients with diabetes mellitus. DIGAMI (Diabetes Mellitus, Insulin Glucose Infusion in Acute Myocardial Infarction) Study Group. *BMJ* 1997;314:1512.
141. Malmberg K et al. Intense metabolic control by means of insulin in patients with diabetes mellitus and acute myocardial infarction (DIGAMI-2): effects on mortality and morbidity. *Eur Heart J* 2005;26:650.
142. Metha SR et al. Effect of glucose-insulin-potassium infusion on mortality in patients with acute ST-segment elevation myocardial infarction: the CREATE-ECLA randomized controlled trial. *JAMA* 2005;293:437.
143. Cheung NW et al. The hyperglycemia intensive insulin infusion in infarction (HI-5) study: a randomized controlled trial of insulin infusion therapy for myocardial infarction. *Diabetes Care* 2006;29:765.
144. van den Berghe G et al. Intensive insulin therapy in the critically ill patients. *N Engl J Med* 2001;345:1359.
145. van den Berghe G et al. Intensive insulin therapy in the medical ICU. *N Engl J Med* 2006;449.
146. Krinsley J. Glycemic control in critically ill patients: Leuven and beyond. *Chest* 2007;132:1.
147. Pittas AG et al. Insulin therapy for critically ill hospitalized patients: a meta-analysis of randomized controlled trials. *Arch Intern Med* 2004;164: 2005.
148. Krinsley J. Severe hypoglycemia in critically ill patients: risk factors and outcomes. *Crit Care Med* 2007;35:2262.
149. Clement S et al. Management of diabetes and hyperglycemia in hospitals. *Diabetes Care* 2004;27:553.
150. Goldberg PA et al. Implementation of a safe and effective insulin infusion protocol in a medical intensive care unit. *Diabetes Care* 2004;27:461.
151. Markovitz LJ et al. Description and evaluation of a glycemic management protocol for patients with diabetes undergoing heart surgery. *Endocr Pract* 2002;8:10.
152. Saudek CD. Novel forms of insulin delivery. *Endocrinol Metab Clin North Am* 1997;26:599.
153. Cryer PE, Gerich J. Hypoglycemia in insulin-dependent diabetes mellitus: interplay of insulin excess and compromised glucose regulation. In: Porte D Jr et al., eds. *Ellenberg's and Rifkin's Diabetes Mellitus*. 6th ed. New York: McGraw-Hill; 2003: 523.
154. Pramming S et al. Symptomatic hypoglycaemia in 411 type 1 diabetic patients. *Diabet Med* 1991; 8:217.
155. Ennis E et al. Diabetic ketoacidosis. In: Porte D Jr, Sherwin R, eds. *Ellenberg's and Rifkin's Diabetes Mellitus*. 5th ed. Stamford, CT: Appleton & Lange; 1997:827.

156. Viallon A et al. Does bicarbonate therapy improve the management of severe diabetic ketoacidosis? *Crit Care Med* 1999;27:2690.
157. Kirpichnikov D et al. Metformin: an update. *Ann Intern Med* 2002;137:25.
158. Bristol-Myers Squibb Company. Glucophage and Glucophage XR Package Insert. June 2006.
159. UKPDS 28: a randomized trial of efficacy of early addition of metformin in sulfonylurea-treated type 2 diabetes. U.K. Prospective Diabetes Study Group. *Diabetes Care* 1998;21:87.
160. Sambol NC et al. Kidney function and age are both predictors of pharmacokinetics of metformin. *J Clin Pharmacol* 1995;35:1094.
161. Tahrani AA et al. Metformin, heart failure, and lactic acidosis: is metformin absolutely contraindicated? *BMJ* 2007;335:508.
162. Salpeter SR et al. Risk of fatal and nonfatal lactic acidosis with metformin use in type 2 diabetes mellitus. *Arch Intern Med* 2003;163:2594.
163. Shu Y et al. Effect of genetic variation in the organic cation transporter 1 (OCT1) on metformin action. *J Clin Invest* 2007;117:1422.
164. Novo Nordisk Pharmaceuticals, Inc. Prandin Package Insert. June 19, 2006.
165. Novartis Pharmaceuticals Corporation. Starlix Package Insert. November 2006.
166. Nan DN, Fernandez-Ayala M. Acute hepatotoxicity caused by repaglinide. *Ann Intern Med* 2004;141:823.
167. Scheen AJ. Drug-drug and drug-food pharmacokinetic interactions with new insulinotropic agents repaglinide and nateglinide. *Clin Pharmacokinet* 2007;46:93.
168. Black C et al. Meglitinide analogues for type 2 diabetes mellitus. Cochrane Database of Systematic Reviews 2007, Issue 2. Art. No.: CD004654. DOI: 10.1002/14651858.CD004654.pub2.
169. Inzucchi SE. Oral antihyperglycemic therapy for type 2 diabetes. *JAMA* 2002;287:360.
170. Groop LC. Sulfonylureas in NIDDM. *Diabetes Care* 1992;15:737.
171. Groop LC et al. Effect of sulphonylurea on glucose-stimulated insulin secretion in healthy and non-insulin dependent diabetic subjects: a dose-response study. *Acta Diabetol* 1991;28:162.
172. Wahlin-Boll E et al. Impaired effect of sulfonylurea following increased dosage. *Eur J Clin Pharmacol* 1982;22:21.
173. Stenman S et al. What is the benefit of increasing the sulfonylurea dose? *Ann Intern Med* 1993;118:169.
174. Marchetti P, Navalesi R. Pharmacokinetic-pharmacodynamic relationships of oral hypoglycaemic agents. An update. *Clin Pharmacokinet* 1989;16:100.
175. Jaber LA et al. Comparison of pharmacokinetics and pharmacodynamics of short- and long-term glyburide therapy in NIDDM. *Diabetes Care* 1994;17:1300.
176. Feldman JM. Glyburide: a second-generation sulfonylurea hypoglycemic agent. History, chemistry, metabolism, pharmacokinetics, clinical use and adverse effects. *Pharmacotherapy* 1985;5:43.
177. Sanofi-Aventis. Amaryl package insert. February 2006.
178. Sulfonylurea monograph. Drug Facts and Comparisons. Version 4.0
179. Donath MY et al. Mechanisms of beta-cell death in type 2 diabetes. *Diabetes* 2005;54(Suppl 2):S108.
180. Yki-Jaervinen H. Thiazolidinediones. *N Engl J Med* 2004;351:1106.
181. GlaxoSmithKline. Avandia Package Insert. November 2007.
182. Takeda Pharmaceuticals America, Inc. Actos Package Insert. September 2007.
183. Hanefeld M. Pharmacokinetics and clinical efficacy of pioglitazone. *Int J Clin Pract Suppl* 2001; 121:19.
184. Murphy EJ et al. Troglitazone-induced fulminant hepatic failure. *Dig Dis Sci* 2000;45:549.
185. Al-Salman J et al. Hepatocellular injury in a patient receiving rosiglitazone. *A case report. Ann Intern Med* 2000;132:121.
186. Su DH, Lai MY, Wu HP. Liver failure in a patient receiving rosiglitazone therapy. *Diab Med* 2006;23:105.
187. Farley-Hills E, Sivasankar R, Martin M. Fatal liver failure associated with pioglitazone. *BMJ* 2004;329:429.
188. Lipscombe LL et al. Thiazolidinediones and cardiovascular outcomes in older patients with diabetes. *JAMA* 2007;298:2634.
189. Singh S et al. Long-term risk of cardiovascular events with rosiglitazone. A meta-analysis. *N Engl J Med* 2007;298:1189.
190. Nissen SE, Wolski K. Effect of rosiglitazone on the risk of myocardial infarction and death from cardiovascular causes. *N Engl J Med* 2007;356:2457.
191. Richter B et al. Rosiglitazone for type 2 diabetes mellitus. Cochrane Database of Systematic Reviews 2007, Issue 3. Art. No.: CD006063. DOI: 10.1002/14651858.CD006063.pub2.
192. Lincoff AM et al. Pioglitazone and risk of cardiovascular events in patients with type 2 diabetes mellitus. A meta-analysis of randomized trials. *JAMA* 2007;298:1180.
193. Richter B et al. Pioglitazone for type 2 diabetes mellitus. Cochrane Database of Systematic Reviews 2006, Issue 4. Art. No.: CD006060. DOI: 10.1002/14651858.CD006060.pub2.
194. Ryan EH Jr et al. Diabetic macular edema associated with glitazone use. *Retina* 2006;26:562.
195. Schwartz AV, Sellmeyer DE. Thiazolidinedione therapy gets complicated. Is bone loss the price of improved insulin resistance? *Diab Care* 2007;30: 1670.
196. Scheen AJ. Pharmacokinetic interactions with thiazolidinediones. *Clin Pharmacokinet* 2007;46:1.
197. Bayer Corporation. Precose Package Insert. November 2004.
198. Pharmacia and Upjohn Company. Glyset Package Insert. February 2006.
199. Van de Laar FA et al. Alpha-glucosidase inhibitors for type 2 diabetes mellitus. Cochrane Database of Systematic Reviews 2005, Issue 2. Art. No.: CD003639. DOI: 10.1002/14651858. CD003639.pub2.
200. Drucker DJ, Nauck MA. The incretin system: glucagon-like peptide-1 receptor agonists and dipeptidyl peptidase-4 inhibitors in type 2 diabetes. *Lancet* 2006: 368:1696.
201. Vilsboll T. Liraglutide: a once-daily GLP-1 analogue for the treatment of type 2 diabetes mellitus. *Expert Opin Invest Drugs* 2007;16:231.
202. Amylin Pharmaceuticals, Inc. Byetta Package Insert. October 2007.
203. Vilsboll T et al. Liraglutide, a long-acting human glucagon-like peptide-1 analog, given as monotherapy significantly improves glycemic control and lowers body weight without risk of hypoglycemia in patients with type 2 diabetes. *Diab Care* 2007;30:1608.
204. Langley AK et al. Dipeptidyl peptidase IV inhibitors and the incretin system in type 2 diabetes mellitus. *Pharmacotherapy* 2007;27:1163.
205. Merck and Co., Inc. Januvia Package Insert. October 2007.
206. He YL et al. Pharmacokinetics and pharmacodynamics of vildagliptin in patients with type 2 diabetes mellitus. *Clin Pharmacokinet* 2007;46: 577.
207. He YL et al. The absolute oral bioavailability and population-based pharmacokinetic modelling of a novel dipeptidyl peptidase-IV inhibitor, vildagliptin, in healthy volunteers. *Clin Pharmacokinet* 2007;46:787.
208. Sunkara G et al. Dose proportionality and the effect of food on vildagliptin, a novel dipeptidyl peptidase-IV inhibitor, in healthy volunteers. *J Clin Pharmacol* 2007;47:1152.
209. Amori RE et al. Efficacy and safety of incretin therapy in type 2 diabetes. A systematic review and meta-analysis. *JAMA* 2007: 298:194.
210. Kleppinger EL, Helms K. The role of vildagliptin in the management of type 2 diabetes mellitus. *Ann Pharmacother* 2007;41:824.
211. He YL et al. Evaluation of pharmacokinetic interactions between vildagliptin and digoxin in healthy volunteers. *J Clin Pharmacol* 2007;47:998.
212. Singh-Franco D et al. Pramlintide acetate injection for the treatment of type 1 and type 2 diabetes mellitus. *Clin Therapeutics* 2007;29:535.
213. Amylin Pharmaceuticals, Inc. Symlin Package Insert. December 2007.
214. American Diabetes Association (ADA) Position Statement. Implications of the Diabetes Control and Complications Trial. *Diabetes Care* 2003;24(Suppl 1):S28.
215. Efficacy of atenolol and captopril in reducing risk of macrovascular and microvascular complications in type 2 diabetes: UKPDS 39. UK Prospective Diabetes Study Group. *Br Med J* 1998;317:713.
216. Tight blood pressure control and risk of macrovascular and microvascular complications in type 2 diabetes: UKPDS 38. UK Prospective Diabetes Study Group. *Br Med J* 1998;317:703.
217. Colwell JA. DCCT findings. Applicability and implications for NIDDM. *Diabetes Res* 1994:277.
218. Colwell JA. Should we use intensive insulin therapy after oral agent failure in type II diabetes? *Diabetes Care* 1996;19:896.
219. Henry RR, Genuth S. Forum one: current recommendations about intensification of metabolic control in non-insulin-dependent diabetes mellitus. *Ann Intern Med* 1996;124:175.
220. Nathan DM et al. Management of hyperglycemia in type 2 diabetes: a consensus algorithm for the initiation and adjustment of therapy. A consensus statement from the American Diabetes Association and the European Association for the Study of Diabetes. *Diabetes Care* 2006;29:1963.
221. Effect of intensive blood-glucose control with metformin on complications in overweight patients with type 2 diabetes (UKPDS 34). UK Prospective Diabetes Study (UKPDS) Group. *Lancet* 1998;352:854.
222. Feher MD et al. Tolerability of prolonged-release metformin (Glucophage) in individuals intolerant to standard metformin—results from four UK centres. *Br J Diabetes Vasc Dis* 2007;7:225.
223. Welschen LM et al. Self-monitoring of blood glucose in patients with type 2 diabetes who are not using insulin: a systematic review. *Diabetes Care* 2005;28:1510.
224. Avignon A et al. Nonfasting plasma glucose is a better marker of diabetic control than fasting plasma glucose in type 2 diabetes. *Diabetes Care* 1997;20:1822.
225. Turner R et al. United Kingdom Prospective Diabetes Study 17: a 9-year update of a randomized, controlled trial on the effect of improved metabolic control on complications in non-insulin-dependent diabetes mellitus. *Ann Intern Med* 1996;124:136.
226. Nathan DM et al. Management of hyperglycaemia in type 2 diabetes mellitus: a consensus algorithm for the initiation and adjustment of therapy. *Diabetologia* 2008;51:8.
227. Bolen S et al. Systematic review: comparative effectiveness and safety of oral medications for type 2 diabetes mellitus. *Ann Intern Med* 2007;147:386.
228. Charpentier G. Oral combination therapy for type 2 diabetes. *Diabetes Metab Res Rev* 2002;18(Suppl 3):S70.
229. Gavin LA et al. Troglitazone add-on therapy to a combination of sulfonylureas plus metformin achieved and sustained effective diabetes control. *Endocr Pract* 2000;6:305.
230. Bell DS, Ovalle F. Long-term efficacy of triple oral therapy for type 2 diabetes mellitus. *Endocr Pract* 2002;8:271.
231. Kaye TB. Triple oral antidiabetic therapy. *J Diabetes Complications* 1998;12:311.
232. Rosenstock J et al. Triple therapy in type 2 diabetes: insulin glargine or rosiglitazone added to combination therapy of sulfonylurea plus metformin in insulin-naive patients. *Diabetes Care* 2006;29:554.
233. Schwartz S et al. Insulin 70/30 mix plus metformin versus triple oral therapy in the treatment of type 2 diabetes after failure of two oral drugs:

efficacy, safety, and cost analysis. *Diabetes Care* 2003;26:2238.
234. Wright A et al. Sulfonylurea inadequacy: efficacy of addition of insulin over 6 years in patients with type 2 diabetes in the U.K. Prospective Diabetes Study (UKPDS 57). *Diabetes Care* 2002;25: 330.
235. Kahn SE et al for the ADOPT Study Group. Glycemic durability of rosiglitazone, metformin, or glyburide monotherapy. *N Engl J Med* 2006;355: 2427.
236. GlaxoSmithKline. Advisory committee briefing document: cardiovascular safety on rosiglitazone. GlaxoSmithKline, Philadelphia; 2007:40. Available at: http://www.fda.gov/ohrms/dockets/ac/07/briefing/2007-4308b1–01-sponsor-backgrounder.pdf. Accessed March 30, 2008.
237. U.S. Food and Drug Administration briefing document. Rockville, MD: U.S. Food and Drug Administration; 2007:13. Available at: http://www.fda.gov/ohrms/dockets/ac/07/briefing/2007-4308b1-02-fda-backgrounder.pdf. Accessed March 30, 2008.
238. Lago RM et al. Congestive heart failure and cardiovascular death in patients with prediabetes and type 2 diabetes given thiazolidinediones: a meta-analysis of randomized clinical trials. *Lancet* 2007;370:1129.
239. Home PD et al; for the RECORD Study Group et al. Rosiglitazone evaluated for the cardiovascular outcomes-an interim analysis. *N Engl J Med* 2007;357:28.
240. Singh S et al. Thiazolidinediones and heart failure: a teleo-analysis. *Diabetes Care* 2007;30:2248.
241. Schwartz AV et al. Thiazolidinedione use and bone loss in older diabetic adults. *J Clin Endocrinol Metab* 2006;91:3349.
242. Ali AA et al. Rosiglitazone causes bone loss in mice by suppressing osteoblast differentiation and bone formation. *Endocrinology* 2005;146:1226.
243. Faber OK et al. Acute actions of sulfonylurea drugs during long-term treatment of NIDDM. *Diabetes Care* 1990;13(Suppl 3):26.
244. Kradjan WA et al. Pharmacokinetics and pharmacodynamics of glipizide after once-daily and divided doses. *Pharmacotherapy* 1995;15:465.
245. Leahy JL. Natural history of beta-cell dysfunction in NIDDM. *Diabetes Care* 1990;13:992.
246. DeFronzo RA, Goodman AM. Efficacy of metformin in patients with non-insulin-dependent diabetes mellitus. The Multicenter Metformin Study Group. *N Engl J Med* 1995;333:541.
247. Fonseca V et al. Effect of metformin and rosiglitazone combination therapy in patients with type 2 diabetes mellitus: a randomized controlled trial. *JAMA* 2000;283:1695.
248. Charbonnel B et al. Efficacy and safety of the dipeptidyl peptidase-4 inhibitor sitagliptin added to ongoing metformin therapy in patients with type 2 diabetes inadequately controlled on metformin alone. *Diabetes Care* 2006;29:2638.
249. Defronzo RA et al. Effects of exenatide (exendin-4) on glycemic control and weight over 30 weeks in metformin-treated patients with type 2 diabetes. *Diabetes Care* 2005;28:1092.
250. Langtry HD, Balfour JA. Glimepiride. A review of its use in the management of type 2 diabetes mellitus. *Drugs* 1998;55:563.
251. Kendall DM et al. Effects of exenatide (exendin-4) on glycemic control over 30 weeks in patients with type 2 diabetes treated with metformin and a sulfonylurea. *Diabetes Care* 2005;28:1083.
252. Klonoff DC et al. Exenatide effects on diabetes, obesity, cardiovascular risk factors and hepatic biomarkers in patients with type 2 diabetes treated for at least 3 years. *Curr Med Res Opin* 2008;24:275.
253. Kim D et al. Effects of once-weekly dosing of a long-acting release formulation of exenatide on glucose control and body weight in subjects with type 2 diabetes. *Diabetes Care* 2007;30:1487.
254. DeWitt DE, Hirsch IB. Outpatient insulin therapy in type 1 and type 2 diabetes mellitus: scientific review. *JAMA* 2003;289:2254.
255. Giugliano D et al. Metformin for obese, insulin-treated diabetic patients: improvement in glycaemic control and reduction of metabolic risk factors. *Eur J Clin Pharmacol* 1993;44:107.
256. McNulty et al. Comparison of metformin and sulfonylurea (glicazide) in combination with daily NPH insulin in type 2 diabetic patients inadequately controlled on maximal oral therapy [Abstract #0622]. *Diabetes* 1997:161A.
257. Yki-Jarvinen H et al. Comparison of bedtime insulin regimens in patients with type 2 diabetes mellitus. A randomized, controlled trial. *Ann Intern Med* 1999;130:389.
258. Rosenstock J et al. Efficacy and safety of pioglitazone in type 2 diabetes: a randomised, placebo-controlled study in patients receiving stable insulin therapy. *Int J Clin Pract* 2002;56:251.
259. Riddle MC. Tactics for type II diabetes. *Endocrinol Metab Clin North Am* 1997;26:659.
260. Genuth S. Management of the adult onset diabetic with sulfonylurea drug failure. *Endocrinol Metab Clin North Am* 1992;21:351.
261. DeWitt DE, Dugdale DC. Using new insulin strategies in the outpatient treatment of diabetes: clinical applications. *JAMA* 2003;289:2265.
262. Arshag D et al. Narrative review: a rational approach to starting insulin therapy. *Ann Intern Med* 2006;145:125.
263. Riddle MC et al. The treat-to-target trial: randomized addition of glargine or human NPH insulin to oral therapy of type 2 diabetic patients. *Diabetes Care* 2003;26:3080.
264. Anderson JH Jr et al. Mealtime treatment with insulin analog improves postprandial hyperglycemia and hypoglycemia in patients with non-insulin-dependent diabetes mellitus. Multicenter Insulin Lispro Study Group. *Arch Intern Med* 1997;157:1249.
265. Jain R et al. Efficacy of biphasic insulin aspart 70/30 in patients with T2DM not achieving glycemic targets on OADS with/without basal insulin therapy. *Diabetes* 2005;54:A69.
266. Misbin RI et al. Lactic acidosis in patients with diabetes treated with metformin. *N Engl J Med* 1998;338:265.
267. Cusi K, DeFronzo R. Metformin: a review of its metabolic effects. *Diabetes Review* 1998;6: 89.
268. University Group Diabetes Program. A study of the effects of hypoglycemic agents on vascular complications in patients with adult-onset diabetes I. Design, methods, and baseline results. *Diabetes* 1970: 747.
269. Kilo C et al. The Achilles heel of the University Group Diabetes Program. *JAMA* 1980;243:450.
270. Gan SC et al. Biguanide-associated lactic acidosis. Case report and review of the literature. *Arch Intern Med* 1992;152:2333.
271. Misbin RI. Phenformin-associated lactic acidosis: pathogenesis and treatment. *Ann Intern Med* 1977;87:591.
272. Phenformin: removal from the general market. *FDA Drug Bull* 1977;19.
273. Stang M et al. Incidence of lactic acidosis in metformin users. *Diabetes Care* 1999;22:925.
274. Emslie-Smith AM et al. Contraindications to metformin therapy in patients with type 2 diabetes—a population-based study of adherence to prescribing guidelines. *Diabet Med* 2001;18:483.
275. Calabrese AT et al. Evaluation of prescribing practices: risk of lactic acidosis with metformin therapy. *Arch Intern Med* 2002;162:434.
276. Horlen C et al. Frequency of inappropriate metformin prescriptions. *JAMA* 2002;287:2504.
277. Masoudi FA et al. Metformin and thiazolidinedione use in Medicare patients with heart failure. *JAMA* 2003;290:81.
278. Swedko PJ et al. Serum creatinine is an inadequate screening test for renal failure in elderly patients. *Arch Intern Med* 2003;163:356.
279. Seltzer HS. Drug-induced hypoglycemia. A review of 1418 cases. *Endocrinol Metab Clin North Am* 1989;18:163.
280. Pearson JG et al. Pharmacokinetic disposition of 14C-glyburide in patients with varying renal function. *Clin Pharmacol Ther* 1986;39:318.
281. Gulati P et al. A double-blind trial of tolbutamide in cirrhosis of the liver. *Am J Dig Dis* 1967:42.
282. Ueda H et al. Disappearance rate of the tolbutamide in normal subjects and in diabetes mellitus, liver cirrhosis, and renal disease. *Diabetes* 1963:414.
283. Gambert SR. Atypical presentation of diabetes mellitus in the elderly. *Clin Geriatr Med* 1990;6:721.
284. Morley JE, Perry HM 3rd. The management of diabetes mellitus in older individuals. *Drugs* 1991; 41:548.
285. Carlisle B. Diabetes in the elderly: factors to consider. *Pharm Times* 1992:130.
286. Matz R. Hyperosmolar syndrome. In: Porte D Jr et al., eds. *Ellenberg's and Rifkin's Diabetes Mellitus*. 6th ed. New York: McGraw-Hill; 2003:587.
287. Silver AJ, Morley JE. Role of the opioid system in the hypodipsia associated with aging. *J Am Geriatr Soc* 1992;40:556.
288. Morley JE et al. Diabetes mellitus in elderly patients. Is it different? *Am J Med* 1987;83:533.
289. Brown AF et al. Guidelines for improving the care of the older person with diabetes mellitus. *J Am Geriatr Soc* 2003;51:S265.
290. Mokdad AH et al. Prevalence of obesity, diabetes, and obesity-related health risk factors, 2001. *JAMA* 2003;289:76.
291. Hogikyan R, Halter J. Aging and diabetes. In: Porte DS et al., eds. *Ellenberg and Rifkin's Diabetes Mellitus*. 6th ed. New York: McGraw Hill, 2003: 415.
292. Greenblatt DJ. Reduced serum albumin concentration in the elderly: a report from the Boston Collaborative Drug Surveillance Program. *J Am Geriatr Soc* 1979;27:20.
293. Shorr RI et al. Individual sulfonylureas and serious hypoglycemia in older people. *J Am Geriatr Soc* 1996;44:751.
294. Hasslacher C. Safety and efficacy of repaglinide in type 2 diabetic patients with and without impaired renal function. *Diabetes Care* 2003;26:886.
295. Fajans S. Classification and diagnosis of diabetes. In: Porte D et al., eds. *Ellenberg's and Rifkin's Diabetes Mellitus*. 5th ed. Stamford, CT: Appleton & Lange; 1997:357.
296. Fajans SS et al. Molecular mechanisms and clinical pathophysiology of maturity-onset diabetes of the young. *N Engl J Med* 2001;345:971.
297. American Diabetes Association. Hypertension management in adults with diabetes. *Diab Care* 2004;27(Suppl 1):S65.
298. American Diabetes Association. Position statement. Nephropathy in Diabetes. *Diabetes Care* 2004;27(Suppl 1):S79.
299. DeFronzo RA. Diabetic nephropathy. In: Porte D, Jr et al., eds. *Ellenberg and Rifkin's Diabetes Mellitus*. 6th ed. Stamford, CT: Appleton & Lange; 2003: 723.
300. Lteif AA et al. Diabetes and heart disease an evidence-driven guide to risk factors management in diabetes. *Cardiol Rev* 2003;11:262.
301. Young L, Chyun D. Heart disease in patients with diabetes. In: Porte DS et al., eds. *Ellenberg and Rifkin's Diabetes Mellitus*. 6th ed. New York: McGraw-Hill; 2003:823.
302. Haffner SM. Dyslipidemia management in adults with diabetes. *Diabetes Care* 2004;27(Suppl 1):S68.
303. Consensus development conference on the diagnosis of coronary heart disease in people with diabetes: 10–11 February 1998, Miami, Florida. American Diabetes Association. *Diabetes Care* 1998;21:1551.
304. Elam MB et al. Effect of niacin on lipid and lipoprotein levels and glycemic control in patients with diabetes and peripheral arterial disease: the ADMIT study: a randomized trial. Arterial Disease Multiple Intervention Trial. *JAMA* 2000;284:1263.
305. Grundy SM et al. Efficacy, safety, and tolerability of once-daily niacin for the treatment of dyslipidemia associated with type 2 diabetes: results of

the assessment of diabetes control and evaluation of the efficacy of niaspan trial. *Arch Intern Med* 2002;162:1568.

306. Aiello LP et al. Diabetic retinopathy. *Diabetes Care* 1998;21:143.
307. Fong DS et al. Diabetic retinopathy. *Diabetes Care* 2004;27(Suppl 1):S84.
308. Vinik A et al. Diabetic autonomic neuropathy. *Diabetes Care* 2003;26:1553.
309. Vinik A et al. Gastrointestinal, genitourinary, and neurovascular disturbances in diabetes. *Diabetes Review* 1999:358.
310. Patterson D et al. A double-blind multicenter comparison of domperidone and metoclopramide in the treatment of diabetic patients with symptoms of gastroparesis. *Am J Gastroenterol* 1999;94:1230.
311. Boulton AJ et al. Diabetic neuropathies: a statement by the American Diabetes Association. *Diabetes Care* 2005;28:956.
312. Malik R. Pathology and pathogenesis of diabetic neuropathy. *Diabetes Review* 1999:253.
313. Backonja M, Glanzman RL. Gabapentin dosing for neuropathic pain: evidence from randomized, placebo-controlled clinical trials. *Clin Ther* 2003;25:81.
314. Backonja M et al. Gabapentin for the symptomatic treatment of painful neuropathy in patients with diabetes mellitus: a randomized controlled trial. *JAMA* 1998;280:1831.
315. Freeman R et al. Efficacy, safety and tolerability of pregabalin treatment of painful diabetic peripheral neuropathy: findings from 7 randomized, controlled trials across a range of doses. *Diabetes Care* 2008; Mar 20 [Epub ahead of print].
316. Eisenberg E et al. Lamotrigine reduces painful diabetic neuropathy: a randomized, controlled study. *Neurology* 2001;57:505.
317. Kline KM et al. Painful diabetic peripheral neuropathy relieved with use of oral topiramate. *South Med J* 2003;96:602.
318. Harati Y et al. Double-blind randomized trial of tramadol for the treatment of the pain of diabetic neuropathy. *Neurology* 1998;50:1842.
319. Harati Y et al. Maintenance of the long-term effectiveness of tramadol in treatment of the pain of diabetic neuropathy. *J Diabetes Complications* 2000;14:65.
320. Kajdasz DK et al. Duloxetine for the management of diabetic peripheral neuropathic pain: evidence-based findings from post-hoc analysis of three multicenter, randomized, double-blind, placebo-controlled, parallel-group studies. *Clin Ther* 2007;29(Suppl 1):2536.
321. Smith T, Nicholson RA. Review of duloxetine in the management of diabetic peripheral neuropathic pain. *Vasc Health Risk Manag* 2007;3:833.
322. Mendell JR, Sahenk Z. Clinical practice. Painful sensory neuropathy. *N Engl J Med* 2003;348: 1243.
323. Luscher TF et al. Diabetes and vascular disease: pathophysiology, clinical consequences, and medical therapy: part II. *Circulation* 2003;108:1655.
324. Mayfield JA et al. Preventive foot care in diabetes. *Diabetes Care* 2004;27(Suppl 1):S63.
325. Shilling F. Foot care in patients with diabetes. *Nurs Stand* 2003;17:61, 66, 68.
326. Bressler P, DeFronzo RA. Drugs and diabetes. *Diabetes Review* 1994:53.
327. Gomez EC, Frost P. Induction of glycosuria and hyperglycemia by topical corticosteroid therapy. *Arch Dermatol* 1976;112:1559.
328. McMahon M et al. Effects of glucocorticoids on carbohydrate metabolism. *Diabetes Metab Rev* 1988;4:17.
329. Davies D, ed. *Textbook of Adverse Drug Reactions*. 3rd ed. Oxford: Oxford University Press; 1985.
330. Baker L et al. Hyperglycemia and acetonuria simulating diabetes. Phenylephrine associated hyperglycemia and acetonuria simulating diabetes mellitus. *Am J Dis Child* 1966;111:59.
331. Porte D Jr. Sympathetic regulation of insulin secretion. Its relation to diabetes mellitus. *Arch Intern Med* 1969;123:252.
332. McDonald J. Alcohol and diabetes. *Diabetes Care* 1980;3:629.
333. Franz MJ. Diabetes mellitus: considerations in the development of guidelines for the occasional use of alcohol. *J Am Diet Assoc* 1983;83:147.
334. Mitrakou A et al. Long-term effectiveness of a new alpha-glucosidase inhibitor (BAY m1099-miglitol) in insulin-treated type 2 diabetes mellitus. *Diabet Med* 1998;15:657.
335. Wildasin EM et al. Metformin, a promising oral antihyperglycemic for the treatment of noninsulin-dependent diabetes mellitus. *Pharmacotherapy* 1997;17:62.
336. Bell PM, Hadden DR. Metformin. *Endocrinol Metab Clin North Am* 1997;26:523.
337. Bailey CJ, Turner RC. Metformin. *N Engl J Med* 1996;334:574.
338. Novartis Pharmaceuticals Corporation. Starlix Package Insert. November 2002.
339. Van Haeften TW. Clinical significance of insulin antibodies in insulin-treated diabetic patients. *Diabetes Care* 1989;12:641.
340. Novo Nordisk Pharmaceuticals, Inc. Prandin Package Insert. October 2002.
341. Eli Lilly & Company. Originally in Galloway JA et al., eds. *Diabetes Mellitus*. 9th ed. Indianapolis, In: Eli Lilly & Company; 1988.
342. Farkas-Hirsch R. Intensive Diabetes Management. Alexandria, VA: American Diabetes Association; 1995:57.
343. How to inject your insulin. Patient education pamphlet #000-180pl. Novo Nordisk Pharmaceuticals; 1995.
344. Gabbe SC et al. New strategies for glucose control in patients with type 1 and type 2 diabetes mellitus in pregnancy. *Clin Obstet Gynecol* 2007;50: 1014.

SECTION THIRTEEN

EYE DISORDERS

Lloyd Young
SECTION EDITOR

CHAPTER 51

Eye Disorders

Steven R. Abel and Suellyn J. Sorensen

The eye is a highly complex organ composed of various parts, all of which must function in integration to permit vision. A brief overview of the anatomy and physiology of the eye prefaces the presentation of specific eye disorders. Readers should consult an ophthalmology textbook for an understanding of ocular anatomy, physiology, and general ophthalmology (e.g., Vaughn and Asbury's General Ophthalmology).[1]

OCULAR ANATOMY AND PHYSIOLOGY

The eyeball is approximately 1 inch wide and is housed in a cavity (i.e., eye socket) formed by two bony orbits that are lined with fat, which serves to protect the eyeball. Six ocular muscles facilitate movement of the eyeball (Fig. 51-1).

The outer coat of the eye is made up of the sclera, conjunctiva, and cornea. The *sclera* is the white, dense, fibrous protective coating. The episclera, a thin layer of loose connective tissue, contains blood vessels that cover and nourish the sclera. The *conjunctiva* is a mucous membrane that covers the anterior portion of the eye and lines the eyelids. The *cornea* is the transparent, avascular tissue that functions as a refractive and protective window membrane through which light rays pass en route to the retina. The corneal epithelium and endothelium are lipophilic, and the centrally located stroma is hydrophilic.

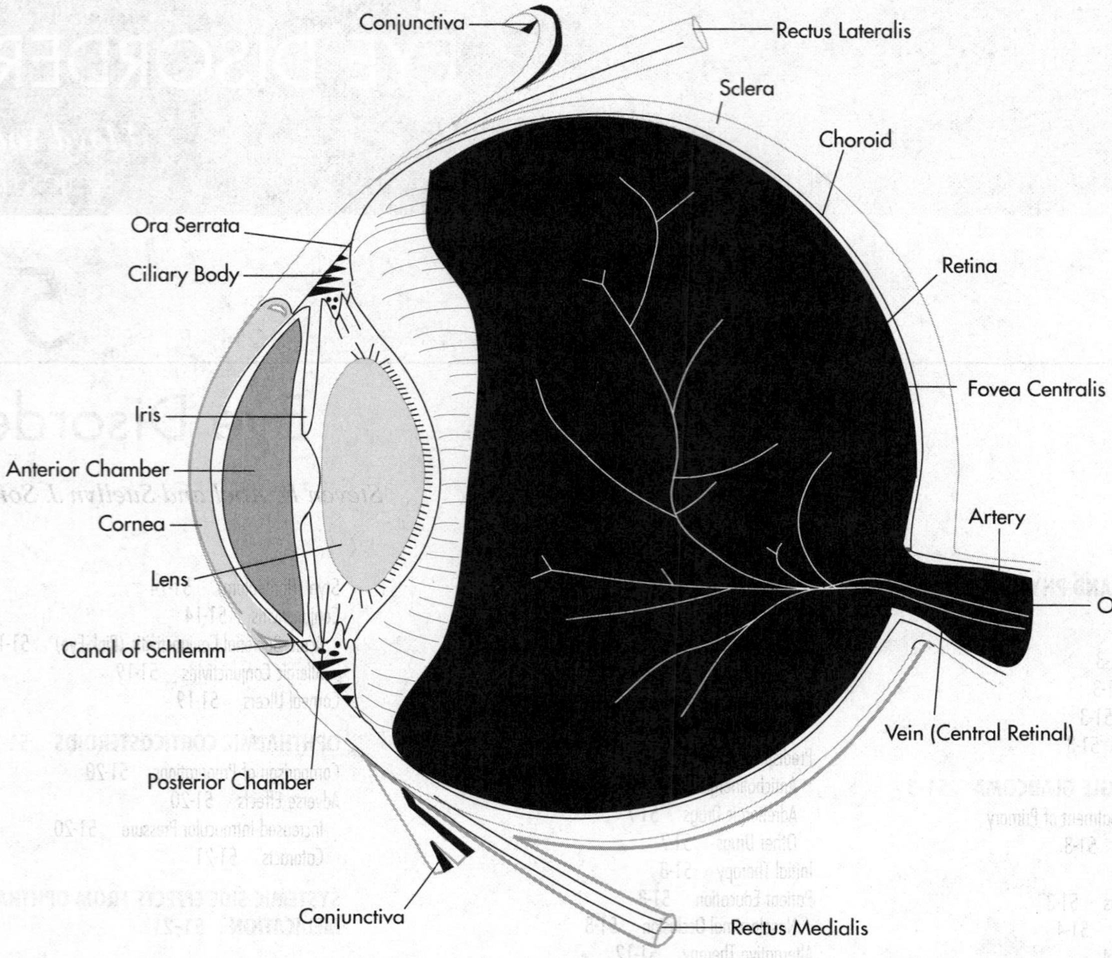

FIGURE 51-1 Anatomy of the human eye. (Adapted from artwork courtesy of Burroughs Wellcome.)

These three corneal layers are particularly important because they affect drug penetration through the cornea. Ophthalmic medications, which are both fat- and water-soluble, are best able to penetrate through the intact cornea.

The iris, choroid, and ciliary body are known collectively as the uveal tract. The *iris* is a colored, circular membrane suspended between the cornea and the crystalline lens. It controls the amount of light that enters the eye. The *choroid*, located between the sclera and retina, is largely made up of blood vessels, which nourish the retina. The *ciliary body* is adherent to the sclera and contains the ciliary muscle and ciliary processes. The ciliary muscle contracts and relaxes the zonular fibers, which hold the crystalline lens in place. The ciliary processes are responsible for the secretion of aqueous humor, a clear liquid that occupies the anterior chamber. The anterior chamber is bounded anteriorly by the cornea and posteriorly by the iris. The posterior chamber lies between the iris and the crystalline lens.

The inner segment of the eye contains the retina with the optic nerve. The *retina*, the light-sensitive tissue at the back of the eye, contains all of the sensory receptors for light transmission. The *optic nerve*, a bundle of more than a million nerve fibers, transmits visual impulses from the retina to the brain.

The crystalline lens, aqueous humor, and vitreous humor assist the cornea with the refraction of light. The *lens*, located behind the iris, functions to focus light onto the retina by changing its shape to accommodate near or distant vision. The innermost part of the lens (i.e., the nucleus) is surrounded by the softer material of the cortex. The *aqueous humor*, the thin watery fluid that fills the anterior chamber (i.e., the space between the cornea and the iris) and posterior chamber of the eye, functions to provide nourishment to the cornea and lens. Disorders involving the aqueous humor are presented in the section on glaucoma. The primary function of the *vitreous humor* (i.e., the jelly-like substance between the lens and the retina) is to maintain the shape of the eye and allow the transmission of light to the retina.

The eyelids and eyelashes are the outermost means of protection for the eye. The eyelids contain various sebaceous and sweat glands, which may become infected or inflamed, contributing to many ocular disorders.

The eye is innervated by both the sympathetic and parasympathetic nervous systems. Parasympathetic fibers, originating from the oculomotor nerve in the brain, innervate the ciliary muscle and sphincter pupillae muscle that constrict the pupil. As a result, parasympathomimetic (cholinergic) medications generally are associated with *miosis* (pupillary contraction), and parasympatholytic (anticholinergic) agents with *mydriasis* (pupillary dilation) and cycloplegia. The term, *cycloplegia*, refers to a paralysis of the ciliary muscle and zonules (fibrous strands connecting the ciliary body to the lens) that results in decreased accommodation (adjustment of the lens curvature for various distances) and blurred vision. Tear secretion by the lacrimal glands also is a parasympathetic function.

Sympathetic fibers from the superior cervical ganglion in the spinal cord innervate the dilator pupillae muscle, the blood vessels of the ciliary body, the episclera, and the extraocular muscles. Sympathomimetics cause mydriasis without affecting accommodation.

GLAUCOMA

Glaucoma, a leading cause of blindness worldwide, is a nonspecific term used for a group of diseases that can irreversibly damage the optic nerve resulting in visual field loss. Increased intraocular pressure (IOP) is the most common risk factor for the development of glaucoma; however, even people with "normal" IOPs can experience vision loss from glaucoma. Generally, the higher the IOP, the greater the risk for developing glaucoma. Increasing age, African American race, family history, thinner central corneas, and larger vertical cup–disk ratios are other risk factors for glaucoma.[1,2]

Intraocular Pressure

The inner pressure of the eye (i.e., IOP) is influenced by the production of aqueous humor by the ciliary processes and the outflow of aqueous humor through the trabecular meshwork. The tonometry test to measure the IOP is based upon the pressure required to flatten a small area of the central cornea. Generally, an IOP of 10 to 20 mmHg is considered normal. An IOP of 22 mmHg or higher should arouse suspicion of glaucoma, although a more rare form of glaucoma is associated with a low IOP.

Ocular Hypertension

Ocular hypertension has been defined as an IOP >21 mmHg, normal visual fields, normal optic discs, open angles, and the absence of any ocular disease contributing to the elevation of IOP. Only a small percentage of patients with ocular hypertension develop open-angle glaucoma. An ophthalmoscope can examine the inside of the eye, especially the optic nerve, and a diagnosis of glaucoma can be applied when pathologic cupping of the optic nerve is observed.

Open-Angle Glaucoma

Primary open-angle glaucoma occurs in about 1.8% of people older than 40 years of age in the United States; however, glaucoma can affect other age groups, including children.[1–3] About 2.2 million people in the United States have glaucoma and this number likely will increase to about 3.3 million by the year 2020 as the population ages.[3] In patients with primary open-angle glaucoma (POAG), aqueous humor outflow from the anterior chamber is continuously subnormal primarily because of a degenerative process in the trabecular meshwork. The IOP can vary in the course of a day from normal to significantly high pressures.[1] The decreased outflow appears to be caused by degenerative changes in outflow channels (i.e., the trabecular meshwork and Schlemm's canal) and tends to worsen with the passage of time.[1] In rare cases, the outflow is normal even during a phase of elevated IOP, and the elevation appears to be to the result of hypersecretion of aqueous humor.[1]

The onset of POAG usually is gradual and asymptomatic. A defect in the visual field examination may be present in early glaucoma, but loss of peripheral vision usually is not seen until late in the course of the disease. Visual field defects correlate well with changes in the optic disc and help differentiate glaucoma from ocular hypertension in patients with increased IOP. Patients with normal visual fields and an IOP of 24 mmHg or greater have a 10% likelihood of developing glaucoma in 5 years.[3]

Angle-Closure Glaucoma

Examination of the anterior chamber angle by gonioscopy, using a corneal contact lens, a magnifying device (e.g., a slit-lamp microscope), and a light source, assists in differentiating between open-angle glaucoma and angle-closure glaucoma. Angle-closure glaucoma accounts for approximately 5% to 10% of all primary glaucoma cases. The sole cause of the elevated IOP in angle-closure glaucoma is closure of the anterior chamber angle.[1,4]

Angle-closure glaucoma, which is a medical emergency, usually presents as an acute attack with a rapid increase in IOP, blurring or sudden loss of vision, appearance of haloes around lights, and pain that is often severe. When patients are predisposed to angle-closure glaucoma, their pupils should not be dilated (e.g., during an ophthalmic examination) and they should be taught the signs and symptoms of angle closure. Acute attacks can terminate without treatment, but if the IOP remains high, the optic nerve can be irreparably damaged.[1] Patients with chronic angle closure generally experience a gradual closure of aqueous humor outflow channels, and patients can be asymptomatic until the glaucoma is in an advanced stage.[1] Permanent medical management of acute or chronic angle closure glaucoma is difficult: surgical procedures (e.g., peripheral iridectomies) often are needed.

PRIMARY OPEN-ANGLE GLAUCOMA

Therapeutic Agents for Treatment of Primary Open-Angle Glaucoma

Initial Therapy

β-ADRENERGIC BLOCKERS

All of the ocular β-adrenergic blockers (e.g., timolol, levobunolol, metipranolol, carteolol, betaxolol, levobetaxolol) have the same basic mechanism of action. Ophthalmic β-blockers block the β-adrenergic receptors in the ciliary epithelium of the eye and lower IOP primarily by decreasing aqueous humor production. β-adrenergic blockers have been the most commonly prescribed first-line agents for the treatment of POAG.

Timolol (Timoptic)

Timolol, a nonselective β_1- and β_2-adrenergic antagonist, is one of the most commonly prescribed glaucoma medications. Because timolol was the first ocular β-adrenergic blocker marketed, subsequently marketed ophthalmic β-blockers usually are compared with timolol for safety and effectiveness. Concentrations or dosages exceeding one drop of timolol 0.5% BID do not produce further significant decreases in IOP.[5] Therapy usually is initiated with a 0.25% solution administered as one drop BID. Monocular administration of timolol has resulted in equal bilateral IOP reduction and can reduce the cost of therapy and side effects for some patients.[6] An escape phenomenon, or tachyphylaxis, can occur with timolol.

If a patient has a large initial decrease in IOP, the IOP often stabilizes at a lesser reduction in about 4 to 6 weeks.[7,8] Timolol, safe and effective in adult and pediatric patients, is at least as effective as pilocarpine and epinephrine and can be more efficacious in daily IOP control.[9–12]

Timolol has been associated with a modest reduction of resting pulse rate (5–8 beats/minute)[13,14], worsening of congestive heart failure, and adverse pulmonary effects (e.g., dyspnea, airway obstruction, pulmonary failure).[15,16] After chronic administration in susceptible individuals, timolol can cause corneal anesthesia.[17,18] Although uveitis has been reported in patients receiving ophthalmic timolol, a cause-and-effect relationship has not been established.[19,20]

In one study, plasma levels after ophthalmic administration of timolol were not detected in all but one human subject, who had a level of 9.6 ng/mL.[21,22] In another study, the baseline mean plasma timolol level was 0.34 ng/mL in 10 patients, who were more than 60 years of age and receiving chronic timolol. In these patients, the plasma timolol concentration increased to 1.34 ng/mL 1 hour after administration of one drop of 0.5% timolol, and the mean 1-hour plasma timolol level decreased to 0.9 ng/mL with punctal occlusion.[23] The β-blocking plasma concentration of timolol has been estimated to be about 5 to 10 ng/mL.[8]

Although systemic absorption after topical administration does not appear to be significant in most cases, care should be taken when timolol is used in patients with sinus bradycardia, CHF (Chapter 18: Heart Failure), or pulmonary disease. Systemic side effects could be exaggerated in elderly patients secondary to inadvertent overdosing associated with poor administration technique (see Question 3).

A breast milk sample from a nursing mother, obtained 1.5 hours after administration of one drop of 0.5% topical timolol, resulted in a timolol concentration in the breast milk of 5.6 ng/mL and a concomitant plasma concentration of 0.93 ng/mL.[24] Timolol should be used cautiously in nursing mothers.

Timoptic XE

Timoptic XE, a timolol ophthalmic gel-forming solution, is administered once daily. The ophthalmic vehicle, gellan gum (Gelrite), is a solution that forms a clear gel in the presence of mono or divalent cations.[25] This ion-activated gelation prolongs precorneal residence time and increases ocular bioavailability, allowing timolol to be administered once daily.[25] In a 24-week study, Timoptic XE 0.5% once daily and Timoptic solution 0.5% BID were equally effective in lowering IOP.[26]

Levobunolol (Betagan)

Levobunolol, another nonselective β-adrenergic antagonist, can decrease IOP on average about 9 mmHg with either the 0.5% or 1% solutions and is approved for both once daily or BID administration.[27,28] When levobunolol 0.5% once daily was compared with BID administration, both regimens reduced IOP similarly.[29] When levobunolol 0.5% and 1% BID were compared with timolol 0.5% BID, ocular hypotensive effects, incidence of adverse reactions, and slight to significant decreases in heart rate were noted for both agents.[30,31] In one 3-month study, levobunolol once daily was more effective than timolol at various concentrations;[32] however, in another study, both timolol 0.25% and levobunolol 0.25% once daily were equally effective.[33] Levobunolol can be more expensive than timolol (depending on negotiated contract purchase prices) whether it is administered once or BID.[34]

Metipranolol (Optipranolol)

Another nonselective β-adrenergic blocking agent, metipranolol 0.1% to 0.6%, is comparable to timolol 0.25% to 0.5% in reducing IOP in patients with open-angle glaucoma.[35,36] Single-dose metipranolol 0.1% and 0.3% and timolol 0.25% did not significantly change resting heart rate or the resting or exercise mean blood pressure,[37] but timolol significantly reduced exercise tachycardia. Metipranolol 0.6% and levobunolol 0.5% BID reduced IOP by about 7 mmHg (29%), and neither significantly reduced heart rate or blood pressure[38] Metipranolol is associated with a greater incidence of stinging or burning upon administration than other ophthalmic β-adrenergic blockers. Topical metipranolol appears to offer no advantage over timolol or levobunolol in the treatment of glaucoma.

Like timolol, metipranolol produces corneal anesthesia, which occurs within 1 minute of instillation and returns to baseline after 10 minutes.[18] Metipranolol has been withdrawn from clinical use in the United Kingdom because it has been associated with granulomatous anterior uveitis. Although this adverse effect was initially attributed to its irradiated plastic containers,[39] metipranolol subsequently was deemed to be the responsible agent for these inflammatory reactions.[40] A significant secondary elevation (57.6%) in IOP occurred in patients with metipranolol-associated adverse reactions.[41] Although metipranolol may be cost-effective, its higher association with ocular burning and stinging and granulomatous anterior uveitis limit its use.

Carteolol (Ocupress)

Carteolol, a nonselective β-adrenergic blocking agent with partial β-adrenergic agonist activity, theoretically, should minimize the bronchospastic, bradycardic, and hypotensive effects associated with other ocular β-adrenergic blockers.[37] However, no clinical difference was noted when the cardiovascular and pulmonary function effects of carteolol were compared with timolol. Carteolol 1% and timolol 0.25% administered BID are equally effective in reducing IOP.[43–45]

Betaxolol (Betoptic) and Levobetaxolol (Betaxon)

In contrast to other β-adrenergic blocking ophthalmic agents, betaxolol and levobetaxolol are selective β_1-adrenergic blockers. Although levobetaxolol, the S-isomer of betaxolol, is more active than the racemic mixture of betaxolol, its pharmacological and toxicological effects are similar. Betaxolol 0.125% to 0.5% can reduce IOP up to 35%.[46] In comparative studies, betaxolol 0.5% and timolol 0.5% BID decreased IOP with similar side-effect profiles including slight, but insignificant, decreases in systolic and diastolic blood pressure (BP).[46–48] In these studies, timolol was slightly, but not significantly, more effective in decreasing IOP, with fewer patients requiring adjunctive therapy for adequate IOP control. In another study, timolol 0.25% and 0.5% consistently and significantly decreased median IOP more than comparable doses of betaxolol and more of the betaxolol-treated patients required adjunctive therapy.[49] These two cardioselective β-blockers, betaxolol and levobetaxolol, would be expected to have less adverse effect on pulmonary function than nonselective β-adrenergic blockers in some patients with reactive airway disorders; however, the practical significance of this pharmacological expectation needs validation.

PROSTAGLANDIN ANALOGS

Latanoprost (Xalatan), travoprost (Travatan), and bimatoprost (Lumigan), are all prostaglandin analogs. Latanoprost and travoprost are analogs of prostaglandin F_{α}, and they lower intraocular pressure by serving as selective prostaglandin $F_{2\alpha}$-receptor agonists. Bimatoprost is a synthetic prostamide analog. The prostaglandin analogs (PGAs) increase uveoscleral outflow of aqueous humor and, thereby, decrease IOP.[50] These agents often are prescribed as first-line agents for the treatment of POAG, because they are at least as effective as the β-blockers, can be administered once a day, and are associated with minimal adverse effects. Unlike the β-blockers, generic versions of these drugs are not yet available and cost can be a consideration in elderly patients who are on a fixed income.

Latanoprost

Latanoprost (Xalatan) is approved for the initial treatment of POAG or ocular hypertension.[51] When administered once daily in the evening, latanoprost is at least as effective as timolol in decreasing IOP. When the effectiveness of latanoprost 0.005% once daily was compared with timolol 0.5% BID, the IOP-lowering effects of latanoprost were superior to timolol.[52,53] In addition, the nocturnal control of IOP with latanoprost was superior to that with timolol. Latanoprost 0.005% should be dosed once daily in the evening because the IOP-lowering effects of latanoprost might actually be inferior when administered more frequently.

Systemic side effects are minimal with latanoprost, but local reactions (e.g., iris pigmentation; eyelid skin darkening; eyelash lengthening, thickening, pigmentation, and misdirected growth; conjunctival hyperemia; ocular irritation; superficial punctate keratitis) are relatively common. Latanoprost can gradually increase the amount of brown pigment in the iris by increasing the melanin content in the stromal melanocytes of the iris. This pigment change occurs in 7% to 22% of patients and is most noticeable in those with green-brown, blue/gray-brown, or yellow-brown eyes.[51,52] The onset of increased iris pigmentation usually is noticeable within the first year of treatment and can be permanent. The nature or severity of adverse events are not affected by the increased pigmentation of the iris.

Latanoprost has additive effects when administered with β-blockers (e.g., timolol), carbonic-anhydrous inhibitors (e.g., dorzolamide), α_2-adrenergic agonists (e.g., brimonidine, apraclonidine), and dipivefrin. When added to existing therapy, latanoprost decreases IOP an additional 2.9 to 6.1 mmHg. As a result, latanoprost is a good adjunctive ophthalmic for patients who are unable to adequately lower their IOP with single-agent therapy. Although the complementary IOP-lowering effects of latanoprost are comparable to those of brimonidine (at least a 15% reduction in IOP) in patients inadequately controlled on β-adrenergic blocking agents, brimonidine (an α_2-adrenergic agonist) has been associated with fewer adverse effects on the quality of life. For example, watery or teary eyes and cold hands and feet were reported more frequently in latanoprost-treated patients.[54] The effectiveness of latanoprost when used once a day alone or as an adjunct to other IOP-lowering drugs, and its relative tolerability make it an important treatment option for POAG and ocular hypertension.[53,55–57]

Travoprost

Travoprost (Travatan) is FDA approved for the reduction of elevated IOP and ocular hypertension in patients who are intolerant, or who fail to respond to other agents. Travoprost is used as a first-line agent in clinical practice because it is more effective than timolol and at least as effective as latanoprost. The mean IOP reduction with travoprost in African American patients was 1.8 mmHg greater than in non–African American patients. Travoprost, as adjunctive therapy to timolol in patients not responding adequately to timolol alone, reduced IOP an additional 6 to 7 mmHg. The side-effect profile of travoprost is similar to latanoprost including increased iris pigmentation and eyelash changes.[58–60] Local irritation from travoprost may be less with the new formulation (i.e., Travatan Z) which replaced the preservative, benzalkonium chloride.

Bimatoprost

Like travoprost, bimatoprost (Lumigan) once daily or BID achieved lower target IOPs than did timolol BID. Bimatoprost BID, however, was less effective than bimatoprost once-a-day. Iris pigmentation changed in 1.1% of bimatoprost-treated patients. In a 6-month randomized multicenter study, bimatoprost once a day lowered IOP more effectively than latanoprost once a day. Side effects were similar between treatment groups; however, conjunctiva hyperemia was more common ($p < 0.001$) in bimatoprost treated patients. Overall, the side effect profile of bimatoprost appears to be similar to latanoprost and travoprost.[61–63]

α_2-ADRENERGIC AGONISTS

Apraclonidine (Iopidine) and brimonidine (Alphagan) are selective α_2-adrenergic agonists similar to clonidine. Apraclonidine is less lipophilic than clonidine and brimonidine; does not cross the blood-brain barrier as readily; and, theoretically, has less systemic side effects (e.g., hypotension, decreased pulse, dry mouth). Brimonidine is more highly selective for α_2-adrenergic receptors than clonidine or apraclonidine and, theoretically, should be associated with less ocular side effects. α_2-adrenergic agonists appear to lower IOP by decreasing the production of aqueous humor and by increasing uveoscleral outflow.[64]

Brimonidine is an alternative first-line agent in the treatment of POAG. It may also be used as adjunctive therapy in patients not responding to other agents. Apraclonidine 1% is indicated to control or prevent postsurgical elevations in IOP after argon laser trabeculoplasty or iridotomy. The 0.5% apraclonidine solution is indicated for short-term adjunctive therapy in patients on maximally tolerated medical therapy. Long-term IOP control should be monitored closely in patients on α_2-adrenergic agonists because tachyphylaxis can occur. Common ocular side effects include burning, stinging, blurring, conjunctival follicles, and an allergic-like reaction consisting of hyperemia, pruritus, edema of the lid and conjunctiva, and foreign body sensation. Although, ocular side effects are less common with brimonidine than with apraclonidine, systemic side effects (e.g., dry nose and mouth, mild hypotension, decreased pulse, and lethargy) are more common with brimonidine. α_2-adrenergic agonists should be used with caution in patients with cardiovascular disease, orthostatic hypotension, depression, and renal or hepatic dysfunction.[64,65] Brimondine (Alphagan P) is now available with purite as a preservative which facilitates drug delivery into the eye allowing use of a lower drug concentration.[65]

The IOP-reduction effects (peak and trough) of brimonidine 0.2% BID is 14% to 28%. Although the approved dosing schedule of brimonidine is TID, brimonidine 0.2% BID lowers IOP comparably to timolol 0.5% BID, and both are slightly better than betaxolol 0.25% BID.[65–67] The IOP-lowering effect of brimonidine also may be comparable to that of latanoprost; however, conflicting efficacy and tolerability results in clinical studies may be related to differences in study design.[68] The combination of brimonidine and timolol is equally tolerable and effective as the combination of dorzolamide and timolol.[69] The FDA-approved Combigan ophthalmic solution combines a β-adrenergic agonist (brimonidine tartrate 0.2%) with a β-adrenergic blocker (timolol maleate 0.5%).

TOPICAL CARBONIC ANHYDRASE INHIBITORS

Carbonic anhydrase occurs in high concentrations in the ciliary processes and retina of the eye. Carbonic anhydrase inhibitors (CAIs) lower IOP is by decreasing bicarbonate production and, therefore, the flow of bicarbonate, sodium, and water into the posterior chamber of the eye resulting in a 40% to 60% decrease in aqueous humor secretion.

Although CAIs have been used orally for many years in the treatment of elevated IOPs, they have been replaced by the topical ophthalmic CAIs, dorzolamide (Trusopt) and brinzolamide (Azopt), which are safer and better tolerated. Topical CAIs are excellent alternatives to β-blockers in the initial management of elevated IOPs, and are effective as adjunctive agents. Brinzolamide 1% TID reduces IOP comparably to that achieved with dorzolamide 2% TID and to betaxolol 0.5% BID, but slightly less than timolol 0.5% BID. The IOP-reduction effects (peak and trough) of dorzolamide 2% TID is 16% to 25%. Brinzolamide and dorzolamide are approved for TID dosing; however, BID dosing may be adequate. Dorzolamide provides additional IOP-lowering effects when added to existing β-blocker therapy.[70,71] An ophthalmic solution of dorzolamide hydrochloride and timolol maleate is marketed as Cosopt. The combined use of topical dorzolamide and oral acetazolamide does not result in additive effects and might increase the risk of toxicity. Therefore, the concomitant use of topical and oral CAIs is not advised.[72–74]

The topical CAIs are well tolerated with few systemic side effects. The most common adverse effects reported with dorzolamide are ocular burning, stinging, discomfort and allergic reactions, bitter taste, and superficial punctate keratitis. Brinzolamide causes less burning and stinging of the eyes than dorzolamide, because its pH more closely resembles that of human tears. Dorzolamide and brinzolamide are sulfonamides and may cause the same types of adverse reactions attributable to sulfonamides. These drugs should not be used in patients with renal or hepatic impairment.

PILOCARPINE

Pilocarpine (IsoptoCarpine) historically was an initial treatment of choice, but with the introduction and widespread use of newer agents, pilocarpine has fallen out of favor as an initial treatment. Therapy usually is begun using lower concentrations (0.5%–1%), such as one drop QID. Pilocarpine is a direct-acting cholinergic (parasympathomimetic) that causes contraction of ciliary muscle fibers attached to the trabecular meshwork and scleral spur. This opens the trabecular meshwork to enhance aqueous humor outflow. There also may be a direct effect on the trabecular meshwork. Pilocarpine causes miosis by contraction of the iris sphincter muscle, but the miosis is not related to the decrease in IOP.

EPINEPHRINE

Epinephrine (Glaucon, Eppy/N, Epitrate) is a sympathomimetic that stimulates both

α-and β-receptors. The β-adrenergic stimulation is responsible for increasing aqueous humor outflow and is the probable basis of epinephrine's ability to lower IOP.[75,76] In contrast, the β-adrenergic blockers decrease aqueous humor production. The α-adrenergic effect of epinephrine predominantly decreases the inflow of aqueous humor, which is not as significant as the increase in aqueous humor outflow.[75,76] Patients in whom systemic effects of this drug could potentiate preexisting problems should be monitored closely. Dipivefrin is an epinephrine prodrug that is better tolerated and absorbed than epinephrine. It is usually the preferred product when agents from this class are indicated. Dipivefrin or epinephrine is often used in younger patients or patients with cataracts in which miosis and the resultant decreased vision from cholinergic agents are a problem. Both are second or third-line drugs in the therapy of POAG and are used most often as second agents in combination regimens rather than as monotherapy.

CARBACHOL

Carbachol (Isopto-Carbachol) is reserved as a third-line agent in patients who are unresponsive or intolerant to initial medications. In addition to having direct cholinergic effects, carbachol is more resistant to cholinesterase than pilocarpine. Added benefits include increased release of acetylcholine from parasympathetic nerve terminals and a weak anticholinesterase effect. Carbachol is administered TID.

ANTICHOLINESTERASE AGENTS

If control of IOP is not achieved with optimal use of other topical monotherapy and combination therapy agents, then anticholinesterase agents may be prescribed as a last topical therapy option. Anticholinesterase agents inhibit the enzyme cholinesterase, thereby increasing the amount of acetylcholine and its naturally occurring cholinergic effects.

ECHOTHIOPHATE IODIDE

Echothiophate iodide (Phospholine Iodide), an irreversible cholinesterase inhibitor, primarily inactivates pseudocholinesterase and secondarily inhibits true cholinesterase. Echothiophate iodide is the most widely used cholinesterase inhibitor for open-angle glaucoma and can be used if maximal doses of other agents and combination therapy are ineffective. Echothiophate iodide has a long duration of action that affords good control of IOP; however, miosis and myopia are significant side effects. Concentrations higher than 0.06% are associated with a significant increase in subjective complaints (e.g., brow ache).[77]

Combination Therapy

In general, drugs with different pharmacologic actions have at least partially additive effects in lowering IOP in the treatment of glaucoma. Drugs with similar pharmacologic actions (i.e., from the same pharmacologic class) should not be combined because dose-related adverse effects are more likely and the incremental increase in benefits is likely to be more modest.

Timolol and other β-adrenergic blocking drugs have additive IOP-lowering effects when used in combination with epinephrine,[78] dipivefrin,[78,79] miotics, prostaglandin analogs,[54,80] α_2-agonists,[81] and CAIs.[82–84] For example, the IOP-lowering effect is greater when timolol is used in combination with pilocarpine,[53,85] dorzolamide,[85] brimonidine, [54,81,86] and travoprost.[53,56] Likewise, for example, latanoprost has additive effects when administered with timolol,[53,58] dorzolamide,[55,56] α_2-adrenergic agonists,[54,55,86] and dipivefrin.[53,55–57] Other combinations of drugs also provide additive effects when used in combination for the management of increased intraocular pressure.

The trend toward the development of fixed-combination products offers many advantages in the treatment of POAG. These advantages include: improved adherence due to a reduction in the number of dosages and bottles, eliminating the need to instill two separate drugs 5 to 10 minutes apart to prevent a washout effect from the second medication; improving safety and tolerability by limiting the exposure to the benzalkonium chloride preservative; and a cost savings for the patient by potentially eliminating a co-pay for one of the medications. Currently, timolol/dorzolamide (Cosopt) is the only topical β-blocker combination product. The IOP lowering effects of Cosopt are comparable to or greater than latanoprost monotherapy.[87] Several other combination products are under investigation for POAG that will offer a wide range of options for patients. These investigational agents include timolol/latanoprost (Xalacom), timolol/travoprost (DuoTrav, Extravan), and timolol/bimatoprost.[88,89]

Predisposing Factors

1. M.H., a 52-year-old African American woman with brown eyes, presented for routine ophthalmic examination. Visual acuity without correction was 20/40 right eye and 20/80 left eye. Tonometry measured an IOP of 36 mmHg in both eyes. Ophthalmoscopy revealed physiologic cupping of the optic discs in both eyes, and visual field examination revealed a nerve fiber bundle defect consistent with glaucoma. Pupils were normal both eyes, and gonioscopy indicated that anterior chamber angles were open in both eyes. There were no signs of cataract formation. M.H. related a positive family history for glaucoma and presently is being treated for hypertension, CHF, and asthma. Her medications include the following:

Amitriptyline	75 mg at bedtime
Chlorpheniramine	4 mg Q 6 hr PRN
Digoxin	0.25 mg daily
Furosemide	40 mg BID
Nitroglycerin	1/150 g SL PRN
Theophylline SR	300 mg Q 12 hr

Findings on examination indicate that M.H. has POAG. What other factors may predispose M.H. to an increased IOP?

POAG is thought to be determined genetically, and M.H. has a positive family history. The disease is more prevalent and aggressive in African Americans.[1] In addition, she is taking several medications that have been associated with increases in IOP.

Anticholinergic Drugs

Most reports dealing with drug-induced increases in IOP center around precipitation of angle-closure glaucoma by topical mydriatic/cycloplegic agents (anticholinergics). In patients with open-angle glaucoma, topical anticholinergics can significantly increase resistance to aqueous humor outflow and elevate IOP while the anterior chamber remains grossly open.[2] As part of any routine ophthalmic examination, the pupils are dilated with a mydriatic/cycloplegic (unless otherwise contraindicated). The IOP is always measured before this procedure, so the use of these agents would not have influenced the IOP readings in M.H.

If systemic anticholinergic agents are administered in doses sufficient to cause pupillary dilation, the risk of precipitating angle-closure increases. However, it is unlikely that these agents will aggravate open-angle glaucoma unless the amount reaching the eye is sufficient to cause cycloplegia.[2] Although literature documentation of POAG exacerbation by these agents is scarce, medications with anticholinergic side effects (antihistamines, benzodiazepines, disopyramide, phenothiazines, tricyclic antidepressants) should be considered. M.H. is receiving chlorpheniramine as needed (PRN) and amitriptyline at bedtime, but her pupil examination is normal with no evidence of mydriasis or cycloplegia. Therefore, it is highly unlikely that these medications contributed to her increased IOP.

Adrenergic Drugs

Adrenergic agents, such as central nervous system (CNS) stimulants, vasoconstrictors, appetite suppressants, and bronchodilators, may produce minimal pupillary dilation. These have no proven adverse influences on IOP in patients with either normal eyes or eyes with open-angle glaucoma. Consequently, the use of theophylline in M.H. is also an unlikely source of the increased IOP.

Other Drugs

Conclusive evidence for the production of angle-closure glaucoma by vasodilators is lacking, although slight increases in IOP have been reported. Use of nitroglycerin (NTG) as needed in M.H. is not a cause for concern. There have been isolated reports of other medications causing mydriasis in glaucoma patients. These include muscle relaxants (carisoprodol), monoamine oxidase inhibitors, fenfluramine, ganglionic blocking agents, salicylates, oral contraceptives, and chlorpropamide. Succinylcholine, ketamine, and caffeine have been associated with increases in IOP. α-chymotrypsin has been reported to increase IOP in patients who have received the medication during operative procedures; these patients' outflow channels probably were obstructed by debris generated from use of the enzyme.[68] Corticosteroid-induced IOP elevation is presented in Question 14. If M.H. requires administration of any other medications associated with increases in IOP, the risk of potential adverse effects can be minimized by routine follow-up.

Initial Therapy

2. What is the best initial therapeutic treatment in M.H.?

Topical β-blockers or prostaglandin analogs (PGAs) are the initial agents of choice in the treatment of POAG (Fig. 51-2). Their efficacy is well documented in numerous studies, and side effects are well characterized. Brimonidine (Alphagan) and topical carbonic-anhydrase inhibitors (CAIs) are alternative first-line agents. Table 51-1 lists the common topical agents used in the treatment of primary open angle glaucoma.

Timolol or other nonselective β-adrenergic blockers should not be initiated for M.H. because of her history of asthma (the indications and use of β-blockers for patients with heart failure are described in Chapter 18, Heart Failure). Betaxolol, a β_1-adrenergic blocker, is better tolerated than the nonselective β-adrenergic blocker, timolol, in patients with reactive airway disease and should be considered when topical β-blocker therapy is indicated in patients such as M.H.[46–48] Betaxolol 0.25% suspension BID would be reasonable for the initial treatment of M.H.'s glaucoma. Nevertheless, adverse pulmonary and cardiac side effects can occur with betaxolol: M.H. should be followed-up closely for these adverse effects. Although ocular burning and stinging have been associated more frequently with betaxolol and metipranolol than with other topical β-blockers, the 0.25% suspension is better tolerated than the 0.5% solution and is as effective.[49] Brimonidine, a topical CAI, or a prostaglandin analog (e.g., latanoprost) are acceptable alternatives to betaxolol as initial therapy. Although brimonidine, topical CAIs, and latanoprost may not exacerbate her asthma or CHF, they can cause localized side effects and brimonidine can cause systemic hypotension and lethargy.

Patient Education

3. Betaxolol 0.25% suspension, one to two drops both eyes BID, is ordered for M.H. How should M.H. be instructed regarding the proper use of her betaxolol and expected therapeutic side effects?

M.H. should be instructed to hold the inverted betaxolol bottle between her thumb and middle finger and to rest this hand on her forehead to minimize the risk of inadvertent eye injury caused by sudden unexpected movement of the hand. The index finger is left free to depress the bottom of the container, releasing one drop for the dose. With a little practice, this technique is easy to master. The lower eyelid should be drawn downward with the index finger of the opposite hand or pinched between the thumb and index finger to form a pouch. The patient should look up and administer the drug into the pouch of the eye.

Patients must be encouraged to continue regular use of their medications for effective treatment of glaucoma. Chronic glaucoma is a silent disease and often not associated with symptoms; therefore, the continuation of therapy should be encouraged continuously in patients, especially when side effects to drug therapy can be encountered. Betaxolol is best administered Q 12 hr, because this schedule of administration is consistent with its duration of action (see Table 51-1).

Systemic side effects (e.g., bradycardia, heart block, CHF, pulmonary distress, CNS) are rare with betaxolol, but M.H. should be instructed to report any of these effects to her primary care provider.

Nasolacrimal Occlusion

4. How much would occlusion of the nasolacrimal ducts (punctal occlusion) by M.H. influence systemic absorption or alter the therapeutic effects of betaxolol?

Nasolacrimal, or punctal, occlusion is a technique that can decrease the amount of drug absorbed systemically.[90] Occlusion of the puncta (through the application of slight pressure with the finger to the inner corner of the eye closest to the nose for 3 to 5 minutes during and after drug instillation) can minimize systemic absorption of ophthalmic medications (e.g., betaxolol) and decrease the incidence of side effects and improve medication effectiveness.[90–92] When a single drop of ophthalmic timolol 0.5% was instilled into the eyes of patients at various times before cataract surgery and the nasolacrimal duct occluded for 5 minutes, drug levels in the aqueous humor were significantly greater in patients who had their nasolacrimal ducts occluded than those who did not.[91] The average measured maximum aqueous humor timolol concentration of 1.66 mcg/mL in the occlusion group was significantly greater than 0.85 mcg/mL in the nonocclusion group. The area under the curve was 1.7 times greater in patients who used the technique of nasolacrimal occlusion, and the duration of action was prolonged.[91]

Nasolacrimal occlusion is effective and can maximize drug benefits because a lower concentration of an ophthalmic formulation can be used and the dose administered less frequently. Pilocarpine 1% and 2% significantly decreased IOP at 6, 8, and 12 hours after instillation when the technique of nasolacrimal occlusion was applied.[90] Similarly, carbachol 1.5%, 3%, and the combination of carbachol 1.5% with timolol 0.25% Q 12 hr also were maximally beneficial with nasolacrimal occlusion.[90] Timolol reduced IOP by 15% and maintained this reduction of IOP at 24 hours in 92% of patients when nasolacrimal occlusion was used; in comparison, only 55% achieved comparable IOP reductions when nasolacrimal ducts were not occluded.[90] When nasolacrimal occlusion is used, pilocarpine 2% and carbachol 1.5% can be administered Q 12 hr rather than the usual TID or QID regimens needed when the technique of nasolacrimal occlusion is not applied.[90] The Q 12-hr regimen of treatment then can be adjusted according to the patient's response. Timolol can be administered Q 24 hr, if the nasolacrimal occlusion technique is used.[85] If nasolacrimal occlusion is used consistently and properly, maximal drug effect can be achieved with a reduced frequency of administration

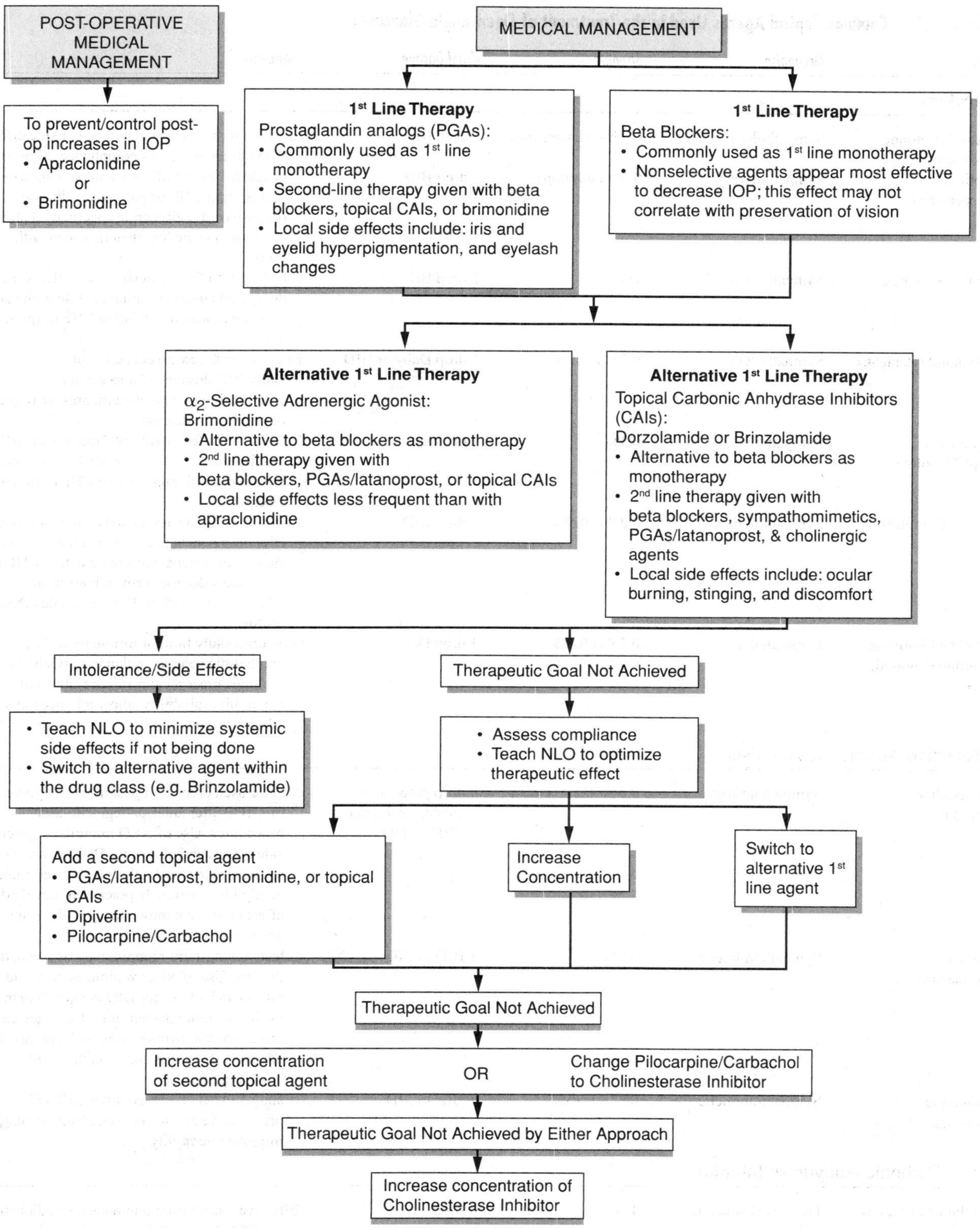

FIGURE 51-2 Medical management of glaucoma. IOP, intraocular pressure; NLO, nasolacrimal occlusion.

Table 51-1 Common Topical Agents Used in the Treatment of Open-angle Glaucoma

Generic	Mechanism	Strength	Usual Dosage	Comments
β-Blockers				
Betaxolol (Betoptic [solution],	Sympatholytic	0.25% (suspension)	1 drop BID	Effective with few associated ocular side effects. BID dosage enhances compliance. May be the ocular β-blocker of choice in patients with pre-existing CHF or pulmonary disease, because of β_1-adrenergic specificity. Patient response may be less than that seen with timolol.
Betoptic S [suspension])	Sympatholytic	0.5% (solution)	1 drop BID	
Carteolol (Ocupress)	Sympatholytic	1%	1 drop BID	Effective with few associated side effects. BID dosage enhances compliance. Use with caution in patients with pre-existing CHF or pulmonary disease.
Levobunolol (Betagan)	Sympatholytic	0.25%–0.5%	1 drop Daily or BID	Effective with few associated ocular side effects. Daily BID dosage enhances compliance. Use with caution in patients with pre-existing CHF or pulmonary disease.
Metipranolol (OptiPranolol)	Sympatholytic	0.3%	1 drop BID	Effective with few associated side effects. BID dosage enhances compliance. Use with caution in patients with pre-existing CHF or pulmonary disease.
Timolol (Timoptic)	Sympatholytic	0.25%–0.5%	1 drop BID	Effective with few associated ocular side effects. BID dosage enhances compliance. Use with caution in patients with pre-existing CHF or pulmonary disease. Proven long-term effectiveness, with well-defined side effect profile.
Timolol Gel Forming Solution (Timoptic XE)	Sympatholytic	0.25%–0.5%	1 drop Daily	New once-daily timolol formulation. The ophthalmic vehicle, gellan gum (Gelrite), prolongs precorneal residence time and ↑ ocular bioavailability, allowing once daily administration.
α_2-Selective Adrenergic Agonists				
Apraclonidine (Iopidine)	Sympathomimetic	0.5%–1%	1 drop preop and postop or 1 drop BID to TID	May be used preop and postop for the prevention of ↑ IOP after anterior-segment laser procedures. Use of NLO minimizes systemic side effects and allows for BID dosing. Does not penetrate the blood–brain barrier; therefore, negligible systemic hypotension. Local adverse effects fairly common. Tachyphylaxis may be observed.
Brimonidine (Alphagan)	Sympathomimetic	0.2%	1 BID to TID	Effective long-term monotherapy or adjunctive therapy. Use of NLO minimizes systemic side effects and allows for BID dosing. Penetrates the blood–brain barrier; therefore, may cause mild systemic hypotension, and lethargy. Local adverse effects less common than with apraclonidine.
Brimonidine (Alphagan P)	Sympathomimetic	0.1%–0.15%	1 BID to TID	Contains PURITE preservative. PURITE preservative and lower concentrations may improve tolerability.
Topical Carbonic Anhydrase Inhibitor				
Brinzolamide (Azopt)	Decreased aqueous humor production	1%	1 drop TID	Effective long-term monotherapy or adjunctive therapy. Well tolerated with few systemic side effects. Less burning and stinging compared to dorzolamide.
Dorzolamide (Trusopt)	Decreased aqueous humor production	2%	1 drop TID	Effective long-term monotherapy or adjunctive therapy. Well tolerated with few systemic side effects.

Table 51-1 Common Topical Agents Used in the Treatment of Open-angle Glaucoma *(Continued)*

Generic	*Mechanism*	*Strength*	*Usual Dosage*	*Comments*
Prostaglandin Analogs				
Latanoprost (Xalatan)	Prostaglandin $F_{2\alpha}$ agonist	0.005%	1 drop once a day at bedtime	BID dosing may be less effective than once a day at bedtime dosing. May cause increased pigmentation of the iris. Systemic side effects are rare, but may cause muscle, joint, back pain, headaches, migraines, and skin rash. Effective monotherapy or adjunctive therapy. May cause increased pigmentation of the iris and eyelid. Store unopened bottles in refrigerator. Opened bottles may be stored at room temperature up to 6 weeks.
Travoprost (Travatan)	Prostaglandin $F_{2\alpha}$ agonist	0.004%	1 drop once a day at bedtime	BID dosing may be less effective than once a day at bedtime dosing. May cause increased pigmentation of the iris and eyelid. Systemic side effects are rare, but may include colds and upper tract infections. Effective monotherapy or adjunctive therapy with timolol. May be more effective than timolol and latanoprost and more effective in African Americans.
Travoprost (Travatan Z)	Prostaglandin $F_{2\alpha}$ agonist	0.004%	1 drop once a day at bedtime	Benzalkonium chloride preservative replaced with a preservative that may be better tolerated.
Bimatoprost (Lumigan)	Prostamide	0.03%	1 drop once a day at bedtime	BID dosing may be less effective than QHS dosing. May cause increased pigmentation of the iris and eyelid. Systemic side effects are rare but include colds and upper respiratory tract infections and headache. May be more effective than timolol and latanoprost.
Miotics				
Pilocarpine (Isopto-Carpine)	Parasympathomimetic	0.25%–10% 4% (ointment) 20–40 mcg/hr (Ocusert)	1–2 drops TID or QID 1/2 inch in cul-de-sac daily Weekly	Long-term proven effectiveness. Little rationale for use of concentrations >4% or administration more frequently than Q 4 hr. Side effects of miosis with decreased vision and brow ache are common sources of patient complaints. Once-daily administration of ointment may increase compliance. Effectiveness over 24 hours should be assessed in patients receiving the ointment. Ointment may cause a visual haze and blurred vision.
Carbachol (Isopto-Carbachol)	Parasympathomimetic	0.75–3%	1–2 drops TID–QID	Used in patients allergic to or intolerant of other miotics. May be used as frequently as Q 4 hr. Corneal penetration is enhanced by benzalkonium chloride in commercial preparations. Side effects are similar to those of pilocarpine.
Echothiophate Iodide (Phospholine Iodide)	Anticholinesterase	0.03%–0.25%	1 drop BID	Most used anticholinesterase agent. Long duration, although usually dosed BID, which enhances compliance. Available as powder + diluent, following reconstitution stable 30 days room temp, 6 months refrigerated. Side effects similar to those of pilocarpine, especially in concentrations >0.06%. Increased cataract formation has been associated with its use.

(continued)

Table 51-1 Common Topical Agents Used in the Treatment of Open-angle Glaucoma *(Continued)*

Generic	*Mechanism*	*Strength*	*Usual Dosage*	*Comments*
Mydriatics				
Epinephrine (Glaucon, Eppy/N, Epitrate)	Sympathomimetic	0.25%–2%	1 drop BID	Good response often seen with use of lower concentrations (0.5%–1%). Bitartrate salt contains half-labeled strength in epinephrine-free base equivalent. BID dosage enhances compliance. Cosmetic complaints associated with use include hyperemia and pigment deposits on the cornea and conjunctiva. Not recommended for use in aphakic patients because of 20%–30% incidence of cystoid macular edema.
Dipivefrin (Propine)	Sympathomimetic	0.1%	1 drop BID	Prodrug of epinephrine associated with increase in systemic side effects if absorbed. BID dosage enhances compliance.

CHF, congestive heart failure; NLO, nasolacrimal occlusion.

and at about half of the drug concentrations typically used. Nasolacrimal occlusion should be incorporated into patient counseling for instillation of all eye drops.[90]

Alternative Therapy

5. Two weeks after initiation of therapy, M.H. returns to clinic for a follow-up evaluation. Her IOP measures 32 mmHg right eye and 30 mmHg left eye. She denies noncompliance and has no complaints of intolerable side effects. How should therapy be altered? Are there alternative dosage forms or drugs that can be used?

Betaxolol may not be as effective as other ocular β-blockers. Therefore, adjunctive therapy may be required. However, M.H. should be evaluated to determine whether she has been using the technique of nasolacrimal occlusion. If not, M.H. should be again instructed on the technique of nasolacrimal occlusion and the importance of this technique in achieving the maximum therapeutic effect of her therapy (see previous question).

After the initiation of therapy, patients should be seen for a follow-up evaluation within about 2 weeks. If M.H. has been adherent to therapy and has been occluding her nasolacrimal ducts, a new course of action is needed because her intraocular pressure still is elevated. When the goal of therapy has not been achieved, the drug concentration of the ophthalmic formulation can be increased; adjunctive therapy (e.g., brimonidine, a topical CAI, a PGA) can be initiated; or an alternative first-line agent can be selected. Patients who are experiencing unstable reductions of IOP should be followed up within 4 months.[3] Stable patients usually are evaluated every 6 to 12 months.[3]

Adverse Effects

6. Several weeks later, dorzolamide 2% solution, one drop both eyes BID is added to M.H.'s betaxolol therapy. Two weeks later, M.H. returns for a follow-up evaluation and complains of bilateral stinging and foreign body sensation. Her IOP measures 30 mmHg in the right eye and 29 mmHg in the left eye. What are the possible causes of her side effects and poor response to therapy?

The exposure of dorzolamide to the outside environment may result in the aggregation of dry white granules on the tip of the dorzolamide bottle. These granules can drop into a patient's eyes when instilling the medication, leading to local side effects, such as stinging and foreign body sensation. Such foreign bodies may cause enough discomfort to induce noncompliance, resulting in a poor response to therapy. M.H. should be questioned about the presence of dry white granules on the tip of her dorzolamide bottle.[93]

These complaints may also be a side effect from the medications, regardless of the granule presence. Ocular burning, stinging, and discomfort were reported in one-third of patients in dorzolamide clinical trials. M.H.'s administration technique should also be assessed to determine whether she is administering the two drugs at least 5 to 10 minutes apart so that the first drug is not washed away by the second drug. This should be a consideration when assessing her response to therapy.[5]

7. After further discussions with M.H., it is determined that she has not been adherent to her dorzolamide therapy because of intolerable side effects. The dorzolamide is discontinued and replaced with travoprost 0.004% one drop both eyes once a day at bedtime. Why might this drug selection be especially appropriate for M.H.? What patient education information should be provided to M.H. about travoprost side effects?

Prostaglandin analogs are first-line agents and are appropriate in patients who are not responding or having intolerable side effects from other medications. Travoprost is an ideal choice for M.H., because African Americans respond especially well to travoprost.[58] M.H. still needs to be informed about the PGA-induced potential for hyperpigmentation of the iris, which may be permanent. She also needs to be educated on the possibility of eyelid skin darkening and increased thickness, length, and pigmentation of her eyelashes, which all may be reversible. These side effects might not be as cosmetically concerning to M.H., because she has brown eyes and will be instilling travoprost eye drops into both eyes.

Table 51-2 CAIs Used in Treatment of Glaucoma

Agent	Strength	Onset (min)	Peak (hr)	Duration (hr)	Usual Dose
Acetazolamide injection	500 mg	5–10		2	500 mg
Acetazolamide tablets	125 mg 250 mg	120	4	6–8	250 mg QID
Acetazolamide sequels	500 mg	120	8–18	22–30	500 mg BID
Dichlorphenamide	50 mg	30	2–4	6–12	50 mg TID
Methazolamide	50 mg	120	4–8	10–12	50 mg TID

CAIs, carbonic anhydrase inhibitors.

ANGLE-CLOSURE GLAUCOMA

Treatment

8. D.H., a 72-year-old man, presents to the emergency department (ED) with an intensely red right eye, a "steamy" appearing cornea, complaints of haloes around lights, and extreme pain. A diagnosis of acute angle-closure glaucoma is made. How should D.H. be managed?

D.H. should be seen by an ophthalmologist, because acute angle-closure glaucoma is a medical emergency. Medical treatment usually consists of pilocarpine 2% to 4%, one drop every 5 minutes for four to six administrations. It is recommended that the puncta be covered during administration to decrease the possibility of systemic absorption. Stronger miotics are contraindicated, because they may potentiate angle closure. Topical timolol also has been used in acute angle-closure glaucoma, commonly in combination with pilocarpine. However, drugs that decrease aqueous humor production may be ineffective in this situation, because they have a decreased ability to reduce aqueous production if the ciliary body is ischemic.[4]

Hyperosmotic Agents

Hyperosmotic agents act by creating an osmotic gradient between the plasma and ocular fluids.[94] Agents that are confined to the extracellular fluid space (e.g., mannitol) provide a greater effect on blood osmolality at the same dosage than do agents distributed in total body water.[94] Intravenously administered drugs provide a faster, somewhat greater effect than oral agents. Palatability may be a problem with oral agents and can be improved by serving these agents over crushed ice or with lemon juice or cola flavoring.

Orally, 50% glycerin is the usual drug of choice and is administered in dosages of 1 to 1.5 g/kg.[95] Isosorbide is an alternative, especially in diabetic patients because it is not metabolized to provide calories.[96] Ethyl alcohol (2–3 mL/kg) is effective and can be helpful in emergency situations when other agents are unavailable.[97] Parenterally, mannitol is the drug of choice. It is administered in doses of 1 to 2 g/kg, is not metabolized to provide calories, and may be used in patients with renal failure.[98,99]

Primary side effects of hyperosmotic agents include headache, nausea, vomiting, diuresis, and dehydration. It is important that the patient not be allowed to drink because this will counteract the osmotic effects of these agents. Precipitation of pulmonary edema and CHF has been reported with hyperosmotic agents, and an allergic reaction has been reported with mannitol.[99,100]

Acetazolamide (Diamox) 500 mg intravenously is often administered in addition to hyperosmotic agents (Tables 51-2 and 51-3).

OCULAR SIDE EFFECTS OF DRUGS

9. B.C., a 64-year-old man, has a history of hypertension managed with hydrochlorothiazide 25 mg/day. He takes amiodarone 800 mg/day for cardiac arrhythmia, and chlorpheniramine 12 mg BID PRN for allergies. Four weeks ago, risperidone 1 mg BID was added to his medication regimen. He also takes sildenafil 100 mg an average of twice weekly. He complains of occasional blurred vision. Could these symptoms be related to his medications?

All the drugs that B.C. is taking have been associated with ocular side effects. Thiazide diuretics have been associated with acute myopia that may last from 24 to 48 hours.[101,102] However, hydrochlorothiazide is an unlikely cause of B.C.'s blurred vision considering its recent onset.

Amiodarone can cause keratopathy, but it is asymptomatic.[103,104] A high percentage of patients who receive this drug develop microdeposits within the corneal epithelium that resemble the verticillate keratopathy induced by chloroquine.[103] These corneal deposits are bilateral, dose and

Table 51-3 Hyperosmotic Agents

Generic	Mode of Administration	Strength	Onset	Peak	Duration	Dose	Ocular Penetration	Distribution
Mannitol	IV	5%, 10%, 15%, 20%	30–60 min	1 hr	6–8 hr	1–2 g/kg	Very poor	E
Glycerin	PO	50%	10–30 min	30 min	4–5 hr	1–1.5 g/kg	Poor	E
Isosorbide	PO	45%	10–30 min	1 hr	5 hr	1.5–2 g/kg	Good	TBW
Ethyl alcohol	PO	50%				2–3 mL/kg	Good	TBW

E, Extracellular water; TBW, total body water.

duration related, reversible, and unassociated with visual symptoms.

Risperidone has been associated with disturbances of accommodation and blurred vision.[104,105]

B.C. may be one of the approximately 1% of the population who experiences blurred vision with chlorpheniramine. This effect has been seen in patients receiving 12 to 14 mg/day.[100,101]

Sildenafil has been associated with change in color and light perception as well as blurred vision.[106] These effects generally subside within 4 hours of the dose.

Table 51-4 outlines some of the more common ocular side effects associated with systemic medications. Each case should be evaluated individually and alternative therapy considered in intolerant patients.

OCULAR EMERGENCIES

Chemical Burns

10. S.J., a 24-year-old construction worker, has splashed an unidentified chemical in his eyes and runs into a nearby pharmacy complaining of burning in both eyes. Should the pharmacist attempt to treat S.J. or refer him to the ED?

Chemical burns require immediate attention. The immediate treatment is copious irrigation using the most accessible source of water (e.g., shower, faucet, drinking fountain, hose, bathtub). After at least 5 minutes of initial irrigation, S.J. should be taken immediately to the ED. A water-soaked towel or cloth should be kept on his eyes during transport.

Other Ocular Emergencies

When health care professionals are approached by patients with acute ocular emergencies (e.g., chemical burns, corneal trauma, corneal ulcers, acute angle-closure glaucoma), patients require immediate treatment and should be referred to an ophthalmologist if the practitioner has even the slightest doubt about appropriate therapy. It is difficult to effectively evaluate the severity of ocular disorders without the benefit of a thorough ophthalmologic workup and specialized training. In situations of corneal trauma from abrasion or foreign bodies, the patient often complains of a gritty, scratchy feeling and can be aware of a foreign body's presence. The corneal tissue is an excellent culture medium for bacteria (e.g., *Pseudomonas aeruginosa),* and therapy should be initiated as soon as possible to avoid corneal perforation and possible blindness.[1] Signs and symptoms of acute angle-closure glaucoma are reviewed in Question 8.

Gonococcal conjunctivitis is an ocular emergency and patients should be referred immediately to an ophthalmologist to minimize the potential of corneal perforation.[1] These patients, who can present with symptoms of red, tender, swollen eyelids with exophthalmos and mild pain, may be suffering from orbital cellulitis or endophthalmitis, which require immediate treatment with systemic antibiotics. Conjunctivitis of other origins (see Bacterial and Allergic Conjunctivitis sections later in this chapter) generally are not ocular emergencies.

Any loss of vision (whether sudden, complete, or transient), flashes of light, pain, or photophobia can signify potentially damaging ocular disorders (e.g., retinal artery occlusion, optic neuritis, amaurosis fugax, retinal detachment) and an ophthalmologist should evaluate the patient as soon as possible. Referral also is recommended for patients with blurred vision, pupil disorders, diplopia, nystagmus, or ocular hemorrhage.

COMMON OCULAR DISORDERS

Stye (Hordeolum)

Sties are infections of the hair follicles or sebaceous glands of the eyelids. The most common infecting organism is *Staphylococcus aureus.* Treatment consists of hot, moist compresses and topical antibiotics (e.g., sulfacetamide). Over-the-counter products should not be recommended. Sties that do not respond to warm compresses within a few days should be evaluated by an ophthalmologist.

Conjunctivitis

Conjunctivitis, a common external eye problem that involves inflammation of the conjunctiva, usually is associated with symptoms of a diffusely reddened eye with purulent or serous discharge accompanied by itching, smarting, stinging, or a scratching, and foreign-body sensation. Patients with pain, decreased vision, unequal distribution of redness, irregular pupils, or opacity should be referred immediately to an ophthalmologist, because these are signs of more serious eye disease.

Conjunctivitis can be bacterial, fungal, parasitic, viral, or allergic in origin. Most cases of bacterial conjunctivitis are caused by *S. aureus, S. pneumococcus* (in temperate climates), or *Haemophilus aegyptius* (in warm climates), although a number of other organisms may be responsible. The infection usually starts in one eye and is spread to the other by the hands. It also may be spread to other persons. Unlike bacterial conjunctivitis, corneal infections can obliterate vision rapidly; therefore, accurate diagnosis is important.

Acute Bacterial Conjunctivitis (Pink-Eye)

11. L.T. is a 6-year-old boy with diffuse bilateral conjunctival redness that has been present for 2 days. A crusting discharge is deposited on his lashes and the corners of his eyes. His vision is normal, and his pupils are round and equal. The diagnosis of acute bacterial conjunctivitis is made, and sodium sulfacetamide 10% ophthalmic drops, two drops in both eyes Q 2 hr while awake, are prescribed. What other measures should be used? What instructions should his caregivers receive?

Although treatment of typical bacterial conjunctivitis such as this is empirical, a culture should be obtained. Other ophthalmic antibiotic drops or ointments, such as neomycin-polymyxin-B-gramicidin combination (Neosporin), also are used in these situations. Although other antimicrobials, such as the ocular quinolones may be used for bacterial conjunctivitis, these agents should be reserved as second-line therapies, because of cost and the potential development of resistance. Proper management of this infection also includes mechanical cleaning of the eyelids and hygienic measures that prevent spreading the infection to other children. The deposits should be removed as often as possible with moist cotton swabs or cotton-tipped applicators. A mild baby shampoo can be used to moisten the applicator. Firm adherent crusts may be softened with warm, moist compresses. Because this material is

Table 51-4 Ocular Side Effects of Systemic Medications

Drug Class	*Effect(s)*	*Clinical Remarks*
Analgesics		
Ibuprofen	Reduced vision	Rare; blurred vision reported in patients taking from four 200 mg tablets/wk to six tablets/day; changes in color vision rarely reported.[157]
Narcotics, including pentazocine	Miosis	Miosis often with morphine in normal doses: slight with other agents; effect secondary to CNS action on the pupilloconstrictor center.[101,102]
	Tearing Irregular pupils Paresis of accommodation Diplopia	Effects associated with narcotic withdrawal.[101,102]
Antiarrhythmics		
Amiodarone	Keratopathy	Dose and duration related; resembles chloroquine keratopathy. Corneal deposits are bilateral, reversible, and unassociated with visual symptoms. Patients taking 100–200 mg/day have only minimal deposits. Deposits occur in almost 100% of patients receiving 400 mg/day.[101–104]
	Cataracts Optic neuropathy	Previously reported as insignificant, anterior subcapsular lens opacities have been associated with amiodarone therapy. Rarely, such opacities may progress, increasing in density and in the diffuse distribution of the deposits, ultimately covering an area somewhat larger than the undilated pupil's aperture. The mechanism for this effect is unclear, but like chlorpromazine, amiodarone is a photosensitizing agent. Given that the lens changes are limited largely to the pupillary aperture, light exposure may result in the lens changes.[101–104] Approximately 2% of patients experience optic neuropathy.[106]
Anticholinergics		
Atropine Dicyclomine Glycopyrrolate Propantheline Scopolamine Trihexyphenidyl	Mydriasis Cycloplegia with ↓ accommodation Photophobia	Systemic and transdermal anticholinergic agents may cause mydriasis and, less frequently, cycloplegia. Mydriasis may precipitate angle-closure glaucoma. Photophobia is related to the mydriasis. Accommodation for near objects.[101,102,158]
Anticonvulsants		
Carbamazepine	Diplopia Blurred vision	Ocular adverse reactions when dosage >1–2 g/day; disappear when dosage is reduced.[101]
Phenytoin	Nystagmus Cataracts	Nystagmus in patients with high blood levels (>20 mcg/mL); rarely occurs with other hydantoins. Cataracts may occur rarely with prolonged therapy.[101,102,159]
Topiramate	Acute myopia Secondary angle closure glaucoma	Topiramate has been associated with angle-closure glaucoma. Symptoms including ocular pain, headache, nausea, vomiting, hyperemia, visual field defects, and blindness have been reported. This process is usually bilateral, but if symptoms are recognized and the drug is stopped in a timely manner, adverse outcomes may be minimized.[106]
Trimethadione	Visual glares	A prolonged glare or dazzle occurs when eyes are exposed to light. The glare is reversible, occurs at the retinal level, and is more common in adolescents and adults; rarely in young children.[101,102]
Vigabatrin	Visual field abnormalities	Visual field abnormalities including bilateral, symmetrical, and irreversible peripheral constriction occur in up to 30% of patients. Most patients are asymptomatic and <0.1% of patients are clinically affected.[106]
Anesthetics		
Propofol	Inability to open eyes	6 of 50 patients undergoing ENT procedures using standardized anesthesia with propofol were unable to open their eyes either spontaneously or in response to verbal commands. This effect lasted from 3–20 min after the end of anesthetic administration. Two patients showed complete loss of ocular motility. This was a transient, myastheniclike weakness.[160]

(continued)

Table 51-4 Ocular Side Effects of Systemic Medications *(Continued)*

Drug Class	*Effect(s)*	*Clinical Remarks*
Antidepressants		
Tricyclic antidepressants (TCAs)		Mydriasis is most common ocular side effect of TCAs. Cycloplegia is rare. Reports of precipitation of angle-closure glaucoma.[101,102]
Fluoxetine	Mydriasis Cycloplegia Eye tics	Administration of fluoxetine 20–40 mg/day has been associated with paroxysmal contractions of the muscles around the lateral aspect of the eye. This effect occurred 3–4 wk after initiation of fluoxetine therapy and resolved within 2 wk of discontinuation.[161]
Antihistamines		
Chlorpheniramine	Blurred vision	Blurred vision occurs rarely (about 1% of patients taking 12–14 mg/day).[101,102]
	Mydriasis, decreased lacrimal secretions	Rare[101,102]
Antihypertensives		
Clonidine	Miosis	Miosis is seen in overdose.[102]
	Dry itchy eyes	Rare[102]
Diazoxide	Lacrimation	About 20% experience lacrimation, which may continue after drug is discontinued.[101]
Guanethidine	Miosis Ptosis Conjunctivitis Blurred vision	Sporadically documented. One study reported a 17% incidence of blurred vision in patients taking guanethidine 70 mg/day.[101,102]
Reserpine	Miosis	Miosis is slight, but can last up to 1 wk after a single dose[101,102]
	Conjunctivitis	Common, secondary to dilation of conjunctival blood vessels[101,102]
Anti-Infectives		
Amantadine	Corneal lesions	Diffuse, white punctate subepithelial corneal opacities have been reported, occasionally associated with superficial punctate keratitis. Onset has been 1–2 wk after initiation of therapy with dosages of 200–400 mg/day. Resolves with drug discontinuation.[162]
Chloramphenicol	Optic neuritis	Rare unless a total dose of 100 g and duration >6 wk are exceeded. Vision usually improves after the drug is discontinued.[101,102]
Chloroquine	Corneal deposits	Some patients using ordinary doses may develop corneal deposits in a few months. The deposits are visible with use of a biomicroscope, appear as white-yellow in color, but are of no consequence.[101,102]
	Retinopathy (macular degeneration)	Serious retinopathy when total dose >100 g. Usually develops after 1–3 yr; can occur in 6 mon. Visual loss may be peripheral, with progression to central vision loss and disturbance of color vision. Rarely, effects such as blurred vision are seen earlier when larger doses (500–700 mg/day) are used. Macular changes may progress after drug is discontinued. These agents concentrate in pigmented tissue.[101,102]
Ethambutol	Retrobulbar neuritis	At dosages of 15 mg/kg/day, virtually void of ocular side effects. Such effects are rare at dosages of 25 mg/kg/day for a duration of a few months. Patients treated for prolonged periods should have routine visual examinations including visual fields. Most effects are reversible after the drug is discontinued, but optic neuritis may continue to progress for 1–2 mon after the drug has been discontinued.[101,102,106]
Gentamicin	Pseudotumor cerebri	Rare, but has been well documented with secondary papilledema and visual loss[101,102]
Isoniazid	Optic neuritis	Prevalence not well defined, but appears to be significantly less than peripheral neuritis. Evaluation difficult because most patients malnourished, chronic alcoholics, or receiving multiple medications. Pre-existing eye disease does not appear to be a predisposing factor.[101,102]
Nalidixic acid	Visual sensations	Most common ocular side effect. Main feature a brightly colored appearance of objects; occurs soon after the drug is taken. Although quinolone antibiotics are nalidixic acid derivatives, they have rarely been associated with these ocular side effects.[101,102]
	Visual loss	Temporary effect (30 min–3 days.)
	Papilledema	Primarily in infants and young children and secondary to intracranial pressure; reversible upon withdrawal of the drug.
Sulfonamides	Myopia	Acute and reversible; most common ocular side effect.[101,102]
	Conjunctivitis	Primarily with topical sulfathiazole, 4% incidence between the fifth and ninth days of therapy.[101,102]
	Optic neuritis	Even in low dosages. Usually reversible with complete recovery of vision.[101,102]

Table 51-4 Ocular Side Effects of Systemic Medications *(Continued)*

Drug Class	*Effect(s)*	*Clinical Remarks*
	Photosensitivity	Associated with use of sulfisoxazole lid margin therapy.[163,164]
Tetracyclines	Myopia	Appears to be acute, transient, and rare.[101,102]
	Papilledema	More common in children and infants than adults; rare.[101,102]
Voriconazole	Altered visual perception Blurred vision	May be associated with higher doses or plasma concentrations.[165]
Anti-Inflammatory Agents (also see Analgesics; Corticosteroids)		
Cyclo-oxygenase-2 inhibitors	Blurred vision Conjunctivitis	Discontinuation of therapy leads to resolution without long-term effects.[106]
Gold	Corneal Conjunctival deposits	Deposition in the conjunctiva and superficial cornea more common than in the lens or deep cornea. Incidence in cornea of 40%–80% in total doses of 1.5 g; visual acuity is unaffected. One reported case after oral therapy.[101]
Indomethacin	Decreased vision	Rare; also changes in color vision have been rarely reported.[101,102]
Phenylbutazone	Decreased vision	Most common ocular side effect with this drug may be caused by lens hydration.[101,102]
	Conjunctivitis Retinal hemorrhage	Occurs less often than vision. The conjunctivitis may be associated with development of Stevens-Johnson syndrome or an allergic reaction.[101,102]
Antilipemic Agents		
Lovastatin	Cataracts	The crystalline lenses of hypercholesteremic patients were assessed before and after 48 wk of treatment with lovastatin 20–80 mg/day. Statistical analyses of the distribution of cortical, nuclear, and subcapsular opacities at 48 wk showed no significant differences between placebo-treated and lovastatin-treated groups. Visual acuity assessments also were not significantly different among the groups.[166]
Antineoplastic Agents		
Busulfan	Cataracts	Reported with high dosages.[101,102]
Carmustine	Arterial narrowing Nerve fiber-layer infarcts Intraretinal hemorrhages	These ocular side effects are not well established. Evidence of delayed bilateral ocular toxicity developed in 2 of 50 patients treated with high-dose IV carmustine (800 mg/m^2). Symptoms of ocular toxicity became evident 4 wk after IV treatment. Evidence of delayed ocular toxicity (mean onset 6 wk) ipsilateral to the site of infusion developed in 7 of 10 patients treated with intra-arterial carotid doses of carmustine to a cumulative minimum of 450 mg/m^2 in two treatments.[162]
Cytarabine	Keratoconjunctivitis Ocular burning Photophobia Blurred vision	Corneal toxicity and conjunctivitis have been reported with high-dose (3 g/m^2) therapy.[168,169]
Doxorubicin	Conjunctivitis Excessive tearing	May last for several days after treatment[101,102]
Fluorouracil	Ocular irritation Lacrimation	Reversible and seldom interfere with continued therapy.[101,102]
Tamoxifen	Corneal opacities Decreased vision Retinopathy	Generally occurs in patients receiving more than 1 year of treatment with a total dose exceeding 100 g has been taken.[101]
Vinca alkaloids (especially vincristine)	Extraocular muscle paresis (EMP) Ptosis	The onset of EMP or paralysis may be seen as early as 2 wk. Dose related. Most recover fully when drug is discontinued.[101,102]
Barbiturates		
	Miosis Mydriasis Disturbances in ocular movement Ptosis	Most significant ocular side effects occur in chronic users or in toxic states. Pupillary responses are variable; miosis seen most frequently except in toxicity when mydriasis predominates. Nystagmus and weakness in extraocular muscles may be seen. Chronic abusers have a characteristic ptosis.[101,102]
Bisphosphonates (alendronate, etidronate, pamidronate, risedronate)		
	Blurred vision, pain, photophobia, conjunctivitis, scleritis, uveitis	Adverse events more common with pamidronate. Scleritis and uveitis are of greatest concern. Following persistent reduction in vision of sustained ocular pain, refer patient to an ophthalmologist. Ocular NSAID treatment may be of symptomatic benefit.[106]

(continued)

Table 51-4 Ocular Side Effects of Systemic Medications *(Continued)*

Drug Class	*Effect(s)*	*Clinical Remarks*
Calcium Channel Blockers		
	Blurred vision Transient blindness	Primarily blurred vision; transient blindness at peak concentrations has been observed in several patients.[202]
Corticosteroids		
	Cataracts	Posterior subcapsular cataracts have been associated with systemic corticosteroids in patients who have received >15 mg/day of prednisone or its equivalent daily for periods >1 year.[101,102] Rare reports of bilateral posterior subcapsular cataracts associated with nasal aerosol or inhalation of beclomethasone dipropionate have been received. Most patients had received therapy for >5 year, often in higher than the recommended dosage. Approximately 40% of patients also were receiving systemic corticosteroids.[170] (Also see Question 14.)
	↑ intraocular pressure	More common with topical corticosteroids than with systemic therapy. Of little consequence in patients without pre-existing glaucoma. Glaucoma patients should be monitored routinely if receiving systemic corticosteroids.[101,102] (See Question 13.)
	Papilledema	Intracranial hypertension or pseudotumor cerebri from systemic corticosteroids has been well documented. The incidence appears to be greater in children than in adults; primarily associated with chronic therapy.
Digitalis		
	Altered color vision, visual acuity	Changes in color vision. A glare phenomenon and a snowy appearance in objects have been associated primarily with digitalis intoxication. In a small number of cases, reversible reduction in visual acuity has been noted. Also associated with changes in the visual fields.[101,102]
	Decreased intraocular pressure	Digitalis derivatives can intraocular pressure, but clinical use for glaucoma is not practical because the therapeutic systemic dose for this effect is very near the toxic dose.[101,102]
Diuretics		
Carbonic anhydrase inhibitors Thiazides	Myopia	Acute myopia that may last from 24–48 hr. Probably caused by an in the anteroposterior diameter of the lens, which may be reversible even if drug use is continued.[101,102]
Estrogens		
Clomiphene	Blurred vision Mydriasis Visual field changes Visual sensations	5%–10% experience ocular side effects. Blurred vision is the most common effect, although visual sensations such as flashing lights, distortion of images, and various colored lights (primarily silver) may occur.[101,102]
Oral contraceptives (OCs)	Optic neuritis Pseudotumor cerebri Retrobulbar neuritis	Quite rare. In patients with retinal vascular abnormalities, use of OCs is questionable. Numerous other possible ocular side effects are associated with these agents, and further documentation is required.[101,102]
Hypouricemics		
Allopurinol	Cataracts	Conflicting reports have suggested allopurinol may be associated with anterior and posterior lens capsule changes and with anterior subcapsular vacuoles; 42 cases of cataracts have been reported; these have been observed primarily in age groups in whom normal lens aging changes would not be expected. No cause-and-effect relationship has been proven.[101,171]
Immune Modulators		
Interleukin-2	Visual deficits	Interleukin-2 visual complications have occurred during the first or second treatment cycle, usually within 5–6 days of initiation of therapy. Ocular symptoms included diplopia, binocular negative scotomata (isolated areas of varying size and shape in which vision is absent or depressed. These are not perceived ordinarily, but would be apparent upon completion of a visual field examination), and palinopsia (abnormal recurring visual imagery). In most cases, treatment was continued for the entire planned duration of therapy. Symptoms resolved after discontinuation.[174]

Table 51-4 Ocular Side Effects of Systemic Medications *(Continued)*

Drug Class	*Effect(s)*	*Clinical Remarks*
Phenothiazines		
Chlorpromazine	Deposits on the lens	Rare when total dose <0.5 kg. Visible after a total dose of 1 kg in most cases; incidence may increase to 90% after ≥2.5 kg. Usually, deposits do not affect vision appreciably. The cornea and conjunctiva may be affected after the lens shows pigment changes.[101,102]
	Retinal pigment deposits	The number of reported cases is small; further documentation is necessary.[101,102]
Thioridazine	Pigmentary retinopathy	Primarily associated with maximal daily dosages or average doses more than 1,000 mg. Daily dosages up to 600 mg are relatively safe; 600–800 mg is uncertain, but rarely suspect. If more than 800 mg/day is used, periodic ophthalmoscopic examinations may uncover problems before visual acuity is compromised.[101,102]
Therapy for Erectile Dysfunction		
Sildenafil Tadalafil Vardenafil	Changes in color and/or light perception, blurred vision, conjunctival hyperemia, ocular pain, photophobia	Color vision alterations are mild to moderate. Blurred vision does not impair visual acuity. Visual alterations usually subside within 4 hr after the dose.[172,173,184] Ocular adverse effects are uncommon, dose dependent, and fully reversible to date. Incidence is not related to age, but is related to blood concentration. Peak visual effects usually occur within 60 min following ingestion[106]
α-Blockers		
Tamsulosin	Floppy iris	Approximately 3% of patients taking tamsulosin for benign prostatic hypertrophy (BPH) experience floppy iris during cataract surgery. Modification of the surgical procedure usually results in successful surgery.[175]

CNS, central nervous system; ENT, ear, nose, and throat.

infectious, it should be disposed of in a sanitary fashion. The common use of washcloths by several individuals will spread bacterial conjunctivitis.

Allergic Conjunctivitis

12. N.V., a 10-year-old girl, has experienced redness in both eyes accompanied by "hay fever" for the past 2 months (June and July). There is no crusting on her eyelids, and her vision is normal; she rubs her eyes often because they itch. What treatment is best for N.V.'s allergic conjunctivitis?

Topical vasoconstrictors (e.g., naphazoline, tetrahydrozoline) with or without antihistamines (e.g., antazoline, pheniramine) may be used to treat hyperemia, but they should not be used excessively because rebound congestion can occur secondary to the vasoconstrictors. Antihistamine tablets or syrup can provide considerable, but temporary, relief. Several ophthalmic histamine H_1-receptor antagonists are effective in the treatment of allergic conjunctivitis. Levocabastine 0.05% is administered BID to QID, olopatadine 0.1% BID (separating doses by 6–8 hours) or 0.2% once daily, emedastine 0.05% QID, and ketotifen 0.025% BID to QID.[107–109] Ketotifen, olopatadine, azelastine, and epinastine exhibit both antihistamine and mast cell stabilizing effects. Olopatadine inhibits the release of other mast cell inflammatory mediators such as tryptase and prostaglandin. Ketotifen and azelastine suppress the release of mediators from cells involved in hypersensitivity reactions and decrease chemotaxis and activation of eosinophils. Azelastine inhibits other mediators involved in allergic reactions such as leukotrienes and platelet activating factor. Epinastine produces antileukotriene, anti-platelet activating factor and antibradykinin effects. Emedastine was more efficacious than levocabastine when used BID for 6 weeks in adult and pediatric patients with seasonal allergic conjunctivitis.[110] Olopatadine provided superior efficacy and a more rapid resolution of the signs and symptoms of allergic conjunctivitis when compared with ketotifen in a small trial involving adult patients.[111] Azelastine has a slightly quicker onset of therapeutic effect when compared to olopatadine and placebo.[112] Information to date is insufficient to definitively recommend one of these products as superior to the others. The ideal treatment would be removal of the allergen, but this usually is impossible when the conjunctivitis is secondary to seasonal allergies. Topical corticosteroids provide dramatic relief, but their use must be limited because of potential adverse effects (see the Ophthalmic Corticosteroids section subsequently).

Sodium cromoglycate, a drug that inhibits the release of histamine in response to antigen, may be effective as an alternative for patients who fail to respond to more conservative measures. Lodoxamide, pemirolast, and nedocromil have a similar mechanism of action to sodium cromoglycate, but these agents also decrease chemotaxis and activation of eosinophils. In comparative studies, lodoxamide tromethamine 0.1% is at least as effective as sodium cromoglycate 2% to 4% in treating allergic ocular disorders, including vernal keratoconjunctivitis.[113,114] Patients in these studies demonstrated more rapid and greater response when treated with lodoxamide, one drop QID. In a 2-week crossover study of nedocromil and olopatadine involving 28 patients aged 7 years and older, patient acceptance of nedocromil BID was better than for olopatadine BID, but treatment outcomes were essentially equal.[114,115]

Corneal Ulcers

13. T.S. presents with a diagnosis of bacterial corneal ulcer right eye and prescriptions for "fortified gentamicin" and cefazolin eye

Table 51-5 Ophthalmic Corticosteroids

Low Potency	*Intermediate Potency*	*High Potency*
Dexamethasone 0.05% (Decadron Phosphate)	Clobetasone 0.1%[a]	Clobetasone 0.5%[a]
Dexamethasone 0.1% (Decadron Phosphate)	Dexamethasone Alcohol 0.1% (Maxidex)	Fluorometholone Acetate 0.1% (Flarex)
Medrysone 1% (HMS)	Fluorometholone 0.1% (FML)	Prednisolone Acetate 1% (Pred Forte)
	Fluorometholone 0.25% (FML Forte)	Rimexolone 1% (Vexol)
	Loteprednol 0.2% (Lotemax)	
	Loteprednol 0.5% (Alrex)	
	Prednisolone Acetate 0.12% (Pred Mild)	
	Prednisolone Sodium Phosphate 0.125% (Inflamase Mild)	
	Prednisolone Sodium Phosphate 1% (Inflamase Forte)	

[a]Not commercially available in the United States.

drops, which are not commercially available. What is the rationale for this therapy?

The initial choice of therapy for bacterial corneal ulcers commonly is based on a Gram's stain and clinical impression of the severity of the ulcer. Single or combination antimicrobial therapy can be prescribed. Although commercial antimicrobial ophthalmic formulations are available, the antimicrobial concentrations in these products might be inadequate to effectively treat bacterial corneal ulcers.[116,117]

Topical antimicrobials for the treatment of bacterial corneal ulcers can be prepared from parenteral antimicrobials or by the addition of parenteral antimicrobials to "fortify" commercially available products. Commonly prescribed products include bacitracin 5,000 to 10,000 U/mL, cefazolin 33 to 100 mg/mL, gentamicin or tobramycin 9.1 to 13.6 mg/mL, and vancomycin 25 to 50 mg/mL. Fortified gentamicin has been prepared by adding 80 mg of parenteral gentamicin to the commercially available gentamicin ophthalmic solution. The final concentration of this solution is 13.6 mg/mL. Cefazolin ophthalmic solution is prepared by reconstituting 500 mg parenteral cefazolin with 2 mL sterile normal saline. Two milliliters of artificial tears solution are removed from a commercially available 15-mL bottle and replaced with the 2-mL reconstituted cefazolin solution (resulting in a final cefazolin concentration of 33 mg/mL). Therapy initially can be administered as frequently as every 15 to 30 minutes with extension of intervals as the ulcer resolves.[118,119] The preparation of extemporaneously compounded ophthalmic products must adhere to established federal and state agency guidelines, and must address quality control concerns (e.g., pH, tonicity, sterility, particulate matter). The formulation of sterile products should not be undertaken without due consideration of well-established practice standards.

OPHTHALMIC CORTICOSTEROIDS

Comparison of Preparations

The topical ophthalmic corticosteroid preparations are described in Table 51-5. The salt form affects the ability of the preparation to penetrate the cornea. For example, biphasic salts penetrate the intact cornea better than water-soluble salts. The ability of a formulation to penetrate the cornea, however, does not indicate increased therapeutic effectiveness. Prednisolone acetate 1% and fluorometholone acetate 0.1% have the best anti-inflammatory effects.[120–121]

Adverse Effects

Increased Intraocular Pressure

14. L.P. has been treated with topical prednisolone acetate 1%, one drop in each eye QID for 8 weeks. Before therapy, the IOPs in both eyes were 16 mmHg, but on the last follow-up visit, his IOP was 26 mmHg in the right eye and 22 mmHg in the left eye. Assess these observations.

L.P.'s elevated IOP could be related to topical steroid therapy. In one study, the ophthalmic administration of corticosteroid preparations (Table 51-6) increased intraocular pressure in three genetically distinct subgroups.[122,123] Fluorometholone acetate increased IOP by more than 10 mmHg in known steroid responders in 29.5 days (median), whereas dexamethasone did the same in 22.7 days (median).[124]

Table 51-6 Intraocular Pressure Response to Topical Steroids in Random Populations

Author	*Parameter of Response*	*No. of Subjects*	*Low*	*Medium*	*High*	*Mean*
Armalay[122]	Increase of pressure in eye medicated with 0.1% dexamethasone	80	<5 mmHg 66%	6–15 mmHg 29%	>16 mmHg 5%	5.5 mmHg
Becker et al.[123]	Final pressure in eye medicated for 6 wk with 0.1% betamethasone	50	<19 mmHg 70%	20–30 mmHg 26%	>32 mmHg 4%	17.0 mmHg
	Time to maximum response		2 wk	4 wk	4 wk	

In a retrospective follow-up, 13% of high-corticosteroid responders developed POAG and 63.8% developed ocular hypertension. No low responders developed POAG, and only 2.4% developed ocular hypertension.[124] Although corticosteroid-induced increases in IOP are associated most frequently with topical ophthalmic preparations, systemic corticosteroids may cause a similar response, although the magnitude is somewhat less.[125] The risk for corticosteroid-induced ocular hypertension is greater in patients with high myopia, diabetes mellitus, or connective tissue disease (particularly rheumatoid arthritis).

Topical corticosteroids exert their effects by decreasing aqueous humor outflow, whereas systemic corticosteroids may increase aqueous humor production.[125] The effects on IOP apparently are unrelated to the corticosteroid's ability to penetrate the cornea. Dexamethasone has been associated with the greatest IOP increase.[126] Fluorometholone, medrysone, rimexolone, and loteprednol have been associated with lower, although sometimes significant, increases in IOP.[127–130] The pressure response often is reversible when the offending agent is discontinued. In subjects with prolonged IOP elevation, glaucomatous field defects are more likely to develop in corticosteroid-responsive patients.[131]

Cataracts

15. G.A., who had asthma, has been taking prednisone 10 mg/day for 1 year. A routine ophthalmic examination revealed early cataract formation. Why could this be related to the prednisone?

Systemic and topical ophthalmic corticosteroids have been associated with the development of cataracts. About 23% of patients treated with 10 to 16 mg/day of prednisone orally (or its equivalent dose) for 1 year or more developed posterior subcapsular cataracts (PSC).[132,133] The estimated occurrence of PSC in patients treated with more than 16 mg/day of prednisone for more than a year increased to more than 70% over the same time period. Patients receiving <10 mg/day prednisone or its equivalent are unlikely to develop PSC, although some contend that the concept of a "safe" dosage should be abandoned because of variable patient sensitivity to this side effect.[134] As illustrated by G.A., the cataracts cause few subjective complaints and little measurable decrease in visual acuity. Although systemic corticosteroids primarily are implicated, use of topical corticosteroids also has been associated with PSC formation.[135] Patients treated with alternate-day dosing of oral corticosteroids may be at lower risk for PSC formation.[136] Any patient receiving long-term corticosteroids should receive routine ophthalmic follow-up.

SYSTEMIC SIDE EFFECTS FROM OPHTHALMIC MEDICATION

16. J.F., a 62-year-old woman, received one drop of phenylephrine 10% in each eye to dilate the pupils. Shortly after administration, her BP increased to 210/130 mmHg for 5 minutes, and she became confused. How common is this type of reaction in patients receiving topical phenylephrine? What other topical ophthalmic medications been associated with systemic effects?

In 33 cases, possible adverse effects had been associated with topical phenylephrine 10%.[137] In a double-blind study, no statistically significant differences were observed in BP or pulse rate between experimental and control groups when phenylephrine 10% or tropicamide (Mydriacyl) 1% was administered to 150 patients.[138] Nevertheless, care should be taken when phenylephrine 10% is administered in patients with hypertension or cardiac abnormalities in whom systemic absorption could be hazardous. No similar reports have been associated with topical use of phenylephrine 2.5%.

In addition to the systemic effects from topical administration of cholinergic agents, epinephrine, and timolol that were previously described, topical atropine, cyclopentolate (Cyclogyl), and scopolamine have been associated with psychosis.[139–141] Fatalities have been associated with topical atropine,[142] ataxia with topical homatropine, and one case of unconsciousness with tropicamide.[142,143]

Topical chloramphenicol-polymyxin-B sulfate ophthalmic ointment has been associated with bone marrow aplasia after intermittent use for 4 months.[144] A cushingoid reaction has been reported in a 30-month-old baby girl treated with dexamethasone alcohol (Maxidex) four times a day in both eyes for 14 months.[145]

OCULAR NONSTEROIDAL ANTI-INFLAMMATORY DRUGS

17. W.A. is scheduled to undergo cataract extraction with implantation of an intraocular lens. Preoperative orders include administration of flurbiprofen 0.03% to inhibit intraoperative miosis. The formulary includes only diclofenac 0.1%. Is this a suitable alternative to flurbiprofen?

The administration of ophthalmic prostaglandins and prostaglandin analogs are associated with some systemic effects (Table 51-1), and ocular instillation of nonsteroidal anti-inflammatory drugs (NSAIDs) can inhibit prostaglandin synthesis and reduce prostaglandin-mediated ocular effects.[146] Commercially available ophthalmic NSAIDs (e.g. bromfenac, diclofenac, flurbiprofen, ketorolac and nepafenac) are well tolerated, but can cause transient burning and stinging upon instillation. Although the ocular NSAIDs share a similar mechanism of action, minor clinical differences, which probably are insignificant, exist and approved indications differ. (Table 51-7).

OCULAR HERPES SIMPLEX VIRUS INFECTIONS

18. P.B., a 34-year-old man, presents with a 2-week history of a red, irritated left eye with watery discharge. Recently, vision in his left eye became blurred, and he complained of light sensitivity. A slit-lamp examination with rose Bengal stain revealed a multibranched corneal epithelial defect. This dendritic ulcer is the hallmark of ocular herpes simplex (type I) infection. What is the therapy of choice?

Ocular herpes is common, and can be caused by herpes simplex virus, or less commonly, by the varicella-zoster virus (herpes zoster ophthalmicus). Herpes simplex of the eye typically affects the eyelids, conjunctiva, and cornea and patients often present with symptoms of pain, tearing, eye redness, sensitivity to light, and irritation or a foreign body sensation. When herpes affects the epithelium of the cornea (herpes keratitis), it generally heals without scarring. Occasionally, deeper layers of the cornea are affected (stromal keratitis) and scarring can lead to blindness.

Table 51-7 Ocular Nonsteroidal Anti-Inflammatory Drugs

Indication	Drug/Approval Status for Indication	Dosage(s)
Inhibition of intraoperative miosis	Diclofenac 0.1% (Voltaren, U)[176]	Three reported regimens; 1 drop Q 15–30 min for four doses; 1 drop TID for 2 preoperative days; 1 drop at 2 hr, 1 hr, and 15 min before surgery.
	Flurbiprofen 0.03% (Ocufen, A)[177]	One drop Q 30 min for 2 hr before surgery.
	Ketorolac 0.5% (Acular, U)	One drop Q 15 min beginning 1 hr before surgery.
Anti-inflammatory postcataract surgery	Bromfenac 0.09% (Xibrom, A)	One drop BID beginning 24 hr after surgery and continuing through the 2 wk of the postoperative period.
	Diclofenac 0.1% (A)[174,178]	One drop BID to QID, including 24 hr preoperative administration.
	Nepavanac 0.1% (Nevanac, A)	One drop 3 times daily beginning 1 day prior to cataract surgery, continued on the day of surgery and through the first 2 wk of the postoperative period. (Nevanac prescribing information. Alcon Laboratories, November 2006)
	Flurbiprofen 0.03% (U)	One drop 4–5 times daily.
	Ketorolac 0.5% (A)[179]	One drop TID, including 24 hr preoperative administration.
Prevention/treatment of cystoid macular edema	Diclofenac 0.1% (U)[180]	Two drops 5 times preoperatively followed by one drop 3–5 times daily
	Ketorolac 0.5% (U)[179,181]	One drop TID or QID, including 24 hr preoperative administration.
Ocular inflammatory conditions (iritis, iridocyclitis, episcleritis)	Diclofenac 0.1% (U)	One drop QID.
Seasonal allergic/vernal conjunctivitis	Bromfenac 0.1% (U)	One drop BID
	Diclofenac 0.1% (U)	One drop Q 2 hr for 48 hr; then QID
	Ketorolac 0.5% (A)[182,183]	One drop QID

A, approved use; U, unapproved use.

Trifluridine

In-vitro, trifluridine's mechanism of action is similar to that of idoxuridine (IDU). Trifluridine also inhibits thymidylate synthase, an enzyme required for DNA synthesis. The actual in-vivo antiviral effects of trifluridine have not been determined.

For the treatment of ocular herpes, one drop of trifluridine 1% ophthalmic solution should be instilled into the affected eye every 2 hours while awake with a maximum daily dose of nine drops. Following re-epithelialization, application of trifluridine should be continued for an additional 7 days at a reduced dosage of one drop every 4 hours while awake with a minimum of five drops daily. Continuous administration for periods exceeding 21 days is not recommended because of potential ocular toxicity.

Approximately 96% of treated herpetic corneal ulcers heal within 2 weeks.[147] Therapeutic levels of trifluridine can be found in the aqueous humor after topical administration of a 1% solution, enhancing its possible effectiveness in the treatment of stromal keratitis and uveitis. Trifluridine also is effective in treating HSV infections resistant to IDU and/or vidarabine.

Despite the apparent superiority of trifluridine over its antiviral predecessors (IDU, vidarabine), it is not without disadvantages. Trifluridine is activated by noninfected corneal cells and is incorporated into cellular as well as viral DNA. Punctate lesions in the corneal epithelium are clinical manifestations of trifluridine cytotoxicity.[148] Yet these effects seem to occur less often than with IDU and vidarabine.

Acyclovir

Acyclovir in in vitro plaque inhibition assays have 5 to 10 times the activity of IDU and trifluridine and more than 100 times the activity of vidarabine against strains of type I and type II HSV.[149] Acyclovir's apparent superiority lies in its lack of toxicity to normal host cells.[155] In rabbits (rabbit eyes are similar to human eyes), acyclovir 3% ointment healed established herpes simplex epithelial ulcerations at a faster rate and eliminated the virus more effectively than 0.5% IDU, and 3% vidarabine ointments.[150,152] In humans, ulcerative corneal epithelial lesions appear to respond similarly to acyclovir and IDU.[153] In comparison to idoxuridine, the topical application of acyclovir or trifluridine resulted in a greater proportion of subjects healing within 1 week and neither was superior for the treatment of dendritic epithelial keratosis.[199] The dose usually is a 1-cm ribbon of ointment instilled five times a day at four-hour intervals for 14 days or at least for 3 days after healing is completed, whichever is shorter. Detailed dosing instructions are available in product literature of specific manufacturers, and brief reviews of acyclovir and acyclovir resistance in Chapter 70: Opportunistic Infections in HIV-Infected Patients; and Chapter 72: Viral Infections.

Other Drugs

Ganciclovir 0.05% and 0.15% gel has been shown to be equivalent to 3% acyclovir ointment in the treatment of superficial herpes simplex keratitis.[155] Cidofovir 1% ointment administered BID was equivalent to trifluridine administered five times daily in the rabbit model.[156] Cidofovir was more efficacious than 3% penciclovir ointment administered two or four times a day.[156]

AGE-RELATED MACULAR DEGENERATION

Age-related macular edema is the leading cause of blindness in Americans of European descent who are 55 years of age and older.[191] There are two forms of macular degeneration, wet and dry. The dry form, affecting about 85% of patients, develops as a result of the breakdown of light-sensitive cells in the macula.[192] The most common symptom associated with dry macular degeneration is blurred vision. In this situation, details (e.g., faces, words in a book) are seen less clearly. Wet macular degeneration occurs in 15% of patients and is the more serious form, responsible for the most cases of vision loss. Wet macular degeneration is associated with abnormal growth of blood vessels behind the retina, known as choroidal neovascularization. Vascular endothelial growth factor (VEGF) is associated with the pathogenesis of choroidal neovascularization. VEGF may stimulate neovascularization by influencing endothelial cell proliferation, vascular permeability, and ocular inflammation.[193] The correlation between VEGF and wet age-related macular degeneration has led to interest in VEGF inhibitors (pegaptanib, bevacizumab, ranibizumab) as treatment agents.

Pegaptanib

Pegaptanib inhibits angiogenesis, decreases permeability of the vascular bed and decreases inflammation. The efficacy of pegaptanib has been evaluated in two concurrent, prospective, randomized, double-blind trials involving 1,208 patients. A total of 1,190 patients received at least one study treatment, with four subjects being excluded from the efficacy analysis due to insufficient assessment of visual acuity at baseline. A combined analysis of 1,186 patients at week 54 showed a statistically significant reduction in vision loss associated with pegaptanib, realized as early as week 6 and continued through week 54.[196] The FDA-approved dose of pegaptanib (0.3 mg IV Q 6 weeks) is no less effective than 1 mg or 3 mg doses and the most serious injection-related adverse events were endophthalmitis (12 patients), traumatic injury to the lens (five patients), and retinal detachment (six patients).[196] Patients should be monitored for elevations in IOP following injection; increases in IOP have been seen within 30 minutes of injection and should be monitored within 2 to 7 days following the injection.

Bevacizumab

Bevacizumab is a recombinant humanized monoclonal immunoglobulin G1 antibody approved for intravenous use for first- or second-line treatment of metastatic colorectal cancer. This product has been used off-label via the IV and intravitreal route for the treatment of neovascular ocular disorders in more than 3,500 patients.[193] Intravenous bevacizumab 5 mg/kg was administered every 2 weeks for two or three infusions in 18 patients for whom 12- and 24-week results on subfoveal choroidal neovascularization were published separately. Therapy was associated with improved visual acuity. No serious ocular or systemic adverse effects were noted, although a statistically significant increase in blood pressure was noted at week 3. Nineteen published, uncontrolled case series studies have evaluated the use of intravitreal bevacizumab for the treatment of wet macular degeneration as well as other conditions associated with neovascularization. The most common intravitreal dose was 1.25 mg, usually administered every 4 to 6 weeks. Doses could be repeated if signs of progression occurred. The longest period of study for intravitreal use was 1 year. The majority of patients in these open-label trials were followed for 3 months. Mean visual acuity improved and no serious ocular effects were noted.

Ranibizumab

Ranibizumab is a Fab fragment of bevacizumab approved in June 2006 for the intravitreal treatment of wet macular degeneration. Ranibizumab is approximately one-third the size of bevacizumab. Its size may facilitate retinal penetration following intravitreal injection. Ranibizumab has a shorter-systemic half life and higher VEGF binding affinity than bevacizumab, but bevacizumab has two binding sites per molecule versus one for ranibizumab. The clinical relevance of these pharmacokinetic and pharmacodynamic differences is not known.[193] The recommended dosage of ranibizumab is 0.5 mg via the intravitreal route administered every 4 weeks. This treatment has been associated with maintenance or improvement of vision for 12 to 24 months.[197] The primary ocular side effects associated with ranibizumab administration include conjunctival hemorrhage, eye pain, and increased IOP.

REFERENCES

1. Riordan-Eva P, Whitcher JP. Vaughn and Ashbury's General Ophthalmology, 16th ed. New York, NY: McGraw-Hill Professional; 2004.
2. Gordon MO et al. The ocular hypertension treatment study: baseline factors that predict the onset of primary open-angle glaucoma. *Arch Ophthalmol* 2002;120:714.
3. American Academy of Ophthalmology. Primary open-angle glaucoma, preferred practice pattern. San Francisco: American Academy of Ophthalmology, 2005. Available at: http://www.aao.org/ppp. Accessed July 11, 2007.
4. American Academy of Ophthalmology. Primary angle closure glaucoma, preferred practice pattern. San Francisco: American Academy of Ophthalmology, 2005. Available at: http://www.aao.org/ppp. Accessed July 11, 2007.
5. Zimmerman TJ et al. Timolol: dose response and duration of action. *Arch Ophthalmol* 1977;95:605.
6. Kwitko GM et al. Bilateral effects of long-term monocular timolol therapy. *Am J Ophthalmol* 1987;104:591.
7. Boger WP et al. Long-term experience with timolol ophthalmic solution in patients with open-angle glaucoma. *Ophthalmology* 1978;85:259.
8. Heel RC et al. Timolol: a review of its therapeutic efficacy in the topical treatment of glaucoma. *Drugs* 1979;17:38.
9. Goethals M. Ten-year follow-up of timolol-treated open-angle glaucoma [summary]. *Surv Ophthalmol* 1989;33:S463.
10. Zimmerman TJ et al. Safety and efficacy of timolol in pediatric glaucoma. *Surv Ophthalmol* 1983;28:262.
11. Boger WP et al. Clinical trials comparing timolol ophthalmic solution to pilocarpine in open-angle glaucoma. *Am J Ophthalmol* 1978;86:8.
12. Moss AP et al. A comparison of the effects of timolol and epinephrine on intraocular pressure. *Am J Ophthalmol* 1978;86:489.
13. Britman NA. Cardiac effects of topical timolol. *N Engl J Med* 1979;300:566.
14. Kim JW et al. Timolol-induced bradycardia. *Anesth Analg* 1980;59:301.
15. McMahon CD et al. Adverse effects experienced by patients taking timolol. *Am J Ophthalmol* 1979;88:736.
16. Jones FC et al. Exacerbation of asthma by timolol. *N Engl J Med* 1979;301:270.
17. Van Buskirk EM. Corneal anesthesia after timolol maleate therapy. *Am J Ophthalmol* 1979;88: 739.
18. Draeger J, Winter R. The local anaesthetic action of metipranolol versus timolol in patients with healthy eyes. In: Merte HJ, ed. *Metipranolol.* New York: Springer-Verlag Wien; 1983:76.
19. Akingbehin T, Villada JR. Metipranolol-associated granulomatous anterior uveitis. *Br J Ophthalmol* 1991;75:519.
20. Zimmerman TJ et al. Side effects of timolol. *Surv Ophthalmol* 1983;28(Suppl):243.
21. Schmitt CJ et al. Penetration of timolol into the rabbit eye. *Arch Ophthalmol* 1980;98:547.
22. Affrime MD et al. Dynamics and kinetics of ophthalmic timolol. *Clin Pharmacol Ther* 1980;27:471.
23. Passo MS et al. Plasma timolol in glaucoma patients. *Ophthalmology* 1984;91:1361.
24. Lustgarten JS, Podos SM. Topical timolol and the nursing mother. *Arch Ophthalmol* 1983;101:1381.
25. Rozier A et al. Gelrite: a novel, ion-activated, in situ gelling polymer for ophthalmic vehicles. Effect on bioavailability of timolol. *Int J Pharm* 1989;57: 163.
26. Shedden AH et al. Multiclinic, double-masked study of 0.5% Timoptic-XE once daily versus

0.5% Timoptic twice daily. *Ophthalmology* 1993; 100:111.
27. Partamian LG et al. A dose-response study of the effect of levobunolol on ocular hypertension. *Am J Ophthalmol* 1983;95:229.
28. Bensinger RE et al. Levobunolol: a three-month efficacy study in the treatment of glaucoma and ocular hypertension. *Arch Ophthalmol* 1985;103:375.
29. Rakofsky SI et al. A comparison of the ocular hypotensive efficacy of once-daily and twice-daily levobunolol treatment. *Ophthalmology* 1989;96:8.
30. Berson FG. Levobunolol compared with timolol for the long-term control of elevated intraocular pressure. *Arch Ophthalmol* 1985;103:379.
31. Berson FG et al. Levobunolol: a β-adrenoreceptor antagonist effective in the long-term treatment of glaucoma. *Ophthalmology* 1985;92:1271.
32. Wandel T et al. Glaucoma treatment with once-daily levobunolol. *Am J Ophthalmol* 1986;101:298.
33. Silverstone D et al. Evaluation of once-daily levobunolol 0.25% and timolol 0.25% therapy for increased pressure. *Am J Ophthalmol* 1991;112:56.
34. Ball SF, Scheider E. Cost of β-adrenergic receptor blocking agents for ocular hypertension. *Arch Ophthalmol* 1992;110:654.
35. Battershill PE, Sorkin EM. Ocular metipranolol: a preliminary review of its pharmacodynamic and pharmacokinetic properties, and therapeutic efficacy in glaucoma and ocular hypertension. *Drugs* 1988;36:601.
36. Mills KB, Wright G. A blind randomized crossover trial comparing metipranolol 0.3% with timolol 0.25% in open-angle glaucoma: a pilot study. *Br J Ophthalmol* 1986;70:39.
37. Bacon PJ et al. Cardiovascular responses to metipranolol and timolol eyedrops in healthy volunteers. *Br J Clin Pharmacol* 1989;27:1.
38. Krieglstein GK et al. Levobunolol and metipranolol: comparative ocular hypotensive efficacy, safety, and comfort. *Br J Ophthalmol* 1987;71:250.
39. Anon. Dr. Mann on metipranolol difference. *Scrip* 1991;1601:26.
40. Akingbehin T et al. Metipranolol-induced adverse reactions: I. The rechallenge study. *Eye* 1992;6:277.
41. Akingbehin T, Villada JR. Metipranolol-induced adverse reactions: II. Loss of intraocular pressure control. *Eye* 1992;6:280.
42. James IM. Pharmacologic effects of β-blocking agents used in the management of glaucoma. *Surv Ophthalmol* 1989;33(Suppl):453.
43. Scoville B et al. A double-masked comparison of carteolol and timolol in ocular hypertension. *Am J Ophthalmol* 1988;105:150.
44. Stewart WC et al. A 3-month comparison of 1% and 2% carteolol and 0.5% timolol in open-angle glaucoma. *Graefes Arch Clin Exp Ophthalmol* 1991; 229:258.
45. Brazier DJ, Smith SE. Ocular and cardiovascular response to topical carteolol 2% and timolol 0.5% in healthy volunteers. *Br J Ophthalmol* 1988;72:101.
46. Levy NS et al. A controlled comparison of betaxolol and timolol with long-term evaluation of safety and efficacy. *Glaucoma* 1985;7:54.
47. Berry DP et al. Betaxolol and timolol: a comparison of efficacy and side effects. *Arch Ophthalmol* 1984;102:42.
48. Stewart RH et al. Betaxolol vs. timolol: a six-month double-blind comparison. *Arch Ophthalmol* 1986;104:46.
49. Allen RC et al. A double-masked comparison of betaxolol vs. timolol in the treatment of open-angle glaucoma. *Am J Ophthalmol* 1986;101:535.
50. Alexander CL et al. Prostaglandin analog treatment of glaucoma and ocular hypertension. *Ann Pharmacother* 2002;36:504.
51. Xalatan [package insert]. Kalamazoo, MI: Pharmacia and Upjohn Company; 2006.
52. Camras CB et al. Latanoprost treatment for glaucoma: effects of treating for 1 year and of switching from timolol. United States Latanoprost Study Group. *Am J Ophthalmol* 1998;126:390.
53. Bucci MG. Intraocular pressure-lowering effects of latanoprost monotherapy versus latanoprost or pilocarpine in combination with timolol: a randomized, observer-masked multicenter study in patients with open-angle glaucoma. Italian Latanoprost Study Group. *J Glaucoma* 1999;8:24.
54. Simmons ST et al. Three-month comparison of brimonidine and latanoprost as adjunctive therapy in glaucoma and ocular hypertension patients uncontrolled on β-blockers: tolerance and peak intraocular pressure lowering. *Ophthalmology* 2002;109:307.
55. Hoyng PF et al. The additive intraocular pressure-lowering effects of latanoprost in combined therapy with other ocular hypotensive agents. *Surv Ophthalmol* 1997;41:S93.
56. Kimal Arici M et al. Additive effect of latanoprost and dorzolamide in patients with elevated intraocular pressure. *Int Ophthalmol* 1998;22:37.
57. Smith SL et al. The use of latanoprost 0.005% once daily and its effects on intraocular pressure as primary or adjunctive therapy. *J Ocular Pharm Ther* 1999;15:29.
58. Netland PA et al. Travoprost compared with latanoprost and timolol in patients with open-angle glaucoma or ocular hypertension. *Am J Ophthalmol* 2001;132:472.
59. Goldberg I et al. Comparison of topical travoprost eye drops given once daily and timolol 0.5% given twice daily in patients with open-angle glaucoma or ocular hypertension. *J Glaucoma* 2001;10: 414.
60. Travatan [package insert]. Fort Worth, TX: Alcon Pharmaceuticals; 2004.
61. Sherwood M et al. Six-month comparison of bimatoprost once-daily and twice daily with timolol twice daily in patients with elevated intraocular pressure. *Surv Ophthalmol* 2001;45(Suppl 4):S361.
62. Noecker RS et al. A six-month randomized clinical trial comparing the intraocular pressure-lowering of bimatoprost and latanoprost in patients with ocular hypertension or glaucoma. *Am J Ophthalmol* 2003;135:55.
63. Lumigan [package insert]. Irvine, CA: Allergan; 2006.
64. Toris CB et al. Effects of brimonidine on aqueous humor dynamics in human eyes. *Arch Ophthalmol* 1995;113:1514.
65. Alphagan P [package insert]. Irvine, CA: Allerhan P; 2005.
66. Meland S et al. Ongoing clinical assessment of the safety profile and efficacy of brimonidine compared with timolol: year-three results. Brimonidine Study Group II. *Clin Ther* 2000;22:103.
67. Serle JB et al. A comparison of the safety and efficacy of twice daily brimonidine 0.2% versus betaxolol 0.25% in subjects with elevated intraocular pressure. *Surv Ophthalmol* 1996;41:S39.
68. DuBiner HB et al. A comparison of the efficacy and tolerability of brimonidine and latanoprost in adults with open-angle glaucoma or ocular hypertension: a three-month, multicenter, randomized, double-masked, parallel-group trial. *Clin Ther* 2001;23: 1969.
69. Sall KN et al. Dorzolamide/timolol combination verses concomitant administration of brimonidine and timolol: six-month comparison of efficacy and tolerability. *Ophthalmology* 2003;110:615.
70. Strahlman E et al. A double-masked, randomized 1-year study comparing dorzolamide, timolol, and betaxolol. *Arch Ophthalmol* 1995;113:1009.
71. Wayman L et al. Comparison of dorzolamide and timolol as suppressors of aqueous humor flow in humans. *Arch Ophthalmol* 1997;115:1368.
72. Azopt [package insert]. Fort Worth, TX: Alcon Laboratories; 2003.
73. Trusopt [package insert]. Whitehouse Station, PA: Merck & Co.; 2005.
74. Rosenburg LF et al. Combination of systemic acetazolamide and topical dorzolamide in reducing intraocular pressure and aqueous humor formation. *Ophthalmology* 1998;105:88.
75. Polansky JR. β-adrenergic therapy for glaucoma. *Int Ophthalmol Clin* 1990;20:219.
76. Allen RC, Epstein DL. Additive effect of betaxolol and epinephrine in primary open angle glaucoma. *Arch Ophthalmol* 1986;104:1178.
77. Harris LS. Dose response analysis of echothiophate iodide. *Arch Ophthalmol* 1971;86:502.
78. Keates EU, Stone RA. Safety and effectiveness of concomitant administration of dipivefrin and timolol. *Am J Ophthalmol* 1981;91:243.
79. Cebon L et al. Experience with dipivalyl epinephrine: its effectiveness alone or in combination and its side effects. *Aust J Ophthalmol* 1983;11: 159.
80. Nordmann JP et al. A double-masked randomized comparison of the efficacy and safety of unoprostone and timolol and betaxolol in patients with primary open-angle glaucoma including pseudoexfoliation glaucoma or ocular hypertension. *Am J Ophthalmol* 2002;133:1.
81. Yuksel N et al. The short-term effect of adding brimonidine 0.2% to timolol treatment in patients with open-angle glaucoma. *Ophthalmologica* 1999; 213:228.
82. VanBuskirk EM et al. Betaxolol in patients with glaucoma and asthma. *Am J Ophthalmol* 1986;101:531.
83. Sorensen SJ, Abel SR. Comparison of the ocular β-blockers. *Ann Pharmacother* 1996;30:43.
84. Berson FG, Epstein DL. Separate and combined effects of timolol maleate and acetazolamide in open-angle glaucoma. *Am J Ophthalmol* 1981;92: 788.
85. Strahlman ER et al. The use of dorzolamide and pilocarpine as adjunctive therapy to timolol in patients with elevated intraocular pressure. *Ophthalmology* 1996;103:1283.
86. thoe Schwartzenberg GW, Buys YM. Efficacy of brimonidine 0.2% as adjunctive therapy for patients with glaucoma inadequately controlled with otherwise maximal medical therapy. *Ophthalmol* 1999;106:1616.
87. Orzalesi N et al. The effect of latanoprost, brimonidine, and a fixed combination of timolol and dorzolamide on circadian intraocular pressure in patients with glaucoma or ocular hypertension. *Arch Ophthalmol* 2003;121:453.
88. Stewart WC. Combination therapy: is the whole greater? Review of Ophthalmology e-Newsletter 2005;12:06 Issue 6/15/2005. http://www.revophth.com
89. Hoy SM et al. Travoprost/timolol. *Drugs Aging* 2006;23:587.
90. Zimmerman TJ et al. Therapeutic index of pilocarpine, carbachol, and timolol with nasolacrimal occlusion. *Am J Ophthalmol* 1992;114:1.
91. Ellis PP et al. Effect of nasolacrimal occlusion on timolol concentrations in the aqueous humor of the human eye. *J Pharm Sci* 1992;81:219.
92. Urtti A, Salminen L. Minimizing systemic absorption of topically administered ophthalmic drugs. *Surv Ophthalmol* 1993;37:435.
93. Zambarakji HJ et al. An unusual side effect of dorzolamide. *Eye* 1997;11:418.
94. Galin MA et al. Ophthalmological use of osmotic therapy. *Am J Ophthalmol* 1966;62:629.
95. Drance SM. Effect of oral glycerol on intraocular pressure in normal and glaucomatous eyes. *Arch Ophthalmol* 1964;72:491.
96. Becker B et al. Isosorbide: an oral hyperosmotic agent. *Arch Ophthalmol* 1967;78:147.
97. Obstbaum SA et al. Low-dose oral alcohol and intraocular pressure. *Am J Ophthalmol* 1973;76:926.
98. Adams RE et al. Ocular hypotensive effect of intravenously administered mannitol. *Arch Ophthalmol* 1963;69:55.
99. D'Alena P et al. Adverse effects after glycerol orally and mannitol parenterally. *Arch Ophthalmol* 1966;75:201.
100. Spaeth GL et al. Anaphylactic reaction to mannitol. *Arch Ophthalmol* 1967;78:583.
101. Fraunfelder FT. Drug-Induced Ocular Side Effects and Drug Interactions. Philadelphia: Lea & Febiger; 1976.
102. Grant WM. Toxicology of the Eye. 2nd ed. Springfield, IL: Charles C Thomas; 1974.

103. D'Amico DJ et al. Amiodarone keratopathy: drug-induced lipid storage disease. *Arch Ophthalmol* 1981;99:257.
104. Kaplan LJ, Cappaert WE. Amiodarone keratopathy: correlation to dosage and duration. *Arch Ophthalmol* 1982;100:601.
105. Risperidone [package insert]. Janssen: Risperdal; 1997.
106. Santaella RM, Fraunfelder, FW. Ocular adverse effects associated with systemic medications. *Drugs* 2007;67:75.
107. Abelson MB, Spitalny L. Combined analysis of two studies using the conjunctival allergen challenge model to evaluate olopatadine hydrochloride, a new ophthalmic antiallergic agent with dual activity. *Am J Ophthalmol* 1998;125:797.
108. Emadine [package insert]. Fort Worth, TX: Alcon Laboratories; 1999.
109. Zaditor [package insert]. Duluth, GA: CIBA Vision; 1999.
110. Yanni JM et al. Preclinical efficacy of emedastine, a potent selective histamine H1 antagonist for topical ocular use. *J Ocular Pharmacol* 1994;10:665.
111. Aguilar A. Comparative study of clinical efficacy and tolerance in seasonal allergic conjunctivitis management with 0.1% olopatadine hydrochloride versus ketotifen fumarate. *Acta Ophthalmol Scand Suppl* 2000;230:52.
112. Spangler SL et al. Evaluation of the efficacy of olopatadine hydrochloride 0.1% ophthalmic solution and azelastine hydrochloride 0.05% ophthalmic solution in the conjunctival allergen challenge model. *Clin Ther* 2001;23:1272.
113. Caldwell DR et al. Efficacy and safety of lodoxamide 0.1% vs cromolyn sodium 4% in patients with vernal keratoconjunctivitis. *Am J Ophthalmol* 1992;113:632.
114. Fahy GT et al. Randomized double-masked trial of lodoxamide and sodium cromoglycate in allergic eye disease. A multicentre study. *Eur J Ophthalmol* 1992;2:144.
115. Butrus S et al. Comparison of the clinical efficacy and comfort of olopatadine hydrochloride 0.1% ophthalmic solution and nedocromil sodium 2% solution in the human conjunctival allergen challenge model. *Clin Ther* 2000;22:1462.
116. Baum JL. Initial therapy of suspected microbial corneal ulcers: antibiotic therapy based on prevalence of organisms. *Surv Ophthalmol* 1979; 24:97.
117. Jones DB. Initial therapy of suspected microbial corneal ulcers: specific antibiotic therapy based on corneal smears. *Surv Ophthalmol* 1979;24: 97.
118. Leibowitz H et al. Bioavailability and effectiveness of topically administered corticosteroids. *Trans Am Acad Ophthalmol Otolaryngol* 1975;79:78.
119. Leibowitz H et al. Anti-inflammatory effectiveness in the cornea of topically administered prednisolone. *Invest Ophthalmol Vis Sci* 1974;13: 757.
120. Kupferman A et al. Therapeutic effectiveness of fluorometholone in inflammatory keratitis. *Arch Ophthalmol* 1975;93:1011.
121. Leibowitz HM et al. Comparative anti-inflammatory efficacy of topical corticosteroids with low glaucoma-inducing potential. *Arch Ophthalmol* 1992;110:118.
122. Armalay MF. Statistical attributes of the steroid hypertensive response in the clinically normal eye. *Invest Ophthalmol* 1965;4:187.
123. Becker B et al. Glaucoma and corticosteroid provocative testing. *Arch Ophthalmol* 1965;74:621.
124. Lewis JM et al. Intraocular pressure response to topical dexamethasone as a predictor for the development of primary open-angle glaucoma. *Am J Ophthalmol* 1988;106:607.
125. Godel V et al. Systemic steroids and ocular fluid dynamics II: systemic versus topical steroids. *Acta Ophthalmol (Copenh)* 1972;50:664.
126. Cantrill HL et al. Comparison of *in vitro* potency of corticosteroids with ability to raise intraocular pressure. *Am J Ophthalmol* 1975;79:1012.
127. Stewart RH, Smith JP, Rosenthal AL. Ocular pressure response to fluorometholone acetate and dexamethasone phosphate. *Curr Eye Res* 1984;3:835.
128. Stewart RH et al. Intraocular pressure response to topically administered fluorometholone. *Arch Ophthalmol* 1979;97:2139.
129. Leibowitz HM et al. Intraocular-pressure raising potential of 1.0% rimexolone in patients responding to corticosteroids. *Arch Ophthalmol* 1996;114:933.
130. Dell SJ et al. A controlled evaluation of the efficacy and safety of loteprednol etabonate in the prophylactic treatment of seasonal allergic conjunctivitis. *Am J Ophthalmol* 1997;123:791.
131. Kitazawa Y, Horie T. The prognosis of corticosteroid-responsive individuals. *Arch Ophthalmol* 1981;99:819.
132. Oglesby RB et al. Cataracts in rheumatoid arthritis patients treated with corticosteroids: description and differential diagnosis. *Arch Ophthalmol* 1961;66:519.
133. Oglesby RB et al. Cataracts in patients with rheumatic diseases treated with corticosteroids: further observations. *Arch Ophthalmol* 1961;66:625.
134. Skalka HW, Prchal JT. Effect of corticosteroids on cataract formation. *Arch Ophthalmol* 1980;98:1773.
135. Yablonski MF et al. Cataracts induced by topical dexamethasone in diabetics. *Arch Ophthalmol* 1975;94:474.
136. Sevel D et al. Lenticular complications of long-term steroid therapy in children with asthma and eczema. *J Allergy Clin Immunol* 1977;60:215.
137. Fraunfelder FT et al. Possible adverse effects from topical ocular 10% phenylephrine. *Am J Ophthalmol* 1978;85:447.
138. Brown MN et al. Lack of side effects from topically administered 10% phenylephrine eye drops: a controlled study. *Arch Ophthalmol* 1980;98: 487.
139. Morton HG. Atropine intoxication: its manifestations in infants and children. *J Pediatr* 1939;14:755.
140. Marks HH. Psychotogenic properties of cyclopentolate. *JAMA* 1963;186:430.
141. Freund M et al. Toxic effects of scopolamine eye drops. *Am J Ophthalmol* 1970;70:637.
142. Hoefnagel D. Toxic effects of atropine and homatropine eye drops in children. *N Engl J Med* 1961;264:168.
143. Wahl JW. Systemic reaction to tropicamide. *Arch Ophthalmol* 1969;82:320.
144. Abrams SM et al. Marrow aplasia following topical application of chloramphenicol eye ointment. *Arch Intern Med* 1980;140:576.
145. Musson K. Cushingoid status: induced by topical steroid medication. *J Pediatr Ophthalmol Strabismus* 1968;5:33.
146. Flach AJ. Cyclo-oxygenase inhibitors in ophthalmology. *Surv Ophthalmol* 1992;36:259.
147. Pavan-Langston DR, Foster CS. Trifluorothymidine and idoxuridine therapy of ocular herpes. *Am J Ophthalmol* 1977;84:818.
148. McGill J et al. Some aspects of the clinical use of trifluorothymidine in the treatment of herpetic ulceration of the cornea. *Trans Ophthalmol Soc U K* 1974;94:342.
149. Collins P, Bauer DJ. The activity in vitro against herpes virus of 9-(2-hydroxyethoxymethyl) guanine (acycloguanosine), a new antiviral agent. *J Antimicrob Chemother* 1979;5:431.
150. Pavan-Langston DR et al. Acyclic antimetabolite therapy of experimental herpes simplex keratitis. *Am J Ophthalmol* 1978;86:618.
151. Falcon MG, Jones BR. Acycloguanosine: antiviral activity in the rabbit cornea. *Br J Ophthalmol* 1979;63:422.
152. Shiota J et al. Efficacy of acycloguanosine against herpetic ulcers in rabbit cornea. *Br J Ophthalmol* 1979;63:425.
153. Coster DJ et al. A comparison of acyclovir and idoxuridine as treatment for ulcerative herpetic keratitis. *Br J Ophthalmol* 1980;64:763.
154. Kaufman HE. Antimetabolite drug therapy in herpes simplex. *Ophthalmology* 1980;87:135.
155. Colin J et al. Ganciclovir ophthalmic gel in the treatment of herpes simplex keratitis. *Cornea* 1997; 16:393.
156. Kaufman HE et al. Trifluridine, cidofovir, and penciclovir in the treatment of experimental herpetic keratitis. *Arch Ophthalmol* 1998;116:777.
157. Nicastro NJ. Visual disturbances associated with over-the-counter ibuprofen in three patients. *Ann Ophthalmol* 1989;29:447.
158. Hamill MB et al. Transdermal scopolamine delivery system and acute angle-closure glaucoma. *Ann Ophthalmol* 1983;1:1011.
159. Bar S et al. Presenile cataracts in phenytoin-treated epileptic patients. *Arch Ophthalmol* 1983;101:422.
160. Marsch SCU, Schaefer HG. Problems with eye opening after propofol anesthesia. *Anesth Analg* 1990;70:115.
161. Cunningham M et al. Eye tics and subjective hearing impairment during fluoxetine therapy. *Am J Psychiatry* 1990;147:947.
162. Fraunfelder FT, Meyer SM. Amantadine and corneal deposits. *Am J Ophthalmol* 1990;110:96.
163. Flach A. Photosensitivity to sulfisoxazole ointment. *Arch Ophthalmol* 1981;99:609.
164. Flach AJ et al. Photosensitivity to topically applied sulfisoxazole ointment. *Arch Ophthalmol* 1982;100:1286.
165. VFEND [package insert]. New York, NY: Pfizer Roerig Pharmaceuticals; 2003.
166. Laties AM et al. Expanded clinical evaluation of lovastatin (EXCEL) study results. II. Assessment of the human lens after 48 weeks of treatment with lovastatin. *Am J Cardiol* 1991;67:447.
167. Shingleton BJ et al. Ocular toxicity associated with high-dose carmustine. *Arch Ophthalmol* 1981;100:1766.
168. Hopen G et al. Corneal toxicity with systemic cytarabine. *Am J Ophthalmol* 1981;91:500.
169. Smollen KW et al. Non-hematologic toxicities from high-dose cytarabine: analysis of seven patients and development of a monitoring guide. *PharmFax* 1984;13:4.
170. Franufelder FT, Meyer SM. Posterior subcapsular cataracts associated with nasal or inhalation corticosteriods. *Am J Ophthalmol* 1990;109:489.
171. Jick H, Brandt DE. Allopurinol and cataracts. *Am J Ophthalmol* 1984;98:355.
172. Cialis [package insert]. Indianapolis, IN: EliLilly & Company; 2003.
173. Levitra [package insert]. West Haven, CT: Bayer Health Care; 2003.
174. Friedman DI et al. Neuro-ophthalmic complications of interleukin 2 therapy. *Arch Ophthalmol* 1991;109:1679.
175. Chang DF, Campbell JR. Intraoperative floppy iris syndrome associated with tamsulosin. *J Cataract Refractive Surg* 2005;31:664.
176. Goa KL, Chrisp P. Ocular diclofenac: a review of its pharmacology and clinical use in cataract surgery, and potential in other inflammatory ocular conditions. *Drugs Aging* 1992;2:473.
177. Ocufen [package insert]. Hormigueros, PR: Allergan America; 1992.
178. Voltaren Ophthalmic [package insert]. Atlanta, GA: CIBA Vision Ophthalmics; 1991.
179. Flach AJ et al. The effect of ketorolac tromethamine solution in reducing postoperative inflammation after cataract extraction and intraocular lens implantation. *Ophthalmology* 1988;95:1279.
180. Flach AJ et al. Prophylaxis of aphakic cystoid macular edema without corticosteroids. *Ophthalmology* 1990;97:1253.
181. Flach AJ et al. Improvement in visual acuity in chronic aphakic and pseudophakic cystoid macular edema after treatment with topical 0.5% ketorolac tromethamine. *Am J Ophthalmol* 1991;112: 514.
182. Tinkelman DG et al. Double-masked, paired-comparison clinical study of ketorolac tromethamine 0.5% ophthalmic solution compared with placebo eyedrops in the treatment of seasonal allergic conjunctivitis. *Surv Ophthalmol* 1993;38(Suppl):133.

183. Ballas Z et al. Clinical evaluation of ketorolac tromethamine 0.5% ophthalmic solution for the treatment of seasonal allergic conjunctivitis. *Surv Ophthalmol* 1993;38(Suppl):141.
184. Viagra [package insert]. New York, NY: Pfizer, Inc.; October 2007.
185. Bauer DJ et al. Treatment of experimental herpes simplex keratitis with acycloguanosine. *Br J Ophthalmol* 1979;63:429.
186. Tinkelman DG et al. Double-masked, paired-comparison clinical study of ketorolac tromethamine 0.5% ophthalmic solution compared with placebo eyedrops in the treatment of seasonal allergic conjunctivitis. *Surv Ophthalmol* 1993; 38(Suppl):133.
187. Flach AJ et al. Effectiveness of ketorolac tromethamine 0.5% ophthalmic solution for chronic aphakic and pseudophakic cystoid macular edema. *Am J Ophthalmol* 1987;103:479.
188. Flach AJ et al. Improvement in visual acuity in chronic aphakic and pseudophakic cystoid macular edema after treatment with topical 0.5% ketorolac tromethamine. *Am J Ophthalmol* 1991;112:514.
189. Topamax [package insert]. Raritan, NJ: Ortho McNeil Pharmaceuticals Inc.; 2003.
190. Flach AJ, Bolan BJ. Amiodarone-induced lens opacities: an 8-year follow-up study. *Arch Ophthalmol* 1996;108:1668.
191. The Eye Diseases Prevalence Research Group. Causes and prevalence of visual impairment among adults in the United States. *Arch Ophthalmol* 2004; 122:477.
192. Age-related macular degeneration: what you should know. Washington, DC: U.S. Dept of Health and Human Services, National Institutes of Health, National Eye Institute; 2003. Publication no. 03-2294.
193. Lynch SS, Chent CM. Bevacizumab for neovascular ocular diseases. *Ann Pharmacother* 2007;41:14.
194. Lynch SS, Cheng CM. Bevacimab for neovascular ocular diseases. *Ann Pharmacother* 2007;41: 614.
195. Wilhermus KR. Therapeutic interventions for herpes simplex virus epithelial keratitis. *Cochrane Databse Syst Rev* 2007;Jan 24;(1):CD002898.
196. Chapman JA, Beckey C. Pegaptanib: a novel approach to ocular neovascularization. *Ann Pharmacother* 2006;40:1322.
197. Anon. Lucentis prescribing information. San Francisco, CA: Genentech; 2007.
198. Pitlik S et al. Transient retinol ischaemia induced by nifedipine. *Br Med J* (Clin Res Ed). 1983;287:1845.

SECTION FOURTEEN

NEUROLOGIC DISORDERS

Brian K. Alldredge

SECTION EDITOR

CHAPTER 52

Headache

Brian K. Alldredge

Clinical features and drug therapy of the common headache syndromes are presented in this chapter. Proposed pathophysiologic features of the major headache types also are presented to provide the reader with an understanding of the rationale for current and future therapies.

Prevalence

In the United States, migraine headache affects approximately 23 million persons, and 11 million experience significant headache-related disability.[1] Headache is the fourth most common symptom reported at outpatient medical visits,[2] and the associated economic costs in America are estimated to be between $1 billion and $17 billion dollars annually.[3] Overall, the prevalence of headache is highest in adolescence and early adulthood and declines with age through the elderly years.[4,5] Despite numerous potential causes of headaches, more than 90% of patients with a chief complaint of continuous or sporadically recurring headaches are eventually diagnosed as having either tension-type or migraine headache.[6]

Classification

Headache is a symptom that can be caused by many disorders. For example, head pain can result from traction, displacement, or inflammation of pain-sensitive structures within the head, or it can be due to disorders of extracranial structures such as the eyes, ears, or sinuses. For diagnostic and therapeutic purposes, it is useful to categorize headache into one of two major types (*primary* and *secondary*) on the basis of the underlying etiology. *Primary headache disorders* are characterized by the lack of an identifiable and treatable underlying cause. Migraine, tension-type, and cluster headaches are examples of primary headache disorders. *Secondary headache disorders* are those associated with a variety of organic causes such as trauma, cerebrovascular malformations, and brain tumors. Depending on the cause, headache may manifest in a variety of ways or may be accompanied by other associated signs or symptoms. A comprehensive classification scheme of the different types of headaches, modified from the International Headache Society (IHS) is shown in Table 52-1.[7] Readers are referred to the IHS classification report for the comprehensive headache classification scheme and a detailed description of the specific diagnostic features of each headache type. This classification scheme is useful for grouping headaches with similar clinical features or etiologies. Headache must be accurately evaluated and classified because this symptom may reflect an ominous problem such as the presence of a brain tumor or a much more benign process such as muscle tension. Moreover, effective intervention depends on a correct diagnosis.

Primary Headache Disorders

MIGRAINE HEADACHES

Migraine headaches usually develop over a period of minutes to hours, progressing from a dull ache to a more intense pulsating pain that worsens with each pulse. The headache usually begins in the frontotemporal region and may radiate to the occiput and neck; it may occur unilaterally or bilaterally. Migraine headaches often are accompanied by nausea and vomiting and may last for up to 72 hours. These headaches usually are alleviated by relaxation in a dark room and sleep. Migraine is more common in females than males. Migraine headaches are divided into those with and without an aura. The term, *aura,* refers to the complex of focal neurologic symptoms (e.g., alterations in vision or sensation) that initiate or accompany a migraine attack. Migraine may be precipitated by a variety of dietary, pharmacologic, hormonal, or environmental factors.

CLUSTER HEADACHES

Cluster headaches derive their name from a characteristic pattern of recurrent headaches that are separated by periods of remission that last from months to even years. During those periods when clusters of headaches are experienced, the

Table 52-1 Classification of Headache[7]

Migraine
Migraine without aura
Migraine with aura
Complicated migraine (see Table 52-2)
Tension-Type Headache
Episodic tension-type headache
Chronic tension-type headache
Cluster Headache
Episodic cluster headache
Chronic cluster headache
Miscellaneous Headaches Unassociated with Structural Lesion (e.g., cold stimulus headache, benign exertional headache)
Headache Associated with Head Trauma
Acute post-traumatic headache
Chronic post-traumatic headache
Headache Associated with Vascular Disorders
Acute ischemic cerebrovascular disease (TIA or stroke)
Intracranial hematoma
Subarachnoid hemorrhage
Unruptured vascular malformation
Arteritis
Carotid or vertebral artery pain
Venous thrombosis
Arterial hypertension
Headache Associated with Nonvascular Intracranial Disorder (e.g., high or low CSF pressure, intracranial infection, or neoplasm)
Headache Associated with Substances or their Withdrawal (e.g., withdrawal from alcohol, caffeine, ergotamine, narcotics; also see Table 52-3).
Headache Associated with Noncephalic Infection (e.g., viral or bacterial infection)
Headache Associated with Metabolic Disorder (e.g., hypoxia, hypercapnia, hypoglycemia, dialysis)
Headache or Facial Pain Associated with Disorder of Cranium, Neck, Eyes, Ears, Nose, Sinuses, Teeth, Mouth, or Other Facial or Cranial Structures (e.g., cervical spine, acute glaucoma, refractive errors, acute sinus headache)
Cranial Neuralgias, Nerve Trunk Pain and Deafferentation Pain (e.g., compression, demyelination, infarction, or inflammation of cranial nerves)
Headache Not Classifiable

CSF, cerebrospinal fluid; TIA, transient ischemic attacks.

headaches usually occur at least once daily. The headache generally is unilateral, occurs behind the eye, reaches maximal intensity over several minutes, and lasts for <3 hours. Unilateral lacrimation, rhinorrhea, and facial flushing may accompany the cluster headache. During cluster periods, headache is commonly precipitated by alcohol, naps, and vasodilating drugs. In contrast to migraine headaches, cluster headaches are more common in males than females.

TENSION-TYPE HEADACHES

A dull, persistent headache, occurring bilaterally in a hatband distribution around the head is characteristic of tension-type headaches. The headache is usually not debilitating and may fluctuate in intensity throughout the day. Tension-type headaches often occur during or after stress, but chronic tension-type headaches may persist for months even in the absence of recognizable stress. Skeletal muscle overcontraction, depression, and occasionally nausea may accompany the headache. Prodrome neurologic symptoms do not occur in association with tension-type headache. More detailed descriptions of migraine, cluster, and tension-type headaches appear in following sections of this chapter.

Secondary Headache Disorders

In addition to migraine, cluster, and tension-type headaches, patients may also experience headache associated with head trauma, vascular disorders, central nervous system (CNS) infection (including HIV), or metabolic disorders. More than 300 disorders capable of producing headache have been identified.[8] Examples of secondary headache disorders are given in Table 52-1.

The length of time that a patient has experienced headaches provides highly useful information for assessing the nature and etiology of the headaches. A new severe headache in a patient without a previous history is the most useful single piece of information for identifying potentially destructive intracranial or extracranial causes of headache. Such headaches may develop suddenly, over a period of hours to days (acute headache), or more gradually over days to months (subacute headache).

Acute Headaches

Acute headaches can be symptomatic of subarachnoid hemorrhage, stroke, meningitis, or intracranial mass lesion (e.g., brain tumor, hematoma, abscess). The headache that accompanies subarachnoid hemorrhage is typically severe (often described by the patient as the "worst headache of my life") and may occur in conjunction with alteration of mental status and focal neurologic signs. The headache of meningitis is usually bilateral and develops gradually over hours to days; symptoms such as fever, photophobia, and positive meningeal (Kernig's and Brudzinski's) signs often accompany the meningeal headache. Although the acute onset of headache associated with coughing, sneezing, straining, or change in head position is commonly thought to indicate a cranial mass lesion with cerebrospinal fluid (CSF) pathway obstruction, several varieties of exertional headache are benign (see Table 52-1).

Subacute Headaches

Subacute headaches may be a sign of increased intracranial pressure, intracranial mass lesion, temporal arteritis, sinusitis, or trigeminal neuralgia (i.e., tic douloureux). Trigeminal neuralgia usually occurs after the age of 40 and is more common in women than men. The pain usually occurs along the second or third divisions of the trigeminal (facial) nerve and lasts only moments. Trigeminal neuralgia is characterized by sudden, intense pain that recurs paroxysmally, often in response to triggers such as talking, chewing, or shaving.

The clinical manifestations of headache, as described previously, focus on the onset, frequency, duration, site, gender of the patient, distribution, and other unique characteristics of the head pain. A comprehensive medical history and physical examination of the patient often provide sufficient information to make an adequate assessment of a patient's headache complaint, and may enable the practitioner to rule out headache as a manifestation of more serious illness. Physical examination of the patient suffering from the common, benign forms of headache (e.g., migraine, cluster, and tension-type headaches) is usually normal. When the medical history of the patient is suggestive of a secondary cause of headache, a more extensive evaluation with referral to or consultation by a neurologist is necessary.

Pathophysiology

Intracranially, only a limited number of structures are sensitive to pain. The most important pain-sensitive structures within the cranium are the proximal portions of the cerebral arteries, large veins, and the venous sinuses.[9] Headache may result from dilation, distention, or traction of the large intracranial vessels. The brain itself is insensitive to pain. Referred pain from inflammation of frontal or maxillary sinuses or refractive errors of the eye are potential, although overdiagnosed, causes of headache.[10] Scalp arteries and muscles are also capable of registering pain and have been implicated in the pathophysiology of migraine and tension-type headache. Extracranially, most of the structures outside the skull (e.g., periosteum, eye, ear, teeth, skin, deeper tissues) have pain afferents. In general, pain can be produced by activation of peripheral pain receptors (nociceptors), injury to CNS or peripheral nervous system, or displacement of the pain-sensitive structures mentioned earlier.

Historically, the primary headache disorders have been thought to be related either to vascular disturbances (migraine and cluster headache) or muscular tension (tension-type headache). However, clinical and experimental evidence now suggests that these headaches have their origin in an underlying disturbance in brain function.[11] Evidence in this regard is particularly strong for migraine and cluster headache. Many authors now hold the opinion that these clinically dissimilar primary headache syndromes represent variable manifestations of a common pathogenetic phenomenon that involves neural innervation of the cranial circulation. The specific mechanisms that lead to primary headaches have not been identified. However, a *neurovascular hypothesis* has been proposed in which headache is triggered by disturbances in central pain processing pathways (the trigeminocervical complex) leading to the release of potent neuropeptides (calcitonin gene-related peptide [CGRP], substance P, and neurokinin A) and subsequent vasodilation.[12] Serotonin, a vasoactive neurotransmitter released by brainstem nuclei of the trigeminovascular system, likely plays a role in migraine pathogenesis.[13] Furthermore, drugs that alter serotonergic function are highly effective for the symptomatic treatment of migraine and cluster headache.

Drug Therapy

Drug therapy for headache is divided into two major categories: (a) abortive therapy to provide relief during an acute headache attack and (b) prophylactic therapy to prevent or reduce the severity of recurrent headaches. Most people with infrequent tension-type headaches self-medicate with over-the-counter (OTC) analgesics to abort the acute event and do not require prophylactic therapy. By contrast, migraine and cluster headache sufferers who experience frequent headaches and who respond poorly to abortive measures are good candidates for preventive therapy.

Although analgesics are often useful for the treatment of episodic tension-type headaches, most patients with migraine and all patients with cluster headaches require other abortive measures. Until recently, ergot alkaloids (e.g., ergotamine and dihydroergotamine) were the most commonly prescribed agents for relief of migraine and cluster headaches. Now, the triptan class of agents (e.g., sumatriptan, zolmitriptan, naratriptan, rizatriptan, almotriptan, frovatriptan and eletriptan) is often preferred because of their favorable efficacy and tolerable adverse effect profiles.[14] However, the greater expense of the triptans limits the availability of these drugs for some patients.

Antidepressant agents (e.g., amitriptyline) are useful for prophylactic treatment of migraine and tension-type headaches. Because many patients suffer from mixed headache types, these agents can be useful for patients who might otherwise require preventive polytherapy. Other agents useful for migraine headache prophylaxis include β-blocking agents (e.g., propranolol), valproate, calcium channel blocking agents (particularly verapamil), and nonsteroidal anti-inflammatory drugs (NSAIDs). Among the agents effective for prophylaxis against episode cluster headaches, verapamil, corticosteroids (e.g., prednisone) and lithium are usually preferred.

MIGRAINE HEADACHE

The word *migraine* comes from the Greek "hemicrania" and historically was used to describe unilateral headaches with associated symptoms. More recently, the IHS described migraine as follows. Migraine is an "idiopathic, recurring headache disorder manifesting in attacks lasting 4 to 72 hours. Typical characteristics of [migraine] headache are unilateral location, pulsating quality, moderate or severe intensity, aggravation by routine physical activity, and association with nausea, photo- and phonophobia."[7] Migraine headaches are subclassified according to the presence or absence of aura symptoms. Most persons who suffer from migraine do not experience aura symptoms. In patients with aura, visual symptoms are most common. Complicated migraine is a less common type of migraine in which the neurologic symptoms are more pronounced or disabling; in some cases the aura symptoms may outlast the headache itself. Table 52-2 outlines the predominant types of complicated migraine. Although patients with persistent symptoms should be thoroughly evaluated by a neurologist, permanent neurologic sequelae after migraine are rare even for patients with complicated migraine.

Pathophysiology

Past theories of pathogenesis have focused on alterations in cranial vessel diameter and blood flow as the primary cause of migraine. In this "vascular hypothesis," it was thought that focal neurologic symptoms preceding or accompanying the headache were caused by vasoconstriction and reduction in cerebral blood flow. The headache was thought to be caused by a compensatory vasodilation with displacement of pain-sensitive intracranial structures. Although blood flow is decreased during the aura of migraine,[15] other observations do not support the vascular hypothesis. The headache phase of migraine with aura has been shown to begin while blood flow is reduced,[15] and migraine without aura is not associated with alterations in regional cerebral blood flow.[16] Furthermore, the therapeutic effect of sumatriptan, a drug highly specific for neurovascular headaches, is not temporally related to its vasoconstrictive effect.[17] More recent evidence suggests that the pain of migraine is generated centrally and involves episodic dysfunction of neural structures that control the cranial circulation (the *trigeminovascular system*). The availability of functional brain imaging has had a dramatic effect on the ability to visualize the pathophysiologic events of a migraine attack.[12] The trigeminovascular system consists of neurons, originating in the trigeminal ganglion, which innervate the cerebral circulation. Several potent vasodilator neuropeptides are contained within these trigeminal neurons, including calcitonin gene-related peptide, substance P, and neurokinin A. In animals, stimulation of the trigeminal ganglion significantly alters regional brain blood flow.[12] Stimulation of the trigeminal ganglion in humans causes facial flushing, an increase in facial temperature,[18] and increases in extracerebral venous concentrations of calcitonin gene-related peptide and substance P.[19] The specific events leading to trigeminovascular dysfunction in migraine are unknown. However, evidence from positron emission tomography (PET) scanning (a technique to measure regional cerebral blood flow as an index of neuronal activity)

Table 52-2 Types of Complicated Migraine[7]

Type	Description
Migraine with Prolonged Aura	Aura symptoms lasting >60 min but <1 wk
Familial Hemiplegic Migraine	Aura with hemiparesis; identical attacks in a first-degree relative
Basilar Migraine	Aura symptoms arising from brainstem or occipital lobes (e.g., dysarthria, vertigo, ataxia, decreased level of consciousness)
Ophthalmoplegic Migraine	Paresis of one or more ocular cranial nerves
Retinal Migraine	Aura symptoms with monocular scotoma or blindness lasting <1 hr
Status Migrainosus	Migraine headache lasting >72 hr despite treatment
Migrainous Infarction	Aura symptoms lasting longer than 7 days.

suggests that episodic dysfunction of the brainstem, with corresponding effects on the trigeminal system, are involved. Using PET, Weiller and et al.[20] found activation of the brainstem (periaqueductal gray, dorsal raphe nucleus, and locus ceruleus) at the onset of migraine headaches in nine patients. This area may represent an endogenous "migraine generator." Sporadic dysfunction of the nociceptive system (periaqueductal gray and dorsal raphe nucleus) and the neural control of cerebral blood flow (dorsal raphe nucleus and locus ceruleus) is hypothesized to trigger migraine headache via their effects on the trigeminovascular system. Further support for a trigeminovascular mechanism for migraine comes from studies that demonstrate inhibition of trigeminal neurons and associated nociceptive responses by various antimigraine drugs such as dihydroergotamine,[21] rizatriptan,[22] and zolmitriptan.[23] Abnormalities in serotonin (5-HT) activity are also thought to play a role in migraine headache. Plasma 5-HT levels decrease by nearly half during a migraine attack,[24] with a corresponding rise in the urinary excretion of 5-hydroxyindoleacetic acid,[25] the primary metabolite of 5-HT. Also, reserpine, a drug that depletes 5-HT from body stores, has been found to induce a stereotypical headache in migraineurs and a dull discomfort in patients not prone to migraine.[24,26] An intravenous (IV) injection of 5-HT effectively relieved both reserpine-induced and spontaneous migraine headache.[24,26] The therapeutic effects of drugs that stimulate 5-HT_1 receptors (e.g., dihydroergotamine, sumatriptan), antagonize 5-HT_2 receptors (e.g., methysergide, cyproheptadine), prevent 5-HT reuptake (e.g., amitriptyline) or release (e.g., calcium channel blockers), or inhibit brainstem serotonergic raphe neurons (e.g., valproate) all lend support to the hypothesis that 5-HT is an important mediator of migraine. Furthermore, brainstem nuclei activated during migraine have high densities of serotonergic neurons. Specific 5-HT receptor subtypes, 5-HT_{1B} and 5-HT_{1D}, are largely distributed in blood vessels[27] and nerves,[28] respectively. These same 5-HT receptor subtypes are the targets of antimigraine drugs such as the triptans and ergot alkaloids.

Genetics

A familial predisposition for migraine has been well recognized, although not until recent advances in gene mapping techniques has the genetic basis of a specific migraine disorder been discovered. The first identified migraine gene was found among several unrelated families with familial hemiplegic migraine. The mutations involved a gene encoding the α_1 subunit of a voltage-gated P/Q-type neuronal calcium channel.[29] The relevance of this discovery to other migrainous disorders is unknown, but it suggests that some forms of migraine may be fundamentally related to other episodic disorders of neurologic dysfunction known as "channelopathies."[11] Recently, genomewide linkage analysis in families with migraine (both with and without aura) have identified susceptibility loci on chromosomes 4 and 14.[30,31] An improved understanding of the genetics of migraine is likely to improve our understanding of the pathophysiology of the disorder as well as to hold promise for the identification of homogenous subgroups of patients in whom targeted drug (or other) interventions are likely to be highly effective.

In summary, the pathophysiology of migraine probably involves dysfunction of the trigeminal neurons that provide sensory innervation and modulate blood flow for intracranial blood vessels. The endogenous stimulus causing this dysfunction may arise from a "migraine generator" in the brainstem. Disturbances in 5-HT activity are also probably involved and it is this feature that serves as the target for many migraine-specific therapies.

Signs and Symptoms

Migraine With and Without Aura

1. K.L., a 29-year-old woman, presents to the clinic with a 5-month history of left-sided pulsatile head pain recurring on a weekly basis. Her headaches are usually preceded by unformed flashes of light bilaterally and a sensation of light-headedness. The ensuing pain is always unilateral and is commonly associated with nausea, vomiting, and photophobia. The headache is not relieved by two tablets of either aspirin 325 mg or ibuprofen 200 mg and generally lasts all day unless she is able to lie in a dark room and sleep. The headaches usually interfere with her ability to continue work. K.L. is unable to identify any external factors that precipitate a migraine attack. Both K.L.'s mother and grandmother also were affected by migraine headaches. Medical history is unremarkable, and K.L. denies any other medical problems. Current medications include only the OTC analgesics for headache and the contraceptive, Ortho-Novum 7/7/7. General physical and neurologic examinations are within normal limits. What subjective and objective data from the above description are consistent with a diagnosis of migraine with aura?

Given K.L.'s headache description, normal physical examination, and age of onset, she is most likely suffering from migraine with aura; a benign, though often disabling, disorder.

Approximately 17% of females and 6% of males in the United States suffer from migraine headaches,[1] and the incidence and prevalence of migraine has increased in recent decades.[32,33] The typical age of onset of migraine headaches is 15 to 35 years; after the age of 50, the onset of new migraine headaches is less common and is suggestive of a secondary cause. Although influenced by physiologic and environmental factors, migraine headaches occur more frequently among first-degree relatives, suggesting a genetic basis for this disorder.[33] K.L.'s gender (female), age (29 years), and positive family history are compatible with these aspects of migraine.

In the assessment of headache, the site or location of the pain, the quality of the pain, the duration and time course of the pain, and the conditions that provoke or palliate the pain should be considered.

The site or location of head pain can provide the clinician with clues as to the potential for secondary causes (e.g., lesions in the frontal sinuses, eyes, ears, teeth, or cerebral arteries). However, pain often is referred from other regions and the location of pain can provide misleading information. Thus, the site of head pain need not be related to the apparent site of the focal neurologic symptoms that accompany migraine with aura. Head pain may be either unilateral or bilateral, and the pain need not recur on the same side if unilateral. In fact, 50% of patients with unilateral headache report that either side of the head may be affected during any individual migraine attack.[34]

The quality of migraine head pain usually begins as a dull ache that intensifies over a period of minutes or hours to a throbbing headache, which worsens with each arterial pulse. If untreated, the headache lasts from several hours to as long as 3 days or until the patient goes to sleep. The pain usually is intense enough to interfere with daily activities. Although migraine headaches seldom occur more often than once every few weeks, there is great interpatient variability in the frequency of occurrence. A patient may experience only several migraines in a lifetime, whereas others may suffer several headaches weekly on a chronic basis. K.L., like half of all patients with migraine, describes headaches that recur between one to four times monthly.[34] In this patient, the quality of the pain (i.e., interferes with K.L.'s ability to continue work); the duration and the time course of the pain (i.e., usually lasts all day); and the conditions that palliate the pain (i.e., lie in a dark room and sleep) are all compatible with the description of migraine headaches.

Aura symptoms are focal neurologic features that precede or accompany the headache in up to 30% of migraine sufferers.[35] When they precede the headache, aura symptoms usually begin 10 minutes to 1 hour before the onset of head pain. Lightheadedness and photopsia (unformed flashes of light) are frequently reported and were described by K.L. before the onset of her head pain. Visual disturbances, such as scotoma (an isolated area within the visual field where vision is absent), occur in 30% of migraine patients.[35] At times, the scotoma is preceded only by a sensation that something is wrong with vision that cannot be more specifically characterized. At other times, the scotoma may be preceded by other visual distortions (e.g., the "halves of peoples' faces were vertically displaced in such a way that one eye appeared to be 1 or 2 cm lower than the other").[36] When scotomata are surrounded by a shiny pattern, they are termed *scintillating scotomata.* These scintillating scotomata can have "the visual quality of images in the kaleidoscopes we looked into as children, with the difference that the scotoma are silvery instead of multicolored as in the toy."[36] Other neurologic symptoms of cortical origin (e.g., paresthesias, temporal lobe symptoms) occur less commonly in patients who suffer from migraine with aura. K.L.'s physical and neurologic examinations were within normal limits. The nausea and vomiting that were experienced by K.L. accompany migraine headaches (with or without aura) in 90% of patients. Vomiting is occasionally followed by a gradual resolution of migraine symptoms. Diarrhea may also occur.

In summary, K.L.'s history and relative lack of important physical findings are compatible with a diagnosis of migraine with aura.

Diagnostic Tests

2. What further laboratory or diagnostic tests should be ordered for K.L.?

Headaches are common medical complaints and evaluation of these headaches with sophisticated diagnostic procedures (e.g., computed tomography [CT], magnetic resonance imaging [MRI] scans) are generally unnecessary in the uncomplicated migraine patient. Because K.L.'s headaches are not of recent origin, not progressive, and unassociated with traumatic injury or persistent neurologic deficits, CT or MRI scanning procedures should be unnecessary. Her headaches are unaccompanied by fever or nuchal rigidity, and she does not present with headache described as being "the worst headache of my life." Therefore, a lumbar puncture would not likely be of diagnostic value because meningitis or subarachnoid hemorrhage is unlikely. The signs and symptoms experienced by K.L., as described in the answer to Question 1, are typical of migraine with aura. The most important diagnostic evaluations of patients presenting with headache should be based on a thorough medical history and physical examination. The role of costly or invasive diagnostic procedures is limited to their usefulness in detecting other more serious disorders that may manifest as migrainous headache.

Therapeutic Considerations

3. What should be the general approach to the treatment of K.L.'s headache attacks?

The concept that moderate to severe headaches can be classified into distinct types with unrelated pathophysiologic features is probably incorrect. Patients commonly complain of more than one type of headache or report symptoms or recurrence patterns that are inconsistent with a single diagnosis. Because the selection of therapy is based primarily on the characteristics of headache gathered from the history, the practitioner needs to be flexible in the choice of treatments when the features do not fit within classic definitions. Even for patients with well-defined headache types, specific therapies may alleviate pain in only 50% to 80% of patients. Still, with careful monitoring of therapeutic response and optimization of effective treatments, patients with a wide variety of headache complaints can be successfully managed with relatively few drugs.

Abortive Therapy

The general approach to treatment of acute migraine headache attacks is one of pharmacotherapy aimed at relieving migraine headache pain and associated symptoms. Such a treatment plan may include (a) 5-HT receptor agonists (e.g., triptans or ergot derivatives), (b) analgesics, (c) sedatives, and (d) antiemetic drug therapy, depending on the exact nature of the patient's complaint. The selection of a specific treatment should be based on the level of disability and associated symptoms such as nausea and vomiting. This "stratified care" approach is preferred over a "step care" approach that may begin with agents that are likely to be ineffective for the patient's headache.[37] This latter approach, when applied to all patients regardless of headache severity, only serves to delay effective therapy in many people.[38]

Aggravating Factors

Clinicians should always search for factors that might precipitate migraine attacks in their patients before initiating drug therapy. Although K.L. could not associate her migraine attacks with any external events, the factors listed in Table 52-3 should be discussed with her in hopes that their elimination or avoidance may improve her headaches. However, complete relief, even in patients who can clearly identify such precipitants, is unlikely.

ORAL CONTRACEPTIVES

4. K.L. recalls being told by her gynecologist that headaches are a possible side effect of oral contraceptive use. She initially started oral contraceptives 2 years ago and did not associate the

Table 52-3 Factors That May Precipitate Migraine Headache

Stress
Emotion
Glare
Hypoglycemia
Altered sleep pattern
Menses
Exercise
Alcohol
Carbon monoxide
Excess caffeine use or withdrawal
Foods containing:
MSG (e.g., Chinese food, canned soups, seasonings)
Tyramine (e.g., red wine, ripened cheeses)
Nitrites (e.g., cured meat products)
Phenylethylamine (e.g., chocolate, cheese)
Aspartame (e.g., artificial sweeteners, diet sodas)
Drugs
Excess use or withdrawal (ergots, triptans, analgesics)
Estrogens (e.g., oral contraceptives)
Cocaine
Nitroglycerin

MSG, monosodium glutamate.

medication with the recent onset of migraine attacks. Why should the discontinuation of Ortho-Novum 7/7/7 be considered in K.L.?

Oral contraceptives may either worsen or precipitate migraine attacks in women without a previous history of this problem.[39] Although headaches usually arise within the first few months of oral contraceptive use, headaches developing after several years have been described.[40] The adverse effect of oral contraceptives on migraine headaches is likely related to the estrogen content. The use of a lower-potency estrogen product decreases the frequency of migraine attacks in some women. Migraine with aura is an independent risk factor for stroke in women, with the highest risk found among those younger than 45 years of age.[41] No consistent increased risk for stroke has been found among men, women older than 45 years old, and women who have migraine without aura.[39] Use of oral contraceptives increases the risk of stroke even further. Adjusted odds ratios for stroke risk in women with migraine are 4 for oral contraceptives containing >50 mcg estrogen and 2 for oral contraceptives containing <50 mcg estrogen.[39] Several groups recommend against the use of estrogen-containing contraceptives in many women with migraine.[39a] K.L. should be counseled about her increased risk for stroke and the options for alternative birth control methods. She can then make an informed decision regarding whether or not to continue oral contraceptives. When oral contraceptives are discontinued, 30% to 40% of women[42] notice an improvement in their headaches, although several months may elapse before a benefit is realized.[43] If K.L. elects to discontinue oral contraceptives an alternative form of birth control should be recommended, and the frequency of her headaches should be monitored to detect an improvement in this problem.

Abortive Therapy Triptans (5-HT$_{1B/1D}$ Receptor Agonists)

5. What would be an appropriate drug of first choice for the treatment of K.L.'s acute headaches?

Agents in the triptan class (sumatriptan, zolmitriptan, naratriptan, rizatriptan, almotriptan, frovatriptan and eletriptan) are effective and well tolerated relative to other agents used for the abortive treatment of acute migraine headaches. Consequently, triptans are appropriate initial therapy for patients with moderate to severe migraine headaches who have no contraindications to their use. Introduction of these agents has had a dramatic effect on the successful relief of disabling headache in many patients. Before this, ergot alkaloids (e.g., ergotamine tartrate) were the preferred agents for migraine headaches when non-narcotic analgesics were ineffective.

Unlike ergotamine, which needs to be taken at the earliest sign of a migraine attack for maximal benefit, the triptans are effective when given 4 hours or longer after the onset of headache.[44] However, they are more expensive than ergotamine. For this reason, some prescribers and health plans reserve the triptans for patients who are unresponsive or intolerant to less expensive alternatives (e.g., ergotamine, NSAIDs). Pharmacoeconomic studies have suggested an advantage of triptan agents over nontriptan medications when costs are considered from a societal perspective (i.e., take into account lost work productivity in addition to health care costs).[45]

Unlike the ergot alkaloids, which stimulate serotonergic, dopaminergic, and noradrenergic receptors, the triptans have selective agonist activity at 5-HT$_{1B/1D}$ subtype receptors. This feature is likely responsible for the improved tolerability profile for these agents. There are three proposed mechanisms for the effectiveness of the triptans in acute migraine headache: (a) reducing the excitability of neurons in the trigeminovascular system via stimulation of brainstem 5-HT$_{1B/1D}$ receptors, (b) attenuating the release of neuropeptides with inflammatory and vasodilating properties (e.g., CGRP, substance P, and neurokinin A) via a presynaptic 5-HT$_{1D}$ receptor effect, and (c) vasoconstriction of cerebral and extracerebral vessels by stimulation of vascular 5-HT$_{1B}$ receptors.[35] The coronary vasculature also contains 5-HT$_{1B}$ receptors; thus, these agents have the potential to cause coronary artery vasoconstriction. For this reason, patients with coronary artery disease and uncontrolled hypertension were excluded from premarketing clinical trials, and the triptans are contraindicated in these patients. Sumatriptan (Imitrex) was the first triptan approved for use, and it is the prototype against which the other "second-generation" triptans are compared. Table 52-4 compares the triptans with regard to selected clinical and pharmacokinetic features.

SUMATRIPTAN

Sumatriptan (Imitrex) is a structural analog of 5-HT that was introduced in 1993 for the abortive treatment of migraine headache (Fig. 52-1). Available formulations include an injection pen device for subcutaneous self-administration, oral tablets, and a nasal spray. All of these formulations (including a rectal formulation not available in the United States) reduce the severity of migraine headache and improve associated symptoms such as nausea, vomiting, photophobia, and phonophobia.[45] The choice of dosage form depends on the intensity of the headache and the presence of severe nausea. For patients who are nauseated and prone to vomit during an acute attack, the subcutaneous and intranasal dosage forms are preferred. Both formulations have a rapid onset of effect. Reduction in headache intensity is reported within 10 minutes after subcutaneous injection and within 15 minutes after administration of the nasal spray.[46] Clinical response is delayed after oral administration of sumatriptan tablets,[46] but this dosage

Table 52-4 Clinical and Pharmacokinetic Features of the Triptans for Acute Migraine Headache[60]

Drug	Route	Bioavailability (%)	T-max (hr)	Half-Life (hr)	Response Rate at 2 hr (%)	HA Recurrence Within 24–48 hr (%)	Dose/ Attack (mg)	Maximum Dose in 24 hr (mg)
Sumatriptan (Imitrex)	PO	14	1.2–2.3	2	50–69	25–41	25–100	200
	IN	–	1–1.5	2	62–78	10–40	20–40	40
	SC	96	0.2	2	63–82	10–40	6–12	12
Zolmitriptan (Zomig)	PO	40–46	1.5	2.5–3	62–67	22–37	2.5–10	10
	IN	100	3	2.5–3	69		5–10	10
Naratriptan (Amerge)	PO	60–70	3–5	6	43–49	17–28	1–5	5
Rizatriptan (Maxalt)	PO	40–45	1.3	1.8	60–77	35–47	5–20	30
Almotriptan (Axert)	PO	70	1–3	3–4	55–65	18–30	6.25–25	25
Frovatriptan (Frova)	PO	20–30	2–4	26	37–46	7–25	2.5–5	7.5
Eletriptan (Relpax)	PO	50	2	4	47–65	6–34	20–40	80

HA, headache; IN, intranasal; PO, oral; SC, subcutaneous.
Adapted from reference 60.

form is more convenient and preferred by many patients. During migraine attacks, the gastrointestinal absorption of many drugs is delayed.[47] This may contribute to the faster onset of action of the nonoral dosage forms of sumatriptan and other drugs.

The efficacy of the triptans has been evaluated using the primary endpoint of headache response (reduction in headache intensity to mild pain or no pain) at 2 hours. Response rates for sumatriptan vary from 50% to 82% (see Table 52-4). Subcutaneous injection is associated with higher response rates than non-parenteral routes of administration. Comparative trials with other antimigraine therapies also support the efficacy of sumatriptan. Subcutaneous sumatriptan is more effective and faster acting than dihydroergotamine (DHE) nasal spray.[48] When compared with subcutaneous DHE, subcutaneous sumatriptan is more effective at 1 and 2 hours, but the two treatments are equally effective at 3 and 4 hours.[49] In this trial, headache recurrence rates at 24 hours favored subcutaneous DHE.[49] Studies of oral sumatriptan show this treatment is more effective than both ergotamine 2 mg with caffeine 200 mg[50] and aspirin 900 mg plus metoclopramide 10 mg.[51]

Adverse Effects

Sumatriptan is usually well tolerated, and this feature offers a significant advantage over ergot alkaloids in many patients.

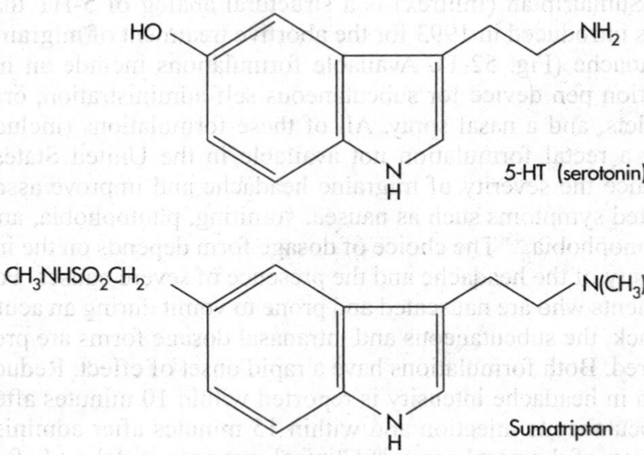

FIGURE 52-1 Structures of 5-HT (serotonin) and sumatriptan.

After oral administration, the most common adverse effects of sumatriptan include nausea and vomiting (which could be related to the migraine itself), malaise, and dizziness. Intranasal sumatriptan is associated with a bitter, unpleasant taste in most patients. Adverse effects following subcutaneous sumatriptan are more common and more uncomfortable than those following oral or intranasal administration. The most common adverse events after subcutaneous administration are mild pain or redness at the site of injection.[52] These injection site reactions occur in 40% of patients and usually resolve within 60 minutes.[52] Symptoms of chest pressure or tightness (sometimes extending to the throat) have been reported in 3% to 5% of patients treated with oral or subcutaneous sumatriptan in controlled trials.[52] However, a questionnaire-based study of 453 users of sumatriptan found a much higher incidence—42% of subcutaneous sumatriptan users and 26% of oral sumatriptan users reported chest symptoms in almost all of their sumatriptan-treated migraine attacks.[53] These symptoms are usually mild, resolve within 2 hours, and are unrelated to cardiac ischemia. However, they are uncomfortable enough that 7% to 12% of patients discontinue the drug based on these symptoms.[53] Although chest symptoms are rarely serious, sumatriptan has been associated with vascular events, including coronary vasospasm,[54] angina,[55] myocardial infarction,[56] and stroke.[57] These adverse events usually occur in patients with coronary artery disease or significant risk factors. However, myocardial infarction was reported in one otherwise healthy young woman after sumatriptan.[58] Because of potential vasoconstrictive effects, sumatriptan should not be used in patients with uncontrolled hypertension, peripheral or cerebral vascular disease, coronary artery disease, previous myocardial infarction, Prinzmetal's angina, or coronary vasospasm. For patients with risk factors of coronary artery disease but who are otherwise deemed appropriate for sumatriptan, the first dose should be administered in a physician's office or an area in which medical support in available.

Headache Recurrence

Another complication of sumatriptan use is recurrent migraine headache. In 25% to 40% of patients, migraine headache recurs within 24 hours after initial successful treatment with sumatriptan.[59] This phenomenon may be related to the short half-life of the drug, and the recurrent headache often responds to a repeat dose of sumatriptan.[60]

Drug Interactions

Although few drug interactions have been reported with sumatriptan, concomitant use with ergot alkaloids, lithium, serotonin-specific reuptake inhibitors (SSRIs), other triptans, and monoamine oxidase (MAO) inhibitors is not recommended because of the potential for precipitating the serotonin syndrome.[45] However, several reports describe the safe use of sumatriptan in conjunction with MAO-B inhibitors, SSRIs, and lithium, and clinical evidence of adverse effects is minimal.[61–63] The potential risks and benefits should be considered when these therapies are used in combination.

Dosing

The recommended dosage of sumatriptan varies according to the route of administration. The initial dose of subcutaneous sumatriptan is 6 mg. If there is no relief within 1 hour, the dose can be repeated. Initial doses of oral and intranasal sumatriptan are 25 to 100 mg and 5 to 20 mg, respectively. These doses may be repeated if there is no relief within 2 hours. When migraine headache recurs after an initial positive response, a repeat dose is often effective. However, the maximum doses in a 24-hour period listed in Table 52-4 should not be exceeded.

SECOND-GENERATION TRIPTANS (ZOLMITRIPTAN, NARATRIPTAN, RIZATRIPTAN, ALMOTRIPTAN, FROVATRIPTAN, ELETRIPTAN)

Since the introduction of sumatriptan, several second-generation triptan agents have been approved for the acute treatment of migraine. In general, these agents have similar pharmacologic features (all are 5-$HT_{1B/1D}$ receptor agonists), and improved oral bioavailability over sumatriptan. Although these agents have similar pharmacologic effects on 5-HT receptors, patients who fail to respond to one triptan may respond to another agent in this class. Like sumatriptan, second-generation triptans also have potential vasoconstrictive effects on coronary arteries. The pharmacokinetic and clinical effects of the second-generation triptans are shown in Table 52-4.

All second-generation triptans have been shown to be superior to placebo for acute migraine relief. Fewer studies compare one agent to another. A recent meta-analysis of 53 controlled clinical trials compared the second-generation triptans with sumatriptan 100 mg orally with regard to efficacy, consistency of relief, and tolerability.[44,64] Rizatriptan (Maxalt) 10 mg and eletriptan (Relpax) 80 mg were significantly more effective than sumatriptan 100 mg in headache response at 2 hours; naratriptan (Amerge) 2.5 mg, eletriptan 20 mg and frovatriptan (Frova) 2.5 were significantly less effective. Agents were also compared with regard to the percentage of patients with sustained freedom from headache (i.e., no pain at 2 hours, no requirement for rescue medication, and no headache recurrence within 24 hours). Compared with sumatriptan 100 mg, response rates were higher for rizatriptan 10 mg, eletriptan 80 mg and almotriptan (Axert) 12.5 mg, and lower for eletriptan 20 mg. The consistency of therapeutic effect across multiple attacks was also compared. Rizatriptan 10 mg provided more consistent relief than sumatriptan 100 mg. Differences between the triptans in tolerability were generally small. However, the adverse effect rates of naratriptan 2.5 mg and almotriptan 12.5 mg were lower than that for sumatriptan 100 mg.[44,64] Although comparison of drugs based on results from different trials may not be reliable, the results of head-to-head comparison studies were consistent with those from single triptan studies when results were pooled for meta-analysis.[64]

Drug Interactions

The metabolism of rizatriptan and zolmitriptan (Zomig) is reduced by MAO inhibitors (particularly MAO-A inhibitors). Thus, like sumatriptan, rizatriptan and zolmitriptan should be avoided in patients taking MAO inhibitors. Propranolol reduces the metabolic clearance of frovatriptan, zolmitriptan, rizatriptan and eletriptan to varying extents. The clinical significance of these interactions is unknown but increased exposure to these triptans should be considered in patients concomitantly receiving propranolol. Inhibitors of CYP3A4 reduce the clearance of almotriptan and eletriptan. For almotriptan, increased exposure to triptans should be anticipated, however no specific dosing adjustments are proposed. The interaction between eletriptan and CYP3A4 inhibitors is more significant, and particular precautions are necessary. Eletriptan should not be used within 72 hours of treatment with potent CYP3A4 inhibitors (e.g., ketoconazole, itraconazole, nefazodone, troleandomycin, clarithromycin, ritonavir and nelfinavir). As with sumatriptan, there is potential concern regarding the coadministration of second generation triptans and SSRIs. Weakness, hyperreflexia and incoordination have been reported when 5-$HT_{1B/1D}$ agonists are administered to patients taking SSRIs. These potential adverse effects should be considered in patients who require both classes of medication.

Precautions regarding the use of second generation triptans in patients with known or suspected cardiovascular disease are similar to those for sumatriptan and should be strictly followed (see Sumatriptan, Adverse Effects).

All second-generation triptans are available as oral tablets. Rizatriptan and zolmitriptan are also available as oral disintegrating tablets that are placed on the tongue where they dissolve and are swallowed with saliva. Patients who receive these formulations (Maxalt-MLT, Zomig-ZMT) should be told to handle the tablet with dry hands. Zolmitriptan is also available as a nasal spray.

K.L.'s migraine headaches are of moderate to severe intensity (her activities of daily living are negatively affected) and do not respond to moderate doses of aspirin and ibuprofen. Triptans (including sumatriptan and second-generation agents) are appropriate initial antimigraine agents for patients such as K.L. Although her headaches are frequently associated with nausea and vomiting, it is not clear whether these symptoms occur soon after the onset of the attack or whether they evolve gradually as the migraine progresses. If vomiting occurs early, a nonoral route of administration should be considered. Subcutaneous or intranasal sumatriptan are appropriate therapy options. If K.L.'s migraines evolve gradually after the onset of her aura symptoms, then an oral triptan may provide sufficiently rapid relief to be effective. Most patients prefer the convenience of oral dosing. The initial choice of a triptan for oral administration can be made based on cost, pharmacokinetic features and familiarity of the prescriber.

6. Ortho-Novum 7/7/7 was discontinued, and K.L. was fitted for a diaphragm and given instructions on its proper use. She was also given a prescription for sumatriptan 50 mg and told to

take one tablet at the onset of her aura symptoms. At her follow-up clinic visit 2 months later, K.L. reported inconsistent relief from migraine headache with sumatriptan. She experienced six headaches over the past 2 months. The first attack responded to a single dose of sumatriptan 50 mg. The next three migraine attacks failed to respond to the first dose, but responded when she took another 50-mg tablet of sumatriptan 2 hours after the first. However, K.L. is concerned that she is becoming "tolerant" to this medication and has been hesitant to take more than one tablet of sumatriptan for subsequent migraines. Is tolerance a concern with the triptan agents? Should K.L. be changed to another triptan for acute relief of her migraine headaches?

Although there can be some inconsistency in response when triptans are used to treat multiple migraine attacks, the gradual development of tolerance in patients who experience an initial favorable effect is uncommon and not expected. Patients who experience relief after treatment of several migraines with the same dose of a triptan usually continue to experience similar relief over long periods of time.[53] Thus, K.L. need not avoid taking sumatriptan (at an effective dosage) because of concerns regarding headache tolerance. In those instances when K.L. experienced adequate relief of her migraine attacks, she usually required two doses of sumatriptan 50 mg. Given this response pattern, she should be encouraged to take 100 mg of sumatriptan at the onset of her migraines in the future. Potential adverse effects should again be discussed with K.L., and she should be informed that these side effects might be more significant with the higher initial dose. However, most patients who tolerate an initial dose of sumatriptan 50 mg are able to tolerate 100 mg as well. At this time, there is no need to consider an alternate triptan for K.L. However, if she is intolerant of sumatriptan 100 mg, then alternate agents such as naratriptan or almotriptan could be considered. However, naratriptan generally has a slower onset of effect than other triptans, and this may be a disadvantage for K.L. If, at a future visit, K.L. is not obtaining adequate relief from sumatriptan 100 mg (followed by an additional dose at 2 hours), then rizatriptan 10 mg should be considered as initial treatment for her migraines. Although eletriptan 80 mg also was superior to sumatriptan 100 mg for migraine response at 2 hours in the meta-analysis discussed above, this dose of eletriptan is higher than that recommended by the manufacturer for initial treatment.[44]

Ergotamine Tartrate

7. What is the role of ergotamine tartrate in the acute treatment of migraine headaches?

Ergotamine tartrate (Bellergal-S, Cafergot) has been used since 1925 for the acute treatment of migraine headaches. Before the availability of agents in the triptan class, ergotamine was widely considered the drug of choice when non-narcotic analgesics were ineffective. The major advantages of this agent are low cost and long history of experience with its use. However, adverse effects of ergotamine are common and potentially serious, particularly when the drug is used in excessive doses or for prolonged periods.[42] Furthermore, the strength and quality of evidence for ergotamine in acute migraine therapy is less than that for the triptans.[38] For these reasons, triptans are often preferred as initial therapy. About 50% to 70% of migraine sufferers benefit from ergotamine given during an acute attack.[65] Ergotamine is highly specific for migraine and cluster headaches; only occasionally are other types of headaches affected by this drug.

Ergotamine and other ergot derivatives (e.g., dihydroergotamine [DHE]) have numerous pharmacologic effects. However, their precise mechanism of action in migraine is unknown. These drugs are agonists at numerous 5-HT_1 receptor subtypes (5-HT_{1A}, 5-HT_{1B}, 5-HT_{1D}, 5-HT_{1F}), 5-HT_2, adrenergic, and dopaminergic receptors.[42] Ergotamine has both venous and arterial vasoconstrictive effects. Although it has been presumed that ergot alkaloids relieve migraine by their cerebral vasoconstrictive effects, experimental evidence does not support this as the sole mechanism.[66] Ergotamine and dihydroergotamine block inflammation of the trigeminal neurovascular system, presumably by inhibiting the release of the neuropeptides discussed above (see Pathophysiology). This action, possibly mediated by 5-HT receptor effects, may be responsible for both the pain-relieving and vasoconstrictive effects of the ergot alkaloids.

Ergotamine should be given at the first sign of a migraine attack in a dosage that is effective and acceptable to the patient. If administration is delayed until the headache is firmly established, ergotamine is rarely effective and other therapies (e.g., DHE, triptans, or narcotic analgesics) are usually required.

CAFFEINE

8. Why is caffeine added to some ergotamine products (e.g., Cafergot)?

Caffeine is combined with ergotamine in several preparations and was originally added to potentiate the vasoconstrictive properties of ergotamine.[67] Subsequent studies have shown that caffeine improves intestinal ergotamine absorption[68] and potentiates the pain relief properties of analgesics.[69] However, it should be kept in mind that caffeine's stimulant effect may prevent sleep, which is beneficial to many migraine sufferers.

9. How do different ergotamine dosage forms compare with each other? What is the usual dosage of ergotamine for acute migraine?

ROUTE OF ADMINISTRATION

Ergotamine tartrate is available for oral, sublingual, rectal, or parenteral use. The rate and extent of drug absorption are erratic following oral, sublingual, and rectal administration. The rectal and sublingual routes of administration bypass the portal circulation, avoid first-pass metabolism, and are more bioavailable than the oral route of administration. However, documentation of improved efficacy is lacking.[70,71] A metered-dose inhaler containing ergotamine tartrate was previously marketed in the United States, but this product has been withdrawn.

When ergotamine is prescribed, the sublingual preparation is often preferred because it is convenient to use and has a faster onset of action than oral ergotamine.[72] Acute migraine attacks also are associated with decreased gastric motility.[73] This phenomenon is presumably responsible for the impaired oral absorption of aspirin and ergotamine when given during an acute migraine attack.[47,74] Delayed drug absorption during a migraine attack occurs independent of associated nausea or vomiting and is primarily related to headache severity.[75] In patients who do not respond to oral or sublingual dosage forms, a trial with ergotamine rectal suppositories may be successful.[75]

Some studies report higher rates of success with rectal administration of ergotamine (i.e., about 70%) than with the oral or sublingual routes of administration (about 50%–60% effective).[76] This difference may be due to improved bioavailability of ergotamine when administered rectally.[77] The usual ergotamine dosage (when given by either oral, sublingual, or rectal routes) is 1 to 4 mg given immediately and followed by 1 to 2 mg at 30-minute intervals to a maximum of 6 mg/attack or 10 mg/week. Also, the use of ergotamine should be limited to no more than twice per week to reduce the risk of chronic ergot-related adverse effects (see Question 11).[42]

CONTRAINDICATIONS

10. What are the contraindications to the use of an ergotamine-containing product?

Contraindications to the use of ergot alkaloids include cardiac, peripheral, and cerebral vascular disease; sepsis; liver and kidney disease; pregnancy; breast-feeding; and concomitant use of triacetyloleandomycin or erythromycin.[65] The latter drugs can inhibit the metabolism of ergotamine and may potentiate the toxicity of this agent.[78] The vasoconstrictive effects of ergotamine can be particularly harmful to the patient with these pre-existing conditions. Some sources cite hypertension as a contraindication to ergotamine use, but this is controversial. The usual therapeutic doses of ergotamine used for migraine therapy have minimal effects on blood pressure, and hypertension need not be a strict contraindication to its occasional use.[79]

Concerns about using ergotamine during the aura of migraine when focal neurologic deficits may be due to cerebral ischemia have not been validated. Human studies have found no alteration in regional cerebral blood flow after parenteral administration of either ergotamine or dihydroergotamine and their use during the prodrome is not contraindicated.[66,80,81] Occasionally, patients experience a prolonged aura or more prominent neurologic symptoms with ergotamine use. In these individuals, ergotamine use should not be continued.[42]

ADVERSE EFFECTS

11. What adverse effects should be monitored for in patients who receive ergotamine?

Gastrointestinal (GI) disturbances can be a limiting factor to the use of ergotamine for headache therapy. Nausea, vomiting, and anorexia are common, dose-dependent ergotamine adverse effects, which may worsen the GI symptoms that commonly accompany acute migraine headaches. These GI symptoms after ergotamine use are likely the result of central dopamine receptor agonism at the chemoreceptor trigger zone. Because these effects are centrally mediated, they can occur after administration of ergotamine by any bioavailable route. Patients are reluctant to continue therapy if their initial experience with the medication has been unpleasant. Therefore, patients should be educated as to the potential for this adverse effect.

Clinicians can also take measures to minimize migraine-associated and ergotamine-induced GI upset. One useful technique is to determine the smallest dose of ergotamine that will elicit GI distress in a patient during a headache-free interval. For example, if the suppository form of ergotamine is being used, the patient can be instructed to insert one-fourth of a suppository at hourly intervals until nausea develops. The total dosage is then reduced by one-fourth of a suppository and used as the initial dose for subsequent migraine attacks.[79] The same technique can be used for patients using oral or sublingual ergotamine by splitting the tablets in half.

The peripheral vasoconstrictive effects of ergotamine most commonly involve the lower extremities and are often characterized by coldness, decreased distal pulses, and a tingling sensation. Continuous paresthesias, limb pain, venous thrombosis, or gangrene necessitating amputation are more severe consequences of ergotamine therapy.[82] Although some of these symptoms may occur with therapeutic doses in hypersensitive individuals, they are most commonly associated with overdose or excessive therapeutic use of ergotamine. Beta-adrenergic receptor blocking agents, commonly used in migraine prophylaxis, occasionally can potentiate the vasoconstrictive effects of ergotamine.[83,84] Their concomitant use is not contraindicated, but patients should be closely monitored for the signs and symptoms of peripheral vasoconstriction.

Rebound headache after discontinuation of long-term, daily ergotamine use is another common adverse effect. These rebound headaches respond to larger ergotamine doses, but ultimately the headaches become more frequent and other symptoms of ergotamine overuse become apparent (e.g., symptoms of peripheral vascular insufficiency). This cycle of overmedication and resultant headaches can render patients refractory to other forms of headache treatment.[85]

ANTIEMETICS

12. What is the role of antiemetic therapy for the outpatient treatment of migraine-associated nausea and vomiting?

In most patients, triptan agents provide effective relief of migraine-associated nausea. Therefore, specific antiemetic therapy usually is not required. However, as mentioned above, persistent nausea is more common in patients who use ergotamine for acute migraine therapy. In these patients, and in triptan-treated patients who experience incomplete nausea relief, adjunctive antiemetic therapy should be considered. Phenothiazine antiemetics can provide symptomatic relief from nausea; however, they can also reduce GI motility and further impair absorption of medication taken orally.[86] Metoclopramide (Reglan) is the antiemetic of choice in migraine.[87] The recommended dose is 10 mg taken orally as soon as possible. Although the drug has no direct antimigraine effect,[88] it does provide symptomatic relief from nausea and vomiting while enhancing the oral absorption of medications taken during the migraine attack.[86] Unfortunately, metoclopramide is not available in a suppository dosage form.

13. In addition to the triptans and ergotamine tartrate, what other abortive agents are available for outpatient treatment of acute migraine headache?

In the stratified care approach, isometheptene compound, NSAIDs, and combination analgesics are reasonable treatment options for patients with mild-to-moderate migraine headaches or those with severe attacks that have responded to these agents in the past.[38] Dihydroergotamine nasal spray is indicated for moderate-to-severe migraine headache.[38]

Isometheptene Compound

Isometheptene, a sympathomimetic amine, is combined with acetaminophen and a sedative (dichloralphenazone) in the product of Midrin. This combination is as effective as oral ergotamine in the treatment of acute migraine headaches[89,90] and, in many patients, better tolerated. Although the contraindications to Midrin are similar to those of ergotamine, severe adverse effects are less common. Patients unresponsive to ergotamine products occasionally respond to Midrin. In patients with mild to moderate migraine, isometheptene compound provides comparable relief to sumatriptan 25 mg given orally.[91] The usual dosage of Midrin is two capsules taken immediately followed by one additional capsule every hour until the headache is relieved. Subsequent migraine attacks can be managed by administering the same total dose of Midrin that was effective in treating the previous headache, but no more than five Midrin capsules should be taken within a 12-hour period.[89]

Nonsteroidal Anti-Inflammatory Drugs and Combination Analgesics

Many NSAIDs and combination analgesics containing caffeine have been shown to be effective for the acute treatment of migraine headache.[92] Significant clinical benefit in double-blind, placebo-controlled trials has been shown for aspirin, ibuprofen, naproxen sodium, and combination analgesics containing acetaminophen, aspirin, and caffeine.[38] Selected NSAIDs (e.g., naproxen sodium, ketoprofen, diclofenac potassium) are as effective as ergotamine[93–95] or sumatriptan[93] in the relief of migraine headache. However, consistent differences among NSAIDs in migraine therapy have not been demonstrated. If NSAIDs are to be used in the abortive treatment of migraine, the concomitant administration of metoclopramide can enhance their absorption, providing more effective and rapid pain relief.[47,96]

Dihydroergotamine Nasal Spray

A nasal spray formulation of dihydroergotamine (DHE) (Migranal) is available for abortive therapy of migraine. Previously, this agent was available for parenteral use only and was usually restricted to use in clinic and emergency department (ED) settings (see Intractable Migraine). DHE is less likely than ergotamine to cause severe nausea and vomiting, and it is a less potent arterial vasoconstrictor.[97] In clinical trials, DHE nasal spray is more effective than placebo in relieving pain (beginning as early as 30 minutes after treatment) and reducing post-treatment nausea.[98–100] In an unpublished, active control trial, DHE nasal spray was equally effective and better tolerated than an ergotamine/caffeine combination product (Cafergot).[101] Patients given this treatment should self-administer one spray (1 mg) into each nostril followed in 15 minutes by an additional spray in each nostril for a total of four sprays (4 mg). DHE nasal spray is reasonable to consider as an initial agent for moderate to severe migraine headache.[38]

Intractable Migraine

14. K.L. used sumatriptan 100 mg PO for her next two migraine headache attacks and obtained good relief. K.L. experienced another headache with severe nausea. She took sumatriptan 100 mg PO but vomited immediately thereafter, and the headache continued to worsen throughout the day until she could no longer work. K.L. was taken to the ED by a friend. The diagnosis of intractable migraine was made. How should K.L. be treated?

Dihydroergotamine

Intractable migraine with associated vomiting usually requires parenteral therapy with ergot derivatives, sumatriptan, or potent narcotic analgesics. DHE-45, 1 mg subcutaneously[102] or intramuscularly[103] or 0.75 mg intravenously,[104] is particularly effective in the treatment of acute and intractable migraine headaches and thereby reduces the necessity for narcotic analgesics. If ineffective, a second dose of DHE should be administered 30 to 45 minutes later. An IV antiemetic (prochlorperazine 5 to 10 mg or metoclopramide 10 mg) should be administered 15 to 30 minutes before DHE to minimize the GI side effects of this agent. Intramuscular administration of ergotamine tartrate 0.5 mg is also effective, but ergot-related side effects are more severe with ergotamine tartrate than with DHE. Ergotamine tartrate administered by the oral, sublingual, or rectal routes is unlikely to be effective in this setting.

Sumatriptan

Sumatriptan 6 mg subcutaneously is also effective for the treatment of established migraine.[53] If the first injection does not provide relief at 1 hour, a second injection may be administered. However, the daily dosage should not exceed 12 mg. Sumatriptan should not be administered within 24 hours of ergot alkaloids because of the potential for prolonged vasospastic reactions.

Prochlorperazine

Prochlorperazine (Compazine) is an antiemetic agent often used as an adjunct for patients with migraine-associated nausea and vomiting. However, when given by IV route prochlorperazine is also a nonspecific yet highly effective agent for aborting intractable migraine.[38] In randomized, controlled trials, prochlorperazine 10 mg IV was more effective than placebo, IV metoclopramide, IV ketorolac, and IV valproate for the treatment of acute migraine in the emergency department.[105–107]

Chlorpromazine

Like prochlorperazine, chlorpromazine (Thorazine) given parenterally has both antimigraine and antiemetic properties and has gained increased acceptance in EDs as a pharmacologic alternative to potent narcotic analgesics such as meperidine. In a double-blind, controlled trial, IV chlorpromazine (0.1 mg/kg) provided more effective pain relief from intractable migraine than meperidine (0.4 mg/kg) plus dimenhydrinate.[108] Chlorpromazine 1 mg/kg intramuscularly has also been shown to relieve migraine headache more effectively than placebo.[109]

Narcotic Analgesics

Parenteral narcotic analgesics also effectively relieve intractable migraine headache pain, but they should generally be reserved for second- or third-line therapy after patients have failed to respond to parenteral sumatriptan, DHE, prochlorperazine or chlorpromazine. ED treatment of headache with narcotics is a common antecedent to iatrogenic drug addiction.[110] In some EDs that deal with a large number of drug-seeking patients, the use of synthetic narcotic agonist/antagonists (e.g., butorphanol, nalbuphine) has been advocated for treatment of intractable migraine.[111,112] Butorphanol is also available as a

Table 52-5 Drug Treatment of Acute Migraine Headache[a]

Drug	Route	Dose	Contraindications	Adverse Effects	Comments
Sumatriptan (Imitrex)	PO IN SC	6 mg SC stat; may repeat in 1 hr	Ischemic heart disease, within 24 hr of ergot alkaloids	Heavy sensation in head or chest, tingling, pain at injection site	First-line therapy for moderate-to-severe headaches; SC for intractable migraine
Ibuprofen (Motrin) or other NSAIDs	PO	400–800 mg	Aspirin or NSAID-related bronchospasm	N, V, bleeding, renal dysfunction	First-line therapy for mild-to-moderate headaches
Dihydroergotamine (Migranal)	IN IM IV	2 mg IN stat; repeat in 15 min	See Ergotamine	Rhinitis, dizziness, N, V	For moderate-to-severe headaches; parenteral use for intractable migraine
Ergotamine tartrate (Cafergot, Ergostat)	PO SL PR	1–4 mg stat, then 1–2 mg Q 30 min to max of 6 mg/attack or 10 mg/wk	CV disease, sepsis, liver or kidney disease, arterial insufficiency, pregnancy, breast feeding, concomitant macrolide use	N, V, anorexia, limb paresthesias or pain	Use at HA onset for max effect; ↓ N and V by using smallest effective dose
Isometheptene/ dichloralphenazone/ acetaminophen (Midrin)	PO	2 cap stat, then 1 cap Q hr to max 5 cap/12 hr	See Ergotamine tartrate; avoid in patients taking MAOIs	N, V, dizziness, drowsiness	As effective as ergotamine tartrate
Prochlorperazine (Compazine)	IM IV	10 mg stat	CV disease	Extrapyramidal reactions, sedation, dizziness	IV/IM for adjunctive antiemetic therapy; IV for antimigraine effect in intractable migraine
Chlorpromazine (Thorazine)	IM	1 mg/kg	CV disease, history of seizures	Extrapyramidal reactions, sedation, hypotension	For intractable migraine; also has antiemetic properties
Morphine (or meperidine)	IM	5–10 mg	↑ ICP or head trauma with funduscopic changes	Sedation, hypoventilation	For intractable migraine
Metoclopramide (Reglan)	PO IM	10 mg stat	GI hemorrhage or obstruction; pheochromocytoma	Extrapyramidal reactions, sedation, restlessness	For adjunctive antiemetic therapy; prochlorperazine also effective

[a]See text for references and additional details. See Table 52-4 for additional information on sumatriptan and other triptan agents.
CV, cardiovascular; GI, gastrointestinal; HA, headache; ICP, intracranial pressure; IM, intramuscular; IN, intranasal; MAOIs, monoamine oxidase inhibitors; N, nausea; NSAID, nonsteroidal anti-inflammatory drug; PO, oral; PR, rectal; SC, subcutaneous; SL, sublingual; V, vomiting.

nasal spray for self-administration during migraine headache. Although this product was initially thought to have a low addiction liability, subsequent experience suggests that the product is often misused or diverted for misuse purposes.[113] Patients receiving this medication should be monitored for excessive use. In a comparison with intramuscular butorphanol and intramuscular meperidine plus hydroxyzine, the superiority of IV DHE plus metoclopramide was clearly demonstrated.[111]

In general, narcotic analgesics can be highly effective therapies for acute and intractable migraine. However, these agents often cause or exacerbate nausea and vomiting. Also, excessive use should be monitored closely because of the risk of addiction and dependence. Alternative symptomatic therapies should be pursued for those patients who require frequent use of narcotic analgesics (usually defined as two or more treatments per week).[44]

Corticosteroids

Prednisone 40 to 60 mg orally for 3 to 5 days or dexamethasone 4 to 16 mg intramuscularly may be used as alternative treatments for intractable migraine and presumably work by suppressing the sterile perivascular inflammation of resistant headache.[114] Table 52-5 summarizes the agents commonly used for the treatment of acute migraine headaches.

Appropriate treatments for K.L.'s current headache include DHE (by subcutaneous, intramuscular, or IV route), subcutaneous sumatriptan, or intravenous prochlorperazine. Each of these treatments has proved effective in at least two double-blind trials.[44] Although ergot alkaloids should not be administered within 24 hours of sumatriptan, K.L. vomited immediately after taking sumatriptan and it is unlikely that she absorbed the drug. Thus, DHE is not contraindicated. Since K.L. has responded to oral sumatriptan in the past, subcutaneous administration of this drug would be appropriate initial therapy at this time. Adjunctive therapy with prochlorperazine (5 mg intramuscularly or intravenously) would provide relief from nausea and vomiting, and may also contribute to a reduction in headache severity. If K.L.'s headache persists after 6 mg subcutaneous sumatriptan, a second injection can be given 1 hour after the first.

Prophylactic Therapy

15. K.L. returns to the clinic 6 weeks later for follow-up. Her current medications include oral sumatriptan and acetaminophen with codeine. Acetaminophen with codeine 30 mg (#20) was prescribed by the ED physician who treated her single episode of intractable migraine. Since that episode, about 75% of her headaches have responded to sumatriptan 100 mg orally. The remainder of her attacks have been aborted with two acetaminophen with codeine tablets and rest. Her concern is that these resistant headaches occur as often as once or twice monthly and necessitate her taking the rest of the day off from work. K.L. reports no adverse effects from sumatriptan.

K.L.'s primary care physician wants to initiate treatment to reduce the frequency and severity of K.L.'s migraine attacks and chooses propranolol as the initial agent. When should prophylactic therapy of migraine be considered? Is propranolol a reasonable choice for K.L.?

Criteria for Use

K.L.'s present drug regimen is effectively aborting about 75% of her migraine attacks. The frequency of her disabling, drug-resistant headaches, however, is sufficient to warrant additional therapy that is directed toward preventing migraine attacks. Prophylactic migraine treatment not only reduces the frequency of migraine attacks, but also may reduce the severity of ensuing headaches, render them more responsive to abortive measures, or reduce the duration of headaches. The usual criteria for migraine prophylaxis are (a) headaches that impact a patient's life despite the use of abortive treatments (e.g., twice monthly or more), (b) headaches occurring so frequently that acute medications are overused, (c) disabling headaches that are unresponsive to abortive treatments, (d) patients in whom abortive agents are contraindicated, and (e) headaches that present a significant risk for future morbidity or mortality (e.g., hemiplegic migraine, migraine with prolonged aura, basilar migraine, or migraines associated with stroke).[115] Given the frequency with which K.L. continues to experience migraine headaches and the detrimental effect they have on her job performance, prophylactic migraine therapy is warranted.

Various prophylactic agents have been advocated to reduce the frequency and severity of migraine headaches. For many of these drugs, it is difficult to make an adequate assessment of relative efficacy based on the available literature. Therapeutic trials often are not optimally designed to establish the relative usefulness of a given drug relative to other prophylactic agents. For example, the efficacy of newer therapies may be repeatedly compared with placebo rather than with other agents whose effectiveness is well documented, whose dosages are often suboptimal, or whose duration of therapy may be insufficient to document maximal efficacy. Ideally, the evaluation of migraine drug therapy should be based on double-blind, controlled, crossover trials with optimal dosage titration (to effect, toxicity, or established maximum dosing recommendations) and with sufficient wash-out periods to minimize ambiguous results. Many prophylactic therapy recommendations are not so well grounded. Recently, a structured, evidence-based guideline for prophylactic treatment of migraine headache was published.[115,116] Recommendations given below are based on these guidelines, which represent a synthesis of the results from published trials and expert opinion. Generally, the preferred agents for prophylaxis of migraine headache are propranolol, timolol, amitriptyline, and valproate (including divalproex sodium). The use of these agents is supported by multiple randomized controlled trials and mild-to-moderate adverse effects. Other agents discussed below either have less evidence basis for a strong recommendation (i.e., few or no randomized controlled trials), or have been associated with significant adverse effects that limit their usefulness. In the United States, the only agents approved by the FDA for migraine prophylaxis are propranolol, timolol, valproate, topiramate and methysergide. Table 52-6 contains a list of the more well-established drugs used for migraine headache prophylaxis.

Propranolol

K.L.'s primary care physician has chose propranolol for prophylactic therapy of migraine. This is an appropriate choice. Propranolol (Inderal) is a first-line agent for migraine prophylaxis because of its safety, efficacy, favorable adverse effect profile, and the large number of studies that support its effectiveness.[117,118] Although the effectiveness of propranolol in the prophylaxis of migraine is well established, not all individuals respond to this treatment.[118–124] When propranolol is used, approximately 50% to 80% of patients obtain complete or partial relief from migraine attacks[118,124,125]; most patients who initially respond to propranolol continue to benefit without any evidence of drug tolerance.[124]

The mechanism by which propranolol exerts its antimigraine effects is unknown. It was generally assumed, without evidence to support the hypothesis, that β-receptor blockade prevented the vasodilatory phase of migraine; however, propranolol has no significant effect on cerebral blood flow.[126] The mechanism of action may be related to the drug's effects on the serotonergic system.[127,128] Propranolol has a high affinity for serotonin receptors[128] and has been shown to inhibit platelet uptake of serotonin in vivo and in vitro.[129]

Other β-adrenergic blocking drugs such as timolol[134] and the cardioselective agents, metoprolol[130] and atenolol,[131,132] appear to be as efficacious as propranolol in double-blind, crossover trials. However, besides propranolol, timolol is the only β-blocker with FDA approval for this indication. Atenolol is an appropriate therapeutic alternative for patients who cannot tolerate propranolol's CNS adverse effects. The lack of efficacy demonstrated for pindolol,[133] acebutolol,[134] alprenolol,[135] and oxprenolol[136] may be related to their intrinsic sympathomimetic activity, and these agents should not be used.

DOSING

16. What dose of propranolol should be prescribed for K.L.? When can she expect a response?

Propranolol 80 to 240 mg/day in two to four divided doses is effective in the prophylaxis of migraine headaches.[115,118] Because the dosage range is wide, propranolol therapy should be initiated with 20 mg two or three times a day; this dose can be increased gradually at weekly intervals according to patient tolerability or to a maximum of 320 mg/day.[117] Once the daily dosage of propranolol required to control headaches is established, patient adherence may be improved by changing to a long-acting oral dosage form (e.g., Inderal LA). Although the

Table 52-6 Drugs Useful for Migraine Headache Prophylaxis[a]

Drug	Dose	Dosage Forms/Strengths	Effectiveness	Comments
Propranolol (Inderal)	20 mg BID–TID; gradually ↑ dose at weekly intervals to effect or max of 320 mg/day	Tab: 10, 20, 40, 60, 80, 90 mg ER Cap: 60, 80, 120, 160 mg	50–80% obtain complete or partial relief; comparable to methysergide	First line therapy; atenolol, metoprolol, and timolol also effective
Amitriptyline (Elavil)	10–25 mg HS; ↑ by 10–25 mg/day at weekly intervals to max 150 mg/day; most should benefit from 50–75 mg/day	Tab: 10, 25, 50, 75, 100, 150 mg	Effectiveness comparable to propranolol and methysergide	First line therapy effective for prophylaxis of migraine and tension-type headache
Valproate (Depakote)	250 mg BID; ↑ by 250 mg/day at weekly intervals to effect or adverse effects; most should benefit from 1,000–2,000 mg/day	Cap[b]: 250 mg DR Tab[c]: 125, 250, 500 mg ER Tab: 250,500 mg SCaps: 125 mg	50% obtain complete or partial relief	First line therapy
Verapamil (Isoptin, Calan)	80 mg TID. If needed, ↑ dose gradually to max of 480 mg/day	Tabs: 40, 80, 120 mg ER Cap: 120, 240 mg ER Tab: 180, 240 mg	50% obtain complete or partial relief	Second line therapy Delay of 1–2 months for maximal effect; efficacy of nifedipine and diltiazem questionable
Methysergide (Sansert)	2–8 mg/day in 3–4 divided daily doses to be taken with food	Tab: 2 mg	60–70% obtain complete or partial relief	Use limited by propensity for frequent and sometimes severe adverse effects; drug holidays should be planned every 6 mo. Rarely used
Naproxen sodium	550 mg BID	Tab: 220, 275, 550 mg	30% obtain complete or partial relief	Second line therapy Modest efficacy; effective for menstrual migraine; naproxen, flurbiprofen, ketoprofen, mefenamic acid also effective

[a] See text for references and additional details.
[b] Valproic acid capsules.
[c] Divalproex sodium delayed-release tablets.
Cap, capsules; DR, delayed release; ER, extended release; SCap, sprinkle capsules containing coated particles; Tab, tablets.

usual dosage for migraine prophylaxis is 80 to 240 mg/day, up to 30% of patients prophylactically treated with propranolol would not have benefited in one clinical study of 865 patients if the propranolol dosage had not been titrated to a maximum of 320 mg/day.[125] Most propranolol responders will experience relief within 4 to 6 weeks of beginning therapy.[79] However, in unusual circumstances, 3 to 6 months may be required before maximal benefit is realized.[125] Tolerance to the antimigraine effects of propranolol over long-term therapy does not occur.[124]

Because propranolol is highly effective and well tolerated in most patients, it is an appropriate prophylactic agent for K.L. She has no pre-existing disease states that would prohibit its use. K.L. should be started at a low dosage with gradual titration to either therapeutic response, side effects, or a maximum dose of 320 mg/day. Six weeks or longer may be required before optimal results are achieved.

Methysergide

17. G.W., a 46-year-old man with an 11-year history of migraine without aura, comes to a clinic with a complaint of epigastric distress for the past 2 days. Current medications include Fiorinal (aspirin 325 mg, butalbital 50 mg, caffeine 40 mg) two capsules PO at headache onset, methysergide (Sansert) 2 mg PO TID, salmeterol inhaler 1 puff every 12 hours, fluticasone (44 mcg/puff) 2 puffs every 12 hours, albuterol metered-dose inhaler 2 puffs as needed for shortness of breath, and Theo-Dur 300 mg PO BID. G.W.'s headaches are notable for bilateral, throbbing, temporal head pain and the absence of associated GI or focal neurologic symptoms. Migraine prophylaxis with methysergide has reduced his headache frequency from three headaches monthly to about one headache every 2 to 3 months. A review of G.W.'s medical record reveals that methysergide therapy was initiated 2 years ago and that a drug holiday was not taken. Past medical history includes asthma since adolescence, with frequent ED visits for exacerbation of symptoms and a 3-year history of painful lower extremity peripheral vascular disease (PVD). Why is methysergide an inappropriate alternative to propranolol prophylaxis of migraine in this asthmatic patient with PVD?

Methysergide, a semisynthetic ergot alkaloid with 5-HT_2-receptor antagonist properties, is one of the most effective agents for migraine prophylaxis;[137] in past decades, it was the standard by which newer therapies were often judged. However, its use is limited by a propensity for frequent, and sometimes severe, side effects. For this reason, methysergide is considered a fourth-line agent for migraine prophylaxis.[115]

Within the usual dosage range of 2 to 8 mg in three to four daily divided doses, as many as 40% of patients treated with methysergide will experience side effects. Adverse effects are severe enough to require discontinuation in 10% of patients.

CONTRAINDICATIONS

Like other ergot alkaloids, methysergide has peripheral vasoconstrictive properties that may preclude its use in some patients. Contraindications to methysergide use include PVD, coronary artery disease, thrombophlebitis, and pregnancy. Even when such precautions are kept in mind, some patients experience side effects attributable to the drug's vasoconstrictive properties (e.g., coldness, numbness, and tingling of the extremities or even anginal pain).

Given G.W.'s history of PVD, methysergide is not an appropriate agent for migraine prophylaxis. Although he had a history of PVD before methysergide was initiated, the continued use of this drug may have aggravated his condition. G.W.'s methysergide should be tapered immediately and an alternative treatment regimen initiated.

ADVERSE EFFECTS

18. In addition to G.W.'s history of PVD, what is another reason for discontinuing his methysergide therapy, and how should it be tapered?

Retroperitoneal, endocardial, and pleuropulmonary fibrosis are severe complications of methysergide. Fibrosis has developed after 7 to 79 months of methysergide therapy and has been associated with dosages in excess of 8 mg/day.[79] Because most fibrotic complications have been reported following long-term, uninterrupted use of methysergide,[138] drug-free holidays of 3 to 4 weeks are recommended after each 6-month treatment period to minimize this risk. However, the discontinuation of methysergide should be gradual to avoid the rebound vascular headache that can occur after abrupt discontinuation. Patients receiving long-term therapy should be counseled to report any flank pain, dysuria, or chest pain to their physician. During each patient visit, cardiac auscultation should be performed. An IV pyelogram and chest radiograph also should be obtained after 6 months of therapy to monitor for the development of fibrosis. When the therapeutic benefits of methysergide become evident (~3 to 4 weeks after initiation of therapy), the dose of this drug should be reduced to the minimum effective amount.[79]

Because G.W. has received methysergide continuously for 2 years without a drug holiday, he is at risk for developing methysergide fibrosis. The methysergide should be discontinued in G.W. because of the risk of drug-induced fibrosis and because of his history of PVD. His methysergide therapy should be gradually tapered to discontinuation over a 3-week period to avoid migraine headache rebound. Subsequently, another form of prophylactic therapy should be initiated for G.W.

19. G.W. has been experiencing nausea for the past 2 days. What is one approach to resolving these GI complaints?

GI distress is the most common side effect to methysergide therapy. However, the discomfort is usually mild and disappears within the first several days to weeks of therapy. GI distress can be minimized by administering methysergide doses with food and by avoiding rapid increases in dose. Because G.W. has received methysergide therapy for 2 years and his GI complaints appear to be of recent origin, other potential causes for GI distress should be investigated. Methysergide can also activate latent peptic ulcer disease,[139] presumably by increasing gastric acid secretion.[140] However, G.W. has no known history of ulcer disease and his GI complaint does not specifically suggest this complication.

G.W.'s GI distress may be the result of gastritis or peptic ulcer disease caused by the aspirin component in Fiorinal (G.W. receives 650 mg aspirin with each two capsule Fiorinal dose). The nausea also could be due to theophylline toxicity. These potential causes of G.W.'s nausea should be evaluated. A laboratory determination of G.W.'s hemoglobin (Hgb) concentration and evaluation of his stools for occult blood would be helpful in assessing aspirin-induced gastritis with blood loss. A serum theophylline concentration also should be obtained. A more detailed history that focuses on the relation between nausea and medication use or other concurrent illness may also provide useful information for assessing G.W.'s GI distress.

20. What drug should be prescribed in place of methysergide to prevent G.W.'s migraine attacks?

Along with propranolol, amitriptyline and valproate are effective first-line therapies for prevention of migraine headache. The effectiveness of these agents is supported by randomized controlled trials, and adverse effects are generally mild-to-moderate in severity.

Amitriptyline

Amitriptyline (Elavil) is effective for prevention of both migraine and tension-type headaches. It may be the drug of choice for patients whose symptoms suggest features of both headache types (i.e., mixed tension-type/migraine headaches), and for those with coexisting depression. Along with propranolol and valproate, amitriptyline is considered a first-line therapy for migraine prophylaxis.[115]

In a double-blind, placebo-controlled, cross-over study, amitriptyline was as effective as propranolol.[141] It also was as effective as methysergide based on comparative results from previous studies.[142] The mechanism of amitriptyline's antimigraine effect is independent of its antidepressant activity[141,143] and may be related to its ability to block the reuptake of serotonin at central sites.[144] However, other antidepressant agents that block 5-HT reuptake (e.g., clomipramine) have been ineffective for migraine prophylaxis.[145] Amitriptyline and other antidepressants have been reported to down-regulate 5-HT receptors, although this effect has been inconsistent in published reports.[146]

DOSING

The initial dose of amitriptyline is 10 to 25 mg at bedtime. This nightly dose can be increased at weekly intervals by 10 to 25 mg until the maximum dose of 150 mg/day is reached. Most patients achieve optimal benefit from 50 to 75 mg/day of amitriptyline; doses greater than 150 mg/day are unlikely to produce better results.[79] Two-thirds of patients note a decrease in the number of headaches within 7 days of starting amitriptyline therapy, but a 6-week trial is warranted before the drug should be considered ineffective.[142,143]

No other antidepressant agents have been studied as extensively as amitriptyline for migraine prophylaxis and their efficacy remains unproven. Fluoxetine (Prozac) was effective in one small trial.[147] However, the favorable results were not reproduced in a larger, subsequent study.[148] A study of amitriptyline 25 mg/day and fluvoxamine 50 mg/day demonstrated reductions in headache frequency for both drugs when pretreatment and post-treatment periods were compared.[149]

Valproate

The antiepileptic drug valproate (and divalproex sodium, Depakote) is also approved for the prevention of migraine headaches and is useful as a first-line agent in this regard.[115,150] In a randomized, double-blind, parallel treatment comparison of valproate (titrated to trough serum concentrations of 70 to 120 mcg/mL) and placebo, 48% of valproate-treated patients had a 50% or greater reduction in the frequency of migraine.[151] In a single-blind comparison of valproate and propranolol, both agents were equally effective as prophylaxis for migraine without aura.[152]

DOSING

The initial dose of valproate is 250 mg PO BID. The dose can be increased in 250- to 500-mg/day increments at weekly intervals. The usual range of effective doses is 500 to 1,500 mg/day. Serum levels of valproate may be useful to monitor therapy; however, a clear relation between concentration and antimigraine effect has not been established. Enteric-coated products (e.g., Depakote) are preferred over immediate release products (e.g., Depakene) to minimize gastrointestinal upset. An extended-release dosage form (Depakote ER) is approved for once-daily dosing and may be useful to improve medication adherence.

Either amitriptyline or valproate would be reasonable choices for prevention of migraine headaches in G.W. Although direct comparative trials have not been performed, these agents appear to be equally effective. Thus, the choice can be made on the basis of the adverse effect profile of these agents. The most common adverse effects of amitriptyline include dry mouth, reflex tachycardia, blurred vision, weight gain, and difficulty with cognition. The most common adverse effects of valproate include nausea, alopecia, tremor, and weight gain. The adverse effect profiles of each agent should be discussed with G.W., and, on the basis of his preference, a choice between these agents should be made.

21. S.A. is a 31-year old woman with a 4-year history of disabling migraine headaches (with aura) occurring two to three times weekly. She is currently using zolmitriptan (Zomig) 5 mg for abortive therapy, and the clinic physician is concerned about overuse of this agent. Medical history includes bipolar affective disorder and a history of polydrug abuse. S.A. has failed prophylactic therapy with propranolol (ineffective) and valproate (modestly effective, but caused unacceptable weight gain). She is currently taking lithium for her bipolar disorder, and her serum levels have been stable at 0.8 mEq/L. Her physician wishes to avoid antidepressants because of her psychiatric history. What other prophylactic therapies are available?

Nonsteroidal Anti-Inflammatory Drugs

In addition to being effective as symptomatic therapy for migraine, selected NSAIDs are also effective as prophylactic agents. However, their effectiveness as preventive therapy is considered to be modest compared with the first-line agents, propranolol, amitriptyline, and valproate.[115] The rationale for their use is that inhibition of prostaglandin and leukotriene synthesis might inhibit the neurogenic inflammation of migraine. However, their actual mechanism of action is unknown. Placebo-controlled trials have documented the effectiveness of naproxen,[153] naproxen sodium,[154,155] ketoprofen,[156] flurbiprofen,[157] and mefenamic acid.[158] A comparative study of naproxen sodium 1,100 mg/day and propranolol 120 mg/day found a trend favoring propranolol, although the difference in response between the two treatments was not significant.[159] Given the favorable trend toward propranolol and the use of a suboptimal dose of the drug in this trial, it is unlikely that naproxen sodium is a superior agent for migraine prophylaxis. The NSAIDs mentioned above may be effective as short-term therapy for menstruation-associated migraine.[115]

Calcium Channel Blockers

VERAPAMIL

Calcium channel blockers influence the final common pathway of vascular reactivity by altering calcium flux across smooth muscle. Hormone and neurotransmitter secretion are also calcium-dependent processes that can be altered by calcium channel blockers.[160] Whether the efficacy of calcium antagonists in migraine therapy is due to their vasoactive properties, modulation of neurotransmitter release, or a serotonergic effect is unknown.

Verapamil (Isoptin, Calan, Verelan) is the calcium channel blocker of choice for preventive migraine therapy because it is effective and has been most extensively studied in randomized controlled trials. Most patients respond to verapamil at doses of 240 to 320 mg/day. Therefore, treatment can be initiated with an 80-mg dose three times a day and increased to 80 mg four times a day after 1 week. Observable benefits from this treatment may not be apparent for 3 to 8 weeks; as a result, verapamil should be continued for at least 2 months to properly evaluate response to therapy. This is one of the limiting properties of calcium channel antagonists. If an adequate response is not achieved in this interval, the verapamil dose can be increased weekly by increments of 80 mg to a maximum of 480 mg/day. Sustained-release (SR) formulations (Calan SR, Isoptin SR) and extended-release formulations (Covera-HS, Verelan) of verapamil, are available and are often useful in improving patient adherence with long-term therapy. Headache frequency, intensity, and duration are reduced in 50% of patients treated with verapamil.[161–163] Patients who suffer from migraine with or without aura respond equally well.[161,162] Verapamil may be particularly effective for patients with a prolonged or atypical migraine aura.[116] Although there are few comparative studies, most practitioners consider the benefits of calcium channel blockers to be modest relative to β-blockers, valproate, and amitriptyline. For this reason, verapamil is usually considered when these agents fail or are contraindicated.[8,117]

NIFEDIPINE, DILTIAZEM AND NIMODIPINE

Nifedipine (Procardia) and diltiazem (Cardizem) are other calcium antagonists that have been used to treat migraine.[164–166] Although preliminary experience suggested that nifedipine was effective, a double-blind, crossover study found nifedipine to be no more effective than placebo for preventing migraine headaches with aura. This study was designed to detect a 50% reduction in migraine frequency during treatment.[167] The effectiveness of diltiazem is based on two open-label studies with no control treatment.[166,168] As yet, no placebo-controlled, crossover studies have been reported. On the basis of current evidence, neither nifedipine nor diltiazem can be recommended for prophylaxis of migraine headache until other, better-established therapies (see Table 52-6) have been adequately tried and yielded unsatisfactory results.

Nimodipine (Nimotop) is a calcium antagonist with marked selectivity for the cerebral vasculature.[169] The drug is approved only to improve neurologic deficits after aneurysmal subarachnoid hemorrhage. Results from double-blind, placebo-controlled trials have been inconsistent in showing a benefit of nimodipine for preventing migraine headaches.[170–173]

In most studies, the dose of oral nimodipine was 40 mg given three times daily.[171–173] Unfortunately, no adequate studies are available that compare nimodipine to other first-line preventative therapies. In light of the inconsistent results from placebo-controlled trials and the high cost of this drug, nimodipine appears to have little utility as a prophylactic agent.

Other Prophylactic Therapies

Some of the less established therapies occasionally recommended for migraine prophylaxis are listed in Table 52-7.[79,115,174–177] Evaluative reports for some of these agents do not meet the criteria for establishing a clear benefit in migraine. In general, a significant reduction of headache frequency in 50% of patients should be demonstrated before a drug can be said to be more effective than placebo. Placebo response rates for migraine and other painful conditions range from 30% to 50%[10,178,179] and may be maintained over several months.[179] This significant effect should also be considered when evaluating studies of migraine therapy.

On the basis of efficacy, either NSAIDs (i.e., naproxen, naproxen sodium, flurbiprofen, ketoprofen or mefenamic acid) or verapamil could be considered for prophylactic therapy to reduce the frequency of S.A.'s migraine headaches. However, NSAIDs are likely to interact with her lithium therapy, resulting in an increase in serum concentration and risk for adverse effects. For this reason, NSAIDs are best avoided at this time. S.A. should be started on verapamil 80 mg three times a day with gradual dosage titration to side effects, cessation of migraine attacks, or a maximum dose of 480 mg/day. She should be counseled regarding the possible occurrence of constipation and the appropriate management of this common side effect of verapamil. A 2-month trial may be necessary to demonstrate optimal therapeutic effect. Prophylactic therapy for migraine should be continued for 3 to 6 months. If a satisfactory response is achieved, the prophylactic agent should be gradually discontinued over several weeks to assess the continued need for this mode of therapy.

Analgesic Overuse

22. L.D. is a 39-year-old woman with a 7-year history of migraine (without aura) and tension-type headache who comes to clinic requesting a refill of her Fiorinal (aspirin, butalbital, and caffeine) and acetaminophen with codeine (30 mg). She reports an increase in the frequency of both her "throbbing" and "dull, pressure-sensation" headaches over the past year, and lately she has had difficulty distinguishing the two types. Over the past 2 months, she has had only 5 days with no headache, and she has been much less productive in her work as a magazine editor. A review of her medication refill records indicates that she has had four refills of Fiorinal (#30) and three refills of acetaminophen with codeine (#20) in the past 2 months and that her use of these drugs has increased over the past year. During the visit, she also indicates that she uses OTC acetaminophen and naproxen sodium on an "as-needed" basis. Although L.D. had experienced relief of mild headaches in the past with the use of OTC analgesics, these medications no longer reduce the intensity of her pain. What is the potential role of analgesic overuse in the worsening of L.D.'s headaches? How should her condition be managed?

Narcotics, NSAIDs, and other analgesics can be very effective for the treatment of infrequent, episodic migraine and other headache types. However, the use of these agents in patients with frequent headaches should be undertaken with caution. Analgesic overuse is common in these patients and associated with a gradual worsening of the headache symptoms. Any type of headache syndrome (e.g., migraine, tension-type, and other headaches) can be worsened by analgesic overuse.[180] This exacerbation is termed *analgesic-induced headache* (also, *analgesic rebound headache*) and is characterized by an increase in the use of analgesics, development of tolerance to the pain-relieving effect of these drugs, an increase in headache intensity, and an increase in headache frequency. In severe circumstances, a pattern of chronic daily headache can emerge. These chronic daily headaches often have features of both migraine and tension-type headaches.[181] The mechanism of analgesic rebound headache is unknown. However, alterations in serotonergic transmission are suspected.[182,183] L.D. displays many of the features of analgesic-induced headache. She reports an increase in the frequency of headaches to a near-daily pattern and she is no longer able to distinguish between migrainous

Table 52-7 Other Drugs for Migraine Headache Prophylaxis[a]

Drug	Dose/Day (Oral)	Comments
Clonidine	0.1–0.2 mg BID–TID	No benefit found in some studies
Cyproheptadine	4–8 mg TID–QID (adults)	Particularly useful for migraine in children
Ergonovine maleate	0.2 mg TID–QID during menses or continuously	Effective for menstrual migraine and when other prophylactic agents contraindicated; recommended by some authors as a first-line prophylactic agent
Feverfew	Variable	Demonstrated effective in randomized, controlled trial though additional study needed
Phenelzine	15 mg TID–QID	Caution when used simultaneously with antidepressants and β-blockers
Phenytoin	200–400 mg QD	Benefits in children and adults established by uncontrolled studies
Riboflavin	400 mg QD	Demonstrated effective in a randomized, controlled trial though additional study needed
Topiramate	100 mg/day (given BID)	Effective in three randomized controlled trials
Gabapentin	900–2400 mg/day (given TID)	Effective in one randomized controlled trial

and tension-type headaches. Furthermore, the exacerbation of her headaches appears to coincide with the escalating use of analgesics. L.D. should be questioned carefully to determine the total amount of acetaminophen, naproxen sodium, and aspirin that she consumes daily and weekly. Daily users of analgesics are at increased risk for chronic renal disease, chronic liver disease, and acute GI bleeding.[183–185] Laboratory tests should be ordered to assess L.D.'s renal and hepatic function, and she should be questioned regarding the occurrence of GI discomfort, acute bleeding, or a change in her stool color.

In general, patients who receive analgesics for headache treatment should be counseled to restrict their use of these agents to no more than twice per week.[44] However, in patients with analgesic-induced headache, a reduction in the use of these drugs will likely worsen their headache condition. The management of analgesic-induced headache is a challenge to clinicians and the patients who suffer from them. These headaches are often unresponsive to the usual abortive and prophylactic therapy measures discussed in earlier sections of this chapter. Successful management requires gradual withdrawal from the overused drugs. This process can be protracted and made even more difficult when barbiturate, codeine, or ergotamine-containing drugs are involved.[181] Withdrawal can usually be accomplished on an outpatient basis although in some patients, inpatient detoxification is required. Once the frequency and quantity of analgesic use by L.D. have been adequately quantified, a process of gradual drug removal should be initiated. Medications taken on an infrequent basis (e.g., fewer than two times per week) can be abruptly stopped. For medications currently taken on a daily basis, L.D. should be counseled to reduce the medication by one tablet per day at 3-day intervals.[181] She should be informed that her headaches may worsen during this period but that symptoms will gradually improve as she proceeds through the detoxification process.

L.D.'s use of acetaminophen with codeine does not appear to be frequent enough to place her at risk for the development of opiate withdrawal symptoms. However, she should be counseled to report symptoms such as anxiety, tremulousness, insomnia, or diarrhea. If these symptoms occur, the rate of drug withdrawal should be reduced. Some clinicians prescribe a tricyclic antidepressant such as amitriptyline during the withdrawal period.[181] These agents can be useful for their central pain-relieving properties, antidepressant effects, and for their effect as preventative therapy for both migraine and tension-type headaches. Even if a tricyclic antidepressant is not prescribed during the withdrawal period, L.D. should be considered as a candidate for prophylactic headache therapy once analgesic withdrawal has been accomplished. If prophylaxis of both migraine and tension-type headache is necessary, amitriptyline would be an appropriate choice for L.D. After withdrawal is complete, L.D. should be educated regarding the future risk of analgesic-induced headache. A medication other than the withdrawn drugs should be prescribed for treatment of her acute attacks. For example, a triptan agent may be useful for abortive treatment of her migraine headaches. An NSAID may be considered for acute treatment of her tension-type headaches. L.D. must clearly understand that these agents should not be used more than twice per week, and her use of all abortive or symptomatic therapies should be monitored closely.

In extreme circumstances, analgesic abuse can precipitate chronic daily headache. In addition, analgesic abuse is a common cause of failure of the usual abortive treatment measures (e.g., sumatriptan and ergotamine). Successful abortive and prophylactic treatment of migraine headache in patients with a history of analgesic overuse necessitates detoxification from the abused agents.[186] Headaches often worsen during the withdrawal period, but within several weeks the headache characteristics return to baseline and responsiveness to traditional pharmacotherapy is restored. To minimize the risk of analgesic abuse and rebound headaches, patients should restrict their use of these agents to no more than twice per week.[44]

CLUSTER HEADACHE

Cluster headache is a relatively infrequent headache disorder (estimated prevalence 0.07–0.4%) that derives its name from the characteristic pattern of headache recurrence–headaches tend to occur nightly over a relatively short period of time (i.e., several weeks or months), followed by a long period of complete remission.[187] Cluster headaches occur more commonly in males than females. There may be a seasonal predilection to cluster attacks with the spring and fall being common times for headache recurrence. Headaches are usually of short duration and present as severe, unrelenting, unilateral pain occurring behind the eye with radiation to the territory of the ipsilateral trigeminal nerve (temple, cheek, or gum).

The different clinical characteristics between cluster and migraine headaches (e.g., sex ratio, periodicity of attacks, duration of headaches, aura symptoms) suggest that these two types of vascular headaches are different clinical entities.[188]

Pathophysiology

The pathophysiology of cluster headache is undetermined. As in migraine, vascular, neurogenic, metabolic, and humoral factors have been proposed to play a role in cluster headache pathogenesis. Precipitation of headaches during a cluster period by vasodilators and response to vasoconstrictors suggests an underlying vascular component. During a cluster headache, thermography shows increased periorbital heat emission ipsilateral to the head pain.[189] Also, patients commonly report flushing in the same area, and these observations suggest that extracranial vasodilation occurs in cluster headache. However, intracranial blood flow studies fail to show consistent changes during a cluster attack,[190–192] and the alterations in extracranial blood flow follow the onset of head pain,[193] suggesting that vasodilation occurs in response to some other initiating stimulus. Abnormal plasma levels of melatonin, growth hormone, testosterone, and prolactin have been reported in patients with cluster headache. These findings, along with the cyclic recurrence pattern of the disorder suggest a disturbance in hypothalamic function.[194]

Observations that suggest a neural component to cluster headache include the occurrence of headache in the distribution of the trigeminal nerve, accompanying autonomic symptoms, and the fact that headache precedes extracranial vasodilation. Stimulation of the trigeminal nerve results in the release of substance P and vasoactive polypeptides, vasodilation, and pain.[195] These features implicate the trigeminovascular system in cluster headache pathogenesis. However, a coherent theory to explain the symptoms, periodicity, and circadian regularity of cluster headaches remains elusive.

In recent years, the role of heredity in cluster headache has been appreciated.[187] Cluster headache has been reported in monozygotic twins,[196] and first-degree relatives of individuals with cluster headache have a 14-fold higher risk of also having cluster headaches.[197] However, a specific genetic basis for the disorder remains elusive.[198]

Signs and Symptoms

23. R.H. is a 31-year-old man with a 3-year history of episodic cluster headache. He has been headache free for the past year but today states that the headaches are returning in their characteristic fashion. He reports abrupt onset of right-sided retro-orbital pain with occasional superimposed knifelike "jabs" that increase in intensity over several minutes to a severe, unrelenting pain lasting about 90 minutes. The headache then gradually subsides. Associated symptoms include right-sided lacrimation, conjunctival injection, and rhinorrhea. He denies any premonition of ensuing headache or GI upset during the attacks. Physical examination during a cluster headache shows right eyelid droop and pupillary miosis. R.H.'s cluster periods characteristically last about 2 months and usually recur once or twice yearly. The first headache of the current bout awoke him from a short nap. R.H. expects to suffer one or two such headaches daily because this has been the usual pattern during each cluster period. Previous cluster headaches have been symptomatically treated with aspirin and codeine 30 mg. However, R.H. reports only modest relief with this treatment approach.

R.H.'s medical history is unremarkable. He does not use tobacco but admits to occasional social drinking. What subjective and objective evidence in this case is consistent with a diagnosis of cluster headaches?

R.H.'s gender, age of onset, quality and intensity of headache pain, periodicity of headache attacks, and associated symptoms all support the diagnosis of cluster headaches.

Cluster headaches affect men more commonly than women by a ratio of 5:1,[189,199] and have their usual onset between the second and fourth decades of life.[199] R.H.'s gender (male) and age of onset (28 years) are compatible with these aspects of cluster headaches.

Recurrent cluster headaches are usually severe and throbbing and affect the same side of the head. Occasionally, cluster headaches may involve the entire hemicranium. The pain starts abruptly, often waking the patient from sleep, reaches maximum intensity over 5 to 15 minutes, and usually lasts 45 to 60 minutes.[189] Unlike migraine, cluster headache is not preceded by an aura. Thus, patients have no warning before onset of head pain. Cluster periods often last from 2 to 3 months and recur once or twice yearly.[189] Patients suffering from chronic cluster headaches have bouts that last 12 months or longer. R.H.'s headache quality (severe, unrelenting pain), site (unilateral), evolution and resolution pattern (worsens over several minutes and resolves within 90 minutes), and periodicity of attacks (one or two headaches occurring daily for about 2 months followed by a period of remission that lasts about 1 year) are all compatible with the usual character of cluster headaches.

Associated features may include ipsilateral lacrimation, injected conjunctiva, and rhinorrhea or blocked nasal passage. A partial Horner's syndrome (ptosis with miosis) occurs in one-third of patients and is often the only abnormal physical finding during a cluster headache. Nausea, vomiting, and focal neurologic symptoms are often absent. Associated symptoms reported by R.H. during headache attacks (e.g., lacrimation, rhinorrhea, conjunctival injection) and the absence of GI or neurologic disturbances are also compatible with the diagnosis of cluster headaches.

During a cluster period, headaches may be precipitated by alcohol (even in small amounts), vasodilators, stress, warm weather, missed meals, and excessive sleep. Therefore, during the current cluster period, R.H. should be counseled to avoid all alcohol and daytime naps.

Abortive Therapy

24. What abortive measures are available for symptomatic treatment of individual headaches during R.H.'s current cluster period?

The treatments of choice for abortive treatment of cluster headaches are sumatriptan by subcutaneous injection and oxygen inhalation.[187,198] The expense and inconvenience of having oxygen inhalation apparatus close at hand limit the usefulness of this treatment for many patients. A recent community-based study found that most patients suffering from cluster headaches do not receive optimal treatment for their condition.[200] Table 52-8 is a summary of drugs commonly used for the acute treatment of cluster headache.

Sumatriptan

Sumatriptan 6 mg subcutaneously has been shown to effectively relieve cluster headache in randomized, double-blind, placebo-controlled trials. Cluster headaches are reduced in severity in 74% of attacks within 15 minutes, compared with 26% of attacks treated with placebo.[187] An additional injection of 6 mg does not appear to give additional headache relief.[201] However, in patients who experience a recurrent headache after initial relief with sumatriptan, a second injection is often useful.[194] Sumatriptan should not be used more often than twice daily during cluster bouts. For patients who experience more than two attacks per day, adjunctive therapy with oxygen inhalation should be considered.[187]

Intranasal and oral sumatriptan have also been evaluated in patients with cluster headache. A randomized, open-label comparison of sumatriptan by intranasal (20 mg) and subcutaneous (6 mg) routes found a much higher response with the injectable form of the drug at 15 minutes post-treatment (94% versus 13%, respectively). Patients included in this study indicated a clear preference for the subcutaneous dosage form.[202] Oral sumatriptan (100 mg three times a day) was studied as a prophylactic agent during cluster headache bouts and found to be ineffective.[203]

Oxygen

Oxygen inhalation is preferred not only for in-hospital treatment of cluster headache but also for use by some patients at home or at work. Oxygen is also useful for patients with frequent cluster headaches who would otherwise exceed maximum dosing restrictions of sumatriptan.[187] The benefits of oxygen inhalation at 7 L/minute for 15 minutes, are superior

Table 52-8 Drugs Commonly Used for Acute Treatment of Cluster Headache[a]

Drug	Route	Dose	Contraindications	Adverse Effects	Comments
Sumatriptan (Imitrex)	SC	6 mg at HA onset	Ischemic heart disease, within 24 hr of ergot alkaloids	Heavy sensation in head or chest, tingling, pain at injection site	Not an FDA-approved indication; costly but well tolerated
Oxygen	Inhalation	7 L/min for 15 min			Fast onset of effect; equally effective as ergotamine tartrate
Ergotamine tartrate (Ergostat, Cafergot)	SL, PR	1–2 mg at HA onset; may repeat in 5 min (SL only); do not exceed 6 mg/attack or 10 mg/wk	CV disease, sepsis, liver or kidney disease, arterial insufficiency, pregnancy, breast feeding, concomitant macrolide use	N, V, anorexia, limb paresthesias or pain	SL ergotamine may have faster onset of effect; ↓ N and V by using smallest effective dose
DHE-45	SC, IM, IV	1 mg (SC, IM) or 0.75 mg (IV) stat; may repeat in 45 min	CV disease, sepsis, liver or kidney disease, arterial insufficiency, pregnancy, breast feeding	N, V, limb paresthesias or pain	More effective and faster onset than SL or PR ergotamine. Premedicate with antiemetic (e.g., metoclopramide or prochlorperazine)

[a] See text for references and additional details.
CV, cardiovascular; HA, headache; IM, intramuscular; IV, intravenous; N, nausea, PR, rectal; SC, subcutaneous; SL, sublingual; V, vomiting.

to placebo[204] and equal to those of ergotamine[205] in relieving cluster headaches. In addition, oxygen is very fast-acting, with most patients experiencing headache relief within 7 minutes of beginning inhalation.[205] The mechanism of oxygen's effect is unknown but may be related to a direct vasoconstrictive action.[187]

Ergotamine Tartrate

Inhalational, sublingual, and parenteral routes of ergotamine administration have a rapid onset of action and are effective for aborting acute cluster headaches.[206] Ergotamine by inhalation or sublingual administration is effective in 70% to 80% of patients,[207,208] and traditionally these routes of administration have been preferred. Unfortunately, no inhaled ergotamine product is currently marketed in the United States, and the product is likely to remain unavailable. Ergotamine tartrate 2 mg given rectally also can be effective if given early in the attack.[207] Ergotamine tartrate 0.5 mg and DHE 1 mg given intramuscularly are equally effective; DHE is better tolerated and less likely to cause vasoconstrictive adverse effects.[207]

Other Therapeutic Interventions

Cluster headaches also can be relieved by less commonly used therapeutic interventions such as intranasal capsaicin,[209] dexamethasone 8 mg orally,[194] methoxyflurane inhalation (10–15 drops applied to a handkerchief and inhaled for several seconds),[79] somatostatin IV infusion (25 mcg/minute for 20 minutes),[210] and local anesthesia with either intranasal application of 1 mL of 4% lidocaine hydrochloride[211] or 0.3 mL of a 5% to 10% solution of cocaine hydrochloride[212] to the ipsilateral sphenopalatine fossa.

Orally administered narcotic analgesics are usually ineffective in cluster headache,[189] and R.H. has suffered several cluster periods with inadequate therapy. Improved response can be expected with the use of a more effective agent that has a faster onset of action. Reasonable options for the acute treatment of R.H.'s acute cluster headaches include subcutaneous sumatriptan or oxygen inhalation. The success rate with each of these therapies is high. For many patients, oxygen is a less convenient therapy since the equipment is not easily portable and the patient must sit still during the treatment. The choice can be made on the basis of patient preference or cost.

Prophylactic Therapy

25. What therapeutic agents are available for headache prophylaxis during an active cluster period?

Pharmacotherapy aimed at preventing cluster headaches during an active period should be considered if symptomatic therapy is ineffective, intolerable, or if headaches occur more frequently than twice daily. Table 52-9 contains a list of available drugs for cluster headache prophylaxis.

Verapamil

Verapamil is effective for the prevention of cluster headaches,[165,213,214] and many authors now considered this agent to be the prophylactic agent of choice.[187,189] The usual effective daily dose is 240 to 480 mg/day and approximately two-thirds of patients have a 50% or greater reduction in headache frequency. Verapamil can be combined with lithium for prophylaxis in patients with chronic cluster headaches.[187]

Prednisone

Prednisone 40 to 80 mg daily provides relief from episodic cluster headache in 50% to 75% of patients[215,216] and is superior to methysergide in both episodic and chronic cluster types.[216] Prednisone also has a faster onset of action than many other agents used for cluster headache prophylaxis. The beneficial effect is usually evident within 48 hours of initiating treatment.[79] Corticosteroids are best used for short bouts of cluster headaches (1–2 months or less) because of the side effects associated with prolonged use.

Ergotamine

Ergotamine's use as a prophylactic agent is particularly attractive when headache recurrence follows a predictable pattern (e.g., nocturnal attacks). Prophylactic administration at

Table 52-9 Drugs for Prophylaxis of Cluster Headache[a]

Drug	Dose/Day	Route	Comments
Ergotamine tartrate (Cafergot, Ergostat)	0.25–0.5 mg BID–TID 5 days/wk 1–2 mg BID or HS for nocturnal HA; max 12 mg/wk	SC, PO, SL, PR	Effective when given 30 min before anticipated cluster HA
Indomethacin (Indocin)	50 mg TID	PO	Effective for chronic cluster HA
Lithium carbonate	600–1,500 mg	PO	Effective for chronic cluster HA; effective in 80% of patients
Melatonin	10 mg QD	PO	Efficacy demonstrated in 1 randomized controlled trial; patients with chronic cluster headache did not respond
Methylergonovine maleate	0.2 mg TID–QID	PO	Effective in 75% of patients in one retrospective study
Methysergide (Sansert)	2 mg TID–QID	PO	Effective in 65–70% of patients with episodic cluster HA; less effective for chronic cluster HA
Prednisone	40 mg QID × 2 days, then taper by 5 mg/day to maintenance dose of 15–30 mg QID	PO	A first-line agent for episodic cluster HA; more effective and faster-acting than methysergide; benefits usually within 48 hr; best for short bouts of cluster HA because of long-term adverse effects
Triamcinolone (Aristocort)	4–8 mg QID	PO	May be useful in patients unresponsive to prednisone
Valproate (Depakote)	600–2,000 mg/day divided TID–QID	PO	Effective in 73% of patients in 1 open trial
Verapamil (Isoptin, Calan)	240–480 mg/day divided TID–QID	PO	Drug of choice for prophylaxis

[a] See text for references and additional details.
HA, headache; PO, oral; PR, rectal; SC, subcutaneous; SL, sublingual.

bedtime or at least 30 minutes before the anticipated headache often will prevent the attack.[189]

Methysergide

Methysergide is effective in 65% to 70% of patients with episodic cluster headache and can be used for cluster periods of less than 3 months' duration without the same degree of concern for fibrotic complications because of the anticipated shorter period of drug exposure.[207,216] A limitation to the use of methysergide as the sole prophylactic agent for cluster headache is the delay in symptomatic response, which may be up to 2 weeks in some patients. Chronic cluster headache responds less dramatically to methysergide and other agents (e.g., lithium) are preferred.[207]

Lithium Carbonate

Lithium carbonate is effective in preventing episodic and chronic cluster headache.[207,217,218] Benefits from lithium prophylaxis are observable 1 to 2 weeks after initiation of therapy[79,217,218] and are maintained with long-term use.[219] Lithium serum levels associated with efficacy in cluster headache prophylaxis are usually between 0.6 and 1.2 mEq/L.[189] However, lower levels (0.3–0.8 mEq/L) may also be effective.[187] Adverse effects from long-term lithium use (e.g., renal toxicity) are discussed in Chapter 80, Mood Disorders II: Bipolar Disorders.

Other Therapies

Valproate has not been adequately studied, but one open trial reported that 73% of patients with cluster headache responded to this treatment.[220] In a recent pilot study, melatonin was superior to placebo for prophylaxis of cluster headache.[221] β-Blockers, antidepressants, and carbamazepine have no proven usefulness in the treatment of cluster headaches.[79]

R.H. should be evaluated at his next clinic visit for response to abortive sumatriptan or oxygen therapy. Prompt consideration should be given to the aforementioned additional treatments if suppression of headaches during the cluster period is warranted. In general, after response to a prophylactic agent has been established and maintained for at least 2 weeks, attempts can be made to discontinue the drug. Treatment should be reinstituted if headaches recur.

TENSION-TYPE HEADACHE

Tension-type headache is the most common headache type with a lifetime prevalence of 88% in women and 69% in men.[222] In a population-based study, the 1-year prevalence of tension-type headache was 38%. Highest prevalence rates were found in women between 30 and 39 years of age and, in both sexes, those with higher education levels.[223] Tension-type headaches (previously known as *tension* or *muscle contraction* headaches) are usually characterized by a dull aching sensation bilaterally that occurs in a hatband distribution around the head. The pain is usually mild to moderate in severity and has a nonpulsating quality.[224] Tension-type headaches are not associated with aura symptoms, nor are they accompanied by nausea, vomiting, or photophobia. The headache is usually not of sufficient intensity to interfere with daily activities but may be a nuisance by virtue of its persistent nature. Headache frequency varies widely between patients. Chronic tension-type headache occurs in approximately 2% of the population (1-year prevalence rate) and sufferers may have headache continuously for months or even years.[223]

Pathophysiology

The throbbing pain associated with migraine headaches is not characteristic of tension-type headaches, although it may occur in 25% of tension-type headache sufferers when the pain becomes severe.[79] Such patients may be diagnosed more appropriately as having a mixed tension-type/migraine headache disorder.[225] Indeed, in recent years the traditional boundaries distinguishing migraine from tension-type headaches have become less clear. Headache features such as neck muscle contraction and precipitation by stress were previously thought to be specific for tension-type headaches but are now recognized to occur in migraine as well.

For many years, excessive muscle contraction with constriction of pain-sensitive extracranial structures was thought to be the cause of tension-type headache.[226] More recent evidence shows no correlation between muscle contraction and the presence of tension-type headache.[227] Abnormal vascular reactivity was also thought to play a role in tension-type headache, but temporal muscle blood flow is unaltered compared with controls.[227] Platelet 5-HT content is lower in patients with chronic tension-type headache suggesting that migraine and tension-type headaches share some pathophysiologic features.[224]

Tension-type headaches also may be associated with depression,[225] repressed hostility, or resentment.[228] However, these psychological associations may be the result of the chronic pain syndrome rather than a cause or feature of the headache disorder. Patients with recurrent tension-type headaches probably do not experience more frequent stressful events, but may use less effective coping strategies in stressful situations.[229]

General Management and Abortive Therapy

26. K.B., a 27-year-old female financial analyst, presents to her general practitioner with a complaint of recurring headaches that worsened when she started her current job. Before this time, she had experienced infrequent headaches, which she associated with periods of stress. The headaches would occur three to four times yearly, were of a constant, dull, or "pressing" character and were present around the entire head. Recently, headaches of similar character have been occurring about one to two times weekly, usually toward the end of her work day. The pain usually lasts the rest of the day but varies in intensity. Occasionally, a headache is present when she wakes up in the morning as well. K.B. denies GI and aura symptoms associated with her headaches. She has noticed that relaxation and alcohol ingestion seem to relieve these headaches, but aspirin and acetaminophen have been ineffective. Her blood pressure is 120/74 mmHg; her physical and neurologic examinations are completely normal. What measures should be taken to relieve K.B.'s headaches? What is an appropriate goal for treatment?

As in the treatment of other chronic headache disorders, a cure for recurrent tension-type headache is unlikely. K.B. should clearly understand that the goal of treatment is a reduction in the frequency and severity of headache. Drug therapy and relaxation techniques are the primary means by which tension-type headaches are treated.

Analgesics

Analgesics are the drugs of choice for treatment of acute tension headache attacks.[224] The initial choice of an analgesic should be based on the severity of the pain. Acetaminophen, aspirin, and NSAIDs are often effective, although their benefits may be short lived. Acetaminophen 1,000 mg provides equal relief from moderately severe tension-type headache when compared with 650 mg aspirin; both are superior to placebo.[230] Ibuprofen is as effective as aspirin for relief from tension headache discomfort, and side effects with both 400 and 800 mg ibuprofen are less common than with aspirin.[231] Ibuprofen 400 mg is superior to acetaminophen 1,000 mg for relief of tension-type headache pain.[232] Naproxen sodium 550 mg is more effective than placebo and acetaminophen 650 mg for relieving the pain of tension-type headache.[224] The potency of some analgesics may be enhanced by combination with an antihistamine (e.g., doxylamine).[233] Because the relative potencies of non-narcotic analgesics are equivalent, the choice between agents should be guided by cost and patient preference.

Sedatives (e.g., butalbital),[79] anxiolytics (e.g., meprobamate,[234] diazepam[235]), and skeletal muscle relaxants (e.g., orphenadrine) have also been used to treat tension-type headache and occasionally, patients respond to their concomitant use when an analgesic alone affords insufficient relief.

Nondrug Techniques

Nondrug techniques such as massage, hot baths, acupuncture, and various relaxation methods can provide relief from tension headache and are often effective adjuncts to drug therapy.[236] The literature both supports and refutes the effectiveness of acupuncture,[10,237] EMG (electromyography) biofeedback,[238–240] and other relaxation techniques in the therapy of tension-type headache. The utility of biofeedback and other relaxation techniques is based on the premise that voluntary control of muscle contraction could benefit the headache sufferer. These techniques are most successful in young, episodic headache sufferers who are motivated to apply the techniques as instructed.[241] A randomized, controlled trial of spinal manipulation for the treatment of tension-type headache failed to demonstrate a benefit of this approach.[242]

An NSAID (e.g., ibuprofen or naproxen) would be an appropriate recommendation for therapy of K.B.'s tension-type headaches because of her previous inadequate responses to aspirin and acetaminophen. Drug use should be carefully monitored because analgesic abuse in patients with frequently recurring tension headache is a primary factor in the perpetuation of chronic pain syndromes.[243]

Prophylactic Therapy

27. Ibuprofen 400 mg Q 4 to 6 hr as needed for headache was prescribed for acute relief of K.B.'s recurrent tension-type headaches. At her next scheduled follow-up visit, K.B. reported moderate relief with ibuprofen but complained of GI upset with each dose, even when taken with food. Because headaches have been occurring more frequently, her use of ibuprofen has also increased. What prophylactic agents are available for continuous suppression of K.B.'s tension-type headaches?

Antidepressants are the most useful group of agents in the prophylaxis of tension-type and mixed-type headaches. Amitriptyline (Elavil) is considered the drug of choice because it is most effective[244,245]; 65% of patients improved by more than 50% and 25% became headache-free in an early report.[225] The effective daily dose of amitriptyline for most patients is 10 to 75 mg,[244] although up to 300 mg/day may be required.[79] Response to amitriptyline does not require a history of depressive symptoms, and benefit to the tension-type headache sufferer is usually evident within 2 to 10 days.[79] Amitriptyline should be initiated at a dose of 10 to 25 mg/day at bedtime and increased gradually as needed to allow for the development of tolerance to the sedative and anticholinergic side effects of this drug. About 7% of patients discontinue amitriptyline because of side effects.[10] Although there is less experience with their use, doxepin (Sinequan),[246] imipramine (Tofranil),[6,225] maprotiline (Ludiomil),[247] and protriptyline (Vivactil)[248] are also effective in tension-type headache prophylaxis. Like amitriptyline, these agents have significant anticholinergic activity. If an agent with less anticholinergic activity is desired, desipramine (Norpramin) may be used. Although fluoxetine has been suggested as an alternative for the treatment of tension-type headache,[249] its effectiveness has not been established in a randomized, controlled trial. A randomized placebo-controlled trial comparing citalopram (an SSRI) with amitriptyline found that citalopram was not effective for prophylaxis of chronic tension-type headache.[250] At this time, SSRI antidepressants are not recommended for tension-type headache prophylaxis.[244] Given K.B.'s increasing frequency of tension-type headache and her intolerance to moderate doses of ibuprofen, prophylactic treatment with amitriptyline would be appropriate. A starting dose of amitriptyline 10 mg nightly, increasing by 10 to 25 mg at 1-week intervals to a maintenance dose of 50 mg/day should be prescribed, at which time headache response can be assessed and the dose increased or decreased as necessary. If effective, amitriptyline should be continued for 3 to 4 months before gradually decreasing the dose until the drug is completely discontinued. Therapy should be reinstituted if headaches return.

Because the dividing line between migraine and tension-type headache is often vague, the entire range of migraine drugs may be tried in refractory cases of tension-type headache or when symptoms suggest a mixed tension-type/migraine headache disorder.

REFERENCES

1. Stewart WF et al. Prevalence of migraine headache in the United States. Relation to age, income, race, and other sociodemographic factors. *JAMA* 1992;267:64.
2. Kroenke K, Mangelsdorff AD. Common symptoms in ambulatory care: incidence, evaluation, therapy, and outcome. *Am J Med* 1989;86:262.
3. Stang PE, Osterhaus JT. Impact of migraine in the United States: data from the National Health Interview Survey. *Headache* 1993;33:29.
4. Cook NR et al. Correlates of headache in a population-based cohort of elderly. *Arch Neurol* 1989;46:1338.
5. Linet MS et al. An epidemiologic study of headache among adolescents and young adults. *JAMA* 1989;261:2211.
6. Lance JW et al. Investigations into the mechanism and treatment of chronic headache. *Med J Aust* 1965;2:909.
7. Classification and diagnostic criteria for headache disorders, cranial neuralgias and facial pain. Headache Classification Committee of the International Headache Society. *Cephalalgia* 1988; 8(Suppl 7):1.
8. Saper JR. Headache disorders. *Med Clin North Am* 1999;83:663.
9. Ray B, Wolff HG. Experimental studies on headache. Pain sensitive structures of the head and their significance in headache. *Arch Surg* 1940; 41:813.
10. Lance JW. *Mechanism and Management of Headache,* 4th Ed. London: Butterworths Scientific; 1982
11. Welch KM. Current opinions in headache pathogenesis: introduction and synthesis. *Curr Opin Neurol* 1998;11:193.
12. May A, Goadsby PJ. The trigeminovascular system in humans: pathophysiologic implications for primary headache syndromes of the neural influences on the cerebral circulation. *J Cereb Blood Flow Metab* 1999;19:115.
13. Silberstein SD. Serotonin (5-HT) and migraine. *Headache* 1994;34:408.
14. Goadsby PJ. Mechanisms and management of headache. *J R Coll Physicians Lond* 1999;33:228.
15. Olesen J et al. Timing and topography of cerebral blood flow, aura, and headache during migraine attacks. *Ann Neurol* 1990;28:791.
16. Olesen J et al. The common migraine attack may not be initiated by cerebral ischaemia. *Lancet* 1981;2:438.
17. Limmroth V et al. Changes in cerebral blood flow velocity after treatment with sumatriptan or placebo and implications for the pathophysiology of migraine. *J Neurol Sci* 1996;138:60.
18. Drummond PD et al. Facial flushing after thermocoagulation of the Gasserian ganglion. *J Neurol Neurosurg Psychiatry* 1983;46:611.
19. Goadsby PJ et al. Release of vasoactive peptides in the extracerebral circulation of humans and the cat during activation of the trigeminovascular system. *Ann Neurol* 1988;23:193.
20. Weiller C et al. Brain stem activation in spontaneous human migraine attacks. *Nat Med* 1995;1: 658.
21. Hoskin KL et al. Central activation of the trigeminovascular pathway in the cat is inhibited by dihydroergotamine. A c-Fos and electrophysiological study. *Brain* 1996;119(Pt 1):249.
22. Cumberbatch M et al. Rizatriptan inhibits central trigeminal nociceptive responses in an electrophysiological assay in the anaesthetized rat [Abstract]. In: Elesen J, Edvinsson L, eds. Messenger Molecules in Headache Pathogenesis: Monoamines, Neuropeptides, Purines and Nitric Oxide. Proceedings of the 7th International headache research seminar. Copenhagen; 1996:18.
23. Goadsby PJ, Hoskin KL. Inhibition of trigeminal neurons by intravenous administration of the serotonin (5HT)1B/D receptor agonist zolmitriptan (311C90): are brain stem sites therapeutic target in migraine? *Pain* 1996;67:355.
24. Anthony M et al. Plasma serotonin in migraine and stress. *Arch Neurol* 1967;16:544.
25. Curran DA et al. Total plasma serotonin, 5-hydroxyindoleacetic acid and p-hydroxy-m-methoxymandelic acid excretion in normal and migrainous subjects. *Brain* 1965;88:997.
26. Kimball RW et al. Effect of serotonin in migraine patients. *Neurology* 1960;10:107.
27. Hamel E et al. Expression of mRNA for the serotonin 5-hydroxytryptamine1D beta receptor subtype in human and bovine cerebral arteries. *Mol Pharmacol* 1993;44:242.
28. Rebeck GW et al. Selective 5-HT1D alpha serotonin receptor gene expression in trigeminal ganglia: implications for antimigraine drug development. *Proc Natl Acad Sci U S A* 1994;91:3666.
29. Ophoff RA et al. Familial hemiplegic migraine and episodic ataxia type-2 are caused by mutations in the Ca2+ channel gene CACNL1A4. *Cell* 1996;87:543.
30. Wessman M et al. A susceptibility locus for migraine with aura, on chromosome 4q24. *Am J Hum Genet* 2002;70:652.
31. Soragna D et al. A locus for migraine without aura maps on chromosome 14q21.2-q22.3. *Am J Hum Genet* 2003;72:161.
32. Rozen TD et al. Increasing incidence of medically recognized migraine headache in a United States population. *Neurology* 1999;53:1468.
33. Russell MB et al. Familial occurrence of migraine without aura and migraine with aura. *Neurology* 1993;43:1369.
34. Selby G, Lance JW. Observations on 500 cases of migraine and allied vascular headache. *J Neurol Neurosurg Psychiatry* 1960;23:23.
35. Ferrari MD. Migraine. *Lancet* 1998;351:1043.
36. Creditor MC. Me and migraine. *N Engl J Med* 1982;307:1029.
37. Lipton RB et al. Stratified care vs step care strategies for migraine: the Disability in Strategies of Care (DISC) Study: A randomized trial. *JAMA* 2000;284:2599.
38. Silberstein SD. Practice parameter: evidence-based guidelines for migraine headache (an evidence-based review): report of the Quality Standards Subcommittee of the American Academy of Neurology. *Neurology* 2000;55:754.
39. Becker WJ. Use of oral contraceptives in patients with migraine. *Neurology* 1999;53:S19.
39a. Loder EL et al. Hormonal management of migraine associated with menses and menopause: a clinical review. *Headache* 2007;47:329.
40. Ryan RE. A controlled study of the effect of oral contraceptives on migraine. *Headache* 1978;17: 250.
41. Tzourio C et al. Case-control study of migraine and risk of ischaemic stroke in young women. *Br Med J* 1995;310:830.
42. Silberstein SD, Young WB. Safety and efficacy of ergotamine tartrate and dihydroergotamine in the treatment of migraine and status migrainosus. Working Panel of the Headache and Facial Pain Section of the American Academy of Neurology. *Neurology* 1995;45:577.
43. Bousser MG, Massiou H. Migraine in the reproductive cycle. In: Olesen J et al., eds. The Headaches. New York: Raven Press; 1993:313.
44. Goadsby PJ et al. Migraine-current understanding and treatment. *N Engl J Med* 2002;346:257.
45. Perry CM, Markham A. Sumatriptan. An updated review of its use in migraine. *Drugs* 1998;55:889.
46. O'Quinn S et al. Sumatriptan injection and nasal spray: onset of efficacy in the acute treatment of migraine [Abstract]. *Neurology* 1998;50:A264.
47. Volans GN. Absorption of effervescent aspirin during migraine. *Br Med J* 1974;4:265.
48. Touchon J et al. A comparison of subcutaneous sumatriptan and dihydroergotamine nasal spray in the acute treatment of migraine. *Neurology* 1996;47:361.
49. Winner P et al. A double-blind study of subcutaneous dihydroergotamine vs. subcutaneous

sumatriptan in the treatment of acute migraine. *Arch Neurol* 1996;53:180.
50. A randomized, double-blind comparison of sumatriptan and Cafergot in the acute treatment of migraine. The Multinational Oral Sumatriptan and Cafergot Comparative Study Group. *Eur Neurol* 1991;31:314.
51. A study to compare oral sumatriptan with oral aspirin plus oral metoclopramide in the acute treatment of migraine. The Oral Sumatriptan and Aspirin plus Metoclopramide Comparative Study Group. *Eur Neurol* 1992;32:177.
52. Brown EG et al. The safety and tolerability of sumatriptan: an overview. *Eur Neurol* 1991;31:339.
53. Visser WH et al. Sumatriptan in clinical practice: a 2-year review of 453 migraine patients. *Neurology* 1996;47:46.
54. Lippolis A et al. [Coronary vasospasm secondary to subcutaneous administration of sumatriptan.] *G Ital Cardiol* 1994;24:883.
55. Walton-Shirley M et al. Unstable angina pectoris associated with Imitrex therapy. *Cathet Cardiovasc Diagn* 1995;34:188.
56. Mueller L et al. Vasospasm-induced myocardial infarction with sumatriptan. *Headache* 1996;36:329.
57. Cavazos JE et al. Sumatriptan-induced stroke in sagittal sinus thrombosis. *Lancet* 1994;343:1105.
58. Ottervanger JP et al. Transmural myocardial infarction with sumatriptan. *Lancet* 1993;341:861.
59. Saxena P, Tfelt-Hansen P. Sumatriptan. In: Olesen J, ed. *The Headaches.* New York: Raven Press; 1993:329.
60. Geraud G et al. Migraine headache recurrence: relationship to clinical, pharmacological, and pharmacokinetic properties of triptans. *Headache* 2003;43:376.
61. Diamond S. The use of sumatriptan in patients on monoamine oxidase inhibitors. *Neurology* 1995; 45:1039.
62. Blier P, Bergeron R. The safety of concomitant use of sumatriptan and antidepressant treatments. *J Clin Psychopharmacol* 1995;15:106.
63. Gardner DM, Lynd LD. Sumatriptan contraindications and the serotonin syndrome. *Ann Pharmacother* 1998;32:33.
64. Ferrari MD et al. Oral triptans (serotonin 5-HT(1B/1D) agonists) in acute migraine treatment: a meta-analysis of 53 trials. *Lancet* 2001;358:1668.
65. Tfelt-Hansen P, Johnson ES. Ergotamine. In: Olesen J et al, eds. *The Headaches.* New York: Raven Press; 1993:313.
66. Hachinski V et al. Ergotamine and cerebral blood flow. *Stroke* 1978;9:594.
67. Moyer JH et al. The effect of theophylline with ethylenediamine (aminophylline) and caffeine on cerebral hemodynamics and cerebrospinal fluid pressure in patients with hypertensive headaches. *Am J Med Sci* 1952;224:377.
68. Schmidt R, Fanchamps A. Effect of caffeine on intestinal absorption of ergotamine in man. *Eur J Clin Pharmacol* 1974;7:213.
69. Laska EM et al. Caffeine as an analgesic adjuvant. *JAMA* 1984;251:1711.
70. Sutherland JM et al. Buccal absorption of ergotamine. *J Neurol Neurosurg Psychiatry* 1974;37: 1116.
71. Tfelt-Hansen P et al. Clinical pharmacology of ergotamine studied with a high performance liquid chromatographic method. In: Rose FC, ed. *Advances in Migraine Research and Therapy.* New York: Raven Press; 1982:173.
72. Crooks J et al. Clinical Trial of Inhaled Ergotamine Tartrate in Migraine. *Br Med J* 1964;5377:221.
73. Carstairs LS. Headache and gastric emptying time. *Proc R Soc Med* 1958;51:790.
74. Orton D. Ergotamine tartrate levels in migraine, ergotamine tartrate overdose, and normal subjects using a rasioimmunoassay. Proceedings of the Migraine Trust International Symposium. London; 1976
75. Raskin NH. Acute and prophylactic treatment of migraine: practical approaches and pharmacologic rationale. *Neurology* 1993;43:S39.
76. Saper J. *Headache Disorders: Current Concepts and Treatment Strategies.* Littleton, MA: Wright-PSG Publishers; 1983.
77. Ala-Hurula V et al. Systemic availability of ergotamine tartrate after oral, rectal and intramuscular administration. *Eur J Clin Pharmacol* 1979; 15:51.
78. Krupp P, Haas G. Effects indesirables et interactions medicamenteuse des alcaloides de l'ergot de seigle. *J Pharmacol* 1979;10:401.
79. Raskin NH. *Headache,* 2nd Ed. New York: Churchill Livingstone; 1988.
80. Andersen AR et al. The effect of ergotamine and dihydroergotamine on cerebral blood flow in man. *Stroke* 1987;18:120.
81. Edmeads J. Ergotamine and the cerebral circulation. *Hemicrania* 1976;7:6.
82. Blau JN et al. Ergotamine tartrate overdosage. *Br Med J* 1979;1:265.
83. Baumrucker JF. Drug interaction-propranolol and cafergot. *N Engl J Med* 1973;288:916.
84. Venter CP et al. Severe peripheral ischaemia during concomitant use of beta blockers and ergot alkaloids. *Br Med J (Clin Res Ed)* 1984;289:288.
85. Saper JR, Jones JM. Ergotamine tartrate dependency: features and possible mechanisms. *Clin Neuropharmacol* 1986;9:244.
86. Tokola RA. The effect of metoclopramide and prochlorperazine on the absorption of effervescent paracetamol in migraine. *Cephalalgia* 1988;8:139.
87. Tfelt-Hansen P, Johnson ES. Antiemetic and prokinetic drugs. In: Olesen J, ed. *The Headaches.* New York: Raven Press; 1993:343.
88. Tfelt-Hansen P et al. A double blind study of metoclopramide in the treatment of migraine attacks. *J Neurol Neurosurg Psychiatry* 1980;43:369.
89. Diamond S. Treatment of migraine with isometheptene, acetaminophen, and dichloralphenazone combination: a double-blind, crossover trial. *Headache* 1976;15:282.
90. Yuill GM et al. A double-blind crossover trial of isometheptene mucate compound and ergotamine in migraine. *Br J Clin Pract* 1972;26:76.
91. Freitag FG et al. Comparative study of a combination of isometheptene mucate, dichloralphenazone with acetaminophen and sumatriptan succinate in the treatment of migraine. *Headache* 2001;41:391.
92. Deleu D et al. Symptomatic and prophylactic treatment of migraine: a critical reappraisal. *Clin Neuropharmacol* 1998;21:267.
93. McNeely W, Goa KL. Diclofenac-potassium in migraine: a review. *Drugs* 1999;57:991.
94. Pradalier A et al. Acute migraine attack therapy: comparison of naproxen sodium and an ergotamine tartrate compound. *Cephalalgia* 1985;5:107.
95. Kangasniemi P, Kaaja R. Ketoprofen and ergotamine in acute migraine. *J Intern Med* 1992;231: 551.
96. Volans GN. Migraine and drug absorption. *Clin Pharmacokinet* 1978;3:313.
97. Goldstein J. Ergot pharmacology and alternative delivery systems for ergotamine derivatives. *Neurology* 1992;42:45.
98. Ziegler D et al. Dihydroergotamine nasal spray for the acute treatment of migraine. *Neurology* 1994; 44:447.
99. Efficacy, safety, and tolerability of dihydroergotamine nasal spray as monotherapy in the treatment of acute migraine. Dihydroergotamine Nasal Spray Multicenter Investigators. *Headache* 1995;35:177.
100. Gallagher RM. Acute treatment of migraine with dihydroergotamine nasal spray. Dihydroergotamine Working Group. *Arch Neurol* 1996;53:1285.
101. Hirt D. A comparison of DHE nasal spray and Cafegot in acute migraine [Abstract]. *Cephalalgia* 1989;9(Suppl 10):410.
102. Klapper JA, Stanton J. Clinical experience with patient administered subcutaneous dihydroergotamine mesylate in refractory headaches. *Headache* 1992;32:21.
103. Saadah HA. Abortive headache therapy with intramuscular dihydroergotamine. *Headache* 1992;32: 18.
104. Callaham M, Raskin N. A controlled study of dihydroergotamine in the treatment of acute migraine headache. *Headache* 1986;26:168.
105. Coppola M et al. Randomized, placebo-controlled evaluation of prochlorperazine versus metoclopramide for emergency department treatment of migraine headache. *Ann Emerg Med* 1995;26:541.
106. Seim MB et al. Intravenous ketorolac vs intravenous prochlorperazine for the treatment of migraine headaches. *Acad Emerg Med* 1998;5:573.
107. Tanen DA et al. Intravenous sodium valproate versus prochlorperazine for the emergency department treatment of acute migraine headaches: a prospective, randomized, double-blind trial. *Ann Emerg Med* 2003;41:847.
108. Lane PL et al. Comparative efficacy of chlorpromazine and meperidine with dimenhydrinate in migraine headache. *Ann Emerg Med* 1989;18:360.
109. McEwen JI et al. Treatment of migraine with intramuscular chlorpromazine. *Ann Emerg Med* 1987;16:758.
110. Lane PL, Ross R. Intravenous chlorpromazine-preliminary results in acute migraine. *Headache* 1985;25:302.
111. Belgrade MJ et al. Comparison of single-dose meperidine, butorphanol, and dihydroergotamine in the treatment of vascular headache. *Neurology* 1989;39:590.
112. Tek D, Mellon M. The effectiveness of nalbuphine and hydroxyzine for the emergency treatment of severe headache. *Ann Emerg Med* 1987;16:308.
113. Fisher MA, Glass S. Butorphanol (Stadol): a study in problems of current drug information and control. *Neurology* 1997;48:1156.
114. Rapoport AM, Silberstein SD. Emergency treatment of headache. *Neurology* 1992;42:43.
115. Silberstein SD, Freitag FG. Preventative treatment of migraine. *Neurology* 2003;60(Suppl 2):S38.
116. Ramadan NM et al. Evidence-based guidelines for migraine headache in the primary care setting: pharmacological management for prevention of migraine. http://www.aan.com 2000.
117. Tfelt-Hansen P. Prophylactic pharmacotherapy of migraine. Some practical guidelines. *Neurol Clin* 1997;15:153.
118. Holroyd KA et al. Propranolol in the management of recurrent migraine: a meta-analytic review. *Headache* 1991;31:333.
119. Weber RB, Reinmuth OM. The treatment of migraine with propranolol. *Neurology* 1972;22:366.
120. Wideroe TE, Vigander T. Propranolol in the treatment of migraine. *Br Med J* 1974;2:699.
121. Diamond S, Medina JL. Double blind study of propranolol for migraine prophylaxis. *Headache* 1976;16:24.
122. Forssman B et al. Propranolol for migraine prophylaxis. *Headache* 1976;16:238.
123. Stensrud P, Sjaastad O. Short-term clinical trial of phopranolol in racemic form (Inderal), D-propranolol and placebo in migraine. *Acta Neurol Scand* 1976;53:229.
124. Diamond S et al. Long-term study of propranolol in the treatment of migraine. *Headache* 1982;22:268.
125. Rosen JA. Observations on the efficacy of propranolol for the prophylaxis of migraine. *Ann Neurol* 1983;13:92.
126. Olesen J et al. Isoproterenol and propranolol: ability to cross the blood-brain barrier and effects on cerebral circulation in man. *Stroke* 1978;9:344.
127. Middlemiss D. Direct evidence for an interaction of beta-adrenergic blockers with the 5-HT receptor. *Nature* 1977;267:289.
128. Hiner BC et al. Antimigraine drug interactions with 5-hydroxytryptamine1A receptors. *Ann Neurol* 1986;19:511.

129. Lingjaerde O. Platelet uptake and storage of serotonin. In: Essman W, ed. *Serotonin in Health and Disease.* New York: Spectrum; 1977:139.
130. Olsson JE et al. Metoprolol and propranolol in migraine prophylaxis: a double-blind multicentre study. *Acta Neurol Scand* 1984;70:160.
131. Stensrud P, Sjaastad O. Comparative trial of Tenormin (atenolol) and Inderal (propranolol) in migraine. *Headache* 1980;20:204.
132. Forssman B et al. Atenolol for migraine prophylaxis. *Headache* 1983;23:188.
133. Sjaastad O, Stensrud P. Clinical trial of a beta-receptor blocking agent (LB 46) in migraine prophylaxis. *Acta Neurol Scand* 1972;48:124.
134. Nanda RN et al. A double blind trial of acebutolol for migraine prophylaxis. *Headache* 1978;18:20.
135. Ekbom K. Alprenolol for migraine prophylaxis. *Headache* 1975;15:129.
136. Ekbom K, Zetterman M. Oxprenolol in the treatment of migraine. *Acta Neurol Scand* 1977;56:181.
137. Curran DA, Lance JW. Clinical Trial of Methysergide and Other Preparations in the Management of Migraine. *J Neurol Neurosurg Psychiatry* 1964;27:463.
138. Graham JR et al. Inflammatory fibrosis associated with methysergide therapy. *Res Clin Stud Headache* 1967;1:123.
139. Curran DA et al. Methysergide. *Res Clin Stud Headache* 1967;1:74.
140. Caldara R et al. Effect of two antiserotoninergic drugs, methysergide and metergoline, on gastric acid secretion and gastrin release in healthy man. *Eur J Clin Pharmacol* 1980;17:13.
141. Ziegler DK et al. Migraine prophylaxis. A comparison of propranolol and amitriptyline. *Arch Neurol* 1987;44:486.
142. Couch JR, Hassanein RS. Amitriptyline in migraine prophylaxis. *Arch Neurol* 1979;36:695.
143. Couch JR et al. Amitriptyline in the prophylaxis of migraine. Effectiveness and relationship of antimigraine and antidepressant effects. *Neurology* 1976;26:121.
144. Pringsheim T et al. Selective decrease in serotonin synthesis rate in rat brainstem raphe nuclei following chronic administration of low doses of amitriptyline: an effect compatible with an antimigraine effect. *Cephalalgia* 2003;23:367.
145. Langohr HD et al. Clomipramine and metoprolol in migraine prophylaxis-a double-blind crossover study. *Headache* 1985;25:107.
146. Heninger G, Charney D. Mechanism of action of antidepressant treatments: implications for the etiology and treatment of depressive disorders. In: Meltzer H, ed. *Psychopharmacology: The Third Generation of Progress.* New York: Raven Press; 1987:535.
147. Adly C et al. Fluoxetine prophylaxis of migraine. *Headache* 1992;32:101.
148. Saper JR et al. Double-blind trial of fluoxetine: chronic daily headache and migraine. *Headache* 1994;34:497.
149. Bank J. A comparative study of amitriptyline and fluvoxamine in migraine prophylaxis. *Headache* 1994;34:476.
150. Hering R, Kuritzky A. Sodium valproate in the prophylactic treatment of migraine: a double-blind study versus placebo. *Cephalalgia* 1992;12:81.
151. Mathew NT et al. Migraine prophylaxis with divalproex. *Arch Neurol* 1995;52:281.
152. Kaniecki RG. A comparison of divalproex with propranolol and placebo for the prophylaxis of migraine without aura. *Arch Neurol* 1997;54:1141.
153. Lindegaard KF et al. Naproxen in the prevention of migraine attacks. A double-blind placebo-controlled cross-over study. *Headache* 1980;20:96.
154. Bellavance AJ, Meloche JP. A comparative study of naproxen sodium, pizotyline and placebo in migraine prophylaxis. *Headache* 1990;30:710.
155. Sances G et al. Naproxen sodium in menstrual migraine prophylaxis: a double-blind placebo controlled study. *Headache* 1990;30:705.
156. Stensrud P, Sjaastad O. Clinical trial of a new antibradykinin, anti-inflammatory drug, ketoprofen (19.583 r.p.) in migraine prophylaxis. *Headache* 1974;14:96.
157. Solomon GD, Kunkel RS. Flurbiprofen in the prophylaxis of migraine. *Cleve Clin J Med* 1993;60:43.
158. Johnson RH et al. Comparison of mefenamic acid and propranolol with placebo in migraine prophylaxis. *Acta Neurol Scand* 1986;73:490.
159. Sargent J et al. A comparison of naproxen sodium to propranolol hydrochloride and a placebo control for the prophylaxis of migraine headache. *Headache* 1985;25:320.
160. Reuter H. Calcium channel modulation by neurotransmitters, enzymes and drugs. *Nature* 1983;301:569.
161. Markley HG et al. Verapamil in prophylactic therapy of migraine. *Neurology* 1984;34:973.
162. Solomon GD et al. Verapamil prophylaxis of migraine. A double-blind, placebo-controlled study. *JAMA* 1983;250:2500.
163. Solomon GD. Comparative efficacy of calcium antagonist drugs in the prophylaxis of migraine. *Headache* 1985;25:368.
164. Meyer JS et al. Migraine and cluster headache treatment with calcium antagonists supports a vascular pathogenesis. *Headache* 1985;25:358.
165. Meyer JS, Hardenberg J. Clinical effectiveness of calcium entry blockers in prophylactic treatment of migraine and cluster headaches. *Headache* 1983;23:266.
166. Smith R, Schwartz A. Diltiazem prophylaxis in refractory migraine. *N Engl J Med* 1984;310:1327.
167. McArthur JC et al. Nifedipine in the prophylaxis of classic migraine: a crossover, double-masked, placebo-controlled study of headache frequency and side effects. *Neurology* 1989;39:284.
168. Riopelle R, McCans J. A pilot study of the calcium antagonist diltiazem in migraine syndrome prophylaxis. *J Can Sci Neurol* 1982;9:269.
169. Flaim S. Comparative pharmacology of calcium blockers based on studies of vascular smooth muscle. In: Flaim S, Zelig R, eds. *Calcium Blockers: Mechanism of Action and Clinical Applications.* Baltimore: Urban & Schwarzenberg; 1982:155.
170. Havanka-Kanniainen H et al. Efficacy of nimodipine in the prophylaxis of migraine. *Cephalalgia* 1985;5:39.
171. Gelmers HJ. Nimodipine, a new calcium antagonist, in the prophylactic treatment of migraine. *Headache* 1983;23:106.
172. Stewart DJ et al. Effect of prophylactic administration of nimodipine in patients with migraine. *Headache* 1988;28:260.
173. Ansell E et al. Nimodipine in migraine prophylaxis. *Cephalalgia* 1988;8:269.
174. Stensrud P, Sjaastad O. Clonidine (Catapresan)-double-blind study after long-term treatment with the drug in migraine. *Acta Neurol Scand* 1976;53:233.
175. Vogler BK et al. Feverfew as a preventive treatment for migraine: a systematic review. *Cephalalgia* 1998;18:704.
176. Anthony M, Lance JW. Monoamine oxidase inhibition in the treatment of migraine. *Arch Neurol* 1969;21:263.
177. Schoenen J et al. Effectiveness of high-dose riboflavin in migraine prophylaxis. A randomized controlled trial. *Neurology* 1998;50:466.
178. Beecher HK. The powerful placebo. *J Am Med Assoc* 1955;159:1602.
179. Couch JR et al. The long-term effect of placebo on migraine [Abstract]. *Neurology* 1987;27(Suppl 1):238.
180. Sandrini G et al. An epidemiological approach to the nosography of chronic daily headache. *Cephalalgia* 1993;13(Suppl 12):72.
181. Martignoni E, Solomon S. The complex chronic headache: mixed headache and drug overuse. In: Olesen J et al, eds. The Headaches. New York: Raven Press; 1993:849.
182. Srikiatkhachorn A, Anthony M. Serotonin receptor adaptation in patients with analgesic-induced headache. *Cephalalgia* 1996;16:419.
183. Sandler DP et al. Analgesic use and chronic renal disease. *N Engl J Med* 1989;320:1238.
184. McGoldrick MD, Bailie GR. Nonnarcotic analgesics: prevalence and estimated economic impact of toxicities. *Ann Pharmacother* 1997;31:221.
185. Tolman KG. Hepatotoxicity of non-narcotic analgesics. *Am J Med* 1998;105:13S.
186. Hering R, Steiner TJ. Abrupt outpatient withdrawal of medication in analgesic-abusing migraineurs. *Lancet* 1991;337:1442.
187. Ekbom K, Hardebo JE. Cluster headache: aetiology, diagnosis and management. *Drugs* 2002;62:61.
188. Ekbom K. A clinical comparison of cluster headache and migraine. *Acta Neurol Scand* 1970; (Suppl) 41:1.
189. Mathew NT. Cluster headache. *Neurology* 1992; 42:22.
190. Sakai F, Meyer JS. Regional cerebral hemodynamics during migraine and cluster headaches measured by the 133Xe inhalation method. *Headache* 1978;18:122.
191. Sakai F, Meyer JS. Abnormal cerebrovascular reactivity in patients with migraine and cluster headache. *Headache* 1979;19:257.
192. Krabbe AA et al. Tomographic determination of cerebral blood flow during attacks of cluster headache. *Cephalalgia* 1984;4:17.
193. Drummond PD, Lance JW. Thermographic changes in cluster headache. *Neurology* 1984;34:1292.
194. Mendizabal JE et al. Cluster headache: Horton's cephalalgia revisited. *South Med J* 1998;91:606.
195. Buzzi M et al. Morphological effects of electrical trigeminal ganglion stimulation on intra and extracranial vessels [Abstract]. *Soc Neurosci* 1990;16:591.
196. Sjaastad O et al. Cluster headache in identical twins. *Headache* 1993;33:214.
197. Russell MB et al. Familial occurrence of cluster headache. *J Neurol Neurosurg Psychiatry* 1995;58:341.
198. May A, Leone M. Update on cluster headache. *Curr Opin Neurol* 2003;16:333.
199. Manzoni GC et al. Lithium carbonate in cluster headache: assessment of its short- and long-term therapeutic efficacy. *Cephalalgia* 1983;3:109.
200. Riess CM et al. Episodic cluster headache in a community: clinical features and treatment. *Can J Neurol Sci* 1998;25:141.
201. Ekbom K, Sakai F. Tension-type headache, cluster headache and miscellaneous headaches; management. In: Olesen J, ed. *The Headaches.* New York: Raven Press; 1993:591.
202. Hardebo JE, Dahlof C. Sumatriptan nasal spray (20 mg/dose) in the acute treatment of cluster headache. *Cephalalgia* 1998;18:487.
203. Monstad I et al. Preemptive oral treatment with sumatriptan during a cluster period. *Headache* 1995;35:607.
204. Fogan L. Treatment of cluster headache. A double-blind comparison of oxygen v air inhalation. *Arch Neurol* 1985;42:362.
205. Kudrow L. Response of cluster headache attacks to oxygen inhalation. *Headache* 1981;21:1.
206. Ekbom K et al. Optimal routes of administration of ergotamine tartrate in cluster headache patients. A pharmacokinetic study. *Cephalalgia* 1983; 3:15.
207. Kudrow L. *Cluster Headache: Mechanisms and Management.* Oxford: Oxford University Press; 1980.
208. Graham JR et al. Aerosol ergotamine tartrate for migraine and Horton's syndrome. *N Engl J Med* 1960;263:802.
209. Marks DR et al. A double-blind placebo-controlled trial of intranasal capsaicin for cluster headache. *Cephalalgia* 1993;13:114.
210. Sicuteri F et al. Pain relief by somatostatin in attacks of cluster headache. *Pain* 1984;18:359.

211. Kittrelle JP et al. Cluster headache. Local anesthetic abortive agents. *Arch Neurol* 1985;42:496.
212. Barre F. Cocaine as an abortive agent in cluster headache. *Headache* 1982;22:69.
213. de Carolis P et al. Nimodipine in episodic cluster headache: results and methodological considerations. *Headache* 1987;27:397.
214. Meyer JS et al. Clinical and hemodynamic effects during treatment of vascular headaches with verapamil. *Headache* 1984;24:313.
215. Couch JR, Jr., Ziegler DK. Prednisone therapy for cluster headache. *Headache* 1978;18:219.
216. Kudrow L. Comparative results of prednisone, methysergide, and lithium therapy in cluster headache. In: Greene R, ed. *Current Concepts in Migraine Research.* New York: Raven Press; 1978: 159.
217. Damasio H, Lyon L. Lithium carbonate in the treatment of cluster headaches. *J Neurol* 1980; 224:1.
218. Ekbom K. Lithium for cluster headache: review of the literature and preliminary results of long-term treatment. *Headache* 1981;21:132.
219. Savoldi F et al. Lithium salts in cluster headache treatment. *Cephalalgia* 1983;3(Suppl 1):79.
220. Hering R, Kuritzky A. Sodium valproate in the treatment of cluster headache: an open clinical trial. *Cephalalgia* 1989;9:195.
221. Leone M et al. Melatonin versus placebo in the prophylaxis of cluster headache: a double-blind pilot study with parallel groups. *Cephalalgia* 1996; 16:494.
222. Rasmussen BK et al. Epidemiology of headache in a general population-a prevalence study. *J Clin Epidemiol* 1991;44:1147.
223. Schwartz BS et al. Epidemiology of tension-type headache. *JAMA* 1998;279:381.
224. Silberstein SD. Tension-type and chronic daily headache. *Neurology* 1993;43:1644.
225. Lance JW, Curran DA. Treatment of chronic tension headache. *Lancet* 1964;42:1236.
226. Tunis MM, Wolff HG. Studies on headache; cranial artery vasoconstriction and muscle contraction headache. *AMA Arch Neurol Psychiatry* 1954;71:425.
227. Langemark M et al. Temporal muscle blood flow in chronic tension-type headache. *Arch Neurol* 1990;47:654.
228. Kolb LC. Psychiatric aspects of the treatment of headache. *Neurology* 1963;2:34.
229. Holm JE et al. The role of stress in recurrent tension headache. *Headache* 1986;26:160.
230. Peters BH et al. Comparison of 650 mg aspirin and 1,000 mg acetaminophen with each other, and with placebo in moderately severe headache. *Am J Med* 1983;74:36.
231. Diamond S. Ibuprofen versus aspirin and placebo in the treatment of muscle contraction headache. *Headache* 1983;23:206.
232. Schachtel BP et al. Nonprescription ibuprofen and acetaminophen in the treatment of tension-type headache. *J Clin Pharmacol* 1996;36:1120.
233. Gawel MJ et al. Evaluation of analgesic agents in recurring headache compared with other clinical pain models. *Clin Pharmacol Ther* 1990;47:504.
234. Friedman AP. The treatment of chronic headache with meprobamate. *Ann N Y Acad Sci* 1957;67:822.
235. Weber MB. The treatment of muscle contraction headaches with diazepam. *Curr Ther Res Clin Exp* 1973;15:210.
236. Jay GW et al. The effectiveness of physical therapy in the treatment of chronic daily headaches. *Headache* 1989;29:156.
237. Hansen PE, Hansen JH. Acupuncture treatment of chronic tension headache-a controlled cross-over trial. *Cephalalgia* 1985;5:137.
238. Nuechterlein KH, Holroyd JC. Biofeedback in the treatment of tension headache. Current status. *Arch Gen Psychiatry* 1980;37:866.
239. Bakal DA, Kaganov JA. Muscle contraction and migraine headache: psychophysiologic comparison. *Headache* 1977;17:208.
240. Andrasik F, Holroyd KA. Specific and nonspecific effects in the biofeedback treatment of tension headache: 3-year follow-up. *J Consult Clin Psychol* 1983;51:634.
241. Solbach P et al. An analysis of home practice patterns for non-drug headache treatments. *Headache* 1989;29:528.
242. Bove G, Nilsson N. Spinal manipulation in the treatment of episodic tension-type headache: a randomized controlled trial. *JAMA* 1998;280: 1576.
243. Black RG. The chronic pain syndrome. *Surg Clin North Am* 1975;55:999.
244. Jensen R, Olesen J. Tension-type headache: an update on mechanisms and treatment. *Curr Opin Neurol* 2000;13:285.
245. Diamond S, Baltes BJ. Chronic tension headache-treated with amitriptyline-a double-blind study. *Headache* 1971;11:110.
246. Morland TJ et al. Doxepin in the prophylactic treatment of mixed 'vascular' and tension headache. *Headache* 1979;19:382.
247. Fogelholm R, Murros K. Maprotiline in chronic tension headache: a double-blind cross-over study. *Headache* 1985;25:273.
248. Diamond S. Management of headaches. Focus on new strategies. *Postgrad Med* 1990;87:189.
249. Diamond S, Freitag FG. The use of fluoxetine in the treatment of headache. *Clin J Pain* 1989;5:200.
250. Bendtsen L et al. A non-selective (amitriptyline), but not a selective (citalopram), serotonin reuptake inhibitor is effective in the prophylactic treatment of chronic tension-type headache. *J Neurol Neurosurg Psychiatry* 1996;61:285.

CHAPTER 53

Parkinson's Disease and Other Movement Disorders

Michael E. Ernst and Mildred D. Gottwald

PARKINSON'S DISEASE

Incidence, Prevalence, and Epidemiology

Parkinson's disease (PD) is a chronic, progressive movement disorder in which drug therapy plays a central role. Nearly 200 years have elapsed since Dr. James Parkinson published his case series "An Essay on the Shaking Palsy" in 1817, becoming the first to describe features of the disease that bears his name. Since then, the term *parkinsonism* has come to refer to any disorder associated with two or more features of tremor, rigidity, bradykinesia, or postural instability.[1] Most cases of PD are of unknown cause, and referred to as *idiopathic parkinsonism*; however, viral encephalitis, cerebrovascular disease, and hydrocephalus have symptoms similar to PD as part of their clinical presentation.[1] Unless otherwise stated, all references to PD in this chapter refer to the idiopathic type.

The age at onset of PD is variable, usually between 50 and 80 years, with a mean onset of 55 years.[2] The prevalence of PD is about 100 cases per 100,000 population, and the incidence is estimated at 20 cases per 100,000 people annually.[3] An estimated 1 million Americans, or 1% of the population age >65 years, have PD.[4] Men are affected slightly more frequently than women.[5] Despite the availability of effective symptomatic treatments to improve both quality of life and life expectancy, no cure exists and the disease is associated with increased morbidity and mortality.[6] The symptoms of PD are progressive and, within 10 to 20 years, total immobility results for most PD patients.[7] The patient's age at the time of onset of clinically recognizable disease may significantly influence the rate of disease progression. A more rapid rate of progression has been observed in elderly patients and may be associated with a greater degree of motor disability.[8] Death is not usually caused by the disease itself, but rather by complications related to immobility (e.g., aspiration pneumonia, cardiovascular, and cerebrovascular disease).[7]

Several organizations provide services for persons with PD (as well as other movement disorders) and their families. Valuable information in the form of internet monographs, books, newsletters, videos, and audiotapes in addition to information

Table 53-1 Service Organizations for Patients with Parkinson's Disease and Other Movement Disorders

American Parkinson Disease Association, Inc. 135 Parkinson Avenue Staten Island, NY 10305 1-800-223-2732 Website: http://www.apdaparkinson.com
National Parkinson Foundation, Inc. 1501 NW Ninth Avenue NW/Bob Hope Road Miami, FL 33136-1494 1-800-327-4545 Website: http://www.parkinson.org
The Parkinson's Disease Foundation 1359 Broadway, Suite 1509 New York, NY 10018 1-800-457-6676 Website: http://www.pdf.org
Parkinson's Action Network 1025 Vermont Avenue, NW Suite 1120 Washington, DC 20005 1-800-850-4726 Website: http://www.parkinsonaction.org
WE MOVE 204 West 84th Street New York, NY 10024 1-800-437-6682 Website: http://www.wemove.org
The Michael J. Fox Foundation for Parkinson's Research Grand Central Station, P.O. Box 4777 New York, NY 10163 1-800-708-7644 Website: http://www.michaeljfox.org
International Essential Tremor Foundation 11111 West 95th Street, Suite 260 Lenexa, Kansas 66214-1824 1-888-387-3667 Website: http://www.essentialtremor.org
Restless Legs Syndrome Foundation 1610 14th Street NW, Suite 300 Rochester, MN 55901 1-877-463-6757 Website: http://www.rls.org

about local support groups is available from the organizations listed in Table 53-1.

Etiology

Many theories have been advanced regarding the origin of PD. Environmental factors have been implicated since it was discovered that many patients developed a parkinsonian syndrome following the epidemic of encephalitis lethargic in the United States between 1919 and the early 1930s.[9] Attempts to isolate a virus as a causative agent of the disease have been unsuccessful, however. Renewed interest in environmental factors resurfaced with the discovery that ingestion of a meperidine analog, 1-methyl-4-phenyl-1,2,3,6-tetrahydropyridine (MPTP), causes irreversible parkinsonism.[10] The discovery of an autosomal dominant familial form of PD caused by a mutation in the α-synuclein gene has sparked interest in genetic constitution as a factor explaining the development of PD.[11] In addition to environment and genetics, it has also been reported that byproducts of normal dopamine metabolism (e.g., hydrogen peroxide) can lead to the production of free radicals that cause peroxidation of cell membranes and cell death. Thus, the most attractive hypothesis for the etiology of PD is that the disease results from a complex interplay of age-related changes to the nigrostriatal tract, genetic predisposition, and toxin exposure.

Pathophysiology

Parkinson's disease is a disorder of the extrapyramidal system of the brain involving the basal ganglia. The extrapyramidal system is involved with maintaining posture and muscle tone and with regulating voluntary smooth motor activity. For reasons not understood, melanin-containing cells within the substantia nigra are lost in PD. The pigmented neurons within the substantia nigra have dopaminergic fibers that project into the neostriatum and globus pallidus. Together, the substantia nigra, neostriatum, and globus pallidus make up the basal ganglia. In PD, dopamine (the inhibitory neurotransmitter) is progressively lost in the nigrostriatal tracts, and acetylcholine (the excitatory neurotransmitter) is relatively increased. It is generally believed that a 70% to 80% loss of nigral neurons must occur before PD becomes clinically recognizable.[1] On pathologic examination of postmortem basal ganglia, the presence of Lewy bodies (spherical, abnormal intraneuronal protein aggregates) are noted within the remaining dopaminergic cells of the substantia nigra.[12] The presence of Lewy bodies is considered pathognomic for the disease.

Overview of Drug Therapy

Because the salient pathophysiologic feature of PD is the progressive loss of dopamine from the nigrostriatal tracts in the brain, drug therapy for the disease is aimed primarily at replenishing the supply of dopamine (Table 53-2). This is accomplished through one, or a combination, of the following methods: (a) administering exogenous dopamine in the form of a precursor, levodopa; (b) stimulating dopamine receptors within the corpus striatum through the use of dopamine agonists (e.g., pramipexole, ropinirole); or (c) inhibiting the major metabolic pathways within the brain that are responsible for the degradation of levodopa and its metabolites. This latter effect is achieved through the use of aromatic L-amino acid decarboxylase (AAD) inhibitors (e.g., carbidopa), catechol-O-methyltransferase (COMT)-inhibitors (e.g., entacapone), or monoamine oxidase type B (MAO-B) inhibitors (e.g. selegiline, rasagiline). Additional therapies, such as anticholinergics, may occasionally be used to counterbalance the negative effects of the relative increase in acetylcholine activity and improve tremor symptoms.

Parkinson's disease is a debilitating disorder that affects both physical and mental functions of the body. Despite our best treatment efforts to restore dopaminergic function and preserve dopamine production, the disease will invariably progress. In many instances, adverse effects of the medications themselves can lead to additional problems. Supportive drug treatment of the complications of PD is also necessary. These complications include neuropsychiatric problems (cognitive impairment

Table 53-2 Medications Used for the Treatment of Parkinson's Disease

Generic (Trade) Name	*Dosage Unit*	*Titration Schedule*	*Usual Daily Dose*	*Adverse Effects*
Amantadine (Symmetrel)	100-mg capsule Liquid: 50 mg/5 mL	100 mg QD; increased by 100 mg 1–2 wk	100–300 mg	Orthostatic hypotension, insomnia, depression, hallucinations, livedo reticularis, xerostomia
Anticholinergic Agents				
Benztropine (Cogentin)	0.5-, 1-, and 2-mg tablets Injection: 2 mL (1 mg/mL)	0.5 mg/day increased by 0.5 mg Q 3–5 days	1–3 mg given QD to BID	Constipation, xerostomia, dry skin, dysphagia, confusion, memory impairment
Trihexyphenidyl (Artane)	2- and 5-mg tablets Liquid: 2 mg/5 mL	1–2 mg/day increased by 1–2 mg Q 3–5 days	6–15 mg divided TID to BID	Constipation, xerostomia, dry skin, dysphagia, confusion, memory impairment
Combination Agents				
Carbidopa-Levodopa (immediate release)/ entacapone (Stalevo)	12.5/50/200, 25/100/200, and 37.5/150/200 mg tablets	Titrate with individual dosage forms (carbidopa/levodopa and entacapone) first, then switch to combination tablet	Varies (see listings for individual drugs)	See listing for individual drugs
Dopamine Replacement				
Carbidopa-Levodopa (Regular) (Sinemet)	10/100, 25/100, and 25/250 tablets	25/100 mg BID, increased by 25/100 weekly to effect and as tolerated	30/300 to 150/1,500 divided TID to QID	Nausea, orthostatic hypotension, confusion, dizziness, hallucinations, dyskinesias, blepharospasm
Carbidopa-Levodopa (CR) (Sinemet CR)	25/100 and 50/200 tablets	25/100 mg BID (spaced at least 6 hr apart), increased Q 3–7 days	50/200 to 500/2,000 divided QID	Same as regular Sinemet
Carbidopa-Levodopa ODT (Parcopa)	10/100, 25/100, and 25/250 mg tablets	25/100 BID, increased Q 1–2 days; if transferring from regular levodopa <1,500 mg/day) start 25/100 mg TID to QID (start 25/250 mg TID to QID if already on >1,500 mg/day of regular levodopa)	25/100 to 200/2,000 divided TID to QID	Same as regular Sinemet; may occur more rapidly than with regular Sinemet
Dopamine Agonists				
Bromocriptine (Parlodel)	2.5-mg tablet, 5-mg capsule	1.25 HS, titrate slowly as tolerated over 4–6 weeks	10–40 mg divided TID	Orthostatic hypotension, confusion, dizziness, hallucinations, nausea, leg cramps; retroperitoneal, pleural, pericardial fibrosis; cardiac valve thickening
Pramipexole (Mirapex)	0.125-, 0.25-, 0.50-, 1-, 1.5-mg tablets	0.375 divided TID; titrate weekly by 0.125–0.25 mg/dose	1.5–4.5 mg divided TID	Orthostatic hypotension, confusion, dizziness, hallucinations, nausea, somnolence
Ropinirole (Requip)	0.25-, 0.5-, 1-, 2-, 4-, 5-mg tablet	Titrate weekly by 0.25 mg/dose	3–12 mg divided TID	Orthostatic hypotension, confusion, dizziness, hallucinations, nausea, somnolence
Apomorphine (Apokyn)	10 mg/mL injection	Initial 2-mg test dose, then begin 1 mg less than tolerated test dose; increase by 1 mg every few days; approved for "rescue" during periods of hypomobility	2–6 mg TID	Nausea, vomiting; administer with trimethobenzamide (not 5-hydroxytryptamine-3 [5HT3] antagonists)
Rotigotine (Neupro)	2-, 4-, 6-mg/24 hr transdermal delivery system	2 mg/24 hr; titrate weekly by 2 mg/24 hr until response noted or maximal dose of 6 mg/24 hrs reached. Application site should be rotated daily between abdomen, thigh, hip, flank, shoulder, or upper arm	4–6 mg/24 hr	Hallucinations, abnormal dreaming, insomnia, somnolence, nausea, vomiting, application site reactions; avoid in patients with known sulfite sensitivity

(continued)

Table 53-2 Medications Used for the Treatment of Parkinson's Disease *(Continued)*

Generic (Trade) Name	*Dosage Unit*	*Titration Schedule*	*Usual Daily Dose*	*Adverse Effects*
COMT Inhibitors				
Entacapone (Comtan)	200-mg tablet	One tablet with each administration of levodopa/carbidopa, up to 8 tablets daily	3–8 tablets daily	Diarrhea, dyskinesias, abdominal pain, urine discoloration
Tolcapone (Tasmar)	100-, 200-mg tablet	100–200 mg TID	300–600 mg divided TID	Diarrhea, dyskinesias, abdominal pain, urine discoloration, hepatotoxicity
MAO-B Inhibitors				
Selegiline (Eldepryl)	5-mg tablet, capsule	5 mg AM; may increase to 5 mg BID	5–10 mg (take 5 mg with breakfast and 5 mg with lunch)	Insomnia, dizziness, nausea, vomiting, xerostomia, dyskinesias, mood changes; use caution when coadministered with sympathomimetics or serotoninergic agents (increased risk of serotonin syndrome); avoid tyramine-containing foods
Selegiline ODT (Zelapar)	1.25-mg tablet	1.25 mg QD; may increase to 2.5 mg QD after 6 wk	1.25–2.5 mg QD	Insomnia, dizziness, nausea, vomiting, xerostomia, dyskinesias, mood changes; use caution when coadministered with sympathomimetics or sertoninergic agents (increased risk of serotonin syndrome); avoid ingestion large amounts of tyramine-containing foods
Rasagiline (Azilect)	0.5 mg tablet	0.5 mg QD; may increase to 1 mg QD	0.5–1 mg/day	Similar to selegiline

BID, twice daily; COMT, catechol-O-methyltransferase; HS, bedtime; ODT, orally disintegrating tablet; QD, every day.; QID, four times daily; TID, three times daily.

and dementia, hallucinations and delirium, depression, agitation, anxiety), autonomic dysfunction (constipation, urinary problems, sexual problems, orthostasis, thermoregulatory imbalances), falls, and sleep disorders (insomnia or sleep fragmentation, nightmares, restless leg syndrome).

CLINICAL PRESENTATION OF PARKINSON'S DISEASE

1. L.M., a 55-year-old, right-handed male artist, presents to the neurology clinic complaining of difficulty painting because of unsteadiness in his right hand. He also complains of increasing difficulty getting out of chairs and tightness in his arms and legs. His wife claims that he has become more "forgetful" lately, and L.M. admits that his memory does not seem to be as sharp. His medical history is significant for depression for the past year, gout (currently requiring no treatment), constipation, benign prostatic hypertrophy, and aortic stenosis. On physical examination, L.M. is noted to be a well-developed, well-nourished man who displays a notable lack of normal changes in facial expression and speaks in a soft, monotone voice. A strong body odor is noted. Examination of his extremities reveals a slight "ratchetlike" rigidity in both arms and legs, and a mild resting tremor is present in his right hand. His gait is slow, but otherwise normal, with a slightly bent posture. His balance is determined to be normal, with no retropulsion or loss of righting reflexes after physical threat. His genitourinary examination is remarkable only for prostatic enlargement. The remainder of L.M.'s physical examination and laboratory studies are within normal limits. What signs and symptoms suggestive of PD are present in L.M.? Which of these symptoms are among the classic symptoms for diagnosing PD and which are considered "associated" symptoms? How should L.M.'s PD and associated symptoms be treated?

Establishing the diagnosis of PD is based on careful history taking and physical examination.[12] No laboratory or radiological tests have demonstrated consistent benefit in diagnosing the disease.[8] The four classic features of PD—tremor, rigidity, bradykinesia, and postural disturbances—are easily recognized. Tremor, which is most often the first symptom observed, is usually unilateral on initial presentation. Frequently, the tremor is of a "pill-rolling" type involving the thumb and index finger; it is present at rest, worsens under fatigue or stress, and is absent with purposeful movement or when asleep.[1] These features help distinguish it from essential tremor, which usually causes a symmetric tremor in the hands and is often accompanied by head and voice tremor.[12] Muscular rigidity resulting from increased muscle tone often manifests as a "cogwheel" or "ratchet" (catch-release) type of motion when an extremity is moved passively.[1] Rigidity may also be experienced as stiffness or vague aching or limb discomfort.[12] Bradykinesia refers to an overall slowness in initiating movement. Early in the disease, patients may describe this as weakness or clumsiness of a hand or leg.[12] As the disease progresses, difficulty initiating and terminating steps results in a hurried or festinating gait;

the posture becomes stooped (simian posture), and postural reflexes are impaired.[1] Symptoms that were unilateral on initial presentation progress asymmetrically and often become bilateral and more severe with disease progression.[1] Patients with PD develop "masked facies," or a blank stare with reduced eye blinking.

Patients with PD are often misdiagnosed, leading to inappropriate, ineffective, or delayed treatment.[1] It is important to note that all four symptoms do not need to be present to make the diagnosis of PD. For example, unilateral tremor (frequently on the right side) is one of the most common initial presenting symptoms, but approximately 30% of patients with idiopathic PD do not present with tremor.[13] Patients with PD may have an insidious onset of nonspecific symptoms such as generalized malaise and fatigue.[1] Several conditions can be mistaken for PD, and include multiple system atrophy (formerly known as Shy-Drager syndrome), progressive supranuclear palsy, and normal pressure hydrocephalus. These conditions are referred to as "parkinson-plus" syndromes and are important to distinguish from PD because they respond poorly to antiparkinsonian medications and are associated with worse prognosis.[12] Magnetic resonance imaging can be useful in some situations to exclude these conditions, particularly when clinical signs suggest an alternate diagnosis. Falls or dementia early in the disease, symmetric parkinsonism, wide-based gait, abnormal eye movements, marked orthostatic hypotension, urinary retention, and marked disability within 5 years after the onset of symptoms suggest alternate diagnoses other than PD.[12] Drugs with strong antidopaminergic activity (e.g., neuroleptics, prochlorperazine, and metoclopramide), and other drugs, such as valproate, amiodarone, phenytoin, and lithium, may also cause a state of drug-induced parkinsonism that mimics idiopathic PD. It is important to rule out drugs as a cause of symptoms before the diagnosis of PD is established. Although reversible, symptoms may persist for weeks or months after discontinuation of the offending agent.[12]

L.M. presents with many of the classic symptoms of PD. A noticeable unilateral resting tremor is present along with decreased manual dexterity, as evidenced by his difficulty handling a paintbrush. Rigidity ("ratcheting" of the arms), bradykinesia (slowness of movement), and a masklike facial expression also are present. Although he has a partially stooped posture, it is difficult to attribute this entirely to the disease because postural changes commonly occur with advancing age and, on physical examination, his balance was normal. To confirm the diagnosis of PD, a therapeutic trial of levodopa may be considered. A resulting improvement in motor or cognitive function in response to levodopa therapy suggests the diagnosis of PD. Patients with the tremor-predominant form of the disease may, however, not respond to levodopa, especially in the early stages of the disease.[13] In addition, lack of a positive response to an acute dopaminergic challenge may not exclude a positive response to chronic therapy. At least 30% of patients with PD will not respond to an acute dopaminergic challenge (false–negative response).[8] Therefore, this approach would not be routinely recommended in a patient such as L.M.

In choosing when to treat the symptoms of PD and which therapy to use, care must be exercised to approach each patient individually. Although no consensus has been reached about when to initiate symptomatic treatment, most health care professionals agree that treatment should begin when the patient begins to experience functional impairment as defined by (a) threat to employment status; (b) symptoms affecting the dominant side of the body; or (c) bradykinesia or rigidity. Individual patient preferences also should be considered. Judging by the symptoms L.M. is displaying, he would likely benefit from immediate treatment. His symptoms are unilateral but are occurring on his dominant side and are interfering with his ability to paint, thus affecting his livelihood. He is also showing signs of rigidity and bradykinesia but can otherwise live independently.

Numerous features are associated with PD. Handwriting abnormalities occur frequently, particularly micrographia, a symptom of bradykinesia. Because L.M. is an artist, this abnormality would be particularly troublesome. He also is showing signs of autonomic nervous system dysfunction, such as drooling (sialorrhea), seborrhea, and constipation, all of which can be particularly embarrassing to the patient. Drooling also may be a consequence of impaired swallowing.[13] The foul body odor exhibited by L.M. could be ascribed to excess sebum production. L.M.'s seborrhea can be treated with coal tar or selenium-based shampoos twice weekly, topical hydrocortisone, or topical ketoconazole.[13] His constipation should be managed first by evaluating his diet and exercise level, by stopping all medications such as anticholinergics (including over-the-counter cold and sleep medications) that may exacerbate constipation, and by trying a stool softener such as sodium or calcium docusate. In more severe cases, lactulose, mild laxatives, or enemas may be required.

L.M. should also be evaluated for other manifestations of dysautonomia, including urinary problems, increased sweating, orthostatic hypotension, erectile dysfunction, pain or dysesthesias, and problems swallowing. L.M. has benign prostatic hypertrophy; therefore, a urologic workup may be necessary. He also should be counseled to avoid anticholinergic agents that may exacerbate this problem. Anticholinergic agents also should not be used to treat his hypersalivation, but he should be referred to a speech and swallowing expert because dysphagia can result in impaired absorption and lead to aspiration.[13] A soft diet may be indicated. L.M.'s soft, mumbled, or monotone voice is also consistent with the disease and is often one of the first symptoms noted. Speech therapy is often beneficial for managing this problem.[14]

Psychiatric disturbances, such as nervousness, anxiety, and depression, occur commonly in patients with PD and they should be screened regularly for these conditions.[13,15] L.M. has a history of depression that could be attributable to PD. Finally, the prevalence of cognitive decline and dementia among parkinsonian patients ranges from 10% to 30% and may be associated with a more rapid progression of disease-related disability.[8] The development of hallucinations in patients with PD with dementia is a poor prognostic sign.[16] The "forgetfulness" and decreased memory described by L.M. could be early signs of dementia and warrant close observation.

Staging of Parkinson's Disease

2. What are the stages of PD? In what stage of the disease is L.M.?

The symptomatology and progression of symptoms among parkinsonian patients is tremendously variable. To assess the

Table 53-3 Staging of Disability in Parkinson's Disease

Stage I	Unilateral involvement only; minimal or no functional impairment
Stage II	Bilateral involvement, without impairment of balance
Stage III	Evidence of postural imbalance; some restriction in activities; capable of leading independent life; mild to moderate disability
Stage IV	Severely disabled, cannot walk and stand unassisted; significantly incapacitated
Stage V	Restricted to bed or wheelchair unless aided

From reference 2, with permission.

degree of disability and determine the rate of disease progression relative to treatment, various scales have been developed. The most common of these is the Hoehn and Yahr scale (Table 53-3).[2] In general, patients in Hoehn and Yahr stage I or II of PD have mild disease that does not interfere with activities of daily living or work and usually requires minimal or no treatment. In stage III disease, daily activities are restricted and employment may be significantly affected unless effective treatment is initiated.

With advanced-stage disease (III to IV), most patients require levodopa therapy (with a peripheral decarboxylase inhibitor such as carbidopa [Sinemet]) and often in combination with a COMT inhibitor such as entacapone or a dopamine agonist such as pramipexole (Mirapex), or ropinirole (Requip). In some cases, selegiline (Eldepryl), rasagiline (Azilect), or amantadine may provide further symptomatic relief. Patients with end-stage disease (stage V) are severely incapacitated and, because of extended disease progression, often do not respond well to drug therapy.

TREATMENT OF PARKINSON'S DISEASE

An algorithm for the management of cases of PD is presented in Figure 53-1. No cure is known for PD; therefore, treatment is symptomatic only. The long-term, individualized treatment plan is usually characterized by frequent dosage adjustments over time because of the chronic and progressive nature of this disease. Although most of this chapter is devoted to the drug therapy of PD, the importance of supportive care cannot be overemphasized. Exercise, physiotherapy, and good nutritional support can be beneficial at the earlier stages to improve mobility, increase strength, and enhance well-being and mood.[13] Speech therapy may be helpful, and psychological support is often necessary in dealing with depression and other related problems. Newly diagnosed patients need to be educated about what to expect from the disease and the various forms of treatment available. In addition, enlisting the support of family members is vital in establishing an overall effective therapeutic plan.

Dopamine Agonists

Initial Therapy

3. The decision is made to begin drug therapy for L.M. Should therapy be initiated with a dopamine agonist or levodopa?

Levodopa, without question, has revolutionized the treatment of PD. It is considered to be the most effective antiparkinsonian agent.[12] Declining efficacy and response fluctuations encountered with long-term levodopa therapy, as well as a high frequency of undesirable side effects, prompted investigators to search for agents that could directly stimulate dopamine receptors. This led to the development of the dopamine agonists.

In clinical trials comparing dopamine agonists and levodopa, activities of daily living and motor features are improved 40% to 50% with levodopa compared with 30% with dopamine agonists.[17–19] Although they are not as effective as levodopa, the dopamine agonists have a number of potential advantages over levodopa. Because they act directly on dopamine receptors, they do not require metabolic conversion to an active product and therefore act independently of degenerating dopaminergic neurons.[13] Unlike levodopa, circulating plasma amino acids do not compete with dopamine agonists for absorption and transport into the brain. Dopamine agonists have a longer half-life than levodopa formulations, reducing the need for multiple daily dosing. Initial therapy with dopamine agonists is associated with fewer motor complications and can delay the need for levodopa.[17,18,20] As a class, dopamine agonists provide adequate control of symptoms when given as monotherapy in up to 80% of patients with early-stage disease. These benefits are sustained for 3 years or more in most patients. With disease progression, levodopa therapy will eventually be necessary, however.

Guidelines from the American Academy of Neurology support either dopamine agonists or levodopa as initial therapy for PD.[21] In younger patients (e.g., age <65 years) with milder disease, such as L.M., the initiation of a dopamine agonist as a first-line agent is a strategy used to delay the introduction of levodopa. This levodopa-sparing effect, as well as the reduction in motor complications observed with early dopamine agonist therapy, is the reason why many clinicians opt for using this class of drugs as initial treatment for PD in younger patients who would be expected to live many years with the disease.[13] In older patients (e.g., age >65 years) with PD, it may be more appropriate to initiate treatment with levodopa instead of a dopamine agonist, because these patients are less likely to live sufficiently long with the disease to experience the levodopa-related motor complications that occur after prolonged therapy with the drug.[13] An additional consideration is that dopamine agonist therapy is more costly than levodopa.[21]

In the case of L.M., his relatively young age (<65 years) and mild disease make him a good candidate for initial therapy with a dopamine agonist. L.M. will certainly require levodopa therapy later, when he reaches more advanced stages of the disease. By initiating therapy first with a dopamine agonist, rescue levodopa therapy can likely be started at smaller doses, and the onset of motor complications that often occur with escalating doses and extended therapy with levodopa may be delayed.

Selection of Agents

4. L.M. is to be started on a dopamine agonist. Which agent should be selected?

Two generations of dopamine agonists have been used for the treatment of idiopathic, early-stage PD as monotherapy, or as an adjunct to levodopa in patients with advanced disease.

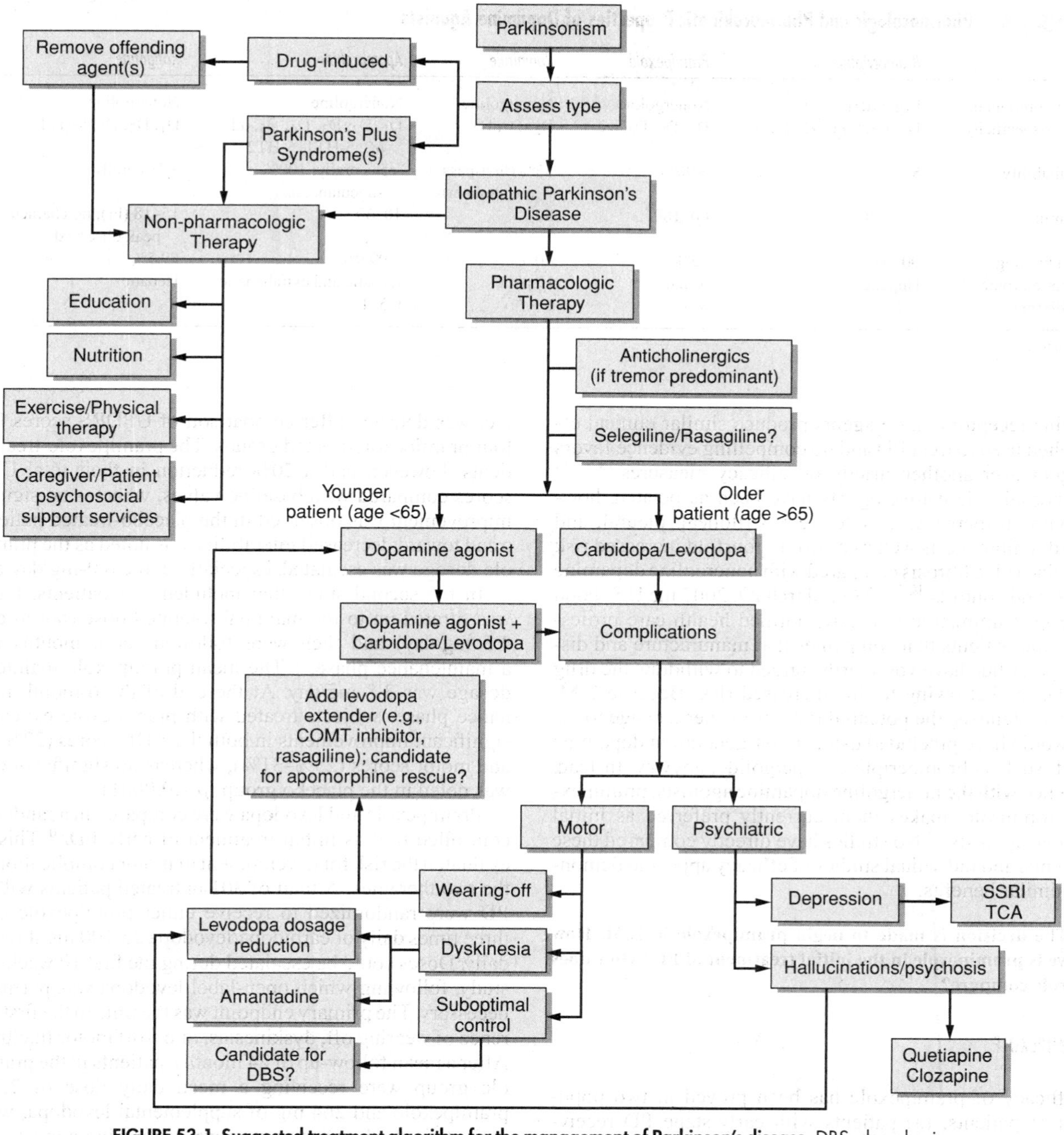

FIGURE 53-1 Suggested treatment algorithm for the management of Parkinson's disease. DBS, deep brain stimulation. (Modified with permission from the American College of Clinical Pharmacy. Michael E. Ernst. Parkinson's Disease. In: Dunsworth T et al, eds. Pharmacotherapy Self-Assessment Program, 6th ed., Neurology and Psychiatry module. Lenexa, KS: American College of Clinical Pharmacy; 2007:22.)

The comparative pharmacologic and pharmacokinetic properties of these agents are shown in Table 53-4. The first generation, ergoline-class dopamine agonists, which are derived from ergot alkaloids, include bromocriptine, pergolide, and cabergoline. Although cabergoline is widely used in Europe, it is only indicated in the United States for treating hyperprolactinemia. Pramipexole, ropinirole, apomorphine, and rotigotine are newer, nonergoline dopamine agonists. Apomorphine is only available in injectable form, and is used as a rescue agent approved for the treatment of hypomobility or "off" episodes in patients with PD. Rotigotine is the newest dopamine agonist approved for use in PD, and is formulated in a once-daily transdermal delivery system.

The dopamine agonists work by directly stimulating postsynaptic dopamine receptors within the corpus striatum.[22] The two families of dopamine receptors are D_1 and D_2. The D_1 family includes the D_1 and D_5 dopamine subtype receptors and the D_2 family includes D_2, D_3, and D_4 dopamine subtype receptors. Stimulation of D_2 receptors is largely responsible for reducing rigidity and bradykinesia, whereas the precise role of the D_1 receptors remains uncertain.[22] Although the dopamine agonists differ slightly from each other in terms of their affinities for

Table 53-4 Pharmacologic and Pharmacokinetic Properties of Dopamine Agonists

	Bromocriptine	*Pramipexole*	*Ropinirole*	*Apomorphine*	*Rotigotine*
Type of compound	Ergot derivative	Nonergoline	Nonergoline	Nonergoline	Nonergoline
Receptor specificity	D_2, D_1,[a] $\alpha1$, $\alpha2$, 5-HT	D_2, D_3, D_4, $\alpha2$	D_2, D_3, D_4	D_1, D_2, D_3, D_4, D_5, $\alpha1$, $\alpha2$, 5-HT1, 5-HT2	D_1, D_2, D_3, 5-HT1
Bioavailability	8%	>90%	55% (first-pass metabolism)	<5% orally; 100% subcutaneous	<1% orally
T_{max} (min)	70–100	60–180	90	10–60	15–18 (hr); no characteristic peak observed
Protein binding	90–96%	15%	40%	>99.9%	89.5%
Elimination route	Hepatic	Renal	Hepatic	Hepatic and extrahepatic	Hepatic
Half-life (hr)	3–8	8–12	6	0.5–1	3

[a] Antagonist.

dopamine receptors, these agents produce similar clinical effects when used to treat PD and no compelling evidence favors one agent over another strictly on efficacy measures.[13,22,23] Older ergoline derivative agents have been associated, however, with an increased risk for retroperitoneal, pleural, and pericardial fibrosis, as well as a two- to fourfold increased risk for cardiac valve fibrosis compared with nonergoline dopamine agonists and controls.[12,24,25] On March 29, 2007 the U.S. Food and Drug Administration (FDA) notified health care professionals and patients that companies that manufacture and distribute pergolide have voluntarily agreed to withdraw the drug from the market owing to this increased risk. Because L.M. has aortic stenosis, the potential risk for further damage to his valve would have precluded using a first-generation dopamine agonist, such as bromocriptine or pergolide, anyway. Instead, experience with the nonergoline dopamine agonists, pramipexole or ropinirole, makes them currently preferred as initial dopamine agonists.[12] No studies have directly compared these two agents, and individual studies of efficacy appear to demonstrate similar benefits.

5. The decision is made to begin pramipexole in L.M. How effective is pramipexole in the initial treatment of PD? How does ropinirole compare?

PRAMIPEXOLE

Efficacy

The efficacy of pramipexole has been proved in two populations of patients: (a) patients with early-stage PD receiving pramipexole as monotherapy[26–29] and (b) patients with advanced-stage disease receiving pramipexole as an adjunct to levodopa therapy.[30,31] These trials were multicenter, placebo-controlled, parallel-group studies, and the primary outcome measures included improvement in activities of daily living (ADL, part II) and motor function scores (part III) as measured by the Unified Parkinson Disease Rating Scale (UPDRS).[32] Each evaluation on the UPDRS is rated on a scale of 0 (normal) to 4 (can barely perform). Lower scores on the UPDRS after treatment indicate an improvement in overall performance.

Two large-scale, double-blind, placebo-controlled studies were performed that included a total of 599 patients with early-stage PD (mean disease duration of 2 years). In the first study, 264 patients were randomized to receive one of four fixed doses (1.5, 3.0, 4.5, or 6.0 mg/day) or placebo.[28] At the end of the 4-week maintenance period, no significant dose-response effect was detected after comparison of UPDRS scores for the four pramipexole-treated groups. The pramipexole-treated patients, however, had a 20% reduction in their total UPDRS scores compared with baseline values, whereas no significant improvement was observed in the placebo-treated patients. A trend toward decreased tolerability was noted as the pramipexole dosage was escalated, especially in the 6.0-mg/day group.

In the second study that included 335 patients, the dose was titrated up to the maximal tolerated dose (not to exceed 4.5 mg/day) and then were followed for 6 months during a maintenance phase.[29] The mean pramipexole maintenance dosage was 3.8 mg/day. At the end of the 6-month maintenance phase, subjects treated with pramipexole experienced significant improvements in both the ADL scores (22%–29%) and motor scores (25%–31%), whereas no significant change was noted in the placebo group ($p < 0.0001$).

Pramipexole and levodopa were compared in a randomized, controlled trial as initial treatment of early PD.[20] This study evaluated the risk for development of motor complications with the two therapies. A total of 301 untreated patients with early PD were randomized to receive either pramipexole 0.5 mg three times daily or carbidopa/levodopa 25/100 mg three times daily. Doses could be escalated during the first 10 weeks of the study, following which open-label levodopa was permitted if necessary. The primary endpoint was the time to the first occurrence of wearing off, dyskinesias, or on-off motor fluctuations. After a mean follow-up of 24 months, patients in the pramipexole group were receiving a mean daily dose of 2.78 mg pramipexole and 264 mg of supplemental levodopa, whereas patients in the levodopa group were receiving a mean total of 509 mg/day levodopa. Fewer pramipexole-treated patients reached the primary endpoint (28% vs. 51%; $p < 0.001$) than the patients initially randomized to levodopa therapy. Dyskinesias were noted in only 10% of pramipexole-treated patients compared with 31% of levodopa-treated patients ($p < 0.001$), and fewer wearing-off effects were reported with pramipexole (24% vs. 38%; $p = 0.01$).

ROPINIROLE

Efficacy

Ropinirole is a synthetic nonergoline aminoindolone and a full dopamine agonist with selectivity for D_2 receptors; as with pramipexole, however, it has no significant affinity for D_1 receptors.[33] Although the drug is pharmacologically similar to pramipexole, it has some distinct pharmacokinetic properties, as shown in Table 53-4. Unlike pramipexole, which is primarily eliminated by renal excretion, ropinirole is metabolized by the cytochrome P450 (primarily CYP1A2) oxidative pathway and undergoes significant first-pass hepatic metabolism.[34] Ropinirole is approved for use as monotherapy in early-stage idiopathic PD and as an adjunct to levodopa therapy in patients with advanced-stage disease.

The efficacy of ropinirole as monotherapy in patients with early PD has been evaluated in several randomized, double-blind, multicenter, parallel group studies.[35–37] One study was placebo-controlled, another study compared ropinirole with bromocriptine, and the third study compared initial therapy with ropinirole versus levodopa in early PD. After 6 months of maintenance therapy with ropinirole, all three studies showed a significant improvement in UPDRS motor scores compared with baseline values (20%–30%). In the placebo-controlled study, ropinirole-treated patients had a 24% reduction in their UPDRS motor scores compared with their baseline values, whereas the placebo-treated patients decreased their scores by only 3%.[36] In the study comparing the effectiveness of ropinirole with bromocriptine, a significantly greater number of ropinirole-treated patients (58%) experienced a 30% reduction in their UPDRS scores compared with bromocriptine-treated patients (43%).[37] A 6-month interim analysis of the third study, which compared the efficacy of ropinirole (mean dosage, 9 mg/day) with levodopa (mean dosage, 464 mg/day), reported that the levodopa-treated patients had a 44% improvement in their UPDRS motor scores compared with a 32% improvement in the ropinirole-treated patients.[35] When the two treatments were stratified for disease stage, however, the two treatments were equally effective in patients with mild PD.

After 5 years of follow-up, ropinirole-treated patients had a reduced risk for developing dyskinesias compared with initial therapy with levodopa.[18] At the end of the study, the mean daily dose of ropinirole was 16.5 mg plus 427 mg of open-label levodopa, compared with a mean daily dose of 753 mg of levodopa for the levodopa group. Of patients in the ropinirole group, 66% required open-label levodopa supplementation compared with 36% in the levodopa group. Dyskinesias developed in 20% of the ropinirole-treated patients compared with 45% of the levodopa-treated patients (hazard ratio for remaining free of dyskinesia in the ropinirole group, compared with the levodopa group, 2.82; $p < 0.001$). This difference between the two groups was not dependent on whether the patient received open-label levodopa supplementation. For ropinirole-treated patients who were able to remain on monotherapy without open-label levodopa supplementation, only 5% developed dyskinesia, compared with 36% of those receiving levodopa monotherapy.

DOSING

6. What is the most effective way to dose pramipexole or ropinirole?

Pramipexole should always be initiated at a low dosage and gradually titrated to the maximal effective dose, as tolerated. This approach minimizes adverse effects that may result in noncompliance or discontinuation of the drug. In clinical trials, the maximal effective dose was variable and correlated with disease severity and tolerability. One fixed-dose study in early PD showed, however, that most patients responded maximally at a dosage of 0.5 mg three times daily.[28] In patients with advanced-stage disease, an average of 3.4 mg/day is usually required to reach the maximal effect of pramipexole.[31] Studies have shown that pramipexole is nearly equipotent with pergolide, about tenfold more potent than bromocriptine, and about threefold more potent than ropinirole.[38]

L.M. has normal renal function and therefore should be started at an initial dosage of 0.125 mg three times daily for 5 to 7 days. At week 2, the dosage should be increased to 0.25 mg three times daily. Thereafter, his dosage may be increased weekly by 0.25 mg/dose (0.75 mg/day) as tolerated and up to the maximal effective dose, not to exceed 1.5 mg three times daily.[39] The titration period usually takes about 4 to 7 weeks, depending on the optimal maintenance dose.

Patients with a creatinine clearance of <60 mL/minute should be dosed less frequently than those with normal renal function.[39] Patients with a creatinine clearance of 35 to 59 mL/minute should receive a starting dose of 0.125 mg twice daily up to a maximal dose of 1.5 mg twice daily; patients with a creatinine clearance of 15 to 34 mL/minute should receive a starting dose of 0.125 mg daily up to a maximal dose of 1.5 mg daily. Pramipexole has not been studied in patients with a creatinine clearance of <15 mL/minute or those receiving hemodialysis.

Ropinirole should be initiated at a dosage of 0.25 mg three times daily with gradual titration in weekly increments of 0.25 mg/dose over 4 to 6 weeks.[13] Clinical response to ropinirole is usually observed at a daily dose of 9 to 12 mg given in three divided doses. No dosage adjustments are necessary with renal dysfunction.

ADVERSE EFFECTS

7. What are the adverse effects of pramipexole and ropinirole? How can these be managed?

Because pramipexole and ropinirole are approved for use as both monotherapy in early-stage disease and as adjunctive therapy in advanced-stage disease, the adverse events of these agents have been evaluated as a function of disease stage. In studies of pramipexole-treated patients with early-stage disease, the most common adverse effects were nausea (28%–44%), dizziness (25%), somnolence (22%), insomnia (17%), constipation (14%), asthenia (14%), and hallucinations (9%).[26–29,39,35–37,40] Nausea, with or without vomiting, can be a significant problem, particularly with higher doses.[39] Administering the drug with food may partially alleviate this problem. With continued use, many patients develop tolerance to the gastrointestinal side effects of pramipexole. Mental changes were the most common reason for discontinuation of pramipexole in both patient populations. Patients >65 years of age are threefold more likely to experience hallucinations with dopamine agonists.[41] The incidence of orthostatic hypotension was relatively low (1%–9%) and may in part reflect the exclusion of patients with underlying cardiovascular disease in several of the studies.[39]

In advanced-stage disease, the most common adverse events of dopamine agonists were nausea (25%), orthostatic hypotension (10–54%), dyskinesias (26%–47%), insomnia (27%), somnolence (11%), confusion (10%), and hallucinations (11% to 17%).[31,39,40,42] As expected, in patients with advanced-stage disease, the most common reasons for discontinuing these agents are mental disturbances (nightmares, confusion, hallucinations, insomnia) and orthostatic hypotension. Dyskinesias experienced when pramipexole is used in combination with levodopa in advanced-stage disease may be managed by first lowering the daily dose of levodopa. If unsuccessful, the dopamine agonist dose can be lowered; however, parkinsonian symptoms may worsen.

Excessive daytime somnolence during ADL, including driving, has been reported with dopamine agonists and has resulted in accidents.[43,44] Affected patients have not always reported warning signs before falling asleep and believed they were alert immediately before the event. Labeling for these drugs has since been changed to warn that patients should be alerted to the possibility of falling asleep while engaged in ADL. Patients should be advised to refrain from driving or engaging in other potentially dangerous activities until they have gained sufficient experience with pramipexole to determine whether it will hinder their mental and motor performance. Caution should be advised when patients are taking other sedating medications or alcohol in combination with pramipexole and ropinirole. If excessive daytime somnolence does occur, patients should be advised to contact their physician.

Recently, several reports of compulsive gambling and other impulse control disorders (hypersexuality, alcoholism, kleptomania) have been reported with dopamine agonist use.[45–48] In one study, a prevalence of 6.1% was noted for pathologic gambling in patients with PD compared with 0.25% for age and sex-matched controls.[48] These cases may represent variations of a behavioral syndrome termed "hedonistic homeostatic dysregulation" or "dopamine dysregulation syndrome."[49] Other features of the syndrome have been reported, including punding (carrying out repetitive, purposeless motor acts), hypersexuality, walkabout (having the urge to walk great distances during "on" times, often with no purpose or destination, and abnormalities in time perception), pathologic gambling and shopping, alterations in appetite, drug hoarding, and social independence or isolation.[49] The syndrome appears to be more common among younger, male patients with early onset PD, as well as those having "novelty seeking" personality traits, depressive symptoms, and increased alcohol intake.[50]

Although L.M. is <65 years of age, he is experiencing memory difficulty and may be at increased risk for visual hallucinations and cognitive problems from dopamine agonist therapy. He should be monitored closely for occurrence or exacerbation of these problems. He should also be evaluated for lightheadedness before initiation of pramipexole and counseled to report dizziness or unsteadiness, because this may lead to falls. He should also be reassured that if these effects are caused by pramipexole, they should subside with time and that he should not drive or operate complex machinery until he can assess the drug's effect on his mental status. L.M. should be counseled about the possibility of excessive, and potentially unpredictable, daytime somnolence as pramipexole is introduced. L.M. and his family should be educated about the reports of pathologic gambling and advised to report any unusual or uncharacteristic behaviors.

ROTIGOTINE

8. What type of dopamine agonist is rotigotine? How is it used?

Rotigotine is a new nonergolinic dopamine receptor agonist approved in May 2007 for the treatment of early stage idiopathic PD. It has previously been available only in Europe. Rotigotine is unique among PD medications because it is formulated in a transdermal patch delivery system designed for once a day application.[51] Other dopamine agonists currently available offer longer half-lives that levodopa; however, they do not provide a truly continuous stimulation of dopamine receptors and must be dosed multiple times daily. In theory, the transdermal application system may provide a more continuous stimulation of dopamine receptors than traditional oral formulations, which may translate into improved efficacy. Three strengths are available, based on drug delivery rate (total rotigotine content per system): 2 mg/24 hours (4.5 mg), 4 mg/24 hours (9 mg), and 6 mg/24 hours (13.5 mg).

Rotigotine has been studied in both early and advanced stages of disease, although it is currently indicated for use in the United States only as monotherapy in early stage PD. As monotherapy in clinical trials of patients with early-stage PD, rotigotine has been dosed in a range of 2 mg/24 hours up to 18 mg/24 hours.[52–54] In the 2 to 8 mg/24 hour dosing range, mean differences from placebo in the UPDRS ranged from −2.1–−5.0. Rotigotine is initiated at 2 mg/24 hours and titrated each week by 2 mg/24 hours until response is noted. The maximal recommended dose is 6 mg/24 hours.[55] Doses beyond 6 mg/24 hours did not result in additional improvement in the UPDRS and resulted in an increased incidence of adverse effects.

Rotigotine has also been studied in slightly higher doses as adjunctive therapy to levodopa in patients with advanced stages of PD. In one 6-month trial that included 351 patients, 8 mg/24 hours and 12 mg/24 hours reduced "off" time an average of 2.1 and 2.7 hours, respectively, from baseline compared with a 0.9-hour decrease in the placebo group.[56] Adverse events with rotigotine appear similar to those observed with other dopamine agonists (nausea, vomiting, somnolence, dizziness). As with other dopamine agonists, patients should be warned about the possibility of sudden sleep attacks. Transient application site reactions, including mild skin irritation, erythema, and rash at the patch site are also reported.[52,53,55] Rotigotine contains sodium metabisulfite and should not be used by patients with known sulfite sensitivity owing to the risk for anaphylaxis. If rotigotine is discontinued, it should be done so gradually by 2 mg/24 hours every other day to reduce the possibility of a neuroleptic malignant syndrome that has been reported with rapid dose reduction or withdrawal of other anti-parkinsonian therapies. The pharmacokinetic profile of rotigotine reveals an initial half-life of 3 hours, and after removal of the patch, plasma levels decreased with a terminal half-life of 5 to 7 hours.[55]

Although clinical experience with rotigotine in the United States is limited, the encouraging study results and unique drug delivery system appear poised to place rotigotine as an important addition to the dopamine agonist class of medications. Only the results of future studies will determine how well the agent compares with existing first-line dopamine agonists, ropinirole and pramipexole, in delaying the eventual need for levodopa and in reducing the risk for dyskinesias.

Levodopa

Timing of Initiation of Therapy

9. L.M. has responded well to pramipexole 1.0 mg three times daily (TID) for the past 18 months, with an increased ability to paint and carry out ADLs. Over the past few weeks, however, he

has noticed a gradual worsening in his symptoms and once again is having difficulty holding a paintbrush. He currently complains of feeling more "tied up," he has more difficulty getting out of a chair, and his posture is slightly more stooped. Otherwise, he can carry out most of his ADLs without great difficulty. Should levodopa be considered for the treatment of L.M.'s PD at this time?

For patients with advancing PD, levodopa remains the mainstay of treatment. Nearly all patients will eventually require treatment with the drug, regardless of initial therapy. Because PD is characterized by the absence of dopamine in the brain, the most rational approach to treatment is to replenish the depleted dopamine. Dopamine itself does not cross the blood—brain barrier, however. In high doses, levodopa, a dopamine precursor with no known pharmacologic action of its own, penetrates into the brain, where it is converted by aromatic amino acid (dopa) decarboxylase to dopamine.[57] Early trials by Cotzias et al.[57,58] and Barbeau[59] demonstrating significant and dramatic improvement in the classic features of the disease soon led to further studies, which clearly established levodopa as the drug of choice for long-term treatment of PD. Although levodopa is the most effective therapy for treating the rigidity and bradykinesia of PD, as with other dopaminergic agents, it does not effectively improve postural instability, or reduce dementia, autonomic dysfunction, or "freezing," an extreme type of akinesia that often occurs in advanced-stage disease.[60]

The question of when to begin levodopa in the treatment of PD has been historically debated. With long-term use, the efficacy of levodopa decreases, and the development of motor fluctuations and dyskinesias occurs. These observations led to the belief that chronic levodopa therapy may actually accelerate the neurodegenerative process through formation of free radicals via dopamine metabolism.[61,62] The Earlier versus Later Levodopa Therapy in Parkinson's Disease (ELLDOPA) study was designed to answer the question of whether long-term use of levodopa accelerates neurodegeneration and paradoxically worsens PD.[63] The investigators of this study randomized 361 patients with early PD to either carbidopa/levodopa 37.5/150 mg, 75/300 mg or 150/600 mg/day or placebo for 40 weeks followed by a 2 week withdrawal of treatment. After 42 weeks, the severity of symptoms as measured by changes in the total UPDRS score increased more in the placebo group than in all of the groups receiving levodopa. The findings of this study provide assurance that early levodopa use does not result in accelerated progression of the disease based on clinical evaluations.

The optimal time to initiate levodopa therapy must be individualized. Most clinicians agree that there is little reason to start levodopa until the patient reports worsening of functionality (socially, vocationally, or otherwise). Before levodopa is started, patients must fully understand the nature of the disease and what to expect with long-term therapy. L.M. should be considered for levodopa therapy because his disease has progressed sufficiently to threaten his job performance, and his symptoms have progressed despite therapy with a dopamine agonist.

Sinemet: Advantages and Disadvantages

10. What are the advantages and disadvantages of Sinemet over levodopa alone?

Although levodopa is highly effective, its use is not without problems including many undesirable side effects, such as nausea, vomiting, and anorexia (50% of patients); postural hypotension (30% of patients); and cardiac arrhythmias (10% of patients).[59,60,64] In addition, mental disturbances (see Question 12) are encountered in 15% of patients, and abnormal involuntary movements (dyskinesias) can be seen in up to 55% of patients during the first 6 months of levodopa treatment.[59,60,64,65] Because significant amounts of levodopa are peripherally (extracerebrally) metabolized to dopamine by the enzyme aromatic amino acid (dopa) decarboxylase, extremely high doses would be necessary if administered alone. For this reason, levodopa is always administered with a dopa decarboxylase inhibitor.

By combining levodopa with a dopa decarboxylase inhibitor that does not penetrate the blood–brain barrier, a decrease in the peripheral conversion of levodopa to dopamine can be achieved, while the desired conversion within the basal ganglia remains unaffected (Fig. 53-2).[66] The two peripheral decarboxylase inhibitors in clinical use are benserazide (unavailable in the United States) and carbidopa (Lodosyn).[13] Sinemet is the fixed combination of carbidopa and levodopa and is available in ratios of 1:4 (Sinemet 25/100) and 1:10 (Sinemet 10/100 and 25/250).[13] A controlled-release product (Sinemet CR) is available in a ratio of 25/100 and 50/200. In addition, carbidopa/levodopa is also available as an orally disintegrating tablet.

Combining levodopa with carbidopa enhances the amount of dopamine available to the brain and thereby allows the dose of levodopa to be decreased by 80%.[67] This combination also shortens by several weeks the time needed to increase the levodopa dose to achieve maximal effects because carbidopa substantially decreases levodopa-induced nausea and vomiting.[13,60]

CARBIDOPA/LEVODOPA (SINEMET) DOSING

11. The decision is made to begin L.M. on carbidopa/levodopa (Sinemet). How is Sinemet dosed?

About 75 to 100 mg/day of carbidopa is necessary to saturate peripheral dopa decarboxylase.[13] It is usually unnecessary and more costly to give higher amounts of carbidopa than this. Therapy should be initiated with Sinemet 25/100 (carbidopa/levodopa) at a dosage of one tablet three times a day. The dosage can then be increased by 100 mg levodopa every day or every other day up to eight tablets (800 mg) or to the maximal effective dose, to individual requirements, or as tolerated. If troublesome dyskinesias occur at dosages needed for maximal response (as is frequently the case), the levodopa dose can be decreased in approximately 25-mg increments while monitoring for recurrence of symptoms. If the dyskinesias occur only at the peak plasma concentration of levodopa, the dose can be lowered and given more frequently. Alternatively, a levodopa-extender such as a COMT inhibitor, dopamine agonist, or rasagiline can be added and the levodopa dose decreased. The goal of optimizing therapy lies in balancing the most therapeutic dose with that which does not produce unacceptable side effects.

Because L.M. is currently treated with a dopamine agonist, he may respond to lower doses of levodopa than patients who are naïve to dopaminergic therapy. He must also be monitored

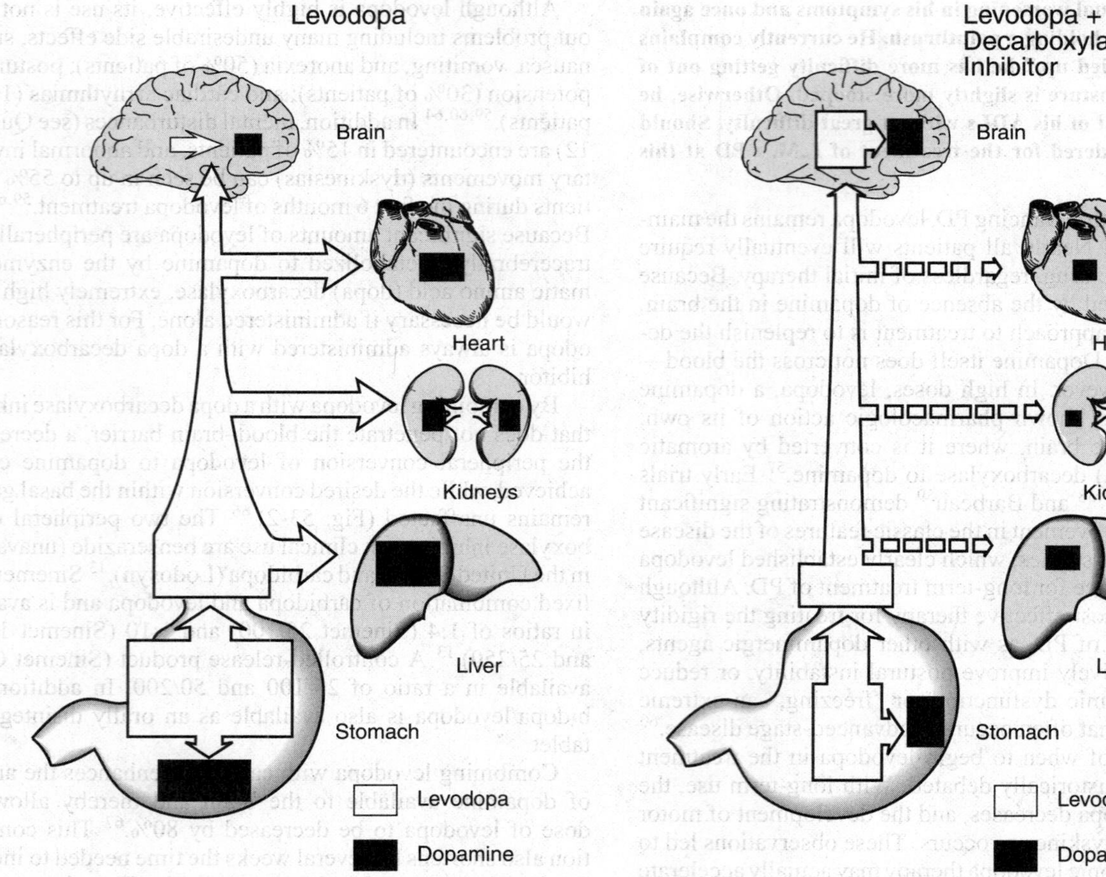

FIGURE 53-2 Peripheral decarboxylation of levodopa when given alone (*left*) and with a peripheral decarboxylase inhibitor (*right*). When combined with a decarboxylase inhibitor, less drug is required and more levodopa reaches the brain. (Reproduced with permission from Pinder RM et al. Levodopa and decarboxylase inhibitors: a review of their clinical pharmacology and use in the treatment of parkinsonism. *Drugs* 1976;11:329.)

closely for the development of motor complications with the addition of levodopa. Therefore, for best results, long-term follow-up with frequent subtle dosage adjustments is the preferred approach.

Most patients respond to levodopa dosages of 750 to 1,000 mg/day when given with carbidopa.[13] When levodopa dosages exceed 750 mg/day, patients such as L.M. can be switched from the 1:4 ratio of carbidopa/levodopa to the 1:10 ratio to prevent providing excessive amounts of decarboxylase inhibitor. For example, if L.M. needed 800 mg/day of levodopa, two Sinemet 10/100 tablets four times daily could be given. If L.M. had not been initially treated with a dopamine agonist, some clinicians would consider adding a dopamine agonist after the daily levodopa dose has been increased to >600 mg because dopamine agonists directly stimulate dopamine receptors, have longer half-lives, and result in a lower incidence of dyskinesias, thus providing a smoother dopaminergic response.[13,41]

Clinical response to L.M.'s levodopa therapy may be improved by modifying dietary protein ingestion.[13,68] Levodopa is actively transported across the blood–brain barrier by a large neutral amino acid transport system. This transport system also facilitates the blood-to-brain transport of amino acids such as L-leucine, L-isoleucine, L-valine, and L-phenylalanine. Levodopa and these neutral amino acids compete for transport mechanisms, and high plasma concentrations of these amino acids can decrease brain concentration of levodopa.[68] Patients are generally instructed to take immediate-release Sinemet 30 minutes before or 60 minutes after meals for maximal effect.

ADVERSE EFFECTS: MENTAL CHANGES

12. Since initiating carbidopa/levodopa, L.M. reports he feels confused at times and has trouble remembering things that happened recently. To what extent is levodopa contributing to these mental problems? How should they be managed?

Several psychiatric side effects have been associated with levodopa therapy. These include confusion, depression, restlessness and overactivity, psychosis, hypomania, and vivid dreams.[69] Mental side effects occur in approximately 20% of patients receiving levodopa, but the incidences vary. The combination of levodopa and a decarboxylase inhibitor has little effect on the incidence of mental disturbances.[70] Patients predisposed to levodopa-induced mental disturbances include those with underlying or pre-existing psychiatric disorders and those receiving high doses for prolonged periods.[69]

An organic confusional state with disorientation, which may progress to delirium, is the most commonly observed mental side effect.[69] This side effect can be exacerbated by concurrent anticholinergic or amantadine therapy. Because of its ability to improve disease symptoms and profoundly affect neurologic function, levodopa often produces an elevation in mood, but this is not always the case. Depression, often out of proportion to the degree of neurologic impairment, is another commonly observed finding and may precede motor dysfunction.[69]

Some patients receiving levodopa experience psychomotor excitation. Symptoms associated with psychomotor activation include overactivity, restlessness, and agitation. Similarly, hypomania has been reported in up to 8% of patients and is characterized by grandiose thinking, flight of ideas, tangential thinking, and poor social judgment. Normal sexual activity often is restored with improved motor function; however, hypersexuality and libido are increased in about 1% of levodopa-treated patients.[69] Hypersexuality is most likely an associated feature of levodopa-induced hypomania.

In general, most of the mental disturbances are dose related and can be lessened by reducing the dosage of levodopa. In patients such as L.M who are concurrently receiving levodopa and a dopamine agonist, the dosage reduction should be attempted first with levodopa. If symptoms do not improve, a reduction in the dosage of the dopamine agonist may also be warranted. These dosage reductions may, however, be impractical for L.M. because a return of parkinsonian symptoms is likely, and the benefits of levodopa therapy may outweigh the risk for mental disturbances.

Motor Complications

13. L.M. had a dramatic improvement in all of his parkinsonian symptoms with the initiation of levodopa therapy after being maintained on 25/250 regular Sinemet four times a day. After 6 months of treatment, he began to experience dyskinesias. These usually occurred 1 to 2 hours after a dose and were manifested by facial grimacing, lip smacking, tongue protrusion, and rocking of the trunk. These dyskinetic effects were lessened by decreasing his pramipexole dose to 0.5 mg TID and gradually decreasing his dosage of Sinemet to 25/250 TID, but the effects have not totally cleared.

After 3 years of levodopa therapy, more serious problems have begun to emerge. In the mornings, L.M. often experiences immobility. Nearly every day, he has periods (lasting for a few minutes) in which he cannot move, followed by a sudden switch to a fluid-like state, often associated with dyskinetic activity. He continues to take Sinemet (25/250 TID), but gains symptomatic relief only for about 3 to 4 hours after a dose. Also, the response to a given dose varies and is often less in the afternoon. At times, he becomes "frozen," particularly when he needs to board an elevator or is required to move quickly. What are possible explanations for these alterations in clinical response?

For most patients, the initial response to levodopa is favorable, and this early phase is called the "honeymoon period." Although variable, the honeymoon period can last for up to 5 years. After an initial period of stability, however, 50% to 90% of patients with PD will experience motor complications after receiving levodopa for 5 or more years.[13] In attempting to describe response fluctuations, it is important to separate those effects attributable to the disease and those attributable to the drug. Levodopa-induced dyskinesias often appear concurrently with the development of motor fluctuations.[13,71] Reducing the levodopa dosage will often reverse these symptoms. The reduction in levodopa dosage usually results, however, in deterioration in the control of the disease.

Because levodopa is a short-acting agent with an elimination half-life of about 1.5 hours, much of the effect from the evening dose has dissipated by morning.[67] For this reason, it is not surprising that L.M. is experiencing a period of immobility on arising. This is alleviated in most patients shortly after taking the morning dose.[72,73]

Two of the more common motor complications are the true "on-off" effect and the "wearing off," or "end-of-dose deterioration" effect.[71,72] The true "on-off" effect is described as random fluctuations from mobility to the parkinsonian state, which appears suddenly as if a switch has been turned. These fluctuations can last from minutes to hours and increase in frequency and intensity with time. Although most patients prefer to be *on* with dyskinesias rather than *off* with akinesis, dyskinesias in some patients can be more disabling than the parkinsonism.[13] Early in the course of disease, it is usually possible to adjust the amount and timing of the doses of levodopa to control parkinsonian symptoms without inducing dyskinesias; however, as the disease advances and the therapeutic window narrows, cycling between *on* periods complicated by dyskinesia and *off* periods with resulting immobility is common.[13]

Eventually, despite adjustments in levodopa dosage, many patients with end-stage PD experience either mobility with severe dyskinesias or complete immobility.[74,75] In most patients, this effect bears no clear-cut relation to the timing of the dose or levodopa serum levels.[76–78] The *wearing off* or *end-of-dose* effect is a more predictable effect that occurs at the latter part of the dosing interval following a period of relief; it can be improved by various means such as shortening the dosing interval or by adjunctive dopamine agonist or adding a levodopa extender such as a COMT inhibitor.

The reasons for these motor complications are not entirely clear, but incomplete delivery of dopamine to central receptors is at least partially responsible. As the disease progresses, dopamine terminals are lost and the capacity to store dopamine presynaptically is diminished.[79] This can impair buffering of the rising and falling concentrations of levodopa. Consequently, dopamine receptors are subject to intermittent or phasic stimulation rather than by physiologic tonic stimulation. Variations in the rate and extent of levodopa absorption, dietary substrates (e.g., large neutral amino acids) that compete with cerebral transport mechanisms, levodopa drug–drug interactions (Table 53-5), and competition for receptor binding by levodopa metabolites can explain these variable responses to levodopa.[71,76] Furthermore, early in the course of the disease, sufficient dopaminergic neurons remain that can store dopamine derived from levodopa administration and release it in a more physiologic manner. These neurons act as a buffer against fluctuating levodopa concentrations. With disease progression, the buffering capacity of these neurons is diminished and motor response becomes more dependent on fluctuations in synaptic dopamine concentrations.[72,76,77,79]

14. What options are available to reduce L.M.'s motor fluctuations?

Table 53-5 Levodopa Drug Interactions

Drug	*Interaction*	*Mechanism*	*Comments*
Anticholinergics	↓ Levodopa effect	↓ Gastric emptying, thus ↑ degradation of levodopa in gut, and ↓ amount absorbed	Watch for ↓ levodopa effect when anticholinergics used in doses sufficient to ↓ GI motility. When anticholinergic therapy discontinued in a patient on levodopa, watch for signs of levodopa toxicity. Anticholinergics can relieve symptoms of parkinsonism and might offset the reduction of levodopa bioavailability. Overall, interaction of minor significance.
Benzodiazepines	↓ Levodopa effect	Mechanism unknown	Use together with caution; discontinue if interaction observed.
Ferrous sulfate	↓ Levodopa oral absorption by 50%	Formation of chelation complex	Avoid concomitant administration.
Food	↓ Levodopa effect	Large, neutral amino acids compete with levodopa for intestinal absorption	Although levodopa usually taken with meals to slow absorption and ↓ central emetic effect, high-protein diets should be avoided.
MAOI (e.g., phenelzine, tranylcypromine)	Hypertensive crisis	Peripheral dopamine and norepinephrine	Avoid using together; selegiline and levodopa used successfully together. Carbidopa might minimize hypertensive reaction to levodopa in patients receiving an MAOI.
Methyldopa	↑ or ↓ levodopa effect	Acts as central and peripheral decarboxylase inhibitor	Observe for response; may need to switch to another antihypertensive.
Metoclopramide	↓ Levodopa effect	Central dopamine blockade	Avoid using together
Neuroleptics (e.g., butyrophenones, phenothiazines)	↓ Levodopa effect	Central blockade of dopamine neurotransmission	Important interaction; avoid using these drugs together.
Phenytoin	↓ Levodopa effect	Mechanism unknown	Avoid using together if possible.
Pyridoxine	↓ Levodopa effect	Peripheral decarboxylation of levodopa	Not observed when levodopa given with carbidopa
TCA	↓ Levodopa effect	Levodopa degradation in gut because of delayed emptying	TCA and levodopa have been used successfully together; use with caution

MAO-A, monoamine oxidase A; MAO-B, monoamine oxidase B; MAOI, monoamine oxidase inhibitor; TCA, tricyclic antidepressants.

Controlled-Release Sinemet

The ability to partially alleviate response fluctuations by using continuous infusions of levodopa prompted the development of slow-release carbidopa/levodopa formulations in an attempt to ensure a smoother, more sustained delivery of drug.[80] Sinemet CR contains 25 mg carbidopa and 100 mg levodopa or 50 mg carbidopa and 200 mg levodopa in an erodible polymer matrix that retards dissolution in gastric fluids. By gradually dissolving, Sinemet CR may provide a more gradual absorption of levodopa and more sustained plasma concentrations of levodopa compared with standard Sinemet.[80] While *off* time should theoretically be reduced by the slower rate of plasma levodopa decline, clinical studies have generally not found a difference in *off* time with the controlled-release preparation compared with the immediate-release preparation. As a result, the American Academy of Neurology Practice Parameter for treatment of motor fluctuations and dyskinesias does not recommend switching to controlled-release carbidopa/levodopa as a primary strategy to reduce off time.[81]

Controlled-release Sinemet is about 30% less bioavailable than immediate-release Sinemet. Patients converted from standard Sinemet should receive a dose of Sinemet CR that will provide 10% more levodopa, and then the dose should be titrated upward to clinical reponse.[13] If L.M. were converted to Sinemet CR, the dosage of Sinemet CR would need to be increased about 10% (100 mg) to offset the relative decrease in bioavailability.

Assuming L.M. prefers not to convert to Sinemet CR, his condition may be improved by taking his daily doses of immediate-release Sinemet at shorter dosing intervals while avoiding substantial increases in the daily dosage, which could worsen his dyskinesias. Taking his morning dose before arising from bed may help with his early morning problems and prevent other response fluctuations.

Other means for reducing motor fluctuations include the use of adjunctive agents such as the dopamine agonists, apomorphine rescue, COMT inhibitors, and MAO-B inhibitors, such as selegiline or rasagiline. In severe cases, continuous duodenal infusion of levodopa or administration of liquid levodopa has been useful in managing motor fluctuations (wearing off, unpredictable on and off times, and dyskinesias).[82,83] Liquid levodopa is administered by crushing 10 immediate-release 25/100 tablets and dissolving them in 1 L of tap water, ginger ale, juice, or lemon-lime soda (final concentration is 1 mg/L levodopa). Vitamin C (four 500-mg tablets or 2 g of powder) should be added as a preservative and the mixture shaken well. This provides a solution that is stable for 24 hours at room temperature or 3 days refrigerated. Although this is an effective means for achieving fine titration increments and managing dyskinesias, the duration of effect is extremely short (60–90 minutes), and frequent administration is needed.[13,83]

Dopamine Agonists

The effectiveness of pramipexole as an adjunct to levodopa therapy was evaluated in one large multicenter, placebo-controlled study of 360 patients with a mean disease duration of 9 years and an average duration of levodopa therapy of 8 years.[31] Doses were titrated gradually to their maximal effective dosage as tolerated and not >4.5 mg/day in three divided doses. At the end of a 6-month maintenance period, the patients treated with pramipexole had a 22% improvement in their ADL ($p < 0.0001$) and a 25% improvement in their motor scores ($p < 0.01$) compared with baseline values. Patients treated with pramipexole also had a 31% improvement in the mean off time, compared with a 7% improvement in the placebo-treated group ($p < 0.0006$). Levodopa dose reduction was permitted for increased dyskinesias or hallucinations and occurred in 76% of the pramipexole group compared with 54% in the placebo group. The total daily levodopa dose was decreased by 27% in those treated with pramipexole compared with 5% in the placebo group.

Ropinirole has also shown efficacy in improving motor scores when added to levodopa therapy in patients with advanced-stage disease.[42] In a multicenter, double-blind, randomized parallel-group study, patients treated with ropinirole experienced an average *off* time that was decreased by 1.9 hours daily. In those treated with ropinirole, the total daily levodopa dose was decreased by an average of 19%. Of patients, 28% experienced at least a 35% reduction in both *off* time and in their levodopa dose, compared with 13% of the those in the placebo group. After 1 year of treatment, 47.5% of patients (n = 865) continued treatment with ropinirole as an adjunct to levodopa therapy in advanced-stage disease.

APOMORPHINE

Apomorphine is a dopamine agonist that is approved as rescue therapy for treatment of hypomobility or *off* episodes in patients with PD. It is available only in injectable form. In a randomized, double-blind, parallel-group study of 29 patients, rescue treatment with apomorphine resulted in a 34% reduction (~2 hours) in *off* time compared with 0% in the placebo group ($p = 0.02$).[84] Mean UPDRS motor scores were reduced by 23.9 points (62%) in the those treated with apomorphine, compared with 0.1 (1%) in those receiving placebo ($p < 0.001$). Adverse events in the apomorphine group included yawning (40%), dyskinesias (35%), drowsiness or somnolence (35%), nausea or vomiting, (30%), and dizziness (20%), although only yawning was statistically different than placebo (40% vs. 0%; $p = 0.03$).

Because nausea and vomiting frequently occur with apomorphine treatment, it should be administered with an antiemetic such as trimethobenzamide. The antiemetic should be started 3 days before initiating apomorphine and continued for the first 2 months of treatment. Apomorphine should not be used with ondansetron and other serotonin antagonists used to treat nausea because the combination may cause severe hypotension. In addition, other antiemetics, such as prochlorperazine and metoclopramide, should not be given concurrently with apomorphine because they are dopamine antagonists and can decrease the effectiveness of apomorphine.

Doses of apomorphine range from 2 to 6 mg per subcutaneous injection. A 2-mg test dose is recommended while monitoring blood pressure. If tolerated, the recommendation is to start with a dose of 1 mg less than the tolerated test dose, and increase the dose by 1-mg every few days if needed. Peak plasma levels are observed within 10 to 60 minutes after dosing, so the onset of therapeutic effect is rapid. Two main disadvantages of apomorphine are that the test dose and titration are time-consuming and must be done under physician supervision; and, secondly, patients may require someone else to inject the drug once hypomobility has occurred.

Catechol-O-Methyltransferase (COMT) Inhibitors

Although levodopa has been the mainstay of symptomatic treatment of PD, the increased incidence of motor complications and mental disturbances that occur after prolonged therapy prompted the development of therapies other than replenishment of dopamine. One of these strategies is to prevent the peripheral degradation of levodopa by metabolizing enzymes. COMT is an enzyme found in many body tissues, especially the liver, kidney, and intestines.[85] COMT, which catalyzes the transfer of a methyl group of S-adenosyl-L-methionine to a phenolic group of the catechol, is responsible for the biotransformation of many catechols and hydroxylated metabolites.[86] Carbidopa, an inhibitor of aromatic AAD, prevents the peripheral conversion of levodopa to dopamine. With AAD inhibitors, such as carbidopa or benserazide, the conversion of levodopa to 3-O-methyldopa (3-OMD) by COMT becomes a major metabolic pathway and is increased.[85] The metabolite 3-OMD lacks antiparkinsonian activity and may compete with levodopa for transport into the circulation and brain.

Entacapone and tolcapone are selective, reversible, and potent COMT inhibitors that increase the amount of levodopa available for transport across the blood–brain barrier (Fig. 53-3).[87–89] This effect improves and prolongs the response to levodopa as measured by an increase in the amount of time spent *on* and a decrease in the daily levodopa dosage.[85] The pharmacologic and pharmacokinetic effects of entacapone and tolcapone are compared in Table 53-6. Tolcapone is slightly more potent and has a longer duration of action than entacapone.[90,91] Unlike entacapone, which is usually given with every administration of carbidopa/levodopa (up to eight tablets per day), tolcapone is dosed three times daily. Tolcapone, however, is associated with cases of fatal, acute fulminant liver failure which have led to stringent liver function monitoring requirements.[92] It is recommended for use only in patients taking levodopa who are experiencing motor fluctuations and are not responding adequately to, or are not appropriate candidates for, other adjunctive therapy.[81] When initiated, liver function monitoring should be performed at baseline and every 2 to 4 weeks for the first 6 months, followed periodically thereafter as clinically necessary.[93] Because of the risks for hepatotoxicity associated with tolcapone, entacapone is the preferred COMT inhibitor.[81]

ENTACAPONE

15. Six months after adjusting the frequency of his carbidopa/levodopa, L.M. reports that his dyskinetic activity is not too bothersome, but he is having increased periods (lasting a few minutes) in which he cannot move. He is currently taking pramipexole 0.5 mg TID, immediate-release carbidopa/levodopa 25/250 five times a day, but "even on a good day" gains symptomatic relief for only about 2 to 3 hours following a dose. The decision is made to initiate entacapone therapy and gradually discontinue pramipexole as symptoms or side effects demand. How effective is entacapone for reducing the symptoms of PD?

Efficacy

Several trials have investigated the efficacy and safety of entacapone as an adjunct to levodopa therapy. The Nordic Multicenter Study on Entacapone, The COMT Inhibitor Trial (NOMECOMT) study was conducted in the Nordic

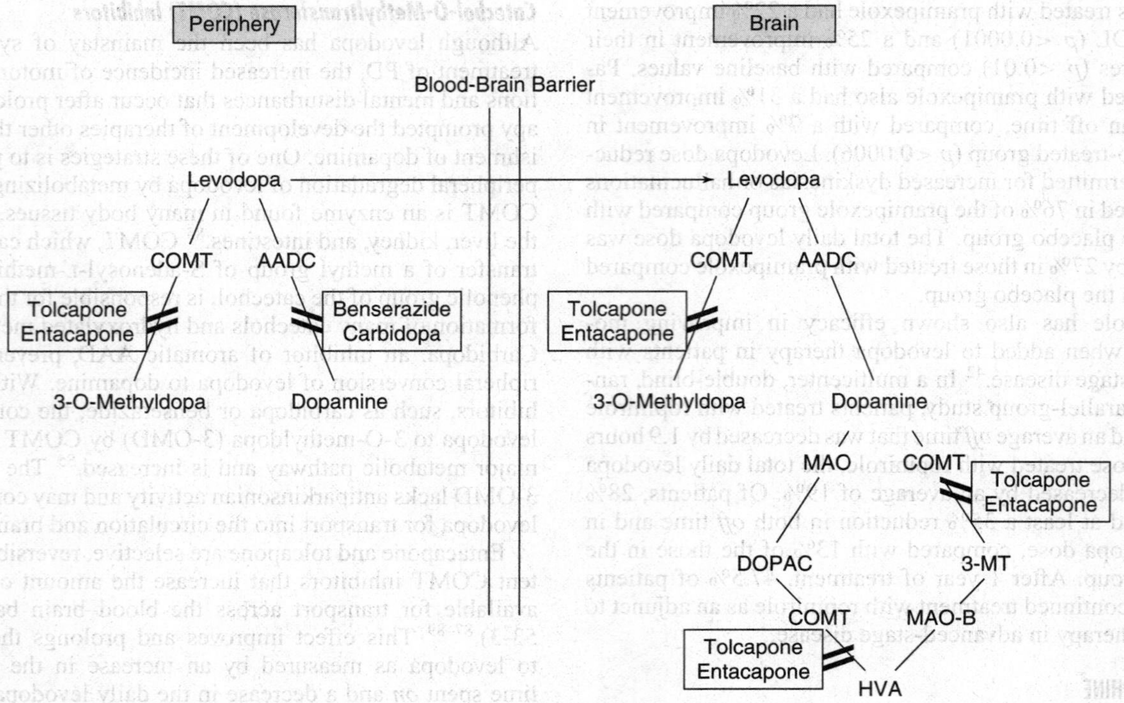

FIGURE 53-3 Levodopa metabolism in the human body. COMT, catechol-O-methyltransferase; AADC, aromatic amino acid decarboxylase; DOPAC, dihydroxyphenylacetic acid; 3-MT, 3-methoxytyramine; MAO, monoamine oxidase.

countries[94]; the Safety and Efficacy Study of Entacapone Assessing Wearing Off (SEESAW) study[95] was conducted in North America. Both trials were multicenter, randomized, double-blind, placebo-controlled, parallel-group studies. Subjects for both studies had idiopathic PD with motor fluctuations, including *wearing off* phenomena, despite maximal tolerated doses of levodopa.

In the NOMECOMT study, 171 patients were randomized to receive either entacapone 200 mg or placebo (4–10 doses per day) with each dose of carbidopa/levodopa. After 6 months, the mean *on* time per 18-hour period increased by 1.5 hours in the entacapone-treated group compared with the placebo-treated group ($p < 0.001$). Withdrawal of entacapone resulted in a return to baseline *on time* levels. Mean *off time* over an 18-hour day decreased by 1.2 hours in the entacapone-treated group compared with the placebo-treated group ($p < 0.001$). Motor scores on the UPDRS decreased by about 10% from baseline in the entacapone-treated group compared with the placebo group ($p < 0.01$). Improvements of approximately 10% to 20% in these motor scores usually produce clinically significant improvements as indicated by increased functional capacity and decreased parkinsonian symptoms (bradykinesia and rigidity).[13] Patients who received entacapone could also lower their levodopa daily dose by an average of 79 mg, whereas placebo-treated subjects required an increase of 12 mg in their average daily levodopa dose ($p < 0.001$). A 3-year open-label extension of this trial demonstrated continued efficacy and tolerability of entacapone.[96]

Table 53-6 Pharmacologic and Pharmacokinetic Properties of Catechol-O-Methyltransferase Inhibitors

	Tolcapone	*Entacapone*
Bioavailability	65%	30–46%
T_{max} (hr)	2.0	0.7–1.2
Protein binding	99.9%	98%
Metabolism	Glucuronidation; CYP 3A4, 2A6 Acetylation; methylated by COMT	Glucuronidation
Half-life (hr)	2–3	1.6–3.4
Time to reverse COMT inhibition (hr)	16–24	4–8
Maximum COMT inhibition at 200-mg dose	80%–90%	60%
Increase in levodopa AUC	100%	30%–45%
Increase in levodopa half-life	75%	60%–75%
Dosing method	TID, spaced 6 hrs apart	With every administration of levodopa

COMT, catechol-O-methyltransferase; TID, three times daily.

In the SEESAW study, 205 patients were randomized to receive either entacapone 200 mg or placebo (up to 10 doses per day) with each dose of carbidopa/levodopa. At baseline, patients had experienced about 4 years of motor fluctuations and had been taking levodopa for about 9 years. Approximately 80% of the study subjects continued to take other antiparkinsonian therapies, including anticholinergic agents, selegiline, dopamine agonists, and amantadine. Compared with placebo over 8 to 24 weeks, daily, *on time* increased by about 1 hour ($p < 0.05$) in patients treated with entacapone, with the greatest improvements observed in those who had a smaller percentage of *on time* at baseline. Those treated with entacapone also had about a 10% reduction in their total UPDRS scores, and they decreased their daily levodopa dose by about 100 mg (13%).

Dosing

16. When should entacapone be initiated, and what is the most effective method for dosing the drug?

Both COMT inhibitors available in the United States are approved for use as adjunctive therapy to levodopa for the treatment of PD in patients experiencing "wearing-off" or "end-of-dose deterioration." No studies have yet examined the effect of early initiation of a COMT inhibitor from the time levodopa is first introduced. This strategy has been proposed as a way of reducing the risk for levodopa-induced motor complications, because the administration of a COMT inhibitor results in a functional extension in the half-life of levodopa.[97] The more stable plasma levels of levodopa resulting from the coadministration of the three-drug combination (levodopa, carbidopa, COMT inhibitor) may lessen levodopa-induced pulsatile stimulation of striatal dopamine receptors and consequently delay motor complications.[13]

Entacapone should not be titrated. It should be given as one 200-mg tablet with each carbidopa/levodopa administration, up to eight tablets per day. It is available in a combination tablet (Stalevo) with a 1:4 ratio of immediate-release carbidopa/levodopa that patients can be switched to once they are stabilized individually on carbidopa/levodopa and entacapone. If dyskinesias occur, it may be necessary to lower the levodopa dose by approximately 10% to 25%, particularly if the patient is receiving >800 mg/day of levodopa. L.M. should be monitored for dyskinesias, especially during the first few weeks of therapy, to determine the need for lowering his carbidopa/levodopa dose.

Adverse Effects

17. What are the adverse effects of entacapone, and how should they be managed?

Most entacapone-induced adverse effects are consistent with increased levodopa exposure. They include dyskinesias (50%–60%), nausea (15%–20%), dizziness (10%–25%), and hallucinations (1%–14%).[94,95] Reducing the levodopa dosage by 10% to 15% as a strategy for circumventing these effects was successful in about one-third of patients experiencing dyskinesias. One study evaluated the incidence of dyskinesias compared with baseline frequency and found an increase of 8% in the entacapone-treated group.[94] Adverse effects related to entacapone include urine discoloration (11%–40%), abdominal pain (6%), and diarrhea (10%).[94,95] Urine discoloration (brownish-orange) is attributed to entacapone and its metabolites and is considered benign, but patients should be counseled regarding this effect to avoid undue concern. The most common reason for withdrawal from clinical studies and discontinuation of therapy was severe diarrhea (2.5%). No monitoring of liver function tests is required during entacapone therapy.

Monoamine Oxidase-B (MAO-B) Inhibitors

Selegiline and Rasagiline

18. What type of antiparkinsonian drugs are selegiline and rasagiline, and what place do they have in the treatment of PD?

SELEGILINE

Selegiline (also referred to as deprenyl) is an MAO inhibitor that irreversibly inhibits MAO type B. Two types of MAO enzymes are present: type A (MAO-A) oxidatively deaminates catecholamines, such as serotonin, norepinephrine, and tyramine, and MAO-B, among other actions, is responsible for the metabolism of dopamine.[13,98] Within the brain, approximately 80% of MAO activity is attributable to MAO-B.[98] The antiparkinsonian activity of selegiline presumably lies in its ability to act centrally to prevent the destruction of endogenous and exogenously administered dopamine.[98] Because selegiline selectively binds to MAO-B, in usual doses (≤10 mg/day), it does not produce a hypertensive reaction ("cheese effect") with dietary tyramine or other catecholamines.[98] It is still recommended, however, that patients be counseled regarding this potential risk.

Selegiline is available in a 5-mg capsule or tablet, and as a 1.25-mg orally disintegrating tablet. The bioavailability of conventional selegiline is low, however, and it undergoes extensive hepatic first-pass metabolism into amphetamine-based metabolites.[99] The usual dosage of conventional selegiline is 10 mg/day given in 5-mg doses in the morning and early afternoon. It is not given in the evening, because excess stimulation from metabolites (L-methamphetamine and L-amphetamine) can cause insomnia and other psychiatric side effects.[98] The orally disintegrating tablet formulation dissolves in the mouth on contact with saliva and undergoes pregastric absorption. This minimizes the effect of first-pass metabolism and results in higher plasma concentrations of selegiline and reductions in the amphetamine-based metabolites.[100]

Efficacy

Selegiline has been studied in PD since the 1970s. Attention initially focused on the potential of selegiline as a "neuroprotective" agent that could conceivably slow the progression of PD.[98,101] With the discovery of parkinsonism developing in addicts who injected MPTP, a synthetic meperidine analog, new information regarding the pathophysiology of PD and the potential for new forms of treatment began to emerge.[102,103] The isolation and identification of this compound fostered the development of superior animal models in which it was found that the neurotoxicity associated with MPTP is not caused by MPTP itself, but rather the oxidized product, L-methyl-4-phenylpyridinium (MPP) ion, a compound that can persist for long periods in the brain.[103] The conversion of MPTP to its neurotoxic metabolite MPP is a two-step process mediated in part by MAO-B.[103,104] Inhibition of MAO-B can inhibit the oxidative conversion of dopamine to potentially reactive peroxides. In animals, pretreatment with selegiline protects against neuronal damage following the administration of MPTP.[101]

The Deprenyl and Tocopherol Antioxidative Therapy of Parkinsonism (DATATOP) study was designed to test the hypothesis that the combined use of both an MAO-B inhibitor (selegiline) and an antioxidant (α-tocopherol) early in the course of the disease may slow disease progression.[105] The primary outcome was the length of time that patients could be sustained without levodopa therapy (an indication of disease progression). Results of this study demonstrated that early treatment with selegiline 10 mg/day delayed the need to start levodopa therapy by approximately 9 months compared with patients given placebo.[105] Long-term observation demonstrated, however, that the benefits of selegiline diminished over time. During an additional year of observation, patients originally randomized to selegiline tended to reach the endpoint of disability more quickly than did those not assigned to receive selegiline. Initial selegiline treatment also did not alter the development of levodopa's adverse effects such as dyskinesias and "wearing-off" and "on-off" phenomena. In other words, early treatment with this agent did not produce a sustained benefit.[106] The finding that selegiline as initial therapy does not alter the development of motor fluctuations was corroborated in a study by Caraceni et al.[107]

Selegiline has also been studied as a symptomatic adjunct to levodopa in more advanced disease. Early studies found improvement in the "wearing off" effect of levodopa in 50% to 70% of patients treated with selegeline and a reduction in as much as 30% in the total daily dose of levodopa.[108,109] The *on-off* effect was less responsive to the addition of selegiline. A second follow-up study involving the original DATATOP cohort randomized patients who had been treated with selegiline initially whose disease had advanced to their requiring levodopa to continue selegiline or switch to placebo. After 2 years, no significant difference was found in the primary outcome events of *wearing off*, dyskinesias, or *on-off* motor fluctuations between the groups.[110] In contrast, the orally disintegrating tablet has been shown to reduce *off* time by 32% (2.2 hours) compared with 9% (0.6 hours) for placebo in a 12-week, randomized, multicenter, parallel group, double-blind study.[111] This, in part, may be owing to the improved bioavailability and increased plasma concentrations of selegiline that are observed with the orally disintegrating tablet formulation.

In summary, no convincing evidence indicates that selegiline offers neuroprotection in patients with PD.[112] The benefits of selegiline are modest in early disease, and tolerance to the beneficial effects is seen with long-term use. In more advanced disease, selegiline (particularly the orally disintegrating tablet formulation) could be considered for adjunctive therapy.[81] Its efficacy in reducing the *wearing off* effect is modest at best, and insufficient evidence exists to determine whether it would be effective in controlling the *on-off* effect that L.M. has been experiencing. Thus, for L.M., selegiline does not appear to offer any advantages at this time.

RASAGILINE

Rasagiline is a new, second-generation, propargylamine-type irreversible selective inhibitor of MAO-B. It is indicated as monotherapy in early disease or as adjunct therapy to levodopa in advanced disease. Rasagiline is differentiated from selegiline primarily in that it is a more potent inhibitor of MAO-B, and it is not metabolized into amphetamine-based metabolites.[113] Rasagiline has been found to protect from MPTP-induced parkinsonism in animal models, possibly through a multifactorial process that includes suppression of oxidant stress and stabilization of mitochondrial apoptosis.[114] Rasagiline is approximately 60 to 100 times more selective in inhibiting MAO-B than MAO-A.[113]

Rasagiline is available in 0.5- and 1-mg tablets. When used as monotherapy, it is initiated at 1 mg daily. When combined with levodopa, the initial dose is lowered to 0.5 mg daily, and can be increased to 1 mg daily based on response. Although tyramine-challenge studies have not demonstrated any clinically significant reactions, the product labeling still contains a warning that patients should be advised to restrict tyramine intake.[115,116]

Efficacy

Rasagiline was studied as monotherapy in early PD in a randomized, double-blind, placebo-controlled trial comparing rasagiline 1 mg (n = 134) or 2 mg (n = 132) daily with placebo (n = 138). After 6 months of therapy, the mean adjusted change in UPDRS score was −4.2 and −3.56 in the 1- and 2-mg groups, respectively, compared with placebo ($p < 0.001$ for both).[117] These changes are quantitatively similar to those observed with levodopa therapy. Quality-of-life measurements were significantly improved in both rasagiline groups compared with placebo; however, the time to requiring levodopa did not differ between groups. At the end of the initial 6 months of treatment, patients who received placebo were then switched over to receive active treatment with rasagiline, while the rasagiline-treated patients continued on therapy. After an additional 6 months of study, it was found that patients receiving rasagiline for all 12 months had less functional decline than patients in whom rasagiline was delayed.[118] The mean adjusted difference at 12 months for patients receiving rasagiline 2 mg/day for all 12 months was −2.29 compared with the delayed-start rasagiline 2 mg group ($p = 0.01$). In an ongoing, open-label extension, the advantage of earlier treatment appears to persist even after 5 years of treatment.[119] Further human studies are ongoing to investigate the potential disease-modifying effects of rasagiline.

In advanced disease, rasagiline added to levodopa therapy appears to improve motor fluctuations, reducing *off* time by 1.4 hours and 1.8 hours compared with 0.9 hours for placebo ($p = 0.02$ and $p < 0.0001$ for 0.5- and 1-mg/day groups, respectively).[120] Significant improvements were reported in the UPDRS subscores for ADL in the *off* state and motor performance in the on state, as well as clinician global assessments. Dyskinesias were slightly worsened in the 1-mg/day group. As adjunctive therapy to levodopa, rasagiline appears to provide similar benefit to entacapone. When compared with entacapone 200 mg administered with each levodopa dose, rasagiline 1 mg/day reduced total daily *off* time in a similar manner (decrease of 21% or 1.18 hours for rasagiline and 21% or 1.2 hours for entacapone).[121]

Rasagiline is well-tolerated. Headache, dizziness, and nausea appear to be the most common adverse effects when rasagiline is given as monotherapy.[116] When administered in combination with levodopa, treatment-emergent dyskinesias and orthostasis also occur. Reduction of levodopa dose may be necessary if dyskinesias occur when rasagiline is added. Similar precautions regarding drug interactions exist with rasagiline as selegiline; that is, sympathomimetics, meperidine, dextromethrophan, other MAO inhibitors, and serotonin reuptake inhibitors (SSRI) should be avoided or used with caution. Because rasagiline is metabolized by CYP1A2, inhibitors such as ciprofloxacin may increase plasma concentrations of rasagiline.

Because L.M. is currently receiving entacapone, administration of rasagiline is not indicated. In patients with early disease, rasagiline is as effective as monotherapy in reducing symptoms; and in patients with advanced disease, consensus recommendations support the use of either entacapone or rasagiline as treatments of choice to reduce *off time*.[81,112]

Anticholinergics

19. What role do anticholinergic drugs play in the treatment of PD?

Anticholinergic drugs have been used to treat PD since the mid-1800s, when it was discovered that symptoms were reduced by the belladonna derivative hyoscyamine sulfate (scopolamine).[13] These drugs remained the mainstay of treatment until the late 1960s, when amantadine and levodopa were introduced. Because of their undesirable side effect profile and poor efficacy, anticholinergic agents have been abandoned as first-line agents.

In PD, the loss of dopamine-producing neurons results in a loss of the balance that normally exists between acetylcholine and dopamine-mediated neurotransmission. The anticholinergic agents work by blocking the excitatory neurotransmitter acetylcholine in the striatum, thereby minimizing the effect of the relative increase in cholinergic sensitivity. This form of therapy is usually reserved for the treatment of resting tremor early in the disease, particularly in younger patients with preserved cognitive function. Anticholinergic agents are considered less effective than carbidopa/levodopa and dopamine agonists for the treatment of bradykinesia and rigidity.[13] Overall, only a mild reduction in symptoms can be expected with anticholinergic therapy, and the risk for side effects would probably outweigh any benefit in L.M.[13,41]

Anticholinergic drugs produce both peripherally and centrally mediated adverse effects. Peripheral effects, such as dry mouth, blurred vision, constipation, and urinary retention, are common and bothersome.[13] Anticholinergic agents can increase intraocular pressure and should be avoided in patients with angle-closure glaucoma. Central nervous system effects can include confusion, impairment of recent memory, hallucinations, and delusions.[13] Patients with PD are more susceptible to these central effects because of advanced age, intercurrent illnesses, and impaired cognition.[13]

Given his history and clinical presentation, L.M. probably should not be given an anticholinergic drug. He originally presented with signs of intellectual impairment and subsequently developed hallucinations. These symptoms may worsen on anticholinergic therapy. L.M. also has prostatic hyperplasia and his symptoms of urinary retention may be exacerbated by anticholinergic drugs. The mydriasis and cycloplegia associated with these drugs could interfere with his ability to paint. Finally, anticholinergic drugs also could aggravate his constipation.

Amantadine

20. How does amantadine work in PD, and what place does it have in treatment of the disease?

Efficacy and Dosing

Amantadine, an antiviral agent, was discovered serendipitously to have antiparkinsonian activity when a patient given the drug for influenza experienced a remission in her tremor, rigidity, and bradykinesia.[122] Shortly thereafter, clinical trials documented its effectiveness when used alone and in combination with levodopa to treat mild forms of PD.[123–125] The mechanism of action of amantadine for PD treatment is not entirely understood, but it probably augments dopamine release from presynaptic nerve terminals and possibly inhibits dopamine reuptake into storage granules.[126] Others have suggested an anticholinergic mechanism of action because certain anticholinergic-type side effects are caused by the drug.[123]

Amantadine reduces all the symptoms of parkinsonian disability in about 50% of patients, usually within days after starting therapy; however, a substantial number of patients develop tachyphylaxis within 1 to 3 months. Temporary withdrawal, discontinuation, and subsequent reinstitution of amantadine at a later date can be beneficial in some patients.[125] In addition, amantadine is associated with neuropsychiatric side effects, which limits its use.

More recently, amantadine has been found to be an antagonist at *N*-methyl-D-aspartate (NMDA) receptors; therefore, it may block glutamate transmission and attention dyskinesias.[127] This finding has been corroborated in studies of patients with PD with levodopa-induced dyskinesias, which have found a reduction in dyskinesia scores with amantadine.[124,128–130] With more effective agents available for use in early disease, the main role of amantadine in the treatment of PD appears limited to add-on therapy for treating levodopa-induced dyskinesias.

When used, amantadine should be started with one 100-mg capsule taken with breakfast; an additional 100-mg capsule can be taken with lunch 5 to 7 days after the initiation of the drug.[123] The dosage can be increased to a maximum of 300 mg/day; however, doses >200 mg/day are rarely necessary and pose a greater risk of adverse effects. The second dose is best taken in the early afternoon to minimize the likelihood of insomnia. Amantadine also is available in a liquid preparation, which is advantageous for patients with dysphagia. Amantadine is renally excreted and the dosage needs to be reduced in patients with renal impairment.[131]

Adverse Effects

Side effects of amantadine mainly involve the gastrointestinal, cardiovascular, and central nervous systems. In one large-scale study, at least one side effect was experienced by 15% of patients, whereas 9% had two or more adverse effects.[123] Seen most frequently are neuropsychiatric complaints, which include dizziness, confusion, disorientation, depression, nervousness, irritability, insomnia, nightmares, and hallucinations.[60,123,124] Convulsions have been observed on rare occasions with high dosages (>800 mg/day), particularly in patients with renal impairment.[60] Amantadine does have some anticholinergic properties, and patients concomitantly receiving anticholinergic agents appear to experience more prominent central nervous system side effects.[60,123,124] Dry mouth, nausea, vomiting, cramps, diarrhea, and constipation are less frequently encountered. Ankle edema occurs in up to 10% of patients and is usually seen in association with livedo reticularis.[60] Elevation of the legs, diuretic therapy, and dosage reduction often alleviate the edema.

Livedo reticularis is a rose-colored mottling of the skin, usually involving the lower extremities (but can involve the upper extremities as well), that occurs in up to 80% of patients receiving amantadine.[60,124,125,132] It can be observed as early as 2 weeks after initiating amantadine therapy and persists until therapy is discontinued, often intensifying to a blackish-purple color.[124] It is more commonly observed in women taking higher dosages (>200 mg/day) and is worse on standing and in colder climates.[60,124] Livedo reticularis is believed to be caused by local release of catecholamines, which cause vasoconstriction and alter the permeability of cutaneous blood vessels.[132] The consequences of livedo reticularis are entirely cosmetic; therefore, discontinuation of therapy is unnecessary.

Investigational Pharmacotherapy

21. What antioxidants, dietary supplements, or other investigational therapies have been evaluated in the treatment of PD?

Antioxidants

If free radical generation is important in the pathophysiology of PD, then adjunctive therapy with antioxidant drugs early in the course of disease should theoretically provide benefit.[133] The most comprehensive evaluation of antioxidant therapy for PD has come from the DATATOP study.[105,134,135] In this study, patients were assigned to one of four treatment regimens: α-tocopherol (2,000 IU/day) and selegiline placebo; selegiline 10 mg/day and α-tocopherol placebo; selegiline and α-tocopherol active treatments; or placebos. The primary endpoint was time to requirement of levodopa therapy. After approximately 14 months of follow-up, no difference was seen between the α-tocopherol group and placebo group in time to require levodopa.[135] Thus, despite the theoretic benefit, clinical data are lacking to support the routine use of α-tocopherol and it is not recommended.[14]

Coenzyme Q10

Coenzyme Q10 (CoQ_{10}), also known as ubiquinone, is an antioxidant involved in the mitochondrial electron transport chain that has been shown to have reduced activity in patients with PD.[136] The finding that MPTP can induce parkinsonism through inhibition of complex I in the mitochondrial electron transport chain and result in injury of nigral dopaminergic neurons, led investigators to evaluate whether supplementation with CoQ_{10} could restore dysfunctional mitochondria.[137] In a randomized, placebo-controlled trial, 80 patients with early untreated PD were randomly assigned to placebo or CoQ_{10} at dosages of 300, 600, or 1,200 mg/day in four divided doses.[138] Subjects were followed for up to 16 months or until therapy with levodopa was required. The primary outcome was a change in total score on the UPDRS from baseline to the last visit. Total UPDRS scores increased (indicating worsening of symptoms) to a greater extent in placebo-treated patients than in those treated with CoQ_{10} (+11.99 for placebo, +8.81 for 300 mg/day, +10.82 for 600 mg/day, and +6.69 for 1,200 mg/day). These results indicated a linear trend between CoQ_{10} dosage and changes in UPDRS scores. Time to requirement of levodopa, however, did not differ among the groups. Side effects of CoQ_{10} were minimal and not different than placebo.

In a larger, National Institute of Health-sponsored futility-design study, CoQ_{10} 600 mg four times daily was compared with placebo in 213 patients with early PD not requiring medications.[139] This was a randomized, double-blind, placebo-controlled trial. The primary outcome measure was the mean change in total UPDRS score from baseline to either the time required for symptomatic therapy or 12 months, whichever came first. The threshold value for futility of CoQ_{10} was defined as 30% less progression on the total UPDRS than the 10.65 unit change observed historically in the placebo arm of the DATATOP trial, or 7.46. After 12 months of therapy, the mean change in the CoQ_{10} group was 7.52 compared with 6.31 in the placebo group. Based on the prespecified criteria, although CoQ_{10} did not meet the prespecified endpoint of a change of 7.46 or less, it could not be rejected as futile and met criteria for further clinical testing. At this time, it is premature to recommend routine use of CoQ_{10} in PD. Future studies should focus on clinically meaningful outcomes to prove or disprove the clinical efficacy of CoQ_{10}.

Creatine and Minocycline

Creatine is a dietary supplement marketed for performance enhancement. Similar to the theory for efficacy of CoQ_{10}, creatine plays a role in mitochondrial energy production and has been shown to protect from MPTP-induced dopamine depletion in animal models.[140] Minocycline is a second-generation tetracycline used to treat various infections, but has also been shown to display anti-inflammatory effects, which have resulted in improvements in chronic inflammatory conditions such as rheumatoid arthritis.[141] An inflammatory response occurs with loss of dopaminergic neurons in PD, and minocycline has been shown to be protective in MPTP animal models of PD.[142]

Both creatine and minocycline were examined for use in PD in a futility study that was similar in design to that conducted with CoQ_{10}. In this randomized, double-blind, placebo-controlled trial, 200 patients with early PD not requiring therapy were randomized to receive creatine (n = 67) 10 g/day, minocycline 200 mg/day (n = 66), or placebo (n = 67).[143] The primary outcome measure was the mean change in total UPDRS score from baseline to either the time required for symptomatic therapy or 12 months, whichever came first. The threshold value for futility of creatine or minocycline use was defined as 30% less progression on the total UPDRS (≤7.46 units) than the historical DATATOP trial cohort (10.46 units). After 12 months, the mean change in the total UPDRS was 5.6 units in the creatine group, 7.09 in the minocycline group, and 8.39 in the placebo group. Based on the prespecified criteria, neither creatine nor minocycline could be rejected as futile and met criteria for further clinical testing. Although it is too early to recommend either agent for use, future studies will likely proceed based on the encouraging results of this study.

Surgery

22. L.M. has gained additional improvement in rigidity, bradykinesia, and posture, as well as improvement in the "on-off" and "wearing off" effects, with the combination of Sinemet (carbidopa/levodopa) and entacapone. He has experienced little if any reduction in his tremor, which is one of the most debilitating symptoms of his disease. What are other therapies for severe parkinsonian tremor?

Parkinsonian tremor is often less responsive to dopaminergic therapy than other symptoms. There can be considerable interpatient variability in the frequency and amplitude of parkinsonian tremor. Tremor can be worsened by peripheral factors, such as catecholamine release, often in association with stress or anxiety, as well as central factors inherent to the disease.[144]

Surgery has played a role in the treatment of PD, particularly in patients who cannot achieve a satisfactory response to available medications. Before the introduction of levodopa, PD was primarily viewed as a surgically treated condition. With the availability of effective drug therapies, the importance of surgical intervention lessened. Posteroventral pallidotomy is an effective method for reducing dyskinesias on the contralateral side and may permit the use of higher dosages of levodopa for managing rigidity and bradykinesia.[145,146] One of its disadvantages is the need to make a lesion near the optic tract; however, studies have shown significant improvements in rigidity and bradykinesia and also relief from tremor following posteroventral pallidotomy. The risks of pallidotomy include visual loss; weakness, including paralysis; and hemorrhage that can cause stroke and speech difficulty.

In patients with mild forms of parkinsonism in which bradykinesia and gait disturbances are absent, symptoms of debilitating tremor and rigidity can benefit from stereotaxic thalamotomy. This intervention has eliminated contralateral tremor in 80% of patients, and improvement has been sustained for up to 10 years.[146,147] A disadvantage of both pallidotomy and thalamotomy is the need to make an irreversible lesion in the basal ganglia that may limit the effectiveness of newer procedures as they become available.

Deep brain stimulation (DBS) is a method that uses an implanted electrode in the brain (either the subthalamic nucleus [STN] or the globus pallidus interna [GPi]) with a lead connected to a subcutaneously implanted pacemaker.[148,149] This permits delivery of a high-frequency stimulation to the desired target. Advantages of DBS include no need for an irreversible brain lesion, and it provides flexibility for altering the target site and program stimulation parameters. Candidates for DBS should have idiopathic PD and be levodopa-responsive, but continue to experience motor complications or tremor despite optimal pharmacotherapeutic regimens.[81] It should be avoided in patients with pre-existing cognitive or psychiatric problems owing to a slight risk of decline in cognition. No strict age limitation for DBS exists, but patients <70 years of age appear to recover from surgery more quickly and show greater motor improvements. Although studies have shown that both DBS of the GPi and STN improve tremor, bradykinesia, and rigidity in patients with PD, DBS of the STN is currently the preferred approach as the available data consistently demonstrate marked reduction in the need for escalating levodopa dosages compared with DBS of the GPi.[81,150,151]

Attention also has been directed toward surgical treatment of PD by transplanting fetal dopaminergic neurons directly into dopamine-depleted regions of the basal ganglia in the hopes of providing a localized infusion of dopamine from these cells.[149,152] The observed benefits from this procedure have included improved motor response while lowering the incidence and severity of dyskinesias.[149] Research efforts also include transplanting genetically engineered cell lines such as those capable of overexpressing tyrosine hydroxylase or neurotrophic factors. All of these methods are considered experimental, however, and are not routinely available.[149]

Other Treatment Considerations in Parkinson's Disease

Dementia

23. As L.M.'s disease has progressed, he has become increasingly demented and reliant on family members for help in performing ADL. He scored 16 (below normal) on his most recent Mini-Mental Status Examination, and his family describes periodic episodes of confusion and agitation. Neuropsychiatric testing is performed to help distinguish whether his confusion and agitation are caused by his progressing dementia or whether depression is contributory. Subsequent recommendations from the neuropsychiatrist are that he avoid driving and receive 24-hour supervision, along with participation in structured leisure activities such as adult daycare several hours per week to help relieve his wife's caregiver burden. In addition, he has a significant depressive component to his dementia that should be treated. How should L.M.'s progressive cognitive decline and depression be treated?

Cognitive impairment, manifested by bradyphrenia (slowed mental processes), altered executive functions, memory loss, decreased attention span, or inappropriate behavior, is common in patients with PD. The prevalence of dementia in patients with PD increases with age and duration of disease and is approximately 6- to 12-fold greater than in age-matched controls.[13] Successful management of cognitive impairment in patients with PD requires first that all potentially reversible causes or contributing factors be addressed. These include treating infections, dehydration, and metabolic abnormalities, as well as eliminating unnecessary medications (particularly anticholinergics, sedatives, anxiolytics) that can exacerbate dementia or delirium.

Experience with cholinesterase inhibitors such as donepezil (Aricept) and rivastigmine (Exelon) for treating cognitive impairment in PD is limited, but preliminary studies suggest that some improvement may occur with their use.[153–156] Outcomes of these studies are usually measured using different scales, such as the Mini Mental Status Examination, the Alzheimer's Disease Assessment Scale-Cognitive Subscale, the Alzheimer's Disease Assessment Scale-Clinicians Global Impression of Change, and the Clinicians Interview Based Impression of Change Plus Caregiver Input. Compared with placebo, the cholinesterase inhibitors often result in a marginal change of a couple of points in these scales that is statistically significant. It is unclear, however, to what extent the changes in the scores of these outcome measures are clinically relevant in such areas as ability to perform ADL without assistance, and delay in nursing home placement.

Although donepezil or rivastigmine can be considered for demented patients with PD such as L.M., they are expensive, and he must be monitored closely for signs of deterioration of motor function such as worsening of tremor.[15] Cholinesterase inhibitors are also associated with adverse events that may be overlooked and attributed to the disease itself in patients with PD, including sialorrhea, excessive lacrimation, incontinence, nausea, vomiting, and orthostasis. More importantly, adequate supportive home care for L.M. should be ensured. As he becomes further dependent on family members for assistance with ADL, the increased needs of the caregiver(s) should also be considered. In L.M.'s case, attending adult daycare several times weekly if available, would provide a structured, supervised environment for interaction with others, as well as providing a rest period for his caregiver. When severe, dementia is a leading cause of nursing home placement for patients with PD.[13]

Depression

Depression occurs frequently in patients with PD. The physical appearance of the patient may, however, make it difficult to determine whether the symptoms are attributed to depression or to the PD.[13] Patients manifesting symptoms of hypomimia (facial masking), hypophonia (weak voice), psychomotor retardation, and a stooped posture may be incorrectly diagnosed with depression if these features are solely the result of the PD. In contrast, depression in patients with loss of energy, decreased appetite, reduced libido, and insomnia may go unrecognized, because the symptoms are often attributed to the PD.[13]

Treatment of the depressed patient with PD should first focus on providing adequate treatment of the symptoms of PD through restoring mobility and independence, particularly in patients whose depression can be attributed to lengthy *off* periods. Antiparkinson drugs, such as pramipexole, can be associated with mood-enhancing effects independent of their ability to reduce time in the *off* state.[157] Depression in patients with PD can be successfully treated with antidepressant drugs, although controlled research trials in this area are lacking.[158] SSRI are often considered for prolonged bouts of depression, but other classes of antidepressants, such as tricyclic antidepressants, may also be effective.[15] Bupropion, a dopamine reuptake inhibitor, should theoretically reduce PD symptoms as well; however, limited evidence supports this hypothesis.[159] It is important to note that some SSRI, such as fluoxetine, can be activating. Although this may be beneficial in patients who are apathetic or withdrawn, it may worsen symptoms in agitated patients.[13] Fluoxetine also has a prolonged elimination half-life and is metabolized to an active metabolite, which can increase the risk for side effects even after the drug is withdrawn. With tricyclic antidepressants, care must be taken to observe for anticholinergics side effects that may worsen PD symptoms, such as delayed gastric emptying (which may reduce levodopa effectiveness by increasing levodopa degradation in the gut), orthostatic hypotension, and a subsequent increased risk for falls. Psychotherapy can also be considered in patients with PD who are depressed. Lastly, electroconvulsive therapy may be beneficial if medications fail.

Based on L.M.'s symptoms, it is reasonable to start him on an antidepressant. Regardless of which agent or class of antidepressant is selected, therapy should be started at the lowest dose and gradually titrated to effect. He should be monitored closely for side effects, particularly anticholinergic symptoms with tricyclic antidepressants, and for any adverse effects on mobility. He should be observed carefully for changes in parkinsonian symptoms, including development of extrapyramidal symptoms, as well as any signs of psychomotor agitation.[160]

Psychomotor Agitation

The incidence of hallucinations and delirium increases with age and cognitive impairment in patients with PD. These symptoms are often caused or exacerbated by medications.[13] Symptoms are often more pronounced at night (the "sundowning" effect), and hallucinations are typically visual. As with the management of cognitive impairment, it is important to eliminate or minimize any potential causative factors, particularly anticholinergic medications that could be contributing to the hallucinations or delirium. In some patients, reducing the dose of levodopa improves mental function and also provides satisfactory control of motor features (see Question 12). If it is not possible to achieve a balance between preserving motor control and decreasing neuropsychiatric symptoms through reduction in levodopa dosage, antipsychotics may be considered.

Older antipsychotic medications, such as haloperidol, perphenazine, and chlorpromazine, block striatal dopamine D_2 receptors and may exacerbate parkinsonian symptoms. Therefore, these agents are not recommended.[13] Newer "atypical" antipsychotics are more selective for limbic and cortical D_3, D_4, D_5 receptors; they have minimal activity at D_2 receptors and can control symptoms without worsening parkinsonism. Of these agents, clozapine has the best evidence of efficacy in patients with PD.[15,161] Its use is limited, however, by the need for frequent monitoring of white blood cell counts owing to the risk of agranulocytosis. Other newer agents, particularly quetiapine (Seroquel), appear promising and have controlled psychosis without worsening parkinsonism.[162,163] Risperdal (Risperdal) and olanzapine (Zyprexa) have also been studied, but both worsened parkinsonism and were inferior to clozapine in patients with PD.[164–167]

Agitation, characterized by restlessness, irritability, apprehension, and dysphoria, occurs commonly in patients with PD.[13] These symptoms often occur during off periods and may be a manifestation of underlying anxiety. Treatment should begin by ensuring optimal control of motor fluctuations, followed by discontinuation or reduction in dosage of any antiparkinsonian drugs, particularly anticholinergic agents that might exacerbate the symptoms. Short-term use of short-acting benzodiazepines, such as lorazepam or alprazolam, may also provide relief.[13]

Autonomic Dysfunction

Patients with PD also experience symptoms of dysautonomia, including orthostasis, erectile dysfunction, constipation, nocturia, sensory disturbances, dysphagia, seborrhea, and thermoregulatory imbalances.[13] Management of these symptoms is generally supportive, and appropriate medical interventions similar to those used in other geriatric patients can be used to treat these symptoms whenever encountered. In some cases, fludrocortisone or midodrine can be considered if orthostatic hypotension is severe.

Falls

Patients with PD and their caregivers should be counseled on the prevention of falls, because they can result in serious morbidity and mortality. Falls generally result from one of several factors, including postural instability, freezing and festination, levodopa-induced dyskinesia, symptomatic orthostatic hypotension, coexisting neurologic or other medical disorders, and environmental factors.[13] Prevention remains the best strategy and includes environmental precautions, such as proper lighting, use of handrails, removing tripping hazards, and incorporating physical and occupational therapy. Reversible causes of postural or gait instability should be addressed whenever suspected.

Sleep Disorders

The sleep disorders often experienced by elderly persons are accentuated in PD patients.[13] Insomnia, sleep fragmentation owing to PD symptoms, restless legs syndrome, and nightmares are common and a source of decreased quality of life. When sleep dysfunction can be directly attributed to PD symptoms, such as akinesia, tremor, dyskinesia, or nightmares, dosage adjustment of dopaminergic medications is indicated. Proper sleep hygiene should be encouraged. Short-acting benzodiazepines can be used if insomnia occurs; however, a longer-acting agent or controlled-release formulation may be preferred if the patient wakes early and is unable to return to sleep. If excessive daytime drowsiness occurs, modafinil may be considered. Similar to dysautonomia, management of sleep disorders that are not directly attributable to PD symptoms can be managed supportively, as in other geriatric patients.

RESTLESS LEGS SYNDROME

Clinical Presentation

24. J.J., a 42-year-old woman, presents to her family physician complaining of intermittent difficulty sleeping at night because of "jumpy legs." Her symptoms bother her most in the evening, and she reports being able to sleep only 4 to 5 hours per night because of the accompanying restlessness. On further questioning, she describes the sensation in her legs as being like "bugs crawling under the skin." The sensation is not painful. She explains that the symptoms worsen in the evening and at night and are partially relieved with walking. She recalls that her mother had similar symptoms. J.J.'s spouse notes that she often "kicks" him in her sleep. Review of her medical history shows an otherwise healthy postmenopausal female. What signs and symptoms are suggestive of restless legs syndrome (RLS) in J.J.? What laboratory tests or diagnostic procedures should be performed in J.J. to evaluate her condition?

Restless legs syndrome is an increasingly recognized and disabling sensorimotor disorder estimated to affect approximately 10% of the adult population.[168] Although most patients with mild symptoms will not require treatment, RLS can be associated with adverse health outcomes, including sleep onset insomnia, missed or late work, anxiety, depression, marital discord, and even suicide in severe cases.

Four essential criteria have been established by the International Restless Legs Syndrome Study Group to diagnose RLS (Table 53-7).[169] The pathognomonic trait of RLS is an almost irresistible urge to move the legs (akathisia), often associated with uncomfortable paresthesias or dysesthesias felt deep inside the limbs. Patients describe the sensation as "creepy-crawly" or "like soda water in the veins."[170] The symptoms may occur unilaterally or bilaterally, affecting the ankle, knee, or entire lower limb. With progressive disease, symptoms can begin earlier in the day, and progressive involvement of the arms or trunk may occur.[171] Temporary or partial relief of symptoms can be achieved with movement. If patients attempt to ignore the urge to move the legs, akathisia will progressively intensify until they either move their legs or the legs jerk involuntarily.[170] Symptoms usually manifest in a circadian pattern with onset or worsening during nighttime hours (usually between 6 PM and 4 AM, with peak symptoms between midnight and 4 AM). The circadian pattern persists even in patients with inverted sleep–wake cycles. As a result of their symptoms, patients with RLS become "nightwalkers," spending significant time walking, stretching, or bending the legs in an effort to relieve symptoms.

Table 53-7 Clinical Features of Restless Legs Syndrome

Essential Criteria
Urge to move legs, associated with parethesias or dysesthesias
Relief of symptoms with movement
Onset or exacerbation of symptoms at rest
Onset or worsening of symptoms during nighttime
Supportive Clinical Features
Accompanying sleep disturbance (sleep onset insomnia)
Periodic leg movements
Positive response to dopaminergic therapy
Positive family history of RLS
Otherwise normal physical exam

J.J.'s case is an example of a classic presentation of RLS. The prevalence of RLS increases with age and appears to be slightly more common in females.[172] She describes "creepy-crawly" sensations that are relieved partially with walking, a core feature of RLS. Her symptoms are worse during the evening hours. J.J. reports her mother suffered from similar symptoms. The observation of a familial tendency suggests a genetic component and several chromosomal loci have been linked to the disease.[173] A strong family history of RLS appears to correlate with an early age of onset (<45 years), whereas presentation at a later age is associated with more neuropathy and accelerated disease progression.[170] J.J.'s spouse has noticed what are likely periodic limb movements of sleep (PLMS). Approximately 80% of patients with RLS will also have PLMS, but their clinical significance is uncertain because they are not definitively linked to poor sleep quality.[174] Furthermore, not all patients with PLMS have associated RLS, further questioning their value in the diagnosis.

Most cases of RLS are considered primary or idiopathic; therefore, the diagnosis does not require elaborate laboratory tests or diagnostic procedures. Several conditions are known to be associated with RLS, and include iron deficiency, pregnancy, and end-stage renal disease. A thorough medical history should be taken in J.J. to rule reversible causes of RLS or other conditions with similar characteristics. It should be relatively straightforward to rule out other disorders of the RLS differential if the diagnostic criteria and characteristics of the patient's complaint are kept in mind.[173] Several medications and substances are known aggravators of RLS, including medications with antidopaminergic properties, such as metoclopramide and prochlorperazine. Nicotine, caffeine, and alcohol can aggravate RLS, through their own ability to interfere with quality of sleep. Additionally, SSRI, tricyclic antidepressants, and commonly used over-the-counter antihistamines, such as diphenhydramine, can trigger or worsen RLS symptoms.[173] Hypotensive akathesia, leg cramps, and other conditions such as arthritis which can cause positional discomfort with extended periods of sitting in one position can mimic RLS. These conditions are easily distinguished from RLS, because they are usually localized to certain joints or muscles, do not have a circadian pattern, and are not associated with an uncontrollable urge to move.

With an otherwise unremarkable physical examination and medical history, specific laboratory tests that should be performed in J.J. are limited to serum ferritin and percent transferrin saturation (total iron-binding capacity) to rule out iron deficiency anemia. It is important to note that ferritin is an acute phase reactant and may be artificially elevated owing to inflammatory or infectious comorbid conditions. Therefore, the ferritin level should always be accompanied by the percent transferrin saturation. Several studies have documented a relationship between low ferritin concentrations and increased symptom severity.[175,176] J.J. is postmenopausal, so a pregnancy test is not necessary. Polysomnography is not usually indicated unless there is clinical suspicion for sleep apnea or if sleep remains disrupted despite treatment of RLS. When clinical suspicion from the physical examination or medical history suggests a possible peripheral nerve or radiculopathy cause, a routine neurologic panel, including thyroid function tests, fasting glucose, vitamins B_6 and B_{12}, and folate, should be obtained.[173] Renal function tests (serum creatinine and blood urea nitrogen) can be obtained to screen for uremia, although RLS does not usually occur in this situation until the patient has reached end-stage renal failure.

Treatment

25. The decision is made to treat J.J.'s symptoms with medication. What pharmacologic therapy should be selected? What nonpharmacologic therapies should be recommended?

Figure 53-4 presents an approach to the treatment of RLS. Iron supplements can potentially cure RLS symptoms in patients found to be iron deficient.[173] If J.J. is iron-deficient, she should be prescribed supplemental iron 50 to 65 mg of elemental iron one to three times daily on an empty stomach with 200 mg of vitamin C to enhance absorption. After ruling out possible reversible causes of RLS, it is important to establish the frequency of J.J.'s symptoms and whether or not they are associated with pain. This information will help determine appropriate therapy.

Several classes of medications are effective for treating RLS, including dopaminergics, benzodiazepines, anticonvulsants,

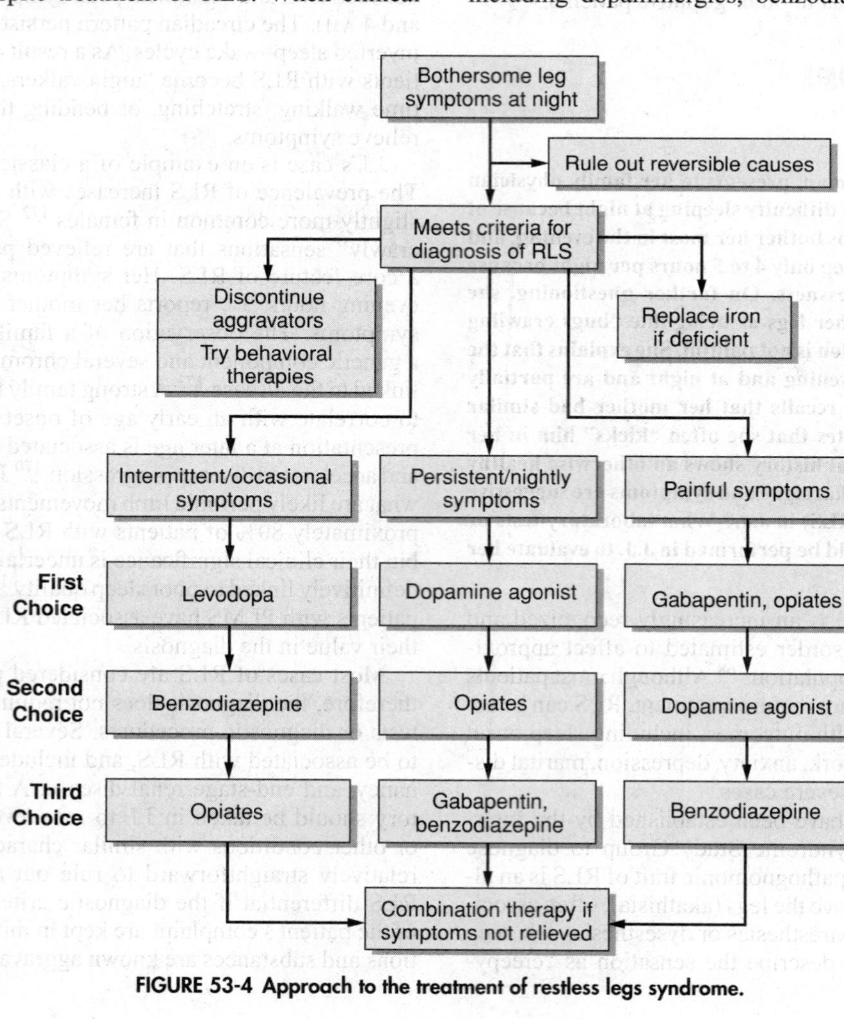

FIGURE 53-4 Approach to the treatment of restless legs syndrome.

and opiates. Dopaminergic therapies have demonstrated the most consistent efficacy in most patients for relieving RLS symptoms, improving sleep, and reducing leg movements.[177] The available dopaminergic therapies that have been evaluated in RLS are carbidopa/levodopa, pramipexole, ropinirole, and pergolide.[177] In addition, amantadine and selegiline have also been studied. The earliest clinical trials of dopaminergic therapies for RLS were of carbidopa/levodopa, which demonstrated improvement in both subjective and objective quality of sleep measures in patients with idiopathic or uremic disease.[178,179] Carbidopa/levodopa is usually recommended as initial therapy in patients with mild, intermittent, nonpainful symptoms.[173,170] Because J.J.'s symptoms are mostly intermittent at the present time and do not cause her pain, carbidopa/levodopa would be an appropriate initial therapy. It should be initiated at one-half of a 25/100 mg tablet, administered 1 or 2 hours before bedtime. The dose can be titrated according to symptoms up to a usual daily dose range of 100 to 250 mg of levodopa. With the immediate-release formulation, relief of symptoms occurs in as little as 20 minutes. Because levodopa has a short half-life, patients may wake from their sleep with rebound symptoms and require an additional dose of carbidopa/levodopa.[180] Two studies have demonstrated that a combination of slow-release and immediate-release carbidopa/levodopa may be superior to the immediate-release product used alone.[181,182]

Benzodiazepines have been shown to relieve RLS symptoms in small, open-label studies; however, controlled clinical trials have yielded less promising results.[180] They are recommended as an alternate to carbidopa/levodopa if the RLS symptoms are intermittent, or as add-on therapy in patients refractory to other treatments.[173] The dosing and adverse effects of the benzodiazepines used in RLS are similar to their use in the general population. No evidence suggests that one benzodiazepine is more effective than another for RLS, and selection should be based on the patient's primary sleep disorder complaint. For example, a newer short-acting benzodiazepine with quick onset of action may be preferred in a patient whose primary problem is getting to sleep. Because benzodiazepines appear to be less effective overall than dopaminergics, they would probably not be a first-line choice in J.J.

If J.J. experienced her symptoms on a nightly basis or during the day, a dopamine agonist should be recommended.[177,180] They are longer acting than levodopa, which allows for more sustained efficacy.[173] Ropinirole (0.25 mg initially, up to 0.5–8.0 mg/day) and pramipexole (0.125 mg initially, up to 0.5–1.5 mg/day) are both FDA-approved for treating RLS. Several randomized, controlled clinical trials have documented efficacy of these agents in both objective and subjective ratings of improvement by patients and clinicians with either short- or long-term use.[177,183–187] Between ropinirole and pramipexole, there does not appear to be greater efficacy or fewer adverse effects with one agent over the other. An older dopamine agonist, pergolide, has also demonstrated efficacy in RLS; however, the increased risk for pulmonary fibrosis and cardiac valvulopathy with this ergot derivative precludes its routine use when dopamine agonists are indicated.[24,25] When used for RLS, ropinirole and pramipexole should be administered 2 hours before bedtime. Adverse effects are similar to those seen with their use in PD and patients should be counseled accordingly (see Question 7).

In addition to her carbidopa/levodopa, nonpharmacologic therapies and behavioral techniques should also be recommended for J.J. Most important among these include discontinuing all RLS aggravators, and practicing good sleep hygiene. Physical and mental activity (e.g., reading, playing card games, or working on the computer) if patients are unable to sleep can reduce symptoms.[173] Counter stimuli such as massage or hot baths have also been helpful.[173]

26. After careful consideration, J.J. and her doctor choose levodopa to treat her RLS. She initially responds well to the therapy. One year later, J.J. returns for follow-up. Her dose of carbidopa/levodopa has progressively increased to three 25/100 mg tablets at bedtime. She describes continued worsening of her symptoms and they do not seem to be relieved with increasing doses of carbidopa/levodopa. Her symptoms are now starting earlier in the evening, occur almost every night, and are now painful. How should J.J.'s therapy be further adjusted?

J.J. is likely experiencing augmentation, a common problem with long-term use of dopaminergic drugs. Augmentation is described as a progressive symptomatic worsening of RLS symptoms after an initial improvement.[173] It is the most common side effect occurring with long-term use (>3 months) of dopaminergic agents. It usually occurs 6 to 18 months after therapy is initiated.[173] The most common presentation of augmentation is that RLS symptoms become more intense, occurring earlier in the evening, with movements spreading to other parts of the body. Increasing doses of dopaminergic agents will initially relieve symptoms; however, with each incremental dose increase symptoms progress more rapidly until they may occur continuously throughout the day.[173] The highest risk for augmentation is with levodopa. An estimated 50% to 85% of patients on levodopa will develop augmentation, compared with only 20% to 30% with dopamine agonists.[180] The primary treatment strategy in dealing with augmentation is to withdraw the dopaminergic agent and substitute other agents. Given her presentation, J.J. should have her carbidopa/levodopa discontinued. She should be counseled that her symptoms will likely rebound severely for 48 to 72 hours, but approximately 4 to 7 days later her symptoms should gradually return to baseline or pretreatment state.[173]

With the discontinuation of carbidopa/levodopa in J.J., an alternate therapy should be selected. Anticonvulsants (particularly gabapentin, lamotrigine, and carbamazepine), and opiates have also been studied for treatment of RLS and are particularly useful if patients have pain with their symptoms. Gabapentin in a dose of 600 to 2,400 mg/day has demonstrated relief in subjective symptoms as well as PLMS and sleep architecture in 50% to 90% of patients in open-label and controlled trials.[180,188,189] Lamotrigine (25 mg/day up to 200 mg/day) and carbamazepine (100–400 mg/day) have also demonstrated efficacy, mostly in open-label studies.[180] Because of its high efficacy and more favorable risk profile, gabapentin is preferred as first-line therapy in patients with RLS who have coexisting neuropathy or associated pain.[170] Because J.J. describes increasing pain from her RLS, after discontinuation of her carbidopa/levodopa it would be appropriate to initiate gabapentin. If necessary, a dopamine agonist could be added at a later time if her symptoms are not completely controlled on gabapentin. If gabapentin is ineffective or not tolerated, J.J. could be prescribed an opiate, which is also an acceptable choice in patients with RLS who have neuropathy or painful dysethesias.[173] Hydrocodone, oxycodone, methadone, codeine, and tramadol have all demonstrated efficacy in RLS.[173] For intermittent symptoms, it is recommended to use short-acting agents. If symptoms extend beyond 8 hours, patients may require twice daily dosing or a switch to a longer acting agent.[173]

ESSENTIAL TREMOR

Clinical Presentation

27. K.H. is a 52-year-old white female office manager who was referred to a neurologist for evaluation of tremor. She is otherwise healthy and reports not taking any regularly prescribed medications. She describes her tremor as being present mainly when she performs voluntary movements. The tremor is not noticeable during rest. She also notices the tremor seems to disappear in the evening after drinking a couple of glasses of wine. The tremor interferes with several of her ADL, including writing, eating, drinking from a cup, and inserting her keys into the ignition. She reports mild interference with her job function and some social embarrassment. No bradykinesia or rigidity is elicited on physical examination. A handwriting sample reveals large characters that are difficult to decipher. Family history reveals that her maternal grandmother and mother both had similar symptoms. What signs and symptoms are consistent with essential tremor in K.H.?

Essential tremor (ET) is a common neurologic disorder that has been written about since ancient times.[190] Beginning in the mid-20th century, the term essential tremor has been consistently used to describe this form of kinetic tremor for which no definite cause has been established.[190] ET has traditionally been viewed as a monosymptomatic disorder of little consequence, but more recently it is recognized to be complex and progressive and to result in significant disability in ADL and job performance, and is a cause of social embarassment.[190] The incidence of ET is estimated to be approximately 616 cases per 100,000 person-years, and the prevalence rate ranges from 6% to 9%.[191,192] Both incidence and prevalence of ET increase with age. In addition, ethnicity and family history of ET are consistently identified risk factors; it is approximately five times more common in whites than blacks, and approximately 50% of patients report a positive family history. The latter finding suggests that genetic predisposition may play a role in ET; however, differences in intrafamilial onset and severity suggest environmental factors may also influence underlying susceptibility to the disease.[190] Several environmental toxins have been proposed as causes of ET, including β-carboline alkaloids (e.g., harmane and harmine) and lead, both of which have been found in elevated concentrations in patients with ET compared with normal controls.[193,194]

Because parkinsonian tremor and ET are the most common forms of tremor observed in practice, it is important to distinguish between the two because the treatments are very different. Diagnostic criteria for ET developed by the Movement Disorder Society are shown in Table 53-8.[195] Tremor should first be identified as either an action or resting tremor. Action tremors include kinetic, postural, and isometric tremors. The defining feature of ET is kinetic tremor of the arms. The tremor can also affect head or voice. Kinetic tremor can be elicited in patients during voluntary movement, such as finger-to-nose test, signing their name, drawing spirals, or drinking water from a cup. Postural tremor occurs during sustained arm extension. Although both types of action tremors (kinetic or postural) can be present in ET and PD, the presence of resting tremor is much more common in PD.[190] Lack of resting tremor and absence of bradykinesia or rigidity in K.H. suggest the tremor is not parkinsonian. She describes interference of her tremor occurring with voluntary movement, such as her ADL and drinking from a cup. Other signs and symptoms that support a diagnosis of ET include her age, family history, large and tremulous handwriting (as opposed to micrographia in PD), and improvement in tremor with alcohol consumption. Table 53-9 summarizes the similarities and differences of ET and parkinsonian tremor.

Table 53-8 Diagnostic Criteria for Essential Tremor

Inclusion Criteria
Bilateral postural tremor with or without kinetic tremor, involving hands and forearms, that is visible and persistent
Duration >5 yr
Exclusion Criteria
Other abnormal neurological signs (except Froment's sign)
Presence of known causes of increased physiological tremor
Concurrent or recent exposure to tremorogenic drugs or the presence of a drug withdrawal state
Direct or indirect trauma to the nervous system within 3 mo before the onset of tremor
Historical or clinical evidence of psychogenic origins
Convincing evidence of sudden onset or evidence of stepwise deterioration

Several medications and substances are known to be tremorogenic. All patients with tremor should have thorough medication history to rule out these possible causes. Medications commonly implicated include corticosteroids, metoclopramide, valproate, sympathomimetics (e.g. albuterol, amphetamines, pseudoephedrine), SSRI, tricyclic antidepressants, theophylline, and thyroid preparations.[190] In addition, caffeine, tobacco, and chronic alcohol use can cause tremor that resembles ET. K.H. does not report taking any regularly prescribed medications; however, she should be questioned regarding any over-the-counter medication use as well as her caffeine and smoking habits if applicable.

The final step in evaluating K.H.'s tremor should include laboratory analysis to rule out possible medical conditions associated with tremor. If clinical signs suggest the possibility of hyperthyroidism, thyroid function tests should be performed. In patients <40 years of age who present with action tremor, serum ceruloplasmin can be tested to evaluate for possible Wilson's disease.[190] Neuroimaging tests are not useful in the diagnosis and evaluation of ET.

Treatment

28. What therapies are effective in treating essential tremor? How should KH be treated?

Patients with ET who have mild disability that does not cause dysfunction or social embarrassment can go without

Table 53-9 Differentiation of Essential Tremor and Parkinson's Disease

Characteristic	Essential Tremor	Parkinson's Disease
Kinetic tremor in arms, hands, or head	++	++
Hemibody (arm and leg) tremor	0	++
Kinetic tremor > resting tremor	++	+
Resting tremor > kinetic tremor	0	++
Rigidity or bradykinesia	0	++
Postural instability	0	++
Usual age of onset (yr)	15–25, 45–55	55–65
Symmetry	Bilateral	Unilateral > Bilateral
Family history of tremor	+++	+
Response to alcohol	+++	0
Response to anticholinergics	0	++
Response to levodopa	0	+++
Response to primidone	+++	0
Response to propranolol	+++	+
Handwriting analysis	Large, tremulous script	Micrographia

0, not observed; +, rarely observed; ++, sometimes observed; +++, often observed.

treatment.[196] It is estimated that 15% to 25% of patients with ET will retire prematurely, and 60% will not apply for a job or promotion because of their tremor.[197] Because K.H. is experiencing tremor that is causing both significant functional disability in her occupation and social embarrassment, she should be considered for pharmacotherapy (Table 53-10). It is important to note that, although effective treatments exist, tremor is rarely eliminated completely.[190] Factors predicting lack of response have not been readily identified.[190]

Propranolol, a nonselective β-adrenergic receptor blocker, or primidone, an anticonvulsant, are recommended as first-line agents to treat ET.[196,198] Propranolol is typically effective in doses of at least 120 mg/day, with 45% to 75% of patients reporting benefit.[196] Long-acting propranolol is as effective as the regular-release formulation.[199] Other β_1-selective blockers such as atenolol and metoprolol, have also been studied, but with mixed findings.[200] Propranolol has demonstrated greater efficacy than these B_1 selective agents,[201] suggesting

Table 53-10 Pharmacotherapy for Essential Tremor

Drug	Initial Dose	Usual Therapeutic Dose	Adverse Effects
β-Blockers			
Propranolol	10 mg QD-BID	160–320 mg divided QD-BID	Bradycardia, fatigue, hypotension, depression, exercise intolerance
Atenolol	12.5–25 mg QD	50–150 mg QD	Bradycardia, fatigue, hypotension, exercise intolerance
Nadolol	40 mg QD	120–240 mg QD	Bradycardia, fatigue, hypotension, exercise intolerance
Anticonvulsants			
Primidone	12.5 mg QD	50–750 mg divided QD-TID	Sedation, fatigue, nausea, vomiting, ataxia, dizziness, confusion, vertigo
Gabapentin	300 mg QD	1,200–3,600 mg divided TID	Nausea, drowsiness, dizziness, unsteadiness
Topiramate	25 mg QD	200–400 mg divided BID	Appetite suppression, weight loss, paresthesias, concentration difficulties
Benzodiazepines			
Alprazolam	0.125 mg QD	0.75–3 mg divided TID	Sedation, fatigue, potential for abuse
Clonazepam	0.25 mg QD	0.5–6 mg divided QD-BID	Sedation, fatigue, ataxia, dizziness, impaired cognition
Miscellaneous			
Botulinum toxin A	Varies by injection site: 50–100 U/arm for hand tremor; 40–400 U/neck for head tremor; 0.6–15 U/vocal cords for voice tremor; retreat no sooner than every 3 mo (extend as long as possible)		Hand weakness (with wrist injection); dysphagia, hoarseness, breathiness (with neck or vocal cord injection)

BID, two times daily; QD, every day; TID, three times daily.

that blockade of β_2 receptors is of importance. β-adrenergic receptor blockers with intrinsic sympathomimetic activity, such as pindolol, appear ineffective in ET.[202] Caution should be exercised with propranolol in patients with asthma, congestive heart failure, diabetes mellitus, and atrioventricular block.[196]

Several studies have compared propranolol and primidone in ET,[203,204] and they are considered to have similar efficacy.[198] Primidone is metabolized to a phenobarbital-based metabolite; however, phenobarbital is inferior to primidone in treating ET.[205] Acute adverse effects of primidone include nausea, vomiting, and ataxia, which can occur in up to one-quarter of patients often limiting its use.[190] Long-term tolerability of primidone is very good, however, and may actually be superior to propranolol.[204] Primidone should be initiated at 12.5 mg/day, administered at bedtime, to reduce the occurrence of acute side effects. It can be titrated gradually as tolerated up to 750 mg/day in divided doses.

Other agents that have demonstrated variable efficacy in ET include gabapentin,[206] topiramate,[207] and benzodiazepines (specifically, alprazolam[208] and clonazepam[209]). They are generally considered to be less-proven, second-line therapies, however.[196,198] Adverse effects and potential for abuse (specifically with benzodiazepines) should be considered when an agent is selected.

If oral pharmacotherapy options for ET are not beneficial, intramuscular injections of botulinum toxin A or surgical treatments can be used in selected patients. Targeted botulinum toxin A injections can reduce hand, head, and voice tremor; however, they are associated with focal weakness of the adjacent areas. Injections in the wrist can cause hand weakness, and dysphagia; hoarseness and breathiness can occur with injections into the neck or vocal cords.[198] Treatment should occur with the lowest dose and the interval should be as long as possible between injections. Deep brain stimulation of the ventral intermediate nucleus of the thalamus or unilateral thalamotomy is highly efficacious in reducing ET.[198] Greater improvement in self-reported measures of function and fewer adverse events make DBS the preferred surgical option of the two.[196,210]

Because K.H. is otherwise healthy, she is a good candidate for propranolol therapy. Propranolol can be initiated as needed or on a scheduled basis depending on the degree of impairment and desire of the patient. If the decision is made with K.H. to use propranolol on an as-needed basis, she should begin with one-half of a 20-mg tablet administered 30 minutes to 1 hour before the desired effect. The dose can be increased from one-half to two tablets. An example of a situation where this may occur is if she wants to avoid embarrassment with attending a social activity or before certain tasks requiring manual dexterity at work. Given the degree of her impairment, she is probably a better candidate for chronic suppressive therapy with propranolol. In this situation, she can be prescribed 10 mg twice daily and titrated every few days up to 120 to 360 mg/day in divided doses.

REFERENCES

1. Rao G et al. Does this patient have Parkinson disease? *JAMA* 2003;289:347.
2. Hoehn MM et al. Parkinsonism: onset, progression, and mortality. *Neurology* 1967;17:427.
3. Barbosa ER et al. Parkinson's disease. *Psychiatr Clin North Am* 1997;20:769.
4. de Rijk MC et al. Prevalence of Parkinson's disease in the elderly: the Rotterdam Study. *Neurology* 1995;45:2143.
5. Wooten GF et al. Are men at greater risk for Parkinson's disease than women? *J Neurol Neurosurg Psychiatry* 2004;75:637.
6. Fall PA et al. Survival time, mortality, and cause of death in elderly patients with Parkinson's disease: a 9-year follow-up. *Mov Disord* 2003;18:1312.
7. Hoehn MM. The natural history of Parkinson's disease in the pre-levodopa and post-levodopa eras. *Neurol Clin* 1992;10:331.
8. Suchowersky O et al. Practice parameter: diagnosis and prognosis of new-onset Parkinson disease (an evidence-based review). Report of the Quality Standards Subcommittee of the American Academy of Neurology. *Neurology* 2006;66:968.
9. Duvoisin R. History of parkinsonism. *Pharmacol Ther* 1987;32:1.
10. Ballard PA et al. Permanent human parkinsonism due to 1-methyl-4-phenyl- 1,2,3,6-tetrahydropyridine (MPTP): seven cases. *Neurology* 1985;35:949.
11. Polymeropoulos MH et al. Mutation in the α-synuclein gene identified in families with Parkinson's disease. *Science* 1997;276:2045.
12. Nutt JG et al. Diagnosis and initial management of Parkinson's disease. *N Engl J Med* 2005;353:1021.
13. Olanow CW et al. An algorithm (decision tree) for the management of Parkinson's disease: treatment guidelines. *Neurology* 2001;56(Suppl 5):S1.
14. Suchowersky O et al. Practice parameter: neuroprotective strategies and alternative therapies for Parkinson disease (an evidence-based review). Report of the Quality Standards Subcommittee of the American Academy of Neurology. *Neurology* 2006;66:976.
15. Miyasaki JM et al. Practice parameter: evaluation and treatment of depression, psychosis, and dementia in Parkinson's disease (an evidence-based review). Report of the Quality Standards Subcommittee of the American Academy of Neurology. *Neurology* 2006;66:996.
16. Goetz CG et al. Mortality and hallucinations in nursing home patients with advanced Parkinson's disease. *Neurology* 1995;45:669.
17. Lees AJ et al. Ten-year follow-up of three different initial treatments in de novo PD: a randomized trial. *Neurology* 2001;57:1687.
18. Rascol O et al. A five-year study of the incidence of dyskinesia in patients with early Parkinson's disease who were treated with ropinirole or levodopa. *N Engl J Med* 2000;342:1484.
19. Holloway RG et al. Pramipexole vs levodopa as initial treatment for Parkinson's disease: a 4-year randomized controlled trial. *Arch Neurol* 2004;61:1044.
20. Parkinson Study Group. Pramipexole vs. levodopa as initial treatment for Parkinson disease: a randomized controlled trial. *JAMA* 2000;284:1931.
21. Miyasaki JM et al. Practice parameter: initiation of treatment for Parkinson's disease: an evidence-based review. Report of the Quality Standards Subcommittee of the American Academy of Neurology. *Neurology* 2002;58:11.
22. Piercy MF et al. Functional roles for dopamine-receptor subtypes. *Clin Neuropharmacol* 1995;18:34.
23. Uitti RJ et al. Comparative review of dopamine receptor agonists in Parkinson's disease. *Drugs* 1996;5:369.
24. Schade R et al. Dopamine agonists and the risk of cardiac-valve regurgitation. *N Engl J Med* 2007;356:29.
25. Zanettini R et al. Valvular heart disease and the use of dopamine agonists for Parkinson's disease. *N Engl J Med* 2007;356:39.
26. Dooley M et al. Pramipexole. A review of its use in the management of early and advanced Parkinson's disease. *Drugs Aging* 1998;6:495.
27. Hubble JP et al. Pramipexole in patients with early Parkinson's disease. *Clin Neuropharmacol* 1995;18:338.
28. Parkinson Study Group. Safety and efficacy of pramipexole in early Parkinson's disease. A randomized dose-ranging study. *JAMA* 1997;278:125.
29. Shannon KM et al. Efficacy of pramipexole, a novel dopamine agonist, as monotherapy in mild to moderate Parkinson's disease. The Pramipexole Study Group. *Neurology* 1997;49:724.
30. Molho ES et al. The use of pramipexole, a novel dopamine agonist, in advanced Parkinson's disease. *J Neural Transm* 1995;45(Suppl):225.
31. Lieberman A et al. Clinical evaluation of pramipexole in advanced Parkinson's disease: results of a double-blind, placebo-controlled, parallel-group study. *Neurology* 1997;49:162.
32. Fahn S et al. Unified Parkinson's Disease Rating Scale. In: Fahn S et al., eds. *Recent Developments in Parkinson's Disease. Vol. II*. Florham Park: Macmillan Health Care Information; 1987:153.
33. Tulloch IF. Pharmacologic profile of ropinirole: a nonergoline dopamine agonist. *Neurology* 1997;49(Suppl 1):S58.
34. Bloomer JC et al. In vitro identification of the P450 enzymes responsible for the metabolism of ropinirole. *Drug Metab Disp* 1997;25:840.
35. Rascol O et al. Ropinirole in the treatment of early Parkinson's disease: a 6-month interim report of a 5-year levodopa-controlled study. *Move Disord* 1998;13:39.
36. Adler CH et al. Ropinirole for the treatment of early Parkinson's disease. *Neurology* 1997;49:393.
37. Korczyn AD et al. Ropinirole versus bromocriptine in the treatment of early Parkinson's disease: a 6-month interim report of a 3-year study. *Move Disord* 1998;13:46.
38. Watts RL. The role of dopamine agonists in early Parkinson's disease. *Neurology* 1997;49(Suppl 1):S2.

39. Mirapex package insert. Ridgefield, CT: Boehringer Ingelheim Pharmaceuticals, Inc.; November 2006.
40. Schrag AE et al. The safety of ropinirole, a selective nonergoline dopamine agonist, in patients with Parkinson's disease. *Clin Neuropharmacol* 1998;21:169.
41. Stern MB. Contemporary approaches to the pharmacotherapeutic management of Parkinson's disease: an overview. *Neurology* 1998;49(Suppl 1):S2.
42. Lieberman A et al. A multicenter trial of ropinirole as adjunct treatment for Parkinson's disease. *Neurology* 1998;51:1057.
43. Frucht S et al. Falling asleep at the wheel: motor vehicle mishaps in persons taking pramipexole and ropinirole. *Neurology* 1999;52:1908.
44. Boehringer Ingelheim Pharmaceuticals. Dear Health Care Professional advisory letter, September 21, 1999.
45. Dodd ML et al. Pathological gambling caused by drugs used to treat Parkinson disease. *Arch Neurol* 2005;62:1377.
46. Driver-Dunckley E et al. Pathological gambling associated with dopamine agonist therapy in Parkinson's disease. *Neurology* 2003;61:422.
47. Weintraub D et al. Association of dopamine agonist use with impulse control disorders in Parkinson disease. *Arch Neurol* 2006;63:969.
48. Avanzi M et al. Prevalence of pathological gambling in patients with Parkinson's disease. *Mov Disord* 2006;21:2068.
49. Giovannoni G et al. Hedonistic homeostatic dysregulation in patients with Parkinson's disease on dopamine replacement therapies. *J Neurol Neurosurg Psychiatry* 2000;68:423.
50. Evans AH et al. Factors influencing susceptibility to compulsive dopaminergic drug use in Parkinson's disease. *Neurology* 2005;65:1570.
51. Reynolds NA et al. Rotigotine. In Parkinson's disease. *CNS Drugs* 2005;19:973.
52. The Parkinson Study Group. A controlled trial of rotigotine monotherapy in early Parkinson's disease. *Arch Neurol* 2003;60:1721.
53. Guidenpfennig WM et al. Safety, tolerability, and efficacy of continuous transdermal dopaminergic stimulation with rotigotine patch in early-stage idiopathic Parkinson's disease. *Clin Neuropharmacol* 2005;28:106.
54. Watts RL et al. Randomized, blind, controlled trial of transdermal rotigotine in early Parkinson disease. *Neurology* 2007;68:272.
55. Neupro package insert. Mequon, WI: Schwarz Pharma, LLC; July 2004.
56. LeWitt PA et al. Rotigotine transdermal system in treatment of patients with advanced-stage Parkinson's disease. *Eur J Neurol* 2005;12(Suppl. 2):15. Abstract.
57. Cotzias GC et al. Aromatic amino acids and modification of parkinsonism. *N Engl J Med* 1967;267:374.
58. Cotzias GC et al. Modification of parkinsonism—chronic treatment with L-dopa. *N Engl J Med* 1969;280:337.
59. Barbeau A. L-dopa therapy in Parkinson's disease. *Can Med Assoc J* 1969;101:791.
60. Parkes JD. Adverse effects of antiparkinsonian drugs. *Drugs* 1981;21:341.
61. Melamed E. Initiation of levodopa therapy in parkinsonian patients should be delayed until advanced stages of the disease. *Arch Neurol* 1986;43:402.
62. Olanow CW. An introduction to the free radical hypothesis in Parkinson's disease. *Ann Neurol* 1992;32:S2.
63. The Parkinson Study Group. Levodopa and the progression of Parkinson's disease. *N Engl J Med* 2004;351:2498.
64. McDowell F et al. Treatment of Parkinson syndrome with L-dihydroxyphenyl-alanine (levodopa). *Ann Intern Med* 1970;72:29.
65. Riley DE et al. The spectrum of levodopa-related fluctuations in Parkinson's disease. *Neurology* 1993;43:1459.
66. Papavasiliou PS et al. Levodopa in parkinsonism: potentiation of central effects with a peripheral inhibitor. *N Engl J Med* 1972;285:8.
67. Nutt JC et al. Pharmacokinetics of levodopa. *Clin Neuropharmacol* 1984;7:35.
68. Braco F et al. Protein redistribution diet and antiparkinsonian response to levodopa. *Eur Neurol* 1991;31:68.
69. Goodwin FK. Psychiatric side effects of levodopa in man. *JAMA* 1971;218:1915.
70. Koller WC et al. Levodopa therapy in Parkinson's disease. *Neurology* 1990;40(Suppl 3):S40.
71. Wooten GF. Progress in understanding the pathophysiology of treatment-related fluctuations in Parkinson's disease. *Ann Neurol* 1988;24:363.
72. Obeso JA et al. Complications with chronic levodopa therapy in Parkinson's disease. In: Olanow CW et al., eds. *Dopamine Agonists in Early Parkinson's Disease*. Kent: Wells Medical Limited; 1997:11.
73. Nutt JG et al. The response to levodopa in Parkinson's disease: imposing pharmacological law and order. *Ann Neurol* 1996;39:561.
74. Luquin MR et al. Levodopa-induced dyskinesias in Parkinson's disease: clinical and pharmacological classification. *Move Disord* 1992;7:117.
75. Nutt JG. Levodopa-induced dyskinesia: review, observations, and speculations. *Neurology* 1990; 40:340.
76. Harder S et al. Concentration—effect relationship of levodopa in patients with Parkinson's disease. *Clin Pharmacokinet* 1995;29:243.
77. Mouradian MM et al. Motor fluctuations and Parkinson's disease: pathogenetic and therapeutic studies. *Ann Neurol* 1987;22:475.
78. Mouradian MM et al. Motor fluctuations in Parkinson's disease: central pathophysiology mechanisms, Part II. *Ann Neurol* 1988;24:372.
79. Stocchi F et al. Motor fluctuations in levodopa treatment: clinical pharmacology. *Eur Neurol* 1996;36(Suppl 1):38.
80. LeWitt PA. Clinical studies with and pharmacokinetic considerations of sustained-release levodopa. *Neurology* 1992;42(Suppl 1):29.
81. Pahwa R et al. Practice parameter: treatment of Parkinson disease with motor fluctuations and dyskinesia (an evidence-based review). Report of the Quality Standards Subcommittee of the American Academy of Neurology. *Neurology* 2006; 66:983.
82. Kurth MC et al. Double-blind, placebo-controlled, crossover study of duodenal infusion of levodopa/carbidopa in Parkinson's disease patients with "on-off" fluctuations. *Neurology* 1993;43:1698.
83. Pappert E et al. Liquid levodopa/carbidopa produces significant improvement in motor function without dyskinesia exacerbation. *Neurology* 1996;47:1493.
84. Dewey RB et al. A randomized, double-blind, placebo-controlled trial of subcutaneously injected apomorphine for parkinsonian off-state events. *Arch Neurol* 2001;58:1385.
85. Bonifati V et al. New, selective catechol-O-methyltransferase inhibitors as therapeutic agents in Parkinson's disease. *Pharmacol Ther* 1999; 81:1.
86. Backstrom R et al. Synthesis of some novel potent and selective catechol-O-methyltransferase inhibitors. *J Med Chem* 1989;32:841.
87. De Santi C et al. Catechol-O-methyltransferase: variation in enzyme activity and inhibition by entacapone and tolcapone. *Eur J Pharmacol* 1998;54:215.
88. Keranen T et al. Inhibition of soluble catechol-O-methyltransferase and single-dose pharmacokinetics after oral and intravenous administration of entacapone. *Eur J Pharmacol* 1994;46:151.
89. Micek ST et al. Tolcapone: a novel approach to Parkinson's disease. *Am J Health Syst Pharm* 1999;56:2195.
90. Dingemanse J et al. Integrated pharmacokinetics and pharmacodynamics of the novel catechol-O-methyltransferase inhibitor tolcapone during first administration to humans. *Clin Pharmacol Ther* 1995;57:508.
91. Jorga KM et al. Effect of liver impairment on the pharmacokinetics of tolcapone and its metabolites. *Clin Pharmacol Ther* 1998;63:646.
92. Olanow CW. Tolcapone and hepatotoxic effects. Tasmar Advisory Panel. *Arch Neurol* 2000;57: 263.
93. Tasmar package insert. Aliso Viejo, CA: Valeant Pharmaceuticals Int.; December 2006.
94. Rinne UK et al. Entacapone enhances the response to levodopa in parkinsonian patients with motor fluctuations. *Neurology* 1998;51:1309.
95. Parkinson Study Group. Entacapone improves motor fluctuations in levodopa-treated Parkinson's disease patients. *Ann Neurol* 1997;42:747.
96. Larsen JP et al. The tolerability and efficacy of entacapone over 3 years in patients with Parkinson's disease. *Eur J Neurol* 2003;10:137.
97. Schrag A. Entacapone in the treatment of Parkinson's disease. *Lancet Neurol* 2005;4:366.
98. Tetrud JW et al. The effect of deprenyl (selegiline) on the natural history of Parkinson's disease. *Science* 1989;245:519.
99. Mahmood I. Clinical pharmacokinetics and pharmacodynamics of selegiline. An update. *Clin Pharmacokinet* 1997;33:91.
100. Seager H. Drug-delivery products and the Zydis fast-dissolving dosage form. *J Pharm Pharmacol* 1998;50:375.
101. Heikkila TE et al. Protection against the dopaminergic neurotoxicity of l-methyl-4-phenyl-1,2,5,6-tetrahydropyridine by monoamine oxidase inhibitors. *Nature* 1984;311:467.
102. Langston JW. MPTP: insights into the etiology of Parkinson's disease. *Eur Neurol* 1987;26(Suppl 1):2.
103. Snyder SH et al. MPTP: a neurotoxin relevant to the pathophysiology of Parkinson's disease. *Neurology* 1986;36:250.
104. Markey SP et al. Intraneuronal generation of a pyridinium metabolite may cause drug-induced parkinsonism. *Nature* 1984;311:464.
105. Parkinson Study Group. Effect of deprenyl on the progression of disability in early Parkinson's disease. *N Engl J Med* 1989;321:1364.
106. Parkinson Study Group. Impact of deprenyl and tocopherol treatment on Parkinson's disease in DATATOP subjects not requiring levodopa. *Ann Neurol* 1996;39:29.
107. Caraceni T et al. Levodopa or dopamine agonists, or deprenyl as initial treatment for Parkinson's disease. A randomized multicenter study. *Parkinsonism and Relat Disord* 2001;7:107.
108. Golbe LI. Deprenyl as symptomatic therapy in Parkinson's disease. *Clin Neuropharmacol* 1988; 11:387.
109. Elizam TS et al. Selegiline as an adjunct to conventional levodopa therapy in Parkinson's disease. *Arch Neurol* 1989;46:1280.
110. Shoulson I et al. Impact of sustained deprenyl (selegiline) in levodopa-treated Parkinson's disease: a randomized, placebo-controlled extension of the deprenyl and tocopherol antioxidative therapy of parkinsonism trial. *Ann Neurol* 2002;51:604.
111. Waters CH et al. Zydis selegiline reduces off time in Parkinson's disease patients with motor fluctuations: a 3-month, randomized, placebo-controlled study. *Mov Disord* 2004;19:426.
112. Goetz CG et al. Evidence-based medical review update: pharmacological and surgical treatments of Parkinson's disease: 2001 to 2004. *Mov Disord* 2005;20:523.
113. Youdim MB et al. Rasagiline [N-propargyl-1R(+)-aminoindan], a selective and potent inhibitor of mitochondrial monoamine oxidase B. *Br J Pharmacol* 2001;132:500.
114. Kupsch A et al. Monoamine oxidase-inhibition and MPTP-induced neurotoxicity in the non-human primate: comparison of rasagiline (TVP1012) with selegiline. *J Neural Transm* 2001;108:985.
115. deMarcaida JA et al. Effects of tyramine administration in Parkinson's disease patients treated with

selective MAO-B inhibitor rasagiline. *Mov Disord* 2006;21:1716.
116. Azilect package insert. Kansas City, MO: Teva Neuroscience, Inc.; May 2006.
117. Parkinson Study Group. A controlled trial of rasagiline in early Parkinson disease: the TEMPO study. *Arch Neurol* 2002;59:1937.
118. Parkinson Study Group. A controlled, randomized, delayed-start study of rasagiline in early Parkinson disease. *Arch Neurol* 2004;61:561.
119. Hauser RA et al. Early treatment with rasagiline is more beneficial than delayed treatment start in the long-term management of Parkinson's disease [Abstract]. *Mov Disord* 2005;20(Suppl 10):S75.
120. Parkinson Study Group. A randomized placebo-controlled trial of rasagiline in levodopa-treated patients with Parkinson disease and motor fluctuations: the PRESTO study. *Arch Neurol* 2005;62:241.
121. Rascol O et al. Rasagiline as an adjunct to levodopa in patients with Parkinson's disease and motor fluctuations (LARGO, Lasting effect in Adjunct therapy with Rasagiline Given Once daily, study): a randomised, double-blind, parallel-group trial. *Lancet* 2005;365:947.
122. Schwab RS et al. Amantadine in the treatment of Parkinson's disease. *JAMA* 1969;208:1168.
123. Schwab RS et al. Amantadine in Parkinson's disease. *JAMA* 1972;222:792.
124. Verhagen ML et al. Amantadine as treatment for dyskinesias and motor fluctuations in Parkinson's disease. *Neurology* 1998;50:1323.
125. Fahn S et al. Long-term evaluation of amantadine and levodopa combination in parkinsonism by double-blind crossover analyses. *Neurology* 1975;25:695.
126. Bailey EV et al. The mechanism of action of amantadine in parkinsonism: a review. *Arch Int Pharmacodyn Ther* 1975;216:246.
127. Greenamayre JT et al. *N*-methyl-D-aspartate antagonists in the treatment of Parkinson's disease. *Arch Neurol* 1991;48:977.
128. Metman LV et al. Amantadine for levodopa-induced dyskinesias: a 1-year follow-up study. *Arch Neurol* 1999;56:1383.
129. Snow BJ et al. The effect of amantadine on levodopa-induced dyskinesias in Parkinson's disease: a double-blind, placebo-controlled study. *Clin Neuropharmacol* 2000;23:82.
130. Thomas A et al. Duration of amantadine benefit on dyskinesia of severe Parkinson's disease. *J Neurol Neurosurg Psychiatry* 2004;75:141.
131. Aoki FY et al. Clinical pharmacokinetics of amantadine hydrochloride. *Clin Pharmacokinetics* 1988;14:35.
132. Kulisevsky J et al. Amantadine in Parkinson's disease. In: Koller WC et al., eds. *Therapy of Parkinson's Disease*. New York: Marcel Dekker; 1990:143.
133. Dexter D et al. Alpha-tocopherol levels in brain are not altered in Parkinson's disease. *Ann Neurol* 1992;32:591.
134. Parkinson Study Group. DATATOP: a multicenter controlled clinical trial in early Parkinson's disease. *Arch Neurol* 1989;46:1052.
135. Parkinson Study Group. Effects of tocopherol and deprenyl on the progression of disability in early Parkinson's disease. *N Engl J Med* 1993;328:176.
136. Shults CW et al. Coenzyme Q10 levels correlate with the activities of complexes I and II/III in mitochondria from parkinsonian and non-parkinsonian subjects. *Ann Neurol* 1997;42:261.
137. Weber CA et al. Antioxidants, supplements, and Parkinson's disease. *Ann Pharmacother* 2006;40:935.
138. Shults CW et al. Effects of coenzyme Q10 in early Parkinson's disease: evidence of slowing of the functional decline. *Arch Neurol* 2002;59:1541.
139. The NINDS NET-PD Investigators. A randomized clinical trial of coenzyme Q10 and GPI-1485 in early Parkinson disease. *Neurology* 2007;68:20.
140. Matthews RT et al. Creatine and cyclocreatine attenuate MPTP neurotoxicity. *Exp Neurol* 1999;157:142.
141. Tilley BC et al. Minocycline in rheumatoid arthritis. A 48-week, double-blind, placebo-controlled trial. MIRA Trial Group. *Ann Intern Med* 1995;122:81.
142. Du Y et al. Minocycline prevents nigrostriatal dopaminergic neurodegeneration in the MPTP model of Parkinson's disease. *Proc Natl Acad Sci U S A* 2001;98:14669.
143. The NINDS NET-PD Investigators. A randomized, double-blind, futility clinical trial of creatine and minocycline in early Parkinson disease. *Neurology* 2006;66:664.
144. Owen DAL et al. Effect of adrenergic beta-blockade on parkinsonian tremor. *Lancet* 1965;2:1259.
145. Lang AE et al. Posteroventral medial pallidotomy in advanced Parkinson's disease. *N Engl J Med* 1997;337:1036.
146. Jankovic J et al. Outcome after stereotactic thalamotomy for parkinsonian, essential and other types of tremor. *Neurosurgery* 1995;37:680.
147. Kelly PJ et al. The long-term results of stereotaxic surgery and l-dopa therapy in patients with Parkinson's disease. *J Neurosurg* 1980;53:332.
148. Olanow CW et al. Deep brain stimulation of the subthalamic nucleus for Parkinson's disease. *Move Disord* 1996;11:598.
149. Pollak P et al. New surgical treatment strategies. *Eur Neurol* 1996;36:396.
150. Krack P et al. Five-year follow-up of bilateral stimulation of the subthalamic nucleus in advanced Parkinson's disease. *N Engl J Med* 2003;349:1925.
151. Rodriguez-Oroz MC et al. Bilateral deep brain stimulation in Parkinson's disease: a multicentre study with 4 years follow-up. *Brain* 2005;128:2240.
152. Ahlskog JE. Cerebral transplantation for Parkinson's disease: current progress and future prospects. *Mayo Clin Proc* 1993;68:578.
153. Aarsland D et al. Donepezil for cognitive impairment in Parkinson's disease: a randomized controlled study. *J Neurol Neurosurg Psychiatry* 2002;72:708.
154. Bergman J et al. Successful use of donepezil for the treatment of psychotic symptoms in patients with Parkinson's disease. *Clin Neuropharmacol* 2002;25:107.
155. Fabbrini G et al. Donepezil in the treatment of hallucinations and delusions in Parkinson's disease. *Neurol Sci* 2002;23:41.
156. Emre M et al. Rivastigmine for dementia associated with Parkinson's disease. *N Engl J Med* 2004;351:2509.
157. Barone P et al. Pramipexole versus sertraline in the treatment of depression in Parkinson's disease. A national multicenter parallel-group randomized study. *J Neurol* 2006;253:601.
158. Weintraub D et al. Antidepressant studies in Parkinson's disease: a review and meta-analysis. *Mov Disord* 2005;20:1161.
159. Leentjens AFG. Depression in Parkinson's disease: conceptual issues and clinical challenges. *J Geriatr Psychiatry Neurol* 2004;17:120.
160. Leo RJ. Movement disorders associated with the serotonin selective reuptake inhibitors. *J Clin Psychol* 1996;57:449.
161. The Parkinson Study Group. Low-dose clozapine for the treatment of drug-induced psychosis in Parkinson's disease. *N Engl J Med* 1999;340:757.
162. Morgante L et al. Quetiapine versus clozapine: a preliminary report of comparative effects on dopaminergic psychosis in patients with Parkinson's disease. *Neurol Sci* 2002;23:S89.
163. Juncos JL, et al. Quetiapine improves psychotic symptoms and cognition in Parkinson's disease. *Mov Disord* 2004;19:29.
164. Fernandez HH et al. Quetiapine for the treatment of drug-induced psychosis in Parkinson's disease. *Mov Disord* 1999;14:484.
165. Wolters EC et al. Olanzapine in the treatment of dopaminomimetic psychosis in patients with Parkinson's disease. *Neurology* 1996;47:1085.
166. Goetz CG et al. Olanzapine and clozapine: comparative effects on motor function in hallucinating Parkinson's disease patients. *Neurology* 2000;55:789.
167. Rich SS et al. Risperidone versus clozapine in the treatment of psychosis in six patients with Parkinson's disease and other akinetic-rigid syndromes. *J Clin Psychol* 1995;56:556.
168. Hogl B et al. Restless legs syndrome: a community-based study of prevalence, severity, and risk factors. *Neurology* 2005;64:1920.
169. Allen RP et al. Restless legs syndrome: diagnostic criteria, special considerations, and epidemiology; a report from the restless legs syndrome diagnosis and epidemiology workshop at the National Institutes of Health. *Sleep Med* 2003;4:101.
170. Earley CJ. Restless legs syndrome. *N Engl J Med* 2003;348:2103.
171. Trenkwalder C et al. The restless legs syndrome. *Lancet Neurol* 2005;4:465.
172. Berger K et al. Sex and the risk of restless legs syndrome in the general population. *Arch Intern Med* 2004;164:196.
173. Gamaldo CE et al. Restless legs syndrome. A clinical update. *Chest* 2006;130:1596.
174. Montplaisir J et al. Clinical, polysomnographic, and genetic characteristics of restless legs syndrome: a study of 133 patients diagnosed with new standard criteria. *Mov Disord* 1997;12:61.
175. Kryger MH et al. Low body stores of iron and restless legs syndrome: a correctable cause of insomnia in adolescents and teenagers. *Sleep Med* 2002;3:127.
176. Earley CJ et al. The treatment of restless legs syndrome with intravenous iron dextran. *Sleep Med* 2004;5:231.
177. Hening WA et al. An update on the dopaminergic treatment of restless legs syndrome and periodic limb movement disorder. *Sleep* 2004;27:560.
178. Brodeur C et al. Treatment of restless legs syndrome and periodic movements during sleep with L-dopa: a double-blind, controlled study. *Neurology* 1988;38:1845.
179. Trenkwalder C et al. L-dopa therapy of uremic and idiopathic restless legs syndrome: a double-blind, crossover trial. *Sleep* 1995;18:681.
180. Schapira AHV. Restless legs syndrome. An update on treatment options. *Drugs* 2004;64:149.
181. Collado-Seidel V et al. A controlled study of additional SR-L-dopa in L-dopa responsive restless legs syndrome with late-night symptoms. *Neurology* 1999;52:285.
182. Saletu M et al. Acute double-blind, placebo-controlled sleep laboratory and clinical follow-up studies with a combination treatment of rr-L-dopa and sr-L-dopa in restless legs syndrome. *J Neural Transm* 2003;110:611.
183. Montplaisir J et al. Restless legs syndrome improved by pramipexole: a double-blind randomized trial. *Neurology* 1999;52:938.
184. Winkelman JW et al. Efficacy and safety of pramipexole in restless legs syndrome. *Neurology* 2006;67:1034.
185. Montplaisir J et al. Ropinirole is effective in the long-term management of restless legs syndrome: a randomized controlled trial. *Mov Disord* 2006;21:1627.
186. Trenkwalder C et al. Ropinirole in the treatment of restless legs syndrome: results from the TREAT RLS 1 study, a 12 week, randomised, placebo controlled study in 10 European countries. *J Neurol Neurosurg Psychiatry* 2004;75:92.
187. Walters AS et al. Ropinirole is effective in the treatment of restless legs syndrome: TREAT RLS 2: a 12-week, double-blind, randomized, parallel-group, placebo-controlled study. *Mov Disord* 2004;19:1414.
188. Garcia-Borreguero D et al. Treatment of restless legs syndrome with gabapentin: a double-blind, cross-over study. *Neurology* 2002;59:1573.
189. Happe S et al. Gabapentin versus ropinirole in the treatment of idiopathic restless legs syndrome. *Neuropsychobiology* 2003;48:82.

190. Louis ED. Essential tremor. *Clin Geriatr Med* 2006;22:843.
191. Benito-Leon J et al. Incidence of essential tremor in three elderly populations of central Spain. *Neurology* 2005;64:1721.
192. Louis ED et al. How common is the most common adult movement disorder?: Estimates of the prevalence of essential tremor throughout the world. *Mov Disord* 1998;13:5.
193. Louis ED et al. Elevation of blood beta-carboline alkaloids in essential tremor. *Neurology* 2002;59:1940.
194. Louis ED et al. Association between essential tremor and blood lead concentration. *Environ Health Perspect* 2003;111:1707.
195. Deuschl G et al. Consensus statement of the Movement Disorder Society on Tremor. *Mov Disord* 1998;13(Suppl 3):2.
196. Louis ED. Essential tremor. *N Engl J Med* 2001; 345:887.
197. Bain PG et al. A study of hereditary essential tremor. *Brain* 1994;117:805.
198. Zesiewicz TA et al. Practice parameter: therapies for essential tremor. Report of the Quality Standards Subcommittee of the American Academy of Neurology. *Neurology* 2005;64:2008.
199. Cleeves L et al. Propranolol and propranolol-LA in essential tremor: a double blind comparative study. *J Neurol Neurosurg Psychiatry* 1988;51: 379.
200. Dietrichson P et al. Effects of timolol and atenolol on benign essential tremor: placebo-controlled studies based on quantitative tremor recording. *J Neurol Neurosurg Psychiatry* 1981;44:677.
201. Jefferson D et al. Beta-adrenoceptor antagonists in essential tremor. *J Neurol Neurosurg Psychiatry* 1979;42:904.
202. Teravainen H et al. Comparison between the effects of pindolol and propranolol on essential tremor. *Neurology* 1977;27:439.
203. Gorman WP et al. A comparison of primidone, propranolol, and placebo in essential tremor, using quantitative analysis. *J Neurol Neurosurg Psychiatry* 1986;49:64.
204. Koller WC et al. Acute and chronic effects of propranolol and primidone in essential tremor. *Neurology* 1989;39:1587.
205. Sasso E et al. Double-blind comparison of primidone and phenobarbital in essential tremor. *Neurology* 1988;38:808.
206. Gironell A et al. A randomized placebo-controlled comparative trial of gabapentin and propranolol in essential tremor. *Arch Neurol* 1999;56: 475.
207. Connor GS. A double-blind placebo-controlled trial of topiramate treatment for essential tremor. *Neurology* 2002;59:132.
208. Huber SJ et al. Efficacy of alprazolam for essential tremor. *Neurology* 1988;38:241.
209. Biary N et al. Kinetic predominant essential tremor: successful treatment with clonazepam. *Neurology* 1987;37:471.
210. Schuurman PR et al. A comparison of continuous thalamic stimulation and thalamotomy for suppression of severe tremor. *N Engl J Med* 2000;342: 461.

CHAPTER 54

Seizure Disorders

James W. McAuley and Rex S. Lott

Incidence, Prevalence, and Epidemiology

Approximately 10% of the population will experience a seizure at some time. Up to 30% of all seizures are provoked by central nervous system (CNS) disorders or insults (e.g., meningitis, trauma, tumors, and exposure to toxins); these seizures may become recurrent and require chronic treatment with antiepileptic drugs (AED). Reversible conditions such as alcohol withdrawal, fever, and metabolic disturbances may provoke acute, isolated seizures. These seizures are not considered to be epilepsy and usually do not require long-term AED therapy. Approximately 1% of the general population has epilepsy.[1]

Terminology, Classification, and Diagnosis of Epilepsies

Classification of Seizures and Epilepsies

A seizure is the "clinical manifestation presumed to result from an abnormal and excessive discharge of a set of neurons in the brain. The clinical manifestation consists of sudden and

Table 54-1 International Classification of Epileptic Seizures

Partial Seizure (Local or Focal)
Simple Partial Seizures (Without Impairment of Consciousness)
Motor symptoms
Special sensory or somatosensory symptoms
Autonomic symptoms
Psychic symptoms
Complex[a] Partial Seizures (With Impairment of Consciousness)
Progressing to impairment of consciousness
With no other features
With features as in simple partial seizures
With automatisms
With impaired consciousness at onset
With no other features
With features as in simple partial seizures
With automatisms
Partial Seizures That Evolve to Generalized Seizures
Simple partial seizures evolving to generalized seizures
Complex partial seizures evolving to generalized seizures
Simple partial seizures evolving to complex partial seizures to generalized seizures
Generalized Seizures (Convulsive or Nonconvulsive)
Absence Seizures
Typical seizures (impaired consciousness only)
Atypical absence seizures
Myoclonic Seizures
Clonic Seizures
Tonic Seizures
Tonic-Clonic Seizures
Atonic (Astatic or Akinetic) Seizures
Unclassified Epileptic Seizures
All seizures that cannot be classified because of inadequate or incomplete data and some that cannot be classified in previously described categories

[a]Complex implies organized, high-level activity.
From references 1 and 3, with permission.

transitory abnormal phenomena that may include alterations of consciousness, motor, sensory, autonomic, or psychic events perceived by the patient or observer."[1] Epilepsy is a "condition characterized by recurrent (≥2) epileptic seizures, unprovoked by any immediate identified cause."[1] The current International Classification of Epileptic Seizures is shown in Table 54-1.[2,3] Older terms such as "grand mal" and "petit mal" should not be used, because their use may create confusion in the clinical setting. For example, it is common for patients or caregivers to identify any seizure other than a generalized tonic-clonic seizure as a "petit mal" seizure. This labeling may result in the selection of an inappropriate medication.

Generalized tonic-clonic (grand mal) seizures are common. The patient loses consciousness and falls at the onset. Simultaneously, tonic muscle spasms begin and may be accompanied by a cry that results from air being forced through the larynx. Bilateral, repetitive clonic movements follow. After the clonic phase, patients return to consciousness but remain lethargic and may be confused for varying periods of time (postictal state). Urinary incontinence and tongue biting is common. Primary generalized tonic-clonic seizures affect both cerebral hemispheres from the outset. Secondarily generalized tonic-clonic seizures begin as either simple or complex partial seizures. The aura described by some patients before a generalized tonic-clonic seizure actually represents an initial partial seizure that spreads to become a secondarily generalized seizure. Identification of secondarily generalized tonic-clonic seizures is important because some AED are more effective at controlling primary generalized seizures than secondarily generalized seizures, and partial seizures are often more difficult to control with AED.[4–6]

Absence (petit mal) seizures occur primarily in children and often remit during puberty; affected patients may develop a second type of seizure. Absence seizures consist of a brief loss of consciousness, usually lasting several seconds. Simple (typical) absence seizures are not accompanied by motor symptoms; automatisms, muscle twitching, myoclonic jerking, or autonomic manifestations may accompany atypical (complex) absence seizures. Although consciousness is lost, patients do not fall during absence seizures. Patients are unaware of their surroundings and will have no recall of events during the seizure. Consciousness returns immediately when the seizure ends, and postictal confusion is not seen. Differentiation of atypical absence seizures from complex partial seizures may be difficult if only a second-hand account of the episodes is available; identification of a focal abnormality by an electroencephalogram (EEG) often is necessary to identify complex partial seizures. This distinction is important for the proper selection of AED.

Simple partial (focal motor or sensory) seizures are localized in a single cerebral hemisphere or portion of a hemisphere. No loss of consciousness is experienced. Various motor, sensory, or psychic manifestations may occur depending on the area of the brain that is affected. A single part of the body may twitch, or the patient may experience only an unusual sensory experience.

Complex partial (psychomotor or temporal lobe) seizures result from the spread of focal discharges to involve a larger area. Consciousness is impaired and patients may exhibit complex but inappropriate behavior (automatisms) such as lip smacking, picking at clothing, or aimless wandering. A period of brief postictal lethargy or confusion is common.

Epileptic Syndromes

Epilepsy can be classified based on seizure type as shown in Table 54-1. Epilepsy syndromes can be defined on the basis of seizure type as well as cause (if known), precipitating factors, age of onset, characteristic EEG patterns, severity, chronicity, family history, and prognosis. Accurate diagnosis of epilepsy syndromes may better guide clinicians regarding the need for drug therapy, the choice of appropriate medication, and the likelihood of successful treatment.[1,4,5] Many epilepsy syndromes have been defined; a complete listing is beyond the scope of this chapter. Several are of interest with respect to pharmacotherapy and are described in (Table 54-2).[5]

Diagnosis

Optimal treatment of seizure disorders requires accurate classification (diagnosis) of seizure type and appropriate choice and use of medications. Seizure classification may be straightforward if an adequate history and description of the clinical

Table 54-2 Selected Epilepsy Syndromes

Syndrome	Seizure Patterns and Characteristics	Preferred Antiepileptic Drug (AED) Therapy	Comments
Juvenile myoclonic epilepsy	Myoclonic seizures often precede generalized tonic-clonic seizures. Myoclonic and generalized tonic-clonic episodes on awakening. Absence seizures also common. ↓ sleep, fatigue, and alcohol commonly precipitate seizures.	Valproate. Levetiracetam FDA-approved as adjunct for myoclonic seizures. Phenytoin possibly an adjunct to valproate in resistant cases. Carbamazepine reported to exacerbate seizures in some patients.	5% to 10% of all epilepsies; 85%–90% response to valproate. Lifelong therapy usually needed. High relapse rate with attempts to discontinue AED therapy.
Lennox-Gastaut syndrome	Generalized seizures: atypical absence, atonic/akinetic, myoclonic, and tonic most common. Abnormal interictal EEG with slow spike-wave pattern. Cognitive dysfunction and mental retardation. Status epilepticus common.	Valproate and benzodiazepines may be effective. Lamotrigine and topiramate FDA-approved. Felbamate also may be effective, but potential hematologic toxicity limits use. Poorly responsive to AED.	Oversedation with aggressive AED trials may ↑ seizure frequency. Tolerance to benzodiazepines limits their usefulness.
Childhood absence epilepsy (true petit mal)	Typical absences often in clusters of multiple seizures (pyknolepsy). Tonic-clonic seizures in ~40%. Onset usually between ages 4 and 8. Significant genetic component. EEG shows classic 3-Hz spike-wave pattern.	Ethosuximide or valproate. Lamotrigine probably effective.	80%–90% response rate to AED therapy. Good prognosis for remission. Tonic-clonic seizures may persist.
Reflex epilepsy	Tonic-clonic seizures most common. Induced by flicker or patterns (photosensitivity) most commonly. Reading also may precipitate partial seizures affecting the jaw, which may generalize. Some cases involve precipitation of underlying seizures; some seem primary.	AED specific to underlying seizures. Avoidance of precipitating stimuli when possible. Valproate usually effective for cases of spontaneous seizures precipitated by photosensitivity.	Relatively rare; seizures may be precipitated by television or video games.
Temporal lobe epilepsy	Complex partial seizures with automatisms. Simple partial seizures (auras) common; secondary generalized seizures occur in 50%.	Carbamazepine, phenytoin, valproate, gabapentin, lamotrigine, topiramate, tiagabine, levetiracetam, oxcarbazepine, zonisamide, pregabalin	Often incompletely controlled with current AED. Emotional stress may precipitate seizures; psychiatric disorders seen with temporal lobe epilepsy; surgical resection can be effective when patient is identified as a good surgical candidate.

EEG, electroencephalogram; FDA, U.S. Food and Drug Administration.
From references 5, 266–270, with permission.

seizure are available. Physicians often do not observe patients' seizures; thus, family members, teachers, nurses, and others who have frequent direct contact with patients should learn to observe accurately and objectively describe and record these events. The onset, duration, and characteristics of a seizure should be described as completely as possible. Several aspects of the events surrounding a seizure may be especially significant: the patient's behavior before the seizure (e.g., did the patient complain of feeling ill or describe an unusual sensation?), deviation of the eyes or head to one side or localization of convulsive activity to one portion of the body, impaired consciousness, loss of continence, and the patient's behavior after the seizure (e.g., was there any postictal confusion?). In addition, it is helpful if the observer can record the length of the event and how long it took for the patient to return to baseline. The patient and caregivers should have a seizure calendar or diary to record events. Those who observe a seizure should not try to label the seizure but should be encouraged to describe the event fully and objectively.

Accurate seizure diagnosis and identification of the type of epilepsy or epilepsy syndrome also depend on neurologic examination, medical history, and diagnostic techniques, such as EEG, computed tomography (CT), and magnetic resonance imaging (MRI). The EEG often is critical for identifying specific seizure types. CT scanning may help assess newly diagnosed patients, but MRI is preferred. MRI may locate brain lesions or anatomic defects that are missed by conventional radiographs or CT scans.[6]

Treatment

Early control of epileptic seizures is important because it allows normalization of patients' lives and prevents acute physical harm and long-term morbidity associated with recurrent seizures. In addition, early control of tonic-clonic seizures is associated with a reduced likelihood of seizure recurrence.[51] Early control of epileptic seizures also correlates with successful discontinuation of AED treatment after long-term seizure control.[7–9]

Nonpharmacologic Treatment of Epilepsy

Alternatives or adjuncts to pharmacotherapy may be helpful in some patients. Surgery is an extremely useful form of treatment in selected patients. Depending on the epilepsy syndrome and procedure performed, up to 90% of patients treated surgically may improve or become seizure free. A study of 80 patients with medically refractory temporal lobe epilepsy randomized to either surgery or continued medical treatment showed that after 1 year, patients were more likely to be seizure free after surgery.[10] Surgery is advocated as early therapy for some patients with specific epilepsy syndromes, such as mesial temporal sclerosis. Early surgical intervention may prevent or lessen neurologic deterioration and developmental delay.

Dietary modification may be used for patients who cannot tolerate AED or to treat seizures that are not completely responsive to AED. In most circumstances, dietary modification consists of a ketogenic diet. This low-carbohydrate, high-fat diet results in persistent ketosis, which is believed to play a major role in the therapeutic effect. Ketogenic diets are most commonly used and seem to be most beneficial in children; they are also used as adjuncts to ongoing AED treatment.[11,12]

The vagus nerve stimulator (VNS) is approved for treatment of intractable partial seizures. This device uses electrodes attached around the left branch of the vagus nerve. The electrodes are attached to a programmable stimulator that delivers stimuli on a regular cycling basis; patients can also use "on demand" stimulation at the onset of seizures by placing a magnet next to the subcutaneously implanted stimulator. Approximately 30% to 40% of patients who are so treated have a positive response (50% reduction in seizures).[13,14] The primary side effect of this device is hoarseness during stimulation; infrequently, this is accompanied by left vocal cord paralysis.

AVOIDANCE OF POTENTIAL SEIZURE PRECIPITANTS

It is impossible to generalize about environmental and lifestyle precipitants of seizure activity in persons with epilepsy. Individual patients or caregivers may identify specific circumstances, such as stress, sleep deprivation, or ingestion of excessive amounts of caffeine or alcohol, which can increase the likelihood of a seizure. Some women experience an increase in the frequency and severity of seizures around the time of menstruation or ovulation. Patients with epilepsy should avoid activities that seem to precipitate seizures; as always, the goal is complete seizure control with as little alteration in quality of life as possible.

Antiepileptic Drug Therapy

Pharmacotherapy is the mainstay of treatment for epilepsy. Therefore, patient education regarding medications and consultation among health care professionals regarding the optimal use of AED are essential to quality patient care. Optimal AED therapy completely controls seizures in 60% to 95% of patients.[4,15–17] Optimization of drug therapy depends on several factors; with the choice of appropriate AED, individualization of dosing, and adherence being the most important.

CHOICE OF ANTIEPILEPTIC DRUG

Many AED have a relatively narrow spectrum of efficacy; therefore, choice of appropriate drug therapy for a specific patient depends on an accurate diagnosis of epilepsy. In addition, toxicity must be considered when selecting an AED. Preferred drugs for specific types of seizures and common epileptic syndromes are listed in Tables 54-2 and 54-3. Although certain drugs are preferred, the identification of the most effective drug for a particular patient may be a process of trial and error; several medication trials may be necessary before success is achieved. The consensus method was used to analyze expert opinion on treatment of three epilepsy syndromes and status epilepticus.[18] The experts recommended monotherapy first, followed by a second monotherapy agent if the first failed. If the second monotherapy failed, the experts were not in agreement on whether to try a third monotherapy agent or to combine two therapies. The experts recommended epilepsy surgery evaluation after the third failed AED for patients with symptomatic localization-related epilepsies.

To assess the evidence on efficacy, tolerability, and safety of many of the new AED in treating children and adults with new-onset and refractory partial and generalized epilepsies, a panel evaluated the available evidence.[19,20] They concluded that the AED choice depends on seizure and syndrome type, patient age, concomitant medications, and AED tolerability, safety, and efficacy. The results of these two evidence-based assessments provide guidelines for the use of newer AED in patients with new-onset and refractory epilepsy.

THERAPEUTIC ENDPOINTS

The individual patient's response to AED treatment (i.e., seizure frequency and severity, and symptoms of toxicity) must be the major focus for therapy assessment. In general, the goal of AED treatment is administration of sufficient medication to completely prevent seizures without producing significant toxicity.[21] Realistically, this goal may be compromised for many patients; it may not be possible to completely prevent seizures without producing intolerable adverse effects. Thus, the therapeutic endpoints achieved can vary among patients; optimization of AED therapy for a specific person depends on tailoring therapy to the patient's needs and lifestyle. It is rarely optimal to administer "standard" or "usual" doses of an AED to a patient or to adjust doses to achieve a "therapeutic blood level" without paying consideration to the effect of the dose or serum concentration on the patient's condition and quality of life. As with many conditions requiring chronic drug therapy, patient participation in developing and evaluating a therapeutic plan is extremely important. Patients should be educated regarding the expected positive and negative effects of their AED therapy, and they must be encouraged to communicate with their health care provider regarding their responses to prescribed AED.

SERUM DRUG CONCENTRATIONS

Relation to Dosage

For some AED, although not all, a good correlation exists between serum concentrations and both therapeutic response and toxicity. For these agents, the wide availability of AED serum concentration determinations has had a significant impact on the treatment of seizure disorders. The correlation between the administered maintenance dose of an AED and the resulting steady-state serum concentration is poor. Administration of "usual therapeutic doses," even when calculated on the basis of body weight, is equally likely to produce subtherapeutic, therapeutic, or potentially intoxicating serum concentrations. Interindividual variation in hepatic metabolic capacity probably accounts for most of this variability.

Relation to Clinical Response

For selected AED, proper use and interpretation of serum concentrations are important for optimizing treatment regimens in

Table 54-3 Antiepileptic Drugs (AED) Useful for Various Seizure Types[a]

Primary Generalized Tonic-Clonic	*Secondarily Generalized Tonic-Clonic*	*Simple or Complex Partial*	*Absence*	*Myoclonic, Atonic/Akinetic*
Most Effective With Least Toxicity				
Valproate	Carbamazepine	Carbamazepine	Ethosuximide	Valproate
Phenytoin	Oxcarbazepine	Oxcarbazepine	Valproate	Clonazepam
Carbamazepine	Phenytoin	Phenytoin	Lamotrigine[b]	Lamotrigine[b]
(Lamotrigine)[b]	Valproate	Valproate		(Topiramate)[b]
(Levetiracetam)[b]	(Gabapentin)[b]	Lamotrigine		
(Oxcarbazepine)[b]	(Lamotrigine)[b]	(Gabapentin)[b]		
(Topiramate)[b]	(Topiramate)[b]	(Levetiracetam)[b]		
(Zonisamide)[b]	(Tiagabine)[b]	(Topiramate)[b]		
	(Zonisamide)[b]	(Tiagabine)[b]		
	(Levetiracetam)[b]	(Pregabalin)[b]		
	(Pregabalin)[b]	(Zonisamide)[b]		
Effective, But Often Cause Unacceptable Toxicity				
Phenobarbital	Phenobarbital	Clorazepate	Clonazepam	(Felbamate)[c]
Primidone	Primidone	Phenobarbital	Trimethadione	
(Felbamate)[c]	(Felbamate)[c]	Primidone		
		(Felbamate)[c]		
Of Little Value				
Ethosuximide	Ethosuximide	Ethosuximide	Phenytoin	
Trimethadione	Trimethadione	Trimethadione	Carbamazepine	
			Phenobarbital	
			Primidone	

[a] Drugs are listed in general order of preference within each category. Recommendations by various authorities may differ, especially regarding the relative place of valproate and the role of phenytoin as a first-line AED. Many authorities now discourage the use of phenobarbital and primidone.

[b] The place of gabapentin, lamotrigine, oxcarbazepine, levetiracetam, topiramate, tiagabine, and zonisamide is yet to be determined. They are placed on this table only to indicate the types of seizures for which they appear to be effective. Much more clinical experience is needed before their roles as possible primary AED are clarified.

[c] The place of felbamate is yet to be determined. It is placed on this table only to indicate the types of seizures for which it appears to be effective. Felbamate has been associated with aplastic anemia and hepatic failure; until a possible causative role is clarified, felbamate cannot be recommended for treatment of epilepsy unless all other, potentially less toxic treatment options have been exhausted.

From references 16, 53, 54, 271, with permission.

epilepsy.[14,22] An individual patient's clinical response to AED treatment must be the major focus for therapy assessment. Neither therapeutic effects nor toxic symptoms are "all or none"; in most situations, there are gradations of efficacy and toxicity. Dosage increases and titration to AED serum concentrations within and occasionally above the "therapeutic range" may significantly improve therapeutic responses without producing significant toxicity.[22] Individual patients often differ dramatically in their response to a particular serum drug concentration; therefore, therapeutic serum concentrations should be considered only as guidelines for treatment. Many patients condition may be controlled with serum drug concentrations below the usual therapeutic range.[23] In these patients, dosage adjustment to increase the serum drug concentration is not warranted. In this case, it is better to "treat the patient, not the level."

Interestingly, a recent Cochrane Review found no evidence to indicate that the use of measuring AED concentrations routinely to inform dose adjustments is superior to dose adjustments based on clinical information.[24] Only one study fit their evaluation criteria and that was done in patients newly diagnosed with epilepsy treated with a single older AED: carbamazepine, valproate, phenytoin, phenobarbital, or primidone. The authors do state that their review does not exclude the possibility that AED serum concentration might be useful in special situations or in selected patients.

Indications for Use

Measurement of serum drug concentrations may provide clinically useful information in the following situations:

- Uncontrolled seizures despite administration of greater-than-average doses: Serum concentrations of AED may help distinguish drug resistance from subtherapeutic drug concentrations caused by malabsorption, noncompliance, or rapid metabolism.
- Seizure recurrence in a patient whose seizures were previously controlled: This often is owing to noncompliance with the prescribed medication regimen.
- Documentation of intoxication: In patients who develop signs or symptoms of dose-related AED toxicity, documentation of the dose and serum concentration of the responsible drug is helpful.
- Assessment of patient compliance: Although monitoring AED serum concentrations can be used to assess patient

Table 54-4 Pharmacokinetic Properties of Antiepileptic Drugs

Drug	Oral Absorption (%)	Half-Life (hr)	Time to Steady State[a]	Dosage Schedule	Usual Therapeutic Serum Concentration	Plasma Protein Binding (%)	Volume of Distribution (L/kg)
Carbamazepine	90–100	*Chronic:* 5–25	2–4 day	BID to TID	5–12+ mcg/mL	75 (50–90)	0.8–1.6
Ethosuximide	90–100	*Pediatric:* 30 *Adult:* 60	5–10 day	QD (BID)	40–100 mcg/mL	0	0.7
Gabapentin	40–60; ↓ with ↑ dose	*Normal renal function:* 5–9; ↑ with ↓ renal function	*Normal renal function:* 1–1.5 day	TID to QID (every 6–8 hr)	>2 mcg/mL (proposed)	0	≈0.8
Lamotrigine	90–100	*Monotherapy:* 24–29 *Enzyme inducers:* 15 *Enzyme inhibitor (VPA):* 59	4–9 day	BID	4–18 mcg/mL (proposed)	55	0.9–1.2
Levetiracetam	100	*Normal renal function:* 6–8; ↑ with ↓ renal function	*Normal renal function:* 1–1.5 day	BID	Not determined	<10	≈0.7
Oxcarbazepine	100	8–13	2–3 day	BID to TID	Not determined	40	
Phenobarbital	90–100	2–4 day	8–16 day	QD	15–40 mcg/mL	50	0.5–0.6
Phenytoin	90–100	Varies with dose	5–30+ day	QD to BID	10–20 mcg/mL	95	0.5–0.7
Pregabalin	≥90	*Normal renal function:* 6; ↑ with ↓ renal function	24 hr	BID to TID	Not determined	0	0.5
Tiagabine	90	*Monotherapy:* 7–9 *Enzyme inducers:* 4–7	1–2 day	BID to QID	Not determined	96	1.1
Topiramate	≥80	12–24	3–4 day	BID	Not determined	10–15	0.7
Valproate	100	10–16	2–3 day	BID to QID	50–150+ mcg/mL	90+	0.09–0.17
Zonisamide	≈80	*Monotherapy:* ≈60 *Enzyme inducers:* 27–36	2 wk	QD to BID	Not determined	50–60	1.3

[a] Based on four half-lives. This lag time should allow determination of steady-state serum concentrations within limits of most assay sensitivities.
BID, twice daily, QD, every day; QID, four times daily; VPA, valproic acid.

compliance with therapy, conclusions must be based on comparisons with previous steady-state serum concentrations that reflected reliable intake of a given dose of AED.

- Documentation of desired results from a dose change or other therapeutic maneuver (e.g., administration of a loading dose): When patients are receiving multiple AED, serum concentrations of all drugs should be measured following a change in the dose of one drug because changes in the serum concentration of one drug frequently change the pharmacokinetic disposition of other drugs.
- When precise dosage changes are required: On occasion, small changes in the dose of a drug (e.g., phenytoin) can result in large changes in both the serum concentration and clinical response. In addition, cautious titration of dosage and serum concentration may be necessary to avoid intoxication. Knowledge of the serum drug concentration before the dosage change may allow the clinician to select a more appropriate new maintenance dose.

Frequent, "routine" determinations of serum AED concentrations are costly and not warranted for patients whose clinical status is stable. Clinicians may tend to focus attention on normal variability in serum concentrations rather than on the patient's clinical status; as a result, unnecessary dosage adjustments may be made to make serum concentrations fit the "normal range." A plan of action for what the clinician is going to do with the information once it is obtained should be in place before obtaining the sample. Therefore, the results of individual serum concentration determinations must be evaluated carefully to decide whether a significant, clinically meaningful change has occurred.[25]

Interpretation of Serum Concentrations

Several factors can alter the relationship between AED serum concentration and the patient's response to the drug. Whenever a change in serum concentration is apparent, pharmacokinetic factors (Table 54-4) should be considered (along with the patient's clinical status) before a decision is made to adjust the AED dosage. Laboratory variability can cause minor fluctuations in reported AED serum concentrations. Under the best conditions, reported values for serum concentrations may be within ±10% of "true" values.[26,27] Therefore, the magnitude of any apparent change must be considered. Therapeutic ranges are not well established for some drugs (e.g., valproate and the newer AED, such as lamotrigine, topiramate, and tiagabine). Published *therapeutic ranges* may have been determined in small numbers of patients or may more accurately represent *average serum concentrations* at *usual doses*. As an example, many clinicians agree that "pushing" valproate serum concentrations up to 150 to 200 mcg/mL may be beneficial for some patients; these higher concentrations are not consistently associated with specific toxicity symptoms.[28–31] Nevertheless, most laboratories report 50 to 100 g/mL as a therapeutic range for valproate. Inappropriate sample timing can result in inconsistent and clinically meaningless changes in AED serum concentrations.[14] Generally, serum concentrations of AED should not be measured until a minimum of four to five half-lives have elapsed since initiation of therapy or a dosage change. Blood samples should be obtained in the morning, before any doses of the AED have been taken; this practice provides reproducible, postabsorptive (i.e., "trough") serum concentrations. On occasion, especially for rapidly absorbed drugs with short half-lives (e.g., valproate), determination of peak serum concentrations may help assess possible toxic symptoms. Interindividual variability in response to a given serum concentration of medication is common. Excellent therapeutic response or even symptoms of intoxication may be associated with AED serum concentrations that are classified as "subtherapeutic."[32] Active metabolites of AED usually are not measured when serum concentrations are determined.[27,33] Alterations in the relative proportion of parent drug and active metabolite may result in an apparent alteration in the relationship between the serum concentration of the parent drug and the patient's response. Binding to serum proteins is significant for some AED (e.g., phenytoin, valproate, tiagabine). Changes in protein binding can result from drug interaction, renal failure, pregnancy, or changes in nutritional status. These changes can alter the usual relationship between the measured total drug concentration (bound and unbound to plasma proteins) and the unbound (pharmacologically active) drug concentration. This change may not be apparent when only total serum concentrations are measured. Determination of serum concentrations of free (i.e., unbound) AED is available from many commercial laboratories; these determinations are expensive and results may not be available for several days. If significant changes in protein binding are suspected, measurement of free concentrations of AED may provide additional information useful for adjustment of doses or interpretation of the patient's symptoms.[26,27,33]

MONOTHERAPY VERSUS POLYTHERAPY

Decades ago, seizure disorders were often treated with multiple AED (polytherapy). A second, third, or even fourth drug was added when seizures were incompletely controlled with a single AED. Evaluation of the effectiveness of polytherapy in recent years has shown little advantage for most patients. Use of a single drug at optimal tolerated serum concentrations produces excellent therapeutic results and minimal side effects in up to 80% of patients. Addition of a second AED significantly improves seizure control in only 10% to 20% of patients.[34,35] Reduction or elimination of existing polytherapy in patients with longstanding seizure disorders often lessens or eliminates cognitive impairment and other side effects: seizure control actually may improve.[34,36–39]

Most experts advocate the use of monotherapy (i.e., use of a single AED) whenever possible. Successful monotherapy may require higher-than-usual AED doses or serum concentrations above the upper limit of the usual therapeutic range.[16,40] Addition of a second drug may be necessary in some patients; however, polytherapy should be reserved for patients with multiple seizure types or for patients in whom first-line AED have failed to control seizures when titrated to maximal tolerated doses.[16,37] When a new AED is added to a patient's regimen with the goal of improving seizure control, the existing AED regimen should be scrutinized for continued value. In some cases, a patient's AED regimen can accumulate drugs that may be unnecessary because they were started and never re-evaluated. Continued vigilance and critical assessment of every drug in a patient's regimen is important.

Use of polytherapy creates several disadvantages that must be weighed against possible benefits. Seizure control may not significantly improve; in fact, these authors' experience and information from studies in which patients were converted from polytherapy to monotherapy indicate that even with use of an optimal AED, seizure control may be worsened in some patients by polytherapy regimens.[39] Patient expenses for medications and for increased laboratory monitoring may increase significantly with polytherapy. In addition, drug interactions among AED can complicate assessment of the patient's response and serum concentrations. Patient compliance often is worsened when multiple medications are prescribed, and adverse effects often increase because the side effects of many AED are additive.

Although AED monotherapy is preferred whenever feasible, the recent introduction of several new AED has increased the use of polytherapy.[40] Owing to limitations on the patient populations used for clinical trials of new drugs (i.e., patients with seizure disorders not completely controlled by previous medications), most new AED are labeled only for use as add-on therapy. Although reports exist on the efficacy of the new AED as monotherapy,[41–44] only lamotrigine, topiramate, oxcarbazepine, and felbamate are U.S. Food and Drug Administration (FDA) approved for monotherapy. Lamotrigine is indicated for conversion to monotherapy in adults with partial seizures who are receiving treatment with carbamazepine, phenytoin, phenobarbital, primidone, or valproate as the single AED.[45] Topiramate is approved as initial monotherapy in patients 10 years of age and older with partial-onset or primary generalized tonic-clonic seizures.[46] Felbamate should be considered (as monotherapy or polytherapy) only when other AED have failed. Other AED will undoubtedly follow with monotherapy indications. At present, data concerning the use of these new drugs as single agents are limited.

DURATION OF THERAPY AND DISCONTINUATION OF ANTIEPILEPTIC DRUGS

A diagnosis of epilepsy may not necessitate lifelong drug therapy. Several long-term studies have examined the prognosis of epilepsy following drug discontinuation; AED therapy may be successfully withdrawn from some patients after a seizure-free period of 2 to 5 years.[7–9] Seizures recurred in only 12% to 36% of patients who were followed for up to 23 years after AED withdrawal. Therefore, many patients whose epilepsy is completely controlled with medication can stop therapy after a seizure-free period of at least 2 years.

Discontinuation of medications is advantageous for economic, medical, and psychosocial reasons. Costs associated with physician visits, serum concentration determinations, and the medications themselves are eliminated. The risk of adverse effects from long-term medication use is eliminated, and patients can expect fewer lifestyle restrictions. Attempts to withdraw AED therapy are associated with risks, however: reappearance of seizure activity can result in status epilepticus, loss of driving privileges, employment difficulties, or physical injury.

Risk factors for seizure recurrence following discontinuation of AED have been identified in observational studies; complete agreement, however, is not found among studies regarding the nature and importance of specific risk factors. Opinions and data also differ regarding the optimal duration of the seizure-free period before discontinuation of AED is

Table 54-5 Risk Factors Possibly Predicting Seizure Recurrence Following AED Withdrawal

- <2 yr seizure free before withdrawal
- Onset of seizures after age 12
- History of atypical febrile seizures
- Family history of seizures
- >2–6 yr before seizures controlled
- Large number of seizures (>30) before control or total of >100 seizures
- Partial seizures (simple or complex)
- History of absence seizures
- Abnormal EEG persisting throughout treatment
- Slowing on EEG before medication withdrawal
- Organic neurologic disorder
- Moderate to severe mental retardation
- Withdrawal of valproate or phenytoin (higher rate of recurrence than withdrawal of other AED)

AED, antiepileptic drug; EEG, electroencephalogram.
From references 7–9, 47, and 48, with permission.

attempted. Nevertheless, at least some consensus has been reached regarding certain factors that may predict a higher risk of seizure recurrence (Table 54-5).[7–9,47,48]

In nonemergency situations, AED should be withdrawn slowly; if a patient receives multiple drugs, each drug should be withdrawn separately. Too-rapid withdrawal can result in status epilepticus. Clinical studies of AED discontinuation usually used a 2- to 3-month withdrawal schedule for each drug. The optimal rate of withdrawal of AED has not been identified. One study compared withdrawal of individual drugs over a 6-week and a 9-month period and found no difference in seizure recurrence between the groups.[49] Another study compared seizure frequencies in patients withdrawn from carbamazepine rapidly (over 4 days) and in patients withdrawn more slowly (over 10 days).[50] Significantly more generalized tonic-clonic seizures occurred when carbamazepine was withdrawn rapidly; complex partial seizures, however, did not occur at a higher rate with rapid withdrawal. Therefore, withdrawal of each AED over at least 6 weeks would seem to be a safe approach. Gradual withdrawal is recommended even for medications such as phenobarbital that have long half-lives and should theoretically be "self-tapering." In these authors' experience, gradual reduction of medications such as phenobarbital is associated with a significantly higher success rate. Appearance of seizures during medication withdrawal is not necessarily an indication for reinstitution of maintenance therapy; many patients who experience seizures during drug withdrawal remain seizure free after complete withdrawal.[51]

CLINICAL ASSESSMENT AND TREATMENT OF EPILEPSY

Complex Partial Seizures with Secondary Generalization

Diagnosis

1. A.R. is a 14-year-old, 40-kg, female high school student. A.R. had three febrile seizures when she was 3 years old. She received phenobarbital prophylaxis "off and on," according to her parents, for about 6 months following her second febrile seizure. Since then, she had no reported seizures until 24 hours before admission. At that time she had a "convulsion" shortly after arriving at school in the morning. A teacher who witnessed the episode describes her as behaving "oddly" before the seizure. She abruptly got up from her desk and began to walk clumsily toward the door; she bumped into several desks and did not respond to the teacher's attempts to redirect her back to her seat. After approximately 1 minute of this behavior, she fell to the floor and experienced an apparent generalized tonic-clonic seizure that lasted approximately 90 seconds. During the episode, she was incontinent of urine and was described as "turning kind of blue." Following this episode, A.R. was transported to the hospital.

On arrival at the hospital, A.R. appeared drowsy and confused. Laboratory studies—a complete blood count (CBC), serum glucose, electrolytes, drug and alcohol screen, and lumbar puncture—were normal. Physical examination and a complete neurologic evaluation were normal. An EEG showed diffuse slowing with focal epileptiform discharges in the left temporal area; it was interpreted as abnormal. There was no history of recent illness or injury, although A.R. had stayed up late several nights recently studying for an examination.

A second seizure occurs in the hospital. The nursing staff's description of the episode is similar to that provided by the observers at school. After recovery from each episode, A.R. has no memory of events during the seizures; she only remembers a "funny feeling" in her stomach and a "buzzing" in her head before she lost consciousness. She describes having these feelings "a couple of times" in the past; she attributed them to "just getting dizzy" and had not reported them to her parents. After these previous episodes, A.R. described feeling "mixed up" and groggy for a few minutes. What subjective and objective features of A.R.'s seizures are consistent with a diagnosis of complex partial seizures with secondary generalization?

A.R.'s clinical pattern of observed seizure activity (an apparent aura preceding her loss of consciousness), her history of apparent complex partial seizures not accompanied by generalized seizures, and the findings of focal abnormal activity on EEG are all concordant of this diagnosis. Postictal confusion and grogginess are also common after both generalized tonic-clonic and complex partial seizures. Her unusual or inappropriate behavior represents a complex partial seizure that subsequently generalized. The clinical features, accompanied by her EEG findings, also help rule out possible atypical absence seizures, which can be confused with complex partial epileptic syndromes based on only clinical presentation. In both syndromes, patients may briefly appear to lose contact with their surroundings and display automatisms and mild clonic movements during seizure activity. In A.R.'s case, the EEG and the generalized tonic-clonic seizures during her episodes would rule out atypical absence as a likely possibility.

Decision to Use Antiepileptic Drug Therapy

2. What factors should be considered in a decision to treat A.R.'s seizures with AED therapy?

Once a diagnosis of epilepsy is established, the decision to treat the patient with medication is based on the likelihood of recurrence. The need for AED therapy after a single seizure is controversial; however, recurrence of generalized tonic-clonic seizures is less likely if AED therapy is initiated after the first generalized tonic-clonic seizure.[52] Therefore, at least for this one specific seizure type, early use of AED is supported. Whether this information applies to other types of seizures is not known. Clinical wisdom, however, holds that "seizures beget seizures," and most experts advocate early treatment of epilepsy (i.e., after a first or second unprovoked seizure).

In A.R.'s case, the potential benefits of immediate introduction of AED therapy appear to outweigh potential risks. She experienced complex partial seizures followed by secondarily generalized tonic-clonic seizures. Recurrences of seizure activity are likely to result in physical injury, social embarrassment, and interference with her participation in activities typical of a person her age. If her seizures are not controlled, she faces future limitation of her driving privileges and may face barriers to employment. Although AED therapy is associated with risks, they probably are outweighed by the potential benefits.

Choice of Antiepileptic Drug

3. Discuss the AED commonly used for A.R.'s seizure type. Based on the subjective and objective data available, recommend a first-choice AED for A.R. and a plan for initial dosing of this medication.

Many AED would be appropriate choices for A.R.'s complex partial seizures that can secondarily generalize (Table 54-3).[35,53,54] Some AED are not FDA approved as initial monotherapy. Though valproate (Depakene/Depakote) is effective for treating both generalized and complex partial seizures,[55] it would not be a good initial choice for this patient owing to the increased risks in a woman of childbearing age (see Women's Issues section below).

Felbamate (Felbatol), gabapentin (Neurontin), lamotrigine (Lamictal), topiramate (Topamax), tiagabine (Gabitril), levetiracetam (Keppra), oxcarbazepine (Trileptal), zonisamide (Zonegran), and pregablin (Lyrica) are effective for control of partial seizures with or without secondary generalization. Most experience with these drugs was obtained when they were used as adjunctive agents when previous AED therapies were unsuccessful. Initial clinical trials with these newer medications indicate that several of them may be useful as single agents. As mentioned previously, lamotrigine, oxcarbazepine, and topiramate have monotherapy indications. Most of these more recent medications appear to be safe and are usually well tolerated. The usefulness of felbamate is, however, limited owing to its potential for serious hematologic and hepatic toxicity.

Carbamazepine has several advantages that make it a preferred first-choice agent in the opinion of many clinicians. In comparison with phenytoin, carbamazepine is less sedating and is not associated with dysmorphic effects, such as hirsutism, acne, gingival hyperplasia, and coarsening of facial features. Carbamazepine's pharmacokinetic profile also makes dosage adjustment easier. In A.R.'s case, the lack of cosmetic side effects may be especially significant because she may be taking medication for many years. In addition, reduced sedation may be important with respect to her school performance.

Carbamazepine Therapy

INITIATION AND DOSAGE

Initiation of treatment with full therapeutic maintenance doses of carbamazepine often causes excessive side effects such as nausea, vomiting, diplopia, and significant sedation. Therefore, carbamazepine therapy should be initiated gradually and patients should be allowed time to acclimate to the effects of the drug. Final dosing requirements are difficult to anticipate in individual patients. A reasonable starting dosage of carbamazepine for A.R. would be 100 mg twice a day; her dosage could be increased by 100 to 200 mg/day every 7 to 14 days. The rapidity of increases will depend on A.R.'s tolerance for the drug and the frequency of seizures.

HEMATOLOGIC TOXICITY

4. Carbamazepine has been associated with hematologic and hepatic toxicities. What is the incidence and significance of these toxicities? How should A.R. be monitored for them?

Aplastic anemia and agranulocytosis have occurred in association with carbamazepine therapy.[56] Several cases have been fatal; however, most cases occurred in older patients treated for trigeminal neuralgia. Many patients were receiving other medications, and occasionally the reports were incomplete; thus, assessment of a causal role for carbamazepine is difficult.[57] Severe blood dyscrasias from carbamazepine seem rare (estimated prevalence of <1/50,000) and have predominantly occurred in nonepileptic patients. The lack of severe hematologic toxicity in various published series and clinical trials in patients with epilepsy has been notable.[58,59]

Leukopenia is relatively common in patients taking carbamazepine. It is usually mild and often reverses despite continued administration of the drug.[58] Total leukocyte counts may fall to <4,000 cells/mm^3 in some patients, but differentials and platelet and erythrocyte counts remain normal. Symptoms (e.g., fever, sore throat) that might suggest early stages of agranulocytosis do not occur. Carbamazepine-associated hematologic disorders occur independent of drug dosage; thus, these reactions appear to be idiosyncratic.

Routine Hematologic Testing

Laboratory monitoring of A.R.'s hematologic status is recommended during carbamazepine therapy. The likelihood of early detection of aplastic anemia or agranulocytosis through frequent blood counts is low, however, and such monitoring is costly.[58,60] Because hematologic toxicity from carbamazepine primarily occurs early in therapy, CBC can be obtained before therapy and at monthly intervals during the first 2 to 3 months of therapy; thereafter, a yearly or every-other-year CBC, white blood cell (WBC) count with differential, and platelet count should be sufficient.

HEPATOTOXICITY

Carbamazepine-related liver damage appears to be extremely rare despite its being frequently mentioned as a potential problem and strong warnings are in the package insert.[61,62] Hepatic adverse reactions are believed to be idiosyncratic or immunologically based. Aggressive laboratory monitoring of liver function tests (LFT) probably is unnecessary.[60] Alkaline phosphatase and γ-glutamyl-transferase (GGT) concentrations often are elevated in patients taking carbamazepine (and other AED). This is believed to result from hepatic enzyme induction and is not necessarily evidence for hepatic disease.[63]

In summary, hepatic and hematologic toxicities of carbamazepine are rare. Although potentially serious, they are best monitored on clinical grounds rather than by ongoing, intensive laboratory testing. Patients, families, or caregivers should be aware that the appearance of unusual symptoms (e.g., jaundice, abdominal pain, excessive bruising and bleeding, or sudden onset of severe sore throat with fever) should be reported to a health care professional. Baseline (pretreatment) determination of A.R.'s hepatic and hematologic status, possibly with monthly follow-up testing for 2 to 3 months, probably will be sufficient.[59,60] Thereafter, a CBC and a liver function battery should probably be evaluated only every 1 to 2 years, unless signs or symptoms of hepatic or hematologic disorders are observed.

PHARMACOKINETICS AND AUTOINDUCTION OF METABOLISM

5. Over the following 6 weeks, A.R.'s carbamazepine dosage was gradually increased to 400 mg twice daily (BID) (20 mg/kg/day). Until the last dose increase, she had been experiencing one or two complex partial seizures weekly; she had had only one generalized tonic-clonic seizure since her hospitalization. One week following the increase to 20 mg/kg/day, her serum carbamazepine concentration was 9 mcg/mL just before her first dose of the day. No seizures occurred for 4 weeks, and she tolerated the medication well. Subsequent to the 4-week seizure-free period, she again began experiencing one seizure weekly. What factor(s) might be responsible for this reversal of seizure control?

Several factors may account for this change. It is important always to consider the possibility of poor medication adherence when clinical response changes unexpectedly. This should be investigated, and A.R. and her family should be educated regarding the importance of regular medication intake if necessary.

The observed changes in A.R.'s seizure control may also be owing to unique features of carbamazepine pharmacokinetics. Carbamazepine is a potent inducer of hepatic cytochrome P450 (CYP3A4). The drug is also a substrate for this enzyme. As a result, carbamazepine not only stimulates the metabolism of other CYP3A4 substrates but also induces its own metabolism by autoinduction. Carbamazepine's half-life following single acute doses is approximately 35 hours; with chronic dosing, its half-life decreases to 15 to 25 hours. This induction of metabolism may be enhanced by combined administration of carbamazepine and other enzyme-inducing AED; with polytherapy, carbamazepine's half-life may be as short as 6 to 10 hours.[27] This increase in clearance necessitates increased doses, increased frequency, or both of carbamazepine administration. Autoinduction of carbamazepine metabolism appears to be related to dose and serum concentration. Approximately 1 month may be required for the autoinduction process to reach completion after each increase in carbamazepine dose.[64]

Assuming that adherence was not the main problem, A.R.'s carbamazepine dose should be increased. The drug's pharmacokinetics are generally linear with respect to acute dosage changes.[65] A 50% increase in dosage to 1,200 mg/day should re-establish seizure control. Depending on A.R.'s clinical status, further increases in dosage may be necessary.

BIOEQUIVALENCE OF GENERIC DOSAGE FORMS AND EFFECTS OF STORAGE ON BIOEQUIVALENCE

6. A.R.'s dosage was increased to 600 mg BID. Four weeks later, she was still experiencing approximately one complex partial seizure weekly. A repeat trough serum carbamazepine concentration was 6.5 mcg/mL. On questioning, A.R. denied missing doses of medication, and a tablet count confirmed apparently accurate drug intake. A.R. relates that she experiences some mild nausea following her doses, but she has not vomited. It is noted that her pharmacist has begun substituting generic carbamazepine tablets for the Tegretol that was previously dispensed. What role, if any, might this change in carbamazepine tablet brand have played in the failure of A.R.'s serum concentrations to increase as expected? What other factors might be considered in explaining this situation?

Several manufacturers market generic carbamazepine tablets. Bioavailability data supplied by the manufacturers are based on single-dose or short multiple-dose studies in healthy subjects. Therefore, it is impossible to completely predict the results of a change from Tegretol to generic carbamazepine for maintenance therapy in an individual patient.[66] Because of variations in amount of drug available from different products, some patients with epilepsy cannot tolerate changes in formulations between brand to generic, generic to generic, or generic to brand.[67] Changes in seizure control from too little drug or toxicity from too much drug have been reported. Bioavailability data and the author's (R.L.) experience with institutionalized patients with severe seizure disorders suggest that the generic carbamazepine preparations currently on the market may be substituted for Tegretol with little need for dosage adjustment. In A.R.'s case, substitution of generic carbamazepine may be a possible cause for the loss of seizure control. Readjustment of her dose to gain seizure control and consistent use of one manufacturer's product might alleviate this problem.

Three extended-release forms of carbamazepine (Tegretol XR, Carbatrol and Equetro) available and may provide an alternative for A.R. These formulations allow more reliable absorption of drug when administered on a twice-daily dosing schedule. Many patients can better tolerate carbamazepine when these forms are used because large fluctuations in plasma concentrations are avoided. Use of Tegretol XR to avoid three-times-daily or four-times-daily dosing schedules has been shown to increase adherence for many patients.[68] It is important to counsel patients on the fact that the empty Oros tablet shell from the Tegretol XR dose does not dissolve as it passes through the gastrointestinal (GI) tract, and it may be visible in the stool. Patients need to understand that the carbamazepine has been absorbed, and that this is an empty shell. Tegretol XR tablets lose their extended-release properties when broken or crushed; Carbatrol beads may be emptied onto food or administered via feeding tube.[69] Equetro is not FDA approved for epilepsy, it is indicated for the treatment of acute manic and mixed episodes associated with bipolar I disorder.

In conclusion, it may be impossible to identify a single cause for the unexpected change in A.R.'s seizure control. Common reasons for loss of seizure control include sleep deprivation, increased stress, acute infection, and medication nonadherence.

Treatment Failure and Alternative Antiepileptic Drugs

7. R.H., a 19-year-old, 64-kg young woman, has experienced simple partial seizures, complex partial seizures, and secondarily generalized tonic-clonic seizures for the past 2 years. She could not tolerate treatment with phenytoin (severe gingival hyperplasia and mental "dullness") or valproate (hair loss, tremor, and a weight gain of 8 kg). In addition, neither phenytoin nor valproate

was dramatically effective in reducing her seizures. She currently receives carbamazepine 600 mg three times daily (TID). Over the past 3 months, while being treated with carbamazepine, she has had approximately five simple partial seizures, three complex partial seizures, and one generalized tonic-clonic seizure. This represents an approximate 30% reduction in her frequency of seizures. She tolerates her present dose of carbamazepine but has experienced significant drowsiness, incoordination, and mental confusion at higher doses. What are possible therapeutic options for R.H.? Evaluate the newer AED and their possible usefulness for R.H.

R.H. is exhibiting a partial response to maximally tolerated doses of carbamazepine. An alteration in her current AED regimen is indicated. She has not tolerated other AED because of side effects. Although valproate is effective for control of partial seizures, it is not considered an alternative in a woman of childbearing age. R.H.'s CNS side effects (e.g., persistent drowsiness) with other AED would make many clinicians reluctant to consider medications such as phenobarbital or primidone as either alternatives or adjunctive agents to her current carbamazepine regimen. Use of one of the newer AED as adjunctive medication may be of value for R.H.

Many new AED marketed in the United States since 1993 for maintenance treatment of epilepsy include the following: felbamate (Felbatol), gabapentin (Neurontin), lamotrigine (Lamictal), levetiracetam (Keppra), oxcarbazepine (Trileptal), topiramate (Topamax), tiagabine (Gabitril), zonisamide (Zonegran) and pregabalin (Lyrica) (Table 54-6).[70–81,82] Clinical trials for new AED are most often carried out in patients with partial seizures refractory to standard AED. Most of these newer or "second-generation" AED were initially FDA approved as "add-on" or adjunctive treatment in patients with partial seizures with or without secondary generalization. At the time of this writing, oxcarbazepine, felbamate, lamotrigine, and topiramate have FDA-approved monotherapy indications. Also, consensus is that some of these AED may be effective as broad-spectrum agents; for example, lamotrigine appears to be a useful treatment in absence seizures.

SIDE EFFECTS

Common side effects for the newer AED are described in Table 54-6. Most of the newer AED are less sedating than older medications such as phenobarbital or phenytoin. Felbamate causes insomnia and irritability in a significant proportion of treated patients. Other side effects that may be prominent during felbamate therapy include headaches, weight loss, and GI effects, such as nausea, vomiting, and anorexia. Felbamate's usefulness is seriously limited by its association with aplastic anemia and hepatic failure. Some cases of felbamate-associated aplastic anemia and hepatotoxicity were fatal. A conservative estimate of the occurrence rate is 1 case per 2,000 to 5,000 patients treated.[83] Too few cases of hepatic failure associated with felbamate therapy have been reported to allow conclusions to be drawn regarding characteristics of this potential adverse effect and risk factors for its development. Routine hematologic studies and LFT should be performed and patients and their families should be fully informed of the potential risks. Written consent is recommended. Patients must be educated about the symptoms of hematologic and hepatic toxicity. Because of the relationship between felbamate therapy and aplastic anemia and hepatic failure, the place of felbamate in the treatment of epilepsy is uncertain.

Topiramate can cause cognitive disturbances, lethargy, and impaired mental concentration when given in large daily doses (especially in combination with other AED) or when the dosage is titrated too aggressively.[84] Topiramate has caused nephrolithiasis in approximately 1.5% of treated patients. This adverse effect is believed to be related to inhibition of carbonic anhydrase by topiramate, with resulting increased urinary pH and decreased citrate excretion. Topiramate can also cause dose-related weight loss.

Gabapentin and tiagabine have not been associated with serious side effects; gabapentin has caused weight gain and tiagabine has caused nonspecific dizziness relatively frequently.[85,86]

Levetiracetam is generally well tolerated with the most common adverse events in clinical trials being asthenia, vertigo, flu-syndrome, headache, rhinitis, and somnolence. The most serious adverse effects are behavioral and are more common in patients with a history of behavioral problems.[87] Levetiracetam should be used with caution in patients with a history of suicidal ideations.

The most serious adverse effect associated with lamotrigine is skin rash. Rashes occur in approximately 10% of treated patients, usually in the first 8 weeks.[88] Rashes leading to hospitalization occurred in 1 of 300 adults and 1 of 100 children. Widespread, maculopapular rashes usually appear and may progress to erythema multiforme or toxic epidermal necrolysis. Lamotrigine-related rashes may resolve rapidly when lamotrigine is discontinued. Coadministration of valproate with lamotrigine may increase the likelihood of dermatologic reactions; it is partly for this reason that more conservative dosage titration and lower maintenance doses of lamotrigine are recommended for patients receiving concomitant valproate. Higher starting doses and more rapid dose escalation than those recommended by the manufacturer also increase the risk of skin rash.

Oxcarbazepine, a keto-derivative of carbamazepine, is essentially a prodrug for the monohydroxy active metabolite.[89] Oxcarbazepine probably causes less frequent, less severe adverse effects compared with carbamazepine, with the exception of hyponatremia. An exception is hyponatremia, which is more common with oxcarbazepine than with carbamazepine. Baseline and periodic serum sodium monitoring is indicated during oxcarbazepine therapy. The most commonly reported side effects of oxcarbazepine in clinical trials include ataxia, dizziness, fatigue, nausea, somnolence, and diplopia.

Zonisamide is a potent broad-spectrum AED.[90] Zonisamide is a sulfonamide derivative and thus is contraindicated in patients allergic to sulfonamides. The most commonly reported adverse events include ataxia, somnolence, agitation, and anorexia. Kidney stones have developed in 3% to 4% of patients, some of whom had a family history of nephrolithiasis.

Adverse effects of pregabalin are dose-dependent and usually occur within the first 2 weeks of treatment.[82] Somnolence, dizziness, and ataxia are most common. Pregabalin also appears to be associated with a dose-related weight gain. It should not be discontinued rapidly.

PHARMACOKINETICS

The newer AED have somewhat different pharmacokinetic profiles from those of older agents. They also differ in their

Table 54-6 Drugs Used for the Treatment of Partial and Generalized Tonic-Clonic Seizures

AED	Regimen	Adverse Effects	Comments
Carbamazepine (Tegretol, Tegretol XR, Carbatrol, Equetro)	Initial 200 mg BID (adults) or 100 mg BID (children) and weekly until therapeutic response or target serum concentrations. Usual maintenance doses 7–15 mg/kg/day in adults; 10–40 mg/kg/day in children.	Sedation, visual disturbance may limit dosage. Severe blood dyscrasias extremely rare. Mild leukopenia more common. Laboratory monitoring of little value. Hepatotoxicity rare. May cause SIADH. Long-term use may cause osteomalacia.	Usually little sedation and minimal interference with cognitive function or behavior. Preferred by most for partial or secondarily generalized seizures. Extended-release products may allow less frequent dosing with fewer peak serum concentration-related side effects. These products may also facilitate adherence.
Phenytoin (Dilantin, Phenytek)	Initiate at maintenance dose of 4–5 mg/kg/day (300–400 mg/day). Titrate on basis of clinical response and target serum concentration. 3–4 wk between dose ↑ recommended because of potentially slow accumulation.	Nystagmus, ataxia, sedation may limit dosage. Gum hyperplasia, hirsutism common. Long-term use may cause osteomalacia. Peripheral neuropathy, hypersensitivity with liver damage rare.	Clearance and half-life change with dose. Small ↑ in dose (30 mg capsule) recommended as dose reaches 300 or 400 mg/day. Cautious use of suspension; dose measurement and potential mixing difficulties. IM administration not recommended. Potential precipitation in IV solutions. Fosphenytoin (Cerebyx) recommended for IM and IV use. Due to faster administration rate, admixture compatibility and lower rate of injection site complications.
Valproate (Depakene, Depakote, Depakote-ER)	See Table 52-7.	—	—
Phenobarbital	Initial 1 mg/kg/day; titrate to therapeutic response. 2–3 wk between dose ↑	Sedation (chronic), behavior disturbances common, especially in children. Possibly impairs learning and intellectual performance. Long-term use may cause osteomalacia	Considered outmoded for AED therapy in most patients; adverse effects outweigh benefits. IV use for refractory status epilepticus.
Pregabalin (Lyrica)	Initial 50 mg BID then titrate to therapeutic response with maximal daily dose at 600 mg/day in BID or TID frequency	Potential side effects include dizziness, blurred vision and weight gain.	At the time of this writing, this is the most recently approved AED. Its place in therapy is emerging. No significant interactions with other AED. Can be useful for patients with concomitant pain disorders.
Gabapentin (Neurontin)	Initial 300 mg/day with titration to 900–1,800 mg/day over 1–2 wk. Up to 2,400 mg/day or higher may be needed for some patients. Owing to short half-life, TID or QID dosing recommended.	Sedation, dizziness, and ataxia relatively common with initiation of therapy. Gabapentin therapy usually not associated with prominent side effects.	Primarily excreted unchanged by kidneys. No significant interactions with other AED or other drugs identified to date. Absorption may be dose dependent; fraction absorbed ↓ as size of individual dose ↑
Lamotrigine (Lamictal)	*When added to enzyme inducers alone:* Initiate at 50 mg QD HS. May start at 50 mg BID. Daily dose can be ↑ by 50–100 mg Q 7–14 days. Usual maintenance doses of 400–500 mg/day. BID dosing may be necessary with enzyme inducer cotherapy. *When added to valproate alone:* Initiate at 25 mg QOD HS. Daily dose can be ↑ by 25 mg Q 14 days. Usual maintenance doses of 100–200 mg/day. *When added to valproate and enzyme inducers:* Initiate at 25 mg QOD HS. Daily dose can be ↑ by 25 mg Q 14 days. Usual daily doses of 100–200 mg/day.	Dizziness, diplopia, sedation, ataxia, and blurred vision can be common with initiation of therapy; limit speed of titration. Incidence of serious rash ranges from 0.8–8.0 per 1,000.	Significant ↑ in clearance of lamotrigine when coadministered with enzyme inducers. Significant ↓ in clearance when coadministered with valproate. Slow, gradual titration of dose may reduce risk of skin rash. Hormones can influence clearance.

(continued)

Table 54-6 Drugs Used for the Treatment of Partial and Generalized Tonic-Clonic Seizures *(Continued)*

AED	Regimen	Adverse Effects	Comments
Tiagabine (Gabitril)	Initial 4 mg/day. ↑ by 4 mg/day at 7 days. Then ↑ daily dose by 4–8 mg Q wk. Maximal recommended dose of 32 mg/day in adolescents or 56 mg/day in adults. BID to QID dosing recommended.	Drowsiness, nervousness, difficulty with concentration or attention, tremor. Nonspecific dizziness described by some patients.	Increased clearance when given with enzyme inducers. TID or QID doses probably needed. Potential for protein-binding displacement interactions with other highly protein bound drugs (e.g., valproate). Significance of protein-binding displacement not known. Substrate for CYP 3A.
Topiramate (Topamax)	Initial 50 mg HS. ↑ daily dose by 50 mg Q 7 days. 200–400 mg/day recommended as target dosage range. Larger daily doses associated with increased CNS side effects. BID dosing recommended.	Sedation, dizziness, difficulty concentrating, confusion. May be dose related. Possible weight loss. Weak carbonic anhydrase (CA) inhibitor; may cause or predispose to kidney stones; CA inhibition also possibly related to paresthesias in up to 15%.	Approximately 70% renal elimination. Phenytoin and carbamazepine may reduce topiramate plasma concentrations and potentially increase dosage requirements. Topiramate may cause small ↑ in phenytoin plasma concentration. Advise patients to drink plenty of fluids. May affect oral contraceptives above 200 mg/day.
Levetiracetam (Keppra)	Initial 250–500 mg BID. ↑ by 500–1,000 mg/day Q 2 wk. Usual maximal dose is 3,000 mg/day. Doses up to 4,000 mg/day have been used. BID dosing recommended.	Somnolence, dizziness, asthenia are commonly reported. Behavioral symptoms (agitation, emotional lability, hostility, depression, and depersonalization) reported.	No hepatic (CYP450 or UGT) metabolism. 66% excreted unchanged in urine. Less than 10% protein bound. No significant drug interactions reported.
Oxcarbazepine (Trileptal)	*Monotherapy:* Initial 300 mg BID. ↑ weekly up to 1,200 mg/day. Can go up to 2,400 mg/day. *Adjunctive therapy:* Initial 300 mg BID. ↑ weekly up to 1,200 mg/day.	Dizziness, somnolence, diplopia, nausea, and ataxia are commonly reported. Hyponatremia is described with the administration of this drug; most cases asymptomatic, more common in elderly. A 25% cross-sensitivity reported between oxcarbazepine and carbamazepine.	Parent is a prodrug; the monohydroxy derivative (MHD) is the active component. It is readily converted to MHD via omnipresent cytosolic enzymes. Lacks autoinduction properties. Many years of experience with this drug in Europe before U.S. approval. In doses above 1,200 mg/day, may affect oral contraceptives.
Zonisamide (Zonegran)	Initial 100 mg QD. ↑ by 100 mg/day Q 2 wks. General 200–400 mg/day; maximum 600 mg/day.	Somnolence, nausea, ataxia, dizziness, headache, and anorexia are common. Also reported are weight loss, and nephrolithiasis. Serious skin eruptions, oligohidrosis, and hyperthermia have also occurred.	Broad spectrum, long half-life. 35% of dose is excreted unchanged in the urine. Advise patients to drink plenty of fluids. Many years of experience with this drug in Korea and Japan before U.S. approval.

AED, antiepileptic drugs; BID, twice daily; CNS, central nervous system; GI, gastrointestinal; HS, at bedtime; PE, phenytoin sodium equivalent; QD, every day; QID, four times daily; QOD, every other day; SIADH, syndrome of inappropriate antidiuretic hormone secretion; TID, three times daily.

tendency to interact with other AED. Gabapentin is excreted entirely by the kidneys as unchanged drug and is not significantly bound to plasma protein. Gabapentin has a relatively short half-life and should be administered three times daily.[91]

Topiramate has a half-life of approximately 20 hours, which allows twice-daily administration. It is only partially excreted by hepatic metabolism; approximately 70% of the drug is excreted unchanged by the kidneys. Topiramate is minimally protein bound (~10%–15%). When topiramate is coadministered with enzyme-inducing agents, such as carbamazepine, hepatic metabolism is increased and topiramate clearance is increased. This interaction may necessitate titration to somewhat higher doses when topiramate is used with enzyme-inducing drugs. Inconsistently, topiramate can cause a small and often nonsignificant decrease in phenytoin plasma concentrations.

Tiagabine has a relatively short half-life (4–7 hours). It should be administered at least twice daily.[92] Concurrently administered enzyme-inducing AED may reduce tiagabine's half-life to 2 to 3 hours and necessitate use of larger daily doses and, possibly, more frequent dosing intervals. Tiagabine is highly protein bound (96%), and it is displaced from protein-binding sites by valproate, salicylate, and naproxen. The clinical significance of these protein-binding interactions is unknown.

Felbamate undergoes both hepatic metabolism and renal excretion as unchanged drug. Phenytoin and carbamazepine induce the hepatic metabolism of felbamate and lower steady-state felbamate concentrations.[70] Interactions between felbamate and other AED may make therapeutic monitoring difficult. Felbamate reduces the clearance of phenytoin, valproate, and probably phenobarbital; it also reduces the clearance of carbamazepine-10,11-epoxide (CBZ-E) while apparently increasing the conversion of carbamazepine to the epoxide metabolite.[93,94] Clinically, this latter effect may create a somewhat paradoxical situation: patients may experience symptoms of carbamazepine intoxication (including increased seizure activity)[95] with carbamazepine serum concentrations lower than those found before the addition of felbamate. CBZ-E serum concentrations are often elevated in these situations.

Lamotrigine is primarily eliminated by hepatic glucuronidation and excretion of metabolites in the urine. Other AED, such as carbamazepine and phenytoin, induce lamotrigine's hepatic metabolism. When lamotrigine is coadministered with enzyme-inducing drugs, its half-life decreases from approximately 24 hours to 15 hours. Valproate inhibits lamotrigine metabolism, causing increases in half-life and serum concentrations.[96,97] Patients treated with both lamotrigine and carbamazepine may experience more nausea, drowsiness, and ataxia. Although this interaction has been attributed to lamotrigine-induced increases in serum concentrations of CBZ-E in some patients,[98] lamotrigine does not consistently produce increases in this metabolite. It appears more likely that this interaction represents a pharmacodynamic interaction between lamotrigine and carbamazepine.[99]

Levetiracetam has a short half-life and is eliminated primarily by renal mechanisms. Dosage reductions are warranted for patients with renal impairment (creatinine clearance <80 mL/minute). The drug has a low potential for interactions with other drugs.[100]

Zonisamide has a long half-life and low protein binding. It is eliminated by both liver metabolism and renal excretion. The average half-life of zonisamide is 63 hours, but there is wide interpatient variation. Serum levels of zonisamide are reduced by enzyme-inducing AED.[90]

Oxcarbazepine is a prodrug that is converted to the monohydroxy derivative (MHD), its primary active metabolite. It may cause less hepatic enzyme induction than carbamazepine and may therefore be less likely to interact with other medications. Oxcarbazepine, however, does increase the metabolism of oral contraceptive hormones.[101] Because oxcarbazepine probably has a similar mechanism of action to that of carbamazepine, it is unlikely that it would offer significant benefits to R.H. because she has not responded to maximal tolerated doses of carbamazepine.[89]

Pregabalin is excreted entirely by the kidneys as unchanged drug and is not significantly bound to serum proteins. Unlike gabapentin, pregabalin can be administered two or three times daily.[82]

On the basis of efficacy and side effect characteristics, gabapentin, lamotrigine, topiramate, tiagabine, levetiracetam, zonisamide, or pregabalin could be considered for use as adjunctive therapy for R.H. In young, active patients such as R.H., sedation might prove to be a problem; however, it is not clear that any of these drugs predictably causes more initial or long-term sedation. The short half-lives of gabapentin and tiagabine and the associated need for R.H. to take several doses during the day might decrease her adherence. Therefore, topiramate, lamotrigine, levetiracetam, zonisamide, or pregabalin would be reasonable choices on the basis of convenience.

POTENTIAL THERAPIES

Other AED that may become available in the near future include brivaracetam, remacemide, rufinamide, fluorofelbamate, and harkoseride.[102] These drugs may become useful as alternatives or adjuncts to established and newer medications in the future.

With advancing technology and knowledge about genes and brain networks, future treatment strategies should move from controlling symptoms of epilepsy with AED to prevention and cure.[103] For AED-resistant epilepsy, much research is examining the role of multidrug transporters (e.g., P-glycoprotein) at the blood–brain barrier. These proteins may act as a defense mechanism by limiting the accumulation of AED in the brain.[104] Although it has not yet had an impact on the clinical care of patients with epilepsy, pharmacogenetics of AED therapy is continually advancing.[105]

Lamotrigine Therapy

INITIATION AND DOSAGE TITRATION

8. R.H. is to be started on lamotrigine as adjunctive therapy to her carbamazepine. Outline a treatment plan for initiating and monitoring therapy for R.H. What should R.H. and her family be told about this medication and how to use it?

Lamotrigine therapy should be initiated in R.H. with slow upward dosage titration to minimize early sedative effects and reduce the likelihood of skin rash. An initial dosage of 50 mg/day given at bedtime is recommended; the daily dose can be increased by 50 mg every 1 to 2 weeks. Because R.H. is currently receiving carbamazepine, induction of liver enzymes is likely to increase her dosage requirements for lamotrigine and allow a less conservative dosage titration. A twice-daily schedule is recommended for maintenance therapy. Usual maintenance dosages of lamotrigine are approximately 300 to 500 mg/day, although there is some experience with dosages of up to 700 mg/day. A patient's ability to tolerate this medication ultimately determines dosage limitations. Onset of side effects (e.g., nausea, diplopia, ataxia, and dizziness) may prevent further dosage increases. Lower initial dosages of lamotrigine (25 mg every other day) with more conservative increases (i.e., by 25 mg/day every 2 weeks) have been recommended for patients who also are receiving valproate. Valproate's inhibition of lamotrigine metabolism results in significantly lower lamotrigine dosage requirements; side effects appear to be much more common with lamotrigine doses >200 mg when it is administered with valproate.

R.H. should be told that she may feel drowsy and possibly experience headache and upset stomach, but that these side effects usually disappear with ongoing therapy. She should contact her physician or other health care professional if severe side effects occur that make it difficult to take the medication; this is especially important if she develops a skin rash.

SIDE EFFECTS AND POSSIBLE INTERACTION WITH CARBAMAZEPINE

9. Two days after her dosage of lamotrigine was increased to 300 mg/day (12 weeks after beginning therapy), R.H. noticed that her vision was blurring; she also complained of feeling dizzy and having difficulty maintaining her balance. Previously, she had experienced only mild, occasional nausea. She had continued to experience seizures at approximately the same frequency she had before the initiation of lamotrigine. Her physician had encouraged her to continue taking the medication and explained that it would take time to increase the dose to possibly effective levels. Her

current carbamazepine serum concentration is essentially unchanged when compared with when she was taking it in monotherapy. Do these new side effects represent treatment failure with lamotrigine? If not, how might these new side effects be managed?

R.H.'s seizure disorder may be unresponsive to lamotrigine therapy, and her side effects may limit further dosage increases. Her current side effects might represent carbamazepine intoxication, lamotrigine side effects, or an interaction between these two medications. Because R.H. tolerated the same carbamazepine dose previously, carbamazepine "intoxication" seems a less likely cause. Assessing the role of lamotrigine as a single agent is difficult. Obtaining a lamotrigine serum concentration to aid in assessing her adverse effects is not likely to be helpful. A usual "therapeutic range" for lamotrigine serum concentrations has not been established. Clinical studies have failed to demonstrate a significant correlation between lamotrigine serum concentrations and either therapeutic or adverse responses.[106,107] Her symptoms may also be related to an apparent pharmacodynamic interaction between lamotrigine and carbamazepine reported by some authors.[99] The effects experienced by some patients taking both drugs can be relieved by reducing the carbamazepine dosage. Subsequently, it may be possible to further increase her lamotrigine dosage to improve seizure control. This situation also should be assessed and possibly managed by empirically decreasing R.H.'s carbamazepine dosage by 200 to 400 mg/day and observing the effect on her current symptoms.

Levetiracetam Therapy

INITIATION AND DOSAGE TITRATION

10. R.H.'s carbamazepine dosage was reduced to 1,400 mg/day. After 5 days, her symptoms persisted and her seizure frequency appeared to be increasing. The clinician decides to abandon lamotrigine therapy and institute treatment with levetiracetam. Recommend a plan for initiating R.H.'s levetiracetam treatment.

R.H. previously tolerated and had a better therapeutic response to a higher carbamazepine dose. Therefore, the dosage of carbamazepine should be returned to 1,800 mg/day before levetiracetam therapy is initiated. Little specific information is available to help determine how lamotrigine can be safely discontinued. As a general rule, rapid discontinuation of AED is not recommended in other than emergency situations. Therefore, immediate reduction of R.H.'s lamotrigine dosage to 200 mg/day would seem reasonable. This dosage could then be reduced by 50 to 100 mg every week until lamotrigine was discontinued.

Levetiracetam treatment should be instituted immediately for R.H. because of her continuing seizures. Levetiracetam does not interact with other AED. Therefore, discontinuing lamotrigine during initiation of levetiracetam should not create difficulties in assessing R.H.'s response. Levetiracetam should be initiated at a dosage of 250 to 500 mg two times daily.[81,100] Although the manufacturer recommends initiating treatment at 500 mg twice daily, patients may better tolerate lower initial doses and more gradual titration.[100] R.H.'s daily levetiracetam dose can be increased by 500 to 1,000 mg every 2 or 3 weeks, according to her tolerance of side effects and her change in seizure frequency. Although the drug reaches steady state quickly, allowing at least 2 weeks for observation before dosage increases may improve patient tolerability and allow for a more thorough evaluation of therapeutic response. At present, the relationship between serum concentrations of levetiracetam and therapeutic response or symptoms of intoxication is not well defined. Therefore, R.H.'s dose should be titrated to the maximal tolerated amount required to control her seizures. There is limited published experience with levetiracetam dosages as high as 4,000 mg/day.

PATIENT EDUCATION

R.H. should be informed that with levetiracetam she may experience side effects similar to those she had with lamotrigine, but that they are less likely and should be temporary. Much reassurance and encouragement may need to be given along with this information to help ensure that R.H. adheres to her treatment regimen. Many patients become discouraged when multiple trials of medication are necessary and side effects are prominent. They may express feelings of being "guinea pigs" and may become uncooperative with the therapeutic plan.

Phenytoin Therapy

INITIATION AND DOSAGE

11. J.N., an 18-year-old, 88-kg male college student, was diagnosed with epilepsy. He experiences generalized tonic-clonic seizures that last 2 minutes approximately three times monthly. J.N. describes a "churning" feeling in his abdomen before his seizures; this is followed by involuntary right-sided jerking of his upper extremities, during which J.N. is awake and aware of his surroundings. His seizures have been observed and described well both by his family and by nursing staff who cared for him during a brief hospitalization following his first seizure. An EEG showed diffuse slowing with focal epileptiform discharges in the left temporal area; it was interpreted as abnormal. No correctable cause for his seizure disorder was identified despite a thorough workup. He has no other medical conditions and takes no routine medications. He was treated initially with carbamazepine up to 600 mg/day. He could not tolerate the medication because of nausea and diplopia despite relatively low doses. His physician has elected to implement a therapeutic trial of phenytoin for J.N. Recommend an initial dosage. What information should be provided to J.N. about his new medication?

Selecting a nontoxic, therapeutic dose of any AED is difficult without having information about the drug's disposition in the individual patient (i.e., prior dosages and clinical response). Although "average" dosages and resulting serum concentrations for phenytoin often are quoted, interpatient variability is significant. An initial phenytoin dosage of 400 mg/day would be appropriate for J.N. This represents a dosage of approximately 4.5 mg/kg/day. To avoid patient nonadherence because of transient side effects, J.N. could be instructed to take 100 mg in the morning and 100 mg 12 hours later for 1 week. The following week he could take 100 mg in the morning and 200 mg 12 hours later. If he can tolerate this regimen, he could then take 200 mg every 12 hours.

PATIENT EDUCATION

In addition to the name and strength of the medication and instructions for when and how it should be taken, J.N. should be informed that he may experience initial mild sedation from phenytoin. He should be cautioned that symptoms such as blurred or double vision, dysarthria ("thick" tongue), dizziness, or staggering may indicate that his dosage is too high; he should be instructed to notify his physician, pharmacist, or other health care professional of these symptoms. It is also a good idea to inform patients, at the beginning of therapy, that adjustments of medication dosage and possibly medication changes may be necessary before the medication regimen is stabilized.

ACCUMULATION PHARMACOKINETICS

12. What are the characteristics of phenytoin accumulation pharmacokinetics?

Phenytoin exhibits dose-dependent (Michaelis-Menten or capacity-limited) pharmacokinetics; therefore, the usual pharmacokinetic concepts of "clearance" and "half-life" are meaningless. The apparent half-life of phenytoin changes with the dose and serum concentration. Thus, the time required to reach a new steady state after dose alteration is difficult to predict because it depends on the dose itself and the patient's pharmacokinetic parameters, V_{max} and K_m.[108] V_{max} is a kinetic constant representing the maximal rate of phenytoin elimination from the body. K_m is the Michaelis constant, the serum concentration at which the rate of elimination is 50% of V_{max}. Values for these parameters vary widely among patients; as a result, patterns of phenytoin accumulation and the time required to achieve steady state also are variable.

Many clinicians assume that phenytoin's apparent half-life is approximately 24 hours, and they wait 5 to 7 days before assessing the patient's clinical response and measuring serum phenytoin concentrations. Both clinical studies[109] and model simulations[110] using observed values for K_m and V_{max} indicate that up to 30 days may be required for serum concentrations to reach 90% of the steady state resulting from a dosage of 4 mg/kg/day. Occasionally, such a dose may exceed a patient's V_{max}; the result is extremely high serum phenytoin concentrations, with probable intoxication. If doses sufficient to produce steady-state serum concentrations of 10 to 15 mcg/mL are given, 5 to 30 days may be required to achieve 90% of these concentrations.[108,111] It is important not assume that steady state has been reached unless widely spaced, serial serum concentrations indicate that accumulation has ceased. Alterations in phenytoin dosage before steady state has been reached can result in significant fluctuations in serum concentrations and the patient's clinical status. Such situations occur frequently and result in unnecessary confusion and expense. As always, serum concentrations in J.N. must be interpreted in the context of his clinical response.

ORAL LOADING DOSES

13. Would a loading dose be of value for J.N. to reduce the potential delay in achieving a "therapeutic" serum concentration of phenytoin? How large a loading dose should be used, and how should it be administered?

Administration of a loading dose would allow therapeutic serum concentrations of phenytoin to be achieved more rapidly, and more rapid control of J.N.'s seizure activity also would result. Because he is active and pursuing an education, more rapid seizure control may be a significant therapeutic goal. Studies of oral phenytoin loading indicate that doses of approximately 18 mg/kg will achieve serum concentrations approaching the usual therapeutic range after approximately 8 hours in most patients.[112,113] Oral loading doses appear to be better tolerated when administered in divided doses over 4 or more hours. GI upset appears to be the most common side effect related to this procedure. Cardiac side effects (e.g., sinus bradycardia, shortened PR intervals) have been observed rarely; they were not related to serum phenytoin concentrations, and their significance is uncertain.[110]

Oral phenytoin absorption after large doses is unpredictably slow, and it may be less complete than after smaller doses.[114] Although potentially therapeutic serum concentrations usually are seen after approximately 8 hours, peak concentrations may not occur for up to 60 hours after administration of large single doses.[108,110,114] Record et al.[115] estimated that 18 mg/kg given in three doses over 6 hours would produce serum concentrations of 13 to 20 mcg/mL 12 hours after completion of loading. No rigorous clinical evaluations of this recommendation are available, although these suggested doses compare well with intravenous (IV) loading regimens. IV loading doses of 18 mg/kg will maintain phenytoin serum concentrations >10 mcg/mL for 24 hours.[116]

Although administration of an oral loading dose to J.N. is pharmacokinetically sound and has certain therapeutic advantages, practical difficulties in monitoring an ambulatory patient for potential complications may indicate caution in recommending such a procedure. In addition, because J.N. had difficulty tolerating carbamazepine, it may be difficult to justify exposing him to the potential neurologic side effects of a phenytoin loading dose. A more practical approach with a lower risk of complications involves giving one and a half to two times the prescribed maintenance dose for the first 2 or 3 days of treatment. J.N. should be checked for dose-related adverse effects of phenytoin on the day after completion of such a "miniloading" and routinely thereafter.

PHENYTOIN INTOXICATION

14. J.N. was given phenytoin 200 mg AM and 400 mg PM for 3 days. No seizures had occurred, and J.N. experienced no side effects other than mild morning sedation. He was then instructed to take 200 mg every 12 hours. One week later, mild lateral gaze nystagmus was noted, but J.N. had no subjective complaints and remained seizure free. After 3 weeks, J.N. complained of double vision and feeling "drunk" and "unsteady." Significant nystagmus was present. How should J.N.'s phenytoin dosage be altered?

J.N.'s signs and symptoms indicate mild phenytoin intoxication. Dosage reduction is indicated. Reducing J.N.'s dosage to 360 or 330 mg/day would be reasonable. This dosage reduction can be accomplished using 30-mg phenytoin capsules along with the usual 100-mg capsules. A larger reduction may result in a loss of seizure control. Many clinicians also would have J.N. omit one day's dose of phenytoin before beginning the new maintenance dosage. This would accelerate the decline in phenytoin serum levels. Following this dosage change, clinical response should be monitored closely. The new maintenance dose may still be excessive; if J.N.'s V_{max} for phenytoin is low. If this were the case, continued accumulation of drug would occur despite the dosage reduction.[108]

INTRAMUSCULAR PHENYTOIN AND FOSPHENYTOIN (PHENYTOIN PRODRUG)

15. S.D. is a 24-year-old, male state hospital patient with a history of complex partial and secondarily generalized tonic-clonic

seizures. Within the past year, his phenytoin formulation was switched from Dilantin Kapseals to phenytoin suspension because S.D. was suspected of "cheeking" his medicines and not swallowing the capsules properly. He has had no seizures in the past 3 months on 275 mg/day of phenytoin suspension. S.D. has now been transferred to the acute medical unit following a 2-day history of anorexia, nausea, occasional vomiting, and abdominal pain accompanied by diarrhea. He is now "nothing per os" (NPO). Intramuscular (IM) fosphenytoin, 275 mg (phenytoin sodium equivalents [PE]) per day, has been ordered. Discuss the use of IM fosphenytoin, and devise a dosage regimen for S.D.

S.D. is a candidate for parenteral administration of his AED. If placement of an IV line for fluid administration is not planned, then IM administration is probably an acceptable approach to treatment. Previously, sodium phenytoin (Dilantin) injection was the only parenteral preparation available for replacement of oral phenytoin. Fosphenytoin sodium (Cerebyx) injection is available, and Dilantin injection has been discontinued. Preparations of sodium phenytoin injection are still available. IM administration of sodium phenytoin is not recommended. Injectable phenytoin is highly alkaline (pH 12) and extremely irritating to tissue. Following IM injection, the drug may precipitate at the injection site because of the change in pH. As a result, phenytoin crystals form a repository or depot from which the drug is slowly absorbed.[117–119] Often injection site discomfort is noted, although severe muscle damage does not seem to occur.[119]

Fosphenytoin, a phosphate ester prodrug of phenytoin, is highly water soluble. Its solubility allows this preparation to be administered parenterally without the need for solubilization using propylene glycol or the adjustment of pH to nonphysiologic levels. Therefore, fosphenytoin may be administered either IM or IV with less risk of tissue damage and venous irritation than with parenteral administration of phenytoin.[120–122] (See later discussion of IV administration of phenytoin and fosphenytoin.) After administration, the prodrug is rapidly absorbed and converted to phenytoin by phosphatase enzymes. Ultimately, the bioavailability of phenytoin from IM fosphenytoin administration is 100%.

Fosphenytoin is available as a solution containing 50 mg PE/mL, where PE equals phenytoin sodium equivalents. By labeling fosphenytoin this way, no dosing adjustments are necessary when converting from phenytoin sodium to fosphenytoin or vice versa. Although the prescriber ordered 275 mg PE, S.D. may be underdosed. His dosage of phenytoin suspension is providing the equivalent of 300 mg/day of sodium phenytoin. Phenytoin suspension and chewable tablets contain free acid, whereas capsules contain sodium phenytoin. Therefore, phenytoin capsule products contain only 92% of the labeled content as phenytoin acid (i.e., a 100-mg sodium phenytoin capsule contains only 92 mg of phenytoin acid). He should receive a 300-mg dose of fosphenytoin daily to fully replace his current dosage of phenytoin suspension.[122]

Assuming that S.D. will be given 300 mg PE of fosphenytoin daily, he will require a total of 6 mL of this injection given IM. This medication is well tolerated when it is given IM, and S.D.'s full daily dose can probably be given in a single injection site without causing excessive discomfort. Some clinicians report administering IM injections of fosphenytoin as large as 20 mL in a single site without adverse consequences or serious discomfort.[123] It is also possible to divide his daily dosage into two injections given in two different sites, although many patients prefer to receive fewer injections.

ADVERSE EFFECTS

16. M.N., a 10-year-old boy receiving 150 mg/day of phenytoin as chewable tablets, is to be fitted with orthodontic braces. He exhibits moderate gingival hyperplasia resulting in difficulty maintaining oral hygiene and halitosis. Discuss phenytoin-related gingival hyperplasia and management techniques that may be helpful for M.N.

Gingival Hyperplasia

Gum hyperplasia related to phenytoin is common and troublesome. Prevalence is estimated at up to 90%,[124] depending on the rating system used and the degree of gum change rated as hyperplastic. A realistic prevalence estimate is probably 40% to 50% of treated patients.[125] Prevalence and incidence rates, however, are misleading because the occurrence and severity of hyperplasia are related to the dose and serum concentration of phenytoin.[125,126] Gingival hyperplasia is of obvious cosmetic importance. Also, as in M.N., formation of pockets of tissue leads to difficulties with oral hygiene, and severe halitosis may result.

The mechanism of phenytoin-induced gingival hyperplasia is not well understood. The drug is excreted in saliva and saliva phenytoin concentrations and hyperplasia are correlated; however, this correlation may simply reflect higher serum concentrations producing a greater pharmacologic effect. Phenytoin may stimulate gingival mast cells to release heparin and other mediators. These mediators may encourage the synthesis of excessive amounts of new connective tissue by fibroblasts. Local irritation caused by dental plaque and food particles may further stimulate this process. Some patients may be predisposed to gum hyperplasia because they accumulate higher concentrations of phenytoin in gum tissue.[125,126]

The three approaches to the treatment of existing hyperplasia[126] are (a) dosage reduction or replacement of phenytoin with an alternative AED, if possible, will permit partial or complete reversal of hyperplasia; (b) surgical gingivectomy will correct the problem temporarily, but hyperplasia eventually recurs; and (c) oral physiotherapy (periodontal treatment) eliminates local irritants and maintains oral hygiene. Because M.N. is to be fitted with braces, oral hygiene will be further complicated. Some form of treatment for existing hyperplasia and prevention of further tissue enlargement is important. Assuming that phenytoin is producing adequate seizure control, a combination of gingivectomy and follow-up periodontal treatment may be the best approach.

Theoretically, the use of chewable phenytoin tablets in M.N. may aggravate hyperplasia. Exposure of the gingiva to high localized concentrations of phenytoin may result from braces holding tablet fragments in close physical contact with gum tissue. The significance of this relationship, however, is questionable. If M.N. can swallow capsules, a change to this dosage form may be beneficial and is usually less expensive. The most appropriate dosage of phenytoin sodium capsules for M.N. would be 160 mg/day. If chewable tablets are used, having M.N. rinse and swallow after each dose may eliminate problems. Use of phenytoin suspension also may be a useful option.

Drug particles, however, may still be retained by the braces, and maintenance of uniform dosage may be more difficult.

Oral hygiene programs appear to reduce the degree and severity of gingival hyperplasia when they are initiated before phenytoin therapy is started.[126] Patients who are beginning phenytoin therapy should be educated about the role of oral hygiene in diminishing this side effect. The use of dental floss, gum stimulators, and Water Pik-type appliances may be beneficial adjuncts to other oral hygiene techniques.

17. G.R. is a 53-year-old man with primary generalized epilepsy characterized by occasional tonic-clonic seizures. He was started on phenytoin when he was 25 years of age. His dosage of phenytoin was recently reduced from 400 mg/day to 360 mg/day because of symptoms of AED intoxication. Mild confusion, occasional diplopia, ataxia, and lateral gaze nystagmus were present at the 400 mg/day dose. After the dose was reduced to 360 mg/day, his confusion and diplopia decreased significantly. The neurologic evaluation at the lower dose was within normal limits. No seizures occurred during the following 8 weeks. He continued to complain of being mildly "unsteady" on his feet. Because G.R.'s seizures are apparently under complete control, is there any problem maintaining him on this dose of phenytoin?

Neurotoxicity

Patients chronically maintained on intoxicating doses of phenytoin appear to be at some risk for developing irreversible cerebellar damage or peripheral neuropathy. Cerebellar degeneration, resulting in symptoms such as dysarthria, ataxic gait, intention tremor, and muscular hypotonia, is of particular concern; this complication has been observed following episodes of acute phenytoin intoxication.[127,128] Generalized seizures also can cause cerebellar degeneration secondary to hypoxia. For this reason, the relative importance of phenytoin in the development of this condition is controversial. Nevertheless, cerebellar degeneration has been reported in several patients without hypoxic seizures.[128,129]

Symptomatic phenytoin-related peripheral neuropathy is rare, although electrophysiologic evidence of impaired neuronal conduction may be found in many patients.[127,130] Symptomatic patients may complain of paresthesias, muscle weakness, and occasional muscle wasting. Knee and ankle tendon reflexes are absent in 18% of patients on long-term phenytoin therapy; the upper limbs are affected rarely. Although areflexia may be irreversible,[131] electrophysiologic abnormalities may be closely related to excessive serum phenytoin concentrations and are reversible following dosage reduction or discontinuation.[129]

In G.R., the general discomfort of mild phenytoin intoxication and the potential for producing cerebellar degeneration necessitates a therapy alteration. The phenytoin dose should be reduced to 330 mg/day because it may produce adequate seizure control without toxic symptoms. Should seizures recur at this lower dosage, it may be advisable to consider an alternative AED.

ANTIEPILEPTIC DRUG IMPACT ON BONE

Some AED have a negative impact on bone density.[132] Although bone disorders are more common in women, the negative impact of AED on bone is not gender specific. Longer duration of AED therapy and exposure to multiple AED are thought to be predictors of bone loss. The enzyme-inducing AED (carbamazepine, phenytoin, and phenobarbital) have been associated with bone loss and an increased risk for fracture. Valproate, although not an enzyme inducer, is associated with decreased bone mineral density in children.[133] Less is known about the impact of the second-generation AED on bone mineral metabolism, although a recent report suggests lamotrigine has no effect.[134] Because of the length of phenytoin use, G.R. is at risk. His bone health should be further evaluated by his primary care physician. Minimally, oral calcium and vitamin D supplementation should be implemented. Depending on the outcome of evaluation, a therapy alteration from phenytoin to an AED with less or no effect on bone should be considered.

NEW ONSET SEIZURES IN THE ELDERLY

18. J.R., a 74-year-old man with newly diagnosed partial seizures, is referred to the neurology clinic for evaluation and treatment. The etiology of his new-onset seizures is presumed to be a recent cerebral infarct. His seizures are complex partial seizures where he "blacks out" and loses track of time. He has no history of secondarily generalized tonic-clonic convulsions. He has had three seizures in the last 4 weeks. His last seizure occurred 1 week ago, which resulted in a fall down a flight of stairs. His wife reports that he is more likely to have a seizure if he gets "overtired" or "stressed-out". He is also being treated for hypertension and diabetes. What options are available for the treatment of J.R.'s epilepsy?

In general, head-to-head comparative studies of AED are rare in patients with epilepsy. Even fewer studies address the comparative efficacy of AED in elderly patients. Two studies, in particular, are important when discussing AED treatment elderly persons with epilepsy.

Brodie et al.[135] compared lamotrigine (n = 102) with carbamazepine (n = 48) in elderly patients with newly diagnosed epilepsy via a double-blind, randomized, parallel study. Discontinuation rates because of adverse effects (the primary outcome parameter) were higher for carbamazepine (42%) than for lamotrigine (18%). Using time to first seizure as a measure of efficacy, no differences were found between the two AED, thus allowing the authors to suggest that lamotrigine is "acceptable" as initial treatment in elderly patients with newly diagnosed epilepsy.

More recently, in a randomized, parallel study, carbamazepine (600 mg/day), gabapentin (1,500 mg/day), and lamotrigine (150 mg/day) were compared for efficacy and tolerability in 593 patients >55 years of age (mean age = 72 years).[136] Although efficacy was similar in all three groups, study termination for adverse events varied between treatment groups. Carbamazepine had the highest termination rate (31%), followed by gabapentin (21.6%), and then lamotrigine (12.1%) ($p = 0.001$). The authors concluded that lamotrigine and gabapentin should be considered as initial therapy for new-onset seizures in older patients with epilepsy.

Evaluating the results from these two studies in elderly patients with epilepsy alone, it would suggest that either gabapentin or lamotrigine would be very good choices for initial treatment of J.R.'s epilepsy. It is noteworthy that neither AED is FDA approved for newly diagnosed epilepsy.

It is also important to consider drug-interaction profile, dosing frequency, and drug costs when selecting AED therapy. Generally, elderly persons take more medicines than younger individuals. For example, the average number of concomitant medications in the study by Rowan et al.[136] was seven. In J.R.'s case, he is likely to be taking other medicines for diabetes and hypertension. Neither gabapentin, nor lamotrigine cause drug–drug interactions, although lamotrigine is influenced more so than gabapentin by other medicines. When evaluating dosing frequency, gabapentin will probably have to be dosed more frequently than lamotrigine. From a cost perspective, gabapentin is currently available as a generic product; lamotrigine is soon to follow.

ADVERSE EFFECTS

Interestingly, in both of the comparative studies cited above, minimal differences were found in efficacy, but the newer AED showed better tolerability than the older AED. In general, elderly patients not only respond to AED at lower doses and concentrations, but they also develop toxicity symptoms at lower doses than do younger patients. Age-related declines in renal and hepatic function may account for those observations. The pharmacokinetics of most AED have been studied in the elderly and a decrease in clearance is noted as compared with the young.[137]

The impact of AED on cognition is an important issue for all patients with epilepsy and perhaps it is an even greater issue in elderly patients. Martin et al.,[138] evaluated cognitive functioning using a number of standardized measures in 25 older adults with epilepsy (>60 years of age) and compared them with healthy older adults (n = 27). The patients with epilepsy faired worse than their healthy counterparts, especially if they were receiving AED polytherapy. Piazzini et al.,[139] found very similar results in 40 patients >60 years of age compared with 40 controls. Additionally, Bambara et al.[140] reported that 20 older adults (>60 years) with epilepsy demonstrated deficits in their ability to provide informed consent for medical treatment. These authors expressed concern over their patients' medical decision-making abilities.

As evidenced from the study by Rowan et al.[136] mentioned above, CNS toxicities such as dizziness, unsteady gait, and ataxia are common adverse effects of AED. These symptoms may increase the risk of falls, which are of particular concern in light of the potential negative effects of AED on bone mineral density. In an effort to prospectively compare the impact of AED on balance, Fife et al.[141] reported their findings on three AED in patients with epilepsy >50 years of age. Ten patients each on monotherapy with carbamazepine, gabapentin, or lamotrigine underwent extensive testing in this cross-sectional study. The finding was that older epilepsy patients on lamotrigine monotherapy exhibited better scores on select measures of balance as compared with carbamazepine. Although not statistically significant, perhaps owing to a small sample size, gabapentin showed a trend toward better balance scores than carbamazepine.

J.R. and his family should be informed about the benefits and risks associated with each AED and they should also be incorporated into the decision-making. AED therapy in the elderly should follow the "start low and go slow" adage and elderly patients should be monitored for both efficacy (via a seizure calendar) and toxicity (reporting any intolerable side effects).

Absence Seizures

Choice of Medication and Initiation of Ethosuximide Therapy

19. T.D., a 7-year-old, 25-kg girl, is reported by her teacher to have three or four episodes of "staring" daily. Each spell lasts 5 to 10 seconds. Although no convulsive movements occur, her eyelids appear to flutter during the episodes. She is fully alert afterward. T.D.'s school performance is somewhat below average, despite an IQ of 125. An EEG shows 3/second spike-wave activity. Typical absence epilepsy is diagnosed. Physical examination and laboratory evaluation findings are normal, and no other positive findings are evident on the neurologic examination. What drug should be prescribed for T.D., and how should therapy with this drug be initiated?

Ethosuximide (Zarontin) and valproate are commonly used to treat absence epilepsy in the United States. Both drugs are equally effective. Lamotrigine is also effective and has been recommended as an initial monotherapy agent for treatment of absence epilepsy, although it is not FDA approved for this indication[17,142–144] (Tables 54-2 and 54-7). Valproate was more efficacious than lamotrigine for treatment of idiopathic generalized seizures (including absence) in the SANAD (Standard and New Antiepileptic Drugs) trial.[145] Trimethadione (Tridione), which is less effective than other agents, is associated with a high rate of neurologic side effects and a risk of hematologic toxicity.[146] At present, most authorities consider ethosuximide the drug of first choice for treatment of absence seizures. In comparison to ethosuximide, valproate is more likely to cause significant nausea and initial drowsiness, and it is more likely to interact with other AED. Valproate usually is reserved for patients whose absence seizures do not respond to ethosuximide.[147] Clonazepam (Klonopin), a benzodiazepine, often is effective for control of absence seizures. Therapy with this drug is limited by prominent CNS side effects (sedation, ataxia, and mood changes) and development of tolerance to its antiepileptic effect after long-term use.[148] Most authorities consider clonazepam a fourth-choice drug for treatment of absence seizures.

T.D. should be started on ethosuximide at a dosage of 15 to 20 mg/kg/day or 250 mg twice daily. The daily dose can be increased by 250 mg every 10 to 14 days as necessary to control seizures. Because the average half-life of ethosuximide in children is ~30 hours, a delay of 10 to 14 days between dosage increments allows ~7 days for achievement of steady state and 7 days for assessment of response.[27]

PATIENT OR CAREGIVER EDUCATION

Educating T.D. and her parents regarding the importance of regular drug administration is extremely helpful in ensuring successful therapy. Noncompliance is common in patients taking AED, and rapid discontinuation of these drugs (often secondary to noncompliance) may precipitate status epilepticus. The concept that medication controls rather than cures the seizure disorder should be strongly reinforced. It is also critical to inform both the parents and T.D. that a therapeutic response may not occur immediately and that dosage adjustments may

Table 54-7 Common Drugs for the Treatment of Absence Seizures

AED	*Regimen*	*Adverse Effects*	*Comments*
Valproate (Depakene, Depakote, Depakote ER)	Initial 5–10 mg/kg/day (sprinkle caps or syrup); then ↑ by 5–10 mg/kg/day weekly to therapeutic effect or target serum concentration. Manufacturer's recommended usual maximal dose of 60 mg/kg/day often must be exceeded clinically (especially for patients receiving enzyme-inducing AED) to achieve optimal clinical results. QD dosing recommended for extended-release (ER) product; doses should be 8%–20% higher than non-ER products.	GI upset, hair loss, appetite stimulation, and weight gain common. Tremor may occur. Serious hepatotoxicity extremely rare with monotherapy and in patients >2 yr.	Enteric-coated tablets or capsules or extended release tablets may ↓ GI toxicity. Time to peak serum concentrations delayed for 3–8 hr with enteric coating; longer delay if given with food; serum concentrations must be interpreted carefully. Also effective against primarily generalized tonic-clonic seizures.
Lamotrigine (Lamictal)	See Table 54-6		
Ethosuximide (Zarontin)	Initial 20 mg/kg/day or 250 mg QD or BID; then ↑ by 250 mg/day Q 2 wks to therapeutic effect or target serum concentration.	GI upset and sedation common with large single dose, especially on initiation. Daily divided doses may be necessary despite long half-life. Leukopenia (mild, transient) in up to 7%; serious hematologic toxicity extremely rare.	Parents/patient should be informed that GI effects and sedation may occur but tolerance usually develops. No good evidence it precipitates tonic-clonic seizures. Up to 50% of patients with absence may develop tonic-clonic seizures independent of ethosuximide.

AED, antiepileptic drug; BID, twice daily; GI, gastrointestinal; QD, every day.

be necessary to establish an effective dose with minimal side effects.

THERAPEUTIC MONITORING

20. What subjective or objective clinical data should be monitored in T.D. for evidence of ethosuximide's therapeutic and adverse effects?

T.D.'s seizure frequency and the side effects she experiences are the primary monitoring parameters. If ethosuximide serum concentrations are used to assist in dosing, 40 to 100 mcg/mL is the usual target range; however, a clearly defined toxicity syndrome does not seem to develop when ethosuximide serum concentrations exceed 100 mcg/mL. Gradual and cautious increases in ethosuximide dosage when serum concentrations are beyond the upper limits of the "usual therapeutic range" may improve response in resistant patients. Although ethosuximide traditionally is administered in divided doses, its long half-life allows successful use of single daily doses for many patients. Clinicians should be alert to acute side effects of nausea and vomiting that are associated with large single doses of ethosuximide; should these occur, divided daily doses may be necessary.[27]

Laboratory monitoring for idiosyncratic hematologic toxicity from ethosuximide often is recommended. Ethosuximide causes neutropenia in approximately 7% of patients. Although this reaction often is transient even if the drug is continued, rare patients may develop fatal pancytopenia. Presumably, early detection of neutropenia by means of periodic CBC will allow discontinuation of the drug and potential reversal of this adverse effect.[149] These hematologic reactions, however, can occur unpredictably at any time during therapy and often are missed by routine laboratory monitoring. Patient or caregiver education regarding signs and symptoms associated with leukopenia and pancytopenia (e.g., sudden onset of severe sore throat with oral lesions, easy bruisability, increased bleeding tendency) and instructions to consult the physician if these symptoms occur may be more important than laboratory monitoring.[60]

T.D.'s parents should be informed that nausea or sedation may occur with initiation of ethosuximide. Tolerance to these effects usually develops, although temporary dose reductions may be necessary. Subtle degrees of sedation may persist throughout therapy and may not be recognized until the drug has been discontinued and alertness improves.

Generalized Tonic-Clonic Seizures Accompanying Absence Seizures

21. Three months later, T.D.'s absence seizures have been reduced to a frequency of one every 2 weeks with an ethosuximide dosage of 750 mg/day. Her initial drowsiness has almost disappeared, and nausea was alleviated by administering doses with food. She has, however, experienced two tonic-clonic convulsions in the past month. Both seizures were witnessed by her parents and were well described: no auras or signs of focal seizure activity were apparent, and each episode lasted 3 to 4 minutes and apparently consisted of typical tonic-clonic activity. T.D. was incontinent of urine on both occasions, and postictal confusion and drowsiness were significant. Physical examination and laboratory testing showed no abnormalities. A repeat EEG continued to show infrequent 3/second spikes and waves; no abnormal focal discharges were noted. What is the relationship between T.D.'s tonic-clonic seizures and ethosuximide therapy?

It is commonly believed, and often stated in the literature, that ethosuximide may precipitate or worsen tonic-clonic seizures; however, this effect has not been clearly demonstrated. As many as 50% of patients who initially present with absence seizures also develop tonic-clonic seizures.[150] It had been common practice to add phenobarbital or phenytoin to ethosuximide therapy to prevent this. Livingston et al.[151] found that 80.5% of their patients treated with a drug specific for absence seizures developed "grand mal" seizures, whereas only 36% did so while receiving combined therapy. On the other hand, Browne et al.[150] pointed out that a child with absence seizures who has not yet had a tonic-clonic seizure has only a 25% chance of doing so in the future. In addition, routine use of drugs for prophylaxis of tonic-clonic seizures may increase the risk of toxicity and potentially reduce adherence with medication regimens. Sedative drugs, especially phenobarbital, actually may aggravate absence seizures in some patients.[152]

In summary, subsequent generalized tonic-clonic seizures are common in patients who initially develop absence spells. It is not possible to assess the causative role of ethosuximide for this development in T.D.

Assessment Regarding Need for Alteration in Antiepileptic Drug Therapy and Choice of Alternative Antiepileptic Drug

22. What alterations are indicated in T.D.'s drug therapy because of the appearance of generalized tonic-clonic seizures?

Drug therapy for prevention of further tonic-clonic seizures is indicated. Phenobarbital, phenytoin, carbamazepine, or valproate might be considered for use in T.D. Owing to her age and sex, many clinicians would avoid using phenytoin because of its dysmorphic and cosmetic side effects. Phenobarbital can cause sedation and behavioral disturbances (see below) and may aggravate coexisting absence seizures. Carbamazepine is widely used for secondarily generalized tonic-clonic seizures and some cases of primary tonic-clonic seizures in children. It lacks many of the troublesome, common side effects associated with phenobarbital and phenytoin. In young children with primary generalized tonic-clonic seizures, carbamazepine may be preferred over valproate because it is less likely to induce serious hepatotoxicity.[153] Carbamazepine, however, is not effective for control of absence seizures. Therefore, it is likely that both ethosuximide and carbamazepine would be needed by T.D. Carbamazepine also has been occasionally associated with exacerbation of seizures (including atonic, myoclonic, and absence seizures) in children with mixed seizure disorders who exhibit bilaterally synchronous 2.5- to 3-cycle/second discharges on the EEG.[154,155] The need for polytherapy and the possible risk of seizure exacerbation make carbamazepine a less attractive treatment option for T.D.

Valproate is effective for controlling both absence and primary generalized tonic-clonic seizures.[16,54] T.D. appears to have primary generalized tonic-clonic convulsions; focal signs (e.g., unilateral or single limb involvement) were not observed, and focal discharges (e.g., isolated abnormal electrical activity localized to one portion of the brain) were not found on the EEG. Although neither observation completely rules out secondarily generalized tonic-clonic seizures, the likelihood seems low. Therefore, valproate may offer some advantages over carbamazepine in terms of efficacy. In addition, both of T.D.'s seizure types potentially could be controlled with a single medication.

Valproate Therapy

INITIATION AND DOSAGE

23. T.D.'s physician elects to use valproate. The therapeutic goal is control of her seizures with valproate alone. What procedure should be followed regarding discontinuation of ethosuximide and initiation of valproate?

Techniques used by clinicians to substitute one AED for another depend largely on experience and judgment. Generally, it is best to attain a potentially therapeutic dose of a new medication before attempting to discontinue the previous drug. Serum concentration monitoring may be helpful. Ethosuximide has a relatively long half-life, whereas valproate's half-life is short. Therefore, if necessary, steady-state serum concentrations of valproate can be established and evaluated rapidly; evaluation of the effect of decreases in the ethosuximide dosage must await the prolonged elimination of this drug. Once a desired valproate dose or serum concentration has been achieved, the ethosuximide dosage can be reduced gradually by 250 mg/day every 2 to 4 weeks.

Valproate should be initiated at 125 to 250 mg twice daily. Valproic acid syrup or capsules or divalproex sodium (Depakote tablets or Depakote Sprinkle capsules) can be used. Divalproex often is preferred because it is enteric coated and may cause fewer GI side effects than valproic acid. Generic formulations of valproic acid capsules are available; they are often tolerated well and are inexpensive. Syrup forms of valproate probably should be avoided unless extremely small doses are required (e.g., infants) or patients cannot swallow. Valproate syrup has an unpleasant taste, and its rapid absorption increases the likelihood of acute, dose-related side effects such as nausea. Lower initial doses are less likely to cause acute side effects (e.g., drowsiness and GI upset). Weekly dosage increases of 5 to 10 mg/kg/day of valproate usually are well tolerated and would be appropriate for T.D. More rapid increases may be desirable if tonic-clonic seizures are occurring frequently. The maximal recommended dosage of valproate is 60 mg/kg/day. Many patients, especially those receiving enzyme-inducing drugs, require higher-than-recommended doses to achieve adequate clinical effect; other patients may respond at much lower doses. Valproate can be titrated in T.D. to produce a "target" serum concentration of approximately 75 mcg/mL. As ethosuximide is withdrawn, the valproate dose can be further adjusted on the basis of seizure frequency and side effects.

DOSAGE FORMS

24. T.D. has been taking valproic acid capsules, 250 mg TID, for 3 weeks. Ethosuximide was discontinued 2 weeks ago; at that time, a valproate serum level just before her morning dose was 68 mcg/mL. She has not experienced generalized tonic-clonic seizures for 6 weeks but continues to have an absence seizure every 2 to 3 weeks. T.D. complains of nausea, epigastric burning pain, and occasional vomiting lasting approximately 1 hour following her doses of valproate. All recent laboratory tests were within normal limits. Administration of the drug with meals is only partially helpful. What alterations can be made in T.D.'s dosing regimen to relieve these symptoms and possibly improve seizure control?

T.D. appears to be a candidate for the use of divalproex (Depakote), an enteric-coated preparation of a complex salt of valproic acid. Capsules containing enteric-coated beads of divalproex (Depakote Sprinkles 125 mg) also are available; the capsule contents can be dispersed in food for administration to children or others who have difficulty swallowing tablets or capsules. In addition, use of the "cap" end of the capsule to measure half of the contents can approximate doses of

62.5 mg. Patients with feeding tubes in place may be given opened Depakote Sprinkles through their feeding tubes; however, patients with certain types of feeding gastrostomies should be assessed frequently for possible leakage at the insertion point. This complication may occur because of adherence of undissolved medication beads to the exterior of the feeding tube. This complication seems more likely when the sprinkle formulation is administered through a *button-type* gastrostomy feeding tube; use of divalproex sprinkles should be avoided in such patients.[156] The beads contained in Depakote Sprinkles may also clog the lumen of smaller-bore feeding tubes.

Administration of divalproex tablets results in delayed rather than prolonged absorption of valproate; therefore, these tablets are not a sustained-release product formulation. When patients are switched from nonenteric-coated formulations to divalproex tablets, the frequency of administration should not be decreased. Divalproex sodium extended release (Depakote ER) is also available. This form of divalproex can be administered as a single daily dose. All older dosage forms of valproate are completely absorbed and can be interconverted at the same total daily dose of medication.[157,158] Depakote ER, however, is not bioequivalent to other dosage forms of valproate.[159] When equal doses are administered, Depakote ER achieves serum concentrations that are approximately 89% of those produced by other valproate dosage forms. Accordingly, when patients are converted to Depakote ER from other forms of valproate, the manufacturer recommends an increase of 8% to 20% in the administered dose. T.D.'s valproic acid capsules can be replaced with an equal daily dose of divalproex tablets. Divalproex should be administered on a three-times-daily dosing schedule. Alternatively, T.D. could be given 1,000 mg of Depakote ER once daily. The results of this change should be apparent within approximately 1 week. By that time, significant relief from GI side effects should have occurred. It may then be possible to increase the dose of divalproex in an effort to improve control of both absence and generalized tonic-clonic seizures.

PHARMACOKINETICS AND SERUM CONCENTRATION MONITORING

25. Two weeks later, T.D. returns for follow-up. Her GI symptoms have almost completely disappeared. She has been taking divalproex tablets 250 mg with breakfast and lunch and 375 mg with a bedtime snack for the past week. She has had no seizures in the past 2 weeks and complains of no side effects. A valproate serum level before her morning dose today was 117 mcg/mL (considerably higher than her previous valproate level of 68 mcg/mL). The laboratory reports that duplicate determinations of this level agreed within 5 mcg/mL. T.D. denies taking her medication incorrectly; her parents support this, and the tablet count in her prescription bottle is correct. She has taken no other drugs except a multivitamin. How can this disproportionate increase in her valproate serum concentration be explained, and what is its clinical significance? Does valproate exhibit dose-dependent pharmacokinetics?

Changes in valproate serum concentrations of this nature are, in this author's experience (R.L.), relatively common with divalproex. They are probably not the result of saturable, dose-dependent metabolism as is seen with phenytoin; instead, these changes are more readily explained by the absorption characteristics of divalproex tablets. Peak serum concentrations of valproate after administration of divalproex may be delayed for 3 to 8 hours, and administration of food may further delay absorption.[160] In addition, diurnal fluctuation in both the rate and extent of absorption of divalproex may be significant. Absorption may be reduced by approximately one-third and peak plasma concentrations may be delayed for up to 12 hours for divalproex doses administered in the evening.[33] Twelve to 15 hours probably elapsed between the administration of T.D.'s last dose and blood sampling; therefore, the currently reported blood level may more closely approximate a peak concentration. Previous blood levels, determined while she was receiving rapidly absorbed valproate syrup, are more likely to have been trough concentrations. T.D.'s adherence to her prescribed dosage regimen also may have increased because of the change in dosage form and reduced side effects; her previous serum concentrations may not have reflected administration of the prescribed dose.

Other pharmacokinetic factors may have actually moderated this unusual increase in valproate concentrations. Fluctuation in valproate concentrations occurs throughout the day in a pattern that does not reflect the timing of doses.[161] This fluctuation may be partially related to changes in serum concentrations of endogenous fatty acids that displace valproate from protein-binding sites.[28] Valproate's hepatic clearance is restrictive (i.e., valproate has a low extraction ratio and its clearance is limited by the free fraction of drug in blood); therefore, protein-binding displacement increases plasma concentration of free drug and clearance. As a result, total serum concentrations decrease. Valproate also exhibits dose dependency in its binding to serum proteins. As concentrations approach 70 to 80 mcg/mL, binding sites on albumin molecules become saturated, and the free fraction of drug in plasma increases.[27,157] This effect also increases valproate clearance and reduces total serum concentrations. Both of these effects may actually "dampen" the apparent increase in plasma concentrations seen in T.D. When also considering the poorly established "therapeutic range" for this drug, it becomes apparent that monitoring serum concentrations is a less useful tool in valproate therapy than with other AED.[28,157]

The clinical significance of T.D.'s elevated valproate serum concentrations is minimal. She is not experiencing any symptoms suggestive of valproate toxicity, and it is too soon following the dosage increase to assess the effect of this change on her seizure frequency. Therefore, alteration in her drug therapy is unnecessary at present and might only confuse evaluation of her response to this drug. She should be observed for an additional 4 to 6 weeks to evaluate seizure frequency before further alterations in her dosing regimen are considered. These apparently elevated valproate levels should not discourage further increases in her dosage as long as she is tolerating the medication and such increases are justified on the basis of seizure frequency. This case illustrates what can happen if too much attention is paid to serum concentrations.

HEPATOTOXICITY

26. Two months later, T.D. is taking 375 mg of divalproex TID with meals. She has had no absence seizures for 5 weeks and no generalized tonic-clonic seizures for 10 weeks. Yesterday, her valproate plasma concentration was 132 mcg/mL. In addition, her alanine aminotransferase (ALT) was 32 IU/mL (normal,

6–14) and her aspartate aminotransferase (AST) was 41 IU/mL (normal, 7–17). All other laboratory tests (bilirubin, alkaline phosphatase, lactate dehydrogenase [LDH], prothrombin time, and serum albumin) were normal. T.D.'s LFT have been monitored monthly since she began taking valproate, and they were previously normal. Physical examination was negative for scleral icterus, abdominal pain, or other signs of liver disease. Discuss these laboratory abnormalities and physical findings in relation to possible valproate-induced hepatotoxicity in T.D.

Liver damage related to valproate therapy appears to be caused by accumulation of directly hepatotoxic metabolites of valproate (probably 4-en-valproate) in certain patients.[162,163] These metabolites may be formed in larger quantities in patients who also receive enzyme-inducing drugs such as phenobarbital. Most cases of fatal hepatotoxicity have occurred in young (<2 years of age) patients with neurologic and metabolic abnormalities who also had severe, difficult-to-control seizures and who were taking multiple AED.[162–167] It is important to recognize, however, that severe hepatotoxicity is not limited to this population.[168] Liver damage occurs early in therapy and symptomatically resembles fulminant hepatitis with hepatic failure. Patients may experience vomiting, drowsiness, lethargy, anorexia, edema, and jaundice; these symptoms often precede laboratory evidence of hepatic damage. Liver biopsies in affected patients show evidence of hepatic necrosis and steatosis. Laboratory findings consist of dramatic elevations of AST, total bilirubin, and serum ammonia; coagulation disturbances accompanied by prolonged prothrombin times, low fibrinogen concentrations, and thrombocytopenia also may be observed. Death results from hepatic failure or a Reye's-like syndrome.[163,165,169]

Asymptomatic elevations in liver enzymes (such as those found in T.D.) occur commonly during the first 6 months of treatment with valproate and usually are not associated with severe or potentially fatal valproate-induced hepatotoxicity. These changes in aminotransferase usually disappear without alteration in therapy; in some cases, temporary dosage reduction is followed by normalization of laboratory tests within 4 to 6 weeks.[163,165] Without systemic symptoms or other signs of significant liver damage, it is unlikely that the laboratory abnormalities observed in T.D. represent severe liver toxicity from valproate. Because T.D. is responding well to valproate therapy, no change in therapy is warranted at this time. Laboratory testing probably can be repeated in 4 to 6 weeks. T.D. and her family should be educated regarding the possible signs and symptoms of valproate-induced liver damage and instructed to consult their physician if these symptoms are noted.

Routine Liver Function Tests

27. What is the usefulness of routinely monitoring LFT in patients receiving valproate?

Serious hepatotoxicity related to valproate therapy is extremely rare. Dreifuss et al.[163,166] estimated that <0.002% of patients treated with valproate developed fatal hepatotoxicity between 1985 and 1986. This compares with an incidence of 0.01% between 1978 and 1984.[164] The lower recent incidence (despite much wider use of valproate) is attributed to increased valproate monotherapy and reduced use of this drug in high-risk patients such as the very young (Table 54-7). Most cases of fatal hepatotoxicity occur in children <10 years of age. In children <2 years of age who receive AED polytherapy, the incidence of this complication is 1 in 500 to 1 in 800. Because asymptomatic, apparently benign elevations in liver enzymes are common early in therapy with valproate and symptoms of liver damage often precede laboratory changes, frequent LFT during early valproate therapy are unlikely to detect serious hepatotoxicity.[60,163–165,170] In addition, this type of laboratory monitoring adds significant cost while providing little benefit for patients. Education of caregivers or patients regarding potential symptoms of hepatotoxicity, with careful observation and follow-up by health care professionals, is recommended as the most effective method for monitoring for this drug-induced illness.

Especially careful monitoring should be provided for predisposed patients (i.e., very young children with associated neurologic abnormalities and those receiving polytherapy). In predisposed patients, significant increases in LFT values that are noted early in therapy may be clinically significant. At the onset of symptoms suggesting this condition, laboratory testing may help confirm its presence. Practitioners who feel compelled to perform frequent laboratory testing for liver dysfunction on the basis of manufacturer's package insert recommendations should be cautious not to overinterpret common, transient, and apparently benign elevations in aminotransferases or ammonia levels.

Acute Repetitive ("Cluster") Seizures

Rectal Diazepam Gel

28. B.N., a 7-year-old, 28-kg boy, has had seizures since age 3 months. He suffered anoxia at birth. His seizures usually involve initial confusion and disorientation, shortly followed by generalized tonic-clonic convulsive activity. Despite treatment with carbamazepine at maximal tolerated doses and serum concentrations (300 mg TID; 9–11 mcg/mL), he continues to have approximately two seizures monthly. Recent trials of topiramate and tiagabine as additions to his carbamazepine were unsuccessful and caused intolerable sedation and lethargy. During the past year, he has been admitted to the emergency department (ED) five times because of seizure "flurries" consisting of three to six seizures occurring over a period of 12 or fewer hours. While he regains consciousness between these "flurry" seizures, he becomes lethargic. During ED admissions, IV diazepam was administered. This was rapidly successful in terminating seizure activity. B.N.'s mother relates that she usually can identify the onset of seizure flurries; B.N.'s behavior changes and he becomes "clinging" and "whiny" and hyperactive. She also indicates that the initial seizure in a flurry differs from B.N.'s typical episodes. Before the onset of generalized seizure activity, he experiences much briefer periods of confusion. In addition, the generalized seizures are longer and more severe (often with dramatic cyanosis) at the beginning of a "flurry."

Why is prophylactic or abortive therapy for B.N.'s seizure flurries indicated? What factors about B.N. predict successful use of such treatment, and how can it be administered?

B.N.'s relatively frequent flurries or clusters of seizures are causing him and his family significant difficulty. Frequent ED visits are expensive and frightening for many patients and their families. B.N. continues to experience seizure flurries despite carbamazepine therapy. He responds well to IV diazepam and has a caregiver who can identify the onset of seizure clusters. His seizure clusters appear to be distinct from the other seizures that he experiences. All of these factors indicate that a trial of home-administered treatment to abort these cluster episodes is likely to be helpful and should be initiated.

Rectal diazepam gel (Diastat) is available for home administration to patients with acute episodes of repetitive seizure activity.[171] When diazepam gel is administered rectally, it is absorbed relatively rapidly (peak plasma concentrations occur in approximately 1.5 hours),[172] and is often effective in terminating cluster seizures within 15 or fewer minutes. Use of diazepam rectal gel is recommended only when caregivers can recognize the onset of cluster seizures, which are different from a patient's usual seizure activity, and when the caregivers can be trained to administer the preparation safely and to monitor the patient's response (e.g., respiratory status) following administration. Caregivers should be informed that this preparation is not for as needed (PRN) use with every seizure; it should be used only for identifiable cluster seizures or prolonged seizures. Home use of rectal diazepam may result in significant reduction in the costs of treating these events and may decrease ED visits.[173]

B.N.'s mother should administer rectal diazepam gel at the onset of identifiable cluster seizure activity. A dose of approximately 0.3 mg/kg (10 mg) should be given and repeated, if necessary, within 4 to 12 hours of the first dose. B.N.'s mother should be counseled on the administration of this product and given the patient package insert, which gives complete instructions for the administration of rectal diazepam. After administration, B.N. should be monitored for at least 4 hours to ensure that no respiratory depression or other adverse side effects are occurring and to assess the effect of the medication on his seizures. The most common adverse effect seen with rectal diazepam is somnolence, occasionally accompanied by dizziness and ataxia. Respiratory depression is very uncommon.

Febrile Seizures

Incidence and Classification

29. J.J., a 14-month-old girl, is brought to the ED after having a generalized tonic-clonic convulsion lasting approximately 5 minutes. The episode occurred in association with an upper respiratory infection. On arrival in the ED, her temperature was 39.5°C rectally. She was alert at that time; all laboratory and neurologic findings, including lumbar puncture, were normal. J.J. has no history of neurologic abnormality. Her 7-year-old brother suffers from both absence and generalized tonic-clonic seizures. What is the relationship between febrile seizures and epilepsy? How may J.J.'s convulsion be classified on the basis of the data available?

Up to 5% of children have a febrile seizure between 6 months and 6 years of age.[174] Simple febrile seizures occur with a fever of $\geq$38°C in previously normal children <5 years of age. They last <15 minutes and have no focal features. The associated seizure does not arise from CNS pathology. Complex febrile seizures show focal characteristics or are prolonged. The child may or may not have previous neurologic abnormalities. The risk of occurrence of unprovoked afebrile seizures following a febrile seizure is four times greater than in the general population. A family history of afebrile seizures, a complicated initial seizure, and pre-existing neurologic abnormality are risk factors associated with the later development of chronic epilepsy.[174,175]

J.J.'s seizure appears to be a typical simple febrile seizure that developed in association with her upper respiratory tract infection. The lack of previous neurologic abnormality and normal findings on lumbar puncture and laboratory evaluation help confirm this assessment.

Treatment of Acute Seizure

30. How should J.J.'s febrile seizures be treated?

Because J.J. is not having a seizure at present, AED therapy is not required. Measures to reduce her elevated temperature should be initiated; however, these measures may not reduce the risk of further seizures. Acetaminophen and tepid sponge baths usually are helpful.

If patients experience prolonged or repeated febrile seizures, either diazepam or, less commonly, phenobarbital may be administered.[175] Rectal diazepam gel can be used for this purpose.

Prophylaxis and Choice of Antiepileptic Drug

31. On the basis of the subjective and objective data available for J.J., is AED therapy indicated on a long-term basis? What are the benefits and risks of AED prophylaxis for febrile seizures?

Long-term treatment or prophylaxis with AED for simple febrile seizures is not recommended. Up to 54% of affected patients will have recurrent febrile seizures, and the risk of recurrence is even greater when the first episode occurs before 13 months of age. Nonetheless, recurrent febrile seizures are not associated with brain damage or development of epilepsy.[174] The efficacy of prophylactic AED for prevention of chronic epilepsy following febrile seizures has not been evaluated.[176] Thus, the primary potential benefit of long-term AED therapy would be prevention of recurrent febrile seizures.

Phenobarbital and, occasionally, valproate used to be used as prophylaxis in patients with febrile seizures.[177] A reanalysis of published British trials of both valproate and phenobarbital for febrile seizure prophylaxis found that neither drug was reliably effective.[178] Although phenobarbital had been considered at least partially effective, the high rate of side effects (40%) preclude recommending its use. When the effects on intelligence of phenobarbital versus placebo prophylaxis for febrile seizures in young children were evaluated, IQ scores were significantly lower in children treated with phenobarbital.[179] This effect persisted for at least 6 months after discontinuation of drug therapy. In addition, reduction in the recurrence rate of febrile seizures in children treated with phenobarbital was not statistically significant, although approximately one-third of patients who experienced recurrent febrile seizures were noncompliant with phenobarbital therapy. This study's design and findings have been criticized on the basis of patient selection and "crossing over" of patients from the control group to the study group.[180] Nevertheless, on retesting after 3 to 5 years, phenobarbital-treated children scored significantly lower on the Wide Range Achievement Test. Their mean IQ were 3.71 points lower than those of placebo-treated children, although this difference was not statistically significant. Therefore, phenobarbital has no beneficial effect on preventing febrile seizure recurrence and may adversely affect cognitive function.[181]

Antiepleptic drug prophylaxis for febrile seizures is probably not warranted for J.J., even though she is at risk for both development of epilepsy and recurrence of febrile seizures. No evidence supports that medication will significantly affect her later development of epilepsy. Phenobarbital's use for this purpose is difficult to justify when considering the risk of learning impairment. In addition, phenobarbital therapy is associated with hyperactivity and behavioral disturbance in up to 75% of children receiving the drug.[182–184] J.J.'s age places her at higher risk of valproate-related hepatotoxicity, and this risk probably outweighs any potential benefit from treatment with this drug. Close medical follow-up of J.J. is warranted. In addition, her parents should be instructed to institute antipyretic measures (i.e., acetaminophen and tepid sponge baths) at the onset of any febrile illness. Many febrile seizures occur early in the course of an illness before fever is detected[175]; nevertheless, vigilance by her parents and early antipyretic therapy may help prevent further febrile seizures. The intermittent administration of oral diazepam (Valium) at the onset of a febrile illness also may be of value. A dosage of 0.33 mg/kg orally given every 8 hours appears to be effective in reducing the recurrence rate of febrile seizures.[185] Diazepam should be initiated as soon as a febrile illness appears and continued until J.J. has been afebrile for 24 hours. Side effects are common when diazepam is used in this manner; approximately one-third of patients will experience ataxia, lethargy, or irritability. These and other common CNS side effects, such as dysarthria and insomnia, may confuse assessment of the condition of children with febrile illnesses.[174]

Seizures Secondary to Toxic Exposures: Nerve Gas

32. How likely are seizures to result from exposure to chemical warfare agents such as sarin nerve gas, and how are these seizures treated?

Nerve agents that may be used in chemical warfare or terrorist attacks can cause seizures. These agents include tabun (synonym, GA), sarin (GB), soman (GD), and VX. At normal environmental temperatures, all of these agents except VX are volatile and therefore become "nerve gases." VX is a viscous liquid. Nerve agents are both lipophilic and hydrophilic and therefore can rapidly penetrate clothing, skin, and mucous membranes and be absorbed systemically.[186,187] Nerve agents are closely related to organophosphate insecticides, and their toxic effects result from their actions as acetylcholinesterase (AChE) inhibitors. The toxins bind to the active site of AChE and prevent hydrolysis of acetylcholine (ACh). Excessive quantities of ACh then accumulate, causing excessive stimulation of muscarinic and nicotinic receptors. Manifestations of nerve agent exposure can be broadly described as muscarinic (ophthalmic symptoms such as miosis, lacrimation, and blurred vision; respiratory symptoms such as severe rhinorrhea, wheezing, and dyspnea; cardiovascular symptoms such as bradydysrhythmia, atrioventricular (A-V) block and hypotension; and GI symptoms such as salivation, nausea, vomiting, and severe diarrhea), nicotinic (cardiovascular symptoms such as tachydysrhythmia and hypertension; fasciculation of voluntary muscles; and metabolic symptoms such as hyperglycemia, metabolic acidosis, and hypokalemia), and CNS symptoms (anxiety, agitation, vertigo, ataxia, central respiratory depression, convulsions, and coma). The likelihood and the severity of CNS toxicity and seizures will depend on the amount of nerve agent and the route of exposure. CNS symptoms are associated with severe exposure to nerve agents. When seizures occur, they are usually generalized; the exact mechanism of seizure induction by these agents has not been identified.[187]

Following exposure to nerve agents, early treatment with antidotes may prevent severe toxic manifestations. Large doses of IM atropine (2–6 mg) should be given; dosing is based on respiratory symptoms. Therapeutic endpoints are drying of respiratory secretions and relief of dyspnea.[186,187] Pralidoxime (Protopam) is an AChE reactivator. This antidote binds nerve agents and removes them from binding sites on AChE. Pralidoxime is useful only if given before the bond between the nerve agent and AChE becomes permanent. This time interval varies from minutes to hours after exposure, depending on the nerve agent.[188] Pralidoxime is a quaternary agent, and it is not clear to what extent it enters the CNS. The effects of pralidoxime are most dramatically seen on skeletal muscle symptoms. Pralidoxime should be given along with the antimuscarinic agent atropine.

Few published data exist regarding the use of anticonvulsant drugs for treatment of nerve agent exposure. It is claimed that early administration of 10 mg IM diazepam may prevent permanent CNS damage in patients with severe nerve agent toxicity.[186] In situations of severe exposure with CNS manifestations and seizures, use of a more rapidly absorbed IM agent such as lorazepam would be expected to produce a more rapid and reliable response; IV administration of diazepam or lorazepam, if feasible, would be more likely to rapidly control seizure activity. If necessary, rectal administration of diazepam gel would be an option (see Question 28).

ANTIEPILEPTIC DRUG INTERACTIONS AND ADVERSE EFFECTS

Carbamazepine–Erythromycin Interaction

33. J.N., a 17-year-old boy, is treated with carbamazepine 600 mg/day for complex partial seizures. His seizures are well controlled with serum carbamazepine concentrations of 8 mcg/mL. He developed an upper respiratory infection, assessed as probable streptococcal pharyngitis. Because J.N. is allergic to penicillin, erythromycin 333 mg TID with meals for 10 days was prescribed. Four days after beginning erythromycin therapy, J.N. complains that, although his upper respiratory symptoms are abating, he is constantly drowsy and is experiencing dizziness and double vision. He also complains of nausea and has vomited once this morning. He receives no other routine medication, although he did take approximately five doses of two tablets of Extra-Strength Tylenol (acetaminophen 500 mg/tablet) during the initial stage of his current illness for fever and general discomfort. What is the relationship between J.N.'s symptoms and the potential interaction between carbamazepine and erythromycin? How might this interaction be further assessed and managed at this point?

Inhibition of CYP3A4 by erythromycin can result in dramatic elevations in carbamazepine serum concentrations and precipitation of intoxication.[189,190] J.N.'s symptoms are consistent with carbamazepine toxicity, although erythromycin therapy may be contributing to his GI symptoms. Although dramatic elevation of carbamazepine serum concentrations is not consistently seen, susceptible patients may exhibit a twofold increase in serum levels. Determination of a carbamazepine serum concentration may help confirm probable toxicity and assess the magnitude of the interaction.

Management of this interaction at this point is somewhat difficult; prevention of the interaction by avoiding the use of erythromycin whenever possible is usually the best clinical strategy. Replacement of erythromycin with azithromycin or, possibly, clindamycin should provide adequate antibiotic therapy with no risk of further interaction with carbamazepine. Other macrolide antibiotics (e.g., clarithromycin, triactyloleandomycin, and telithromycin) are likely to cause significant inhibition of carbamazepine metabolism. One or two doses of carbamazepine could be held to allow carbamazepine serum concentrations to decrease to pre-erythromycin levels and correct J.N.'s present intoxication. An alternative approach would be to reduce J.N.'s carbamazepine dose, based on his present serum level, for the duration of erythromycin therapy. This approach may be more difficult to manage; the time required for erythromycin-induced metabolic inhibition to subside when the antibiotic is stopped is unpredictable. With either approach to management of this interaction, J.N.'s clinical status will need to be monitored carefully. Further adjustment of carbamazepine dosage may be required, and repeat serum level determinations may be helpful.

Valproate–Carbamazepine Interaction

34. D.H., a 21-year-old, 84-kg man, was taking carbamazepine 1,400 mg/day (600 mg every AM and 800 mg at bedtime [HS]) for treatment of generalized tonic-clonic seizures. Despite carbamazepine serum concentrations of 14 mcg/mL, he continued to have a seizure every 6 to 8 weeks. Higher serum levels were associated with toxicity symptoms. Valproate (divalproex) was recently added and gradually increased to a dosage of 1,000 mg TID; the therapeutic goal is replacement of carbamazepine with valproate. At this dose, D.H. again experienced symptoms of carbamazepine intoxication (double vision, unsteady gait, and drowsiness), although his carbamazepine serum concentration was 12 mcg/mL. Valproate serum levels were 40 mcg/mL and 43 mcg/mL on two occasions. D.H. has continued to experience seizures at his previous rate. He appears to be adherent with his prescribed medication regimen. How can D.H.'s symptoms and low valproate levels be explained on the basis of an interaction between his two AED?

Difficulty in achieving serum valproate concentrations adequate for improvement in seizure control frequently is encountered in patients who receive concomitant therapy with potent enzyme inducers such as carbamazepine. Clinicians frequently note that it is difficult to administer doses of valproate sufficiently large to achieve desired serum levels under these circumstances.[27,191] Serum concentrations of valproate in patients receiving carbamazepine may be only approximately 50% of those expected on the basis of single-dose valproate pharmacokinetic studies.

D.H.'s symptoms of carbamazepine intoxication at plasma levels that were previously tolerated suggest possible accumulation of CBZ-10,11-epoxide (CBZ-E). This compound is an active metabolite of carbamazepine. Valproate may inhibit epoxide hydrolase and cause accumulation of CBZ-E sufficient to exert significant pharmacologic effects, including intoxication. This author (R.L.) has observed a patient receiving both valproate and carbamazepine who developed serum concentrations of CBZ-E equal to the concentration of carbamazepine itself (both compounds were measured at ~12 mcg/mL) and experienced significant intoxication. Determination of the serum concentration of carbamazepine and CBZ-E could help confirm the clinical impression. Unfortunately, the assay for CBZ-E is not readily available in many clinical laboratories.

35. What recommendations can be made for alteration in D.H.'s drug therapy regimen to alleviate the effects of this drug interaction and enhance his therapeutic response to the medication?

On clinical and empiric grounds, D.H.'s dosage of carbamazepine should be reduced; this would seem especially appropriate because the therapeutic goal was replacement of carbamazepine with valproate. Dosage reduction will result in a decrease in serum concentrations of both carbamazepine and CBZ-E and a reduction in symptoms of intoxication. An initial decrease of 10% to 20% (200 mg) of D.H.'s daily carbamazepine dose would be reasonable. Subsequently, his carbamazepine dose can be tapered using reductions of 200 mg every 1 to 2 weeks. During tapering of carbamazepine, D.H. should be monitored carefully for increased seizure activity.

Valproate-Related Thrombocytopenia

36. D.H.'s symptoms abated significantly within 3 days of reduction of his carbamazepine dosage to 1,200 mg/day. A CBZ-E serum concentration was not determined. His carbamazepine dosage was reduced by 200 mg/day in weekly steps, with no increase in seizure activity. A serum valproate concentration after his carbamazepine dosage reached 600 mg/day was 53 mcg/mL. At that time, he had not had a seizure in approximately 6 weeks. A serum valproate concentration was repeated when his carbamazepine dosage reached 200 mg/day and it was 58 mcg/mL. Three weeks following discontinuation of carbamazepine, D.H. noted the onset of tremor affecting his hands and a "fuzzy sensation in my head" accompanied by difficulty concentrating on tasks. His serum valproate concentration was 126 mcg/mL. In addition, a CBC showed a platelet count of 60,000/mm^3 cells; no other abnormalities were seen. No bleeding tendencies were noted, and D.H. denied easy bruisability or unusual bleeding. Previous CBC had been normal. Is this pattern of increase in valproate serum concentrations consistent with the loss of carbamazepine-related enzyme induction? What is the relationship between D.H.'s new symptoms, his reduced platelet count, and the elevation in his valproate serum concentration?

[SI unit: 60×10^5/L]

D.H.'s valproate serum concentrations were expected to increase with "deinduction" of hepatic microsomal enzymes while carbamazepine was being discontinued. The pattern and timing of deinduction are not consistently predictable. Although a somewhat linear increase in valproate concentrations might be anticipated as enzyme inducers such as carbamazepine are gradually reduced, it is not unusual for valproate levels to remain relatively constant until 1 to 2 weeks after discontinuation of enzyme inducers.[191] Therefore, patients should be monitored for signs or symptoms of possible valproate intoxication during and for several weeks after such a discontinuation process; clinicians and patients should be aware that dosage adjustment may not be required until the enzyme-inducing drug has been completely discontinued.

D.H.'s new symptoms appear to be consistent with mild to moderate intoxication with valproate. Tremor is a relatively common side effect of valproate that is likely to appear as serum concentrations exceed approximately 80 mcg/mL.[27] This side effect may be troublesome for some patients because the tremor is usually an intention tremor, which worsens with physical activity. In most patients, dose reduction will improve or eliminate tremor. Some practitioners counter this side effect with propranolol therapy in doses similar to those used to treat essential tremor.[192] The neurologic symptoms exhibited by D.H. also are typically seen with valproate intoxication. All of these symptoms are reversible with dosage reduction.

Reductions in platelet counts are not rare in patients treated with valproate. Significant thrombocytopenia with bleeding manifestations is extremely uncommon, although measurable changes in platelet function may occur.[193,194] The mechanism underlying thrombocytopenia is not known; evidence exists for both a dose- or serum concentration-related effect[194] and an immunologic mechanism.[195] Affected patients usually can be continued on valproate therapy at reduced doses without adverse effects. The author (R.L.) has observed two patients who developed significant valproate-related thrombocytopenia without bleeding complications; both cases were associated with dramatic increases in valproate serum concentrations following discontinuation of enzyme-inducing drugs.

Both the neurologic symptoms and thrombocytopenia exhibited by D.H. probably can be corrected by reducing his dose of divalproex. The magnitude of dose reduction should be determined by titration using symptom remission and normalization of his platelet count as endpoints. Periodically rechecking valproate serum concentrations can help establish a safe upper limit dose and serum levels for D.H. Ongoing monitoring also will be important for several weeks because the process of deinduction of hepatic enzymes may not yet be complete. Further dose reductions may be necessary as this process reaches completion and D.H.'s valproate clearance gradually decreases. Reduction of D.H.'s dosage to 2,000 mg/day should approximate serum concentrations between those that were previously subtherapeutic and those that are causing his current adverse effects.

Skin Rash: Hypersensitivity Reactions to Antiepileptic Drugs

37. R.S., a 34-year-old man, has been taking phenytoin 200 mg BID for the past 7 weeks to control complex partial and secondarily generalized tonic-clonic seizures. Seizures began approximately 4 months ago following surgical evacuation of a subdural hematoma. Today he appeared at the walk-in clinic and complained of an "itchy rash" that had begun 2 days ago. He described "feeling lousy" for the past week. On examination he is febrile (38.5°C orally). A maculopapular, scaly, erythematous rash covered his upper extremities and torso, and the mucous membranes of his mouth appeared to be mildly inflamed. Cervical lymphadenopathy was noted, and the liver was found to be enlarged and tender. R.S. also related that his urine had become very dark in the past 2 days and that his stools were light colored. What is the significance of R.S.'s skin rash and other signs and symptoms? Are these likely to be related to his phenytoin therapy?

Skin rash is a relatively common (2%–3% of patients) side effect related to AED therapy. It is most commonly associated with phenytoin, lamotrigine, carbamazepine, and phenobarbital. Most cases are relatively mild, but severely affected patients may develop Stevens-Johnson syndrome or a systemic hypersensitivity syndrome accompanied by severe hepatic damage. In R.S.'s case, signs and symptoms suggesting hepatic involvement accompany the skin rash. Fever, lymphadenopathy, and apparent inflammation of mucous membranes also suggest a hypersensitivity reaction to phenytoin with multisystem involvement and the potential for progression to Stevens-Johnson syndrome. Viral infection (e.g., hepatitis, influenza, infectious mononucleosis) should be considered and ruled out as a possible cause of R.S.'s symptoms before they are attributed to phenytoin therapy.[124,196–199]

Phenytoin hypersensitivity syndrome is most commonly seen in adults and is more likely to affect blacks.[197] Typically, patients with this syndrome present with complaints of fever, skin rash, and lymphadenopathy during the first 2 months of phenytoin therapy. Hepatomegaly, splenomegaly, jaundice, and bleeding manifestations such as petechial hemorrhage also are relatively common. Laboratory manifestations usually include leukocytosis with eosinophilia, elevated serum bilirubin, and elevated AST and ALT. When a phenytoin hypersensitivity reaction includes significant hepatotoxicity, fatality may occur in as many as 38% of affected patients.[196]

A high likelihood exists that R.S. has developed a severe reaction to phenytoin; the clinical manifestations and the timing of their appearance are typical of this reaction. Phenytoin should be discontinued immediately pending diagnostic clarification (i.e., evaluation for other possible causes of his symptoms such as viral illness). R.S. should be hospitalized for further diagnostic evaluation and treatment. Treatment of phenytoin-related hypersensitivity and hepatotoxicity is symptomatic and supportive. Intensive therapy with corticosteroids has commonly been used, although little objective evidence exists for beneficial effects of this treatment. Potential complications of this reaction include sepsis and hepatic failure; these conditions should be treated specifically.

38. R.S. was hospitalized and treated with oral prednisone and topical corticosteroids. Other potential causes for his condition were ruled out, and his signs and symptoms were attributed to phenytoin hypersensitivity. His fever resolved within 5 days; the skin rash became exfoliative but resolved without infectious complications. Laboratory parameters began to normalize after 10 days. While he was hospitalized, R.S. experienced three episodes of generalized seizure activity that were treated with acute administration of IV lorazepam. R.S. was afebrile at the time these episodes occurred. What information regarding the pathogenesis of phenytoin hypersensitivity and hepatotoxicity can be used to guide selection of an alternative AED for R.S.?

Further administration of phenytoin to R.S. is contraindicated on the basis of his history of a severe hypersensitivity reaction to this drug. Readministration of phenytoin is likely to result in rapid recurrence of severe symptoms of this syndrome. Although the mechanism of this reaction is not fully understood, research implicates reactive arene oxide metabolites of phenytoin (and other chemically similar AED) as possible causative agents for hypersensitivity reactions. Affected patients purportedly are predisposed genetically to the development of hypersensitivity, possibly because a relative deficiency of epoxide hydrolase enzymes allows the accumulation of toxic concentrations of reactive epoxide metabolites, which are believed to exert a direct cytotoxic effect and to interact with cellular macromolecules, thereby functioning as haptenes that stimulate an immunologic reaction.[200,201] Carbamazepine, phenytoin, and phenobarbital all are metabolized by similar pathways and converted to reactive arene oxides. It is hypothesized that carbamazepine-induced liver damage also may result from the effects of accumulation of reactive epoxide metabolites; these reactive metabolites differ from the 10,11-epoxide metabolite that accumulates during carbamazepine therapy. For this reason, these drugs potentially cross-react in susceptible patients. Cases of apparent cross-reactivity between phenytoin and phenobarbital or carbamazepine have been documented.[202–204] In addition, both carbamazepine and phenobarbital can produce hypersensitivity reactions similar to those seen with phenytoin. This potential for cross-reactivity should be considered when an alternative AED is selected for R.S. An analysis of cases of AED-related skin rashes found that the most significant nondrug predictor of skin rash was the occurrence of a rash with another AED.[205]

Valproate has been suggested as the preferred alternative AED for patients who have developed hypersensitivity reactions to phenytoin.[203] Valproate is not metabolized to arene oxides and also is chemically dissimilar to all other AED. Because valproate often shows good efficacy for complex partial seizures with secondary generalization, it would seem to be a safe and potentially effective alternative AED for R.S. Of the newer AED, lamotrigine should probably be avoided in R.S. because of its likelihood of causing skin rash and apparent hypersensitivity reactions. Oxcarbazepine is potentially an alternative AED for R.S. because it is not metabolized through the arene oxide pathway. Nevertheless, 25% to 30% of patients who develop a rash in response to carbamazepine will also develop a rash with oxcarbazepine.[206] Therefore, many clinicians would avoid oxcarbazepine. Topiramate, tiagabine, levetiracetam, gabapentin, pregabalin, or zonisamide could be considered as alternative medications for R.S. These medications appear less likely to cause skin rash or hypersensitivity reactions.[205,207]

WOMEN'S ISSUES IN EPILEPSY

Although epilepsy affects men and women equally, many health issues are of specific importance to women, such as contraceptive interactions with AED, teratogenicity, pharmacokinetic changes during pregnancy, breast-feeding, menstrual cycle influences on seizure activity (catamenial epilepsy), AED impact on bone, and sexual dysfunction.[208] A great need exists to educate both health care professionals and patients about the many complex issues facing women with epilepsy.

For women of child-bearing potential, prepregnancy planning and counseling are important, because significant AED exposure of the fetus often occurs by the time the pregnancy is confirmed. This is especially important because of the potential for unplanned pregnancies from the AED–contraceptive drug interactions. Prepregnancy counseling also should include the importance of folic acid supplementation and medication adherence. Patients should be informed about the risk of teratogenicity and the importance of prenatal care.

Although complete seizure control is desirable for all patients with epilepsy, it is especially favorable for a woman's seizures to be well controlled before conception. Monotherapy is preferred whenever possible, because the relative risk of birth defects dramatically increases with AED polytherapy.[209,210] Monotherapy also improves patient adherence. The AED should be given at the lowest effective dose to reduce the possibility of birth defects.[211] The gradual discontinuation of AED may be considered if a woman has been seizure-free for 2 years or longer.

Antiepileptic Drug–Oral Contraceptive Interaction

39. P.Z., a 26-year-old woman, experiences complex partial and secondarily generalized tonic-clonic seizures. She is taking phenytoin 400 mg/day and divalproex 2,000 mg/day. She reports having two or three partial seizures and one generalized seizure every 3 to 4 months. Despite treatment with Lo/Ovral (norgestrel 0.3 mg with ethinyl estradiol 30 mcg), she has just learned she is pregnant. Her last menstrual period was 6 weeks ago. What is the relationship between P.Z.'s apparent contraceptive failure and her antiepileptic drug therapy?

There have been several reports of reduced efficacy of oral contraceptives in patients receiving various AED.[212,213] These reports describe both breakthrough bleeding and pregnancy. Phenobarbital, phenytoin, carbamazepine, oxcarbazepine, and felbamate have been shown to increase the metabolism of ethinylestradiol and progestogens.[214] This effect is not associated with valproate, lamotrigine, gabapentin, tiagabine, zonisamide, levetiracetam, or pregabalin.[82,208,215] Topiramate in polytherapy and at high dosages (200–800 mg/day) appears to have a mild though measurable effect on oral contraceptive pharmacokinetics; apparent clearance of the estrogen component of combined oral contraceptives is increased in patients taking topiramate.[216] In contrast, topiramate monotherapy in lower dosages (50–200 mg/day) has a lesser impact on the pharmacokinetics of the oral contraceptive.[217]

A different drug interaction exists between oral contraceptives and lamotrigine. It is currently thought that the estrogen component in oral contraceptives increases the clearance of lamotrigine. Lamotrigine concentrations may increase twofold when contraceptive steroids are begun and fall by 50% when contraceptive steroids are discontinued. Changes in lamotrigine levels associated with initiation and discontinuation of contraceptive steroids can result in increased seizure activity in some patients and toxicity in others.[218] Within a 28-day cycle of oral contraceptives, lamotrigine concentrations decrease during the 21 days of steroid hormone and fairly rapid increases in concentrations during the 'pill-free' week.

A lack of contraceptive efficacy may present as irregular or breakthrough menstrual bleeding. Decreased efficacy is not always associated with breakthrough bleeding, however. Oral contraceptive doses can be increased to compensate for the effect of an AED.[219] Estrogens also may exacerbate seizures in some women.[220] Women >35 years of age or those who smoke must consider the risk of thromboembolic complications associated with higher doses of contraceptives. A second contraceptive method (e.g., condoms, intrauterine devices, or spermicide) is recommended to avoid contraceptive failure.[207] Tubal ligation is also an alternative.

Assuming P.Z. was taking her contraceptive pills on a regular basis, it is possible that her enzyme-inducing AED (phenytoin) is responsible for their failure. Patients receiving AED should be prospectively informed that this interaction can occur and advised concerning the use of alternative contraceptives (see Chapter 45, Contraception).

Teratogenicity

40. What are the risks of teratogenic effects from P.Z.'s medications? What steps might be taken to minimize these risks?

P.Z.'s child is at a relatively high risk of congenital malformations because of exposure to several potentially teratogenic drugs: estrogen–progestin combination oral contraceptives, valproate and phenytoin (also see Chapter 46, Obstetric Drug Therapy).

Many AED have teratogenic effects.[221] Animal data regarding the teratogenic potential of lamotrigine, felbamate, gabapentin, topiramate, tiagabine, levetiracetam, oxcarbazepine, pregabalin, and zonisamide are encouraging, but conclusions regarding the teratogenic potential of these recently marketed AED cannot be made because of limited experience in pregnant women. Controversy has been significantly reduced regarding the relative contributions of parental epilepsy itself, genetic influences, and drug therapy since recent data have shown that the infants of untreated women with epilepsy had fewer abnormalities compared with those born to women with epilepsy who were taking AED.[222] The risk of major congenital malformations (e.g., facial clefts, cardiac septal defects) in children exposed to AED in utero may be as high as two to three times the baseline risk in the general population.[223] In addition, maternal epilepsy increases the risk of complications of pregnancy, prenatal or postnatal infant mortality, premature birth, and low infant birth weight.

Most AED, with the exception of valproate, are believed to exert their teratogenic effects (and possibly other adverse effects such as hepatotoxicity) partly via reactive epoxide metabolites.[223] Enhancement of the formation of these metabolites via hepatic enzyme induction (e.g., by carbamazepine or phenobarbital) or inhibition of their breakdown (e.g., through inhibition of epoxide hydrolase by valproate) would increase the risk of teratogenicity. Combined administration of enzyme inducers and valproate (specifically the combination of carbamazepine, phenobarbital, and valproate with or without phenytoin) is associated with an especially high risk of teratogenicity.[224] In addition, each of the present major AED has been associated with congenital malformations when administered alone. Meador et al.[225] have recently provided data from 333 pregnancies in women with epilepsy taking an AED in monotherapy and enrolled in the Neurodevelopmental Effects of Antiepileptic Drugs (NEAD) study. Serious adverse outcomes (major malformations and fetal death) were significantly more likely to occur with exposure to valproate (20.3%), than with carbamazepine (8.2%), phenytoin (10.7%), or lamotrigine (1%).

The NEAD study included one second-generation AED, lamotrigine. The North American AED Pregnancy Registry recently reported that the risk for a major malformation after first trimester monotherapy exposure to lamotrigine was not increased compared with the risk for the nonexposed control population. The risk for nonsyndromic cleft lip or palate was increased in the babies exposed to lamotrigine,[226] although this has not been identified in other registries.[227] The reason for this incongruence is not known.

In addition to malformations, AED exposure in utero may have an effect on neurodevelopment. An interim analysis of the NEAD study raised concerns about the effects of in utero exposure to valproate on neurodevelopment.[228] It was found that valproate-exposed children have low scores (mean = 85) on the Children's Mental Development Index (MDI), even after controlling for the mother's IQ and seizure type. The MDI scores were significantly lower for children exposed in utero to valproate compared with scores of children exposed to carbamazepine (mean, 94), phenytoin (mean, 90), and lamotrigine (mean, 97) monotherapy.

Several strategies can be used to reduce the potential adverse effects of AED on pregnancy outcomes.[228,229] If feasible, before conception, seizure control should be optimized using the AED of first choice for the prospective mother's seizure type or epilepsy syndrome. Monotherapy at the lowest effective dose is the goal. Maintenance of adequate folic acid stores before conception and during fetal organogenesis is also important. Folic acid supplementation can reduce the risk of congenital neural tube malformations in infants at risk who are born to women without epilepsy, but folate supplementation does not reliably reduce the teratogenic effects of AED. Nevertheless, supplementation of folic acid (and ensuring adequate folate levels) is recommended. Because about half of pregnancies are unplanned and not evident until weeks after conception, folate supplementation should be routinely given to women of child-bearing age with epilepsy. No study has been conducted to determine the optimal dose of folic acid supplementation in patients taking AED. Clinicians engage in much discussion of this topic, but the current practices are not evidence based. Even though this is the case, P.Z. should start taking 4 mg of folic acid supplementation each day.

Physiologic changes in pregnant women may affect the pharmacokinetics of AED.[206] Absorption can be influenced by nausea and vomiting. Hepatic metabolism and renal function both increase during pregnancy. The binding capacity of albumin is decreased during pregnancy, resulting in decreased protein binding for highly bound drugs. Unbound fractions of phenobarbital, phenytoin, and valproate increase with decreased concentrations of albumin.[229–231] For drugs predominately metabolized by the liver with a restrictive clearance (e.g., carbamazepine and valproate), decreased protein binding without changes in intrinsic clearance should result in a decrease in total drug concentrations; unbound drug concentrations should remain unchanged. For drugs with both increased hepatic metabolism and decreased protein binding (e.g., phenytoin and phenobarbital), both total and unbound plasma concentrations decrease, but not necessarily proportionately.

The clearance of lamotrigine increases as pregnancy progresses, presumably related to the impact of estrogen on lamotrigine metabolism as mentioned above.[232] This alteration in clearance changes immediately postpartum. Preliminary data suggest that oxcarbazepine concentrations may also decrease as pregnancy progresses.[232]

The effects of changes in renal function during pregnancy on AED concentrations are not well known.[232] Renal blood flow and glomerular filtration rate increase during pregnancy. Thus, the pharmacokinetics of drugs that are predominately excreted through the kidneys, such as gabapentin, levetiracetam, and pregabalin, could change during pregnancy.

During pregnancy, serum levels of AED (including free serum levels for highly protein-bound drugs) can be monitored. Dosage adjustments may help to prevent the increase in seizure frequency that is seen in approximately 25% of pregnant women with epilepsy. Because falls and anoxia associated with uncontrolled seizures may increase the risk to the unborn baby, P.Z. should be educated on the value of adherence to her AED regimen.

For P.Z., it can be presumed that significant exposure of the fetus to any teratogenic influence of AED has already occurred. Optimization of seizure control is a primary concern for this woman. Any major alterations in P.Z.'s AED regimen should be made cautiously to avoid precipitating seizures. In addition, she should be instructed to contact the AED pregnancy registry at Massachusetts General Hospital (1-888-233-2334). Information provided to the registry will aid in the ongoing monitoring of outcomes of babies born to mothers taking AED. Reports from this registry have provided risk information on two of the older AED (phenobarbital and valproate). In utero exposure to either of these AED in monotherapy caused a significantly increased incidence of major birth defects compared with controls.

Vitamin K Supplementation

Babies born to women with epilepsy who are taking enzyme-inducing AED are at risk of hemorrhage owing to decreased vitamin K-dependent clotting factors. Although some question the evidence, women taking carbamazepine, phenobarbital, primidone, or phenytoin should receive vitamin K 10 mg orally every day from 36 weeks of gestation until delivery, and babies should also receive vitamin K 1 mg IM at birth.[233]

Breast-Feeding

In a lactating woman who is taking medications, the risk of drug exposure to the infant needs to be weighed against the benefits of breast-feeding.[234] All drugs transfer into milk to some extent. The extent of protein binding of the drug is the most important predictor of drug passage into milk.[235,236] For the AED, a large intersubject variability in the milk:plasma ratio (M:P) is seen, presumably owing to a difference in volume and composition of the milk. Thus, the M:P ratio is not useful for predicting infant AED exposure. Two recent reviews on AED and breast-feeding are available.[237,238] For most first-generation AED (carbamazepine, phenytoin, valproic acid), breast-feeding results in negligible AED plasma concentrations in the infants. For the second-generation AED, breast-feeding should be done cautiously and the infant should be monitored for excess AED plasma concentrations and toxicity, if possible. This information should be presented to P.Z. in an appropriate manner. Once she delivers her baby, re-evaluation and optimization of P.Z.'s AED therapy should occur.

STATUS EPILEPTICUS

Characteristics and Pathophysiology

41. V.S., a 22-year-old, 85-kg man, was recently diagnosed as having idiopathic epilepsy with generalized tonic-clonic seizures. For the past 3 months, he has been treated with 600 mg/day of carbamazepine, which completely eliminated his seizures. His steady-state carbamazepine serum concentration was 10 mcg/mL. While at his parents' home, he had two tonic-clonic seizures, each lasting 3 to 4 minutes. On arrival at the hospital (~30 minutes after the first seizure began), he was noted to be only semiconscious. His blood pressure was 197/104 mmHg, his pulse was 124 beats/minute, respirations were 23 breaths/minute, and his body temperature was 37.5°C rectally. Shortly after his arrival, another generalized tonic-clonic seizure began. How does V.S.'s current condition meet accepted diagnostic criteria for status epilepticus? What risks are associated with status epilepticus?

Status epilepticus (SE) exists if "recurrent seizures occur without complete recovery of consciousness between attacks or virtually continuous seizure activity for >30 minutes, with or without impaired consciousness."[239] Because V.S. has had three seizures within slightly more than 30 minutes and remains unconscious, his present condition meets this definition. V.S. is experiencing generalized convulsive SE; this is the most common type and it is associated with the greatest risk of physical and neurologic damage. SE also may be characterized by nonconvulsive seizures that produce a persistent state of impaired consciousness or by partial seizures (motor or sensory) that may not interfere with consciousness.

Uncontrolled, convulsive SE can cause severe metabolic and hemodynamic alterations. V.S.'s vital signs (tachycardia, elevated blood pressure, increased respiratory rate, and elevated body temperature) are typical for a patient in SE. Prolonged, severe muscle contractions and CNS dysfunction from uncontrolled seizure discharges result in hyperthermia, cardiorespiratory collapse, myoglobinuria, renal failure, and neurologic damage. Neurologic damage also may occur with nonconvulsive SE; the neurologic sequelae of SE are related to the excessive electrical activity and resulting alterations in brain metabolism. When seizure activity persists longer than approximately 30 minutes, failure of mechanisms that regulate cerebral blood flow is more likely; this failure accompanies dramatic increases in brain metabolism and demand for glucose and oxygen. Failure to meet the metabolic demands of brain tissue results in accumulation of lactate and cell death. Peripherally, lactate accumulates and serum glucose and electrolytes are altered. After 30 minutes of seizure activity, the body often fails to compensate for increased metabolic demands, and cardiovascular collapse can occur.[240,241] For these reasons, SE is considered a medical emergency that requires immediate treatment to prevent or lessen both physical and neurologic damage. Mortality in SE may be 20% or higher[239]; fatal outcome is often the result of the injury or condition that precipitated SE (e.g., cardiopulmonary arrest, stroke). Long-term neurologic consequences of severe SE may include cognitive impairment, memory loss, and worsening of seizure disorders. The effect of SE on cognitive function is not clearly established, however; cognitive impairment may result from the neurologic disorder underlying SE rather than from SE itself.[242]

General Treatment Measures and Antiepileptic Drug Therapy

42. Describe a general treatment plan for V.S.'s episode of status epilepticus.

The immediate therapeutic concern in V.S. is to ensure ventilation and terminate current seizure activity. If possible, an airway should be placed; however, this may not be possible while he is convulsing. Objects (e.g., spoons, tongue blades) should never be placed into the mouth of a seizing patient. If airway placement is impossible, V.S. should be positioned on his side to allow drainage of saliva and mucus from the mouth and prevent aspiration. An IV line should be established using normal saline, and blood should be obtained for serum chemistries (especially glucose and electrolytes), AED serum concentrations, and toxicology screens. Glucose, 25 g (50 mL of 50% dextrose solution) by IV push should be administered to correct any hypoglycemia, which may be responsible for SE. Glucose administration should be preceded by IV thiamine 100 mg or vitamin B complex to prevent Wernicke's encephalopathy.[239]

Intravenous administration of rapidly effective anticonvulsant medication should begin as soon as possible to terminate V.S.'s seizure activity. IM or rectal administration of medication is not recommended in the initial treatment of this condition unless IV access is impossible. IM medications are unlikely to be absorbed sufficiently rapidly to achieve the CNS concentrations needed to terminate status seizures.

43. Which anticonvulsants are available for IV administration? Evaluate the available drugs and recommend a drug, dosage, and regimen for initial treatment of status epilepticus in V.S.

Lorazepam (Ativan), diazepam (Valium), phenytoin (Dilantin), and fosphenytoin (Cerebyx) are the agents most commonly employed as IV therapy in the initial treatment of SE.[243] Phenytoin and fosphenytoin are indicated for treatment of SE, but owing to limitations on their rates of infusion, the onset of their peak effect may be delayed. Therefore, phenytoin or fosphenytoin are usually used following initial treatment with lorazepam or diazepam.

Intravenous sodium valproate (Depacon) is available, but it is not indicated for the treatment of SE. Although the manufacturer only recommends Depacon be administered slowly (<20 mg/minute), it has been administered safely at higher doses and rates.[244] Currently, IV valproate is indicated only for use in patients who cannot take oral dosage forms of valproate. An IV form of levetiracetam is now available. This drug also is indicted only for patients who cannot receive oral dosage forms of levetiracetam. Rapid IV administration of levetiracetam has been used, however, in the treatment of SE in Europe.[245] IV phenobarbital is usually reserved for SE that does not respond to benzodiazepines and phenytoin.

Four IV regimens for generalized convulsive SE have been directly compared.[246] The trial evaluated diazepam (0.15 mg/kg) followed by phenytoin (18 mg/kg), lorazepam (0.1 mg/kg) alone, phenobarbital (15 mg/kg) alone, and phenytoin (18 mg/kg) alone. For initial IV treatment of overt generalized SE, lorazepam was more effective than phenytoin alone. Lorazepam was as effective as the other two regimens, and it was easier to use.

Intravenous administration of either diazepam or lorazepam is usually effective for rapid termination of seizure activity in SE.[247] Owing to diazepam's higher lipid solubility, it redistributes from the CNS to peripheral tissues rapidly after administration; this results in a short duration of action (<60 minutes).[248] Lorazepam's lower lipid solubility prevents rapid redistribution and accounts for its longer duration of action.[248] Lorazepam may be effective for up to 72 hours.[249,250] Owing to this longer duration, lorazepam is now the preferred benzodiazepine for immediate treatment of SE in many centers.[239] Repeated doses of lorazepam have been associated with development of tachyphylaxis, and lorazepam may be less effective for patients who have received chronic maintenance doses of benzodiazepines.[251,252] At adequate doses, the onset of antiepileptic activity and efficacy of lorazepam and diazepam are equal.[247]

Either 0.1 mg/kg of lorazepam at 2 mg/minute or 0.2 mg/kg of diazepam at 5 mg/minute by IV is administered to stop SE.[239] Lorazepam may cause significant venous irritation, and the manufacturer recommends dilution with an equal volume of normal saline solution or water for injection before IV administration. Doses of either lorazepam or diazepam should be repeated after 5 to 10 minutes if seizure activity has not stopped. The efficacy of either drug depends on rapid achievement of high serum and CNS concentrations. Although both diazepam and lorazepam can be administered IM, this route should not be used for treatment of SE because it is unlikely that either drug would achieve serum concentrations necessary for termination of seizure activity. This is especially true for diazepam, which is absorbed slowly and erratically from gluteal IM injection sites.[248] Both lorazepam and diazepam are relatively safe drugs. Their primary adverse effects are sedation, hypotension, and respiratory arrest.[248] These side effects are usually short-lived and, when adequate facilities are available for assisted ventilation and administration of fluids, they usually can be managed without major risk to the patient. Respiratory depression occurs most commonly in patients who receive multiple IV medications for control of SE.

Intravenous Phenytoin and Fosphenytoin

44. V.S. was given lorazepam 8 mg IV. Seizure activity ceased 5 minutes after the injection was completed. What drug should be administered to V.S. for prolonged control of seizures? Recommend a dose, route, and method of administration.

Continued effective seizure control is important for patients who experience SE. Previously, when diazepam was the benzodiazepine predominantly used for immediate control of SE, a long-acting AED such as phenytoin was routinely administered at the same time to ensure continued suppression of seizure activity. Routine use of phenytoin has been somewhat de-emphasized with increased use of lorazepam[239]; lorazepam's apparent longer duration of effect may make routine use of IV phenytoin less necessary. Nevertheless, many centers still use phenytoin in conjunction with both lorazepam and diazepam.

The availability of fosphenytoin (Cerebyx) for IV administration has provided an additional option for administration of phenytoin in the treatment of SE. Use of this phenytoin prodrug allows more rapid administration of large IV loading doses of phenytoin with less risk of injection site complications and potentially fewer cardiovascular adverse effects. Fosphenytoin itself is inactive; the therapeutic effect results from its conversion to phenytoin.[121,122] Because fosphenytoin is more expensive, many facilities have been reluctant to place this product on their formularies. Pharmacoeconomic studies, however, seem to indicate that, although it is initially more expensive, fosphenytoin may be more economical because it causes fewer adverse effects than phenytoin.[253] Generic formulations of injectable sodium phenytoin are still available; nevertheless, when the safety profile of fosphenytoin is considered, fosphenytoin may ultimately replace parenteral sodium phenytoin injection.

Phenytoin (administered as either sodium phenytoin injection or as sodium fosphenytoin injection) is presently considered the long-acting anticonvulsant of choice for most patients with generalized convulsive SE.[243] Extensive clinical experience with the use of IV loading doses of phenytoin has established its efficacy and general safety. Phenytoin causes much less sedation and respiratory depression than drugs such as phenobarbital when it is used in conjunction with IV benzodiazepines.[239] V.S.'s maintenance carbamazepine therapy produced moderate serum concentrations and was previously effective. Without obvious precipitating factors such as head trauma, CNS infection, and drug or alcohol abuse, SE, in a patient with a history of epilepsy, most commonly results from poor compliance with maintenance medication. Therefore, IV use of either phenytoin or fosphenytoin is a good choice for re-establishing effective AED therapy for V.S.

LOADING DOSE

Whether or not V.S. has a detectable serum concentration of carbamazepine, he should be given an IV loading dose of either phenytoin (20 mg/kg IV at 50 mg/minute) or fosphenytoin (20 mg/kg PE IV at 150 mg/minute). After administration of either of these loading doses, serum phenytoin concentrations should remain >10 mcg/mL for approximately 24 hours; this will allow time for determination of V.S.'s serum carbamazepine concentration and estimation of an appropriate maintenance dose of oral carbamazepine. In this setting, the use of IV phenytoin or fosphenytoin is a temporary measure. V.S.'s previous positive response to carbamazepine indicates that he should continue to receive this drug as oral maintenance medication.

Intravenous phenytoin can be administered by direct injection into a running IV line. The rate of administration should be no faster than 50 mg/minute to minimize the risk of hypotension and acute cardiac arrhythmias. Cardiovascular status (blood pressure, electrocardiogram) should be monitored closely during administration. Hypotension or electrocardiographic abnormalities usually reverse if the administration of phenytoin is slowed or stopped temporarily. If fosphenytoin is administered, it can be given by either direct IV injection or, after dilution in any suitable IV solution, by infusion at up to 150 mg PE/minute.[121] Absence of propylene glycol as a diluent renders fosphenytoin potentially less likely than phenytoin to cause cardiovascular adverse effects; however, clear documentation of this effect is lacking. Electrocardiographic and blood pressure monitoring is recommended when this drug is given IV. Pruritus and paresthesias, usually localized to the face and groin, are relatively common side effects during IV fosphenytoin administration. These sensations are not allergic reactions to the medication. Their occurrence is related to the administration rate, and they are reversible with temporary discontinuation or slowing of the injection.[121] These side effects are thought to be related to the phosphate component of fosphenytoin.

INTRAVENOUS INFUSION

45. V.S.'s physician is reluctant to administer this dose of either phenytoin or fosphenytoin by direct IV injection. What are the guidelines for administration of phenytoin and fosphenytoin by IV infusion?

Practical difficulties associated with administration of phenytoin by direct IV push undoubtedly have contributed to its low usage rate. In many hospitals or other facilities, direct IV injections must be administered by a physician, and many physicians would be unwilling to commit the 30 to 45 minutes necessary to administer V.S.'s loading dose at a safe rate. In addition, the rate of direct IV administration is difficult to control, and too-rapid administration resulting in cardiac toxicity is a risk. Although fosphenytoin can be given at a faster injection rate with a lower risk of complications, direct IV administration of this drug still presents practical difficulties.

The compatibility of phenytoin injection with IV solutions has been controversial. Phenytoin's chemical properties (weakly acidic with a pKa of 8 and low water solubility) require that the commercial injectable dosage form of sodium phenytoin be dissolved in a mixture of 40% propylene glycol and 10% alcohol; the pH of the final product is adjusted to approximately 12 with sodium hydroxide. Addition of the preparation to IV fluids dilutes the drug's solvent system and reduces pH. A possible result would be precipitation of free phenytoin. Several studies indicate, however, that phenytoin can be diluted, preferably in small total volumes, with saline solution.[254,255] Despite the formation of crystals in many solutions, measured phenytoin concentrations are essentially identical to those predicted. Thus, dilution of the required volume of phenytoin injection in approximately 100 to 500 mL of 0.45% or 0.9% saline should provide an appropriate solution for IV administration. An in-line filter of 0.45 to 0.22 micron pore size may be used to prevent the infusion of crystals.[253] The administration rate should be no faster than 50 mg/minute. This method of administration is both safe and effective when the infusion rate is monitored carefully. Burning pain at the IV infusion site, hypotension, and cardiac arrhythmias can occur during the infusion and appear to be related to the infusion rate. Either slowing or temporarily stopping the infusion may relieve these side effects.[256,257] IV administration of phenytoin is also associated with phlebitis; extravasation has resulted in chemical cellulitis and tissue necrosis.[258]

Intravenous infusion of fosphenytoin is less troublesome. Fosphenytoin is compatible with virtually all IV fluids because of its high water solubility and the lower pH required to maintain the drug in solution. Hypotension can occur during fosphenytoin infusion, and cardiovascular status should still be monitored closely. Fosphenytoin should not be infused at a rate >150 mg PE/minute. Injection site complications and phlebitis are significantly less likely with administration of fosphenytoin.[120]

Maintenance Therapy

46. Following administration of IV phenytoin, no further seizures occurred. The laboratory reported that serum chemistries were all normal. The carbamazepine serum concentration was 5 mcg/mL on admission. A serum phenytoin concentration determined 1 hour after administration of the IV loading dose was 24 mcg/mL. How should V.S.'s maintenance AED therapy be altered?

The reduced serum concentration of carbamazepine appears to confirm the role of nonadherence in this episode of SE. As V.S. was previously well controlled on 600 mg/day, this also would be a reasonable maintenance dosage at this time. Administration of maintenance doses should be resumed as soon as V.S. can take oral medication. V.S. should be counseled regarding the importance of taking his medication according to directions.

Alternative Therapies for Refractory Status Epilepticus

47. What other medications are options for treatment of SE that does not respond to benzodiazepines or phenytoin?

Phenobarbital may be useful for treatment of SE if the patient cannot tolerate phenytoin or when seizures continue following administration of appropriate loading doses of phenytoin. Patients who receive phenobarbital after being treated with IV benzodiazepines should be monitored closely for respiratory depression because this effect may be additive. Equipment and personnel to provide ventilatory assistance should be available.[239] Administration of IV phenobarbital can cause hypotension, which may necessitate discontinuation of the drug or the use of pressor agents. An initial dose of 20 mg/kg given IV at a rate no faster than 100 mg/minute is recommended.[239] IM administration of phenobarbital results in slow absorption, and this route of administration is not recommended for treatment of SE.

Pentobarbital or other anesthetic barbiturates are administered for treatment of SE that has not responded to more conservative measures, including phenobarbital. Significant respiratory depression is expected with this therapy; patients will require intubation and mechanical ventilation. In addition, vasopressors, such as dopamine or dobutamine, may be required to control hypotension. Constant EEG monitoring also is required to assess the effect of the drug.

Pentobarbital is given as a loading dose of 5 mg/kg IV and is followed by an IV infusion of 0.5 to 3 mg/kg/hour.[239] The dose and infusion rate are adjusted to produce either a flat or a burst-suppression EEG pattern.[259] Most protocols for pentobarbital coma recommend attempts at gradually reducing the dose of medication after 12 to 24 hours of treatment. If clinical or EEG seizure activity recurs, the dose is increased again to produce continued EEG suppression. Pentobarbital coma may be continued for several days in some patients.

Several other drugs have been used for treatment of refractory SE, but experience with these agents is somewhat limited. Midazolam (Versed), a short-acting anesthetic benzodiazepine, has been used by IV infusion.[260–262] Valproate has been used for treatment of refractory SE. Because no parenteral form of this drug has been available until recently, the syrup form has been administered either rectally or via nasogastric tube. At present, information regarding the IV use of valproate for SE is largely anecdotal.[263] Other drugs that have been used for refractory SE include lidocaine (Xylocaine), general anesthetics (halothane or isoflurane), and propofol.[243,264,265]

REFERENCES

1. Commission on Epidemiology and Prognosis, International League Against Epilepsy. Guidelines for epidemiologic studies on epilepsy. *Epilepsia* 1993;34:592.
2. Annegers JF. The epidemiology of epilepsy. In: Wyllie E, ed. *The Treatment of Epilepsy: Principles and Practice*. 3rd ed. Philadelphia: Lippincott Williams & Wilkins; 2001:131.
3. Luders HO et al. Classification of seizures. In: Wyllie E, ed. *The Treatment of Epilepsy: Principles and Practice*. 3rd ed. Philadelphia: Lippincott Williams & Wilkins; 2001:287.
4. Dreifuss FE. Classification of epileptic seizures and the epilepsies. *Pediatr Clin North Am* 1989;36:265.
5. Dreifuss FE. The epilepsies: clinical implications of the international classification. *Epilepsia* 1990;31(Suppl 3):S3.
6. Holmes GL. Electroencephalographic and neuroradiologic evaluation of children with epilepsy. *Pediatr Clin North Am* 1989;36:395.
7. Berg AT et al. Discontinuing antiepileptic drugs. In: Engel J et al., eds. *Epilepsy: A Comprehensive Textbook*. Philadelphia: Lippincott-Raven; 1998:1275.
8. Callaghan N et al. Withdrawal of anticonvulsant drugs in patients free of seizures for two years: a prospective study. *N Engl J Med* 1988;318:942.
9. Matricardi M et al. Outcome after discontinuation of antiepileptic drug therapy in children with epilepsy. *Epilepsia* 1989;30:582.
10. Wiebe S et al. A randomized, controlled trial of surgery for temporal-lobe epilepsy. *N Engl J Med* 2001;345:311.
11. Bainbridge JL et al. The ketogenic diet. *Pharmacotherapy* 1999;19:782.
12. Hassan AM et al. Ketogenic diet in the treatment of refractory epilepsy in childhood. *Pediatr Neurol* 1999;21:548.
13. Tecoma ES et al. Vagus nerve stimulation use and effect in epilepsy: what have we learned? *Epilepsy Behav*. 2006;8:127.
14. Schoenenberger RA et al. Appropriateness of antiepileptic drug level monitoring. *JAMA* 1995; 274:1622.
15. Reynolds EH. Early treatment and prognosis of epilepsy. *Epilepsia* 1987;28:97.
16. Pellock JM. Efficacy and adverse effects of antiepileptic drugs. *Pediatr Clin North Am* 1989;36: 435.
17. Devinsky O. Patients with refractory seizures. *N Engl J Med* 1999;340:1565.
18. Karceski S et al. The expert consensus guideline series: the treatment of epilepsy. *Epilepsy Behav* 2001;2:A1.
19. French JA et al. Efficacy and tolerability of the new antiepileptic drugs. I: Treatment of new onset epilepsy: report of the Therapeutics and Technology Assessment Subcommittee and Quality Standards Subcommittee of the American Academy of Neurology and the American Epilepsy Society. *Neurology*. 2004;62:1252.
20. French JA et al. Efficacy and tolerability of the new antiepileptic drugs. II: Treatment of refractory epilepsy: report of the Therapeutics and Technology Assessment Subcommittee and Quality Standards Subcommittee of the American Academy of Neurology and the American Epilepsy Society. *Neurology*. 2004;62:1261.
21. Garnett WR. Antiepileptic drug treatment: outcomes and adherence. *Pharmacotherapy*. 2000;20: 191S.
22. Choonara IA et al. Therapeutic drug monitoring of anticonvulsants: state of the art. *Clin Pharmacokinet* 1990;18:318.
23. Hayes G et al. Reassessing the lower end of the phenytoin therapeutic range: a review of the literature. *Ann Pharmacother* 1993;27: 1389.
24. Tomson T et al. Therapeutic monitoring of antiepileptic drugs for epilepsy. *Cochrane Database of Syst Rev* 2007;2. Art. No.:CD002216. DOI: 10.1002/14651858.CD002216.pub2.
25. Commission on Antiepileptic Drugs, International League Against Epilepsy. Guidelines for therapeutic monitoring on antiepileptic drugs. *Epilepsia* 1993;34:585.
26. Tozer TN et al. Phenytoin. In: Evans WE et al., eds. *Applied Pharmacokinetics: Principles of*

Therapeutic Drug Monitoring. 3rd ed. Vancouver: Applied Therapeutics; 1992:25.
27. Levy RH et al. Carbamazepine, valproic acid, phenobarbital, and ethosuximide. In: Evans WE et al., eds. *Applied Pharmacokinetics: Principles of Therapeutic Drug Monitoring*. 3rd ed. Vancouver: Applied Therapeutics; 1992:26.
28. Chadwick DW. Concentration-effect relationships of valproic acid. *Clin Pharmacokinet* 1985;10:155.
29. Bourgeois BFD. Valproic acid: clinical efficacy and use in epilepsy. In: Levy RH et al., eds. *Antiepileptic Drugs*. 5th ed. Philadelphia: Lippincott Williams & Wilkins; 2002:808.
30. Ohtsuka Y et al. Treatment of intractable childhood epilepsy with high-dose valproate. *Epilepsia* 1992;33:158.
31. Hurst DL. Expanded therapeutic range of valproate. *Pediatr Neurol* 1987;3:342.
32. Woo E et al. If a well-stabilized epileptic patient has a subtherapeutic antiepileptic drug level, should the dose be increased? A randomized prospective study. *Epilepsia* 1988;29:129.
33. Cloyd JC. Pharmacokinetic pitfalls of present antiepileptic medications. *Epilepsia* 1991;32(Suppl 5):S53.
34. Schmidt D. Reduction of two-drug therapy in intractable epilepsy. *Epilepsia* 1983;24:368.
35. Smith DB et al. Results of a nationwide Veterans Administration Cooperative Study comparing the efficacy and toxicity of carbamazepine, phenobarbital, phenytoin, and primidone. *Epilepsia* 1987;28(Suppl 3):S50.
36. Thompson PJ et al. Anticonvulsant drugs and cognitive functions. *Epilepsia* 1982;23:531.
37. Albright P et al. Reduction of polypharmacy in epileptic patients. *Arch Neurol* 1985;42:797.
38. Prevey ML et al. Improvement in cognitive functioning and mood state after conversion to valproate monotherapy. *Neurology* 1989;39:1640.
39. Mirza WU et al. Results of antiepileptic drug reduction in patients with multiple handicaps and epilepsy. *Drug Invest* 1993;5:320.
40. Guberman A. Monotherapy or polytherapy for epilepsy? *Can J Neurol Sci* 1998;25:S3.
41. Chadwick DW et al. A double-blind trial of gabapentin monotherapy for newly diagnosed partial seizures. International Gabapentin Monotherapy Study Group 945-77. *Neurology* 1998;51:1282.
42. Devinsky O et al. Efficacy of felbamate monotherapy in patients undergoing presurgical evaluation of partial seizures. *Epilepsy Res* 1995;20:241.
43. Sachdeo RC et al. Topiramate monotherapy for partial seizures. *Epilepsia* 1997;38:294.
44. Schacter SC. Tiagabine monotherapy in the treatment of partial epilepsy. *Epilepsia* 1995;36:S2.
45. Gilliam F et al. An active-control trial of lamotrigine monotherapy for partial seizures. *Neurology* 1998;51:1018.
46. Arroyo S et al. Randomized dose-controlled study of topiramate as first-line therapy in epilepsy. *Acta Neurol Scand* 2005;112:214.
47. Shinnar S et al. Discontinuing antiepileptic drugs in children with epilepsy: a prospective study. *Ann Neurol* 1994;35:534.
48. Berg AT et al. Relapse following discontinuation of antiepileptic drugs: a meta-analysis. *Neurology* 1994;44:601.
49. Tennison M et al. Discontinuing antiepileptic drugs in children: a comparison of a six-week and a nine-month taper period. *N Engl J Med* 1994;330:1407.
50. Malow BA et al. Carbamazepine withdrawal: effects of taper rate on seizure frequency. *Neurology* 1993;43:2280.
51. Todt H. The late prognosis of epilepsy in childhood: results of a prospective follow-up study. *Epilepsia* 1984;25:137.
52. First Seizure Trial Group. Randomized clinical trial on the efficacy of antiepileptic drugs in reducing the risk of relapse after a first unprovoked tonic-clonic seizure. *Neurology* 1993;43:478.
53. Mattson RH et al. Comparison of carbamazepine, phenobarbital, phenytoin, and primidone in partial and secondarily generalized tonic-clonic seizures. *N Engl J Med* 1985;313:145.
54. Mattson RH et al. A comparison of valproate with carbamazepine for the treatment of complex partial seizures and secondarily generalized tonic-clonic seizures in adults. *N Engl J Med* 1992;327:765.
55. Beydoun A et al. Safety and efficacy of divalproex sodium monotherapy in partial epilepsy: a double-blind, concentration-response design clinical trial. *Neurology* 1997;48:182.
56. Franceschi M et al. Fatal aplastic anemia in a patient treated with carbamazepine. *Epilepsia* 1988;29:582.
57. Pisciotta AV. Carbamazepine: hematological toxicity. In: Woodbury DM et al., eds. *Antiepileptic Drugs*. 2nd ed. New York: Raven Press; 1982:533.
58. Pellock JM. Carbamazepine side effects in children and adults. *Epilepsia* 1987;28(Suppl 3):S64.
59. Holmes GL. Carbamazepine: adverse effects. In: Levy RH et al., eds. *Antiepileptic Drugs*. 5th ed. Philadelphia: Lippincott Williams & Wilkins; 2002:285.
60. Camfield C et al. Asymptomatic children with epilepsy: little benefit from screening for anticonvulsant-induced liver, blood, or renal damage. *Neurology* 1986;36:838.
61. Horowitz S et al. Hepatotoxic reactions associated with carbamazepine therapy. *Epilepsia* 1988;29:149.
62. Hadzic N et al. Acute liver failure induced by carbamazepine. *Arch Dis Child* 1990;65:315.
63. Livingston S et al. Carbamazepine (Tegretol) in epilepsy: nine-year follow-up study with special emphasis on untoward reactions. *Dis Nerv System* 1974;35:103.
64. Tomson T et al. Relationship of intraindividual dose to plasma concentration of carbamazepine: indication of dose-dependent induction of metabolism. *Ther Drug Monit* 1989;11:533.
65. Sanchez A et al. Steady-state carbamazepine concentration-dose ratio in epileptic patients. *Clin Pharmacokinet* 1986;11:41.
66. Oles KS et al. Bioequivalency revisited: Epitol versus Tegretol. *Neurology* 1993;43:2435.
67. Crawford P et al. Are there potential problems with generic substitution of antiepileptic drugs? A review of issues. *Seizure*. 2006;15:165.
68. The Tegretol Oros Osmotic Release Delivery System Study Group. Double-blind crossover comparison of Tegretol-XR and Tegretol in patients with epilepsy. *Neurology* 1995;45:1703.
69. Riss JR et al. Administration of Carbatrol to children with feeding tubes. *Pediatr Neurol* 2002; 27:193.
70. Graves NM. Felbamate. *Ann Pharmacother* 1993; 27:1073.
71. Sachdeo R et al. Felbamate monotherapy: controlled trial in patients with partial onset seizures. *Ann Neurol* 1992;32:386.
72. U.S. Gabapentin Study Group No. 5. Gabapentin as add-on therapy in refractory partial epilepsy: a double-blind, placebo-controlled, parallel-group study. *Neurology* 1993;43:2292.
73. U.S. Gabapentin Study Group. The long-term safety and efficacy of gabapentin (Neurontin) as add-on therapy in drug-resistant partial epilepsy. *Epilepsy Res* 1994;18:67.
74. UK Gabapentin Study Group. Gabapentin in partial epilepsy. *Lancet* 1990;335:1114.
75. Matsuo F et al. Placebo-controlled study of the efficacy and safety of lamotrigine in patients with partial seizures. *Neurology* 1993;43:2284.
76. Messenheimer J et al. Lamotrigine therapy for partial seizures: a multicenter, placebo-controlled, double-blind, cross-over trial. *Epilepsia* 1994;35:113.
77. Sachdeo RC et al. Tiagabine therapy for complex partial seizures. A dose-frequency study. *Arch Neurol* 1997;54:595.
78. Ben-Menachem E et al. Double-blind, placebo-controlled trial of topiramate as add-on therapy in patients with refractory partial seizures. *Epilepsia* 1996;37:539.
79. Sharief M et al. Double-blind, placebo-controlled study of topiramate in patients with refractory partial epilepsy. *Epilepsy Res* 1996;25:217.
80. Faught E. Efficacy of topiramate as adjunctive therapy in refractory partial seizures: United States trial experience. *Epilepsia* 1997;38(Suppl 1):S24.
81. McAuley JW et al. Newer therapies in the drug treatment of epilepsy. *Ann Pharmacother* 2002;36:119.
82. Shneker BF et al. Pregabalin: a new neuromodulator with broad therapeutic indications. *Ann Pharmacother* 2005;39:2029.
83. Pellock JM et al. Felbamate: 1997 update. *Epilepsia* 1997;38:1261.
84. Jones MW. Topiramate: safety and tolerability. *Can J Neurol Sci* 1998;25:S13.
85. McLean MJ et al. Safety and tolerability of gabapentin as adjunctive therapy in a large, multicenter study. *Epilepsia* 1999;40:965.
86. Leppik IE et al. Safety of tiagabine: summary of 53 trials. *Epilepsy Res* 1999;33:235.
87. Sirsi D et al. The safety of levetiracetam. *Expert Opinion on Drug Safety* 2007;6:241.
88. Guberman AH et al. Lamotrigine-associated rash: risk/benefit considerations in adults and children. *Epilepsia* 1999;40:985.
89. Tecoma ES. Oxcarbazepine. *Epilepsia* 1999;40 (Suppl 5):S37.
90. Oommen KJ et al. Zonisamide: a new antiepileptic drug. *Clin Neuropharmacol* 1999;22:192.
91. Goa KL et al. Gabapentin: a review of its pharmacological properties and clinical potential in epilepsy. *Drugs* 1993;46:409.
92. Luer MS et al. Tiagabine: a novel antiepileptic drug. *Ann Pharmacother* 1998;32:1173.
93. Sachdeo R et al. Coadministration of phenytoin and felbamate: evidence of additional phenytoin dose-reduction requirements based on pharmacokinetics and tolerability with increasing doses of felbamate. *Epilepsia* 1999;40:1122.
94. Albani F et al. Effect of felbamate on plasma levels of carbamazepine and its metabolites. *Epilepsia* 1991;32:130.
95. So EL et al. Seizure exacerbation and status epilepticus related to carbamazepine-10,11-epoxide. *Ann Neurol* 1994;35:743.
96. Yuen AWC et al. Sodium valproate acutely inhibits lamotrigine metabolism. *Br J Clin Pharmacol* 1992;33:511.
97. Anderson GD et al. Bidirectional interaction of valproate and lamotrigine in healthy subjects. *Clin Pharmacol Ther* 1996;60:145.
98. Warner T et al. Lamotrigine-induced carbamazepine toxicity: an interaction with carbamazepine-10,11-epoxide. *Epilepsy Res* 1992;11:147.
99. Besag FM et al. Carbamazepine toxicity with lamotrigine: pharmacokinetic or pharmacodynamic interaction? *Epilepsia* 1998;39:183.
100. Welty TE et al. Levetiracetam: a different approach to the pharmacotherapy of epilepsy. *Ann Pharmacother* 2002;36:296.
101. Fattore C et al. Induction of ethynylestradiol and levonorgestrel metabolism by oxcarbazepine in healthy women. *Epilepsia* 1999;40:783.
102. Bialer M et al. Progress report on new antiepileptic drugs: a summary of the Eighth Eilat Conference (EILAT VIII). *Epilepsy Res* 2007;73:1.
103. Jacobs MP et al. Future directions for epilepsy research. *Neurology* 2001(13);57:1536.
104. Loscher W et al. Role of multidrug transporters in pharmacoresistance to antiepileptic drugs. *J Pharmacol Exp Ther* 2002;301:7.
105. Mann MW et al. Various pharmacogenetic aspects of antiepileptic drug therapy: a review. *CNS Drugs*. 2007;21:143.
106. Fitton A et al. Lamotrigine: an update of its pharmacology and therapeutic use in epilepsy. *Drugs* 1995;50:691.
107. Kilpatrick ES et al. Concentration-effect and concentration-toxicity relations with lamotrigine: a prospective study. *Epilepsia* 1996;37:534.

108. Tozer TN et al. Phenytoin. In: Evans WE et al., eds. *Applied Pharmacokinetics: Principles of Therapeutic Drug Monitoring*. 3rd ed. Vancouver: Applied Therapeutics; 1992:25.
109. Allen JP et al. Phenytoin cumulation kinetics. *Clin Pharmacol Ther* 1979;26:445.
110. Evans RP et al. Phenytoin toxicity and blood levels after a large oral dose. *Am J Hosp Pharm* 1980;37:232.
111. Ludden TM et al. Rate of phenytoin accumulation in man: a simulation study. *J Pharmacokinetics Biopharm* 1978;6:399.
112. Osborn HH et al. Single-dose oral phenytoin loading. *Ann Emerg Med* 1987;16:407.
113. Goff DA et al. Absorption characteristics of three phenytoin sodium products after administration of oral loading doses. *Clin Pharm* 1984;3:634.
114. Jung D et al. Effect of dose on phenytoin absorption. *Clin Pharmacol Ther* 1980;28:479.
115. Record KE et al. Oral phenytoin loading in adults: rapid achievement of therapeutic plasma levels. *Ann Neurol* 1979;5:268.
116. Cranford RE et al. Intravenous phenytoin: clinical and pharmacokinetic aspects. *Neurology* 1978;28:874.
117. Kostenbauder HB et al. Bioavailability and single-dose pharmacokinetics of intramuscular phenytoin. *Clin Pharmacol Ther* 1975;18:449.
118. Serrano EE et al. Plasma diphenylhydantoin values after oral and intramuscular administration of diphenylhydantoin. *Neurology* 1973;23:311.
119. Serrano EE et al. Intramuscular administration of diphenylhydantoin: histologic follow-up studies. *Arch Neurol* 1974;31:276.
120. Jamerson BD et al. Venous irritation related to intravenous administration of phenytoin versus fosphenytoin. *Pharmacotherapy* 1994;14:47.
121. Fischer JH et al. Fosphenytoin: clinical pharmacokinetics and comparative advantages in the acute treatment of seizures. *Clin Pharmacokinet* 2003;42:33.
122. Boucher BA. Fosphenytoin: a novel phenytoin prodrug. *Pharmacotherapy* 1996;16:777.
123. Ramsay RE et al. Intramuscular fosphenytoin (Cerebyx) in patients requiring a loading dose of phenytoin. *Epilepsy Res* 1997;28:181.
124. Silverman AK et al. Cutaneous and immunologic reactions to phenytoin. *J Am Acad Dermatol* 1988;18:721.
125. Butler RT et al. Drug-induced gingival hyperplasia: phenytoin, cyclosporine, and nifedipine. *J Am Dent Assoc* 1987;114:56.
126. Stinnett E et al. New developments in understanding phenytoin-induced gingival hyperplasia. *J Am Dent Assoc* 1987;114:814.
127. Bruni J. Phenytoin: adverse effects. In: Levy RH, et al., eds. *Antiepileptic Drugs*. 5th ed. Philadelphia: Lippincott Williams & Wilkins; 2002:605.
128. Kuruvilla T et al. Cerebellar atrophy after acute phenytoin intoxication. *Epilepsia* 1997;38:500.
129. Rapport RL et al. Phenytoin-related cerebellar degeneration without seizures. *Ann Neurol* 1977;2:437.
130. So EL et al. Adverse effects of phenytoin on peripheral nerves and neuromuscular junction: a review. *Epilepsia* 1981;22:467.
131. Lovelace RE et al. Peripheral neuropathy in long-term diphenylhydantoin therapy. *Arch Neurol* 1968;18:69.
132. Pack AM et al. Adverse effects of antiepileptic drugs on bone structure: epidemiology, mechanisms and therapeutic implications. *CNS Drugs*. 2001;15:633.
133. Sheth RD. Bone health in pediatric epilepsy. *Epilepsy Behav* 2004;5(Suppl 2):S30.
134. Pack AM et al. Bone mass and turnover in women with epilepsy on antiepileptic drug monotherapy. *Ann Neurol* 2005;57:252.
135. Brodie MJ et al. The UK lamotrigine elderly study group. Multicentre, double-blind, randomised comparison between lamotrigine and carbamazepine in elderly patients with newly diagnosed epilepsy. *Epilepsy Res* 1999;37:81.
136. Rowan AJ et al. New onset geriatric epilepsy: a randomized study of gabapentin, lamotrigine, and carbamazepine. *Neurology* 2005;64:1868.
137. Perucca E. Clinical pharmacokinetics of new-generation antiepileptic drugs at the extremes of age. *Clin Pharmacokinet* 2006;45:351.
138. Martin R et al. Cognitive functioning in community dwelling older adults with chronic partial epilepsy. *Epilepsia* 2005;46:298.
139. Piazzini A et al. Elderly people and epilepsy: cognitive function. *Epilepsia* 2006;47(Suppl 5):82.
140. Bambara JK et al. Medical decision-making abilities in older adults with chronic partial epilepsy. *Epilepsy Behav* 2007;10:63.
141. Fife TD et al. Measuring the effects of antiepileptic medications on balance in older people. *Epilepsy Res* 2006;70:103.
142. Coppola G et al. Lamotrigine versus valproic acid as first-line monotherapy in newly diagnosed typical absence seizures: an open-label, randomized parallel-group study. *Epilepsia* 2004;45:1053
143. Frank LM et al. Lamictal (lamotrigine) monotherapy for typical absence seizures in children. *Epilepsia* 1999;40:973.
144. Beran RG et al. Double-blind, placebo-controlled, crossover study of lamotrigine in treatment-resistant generalised epilepsy. *Epilepsia* 1998;39:1329.
145. Marson AG et al. The SANAD study of effectiveness of valproate, lamotrigine, or topiramate for generalised and unclassifiable epilepsy: an unblinded randomised controlled trial. *Lancet* 2007;369:1016.
146. Pellock JM et al. Trimethadione. In: Levy RH et al., eds. *Antiepileptic Drugs*. 4th ed. New York: Raven Press; 1995:689.
147. Mattson RH. Antiepileptic drug monotherapy in adults: selection and use in new-onset epilepsy. In: Levy RH et al., eds. *Antiepileptic Drugs*. 5th ed. Philadelphia: Lippincott Williams & Wilkins; 2002:72.
148. Sato S et al. Benzodiazepines: clonazepam. In: Levy RH et al., eds. *Antiepileptic Drugs*. 4th ed. New York: Raven Press; 1995:725.
149. Glauser TA. Succinimides: adverse effects. In: Levy RH et al., eds. *Antiepileptic Drugs*. 5th ed. Philadelphia: Lippincott Williams & Wilkins; 2002:658.
150. Browne TR et al. Absence (petit mal) seizures. In: Browne TR et al., eds. *Epilepsy: Diagnosis and Management*. Boston: Little Brown; 1983:61.
151. Livingston S et al. Petit mal epilepsy: results of a prolonged follow-up study of 117 patients. *JAMA* 1965;194:227.
152. Penry JK et al. Refractiveness of absence seizures and phenobarbital. *Neurology* 1981;31:158.
153. Scheuer ML et al. The evaluation and treatment of seizures. *N Engl J Med*. 1990;323:1468.
154. Snead OC et al. Exacerbation of seizures in children by carbamazepine. *N Engl J Med* 1985;313:916.
155. Shields WD et al. Myoclonic, atonic and absence seizures following institution of carbamazepine therapy in children. *Neurology* 1983;33:1487.
156. Jones-Saete C et al. External leakage from feeding gastrostomies in patients receiving valproate sprinkle. *Epilepsia* 1992;33:692.
157. Zaccara G et al. Clinical pharmacokinetics of valproic acid, 1988. *Clin Pharmacokinet* 1988;15:367.
158. Cloyd JC et al. Comparison of sprinkle versus syrup formulations of valproate for bioavailability, tolerance, and preference. *J Pediatr* 1992;120:634.
159. Dutta S et al. Comparison of the bioavailability of unequal doses of divalproex sodium extended-release formulation relative to the delayed-release formulation in healthy volunteers. *Epilepsy Res* 2002;49:1.
160. Fischer JH et al. Effect of food on the serum concentration profile of enteric-coated valproic acid. *Neurology* 1988;38:1319.
161. Bauer LA et al. Valproic acid clearance: unbound fraction and diurnal variation in young and elderly adults. *Clin Pharmacol Ther* 1985;37:697.
162. Tennison MB et al. Valproate metabolites and hepatotoxicity in an epileptic population. *Epilepsia* 1988;29:543.
163. Eadie MJ et al. Valproate-associated hepatotoxicity and its biochemical mechanisms. *Medical Toxicology* 1988;3:85.
164. Dreifuss FE et al. Valproic acid hepatic fatalities: a retrospective review. *Neurology* 1987;37:379.
165. Dreifuss FE et al. Valproic acid hepatic fatalities. II. U.S. experience since 1984. *Neurology* 1989;39:201.
166. Dreifuss FE. Valproic acid hepatic fatalities: revised table [Letter]. *Neurology* 1989;39:1558.
167. Scheffner E et al. Fatal liver failure in 16 children with valproate therapy. *Epilepsia* 1988;29:530.
168. Koenig SA et al. Valproic acid-induced hepatopathy: nine new fatalities in Germany from 1994 to 2003. *Epilepsia*. 2006;47:2027.
169. Willmore LJ. Clinical manifestations of valproate hepatotoxicity. In: Levy RH et al, eds. *Idiosyncratic Reactions to Valproate: Clinical Risk Patterns and Mechanisms of Toxicity*. New York: Raven Press; 1991:3.
170. Willmore LJ et al. Valproate toxicity: risk-screening strategies. *J Child Neurol* 1991;6:3.
171. Kriel RL et al. Rectal diazepam gel for treatment of acute repetitive seizures. The North American Diastat Study Group. *Pediatr Neurol* 1999;20:282.
172. Cloyd JC et al. A single-blind, crossover comparison of the pharmacokinetics and cognitive effects of a new diazepam rectal gel with intravenous diazepam. *Epilepsia* 1998;39:520.
173. Kriel RL et al. Home use of rectal diazepam for cluster and prolonged seizures: efficacy, adverse reactions, quality of life, and cost analysis. *Pediatr Neurol* 1991;7:13.
174. Waruiru C et al. Febrile seizures: an update. *Arch Dis Child*. 2004;89:751.
175. Duchowny M. Febrile seizures. In: Wyllie E, ed. *The Treatment of Epilepsy: Principles and Practice*. 3rd ed. Philadelphia: Lippincott Williams & Wilkins; 2001:601.
176. Berg AT et al. Predictors of recurrent febrile seizures: a metaanalytic review. *J Pediatr* 1990;116:329.
177. Fischbein CA et al. Diazepam to prevent febrile seizures [Letter]. *N Engl J Med* 1993;329:2033.
178. Newton RW. Randomized controlled trials of phenobarbitone and valproate in febrile convulsions. *Arch Dis Child* 1988;63:1189.
179. Farwell JR et al. Phenobarbital for febrile seizures: effects on intelligence and on seizure recurrence. *N Engl J Med* 1990;322:364.
180. Holmes GL et al. Panel discussion. *Epilepsia* 1991;32(Suppl 5):S80.
181. Sulzbacher S et al. Late cognitive effects of early treatment with phenobarbital. *Clin Pediatr* 1999;38:387.
182. Meador KJ. Cognitive effects of epilepsy and of antiepileptic medications. In: Wyllie E, ed. *The Treatment of Epilepsy: Principles and Practice*. 3rd ed. Philadelphia: Lippincott Williams & Wilkins; 2001:1215.
183. Committee on Drugs. Behavioral and cognitive effects of anticonvulsant therapy. *Pediatrics* 1985;76:644.
184. Hanzel TE et al. A case of phenobarbital exacerbation of a preexisting maladaptive behavior partially suppressed by chlorpromazine and misinterpreted as chlorpromazine efficacy. *Res Dev Disabil* 1992;13:381.
185. Rosman NP et al. A controlled trial of diazepam administered during febrile illnesses to prevent recurrence of febrile seizures. *N Engl J Med* 1993;329:79.
186. Prevention and treatment of injury from chemical warfare agents. *Med Letter Drugs Ther* 2002;44:1.
187. Holstege CP et al. Chemical warfare: nerve agent poisoning. *Crit Care Clin* 1997;13:923.
188. Leikin JB et al. A review of nerve agent exposure for the critical care physician. *Crit Care Med* 2002;30:2346.

189. Wroblewski BA et al. Carbamazepine–erythromycin interaction: case studies and clinical significance. *JAMA* 1986;255:1165.
190. Miles MV et al. Erythromycin effects on multiple-dose carbamazepine pharmacokinetics. *Ther Drug Monit* 1989;11:47.
191. Scheyer RD. Valproate: drug interactions. In: Levy RH et al., eds. *Antiepileptic Drugs*. 5th ed. Philadelphia: Lippincott Williams & Wilkins; 2002:801.
192. Genton P et al. Valproate: adverse effects. In: Levy RH et al., eds. *Antiepileptic Drugs*. 5th ed. Philadelphia: Lippincott Williams & Wilkins; 2002:837.
193. Blackburn SC et al. Antiepileptics and blood dyscrasias: a cohort study. *Pharmacotherapy* 1998; 18:1277.
194. Gidal B et al. Valproate-mediated disturbances of hemostasis: relationship to dose and plasma concentration. *Neurology* 1994;44:1418.
195. Barr RD et al. Valproic acid and immune thrombocytopenia. *Arch Dis Childhood* 1982;57:681.
196. Dreifuss FE et al. Hepatic considerations in the use of antiepileptic drugs. *Epilepsia* 1987;28(Suppl 2):S23.
197. Smythe MA et al. Phenytoin hepatotoxicity: a review of the literature. *Drug Intell Clin Pharm* 1989;23:13.
198. Howard PA et al. Phenytoin hypersensitivity syndrome: a case report. *Drug Intell Clin Pharm* 1991;25:929.
199. Pelekanos J et al. Allergic rash due to antiepileptic drugs: clinical features and management. *Epilepsia* 1991;32:554.
200. Shear NH et al. Anticonvulsant hypersensitivity syndrome: in vitro assessment of risk. *J Clin Invest* 1988;82:1826.
201. Pirmohamed M et al. Detection of an autoantibody directed against human liver microsomal protein in a patient with carbamazepine hypersensitivity. *Br J Clin Pharmacol* 1992;33:183.
202. Engel JN et al. Phenytoin hypersensitivity: a case of severe acute rhabdomyolysis. *Am J Med* 1986;81:928.
203. Reents SB et al. Phenytoin-carbamazepine cross-sensitivity. *Drug Intell Clin Pharm* 1989;23: 235.
204. Ettinger AB et al. Use of ethotoin in phenytoin-related hypersensitivity reactions. *J Epilepsy* 1993;6:29.
205. Arif H et al. Comparison and predictors of rash associated with 15 antiepileptic drugs. *Neurology* 2007;68:1701.
206. Beran RG. Cross-reactive skin eruption with both carbamazepine and oxcarbazepine. *Epilepsia*. 1993;34:163.
207. Asconape JJ. Some common issues in the use of antiepileptic drugs. *Semin Neurol* 2002;22:27.
208. McAuley JW et al. Treatment of epilepsy in women of reproductive age: pharmacokinetic considerations. *Clin Pharmacokinet* 2002;41:559.
209. Dansky LV. The teratogenic effects of epilepsy and anticonvulsant drugs. In: Hopkins A et al., eds. *Epilepsy*. New York: Demos; 1995:535.
210. Yerby MS et al. Antiepileptics and the development of congenital anomalies. *Neurology* 1992;42 (Suppl 5):132.
211. Delgado-Escueta AV et al. Consensus guidelines: preconception counseling, management, and care of the pregnant woman with epilepsy. *Neurology* 1992;42(Suppl 5):149.
212. Mattson RH et al. Use of oral contraceptives by women with epilepsy. *JAMA* 1986;256:238.
213. Back DJ et al. Evaluation of Committee on Safety of Medicines yellow card reports on oral contraceptive-drug interactions with anticonvulsants and antibiotics. *Br J Clin Pharmacol* 1988;25:527.
214. Crawford P. Interactions between antiepileptic drugs and hormonal contraception. *CNS Drugs* 2002;16:263.
215. Sills G et al. Pharmacokinetics and drug interactions with zonisamide. *Epilepsia*. 2007;48:435.
216. Rosenfeld WE et al. Effect of topiramate on the pharmacokinetics of an oral contraceptive containing norethindrone and ethinyl estradiol in patients with epilepsy. *Epilepsia* 1997;38:317.
217. Doose DR. Oral contraceptive–AED interactions: no effect of topiramate as monotherapy at clinically effective dosages of 200 mg or less. *Epilepsia* 2002;43(Suppl 7):205.
218. Christensen J et al. Oral contraceptives induce lamotrigine metabolism: evidence from a double-blind, placebo-controlled trial. *Epilepsia*. 2007;48: 484.
219. Krauss GL et al. Antiepileptic medication and oral contraceptive interactions: a national survey of neurologists and obstetricians. *Neurology* 1996;46:1534.
220. Morrell MJ. Catamenial epilepsy and issues of fertility, sexuality, and reproduction. In: Wyllie E, ed. *The Treatment of Epilepsy: Principles and Practice*. 3rd ed. Philadelphia: Lippincott Williams & Wilkins; 2001:671.
221. Zahn CA et al. Management issues for women with epilepsy: a review of the literature. *Neurology* 1998;51:949.
222. Holmes LB et al. The teratogenicity of anticonvulsant drugs. *N Engl J Med* 2001;344:1132.
223. Yerby MS et al. Teratogenicity of antiepileptic drugs. In: Engel J et al., eds. *Epilepsy: A Comprehensive Textbook*. Philadelphia: Lippincott-Raven; 1998:1195.
224. Kaneko S et al. Teratogenicity of antiepileptic drugs: analysis of possible risk factors. *Epilepsia* 1988;29:459.
225. Meador KJ et al. NEAD Study Group. In utero antiepileptic drug exposure: fetal death and malformations. *Neurology* 2006;67:407.
226. Holmes LB et al. Increased risk for non-syndromic cleft palate among infants exposed to lamotrigine during pregnancy [Abstract]. *Birth Defects Research* 2006;76:5.
227. FDA/CFSAN resources page. U.S. Food and Drug Administration Web site. Available at: http://www.fda.gov/cder/drug/InfoSheets/HCP/lamotrigineHCP.htm. Accessed March 22, 2007.
228. Meador KJ et al. In utero antiepileptic drugs: differential cognitive outcomes in children of women with epilepsy [Abstract]. *Epilepsia* 2006;47(Suppl 4):2.
229. Chen SS et al. Serum protein binding and free concentration of phenytoin and phenobarbitone in pregnancy. *Br J Clin Pharmacol* 1982;13:547.
230. Perucca E et al. Plasma protein binding of drugs in pregnancy. *Clin Pharmacokinet* 1982;7: 336.
231. Patel IH et al. Valproic acid binding to human serum albumin and determination of free fractions in the presence of anticonvulsants and free fatty acids. *Epilepsia* 1979;20:85.
232. Tomson T et al. Pharmacokinetics and therapeutic drug monitoring of newer antiepileptic drugs during pregnancy and the puerperium. *Clin Pharmacokinet*. 2007;46:209.
233. Pack AM. Therapy Insight: clinical management of pregnant women with epilepsy. *Nature Clinical Practice Neurology* 2006;2:190.
234. American Academy of Pediatrics Committee on Drugs. The transfer of drugs and other chemicals into human milk. *Pediatrics* 1994;93:137.
235. Begg EJ et al. Prospective evaluation of a model for the prediction of milk:plasma drug concentratoins from physiochemical characteristics. *Br J Clin Pharmacol* 1992;33:501.
236. Notarianni LJ et al. An in vitro technique for the rapid determination of drug entry into breast milk. *Br J Clin Pharmacol* 1995;40:333.
237. Hagg S et al. Anticonvulsant use during lactation. *Drug Saf* 2000;22:425.
238. Bar-Oz B et al. Anticonvulsants and breastfeeding: a critical review. *Pediatr Drugs* 2000; 2:113.
239. Treiman DM. Status epilepticus. In: Wyllie E, ed. *The Treatment of Epilepsy: Principles and Practice*. 3rd ed. Philadelphia: Lippincott Williams & Wilkins; 2001:681.
240. Wasterlain CG et al. Pathophysiologic mechanisms of brain damage from status epilepticus. *Epilepsia* 1993;34(Suppl 1):S37.
241. Lothman E. The biochemical basis and pathophysiology of status epilepticus. *Neurology* 1990; 40(Suppl 2):13.
242. Dodrill CB et al. Intellectual impairment as an outcome of status epilepticus. *Neurology* 1990;40.
243. Lowenstein DH et al. Status epilepticus. *N Engl J Med* 1998;338:970.
244. Ramsay RE et al. Safety and tolerance of rapidly infused Depacon. A randomized trial in subjects with epilepsy. *Epilepsy Res* 2003;52:189.
245. Besser R et al. Rapid intravenous infusion of levetiracetam: tolerability and pharmacokinetics in elderly epileptic patients [Abstract]. *Epilepsia*. 2007;48 (Suppl 3):40.
246. Treiman DM et al. A comparison of four treatments for generalized convulsive status epilepticus. Veterans Affairs Status Epilepticus Cooperative Study Group. *N Engl J Med* 1998;339:792.
247. Leppik IE et al. Double-blind study of lorazepam and diazepam for status epilepticus. *JAMA* 1983;249:1452.
248. Rey E et al. Pharmacokinetic optimization of benzodiazepine therapy for acute seizures. Focus on delivery routes. *Clin Pharmacokinet* 1999;36:409.
249. Levy RJ et al. Treatment of status epilepticus with lorazepam. *Arch Neurol* 1984;41:605.
250. Lacey DJ et al. Lorazepam therapy of status epilepticus in children and adolescents. *J Pediatr* 1986;108:771.
251. Treiman DM. The role of benzodiazepines in the management of status epilepticus. *Neurology* 1990;40(Suppl 2):32.
252. Crawford TO et al. Lorazepam in childhood status epilepticus and serial seizures: effectiveness and tachyphylaxis. *Neurology* 1987;37:190.
253. Armstrong EP et al. Phenytoin and fosphenytoin: a model of cost and clinical outcomes. *Pharmacotherapy* 1999;19:844.
254. Cloyd JC et al. Concentration-time profile of phenytoin after admixture with small volumes of intravenous fluids. *Am J Hosp Pharm* 1978;35:45.
255. Salem RB et al. Investigation of the crystallization of phenytoin in normal saline. *Am J Hosp Pharm* 1980;14:605.
256. DelaCruz FG et al. Efficacy of individualized phenytoin sodium loading doses administered by intravenous infusion. *Clin Pharm* 1988;7:219.
257. Vozeh S et al. Intravenous phenytoin loading in patients after neurosurgery and in status epilepticus: a population pharmacokinetic study. *Clin Pharmacokinet* 1988;14:122.
258. Spengler RF et al. Severe soft-tissue injury following intravenous infusion of phenytoin. Patient and drug administration risk factors. *Arch Intern Med* 1988;148:1329.
259. Yaffe K et al. Prognostic factors of pentobarbital therapy for refractory generalized status epilepticus. *Neurology* 1993;43:895.
260. Lal-Koul R et al. Continuous midazolam infusion as treatment of status epilepticus. *Arch Dis Child* 1997;76:445.
261. Denzel D et al. Midazolam in re-fractory status epilepticus. *Ann Pharmacother* 1996;30:1481.
262. Lowenstein DH et al. Treatment of refractory generalized status epilepticus with continuous infusion of midazolam. *Neurology* 1994;44:1837.
263. Hovinga CA et al. Use of intravenous valproate in three pediatric patients with nonconvulsive or convulsive status epilepticus. *Ann Pharmacother* 1999;33:579.
264. van Gestel JPJ et al. Propofol and thiopental for refractory status epilepticus in children. *Neurology* 2005;65:591.
265. Claassen J et al. Treatment of refractory status epilepticus with pentobarbital, propofol, or midazoloam: a systematic review. *Epilepsia* 2002;43:146.
266. Serratosa JM. Juvenile myoclonic epilepsy. In: Wyllie E, ed. *The Treatment of Epilepsy: Principles and Practice*. 3rd ed. Philadelphia: Lippincott Williams & Wilkins; 2001:491.

267. Farrell K. Secondary generalized epilepsy and Lennox-Gastaut syndrome. In: Wyllie E, ed. *The Treatment of Epilepsy: Principles and Practice*. 3rd ed. Philadelphia: Lippincott Williams & Wilkins; 2001:525.
268. Kotagal P. Complex partial seizures. In: Wyllie E, ed. *The Treatment of Epilepsy: Principles and Practice*. 3rd ed. Philadelphia: Lippincott Williams & Wilkins; 2001:309.
269. Berkovic SF et al. Absence seizures. In: Wyllie E, ed. *The Treatment of Epilepsy: Principles and Practice*. 3rd ed. Philadelphia: Lippincott Williams & Wilkins; 2001:357.
270. Zifkin BG et al. Epilepsy with reflex seizures. In: Wyllie E, ed. *The Treatment of Epilepsy: Principles and Practice*. 3rd ed. Philadelphia: Lippincott Williams & Wilkins; 2001:537.
271. Fisch BJ et al. Generalized tonic-clonic seizures. In: Wyllie E, ed. *The Treatment of Epilepsy: Principles and Practice*. 3rd ed. Philadelphia: Lippincott Williams & Wilkins; 2001:369.

CHAPTER 55

Cerebrovascular Disorders

Timothy E. Welty

TRANSIENT ISCHEMIC ATTACKS

Cerebrovascular disease is a broad term encompassing many disorders of the blood vessels of the central nervous system (CNS). These disorders result from either inadequate blood flow to the brain (i.e., cerebral ischemia) with subsequent infarction of the involved portion of the CNS or from hemorrhages into the parenchyma or subarachnoid space of the CNS and subsequent neurologic dysfunction. This group of disorders is the third leading cause of deaths among adults in the United States.[1]

Definitions

Transient Ischemic Attack

A transient ischemic attack (TIA) describes the clinical condition in which a patient experiences a temporary focal neurologic deficit such as slurred speech, aphasia, weakness or paralysis of a limb, or blindness. These symptoms appear rapidly and are temporary, lasting <24 hours (usually only 2–15 minutes). The exact clinical presentation depends on the portion of the cerebrovascular tree (e.g., carotid artery, vertebrobasilar artery, or both) affected by diminished or absent blood flow. TIAs frequently result from small clots breaking away from larger, distant blood clots. These emboli are then dissolved by the fibrinolytic system, allowing re-establishment of blood flow and return of neurologic function.

Cerebral Infarction

A cerebral infarction is a permanent neurologic disorder characterized by symptoms similar to a TIA. The patient with a cerebral infarction presents with neurological deficits caused by the death of neurons in a focal area of the brain. The two primary causes of infarction and persistent ischemia are atherosclerosis of cerebral blood vessels, or an embolus to cerebral arteries from a distant clot. Cerebral infarctions can present in three forms: stable, improving, or progressing. A *stable infarction* describes the condition when the neurologic deficit is permanent, will not improve, and will not deteriorate. An *improving infarction* is marked by return of previously lost neurologic function over several days or weeks. A *progressing infarction* is one in which the patient's neurologic status continues to deteriorate following the initial onset of focal deficits.

Cerebral Hemorrhage

Cerebral hemorrhage is a cerebrovascular disorder that involves escape of blood from blood vessels into the brain and its surrounding structures. The leakage of blood causes clinical symptoms similar to those associated with a TIA or infarction. The neurologic dysfunction that is associated with TIAs or cerebral infarction results from the lack of blood flow to a given portion of the brain. In a cerebral hemorrhage, the initial neurologic deficits are due to the direct irritant effects of blood that is in direct contact with brain tissue. Primary causes of a cerebral hemorrhage include cerebral artery aneurysm, arteriovenous malformation, hypertensive hemorrhage, and trauma.

The terms *apoplexy, stroke,* and *paralytic stroke* are commonly used by lay persons to describe a sudden neurologic affliction that usually is related to the cerebral blood supply. The term *stroke* is used to describe a cerebral vascular event when neurologic deficits persist for at least 24 hours.

Epidemiology

Annually, approximately 700,000 individuals in the United States experience a cerebral infarction, and approximately 160,000 will die as a result of the stroke.[2] Of the 700,000 strokes annually, 500,000 are first-ever strokes and 200,000 are recurrent events.[3] Cerebrovascular disease is the third most common cause of death in adults and is one of the more commonly encountered causes of neurologic dysfunction. Nevertheless, this represents a dramatic decrease in the mortality rate of ischemic stroke from 88.8 per 100,000 population in 1950 to 54.3 per 100,000 in 2003. There are important racial and ethnic differences in incidence and mortality rates for ischemic stroke as shown in Table 55-1. The precise reasons for these differences are unclear, but genetic, geographic, dietary, and cultural factors have been considered.[4] In addition, the incidence of risk factors for stroke such as hypertension, diabetes, and hypercholesterolemia differ between racial groups.[4]

In the United States, ischemic stroke is the most common type of infarction (Fig. 55-1). Atherothrombotic disease of the large cerebral blood vessels is responsible for the majority of cerebral ischemic events and infarctions. Disease of penetrating arteries that are responsible for oxygenation and nutrition of the CNS, thromboembolic causes (e.g., atrial fibrillation), and other causes such as infection or inflammation of arteries are also responsible for ischemic stroke.[1,2]

There is a strong relationship between the occurrence of TIA and an increased risk for subsequent cerebral infarction.[1] The risk of an ischemic stroke is highest in the first 30 days after a TIA and the risk within 90 days of a TIA is 3% to 17.3%. Additionally, nearly 25% of patients who suffer a TIA will die within a year.[1]

Definite risk factors for cerebral infarction are listed in Table 55-2. A key element in the prevention of stroke is the elimination or modification of risk factors.[5,6] The control of risk factors is of primary importance in managing a patient with a TIA or cerebral infarction.

Table 55-1 Epidemiology of Stroke by Race or Ethnic Group

Ethnic/Racial Group	First-ever Age-adjusted Stroke Incidence (per 100,000 people)	Death Rate (per 100,000 people)
Overall	208	54.3
Black Men	323	78.8
Black Women	260	69.1
White Men	167	51.9
White Women	138	50.5
Hispanic Men		44.3
Hispanic Women		38.6
Asian Men		50.8
Asian Women		45.4
Native American Men		37.1
Native American Women		38

Adapted from references 129, 130, 131.

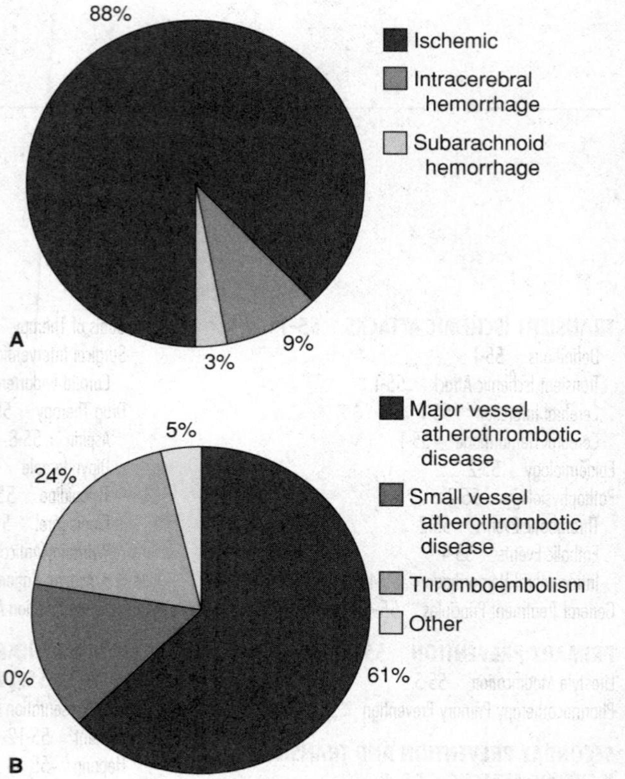

FIGURE 55-1 Etiology of Strokes (A) Causes of All Strokes (B) Causes of Ischemic Strokes

Hemorrhage into the brain accounts for 12% of all strokes in North America. Hypertensive hemorrhage is the most common cause of intracerebral hemorrhages (ICHs), with 46% of ICHs resulting from hypertension.[7] Subarachnoid hemorrhage is the second most common cause of hemorrhagic stroke and has a mortality rate of approximately 50%. Patients with subarachnoid hemorrhage are usually 20 to 70 years old, and the majority of survivors suffer permanent neurologic deficits. A less common cause of ICH is an arteriovenous malformation (AVM), which is a clump of arteries and veins that are intertwined, resulting in weakened blood vessel walls. AVMs usually result from a congenital defect or trauma.

Pathophysiology

Thrombotic Events

The neurologic sequelae of cerebral ischemia or infarction directly result from an embolic or thrombotic source. A clot may form in the heart, along the wall of a major blood vessel (e.g., aorta, carotid, or basilar artery), or in small arteries penetrating deep into the brain. If the clot is located near the infarction, it is considered to be a thrombus; however, when the clot has migrated to the brain from a distant source, it is considered an embolus. Either can diminish or block blood flow to the affected area of the brain.

Table 55-2 Risk Factors for Ischemic Stroke

Modifiable	*Potentially Modifiable*	*Nonmodifiable*
Cardiovascular disease (coronary heart disease, heart failure, peripheral arterial disease)	Metabolic syndrome	Age (doubling each 10 years over age 55)
Hypertension	Alcohol abuse (≥5 drinks daily)	Race (blacks>Hispanics>whites)
Cigarette smoking	Hyperhomocysteinemia	Sex (men>women)
Diabetes	Drug abuse (e.g., cocaine, amphetamine, methamphetamine)	Low birth weight (<2,500 g)
Asymptomatic carotid stenosis	Hypercoagulability (e.g., anticardiolipin, Factor V Leiden, protein C deficiency, protein S deficiency, antithrombin III deficiency)	Family history of stroke (paternal>maternal)
Atrial fibrillation	Oral contraceptive use (women 25–44 years old)	
Sickle cell disease	Inflammatory processes (e.g., periodontal disease, Cytomegalovirus, *Helicobacter pylori* seropositive)	
Dyslipidemia (high total cholesterol, low HDL)	Acute infection (e.g., respiratory infection, urinary tract infection)	
Dietary factors (sodium intake <2,300 mg/day; potassium intake <4,700 mg/day)	CD 40 ligand >3.71 ng/mL in women free of cardiovascular disease	
Obesity	IL-18 upper tertile	
Physical inactivity	hs-CRP >3 mg/L in women 45 years or older	
Postmenopausal hormone therapy (women 50–74 years old)	Migraine headaches	
	High Lp(a)	
	High Lp-PLA$_2$	
	Sleep-disordered breathing	

Adapted from reference 5.

Clots, both embolic and thrombotic, affecting the cerebral vasculature are typically arterial in origin and are formed primarily by fibrin. Tissue injury or turbulent blood flow causes the release of adenosine diphosphate (ADP), thrombin, epinephrine, and a variety of other substances to stimulate platelet migration. Exposure of collagen and other subendothelial surfaces of the blood vessel wall cause adhesion of platelets to the damaged vessel wall. As platelets adhere and aggregate, phospholipase is activated, leading to the splitting of arachidonic acid from platelet membrane phospholipid. This begins a cascade of events ultimately ending in the formation of thromboxane A_2 (TXA_2) and prostacyclin. Prostacyclin inhibits platelet aggregation and is a powerful vasodilator, whereas TXA_2 is a potent inducer of platelet release and aggregation. Prostacyclin is formed in and released from arterial and venous walls. TXA_2 is formed in and released from platelets. The delicate balance between the actions of these two compounds controls thrombogenesis. When a clot is formed, it can either embolize to the cerebral vasculature or occlude a cerebral artery.

Inflammatory mechanisms also contribute to the development of ischemia, especially thrombotic lesions. Substances like C-reactive protein, a mediator of inflammation, are elevated in patients with an acute stroke. Inflammation is thought to enhance the development of thrombotic lesions and result in sudden, intermittent occlusion of blood vessels.

Cerebral blood flow in the normal adult brain is 30 to 70 mL/100 g/minute. When a thrombotic or embolic clot partially occludes a cerebral artery, causing a reduction in blood flow to <20 mL/100 g/minute, various compensatory mechanisms are activated. These include vasodilation and increased oxygen extraction. If the artery is further occluded and cerebral blood flow is reduced to <12 mL/100 g/minute, the affected neurons become sufficiently anoxic to die within minutes (Fig. 55-2).[8] Rapid re-establishment of blood flow to the ischemic area can delay, prevent, or limit the onset of infarction, improving the outcome of the acute stroke.

Ischemia in the brain usually involves a core or focal region of profound ischemia that results in neuronal death. The extent of this region is dependent on the amount of brain that is perfused directly by the blood vessel that becomes occluded. There is a surrounding area of brain that becomes marginally ischemic with normal function being disrupted. This region of marginal ischemia is frequently called the *ischemic penumbra.* If ischemia continues, neurons in this region will die. However, if normal blood flow is restored quickly, neurons in this area will survive.

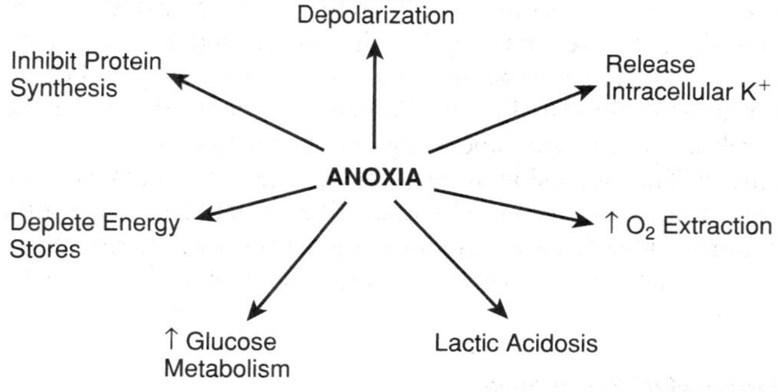

FIGURE 55-2 Physiologic effects of cerebral anoxia.

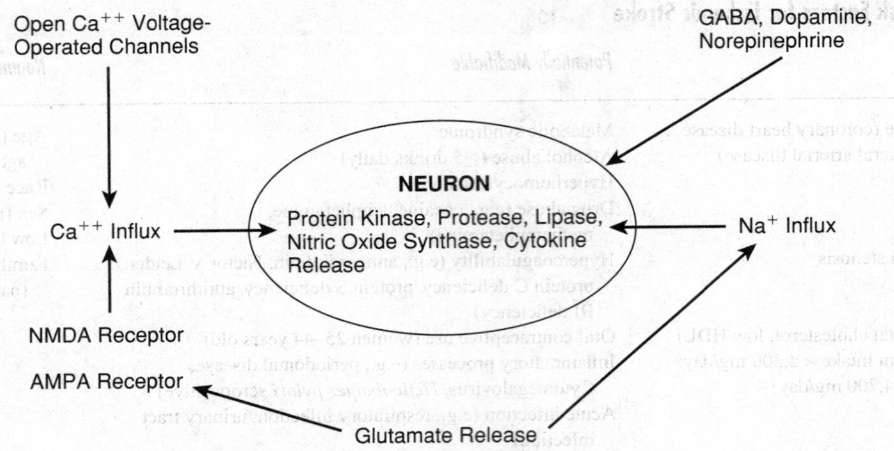

FIGURE 55-3 The effects of membrane depolarization.

When neurons become ischemic, excitatory neurotransmitters are released, causing neurons to rapidly and repeatedly discharge. This compromises the survival of damaged neurons around the area of infarction. Increased neuronal activity results in extreme metabolic demands, disrupts neuronal homeostasis, and synergistically increases the effects of hypoxia. Especially vulnerable to ischemic effects are neurons in the middle layers of the cerebral cortex; portions of the hippocampus (CA-1 and subiculum regions), a structure running parallel to the parahippocampal gyrus; and Purkinje cells in the cerebellum.[9] There is also a rapid intracellular influx of calcium. Both voltage-dependent and chemical-dependent calcium channels are unable to act as a gate to prevent the movement of calcium, due to depletion of cellular energy sources. Intracellular stores of calcium ions also are disrupted, causing release of calcium into the cytoplasm. Increased concentration of calcium ions enhances phospholipase and protease activity and increased reactive metabolites, such as $-O_2$, $-OH$, and nitric oxide (Fig. 55-3). This eventually causes neuronal death.[8,9] In addition, lipolysis of cell membranes occurs in the presence of an accumulation of neurotoxic free radicals.

Immediate therapeutic intervention is needed to limit and prevent permanent neurologic damage from these rapidly occurring events.

Embolic Events

The pathophysiology of infarction of brain tissue and neuronal death is similar for both embolic and thrombotic events. However, rather than forming locally in the vasculature of the brain, embolic events result from clots that are formed in distant parts of the body. Portions of these clots may break away and travel through the blood to the brain. When they become lodged in the cerebral vasculature, blood flow will be partially or totally occluded. This occlusion initiates the cascade of ischemic events in the brain and neurons. Disorders like atrial fibrillation, mitral or aortic valve disease, patent foramen ovale, or coagulopathies are associated with formation of clots that may embolize to the brain.

Intracerebral Hemorrhage

Cerebral aneurysms, AVMs, hypertension, and adverse drug reactions are the primary causes of ICH. One type of ICH, subarachnoid hemorrhage, can result from weakened blood vessel walls (i.e., aneurysms) caused by congenital defects, trauma, infection, and hypertension. Blood slowly leaks from the involved vessel or the aneurysm may rupture suddenly. In this type of hemorrhage, blood typically is released into the subarachnoid space and, depending on the severity of the hemorrhage, into the ventricles of the brain. Direct contact of blood with brain tissue irritates and damages brain cells. Rebleeding, hydrocephalus, and delayed cerebral ischemia frequently occur after the aneurysm ruptures, further worsening the patient's neurologic function.

AVMs due to congenital causes or traumatic injury, and uncontrolled hypertension also can cause devastating intracerebral bleeding. In these patients, blood is usually released directly into the brain parenchyma. In more severe cases blood is released into the surrounding brain structures. ICHs can be the result of adverse reactions to drugs, such as anticoagulants, thrombolytics, and sympathomimetics.

General Treatment Principles

Rapid recognition of stroke symptoms and immediate initiation of treatment are essential to the management of ischemic or hemorrhagic stroke. Appropriate pharmacotherapy of cerebrovascular disease requires a precise diagnosis. It is vital to differentiate between an ischemic stroke and a hemorrhagic stroke, because an inaccurate diagnosis can lead to the use of drugs that may cause severe morbidity or mortality. Interventions to prevent and treat ischemic strokes are directed at reducing risk factors, eliminating or modifying the underlying pathologic process, reducing secondary brain damage, and rehabilitation.

Treatments for ischemic stroke and hemorrhagic stroke vary. In ischemic stroke, treatment involves acute management, chronic management of the effects of the stroke, and prevention of further events. In acute management, the only effective treatment is the use of tPA in combination with supportive measures. Chronic management of the effects of a stroke focus primarily on treating depression, spasticity, possible neurogenic bowel or bladder, and self-care issues. Antiplatelet agents, especially, aspirin, clopidogrel, and aspirin/dipyridamole combination, form the cornerstone of prevention.

In hemorrhagic stroke, the emphasis of treatment is on supportive therapy to maximize neurological function, prevention of further hemorrhagic events, and management of complications. This involves wise management of blood pressure, pulmonary function, fluid and electrolytes, and elimination of drugs that inhibit coagulation. There are no proven direct therapies for hemorrhagic events.

PRIMARY PREVENTION

Lifestyle Modification

1. R.B. is a 60-year-old, 5 feet 6 inches tall, 85-kg woman who is concerned about having a stroke. Her father died from a stroke and her 85-year-old mother has had several episodes diagnosed as TIA. R.B.'s blood pressure is 140–150/90–100 mmHg, and she was recently diagnosed with diabetes mellitus. She does not have a history of TIA or stroke. Additionally, she smoked for 25 years, but has not used tobacco for the past 10 years. Her current medications include lisinopril, metformin, conjugated estrogen/medroxyprogesterone, and acetaminophen. She approaches her pharmacist because of concerns about having a stroke and being "like her parents." What are the first things she can do to limit her risk of stroke?

Any plan for *primary prevention* (i.e., orevebtuib if a first event) of TIA or stroke must address the control or reduction of risk factors (Table 55-3).

For R.B., hypertension is a risk factor that requires immediate attention. Nearly 70% of strokes result from hypertension and blood pressure control is vital for stroke prevention. Both systolic and diastolic hypertension increases the risk of stroke.[10,11] Adequate control of her blood pressure should reduce R.B.'s risk of stroke by 35% to 44%.[12] Based upon JNC 7 guidelines, R.B.'s blood pressure goal should be <130/80 mmHg due to the additional risk factor of diabetes.[13] Because she is already receiving lisinopril and her blood pressure is poorly controlled, it is likely that combination therapy is needed. Addition of hydrochlorthiazide 25 mg/day is advisable.[5]

Diabetes is another important risk factor for stroke. In older women, diabetes is a more significant risk factor for stroke than for men.[14] There is controversy regarding the intensity of glucose control that optimally reduces stroke risk. Clearly, good control of diabetes results in better control of hypertension and other risk factors for stroke.[15] Additionally, use of oral hypoglycemics may reduce the risk of stroke through mechanisms other than glycemic control. However, strict control of blood glucose did not reduce the risk of stroke over 9 years in one study.[15] There is evidence that angiotensin converting enzyme inhibitors (ACEI) and angiotensin receptor blockers (ARB) reduce the risk of stroke in diabetics, with or without hypertension.[16,17] For diabetic patients with at least one additional risk factor for cardiovascular disease, taking a HMG-CoA reductase inhibitor appears to reduce the risk of stroke by approximately 24% even in the absence of hypercholesterolemia.[18,19] For RB, she should maintain tight control of her diabetes, continue her lisinopril, and start a HMG-CoA reductase inhibitor, such as simvastatin or atorvastatin.

The body mass index (BMI) for R.B. is 30.2, placing her in the obese category. Multiple large studies have demonstrated a direct relationship between increased body weight and an increased risk of stroke.[20,21] There are no data available to establish the precise effect of weight reduction on reducing the risk of stroke. Data are available to show that an average weight reduction of 5.1 kg results in a reduction in systolic blood pressure of 4.4 mmHg and a reduction in diastolic pressure of 3.6 mmHg.[22] In addition to weight loss, a proper diet and exercise are important for controlling risk factors. A diet high in sodium is associated with an increased risk in stroke, whereas a diet high in potassium appears to reduce the risk of stroke.[23,24] Current recommendations for diet are for sodium intake of ≤2.3 g/day and potassium intake of ≥4.7 g/day.[5] Several studies have shown an inverse relationship between physical activity and risk of stroke.[25,26] At least 30 minutes of moderate intensity exercise daily is recommended.[5] Based upon these data, R,B. should initiate a weight reduction program that includes a low-sodium and high-potassium diet with an exercise program.

Table 55-3 Primary Prevention of Ischemic Stroke

Factor	*Goal*	*Recommendation*
Hypertension	Blood Pressure <140/90 mmHg; with diabetes <130/80	Follow JNC 7 guidelines; after lifestyle modification thiazide-type diuretic, angiotensin converting enzyme inhibitor, or angiotensin receptor blocker
Atrial fibrillation	When warfarin is used INR 2–3	Aspirin 75–325 mg/day or warfarin as determined by the use of the $CHADS_2$ score
Dyslipidemia	National Cholesterol Education Program III goals	Lifestyle modification, HMG CoA reductase inhibitor
Women (>65 years, history of hypertension, hyperlipidemia, diabetes, or 10-year cardiovascular risk ≥10%)	Reduce risk without bleeding complications	Aspirin 75–325 mg/day; use the lowest possible dose
Cigarette smoke	Elimination of cigarette smoke	Smoking cessation; avoidance of environmental tobacco smoke
Physical inactivity	≥30 minutes daily of moderate intensity activity	Establish exercise program of aerobic activity
Excessive alcohol intake	Moderation	≤2 drinks/day for men or ≤1 drink/day for nonpregnant women
Diet and nutrition	≤2.3 g/day of sodium; ≥4.7 g/day of potassium	Institute a diet that is high in fruits and vegetables and low in saturated fats
Elevated lipoprotein(a)	Reduction of lipoprotein(a) by ≥25%	Niacin 2,000 mg/day as tolerated

Adapted from reference 5.

Cigarette smoking is an independent risk factor for stroke and potentiates other risk factors. In addition to active smoking, passive inhalation of cigarette smoke also appears to be a risk factor for stroke.[27] Smoking cessation does result in a rapid reduction in the risk of stroke, but the risk never returns to levels seen in individuals who have never smoked.[28] R.B. should be encouraged to avoid passive smoke and to continue avoiding the use of tobacco.

Previously, treatment guidelines suggested that hormone replacement therapy was at least neutral in its effects on the risk of stroke and perhaps beneficial. However, three subsequent studies have specifically investigated the effect of hormone replacement on stroke risk. The Women's Estrogen for Stroke Trial (WEST) investigated the effect of hormonal therapy on the secondary prevention of stroke.[29] In the first 6 months of the study, those randomized to receive estradiol had a significantly higher risk of recurrent stroke and were less likely to recover if they had a stroke. A second study, the Heart and Estrogen/Progesterone Replacement Study (HERS) evaluated the effect of hormone therapy on the secondary prevention of MI in postmenopausal women.[30] In a posthoc analysis, hormone replacement therapy had no effect on stroke risk.[31] The Women's Health Initiative (WHI) study specifically evaluated the effect of conjugated estrogens and medroxyprogesterone on primary prevention of cardiovascular events, including stroke, in women who were postmenopausal.[32] The study was terminated early due to a significant increase in stroke rates and other cardiovascular events in women receiving hormone replacement therapy. Similar findings were seen in a parallel group of women who were surgically postmenopausal.[33] Based upon results from these studies, R,B. should discontinue the conjugated estrogen/medroxyprogesterone product, unless she is taking this medication for a specific reason other than control of menopausal symptoms or prevention of cardiovascular events.

Pharmacotherapy Primary Prevention

2. Are there specific pharmacotherapeutic treatments to reduce the risk of stroke for R.B.?

Aspirin has been carefully investigated for primary prophylaxis of stroke. Although aspirin is recommended in the primary prevention of coronary heart disease, it is not generally recommended for the primary prevention of stroke. In a study of 22,071 male physicians who took 325 mg of aspirin or placebo every other day for 5 years, there was not a reduced incidence of stroke.[34] This group of individuals who had no previous history of cerebrovascular disease experienced 217 strokes, 119 in the aspirin group and 98 in the placebo group. In addition, there was an increased risk of cerebrovascular events due to hemorrhage in the aspirin group. Chen et al. reported a meta-analysis of 40,000 patients randomly assigned to aspirin and found a reduction from 47% to 45.8% in death and disability due to stroke.[35] Another study considered the role of aspirin for primary stroke prevention in women.[36] Women who took one to six aspirin per week had a slightly reduced risk of stroke and a lower risk of large-artery occlusive disease (relative risk, 59%; 95% confidence level (CI), 0.29–0.85, $p = 0.01$). An increased risk of stroke was seen in women who took >7 aspirin weekly and an excess risk of subarachnoid hemorrhage was seen for those taking >15 aspirin a week. The Women's Health Study also investigated the use of 100 mg/day in asymptomatic women and followed them for 10 years, monitoring for nonfatal cardiovascular events including stroke.[37] In this study there was a 17% reduction in the risk for all strokes and a 24% reduction in the risk for ischemic stroke, while there was a nonsignificant increase in the risk for hemorrhage. Women 65 years of age and older at entry into the trial showed the most consistent risk reduction, but hemorrhagic strokes negated some of the benefit. Additionally, women with a history of hypertension, hyperlipidemia, or diabetes, or a 10-year cardiovascular risk of ≥10% had the most benefit. Thus, aspirin should only be considered in women who are 65 years or older, or have other important risk factors for stroke. There are very limited data currently available regarding the use of other antiplatelet drugs for primary prevention of stroke.

Although oral anticoagulants are not generally considered safe for primary prevention of stroke, a major exception is patients with atrial fibrillation. These individuals are at risk for an embolic event arising from clot formation in the atrium of the heart. Numerous studies have clearly shown that warfarin prevents embolic cerebrovascular events for patients with nonvalvular atrial fibrillation.[38–42] In these studies, the warfarin dose was adjusted to maintain an INR of 1.5 to 4.5. The Stroke Prevention in Atrial Fibrillation (SPAF) trial included aspirin combined with warfarin in one study arm and indicated that some benefit may be derived by combining antiplatelet agents with anticoagulants.[38] A follow-up study was performed and showed no difference between warfarin and aspirin in preventing stroke in atrial fibrillation.[42] Aspirin can be used as an alternative to warfarin in patients with atrial fibrillation, based upon the $CHADS_2$ score (Table 55-4).[5,43,44] Additionally, warfarin may be used in primary prevention of embolic stroke due to a patent foramen ovale.

For R.B., primary prevention of stroke with aspirin 81 mg/day can be considered due to her history of hypertension and diabetes.

SECONDAY PREVENTION AND TRANSIENT ISCHEMIC ATTACKS

Clinical Presentation

3. J.S., a 55-year-old, 5 feet 11 inches tall, 120-kg man, experienced a rapidly progressive paralysis of his right arm and slurred speech yesterday. These symptoms lasted for 15 to 20 minutes and resolved rapidly. His neurologic examination is entirely

Table 55-4 $CHADS_2$ Score: Primary Stroke Prevention in Atrial Fibrillation

Add points for the following items. If score is <2, aspirin can be considered. If score is ≥2, then warfarin is recommended.
Congestive heart failure = 1 point
Hypertension = 1 point
Age >75 years = 1 point
Diabetes mellitus = 1 point
Prior stroke or TIA = 2 points

Adapted from references 43 and 44.

normal, and he denies any feeling of weakness. He smokes two packs of cigarettes daily and drinks three to six cans of beer each evening. His physical examination is entirely normal except for a left carotid bruit, which was first noted 2 years ago. His blood pressure (BP) is 165/100 mmHg, and he has a long history of hypertension. His hemoglobin (Hgb) is 16.5 g/dL (normal, 12–16 g/dL), his hematocrit (Hct) is 51% (normal, 42%–52%), and his total serum cholesterol concentration is 275 mg/dL (normal, <200 mg/dL). A Doppler examination of his carotid arteries shows a 90% stenosis on the left and a 40% stenosis on the right. What subjective and objective data in J.S.'s history are consistent with a TIA?

[SI units: Hgb, 165 g/L (normal, 120–160); Hct, 0.51 (normal, 0.42–0.52); cholesterol, 7.11 mmol/L]

A TIA can present with any type of neurologic symptoms. The presentation is determined entirely by the location of the involved arteries and the portion of the brain that they supply. For example, if the affected artery provides circulation to the motor area in the left hemisphere of the brain, the expected result would be impairment of muscle strength on the right side of the body. Symptoms of TIA may include paresis or paralysis of one or more limbs, paraesthesia, slurred speech, blurred vision, blindness (amaurosis fugax), facial droop, dizziness, or difficulty in swallowing (Table 55-5). Patients rarely lose consciousness. Symptoms always resolve within 24 hours, and there is no residual clinical focal neurologic deficit. Most often, the neurologic deficits last for only 2 to 15 minutes, and neurologic function rapidly returns to normal. However, with newer imaging techniques small areas of permanent ischemic damage may be seen, even in the absence of neurologic deficits.

J.S.'s rapid onset of right arm paralysis and slurred speech suggest involvement of the left cerebral cortex. The 15- to 20-minute duration of these symptoms and the entirely normal neurologic examination on the day after these symptoms also are compatible with a TIA. The left carotid bruit heard on physical examination suggests a left-sided process.

Right-sided neurologic deficits generally suggest left-sided cerebral dysfunction because motor and sensory neuronal tracts cross over in the midbrain. Thus, the left hemisphere of the cerebral cortex controls the right or contralateral side of the body. CNS lesions occurring below the midbrain will cause ipsilateral neurologic deficits. Therefore, J.S.'s right arm paralysis suggests a left-sided cerebral lesion above the midbrain.

Table 55-5 Symptoms Associated With Transient Ischemic Attacks

Symptom	Right Carotid	Left Carotid	Vertebrobasilar
Aphasia	Possible	Yes	No
Ataxia	No	No	Yes
Blindness	Right	Left	Right or left side
Clumsiness	Yes	Yes	Yes
Diplopia	No	No	Yes
Dysarthria	Yes	Yes	No
Paralysis	Left side	Right side	Any limb
Paresthesia	Left side	Right side	Any limb
Vertigo	No	No	Yes

Risk Factors

4. How can another TIA be prevented?

As with primary prevention, the initial interventions for secondary prevention of stroke are reduction of the risk factors. J.S. has several risk factors for TIA and ischemic stroke (Table 55-2): a smoking history, excessive alcohol consumption, obesity, older age, male gender, hypercholesterolemia, and hypertension. He should be instructed and counseled to change his lifestyle by discontinuing his smoking, limiting his alcohol consumption, reducing his weight, and increasing his physical exercise. Hypoxia and hypercarbia induced by cigarette smoking may have caused his increased hematocrit, and his high serum cholesterol and obesity suggest the need for dietary changes. The goal of a weight control program should be for his body mass index (BMI) to be 18.5–24.9 kg/m^2, and a waist circumference of <40 inches.[6] A smoking cessation program, substance abuse program, and consultation with a dietitian should be useful in reducing his risk factors. Additionally, steps should be taken to ensure at least 30 minutes of moderate intensity physical activity for 5 to 7 days of the week.[6]

The goals of antihypertensive therapy should be individualized. A mean blood pressure reduction of approximately 10/5 mmHg has been associated with risk reduction for stroke.[6] Further reductions may be useful, but in managing his blood pressure all reductions should be gradual. A sudden or dramatic decrease in blood pressure could compromise cerebral perfusion and result in a decreased level of consciousness or cerebral infarction. The degree of his carotid artery stenosis will contribute to the problem of decreased perfusion if the blood pressure is decreased rapidly. A mild degree of hypertension may be temporarily acceptable because of the extent of carotid stenosis. Data are lacking to indicate an optimal treatment regimen, and pharmacotherapy plans should be individualized to the patient. The use of a diuretic or a diuretic combined with an angiotensin converting enzyme inhibitor (ACEI) is supported by available literature.[6] Initiation of hydrochlorothiazide at a dosage of 12.5 mg/day or a combination of hydrochlorothiazide with an ACEI should be considered.

Reduction of serum cholesterol is important for J.S. The first step in managing his cholesterol is to institute lifestyle and dietary modifications. Several placebo controlled studies have shown that HMG-CoA reductase inhibitors significantly reduce the risk of stroke and TIA.[45–49] For example, individuals with coronary disease who received pravastatin had a 20% to 40% reduction in the risk of stroke. A study of atorvastatin showed similar risk reductions.[50] These findings are reinforced by two meta-analyses that reported a 25% to 32% reduction in the risk of stroke.[51,52] It is known that HMG-CoA reductase inhibitors have anti-inflammatory activity that may influence the development of atherosclerotic plaques and cerebral ischemic processes.[53–55] Because of these effects of HMG-CoA reductase inhibitors, these drugs should be started following a TIA or stroke even in patients who do not have dyslipidema.[56] Targets for managing cholesterol in patients with atherosclerotic disease are a LDL-C of <100 mg/dL or, in extremely high risk patients, a LDL-C of <70 mg/dL.[6] Niacin or gemfibrozil can be considered for patients with low HDL-C concentrations. Based on these data, J.S. should receive a HMG-CoA reductase inhibitor. The benefits of HMG-CoA reductase inhibitors appear to be a class effect, so selection of a specific agent should be based on the individual characteristics of the patient.

Treatment

Goals of Therapy

5. What are the initial and long-term goals in treating J.S.?

The immediate goal is to re-establish adequate blood flow in his diseased cerebral vessels. Longer-range objectives are to prevent reocclusion, decrease the risk of future symptomatic TIAs, and ultimately, prevent a cerebral infarction.[57]

Surgical Interventions

6. What nonpharmacologic interventions might be available to prevent another TIA? What would be the best choice for J.S.?

Various surgical interventions are available to prevent TIA or infarction. These are designed to either remove the source for an embolism or improve circulation to ischemic areas of the brain.

CAROTID ENDARTERECTOMY

Carotid endarterectomy (CEA) is a common surgical procedure for correcting atheromatous lesions responsible for causing a TIA. In this procedure, the carotid artery is surgically exposed, and the atheromatous plaque is excised. Balloon angioplasty and placement of stents also can improve blood flow through a stenosed artery. During this procedure, a catheter with a small, deflated balloon is placed in the stenosed artery and the atherosclerotic lesion is pressed into the arterial wall when the balloon is inflated. A small, plastic tube stent is placed in the artery to prevent the vessel from collapsing at the site of the lesion.

CEA is most effective for patients with an ulcerated lesion or stenotic clot that occludes >70% of blood flow in the ipsilateral carotid artery and who experience symptoms of a TIA or stroke. Use of CEA in these patients may result in a 60% reduction in stroke risk over the subsequent 2 years.[58] Of six to eight patients treated with CEA, one stroke will be prevented within 2 years.[59] The use of CEA in other patient groups must be balanced with the risk of the procedure and life expectancy.[60] CEA is beneficial in patients with 50% to 69% stenosis of the carotid artery.[6] Surgery should be done within 2 weeks of a TIA or stroke. In other patients, the benefits of CEA are questionable. Generally, CEA is not indicated in patients who have permanent neurologic deficits or total occlusion of the carotid artery.[58] CEA should be done by a surgeon with <6% morbidity and mortality rates.[6]

Carotid artery angioplasty and stenting (CAS) is another alternative. The initial study of this procedure was halted due to poor outcomes.[61] Subsequently, two studies have shown that CAS is not inferior to CEA, but further study is underway to determine if CAS is more beneficial than CEA.[62,63] CAS can be used in patients who are not candidates for CEA.

J.S. should undergo CEA for his left carotid lesion as soon as possible. The lesion on the right should be monitored closely for continued progression. If further TIAs occur or the right carotid stenosis is >60%, he should have a CEA performed on the right carotid artery.

Drug Therapy

ASPIRIN

7. What role does aspirin have in preventing the occurrence of ischemic stroke in patients who have experienced a TIA?

Because platelets play a key role in the formation of atheromatous clots (see Fig. 55-4), various antiplatelet drugs, such as aspirin, sulfinpyrazone, dipyridamole, ticlopidine, and clopidogrel have been tried to prevent ischemic strokes. These agents generally work by either preventing the formation of TXA_2 or increasing the concentration of prostacyclin. These actions seek to re-establish the proper balance between these two substances, thus preventing the adhesion and aggregation of platelets (Table 55-6).

Aspirin has been the most widely tested agent for use in preventing TIA and ischemic stroke. It acts primarily by irreversibly inactivating platelet cyclooxygenase.[64] Inactivation of cyclooxygenase decreases platelet aggregation, prevents release of vasoactive substances, and prolongs the bleeding time. Because binding of cyclooxygenase by the acetyl component of acetylsalicylic acid ([ASA] aspirin) is irreversible and the platelet cannot synthesize new protein, platelet function is altered for the duration of the platelet's life, usually 5 to 7 days. Aspirin's ability to prevent clot formation and subsequent embolic or thrombotic events also can be attributed to an inhibition of TXA_2-mediated vasoconstriction, activation of fibrinolysis, inhibition of synthesis of vitamin K–dependent clotting factors, and inhibition of lipoxygenase pathways.

In addition to its action on platelet cyclooxygenase, high concentrations of aspirin also inhibit prostacyclin synthesis in the walls of blood vessels. Because prostacyclin inhibits platelet aggregation, depletion of prostacyclin could result in an undesirable increase in aggregation of platelets. However, depletion of prostacyclin is not prolonged because the vascular endothelium is able to synthesize new enzymes. Higher dosages of aspirin (1.3 g/day) also may decrease vascular plasminogen activator, thereby enhancing thrombus formation.[65] Therefore, aspirin should be dosed carefully.

At least 15 randomized trials, with 7 being placebo-controlled, have studied aspirin alone or in combination with other antiplatelet drugs in the prevention of vascular events.[36,66–70] Patients were enrolled in these studies for as long as 5 years after experiencing a vascular event (i.e., TIA, stroke, unstable angina, or myocardial infarction). Follow-up periods lasted from 1 to 6 years. The incidence of ischemic stroke or TIA ranged from 7% to 23%: the aspirin-treated patients experienced an average 22% decrease in relative risk of a stroke compared with those receiving placebo. In 10 trials that considered only TIA or stroke patients, there was a 24% relative risk reduction in the incidence of nonfatal stroke associated with the use of aspirin.

In initial studies of aspirin in stroke prevention, the positive effects were seen primarily in men. However, the European Stroke Prevention Study and a French study included an equal balance of men and women.[66,71] In both studies, the risk reduction rate was equal for men and women, indicating that the benefit of aspirin in stroke prevention extends to both sexes.

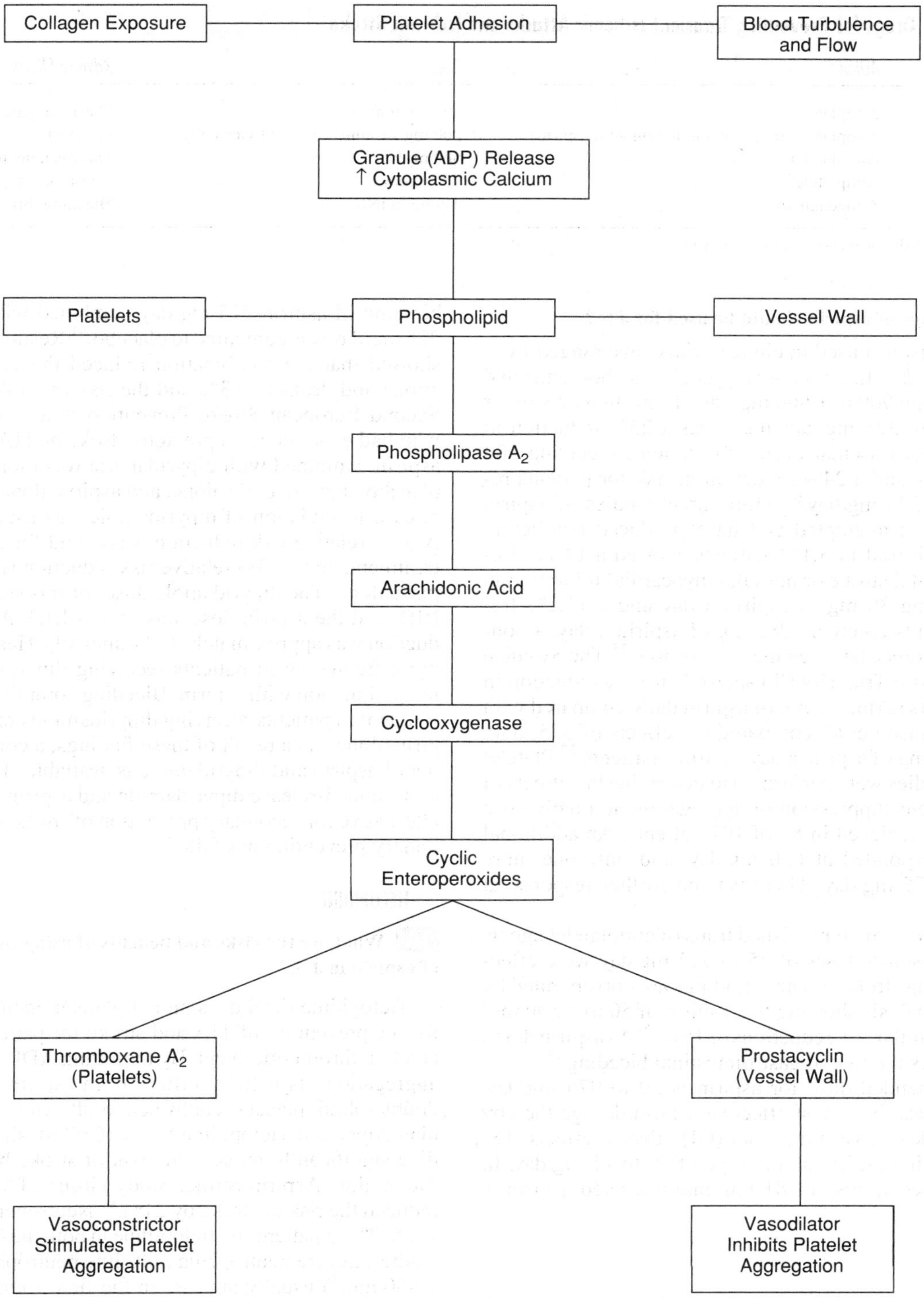

FIGURE 55-4 Arachidonic acid cascade and platelet plug formation.

Aspirin also has been used for prevention of restenosis following CEA. Over the first year after CEA, 25% of patients will redevelop a stenotic lesion, with more than half of these causing a >50% reduction in carotid blood flow.[72] Stent placement is useful in preventing restenosis. Initial studies indicated that combination therapy with aspirin 325 mg/day and dipyridamole 75 mg TID would decrease the rate of restenosis. However, a subsequent randomized, placebo-controlled study using this regimen in post-CEA patients did not substantiate the earlier findings.[73] A combination of clopidogrel with aspirin has been shown to reduce postoperative ischemic events.[74] Stents impregnated with anticoagulants are being evaluated.

Table 55-6 Drugs for Preventing Transient Ischemic Attacks and Ischemic Stroke

Drug	Action	Dose	Adverse Effects
Aspirin	Antiplatelet	50–1,300 mg/day	Diarrhea, gastric ulcer, GI upset
Dipyridamole	Antiplatelet (use in combination with aspirin)	200 mg sustained release twice daily	GI upset
Ticlopidine	Antiplatelet	500 mg/day	Diarrhea, neutropenia, rash
Clopidogrel	Antiplatelet	75 mg/day	Thrombocytopenia, neutropenia
Warfarin	Anticoagulant	Titrate to INR 2–3	Bleeding, bruising, petechiae

GI, gastrointestinal; INR, international normalized ratio.

8. What dosage of aspirin should be used for J.S.?

Dosages of aspirin used in clinical trials have ranged from 30 to 1,500 mg/day. In a meta-analysis of placebo-controlled studies comparing 900 to 1,500 mg/day of aspirin with similar studies of 300 to 325 mg/day, there was a 23% reduction in the risk of cerebrovascular events for patients receiving 900 to 1,500 mg/day and a 24% reduction in risk for patients receiving 300 to 325 mg/day.[68] More direct studies of aspirin dosing have been attempted and have produced conflicting results. A Dutch trial in 3,131 patients showed a 14.7% frequency of nonfatal stroke or nonfatal myocardial infarction in patients receiving 30 mg of aspirin a day and a 15.2% frequency in patients receiving 283 mg of aspirin a day, a nonsignificant difference between these two doses.[75] The Swedish Aspirin Low-Dose Trial (SALT) showed an 18% reduction in stroke in patients taking 75 mg of aspirin daily compared with placebo.[76] Helgason et al. compared the effects of 325, 650, 975, and 1,300 mg of aspirin a day in stroke patients.[77] Platelet aggregation studies were performed to determine the effects of aspirin. Complete suppression of aggregation at a daily dose of 325 mg was achieved in 85 of 107 patients. An additional five patients responded at 650 mg/day, and only one more responded at 975 mg/day. There was no further response at 1,300 mg.

A meta-analysis of all published trials of antiplatelet agents did show that aspirin doses of 75 to 325 mg/day were effective in preventing stroke.[78] These findings are corroborated by another meta-analysis showing that aspirin of 50 to 1,500 mg/day produced similar risk reductions of 15%.[79] As aspirin doses increase, so does the risk of gastrointestinal bleeding.[80]

The recommended dose for aspirin is 50 to 975 mg/day. The goal is to use the lowest effective aspirin dosage thereby limiting the risk of gastrointestinal (GI) adverse effects. J.S. should start taking aspirin at a dosage of 50 to 75 mg/day. In the United States, a dose of 81 mg enteric-coated aspirin is usually started.

DIPYRIDAMOLE

9. Should dipyridamole be used alone or in combination with aspirin for J.S.?

Two pharmacologic actions of dipyridamole prompted investigations into its use in preventing TIAs and ischemic stroke. Dipyridamole weakly inhibits platelet aggregation and platelet phosphodiesterase and has potential vasodilating properties through its inhibition of adenosine uptake in vascular smooth muscle.[64]

Two European studies have shown benefit with a combination of aspirin and dipyridamole. In the first study, a combination of aspirin 975 mg/day combined with dipyridamole 225 mg/day was compared to placebo.[81] Results from this study showed that the combination reduced the combined risk of stroke and death by 33% and the risk of stroke by 38%. The Second European Stroke Prevention Study enrolled patients who had experienced a previous stroke or TIA and found that aspirin combined with dipyridamole was more effective than placebo, dipyridamole alone, and aspirin alone.[82] A sustained-release formulation of dipyridamole was used for this study. A 37% relative-risk reduction was found for the combination treatment, and a 23% relative risk reduction was found for aspirin alone. The dipyridamole dose for this study was 200 mg BID, and the aspirin dose was 25 mg BID. Absolute risk reduction was approximately 1.5% annually. Headache occurred more frequently in patients receiving dipyridamole alone or in combination with aspirin. Bleeding complications were less frequent in patients receiving dipyridamole compared with aspirin alone. As a result of these findings, a combination product of aspirin and dipyridamole is available. The combination of sustained-release dipyridamole and aspirin is an acceptable alternative for secondary prevention of stroke when initial secondary prevention has failed.

TICLOPIDINE

10. What are the risks and benefits of using ticlopidine instead of aspirin in J.S.?

Ticlopidine (Ticlid) is an antiplatelet agent approved only for the prevention of TIA and stroke for patients with a prior cerebral thrombotic event. By inhibiting ADP-induced platelet aggregation, its activity differs from aspirin. A randomized, double-blind, placebo-controlled, multicenter trial, the Canadian American Ticlopidine Study (CATS), shows that ticlopidine significantly reduces the risk of stroke by 33.5.[83] In the Ticlopidine Aspirin Stroke Study Group (TASS), ticlopidine reduced the risk of stroke by 21%.[84] Neutropenia developed in 1% to 2% of patients on ticlopidine in both the CATS and TASS studies. Severe neutropenia (absolute neutrophil count [ANC] $<450/mm^3$) usually appears in the first 3 months of therapy and is reversible when the drug is discontinued. One episode of neutropenia-associated infection was reported in the CATS study. Because of the rather high potential for this adverse reaction, a complete blood count should be performed at baseline and every 2 weeks for the first 3 months of therapy. Additional data have shown that severe bone marrow depression is fatal in 16% of patients who develop this complication.[85] Thrombotic thrombocytopenia purpura has also been associated with ticlopidine and proved fatal in 33% of 60 patients.[86] Additionally, nearly 25% of patient will experience gastrointestinal adverse events, especially diarrhea, with around 10% requiring discontinuation of ticlopidine.

Ticlopidine is more effective in the secondary prevention of stroke and less likely to cause GI bleeding when compared with aspirin. However, hematologic and gastrointestinal adverse effects severely limit its use.

CLOPIDOGREL

11. Is clopidogrel a reasonable alternative for J.S.?

Clopidogrel (Plavix) is chemically related to ticlopidine and works by inhibiting platelet aggregation induced by ADP. A randomized, double-blind, international trial (Clopidogrel vs. Aspirin in Patients at Risk of Ischaemic Events [CAPRIE]) compared clopidogrel 75 mg/day with aspirin 325 mg/day.[87] Patients enrolled in the study had a history of atherosclerotic vascular disease manifested by recent ischemic stroke, myocardial infarction, or symptomatic peripheral vascular disease. Using intention-to-treat analysis, a 5.3% risk of an event in patients receiving clopidogrel and a 5.83% risk in patients receiving aspirin was observed. This represents a statistically significant relative risk reduction of 8.7%, favoring clopidogrel. On-treatment analysis showed a relative risk reduction of 9.4%, again in favor of clopidogrel. For patients whose primary condition for entry into CAPRIE was stroke, the relative risk reduction was 7.3%, however this difference was not statistically significant. Patients receiving clopidogrel more frequently experienced rash and diarrhea compared with those receiving aspirin. Patients receiving aspirin were more frequently affected by upper GI distress, intracranial hemorrhage, and GI hemorrhage. Significant reductions in neutrophils occurred in 0.10% of patients on clopidogrel and in 0.17% of patients on aspirin. Some cases of thrombocytopenia purpura are reported in the literature.[88]

Clopidogrel is as effective and safe as aspirin. Clopidogrel is an alternative to aspirin in secondary prevention of stroke.

WARFARIN/ANTICOAGULANTS

12. Is an anticoagulant such as warfarin an alternative instead of aspirin for a patient such as J.S.? What situations make anticoagulants more desirable?

Large randomized trials have compared oral anticoagulants to aspirin in the secondary prevention of stroke and TIA. In one study, aspirin 30 mg/day was compared to oral anticoagulants in doses adjusted to maintain an International Normalized Ratio (INR) between 3.0 and 4.5.[89] This study was terminated early when the mortality rate due to major bleeding events in the anticoagulant group was double the rate in the aspirin group. In this study, there was no difference between anticoagulants and aspirin in the frequency of stroke. A second study compared warfarin, dosed to maintain the INR between 1.4 and 2.8, and aspirin 325 mg/day.[90] Results from this study did not demonstrate a significant difference between aspirin and warfarin with regard to the prevention of stroke or major hemorrhagic events. However, minor hemorrhages were significantly more frequent among patients receiving warfarin. A third study was terminated early due to safety concerns in the warfarin arm of the study.[91] The target INR for this study was 2 to 3 in the warfarin arm compared to aspirin. The study was stopped due to significantly higher rates of adverse events in individuals receiving warfarin and no difference in the risk of stroke. Events including major hemorrhage, myocardial infarction or sudden death, and overall death were increased in those receiving warfarin. Warfarin is not generally recommended for secondary prevention of stroke.

J.S. is clearly at risk for additional TIAs or an ischemic stroke. The most important step in reducing this risk is to change his lifestyle. However, because J.S. has experienced a TIA, he also should be placed on an antiplatelet agent. Aspirin, dipyridamole combined with aspirin, or clopidogrel are acceptable alternatives for J.S. Warfarin is not an acceptable alternative in J.S. for initial, secondary prevention of TIA or stroke. Considering the overall costs of therapy and that he does not have any definite contraindications to aspirin, J.S. should be started on aspirin 81 mg/day. Clopidogrel or a combination of aspirin and dipyridamole can be used if J.S. is unable to tolerate aspirin or he experiences a recurrent TIA or a stroke while taking aspirin (Table 55-6).

Aspirin: Patient Education

13. The physician decides to begin J.S. on aspirin 81 mg/day. How should he be counseled on the use of aspirin? Should J.S. be advised to discontinue aspirin before surgical and dental procedures?

Even low dosages of aspirin may cause gastric erosions and gastric ulcers. J.S. should be instructed to take aspirin with the largest meal of the day, inform his physician of any epigastric pain, and seek medical attention at the first sign of any gastric bleeding (e.g., dark stools). Enteric-coated aspirin may cause less gastric upset than uncoated aspirin formulations.

J.S. should inform all of his healthcare providers, especially his physicians, pharmacist, and dentist, that he is taking aspirin daily. The decision to discontinue aspirin is at the discretion of his physician or dentist. This decision is based on the possibility of bleeding complications from the procedure and the risk of J.S. having a TIA while off aspirin. If aspirin is to be temporarily discontinued, it should be stopped at least 5 to 7 days before the procedure and restarted several days after the procedure.

Combination Antiplatelet Pharmacotherapy

14. Six months later J.S. has another TIA, despite taking aspirin. What is an appropriate intervention to prevent further TIA or stroke?

Possible interventions at this point are to switch to a different antiplatelet therapeutic regimen, to add clopidogrel to aspirin, or to increase the aspirin dose. A major study has compared clopidogrel 75 mg/day to the combination of clopidogrel 75 mg/day and aspirin 75 mg/day.[92] There was no difference in the risk of recurrent stroke or other cardiovascular outcomes between the groups, but the combination therapy group had a significant increase in life-threatening bleeding. Some individuals may be resistant to aspirin's effects on platelets.[64] Although poorly understand and studied, aspirin resistance may be due to the presence of extra-platelet sources of thromboxane A_2 and an interaction with over the counter nonsteroidal anti-inflammatory drugs or high levels of circulating 11-dehydro-thromboxane B_2.[93–95] There are no data to suggest that increasing the aspirin dose will overcome possible resistance to the antiplatelet effects of aspirin, but it is clear that an increased dose of aspirin increases his risk of major bleeding.

Based upon available data, the antiplatelet therapy for J.S. should be switched to clopidogrel monotherapy or the combination product of aspirin with dipyridamole.

CEREBRAL INFARCTION AND ISCHEMIC STROKE

Clinical Presentation and Diagnostic Tests

15. P.C., a 65-year-old man, is admitted through the emergency department (ED) after collapsing to the ground and experiencing a brief loss of consciousness. He regained consciousness by the time he arrived in the ED, 1 hour after the initial event. Both right extremities are flaccid. He is unable to speak but is capable of understanding instructions (i.e., expressive aphasia). Gross ophthalmologic examination indicates right-sided neglect (inability of his eyes to track to the right or acknowledge the right side of his body). His BP is 175/105 mmHg; other vital signs are normal. Laboratory studies are all within normal limits. By the next day, his neurologic status is unchanged and he is diagnosed as having an ischemic stroke. What interventions should be initiated prior to arrival in the ED?

Immediate recognition of and response to stroke symptoms are essential to an optimal outcome. As soon as stroke symptoms are recognized, the emergency medical system should be activated. Emergency medical personnel should be trained to gather important historical information, especially when the symptoms started. Use of a standardized evaluation tool like the Cincinnati Prehospital Stroke Scale or Los Angeles Prehospital Stroke Screen are useful in distinguishing stroke symptoms from other disorders like conversion disorder, hypertensive encephalopathy, hypoglycemia, complicated migraine, or seizures.[96] General supportive care for respiratory and cardiovascular function should be initiated prior to transporting the patient to the ED. An important key to effectively managing acute stroke patients is to have a well designed evaluation and treatment algorithm that addresses assessment and care of the patient from initial onset of symptoms through rehabilitation (Fig. 55-5).[96]

16. What diagnostic tests and evaluations will be helpful in guiding P.C.'s therapy?

Basic laboratory and diagnostic tests should be quickly performed to exclude noncerebrovascular causes, such as metabolic or toxicologic derangement, or infections for the neurologic compromise that P.C. has experienced. These tests include a routine serum chemistry profile (electrolytes, blood urea nitrogen [BUN], serum creatinine [SrCr], hepatic enzymes, calcium, phosphorus, magnesium, albumin), complete blood count, and toxicology screen. Coagulation studies, including a prothrombin time with INR and partial thromboplastin time (PTT), should be performed to provide baseline values for potential anticoagulation or thrombolytic therapy. In addition, a thorough physical, neurologic, cardiovascular, and mental status examination should be performed. The neurologic examination will allow a localization of the lesion in the CNS. The physical examination should include use of the National Institutes of Health Stroke Scale.[97] In addition to providing important information for diagnosis of his neurologic compromise, these tests will provide baseline data for ongoing assessment of P.C.'s progress and recovery.

The etiology of a stroke is difficult to discern based solely on a physical and neurologic examination. As a result, CT or magnetic resonance imaging (MRI) is valuable in the evaluation of these patients. An MRI is preferred to a CT due to its superior tissue contrast, ability to obtain images in multiple planes, absence of artifacts caused by bone, vascular imaging capabilities, absence of ionizing radiation, and safer contrast medium. MRI also allows for a magnetic resonance angiogram to be performed, allowing visualization of the cerebrovasculature and possible identification of the precise location of the thrombus or embolus. Within the first 24 hours of an ischemic stroke, an MRI is clearly more sensitive than a CT. After 48 hours, the MRI and CT are equally effective in detecting ischemic infarcts. The primary disadvantage of the MRI is that it is more sensitive to artifacts and less practical in unstable patients.

P.C. must have either a CT or an MRI before initiation of anticoagulation, thrombolytic agents, or other therapies for stroke. A follow-up CT or MRI in 5 to 7 days is useful to determine the extent of neurologic damage resulting from the ischemic stroke.

Angiographic, Doppler, or sonographic examination of the cerebral vasculature may be helpful in identifying the location of the vascular lesion. These tests usually are performed after the patient has been stabilized, unless angioplasty with stents or use of intra-arterial fibrinolytics are anticipated. A lumbar puncture with collection of cerebrospinal fluid (CSF) for evaluation may be helpful in identifying the presence of blood in the CNS. In the presence of suspected increased intracranial pressure, a lumbar puncture must be avoided because of the potential for tentorial herniation. Tentorial herniation occurs when the ventral half of the midbrain (i.e., the cerebral peduncles) pass through the tentorial notch (i.e., a portion of the dura mater that provides support for the occipital lobe and covers the cerebellum). This causes pressure on blood vessels that supply the cerebral cortex, resulting in restricted blood flow.

Treatment

17. What general treatment interventions should be made for P.C.?

In addition to the general supportive therapy needed for a hospitalized patient, several issues are important to the proper management of a stroke patient. Careful attention should be given to fluid and electrolyte control. Excessive hydration or inadequate sodium supplementation may result in hyponatremia, thereby forcing fluid into neurons to further increase the damage from ischemia. In addition, hyponatremia can produce seizures, which increases the metabolic demand on compromised neurons. Thus, it is advisable to initiate fluid therapy with a solution containing at least 0.45% saline and preferably 0.9% saline.

Attention to body temperature needs to be given. Studies have shown that even small increases in temperature are associated with worse outcomes.[98,99] Hypothermia is neuroprotective and some studies indicate that even a reduction in body

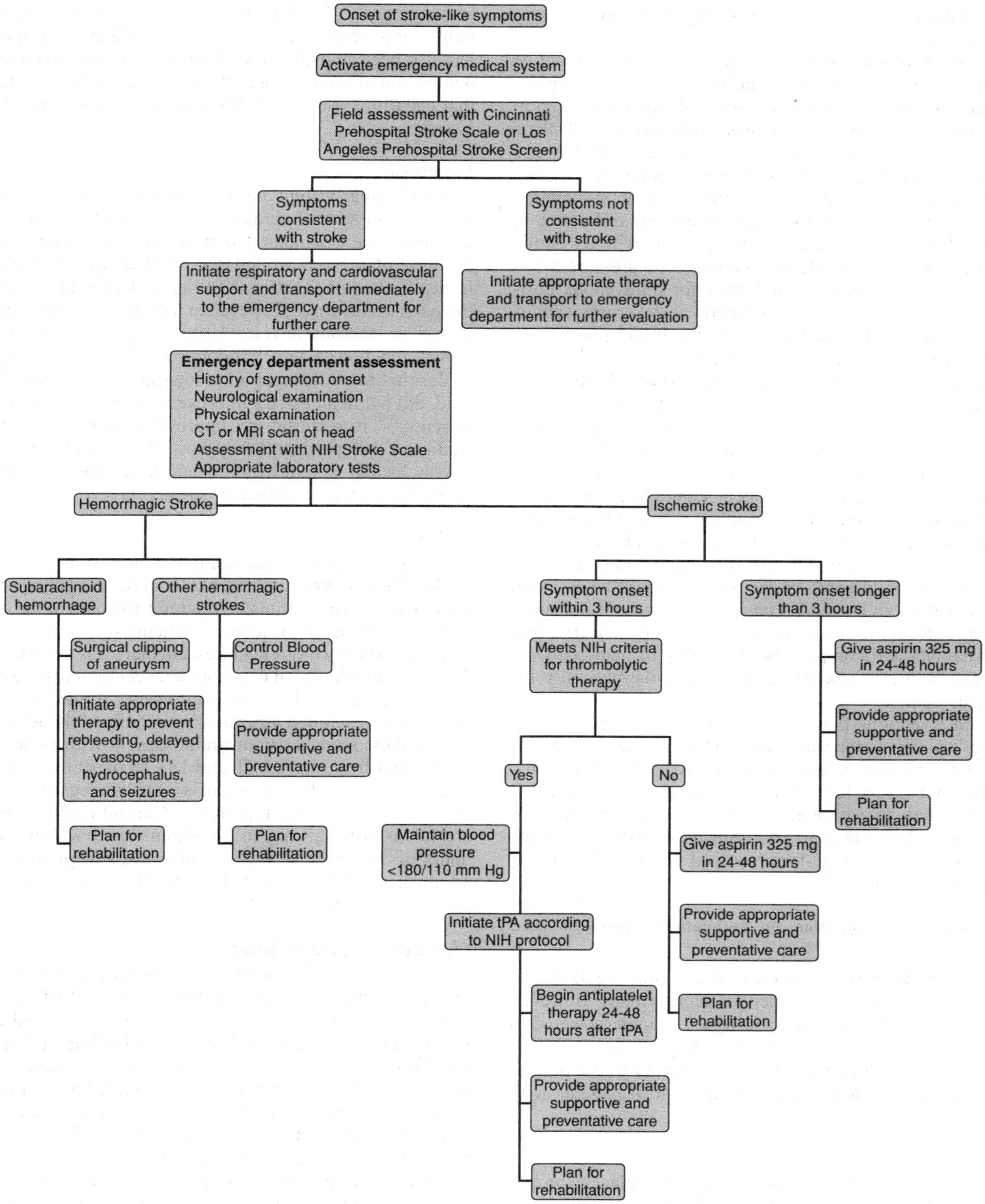

FIGURE 55-5 Treatment algorithim for management of patient with acute stroke-like symptoms (Adapted from Adams HP et al.)

temperature of 0.26°F can be beneficial in stroke patients.[96,100] Use of antipyretics, like acetaminophen, are advised to maintain normal or slightly subnormal body temperatures.

Another metabolic parameter that must be followed carefully is the serum glucose concentration, because hyperglycemia may adversely affect ischemic infarction outcomes. A review of multiple studies on the effects of hyperglycemia in acute stroke concluded that hyperglycemia results in poor outcomes and increased mortality.[101] If hyperglycemia is detected, appropriate insulin therapy should be initiated to keep the serum glucose concentration <140 mg/dL without causing hypoglycemia.[96]

Caution should be exercised in the acute management of P.C.'s blood pressure. Decreasing the blood pressure too rapidly will compromise cerebral blood flow and expand the region of ischemia and infarction, whereas hypertension will place him at a greater risk for cerebral hemorrhage, especially if a thrombolytic agent is used. However, a study comparing treated and untreated patients who were hypertensive in association with an acute stroke failed to demonstrate any difference in outcomes between the groups.[102] For patients with a systolic blood pressure >185 mmHg or diastolic blood pressure >110 mmHg, who are otherwise candidates for intravenous fibrinolytic treatment, labetalol, nitroglycerin paste, or intravenous nicardipine should be used to reduce the blood pressure to these goals prior to starting tPA.[96] After administration with tPA, blood pressure should be kept below 180/105 mmHg. In other patients, the only consensus on blood pressure control is that treatment is required when pressures exceed 220/120 mmHg.[96] If there is a clinical deterioration of neurologic function associated with the reduction of blood pressure, the infusion rate of the antihypertensive agent should be slowed or the drug discontinued. Maintenance antihypertensive therapy can then be initiated using an oral agent, such as a calcium channel antagonist or angiotensin-converting enzyme inhibitor.

The general daily needs of the patient should be assessed and provided on an as-needed basis. These include nutrition, urination, defecation, and prevention of decubitus ulcers. Neurologic deficits will compromise the ability of many patients to adequately meet these needs, increasing the necessity for medical assistance.

Two interventions that have been shown to improve outcomes of ischemic stroke are reducing the time to treatment of stroke and admitting patients to specialized stroke care units. Reduction of the time to treatment permits the use of interventions shown only to work within the first 2 hours of a stroke.[103] In addition, Indredavik et al. have shown that stroke care units significantly improve long-term survival and functionality of patients after a stroke.[104]

18. Should anticoagulation or antiplatelet agents be used acutely in P.C.?

Several studies have evaluated the use of anticoagulants and antiplatelet agents in the treatment of acute strokes. However, most of these studies are poorly designed or underpowered to determine the efficacy of these agents. Despite these problems with published studies, many physicians prefer to use anticoagulants or antiplatelets in the management of patients with acute stroke.

Heparin

Duke et al. compared intravenous heparin to placebo in patients with acute partially stable stroke.[105] In this double-blind study, heparin doses were adjusted to maintain the PTT at 1.5 to 2 times control and continued for 7 days. There were no significant differences in death at 7 days, and no differences in functional ability were observed to 1 year following the stroke. At 1 year there was a significantly greater mortality rate in heparin-treated patients. The International Stroke Trial compared aspirin, subcutaneous heparin (5,000 IU or 12,500 IU BID), both and neither treatments for patients with acute ischemic stroke.[106] There was no reduction of mortality or morbidity for patients receiving either dose of heparin. Heparin use has also been studied in progressing stroke and no benefit was demonstrated with its use.[107] No studies have demonstrated that heparin is useful in mitigating the neurological effects of a stroke.

Heparinoids

Low-molecular-weight heparins and heparinoids have been evaluated in several studies for acute stroke. Two doses of nadroparin were compared to placebo in one randomized, double blind, placebo controlled trial.[108] There were no differences in death rates or functional ability at 3 months between the three treatment arms. However, at 6 months, patients receiving high-dose nadroparin (i.e., 4,100 anti-Xa IU BID) had improved function. A large randomized, placebo controlled trial of dose-adjusted danaparoid, a low-molecular-weight heparinoid, did not demonstrate improvement in danaparoid-treated patients.[109] In addition, no improvements were observed in studies of dalteparin and certoparin.[110,111] Similar to heparin, low-molecular-weight heparins and heparinoids are not indicated in the acute treatment of stroke.

Aspirin

One study evaluated early administration of aspirin in acute stroke. The Chinese Acute Stroke Trial (CAST) compared 160 mg/day of aspirin administered within 48 hours of the onset of stroke symptoms to placebo.[112] Patients who received aspirin had reduced early mortality rates, but there was no difference in the primary endpoint of death or dependency at discharge from the hospital. The IST and the Multicenter Acute Stroke Trial-Italy studies included aspirin arms in their study design. Neither of these studies demonstrated benefit with aspirin.[106,113] When data from the CAST and IST studies are combined, a slight beneficial effect of aspirin is seen with regard to reducing the risk of early stroke recurrence. Current recommendations are for aspirin 325 mg to be administered within 24 to 48 hours of the onset of stroke symptoms, except when tPA is administered.[96] If tPA is used, aspirin should not be given until 24 to 48 hours after the tPA infusion.

Glycoprotein IIb/IIIa Inhibitors

Platelet glycoprotein IIb/IIIa inhibitors have also been studied in acute stroke. A placebo controlled Phase II trial of abciximab given within 24 hours of acute stroke showed a trend toward improved functionality in abciximab-treated patients, but the study was not powered to show significance for this outcome.[114] In another placebo controlled, Phase II study of patients with acute stroke the direct thrombin inhibitor, argatroban, was associated with statistically significant improvements in neurologic symptoms and daily living activities.[115] The number of patients enrolled in this study was small, but the results show promise. Currently, the use of these agents is limited to clinical trials.

Ancrod

Derived from the venom of the Malayan pit viper snake, ancrod cleaves fibrinogen in a way similar to thrombin. Ancrod leads to fibrinolysis soon after its administration and is rarely associated with significant bleeding complications. This low risk of hemorrhagic complications makes ancrod especially attractive for use in ischemic stroke. The Stroke Treatment with Ancrod Trial (STAT) compared a continuous 72-hour infusion of ancrod dosed to decrease fibrinogen levels to 1.18 to 2.03 mU/L to receive placebo.[116] This infusion was followed by 1-hour infusions at approximately 96 and 120 hours after treatment was started. Ancrod infusion rates of 0.167, 0.125, and 0.082 IU/kg/hour were used based on pretreatment fibrinogen concentrations. Significantly more patients treated with ancrod achieved favorable functional status and had fewer disabilities, with no difference in mortality rates. Due to the lack of additional data, the use of ancrod is limited to clinical trials.

19. When might anticoagulants be used in the treatment of acute stroke?

Deep vein thrombosis and pulmonary embolism are common complications in patients following a stroke. The incidence of deep vein thrombosis (DVT) and pulmonary embolus (PE) were reduced in most studies where patients received heparin, low-molecular-weight heparins, or heparinoids.[117]

Two systematic reviews of the literature in this area resulted in the following recommendations and guidelines[96,117]:

1. Aspirin 325 mg/day should be initiated within 48 hours of the onset of stroke symptoms, unless tPA is used. If tPA is used, aspirin should not be started until 24 to 48 hours after tPA administration.
2. Heparin, low-molecular-weight heparins, and heparinoids may be considered for prevention of DVT and PE. Use of these agents must be weighed against the risk of hemorrhagic complications.
3. Fixed dose heparin may have some early benefit in the treatment of acute stroke, but this benefit is negated by an increased risk of hemorrhage and is not recommended.
4. Dose-adjusted heparin is associated with increased bleeding complications and is not recommended.
5. Low-molecular-weight heparins and heparinoids at high doses are not recommended in patients with acute stroke.
6. Intravenous heparin, high-dose low-molecular-weight heparins, or heparinoids are not recommended for any subgroup or specific type of stroke.

On the basis of these recommendations, P.C. should receive 325 mg/day of aspirin to be started within 24 to 48 hours of onset of his stroke symptoms, unless tPA is administered. If tPA is used, then aspirin should be started 24 to 48 hours after the tPA infusion. Use of other anticoagulants is not recommended.

Thrombolytics

20. Would thrombolytic agents be useful to treat P.C.'s acute ischemic stroke?

The critical primary event in a thromboembolic stroke is the development of an acute thrombus. Prospective cerebral angiography has demonstrated an arterial occlusion corresponding to the area of acute neurologic deficit in >90% of cases.[118] Occlusion of cerebral arteries does not cause complete ischemia because collateral circulation from other arterial sources provides unstable and incomplete circulation to the ischemic region of the brain.[119] When blood flow is sustained in the range of 10 to 18 mL/100 g per minute, irreversible cellular damage may occur. Blood flow must be restored quickly after the event. Experimental studies in dogs and cats have shown that when blood flow is restored within 2 to 3 hours, neurologic deficits are prevented.[120,121] Thrombolytic agents can reestablish blood flow to ischemic regions of the brain.

A total of five large, placebo-controlled trials using either tPA or streptokinase for acute stroke have been published. In three studies, streptokinase was used as the thrombolytic and all of these studies were terminated early due to high rates of mortality and intracranial hemorrhage associated with streptokinase.[113,122,123] These trials clearly demonstrate that streptokinase is associated with increased mortality and disability. The rates of intracranial hemorrhage ranged from 6% to 17% for patients receiving streptokinase compared with 0.6% to 3% for patients receiving placebo. In all three trials the mortality rates were significantly greater for patients receiving streptokinase. Streptokinase should not be used for P.C.

Studies with tPA demonstrate some benefit associated its use.[124,125] The National Institute of Neurological Disorders and Stroke (NINDS) tPA trial and the European Cooperative Acute Stroke Study (ECASS) used different doses, inclusion criteria, and treatment protocols. Both trials showed the benefit of tPA in at least some outcome parameters. In the NINDS tPA study, patients were enrolled using strict inclusion and exclusion criteria (Table 55-7). All patients were within 3 hours of symptom onset and had to undergo a CT scan before enrollment. When enrolled, patients received either tPA 0.9 mg/kg (maximum dose, 90 mg), with 10% of the dose given as a bolus over 1 minute and the remainder infused over 60 minutes, or placebo. Patients were divided into two groups for the purpose of analysis. One group consisted of 291 patients whose early neurologic recovery was assessed 24 hours after enrollment. The second group of 333 patients had neurologic outcomes evaluated at 3 months. In the first group, there was

Table 55-7 Criteria for Alteplase Use in Treatment of Acute Stroke

Inclusion Criteria	*Exclusion Criteria*
18 years of age or older	Minor or rapidly improving symptoms
Clinical diagnosis of stroke with clinically meaningful neurologic deficit	CT signs of intracranial hemorrhage
Clearly defined onset within 180 minutes before treatment	History of intracranial hemorrhage
Baseline CT with no evidence of intracranial hemorrhage	Seizure at onset of stroke
	Stroke or serious head injury within 3 months
	Major surgery or serious trauma within 2 weeks
	GI or urinary tract hemorrhage within 3 weeks
	Systolic BP >185 mmHg, diastolic BP >110 mmHg
	Aggressive treatment to lower BP
	Glucose 400 mg/dL
	Symptoms of subarachnoid hemorrhage

BP, blood pressure; CT, computed tomography; GI, gastrointestinal.

no difference in positive responses between patients receiving tPA or placebo. However, a secondary analysis showed that National Institutes of Health Stroke Scale scores were significantly greater at 24 hours for patients receiving tPA. Results in the second group were favorable for tPA. At 3 months, patients who received tPA were 30% more likely to have minimal or no disability and there was an 11% to 13% absolute increase in the number of patients with excellent outcomes. There was a corresponding decrease in the number of patients with severe neurologic impairment or death at 3 months. Improvements associated with tPA were seen across age groups, stroke subtypes, stroke severity, and status of aspirin use before the stroke. Intracranial hemorrhage occurred more frequently among patients receiving tPA (6.4%) than in patients receiving placebo (0.6%). Despite the increased incidence of ICH, outcomes remained better for patients receiving tPA.

For the ECASS I trial, patients with the onset of a stroke were enrolled within 6 hours of the onset of symptoms.[125] The treatment protocol consisted of IV tPA 1.1 mg/kg (maximum, 100 mg) or placebo. Using intention-to-treat analysis, there was no difference in the primary outcome measures of functionality at 3 months. However, with target population analysis, there was a significant difference favoring tPA. Of tPA-treated patients, 41% had minimal or no disability compared with 29% of placebo-treated patients. A variety of secondary outcome measures favored tPA. There was no difference in 30-day mortality rates, but 19.8% of tPA-treated patients had major parenchymal hemorrhages compared with 6.5% of placebo-treated patients. A more recent trial, ECASS II, used a tPA dose of 0.9 mg/kg and was designed to replicate the NINDS trial.[126] However, patients were enrolled up to 6 hours after the onset of stroke symptoms. This study found no difference between tPA and placebo. Too few patients were enrolled with stroke symptoms <3 hours to reliably evaluate the influence of this variable on outcome.

The Cochrane Stroke Review Group performed a meta-analysis of 17 thrombolytic trials.[127] In this analysis, thrombolytic therapy was associated with an excess of early deaths (odds ratio, 1.85; 95% CI, 1.48–2.32) and early symptomatic hemorrhages (odds ratio, 3.53; 95% CI, 2.79–4.45). However, thrombolytic therapy initiated within 6 hours of symptom onset reduced the proportion of patients who were dead or dependent at the end of follow-up (odds ratio, 0.83; 95% CI, 0.73–0.94). Similar results were obtained when the analysis included patients treated within 3 hours of symptom onset (odds ratio, 0.58; 95% CI, 0.46–0.74). About half of the data included in these analyses came from trials of tPA and the results support the use of tPA in the treatment of acute ischemic stroke. This analysis substantiates the use of tPA in the treatment of ischemic stroke.

Several studies have reported the use of intra-arterial thrombolytic therapy. In one trial, patients were randomized to receive either 6 mg of recombinant prourokinase or placebo over 120 minutes.[128] All patients received IV heparin. Patients who were randomized received treatment at a median of 5.5 hours from symptom onset. Recanalization was significantly greater in the prourokinase group. However, hemorrhagic transformation occurred in 15.4% of prourokinase-treated patients compared with 7.1% of placebo-treated patients. Hemorrhage frequencies and recanalization rates were influenced by heparin dose. A second trial has confirmed these findings, showing significantly improved outcomes with intra-arterial prourokinase, despite increased intracranial hemorrhage.[129] Although useful in major medical centers, intra-arterial prourokinase presents major technical obstacles that limit its use in most emergency departments.

The only study that has clearly shown benefit associated with systemic tPA use for acute stroke is the NINDS tPA trial. If tPA is to be used for acute stroke, the NINDS inclusion and exclusion criteria and treatment protocol should be used.

Because P.C. presented to the ED within 1 hour of the onset of his stroke symptoms, he is a candidate for tPA therapy in accordance with the NINDS study protocol. A thorough history and CT scan must be performed before initiation of tPA to ensure compliance with inclusion and exclusion criteria.

Preservation of CNS Function

Preservation of marginally ischemic regions of the brain is an active area of investigation. Hemodilution, corticosteroids, calcium channel blockers, 21-aminosteroids, NMDA receptor antagonists, lubeluzole, citicoline, anti-intercellular adhesion molecule (ICAM)-1 antibody, clomethiazole, fosphenytoin, piracetam, ebselen, and ganglioside GM-1 are therapeutic interventions that have been studied to retain CNS function in the ischemic penumbra. None of these interventions has been clearly shown to preserve neurologic function. Because the events leading to neuronal death involve numerous pathways, it is possible that a combination of some of these agents will prove to be most effective.

Hemodilution

21. What is the rationale for hemodilution therapy in ischemic stroke? Should this therapeutic approach be recommended for P.C.?

Based on a direct relationship between a lowered hematocrit and decreased blood viscosity, various colloid and crystalloid solutions have been administered to ischemic stroke patients. Initial studies indicated that volume expansion might be useful, but larger trials have not supported the original findings.[130,131] A more recent trial failed to show any benefit from hemodilution, but found this practice to be as safe as regular hydration therapy.[132] None of the studies have shown a benefit as measured by a reduction in mortality rates. Hemodilution is not recommended in P.C.'s management.

Corticosteroids

22. Should corticosteroids be used in P.C.?

Corticosteroids have been used to treat stroke on the theory that decreasing edema and swelling of the brain will increase cerebral blood flow to ischemic regions. Dexamethasone (4–20 mg Q 6 hr) was commonly used because it has substantial anti-inflammatory effects without mineralocorticoid activity; however, multiple studies have shown that corticosteroids are ineffective in treating cerebral infarction or hemorrhagic stroke.[133–138] The lack of efficacy of steroids might be explained by inflammation of dead neurons rather than in marginally ischemic neurons. The use of corticosteroids is relatively contraindicated in these patients because of possible increases in morbidity and mortality.[133] Corticosteroids are ineffective in the treatment of cerebral infarction or hemorrhagic stroke.

Calcium Channel Blockers

23. What is the rationale for using calcium channel blockers in ischemic stroke? Are they indicated for use in P.C.?

Calcium influx into neurons coincides with much of the cellular destruction associated with ischemia. Because calcium influx into the neuron is modulated by both voltage-dependent channels and neurotransmitter-dependent channels, calcium channel blockers that penetrate the CNS could be useful for limiting the neurologic damage associated with an ischemic stroke. In addition, the calcium channel blockers have been shown to increase blood flow into ischemic regions of the brain.

Initial studies of nimodipine for ischemic stroke indicated that treatment positively improved outcomes. A study of 186 patients showed an 8.6% mortality rate in the nimodipine-treated group compared with a 20.4% mortality rate in the placebo-treated group.[139] Stratification according to gender indicated a significant difference in males but not in females.

Eight other studies failed to substantiate this first study. One study evaluated nimodipine 120 mg/day in a double blind, randomized trial.[140] Based on two stroke rating scales and mortality rates, there was no difference between nimodipine and placebo. Another randomized, double blind, placebo-controlled study of nimodipine showed no improvement with nimodipine.[141] A meta-analysis of nimodipine use in 3,719 patients showed a benefit only for patients who were treated with 30 mg Q 6 hr beginning within 12 hours of symptom onset.[142] A second systematic review came to a similar conclusion and effectively ruled out a clinically significant benefit of calcium channel blockers in acute ischemic stroke.[143]

Calcium channel blockers are not indicated in P.C. Their use in subarachnoid hemorrhage is discussed in Question 30.

Stroke Education

24. What information and instruction should be given to P.C. regarding future stroke symptoms?

Early treatment of acute stroke with available or investigational drugs appears to be the most important factor in determining optimal outcome. Nearly every clinical trial demonstrating some benefit of pharmacotherapy for acute stroke has shown the greatest effect for patients who are treated within a few hours of the onset of stroke symptoms. Immediate detection of stroke symptoms and initiation of treatment are imperative. The primary rate-limiting step in diagnosis and provision of medical care is recognition by the patient of stroke symptoms. Every patient who is at increased risk of stroke should be carefully instructed to seek emergent medical attention if they experience any weakness or paralysis, speech impairment, numbness, blurred vision or sudden loss of vision, or altered level of consciousness. These symptoms should be handled with the same urgency as the symptoms of a myocardial infarction. The pharmacist should ensure that P.C. and his caregivers know the symptoms of stroke and understand what to do if they occur.

Complications

25. What complications associated with stroke might P.C. experience?

Agitation, delirium, stupor, coma, cerebral edema, and/or increased intracranial pressure are other symptoms that can be associated with ischemic stroke. These symptoms correlate with the specific blood vessels that are affected, and the development of these complications in P.C. would depend on the progression of his stroke.

Seizures may occur in up to 20% of stroke patients. Pneumonia, pulmonary edema, cardiac arrest, deep vein thrombosis, and arrhythmias commonly are associated with ischemic stroke and should be managed as they occur. In P.C., these may occur soon after his stroke or be related to a rapidly developing neurologic event such as further infarction, hemorrhage, or severe cerebral edema. Pneumonia or deep venous thrombosis are related primarily to inactivity, and the risk of these events will increase the longer P.C. remains immobile.

Stroke patients frequently experience psychologic reactions. The most common psychiatric complication is depression, occurring in 30% to 50% of patients.[145] The severity of depression varies from mild to major depressive episodes. If the depression interferes with recovery and the rehabilitative process, it should be managed with the use of a selective serotonin reuptake inhibitor (SSRI) or other appropriate agent. Severe psychomotor depression may respond to CNS stimulants, such as methylphenidate or dextroamphetamine. Because of P.C.'s hypertension, stimulants only should be used with careful blood pressure monitoring.

Prognosis

26. After 4 days in the hospital, P.C.'s neurologic status is stabilized. Will further neurologic improvements be realized?

Neurologic deficits in stroke patients are not considered stable or fixed until at least 8 to 12 months have elapsed. During this time, neurologic function may return, but rarely to normal. The prognosis following ischemic stroke depends on a variety of factors including age, hypertension, coma, cardiopulmonary complications, hypoxia, and neurogenic hyperventilation. However, infarction of the middle cerebral artery is associated with a poor chance for recovery. Therefore, it is possible that P.C. will experience further neurologic improvement.

Rehabilitation

27. As P.C. enters rehabilitation, what interventions will aid his recovery?

Rehabilitation for P.C. is directed at managing daily functions, enhancing existing neurologic function, and attempting to regain lost function. Considerations for daily functions include activities of daily living and bowel and bladder management through balanced pharmacologic interventions. Efforts should be made to allow P.C. to function independently with activities of daily living and manage the psychologic effects of stroke. Enhancement of current neurologic function and minimizing depression includes elimination of drugs that may compromise P.C.'s memory and mental function. These include benzodiazepines, major tranquilizers, and sedating antiepileptic drugs.

Spasticity of the affected limb may present a problem for P.C. Because spasticity often is localized to a single limb after ischemic stroke, it frequently responds to regional motor nerve blocks with botulinum toxin. Aggressive physical therapy also is essential to the management of spasticity. Systemic antispasticity agents such as diazepam, baclofen, or dantrolene sodium are not used routinely because of the risk for toxicity. They are used only when spasticity involves multiple parts of the body or is unresponsive to other therapies.

Other less common impediments to P.C.'s recovery include decubitus ulcers, hypercalcemia, and heterotopic ossification (e.g., the laying down and calcification of a bone matrix in muscle surrounding major joints). Prevention through meticulous skin care is the key to the management of pressure ulcers. Mobilizing P.C. as soon as possible after the stroke can prevent hypercalcemia and heterotopic ossification. If necessary, these complications may be treated with etidronate (Didronel).

SUBARACHNOID HEMORRHAGE

Clinical Presentation and Treatment

28. R.A., a 65-year-old woman, suddenly collapsed in the bathroom of her home. An ambulance was immediately called, and on arrival at the ED she had regained consciousness. She complained of a severe headache and kept dropping off to sleep during the examination. Nuchal rigidity (i.e., a stiff and painful neck when flexed) and mild mental confusion with regard to place also were observed. A CT scan demonstrated blood in the subarachnoid space and in her ventricles. A cerebral angiogram demonstrated a posterior communicating artery aneurysm. Electrolytes, coagulation studies, and blood counts were within normal limits. What pharmacotherapy is used for subarachnoid hemorrhage?

R.A.'s neurologic symptoms and the appearance of blood on her CT scan are consistent with a diagnosis of subarachnoid hemorrhage. Unfortunately, there are no direct pharmacotherapeutic interventions that are effective for subarachnoid hemorrhage. Surgical repair and clipping of the aneurysm is the definitive intervention. Pharmacotherapy is directed at preventing or managing complications of SAH (Fig. 55-5).

Complications

29. R.A.'s neurologic status deteriorated approximately 3 days after admission. What complications may be responsible for these changes?

Following the initial hemorrhagic event, there are three major complications that usually are responsible for neurologic changes (Table 55-8). *Rebleeding* from an aneurysm occurs in 20% of patients, usually within the first 48 hours after the initial event. In some cases, rebleeding can happen as long as 14 days later. From 24 hours to weeks after the hemorrhage, *hydrocephalus* (i.e., accumulation of excessive CSF within the ventricular system of the brain) may be caused by blood interrupting CSF flow through the ventricles and reabsorption of CSF through the arachnoid villa. Another 20% to 40% of

Table 55-8 Therapy for Subarachnoid Hemorrhage Complications

Rebleeding	*Hydrocephalus*	*Delayed Ischemia*
Surgical clip	Ventricular drain	Nimodipine 60 mg Q 4 hr for 21 days
Aminocaproic acid 5 g loading dose and 1 to 2 g/hr	Ventricular-peritoneal shunt	Hypervolemia PCWP 12–15 mmHg
		Hypertension Systolic BP 170–220 mmHg

BP, blood pressure; PCWP, pulmonary capillary wedge pressure.

patients will develop *delayed cerebral ischemia,* usually within 5 to 12 days following the initial hemorrhage. Delayed ischemia caused by vasospasm of the cerebral vessels is evidenced by development of new neurologic deficits and confirmed by a cerebral angiogram. At least half of these individuals will die or experience permanent neurologic damage. Approximately 5% to 15% of patients have seizures.

30. How should each of these complications (rebleeding, hydrocephalus, vasospasm, seizures) be managed in R.A.? Are calcium channel blockers more effective in treating subarachnoid hemorrhage than ischemic stroke?

Rebleeding

Surgical clipping of the aneurysm is the best method to prevent rebleeding. If early surgery is contraindicated or unavailable, antifibrinolytic therapy with epsilon aminocaproic acid (EACA) may be instituted. EACA blocks the activation of plasminogen and inhibits the action of plasmin on the fibrin clot. EACA enhances hemostasis when fibrinolysis contributes to bleeding and stabilizes the clot that has formed around the ruptured aneurysm. The incidence of rebleeding is decreased from 20% to 30% to 10% to 15% by EACA.[146,147] However, delayed cerebral ischemia occurs more frequently in patients receiving EACA.[146] It is unclear whether this is a direct effect of EACA or whether more individuals survive to experience delayed cerebral ischemia. EACA usually is given as a 5-g IV bolus followed by a continuous infusion of 1 to 2 g/hour. Dosages can be adjusted to maintain serum concentrations of 200 to 400 mg/mL. R.A. may benefit from receiving EACA as soon as a subarachnoid hemorrhage is diagnosed, and it should be continued until surgical clipping can be performed or for at least 2 weeks after the initial hemorrhage. It is preferable to surgically repair the aneurysm as soon as possible after R.A. is admitted to the hospital.

Hydrocephalus

The only effective treatment for hydrocephalus is surgical intervention. If a CT scan demonstrates hydrocephalus, a ventricular drain should be surgically placed after the aneurysm has been clipped. When hydrocephalus becomes a chronic problem, the drain can be replaced with a permanent ventriculoperitoneal shunt.

Ventriculitis is a common complication of a ventricular drain and is most likely caused by staphylococci or Gram-negative bacteria. Antibiotic therapy for this complication should consist of an IV agent (e.g., chloramphenicol, ceftriaxone, ampicillin, penicillin, vancomycin, ceftazidime, cefuroxime, nafcillin, rifampin) that readily crosses the blood–brain barrier with inflamed meninges. Alternatively, gentamicin and vancomycin can be instilled through the ventricular drains directly to the site of infection.[148] The antibiotic solution is prepared using a preservative-free sterile powder for injection. Gentamicin 4 to 8 mg or vancomycin 5 to 20 mg is instilled once a day. Systemic and intraventricular antibiotics should be continued until three consecutive CSF cultures are free of bacterial growth.

Delayed Cerebral Ischemia (Vasospasm)

The occurrence of delayed cerebral ischemia probably is due to vasospasm of the cerebral blood vessels. Current therapy for delayed ischemia is not optimal and is rather confusing. Volume expansion with normal saline or plasma protein fraction usually is initiated when focal neurologic changes develop, with the goal of maintaining a pulmonary capillary wedge pressure of 15 to 20 mmHg.[149–152] Some clinicians may institute hypervolemia therapy in anticipation of delayed cerebral ischemia. If the neurologic deficits are not reversed with hypervolemia, systolic blood pressure can be increased to as high as 200 to 220 mmHg using dopamine or norepinephrine. A high systolic pressure allows the brain to redirect flow to ischemic areas, and such therapy is often continued for 7 to 14 days.

CALCIUM CHANNEL BLOCKERS

Nimodipine

Nimodipine also is indicated for the prevention of delayed cerebral ischemia for patients with a subarachnoid hemorrhage. Its mechanisms of action may include preventing cerebral vasospasm that is responsible for delayed ischemia, inhibiting calcium influx into ischemic neurons, or re-establishing cerebrovascular autoregulation (i.e., the ability of the brain to control blood flow in accordance with metabolic needs).

Nimodipine has been administered in clinical studies intravenously, orally, or topically (i.e., direct application to the brain's surface and the cerebral vasculature during surgery). Several studies of nimodipine in subarachnoid hemorrhage have used oral formulations. In these studies, a total of 1,038 patients were given nimodipine prophylactically according to double-blind, placebo-controlled, randomized protocols.[153–156] Angiographic improvement was not significantly different in patients treated with nimodipine or placebo, but neurologic outcomes improved significantly in nimodipine-treated patients who presented with a mild to moderately severe subarachnoid hemorrhage. In another study, nimodipine significantly benefited patients with severe hemorrhage. Nimodipine 60 to 90 mg Q 4 hr for 21 days was initiated within the first 96 hours after the original subarachnoid hemorrhage in these patients. No trial has compared the efficacy of nimodipine with hypervolemia therapy and interventions to increase systolic blood pressure. Nimodipine's approved dose is 60 mg PO Q 6 hr.

R.A. should receive nimodipine 60 mg PO Q 4 hr for 21 days, because she was diagnosed within several hours of her subarachnoid hemorrhage.

Seizures

PHENYTOIN

Seizures occur in approximately 9% of patients experiencing a subarachnoid hemorrhage. Only two factors associated with subarachnoid hemorrhage have been identified as predictive of seizures: rebleeding or large amounts of cisternal blood on CT scan.

Phenytoin often is used for seizure prophylaxis. However, no trials have investigated the efficacy of phenytoin in preventing seizure in patients with subarachnoid hemorrhage. The usual dose of phenytoin is 15 to 20 mg/kg administered as an IV bolus at a rate <50 mg/minute. A maintenance dose of 5 to 7 mg/kg/day either orally or intravenously is titrated to maintain steady-state serum concentrations of 10 to 20 mg/mL. Alternatively, fosphenytoin, a phenytoin prodrug, can be administered intravenously or intramuscularly at a loading dose of 15 to 20 mg phenytoin equivalents (PE)/kg and a maintenance dose of 5 to 7 mg PE/kg/day. Infusion rates of fosphenytoin should be <150 mg PE/minute. Maintenance phenytoin usually is continued for 1 to 2 years or longer if the patient experiences seizures. Because there is a 5% to 20% risk of seizures for R.A., she should receive phenytoin prophylactically. Valproic acid (Depacon) and levetiracetam (Keppra) are available in intravenous formulations; however there is little experience with the use of these agents for seizures in the setting of subarachnoid hemorrhage.

REFERENCES

1. Rosamond W et al. Heart disease and stroke statistics-2007 update: a report from teh American Heart Association Statistics Committee and Stroke Statistics Subcommittee. *Circulation* 2007; 115:69.
2. Thom T et al. Heart disease and stroke statistics–2006 update: a report from the American Heart Association Statistics Committee and Stroke Statistics Subcommittee. *Circulation* 2006;113:85.
3. Williams GR. Incidence and characteristics of total stroke in the United States. *BMC Neurology* 2001; 1:2.
4. Howard G et al. Decline in U.S. stroke mortality an analysis of temporal patterns by sex, race, and geographic region. *Stroke* 2001;32:2213.
5. Goldstein LB et al. Primary prevention of ischemic stroke: a guideline from the American Heart Association/American Stroke Council: cosponsored by the Atherosclerotic Peripheral Vascular Disease Interdisciplinary Working Group; Cardiovascular Nursing Council; Clinical Cardiology Council; Nutrition Physical Activity, and Metabolism Council; and the Quality of Care and Outcomes Research Interdisciplinary Working Group: The American Academy of Neurology affirms the value of this guideline. *Stroke* 2006;37:1583.
6. Sacco RL et al. Guidelines for the prevention of stroke in patients with ischemic stroke or transient ischemic attack: a statement for healthcare professionals from the American Heart Association/American Stroke Association Council on Stroke: co-sponsored by the Council on Cardiovascular Radiology and Intervention: The American Academy of Neurology affirms the value of this guideline. *Stroke* 2006;37:577.
7. Woo D et al. Genetic and environmental risk factors for intracerebral hemorrhage: preliminary results of a population-based study. *Stroke* 2002;33:1190.
8. Astrup J. Cortical evoked potential and extracellular K^+; and H^+; at critical levels of brain ischemia. *Stroke* 1977;8:51.
9. Hickenbottom SL et al. Neuroprotective therapy. *Semin Neurol* 1998;18:485.
10. Prospective Studies Collaboration. Cholesterol, diastolic blood pressure, and stroke: 13,000 strokes in 450,000 people in 45 prospective cohorts. *Lancet* 1995;346:1647.
11. Dunbalin DW et al. Preventing stroke by the modification of risk factors. *Stroke* 1990;21(Suppl IV): IV–36.
12. Neal B et al. Blood Pressure Lowering Treatment Trialists' Collaboration. Effects of ACE inhibitors, calcium antagonists, and other blood-pressure-lowering drugs: results of prospectively

designed overviews of randomised trials. Blood Pressure Lowering Treatment Trialists' Collaboration. *Lancet* 2000;356:1955.
13. Chobanian AV et al. National Heart, Lung, and Blood Institute Joint National Committee on Prevention, Detection, Evaluation, and Treatment of High Blood Pressure; National High Blood Pressure Education Program Coordinating Committee. The Seventh Report of the Joint National Committee on Prevention, Detection, Evaluation, and Treatment of High Blood Pressure: the JNC 7 report. *JAMA* 2003;289:2560.
14. Kannel WB, McGee DL. Diabetes and cardiovascular disease: the Framingham Study. *JAMA* 1979;241:2035.
15. Effect of intensive blood-glucose control with metformin on complication in overweight patients weight type 2 diabetes (UKPDS 34). *UK Prospective Diabetes Study (UKPDS) Group Lancet* 1998;352:854.
16. Lindholm LH et al. Cardiovascular morbidity and mortality in patients with diabetes in the Losartan Intervention for Endpoint reduction in hypertension study (LIFE): a randomised trial against atenolol. *Lancet* 2002;359:1004.
17. Heart Outcomes Prevention Evaluation Study Investigators. Effects of ramipril on cardiovascular and microvascular outcomes in people with diabetes mellitus: results of the HOPE study and MICRO-HOPE substudy. *Lancet* 2000;355:253.
18. Collins R et al. MRC/BHF Heart Protection Study of cholesterol-lowering with simvastatin in 5,963 people with diabetes: a randomised placebo-controlled trial. *Lancet* 2003;361:2005.
19. Colhoun HM et al. Primary prevention of cardiovascular disease with atorvastatin in type 2 diabetes in the Collaborative Atorvastatin Diabetes Study (CARDS): multicentre randomised placebo-controlled trial. *Lancet* 2004;364:685.
20. Rexrode KM et al. A prospective study of body mass index, weight change, and risk of stroke in women. *JAMA* 1997;277:1539.
21. Kurth T et al. Body mass index and the risk of stroke in men. *Arch Intern Med* 2002;162:2557.
22. Neter JE et al. Influence of weight reduction on blood pressure: a meta-analysis of randomized controlled trials. *Hypertension* 2003;42:878.
23. He J et al. Dietary sodium intake and subsequent risk of cardiovascular disease in overweight adults. *JAMA* 1999;282:2027.
24. Khaw KT, Barrett-Connor E. Dietary potassium and stroke-associated mortality. A 12-year prospective population study. *N Engl J Med* 1987;316:235.
25. Fletcher GF. Exercise in the prevention of stroke. *Health Rep* 1994;6:106.
26. Lindenstrom E et al. Lifestyle factors and risk of cerebrovascular disease in women. The Copenhagen City Heart Study. *Stroke* 1993;24:1468.
27. Bonita R et al. Passive smoking as well as active smoking increases the risk for acute stroke. *Tob Control* 1999;8:156.
28. Robbins AS et al. Cigarette smoking and stroke in a cohort of U.S. male physicians. *Ann Intern Med* 1994;120:458.
29. Viscoli CM et al. A clinical trial of estrogen-replacement therapy after ischemic stroke. *N Engl J Med* 2001;345:1243.
30. Hulley S et al. Randomized trial of estrogen plus progestin for secondary prevention of coronary heart disease in postmenopausal women. Heart and Estrogen/progestin Replacement Study (HERS) Research Group. *JAMA* 1998;280:605.
31. Simon JA et al. Postmenopausal hormone therapy and risk of stroke: the Heart and Estrogen-progestin Replacement Study (HERS). *Circulation* 2001;103:638.
32. Rossouw JE et al. Risks and benefits of estrogen plus progestin in healthy postmenopausal women: principal results from the Women's Health Initiative randomized controlled trial. *JAMA* 2002;288:321.
33. Anderson GL et al. Effects of conjugated equine estrogen in postmenopausal women with hysterectomy: The Women's Health Initiative randomized controlled trial. *JAMA* 2004;291:1701.
34. Steering Committee of the Physicians' Health Study Research Group. Final report on the aspirin component of the ongoing physicians' health study. *N Engl J Med* 1989;321:129.
35. Chen ZM et al. Indications for early aspirin use in acute ischemic stroke: a combined analysis of 40,000 randomized patients from the Chinese acute stroke trial and the international stroke trial. On behalf of the CAST and IST collaborative groups. *Stroke* 2000;31:1240.
36. Hiroyasu I et al. Prospective study of aspirin use and risk of stroke in women. *Stroke* 1999;30:1764.
37. Ridiker PM et al. A randomized trial of low-dose aspirin in the primary prevention of cardiovascular disease in women. *N Engl J Med* 2005;352:1293.
38. Stroke Prevention in Atrial Fibrillation Study Group Investigators. The Stroke Prevention in Atrial Fibrillation study: patient characteristics and final results. *Circulation* 1991;84:527.
39. Peterson P et al. Placebo-controlled, randomized trial of warfarin and aspirin for prevention of thromboembolic complications in chronic atrial fibrillation: the Copenhagen AFASAK study. *Lancet* 1989;1:175.
40. The Boston Area Anticoagulation Trial for Atrial Fibrillation Investigators. The effect of low-dose warfarin on the risk of stroke in patients with nonrheumatic atrial fibrillation. *N Engl J Med* 1990;323:1505.
41. Connolly SJ et al. Canadian atrial fibrillation anticoagulation (CAFA) study. *J Am Coll Cardiol* 1991;18:349.
42. Stroke Prevention in Atrial Fibrillation Investigators. Warfarin versus aspirin for prevention of thromboembolism in atrial fibrillation: Stroke Prevention in Atrial Fibrillation II study. *Lancet* 1994;343:687.
43. Gage BF et al. Validation of clinical classification schemes for predicting stroke: results from the National Registry of Atrial Fibrillation. *JAMA* 2001;285:2864.
44. Gage BF et al. Selecting patients with atrial fibrillation for anticoagulation: stroke risk stratification in patients taking aspirin. *Circulation* 2004;110:2287.
45. Plehn JF et al. Reduction of stroke incidence after myocardial infarction with pravastatin the Cholesterol and Recurrent Events (CARE) study. *Circulation* 1999;99:216.
46. The Long-Term Intervention with Pravastatin in Ischaemic Disease (LIPID) Study Group. Prevention of cardiovascular events and death with pravastatin in patients with coronary heart disease and a broad range of initial cholesterol levels. *N Engl J Med* 1998;339:1349.
47. White HD et al. Pravastatin therapy and the risk of stroke. *N Engl J Med* 2000;343:317.
48. Shepherd J et al. Pravastatin in elderly individuals at risk of vascular disease (PROSPER): a randomized controlled trial. *Lancet* 2002;360:1623.
49. Hunt D et al. Benefits of pravastatin on cardiovascular events and mortality in older patients with coronary heart disease are equal to or exceed those seen in younger patients: results from the LIPID trial. *Ann Intern Med* 2001;134:931.
50. Sever PS et al. Prevention of coronary and stroke events with atorvastatin in hypertensive patients who have average or lower-than-average cholesterol concentrations, in the Anglo-Scandinavian Cardiac Outcomes Trial–Lipid Lowering Arm (ASCOT-LLA): a multicentre randomised controlled trial. *Lancet* 2003;361:1149.
51. Byington RP et al. Reduction of stroke events with pravastatin The Prospective Pravastatin Pooling (PPP) Project. *Circulation* 2001;103:387.
52. Ross SD et al. Clinical outcomes in statin treatment trials a meta-analysis. *Arch Intern Med* 1999;159:1793.
53. Blake GJ et al. Projected life-expectancy gains with statin therapy for individuals with elevated C-reactive protein levels. *J Am Coll Cardiol* 2002;40:49.
54. Vaughan CJ et al. Do statis afford neuroprotection in patients with cerebral ischaemia and stroke? *CNS Drugs* 2001;15:589.
55. Gil-Nunez AC et al. Advantages of lipid-lowering therapy in cerebral ischemia: role of HMG-CoA reductase inhibitors. *Cerebrovasc Dis* 2001;11(Suppl 1):85.
56. The Stroke Council. Statins after ischemic stroke and transient ischemic attack: an advisory statement from the Stroke Council, American Heart Association and American Stroke Association. *Stroke* 2004;35:1023.
57. Albers GW et al. Supplement to the guidelines for the management of transient ischemic attacks a statement from the Ad Hoc Committee on Guidelines for the Management of Transient Ischemic Attacks, Stroke Council, American Heart Association. *Circulation* 1999;30:2502.
58. North American Symptomatic Carotid Endarterectomy Trial Collaborators. Beneficial effect of carotid endarterectomy in symptomatic patients with high-grade stenosis. *N Engl J Med* 1991; 325:445.
59. Barnett HJM et al. Prevention of ischemic stroke. *Br Med J* 1999;318:1539.
60. Biller J et al. Guidelines for carotid endarterectomy a statement for healthcare professionals from a special writing group of the Stroke Council, American Heart Association. *Circulation* 1998;97:501.
61. Alberts MK. Results of a multicenter prospective randomized trial of carotid artery stenting vs. carotid endarterectomy. *Stroke.* 2001;32:325.
62. Endovascular versus surgical treatment in patients with carotid stenosis in the Carotid and Vertebral Artery Transluminal Angioplasty Study (CAVATAS): a randomised trial. *Lancet* 2001; 357:1729.
63. Yadav JS et al. Protected carotid stenting versus endarterectomy in high risk patients. *N Engl J Med* 2004;351:1493.
64. Patrono C et al. Platelet-active drugs: the relationships among does, effectiveness, and side effects: The Seventh ACCP Conference on Antithrombotic and Thrombolytic Therapy. *Chest* 2004;126: 234.
65. Levin RI et al. Aspirin inhibits vascular plasminogen activity in vivo. *J Clin Invest* 1984;74:571.
66. Bousser MG et al. "AICLA" controlled trial of aspiring and dipyridamole in the secondary prevention of Atherothrombotic cerebral ischemia. *Stroke* 1983;14:5.
67. Sorenson PS et al. Acetylsalicylic acid in the prevention of stroke in patients with reversible cerebral ischemic attacks. A Danish Cooperative Study. *Stroke* 1983;14:15.
68. Antiplatelet Trialists' Collaboration. Secondary prevention of vascular disease by prolonged antiplatelet treatment. *Br Med J (Clin Res Ed)* 1988;290:320.
69. Swedish Cooperative Study. High-dose acetylsalicylic acid after cerebral infarction. *Stroke* 1987; 18:325.
70. UK-TIA Study Group. The United Kingdom transient ischemic attack (UK-TIA) aspirin trial: final results. *J Neurol Neurosurg Psychiatry* 1991;54: 1044.
71. Sivenius J et al. Antiplatelet therapy is effective in the prevention of stroke or death in women: subgroup analysis of the European Stroke Prevention Study (ESPS). *Acta Neurol Scand* 1991;84:286.
72. Bernstein EF et al. Life expectancy and late stroke following carotid endarterectomy. *Ann Surg* 1983; 198:80.
73. Harker LA et al. Failure of aspirin plus dipyridamole to prevent restenosis after carotid endarterectomy. *Ann Intern Med* 1992;116:731.
74. Bhatt DL et al. Dual antiplatelet therapy with clopidogrel and aspirin after carotid artery stenting. *J Invasive Cardiol* 2001;13:767.
75. The Dutch TIA Trial Study Group. A comparison of two doses of aspirin (30 mg vs. 283 mg a day) in patients after a transient ischemic attack or minor ischemic stroke. *N Engl J Med* 1991;325:1261.

76. The SALT Collaborative. Swedish aspirin low-dose trial (SALT) of 75 mg aspirin as secondary prophylaxis after cerebrovascular ischemic events. *Lancet* 1991;338:1345.
77. Helgason CM et al. Aspirin response and failure in cerebral infarction. *Stroke* 1993;24:345.
78. Antiplatelet Trialists' Collaboration. Collaborative overview of randomized trials of antiplatelet therapy. I: prevention of death, myocardial infarction, and stroke by antiplatelet therapy in various categories of patients. *Br Med J* 1994;308:83.
79. Johnson ES et al. A meta-regression analysis of dose-response effect of aspirin in stroke. *Arch Intern Med* 1999;159:1258.
80. Hansson L et al. Effects of intensive blood-pressure lowering and low-dose aspirin in patients with hypertension: principal results of the Hypertension Optimal Treatment (HOT) randomised trial: HOT Study Group. *Lancet* 1998;351:1755.
81. The ESPS Group. The European Stroke Prevention Study (ESPS): principal end-points. *Lancet* 1987;2:1351.
82. Diener HC et al. European stroke prevention study 2. Dipyridamole and acetylsalicylic acid in the secondary prevention of stroke. *J Neurol Sci* 1996;143:1.
83. Gent M et al. The Canadian-American ticlopidine study (CATS) in thromboembolic stroke. *Lancet* 1989;2:1215.
84. Hass WK et al. A randomized trial comparing ticlopidine hydrochloride with aspirin for the prevention of stroke in high risk patients. *N Engl J Med* 1989;321:501.
85. Barnett HJM et al. Prevention of ischemic stroke [letter]. *N Engl J Med* 1995;333:460.
86. Bennett CL et al. Thrombotic thrombocytopenia purpura associated with ticlopidine. *Ann Intern Med* 1998;128:541.
87. CAPRIE Steering Committee. A randomized, blinded, trial of clopidogrel versus aspirin in patients at risk of ischaemic events (CAPRIE). *Lancet* 1996;348:1329.
88. Bennett CL et al. Thrombotic thrombocytopenia purpura associated with clopidogrel. *N Engl J Med* 2000;342:1773.
89. The Stroke Prevention in Reversible Ischemia Trial (SPIRIT) Study Group. A randomized trial of anticoagulants versus aspirin after cerebral ischemia of presumed arterial origin. *Ann Neurol* 1997;42:857.
90. Mohr JP et al. A comparison of warfarin and aspirin for the prevention of recurrent ischemic stroke. *N Engl J Med* 2001;345:1444.
91. Chimowtiz MLM et al. Warfarin-Aspirin Symptomatic Intracranial Disease (WASID) Trial: final results. *Stroke* 2004;35:235.
92. Diener HC et al. Aspirin and clopidogrel compared with clopidogrel alone after recent ischaemic stroke or transient ischaemic attack in high-risk patients (MATCH): randomised, double-blind, placebo-controlled trial. *Lancet* 2004;364:331.
93. Rocca B et al. Clyclooxygenase-2 expression is induced during human megakaryopoesis and characterizes newly formed platelets. *Proc Natl Acad Sci U S A* 2002;99:7634.
94. Catella-Lawson R et al. Cyclooxygenase inhibitors and the antiplatelet effects of aspirin. *N Engl J Med* 2001;345:1809.
95. Eikelboom JW et al. Aspirin-resistant thromboxane biosynthesis and the riks of myocardial infarction, stroke, or cardiovascular death in patients at high risk for cardiovascular events. *Circulation* 2002;105:1650.
96. Adams HP et al. Guidelines for the early management of adults with ischemic stroke. *Stroke* 2007;38:1655.
97. National Institute of Neurological Disorders and Stroke. NIH Stroke Scale. Availble at: http://www.ninds.nih.gov/doctors/NIH_Stroke_Scale_Booklet.pdf. Accessed 23 May 2007.
98. Kammersgaard LP et al. Admission body temperature predicts long-term mortality after acute stroke, the Copenhagen Stroke Study. *Stroke* 2002; 33:1759.
99. Zaremba J. Hyperthermia in ischemic stroke. *Med Sci Monit* 2004;10:RA148.
100. Dippel DW, et.al. Effect of paracetamol (acetaminophen) and ibuprofen on body temperature in acute ischemic stroke: PISA, a phase II double-blind randomized, placebo-controlled trial [ISRCTN98608690]. *BMC Cardivasc Disord* 2003;3:2.
101. Kagansky N et al. The role of hyperglycemia in acute stroke. *Arch Neurol* 2001;58:1209.
102. Brott T et al. Hypertension and its treatment in the NINDS rt-PA stroke trial. *Stroke* 1998;29:1504.
103. Tilley BC et al. Total quality improvement method for reduction of delays between emergency department admission and treatment of ischemic stroke. *Arch Neurol* 1997;54:1466.
104. Indredavik B et al. Stroke unit care improved survival and function for 5 years after an acute stroke. *Stroke* 1997;28:1861.
105. Duke RJ et al. Intravenous heparin for the prevention of stroke progression in acute partial stable stroke. *Ann Intern Med* 1986;105:825.
106. International Stroke Trial Collaboration Group. The International Stroke Trial (IST): a randomized trial of aspirin, subcutaneous heparin, both or neither among 19435 patients with acute stroke. *Lancet* 1997;349:1569.
107. Roden-Jullig A et al. Effectiveness of heparin treatment of progressing ischaemic stroke: before and after study. *J Intern Med.* 2000;248:287.
108. Kay R et al. Low molecular weight heparin for the treatment of acute ischemic stroke. *N Engl J Med* 1995;333:1588.
109. The Publications Committee for the Trial of ORG 10172 in Acute Stroke Treatment (TOAST) Investigators. Low molecular weight heparinoid, ORG 10172 (danaparoid), and outcome after acute ischemic stroke: a randomized controlled trial. *JAMA* 1998;279:1265.
110. Berge E et al. Low molecular-weight heparin versus aspirin in patients with acute ischaemic stroke and atrial fibrillation: a double-blind randomised study. HAEST Study Group. Heparin in Acute Embolic Stroke Trial. *Lancet* 2000;355:1205.
111. Diener HC et al. Treatment of acute ischemic stroke with the low-molecular-weight heparin Certoparin: results of the TOPAS trial. Therapy of Patients with Acute Stroke (TOPAS) Investigators. *Stroke* 2001;32:22.
112. CAST (Chinese Acute Stroke Trial) Collaboration Group. CAST: randomized placebo-controlled trial of early aspirin use in 20,000 patients with acute ischaemic stroke. *Lancet* 1997;349:1641.
113. Multicentre Acute Stroke Trial-Italy (MAST-I) Group. Randomised controlled trial of streptokinase, aspirin, and combination of both in treatment of acute ischaemic stroke. *Lancet* 1995;346:1509.
114. The Abciximab in Ischemic Stroke Investigators. Abciximab in acute ischemic stroke: a randomized, double-blind, placebo-controlled, dose-escalation study. *Stroke* 2000;31:601.
115. Kobayashi S et al. Effect of the thrombin inhibitor argatroban in acute cerebral thrombosis. *Semin Thromb Hemost* 1997;23:531.
116. Sherman DG et al. Intravenous ancrod for treatment of acute ischemic stroke: the STAT study: a randomized controlled trial. *JAMA* 2000;283:2395.
117. Coull BM et al. Anticoagulants and antiplatelet agents in acute ischemic stroke report of the Joint Stroke Guideline Development Committee of the American Academy of Neurology and the American Stroke Association (a division of the American Heart Association). *Neurology* 2002;59:13.
118. Solis OJ et al. Cerebral angiography in acute cerebral infarction. *Rev Interam Radiol* 1977;2:19.
119. Symon L et al. The concept of thresholds of ischaemia in relation to bring structure and function. *J Clin Pathol Suppl (R Coll Pathol)* 1977;30(Suppl II):149.
120. Sharbrough FW et al. Correlation of continuous electroencephalograms with cerebral blood flow measurements during carotid endarterectomy. *Stroke* 1973;4:674.
121. Sundt TM Jr et al. Restoration of middle cerebral artery flow in experimental infarction. *J Neurosurg* 1969;31:311.
122. The Multicenter Acute Stroke Trial-Europe Study Group. Thrombolytic therapy with streptokinase in acute ischemic stroke. *N Engl J Med* 1996;335: 145.
123. Donnan GA et al. Streptokinase for acute ischemic stroke with relationship to time of administration. *JAMA* 1996;276:961.
124. The National Institute of Neurological Disorders and Stroke rt-PA Stroke Study Group. Tissue plasminogen activator for acute ischemic stroke. *N Engl J Med* 1995;333:1581.
125. Hacke W et al. Intravenous thrombolysis with recombinant tissue plasminogen activator for acute hemispheric stroke. *JAMA* 1995;274:1017.
126. Hacke W et al. Randomised double-blind placebo-controlled trial of thrombolytic therapy with intravenous alteplase in acute ischemic stroke. *Lancet* 1998;352:1245.
127. Wardlaw JM et al. Thrombolysis for acute ischaemic stroke. *Cochrane Database of Systemic Reviews* 1995;2:CDOOO213.
128. Del Zoppo GJ et al. PROACT: a phase II randomized trial of recombinant pro-urokinase by direct arterial delivery in acute middle cerebral artery stroke. *Stroke* 1998;29:4.
129. Furlan A et al. Intra-arterial prourokinase for acute ischemic stroke. *JAMA* 1999;282:2003.
130. Scandinavian Stroke Study Group. Multicenter trial of hemodilution in acute ischemic stroke. *Stroke* 1987;18:691.
131. Strand T et al. A randomized controlled trial of hemodilution therapy in acute ischemic stroke. *Stroke* 1984;15:980.
132. Aichner FT et al. Hypervolemic hemodilution in acute ischemic stroke. *Stroke* 1998;29:743.
133. Bauer RB et al. Dexamethasone as treatment in cerebrovascular disease. A controlled study in acute cerebral infarction. *Stroke* 1973;4:547.
134. Norris JW. Steroid therapy in acute cerebral infarction. *Arch Neurol* 1976;33:69.
135. Dyken M et al. Evaluation of cortisone in the treatment of cerebral infarction. *JAMA* 1956;162:1531.
136. Mulley G et al. Dexamethasone in acute stroke. *Br Med J* 1978;2:994.
137. Norris JW et al. High-dose steroid treatment in cerebral infarction. *Br Med J (Clin Res)* 1986; 292:21.
138. Poungvarin N et al. Effects of dexamethasone in primary supratentorial intracerebral hemorrhage. *N Engl J Med* 1987;315:1229.
139. Gelmers HJ et al. A controlled trial of nimodipine in acute ischemic stroke. *N Engl J Med* 1988;318:203.
140. TRUST Study Group. Randomized, double-blind, placebo-controlled trial of nimodipine in acute stroke. *Lancet* 1990;336:1205.
141. Kaster M et al. A randomized, double-blind, placebo-controlled trial of nimodipine in acute ischemic stroke. *Stroke* 1994;25:1348.
142. Mohr J et al. Meta-analysis of oral nimodipine in acute ischemic stroke. *Cerebrovasc Dis* 1994; 4:197.
143. Horn J et al. Calcium antagonists for ischemic stroke: a systematic review. *Stroke* 2001;32:570.
144. Ovbiagele B et al. Neuroprotective agents for the treatment of acute ischemic stroke. *Curr Neurol Neurosci Rep* 2003;3:9.
145. Robinson RG. Treatment issues in poststroke depression. *Depress Anxiety* 1998;8:85.
146. Vermeulen M et al. Antifibrinolytic treatment in subarachnoid hemorrhage. *N Engl J Med* 1984; 311:432.
147. Adams HP et al. Antifibrinolytic therapy in patients with aneurysmal subarachnoid hemorrhage: a report of the cooperative aneurysmal study. *Arch Neurol* 1981;38:25.
148. Baystone R et al. Intraventricular vancomycin in the treatment of ventriculitis associated with cerebrospinal fluid shunting and drainage. *J Neurol Neurosurg Psychiatry* 1987;50:1419.
149. Kassell NJ et al. Treatment of ischemic deficits from

vasospasms with intravascular volume expansion and induced arterial hypertension. *Neurosurgery* 1982;11:337.
150. Kosnik EJ et al. Postoperative hypertension in the management of patients with intracranial arterial hypertension. *J Neurosurg* 1976;45:148.
151. Awad IA et al. Clinical vasospasm after subarachnoid hemorrhage: response to hypervolemic hemodilution and arterial hypertension. *Stroke* 1987;18:365.
152. Otsubo H et al. Normovolemic induced hypertension therapy for cerebral vasospasm after subarachnoid hemorrhage. *Acta Neurochi (Wien)* 1990; 103:18.
153. Allen GS et al. Cerebral arterial spasm—a controlled trial of nimodipine in patients with subarachnoid hemorrhage. *N Engl J Med* 1983;308: 619.
154. Petruk KC et al. Nimodipine treatment in poor-grade aneurysm patients-results of a multicenter double-blind placebo-controlled trial. *J Neurosurg* 1988;68:505.
155. Phillippon J et al. Prevention of vasospasm in subarachnoid hemorrhage: a controlled study with nimodipine. *Acta Neurochir (Wien)* 1986;82: 110.
156. Pickard JD et al. Effect of oral nimodipine on cerebral infarction and outcome after subarachnoid hemorrhage: British Aneurysm Nimodipine Trial. *Br Med J (Clin Res Ed)* 1989;289:636.

INFECTIOUS DISORDERS

B. Joseph Guglielmo
SECTION EDITOR

CHAPTER 56

Principles of Infectious Diseases

B. Joseph Guglielmo

APPROACHING THE PROBLEM

The proper selection of antimicrobial therapy is based on several factors. Before initiating therapy, it is important first to clearly establish the presence of an infectious process because several disease states (e.g., malignancy, autoimmune disease) and drugs can mimic infection. Once infection has been documented, its most likely site must be identified. Signs and symptoms (e.g., erythema associated with cellulitis) direct the clinician to the likely source. Because certain pathogens are known to be associated with a specific site of infection, therapy often can be directed against these organisms. Additional laboratory tests, including the Gram stain, serology, and antimicrobial susceptibility testing, generally identify the primary pathogen. Although several antimicrobials potentially can be considered, their spectrum of activity, clinical efficacy, adverse effect profile, pharmacokinetic disposition, and cost considerations ultimately guide the choice of therapy. Once an agent has been selected, the dosage must be based on the size of the patient, site of infection, route of elimination, and other factors.

ESTABLISHING THE PRESENCE OF AN INFECTION

1. R.G., a 63-year-old man in the intensive care unit, underwent emergency resection of his large bowel. He has been intubated throughout his postoperative course. On day 20 of his hospital stay, R.G. suddenly becomes confused; his blood pressure (BP) drops to 70/30 mmHg, with a heart rate of 130 beats/minute. His extremities are cold to the touch, and he presents with circumoral pallor. His temperature increases to 40°C (axillary) and his respiratory rate is 24 breaths/minute. Copious amounts of yellow-green secretions are suctioned from his endotracheal tube.

Physical examination reveals sinus tachycardia with no rubs or murmurs. Rhonchi with decreased breath sounds are observed on auscultation. The abdomen is distended and R.G. complains of new abdominal pain. No bowel sounds can be heard and the stool is guaiac positive. Urine output from the Foley catheter has been 10 mL/hour for the past 2 hours. Erythema is noted around the central venous catheter.

A chest radiograph reveals bilateral lower lobe infiltrates, and urinalysis reveals >50 white blood cells/high-power field

(WBC/HPF), few casts, and a specific gravity of 1.015. Blood, tracheal aspirate, and urine cultures are pending. Other laboratory values include sodium (Na), 131 mEq/L (normal, 135 to 147); potassium (K), 4.1 mEq/L (normal, 3.5 to 5); chloride (Cl), 110 mEq/L (normal, 95–105); CO_2, 16 mEq/L; blood urea nitrogen (BUN), 58 mg/dL (normal, 8–18); creatinine, 3.8 mg/dL (increased from 0.9 mg/dL at admission) (normal, 0.6–1.2); glucose 320 mg/dL (normal, 70–110); serum albumin, 2.1 g/dL (normal, 4–6); hemoglobin (Hgb), 10.3 g/dL; hematocrit (Hct), 33% (normal, 39%–49% [male patients]); WBC count, 15,600/mm^3 with bands present; platelets, 40,000/mm^3 (normal, 130,000–400,000); prothrombin time (PT), 18 seconds (normal, 10–12); erythrocyte sedimentation rate (ESR), 65 mm/hour (normal, 0–20). Which of R.G.'s signs and symptoms are consistent with infection?

[SI units: Na, 131 mmol/L; K, 4.1 mmol/L; Cl, 110 mmol/L; CO_2, 16 mmol/L; BUN, 20.71 mmol/L of urea; creatinine, 335.92 and 7.56 mmol/L, respectively; glucose, 17.76 mmol/L; albumin, 235.62 mmol/L; Hgb, 103 g/L; Hct, 0.33; WBC, 15.6 × 10^9; platelets, 40 × 10^9; ESR 65 mm/hour]

R.G. has numerous signs and symptoms consistent with an infectious process. He has both an increased WBC count (15,600/mm^3) and a "shift to the left" (bands are present on the differential). An increased WBC count commonly is observed with infection, particularly with bacterial pathogens. The WBC differential in patients with a bacterial infection often demonstrates a shift to the left (i.e., presence of immature neutrophils), suggesting that the bone marrow is responding to an infectious insult. Infection is not always associated with leukocytosis, however. Overwhelming sepsis can cause a decreased WBC count; some patients become neutropenic secondary to infection. In less acute infection (e.g., uncomplicated urinary tract infection, abscess), the WBC count may remain within the normal range. Because the abscess is a localized lesion, less bone marrow response would be anticipated; thus, the WBC count may not increase in these patients.

R.G.'s temperature is 40°C by axillary measurement. Fever is a common manifestation of infection, with oral temperatures generally >38°C. Oral and axillary temperatures tend to be approximately 0.4°C lower compared with rectal measurement.[1] As a result, R.G.'s temperature would be expected to be 40.4°C if his temperature had been taken rectally. In general, rectal measurement of temperature is a more reliable determination of fever. Some patients with overwhelming infection, however, may present with hypothermia and temperatures <36°C. Furthermore, patients with localized infections (e.g., uncomplicated urinary tract infection, chronic abscesses) may be afebrile.

The bilateral lower lobe infiltrates on R.G.'s chest radiograph, the presence of copious amounts of yellow-green secretions from his endotracheal tube, and the erythema surrounding his central venous catheter also are compatible with an infectious process. Furthermore, R.G. has the signs and symptoms that also are consistent with sepsis, which are discussed next.

ESTABLISHING THE SEVERITY OF AN INFECTION

2. What signs and symptoms manifested by R.G. are consistent with a serious systemic infection?

The term *sepsis* is used to describe a poorly defined syndrome; however, sepsis generally suggests more systemic infection associated with the presence of pathogenic microorganisms or their toxins in the blood. A uniform system for defining the spectrum of disorders associated with sepsis has been established.[2]

The pathogenesis of sepsis is complex (Fig. 56-1) and only partially understood.[2–4] Gram-negative aerobes produce

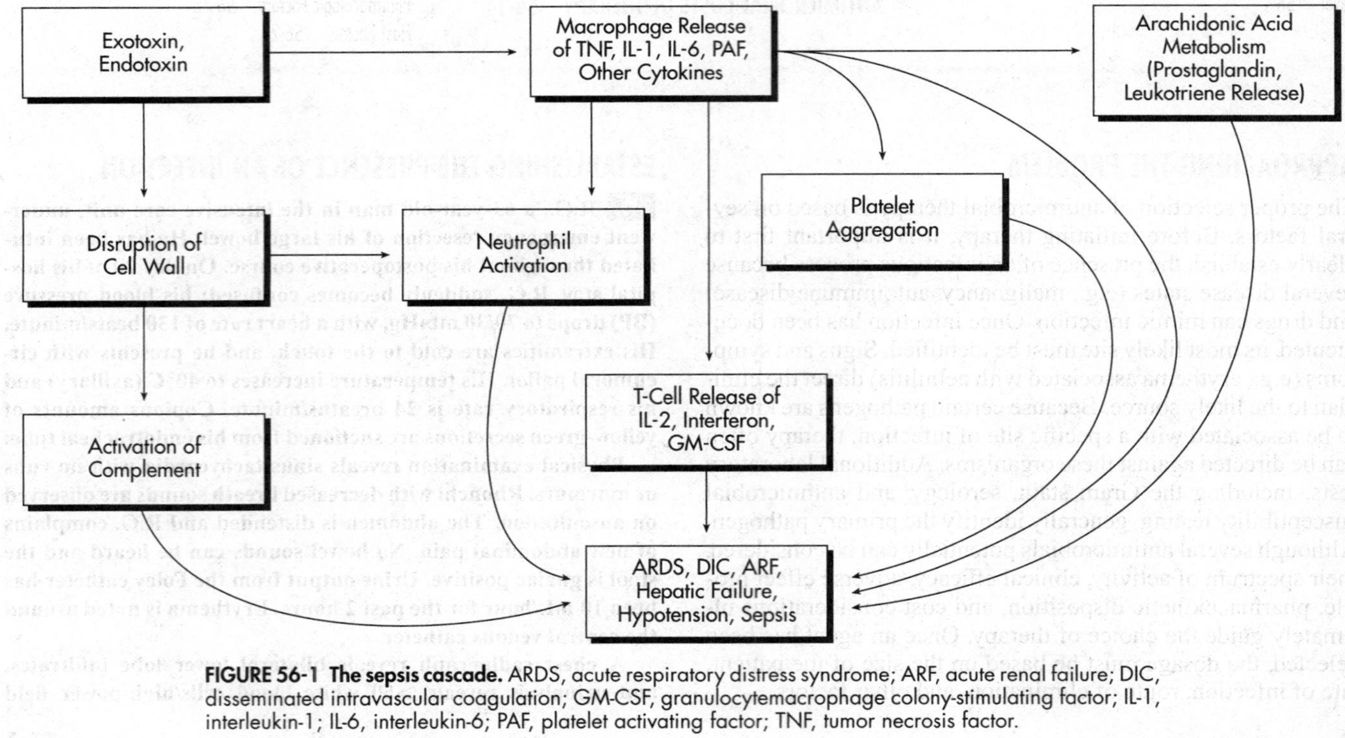

FIGURE 56-1 The sepsis cascade. ARDS, acute respiratory distress syndrome; ARF, acute renal failure; DIC, disseminated intravascular coagulation; GM-CSF, granulocytemacrophage colony-stimulating factor; IL-1, interleukin-1; IL-6, interleukin-6; PAF, platelet activating factor; TNF, tumor necrosis factor.

endotoxin that results in a cascade of endogenous mediator release, including tumor necrosis factor (TNF), interleukin-1 (IL-1) and interleukin-6 (IL-6), platelet activating factor (PAF), and various other substances, from mononuclear phagocytes and other cells. Although this initial stimulus commonly is associated with gram-negative endotoxin, other substances, including gram-positive exotoxin and fungal cell wall constituents, also may be associated with cytokine release. After release of TNF, IL-1, and PAF, arachidonic acid is metabolized to form leukotrienes, thromboxane A_2, and prostaglandins, particularly prostaglandin E_2 and prostaglandin I_2. IL-1 and IL-6 activate the T cells to produce interferon, IL-2, IL-4, and granulocytemacrophage colony-stimulating factor (GM-CSF). Increased endothelial permeability ensues. Subsequently, the endothelium releases two hemodynamically active substances: endothelium-derived relaxing factor (EDRF) and endothelin-1. Activation of the complement cascade (fragments C3a and C5a) follows with additional vascular abnormalities and neutrophil activation. Other potentially important agents in this cascade include adhesion molecules, kinins, thrombin, myocardial depressant substance, endorphins, and heat shock protein. The net result of this cascade involves several hemodynamic, renal, acid base, and other disorders. Uncontrolled inflammation and coagulation also have an important role in this sepsis cascade.[4]

Hemodynamic Changes

Critically ill patients often have central intravenous (IV) lines in place for measuring cardiac output and systemic vascular resistance (SVR). A normal SVR of 800 to 1,200 dyne.sec.cm^{-5} may fall to 500 to 600 dyne.sec.cm^{-5} with septic shock because of intense vasodilation. In response to this vasodilation, the heart reflexively increases cardiac output from its normal 4 to 6 L/minute to as much as 11 to 12 L/minute in septic patients. This increase in cardiac output primarily is caused by an increased heart rate; stroke volume is unchanged or decreased because of the hypovolemic state. Although the heart rate is increased on the basis of reflex tachycardia, a chronotropic response also takes place as a result of stress-induced catecholamine release (norepinephrine, epinephrine). Thus, the cardiac output increases in response to arterial vasodilation; however, this increase generally is insufficient to overcome the vasodilatory state, and hypotension ensues. In overwhelming septic shock, myocardial depression results in a decreased cardiac output. The combination of decreased cardiac output and decreased SVR results in hypotension unresponsive to pressors and IV fluids. R.G. has hemodynamic evidence of septic shock. He is hypotensive (BP 70/30 mmHg) and tachycardic (130 beats/minute), presumably in response to significant vasodilation and catecholamine release.

Although vasodilation commonly occurs in sepsis, hemodynamic changes are not equal throughout the vasculature. Some vascular beds constrict, resulting in maldistribution of blood flow. Significant amounts of blood are shunted away from the kidneys, mesentery, and extremities.

Normal urine output of approximately 0.5 to 1.0 mL/kg/hour (30–70 mL/hour for a 70-kg patient) can decrease to <20 mL/hour in sepsis. The urine output for R.G. has decreased to 10 mL/hour, consistent with sepsis-induced perfusion abnormalities. Decreased blood flow to the kidney as well as mediator-induced microvascular failure can cause acute-tubular necrosis (ATN). R.G.'s uremia (BUN 58 mg/dL) and increased serum creatinine concentration (3.8 mg/dL) are consistent with decreased renal perfusion secondary to sepsis. When sepsis has progressed to septic shock, blood flow to most major organs is decreased. Decreased blood flow to the liver may result in "shock liver," in which liver function tests, including alanine aminotransferase (ALT), aspartate aminotransferase (AST), and alkaline phosphatase, become elevated. The liver function tests for R.G. are not available; however, his serum albumin concentration is low (2.1 g/dL) and his PT of 18 seconds is prolonged. Decreased blood flow to the musculature classically is characterized by cool extremities, and decreased blood flow to the brain can result in decreased mentation. R.G. is confused, his extremities are cold, and the area around his mouth appears pale. All these signs and symptoms provide strong evidence that he is in septic shock.

Cellular Changes

The sepsis syndrome is associated with significant abnormalities in cellular metabolism. Glucose intolerance commonly is observed in sepsis, and patients with previously normal blood glucose levels may experience sudden increases in blood sugar. In some cases, an increase in glucose is one of the first signs of an infectious process. R.G.'s increased blood glucose concentration (320 mg/dL) is, therefore, consistent with sepsis. Other sensitive indicators of sepsis-associated inflammation include the ESR and C-reactive protein, nonspecific tests that are commonly elevated in various inflammatory states, including infection. The ESR or C-reactive protein can be used to follow the progression of infection; currently, R.G.'s ESR is elevated at 65 mm/hour. With appropriate management of infection, the ESR would be expected to decrease; inadequate treatment would be associated with persistent elevation of the ESR and C-reactive protein.

Respiratory Changes

Production of organic acids, such as lactate, increased glycolysis, decreased fractional extraction of oxygen, and abnormal delivery-dependent oxygen consumption are observed.[4] This increase in lactic acid results in metabolic acidosis, with accompanying decreased serum bicarbonate levels. The lungs normally respond in a compensatory manner with an increased respiratory rate (tachypnea), resulting in an increased elimination of arterial carbon dioxide. R.G.'s acid-base status is consistent with sepsis-associated metabolic acidosis (CO_2 16 mEq/L) and compensatory respiratory alkalosis (respiratory rate 24 breaths/minutes).

Although not currently present in R.G., a late complication of the above-mentioned sepsis cascade is acute respiratory distress syndrome (ARDS). ARDS initially was described as noncardiogenic pulmonary edema with severe hypoxemia caused by right-to-left intrapulmonary shunting resulting from atelectasis and edema-filled alveoli. The primary pathophysiology of ARDS is a breakdown in the natural integrity of the alveolar capillary network in the lung.[5] In the early phase of ARDS, patients have severe alveolar edema with large numbers of inflammatory cells, primarily neutrophils. The chronic phase of ARDS (10–14 days after development of the syndrome) is associated with significant lung destruction. Emphysema, pulmonary vascular obliteration, and fibrosis commonly are observed. Severe ARDS is associated with arterial oxygen level/fraction of inspired oxygen (Pao_2/Fio_2) ratios of <100, low lung compliance, a need for high positive end-expiratory pressure (PEEP), and other respiratory maneuvers. At present, the treatment for this syndrome primarily is supportive, including mechanical ventilation, high inspired oxygen, and PEEP. If patients fail to show improved gas exchange by day 7, the mortality associated with ARDS is high (>80%).[6] Although R.G. currently does not have ARDS, the severity of his septic episode strongly suggests he may develop this complication in the next few days.

Hematologic Changes

Disseminated intravascular coagulation (DIC) is a well-recognized sequel of sepsis. Huge quantities of clotting factors and platelets are consumed in DIC as widespread clotting takes place throughout the circulatory system. As a result, the PT and the activated partial thromboplastin time (aPTT) are prolonged and the platelet count commonly is decreased in sepsis. Decreased fibrinogen levels and increased fibrin split products generally are diagnostic for DIC. The PT of 18 seconds and the decreased platelet count of 40,000/mm^3 in R.G. are consistent with sepsis-induced DIC.

Neurologic Changes

Central nervous system (CNS) changes, including lethargy, disorientation, confusion, and psychosis, predominate in sepsis. Altered mental status is well recognized as a symptom associated with infections of the CNS, such as meningitis and brain abscess. These changes, however, also are common with other sites of sepsis. On day 20 of his hospital stay, R.G. suddenly became confused, his BP dropped, and his heart rate increased. Thus, R.G.'s CNS effects as well as his hematologic, respiratory, hemodynamic, and cellular effects all provide substantial evidence of septic shock.

PROBLEMS IN THE DIAGNOSIS OF AN INFECTION

3. R.G.'s medical history includes temporal arteritis and seizures chronically treated with corticosteroids and phenytoin. Perioperative "stress doses" of hydrocortisone recently were administered because of his surgical procedure. What medications or disease states confuse the diagnosis of infection?

Confabulating Variables

Various factors, including major surgery, acute myocardial infarction, and initiation of corticosteroid therapy are associated with an increased WBC count. Unlike infection, however, a shift to the left does not occur with these disease states. In R.G., the stress dose of hydrocortisone and his recent surgical procedure might have contributed to the increased WBC count. The presence of bands in R.G., however, strongly suggests an infectious process.

Drug Effects

The ability of corticosteroids to mimic or mask infection is noteworthy. Corticosteroids are associated with an increased WBC count and glucose intolerance when therapy is initiated or when doses are increased. Furthermore, some patients experience corticosteroid-induced mental status changes that may complicate the diagnosis of a septic infection. Although corticosteroids mimic infection, they also have the ability to mask infection. Bowel perforation in a patient with ulcerative colitis would result in significant peritoneal contamination. Concomitant corticosteroids, because of their potent anti-inflammatory effects, may, however, reduce the classic findings of peritonitis. Furthermore, corticosteroids can reduce and sometimes ablate the febrile response. Thus, these corticosteroid-treated patients may be asymptomatic but at great risk for gram-negative septic shock.

Another example of the influence of corticosteroids on the diagnosis of infection relates to neurosurgical procedures. Dexamethasone is a corticosteroid commonly used to reduce the inflammation and swelling associated with neurosurgical procedures. Certain neurosurgical procedures are associated with significant trauma to the meninges; however, the patient often is asymptomatic while receiving high-dose dexamethasone. When the dexamethasone dose is decreased, the patient subsequently may experience classic meningismus, including stiff neck, photophobia, and headache. The lumbar puncture may demonstrate cloudy cerebrospinal fluid (CSF), an elevated WBC count, high CSF protein, and low CSF glucose. Although the signs and symptoms are consistent with infectious meningitis, this disease state is considered aseptic meningitis (i.e., inflammation of the meninges without an infectious origin).[7] Certain drugs may cause aseptic meningitis, including OKT3,[8] nonsteroidal anti-inflammatory agents, and sulfonamides.

Fever

Fever also is consistent with autoimmune diseases, such as lupus erythematosus and temporal arteritis.[9,10] Neoplasms, such as leukemia and lymphoma, also may present with low-grade fevers, similar to those observed in an infectious process. One evaluation of fever of unknown origin (FUO) in community hospitals demonstrated a 25% incidence of FUO caused by cancer.[10] Other diseases associated with fever include sarcoidosis, chronic liver disease, and familial Mediterranean fever. Acute myocardial infarction, pulmonary embolism, and postoperative pulmonary atelectasis are commonly associated with an elevated temperature. Factitious fever or self-induced disease must be considered in certain patients. After infection, autoimmune disease, and malignancy have been ruled out, drug fever should be considered. Drugs, including certain antimicrobials (e.g., amphotericin B) and phenytoin, have been associated with drug fever. Drug fever generally occurs after 7 to 10 days of therapy and resolves within 48 hours of the drug's discontinuation.[11] Some clinicians claim that patients with drug fever generally feel "well" and are unaware of their fever. Rechallenge with the offending agent usually results in recurrence of fever within hours of administration. Drug fever should be considered a diagnosis of exclusion, however, and should be considered only after eliminating the presence of other disease states (also see Chapter 4, Anaphylaxis and Drug Allergies).

Neoplasms may be radiographically indistinguishable from an abscess. An example of this dilemma is the differential diagnosis of toxoplasmosis versus lymphoma in patients with human immunodeficiency virus (HIV) with brain lesions documented by a computed axial tomography scan. One method for diagnosis is to use empiric therapy against *Toxoplasma gondii*. If the lesions are unresponsive to therapy, the presumptive diagnosis of malignancy can be made.

In summary, R.G. has an autoimmune disease, temporal arteritis, which has been associated with fever. Similarly, his corticosteroid administration and phenytoin use may confound the diagnosis of infection. His other signs and symptoms, however, strongly suggest that R.G.'s problems are of an infectious origin.

ESTABLISHING THE SITE OF THE INFECTION

4. What are the most likely sources of R.G.'s infection?

Independent of the presumed site of infection, a blood culture should be drawn to demonstrate the presence of bacteremia. After blood cultures are sampled, a thorough physical examination generally documents the source of infection. Urosepsis, the most common cause of nosocomial infection, may be associated with dysuria, flank pain, and abnormal urinalysis.[12] Tachypnea, increased sputum production, altered chest radiograph, and hypoxemia may direct the clinician toward a pulmonary source. Evidence for an infected IV line would include pain, erythema, and purulent discharge around the IV catheter. Other potential sites of infection include the peritoneum, pelvis, bone, and CNS.

R.G. is demonstrating several possible sites of infection. The copious production of yellow-green sputum, tachypnea, and the altered chest radiograph suggest the presence of pneumonia. The abdominal pain, absent bowel sounds, and recent surgical procedure, however, require evaluation for an intra-abdominal source.[13] Lastly, the abnormal urinalysis (>50 WBC/HPF) and the erythema around the central venous catheter suggest other sites of infection.

DETERMINING LIKELY PATHOGENS

5. What are the most likely pathogens associated with R.G.'s infection(s)?

R.G. has several possible sources of infection. The suspected pathogens depend on the presumed site of infection. Table 56-1 provides a classification of infectious organisms (e.g., gram-positive, gram-negative, aerobic, anaerobic),

Table 56-1 Classification of Infectious Organisms

1. Bacteria
   - *Aerobic*
     - ***Gram-positive***
       - *Cocci*
         - Streptococci: pneumococcus, viridans streptococci; group A streptococci
         - *Enterococcus*
         - Staphylococci: *Staphylococcus aureus, Staphylococcus epidermidis*
       - *Rods (bacilli)*
         - *Corynebacterium*
         - *Listeria*
     - ***Gram-negative***
       - *Cocci*
         - *Moraxella*
         - *Neisseria (Neisseria meningitides. Neisseria gonorrhoeae).*
       - *Rods (bacilli)*
         - Enterobacteriaceae *(Escherichia coli, Klebsiella, Enterobacter, Citrobacter, Proteus, Serratia, Salmonella, Shigella, Morganella, Providencia)*
         - *Campylobacter*
         - *Pseudomonas*
         - *Helicobacter*
         - *Haemophilus (coccobacilli morphology)*
         - *Legionella*
   - *Anaerobic*
     - ***Gram-positive***
       - *Cocci*
         - *Peptococcus*
         - *Peptostreptococcus*
       - *Rods (bacilli)*
         - Clostridia *(Clostridium perfringens, Clostridium tetani, Clostridium difficile)*
         - *Propionibacterium acnes*
     - ***Gram-negative***
       - *Cocci*
         - None
       - *Rods (bacilli)*
         - Bacteroides *(Bacteroides fragilis, Bacteroides melaninogenicus)*
         - Fusobacterium
         - Prevotella
2. Fungi
   - *Aspergillus, Candida, Coccidioides, Cryptococcus, Histoplasma, Mucor, Tinea, Trichophyton*
3. Viruses
   - Influenza, hepatitis A, B, C, D, E; human immunodeficiency virus; rubella; herpes; cytomegalovirus; respiratory syncytial virus; Epstein-Barr virus, severe acute respiratory syndrome (SARS) virus
4. Chlamydiae
   - *Chlamydia trachomatis*
   - *Chlamydia psittaci*
   - *Chlamydia pneumoniae*
   - Lymphogranuloma venereum (LGV) disease caused by *Chlamydia trachomatis* of immunotype L1–L3
5. Rickettsiae
   - Rocky Mountain spotted fever, Q fever
   - Ureaplasma
6. Mycoplasmas
   - *Mycoplasma pneumoniae, Mycoplasma hominis*
7. Spirochetes
   - *Treponema pallidum, Borrelia burgdorferi* (Lyme disease)
8. Mycobacteria
   - *Mycobacterium tuberculosis*
   - *Mycobacterium avium intracellulare*

Table 56-2 Site of Infection: Suspected Organisms

Site/Type of Infection	*Suspected Organisms*
1. Respiratory	
Pharyngitis	Viral, group A streptococci
Bronchitis, otitis	Viral, *Haemophilus influenzae, Streptococcus pneumoniae, Moraxella catarrhalis*
Acute sinusitis	Viral, *Streptococcus pneumoniae, Haemophilus influenzae, Moraxella catarrhalis*
Chronic sinusitis	*Anaerobes, Staphylococcus aureus* (as well as suspected organisms associated with acute sinusitis)
Epiglottitis	*Haemophilus influenzae*
Pneumonia	
Community-Acquired	
Normal host	*Streptococcus pneumoniae,* viral, mycoplasma
Aspiration	Normal aerobic and anaerobic mouth flora
Pediatrics	*Streptococcus pneumoniae, Haemophilus influenzae*
COAD	*Streptococcus pneumoniae, Haemophilus influenzae, Legionella, Chlamydia, Mycoplasma*
Alcoholic	*Streptococcus pneumoniae, Klebsiella*
Hospital-Acquired	
Aspiration	Mouth anaerobes, aerobic gram-negative rods, *Staphylococcus aureus*
Neutropenic	Fungi, aerobic Gram-negative rods, *Staphylococcus aureus*
HIV	Fungi, *Pneumocystis, Legionella, Nocardia, Streptococcus pneumoniae, Pseudomonas*
2. Urinary Tract	
Community-Acquired	*Escherichia coli,* other gram-negative rods, *Staphylococcus aureus, Staphylococcus epidermidis,* enterococci
Hospital-Acquired	Resistant aerobic Gram-negative rods, enterococci
3. Skin and Soft Tissue	
Cellulitis	Group A streptococci, *Staphylococcus aureus*
IV catheter site	*Staphylococcus aureus, Staphylococcus epidermidis*
Surgical wound	*Staphylococcus aureus,* Gram-negative rods
Diabetic ulcer	*Staphylococcus aureus,* Gram-negative aerobic rods, anaerobes
Furuncle	*Staphylococcus aureus*
4. Intra-abdominal	*Bacteroides fragilis, Escherichia coli,* other aerobic Gram-negative rods, enterococci
5. Gastroenteritis	*Salmonella, Shigella, Helicobacter, Campylobacter, Clostridium difficile,* amoeba, Giardia, viral, enterotoxigenic-hemorrhagic *Escherichia coli*
6. Endocarditis	
Pre-existing valvular disease	*Streptococcus viridans*
IV drug abuser	*Staphylococcus aureus,* aerobic Gram-negative rods, enterococci, fungi
Prosthetic valve	*Staphylococcus epidermidis*
7. Osteomyelitis and Septic Arthritis	*Staphylococcus aureus,* aerobic Gram-negative rods
8. Meningitis	
<2 months	*Escherichia coli,* group B streptococci, *Listeria*
2 months–12 years	*Streptococcus pneumoniae, Neisseria meningitides, Haemophilus influenzae*
Adults	*Streptococcus pneumoniae, Neisseria meningitides*
Hospital-acquired	*Streptococcus pneumoniae, Neisseria meningitides,* aerobic Gram-negative rods
Post-neurosurgery	*Staphylococcus aureus,* aerobic Gram-negative rods

COAD, chronic obstructive airways disease; IV, intravenous.

and Table 56-2 lists the most likely organisms associated with sites of infection. Determining the most likely infectious agent depends not only on the site of infection but also on host factors. For example, bacterial pneumonia can be caused by various pathogens, including *Streptococcus pneumoniae, Enterobacteriacae*, and atypical pathogens (e.g., *Legionella pneumophila*).[14] Empiric antimicrobial therapy directed against all the above organisms, however, is unnecessary. Several host factors must be evaluated to streamline therapy against the most likely pathogens. If the pneumonia is community acquired, *S. pneumoniae, Haemophilus influenzae, Moraxella catarrhalis,* and "atypical" bacterial pathogens may predominate.[15] In nosocomial (hospital, nursing home) pneumonia, however, gram-negative enterics (e.g., *Escherichia coli, Klebsiella* species, *Enterobacter* species, and *Pseudomonas aeruginosa*) become more significant pathogens. If the pneumonia is a result of a gastric aspiration, mouth anaerobes should probably be covered empirically; however, the true pathogenicity of these anaerobes in aspiration pneumonia is not clear. In nosocomial pneumonia, knowledge of the hospital-specific flora is important. If *E. coli* is the most commonly isolated pathogen at a given institution, antimicrobials, such as first- or second-generation cephalosporins, can be used. If *P. aeruginosa* or *Enterobacter cloacae* predominate, then alternative, broader-spectrum therapy is necessary. A thorough evaluation of antimicrobial exposure also is necessary. Recent use of antimicrobials clearly predisposes to subsequent infection caused by resistant gram-negative organisms.

The patient's age is also an important determinant in the epidemiology of infection. For example, meningitis in a neonate is commonly caused by group B streptococci, *E. coli,* and *Listeria monocytogenes,* whereas these bacteria are uncommon pathogens in normal adults. The presence of concomitant diseases, such as chronic obstructive airways disease (COAD) or alcohol and IV drug abuse, also can help determine the pathogen. For example, patients with COAD-associated pneumonia are more likely to be infected by *S. pneumoniae, H. influenzae,* and *M. catarrhalis.* Chronic alcoholics are more likely to have infection caused by enteric gram-negative pathogens, such as *Klebsiella* species.

Immune status is an important predictor of likely pathogens. HIV-positive patients or those receiving cyclosporine (or tacrolimus) and corticosteroids have lymphocyte deficiency-associated infections, including those caused by cytomegalovirus, *Pneumocystis carinii,* atypical mycobacteria, and *Cryptococcus neoformans.* Patients with leukemia and neutropenia are at risk for infection caused by aerobic gram-negative bacilli, including *P. aeruginosa* and fungi.

In R.G., the abdomen, respiratory tract, urinary tract, and IV catheter are all potential sites of infection. Intra-abdominal infection is likely caused by gram-negative enterics and *Bacteroides fragilis;* nosocomial urinary tract infection is usually secondary to aerobic gram-negative rods. R.G.'s pneumonia possibly is caused by gram-negative bacilli, staphylococci, and various other organisms. Furthermore, his use of corticosteroids may predispose him to infection caused by more opportunistic organisms, including *Legionella, P. carinii,* and fungi. Lastly, his IV catheter infection suggests infection caused by staphylococci, including *Staphylococcus epidermidis* and *Staphylococcus aureus.*

MICROBIOLOGIC TESTS AND SUSCEPTIBILITY OF ORGANISMS

6. A Gram stain of R.G.'s tracheal aspirate shows gram-negative bacilli. What tests may assist with the identification of the pathogen(s)?

Once the site of infection has been determined and host defense and other epidemiologic factors have been evaluated, additional tests can be performed to identify the pathogen. Some tests that provide immediate information to guide selection of the initial antimicrobial regimen can be performed. The Gram stain uses crystal violet solution and iodine, which results in bacteria staining gram positive or gram negative; some organisms are gram variable. In addition, the shape of the organism (cocci, bacilli) is readily apparent with the use of the Gram stain. Streptococci and staphylococci are gram-positive cocci, whereas *E. coli, E. cloacae,* and *P. aeruginosa* appear as gram-negative bacilli (Table 56-1).[16] If the Gram stain of the tracheal aspirate demonstrates gram-positive cocci in clusters, empiric antistaphylococcal therapy is indicated. In contrast, if the Gram stain shows gram-negative rods, antimicrobials with activity against these pathogens are indicated.

Similar to the Gram stain in bacterial infection, the India ink and potassium hydroxide (KOH) stains are helpful in the identification of certain fungi. The acid-fast bacilli (AFB) stain is critical in the diagnosis of infection caused by *Mycobacterium tuberculosis* or atypical mycobacteria.

In R.G., the Gram stain suggests that antimicrobials active against gram-negative bacilli should be used. Table 56-3 provides a classification of antibacterials (e.g., different generations of cephalosporins). Tables 56-4, 56-5, and 56-6 list in vitro susceptibilities of aerobic gram-positive organisms, gram-negative aerobes, and anaerobic organisms, respectively.

Culture and Susceptibility Testing

Culture and susceptibility testing provides final identification of the pathogen, as well as information regarding the effectiveness of various antimicrobials. Although these tests provide more information than the Gram stain, they generally require 18 to 24 hours to complete. After the pathogen has been identified, Table 56-7 can be used in conjunction with an institution's specific susceptibility studies to select the most appropriate antimicrobial.

Disk Diffusion

The most widely used tests for bacterial susceptibility are the disk diffusion and the broth dilution methods. The disk diffusion (Kirby-Bauer) technique uses an agar plate on which an inoculum of the organism is placed. After inoculation, several antimicrobial-laden disks are placed on the plate, and evidence of bacterial growth is observed after 18 to 24 hours. If the antimicrobial is active against the pathogen, a zone of growth inhibition is observed around the disk. Based on guidelines provided by the Clinical Laboratory Standards Institute (CLSI), the diameter of inhibition is reported as susceptible, intermediate, or resistant.

Broth Dilution

The broth dilution method involves placing a bacterial inoculum into several tubes or wells filled with broth. Serial dilutions of antimicrobials (e.g., nafcillin 0.5, 1.0, and 2.0 g/mL) are placed in the respective wells. After bacteria are allowed to incubate for 18 to 24 hours, the wells are examined for bacterial growth. If the well is cloudy, bacterial growth has occurred, suggesting resistance to the antimicrobial at that concentration.

Table 56-3 Classification of Antibacterials

β-Lactam Antibiotics
Cephalosporins
First-generation
Cefadroxil (Duricef)
Cefazolin (Ancef)
Cephalexin (Keflex)
Second-generation
Cefaclor (Ceclor)
Cefamandole (Mandol)
Cefonicid (Monocid)
Ceforanide (Precef)
Cefotetan (Cefotan)
Cefoxitin (Mefoxin)
Cefprozil (Cefzil)
Cefuroxime (Zinacef)
Cefuroxime axetil (Ceftin)
Third-generation
Cefdinir (Omnicef)
Cefditoren (Spectracef)
Cefixime (Suprax)
Cefotaxime (Claforan)
Cefpodoxime proxetil (Vantin)
Ceftazidime (Fortaz)
Ceftibuten (Cedax)
Ceftizoxime (Cefizox)
Ceftriaxone (Rocephin)
Fourth-generation
Cefepime (Maxipime)
Carbacephems
Loracarbef (Lorabid)
Monobactams
Aztreonam (Azactam)
Penems
Doripenem (Doribax)
Ertapenem (Invanz)
Imipenem (Primaxin)
Meropenem (Merem)
Penicillins
Natural Penicillins
Penicillin G
Penicillin V
Aminopenicillins
Ampicillin (Omnipen)
Amoxicillin (Amoxil)

β-Lactam Antibiotics
Bacampicillin (Spectrobid)
Penicillinase-Resistant Penicillins
Isoxazolyl penicillins (dicloxacillin, oxacillin, cloxacillin)
Nafcillin (Unipen)
Combination with β-lactamase Inhibitors
Augmentin (amoxicillin plus clavulanic acid)
Unasyn (ampicillin plus sulbactam)
Zosyn (piperacillin plus tazobactam)
Aminoglycosides
Amikacin (Amikin)
Gentamicin (Garamycin)
Neomycin (Mycifradin)
Netilmicin (Netromycin)
Streptomycin
Tobramycin (Nebcin)
Protein Synthesis Inhibitors
Azithromycin (Zithromax)
Clarithromycin (Biaxin)
Clindamycin (Cleocin)
Chloramphenicol (Chloromycetin)
Dalfopristin/Quinupristin (Synercid)
Dirithromycin (Dynabac)
Erythromycin (Erythrocin)
Linezolid (Zyvox)
Telithromycin (Ketek)
Tetracyclines (doxycycline, minocycline, tetracycline)
Folate Inhibitors
Sulfadiazine
Sulfadoxine (Fansidar)
Trimethoprim (Trimpex)
Trimethoprim-sulfamethoxazole (Bactrim, Septra)
Quinolones
Ciprofloxacin (Cipro)
Gemifloxacin (Factive)
Levofloxacin (Levoquin)
Moxifloxacin (Avelox)
Norfloxacin (Noroxin)
Ofloxacin (Floxin)
Daptomycin (Cubicin)
Vancomycin (Vancocin)
Metronidazole (Flagyl)

As an example, if bacterial growth is observed with *S. aureus* at 0.5 g/mL of nafcillin but not at 1.0 g/mL, then 1.0 g/mL would be considered the minimum inhibitory concentration (MIC) for nafcillin against *S. aureus*.

Similar to the disk diffusion method, the CLSI provides guidelines[17] that also take into account the pharmacokinetic characteristics of an antimicrobial to determine whether the MIC should be reported as susceptible, moderately susceptible, or resistant. MIC interpretations are specific to both the organism and the antimicrobial. For example, ciprofloxacin achieves serum concentrations of 1–4 mcg/mL and ceftriaxone achieves peak serum concentrations of 100–150 mcg/mL; an MIC of 4 g/mL for *E. coli* would be interpreted as resistant to ciprofloxacin and susceptible to ceftriaxone.

Although these tests provide an accurate assessment of *in vitro* susceptibility, the time delay (18–24 hours) can hinder streamlining of therapy. An alternative efficient but more expensive MIC test is the E test, which uses an antibiotic-laden plastic strip with increasing concentration of a specific antimicrobial from one end to the other. The strip is placed on an agar plate with the actively growing pathogen. Inhibition of growth observed at specific marks on the strip coincides with

Table 56-4 In Vitro Antimicrobial Susceptibility: Aerobic Gram-Positive Cocci

Drugs	*Staphylococcus aureus*	*Staphylococcus aureus* (MR)	*Staphylococcus epidermidis*	*Staphylococcus epidermidis* (MR)	*Streptococci*[a]	*Enterococci*[b]	*Pneumococci*
Ampicillin	+		+		++++	++	+++
Augmentin	++++	+	++++		++++	++	++++
Aztreonam							
Cefazolin	++++		++++		++++		++
Cefepime	++++		++++		++++		+++
Cefoxitin/Cefotetan	++		++		++		+
Cefuroxime	++++		++++		++++		+++
Ciprofloxacin[c]	+++	++	+++	++	+	+	++
Clindamycin	++++	+	++++	+	+++		+++
Cotrimoxazole	++++	+++	++	+	++	+	+
Daptomycin[f]	++++	++++	++++	++++	++++	++++	++++
Erythromycin (azithromycin/ clarithromycin)	++		+		+++		++
Imipenem	++++		++++		++++	++	+++
Levofloxacin (gemifloxacin, moxifloxacin)	++++	++	+++	++	+++	++	++++
Linezolid[f]	++++	++++	++++	++++	++++	++++	++++
Nafcillin	++++		++++		++++		++
Penicillin	+		+		++++	++	+++
Quinupristin/ dalfopristin[d,f]	++++	++++	++++	++++	++++	++++	++++
TGC[e]	+++		++		++++		+++
Tigecycline	++++	++++	++++	++++	++++	++++	++++
Timentin	++++		++++		++++	+	+
Unasyn	++++		++++		++++	++	+++
Vancomycin	++++	++++	++++	++++	++++	+++	++++
Zosyn	++++		++++		++++	++	+++

[a] Nonpneumococcal streptococci.
[b] Usually requires combination therapy (e.g., ampicillin and an aminoglycoside) for serious infection.
[c] Levofloxacin (gatifloxacin, gemifloxacin, moxifloxacin) is more active than ciprofloxacin against staphylococci and streptococci.
[d] Active against *E. faecium* but unpredictable against *E. faecalis*.
[e] TGC, cefotaxime, ceftizoxime, ceftriaxone, cefoperazone. Ceftazidime has comparatively inferior antistaphylococcal and antipneumococcal activity. Cefotaxime and ceftriaxone are the most reliable cephalosporins versus *S. pneumoniae*.
[f] Active versus vancomycin-resistant *Enterococcus faecium*.
MR, methicillin resistant.

the MIC of the organism. Numerous studies have confirmed that the E test is as effective as traditional susceptibility testing. Some rapid diagnosis culture and susceptibility tests may provide similar information within hours, potentially resulting in more rapid selection of appropriate antimicrobial therapy.

Although susceptibility testing is relatively well standardized for aerobic gram-negative and gram-positive organisms, its utility continues to evolve for anaerobes[18] and fungi.[19] In general, despite improvements in the standardization of testing in anaerobes, most institutions do not routinely perform susceptibility testing for these bacteria. In contrast, susceptibility testing is now available for yeast, and these in vitro data have been demonstrated to predict clinical success in the patient care setting.

The consensus of the CLSI and other experts is that anaerobic isolates from blood, bone, and joint sources, brain abscesses, empyemic fluid, and other body fluids that are normally sterile should be considered for susceptibility testing. Isolates from other sources should be considered for testing only if the physician believes the test is clearly indicated in the given patient.[18] Although progress has been made in developing a standardized test for determining fungal susceptibility, the primary emphasis has been on the susceptibility of *Candida* species and other yeasts to azoles in oropharyngeal candidiasis. Standardized susceptibility testing for molds recently has been established by the CLSI; however, this testing is rarely performed in the clinical setting.[19]

The MIC is the minimum concentration at which an antimicrobial inhibits the growth of the organism; the test does not provide information regarding whether the organism is actually killed. In some disease states (e.g., endocarditis, meningitis), bactericidal therapy may be necessary. The minimum bactericidal concentration (MBC) is the test that can be used to determine the killing activity associated with an antimicrobial. The MBC is determined by taking an aliquot from each clear MIC tube for subculture onto agar plates. The concentration at which no significant bacterial growth is observed on these plates is considered the MBC.

Table 56-5 In Vitro Antimicrobial Susceptibility: Gram-Negative Aerobes

Drugs	*Escherichia coli*	*Klebsiella pneumoniae*	*Enterobacter cloacae*	*Proteus mirabilis*	*Serratia marcescens*	*Pseudomonas aeruginosa*	*Haemophilus influenzae*	*Haemophilus influenzae*[a]
Ampicillin	++			+++			++++	
Augmentin	+++	++		++++			++++	++++
Aztreonam	++++	++++	+	++++	++++	++++	++++	++++
Cefazolin	+++	+++		++++			++	
Cefepime	++++	++++	+++	++++	++++	++++	++++	++++
Ceftazidime	++++	++++	+	++++	++++	++++	++++	++++
Cefuroxime	+++	+++		++++	+		++++	++++
Cotrimoxazole	++	+++	+++	++++	+++		++++	++++
Ertepenem	++++	++++	++++	++++	++++	+	++++	++++
Gentamicin	++++	++++	++++	++++	++++	+++	++	++
Imipenem/ Meropenem/ Doripenem	++++	++++	++++	+++	++++	++++	++++	++++
Quinolones	+++	++++	+++	++++	++++	++	++++	++++
TGC	++++	++++	+	++++	++++	+	++++	++++
Tigecycline	++++	++++	++++	++	++++	−	++++	++++
Timentin	+++	++	+	++++	+++	+++	++++	++++
Tobramycin	++++	++++	++++	++++	+++	++++	++	++
Unasyn	+++	+++		++++	++		++++	++++
Zosyn	++++	++++	++	++++	++++	++++	++++	++++

TGC, cefataxime, ceftizoxime, ceftriaxone.
[a] β-Lactamase-producing strains.

The serum bactericidal test (SBT) occasionally is used as an in vivo test of antimicrobial activity.[20] The test may have utility in assessing the treatment of more severe infections, such as endocarditis (see Chapter 59, Endocarditis) and osteomyelitis. A blood sample taken from a patient receiving an antibiotic is serially diluted using Mueller-Hinton broth (e.g., 1:2, 1:4, 1:8, 1:16) and then inoculated with the infecting organism. After 18 to 24 hours, the samples are visually inspected for evidence of bacterial growth. If no growth is observed at dilutions of 1:8 and 1:16 but growth is seen at 1:32 and above, the serum is considered inhibitory at 1:16. Similar to the MIC methodology, the clear tubes define the inhibitory titers; however, it is unknown whether bactericidal concentrations have been achieved. As a result, aliquots of each of the clear tubes are plated onto agar. If significant bacterial growth is observed at 1:16 but not at 1:8 or less, the serum is considered bactericidal at 1:8. The CLSI considers as appropriate "peak," an SBT of 1:8 to 1:16 and a "trough" SBT of 1:4 to 1:8. Although the SBT provides an

Table 56-6 Antimicrobial Susceptibility: Anaerobes

Drugs	*Bacteroides fragilis*	*Peptococcus*	*Peptostreptococcus*	*Clostridia*
Ampicillin	+	++++	++++	+++
Aztreonam				
Cefazolin		+++	+++	
Cefepime	+	+++	+++	+
Cefotaxime	++	+++	+++	+
Cefoxitin	+++	+++	++++	+
Ceftazidime		+	+	+
Ceftizoxime	+++	+++	+++	+
Ciprofloxacin	+	+	+	+
Clindamycin	+++	++++	++++	++
Moxifloxacin	+++	+++	+++	++
Imipenem (Doripenem/ Ertapenem/Meropenem)	++++	++++	++++	++
Metronidazole	++++	+++	+++	+++
Penicillin	+	++++	++++	++++
Timentin	++++	+++	+++	+++
Unasyn	++++	++++	++++	++++
Vancomycin		+++	+++	+++
Zosyn	++++	++++	+++	+++

Table 56-7 Antimicrobials of Choice in the Treatment of Bacterial Infection

Organism	*Drug of Choice*	*Alternatives*	*Comments*
Aerobes			
Gram-positive cocci			
Streptococcus pyogenes (group A streptococci)	Penicillin	Clindamycin, macrolide, cephalosporin	Clindamycin is the most reliable alternative for penicillin-allergic patients.
Streptococcus pneumoniae	Penicillin, amoxicillin	Macrolide, cephalosporin, doxycycline	Although the incidence of penicillin nonsusceptible pneumococci continues to increase, high-dose penicillin or amoxicillin is active against most of these isolates. Penicillin-resistant pneumococci commonly demonstrate resistance to other agents, including erythromycin, tetracyclines, and cephalosporins. Antipneumococcal quinolones (gemifloxacin, levofloxacin, moxifloxacin), ceftriaxone, cefotaxime, and telithromycin are options for treatment of high-level penicillin-resistant isolates.
Enterococcus faecalis	Ampicillin ± gentamicin	Vancomycin gentamicin; daptomycin, linezolid	Most commonly isolated enterococcus (80%–85%). Most reliable antienterococcal agents are ampicillin (penicillin, piperacillin-tazobactam), vancomycin, daptomycin and linezolid. Monotherapy generally inhibits but does not kill the enterococcus. Daptomycin is unique in its bactericidal activity against Enterococci. Aminoglycosides must be added to ampicillin or vancomycin to provide bactericidal activity. Ampicillin resistance and high-level aminoglycoside resistance takes place commonly.
Enterococcus faecium	Vancomycin ± gentamicin	Daptomycin, dalfopristin/quinupristin (D/Q), linezolid	Second most common enterococcal organism (10–20%) and is more likely than *E. faecalis* to be resistant to multiple antimicrobials. Most reliable agents are daptomycin, D/Q and linezolid. Monotherapy generally inhibits but does not kill the enterococcus. Aminoglycosides must be added to cell wall active agents to provide bactericidal activity. Ampicillin and vancomycin resistance is common. Daptomycin, D/Q, and linezolid are drugs of choice for vancomycin-resistant isolates.
Staphylococcus aureus	Nafcillin	Cefazolin, vancomycin, clindamycin, trimethoprim-sulfamethoxazole linezolid,	10%–15% of isolates inhibited by penicillin. Most isolates susceptible to nafcillin, cephalosporins, trimethoprim-sulfamethoxazole, and clindamycin. First-generation cephalosporins are equal to nafcillin. Most second- and third-generation cephalosporins adequate in the treatment of infection (exceptions include ceftazidime and cefonicid). Methicillin-resistant *S. aureus* must be treated with vancomycin; however, trimethoprim-sulfamethoxazole, daptomycin, D/Q, linezolid, or minocycline can be used.
(Nafcillin-resistant)	Vancomycin	trimethoprim-sulfamethoxazole, minocycline, daptomycin	
Staphylococcus epidermidis	Nafcillin	Cefazolin, vancomycin, clindamycin	Most isolates are Most isolates are β-lactam-, clindamycin-, and trimethoprim-sulfamethoxazole-resistant. Most reliable agents are vancomycin, daptomycin, D/Q, and linezolid. Rifampin is active and can be used in conjunction with other agents; however, monotherapy with rifampin is associated with development of resistance.
(Nafcillin-resistant)	Vancomycin	Daptomycin, linezolid, D/Q	
Gram-positive Bacilli			
Diphtheroids	Penicillin	Cephalosporin	
Corynebacterium jeikeium	Vancomycin	Erythromycin, quinolone	
Listeria monocytogenes	Ampicillin (± gentamicin)	Trimethoprim-sulfamethoxazole	

(continued)

Table 56-7 Antimicrobials of Choice in the Treatment of Bacterial Infection *(Continued)*

Organism	Drug of Choice	Alternatives	Comments
Gram-negative Cocci			
Moraxella catarrhalis	Trimethoprim-sulfamethoxazole	Amoxicillin-clavulanic acid, erythromycin, doxycycline, second- or third-generation cephalosporin	
Neisseria gonorrhoeae	Cefixime	Ceftriaxone	
Neisseria meningitides	Penicillin	Third-generation cephalosporin	
Gram-negative Bacilli			
Campylobacter fetus	Imipenem	Gentamicin	
Campylobacter jejuni	Quinolone, erythromycin	A tetracycline, amoxicillin-clavulanic acid	
Enterobacter	Trimethoprim-sulfamethoxazole	Quinolone, imipenem, aminoglycoside	Not predictably inhibited by most cephalosporins. Imipenem, quinolones, trimethoprim-sulfamethoxazole, cefepime, and aminoglycosides are most active agents.
Escherichia coli	Third-generation cephalosporin	First- or second-generation cephalosporin, gentamicin	Extended spectrum β-lactamase (ESBL)-producers should be treated with a carbapenem.
Haemophilus influenzae	Third-generation cephalosporin	β-lactamase inhibitor combinations, second-generation cephalosporin, trimethoprim-sulfamethoxazole	
Helicobacter pylori	Amoxicillin + clarithromycin + omeprazole	Tetracycline + metronidazole + bismuth subsalicylate	
Klebsiella pneumoniae	Third-generation cephalosporin	First- or second-generation cephalosporin, gentamicin, trimethoprim-sulfamethoxazole	Extended spectrum β-lactamase (ESBL)-producers should be treated with a carbapenem.
Legionella	Fluoroquinolone	Erythromycin ± rifampin, doxycycline	
Proteus mirabilis	Ampicillin	First-generation cephalosporin, trimethoprim-sulfamethoxazole	
Other *Proteus*	Third-generation cephalosporin	β-lactamase inhibitor combination, aminoglycoside, trimethoprim-sulfamethoxazole	
Pseudomonas aeruginosa	Antipseudomonal penicillin (or ceftazidime±) aminoglycoside (or quinolone)	Quinolone or imipenem ± aminoglycoside	Most active agents include aminoglycosides, doripenem, imipenem, meropenem, ceftazidime, cefepime, aztreonam and the extended-spectrum penicillins. Monotherapy is adequate for most pseudomonal infections.
Salmonella typhi	Quinolone	Ceftriaxone	
Serratia marcescens	Third-generation cephalosporin	Trimethoprim-sulfamethoxazole, aminoglycoside	
Shigella	Quinolone	Trimethoprim-sulfamethoxazole, ampicillin	
Stenotrophomonas maltophilia	Trimethoprim-sulfamethoxazole	Ceftazidime, minocycline, β-lactamase inhibitor combination (Timentin)	

Anaerobes			
Bacteroides fragilis	Metronidazole	β-lactamase inhibitor combinations, penems	Most active agents (95%–100%) include metronidazole, the β-lactamase inhibitor combinations (ampicillin-sulbactam, piperacillin-tazobactam, ticarcillin-clavulanic acid), and penems. Clindamycin, cefoxitin, cefotetan, cefmetazole, ceftizoxime have good activity but not to the degree of metronidazole. Aminoglycosides and aztreonam are inactive.
Clostridia difficile	Metronidazole	Vancomycin	
Fusobacterium	Penicillin	Metronidazole, clindamycin	
Other Oropharyngeal			
Prevotella	β-lactamase inhibitor combination	Metronidazole, clindamycin	
Peptostreptococcus	Penicillin	Clindamycin, cephalosporin	Most β-lactams active (exceptions include aztreonam, nafcillin, ceftazidime).
Other			
Actinomycetes			
Actinomyces israelii	Penicillin	Tetracyclines	
Nocardia	Trimethoprim-sulfamethoxazole	Amikacin, minocycline, imipenem	
Chlamydiae	Doxycycline		
Chlamydia trachomatis	Doxycycline	Azithromycin	
Chlamydia pneumoniae		Azithromycin, clarithromycin	
Mycoplasma			
Mycoplasma pneumoniae	Doxycycline	Azithromycin, clarithromycin	
Spirochetes			
Borrelia burgdorferi	Doxycycline	Ampicillin, second- or third-generation cephalosporin	
Treponema pallidum	Penicillin	Doxycycline	

in vivo test of antibacterial activity, the practical utility of the test is limited.

DETERMINATION OF ISOLATE PATHOGENICITY

7. *Serratia marcescens* grows from a culture of R.G.'s tracheal aspirate, and the decision to treat this organism is based on whether the isolate is a true pathogen. How can the difference between true bacterial infection and colonization or contamination be determined?

A positive culture may represent colonization, contamination, or infection. Colonization indicates that bacteria are present at the site but are not actively causing infection. Poor sampling techniques or inappropriate handling of specimens can result in contamination. Infection, colonization, and contamination might all be applicable to R.G. If a suction catheter was used for a sample of R.G.'s tracheal aspirate, the infecting organism likely would be cultured; however, other flora present in the oropharynx (but not associated with infection) would also appear in the culture medium (colonization). Furthermore, if the sample is not handled aseptically by the clinician or the microbiology laboratory, bacterial contamination is possible.

In summary, culture results do not necessarily identify only the actual pathogens. In R.G., the *Serratia* may be a pathogen, contaminant, or colonizer. Nevertheless, considering the severity of R.G.'s illness, treatment directed against this pathogen is necessary.

ANTIMICROBIAL TOXICITIES

8. In light of the positive culture for *Serratia,* his increased respiratory secretions, and a worsening chest radiograph, R.G.'s lungs are considered a source of infection. Pending susceptibility results, R.G. is started on combination imipenem and gentamicin. Are there equally effective, less toxic options for this patient?

Adverse Effects and Toxicities

Before therapy is started, it is important to elicit an accurate drug and allergy history. When "allergy" has been reported by the patient, it is necessary to determine whether the reaction was intolerance, toxicity, or true allergy (see Chapter 4 Anaphylaxis and Drug Allergies). Table 56-8 lists the most common adverse effects and toxicities associated with antimicrobial therapy. For example, gastric intolerance caused by oral erythromycin is common; however, this adverse effect does not represent an allergic manifestation or toxicity caused by the drug. In R.G.'s case, neither imipenem nor gentamicin is an optimal choice. Imipenem is known to be associated with seizures, particularly in patients with renal failure and in doses in excess of 50 mg/kg/D. Considering R.G.'s acute onset of renal failure and his history of seizures, other carbapenems, such as meropenem, would be preferable. Gentamicin similarly may not be a good choice in R.G. His increased age and changing renal function predispose him to aminoglycoside nephrotoxicity and ototoxicity (cochlear and vestibular).[21] A reasonable recommendation would be to discontinue imipenem and gentamicin and treat with meropenem with or without a fluoroquinolone.

Concomitant Disease States

Concomitant disease states also should be considered in the selection of therapy. As discussed above, older patients with hearing deficits are poor candidates for potentially ototoxic aminoglycoside therapy. Diabetics or patients with kidney transplants may be better treated with IV fluconazole than nephrotoxic amphotericin B products in candidemia. Patients with a preexisting seizure history should not receive imipenem if less toxic therapy can be used. In summary, the toxicologic profile must be taken into account in the selection of antimicrobial therapy.

ANTIMICROBIAL COSTS OF THERAPY

9. What factors should be included in calculating the cost of R.G.'s antimicrobial therapy?

The true cost of antimicrobial therapy is difficult to quantitate.[22] Although acquisition cost traditionally has been the primary factor in the overall cost of therapy, drug administration labor costs (i.e., nursing and pharmacy) and the use of IV sets, piggyback bags, and infusion control devices must be included in the analysis. As a result, a drug that must be administered several times daily, such as penicillin, will incur increased administration costs compared with one that requires once-a-day dosing.

Some drugs, such as aminoglycosides, are associated with increased laboratory costs (e.g., aminoglycoside serum concentrations, serum creatinine, audiometry) that are not required for other agents,[23] such as the third-generation cephalosporins and quinolones. Similarly, drugs with a high potential for misuse or toxicity can be associated with increased costs because of monitoring (e.g., drug use evaluation, pharmacokinetic monitoring). If meropenem with or without ciprofloxacin had been selected for R.G., this therapy would be expected to be associated with relatively few laboratory costs. The broad spectrum of activity[24] and potential for misuse and development of resistance might, however, result in increased monitoring costs and overall cost to society.

Costs that are difficult to quantitate include that of both therapy failure and antimicrobial toxicity. Ineffective or toxic therapy can prolong hospitalization and may require expensive interventions, such as hemodialysis,[23] mechanical ventilation, and intensive care unit admission. The net effect of these latter costs can be significantly greater than the acquisition and administration costs of antimicrobial therapy.

In summary, determining the true cost of antimicrobial therapy is complex. Acquisition cost, IV bags, infusion controllers, and labor must be incorporated into the analysis. Although they are difficult to estimate, other costs, including antibiotic toxicity and failure of therapy, also should be included.

ROUTE OF ADMINISTRATION

10. The *Serratia* was determined to be susceptible to ciprofloxacin. Oral ciprofloxacin was considered for the treatment of R.G.'s presumed *Serratia* pneumonia, but the IV route was prescribed. Why is the oral administration of ciprofloxacin reasonable (or unreasonable) in R.G.?

Table 56-8 Antibiotic Adverse Effects and Toxicities

Antibiotic	Side Effects	Comments
β-Lactams, (penicillin, cephalosporins, monobactams, penems)	*Allergic:* anaphylaxis, urticaria, serum sickness, rash, fever	Many patients will have "ampicillin rash" with no cross-reactivity with any other penicillins. Most common in patients with mononucleosis or those receiving allopurinol. Likelihood of IgE-mediated cross-reactivity between penicillins and cephalosporins approximately 37%. Recently documented is minimal cross-reactivity between penicillins and imipenem/meropenem. No IgE cross-reactivity between aztreonam and penicillins.
	Diarrhea	Particularly common with ampicillin, Augmentin, ceftriaxone, and cefoperazone. Antibiotic-associated colitis can occur with most antimicrobials
	Hematologic: anemia, thrombocytopenia, antiplatelet activity, hypothrombinemia	Hemolytic anemia more common with higher doses. Antiplatelet activity (inhibition of platelet aggregation) most common with the antipseudomonal penicillins and high serum levels of other lactams. Hypothrombinemia more often associated with those cephalosporins with the methyltetrazolethiol side chain (cefamandole, cefotetan). Reaction preventable and reversible with vitamin K.
	Hepatitis or biliary sludging	Most common with oxacillin. Biliary sludging and stones reported with ceftriaxone.
	Phlebitis	
	Seizure activity	Associated with high levels of β-lactams, particularly penicillins and imipenem
	Potassium load	Penicillin G (K^+)
	Nephritis	Most common with methicillin; however, occasionally reported for most other β-lactams
	Neutropenia	Nafcillin
	Disulfiram reaction	Associated with cephalosporins with methyltetrazolethiol side chain (cefamandole, cefotetan)
	Hypotension, nausea	Associated with fast infusion of imipenem
Aminoglycosides (gentamicin, tobramycin, amikacin, netilmicin)	Nephrotoxicity	Averages 10%–15% incidence. Generally reversible, usually occurs after 5–7 days of therapy. *Risk factors:* dehydration, age, dose, duration, concurrent nephrotoxins, liver disease.
	Ototoxicity	1–5% incidence, often irreversible. Both cochlear and vestibular toxicity occur.
	Neuromuscular paralysis	Rare, most common with large doses administered via intraperitoneal instillation or in patients with myasthenia gravis
Macrolides (erythromycin, azithromycin, clarithromycin)	Nausea, vomiting, "burning" stomach	Oral administration. Azithromycin and clarithromycin associated with less nausea than erythromycin.
	Cholestatic jaundice	Reported for all erythromycin salts, most common with estolate
	Ototoxicity	Most common with high doses in patients with renal or hepatic failure
Clindamycin	Diarrhea	Most common adverse effect. High association with antibiotic-associated colitis.
Tetracyclines (including tigecycline)	Allergic	
	Photosensitivity	
	Teeth and bone deposition and discoloration	Avoid in pediatrics, pregnancy, and breast-feeding.
	GI	Upper GI predominates.
	Hepatitis	Primarily in pregnancy or the elderly
	Renal (azotemia)	Tetracyclines have antianabolic effect and should be avoided in patients with ↓ renal function. Less problematic with doxycycline.
	Vestibular	Associated with minocycline, particularly high doses
Vancomycin	Ototoxicity	Only with receipt of concomitant ototoxins such as aminoglycosides or macrolides
	Nephrotoxicity	Nephrotoxic only with high doses or in combination with other nephrotoxins.
	Hypotension, flushing	Associated with rapid infusion of vancomycin. More common with increased doses.
	Phlebitis	Needs large volume dilution
Dalfopristin/Quinupristin	Phlebitis	Generally requires central line administration
	Myalgia	Moderate to severe in many patients
	Increased bilirubin	

(continued)

Table 56-8 Antibiotic Adverse Effects and Toxicities *(Continued)*

Antibiotic	Side Effects	Comments
Daptomycin	Myalgia	Primarily at high doses and reversible
Linezolid	Thrombocytopenia, neutropenia, anemia, MAO inhibition, tongue discoloration	
Sulfonamides	GI	Nausea, diarrhea
	Hepatic	Cholestatic hepatitis, ↑ incidence in HIV.
	Rash	Exfoliative dermatitis, Stevens-Johnson syndrome. More common in HIV.
	Bone marrow	Neutropenia, thrombocytopenia. More common in HIV.
	Kernicterus	Caused by unbound drug in the neonate. Premature liver cannot conjugate bilirubin. Sulfonamide displaces bilirubin from protein, resulting in excessive free bilirubin and kernicterus.
Chloramphenicol	Anemia	Idiosyncratic irreversible aplastic anemia (rare) Reversible dose-related anemia
	Gray syndrome	Caused by inability of neonates to conjugate chloramphenicol
Quinolones	GI	Nausea, vomiting, diarrhea
	Prolonged QT	Moxifloxacin; possibly all quinolones as a class
	Drug interactions	↓ Oral bioavailability with multivalent cations
	CNS	Altered mental status, confusion, seizures
	Cartilage toxicity	Toxic in animal model. Despite this toxicity, appears safe in children including patients with cystic fibrosis.
	Tendonitis or tendon rupture	Common in elderly, renal failure, concomitant glucocorticoids
Antifungals		
Amphotericin B products	Nephrotoxicity	Common. May depend on patient Na load. Caution with concomitant nephrotoxins (e.g., aminoglycosides, cyclosporine).
	Hypokalemia	Predictable. Probably caused by renal tubular excretion of potassium. More common in patients receiving concomitant piperacillin-tazobactam.
	Hypomagnesemia	Less commonly observed than hypokalemia
	Anemia	Long-term adverse effect. Similar to anemia of chronic disease.
Caspofungin, micafungin, anidulofungin	Mild LFT increase with concomitant cyclosporine Anidulofungin is reconstituted with alcohol (about the equivalent of a beer).	
Flucytosine	Neutropenia, thrombocytopenia	Secondary to metabolism of flucytosine to fluorouracil. More commonly observed with flucytosine levels >100 mg/mL. More common in patients with HIV.
	Hepatitis	Usually moderate ↑ in LFT. Rarely clinical hepatitis.
Ketoconazole (fluconazole, itraconazole, posaconazole, voriconazole)	Drug interactions	↓ Oral bioavailability of ketoconazole tablet, and itraconazole capsules with ↑ gastric pH. Azoles are CYP450 substrates and also inhibitors of CYP450 3A4 and other CYP isoenzymes
	Hepatitis	Ranges from mild ↑in LFT to occasional fatal hepatitis.
	Gynecomastia, ↓ libido	More common with high-dose ketoconazole (>400 mg/day). Less common with other azoles.
	Visual disturbance	Unique to voriconazole, particularly first week of therapy

Antivirals (excluding antiretrovirals)		
Acyclovir	Phlebitis	Caused by poor solubility of IV preparation. Reported in 1–20% of cases.
	Renal failure	Low solubility of acyclovir associated with renal failure. Dehydrated patients, as well as rapid infusions, predispose to toxicity.
	CNS	1% incidence in AIDS. ↑ Incidence with dose in >10 mg/kg/day.
Foscarnet	Nephrotoxicity	Occurs in up to 60% of patients. May be prevented with normal saline bolus before dose. Frequent monitoring of renal function imperative.
	Mineral and electrolyte abnormalities	↑ and ↓ calcium or phosphate may be observed. Hypocalcemia, hypo- and hyperphosphatemia, hypo-magnesemia, hypokalemia. ↑ Risk of cardiomyopathy and seizures.
	Anemia	Anemia in 33%; usually manageable with transfusions and discontinuation of foscarnet
	Nausea, vomiting	
Ganciclovir	Neutropenia, thrombocytopenia	↑ Incidence in AIDS. ↑Incidence with doses in excess of 10 mg/kg/day.
	Hepatitis	Usually mild to moderate in LFT
Oseltamavir	Nausea	

AIDS, acquired immunodeficiency syndrome; CNS, central nervous system; GI, gastrointestinal; HIV, human immunodeficiency virus; IV, intravenous; LFT, liver function tests; MAO, monoamine oxidase; MCV, mean corpuscular volume; Na, sodium.

The proper route of antibiotic administration depends on many factors, including the infection severity, bioavailability, and other patient factors. In patients who appear "septic," blood flow often is shunted away from the mesentery and extremities, resulting in unreliable bioavailability from the GI tract or muscles. Therefore, hemodynamically unstable patients should receive antimicrobials by the IV route to ensure therapeutic antimicrobial levels. Furthermore, some drug interactions can result in subtherapeutic serum concentrations (e.g., reduced bioavailability associated with concomitant quinolone and antacid administration and the decreased absorption of ketoconazole or itraconazole with concurrent H_2-blocker therapy).

R.G. is clinically septic with a possible *Serratia* pneumonia. Considering his unstable state, the bioavailability of oral ciprofloxacin cannot be guaranteed; thus, he should be treated with IV antimicrobials.

ANTIMICROBIAL DOSING

11. What dose of IV ciprofloxacin should be given to R.G.? What factors must be taken into account in determining a proper antimicrobial dose?

The choice of dosing regimen is based on many factors. Table 56-9 provides a guide for the dosing of more commonly administered antimicrobials. Selection of the appropriate dosage should be based on information that documents the efficacy of the dosage in the treatment of infection. Patient-specific factors, including weight, infection site, and route of elimination, also must be considered in dosage selection. The patient's weight is important, particularly for agents with a low therapeutic index (e.g., aminoglycosides, imipenem, flucytosine); these drugs should be dosed on a mg/kg/day basis. Other agents with a more favorable adverse effect profile, such as cephalosporins, are less likely to require weight-specific dosing.

Site of Infection

The infection site also requires differing dosage requirements. An uncomplicated urinary tract infection requires low antimicrobial doses because of the high urinary drug concentrations that are achieved. In contrast, a more serious systemic infection, such as pyelonephritis, requires increased antimicrobial dosages to achieve therapeutic drug levels in tissue and in serum.

Anatomic and Physiologic Barriers

Anatomic and physiologic barriers also must be considered in evaluating a dosing regimen. For example, penetration into the CNS necessitates high doses to ensure adequate antimicrobial concentrations at the infection site.[25] Vitreous humor[26] and the prostate gland[27] are additional sites in which therapeutic antimicrobial concentrations are more difficult to achieve.

Route of Elimination

Route of elimination must also be considered in the dosage calculation. In general, antimicrobials are eliminated via the kidney or nonrenally (metabolic or biliary). Renal function can be estimated via 24-hour urine collection or with equations such as the Cockcroft and Gault equation[28]:

$$\text{Creatinine clearance} = ([140 - \text{age}]^*[\text{weight in kg}])/(72^*\text{SrCr})$$

Several anti-infectives are eliminated renally (Table 56-10). Most β-lactams are eliminated by the kidney. Ceftriaxone, cefoperazone, and most antistaphylococcal penicillins (e.g., nafcillin, oxacillin, dicloxacillin) are eliminated both renally and nonrenally. Aminoglycosides, vancomycin, acyclovir, and ganciclovir are cleared extensively by the kidney. Thus, dosage adjustment is recommended for these drugs in patients with renal failure (Table 56-9 and). Since azithromycin, clindamycin, and metronidazole are primarily eliminated by the liver, no dose reduction is required in renal failure.

Although renal function can be approximated with the use of the Cockcroft and Gault equation (or a similar equation), hepatic function is more difficult to evaluate. No standard liver function test (AST, ALT, alkaline phosphatase) has been demonstrated to correlate well with hepatic drug clearance. Some tests, such as PT and albumin, are markers of hepatic function, but even these tests do not clearly predict drug clearance. Patients receiving hemodialysis or continuous hemofiltration provide additional dosing challenges. Table 56-10 provides dosing recommendations in patients receiving hemodialysis or continuous hemofiltration.

Patient Age

Most dosing information has been derived from a young, relatively healthy patient population, so total drug clearance for several antimicrobials may be decreased in neonatal and geriatric patients. As a result, the age of the patient may be an important factor in the selection of a proper dose.

Fever and Inoculum Effect

The impact of other factors on the selection of an antimicrobial dose is less clear. Fever increases and decreases blood flow to mesenteric, hepatic, and renal organ systems[29] and can either increase or decrease drug clearance. Inoculum effect also may be a factor in the selection of a dosing regimen because it is associated with an increase in the MIC of the organism in response to increasing bacterial concentrations.[30] For example, piperacillin may demonstrate an MIC of 8.0 g/mL against *P. aeruginosa* at a concentration of 10^5 colony-forming units/mL (CFU/mL); however, at 10^9 CFU/mL, the MIC may increase to 32 to 64 g/mL. This phenomenon is well recognized, particularly with β-lactamase–producing bacteria treated with β-lactam antimicrobials. The more stable the antimicrobial is to β-lactamase, the less the influence is the inoculum effect. Aminoglycosides, quinolones, and imipenem appear to be less affected by the inoculum effect than β-lactams. The inoculum effect probably is most relevant in the treatment of a bacterial abscess, in which extremely high concentrations of bacteria would be expected. As a result, antimicrobials that are more susceptible to the inoculum effect may require increased drug dosages for optimal outcome in the treatment of abscesses.

In summary, R.G. normally would be given an IV dosage of ciprofloxacin at 400 mg every 12 hours. His reduced renal function suggests, however, that his dosage should be decreased to 200 to 300 mg every 12 hours.

Table 56-9 University of California San Francisco/Mt. Zion Medical Center Adult Antimicrobial Dosing Guidelines*

Approved by the Antibiotic Advisory Subcommittee (3/13/91) and the Pharmacy and Therapeutics Committee (4/11/91) Rev 2007.

Drug	CrCl > 50 mL/min	CrCl 10–50 mL/min	CrCl < 10 mL/min (ESRD not on HD)
Acyclovir	Herpes simplex infections 5 mg/kg/dose Q 8 hr	5 mg/kg/dose Q 12–24 hr	2.5 mg/kg Q 24 hr
	herpes simplex virus encephalitis/herpes zoster 10 mg/kg/dose Q 8 hr	10 mg/kg/dose Q 12–24 hr	5 mg/kg Q 24 hr
Amphotericin B	0.3–1.0 mg/kg	No change	No change
Dosage reductions in renal disease are not necessary. Because of the nephrotoxic potential of the drug, reducing the dose or holding the drug in the setting of a rising serum creatinine may be warranted.			
Ampicillin	1–2 g Q 4–6 hr	1–1.5 g Q 6 hr	1 g Q 8–12 hr
Cefazolin	1–2 g Q 8 hr	1–2 g Q 12 hr	0.5–1.0 g Q 24 hr
Caspofungin	LD = 70 mg × 1, then 50 mg Q 24 hr	No change	No change
Cefepime	>60 mL/min 1–2 g Q 12 hr Febrile neutropenia: 2 g Q 8 hr	30–60 mL/min: 1–2 g Q 24 hr 10–30 mL/min: 0.51 g Q 24 hr	0.25–0.5 g Q 24 hr
Ceftazidime	1–2 g Q 8 hr	1–2 g Q 12–24 hr	0.5 g Q 24 hr
Ceftriaxone	1 g Q 24 hr Meningitis: 2 g Q 12 hr	No change Endocarditis and osteomyelitis: 2 g Q 24 hr	No change
Cefuroxime	0.75–1.5 g Q 8 hr	0.75–1.5 g Q 12–24 hr	0.5 g Q 24 hr
Ciprofloxacin	400 mg Q 12 hr* (500–750 mg PO Q12 hr)	200–400 mg Q12 hr (250–500 mg PO Q12 hr)	200 mg Q12 hr (250 mg PO Q12 hr)
The use of every (Q) 12-hour dosing intervals is recommended in ESRD because of the variability in half-life data observed in anephric patients. *Note: Higher doses, increased frequency, or both may be necessary in the treatment of serious pseudomonal infections.			
Clindamycin	600–900 mg Q 8 hr	No change	No change
Ethambutol	15 mg/kg QD	7.5–10 mg/kg QD	5 mg/kg QD
Fluconazole	100–400 mg Q 24 hr	50–200 mg Q 24 hr	50–100 mg Q 24 hr
Flucytosine (PO)	12.5–37.5 mg/kg/dose Q 6 hr	25–50 mL/min: 12.5–37.5 mg/kg/dose Q 12 hr 10–25 mL/min: 12.5–37.5 mg/kg/dose Q 24 hr	12.5–25 mg/kg/dose Q 24 hr
Steady-state serum 5-FC level measurements are difficult to obtain. However, they may be useful in guiding dosing of 5-FC in anuria. Bone marrow suppression has been associated with 2-hour postdose 5-FC peaks of >100 mg/L.			
Ganciclovir	30–60 mL/min: 5 mg/kg/dose 50–69 mL/min: 2.5 mg/kg/dose Q 12 hr	25–49 mL/min: 2.5 mg/kg/dose Q 24 hr	10–24 mL/min: 0.625–1.25 mg/kg/dose Q 24 hr 1.25 mg/kg/dose Q 24 hr
Gentamicin	5 mg/kg/dose Q 24 hr	See below	See below
The total daily dose of gentamicin can be administered as a single daily dose in patients with normal renal function (CrCl 60 mL/minute). Patients with decreased renal function or abnormal body composition should have their doses adjusted according to the recommendations below. All patients who are anticipated to receive aminoglycosides for ≥7 days should be monitored with gentamicin levels. Peak levels are not useful with this dosing regimen; however, trough levels are recommended and in most cases will be nondetectable.			
		40–60 mL/min: 1.2–1.5 mg/kg Q 12 hr 20–40 mL/min: 1.2–1.5 mg/kg Q 12–24 hr	<20 mL/min 2 mg/kg loading dose (consult pharmacy for maintenance dose)
With traditional dosing of gentamicin, peak (5–8 mg/L) and trough (<2 mg/L) levels are recommended in patients anticipated to receive aminoglycosides for ≥7 days for severe gram-negative infection. Lower doses (1 mg/kg/dose Q 8 hrs) are suggested when aminoglycosides are used synergistically in gram-positive infections. Those patients with CrCl <60 mL/minute, obesity, or increased fluid volume should be monitored with serum gentamicin levels.			

(continued)

Table 56-9 University of California San Francisco[a]/Mt. Zion Medical Center Adult Antimicrobial Dosing Guidelines[a] *(Continued)*

Drug	*CrCl > 50 mL/min*	*CrCl 10–50 mL/min*	*CrCl < 10 mL/min (ESRD not on HD)*
Imipenem	500 mg Q 6–8 hr; *maximum, 50 mg/kgday*	500 mg Q 8 hr	<20 mL/min 250–500 mg Q 12 hr (or consider meropenem)
Isoniazid	300 mg QD	No change	No change
Levofloxacin	250–500 mg Q 24 hr	LD = 500 mg × 1, then 250 mg Q 24 hr	LD = 500 mg × 1, then 250 mg Q 48 hr
Meropenem	0.5–1 g Q 8 hr Meningitis: 2 g Q 8 hr	25–50 mL/min: 0.5–1 g Q 12 hr 10–25 mL/min: 0.5 g Q 12 hr	0.5 g Q 24 hr
Metronidazole	500 mg Q 8 hr	500 mg Q 8 hr	500 mg Q 12 hr; metabolites accumulate in ESRD
Nafcillin	1–2 g Q 4–6 hr	No change	No change
Penicillin G	2–3 MU Q 4–6 hr	1–2 MU Q 4–6 hr	1 MU Q 6 hr
Piperacillin/Tazobactam (Zosyn)	3.375–4.5 g Q 6–8 hr *Pseudomonas:* 4.5 g Q 6 hr for ClCr >20 mL/min	3.375–4.5 g Q 6–8 hr	2.25–3.375 g Q 8 hr
Pyrazinamide	20–25 mg/kg/day	No change	No change
Rifampin	600 mg QD	No change	No change
Tobramycin	See Gentamicin	See Gentamicin	See Gentamicin
TMP-SMX	*Systemic GNR infections* 10 mg TMP/kg/day divided Q 6–12 hr	5–7.5 mg TMP/kg/day divided Q 12–24 hr	2.5–5.0 mg TMP/kg Q 24 hr
	Pneumocystis carinii pneumonia 15–20 mg TMP/kg/day divided Q 6–12 hr	10–15 mg TMP/kg/day divided Q 12–24 hr	5–10 mg TMP/kg Q 24 hr
Voriconazole	LD = 400 mg Q 12 hr × 1 day, then 200 mg Q 12 hr (PO)	No change	No change
By mouth (PO) should be used when possible, as oral bioavailability >95%. IV dose: LD = 6 mg/kg/dose Q 12 hr × 1 day, then 4 mg/kg/dose Q 12 hr. The use of IV should be avoided in patients with CrCl <50 mL/min owing to the accumulation of the IV vehicle and it is contraindicated in ESRD.			
Vancomycin	>60 mL/min: 10–15 mg/kg Q 12 hr 40–60 mL/min: 10–15 mg/kg Q 12–24 hr	20–40 mL/min: 10–15 mg/kg Q 24–48 hr	10–20 mL/min: 10–15 mg/kg Q 48–72 hr <10 mL/min: 10–15 mg/kg Q 4–7 days
Vancomycin dosing should be guided by serum level measurements in patients with decreased renal function or abnormal body composition. Peak levels are not recommended. Trough levels (30 minutes before next dose) should be 5–15 mg/L.			

[a] Doses are those recommended for systemic infections commonly treated with these agents. Infections involving the urinary tract may require lower doses. Infections involving the central nervous system may require higher doses. Estimate of renal function using Cockcroft and Gault equation:

$$\text{CrCl (mL/min)} = \frac{(140 - \text{age})^{*}\text{Wt (kg)}}{72^{*}\text{SCr (mg/dL)}} \quad \text{(for females multiply by 0.85)}$$

PHARMACOKINETICS/PHARMACODYNAMICS

12. R.G.'s respiratory status remains unchanged; thus, the ciprofloxacin is discontinued and cefotaxime and gentamicin are started empirically. The use of a constant IV infusion of cefotaxime is being considered in R.G. In addition, the use of single daily dosing of gentamicin is being discussed. What is the rationale for these approaches, and would either be advantageous for R.G.?

β-lactams, such as cefotaxime, are not associated with increased bacterial killing with increasing drug concentrations. Pharmacodynamic activity best correlates with the duration of time that antimicrobial levels are maintained above the MIC.[31] The animal model suggests that β-lactam antimicrobials should be dosed such that their serum levels exceed the MIC of the pathogen as long as possible.[32] This observation appears to be most important in the neutropenic model, in which the use of a constant infusion more reliably inhibits bacterial

Table 56-10 University of California San Francisco Medical Center

Adult Antimicrobial Dosing Card for Continuous Renal Replacement Therapy (CRRT) and Hemodialysis (HD)[a]
Department of Clinical Pharmacy, Division of Infectious Diseases and Division of Nephrology University of California, San Francisco Medical Center (6/03)

CRRT: This assumes an ultrafiltration (UF) rate of 2 L/hr with continuous venous-venous hemofiltration (CVVH) and a UF rate of 1 L/hr and dialysate flow rate of 1 L/hr with continuous veno-venous hemodiafiltration (CVVHDF) and residual native glomular filtration rate (GFR) <10 mL/min.

Drug	CRRT	HD
Acyclovir	**Herpes simplex infections** 2.5–5.0 mg/kg Q 24 hr **HSV Encephalitis/ Herpes Zoster** 5–7.5 mg/kg Q 24 hr	**Herpes simplex infections** 2.5 mg/kg Q 24 hr and post HD **HSV Encephalitis/ Herpes Zoster** 5 mg/kg Q 24 hr and post HD
Ampicillin	1 g Q 6 hr	1 g Q 12 hr
Ampicillin/Sul (Unasyn)	1.5 g Q 6 hr	1.5 g Q 12 hr
Cefazolin	1 g Q 12 hr	2 g post HD only
Cefepime	2 g Q 12 hr	2 g post HD only
Cefotetan	1 g Q 12 hr	2 g post HD only
Ceftazidime	2 g Q 12 hr	1 g post HD
Ciprofloxacin	400 mg IV Q 12 hr	200 mg IV Q12 hr or 250 mg PO Q 12 hr
Fluconazole	400 mg PO Q 24 hr	200 mg PO post HD only
Ganciclovir	2.5–5.0 mg/kg Q 24 hr	1.25 mg/kg post HD only
Gentamicin	Gram-negative infections: 2 mg/kg loading dose *then* 1.5 mg/kg Q 24 hr Monitoring of serum levels is recommended; trough <2 mcg/mL	Gram-negative infections: 2 mg/kg loading dose *then* 1 mg/kg post HD Monitoring of serum levels is recommended; trough <2 mcg/mL
Imipenem	500 mg Q 8 hr	250 mg Q 12 hr
Levofloxacin	500 mg loading dose *then* 250 mg IV/PO Q 24 hr	500 mg loading dose *then* 250 mg IV/PO Q 48 hr
Meropenem	1 g Q 12 hr	500 mg Q 24 hr and post HD
Penicillin G	2 MU Q 4–6 hr	1 MU Q 6 hr
Piperacillin/Tazobactam (Zosyn)	3.375 g Q 6 hr or 4.5 g Q 8 hr	2.25 g Q 8 hr
Tobramycin	Gram-negative infections: 2 mg/kg loading dose *then* 1.5 mg/kg Q 24 hr Monitoring of serum levels is recommended; trough <2 mcg/mL	Gram-negative infections: 2 mg/kg loading dose *then* 1 mg/kg post HD Monitoring of serum levels is recommended; trough <2 mcg/mL
TMP-SMX	5–7.5 mg TMP/kg per day divided Q 12–24 hr	2.5–5.0 mg TMP/kg Q 24 hr
Vancomycin	7.5–15 mg/kg Q 24 hr Monitoring of serum levels is recommended; trough 10–15 mg/mL	Loading dose 15–20 mg/kg *then* 500 mg post HD only Monitoring of serum levels is recommended; trough 10–15 mg/mL

(continued)

Table 56-10 University of California San Francisco Medical Center (*Continued*)

Drug	*CRRT*	*HD*
Voriconazole	**ORAL** formulation should be administered when possible, as oral bioavailability 95%. The use of IV should be avoided in patients with CrCl <50 mL/min due to the accumulation of the IV vehicle (cyclodextran) and is contraindicated in ESRD. LD: 400 mg PO Q 12 hr × 2 doses only [40 kg] MD: 200 mg PO Q 12 hr [40 kg]	

[a] Recommended doses are for critically ill patients with serious systemic infection. Lower doses may be used for less serious infections.
STANDARD DOSING for the following:
Amphotericin B, Caspofungin, Ceftriaxone, Clindamycin, Erythromycin, Metronidazole, Nafcillin
Please refer to Table 57-9 for additional information.

growth compared with traditional intermittent dosing. An additional benefit of the use of constant infusions of β-lactams is that smaller daily doses appear to be as effective as higher doses administered intermittently. Other than this latter outcome, it is unclear, however, whether constant infusions have any distinct advantages or disadvantages compared with usual dosing of β-lactams. The efficacy of quinolone antimicrobials appears to correlate with the peak plasma concentration to MIC ratio or area under the curve (AUC) to MIC ratio.[33] In light of this pharmacodynamic principle, it is possible that ciprofloxacin was underdosed in this patient, contributing to the therapeutic failure, particularly if the MIC was in the upper range of susceptibility for this agent.

Aminoglycosides traditionally have been administered every 8 to 12 hours to achieve peak serum gentamicin levels of 5 to 8 g/mL to ensure efficacy in the treatment of serious gram-negative infection.[34,35] Gentamicin troughs of >2 g/mL have been associated with an increased risk for nephrotoxicity.[35,36] These studies attempting to correlate efficacy and toxicity with serum levels and the association of peaks or troughs with clinical outcomes have been questioned.[37] Vancomycin peaks generally have been recommended to be <50 g/mL and troughs 5 to 10 g/mL[38,39]; however, the validity of these recommendations has also been questioned.[40]

Several antimicrobials (e.g., aminoglycosides) have been associated with a pharmacodynamic phenomenon known as a postantibiotic effect (PAE). PAE is delayed regrowth of bacteria following exposure to an antibiotic[41,42] (i.e., continued suppression of normal growth in the absence of antibiotic levels above the MIC of the organism). As an example, if *P. aeruginosa* is cultured in broth, it will multiply to a concentration of 10^9 CFU/mL. If piperacillin is added in a concentration above the MIC for the organism, a reduction in the bacterial concentration is observed. When piperacillin is removed from the broth, immediate bacterial growth takes place. As described, β-lactam antibiotics should be present in concentrations above the MIC to optimize its time-dependent killing. If the above experiment is repeated with gentamicin, a reduction in bacterial CFU is observed. In contrast to that observed with β-lactam antibiotics, if the gentamicin is removed from the system, a lag period of 2 to 6 hours takes place before characteristic bacterial growth occurs. This lag period is defined as the PAE. A PAE also has been observed with quinolones and imipenem against gram-negative organisms. Although most β-lactam antibiotics, such as antipseudomonal penicillins or cephalosporins, do not exhibit PAE with gram-negative organisms, PAE has been demonstrated with gram-positive pathogens such as *S. aureus*.

Once-Daily Dosing of Aminoglycosides

As a result of PAE and other pharmacodynamic factors, certain antimicrobials may be dosed less frequently. The greatest clinical experience has been with the aminoglycosides in the treatment of gram-negative infection.[43,44] Earlier data suggested that the maximal aminoglycoside peak level:MIC ratio correlates well with clinical response. Thus, the higher the achievable peak, the greater likelihood of a favorable outcome. Once-daily dosing of aminoglycosides in the treatment of gram-negative infection is as efficacious as traditional multiple daily dosing.[45]

Single daily dosing of aminoglycosides has been investigated primarily in patients with normal renal function, and few critically ill patients have been treated with this nontraditional regimen. Thus, patients in septic shock are not candidates for once-daily dosing. The utility and proper timing of serum aminoglycoside concentrations and association with clinical outcomes are debatable with nontraditional once-daily aminoglycosides.

In summary, the use of a constant IV infusion of cefotaxime is possible in R.G., but the benefit of this mode of administration is not clear. Considering the severity of R.G.'s infection and his elevated creatinine level, he is not a candidate for single daily dosing of aminoglycosides (i.e., 5–6 mg/kg every 24 hours). Independent of the aminoglycoside-associated PAE, his current renal function requires a reduced gentamicin dose to treat his infection.

Antimicrobial Protein Binding

13. Ceftriaxone (Rocephin), rather than cefotaxime (Claforan), is being considered for the treatment of R.G.'s infection. Ceftriaxone is more highly protein bound than cefotaxime. Why is protein binding important in the selection of therapy?

Free (i.e., unbound) rather than total drug levels are best correlated with antimicrobial activity,[46] and the degree of protein binding may have important clinical consequences in some patients. Chambers et al.[47] reported treatment failures with the highly protein-bound cefonicid (98% protein bound) in patients with endocarditis caused by *S. aureus*. Despite achievable serum drug concentrations well above the MIC of the organism, breakthrough bacteremia occurred in three of four patients. Although total drug concentrations greatly exceeded the MIC of the pathogen, free concentrations were consistently below the level necessary to inhibit bacterial growth. Similar experiences have been reported with teicoplanin (98% protein bound).[48] Thus, clinical cure appears to be more likely if unbound antibiotic concentrations exceed the MIC of the infecting organism. Although ceftriaxone is 85% to 90% protein bound, the free concentrations probably remain far above the MIC of the *Serratia*. Therefore, protein-binding considerations are unlikely to be important in the treatment of R.G.'s infection.

ANTIMICROBIAL FAILURE

Antibiotic-Specific Factors

14. Despite "appropriate" treatment, R.G. is unresponsive to antimicrobial therapy. What antibiotic-specific factors may contribute to "antimicrobial failure"?

Antimicrobials may fail for various reasons, including patient-specific host factors, drug or dosage selection, and concomitant disease states. One of the most common reasons for antimicrobial failure is drug resistance.[49–51] Several clinically important pathogens have been associated with emergence of resistance over the past decade, including *M. tuberculosis,*[52] enterococci,[53] gram-negative rods,[54] *S. aureus,*[55] *S. pneumoniae,*[56] and others. Of particular concern is the isolation of glycopeptide-resistant *S. aureus*[55] and vancomycin-tolerant pneumococci.[57] Considering the common prevalence of these two gram-positive pathogens and the role of vancomycin as the last-line therapy for these organisms, these findings are worrisome. Development of resistance, although less common than initial resistance, may also account for failure to respond to therapy. Cephalosporin-susceptible *E. cloacae* may appear to be susceptible to a cephalosporin; however, β-lactamase production can result in development of resistance to the agent.[58]

Superinfection also may play a role in the unsuccessful treatment of infection. Superinfection is isolation of a new pathogen resistant to the previous antimicrobial regimen. If R.G.'s ceftriaxone-treated *Serratia* pneumonia subsequently worsens and a tracheal aspirate is positive for *P. aeruginosa,* then supercolonization and, perhaps, superinfection has occurred.

Concurrent Therapy

Most infections can be treated with monotherapy (e.g., an *E. coli* wound infection is treatable with a cephalosporin). Some infections, however, require two-drug therapy, including most cases of enterococcal endocarditis and certain *P. aeruginosa* infections. Hilf et al.[59] studied 200 consecutive patients with *P. aeruginosa* bacteremia and demonstrated a 47% mortality in those receiving monotherapy (antipseudomonal β-lactam or aminoglycoside) versus 27% in those in whom two-drug therapy was used. Thus, monotherapy can contribute to antimicrobial failure in certain infections.

In contrast to these findings, most current investigations do not support the use of two drugs over monotherapy in the treatment of serious gram-negative infection.[60–62] An exception to this rule is bacteremia caused by *P. aeruginosa* in neutropenic patients.[62]

If two antimicrobials are used in the treatment of infection, one of three sequelae will result: indifference, synergism, or antagonism.[63] Indifference occurs when the antimicrobial effect of drug A plus that of drug B equals the anticipated sum activity of drug A plus drug B. Although numerous definitions exist, synergism generally occurs when the addition of drug A to drug B results in a total antibiotic activity greater than the expected sum of the two agents. Antagonism occurs if the addition of drug A to drug B results in a combined activity less than the sum of drug A plus drug B. An example of antagonism is the combination of imipenem with a less β-lactamase stable β-lactam, such as piperacillin.[64] Certain organisms, including *P. aeruginosa* and *E. cloacae,* can be induced to produce β-lactamases.[51] If *P. aeruginosa* is exposed to imipenem and piperacillin, the β-lactamase degrades and inactivates piperacillin, and antagonism have resulted. Antagonism is not unique to antibacterials; itraconazole may antagonize amphotericin B in the treatment of certain infections.[65]

Pharmacologic Factors

15. What pharmacologic or pharmaceutic factors may be implicated in failure of therapy?

Subtherapeutic dosing regimens are common, especially for agents with a low therapeutic index, such as the aminoglycosides. For example, a serious gram-negative pneumonitis may not respond to therapy if the achievable peak gentamicin serum levels are only 3 to 4 mcg/mL.[34] Considering that only 20% to 30% of the aminoglycoside penetrates into bronchial secretions, only 0.5 to 1.0 mcg/mL may exist at the site of infection,[66] a level that may be inadequate to treat pneumonia. As another example, the use of an aminoglycoside loading dose is particularly important in patients with renal failure because it may otherwise take several days before a therapeutic level is achieved. Yet another reason for subtherapeutic levels is reduced oral absorption secondary to drug interactions (e.g., ciprofloxacin with antacids or sucralfate).

An emerging problem relates to the use of vancomycin in the treatment of serious methicillin-resistant *S. aureus* infection (MRSA). By CLSI standards, an isolate of MRSA with an MIC of 2 mcg/mL is considered susceptible. Retrospective analyses have, however, demonstrated high failure rate associated with vancomycin in the treatment of MRSA isolates with MIC of 2 mcg/mL.[67,68] Hidayat et al.[67] observed that an MIC of 2 mcg/mL was associated with a greater rate of vancomycin nonresponse. Achievement of therapeutic to supratherapeutic vancomycin trough levels had no influence on efficacy.[67] Similarly, in another retrospective analysis of MRSA bacteremia, investigators noted that a vancomycin MIC of 2 mcg/mL was an independent risk factor for increased mortality.[68] The pharmacodynamic parameter which serves as the best predictor of vancomycin activity against *S. aureus* is the AUC:MIC ratio, with a value >350 independently associated with success. The probability of attaining this value with isolates with an MIC of 2 mcg/mL is 0%, even when achieving vancomycin trough concentrations of 15 mcg/mL.[69]

The infection site also potentially contributes to antimicrobial failure. Most antimicrobials concentrate in the urine, resulting in therapeutic levels even with low doses. In some infections, such as meningitis, prostatitis, and endophthalmitis, antimicrobial penetration to the site of infection may be inadequate. Agents that have been proved to penetrate into these infected sites are required for a favorable outcome.

Another potential reason for antimicrobial failure is inadequate therapy duration. A woman with a first-time uncomplicated cystitis may respond adequately to a 3-day course of an antibiotic. Patients with recurrent urinary tract infections are not candidates for this therapy, however, and failure would be expected with short-course therapy.

Host Factors

16. What host factors may contribute to the failure of antimicrobial therapy?

Several host factors may limit the ability of an antibiotic to cure infection. Infection of prosthetic material (e.g., IV catheters, prosthetic hip replacement, mechanical cardiac valves, and vascular grafts) is difficult to eradicate without removal of the hardware. In most cases, surgical intervention is necessary. To treat R.G.'s IV catheter infection adequately, removal of his central line probably would be required. Similar to removal of prostheses, large undrained abscesses are difficult, if not impossible, to treat with antimicrobial therapy. These infections generally require surgical drainage for successful outcome.

Diabetic foot ulcer cellulitis may not respond adequately to antimicrobial therapy. Reasons for antimicrobial failure in patients with diabetes include poor wound healing as well as significant peripheral vascular disease that reduces the delivery of antibiotics to the infection site.

Immune status, particularly neutropenia or lymphocytopenia, also affects the outcome in the treatment of infection. Profoundly neutropenic patients with disseminated *Aspergillus* infections are unlikely to respond to amphotericin B therapy. Similarly, patients with acquired immunodeficiency syndrome (AIDS) who have low CD4 lymphocyte counts cannot eradicate various infections, including cytomegalovirus, atypical mycobacteria, and cryptococci.

Once these factors have been eliminated as causes for antimicrobial failure, noninfectious sources must be ruled out. As discussed, malignancy, autoimmune disease, drug fever, and other diseases must be evaluated.

17. Other than initiation of adequate antimicrobial therapy, what adjunct measures can be considered in this patient with septic shock?

The 2008 Surviving Sepsis Campaign: International Guidelines for Management of Severe Sepsis and Septic Shock consultants developed key recommendations toward the early goal-directed resuscitation of the septic patient. Key recommended adjuncts include administration of broad-spectrum antibiotics within 1 hour of diagnosis of septic shock, administration of either crystalloid or colloid fluid resuscitation, norepinephrine or dopamine to maintain mean arterial pressure $\geq$65 mmHg. In addition, stress-dose steroid therapy can be given in those patients whose blood pressure is poorly responsive to fluid resuscitation and vasopressors. Recombinant activated protein C (rhAPC) is controversial, but may be considered in those patients at high risk of death as documented by Acute Physiology and Chronic Health Evaluation (APACHE) II scores of $\geq$25 or multiple organ failure; however, those patients with severe sepsis and low risk of death, as measured by APACHE II scores of <25 or one organ failure should not receive rhAPC. Contraindications, including recent major surgery and other bleeding disorders, must also be evaluated before administering rhAPC. Other adjuncts include targeting lower blood glucose levels, stress ulcer prophylaxis, and prevention of DVT in septic patients.[70]

REFERENCES

1. Cranston WI et al. Oral, rectal and esophageal temperatures and some factors affecting them in man. *J Physiol* 1954;126:347.
2. Bone RC et al. Definitions for sepsis and organ failure and guidelines for the use of innovative therapies in sepsis. *Chest* 1992;101:1644.
3. Nystrom P-O. The systemic inflammatory response syndrome: definitions and aetiology. *J Antimicrob Chemother* 1998;41(Suppl A):1.
4. Hotchkiss RS et al. The pathophysiology and treatment of sepsis. *N Engl J Med* 2003;348:138.
5. Kollef MH et al. The acute respiratory distress syndrome. *N Engl J Med* 1995;332:27.
6. Headley AS et al. Infections and the inflammatory response in acute respiratory distress syndrome. *Chest* 1997;111:1306.
7. Forgacs P et al. Characterization of chemical meningitis after neurological surgery. *Clin Infect Dis* 2001;32:179.
8. Hasbun R. The acute aseptic meningitis syndrome. *Current Infectious Diseases Report* 2000;2:345.
9. Vanderschueren S et al. From prolonged febrile illness to fever of unknown origin: the challenge continues. *Arch Intern Med* 2003;163:1033.
10. Mourad O et al. A comprehensive evidence-based approach to fever of unknown origin. *Arch Intern Med* 2003;163:545.
11. Lipsky BA et al. Drug fever. *JAMA* 1981;245:851.
12. Bent S et al. Does this woman have an acute uncomplicated urinary tract infection? *JAMA* 2002;287:2701.
13. Podnos YD et al. Intra-abdominal sepsis in elderly persons. *Clin Infect Dis* 2002;35:62.
14. Benin AL et al. Trends in Legionnaires' disease, 1980–1998: declining mortality and new patterns of diagnosis. *Clin Infect Dis* 2002;35:1039.
15. Mandell LA et al. Infectious Diseases Society of America/American Thoracic Society Consensus Guidelines on the Management of Community-Acquired Pneumonia in Adults. *Clin Infect Dis* 2007;44:S27.
16. Mandell GL et al., eds. *Principles and Practice of Infectious Diseases.* 6th ed. Churchill Livingstone; 2005.
17. Clinical Laboratory Standards Institute (CLSI). Performance standards for antimicrobial susceptibility testing; sixteenth informational supplement. CLSI document M100-S16. Wayne, PA: CLSI; 2006.
18. Hecht DW. Evolution of anaerobe susceptibility testing in the United States. *Clin Infect Dis* 2002;35(Suppl 1):S28.
19. Rex JH et al. Has antifungal susceptibility testing come of age? *Clin Infect Dis* 2002;35:982.
20. Wolfson JS et al. Serum bactericidal activity as a monitor of antibiotic therapy. *N Engl J Med* 1985;312:968.
21. Drusano GL et al. Back to the future: using aminoglycosides again and how to dose them optimally. *Clin Infect Dis* 2007;45:753.
22. Guglielmo BJ et al. Antimicrobial therapy. Cost-benefit considerations. *Drugs* 1989;38:473.
23. Eisenberg JM et al. What is the cost of nephrotoxicity associated with aminoglycosides? *Ann Intern Med* 1987;107:900.
24. Spellberg B et al. The epidemic of antibiotic-resistant infections: a call to action for the medical community from the Infectious Diseases Society of America. *Clin Infect Dis* 2008;46:155.
25. Lutsar I et al. Antibiotic pharmacodynamics in cerebrospinal fluid. *Clin Infect Dis* 1998;27:1117.
26. Papastamelos AG et al. Antibacterial agents in infections of the central nervous system and eye. *Infect Dis Clin North Am* 1995;9:615.
27. Schaeffer AJ et al. Overview summary statement. Diagnosis and management of chronic prostatitis/chronic pelvic pain syndrome (CP/CPPS). *Urology* 2002;60(6 Suppl):1.

28. Cockcroft DW et al. Prediction of creatinine clearance from serum creatinine. *Nephron* 1976;16:31.
29. Mackowiak PA. Influence of fever on pharmacokinetics. *Rev Infect Dis* 1989;11:804.
30. Brook I. Inoculum effect. *Rev Infect Dis* 1989;11:361.
31. Craig WA. Pharmacokinetic/pharmacodynamic parameters: rationale for antibacterial dosing of mice and men. *Clin Infect Dis* 1998;26:1.
32. Roosendaal R et al. Continuous infusion versus intermittent administration of ceftazidime in experimental *Klebsiella pneumoniae* pneumonia in normal and leukopenic rats. *Antimicrob Agents Chemother* 1986;30:403.
33. Preston SL et al. Pharmacodynamics of levofloxacin. A new paradigm for early clinical trials. *JAMA* 1998;279:125.
34. Moore RD et al. Association of aminoglycoside levels with therapeutic outcome in gram-negative pneumonia. *Am J Med* 1984;77:657.
35. Mattie H. Determinants of efficacy and toxicity of aminoglycosides. *J Antimicrob Chemother* 1989;24:281.
36. Matske GR et al. Controlled comparison of gentamicin and tobramycin nephrotoxicity. *Am J Nephrol* 1983;3:11.
37. McCormack JP et al. A critical reevaluation of the "therapeutic range" of aminoglycosides. *Clin Infect Dis* 1992;14:320.
38. Begg EG et al. The therapeutic monitoring of antimicrobial agents. *Br J Clin Pharmacol* 2001;52(Suppl 1):35S.
39. MacGowan AP. Pharmacodynamics, pharmacokinetics, and therapeutic drug monitoring of glycopeptides. *Ther Drug Monit* 1998;20:473.
40. Cantu TG et al. Serum vancomycin concentrations: reappraisal of their clinical value. *Clin Infect Dis* 1994;18:533.
41. MacKenzie FM et al. The post-antibiotic effect. *J Antimicrob Chemother* 1993;32:519.
42. Andes DA et al. Animal model pharmacokinetics and pharmacodynamics: a critical review. *Int J Antimicrob Agents* 2002;19:261.
43. Hatala R et al. Single daily dosing of aminoglycosides in immunocompromised adults: a systematic review. *Clin Infect Dis* 1997;24:810.
44. Ferriols-Lisart R. Effectiveness and safety of once-daily aminoglycosides: a meta-analysis. *Am J Health Syst Pharm* 1996;53:1141.
45. McCormack JP. An emotional-based medicine approach to monitoring once-daily aminoglycosides. *Pharmacol* 2000;20:1524.
46. Lam YWF et al. Effect of protein binding on serum bactericidal activities of ceftazidime and cefoperazone in healthy volunteers. *Antimicrob Agents Chemother* 1988;32:298.
47. Chambers HF et al. Failure of a once-daily regimen of cefonicid for treatment of endocarditis due to *Staphylococcus aureus*. *Rev Infect Dis* 1984;6(Suppl 4):S870.
48. Greenberg RN. Treatment of bone, joint, and vascular-access-associated gram-positive bacterial infections with teicoplanin. *Antimicrob Agents Chemother* 1990;34:2392.
49. McGowan JE Jr. Resistance in nonfermenting gram-negative bacteria: multidrug resistance to the maximum. *Am J Med* 2006;119 (6 Suppl 1):S29.
50. McDonald AC. Trends in antimicrobial resistance in health care-associated pathogens and effect on treatment. *Clin Infect Dis* 2006;42 (Suppl 2):S65.
51. Acar JF et al. Consequences of increasing resistance to antimicrobial agents. *Clin Infect Dis* 1998;27(Suppl 1):S125.
52. Small PM et al. Management of tuberculosis in the United States. *N Engl J Med* 2001;345:189.
53. Harbarth S et al. Effects of antibiotics on nosocomial epidemiology of vancomycin-resistant enterococci. *Antimicrob Agents Chemother* 2002;46:1619.
54. Neuhauser MM et al. Antibiotic resistance among gram-negative bacilli in U.S. intensive care units: implications for fluoroquinolone use. *JAMA* 2003;289:885.
55. Sievert DM et al. Vancomycin-resistant Staphylococcus aureus in the United States, 2002–2006. *Clin Infect Dis* 2008;46:668.
56. Butler JC et al. Pneumococcal drug resistance: the new "special enemy of old age." *Clin Infect Dis* 1999;28:730.
57. Novak R et al. Emergence of vancomycin tolerance in *Streptococcus pneumoniae*. *Nature* 1999;399:590.
58. Chow JW et al. Enterobacter bacteremia: clinical features and emergence of antibiotic resistance during therapy. *Ann Intern Med* 1991;115:585.
59. Hilf M et al. Antibiotic therapy for *Pseudomonas aeruginosa* bacteremia: outcome correlations in a prospective study of 200 patients. *Am J Med* 1989;87:540.
60. Vidal F et al. Epidemiology and outcome of *Pseudomonas aeruginosa* bacteremia, with special emphasis on the influence of antibiotic treatment. *Arch Intern Med* 1996;156:2121.
61. Siegman-Igra Y et al. Pseudomonas aeruginosa bacteremia: an analysis of 123 episodes, with particular emphasis on the effect of antibiotic therapy. *Int J Infect Dis* 1998;2:211.
62. Leibovici L et al. Monotherapy versus β-lactam-aminoglycoside combination treatment for gram-negative bacteremia: a prospective, observational study. *Antimicrob Agents Chemother* 1997;41:1127.
63. Fantin B et al. *In vivo* antibiotic synergism: contribution of animal models. *Antimicrob Agents Chemother* 1992;36:907.
64. Bertram MA et al. Imipenem antagonism of the in vitro activity of piperacillin against *Pseudomonas aeruginosa*. *Antimicrob Agents Chemother* 1984;26:272.
65. Sugar AM et al. Interactions of itraconazole with amphotericin B in the treatment of murine invasive candidiasis. *J Infect Dis* 1998;177:1660.
66. Bergogne-Berezin E. New concepts in the pulmonary disposition of antibiotics. *Pulm Pharmacol* 1995;8:65.
67. Hidayat LK et al. High-dose vancomycin therapy for methicillin-resistant *Staphylococcus aureus* infections: efficacy and toxicity. *Arch Intern Med* 2006;166:2138.
68. Soriano A et al. Influence of vancomycin minimum inhibitory concentration on the treatment of methicillin-resistant *Staphylococcus aureus* bacteremia. *Clin Infect Dis* 2008;46:193.
69. Jeffres MN et al. Predictors of mortality for methicillin-resistant *Staphylococcus aureus* health-care-associated pneumonia: specific evaluation of vancomycin pharmacokinetic indices. *Chest* 2006;130:947.
70. Dellinger RP et al. Surviving sepsis campaign: international guidelines for management of severe sepsis and septic shock. *Crit Care Med* 2008;36:296.

CHAPTER 57

Antimicrobial Prophylaxis for Surgical Procedures

Daniel J. G. Thirion and B. Joseph Guglielmo

Prophylactic antibiotics are widely used in surgical procedures and account for substantial antibiotic use in many hospitals.[1] The purpose of surgical antibiotic prophylaxis is to reduce the prevalence of postoperative wound infection (about 5% of surgical cases overall) at or around the surgical site.[2] Such surgical site infections reportedly increase morbidity and extend the duration of hospitalization by at least 1 week, at an annual cost of up to $10 billion nationwide.[3–7] By preventing surgical site infections, prophylactic antimicrobial agents have the potential to decrease patient morbidity and hospitalization costs for many surgical procedures that pose significant risk of infection (e.g., appendectomy); however, the benefits of prophylaxis are controversial, and prophylaxis is not justified for some surgical procedures (e.g., urologic operations in patients with sterile urine).[8] Consequently, the inappropriate or indiscriminate use of prophylactic antibiotics can increase the risk of drug toxicity, selection of resistant organisms, and costs.

RISK FACTORS FOR INFECTION

The development of postoperative site infection is related to the degree of bacterial contamination during surgery, the virulence of the infecting organism, and host defenses. Risk factors for postoperative site infection can be classified according to operative and environmental factors, and patient characteristics.[9,10]

Bacterial contamination can occur from exogenous sources (e.g., the operative team, instruments, airborne organisms) or from endogenous sources (e.g., the patient's microflora of the skin, respiratory, genitourinary, or gastrointestinal [GI] tract).[9,11] Infection control procedures to minimize all sources of bacterial contamination, including patient and surgical team preparation, operative technique, and incision care, are compiled in Centers for Disease Control and Prevention guidelines for surgical site infection.[9]

The risk of postoperative site infection is affected by host factors such as extremes of age, obesity, cigarette smoking, malnutrition, and comorbid states, including diabetes mellitus, remote infection, ischemia, colonization with microorganisms, and immunosuppressive therapy.[11,12] In addition, the longer the preoperative hospital stay and the surgical procedure, the greater the likelihood of developing a postoperative wound infection, presumably as a result of nosocomial bacterial acquisition in the former and the greater amount of bacterial contamination occurring over time in the latter.[11]

Another major risk factor for infection is the skill of the surgeon. In one study,[13] postoperative wound infection rates were related inversely to the frequency of performing a surgical procedure; thus, hospitals with the highest frequency of surgical procedures have the lowest incidence of postoperative infection.

Based on these risk factors for infection, the decision whether a given patient should receive antimicrobial prophylaxis is multifactorial. Many experts recommend that antimicrobial prophylaxis should be given for surgical procedures (*a*) with a high rate of infection, (*b*) involving the implantation of prosthetic materials, or (*c*) those in which an infection would have catastrophic consequences.[12] A widely used surgical wound classification system to assist in this decision-making process follows.

CLASSIFICATION OF SURGICAL SITE INFECTIONS

From 1960 to 1964, the National Academy of Sciences National Research Council conducted a landmark study of surgical site infections and formulated a widely used standard classification based on the risk of intraoperative bacterial contamination (Table 57-1).[11] Current recommendations for surgical prophylaxis pertain to clean surgeries involving implantation of prosthetic material, clean-contaminated surgeries, and select contaminated wounds. Antimicrobial therapy for most contaminated and all dirty surgeries in which infection already is established is considered treatment instead of prophylaxis and is not discussed further in this chapter. Table 57-2 lists suspected pathogens and recommendations for site-specific prophylactic antimicrobial regimens; a detailed examination of clinical trials supporting these recommendations is presented elsewhere.[8,14]

Table 57-1 National Research Council Wound Classification

Classification	Criteria	Infection Rate (%)
Clean	No acute inflammation or entry into GI, respiratory, GU, or biliary tracts; no break in aseptic technique occurs; wounds primarily closed	<5
Clean-contaminated	Elective, controlled opening of GI, respiratory, biliary, or GU tracts without significant spillage; clean wounds with major break in sterile technique	<10
Contaminated	Penetrating trauma (<4-hr old); major technique break or major spillage from GI tract; acute, nonpurulent inflammation	15–20
Dirty	Penetrating trauma (>4-hr old); purulence or abscess (active infectious process); preoperative perforation of viscera	30–40

GI, gastrointestinal; GU, genitourinary.
From reference 11.

Table 57-2 Suggested Prophylactic Antimicrobial Regimens for Surgical Procedures

Procedure	Predominant Organism(s)	Antibiotic Regimen (Alternative)	Adult Preoperative IV Dose (Alternative)[a]
Clean			
Cardiac (all with sternotomy, cardio-pulmonary bypass)	*Staphylococcus aureus, Staphylococcus epidermidis*	Cefazolin (Vancomycin)	1 g (1 g)
Thoracic	*S. aureus, S. epidermidis,* gram-negative enterics	Cefazolin (Vancomycin)	1 g (1 g)
Vascular (aortic resection, groin incision, prosthesis)	*S. aureus, S. epidermidis,* gram-negative enterics	Cefazolin (Vancomycin)	1 g (1 g)
Orthopedic (total joint replacement, internal fixation of fractures)	*S. aureus, S. epidermidis*	Cefazolin (Vancomycin)	1 g (1 g)
Neurosurgery	*S. aureus, S. epidermidis*	Cefazolin (Vancomycin)	1 g (1 g)
Clean-Contaminated			
Head and neck	*S. aureus,* oral anaerobes, streptococci	Cefazolin (clindamycin-gentamicin)	2 g (600 mg clindamycin-1.5 mg/kg gentamicin)
Gastroduodenal (only for procedures entering stomach)	Gram-negative enterics, *S. aureus,* mouth flora	Cefazolin	1 g
Colorectal	Gram-negative enterics, anaerobes (*Bacteroides fragilis*), enterococci	Oral neomycin-erythromycin base (IV Cefoxitin)	1 g each at 1 PM, 2 PM, and 11 PM day before surgery (1 g)
Appendectomy (uncomplicated)	Gram-negative enterics, anaerobes (*B. fragilis*)	Cefoxitin	1–2 g
Biliary tract (only for high-risk procedures)	Gram-negative enterics, *Enterococcus faecalis, Clostridia*	Cefazolin	1 g
Cesarean section	Group B streptococci, enterococci, anaerobes, gram-negative enterics	Cefazolin	2 g after umbilical cord clamped
Hysterectomy	Group B streptococci, enterococci, anaerobes, gram-negative enterics	Cefazolin or cefoxitin	1 g
Abortion (only for high-risk in first trimester)	Group B streptococci, enterococci, anaerobes, gram-negative enterics	Aqueous penicillin G (doxycycline) (first trimester) Cefazolin (second trimester)	2 million units (100 mg PO before and 200 mg PO after) 1 g
Genitourinary (only for high-risk procedures)	Gram-negative enterics, enterococci	Ciprofloxacin	400 mg

[a]Cefazolin should be dosed at 2 g in patients >80 kg.

PRINCIPLES OF SURGICAL ANTIMICROBIAL PROPHYLAXIS

Decision to Use Antimicrobial Prophylaxis

1. M.R., a 72-year-old woman, is admitted to the hospital with severe abdominal pain, nausea and vomiting, and temperature of 39.3°C. A diagnosis of acute cholecystitis is made, and M.R. is scheduled for biliary tract surgery (cholecystectomy). Why is antimicrobial prophylaxis warranted for M.R.?

Biliary tract surgery is considered a clean-contaminated procedure and, therefore, carries a risk of surgical wound infection approaching 10% (Tables 57-1 and 57-2). Prophylaxis for biliary tract surgery is limited to "high-risk" procedures, which include obesity, age >70 years, diabetes mellitus, acute cholecystitis, obstructive jaundice, or common duct stones.[8,12,15] Thus, prophylaxis is warranted in M.R., who falls into at least two high-risk categories (age >70 years and acute cholecystitis).

2. An order for intravenous (IV) cefazolin 1 g on call to the operating room (OR) is written for M.R. Why is this an appropriate (or inappropriate) antibiotic selection?

The selected prophylactic agent should be directed against likely infecting organisms (Table 57-2), but need not eradicate every potential pathogen. Cefazolin has been proved effective for most surgical procedures, including biliary tract surgery, given that the goal of prophylaxis is to decrease bacterial counts below critical levels necessary to cause infection. Broad-spectrum agents, such as third-generation cephalosporins, should be avoided for prophylaxis because they are no more effective than cefazolin and may alter microbial flora, increasing the emergence of microbial resistance to these otherwise valuable agents.

Timing of Antimicrobial Administration

3. Why is the administration time for this antimicrobial appropriate (or inappropriate) for M.R.?

Classic animal studies conducted by Burke[16] and others[17] clearly demonstrated the need for therapeutic antibiotic concentrations in the bloodstream and in vulnerable tissue at the time of wound contamination. Bacteria were most likely to enter the tissue beginning with the initial surgical incision and continuing until the wound was closed; antibiotics administered >3 hours after bacterial contamination were ineffective in minimizing the development of wound infection.[16,17] This 2- to 3-hour period after the surgical incision was deemed the "effective" or "decisive" period for prophylaxis, when the animal wound was most susceptible to the beneficial effects of the antibiotic. This decisive period for administration of prophylactic antibiotics has been confirmed in humans.[18,19]

For maximal efficacy, an antibiotic should be present in therapeutic concentrations at the incision site as early as possible during the decisive period and continuing until the wound is closed. Because an antibiotic administered postoperatively cannot achieve therapeutic concentrations during the decisive period, such timing of surgical "prophylaxis" is of no benefit in preventing postoperative wound infections, and infection rates are similar to those in patients who receive no antibiotics.[19]

An exception in which postincision administration sometimes is justified is in cesarean sections, because the incidence of endometritis after cesarean section is decreased significantly by postoperative administration of antibiotics.[8]

Based on these study results, prophylactic antibiotics should be administered before the surgical procedure in the OR before the induction of anesthesia.[14] Prophylactic antibiotics are most effective when given during the 1-hour period before the surgical incision is made, and rates of infection increase significantly if antibiotics are administered >1 hour preoperatively or any time postoperatively.[20,21] If a tourniquet is required, then the entire antibiotic dose should be administered before inflation of the tourniquet.

The "on call" prescribing practice for surgical prophylaxis, as with M.R., has fallen into disfavor because the time between antibiotic administration and the actual incision may exceed 1 hour and, therefore, may result in subtherapeutic antibiotic concentrations during the decisive period.[14,22] M.R.'s cefazolin should be ordered preoperatively and should be administered in the OR no earlier than 1 hour before the operative procedure.

4. Will M.R. require a second dose of cefazolin during the surgical procedure?

The duration of the surgical procedure and the half-life of the administered antibiotic should be considered when determining whether an additional dose is necessary to maintain adequate antibiotic concentrations at the operative site. Studies have indicated an inverse relationship between the efficacy of short-acting antibiotics and the duration of the surgical procedure; as operative time increases, so does the incidence of postoperative infection.[23] Cefazolin, with a half-life of ~1.8 hours, is effective in a single preoperative dose for most surgical procedures. For procedures lasting >2 hours, or those with major blood loss, additional intraoperative doses should be administered every one to two times the half-life of the drug during the procedure.[14,23] M.R. should require an additional intraoperative cefazolin dose only if the surgical procedure is prolonged (>3 hours).[23]

Route of Administration

5. G.B., a 55-year-old woman recently diagnosed with carcinoma of the large bowel, is admitted to the hospital for an elective colorectal surgical resection; the surgery is expected to last 5 hours. Physical examination reveals a cachectic woman with a 9-kg weight loss over the previous 3 months (current weight, 60 kg). Increased frequency of bowel movements and chronic fatigue are noted; all other systems are normal. Laboratory data include hemoglobin (Hgb), 10.4 g/dL (normal, 11.5–15.5); hematocrit (Hct), 29.7% (normal, 33%–43%); and prothrombin time (PT), 15 secs (normal, 11–13). Stool guaiac is positive. Vital signs are within normal limits. G.B. is taking no medications and has no history of drug allergies. The following orders are written to begin at home on the day before surgery: (*a*) Clear liquid diet; (*b*) mechanical bowel cleansing with polyethylene glycol-electrolyte lavage solution (CoLYTE, GoLYTELY); and (*c*) neomycin sulfate 1 g and erythromycin 1 g PO at 1 PM, 2 PM, and 11 PM, Comment on the appropriateness of the oral route of administration of antibiotic prophylaxis for G.B.

[SI units: Hgb, 104 g/L; Hct, 0.297]

In general, oral administration of surgical antimicrobial prophylaxis is not recommended because of unreliable or poor absorption of oral agents in the anesthetized bowel. Oral agents, however, function effectively as GI decontaminants because high intraluminal drug concentrations are sufficient to decrease bacterial counts.[24] The concentration of bacteria in the colon may approach 10^{16} bacteria/mm^3 and colorectal procedures, such as the one G.B. will undergo, carry a relatively high risk of postoperative infection. Antimicrobial regimens with activity against the mixture of aerobic and anaerobic bacteria that make up the fecal flora (*Escherichia coli* and other Enterobacteriaceae and *Bacteroides fragilis*) are effective in preventing postoperative wound infections.[25]

The most widely used oral antimicrobial regimen directed against the fecal flora is 1 g each of the nonabsorbable antibiotics neomycin sulfate (for gram-negative aerobes) and erythromycin base (for anaerobes), given 1 day before surgery at the times indicated for G.B.[19,25] Mechanical bowel cleansing, such as with polyethylene glycol-electrolyte or sodium phosphate lavage solution, should precede this regimen; the purpose of such bowel purging is to evacuate the colonic contents as completely as possible to decrease colonic bacterial counts. Effective oral alternatives to neomycin plus erythromycin include metronidazole with or without neomycin or with kanamycin, or kanamycin plus erythromycin[26]; however, clinical situations warranting the use of such alternatives over the well-established neomycin-erythromycin regimen are practically nonexistent. Thus, the regimen selected for G.B. is highly appropriate.

6. The surgical resident has canceled the oral neomycin-erythromycin bowel regimen for G.B. Instead, he orders cefoxitin (Mefoxin) 1 g IV preoperatively. Why is (or is not) this change in therapy an effective and rational choice for G.B.?

Numerous parenteral regimens, specifically with agents that possess both aerobic and anaerobic activity, are effective as surgical prophylaxis in colorectal procedures. The second-generation cephalosporins with significant anaerobic activity (e.g., cefoxitin) are superior to first-generation cephalosporins, which lack sufficient anaerobic activity.[27] At present, it is not clear whether oral antimicrobial prophylaxis is superior to parenteral therapy in preventing infection after colorectal surgery.[28]

Thus, although both IV and oral regimens are effective for prophylaxis before colorectal surgery, the parenteral route of administration, selected because of physician preference, may be less effective.[12] Furthermore, the cefoxitin order for G.B. would be unacceptable if the surgery lasts >3.5 hours (the relatively short half-life of cefoxitin could render G.B. antibiotic-free and predispose her to infection).[29] For prolonged procedures (>3 hours) such as anticipated for G.B., an alternative agent with a longer half-life, such as ertapenem, or a second dose of cefoxitin should be considered. Ertapenem has been found to be superior to cefotetan in preventing infection after colorectal surgery.[30] This improved efficacy may be because of the long half life or more broad antibacterial activity.[31] Whereas ertapenem may offer certain advantages as a prophylactic antibiotic, its use in this indication is discouraged by some clinicians. Although unproved, the potential impact of widespread ertapenem utilization on subsequent carbapenem resistance is of concern. The higher acquisition cost of ertapenem also needs to be considered.[12] Thus, for G.B., the importance and efficacy of established oral prophylactic regimens (plus bowel cleansing) should be stressed to the resident.

7. The surgical resident has reconsidered the cefoxitin order and decided to prescribe both the oral and parenteral prophylactic regimens for G.B. Will the combination significantly reduce the rate of postoperative wound infection compared with either regimen administered singly?

Although the coadministration of both oral and parenteral prophylactic regimens occurs commonly in practice (75% of one survey's respondents),[32] data in support of this practice are conflicting.[26,33] Oral plus parenteral antimicrobial prophylaxis combination is equivalent or superior to either regimen administered alone in reducing infection rates.[26,33,34] As a result, a combination of oral and parenteral antimicrobial prophylaxis is recommended for colorectal surgery.[8,12]

Duration of Administration

8. L.G., a 28-year-old man with a history of rheumatic heart disease, has a 12-year history of a heart murmur consistent with mild mitral stenosis and mitral regurgitation. Over the past 4 months his murmur has become much more prominent. In addition, he has developed severe dyspnea with light physical activity and 3+ pitting edema over both lower legs. Physical examination is notable for coarse rales and an S_3 gallop. For the past 6 weeks he has been maintained on digoxin and diuretics without significant relief of his shortness of breath (SOB). The cardiothoracic surgeon recommends mitral valve replacement and orders the following surgical antibiotic prophylaxis regimen: cefazolin 1 g IV preoperatively, then Q 8 hr for 48 hrs. Why is cefazolin the most appropriate antimicrobial for L.G.? Why was prophylaxis ordered for only 48 hrs?

Although the incidence of postoperative wound infection for cardiothoracic procedures is low (<5%), the devastating consequences of a postoperative endocarditis (following valve replacement) and mediastinitis or sternal osteomyelitis (following sternotomy) warrant careful antimicrobial prophylaxis.[35–46] Organisms of concern for cardiothoracic surgery include *Staphylococcus aureus* and *Staphylococcus epidermidis* (Table 57-2); based on these potential pathogens, successful prophylactic regimens include cefazolin (Ancef), cefamandole (Mandol), and cefuroxime (Zinacef). When cefazolin has been compared with cefuroxime or cefamandole, a statistical trend in favor of the second-generation cephalosporins has been noted, and collective wound infection rates were slightly higher in the cefazolin group.[37–39] In contrast, a comparison of prophylactic cefazolin and cefuroxime in patients having open heart surgery noted a significantly greater incidence of sternal wound infection and mediastinitis in the cefuroxime group.[40] Furthermore, equal efficacy between the two agents was noted in yet another study.[43] In conclusion, cefazolin probably is at least as effective as second-generation cephalosporins; therefore, the choice of agent should be based on an institution's antimicrobial susceptibility and cost data. Hospital-specific antimicrobial resistance patterns are especially important in determining the incidence of methicillin-resistant *S. aureus* (MRSA) or methicillin-resistant

S. epidermidis (MRSE) surgical site infection rates is important, although evidence does not support the use of vancomycin at large in hospitals with high prevalence.[47] Vancomycin is the drug of choice for prophylaxis in patients known to be colonized with such organisms.[14,47]

Meta-analyses of the use of prophylactic antibiotics in cardiac surgery demonstrated no significant differences in the rate of surgical site infection between first- and second-generation cephalosporins and between β-lactams and glycopeptides.[41,46,48] Thus, the cefazolin prophylaxis selected for L.G. is acceptable, provided the patient is not colonized with MRSA or MRSE.

With regard to duration, the shortest effective prophylactic course of antibiotics should be used (i.e., single dose preoperatively or not more than 24 hours postoperatively for most procedures).[45] Postoperative doses after wound closure are usually not required and may increase the risk of resistance. Single-dose prophylaxis, a viable option for many surgical procedures (see Question 9), is controversial for cardiac procedures.[49] In practice, cardiothoracic antimicrobial prophylaxis often is continued 48 hours after surgery,[12] as in L.G. No benefit is seen to prolonging prophylaxis to >48 hours, and such use should be discouraged. The duration of antimicrobial prophylaxis ordered for L.G. is appropriate.

9. G.J., a 27-year-old woman, is admitted to the obstetrics unit at term with her first pregnancy. She is scheduled for a cesarean section because the baby is breech. Cefazolin 1 g IV to be administered after the cord is clamped and Q 8 hr for 24 hrs is ordered. Why is this surgical prophylaxis inappropriate?

As noted previously, the shortest effective duration of prophylaxis is desired. In the past, 5- or 6-day antimicrobial regimens were used for cesarean section, but 24-hour regimens have since been proved as effective as these longer regimens.[50] Faro et al.[50] demonstrated that a single 2-g dose of cefazolin was superior to either a single 1-g dose or to a three-dose, 1-g prophylactic regimen. Others have noted similar results (i.e., a single cefazolin dose administered after the umbilical cord is clamped seems to be sufficient in preventing postoperative wound infections in cesarean section).[51–53] Single-dose prophylaxis is less costly[54] and minimizes the development of bacterial resistance.[55] Thus, G.J. should receive a single 2-g dose of cefazolin after the cord has been clamped, without the three additional doses.

Single-dose prophylaxis also is effective in a variety of GI tract, orthopedic, and gynecologic procedures.[23] A single dose of an antibiotic with a short half-life, however, may provide insufficient antimicrobial coverage during a prolonged surgical procedure, and repeated intraoperative dosing or selection of an agent with a longer half-life is recommended when the duration of surgery is long.[14]

Signs of Surgical Site Infection

10. G.J. is discharged on the fifth hospital day and instructed to observe her incision site carefully for signs of infection. What are the typical signs of site infection? What is the typical time course for signs of site infection to become manifest?

Most surgical site infections involve the incision site and are defined as either *superficial* (involving the skin and subcutaneous fat) or *deep incisional* (involving fascia and muscle). Typically, an infected incision site wound is red, inflamed, and purulent. The purulent drainage should be cultured to identify the causative pathogen and to direct antimicrobial therapy. Empiric therapy directed against the most likely pathogens should be instituted while awaiting culture and sensitivity test results. Although most incision site infections are clinically apparent shortly after surgery (within 30 days), some deep-seated infections present indolently over weeks to months, by which time an abscess may have developed.[11] When implants are involved, infections occurring up to a year after surgery may be related to the operation.[56]

Selection of an Antimicrobial Agent

11. L.T., a 46-year-old woman, has a recent history of abnormal uterine bleeding and vaginal discharge. Endometrial biopsy is positive for squamous cell carcinoma. Invasive disease is not evident. The diagnosis is carcinoma in situ, and a vaginal hysterectomy is scheduled. What would be a good surgical prophylaxis antimicrobial regimen for L.T.?

The selection of a prophylactic regimen should incorporate such factors as the agent's microbiologic activity against the most likely potential pathogens encountered during the surgical procedure (Table 57-2), pharmacokinetic characteristics (e.g., half-life), inherent toxicity, potential to promote the emergence of resistant strains of bacteria, and cost.

The usefulness of antimicrobial prophylaxis in vaginal hysterectomies is well established and is directed against vaginal microflora, including gram-positive and gram-negative aerobes and anaerobes (Table 57-2). The narrowest-spectrum agent that is efficacious is desired, given that the goal of prophylaxis is not to eradicate every potential pathogen, but to reduce bacterial counts below a critical level necessary to cause infection. Cefazolin has been proved to be an effective prophylactic agent for vaginal hysterectomy when compared with broad-spectrum agents such as ceftriaxone (Rocephin).[57] This indicates that a broader-spectrum agent with anaerobic activity (which cefazolin lacks) is unwarranted.

Similar to vaginal hysterectomy, cefazolin and numerous agents have been documented to reduce the incidence of postoperative surgical infection via the abdominal approach.[58,59] As with vaginal hysterectomy, most trials have not documented significant differences between first- and second-generation cephalosporins.[58] In contrast, Hemsell et al.[60] observed a significantly higher incidence of major postoperative surgical infections in patients receiving the first-generation agent cefazolin when compared with cefotetan. Cefazolin exhibits a favorable toxicity profile and has a relatively long half-life (~1.8 hours) such that a single dose has proven prophylactic efficacy.[57] Cefazolin also is considerably less expensive than broader-spectrum agents and is currently recommended by the American College of Obstetricians and Gynecologists.[61] Although it has a broader spectrum of coverage, a single dose of cefoxitin would also be an appropriate choice for this patient.

12. Because cefoxitin has an increased spectrum of activity against the anaerobe *B. fragilis*, it is being considered as an alternative to cefazolin prophylaxis for L.T. Comment on the appropriateness of this proposed change in prophylaxis.

The second- and third-generation cephalosporins and ampicillin-sulbactam generally are not more effective than the first-generation cephalosporins for surgical prophylaxis in vaginal hysterectomy or gastroduodenal, biliary, and clean surgical procedures.[8] One clear exception to these findings is in the prevention of infection after colorectal procedures and perhaps hysterectomy. Several investigations have documented the failure of first-generation agents when used as prophylaxis in colorectal procedures, probably a consequence of their weak anaerobic coverage.[27] As stated previously, second- and third-generation agents and ampicillin-sulbactam generally are no more efficacious than cefazolin and should not be used for surgical prophylaxis in most procedures. Cefoxitin, however, would be a reasonable choice in colorectal surgery or hysterectomy. Considering that this patient is having a hysterectomy, either cefazolin or cefoxitin is appropriate.

13. S.N., a 57-year-old woman with rheumatoid arthritis and degenerative joint disease, has been admitted for total hip arthroplasty. She had an anaphylactic reaction to penicillin in the past. What should be prescribed for S.N. for surgical prophylaxis?

Cefazolin is the preferred prophylactic agent for most clean procedures, including cardiac, vascular, and orthopedic procedures[8] (Table 57-2). Although the risk of cefazolin cross-allergenicity to penicillin is minimal, S.N. experienced a significant penicillin allergy (hives, SOB); therefore, an alternative prophylactic agent definitely is appropriate. The organisms most likely to cause postoperative infection after total hip replacement are *S. aureus* and *S. epidermidis* (Table 57-2). Nafcillin, cefazolin, and vancomycin possess excellent activity against *S. aureus,* however, the β-lactams have only marginal activity against *S. epidermidis.* Regardless, nafcillin clearly must be avoided because of the penicillin allergy. Thus, the preferred agent for S.N. is vancomycin.

Preoperative vancomycin 1 g should be administered IV slowly, over at least 60 minutes. This slow rate of infusion is necessary to reduce the risk of infusion-related hypotension, which poses a particular danger during anesthesia induction and has been reported to cause cardiac arrest.[62]

14. B.K., an 18-year-old woman, complains of severe acute abdominal pain and nausea; the pain is localized to the periumbilical region. B.K. has a temperature of 39.5°C. After initial examination by her pediatrician, she is admitted to the hospital with presumed appendicitis and an exploratory laparotomy is scheduled. What surgical antimicrobial prophylaxis should be ordered for B.K.?

As with colorectal surgery, the most likely infecting organisms in appendectomy are *Bacteroides* species and gram-negative enterics (Table 57-2). On surgical inspection, if the appendix appears normal (uninflamed, without perforation), then antimicrobial prophylaxis is unnecessary.[63] If the appendix is inflamed without perforation, a single preoperative antibiotic dose is necessary. If the appendix is perforated or gangrenous (complicated), infection is already established and postoperative treatment is warranted. The status of the appendix, however, cannot be determined before surgery; therefore, all patients should receive at least one dose of an appropriate antibiotic preoperatively.[64] After surgical inspection of the appendix, the need for postoperative antibiotic therapy can be determined.

Based on the pathogens likely to be encountered, an antimicrobial agent with both aerobic and anaerobic activity is desired for surgical prophylaxis in this situation. Consequently, cefoxitin (Mefoxin), ceftizoxime (Cefizox), or cefotaxime (Claforan) are acceptable choices for prophylaxis.[65]

Risks of Indiscriminate Antimicrobial Use

15. On surgical exploration, B.K. was found to have uncomplicated (nonperforated, nongangrenous) appendicitis; however, cefoxitin therapy was continued for 3 days for unclear reasons. What are the risks of indiscriminate use of antimicrobials for surgical prophylaxis?

The risks of indiscriminate use of antimicrobials to a given patient include the potential for adverse effects and superinfection. The administration of any β-lactam agent poses the risk of a hypersensitivity reaction, and many antibiotics, including cefoxitin, such as in B.K., are known to predispose patients to *Clostridium difficile*-associated disease. The risk of developing this superinfection increases with duration of antibiotic exposure.[66] Avoiding unnecessary initial and prolonged exposure may help reduce the risk to patients of contracting this emerging disease and its associated complications.[67] In addition, widespread or prolonged use of antimicrobial agents increases the potential for the development or selection of resistant organisms in a given patient or other patients who may acquire a pathogen nosocomially.[68]

OPTIMIZING SURGICAL ANTIMICROBIAL PROPHYLAXIS

Antibiotic control strategies have improved the appropriate use of antimicrobial agents for surgical prophylaxis. The implementation of an automatic stop-order policy for surgical prophylaxis has reduced the duration of antimicrobial prophylaxis dramatically. These stop-order policies can be printed directly onto an antibiotic order form.[69] Reviewing the process can help improve antibiotic appropriateness and timing of administration. This was achieved in one study by redesign of the process and education of medical staff by a multidisciplinary quality-improvement team and it resulted in substantial cost avoidance.[70] In a second study, a multidisciplinary team generated electronic quick orders allowing for a computer-enhanced decision-making process and developed an antibiotic administration protocol. Appropriate antibiotics administered increased from 78% to 94%, timely administration improved from 51% to 98%, and clean wound infection rate decreased from 2.7% to 1.4%.[71]

In collaboration with other health care providers, the pharmacy department of health care organizations is responsible for optimizing the timing, choice, and duration of antimicrobial surgical prophylaxis.[72] Education of surgical, anesthesia, and nursing staff, supported by hospital policy changes initiated by pharmacists improved appropriate timing from 68% to 97% and resulted in significant cost avoidance.[72] More recently, a quality improvement approach developed by a national collaborative involving multidisciplinary teams achieved a decrease in the surgical infection rate from 2.3% to 1.7% over a 1-year period.[14,73] Postdischarge surveillance can also help in reducing surgical site infections.[74]

REFERENCES

1. Shapiro M et al. Use of antimicrobial drugs in general hospitals: patterns of prophylaxis. *N Engl J Med* 1979;301:351.
2. Khuri SF et al. The National Veterans Administration Surgical Risk Study: risk adjustment for the comparative assessment of the quality of surgical care. *J Am Coll Surg* 1995;180:519.
3. Coello R et al. Adverse impact of surgical site infections in English hospitals. *J Hosp Infect* 2005;60:93.
4. Wong ES. Surgical Site Infection. In: Mayhall CG, ed. *Hospital Epidemiology and Infection Control.* 2nd ed. Philadelphia: Lippincott; 1999;189.
5. Whitehouse JD et al. The impact of surgical-site infections following orthopedic surgery at a community hospital and a university hospital: adverse quality of life, excess length of stay, and extra cost. *Infect Control Hosp Epidemiol* 2002;23:183.
6. McGarry SA et al. Surgical-site infection due to Staphylococcus aureus among elderly patients: mortality, duration of hospitalization, and cost. *Infect Control Hosp Epidemiol* 2004;25:461.
7. Kirkland KB et al. The impact of surgical-site infections in the 1990s: attributable mortality, excess length of hospitalization, and extra costs. *Infect Control Hosp Epidemiol* 1999;20:725.
8. Anonymous. Antimicrobial prophylaxis for surgery. *Med Lett Drugs Ther* 2006;52:83.
9. Mangram AJ et al. Guideline for prevention of surgical site infection, 1999. Hospital Infection Control Practices Advisory Committee. *Infect Control Hosp Epidemiol* 1999;20:250.
10. Belda FG et al. Supplemental perioperative oxygen and the risk of surgical wound infection: a randomized controlled trial. *JAMA* 2005;294:2035.
11. Ad Hoc Committee of the Committee on Trauma, Division of Medical Sciences. National Academy of Sciences/National Research Council. Postoperative wound infections: the influence of ultraviolet irradiation of the operating room and various other factors. *Ann Surg* 1964;160(Suppl 2):1.
12. American Society of Health-System Pharmacists. ASHP Therapeutic Guidelines on Antimicrobial Prophylaxis in Surgery. *Am J Health Syst Pharm* 1999; 56:1839.
13. Farber BF et al. Relation between surgical volume and incidence of postoperative wound infection. *N Engl J Med* 1981;305:200.
14. Bratzler DW et al. Antimicrobial prophylaxis for surgery: an advisory statement from the National Surgical Infection Prevention Project. *Clin Infect Dis* 2004;38:1706.
15. Dervisoglou A et al. The value of chemoprophylaxis against Enterococcus species in elective cholecystectomy: a randomized study of cefuroxime vs. ampicillin-sulbactam. *Arch Surg* 2006;141: 1162.
16. Burke JF. Effective period of preventive antibiotic action in experimental incisions and dermal lesions. *Surgery* 1961;50:161.
17. Miles AA et al. The value and duration of defence reactions of the skin to the primary lodgement of bacteria. *Br J Exp Pathol* 1957;38:79.
18. van Kasteren ME et al. Antibiotic prophylaxis and the risk of surgical site infections following total hip arthroplasty: timely administration is the most important factor. *Clin Infect Dis* 2007;44:928.
19. Stone HH et al. Antibiotic prophylaxis in gastric, biliary and colonic surgery. *Ann Surg* 1976;184:443.
20. Classen DC et al. The timing of prophylactic administration of antibiotics and the risk of surgical-wound infection. *N Engl J Med* 1992;326:281.
21. Garey KW et al. Timing of vancomycin prophylaxis for cardiac surgery patients and the risk of surgical site infections. *J Antimicrob Chemother* 2006; 58:645.
22. Wong-Beringer A et al. Influence of timing of antibiotic administration on tissue concentrations during surgery. *Am J Surg* 1995;169:379.
23. Scher KS. Studies on the duration of antibiotic administration for surgical prophylaxis. *Am Surg* 1997;63:59.
24. Bartlett JG et al. Veterans Administration Cooperative Study on bowel preparation for elective colorectal operations. *Ann Surg* 1978;188:249.
25. Nichols RL et al. Effect of preoperative neomycin-erythromycin intestinal preparation on the incidence of infectious complications following colon surgery. *Ann Surg* 1973;178:453.
26. Lewis RT. Oral versus systemic antibiotic prophylaxis in elective colon surgery: a randomized study and meta-analysis send a message from the 1990s. *Can J Surg* 2002;45:173.
27. Condon RE et al. Preoperative prophylactic cephalothin fails to control septic complications of colorectal operations: results of a controlled clinical trial. *Am J Surg* 1979;137:68.
28. Song F et al. Antimicrobial prophylaxis in colorectal surgery: a systematic review of randomised controlled trials. *Health Technol Assess* 1998;2(7).
29. Morita S et al. The significance of the intraoperative repeated dosing of antimicrobials for preventing surgical wound infection in colorectal surgery. *Surg Today* 2005;35:732.
30. Itani KM et al. Ertapenem versus cefotetan prophylaxis in elective colorectal surgery. *N Engl J Med* 2006;355:2640.
31. Weigelt JA et al. Abdominal surgical wound infection is lowered with improved perioperative enterococcus and bacteroides therapy. *J Trauma* 1993; 34:579.
32. Zmora O et al. Trends in preparation for colorectal surgery: survey of the members of the American Society of Colon and Rectal Surgeons. *Am Surg* 2003; 69:150.
33. Espin-Basany E et al. Prospective, randomised study on antibiotic prophylaxis in colorectal surgery. Is it really necessary to use oral antibiotics? *Int J Colorectal Dis* 2005;20:542.
34. Shoetz DJ Jr et al. Addition of parenteral cefoxitin to regimen of oral antibiotics for elective colorectal operations. A randomized prospective study. *Ann Surg* 1990;212:209.
35. Ariano RE et al. Antimicrobial prophylaxis in coronary bypass surgery: a critical appraisal. *DICP* 1991;25:478.
36. Gelfand MS et al. Cefamandole versus cefonicid prophylaxis in cardiovascular surgery: a prospective study. *Ann Thorac Surg* 1990;49:435.
37. Slama T et al. Randomized comparison of cefamandole, cefazolin and cefuroxime prophylaxis in open-heart surgery. *Antimicrob Agents Chemother* 1986;29:744.
38. Kaiser A et al. Efficacy of cefazolin, cefamandole, and gentamicin as prophylactic agents in cardiac surgery. *Ann Surg* 1987;206:791.
39. Geroulanos S et al. Antimicrobial prophylaxis in cardiovascular surgery. *Thorac Cardiovasc Surg* 1987;35:199.
40. Doebbeling B et al. Cardiovascular surgery prophylaxis: a randomized, controlled comparison of cefazolin and cefuroxime. *J Thorac Cardiovasc Surg* 1990;99:981.
41. Kreter B et al. Antibiotic prophylaxis for cardiothoracic operations. Meta-analysis of thirty years of clinical trials. *J Thorac Cardiovasc Surg* 1992;104:590.
42. Townsend TR et al. Clinical trial of cefamandole, cefazolin, and cefuroxime for antibiotic prophylaxis in cardiac operations. *J Thorac Cardiovasc Surg* 1993;106:664.
43. Curtis JJ et al. Randomized, prospective comparison of first- and second-generation cephalosporins as infection prophylaxis for cardiac surgery. *Am J Surg* 1993;166:734.
44. Da Costa A et al. Antibiotic prophylaxis for permanent pacemaker implantation. *Circulation* 1998; 97:1796.
45. Bucknell SJ et al. Single-versus multiple-dose antibiotics prophylaxis for cardiac surgery. *Aust N Z J Surg* 2000;70:409.
46. Kriaras I et al. Evolution of antimicrobial prophylaxis in cardiovascular surgery. *Eur J Cardiothorac Surg* 2000;18:440.
47. Finkelstein R et al. Vancomycin versus cefazolin prophylaxis for cardiac surgery in the setting of a high prevalence of methicillin-resistant staphylococcal infections. *J Thorac Cardiovasc Surg* 2002; 123:326.
48. Bolon MK et al. Glycopeptides are no more effective than beta-lactam agents for prevention of surgical site infection after cardiac surgery: a meta-analysis. *Clin Infect Dis* 2004;38:1357.
49. Edwards FH et al. The Society of Thoracic Surgeons Practice Guideline Series: Antibiotic Prophylaxis in Cardiac Surgery, Part I: Duration. *Ann Thorac Surg* 2006;81:397.
50. Faro S et al. Antibiotic prophylaxis: is there a difference? *Am J Obstet Gynecol* 1990;162:900.
51. Jacobi P et al. Single-dose cefazolin prophylaxis for cesarean section. *Am J Obstet Gynecol* 1988; 158:1049.
52. Crombleholme WR. Use of prophylactic antibiotics in obstetrics and gynecology. *Clin Obstet Gynecol* 1988;31:466.
53. Chelmow D et al. Prophylactic use of antibiotics for nonlaboring patients undergoing cesarean delivery with intact membranes: a meta-analysis. *Am J Obstet Gynecol* 2001;184:656.
54. Smith KS et al. Multidisciplinary program for promoting single prophylactic doses of cefazolin in obstetrical and gynecological surgical procedures. *Am J Hosp Pharm* 1988;45:1338.
55. Kaiser AB. Antimicrobial prophylaxis in surgery. *N Engl J Med* 1986;315:1129.
56. Horan TC et al. CDC definitions of nosocomial surgical site infections, 1992: a modification of CDC definitions of surgical wound infections. *Am J Infect Control* 1992;20:271.
57. Hemsell D et al. Ceftriaxone or cefazolin prophylaxis for the prevention of infection after vaginal hysterectomy. *Am J Surg* 1984;148(4A):22.
58. Mittendorf R et al. Avoiding serious infections associated with abdominal hysterectomy: a meta-analysis of antibiotic prophylaxis. *Am J Obstet Gynecol* 1993;169:1119.
59. Kamat AA et al. Wound infection in gynecologic surgery. *Infect Dis Obstet Gynecol* 2000;8:230.
60. Hemsell DL et al. Cefazolin is inferior to cefotetan as single-dose prophylaxis for women undergoing elective total abdominal hysterectomy. *Clin Infect Dis* 1995;20:677.
61. American College of Obstetricians and Gynecologists (ACOG). Antibiotic prophylaxis for gynecologic procedures. *ACOG Practice Bulletin* 2006;108: 225.
62. Dajee H et al. Profound hypotension from rapid vancomycin administration during cardiac operation. *J Thorac Cardiovasc Surg* 1984;87:145.
63. Gorecki WJ et al. Are antibiotics necessary in nonperforated appendicitis in children? A double-blind randomized controlled trial. *Med Sci Monit* 2001; 7:289.
64. Andersen BR et al. Antibiotics versus placebo for prevention of postoperative infection after appendectomy. *Cochrane Database Syst Rev* 2005;3: CD001439.
65. Liberman MA et al. Single-dose cefotetan or cefoxitin versus multiple-dose cefoxitin as prophylaxis in patients undergoing appendectomy for acute nonperforating appendicitis. *J Am Coll Surg* 1995; 180:77.
66. Pepin J et al. Emergence of fluoroquinolones as the predominant risk factor for *Clostridium difficile*-associated diarrhea: a cohort study during an epidemic in Quebec. *Clin Infect Dis* 2005;41:1254.
67. Loo VG et al. A predominantly clonal multi-institutional outbreak of *Clostridium difficile*-associated diarrhea with high morbidity and mortality. *N Engl J Med* 2005;353:2442.
68. Crtistino JM. Correlation between consumption of antimicrobials in humans and development of resistance in bacteria. *Int J Antimicrob Agents* 1999; 12:199.
69. Lipsy RJ et al. Design, implementation, and use of

a new antimicrobial order form: a descriptive report. *Ann Pharmacother* 1993;27:856.
70. Welch L et al. A quality management approach to optimizing delivery and administration of preoperative antibiotics. *Clinical Performance and Quality Health Care* 1998;6:168.
71. Webb ALB et al. Reducing surgical site infections through a multidisciplinary computerized process for preoperative prophylactic antibiotic administration. *Am J Surg* 2006;192:663.
72. Frighetto L et al. Economic impact of standardized orders for antimicrobial prophylaxis program. *Ann Pharmacother* 2000;34:154.
73. Dellinger EP et al. Hospitals collaborate to decrease surgical site infections. *Am J Surg* 2005; 190:9.
74. Brandt C et al. Reduction of surgical site infection rates associated with active surveillance. *Infect Control Hosp Epidemiol Infect Control Hosp Epidemiol* 2006;27:1347.

CHAPTER 58

Central Nervous System Infections

Vicky Dudas

The pharmacotherapy of central nervous system (CNS) infections presents a tremendous challenge to the clinician. CNS infections often are caused by virulent pathogens. These infections occur in an area of the body in which antibiotic penetration often is limited and where host defenses are absent or inadequate. Thus, morbidity and mortality from infections of the CNS remain high despite the availability of highly potent, bactericidal antibiotics. In a review of 493 adult patients treated for bacterial meningitis at the Massachusetts General Hospital between 1962 and 1988, the mortality rates were 25% and 35% for community-acquired and hospital-acquired cases, respectively.[1] The overall case fatality rate of 25% did not change significantly over the 27-year period of the study. Although eradication of bacteria is essential, it is only one of the variables that affect mortality from CNS infections. In an attempt to improve morbidity and mortality statistics, the pathophysiologic mechanisms of CNS infections continue to be further scrutinized.[2–4] In addition, the beneficial effects of corticosteroids in bacterial meningitis continue to be evaluated.[5]

A number of infectious processes can occur within the CNS (e.g., meningitis, encephalitis, meningoencephalitis, brain abscess, subdural empyema, and epidural abscess).[6,7] In addition, prosthetic devices placed into the CNS (e.g., cerebrospinal fluid [CSF] shunts for management of hydrocephalus) often are complicated by infection.[8] Many etiologic agents are capable of inducing CNS infections, including bacteria, viruses, fungi, and certain parasites. This chapter focuses primarily on bacterial infections of the CNS, with an emphasis on the pharmacotherapy of bacterial meningitis and brain abscess. (Also see Chapter 69, Pharmacotherapy of Human Immunodeficiency Virus Infection, and Chapter 70, Opportunistic Infection in HIV-Infected Patients, for presentations pertaining to CNS infections in these populations.)

REVIEW OF CENTRAL NERVOUS SYSTEM

Anatomy and Physiology

Meninges

Proper therapy of CNS infections first requires an understanding of the anatomic and physiologic characteristics of this region. The brain and spinal cord are ensheathed by a protective covering known as the meninges and suspended in CSF, which acts as a "shock absorber" to outside trauma.[9,10] The meninges consist of three layers of fibrous tissue: the *pia mater, arachnoid,* and *dura mater.* The pia mater, the innermost layer of the meninges, is a thin, delicate membrane that closely adheres to the contours of the brain. Separating the pia mater from the more loosely enclosed arachnoid membrane is the subarachnoid space, where the CSF resides. The pia mater and arachnoid, known collectively as the *leptomeninges*, lie interior to the dura mater, a tough outer membrane that adheres to the periosteum and vertebral column.[9,11] *Meningitis* is a term describing inflammation (often the result of infection) of the subarachnoid space, whereas *subdural empyema* refers to a collection of purulent material (pus) in the region separating the dura and arachnoid.[7,9] Abscesses also can form outside the dural space (epidural abscess), often with devastating consequences.[7]

Cerebrospinal Fluid

The CSF is produced and secreted by the choroid plexus in the lateral ventricles and, to a lesser extent, by the choroid plexuses within the third and fourth ventricles.[10,12] The choroid plexus is histologically similar to the renal tubules and removes organic acids (including penicillins) from the CSF via active transport mechanisms. These transport processes can be inhibited by probenecid (Benemid) administration.[12] CSF flows unidirectionally from the lateral ventricles through the foramina of the third and fourth ventricles into the subarachnoid space, then over the cerebral hemispheres and downward into the spinal canal. CSF is absorbed through villous projections (arachnoid villi) into veins, primarily the cerebral venous sinuses.[10,12] About 550 mL/day of CSF is produced, with complete exchange occurring every 3 to 4 hours.[10,12] The flow of CSF is unidirectional from the ventricles to the intralumbar space. Therefore, intrathecal injection of antibiotics results in little, if any, antibiotic reaching the cerebral ventricles.[13,14] This unidirectional flow of CSF presents a problem because ventriculitis commonly occurs in conjunction with bacterial meningitis. Direct intraventricular instillation of antibiotics, usually by means of a reservoir, is preferable in the setting of ventriculitis (see Question 21).[13,14]

In adults, children, and infants the volume of CSF is approximately 150 mL, 60 to 100 mL, and 40 to 60 mL, respectively.[10,12] Knowledge of approximate CSF volume facilitates estimation of the CSF concentration of a drug subsequent to intrathecal administration. For example, administration of gentamicin 5 mg (5,000 mcg) intrathecally should result in a CSF concentration of roughly 33 mcg/mL in an adult shortly after administration.

The composition of CSF differs from other physiologic fluids. The pH of CSF is slightly acidic (normal pH, 7.3) and, with the exception of chloride ion, electrolyte concentrations are slightly less than those in serum.[10,12] Under normal conditions, the protein concentration in CSF is <50 mg/dL, CSF glucose values are approximately 60% those of plasma, and few if any white blood cells (WBC) are present (<5 cells/mm^3).[10,12] When the meninges become inflamed (i.e., in meningitis), the composition of the CSF is altered. In particular, the protein concentration in the CSF increases, and the glucose concentration in the CSF usually declines with meningitis. Therefore, careful evaluation of CSF chemistries is useful when establishing a diagnosis of meningitis.

Blood–Brain Barrier

The blood–brain barrier plays a crucial role in protecting the brain and maintaining homeostasis within the CNS.[10,15,16] Actually, two distinct barriers exist within the brain: the blood–CSF barrier and the blood–brain barrier.[15,16] The blood–CSF barrier is located in the choroid plexus and circumventricular organs (e.g., area postrema) and is characterized morphologically by fenestrated (porous) capillaries (Fig. 58-1).[15] This arrangement allows proteins and other molecules (including antibiotics) to pass freely into the immediate interstitial space. Diffusion of substances into the CSF is restricted by tightly fused ependymal cells lining the ventricular side of the choroid plexus (Fig. 58-1).[15] Cerebral capillary endothelial cells make up the blood–brain barrier, which separates blood from the interstitial fluid of the brain. Unlike capillaries in other areas of the body, the capillary endothelia of the brain are packed closely together, forming tight junctions that in effect produce a barrier physiologically similar to a continuous lipid bilayer.[15]

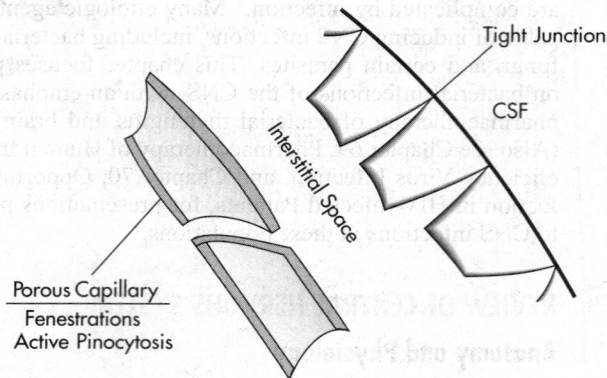

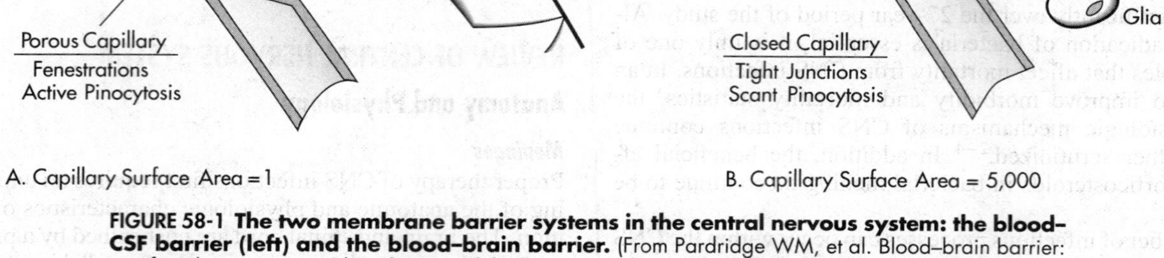

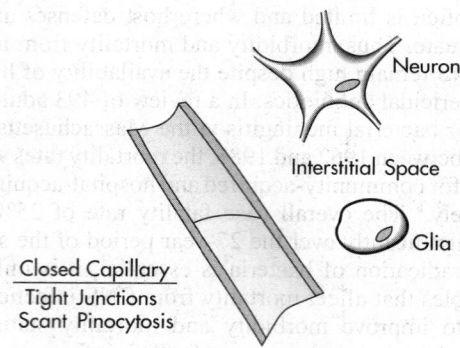

FIGURE 58-1 The two membrane barrier systems in the central nervous system: the blood–CSF barrier (left) and the blood–brain barrier. (From Pardridge WM, et al. Blood–brain barrier: interface between internal medicine and the brain. *Ann Intern Med* 1986;105:82, with permission.)

The surface area of the blood–brain barrier is >5,000 times greater than that of the blood–CSF barrier; thus, the blood–brain barrier plays a more important role in protecting the brain and regulating its chemical composition.[12,15] Many antimicrobials traverse the blood–brain barrier with difficulty, particularly agents having low lipid solubility (see the following discussion).[16]

MENINGITIS

Meningitis is the most common type of CNS infection. The signs and symptoms associated with bacterial meningitis usually are acute in onset, evolving over a few hours.[6] Prompt recognition and early institution of therapy are essential to ensuring beneficial outcomes. In contrast, a diverse group of infectious (e.g., viruses, fungi, and mycobacteria) and noninfectious (e.g., chemical irritants) agents produce a meningitic picture often of a less acute or chronic nature.[17] On occasion, such "aseptic" causes can produce signs and symptoms nearly indistinguishable from those of acute bacterial meningitis.[6,17] Drugs that can induce aseptic meningitis include trimethoprim-sulfamethoxazole (TMP-SMX), the antirejection monoclonal antibody muromonab (OKT3), azathioprine, and nonsteroidal anti-inflammatory drugs (NSAID) such as ibuprofen, naproxen, and sulindac.[18]

Microbiology

The bacterial causes of meningitis correlate well with age and underlying conditions, such as head trauma or recent neurosurgery (Table 58-1).[19–22] Generally, meningitis is a disease of the very young and very old: most cases occur in children <2 years of age and in elderly adults.[19,20]

Neonates (infants <1 months) are at an especially high risk of developing meningitis. Meningitis in neonates most often is caused by group B streptococci (*Streptococcus agalactiae*) or coliform organisms such as *Escherichia coli*.[19,20,23] These highly virulent pathogens usually are acquired during passage through the birth canal or from the hospital environment and are associated with significant morbidity and mortality, particularly in premature infants.[19,20,23] Case fatality rates of >20% and 30% have been reported for meningitis caused by group B streptococci and gram-negative bacilli, respectively.[19] *Listeria monocytogenes* is another important and often overlooked pathogen in neonates.[19,20,24] Because *L. monocytogenes* is resistant to many antimicrobial agents, including third-generation cephalosporins, selection of initial (empiric) therapy in neonates must be approached with this pathogen in mind.[24]

Infants >1 month of age and children <4 years of age are at the highest risk for meningitis. Dramatic changes have occurred in the epidemiology of bacterial meningitis in this age group over the past several years. Historically, in this age group, the disease was caused predominantly by three pathogens: *Haemophilus influenzae, Streptococcus pneumoniae,* and *Neisseria meningitidis*.[19,20] Up to 45% of all cases of meningitis in the United States before 1985 were caused by *H. influenzae* type b (Hib).[20] From 1987 through 1997, however, Hib meningitis cases in children <5 years of age decreased by 97%.[25,26] This reduction in *H. influenzae*-induced meningitis correlates with the widespread vaccination of children against invasive *H. influenzae* disease with the Hib polysaccharide–protein conjugate vaccines. Invasive *H. influenzae* infection now is considered a vaccine-preventable disease in the United States as well as in other countries, highlighting the importance of vaccinating children against Hib invasive disease.[27] Further follow-up from 1998 to 2000 indicates that the incidence of Hib has remained extremely low. One of the national health objectives in *Healthy People 2010* is to reduce the incidence of Hib to zero.[26] In addition, widespread vaccination has caused a shift in the age distribution of bacterial meningitis. Before the Hib vaccine was available, more than two-thirds of cases occurred in children <5 years of age. With the dramatic reduction of Hib cases in this age group, most cases now are observed in adults.[27,28]

In adults and children who have received the conjugated Hib vaccine, community-acquired meningitis most often is caused by *S. pneumoniae* (the pneumococcus) and *N. meningitidis* (the meningococcus).[4,19,20] Meningococci more commonly are implicated in individuals ages 5 to 30 years, whereas pneumococci are the predominant pathogens in adults >30 years of age.[19] In the past several years, meningococcal meningitis has been occurring in clusters within the general population with increased frequency. The observed clusters, defined as two or more cases of the same serogroup that are closer in time or

Table 58-1 Microbiology of Bacterial Meningitis

Age Group or Predisposing Condition	Most Likely Organisms[a]
Neonates (<1 mo)	Group B streptococcus (*Streptococcus agalactiae*), *Escherichia coli,* and other gram-negative bacilli (*Klebsiella, Serratia* species), *Listeria monocytogenes*
Infants and children (2–23 mons)	*Streptococcus pneumoniae, Neisseria meningitidis, S. agalactiae, Haemophilus influenzae*,[b] *E. coli*
Children and adults (2–50 yrs)	*N. meningitidis, S. pneumoniae*
Adults (>50 yr)	*S. pneumoniae, N. meningitidis, L. monocytogenes, E. coli, Klebsiella* species, and other gram-negative bacilli
Postneurosurgical	*Staphylococcus aureus,* gram-negative bacilli (e.g., *E. coli, Klebsiella* * species, *Pseudomonas aeuruginosa*), *Staphylococcus epidermidis*[c]
Closed head trauma	*S. pneumoniae, H. influenzae,* group A β-hemolytic streptococci
Penetrating trauma	*S. aureus, S. epidermidis,* gram-negative bacilli (e.g., *E. coli, Klebsiella* * species, *P. aeuruginosa*)
Presence of risk factor (alcoholism and altered immune status)	*S. pneumoniae, L. monocytogenes, H. influenzae, N. meningitidis*

[a]Organisms listed in descending order of frequency.
[b]Need to consider this pathogen only in children not vaccinated with Hib.
[c]Most commonly seen in association with prosthetic devices (e.g., cerebrospinal fluid shunts).

space than expected, usually occur in secondary schools or university settings.[28]

Traditionally, pneumococci and meningococci have been highly susceptible to penicillin G (minimum inhibitory concentration [MIC] <0.1 mcg/mL). Pneumococcal strains showing intermediate penicillin resistance (MIC 0.1 to 1.0 mcg/mL) and high resistance (MIC ≥2.0 mcg/mL), however, are a problem in many areas of the world, including the United States. Penicillin-resistant pneumococci are of particular concern in relation to meningitis because there is the additional challenge of delivering adequate levels to the site of infection, the CSF.[2,29] Optimal therapy for resistant pneumococci is controversial and is discussed in greater detail in Question 14.

The elderly also are susceptible to developing meningitis, and the infection-related mortality in this population often is higher than in other age groups.[19,20,30] For example, the case-fatality rate for pneumococcal meningitis is 5% in children <5 years of age but 19% to 37% in adults.[20,31] Patients of advanced age are most susceptible to meningitis from pneumococci and meningococci. Enteric gram-negative bacilli (e.g., *E. coli, Klebsiella pneumoniae*) also are occasionally isolated.[19,20,30] Furthermore, *L. monocytogenes* is a problem pathogen in the elderly, especially in immunocompromised patients.[19,20,24,30,32]

Meningitis after neurosurgical procedures or open trauma to the head most often is caused by enteric gram-negative bacilli (predominantly *E. coli* and *K. pneumoniae*) and, to a lesser extent, staphylococci, particularly *Staphylococcus aureus*.[1,21,32] Meningitis that occurs after neurosurgery is occasionally caused by resistant pathogens, such as *Enterobacter* species and *Pseudomonas aeruginosa,* often with devastating consequences.[21,33–35] In addition, patients requiring ventriculostomy or placement of CSF shunts can develop infections of these prosthetic devices by coagulase-negative staphylococci (e.g., *S. epidermidis*) or diphtheroids.[8,21] Closed head trauma, particularly when associated with CSF rhinorrhea or otorrhea, can lead to pneumococcal meningitis or, to a lesser extent, *H. influenzae* meningitis.[21]

Pathogenesis and Pathophysiology

The steps leading to the development of meningitis and the underlying pathophysiologic processes involved have become more clearly understood in the past few years.[2,4] In general, meningitis can develop from *hematogenous* spread of organisms (the most common mechanism), by *contiguous* spread from a parameningeal focus (e.g., sinusitis or otitis media), or by direct bacterial *inoculation,* as occurs with head trauma or neurosurgery.

The list of pathogens causing bacterial meningitis is relatively short because only bacteria possessing certain virulence factors are capable of invading the meninges. Specifically, the presence of a polysaccharide capsule and other cell surface structures (e.g., pili) are necessary for bacteria to evade host defenses and gain entry into the subarachnoid space.[2–4] Once in the CSF, virulence factors contained within the cell wall (e.g., lipopolysaccharide or endotoxin in the case of *H. influenzae*) initiate a complex cascade of events culminating in neurologic damage.[2,3] These cell wall substances trigger the release of various cytokines, which act as mediators of the inflammatory response.[2–4]

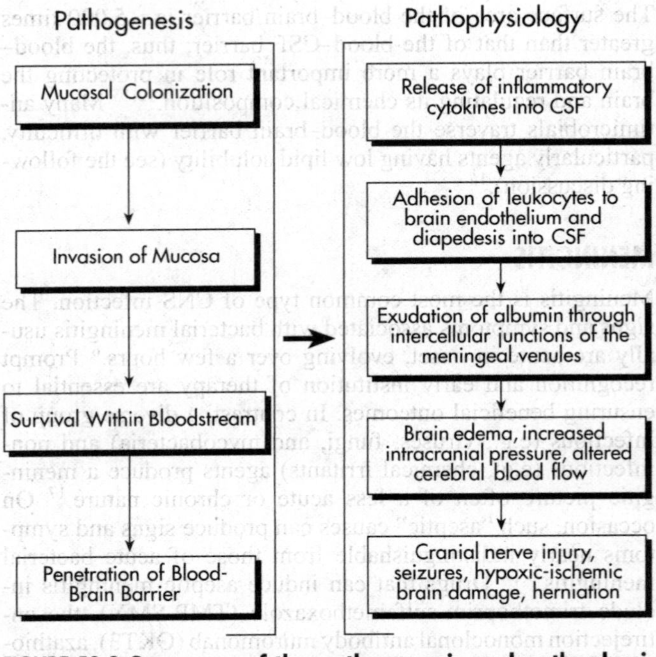

FIGURE 58-2 Summary of the pathogenesis and pathophysiology of bacterial meningitis. (Adapted from Quagliarello VJ, et al. New perspectives on bacterial meningitis. *Clin Infect Dis* 1993;17:603; and Quagliarello VJ, et al. Bacterial meningitis: pathogenesis, pathophysiology, and progress. *N Engl J Med* 1992;327:864, with permission.)

Colonization of mucosal surfaces is a necessary first step in the pathogenesis of meningitis (Fig. 58-2).[3,4] The polysaccharide capsule and pili or fimbriae on the bacterial cell surface allow attachment to oropharyngeal or nasopharyngeal mucosa.[2–4] Secretion of protease enzymes that neutralize the protective activity of mucosal IgA and intrinsic resistance to ciliary clearance mechanisms allow meningeal pathogens to adhere to, and penetrate through, the epithelial surface and enter the intravascular space.[3] The presence of a capsule prevents binding by the alternative complement pathway and prolongs survival within the bloodstream.[3,4] Eventually, organisms multiply to sufficient numbers that allow invasion of the blood–brain barrier. The exact mechanism by which bacteria invade the blood–brain barrier is not well understood. Bacteria, however, probably adhere to cerebral capillary endothelia or perhaps the epithelium of the choroid plexus.[3,4]

Once bacteria gain entry into the CSF, host defenses are inadequate to contain the infection, and bacteria replicate rapidly. Humoral immunity (both complement and immunoglobulin) essentially is absent within the CSF.[2–4] In addition, opsonic activity in CSF is negligible, and although leukocytosis ensues shortly after bacterial invasion, phagocytosis also is inefficient.[3,4] Therefore, this relative immunodeficiency state necessitates the initiation of bactericidal therapy.[2]

Inflammation of the meninges is initiated by contents within the bacterial cell wall.[2–4] Specifically, gram-negative bacteria possess lipopolysaccharide, or endotoxin, and gram-positive bacteria contain teichoic acid in their cell walls. Release of lipopolysaccharide (or teichoic acid) induces the production and secretion of inflammatory cytokines such as interleukin-1 (IL-1), interleukin-6 (IL-6), prostaglandin E_2, and tumor necrosis factor (TNF) from astrocytes, endothelial cells, and circulating monocytes.[3,4] These cytokines play an essential role in promoting the adherence of leukocytes to cerebral capillary endothelial cells, and they also facilitate the migration of leukocytes into the CSF.[2,3] On attachment to brain endothelium, leukocytes release toxic oxygen products that damage endothelial cells. This increases pinocytotic activity, widens tight junctions, and eventually increases blood–brain barrier permeability (Fig. 58-2).[2–4]

Inflammation of the blood–brain barrier allows the influx of albumin and, consequently, vasogenic cerebral edema.[2,3] The brain edema combined with obstruction of CSF outflow increases intracranial pressure and alters cerebral blood flow.[3] Altered cerebral blood flow is a problem because it often is coupled with a loss of cerebrovascular autoregulation. Hyperperfusion or hypoperfusion of the brain secondary to increases or decreases in systemic blood pressure, respectively, ultimately can result in neuronal injury, cerebral ischemia, and irreversible brain damage.[3] The use of adjunctive corticosteroids in certain patient populations can substantially reduce inflammation and the subsequent neurologic sequelae of meningitis.[2,5]

The inflammatory response in meningitis also can be aggravated by some antibiotics, notably the penicillins and cephalosporins.[2,35] When the β-lactam antibiotics lyse bacterial cell walls, large amounts of cell wall products are liberated early in the course of disease, and these contents of bacterial cell walls amplify the inflammatory response.[35] The long-term benefits of β-lactam therapy far outweigh such transient detrimental effects. The use of less rapidly bacteriolytic agents, however, may be theoretically advantageous.[2] The proinflammatory effect of β-lactam antibiotics is attenuated by concomitant corticosteroid therapy.[2,5]

Neurologic sequelae develop in one-third to one-half of patients with bacterial meningitis.[31,36–38] The type and severity of neurologic complications vary with the specific infecting organism, the severity of the infection, and the susceptibility of the host. In children, pneumococcal meningitis carries the highest risk of permanent neurologic sequelae, particularly sensorineural hearing loss.[6,38] In a long-term prospective study of 185 children with acute bacterial meningitis, permanent hearing loss occurred in 6%, 10.5%, and 31% of children with meningitis caused by *H. influenzae, N. meningitidis,* and *S. pneumoniae,* respectively.[38] Although seizures are fairly common on initial presentation, long-term epilepsy occurs in approximately 7% of patients.[36] Other important long-term complications include spastic paraparesis, behavioral disorders, and learning deficits.[36]

Diagnosis and Clinical Features

Clinical and Laboratory Features of Bacterial Meningitis

1. S.C., a 5-year-old boy, is brought to the emergency department (ED) by his mother, who says her son has a temperature of 39°C, is irritable and lethargic, and has a rash. S.C. was in his usual state of good health until last night, when he awoke crying. When she went to investigate, her son began to stiffen up and rock back and forth in his bed. Because he was unarousable, S.C.'s mother rushed him to the hospital. S.C.'s medical history is noncontributory except for an allergy to amoxicillin described as a skin rash. S.C., his mother and father, and his 7-year-old brother recently moved to the United States. S.C.'s vaccination history currently is unknown. S.C. and his brother currently attend a community day care center.

On physical examination, S.C. was in marked distress, with a temperature of 40 °C, blood pressure (BP) of 90/60 mmHg, and a respiratory rate of 32 breaths/minute. His weight on admission was 20 kg. Neurologic examination showed evidence of nuchal rigidity; he was lethargic and difficult to arouse. Brudzinski's and Kernig's signs were positive. On head, eyes, ears, nose, and throat examination, S.C. demonstrated photophobia (he squinted severely when the examiner shined a light in his eyes), but no evidence was noted of papilledema. A petechial rash was visible on his extremities. The remainder of S.C.'s examination was essentially normal.

Blood drawn for laboratory tests revealed sodium (Na), 128 mEq/L (normal, 135–145); potassium (K), 3.2 mEq/L (normal, 3.5–5); chloride (Cl), 100 mEq/L (normal, 95–105); bicarbonate (HCO_3), 25 mEq/L (normal, 22–28); blood urea nitrogen (BUN), 16 mg/dL (normal, 8–18); serum creatinine (SrCr), 0.6 mg/dL (normal, 0.6–1.2); and serum glucose, 80 mg/dL (normal, 70–110). The WBC count was 18,000 cells/mm^3 with 95% polymorphonuclear (PMN) cells (normal, 54%–62%); the hemoglobin (Hgb), hematocrit (Hct), and platelet count all were within normal limits.

What clinical and laboratory features does S.C. display that are suggestive of meningitis?

[SI units: Na, 128 mmol/L; K, 3.2 mmol/L; Cl, 100 mmol/L; 25, mmol/L; BUN, 5.7 mmol/L; SrCr, 53.04 μmol/L; serum glucose, 4.44 mmol/L; WBC count, 18×10^9/L]

S.C.'s presentation contains many features typical of acute bacterial meningitis. For example, the boy was in good health until he awoke at night confused and disoriented. When symptoms present abruptly and evolve quickly over a period of several hours, an acute bacterial process is a strong possibility.[39,40] S.C. has several predisposing factors for the development of meningitis: young age, an unknown vaccination history, and day care exposure.[1,37]

The clinical features of bacterial meningitis are summarized in Table 58-2.[1,6,21,39,40] The most common symptoms include the triad of fever, stiff neck (nuchal rigidity), and altered mental status.[1,6,39] When all three of these features are present, as is S.C.'s case, meningitis should be strongly suspected. Other less common signs and symptoms include headache, photophobia (unusual intolerance to light), and focal neurologic deficits, including cranial nerve palsies.[1,6,39,40] A positive Brudzinski's sign (reflex flexion of the hips and knees produced on flexion

Table 58-2 Signs and Symptoms of Acute Bacterial Meningitis

Fever	Anorexia
Nuchal rigidity (stiff neck)	Headache
Altered mental status	Photophobia
Seizures	Nausea and vomiting
Brudzinski's sign[a]	Focal neurologic deficits
Kernig's sign[a]	Septic shock
Irritability[b]	–

[a] See text for description of sign.
[b] Symptoms seen in infants with meningitis.

of the neck when lying in the recumbent position), and Kernig's sign (pain on extension of the hamstrings when lying supine with the thighs perpendicular to the trunk) provide physical evidence of meningeal irritation.[41] Brudzinski's and Kernig's signs both were positive in S.C. Seizures occur on initial presentation in 15% to 30% of patients and may be focal or generalized.[1,6,36] The presence of seizures or a severely depressed mental status (i.e., obtundation or coma) generally is associated with a poorer prognosis.[1,6,36] Headache, nausea, vomiting, photophobia, and papilledema on eye examination all suggest increased intracranial pressure.[6,39,40] When these symptoms or focal neurologic deficits are present, a computed tomographic (CT) scan is recommended before lumbar puncture to rule out an intracranial mass.[6,39,40] Although controversial, brain herniation can occur when lumbar puncture is performed in such patients because of the pressure changes induced within the cranial vault.[42]

As is clearly evident, S.C. has many of the clinical features associated with acute bacterial meningitis. High fever, stiff neck, altered mentation, photophobia, and positive Kernig's and Brudzinski's signs all are consistent with bacterial meningitis. Furthermore, the low blood pressure (hypotension) and increased respiratory rate are characteristic findings in severe, life-threatening types of bacterial infection (e.g., septic shock, meningitis) and are likely the result of endotoxin release.

The signs and symptoms of meningitis in the very young and very old differ from those in older children and adults.[6,23,30,37] In neonates, signs of meningeal irritation may be absent; fever, irritability, and poor feeding are often the only symptoms manifested.[6,23] Fullness of the fontanel in infants also may reflect the increased intracranial pressure that occurs with meningitis.[6,38] Because S.C. is 5 years of age, accurate assessment of his mental status is challenging. Irritability (crying), as was manifested by S.C., is an important finding that suggests an altered mental status.

In elderly patients, many of the classic signs of meningeal irritation are absent as well, and the disease presentation can be subtler.[6,30,39] Therefore, given the grave consequences of a misdiagnosis, clinicians caring for infants and elderly patients must have a particularly high index of suspicion for meningitis.

Laboratory evaluation of meningitis should include serum chemistries and a hemogram as well as a detailed examination of the CSF.[6,12,39] The peripheral WBC count often is markedly elevated in acute bacterial meningitis, usually with a left shift evident on the differential. This finding, however, is nonspecific and occurs in many acute inflammatory and infectious diseases. S.C. has a marked leukocytosis with a predominance of PMN cells on the differential. A low serum sodium value, which is present in S.C., reflects the syndrome of inappropriate secretion of antidiuretic hormone (SIADH), a frequent complication of acute bacterial meningitis.[4,6] SIADH is an important finding in meningitis because it worsens cerebral edema.[4,6]

The abrupt onset of S.C.'s clinical symptoms is consistent with an acute bacterial process rather than a fungal or viral etiology. Given his age (5 years) and the community-acquired nature of the infection, the most likely pathogens for his meningitis are *H. influenzae, N. meningitidis,* and *S. pneumoniae.* The presence of maculopapular lesions argues for *N. meningitidis* as the causative pathogen because this is a common finding in cases of meningococcemia or meningococcal meningitis.[3] To make an accurate clinical and microbiologic diagnosis in S.C., it is necessary to obtain CSF for analysis. Thus, a lumbar puncture is required as soon as possible.

Cerebrospinal Fluid Examination

2. The resident in the ED performs a lumbar puncture, which yielded the following: opening pressure, 300 mm CSF (normal, <20); CSF glucose, 20 mg/dL (normal, 60% of plasma glucose); protein, 250 mg/dL (normal, <50); WBC count, 1,200 cells/mm^3 (normal, <5), with 90% PMN, 4% monohistiocytes, and 6% lymphocytes. The CSF red blood cell (RBC) count was 50/mm^3. A stat gram's stain of CSF revealed numerous WBC but no organisms. CSF, blood, and urine cultures are pending. What CSF findings in S.C. are consistent with a diagnosis of bacterial meningitis?

[SI units: CSF glucose, 1.1 mmol/L; protein, 2.5 g/L; WBC count, 1,200 × 10^6 cells/L; RBC count, 5 × 10^6/L]

Careful examination of the CSF is essential to confirm the diagnosis of meningitis.[10] Table 58-3 compares the typical findings in CSF obtained from patients with acute bacterial meningitis with those seen with fungal or viral causes.[6,17,39] In acute bacterial meningitis, the CSF is purulent, containing numerous WBC (usually >500 cells/mm^3) with a predominance of PMN, and often is turbid.[12,39] CSF protein nearly always is elevated, usually >100 mg/dL, and the CSF glucose concentration is low, either <50 mg/dL or <50% of a simultaneously obtained serum glucose value.[10,13] In contrast, CSF obtained in viral and fungal cases of meningitis usually is clear and characterized by a much lower WBC count (<100 cells/mm^3), with a mononuclear or lymphocyte predominance.[17,39] Although the CSF protein concentration often is elevated, it may be normal.[17] A variable effect is observed with CSF glucose.[17]

Microbiologic Evaluation

Microbiologic evaluation should include examination of CSF by Gram stain and culture as well as cultures obtained from other potential sites of infection (e.g., blood, sputum, urine).[6,39] Gram stain of the CSF is positive in >50% of acute bacterial meningitis cases and is an extremely useful test to help direct initial (empiric) antimicrobial therapy.[6,10,39] The presence of organisms on smear is indicative of a high bacterial inoculum (i.e., inoculum >10^5 colony-forming units/mL) and is associated with more fulminant disease.[2] The absence of organisms on Gram stain by no means rules out infection but does make selection of empiric therapy more difficult.

S.C. has a negative Gram stain, which may be the result of previous antibiotic therapy or the early detection of disease. Given the negative CSF Gram stain result, S.C. must

Table 58-3 CSF Findings in Various Types of Meningitis

Microbial Etiology	*WBC Count (cells/mm³)*	*Predominant Cell Type*	*Protein*	*Glucose*
Bacterial	>500	PMN	Elevated	—
Fungal	10–500	MN	Elevated	Variable
Viral	10–200	PMN or MN	Variable	Normal

CSF, cerebrospinal fluid; MN, mononuclear cells; PMN, polymorphonuclear neutrophils; WBC, white blood cell.

receive antibacterial therapy sufficiently broad to cover all pathogens associated with meningitis in his age group until the results from his CSF culture are available (usually within 24 to 48 hours). The CSF culture nearly always is positive in purulent meningitis, and the presence of any organism in this normally sterile fluid must always be taken seriously.[6,39,43] In a few instances, particularly when prior antibiotic therapy has been given, CSF cultures are negative in a patient who clearly appears to have meningitis.[10,37,43] In this setting, newer diagnostic tests, such as latex particle agglutination, which reliably detect antigens of *H. influenzae, S. pneumoniae, N. meningitidis, E. coli* (K-1 capsular antigen), and group B streptococci in CSF, are available. Latex particle agglutination should be considered for S.C., especially if his cultures fail to yield any growth. Finally, results from cultures of other sites, such as the blood, urine, and sputum (when appropriate), can yield very useful microbiologic information.[39,43]

The CSF findings in S.C. also strongly support the diagnosis of bacterial meningitis. He has a markedly elevated opening CSF pressure, CSF leukocytosis (with a predominance of PMN), an elevated CSF protein concentration, and a depressed CSF glucose value. A few RBC are present in the CSF, which suggests contamination with peripheral blood caused by the traumatic nature of the lumbar puncture. Precise identification of the offending organism is not possible until CSF culture results are available.

Table 58-4 CSF Penetration Characteristics of Various Antimicrobials

Very Good[a]
Chloramphenicol, metronidazole, TMP-SMX, linezolid
Good[b]
Penicillins: Penicillin G, ampicillin, nafcillin, piperacillin, ticarcillin
Other β-lactams: Aztreonam, clavulanic acid, imipenem, meropenem, sulbactam
Cephalosporins: Cefepime, cefotaxime, cefazidime, ceftizoxime, ceftriaxone, cefuroxime
Fluoroquinolones: Ciprofloxacin
Other agents: Rifampin
Fair to Poor[c]
Aminoglycosides: Amikacin, gentamicin, tobramycin
Other agents: Azithromycin, clarithromycin, clindamycin, erythromycin, vancomycin, daptomycin

[a]Penetrate CSF well regardless of meningeal inflammation.
[b]Adequate CSF penetration achieved when the meninges are inflamed.
[c]Penetration often inadequate even when the meninges are inflamed.
CSF, cerebrospinal fluid; TMP-SMX, trimethoprim-sulfamethoxazole.

Treatment Principles

Prompt institution of appropriate antimicrobial therapy is essential when treating meningitis.[39] Delay in antibiotic administration is associated with increased morbidity and mortality.[44] When choosing antimicrobial therapy, a number of factors must be considered. First, the antibiotics selected must penetrate adequately into the CSF.[13,16,45] In addition, the regimen chosen must have potent activity against known or suspected pathogens and exert a bactericidal effect.[16,42–44]

Antimicrobial Penetration Into the Cerebrospinal Fluid

In cases of purulent meningitis, the amount of bacteria in the CSF often is much higher than the standard inoculum (~10^5 colony-forming units per milliliter) used in routine antimicrobial susceptibility testing.[16,46] As a result, extrapolation of in vitro sensitivity results to clinical efficacy is difficult, particularly for antimicrobials susceptible to an inoculum effect (i.e., an increase in the MIC with an increase in inoculum size). Cefuroxime (Zinacef), for example, is affected by an inoculum effect against *H. influenzae,* and extended-spectrum penicillins (e.g., piperacillin and mezlocillin) are affected similarly by enteric gram-negative bacilli.[16,47] In addition, some antimicrobials (e.g., aminoglycosides, fluoroquinolones) have reduced bactericidal activity in the acidic milieu of purulent CSF.[16,45,48,49] For example, gentamicin has a minimum bactericidal concentration (MBC) of 1 mcg/mL against *E. coli* at a pH of 7.35, and a decrease in the pH to 7.0 results in an eightfold increase in MBC.[49] This may partially explain why aminoglycoside therapy for gram-negative bacillary meningitis is suboptimal, even when direct intrathecal therapy is given.[32,35] The ability of antimicrobials to penetrate into CSF is affected by lipid solubility, degree of ionization, molecular weight, protein binding, and susceptibility to active transport systems operative within the choroid plexus.[13,16,46,50] In general, the penetration of most antibiotics into the CSF is increased when the meninges are inflamed. Although the optimal degree of CSF penetration has not been elucidated entirely, experiments in the rabbit meningitis model indicate that bactericidal effects are maximal when CSF antibiotic concentrations exceed the MBC of the infecting pathogen by 10- to 30-fold.[16,45,51] Antimicrobial penetration into CSF is most commonly reported as a ratio of CSF to serum antimicrobial levels. Table 58-4 summarizes the CSF penetration characteristics of various antimicrobials during acute bacterial meningitis.[13,14,45,51,52] Chloramphenicol, metronidazole, and trimethoprim are highly lipophilic compounds and penetrate into the CSF extremely well, achieving high concentrations even when meningeal inflammation is absent.[13,45,53] Rifampin also has good CSF penetration; because of this, it often is combined with vancomycin to treat coagulase-negative staphylococcal infections in the CNS.[8,45,53] Because β-lactams and aminoglycosides usually are ionized at physiologic pH, they are more polar and do not penetrate into the CSF as well. β-Lactams penetrate poorly when the meninges are intact, but when the meninges are inflamed, most penicillins and the third-generation cephalosporins achieve CSF concentrations sufficient to treat meningitis (~10%–30% of simultaneously obtained serum concentrations).[13,45,50,52,53] An additional factor working against maintenance of therapeutic concentrations of β-lactams in the CSF is the active transport system of the choroid plexus, which pumps these organic acids out of the CSF.[16] Carbapenems, namely meropenem, attain CSF levels that are 10% to 40% of serum levels.[51]

The aminoglycosides have a low therapeutic index, and adequate CSF concentrations are difficult to achieve with intravenous (IV) dosing alone without risking significant toxicity.[14,45] Furthermore, the acidic nature of purulent CSF

Table 58-5 Empiric Therapy for Bacterial Meningitis

Age Group or Predisposing Condition	Recommended Therapy	Alternative Therapy
Neonates (<1 mo)	Ampicillin + cefotaxime	Ampicillin + gentamicin
Infants and children (1–23 mons)	Cefotaxime or ceftriaxone + vancomycin	Vancomycin + rifampin + aztreonam
Older children and adults (2–50 yr)	Cefotaxime or ceftriaxone + vancomycin	Vancomycin + rifampin + aztreonam
Elderly (>50 yr)	Ampicillin, cefotaxime, or ceftriaxone + vancomycin	Vancomycin + TMP-SMX + aztreonam
Postneurosurgical	Vancomycin + ceftazadime	Vancomycin + cefepime or meropenem
Closed head trauma	Cefotaxime or ceftriaxone + vancomycin	Vancomycin + rifampin + aztreonam
Penetrating head trauma	Vancomycin + ceftazadime	Vancomycin + cefepime or meropenem
Presence of risk factor (alcoholism and altered immune status)	Vancomycin + ceftriaxone or cefotaxime + ampicillin	Vancomycin + TMP-SMX + aztreonam

reduces the antimicrobial activity of the aminoglycosides.[49] Thus, when aminoglycoside therapy is initiated for adults with CNS infections, concomitant intrathecal therapy is required.[14,54] Direct instillation of aminoglycosides into the ventricles is preferred, but this approach requires the surgical insertion of a reservoir (e.g., Ommaya reservoir), which often is not possible, particularly in the early stages of bacterial meningitis.[16,45] Thus, at the very least, patients requiring aminoglycosides for meningitis should receive daily intralumbar injections until clinical improvement is seen and CSF cultures are sterilized.[14,16]

The degree of serum protein binding correlates well with the extent of CSF penetration.[16,50] Ceftriaxone is highly bound to serum proteins and, thus, they are more confined to the intravascular space and not as readily available for CSF penetration as cefotaxime and ceftazidime, which are protein bound to a lesser extent. Ceftriaxone achieves sustained, reliable bactericidal activity within the CSF despite its high protein binding.[45,52] Ceftriaxone has been used successfully to treat meningitis in both children and adults for many years.[5,52,55]

Vancomycin and polymyxin B do not diffuse well across the blood–CSF barrier, primarily because of their large molecular size.[13,16,45,53] Therapeutic concentrations in the CSF (up to 22% of serum concentrations) are attained with systemic vancomycin therapy when the meninges are inflamed. In selected circumstances, however, concomitant intralumbar or intraventricular therapy also may be necessary.[8,45] The commonly prescribed antimicrobials, clindamycin and erythromycin, penetrate the CSF poorly,[13,45,53] and they have limited usefulness because of their bacteriostatic mode of action.

Finally, fluoroquinolones, such as ciprofloxacin and ofloxacin, penetrate reasonably well into the CSF on a percentage basis (~20%–30%); however, the concentrations attained are fairly low (≤1 mcg/mL) when standard doses are administered.[45,48] Given the potential neurotoxicity and the limited amount of clinical data, the quinolones have limited use in treating meningitis.

Empiric Therapy for Childhood Meningitis

3. A detailed medication and vaccination history reveals that S.C. and his brother appropriately received vaccination for Hib when they were 2 months of age. What constitutes appropriate empiric therapy for childhood meningitis? Which antibiotic would be appropriate for S.C.? What dose and route of administration should be used?

Because results from culture and sensitivity testing of CSF will not be available for >24 hours, empiric therapy must be instituted promptly to provide coverage of potential pathogens. The initial antimicrobial regimen should take into consideration the patient's age, any predisposing conditions that might make the patient vulnerable to increased morbidity and mortality, results from the CSF Gram stain, history of allergy, and the presence of organ dysfunction. Table 58-5 gives recommendations for empiric antimicrobial therapy for acute bacterial meningitis.[4,6,20,22,39,40,54–56]

S.C. is 5 years of age and has a negative CSF Gram stain. Therefore, therapy with a third-generation cephalosporin, such as ceftriaxone (Rocephin) or cefotaxime (Claforan), is preferred. Either of these two agents will provide excellent coverage of the most likely pathogens in this age group (*S. pneumoniae* and *N. meningitidis*).[19,20,56] Of these two pathogens, S.C.'s rash suggests that *N. meningitidis* is likely.[39] *H. influenzae* is not very likely because he was vaccinated against Hib. Thus, initiation of ceftriaxone would be appropriate for S.C. at this time.

Use of a cephalosporin in this case is appropriate even though S.C. may be allergic to amoxicillin (history of skin rash). Patients with penicillin allergy carry a 5% to 12% risk of cross-reactivity when cephalosporins are prescribed.[57] In this setting, the type of reaction to penicillin is important to consider.[57] Patients with a history of accelerated hypersensitivity reactions (e.g., hives, shortness of breath [SOB], or anaphylaxis) to penicillins should not be given cephalosporins because the risk of cross-reactivity is too high. Conversely, a benign skin rash would not contraindicate use of a cephalosporin. If S.C. had experienced an accelerated reaction to penicillin, vancomycin plus aztreonam would be the best alternative choice (Table 58-5).[4,6,22]

Dosing Considerations

In general, therapy of meningitis requires the use of high dosages of antimicrobials administered by the IV route. Table 58-6 lists the recommended dosing regimens for the treatment of CNS infections.[4,6,8,14,54,56,58]

S.C. should receive ceftriaxone in a dosage of 100 mg/kg/day given in one or two doses.[6,55,56] A ceftriaxone regimen of 1,000 mg IV Q 12 hours is reasonable for S.C. The elimination half-life of ceftriaxone is long (usually 6–8 hours), and once-daily dosing is feasible. Many clinicians, however, prefer to administer ceftriaxone on a twice-daily schedule[4,56] because most published trials used the twice-daily regimen

Table 58-6 Suggested Antibiotic Dosing Regimens for Treatment of Central Nervous System Infections

	Daily Dose[a]			Dosing Interval (hr)	
Antibiotic	Neonates[b]	Children	Adults	Neonates	Children/Adults
Penicillins					
Ampicillin	100–200 mg/kg	200–300 mg/kg	12 g	8–12	4–6
Nafcillin	100–150 mg/kg	150–200 mg/kg	12 g	8–12	4–6
Penicillin G	0.1–0.2 million units/kg	0.15–0.2 million units/kg	20–24 million units	8–12	4–6
Meropenem	20 mg/kg	120 mg/kg	6 g	8–12	8
Cephalosporins					
Cefotaxime	100–150 mg/kg	200–300 mg/kg	12 g	9–12	4–6
Ceftizoxime	100–150 mg/kg	200 mg/kg	12 g	8–12	6–8
Ceftriaxone	NR	100 mg/kg	4 g	—	12–24
Cefazidime	100–150 mg/kg	150–200 mg/kg	8–12 g	8–12	6–8
Cefepime	100 mg/kg	150 mg/kg	6 g	1–2	8
Aminoglycosides					
Gentamicin	5–7.5 mg/kg[d,e]	—	5–6 mg/kg[d,e]	12	8–12
Tobramycin	5–7.5 mg/kg[d,e]	—	5–6 mg/kg[d,e]	12	8–12
Amikacin	15–30 mg/kg[d,e]	—	15–25 mg/kg[d,e]	12	8–12
Chloramphenicol	NR	75–100 mg/kg	4–6 g	—	6
Metronidazole	—	30 mg/kg	1.5–2 g	—	6–8
TMP-SMX	—	12–15 mg/kg[f]	12–15 mg/kg[f]	—	8
Vancomycin	20–30 mg/kg	40–60 mg/kg[g]	2–3 g[g] or 20–30 mg/kg[g]	12	8–12

[a] Recommended daily dose when renal and hepatic functions are normal.
[b] Infants <1 month of age; lower end of dosage range applies to neonates <7 days of age.
[c] Concurrent intraventricular doses of 5–10 mg (gentamicin, tobramycin), or 20 mg (amikacin) often required when treating gram-negative bacillary meningitis.
[d] Dose should be individualized based on serum level monitoring.
[e] Concurrent intraventricular therapy not recommended for neonatal meningitis.
[f] Dose is based on the trimethoprim component.
[g] Concurrent intraventricular doses of 5–20 mg recommended if response to intravenous therapy is inadequate.
NR, not recommended.

and such a schedule reduces the potential for prolonged periods of subtherapeutic CSF concentrations if a dose is delayed or missed.[4] Nevertheless, the U.S. Food and Drug Administration (FDA) has approved the use of the once-daily dosing regimen of ceftriaxone for treatment of pediatric meningitis.[59]

Adjunctive Corticosteroid Therapy

4. What is the rationale for adjunctive corticosteroid therapy in acute bacterial meningitis, and would it be appropriate for S.C.? How should dexamethasone be dosed and monitored for S.C.?

Corticosteroids, particularly dexamethasone, can reduce cerebral edema and lower intracranial pressure.[60] Before 1988, however, studies that evaluated the efficacy of corticosteroids in bacterial meningitis failed to demonstrate any beneficial effects.[61,62] These studies were not designed very well, and importantly, hearing loss was not a routinely monitored complication. Given the recent elucidation of the pathophysiologic mechanisms of meningeal inflammation and the important role of cytokine mediators in this process, attention has been refocused on adjunctive corticosteroid therapy for meningitis.

The rationale for steroid therapy in meningitis stems from the fact that steroids reduce the synthesis and release of the proinflammatory cytokines TNF-α and IL-1β from monocytes and astrocytes.[3–5] These two cytokines play a central role in initiating the cascade of events that lead to neuronal tissue damage and neurologic sequelae. Early use of steroids now has been shown in several studies to reduce neurologic complications, particularly sensorineural hearing loss.[5,63–66]

Despite these studies, controversy remains regarding the efficacy and safety of adjunctive dexamethasone therapy in the treatment of bacterial meningitis. Several prospective placebo-controlled, randomized trials have demonstrated that adjunctive dexamethasone therapy significantly reduces audiologic and neurologic sequelae in children >2 months of age. *H. influenzae*, however, was the causative pathogen in most of these meningitis cases, whereas the number of children with streptococcal and meningococcal meningitis in these trials was small.[5,63–67] As previously mentioned, the number of Hib cases has decreased dramatically in recent years and the rate of resistant streptococci has increased, making the data from these trials difficult to apply to other pathogens. In one small study, 29 of 56 children were randomized to receive dexamethasone for the management of pneumococcal meningitis.[68] Few audiologic and neurologic sequelae were observed in the dexamethasone-treated group compared with the placebo group, but the difference did not reach statistical significance.[68]

Other studies have demonstrated the critical importance of the timing of dexamethasone dosing with respect to antimicrobial therapy. Significant differences in outcome have been observed when dexamethasone was given only before or at the time of administration of the first dose of parenteral antibiotic, as opposed to several hours after antibiotic administration.[5,67]

A meta-analysis by McIntyre et al.[5] was designed to address important issues regarding the concomitant use of dexamethasone, including the value of dexamethasone for organisms other than Hib, the importance of the nature and timing of antibiotic therapy, the effect of dexamethasone on neurologic deficits other than hearing loss, and the frequency of adverse events. Eleven randomized studies published between 1988 through 1996 were eligible for this analysis. One of the most significant findings of this analysis was that the administration of dexamethasone significantly reduced severe hearing loss in Hib meningitis. In pneumococcal meningitis, severe hearing loss was reduced in patients who received dexamethasone early (with or before parenteral antibiotics).[5] Significant variation was seen in hearing loss, depending on the causative pathogen. In patients with meningococcal meningitis, only 1 child of 61 randomized to dexamethasone and none of the 50 controls had severe hearing loss. Although the efficacy of shorter treatment duration has not been extensively studied, similar outcomes were observed with 2 versus 4 days of therapy. Although not statistically significant, a trend was noted toward less gastrointestinal (GI) bleeding in patients who were treated for only 2 days compared with patients who received 4 days of therapy (0.8% vs. 3.0%, respectively).[5]

These studies, taken together, provide convincing evidence for the beneficial effects of adjunctive dexamethasone therapy. The risks associated with short-term steroid therapy are low and are far outweighed by the benefit of a reduction in neurologic complications. Therefore, children with bacterial meningitis should receive concomitant dexamethasone therapy.[2,4,63]

Thus, S.C. should receive dexamethasone therapy, 0.15 mg/kg/dose given IV Q 6 hours for 2 to 4 days. For S.C., who is 20 kg, this would be 3 mg Q 6 h, with the first dexamethasone dose given 15 minutes before initiating ceftriaxone therapy.

The benefit of corticosteroid therapy in adults has recently been studied in a prospective, randomized, double-blind multicenter trial.[69] A total of 301 patients with acute bacterial meningitis were randomized to receive dexamethasone or placebo 15 to 20 minutes before or with the first dose of antibiotic every 6 hours for 4 days. Dexamethasone reduced the risk of unfavorable outcome, defined as a Glasgow Coma Scale score of 1 to 4 at 8 weeks (relative risk, 0.59; $P = 0.03$), and of death (relative risk, 0.48; $P = 0.04$). Among the patients with pneumococcal meningitis, 26% in the dexamethasone group and 52% in the placebo group had unfavorable outcomes (relative risk, 0.5; $P = 0.06$). Although this was not statistically significant, patients with pneumococcal meningitis appeared to receive the most benefit from steroids. Neither GI bleeding nor other adverse effects were increased in the dexamethasone group.

In addition, in a recent Cochrane review of this topic,[70] treatment with corticosteroids was associated with reduced mortality and neurologic sequelae in adults. Regardless of the pathogen or clinical severity of illness, dexamethasone should be continued for 4 days in patients with bacterial meningitis.[31,70,71] For such patients, the risk of neurologic complications is much greater than the potential for adverse drug effects. In some adults, such as those with septic shock and adrenal insufficiency with suspected meningitis, adjunctive dexamethasone may be harmful, however.[31] The data evaluating patients with septic shock and meningitis are lacking, therefore, dexamethasone cannot be recommended. Although the use of low doses of hydrocortisone 50 mg every 6 hours or fludrocortisone 50 mcg daily seems reasonable.[31]

Potential adverse effects associated with dexamethasone include GI bleeding, mental status changes (e.g., euphoria or encephalopathy), increases in blood glucose, and possibly elevations in blood pressure.[5,60–65] For S.C., the complete blood count (CBC), serum chemistries, and stool guaiac should be monitored daily while he is receiving dexamethasone. He also should be questioned about possible GI upset and assessed for changes in mental status (e.g., confusion, combativeness). Given the short duration of corticosteroid therapy, dexamethasone can be discontinued abruptly without tapering after 2 days.

Effect on Central Nervous System Penetration of Antibiotics

Another important issue to consider is whether dexamethasone, a potent anti-inflammatory agent, reduces the ability of some antimicrobials (e.g., the β-lactams) to penetrate across the blood–brain barrier into CSF. Because CSF penetration of the penicillins, cephalosporins, and other β-lactams is greatest when the meninges are inflamed, a hypothetical concern is that concomitant dexamethasone may reduce CSF concentrations of these agents, resulting in reduced efficacy. Data to support or refute this hypothesis are limited. In animal models of pneumococcal meningitis, vancomycin penetration into the CSF was reduced in dexamethasone-treated animals compared with animals not treated with steroids.[72–74] Unlike vancomycin, ceftriaxone penetration was not reduced in these animal models. Decreased bactericidal activity, however, was reported with cephalosporin- and penicillin-resistant *S. pneumoniae* isolates. Furthermore, only the combination of ceftriaxone and rifampin sterilized the CSF when dexamethasone was given in cases of highly resistant strains of *S. pneumoniae.*[73] In another cephalosporin-resistant pneumococcal meningitis animal model, dexamethasone did not decrease ceftriaxone levels in the CSF, but concomitant use of dexamethasone resulted in a higher number of failures owing to decreased bacterial killing and bactericidal effect.[75] Although McIntyre et al. did not directly measure antibiotic concentrations in the CSF, they did not observe any significant differences in CSF bactericidal activity (a test in which CSF is serially diluted and tested for activity against the infecting pathogen) in steroid-treated versus placebo-treated children.[5] Furthermore, children given dexamethasone had similar, if not better, clinical responses (e.g., shorter duration of fever) than placebo controls,[5] and the rate of CSF sterilization did not differ.[5,63,65] A recent study evaluated vancomycin levels in CSF in 14 adult patients receiving adjunctive corticosteroids to treat pneumococcal meningitis.[76] Vancomycin was administered by continuous infusion at 60 mg/kg/day. In this small observational study, vancomycin concentrations in the CSF were therapeutic even in the setting of dexamthasone.[76] Therefore, based on current evidence, vancomycin penetration into CSF does not appear to be reduced by dexamethasone administration in children, but decreased penetration of vancomycin is observed in adults.[67,72,73] In a rabbit meningitis model, the coadministration of dexamethasone and vancomycin resulted in 29% less penetration of vancomycin into the CSF. By increasing the daily dose of vancomycin in these rabbits, therapeutic CSF levels were achieved, however, suggesting that giving larger daily doses of vancomycin circumvents the steroid effect on CNS penetration.[77] Currently, it is unknown whether the decreased penetration of antibiotics secondary to dexamethasone administration is of clinical significance, especially in this era of penicillin- and cephalosporin-resistant pneumococcal isolates.[51,67] In adults receiving concomitant dexamethasone, experts suggest using the combination of ceftriaxone, vancomycin, and rifampin.[46,67]

Neisseria meningitidis Meningitis

Definitive Therapy

5. Twenty-four hours after admission, S.C.'s culture results from his blood and CSF samples are available. The CSF culture is growing * *N. meningitidis* (penicillin MIC 0.06), also present in both of the two collected blood cultures. What modification in S.C.'s antimicrobial therapy is necessary at this time?

Once culture and sensitivity results become available, definitive therapy can be instituted, often with a single agent (Table 58-7).[4,6,33–35,56] As suspected, S.C.'s CSF culture is positive for *N. meningitidis*. Cefuroxime, a second-generation cephalosporin, also has activity against *N. meningitidis*. However, cefuroxime is less effective for meningitis than third-generation cephalosporins.[78,79] In a prospective, randomized trial involving 106 children with acute bacterial meningitis, 12% of the patients receiving cefuroxime had positive CSF cultures after 18 to 24 hours versus 2% of those who received ceftriaxone ($p = 0.11$), and 17% of cefuroxime-treated patients developed moderate to severe hearing loss compared with only 4% of those receiving ceftriaxone ($p = 0.05$).[78] Nearly identical findings to these also were noted in a retrospective analysis of four comparative trials of children treated with cefuroxime (159 patients) and ceftriaxone (174 patients) for bacterial meningitis.[79] The reason for the inferiority of cefuroxime relative to ceftriaxone most likely is related to reduced potency and the presence of an inoculum effect (described earlier).[47]

Because *N. meningitidis* is susceptible to penicillin and ampicillin currently, penicillin is the drug of choice. However, S.C.'s questionable history of amoxicillin rash makes the use of penicillin worrisome, and therapy previously begun with ceftriaxone should be continued.

Monitoring Therapy

6. What subjective and objective data should be monitored to evaluate the efficacy and toxicity of treatment of patients with meningitis, and what specifically should be monitored in S.C.?

Monitoring of patients with meningitis is similar in many respects to monitoring patients with other infectious diseases. Clinical signs and symptoms attributable to the disease, such as fever, altered mental status, and stiff neck, need to be checked

Table 58-7 Definitive Therapy for Bacterial Meningitis

Pathogen	Recommended Treatment	Alternative Agents
Haemophilus influenzae		
β-Lactamase-negative	Ampicillin	Cefotaxime or ceftriaxone
β-Lactamase-positive	Cefotaxime or ceftriaxone	Chloramphenicol
Neisseria meningitidis	Penicillin G or ampicillin	Cefotaxime or ceftriaxone or chloramphenicol
Streptococcus pneumoniae	*Penicillin-sensitive*[a] Penicillin G or ampicillin	
	Intermediately penicillin-resistant[a]: Vancomycin + cefotaxime or ceftriaxone[e]	Cefotaxime or ceftriaxone or chloramphenicol
	Highly penicillin-resistant[a]: Vancomycin + cefotaxime or ceftriaxone[d] ± rifampin	Cefotaxime or ceftriaxone and rifampin
Streptococcus agalactiae	Penicillin G or ampicillin + gentamicin	Cefotaxime or ceftriaxone and rifampin
Listeria monocytogenes	Ampicillin ± gentamicin	TMP-SMX
Enterobacteriaceae		
Escherichia coli, Klebsiella species	Cefotaxime or ceftriaxone	Cefepime + gentamicin[b]
Enterobacter, Serratia species	TMP-SMX	Cefepime + gentamicin,[b] or ciprofloxacin,[c] or meropenem, cefepime[c]
Pseudomonas aeruginosa	Ceftazidime + tobramycin[b]	Cefepime + tobramycin, or ciprofloxacin,[c] meropenem
Staphylococcus aureus		
Methicillin-susceptible (MSSA)	Nafcillin or oxacillin	Vancomycin[b]
Methicillin-resistant (MRSA)	Vancomycin[c] ± rifampin	TMP-SMX[c] ± rifampin
Staphylococcus epidermidis	Vancomycin[b] ± rifampin	TMP-SMX[c] ± rifampin

[a] Penicillin-sensitive strains defined as having MIC ≤0.1 mcg/mL; intermediately resistant strains MIC >0.1–1.0 mcg/mL; highly resistant strains MIC ≥2.0 mcg/mL.
[b] Concomitant intrathecal therapy often required for optimal response.
[c] Limited experience or efficacy data for the agent against with this pathogen.
[d] Check cefotaxime or ceftriaxone if MIC ≤0.5; then susceptible in CSF isolates.
MIC, minimum inhibitory concentration; TMP-SMX, trimethoprim-sulfamethoxazole.

periodically throughout the day and monitored for resolution. S.C.'s temperature and mental status should be assessed at least four times a day. Accurate assessment of S.C.'s mental status can be difficult because of his young age. Thus, his baseline level of mental status should be evaluated (e.g., whether he is awake and alert, or lethargic and difficult to arouse). If awake and alert, S.C. should be observed for irritability, because this often is the only sign of altered mentation. Questions can be used to assess his orientation: Does he know where he is? Does he know his name? Can he recognize his mother or other family members? In general, signs of clinical improvement should be evident within 24 to 48 hours for most uncomplicated cases of acute bacterial meningitis,[5,6,39,78] and the corticosteroid therapy that S.C. is receiving may accelerate the clinical response.[5,64]

Laboratory tests should be monitored as well. A CBC with differential, serum electrolytes (e.g., Na, K, Cl, HCO_3), blood glucose, and renal function tests (e.g., BUN, SrCr) should be performed daily. Abnormal electrolyte results may require more frequent monitoring. Laboratory abnormalities, such as leukocytosis and hyponatremia, may take longer to normalize than clinical symptoms. If S.C. develops severe SIADH, as manifested by serum sodium values up to 120 mEq/L with altered mental status or seizures, fluid restriction and short-term (i.e., 6–12 hours) IV administration of 3% sodium chloride may be necessary.

Cerebrospinal fluid chemistries usually normalize after several days, although CSF protein may remain elevated for a week or more.[6,39] With effective therapy, the CSF culture usually is sterile after about 18 to 24 hours of therapy.[5,64,78] Delays in CSF sterilization are associated with a higher propensity for neurologic complications.[4,35] If S.C. responds to therapy in a straightforward manner, he need not have a repeat lumbar puncture. If the response is inadequate, as evidenced by persistent fever or deteriorating mental status, S.C. will require a repeat lumbar puncture to re-examine the CSF parameters.[6,39]

In addition to monitoring the therapeutic response, side effects of the antimicrobial regimen also need to be assessed frequently. Meningitis requires high-dose therapy, making the likelihood of adverse effects much greater. Currently, S.C. is being treated with ceftriaxone, a cephalosporin antibiotic. The adverse effects most often associated with ceftriaxone include hypersensitivity reactions, mild pain and phlebitis at the injection site, and GI complaints.[80] S.C. should be observed for the formation of an antibiotic-related skin rash or evidence of an accelerated allergic reaction (e.g., hives, wheezing). The IV catheter site should be observed daily for redness, tenderness, or pain on palpation of the vein. S.C. should be watched closely for loose stools or diarrhea. Although diarrhea is a common side effect of most antimicrobials, this adverse effect is more likely to occur with ceftriaxone because approximately 40% to 50% of the dose is excreted unchanged into the bile. Mild diarrhea, which usually does not require discontinuation of therapy, occurs in 23% to 41% of children receiving ceftriaxone for meningitis therapy.[55,78] Less common but of concern is the potential for antibiotic-associated colitis.[80,81] If S.C. experiences diarrhea that is persistent, accompanied by fever and abdominal cramping, a stool sample should be tested for *Clostridium difficile* toxin. If positive, oral antibiotic therapy, preferably with metronidazole, should correct the problem (see Chapter 62, Infectious Diarrhea).

Ceftriaxone-Induced Biliary Pseudolithiasis

7. After 5 days of treatment, the nurse caring for S.C. notes that his appetite is markedly diminished, and he complains of an upset stomach. S.C. was afebrile and alert and oriented, but abdominal examination revealed "guarding," with pain localized in the right upper quadrant area. Laboratory data at this time are WBC count, 6,000 cells/mm^3 (normal, 3,200–9,800); Hgb, 12.5 g/dL (normal, 14–19); Hct, 34% (normal, 39%–49%); platelets, 120,000/mm^3 (normal, 130,000 to 400,000); Na, 135 mEq/L; K, 3.6 mEq/L; Cl, 98 mEq/L; aspartate aminotransferase (AST), 35 U/L (normal, 0–35); alanine aminotransferase (ALT), 33 U/L (normal, 0–3.5); alkaline phosphatase, 110 MU/dL (normal, 30–120); total bilirubin, 1.2 mg/dL (normal, 0.1–1.0); and amylase 70 U/L. A stool guaiac is negative. What are possible causes of S.C.'s abdominal discomfort?

[SI units: WBC count, 6 × 10^9 cells/L; Hgb, 125 g/L; Hct, 0.34; platelets, 120 × 10^9/L; Na, 135 mmol/L; K, 3.6 mmol/L; Cl, 98 mmol/L; AST, 33 U/L; ALT, 33 U/L; alkaline phosphatase, 110 U/L; total bilirubin, 20.5 μmol/L; amylase, 70 U/L]

A number of possible causes exist for S.C.'s abdominal discomfort. His corticosteroid therapy may have caused acute GI bleeding. This is unlikely because the dexamethasone was discontinued 3 days ago and S.C.'s hemoglobin and hematocrit values are in the low-normal range. The negative stool guaiac result also argues strongly against a GI bleed. Acute pancreatitis is unlikely given the normal amylase result. Viral or drug-induced hepatitis is another possibility but also is unlikely given his normal AST, ALT, and bilirubin results. An intra-abdominal infection also is possible, but this is improbable because he is afebrile and has a normal WBC count. Other causes, such as acute cholecystitis or appendicitis, require further diagnostic evaluation.

8. An abdominal ultrasound reveals sludge in the gallbladder. What is the significance of this finding in S.C., and how should this abnormality be managed?

The abnormality on S.C.'s abdominal ultrasound explains his right upper quadrant pain. S.C. has what appears to be a condition known as biliary pseudolithiasis (i.e., biliary "sludging"). Biliary sludging can occur in conditions of gallbladder hypomotility (e.g., recent surgery, burns, total parenteral nutrition) and, in some instances, can be drug induced. S.C. has been receiving ceftriaxone for treatment of his meningitis, and this drug can cause biliary pseudolithiasis.[82–85]

Antibiotic-associated biliary pseudolithiasis is seen almost exclusively with ceftriaxone.[80] The predominance of biliary excretion that occurs with ceftriaxone results in very high concentrations of the drug in gallbladder bile.[82] In selected circumstances, the biliary concentration of ceftriaxone may exceed solubility limits, resulting in formation of a fine, granular precipitate (i.e., sludge),[82] which differs in composition and ultrasound features from true gallstones.[78,83] The precipitate is composed of a ceftriaxone–calcium complex, the formation of which is dose dependent.[82,84] Given the high dosages required for meningitis therapy, it is not surprising that this adverse effect has occurred in S.C.[78,83] In the comparative randomized trial between ceftriaxone and cefuroxime cited previously, evidence of biliary pseudolithiasis on abdominal ultrasonography was observed in 16 of 35 (46%) patients who received ceftriaxone and in none of 35 patients receiving cefuroxime.[78] Pseudolithiasis usually appears 3 to 10 days following the start of therapy and, in most instances, it is clinically asymptomatic. Symptoms similar to acute cholecystitis are evident in some individuals and include nausea with or without vomiting and abdominal right upper quadrant pain. Although he has not vomited yet, S.C.'s symptoms fit this description. Approximately 10% to 20% of patients with evidence of biliary sludging on ultrasound are symptomatic.[83,85]

Prompt recognition of this adverse effect and discontinuation of ceftriaxone therapy are required to effectively manage biliary pseudolithiasis. Before this complication was recognized, a few patients underwent cholecystectomies, but this intervention is rarely necessary because the condition nearly always is reversible. Once S.C.'s ceftriaxone is discontinued, the condition should resolve gradually over a period of weeks to months; the clinical symptoms should disappear within a few days.[83,85] Cefotaxime can be substituted for ceftriaxone; cefotaxime is not associated with biliary complications, and the efficacy of these two agents is equivalent.[64,80] For S.C., the cefotaxime dosage would be 1,000 mg IV every 6 hours (Table 58-6).

Duration of Therapy

9. What is the recommended duration of antimicrobial therapy for *N. meningitidis* meningitis, and for how long should S.C. be treated?

The optimal duration of therapy for meningitis is difficult to ascertain because few trials have been designed to address this issue.[86] Although general guidelines exist, the decision to discontinue therapy should be individualized based on the response to therapy, the presence of complicating factors (e.g., immunosuppression), and the specific causative pathogen. Table 58-8 lists the recommended treatment durations for uncomplicated cases of bacterial meningitis according to the specific pathogen.[6,22,56,58,86] Patients such as S.C. with meningitis caused by *N. meningitidis* should be treated for 7 days.[22,79] Complicated cases, such as those with delayed CSF sterilization, require therapy for longer periods (up to 2 weeks or more).

S.C. had been responding well to the ceftriaxone therapy, and if he continues to respond well to the cefotaxime regimen outlined previously, there is no need for additional oral antibiotics when he is discharged from the hospital. An oral second- or third-generation cephalosporin cannot be recommended in the treatment of meningitis because insufficient concentrations are achieved in the CSF. S.C. should be watched carefully for a possible relapse (e.g., the reappearance of signs and symptoms of meningitis), which would require readmission to the hospital for further evaluation and IV antibiotic therapy.

Table 58-8 Duration of Therapy for Bacterial Meningitis

Etiology	*Duration of Therapy (0 days)*
Haemophilus influenzae	7
N. meningitidis	7
Streptococcus pneumoniae	10–14
Group B streptococci (*Streptococcus agalactiae*)	14–21
Listeria monocytogenes	14–21
Gram-negative bacilli	21

Prevention of Neisseria meningitidis Meningitis

10. S.C. is ready to be discharged home. How can the potential spread of meningococcal disease be prevented in persons with whom S.C. has contact?

CHEMOPROPHYLAXIS OF CLOSE CONTACTS

Despite an excellent response to therapy, S.C. still may harbor *N. meningitidis* in his nasopharynx and could transmit this organism to individuals with whom he has close contact.[88,89] Therefore, chemoprophylaxis to reduce nasopharyngeal carriage of *N. meningitidis* is indicated for S.C. and his close contacts.[87,89] In this context, close contacts are defined as individuals who frequently sleep and eat in the same dwelling with an index case: a household member, day care center contacts, and any person directly exposed to the patient's oral secretions (e.g., boyfriend or girlfriend, mouth-to-mouth resuscitation, or endotracheal intubation).[87,89] The potential for a close contact to become infected with *N. meningitidis* is 500 to 800 times greater than for the total population.[87] S.C.'s 7-year-old brother, who is at risk for invasive *N. meningitidis* disease, should receive chemoprophylaxis. Also, the children at the day care center or close contacts at the hospital who have been caring for S.C. may benefit from chemoprophylaxis. Because the risk of secondary disease is greatest within 2 to 5 days after exposure to the index case, chemoprophylaxis should be instituted as soon as possible and ideally within 24 hours.[87] Administering chemoprophylaxis 14 days or more after identification of the index case is probably of little value. The most frequently used regimen to reduce nasopharyngeal carriage of *N. meningitidis* for children >1 month is rifampin, given once daily in a dosage of 10 mg/kg/day for 2 days.[87,89] A suspension containing 10 mg/mL of rifampin (which requires extemporaneous compounding) is available; 20 mL will provide a 200-mg dose. The index patient should also receive prophylaxis if he or she was treated with penicillin or chloramphenicol as soon as he or she is able to tolerate oral medications. Because S.C. is receiving ceftriaxone, he does not need chemoprophylaxis. For adult close contacts, rifampin 600 mg twice a day for 2 days should be administered. Thus, S.C.'s brother, parents, and day care contacts should be treated with appropriate doses of rifampin as soon as he is diagnosed. Alternative chemoprophylactic regimens shown to be effective for reducing nasopharyngeal carriage of *N. meningitidis* are ceftriaxone 250 mg or 125 mg intramuscularly in adults and children, respectively, and ciprofloxacin 500 mg orally as a single dose in adults. Because rifampin is not recommended for pregnant women, ceftriaxone would be a viable alternative.[87,89]

Prevention of Haemophilus influenzae Type b Meningitis

HIB VACCINATION RECOMMENDATIONS

11. S.C. and his brother were vaccinated for Hib. Are these vaccinations now routinely recommended?

Yes. S.C. appropriately received one of the Hib protein conjugate vaccines when he was 2 months of age.[91] Given the tremendous success that conjugated Hib vaccines have had on

Table 58-9 Recommended Vaccination Schedule for *Haemophilus influenzae* Protein Conjugated Vaccines

	Schedule				
Vaccine (Trade Name)	*2 Months*	*4 Months*	*6 Months*	*12 Months*	*15 Months*
HbOC (HibTITER)	Dose 1	Dose 2	Dose 3	—	Booster
PRP-T (ActHIB)	Dose 1	Dose 2	Dose 3	—	Booster
PRP-OMP (PedvaxHIB)	Dose 1	Dose 2	—	Booster	

reducing the incidence of Hib meningitis in the United States, all children >2 months of age should receive the vaccination series with one of the three commercially available products.[91] HbOC (HibTITER) is a product that links polyribosylribitol phosphate (PRP), the antigen derived from Hib purified capsular polysaccharide, with a carrier protein (CRM_{197}) derived from a mutated variant of the diphtheria toxin protein, whereas PRP-OMP (PedvaxHIB) links PRP with the outer membrane complex protein of *N. meningitidis*.[87,90] The third product, PRP-T (ActHIB), is a PRP–tetanus toxoid conjugate. The linkage of PRP with a carrier protein is necessary to elicit an adequate immune response in children <15 months of age.[87,91] HbOC and PRP-OMP have been licensed since 1988 and 1989, respectively. In 1990, both products received FDA approval for use in infants 2 months of age or older. PRP-T was approved for use in infants 2 months of age or older by the FDA in early 1993. All three of these conjugate vaccines are equally effective.[25,26,90,91] Table 58-9 outlines the vaccination schedule for HbOC, PRP-OMP, and PRP-T as recommended by the Centers for Disease Control and Prevention Advisory Committee on Immunization Practices.[90] In general, the vaccines are well tolerated; fever, redness, and swelling at the injection site are the most common adverse effects and occur in <4% of patients.[26,89,91]

Neisseria meningitidis VACCINATION RECOMMENDATIONS

12. A 21-year-old college student who lives in a dormitory dies of *N. meningitidis* meningitis. Two additional cases are diagnosed in students living in the same dormitory. Should all individuals living in the dormitory be vaccinated? What are the current recommendations for the use of meningococcal vaccine?

Neisseria meningitidis is responsible for causing both outbreaks (clusters of cases) as well as epidemics. Currently, two meningococcal vaccines are available in the United States. MPSV4 or Menomune, a quadrivalent (Men A,C,Y,W-135) polysaccharide vaccine, has been available for over 25 years and is approved for all age groups. Meningococcal conjugate vaccine (MCV4 or Menactra) was approved in January 2005 for use in persons 11 to 55 years of age. Unlike MPSV4, the new vaccine elicits a more durable initial antibody response and it will also reduce nasopharyngeal carriage. Meningococci serogroups A, B, and C are responsible for causing >90% of cases. After vaccination, protective levels of antibody are usually achieved within 7 to 10 days. Neither vaccine has activity against meningococci serogroup B.[87–89]

With the advantages of the second vaccine, the Advisory Committee on Immunization Practices (ACIP) of the CDC extensively revised its recommendations for use of meningococcal vaccines. ACIP recommends routine vaccination of young adolescents (age 11 to 12 years) with MCV4.[89] If persons have not received the vaccine before entering high school, ACIP recommends vaccination before high-school entry. By 2008, all adolescents, beginning at the age of 11 years, will have routine vaccination with MCV4. In addition, routine vaccination with meningococcal vaccine is recommended for college freshman living in dormitories and for other populations at increased risk (i.e., military recruits, travelers to areas in which menigococcal disease is hyperendemic or epidemic, microbiologists who are routinely exposed to meningococcal isolates, patients with anatomic or functional asplenia and patients with terminal complement deficiency).[88,89] Therefore, all students living in the dormitory should be vaccinated. Other college students may elect to receive vaccination as well.

Streptococcus pneumoniae Meningitis

Clinical Features, Predisposing Factors, and Diagnosis

13. A.L., a 58-year-old man with a long history of alcohol abuse, is admitted to the ED febrile and unresponsive. Over the past several days, A.L. has experienced intermittent episodes of fever, chills, SOB, and a worsening productive cough. A friend visiting A.L. called 911 when he could not arouse him. A.L.'s medical records indicate that he has hypertension, adult-onset diabetes mellitus, peptic ulcer disease (PUD), and chronic obstructive airways disease (COAD). A splenectomy was performed 10 years ago after trauma to the abdomen. A.L. is divorced and lives alone in a low-income apartment. He has no known drug allergies. His records show him to be a smoker for >30 years. Current medications include hydrochlorothiazide 50 mg QOD, sustained-release theophylline (Theo-Dur) 300 mg PO TID, glipizide 5 mg PO BID, famotidine 20 mg PO HS, and ciprofloxacin 250 mg PO BID PRN for cough and increased sputum production.

On admission to the ED, A.L. had a temperature of 40°C, BP of 90/50 mmHg, and pulse and respiratory rates of 115 beats/minute and 25 breaths/min, respectively. His weight is 59 kg. A.L. was unresponsive but withdrew all extremities to painful stimuli. His pupils were equal and sluggishly reactive to light; papilledema and evidence of meningismus were present. Wheezes and crackles were heard throughout both lung fields, with dense consolidation noted in the left lower lobe. The remainder of his physical examination was noncontributory.

Stat laboratory tests revealed a WBC count of 18,000 cells/mm^3 (normal, 3,200–9,800), with 80% PMN, 15% bands, 3% lymphocytes, and 2% basophils; Hgb and Hct of 10.5 g/dL (normal, 14–18) and 34% (normal, 39–49%), respectively; and a platelet count of 250,000/mm^3 (normal, 130,000–400,000). Serum chemistries were significant for K, 3.0 mEq/L (normal, 3.5–5.0); glucose, 250 mg/dL (normal, 70–110); AST and ALT, 190 mg/dL (normal, 0–35) and 140 mg/dL (normal, 0–3.5), respectively; BUN,

35 mg/dL (normal, 8–18); and SrCr, 2.4 mg/dL (normal, 0.6–1.2). The prothrombin time was high-normal, and albumin was 3.1 mg/dL (normal, 4–6). A stat blood alcohol level of 100 mg/dL was reported, and a urine toxicology screen was negative. A.L.'s serum theophylline concentration was 18 mg/dL. Stool guaiac was positive.

A CT scan showed no evidence of mass lesions or cerebral hematoma. Lumbar puncture yielded CSF opening pressure, 200 mmHg (normal, <20); protein, 120 mg/dL (normal, <50); glucose, 100 mg/dL (normal, 60% of plasma glucose); WBC count, 8,500 cells/mm^3 (normal, <5 cells/mm^3), 92% PMN, 4% monohistiocytes, and 4% lymphocytes; and RBC count, 400/mm^3. Gram-positive, lancet-shaped diplococci were visible on CSF Gram stain. In addition, a sputum Gram stain revealed numerous WBC, few epithelial cells, and numerous gram-positive cocci in pairs and in short chains. Blood, CSF, urine, and sputum cultures are pending.

What are the clinical and laboratory features of pneumococcal meningitis? What features of pneumococcal meningitis are present in A.L.?

[SI units: WBC count, 18 × 10^9 cells/L with 0.8 PMN, 0.15 bands, 0.03 lymphocytes, and 0.02 basophils; Hgb, 105 g/L; platelets, 250 × 10^9/L; K, 3.0 mmol/L; glucose, 13.9 mmol/L; BUN, 12.5 mmol/L urea; SrCr, 212 mmol/L; glucose, 5.5 mmol/L; WBC count, 8,500 × 10^6 cells/L; RBC count, 400 × 10^6/L]

A.L. presents to the ED with many signs and symptoms suggestive of pneumococcal meningitis. He is 56 years of age, and *S. pneumoniae* is the most common bacterial etiology for meningitis in adults >30 years of age (Table 58-1).[19,20] As is evidenced by A.L.'s presentation, invasive pneumococcal disease often is associated with significant morbidity, and mortality rates remain high.[20] Over the past several years, the incidence of *S. pneumoniae* meningitis in the United States has consistently ranged between 1.2 and 2.8 cases per 100,000 population per year.[19,20,25] Predisposing factors to invasive pneumococcal disease include advanced age, alcoholism, chronic pulmonary disease, and sickle cell disease.[6,39,87] In addition, individuals infected with the human immunodeficiency virus (HIV), those with Hodgkin's disease, and patients who have undergone kidney, liver, or bone marrow transplantation also appear to be at higher risk.[6,88,92,93] Patients with CSF otorrhea or rhinorrhea induced by closed head trauma or neurosurgical procedures are more susceptible to develop pneumococcal meningitis as well.[20,87,93]

A.L. has many predisposing factors for pneumococcal meningitis. He has a low socioeconomic status, smokes, has a long history of alcohol abuse, has had a splenectomy, and has diabetes and COAD. Underlying COAD is an important predisposing factor in that chronic colonization with pneumococci occurs in such patients. Intermittent use of ciprofloxacin by A.L. for acute exacerbations of COAD is unjustified. The poor activity of this antibiotic against *S. pneumoniae* is likely to select out this organism for infection. Furthermore, ciprofloxacin can increase serum theophylline concentrations by inhibiting its metabolism, another important reason why this agent is not a good therapeutic choice for productive cough in A.L.[94]

A diagnosis of pneumococcal meningitis in A.L. is supported by the high fever, stiff neck (meningismus), and altered mental status. He is unresponsive, which is a definite negative prognostic factor.[1,6] Results from CSF chemistries and microbiologic analysis are highly suggestive of pneumococcal meningitis. A.L. has an elevated opening CSF pressure and a markedly elevated CSF protein and WBC count with a predominance of neutrophils on differential examination. The normal CSF glucose level (100 g/dL) is misleading because A.L. is diabetic. The calculated ratio of CSF-to-serum glucose for A.L. is <50%, which is consistent with acute bacterial meningitis (Table 58-3). The presence of gram-positive, lancet-shaped diplococci in pairs on the CSF Gram stain strongly supports the diagnosis of pneumococcal disease. The signs and symptoms of pneumococcal pneumonia (cough, SOB, increased sputum production, and pulmonary consolidation) as well as the sputum Gram stain result also lend support to a diagnosis of invasive pneumococcal infection.

Empiric Therapy in Adults

14. What empiric therapy is appropriate for A.L. at this time?

Resistance among pneumococci to penicillin G has become an important concern worldwide and in the United States.[2,29,96] For this reason, susceptibility testing should be performed on all pneumococcal isolates obtained from sterile sites (e.g., blood, CSF).[2,95] For treatment of meningitis caused by strains intermediately resistant to penicillin, ceftriaxone and cefotaxime are the most useful agents because many of these isolates retain cephalosporin sensitivity.[2,8,95] Management of invasive pneumococcal infections in sites other than CSF (e.g., lungs, bloodstream) usually can be accomplished by increasing the dose of penicillin G to 20 to 24 million units/day. This approach is not possible with meningitis caused by intermediately resistant strains because further increases in the penicillin dose are likely to produce unacceptable neurotoxicity. Vancomycin and chloramphenicol are potential options, but relapses and clinical failures have been reported with both of these agents when given alone.[95,96,97] Many penicillin-resistant pneumococcal isolates also are resistant to chloramphenicol (defined as an MIC >4 mcg/mL), and even against susceptible isolates, chloramphenicol may fail to elicit a bactericidal effect.[2] Third-generation cephalosporins cannot be relied on for treatment of meningitis caused by strains fully resistant to penicillin (MIC ≥2.0 mcg/mL) because reduced cephalosporin sensitivity often occurs (MIC range from 2–8 mcg/mL to both cefotaxime and ceftriaxone). *S. pneumoniae* strains in CSF with MIC >0.5 mcg/mL to cefotaxime or ceftriaxone are considered resistant.[98] Reduced activity of ceftriaxone and cefotaxime against penicillin-resistant pneumococci affects the therapeutic ratio achieved in CSF and is the likely explanation for reports of clinical failure.[95] Optimal therapy for fully penicillin-resistant pneumococcal meningitis is unclear. Vancomycin alone in high dosage (3–4 g/day in adults) has been suggested.[2,95,96] The combination of vancomycin and ceftriaxone was superior to either agent given alone in a rabbit model of penicillin-resistant pneumococcal meningitis.[99] Ceftriaxone or vancomycin combined with rifampin also may be superior to either drug given alone.[95,96] Animal data suggest that the use of rifampin reduces early mortality in pneumococcal meningitis by reducing the release of proinflammatory bacterial cell components.[100] Thus, until more information is available, the combination of ceftriaxone or cefotaxime with vancomycin represents the most reasonable approach to empiric therapy for potential penicillin-resistant pneumococcal meningitis.

Until culture and susceptibility results are available, the recommended antibiotic in this situation is ceftriaxone 2 g given IV Q 12 h and vancomycin 500 mg given IV Q 12 h. A.L. weighs 59 kg, and because his renal function is not normal (SrCr, 2.4 mg/dL; creatinine clearance, 30 mL/minute), a dosage adjustment was made. (See Question 23 for vancomycin dosing in CNS infections.)

Corticosteroid Therapy for Adult Meningitis

15. Should A.L. receive corticosteroid therapy in addition to his antibiotic therapy?

The issue of adjunctive corticosteroid therapy for A.L. needs to be addressed. As previously stated, the efficacy of dexamethasone in adults with meningitis has recently been studied.[69] Clearly, A.L. presents with profoundly altered mental status, and his signs and symptoms are consistent with a fulminant course of disease. Given that he is unarousable, hypotensive, and tachycardic, A.L. likely will be admitted to the intensive care unit. Thus, his age, underlying medical problems, likely streptococcal meningitis, and deteriorating clinical status all point to a poor prognosis and argue for the use of adjunctive dexamethasone. On the other hand, A.L. is diabetic and has an elevated glucose concentration. He also has PUD, which may be active given that he is anemic and has a positive stool guaiac result. High-dose dexamethasone therapy may cloud A.L.'s sensorium, making mental status assessment even more difficult. Although each of these issues is a concern, none appears to be so critical as to preclude the use of corticosteroids.[69] Therefore, dexamethasone given in a dosage of 10 mg IV Q 6 h could be instituted before starting ceftriaxone therapy and continued for up to 4 days, provided that the diagnosis of bacterial meningitis is confirmed. If corticosteroids are administered, the addition of rifampin to ceftriaxone is recommended.[46] To control blood glucose, a sliding-scale dosing schedule of regular insulin is recommended. A.L.'s PUD should be properly worked up and treated if necessary.

Treatment of Penicillin-Susceptible Pneumococcal Meningitis

16. Results from A.L.'s CSF, blood, and sputum cultures are available and are positive for *S. pneumoniae* at each site. Sensitivity testing in CSF revealed an MIC of 0.06 mcg/mL to penicillin, 0.25 mcg/mL to cefotaxime and ceftriaxone, 0.25 mcg/mL to vancomycin, and 8 mcg/mL to chloramphenicol. What therapy is indicated for A.L.?

A.L. has become infected with a strain of *S. pneumoniae* that is susceptible to penicillin G (Table 58-5).[4,6,39] The dosage usually is 20 to 24 million units/day in adults with normal renal function (Table 58-6). A.L. has renal impairment, however, which means he should receive a reduced penicillin dosage. One of the most useful methods for calculating the dose of penicillin G when renal function is compromised is the following equation[101]:

$$\text{Dose (in million units/days)} = (\text{Calculated creatinine clearance}/7) + 3.2$$

This equation should be used only when the calculated creatinine clearance is <40 mL/minute.[101] For A.L., who has a calculated creatinine clearance of 30 mL/minute (according to the method of Cockcroft and Gault), the daily dose would be approximately 8 million units, or 2 million units Q 6 hours. This revised regimen should provide penicillin serum concentrations similar to those achieved with high-dose therapy when kidney function is normal. Failure to adjust the dosage appropriately is equivalent to providing massive doses of penicillin, which may result in hyperkalemia (if the potassium-containing preparation is used), seizures, and encephalopathy.[101]

In patients unable to tolerate penicillin G, the best alternatives are ceftriaxone or cefotaxime (Table 58-5).[4,6] First-generation cephalosporins (e.g., cefazolin) have good activity against pneumococci, but their limited CSF penetration makes these agents poor choices for therapy.[45,52] Conversely, the third-generation agent, ceftazidime, penetrates well into CSF, but its usefulness is limited by reduced activity against pneumococci in comparison to other third-generation agents.[50,52] Cefuroxime also has good pneumococcal activity but, as previously mentioned, is inferior to ceftriaxone and cefotaxime.[78] Vancomycin has more limited and variable CSF penetration.[45,102] Therefore, vancomycin should be reserved for situations in which there is bacterial resistance or penicillin intolerance. TMP-SMX has excellent CSF penetration characteristics but is not active against many strains of *S. pneumoniae.* Limited experience exists with this product for the treatment of pneumococcal meningitis, however.[45,103]

Prevention of Meningitis

17. Should A.L. have received pneumococcal vaccine? How effective is vaccination in preventing invasive pneumococcal disease?

Yes, he should receive this vaccine. The pneumococcal vaccine (Pneumovax 23, Pnu-Immune 23) provides protection against invasive pneumococcal disease.[87,89,93] The vaccine is composed of purified capsular polysaccharide antigens of 23 serotypes of *S. pneumoniae,* which are responsible for causing approximately 88% of the bacteremic pneumococcal disease in the United States.[87,93] Individuals such as A.L. who are at high risk for pneumococcal infection should be given the vaccine. Persons with chronic cardiopulmonary diseases, diabetes, alcoholism, cirrhosis, CSF leaks, and asplenia, and those >65 years of age should be vaccinated with the pneumococcal vaccine.[93] Immunocompromised patients, such as those with Hodgkin's disease, lymphoma, multiple myeloma, and chronic renal failure; patients who have undergone organ transplantation and HIV-infected individuals also are at high risk for pneumococcal disease and should receive the vaccine.[93] Immunocompromised patients, however, often fail to mount a sufficient immune response to the vaccine to fully protect them against infection.[87,93,104] Patients with asymptomatic HIV disease respond more favorably to the vaccine than those with advanced acquired immunodeficiency syndrome (AIDS).[104] The antibody response in children <2 years of age also is poor or absent, and the vaccine is not recommended for these young children.[87]

Thus, given his underlying medical condition (splenectomy) and history of alcoholism, A.L. should receive the pneumococcal vaccine. A single dose is all that is required; subsequent doses may be necessary in ≥5 years.

Gram-Negative Bacillary Meningitis

18. R.R., a 40-year-old, 80-kg man, is admitted to the hospital for a cervical laminectomy with vertebral fusion. His surgical procedure was complicated by a dural tear. On the third postoperative day, drainage at his surgical excision site was noted, and R.R. was febrile to 38.2°C. A Gram stain of the drainage revealed few gram-positive cocci and moderate gram-negative bacilli. Therapy with IV cefazolin 1 g Q 8 h was begun. The following morning, R.R. was oriented to person, place, and time, but he was slightly obtunded and had a temperature of 40°C. Neck stiffness could not be assessed because of his recent surgery. A magnetic resonance imaging (MRI) scan of the head and neck was negative, and lumbar puncture yielded a CSF WBC count of 3,000 cells/mm^3 (normal, <5 cells/mm^3), with 95% PMN; glucose of 20 mg/dL (normal, 60% of plasma glucose); and protein of 280 mg/dL (normal, <50). CSF Gram stain showed numerous gram-negative rods. What important clinical and laboratory features of gram-negative bacillary meningitis are manifested in R.R.?

[SI units: WBC count, 3×10^9 cells/L; glucose, 1.11 mmol/L; protein, 2.8 g/L]

Epidemiology

R.R. has developed gram-negative meningitis as a complication of his recent neurosurgical procedure. Although gram-negative bacilli do not cause meningitis nearly as often as *H. influenzae, S. pneumoniae,* and *N. meningitidis,* they remain important pathogens in both the community and hospital setting.[1,19,20,32,35,58] During an 8-year period covering 1972 to 1979, 158 cases of gram-negative bacillary meningitis were reported to the New York City Health Department, or approximately 20 cases per year for the population of 8 million.[32] Of 493 episodes of meningitis occurring over a 27-year period (1962–1988) at the Massachusetts General Hospital, enteric gram-negative bacilli accounted for 33% of all nosocomial episodes and 3% of community-acquired cases.[1] Historically, mortality rates from gram-negative bacillary meningitis have been extremely high, ranging from 40% to 70%. With the availability of newer antimicrobials such as third-generation cephalosporins, fatalities have declined to <40%.[19,32,35,58] Increasing resistance among certain gram-negative bacilli, such as *Enterobacter* species and *P. aeruginosa,* presents a therapeutic dilemma in that mortality associated with these pathogens is high and therapeutic options are fewer.[33,34]

Predisposing Factors

Individuals at greatest risk for gram-negative bacillary meningitis include neonates, the elderly, debilitated individuals, patients with open trauma to the head, and individuals such as R.R. undergoing neurosurgical procedures.[19–21,32,58] Although meningitis is a rare complication of clean neurosurgical procedures (e.g., craniotomy, laminectomy), the consequences can be devastating when it does happen.[1,21,105]

Microbiology

Escherichia coli and *K. pneumoniae* are the most common gram-negative bacteria causing meningitis and they represent about two-thirds of all cases.[35,58,105] *E. coli* is the most common gram-negative cause of neonatal meningitis, whereas *K. pneumoniae* is isolated more often in the adult population.[23,35,58,105] The remaining one-third of cases are divided evenly among *Proteus, Serratia, Enterobacter,* and *Salmonella* species, *P. aeruginosa,* and other less common bacilli.[35,58,105]

Clinical Features

In general, clinical laboratory features of gram-negative bacillary meningitis are similar to other types of bacterial meningitis.[23,39,58,98] Because of high virulence, gram-negative bacillary meningitis often is a fulminant, rapidly progressive disease. An exception to this rule is meningitis after neurosurgery.[21] As is evidenced by R.R.'s clinical presentation, postneurosurgical gram-negative bacillary meningitis can present in a more subtle fashion. In such patients, many of the symptoms of meningitis (e.g., altered mental status, stiff neck) are masked by underlying neurologic disease. Thus, a high index of suspicion is warranted in the postsurgical setting. In addition to gram-negative bacilli, staphylococci also are associated with postneurosurgical meningitis.[21] The presence of what looks like staphylococci on R.R.'s wound drainage fluid is of concern, but the abundance of gram-negative rods on his CSF Gram stain supports the latter as being the most likely causative pathogen.

Treatment of Gram-Negative Bacillary Meningitis

19. What would be appropriate therapy for gram-negative bacillary meningitis in R.R.?

Fewer choices are available for treatment of gram-negative bacillary meningitis than for other meningitides. Ampicillin is active against only *E. coli, P. mirabilis,* and *Salmonella* species, but its low potency and a high likelihood of resistance severely limit its use.[35,58,105] Chloramphenicol has mediocre gram-negative activity (except against *P. aeruginosa*), but it is only bacteriostatic in activity against enteric bacilli.[35] Chloramphenicol treatment of gram-negative bacillary meningitis historically has been associated with excessively high mortality.[32,35,58,105] Aminoglycosides are limited by their inability to achieve therapeutic CSF concentrations, as well as reduced activity in the acidic milieu of purulent CSF.[14,16,35,54] Intrathecal administration will produce therapeutic CSF concentrations, but repeated administration often is complicated by painful arachnoiditis. Even with this approach, mortality rates are high (>40%).[14,58] Unlike intrathecal administration, lumbar injections will not result in therapeutic CSF concentrations in the ventricle. Extended-spectrum penicillins (e.g., piperacillin) are active against most gram-negative rods but require combination therapy with aminoglycosides for optimal results.[58] The third-generation cephalosporins represent by far the most useful group of agents for treating gram-negative bacillary meningitis, given their high potency against many enteric gram-negative bacilli and good CSF penetration. Experience with these agents spanning over a decade has resulted in the third-generation cephalosporins becoming the drugs of choice for gram-negative bacillary meningitis.[4,35,106]

Empiric therapy for R.R. should include an antipseudomonal β-lactam such as cefepime (Table 58-5).[4,21,56] Cefepime has excellent activity against *E. coli* and *K. pneumoniae* and is active against other enteric gram-negative bacilli as well[35,106] (Table 58-7). Resistance to third-generation cephalosporins among species of *Enterobacter, Citrobacter,* and *Serratia* is so problematic that these drugs cannot be relied on for the treatment of meningitis caused by these pathogens.[33–35,107,108] With this in mind, therapy of gram-negative meningitis in situations in which resistance is more likely to be encountered (e.g., nosocomial or postneurosurgical meningitis) also may include an aminoglycoside based on susceptibility results. Of the third-generation cephalosporins currently available, the most experience has been accumulated with cefotaxime; success rates are >80% for treatment of gram-negative bacillary meningitis caused by *E. coli* or *K. pneumoniae.*[35,106,108] Ceftriaxone has comparable efficacy to cefotaxime and is considered a good alternative.[35] Ceftizoxime penetrates CSF to about the same extent as cefotaxime and has virtually the same spectrum of activity, but published experience with this agent is limited.[35,109] Nonetheless, no compelling evidence suggests that ceftizoxime is inferior to cefotaxime or ceftriaxone.

For R.R., cefazolin should be discontinued, and treatment with cefepime (2 g IV Q 8 h) should be instituted. The choice of cefepime for empiric therapy is appropriate while waiting for results from culture and sensitivity testing. Until these results are available, combination therapy with cefotaxime and an aminoglycoside (gentamicin) is not unreasonable. The dosage of IV gentamicin should be designed to achieve high peak serum concentrations (i.e., >6 mcg/mL) while maintaining trough concentrations <2 mcg/mL (Table 58-6). If intrathecal administration is indicated based on culture and susceptibility data, a 5- to 10-mg intrathecal dose of gentamicin also may be administered daily until clinical improvement is noted.[13,14,58] Gentamicin is commercially available in a 2-mg/mL, preservative-free solution for intrathecal use. The most practical way to provide intrathecal gentamicin to R.R. is by performing a lumbar puncture each day and administering the drug by intralumbar injection. This also will allow daily sampling of CSF for cultures and chemistries. Although intraventricular administration of gentamicin is ideal, insertion of a ventricular reservoir (e.g., Ommaya reservoir) is not appropriate at this time because R.R. has just had major spinal surgery, and it is not clear yet whether prolonged therapy is required.

It is important to make the distinction between aminoglycoside therapy for gram-negative bacillary meningitis in neonates versus adults. In adults, results from clinical trials support the use of combined IV and intrathecal therapy for reasons described previously.[35,58] In neonates, however, combined intraventricular and IV gentamicin produces higher mortality rates than IV gentamicin alone.[110] The reason for the poor clinical outcomes associated with direct instillation of gentamicin into ventricular fluid is unclear. Initially, the increased mortality was attributed to increased trauma related to repeated insertion of the intrathecal needle into the infant's fontanel. More recent evidence suggests that the direct intraventricular injection of aminoglycoside can cause an abrupt release of inflammatory cytokines (TNF and IL-1) from mononuclear cells that could have led to enhanced neurologic sequelae.[111] Whatever the reason, intraventricular and intrathecal therapy should not be given to neonates with gram-negative bacillary meningitis (Tables 58-5 and 58-6)[56] without due consideration of this increased risk.

Treatment of Enterobacter Meningitis

20. Culture results from R.R.'s wound drainage and CSF both are positive for *Enterobacter cloacae.* Sensitivity data reveal resistance to ceftriaxone, cefepime, ceftazidime, piperacillin, aztreonam, and chloramphenicol. Drugs to which the isolate is sensitive include imipenem, TMP-SMX, gentamicin, tobramycin, and ciprofloxacin. What alteration in antimicrobial therapy is most appropriate for R.R. at this time?

Treatment of meningitis caused by *Enterobacter* and related species (e.g., *Serratia, Citrobacter* species) presents a challenge in that resistance is encountered more commonly.[33,35,106] Furthermore, some isolates that are sensitive to third-generation cephalosporins can become resistant during therapy by virtue of possessing inducible, type I β-lactamases.[33] Thus, in contrast to gram-negative bacillary meningitis caused by *E. coli* and *Klebsiella* species, alternative therapies are needed when treating meningitis caused by *Enterobacter, Serratia, Citrobacter,* and *Pseudomonas* species. Based on the sensitivity profile of R.R.'s infecting strain, it is apparent that an extended-spectrum penicillin (e.g., piperacillin) would not be appropriate. Aztreonam, a monobactam antibiotic with good CSF penetration and gram-negative activity comparable to ceftazidime, also is inactive against R.R.'s infecting strain.[112] The isolate is sensitive to imipenem, but the higher propensity for seizures compared with other β-lactams (including penicillin G) argues against its use in R.R.[113–115] Meropenem is not considered to be epileptogenic and is an alternative to imipenem for meningitis.[67,116] Clinical trials have evaluated the efficacy and safety of meropenem versus cefotaxime in the treatment of meningitis in children. Clinical outcomes were similar among the patients randomized to either group, and the incidence of seizures was similar in the treatment groups.[116,117] Ciprofloxacin, a fluoroquinolone antibiotic, offers the attractive features of excellent in vitro potency against gram-negative bacilli (including *Enterobacter* and *Pseudomonas* species).[48,118] Experience with ciprofloxacin in meningitis is limited, however, and achievable CSF levels are relatively low despite reasonable CSF penetration.[48] Furthermore, fluoroquinolones are associated with adverse CNS effects, including the potential to cause seizures.[119] Because limited clinical data exist on the use of meropenem and fluoroquinolones in adults, these agents should be reserved for the treatment of multiresistant isolates.[46,67] TMP-SMX has excellent activity against most gram-negative bacteria, with the exception of *P. aeruginosa,* and penetrates into the CSF especially well.[46,53,103]

Thus, after consideration of the aforementioned options, TMP-SMX appears to be the best choice of therapy for R.R. Cefepime should be discontinued and therapy started with TMP-SMX 15 mg/kg/day (based on the trimethoprim component) given IV in three divided doses.[4,58,103] For R.R., this would be a dosage of 400 mg (trimethoprim component) Q 8 h. Because of poor aqueous solubility, IV TMP-SMX must be prepared such that each 80 mg (5 mL) of TMP-SMX injectable solution is diluted with 75 to 125 mL of 5% dextrose in water. For R.R., 400 mg of TMP-SMX would be administered in approximately 500 mL of D_5W and each dose infused over 1 hour. Whether or not to discontinue gentamicin in R.R. at this time is less clear. Although no data demonstrate superiority of TMP-SMX combined with aminoglycosides over TMP-SMX alone, in vitro evidence is found of synergy, which may be of theoretic advantage.[120]

A review of antibiotic therapy for *Enterobacter* meningitis supports the contention that TMP-SMX is the most useful therapy currently available.[33] Although the study was uncontrolled and retrospective in design, infection was cured in all 7 patients receiving TMP-SMX, compared with 21 of 32 (65%) patients treated solely with third-generation cephalosporins. In all 11 instances of clinical failure, resistance developed during therapy.[33] In an earlier report describing TMP-SMX treatment of bacterial meningitis, including eight cases of gram-negative bacillary meningitis caused by organisms known to be moderately susceptible to third-generation cephalosporins, clinical and bacteriologic cures were observed in all instances (two cases each of *E. cloacae, Serratia marcescens,* and *C. diversus;* one case each of *Proteus vulgaris* and *Morganella morganii*).[103] In contrast, TMP-SMX therapy failed to cure six cases of gram-negative bacillary meningitis caused by *E. coli* (four cases) and *K. pneumoniae* (two cases) despite documented sensitivity to the drug combination. Thus, TMP-SMX appears to be most useful for treatment of gram-negative bacillary meningitis caused by organisms that are only moderately susceptible to third-generation agents, whereas cefotaxime and ceftriaxone remain the drugs of choice for meningitis caused by *E. coli* and *K. pneumoniae* (Table 58-7).

Duration of Therapy

The optimal duration of therapy for gram-negative bacillary meningitis has not been clearly established. Because of the high mortality and morbidity associated with these pathogens and the reduced susceptibility of enteric pathogens to antimicrobial agents, 21 days has been suggested (Table 58-8).[46,56,58] Although R.R. does not appear to have a fulminant case of gram-negative meningitis, a 21-day course of therapy is recommended with close follow-up.

Staphylococcus epidermidis Meningitis/Ventriculitis

Clinical Presentation of CSF Shunt Infections

21. T.A., a 21-year-old woman with a history of congenital hydrocephalus, is admitted to the neurosurgery unit for worsening mental status and fever. T.A. has a history of multiple revisions and placements of intraventricular shunts for control of hydrocephalus. Currently, she has a ventriculoperitoneal (VP) shunt, which was placed 1 month ago and previously had been functioning normally. Over the past few days, T.A. has developed worsening obtundation, stiff neck, and a temperature of 39.5°C. A CT scan performed today reveals enlarged ventricles consistent with acute hydrocephalus.

T.A.'s medical history is noncontributory except for a seizure disorder for which she takes phenytoin 400 mg PO QHS. She also takes Lo-Ovral for birth control. T.A. is allergic to sulfa drugs (severe skin rash). Her weight on admission is 60 kg.

Laboratory analysis was significant for a WBC count of 14,000 cells/mm^3 (normal, 3,200–9,800), with a differential of 85% PMN and 10% lymphocytes; BUN and SrCr values were within the normal range at 19 mg/dL and 0.9 mg/dL, respectively.

A tap of T.A.'s shunt was performed, and the ventricular fluid was notable for total protein of 150 mg/dL (normal, <50), glucose of 40 mg/dL (normal, 60% of serum glucose), and a WBC count of 200 cells/mm^3 (normal, <5 cells/mm^3), with 85% PMNs and 10% lymphocytes. Gram stain of the ventricular fluid showed numerous gram-positive cocci in clusters. What are the subjective and objective findings of CSF shunt infections, and what manifestations of this type of infection are present in T.A.?

[SI units: WBC count, 14 × 10^9 cells/L with 0.85 PMN and 0.1 lymphocytes; BUN, 6.8 mmol/L urea; SrCr, 80 μmol/L; total protein, 1.0 g/L; glucose, 2.2 mmol/L; WBC count, 200 × 10^6 cells/L with 0.85 PMN and 0.1 lymphocytes]

T.A. appears to have meningitis with ventriculitis secondary to infection of her VP shunt. The most important way to manage hydrocephalus involves the use of devices that divert (shunt) CSF from the cerebral ventricles to other areas of the body such as the peritoneum (VP shunts) or atrium (VA shunts).[8,121,122] This approach alleviates increased CSF pressure and substantially reduces morbidity and mortality.[121,122] Infection of these devices, however, is a common cause of shunt malfunction, as seen in T.A. The reported incidence of CSF shunt infections varies from 2% to 39% (usually between 10% and 11%) and depends on patient factors, surgical technique, and the type and duration of the procedure performed (i.e., shunt revision versus placement of a new device).[121,122] T.A., who has been hydrocephalic since birth and has a history of multiple shunt procedures, is at high risk for such an infection.

Clinical symptoms associated with infected CSF shunts vary widely from asymptomatic colonization to fulminant ventriculitis with meningitis.[121–123] Fever is common and, in many instances, is the only presenting symptom.[121] CSF findings also are slightly different in shunt infection compared with acute meningitis: the WBC count usually is not as elevated, the decrease in CSF glucose is less pronounced, and the protein value may be normal or slightly elevated.[121,122] CSF culture is positive in most patients not receiving concurrent antibiotics.[123,124] T.A.'s clinical presentation, CSF findings, and radiographic evidence of hydrocephalus are highly suggestive of a VP shunt infection. She is febrile and has altered mental status. The presence of a stiff neck strongly suggests meningeal involvement. Evaluation of T.A.'s ventricular fluid reveals a slightly elevated WBC count, with a predominance of polymorphonuclear neutrophils, an elevated protein concentration, and a slightly lower than normal glucose concentration.

Skin microflora are the most common causes for CSF shunt infections.[121–124] Staphylococci account for 75% of all cases, with two-thirds of these caused by coagulase-negative staphylococci (usually *S. epidermidis*) and one-third by *S. aureus.*[123,124] Other less common pathogens include diphtheroids, enterococci, and *Propionibacterium acnes* (an anaerobic diphtheroid). Enteric gram-negative bacilli are responsible for a small percentage of cases; these cases usually occur when the distal end of the shunt is inserted improperly into the peritoneal cavity.[123,124] The gram-positive cocci in clusters on Gram stain of T.A.'s CSF strongly suggest a staphylococcal shunt infection. Determining the coagulase status of the isolate will allow differentiation between *S. aureus* and *S. epidermidis.*

Treatment of CSF Shunt Infections

22. Culture and sensitivity tests of T.A.'s ventricular fluid are positive for *S. epidermidis.* The isolate is resistant to nafcillin but sensitive to vancomycin, rifampin, and TMP-SMX. How should T.A.'s CSF shunt infection be treated?

For T.A.'s CSF shunt infection to be optimally treated, a combined medical and surgical approach is required.[117,118,125] Antibiotic therapy directed against the causative organism, although essential, often is inadequate by itself. On average, antibiotic therapy by itself produces cure rates of <40%.[124] In contrast, antibiotic therapy plus surgical removal of the infected device produces clinical cure rates of >80%.[124] Because many patients cannot tolerate the complete removal of their shunt for long, externalization of the distal end of the shunt, or shunt removal and placement of an external drainage device, often is necessary during systemic antibiotic therapy. The presence of an externalized device permits sequential sampling of ventricular fluid and also provides a convenient way to administer antibiotic intraventricularly (see the following discussion).

GLYCOCALYX

Although *S. epidermidis* is not as virulent a pathogen as *S. aureus,* it is extremely difficult to eradicate this organism from prosthetic devices such as CSF shunts. This is because many strains of *S. epidermidis* produce a mucous film or slime layer known as *glycocalyx*, which allows the staphylococci to adhere tightly to the Silastic shunt material, protecting them against phagocytosis.[126,127] As expected, antibiotic failures are much more likely with slime-producing strains of *S. epidermidis.*

Vancomycin is the drug of choice for treatment of shunt infections caused by *S. epidermidis* and should be instituted immediately in T.A.[8,121,127] This is because a high percentage (>60%) of coagulase-negative staphylococci are resistant to methicillin (e.g., methicillin-resistant *S. epidermidis* [MRSE]). Furthermore, methicillin-resistant staphylococci (both methicillin-resistant *S. aureus* [MRSA] and MRSE) also are resistant to cephalosporins. T.A.'s isolate also is sensitive to TMP-SMX, as is the case with many strains of MRSE (and also MRSA),[8] and it must be avoided because T.A. is allergic to this drug combination. Although many staphylococcal isolates (both *S. epidermidis* and *S. aureus*) are susceptible to rifampin, monotherapy with this drug is not recommended because of rapid emergence of resistance. Combination therapy with vancomycin and rifampin may be synergistic and sometimes is used.

VANCOMYCIN THERAPY

23. What would be an appropriate dosage of vancomycin therapy in T.A.? What subjective or objective data should be monitored to evaluate the efficacy and toxicity of the treatment?

Vancomycin therapy for T.A.'s CSF shunt infection requires the use of higher than usual doses, which is true for the treatment of other types of staphylococcal CNS infections as well.[8,56,128] For adults such as T.A., vancomycin dosages of 20 to 30 mg/kg/day to a maximum of 2 g/day have been suggested. Even higher dosages, however, may be required in patients with fulminant disease (Table 58-6).[8,56,96,128] For children with meningitis or infected shunts, the recommended dosage of vancomycin is 40 to 60 mg/kg/day, given IV in two to four divided doses (Table 58-6).[8,56] Although specific recommendations are lacking, it is reasonable to target serum trough concentrations of vancomycin toward the higher end of the target range (i.e., ~15 to 20 mcg/mL). With an every-12-hour dosing schedule, peak serum levels will approach or possibly exceed 40 mcg/mL. It is unlikely, however, that peak serum concentrations of >60 mcg/mL will be observed. Although the potential for toxicity may be greater, higher than usual vancomycin serum concentrations are warranted to ensure adequate penetration into the CSF.[96,128]

T.A., who weighs 60 kg, should be started on a vancomycin regimen of 1 g IV Q 12 h (~30 mg/kg/day) because her renal function is normal. Alternatively, the dose could be calculated using population estimates of vancomycin pharmacokinetic parameters to achieve a trough serum concentration of 15 mcg/mL. In either case, trough serum concentrations should be obtained at steady-state to assess whether the initial dosing regimen is adequate.

Anecdotal evidence suggests that very high dosages of vancomycin (≥3 g/day in adults with normal renal function) are associated with an increased risk of ototoxicity.[96,129] This observation is difficult to verify because hearing loss also is a potential sequelae of meningitis. High-dose vancomycin therapy also has a greater likelihood of inducing the "red man syndrome."[130,131] This adverse effect, manifested by flushing and pruritus, with or without hypotension, is related directly to the amount of drug infused over a given period of time.[130] It usually can be avoided or minimized by infusing vancomycin doses of 1,000 mg in ≥250 mL of solution (either D_5W or normal saline) over at least 1 hour. If red man syndrome is observed, slowing the infusion rate often ameliorates symptoms.[130] Pretreatment with antihistamines (diphenhydramine or hydroxyzine) may also minimize the reaction because the proposed mechanism partially involves histamine release.[131]

Another consideration for T.A. is the addition of rifampin to her vancomycin regimen. This is based on the excellent staphylococcal activity of rifampin, its good CSF penetration, and the potential for synergy between these two agents.[8,121] Whether rifampin plus vancomycin is superior to vancomycin alone has not been determined. For T.A., it is best to avoid rifampin because evidence supporting its efficacy is weak, and she currently is taking phenytoin and birth control pills. Rifampin is a potent inducer of hepatic microsomal enzymes, which can lower serum phenytoin concentrations (possibly resulting in seizure activity) and increase the possibility of an unplanned pregnancy (from reduced effectiveness of the birth control pill).

Intraventricular and Intravenous Dosing of Vancomycin

24. Should T.A. receive intraventricular vancomycin? If so, what would be an appropriate dosage?

T.A. has a long history of hydrocephalus and will require placement of an external drainage device after removal of her VP shunt. This makes intraventricular administration of vancomycin possible, and such treatment should be instituted promptly. The dosages used in the literature vary from 5 to 20 mg/day. Experts recommend 20 mg/day of intraventricular vancomycin; therefore, an intraventricular vancomycin dosage of 20 mg/day is recommended for T.A. Also, serial (daily) cultures of CSF are recommended to monitor her response to therapy. Some authors suggest adjusting intraventricular vancomycin doses to achieve trough CSF vancomycin concentrations of at least 5 mcg/mL or CSF bactericidal activity of at least 1:8 against the infecting strain.[8,121] Until more information is available, monitoring serial CSF trough concentrations is more appropriate than CSF bactericidal titers, and serial trough levels should be obtained in T.A. To summarize, T.A. should receive combined IV and intraventricular vancomycin therapy as described previously. Therapy should be continued for at least 10 days after sterilization of her ventricular fluid is documented, at which time a new VP shunt can be placed.[121,124,132]

In contrast to T.A.'s situation, vancomycin therapy for patients with staphylococcal meningitis not associated with a CSF shunt or indwelling ventricular catheter is more problematic. Because of this, therapy often is instituted with IV vancomycin alone.[96,128] Intrathecal vancomycin, although preferable, requires either daily lumbar puncture (for intralumbar therapy) or surgical placement of an intraventricular reservoir. If the response to therapy is inadequate within the first 24 to 48 hours, the addition of intrathecal vancomycin therapy (5 to 20 mg/day) is recommended.[96,128] In fulminant cases of staphylococcal meningitis, however, intrathecal vancomycin should be instituted as quickly as possible (i.e., with the first lumbar puncture) to optimize the response to therapy.

BRAIN ABSCESS

Epidemiology

Although not nearly as common as meningitis, abscesses of the brain parenchyma (brain abscess) remain an important type of CNS infection. The incidence of brain abscess has not varied since the preantibiotic era and is estimated to account for 1 in 10,000 hospital admissions.[133] On a busy neurosurgical service, 4 to 10 cases a year typically are seen.[133,134] For reasons that are not entirely clear, men are more likely to develop abscesses within the brain than women.[133,135] Brain abscess can occur at any age, but the median age is 30 to 40 years, with approximately 25% of cases occurring in children.[133,136,137]

Despite advances in antimicrobial therapy over the past several decades, mortality rates from brain abscess has remained above 40% until just recently. Developments in imaging techniques (e.g., CT and MRI scanning), which allow early recognition of abscesses and the ability to serially monitor the radiographic response to antimicrobial therapy, have had the most profound impact on reducing morbidity and mortality from brain abscess.[133,134,138] In a review of 102 cases of bacterial abscesses occurring over a 17-year period, mortality was 41% in the period before 1975 (pre-CT scan era), compared with 6% during 1975 to 1986, when CT scanning became routinely available.[134] With the combined medical and surgical approach currently recommended, mortality rates continue to average <10%.[133,134,138]

Predisposing Factors

Brain abscesses most commonly arise from a contiguous suppurative source of infection (e.g., sinusitis, otitis, mastoiditis, or dental infections).[133,135,139] In the United States, abscesses occurring as a complication of sinusitis are more common than abscesses arising from otitic or dental sources.[133] The formation of a single abscess cavity usually is found when infection develops from a contiguous source. In addition, the abscess nearly always is formed in close proximity to the primary focus of infection (Table 58-10).[133,139] For example, abscesses of sinusitic origin more commonly involve the frontal lobe, whereas otitic infections often lead to temporal lobe abscess formation.[139] Brain abscess also occurs as a consequence of metastatic spread of organisms from a primary site of infection (e.g., lung abscess, endocarditis, osteomyelitis, pelvic, and intra-abdominal infections).[129,131] In children, cyanotic congenital heart disease is a common predisposing factor for brain abscess.[136,137] Multiple abscesses suggest a metastatic source of infection.[133] As with meningitis, brain abscess occurs as an infrequent complication of head trauma or neurosurgery.[11,133,139] No identifiable source (cryptogenic abscess) is detected in as many as 30% of cases.[133,139]

Staging

Once an intracranial focus of infection is established, the evolution of brain abscess involves two distinct stages: cerebritis and capsule formation.[136,138] The cerebritis stage evolves gradually over the first 9 to 10 days of infection and is characterized by an area of marked inflammatory infiltrate that contains a necrotic center surrounded by an area of cerebral edema.[136,138] Capsule formation occurs about 10 to 14 days after the initiation of infection, and once formed, the capsule continues to thicken over a period of weeks.[136,138] The stage of abscess development has important implications for therapy. Although it is best to wait until the capsule is fully formed before attempting any type of surgical intervention, antimicrobial therapy alone may resolve the infection if discovered in the early cerebritis stage.[138]

Table 58-10 Predisposing Conditions, Microbiology, and Recommended Therapy for Bacterial Brain Abscess

Predisposing Condition	*Usual Location of Abscess*	*Most Likely Organisms*	*Recommended Therapy*
Contiguous Site			
Otitic infection	Temporal lobe or cerebellum	Streptococci (anaerobic and aerobic), *Bacteroides fragilis*, gram-negative bacilli	Penicillin G + metronidazole + cefotaxime or ceftriaxone
Sinusitis	Frontal lobe	Streptococci (predominantly), *Bacteroides* species, gram-negative bacilli, *Staphylococcus aureus*, *Haemophilus* species	Penicillin G + metronidazole + cefotaxime or ceftriaxone
Dental infection	Frontal lobe	*Fusobacteria* species, *Bacteroides* species, and streptococci	Penicillin G + metronidazole
Primary Infection			
Head trauma or neurosurgery	Related to site of wound	Gram-negative bacilli, staphylococci, streptococci, diphtheroids	Vancomycin + ceftazidime

Microbiology

The microbiology of brain abscess is distinctly different from that of meningitis. Streptococci are implicated in 60% to 70% of cases and include anaerobic as well as microaerophilic streptococci of the *S. milleri* group.[133,139,140] Other anaerobes, particularly *Bacteroides* species (including *B. fragilis*) and *Prevotella* species, are found in up to 40% of cases, usually in mixed culture.[133,139] In recent years, staphylococci appear to be decreasing and enteric gram-negative bacteria increasing as etiologic agents of bacterial brain abscess.[123] Although somewhat imprecise, a reasonable correlation exists between the various predisposing conditions and the microbiologic etiology of brain abscess (Table 58-10).[133,135,137,138]

In the immunocompromised patient, a diverse group of microorganisms can induce abscesses within the brain. In patients with AIDS, *Toxoplasma gondii* is by far the most common infectious cause of focal brain lesions.[141] Transplant recipients and those receiving immunosuppressive therapy are susceptible to infection from *Nocardia* species.[142] In Mexico and other Central American countries, cysticercosis remains a common cause of intracerebral infection.[143]

Clinical and Radiologic Features

25. **L.Y., a 40-year-old man, is brought to the ED by a friend. L.Y. complains of severe headache, fever, weakness in his left arm and leg, and increasing drowsiness. Over the past week, L.Y. has suffered from headaches, which have gradually worsened in intensity, and from intermittent episodes of fever. Despite getting plenty of sleep, L.Y. has been feeling increasingly drowsy over the past several days. When he noticed weakness in his left arm and difficulty concentrating this morning, he called a friend and asked to be taken in for evaluation.**

L.Y. has a history of chronic sinusitis that has been treated with a variety of oral antibiotics. His last episode of sinusitis, which occurred about 1 month ago, was treated with a 10-day course of cephalexin. He denies any nausea or vomiting and has not experienced any seizures in the recent past. L.Y. was tested for HIV 6 months ago, and the result of his antibody test was negative. He takes no current medications, denies smoking and use of recreational drugs, and drinks alcohol only on social occasions a few times a month. L.Y. has no known drug allergies.

Physical examination reveals L.Y. to be in mild distress, with a temperature of 38.2°C. He is slightly lethargic and is oriented to person and place but not time (0 × 2). The strength in L.Y.'s left arm is 3/5; the strength in his left leg is 4/5. The remainder of his neurologic examination is grossly normal. L.Y. described moderate pain on palpation of his frontal sinuses, and a purulent discharge is noted.

Laboratory evaluation shows a WBC count of 8,000 cells/mm^3 (normal, 3,200–9,800), with 70% PMN, 25% lymphocytes, and 5% monocytes; Hgb, Hct, platelets, and serum chemistries are within normal limits; and his BUN and SrCr are 16 mg/dL (normal, 8 to 18) and 1.2 mg/dL (normal, 0.6 to 1.2), respectively. L.Y.'s erythrocyte sedimentation rate (ESR) is 40 mm/hour (normal, 0 to 20).

A CT scan with contrast dye reveals a right frontal ring-enhancing lesion with a small amount of surrounding cerebral edema. L.Y. is admitted to the neurosurgery unit for further evaluation and treatment. What clinical signs and symptoms does L.Y. display that are suggestive of bacterial brain abscess? How can brain abscess be diagnosed in L.Y.?

[SI units: WBC count, 8 × 10^9 cells/L with 0.7 PMN, 0.25 lymphocytes, and 0.05 monocytes; Hgb, 145 g/L; Hct, 0.4; platelets, 120 × 10^9/L; BUN, 5.7 mmol/L urea; SrCr, 106.1 μmol/L; ESR 40 mm/hr]

L.Y. has presented to the ED with many signs and symptoms suggestive of bacterial brain abscess. He is 40 years of age and a man, both of which place him in a group with the highest likelihood of having a brain abscess. In contrast to the diffuse nature of meningitis, brain abscess presents as a focal neurologic process.[133,134] Notable in L.Y.'s presentation is left-sided (arm and leg) weakness. Symptoms of brain abscess range in severity from indolent to fulminant and, in most patients, the duration of symptoms at the time of presentation is ≤2 weeks.[133,134,136] Headache is the most common symptom of brain abscess, occurring in approximately 70% of cases. L.Y.'s clinical manifestations have become gradually worse over the past week, and his worsening headaches, increasing drowsiness, and difficulty in concentrating all are consistent with bacterial brain abscess.

L.Y. presents with the classic triad of fever, headache, and focal neurologic deficits. Although this triad should always be looked for, fewer than half of patients with confirmed bacterial brain abscess present in this manner.[133,134,135] The absence of fever does not rule out infection because fever is found in <50% of patients.[133,134] Focal neurologic deficits are present in approximately 50% of patients and vary in nature and severity in relation to the location and size of the abscess and surrounding cerebral edema.[133,134,137] Although L.Y. does not have a history of seizure activity, approximately one-third of patients experience partial seizures that often become generalized.[133,137] Papilledema and nuchal rigidity occur in ≤25% of cases and often are not useful in confirming the diagnosis. Symptoms associated with a contiguous focus of infection should always be sought and, in some situations, they may dominate the clinical picture.[133,134] L.Y. has a history of sinus infection, and the pain on palpation of his sinuses coupled with the purulent sinus drainage suggests active infection at this site.

As can be seen from L.Y.'s test results, laboratory evaluation usually is not very helpful when diagnosing brain abscess. L.Y. does not have a peripheral leukocytosis, but he does have an elevated ESR. A normal peripheral WBC count is not unusual in patients with intracranial suppuration. The ESR often is elevated in brain abscess, but this test is nonspecific and only indirectly supports the diagnosis.

L.Y. did not have a lumbar puncture because this procedure is contraindicated for diagnosing brain abscess.[42,133,134] The diagnostic yield from CSF is low because chemistries (e.g., protein, glucose, WBC) usually are normal and culture of the CSF in patients with brain abscess is unlikely to yield the causative pathogen. More important, performing a lumbar puncture in patients with space-occupying lesions of the brain can produce cerebral herniation as a consequence of the shifting pressure gradient induced within the cranial vault after insertion of the lumbar puncture needle.[42]

Of paramount importance is the abnormality detected on the CT scan of L.Y.'s brain. When dye is injected before the CT scan, brain abscesses will appear to "ring enhance." Furthermore, cerebral edema can be identified as a variable hypodense region immediately surrounding the abscess cavity. As stated earlier, CT and MRI scanning techniques have revolutionized the diagnosis and treatment of brain abscess.[133,134,138] The superiority of CT versus MRI is unclear. MRI, however, is more sensitive in detecting cerebritis than CT, and it can be helpful in ruling out (or ruling in) an abscess when the CT scan is negative.[133,138] Assessment of the size and location of the lesion is possible with both techniques, which is invaluable in deciding which surgical intervention is indicated. In addition, serial radiographic studies can be used to evaluate antimicrobial response over time.[134,138] In general, a good correlation exists between the clinical and radiologic response to therapy of bacterial brain abscess.

Treatment

26. **How should L.Y.'s brain abscess be treated?**

Surgical Techniques

A combined medical and surgical approach is the best form of therapy for L.Y.'s brain abscess.[133,138] Response rates to antimicrobial therapy alone have been disappointing and, with a few exceptions, surgical intervention is necessary to ensure optimal results. Medical therapy is indicated when multiple abscesses are present, when the abscess cavity is inaccessible surgically, for patients who are poor surgical candidates, and when the abscess is small (<4 cm).[133,138,144]

The two types of surgical approaches for brain abscess are (a) stereotactic needle aspiration and (b) craniotomy for abscess excision.[138] Stereotactic aspiration of abscess contents can be performed under local anesthesia and produces lower morbidity and mortality than craniotomy.[19] Such an approach is highly effective, except when multiloculated abscesses are present.[138] With craniotomy, the abscess cavity can be excised completely, which often allows a shorter duration of antimicrobial therapy. Both techniques are effective, and the decision regarding which procedure is most appropriate must be individualized.

Antimicrobial Penetration Into Brain Abscess

Antimicrobial therapy is an essential component of brain abscess therapy.[139] Penetration of antibiotics into brain abscess fluid has not been studied as carefully as penetration into CSF, and as discussed earlier, the barrier involved is different (Fig. 58-1).[15] Penicillins and cephalosporins penetrate adequately into abscess fluid, but certain agents (e.g., penicillin G) may be susceptible to degradation by enzymes present within the abscess milieu.[133,139,145–147] Third-generation cephalosporins (e.g., cefotaxime, ceftriaxone, and ceftizoxime) are believed to penetrate sufficiently into the abscess and are good choices when gram-negative bacteria are present.[133,147] Chloramphenicol penetrates very well into brain abscesses and has been used extensively.[133,139,145] It has excellent anaerobic activity, but also can be degraded (deacetylated) in purulent abscess fluid.[133] Metronidazole achieves abscess fluid concentrations equal to or in excess of serum levels and is bactericidal against strict anaerobes. The unique mechanism of action of metronidazole makes it particularly useful in the necrotic core of the cavity, where the oxidation-reduction potential is low and bacteria replicate slowly or are dormant. For these reasons, metronidazole has supplanted chloramphenicol for treatment of bacterial brain abscess.[133] Although data are limited, vancomycin and carbapenems appear to penetrate sufficiently into brain abscess fluid.[133,148] Although specific abscess-penetration data are unavailable, successful treatment of cerebral nocardiosis with TMP-SMX and CNS toxoplasmosis with clindamycin suggests that these compounds also achieve adequate penetration into cerebral abscess cavities.[141,143]

Antibiotic Therapy

When antibiotic therapy should be instituted depends on the status of the patient and the stage of abscess development. For patients diagnosed during the cerebritis stage, before formation of a well-circumscribed capsule, surgery should be delayed and antimicrobial therapy begun in patients with significant symptoms.[133,138] If capsule formation already has taken place, it is better to delay initiation of antibiotics until after surgery to increase the microbiologic yield from tissue and fluid samples. If the disease is fulminant, antibiotics must be instituted promptly and surgical intervention performed as quickly as possible.[133,138]

L.Y.'s clinical presentation suggests an advanced brain abscess. The presence of ring enhancement on CT and the onset of symptoms over 2 weeks support this. Because he is not critically ill, antibiotic therapy should be delayed until surgery is performed. Specimens obtained from the surgical procedure should be sent for aerobic and anaerobic culture and a stat Gram stain.

Initial antibiotic therapy for brain abscess needs to be sufficiently broad to cover the most likely pathogens (Table 58-10).[133,135,137,139] In most cases, a combination of high-dose penicillin G and metronidazole is indicated. Penicillin will cover aerobic, anaerobic, and microaerophilic streptococci, whereas metronidazole will provide coverage for strict anaerobes, including *Bacteroides* and *Prevotella* species. If gram-negative bacilli are suspected or documented, as in abscesses related to otitis, head trauma, or neurosurgery, a third-generation cephalosporin is indicated.[133] Staphylococcal abscesses should be treated with nafcillin or vancomycin.[133,135,149]

For L.Y., therapy with penicillin G 4 million units IV Q 4 h and metronidazole 500 mg IV Q 8 hours should be started postoperatively (Table 58-6). Because his abscess appears to originate from the sinus, the likelihood of gram-negative infection is reduced. With evidence of gram-negative bacteria on the Gram stain of abscess fluid, therapy with cefotaxime 3 g IV Q 6 h also should be included. Ceftriaxone 2 g IV Q 12 h is a viable alternative to cefotaxime, particularly if the patient is going to be discharged to home on a prolonged course of therapy. Outpatient therapy is appropriate for CNS infections as long as patients are carefully selected and monitored, as described in a recent report.[150] Of interest, of the 24 patients treated on an outpatient basis, 46% received ceftriaxone 2 g IV once daily with a cure.[150] TMP-SMX is an alternative if the organism is resistant to cefotaxime. The large fluid volume required (particularly when 5% dextrose in water is used) for IV TMP-SMX administration may contribute, however, to worsening cerebral edema.[129] Antimicrobial therapy for L.Y. should be revised once results from culture and sensitivity testing are available.

Adjunctive Corticosteroid Therapy

Adjunctive corticosteroid therapy for bacterial brain abscess is controversial.[133,138] Steroids can interfere with antibiotic penetration into abscesses and obscure the interpretation of serial CT scans when assessing response to therapy.[133,138] Therefore, steroids are indicated only if significant cerebral edema is present, particularly if it is accompanied by rapid neurologic deterioration.[133,138] L.Y. should not receive dexamethasone because his mental status is only mildly depressed and the cerebral edema seen on CT scan is not massive.

Adjunctive Anticonvulsant Therapy

L.Y. has shown no signs of seizure activity thus far and, therefore, does not require anticonvulsant therapy. Anticonvulsants should be used in the acute setting when seizures are present, however.[133,138] Agents with activity against partial and complex partial seizures are preferred (e.g., phenytoin, carbamazepine). The long-term use of anticonvulsants depends on whether seizure activity persists. Insufficient information exists regarding how long to continue anticonvulsants in such cases. Therefore, discontinuation of these agents must be individualized.

No formal guidelines are available regarding the optimal duration of therapy for bacterial brain abscess. Given the serious nature of the infection and the difficulty associated with antibiotic penetration, therapy with high-dose IV therapy should continue for at least 6 to 8 weeks.[133,138] The duration of therapy should be evaluated on a case-by-case basis. In an attempt to ensure complete eradication of infection, some experts recommend long-term (2–6 months) oral antibiotics after the IV course, provided agents with good oral absorption and activity against the offending pathogens are available.[133]

Monitoring Therapy

27. How should L.Y. be monitored for therapeutic response and toxicity?

Although L.Y. is on antibiotic therapy, weekly or biweekly CT scans should be obtained to evaluate abscess resolution. His clinical response to therapy also should be assessed daily. If therapy is effective, L.Y.'s mental status should improve gradually (e.g., he will become more alert and oriented) over a period of several days. L.Y.'s headaches and hemiparesis (weakness in his arm and leg) also should resolve eventually. It may take a week or longer, however, to see a complete resolution of symptoms.[133,135] In general, radiologic improvement (i.e., reduction in abscess size) correlates reasonably well with clinical response, but not always.[133,135,138] Persistent symptoms or failure to detect a reduction in abscess size on CT scan or the appearance of new abscesses may indicate improper antimicrobial therapy or the need for more surgery.[133,138] Repeated surgical intervention with appropriate reculturing may be required in some instances to optimize therapy.

Adverse effects associated with the penicillin G therapy that L.Y. is receiving are similar to those of other β-lactam antibiotics. Seizures are a potential complication when high doses of penicillin are used in the presence of a mass lesion in the brain.[6,101,115,151] L.Y. should be observed closely by those providing care and questioned regularly for any evidence of seizure activity. Metronidazole usually is well tolerated, but may also cause neurotoxicity,[133,148,151,152] most commonly peripheral neuropathy.[152] L.Y. should be assessed for the presence of numbness or tingling in his hands or feet. Seizures, although uncommon, occasionally occur with metronidazole.[152] If L.Y. experiences peripheral neuropathy or seizures, a switch to chloramphenicol would be appropriate. Other adverse effects associated with metronidazole include mild nausea, brownish discoloration of the urine, and the potential for a disulfiramlike reaction with concomitant ethanol ingestion.[148] L.Y. should be counseled regarding the possibility of gastric upset and discoloration of the urine, and he should be strongly cautioned to avoid alcoholic beverages while receiving metronidazole. Given his young age, the absence of significant underlying diseases, and the relative early detection of his brain abscess, there is every reason to expect a good response to his treatment and, eventually, a complete resolution of his abscess.

REFERENCES

1. Durand ML et al. Acute bacterial meningitis in adults. *N Engl J Med* 1993;328:21.
2. Quagliarello VJ et al. New perspectives on bacterial meningitis. *Clin Infect Dis* 1993;17:603.
3. Quagliarello VJ et al. Bacterial meningitis: pathogenesis, pathophysiology, and progress. *N Engl J Med* 1992;327:864.
4. Scheld WM et al. Pathophysiology of bacterial meningitis: mechanism(s) of neuronal injury. *J Infect Dis* 2002;186(Suppl 2):S225.
5. McIntyre PB et al. Dexamethasone as adjunctive therapy in bacterial meningitis. A meta-analysis of randomized clinical trials since 1988. *JAMA* 1997;278:925.
6. Overturf GD. Pyogenic bacterial infections of the CNS. *Neurol Clin* 1986;4:69.
7. Silverberg AL et al. Subdural empyema and cranial epidural abscess. *Med Clin North Am* 1985;69:361.
8. Morris A et al. Nosocomial bacterial meningitis, including central nervous system shunt infections. *Infect Dis Clin North Am* 1999;13:735.
9. Romanes GJ. *Cunningham's Textbook of Anatomy.* 12th ed. New York: Oxford University Press; 1981:28.
10. Bonadio WA. The cerebrospinal fluid: physiologic aspects and alterations associated with bacterial meningitis. *Pediatr Infect Dis J* 1992;11:423.
11. Tunkel AR. Approach to the patient with central nervous system infections. In: Mandell GL et al., eds. *Principles and Practice of Infectious Diseases.* 6th ed. New York: Churchill Livingstone; 2005:1079.
12. Gagnong WF. *Review of Medical Physiology.* 16th ed. Norwalk, CT: Appleton & Lange; 1993:551.
13. Allinson RR et al. Intrathecal drug therapy. *Drug Intell Clin Pharm* 1978;12:347.
14. Kaiser AB et al. Aminoglycoside therapy of gram-negative bacillary meningitis. *N Engl J Med* 1975;293:1215.
15. Pardridge WM et al. Blood–brain barrier: interface between internal medicine and the brain. *Ann Intern Med* 1986;105:82.
16. Scheld WM. Drug delivery to the central nervous system: general principles and relevance to therapy for infections of the central nervous system. *Rev Infect Dis* 1989;11(Suppl 7):S1669.
17. Behlau I et al. Chronic meningitis. In: Mandell GL et al., eds. *Principles and Practice of Infectious Diseases.* 6th ed. New York: Churchill Livingstone; 2005:1132.
18. Moris G et al. The challenge of drug-induced aseptic meningitis. *Arch Intern Med* 1999;159:1185.
19. Fitch MT. Emergency diagnosis and treatment of adult meningitis. *Lancet Infect Dis* 2007;7:191.
20. Wenger JD et al. Bacterial meningitis in the United States, 1986: report of a multistate surveillance study. *JAMA* 1990;162:1316.
21. Tenney JH. Bacterial infections of the central nervous system in neurosurgery. *Neurol Clin* 1986;4:91.
22. Tunkel AR. et al. Practice guidelines for the management of bacterial meningitis. *Clin Infect Dis* 2004;39:1267.
23. Unhanand M et al. Gram-negative enteric bacillary meningitis: a twenty-one-year experience. *J Pediatr* 1993;122:15.
24. Gellin BG et al. Listeriosis. *JAMA* 1989;261:1313.
25. Adams WG et al. Decline of childhood *Haemophilus influenzae* type b (Hib) disease in the Hib vaccine era. *JAMA* 1993;269:221.
26. Progress toward elimination of *Haemophilus influenzae* type b invasive disease among infants

and children, United States, 1998–2000. *MMWR* 2002;51:234.
27. Schuchat A et al. Bacterial meningitis in the United States in 1995. *N Engl J Med* 1997;337:970.
28. Gold R. Epidemiology of bacterial meningitis. *Infect Dis Clin North Am* 1999;13:515.
29. Doern GV et al. Antimicrobial resistance among clinical isolates of *Streptococcus pneumoniae* in the United States during 1999–2000, including a comparison of resistance rates since 1994–1995. *Antimicrob Agents Chemother* 2001;45:1721.
30. Choi C. Bacterial meningitis. *Clin Geriatr Med* 1992;8:889.
31. van de Beek D et al. Community-acquired bacterial meningitis in adults. *N Engl J Med* 2006;354:44.
32. Cherubin CE et al. Listeria and gram-negative bacillary meningitis in New York City, 1972–1979. *Am J Med* 1981;71:199.
33. Wolff MA et al. Antibiotic therapy for *Enterobacter* meningitis: a retrospective review of 13 episodes and review of the literature. *Clin Infect Dis* 1993;16:772.
34. Fong IW et al. Review of *Pseudomonas aeruginosa* meningitis with special emphasis on treatment with ceftazidime. *Rev Infect Dis* 1985;7:604.
35. Cherubin CE et al. Treatment of gram-negative bacillary meningitis: role of the new cephalosporin antibiotics. *Rev Infect Dis* 1982;4(Suppl):S453.
36. Pomeroy SL et al. Seizures and other neurologic sequelae of bacterial meningitis in children. *N Engl J Med* 1990;323:1651.
37. Taylor HG et al. The sequelae of *Haemophilus influenzae* meningitis in school-age children. *N Engl J Med* 1990;323:1657.
38. Dodge PR et al. Prospective evaluation of hearing impairment as a sequelae of acute bacterial meningitis. *N Engl J Med* 1984;311:869.
39. Aronin SI et al. Community-acquired bacterial meningitis: risk stratification for adverse clinical outcomes and effect of antibiotic timing. *Ann Intern Med* 1998;129:862.
40. Keroack MA. The patient with suspected meningitis. *Emerg Med Clin North Am* 1987;5:807.
41. Verghese A et al. Kerning's and Brudzinski's signs revisited. *Rev Infect Dis* 1987;9:1187.
42. Addy DP. When not to do a lumbar puncture. *Arch Dis Child* 1987;62:873.
43. Edberg SC. Conventional and molecular techniques for the laboratory diagnosis of infections of the central nervous system. *Neurol Clin* 1986;4:13.
44. Proulx N et al. Delays in the administration of antibiotics are associated with mortality from adult acute bacterial meningitis. *QJM* 2005;98:291.
45. Lutsar I et al. Antibiotic pharmacodynamics in cerebrospinal fluid. *Clin Infect Dis* 1998;27:1117.
46. Quagliarello VJ et al. Treatment of bacterial meningitis. *N Engl J Med* 1997;336:708.
47. Arditi M et al. Cefuroxime treatment failure and *Haemophilus influenzae* meningitis: case report and review of the literature. *Pediatrics* 1989;84:132.
48. Scheld WM. Quinolone therapy for infections of the central nervous system. *Rev Infect Dis* 1989;11(Suppl 5):S1194.
49. Scheld WM et al. Comparison of netilmicin with gentamicin in the therapy of experimental *Escherichia coli* meningitis. *Antimicrob Agents Chemother* 1978;13:899.
50. Norrby SR. Role of cephalosporins in the treatment of bacterial meningitis. *Am J Med* 1985;79(Suppl 2A):56.
51. Andes DR et al. Pharmacokinetics and pharmacodynamics of antibiotics in meningitis. *Infect Dis Clin North Am* 1999;13:595.
52. Lutsar I et al. Pharmacokinetics and pharmacodynamics of cephalosporins in cerebrospinal fluid. *Clin Pharmacokinet* 2000:39:335.
53. Norrby SR. A review of the penetration of antibiotics into CSF and its clinical significance. *Scand J Infect Dis* 1978(Suppl);14:296.
54. Bolan G et al. Acute bacterial meningitis in children and adults. *Med Clin North Am* 1985;69:231.
55. Del Rio M et al. Ceftriaxone versus ampicillin and chloramphenicol for treatment of bacterial meningitis in children. *Lancet* 1983;1:1241.
56. Plotkin SA et al. Treatment of bacterial meningitis. *Pediatrics* 1988;81:904.
57. Saxon A et al. Immediate hypersensitivity reactions to beta-lactam antibiotics. *Ann Intern Med* 1987;107:204.
58. Rahal JJ et al. Host defense and antimicrobial therapy in adult gram-negative bacillary meningitis. *Ann Intern Med* 1982;96:468.
59. Roche Laboratories. Rocephin package insert. Nutley, NJ: January 1994.
60. Fishman R. Steroids in the treatment of brain edema. *N Engl J Med* 1982;306:359.
61. deLemos RA et al. Corticosteroids as an adjunct to treatment in bacterial meningitis. *Pediatrics* 1969;44:30.
62. Belsey MA et al. Dexamethasone in the treatment of acute bacterial meningitis: the effect of study design on the interpretation of results. *Pediatrics* 1969;44:503.
63. Syrogiannopoulos GA et al. Dexamethasone therapy for bacterial meningitis in children: 2- versus 4-day regimen. *J Infect Dis* 1994;169:853.
64. Odio CM et al. The beneficial effects of early dexamethasone administration in infants and children with bacterial meningitis. *N Engl J Med* 1991;324:1525.
65. Schaad UB et al. Dexamethasone therapy for bacterial meningitis in children. *Lancet* 1993;342:457.
66. Girgis NI et al. Dexamethasone treatment for bacterial meningitis in children and adults. *Pediatr Infect Dis J* 1989;8:848.
67. Saez-Lloren X et al. Antimicrobial and anti-inflammatory treatment of bacterial meningitis. *Infect Dis Clin North Am* 1999;13:619.
68. Kanra GY et al. Beneficial effects of dexamethasone in children with pneumococcal meningitis. *Pediatric Infect Dis J* 1995;14:490.
69. de Gans J et al. Dexamethasone in adults with bacterial meningitis. *N Engl J Med* 2002;347:1549.
70. van de Beek D et al. Corticosteroids for acute bacterial meningitis. *Cochrane Database Syst Rev* 2007;1:CD004405.
71. van de Beek D et al. Dexamethasone in adults with community-acquired bacterial meningitis. *Drugs* 2006;66:415.
72. Cabellos C et al. Influence of dexamethasone on efficacy of ceftriaxone and vancomycin therapy in experimental meningitis. *Antimicrob Agents Chemother* 1995;39:2158.
73. Paris MM. Effect of dexamethasone on therapy of experimental penicillin and cephalosporin resistant pneumococcal meningitis. *Antimicrob Agents Chemother* 1994;38:1320.
74. Martinez-Lacasa J et al. Experimental study of the efficacy of vancomycin, rifampicin and dexamethasone in the therapy of pneumococcal meningitis. *J Antimicrob Chemother* 2002;49:507.
75. Cabellos C et al. Evaluation of combined ceftriaxone and dexamethasone therapy in experimental cephalosporin-resistant pneumococcal meningitis. *J Antimicrob Chemother* 2000;45:315.
76. Ricard J-D et al. Levels of vancomycin in cerebrospinal fluid of adult patients receiving adjunctive corticosteroids to treat pneumococcal meningitis: a prospective multicenter observational study. *Clin Infect Dis* 2007;44:250.
77. Ahmed A et al. Pharmacodynamics of vancomycin for the treatment of experimental penicillin- and cephalosporin-resistant pneumococcal meningitis. *Antimicrob Agents Chemother* 1999;43:876.
78. Schaab UB et al. A comparison of ceftriaxone and cefuroxime for the treatment of bacterial meningitis in children. *N Engl J Med* 1990;322:141.
79. Lebel MH et al. Comparative efficacy of ceftriaxone and cefuroxime for treatment of bacterial meningitis. *J Pediatr* 1989;114:1049.
80. Neu HC. Third-generation cephalosporins: safety profiles after 10 years of clinical use. *J Clin Pharmacol* 1990;30:396.
81. Kelly CP et al. Clostridium difficile colitis. *N Engl J Med* 1994;330:257.
82. Shiffman ML et al. Pathogenesis of ceftriaxone-associated biliary sludge. *Gastroenterology* 1990;99:1772.
83. Schaad UB et al. Reversible ceftriaxone-associated biliary pseudolithiasis in children. *Lancet* 1988;2:1411.
84. Park HZ et al. Ceftriaxone-associated gallbladder sludge. *Gastroenterology* 1991;100:1665.
85. Heim-Duthoy KL et al. Apparent biliary pseudolithiasis during ceftriaxone therapy. *Antimicrob Agents Chemother* 1990;34:1146.
86. Radetsky M. Duration of treatment in bacterial meningitis: a historical inquiry. *Pediatr Infect Dis J* 1990;9:2.
87. Peltola H. Prophylaxis of bacterial meningitis. *Infect Dis Clin North Am* 1999;13:685.
88. Gardner P. Prevention of meningococcal disease. *N Engl J Med* 2006;355:14.
89. Prevention and control of meningococcal disease: recommendations of the Advisory Committee on Immunization Practices (ACIP). *MMWR* 2005;54:1–21.
90. Immunization Practices Advisory Committee. Haemophilus b conjugate vaccines for prevention of Haemophilus influenzae type b disease among infants and children two months of age and older. *MMWR* 1991;40:1.
91. Ward JI et al. Haemophilus influenzae type b vaccines: lessons for the future. *Pediatrics* 1988;81:886.
92. Redd SC et al. The role of human immunodeficiency virus infection in pneumococcal bacteremia in San Francisco residents. *J Infect Dis* 1990;162:1012.
93. Prevention of pneumococcal disease: recommendations of the Advisory Committee on Immunization Practices (ACIP). *MMWR* 1997;46:1
94. Polk RE. Drug–drug interactions with ciprofloxacin and other fluoroquinolones. *Am J Med* 1989;87 (Suppl 5A):76S.
95. Kaplan SL et al. Management of infections due to antibiotic-resistant Streptococcus pneumoniae. *Clin Micro Rev* 1998;11:628.
96. John CC. Treatment failure with use of a third-generation cephalosporin for penicillin-resistant pneumococcal meningitis: case report and review. *Clin Infect Dis* 1994;18:188.
97. Viladrich PF et al. Evaluation of vancomycin therapy for therapy of adult pneumococcal meningitis. *Antimicrob Agents Chemother* 1991;35:2467.
98. Friedland IR et al. Failure of chloramphenicol therapy in penicillin-resistant pneumococcal meningitis. *Lancet* 1992;339:405.
99. NCCLS. Performance standards for antimicrobial susceptibility testing. Document M100-S5. 1995;15 NCCLS, Wayne, PA.
100. Friedland IR et al. Evaluation of antimicrobial regimens for treatment of experimental penicillin- and cephalosporin-resistant pneumococcal meningitis. *Antimicrob Agents Chemother* 1993;37:1630.
101. Nau R et al. Rifampin reduces early mortality in experimental Streptococcus pneumoniae meningitis. *J Infect Dis* 1999;179:1557.
102. Bryan SC et al. "Comparably massive" penicillin G therapy in renal failure. *Ann Intern Med* 1975;82:189.
103. Farber BF et al. Retrospective study of the toxicity of preparations of vancomycin from 1974 to 1981. *Antimicrob Agents Chemother* 1983;23:138.
104. Levitz RE et al. Trimethoprim-sulfamethoxazole for bacterial meningitis. *Ann Intern Med* 1984;100:881.
105. Rodriguez-Barradas MC et al. Antibody to capsular polysaccharides of Streptococcus pneumoniae after vaccination of human immunodeficiency virus-infected subjects with 23-valent pneumococcal vaccine. *J Infect Dis* 1992;165:553.
106. Berk SL et al. Meningitis caused by gram-negative bacilli. *Ann Intern Med* 1980;93:253.
107. Corrado ML et al. Designing appropriate therapy in the treatment of gram-negative bacillary meningitis. *JAMA* 1982;248:71.
108. Tauber MG et al. Antibiotic therapy, endotoxin

concentrations in cerebrospinal fluid, and brain edema in experimental *Escherichia coli* meningitis in rabbits. *J Infect Dis* 1987;156:456.
109. Cherubin CE et al. Experience with the use of cefotaxime in the treatment of bacterial meningitis. *Am J Med* 1986;80:398.
110. Overturf GD et al. Treatment of bacterial meningitis with ceftizoxime. *Antimicrob Agents Chemother* 1984;25:258.
111. McCracken GH et al. Intraventricular gentamicin therapy in gram-negative bacillary meningitis in infancy. *Lancet* 1980;1:787.
112. Swartz MN. Intraventricular use of aminoglycosides in the treatment of gram-negative bacillary meningitis: conflicting views. *J Infect Dis* 1981;143:293.
113. Lentnek AL et al. Aztreonam in the treatment of gram-negative bacterial meningitis. *Rev Infect Dis* 1991;13(Suppl 7):S586.
114. Wong VK et al. Imipenem/cilastatin treatment of bacterial meningitis in children. *Pediatr Infect Dis J* 1991;10:122.
115. Calandra G et al. Factors predisposing to seizures in seriously ill infected patients receiving antibiotics: experience with imipenem/cilastatin. *Am J Med* 1988;84:911.
116. Eng RHK et al. Seizure propensity with imipenem. *Arch Intern Med* 1989;149:1881.
117. Klugman K et al. Randomized comparison of meropenem with cefotaxime for treatment of bacterial meningitis. *Antimicrob Agents Chemother* 1995;39:1140.
118. Odio CM et al. Prospective, randomized, investigator-blinded study of the efficacy and safety of meropenem vs. cefotaxime therapy in bacterial meningitis in children. *Pediatric Infect Dis J* 1999;18:581.
119. Wolff M et al. Penetration of ciprofloxacin into cerebrospinal fluid of patients with bacterial meningitis. *Antimicrob Agents Chemother* 1987;31:899.
120. Hooper DC et al. Fluoroquinolone antimicrobial agents. *N Engl J Med* 1991;324:384.117.
121. Parsley TL et al. Synergistic activity of trimethoprim and amikacin against gram-negative bacilli. *Antimicrob Agents Chemother* 1977;12:349.
122. Gardner P et al. Infections of central nervous system shunts. *Med Clin North Am* 1985;69:297.
123. Yogev R et al. Neurosurgical shunt infections. A review. *Childs Brain* 1980;6:74.
124. Schoenbaum SC et al. Infections of cerebrospinal fluid shunts: epidemiology, clinical manifestations, and therapy. *J Infect Dis* 1975;131:543.
125. Yogev R. Cerebrospinal fluid shunt infections: a personal view. *Pediatr Infect Dis J* 1985;4:113.
126. Walters BC et al. Cerebrospinal fluid shunt infection. *J Neurosurg* 1984;60:1014.
127. Younger JJ et al. Coagulase-negative staphylococci isolated from cerebrospinal fluid shunts: importance of slime production, species identification, and shunt removal to clinical outcome. *J Infect Dis* 1987;156:548.
128. Shapiro S et al. Origin of organisms infecting ventricular shunts. *Neurosurgery* 1988;22:868.
129. Gump DW. Vancomycin for treatment of bacterial meningitis. *Rev Infect Dis* 1981;3(Suppl):S289.
130. Brummett RE et al. Vancomycin- and erythromycin-induced hearing loss in humans. *Antimicrob Agents Chemother* 1989;33:791.
131. Polk RE et al. Vancomycin and the red-man syndrome: pharmacodynamics of histamine release. *J Infect Dis* 1988;157:502.
132. Sahai J et al. Influence of antihistamine pretreatment on vancomycin-induced red-man syndrome. *J Infect Dis* 1989;160:876.
133. Bayston R. Epidemiology, diagnosis, treatment and prevention of cerebrospinal fluid shunt infections. *Neurosurg Clin North Am* 2001;36:703.
134. Mathisen GE et al. Brain abscess. *Clin Infect Dis* 1997;25:763.
135. Mampalam TJ et al. Trends in the management of bacterial brain abscesses: a review of 102 cases over 17 years. *Neurosurgery* 1988;23:451.
136. Yoshikawa TT et al. The aching head. Intracranial suppuration due to head and neck infections. *Infect Dis Clin North Am* 1988;2:265.
137. Patrick CC et al. Current concepts in the pathogenesis and management of brain abscesses in children. *Pediatr Clin North Am* 1988;35:625.
138. Saez-Llorens X et al. Brain abscess in infants and children. *Pediatr Infect Dis J* 1989;8:449.
139. Rosenblum ML et al. Controversies in the management of brain abscesses. *Clin Neurosurg* 1986;33:603.
140. de Louvois J. The bacteriology and chemotherapy of brain abscess. *J Antimicrob Chemother* 1978;4:395.
141. Gossling J. Occurrence and pathogenicity of the Streptococcus milleri group. *Rev Infect Dis* 1988;10:257.
142. Luft BJ et al. Toxoplasmic encephalitis in AIDS. *Clin Infect Dis* 1992;15:211.
143. Simpson GL et al. Nocardial infections in the immunocompromised host: a detailed study in a defined population. *Rev Infect Dis* 1981;3:492.
144. Del Brutto OH et al. Therapy for neurocysticercosis: a reappraisal. *Clin Infect Dis* 1993;17:730.
145. Rosenblum ML et al. Nonoperative treatment of brain abscesses in selected high-risk patients. *J Neurosurg* 1980;52:217.
146. Black P et al. Penetration of brain abscess by systemically administered antibiotics. *J Neurosurg* 1973;38:705.
147. de Louvois J et al. Inactivation of penicillin by purulent exudates. *BMJ* 1977;1:998.
148. Yamamoto M et al. Penetration of intravenous antibiotics into brain abscesses. *Neurosurgery* 1993;33:44.
149. Warner JF et al. Metronidazole therapy of anaerobic bacteremia, meningitis, and brain abscess. *Arch Intern Med* 1979;139:167.
150. Levy RM et al. Vancomycin penetration of a brain abscess: case report and review of the literature. *Neurosurgery* 1986;18:632.
151. Tice AD et al. Outpatient parenteral antimicrobial therapy for central nervous system infections. *Clin Infect Dis* 1999;29:1394.
152. Snavely SR et al. The neurotoxicity of antibacterial agents. *Ann Intern Med* 1984;101:92.
153. Smilack JD et al. Tetracyclines, chloramphenicol, erythromycin, clindamycin, and metronidazole. *Mayo Clin Proc* 1991:66:1270.
154. Lorber B. Listeriosis. State-of-the-art clinical article. *Clin Infect Dis* 1997; 24:1.
155. Spitzer PG et al. Treatment of Listeria monocytogenes infection with trimethoprim-sulfamethoxazole: case report and review of the literature. *Rev Infect Dis* 1986;8:427.
156. Tuomanen E et al. Nonsteroidal anti-inflammatory agents in the therapy for experimental pneumococcal meningitis. *J Infect Dis* 1987;155:985.
157. Cartwright KA. Early management of meningococcal disease. *Infect Dis Clin North Am* 1999;13:661.
158. van de Beek D et al. Clinical features and prognostic factors in adults with bacterial meningitis. *N Engl J Med* 2004;352:1849.

CHAPTER 59

Endocarditis

Annie Wong-Beringer and Michelle Lee

INFECTIVE ENDOCARDITIS

Infective endocarditis (IE), a microbial infection of the heart valves or other endocardial tissue, usually is associated with an underlying cardiac defect. IE used to be classified as either "acute bacterial endocarditis" or "subacute bacterial endocarditis," based on the clinical presentation and course of the untreated disease. This classification system is nonspecific, however, and it does not account for many nonbacterial causes of endocarditis, such as chlamydiae, rickettsiae, and fungi. Hence, the current system based on the causative organism is preferred because it provides information regarding the probable course of the disease, the likelihood of underlying heart disease, and the appropriate antimicrobial regimens.[1]

Pathogenesis[1,2]

The pathogenesis of endocarditis involves a complex series of events that ultimately results in the formation of an infected platelet β fibrin thrombus on the valve surface. This thrombus is called a *vegetation.*

The first step in the formation of the vegetation involves modification of the endocardial surface, which is normally nonthrombogenic. In patients with rheumatic heart disease, endocardial injury occurs as a result of immune complex deposition or hemodynamic disturbances. Valvular insufficiency caused by aortic stenosis or ventricular septal defects can produce regurgitant blood flow, high-pressure gradients, or narrow orifices, resulting in turbulence and endocardial damage.

Once the endocardial surface of the valve is traumatized, small, sterile thrombi consisting of platelets and fibrin are deposited, forming the lesion called *nonbacterial thrombotic endocarditis* (NBTE). NBTE occurs most commonly on the atrial surfaces of the mitral and tricuspid valves and on the ventricular surface of the aortic valve.

NBTE serves as a nidus for microbial colonization during periods of bacteremia. Table 59-1 lists procedures that

Table 59-1 Cardiac Conditions for Which Prophylaxis is Recommended

Cardiac Conditions
Prophylaxis Recommended
• Prosthetic cardiac valves
• Previous bacterial endocarditis
• Congenital heart disease (CHD)
– Unrepaired cyanotic CHD, including palliative shunts and conduits
– Completely repaired congenital heart defect with prosthetic material device during the first 6 months after the procedure
– Repaired CHD with residual defects at or adjacent to the site of the prosthetic device or patch
– Mitral valve prolapse with valvular regurgitation and/or thickened leaflets
• Cardiac transplantation recipients who develop cardiac valvulopathy

Adapted from reference 230, with permission.

cause bacteremia. Organisms such as *Streptococcus viridans, Enterococcus* species, *Staphylococcus aureus, Staphylococcus epidermidis, Pseudomonas aeruginosa,* and *Candida albicans* possess adherence factors that facilitate their colonization. In particular, platelet aggregation has been shown to be an important virulence factor in experimental streptococcal endocarditis; larger vegetations and multifocal embolic spread have been associated with strains that aggregate platelets.[3] Once the NBTE lesion becomes colonized by microorganisms, the surface is rapidly covered with a sheath of fibrin and platelets. This avascular encasement provides an environment protected from host defenses and is conducive to further bacterial replication and vegetation growth. Progression of the infection can be interrupted at any time by various host defense mechanisms, including blocking antibodies that interfere with bacterial adherence, serum bactericidal complement activity, hemodynamic forces that dislodge poorly adherent bacteria, and circulating prophylactic antibiotics.

The vegetation is thought to propagate by continuous reseeding of the thrombus by circulating organisms. As the vegetation enlarges, it takes on a laminar appearance caused by the alternating layers of bacteria and platelet βfibrin deposits. The bacterial colony count can be as high as 10^4 to 10^5 bacteria per gram of valvular vegetation.

Endocarditis can result in life-threatening hemodynamic disturbances and embolic episodes. Without antimicrobial therapy and surgical intervention, IE is virtually 100% fatal. Because of bacterial proliferation to high densities in the fibrin mesh protected from normal host defenses, cure of infection requires prolonged therapy of 4 to 6 weeks with relapse not uncommon.

Epidemiology

Among the leading causes of life-threatening infectious disease syndromes, IE accounts for approximately 15,000 to 20,000 new cases per year in the United States.[6] The overall incidence appears to have remained stable over time; however, health care-associated IE has emerged as a result of increased use of invasive medical devices and procedures (e.g., intravenous catheters, hyperalimentation lines, pacemakers, dialysis shunts) and will undoubtedly contribute to an increase in IE.[1] The mean patient age reportedly has shifted from <30 years in the 1920s to above 55 years today.[6,7] This increase in age is thought to be related to (a) a decline in the incidence of acute rheumatic fever and rheumatic heart disease counterbalanced by degenerative valvular disease in an increasing elderly population, (b) the increasing longevity of the general population, and (c) increased exposure to more intense and invasive medical procedures in both the overall and the aging populations. Men are affected more often than women (roughly 2:1), and the disease remains uncommon in children, primarily in association with underlying congenital cardiac defect and nosocomial catheter-related bacteremia in infants.[1]

Predisposing Factors

In general, any structural cardiac defect that leads to the turbulence of blood flow predisposes to the development of IE. Rheumatic heart disease was at one time the most common underlying cardiac defect associated with endocarditis; however, the proportion of cases related to rheumatic heart disease have declined substantially to 25% or less in developed countries while remaining the predominant defect among patients in developing countries. Mitral valve prolapse with thickened leaflets and valvular redundancy is a recognized predisposing risk to IE, with a documented occurrence rate of 10%. Clinical presentation is often subtle with lower associated mortality in these individuals compared with left-sided IE of other types. In the absence of underlying valvular defects, degenerative cardiac lesions, such as calcified mitral annulus secondary to atherosclerotic cardiovascular disease and postmyocardial infarction thrombus, may be a significant risk factor predisposing the elderly to IE. In one series of native valve endocarditis cases, 50% of patients aged 60 years and above had degenerative cardiac lesions; however, the actual contribution of these lesions is unknown.[8] The intravenous (IV) drug users constitute a unique population at greatest risk for recurrent and polymicrobial IE. In addition, health care-related IE occurs with increasing frequency among hospitalized critically ill patients and others who are subjected to IV access procedures or invasive medical device placement (hemodialysis shunts or fistulas, intracardiac prosthesis, central venous pressure monitoring lines, hyperalimentation lines, defibrillators, permanent cardiac pacemakers).[1]

In a prospective cohort of 1,779 patients with IE, hemodialysis-dependency (8%) and diabetes mellitus (16%) were identified as the two most common demographic characteristics besides a history of congenital heart disease (12%).[7] Up to 25% of all cases were acquired in health care-related settings. Notably, in the United States, health care-associated IE was more likely to occur compared with community acquisition.

Bacteriology

Overall, streptococci and staphylococci are identified as the cause of 80% to 90% of cases of IE. Historically, viridans streptococci have been the predominant causative pathogens in IE, accounting for 60% to 80% of all cases.[1] When comparing epidemiologic studies in the aggregate over the past decades, however, staphylococci have assumed increased importance as a cause of IE. Viridans streptococci remain the predominant cause of IE in children and in young women with isolated mitral valve involvement.[1]

Staphylococcus aureus is identified as the leading cause of IE (40%) in one US study and confirmed in another large multinational study at 32%.[6,7] Acquisition of IE in nearly half was presumed to be health care-related, supporting a low threshold to evaluate underlying IE in the setting of health care-related *S. aureus* bacteremia. More importantly, strains exhibiting methicillin-resistance account for up to 40% of IE cases involving *S. aureus*.[6,7]

Endocarditis in IV drug users often is caused by *S. aureus*, whereas prosthetic valve endocarditis is more commonly caused by coagulase-negative staphylococci, such as *S. epidermidis*. Gram-negative bacilli and fungi together account for <10% of all endocarditis cases, which usually are associated with IV drug use, valvular prostheses, and hospital IV access procedures. Endocarditis caused by anaerobes and other organisms is rare. Polymicrobial infective endocarditis (caused by at least two organisms), although uncommon in the typical patient, is being recognized more frequently in IV drug users and postoperative patients. Candida species, *S. aureus*, *P. aeruginosa*, *Serratia marcescens*, and nonβgroup D streptococci are the organisms involved most frequently.

Site of Involvement

The site of heart valve involvement is determined by the underlying cardiac defect and the infecting organism.[1,2,6,9] The mitral valve is affected in >85% of cases caused by viridans streptococci when rheumatic heart disease is the underlying abnormality. The tricuspid valve is the common site of involvement in staphylococcal endocarditis associated with IV drug use. In addition, more than one heart valve may be affected simultaneously. Overall, the mitral valve is affected slightly more often than the aortic (55%), followed by the tricuspid (20%) and the pulmonic (1%) valves. Some studies have shown that aortic valve involvement is increasing in frequency and is associated with higher morbidity and mortality.

STREPTOCOCCUS VIRIDANS ENDOCARDITIS

Clinical Presentation

1. A.G., a 57-year-old, 60-kg man with chief complaints of fatigue, a persistent low-grade fever, night sweats, arthralgias, and a 7-kg unintentional weight loss, is admitted to the hospital for evaluation. Visual inspection reveals a cachectic, ill-appearing man in no acute distress. Physical examination on admission is significant for a grade III/IV diastolic murmur with mitral regurgitation (insufficiency) that has increased from pre-existing murmur, a temperature of 100.5F, petechial skin lesions, subungual splinter hemorrhages, and Janeway lesions on the soles of both feet (Figs. 59-1, 59-2, and 59-5). Nail clubbing, Roth spots, or Osler's nodes are not evident (Figs. 59-3 and 59-4). The remainder of his physical examination is unremarkable. A.G.'s medical history is significant for mitral valve prolapse and, more recently, a dental procedure involving the extraction of four wisdom teeth. The history of his present illness is noteworthy for the development of the aforementioned symptoms about 2 weeks after the dental procedure (about 2 months before admission). His only current medication is ibuprofen 600 mg QID.

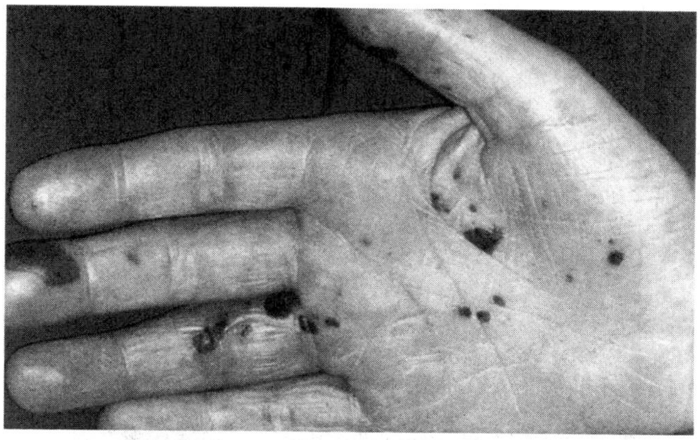

FIGURE 59-1 Janeway lesions. Extensive ecchymotic embolic lesions in a case of acute bacterial endocarditis.

Relevant laboratory results include hemoglobin (Hgb), 11.4 g/dL; hematocrit (Hct), 34%; reticulocyte count, 0.5%; white blood cell (WBC) count, 85,000/mm^3 with 65% polys and 1% bands; blood urea nitrogen (BUN), 21 mg/dL; and serum creatinine (SrCr), 1.8 mg/dL. A urinalysis (UA) reveals 2+ proteinuria and 10 to 20 red blood cells (RBC) per high-power field (HPF). The erythrocyte sedimentation rate (ESR) on admission is elevated at 66 mm/hr and the rheumatoid factor (RF) is positive. Results from a transthoracic echocardiogram (ECG) were unrevealing.

To establish the diagnosis of IE, three blood cultures were obtained over 24 hours. All cultures obtained on day 1 are reported to be growing α-hemolytic streptococci. While confirmation and speciation of the organism is being performed, A.G. is started on penicillin G, 2 million units IV Q 4 hr (12 million U/day), and gentamicin, 120 mg (loading dose) followed by 60 mg Q 12 hr. Antimicrobial susceptibility results are pending. What clinical manifestations and laboratory abnormalities in A.G. are consistent with IE?

[SI units: Hgb, 114 g/L (normal, 140–180); Hct, 0.34 (normal, 0.39–0.49); reticulocyte count, 0.005 (normal, 0.001–0.024); WBC count, 85 × 10/L

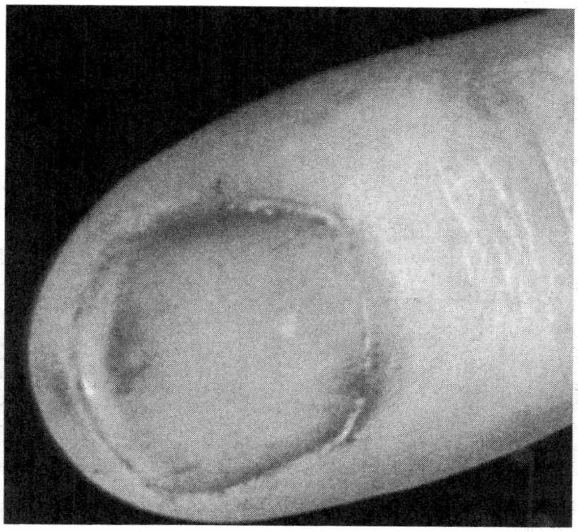

FIGURE 59-2 Splinter hemorrhages in the nailbed.

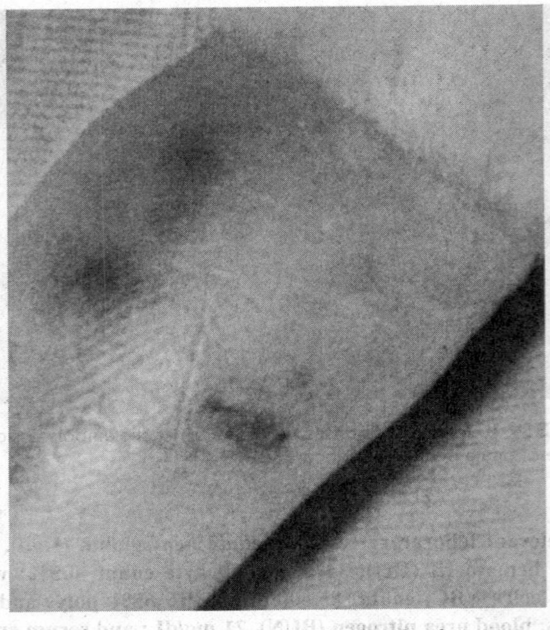

FIGURE 59-3 Osler's nodes on the tip of the index finger in a case of endocarditis caused by *Staphylococcus aureus.*

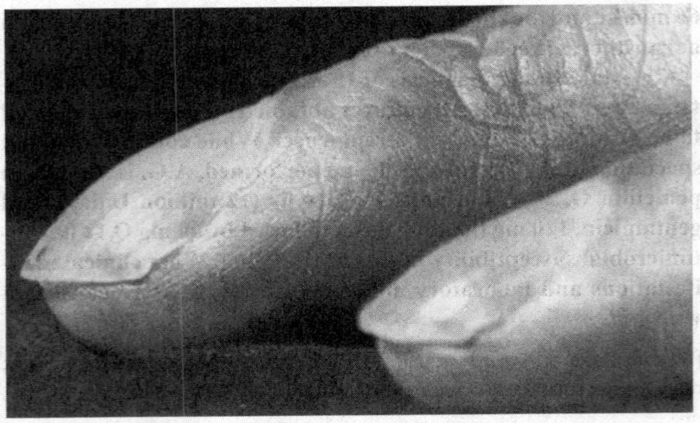

FIGURE 59-4 Clubbing of the fingers in longstanding subacute bacterial endocarditis.

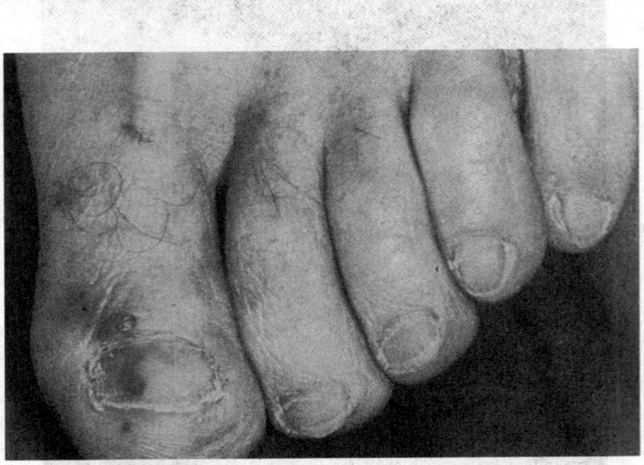

FIGURE 59-5 Petechial skin lesions in a case of acute staphylococcal endocarditis.

with 0.65 polys and 0.01 bands (normal, 3.2–9.8 with 0.54–0.62 polys and 0.03–0.05 bands); BUN, 7.5 mmol/L of urea (normal, 2.9–8.9); and SrCr, 159 mmol/L (normal, 53–133)]

The clinical presentation of IE is highly variable and can involve almost any organ system.[1] A.G. appears pale and chronically ill and represents the typical patient with subacute disease (e.g., that caused by viridans streptococci). Nonspecific complaints consistent with endocarditis in A.G. include fatigue, weight loss, fever, night sweats, and arthralgias. Only fever is present in most (90%) patients with endocarditis. The fever is characteristically low grade and remittent, with peaks in the afternoon and evening. The temperature rarely exceeds 103°F in subacute disease.[1] Fever may be absent or minimal in patients with congestive heart failure (CHF), chronic renal and liver failure, prior use of antimicrobial agents, or IE caused by less virulent organisms.[1] Musculoskeletal complaints (e.g., arthralgias, myalgias, and back pain) are common and may mimic rheumatic disease. Other symptoms can include lethargy, anorexia, malaise, nausea, and vomiting.[1] Because signs and symptoms are nonspecific and subtle, diagnosis often is difficult. In addition, the time from bacteremia to diagnosis often is prolonged because of the insidious progression of symptoms.[1] In particular, delayed diagnosis occurs more commonly in the elderly. Fever may be absent in 30% to 40% of patients >60 years of age, whereas it can be present in >90% of patients <40 years of age. Fewer of these patients have new or changed heart murmurs. The most common presenting complaints in the elderly with endocarditis are confusion, anorexia, fatigue, and weakness, which may be readily attributable to stroke, heart failure, or syncope.

The temporal relationship between A.G.'s dental procedure and the onset of symptoms makes it the most obvious cause of bacteremia and subsequent endocarditis. Although it is assumed that prophylactic antibiotics were administered before the procedure, endocarditis can develop despite apparently adequate chemoprophylaxis.[10]

A.G. is noted to have an increase in his pre-existing diastolic murmur with mitral insufficiency, a finding consistent with endocarditis. Cardiac murmurs are present in >85% of patients with endocarditis. Murmurs frequently are absent, however, in patients with acute disease (e.g., staphylococcal endocarditis), right-sided disease (e.g., endocarditis in IV drug users), or mural infection.[1]

A.G. exhibits several peripheral manifestations of infective endocarditis, including conjunctival petechiae, Janeway lesions, and splinter hemorrhages. Overall, peripheral manifestations are found in 10% to 50% of cases, but none of these is pathognomonic for IE. These manifestations are usually a result of septic embolization of vegetations to distal sites or immune complex deposition. Mucocutaneous petechial lesions of the conjunctiva, mouth, or pharynx are present in 20% to 40% of patients, especially those with longstanding disease. These lesions generally are small, nontender, and hemorrhagic in appearance and occur as a result of vasculitis or peripheral embolization. Janeway lesions are painless, hemorrhagic, macular plaques most commonly found on the palms and soles (Fig. 59-1). Splinter hemorrhages are nonspecific findings that appear as red to brown linear streaks in the proximal portion of the fingers or toenails (Fig. 59-2). Other findings can include

Roth spots (small, flame-shaped retinal hemorrhages with pale white centers found near the optic nerve) and Osler's nodes (purplish, nonhemorrhagic, painful nodules that develop on the subcutaneous pads of the fingers and toes or on palms and soles) (Fig. 59-3). Clubbing (broadening and thickening) of the nails also may be observed in patients with prolonged disease[1,11] (Fig. 59-4). Petechial skin lesions also are seen (Fig. 59-5).

Several laboratory findings are consistent with IE in A.G. A low Hgb and Hct with normal red cell indices suggest anemia of chronic disease. Of patients with subacute disease, 70% to 90% will have a normochromic, normocytic anemia as part of their initial presentation. Leukocytosis with a left shift, although not evident in A.G., commonly is seen in those with acute, fulminant disease such as staphylococcal endocarditis. The ESR nearly always is elevated in IE, but this finding is nonspecific and can be associated with several other disease entities. Rheumatoid factor (an IgM antiglobulin) and circulating immune complexes can be detected in most patients with longstanding disease, but both are nonspecific findings.[1]

Major embolic episodes and infarction involving the kidney, spleen, lung, and brain develop as secondary complications in up to one-third of cases.[1] A.G. exhibits some degree of renal damage, as evidenced by moderate hematuria and proteinuria. Erythrocyte and leukocyte cast formation also may be present. Alterations in A.G.'s renal function (increased BUN and creatinine) probably are a result of immune complex deposition (diffuse glomerulonephritis) or secondary to renal embolization (focal glomerulonephritis). Renal impairment, however, usually is reversible with the institution of effective antimicrobial therapy.[1,11]

Cardiac complications occur most frequently. CHF, the most common cause of death in IE, is the most compelling indication for surgery. Infection-induced valvular damage is responsible for valvular insufficiency causing heart failure.[1,11] As many as two-thirds of patients with endocarditis develop CHF. Aortic valve infection is more frequently associated with CHF than that of mitral valve infection. Other manifestations include paravalvular abscesses, pulmonary edema, and pericarditis.[11] Mitral valve injury caused by viridans streptococci generally is better tolerated hemodynamically than aortic valve injury caused by staphylococci. Although A.G. has no apparent signs of overt heart failure, he should be monitored closely for the development of hemodynamic instability.

Neurologic complications rank second to cardiac complications in frequency, but they may be the leading cause of death in patients with endocarditis. Stroke is the most common neurologic complication of IE.[11] A stroke syndrome in a patient with underlying valvular abnormalities should prompt the clinician to rule out IE. Other clinical manifestations include headache, mental status change, stroke or transient ischemic attack, seizures, brain abscess, or intracranial mycotic aneurysms.[1,11] Neurologic symptoms were noted in as many as 35% of patients in a study of *S. aureus* endocarditis in patients who were not drug addicts. A mortality rate of 74% was found for those with major neurologic manifestations compared with 56% in those without.[12]

Splenomegaly, although not part of A.G.'s findings, occurs in 20% to 60% of all cases and is more common in patients with a prolonged subacute presentation. In addition, metastatic abscesses can develop in virtually any organ secondary to systemic septic embolization. The most commonly involved metastatic foci are the spleen, kidney, liver, and iliac and mesenteric arteries.[11]

Diagnosis

2. How was the diagnosis of IE established in A.G.?

Blood Cultures

Although A.G.'s medical history (mitral valve prolapse, recent dental procedure) and clinical presentation are highly suggestive of IE, blood culture is the single most important diagnostic workup of a patient suspected to have IE.[1] Bacteremia secondary to endocarditis is continuous and low grade; >50% of the cultures have only 1 to 30 bacteria/mL. Despite the low concentration of organisms, bacteremia (when present) results in at least one of the first two blood cultures being positive in 95% of cases.[1] Administration of antibiotics within the previous 2 weeks may significantly decrease this yield.[13]

At least three sets of blood cultures collected by separate venipunctures should be obtained over the first 24 hours of presentation.[1] In a "stable" patient such as A.G. who has had the disease for several weeks or months, it is important to establish the exact microbiologic cause before initiating antimicrobial therapy. Patients who are acutely ill should have empiric therapy started as soon as the appropriate cultures are obtained to avoid further valvular damage or other complications.[1]

Echocardiography

Echocardiography is a valuable tool in establishing early diagnosis, identifying patients at high risk for complications, and optimizing the timing and mode of surgical intervention by detecting and monitoring associated pathologic changes such as valvular abscess, as well as the presence and size of vegetations.[1,14,15] In an ECG, high-frequency sound waves are applied, and the reflection by body tissues is processed by a transducer to create images. The transducer may be placed on the chest (transthoracic echocardiogram [TTE]) or in the esophagus (transesophageal echocardiogram [TEE]).[14] TTE is a rapid and noninvasive procedure with a 98% specificity for vegetations. Sensitivity for vegetations may be <60% to 70%, however, for adult patients with obesity, hyperinflated lungs caused by emphysema, or a prosthetic valve. TEE is more costly and invasive, but is significantly more sensitive in detecting vegetations while maintaining high specificity. All patients with suspected IE should have an ECG on admission and repeated during their course, as necessary.[14] Two cost-effective analyses support the increased use of TEE to define antibiotic therapy duration for intravascular catheter-related *S. aureus* bacteremia (2 vs. 4 weeks)[16,18] In particular, compared with TTE, TEE is superior in the diagnosis of pacemaker IE and IE in the elderly, and should be performed in all patients with a complicated course in whom perivalvular extension is suspected unless contraindicated by underlying esophageal disease.[1] A.G. has a negative TTE result on admission. Given the high clinical suspicion for IE in A.G., a follow-up TEE is recommended to rule out a false–negative result because TTE is less sensitive than TEE and that initial perivalvular abscesses may be missed by both TTE and TEE when performed early in a patient's illness. Documentation of valvular morphology, the presence and size of vegetations, ventricular function, and valvular insufficiency is important to establish a baseline and, on completion of therapy, to guide future medical management and appropriate timing of intervention.[9]

In summary, IE should be suspected in any patient who has a documented fever and heart murmur. Prior cardiac disease, peripheral manifestations, splenomegaly, various laboratory abnormalities, and a positive ECG strengthen the diagnosis, but microbiologic documentation is the most important factor in confirming IE. Disease entities with overlapping clinical presentation and laboratory abnormalities should be excluded using the appropriate tests.[1]

Standardized criteria (Duke criteria) for the clinical assessment of patients suspected of having IE were proposed by a group at Duke University in 1994.[19] Limitations of the Duke criteria, such as misclassification of culture-negative endocarditis and the overly broad categorization of "possible" causes as well as the increasing role of TEE and the relative risk of IE with *S. aureus* bacteremia, were addressed in a modified version.[20] Diagnostic criteria for IE are listed in Table 59-2 and Table 59-3, which integrate clinical, laboratory, microbiologic, and echocardiographic data.[9,20] Based on published evidence involving nearly 2,000 patients, the American Heart Association (AHA) recommends in its 2005 statement that the modified Duke criteria be used as the primary diagnostic schema to evaluate patients suspected of IE.[9]

A.G. possesses one major criterion (positive blood cultures) and three minor criteria (fever, predisposing heart condition, vascular and immunologic phenomena); therefore, he meets the diagnostic criteria for definite IE.[20]

Table 59-2 Definition of Infective Endocarditis (IE) According to the Modified Duke Criteria

Definite Infective Endocarditis

PATHOLOGIC CRITERIA

Microorganisms: Demonstrated by culture or histology examination of a vegetation, a vegetation that has embolized, or an intracardiac abscess specimen, or

Pathologic lesions: Vegetation or intracardiac abscess confirmed by histologic examination showing active endocarditis

CLINICAL CRITERIA

Using specific definitions listed in Table 59-3; two major criteria *or* one major and three minor criteria *or* five minor criteria

Possible Infective Endocarditis

One major criterion and one minor criterion; or three minor criteria

Rejected

Firm alternative diagnosis explaining evidence of IE; *or*

Resolution of IE syndrome with antibiotic therapy for <4 days; *or*

No pathologic evidence of infective endocarditis at surgery or autopsy, with antibiotic therapy for <4 days; or not meet criteria for possible IE as above

Modifications shown in bold.
From reference 20, with permission.

Table 59-3 Definitions of Terminology Used in the Modified Duke Criteria for the Diagnosis of Infective Endocarditis (IE)

Major Criteria

Blood culture positive for infective endocarditis

- Typical microorganisms consistent with IE from two separate blood cultures
  1. *Viridans streptococci, Streptococcus bovis,* HACEK group, *or*
  2. ***Staphylococcus aureus*** or community-acquired enterococci in the absence of a primary focus, *or*
- Microorganisms consistent with IE from persistently positive blood cultures defined as follows:
  1. At least two positive blood cultures drawn >12 hr apart, *or*
  2. All of three or a majority of four separate cultures of blood (with first and last sample drawn at least 1 hr apart)
- **Single positive blood culture for *Coxiella burnetti* or antiphase 1 IgG antibody titer > 1:800**

Evidence of endocardial involvement

- Echocardiogram positive for IE **(TEE recommended for patients with prosthetic valves, rated at least "possible IE" by clinical criteria or complicated IE [paravalvular abscess]; TEE as first test in other patients)** defined as follows:
  1. Oscillating intracardiac Masson valve or supporting structures, in the path of regurgitant jets, or on implanted material in the absence of an alternative anatomic explanation; *or*
  2. Abscess, *or*
  3. New partial dehiscence of prosthetic valve
- New valvular regurgitation (worsening or changing of pre-existing murmur not sufficient)

Minor Criteria

- Predisposition: Predisposing heart condition or intravenous drug use
- Fever >38°C (100.4°F)
- *Vascular Phenomena:* Major arterial emboli, septic pulmonary infarcts, mycotic aneurysm, intracranial hemorrhage, conjunctival hemorrhages, Janeway lesions
- *Immunologic Phenomena:* Glomerulonephritis, Osler's nodes, Roth spots, rheumatoid factor
- *Microbiologic Evidence:* Positive blood culture but not meeting major criterion as noted above or serologic evidence of active infection with organism consistent with IE
- **Echocardiographic minor criteria eliminated**

Modifications shown in bold.
Excludes single positive cultures for coagulase-negative staphylococci and organisms that do not cause endocarditis.
HACEK, *Haemophilus species, Actinobacillus actinomycetemcomitans, Cardiobacterium hominis, Eikenella* species, and *Kingella kingae*; TEE, transesophageal echocardiography
From reference 20, with permission.

Antimicrobial Therapy

General Principles

3. What would be a reasonable duration of antibiotic therapy for A.G.? When are serum bactericidal titers (SBT) useful in treating bacterial endocarditis?

The avascular nature of the vegetation results in an environment that is devoid of normal host defenses (e.g., phagocytic cells and complement); this permits uninhibited growth of bacteria.[2] Therefore, to eradicate the causative organism, high doses of a parenterally administered, bactericidal antibiotic generally are administered for 4 to 6 weeks.[1,21] For some infections, it may be necessary to use two antibiotics to achieve synergistic activity against the organism.[22] For example, the addition of an aminoglycoside to penicillin results in a more rapid and complete bactericidal effect against enterococci.[23]

Once an organism has been identified, its in vitro susceptibility pattern is determined by the minimum inhibitory concentration (MIC) for various antibiotics. Standard Kirby-Bauer disk testing is inadequate in the setting of IE to aid in selection of antibiotics without the quantitative information provided by the MIC.[1] In addition, the minimum bactericidal concentration (MBC) may be useful in detecting tolerant strains, particularly in the setting of unexplained slow response or treatment failure. Routine MBC determination is not recommended, however.[1] Treatment of endocarditis requires antibiotics with bactericidal activity; therefore, the serum concentration of the antibiotic must greatly exceed the MBC for the particular organism. For endocarditis caused by viridans streptococci acquired from the community, this usually is achieved without much difficulty because most isolates are sensitive to penicillin at an MIC of <0.125 mcg/mL; corresponding MBC are, at most, one or two tube dilutions higher.[24] The emergence of strains demonstrating resistance to penicillin and related β-lactams, such as ceftriaxone, is a significant problem, particularly among bloodstream isolates obtained from the nosocomial setting and neutropenic cancer patients.[24–27] The increasing prevalence of β-lactam-resistant clinical isolates highlights the importance of determining the MIC and continued close monitoring of the antibiotic susceptibility of viridans streptococci. An increasing number of reports have described suboptimal response to vancomycin therapy for the treatment of invasive infection caused by methicillin-resistant *Staphylococcus aureus* (MRSA) strains showing borderline susceptibility (MIC 2 mcg/mL).[28] Many such strains demonstrated tolerance to vancomycin as defined by a high MBC-to-MIC ratio (≥32).[29] Thus, these data support the need to determine MBC and possibly SBT (see below) in the setting where the treatment option for IE caused by *S. aureus* is limited to vancomycin and suboptimal response is observed.[29]

The SBT, commonly called a Schlichter test, is an in vitro modification of the MBC test. It measures the killing activity of the patient's serum (containing antibiotic) against the isolated organism.[30] To perform the test, a known inoculum of the patient's organism is added to serial dilutions of the patient's serum. The SBT is the highest dilution that kills 99% to 100% of the inoculum.

Much controversy surrounds the value of the SBT in monitoring therapy for IE, the usefulness of peak versus trough SBT, and the appropriate SBT endpoint required for successful treatment of bacterial endocarditis.[1,31] The lack of agreement is partly because of the nonstandardized method for performing SBT, such as the inoculum size used and the timing of SBT samples, which leads to difficulty in test interpretation and correlation with clinical outcome.[1,31] In one large, multicenter study using a standardized method, peak titers (dilutions) of ≥1:64 and trough titers of ≤1:32 were needed to predict bacteriologic cure in all patients.[31] On the other hand, the SBT was a poor predictor of failure, because many patients who were cured had much lower SBT (e.g., <1:8). Until an accepted, standardized method is established, routine performance of SBT is not recommended. The SBT test may be useful in the following situations: (a) when endocarditis is caused by relatively resistant organisms (e.g., relatively penicillin-resistant viridans streptococci, MIC 0.1–0.5 mcg/mL) when a synergistic combination of antibiotics might be beneficial; (b) when response to therapy has been suboptimal; and (c) when less well-established regimens are used for treatment.[1,30] Alternatively, in vitro synergy studies using the standard microtiter checkerboard tests or time-kill curves in broth may be performed to evaluate the synergistic potential of combination therapy in the above situations.[1]

4. What antibiotic regimens are most useful for the treatment of viridans streptococci endocarditis?

Patients with endocarditis caused by penicillin-sensitive strains of viridans streptococci and nonenterococcal group D streptococci (e.g., *S. bovis;* MIC <0.1 mcg/mL) can be treated with any one of three regimens as outlined in the 1995 AHA treatment guidelines.[21] The suggested regimens (Table 59-4) are associated with cure rates of up to 98% and include (a) high-dose parenteral penicillin for 4 weeks; (b) high-dose parenteral ceftriaxone for 4 weeks; and (c) 2 weeks of combined therapy with high-dose parenteral penicillin and an aminoglycoside.[4,21,32–37] Studies also indicate that combined therapy with once-daily dosing of ceftriaxone and an aminoglycoside for 2 weeks demonstrate comparable efficacy for selected patients.[38,39]

High-Dose Penicillin for 4 Weeks

The IV administration of 10 to 20 million units/day of penicillin G for 4 weeks resulted in a cure rate of 100% for 66 patients with nonenterococcal streptococcal endocarditis.[33] Another study using penicillin alone reported relapse in only 2 of 49 patients; however, both of these patients received <4 weeks of therapy.[37] The large range of 12 to 18 million units/day of penicillin is recommended to allow flexibility in dosing based on the patient's renal function and disease severity.

Single Daily Ceftriaxone for 4 Weeks

Ceftriaxone has been shown to have excellent in vitro activity against viridans streptococcal strains isolated from patients with endocarditis. In one study, all 49 strains of viridans streptococci and 11 strains of *S. bovis* were inhibited at a concentration of <0.125 mcg/mL of ceftriaxone; one strain of *S. sanguis* was inhibited at an MIC of 0.25 mcg/mL.[40] Although no direct comparative trials have been performed evaluating ceftriaxone against high-dose penicillin for the treatment of streptococcal endocarditis, current data (based on open-label studies of ceftriaxone) indicate an efficacy rate comparable to that of high-dose penicillin when treatment is given for 4 weeks.[41–42] Of the 70 assessable patients who received ceftriaxone 2 g as a single daily dose for 4 weeks, all were cured, except for 1 patient who had a probable relapse 3 months after completion of therapy. All strains of viridans streptococci were inhibited by ceftriaxone at an MIC of 0.25 mcg/mL in both studies. One study included only patients without cardiovascular risk factors or complications. Although the simplicity of single daily treatment with ceftriaxone is attractive for outpatient use, careful patient selection based on microbiologic, clinical, and host factors is critical to the success of treatment and the proper and

Table 59-4 Suggested Regimens for Therapy of Native Valve Endocarditis Caused by *Streptococcus viridans* and *Streptococcus bovis*

Antibiotic	*Dose[a,b] and Route*	*Duration*
Penicillin-Susceptible (Minimum Inhibitory Concentration = 0.12 mcg/mL)		
Aqueous crystalline penicillin G[c]	*Adult:* 12–18 million units/24 hr intravenously (IV) either continuously or in four to six equally divided doses *Pediatric:* 200,000 units/kg/24 hr IV (max: 20 million units/24 hr) either continuously or in four to six equally divided doses	4 wk
Ceftriaxone sodium[c]	*Adult:* 2 g once daily IV or intramuscularly (IM) *Pediatric:* 100 mg/kg once daily IV or IM	4 wk
Aqueous crystalline penicillin G	*Adult:* 12–18 million units/24 hr IV either continuously or in six equally divided doses *Pediatric:* 200,000 units/kg/24 hr IV (max: 20 million units/24 hr) either continuously or in six equally divided doses	2 wk
Ceftriaxone sodium	*Adult:* 2 g once daily IV or IM *Pediatric:* 100 mg/kg once daily IV or IM	
With gentamicin sulfate[d]	*Adult:* 3 mg/kg once daily IV or IM *Pediatric:* 3 mg/kg once daily IV or IM or in three equally divided doses	2 wk
Relatively Penicillin G Resistant (Minimum InhibitoryConcentration >0.1 mcg/mL and <0.5 mcg/mL)		
Aqueous crystalline penicillin G[e]	*Adult:* 24 million units/24 hr IV either continuously or in four to six equally divided doses *Pediatric:* 200,000–300,000 units/kg/24 hr IV (max: 20 million units/24 hr) either continuously or in four to six equally divided doses	4 wk
Ceftriaxone sodium	*Pediatric:* 100 mg/kg once daily IV or IM	
With gentamicin sulfate[d]	*Adult:* 3 mg/kg once daily IV or IM *Pediatric:* 3 mg/kg once daily IV or IM or in three equally divided doses	2 wk
β-Lactam Allergic Patients		
Vancomycin hydrochloride[f]	*Adult:* 30 mg/kg/24 hr IV in two equally divided doses (max: 2 g/24 hr unless serum concentrations are monitored) *Pediatric:* 40 mg/kg/24 hr IV in two or three equally divided doses (max: 2 g/24 hr unless serum concentrations are monitored)	4 wk

[a] Pediatric doses should not exceed that of a normal adult.
[b] Antibiotic doses for patients with impaired renal function should be modified appropriately. Vancomycin dosage should be reduced in patients with renal dysfunction; cephalosporin dosage may need to be reduced in patients with moderate to severe renal dysfunction.
[c] Preferred in most patients >65 years of age and in those with impairment of the eighth nerve or renal function.
[d] Two-week regimen not intended for patients with known cardiac or extracardiac abscess or for those with creatinine clearance of <20 mL/min, impaired eighth cranial nerve function or *Abiotrophia, Granullicatella, or Gemelia infection. Gentamicin dosage should be adjusted to achieve peak serum concentrations of 3–4 mcg/mL and trough serum concentrations of <1 mcg/mL when three divided doses are used; nomogram used for single daily dosing. Other potential nephrotoxic drugs should be used with caution in patients receiving gentamicin therapy.*
[e] Cefazoilin or other first-generation cephalosporins may be substituted for penicillin in patients whose penicillin hypersensitivity is not of the immediate type.
[f] Vancomycin dosage should be reduced in patients with impaired renal function. Vancomycin given on a mg/kg basis produces higher serum concentrations in obese patients than in lean patients. Therefore, in obese patients, dosing should be based on ideal body weight. Each dose of vancomycin should be infused over at least 1 hr to reduce the risk of the histamine-release red man syndrome. Peak serum concentrations of vancomycin should be obtained 1 hr after completion of the infusion and should be in the range of 30–45 mg/mL. Trough concentrations should be obtained within half an hour of the next dose and be in the range of 10–15 mcg/mL.
Adapted from reference 9, with permission.

timely management of potential complications. (See Question 32 for a detailed discussion of outpatient therapy.)

High-Dose Penicillin or Ceftriaxone Plus an Aminoglycoside for 2 Weeks

The combination of 2 weeks of streptomycin (or gentamicin) with 4 weeks of penicillin is synergistically bactericidal for most streptococci, including enterococci (see Question 16).[22,35] This in vitro synergy also has been correlated with a more rapid rate of eradication of viridans streptococci from cardiac vegetations in the rabbit model of endocarditis.[4] A shortened combination regimen consisting of high-dose penicillin G and streptomycin for 2 weeks is an effective alternative to the previously described regimens. The reported cure rate in 104 patients treated at the Mayo Clinic with this regimen was 99%.[34,35]

Although clinical experience with combination therapy has been primarily with penicillin and streptomycin, in vitro and animal data support that streptomycin and gentamicin are reasonably interchangeable. Gentamicin is more widely used in clinical practice and serum concentrations are more readily available to monitor efficacy and toxicities. Experimental data suggest that a gentamicin dosing interval of once versus thrice daily does not affect the relative efficacy of penicillin plus gentamicin for treatment of viridans streptococcal endocarditis.[36]

Combination therapy with ceftriaxone and an aminoglycoside for 2 weeks has also been evaluated in two studies.[37,38] In a noncomparative, open-label study, a 2-week course of ceftriaxone 2 g plus netilmicin (3 mg/kg) (both given once daily) resulted in a clinical cure of 87% in 48 evaluable patients.[38] A second open-label study compared ceftriaxone 2 g alone versus the combination of ceftriaxone 2 g plus gentamicin (3 mg/kg), both given once daily, for the treatment of endocarditis caused by penicillin-susceptible streptococci.[39] Patients were randomized to either regimen; 26 monotherapy recipients and 25 combination therapy recipients were evaluable. Clinical cure was observed in 96% of the patients in both groups at completion of therapy and at 3-month follow-up. This study excluded patients with suspected or documented cardiac or extracardiac abscesses and those with prosthetic valve endocarditis. Although the aminoglycoside agent (netilmicin or gentamicin) was administered as a single daily dose in both studies, all of the patients had measurable serum trough levels. Therefore, the efficacy of "extended-interval dosing" of aminoglycoside (whereby trough levels are not detectable, allowing a drug-free interval) in short-course combination therapy will need to be confirmed in future studies.

Based on available data, the 2-week regimen of penicillin or ceftriaxone plus an aminoglycoside appears to be efficacious for uncomplicated cases of penicillin-susceptible viridans streptococci endocarditis. It is not currently recommended for patients with extracardiac complications or intracardiac abscesses. Patients infected with *Abiotrophia* species (formerly known as nutritionally variant viridans streptococci) or viridans streptococci who have a penicillin MIC >0.1 mcg/mL, or patients who have prosthetic valve infections should not receive short-course therapy.[21]

Special Considerations

The risk of relapse may be higher in patients who have had symptoms for >3 months before the initiation of treatment.[1,21,42] These patients should be treated with 4 to 6 weeks of penicillin combined with an aminoglycoside for the first 2 weeks.[1,21,42]

Nutritionally deficient or variant streptococci (NVS) have been reclassified into a new genus, *Abiotrophia,* which includes *A. defectiva, A. adjacens* (renamed again as *Granulicatella adjacens*), and *A. elegans. Abiotrophia* species are slow-growing, fastidious organisms that are responsible for approximately 5% of IE cases. Previously, NVS was the cause of most of the cases of endocarditis diagnosed as "culture-negative" initially owing to its requirement for the addition of vitamin B_6 (pyridoxal HCl) to the culture media for laboratory growth. Laboratory identification is no longer a significant problem, however, because of current culture media and laboratory techniques.[24]

Nutritionally deficient or variant streptococci are less susceptible to penicillin when compared with other streptococci. Up to two-thirds of NVS organisms have relatively high MIC to penicillin (0.2–2.0 mcg/mL), and some show high-level resistance to penicillin (MIC >4 mcg/mL).[24] In addition, tolerance to penicillin has been described in many strains.[24] An animal model of endocarditis indicates that a penicillin–aminoglycoside (streptomycin or gentamicin) combination is significantly better than penicillin alone in reducing bacterial counts of these organisms.[43] More importantly, endocarditis caused by NVS is associated with greater morbidity and mortality compared with IE caused by other streptococci. Higher mortality rate (14% vs. 5%), more frequent complications of embolization (33% vs. 11%) and CHF (33% vs. 18%), and an increased rate of surgical intervention (33% vs. 18%) were observed in a study comparing 49 patients with NVS endocarditis versus 130 patients infected with other oral streptococci.[24] High rates of bacteriologic failure and relapse may be expected in patients despite completion of the treatment course for strains highly susceptible to penicillin.[24] All patients infected with NVS or *Abiotrophia* should receive 4 to 6 weeks of penicillin (or ampicillin) in combination with gentamicin.[21] A 6-week course of combination therapy with penicillin and gentamicin is recommended for patients with symptoms >3 months in duration and those with prosthetic valve endocarditis caused by these strains.[21,24] Patients with endocarditis caused by relatively resistant viridans streptococci with penicillin MIC of >0.5 mcg/mL or enterococci should receive a similar treatment regimen, as described above.[21]

Patients allergic to β-lactams should receive vancomycin 30 mg/kg/day divided into two doses for 4 to 6 weeks. In patients who have had minor reactions to penicillins (e.g., a delayed rash), a first-generation cephalosporin, such as cefazolin (1–2 g Q 6–8 hr), may be cautiously substituted. Although the addition of an aminoglycoside to a cephalosporin or vancomycin enhances bactericidal activity in vitro, it is unknown whether the addition of an aminoglycoside confers any additional clinical benefit.[21]

Regimen Selection

5. What factors must be considered in selecting a regimen for A.G.? Which regimen should be used for A.G.?

For most cases of endocarditis caused by penicillin-sensitive viridans streptococci (in patients not allergic to penicillin), all three of the aforementioned regimens are equally acceptable; therefore, the choice should be based on their relative advantages and disadvantages. The 2-week regimen requires the shortest hospital stay, but it has the disadvantage of possible ototoxicity and nephrotoxicity secondary to aminoglycoside administration. Therefore, it may be prudent to consider the use of penicillin or ceftriaxone alone for 4 weeks in older persons (>65 years) and those with impaired renal or vestibular function. For those with uncomplicated viridans streptococci endocarditis who can manage the technical aspects of outpatient therapy, ceftriaxone monotherapy offers the convenience of single daily administration. The combined regimen consisting of penicillin (or ampicillin) and an aminoglycoside for 4 to 6 weeks can be used for patients infected with NVS or relatively penicillin-resistant strains, those with prosthetic valve infections, and those with longstanding disease (symptoms >3 months).[21,24,42]

Assuming the viridans streptococci isolated from A.G. is not resistant to penicillin and he has no other complicating factors, any of the suggested regimens would be appropriate. Because no compelling reason exists to use the 4-week regimens, the 2-week penicillin–aminoglycoside regimen is the most economic choice. Although A.G. has mild renal impairment, this is most likely secondary to the endocarditis and should improve once adequate antimicrobial therapy has been instituted. A.G. was begun on 12 million units/day of penicillin G, which would be reasonable for his age and mild renal impairment. If nephrotoxicity were a major concern in A.G., penicillin or ceftriaxone alone for 4 weeks would be reasonable. If gentamicin is used, A.G.'s dose should be adjusted appropriately and he should be evaluated frequently for signs of toxicity. Periodic peak and trough aminoglycoside concentrations should be monitored.

STAPHYLOCOCCUS EPIDERMIDIS: PROSTHETIC VALVE ENDOCARDITIS

Etiology

6. F.T., a 65-year-old man, presents with chief complaints of anorexia, fever, chills, and weight loss. His medical history is significant for replacement of his mitral and aortic heart valves (both porcine) 1 year ago for aortic stenosis, mitral regurgitation, and mitral stenosis secondary to rheumatic heart disease. One month later he was readmitted with fever, a right pleural effusion, a pericardial friction rub, and pericarditis. The impression at that time was either postpericardiotomy or Dressler's syndrome. F.T. was sent home on anti-inflammatory agents but failed to improve. After continued complaints of anorexia, nausea, chills, and fever to 101°F, he returned to the hospital. On readmission, his physical examination was noteworthy for a systolic ejection murmur at the left sternal border and 3+ pedal edema. Blood cultures were obtained and routine laboratory studies were performed. His history and clinical presentation were strongly suggestive of prosthetic valve endocarditis (PVE). What are the most likely agents responsible for PVE in F.T.?

Prosthetic valve endocarditis is a life-threatening infectious complication of artificial heart valve implantation that accounts for 7% to 25% of cases of IE in developed countries.[44] The prevalence of complications resulting in death has been as high as 20% to 40%.[45] The risk of PVE after surgery is approximately 1% at 12 months and 2% to 3% at 60 months. PVE is categorized as early or late, depending on the onset of clinical manifestations following cardiac surgery.[45,44] Early PVE occurs within 2 months following surgery and is thought to represent infection acquired during valve placement. It usually is caused by skin organisms that were implanted into the valve annulus (suture site where the valve is attached to cardiac muscle) at the time of surgery.[44,45] The most common organisms cultured from patients such as F.T. with early PVE are coagulase-negative staphylococci (primarily *S. epidermidis* [>30%], most of which are resistant to methicillin), followed by *S. aureus* (20%), and gram-negative bacilli (10%–15%). Miscellaneous organisms, such as diphtheroids and fungi, account for the remainder.[44,45] On the other hand, streptococci are a more common cause of late PVE (>2 months after surgery).[44,45]

Nosocomial bacteremia and fungemia in a patient with prosthetic heart valves contribute to a significant risk for the development of PVE. One study noted that bacteremia caused by staphylococci and gram-negative bacilli resulted in 55% and 33% of subsequent PVE cases, respectively.[46] Another study observed the development of PVE in 25% (11 of 44) of patients following nosocomial candidemia.[47]

Prophylaxis

7. What measures can be taken to prevent early PVE?

The overall frequency of early PVE, despite antibiotic prophylaxis, is 1% to 4%.[48] Complications are severe and include valve dehiscence, acute heart failure, arrhythmias, and outflow obstruction. Although antibiotic prophylaxis before valve surgery (a "clean" procedure) has not been proved to reduce the frequency of early PVE, it is indicated nevertheless because the complications of infection are catastrophic. Animal data indicate that antibiotic prophylaxis reduces the infection rate.[48]

Cephalosporins

The antimicrobial regimen used most commonly for cardiac surgery prophylaxis consists of an antistaphylococcal cephalosporin, such as cefazolin, given in the operating room at the time of induction of anesthesia or within 60 minutes before the procedure. Drug administration should be timed to produce peak concentrations at the time when bacteremia may result from the procedure. Cephalosporins are frequently selected because they are active against most strains of *S. aureus*. The prevalence of methicillin- (and cephalosporin-) resistant strains is increasing, however, exceeding 50% in many centers.

Most strains (87%) of coagulase-negative staphylococci are also methicillin- (and cephalosporin-) resistant.[45,49]

Resistance is thought to be caused by an altered penicillin binding protein (PBP 2a); thus, cross-resistance to all other β-lactams is expected.[50]

Vancomycin

Vancomycin has been used as the alternative prophylactic agent of choice when a first-generation cephalosporin cannot be used. Given its demonstrated efficacy, vancomycin could be considered the prophylactic agent of choice for cardiovascular procedures, including prosthetic valve replacement and implantation of prosthetic grafts, if (a) the patient recently has received broad-spectrum antimicrobial therapy and is likely to be colonized with cephalosporin-resistant staphylococci or enterococci, or (b) the procedure is performed in a center experiencing outbreaks or a high endemic rate of surgical infection with methicillin-resistant staphylococci.[51]

8. What are the disadvantages of the routine use of vancomycin as a prophylactic agent?

Because the frequency of PVE is low, it would be nearly impossible to demonstrate a statistically significant decrease in its incidence following the use of vancomycin compared with conventional agents. Thus, the decision to use vancomycin rests on its superior in vitro activity for methicillin-resistant staphylococci. Arguments against the use of vancomycin in this specific setting are compelling, however. First, the potential for vancomycin-related hypotension is of concern.[51] More importantly, the emergence of vancomycin-resistant enterococci (VRE), glycopeptide-intermediate (GISA) and glycopeptide-resistant *S. aureus* (VRSA) heightens the need to limit vancomycin use, because prior exposure to vancomycin is a recognized predisposing risk for the development of resistance to vancomycin.[52–55]

Of note, ceftobiprole, a novel investigational cephalosporin agent, was shown to be equally effective when compared with vancomycin against MRSA in skin and soft tissue infections in a phase III trial.[56] If proved safe and effective for marketing, this agent holds a promising role for use in this setting.[57]

In summary, the most appropriate prophylactic antibiotic for valve replacement surgery is patient and institution specific.

The decision should be based on the patient's prior exposure to antibiotics and resultant colonization, in addition to the conditions at each institution, such as the infection rate, the types of organisms recovered, the number of procedures performed, and the feasibility of implementing effective infection control measures.

ADVERSE EFFECTS

9. What is the most common infusion-related adverse effect associated with vancomycin, and how can it be minimized?

The most common adverse effect associated with vancomycin administration is the so-called "red man" or "red neck" syndrome,[58,59] which most commonly causes erythema of the head and upper torso, pruritus, urticaria, and in some cases hypotension. It is mediated in part by histamine release, and the severity of the reaction is proportional to the quantity released (see Chapter 4, Anaphylaxis and Drug Allergies). The total dose of vancomycin administered and the rate of infusion are major determinants of the frequency and severity of this reaction. The reaction can be minimized by administering vancomycin over $\geq$1 hour. Cutaneous manifestations of the vancomycin-induced red man syndrome still can occur with a 1-hour infusion, but hypotension is uncommon.[58,59]

Several drugs used perioperatively and in anesthesia also cause histamine release; therefore, the possibility of additive toxicity with vancomycin cannot be dismissed. Most of the serious reactions caused by vancomycin have occurred in patients scheduled for surgery. Vancomycin-induced hypotension occurred in 7% of patients scheduled for cardiothoracic surgery, despite the 1-hour infusion time.[51]

ADMINISTRATION

10. When vancomycin is used to prevent PVE, when should it be administered relative to the time of surgery?

Vancomycin cannot be given in the operating room because it must be administered by infusion over 1 hour, and "on-call" administration right before the procedure may not provide sufficient time for the vancomycin infusion to achieve adequate serum and tissue levels. Therapeutic serum concentrations of vancomycin can be maintained reliably during surgery if the 15 mg/kg dose is infused over 1 hour just before initiation of anesthesia.[51]

Antibiotic-Impregnated Heart Valves

PVE following heart valve replacement surgery is rare, but early-onset infection is associated with a mortality rate of 23% to 41%.[44] Systemically administered antibiotic prophylaxis before surgery does not confer 100% protection. The infectious process typically begins at the sewing ring and extends to involve the adjacent area between the prosthesis and the annulus of the heart valve. Hence, investigators have evaluated the use of antibiotic-impregnated heart valve sewing rings for the prophylaxis and treatment of bacterial endocarditis. Various antibiotics, including rifampin, gentamicin, and clindamycin, have been studied with respect to their diffusion kinetics and duration of antimicrobial activity both in vitro and in animal experiments.[60–62] Whether the combination of "local" and systemic antimicrobial prophylaxis enhances the prophylactic efficacy against PVE will require confirmation, however, from clinical trials involving large number of patients.

Antimicrobial Therapy

11. What are the treatment options for F.T.?

As noted earlier, F.T. most likely is infected with coagulase-negative staphylococci. For those rare coagulase-negative staphylococci that remain sensitive to β-lactams (<20%), a penicillinase-resistant penicillin (nafcillin or oxacillin) is the drug of choice (Table 59-5).[49] For the treatment of PVE caused by methicillin-resistant, coagulase-negative staphylococci, vancomycin remains the cornerstone of therapy.[49] Most of the staphylococci remain sensitive to vancomycin at concentrations of <5 mcg/mL; however, strains of staphylococci with intermediate susceptibility to vancomycin have emerged in the United States and elsewhere and are increasingly reported.[63,64]

The AHA currently recommends the use of triple-drug combination therapy for the treatment of PVE caused by methicillin-resistant, coagulase-negative staphylococci based on experimental models of endocarditis and limited clinical data.[21] In a retrospective review of 75 episodes of PVE caused by methicillin-resistant *S. epidermidis* (MRSE),[65] 21 of 26 patients treated with vancomycin were cured compared with 10 of 20 patients treated with a β-lactam antibiotic ($p = 0.05$); however, the addition of either rifampin or an aminoglycoside to vancomycin appeared to produce superior results (18 of 20 cured) compared with vancomycin alone (3 of 6 cured, $p = 0.06$). A subsequent prospective, multicenter study compared the efficacy of 6 weeks of vancomycin plus rifampin with and without gentamicin for the first 2 weeks for the treatment of PVE caused by MRSE.[45,49] The emergence of rifampin-resistant strains during therapy was reduced by the addition of gentamicin (6 of 15 vs. 0 of 8, $p = 0.04$). Based on current data, a three-drug regimen (vancomycin, gentamicin, and rifampin) appears to be optimal for the medical treatment of PVE caused by MRSE, although toxicity would be expected to be greater. When isolates of MRSE are resistant to all available aminoglycosides, aminoglycoside treatment should be omitted. A fluoroquinolone active against the isolate may be considered as substitute for the aminoglycoside in the three-drug regimen. In addition, most patients who responded to medical treatment also required valve replacement surgery.[44,45]

Although quinupristin/dalfopristin (Synercid), linezolid (Zyvox), and daptomycin (Cubicin) have potent in vitro activity against coagulase-negative staphylococci, clinical experience in the treatment of IE caused by these strains is lacking.[49,66,67]

STAPHYLOCOCCUS AUREUS ENDOCARDITIS

Intravenous Drug Abuser Versus Nonabuser

12. T.J., a 36-year-old human immunodeficiency virus (HIV)-seropositive man with a long history of IV drug abuse, was admitted to the hospital 4 months after being released from the state prison. His chief complaints on admission were fever, night sweats, pleuritic chest pain, shortness of breath (SOB), dyspnea on exertion (DOE), and fatigue. Physical examination was remarkable for a temperature of 101.2°F, splenomegaly, and a pansystolic ejection

Table 59-5 Treatment of Staphylococcal Endocarditis

Antibiotic	*Dosage and Route*	*Duration*
Without Prosthetic Material[a]		
OXACILLIN-SUSCEPTIBLE STAPHYLOCOCCI		
NONPENICILLIN-ALLERGIC PATIENTS		
Nafcillin		
or	*Adult:* 2 g intravenously (IV) Q 4 hr	4–6 wk
	Pediatric: 150–200 mg/kg/24 hr IV (max: 12 g/24 hr) in four to six equally divided doses	
	Adult: 2 g IV Q 4 hr	
Oxacillin	*Pediatric:* 200 mg/kg/24 hr IV (max: 12 g/24 hr) in four to six equally divided doses	4–6 wk
With optional addition	*Adult:* 3 mg/kg IV or intramuscularly (IM) in two or three equally divided doses	3–5 days
of gentamicin[b,c]	*Pediatric:* 3 mg/kg IV or IM in three equally divided doses	
PENCILLIN-ALLERGIC PATIENTS		
1. Cefazolin[d]	*Adult:* 2 g IV Q 8 hr	4–6 wk
	Pediatric: 100 mg/kg/24 hr IV (max: 6 g/24 hr) in equally divided doses Q 8 hr	
With optional addition	*Adult:* See Nonpenicillin-allergic patient	
of gentamicin[b]	*Pediatric:* See Nonpenicillin-allergic patient	
2. Vancomycin[b,e,f]	*Adult:* 30 mg/kg/24 hr IV in two or four equally divided doses (max: 2 g/24 hr unless serum levels monitored)	4–6 wk
	Pediatric: 40 mg/kg/24 hr IV in two or four equally divided doses (max: 2 g/24 hr unless serum levels monitored)	
Methicillin-Resistant Staphylococci		
Vancomycin[b,e,f]	*Adult:* 30 mg/kg/24 hr IV in two or four equally divided doses (max: 2 g/24 hr unless serum levels monitored)	4–6 wk
	Pediatric: 40 mg/kg/24 hr IV in two or four equally divided doses (max: 2 g/24 hr unless serum levels monitored)	
With Prosthetic Valve or Other Prosthetic Material[g]		
Methicillin-Resistant Staphylococci		
Vancomycin[b,e,g]	*Adult:* 30 mg/kg/24 hr IV in two or three equally divided doses (max: 2 g/24 hr unless serum levels monitored)	≥6 wk
	Pediatric: 40 mg/kg/24 hr IV in two or four equally divided doses (max: 2 g/24 hr unless serum levels monitored)	
With rifampin[h]	*Adult:* 300 mg IV/PO Q 8 hr	≥6 wk
and	*Pediatric:* 20 mg/kg/24 hr PO (max: 900 mg/24 hr) in two equally divided doses	
With gentamicin[b,i,j,g]	*Adult:* 3 mg/kg IV or IM in two or three equally divided doses	2 wk
	Pediatric: 3 mg/kg IV or IM in three equally divided doses	
Methicillin-Susceptible Staphylococci		
Nafcillin or oxacillin[k]	*Adult:* 2 g IV Q 4 hr	≥6 wk
	Pediatric: 150–200 mg/kg/24 hr (max: 12 g/24 hr) in four to six equally divided doses	
With rifampin[h]	*Adult:* 300 mg IV/PO Q 8 hr	≥6 wk
and	*Pediatric:* 20 mg/kg/24 hr PO (max: 900 mg/24 hr) in three equally divided doses	
With gentamicin[b,i,j,g]	*Adult:* 3 mg/kg IV or IM in two or three equally divided doses	2 wk
	Pediatric: 3 mg/kg IV or IM in three equally divided doses	

[a] Antibiotic doses should be modified appropriately for patients with impaired renal function. Shorter antibiotic courses have been effective in some drug addicts with right-sided endocarditis caused by *S. aureus.* (See text for comments on the use of daptomycin and rifampin.)
[b] Dosing of aminoglycosides and vancomycin on a mg/kg basis will give higher serum concentrations in obese than in lean patients.
[c] The benefit of additional aminoglycoside has not been established. The risk of toxic reactions because of these agents is increased in patients >65 years of age or those with renal or eighth nerve impairment.
[d] There is potential cross-allergenicity between penicillins and cephalosporins. Cephalosporins should be avoided in patients with immediate-type hypersensitivity to penicillin.
[e] Peak serum concentrations of vancomycin should be obtained 1 hr after infusion and should be in the range of 30–45 mcg/mL for BID dosing and 20–30 mcg/mL for QID dosing. Trough serum concentrations should be obtained within half an hour of the next dose and should be in the range of 10–15 mcg/mL. (See text for detailed discussion on the need for high trough target of 15–20 mcg/mL for strains with reduced susceptibility to vancomycin. Each vancomycin dose should be infused over 1 hr.)
[f] See text for consideration of optional addition of gentamicin.
[g] Vancomycin and gentamicin doses must be modified appropriately in patients with renal failure.
[h] Rifampin is recommended for therapy of infections caused by coagulase-negative staphylococci. Its use in coagulase-positive staphylococcal infections is controversial. Rifampin increases the amount of warfarin sodium required for antithrombotic therapy.
[i] Serum concentration of gentamicin should be monitored and the dose should be adjusted to obtain a peak level of approximately 3 mcg/mL.
[j] Use during initial 2 wk. (See text on alternative aminoglycoside therapy for organisms resistant to gentamicin.)
[k] First-generation cephalosporins or vancomycin should be used in penicillin-allergic patients. Cephalosporins should be avoided in patients with immediate-type hypersensitivity to penicillin and those infected with methicillin-resistant staphylococci.
Adapted from reference 9, with permission.

murmur at the left sternal border, best heard during inspiration. The chest radiograph revealed diffuse nodular infiltrates. TTE was positive for a small vegetation on the tricuspid valve leaflet. Significant laboratory results included WBC count, 14,000/mm^3 with 65% polys and 5% bands; CD4 cell count, 350/mm^3; Hgb, 13.1 g/dL; Hct, 39%; and ESR 55 mm/hour (Westergren). IE was suspected. Blood cultures were obtained and all six samples were positive for coagulase-positive, gram-positive cocci, later identified as methicillin-sensitive *S. aureus* (MSSA). How do the clinical presentation and prognosis of endocarditis in the IV drug abuser

differ from in the nonabuser? What impact does HIV infection have on the risk and outcomes of endocarditis in the IV drug abuser?

[SI units: WBC, 14 × 10/L with 0.65 polys and 0.05 bands (normal, 3.2–9.8 with 0.54–0.62 polys and 0.03–0.05 bands); Hgb, 131 g/L (normal, 140–180); Hct, 0.39 (normal, 0.39–0.49)]

The annual incidence of endocarditis among IV drug users is estimated at 1% to 5%; parenteral cocaine addicts have the highest risk.[68] The presentation, pathophysiology, and prognosis of endocarditis in those who acquire the disease secondary to IV drug abuse differ from those in nonabusers.[1,68,69] IE caused by *S. aureus* is associated with an odds ratio of 9.3 (95% CI, 6.3–13.7) compared with other pathogens in this population.[7] *S. aureus* is part of the normal skin flora and is introduced when the illicit drug is injected. It is hypothesized that insoluble agents used to "cut" the drug damage the normal heart valve, preparing the surface for bacterial adherence and growth.[1]

The following are differences between addicts and nonaddicts with *S. aureus* endocarditis: addicts are significantly younger; they have fewer underlying diseases, more right-sided (tricuspid) involvement (in contrast to the predominance of left-sided disease in the nonaddicts); they are less likely to have heart failure or central nervous system (CNS) complications; they exhibit fewer signs of peripheral involvement and have a lower incidence of death.[69] Among patients without history of IV drug use, MRSA was involved in one-third of a cohort of 424 patients with definite *S. aureus* IE. Clinical features that characterized MRSA IE were persistent bacteremia, chronic immunosuppressive therapy, health care-associated infection, a presumed intravascular device source, and diabetes mellitus.[7]

The prevalence of HIV seropositivity is 40% to 90% among IV drug users with IE.[68,70] One case-control study among an ongoing cohort of IV drug users suggested that HIV-related immunosuppression may be an independent risk factor for the development of endocarditis after controlling for confounding variables such as a history of endocarditis or sepsis before enrollment, injection duration, current injection frequency, and a recent history of abscess at injection sites.[71]

Antimicrobial Therapy

Methicillin-Sensitive Staphylococcus aureus

13. What are the therapeutic options for treating *S. aureus* endocarditis in T.J.?

The susceptibility of *S. aureus* to methicillin is the major determinant of which antibiotic is selected to treat T.J.'s endocarditis. T.J. is infected with MSSA. Therapy of choice for methicillin-sensitive strains is a penicillinase-resistant penicillin, such as nafcillin or oxacillin[21] (Table 59-5). Penicillin G rarely is appropriate because nearly all isolates of *S. aureus* produce penicillinase. Methicillin is no longer used because it is associated with a high incidence of interstitial nephritis.

Prospective, randomized, clinical trials have established that 4 to 6 weeks of therapy with high-dose (12 g/day) nafcillin is effective in most patients.[72,73] Clinical experience and in vitro studies indicate that vancomycin may be less efficacious than nafcillin as an antistaphylococcal agent.[21,73] Therefore, vancomycin should not be used to substitute for nafcillin merely for dosing convenience. IV drug addicts, for the reasons previously identified, have a higher response rate to appropriate therapy compared with nonaddicts, and 4 weeks of therapy is probably adequate. In one study, 31 addicts were successfully treated with 16 days of parenteral therapy followed by 26 days of oral dicloxacillin.[74]

Addicts with uncomplicated right-sided endocarditis caused by MSSA can be treated successfully with a 2-week course of combination therapy with a penicillinase-resistant penicillin and an aminoglycoside.[75–77] In one study, 47 of 50 patients (94%) were cured after treatment with the combination of IV nafcillin (1.5 g Q 4 hr) and tobramycin (1 mg/kg Q 8 hr) for a total of 2 weeks. Notably, two of three patients in this study who were treated with vancomycin relapsed, resulting in early termination of this arm of study. Thus, vancomycin should not be used to substitute for nafcillin in this regimen. In another study, 71 patients who completed the 2-week course of treatment with cloxacillin (2 g IV Q 4 hr) plus amikacin (7.5 mg/kg IV Q 12 hr) had a cure rate of 94%.[76] Of the four patients who failed, the two week treatment period had to be extended to achieve cure. In contrast to the prior study, most (72%) patients had definite endocarditis with echocardiographic vegetations. Overall, none of the patients who responded promptly to treatment relapsed. In addition, the risk of nephrotoxicity secondary to 2 weeks of aminoglycoside therapy was minimal in this selected patient population. Alternatively, Ribera et al. demonstrated in a study that cloxacillin alone was as effective as combination therapy of cloxacillin plus gentamicin for the treatment of right-sided MSSA endocarditis; the treatment response exceeded 90% in the cloxacillin monotherapy arm.[78] Gentamicin administered at 1 mg/kg Q 8 hr for 7 days in the combination group did not improve treatment response.

Clinical studies thus far support the use of an abbreviated course of treatment in a defined group of IV drug users with right-sided endocarditis. These patients should have the following characteristics: (a) clinical and bacteriologic response within 96 hours of initiation of therapy; (b) no evidence of hemodynamic compromise, metastatic infection, or neurologic or systemic embolic complications either at the initiation or completion of 2 weeks of therapy; (c) no echographically demonstrable vegetations >2 cm^3; (d) not infected with MRSA; and (e) not receiving antibiotics other than penicillinase-resistant penicillins, such as first-generation cephalosporins and glycopeptides.[21,77] HIV-seropositive patients (CD4 counts >300 × 10^6 cells) with tricuspid involvement included in the above studies also responded favorably to these short-course regimens, thus short-course regimen is an option for T.J.[78]

Some studies suggest that the addition of an aminoglycoside to the treatment regimen does not appear to improve overall response for patients who meet the above criteria for short-course therapy. Thus, emphasis should be shifted toward careful evaluation of all patients receiving this regimen for evidence of continuing infection or complications at the end of the 2-week treatment course before discontinuing therapy; extension of therapy with a β-lactam agent to at least 4 weeks' duration is prudent for those who demonstrate any evidence of active disease or complications. Although response to antibiotic therapy has been shown to be similar between asymptomatic HIV-seropositive and HIV-seronegative IV drug users, it is prudent to avoid short-course therapy in more immunosuppressed individuals (CD4 cell counts <200 μL) until more definitive outcome data are available in this subgroup.[68]

ORAL REGIMEN

An oral treatment regimen consisting of ciprofloxacin (750 mg Q 12 hr) plus rifampin (300 mg Q 12 hr) has also been evaluated in addicts with uncomplicated right-sided endocarditis. In one small, noncomparative study, 10 addicts were successfully treated with the combination of ciprofloxacin and rifampin for 4 weeks.[79] Ciprofloxacin was given IV (300 mg Q 12 hr) for the first 7 days, followed by oral administration (750 mg Q 12 hr) for the remaining 21 days of therapy. Another study prospectively compared the oral regimen with standard parenteral therapy for this subgroup.[80] Patients were randomized to receive 28 days of therapy with oral ciprofloxacin plus rifampin or oxacillin (2 g IV Q 4 hr) plus gentamicin (2 mg/kg IV Q 8 hr). Vancomycin (1 g IV Q 12 hr) was substituted for oxacillin in the penicillin-allergic patients. A total of 19 patients completed treatment with oral therapy compared with 25 patients with IV therapy. One of 19 patients in the oral group versus 3 of 25 in the IV group failed treatment; however, the difference in cure rates was not statistically significant. Cure was defined by negative blood cultures after 6 and 7 days after treatment. Follow-up 1 month after treatment was available in only 30 patients; no failures were detected. Notably, approximately half of the study patients in either group had possible endocarditis, whereas only 21% versus 31% had definite infections. Given the small number of patients who completed treatment, therapeutic equivalency between the oral and parenteral regimens will need to be confirmed in larger trials. In addition, other issues that may complicate success with this oral regimen are the emerging quinolone resistance in *S. aureus* and the compliance and monitoring required of this regimen when administered in the outpatient setting. Nonetheless, it appears that a 4-week oral regimen with ciprofloxacin and rifampin may be a useful alternative treatment option in addicts with uncomplicated right-sided endocarditis.

PENICILLIN-ALLERGIC PATIENTS

Treatment of penicillin-allergic patients with *S. aureus* endocarditis is somewhat controversial. First-generation cephalosporins have been used with some success for the treatment of patients with mild penicillin allergy, but treatment failures with cefazolin are difficult to explain.[81] The stability of cefazolin when exposed to staphylococcal β-lactamase has been proposed as a mechanism for these failures.[82] Notably, staphylococci are capable of producing four penicillinase subtypes, to which the stability of cefazolin varies. These susceptibility differences are apparent on MIC testing only if a larger-than-usual inoculum is used (i.e., $>10^6$ organisms).[71] It is possible that treatment failures with cefazolin may be caused by a combination of the recalcitrant nature of the infection and the instability of cefazolin against a particular subtype of penicillinase produced by the staphylococcal strain, which is not readily detectable via routine MIC testing. Until further data are available, vancomycin should be used to treat patients with endocarditis caused by *S. aureus* who have immediate-type hypersensitivity to penicillin. Other treatment options include linezolid, quinupristin/dalfopristin, and daptomycin.[57] Selection of agent depends on organism susceptibility, potential of drug-drug interactions, and host predisposition for development of adverse effects.

COMBINATION THERAPY

14. Will the addition of another antibiotic enhance T.J.'s response to nafcillin?

An enhanced response to combination therapy in the experimental animal model of MSSA endocarditis has prompted clinical trials to evaluate whether the addition of gentamicin to nafcillin confers any additional benefit. The combination of nafcillin and gentamicin resulted in more rapid clearing of organisms from the blood, but the response rates were similar to patients treated with nafcillin alone.[81] As expected, the group receiving gentamicin had a higher incidence of nephrotoxicity. Thus, for the routine management of endocarditis caused by MSSA, the addition of a second drug does not appear to offer additional benefit when a penicillinase penicillin is used unless an abbreviated treatment course in a select patient group is desired (see Question 13 above). The addition of rifampin may be indicated in patients who remain bacteremic or who fail to improve clinically (usually nonaddicts).

Methicillin-Resistant Staphylococcus aureus: Vancomycin

15. How would T.J.'s therapy differ if he were infected with MRSA?

Staphylococcus aureus IE involving methicillin-resistant strains has become increasingly common and accounts for up to 40% of cases.[6,7] MRSA-infected patients had more chronic comorbid conditions (e.g., diabetes mellitus, hemodialysis dependency), were more likely to have health care-associated infection (76% vs. 37%) and an indwelling intravascular catheter or hemodialysis fistula as the presumed source of infection (60% vs. 31%) when compared with patients infected with MSSA in a large multinational study.[7] Notably, persistent bacteremia was a distinct feature associated with MRSA IE occurring in 43% versus 9% of patients infected with MSSA. Of interest, in this study, patients with *S. aureus* IE from the United States were significantly more likely to be infected with MRSA, to receive vancomycin therapy, and to develop persistent bacteremia.

In 20% of patients with MRSA IE in the above study, identifiable health care contact was absent. MRSA infection is traditionally associated with health care contact in the nosocomial setting, but is now becoming more prevalent in the community (CA-MRSA).[7] Young and otherwise healthy individuals without the traditional risk factors are affected in the community.[83] CA-MRSA strains are distinct from health care-associated strains in that most possess a distinct exotoxin gene (Panton-Valentine leukocidin [PVL]). Expression of this pore-forming toxin that causes severe necrosis in PMN in a rabbit model has been implicated to cause invasive infections, including necrotizing pneumonia and skin abscesses.[84–90] Specifically, CA-MRSA PVL producing strains causing IE has been reported.[91]

TREATMENT OPTIONS

Vancomycin has been the accepted standard of treatment for MRSA endocarditis. Response to treatment, however, appears to be slower than with semisynthetic penicillins (e.g., nafcillin) for MSSA endocarditis. The mean duration of bacteremia in patients with MSSA endocarditis has been reported to be 3.4 days for nafcillin alone and 2.9 days for the combination of nafcillin and gentamicin.[75] In contrast, the median duration of bacteremia for MRSA endocarditis was 7 days for vancomycin alone. Failure rates of up to 40% have been documented in patients even with right-sided involvement. Of great concern is the emergence of resistant strains of *S. aureus* following repeated and prolonged exposure to vancomycin therapy.[63,91]

Vancomycin 30 mg/kg/day in two divided doses for a total of 4 to 6 weeks is recommended for adults with normal renal function. Ideal body weight should be used to dose vancomycin on a milligram per kilogram basis in obese patients. Dosage adjustment for renal dysfunction is necessary. The prolonged distribution phase of vancomycin may affect the reproducibility of peak levels in general, so they are not practical to obtain. Dosage adjustment of vancomycin therapy based on measured trough levels is more reliable. Published expert recommendations suggest a target trough of 10 to 15 mcg/mL; however, trough levels of 15 to 20 mcg/mL[9,93,94] may be necessary to overcome increasing MIC of clinical strains and limited tissue penetration. Serum vancomycin concentrations have been traditionally targeted for a trough level in the range of 5 to 20 mcg/mL within 30 minutes of the next dose. A dosage regimen of vancomycin aimed to achieve an area under the curve (AUC)-to-MIC ratio of 400 or unbound trough at four to five times MIC of the infected strain have been proposed by different groups as the optimal pharmacodynamic target.[95–98]

16. T.J. has been treated with vancomycin 1 g IV Q 12 hr for 5 days for his MRSA endocarditis, but does not seem to be clinically improving. His blood cultures are still positive and his WBC remains elevated at 12,500/mm^3 with 55% polys and 7% bands. He continues to have a low grade fever since starting vancomycin. His vancomycin trough level on the second day of therapy was 17 mcg/mL. The infected MRSA strain had a vancomycin MIC of 1.5 mcg/mL as determined by Etest. What factors may be contributing to T.J.'s poor response to treatment?

In a large multinational study of nearly 1,800 patients with definite IE, persistent bacteremia, receipt of vancomycin, and health care contact were significantly more likely to be observed in patients with MRSA IE from the United States compared with those from other geographic regions.[7] The authors speculated that the higher rates of persistent bacteremia in U.S. patients may be partly owing to those patients were more likely to have received vancomycin.

Vancomycin MIC against *S. aureus* have been increasing over the years. At one university medical center, vancomycin MIC were determined by broth microdilution for 6,000 nosocomial MRSA isolates collected over a 5-year period. In the year 2000, 80% of the strains had vancomycin MIC of = 0.5 mcg/mL; however, by 2004, 70% of isolates had MICs of 2 mcg/mL.[52] In response to increasing reports of vancomycin failures caused by strains that are in the susceptible range, the vancomycin breakpoint for susceptibility was reduced from 4 to 2 mcg/mL for S. *aureus* in 2005 per the Clinical and Laboratory Standards Institute (CLSI).[99,100]

Widespread use of vancomycin has led to the emergence of *S. aureus* strains with vancomycin intermediate S. aureus (VISA) or heterogeneously expressed resistance to vancomycin (hVISA).[63] Reduced susceptibility to glycopeptides results from an increase in the production of peptidoglycan precursors leading to a thickened cell wall and decreased penetration of glycopeptides into the bacterial cell membrane.[101] In the absence of vancomycin, hVISA strains may revert to glycopeptide susceptibility, making it difficult to detect these strains in vitro. As such, several investigators have found that hVISA strains have an MIC range that overlaps with the currently defined susceptible range and that the prevalence of these strains among hospitalized patients is increasing.[102–104] Of concern is that routine susceptibility testing methods performed in the clinical laboratory are unreliable in detecting MRSA strains with hVISA phenotype.[105] Among the tests performed, MIC determined by Etest appears to be most predictable of treatment outcome with vancomycin.[29,106]

Experts have recommended a target vancomycin trough concentration of 15 to 20 mcg/mL to overcome increasing MIC when treating pneumonia caused by MRSA.[107] A published study of adult infections with MRSA reported that 54% (51 of 95) of clinical isolates had vancomycin MIC of 2 mcg/mL. Notably, invasive infections, such as bacteremia and pneumonia, were linked to higher MIC. Infections caused by those strains were associated with lower end of treatment responses (62% vs. 85%) and increased mortality (24% vs. 10%) compared with strains with MIC of $\leq$1 mcg/mL irrespective of attaining a goal trough of 15 to 20 mcg/mL (achieving the goal of four to five times above MIC of an infected strain that has an MIC of 2 mcg/mL). The study found that borderline susceptibility (MIC 2 mcg/mL) and severity of underlying disease were independent predictors of poor treatment response. Further analysis indicated that a significant proportion of these strains demonstrated tolerance to vancomycin as defined by the MBC-to-MIC ratio of 32 and up to 10% of these invasive strains exhibit heterogeneous vancomycin intermediate resistance phenotype.[29,108] Vancomycin monotherapy was associated with treatment failure of infections caused by these strains, whereas those who received combination therapy responded favorably. Combination regimens included vancomycin plus rifampin, linezolid, or daptomycin. These findings suggest a role for combination therapy or alternative agents when treating invasive infections caused by MRSA strains with borderline susceptibility. Confirmation is required, however, given that the above study was not designed to compare the efficacy of vancomycin monotherapy versus combination therapy for the treatment of MRSA infections and that the sample size of patients infected with hVISA in this study was small. Therefore, the role of vancomycin as the treatment of choice for MRSA IE will need to be re-evaluated against other available treatment options.

Despite attaining a pharmacodynamic goal of unbound vancomycin trough level of at least four times MIC of the infected strain, T.J. fails to clinically improve and has persistent bacteremia. It is possible that T.J. is infected with an hVISA strain, thus, a change in therapy is warranted.

17. What other therapeutic options are available for T.J.?

Trimethoprim-sulfamethoxazole has been used successfully in a limited number of patients with right-sided native valve endocarditis caused by susceptible strains of *S. aureus* and may be an alternative to vancomycin.[109] A study of experimental staphylococcal endocarditis, however, found trimethoprim-sulfamethoxazole to be inferior to cloxacillin, vancomycin, and teicoplanin. Alternatively, minocycline has been shown to be a potential treatment alternative to vancomycin in experimental endocarditis caused by MRSA. Although both drugs are equally effective in decreasing the bacterial density of cardiac vegetations, the penetration of minocycline into vegetation was twice that of vancomycin.[110]

New agents showing promise for the treatment of MRSA IE based on in vitro activity include quinupristin/dalfopristin, linezolid, and daptomycin. Synercid (quinupristin/dalfopristin) used for treatment in animal models of endocarditis have shown successful outcomes. Clinical success has been reported in a limited number of patients with MRSA endocarditis treated with quinupristin/dalfopristin.[111,112] A cure rate of 56% was reported for patients treated with quinupristin/dalfopristin for MRSA endocarditis in an international open trial that evaluated the drug in patients intolerant of or failed prior therapy.[112] Because of a lack of clinical studies establishing the efficacy of this agent, additional data is needed before quinupristin/dalfopristin can be recommended for therapy.

Linezolid (Zyvox), an oxazolidinone, is not U.S. Food and Drug Administration (FDA)-approved for the treatment of endocarditis, but has been used in cases of treatment failures, intolerability to standard therapy, or in infections with multidrug resistant gram-positive cocci.[113] In a review article that included 33 cases reports of endocarditis treated with linezolid, 63.6% of patients had successful outcomes at the end of the follow-up period.[114] MRSA and vancomycin intermediate *S. aureus* were the most common pathogens accounting for 24% and 30% of cases, respectively. Failure with linezolid treatment was documented in seven cases including four deaths attributed to endocarditis and three owing to persistent positive blood cultures Thrombocytopenia was the most common adverse effect occurring in eight of nine patients who reported an adverse effect. In a compassionate use program, linezolid was reported to achieve 50% clinical and microbiologic cure rates at 6-month follow-up in 32 patients with definite IE; MRSA was the causative agent in 7 of those patients. The most common adverse events reported in this group were gastrointestinal system effects and thrombocytopenia, each occurring in 15% of patients.[115] The degree of thrombocytopenia associated with linezolid has been shown to correlate with the extent of drug exposure, as measured by area under the concentration curve and duration of treatment.[116] Of note, treatment failure with linezolid for MRSA endocarditis caused by persistent bacteremia has been described in two patients and in one patient with relapse of infection.[117,119] Thus, additional efficacy data are needed before linezolid can be recommended for the treatment of IE caused by MRSA.

Daptomycin (Cubicin) is a cyclic lipopeptide that has been approved for treatment of *S. aureus* bacteremia and right-sided endocarditis. In vivo, it has a wide spectrum of activity against gram-positive bacteria, including *S. aureus* (including MRSA), *E. faecalis*, *E. faecium*, streptococci, and most other species of aerobic and anaerobic gram-positive bacteria. It was approved for the treatment of *S. aureus* bacteremia/endocarditis in a noninferiority study in patients receiving daptomycin or standard therapy consisting of an antistaphyloccocal penicillin or vancomycin in addition to low-dose gentamicin.[121] Successful outcome was seen in 46% (41 of 90) of patients who had presumed or definite endocarditis at their baseline diagnosis. Of those, MRSA endocarditis was successfully treated in 42% (15 of 36) of cases. In patients with confirmed uncomplicated and complicated right-sided endocarditis, treatment success was similar between the daptomycin group (8 of 18) and the group receiving standard therapy (7 of 16) at 44%. Microbiologic failure occurred in seven patients in the daptomycin group and in five patients receiving standard therapy. Overall, the most common cause of daptomycin failure was persistent or relapsing infections accounting for 16% of failures. In contrast, failure of standard therapy was more often to the result of treatment-limiting adverse events accounting for 15% of failures. Increase in the MIC of the infected strain was observed more often in the daptomycin group compared with standard treatment (six in the daptomycin vs. one patient in the standard therapy group). The use of daptomycin for treatment of left-sided endocarditis is not established because only nine patients were treated and only one had treatment success.

Daptomycin at 6 mg/kg/day for a total duration of 6 weeks should be used for the treatment of endocarditis. Frequency of administration should be increased to every 48 hour for patients with a clearance of creatinine (Clcr) of ≤30 mL/minute. Daptomycin should be dosed based on total body weight because obese patients have a larger volume of distribution as well as increased clearance compared with the nonobese population.[122] Creatinine kinase elevations were more commonly seen in the daptomycin (6.7%) compared with the standard therapy (0.9%) group.[121] Creatinine kinase levels should be obtained at baseline and weekly to monitor for elevations and more frequently in patients who may be at risk for developing skeletal-muscle dysfunction (e.g., concomitant therapy with hydroxymethylglutaryl-coenzyme A (HMG-CoA) reductase inhibitors). In addition, 9% of patients experienced peripheral nervous system-related adverse events (e.g., paresthesia and peripheral neuropathies), which resolved during continued treatment.[121]

Daptomycin at 6 mg/kg daily should be considered as alternative therapy in T.J. Emergence of cross-resistance to daptomycin after vancomycin exposure has been documented, however.[53,117] Similar to a thickened cell wall contributing to decreased susceptibility to vancomycin, the same mechanism is thought to contribute to daptomycin resistance in *S. aureus*.[123–125] As a result, it is important to test for daptomycin susceptibility before initiation of therapy. Until daptomycin susceptibility is documented, rifampin may be added to vancomycin as combination therapy. Linezolid is a potential treatment option for T.J. if his infected MRSA strain demonstrates reduced susceptibility to daptomycin given prior vancomycin exposure; however, clinical experience is limited to case reports and compassionate use.

Once daptomycin therapy is initiated, continued monitoring of clinical response and organism susceptibility to daptomycin is warranted because resistance development has been reported during prolonged therapy.[123–126] Daptomycin MIC increase during therapy for *S. aureus* endocarditis was demonstrated in six patients.[121] Baseline MIC increased from 0.25 to 2 mcg/mL in five isolates and from 0.5 to 4 mcg/mL in one isolate.[121] Five of those six isolates were MRSA.

ENTEROCOCCAL ENDOCARDITIS

Antimicrobial Therapy

Antibiotic Synergy

18. G.S., a 35-year-old woman, has been complaining of anorexia, weight loss, and fever for the past 2 months. Her

medical history is significant for an aortic aneurysm with insufficiency that resulted in an aortic valve replacement (porcine) 3 years before admission. Approximately 2 months before admission, G.S. had a cesarean section followed by a tubal ligation. She did not receive antibiotic prophylaxis for either procedure. Physical examination revealed a thin woman (5 foot 0 inches, 48 kg) in no acute distress with evidence of a systolic heart murmur, splinter hemorrhages, and petechiae on her soft palate. Her temperature was 100.2°F. Her WBC count was 14,000/mm^3 with a slight left shift; all other laboratory results were within normal limits. She was not taking any medications and she has a documented allergy to penicillin (rash, urticaria, and wheezing). The working clinical diagnosis was probable bacterial endocarditis, which was confirmed when four sets of blood cultures grew gram-positive cocci. Biochemical testing subsequently identified the organism as *Enterococcus faecalis,* highly resistant to streptomycin (MIC >2,000 mcg/mL). Antibiotic therapy with gentamicin (50 mg IV Q 8 hr) and vancomycin (1,000 mg IV Q 12 hr) was begun. Why were two antibiotics prescribed for the treatment of enterococcal endocarditis in G.S.?

[SI unit: WBC, 14 × 10/L]

Enterococci, unlike streptococci, are inhibited but not killed by penicillin or vancomycin alone.[22,127] The synergistic combination of penicillin (or ampicillin, piperacillin, or vancomycin) and an aminoglycoside are required to produce the desired bactericidal effect.[22,128] An antibiotic regimen is synergistic when a combination of antibiotics lowers the MIC to at least one-fourth the MIC of either drug alone.[129] The mechanism of synergy against enterococci is caused by an increased cellular uptake of the aminoglycoside with agents that inhibit cell wall synthesis[130] (e.g., β-lactams and vancomycin). Because G.S. is allergic to penicillin, vancomycin was prescribed with an aminoglycoside. Relapse rates are unacceptably high if penicillin is used alone for the treatment of enterococcal endocarditis.[21,23] The addition of an aminoglycoside to penicillin therapy significantly increased the sterilization rate of vegetations in animal studies.[129,130] Numerous clinical studies have confirmed the in vitro synergy for penicillin in combination with streptomycin or gentamicin for enterococcal endocarditis.[131–135]

19. **G.S. has enterococcal endocarditis caused by strains exhibiting high-level resistance to streptomycin. Why would (or would not) treatment with gentamicin achieve the desired synergy with vancomycin in G.S. with enterococcus highly resistant to streptomycin?**

STREPTOMYCIN RESISTANCE

As many as 55% of all enterococcal blood isolates are highly resistant to streptomycin (MIC >2,000 mcg/mL), and the combination of streptomycin with penicillin is not synergistic for those isolates. In contrast, gentamicin in combination with penicillin, ampicillin, or vancomycin is synergistic for most blood isolates of enterococci, regardless of their susceptibility to streptomycin.[1,23,136] In addition, ototoxicity in the form of vestibular dysfunction secondary to streptomycin therapy has been noted in nearly 30% of patients receiving the combination regimen for the treatment of enterococcal endocarditis and is most often irreversible. Maintaining streptomycin peak serum concentrations below 30 mcg/mL reduces the risk of ototoxicity, but laboratory assays for streptomycin levels are not readily available. For these reasons, gentamicin in combination with penicillin (or ampicillin) or vancomycin is recommended by most authorities for the treatment of aminoglycoside-susceptible and, in particular, streptomycin-resistant enterococcal endocarditis, as it was for G.S.[21] Of note, other aminoglycosides cannot be used to substitute for gentamicin or streptomycin because of the uncertain correlation between in vitro synergy and in vivo efficacy.[21] Table 59-6 lists the suggested regimens for the treatment of enterococcal endocarditis.

GENTAMICIN RESISTANCE

About 10% to 25% of the clinical isolates of *E. faecalis* and up to 50% of *E. faecium* are resistant to gentamicin.[136–138] The prevalence of these isolates is expected to continually increase. All available aminoglycosides should be tested with penicillin (or ampicillin) for synergistic bactericidal activity. Without conclusive data, some groups favor long-term (8–12 weeks) therapy with high-dose penicillin (20–40 million units/day IV in divided doses) or ampicillin (2–3 g IV Q 4 hours) for treatment of multiply resistant enterococci. Ampicillin plus the β-lactamase inhibitor sulbactam (Unasyn) would be substituted for β-lactamase producing, high-level gentamicin-resistant enterococci. In light of the increasing prevalence of enterococci with high-level aminoglycoside resistance, the potential synergistic interaction between ampicillin/amoxicillin and a third-generation cephalosporin was explored in vitro and in experimental models of IE[141]. A bactericidal synergistic effect was shown between amoxicillin and cefotaxime against 50 strains of *E. faecalis*. Amoxicillin MIC decreased from 0.25 to 1 mcg/mL to 0.01 to 0.25 mcg/mL for 48 of 50 strains tested.[138] A similar effect was demonstrated by others using the combination of amoxicillin and ceftriaxone. Additionally, Brandt et al.[139] demonstrated a synergistic bactericidal effect for amoxicillin in combination with imipenem against vancomycin-aminoglycoside–resistant *E. faecium* strains. The authors speculated that saturation of different penicillin binding protein (PBP) by different β-lactam agents may be the underlying mechanism for the synergy observed. Limited clinical data on 13 endocarditis cases caused by high-level aminoglycoside-resistant *E. faecalis* treated with the combination of high-dose ceftriaxone (4 g/day) and ampicillin appear to confirm the above synergistic interaction. All 16 evaluable patients were cured by 1 month of double β-lactam therapy with no evidence of relapse during a 3-month follow-up period. Of note, two patients experienced reversible neutropenia and were withdrawn from the study.[140] Double β-lactam therapy appears promising for infections caused by aminoglycoside-resistant *E. faecalis* strains as well as an aminoglycoside-sparing regimen for patients with renal insufficiency, but the above preliminary results need to be confirmed with a larger number of patients.

Gentamicin

DOSING

20. **What is the optimal dosage of gentamicin for G.S.?**

Because patients with enterococcal endocarditis require prolonged therapy with aminoglycosides, the optimal serum concentration should minimize toxicity without jeopardizing

Table 59-6 Therapy for Endocarditis Caused by Enterococci (or *Streptococci viridans* with an MIC ≥0.5 mcg/mL)[a,b]

Antibiotic	*Dose and Route*	*Duration*
Nonpenicillin-Allergic Patient		
1. Aqueous crystalline penicillin G	*Adult:* 18–30 million units/24 hr intravenously (IV) given continuously or in six equally divided doses	4–6 wk
	Pediatric: 300,000 units/kg/24 hr IV (max: 30 million units/24 hr) given continuously or in four to six equally divided doses	4–6 wk
With gentamicin[c,d,e]	*Adult:* 1 mg/kg intramuscularly (IM) or IV Q 8 hr	4–6 wk
or	*Pediatric:* 1 mg/kg IM or IV Q 8 hr	4–6 wk
2. Ampicillin	*Adult:* 12 g/24 hr IV given continuously or in six equally divided doses	4–6 wk
	Pediatric: 300 mg/kg/24 hr IV (max: 12 g/24 hr) in four to six equally divided doses	4–6 wk
With gentamicin[c,d,e]	*Adult:* 1 mg/kg IM or IV Q 8 hr	4–6 wk
or	*Pediatric:* 1 mg/kg IM or IV Q 8 hr	4–6 wk
Penicillin-Allergic Patients[g]		
Vancomycin[e]	*Adult:* 30 mg/kg/24 hr IV in two equally divided doses (max: 2 g/24 hr unless serum levels monitored)	6 wk
	Pediatric: 40 mg/kg/24 hr IV in two to three equally divided doses (max: 2 g/24 hr unless serum levels monitored)	6 wk
With gentamicin[c,d]	*Adult:* 1 mg/kg IM or IV (max: 80 mg) Q 8 hr	6 wk
or	*Pediatric:* 1 mg/kg IM or IV (max: 80 mg) Q 8 hr	6 wk

[a] Antibiotic doses should be modified appropriately in patients with impaired renal function.
[b] Enterococci should be tested for high-level resistance (gentamicin: MIC ≥500 mcg/mL).
[c] Serum concentration of gentamicin should be monitored and dosage adjusted to obtain a peak level of approximately 3 mcg/mL. (For shorter course gentamicin therapy for enterococcal endocarditis see comment in text.)
[d] Dosing of aminoglycosides and vancomycin on a mg/kg basis gives higher serum concentrations in obese than in lean patients.
[e] Peak serum concentrations of vancomycin should be obtained 1 hr after infusion and should be in the range of 30–45 mcg/mL for BID dosing and 20–30 mcg/mL for QID dosing. Trough serum concentrations should be obtained within half an hr of the next dose and should be in the range of 10–15 mcg/mL. Each dose should be infused over 1 hr; 6 weeks of vancomycin therapy recommended because of decreased activity against enterococci.
[f] Desensitization should be considered; cephalosporins are not satisfactory alternatives.
Adapted from reference 9, with permission.

clinical cure. Early in vitro data indicated that the bactericidal activity of gentamicin against enterococci was not significantly different between peak concentrations of 5 mcg/mL and 3 mcg/L; however, the differences between 3 mcg/mL and 1 mcg/mL were significant.[141] In the rat model of endocarditis, the bacterial counts in vegetations at 5 and 10 days were compared between those treated with low-dose (1 mg/kg intramuscularly twice daily) and those treated with high-dose (5 mg/kg intramuscularly twice daily) gentamicin with penicillin[142]. Bacterial counts did not differ at 5 days, but at 10 days they were significantly lower in the rats receiving the high-dose regimen. In contrast, results in the rabbit model showed no difference in the amount of bacteria per gram of vegetation in high- and low-dose gentamicin treatment groups.[143] As for the influence of dosing interval of aminoglycosides on the efficacy of combination regimens in experimental enterococcal endocarditis, studies have demonstrated that multiple daily dosing is more effective in reducing bacterial titers in vegetations than single daily dosing,[144–146] in contrast to that shown with viridans streptococci endocarditis[35] (see Question 4). Thus, extended-interval dosing of aminoglycosides cannot be recommended for the treatment of enterococcal endocarditis at this time.

The only study comparing high-dose (>3 mg/kg/day) and low-dose (<3 mg/kg/day) gentamicin with penicillin in humans with enterococcal endocarditis evaluated 56 patients over a 12-year period (36 with streptomycin-susceptible and 20 with streptomycin-resistant infections).[147] The relapse rate of patients infected with streptomycin-resistant organisms (n = 20) was not significantly different between the high- and low-dose treatment groups (n = 10 each). Furthermore, patients who received the higher doses of gentamicin experienced a greater prevalence of nephrotoxicity (10 of 10 vs. 2 of 10, $p < 0.001$). Mean peak and trough concentrations of gentamicin in the patients who received the high doses were 5 mcg/mL and 2.1 mcg/mL, respectively; corresponding levels for patients receiving the low-dose regimen were 3.1 mcg/mL and 1 mcg/mL.

Based on available data, it would be reasonable to start G.S. on a gentamicin dosage of 1 mg/kg Q 8 hr (assuming her renal function is normal) and to maintain peak concentrations of 3 to 5 mcg/mL and trough concentrations of <1 mcg/mL.

IN COMBINATION WITH VANCOMYCIN

21. Why was vancomycin used in combination with gentamicin in G.S.? Is this combination effective against enterococci?

G.S. has a history of penicillin allergy. Most clinicians favor a combination of vancomycin and gentamicin for penicillin-allergic patients with enterococcal endocarditis, although vancomycin plus streptomycin is a suitable alternative.[21,23,147] The combination of vancomycin and gentamicin demonstrates bactericidal synergy for about 95% of enterococci strains. In contrast, the vancomycin and streptomycin combination demonstrates bactericidal synergy for about 65% of enterococci. Because G.S. has PVE, she should receive approximately 30 mg/kg/day, or roughly 1.5 g/day (750 mg Q 12 hr), of vancomycin in combination with gentamicin (3 mg/kg/day). Serum levels of vancomycin and gentamicin should be monitored as previously discussed.

Duration of Therapy

22. How long should G.S. be treated?

Historically, enterococcal endocarditis has been treated with penicillin plus an aminoglycoside for 6 weeks; the overall cure rate with this regimen is about 85%.[21] Data indicate that 4 weeks of therapy is probably adequate for most patients with enterococcal endocarditis.[21,147,148] One study evaluated the efficacy of a treatment regimen involving shorter course aminoglycoside therapy (median of 15 days) in combination with a cell wall active agent for a median of 42 days in patients with PVE and native valve enterococcal endocarditis.[151] Clinical cure was observed in 75 of 93 (81%) patients overall, 78% of patients with PVE and 82% of patients with native valves. Among those who had a clinical cure, 52% received a β-lactam, 12% received vancomycin and 36% received a combination of both. Ampicillin was given in 88% of patients receiving a β-lactam. The causative organism was *E. faecalis* in 78 patients and *E. faecium* in 5 patients. Clinical success was also achieved in all eight patients with native valve IE who received either vancomycin (50%), ampicillin (25%) or combination of both (25%) without synergistic aminoglycoside therapy.

Patients with complicated courses should receive 6 weeks of therapy, however. These include patients infected with streptomycin-resistant organisms (such as G.S.), those who have had symptoms for >3 months before the initiation of antibiotics, and patients with PVE (such as G.S.).[13,21] Some clinicians recommend 6 weeks of therapy for all patients in whom the duration of illness cannot be firmly established; this accounts for many patients who present with subacute disease.

Increased Nephrotoxicity With Vancomycin Combination Therapy

23. Is the combination of vancomycin and an aminoglycoside more nephrotoxic than either drug alone?

The incidence of nephrotoxicity associated with vancomycin administration (alone) in humans is thought to be minimal or nonexistent.[149] In a three-arm study involving >200 patients, nephrotoxicity was found in 5% of patients who received vancomycin alone, 22% of those receiving vancomycin with an aminoglycoside, and 11% of those receiving an aminoglycoside alone. The study was well designed in that an aminoglycoside control group was included for comparison on the incidence of nephrotoxicity. Patients in whom increases in the serum creatinine concentration may have been a result of clinical conditions and patients who received drugs known to alter renal function were excluded in the analysis of this study. Serial serum vancomycin and aminoglycoside concentrations, as well as duration of therapy, were reported and analyzed. The authors concluded that vancomycin trough concentrations >10 mcg/mL and concurrent therapy with an aminoglycoside were risk factors associated with an increased incidence of nephrotoxicity. Based on the study data, it is difficult to ascertain the precise risk of nephrotoxicity relative to specific vancomycin trough concentrations >10 mcg/mL. Another study specifically evaluated the risk of nephrotoxicity in patients receiving high-dose vancomycin therapy achieving trough concentrations of 15 to 20 mcg/mL for MRSA infections.

Nephrotoxicity occurred in 12% (11 of 95) of patients, significantly predicted by concomitant therapy with other nephrotoxic agents. An incremental increase in the risk of nephrotoxicity was associated with duration of therapy at high trough levels (15–20 mcg/mL): 6.3% for 7 days or less, 21.1% for 8 to 14 days, and 30% for more than 14 days. In a subanalysis that included only patients without receipt of concomitant nephrotoxic agents, nephrotoxicity occurred in only 1 (2%) of 44 high-trough versus 0 of 24 low-trough (<15 mcg/mL) patients. These studies confirm that an increased incidence of nephrotoxicity is likely when vancomycin and an aminoglycoside are given concomitantly.

Glycopeptide Resistance

24. How do enterococci develop vancomycin resistance, and what are the therapeutic implications when treating a patient with glycopeptide-resistant enterococcal endocarditis?

The therapeutic challenges offered by a patient with endocarditis caused by enterococci exhibiting high-level resistance to aminoglycosides are compounded by the acquired resistance of enterococci to glycopeptide antibiotics such as vancomycin. VRE, particularly *E. faecium,* have emerged in the United States since 1987.[150,151] Because the use of prophylactic vancomycin has been increasing steadily since the mid-1980s, it should not be surprising to see increased resistance to this class of compounds. Between 1989 and 1993, the percentage of nosocomial enterococci reported as resistant to vancomycin in the United States rose more than 20-fold, from 0.3% to 7.9%.[151,152] Enterococcal isolates from intensive care units increased even more dramatically, from 0.4% to 13.6%, over the same time. Data from the Centers for Disease Control and Prevention (CDC) National Nosocomial Infections Surveillance (NNIS) system indicate that the rate of increase has slowed down from 31% in 2000 to 12% in 2003.[153] A 12% increase was found in VRE infections in causing infections in intensive care units between 2003 and the prior 5-year period (1998–2002). Nonetheless, epidemiologic studies conducted by the NNIS system as well as others have shown that VRE bacteremia is associated with significantly increased morbidity and mortality.[153,154]

Although *E. faecalis* is responsible for 80% to 90% of infections caused by enterococci, *E. faecium* is more likely to exhibit resistance to glycopeptides compared with *E. faecalis;* more than 95% of VRE recovered in the United States are *E. faecium.* Glycopeptide-resistant enterococci synthesize abnormal peptidoglycan precursors that lower the binding affinity of glycopeptides to peptidoglycans.[150,151] VRE can be broadly classified into three separate phenotypes (A, B, and C), based on three structurally different genes and gene products (e.g., altered ligases).[150] Most (approximately 70%) of resistant enterococci are of the VanA phenotype, which are resistant to high levels of both vancomycin (MIC >256 mcg/mL) and teicoplanin (MIC >16 mcg/mL).[150,151] Expression of resistance is inducible, usually plasmid mediated, and transferable to other organisms via conjugation. The VanB strains exhibit moderate vancomycin resistance (MIC 16–64 mcg/mL), but remain susceptible to teicoplanin (MIC ≤2 mcg/mL). Overall, the VanC isolates are the least resistant (vancomycin MIC 8–16 mcg/mL; teicoplanin MIC ≤2 mcg/mL) because of chromosomal-mediated constitutive expression (i.e., not inducible as are VanA and VanB); however, VanC isolates usually are associated with the much less common *E. gallinarum* and *E. casseliflavus* infections.[150,151]

Several studies have implicated prior use of vancomycin as well as extended-spectrum cephalosporins and drugs with potent antianaerobic activity as risk factors for promoting infection and colonization with VRE.[150,151]

The emergence of VRE causing serious infections is indeed worrisome because few therapeutic alternatives exist for this organism because synergistic combinations are required for bactericidal activity and a clinical cure. As might be anticipated with an organism that is still a relatively uncommon cause of serious infection, well-established guidelines for antimicrobial therapy are not available. To date, no articles have been published in which investigators have demonstrated successful treatment with any particular agent or combination of agents in a large series of patients infected with glycopeptide-resistant enterococci. As a result, practitioners must make decisions using the available data from in vitro synergy studies, experimental models of endocarditis, and scattered case reports. In addition, glycopeptide-resistant isolates often exhibit concomitant high-level resistance to aminoglycosides and high-level resistance to β-lactams (e.g., ampicillin, penicillin) secondary to either β-lactamase production or alteration in the target penicillin-binding proteins.

Several antibiotic combinations appear promising in vitro and in preliminary animal models of endocarditis, but few data are currently available in humans. Those combinations include high-dose ampicillin (20 g/day) or ampicillin/sulbactam plus an aminoglycoside; vancomycin, penicillin or ceftriaxone and gentamicin; ampicillin and imipenem; ciprofloxacin and ampicillin; ciprofloxacin, rifampin, and gentamicin; teicoplanin and gentamicin (teicoplanin is not available in the United States).[150]

STREPTOGRAMIN AND OXAZOLIDINONE

Quinupristin/dalfopristin (Synercid) and linezolid (Zyvox) are two agents with activity and proved efficacy against infections caused by VRE approved for use by the FDA in the United States. Quinupristin/dalfopristin (Synercid), available as a fixed 70:30 combination, is the first drug in the streptogramin class made available in the United States for human use. It belongs to the antibiotic family of macrolides/lincosamides/streptogramins. The agent received accelerated approval by the FDA in late 1999 specifically for the treatment of vancomycin-resistant *E. faecium* bacteremia. The combination is synergistic for glycopeptide-resistant enterococci with an MIC_{90} of 2 mcg/mL. The fixed product is generally bactericidal against susceptible streptococci and staphylococci (including methicillin-resistant strains), but it is bacteriostatic against *E. faecium*. Specifically, *E. faecalis* is not susceptible to the agent because of the presence of an efflux[158,160,161] pump conferring resistance to dalfopristin. Emergence of resistance during therapy has been reported on rare occasions.[156] The recommended dosage is 7.5 mg/kg Q 8 to 12 hr (depending on the severity of infection).[157]

One report describes the largest clinical experience to date on the use of quinupristin/dalfopristin in the treatment of infections caused by multidrug-resistant *E. faecium*.[158] A total of 397 patients were enrolled in two prospective emergency-use studies. Treatment response varied by indication, with an overall success rate of 65%. Of the five clinically evaluable patients who were treated for endocarditis, response occurred in only one (20%). The low response rate observed with endocarditis is likely reflected by the need of bactericidal therapy for treatment success. An additional case of *E. faecium* endocarditis successfully treated by the combination of quinupristin/dalfopristin, doxycycline, and rifampin was reported by Matsumura et al.[159] Arthralgias or myalgias were the most frequently reported events (10%) and also most frequently resulted in drug discontinuation.[158] A higher incidence of arthralgias or myalgias has been reported by others (up to 50%); those patients had significant comorbidities.[160] All cases were reversible on cessation of therapy. Significant venous irritation occurred (46%) when the drug was administered via a peripheral vein. In addition, the dose should be diluted up to 500 to 750 mL, as long as the entire infusion can be given in 1 hour.[158,161] The drug is not compatible with saline solutions. Laboratory abnormalities most frequently observed were increases in total and conjugated bilirubin in up to 34% of patients. As a result, liver function tests should be obtained once a week during therapy. Because quinupristin/dalfopristin is a potent inhibitor of the cytochrome P450 3A4 enzyme system, coadministration of drugs (e.g., cyclosporine, cisapride) metabolized by the same enzyme system should be avoided if possible, or done only with close monitoring of therapeutic levels.[157,160]

Linezolid (Zyvox) is the first drug in the oxazolidinone class to receive FDA approval in 2000 for clinical use. Linezolid has bacteriostatic activity against enterococci, including vancomycin-resistant *E. faecium* and *E. faecalis*. It is also active against other gram-positive cocci, including *S. pneumoniae* and methicillin-resistant staphylococci.[157] Vancomycin-resistant *E. faecium* isolates resistant to linezolid have been encountered in the clinical setting.[162,163] Treatment experience with linezolid under the compassionate use protocol reported clinical and microbiologic cure rates of 50% at 6-month follow-up for patients with endocarditis. Vancomycin-resistant *E. faecium* was the causative organism for 19 of the 32 patients treated. Treatment response was not subgrouped by causative organisms in this report, which was presented in the form of a meeting abstract.[115] Adverse effects associated with linezolid are generally mild in nature and include nausea, headache, diarrhea, rash, and altered taste. Of greater concern is its potential to cause myelosuppression. Thrombocytopenia, leukopenia, anemia, and pancytopenia have all been reported. Up to 30% of patients treated have been reported to experience thrombocytopenia (platelet counts <100,000 platelets/mm^3).[157] In addition, linezolid is a weak monoamine oxidase inhibitor, which may potentiate the adrenergic effects of sympathomimetic agents (i.e., pseudoephedrine, phenylpropanolamine) and precipitate serotonergic syndrome when used concomitantly with selective serotonin reuptake inhibitors. Patients should be advised to avoid tyramine-containing foods (i.e., aged cheese, sausages, sauerkraut, wine) during therapy as well. Linezolid is available both orally and parenterally. Linezolid given orally or via enteral feedings is completely bioavailable.[164] A dosage of 600 mg twice daily is recommended for adults. Persistent MRSA bacteremia caused by suboptimal serum concentrations of linezolid has been described,[120] suggesting a need to obtain serum drug concentrations in patients not responding appropriately to treatment.

DAPTOMYCIN

Daptomycin is active against enterococci in vitro with an MIC range of 0.25 to 4 mcg/mL and a MIC_{90} of 4 mcg/mL for 219 vancomycin resistant *E. faecium* isolates from the United States. For 40 vancomycin-resistant *E. faecalis* isolates,the MIC range is 0.015 to 2 mcg/mL, with an MIC_{90} of 2 mcg/mL.[165] When tested against 20 vancomycin resistant *E. faecium* strain, daptomycin had an MIC_{50} of 2 mcg/mL versus 0.5 mcg/mL and 4 mcg/mL for quinupristin/dalfopristin and linezolid, respectively.[166] Of caution is the emergence of daptomycin resistance during therapy for VRE infections reported in the literature.[167,168] In a case report of a patient with vancomycin resistant *E. faecium* pyelonephritis, the initial isolate had an MIC of 2 mcg/mL; however, after 17 days of treatment, a blood culture yielded growth of vancomycin resistant *E. faecium* with an MIC increase to 32 mcg/mL.[169] Clinical experience with daptomycin for vancomycin resistant *E. faecium* endocarditis is limited to one published case report.[170] The patient received daptomycin 8 mg/kg/day in combination with gentamicin and rifampin for 11 weeks. Subsequent cultures were negative; however, the patient died 4 months after completion of therapy from an unknown cause. Thus, daptomycin's role in treating VRE endocarditis is uncertain at this point.

CONTROL OF GLYCOPEPTIDE RESISTANCE

Considering the continuing rise in prevalence and therapeutic challenges associated with VRE, a control effort involving multiple disciplines is necessary to effect a decrease or prevent an increase in the number of patients colonized or infected by these organisms. The primary focus of control should be on limiting vancomycin use to those indications recommended by the CDC's Hospital Infection Control Practices Advisory Committee in 1994 and enforcing strict adherence to infection control practices to minimize cross-contamination of infected or colonized patients.[150,172]

Selection pressure resulting from continued heavy use of vancomycin is evident with the emergence of vancomycin-intermediate *S. aureus* (VISA) and vancomycin-resistant *S. aureus* (VRSA). Cases of VISA have been reported in the United States and Japan.[63] Although the mechanism of resistance for VISA is unique and does not appear to be mediated by the VanA gene, all patients had prior infections with MRSA and had received repeated and prolonged vancomycin therapy.[63] More alarming is the recovery of a VRSA strain in a patient who had concurrent VRE infections.[92] This case represents the first demonstration of in vivo transfer of *VanA* gene from VRE to *S. aureus,* conferring high-level vancomycin resistance (MIC >1,012 mcg/mL). The isolation of both VISA and VRSA underscores the importance of controlling the spread of vancomycin resistance through proper antibiotic stewardship and infection control practices.

FUNGAL ENDOCARDITIS CAUSED BY *CANDIDA ALBICANS*

Prognosis and Treatment

25. B.G., a 35-yearold male heroin addict, was admitted to the hospital with chief complaints of pleuritic chest pain and DOE. Physical examination revealed a cachectic man with a temperature of 104°F, a diastolic regurgitant heart murmur heard loudest during inspiration, splenomegaly, and pharyngeal petechiae. Funduscopic examination was noncontributory. On the chest radiograph, several pulmonary infiltrates with cavitation were evident. Urinalysis (UA) was significant for microscopic hematuria and RBC casts. An ECG demonstrated vegetations on both the tricuspid and aortic heart valves. B.G. had evidence of moderate heart failure, although his hemodynamic status at that time was "stable." Six sets of blood cultures were drawn over 2 days and broad-spectrum empiric coverage consisting of vancomycin, gentamicin, and ceftazidime was initiated. Two days later, two of the cultures grew *C. albicans,* and a diagnosis of fungal endocarditis was established. What is B.G.'s prognosis, and how should his fungal endocarditis be treated?

Fungal endocarditis is a rare but life-threatening infection with a grave prognosis that is generally difficult to diagnose and even more difficult to treat.[1] Most cases are caused by *Candida* and *Aspergillus* species. Fungal endocarditis occurs primarily in IV drug users, patients with prosthetic heart valves, immunocompromised patients, those with IV catheters, or patients receiving broad-spectrum antibiotics.[172–175]

Management of fungal endocarditis generally requires early valve replacement and aggressive fungicidal therapy with a combination of high-dose amphotericin B (usually 1 mg/kg/day IV) and 5-flucytosine (5-FC; Ancobon) 150 mg/kg/day orally.[1,172–175] These antifungal agents should be prescribed for B.G. and his broad-spectrum antibiotic coverage with vancomycin, gentamicin, and ceftazidime should be discontinued.

B.G.'s clinical presentation and chest radiograph indicate that fragments of vegetation have already embolized to his lungs and possibly to other vital organs (e.g., spleen, kidneys). Because of the morbidity and mortality associated with major emboli and valvular insufficiency, B.G. should undergo surgery within 48–72 hours after antifungal therapy has been initiated. Delaying surgery beyond this time frame can increase B.G.'s risk of mortality.

The prognosis for B.G. is dismal even with proper medical and surgical treatment. In a series analyzing 270 cases of fungal IE occurring over a 30-year period, mortality for those who received combined medical and surgical management was 45%, compared with 64% for those who received antifungal therapy alone.[174] Despite initial response to treatment, the rate of relapse is high (30%–40%), and relapse can occur up to 9 years following the initial episode of infection.[172–175] Most deaths in IV drug users with endocarditis are secondary to heart failure, a finding already evident in B.G.[1] In addition, replacement of a heart valve for fungal endocarditis in a heroin addict carries a significant risk of late morbidity and mortality.[174]

Combination Therapy With 5-Flucytosine and Amphotericin B

26. Why is it important to treat B.G.'s fungal endocarditis with the combination of 5-FC and amphotericin B? What is the optimal duration of therapy?

The importance of adding 5-FC (Ancobon) to amphotericin B (Fungizone) therapy has not been adequately studied; however, the poor prognosis associated with fungal endocarditis warrants the administration of 5-FC, despite its potential for causing bone marrow suppression and hepatotoxicity.[174] (See Chapter 68, Prevention and Treatment of Infections in Neutropenic Cancer Patients, for a discussion of amphotericin B and 5-FC.) The vegetations from his tricuspid or aortic heart valves already have broken off and caused pulmonary cavitation and possibly splenomegaly. His clinical presentation is consistent with a potentially fatal outcome; therefore, his blood isolates should be tested for in vitro susceptibility to amphotericin, to 5-FC, and to both of these drugs in combination. Fungi resistant to 5-FC alone may still be susceptible to the synergistic effect of the 5-FC–amphotericin B combination.[176] If the organism is resistant to 5-FC and in vitro synergy between these two antifungals is lacking, continued treatment with 5-FC is not indicated.

The optimal dose and duration of antifungal therapy for fungal endocarditis have not been determined by clinical studies; however, postoperative treatment with amphotericin B and 5-FC (if it has in vitro activity) for a minimum of 6 weeks (total dose, 1.5–3 g of amphotericin B) is recommended and is supported by the poor penetration of amphotericin B into heart valve tissue.[177] In patients with fungal PVE, some experts advocate secondary prophylaxis for a minimum of 2 years or lifelong suppressive treatment with an oral antifungal agent for nonsurgical candidates in light of the high rates of relapse.[1,174–179]

Nephrotoxicity caused by amphotericin is often a serious dose-limiting factor to completion of therapy, particularly in patients who require a prolonged treatment course (see Chapter 67, Osteomyelitis and Septic Arthritis). Renal dysfunction secondary to the conventional formulation of amphotericin B may stabilize or improve with the switch to lipid-formulated amphotericin B products (i.e., Abelcet).[180] The efficacy of the new formulations in the treatment of endocarditis has been demonstrated only in anecdotal reports,[174–177,181] whereas the drug acquisition cost is substantially higher. Alternative antifungal agents may need to be considered in patients who experience significant renal toxicities.

Alternative Antifungals

27. If B.G. experiences significant toxicities because of prolonged combination treatment with amphotericin and 5-FC, what alternative antifungal agent(s) can be used to treat his fungal endocarditis?

Fluconazole (Diflucan) is a triazole compound active against *Candida* species, particularly *C. albicans* and *C. parapsilosis*. It also has a favorable toxicity profile compared with amphotericin and 5-FC.[182] Prolonged combination treatment with amphotericin and 5-FC often is limited by nephrotoxicity, bone marrow suppression, and hepatic damage. Limited experimental and clinical experience using fluconazole in the treatment of candidal endocarditis has been accumulating.

Fluconazole was effective in eradicating cardiac fungal vegetations caused by *C. albicans* and *C. parapsilosis* in a rabbit model.[183] Successful experience with fluconazole treatment of fungal endocarditis in humans has been described in only a few case reports.[184–189] Patients with endocarditis treated with fluconazole were either intolerant of amphotericin or poor surgical candidates who required suppressive antifungal therapy after completion of a course of amphotericin therapy. Patients with various *Candida* species (i.e., *C. albicans, C. parapsilosis,* and *C. tropicalis)* were treated with 200 to 600 mg of fluconazole daily over 45 days to 6 months or until death. Fluconazole therapy reduced or completely removed all cardiac vegetations and resolved clinical symptoms. Because of the lack of adequate clinical experience, however, the use of fluconazole in treating fungal endocarditis cannot be advocated except in patients who require lifelong therapy because of the following situations: (a) the patient is a poor surgical candidate, (b) the patient has relapsed at least once since the initial infection episode, or (c) the patient has PVE.

Another potential alternative is caspofungin, which is a first-line agent in the echinocandin class.[190] Caspofungin was approved by the FDA for salvage therapy against invasive aspergillosis, esophageal candidiasis, and invasive candidiasis (primarily bloodstream infections and peritonitis). Caspofungin inhibits fungal cell wall synthesis by inhibiting β-1,3 glucan synthesis. It is fungicidal against most *Candida* species (including *C. albicans)*, and its use is not associated with nephrotoxicity. Both characteristics make the drug an attractive treatment option for B.G. should toxicities develop after prolonged therapy with amphotericin B. Limited experience has described successful outcomes associated with caspofungin use in this setting.[191–193] In a patient with *C. glabrata* mitral valve endocarditis without surgical intervention, caspofungin was used successfully as induction therapy in combination with amphotericin B and continued as maintenance therapy for 12 weeks.[194] In a second case report of a patient with prosthetic valve endocarditis caused by *C. glabrata* and *C. krusei*, resolution of vegetation was achieved after 6 weeks of caspofungin therapy alone without valvular replacement. Both patients were deemed to be poor surgical candidates and received medical therapy only[195]. Micafungin and anidulafungin are the latest additions to the echinocandin class; clinical experience in the treatment of endocarditis is currently lacking.

GRAM-NEGATIVE BACILLARY ENDOCARDITIS CAUSED BY *PSEUDOMONAS AERUGINOSA*

Prevalence

28. Fourteen months after completing his course of antifungal therapy, B.G. was readmitted to the hospital with a 48-hour history of fever, shaking chills, rigors, and night sweats. His vital signs at that time were blood pressure, 100/60 mmHg; pulse, 120 beats/minute; respirations, 24/minute; and temperature, 103.7°F. A new-onset systolic murmur was noted on auscultation. Two-dimensional echocardiography revealed two small vegetations on the prosthetic valve. Empiric therapy consisting of amphotericin

B, 5-FC, vancomycin, and gentamicin was initiated. Three blood cultures drawn on the day of admission were positive for *P. aeruginosa* with the following antibiotic susceptibilities (MIC): gentamicin (8 mcg/mL), tobramycin (2 mcg/mL), piperacillin (64 mcg/mL), and ceftazidime (2 mcg/mL). A presumptive diagnosis of PVE caused by *P. aeruginosa* was made. Why was the finding of *pseudomonas* expected in B.G.?

The prevalence of endocarditis caused by gram-negative organisms has increased significantly over the years, especially in IV drug users such as B.G. and patients with prosthetic heart valves. Gram-negative organisms are responsible for about 15% to 20% of endocarditis cases in these populations.[198] Most gram-negative endocarditis cases are caused by *Pseudomonas* species, *S. marcescens,* and *Enterobacter* species, although numerous other gram-negative organisms have been known to cause endocarditis.[196–201] Geographic clustering of certain organisms causing endocarditis in narcotic addicts has been shown in the past, such as the association of *P. aeruginosa* with the Detroit area and *S. marcescens* with San Francisco.[201–204] These past epidemiologic findings are not necessarily true today. In narcotic addicts with gram-negative endocarditis, the tricuspid, aortic, and mitral valves are involved in 50%, 45%, and 40% of cases, respectively.[196]

Antimicrobial Therapy

29. How should B.G.'s gram-negative endocarditis be treated and monitored?

The regimen of amphotericin B, 5-FC, vancomycin, and gentamicin that was initiated empirically for B.G. pending the outcome of culture and sensitivity results should now be discontinued because *P. aeruginosa* has been cultured from B.G.'s blood. Proper antibiotic selection for the treatment of gram-negative endocarditis should be based on antimicrobial susceptibility and synergy testing. A bactericidal combination of antibiotics usually is required to provide in vivo synergy and to prevent resistant subpopulations from emerging during therapy.[1,31] B.G., therefore, should be treated with ceftazidime (2 g IV Q 8 hr) with concurrent high-dose tobramycin (3 mg/kg IV Q 8 hr). The duration of therapy is not well defined, but most authorities recommend 4 to 6 weeks.[1,197,202,204] Despite the problems associated with using the SBT as a monitoring tool (see Question 3), therapy should be tailored to achieve a trough titer of at least 1:8.[22] Because B.G. should be receiving both ceftazidime and tobramycin on the same schedule (Q 8 hr), the trough titer should be drawn just before dose administration. Finally, the infected valve should be surgically excised for the reasons previously discussed.

Endocarditis caused by *P. aeruginosa* (as in B.G.) should be treated for at least 6 weeks with a combination of an aminoglycoside and an antipseudomonal penicillin (ticarcillin or piperacillin) or cephalosporin (ceftazidime).[1,206] The combination of an antipseudomonal penicillin and an aminoglycoside is synergistic in vitro and in the rabbit model of *P. aeruginosa* endocarditis,[205,206] and clinical experience has confirmed this finding in IV drug users. Combination therapy with high dosages of tobramycin or gentamicin (8 mg/kg/day) has been associated with a significantly higher cure rate and lower mortality rate compared with an older, "low-dose" regimen (2.5–5 mg/kg/day).[197,198,202] Aminoglycosides (tobramycin or gentamicin) should be dosed to produce peak and trough serum concentrations of 15 to 20 mcg/mL and <2 mcg/mL, respectively, to ensure maximum efficacy[1]; therefore, high-dose tobramycin should be selected for B.G.

For obvious reasons, peak and trough aminoglycoside concentrations should be routinely monitored in all patients receiving high-dose therapy for gram-negative bacillary endocarditis. Of note, the use of extended-interval dosing of aminoglycoside has not been evaluated for the treatment of endocarditis caused by gram-negative organisms; therefore, this dosing approach cannot be recommended at this time. The choice of aminoglycoside should be based on the in vitro activity of the organism (i.e., MIC), relative toxicity potential, and cost. In B.G.'s case, tobramycin should be selected over gentamicin because the isolated organism exhibited greater susceptibility to this aminoglycoside. Generally, *P. aeruginosa* is more susceptible to tobramycin than to gentamicin. Thus, it is not at all surprising that the *P. aeruginosa* in B.G.'s blood cultures had a 2 mcg/mL MIC for tobramycin compared with the 8 mcg/mL MIC for gentamicin.

Data on the use of ceftazidime for the treatment of *P. aeruginosa* endocarditis are limited; however, it should be preferred over piperacillin for B.G. on the basis of its greater in vitro activity and good penetration into cardiac valvular tissue.[207]

Several compounds such as imipenem (Primaxin), aztreonam (Azactam), and ciprofloxacin (Cipro), have demonstrated excellent in vitro activity against many of the gram-negative organisms causing endocarditis. Clinical data regarding their use in the treatment of endocarditis are very limited, however.[208–211]

CULTURE-NEGATIVE ENDOCARDITIS

30. B.G.'s history, clinical presentation, and imaging studies are strongly suggestive of infective endocarditis. If his blood cultures had been negative after 48 hours of incubation, the working diagnosis would have been culture-negative endocarditis. What are the possible reasons for culture-negative endocarditis, and what measures should be taken to establish a microbiologic etiology?

The proportion of patients with culture-negative endocarditis has diminished considerably, presumably as a result of improved microbiologic culture techniques. Negative blood cultures are present in only 5% to 7% of patients who meet strict criteria for the diagnosis of IE and have not recently received antibiotics.[212]

The prior administration of antimicrobials is thought to account for most cases of culture-negative endocarditis.[213] B.G.'s blood cultures may remain negative for several days to weeks if he has taken antibiotics recently. The use of antibiotic absorbance resins or the addition of β-lactamases to the blood sample may remove or inactivate some antibiotics.[214,215]

Slow-growing and fastidious organisms, such as gram-negative bacilli in the *Haemophilus-Actinobacillus-Cardiobacterium-Eikenella-Kingella* group (HACEK), *Brucella, Coxiella,* chlamydiae, strict anaerobes, and fungi, should be pursued in culture-negative patients. This usually is accomplished by the use of special culture media or by obtaining appropriate serologic acute and convalescent titers. Blood cultures should be saved for at least 3 weeks to detect slow-growing organisms.[213] The use of polymerase chain reaction to identify nonculturable organisms in excised valvular specimens or septic emboli has been helpful in some cases.[216] Of note, previously NVS has been the cause of most of the cases of endocarditis diagnosed as "culture-negative," initially because of its requirement for the addition of vitamin B_6 (pyridoxal HCl) to the culture media for laboratory growth; however, laboratory identification is no longer a significant problem with current culture media and laboratory techniques.[24]

Empiric Therapy

31. Assume that the causative organism remains unidentified. Recommend an antimicrobial regimen for the empiric treatment of B.G.'s presumed culture-negative endocarditis.

In the hemodynamically stable patient, antibiotic therapy should be withheld until positive blood cultures are obtained.[1] Based on B.G.'s clinical presentation and echocardiographic findings, empiric antibiotics should be initiated as soon as necessary cultures have been collected. Because staphylococci and gram-negative bacilli account for most organisms responsible for endocarditis in the narcotic addict with a prosthetic heart valve, B.G. should be started on a regimen consisting of an antistaphylococcal penicillin, such as nafcillin, an aminoglycoside, and a third agent with gram-negative coverage. Because B.G. may be experiencing a relapse caused by *C. albicans,* the addition of amphotericin B and flucytosine would be appropriate. If B.G. is from an area where methicillin-resistant staphylococci are prevalent, vancomycin should be substituted for nafcillin. A third-generation cephalosporin (ceftriaxone or ceftazidime) or piperacillin could be used, depending on the gram-negative pathogens common to the region and their anticipated susceptibilities. This regimen, which contains an aminoglycoside and piperacillin, also will provide coverage for enterococci.

B.G.'s clinical status and the positive ECG indicate that early surgical valve excision and replacement are necessary.[217] Cultures obtained from excised valve may result in identification of the causative organism. His antimicrobial regimen may need to be altered if and when subsequent culture information becomes available. Other noninfective conditions, such as atrial myxoma, marasmic endocarditis, and rheumatic fever, can mimic culture-negative endocarditis and should be excluded from the differential diagnosis with the appropriate tests.[1]

PROPHYLACTIC THERAPY

Rationale and Recommendations

32. B.B., a 74-year-old man with poor dentition, is scheduled to have all of his remaining teeth extracted for subsequent fitting of dentures. His medical history is significant for numerous infections of the oral cavity and prosthetic valve replacement 2 years ago. His only current medications are digoxin (Lanoxin) 0.125 mg/day and furosemide (Lasix) 40 mg every morning. What is the rationale for antibiotic prophylaxis?

Because infective endocarditis is associated with significant mortality and long-term morbidity, prevention in susceptible patients is of paramount importance.[1] Estimates are, however, that <10% of all cases are theoretically preventable.[10,48]

The incidence of endocarditis in patients undergoing procedures known to cause significant bacteremia, even without antibiotic prophylaxis, is low. In addition, endocarditis may develop following the administration of seemingly appropriate chemoprophylaxis. Therefore, it is not surprising that the efficacy of prophylaxis has never been established through placebo-controlled clinical trials. Approximately 6,000 patients would be necessary to demonstrate a statistical difference (if one exists) between untreated controls and a group receiving prophylaxis.[48,218]

Without conclusive clinical data from prospective trials, recommendations for antibiotic prophylaxis have been based largely on in vitro susceptibility data, evaluation of antibiotic regimens using animal models of endocarditis, and anecdotal experiences.[48,218,219,220]

Prophylactic antibiotics are thought to provide protection by decreasing the number of organisms reaching the damaged heart valve from a primary source. Thus, antibiotics theoretically prevent bacterial multiplication on the valve and interfere with bacterial adherence to the cardiac lesion.[48,218]

The 2007AHA recommendations for antibiotic prophylaxis before common medical procedures are outlined in Table 59-7.[218] Compared with the previous (1997) guideline,[218] the current guidelines only recommend the use of prophylaxis in patients with specific cardiac conditions who are undergoing

Table 59-7 Endocarditis Prophylaxis Regimen Indicated for Patients With Cardiac Conditions[a]

Drug	*Dose*
Dental or Upper Respiratory Tract Procedures	Single Dose 30 to 60 Minutes Before Procedure
Standard Regimen	
Amoxicillin (oral)	*Adult:* 2 g
	Pediatric: 50 mg/kg
Allergic to penicillin or ampicillin (oral)	
Clindamycin	*Adult:* 600 mg
or	*Pediatric:* 20 mg/kg
Cephalexin[b,c]	*Adult:* 2 g
or	*Pediatric:* 50 mg/kg
Azithromycin or clarithromycin	*Adult:* 500 mg
	Pediatric: 15 mg/kg
Unable to Take Oral Medications	
Ampicillin	*Adult:* 2 g intramuscularly (IM) or intravenously (IV)
	Pediatric: 50 mg/kg IM or IV
Allergic to penicillin or ampicillin	
Clindamycin	*Adult:* 600 mg (IV)
or	*Pediatric:* 20 mg/kg IV
Cefazolin[b]	*Adult:* 1 g IM or IV
	Pediatric: 50 mg/kg IM or IV

[a] See Table 59-1.
[b] Cephalosporins should not be used in individuals with immediate-type hypersensitivity reaction (e.g., urticaria, angioedema, or anaphylaxis) to penicillins or ampicillin.
[c] Other first- or second-generation oral cephalosporins in equivalent adult or pediatric dose.
Adapted from reference 218, with permission.

only dental or respiratory tract procedures. The use of prophylaxis for patients undergoing gastrourinary or gastrointestinal procedures is no recommended because of a continuing lack of evidence to support efficacy.

Dental and Upper Respiratory Tract Procedures

The new guidelines only recommend prophylaxis in individuals with cardiac conditions associated with the highest risk of adverse outcomes from endocarditis (see Table 59-1). Previous 1997 AHA guidelines listed a substantial number of procedures where prophylaxis is either indicated or not recommended. Analysis of published data shows that viridans streptococci bacteremia can result from any procedure that involves the manipulation of the gingival tissue or the periapical region of the teeth or perforation of the oral mucosa. Placement or removal of prosthodontic or orthodontic appliances, adjustment of orthodontic appliances, taking dental radiographs, bleeding from trauma to the lips or oral mucosa, and so instantaneous shedding of deciduous teeth do not require chemoprophylaxis. Endotracheal intubation also does not require prophylactic therapy.

Antimicrobial prophylaxis should be directed against the viridans group of streptococci because these organisms are the most common cause of endocarditis following dental procedures. Invasive surgical procedures involving the upper respiratory tract, such as incision or biopsy of the respiratory mucosa (e.g., tonsillectomy, adenoidectomy), can cause transient bacteremia with organisms that have similar antibiotic susceptibilities to those that occur after dental procedures; therefore, the same regimens are suggested. Prophylaxis is not recommended for bronchoscopies unless the procedure involves incision of the respiratory mucosa. Amoxicillin is currently recommended for oral prophylaxis in susceptible persons having dental or upper respiratory tract surgery. Oral clindamycin, clarithromycin, or azithromycin is recommended for patients with immediate-type hypersensitivity reaction to penicillins. Unlike past recommendations of the AHA, the current guidelines no longer recommend prophylaxis based on risk stratification and only patients with outlined cardiac conditions should be administered prophylactic antibiotics.

Most cases of endocarditis that are caused by bacterial flora from the mouth do not follow dental procedures but rather are the result of poor oral hygiene. The cumulative exposure to random bacteremias from daily oral activities is estimated to be 5,730 minutes over a 1-month period compared with only 6 to 30 minutes for a dental procedure. Furthermore, it is estimated that the cumulative exposure to bacteremia from routine daily activities may be as high as 5.6 million time greater than a single tooth extraction[218]. Based on the study results, concerns for antimicrobial resistance, and cost, changes to restrict the use of antibiotic prophylaxis to the highest-risk patients before dental procedures may be expected with future guidelines issued by the AHA.

Indications and Choice of Agent

33. Is prophylactic antibiotic therapy indicated for B.B.? If so, which antibiotic(s) should be used?

Based on the current recommendations, B.B. is a candidate for antibiotic prophylaxis. Presence of a prosthetic aortic valve while undergoing multiple tooth extractions places him at risk for developing endocarditis. He also is scheduled to have all of his remaining teeth extracted, a procedure likely to result in bacteremia. According to Table 59-7, B.B. should receive a single 2-g oral dose of amoxicillin 1 hour before the procedure. Previous AHA guidelines recommended a higher dose (3 g) of amoxicillin to be administered before the procedure and followed by a second dose 6 hours after the procedure.[10] When the blood levels and tolerability of 2- and 3-g oral amoxicillin doses were compared in a crossover study involving 30 adult volunteers,[10] the 2-g doses resulted in adequate serum levels; concentrations 6 hours after dosing were well above the MIC for most oral streptococci. Furthermore, no adverse effects were noted with the 2-g dose versus a 10% incidence of gastrointestinal complaints with the 3-g dose.

HOME INTRAVENOUS ANTIBIOTIC THERAPY

34. T.M., a 48-year-old woman, developed viridans streptococci endocarditis following a dental procedure. Her medical history is significant for rheumatic heart disease and chronic renal insufficiency (measured creatinine clearance, 50 mL/minute). She is hemodynamically stable and has no evidence of vegetation on ECG. She is currently on day 7 of therapy with penicillin G, 2 million units IV Q 4 hr. The plan is to continue penicillin therapy for a total of 4 weeks. What are the considerations for using home IV therapy for the treatment of infective endocarditis? Is T.M. a candidate for home antibiotic therapy?

The successful use of home IV antibiotic therapy for the patient with endocarditis has been described, although the number of patients treated is relatively small compared with those treated for osteomyelitis.[220–222] The advantages of home therapy include economic benefits to the hospital for early discharge (the diagnosis-related-group [DRG] allocation for endocarditis is 18.4 days, which is shorter than the usual recommended duration of therapy) and the potential for greater acceptance by the patient.

Home treatment of endocarditis is not without risk, however.[222] Patients must be hemodynamically stable before discharge and free from the risk of sudden valve rupture. The drug abuser is obviously not a candidate for home treatment, nor is the patient receiving frequent doses of medication. The successful management of any infection amenable to home treatment requires careful patient evaluation for suitability and coordination of the health care provided by key personnel.

T.M. represents the typical patient with uncomplicated streptococcal endocarditis. If the sole reason for continued hospitalization is to administer IV antibiotics, she is a potential candidate for home therapy.

Ceftriaxone is an attractive option for outpatient therapy of uncomplicated endocarditis caused by penicillin-susceptible streptococci. The excellent in vitro activity of ceftriaxone and its long half-life of 6 to 9 hours allow once-a-day administration. The feasibility of intramuscular administration of ceftriaxone also obviates the need for IV access, thus avoiding any potential line-related complications when administered in the outpatient setting.

Clinical experience with the use of ceftriaxone in the treatment of patients with penicillin-susceptible streptococcal endocarditis was described in four open-label studies.[38–41] Two of the studies evaluated ceftriaxone monotherapy for 4 weeks; the other two evaluated combination therapy with ceftriaxone and an aminoglycoside for a 2-week duration. All infecting strains of streptococci in the first two studies were inhibited by ceftriaxone at an MIC of <0.25 mcg/mL. In one study, ceftriaxone was given at a dosage of 2 g once daily for 4 weeks to most patients, with 15 receiving ceftriaxone for 2 weeks followed by amoxicillin 1 g four times daily for 2 weeks. Most of the patients received therapy predominantly as outpatients. All patients (N = 30) reported in this study responded favorably to treatment with ceftriaxone or ceftriaxone followed by amoxicillin.[41] Patients with cardiovascular risk factors, such as heart failure, severe aortic insufficiency, or evidence of recurrent thromboembolic events, were excluded from the study. Only one probable relapse was noted at 3 months after therapy with presentation of febrile syndrome, elevated sedimentation rate, and negative bacterial blood culture. An uncontrolled study extended the favorable results of the aforementioned study.[38] Treatment was completed in 55 of 59 patients. Patients were followed for 4 months to up to 5 years after the end of treatment with no clinical signs or laboratory evidence of relapse. Of patients, 71% completed therapy without complications; however, 10 required valve replacement secondary to hemodynamic deterioration or recurrent emboli, whereas 4 required a change in therapy because of drug allergy. Adverse side effects were minor, but 3 patients had neutropenia that resolved after cessation of therapy.

Because of the lack of controlled trials comparing the efficacy of ceftriaxone against penicillin with or without an aminoglycoside in the treatment of penicillin-susceptible streptococcal endocarditis, ceftriaxone should be considered primarily in patients such as T.M. for whom home antibiotic therapy is a treatment option and those who are hemodynamically stable with no evidence of vegetation.

The feasibility of home therapy depends on the following additional factors: (a) patient willingness; (b) adequate venous access; (c) psychosocial stability; (d) access to medical care if an emergency occurs; (e) ability to train T.M. (proper aseptic technique, catheter site care, antibiotic preparation, recognition of untoward effects of the antibiotic, and recognition of symptoms associated with worsening infection); and (f) insurance coverage for home IV therapy. These conditions can be accomplished only with the multidisciplinary involvement of the infectious disease physician, a social worker, a pharmacist, a specialty nurse, and the patient. Home care, outpatient care, and other options will be used increasingly because health care reform mandates the decreased use of tertiary care facilities when possible.

REFERENCES

1. Bayer AS et al. Endocarditis and intravascular infections. In: Mandell GL et al., eds. *Principles and Practice of Infectious Diseases*. 6th ed. New York: Churchill Livingstone; 2005:975.
2. Sullman PM et al. Pathogenesis of endocarditis. *Am J Med* 1985;78:110.
3. Manning JE et al. An appraisal of the virulence factors associated with streptococcal endocarditis. *J Med Microbiol* 1994;40:110.
4. Sande MA et al. Penicillin-aminoglycoside synergy in experimental *Streptococcus viridans* endocarditis. *J Infect Dis* 1974;129:572.
5. Strom BL et al. Dental and cardiac risk factors for infective endocarditis. A population-based, case-control study. *Ann Intern Med* 1998;129:761.
6. Cabell CH et al. Changing patient characteristics and the effect on mortality in endocarditis. *Arch Intern Med* 2002;162:90.
7. Fowler VG, Jr. et al. *Staphylococcus aureus* endocarditis: a consequence of medical progress. *JAMA* 2005:3012.
8. McKinsey DS et al. Underlying cardiac lesions in adults with infective endocarditis: the changing spectrum. *Am J Med* 1987;82:681.
9. Baddour LM et al. Infective endocarditis: diagnosis, antimicrobial therapy, and management of complications: a statement for healthcare professionals from the Committee on Rheumatic Fever, Endocarditis, and Kawasaki Disease, Council on Cardiovascular Disease in the Young, and the Councils on Clinical Cardiology, Stroke, and Cardiovascular Surgery and Anesthesia, American Heart Association: endorsed by the Infectious Diseases Society of America. 2005:e394.
10. Dajani AS et al. Prevention of bacterial endocarditis. Recommendations by American Heart Association (AHA). *JAMA* 1990;264:2919.
11. Sexton DJ et al. Current best practices and guidelines. Assessment and management of complications in infective endocarditis. *Infect Dis Clin North Am* 2002;16:507.
12. Roder BL et al. Neurological manifestations in *Staphylococcus aureus* endocarditis. A review of 260 bacteremic cases in non-drug addicts. *Am J Med* 1997;102:379.
13. Prazin GL et al. Blood culture positivity: suppression by outpatient antibiotic therapy in patients with bacterial endocarditis. *Arch Intern Med* 1982;142:263.
14. Sachdev M et al. Imaging techniques for diagnosis of infective endocarditis. *Infect Dis Clin North Am* 2002;16:319.
15. Cheitlin MD et al. ACC/AHA guidelines for the clinical application of echocardiography: executive summary: a report of the American College of Cardiology/American Heart Association Task Force on Practice Guidelines (Committee on Clinical Application of Echocardiography): developed in collaboration with the American Society of Echocardiography. *J Am Coll Cardiol* 1997;29:862.
16. Rosen AB et al. Cost-effectiveness of transesophageal echocardiography to determine the duration of therapy for intravascular catheter-associated *Staphylococcus aureus* bacteremia. *Ann Intern Med* 1999;130:810.
17. Dajani AS et al. Oral amoxicillin as prophylaxis for endocarditis: what is the optimal dose? *Clin Infect Dis* 1994;18:157.
18. Heidenreich PA et al. Echocardiography in patients with suspected endocarditis: a cost-effective analysis. *Am J Med* 1999;107:198.
19. Durack DT et al. New criteria for diagnosis of infective endocarditis: utilization of specific echocardiographic findings. *Am J Med* 1994;96:200.
20. Li JS et al. Proposed modifications to the Duke criteria for the diagnosis of infective endocarditis. *Clin Infect Dis* 2000;30:63.
21. Wilson WR et al. Antibiotic treatment of adults with infective endocarditis due to streptococci, enterococci, staphylococci, and HACEK microorganisms. *JAMA* 1995;274:1706.
22. Le T et al. Combination antibiotic therapy for bacterial endocarditis. *Clin Infect Dis* 2003;36:615.
23. Watanakunakorn C. Penicillin combined with gentamicin or streptomycin: synergism against enterococci. *J Infect Dis* 1971;124:581.
24. Johnson CC et al. Viridans streptococci and groups C and G streptococci and *Gamelia morbillorum*. In: Mandell GL et al., eds. *Principles and Practice of Infectious Diseases*. 6th ed. New York: Churchill Livingstone; 2005:2434.
25. Alcaide F et al. In vitro activities of 22 β-lactam antibiotics against penicillin-resistant and penicillin-susceptible viridans group streptococci isolated from blood. *Antimicrob Agents Chemother* 1995;39:2243.
26. Carratala J et al. Bacteremia due to *Viridans streptococci* that are highly resistant to penicillin: increase among neutropenic patients with cancer. *Antimicrob Agents Chemother* 1995;20:1169.
27. Doern GV et al. Emergence of high rates of antimicrobial resistance among viridans group streptococci in the United States. *Antimicrob Agents Chemother* 1996;40:891.
28. Hidayat LK et al. High-dose vancomycin therapy for methicillin-resistant *Staphylococcus aureus* infections: efficacy and toxicity. *Arch Intern Med* 2006;166:2138.
29. Hidayat LK et al. Vancomycin (VAN) tolerance in MRSA invasive strains in patients undergoing vancomyin therapy. Abstract L-1210. 46th Interscience Conference on Antimicrobial Agents and Chemotherapy. September 27–30, 2006, San Francisco.
30. Wolfson JS et al. Serum bactericidal activity as a monitor of antibiotic therapy. *N Engl J Med* 1985;312:968.
31. Weinstein MP et al. Multicenter collaborative evaluation of a standardized serum bactericidal test as a prognostic indicator in infective endocarditis. *Am J Med* 1985;78:262.
32. Bisno AL et al. Antimicrobial treatment of infective endocarditis due to viridans streptococci, enterococci and staphylococci. *JAMA* 1989;261:1471.
33. Karchmer AW et al. Single-antibiotic therapy for streptococcal endocarditis. *JAMA* 1979;241:1801.
34. Wilson WR et al. Short-term intramuscular therapy with procaine penicillin plus streptomycin for

infective endocarditis due to viridans streptococci. *Circulation* 1978;57:1158.
35. Wilson WR et al. Short-term therapy for streptococcal infective endocarditis: combined intramuscular administration of penicillin and streptomycin. *JAMA* 1981;245:360.
36. Gavalda J et al. Effect of gentamicin dosing interval on therapy of viridans streptococcal experimental endocarditis with gentamicin plus penicillin. *Antimicrob Agents Chemother* 1995;39:2098.
37. Malacoff RF et al. Streptococcal endocarditis (nonenterococcal, non-group A): single vs. combination therapy. *JAMA* 1979;241:1807.
38. Francioli P et al. Treatment of streptococcal endocarditis with a single daily dose of ceftriaxone and netilmicin for 14 days: a prospective multicenter study. *Clin Infect Dis* 1995;21:1406.
39. Sexton DJ et al. Ceftriaxone once daily for four weeks compared with ceftriaxone plus gentamicin once daily for 2 weeks for treatment of endocarditis due to penicillin-susceptible streptococci. Endocarditis Treatment Consortium Group. *Clin Infect Dis* 1998;27:1470.
40. Francioli P et al. Treatment of streptococcal endocarditis with a single daily dose of ceftriaxone sodium for 4 weeks. *JAMA* 1992;267:264.
41. Stamboulian D et al. Antibiotic management of outpatients with endocarditis due to penicillin-susceptible streptococci. *Rev Infect Dis* 1991;13(Suppl 2):S160.
42. Hoen B. Special issues in the management of infective endocarditis caused by gram-positive cocci. *Infect Dis Clin North Am* 2002;16:437.
43. Henry NK et al. Antimicrobial therapy of experimental endocarditis caused by nutritionally variant viridans group streptococci. *Antimicrob Agents Chemother* 1986;30:465.
44. Karchmer AW et al. Infections of intracardiac devices. *Infect Dis Clin North Am* 2002;16:477.
45. Karchmer AW. Infections of prosthetic valves and intravascular devices. In: Mandell GL et al., eds. *Principles and Practice of Infectious Diseases*. 6th ed. New York: Churchill Livingstone; 2005:903.
46. Fang G et al. Prosthetic valve endocarditis resulting from nosocomial bacteremia: a prospective, multicenter study. *Ann Intern Med* 1993;119:560.
47. Nasser R et al. Incidence and risk of developing fungal prosthetic valve endocarditis after nosocomial candidemia. *Am J Med* 1997;103:25.
48. Durack DT. Prophylaxis of infective endocarditis. In: Mandell GL et al., eds. *Principles and Practice of Infectious Diseases*. 6th ed. New York: Churchill Livingstone; 2005:1044.
49. Archer GL et al. *Staphylococcus epidermidis* and other coagulase-negative staphylococci. In: Mandell GL et al., eds. *Principles and Practice of Infectious Diseases*. 6th ed. New York: Churchill Livingstone; 2005:2352.
50. Hartman B et al. Altered penicillin-binding proteins in methicillin-resistant strains of *Staphylococcus aureus*. *Antimicrob Agents Chemother* 1981;19:726.
51. Maki DG et al. Comparative study of cefazolin, cefamandole, and vancomycin for surgical prophylaxis in cardiac and vascular operations. *J Thorac Cardiovasc Surg* 1992;104:1423.
52. Wang G et al. Increased vancomycin MICs for Staphylococcus aureus clinical isolates from a university hospital during a 5-year period. *J Clin Microbiol* 2006;44:3883.
53. Patel JB et al. An association between reduced susceptibility to daptomycin and reduced susceptibility to vancomycin in *Staphylococcus aureus*. *Clin Infect Dis* 2006;42:1652.
54. Menichetti F. Current and emerging serious gram-positive infections. *Clin Microbiol Infect* 2005;(11 Suppl 3):22.
55. Cosgrove SE. *Staphylococcus aureus* with reduced susceptibility to vancomycin. *Clin Infect Dis* 2004;39:539.
56. Strauss RS et al. Successful treatment of complicated skin infections (cSSSI) due to staphylococci, including MRSA with ceftobiprole. Abstract L-1212, 46th Interscience Conference on Antimicrobial Agents and Chemotherapy. September 17–10, 2006, San Francisco.
57. Drees M et al. New agents for *Staphylococcus aureus* endocarditis. *Curr Opin Infect Dis* 2006; 19:544.
58. Polk RE et al. Vancomycin and the red man syndrome: pharmacodynamics of histamine release. *J Infect Dis* 1988;157:520.
59. Southorn PA et al. Adverse effects of vancomycin administered in the perioperative period. *Mayo Clin Proc* 1986;61:721.
60. Cimbollek M et al. Antibiotic-impregnated heart valve sewing rings for treatment and prophylaxis of bacterial endocarditis. *Antimicrob Agents Chemother* 1996;40:1432.
61. French BG et al. Rifampicin antibiotic impregnation of the St. Jude medical mechanical valve sewing ring: a weapon against endocarditis. *J Thorac Cardiovasc Surg* 1996;112:248.
62. Karck M et al. Pretreatment of prosthetic valve sewing ring with the antibiotic/fibrin sealant compound as a prophylactic tool against prosthetic valve endocarditis. *Eur J Cardiovasc Thorac Surg* 1990;4:142.
63. Fridkin S et al. Epidemiological and molecular characterization of infections caused by *Staphylococcus aureus* with reduced susceptibility to vancomycin, United States, 1997–2001. *Clin Infect Dis* 2003;36:429.
64. Schwalbe RS et al. Emergence of vancomycin resistance in coagulase-negative staphylococci. *N Engl J Med* 1987;316:927.
65. Karchmer AW et al. *Staphylococcus epidermidis* causing prosthetic valve endocarditis: microbiological and clinical observations as guides to therapy. *Ann Intern Med* 1983;98:447.
66. Birmingham MC et al. Linezolid for the treatment of multidrug-resistant, gram-positive infections: experience from a compassionate-use program. *Clin Infect Dis* 2003;36:159.
67. Livermore DM. Quinupristin/dalfopristin and linezolid: where, when, which and whether to use? *J Antimicrob Chemother*. 2000;46:347.
68. Miro JM et al. Infective endocarditis in intravenous drug abusers and HIV-1 infected patients. *Infect Dis Clin North Am* 2002;16:273.
69. Chambers HF et al. The National Collaborative Endocarditis Study Group. *Staphylococcus aureus* endocarditis: clinical manifestations in addicts and nonaddicts. *Medicine (Baltimore)* 1983;62:170.
70. Siddiq S et al. Endocarditis in an urban hospital. *Arch Intern Med* 1996;156:2454.
71. Manoff SB et al. Human immunodeficiency virus infection and infective endocarditis among injecting drug users. *Epidemiology* 1996;7:566.
72. Pulvirenti JJ et al. Infective endocarditis in injection drug users: importance of human immunodeficiency virus serostatus and degree of immunosuppression. *Clin Infect Dis* 1996;22:40.
73. Korzeniowski O et al. The National Collaborative Endocarditis Study Group: combination antimicrobial therapy for *Staphylococcus aureus* endocarditis in patients addicted to parenteral drugs and nonaddicts. *Ann Intern Med* 1982;97:496.
74. Fortun J et al. Short-course therapy for right-sided endocarditis due to *Staphylococcus aureus* in drug abusers: cloxacillin versus glycopeptides in combination with gentamicin. *Clin Infect Dis* 2001;33:120.
75. Chambers HF et al. Right-sided endocarditis in intravenous drug abusers two-week combination therapy. *Ann Intern Med* 1988;104:619.
76. Torres-Tortosa M et al. Prospective evaluation of a two-week course of intravenous antibiotics in intravenous drug addicts with infective endocarditis. *Eur J Clin Microbiol Infect Dis* 1994;13: 559.
77. DiNubile MJ. Short-course antibiotic therapy for right-sided endocarditis caused by *Staphylococcus aureus* in injection drug users. *Ann Intern Med* 1994;121:873.
78. Ribera E et al. Effectiveness of cloxacillin with or without gentamicin in short-term therapy for right-sided *Staphylococcus aureus* endocarditis: a randomized, controlled trial. *Ann Intern Med* 1996;125:969.
79. Dworkin RJ et al. Treatment of right-sided *Staphylococcus aureus* endocarditis in intravenous drug abusers with ciprofloxacin and rifampin. *Lancet* 1989;1071.
80. Heldman AW et al. Oral antibiotic treatment of right-sided staphylococcal endocarditis in injection drug users: prospective randomized comparison with parenteral therapy. *Am J Med* 1996;101:68.
81. Bryant RE et al. Unsuccessful treatment of staphylococcal endocarditis with cefazolin. *JAMA* 1977;237:569.
82. Kernodle DS et al. Failure of cephalosporins to prevent staphylococcal surgical wound infections. *JAMA* 1990;263:961.
83. Gorwitz R. et al. Strategies for clinical management of MRSA in the community: summary of an experts meeting convened by the Center for Disease Control and Prevention. *Center for Disease Control and Prevention*, 2006 (March).
84. Micek S. et al. Pleuropulmonary complications of Panton-Valentine leukocidin-positive community-acquired *Staphylococcus aureus*. *Chest* 2005;128:2732.
85. Boussaud V. et al., Life threatening hemopytsis in adults with community-acquired pneumonia died of Panton-Valentine leukocidin-secreting *Staphylococcal aureus*. *Intensive Care Med* 2003;29: 1840.
86. Francis J. S et al. Severe community-onset pneumonia in healthy adults caused by methicillin-resistant *Staphylococcus aureus* carrying the Panton-Valentine leukocidin genes. *Clin Infect Dis* 2005;40:100.
87. Dufour P et al. Community-acquired methicillin-resistant *Staphylococcus aureus* infections in France: emergence of a single clone that produces Panton-Valentine leukocidin. *Clin Infect Dis* 2002;35:819.
88. Gillet Y et al. Association between *Staphylococcus aureus* strains carrying gene for Panton-Valentine leukocidin and highly lethal necrotising pneumonia in young immunocompetent patients. *Lancet* 2002;359:753.
89. Miller LG et al. Necrotizing fasciitis caused by community-associated methicillin-resistant *Staphylococcus aureus* in Los Angeles. *N Engl J Med* 2005;352:1445.
90. Labandeira-Rey et al. *Staphylococcus aureus* Panton Valentine leukocidin causes necrotizing pneumonia. *Science* 2003;315:1130.
91. Bahrain M et al. Five cases of bacterial endocarditis after furunculosis and the ongoing saga of community-acquired methicillin-resistant *Staphylococcus aureus* infections. *Scand J Infect Dis* 2006;38:702.
92. *Staphylococcus aureus* resistant to vancomycin—United States, 2002. *MMWR Morbid Mortal Wkly Rep* 2002;51:565.
93. Elliott TSJ et al. Guidelines for the antibiotic treatment of endocarditis in adults: report of the Working Party of the British Society for Antimicrobial Chemotherapy. *J Antimicrob Chemother* 2004;54:971.
94. Horstkotte D et al. Guidelines on Prevention, Diagnosis and Treatment of Infective Endocarditis Executive Summary: The Task Force on Infective Endocarditis of the European Society of Cardiology. *Eur Heart J* 2004;25:267.
95. Moise-Broder PA et al. Pharmacodynamics of vancomycin and other antimicrobials in patients with Staphylococcus aureus lower respiratory tract infections. *Clin Pharmacokinet*. 2004;43:925.
96. Larsson AJ et al. The concentration-independent effect of monoexponential and bioexponential decay in vancomycin concentrations on the killing of *Staphylococcus aureus* under aerobic and anaerobic conditions. *J Antimicrob Chemother* 1996;38:589.
97. Zimmermann AE et al. Association of vancomycin serum concentrations with outcomes in patients

with gram-positive bacteremia. *Pharmacotherapy* 1995;15:85.

98. Rybak MJ. The pharmacokinetic and pharmacodynamic properties of vancomycin. *Clin Infect Dis* 2006;42(Suppl 1):S35.
99. Wootton M et al. Evidence for reduction in breakpoints used to determine vancomycin susceptibility in *Staphylococcus aureus*. *Antimicrob Agents Chemother* 2005;49:3982.
100. Clinical and Laboratory Standards Institute. Performance Standards for Antimicrobial Susceptibility Testing: 16th Informational Supplement. Wayne, PA: Clinical and Laboratory Standards Institute; 2006:M100.
101. Howe RA et al. Expression and detection of hetero-vancomycin resistance in *Staphylococcus aureus*. *J Antimicrob Chemother* 1999;44:675.
102. Jones RN. Microbiological features of vancomycin in the 21st century: minimum inhibitory concentration creep, bactericidal/static activity, and applied breakpoints to predict clinical outcomes or detect resistant strains. *Clin Infect Dis* 2006;42:S13.
103. Sancak B et al. Methicillin-resistant *Staphylococcus aureus* heterogeneously resistant to vancomycin in a Turkish university hospital. *J Antimicrob Chemother* 2005;56:519.
104. Charles PG et al. Clinical features associated with bacteremia due to heterogeneous vancomycin intermediate *Staphylococcus aureus*. *Clin Infect Dis* 2004;38:448.
105. Wootton M et al. A multicenter study evaluating the current strategies for isolating *Staphylococcus aureus* strains with reduced susceptibility to glycopeptides. *J Clin Microbiol* 2007;45:329.
106. Hsu DI et al. Correlation of vancomycin (VAN) minimum inhibitory concentration (MIC) using VITEK (VT) versus E Test (ET) with treatment outcomes of methicillin-resistant *Staphylococcus aureus* (MRSA) infections. Abstract D-1734. 45th Interscience Conference on Antimicrobial Agents and Chemotherapy, December 27–30, 2005, Washington, DC.
107. American Thoracic Society; Infectious Diseases Society of America. Guidelines for the management of adults with hospital-acquired, ventilator-associated, and healthcare-associated pneumonia. *Am J Respir Crit Care Med* 2005;171:388.
108. Hidayat LK et al. Detection of hetero-GISA (hGISA) among invasive MRSA and associated clinical features. Abstract C2-1156. 46th Interscience Conference on Antimicrobial Agents and Chemotherapy, September 27–30, 2006, San Francisco, CA.
109. Markowitz N et al. Trimethoprim-sulfamethoxazole compared with vancomycin for the treatment of *Staphylococcus aureus* infection. *Ann Intern Med* 1992;117:390.
110. Nicholau DP et al. Minocycline versus vancomycin for treatment of experimental endocarditis caused by oxacillin-resistant *Staphylococcus aureus*. *Antimicrob Agents Chemother* 1994;38:1515.
111. Anwer S et al. Quinupristin/dalfopristin for treatment of MRSA endocarditis refractory to conventional therapy. *Infect Dis Clin Pract* 1998;7:414.
112. Drew RH et al. Treatment of methicillin-resistant *Staphylococcus aureus* infections with quinupristin-dalfopristin in patients intolerant of or failing prior therapy. *J Antimicrob Chemother* 2000;46:775.
113. Hill EE et al. Infective endocarditis treated with linezolid: case report and literature review. *Eur J Clin Microbiol Infect Dis* 2006;25:202.
114. Falagas ME et al. Linezolid for the treatment of patients with endocarditis: a systematic review of the published evidence. *J Antimicrob Chemother* 2006;58:273.
115. Dresser LD et al. Results of treating infective endocarditis with linezolid (LNZ). Abstract 2239. 40th Interscience Conference on Antimicrobial Agents and Chemotherapy, September 17–20, 2000, Toronto.
116. Forrest A et al. Pharmacostatistical modeling of hematologic effects of linezolid in seriously ill patients. Abstract 283. 40th Interscience Conference on Antimicrobial Agents and Chemotherapy, September 17–20, 2000, Toronto.
117. Cui L et al. Correlation between reduced daptomycin susceptibility and vancomycin resistance in vancomycin-intermediate *Staphylococcus aureus*. *Antimicrob Agents Chemother* 2006;50:1079.
118. Ruiz ME et al. Endocarditis caused by methicillin-resistant *Staphylococcus aureus:* treatment failure with linezolid. *Clin Infect Dis* 2003;35:1018.
119. Corne P et al. Treatment failure of methicillin-resistant *Staphylococcus aureus* endocarditis with linezolid. *Scand J Infect Dis* 2005;37:946.
120. Sperber SJ et al. Persistent MRSA bacteremia in a patient with low linezolid levels. *Clin Infect Dis* 2003;36:675.
121. Fowler VG, Jr. et al. Daptomycin versus standard therapy for bacteremia and endocarditis caused by *Staphylococcus aureus*. *N Engl J Med* 2006: 653.
122. Dvorchik BH et al. The pharmacokinetics of daptomycin in moderately obese, morbidly obese, and matched nonobese subjects. *J Clin Pharmacol* 2005;45:48.
123. Vikram HR et al. Clinical progression of methicillin-resistant *Staphylococcus aureus* vertebral osteomyelitis associated with reduced susceptibility to daptomycin. *J Clin Microbiol* 2005;43: 5384.
124. Mariani PG et al. Development of decreased susceptibility to daptomycin and vancomycin in a *Staphylococcus aureus* strain during prolonged therapy. *J Antimicrob Chemother* 2006;58:481.
125. Kaatz GW et al. Mechanisms of daptomycin resistance in *Staphylococcus aureus*. *Int J Antimicrob Agents* 2006;28:280.
126. Skiest DJ. Treatment failure resulting from resistance of *Staphylococcus aureus* to daptomycin *J Clin Microbiol* 2006;44:655.
127. Wilkowske CJ et al. Antibiotic synergism: enhanced susceptibility of group D streptococci to certain antibiotic combinations. *Antimicrob Agents Chemother* 1970;10:195.
128. Drake TA et al. Studies of the chemotherapy of endocarditis: correlation of in vitro, animal model, and clinical studies. *Rev Infect Dis* 1983;5(Suppl 2):S345.
129. Eliopoulos GM et al. Antimicrobial combinations. In: Lorian V, ed. *Antibiotics in Laboratory Medicine*. Baltimore: Williams & Wilkins; 1996:330.
130. Moellering RC Jr. et al. Studies on antibiotic synergisms against enterococci II: effect of various antibiotics on the uptake of C^{11}-labeled streptomycin by enterococci. *J Clin Invest* 1971;50:2580.
131. Moellering RC Jr. et al. Synergy of penicillin and gentamicin against enterococci. *J Infect Dis* 1971;124(Suppl):S207.
132. Carrizosa J et al. Antibiotic synergism in enterococcal endocarditis. *J Lab Clin Med* 1976;88:132.
133. Mandell GL et al. An analysis of 38 patients observed at New York Hospital–Cornell Medical Center. *Arch Intern Med* 1970;125:258.
134. Serra P et al. Synergistic treatment of enterococcal endocarditis. *Arch Intern Med* 1975;137:1562.
135. Koenig GM et al. Enterococcal endocarditis. Report of nineteen cases with long-term follow-up data. *N Engl J Med* 1961;264:257.
136. Eliopoulos GM. Aminoglycoside-resistant enterococcal endocarditis. *Med Clin North Am* 1993;17: 117.
137. Zervos MJ et al. Nosocomial infection by gentamicin-resistant *Streptococcus faecalis:* an epidemiological study. *Ann Intern Med* 1987;106:687.
138. Mainardi JL et al. Synergistic effect of amoxicillin and cefotaxime against *Enterococcus faecalis*. *Antimicrob Agents Chemother* 1995;39:1984.
139. Brandt CM et al. Effective treatment of multidrug-resistant enterococcal experimental endocarditis with combinations of cell wall-active agents. *J Infect Dis* 1996;173:909.
140. Gavalda J et al. Efficacy of ampicillin (A) plus ceftriaxone (Ctr) or cefotaxime (Cx) in treatment of endocarditis due to *Enterococcus faecalis*. Abstract L1342. In: Programs and Abstracts of the 41st Interscience Conference on Antimicrobial Agents and Chemotherapy (Chicago). Washington, DC: American Society for Microbiology; 2001:3.
141. Matsumoto JY et al. Synergy of penicillin and decreasing concentrations of aminoglycosides against enterococci from patients with infective endocarditis. *Antimicrob Agents Chemother* 1980;18: 944.
142. Carrizosa J et al. Minimal concentrations of aminoglycosides that can synergize with penicillin in enterococcal endocarditis. *Antimicrob Agents Chemother* 1981;20:405.
143. Wright AJ et al. Influence of gentamicin dose size on the efficacies of combinations of gentamicin and penicillin in experimental streptomycin-resistant enterococcal endocarditis. *Antimicrob Agents Chemother* 1982;22:972.
144. Fantin B et al. Importance of the aminoglycoside dosing regimen in the penicillin-netilmicin combination for the treatment of *Enterococcus faecalis*-induced experimental endocarditis. *Antimicrob Agents Chemother* 1990;34: 2387.
145. Marangos MN et al. Influence of gentamicin dosing interval on the efficacy of penicillin-containing regimens in experimental *Enterococcus faecalis* endocarditis. *Antimicrob Agents Chemother* 1997; 39:519.
146. Tam VH et al. Once daily aminoglycosides in the treatment of gram-positive endocarditis. *Ann Pharmacother* 1999;33:600.
147. Wilson WR et al. Treatment of streptomycin-susceptible and streptomycin-resistant enterococcal endocarditis. *Ann Intern Med* 1984;100:816.
148. Olaison L et al. Enterococcal endocarditis in Sweden, 1995–1999: can shorter therapy with aminoglycosides be used? *Clin Infect Dis* 2002;34: 159.
149. Wilhelm MP et al. Vancomycin. *Mayo Clin Proc* 1999;74:928.
150. Murray BE. Vancomycin-resistant enterococcal infections. *N Engl J Med* 2000;342:710.
151. Murray BE. Diversity among multi-drug resistant enterococci. *Emerging Infect Dis* 1998;4:37.
152. Rice LB. Emergence of vancomycin-resistant enterococci. *Emerg Infect Dis* 2001;7:183.
153. Nosocomial enterococci resistant to vancomycin, United States, 1989–1993. *MMWR Morbid Mortal Weekly Report* 1993;42:597.
154. National Nosocomial Infections Surveillance (NNIS) System Report, data summary from January 1992 through June 2004, issued October 2004. *Am J Infect Control* 2004;32:470.
155. Lodise TP et al. Clinical outcomes for patients with bacteremia caused by vancomycin-resistant enterococcus in a level 1 trauma center. *Clin Infect Dis* 2002;34:922.
156. Dowzicky M et al. Characterization of isolates associated with emerging resistance to quinupristin/dalfopristin (Synercid) during the worldwide clinical program. *Diagn Microbiol Infect Dis* 2000;37:57.
157. Eliopoulos GM. Quinupristin-dalfopristin and linezolid: evidence and opinion. *Clin Infect Dis* 2003;36:473.
158. Moellering RC et al. The efficacy and safety of quinupristin/dalfopristin for the treatment of infections caused by vancomycin-resistant *Enterococcus faecium*. Synercid Emergency-Use Study Group. *J Antimicrob Chemother* 1999;44:251.
159. Matsumura S et al. Treatment of endocarditis due to vancomycin-resistant *Enterococcus faecium* with quinupristin/dalfopristin, doxycycline, and rifampin: a synergistic drug combination. *Clin Infect Dis* 1998;27:1554.
160. Olsen KM et al. Arthralgias and myalgias related to quinupristin-dalfopristin administration. *Clin Infect Dis* 2001;32:e83.
161. Fuller RE et al. Treatment of vancomycin-resistant enterococci, with a focus on quinupristin-dalfopristin. *Pharmacotherapy* 1996;16:584.

162. Gonzales RD et al. Infections due to vancomycin-resistant *Enterococcus faecium* resistant to linezolid. *Lancet* 2001;357:1179.
163. Herrero IA et al. Nosocomial spread of linezolid-resistant, vancomycin-resistant *Enterococcus faecium*. *N Engl J Med* 2002;346:867.
164. Beringer P et al. Absolute bioavailabilty and pharmacokinetics of linezolid in hospitalized patients given enteral feeding. *Antimicrob Agents Chemother* 2005;49:3676.
165. Critchley I. Baseline study to determine in vitro activities of daptomycin against gram-positive pathogens isolated in the United States in 2000–2001. *Antimicrob Agents Chemother* 2003; 47:1689.
166. Rybak M. In vitro activities of daptomycin, vancomycin, linezolid, and quinupristin-dalfopristin against staphylococci and enterococci, including vancomycin-intermediate and -resistant strains. *Antimicrob Agents Chemother* 2000;44:1062.
167. Munoz-Price LS. Emergence of resistance to daptomycin during treatment of vancomycin-resistant *Enterococcus faecalis* infection. *Clin Infect Dis* 2005;41:565.
168. Kanafini Z et al. Infective endocarditis caused by daptomycin-resistant *Enterococcus faecalis*: a case report. *Scand J Infect Dis* 2007;39:75.
169. Sabol K et al. Emergence of daptomycin resistance in *Enterococcus faecium* during daptomycin therapy. *Antimicrob Agents Chemother* 2005;49: 1664.
170. Stevens M et al. Endocarditis due to vancomycin-resistant enterococci: a case report and review of the literature. *Clin Infect Dis* 2005;41:1134.
171. Centers for Disease Control and Prevention. Recommendations for preventing the spread of vancomycin resistance. Recommendations of the Hospital Infection Control Practices Advisory Committee (HICPAC). *MMWR Morbid Mortal Wkly Rep* 1995;44:1.
172. Rubinstein E et al. Fungal endocarditis: analysis of 24 cases and review of the literature. *Medicine* 1975;54:331.
173. Melgar GR et al. Fungal prosthetic valve endocarditis in 16 patients. An 11-year experience in a tertiary care hospital. *Medicine* 1997;76:94.
174. Ellis ME et al. Fungal endocarditis: evidence in the world literature, 1965–1995. *Clin Infect Dis* 2001;32:50.
175. Pierrotti LC et al. Fungal endocarditis, 1995–2000. *Chest* 2002;122:302.
176. Shadomy S et al. In vitro studies with combinations of 5-fluorocytosine and amphotericin B. *Antimicrob Agents Chemother* 1975;8:117.
177. Rubinstein E et al. Tissue penetration of amphotericin B in *Candida* endocarditis. *Chest* 1974;66:376.
178. Gilbert HM et al. Successful treatment of fungal prosthetic valve endocarditis: case report and review. *Clin Infect Dis* 1996;22:348.
179. Muehrcke DD et al. Surgical and long-term antifungal therapy for fungal prosthetic valve endocarditis. *Ann Thorac Surg* 1995;60:538.
180. Wong-Beringer A et al. Lipid formulations of amphotericin B: clinical efficacy and toxicities. *Clin Infect Dis* 1998;27:608.
181. Melamed R et al. Successful non-surgical treatment of *Candida tropicalis* endocarditis with liposomal amphotericin B (AmBisome). *Scand J Infect Dis* 2000;32:86.
182. Terrell CL. Antifungal agents. Part II. The azoles. *Mayo Clin Proc* 1999;74:78.
183. Nguyen MH et al. *Candida* prosthetic valve endocarditis: prospective study of six cases and review of the literature. *Clin Infect Dis* 1996;22:262.
184. Isalska BJ et al. Fluconazole in the treatment of candidal prosthetic valve endocarditis. *BMJ* 1988;297:178.
185. Martino P et al. Candidal endocarditis and treatment with fluconazole and granulocyte-macrophage colony-stimulating factor [Letter]. *Ann Intern Med* 1990;112:966.
186. Roupie E et al. Fluconazole therapy of candidal native valve endocarditis [Letter]. *Eur J Clin Microbiol Infect Dis* 1991;10:458.
187. Venditti M et al. Fluconazole treatment of catheter-related right-sided endocarditis caused by *Candida albicans* and associated with endophthalmitis and folliculitis. *Clin Infect Dis* 1992;14:422.
188. Hernandez JA et al. Candidal mitral endocarditis and long-term treatment with fluconazole in a patient with human immunodeficiency virus infection [Letter]. *Clin Infect Dis* 1992;15:1062.
189. Wells CJ et al. Treatment of native valve *Candida* endocarditis with fluconazole. *J Infect* 1995;31:233.
190. Wong-Beringer A et al. Systemic antifungal therapy: new options, new challenges. *Pharmacotherapy* 2003;23:1441.
191. Rajendram R et al. Candida prosthetic valve endocarditis cured by caspofungin therapy without valve replacement. *Clin Infect Dis* 2005;40:e72.
192. Nevado J et al. Caspofungin: a new therapeutic option for fungal endocarditis. *Clin Microbiol Infect* 2005;11:248.
193. Bacak V et al. *Candida albicans* endocarditis treatment with caspofungin in an HIV-infected patient—case report and review of literature. *J Infect* 2006;53:e11.
194. Jimenez-Exposito MJ et al. Native valve endocarditis due to *Candida glabrata* treated without valvular replacement: a potential role for caspofungin in the induction and maintenance treatment. *Clin Infect Dis* 2004;39:70.
195. Rajendram R et al. *Candida* prosthetic valve endocarditis cured by caspofungin therapy without valve replacement. *Clin Infect Dis* 2005;40:272.
196. Watanakunakorn C. Antimicrobial therapy of endocarditis due to less common bacteria. In: Bisno AL, ed. *Treatment of Infective Endocarditis*. New York: Grune and Stratton; 1981:123.
197. Ellner JJ et al. Infective endocarditis caused by slow-growing, fastidious, gram-negative bacteria. *Medicine* 1979;58:145.
198. Cohen PS et al. Infective endocarditis caused by gram-negative bacteria: a review of the literature, 1945–1977. *Prog Cardiovasc Dis* 1980;22:205.
199. von Graevenitz A. Endocarditis due to nonfermentative gram-negative rods. An updated review. *Eur Heart J* 1987;8(Suppl J):331.
200. Tunkel AR et al. Enterobacter endocarditis. *Scand J Infect Dis* 1992;24:233.
201. Reiner NE. Regional pathogens in endocarditis. *Ann Intern Med* 1976;84:613.
202. Reyes MP et al. Current problems in the treatment of infective endocarditis due to *Pseudomonas aeruginosa*. *Rev Infect Dis* 1983;5:314.
203. Mills J et al. *Serratia marcescens* endocarditis: a regional illness associated with intravenous drug abuse. *Ann Intern Med* 1976;84:29.
204. Cooper R et al. *Serratia* endocarditis. A follow-up report. *Arch Intern Med* 1980;140:199.
205. Archer G et al. Experimental endocarditis due to *Pseudomonas aeruginosa*. II. Therapy with carbenicillin and gentamicin. *J Infect Dis* 1977;136: 327.
206. Lerner SA et al. Effect of highly potent antipseudomonal β-lactam agents alone and in combination with aminoglycosides against *Pseudomonas aeruginosa*. *Rev Infect Dis* 1984;6(Suppl 3):S678.
207. Frank U. Penetration of ceftazidime into heart valves and subcutaneous and muscle tissue of patients undergoing open-heart surgery. *Antimicrob Agents Chemother* 1987;31:813.
208. Dickinson G et al. Efficacy of imipenem/cilastatin in endocarditis. *Am J Med* 1985;78:117.
209. Scully BE et al. Use of aztreonam in the treatment of serious infection due to multiresistant gram-negative organisms, including *Pseudomonas aeruginosa*. *Am J Med* 1985;78:251.
210. Strunk RW et al. Comparison of ciprofloxacin with azlocillin plus tobramycin in the therapy of experimental *Pseudomonas aeruginosa* endocarditis. *Antimicrob Agents Chemother* 1985;28:428.
211. Brown NM et al. Ciprofloxacin treatment of bacterial endocarditis involving prosthetic material after cardiac surgery. *Arch Dis Child* 1997;76:68.
212. Brouqui P et al. Endocarditis due to rare and fastidious bacteria. *Clin Microbiol Rev* 2001;14:177.
213. Hoen B et al. Infective endocarditis in patients with negative blood cultures: analysis of 88 cases from a one-year nationwide survey in France. *Clin Infect Dis* 1995;20:501.
214. Washington JA II. The role of the microbiology laboratory in the diagnosis and antimicrobial treatment of infective endocarditis. *Mayo Clin Proc* 1982;57:22.
215. Munro R et al. Is the antimicrobial removal device a cost-effective addition to conventional blood cultures? *J Clin Pathol* 1984;37:348.
216. Goldenberger D et al. Molecular diagnosis of bacterial endocarditis by broad-range PCR amplification and direct sequencing. *J Clin Microbiol* 1997;35:2733.
217. Child JS. Risks for and prevention of infective endocarditis. *Cardiol Clin* 1996;14:327.
218. Wilson W et al. Prevention of infective endocarditis. Guidelines from the American Heart Association Rheumatic Fever, Endocarditis, and Kawasaki Disease Committee, Council on Cardiovascular Disease in the Young, and the Council on Clinical Cardiology, Council on Cardiovascular Surgery and Anesthesia, and the Quality of Care an Outcomes Research Interdisciplinary Working Group. *American Heart Association. Circulation* 2007;116: 1736.
219. Shulman ST et al. Prevention of bacterial endocarditis: a statement for health professionals by the Committee on Rheumatic Fever and Infective Endocarditis of the Council on Cardiovascular Disease in the Young. *Circulation* 1984;70:1123A.
220. Nolet BR. Patient selection in outpatient parenteral antimicrobial therapy. *Infect Dis Clin North Am* 1998;12:835.
221. Huminer D et al. Home intravenous antibiotic therapy for patients with infective endocarditis. *Eur J Clin Microbiol Infect Dis* 1999;18:330.
222. Rehm SJ. Outpatient intravenous antibiotic therapy for endocarditis. *Infect Dis Clin North Am* 1998;12:879.

CHAPTER 60

Respiratory Tract Infections

Steven P. Gelone and Judith O'Donnell

Infection of the respiratory tract continues to be the most common and important cause of short-term illness in the United States. It is typically the first infection to occur after birth, with pneumonia being the sixth leading cause of death and the number one infectious disease cause of death in the United States.[1,2] Respiratory tract infections occur more frequently than they are reported and are responsible for more days of bed disability, restricted activity, and lost time from work and school than any other category of reported acute illness in the United States. Respiratory infections account for >40% of disability days secondary to acute illness,[2] and pneumonia and influenza are among the ten leading causes of death in the overall population, with 80% to 90% of deaths occurring in the elderly (persons >65 years of age).[3,4] In the United States, pneumonia and influenza are in the top ten causes of death in all age groups.[4] The actual number is much larger, because this figure does not include individuals who died of pneumonia who had other diseases (e.g., HIV, tobacco- and alcohol-related diseases).[3]

The financial impact associated with respiratory infections in 1999 was $25.6 billion ($18.6 billion in direct costs and $7 billion in indirect costs).[1] These figures largely underestimate the financial impact of treating ambulatory respiratory infections. Statistics reported by the National Health Interview Survey estimate that 182 million episodes of respiratory infection occur for which no medical attention is sought.[2] Often, individuals with respiratory infections try home remedies or over-the-counter (OTC) medications for relief of their symptoms and only seek medical advice or treatment when these efforts fail. The estimated cost associated with the use of OTC medications in this population will contribute an additional $456 million annually to the treatment of respiratory infections.[1]

This chapter addresses the concepts relevant to the treatment and prevention of lower respiratory tract bacterial infections. Upper respiratory tract infections (see Chapter 96) and respiratory tract infections caused by viruses (with the exception of influenza) (see Chapter 72) and fungi (see Chapter 71) are presented elsewhere in this book, as are the unique features of respiratory tract infections in immunocompromised hosts (see Chapter 68) and *Pneumocystis jirovecii (carinii)* (see Chapter 70).

Bronchial Infections

Acute Bronchitis

1. F.A., a 35-year-old woman, presents with a persistent cough following an acute respiratory viral infection that began 7 days ago. Although the nasal stuffiness and sore throat resolved 3 or 4 days ago, the cough has persisted and her sputum has become

thick and mucoid; a burning, substernal pain is associated with each coughing episode. F.A. is currently afebrile. Coarse rales and rhonchi are heard on physical examination of her chest, and a tentative diagnosis of acute bronchitis (AB) is made. How should F.A. be assessed and managed?

Uncomplicated AB is an isolated event characterized by inflammation of the tracheobronchial tree and clinically presents as cough of <2 to 3 weeks' duration with or without sputum production. Infectious causes of AB are primarily viral and include influenza A and B, rhinovirus, coronavirus, parainfluenza virus 3, and respiratory syncytial virus. As a group, these agents are associated with 5% to 10% of all cases of acute uncomplicated bronchitis in adults. *Streptococcus pneumoniae*, *Haemophilus influenzae*, or *Moraxella catarrhalis* do not produce AB in adults without underlying pulmonary disease.

As in F.A., cough—with or without sputum production—is the most prominent clinical feature of this disease. It usually begins early in the course of the syndrome and may persist after the acute infection is resolved. The initial dry, unproductive cough may progress to one with a productive mucoid sputum.

Most healthy adults with typical symptoms of bronchitis do not require diagnostic evaluation. The presence of a fever (≥38°C), heart rate (HR) >100 beats/minute, respiratory rate (RR) >24 breaths/minute, and signs of focal consolidation on chest examination such as rales, egophony, and fremitus are suggestive of the need for a more thorough diagnostic evaluation. Diagnostic studies to reveal a causative agent are not indicated.

The treatment of AB should be directed at symptom control. The use of antitussive agents to control cough, maintenance of adequate hydration, and the intermittent administration of antipyretics such as acetaminophen or ibuprofen should be employed. On the basis of the microbiology of AB, it is not surprising that randomized controlled clinical trials have failed to support a role for antibiotic therapy. Consistent with this, the U.S. Food and Drug Administration removed uncomplicated AB and secondary bacterial infections of AB as indications for randomized clinical trials in 1998. Meta-analyses confirm no benefit of antibiotic treatment on illness duration, activity limitation, or work loss, and the routine use of antibiotics in adults with AB is not justified. Yet, antibiotics are prescribed for AB commonly in the United States.[5,6] While a reduction in antibiotic use has been confirmed in the recent past, abuse and misuse is still commonplace.[7]

As described above, patients whose coughs are severe or prolonged (≥14 days) or present with the signs and symptoms enumerated above should be evaluated more thoroughly and may be candidates for antibiotic therapy.[8–11] In addition, the one common circumstance for which evidence supports antibiotic therapy in patients with uncomplicated AB is the suspicion of pertussis. Unfortunately, no clinical features allow clinicians to distinguish adults with persistent cough due to pertussis primarily because pertussis in adults with previous immunity does not lead to classic whooping cough seen in patients with primary infection. Therefore, treatment should be limited to adults with a high probability of exposure to pertussis, such as that associated with a documented outbreak. The use of antibiotics in this setting will decrease the shedding of the pathogen and the spread of disease.

Chronic Bronchitis

CLINICAL PRESENTATION

2. M.J., a 54-year-old man with a 40-year, one-pack/day smoking history reports producing two cupfuls of whitish-clear, occasionally mucoid sputum per day over the past several years; he coughs up the largest volumes in the morning on arising. M.J. has a raspy voice and a crackling cough, which often interrupts his talking. Two days ago, he noted that his sputum had increased in volume and had changed in appearance. A sputum sample, which was yellowish-green, tenacious, and purulent, was sent for culture; the Gram stain showed few epithelial cells, moderate white cells, and a few Gram-positive cocci and Gram-negative rods with no predominant organisms. M.J. denies fever or chills and had no signs of pneumonia; a chest radiograph is negative for consolidation. M.J. has experienced similar episodes three or four times per year. What signs and symptoms in M.J.'s history are consistent with chronic bronchitis (CB)?

CB is an inflammatory condition of the tracheobronchial tree in which chronic cough and excessive production of sputum are the prominent features. CB and emphysema are components of chronic obstructive pulmonary disease (COPD). Exacerbations of COPD—which may occur from any of the following: infection, smoking, air pollution, exposure to allergens, occupational exposure, or preclinical or subclinical asthma—are estimated to result in approximately 110,000 deaths and more than 500,000 hospitalizations, with over $18 billion spent in direct costs annually.[12–14] By definition, patients who cough up sputum daily or on most days over 3 or more consecutive months for >2 successive years presumptively have CB.[15] The diagnosis of CB is made only when other etiologies such as bronchiectasis, cardiac failure, and lung cancer have been excluded. M.J. meets these criteria.

Bronchitis is more common in men than women and more common after the age of 40 years than earlier recognized.[16] A genetic basis has been noted with cystic fibrosis (CF), immunoglobulin deficiencies, and primary ciliary dyskinesia. The most common cause of CB is smoking.[17] In M.J., cigarette smoking is an important factor associated with his disease. Smoking is an irritant to the respiratory airways and may stimulate the mucus-secreting goblet cells found in major and smaller bronchi. The increased amount of mucus is not readily cleared from smaller peripheral airways, creating airflow resistance; this accounts for the large volume of sputum cleared from larger airways. However, not all patients with CB have a history of smoking, and 6% to 10% of nonsmoking men will have persistent cough and sputum production.[16]

3. Has M.J.'s bronchitis worsened? What is the likelihood that M.J. has an infection?

Acute exacerbations of chronic bronchitis (AECB) are defined as a worsening of clinical symptoms with increased cough, sputum production, and dyspnea. Some patients report shortness of breath, fatigue, chest tightness, or an increasing cough with dyspnea as their only complaints. Some cases are accompanied by fever, and some patients have symptoms consistent with asthma. Hemoptysis may be seen during acute exacerbations, as CB is the most common cause of hemoptysis in the developed world. As in M.J., the most reliable sign of worsening bronchitis is the patient's observation that his or her

Table 60-1 Most Commonly Identified Bacterial Pathogens Associated With Acute Exacerbations of Chronic Bronchitis

Pathogen	*Incidence (%)*
Haemophilus influenzae	24–26
Haemophilus parainfluenzae	20
Streptococcus pneumoniae	15
Moraxella catarrhalis	15
Klebsiella pneumoniae	4
Serratia marcescens	2
Pseudomonas aeruginosa	2

sputum has changed in amount, color, or consistency. These changes in sputum have been used as presumptive evidence of infection, but similar changes in sputum can be seen without documented infection.[17–19] As illustrated by M.J., patients may present without systemic symptoms of infection such as chills, fever, or leukocytosis.

MICROBIOLOGY

Although infections do not appear to promote the basic disease process or result in deterioration in pulmonary function, they are associated with the majority of exacerbations.[15] The organisms most commonly implicated are viral agents that often cause upper respiratory tract infections. Viruses including influenza A and B, parainfluenza virus 3, coronavirus, and rhinovirus are associated with AECB in 7% to 64% of patients. Gump et al.[19] found viral infections in 32% of patients during AECB compared with 1% of patients during remission periods. The most commonly identified bacterial pathogens associated with acute exacerbations of CB are listed in Table 60-1.

Recent studies with improved molecular and immunologic techniques form the basis for a new model of bacterial exacerbation pathogenesis (Fig. 60-1). In this model, acquisition of new strains from the environment via aerosols or fomites of nontypeable *H. influenzae*, *M. catarrhalis,* and *S. pneumoniae* appears to be the predominant initiating event for an exacerbation.

Treatment of a bronchial infection must be directed at organisms found in the pulmonary tree and not normal flora in the oral cavity. The correct interpretation of a Gram stain of a sputum sample depends on the nature of the sample. Sputum, by definition, represents matter ejected from the lungs or bronchi and should contain, at most, a few white blood cells (WBCs) on microscopic examination. On microscopic evaluation, a good sputum sample should have few epithelial cells. In contrast, saliva often contains large numbers of epithelial cells. The numbers of epithelial cells or WBCs in the sample is important because debilitated patients with pulmonary infection often have difficulty performing the physical maneuvers necessary to eject sputum from the lungs or bronchi. In the case of M.J., the Gram stain would be interpreted as a good specimen (because of the low number of epithelial cells). The presence of moderate amounts of WBCs is consistent with infection, especially considering the recent change in the volume and appearance of M.J.'s sputum. However, using expectorated sputum cytology alone to assess the likelihood of an infection can be misleading, as significant numbers of polymorphonuclear cells can be present throughout the course of CB with or without exacerbation.[20,21]

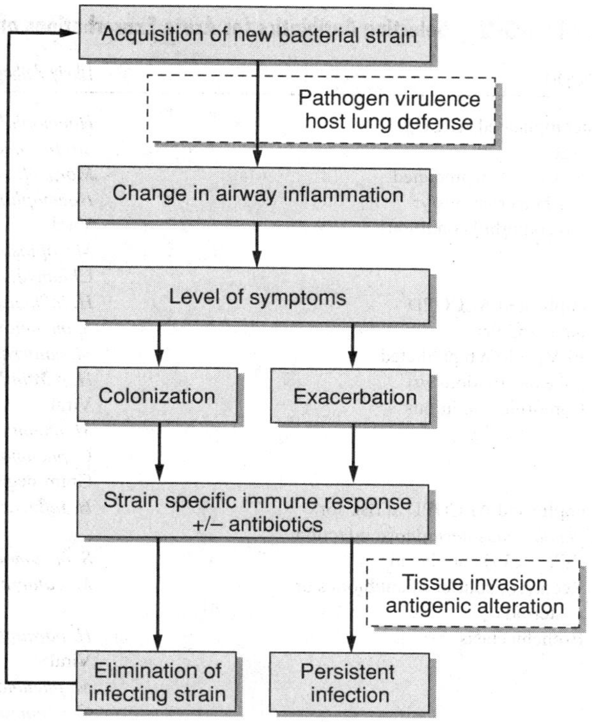

FIGURE 60-1 Model of the pathogenesis of bacterial exacerbations of chronic bronchitis.

Many studies have shown that sputum in patients with CB culture grow potential respiratory pathogens when cultured during periods of exacerbations and remissions. Both *S. pneumoniae* and *H. influenzae* are recovered during periods of exacerbation and remission.[19] Patients with COPD and CB are more likely colonized with these organisms compared with healthy controls.[22] However, a quantitative increase in *S. pneumoniae* during an acute exacerbation is correlated with sputum purulence.[23] This association has not been shown for nontypeable *H. influenzae.*[24] For M.J., the finding of few Gram-positive and Gram-negative organisms with no predominant organism reflects normal oropharyngeal flora and likely colonization with *S. pneumoniae* and *Haemophilus* sp. Consequently, this test result provides little additional information to guide antimicrobial therapy.

ANTIBIOTIC THERAPY

4. Should M.J. be given antibiotic therapy to treat his acute episode?

Mild to moderately ill patients without pneumonia, such as M.J., usually do not require antibiotics to treat exacerbations of CB.[25] Potential occupational and environmental exposures should be conducted. If smoking is identified as the likely irritant (as in M.J.), patients should be encouraged to participate in a comprehensive smoking cessation program. M.J. should be well hydrated and treated with scheduled postural drainage exercises to help mobilize the excessive mucus and improve his pulmonary function. In addition, the use of oral or aerosolized bronchodilators may be of some benefit during acute exacerbations. If his condition does not improve within 3 or 4 days, the initiation of antibiotic therapy should be considered.

Table 60-2 Selecting Antibiotics for Acute Exacerbations of Chronic Obstructive Pulmonary Disease

Category	Likely Pathogens	Antimicrobial Treatment
Uncomplicated AECOPD	*Haemophilus influenzae*	Macrolides[a]
Age <65 yr	*Streptococcus pneumoniae*	Ketolides[b]
FFV_1 >50% predicted	*Moraxella catarrhalis*	Doxycycline
<4 exacerbations/yr	*Haemophilus parainfluenzae*	Second- or third-generation cephalosporin
No comorbid conditions	Viral	Respiratory quinolone[b]
	Mycoplasma pneumoniae	
	Chlamydia pneumoniae	
Complicated AECOPD	*H. influenzae*	Respiratory quinolone[c]
Age >65 yr	*S. pneumoniae*	Amoxicillin/clavulanate
FEV_1 <MWb predicted	*M. catarrhalis*	
≤4 exacerbations/yr	*H. parainfluenzae*	
Comorbid conditions	Viral	
	M. pneumoniae	
	C. pneumoniae	
	Gram-negative enteric bacilli	
Complicated AECOPD at risk for *Pseudomonas aeruginosa* infection	*H. influenzae*	Fluoroquinolone with antipseudomonal activity[c]
FEV_1 <35% predicted	*S. pneumoniae*	
Recurrent courier of antibiotics or steroids	*M. catarrhalis*	
Bronchiectasis	*H. parainfluenzae*	
	Viral	
	M. pneumoniae	
	C. pneumoniae	
	Gram-negative enteric bacilli	
	Pseudomonas aeruginosa	

[a] In active smokers, *H. influenzae* infection is more prevalent—azithromycin and clarithromycin demonstrate improved in vitro activity.
[b] Levofloxacin, moxifloxacin, gatifloxacin, gemifloxacin, and telithromycin have activity against penicillin-resistant *S. pneumoniae*.
[c] Ciprofloxacin and levofloxacin have enhanced antipseudomonal activity.
AECOPD, acute exacerbations of chronic obstructive pulmonary disease; FEV_1, forced expiratory volume at 1 second.
Adapted from references 96 and 11, with permission.

Numerous placebo-controlled trials of antibiotics in AECB have been published, with systematic reviews of these trials suggesting a beneficial treatment effect;[26,27] the latter suggesting a mortality benefit.[27] In the former study, a meta-analysis of nine acceptable studies (of 214 reviewed) addressed the need for antibiotic therapy for AECB.[26] Evaluated agents included tetracyclines, chloramphenicol, ampicillin, and trimethoprim-sulfamethoxazole (TMP-SMX). These studies, conducted between 1957 and 1992, demonstrated benefit of antibiotic therapy especially in those patients requiring hospitalization. Macrolides (e.g., clarithromycin, azithromycin) and fluoroquinolones (including levofloxacin and moxifloxacin) are as efficacious, but not superior, to older therapies.[28–36] While antibiotics offer benefit, identification of those patients most likely to benefit remains elusive. Patients with at least two cardinal symptoms of acute exacerbations of chronic obstructive pulmonary disease (AECOPD; increased dyspnea, increased sputum production, and/or change in sputum color) experience a greater benefit from antibiotic treatment. Table 60-2 serves as a useful guide in selecting antibiotics for AECB.

Independent of selection, predetermined outcome measures should be closely monitored. One of these measures is the infectionfree interval (IFI) when the patient is not taking antibiotics. The IFI is hypothesized to relate to a decrease in colonization of the upper airways with bacteria, reduce cost of treatment of AECB, and decrease antibiotic use.[37] The length of the infectionfree period, number of physician office visits, and hospital admissions associated with a particular antibiotic regimen should be identified in each patient. The longest infectionfree period defines the regimen of choice for that specific patient. Three comparative studies have been conducted with ciprofloxacin to evaluate the IFI as an outcome measure.[38,39] When compared with clarithromycin, the IFI for ciprofloxacin was 142 days versus 52 days ($p = 0.15$); when compared with cefuroxime, the IFI was 146 days versus 178 days ($p = 0.35$); and when compared with amoxicillin/clavulanate, the IFI was 163 days versus 178 days ($p = 0.81$). The infectionfree period is a dynamic outcome measure that needs to be continually evaluated to determine the most appropriate therapy at any point in time in each patient.

ANTIBIOTIC PROPHYLAXIS

5. What strategies should be considered in the use of antibiotic prophylaxis if M.J. develops frequent exacerbations?

Prophylactic antibiotic therapy may decrease the number of acute exacerbations of bronchitis in patients with frequent episodes.[16,40] In patients such as M.J. with infrequent exacerbations, prophylaxis is not beneficial and should be discouraged. Immunization for influenza and pneumococcus and chronic maintenance therapy with bronchodilators or anticholinergic agents preferentially should be used. Antimicrobial prophylaxis should be considered in patients with frequent, severe exacerbations but used only during critical periods when

Table 60-3 Mortality Rates by Pathogen for Community-Acquired Pneumonia

Pathogen	Mortality Rate (%)
Streptococcus pneumoniae	12.0
Haemophilus influenzae	7.4
Staphylococcus aureus	31.8
Klebsiella pneumoniae	35.7
Pseudomonas aeruginosa	61.0
Legionella	14.7
Chlamydia pneumoniae	9.8
Mycoplasma pneumoniae	1.4

patients are most susceptible. For example, daily doses of antibiotics 4 days a week during the winter months[41] or a 7-day course of antibiotics at the first sign of a "chest cold" have been suggested. As mentioned previously, amoxicillin, doxycycline, or TMP-SMX are preferred.[42,43] Antipneumococcal fluoroquinolones should be avoided because of a lack of additional benefit, increased cost, and the concerns regarding selection for bacterial resistance.

PNEUMONIA

Pneumonia is an infectious inflammation of the lung parenchyma. Considering that pneumonia is not a reportable disease and most community-acquired infections are treated on an outpatient basis, it is difficult to determine the true incidence and associated morbidity. Approximately 4 million cases of community-acquired pneumonia (CAP) occur annually, of which almost 1 million occur in those ³65 years of age, with 25% requiring hospitalization.[44] Of those patients hospitalized for pneumonia, the average mortality rate is 10% to 12%, a rate that has not decreased since the introduction of penicillin therapy.[45–47] Associated mortality depends on underlying diseases, age, complications, and pathogen. Table 60-3 summarizes the mortality associated with various bacterial pneumonias. The aggregate cost of care in the United States has been estimated to be in excess of $4.4 billion annually.[45,47–50]

Normal Respiratory Tract Defenses

6. A.T., a 58-year-old man, is admitted to the hospital from home with fever, increased sputum production, tachypnea, and complaints of a knifelike chest pain that is made worse by coughing and breathing. Pertinent medical history includes a 12-year history of CB and chronic renal insufficiency. A.T. regularly produces two cups of sputum per day and continues to smoke two and one-half packs of cigarettes per day. He has been taking amoxicillin 250 mg BID prophylactically for the past 14 months.

Physical examination reveals an elderly man lying restlessly in bed, awake, and oriented to person but not place or time; temperature, 101.5°F (38.6°C), blood pressure (BP), 145/88 mmHg; heart rate (HR), 105 beats/minute; and respiratory rate (RR), 33 breaths/minute. Chest examination reveals slight splinting on the right side with inspiration and fine crackling rales in the lower base of the right lung. Examination of the left lung is normal.

Significant laboratory results include the following: WBC count, 16,200 cells/mm^3 (normal, 5,000–10,000 cells/mm^3); differential polymorphonuclear neutrophils (PMNs), 82% (normal, 45%–79%); bands, 9% (normal, 0%–5%); lymphocytes, 8% (normal, 16%–47%); hematocrit (Hct), 40% (normal, 37%–47%); sodium, 141; potassium, 4.8; blood urea nitrogen (BUN), 32; creatinine, 3.8 mg/dL; glucose 148, mg/dL; arterial blood gases (ABGs), pH 7.46 (normal, 7.38–7.45), Po_2, 68 mmHg (normal, 80–100 mmHg), Pco_2, 36 mmHg (normal, 38–45 mmHg), HCO_3, 24 mEq/L (normal, 22–26 mEq/L); and Gram stain reveals <10 epithelial cells, 20 to 25 PMNs, and predominance of Gram-negative rods.

What are the normal respiratory defenses against infection?

[International System of Units (SI): WBC count, 16.2 –10.0^8/L (normal, 5–10); differential PMNs, 0.82 (normal, 0.45–0.79); bands, 0.09 (normal, 0.00–0.05); lymphocytes, 0.08 (normal, 0.16–0.47); Hct, 0.45 (normal, 0.37); Po_2, 9.06 kPa (normal, 10.66–13.33); Pco_2, 4.8 kPa (normal, 5.07–6.00)]

Preservation of normal respiratory tract function involves a complex system of local pulmonary lung defenses. Anatomic, functional, and mechanical barriers protect the tracheobronchial tree from inert particle and microbial invasion. In addition, an intricate system of cellular and humoral immune host defenses maintain the respiratory tract free of infection. Intrinsic defects in these normal defenses predispose the patient to respiratory infections.[51,52]

The hairs lining the nasal passages, ciliated epithelial cells on mucosal surfaces, production of mucus, salivary enzymes, and the mechanical process of swallowing minimize the passage of foreign material into the lower respiratory tract. Disease states, environmental factors, and age may alter the integrity and function of these barriers.

Alteration in normal oropharyngeal flora by disease or antibiotics permit colonization of the oropharynx with more pathogenic bacteria. Colonization of the oropharynx does not predict infection but predisposes the susceptible patient to aspiration pneumonia.

Neurologic diseases and altered states of consciousness, which result in the loss of control of epiglottal and laryngeal function, predispose the patient to recurrent episodes of aspiration of upper respiratory tract secretions. Without an intact cough or gag reflex, the volume of upper respiratory secretions reaching the lower airways may exceed the local lung defenses, increasing the risk for infection. Patients at risk include any patient with altered consciousness secondary to disease or drugs (e.g., alcoholics, stroke victims, substance abusers, epileptics, surgical patients receiving general anesthesia, head injury patients, patients with any illness associated with obtundation).

A functioning mucociliary transport system, which traps and removes foreign material from the lower respiratory tract, is critical to the protection of the lungs. Diseases that alter mucus production and ciliary function severely compromise the body's ability to defend against infection.

Finally, defects in the cellular and humoral immune response compromise the host to invading pathogens.[53] These defenses include the pulmonary macrophages residing within the alveoli, polymorphonuclear leukocytes, and immunoglobulin and complement present in lung tissue. Deficiency of the latter substances is associated with an increase in the prevalence of infection with encapsulated organisms (i.e., *S. pneumoniae*, *H. influenzae*). These substances enhance the body's defense against bacterial invaders by functioning as opsonins to improve the efficiency of phagocytosis.

In the normal state, the lungs are repeatedly inoculated with microorganisms from the upper airway and inhaled aerosols, but pneumonia rarely occurs.[54] Defects in one or more of the aforementioned mechanisms expose the lung to an increased inoculum of microorganisms for a sufficient period, resulting in pneumonia.

Risk Factors

7. What factors present in A.T. make him susceptible to pulmonary infection?

Most bacterial pneumonias result from the entry of pathogenic bacteria colonizing the mouth and upper respiratory tract into the lung. In the healthy state, the bacterial flora of the oropharynx consists of a mixture of aerobic bacteria (including *Streptococcus* sp., *S. pneumoniae*) and anaerobic bacteria (including *Peptococcus* sp., *Peptostreptococcus* sp., *Fusobacterium* sp., *Prevotella melaninogenica*, and various *Bacteroides* sp.[55] Suppression of normal flora by antibiotics (e.g., amoxicillin in A.T.) and the host's physiologic state can alter oropharyngeal flora.[56,57] These factors facilitate the colonization of the oropharynx with significant numbers of pathogenic Gram-negative aerobic bacteria and staphylococci. Gram-negative rods, including *Klebsiella* sp., are cultured from the sputum in 2% to 18% of healthy individuals, but the concentration of organisms is generally small.[58,59]

Gram-negative bacilli more commonly colonize the oropharyngeal secretions of patients with moderate to severe acute and chronic illnesses, even with no exposure to broad-spectrum antibiotics.[60,61] Patients admitted to the hospital with acute illnesses are rapidly colonized with aerobic Gram-negative bacilli. Approximately 20% are colonized on the first hospital day, and this number increases with the duration of hospitalization and severity of illness.[57] Approximately 35% to 45% of hospitalized patients[57] and up to 100% of critically ill patients[59] will be colonized within 3 to 5 days of admission.

The elderly also have a higher prevalence of oropharyngeal colonization with Gram-negative rods. Level of independent living is a risk factor; Gram-negative bacteria are recovered from the oropharyngeal cultures of only 9% of elderly living in apartments and 60% of elderly in acute hospital wards.[62] Decreased mucociliary transport, decreased cell-mediated immunity, altered immunoglobulin production and antibody response, and increased underlying diseases contribute to increased risk of pneumonia in the elderly.[53,63] Colonization of the upper respiratory tract with Gram-negative bacteria correlates with the development of infection as well.[57,59,60]

Colonization of the lower respiratory tract with potential pathogens is well established in patients with CB such as A.T.[64] Whether a positive sputum culture represents a true pulmonary infection versus colonization is difficult to determine. Additional data from the patient's history, physical examination, and laboratory tests are necessary to appropriately interpret the positive sputum culture.

Clinical Presentation

8. What clinical signs, symptoms, and laboratory tests are consistent with pneumonia in A.T.?

Nearly all patients with pneumonia have fever, cough (with or without sputum production), and a physical examination and chest radiograph finding consistent with consolidation in one or more areas of the lung.[50] Tachypnea, fever, tachycardia, and the chest examination findings represent an acute pulmonary process in this patient.

Although a number of tests are used to document pneumonia, a chest radiograph best distinguishes pneumonia from other disease states. Congestive heart failure, pulmonary embolism, and other diseases may mimic the signs and symptoms of pneumonia. In the majority of cases, a chest radiograph best differentiates between AB, an infection that does not require antibiotics, and pneumonia, one that benefits from antimicrobial therapy. Consequently, a chest radiograph is recommended for all patients hospitalized for presumed pneumonia. The radiograph also may be useful in evaluating the severity of disease (multilobar vs. single lobe involvement). Importantly, A.T. has not received a chest radiograph at this time; thus, a radiograph is recommended to confirm the diagnosis of pneumonia.

Attempts have been made to classify pneumonia as "typical" or "atypical." This categorization originated from the presumption that the presenting symptoms of pneumonia secondary to pathogens such as *S. pneumoniae, H. influenzae, Staphylococcus aureus*, and enteric Gram-negative bacteria ("typical") is different from that observed for Mycoplasma, Legionella, and Chlamydia ("atypical"). However, the Infectious Diseases Society of America (IDSA)/American Thoracic Society (ATS) guidelines caution that this categorization is flawed. *S. pneumoniae* and viruses may cause a syndrome indistinguishable from that caused by *Mycoplasma pneumoniae*. Consequently, reliance on the presence of specific symptoms in the etiology of pneumonia is unreliable. Difficulty with a pathogen-specific diagnosis results in the empiric use of antibacterials active against both "typical" and "atypical" pathogens in the treatment of pneumonia.

A.T. has many signs and symptoms of pneumonia. Fever, tachypnea, tachycardia, a productive cough, and a change in the amount or character of the sputum are common in patients with pneumonia. A.T. gives a history of pleuritic (knifelike) chest pain and examination of the chest shows splinting and an inspiratory lag on the right side during inspiration. All these signs are suggestive of a pneumonic process and usually are present on the affected side. Decreased breath sounds, dullness on chest percussion, and egophony (E – A changes) found during auscultation of the chest are suggestive of consolidation. A.T. is also hypoxemic, as evidenced by his Po_2 of 68 mmHg. A chest radiograph should be performed to identify and/or confirm a pulmonary infiltrate. A.T.'s WBC count is elevated with a left shift (predominance of PMNs and bands), also consistent with bacterial infection.

Determination of Etiologic Agent

9. How can the etiologic organism be determined?

In addition to the clinical and radiographic features noted previously, investigation for specific pathogens should be considered. Such testing may result in changes in antibacterial therapy due to identification of a specific pathogen allowing coverage to be de-escalated or more focused. Correct choice of therapy is critical, since clinical failure and mortality is associated with inappropriate antibiotic therapy. There also are societal benefits associated with establishing an etiologic

Table 60-4 Clinical Indications for More Extensive Diagnostic Testing

Indication	*Blood Culture*	*Sputum Culture*	*Legionella UAT*	*Pneumococcal*	*Other*
ICU admission	X	X	X	X	X[a]
Failure of outpatient antibiotic therapy		X	X	X	—
Cavitary infiltrates	X	X	—	—	X[b]
Leukopenia	X	—	—	X	—
Active alcohol abuse	X	X	X	X	—
Chronic severe liver disease	X	—	—	X	—
Severe obstructive/structural lung disease	—	X	—	—	—
Asplenia (anatomic or functional)	X	—	—	X	—
Recent travel (within past 2 wk)	—	—	X	—	X[c]
Positive *Legionella* UAT result	—	X[d]	NA	—	—
Positive pneumococcal UAT result	X	X	—	NA	—
Pleural effusion	X	X	X	X	X[e]

[a] Endotracheal aspirate if intubated, possibly bronchoscopy or nonbronchoscopic bronchoalveolar lavage.
[b] Fungal and tuberculosis cultures.
[c] See Table 60-10 for details.
[d] Special media for *Legionella*.
[e] Thoracentesis and pleural fluid cultures.
ICU, intensive care unit; NA, not applicable; UAT, urinary antigen test.

diagnosis. For some pathogens, there are important epidemiologic implications. These include severe acute respiratory syndrome (SARS), influenza, Legionnaires disease, and agents of bioterrorism. In addition, empiric treatment guidelines, such as those recently published by the IDSA and ATS, are based on the prevalence of pathogens identified and their in vitro susceptibility patterns.

Adequately and appropriately collected sputum that is Gram stained and cultured remain the mainstays in identifying the etiologic organisms of acute pneumonias. Most often, sputum is collected by having the patient cough and expectorate lower respiratory tract secretions into a collection container; however, because the secretions must pass through the mouth, they may become contaminated with mouth flora. The sputum should be examined macroscopically, and the color, consistency, amount, and odor should be recorded. Appropriately collected specimens should contain 25 PMNs/low-power field (LPF).[65] If there is a predominant organism on Gram stain, empiric therapy can be directed toward the most likely organism. Patients with risk factors for pneumonia (e.g., elderly, hospitalized, chronically ill) often are colonized by multiple pathogens, and a sputum culture is seldom helpful in identifying the specific causative organism.[66] In these cases, physical examination, chest radiograph, and changes in sputum production and quality continue to be the cornerstone for the diagnosis of pneumonia. In patients admitted to the hospital, blood cultures should be evaluated in making a diagnosis, as approximately 12% to 25% will have a positive blood culture with a respiratory pathogen. Empiric antibiotic therapy may be directed based on bacterial morphology or Gram stain while awaiting the culture results to become available 24 to 48 hours later.

If a patient is unable to give an acceptable sputum specimen after three to four attempts, transtracheal aspiration, bronchoscopy, or open lung biopsy can be used to obtain sputum or tissue samples for laboratory analysis. However, these procedures are not without risk and should be used only when the etiology is crucial for diagnosis. Clinical indications for more extensive diagnostic testing are provided in Table 60-4 (from IDSA/ATS guidelines).

Microbiology

The major pathogens for CAP are summarized in Table 60-5. This information is potentially biased, as it is largely based on studies of hospitalized patients, and there is significant variability in the recovery of atypical pathogens, including viruses (influenza A and B), *Legionella* sp., *Chlamydia pneumoniae,* and *M. pneumoniae.* Even with extensive diagnostic studies, the

Table 60-5 Major Pathogens for Community-Acquired Pneumonia

Patient Type	*Etiology*
Outpatient	*Streptococcus pneumoniae*
	Mycoplasma pneumoniae
	Haemophilus influenzae
	Chlamydia pneumoniae
	Respiratory viruses[a]
Inpatient (non-ICU)	*S. pneumoniae*
	M. pneumoniae
	C. pneumoniae
	H. influenzae
	Legionella sp.
	Aspiration
	Respiratory viruses[a]
Inpatient (ICU)	*S. pneumoniae*
	Staphylococcus aureus
	Legionella sp.
	Gram-negative bacilli
	H. influenzae

[a] Influenza A and B, adenovirus, respiratory syncytial virus, and parainfluenza.
ICU, intensive care unit.
Based on collective data from recent studies (reference 174) and adapted from Mandell LA et al. IDSA/ATS guidelines. *Clin Infect Dis* 2007;44:S27–72, and references 52, 55, and 69–72.

causative organism is identified in only 30% to 50% of cases. Several factors contribute to this low yield: (a) 20% to 30% of patients do not provide sputum samples, (b) 20% to 30% have received prior antimicrobial therapy, and (c) some pathogens can only be detected by using specialized techniques.

S. pneumoniae is the most common cause of pneumonia in all age groups and settings, identified in 25% to 60% of all community-acquired bacterial pneumonias.[67] The sudden, rapid onset of dramatic rigors, pleuritic chest pain, a rust-colored sputum with Gram-positive diplococci, and leukocytosis are consistent with pneumococcal pneumonia.

H. influenzae is a significant pulmonary pathogen in infants and children. However, *H. influenzae* also is a significant pulmonary pathogen in adults, particularly those with chronic lung diseases. The high incidence of β-lactamase–producing *H. influenzae* further complicates antimicrobial selection.[68,69]

Gram-negative pneumonia in the community setting is increasing in incidence.[50,70] However, many of these cases are not truly "community acquired," and those cases associated with patients residing in nursing homes and long-term care facilities are now termed *health care–associated facility pneumonia*. In addition, alcoholic individuals are predisposed to Gram-negative pneumonia, often with *Klebsiella pneumoniae*.

The atypical pathogens of CAP are theoretically associated with an atypical clinical presentation, including subacute onset, nonproductive cough, extrapulmonary manifestations, and a chest radiograph that is characteristically worse than the patient's clinical appearance. However, a clear association between these organisms and an atypical presentation has not been established. Atypical pathogens account for 10% to 20% of all cases; however, frequency varies based on temporal and geographic epidemiologic patterns. Diagnostic tests for Legionella include culture, direct fluorescent antigen stain, or urinary antigen assays, which may allow for more directed therapy.

Legionella pneumophila is an important cause of CAP in certain high-risk patients.[70] Patients with altered immunologic function (e.g., elderly) and chronic diseases (e.g., COPD) are most susceptible to infection with this organism. Legionella is more common in middle-age and elderly adults and has the highest mortality rate of the atypical pathogens. Its presentation may be associated with significant gastrointestinal (GI) complaints (nausea, vomiting) and electrolyte abnormalities. Similar to serious pneumococcal pneumonia, the clinical course often is progressive despite administration of appropriate antibiotic therapy. The reported mortality rate is 15% to 25%, even with effective therapy.[47,71]

Mycoplasma (also called *walking pneumonia*) is more common in young adults.[50,72] Diagnostic tests are available (primarily an immunoglobulin M [IgM] enzyme immunoassay), but most laboratories do not provide these tests. Mycoplasma carries virtually no mortality. *C. pneumoniae* reportedly accounts for 5% to 10% of all cases of CAP.[50,73] It has been associated with atherosclerotic disease; however, cause and effect continues to be debated. Diagnostic tests for this pathogen are not offered by most clinical laboratories.

Viral agents account for 2% to 15% of all cases of CAP.[50] Influenza A and B, adenovirus, and parainfluenza virus are most commonly reported in adults, whereas respiratory syncytial virus is most common in the pediatric population.

Epidemiologic factors may favor the presence of certain pathogens.[45] Patients with poor dental hygiene are likely to be infected with anaerobes, whereas HIV-coinfected individuals are more likely to be infected by *P. jirovecii*. A thorough travel and animal-contact history is important. Exposure to birds can be associated with *Chlamydia psittaci* (the cause of psittacosis), exposure to cattle or a parturient cat can be associated with *Coxiella burnetii* (the cause of Q fever), and travel to the southwestern United States can be associated with *Coccidioides immitis* infections. In addition, in the current age of bioterrorism, agents such as *Bacillus anthracis* (anthrax), *Francisella tularensis* (tularemia), and *Yersinia pestis* (plague) may need to be considered as potential causes of pneumonia.

Recently, an increasing incidence of pneumonia due to community-acquired *Staphylococcus aureus* (CA-MRSA) has been observed. These strains are distinct from hospital-acquired strains in that they typically possess a different in vitro susceptibility profile and two unique genes, the SCC*mec* and Panton-Valentine leukocidin (*PVL*) genes. PVL encodes for a toxin that has been associated with necrotizing pneumonia, abscess formation, and empyema. When CA-MRSA has been associated with CAP, it has been most commonly preceded by influenza.

Site of Care for Treatment of Community-Acquired Pneumonia

10. How should A.T. be treated?

The initial management decision after the diagnosis of CAP is to determine the site of care—outpatient, hospitalization in a medical ward, or admission to an intensive care unit (ICU).[47] This is the most costly decision in the management of CAP, as the cost for inpatient care is up to 25 times greater than that for outpatient care and consumes the majority of the estimated $10 billion dollars spent annually on treatment. Severity of illness scores such as the British Thoracic Society (BTS) CURB-65 criteria or prognostic models such as the Pneumonia Severity Index (PSI) can be used to identify patients with CAP who may be candidates for outpatient management.

The PSI and its risk factors for 30-day mortality have been derived by Fine et al.[44,74] by using 20 variables including age, gender, laboratory data on admission, and comorbidities (Fig. 60-2). It stratifies patients in risk categories I to V based on the predicted 30-day mortality. The CURB-65 assigns one point for each of the following criteria: Confusion, Uremia, increased Respiratory rate, low Blood pressure, and age $\geq$65 years). Table 60-6 summarizes the two systems regarding predicted mortality and recommended site of care.

In deciding whether or not to admit to an ICU, one should consider the criteria for severe CAP outlined in Table 60-7, as developed by the IDSA/ATS. The two major criteria or the presence of at least three minor criteria are absolute indications for ICU admission. The use of these criteria allows for appropriate placement of patients and resource utilization, treatment selection, the rapid identification of patients at risk for sepsis, and the availability of ventilator/hemodynamic support.

The use of objective admission criteria such as the PSI or CURB-65 has resulted in a decrease in the number of patients hospitalized with CAP. Whether the PSI or CURB-65 is superior remains unclear, as no randomized trials have compared these methods. The use of objective admission criteria should be supplemented with clinical assessment and determination of

Step 1. Is the patient low risk (class I) based on history and physical examination and not a resident of a nursing home?

- Age 50 years or younger, and
- None of the coexisting conditions or physical examination findings listed in step 2

NO → Go to step 2

YES → Outpatient treatment is recommended

Step 2. Calculate risk score for classes II-V

Patient Characteristics	Points Assigned	Patient's Points
Demographic factors		
Age (in years)		
Males	Age	
Females	Age 2 10	
Nursing home resident	1 10	
Coexisting conditions		
Neoplastic disease	1 30	
Liver disease	1 20	
Congestive heart failure	1 10	
Cerebrovascular disease	1 10	
Renal disease	1 10	
Initial physical examination findings		
Altered mental status	1 20	
Respiratory rate $ 30/min	1 20	
Systolic BP , 90 mmHg	1 20	
Temperature , 35² or $ 40° C	1 15	
Pulse $ 125/min	1 10	
Initial laboratory findings (score zero if not tested)		
ph , 7.35	1 30	
BUN . 30 mg/dl	1 20	
Sodium , 130 mEq/L	1 20	
Glucose $ 250 mg/dl	1 10	
Hematocrit , 30%	1 10	
Po_2 , 60 mmHg or O_2 sat , 90%	1 10	
Pleural effusion	1 10	
Total score (sum of patient's points):		

30-Day Mortality Data by Risk Class

Total Score	Risk Class	Recommended Site of Treatment	Mortality Range Observed in Validation Cohorts. %
None (see step 1)	I	Outpatient	0.1
# 70	II	Outpatient	0.6
71–90	III	Outpatient	0.5–2.8
91–130	IV	Inpatient	8.2–9.3
. 130	V	Inpatient	27.0–29.2

FIGURE 60-2 Model to predict the 30-day mortality in patients with community-acquired pneumonia.

subjective factors including availability of outpatient support resources.

Using the PSI, the scoring for A.T. is as follows: He is a 58-year-old man (58 points), has a history of chronic renal insufficiency (10 points), a RR >30 (20 points), and has an altered mental status (20 points). His score of 108 points places him in risk strata IV, which carries a 30-day mortality risk of 9.3% (Fig. 60-2). Based on A.T.'s PSI assessment and clinical status, he should be admitted to the hospital. Using the CURB-65, A.T. has a score of "3" (30-day mortality of 14.5%–57%) given that he was confused, uremic, and had an increased RR, similarly resulting in the hospital as the preferred site of care.

INITIATION OF ANTIMICROBIAL TREATMENT

Initial antimicrobial therapy is largely empirical and should be guided by the results of the sputum Gram stain, patient age, medical history, concomitant diseases, place of residence, clinical signs and symptoms, and allergy status. An approach to the patient with CAP is presented in Figure 60-3, and antibiotic regimens of choice are provided in Table 60-8 (see below).[45]

If no sputum is available for Gram stain or the microbiologic results do not identify a causative organism, antibiotics active against the most probable bacterial pathogens should be selected (Table 60-9).

Lastly, the underlying conditions that predispose to specific pathogens, such as risks for aspiration, alcohol abuse, smoking, and epidemiologic exposures, also should be considered in the empiric selection of therapy (Table 60-10).

The time to the first dose of antibiotic therapy has been emphasized as a lower mortality, as has been seen in patients with CAP based on the time to first dose received. Those administered their first dose of antibiotic therapy within 4 hours

Table 60-6 Predicted Mortality and Recommended Site of Care

System and Score	Predicted 30-Day Mortality (%)	Recommended Site of Care
PSI strata 1–2	0.1–0.7	Outpatient
PSI strata 3	0.9–2.8	Admit to ward
PSI strata 4–5	9.3–27	Admit; consider ICU
CURB-65 score 0–1	0.7–2.1	Outpatient
CURB-65 score 2	9.2	Admit to ward
CURB-65 score 3	14.5–57.0	Admit; consider ICU

CURB-65, Confusion, Uremia, increased Respiratory rate, low Blood pressure, and age ≥65 years; ICU, intensive care unit; PSI, Pneumonia Severity Index.

have been shown to have a lower mortality compared with those receiving a first dose >4 hours. This has been considered as a potential quality measure to assess the quality of care provided to patients with CAP. However, this recommendation has resulted in administration of antibiotics in many patients who ultimately were determined to not have bacterial pneumonia. One of the consequences of this increased focus on the so-called 4-hour rule has in one center resulted in an increase in cases of *Clostridium difficile*–associated diarrhea (CDAD) with several patients without CAP receiving antibacterials and ultimately succumbing to *C. difficile* disease CDAD. The initiation of antibiotic therapy for patients with suspected CAP should be based on assessment of the patient's clinical presentation rather than achieving an administrative outcome measure.

A.T.'s treatment should be started empirically with antibiotics pending identification of the etiologic bacteria. The choice should be guided by the results of the sputum Gram stain, patient age, medical history, concomitant diseases, place of residence, and clinical signs and symptoms. In A.T.'s case, the Gram stain, which shows a predominance of one organism and many WBCs, should have the greatest influence on initial antimicrobial selection. Because A.T.'s Gram stain shows a predominance of Gram-negative bacilli, empiric therapy should

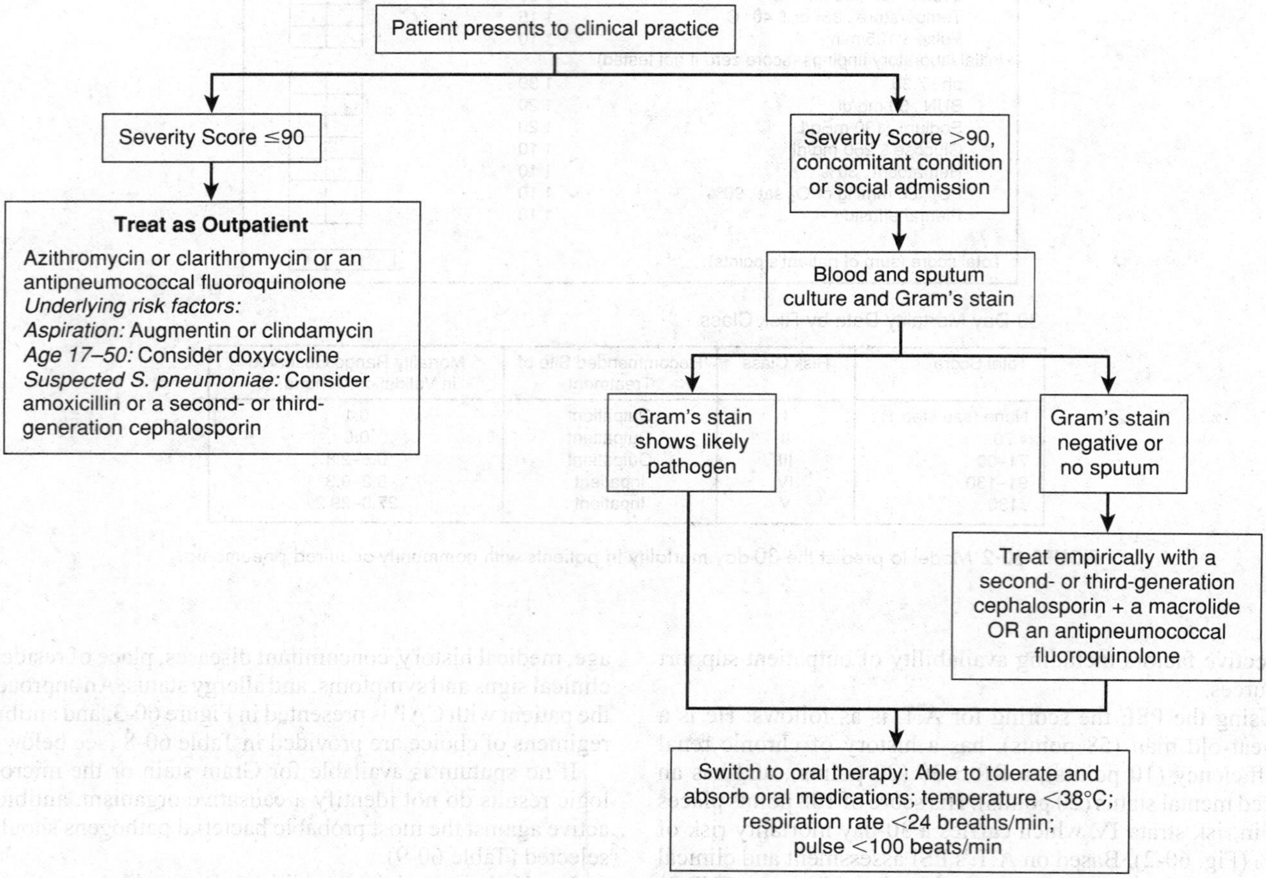

FIGURE 60-3 Application of the Pneumonia Patient Outcomes Research Team Severity Index to determine initial site of treatment. Step 1 identifies patients in risk class 1 on the basis of age ≤50 years and the absence of all comorbid conditions and vital sign abnormalities listed in step 2. For all patients who are not classified at risk class 1, the laboratory data listed in step 2 should be collected to calculate a pneumonia severity score. Risk class and recommended site of care based on the pneumonia severity score listed in the final table. Thirty-day mortality data are based on two independent cohorts of 40,326 patients. For additional information, see reference 98. BP, blood pressure; BUN, blood urea nitrogen. *Source:* Reproduced with permission from Metlay JP, Fine MJ. Testing strategies in the initial management of patients with community-acquired pneumonia. *Ann Intern Med* 2003;138:109.)

Table 60-7 Criteria for Severe Community-Acquired Pneumonia

Minor Criteria[a]
RR[b] ≥30 breaths/minute
PaO_2/FiO_2 ratio[b] ≤250
Multilobar infiltrates
Confusion/disorientation
Uremia (BUN level, ≥20 mg/dL)
Leukopenia[c] (WBC count, <4,000 cells/mm^3)
Thrombocytopenia (platelet count, <100,000 cells/mm^3)
Hypothermia (core temperature, <36°C)
Hypotension requiring aggressive fluid resuscitation
Major Criteria
Invasive mechanical ventilation
Septic shock with the need for vasopressors

[a]Other criteria to consider include hypoglycemia (in nondiabetic patients), acute alcoholism/alcoholic withdrawal, hyponatremia, unexplained metabolic acidosis or elevated lactate level, cirrhosis, and asplenia.
[b]A need for noninvasive ventilation can substitute for a RR >30 breaths/minute or a PaO_2/FiO_2 ratio >250.
[c]As a result of infection alone.
BUN, blood urea nitrogen; PaO_2/FiO_2, arterial oxygen pressure/fraction of inspired oxygen; RR, respiratory rate; WBC, white blood cell.

be directed at *H. influenzae* and other Gram-negative bacilli. Based on A.T.'s age and history of previous amoxicillin prophylaxis, one can assume that the pathogen in question is not susceptible to amoxicillin. Consequently, an antibiotic regimen that is effective against ampicillin-resistant *H. influenzae* and other aerobic Gram-negative bacilli should generally be chosen. A respiratory fluoroquinolone (levofloxacin or moxifloxacin) would be a reasonable selection for empiric treatment of A.T.'s pneumonia.

RESPONSE TO THERAPY

Patient outcomes associated with CAP depend largely on the choice of antimicrobial agent and the patient status at the time of presentation. Poor prognostic factors include age >65 years; coexisting disease such as diabetes, renal failure, heart failure, and COPD; clinical and laboratory findings as outlined in Figure 60-2; and recovery of *S. pneumoniae* or Legionella.[44,45,47]

Most patients with bacterial pneumonia improve clinically (decreased temperature and systemic toxicity) 24 to 48 hours after the initiation of effective antibiotic therapy. Chest radiograph resolution lags, taking 3 weeks in otherwise healthy, young adults and up to 12 weeks in elderly patients and those with complicated infections.[75,76] A subset of patients with bacterial pneumonia can be predicted to do poorly. Factors associated with a poor outcome include multilobar involvement, bacteremia, a history of alcoholism, age >60 years, and neutropenia. Despite the introduction of new anti-infectives, antibiotic therapy has not reduced mortality in pneumococcal pneumonia with bacteremia, which remains at 20% to 30%.[47,77]

When the patient is clinically stable for 24 hours (Table 60-11), conversion to the oral route can be considered. The patient must be able to take oral medications and have adequate GI function. Diarrhea is not a reason to avoid the oral route, because it rarely results in significant reductions in absorption of medications.[45] Selecting an oral agent can be simplified if culture and sensitivity data are available and if the parenteral agent is available in an oral formulation. Patients with CAP should be treated for a minimum of 5 days, should be afebrile for 48 to 72 hours, and should have no more than one CAP-associated sign of clinical instability (Table 60-11) before therapy is discontinued. A longer duration of therapy may be needed if the initial therapy was not active against the identified pathogen or if it was complicated by extrapulmonary infection such as bacteremia.

Table 60-8 Community-Acquired Pneumonia: Antibiotic Regimens of Choice

Outpatient Treatment
1. Previously healthy and no use of antimicrobials within the previous 3 months
A macrolide (strong recommendation; level I evidence)
Doxycyline (weak recommendation; level III evidence)
2. Presence of comorbidities such as chronic heart, lung, liver or renal disease; diabetes mellitus; alcoholism; malignancies; asplenia; immunosuppressing conditions or use of immunosuppressing drugs; or use of antimicrobials within the previous 3 months (in which case an alternative from a different class should be selected)
A respiratory fluoroquinolone (moxifloxacin, gemifloxacin, or levofloxacin [750 mg]) (strong recommendation; level I evidence)
A β-lactam plus a macrolide (strong recommendation; level I evidence)
3. In regions with a high rate (>25%) of infection with high-level (MIC ≥16 mcg/mL) macrolide-resistant *Streptococcus pneumoniae*, consider use of alternative agents listed above in #2 for patients without comorbidities (moderate recommendation; level III evidence)
Inpatients, Non-ICU Treatment
A respiratory fluoroquinolone (strong recommendation; level I evidence)
A β-lactam plus a macrolide (strong recommendation; level evidence)
Inpatients, ICU Treatment
A β-lactam (cefotaxime, ceftriaxone, or ampicilliwsulbactaml plus either azithromycin (level II evidence) or a respiratory fluoroquinolone (level I evidence) (strong recommendation) (for penicillin-allergic patients I a respiratory fluoroquinolone and aztreonam are recommended)
Special Concerns
If *Pseudomonas* is a consideration:
An antipneumococcal, antipseudomonal β-lactim (piperacillintazobactam, cefepirne, irnipenern, or maropenern) plus either ciproflaxacin or levoflaxacin (750 mg)
or
The above β-lactam plus an aminoglycoside and azythromycin
or
The above β-lactam plus an aminoglycoside and an antipneumococcal fluoroquinalone (for penicillin-allergic patients, substitute aztreonam for above β-lactam) (moderate recommendation; level III evidence)
If CA-MRSA is a consideration, add vancomycin or linezolid (moderate recommendation; level III evidence)

CA-MRSA, community-acquired methicillin-resistant *Staphylococcus aureus*; ICU, intensive care unit; MIC, minimum inhibitory concentration.

Table 60-9 Community-Acquired Pneumonia: Preferred Antimicrobial(s) Against Most Probable Bacterial Pathogens

Organism	*Preferred Antimicrobial(s)*	*Alternative Antimicrobial(s)*
Streptococcus pneumoniae		
Penicillin nonresistant; MIC <2 mcg/mL	Penicillin G, amoxicillin	Macrolide, cephalosporins, (or a I [cefpodoxime, cefprozil, cefuroxime, cefdinir, cefditoren] or parenteral [cefuroxime, ceftriaxone, cefotaxime]), clindamycin, doxycyline, respiratory fluoroquinolone[a]
Penicillin resistant; MIC ≥2 mcg/mL	Agents chosen on the basis of susceptibility, including cefotaxime, ceftriaxone, fluoroquinolone	Vancomycin, linezolid, high-dose amoxicillin (3 g/day with penicillin MIC ≤4 mcg/mL)
Haemophilus influenzae		
Non–β-lactamase producing	Amoxicillin	Fluoroquinolone, doxycycline, azithromycin, clarithromycin[b]
β-Lactamase producing	Second- or third-generation cephalosporin, amoxicillin-clavulanate	Fluoroquinolone, doxycycline, azithromycin, clarithromycin[b]
Mycoplasma pneumoniae/ Chlamydia pneumoniae	Macrolide, a tetracycline	Fluoroquinolone
Legionella sp.	Fluoroquinolone, azithromycin	Doxycycline
Chlamydia psittaci	A tetracycline	Macrolide
Coxiella burnetii	A tetracycline	Macrolide
Francisella tularensis	Doxycycline	Gentamicin, streptomycin
Yersinisa pestis	Streptomycin, gentamicin	Doxycyline, fluoroquinolone
Bacillus anthracis (inhalation)	Ciprofloxacin, levofloxacin, doxycycline (usually with second agent)	Other fluoroquinolones; β-lactam, if susceptible; rifampin; clindamycin; chloramphenicol
Enterobacteriaceae	Third-generation cephalosporin, carbapenem[c] (drug of choice if extended-spectrum β-lactamase producer)	β-Lactam/β-Lactamase inhibitor[d] fluoroquinolone
Pseudomonas aeruginosa	Antipseudomonal β-lactam plus ciprofloxacin or levofloxacin[f] or aminoglycoside	Aminoglycoside plus ciprofloxacin or levofloxacin[f]
Burkholderia pseudomallei	Carbapenem, ceftazadime	Fluoroquinolone, TMP-SMX
Acinetobacter sp.	Carbapenem	Cephalosporin-aminoglycoside, ampicillin sulbactam, colistin
Staphylococcus aureus		
Methicillin susceptible	Antistaphylococcal penicillin[g]	Cefazolin, clindamycin
Methicillin resistant	Vancomycin or linezolid	TMP-SMX
Bordetella pertussis	Macrolide	TMP-SMX
Anaerobe (aspiration)	β-Lactam/β-Lactamase inhibitor,[d] clindamycin	Carbapenem
Influenza virus	Oseltamivir or zanamivir	
Mycobacterium tuberculosis	Isoniazid plus rifampin plus ethambutol plus pyrazinamide	Refer to reference 243 for specific recommendations
Coccidioides sp.	For uncomplicated infection in a normal host, no therapy generally recommended; for therapy, itraconazole, fluconazole	Amphotericin B
Histoplasmosis	Itraconazole	Amphotericin B
Blastomycosis	Itraconazole	Amphotericin B

NOTE. Choices should be modified on the basis of susceptibility test results and advice from local specialists. Refer to local references for appropriate doses.

[a] Levofloxacin, moxifloxacin, gemifloxacin (not a first-line choice for penicillin-susceptible strains); ciprofloxacin is appropriate for Legionella and most Gram-negative bacilli (including *H. influenza*).

[b] Azithromycin is more active *in vitro* than clarithromycin for *H. influenza*.

[c] Imipenem-cilastatin, meropenem, ertapenem.

[d] Piperacillin-tazobactam for Gram-negative bacilli, ticarcillin clavulanate, ampicillin-sulbactam or amoxicillin clavulanate.

[e] Ticarcillin, piperacillin, ceftazidime, cefepime, aztreonam, imipenem, meropenem.

[f] 750 mg daily.

[g] Nafcillin, oxacillin, flucloxacillin.

MIC, minimum inhibitory concentration; TMP-SMX, trimethoprim-sulfamethoxazole.

11. What is the impact of drug-resistant *Staphylococcus pneumoniae* (DRSP) in the management of CAP?

Penicillin-Resistant Streptococcus pneumoniae

Despite four decades of using penicillin, only modest rates of reduced susceptibility to penicillin were reported in the 1980s. However, over the past few decades, increased penicillin resistance has been observed. The mechanism by which pneumococci become resistant to β-lactam antibiotics is through alteration in the penicillin binding proteins. This decrease in affinity results in variable increases in the minimum inhibitory concentrations (MICs) of different β-lactams. Strains with MICs of more than 0.1 mcg/mL accounted for 3.8% of isolates in the 1980s; by 1994–1995, the rate was 24%, and by 1997 it was

Table 60-10 Community-Acquired Pneumonia: Underlying Conditions and Commonly Encountered Pathogens

Condition	Commonly Encountered Pathogen(s)
Alcoholism	*Streptococcus pneumoniae*, oral anaerobes, *Klebsiella pneumoniae*, *Acinetobacter* sp., *Mycobacterium tuberculosis*
COPD and/or smoking	*Haemophilus influenzae*, *Pseudomonas aeruginosa*, *Legionella* sp., *S. pneumoniae*, *Moraxella cararrhalis*, *Chlamydia pneumoniae*
Aspiration	Gram-negative enteric pathogens, oral anaerobes
Lung abscess	CA-MRSA, oral anaerobes, endemic fungal pneumonia, *M. tuberculosis*, atypical mycobacteria
Exposure to bat or bird droppings	*Histoplasma capsulatum*
Exposure to birds	*Chlamydia psittaci* (if poultry; avian influenza)
Exposure to rabbits	*Francisella tularensis*
Exposure to farm animals or parturient cats	*Coxiella burnetti* (Q fever)
HIV infection (early)	*S. pneumoniae*, *H. influenzae*, *M. tuberculosis*
HIV infection (late)	The pathogens listed for early infection plus *P. Pneumocystis jirovecii*, *Cryptococcus* sp., *Histoplasma* sp., *Aspergillus* sp., atypical mycobacteria (especially *Mycobacterium kansash*), *P. aeruginosa*, *H. influenzae*
Hotel or cruise ship stay in previous 2 weeks	*Legionella* sp.
Travel to or residence in southwestern United States	*Coccidioides* sp., hantavirus
Travel to or residence in Southeast and East Asia	*Burkholderia pseudomallei*, avian influenza, SARS
Influenza active in community	Influenza, *S. pneumoniae*, *Staphylococcus aureus*, *H. influenzae*
Cough >2 wk with whoop or posttussive vomiting	*Bordetella pertussis*
Structural lung disease (e.g., bronchiectasis)	*P. aeruginosa*, *Burkholderia cepacia*, *S. aureus*
Injection drug use	*S. aureus*, anaerobes, *M. tuberculosis*, *S. pneumoniae*
Endobronchial obstruction	Anaerobes, *S. pneumoniae*, *H. influenzae*, *S. aureus*
In context of bioterrorism	*Bacillus anthracis* (anthrax), *Yersinia pestis* (plague), *Francisella tularensis* (tularemia)

CA-MRSA, community-acquired methicillin-resistant *Staphylococcus aureus*; COPD, chronic obstructive pulmonary disease; SARS, severe acute respiratory syndrome.

43.8%.[78–80] As of 2000, rates of resistance in the United States have reached a plateau at 30% to 35%.

The impact of DRSP on patient outcomes is unclear. Published studies are limited by small sample size, observational design, and the relative infrequency of isolates exhibiting "high-level" resistance. The available data suggest that the clinically relevant level of penicillin resistance is an MIC of at least 4 mg/L. Risk factors for infection with β-lactam-resistant *S. pneumoniae* include age <2 years or >65 years of age, β-lactam therapy in the previous 3 months, alcoholism, medical comorbidities, immunosuppressive illness or therapy, and exposure to a child in a day care center. Although the relative predictive value of these risk factors remains unclear, recent treatment with antimicrobials is likely the most significant risk factor.

Penicillin resistance is also associated with resistance to other antimicrobial classes, including cephalosporins, macrolides, tetracyclines, and TMP-SMZ (Table 60-12). In contrast, vancomycin, the fluoroquinolones, clindamycin, chloramphenicol, and rifampin are less impacted.[78–81] Penicillin susceptibility should be tested for in all significant pneumococcal isolates.[82]

Table 60-11 Criteria for Conversion to Oral Administration of Antibiotics

Temperature ≤37.8°C
HR ≤100 beats/minute
RR ≤24 breaths/minute
Systolic BP ≥90 mmHg
Arterial oxygen saturation ≥90% or Po_2 ≥60 mmHg on room air
Ability to maintain oral intake[a]
Normal mental status[a]

HR, heart rate; RR, respiratory rate; Po_2, oxygen partial pressure.

[a]Important for discharge or oral switch decision but not necessarily for determination of nonresponse.

Adapted from Mandell LA et al. Infectious Diseases Society of America/American Thoracic Society consensus guidelines on the management of community-acquired pneumonia in adults. *Clin Infect Dis* 2007;44(Suppl 2):S2.

Table 60-12 Susceptibility of *Streptococcus pneumoniae* Based on Penicillin Susceptibility

	% Susceptible to Indicated Agent		
Agent	Pen-S	Pen-I	Pen-R
Cefuroxime axetil	99.0	76.3	0.7
Cefpodoxime proxetil	99.5	82.4	0.7
Cefepime	99.7	87.5	3.9
Cefotaxime	100.0	95.7	19.1
Erythromycin	96.6	81.7	50.7
Clarithromycin	94.9	63.5	38.9
Clindamycin	99.2	93.2	86.2
Tetracycline	96.1	86.7	63.2
TMP-SMX	89.0	72.4	23.0
Levofloxacin	97.4	96.9	97.1

Pen-I, penicillin intermediate; Pen-R, penicillin resistant, Pen-S, penicillin sensitive; TMP-SMX, trimethoprim-sulfamethoxazole.

Macrolide-Resistant Streptococcus pneumoniae

Although high rates of in vitro macrolide resistance can coexist with penicillin resistance, there are few reports of macrolide failures in CAP due to drug-resistant pneumococci.[83] Pneumococcal resistance to macrolides is expressed as one of two phenotypes. The first, known as the M phenotype, is an efflux pump associated with the mefE gene that results in the efflux of all 14- and 15-membered macrolides from the cell.[84] M phenotype isolates typically have moderate levels of macrolide resistance (MIC in the range of 1–32 mg/mL) and are almost always susceptible to clindamycin.[85] A second phenotype, called the MLSB phenotype, results from methylation of 23S ribosomal RNA and is encoded by the ermAM gene. Methylation results in blockade of the binding of macrolides, lincosamides, and group B streptogramin agents. The MLSB phenotype is associated with high-level macrolide resistance (MIC >64 mg/mL) as well as resistance to clindamycin.

One investigation demonstrated the following: (a) macrolide use in the United States increased by 13% from 1993 to 1999 (17.7 million prescriptions vs. 21.2 million prescriptions, respectively—the most dramatic increase was in children <5 years of age, a 320% increase over the same time frame); (b) macrolide resistance has doubled from 1995 to 1999 (10.6% in 1995 to 20.4% in 1999), mostly accounted for by increases in the M phenotype; and (c) the median MIC of the M phenotype increased from 4 mcg/mL to 8 mcg/ mL, an MIC associated with treatment failures to clarithromycin and azithromycin.[86] The association between increasing macrolide use and the increasing prevalence of macrolide resistance, and more importantly the shift in the median MIC in M phenotype isolates, is disturbing. As a result, current guidelines recommend macrolide monotherapy only in outpatients who prior to the onset of CAP were otherwise healthy and have no risk factors for DRSP.

Antiviral Agents

12. What treatment options are available for influenza virus infection?

As outlined previously, viruses account for 2% to 15% of all cases of CAP. Influenza represents one organism that commonly may be associated with pneumonia. Influenza is an acute respiratory infection characterized by fever, headache, sore throat, myalgias, and a nonproductive cough. In some cases, it can progress to serious secondary complications such as bacterial and viral pneumonia. In addition to increased health care costs, loss of work days, and unnecessary antibiotics, influenza epidemics are responsible for a large number of deaths each year in the United States. Epidemics occur during the winter months nearly every year, with peak activity between late December and early March. The mainstay of protection against the disease has been the inactivated influenza vaccine. Antiviral agents are important adjuncts to the vaccine but do not serve as a substitute for preseason vaccination.

Both the influenza A and B viruses have two major surface glycoproteins that mediate immunity, hemagglutinin and neuraminidase. These two proteins play a critical role in viral replication. Hemagglutinin attaches virus to cells, whereas neuraminidase has several roles to facilitate the spread of the virus throughout the respiratory tract. The neuraminidase enzyme is responsible for releasing the virus from infected cells, preventing the formation of viral aggregates after the release, and potentially preventing viral inactivation. The active site of neuraminidase is almost identical in both influenza A and B.

Although annual vaccination is the primary strategy for preventing complications of influenza virus infections, antiviral medications with activity against influenza viruses can be effective for the chemoprophylaxis and treatment of influenza. Four licensed influenza antiviral agents are available in the United States: amantadine, rimantadine, zanamivir, and oseltamivir. Influenza A virus resistance to amantadine and rimantadine can emerge rapidly during treatment. Because antiviral testing results indicated high levels of resistance, neither amantadine nor rimantadine should be used for the treatment or chemoprophylaxis of influenza in the United States during the 2007–2008 influenza season. Surveillance demonstrating that susceptibility to these antiviral medications has been reestablished among circulating influenza A viruses will be needed before amantadine or rimantadine can be used for the treatment or chemoprophylaxis of influenza A. Oseltamivir or zanamivir can be prescribed if antiviral treatment of influenza is indicated. Oseltamivir is approved for treatment of persons >1 year of age, and zanamivir is approved for treating persons >7 years of age. Oseltamivir and zanamivir can be used for chemoprophylaxis of influenza; oseltamivir is licensed for use as chemoprophylaxis in persons >1 year of age, and zanamivir is licensed for use in persons >5 years of age.

Antiviral Agents for Influenza

Amantadine and rimantadine are compounds that indirectly interrupt the function of hemagglutinin by blocking the uncoating of the influenza A virus and preventing host penetration. When initiated within 48 hours of the onset of symptoms, both amantadine and rimantadine shorten the clinical course of the illness related to influenza A and enable patients to resume daily activities sooner. Until recently, these agents were the only antiviral agents available for the prevention and treatment of influenza A. However, their use has been limited by lack of activity against influenza B, emergence of resistance, and central nervous system effects, particularly with amantadine. Adamantane resistance among circulating influenza A viruses has increased rapidly worldwide over the past several years. The proportion of influenza A viral isolates submitted from throughout the world to the World Health Organization Collaborating Center for Surveillance, Epidemiology, and Control of Influenza at the Centers for Disease Control and Prevention (CDC) that were adamantane resistant increased from 0.4% during 1994–1995 to 12.3% during 2003–2004. During the 2005–2006 influenza season, the CDC determined that 193 (92%) of 209 influenza A (H3N2) viruses isolated from patients in 26 states demonstrated a change at amino acid 31 in the M2 gene that confers resistance to adamantanes. In addition, two (25%) of eight influenza A (H1N1) viruses tested were resistant (368). All 2005–2006 influenza season isolates in these studies remained sensitive to neuraminidase inhibitors. Preliminary data from the 2006–2007 influenza season indicates that resistance to adamantanes remains high among influenza A isolates, but resistance to neuraminidase inhibitors is extremely uncommon (<1% of isolates) (CDC, unpublished data, 2007). Amantadine or rimantadine should not be used for the treatment or prevention of influenza in the United States

Table 60-13 Comparison of Current Antiviral Agents for Influenza

	Amantadine	Rimantadine	Oseltamivir	Zanamavir
Influenza activity	A	A	A and B	A and B
Route of administration	Oral	Oral	Oral	Oral inhalation
Treatment population	≥1 yr	≥14 yr	≥12 yr	≥18 yr
Prophylaxis population	≥1 yr	≥1 yr	No indication	No indication
Dosage	100 mg PO Q 12 hr	100 mg PO Q 12 hr	75 mg PO BID for 5 days	Two inhalations (5 mg each) PO BID for 5 days
Side effects	CNS, GI	CNS, GI (less than amantadine)	Nasal and throat discomfort, headache, bronchospasm	Nausea, vomiting, headache

BID, twice a day; CNS, central nervous system; GI, gastrointestinal; PO, by mouth.

until evidence of susceptibility to these antiviral medications has been reestablished among circulating influenza A viruses.

Zanamivir and oseltamivir are chemically related antiviral medications known as neuraminidase inhibitors that have activity against both influenza A and B viruses. The two medications differ in pharmacokinetics, adverse events, routes of administration, approved age groups, dosages, and costs.[87] They are sialic acid analogs that work by inhibiting the viral enzyme neuraminidase. The function of neuraminidase is to cleave sialic acid residues on the cell surface, thereby promoting release of virus from infected cells. Blocking the activity of neuraminidase decreases the amount of virus released that can infect other cells. Resistance to the neuraminidase inhibitors can occur but seems to be less common and slower to develop than with the older antivirals amantadine and rimantadine. A comparison of these agents is provided in Table 60-13.

Zanamivir (Relenza) is indicated for the treatment of uncomplicated influenza illness in adults and children >12 years of age who have been symptomatic ≤48 hours.[88–90] Oseltamivir (Tamiflu) is approved for the treatment of uncomplicated influenza infection in adults ≥18 years of age who have been symptomatic ≤48 hours.[91–92] Studies have shown that when administered within 2 days of the onset of symptoms, both zanamivir and oseltamivir reduced the median duration of symptoms by approximately 1 day (6.5–5.0 days and 4.5–3.0 days, respectively). High-risk patients (i.e., the elderly, those with asthma), patients who had a febrile illness, and those treated within 30 hours of symptom onset showed the greatest improvement from zanamivir therapy (8.0–5.5 days). Neither neuraminidase inhibitor is approved for the prevention of influenza, but recent studies have demonstrated both to be approximately 60% to 80% effective when administered prophylactically. Likewise, there are no studies comparing the two neuraminidase inhibitors with each other or with amantadine or rimantadine.

Zanamivir is formulated as a dry powder for oral inhalation; its oral bioavailability is poor. The recommended dosage is two inhalations (5 mg each) twice daily for 5 days. Less than 20% of the inhaled dose is systemically absorbed; 70% to 90% of the inhaled drug deposits in the oropharynx. The half-life of systemically absorbed zanamivir is 3 to 5 hours, and it is excreted unchanged in the urine. The manufacturer does not recommend a dosage adjustment in patients with renal insufficiency. The most common side effects encountered with zanamivir administration are nasal and throat irritation, headache, and bronchospasm.

Oseltamivir, available as a 75-mg oral capsule, is an ester prodrug that is hydrolyzed in the gut and liver to the active form, oseltamivir carboxylate. The recommended dosage is 75 mg twice daily for 5 days. Eighty percent of the drug is absorbed systemically, and the half-life (6–10 hours) of oseltamivir carboxylate is excreted in the urine by glomerular filtration. A dosage reduction to 75 mg daily is recommended in patients with a creatinine clearance <30 mL/minute. The most common side effects experienced are nausea, vomiting, and headache. Food may improve GI tolerance.

Although there is limited clinical experience, no significant drug interactions have been reported with either agent. Neither zanamivir nor oseltamivir are substrates for cytochrome P450 metabolism and are not expected to alter the metabolism of other agents. The cost for 5-day therapy with zanamivir or oseltamivir is approximately $50.

The role of the neuraminidase inhibitors in the prevention and treatment of influenza is not clearly defined. It is widely accepted that influenza vaccination will continue to be the primary method of preventing influenza and its secondary complications. However, the neuraminidase inhibitors may be a reasonable alternative for those who cannot be vaccinated due to true egg allergy, those who are not likely to respond to the vaccination, or those who are at significantly high risk.

Effective treatment of influenza illness with any of the currently available antiviral agents is limited by the need for almost immediate diagnosis and intervention. When these agents are initiated *within 2 days* of the onset of symptoms, they can shorten the duration of the illness. This will require education of both the public and clinicians.[90,92] The role of the pharmacist may be in the early identification of patients who are potential candidates for antiviral therapy. Dialog with patients regarding symptoms and their duration will enable the pharmacist to make appropriate recommendations about the necessity of drug therapy and doctor visits. None of the four agents has been demonstrated to be effective in preventing serious influenza-related complications such as bacterial or viral pneumonia or exacerbation of underlying chronic conditions.

Immunoprophylaxis

13. What agents are available for chemo/immunoprophylaxis against respiratory tract infections?

INFLUENZA VIRUS

In the United States, the primary option for reducing the effect of influenza is immunoprophylaxis with inactivated vaccine. Vaccinating persons at high risk for complications each year before seasonal increases in influenza virus circulation is the most effective means of reducing the effect of influenza. The inactivated influenza vaccines are standardized to contain the hemagglutinins of strains (usually two type A and one type B), representing the influenza viruses likely to circulate in the United States in the upcoming winter. The vaccines are made from highly purified, egg-grown viruses that have been made noninfectious. Because the vaccines are initially grown in embryonated hen eggs, the final product might contain residual egg proteins. In addition, vaccine distributed in the United States might contain the preservative thimerosal, which contains mercury.

The effectiveness of influenza vaccination depends primarily on the age and immunocompetence of the recipient and the degree of similarity between viruses in the vaccine and in circulation. When strains are similar, vaccine prevents influenza illness in 70% to 90% of healthy adults <65 years of age. Children as young as 6 months of age can develop protective levels of antibody after vaccination. Seroconversion rates have been reported to be 44% to 89% and increase with the age of the child. The effectiveness in preventing influenza-related illness in children between 1 to 15 years of age is 77% to 91%. In adults ≥65 years of age, the effectiveness of the vaccine has been reported to be 58%. Importantly, in this population, it has been shown to prevent secondary complications and reduce the risk for influenza-related hospitalization and death.

Influenza vaccination is recommended in the following patients:

- All persons, including school-aged children, who want to reduce the risk of becoming ill with influenza or of transmitting influenza to others
- All children aged 6–59 months (i.e., 6 months–4 years)
- All persons ≥50 years of age
- Children and adolescents (aged 6 months–18 years) receiving long-term aspirin therapy who therefore might be at risk for experiencing Reye syndrome after influenza virus infection
- Women who will be pregnant during the influenza season
- Adults and children who have chronic pulmonary (including asthma), cardiovascular (except hypertension), renal, hepatic, hematologic, or metabolic disorders (including diabetes mellitus)
- Adults and children who have immunosuppression (including immunosuppression caused by medications or by HIV
- Adults and children who have any condition (e.g., cognitive dysfunction, spinal cord injuries, seizure disorders, or other neuromuscular disorders) that can compromise respiratory function or the handling of respiratory secretions or that can increase the risk for aspiration
- Residents of nursing homes and other chronic care facilities
- Health care personnel
- Healthy household contacts (including children) and caregivers of children <5 years of age and adults ≥50 years of age, with particular emphasis on vaccinating contacts of children aged <6 months of age
- Healthy household contacts (including children) and caregivers of persons with medical conditions that put them at higher risk for severe complications from influenza.

The following persons should not be vaccinated:

- Trivalent inactivated influenza vaccine (TIV) should not be administered to persons known to have anaphylactic hypersensitivity to eggs or to other components of the influenza vaccine. Prophylactic use of antiviral agents is an option for preventing influenza among such persons. Information regarding vaccine components is located in package inserts from each manufacturer. Persons with moderate to severe acute febrile illness usually should not be vaccinated until their symptoms have abated. However, minor illnesses with or without fever do not contraindicate use of influenza vaccine. GBS within 6 weeks following a previous dose of TIV is considered to be a precaution for use of TIV.

Live, attenuated influenza vaccine (LAIV) is not currently licensed for use in the following groups, and these persons should not be vaccinated with LAIV:

- Persons with a history of hypersensitivity, including anaphylaxis, to any of the components of LAIV or to eggs
- Persons <5 years of age or those ≥50 years of age
- Persons with any of the underlying medical conditions that serve as an indication for routine influenza vaccination, including asthma, reactive airways disease, or other chronic disorders of the pulmonary or cardiovascular systems
- Other underlying medical conditions, including such metabolic diseases as diabetes, renal dysfunction, and hemoglobinopathies, or known or suspected immunodeficiency diseases or immunosuppressed states
- Children or adolescents receiving aspirin or other salicylates (because of the association of Reye syndrome with wild-type influenza virus infection)
- Persons with a history of Guillain-Barré syndrome
- Pregnant women.

Timing of Vaccination

In general, health care providers should begin offering vaccination soon after vaccine becomes available and if possible by October. To avoid missed opportunities for vaccination, providers should offer vaccination during routine health care visits or during hospitalizations whenever vaccine is available. Vaccination efforts should continue throughout the season, because the duration of the influenza season varies, and influenza might not appear in certain communities until February or March. Providers should offer influenza vaccine routinely, and organized vaccination campaigns should continue throughout the influenza season, including after influenza activity has begun in the community. Vaccine administered in December or later, even if influenza activity has already begun, is likely to be beneficial in the majority of influenza seasons. The majority of adults have antibody protection against influenza virus infection within 2 weeks after vaccination.

Children 6 months to 8 years of age who have not been vaccinated previously or who were vaccinated for the first time during the previous season and received only one dose should receive two doses of vaccine. These children should receive their first dose as soon after vaccine becomes available as is feasible, so both doses can be administered before the onset of influenza activity.

The most common adverse effects of vaccination include local reactions that are typically mild, fever, malaise, myalgia, headache, allergic reaction (in particular in those with an allergy to eggs), and thimerosal-related reactions (usually local, delayed type hypersensitivity reactions).

Chemoprophylaxis

Chemoprophylactic drugs are not a substitute for vaccination, although they are critical adjuncts in the prevention and control of influenza. Both amantadine and rimantadine are indicated for the chemoprophylaxis of influenza A infection but not influenza B. However, as mentioned previously, neither agent should be used for the prevention of influenza. Both drugs are approximately 70% to 90% effective in preventing illness from influenza A infection.[93–95] When used as prophylaxis, these antiviral agents can prevent illness while permitting subclinical infection and development of protective antibody against circulating influenza viruses. Therefore, certain persons who take these drugs will develop protective immune responses to circulating influenza viruses. Amantadine and rimantadine do not interfere with the antibody response to the vaccine.[94] Both drugs have been studied extensively among nursing home populations as a component of influenza outbreak-control programs, which can limit the spread of influenza within chronic care institutions.[94,96–99]

Among the neuraminidase inhibitor antivirals zanamivir and oseltamivir, only oseltamivir has been approved for prophylaxis, but community studies of healthy adults indicate that both drugs are similarly effective in preventing febrile, laboratory-confirmed influenza illness (efficacy: zanamivir, 84%; oseltamivir, 82%).[100–102] Both antiviral agents have also been reported to prevent influenza illness among persons administered chemoprophylaxis after a household member was diagnosed with influenza.[103–105] Experience with prophylactic use of these agents in institutional settings or among patients with chronic medical conditions is limited in comparison with the adamantanes.[106–111] One 6-week study of oseltamivir prophylaxis among nursing home residents reported a 92% reduction in influenza illness.[106,112,113] Use of zanamivir has not been reported to impair the immunologic response to influenza vaccine.[103,114] Data are not available regarding the efficacy of any of the four antiviral agents in preventing influenza among severely immunocompromised persons.

CONTROL OF INFLUENZA OUTBREAKS IN INSTITUTIONS

Chemoprophylactic drugs are not a substitute for vaccination, although they are critical adjuncts in preventing and controlling influenza. In community studies of healthy adults, both oseltamivir and zanamivir had similar efficacy in preventing febrile, laboratory-confirmed influenza illness (efficacy: zanamivir, 84%; oseltamivir, 82%). Both antiviral agents also have prevented influenza illness among persons administered chemoprophylaxis after a household member had influenza diagnosed (efficacy: zanamivir, 72%–82%; oseltamivir, 68%–89%). Experience with prophylactic use of these agents in institutional settings or among patients with chronic medical conditions is limited in comparison with the adamantanes, but the majority of published studies have demonstrated moderate to excellent efficacy. For example, a 6-week study of oseltamivir chemoprophylaxis among nursing home residents demonstrated a 92% reduction in influenza illness. The efficacy of antiviral agents in preventing influenza among severely immunocompromised persons is unknown. A small nonrandomized study conducted in a stem cell transplant unit suggested that oseltamivir can prevent progression to pneumonia among influenza-infected patients.

When determining the timing and duration for administering influenza antiviral medications for chemoprophylaxis, factors related to cost, compliance, and potential adverse events should be considered. To be maximally effective as chemoprophylaxis, the drug must be taken each day for the duration of influenza activity in the community. Currently, oseltamivir is the recommended antiviral drug for chemoprophylaxis of influenza. More details regarding the use of chemoprophylaxis for influenza can be found at www.cdc.gov/flu.

Streptococcus Pneumoniae

S. pneumoniae is the most common bacterial pathogen associated with CAP. Severe infections can result from the dissemination of this organism to the bloodstream and the central nervous system. Pneumococcal infections cause an estimated 40,000 deaths annually in the United States. The currently available pneumococcal vaccine includes 23 purified capsular polysaccharide antigens from serotypes 1–5, 6B, 7F, 8, 9N, 9V, 10A, 11A, 12F, 14, 15B, 17F, 18C, 19A, 19F, 20, 22F, 23F, and 33F. After vaccination, an antigen-specific antibody response develops within 2 to 3 weeks in ≥80% of healthy adults.[115] The levels of antibody to most antigens remains elevated for at least 5 years in healthy adults and decreases to prevaccination levels by 10 years.[116,117]

Pneumococcal vaccine has not been shown to be effective against nonbacteremic pneumococcal disease. Effectiveness against invasive disease is 56% to 81%.[118–121] Pneumococcal polysaccharide vaccine is cost-effective and potentially cost-saving among persons ≥65 years of age for prevention of bacteremia.[122]

The vaccine is both cost-effective and protective against invasive pneumococcal infection when administered to immunocompetent persons ≥2 years of age.[123] Therefore, all persons in the following categories should receive the 23-valent pneumococcal polysaccharide vaccine: patients ≥65 years of age, patients 2 to 64 years of age with chronic illness, patients 2 to 64 years of age with functional or anatomic asplenia, patients 2 to 64 years of age living in special environments or social settings, and immunocompromised patients. If vaccination status is unknown, patients in these categories should be administered pneumococcal vaccine. Children <2 years of age can be administered a conjugated version of the pneumococcal vaccine. The effectiveness and indications are discussed in Chapter 96.

Pneumococcal polysaccharide vaccine generally is considered safe based on clinical experience since 1977, when the pneumococcal polysaccharide vaccine was licensed in the United States. Approximately half of patients who receive pneumococcal vaccine develop mild, local side effects (e.g., pain at the injection site, erythema, and swelling).[124,125] These reactions usually persist <48 hours. Moderate systemic reactions (e.g., fever and myalgias) and more severe local reactions (e.g., local induration) are rare. Intradermal administration may cause severe local reactions and is inappropriate. Severe systemic adverse effects (e.g., anaphylactic reactions) rarely have been reported after administration of pneumococcal vaccine.

Routine revaccination of immunocompetent persons previously vaccinated with 23-valent polysaccharide vaccine is not recommended.[123] However, revaccination is recommended for persons ≥2 years of age who are at highest risk for serious pneumococcal infection and those who are likely to have a rapid decline in pneumococcal antibody levels, provided that 5 years have elapsed since receipt of the first dose of pneumococcal vaccine. Revaccination 3 years after the previous dose may be considered for children at highest risk for severe pneumococcal infection (≤10 years of age at the time of revaccination). These children include those with functional or anatomic asplenia (e.g., sickle cell disease or splenectomy) and those with conditions associated with rapid antibody decline after initial vaccination (e.g., nephrotic syndrome, renal failure, or renal transplantation). Revaccination is contraindicated for persons who had a severe reaction (e.g., anaphylactic reaction or localized arthus-type reaction) to the initial dose.

Chemoprophylaxis

Oral penicillin V (125 mg, twice daily), when administered to infants and young children with sickle cell disease, has reduced the incidence of pneumococcal bacteremia by 84% compared with those receiving placebo.[126] Therefore, daily penicillin prophylaxis for children with sickle cell hemoglobinopathy is recommended before 4 months of age. Consensus on the age at which prophylaxis should be discontinued has not been achieved. However, children with sickle cell anemia who had received prophylactic penicillin for prolonged intervals (but without a prior severe pneumococcal infection or splenectomy) have discontinued penicillin therapy at 5 years of age with no increase in the incidence of pneumococcal bacteremia or meningitis.[104]

Oral penicillin G or V is recommended for prevention of pneumococcal disease in children with functional or anatomic asplenia.[105] Antimicrobial prophylaxis against pneumococcal infection may be particularly useful for asplenic children not likely to respond to the polysaccharide vaccine (e.g., those <2 years of age or those receiving intensive chemotherapy or cytoreduction therapy). However, the impact of this practice on the emergence of DRSP is not known.

The effectiveness of all vaccines depends on administration in those patients at highest risk. Data released from the National Health Interview Survey has shown that for influenza vaccine, persons 50 to 64 years of age were vaccinated 34% of the time and those 65 years and older were vaccinated 65.6% of the time in 2002. For pneumococcal vaccine, those ≥65 years of age were vaccinated 55.7% of the time in 2002.[127] The role of pharmacists in identifying those patients who should be offered vaccination and potentially administering these vaccines may improve in increased rates of vaccination.

Aspiration Pneumonia

Predisposing Factors

14. R.G., a 38-year-old man, was brought to the emergency department (ED) after he was found unconscious, lying on his right side, near a pool of vomitus in a local municipal park. R.G. has a long history of binge drinking and has been admitted to the ED frequently for problems related to his alcoholism. On admission, R.G.'s vital signs were BP, 100/60 mmHg; pulse, 110 beats/minute; respirations, 32 breaths/minute; and temperature, 38.0°C. A strong odor of alcohol and vomitus was noted. R.G.'s overall mental status is depressed; he has intermittent periods of disorientation and uncoordinated motor movements.

Crackling rales were heard in the middle and lower right lung fields; the left fields were clear. An ABG was drawn on room air, with the following results: pH, 7.46 (normal, 7.38–7.45); Po_2, 52 mmHg (normal, 68–100 mmHg); Pco_2, 35 mmHg (normal, 38–45 mmHg); and HCO_3, 24 mEq/L (normal, 22–26 mEq/L). Laboratory data include the following: WBC count, 12,000 cells/mm^3 (normal, 5–10,000 cells/mm^3); differential PMNs, 68% (normal, 45%–79%); bands, 8% (normal, 0%–5%); and lymphocytes, 24% (normal, 16%–47%). During a period of consciousness, the physician obtained a sputum specimen from R.G. for Gram stain and culture. A chest radiograph revealed density changes consistent with interstitial infiltrates in the dependent segments of the middle and lower right lung. A tentative diagnosis of aspiration pneumonitis is made. What factors predispose R.G. to aspiration pneumonitis? How can the aspirated material cause pneumonitis?

[SI units: Po_2, 6.93 kPa; Pco_2, 4.67 kPa; WBC count, 12 10^8/L, with PMNs, 0.68; bands, 0.08; and lymphocytes, 0.24]

Several factors in R.G.'s history make him susceptible to aspiration. Alcohol intoxication has depressed his mental status as well as his cough and gag reflex, which may have led to aspiration of his vomitus. Table 60-14 lists conditions that predispose individuals to aspiration. Those conditions that cause or contribute to an altered state of consciousness are particularly important. The specific effect of the aspirated material on the lungs depends on the quantity and quality of the material aspirated. The latter can be categorized into three types: direct pulmonary toxin, particulate matter, and infected inoculum.[61,128]

Several toxic materials cause pneumonitis, the most common of which is gastric acid. When gastric acid enters the lungs, the sequence of events has been likened to a chemical burn. The aspirated secretions are neutralized rapidly over the first few minutes, and this is accompanied by a shift of fluid into the involved area of the lung. An estimated 96% of patients will demonstrate signs of respiratory compromise within 1 hour of aspiration and 100% within 2 hours. The two immediate

Table 60-14 Predisposing Conditions in Aspiration Pneumonia

Alterations of Consciousness
Alcoholism
Seizure disorders
General anesthesia
Cerebrovascular accident
Drug intoxication
Head injury
Severe illness with obtundation
Impaired swallowing mechanism
Neurologic disorders
Esophageal dysfunction
Nasogastric feeding
Tracheotomy
Endotracheal tube
Periodontal disease

Reprinted with permission from Klein RS, Steigbigel NH. Seminars in Infectious Disease. New York: Thieme Medical Publishers; 1983:5.

consequences of aspiration of gastric acid are rapid, profound hypoxia and shock secondary to massive fluid shifts into lung tissue. In addition, atelectasis, hemorrhage, and pulmonary edema may occur.[61] Approximately 45% of healthy adults aspirate oropharyngeal secretions during deep sleep, and 70% of patients with depressed consciousness aspirate pharyngeal secretions. Gastric juice has a pH ≤ 2.5 and contains few to no bacteria.[129,130] However, after the initial insult, some patients will develop a secondary bacterial pneumonia.[131] The infection is due primarily to aspiration of oropharyngeal contents in a setting of diminished host defenses caused by the chemical pneumonitis.[132] Other toxic materials causing aspiration pneumonitis include hydrocarbons, mineral oil, bile, alcohol, and animal fats.[128]

A second category of aspirated material is fluid containing various amounts of bacteria. Oropharyngeal secretions are the most frequent source of this material. Bacterial pneumonia results when the normal host lung defenses have been damaged or altered and when the bacteria inoculum exceeds the body's ability to contain and eliminate it. Infection due to aspirated bacteria may result in a pneumonia with little or no tissue destruction, necrotizing pneumonia, lung abscess, or empyema.

A third category of aspirated material consists of particulate matter. When relatively large particles are aspirated, sudden aphonia, cyanosis, and respiratory distress occur; the patient can progress rapidly toward death. Smaller particles reaching the lower airways cause local irritation with bronchospasm and infection if they are not removed. Many of these cases occur in young children following the ingestion of coins, peanuts, teeth, vegetables, or other small particles. Rapid removal of these particles usually results in the rapid reversal of symptoms without significant sequelae.

Clinical Course

15. What is the expected clinical course of aspiration pneumonia in R.G.?

The clinical course of a patient such as R.G. who has aspirated gastric contents and/or oropharyngeal secretions is variable; three courses have been identified. Shock will occur in 20% to 30% of patients with documented large volume aspiration[129,133]; respiratory function continues to deteriorate in many of these patients, and approximately 25% die. Mortality rates may be higher in severely ill patients.[134] Early clinical signs and symptoms of gastric aspiration include fever, tachypnea, rales, cough, cyanosis, wheezing, apnea, and shock. A second group of patients will resolve the pneumonitis completely over a few days to weeks without complication. A third group will develop bacterial pneumonia following an initial period of improvement.

Treatment

16. How should R.G. be treated?

R.G.'s initial treatment should primarily consist of supportive measures. Attention should be directed toward respiratory support and correction of his fluid and electrolyte status. In addition, any particulate matter present in the airways should be removed.

Pulmonary edema secondary to massive fluid shifts into the lung can contribute to a decrease in the intravascular volume. If this occurs, aggressive supportive therapy with ventilation, oxygen supplementation, and fluid replacement is indicated.

The use of corticosteroids to reduce inflammation in the setting of aspiration pneumonia is not warranted. There are no well-designed studies, and data supporting their use are anecdotal. In one published report, the use of steroids in the treatment of aspiration in humans was suggested to be harmful.[135] Although no difference was found in mortality, the incidence of Gram-negative pneumonia was more frequent in those patients receiving steroids. Because bacteria play little or no role in the initial events following aspiration, antibiotic therapy should be withheld until bacterial involvement is established.

Prophylactic antibiotics are not beneficial in this setting and may contribute to a change in the oropharyngeal flora that may, in turn, predispose the patient to pneumonia secondary to resistant bacterial organisms. On the other hand, if the patient has been hospitalized for >3 days at the time of aspiration, empiric antimicrobial therapy may be justified, particularly if the patient is elderly, debilitated, or believed to be deteriorating clinically.

Clinical Presentation

17. R.G.'s pulmonary symptoms improved during the next 3 days, but now he has a temperature of 38.5°C with an increase in sputum production. How should he be assessed?

Patients like R.G. with mild aspiration pneumonia usually resolve their respiratory difficulties within a few days following the insult. If an infection occurs, a short period of clinical improvement often takes place before signs and symptoms of bacterial pneumonia present. Criteria used to identify bacterial pneumonia following aspiration include (a) a new fever or a significant rise in temperature from the patient's baseline, (b) a new or extending pulmonary infiltrate after the initial 36- to 48-hour period, (c) an increase in WBCs or a change in the differential WBC count, (d) a change in sputum characteristics with purulence, and (e) the presence of pathogenic bacteria in a transtracheal aspirate.

Microbiology

18. What bacterial organisms are likely to be responsible for R.G.'s infectious pneumonia?

In the setting of aspiration pneumonitis, the bacterial pathogen is difficult to predict because large numbers of potential bacterial pathogens are present in sputum.

Most cases of aspiration pneumonia are caused by a wide spectrum of Gram-positive and Gram-negative anaerobic and aerobic bacteria representing the complex microbial flora of the oropharynx and upper GI tract. When culture technique is utilized, in approximately 50% of cases, aerobic bacteria have been recovered, and in 60% to 90% of cases, anaerobes have been recovered.[57,135] Tables 60-15 and 60-16 list the most common bacteria recovered from patients with aspiration pneumonia. In particular, anaerobes are commonly isolated in patients with a history of alcohol or illicit drug use or other risk factors that impair the gag reflex. In individuals without these risk factors, the most likely pathogens in community-acquired aspiration pneumonia are including *S. pneumoniae*, *S. aureus*, *H. influenzae*, and Enterobacteriaceae. In contrast, a larger percentage of hospital-acquired

Table 60-15 Bacteriology of Aspiration Pneumonia

Community-Acquired Pneumonia
Streptococcus pneumoniae
Peptococcus sp.
Peptostreptococcus sp.
Microaerophilic streptococci
Fusobacterium sp.
Bacteroides melaninogenicus
Bacteroides sp.
Streptococcus sp.
Special Patients (Alcoholics, Diabetics [Nursing Home Residents])
Staphylococcus aureus
Klebsiella pneumoniae
Escherichia coli
Anaerobes included above
Hospital-Acquired Pneumonia
Pseudomonas aeruginosa
S. aureus
S. pneumoniae
Anaerobes included above
E. coli
Enterobacter cloacae
Serratia marcescens
Other Gram-negative bacilli

aspiration pneumonias are caused by aerobic bacteria; they also are usually polymicrobial in nature. The aerobic bacteria recovered from patients with hospital-acquired aspiration pneumonia include *S. aureus*, various Enterobacteriaceae, and *Pseudomonas aeruginosa*. Understanding the differences in the bacterial etiology in these two settings facilitates the selection of antimicrobial therapy. The bacterial etiology of aspiration pneumonia in children is similar to that of adults.[72,137]

When a patient develops aspiration pneumonia in the community setting, mouth anaerobes and Gram-positive aerobic bacteria such as group A streptococcus and *S. pneumoniae* are the most common pathogens. However, some patients with community-acquired aspiration pneumonia are more likely to be infected with *S. aureus* or Gram-negative pathogens because of oropharyngeal colonization. These individuals include alcoholics (as in the case of R.G.), elderly patients housed in long-term care nursing facilities,[63] patients receiving enteral feedings,[138] and patients treated chronically with antacids, proton pump inhibitors, and/or H_2-receptor antagonists. In the latter individuals, Gram-negative flora are recovered from the

Table 60-16 Etiology of Aspiration-Associated Lung Infections

	Number of Patients	Anaerobes Only	Aerobes Only	Mixed
Community acquired	54	32 (59%)	5 (10%)	17 (31%)
Hospital acquired	47	8 (18%)	17 (36%)	22 (47%)

Adapted from references 65 and 159.

stomach because they are better able to survive in a more alkaline pH.[129,139,140] In addition, the oropharynx of these individuals frequently is colonized with the same bacteria found in the gastric flora.[141] Up to 60% of patients colonized with a given Gram-negative pathogen ultimately develop pneumonia due to the same organism. Information suggests that the use of sucralfate reduces bacterial colonization of the stomach of critically ill patients while maintaining adequate stress ulcer prophylaxis and reduced frequency of nosocomial pneumonia.[142,143]

Treatment

ANTIMICROBIAL THERAPY

19. How should antibiotics be used in aspiration pneumonia? How should R.G. be treated?

Antibiotic therapy should be selected on the basis of several criteria: the clinical setting in which the aspiration occurred, knowledge of the patient's medical history, the Gram stain of a reliably obtained sputum, and aerobic and anaerobic culture results of lower respiratory tract secretions. Table 60-17 lists common antibiotics and dosages used to treat aspiration pneumonia.

As noted previously, anaerobes are often the sole or dominant bacteria involved in patients with community-acquired aspiration pneumonia. Preferred therapy for this type of pneumonia is clindamycin. Metronidazole has also been used to treat anaerobic pleuropulmonary infections,[144,145] but the results have been mixed due, in part, to the severity of infections treated (e.g., lung abscess). Metronidazole effectively inhibits Gram-negative obligate anaerobic bacteria, such as *Bacterioides fragilis* and other *Prevotella* sp., but fails to effectively inhibit facultative anaerobic bacteria, such as *Peptococcus* sp. and *Peptostreptococcus* sp.[146] Other agents that can be used intravenously (IV) include a β-lactamase–inhibitor combination or the combination of metronidazole plus penicillin.

Treatment of aspiration pneumonia in the elderly, in patients from extended-care facilities, in patients with extensive medical histories, and in alcoholics (as in the case of R.G.) should include agents with activity against Gram-negative rods. Appropriate therapy choices might be a β-lactamase–inhibitor combination or a fluoroquinolone plus clindamycin.

Due to colonization with more resistant organisms, aspiration pneumonia in the hospital setting should be treated with a regimen active against both Gram-negative pathogens and anaerobes. *P. aeruginosa* should be considered as a possible pathogen in high-risk units (e.g., ICU) or in those patients at high risk (i.e., neutropenic patients or moderate to severe thermal injury patients). Effective regimens include a β-lactamase–inhibitor combination (piperacillin/tazobactam [Zosyn] and ticarcillin/clavulanate [Timentin]), ciprofloxacin, aztreonam or an antipseudomonal cephalosporin plus clindamycin or metronidazole, or a carbapenem. An empiric regimen should be modified when the results of the sputum culture are known. The addition of vancomycin to cover methicillin-resistant *Staphylococcus aureus* (MRSA) should be guided by local epidemiologic data, sputum Gram stain, and culture and sensitivity results. In patients with effusion or an empyema, drainage of the collection will likely be required to achieve a clinical cure.

Parenteral antibiotics should be continued until the patient has responded clinically to the therapy as outlined previously

Table 60-17 Suggested Antimicrobial Dosages for Treatment of Aspiration Pneumonia[a]

Drug	Adult Dose	Adult Interval (hour)	Pediatric[b] Total Daily Dose (mg/kg/24 hr)	Pediatric[b] Interval (hr)
Penicillins				
Ampicillin	1–2 g	Q 4–6	100–200	Q 4–6
Nafcillin	1–2 g	Q 4–6	100–200	Q 4–6
Penicillin (procaine) (IM)	0.6–1.2 million units	Q 12	50,000 units	Q 12
Penicillin G (for anaerobic infection)	1–2 million units	Q 4–6	50,000–100,000 units	Q 4–6
Ticarcillin	2–3 g	Q 4–6	200–300	Q 4–6
Other Antibacterials				
Aztreonam	1–2 g	Q 8–12	50–100	Q 6–8
Chloramphenicol	250–500 mg	Q 6–8	50–100	Q 6–8
Ciprofloxacin	400 mg	Q 12		
Clindamycin	600–900 mg	Q 6–8	25–40	Q 6–8
Doxycycline	100 mg	Q 12		
Erythromycin	250–500 mg	Q 6	40	Q 6
Imipenem	0.5–1 g	Q 6–8	60	Q 6
Metronidazole	500 mg	Q 8	25–60	Q 8–12
TMP-SMX[c]	10 mg/kg	Q 12	10 mg	Q 12
Vancomycin	500–1,000 mg	Q 6–12	40	Q 6–12
Cephalosporins				
Cefamandole	1–2 g	Q 4–6		
Cefazolin	1–2 g	Q 8	50–100	Q 8
Cefotaxime	1–2 g	Q 6–8	50–100	Q 6–8
Cefotetan	1–2 g	Q 8–12		
Cefoxitin	1–2 g	Q 4–6	50–100	Q 4–6
Ceftazidime	1–2 g	Q 8–12	50–100	Q 8–12
Ceftizoxime	1–2 g	Q 8–12	50–100	Q 8–12
Ceftriaxone	1–2 g	Q 12–24	50–75	Q 12–24
Cefuroxime	0.75–1.50 g	Q 6–8	50–100	Q 6–8
Aminoglycosides				
Amikacin	5.0–7.5 mg/kg	Q 8–12	15–30	Q 8–12
Gentamicin	1.7 mg/kg	Q 8	6.0–7.5	Q 8
Tobramycin	1.7 mg/kg	Q 8	6.0–7.5	Q 8

IM, intramuscularly; TMP-SMX, trimethoprim-sulfamethoxazole.
[a] Intravenous doses administered over 30 to 60 minutes; in patients with normal clearance.
[b] Infants and children older than 1 month.
[c] TMP-SMX dosed at 10 mg/kg of TMP.

(Table 60-11). While most patients require 7 days of therapy, patients with lung abscesses, particularly with inadequate drainage, may require weeks of therapy. Oral combination options in treating aspiration pneumonia include amoxicillin/clavulanate or clindamycin or metronidazole plus a fluoroquinolone.

Hospital-Acquired Pneumonia, Health Care-Associated Pneumonia, and Ventilator-Associated Pneumonia

20. A.A., a 68-year-old man, is admitted to the hospital from an extended-care nursing facility because of an acute change in mental status, fever, dyspnea with respiratory difficulty, cough, and sputum production. His medical history is notable for insulin-dependent diabetes mellitus since the age of 10 years, a right-sided cerebrovascular accident that left him with residual weakness, and a recent *Escherichia coli* urinary tract infection that was treated with oral TMP-SMX DS for 10 days. Because of poor nutrition, A.A. has been receiving nutritional supplements through a flexible nasogastric feeding tube for the past 2 months.

Physical examination reveals a restless, elderly man with the following vital signs: BP, 147/87 mmHg; pulse, 110 beats/minute; respirations, 28 breaths/minute; and temperature, 39°C. His head is without obvious trauma, and his neck is supple. Crackling rales with diminished breath sounds are noted in the middle and upper right lung fields. The chest radiograph shows a pulmonary infiltrate involving the right middle and upper lobes of the right lung with lobar consolidation. Because A.A. is relatively uncooperative and cannot give a good sputum specimen, a specimen of lower respiratory tract secretions was collected by transtracheal aspiration. This specimen was sent to the laboratory for Gram stain and culture.

The Gram stain showed Gram-negative rods with 4% neutrophils. ABGs included a Pao_2 of 34 mmHg on room air (normal, 80–100 mmHg); his current Pao_2 is 52 mmHg and 80 to 100 mmHg with 4 L/minute of supplemental oxygen. Other laboratory values include the following: Hct, 39% (normal, 37%–47%); WBC count, 16,000 cells/mm^3 (normal, 5–10,000 cells/mm^3); PMNs, 88% (normal, 45%–79%); bands, 10% (normal, 0%–5%); lymphocytes, 2% (normal, 16%–47%); BUN, 12 mg/dL (normal, 7–20 mg/dL); and creatinine, 1.0 mg/dL (normal, 0.8–1.2 mg/dL).

21. Medications on admission include oral famotidine 20 mg every day (QD). A tentative diagnosis of a hospital-acquired Gram-negative pneumonia is made. A.A. is intubated and placed on a ventilator. In addition, intravenous fluids are started to maintain a urine output of 50 mL/hour. What are the risk factors for pneumonia in A.A.?

[SI units: Pao_2, 4.53 and 6.93 kPa, respectively; Hct, 0.39; WBC count, 16–10^8/L; PMNs, 0.88; bands, 0.1; lymphocytes, 0.02; BUN, 4.28 mmol/L of urea (normal, 2.50–7.14); creatinine 88.4 μmol/L (normal, 70.72–106.08)]

Background

Hospital-acquired pneumonia (HAP), ventilator-associated pneumonia (VAP), and health care-associated pneumonia (HCAP) are important causes of morbidity and mortality despite advances in antimicrobial therapy, better supportive care, and the use of a wide range of preventive measures. HAP is defined as pneumonia that occurs ≥48 hours after admission that was not incubating at the time of admission. VAP refers to pneumonia that arises 48 to 72 hours after endotracheal intubation. HCAP includes any patient who has been hospitalized in an acute care hospital for 2 or more days within 90 days of infection; resided in a nursing home or long-term care facility; received recent intravenous antibiotic therapy, chemotherapy, or wound care within the past 30 days of the current infection; or attended a hospital or hemodialysis clinic.[147]

HAP is the second most common nosocomial infection in the United States. It has been reported to extend hospital stays on average by 7 to 9 days with an associated excess cost >$40,000 per patient. HAP accounts for 25% of all ICU infections and >50% of the antibiotics prescribed. VAP occurs in 9% to 27% of intubated patients, with the highest risk during the first 5 to 10 days of ventilation. The attributable mortality of HAP has been estimated to be 33% to 50%, with the highest mortality rates associated with infection caused by *P. aeruginosa* and *Acinetobacter* sp. and the use of ineffective anti-infective therapy.

Risk Factors

The time of onset of pneumonia is an important epidemiologic variable and risk factor for specific pathogens and outcomes in patients with HAP, VAP, and HCAP. Early-onset HAP and VAP are defined as occurring within the first 4 days of hospitalization, usually carry a better prognosis, and are more likely caused by antibiotic-sensitive bacteria. Late-onset HAP and VAP (those cases occurring ≥5 days of hospitalization) are more likely to be caused by multidrug-resistant (MDR) pathogens and are associated with increased morbidity and mortality.

Several risk factors for HAP have been identified, including intubation and mechanical ventilation, aspiration, a patient's body position, the administration of enteral feeding, prior use of antibacterial agents, bleeding prophylaxis (i.e., histamine type 2 antagonists and proton pump inhibitors), and poor glucose control. Each of the risk factors is potentially modifiable and should be considered as part of the broad management strategy for HAP.

Table 60-18 Risks for Nosocomial Pneumonia

Intubation or tracheostomy
Age >70 years
Chronic lung disease
Poor nutrition status
Depressed consciousness
Thoracic or abdominal surgery
Immunosuppressive therapy

Although A.A. is just now being admitted to the hospital, his diagnosis should be considered HCAP because he resides in a nursing home. Patients residing in nursing homes have an increased incidence of nosocomial pneumonias and oropharyngeal colonization with Gram-negative bacteria. In addition, poor infection control practices contribute to the cross- contamination of patients with pathogenic bacteria.[148] Nursing homes generally have flora similar to a hospital, as reflected by his Gram stain, which is consistent with a Gram-negative pneumonia. Other risk factors associated with developing HAP are listed in Table 60-18. The most significant risk factor is intubation, which increases the risk by 7- to 21-fold. In addition, other risk factors include the use of famotidine, recent antibacterial exposure, and the use of enteral feeding.

An important contributing factor in the cause of a pneumonia is colonization of the oropharynx. Several factors may contribute to the colonization of A.A.'s oropharynx with Gram-negative bacteria.[149] He is disabled because of a cerebrovascular accident, which has left him with right-sided weakness; this chronic condition also may predispose him to changes in oropharyngeal flora. A.A. is prone to aspiration of these secretions because the residual effects of the stroke and nasogastric tube used for nutritional support have decreased his airway protection. Finally, an altered immune response in diabetics and the elderly can further contribute to the establishment of a respiratory infection in A.A. (Table 60-19). The use of drugs that inhibit the production of gastric acid, such as famotidine, increases the possibility of oropharyngeal colonization.[140,141] Finally, the use of broad-spectrum antibiotics may inhibit the

Table 60-19 Conditions Associated With Gram-Negative Colonization

Prolonged hospitalization
Alcoholism
Antibiotic exposure
Diabetes
Advanced age
Coma
Pulmonary disease
Intubation
Azotemia
Major surgery
Neutropenia

Table 60-20 Microbiology of Nosocomial Pneumonia

Pathogen	*Cases (%)*
Gram-Negative Bacilli	50–70
Pseudomonas aeruginosa	
Acinetobacter sp.	
Enterobacter sp.	
Staphylococcus aureus	15–30
Anaerobic bacteria	10–30
Haemophilus influenzae	10–20
Streptococcus pneumoniae	10–20
Legionella	4
Viral	10–20
Cytomegalovirus	
Influenza	
Respiratory syncytial virus	
Fungi	
Aspergillus	<1

growth of many normal flora, which allows Gram-negative bacteria and other multiple-resistant bacteria to colonize the oropharynx.[150–152]

Treatment

22. How does the bacteriology of HAP/HCAP/VAP differ from CAP?

The major difference in the bacteriology between CAP and HAP//HCAP/VAP is a shift to Gram-negative pathogens, MDR pathogens, and MRSA in HAP/HCAP/VAP. Gram-negative bacilli commonly colonize oropharyngeal secretions of patients with moderate to severe acute and chronic illnesses without exposure to broad-spectrum antibiotics.[60,61] Patients admitted to the hospital with acute illnesses are rapidly colonized with Gram-negative organisms. Approximately 20% are colonized on the first hospital day, and this number increases with the duration of hospitalization and severity of illness.[57] Approximately 35% to 45% of hospitalized patients[57] and up to 100% of critically ill patients[59] will be colonized within 3 to 5 days of admission.

Table 60-20 lists the most common bacteria associated with HAP/HCAP/VAP based on the presence of risk factors for MDR pathogens. Virtually all reports indicate that Gram-negative bacteria account for 50% to 70% of all cases.[147,153–157] The most common bacterium within this category is *P. aeruginosa.* In patients who are ventilator dependent, *Acinetobacter* sp. often is reported as the most common Gram-negative pathogen. *S. aureus*, which accounts for 10% to 20% of all cases of HAP, is the most commonly identified Gram-positive organism. Other organisms with special risk factors include Legionella, which is associated with high-dose corticosteroid use and outbreaks secondary to water supplies and cooling systems,[71,158] and Aspergillus, which is associated with neutropenia or organ transplantation.[159] Risk factors for MDR pathogens are listed in Table 60-21.

SELECTING ANTIBIOTIC THERAPY

23. How should antibiotic therapy be started in A.A.?

The IDSA/ATS have published guidelines for the treatment of HAP.[147] The four major principles underlying the management of HAP, HCAP, and VAP include (a) avoid untreated or inadequately treated HAP, VAP, or HCAP, as failure to initiate prompt, appropriate therapy is associated with increased mortality; the variability of bacteriology from one institution to another, as well as within specific sites in a hospital, can be significant; (b) avoid the overuse of antibiotics by focusing on accurate diagnosis; (c) tailor therapy based on lower respiratory tract cultures and shorten the duration of therapy; and (d) apply prevention strategies directed at modifiable risk factors. The likelihood of an infection with a potential pathogen is based largely on the time to onset of HAP (early, <5 days into hospitalization, vs. late, >5 days), severity of the condition, and underlying risk factors. These guidelines are outlined in Figure 60-4 and Tables 60-22 through 60-24.[147] In general, patients with early-onset disease who are not severely ill and have no risk factors can be treated with a single agent, including nonantipseudomonal third-generation cephalosporins or carbapenems, β-lactam–inhibitor combinations, or an antipneumococcal fluoroquinolone. Empiric therapy in those with late-onset or severe disease should include a combination of antibiotics active against *Pseudomonas.* This regimen usually includes an antipseudomonal β-lactam, such as cefepime,

Table 60-21 Risk Factors for Multi-Drug Resistant Pathogens

- Antimicrobial therapy in preceding 90 days
- Current hospitalization of 5 days or more
- High frequency of antibiotic resistance in the community or in the specific hospital unit
- Presence of risk factors for HCAP:
  - Hospitalization for 2 days or more in the preceding 90 days
  - Residence in a nursing home or extended care facility
  - Home infusion therapy (including antibiotics)
  - Chronic dialysis within 30 days
  - Home wound care
  - Family member with multidrug-resistant pathogen
- Immunosuppressive disease and/or therapy

HCAP, health care–associated pneumonia.

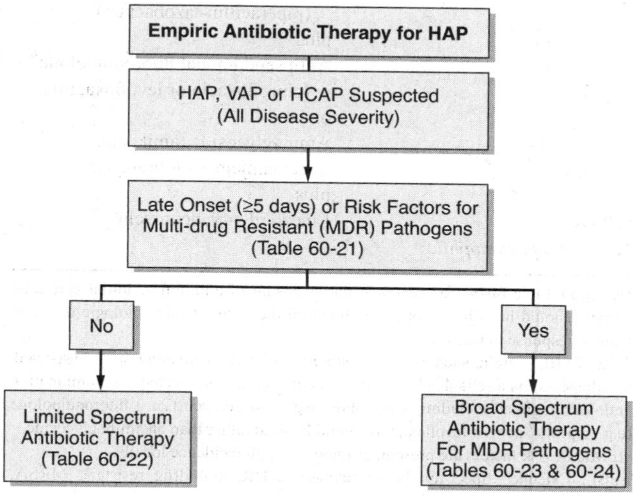

FIGURE 60-4 Approach to empiric antibiotic therapy in patients with healthcare-acquired pneumonia.

Table 60-22 Initial Empiric Antibiotic Therapy for Hospital-Acquired Pneumonia

Potential Pathogen	Recommended Antibiotic
Streptococcus pneumoniae[a]	Ceftriaxone
Haemophilus influenzae	or
Methicillin-sensitive Staphylococcus aureus	
Antibiotic-sensitive enteric Gram-negative bacilli	Levofloxacin, moxifloxacin, or ciprofloxacin
Escherichia coli	or
Klebsiella pneumoniae	
Enterobacter sp.	Ampicillin/sulbactam
Proteus sp.	or
Serratia marcescens	
	Ertapenem

[a] The frequency of penicillin-resistant *S. pneumoniae and* multidrug-resistant *S. pneumoniae is* increasing; levofloxacin or moxifloxacin are preferred to ciprofloxacin, and the role of other new quinolones, such as gatifloxacin, has not been established.

Table 60-23 Initial Empiric Therapy for Hospital-Acquired Pneumonia, Ventilator-Associated Pneumonia, and Health Care-Associated Pneumonia in Patients With Late-Onset Disease or Risk Factors for Multidrug-Resistant Pathogens and All Disease Severity

Potential Pathogens	Combination Antibiotic Therapy[a]
Pathogens listed in Table 60-20 and MDR pathogens	Antipseudomonal cephalosporin (cefepirne, ceftazidime)
Pseudomonas aeruginosa	or
Klebsiella pneumoniae (ESBL$^+$)[b]	Antipseudomonal carbepenem (imipenem or meropenem)
Acinetobacter sp.[b]	or
	β-Lactam/β-Lactamase inhibitor (piperacillin-tazobactam)
	plus
	Antipseudomonal fluoroquinolone[b] (ciprofloxacin or levofloxacin)
	or
	Aminoglycoside (amikacin, gentamicin, or tobramycin)
	plus
MRSA	Linezolid or vancomycin[c]
Legionella pneumophila[c]	

[a] Refer to Table 60-24 for adequate initial dosing of antibiotics. Initial antibiotic therapy should be adjusted or streamlined on the basis of microbiologic data and clinical response to therapy.
[b] If an ESBL$^+$ strain, such as *K. pneumoniae*, or an *Acinetobacter* sp. is suspected, a carbepenem is a reliable choice. If *L. pneumophila* is suspected, the combination antibiotic regimen including a macolide (e.g., azithromycin) or a fluoroquinolone (e.g., ciprofloxacin or levofloxacin) should be used rather than an aminoglycoside.
[c] If MRSA risk factors are present, or there is a high incidence locally.
ESBL, Extended Spectrum beta-lactamase; MDR, multidrug resistant; MRSA, methicillin-resistant *Staphylococcus aureus*.

Table 60-24 Initial Intravenous, Adult Doses of Antibiotics for Empiric Therapy of Hospital-Acquired Pneumonia, Including Ventilator-Associated Pneumonia, and Health Care-Associated Pneumonia, in Patients With Late-Onset Disease or Risk Factors for Multidrug-Resistant Pathogens

Antibiotic	Dosage[a]
Antipseudomonal cephalosporin	
Cefepime	1–2 g Q 8–12 hr
Ceftazidime	2 g Q 8 hr
Carbepenems	
Imipenem	500 mg Q 6 hr or 1 g Q 8 hr
Meropenem	1 g Q 8 hr
β-Lactam/β-Lactamase inhibitor	
Piperacillin-tazobactam	4.5 g Q 6 hr
Aminoglycosides	
Gentamicin	7 mg/kg per day†
Tobramycin	7 mg/kg per day†
Amikacin	20 mg/kg per day†
Antipseudomonal quinolones	
Levofloxacin	750 mg daily
Ciprofloxacin	400 mg Q 8 hr
Vancomycin	15 mg/kg Q 12 hr‡
Linezolid	600 mg Q 12 hr

[a] Dosages are based on normal renal and hepatic function.
† Trough levels for gentamicin and tobramycin should be <1 mcg/mL; for amikacin, they should be <4–5 mcg/mL.
‡ Trough levels for vancomycin should be 15–20 mcg/mL.

imipenem, or piperacillin-tazobactam, plus either an aminoglycoside or ciprofloxacin/levofloxacin. The addition of vancomycin or linezolid should be considered if the Gram stain demonstrates Gram-positive cocci in clusters.[147]

Because delays in the administration of appropriate therapy have been associated with increased hospital mortality from HAP, the prompt administration of empiric therapy is essential. Importantly, changing therapy once culture results are available may not reduce the excess risk of hospital mortality associated with inappropriate initial therapy. To this end, local bacteriologic patterns and in vitro susceptibility results should be made available and updated as frequently as possible. In addition to the selection of an appropriate agent, the selection of adequate dosing regimens is designed to optimize the pharmacodynamic properties of the antibacterial agent(s). The choice of empiric antibiotic therapy should be guided by the results of the Gram stain and an analysis of the patient's risk factors for oropharyngeal colonization or altered pulmonary host factors. When these risk factors are present, as in the case of A.A., coverage for infection due to Gram-negative bacteria is indicated.

Resolution of HAP can be defined both clinically and microbiologically. Clinical improvement usually begins to become apparent after the first 48 to 72 hours of therapy. During this time, the selected antibacterial regimen should not be changed unless progressive deterioration takes place or microbiologic studies confirm the pathogen. Serial quantitative cultures of the lower respiratory tract can also be used to identify microbiologic nonresponse and to modify antimicrobial therapy.

If culture results are negative or inconclusive (because of known specimen contamination with mouth flora), the patient's response to the initial antibiotic therapy should be used to evaluate modification of the antibiotic regimen. If the patient responds to the initial therapy, those antibiotics should be continued with consideration to narrow coverage to the most likely causative pathogens. If the patient is not responding to the initial antibiotic therapy, one should consider whether (a) the pathogen is not covered in the initial choice of antibiotic therapy, (b) the dose of antibiotic is insufficient, and (c) any other factors are responsible for the failure to respond to therapy. Such factors include poor pulmonary clearance of necrotic tissue and cellular debris, lung abscesses, and severely altered host defenses with a rapidly fatal underlying disease.

Of note, if one of the following organisms is isolated (*Serratia*, *Pseudomonas*, indole positive *Proteus*, *Citrobacter*, or *Enterobacter* sp.), in vitro reports indicating susceptibility should be questioned, as these organisms often possess an inducible β-lactamase gene (also referred to as a type I β-lactamase enzyme).[160] In vitro testing may demonstrate susceptibility to third-generation cephalosporins and extended-spectrum penicillins but may not translate to efficacy in the clinical setting. As a possible scenario, after initiation with one of these agents, the patient may initially respond; however, after approximately 1 week, the patient's condition will begin to worsen. Because treatment with the β-lactam agent induces the expression of the type I enzyme, a subsequent specimen sent after approximately 1 week is now likely to demonstrate resistance to the third-generation cephalosporins and extended-spectrum penicillins.[160] Although cefepime is more likely to be active against these isolates, a large inoculum of organisms (e.g., that present in pneumonia) can result in β-lactamase degradation of the cephalosporin.[161] Considering that this phenomenon will not be identified by using usual in vitro testing, cefepime should be used cautiously in these patients.[87] The preferred therapy in these patients includes TMP-SMX, a fluoroquinolone, or a carbapenem.[160] *Acinetobacter* sp. have become resistant to many commonly used antibacterial agents. Treatment of this sometimes multiply-resistant pathogen requires the use of very high doses of ampicillin-sulbactam (up to 24 g/day) or colistin.[162,163]

In summary, A.A. could be started empirically with cefepime or piperacillin-tazobactam, with the addition of gentamicin or ciprofloxacin. When culture results are known, the antibiotic regimen can be modified and individualized for the patient. Therapy is generally continued for 2 weeks, but in some patients, therapy can be shortened to as little as 7 days. A.A.'s clinical response should be monitored to determine whether the selected antibiotics are effective in treating this infection. These parameters include a decrease in temperature and heart rate as well as a decrease in the WBC count with resolution of the left shift. Mental status and sensorium are good monitoring parameters in older individuals.

BROAD-SPECTRUM β-LACTAMS

24. Can the broad-spectrum β-lactam antibiotics be used as monotherapy in the treatment of A.A.'s pneumonia?

In the past, the aminoglycosides were considered the antibiotics of choice in the treatment of nosocomial Gram-negative infections. However, the availability of a large number of relatively nontoxic antibiotics, including β-lactam antibiotics or high-dose ciprofloxacin/levofloxacin has diminished the role of aminoglycosides as the agents of choice for these infections. However, when choosing empiric therapy for a suspected or documented pneumonia caused by *Pseudomonas*, combination therapy is preferred.[147] The potential advantages of combination include an improved likelihood of covering MDR pathogens initially, improved bactericidal activity because of synergy between the agents, and suppression of resistance that may develop to one of the antibiotics.[164]

AMINOGLYCOSIDES

25. What pharmacokinetic and pharmacodynamic characteristics must be considered in the dosing of aminoglycosides in patients with HAP?

Individualization of aminoglycoside dosing is required in patients receiving these drugs.[165–167] The efficacy and toxicity of aminoglycosides correlates with aminoglycoside plasma concentrations and therapeutic outcome in patients with Gram-negative pneumonia.[168] In patients receiving multiple daily doses of gentamicin or tobramycin, achieving a 1-hour postinfusion peak plasma concentration >7 mcg/mL, a successful outcome occurs more often than in those with lower plasma concentrations.

The aminoglycosides are concentration-dependent killing antibiotics. Their rate and extent of killing organisms is maximized by increasing the peak serum concentration relative to the MIC of the pathogen. In addition to maximizing bactericidal activity, in vitro evidence has demonstrated that this concentration goal also minimizes the development of resistance. The use of once-daily dosing strategies to minimize nephrotoxicity of the aminoglycosides has been studied extensively. Single doses of gentamicin and tobramycin (5–7 mg/kg/day) and of amikacin (15–20 mg/kg/day) have been reported to be as effective as standard dosing of these agents in controlled clinical trials. However, none of the trials has enrolled a sufficient number of patients required to demonstrate a difference. There are several advantages of single-dose aminoglycoside therapy: (a) it is no more nephrotoxic than traditional dosing, (b) clinicians are ensured that a therapeutic peak serum level will be achieved with the first dose, (c) it is the only safe and effective way to achieve serum peak levels of 10 to 20 times the MIC for difficult-to-treat organisms such as *P. aeruginosa*, and (d) it is a more efficient dosing regimen (less doses and administration times per day; fewer serum level measurements are required).

Despite the use of individualized aminoglycoside dosing, morbidity and mortality rates due to Gram-negative pneumonia remain high. This is because the success of antibiotic therapy depends on the ability of the antibiotic to reach the site of infection and remain biologically active.[169] Concentrations of the aminoglycosides in bronchial secretions range from 1 to 5 mcg/mL (~30%–40% of serum concentrations) 2 to 4 hours after parenteral administration.[170] These concentrations may be insufficient to inhibit the growth of many Gram-negative organisms, especially *Pseudomonas*.

The bioactivity of the aminoglycosides is influenced by the local tissue pH. In contrast to the penicillins and cephalosporins, whose activities are little affected over a pH range of 6.0 to 8.0, a 2- to 16-fold increase in the aminoglycoside MIC of most Gram-negative bacteria occurs when the pH is decreased from 7.4 to 6.8.[171] The pH of endobronchial fluid in patients with normal lung physiology and pneumonia averages 6.6.

Lastly, aminoglycosides bind to purulent exudates and cellular debris, inactivating these agents.[172–174] In summary, the aminoglycosides penetrate poorly into bronchial secretions and are less active at the site of infection because of local pH effects and binding to cellular debris. These properties may result in the need for increased dosages, placing patients at increased risk for ototoxicity and nephrotoxicity.

BRONCHIAL PENETRATION OF ANTIBIOTICS

26. What factors govern the penetration of antibiotics into bronchial secretions? Is penetration into bronchial secretions critical to the effectiveness of an antibiotic used in the treatment of pneumonia?

An important factor to consider in the selection of an antibiotic used to treat pneumonia is its ability to reach the site of infection (i.e., the lung tissue or bronchopulmonary secretions). Antibiotic concentrations in bronchial secretions do not necessarily reflect the lung tissue concentrations but do represent the ability of the antibiotic to cross the bronchoalveolar barrier.[170]

Many anatomic, physicochemical, and host factors influence drug penetration into respiratory tissue and secretions.[170] Active transport mechanisms for drugs have not been identified in respiratory tissues; therefore, passive diffusion is responsible for the transfer of antibiotics into respiratory tissue. The degree of diffusion is determined by the ability of the antibiotic to reach high free concentrations in the serum. The transfer of an antibiotic into tissue may be slower than its elimination from the serum. Furthermore, elimination of the antibiotic from the tissue site occurs more slowly than from the serum; thus, serum concentrations may not reflect antimicrobial concentrations in lung tissue. The results of studies investigating the penetration of antibiotics into bronchial secretions should be interpreted cautiously because most of these studies have analyzed the amount of antibiotic present in samples of expectorated sputum or saliva, which may significantly underestimate the amount of antibiotic present in respiratory secretions. The use of fiberoptic bronchoscopy with a protected sampling device has been helpful in the study of antibiotic penetration into respiratory secretions, but this procedure is impractical in the routine management of patients with pneumonia. Although some have advocated the use of epithelial lining fluid (ELF) as a surrogate for an antibiotic's ability to be effective in treating patients with pneumonia, ELF may accurately reflect the site of action for antibiotics in the lung.

LOCALLY ADMINISTERED ANTIBIOTICS: PROPHYLAXIS

27. Can locally administered antibiotics be used to prevent Gram-negative pneumonias?

The morbidity and mortality rates from hospital-acquired Gram-negative pneumonia have not been reduced despite aggressive treatment with high-dose parenteral antibiotics. Lack of improved outcomes may be the result of poor antibiotic penetration into the bronchial secretions and the local conditions at the site of infection. Consequently, several investigators have studied the efficacy of endotracheal instillation or aerosolization of antibiotics to prevent Gram-negative pneumonias in patients at risk for oropharyngeal colonization.[175–179] Most patients treated have been seriously ill individuals who were admitted to the ICU unconscious and with tracheotomy to provide long-term ventilatory support. Endotracheal instillation and aerosolization of antibiotics significantly reduced oropharyngeal colonization with Gram-negative pathogens as well as the incidence of pneumonia. However, other investigators have observed the emergence of colonization with antibiotic-resistant Gram-negative organisms and pneumonia caused by these pathogens.[177–179] In summary, endotracheally instilled and aerosolized antibiotics can be used to prevent or reduce oropharyngeal colonization in high-risk patients when used for short periods with close microbiologic monitoring. Routine and long-term use cannot be recommended because of a lack of well-controlled clinical trials and the possible emergence of resistance.[180,181]

AEROSOLIZED ANTIBIOTICS

28. Can aerosolized antibiotics be used to treat patients with Gram-negative pneumonias?

The efficacy of locally administered antibiotics to treat bronchopneumonia has been studied to a limited extent.[180] Klastersky et al.[182] compared the effects of endotracheally instilled gentamicin with intramuscular gentamicin in patients with pneumonia. A favorable outcome occurred in all seven patients receiving endotracheally instilled gentamicin versus only two of eight patients receiving intramuscular gentamicin.

In a second study, these investigators compared the effects of endotracheally instilled sisomicin with placebo in a similar patient population.[183] All patients received systemic antibiotics consisting of parenteral sisomicin and carbenicillin. A more favorable outcome occurred in those patients receiving endotracheally instilled sisomicin versus those receiving a placebo (78% and 45%, respectively). In patients in whom the infecting organism was sensitive to both carbenicillin and sisomicin, a more favorable response occurred in those patients receiving endotracheal sisomicin versus placebo (79% and 54%, respectively). When the infecting organism was sensitive to sisomicin only, a favorable outcome occurred in 79% versus 28%, respectively. The development of resistant organisms was not a problem in either case.

In a third study, these same investigators compared the effects of parenteral mezlocillin and endotracheally administered sisomicin with and without parenteral sisomicin to determine the benefit of concomitant parenteral aminoglycoside.[184] The clinical outcome in both groups was similar; however, resistant bacteria were isolated from the sputum of the groups that were administered endotracheal sisomicin. These findings the need for further investigation into the use of aerosolized antibiotic therapy for HAP/VAP/HCAP.

Administration

29. How is local antibiotic therapy administered?

Local antibiotic therapy may be administered by direct endotracheal instillation or aerosolization. The antibiotic usually is diluted with normal saline before administration. In the case of direct instillation, gentamicin/tobramycin (40–80 mg) or amikacin (500 mg) is diluted in 5 to 10 mL of normal saline and instilled directly into the trachea through a catheter or through an endotracheal tube. The patient is then rotated from side to side to promote distribution. Delivery of the antibiotic into the oropharynx by aerosolization is accomplished by use of an atomizer or nebulizers to deliver the antibiotic to the lungs. The aerosolized route is preferred, and the dosage is 300 to 600 mg every 8 hours for gentamicin and tobramycin diluted in a smaller volume (1–3 mL).[180,181]

Bronchial and Serum Concentrations

30. What concentration of aminoglycoside can be achieved in bronchial secretions by this route of administration, and is any of the antibiotic absorbed?

The concentration of the aminoglycoside in bronchial secretions after parenteral administration (IV or intramuscularly) is low and usually <2 mcg/mL.[170] When the aminoglycosides are delivered by either endotracheal instillation or aerosolization, bronchial fluid antibiotic concentrations are substantially higher.[185–188] Bronchial fluid concentrations are significantly higher when the aminoglycosides are given by endotracheal instillation than by aerosol. These values usually exceed 200 mcg/mL and remain elevated for the dosing interval;[187] when aerosolization is used, bronchial fluid concentrations usually exceed 20 mcg/mL.[186,187]

Absorption of the aminoglycosides from the lung differs with the method of local administration used. Various doses of aminoglycosides have been administered, which makes quantification of the amount of the drug absorbed difficult. When 80 mg of gentamicin is administered by endotracheal instillation, serum concentrations >2.5 mcg/mL are achieved, suggesting that a substantial amount of the administered drug is absorbed.[177,185,186] Approximately 10% to 15% of the dose administered by endotracheal instillation is excreted into the urine.[189] When similar doses of antibiotic are administered by aerosolization, serum concentrations are low or undetectable; approximately 2% to 5% of the dose is excreted into the urine. For this reason, aerosolization is the preferred route of administration. As with parenteral aminoglycoside administration, patients with renal dysfunction should be monitored carefully for drug accumulation.

Adverse Effects

31. What adverse effects are associated with local antibiotic administration?

As noted previously, the emergence of antibiotic-resistant bacteria is of major concern because these may be responsible for subsequent bacterial infections. This phenomenon is more frequently associated with prophylactic aerosolized antibiotics.

Endotracheal instillation or aerosolization of antibiotics may cause cough; bronchial irritation; and in some individuals, bronchospasm. These effects most often have been associated with polymyxin B and have resulted in episodes of acute respiratory failure.[190,191] Polymyxin can stimulate the release of histamine, which is believed to be responsible for these adverse effects; it also can decrease ventilatory function.[190] The aminoglycosides have been relatively well tolerated, although minor alterations in ventilatory function have been reported.[192]

Studies evaluating the incidence of aminoglycoside nephrotoxicity and ototoxicity associated with local antibiotic administration are unavailable; however, the incidence should be low. Patients with renal dysfunction may accumulate this drug, and serum concentrations of the aminoglycoside should be monitored.

32. What preventive measures are effective for hospital-acquired or nosocomial pneumonia?

The substantial risk of pneumonia in the ICU has prompted aggressive methods to prevent this disease.[193,194] As noted previously, several modifiable risk factors have been identified for HAP/VAP/HACP. The most important recommendations include the use of the semiupright position to reduce the risk of aspiration[195] and infection control (including hand washing) to prevent the spread of pathogens from one patient to the next and surveillance for ICU infections. As mentioned in the discussion of aspiration pneumonia, the use of sucralfate in lieu of H_2-antagonists to prevent GI ulcers has been shown to reduce the frequency of nosocomial pneumonia and can be an alternative.[169] The use of "selective decontamination" to decrease the bacterial burden in the GI tract is not advocated. This practice has been extensively studied in >4,000 patients and has been shown to reduce the frequency of pneumonia in the ICU, but it has had no impact on mortality.[196,197] This fact, coupled with the costs of the antibiotic regimens and the potential for the emergence of resistance, makes it difficult to recommend this approach. Finally, as described earlier, the use of inhaled or aerosolized antibiotic therapy requires more data before it can be recommended.[180,181]

Pneumonia in Cystic Fibrosis

Special Treatment Considerations

33. K.P., an 18-year-old man with CF, has been well until 3 days ago when he noted "chest tightness" and a progressive deterioration of pulmonary function requiring supplemental oxygen. Other symptoms include an increased cough with sputum production, decreased appetite, and weight loss.

On physical examination, K.P. is a cachectic young male in moderate respiratory distress. Vital signs include the following: BP, 110/60 mmHg; pulse, 120 beats/minute; respirations, 35 breaths/minute; and temperature, 38.5°C. Examination of the chest reveals an increased chest diameter with diffuse bilateral rales; there are no wheezes. K.P.'s height is 64 inches, weight is 42 kg, and serum creatinine (SrCr) is 1.0 mg/dL. Are there special considerations in the treatment of pneumonia in patients with CF?

[SI unit: SrCr, 88.4 μmol/L]

CF is a genetically linked disease affecting exocrine gland secretions throughout the body (see Chapter 98).[198] Progressive pulmonary disease is the major determinant of the morbidity and mortality of patients with this illness. The presence of airway mucus plugging is likely to contribute to the development of significant respiratory dysfunction and the establishment of infection; recurrent respiratory infections play a major role in the pathogenesis of the chronic pulmonary disease seen in these patients. Symptoms associated with an infectious exacerbation include an increased frequency and duration of cough or increased shortness of breath, increased sputum production, change in the appearance of sputum, decreased exercise tolerance, decreased appetite, and a feeling of increased chest congestion.

MICROBIOLOGY

Early in the disease, *S. aureus* is an important pathogen; but later, colonization and infection with *P. aeruginosa* frequently develops. Multiple bacterial isolates with differing antimicrobial sensitivity patterns often are found.[199] In addition, infection due to *Burkholderia cepacia* is emerging as a significant problem in patients with CF.[200,201] The role of *B. cepacia* as a pathogen in CF patients is difficult to determine because many patients recover from acute infections despite the use of antimicrobials with little activity against this organism. Most strains demonstrate variable sensitivity patterns to many of the presently used antibiotics. Therefore, antibiotic therapy should be based on known in vitro sensitivity testing.

Vigorous chest percussion with postural drainage and systemic antibiotics have been the mainstay of therapy in the prevention and treatment of pulmonary infections in patients with CF. The objectives of antibiotic therapy in CF patients can be divided into three categories: (a) early disease where the goal is to delay chronic colonization with *P. aeruginosa*; (b) once colonization with *S. aureus* and *P. aeruginosa* has occurred, to delay the decline in pulmonary function and reduce frequency and morbidity of exacerbations; and (c) during periodic exacerbations to relieve symptoms and restore pulmonary function to baseline. It is unclear whether combination antibiotic therapy is required to treat these patients, but it frequently is used to treat Gram-negative pulmonary infections in CF patients. Combination therapy usually consists of an aminoglycoside or ciprofloxacin and an antipseudomonal β-lactam (piperacillin-tazobactam, cefepime, aztreonam, imipenem, or meropenem). Therapy generally is continued for 14 to 21 days.

DOSING CONSIDERATIONS

Altered drug elimination in CF patients has been reported for several drugs.[202–205] Jusko et al.[202] studied the pharmacokinetics of dicloxacillin in patients with CF and reported that the total body clearance and renal clearance of this drug were increased. In another study, when specific techniques to assess the glomerular infiltration rate were used, tobramycin renal clearance was not increased out of proportion to the glomerular filtration rate. These results suggest that alterations in the nonrenal clearance are responsible for the increased clearance of the aminoglycosides. The underlying reasons for these changes are unclear. In addition, changes in the pharmacokinetics of antibiotics are neither consistent nor predictable. Patients with CF may require higher dosages to achieve therapeutic plasma concentrations of some antibiotics.[181,205] Therefore, dosages must be carefully individualized, and serum levels (in the case of the aminoglycosides) should be monitored.

LOCAL ANTIBIOTIC ADMINISTRATION

34. Because such high doses of parenteral aminoglycosides are required in CF patients, can aerosolized aminoglycosides be used instead?

Aerosolized antibiotics have been advocated for CF patients with acute pulmonary infections[207–210] because several factors limit the use of IV administration. Because most antibiotics penetrate variably into lung tissue, they usually are administered in maximal doses to facilitate passive diffusion, which also increases the risk of systemic toxicity. In contrast, inhaled antibiotics deliver large concentrations of antibiotics to the site of infection while producing negligible serum concentrations, which should reduce the risk of systemic toxicity.

However, several potential problems are associated with aerosolized antibiotics. Prolonged administration selects out resistant organisms in the bronchial airways, and this may have deleterious consequences because of the recurrent nature of pulmonary infections in CF patients. To be effective, the antibiotic must be delivered to the alveoli. This requires particles $<2\ \mu m$ wide, but most commercially available nebulizers generate particles between 2.5 and 4.5 μm wide,[211] which are deposited primarily in the oropharynx and smaller airways. Also, studies using radioisotope-labeled aerosolized particles have shown that there is a heterogeneous pattern of deposition in CF patients,[212] which may limit the therapeutic effectiveness of this delivery route. Bronchospasm has occurred in patients given aerosolized gentamicin, which also may limit the delivery of antibiotic to the site of infection. Nephrotoxicity and ototoxicity are unlikely with this route of administration.

Stephens et al.[208] administered aerosolized tobramycin along with parenteral antibiotics and reported that the clinical outcomes of those receiving the combination of parenteral and aerosolized antibiotics did not differ from those receiving parenteral antibiotics alone. Steinkamp et al.[210] evaluated the clinical effectiveness of long-term, prophylactic tobramycin aerosol therapy in 14 CF patients. The best clinical outcomes occurred in individuals who were defined as moderately ill and had mild lung disease. Drug toxicity and the emergence of resistant organisms were minimal in the study population. Although aerosolized antibiotics have reportedly slowed the rate of pulmonary function decline in uncontrolled trials,[213] these positive results are difficult to differentiate from the natural course of CF, which is characterized by significant variability in the rate of lung function deterioration. Ramsey et al.[214] conducted a placebo-controlled, parallel-design, cross-over study of 71 patients with stable pulmonary status and *P. aeruginosa* detected in their sputum. Tobramycin 600 mg three times daily or placebo was delivered for 28 days by ultrasonic nebulizer. The dose was based on previous studies showing that sputum tobramycin concentrations >10 times the MIC for *P. aeruginosa* or a minimum sputum concentration of 400 mcg/mL were required to ensure bacterial killing. The results showed a small but significant improvement in pulmonary function in favor of the tobramycin group. They also showed a 100-fold reduction in the density of *P. aeruginosa* in sputum, a modest reduction in PMN count, a reduction in pulmonary exacerbations, and a lower rate of systemic antibiotic use. Similarly, Ramsey et al.[214] conducted two double-blind, placebo-controlled trials of intermittent inhaled tobramycin in patients with CF. These studies used a different formulation of tobramycin for inhalation that is preservative free and less likely to induce local adverse reactions. Patients treated with tobramycin had a statistically significant increase in forced expiratory volume in 1 second (FEV_1), a decrease in the density of *P. aeruginosa*, and a decrease in hospitalization relative to the placebo group. An increase in the percentage of resistant *P. aeruginosa* was noted in the tobramycin-treated patients, but it did not reach statistical significance.[215]

In summary, aerosolized antibiotics provide tangible clinical benefits in this patient population. The development of resistance subsequent to aerosolized therapy is concerning, but the clinical significance of these findings are unknown. This route can be used as an adjunct to parenteral therapy in patients with severe, acute exacerbations of pulmonary infections that are unresponsive to maximal parenteral doses.[206,214–216]

The optimal dose of aerosolized antibiotics is unknown. The regimens found to be most effective include gentamicin or tobramycin, 300 to 600 mg three times daily, administered via a jet nebulizer.[206,215]

REFERENCES

1. Dixon RE. Economic costs of respiratory tract infections in the United States. *Am J Med* 1985; 78(Suppl 6B):45.
2. U.S. Department of Commerce, Bureau of the Census. Statistical Abstract of the United States. 113th ed. Washington, DC: U.S. Government Printing Office; 1993.
3. Centers for Disease Control and Prevention. Trends in morbidity and mortality: pneumonia, influenza, and acute respiratory conditions, January 2001. Available at: http://www.cdc.gov/nchs/about/major/nhis/released200306.htm. Accessed June 30, 2008.
4. Lui KJ, Kendal AP. Impact of influenza epidemics on mortality in the United States from October 1972 to May 1985. *Am J Public Health* 1987;77: 712.
5. Gonzales R et al. What will it take to stop physicians from prescribing antibiotics in acute bronchitis? *Lancet* 1995;345:665.
6. Gonzales R et al. Antibiotic prescribing for adults with colds, upper respiratory tract infections and bronchitis by ambulatory care physicians. *JAMA* 1997;278:901.
7. Steinman MA et al. Changing antibiotic use in community-based outpatient practice, 1991–1997. *Ann Intern Med* 2003;138:523.
8. Franks P et al. The treatment of acute bronchitis with trimethoprim and sulfamethoxazole. *J Fam Pract* 1984;19:185.
9. Verheij TJM et al. Effects of doxycycline in patients with acute cough and purulent sputum: a double-blind placebo-controlled study. *Br J Gen Pract* 1994;44:400.
10. Orr PH et al. Randomized placebo-controlled trials for acute bronchitis: a critical review of the literature. *J Fam Pract* 1993;36:507.
11. Flaherty KR et al. The spectrum of acute bronchitis: using baseline factors to guide empirical therapy. *Postgrad Med* 2001;109:39.
12. National Institutes of Health, National Heart, Lung, and Blood Institute. What is COPD? Available at: http://www.nhlbi.nih.gov/health/public/lung/copd/what-is-copd/index.htm. Accessed June 30, 2008.
13. Mannino DM et al. Surveillance for asthma—United States, 1980–1999. *MMWR Surveill Summ* 2002;51:1.
14. Niederman MS et al. Treatment cost of acute exacerbations of chronic bronchitis. *Clin Ther* 1999;21: 576.
15. Sethi S. Infectious etiology of acute exacerbations of chronic bronchitis. *Chest* 2000;117:380S.
16. Reynolds HY. Chronic obstructive pulmonary disease, chronic bronchitis and acute exacerbations. In: Mandell GL et al., eds. *Principles and Practice of Infectious Diseases*. 6th ed. New York: John Wiley and Sons; 2005.
17. American Thoracic Society. Standards for the diagnosis and care of patients with chronic obstructive pulmonary disease (COPD) and asthma. *Am Rev Respir Dis* 1987;136:225.
18. Burrows B et al. The course and prognosis of different forms of chronic airways obstruction in a sample from the general population. *N Engl J Med* 1987;317:1309.
19. Gump DW et al. Role of infection in chronic bronchitis. *Am Rev Respir Dis* 1976;113:465.
20. Chodosh S. Treatment of acute exacerbations of chronic bronchitis: state of the art. *Am J Med* 1991; 91(Suppl 6A):87S.
21. Chodosh S. Examination of sputum cells. *N Engl J Med* 1970;282:854.
22. Bartlett J. Diagnostic accuracy of transtracheal aspiration bacteriologic studies. *Am Rev Respir Dis* 1977;115:777.
23. Gump DW et al. Role of infection in chronic bronchitis. *Am Rev Respir Dis* 1976;113:465.
24. Pollard JA et al. Incidence of *Moraxellacatarrhalis* in the sputa of patients with chronic lung disease. *Drugs* 1986; 31(Suppl 3):103.
25. Nicotra MB et al. Antibiotic therapy of acute exacerbations of chronic bronchitis: a controlled study using tetracycline. *Ann Intern Med* 1982;97: 18.
26. Saint S et al. Antibiotics in chronic obstructive pulmonary disease exacerbations: a meta-analysis. *JAMA* 1995;273:957.
27. Ram FS et al. Antibiotics for exacerbations of chronic obstructive pulmonary disease. *Cochrane Database Syst Rev*. 200619;(2):CD004403. Review.
28. Anzueto A et al. Etiology, susceptibility, and treatment of acute bacterial exacerbations of complicated chronic bronchitis in the primary care setting: ciprofloxacin 750 mg BID versus clarithromycin 500 mg BID. *Curr Ther* 1998;20:1.
29. Ball P et al. Acute exacerbations of chronic bronchitis: an international comparison. *Chest* 1998; 113(Suppl 3):1995.
30. Chodosh S et al. Efficacy and safety of a 10 day course of 400 mg or 600 mg of grepafloxacin once daily for treatment of acute bacterial exacerbations of chronic bronchitis: comparison with a 10 day course of 500 mg of ciprofloxacin twice daily. *Antimicrob Agents Chemother* 1998;42:114.
31. Rodnick JE et al. The use of antibiotics in acute bronchitis and acute exacerbations of chronic bronchitis. *West J Med* 1988;149:347.
32. Anthonisen NR et al. Antibiotic therapy in exacerbations of chronic obstructive pulmonary diseases. *Ann Intern Med* 1987;106:196.
33. Elmes PC et al. Prophylactic use of oxytetracycline for exacerbations of chronic bronchitis. *BMJ* 1957;2:1272.
34. Nicotra MB et al. Antibiotic therapy of acute exacerbations of chronic bronchitis. *Ann Intern Med* 1982;97:18.
35. Petersen ES et al. A controlled study of the effect of treatment on chronic bronchitis: an evaluation using pulmonary function tests. *Acta Med Scand* 1967;182:293.
36. Jorgensen AF et al. Amoxicillin in treatment of acute uncomplicated exacerbations of chronic bronchitis: a double-blind, placebo-controlled multicentre study in general practice. *Scand J Prev Health Care* 1992;10:7.
37. Anzueto A et al. The infection-free interval: its use in evaluating antimicrobial treatment of acute exacerbation of chronic bronchitis. *Clin Infect Dis* 1999;28:1344.
38. Chodosh S et al. Randomized, double-blind study of ciprofloxacin and cefuroxime axetil for treatment of acute bacterial exacerbations of chronic bronchitis: The Bronchitis Study Group. *Clin Infect Dis* 1999;27:727.
39. Read RC. Infection in acute exacerbations of chronic bronchitis: a clinical perspective. *Respir Med* 1999;93:252.
40. Black P et al. Prophylactic antibiotic treatment for CB. *Cochrane Database Systc Rev* 2003;1: DD004105.
41. Recommendations of the Immunization Practices Advisory Committee (ACIP). Pneumococcal polysaccharide vaccine. *MMWR Morb Mortal Wkly Rep* 1989;38:64.
42. Johnston RN et al. Five year chemoprophylaxis for chronic bronchitis. *BMJ* 1969;4:265.
43. Pridie RB et al. A trial of continuous winter chemotherapy in chronic bronchitis. *Lancet* 1960;2:723.
44. Fine MJ et al. A prediction rule to identify low risk patients with community-acquired pneumonia. *N Engl J Med* 1997;336:243.
45. Bartlett JG et al. Practice guidelines for the management of community-acquired pneumonia in adults. *Clin Infect Dis* 2000;31:347.
46. Garibaldi RA. Epidemiology of community-acquired respiratory tract infections in adults: incidence, etiology, and impact. *Am J Med* 1985;78: 32S.
47. Fine MJ et al. Prognosis and outcomes of patients with community-acquired pneumonia. *JAMA* 1996;275:134.
48. Centers for Disease Control and Prevention. Pneumonia and influenza death rates–United States, 1979–1994. *MMWR Morb Mortal Wkly Rep* 1995; 44:535.
49. Niederman MS et al. The cost of treating community-acquired pneumonia. *Clin Ther* 1998;20:820.
50. Bartlett JG et al. Community-acquired pneumonia. *N Engl J Med* 1995;333:1618.
51. Pennington JE. Respiratory tract infections: intrinsic risk factors. *Am J Med* 1984;76(Suppl 5A):34.
52. Skerett SJ. Host defenses against respiratory infections. *Med Clin North Am* 1994;78:941.
53. Mundy LM et al. Community-acquired pneumonia: impact of immune status. *Am J Respir Crit Care Med* 1995;152:1309.
54. Toews GB. Pulmonary clearance of infectious agents. In: Pennington JE, ed. *Respiratory Infections: Diagnosis and Management*. New York: Raven Press; 1983.
55. Lorber B, Swenson R. Bacteriology of aspiration pneumonia: a prospective study of community- and hospital-acquired cases. *Ann Intern Med* 1974;81: 329.
56. Petersdorf RG et al. A study of antibiotic prophylaxis in unconscious patients. *N Engl J Med* 1957;257:1001.
57. Tillotson JR, Finland M. Bacterial colonization and clinical super-infection of the respiratory tract complicating antibiotic treatment of pneumonia. *J Infect Dis* 1969;119:597.
58. Rosenthal S, Tager IB. Prevalence of Gram-negative rods in the normal pharyngeal flora. *Ann Intern Med* 1975;83:355.
59. Johanson WG et al. Changing pharyngeal bacterial flora of hospitalized patients. *N Engl J Med* 1969;28:1137.
60. Johanson WG et al. Nosocomial respiratory infections with Gram-negative bacilli: the significance of colonization of the respiratory tract. *Ann Intern Med* 1972;77:701.
61. Klein RS, Steigbigel NH. Aspiration pneumonia. *Semin Infect Dis* 1983;5:274.
62. Valenti WM et al. Factors predisposing to oropharyngeal colonization with Gram-negative bacilli in the aged. *N Engl J Med* 1978;298:1108.
63. Verghese A, Berk SL. Bacterial pneumonia in the elderly. *Medicine (Baltimore)* 1983;62:271.
64. Haas H et al. Bacterial flora of the respiratory tract in chronic bronchitis: comparison of transtracheal,

fiberbronchoscopic, and oropharyngeal sampling methods. *Am Rev Respir Dis* 1977;116:41.
65. Murray PR, Washington JA. Microscopic and bacteriologic analysis of expectorated sputum. *Mayo Clin Proc* 1975;50:339.
66. Dal Nogare AR. Nosocomial pneumonia in the medical and surgical patient. *Med Clin North Am* 1994;78:1081.
67. Marrie TJ et al. Community-acquired pneumonia requiring hospitalization: a 5-year prospective study. *Rev Infect Dis* 1989;11:586.
68. Thornsberry C et al. Surveillance of antimicrobial resistance in *Streptococcus pneumoniae, Haemophilus influenzae* and *Moraxella catarrhalis* in the United States in 1996–1997 respiratory season. *Diagn Microbiol Infect Dis* 1997;29:249.
69. Thornsberry C et al. International surveillance of resistance among respiratory tract pathogens in the United States, 1997–1998. 38th Interscience Conference on Antimicrobial Agents and Chemotherapy, San Diego, September 24, 1998. Abstract E-22.
70. Fang GD et al. New and emerging etiologies for community-acquired pneumonia with implications for therapy: a prospective multi-center study of 359 cases. *Medicine* 1990;69:307.
71. Edelstein PH. Legionnaires' disease. *Clin Infect Dis* 1993;16:741.
72. Brook I. Percutaneous transtracheal aspiration in the diagnosis and treatment of aspiration pneumonia in children. *J Pediatr* 1980;96:1000.
73. Grayston JT et al. A new *Chlamydia psittaci* strain, TWAR, isolated in acute respiratory tract infections. *N Engl J Med* 1986;315:161.
74. Metlay SP, Fine MJ. Testing strategies in the initial management of patients with community-acquired pneumonia. *Ann Intern Med* 2003;138:109.
75. Mittl RL Jr et al. Radiographic resolution of community-acquired pneumonia. *Am J Respir Crit Care Med* 1994;149:630.
76. Jay SJ et al. The radiographic resolution of *Streptococcus pneumoniae* pneumonia. *N Engl J Med* 1975;293:798.
77. Austrian R et al. Pneumococcal bacteremia with special reference to bacteremic pneumococcal pneumonia. *Ann Intern Med* 1964;60:759.
78. Thornsberry C et al. Surveillance of antimicrobial resistance in *Streptococcus pneumoniae, Haemophilus influenzae,* and *Moraxella catarrhalis* in the United States in 1996–1997 respiratory season. The Laboratory Investigator Group. *Diagn Microbiol Infect Dis* 1997;29(4):249.
79. Doern GV. Antimicrobial use and the emergence of antimicrobial resistance with *Streptococcus pneumoniae* in the United States. *Clin Infect Dis* 2001; 33(Suppl 3):S187.
80. Doern GV et al. Antimicrobial resistance among clinical isolates of *Streptococcus pneumoniae* in the United States during 1999–2000, including a comparison of resistance rates since 1994–1995. *Antimicrob Agents Chemother* 2001;45(6):1721.
81. Krumpe PE et al. Intravenous and oral mono- or combination-therapy in the treatment of severe infections: ciprofloxacin versus standard antibiotic therapy. Ciprofloxacin Study Group. *J Antimicrob Chemother* 1999;43(Suppl A):117.
82. Whitney CG et al. Increasing prevalence of multidrug resistant *Streptococcus pneumoniae* in the United States. *N Engl J Med* 2003;343:1917.
83. Yu VL et al. An international prospective study of pneumococcal bacteremia: correlation with *in vitro* resistance, antibiotics administered, and clinical outcome. *Clin Infect Dis* 2003;37:230.
84. Lonks JR et al. Failure of macrolide antibiotic treatment in patients with bacteremia due to erythromycin-resistant *Streptococcus pneumoniae*. *Clin Infect Dis* 2002;35:556.
85. Sutcliffe J et al. *Streptococcus pneumoniae* and *Streptococcus pyogenes* resistant to macrolides but sensitive to clindamycin: a common resistance pattern mediated by an efflux system. *Antimicrob Agents Chemother* 1996;40:1817.
86. Johnston NJ et al. Prevalence and characterization of the mechanisms of macrolide, lincosamide, and streptogramin resistance in isolates of *Streptococcus pneumoniae*. *Antimicrob Agents Chemother* 1998;42:2425.
87. Acar J. Rapid emergence of resistance to cefepime during treatment [Letter]. *Clin Infect Dis* 1998;26(6):1484.
88. Monto AS et al. Zanamivir in the prevention of influenza among healthy adults. *JAMA* 1999;282:31.
89. Hayden FG et al. Efficacy and safety of the neuraminidase inhibitor zanamivir in the treatment of influenza virus infections. *N Engl J Med* 1997;337:874.
90. Hayden FG et al. Use of the selective neuraminidase inhibitor oseltamivir to prevent influenza. *N Engl J Med* 1999;341:1336.
91. Treanor JJ et al. Efficacy and of the oral neuraminidase inhibitor oseltamivir in treating acute influenza. *JAMA* 2000;283:1016.
92. Winquist AG et al. Neuraminidase inhibitors for treatment of influenza A and B infections. *MMWR Morb Mortal Wkly Rep* 1999;48(RR-14):1.
93. Demicheli V et al. Prevention and early treatment of influenza in healthy adults. *Vaccine* 2000;18: 957.
94. Uyeki TM et al. Large summertime influenza A outbreak among tourists in Alaska and the Yukon Territory. *Clin Infect Dis* 2003;36:1095.
95. Gross PA et al. Time to earliest peak serum antibody response to influenza vaccine in the elderly. *Clin Diagn Lab Immunol* 1997;4:491.
96. Brokstad KA et al. Parenteral influenza vaccination induces a rapid systemic and local immune response. *J Infect Dis* 1995;171:198.
97. Tominack RL, Hayden FG. Rimantadine hydrochloride and amantadine hydrochloride use in influenza A virus infections. *Infect Dis Clin North Am* 1987;1:459.
98. Nicholson KG. Use of antivirals in influenza in the elderly: prophylaxis and therapy. *Gerontology* 1996;42:280.
99. Wintermeyer SM, Nahata MC. Rimantadine: a clinical perspective. *Ann Pharmacother* 1995;29:299.
100. Gravenstein S et al. Zanamivir: a review of clinical safety in individuals at high risk of developing influenza-related complications. *Drug Saf* 2001;24:1113.
101. Bowles SK et al. Use of oseltamivir during influenza outbreaks in Ontario nursing homes, 1999–2000. *J Am Geriatr Soc* 2002;50:608.
102. Guay DR. Amantadine and rimantadine prophylaxis of influenza A in nursing homes: a tolerability perspective. *Drugs Aging* 1994;5:8.
103. Peters PH Jr et al. Long-term use of oseltamivir for the prophylaxis of influenza in a vaccinated frail older population. *J Am Geriatr Soc* 2001;49:1025.
104. Faletta JM et al. Discontinuing penicillin prophylaxis in children with sickle cell anemia. *J Pediatr* 1995;127:685.
105. American Academy of Pediatrics. *1994 Red Book: Report of the Committee on Infectious Diseases*. Elk Grove Village, IL: Author; 1994:371.
106. Patriarca PA et al. Safety of prolonged administration of rimantadine hydrochloride in the prophylaxis of influenza A virus infections in nursing homes. *Antimicrob Agents Chemother* 1984;26: 101.
107. Arden NH et al. Roles of vaccination and amantadine prophylaxis in controlling an outbreak of influenza A (H3N2) in a nursing home. *Arch Intern Med* 1988;148:865.
108. Monto AS et al. Zanamivir in the prevention of influenza among healthy adults: a randomized controlled trial. *JAMA* 1999;282:31.
109. Hayden FG et al. Use of the selective oral neuraminidase inhibitor oseltamivir to prevent influenza. *N Engl J Med* 1999;341:1336.
110. Monto AS et al. Zanamivir prophylaxis: an effective strategy for the prevention of influenza types A and B within households. *J Infect Dis* 2002;186:1582.
111. Schilling M et al. Efficacy of zanamivir for chemoprophylaxis of nursing home influenza outbreaks. *Vaccine* 1998;16:1771.
112. Lee C et al. Zanamivir use during transmission of amantadine-resistant influenza A in a nursing home. *Infect Control Hosp Epidemiol* 2000;21:700.
113. Shijubo N et al. Experience with oseltamivir in the control of nursing home influenza A outbreak. *Intern Med* 2002;41:366.
114. Parker R et al. Experience with oseltamivir in the control of a nursing home influenza B outbreak. *Can Commun Dis Rep* 2001;27:37.
115. Musher DM et al. Pneumococcal polysaccharide vaccine in young adults and older bronchitics: determination of IgG responses by ELISA and the effect of adsorption of serum with non-type-specific cell wall polysaccharide. *J Infect Dis* 1990;161: 728.
116. Mufson MA et al. G. Long-term persistence of antibody following immunization with pneumococcal polysaccharide vaccine. *Proc Soc Exp Biol Med* 1983;173:270.
117. Mufson MA et al. Pneumococcal antibody levels one decade after immunization of healthy adults. *Am J Med Sci* 1987;293:279.
118. Shapiro ED, Clemens JD. A controlled evaluation of the protective efficacy of pneumococcal vaccine for patients at high risk of serious pneumococcal infections. *Ann Intern Med* 1984;101:325.
119. Sims RV et al. The clinical effectiveness of pneumococcal vaccine in the elderly. *Ann Intern Med* 1988;108:653.
120. Shapiro ED et al. The protective efficacy of polyvalent pneumococcal polysaccharide vaccine. *N Engl J Med* 1991;325:1453.
121. Farr BM et al. Preventing pneumococcal bacteremia in patients at risk: results of a matched case-control study. *Arch Intern Med* 1995;155:2336.
122. Jackson LA, Neuzil KM, Yu O et al. Effectiveness of pneumococcalpolysaccharide vaccine in older adults. *N Engl J Med* 2003;348:1747.
123. Centers for Disease Control and Prevention. Prevention of pneumococcal disease: recommendations from the Committee on Immunization Practices (ACIP). *MMWR Morb Mortal Wkly Rep* 1997; 46(RR-08):1.
124. Centers for Disease Control and Prevention. Recommendations of the Immunization Practices Advisory Committee: pneumococcal polysaccharide vaccine. *MMWR Morb Mortal Wkly Rep* 1989; 38:64.
125. Fedson DS, Musher DM. Pneumococcal vaccine. In: Plotkin SA, Mortimer EA Jr, eds. *Vaccines*. 2nd ed. Philadelphia: WB Saunders; 1994:517.
126. Garner CV, Pier GB. Immunologic considerations for the development of conjugate vaccines. In: Cruse JM, Lewis RE, eds. *Conjugate Vaccines*. Basel, Switzerland: Karger; 1989:11.
127. Centers for Disease Control and Prevention. National Health Interview Survey. Available at: www.cdc.gov/vaccines/stats-surv/imz-coverage.htm#nhis. Accessed June 30, 2008.
128. Bartlett JG, Gorbach SL. The triple threat of aspiration pneumonia. *Chest* 1975;68:560.
129. Gianella RA et al. Gastric acid barrier to ingested microorganisms in man: studies in vivo and in vitro. *Gut* 1972;13:251.
130. Drasar BS et al. Studies on the intestinal flora: I. The bacterial flora of the gastrointestinal tract in health and achlorhydric persons. *Gastroenterology* 1969;56:71.
131. Bynum LJ, Pierce AK. Pulmonary aspiration of gastric contents. *Am Rev Respir Dis* 1976;114: 1129.
132. Huxley EJ et al. Pharyngeal aspiration in normal adults and patients with depressed consciousness. *Am J Med* 1978;64:564.
133. LeFrock JL et al. Aspiration pneumonia: a ten-year review. *Am Surg* 1979;45:305.
134. Landay MJ et al. Pulmonary manifestations of acute aspiration of gastric contents. *Am J Roentgenol* 1978;131:587.
135. Wolfe JE et al. Effects of corticosteroids in the treatment of patients with gastric aspiration. *Am J Med* 1977;63:719.
136. Bartlett JG et al. The bacteriology of aspiration pneumonia. *Am J Med* 1974;56:202.

137. Brook I, Finegold SM. Bacteriology of aspiration pneumonia in children. *Pediatrics* 1980;65:1115.
138. Pingleton SD et al. Enteral nutrition in patients receiving mechanical ventilation: multiple sources of tracheal colonization include the stomach. *Am J Med* 1986;80:827.
139. Drasar BS et al. Studies of the intestinal flora. *Gastroenterology* 1969;56:71.
140. Muscroft TJ et al. The microflora of the postoperative stomach. *Br J Surg* 1981;68:560.
141. DuMoulin GC et al. Aspiration of gastric bacteria in antacid-treated patients: a frequent cause of postoperative colonization of the airway. *Lancet* 1982;1:242.
142. Tryba M. Risk of acute stress bleeding and nosocomial pneumonia in ventilated intensive care unit patients: sucralfate versus antacids. *Am J Med* 1987;83(Suppl 3B):117.
143. Driks MR et al. Nosocomial pneumonia in intubated patients given sucralfate as compared with antacids of histamine type 2 blockers. *N Engl J Med* 1987;317:1376.
144. Sanders CV et al. Metronidazole in the treatment of anaerobic infections. *Am Rev Respir Dis* 1979; 120:337.
145. Perlino CA. Metronidazole vs clindamycin treatment of anaerobic pulmonary infection. *Arch Intern Med* 1981;141:1424.
146. Ingham HR et al. The activity of metronidazole against facultatively anaerobic bacteria. *J Antimicrob Chemother* 1980;6:343.
147. American Thoracic Society. Guidelines for the management of adults with hospital-acquired ventilator-associated, and healthcare-associated pneumonia. *Am Rev Respir Crit Care Med* 2005; 171:388.
148. Garibaldi RA et al. Infections among patients in nursing homes: policies, prevalence, and problems. *N Engl J Med* 1981;305:731.
149. Johanson WG et al. Changing pharyngeal bacterial flora of hospitalized patients: emerging Gram-negative bacilli. *N Engl J Med* 1969;281:1137.
150. Mackowiak PA et al. Pharyngeal colonization by Gram-negative bacilli in aspiration-prone persons. *Arch Intern Med* 1978;138:1224.
151. Johanson WG et al. Association of respiratory tract colonization with adherence of Gram-negative bacilli to epithelial cells. *J Infect Dis* 1979;139:667.
152. Johanson WG et al. Bacterial adherence to epithelial cells in bacillary colonization of the respiratory tract. *Am Rev Respir Dis* 1980;121:55.
153. Rouby JJ et al. Nosocomial bronchopneumonia in the critically ill: histologic and bacteriologic aspects. *Am Rev Respir Dis* 1992;146:1059.
154. Bartlett JG et al. Bacteriology of hospital-acquired pneumonia. *Arch Intern Med* 1986;146:868.
155. Prod'hom G et al. Nosocomial pneumonia in mechanically ventilated patients receiving antacid, ranitidine, or sucralfate as prophylaxis for stress ulcer: a randomized controlled trial. *Ann Intern Med* 1994;120:653.
156. Rello J et al. Impact of previous antimicrobial therapy on etiology and outcome of ventilator-associated pneumonia. *Chest* 1993;104:1230.
157. Fridkin SK et al. Magnitude and prevention of nosocomial prevention infections in the intensive care unit. *Infect Dis Clin North Am* 1997;11:479.
158. Stout JE et al. Ubiquitousness of *Legionella pneumophila* in water supply of a hospital with endemic Legionnaires' diseases. *N Engl J Med* 1982; 306:466.
159. Rhame FS. Prevention of nosocomial aspergillosis. *J Hosp Infect* 1991;18:466.
160. Chow JW et al. Enterobacter bacteremia — clinical features and emergence of antibiotic resistance during therapy. *Ann Intern Med* 1991;115:585.
161. Medeiros AA. Relapsing infection due to Enterobacter species: lessons of heterogeneity [Editorial; Comment]. *Clin Infect Dis* 1997;25:341.
162. Smolyakov R et al. Nosocomial multi-drug resistant Acinetobacter baumannii bloodstream infection: risk factors and outcome with ampicillin-sulbactam treatment. *J Hosp Infect* 2003;54:32.
163. Garnacho-Montero J et al. Treatment of multi-drug-resistant Acinetobactor baumannii ventilator-associated pneumonia (VAP) with intravenous colistin: A comparison with imipenem-susceptible VAP. *Clin Infect Dis* 2003;36:1111.
164. Fagon JY et al. Nosocomial pneumonia in ventilated patients: a cohort study evaluating attributable mortality and hospital stay. *Am J Med* 1993;94:281.
165. Barza M et al. Predictability of blood levels of gentamicin in man. *J Infect Dis* 1975;132:165.
166. Zaske DE et al. Wide interpatient variations in gentamicin dose requirements for geriatric patients. *JAMA* 1982;248:3122.
167. Flint LM et al. Serum level monitoring of aminoglycoside antibiotics. *Arch Surg* 1985;120:99.
168. Moore RD et al. Association of aminoglycoside plasma levels with therapeutic outcome in Gram-negative pneumonia. *Am J Med* 1984;77:657.
169. Moore RD et al. Association of aminoglycoside levels with therapeutic outcome in Gram-negative pneumonia. *Am J Med* 1984;77:657.
170. Bergogne-Berezin E. Pharmacokinetics of antibiotics in respiratory secretion. In: Pennington JE, ed. *Respiratory Infections: Diagnosis and Management*. New York: Raven Press; 1983.
171. Bodem CR et al. Endobronchial pH relevance of aminoglycoside activity in Gram-negative bacillary pneumonia. *Am Rev Respir Dis* 1983;127:39.
172. Vaudaux P. Peripheral inactivation of gentamicin. *J Antimicrob Chemother* 1981;8(Suppl A):17.
173. Levy J et al. Bioactivity of gentamicin in purulent sputum from patients with cystic fibrosis or bronchiectasis: comparison with activity in serum. *J Infect Dis* 1983;148:1069.
174. Mendelman PM et al. Aminoglycoside penetration, inactivation, and efficacy in cystic fibrosis sputum. *Am Rev Respir Dis* 1985;132:761.
175. Greenfield S et al. Prevention of Gram-negative bacillary pneumonia using aerosol polymyxin as prophylaxis: I. Effect on the colonization pattern of the upper respiratory tract of seriously ill patients. *J Clin Invest* 1973;52:2935.
176. Klick JM et al. Prevention of Gram-negative bacillary pneumonia using polymyxin aerosol as prophylaxis: II. Effect on the incidence of pneumonia in seriously ill patients. *J Clin Invest* 1975;55: 514.
177. Klastersky J et al. Endotracheally-administered gentamicin for the prevention of infections of the respiratory tract in patients with tracheostomy: a double-blind study. *Chest* 1974;65:650.
178. Feeley TW et al. Aerosol polymyxin and pneumonia in seriously ill patients. *N Engl J Med* 1975;293: 471.
179. Klastersky J et al. Endotracheal antibiotics for the prevention of tracheobronchial infections in tracheotomized unconscious patients. *Chest* 1975;68: 302.
180. Wood GC et al. Aerosolized antimicrobial therapy in acutely ill patients. *Pharmacotherapy* 2000;20: 166.
181. Ramsey BW et al. Management of pulmonary disease in patients with cystic fibrosis. *N Engl J Med* 1996;335:179.
182. Klastersky J et al. Endotracheal gentamicin in bronchial infections in patients with tracheostomy. *Chest* 1972;61:117.
183. Klastersky J et al. Endotracheally-administered antibiotics for Gram-negative bronchopneumonia. *Chest* 1979;75:586.
184. Sculier JP et al. Effectiveness of mezlocillin and endotracheally-administered sisomicin with or without parenteral sisomicin in the treatment of Gram-negative bronchopneumonia. *J Antimicrob Chemother* 1982;9:63.
185. Lake KB et al. Combined topical pulmonary and systemic gentamicin: the question of safety. *Chest* 1975;68:62.
186. Baran D et al. Concentration of gentamicin in bronchial secretions of children with cystic fibrosis or tracheostomy. *Int J Clin Pharmacol* 1975;12:336.
187. Odio W et al. Concentrations of gentamicin in bronchial secretions after intramuscular and endotracheal administration. *J Clin Pharmacol* 1975;15: 518.
188. Stillwell PC et al. Endotracheal tobramycin in Gram-negative pneumonitis. *Drug Intell Clin Pharm* 1988;22:577.
189. Klastersky J, Thys JP. Local antibiotic therapy for bronchopneumonia. In: Pennington JE, ed. *Respiratory Infections: Diagnosis and Management*. New York: Raven Press; 1983.
190. Dickie KJ, de Groot WJ. Ventilatory effects of aerosolized kanamycin and polymyxin. *Chest* 1974;63:694.
191. Wilson FE. Acute respiratory failure secondary to polymyxin-B inhalation. *Chest* 1981;79:237.
192. Dally MB et al. Cystic fibrosis: ventilatory effects of aerosol gentamicin. *Thorax* 1978;33:54.
193. Craven DE et al. Preventing nosocomial pneumonia: state of the art and perspectives for the 1990s. *Am J Med* 1991;91:44S.
194. Kollef MH. The prevention of ventilator associated pneumonias. *N Engl J Med* 1999;340:627.
195. Torres A et al. Pulmonary aspiration of gastric contents in patients receiving mechanical ventilation: the effect of body position. *Ann Intern Med* 1992;116:540.
196. Gastinne H et al. A controlled trial in intensive care units of selective decontamination of the digestive tract with nonabsorbable antibiotics. *N Engl J Med* 1992;326:594.
197. Selective Decontamination of the Digestive Tract Trialists' Collaborative Group. Meta-analysis of randomized controlled trials of selective decontamination of the digestive tract. *BMJ* 1993;307: 525.
198. Wood RE et al. Cystic fibrosis. *Am Rev Respir Dis* 1976;113:833.
199. Thomassen MJ et al. Multiple isolates of *Pseudomonas aeruginosa* with differing antimicrobial susceptibility patterns from patients with cystic fibrosis. *J Infect Dis* 1979;140:873.
200. Isles A et al. *Pseudomonas cepacia* infection in cystic fibrosis: an emerging problem. *J Pediatr* 1984; 104:206.
201. Tablan OC et al. *Pseudomonas cepacia* colonization in patients with cystic fibrosis: risk factors and clinical outcome. *J Pediatr* 1985;107:382.
202. Jusko WJ et al. Enhanced renal excretion of dicloxacillin in patients with cystic fibrosis. *Pediatrics* 1975;56:1038.
203. Ziemniak JA et al. The bioavailability of pharmacokinetics of cimetidine and its metabolites in juvenile cystic fibrosis patients: age-related differences as compared to adults. *Eur J Clin Pharmacol* 1984; 26:183.
204. Isles A et al. Theophylline disposition in cystic fibrosis. *Am Rev Respir Dis* 1983;127:417.
205. Levy J et al. Disposition of tobramycin in patients with cystic fibrosis: a prospective controlled study. *J Pediatr* 1984;105:117.
206. Beringer PM. New approaches to optimizing antimicrobial therapy in patients with cystic fibrosis. *Curr Opin Pulmon Med* 1999;5:371.
207. Hodson ME et al. Aerosol carbenicillin and gentamicin treatment of *Pseudomonas aeruginosa* infection in patients with cystic fibrosis. *Lancet* 1981; 2:1137.
208. Stephens D et al. Efficacy of inhaled tobramycin in the treatment of pulmonary exacerbations in children with cystic fibrosis. *Pediatr Infect Dis* 1983;2: 209.
209. Cooper DM et al. Comparison of intravenous and inhalation antibiotic therapy in acute pulmonary deterioration in cystic fibrosis. *Am Rev Respir Dis* 1985;131:A242.
210. Steinkamp G et al. Long-term tobramycin aerosol therapy in cystic fibrosis. *Pediatr Pulmonol* 1989; 6:91.
211. Swift DL. Aerosols and humidity therapy: generation and respiratory deposition of therapeutic aerosols. *Am Rev Respir Dis* 1980;122(Suppl):71.
212. Alderson PO et al. Pulmonary disposition of aerosols in children with cystic fibrosis. *J Pediatr* 1974;84:479.

213. MacLusky I et al. Inhaled antibiotics in cystic fibrosis: is there a therapeutic effect? *J Pediatr* 1986; 108:861.
214. Ramsey BW et al. Efficacy of aerosolized tobramycin in patients with cystic fibrosis. *N Engl J Med* 1993;328:1740.
215. Ramsey BW et al. Intermittent administration of inhaled tobramycin in patients with cystic fibrosis. *N Engl J Med* 1999;340:23.
216. Meehan TP et al. Quality of care, process, and outcomes in elderly patients with pneumonia. *JAMA* 1997;278:2080.
217. Centers for Disease Control and Prevention. Health, United States, 2007. Available at: http://www.cdc.gov/nchs/data/hus/hus07.pdf. Accessed June 30, 2008.
218. Celli BR et al. ATS statement: standards for the diagnosis and care of patients with chronic obstructive pulmonary disease. *Am J Respir Crit Care Med* 1995;152(Suppl 2):S77.
219. Adams SG et al. Antibiotics are associated with lower relapse rates in outpatients with acute exacerbations of COPD. *Chest* 2000;117: 1345.
220. Fekety FR Jr et al. Bacteria, viruses, and mycoplasmas in acute pneumonia in adults. *Am Rev Respir Dis* 1971;104:499.
221. Farr BM et al. Predicting death in patients hospitalized with community-acquired pneumonia. *Ann Intern Med* 1991;115:428.
222. Gleason PP et al. Associations between initial antimicrobial therapy and medical outcomes for hospitalized elderly patients with pneumonia. *Arch Intern Med* 1999;159:2562.
223. Mufson MA. Penicillin-resistant *Streptococcus pneumoniae* increasingly threatens the patient and challenges the physician. *Clin Infect Dis* 1998;27: 771.
224. Pallares R et al. Resistance to penicillin and cephalosporin and mortality from severe pneumococcal pneumonia in Barcelona, Spain. *N Engl J Med* 1995;333:474.
225. File T et al. A multicenter, randomized study comparing the efficacy and safety of intravenous and/or oral levofloxacin versus ceftriaxone and/or cefuroxime axetil in the treatment of adults with community-acquired pneumonia. *Antimicrob Agents Chemother* 1997;41:1965.
226. Ortqvist A et al. Oral empiric treatment of community-acquired pneumonia: a multi-center, double blind, randomized study comparing sparfloxacin with roxithromycin: the Scandinavian Sparfloxacin Study Group. *Chest* 1996;110:1499.
227. Dowell ME et al. A randomized, double-blind, multicenter comparative study of gatifloxacin 400 mg IV and PO versus ceftriaxone–erythromycin in treatment of community-acquired pneumonia requiring hospitalization. 39th Interscience Conference on Antimicrobial Agents and Chemotherapy, San Francisco, September 26, 1999. Abstract 2241.
228. Hooper DC. Expanding uses of fluoroquinolones: opportunities and challenges. *Ann Intern Med* 1998; 129:908.
229. Applebaum PC et al. Role of the newer fluoroquinolones against penicillin-resistant *Streptococcus pneumoniae*. *Infect Dis Clin Pract* 1999;8:374.
230. Chen DK et al. Decreased susceptibility of *Streptococcus pneumoniae* to fluoroquinolones in Canada: Canadian Bacterial Surveillance Network. *N Engl J Med* 1999;34:233.
231. Low DE et al. Strategies for stemming the tide of antimicrobial resistance. *JAMA* 1998;273:394.
232. Heffelfinger JD et al. Management of community-acquired pneumonia in the era of pneumococcal resistance: a report from the Drug-Resistant Streptococcus Pneumoniae Therapeutic Working Group. *Arch Intern Med* 2000;160:1399.
233. Webster A et al. Coadministration of orally inhaled zanamivir with inactivated trivalent influenza vaccine does not adversely affect the production of antihaemagglutinin antibodies in the serum of healthy volunteers. *Clin Pharmacokinet* 1999;36(Suppl 1): 51.
234. Patriarca PA et al. Prevention and control of type A influenza infections in nursing homes: benefits and costs of four approaches using vaccination and amantadine. *Ann Intern Med* 1987;107:732.
235. Gomolin IH et al. Control of influenza outbreaks in the nursing home: guidelines for diagnosis and management. *J Am Geriatr Soc* 1995;43:71.
236. Garner JS. Guideline for isolation precautions in hospitals: Hospital Infection Control Practices Advisory Committee. *Infect Control Hosp Epidemiol* 1996;17:53.
237. Paradise JL et al. Otitis media in 2253 Pittsburgh-area infants: prevalence and risk factors during the first two years of life. *Pediatrics* 1997;99:318.
238. Bradley SF. Prevention of influenza in long-term-care facilities. Long-Term-Care Committee of the Society for Healthcare Epidemiology of America. *Infect Control Hosp Epidemiol* 1999;20:629.
239. Centers for Disease Control and Prevention. Prevention and control of influenza: recommendations of the Advisory Committee on Immunization Practices. *MMWR Morb Mortal Wkly Rep* 2003;52(RR-08):1.
240. Celis RT et al. Nosocomial pneumonia: a multivariant analysis of risk and prognosis. *Chest* 1988; 93:318.
241. Hilf M et al. Antibiotic therapy for *Pseudomonas aeruginosa* bacteremia: outcome correlations in a prospective study of 200 patients. *Am J Med* 1989; 87:540.
242. Kollef MH et al. Scheduled change of antibiotic classes: a strategy to decrease the incidence of ventilator associated pneumonia. *Am Rev Respir Crit Care Med* 1997;154(4 Pt 1):1040.
243. Klibanov OM et al. Single versus combined therapy for Gram-negative infections. *Ann Pharmacother* 2004;38:332.

CHAPTER 61

Tuberculosis

Michael B. Kays

History

Tuberculosis (TB) is an ancient disease, and evidence of TB dates back as far as prehistoric times with evidence being found in pre-Columbian and early Egyptian remains. However, TB did not become a problem until the 17th and 18th centuries when crowded living conditions of the industrial revolution contributed to its epidemic numbers in Europe and the United States. Early physicians referred to TB as *phthisis*, derived from the Greek term for wasting, because its clinical presentation consisted of weight loss, cough, fevers, and hemoptysis. Although its characteristics were well known, an etiologic agent was not clearly defined until 1882 when Robert Koch isolated and cultured *Mycobacterium tuberculosis* and demonstrated its infectious nature. With this knowledge, early treatment in the mid-1800s to the early 1900s consisted of removing patients with TB from the community and placing them in a sanatorium for bedrest and fresh air. With the advent of radiographic film, pulmonary cavitary lesions were found to be pivotal in the evolution of the disease. Therapy then included procedures such as pneumoperitoneum, thoracoplasty, and plombage to reduce the size of the cavitary lesion. Some of these therapies may continue to be used for severe and refractory cases.

The modern era of medical therapy for TB began in 1944 with the discovery of streptomycin and, shortly thereafter, para-aminosalicylic acid. The addition of isoniazid (INH) in 1952 and rifampin in the late 1960s greatly increased the hopes for the eventual elimination of TB in the United States.[1] Multidrug-resistant TB (MDR-TB) emerged in the 1990s as a threat to the control of TB in the United States and other countries.[2–4] More recently, TB has once again demanded the attention of national and international medical journals, as well as the lay press, with the emergence of extensively drug-resistant TB (XDR-TB).[5–7] Therefore, a high index of suspicion for TB, rapid pathogen identification, susceptibility testing, patient isolation to prevent dissemination, and aggressive, appropriate antimicrobial therapy are critical to prevent further development and spread of drug-resistant TB.

Incidence and Epidemiology

Assuming life-long infection, approximately 2.0 billion people (30% of the world's population) are infected with *M. tuberculosis*.[8] Tuberculosis is the second most common cause of death from an infectious disease in the world, second only to human immunodeficiency virus (HIV) and acquired immunodeficiency syndrome (AIDS). Globally, an estimated 8.8 million new cases of TB were reported in 2005, which represents an increase of 0.5 million cases compared with 2000.[8] Most (7.4 million) of the new cases in 2005 originated from Asia and sub-Saharan Africa.[9] The countries with the largest number of new cases were India (1.85 million), China (1.32 million), Indonesia (0.53 million), Nigeria (0.37 million), Bangladesh (0.32 million), and Pakistan (0.29 million).[9] Twelve of the 15 countries with the highest incidence rates for TB are located in Africa, a finding which can be explained, at least in part, by the relatively high rates of co-infection with HIV.[9] Countries with the highest rate (per 100,000 population) for new TB cases were Swaziland (1,262), Djibouti (762), Namibia (697), Lesotho (696), Botswana (654), and Kenya (641).[9] Tuberculosis rates have also increased in the former Soviet Union. In Russia, the incidence rate increased from 51 per 100,000 population in 1990 to 119 per 100,000 population in 2005.[9] In 2005, approximately 1.6 million deaths secondary to TB were reported globally, including 195,000 patients infected with HIV.[9]

In the United States, the rate of TB declined from 53.0 per 100,000 population in 1953, when the Centers for Disease Control and Prevention (CDC) began conducting TB surveillance, to 9.1 per 100,000 population in 1988.[10] A resurgence of TB took place in the United States from 1985 to 1992, in large part because of the HIV/AIDS epidemic and the emergence of MDR-TB. At its peak in 1992, 26,673 TB cases (10.5 per 100,000 population) were reported.[10] As a result of this resurgence, an advisory committee was established by the Department of Health and Human Services to provide recommendations for the elimination of TB in the United States. The committee urged the establishment of a national goal of TB elimination (<1 case per million of population) by the year 2010, with an interim target incidence rate of 3.5 per 100,000 population by 2000.[11] The plan incorporated identification of populations more susceptible to TB infection, the use of biotechnology in diagnosis and treatment, and computer telecommunication to track cases.[11] These recommendations, along with strict infection control procedures, prompt initiation of treatment, and ensuring completion of TB therapy, have successfully reduced the TB case rate in the United States. The number of reported TB cases in 2006 was 13,767 cases, which represents an incidence rate of 4.6 per 100,000 population.[12] This incidence rate is the lowest recorded rate since national reporting began over 50 years ago; however, the incidence rate in 2006 remains higher than the interim target goal that was set for 2000.[11,12] TB is more common in patients 25 to 44 years of age (34% of cases), but the highest incidence rate is seen in patients ≥65 years of age (7.7 per 100,000 population).[13]

Although the incidence rate of TB in the United States continues to decline, the rate of decline has slowed since 2000 (Fig. 61-1). From 1993 to 2000, the average annual incidence rate decreased 7.3% per year, but the average annual incidence rate has only decreased 3.8% per year from 2000 to 2006.[12] Foreign-born and ethnic minority populations are disproportionately infected with TB in the United States. The number of TB cases in foreign-born persons increased by 5% from 1993 to 2006, whereas TB cases for persons born in the United States decreased 66% over this time period (Fig. 61-1). In 1993, 69% of reported TB cases were among U.S.-born persons, whereas 29% were among foreign-born persons.[13] In 2006, the total number of TB cases in foreign-born persons was 57% compared with 43% for U.S.-born persons.[12] Stated differently, the rate of TB was 9.5 times greater for foreign-born persons (21.9 per 100,000 population) than for U.S.-born persons (2.3 per 100,000 population).[12] Five countries accounted for over half of TB cases reported in foreign-born persons in 2006: Mexico, Philippines, Vietnam, India, and China.[12] An analysis of the number of TB cases in 2004 found that 50% of cases in foreign-born persons were reported in those who had been in the United States for more than 5 years; however, the incidence rate was highest in persons who had been in the United States for 1 year or less.[14]

In 2006, the TB rates for Hispanics, blacks, and Asians were 7.6, 8.4, and 21.2 times higher, respectively, than the rate for whites.[12] Compared with 2005, 20 states and the District

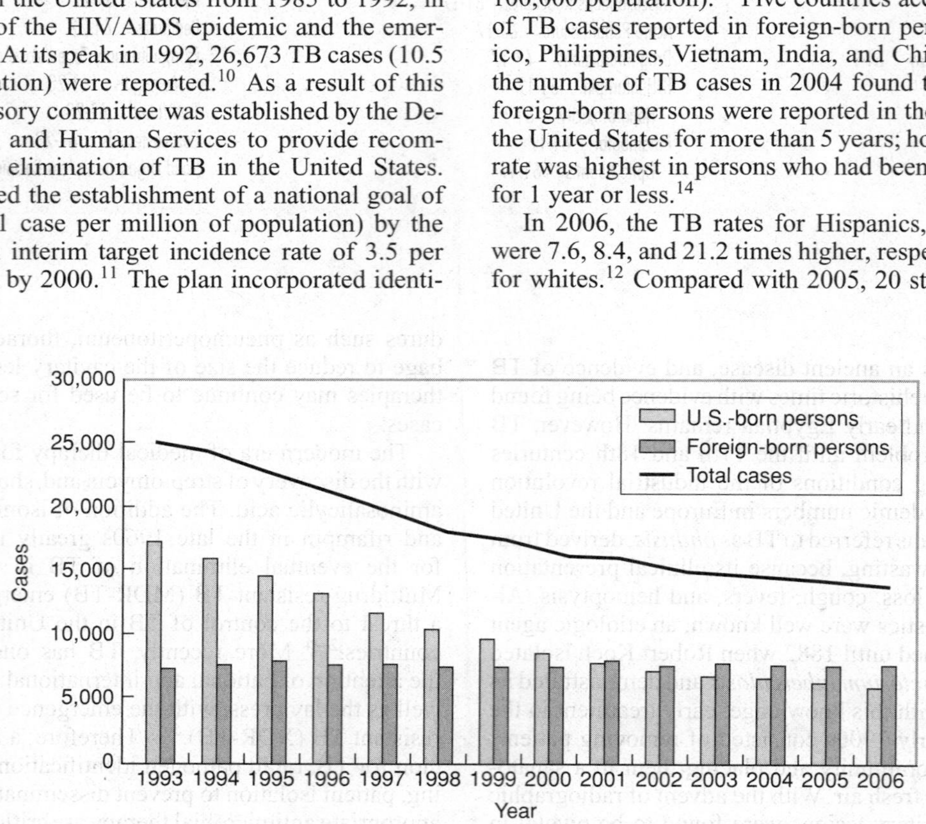

FIGURE 61-1 Reported cases of tuberculosis in the United States, 1993–2006.[12,13]

of Columbia had greater rates in 2006, whereas 30 states had lower rates.[12] Seven states accounted for 60% of all TB cases in the United States in 2006: California (2,781), Texas (1,585), New York (1,274), Florida (1,038), Illinois (569), New Jersey (508), and Georgia (504).[12] In 2005, TB cases were reported in 4.0% of residents in correctional facilities, 6.1% of homeless persons, 2.4% of residents in long-term care facilities, 2.2% of injecting drug users, 7.8% of noninjecting drug users, and 13.9% of persons with excess alcohol use.[13]

In the United States, a total of 124 cases of MDR-TB, defined as resistance to both isoniazid and rifampin, were reported in 2005.[12] The overall proportion of MDR-TB cases remained constant from 2004 to 2005 at approximately 1.2%, which remains lower than the incidence of 2.5% in 1993.[12,13] In recent years, most MDR-TB cases in the United States have been reported in foreign-born persons. In 1993, 410 cases of MDR-TB were reported and 105 (25.6%) were in foreign-born persons.[13] In 2006, 101 (81.5%) of the 124 MDR-TB cases were reported in foreign-born persons.[12]

In the last few years, XDR-TB has emerged as a major threat to global health.[5–7] These extensively resistant strains have been identified in many countries worldwide, including the United States. One of the first reports from South Africa described 53 patients infected with XDR-TB.[15] Of these patients, 55% had no prior history of TB treatment, and 52 (98%) died with a median survival period of only 16 days after the first sputum specimen was collected.[15] HIV testing was performed in 44 of these patients, and 100% of them tested positive.[15]

Evaluation of the incidence of infections caused by XDR-TB has been complicated by recent changes in the definition of XDR-TB. The most recent definition of XDR-TB is resistance to at least isoniazid and rifampin among first-line agents, resistance to any fluoroquinolone, and resistance to at least one second-line injectable drug (amikacin, kanamycin, or capreomycin).[16] Using the revised definition, 49 cases of XDR-TB have been identified in the United States between 1993 and 2006, which represent 3% of evaluable MDR-TB cases.[17] A total of 32 cases were reported between 1993 and 1999, and 17 cases were reported between 2000 and 2006.[17] Overall, 19 cases were reported in New York City, and 11 cases were reported in California. The percentage of XDR-TB cases among foreign-born persons increased from 38% in 1993 to 1999 to 76% in 2000 to 2006.[17] Mortality was strongly associated with concomitant HIV infection; 12 persons died, 10 of whom had HIV infection.[17] The HIV status of the other 2 persons was unknown.

Continued strengthening of TB control and treatment programs remains essential to the goal of TB elimination in the United States. To accomplish this goal, successful strategies for controlling and preventing TB among foreign-born persons must be developed.

Etiology

Tuberculosis is caused by *M. tuberculosis*, an aerobic, non–spore-forming bacillus that resists decolorization by acid alcohol after staining with basic fuchsin. For this reason, the organism is often referred to as an acid-fast bacillus (AFB). It is also different from other organisms in that it replicates slowly once every 24 hours instead of every 20 to 40 minutes as do some other organisms. *M. tuberculosis* thrives in environments where the oxygen tension is relatively high, such as the apices of the lung, the renal parenchyma, and the growing ends of bones.[1]

Transmission

Mycobacterium tuberculosis is transmitted through the air by aerosolized droplet nuclei that are produced when a person with pulmonary or laryngeal TB coughs, sneezes, speaks, or sings. Droplet nuclei can also be produced by other methods, such as aerosol treatments, sputum induction, bronchoscopy, endotracheal intubation, suctioning, autopsy, and through manipulation of lesions or processing of secretions in the hospital or laboratory.[18] These droplet nuclei, which contain one to three *M. tuberculosis* organisms, are small enough (1–5 μg) to remain airborne for long periods of time and reach the alveoli within the lungs when inhaled. Tubercle bacilli are not transmitted on inanimate objects such as dishes, clothing, or bedding, and organisms deposited on skin or intact mucosa do not invade tissue.

Several factors influence the likelihood of transmission of *M. tuberculosis*, including the number of organisms expelled into the air, the concentration of organisms in the air determined by the volume of the space and its ventilation, the length of time an exposed person breathes the contaminated air, and presumably the immune status of the exposed individual.[18] Family household contacts, especially children, and persons working or living in an enclosed environment (e.g., hospitals, nursing homes, prisons) with an infected person are at a significantly increased risk for becoming infected. Individuals with impaired cell-mediated immunity, such as HIV-infected persons or transplant recipients, are thought more likely to become infected with *M. tuberculosis* after exposure than persons with normal immune function.[18]

Several techniques are effective in limiting airborne transmission of *M. tuberculosis*. Adequate room ventilation with fresh air is very important, especially in the health care setting, where six or more room–air exchanges per hour is desirable.[18,19] New construction or renovation of existing facilities should be designed so that airborne infection isolation rooms achieve 12 or more room–air exchanges per hour.[19] Ultraviolet irradiation of air in the upper part of the room can also reduce the number of viable airborne tubercle bacilli. All health care workers and visitors who enter the room of a patient with TB should wear at least N95 disposable respirators, and the mask should be fit tightly around the nose and mouth.[19] Patients with presumed or confirmed infectious TB should wear a protective mask when being transferred to another area of the institution or to another institution.[19] The most important means of reducing transmission of *M. tuberculosis* is by treating the infected patient with effective antituberculosis therapy.

Pathogenesis

Latent Infection versus Active Disease

LATENT INFECTION

A clear distinction should be made between latent infection and active disease (tuberculosis). Latent infection occurs when the tubercle bacilli are inhaled into the body. After inhalation, the droplet nuclei containing *M. tuberculosis* settle into the bronchioles and alveoli of the lungs. Development of infection in the lung is dependent on both the virulence of the organism and the inherent microbicidal ability of the alveolar macrophages.[20,21] In the nonimmune (susceptible) host, the bacilli initially multiply unopposed by normal host defense mechanisms. The organisms are then taken into alveolar macrophages by phagocytosis and may remain viable, multiplying within the cells for extended periods of time. After 14 to 21 days of replication, the tubercle bacilli spread via the lymphatic system to the hilar lymph nodes and through the bloodstream to other organs. Certain organs and tissues in the body, such as the bone marrow, liver, and spleen, are, however, resistant to subsequent multiplication of these bacilli. In contrast, organs with high blood flow and PaO_2, such as the upper lung zones, kidneys, bones, and brain, are particularly favorable for growth of the organisms. The organisms replicate for 2 to 12 weeks until they reach 10^3 to 10^4 in number, then a specific T-lymphocyte–mediated immune response develops. The T cells secrete interferon-γ, interleukin-2, interleukin-10, and other cytokines, and activated macrophages engulf and kill the tubercle bacilli, preventing further replication.[18] At this point, the patient has developed cell-mediated immunity, which can be detected by a reaction to the tuberculin skin test.[18]

In persons with intact cell-mediated immunity, activated T lymphocytes and macrophages may form granulomas that limit multiplication and spread of the bacilli by walling off the infection from the surrounding environment.[18] The organisms tend to localize in the center of the granuloma, which is frequently necrotic. Although small numbers of tubercle bacilli may remain viable within the granuloma, proliferation of *M. tuberculosis* is halted when cell-mediated immunity develops. At this point, most persons with pulmonary tuberculosis infections are clinically asymptomatic and there is no radiographic evidence of the infection.[21] In some patients, there may be a healed, calcified lesion on chest radiograph, but bacteriologic studies are negative. A positive tuberculin skin test is usually the only indication that the person has been infected with *M. tuberculosis*. Individuals with latent TB infection are not infectious and thus cannot transmit the organism.[18]

ACTIVE DISEASE (TUBERCULOSIS)

In most patients, active TB disease results from reactivation of a previously controlled latent infection, termed reactivation tuberculosis. Approximately 10% of individuals who acquire TB infection and do not receive therapy for the latent infection will develop active TB disease. The risk of developing active disease is highest in the first 2 years after infection, when half of the cases occur.[18] The annual and lifetime risks for reactivation TB have been shown, however, to be directly related to the size of the induration on tuberculin skin testing. The risks for reactivation TB were greater in patients with larger induration diameters.[22] The ability of the host to respond to *M. tuberculosis* may also be reduced by certain diseases such as diabetes mellitus, silicosis, chronic renal failure, and diseases or drugs associated with immunosuppression (e.g., HIV infection, antitumor necrosis factor-α agents, organ transplantation, corticosteroids, and other immunosuppressive agents).[18,22] Persons infected with HIV, especially those with low CD4(+) T-cell counts, develop active TB disease rapidly after becoming infected with *M. tuberculosis*; up to 50% of these individuals develop active disease within the first 2 years of infection.[23] In addition, a person with untreated latent TB infection who acquires HIV infection will develop active TB disease at an approximate rate of 5% to 10% per year.[24,25] Physical or emotional stress can destroy the balance between the immune system and the infection, leading to active disease. Other factors that may contribute to developing active disease include gastrectomy, intestinal bypass surgery, alcohol abuse, hematologic disease, reticuloendothelial disease, and intravenous (IV) drug use. The elderly, adolescents, and children <5 years of age also are at an increased risk of developing active disease.[18,26]

DIAGNOSIS

Signs and Symptoms

Subjective Findings

1. M.W., a 36-year-old woman, is admitted to the hospital with a 2-month history of cough, which has recently become productive. She is also experiencing fatigue, night sweats, and has lost 15 pounds. Other medical problems include diabetes mellitus, which is controlled with 10 units of NPH insulin daily, and poor nutritional status secondary to frequent dieting. M.W. works as a volunteer in a nursing home several days a week. Recently, it was discovered that two patients who she had been caring for had undiagnosed active tuberculosis.

M.W.'s physical examination was normal, but her chest radiograph revealed bibasilar infiltrates. A tuberculin purified protein derivative (PPD) skin test, sputum collections for cultures and susceptibility testing, and a sputum AFB smear were ordered as part of M.W.'s diagnostic workup. Initial laboratory test findings were within normal limits.

The result of her tuberculin PPD skin test, read at 48 hours, was a palpable induration of 14 mm. Her sputum smear was positive for AFB, and additional sputum cultures for *M. tuberculosis* were ordered to confirm the diagnosis of active TB disease. What subjective and objective findings does M.W. have that are consistent with active TB disease?

M.W.'s history of cough (which gradually became productive), bibasilar infiltrates, fatigue, and night sweats are consistent with the classic symptoms of active TB.[18] The cough may be nonproductive early in the course of the illness, but with subsequent inflammation and tissue necrosis, sputum is usually produced and is key to most of the diagnostic studies. The sputum may contain blood (hemoptysis) in patients with advanced cavitary disease, which is particularly worrisome because cavitary lesions harbor large numbers of organisms and the pulmonary location allows for airborne transmission. Anorexia from TB, along with frequent dieting, may have resulted in M.W.'s weight loss. Other symptoms of TB can include fever, pleuritic pain secondary to inflammation of lung parenchyma adjacent to the pleural space, and general malaise. Dyspnea is unusual unless there is extensive disease.[18]

Objective Findings

M.W. has a chest radiograph consistent with a lower respiratory tract infection. In pulmonary TB, nodular infiltrates are usually found in the apical or posterior segments of the upper lobes, but markings may be found in any segment. M.W. also has a positive sputum smear for AFB, a positive PPD skin test (14 mm), and diabetes mellitus, which is a risk factor for TB. Although her laboratory test results are within normal limits, peripheral blood leukocytosis and anemia are the most common hematologic manifestations of TB.[18] The white blood cell count is normal or slightly increased, and an increase in monocytes and eosinophils may be observed.

Potential Misdiagnoses

Many patients with active pulmonary TB may have no acute symptoms, and cases are often found following routine chest radiographs for other illnesses. Because many of the symptoms of TB also occur in persons with pre-existing pulmonary disease or pneumonia, they may be overlooked and not attributed to TB.

A lack of clinical symptoms can also contribute to misdiagnosis of TB. Almost 50% of the cases of active TB may be misdiagnosed in the absence of classic symptoms.[27] More than one-third of the patients with active TB may have no sweats, chills, or malaise, and <50% are febrile. Cough may exist in 80% of these patients, and only 25% have hemoptysis. Although dullness over the apices of the lungs and post-tussive rales are expected in TB, less than one-third of these patients may have abnormal pulmonary signs. Reinforcing the need to consider this diagnosis, TB was not suspected in 42% of patients with active disease in a community hospital.[28] The lack of specific clinical symptoms underscores the importance of skin testing, sputum smears for AFB, and chest radiographs as diagnostic tools in those individuals suspected to have TB.

Tuberculin Skin Testing/Whole Blood Interferon-γ Assay

2. What is tuberculin skin testing? How should the results be interpreted in M.W.? What other test may be useful in the diagnostic work-up of M.W.?

The tuberculin skin test (Mantoux method) has been used as a diagnostic tool for infection with *M. tuberculosis* for decades, but a positive skin test is not necessary for the diagnosis of active TB disease.[29] The test is frequently referred to as the PPD test, which contains a protein prepared from a culture of the tubercle bacilli. The skin test is performed by injecting 0.1 mL of solution containing 5-TU PPD *intracutaneously* into the volar or dorsal surface of the forearm.[18,30] The injection is made using a one-quarter to one-half inch, 27-gauge needle and a tuberculin syringe, injected just beneath the surface of the skin, avoiding subcutaneous tissue.[18,31] A discrete, pale elevation of the skin (a wheal) 6 to 10 mm in diameter should be produced when the injection is performed correctly. If the first injection was administered improperly, another test dose can be given at once at a site several centimeters away from the original injection site.[18]

If the patient has previously been infected with *M. tuberculosis*, sensitized T cells are recruited to the skin site where they release cytokines.[32] These cytokines induce an induration (raised area) through local vasodilatation, edema, fibrin deposition, and recruitment of other inflammatory cells to the area.[18] Typically, the reaction to the tuberculin protein begins 5 to 6 hours after injection with maximal induration observed at 48 to 72 hours. Therefore, the test should be read between 48 and 72 hours after injection because tests read after 72 hours tend to underestimate the actual size of the induration.[18] For standardization, the diameter of the induration should be measured transversely to the long axis of the forearm and recorded in millimeters.[18,31] The diameter of the induration should be measured and not the erythematous zone surrounding the induration.

An induration ≥5 mm in diameter read 48 to 72 hours after injection is considered to be a positive reaction in an individual with a recent history of close contact with a person with active TB, a person with fibrotic changes on chest radiograph consistent with previous TB, organ transplant recipients and other immunosuppressed patients (receiving the equivalent of ≥15 mg/day of prednisone for >1 month), or HIV-positive persons.[18,30,33,34] Because M.W. has a history of close contact with two persons with active TB, her tuberculin skin test reaction to the PPD is positive (14 mm).

An induration ≥10 mm in diameter is considered to be a positive reaction in persons with clinical conditions that put them at increased risk for TB, such as diabetes mellitus, silicosis, chronic renal failure, malnutrition, leukemia, lymphoma, gastrectomy, jejunoileal bypass, and weight loss of >10% of ideal body weight.[18,30,34] In addition, an induration ≥10 mm is considered to be positive in recent immigrants (<5 years) from countries with a high prevalence of TB, injection drug users, residents and employees of high-risk congregate settings (e.g., prisons, nursing homes, homeless shelters), health care workers, mycobacteriology laboratory personnel, and children <4 years of age or infants, children, and adolescents exposed to adults in high-risk catgories.[18,30,34] The skin test is also considered positive for persons with an increase in induration diameter of ≥10 mm within a 2-year period.[30,34] For individuals with no risk factors for TB, an induration ≥15 mm is required for a positive reaction.[30,34]

Several limitations are seen when using tuberculin skin testing as a diagnostic tool for the detection of *M. tuberculosis* infection. Most importantly, the sensitivity and specificity of skin testing is poor in certain patients groups who are most at risk for TB infection, especially patients with HIV co-infection or foreign-born persons.[29] False–negative results can occur in patients with impaired cell-mediated immune response. False–positive results can result from infections caused by other mycobacterial species that cross-react with the *M. tuberculosis* antigen, including vaccination with a bacillus of Calmette-Guerin (BCG) vaccine. BCG vaccination increases the likelihood of a false–positive tuberculin skin test result for up to 15 years after administration.[35] False–positive results have been reported with some PPD preparations,[36] and an increase in skin test converters has also been reported after a change in skin testing preparations.[37] Therefore, one preparation should be used consistently in populations undergoing periodic testing.[37] Only experienced persons should read the Mantoux PPD skin tests, because the risk of error in performance and interpretation is high. In a study of 1,036 persons who each received two injections of 5-TU PPD from the same vial (one in each arm), 14.5% had an induration >10 mm in one arm and an induration <10 mm in the other arm, likely because of variability in the reading of the tests.[38]

An *in vitro* enzyme-linked immunosorbent assay (ELISA) test that detects the release of interferon-γ from T cells in whole blood of sensitized patients, QuantiFERON-TB Gold (Cellestis Limited, Carnegie, Victoria, Australia), has been approved by the U.S. Food and Drug Administration (FDA) as an aid in diagnosing *M. tuberculosis* infection, including both active TB disease and latent TB infection.[29,39] Aliquots of fresh (≤12 hours) heparinized whole blood are incubated with the test antigens, early secretory antigenic target-6 (ESAT-6) and culture filtrate protein-10 (CFP-10), for 16 to 24 hours. After incubation, the concentration of interferon-γ released by the T cells is determined by ELISA, and tests results are interpreted.[39] ESAT-6 and CFP-10 are secreted by all *M. tuberculosis* and pathogenic *M. bovis* strains but not from BCG vaccine strains. Therefore, this test is more specific for *M. tuberculosis* infection in BCG-vaccinated persons than tuberculin skin testing.[29] The test depends on adequately functioning T cells, and a negative result may reflect underlying *in vivo* immunosuppression, decreasing *in vitro* stimulation of the T cells.[29] In a study of 294 HIV-infected subjects, indeterminate results were more likely to occur in subjects with a CD4(+) count <100 cells/mm^3 compared with those with a CD4(+) count of ≥100 cells/mm^3.[40] Another study found only 64% sensitivity for detection of active TB disease, suggesting that this interferon-γ assay should not be used alone to exclude active TB.[41] False–negative results were more likely in patients with extrapulmonary TB or in patients who had received antituberculosis therapy for up to 2 weeks.[41]

3. Because M.W.'s Mantoux PPD skin test is positive, does this confirm her diagnosis of active TB?

No. M.W.'s positive reaction to 5-TU PPD alone does not confirm active TB disease. It merely signifies that she has previously been infected with *M. tuberculosis*. To confirm the diagnosis of active TB disease in M.W. and other patients, *M. tuberculosis* must be isolated from sputum, gastric aspirate, spinal fluid, urine, or tissue biopsy, depending on the site of infection.[18] As was done in M.W., the detection of AFB in stained smears is easy and fast, and it can provide the clinician with a preliminary confirmation of the diagnosis. Sputum samples for AFB stain and culture should be obtained early in the morning on at least three separate days.[42] Smears may be prepared directly from clinical specimens or from concentrated preparations.[18] The test is performed by placing the specimen on a glass slide under a microscope with a Ziehl-Neelsen or fluorochrome stain (not a Gram stain). Studies have shown, however, that 5,000 to 10,000 bacilli per milliliter of specimen must be present to allow for detection of AFB in stained smears.[18,43] In 2005, 42% of pulmonary TB cases were sputum smear negative.[13] Therefore, a negative AFB smear does not rule out active TB disease, and patients with active TB and negative AFB smears may play an important role in the ongoing transmission of *M. tuberculosis*.

Additional limitations of the AFB smear include its inability to differentiate among mycobacterial species and between viable and nonviable organisms. *Mycobacterium avium* complex is isolated more frequently from the sputum of patients in whom a diagnosis of TB is highly probable, such as the elderly and patients with HIV infection.[44] This has resulted in a marked decrease in the specificity and positive predictive value of the sputum smear.[45] Nucleic acid amplification (NAA) enhances and expedites the direct identification of *M. tuberculosis*. These technologies amplify specific target sequences of nucleic acids in *M. tuberculosis* that can be detected by a nucleic acid probe *within hours*. In the research laboratory, a positive result can be obtained from specimens containing as few as 10 bacilli, but the sensitivity is somewhat less in the clinical laboratory.[18] The AMPLIFIED *Mycobacterium Tuberculosis* Direct Test (MTD, GenProbe) and Amplicor *Mycobacterium tuberculosis* Test (Roche) are NAA assays available for commercial use in the United States.[44] The AMPLIFIED MTD test is FDA approved for use in both smear-positive and smear-negative specimens whereas the Amplicor test is only approved for smear-positive specimens.

The NAA tests accurately diagnose nearly every case of sputum smear-positive pulmonary TB (sensitivity 95%; specificity 98%); the tests will also diagnose approximately half of the smear-negative, culture-positive pulmonary TB cases and the specificity remains approximately 95%.[18,44] Some investigators suggest that NAA tests should not be performed if sputum smears are negative and if the index of clinical suspicion for active TB is low.[46] The CDC recommends that AFB smear and NAA be performed on the first sputum smear collected.[47] If the AFB smear and NAA are both positive, TB is diagnosed with near total certainty. If the AFB smear is negative and the NAA is positive, additional sputum samples should be obtained, and if positive, the patient can be presumed to have TB. If the AFB smear is positive and the NAA is negative, the patient can be presumed to have nontuberculous mycobacteria. If both AFB smear and NAA are negative, additional samples should be tested by NAA. If negative, the patient can be presumed not to have infectious TB.[44,47] NAA tests should not be used in patients who are being treated because the tests will amplify dead mycobacteria and cannot distinguish viable from nonviable strains.[46]

Some patients may have a negative AFB smear, but a sufficient number of organisms may be present to result in a positive culture. Only 10 to 100 organisms are needed for a positive culture.[18,48] As a result of the limitations of the AFB smear, a positive culture for *M. tuberculosis* is necessary to definitively diagnose TB in M.W. and all patients. In addition, the culture is of paramount importance because it is the only widely available technology that allows for drug susceptibility testing.[44] It is also important to reiterate that *M. tuberculosis* organisms grow slowly (i.e., once every 24 hours). Depending on the type of media and detection system, it may take several weeks for the cultures to become positive.[1,18] Broth-based culture systems, such as BACTEC, MGIT, MB/BacT, Septi-Check, and ESP, when combined with DNA probes, can produce positive results in 2 weeks or less for sputum smear-positive specimens and within 3 weeks for smear-negative specimens.[44]

4. Should M.W. be tested for HIV infection?

Yes, testing should be considered because TB may be the first manifestation of HIV infection.[1,49] Approximately 37% of patients infected with HIV develop active TB disease within 5 months compared with 5% of exposed persons with intact immune defenses.[23,50] A complete discussion of TB and HIV infection can be found in Questions 24 to 28.

5. Would a negative tuberculin skin test have eliminated the possibility of infection with *M. tuberculosis* in M.W.?

No, a negative response to 5-TU PPD in M.W. would not necessarily have excluded infection with *M. tuberculosis*. The

Table 61-1 Factors Associated with False–Negative Tuberculin Skin Tests

Factors related to the person being tested
Bacterial, viral, or fungal infections
Live virus vaccinations (measles, mumps, polio, varicella)
Chronic renal failure
Severe protein depletion
Diseases affecting lymphoid organs (Hodgkin's disease, lymphoma, chronic leukemia)
Corticosteroids, immunosuppressive agents
Age (newborns, elderly)
Factors related to the method of administration
Subcutaneous injection
Injecting too little antigen
Factors related to the tuberculin used
Improper storage (exposure to light and heat)
Improper dilution
Contamination
Factors related to reading the test and recording the results
Inexperienced reader
Error in recording

Adapted from reference 18, with permission.

PPD skin test has a reported false–negative rate of 25% during the initial evaluation of persons with active tuberculosis because of poor nutrition and general health, overwhelming acute illness, or immunosuppression.[18] False–negative results most often occur in persons who (a) have had no prior infection with *M. tuberculosis*, (b) have only recently been infected, or (c) are anergic. Factors that may result in a false–negative tuberculin skin test are shown in Table 61-1.

Anergy (i.e., decreased ability to respond to antigens) can be caused by severe debility, old age, immaturity in newborns, high fever, sarcoidosis, corticosteroids, immunosuppressive drugs, hematologic disease, HIV infections, overwhelming TB, recent viral infection, live-virus vaccinations, and malnutrition.[18] If anergy is suspected, control skin tests (candida, mumps, or trichophyton) should also be placed in the contralateral arm. If the control test results are positive and the PPD test result is negative, infection with *M. tuberculosis* is less likely. The CDC changed its recommendations regarding anergy skin testing in patients infected with HIV with a negative PPD. They cite problems with standardization and reproducibility, a low risk for TB associated with a diagnosis of anergy, and the lack of apparent benefit of therapy for latent TB infection in anergic patients who are infected with HIV. Therefore, the use of anergy testing in conjunction with PPD is no longer routinely recommended in this population or for other patients who are immunocompromised.[33,51,52]

Booster Phenomenon (PPD Skin Test)

6. S.N. is a 50-year-old male hospital employee who had a 7 mm induration after receiving his initial tuberculin skin test (PPD-Mantoux). Because of his age and previous hospital employment, it was decided to retest him 1 week later to rule out any booster effect. The result of the repeated skin test was a 12 mm induration. He denied any known exposure to persons with active TB. What is the significance of this reaction? Should S.N. be placed on INH therapy for latent TB infection?

Some persons experience a significant increase in the size of a tuberculin skin test reaction, which may not be caused by *M. tuberculosis* infection.[18,53] This reaction, or booster phenomenon, is not fully understood but may be caused by the tuberculin skin test itself when tests are performed every 1 to 2 years. It may also be caused by infection with other mycobacteria, remote TB, or prior BCG vaccination. When caused by a previous skin test, the booster phenomenon can occur as soon as 1 week after the previous test. The incidence of this reaction appears to increase with age.[54] Therefore, S.N.'s reaction may not represent infection with *M. tuberculosis*.

Serial, two-step tuberculin testing is recommended for health care workers,[18,55,56] so it is important to distinguish a possible booster reaction from a recent infection with *M. tuberculosis*. Persons who exhibit an increase in the size of the induration from <10 mm to >10 mm, as in the case of S.N., may be mistaken for a recent converter and unnecessarily given INH to treat a latent infection. To determine whether a reaction is caused by boosting rather than an infection, a second identical skin test should be administered 7 to 21 days after the first. The results of this test should be read in 48 to 72 hours. If the repeat test is positive (>10 mm), the reaction should be classified as a booster reaction, and the patient should not be treated with INH. If the repeat test is <10 mm but changes to positive (with a 6-mm increase) after 1 year, the person should be classified as a recent converter and treated accordingly (see Question 15). One report suggested using a 15 mm induration as the appropriate baseline in hospital employees tested annually.[57]

The increase in reaction size in S.N. is most likely caused by the booster phenomenon. Because he is >35 years of age, S.N. would not be an ideal candidate for INH therapy. S.N. should be given a repeat skin test next year and evaluated as previously described. He should not receive a two-step test in the future because this is only done on initial evaluation of an employee.

Bacillus of Calmette-Guerin (BCG) Vaccine

7. C. T., a 25-year-old female refugee from Vietnam, was given a routine physical examination on entering the United States. As part of this examination, she received a tuberculin skin test with 5-TU PPD. The test result was positive with an induration of 12 mm. She denied previous treatment for TB, but she remembered receiving a TB vaccine (BCG) several years ago. What is the BCG vaccine? Does this positive skin test indicate infection with *M. tuberculosis*?

A live vaccine derived from an attenuated strain of *M. bovis*, BCG, is used in many foreign countries with a high prevalence of TB to prevent the disease in persons who are tuberculin negative (no immunity to TB infection). Many different BCG vaccines are available worldwide, and all of them differ with respect to immunogenicity, efficacy, and reactogenicity. Additional factors, such as genetic variability in the subjects vaccinated, the nature of the mycobacteria endemic in different parts of the world, and the use of different doses and different immunization schedules, may contribute to the varied degrees of protection afforded by the vaccine. The protective effect derived from BCG vaccines in case-control studies has ranged from 0 to 80%.[58] Two meta-analyses concerning the efficacy of BCG vaccination for preventing TB attempted to calculate estimates of the protective efficacy of the vaccines. The results of the first meta-analysis indicated an 86% protective effect against meningeal and miliary TB in children in 10 randomized clinical trials and a 75% protective effect in 8 case-control studies.[59] In the second meta-analysis, the overall protective effect of BCG vaccines was 51% in 14 clinical studies and 50% in 12 case-control studies.[60] Vaccine efficacy rates were greater in studies in which persons were vaccinated during childhood compared to those vaccinated at older ages.[60] Neither study, however, was able to determine the vaccine's efficacy for preventing pulmonary TB in adolescents and adults.

Prior vaccination with BCG usually results in a positive tuberculin skin test, but skin test reactivity does not correlate with protection against TB.[18,58] No reliable method exists to distinguish tuberculin reactions caused by BCG vaccination from those caused by natural mycobacterial infections.[18,58] Therefore, it is prudent to consider positive reactions to 5-TU of PPD in BCG-vaccinated persons as indicating infection with *M. tuberculosis*, especially among persons from countries with a high prevalence of TB.[18] As mentioned previously, however, the interferon-γ assay, QuantiFERON-TB Gold, is more specific for *M. tuberculosis* infection in BCG-vaccinated persons than tuberculin skin testing.[29] Therefore, C.T. should have this test performed to determine presence of latent TB. If the interferon-γ assay cannot be performed, C.T. should be treated as though she has a positive tuberculin skin test (see Question 15). Because she is from an area with a high drug-resistance rate, the possibility of infection with organisms that are resistant to INH should also be considered (see Question 22).

Adverse reactions to the BCG vaccine vary according to the type, dose, and age of the vaccine. Osteitis, prolonged ulceration at the vaccination site, lupoid reactions, regional suppurative lymphadenitis, disseminated BCG infection, and death have all been reported.[58]

The BCG vaccine is not recommended for use in the routine prophylaxis of TB in the United States. The risk of exposure to TB in this country is relatively low, and other methods of control (e.g., treatment of high-risk groups) are sufficient. BCG vaccination should be considered for infants or children who are tuberculin negative and are continually exposed to a highly infectious, untreated patient with active TB or if the child is continually exposed to a patient with infectious pulmonary TB caused by *M. tuberculosis* strains resistant to INH and rifampin.[58] BCG vaccination of health care workers should be considered in settings where a high prevalence of patients are infected with MDR-TB, transmission of MDR-TB strains to health care workers and subsequent infection are likely, and comprehensive infection control precautions have been unsuccessful.[58] BCG vaccination is not recommended during pregnancy or for children or adults in the United States infected with HIV.[58]

TREATMENT OF ACTIVE DISEASE

Initial Therapy

Regimens

8. M.W.'s HIV test was negative. How should treatment be initiated in M.W., pending the results of the sputum culture and susceptibility testing? Can she transmit infection during treatment?

The overall goals for the treatment of TB are to cure the patient and to minimize the transmission of *M. tuberculosis* to others. The primary goals of antituberculosis chemotherapy are to kill the tubercle bacilli rapidly, prevent the emergence of drug resistance, and eliminate persistent bacilli from the host's tissues to prevent relapse.[61] To accomplish these goals, it is essential that treatment be tailored and supervision be based on each patient's clinical and social circumstances (patient-centered care). Effective treatment of TB requires a substantial period (minimum 6 months) of intensive drug therapy with at least two bactericidal drugs that are active against the organism. The initial phase of treatment is crucial for preventing the emergence of resistance and for the ultimate outcome of TB therapy.

Four basic regimens are recommended for the treatment of adult patients with TB caused by organisms that are known or presumed to be drug susceptible (Table 61-2).[61] Because M.W. has not been treated previously for TB, she should be started on INH, rifampin, pyrazinamide, and ethambutol. Previous guidelines recommended the addition of ethambutol only if the local prevalence of INH-resistant *M. tuberculosis* was $\geq$4%.[42,62,63] In the United States, however, 7.3% of *M. tuberculosis* isolates recovered from patients with no previous history of TB in 2005 were resistant to INH.[13] The prevalence of INH resistance was higher in foreign-born persons (9.8%) compared with those born in the United States (4.1%).[13] Because of the relatively high likelihood of TB caused by INH-resistant organisms, four drugs are necessary in the initial 8-week treatment phase. The initial four-drug regimen may be administered daily throughout the 8-week period (regimen 1), daily for the first 2 weeks and then twice weekly for 6 weeks (regimen 2), or three times weekly throughout (regimen 3).[61] On the basis of clinical experience, administration of drugs for 5 days/week is considered to be equivalent to 7 days/week administration and either may be considered daily. Five-day-a-week administration should always be given by directly observed therapy (DOT), however.[61] Drug dosages for these recommended regimens are listed in Table 61-3. In addition, two fixed-dose combination preparations are available in the United States: Rifamate, which contains INH 150 mg and rifampin 300 mg per capsule, and Rifater, which contains INH 50 mg, rifampin 120 mg, and pyrazinamide 300 mg per tablet. These formulations are a means of minimizing inadvertent monotherapy, especially when DOT is not possible, and decreasing the risk of acquired drug resistance by reducing the number of capsules or tablets that must be ingested each day.[61] Ethambutol can be discontinued as soon as the results from susceptibility testing demonstrate susceptibility to INH and rifampin. The incidence of streptomycin resistance has increased globally; therefore, streptomycin is no longer recommended as interchangeable with ethambutol unless the organism is known to be susceptible to the drug or the patient is from an area in which streptomycin resistance is unlikely.[61]

The appropriate initial regimen for M.W. may be optimized if drug susceptibility test results are available for the strains recovered from the two patients she had been caring for in the nursing home. M.W., who is diabetic and has a poor nutritional status, should also be given pyridoxine 25 mg/day because she may be at greater risk for the development of INH-induced peripheral neuropathy (see Question 17).

The high risk of transmission of *M. tuberculosis* to other patients and health care workers mandates that hospitalized

Table 61-2 Treatment Regimens for Pulmonary Tuberculosis Caused by Drug-Susceptible Organisms

Initial Phase			Continuation Phase				Rating[a] (Evidence)[b]	
Regimen	Drugs	Interval and Doses (Minimal Duration)	Regimen	Drugs	Interval and Doses[c] (Minimal Duration)	Total Doses (Minimal Duration)	HIV−	HIV+
1	INH, RIF, PZA, EMB	7 days/week for 56 doses (8 weeks) *OR* 5 days/week for 40 doses (8 weeks)[d]	1a	INH/RIF	7 days/week for 126 doses (18 weeks) *OR* 5 days/week for 90 doses (18 weeks)[d]	182–130 (26 weeks)	A (I)	A (II)
			1b	INH/RIF	Twice weekly for 36 doses (18 weeks)	92–76 (26 weeks)	A (I)	A (II)[f]
			1c[e]	INH/RPT	Once weekly for 18 doses (18 weeks)	74–58 (26 weeks)	B (I)	E (I)
2	INH, RIF, PZA, EMB	7 days/week for 14 doses (2 weeks) *then* twice weekly for 12 doses (6 weeks) *OR* 5 days/week for 10 doses (2 weeks)[d] *then* twice weekly for 12 doses (6 weeks)	2a	INF/RIF	Twice weekly for 36 doses (18 weeks)	62–58 (26 weeks)	A (II)	B (II)[f]
			2b[e]	INH/RPT	Once weekly for 18 doses (18 weeks)	44–40 (26 weeks)	B (I)	E (I)
3	INH, RIF, PZA, EMB	Three times weekly for 24 doses (8 weeks)	3a	INH/RIF	Three times weekly for 54 doses (18 weeks)	78 (26 weeks)	B (I)	B (II)
4	INH, RIF, EMB	7 days/week for 56 doses (8 weeks) *OR* 5 days/week for 40 doses (8 weeks)[d]	4a	INH/RIF	7 days/week for 217 doses (31 weeks) *OR* 5 days/week for 155 doses (31 weeks)[d]	273–195 (39 weeks)	C (I)	C (II)
			4b	INH/RIF	Twice weekly for 62 doses (31 weeks)	118–102 (39 weeks)	C (I)	C (II)

EMB, ethambutol; INH, isoniazid; PZA, pyrazinamide; RIF, rifampin; RPT, rifapentine.

[a]Definitions of evidence ratings: A = preferred; B = acceptable alternative; C = offer when A and B cannot be given; E = should never be given.

[b]Definitions of evidence ratings: I = randomized clinical trial; II = data from clinical trials that were not randomized or were conducted in other populations; III = expert opinion.

[c]Patients with cavitation on initial chest radiograph and positive cultures at completion of 2 months of therapy should receive a 7-month continuation phase (31-week; either 217 doses [daily] or 62 doses [twice weekly]).

[d]Five-day-a-week administration is always given by directly observed therapy (DOT). Rating for 5 day/week regimens is A (III).

[e]Options 1c and 2b should be used only in HIV-negative patients who have negative sputum smears at the time of completion of 2 months of therapy and who do not have cavitation on the initial chest radiograph.

[f]Not recommended for HIV-infected patients with CD4+ cell counts <100 cells/mL.

From reference 61, with permission.

persons with suspected or confirmed infectious TB be placed in respiratory isolation until they are determined not to have TB, they are discharged from the hospital, or they are confirmed to be noninfectious.[42] Based on M.W.'s subjective and objective findings, she should be placed in respiratory isolation. M.W.'s symptoms of TB should abate within the first 4 weeks. She would be considered to be noninfectious when she is receiving effective drug therapy, is improving clinically, and has had negative results for three consecutive sputum AFB smears collected on different days.[42] Patients who have responded clinically may be discharged to home despite positive smears if their household contacts have already been exposed and these contacts are not at increased risk of TB (e.g., infants, HIV-positive and immunosuppressed persons). In addition, patients discharged to home with positive smears must agree not to have contact with other susceptible persons.[42]

Fluoroquinolones as Initial Therapy

Interest in the fluoroquinolones for the treatment of TB dates back >20 years with a report describing the use of ofloxacin in 19 patients with chronic, drug-resistant disease.[64] In a more recent study from India, 92% to 98% of patients with newly diagnosed pulmonary TB had negative sputum cultures after 2 months of ofloxacin-containing regimens.[65] This study, however, did not have a standard control for comparison.

Several fluoroquinolones have in vitro activity against *M. tuberculosis*. The most potent activity has been reported with moxifloxacin and gatifloxacin; minimum inhibitory concentrations (MICs) for these agents are 4 to 8 times lower than for levofloxacin.[66] In murine models of TB, moxifloxacin, in combination with rifampin and pyrazinamide, has been shown to reduce the time to negative lung cultures by up to 2 months and produce stable cure compared with isoniazid, rifampin, and pyrazinamide.[67,68] In mice treated for 4 months, no relapses occurred in the moxifloxacin-containing regimen.[68]

In a recent study, moxifloxacin was compared with ethambutol in the first 2 months of treatment in adults with smear-positive pulmonary TB.[69] Patients were randomized to receive moxifloxacin 400 mg daily or ethambutol (based on body weight), and all patients received INH, rifampin, and pyrazinamide. Patients receiving moxifloxacin were more likely to have negative sputum cultures at 4 weeks (37% vs. 26%, $p = 0.05$) and at 6 weeks (54% vs. 42%, $p = 0.06$), but the 2-month conversion rates were 71% in each group.[69] Relapse rates were not evaluated in this study. Nausea was reported more frequently in the moxifloxacin group (22% vs. 9%, $p = 0.002$), but similar proportions of patients in each group

Table 61-3 Drugs Used in the Treatment of Tuberculosis in Adults and Children

Drug	Dosing (Maximal Dose)	Primary Side Effects	Dose Adjustment in Renal Impairment	Comments
First-Line Agents				
Isoniazid	Adults: 5 mg/kg (300 mg) daily; 15 mg/kg (900 mg) once, twice, or thrice weekly. Children: 10–15 mg/kg (300 mg) daily; 20–30 mg/kg (900 mg) twice weekly	Increased aminotransferases (asymptomatic), clinical hepatitis, peripheral neuropathy, CNS effects, lupus-like syndrome, hypersensitivity reactions	No	Peripheral neuropathy preventable with pyridoxine 10–25 mg; increased serum level of phenytoin. Hepatitis more common in older patients and alcoholics
Rifampin	Adults: 10 mg/kg (600 mg) once daily, twice weekly, or thrice weekly. Children: 10–20 mg/kg (600 mg) once daily or twice weekly	Pruritis, rash, hepatotoxicity, GI (nausea, anorexia, abdominal pain), flu-like syndrome, thrombocytopenia, renal failure	No	Orange-red discoloration of body secretions (sweat, saliva, tears, urine). Drug interactions caused by induction of hepatic microsomal enzymes (warfarin, antiretroviral agents, corticosteroids, diazepam, lorazepam, triazolam, quinidine, oral contraceptives, methadone, sulfonylureas)
Rifabutin	Adults: 5 mg/kg (300 mg) once daily, twice weekly, or thrice weekly. Children: unknown	Neutropenia, uveitis, GI symptoms, polyarthralgias, hepatotoxicity, rash	No	Orange-red discoloration of body secretions (sweat, saliva, tears, urine). Weaker inducer of hepatic microsomal enzymes than rifampin.
Rifapentine	Adults: 10 mg/kg (600 mg) once weekly during continuation phase. Children: not approved	Similar to rifampin	Unknown	Drug interactions caused by induction of hepatic microsomal enzymes (see rifampin).
Pyrazinamide	Adults: 20–25 mg/kg (2 g) daily; 40–55 kg: 2 g twice weekly or 1.5 g thrice weekly; 56–75 kg: 3 g twice weekly or 2.5 g thrice weekly; 76–90 kg: 4g twice weekly or 3 g thrice weekly. Children: 15–30 mg/kg (2 g) daily; 50 mg/kg twice weekly (2 g)	Hepatotoxicity, nausea, anorexia, polyarthralgias, rash, hyperuricemia, dermatitis	No	Monitor aminotransferases monthly
Ethambutol	Adults: 15–20 mg/kg (1.6 g) daily: 40–55 kg: 2 g twice weekly or 1.2 g thrice weekly; 56–75 kg: 2.8 g twice weekly or 2 g thrice weekly; 76–90 kg: 4 g twice weekly or 2.4 g thrice weekly. Children: 15–20 mg/kg (1 g) daily; 50 mg/kg (2.5 g) twice weekly	Optic neuritis, skin rash, drug fever	Yes	Routine vision tests recommended; 50% excreted unchanged in urine
Second-Line Agents				
Cycloserine	Adults: 10–15 mg/kg/day (1 g), usually 500–750 mg/day in two divided doses. Children: 10–15 mg/kg/day (1 g)	CNS toxicity (psychosis, seizures), headache, tremor, fever, skin rashes	Yes	May exacerbate seizure disorders or mental illness. Some toxicity preventable by pyridoxine (100–200 mg/day). Monitor serum concentrations (peak 20–35 mg/L desirable)
Ethionamide	Adults: 15–20 mg/kg/day (1 g), usually 500–750 mg/day in one daily dose or 2 divided doses. Children: 15–20 mg/kg/day (1 g)	GI effects (metallic taste, nausea, vomiting, anorexia, abdominal pain), hepatotoxicity, neurotoxicity, endocrine effects (alopecia, gynecomastia, impotence, hypothyroidism), difficulty in diabetes management	Yes	Must be given with meals and antacids. Monitor aminotransferases and thyroid-stimulating hormone monthly.

Table 61-3 Drugs Used in the Treatment of Tuberculosis in Adults and Children *(Continued)*

Drug	Dosing (Maximal Dose)	Primary Side Effects	Dose Adjustment in Renal Impairment	Comments
Second-Line Agents (*Continued*)				
Streptomycin	Adults: 15 mg/kg/day (1 g); ≥60 years, 10 mg/kg/day (750 mg). Children: 20–40 mg/kg/day (1 g)	Vestibular and/or auditory dysfunction of eighth cranial nerve, renal dysfunction, skin rashes, neuromuscular blockade	Yes	Audiometric and neurologic examinations recommended; 60% to 80% excreted unchanged in urine. Monitor renal function
Amikacin	Adults: 15 mg/kg/day (1 g); ≥60 years, 10 mg/kg/day (750 mg). Children: 15–30 mg/kg/day (1 g)	Ototoxicity, nephrotoxicity	Yes	Less vestibular toxicity than streptomycin. Monitoring similar to streptomycin.
Capreomycin	Adults: 15 mg/kg/day (1 g); ≥60 years, 10 mg/kg/day (750 mg). Children: 15–30 mg/kg/day (1 g) as single dose or twice weekly dose	Nephrotoxocity, ototoxicity	Yes	Monitoring similar to streptomycin.
Para-aminosalicylic acid (PAS)	Adults: 8–12 g/day in two to three doses. Children: 200–300 mg/kg/day in two to four divided doses	GI intolerance, hepatotoxicity, malabsorption syndrome, hypothyroidism	Yes	Liver enzymes and thyroid function should be monitored.
Levofloxacin	Adults: 500–1,000 mg/day	Nausea, diarrhea, headache, dizziness	Yes	Do not give with divalent and/or trivalent cations (e.g., aluminum, magnesium, iron)
Moxifloxacin	Adults: 400 mg/day	Nausea, diarrhea, headache, dizziness	No	See levofloxacin
Gatifloxacin	Adults: 400 mg/day	Nausea, diarrhea, headache, headache	Yes	See levofloxacin

CNS, central nervous system; GI, gastrointestinal.
Adapted from reference 61, with permission.

completed study treatment.[69] Controlled studies of other fluoroquinolones have also found sputum conversion earlier in therapy, but no difference in negative cultures at 2 months.[70,71] Lastly, fluoroquinolone resistance in *M. tuberculosis* has been described, occurring more commonly in multidrug-resistant isolates.[72]

Susceptibility Testing

Drug susceptibility testing is essential and should be performed on all initial isolates of *M. tuberculosis*; however, these results may not be available for several weeks after treatment is initiated. The maximal turnaround time for susceptibility testing is ≥30 days from the date of specimen collection.[73] To expedite this process, rapid tests for the detection of drug resistance are being developed, but none of the tests are currently approved by the FDA.[46] Tests using molecular beacons utilize fluorescent-labeled, hairpin-shaped DNA probes in which a fluorophore is adjacent to a molecule which prevents fluorescence.[46] Using a real-time polymerase chain reaction (PCR) assay, fluorescence occurs if the amplified PCR products have the wild-type gene sequence, but fluorescence is not detected if mutations are present in the target sequence. These tests have high sensitivity (89%–98%) and specificity (99%–100%) for rifampin resistance, but sensitivity is lower for detecting INH resistance.[46] Line probe assays and phage-based assays are commercially available, but more data are needed. One of the line probe assay kits, INNO-LiPA Rif. TB, is highly sensitive (>95%) and specific (>99%) for detecting rifampin-resistant *M. tuberculosis* in culture, but more data are needed for application of the test to clinical specimens.[46]

Contact Investigation

9. If M.W. is a risk to the community, does anyone need to know?

Yes! Each case of active TB disease must be reported to the local, state, or both public health departments.[18,42,73] This not only ensures proper therapy by monitoring adherence to therapy, but it also ensures that contact and source case investigations will be performed. They will attempt to evaluate all people who have been in close contact to M.W. so they may be evaluated for latent TB infection or active disease as well. Reporting of cases also permits record-keeping and surveillance to determine if public health TB control efforts are achieving their goal of preventing the spread of TB.[42,73]

Continuation Therapy

Regimens

10. Six weeks later, M.W.'s sputum cultures were positive for *M. tuberculosis*. Drug susceptibility tests demonstrated susceptibility to both INH and rifampin. What drug regimen should be

used for continued therapy of M.W.? How long should treatment be continued?

Successful treatment of uncomplicated TB can now be completed in 6 months (26 weeks) if INH, rifampin, pyrazinamide, and ethambutol are used for the first 2 months (8 weeks) and if patient adherence to the regimen and the organism susceptibility can be assured.[61] Therefore, after 8 weeks of DOT with INH, rifampin, pyrazinamide, and ethambutol, M.W.'s regimen may be reduced to INH and rifampin daily (5 days or 7 days per week) or two to three times per week under continued DOT for an additional 18 weeks (Table 61-2). Because M.W. is HIV-negative and her chest radiograph did not reveal cavitary lesions, she may also be a candidate for once weekly administration of INH and rifapentine, as long as her sputum AFB smear is negative after completing the initial 8 weeks of therapy.[61]

One study of 160 patients with both pulmonary and extrapulmonary TB demonstrated the effectiveness of a primarily twice-weekly treatment regimen. It consisted of INH 300 mg, rifampin 600 mg, pyrazinamide 1.5 to 2.5 g, and streptomycin 750 to 1,000 mg intramuscularly (IM) daily for 2 weeks, followed by the same drugs twice weekly at higher doses (except rifampin) for an additional 6 weeks. The regimen was then reduced to INH and rifampin twice weekly for the remaining 16 weeks (4 months). All doses were administered by DOT. Three months after beginning therapy, 75% of all patients studied had negative sputum cultures, and all patients were culture negative at 20 weeks. A 1.6% relapse rate (two patients) and only minor adverse effects were reported. Another important feature of this regimen is that it is highly cost effective. Among the 6- and 9-month regimens, it is the second lowest in cost, primarily because of the least number of patient–health care worker encounters (62 directly observed doses).[74]

If pyrazinamide cannot be included in the initial regimen, therapy should be initiated with INH, rifampin, and ethambutol for the first 8 weeks. Therapy should be continued with INH and rifampin for 31 weeks given either daily or twice weekly.[61] If drugs other than INH and rifampin are used in the initial phase, treatment must be continued for 18 to 24 months.[62]

Twice weekly administration of INH (900 mg) and rifampin (600 mg) is recommended for M.W. because this approach requires fewer doses and should result in substantial cost savings.[61,74] In addition, the relapse rate for the twice- and thrice-weekly INH and rifampin continuation regimens is significantly lower than the once-weekly regimen of INH and rifapentine 600 mg.[75,76] Five characteristics were identified to be independently associated with increased relapse risk in the INH and rifapentine group: sputum culture positive at 2 months; cavitation on chest radiograph; being underweight; bilateral pulmonary involvement; being a non-Hispanic white person.[76] A potential explanation for these results is the high protein binding of rifapentine (97%). A study evaluated the safety and tolerability of rifapentine 600 mg, 900 mg, and 1,200 mg once weekly (with INH 15 mg/kg) in 150 HIV-negative patients.[77] A trend toward more adverse events was observed in the 1,200 mg treatment arm ($p = 0.051$), but the 900-mg dose was well tolerated.[77] Relapse rates for the higher dose rifapentine regimens were not known, however. A subsequent study demonstrated that low plasma concentrations of INH were associated with failure or relapse with once-weekly INH and rifapentine.[78] Two patients who relapsed with *M. tuberculosis* monoresistant to rifamycin had very low INH concentrations.[78] Rapid acetylation status was a risk factor in those patients who failed or relapsed.[78] Rifamycin pharmacokinetics did not influence patient outcomes, however.[78]

Treatment with INH and rifampin should be continued for a minimum duration of 26 weeks. Recent recommendations suggest that a full course of therapy is determined more accurately by the total number of doses taken, not solely by the duration of therapy.[61] Thus, 26 weeks is the minimum duration of treatment and accurately indicates the amount of time the drugs are given only if there are no interruptions in drug administration.[61] Pyridoxine 10 to 25 mg/day should be continued throughout the treatment period. If M.W. is symptomatic or smear or culture is positive after 3 months of therapy, she should be re-evaluated for possible nonadherence with her therapy or infection with drug-resistant organisms. Evaluation should include a second culture and a second susceptibility test, consideration of DOT (if not already instituted), and consultation with experts in the treatment of TB.[42]

Directly Observed Therapy

11. What exactly is DOT, and why is it important that it be used in M.W.?

Directly observed therapy is the practice of a health care provider or other responsible person observing as the patient ingests and swallows the TB medications. DOT is the preferred core management strategy for *all* patients with TB.[42,46,61] The purpose of DOT is to ensure adherence to TB therapy. DOT not only ensures completion of therapy, but it may also reduce the risk of developing drug resistance. By improving these two factors, it also reduces the risk to the community. DOT can be administered with daily or two- to three-times-per-week regimens. It can be administered to patients in the office or clinic setting, or it be given at the patient's home, school, work, or other mutually agreed on place.[61,62] Often, enablers or incentives, such as food, clothing, or transportation, are used to improve adherence to DOT. A comprehensive review of DOT-related articles by a consensus panel of public health experts found that the completion rate of TB therapy exceeds 90% when DOT, as recommended by the CDC, is used along with enablers.[46,79] A study from San Francisco, California found that culture-positive patients treated for active pulmonary TB with DOT had significantly higher cure rates (97.8% vs. 88.6%, $p < 0.002$) and lower TB-related mortality (0% vs. 5.5%, $p = 0.002$) compared with patients treated using self-administered therapy.[80] Rates of treatment failure and relapse were similar between the two groups.[80] Although DOT is recommended for all patients, public health departments may not provide it for cost reasons. A study reported the cost-to-benefit analysis of DOT versus self-administered therapy. Although the initial cost of DOT is greater, when the costs of relapse and failure were included in the model, DOT was significantly less expensive, with differences up to $3,999.00 versus $12,167.00.[81] When drug resistance develops because DOT was not used, the cost of salvage therapy increases to $180,000.00 per patient![82] It is therefore widely accepted that patients with TB should receive DOT.[81,83]

Multiple Drug Therapy

12. Why is multiple drug therapy indicated for the treatment of active TB disease? What is the role of each drug in the treatment of TB?

The key to treating active TB disease is multiple drug therapy for a sufficient time to kill the organisms and to prevent development of resistant strains of *M. tuberculosis*. Most cavitary lesions contain 10^{9-12} organisms, and the frequency of mutations that confer resistance to a single drug is approximately 10^{-6} for INH and streptomycin, 10^{-8} for rifampin, and 10^{-5} for ethambutol.[61] Considering the many organisms involved, patients with active TB disease likely harbor organisms with random mutations that confer drug resistance to a given drug. If a single drug is given, it would reduce the number of drug-susceptible organisms but leave the drug-resistant organisms to replicate. By using multiple drug therapy, the likelihood of encountering organisms with mutations to multiple drugs is reduced. For example, the frequency of concurrent mutations to INH and rifampin would be 10^{-14} (10^{-6} for INH and 10^{-8} for rifampin), making simultaneous resistance to both drugs an unlikely event in an untreated patient.[61] Therefore, monotherapy has no place in the treatment of active TB disease.[61,82]

Multiple drug therapy also serves to sterilize the sputum and lesions as quickly as possible. The drugs available for the treatment of TB vary in their ability to accomplish this task.[61] Drugs effective against tubercle bacilli can be divided into first-line and second-line agents (Table 61-3). The foundation of treatment should be with first-line agents, such as INH, rifampin, pyrazinamide, and ethambutol. Of the various agents, INH has the most cidal activity versus rapidly multiplying *M. tuberculosis* during the initial phase of therapy (early bactericidal activity), followed by ethambutol, rifampin, and streptomycin.[84–86] Drugs that have potent early bactericidal activity more rapidly decrease the infectiousness of the patient and reduce the likelihood of developing resistance within the bacillary population.[61] Pyrazinamide has weak early bactericidal activity during the first 2 weeks of therapy and is less effective at preventing emergence of drug resistance than INH, rifampin, and ethambutol.[61,84,87] Therefore, pyrazinamide should not be combined with only one other agent when treating active TB disease. Rifampin also has activity against intracellular organisms that are usually dormant but undergo periods of active growth. This ability to penetrate and destroy the persistent intracellular organisms makes rifampin extremely valuable in short-course chemotherapy regimens.[88]

Pyrazinamide is most effective against tubercle bacilli in the acidic environment within the macrophage or areas of tissue necrosis. In addition, it is most effective in sterilizing lesions when used in the first 2 months of treatment, but it does not offer substantial sterilizing activity after 2 months. Pyrazinamide is an essential component of the short-course regimens and must be prescribed for regimens as short as 6 months to be effective.[61,62]

Ethambutol is bacteriostatic at low doses and bactericidal at higher doses. It is moderately effective against the fast-growing bacilli. It has little sterilizing activity and is primarily used to prevent the emergence of drug-resistant organisms.[62]

Streptomycin is bactericidal against the rapidly multiplying extracellular organisms and is effective when given daily for 2 months followed by two to three times weekly administration thereafter. In the past, streptomycin was administered by IM injection, but these IM injections were painful. Therefore, although it is not labeled for IV use, streptomycin may be given in 50 to 100 mL 5% dextrose in water or normal saline and infused over 30 to 60 minutes.[89] Also, as with all aminoglycosides, streptomycin can cause ototoxicity and nephrotoxicity.[62,89]

The other drugs used in the treatment of TB (capreomycin, amikacin, cycloserine, ethionamide, para-aminosalicylic acid) are usually reserved for cases involving drug-resistant organisms, treatment failures, drug toxicity, or patient intolerance to the other agents. Their use is discussed later in the chapter (see Question 23).

Monitoring Drug Therapy

Subjective Symptoms

13. What subjective and objective findings should be followed to ensure therapeutic efficacy and minimize drug toxicity? Should M.W. be followed closely after completion of her treatment regimen?

M.W. should be questioned about the occurrence of adverse reactions secondary to the INH and rifampin (Table 61-3). Specifically, she should be asked about anorexia, nausea, vomiting, or abdominal pain, which may be an indication of possible hepatitis. Because she has diabetes and is at greater risk for the development of peripheral neuropathy, she should be questioned about numbness and tingling in her extremities. INH-induced peripheral neuropathy, however, should not be a problem in M.W. because she is also taking pyridoxine, which should prevent this adverse effect. M.W. also should be examined for, and questioned about, petechiae or bruises, because thrombocytopenia occasionally is seen with intermittent rifampin therapy. This effect purportedly occurs more frequently with intermittent rifampin therapy, but it is rare at the currently recommended intermittent rifampin dose of 10 mg/kg/day (~600 mg).[62]

In a study comparing 6-month versus 9-month antituberculosis therapies of mostly INH and rifampin in 1,451 patients, the incidence of side effects was similar between the two groups. Adverse effects occurred in 7.7% of patients in the 6-month arm compared with 6.4% in the 9-month arm, a difference that was not statistically significant (95% CI, 0.0–4.6%).[90] Hepatic disturbances occurred in 1.6% of patients in the 6-month regimen, a nonsignificant difference from patients in the 9-month regimens (1.2%). Hematologic disturbances were rare at 0.2% and 0.0% in the 6-month and 9-month groups, respectively. Other reported effects, gastrointestinal (GI) problems, rash, and arthralgias, were minor and infrequent in both regimens.[90]

Objective Signs

A pretreatment complete blood count, platelet count, blood urea nitrogen (BUN), hepatic enzymes (serum aminotransferases), bilirubin, and serum uric acid should be evaluated. Baseline visual examination should also be considered for patients receiving ethambutol. These tests are performed to detect any abnormality that may complicate or necessitate modification of the prescribed regimen. They should be repeated if the patient experiences any evidence of drug toxicity or has abnormalities at baseline.[61,62]

M.W. is >35 years of age and at increased risk for development of drug-induced hepatotoxicity. INH can cause asymptomatic increases in serum transaminases as well as clinical hepatitis.[61] Pyrazinamide has also been associated with hepatotoxicity, but the incidence is less common at doses of 25 mg/kg/day. Transient asymptomatic hyperbilirubinemia and typically cholestatic hepatitis can occur in patients receiving rifampin.[61] Therefore, it is important that that patient be instructed about possible symptoms of hepatotoxicity, primarily nausea, vomiting, abdominal pain, anorexia, and jaundice. Monthly serum liver function tests (LFT) are no longer recommended because they are costly, transient, asymptomatic elevations occur, and it may result in discontinuation of optimal therapy. The CDC recommends that medical personnel question the patient about symptoms once monthly.[62]

Sputum cultures and smears for AFB should be ordered every 2 to 4 weeks initially and then monthly after the sputum cultures become negative. With appropriate therapy, sputum cultures should become negative in >85% of patients after 2 months. At this point, they will usually need only one more sputum smear and culture at the completion of therapy. Radiologic examination (chest radiographs) is not as important as sputum examination, but it may be useful at the completion of therapy to serve as a comparison for any future films.

Patients who are culture-positive at 2 months need to be carefully re-examined. Drug susceptibility testing should be performed to rule out acquired drug resistance, and special attention should be given to drug adherence (i.e., DOT should be used). If drug resistance is demonstrated, the regimen should be modified as needed (see MDR-TB, Question 23). Sputum cultures should also be obtained monthly until negativity is achieved.[62]

As was the case for M.W., weight loss and nutritional depletion are common in patients with active TB disease. In a large TB treatment study, 7.1% of patients experienced relapse, with relapse greatest in patients who were underweight at diagnosis (19.1% vs. 4.8%, $p < 0.001$) or with a body mass index < 18.5 kg/m^2 (19.5% vs. 5.8%, $p < 0.001$).[91] In those patients underweight at diagnosis (defined as ≥10% below ideal body weight), weight gain of 5% or less between diagnosis and completion of 2 months of therapy was independently associated with relapse (odds ratio 2.4, $p = 0.03$).[91] In addition, the relapse rate was 50.5% in underweight patients with a cavitary lesion on chest radiograph, positive sputum cultures after 2 months of therapy, and ≤5% weight gain in the first 2 months of therapy.[91] Therefore, it may be prudent to monitor M.W.,'s weight during the initial 2 months of therapy and M.W. may need to receive more intensive therapy or a longer duration of therapy.

Routine follow-up usually is not required after the successful completion of chemotherapy with INH and rifampin. It may be prudent, however to re-examine the patient 6 months after completion of therapy or at the first sign of any symptoms suggestive of active TB. This is especially important in patients who were slow to respond to therapy or who have significant radiologic findings at completion of therapy. These recommendations are only for those patients with organisms fully susceptible to the medications being used.[62]

Patients who are culture negative but have radiographic abnormalities consistent with TB should have an induced sputum or bronchoscopy performed to establish a microbiologic diagnosis and monitored radiographically. Patients with extrapulmonary TB should be evaluated according to the site of involvement.[61,62]

Treatment Failure

14. If M.W. does not respond to her current therapy, should one more drug be added to her regimen?

No! Adding a single drug to a failing regimen is the most common and devastating mistake in TB therapy today. This practice is essentially monotherapy because the assumption is that the organisms are resistant to the medications currently being used. Resistance to the new drug will eventually develop, further reducing the patient's chance of cure. At least two, and preferably three, new drugs to which susceptibility can be inferred should be added to lessen the probability of further acquired drug resistance. Empiric retreatment regimens may include a fluoroquinolone, an injectable agent (e.g., streptomycin, amikacin, or capreomycin), and an additional oral agent (e.g., para-aminosalicylic acid, cycloserine, or ethionamide).[61] New susceptibilities should be obtained and treatment adjusted accordingly.[1,61,82]

TREATMENT OF LATENT TB INFECTION

15. M.W.'s 38-year-old husband, S.W., is skin tested with 5-TU PPD to determine whether he is infected with *M. tuberculosis*. He has a 10 mm reaction to the tuberculin skin test, which is classified as positive. He does not have any clinical symptoms or radiographic findings suggestive of active TB at this time. Is he at risk of developing active disease? What are the current recommendations for drug therapy for persons with latent TB infection? Should S.W. be treated?

Because S.W. is a household contact of a person with active TB disease and has a positive tuberculin skin test, he is at great risk of becoming infected and developing active disease.[33,34] During the first year after infection from the source case, a household contact's risk of developing active disease is 2% to 4%, with persons having a positive skin test at the greatest risk.[62]

Treatment of latent TB infection is effective in preventing active TB disease in persons who have positive tuberculin skin tests and in those at risk for reactivation of active TB; therefore, it is strongly recommended.[33,34,42] Treatment decreases the population of tubercle bacilli and reduces future morbidity from TB in the groups at high risk for developing active disease. In clinical studies, INH prevents TB in up to 93% of persons who receive the drug, depending on the duration of therapy and patient adherence to the prescribed regimen.[33] Although debate regarding the issue continues, the benefits of treating latent TB infection outweigh the risks of INH-induced hepatitis because all persons infected with TB is at risk for developing active disease throughout their lifetime.[2,62]

S.W. is infected with *M. tuberculosis*, but he does not currently have active TB disease. In 2000, the CDC recommended four regimens for the treatment of latent TB infection, and daily

INH for 9 months was the preferred regimen.[33] Studies in HIV-negative persons indicated that 12 months of INH was more effective than 6 months; however, the maximal benefit on INH is likely achieved by 9 months. Daily INH for 6 months and twice weekly INH for 6 or 9 months are also recommended treatment options for latent TB infection.[33] In a population of 3,788 patients beginning INH treatment for latent TB, only 64% of patients completed at least 6 months of therapy.[92] Higher completion rates were associated with younger age, Hispanic ethnicity, and non-U.S. country of birth.[92] Lower completion rates were associated with homelessness, excess alcohol intake, and experiencing an adverse event.[92] One or more adverse event, generally age related, was reported in 18% of patients. INH-associated liver injury was seen in only 0.3% of patients.[92]

Because of concerns about INH toxicity and poor adherence secondary to the relatively long duration of therapy, shorter rifampin-based regimens were also recommended. Rifampin and pyrazinamide, daily for 2 months or twice weekly for 2 to 3 months, and daily rifampin monotherapy for 4 months were recommended alternatives to INH therapy.[33] In 2001, however, severe and fatal hepatitis was reported in two patients receiving rifampin and pyrazinamide for latent TB infection.[93] Both patients developed anorexia and malaise, and liver functions tests revealed an alanine aminotransferase and an aspartate aminotransferase (AST) greater than 20 times the upper limit of normal. The total bilirubin peaked at 17.8 mg/dL and 27.5 mg/dL in the first and second patient, respectively.[93] Later in the same year, the CDC reported an additional 21 cases of liver injury associated with the 2-month rifampin and pyrazinamide regimen.[94] Of these 21 cases, 16 patients recovered and 5 patients died of liver failure. The onset of liver injury occurred during the second month of the 2-month course in those who died.

To reduce the risk of liver injury associated with rifampin and pyrazinamide therapy, the American Thoracic Society and the CDC, with the endorsement of the Infectious Diseases Society of America, have published revised recommendations for the treatment of latent TB infection.[94] For persons not infected with HIV, daily INH therapy for 9 months remains the preferred regimen, and 4 months of daily rifampin is an acceptable alternative. The 2-month rifampin and pyrazinamide regimen should be used with caution, if at all, especially in patients receiving medications associated with liver injury or those with alcoholism. No more than a 2-week supply of INH and pyrazinamide should be dispensed at a time to facilitate periodic clinical assessments of the patient. Serum aminotransferases and bilirubin should be measured at baseline, and at 2, 4, and 6 weeks of treatment in patients receiving the rifampin and pyrazinamide regimen.[94]

Daily rifampin for 4 months was compared with daily INH for 9 months to assess completion of therapy and costs in a relatively small study of patients with latent TB infection.[95] For the patients randomized to rifampin, 91% took 80% of the doses, and 86% took more than 90% of the doses at 20 weeks.[95] For the patients randomized to INH, 76% took 80% of the doses, and only 62% took more than 90% of the doses at 43 weeks.[95] Discontinuation of therapy because of adverse events was more common in the INH group (14%) versus the rifampin group (3%), and the total cost of therapy was significantly less in the rifampin group.[95] Rifampin for 4 months is an effective, safe, and affordable strategy to consider when treating latent TB infection in selected populations of patients.[95,96]

In a study of 399 household contacts of patients with newly diagnosed pulmonary TB with a positive PPD, TB rates, adverse events, and adherence to therapy were compared between weekly rifapentine and isoniazid for 12 weeks and daily rifampin and pyrazinamide for 8 weeks.[97] Adherence to therapy was $\geq$95% in both groups. Four patients developed active TB disease: three in the rifapentine and INH group and one in the rifampin and pyrazinamide group (p = NS).[97] Of patients in the rifapentine and INH group, 1% experienced hepatotoxicity compared with 10% in the rifampin and pyrazinamide group. Although more data are needed, weekly rifapentine and INH may be an alternative for treatment of latent TB infection.

S.W. should be placed on INH 300 mg/day for at least 6 months and preferably up to 9 months or rifampin for 4 months.[33,94] Although at increased risk of developing INH-associated liver damage (2.3%) because of his age, S.W. also has a high risk for developing active TB. In this case, the benefits of treatment outweigh the possible risks of hepatitis. S.W. should be educated and questioned frequently about the clinical symptoms of hepatitis, such as GI complaints. Pretreatment serum aminotransferases and bilirubin should be assessed to rule out pre-existing liver disease. The American Thoracic Society and the CDC do not recommend routine monitoring of LFT unless symptoms suggest hepatotoxicity.[62]

ADVERSE DRUG EFFECTS

Isoniazid

Hepatotoxicity

16. After 2 months of INH therapy, S.W. was found to have an AST of 130 U/L (normal, 7–40). Discuss the presentation, prognosis, and mechanism of INH-induced hepatitis. What are the risk factors for developing hepatitis? Should INH be discontinued to prevent further liver damage?

[SI unit: 130 U/L]

Approximately 10% to 20% of patients treated with INH alone for latent TB infection will develop elevated serum aminotransferases, which are generally transient and asymptomatic.[61,98] Most patients with mild, subclinical hepatic damage do not progress to overt hepatitis and recover completely even while continuing INH. In contrast, continuation of INH in patients with symptoms of hepatitis increased the risk of mortality compared with immediate discontinuation.[61] The risk of death from TB, however, is estimated to be 11 times higher than the risk of death from INH hepatotoxicity.[99]

Isoniazid-induced hepatotoxicity generally occurs within weeks to months of initiating therapy; 60% of cases occur in the first 3 months and 80% occur in the first 6 months.[98] Constitutional symptoms may be seen early and may last from days to months. Nausea, vomiting, and abdominal pain are seen in 50% to 75% of patients with severe hepatotoxicity.[98] Jaundice, dark urine, and clay-colored stools may also be seen. Recovery may take weeks after discontinuing INH therapy. The development of INH hepatotoxicity has been linked to several factors, including acetylator phenotype, age, daily alcohol consumption, and concurrent rifampin use. Additionally, women may be at higher risk of death, especially during the postpartum period.[99]

The mechanisms responsible for INH hepatotoxicity remain unclear. Previously, it was thought that rapid acetylators had a greater risk for INH hepatotoxicity than slow acetylators. Rapid acetylators of INH form monoacetylhydrazine, a compound that can cause liver damage, more rapidly than slow acetylators.[100] Rapid acetylators also would eliminate monoacetylhydrazine at a faster rate, however, and this should equalize the risk of toxicity between slow and fast acetylators.[101] One study demonstrated a different incidence of hepatitis between Asian males and females. Because both groups were fast acetylators, this study suggests that hepatitis is associated with factors other than acetylator phenotype.[102] Acetylator status alone does not explain the development of INH hepatotoxicity. Some evidence supports the theory that INH-induced hepatitis is a hypersensitivity reaction; however, many patients tolerate INH on rechallenge, discounting this theory.[103,104]

Age and concurrent daily alcohol ingestion are the most consistent risk factors for INH hepatitis.[62] Progressive liver damage is rare in persons <20 years of age. It occurs in approximately 0.3% of persons between the ages of 20 and 34 years, 1.2% of those between the ages of 35 and 49 years, and 2.3% of persons >50 years of age.[62] One prospective cohort study, however, demonstrated a low incidence of INH hepatitis. Of 11,141 patients receiving INH alone for the treatment of latent TB infection, only 11 (0.1% of those starting and 0.15% of those completing therapy) developed clinical hepatitis.[105] Previous studies suggested a higher incidence of clinical hepatitis in patients receiving INH alone, and a meta-analysis of six studies estimated the rate to be 0.6%.[61]

High-risk patients should be followed with routine monitoring of LFT. These patients include those who consume alcohol daily, persons >35 years of age, those taking other hepatotoxic drugs, those with pre-existing liver disease, IV drug abusers, black and Hispanic women, and all postpartum women. In these high-risk patients, INH should be discontinued if the AST level exceeds three to five times the upper limit of the normal value.[62] Because S.W.'s AST is three times the upper range of the normal value and he is >35 years of age, INH should be discontinued temporarily until the AST returns to normal. At that time, INH should be resumed, and his LFT rechecked. If the AST increases again, the drug should be discontinued and S.W. should be followed frequently for development of active TB.

17. C.M., a 50-kg, 35-year-old woman, is being treated for active TB disease with INH 1,200 mg and rifampin 600 mg twice weekly. Is 1,200 mg of INH twice weekly an appropriate dose for a 50-kg patient? What INH side effects, other than hepatotoxicity, should be anticipated?

The usual twice-weekly INH dose is 15 mg/kg, with a maximal dose of 900 mg; therefore, C.M. should be receiving no more than 900 mg rather than 1,200 mg of INH. Although high doses or increased serum concentrations have not been linked with hepatitis, elevated serum INH concentrations have been associated with increased central nervous system (CNS) effects, ranging from somnolence to psychosis and seizure. GI complaints are also more commonly observed at doses >20 mg/kg.

Peripheral Neuropathy

Although uncommon at the both the recommended daily and intermittent doses, INH can cause a peripheral neuropathy by interfering with pyridoxine (vitamin B_6) metabolism.[33,61] As many as 20% of patients may experience this problem with INH doses >6 mg/kg/day. Numbness or tingling in the feet or hands is the most common neuropathic symptom. In patients with medical conditions where neuropathy is common, such as diabetes mellitus, alcoholism, HIV infection, malnutrition, and renal failure, supplemental pyridoxine 25 mg/day should be given with INH.[33,61] Women who are pregnant or breastfeeding and persons with seizure disorders should also receive supplemental pyridoxine with INH.[33]

Allergic Reactions

Allergic reactions consisting of arthralgias, skin rash, swelling of the tongue, and fever have also occurred. INH has been associated with arthritic symptoms and systemic lupus erythematosus; approximately 20% of patients receiving INH develop antinuclear antibodies.[61]

Other Reactions

Other reactions that might occur with INH are dry mouth, epigastric distress, CNS stimulation and depression, psychoses, hemolytic anemia, pyridoxine-responsive anemia, and agranulocytosis.[103]

Drug Interactions

In addition to the previously mentioned adverse reactions, INH is a relatively potent inhibitor of several cytochrome P450 isoenzymes (CYP2C9, CYP2C19, CYP2E1), but has minimal effects on CYP3A.[61] INH inhibits the hepatic metabolism of phenytoin and carbamazepine, resulting in increased plasma concentrations of these drugs. Patients receiving either of these two drugs with INH should be observed for signs of phenytoin or carbamazepine toxicity, such as nystagmus, ataxia, headache, nausea, or drowsiness. Plasma phenytoin and carbamazepine concentrations should be monitored periodically so that the doses can be adjusted if necessary. Carbamazepine also may induce INH hepatitis by inducing its metabolism to toxic metabolites.[106] In addition, INH inhibits the metabolism of diazepam and triazolam. It is important to note that rifampin has the exact opposite effect on hepatic metabolism. Rifampin is a stronger inducer than INH is an inhibitor as documented by the fact that INH-rifampin combination therapy induces the metabolism of diazepam, phenytoin, and other agents metabolized by the cytochrome P450 system.[107]

Rifampin

Flu-like Syndrome

18. One month after beginning her twice-weekly DOT regimen, C.M. developed symptoms of myalgias, malaise, and anorexia. Laboratory data were normal except for a slightly decreased platelet count. Could C.M.'s symptoms be related to her drug therapy? What adverse reactions other than hepatotoxicity should be anticipated in a patient receiving rifampin?

A flu-like syndrome has been reported in about 1% of patients receiving intermittent rifampin administration. This syndrome is rarely seen with usual doses of 600 mg twice weekly, but the incidence increases with twice-weekly doses >900 mg. The incidence also increases if the dosage interval is increased to 1 week or longer.[108,109] Unless the symptoms are severe, discontinuation of the drug is unnecessary. Because C.M. is receiving rifampin 900 mg twice weekly, her dose should be reduced to 600 mg and administered daily until the symptoms subside. The temporary administration of a nonsteroidal anti-inflammatory drug (NSAID) has been used to alleviate the flu-like symptoms. Twice-weekly therapy may then be resumed as long as the dose of rifampin dose does not exceed 600 mg.

Hepatotoxicity

Rifampin (rifapentine) is associated with a <1% rate of hepatotoxicity. Therefore, the risk of drug-induced hepatotoxicity is greater with INH than with rifampin. On occasion, rifampin can cause hepatocellular injury and potentiate hepatotoxicity of other antituberculosis drugs.[98] Although elevations of liver enzymes are seen on occasion, rifampin is more likely to produce cholestasis, as manifested by increases in alkaline phosphatase and hyperbilirubinemia without hepatocellular injury.[98] Elevations of all liver function tests may be seen transiently during the first month of rifampin therapy, but they are usually benign.[61]

Thrombocytopenia

Thrombocytopenia is more frequently associated with intermittent or interrupted rifampin administration, likely caused by production of IgG and IgM antibodies to rifampin. These antibodies likely fix complement onto the platelets, resulting in platelet destruction. Hypothetically, intermittent or interrupted rifampin therapy results in increased antibody production resulting in destruction of platelets. Once thrombocytopenia occurs with rifampin, its subsequent use is contraindicated because the problem will likely recur.[110,111]

Miscellaneous Reactions

In addition to the side effects associated with high-dose, intermittent therapy, 3% to 4% of patients taking normal doses of rifampin may experience adverse reactions.[110] The most common of these are nausea, vomiting, fever, and rash. Other reactions to rifampin include the hepatorenal syndrome hemolysis, leukopenia, anemia, and arthralgias as part of a suspected drug-induced lupus syndrome.[61,112] The development of these latter reactions would require discontinuation of the drug.

Acute Renal Failure

Acute renal failure has also occurred rarely with rifampin.[61] This hypersensitivity reaction may occur with both intermittent and daily administration and may last as long as 12 months.[108] Rifampin should be discontinued, and other drugs (e.g., pyrazinamide and ethambutol) should be given. The dose of ethambutol should be adjusted for renal dysfunction. Both rifampin and INH may, however, be given in normal dosages to patients with pre-existing renal failure.[113,114]

Another important characteristic of rifampin relates to its chemical makeup. It is an orange-red crystalline powder that is distributed widely in body fluids. As a result, it can discolor saliva, tears, urine, and sweat.[61] Patients using rifampin should be warned of this effect and cautioned not to use soft contact lenses because of possible discoloration. This effect may also be used to monitor adherence to rifampin therapy.

Drug Interactions

Rifampin is a potent inducer of cytochrome P450 isoenzymes, especially CYP3A4.[61] The rifamycins differ in their ability to induce cytochrome P450 isoenzymes, in which rifampin is the most potent, rifapentine is intermediate, and rifabutin is the least potent enzyme inducer.[61] Rifampin increases the metabolism of protease inhibitors, nonnucleoside reverse transcriptase inhibitors, macrolide antibiotics, azole antifungal agents, corticosteroids, oral contraceptives, warfarin, cyclosporine, tacrolimus, theophylline, phenytoin, quinidine, diazepam, propranolol, metoprolol, sulfonylureas, verapamil, nifedipine, diltiazem, enalapril, and simvastatin.[61,107] While the patient is receiving rifampin, it may be necessary to monitor serum concentrations of the aforementioned drugs, where appropriate, or increase their dosages. Also, women who are taking rifampin and oral contraceptives should use an alternative method of birth control. When treating any patient with rifampin, the health care professional should carefully evaluate all concomitant medications for the possibility of drug–drug interactions.

INH-Rifampin

Hepatotoxicity

19. Does the combination of INH and rifampin cause hepatotoxicity more frequently than either drug alone?

Some initial evidence suggested that the use of INH and rifampin together was associated with a greater incidence of hepatotoxicity. The mechanism was thought to be owing to rifampin induction of the metabolism of INH to either monoacetylhydrazine or to other hepatotoxic products of hydrolysis. Steele et al.[104] performed a meta-analysis reviewing the incidence of hepatitis between 1966 and 1989 using regimens that contained INH without rifampin, rifampin without INH, and regimens containing both drugs. They found the incidence of clinical hepatitis was greater in regimens containing both INH and rifampin (2.7%) versus regimens of INH alone (1.6%), but this effect was additive, not synergistic, and therefore expected.[104] The use of the two drugs together, therefore, is not contraindicated. Caution should be used in high-risk groups such as the elderly, alcoholics, those receiving concomitant hepatotoxic agents, and those with pre-existing liver disease.[98]

Ethambutol

Optic Neuritis

20. S.E., a 65-year-old woman, was placed on INH 300 mg/day, rifampin 600 mg/day, pyrazinamide 900 mg/day, and ethambutol 1,200 mg/day for initial treatment of active pulmonary TB.

Two months after the initiation of therapy, she began to complain of blurred vision. A routine eye examination and visual field tests yielded a diagnosis of optic neuritis. No evidence was seen of glaucoma, cataracts, or retinal damage. Laboratory tests were within normal limits except for an elevated serum uric acid (9.7 mg/dL; normal, 2–8 mg/dL) and a slightly elevated serum creatinine (SrCr) (1.6 mg/dL; normal, 0.6–1.4 mg/dL). No symptoms of joint pain were associated with the elevated serum uric acid, and there was no history of gout. Her calculated creatinine clearance (ClCr) based on her weight of 65 kg was 35 mL/minute. Could the visual problem and increased uric acid levels be related to her medications?

[SI units: uric acid, 576.96 mol/L; SrCr, 123.76 mol/L; ClCr, 0.83 mL/sec]

S.E.'s decrease in visual acuity is compatible with ethambutol-induced optic neuritis. This condition is characterized by central scotomas, loss of red-green color vision, or less commonly, a peripheral vision defect. The intensity of these ocular effects is related to the duration of continued therapy after decreased visual acuity is first noted. The optic neuritis is dose and duration related. The optic neuritis is rare at doses of 15 mg/kg.[115–117] The incidence is estimated to be 6% for doses of 25 mg/kg and increases to 15% for doses >35 mg/kg. Recovery, which may take many months, is usually, but not always, complete when the drug is discontinued.

The optic neuritis manifested in S.E. is probably caused by the use of an increased ethambutol dose (18.5 mg/kg) in a patient with impaired renal function (estimated ClCr 35 mL/minute). Because ethambutol adds no additional benefit to the INH and rifampin regimen after the first 2 months unless drug-resistant organisms are suspected, it can be discontinued. Because ethambutol is excreted by the kidney (50%–80%), her ethambutol dosage interval (or dosage) for ethambutol should have been increased based on the decline in creatinine clearance.[113] Her visual acuity should be monitored closely through periodic eye examinations, and she should be instructed to contact her physician immediately if she experiences any further visual changes.

S.E.'s elevated serum uric acid also may be attributed to her ethambutol as well as a decline in her renal function, but it is more likely caused by pyrazinamide, which decreases the tubular secretion of urate.[90] Asymptomatic hyperuricemia secondary to drugs usually does not require treatment.

SPECIAL TREATMENT CONSIDERATIONS

The Elderly

Incidence

21. G.H., a 75-year-old, 80 kg man who resides in a nursing home, becomes disoriented, refuses to eat, and has a productive cough. Physical examination reveals a thin man who is having slight difficulty breathing. Laboratory findings are essentially normal with the exception of a slightly elevated BUN of 25 mg/dL (normal, 10 to 20 mg/dL) and SrCr of 1.3 mg/dL (normal, 0.6–1.3 mg/dL). A chest radiograph reveals infiltrates in the right lower lobe; he has a history of congestive heart failure, which is well controlled. Blood, urine, and sputum samples are sent for culture and susceptibility testing; the initial Gram stain is negative. Because the nursing home has recently had two cases of active TB, a PPD skin test and sputum smear for AFB are ordered. The PPD skin test induration is 16 mm, and the sputum smear is positive for AFB. G.H.'s admission skin test several months ago was negative. Discuss the presentation of TB in the elderly, and the appropriate treatment of active disease in G.H. Is the incidence of drug side effects higher in the elderly? Should other patients in close contact with G.H. receive INH therapy?

[SI units: BUN, 8.93 mmol/L of urea (normal, 3.57–7.14); SrCr, 114.92 mol/L (normal, 53.04–88.4)]

The case rate of TB in adults ≥65 years is increased over all other age groups (7.7 per 100,000 population).[13] In 2005, 2.4% of TB cases were reported in residents of long-term care facilities,[13] and the case rate for nursing home residents is 1.8 times higher than that for elderly persons living in the community.[118] Active TB disease in the elderly has been attributed to a decrease in the immune system followed by reactivation of an earlier infection, but active disease is a common, endemic infection in nursing home patients with no previous immunity (negative skin test) to *M. tuberculosis*.[118,119] The incidence of positive skin tests increases after patients have been in the nursing home >1 month. Therefore, all patients entering a nursing home should be tested with 5-TU PPD. If the initial test is negative and a source case is present in the nursing home (as illustrated by this case), this test should be repeated in 1 month. The rate of tuberculin skin test conversion (from negative to positive tests) in this population is approximately 5%. If these recent converters are not treated with INH, approximately 17% will develop progressive pulmonary TB.[120]

Diagnosis

The diagnosis of active TB in elderly patients is difficult because the classic symptoms of TB (cough, fever, night sweats, weight loss) are often absent, and elderly patients may describe their symptoms poorly. The chest radiograph and PPD skin test may be the only signs of TB infection.[118,120] Frequently, the chest radiograph is atypical, resembling pneumonia or worsening heart failure. Chest radiographs in the elderly are less likely to have upper lobe infiltration, but more commonly have extensive infiltration of both lungs.[121] If the patient's clinical disease is caused by granuloma breakdown (reactivation), the chest radiograph often shows apical infiltrates or nodules. If the disease is progressing from an initial infection, as in the case of G.H., lower lobe infiltrates may be present.[118] TB in this population may present clinically with changes in activities of daily living, chronic fatigue, cognitive impairment, anorexia, or unexplained low-grade fever. Nonspecific signs and symptoms that range in severity from subacute to chronic and that persist for weeks to months must alert clinicians to the possibility that unrecognized TB is present.[122] Sputum examination for *M. tuberculosis*, and AFB smear and culture should be performed in all patients, including the elderly.

Treatment of Active Disease in the Elderly

The principles of TB treatment are the same for the elderly as for any other age group.[61,118] Because G.H. has clinical symptoms of a respiratory infection, positive sputum smears for AFB, and a positive tuberculin skin test, he should be treated with a four-drug regimen for active TB disease. Most TB cases in elderly patients are caused by drug-susceptible strains of *M. tuberculosis*; however, notable exceptions would be older patients who are from a country or region where the prevalence of drug-resistant strains is high, persons who have been inadequately treated in the past, or persons who acquired the infection from a recent contact known to be infected with drug-resistant *M. tuberculosis*.[122] G.H.'s drug regimen likely would include INH 300 mg, rifampin 600 mg, pyrazinamide 20 to 25 mg/kg daily, and ethambutol 15 to 20 mg/kg daily for 8 weeks followed by INH and rifampin daily or 2 to 3 times a week for 16 weeks (DOT). Another option might be INH, rifampin, pyrazinamide, and ethambutol daily for 2 weeks, followed by twice weekly for 6 weeks, then INH and rifampin twice weekly for 16 weeks.[122] Some clinicians prefer treating the elderly with 9-month regimens of INH and rifampin. G.H. should also receive pyridoxine 10 to 50 mg with each dose.[62]

Adverse Drug Effects

Although INH hepatitis is more common in elderly patients, both INH and rifampin are generally well tolerated within this age group, with major hematologic or hepatic side effects occurring in 3% to 4% of patients.[123] Therefore, serum aminotransferases should be assessed at baseline, and G.H. should be observed monthly for clinical signs of hepatitis. As discussed, routine monitoring of LFT remains controversial because transient, asymptomatic rises do occur among the elderly.[123]

Although uncommon at 600 mg, rifampin given twice weekly may cause a greater incidence of flu-like symptoms. Because potential drug interactions with INH and rifampin are possible, any medication added to the patient's regimen should be carefully evaluated. Considering that G.H. has age-related decreased renal function, signs of ethambutol-induced visual dysfunction should be monitoring carefully.

Treatment of Latent Infection in the Elderly

Treatment of elderly patients with positive tuberculin skin tests but no active TB disease with INH 300 mg daily for 6 to 9 months is essential if a source case is present in the nursing home. Stead et al.[120] reported only one case of active disease in patients receiving therapy for latent TB infection compared with 69 cases in untreated patients. In patients with recently converted skin tests, one patient in the group receiving INH therapy developed active disease compared with 45 who received no treatment.[120] Rifampin for 4 months is also an acceptable regimen in the elderly.[118]

Multidrug-Resistant Organisms

Definition and Etiology

22. **M.S., an ill-appearing 22-year-old Asian man, is admitted to the hospital with signs and symptoms of pneumonia. He is coughing and his chest radiograph indicates bilateral infiltrates. He is placed in respiratory isolation pending the results of sputum testing for *M. tuberculosis*. He states that he was diagnosed with TB 3 months ago and started on a regimen of INH, rifampin, pyrazinamide, and ethambutol. He stopped taking his medication after 1 month, and an HIV test from 3 months ago was negative. What is the likelihood of acquired drug resistance?**

Drug-resistant *M. tuberculosis* became increasingly prevalent in the United States in the late 1980s to early 1990s, although this has decreased in more recent years.[3,4,13,124,125] In 2005, the incidence of INH resistance in the United States was 7.3%, and the incidence of resistance to both INH and rifampin (multidrug-resistance) was 1.0%.[13] These resistance rates have remained stable for the past 10 years.[13] Resistance to *M. tuberculosis* is either primary or acquired. Primary drug resistance occurs when a patient harbors a resistant strain before any drugs have been administered. Acquired drug resistance occurs when resistant subpopulations are selected by inappropriate therapy.[82] The World Health Organization (WHO) conducted a global survey of drug resistance in *M. tuberculosis*, which showed that resistance to at least one antituberculosis drug occurs in a median of 9.9% of strains in patients never having received treatment (primary) and in 36.0% of strains in patients who received treatment for at least 1 month (acquired). Based on these results, acquired drug resistance is a larger problem.[125]

Acquired drug resistance may be the result of treatment errors, such as addition of a single drug to a failing regimen, inadequate primary regimen, failure to recognize resistance, and, most importantly, nonadherence to the prescribed regimen. Sporadic ingestion, inadequate dosages, or malabsorption of medications can cause susceptible *M. tuberculosis* strains to become resistant to multiple drugs within a few months.[76,126,127] These resistant organisms can then be transmitted to persons who have never received treatment and lead to primary resistance in these patients. Patients with MDR-TB are twice as likely to have cavitary lesions on chest radiography ($p < 0.001$) and seven times more likely to have reported prior treatment for TB ($p < 0.001$).[128]

Patterns and prevalence of drug-resistance vary throughout the world, and the highest rates of MDR-TB are in countries of the former Soviet Union and China. As mentioned, the incidence of MDR-TB in the United States has declined from 2.5% in 1993 and has remained stable at 1.0% over the past 10 years.[13] Nonetheless, it is important to note that certain populations are at risk for infections caused by MDR-TB. These include HIV-infected persons and those in groups or institutional settings, such as hospitals, prisons, nursing homes, and homeless shelters.[129]

M.S. is Asian and, therefore, may have primary resistance from his country of origin, making a detailed exposure history essential for the treatment of his infection. M.S. is also an example of the problem of treatment failure caused by nonadherence and the potential development of drug-resistant organisms. Homelessness and lack of awareness of the severity of TB have been shown to be significantly associated with interruptions in TB therapy.[130] Therefore, educational efforts to improve a patient's understanding of TB disease is critical for appropriate treatment of the disease.

Treatment

23. **Can M.S. be cured, and how should he be treated?**

Many factors can affect the outcome of therapy for MDR-TB. These include HIV status, treatment adherence, the number of drugs to which the tubercle bacilli are still susceptible, and the time since the first diagnosis of TB.[131–133] In a recent study, all 11 patients who were HIV-positive died during observation.[132] In another study, 77% of patients with MDR-TB had sputum cultures convert to negative in a median time of 60 days (range, 4–462 days), but 23% of patients never converted to negative cultures.[133] Of the patients who converted, 60% converted after 4 months of therapy.[133] Predictors of a longer time for sputum culture conversion were high initial sputum colony counts, bilateral cavitation on chest radiograph, previous treatment of MDR-TB, and the number of drugs the initial isolate was resistant to at the beginning of therapy.[133]

Because his recent HIV test was negative, M.S. has a high probability of treatment success. In HIV-negative patients, 32 (97%) of 33 patients with MDR-TB were cured, and these patients received an average of five second-line drugs.[132] Only one relapse occurred 5 years after treatment.[132] Therefore, M.S.'s current regimen should be re-evaluated, drug susceptibility testing should be determined, and the patient should be referred to a specialist or consultation at a specialized treatment center.[61] Current drug susceptibility testing in most institutions takes several weeks; however, this can be decreased to 3 weeks with the use of the BACTEC system. When initiating or revising therapy, at least three previously unused drugs to which there is in vitro susceptibility should be employed, and one of these agents should be injectable.[61] A new regimen should contain at least four drugs, possibly more, depending on the severity of the disease and the resistance pattern. If resistance to INH and rifampin is suspected, M.S. should be started on a regimen of pyrazinamide, ethambutol, a fluoroquinolone (levofloxacin, ciprofloxacin, or moxifloxacin), and an injectable agent (streptomycin, amikacin capreomycin), pending the results of susceptibility testing.[61] Treatment should be given by DOT and continued for 18 to 24 months.[61,131]

The fluoroquinolone antibiotics, ciprofloxacin, levofloxacin, and moxifloxacin are active against mycobacteria, including *M. tuberculosis*, and they penetrate rapidly into macrophages and exhibit intracellular mycobactericidal activity.[131] Fluoroquinolones inhibit DNA gyrase in *M. tuberculosis*, but the other molecular target of these agents, topoisomerase IV, is absent.[131] Older studies did not demonstrate cross-resistance between fluoroquinolones and other antimycobacterial drugs[134,135]; however, a recent study found that 76% of ciprofloxacin-resistant strains were resistant to INH and rifampin.[72] Ciprofloxacin, ofloxacin, and levofloxacin have been used long term for the treatment of mycobacterial infections and were well tolerated with few serious adverse effects.[135,136] Of the commercially available fluoroquinolones against *M. tuberculosis,* moxifloxacin is the most potent agent.[66] Limited data suggest that moxifloxacin is an acceptable option in the treatment of MDR-TB.[137] Selection of fluoroquinolone resistance has been observed in vivo, and complete cross-resistance within the class is the accepted rule.[131] Other medications used for MDR-TB include para-aminosalicylic acid, cycloserine, ethionamide, and capreomycin. These are all associated with numerous side effects and should not be prescribed without the guidance of an expert in the treatment of MDR-TB (Table 61-3).

HIV

Treatment of Latent Infection with MDR-TB

24. L.W., the 26-year-old roommate of M.S., was recently found to be HIV-positive. Currently, he does not have symptoms of active TB. His PPD skin test is 6 mm. What is the possibility that M.S. has infected L.W. with drug-resistant *M. tuberculosis*? How should he be managed?

The risk that L.W. is infected with drug-resistant *M. tuberculosis* is high. HIV-infected persons are much more likely to become infected than persons who are immunocompetent. Because L.W. is at high risk of infection with multidrug-resistant organisms, he should be started on two drugs for treatment of latent TB infection.[33] He could be started on pyrazinamide 20 to 25 mg/kg/day and ethambutol 15 to 20 mg/kg/day for 12 months. Another possible regimen would be pyrazinamide and a fluoroquinolone (levofloxacin, moxifloxacin, or ciprofloxacin). The specific regimen for L.W. should also take into consideration the drug susceptibility results of his roommate, M.S.

25. Because he is HIV-positive, what is L.W.'s prognosis?

Mortality in patients with HIV who are infected with MDR-TB remains significantly higher than in HIV-negative patients.[132] If L.W. develops active MDR-TB disease and had acquired immunodeficiency syndrome (AIDS), his risk of death would be >70% even with aggressive multidrug treatment.

26. F.R., a 32-year-old man diagnosed with AIDS 6 months ago, is experiencing mild pleuritic chest pain with a productive cough. He also has experienced weight loss, fatigue, and night sweats over the past 2 weeks. A chest radiograph revealed bilateral infiltrates. Sputum samples are ordered for AFB smear and culture, and a PPD skin test is placed. The AFB smear is positive, and the induration from the PPD is 6 mm. His CD4(+) count is 150/mm^3. He is currently receiving zidovudine, lamivudine, lopinavir, and ritonavir for his HIV disease with no complaints. How does TB present and what is its frequency in a patient with AIDS? How effective is skin testing in the diagnosis of latent TB infection? How should F.R. be treated?

Human immunodeficiency virus infects CD4(+) T cells, leading to a decrease in cell-mediated immunity. This absence of immunity allows the rapid development of active TB disease in a person who is infected with *M. tuberculosis*.[23,49,63,138–140] The lungs are most frequently affected (74%–79% of cases); however, extrapulmonary disease also occurs much more frequently in patients with HIV infection than in patients without HIV infection (45%–72% vs. 17.5%).[138,140] Patients with AIDS have a much greater chance of extrapulmonary disease when compared with an asymptomatic HIV-infected person. Infection with *M. tuberculosis* may be difficult to distinguish from other HIV-related pulmonary opportunistic infections (*Pneumocystis jiroveci*, *M. avium* complex). TB often precedes other opportunistic pulmonary infections and should be ruled out in any patient with HIV infection.[138] Several studies have identified predictors of poor survival in HIV-infected patients. These include low CD4(+) cell counts, MDR-TB, no DOT, and a history of IV drug abuse.[141] New therapies, such as the fluoroquinolones and immunomodulating agents, may improve the outcome in these patients, but more clinical research is needed to assess their value.[142]

PPD and Treatment of Active Disease

A PPD skin test should be applied to HIV-infected patients. Nevertheless, only about 30% to 50% of patients with AIDS and TB will respond to a PPD skin test with an induration >10 mm. Therefore, an induration ≥5 mm is considered to be a positive reaction in this population.[33,62,143] F.R.'s reaction to PPD (6 mm) should be considered positive. Based on his symptoms and positive AFB smear, he should be started on multiple-drug therapy for treatment of active TB disease. Recommendations for the treatment of TB in HIV-infected adults are the same as those for HIV-uninfected persons, with a few important exceptions (Table 61-2).[61] These exceptions include the potential for drug–drug interactions between rifamycins and antiretroviral agents and the potential for the development of acquired rifamycin resistance with intermittent therapy.[61,144,145] Antiretroviral therapy should not be withheld simply because the patient is being treated for TB, and a rifamycin should not be excluded for the treatment regimen for fear of interactions with certain antiretroviral agents.[61,146] Exclusion of a rifamycin will likely delay sputum conversion, prolong the duration of therapy, and possibly result in a poor outcome.

Treatment of active TB in patients with HIV may be complicated by the occurrence of immune reconstitution inflammatory syndrome, which occurs in 30% of patients who begin therapy for both infections in close temporal proximity.[146] This syndrome reflects reconstituted immunity to *M. tuberculosis* and usually occurs in the first 4 to 8 weeks after initiation of antiretroviral therapy.[146] Symptoms include fever, malaise, and local reactions in organs, depending on the location of the mycobacterial infection (e.g., lungs). Immune reconstitution syndrome reactions are best managed with anti-inflammatory agents, including corticosteroids.[146]

As noted earlier, rifampin is a potent inducer of cytochrome P450 isoenzymes (especially CYP3A4), rifapentine is intermediate, and rifabutin is the least potent inducer.[46,61] Rifabutin is highly active against *M. tuberculosis*, so it has been recommended in place of rifampin for the treatment of active TB in HIV-infected patients receiving certain protease inhibitors or nonnucleoside reverse transcriptase inhibitors.[61] Data from clinical trials also suggest that rifabutin- and rifampin-based regimens are equally efficacious.[61] Protease inhibitors and nonnucleoside reverse transcriptase inhibitors may, however, either induce or inhibit cytochrome P450 isoenzymes, depending on the specific drug. As a result, these drugs may alter the serum concentrations of rifabutin.[61,147]

The CDC has published guidelines for the use of rifampin for treatment of TB in HIV-infected patients receiving protease inhibitors and nonnucleoside reverse transcriptase inhibitors.[148] Based on these guidelines, rifampin can be used in the following situations: (a) a patient whose antiretroviral regimen includes the nonnucleoside reverse transcriptase inhibitor efavirenz and two nucleoside reverse transcriptase inhibitors; (b) a patient whose antiretroviral regimen includes the protease inhibitor ritonavir and one or more reverse transcriptase inhibitors; or (c) a patient whose antiretroviral regimen includes the combination of two protease inhibitors.[148] Because F.R. is receiving lopinavir and ritonavir, a potent cytochrome P450 3A4 inhibitor, he could be started on rifampin 600 mg, INH 300 mg, pyrazinamide 20 to 25 mg/kg, and ethambutol 15 to 20 mg/kg daily for the first 8 weeks of therapy. If rifabutin is started in place of rifampin, the dose of rifabutin must be decreased to reduce the likelihood of clinical toxicity associated with increased concentrations of rifabutin (leukopenia, uveitis, arthralgias, skin discoloration).[147] Acquired rifamycin resistance is more common in patients with very low CD4(+) cell counts or who received intermittent dosing in the first 2 months of therapy.[144,145] Therefore, daily administration is necessary during the intensive phase of treatment.

After this initial period, if no drug resistance is evident on susceptibility testing, F.R. can be treated with INH and rifampin (or rifabutin) daily or two to three times a week for a minimum of 26 weeks. Because he is receiving ritonavir, the rifabutin dose for intermittent therapy should be 300 mg.[147] Although not applicable to F.R. because his CD4(+) count is 150 cells/mL, it should be noted that twice weekly continuation therapy with INH and rifampin or INH and rifabutin is not recommended for HIV-infected patients with CD4(+) cell counts <100 cells/mL because of an increased frequency of acquired rifamycin resistance.[61,147,149] In addition, the once weekly continuation regimen of INH and rifapentine is contraindicated in HIV-infected patients because of a high rate of relapse with organisms that have acquired resistance to the rifamycins.[61] Because the margin of error is less in HIV-infected patients, special care to ensure adherence is required. In other words, DOT is highly recommended in this population. Furthermore, if the patient is slow to respond, prolonged therapy (>6 months) should also be considered. In addition to the antituberculosis medications, pyridoxine should be given to prevent peripheral neuropathy.

Drug Interactions

27. Are there any interactions between TB and antiretroviral agents to consider in F.R.'s therapy?

Yes, many! Since 1995, the FDA has approved several products in the protease inhibitor class of antiretroviral drugs: ritonavir (Norvir), saquinavir hard-gel capsule (Invirase), saquinavir soft-gel capsule (Fortovase), indinavir (Crixivan), nelfinavir (Viracept), amprenavir (Agenerase), and lopinavir + ritonavir (Kaletra). These products are the most potent antiretroviral agents available to treat HIV-infected patients, but they have many drug–drug interactions that are important to consider. First, all of the protease inhibitors are cytochrome P450 3A4 inhibitors, and ritonavir is the most potent inhibitor in the class. As a result, drugs affected by this interaction, such as rifabutin, will have elevated concentrations. In addition to their effect on other drugs, the protease inhibitors are affected by other drugs that affect the cytochrome P450 system, such as by rifampin, which is a potent inducer of the cytochrome P450 system. The protease inhibitor concentrations are reduced by 35% to 80% with concomitant rifampin administration. This reduction is somewhat less with rifabutin.[150–152]

The nonnucleoside reverse transcriptase inhibitors, nevirapine (Viramune), delavirdine (Rescriptor), and efavirenz (Sustiva), are metabolized by cytochrome P450, but they affect other drugs metabolized by cytochrome P450 3A4 to varying degrees. Nevirapine is an inducer of CYP 3A4 isoenzymes, delavirdine is an inhibitor of CYP 3A4 isoenzymes, and efavirenz is a mixed inducer–inhibitor. Therefore, their interactions cannot be summarized as a class. The nucleoside reverse transcriptase inhibitors, such as zidovudine and lamivudine, are not metabolized by the cytochrome P450 system, making drug interactions unlikely.[152]

Malabsorption

As mentioned, inadequate therapy of TB is one of the main reasons for treatment failure and development of acquired drug resistance. This can occur in many ways, such as nonadherence to therapy or malabsorption of the TB medications. Malabsorption of TB medications has been documented in HIV-infected patients. In one study, 19 of 20 patients had subtherapeutic serum rifampin concentrations. This phenomenon is particularly common with rifampin and ethambutol and explains, in part, the slow response in HIV-infected patients with TB.[127,153–155] Therefore, serum concentrations of rifampin (or rifabutin) and ethambutol should be monitored in F.R.[127,153–155]

Therapy of Latent Infection in HIV

28. Why should N.M., an HIV-infected person with a positive PPD skin test and no clinical symptoms, receive treatment for his latent TB infection?

The risk of N.M. developing active TB disease is substantial. Pape et al.[156] conducted a randomized, placebo-controlled trial of INH therapy in HIV-infected patients. They found that patients receiving placebo were six times more likely to develop active TB than those receiving INH. The patients receiving INH were also less likely to develop AIDS.[156] INH 300 mg daily for 9 months is, therefore, recommended for N.M.[33] Some clinicians suggest that these patients receive INH for life because eventual failure of the immune system will allow infection to progress to active disease.[138] (Therapy for MDR-TB is addressed in Question 24.) Therapy should also be considered in nonanergic, HIV-infected, PPD-negative patients who have been in recent contact with an infectious TB patient. The effectiveness of INH therapy in anergic, HIV-infected patients has not been established.[51]

Pregnancy

29. E.F. is a 25-year-old Hispanic woman who is being treated with INH 900 mg and rifampin 600 mg twice a week for pulmonary tuberculosis. She completed 2 months of therapy with INH, rifampin, pyrazinamide, and ethambutol, and began the new regimen 2 months ago. She recently became pregnant, and her obstetrician is concerned about the possible teratogenic effects of INH. What are the risks of TB and its treatment to the mother and the fetus? Are these drugs teratogenic?

Risks, Teratogenicity, and Treatment

Although concerns regarding the use of any medication during pregnancy always exist, it is now recognized that untreated TB represents a far greater risk to a pregnant woman and her fetus than does the treatment.[61,62] INH, rifampin, pyrazinamide, and ethambutol are not teratogenic in humans, and the WHO recommends their use in women who are pregnant.[157,158] In the United States, pyrazinamide is not recommended for use during pregnancy because of insufficient safety data.[61] If pyrazinamide is not included in the initial treatment regimen, the minimal duration of therapy is 9 months.[61] All pregnant women receiving INH also should receive pyridoxine 25 mg/day because of the possibility of CNS toxicity.

Streptomycin should not be used during pregnancy except as a last alternative because it has been associated with mild-to-severe ototoxicity in the infant. This ototoxicity can occur throughout the gestational period and is not confined to the first trimester. With the exception of streptomycin ototoxicity, the occurrence of birth defects in women being treated for TB with the above agents is no greater than that of healthy pregnant women.[159,160] Therefore, administration of antituberculosis drugs is not an indication for termination of pregnancy.[61] Because E.F. likely became pregnant after completing the first 2 months of therapy, she should continue her current regimen for a total of 6 months because she received pyrazinamide as part of the initial regimen.

MDR-TB in Pregnancy

Little is known about the efficacy and safety of second-line drugs used to treat MDR-TB during pregnancy. Two reports with small numbers of patients have suggested that treatment is effective with no adverse effects to mother or child.[161,162] In a study of seven women treated for MDR-TB during pregnancy, no obstetrical complications or perinatal transmission of MDR-TB was observed.[161] Five women were cured, one experienced treatment failure, and one stopped therapy prematurely.[161] No evidence of drug toxicity was seen among their children exposed to second-line drugs in utero, although one child was diagnosed with MDR-TB.[162] Clearly, more data are needed, but pregnancy should not be a limitation to the treatment of MDR-TB.

Lactation

When the baby is born, E.F. may breast-feed while continuing her medication. Drug concentrations are minimal and do not provide sufficient quantities for the treatment or prevention of TB in the nursing infant.[61,62,158]

Pediatrics

30. A.M., a 3-year-old black boy, is suspected of having TB. His father has been receiving treatment for TB for the last 2 months. A.M. has a productive cough, fever, and general malaise. His sputum is positive for AFB, and his PPD skin test is positive (10 mm). What is the incidence of TB in children? How should A.M. be treated?

The incidence of TB in children <15 years of age has declined from 1,663 cases (2.9 per 100,000 population) in 1993 to 863 cases (1.4 per 100,000 population) in 2005.[13] Children commonly develop active TB disease as a complication of the initial infection with *M. tuberculosis*, and the disease is characterized by intrathoracic adenopathy, mid and lower lung infiltrates, and the absence of cavitation on chest radiography.[61,163] Because of the high risk of disseminated TB in infants and children, treatment should be started as soon as the diagnosis of TB is suspected. In general, the regimens recommended for adults are also the regimens of choice for infants, children, and adolescents, with the exception that ethambutol is not used routinely in children.[61] Although it is no more toxic, ethambutol is often avoided because it is difficult to assess visual acuity in children. A.M. should be started on INH 10 to 15 mg/kg/day, rifampin 10 to 20 mg/kg/day, and pyrazinamide 15 to 30 mg/kg/day.[61,62,163] Many experts prefer to treat children with three drugs (rather than four) in the initial phase because the bacillary population is usually lower than in an adult and it may be difficult for an infant or child to ingest four drugs. If resistance is suspected, ethambutol 15 to 20 mg/kg/day or streptomycin 20 to 40 mg/kg/day should be added to the regimen until susceptibility of the organism to INH, rifampin, and pyrazinamide is known. Pyridoxine is recommended for infants, children, and adolescents who are receiving INH.[61]

If resistance is not suspected in A.M. and susceptibility is confirmed by testing, he should receive the INH, rifampin, and pyrazinamide daily for 8 weeks. He can then continue to take the INH and rifampin daily or two to three times a week (DOT) for an additional 4 months. The dosage for INH and rifampin in a two to three times a week regimen would be 20 to 30 mg/kg per dose and 10 to 20 mg/kg per dose, respectively (Table 61-3).

A.M. should be examined routinely for signs and symptoms of hepatitis. Although antituberculosis medications are generally well-tolerated in children, LFT two to three times normal are common. These are often benign and transient; however, the incidence of hepatitis in children from INH with rifampin may be four to six times more common than in children receiving INH alone. Most hepatitis occurs within the first 3 months of therapy and generally is associated with more than recommended doses of INH or rifampin.[104,164]

The last guidelines for targeted tuberculin skin testing and treatment of latent TB in children and adolescents were published in 2004.[164] Children and adolescents should be screened for risk factors for TB using a questionnaire, and they should be skin tested with 5 TU PPD if one or more risk factors are present.[164] Insufficient data are available to recommend use of whole blood interferon-γ assays in children. INH for 9 months is recommended for treatment of latent TB in this population.[164] Daily rifampin for 6 months is an acceptable alternative, especially in children who cannot tolerate INH or those exposed to a source case whose isolate was INH-resistant.[165]

Extrapulmonary Tuberculosis and Tuberculous Meningitis

31. R.U. is a 64-year-old man who is brought to the emergency department following a 4-day period during which he became progressively disoriented, febrile to 40.5°C, and obtunded. He also had severe headaches during this time. Physical examination revealed some nuchal rigidity and a positive Brudzinski sign (neck resistant to flexion). An initial diagnosis of possible meningitis was made, and a lumbar puncture ordered. The cerebrospinal fluid (CSF) appeared turbid, and laboratory analysis revealed an elevated protein concentration of 200 mg/dL, a decreased glucose concentration of 30 mg/dL, and a white blood cell (WBC) count of 500/mm^3 (85% lymphocytes). A Gram stain of the spinal fluid and a sputum smear for AFB were negative; other laboratory tests were within normal limits. A diagnosis of tuberculous meningitis was presumed. Discuss the presentation and prognosis of tuberculous meningitis. How should R.U. be treated?

[SI units: WBC count, 500 10^9/L (0.85 lymphocytes)]

Tuberculous meningitis is only one of the extrapulmonary complications of infection with *M. tuberculosis*. Successful treatment of extrapulmonary TB can usually be accomplished in 6 to 9 months with an acceptable relapse rate.[61,62,166] Some forms, such as bone or joint TB, miliary TB, or tuberculous meningitis may require 9 to 12 months of therapy.[61] Because specimens for culture and susceptibility testing may be difficult or impossible to obtain from a site, response to treatment must be based on clinical and radiographic improvement.

Tuberculous meningitis in older persons usually is caused by hematogenous dissemination of the tubercle bacilli from a primary site, usually the lungs. In its early stages, tuberculous meningitis often is confused with aseptic meningitis because the Gram stain is negative. The most common symptoms of tuberculous meningitis are headache, fever, restlessness, irritability, nausea, and vomiting. A positive Brudzinski sign and neck stiffness may be present. As illustrated by R.U., the CSF is usually turbid with increased protein and decreased glucose concentrations. There is an increase in the CSF WBC count with a predominance of lymphocytes. Culture of the CSF for *M. tuberculosis* may not be helpful because rates of positivity for clinically diagnosed cases range from 25% to 70%.[167] Early recognition and treatment is essential for a favorable outcome. Thus, empirical treatment before receipt of confirmatory culture and susceptibility results is common in suspected tuberculous meningitis. Multiple-drug therapy should be used because irreversible brain damage or death can occur as soon as 2 weeks after the onset of infection (not clinical symptoms).[167]

Treatment

Treatment should be initiated in R.U. with daily administration of INH 300 mg, rifampin 600 mg, pyrazinamide 20 to 25 mg/kg, and ethambutol 15 to 20 mg/kg for the first 2 months.[61] After this initial phase of treatment, R.U. should receive daily INH and rifampin treatment for an additional 7 to 10 months, although the optimal duration of therapy is unknown.[61] In addition, because R.U. is older, pyridoxine 10 to 50 mg/day should be given to prevent the occurrence of peripheral neuropathy from INH. It also should be remembered that rifampin may impart a red to orange color to the CSF.

Isoniazid readily penetrates into the CSF, with CSF concentrations reaching up to 100% of those in the serum. Rifampin is often included in tuberculous meningitis regimens and may be associated with reduced morbidity and mortality; however even with inflammation, its CSF concentrations are only 6% to 30% of those found in the serum. Ethambutol should be used in the highest dosage to achieve bactericidal concentrations in the CSF because its CSF concentrations are only 10% to 54% of those in the serum. Streptomycin penetrates into the CSF poorly even with inflamed meninges.[168,169]

Corticosteroids

Corticosteroids in moderate to severe tuberculous meningitis appear to reduce sequelae and prolong survival.[170] The mechanism for this benefit is likely owing to reduction of intracranial pressure. Dexamethasone 8 to 12 mg/day (or prednisone equivalent) for 6 to 8 weeks should be used and then tapered slowly after symptoms subside.[170] Corticosteroids are likely indicated for R.U.

Solid Organ Transplant Recipients

32. M. S. is 66-year-old man with a history of TB as child. He recently underwent a renal transplant. Will he develop TB, and if so, are there any pharmacologic concerns to address in him?

The risk of developing TB is 36 to 74 times greater among solid-organ transplant recipients than in the general population. The overall mortality rate in this population is 29%. The increased risk of developing TB is largely caused by the immunosuppressive therapy given to prevent transplant rejection. Although some patients may acquire the TB nosocomially, most, including possibly M.S., will develop it as reactivation of dormant TB. More than half of the patients will develop pulmonary disease. Many, however, will also develop disseminated or extrapulmonary disease, which is difficult to diagnose and therefore may cause a delay in diagnosis.[171] Patients should be treated with a standard TB regimen.[61,62] Attention should be paid to potential interactions with rifampin, which may increase the metabolism of cyclosporine, tacrolimus, and other medications. In addition, transplant recipients, in particular liver transplant recipients, may be at an increased risk of developing INH hepatitis. It is recommended that all transplant recipients receive a tuberculin skin test and that chemoprophylaxis be offered to all high-risk patients.[171]

REFERENCES

1. Peloquin CA et al. Infection caused by *Mycobacterium tuberculosis*. *Ann Pharmacother* 1994; 28:72.
2. Dooley SW et al. Multidrug-resistant tuberculosis. *Ann Intern Med* 1992;117:257.
3. Freiden TR et al. The emergence of drug-resistant tuberculosis in New York City. *N Engl J Med* 1993;328:521.
4. Riley LW. Drug-resistant tuberculosis. *Clin Infect Dis* 1993;17(Suppl 2):S442.
5. Centers for Disease Control and Prevention. Emergence of *Mycobacterium tuberculosis* with extensive resistance to second-line drugs—Worldwide, 2000–2004. *MMWR* 2006;55:301.
6. Raviglione MC et al. XDR tuberculosis implications for global public health. *New Engl J Med* 2007;356:656.
7. Shah NS et al. Worldwide emergence of extensively drug-resistant tuberculosis. *Emerg Infect Dis* 2007;13:380.
8. Corbett EL et al. The growing burden of tuberculosis. Global trends and interactions with the HIV epidemic. *Arch Intern Med* 2003;163:1009.
9. World Health Organization. WHO Report 2007. Global tuberculosis control surveillance, planning, financing. www.who.int/tb/publications/global_report/2007/pdf/full.pdf. Accessed May 30, 2007.
10. Centers for Disease Control and Prevention. Reported tuberculosis in the United States, 2001. Atlanta, Georgia: US Department of Health and Human Services, CDC, September 2002.
11. Centers for Disease Control and Prevention. A strategic plan for the elimination of tuberculosis in the United States. *MMWR* 1989;38(Suppl S-3):125.
12. Centers for Disease Control and Prevention. Trends in tuberculosis incidence United States, 2006. *MMWR* 2007;56:245.
13. Centers for Disease Control and Prevention. Reported tuberculosis in the United States, 2005. Atlanta, Georgia: U.S. Department of Health and Human Services, CDC, September 2006.
14. Cain KP et al. Tuberculosis among foreign-born persons in the United States. *Am J Respir Crit Care Med* 2007;175:75.
15. Gandhi NR et al. Extensively drug-resistant tuberculosis as a cause of death in patients co-infected with tuberculosis and HIV in a rural area of South Africa. *Lancet* 2006;368:1575.
16. Centers for Disease Control and Prevention. Notice to Readers: Revised definition of extensively drug-resistant tuberculosis. *MMWR* 2006;55:1176.
17. Centers for Disease Control and Prevention. Extensively drug-resistant tuberculosis United States, 1993–2006. *MMWR* 2007;56:250.
18. American Thoracic Society/Centers for Disease Control and Prevention. Diagnostic standards and classification of tuberculosis in adults and children. *Am J Respir Crit Care Med* 2000;161:1376.
19. Centers for Disease Control and Prevention. Guidelines for preventing the transmission of *Mycobacterium tuberculosis* in health-care settings, 2005. *MMWR* 2005;54(RR-17):1.
20. Edwards D et al. The immunology of mycobacterial diseases. *Am Rev Respir Dis* 1986;134:1062.
21. Dannenberg AM. Immune mechanisms in the pathogenesis of pulmonary tuberculosis. *Rev Infect Dis* 1989;11:S369.
22. Horsburgh CR. Priorities for the treatment of latent tuberculosis infection in the United States. *N Engl J Med* 2004;350:2060.
23. Daley CL et al. An outbreak of tuberculosis with accelerated progression among persons infected with the human immunodeficiency virus. *N Engl J Med* 1992;326:231.
24. Selwyn PD et al. A prospective study of the risk of tuberculosis among intravenous drug users with human immunodeficiency virus infection. *N Engl J Med* 1989;320:545.
25. Markowitz N et al. Tuberculin and anergy testing in HIV-seropositive and HIV-seronegative persons. *Ann Intern Med* 1993;119:185.
26. Nelson LJ et al. Epidemiology of childhood tuberculosis in the United States, 1993–2001: the need for continued vigilance. *Pediatrics* 2004;114:333.
27. MacGregor RR. A year's experience with tuberculosis in a private urban teaching hospital in the post-sanatorium era. *Am J Med* 1975;58:221.
28. Counsel SR, et al. Unsuspected pulmonary tuberculosis in a community teaching hospital. *Arch Intern Med* 1989;149:1274.
29. Richeldi L. An update on the diagnosis of tuberculosis infection. *Am J Respir Crit Care Med* 2006; 174:736.
30. Myers JP. New recommendations for the treatment of tuberculosis. *Curr Opin Infect Dis* 2005;18:133.
31. Howard A et al. Bevel-down superior to bevel-up in intradermal skin testing. *Ann Allergy Asthma Immunol* 1977;78:594.
32. Tsicopoulos A et al. Preferential messenger RNA expression of Th1-type cells (IFN-γ+, IL-2+) in classical delayed-type (tuberculin) hypersensitivity reactions in human skin. *J Immunol* 1992;148:2058.
33. Centers for Disease Control and Prevention. Targeted tuberculin testing and treatment of latent tuberculosis infection. *MMWR* 2000;49(RR-6):154.
34. Jasmer RM et al. Latent tuberculosis infection. *N Engl J Med* 2002;347:1860.
35. Wang L et al. A meta-analysis of the effect of Bacille Calmette Guerin vaccination on tuberculin skin test measurements. *Thorax* 2002;57:804.
36. Lanphear BP et al. A high false-positive rate of tuberculosis associated with Aplisol: an investigation among health care workers. *J Infect Dis* 1994;169:703.
37. Gillenwater KA et al. Increase in tuberculin skin test converters among health care workers after a change from Tubersol to Aplisol. *Am J Infect Control* 2006;34:651.
38. Chaparas SD et al. Tuberculin test. Variability with the Mantoux procedure. *Am Rev Respir Dis* 1985;132:175.
39. Centers for Disease Control and Prevention. Guidelines for using the QuantiFERON-TB Gold test for detecting *Mycobacterium tuberculosis* infection, United States. *MMWR* 2005;54(RR-15):49.
40. Luetkemeyer AF et al. Comparison of an interferon-gamma release assay with tuberculin skin testing in HIV-infected individuals. *Am J Respir Crit Care Med* 2007;175:737.
41. Dewan PK et al. Low sensitivity of a whole-blood interferon-γ release assay for detection of active tuberculosis. *Clin Infect Dis* 2007;44:69.
42. Horsburgh CR et al. Practice guidelines for the treatment of tuberculosis. *Clin Infect Dis* 2000; 31:633.
43. Hobby GL et al. Enumeration of tubercle bacilli in sputum of patients with pulmonary tuberculosis. *Antimicrob Agents Chemother* 1973;4:94.
44. Schluger NW. Changing approaches to the diagnosis of tuberculosis. *Am J Respir Crit Care Med* 2001;164:2020.
45. Wright PW et al. Sensitivity of fluorochrome microscopy for detection of *Mycobacterium tuberculosis* versus nontuberculous mycobacteria. *J Clin Microbiol* 1998;36:1046.
46. Nahid P et al. Advances in the diagnosis and treatment of tuberculosis. *Proceedings of the American Thoracic Society* 2006;3:103.
47. Centers for Disease Control and Prevention. Nucleic acid amplification tests for tuberculosis. *MMWR* 2000;49:593.
48. Yeager HJ et al. Quantitative studies of mycobacterial populations in sputum and saliva. *Am Rev Respir Dis* 1967;95:998.
49. Centers for Disease Control. Tuberculosis and human immunodeficiency virus infections: recommendations of the Advisory Committee for the Elimination of Tuberculosis. *MMWR* 1989;38:236.
50. Dooley SW et al. Nosocomial transmission of tuberculosis in a hospital unit for HIV-infected patients. *JAMA* 1992;267:2632.
51. Centers for Disease Control and Prevention. Anergy skin testing and preventive therapy for HIV-infected persons: revised recommendations. *MMWR* 1997;46(RR-15):110.
52. American Thoracic Society/Centers for Disease Control and Prevention. Targeted tuberculin skin testing and treatment of latent tuberculosis infection. *Am J Respir Crit Care Med* 2000;161:S221.
53. Comstock GW et al. Tuberculin conversions: true or false? *Am Rev Respir Dis* 1978;118:215.
54. Thompson NJ et al. The booster phenomenon in serial tuberculin testing. *Am Rev Respir Dis* 1979;119:587.
55. Rosenberg T et al. Two-step tuberculin testing in staff and residents of a nursing home. *Am Rev Respir Dis* 1993;148:1537.

56. Snider DE et al. Tuberculin skin testing of hospital employees: infection, boosting, and two-step testing. *Am J Infect Control* 1984;12:305.
57. Bass JB et al. Choosing an appropriate cutting point for conversion in annual tuberculin skin testing. *Am Rev Respir Dis* 1985;132:379.
58. Centers for Disease Control and Prevention. The role of BCG vaccine in the prevention and control of tuberculosis in the United States. *MMWR* 1996;45(RR-4):118.
59. Rodrigues LC et al. Protective effect of BCG against tuberculous meningitis and miliary tuberculosis: a meta-analysis. *Int J Epidemiol* 1993;22:1154.
60. Colditz GA et al. Efficacy of BCG vaccine in the prevention of tuberculosis: meta-analysis of the published literature. *JAMA* 1994;271:698.
61. American Thoracic Society/Centers for Disease Control and Prevention/Infectious Diseases Society of America. Treatment of tuberculosis. *Am J Respir Crit Care Med* 2003;167:603.
62. Bass JB et al. Treatment of tuberculosis and tuberculosis infection in adults and children. *Am J Respir Crit Care Med* 1994;149:1359.
63. Centers for Disease Control. Initial therapy for tuberculosis in the era of multidrug-resistance: Recommendations of the Advisory Counsel for the elimination of tuberculosis. *MMWR* 1993;42(No. RR-7):18.
64. Tsukamura M et al. Therapeutic effect of a new antibacterial substance ofloxacin (DL8280) on pulmonary tuberculosis. *Am Rev Respir Dis* 1985;131:352.
65. Tuberculosis Research Centre. Shortening short course chemotherapy: a randomized clinical trial for treatment of smear positive pulmonary tuberculosis with regimens using ofloxacin in the intensive phase. *Indian Journal of Tuberculosis* 2002: 49:27.
66. Alvirez-Freites EJ et al. In vitro and in vivo activities of gatifloxacin against *Mycobacterium tuberculosis*. *Antimicrob Agents Chemother* 2002;46: 1022.
67. Nuermberger EL et al. Moxifloxacin-containing regimen greatly reduces time to culture conversion in murine tuberculosis. *Am J Respir Crit Care Med* 2004;169:421.
68. Nuermberger EL et al. Moxifloxacin-containing regimens of reduced duration produce a stable cure in murine tuberculosis. *Am J Respir Crit Care Med* 2004;170:1131.
69. Burman WJ et al. Moxifloxacin versus ethambutol in the first 2 months of treatment for pulmonary tuberculosis. *Am J Respir Crit Care Med* 2006; 174:331.
70. El-Sadr W et al. Evaluation of an intensive intermittent-induction regimen and short course duration of treatment for HIV-related pulmonary tuberculosis. *Clin Infect Dis* 1998;26:1148.
71. Kohno S et al. Prospective comparative study of ofloxacin or ethambutol for the treatment of pulmonary tuberculosis. *Chest* 1992;102:1815.
72. Bozeman L et al. Fluoroquinolone susceptibility among *Mycobacterium tuberculosis* isolates from the United States and Canada. *Clin Infect Dis* 2005;40:386.
73. American Thoracic Society, Centers for Disease Control and Prevention, Infectious Diseases Society of America. Controlling tuberculosis in the United States. *Am J Respir Crit Care Med* 2005; 172:1169.
74. Cohn DL et al. A 62 dose, 6-month therapy for pulmonary and extrapulmonary tuberculosis: a twice-weekly, directly observed and cost-effective regimen. *Ann Intern Med* 1990;112:407.
75. Tam CM et al. Rifapentine and isoniazid in the continuation phase of treating pulmonary tuberculosis. *Am J Respir Crit Care Med* 1998;157:1726.
76. Tuberculosis Trials Consortium. Rifapentine and isoniazid once a week versus rifampicin and isoniazid twice a week for treatment of drug-susceptible pulmonary tuberculosis in HIV-negative patients: a randomised clinical trial. *Lancet* 2002;360:528.
77. Bock NN et al. A prospective, randomized, double-blind study of the tolerability of rifapentine 600, 900, and 1,200 mg plus isoniazid in the continuation phase of tuberculosis treatment. *Am J Respir Crit Care Med* 2002;165:1526.
78. Weiner M et al. Low isoniazid concentrations and outcome of tuberculosis treatment with once-weekly isoniazid and rifapentine. *Am J Respir Crit Care Med* 2003;167:1341.
79. Chaulk CP et al. Directly observed therapy for treatment completion of pulmonary tuberculosis: consensus statement of the Public Health Tuberculosis Guidelines Panel. *JAMA* 1998;279:943.
80. Jasmer RM et al. Tuberculosis treatment outcomes: directly observed therapy compared with self-administered therapy. *Am J Respir Crit Care Med* 2004;170:561.
81. Burman WJ et al. A cost-effectiveness analysis of directly observed therapy vs. self-administered therapy for treatment of tuberculosis. *Chest* 1997;112:63.
82. Mahmoudi A et al. Pitfalls in the care of patients with tuberculosis. Common errors and their association with the acquisition of drug resistance. *JAMA* 1993;270:65.
83. Iseman MD et al. Directly observed treatment of tuberculosis: we can't afford not to try it. *N Engl J Med* 1993;328:576.
84. Jindani A et al. The early bactericidal activity of drugs in patients with pulmonary tuberculosis. *Am Rev Respir Dis* 1980;121:939.
85. Chan SL et al. The early bactericidal activity of rifabutin measured by sputum viable counts in Hong Kong patients with pulmonary tuberculosis. *Tuber Lung Dis* 1992;73:33.
86. Sirgel FA et al. The early bactericidal activity of rifabutin in patients with pulmonary tuberculosis measured by sputum viable counts: a new method of drug assessment. *J Antimicrob Chemother* 1993;32:867.
87. Botha FJH et al. The early bactericidal activity of ethambutol, pyrazinamide, and the fixed combination of isoniazid, rifampicin, and pyrazinamide (Rifater) in patients with pulmonary tuberculosis. *S Afr Med J* 1996;86:155.
88. Dickinson JM et al. Experimental models to explain the high sterilizing activity of rifampin in the chemotherapy of tuberculosis. *Am Rev Respir Dis* 1981;123:367.
89. Peloquin CA et al. Comment: intravenous streptomycin [Letter]. *Ann Pharmacother* 1993;27:1546.
90. Combs DL et al. USPHS tuberculosis short-course chemotherapy trial 21: effectiveness, toxicity, and acceptability: the report of final results. *Ann Intern Med* 1990;112:397.
91. Khan A et al. Lack of weight gain and relapse risk in a large tuberculosis treatment trial. *Am J Respir Crit Care Med* 2006;174:344.
92. LoBue PA et al. Use of isoniazid for latent tuberculosis infection in a public health clinic. *Am J Respir Crit Care Med* 2003;168:443.
93. Centers for Disease Control and Prevention. Fatal and severe hepatitis associated with rifampin and pyrazinamide for the treatment of latent tuberculosis infection New York and Georgia, 2000. *MMWR* 2001;50:289.
94. Centers for Disease Control and Prevention. Update: Fatal and severe liver injuries associated with rifampin and pyrazinamide for latent tuberculosis infection, and revisions in American Thoracic Society/CDC recommendations United States, 2001. *MMWR* 2001;50:733.
95. Menzies D et al. Treatment completion and costs of a randomized trial of rifampin for 4 months versus isoniazid for 9 months. *Am J Respir Crit Care Med* 2004;170:445.
96. Reichman LB et al. Considering the role of four months of rifampin in the treatment of latent tuberculosis infection. *Am J Respir Crit Care Med* 2004;170:832.
97. Schechter M et al. Weekly rifapentine/isoniazid or daily rifampin/pyrazinamide for latent tuberculosis in household contacts. *Am J Respir Crit Care Med* 2006;173:922.
98. Saukkonen JJ et al. An official ATS statement: hepatotoxicity of antituberculosis therapy. *Am J Respir Crit Care Med* 2006;174:935.
99. Moulding T. Isoniazid-associated hepatitis deaths: a review of available information [Letter]. *Am Rev Respir Dis* 1992;146:1643.
100. Ellard GA. Variations between individuals and populations in the acetylation of isoniazid and its significance for the treatment of pulmonary tuberculosis. *Clin Pharmacol Ther* 1976;19:610.
101. Ellard GA et al. The hepatic toxicity of isoniazid among rapid and slow acetylators of the drug. *Am Rev Respir Dis* 1978;118:628.
102. Kopanoff DE et al. Isoniazid-related hepatitis: a U.S. Public Health Service cooperative surveillance study. *Am Rev Respir Dis* 1978;117:991.
103. Girling DJ. Adverse effects of antituberculosis drugs. *Drugs* 1982;23:56.
104. Steele MA et al. Toxic hepatitis with isoniazid and rifampin: a meta-analysis. *Chest* 1991;99:465.
105. Nolan CM et al. Hepatotoxicity associated with isoniazid preventive therapy: a 7-year survey from a public health tuberculosis clinic. *JAMA* 1999;281:1014.
106. Wright JM et al. Isoniazid-induced carbamazepine toxicity and vice versa: a double drug interaction. *N Engl J Med* 1982;307:1325.
107. Strayhorn VA et al. Update on rifampin drug interactions, III. *Arch Intern Med* 1997;157:2453.
108. Sanders WE. Rifampin. *Ann Intern Med* 1976;85: 82.
109. Zierski M et al. Side-effects of drug regimens used in short-course chemotherapy for pulmonary tuberculosis: a controlled clinical study. *Tubercle* 1980;61:41.
110. Girling DJ. Adverse reactions to rifampicin in antituberculosis regimens. *J Antimicrob Chemother* 1977;3:115.
111. Lee CH et al. Thrombocytopenia a rare but potentially serious side effect of initial daily and interrupted use of rifampicin. *Chest* 1989;96:202.
112. Berning SE et al. Rifamycin-induced lupus syndrome. *Lancet* 1997;349(9064):1521.
113. Bennett WM et al. Drug therapy in renal failure: dosing guidelines for adults. *Ann Intern Med* 1980;93:62.
114. Andrew OT et al. Tuberculosis in patients with end-stage renal disease. *Am J Med* 1980;68:59.
115. Citron KM et al. Ocular toxicity from ethambutol. *Thorax* 1986;41:737.
116. Schild HS et al. Rapid-onset reversible ocular toxicity from ethambutol therapy. *Am J Med* 1991; 90:404.
117. Alvarez KL et al. Ethambutol-induced ocular toxicity revisited [Letter]. *Ann Pharmacother* 1993;27: 102.
118. Van den Brande P. Revised guidelines for the diagnosis and control of tuberculosis: impact on management in the elderly. *Drugs Aging* 2005;22: 663.
119. Rajagopalan S et al. Tuberculosis in long-term-care facilities. *Infect Control Hosp Epidemiol* 2000;21:611.
120. Stead WW et al. Tuberculosis as an endemic and nosocomial infection among elderly in nursing homes. *N Engl J Med* 1985;312:1483.
121. Chan CH et al. The effect of age on the presentation of patients with tuberculosis. *Tuber Lung Dis* 1995;76:290.
122. Rajagopalan S. Tuberculosis and aging: a global health problem. *Clin Infect Dis* 2001;33:1034.
123. Van den Brande P et al. Aging and hepatotoxicity of isoniazid and rifampin in pulmonary tuberculosis. *Am J Respir Crit Care Med* 1995;152:1705.
124. Snider DE et al. Drug-resistant tuberculosis. *Am Rev Respir Dis* 1991;144:732.
125. Cohn DL et al. Drug-resistant tuberculosis: review of the worldwide situation and the WHO/IUATLD global surveillance project. *Clin Infect Dis* 1997;24(Suppl 1):S121.
126. Goble M et al. Treatment of 171 patients with pulmonary tuberculosis resistant to INH and rifampin. *N Engl J Med* 1993;328:527.

127. Berning SE et al. Malabsorption of antituberculosis medications by a patient with AIDS. *N Engl J Med* 1992;327:1817.
128. Granich RM et al. Multidrug resistance among persons with tuberculosis in California, 1994–2003. *JAMA* 2005;293:2732.
129. Centers for Disease Control and Prevention. National action plan to combat multidrug-resistant tuberculosis. *MMWR Morbid Mortal Wkly Rep* 1992;41(RR-11):5.
130. Driver CR et al. Factors associated with tuberculosis treatment interruption in New York City. *J Pub Health Management Prac* 2005;11:361.
131. Di Perri G et al. Which agents should we use for the treatment of multidrug-resistant *Mycobacterium tuberculosis*? *J Antimicrob Chemother* 2004;54:593.
132. Burgos M et al. Treatment of multidrug-resistant tuberculosis in San Francisco: an outpatient-based approach. *Clin Infect Dis* 2005;40:968.
133. Holtz TH et al. Time to sputum culture conversion in multidrug-resistant tuberculosis: predictors and relationship to treatment outcome. *Ann Intern Med* 2006;144:650.
134. Ji B et al. In vitro and in vivo activities of levofloxacin against *Mycobacterium tuberculosis*. *Antimicrob Agents Chemother* 1995;39:1341.
135. Berning SE et al. Long-term safety of ofloxacin and ciprofloxacin in the treatment of mycobacterial infections. *Am J Respir Crit Care Med* 1995;151:2006.
136. Peloquin CA et al. Levofloxacin for drug-resistant *Mycobacterium tuberculosis*. *Ann Pharmacother* 1998;32:268.
137. Codecasa LR et al. Long-term moxifloxacin in complicated tuberculosis patients with adverse reactions or resistance to first-line drugs. *Respir Med* 2006;100:1566.
138. Mehta JB et al. Impact of HIV infection on mycobacterial disease. *Am Fam Physician* 1992;45:2203.
139. Snider DE. Recognition and elimination of tuberculosis. *Adv Intern Med* 1993;38:169.
140. Girling DJ, et al. Extrapulmonary tuberculosis. *Br Med Bull* 1988;44:738.
141. Daley CL. Current issues in the pathogenesis and management of HIV-related tuberculosis. *AIDS Clin Rev* 1997;98:289.
142. Schluger NW. Issues in the treatment of active tuberculosis in human immunodeficiency virus-infected patients. *Clin Infect Dis* 1999;28:130.
143. Centers for Disease Control and Prevention. Clinical update: impact of HIV protease inhibitors on the treatment of HIV-infected tuberculosis patients with rifampin. *MMWR* 1996;45:921.
144. Li J et al. Relapse and acquired rifampin resistance in HIV-infected patients with tuberculosis treated with rifampin- or rifabutin-based regimens in New York City, 1997–2000. *Clin Infect Dis* 2005;41:83.
145. Burman W et al. Acquired rifamycin resistance with twice-weekly treatment of HIV-related tuberculosis. *Am J Respir Crit Care Med* 2006;173:350.
146. Hammer SM et al. Treatment for adult HIV infection: 2006 recommendations of the International AIDS Society-USA panel. *JAMA* 2006;296:827.
147. Burman WJ et al. Treatment of HIV-related tuberculosis in the era of effective antiretroviral therapy. *Am J Respir Crit Care Med* 2001;164:712.
148. Centers for Disease Control and Prevention. Updated guidelines for the use of rifabutin and rifampin for the treatment and prevention of tuberculosis among HIV-infected patients taking protease inhibitors or nonnucleoside reverse transcriptase inhibitors. *MMWR* 2000;49:185.
149. Centers for Disease Control and Prevention. Notice to readers: Acquired rifamycin resistance in persons with advanced HIV disease being treated for active tuberculosis with intermittent rifamycin-based regimens. *MMWR* 2002;51:214.
150. Piscitelli SC et al. Drug interactions in patients infected with human immunodeficiency virus. *Clin Infect Dis* 1996;23:685.
151. Antoniskis D et al. Combined toxicity of zidovudine and antituberculosis chemotherapy. *Am Rev Respir Dis* 1992;145:430.
152. Burman WJ et al. Therapeutic implications of drug interactions in the treatment of human immunodeficiency virus-related tuberculosis. *Clin Infect Dis* 1999;28:419.
153. Peloquin CA et al. Malabsorption of antimycobacterial medications. *N Engl J Med* 1993;329:1122.
154. Peloquin CA et al. Low antituberculosis drug concentrations in patients with AIDS. *Ann Pharmacother* 1996;30:919.
155. Peloquin CA. Using therapeutic drug monitoring to dose the antimycobacterial drugs. *Clin Chest Med* 1997;18:79.
156. Pape JW et al. Effect of isoniazid prophylaxis on incidence of active tuberculosis and progression of HIV infection. *Lancet* 1993;342:268.
157. Brost BC et al. The maternal and fetal effects of tuberculosis therapy. *Obstet Gynecol Clin North Am* 1997;24:659.
158. Frieden TR et al. Tuberculosis. *Lancet* 2003;362:887.
159. Vallejo JG et al. Tuberculosis and pregnancy. *Clin Chest Med* 1992;13:693.
160. Bergeron KG et al. Tuberculosis in pregnancy: current recommendations for screening and treatment in the USA. *Expert Review of Anti-infective Therapy* 2004;2:589.
161. Shin S et al. Treatment of multidrug-resistant tuberculosis during pregnancy: a report of 7 cases. *Clin Infect Dis* 2003;36:996.
162. Drobac PC et al. Treatment of multidrug-resistant tuberculosis during pregnancy: long-term follow-up of 6 children with intrauterine exposure to second-line agents. *Clin Infect Dis* 2005;40:1689.
163. Powell DA et al. Tuberculosis in children: an update. *Adv Pediatr* 2006;53:279.
164. Starke JR et al. Management of mycobacterial infection and disease in children. *Pediatr Infect Dis J* 1995;14:455.
165. Pediatric Tuberculosis Collaborative Group. Targeted tuberculin skin testing and treatment of latent tuberculosis infection in children and adolescents. *Pediatrics* 2004;114:1175.
166. Golden MP et al. Extrapulmonary tuberculosis: an overview. *Am Fam Physician* 2005;72:1761.
167. Garg RK. Tuberculosis of the central nervous system. *Postgrad Med J* 1999;75:133.
168. Davidson PT et al. Drug treatment of tuberculosis 1992. *Drugs* 1992;43:651.
169. Holdiness MR. Cerebrospinal fluid pharmacokinetics of the antituberculosis drugs. *Clin Pharmacokinet* 1985;10:532.
170. Dooley DP et al. Adjunctive corticosteroid therapy for tuberculosis: a critical reappraisal of the literature. *Clin Infect Dis* 1997;25:872.
171. Singh N et al. *Mycobacterium tuberculosis* infection in solid-organ transplant recipients: impact and implications for management. *Clin Infect Dis* 1998;27:1266.

CHAPTER 62

Infectious Diarrhea

Gail S. Itokazu, David T. Bearden, and Larry H. Danziger

Infectious diarrhea is caused by the ingestion of food or water contaminated with pathogenic microorganisms or their toxins. The spectrum of infection caused by enteropathogens includes asymptomatic carriage to life-threatening illnesses requiring urgent medical attention. This chapter focuses on the diagnosis and management of the common microbial causes of acute infectious diarrhea.

DEFINITIONS

Diarrhea is often defined as three or more episodes of loose stool or any loose stool with blood during a 24-hour period.[1] The duration of illness is often classified as acute diarrhea if the illness is <2 weeks' duration, persistent diarrhea if the illness lasts >14 days, and chronic diarrhea if the illness lasts >30 days.

The classification of infectious diarrheas as either a noninflammatory or inflammatory diarrheal illness is often used to predict the most likely enteropathgen causing the illness and to guide the overall treatment of this infection. Noninflammatory diarrheas are generally a less severe illness in which patients present with nonbloody, watery stools; patients are afebrile and without significant abdominal pain.[1] Examination of stool specimens does not reveal the presence of fecal white blood cells (WBC) or occult blood. Noninflammatory diarrheas are typically caused by rotaviruses, noroviruses, *Staphylococcus aureus*, *Bacillus cereus*, *Clostridium perfringens*, *Cryptosporidium parvum*, and *Giardia lamblia*.[2] Most patients with noninflammatory diarrheal illnesses require only supportive therapies.

In contrast, inflammatory diarrheas are generally a more severe illness in which patients present with bloody diarrhea, severe abdominal pain, and fever,[2] and examination of stool specimens reveals the presence of large numbers of fecal leukocytes. Inflammatory diarrheas are caused by invasive pathogens including *Campylobacter jejuni*, *Shigella* species, *Salmonella* species, *Clostridium difficile*, *Shiga toxin-producing Escherichia coli* (STEC), and *Entamoeba histolytica*.[2] Selected persons with inflammatory diarrheal illnesses may benefit from antimicrobial therapy directed at the causative pathogen.

PREVALENCE

During the 1990s, worldwide, more than 3 million deaths were attributed to infectious diarrhea, with most deaths occurring in developing countries.[1] The morbidity and mortality from diarrheal illnesses are largely attributed to dehydration,[2] with the very young, the elderly, and the immunocompromised at highest risk for this complication.[2,3] In developing countries, infectious diarrhea is mainly attributed to inadequate disposal of sewage, leading to unsafe drinking water. In developed countries persons at risk for infectious diarrhea include international travelers to underdeveloped countries; and persons in institutional settings where maintenance of good hygiene is often difficult (e.g., day care centers, hospitals, and extended care facilities). Our increasing reliance on foreign food supplies is another means by which exposure to foodborne infections may occur.[1] Finally, the increasing numbers of immunocompromised hosts including human immunodeficiency virus (HIV)-infected persons and organ transplant recipients comprise a population that is more susceptible to intestinal infections.[3]

ETIOLOGY

Microbial causes of infectious diarrhea include bacteria, viruses, protozoa, or fungi (Table 62-1). In developing countries, rotavirus is thought to be responsible for 60% of all diarrheal illnesses,[4] whereas the most common bacterial pathogens include the pathogenic *E. coli*, *Campylobacter*, *Salmonella*, *Shigella*, and *Vibrio* species.[4] In the United States, the FoodNet Surveillance Network also identified these pathogens as the most common causes of bacterial diarrheal illnesses, adding *Cryptosporidium* as a cause of parasitic diarrheal illnesses.[4] Rotavirus infection, which is commonly associated with the hospitalization of children with diarrheal illnesses, is likely to be the causative agent in many cases of community-acquired diarrhea.[4]

PATHOGENESIS

Bacterial Virulence Factors

Enteropathogens possess a number of virulence factors, including toxins, adhesions, and invasive properties that contribute to the organism's pathogenicity.[1] Enterotoxins target the small bowel, causing net movement of fluid into the gut lumen leading to voluminous quantities of watery stools and potentially life-threatening dehydration. Watery diarrhea can also be caused by an alteration in the absorptive function of the villus tip, as seen with rotaviruses and noroviruses.[5] Cytotoxins target the colon, causing direct mucosal damage leading to fever and bloody diarrhea.

The invasive properties identified in *Shigella* species and invasive strains of *E. coli* allow these bacteria to invade and destroy epithelial cells causing bloody or mucoid stools.[5] Some enteropathogens induce a vigorous host response (e.g., release of proinflammatory cytokines from intestinal epithelial cells) that can lead to diarrhea.[5] Adhesions allow enteropathogens to attach to and colonize the gastrointestinal (GI) mucosa, facilitating invasion, dissemination, toxin delivery, or host cell lysis.

Host Defenses

The human gastrointestinal tract possesses numerous defense mechanisms to protect against enteric infection. For example, because many bacteria cannot survive in an acidic environment, the normal gastric acidity of the stomach prevents viable pathogens from passing from the stomach into the small intestine. Intestinal peristalsis moves bacteria and their toxins along and out of the GI tract. Gastrointestinal mucus and mucosal tissue integrity provide physical barriers against infection. Intestinal immunity, including the local production of antibody, contributes to the host's ability to resist enteric infection. Finally, the normal bacterial flora compete for space and nutrients with potentially pathogenic organisms, or produce substances that may be inhibitory to enteropathogens.[5]

Predisposing Factors

Predisposing factors to infectious diarrhea include travel history, compromised immune status, exposure to outbreaks of foodborne or waterborne illnesses, poor personal hygiene, and the use of pharmacologic agents. These predisposing factors also provide clues to the most likely microbes causing the diarrheal illness. For example, a diarrheal illness in the setting of recent travel to a developing country suggests travelers' diarrhea caused by the pathogens endemic to that area. HIV-infected persons are susceptible to infectious diarrhea caused by *Salmonella*, *Cryptosporidium*, and numerous other enteropathogens.[3] Outbreaks of diarrheal illnesses should raise suspicions of illness caused by *S. aureus*, *B. cereus*, *C. perfringens*, *Shigella*, *Salmonella*, *Campylobacter*, or *noncholera Vibrio*.[3] In the day care setting, agents spread by the fecal–oral route, such as *Shigella*, *G. lamblia*, and *Cryptosporidium*, should be considered.[3] Diarrhea in the setting of hospitalization or recent exposure to antibiotics increases the likelihood of *C. difficile* colitis.[1] Drugs that increase gastric pH, such as H_2-receptor antagonists, proton pump inhibitors, or antacids increase the risk for infection with *Salmonella* because these bacteria do not survive well in the normally acidic stomach (Table 62-2).

CLINICAL PRESENTATION

Details of the patient's clinical presentation, such as the specific symptoms, the severity and duration of symptoms, and the

Table 62-1 Predisposing Factors, Symptoms, and Therapy of Gastrointestinal Infections

Pathogen	*Predisposing Factors*	*Symptoms*	*Diagnostic Evaluations*	*Drug of Choice*	*Alternatives*
Salmonella (nontyphoidal)	Ingestion of contaminated poultry, raw milk, custards, and cream fillings; foreign travel	Nausea, vomiting, diarrhea, cramps, fever, tenesmus Incubation: 6–72 hrs	Fecal leukocytes, stool culture	Fluoroquinolone, third-generation cephalosporins	Ampicillin, amoxicillin, TMP-SMX, chloramphenicol, azithromycin
Salmonella (typhoidal)	Ingestion of contaminated food, foreign travel	High fever, abdominal pain, headache, dry cough	Fecal leukocytes, stool culture, blood culture	Fluoroquinolone, third-generation cephalosporins	Chloramphenicol, TMP-SMX, ampicillin, amoxicillin, azithromycin
Shigella	Ingestion of contaminated food, foreign travel.	Fever, dysentery, cramps, tenesmus Incubation: 12–24 hrs	Fecal leukocytes	Fluoroquinolone	Azithromycin, TMP-SMX, ampicillin, ceftriaxone
Campylobacter	Contaminated eggs, raw milk, or poultry; foreign travel	Mild to severe diarrhea; fever, systemic malaise Incubation: 24–72 hrs	Fecal leukocytes, stool culture	Erythromycin, azithromycin	Fluoroquinolone, tetracycline, gentamicin
Clostridium difficile	Antibiotics, antineoplastics	Mild to severe diarrhea, cramps	*C. difficile toxin, C. difficile culture,* colonoscopy	Metronidazole	Vancomycin
Staphylococcal food poisoning	Custard-filled bakery products, canned food, processed meat, ice cream	Nausea, vomiting, salivation, cramps, diarrhea; usually resolves in 8 hrs Incubation: 2–6 hrs	—	Supportive therapy only	—
Travelers' diarrhea *(Escherichia coli)*	Contaminated food (vegetables and cheese), water, foreign travel	Nausea, vomiting, mild to severe diarrhea, cramps	Stool culture	See Table 62-3	—
Shiga toxin-producing *Escherichia coli* (*E. coli* O157:H7)	Beef, raw milk, water	Diarrhea, headache, bloody stools Incubation: 48–96 hrs	Stool cultures on MacConkey's sorbitol	Supportive therapy only	—
Cryptosporidiosis	Immunosuppression, day care centers, contaminated water, animal handlers	Mild to severe diarrhea (chronic or self-limited); large fluid volume	Stool screening for oocytes, PCR, ELISA	See Chapter 71, Opportunistic Infections in HIV-Infected Patients	—
Viral gastroenteritis	Community-wide outbreaks, contaminated food	Nausea, diarrhea (self-limited), cramps Incubation: 16–48 hrs	Special viral studies	Supportive therapy only	—

ELISA, enzyme-linked immunosorbent assay; HAART, highly active antiretroviral therapy; PCR, polymerase chain reaction; TMP-SMX, trimethoprim-sulfamethoxazole.

[a] See text for doses and duration of therapy.

[b] Not all cases require antibiotic therapy. See text for details.

From Hines J et al. Effective use of the clinical microbiology laboratory for diagnosing diarrheal diseases. *Clin Infect Dis* 1996;23:1292, with permission.

Table 62-2 Pharmacologic Agents That May Promote Gastrointestinal Infection

Drug	Mechanism
Antacids, H_2 -receptor antagonists, proton pump inhibitors	Increased gastric pH; viable pathogens passed to lower gut
Antibiotics	Eradication of normal (anaerobic) flora
Antidiarrheals	Decreased gut motility; bacterial growth
Immunosuppressives	Inhibition of gut immune defenses

onset of the illness also help to predict the most likely microbial cause of the diarrheal illness. For example, watery diarrhea associated with nausea and vomiting occurring within hours of exposure to a contaminated food source suggests the ingestion of preformed toxins such as those produced by *S. aureus* or *B. cereus*.[3] Abdominal cramps and diarrhea occurring within 8–16 hours after consumption of contaminated meats and gravies suggests infection with *C. perfringens*.

Bloody diarrhea and fever should raise suspicion of infection with invasive pathogens, such as *Salmonella, Shigella,* and *Campylobacter*. Some invasive enteropathogens, such as *Campylobacter, Aeromonas, Shigella*, and *Vibrio parahaemolyticus,* may, however, initially cause watery diarrhea, which is then followed by bloody diarrhea.[1] In the United States, STEC is the most common cause of bloody diarrhea, and should be suspected, especially if fever is absent.[6]

Persistent diarrhea in travelers is associated with parasites such as *G. lamblia, Cryptosporidium*, or *Isospora belli;* and bacteria such as enteropathogenic *E. coli, enterotoxigenic E. coli*, STEC, *Shigella, C. jejuni*, and *Aeromonas*.[4]

Complications of infectious diarrhea most commonly include dehydration and electrolyte losses. Metabolic alkalosis can result from the severe vomiting associated with staphylococcal food poisoning, or from gastroenteritis caused by rotaviruses or noroviruses. Other complications associated with specific enteropathogens include toxic megacolon and intestinal perforation following *Shigella*, STEC, and *C. difficile* infection; hemolytic uremic syndrome following STEC and *Shigella* infection; a reactive arthritis following *Shigella, Salmonella,* and *Campylobacter* infection; and metastatic infection following *Salmonella* infection.[4]

TREATMENT OF PATIENTS WITH INFECTIOUS DIARRHEA

Infectious diarrhea is generally a self-limiting illness, and most patients never seek medical attention. In many cases, replacement of fluids and electrolytes is all that is required. Medical evaluation is warranted for patients with profuse watery diarrhea with dehydration, six or more unformed stools within a 24-hour period, bloody stools, temperature $>101.3°F$, or illness of >48 hours' duration. Other persons requiring medical evaluation for a diarrheal illness include patients >50 years of age with severe abdominal pain, patients $\geq$70 years of age, and immunocompromised patients (e.g., acquired immunodeficiency syndrome [AIDS], organ transplant recipient, or patients have cancer chemotherapy).[3] The evaluation of any diarrheal illness should also consider the possibility of a noninfectious cause for the illness, such as medications, inflammatory bowel disease, radiation colitis, or malabsorption syndromes.[7]

Rehydration Therapy

Depending on the degree of dehydration and ongoing losses, fluids and electrolytes may be replaced intravenously or orally. The degree of dehydration is assessed by careful physical examination and measurement of vital signs. Severe dehydration is characterized by lethargy and inadequate oral intake; very sunken and dry eyes and a very dry tongue and mouth; and a very fast, weak or nonplapable pulse.[8,9] Other characteristics of dehydration include poor urine output and low blood pressure. Intravenous replacement therapies are warranted for severely dehydrated persons, or persons with intestinal ileus or who are unable to drink on their own.[8]

Mild to moderate dehydration can be treated primarily with oral replacement therapies.[8,9] For adults able to drink normally, beverages containing glucose (e.g., lemonades, sweet sodas, or fruit juices) or soups rich in electrolytes are recommended.[10] In developing countries, oral replacement therapy solutions containing optimal concentrations of glucose, sodium, potassium, chloride, and bicarbonate are responsible for the significant reduction in mortality attributed to dehydration.[9] These oral replacement solutions are effective because sodium absorption is accelerated in the presence of glucose.[9]

Laboratory Tests

Inflammatory diarrheal illnesses are characterized by stool specimens containing large numbers of fecal leukocytes (e.g., more than three leukocytes per high-power microscopic field in four or more fields, or markers of fecal leukocytes such as lactoferrin) or the presence of occult blood.[2,11] Pathogens commonly cultured from these patients include *Shigella, Salmonella, Campylobacter, Aeromonas, Yersinia, noncholera Vibrio*, and *C. difficile*.[3] The absence of leukocytes in a stool specimen, however, does not rule out an inflammatory diarrhea.[11] The mean sensitivity of fecal leukocytes for the prototypical inflammatory diarrheal disease agent *Shigella,* averages 73% (range, 49%–100%).[11] The absence of fecal WBC suggests a noninflammatory diarrhea.

A microbiologic diagnosis of infectious diarrhea from a stool sample is made by culture of the pathogen or isolation of toxins (e.g., *C. difficile*) produced by the organism. Careful selection of patients in whom stool cultures are performed should maximize the cost-effectiveness of performing this test.[11] Stool cultures are recommended for patients with one of the following: severe diarrhea; bloody stools; or stools containing leukocytes, lactoferrin, or occult blood; or an oral temperature $\geq 101.3°F$. Cultures are also recommended in patients with persistent diarrhea who have not been given empiric antimicrobials.[3] Identification of parasitic causes of infectious diarrhea is made by microscopic examination of a stool specimen for ova and parasites. More sensitive tests to diagnose parasitic infections include direct immunofluorescence assay (DFA) to detect *G. lamblia* and *Cryptosporidium*, and enzyme immunoassay (EIA) to detect *G. lamblia* and *Cryptosporidium* antigen.[11]

Enteropathogens may also be isolated from extraintestinal sites such as the blood and bone marrow, or other sites to which infection has spread.

Drug Therapy

Bismuth Subsalicylate

Bismuth subsalicylate is an antidiarrheal agent with antibacterial properties.[12] Adverse effects of bismuth subsalicylate include darkening of the tongue and stools,[4] tinnitus,[13] and encephalopathy when high doses are used.[4] Bismuth subsalicylate can interfere with the absorption of other medications such as doxycycline used in malaria prophylaxis, and fluoroquinolones used in the management of travelers diarrhea.

Loperamide and Diphenoxylate/Atropine

The antimotility agents loperamide and the combination product diphenoxylate/atropine provide symptomatic relief by slowing intestinal transit time.[10] Loperamide is preferred over diphenoxylate/atropine because of its better efficacy, lower potential for adverse effects, and availability as an over-the-counter preparation.[10] Diphenoxylate/atropine can cause drowsiness, dizziness, dry mouth, and urinary retention. Although controversial,[13] experts do not recommend the use of antimotility drugs in persons with fever or bloody diarrhea[14] or when invasive pathogens are suspected, because of concerns that prolonging the clearance of pathogens from the intestinal tract could worsen the severity of illness.[13]

Probiotics

Probiotics are live microbial mixtures of bacteria and yeasts used to restore the normal intestinal flora, thereby reducing intestinal colonization with pathogenic organisms.[15] Probiotics can also produce pathogen-inhibiting substances, inhibit pathogen adhesion to the GI tract, inhibit the action of microbial toxins, and stimulate immune defense mechanisms.[16] Interest in probiotics stems in part from their potential to decrease the use of antibiotics.

Disadvantages of probiotics include the lack of both well-controlled trials supporting their efficacy and quality controls on the manufacturing of these products, and the risk for systemic infection, particularly in the immunocompromised host.[16] Some evidence supports the use of probiotics for the treatment of rotavirus diarrhea in children and as an adjunct for the treatment of recurrent *C. difficile* colitis.[16]

Antimicrobials

Because infectious diarrhea is generally a self-limiting illness, the routine use of antimicrobials is not necessary.[1] In selected individuals antimicrobials are beneficial, however, because they decrease the duration and the severity of illness, prevent invasive infection, and prevent person-to-person transmission of pathogens.[7] In general, antimicrobials are recommended for patients with severe illness, patients with conditions that compromise normal enteric defenses, or for immunocompromised patients. Antibiotics are also necessary to treat extraintestinal complications of enteric infection, such as bacteremia and osteomyelitis.

Trimethoprim-sulfamethoxazole (TMP-SMX), the aminopenicillins, tetracyclines, and nalidixic acid have been used extensively for the treatment of enteric infections because of their ease of administration, relative safety, and low cost. The emergence of enteric pathogens resistant to one or all of these agents is limiting their usefulness for both domestically and internationally acquired infectious diarrhea.[7] Depending on the microbial cause of diarrhea, alternatives to these agents include the fluoroquinolones, selected third-generation cephalosporins (e.g., ceftriaxone, cefotaxime, cefixime), azithromycin, and rifaximin. Because fluoroquinolones have been widely used in humans, and in agriculture and veterinary medicine, increasing resistance to this class of antimicrobials among common bacterial enteropathogens, such *Salmonella, Shigella* and *Campylobacter* species, is not uncommon.

Besides increasing resistance of enteropathogens to fluoroquinolones, another issue with these agents is that they are not approved for use in children because lesions on cartilage tissue have been reported in juvenile animals.[17] Nevertheless, because of the emergence of multidrug-resistant enteropathogens in some geographic areas, clinical trials using fluoroquinolones in children have been performed, and the available data suggest that a short course of these agents is safe.[17,18]

Prevention

Measures to prevent the spread of enteropathogens include good personal hygiene; and proper handling, cooking, and storage of foods. Persons traveling to areas with inadequate sewage and water systems should follow the rule, "boil it, cook it, peel it, or forget it." Vaccines to prevent typhoid fever are available.

TREATMENT OVERVIEW

1. B.K. is a 78-year-old man presenting to his physician with a diarrheal illness of 1 day's duration. His illness began with vomiting, followed by abdominal pain, nausea, and watery diarrhea without blood. He denies any fever. B.K.'s history of present illness is significant for dining with friends at a seafood restaurant 2 nights ago. They all shared an appetizer of raw oysters, and he has since learned his friends are experiencing a similar illness. B.K. has no significant medical history. He denies recent hospitalization, contact with small children, recent travel, or recent use of antimicrobials. On physical examination B.K. is alert and oriented, and is not "toxic" appearing. The remainder of his examination is only significant for decreased skin turgor and dry mucous membranes. What is your general approach to the management of B.K.'s diarrheal illness?

The most common complication of any diarrheal illness is loss of fluids and electrolytes, which in extreme cases can lead to hypovolemia, shock, and death. Once replacement of fluid and electrolyte losses have been addressed, patients are evaluated to determine the need for further medical evaluation and the need for drug therapy to provide symptomatic relief or specific antimicrobial therapy directed at the causative pathogen.

2. What specific plan for rehydration would you recommend for B.K.? Would evaluation of a stool sample for the presence of WBC or blood provide useful information to assist in treating his illness?

B.K.'s clinical presentation is that of a nontoxic-appearing elderly man with signs and symptoms of mild to moderate volume depletion (decreased skin turgor and dry mucous membranes). An oral rehydration solution containing 45 to 90 mEq/L of sodium can be used to manage his fluid and electrolyte losses.[3]

Further medical evaluation to determine if B.K.'s illness is consistent with an inflammatory or noninflammatory diarrheal illness will assist in assessing the role of specific drug therapies. Patients with an inflammatory diarrheal illness may benefit from antimicrobial therapy directed at the causative pathogen, whereas those with a noninflammatory diarrheal illness can generally be treated by fluids and electrolyte replacement. A stool specimen should be sent to the laboratory and examined for the presence of WBC and blood.

VIRAL GASTROENTERITIS

Clinical Presentation and Treatment

3. B.K.'s stool is negative for WBC and blood. In the meantime, because of B.K.'s history of dining with friends with a similar illness, the physician calls the Board of Health to ask about other reports of person with a similar illness, and is told of an outbreak of *Norovirus* (previously called Norwalk-like virus) gastroenteritis associated with food served at the restaurant where B.K had dined. Why are B.K.'s history of present illness and clinical presentation consistent with the presumptive diagnosis of gastroenteritis caused by noroviruses?

Noroviruses are estimated to be responsible for more the two-thirds of pathogen-confirmed, foodborne illnesses.[19] Of the common viral causes of gastroenteritis, B.K.'s history and clinical presentation suggest a *Norovirus* as the likely pathogen. Noroviruses are responsible for major outbreaks of foodborne viral illnesses in both adults and children, usually in association with restaurants, schools, and day care centers.[19] These viruses are spread by (a) the consumption of fecally contaminated water or foods, such as inadequately cooked clams and oysters harvested from contaminated waters, (b) person-to-person contact, or (c) exposure to recreational waters.[19] Illness typically begins within 12–48 hours after exposure to the virus and generally lasts 1–3 days. The gastrointestinal illness is generally mild, with patients reporting nausea, vomiting, diarrhea, abdominal cramps, myalgias, headache, and chills. Fever occurs in one-third to one-half of cases. Prevention of illness is aimed at proper food handling practices.[19]

Rotaviruses and astroviruses are important causes of infectious diarrhea in children, with rotaviruses responsible for 30%–60% of all cases of severe watery diarrhea in this population.[20] Following an incubation period of 1–3 days, patients present with fever, vomiting, and watery but nonbloody diarrhea. In normal hosts, this illness lasts for 5–7 days.[20] Because rotavirus is spread by the fecal–oral route, preventive measures include proper handwashing and disposal of contaminated items. A recently U.S. Food and Drug Administration (FDA)-approved rotavirus vaccine (RotaTeq) is indicated for the prevention of rotavirus gastroenteritis in infants and children caused by selected serotypes. A three-dose series is administered between the ages of 6–32 weeks.[21]

The morbidity and mortality of viral gastroenteritis primarily is caused by fluid and electrolyte losses. Thus, supportive measures to correct these deficits and replace ongoing losses are the mainstay of treatment for viral gastroenteritis. Probiotics have been found to decrease the duration of diarrhea caused by the rotavirus. In young children hospitalized with acute diarrhea primarily caused by rotavirus, a randomized, double-blind placebo-controlled trial demonstrated that a mixture of lactobacillus strains administered early (<60 hours) in the course of illness decreased the duration of the diarrheal illness from 130 hours–80 hours ($p = 0.003$). The lactobacillus strains used in this study were selected for their potential probiotic characteristics.[22]

VIBRIO SPECIES

Vibrio species are curved gram-negative rods whose natural habitats are the environmental waters. Toxigenic *V. cholerae* 01 and 0139 cause epidemic cholera in humans,[23] whereas the *noncholerae Vibrio* species, such as *V. parahaemolyticus,* generally cause gastroenteritis and extraintestinal infection.[24]

Vibrio cholerae

Clinical Presentation

4. M.M., a 50-year-old previously healthy man, is brought to the emergency department (ED) by his family because of severe watery diarrhea, vomiting, and altered mental status. His history of present illness is significant for return 1 day ago from Latin America where he visited with relatives, several of whom were recovering from infection caused by *V. cholerae.* Approximately 24 hours before admission, he noted the onset of watery diarrhea and began drinking the oral rehydrating solution left over from his trip to Latin America. Over the past several hours he has been unable to drink on his own, however, and his family noticed "white flecks" in his stools.

In the ED, M.M.'s vital signs are as follows: temperature 101°F, blood pressure is 70/40 mmHg, and heart rate is 130 beats/minute. His weight is 61 kg, which is 8 kg below his normal weight. Physical examination reveals a critically ill man with sunken eyes, poor skin turgor, and dry mucous membranes. The physician's assessment is severe dehydration, most likely secondary to infection from *V. cholerae.* What are the signs and symptoms suggestive of severe dehydration, and how should M.M.'s dehydration be treated?

M.M. shows signs of severe dehydration as manifested by his altered mental status, sunken eyes, poor skin turgor, dry mucous membranes, low blood pressure, increased heart rate, and weight loss of >10% of his normal body weight.[8] Other complications of severe fluid and electrolyte losses associated with cholera infection include acidosis as a result of bicarbonate losses through stool along with lactic acidosis from shock, and renal failure secondary to hypovolemia.[8]

Fluid and electrolyte replacement is the mainstay of treatment for patients with cholera. The watery stools of patients with cholera contain high concentrations of sodium, potassium, and bicarbonate.[8] In the United States, Ringer's lactate solution is the only readily available intravenous (IV) solution with the electrolyte composition required to treat cholera.[8] Vigorous IV hydration to restore his intravascular volume should be instituted. Monitoring of blood pressure and normalization of heart rate are mandatory. Once M.M. is able to drink fluids, oral rehydration can be started even while rehydration with IV fluids is ongoing. When replacing fluids in patients with cholera, the use of oral replacement solutions containing <75 mEq/L of sodium is inappropriate because of the large amounts of sodium lost through cholera stools.[8]

5. **Why is M.M.'s history of present illness and clinical presentation consistent with a severe diarrheal illness caused by toxin-producing *V. cholerae*?**

The incubation period of *V. cholerae* is typically 1–3 days, but ranges from a few hours to 5 days. The spectrum of illness caused by *V. cholerae* includes asymptomatic carriage (most persons), mild to moderate watery diarrhea, and life-threatening dehydration.[8] M.M. is one of the few (2%–5%) persons with severe dehydration which, within hours, could evolve into hypovolemic shock and death. The watery and colorless stools with "white flecks" of mucus are referred to as *rice-water stools*. Patients can lose up to 1 L/hour of fluid during the first 24 hours and may lose up to 10% of their body weight. The watery diarrhea is caused by the cholera toxin, which promotes the secretion of fluids and electrolytes by the small intestine. Cholera epidemics are caused by toxin-producing strains of *V. cholerae* 01 or 0139.[24] Hypoglycemia can occur in severe cholera, especially in children.[8]

In developing countries with inadequate sanitation facilities, cholera infection is primarily spread by the consumption of contaminated water and foods. Foods that are often contaminated with *V. cholera* include improperly preserved fish, raw oysters, and undercooked shellfish, such as crabs.[8] In the United States and other developed nations, cholera has been virtually eliminated because of modern sewage and water treatment systems. Nevertheless, cases of cholera are still seen in the United States, particularly in persons traveling to parts of Latin America, Africa, or Asia where epidemics of cholera still occur, or in travelers bringing contaminated seafood back to the United States. Domestic cases of cholera arise from the consumption of undercooked seafood harvested from contaminated waters off the Gulf Coast.[23]

Treatment

6. **Would M.M. benefit from the administration of antibiotics?**

Antimicrobials are beneficial in the treatment of patients with cholera because they decrease the volume of diarrheal losses and shorten illness duration.[25] In areas of the world with limited health care resources, shortening the duration of an illness with the use of relatively inexpensive antimicrobials is a means of conserving health care resources because of the shortened hospital stay and less need for intravenous fluids.[25] Because antimicrobial resistance patterns of *V. cholerae* vary in different regions of the world, as well as change over time with antimicrobial resistant strains reverting back to susceptible strains, selection of a specific antimicrobial regimen should consider the susceptibility pattern of the circulating strain.[25] Both single-dose and multiple-dose regimens are clinically effective for the treatment of *V. cholerae* infection caused by susceptible strains; single-dose regimens are preferred because of their ease of administration.[25]

Effective single-dose oral regimens in adults infected with susceptible strains of *V. cholerae* include 300 mg of doxycycline,[25] 1 g of ciprofloxacin,[26] or 1 g of azithromycin.[27] One study illustrated the importance of the need for ongoing surveillance of antimicrobial susceptibility patterns of *V. cholerae* in order to increase the likelihood of clinical success.[27] Although a prior study demonstrated the efficacy of ciprofloxacin for the treatment cholera caused by *V. cholerae*, a more recent study reported that, because resistance to ciprofloxacin had since emerged, a single 1-g dose of ciprofloxacin was less effective than a single 1-g dose of azithromycin.[27]

Effective single-dose, oral regimens for the treatment of cholera in children include ciprofloxacin 20 mg/kg (maximum, 750 mg)[28] or azithromycin 20 mg/kg (maximum, 1 g).[29] These regimens were as effective as the standard treatment with erythromycin 12.5 mg/kg/dose (maximum, 500 mg/dose) Q 6 hr for 3 days. In these studies, single-dose regimens were better tolerated than the multiple-dose regimen using erythromycin. Compared with children treated with erythromycin, children treated with a single dose of ciprofloxacin experienced less vomiting and fewer stools,[28] and those treated with azithromycin also experienced less vomiting.[29]

Effective multiple-dose regimens for cholera include tetracycline (500 mg orally Q 6 hr for 48–72 hours),[25] erythromycin 250 mg orally four times daily for 3 days,[8] and TMP-SMX (adults, 160 mg TMP, 800 mg SMX twice daily for 3 days; children, 5 mg/kg TMP, 25 mg/kg SMX twice daily for 3 days).[8] Although resistance to TMS-SMX had previously been problematic, more recent strains of *V. cholerae* O139 causing infection in Bangladesh are now susceptible to trimethoprim and sulfamethoxazole.[30]

Vibrio parahaemolyticus

Clinical Presentation

7. **C.T. is a 45-year-old man presenting to his family physician with a 1-day history of nonbloody, watery diarrhea. His history is significant for return 2 days ago from the coastal areas of Florida. On the evening before leaving Florida, he and his wife dined at a seafood restaurant where they shared the same meal, with the exception of an appetizer of raw oysters that only C.T. had consumed. His wife is not ill. C.T. has no significant medical history. His physical examination reveals no signs or symptoms of dehydration. Why is C.T.'s history of present illness and clinical presentation consistent with *non-cholerae Vibrio* gastroenteritis?**

A key piece of information from C.T.'s history of present illness, which is consistent with the presumptive diagnosis of *non-cholerae Vibrio* gastroenteritis, is consumption of raw oysters harvested from areas where *V. parahaemolyticus* species have been identified. In a survey of *V. parahaemolyticus* infection in the United States, gastroenteritis accounted for 59% of infections, wound infection accounted for 34% of infections, and septicemia accounted for 5% of infections.[24] Following a median incubation period of 17 hours (range, 4–90 hours),[31] clinical manifestations of gastroenteritis include diarrhea, abdominal cramps, nausea, vomiting, and fever. Bloody diarrhea occurs in 9%–29% of cases.[24,31] In Japan, *V. parahaemolyticus* is a frequent cause of watery diarrhea because of the consumption of raw fish and shellfish.[2]

Treatment

8. **Should a course of antibiotics be prescribed for C.T.?**

In healthy adults, *V. parahaemolyticus* gastroenteritis is usually a mild, self-limiting illness lasting a median of 2.4–6 days.[32] Antibiotics have not been shown to shorten the course of uncomplicated infection,[32] but they may be helpful in patients with severe diarrhea.[24] Antimicrobials are also used to treat wound infections and septicemia.[24] When indicated, ceftazidime with doxycycline, or doxycycline with ciprofloxacin or an aminoglycoside is recommended.[31] Individuals with liver disease or alcoholism are at risk for severe *Vibrio* infections, including septicemia.[24] The risk for infection can be reduced by avoiding the consumption of raw or undercooked shellfish; and avoiding the exposure of wounds to seawater, especially during the warmer months when water temperatures favor the multiplication of *Vibrio*.[31]

STAPHYLOCOCCUS AUREUS, BACILLUS CEREUS, AND CLOSTRIDIUM PERFRINGENS

Clinical Presentation and Treatment

Staphylococcus aureus, B. cereus, and *C. perfringens* are important causes of toxin-mediated foodborne illnesses. Gastrointestinal symptoms typically begin within 24 hours of ingestion of contaminated foods, which is in contrast to the longer incubation periods for illnesses caused by *Salmonella, Shigella,* and *Campylobacter. B. cereus* causes two different intestinal syndromes: the short-incubation disease characterized by vomiting (emetic syndrome) and the long-incubation disease characterized by a diarrheal illness (diarrheal syndrome).[20]

9. T.N., a 30-year-old woman, presents to her family physician with an acute onset of nausea and vomiting. Her history is significant for attending a Chinese buffet 3 hours ago with friends who are experiencing a similar illness. The buffet included a variety of beef, fish, and chicken dishes; fried rice; and desserts, including cream-filled pastries. T.N. is alert and oriented, and her physical examination is normal. Why are T.N.'s history of present illness and clinical presentation consistent with food poisoning caused by *S. aureus,* or short-incubation disease caused by *B. cereus*? Should empiric antibiotics be prescribed?

Foodborne illnesses are often grouped by their usual incubation period: <6 hours, 8–16 hours, and >16 hours. The rapid onset (within 6 hours) of T.N.'s GI symptoms after eating suggests the illness is caused by preformed toxins produced by *S. aureus* or *B. cereus* (short-incubation disease, emetic syndrome). Diarrhea and abdominal cramps may also occur. Although cooking kills the toxin-producing bacteria, it does not destroy toxin that has already been produced. Foods implicated in staphylococcal food poisoning include salads, cream-filled pastries, and meats,[20] whereas foods implicated in *B. cereus* food poisoning include fried rice, dried foods, and dairy products.[20]

In contrast, the features of T.N.'s illness are not consistent with signs and symptoms of toxin-mediated illness caused by *C. perfringens* or *B. cereus* (long-incubation disease, diarrheal syndrome). These bacteria are associated with the onset of diarrhea and abdominal cramps within 8–16 hours after the ingestion of contaminated foods, and vomiting is not a prominent symptom in these illnesses. *C. perfringens* or *B. cereus* causing the long-incubation disease produces heat-labile toxins in vivo after the ingestion of contaminated foods, thus, explaining the longer incubation period compared with illness caused by the ingestion of preformed toxins. Foods implicated in *C. perfringens* food poisoning include improperly stored beef, fish, poultry dishes, pasta salads, and dairy products, whereas foods implicated in long-incubation *B. cereus* food poisoning include meats, vanilla sauce, cream-filled baked goods, and salads.[20]

Illnesses caused by these toxin-producing bacteria usually resolve within 24 hours. Antibiotic therapy is not indicated.[20]

SHIGELLA

Shigella species are gram-negative bacilli that are frequent causes of the dysentery syndrome. Dysentery is a severe manifestation of inflammatory diarrhea characterized by bloody or mucoid stools, abdominal cramps, and tenesmus (painful straining when passing stools). Of the four *Shigella* species, severe dysentery is most likely to be caused by *S. dysenteriae* followed by *S. flexneri,* whereas a milder illness characterized by watery diarrhea with or without blood is generally caused by *S. sonnei* and *S. boydii*.[33,34] In addition to the greater propensity for dysentery to be caused by *S. dysenteriae*, differentiating between the various *Shigella* species (i.e., *S. dysenteriae* versus other *Shigella* species) has implications in terms of the clinical response to the prescribed antimicrobial regimen.

Shigella dysenteriae

Clinical Presentation

10. M.T. is a 60-year-old, ill-appearing man presenting to the hospital because of worsening bloody diarrhea and fever. Two days before admission, he noted the onset of fever, abdominal cramps, and six to seven nonbloody, watery stools. His diarrhea has since worsened to 10–12 small-volume stools with blood and mucus, and he now complains of painful straining while passing his stools. His history of present illness is significant for return 2 days ago from a business trip to Bangladesh. During the business portion of his trip, M.T. remained at the hotel where the meeting was being held and where all of his meals were prepared by the hotel staff. On the day of his departure, however, he decided to consume meals prepared by local street vendors. M.T. lives alone in Florida. He has no significant medical history, has no known drug allergies, and takes no medications. On admission, his temperature is 101°F. Physical examination reveals an acutely ill man with severe abdominal tenderness, and with signs and symptoms of mild dehydration. Why are his history of present illness and clinical presentation consistent with the diagnosis of dysentery, most likely caused by *Shigella dysenteriae*?

A key piece of information from M.T.'s history of present illness that is consistent with his presumptive diagnosis of shigellosis is his recent travel to Bangladesh, where shigellosis is endemic because of the lack of adequate systems for sewage disposal. Epidemics or outbreaks of *S. dysenteriae* have been reported in other areas of the world, including South Asia, India, and Sri Lanka.[34] M.T. probably acquired his infection following the consumption of contaminated foods prepared by local street vendors. Because as few as 10–100 *Shigella* organisms can cause infection in healthy hosts,[34] shigellosis is easily spread by symptomatic persons with diarrhea, by person-to-person contact, by consumption of contaminated food and water, or by asymptomatic persons who continue to excrete shigellae from their stool.[35] Good hygiene and access to clean water and foods are essential to prevent the spread of shigellosis.

As in M.T., symptoms of dysentery begin within 24–48 hours following ingestion of *Shigella* bacteria and include fever, fatigue, malaise, and anorexia.[35] Watery diarrhea generally precedes dysentery, and frequently is the only manifestation of mild infection.[35] Progression to dysentery may follow within hours to days and is characterized by frequent small volume, bloody, and mucoid stools; abdominal cramps; and tenesmus.[35] Of the four *Shigella* species, severe dysentery is most likely to be caused by *S. dysenteriae*.[33,34] Complications of shigellosis include seizures, hemolytic uremic syndrome (HUS), and toxic megacolon.[35]

Treatment

11. Would M.T. benefit from antibiotics to treat his presumed diagnosis of shigellosis?

Effective antimicrobial therapy for shigellosis has several benefits. First, effective therapy reduces the average duration of illness from 5–7 days to about 3 days.[35] Within 48 hours of starting treatment, patients can expect to experience decreases in stool frequency, the volume of bloody stools, and fever, and an improved appetite.[33] Second, effective antimicrobial therapy reduces the risk of death and serious complications associated with shigellosis.[33] Third, effective antimicrobial therapy quickly reduces the carriage and excretion of *Shigella* species, which serves to limit the spread of infection.[36]

Despite the aforementioned benefits of antimicrobial therapy in patients with *S. dysenteriae* type 1 infection, prior case-control studies suggest an association between the development of HUS and antimicrobial use.[37] In contrast, a recent study reported that early administration of effective antimicrobials is associated with a low risk for developing HUS. These authors speculated that the prior association between HUS and antimicrobial use may have been observed because effective antibiotics were given later in the course of the illness. Reasons for the delay in administration of antimicrobials were possibly related to patient's delay in seeking medical care, or because the *Shigella* species were subsequently found to be resistant to the empiric antimicrobials prescribed.[37]

12. What empiric antimicrobial regimens are available for the treatment of shigellosis?

Shigella species are well known for rapidly becoming resistant to antimicrobials following exposure to these drugs.[35] At one time, effective empiric treatments for shigellosis included the following older agents administered orally: TMP-SMX[18] ampicillin (but not amoxicillin),[18,38] or nalidixic acid.[18]

During the 1990s, as multidrug-resistant *Shigella* species (e.g., resistance to ampicillin, TMP-SMX, and chloramphenicol) became more common, fluoroquinolones became the antimicrobials of choice for the empiric treatment of shigellosis.[39] Clinical trials enrolling primarily adults found norfloxacin 400 mg twice daily for 5 days[40] or ciprofloxacin 500 mg twice daily for 3–5 days[39,41] were as effective as the standard therapies used for the treatment of shigellosis. Subsequently, a single dose of ciprofloxacin 1 g[42] or norfloxacin 800 mg[43] were also found to be as effective as longer treatment courses for patients with mild to moderate disease. Although the benefits of the single-dose fluoroquinolone treatments include greater adherence to therapy and less cost, single dose regimens are less effective than the standard 5-day treatment courses in patients with more severe illness[42] and in patients with *S. dysenteriae* type 1 infection.[42]

Since the introduction of fluoroquinolones as the drugs of choice for the empiric treatment of shigellosis, *Shigella* species with reduced susceptibility to ciprofloxacin (i.e., higher ciprofloxacin minimal inhibitory concentrations (MIC) in the range of 0.25–1 mcg/mL) have been identified in England and Wales,[44] and *Shigella* species with even higher MIC to ciprofloxacin (MIC of 8 minimal inhibitory concentration to 32 mcg/mL) have been identified in India.[45] Current alternatives to fluoroquinolones for the empiric treatment of shigellosis include ceftriaxone,[25] and azithromycin,[33,46] although there is no national guideline for in vitro azithromycin susceptibility testing for *Shigella* species.[46]

Besides emerging resistance, also of issue with fluoroquinolones are data citing lesions on cartilage tissue in juvenile animals given these agents.[17] Although fluoroquinolones are not approved for use in children, the emergence of multidrug-resistant enteropathogens in some geographic areas led to clinical trials of the short-term use of fluoroquinolones in children; and the available data suggest that a short course of these agents is safe.[17,47] The World Health Organization's guideline for the control of shigellosis, an infection which is so common in developing countries, note that the risk of fluoroquinolone toxicity in children is outweighed by the benefit of effective therapy.[33] The guideline is intended to assist public health authorities and health care providers with the management of cases shigellosis, and it recommends ciprofloxacin for the treatment of shigellosis in both children (15 mg/kg orally twice daily for 3 days) and adults (500 mg orally twice daily for 3 days).[33]

Azithromycin has been successfully used in the treatment of shigellosis. In adults with moderate to severe shigellosis caused by multidrug-resistant *Shigella* species (e.g., variable resistance to TMP-SMX, ampicillin, and nalidixic acid), clinical success was similar for subjects treated with oral azithromycin (500 mg on day 1, then 250 mg daily for 4 days) or oral ciprofloxacin (500 mg Q 12 hr for 5 days) 89% versus 82%, respectively; $p > 0.2$.[48] Despite in vitro susceptibility to these study antibiotics, both azithromycin and ciprofloxacin, however, were less effective in the subset of patients infected with *S. dysenteriae* type 1 (failure rate of 29% and 17%, respectively) compared with patients infected with other *Shigella* species (failure rate of 6% for either antibiotic).[48]

In the setting of epidemic dysentery caused by *S. dysenteriae* type 1 in which nearly all of the isolates were resistant to ampicillin and TMP-SMX, similar clinical outcomes were observed in adults treated with a single 1-g oral dose of azithromycin or multiple doses of ciprofloxacin 500 mg orally twice daily for 3 days. In this study, the mean number of days until resolution of symptoms after starting therapy was 2.5 days for azithromycin versus 2.3 days of ciprofloxacin.[49]

Ceftriaxone and cefotaxime, which are parenteral third-generation cephalosporins with excellent in vitro activity against *Shigella* species, have been used alone[39] or with amikacin[45] for the treatment of shigellosis in patients failing ciprofloxacin therapy. Of concern are reports of ceftriaxone-resistant *S. dysenteriae* and other *Shigella* species from India, Korea, Taiwan, Argentina, and Turkey. Ceftriaxone resistance in these *Shigella* strains is attributed to the production of extended-spectrum β-lactamases.[50]

Cefixime, an oral third-generation cephalosporin, is unreliable for the treatment of shigellosis with clinical and bacteriologic failures reported in 11%–47% and 22%–60% of patients, respectively.[46] The higher treatment failure rate with cefixime is from a study of adults with illness primarily caused by *S. flexneri* and *S. dysenteriae* type 1, the *Shigella* species that typically cause a more severe illness.[51] When cefixime was compared with azithromycin, a trend toward better clinical outcome and eradication was observed with azithromycin.[52]

13. Should loperamide be started in patients with dysentery?

The use of loperamide in dysentery is controversial.[13] Because of concerns that prolonging the clearance of pathogens from the intestinal tract could worsen the severity of illness, experts do not recommend the use of antimotility drugs in persons with fever or bloody diarrhea[14] or when invasive pathogens are suspected.[13] In adults with bacillary dysentery primarily caused by *Shigella* species but who were not critically ill, however, the combination of ciprofloxacin and loperamide did not prolong fever. Rather, the combination decreased the number of unformed stools and shortened the duration of diarrhea.

14. What would be an appropriate antimicrobial regimen to treat M.T.'s presumed case of shigellosis, likely caused by *S. dysenteriae*?

For persons with mild-to-moderate shigellosis, many authorities recommend treatment with one or two doses of a fluoroquinolone. For more severe shigellosis, such as that displayed by M.T., or for the treatment of proven *S. dysenteriae* type 1 infection, 3–5 days of therapy is recommended.[33,35] Alternatives to fluoroquinolones include ceftriaxone or azithromycin, and, if susceptible, TMP-SMX or ampicillin

Shigella species other than *S. dysenteriae*

Clinical Presentation

15. F.F., a 30-year-old, previously healthy female, presents to her physician with nonbloody, watery diarrhea of 3 days' duration. Her history of present illness is significant for close contact with her 2-year-old nephew who is recovering from shigellosis caused by *S. sonnei*, which he acquired from the day care center he attends. F.F. lives in California and has no significant medical history. Overall, she feels better compared with the previous day. F.F. is afebrile, and her physical examination is completely normal. How does F.F.'s clinical presentation of shigellosis differ from that of M.T. in the previous question?

Unlike the more severe clinical presentation characteristic of shigellosis caused by *S. dysenteriae, S. sonnei* generally causes a mild and self-limited illness for which antimicrobials are not generally required, but are often prescribed to shorten the duration of illness and reduce the infectious period.[53] In industrialized countries, *S. sonnei* is the most common cause of shigellosis, accounting for 90% of infections caused by *Shigella* species.[54]

Treatment

16. Should F.F. receive a course of antibiotics to treat her presumed case of shigellosis?

If prescribed, the antimicrobial choices for F.F. are similar to those discussed in the previous case. Until recently, in the United States multidrug-resistant Shigellae had not been particularly problematic, and therefore TMP-SMX had been recommended for the empiric treatment of shigellosis.[55] In 1995, however, more than 50% of *Shigella* species isolated from persons living in Oregon were reportedly resistant to TMP-SMX or ampicillin.[55] In 2005, outbreaks of shigellosis in United States day care centers reported that 89% of *S. sonnei* was resistant to both ampicillin and TMP-SMX.[53] The origin of multidrug-resistant *Shigella* species in the United States may be related to migrant workers traveling to areas such as Latin American and Mexico where multidrug-resistant *Shigella* species is common.[55]

Because fluoroquinolones are not FDA approved for use in children, in this population, alternatives for the treatment of multidrug-resistant *Shigella* species include azithromycin[46] and ceftriaxone.[33]

SALMONELLA

Salmonellae are often referred to as either nontyphoidal (e.g., *S. typhimurium, S. enteritidis, S. choleraesuis,* and many others) or typhoidal (*S. typhi* and *S. paratyphi*) salmonellae. These enteric gram-negative bacilli are important causes of foodborne illness in humans, causing the clinical syndromes of gastroenteritis, bacteremia, localized infection,[56] typhoid fever (enteric fever) and the chronic carrier state.[57] The role of antimicrobial therapy in the treatment of salmonellosis is based on the severity of the patient's illness, presenting clinical syndrome, and underlying health problems.

Nontyphoidal Salmonellosis

Uncomplicated Gastroenteritis in the Immunocompetent Host

CLINICAL PRESENTATION

17. B.B., a 35-year-old, previously healthy man, presents to his physician with a 1-day history of abdominal pain, nausea, vomiting, and nonbloody stools. One day before the onset of his symptoms, he ate a turkey dinner at the local diner, and was later informed of an outbreak of *Salmonella* gastroenteritis attributed to food served at the restaurant. B.B. has no significant medical history. On physical examination, he is not ill appearing, but is febrile. The rest of his examination is normal. B.B. is given the presumptive diagnosis of mild, uncomplicated nontyphoidal *Salmonella* gastroenteritis. Why is B.B.'s history of present illness and clinical presentation consistent with this diagnosis?

A key piece of information from B.B.'s history of present illness that is consistent with the presumptive diagnosis of foodborne *Salmonella* gastroenteritis is his consumption of foods associated with an outbreak of *Salmonella* gastroenteritis. Salmonellae are widely found in nature, colonizing animal hosts, including mammals, reptiles, and birds. Worldwide, nontyphoidal salmonellae are major causes of foodborne illnesses related to the consumption of contaminated beverages or foods such as poultry (chickens, turkeys, ducks) or poultry products (eggs), and dairy products.[56]

As in B.B., symptoms of *Salmonella* gastroenteritis usually begin 6–72 hours after ingestion of contaminated foods. B.B. displays some of the typical clinical manifestations of *Salmonella* gastroenteritis, including the acute onset of fever, diarrhea, and abdominal cramping. Other manifestations of *Salmonella* gastroenteritis include bloody diarrhea and dehydration.[54]

TREATMENT

18. Should B.B. receive a course of antibiotics to treat his presumed diagnosis of uncomplicated nontyphoidal *Salmonella* gastroenteritis?

In otherwise healthy individuals such as B.B. presenting with a mild episode of uncomplicated gastroenteritis secondary to nontyphoidal *Salmonella* species, antibiotics are not routinely recommended because this is typically a self-limiting illness lasting for 2–5 days. In most instances, persons with uncomplicated nontyphoidal *Salmonella* gastroenteritis require only replacement of fluid and electrolyte losses. When antimicrobials have been prescribed in this setting, they have not reduced the duration or severity of illness.[54] In addition, unnecessary use of antimicrobials may prolong asymptomatic carriage of these organisms,[54] place patients at risk for adverse drug reactions, and promote the emergence of antimicrobial-resistant bacteria.[54] A recent study in children confirmed that antimicrobials are still not mandatory even when nontyphoidal salmonellosis (manifesting primarily with GI symptoms and limited signs of systemic inflammation) is caused by antimicrobial-resistant Salmonellae.[54]

Antimicrobials should be reserved for persons who are severely ill[56] or for persons with risk factors for developing extraintestinal *Salmonella* infection. Antimicrobials can also be used when rapid interruption of fecal excretion of organisms is needed to control outbreaks of salmonellosis in institutionalized persons.[56]

19. Following resolution of B.B.'s acute episode of *Salmonella* gastroenteritis, he is inadvertently found to be still excreting *Salmonella* bacteria from his stool, despite remaining asymptomatic. Should antimicrobials be prescribed to eliminate B.B.'s intestinal carriage of nontyphoidal *Salmonella*?

Antimicrobials provide no benefit to persons such as B.B. who are asymptomatic carriers of nontyphoidal *Salmonella* and, therefore, they are not recommended to eliminate intestinal carriage of these organisms.[58] In healthy, asymptomatic adults living in an area where nontyphoidal salmonellae are endemic, a randomized, double-blind trial concluded that neither norfloxacin nor azthromycin was any better than placebo in eradicating intestinal carriage of these organisms.[58] Although antimicrobials can rapidly convert stool cultures to negative immediately after therapy, a longer follow-up reveals usually no difference in the time to final clearance of *Salmonella* in persons given antimicrobials versus those given placebo.[56] The median duration of fecal shedding of nontyphoidal *Salmonella* is about 1 month in adults and 7 weeks in children <5 years of age.[56]

Adverse consequences of using antimicrobials to eliminate intestinal carriage is the emergence of Salmonellae that are resistant to the antibiotics used,[58] and adverse effects to the antimicrobial.

Gastroenteritis in Patients at Risk for Extraintestinal Salmonella Infection

CLINICAL PRESENTATION

20. W.M., a 75-year-old moderately ill-appearing man, presents to his clinic physician with signs and symptoms of *Salmonella* gastroenteritis. His history of present illness is significant for eating the same turkey dinner as B.B (Question 17). In contrast to B.B., W.M.'s medical history is significant for recently diagnosed leukemia. Would antimicrobial therapy benefit W.M.?

Overall, <5% of patients with nontyphoidal *Salmonella* gastroenteritis become bacteremic, although infections with *S. choleraesuis* and *S. dublin* are more likely to cause bacteremia.[59] Host factors that compromise the body's ability to contain infections increase the risk for extraintestinal *Salmonella* infection. These host factors include a very young age; persons with HIV infection, diabetes, malignancy, rheumatologic disorders, and low gastric pH (e.g., as in infancy, pernicious anemia, or induced by medications); and persons receiving immunosuppressive therapies.[56] Bloodstream infection with *Salmonella* can lead to hematogenous seeding of any body site.[56]

Antimicrobial therapy (usually 3–7 days is reasonable) is recommended for persons such as W.M. who are severely ill, or who have host factors that increase their risk for extraintestinal spread of infection.[56] Additionally, a short course (duration of 48–72 hours or until the patient is afebrile) of antimicrobials is also commonly recommended for persons >50 years of age who may have atherosclerotic lesions which, if bacteremia were to occur, could become hematogenously seeded.[56] Other extraintestinal infections seen in persons with *Salmonella* bacteremia include osteomyelitis, septic arthritis, meningitis, and infectious endarteritis.[59]

TREATMENT

21. What antimicrobials are available for the treatment of nontyphoidal *Salmonella* infection? What empiric antibiotic would be appropriate for W.M.?

Before the 1980s, the drugs of choice for the treatment of nontyphoidal salmonellosis included ampicillin, TMP-SMX, and chloramphenicol.[59] Because it is not uncommon to find that more than 50% of nontyphoidal *Salmonella* are resistant to these antimicrobials, fluoroquinolones are now widely used for the empiric treatment of salmonella infection.[59]

In the 1990s, reports of suboptimal clinical responses in persons with nontyphoidal salmonellosis treated with fluoroquinolones raised questions about the effectiveness of this class of antimicrobials for the treatment of salmonellosis.[60] Microbiologic tests revealed these *Salmonella* strains were resistant to nalidixic acid, a drug which is the prototype for the quinolone group of antimicrobials.[60] Nalidixic acid-resistant salmonellae generally have higher MIC to ciprofloxcin (MIC range of 0.12–0.5 mcg/mL) compared with nalidixic acid-susceptible strains (MIC <0.03 mcg/mL).[60] In the United States, nalidixic acid-resistant, nontyphoidal *Salmonella* species increased from 0.4% in 1996 to 2.3% in 2003.[61]

Infection with antimicrobial-resistant *Salmonella* is associated with suboptimal clinical outcomes. Some evidence suggests that standard, long-course (7–10 days) fluoroquinolone regimens are less effective for the treatment of infection caused by nalidixic acid-resistant *Salmonellae*.[60] In addition, persons with bloodstream infection caused by antimicrobial-resistant nontyphoidal *Salmonella* are more likely to have bloodstream infection and to be hospitalized versus persons with infection caused by pansusceptible *Salmonella*.[62]

With concerns over fluoroquinolone resistance in *Salmonella* species, alternative antimicrobials include the expanded spectrum cephalosporins (cefotaxime or ceftriaxone) and imipenem.[59] Azithromycin has also been used in a limited number of cases of nontyphoidal salmonellosis.[56] Since 1991, however, nontyphoidal *Salmonella* species resistant to extended-spectrum cephalosporins are increasingly being identified in many areas of the world.[59] *Salmonella* resistance to the expanded spectrum cephalosporins is primarily attributed to the production of extended spectrum β-lactamases,[59] and these strains may also exhibit decreased susceptibility to ciprofloxacin.[63] Imipenem has been successfully used for the treatment of invasive infection caused *S. enterica serotype choleraesuis* resistant to both ceftriaxone and ciprofloxacin.[64]

Invasive Nontyphoidal Salmonella Infection

22. B.T., a severely ill-appearing, 70-year-old man, presents to the ED with complaints of severe abdominal pain, bloody diarrhea, new-onset right hip pain, and a temperature of 102°F. His history of present illness is significant for eating the same turkey dinner as B.B. (Question 17) and W.M. (Question 18). His past history is significant for a right hip prosthesis. Would B.T. benefit from antibiotic therapy?

CLINICAL PRESENTATION AND TREATMENT

B.T. is presenting with signs and symptoms of *Salmonella* gastroenteritis, and probable bloodstream infection complicated by localized infection to his prosthetic hip (i.e., new onset right hip pain). Treatment of *Salmonella* bacteremia without other infectious complications is generally successful following 10–14 days of antimicrobial therapy. A longer duration of treatment and surgery may be required for metastatic infections such as osteomyelitis.[56]

Regarding empiric antimicrobial treatment for B.T., the widespread resistance to older agents (e.g., ampicillin and TMP-SMX) makes these agents unsuitable options until susceptibility data are available. Instead, empiric therapy with antimicrobials, such as selected third-generation cephalosporins (cefotaxime or ceftriaxone), or a fluoroquinolone can be used, keeping in mind the possibility of resistance to fluoroquinolones. Selection of a specific antimicrobial should also consider the specific extraintestinal site of infection.

Typhoidal Salmonellosis—Typhoid Fever (Enteric Fever)

Enteric fever is an acute systemic illness caused by typhoidal Salmonellae, most commonly *S. typhi*. Enteric fever caused by *S. typhi* is referred to as "typhoid fever," whereas enteric fever caused by *S. paratyphi* is referred to as "paratyphoid fever."

Clinical Presentation

23. B.C., a 49-year-old obese woman, presents to the ED with a 1-week history of fever, abdominal pain, headache, anorexia, and diarrhea. One day before admission, she noted a new red rash on her chest. Her history of present illness is significant for return 10 days ago from travel to the Indian subcontinent where she stayed with relatives, some of whom were recovering from typhoid fever. B.C.'s medical history is significant for gallstones. She lives in California with her husband. On admission, she is alert and oriented and moderately ill appearing. Vital signs are as follows: temperature is 101 °F and heart rate is 60 beats/minute, blood pressure is stable. Physical examination is significant for splenomegaly and hepatomegaly. Laboratory tests include the following: WBC is $3.0 \times 10^6/mm^3$; liver function tests are mildly elevated and the results of two sets of blood cultures are pending. Why is her history of present illness, clinical presentation, and laboratory findings consistent with the presumed diagnosis of typhoid fever?

B.C.'s recent travel history to the Indian subcontinent and exposure to relatives recovering from typhoid fever are key pieces of information supporting her diagnosis of typhoid fever. Most cases of typhoid fever occur in developing areas of the world, including the Indian subcontinent, Southeast Asia, Africa, and Latin America where the disease is endemic.[57] In developed countries, enteric fever is a sporadic disease occurring mainly in travelers returning from areas where the disease is endemic. In the United States, 74% of cases of typhoid fever are diagnosed in persons reporting recent travel.[57] It is likely that B.C acquired her infection following the consumption of contaminated foods during her trip to the Indian subcontinent.

B.C.'s clinical presentation includes the classic signs and symptoms of enteric fever, such as high fever for >1 week associated with abdominal pain, anorexia, diarrhea or constipation; headache, dry cough, splenomegaly, and hepatomegaly.[57] Other manifestations of severe typhoid fever include GI bleeding, encephalopathy and shock.[57] Laboratory abnormalites consistent with typhoid fever include B.C.'s low WBC count and mildly elevated liver function tests.[57]

The incubation period of B.C.'s illness is consistent with the usual 7–14 days seen in persons with typhoid fever.[57] During the incubation period, Salmonellae multiply within macrophages and monocytes, and systemic manifestations of typhoid fever appear when bacteria are released into the bloodstream.

Treatment

24. Would B.C. benefit from a course of antimicrobials to treat her presumptive diagnosis of typhoid fever? If so, what options are available?

Effective antimicrobials for typhoid fever have several benefits. First, effective therapy reduces fever and other symptoms within 3–5 days, with acceptable regimens clearing all symptoms within 7–10 days.[65] Second, effective antimicrobial therapy decreases mortality–<1%[57] from the 5%–10% mortality rate reported in untreated patients.[65] Third, effective therapy prevents relapse of infection, which generally occurs in 5%–10% of patients, and usually within 2–3 weeks after resolution of fever.[66] Finally, effective therapy eradicates fecal shedding of *S. typhi,* which limits the spread of infection.[65]

Until the late 1980s, the standard treatment for typhoid fever was 14–21 days of chloramphenicol, TMP-SMX, or ampicillin.[66] The subsequent availability of newer, but more costly antimicrobials, including ceftriaxone and azithromycin, provided alternatives for the treatment of typhoid fever. In adults and children with enteric fever caused by *S. typhi* or *S. paratyphi* remaining susceptible to ampicillin, chloramphenicol, and TMP-SMX, clinical cure was achieved in 91% of persons treated with parenteral ceftriaxone (3–4 g/day for 3–7 days), which was similar to the 94% cure rate in persons treated with chloramphenicol.[67] In children and adolescents with uncomplicated typhoid fever caused primarily by antimicrobial-susceptible strains (>90% susceptible to ampicillin, TMP-SMX, chloramphenicol, ciprofloxacin, and ceftriaxone) once daily administration of oral azithromycin (20 mg/kg/day, maximum, 1,000 mg/day for 5 days) or parenteral ceftriaxone (75 mg/kg/day, maximum, 2.5 g/day for 5 days) produced similar clinical cure rates of 94% and 97%, respectively. In this study, although bacteremia was present longer in the azithromycin-treated patients, relapse of infection at day 30 was higher in the ceftriaxone-treated patients versus the azithromycin-treated patients, 6 (19%) versus 0%, respectively. This rate of relapse with the short course of ceftriaxone is consistent with the 5%–15% reported by other investigators.[68]

During the early 1990s, multidrug-resistant (i.e., simultaneous resistance to chloramphenicol, ampicillin, and TMP-SMX) *S. typhi* caused outbreaks of typhoid fever in India, Pakistan, Bangladesh, Vietnam, the Middle East, and Africa, thus, limiting the usefulness of these older antimicrobials for the empiric treatment of typhoid fever.[66] Consequently, the availability of fluoroquinolones, which retained activity against these multidrug-resistant strains,[69,70] and which could be administered orally, made the fluoroquinolones the preferred treatments for enteric fever in both adults and children. In children with uncomplicated typhoid fever in which 86% of isolates were multidrug resistant (i.e., resistant to chloramphenicol, TMP-SMX, ampicillin, and tetracycline), ofloxacin (7.5 mg/kg twice daily for 2–3 days) achieved cure rates of >89%.[70] Likewise, in adults with enteric fever, 63% of whom were infected with multidrug-resistant *S. typhi*, oral ofloxacin (200 mg Q 12 hr for 5 days) was superior to a 5-day course of ceftriaxone (3 g/day) with clinical cure achieved in 22 (100%) versus 18 (75%) patients treated with these respective regimens. In this study, all *S. typhi* isolates were susceptible to the study antimicrobials, and the ceftriaxone failures were successfully treated with ofloxacin.[69]

Azithromycin also has proved to be effective for the treatment of typhoid fever caused by multidrug-resistant strains. In adults (approximately one-third of whom were infected with *Salmonella* resistant to at least two of the following: chloramphenicol, ampicillin, or TMP-SMX, but susceptible to azithromycin and ciprofloxacin), oral azithromycin (1 g on day 1, then 500 mg daily on days 2–6) was as effective as oral ciprofloxacin 500 mg twice daily for 7 days (100% cure rate for both treatment groups).[71] A 7-day course of azithromycin in children (10 mg/kg/day orally once a day; maximum, 500 mg daily) and adults proved effective for the treatment of infection caused by multidrug-resistant and nalidixic acid-resistant *S. typhi*.[72] Finally, in children with typhoid fever, oral azithromycin given once daily (10 mg/kg/day for 7 days; maximum, 500 mg/day) was as effective as ceftriaxone (75 mg/kg/day for 7 days; maximum, 2.5 g/day), with clinical response rates of 91% and 97%, respectively. Despite in vitro susceptibility, relapse of infection was higher in the ceftriaxone versus azithromycin-treated patients, 14% versus 0%, respectively.[73] When a longer course (14 days) of ceftriaxone was used in children with multidrug-resistant *S. typhi* (resistance to ampicillin, chloramphenicol, and TMP-SMX), however, no child experienced a relapse, whereas 14% of children treated with only 7 days of ceftriaxone experienced a relapse.[74] Although ceftriaxone remains very active against *S. typhi*, isolates with high-level resistance to ceftriaxone have been indentifed.[66]

Because the fluoroquinolones have been widely used for the treatment of typhoid fever, increasingly reported are clinical treatment failures when these antimicrobials were used to treat this infection. Microbiologic examination of the strains associated with fluoroquinolone treatment failure reveals these isolates have higher MIC to ciprofloxacin compared with earlier strains. *Salmonella* that are fully susceptible to ciprofloxacin by disc testing generally have a ciprofloxacin MIC of <0.03 mcg/mL and are usually susceptible to nalidixic acid, the prototype drug for the quinolone group of antimicrobials.[65] In contrast, strains with low level ciprofloxacin resistance (intermediate MIC of 0.125–1 mcg/mL) are usually resistant to nalidixic acid, and these strains are associated with unsatisfactory treatment responses to fluoroquinolones (see below).[65] Ciprofloxacin-resistant *S. typhi* have ciprofloxacin MIC >1 mcg/mL and are resistant to nalidixic acid.[64] Fully fluoroquinolone-resistant isolates have been detected in India.[65]

In some regions of the world, clinical failure rates in patients with enteric fever following treatment with fluoroquinolones increased from 9%–35%, in 1997 and 1999, respectively.[75] Following 12–14 days of ciprofloxacin for the treatment of typhoid fever, the overall condition of 32 patients did not improve, and all cases were eventually successfully treated with ceftriaxone.[76] In this report, the ciprofloxacin MIC of *S. typhi* isolates ranged from 0.0625–0.5 mcg/mL, and ceftriaxone MIC were <0.0625 mcg/mL. A retrospective review of persons with infection caused by nalidixic acid-susceptible or nalidixic acid-resistant *S. typhi* and who were treated with a short course of ofloxacin reported more treatment failures in patients infected with the resistant strains versus the susceptible strains, 50% versus <5%, respectively.[77] Short courses of fluoroquinolones are not recommended for the treatment of infections caused by nalidixic acid-resistant *S. typhi*.[65] Recent in vitro data show that the newer fluoroquinolones (gemifloxacin and moxifloxacin) may be the best drugs in this class for the treatment of multidrug-resistant and nalidixic acid-resistant isolates.[78]

Cefixime, an oral third-generation cephalosporin, has been used for the treatment of typhoid fever, although with variable success. In one study, cefixime administered for 12–14 days was effective treatment for typhoid fever; however, when a shorter, 7-day course of cefixime was used, cefixime was less effective than 5 days of ofloxacin.[79] Recent reports from Nepal have shown that cefixime is not an acceptable alternative.[78]

Optimal treatment for fluoroquinolone-resistant isolates has not been determined. Azithromycin, ceftriaxone, or maximal recommended doses of fluoroquinolones for 10–14 days have been recommended.[66]

25. What specific empiric antibiotic regimen would you recommend be initiated for the empiric treatment of B.C.'s typhoid fever?

Uncomplicated cases of typhoid fever can be treated with oral antibiotics, whereas severe cases are treated with parenteral therapy.[66] For the empiric treatment of typhoid fever, ceftriaxone or a fluoroquinolone can be used.[80] Azithromycin is also an alternative agent. When susceptibility data are known, fully susceptible isolates can be treated with a fluoroquinolone for 5–7 days, or with TMP-SMX, ampicillin, or chloramphenicol for 10–14 days.[66] Finally, the re-emergence of *S. typhi* susceptible to TMP-SMX[81] and chloramphenicol[66] may mean these older agents may again be useful and inexpensive alternatives for the treatment of *S. typhi* infection.

Adjunctive Treatment

26. Besides the administration of antibiotics, are there adjunctive therapies from which B.C. could benefit?

For persons with severe typhoid fever (with altered mental status or shock), mortality is decreased to 10% when chloramphenicol is combined with dexamethasone (3 mg/kg IV followed by 1 mg/kg Q 6 hr IV for eight doses) compared with chloramphenicol alone (56% mortality).[82] The benefit of steroids when the more potent fluoroquinolones are used is unknown, however.[83]

Chronic Typhoid Carriers

CLINICAL PRESENTATION

27. Fourteen months following discharge from the hospital, B.C.'s stool is still positive for *S. typhi*. During this time, her husband has had two episodes of typhoid fever. Why is B.C.'s clinical syndrome consistent with the chronic carrier state?

Although most patients excrete *S. typhi* in their stools for 3–4 weeks following recovery from their illness, 1%–3% excrete *Salmonella* from stool or urine for >1 year after infection; and these individuals are referred to as "chronic carriers." B.C.'s risk factor for becoming a chronic carrier is her history of gallstones, which allows the sequestration of organisms in her diseased biliary tract. Although B.C. remains asymptomatic, she serves as a reservoir for spreading infection to others.

TREATMENT

28. What therapeutic options are available to cure B.C.'s chronic carrier state?

Treatment options for chronic *S. typhi* carriers such as B.C. include a prolonged course of antibiotics, cholecystectomy, or suppressive antimicrobial therapy.[66] Of chronic carriers, 50%–90% may be cured following prolonged courses of antibiotics,[84–87] although efficacy may be lessened when anatomic abnormalities (e.g., cholelithiasis) are present.[84] Relapse is usually detected within the first several months after completing antimicrobial therapy,[88] but can occur up to 24 months after completing therapy.[84] If *S. typhi* are susceptible, antimicrobial regimens proved effective in curing chronic carriers include amoxicillin 2 g three times daily for 28 days,[86] ampicillin 1 g four times daily for 90 days,[85] ampicillin 1.5 g four times daily plus probenecid for 6 weeks,[84] TMP-SMX 160/800 mg twice a day for 3 months,[87] ciprofloxacin 500–750 mg twice a day for 3–4 weeks,[88–90] or norfloxacin 400 mg twice daily for 4 weeks.[91] Patient follow-up in these studies ranged from 10–12 months following completion of therapy.

Prevention

29. B.C.'s sister is planning a trip to the Indian subcontinent and is concerned about developing typhoid fever. What can she do to reduce her risk for developing typhoid fever?

In the United States, an intramuscular vaccine that is 51%–77% effective in preventing typhoid fever can be administered to persons >2 years of age. Adverse effects with the parenteral vaccine include local pain and swelling, fever, headache, and malaise.[66] The Ty21a oral vaccine affords a protective efficacy rate ranging from 42%–96%.[66] This oral vaccine is well tolerated and can be administered to persons >6 years of age. B.C.'s sister should consult with her physician regarding the need for typhoid vaccination. She should also be informed that, because the vaccine may not be fully protective, good hygiene and avoiding foods with a high risk for contamination are still necessary to minimize her risk for acquiring typhoid fever.

ESCHERICHIA COLI O157:H7

Epidemiology

30. P.J., a 3-year-old girl, is brought to the ED because of "stomach pains" and nonbloody diarrhea that has progressed to bloody diarrhea over the past 48 hours. Five days before the onset of diarrhea, the family celebrated the Fourth of July at a fast-food restaurant; P.J.'s parents ate fish sandwiches and P.J. ate a hamburger. P.J.'s mother noted that, unlike previous hamburgers eaten at the restaurant, this hamburger was not thoroughly cooked because the juices from the hamburger were still pinkish. P.J. has no significant medical history. During the week, she attends a day care center.

On physical examination P.J. is afebrile, with signs of mild to moderate dehydration. A stool sample is negative for fecal leukocytes. The physician assesses her illness as bloody diarrhea, possibly caused by STEC. The plan is to admit P.J. to the hospital for hydration, observation, and further workup. What clinical and laboratory findings and epidemiologic history are consistent with the diagnosis of STEC as the cause of P.J.'s illness?

Escherichia coli O157:H7 is a strain of *E. coli* that produces Shiga toxins as one of its mechanisms of causing GI illness. A second virulence factor of STEC strains is their ability to attach to and damage the intestinal mucosa.[92] These *E. coli* bacteria cause a spectrum of infection, including asymptomatic carriage, mild and nonbloody diarrhea, bloody diarrhea (hemorrhagic colitis), HUS, and thrombotic thrombocytopenia purpura.[93]

Escherichia coli O157:H7 should be suspected in the setting of abdominal cramps with nonbloody diarrhea that progresses to bloody diarrhea over 1–2 days.[92] Unlike bloody diarrhea associated with *Shigella* species or *Campylobacter* species, fever is often absent or of low grade because this pathogen is not invasive.[94] Patients with severe illness are more likely to have fever, however.[95]

Shiga toxin-producing Escherichia coli is most commonly spread by consumption of undercooked beef products that are contaminated with *E. coli* O157:H7, although other modes of acquiring this infection have been reported (see Question 32). The incubation period for this infection is usually

3–4 days, which is consistent with P.J.'s recent history of eating undercooked hamburger. In most instances, the illness resolves in 5–7 days.[92] Fecal leukocytes may or may not be found in stool samples.[96]

Laboratory Diagnosis

31. How can the diagnosis of *E. coli* O157:H7 infection be confirmed?

In the United States, *E. coli* O157:H7 is the most common STEC serotype identified as causing this infection.[96] Unlike other *E. coli,* O157:H7 does not rapidly ferment sorbitol, thus allowing the use of special culture media (Sorbitol-MacConkey) to help in identifying this organism. Because of sorbitol-fermenting organisms and non-O157 STEC, further testing for Shiga toxins or the genes encoding them is increasingly performed.[92,93,96]

Hemolytic Uremic Syndrome

32. Forty-eight hours after admission to the hospital, P.J. is pale and has developed several "bruises" on her extremities. The nurse recorded only a minimal output of darkened urine during the past 24 hours. New laboratory tests reveal blood urea nitrogen (BUN), 150 mg/dL (normal, 5–25); serum creatinine (SrCr), 6 mg/dL (normal, 0.3–0.7); serum potassium (K), 6.8 mEq/L (normal, 3.5–5.5); WBC count, 20,000 cells/mm^3 (normal, 5,000–15,000); hemoglobin (Hgb), 5 g/dL (normal, 11–13); platelets, 50,000 cells/mm^3 (normal, 150,000–350,000); and urinalysis is positive for blood and protein. The stool specimen sent on admission is positive for *E. coli* O157:H7. What complication of *E. coli* O157:H7 infection does P.J. now display?

[SI units: BUN, 53.55 mmol/L of urea (normal, 1.79–8.93); SrCr, 530.4 μmol/L (normal, 26.52–62.88); K, 6.8 mmol/L (normal, 3.5–5.5); WBC count, 20×10^9/L (normal, 5–15); Hgb, 50 g/L (normal, 110–130); platelets, 50×10^9/L (normal, 150–350)]

The new clinical and laboratory findings support the diagnosis of HUS, a well-known complication of STEC infection. HUS is characterized by the triad of thrombocytopenia, microangiopathic hemolytic anemia, and acute renal failure with oliguria.[97] On physical examination, P.J.'s "bruises" on her extremities are consistent with thrombocytopenia, which is confirmed by the low platelet count. Her pale appearance is consistent with anemia and is confirmed by the low Hgb; the dark urine is caused by the color imparted from bilirubin because of red cell lysis (hemolytic anemia). Finally, P.J.'s decreased urine output and increased serum creatinine and BUN concentrations are consistent with renal failure.[98]

P.J. has several risk factors for HUS: her age (i.e., children aged <5–15 years, median age 4–8 years), fever, increased peripheral WBC count, and the season of the year (i.e., summer).[95,97,99–102] Although not present in this case, another possible risk factor for developing HUS is treatment with antimotility or antidiarrheal agents,[103] although this has not been universally confirmed.[95,100] In addition to young age, age >65 years appears to be a risk factor for HUS.[95] The progression of *E. coli* O157:H7 gastroenteritis to HUS typically becomes apparent about 1 week after the onset of diarrhea.[95,97,99] Of children, 3%–7%[104] may develop HUS, with a mortality rate ranging from 3%–5%. In adults, *E. coli* O157:H7 infection progresses to HUS in as many as 27% of patients, with a higher rate in patients >65 years of age.[95] HUS-related mortality has reached 42% in patients >15 years of age[95]; elderly nursing home patients have a mortality rate of up to 88%.[105]

Treatment

33. Would P.J. benefit from drug therapy, including antimicrobial, antimotility, or antidiarrheal agents?

Other than supportive measures to manage the complications associated with illness caused by *E. coli* O157:H7, no specific drug therapy for this infection exists.[92] In retrospective and prospective studies, antibiotics have not influenced the severity of illness, or the duration of diarrhea or other GI symptoms.[106,107] When TMP-SMX was started a mean of 7 days after the onset of diarrhea, the duration of *E. coli* O157:H7 excretion was not altered.[106]

The effect of antibiotic administration on the risk of *E. coli* O157:H7 complications (e.g., HUS) remains controversial. A prospective cohort study of 71 children with diarrhea caused by *E. coli* O157:H7 found that antibiotic treatment increased the risk of progression to HUS.[100] Previous publications have supported these findings,[104,106,107] whereas others have reported that antibiotics do not increase the risk of progression to HUS.[95,103] A meta-analysis of these and other studies revealed no association between antibiotic administration and development of HUS.[108] Antibiotic selection, timing of administration, STEC strain, and patient selection vary in the selected studies and complicate the analysis. Thus, the role of antibiotics in the treatment of *E. coli* O157:H7 infection remains controversial. Currently, clinicians do not recommend antibiotic treatment for STEC. Clinicians must carefully weigh empiric antibiotic treatment before the organism has been identification.[109]

Antimotility drugs are not recommended for patients with *E. coli* O157:H7 infection because they have been variably associated with an increased risk of progression to HUS,[103,104] although other studies have failed to find an association.[95,100] Although the explanation for the increased risk is unknown, the reduction of bowel motility may decrease the clearance of organisms from the GI tract, thereby increasing the absorption of toxins. Administration of antimotility drugs within the first 3 days of illness has been associated with a longer duration of bloody diarrhea.[110]

Prevention

34. P.J.'s family members want to know what they could have done to prevent this infection. On discharge from the hospital, is it safe for P.J. to return to her day care center?

Shiga toxin-producing Escherichia coli is often spread to humans by consumption of contaminated beef products that are not thoroughly cooked.[93] Because thorough cooking kills this organism, meat should be well cooked (i.e., juices from meat should be clear, not pink). In addition, this infection can be acquired by consuming other contaminated foods, including water, unpasteurized milk, apple cider, lettuce, and sprouts.[92,93]

An experimental *E. coli* O157 O-polysaccharide conjugate vaccine is currently under study by the National Institutes of Health.[111] In a phase II trial, the vaccine was effective in inducing an immune response in the target population of young children and demonstrated no untoward effects.

Finally, because contact with infected persons commonly results in transmission of this infection to others,[104,105,107] P.J. should have two consecutive stool cultures that are negative for *E. coli* O157:H7 before returning to day care.[112]

CAMPYLOBACTER JEJUNI

Campylobacter species are gram-negative bacilli that have a curved or spiral shape. Of the various *Campylobacter* species, *C. jejuni* and *C. fetus* are associated with human illness, with *C. jejuni* accounting for most of *Campylobacter* species isolated.[113]

Clinical Presentation

35. M.U. is a 20-year-old, previously healthy woman presenting to the Student Health Center with the following complaints for the past 24 hours: malaise, fever, diarrhea, abdominal pain, and bloody diarrhea. One day before the onset of her symptoms, she had dinner at a restaurant near campus where she ordered a chicken sandwich, but ate only a portion of it because the chicken was not thoroughly cooked. She has no significant medical history and no recent travel history. On physical examination, M.U. is not ill appearing. The physician tells her that over the past week, several students with gastrointestinal symptoms similar to hers have been diagnosed with *C. jejuni* gastroenteritis, and all had recently eaten at the same restaurant. Why are M.U.'s history of present illness and clinical presentation consistent with *Campylobacter* gastroenteritis?

A key piece of information from M.U.'s history of present illness, which is consistent with her presumptive diagnosis of *Campylobacter* gastroenteritis, is her consumption of undercooked chicken at a restaurant with an ongoing outbreak of *Campylobacter* gastroenteritis. In industrialized nations, the most important risk factor for acquiring *Campylobacter* infection is the consumption of improperly cooked foods such as unpasteurized foods, and contaminated water. Prevention of *Campylobacter* infection involves careful food preparation and cooking practices.[114] Person-to-person transmission is not a major means of spreading this infection.

Symptoms of *Campylobacter* gastroenteritis begin 24–72 hours following exposure to contaminated foods. Clinical manifestations of gastroenteritis include diarrhea and fever (90%), abdominal cramps, and either loose and watery or bloody stools.[113] M.U. does not exhibit signs or symptoms of complications associated with *Campylobacter* infection, such as meningitis, cholecystitis, pancreatitis, peritonitis, gastrointestinal hemorrhage, a reactive arthritis, and bacteremia. Bacteremia occurs in <1% of cases and most commonly in immunosuppressed persons, the very young, or the elderly. Guillain-Barré syndrome is an important but uncommon (<1/1,000 cases of infections) postinfectious complication of *C. jejuni* gastroenteritis.[113]

Treatment

36. Would M.U. benefit from antimicrobial therapy to treat her *Campylobacter* gastroenteritis?

Because *C. jejuni* gastroenteritis is an acute, self-limiting illness that typically resolves within 1 week,[113] antibiotic therapy is usually not necessary.[115] On the other hand, antibiotics are recommended for the treatment of *Campylobacter* infection in patients having symptoms lasting >1 week, high fevers, bloody stools, pregnant women, or immunocompromised hosts.[113] Based on M.U.'s clinical presentation, including fever with bloody stools, antimicrobial therapy is warranted.

When administered early in the course of the illness (i.e., before determining the cause of the diarrhea), antimicrobial therapy shortens the duration and the severity of illness and the duration of fecal excretion of pathogens.[114] In contrast, when antimicrobials are initiated later during the course of the illness (i.e., after determining the cause of the diarrhea), antimicrobials do not alter the clinical course of *Campylobacter* gastroenteritis.[116]

37. What empiric antimicrobial therapies could be initiated to treat M.U.'s presumed case of *C. jejuni* enteritis?

Fluoroquinolones were once considered the drugs of choice for *Campylobacter* infection.[113] Fluoroquinolone-resistance in *Campylobacter* species, *however,* is no longer an uncommon finding. For example, fluoroquinolone-resistant *Campylobacter* in Sweden, the United Kingdom, and The Netherlands ranges from 18%–29%, and is even higher (72%–84%) in Thailand and Spain.[113] In the United States, fluoroquinolone-resistant *Campylobacter* species causing human illness in Minnesota increased from 1.3% in 1992 to 10.2% in 1998, whereas resistance to erythromycin remained low at 2%.[114] This widespread fluoroquinolone resistance is largely attributed to the frequent use of these antimicrobials in veterinary medicine and food animals (e.g., poultry).

In the clinical setting, patients with fluorquinonolone- or erythromycin-resistant *Campylobacter* infection are at increased risk for invasive illness or death.[115] In travelers with *Campylobacter* gastroenteritis, a trend is seen toward a longer duration of illness in patients treated with ciprofloxacin versus azithromycin (52 hours vs. 40 hours, respectively); which may be related to the finding that 50% of the *Campylobacter* isolates were resistant to ciprofloxacin, whereas all isolates were susceptible to azithromycin.[117]

The drug of choice for *C. jejuni* gastroenteritis is erythromycin (adults, 250 mg four times daily; or children, 30–50 mg/kg in divided doses) for 5–7 days[118]; clarithromycin or azithromycin are also effective.[113,117] Based on M.U.'s medical history and clinical presentation, empiric therapy with oral erythromycin can be started.

TRAVELERS' DIARRHEA

Of the more than 50 million persons traveling from industrialized countries to developing countries where individuals are at risk for acquiring travelers' diarrhea (TD), about 40% of travelers will experience a diarrheal illness.[12] Of these travelers, between 5% and 10% will continue to have enteric symptoms for 6 months after the episode of TD, a condition referred to as the *postinfectious irritable bowel syndrome*.[12]

Etiology and Clinical Presentation

38. E.J. and B.R. are healthy 23-year-old women planning a 2-week vacation to Mexico. Before leaving on vacation, they discussed with their physician ways to avoid acquiring travelers' diarrhea. Contrary to their physician's recommendations, on the day of their arrival in Mexico they both began eating fresh fruits and vegetables from street vendors and drinking unbottled water. On the second day of their vacation, B.R. noted the passing of one to two watery stools without blood and without other GI symptoms. In contrast, E.J. felt "feverish" and passed six to seven loose, bloody stools. Neither traveler felt dizzy or thirsty, and both continued drinking adequate amounts of fluids to avoid becoming dehydrated. Why is the history of present illness and clinical presentation of their illnesses consistent with the diagnosis of TD? What risk factors do they have for acquiring TD?

Travelers' diarrhea is defined as three or more loose, unformed stools per day plus at least one symptom of enteric infection, such as abdominal cramps, nausea, vomiting, fever, fecal urgency, tenesmus, or the passage of bloody or mucoid stools.[119] Clinical manifestations of TD typically begin within 24–48 hours after consuming fecally contaminated foods. Of travelers, 40% developing diarrhea have a mild, self-limiting illness of 1–2 days' duration.

The major risk factors these women have for acquiring TD are their destination to a developing country with suboptimal sanitation facilities to manage the disposal of sewage and the consumption of food items with a high likelihood of being contaminated with enteropathogens. These high-risk food items include unbottled water, ice cubes, raw milk, unpeeled fruits and vegetables, uncooked foods, moist foods (e.g., salads served at room temperature), and food from street vendors.[12]

Infectious agents are the major cause of TD, with bacteria representing 80% of the cases in which a pathogen is identified.[12] Overall, *Enterotoxigenic E. coli* (ETEC) and *enteroaggregative E. coli* (EAEC) are the etiologic pathogens identified in 50%–60% of TD cases,[12] and invasive pathogens, such as *Shigella, Campylobacter,* and *Salmonella* species, are responsible for an additional 10%–15% of episodes of TD.[12]

General Management

39. What general approach should B.R. and E.J. take to manage their illnesses?

The general approach to the management of TD includes replenishing fluid and electrolyte losses, avoiding continued ingestion of foods at high risk for being contaminated with enteropathogens, considering the use of specific drug therapy, or seeking medical attention. Neither traveler shows signs and symptoms of dehydration, including thirst, dizziness, and altered mental status, and both are drinking normally. They should continue to drink fluids, such as tea, broth, carbonated beverages, and fruit juices. For travelers able to drink fluids *ad libitum*, a modified World Health Organization oral rehydration solution has not been shown to provide additional benefit over the administration of loperamide alone.[120] Electrolytes can be replaced by eating salted crackers or similar sources of sodium chloride.[120]

Travelers should eat well-cooked foods that are served steaming hot and drink boiled or commercially bottled beverages.[12] Depending on the severity of their illness, travelers can consider the use of antimotility agents alone or in combination with antimicrobials. Self-treatment for TD can be particularly important for persons who become ill in areas where reliable medical care is not available.[12] Of travelers receiving pretravel instructions for the self-medication of TD, 80% report their self-treatment was effective.[121] For severe symptoms, travelers should seek medical attention.

40. What drug therapies could B.R. and E.J. consider using to reduce the duration and severity of travelers' diarrhea?

Bismuth Preparations and Loperamide

Both bismuth subsalicylate and loperamide decrease the number of unformed stools in persons with TD. Concurrent administration of bismuth preparations and fluoroquinolones (antimicrobials commonly used in persons with TD) should be avoided because the chelation of fluoroquinolones by bivalent cations will reduce the bioavailability of these agents.[122,123] Compared with bismuth subsalicylate, loperamide acts more rapidly by exerting an antimotility effect.[13]

Antimicrobials

Effective antimicrobial therapy shortens the duration and severity of TD. Previously effective antimicrobials for the treatment of TD included tetracycline and TMP-SMX, but widespread resistance of enteropathogens to these agents renders them unsuitable for the empiric treatment of this infection. Depending on the most likely pathogen(s) causing TD, the recommended antimicrobial options for the empiric treatment of this infection include the fluoroquinolones, azithromycin, and rifaximin.[13]

Clues to the likely pathogen causing TD include the area of travel and the clinical presentation of the illness. For example, noninvasive pathogens, such as ETEC, are more common causes of TD in Latin America and Africa,[13] and the diarrheal illness caused by these enteropathogens is characterized by a less severe illness in which patients are afebrile, with nonbloody, watery stools, and are without significant abdominal pain.[1] In studies performed in travelers to Mexico[119,124,125] or Kenya,[124] a single dose of an antimicrobial (ciprofloxacin 500 mg,[126] azithromycin 1 g,[119] or levofloxacin 500 mg[119]) decreased the median time to passage of the last unformed stool to 22–33 hours,[119,124] compared with 54–66 hours in travelers given placebo.[119] In some,[127] but not all studies,[128] when ETEC was the most common pathogen identified, the diarrheal illness was shorter in travelers taking loperamide plus an antimicrobial. Specifically, fewer travelers taking ofloxacin plus loperamide passed their last unformed stool at 24 hours compared with travelers treated with ofloxacin alone, 62% versus 91% respectively.[129] A recent study in military personnel stationed in Turkey reported the median time to the passage of the last unformed stool was shortened to as little at 3 hours in recruits given levofloxacin (single 500-mg dose) plus loperamide (4 mg initially, then 2 mg as needed; maximum 16 mg/day); a finding that did not differ significantly from the

13 hours observed in recruits randomized to treatment with azithromycin (single 1-g dose) plus loperamide, $p = 0.2$.[130]

Rifaximin is a poorly absorbed rifamycin derivative that is FDA approved for the treatment of TD caused by noninvasive strains of *E. coli.* In travelers to Mexico and India, oral rifaximin 200 mg three times daily or ciprofloxacin 500 mg twice daily for 3 days significantly reduced the median time to passage of the last unformed stool to 32 hours and 29 hours, respectively, versus 66 hours for travelers given placebo.[131] In this study, rifaximin was as effective as ciprofloxacin against noninvasive bacterial enteropathogens, but was less effective than ciprofloxacin when invasive pathogens were identified. Rifaximin should not be used in patients with diarrhea complicated by fever and bloody stools, or diarrhea caused by pathogens other than *E. coli.*[132]

Invasive pathogens, such as *Shigella, Campylobacter,* and *Salmonella* species, are more common causes of TD in Asia,[12] and the diarrheal illness caused by these pathogens is characterized by a more severe illness in which patients are febrile, with bloody diarrhea, and severe abdominal pain.[2] A recent study enrolling military personnel developing TD while in Thailand reported that most were infected with *Campylobacter* species, of which 50% were resistant to levofloxacin, whereas resistance to azithromycin was not detected. In this study, the cure rate was highest following a single dose of azithromycin 1 g (96%), compared with the cure rates following 3 days of azithromycin 500 mg daily (85%) or levofloxacin 500 mg daily (71%), $p = 0.03$.[133] Levofloxacin was inferior to azithromycin, except when patients were infected with levofloxacin-susceptible *Campylobacter*, or when no pathogen was identified. The highest rate of nausea during the 30 minutes after receiving the first antimicrobial dose was seen in persons given 1 g of azithromycin (14% vs. <6%, respectively, for the other regimens, $p = 0.06$). A prior trial in Thailand also reported a trend toward a shorter duration of illness with azithromycin (40 hours) versus ciprofloxacin (52 hours), which could be related to the slower response in persons infected with ciprofloxacin-resistant strains.[117]

41. Based on the severity of their illnesses, what specific drug therapies could B.R and E.J. consider taking?

Treatment of TD with specific drug therapy is partly based on the severity of the individual's illness and likely enteropathogen. Travelers such as B.R. with a mild diarrheal illness (one to two stools/24 hours) with mild or absent symptoms may forgo specific drug therapy or elect to use bismuth subsalicylate. Patients with a mild to moderate diarrheal illness (more than three stools/24 hours) with no distressing symptoms can consider the use of loperamide or bismuth subsalicylate (Table 62-3), although persons on a short and critical trip (e.g., business) might also consider the addition of an antibiotic. For patients with distressing frequency or symptoms, loperamide plus a fluoroquinolone, azithromycin or rifaximin can be used; they should be reassessed after 24 hours.[13]

For travelers such as E.J., with severe diarrhea or diarrhea with fever or bloody stools, a full 3 days of a fluoroquinolone or azithromycin is recommended. Azithromycin can be considered a first-line agent for TD in areas where fluoroquinolone-resistant *Campylobacter* species is common.[13] Loperamide can be added for severe cramps or fluid losses, although the use loperamide in patients with dysentery is controversial.[13]

Table 62-3 Therapy for Travelers' Diarrhea in Adults

Drug	*Treatment*
Ciprofloxacin	500 mg twice daily for 1–3 days
Ofloxacin	400 mg twice daily for 1–3 days
Levofloxacin	500 mg daily for 1–3 days
Azithromycin	500 mg daily for 1–3 days
Rifaximin	200 mg three times daily for 3 days

Adapted from DuPont HL. Travelers' diarrhea: contemporary approaches to therapy and prevention. *Drugs* 2006;66:303; and Castelli F, et al. Prevention and treatment of traveler's diarrhea. *Digestion* 2006;73(Suppl 1):109, with permission.

Some experts recommend that travelers to high-risk areas for acquiring TD be provided with medications and instructions for the self-treatment of TD, which is particularly important to travelers who become ill in remote areas where reliable medical care is not available.[12] One recommendation is to provide travelers with nine 200-mg tablets of rifaximin for the treatment of nondysenteric illness, and three 500-mg tablets of azithromycin for use in case they develop febrile dysentery.[12]

Prophylaxis

42. On hearing of the travels of B.R. and E.J., classmates J.G. and T.M. begin planning their vacation to Mexico, but want to prevent any diarrheal illness that could interfere with their travel plans. Neither student has any significant medical history. Besides avoiding the consumption of food items with a high likelihood of being contaminated with enteropathogens, what drug therapies can be used to minimize their likelihood of developing TD?

Antimicrobials

A single daily dose of a fluoroquinolone provides a protection rate of 80% against TD.[12] Significantly fewer diarrheal illnesses are reported in patients given norfloxacin 400 mg daily or ciprofloxacin 500 mg daily for 7–15 days (26%–64%) versus travelers given placebo (2%–7%).[127]

Rifaximin provided a protective efficacy of 72%–77% against TD in students traveling from the United States to Mexico. Because ETEC was the main enteropathogen identified in this study, another study is needed to determine if rifaximin can prevent diarrhea caused by invasive bacterial pathogens.[134] Rifaximin is not approved for the prophylaxis of TD.[132]

Miscellaneous Agents

Bismuth subsalicylate, two tablets (524 mg/dose) four times daily for a maximum of 3 weeks, has a protective efficacy of 65% against TD.[12] Probiotics have been studied on the basis of their ability to prevent enteropathogen colonization. To date, the effectiveness of probiotics is conflicting, and the data are not sufficiently strong to recommend their use as the only prophylactic agent for TD.[13]

43. What specific drug therapies would be reasonable for T.M. and J.G. to take as prophylaxis against travelers' diarrhea?

Despite their efficacy in preventing TD, for several reasons many experts[14,135] do not recommend universal antimicrobial prophylaxis against TD. First, most persons will experience a self-limiting illness. Second, if TD should occur effective antimicrobial therapies can reduce the duration of illness to as little as a few hours.[135] Instead, antimicrobials should be reserved for situations where the benefit of preventing illness outweighs the downside of their use, including adverse drug reactions, increased bacterial resistance, and expense.[13] Candidates for prophylactic antimicrobials include travelers in whom a bout of diarrhea would not be well tolerated (e.g., persons with autoimmune disorders, diabetes or chronic cardiac conditions, impaired gastric acid secretion, inflammatory bowel disease, HIV infection or those who are immunosuppressed; or in travelers on short-term critical trips such as diplomats and athletes).[13]

CLOSTRIDIUM DIFFICILE-ASSOCIATED DIARRHEA

Mild to Moderate Infection

Clinical Presentation and Diagnosis

44. B.W., a 35-year-old woman, is admitted to a 10-bed medical ward for the treatment of *Streptococcus pneumoniae* meningitis. On arrival, she is started on ceftriaxone (Rocephin) 2 g IV Q 12 hr and improves over the next few days. On day 7 of antibiotic therapy, she complained of feeling warm, with cramping abdominal pain and diarrhea. She began passing mucoid, greenish, foul-smelling watery stools, and had a temperature of 101°F. Microscopic examination of a stool sample was positive for fecal leukocytes. The physician's assessment of B.W.'s clinical and laboratory findings is antibiotic-associated diarrhea (AAD), most likely caused by *C. difficile*. What is the most likely mechanism for this patient's AAD?

Antibiotic-associated diarrhea is a common complication of antimicrobial therapy.[136] The mechanisms by which antibiotics cause diarrhea include allergic and toxic effects on intestinal mucosa, and alterations of GI motility (e.g., erythromycin), and of normal intestinal flora. Changes in the normal bowel flora can lead to changes in carbohydrate or bile acid metabolism by intestinal bacteria or to overgrowth of pathogenic bacteria, either of which may be followed by diarrhea.[137] Bacteria known to be associated with AAD include *C. perfringens, S. aureus, Klebsiella oxytoca, Candida* species, and *C. difficile.*[137] *C. difficile* infection is most clinically relevant and is the focus of this section.

A spore-forming, gram-positive anaerobic bacillus, *C. difficile* can cause a wide spectrum of syndromes, including asymptomatic carriage, diarrhea of varying severity, colitis with or without formation of pseudomembranes, toxic megacolon, colonic perforation, and death.[136]

The pathogenesis of *C. difficile* infection involves disruption of the normal colonic flora, most commonly by antibiotics; however, antineoplastic drugs[138] and tacrolimus[139] have been implicated as well (Table 62-4). Alteration of the colonic microflora is followed by overgrowth of toxin-producing strains of *C. difficile.*[137] These toxins are responsible for causing colonic inflammation and the clinical manifestations of this infection.[136,139]

Table 62-4 Medications Implicated in Clostridium difficile-Associated Diarrhea

Commonly Implicated	Rarely Implicated
Cephalosporins	Aminoglycosides
Clindamycin	Rifampin
Ampicillin	Tetracycline
Fluoroquinolones	Chloramphenicol
	Vancomycin
Less Commonly Implicated	Metronidazole
Erythromycin	Antineoplastic agents
Clarithromycin	
Azithromycin	
Other penicillins	
Trimethoprim-sulfamethoxazole	

From Fekety R. Guidelines for the diagnosis and treatment of *Clostridium difficile*-associated diarrhea and colitis. *Am J Gastroenterol* 1997;92:739; Johnson S, et al. *Clostridium difficile*-associated diarrhea. *Clin Infect Dis* 1998;26:1027; and Pepin J, et al. Emergence of fluoroquinolones as the predominant risk factor for *Clostridium difficile*-associated diarrhea: a cohort study during an epidemic in Quebec. *Clin Infect Dis* 2005;41:1254, with permission.

45. Why is B.W.'s history and presentation consistent with AAD caused by *C. difficile*?

B.W.'s major risk factor for acquiring *C. difficile*-associated diarrhea (CDAD) is owing to her having received an antibiotic within the last 2 weeks. *C. difficile* is a common cause of nosocomial diarrhea. The clinical and laboratory findings consistent with CDAD include mucoid, greenish, foul-smelling watery stools and crampy abdominal pain. Patients usually present with low-grade fevers, but temperature may be >104°F.[136] Peripheral leukocytosis is common, with CDAD a common cause of WBC >30,000 cells/mm^3.[140,141] Fecal leukocytes are variably present in CDAD and are not clinically useful for diagnosis.[142]

The onset of symptoms of CDAD varies widely from a few days after the start of antibiotic therapy to 8 weeks after the agent is discontinued.[136] Other risk factors for acquiring CDAD are admission to a hospital in which *C. difficile* is endemic or in which there is an ongoing outbreak of *C. difficile* infection.

46. How can the diagnosis of CDAD be confirmed?

Several tests are available to make the diagnosis of *C. difficile* infection. The rapid tests latex agglutination and EIA are commonly used in clinical laboratories. The latex agglutination test detects antigens to *C. difficile*; EIA detects toxins A and B produced by *C. difficile.*[136] Limitations of the latex agglutination test are that it also detects antigens to other intestinal bacteria, and it does not differentiate toxin-producing strains from non–toxin-producing strains.[136] Of the *C. difficile* strains isolated from various populations, 5%–25% do not produce toxins (nontoxigenic) and do not cause colitis or diarrhea.[143]

Colonoscopy with biopsy is used to make the diagnosis of *C. difficile* colitis rapidly. The characteristic colonic changes are raised, yellowish nodules or plaquelike pseudomembranes, often with skip areas of normal mucosa.[136] Because the characteristic pseudomembranes may be scattered throughout the colon, the diagnosis of pseudomembranous colitis can be missed with colonoscopy.

47. How can B.W.'s CDAD be differentiated from enigmatic AAD?

Only 10%–20% of cases of AAD are positive for toxigenic *C. difficile*; the remaining cases have an unknown cause and are referred to as simple, benign, or "nuisance" diarrhea.[136,140] The clinical presentation of benign diarrhea is similar to many cases of CDAD in that it is a self-limited illness that resolves with nonspecific supportive measures and discontinuation of antibiotics.[136] Despite these similarities, these clinical entities can be differentiated from one another by several objective measures. In hospitalized patients, watery diarrhea, low functional capacity, acid suppression, low albumin, and a WBC >13,000 cells/mm^3 were significant predictors of CDAD.[144] Other clinical features that suggest CDAD rather than enigmatic diarrhea are constitutional symptoms, no antibiotic dose relationship to the illness, and hospital-wide epidemics of diarrhea.[140]

Treatment

48. B.W.'s stool sample is positive for *C. difficile* toxin. What is the general plan for treat B.W.'s CDAD?

After replacement of fluids and electrolytes, there are three options to manage B.W.'s diarrhea. The first is to discontinue the offending drug (if possible), which in B.W.'s case is probably the antibiotic ceftriaxone. In approximately 25% of cases, discontinuation of the offending agent with concomitant fluid and electrolyte replacement leads to resolution of symptoms within 48–72 hours.[145] Thus, patients with mild diarrhea may not require any treatment other than discontinuation of the offending agent.[136,143]

Because B.W. is being treated for bacterial meningitis, a life-threatening infection, discontinuing antibiotics is not an option. A second option is to change her antimicrobial therapy to an agent less likely to cause CDAD. B.W. is taking a cephalosporin, which, as with ampicillin, amoxicillin, and clindamycin, is frequently implicated as a cause of *C. difficile* diarrhea (Table 62-4). In contrast, antibiotics, such as TMP-SMX, and aminoglyclosides, are less commonly associated with *C. difficile* infection.[136,143,146] None of these antimicrobials, however, is a suitable alternative for treating *S. pneumoniae* meningitis.

The third and most reasonable option for B.W. is to receive therapy directed against *C. difficile* while continuing to take ceftriaxone for the treatment of her bacterial meningitis.

METRONIDAZOLE AND VANCOMYCIN

49. What antibiotics could be prescribed to treat B.W.'s CDAD?

The oral agents most commonly used to treat CDAD are metronidazole and vancomycin. In a randomized trial that enrolled patients with CDAD and colitis, no significant difference was found in the efficacy of these drugs after 10 days of treatment.[147] Overall, >95% of patients treated for a first episode of CDAD with oral metronidazole or vancomycin is expected to respond to therapy.[147,148] Recent reports have shown increases in *C. difficile* resistance to metronidazole and vancomycin, but the clinical significance in treatment selection is unknown.[149] Antibiotic sensitivities, therefore, are not routinely performed on *C. difficile*.

Metronidazole is well absorbed after oral administration and is excreted through the biliary tract before reaching the colon. Common adverse reactions include nausea, vomiting, diarrhea, dizziness, confusion, and an unpleasant metallic taste.[136] A disulfiramlike reaction can occur when alcohol or alcohol-containing medications are taken concurrently with metronidazole.[150] Because metronidazole is a carcinogen and, in some animal species, a mutagen, it should be used in pregnancy only if clearly needed. Similarly, metronidazole's safety in children has not been proved, and many prefer not to use it in this population if other options exist.[136]

Oral vancomycin produces fecal concentrations that are several hundred times the concentration needed to inhibit toxin-producing strains of *C. difficile*.[148] A 7- to 10-day course of oral vancomycin (125–500 mg orally four times daily) is recommended for the treatment of CDAD, with all dosing regimens equally effective.[136,148,151,152] Because of equal efficacy and high concentrations in the colon with all doses, 125 mg is the most commonly prescribed dose. Although oral vancomycin is not well absorbed, measurable serum concentrations have been found in patients with both normal and compromised renal function.[153–155]

Oral vancomycin is recommended when patients (*a*) fail to respond to metronidazole; (*b*) are infected with *C. difficile* resistant to metronidazole; (*c*) cannot tolerate metronidazole (e.g., allergy, or concurrent use of ethanol-containing products); (*d*) are pregnant or <10 years of age; (*e*) are critically ill because of *C. difficile* infection; or (*f*) have evidence of diarrhea caused by *S. aureus*.[136,156]

50. What antibiotic regimen would you recommend for treatment of B.W.'s CDAD?

When antibiotic therapy is required for patients who are not critically ill as a result of their *C. difficile* infection, metronidazole (250–500 mg orally four times daily or 500–750 mg orally three times daily) for 7–10 days is recommended as first-line treatment.[136,157] Oral metronidazole and oral vancomycin are equally efficacious,[147] but vancomycin use should be limited to prevent emergence of vancomycin-resistant organisms.[157] In addition, oral vancomycin is significantly more expensive than a course of oral metronidazole. Some of this cost differential can be offset by using the IV vancomycin preparation to prepare an oral solution (Table 62-5).

Once therapy directed against *C. difficile* is initiated, diarrhea or cramping should subside within 2–4 days. If B.W.'s symptoms have not resolved, vancomycin can be tried.[140]

51. Following resolution of B.W.'s CDAD, is it necessary to send a follow-up stool sample to determine whether it is negative for *C. difficile* toxin?

After resolution of diarrhea, obtaining a follow-up stool sample to determine whether it is negative for *C. difficile* toxin is not recommended as part of routine practice because most patients with positive tests will not develop a recurrence of their diarrhea.[136] In addition, approximately 5% of healthy adults carry small numbers of *C. difficile* in their feces, whereas colonization rates are much higher (30%–50%) in hospitalized patients and newborns.[136,143]

BACITRACIN

52. What other oral therapies have been used to treat CDAD?

In a randomized, double-blind trial, oral bacitracin (80,000–25,000 U/day) was as effective as oral vancomycin

Table 62-5 Costs of Oral Drug Therapy for *Clostridium difficile*-Associated Diarrhea

Drug	*Regimen*	*Cost*[a]
Metronidazole tablets (generic)	500 mg TID × 10 days	$21.84/10 days
Vancomycin capsules (Vancocin)	125 mg QID × 10 days	$646.40/10 days
Vancomycin solution[b] (generic)	125 mg QID × 10 days	$37.80/10 days
Nitazoxanide (Alinia)	125 mg BID × 10 days	$251.60/10 days

[a] AWP Red Book 2006.
[b] Prepared from intravenous formulation.

(500–2,000 mg/day) in resolving symptoms of CDAD. Although the difference was not statistically significant, however, was a trend was seen toward a slower clinical response with bacitracin. Compared with vancomycin, the clinical response to bacitracin is slower and less certain, possibly because of resistance to bacitracin.[136] The recurrence rate is similar for both antibiotics.[158,159]

NITAZOXANIDE

Nitazoxanide is an oral nitrothiazolide currently FDA approved for the treatment of cryptosporidia and giardia. Nitazoxanide has in vitro activity against *C.difficile* and has been shown to be as effective as metronidazole in the initial treatment of CDAD in a small comparative trial.[160]

RAMOPLANIN

Ramoplanin is a nonabsorbed, investigational, oral glycolipodepsipeptide currently being studied in clinical trials for the treatment of CDAD.[161] Phase II trials have shown similar response rates when compared with vancomycin. In animal models, ramoplanin has been shown to more effectively kill *C. difficile* spores, a potentially important factor in relapse of infection.[162]

TOXIN BINDERS

Anion-binding resins (e.g., cholestyramine, colestipol) are not as reliable or as rapidly effective as oral metronidazole or vancomycin.[136] If prescribed, they are recommended only for mild CDAD.[136,163] The rationale for using exchange resins for CDAD is their ability to bind to toxin B produced by *C. difficile*[163]; however, resins have a limited binding capacity for toxins that is probably inadequate for severe cases.[136] Other limitations of exchange resins include their inability to eradicate the pathogenic organisms responsible for toxin production and their ability to bind to vancomycin, which may reduce the efficacy of the antibiotic.[136] Severe constipation is a side effect of exchange resins.[136]

Tolevamer is an investigational anionic polymer that binds *C. difficile* toxins A and B. In a phase II trial, tolevamer (6 g/d) alone was shown to be as effective as vancomycin for mild to moderate CDAD, and trended toward lower recurrence rates.[164] Further studies of variable doses are ongoing. Toxin binding may also be useful as adjunctive therapy with other antibacterials.

PROBIOTICS

Probiotic microorganisms are introduced into the normal flora to counteract disturbances and reduce the colonization with pathogenic species.[15] Although orally administered *Lactobacillus* species and the yeast *Saccharomyces boulardii* have been used to treat CDAD, no data support the use of probiotics alone to treat CDAD. Adjunctive use, however, has been suggested to prevent CDAD and its recurrences. Reports of isolated adverse effects, including fungemia, with ingestion of viable *S. boulardii* have been reported.[165]

ANTIDIARRHEALS

53. What is the role of antidiarrheal agents in patients with CDAD?

Opiates and other antiperistaltic agents should be avoided in patients with CDAD. Although these types of drugs may relieve diarrheal symptoms, they may also delay toxin removal from the GI tract. Patients with antibiotic-associated pseudomembranous colitis have deteriorated during therapy with antimotility medications.[166]

Transmission

54. H.T., a 76-year-old man with multiple medical conditions, is admitted to the same 10-bed ward as B.W. His medical history is significant for a stroke that has left him bedridden in a nursing home. His only medications are those used to manage his hypertension. On day 4 of his hospitalization, H.T. complained of severe abdominal pain and watery, loose stools with blood. Physical examination revealed a toxic-appearing man with a temperature of 101°F. A stool specimen is positive for *C. difficile* toxin, and colonoscopy reveals pseudomembranes and colitis. A surgical consultant recommends an emergent colectomy because of impending bowel perforation secondary to the *C. difficile* infection. What are H.T.'s risk factors for acquiring *C. difficile*-associated pseudomembranous colitis during his hospitalization?

H.T.'s risk factors for acquiring *C. difficile* infection include his advanced age, bedridden status,[167] underlying diseases,[168] and admission to the hospital. *C. difficile* infection is spread when hospital personnel or equipment contaminated with *C. difficile* spores come into contact with susceptible patients. Physical proximity to an infected patient has been associated with an increased risk of CDAD.[169] Therefore, measures to prevent the spread of *C. difficile* infection include proper handwashing before and after contact with infected patients, and the use of gloves and enteric isolation precautions when in contact with infected patients with diarrhea. Contaminated equipment should be properly disinfected.[136]

Although *C. difficile* is often thought of as a nosocomial pathogen, it is being increasingly isolated in outpatient settings.[170,171] A European study found that up to 28% of all cases occurred without previous hospitalization.[170]

New Epidemic Strain

55. Could there be a strain difference causing the severe CDAD in H.T.?

A highly pathogenic strain of *C. difficile* has recently been described in outbreaks in the United States.[172] This strain, labeled BI/NAP1, causes more severe disease. Among its increased virulence factors are an increased production of both toxins A and B and a binary toxin. These strains are also newly resistant to fluoroquinolones, which may increase the frequency of disease.[146] No current clinical tests exist to distinguish BI/NAP1 from other strains. There are no specific treatment recommendations for this strain.

56. Over the next few days, all 10 patients on the ward with B.W. and H.T. are found to have *C. difficile* toxin in their stools. Five patients have diarrhea and the other five are asymptomatic. What is the role of antibiotic therapy directed at *C. difficile* in controlling this outbreak?

Neither oral metronidazole nor vancomycin is reliably effective in eradicating the carrier state (i.e., asymptomatic, fecal excretion), and neither is recommended for use in this situation.[173] The lack of efficacy of these drugs is probably related because, unlike the vegetative forms of *C. difficile,* the spores of *C. difficile* are resistant to the action of antibiotics.[136] Furthermore, compared with placebo, vancomycin administration is associated with a significantly higher rate of *C. difficile* carriage 2 months after treatment.[173] Restricting the use of clindamycin can be an effective component in efforts to control nosocomial epidemics of CDAD.[167] With the emergence of the BI/NAP1 strain, control of all antibiotic use, including fluoroquinolones, may be important in outbreak control.[174]

57. What effect will the current CDAD outbreak have on the outcomes of the infected patients and on health care costs?

In a prospective study, hospitalized patients who developed CDAD had a 3.6-day increase in length of stay.[175] This increase was accompanied by a doubling of hospital costs. Although 3-month mortality rates were higher in patients with CDAD (48% vs. 22%), no significant differences were observed when adjustments were made for severity of underlying illness. The current outbreak is likely to increase both hospital costs and individual lengths of stay.

Severe *C. difficile* Infection

58. What treatment is recommended for patients such as H.T. who are critically ill from a *C. difficile* infection? What criteria are used to characterize patients as "critically ill"?

Of patients with antibiotic-associated pseudomembranous colitis who require surgical intervention (colectomy), up to 57% die.[176] Although the precise definition of "critically ill" is not clear, it has included patients with pseudomembrane formation, fever >104°F, marked abdominal tenderness, and marked leukocytosis.[157] Limited evidence suggests that vancomycin may be more effective than metronidazole in patients with predefined severe disease, including those admitted to the intensive care unit.[156] H.T. meets these criteria for being critically ill.

Nonoral Treatment

59. Three days after oral vancomycin is initiated, H.T. develops an ileus and cannot take anything by mouth. What therapeutic options are available to treat H.T.'s pseudomembranous colitis?

Adequate antibiotic levels in the colon are necessary to treat *C. difficile*-associated pseudomembranous colitis. If the oral route is not feasible (e.g., patients with an ileus or bowel obstruction), the clinician must choose an agent that is either secreted or excreted into the GI tract in its active form. IV vancomycin is not the most desirable agent in this situation because it is not secreted into the GI tract. In contrast, metronidazole is eliminated by both renal and hepatic routes; bactericidal concentrations are achieved in both serum and bile.[177]

The literature contains few reports of successful attempts to treat CDAD or pseudomembranous colitis with IV metronidazole (500 mg Q 6–8 hr).[178–180] Likewise, unsuccessful attempts to treat CDAD with IV metronidazole have been reported.[178,181] When oral therapy is not feasible in patients with CDAD, some experts recommend IV metronidazole 500–750 mg three or four times daily with concurrent use of enteral vancomycin.[136] The clinical response of *C. difficile* infection to IV vancomycin in a patient who did not survive was difficult to ascertain.[148]

In adults, enteral vancomycin 500 mg four times daily can be given through an ileostomy or colostomy (if present). Several reports of successful outcomes using intercolonic vancomycin (as an adjunct to oral or IV antibiotics) in patients with CDAD have been documented. Rectal doses of vancomycin have varied from 500 mg Q 4–8 hr to 1,000 mg/L Q 8 hr.[182] Because patients with CDAD are at risk for colonic perforation, enteral vancomycin should be administered cautiously.

Relapse

60. One week after discharge from the hospital, B.W. once again developed abdominal pain and diarrhea. Her clinic physician assumed these symptoms could not be related to a relapse of her CDAD because she had responded so well to metronidazole. What is the likelihood that CDAD has recurred?

Regardless of the antibiotic regimen prescribed for CDAD, symptomatic relapse occurs in 5%–30% of patients who respond to their initial treatment regimen.[136,143] Relapses occur 2 weeks to 2 months (median of 7 days) after treatment has been discontinued.[183]

In most instances, relapses are caused by germination of dormant spores that are intrinsically resistant to antibiotics. Reinfection with *C. difficile* from external sources, however, may account for up to half of all second episodes.[184] In rare instances, either vancomycin[185] or metronidazole[186] may have caused CDAD.

Risk factors for recurrent CDAD include increasing age, low quality-of-health score,[183] use of additional antibiotics, spring onset, and multiple prior episodes of *C. difficile* infection.[187] Of patients experiencing their first episode of CDAD, 24% experience a relapse, and 65% of patients with a prior history of CDAD relapse.[188]

Data suggest that patients with a poor immune response to *C. difficile* toxin A are more likely to have a relapse of CDAD.[189] It is not clinically helpful in the case of B.W., because no standard tests are currently available for this immune response. The influence of the immune system, however, has led to the usage of IV immune globulin in refractory or severe cases of CDAD.[190,191] The utility of the usage of immune globulins has been debated in small single institution reviews. Immune globulins would not be the considered the next line of therapy for B.W.

61. How should patients such as B.W. who relapse after therapy for CDAD be treated?

Most infections resulting from relapse are not related to bacterial resistance and they respond to retreatment with the same antibiotic used for initial treatment of the *C. difficile* infection.[143,192] Thus, an appropriate approach for B.W. is to administer another 7- to 10-day course of oral metronidazole.

For patients with multiple recurrences of CDAD, the optimal management plan is unresolved.[136] Different approaches have been tried, including (a) high-dose vancomycin (2,000 mg/day)[193]; (b) a 4- to 6-week course with vancomycin, after which the dose is tapered over a 1- to 2-month period[193,194]; (c) exchange resins[163,195]; (d) "pulse" dosing every 2–3 days[193]; or (e) a combination of vancomycin and rifampin (600 mg orally twice daily).[196] Tapered and pulse therapy with vancomycin were shown to be most effective in a clinical trial comparing multiple strategies.[193] When combined with standard antibiotic therapy, a clinical trial with the probiotic *S. boulardii* for cases of relapsing CDAD noted a 65% response rate versus a 36% response rate for combination therapy with placebo.[188] The relapse rate was reduced to 17% when *S. boulardii* was combined with high-dose vancomycin.[197]

Nitazoxanide had a 74% initial response rate in patients who had previously failed metronidazole therapy.[198] Recurrent relapse was successfully treated with a second course of nitazoxanide in a limited number of individuals, representing an overall 66% response rate in a small difficult-to-treat population.

Following treatment with vancomycin, a 2-week "chaser" course of rifaximin, a poorly absorbed rifamycin derivative, was successful in a case series for seven of eight patients with multiple relapses.[199] Although obviously a small sample, concern must be raised that the single failure occurred in concert with emerging rifaxamin resistance.

Cryptosporidium Parvum

Cryptosporidia are intracellular parasites that infect cells of the GI tract, leading to a watery diarrheal illness. Of the various species, *C. parvum* is the most common cause of human illness. Although *C. parvum* causes an intestinal illness in both healthy and immunocompromised persons; the clinical presentations, the role of antiparasitic agents, and the clinical response to antiparasitic agents differ between these populations.

Clinical Presentation

62. C.K., a 35-year-old, previously healthy man, presents to his family physician with complaints of 15 days of watery diarrhea and a 5-lb weight loss. He heard an announcement by the Board of Health of a community-wide outbreak of cryptosporidiosis from contaminated water supplies, and is concerned that he has this illness. Why are C.K.'s history of present illness and clinical presentation consistent with cryptosporidiosis? Should antiparasitic agents be prescribed to treat cryptosporidiosis in otherwise healthy persons such as C.K.?

A key piece of information from C.K.'s history of present illness that is consistent with the diagnosis of cryptosporidiosis is his exposure to water supplies known to be contaminated with cryptosporidium oocysts, because this is the most important mode of acquiring this infection.[200] Other means of spreading cryptosporidiosis include animal contact (cattle and sheep), and person-to-person contact (e.g., health care workers, day care personnel).[200]

C.K. is presenting with persistent diarrhea, which is defined as diarrhea lasting >14 days. Common microbial causes of persistent watery diarrhea include parasites, such as *Isospora belli, Microsporidia, G. lambli*, and *C. parvum*. The spectrum of infection with *C. parvum* ranges from asymptomatic carriage to a persistent, noninflammatory diarrheal illness.[200] Other manifestations of cryptosporidiosis include nausea, vomiting, abdominal cramps, weight loss, and fever.[200] In immunocompetent patients such as C.K., cryptosporidiosis is generally a self-limiting illness lasting approximately 2 weeks.[200] In contrast, in immunocompromised patients, cryptosporidiosis can be a chronic, debilitating, diarrheal illness associated with malabsorption and significant weight loss.

Treatment

In immunocompetent hosts with a diarrheal illness attributed to *C. parvum* or in asymptomatic persons, other than replacement of fluids and electrolytes, no specific therapy directed at this parasite is generally required.[201] If needed, a 3-day course of nitazoxanide given with food (≥12 years, 500 mg Q 12 hr; 4–11 years, 200 mg Q 12 hr; and 1–3 years, 100 mg Q 12 hr) is approved for the treatment of diarrhea caused by *C. parvum* in persons >1 year of age.[202] A randomized, double-blind, placebo-controlled trial in immunocompetent adults and children found that diarrhea resolved in 80% of those treated with nitazoxanide versus 41% of patients given placebo, $p < 0.0001$; oocyst shedding was also significantly reduced. In this study, diarrhea usually resolved within 3–4 days of starting treatment.[203]

In contrast, for immunocompromised persons, a meta-analysis of treatments for cryptosporidiosis found no evidence to support the role of chemotherapeutic agents for the management of cryptosporidioisis in this population.[201] These findings are consistent with a randomized trial that found a 3-day course of nitazoxanide did not provide any benefit to children who were HIV positive, whereas in children who were HIV negative, nitazoxanide treatment significantly improved the resolution of diarrhea and decreased mortality.[204] In persons who are HIV positive, reconstitution of the immune system is the mainstay of treatment for cryptosporidiosis.[201]

REFERENCES

1. Ilnyckyj A. Clinical evaluation and management of acute infectious diarrhea in adults. *Gastroenterol Clin North Am* 2001;30:599.
2. Turgeon DK et al. Laboratory approaches to infectious diarrhea. *Gastroenterol Clin North Am* 2001;30:693.
3. DuPont HL et al. Guidelines on acute infectious diarrhea in adults. *Am J Gastroenterol* 1997;92:1962.
4. Cheng AC et al. Infectious diarrhea in developed and developing countries. *J Clin Gastroenterol* 2005;39:757.
5. Guerrant RL et al. Principles and syndromes of enteric infection. In: Mandell GL et al., eds. *Principles and Practice of Infectious Diseases.* 6th ed. Philadelphia: Churchill Livingstone; 2005:89.
6. Talan D et al. Etiology of bloody diarrhea among patients presenting to United States emergency departments: prevalence of *Escherichia coli* O157:H7 and other enteropathogens. *Clin Infect Dis* 2001;32:573.
7. Oldfield EC et al. The role of antibiotics in the treatment of infectious diarrhea. *Gastroenterol Clin North Am* 2001;30:817.
8. Swerdlow DL et al. Cholera in the Americas. Guidelines for the clinician. *JAMA* 1992;267:1495.
9. King CK et al. Managing acute gastroenteritis among children: oral rehydration, maintenance, and nutritional therapy. Centers for Disease Control and Prevention. *MMWR Recomm Rep* 2003; 52(RR-16):1.
10. Wingate D et al. Guidelines for adults on self-medication for the treatment of acute diarrhea. *Aliment Pharmacol Ther* 2001;15:773.
11. Hines J et al. Effective use of the clinical microbiology laboratory for diagnosing diarrheal diseases. *Clin Infect Dis* 1996;23:1292.
12. DuPont HL. Travelers' diarrhea: contemporary approaches to therapy and prevention. *Drugs* 2006;66:303.
13. Castelli F et al. Prevention and treatment of traveler's diarrhea. *Digestion* 2006;73(Suppl 1):109.
14. Travelers' diarrhea. www.cdc.gov/ncidod/dbmd/diseaseinfo/travelersdiarrhea_ghtm.
15. Sullivan A et al. Probiotics in human infections. *J Antimicrob Chemother* 2002;50:625.
16. Elmer GW. Probiotics: "living drugs." *Am J Health-Syst Pharm* 2001;58:1101.
17. Thaver D et al. Fluoroquinolones for treating typhoid and paratyphoid fever (enteric fever). *Cochrane Database Syst Rev* 2005;18: CD004530.
18. Alam NH et al. Treatment of infectious diarrhea in children. *Pediatr Drugs* 2003;5:151.
19. Bresee JS et al. Foodborne viral gastroenteritis: challenges and opportunities. *Clin Infect Dis* 2002;35:748.
20. Graman PS et al. Gastrointestinal and intraabdominal infections. In Reese RE et al., eds. *A Practical Approach to Infectious Diseases.* 5th ed. Philadelphia: Lippincott Williams & Wilkins; 2003:403.
21. RotaTeq. [package insert]. Whitehouse Station, NJ: Merck & Co., Inc; 2007.
22. Rosenfeldt V et al. Effect of probiotic lactobacillus strains in young children hospitalized with acute diarrhea. *Pediatr Infect Dis J* 2002;21:411.
23. Steinberg EB et al. Cholera in the United States, 1995–2000: trends at the end of the twentieth century. *J Infect Dis* 2001;184:799.
24. Daniels NA et al. *Vibrio parahaemolyticus* infections in the United States, 1973–1998. *J Infect Dis* 2000;181:1661.
25. Sack DA et al. World Health Organization. Antimicrobial resistance in shigellosis, cholera, and campylobacteriosis. Geneva, Switzerland: World Health Organization, 2001. Available at http://www.who.int/csr/resources/publications/drugresist/WHO_CDS_CSR_DRS_2001_8/en/print.html.
26. Khan WA et al. Randomized controlled comparison of single-dose ciprofloxacin and doxycycline for cholera caused by vibrio cholerae 01 or 0139. *Lancet* 1996;348:296.
27. Saha D et al. Single-dose azithromycin for the treatment of cholera in adults. *N Engl J Med* 2006;354:2452.
28. Saha D et al. Single-dose ciprofloxacin versus 12-dose erythromycin for childhood cholera: a randomized controlled trial. *Lancet* 2005;366: 1085.
29. Khan WA et al. Comparison of single-dose azithromycin and 12-dose, 3-day erythromycin for childhood cholera: a randomized, double-blind trial. *Lancet* 2002;360:1722.
30. Faruque SM et al. Reemergence of epidemic vibrio cholerae 0139, Bangladesh. *Emerg Infect Dis* 2003;9:1116.
31. Daniels NA et al. Emergence of a new *vibrio parahaemolyticus* serotype in raw oysters: a prevention quandary. *JAMA* 2000;284:1541.
32. Potasman I et al. Infectious outbreaks associated with bivalve shellfish consumption: a worldwide perspective. *Clin Infect Dis* 2002;35:921.
33. World Health Organization. Guidelines for the control of shigellosis, including epidemics due to shigella dysenteriae 1. Geneva, Switzerland: World Health Organization, 2005. Available at www.who.int/entity/vaccine_research/documents/Guidelines_Shigellosis.pdf World Health Organization.
34. Sur D et al. Shigellosis: challenges and management issues. *Indian J Med Res* 2004;120:454.
35. Niyogi SK. Shigellosis. *J Microbiol* 2005;43:133.
36. Vinh H et al. Treatment of bacillary dysentery in Vietnamese children: two doses of ofloxacin versus 5-days of nalidixic acid. *Trans R Soc Trop Med Hyg* 2000;94:323.
37. Bennish ML et al. Low risk of hemolytic uremic syndrome after early effective antimicrobial therapy for shigella dysenteriae type 1 infection in Bangladesh. *Clin Infect Dis* 2006;42:356.
38. Nelson JD et al. Amoxicillin less effective than ampicillin against *Shigella* in vitro and in vivo: relationship of efficacy to activity in serum. *J Infect Dis* 1974;129(Suppl):S222.
39. The Zimbabwe, Bangladesh, South Africa (Zimbasa) Dysentery Study Group. *Pediatr Infect Dis J* 2002;21:1136.
40. Rogerie F et al. Comparison of norfloxacin and nalidixic acid for treatment of dysentery caused by *Shigella dysenteriae type 1* in adults. *Antimicrob Agents Chemother* 1986;29:883.
41. Murphy GS et al. Ciprofloxacin and loperamide in the treatment of bacillary dysentery. *Ann Intern Med* 1993;118:582.
42. Bennish ML et al. Treatment of shigellosis, III. Comparison of one- or two-dose ciprofloxacin with standard 5-day therapy. *Ann Intern Med* 1992;117:727.
43. Gotuzzo E et al. Comparison of single-dose treatment with norfloxacin and standard 5-day treatment with trimethoprim-sulfamethoxazole for acute shigellosis in adults. *Antimicrob Agents Chemother* 1989;33:1101.
44. Cheasty T et al. Increasing incidence of resistance to nalidixic acid in shigellas from humans in England and Wales: implications for therapy. *Clin Microbiol Infect* 2004;10:1033.
45. Taneja N et al. Re-emergence of multi-drug resistant Shigella dysenteriae with added resistance to ciprofloxacin in north India and their plasmid profiles. *Indian J Med Res* 2005;122:348.
46. Jain SK et al. Antimicrobial-resistant Shigella sonnei: limited antimicrobial treatment options for children and challenges of interpreting in vitro azithromycin susceptibility. *Pediatr Infect Dis J* 2005;24:494.
47. Salam MA et al. Randomised comparison of ciprofloxacin suspension and pivmecillinam for childhood shigellosis. *Lancet* 1998;352:1313
48. Khan WA et al. Treatment of shigellosis, V. Comparison of azithromycin and ciprofloxacin. *Ann Intern Med* 1997;126:697.
49. Caacas A et al. Single dose of azithromycin or three-day course of ciprofloxacin as therapy for epidemic dysentery in Kenya. *Clin Infect Dis* 1999;29:942.
50. Huang IF et al. Outbreak of dysentery associated with ceftriaxone-resistant *Shigella sonnei*: first report of plasmid-mediated cmy-2-type ampc beta-lactamase resistance in s. sonnei. *J Clin Microbiol* 2005;43:2608.
51. Salam MA et al. Treatment of shigellosis, IV. Cefixime is ineffective in shigellosis in adults. *Ann Intern Med* 1995;123:505.
52. Basualdo W et al. Randomized comparison of azithromycin versus cefixime for treatment of shigellosis in children. *Pediatr Infect Dis J* 2003;22: 374.
53. Centers for Disease Control and Prevention (CDC). Outbreaks of multidrug-resistant *Shigella sonnei* gastroenteritis associated with day care centers—Kansas, Kentucky, and Missouri, 2005. *MMWR Morb Mortal Wkly Rep* 2006;55:1068.
54. Huang IF et al. Nontyphoid salmonellosis in Taiwan children: clinical manifestations, outcome and antibiotic resistance. *J Pediatr Gastroenterol Nutr* 2004;38:518.
55. Replogle ML et al. Emergence of antimicrobial-resistant shigellosis in Oregon. *Clin Infect Dis* 2000;30:515.
56. Hohmann EL. Nontyphoidal salmonellosis. *Clin Infect Dis* 2001;32:263.
57. Basnyat B et al. Enteric (typhoid) fever in travelers. *Clin Infect Dis* 2005;41:1467.
58. Sirinavin S et al. Norfloxacin and azithromycin for treatment of nontyphoidal salmonella carriers. *Clin Infect Dis* 2003;37:685.
59. Chiu CH et al. *Salmonella enterica* serotype choleraesuis: epidemiology, pathogenesis, clinical disease, and treatment. *Clin Microbiol Rev* 2004;17:311.
60. Crump JA et al. Reevaluating fluoroquinolone breakpoints for salmonella enterica serotype typhi and for non-typhi salmonellae. *Clin Infect Dis* 2003;37:75.
61. Stevenson JE et al. Increase in nalidixic acid resistance among non-typhi salmonella isolates in the United States from 1996–2003. *Antimicrob Agents Chemother* 2007;51:195.
62. Varma JK et al. Antimicrobial-resistant nontyphoidal salmonella is associated with excess bloodstream infections and hospitalizations. *J Infect Dis* 2005;191:554.
63. Miriagou V et al. Expanded-spectrum cephalosporin resistance in non-typhoid salmonella. *Int J Antimicrob Agents* 2004;23:547.
64. Ko WC et al. A new therapeutic challenge for old pathogens: community-acquired invasive infections caused by ceftriaxone- and ciprofloxacin-resistant salmonella enterica serotype choleraesuis. *Clin Infect Dis* 2005;40:315.
65. Parry CM. The treatment of multidrug-resistant and nalidixic acid-resistant typhoid fever in Vietnam. *Trans R Soc Trop Med Hyg* 2004;98:413.
66. Parry CM et al. Typhoid fever. *N Engl J Med* 2002;347:1770.
67. Islam A et al. Randomized treatment of patients with typhoid fever by using ceftriaxone or chloramphenicol. *J Infect Dis* 1988;158:742.
68. Frenck RW et al. Short-course azithromycin for the treatment of uncomplicated typhoid fever in children and adolescents. *Clin Infect Dis* 2004;38: 951.
69. Smith M et al. Comparison of ofloxacin and ceftriaxone for short-course treatment of enteric fever. *Antimicrob Agents Chemother* 1994;38: 1716.
70. Ha V et al. Two or three days of ofloxacin treatment for uncomplicated multidrug-resistant typhoid fever in children. *Antimicrob Agents Chemother* 1996;40:958.
71. Girgis NI et al. Azithromycin versus ciprofloxacin for treatment of uncomplicated typhoid fever in a randomized trial in Egypt that included patients with multidrug resistance. *Antimicrob Agents Chemother* 1999;43:1441.

72. Parry CM et al. Randomized controlled comparison of ofloxacin, azithromycin, and an ofloxacin-azithromycin combination for treatment of multidrug-resistant and nalidixic acid-resistant typhoid fever. *Antimicrob Agents Chemother* 2007;51:819.
73. Frenck RW et al. Azithromycin versus ceftriaxone for the treatment of uncomplicated typhoid fever in children. *Clin Infect Dis* 2000;31:1134.
74. Bhutta ZA et al. Failure of short-course ceftriaxone chemotherapy for multidrug-resistant typhoid fever in children: a randomized controlled trial in Pakistan. *Antimicrob Agents Chemother* 2000;44:450.
75. John M. Decreasing clinical response of quinolones in the treatment of enteric fever. *Indian J Med Sci* 2001;55:189.
76. Dutta P. et al. Ceftriaxone therapy in ciprofloxacin treatment failure typhoid fever in children. *Indian J Med Res* 2001;113:210.
77. Wain J et al. Quinolone-resistant *Salmonella typhi* in Vietnam: molecular basis of resistance and clinical response to treatment. *Clin Infect Dis* 1997;25:1404.
78. Farrar J. A personal perspective on clinical research in enteric fever. *Clin Infect Dis* 2007;45:S9.
79. Phuong CX et al. A comparative study of ofloxacin and cefixime for treatment of typhoid fever in children. *Pediatr Infect Dis J* 1999;18:245.
80. Treatment guidelines from the medical letter. *Med Lett* 2007;5:33.
81. Joshi S et al. Fluoroquinolone resistance in salmonella typhi and s. paratyphi a in Bangalore, India. *Trans R Soc Trop Med Hyg* 2007;101:308.
82. Hoffman SL et al. Reduction of mortality in chloramphenicol-treated severe typhoid fever by high-dose dexamethasone. *N Engl J Med* 1984;310:82.
83. Parry CM et al. Typhoid fever [Correspondence]. *N Engl J Med* 2003;348:1182.
84. Kaye D et al. Treatment of chronic enteric carriers of *Salmonella typhosa* with ampicillin. *Ann NY Acad Sci* 1967;145:429.
85. Phillips WE. Treatment of chronic typhoid carriers with ampicillin. *JAMA* 1971;217:913.
86. Nolan CM et al. Treatment of typhoid carriers with amoxicillin. *JAMA* 1978;239:2352.
87. Pichler H et al. Treatment of chronic carriers of *Salmonella typhi* and *Salmonella paratyphi* with trimethoprim-sulfamethoxazole. *J Infect Dis* 1973;128(Suppl):S743.
88. Ferreccio C et al. Efficacy of ciprofloxacin in the treatment of chronic typhoid carriers. *J Infect Dis* 1988;157:1235.
89. Diridl G et al. Treatment of chronic *Salmonella* carriers with ciprofloxacin [Letter]. *Eur J Clin Microbiol* 1986;5:260.
90. Sammalkorpi K et al. Treatment of chronic *Salmonella* carriers with ciprofloxacin [Letter]. *Lancet* 1987;2:164.
91. Gotuzzo E et al. Use of norfloxacin to treat chronic typhoid carriers. *J Infect Dis* 1988;157:1221.
92. Mead PS, Griffin PM. *Escherichia coli* O157:H7. *Lancet* 1998;352:1207.
93. Karch H et al. Epidemiology and diagnosis of Shiga toxin-producing *Escherichia coli* infections. *Diagn Microbiol Infect Dis* 1999;34:229.
94. Ericsson CD et al. Optimal dosing of trimethoprim-sulfamethoxazole when used with loperamide to treat travelers' diarrhea. *Antimicrob Agents Chemother* 1992;36:2821.
95. Dundas S et al. The central Scotland *Escherichia coli* O157:H7 outbreak: risk factors for the hemolytic uremic syndrome and death among hospitalized patients. *Clin Infect Dis.* 2001;33:923.
96. Klein EJ et al. Shiga toxin-producing *Escherichia coli* in children with diarrhea: a prospective point-of-care study. *J Pediatr* 2002;141:172.
97. Banatvala N et al. The United States National Prospective Hemolytic Uremic Syndrome Study: microbiologic, serologic, clinical, and epidemiologic findings. *J Infect Dis* 2001;183:1063.
98. Besbas N et al. A classification of hemolytic uremic syndrome and thrombotic thrombocytopenic purpura and related disorders. *Kidney Int* 2006;70:423.
99. Ikeda K et al. Predictors for the development of haemolytic uraemic syndrome with *Escherichia coli* O157:H7 infections: with focus on the day of illness. *Epidemiol Infect* 2000;124:343.
100. Wong CS et al. The risk of the hemolytic-uremic syndrome after antibiotic treatment of *Escherichia coli* O157:H7 infections. *N Engl J Med* 2000;342:1930.
101. Tserenpuntsag B et al. Hemolytic uremic syndrome risk and *Escherichia coli* O157:H7. *Emerg Infect Dis* 2005;11:1955.
102. Tarr PI et al. Shiga-toxin-producing *Escherichia coli* and haemolytic uraemic syndrome. *Lancet* 2005;365:1073.
103. Cimolai N et al. Risk factors for the progression of *Escherichia coli* O157:H7 enteritis to hemolytic-uremic syndrome. *J Pediatr* 1990;116:589.
104. Slutsker L et al. A nationwide case-control study of *Escherichia coli* O157:H7 infection in the United States. *J Infect Dis* 1998;177:962.
105. Carter AO et al. A severe outbreak of *Escherichia coli* O157:H7-associated hemorrhagic colitis in a nursing home. *N Engl J Med* 1987;317:1496.
106. Proulx F et al. Randomized, controlled trial of antibiotic therapy for *Escherichia coli* O157:H7 enteritis. *J Pediatr* 1992;121:299.
107. Pavia AT et al. Hemolytic-uremic syndrome during an outbreak of *Escherichia coli* O157:H7 infections in institutions from mentally retarded persons: clinical and epidemiologic observations. *J Pediatr* 1990;116:544.
108. Safdar N et al. Risk of hemolytic uremic syndrome after antibiotic treatment of *Escherichia coli* O157:H7 enteritis: a meta-analysis. *JAMA* 2002;288:996.
109. Panos GZ et al. Systematic review: are antibiotics detrimental or beneficial for the treatment of patients with *Escherichia coli* O157:H7 infection? *Aliment Pharmacol Ther* 2006;24:731.
110. Bell BP et al. Prediction of hemolytic uremic syndrome in children during a large outbreak of *Escherichia coli* O157:H7 infections. *Pediatrics* 1997;100:127.
111. Ahmed A et al. Safety and immunogenicity of *Escherichia coli* O157 O-specific polysaccharide conjugate vaccine in 2-5-year-old children. *J Infect Dis* 2006;193:515.
112. Belongia EA et al. Transmission of *Escherichia coli* O157:H7 infection in Minnesota child day-care facilities. *JAMA* 1993;269:883.
113. Allos BM. *Campylobacter jejuni* infections: update on emerging issues and trends. *Clin Infect Dis* 2001;32:1201.
114. Ternhag A et al. A meta-analysis on the effects of antibiotic treatment on duration of symptoms caused by infection with campylobacter species. *Clin Infect Dis* 2007;44:696.
115. Helms M et al. Adverse health events associated with antimicrobial drug resistance in campylobacter species: a registry-based cohort study. *J Infect Dis* 2005;191:1050.
116. Anders BJ et al. Double-blind placebo-controlled study of erythromycin for treatment of *Campylobacter enteritis*. *Lancet* 1982;1:131.
117. Kuschner RA et al. Use of azithromycin for the treatment of *Campylobacter enteritis* in travelers to Thailand, an area where ciprofloxacin resistance is prevalent. *Clin Infect Dis* 1995;21:536.
118. Blaser MJ. Campylobacter jejuni and related species. In: Mandell GL et al, eds. *Principles and Practice of Infectious Diseases.* 6th ed. Philadelphia: Churchill Livingstone; 2005:2548.
119. Adachi JA et al. Azithromycin found to be comparable to levofloxacin for the treatment of us travelers with acute diarrhea acquired in Mexico. *Clin Infect Dis* 2003;37:1165.
120. Caeiro JP et al. Oral rehydration therapy plus loperamide versus loperamide alone in the treatment of traveler's diarrhea. *Clin Infect Dis* 1999;28:1286.
121. Hill DR. Occurrence and self-treatment of diarrhea in a large cohort of Americans traveling to developing countries. *Am J Trop Med Hyg* 2000;62:585.
122. Adachi JA et al. Empirical antimicrobial therapy for traveler's diarrhea. *Clin Infect Dis* 2000;31:1079.
123. Radandt JM et al. Interactions of fluoroquinolones with other drugs: mechanisms, variability, clinical significance, and management. *Clin Infect Dis* 1992;14:272.
124. Steffen R et al. Therapy of travelers' diarrhea with rifaximin in various continents. *Am J Gastroenterol* 2003;98:1073.
125. Infante RM et al. Enteroaggregative *Escherichia coli* diarrhea in travelers: response to rifaximin therapy. *Clin Gastroenterol Hepatol* 2004;2:135.
126. Salam I et al. Randomised trial of single-dose ciprofloxacin for travellers' diarrhoea. *Lancet* 1994;344:1537.
127. Ericsson CD et al. Travelers' diarrhea: approaches to prevention and treatment. *Clin Infect Dis* 1993;16:616.
128. Taylor DN et al. Treatment of travelers' diarrhea: ciprofloxacin plus loperamide compared with ciprofloxacin alone. *Ann Intern Med* 1991;114:731.
129. Ericsson CD et al. Single dose ofloxacin plus loperamide compared with single dose or three days of ofloxacin in the treatment of traveler's diarrhea. *J Travel Med* 1997;4:3.
130. Sanders, et al. Azithromycin and loperamide are comparable to levofloxacin and loperamide for the treatment of traveler's diarrhea in United States military personnel in Turkey. *Clin Infect Dis* 2007;45:294.
131. Taylor DN et al. A randomized, double-blind, multicenter study of rifaximin compared with placebo and with ciprofloxacin in the treatment of travelers' diarrhea. *Am J Trop Med Hyg* 2006;74:1060.
132. Xifaxan. [package insert]. Morrisville, NC: Salix Pharmaceuticals, Inc; 2007.
133. Tribble DR et al. Travelers' diarrhea in Thailand: randomized, double-blind trial comparing single-dose and 3-day azithromycin-based regimens with a 3-day levofloxacin regimen. *Clin Infect Dis* 2007;44:338.
134. DuPont HL et al. A randomized, double-blind, placebo-controlled trial of rifaximin to prevent travelers' diarrhea. *Ann Intern Med* 2005;142:805.
135. Gorbach SL. How to hit the runs for fifty million travelers at risk. *Ann Intern Med* 2005;142:861.
136. Fekety R. Guidelines for the diagnosis and treatment of *Clostridium difficile*-associated diarrhea and colitis. *Am J Gastroenterol* 1997;92:739.
137. Hogenauer C et al. Mechanisms and management of antibiotic-associated diarrhea. *Clin Infect Dis* 1998;27:702.
138. Husain A et al. Gastrointestinal toxicity and *Clostridium difficile* diarrhea in patients treated with paclitaxel-containing chemotherapy regimens. *Gynecol Oncol* 1998;71:104.
139. Sharma AK et al. *Clostridium difficile* diarrhea after use of tacrolimus following renal transplantation. *Clin Infect Dis* 1998;27:1540.
140. Bartlett JG. Antibiotic-associated diarrhea. *Clin Infect Dis* 1992;15:573.
141. Wanahita A et al. Conditions associated with leukocytosis in a tertiary care hospital, with particular attention to the role of infection caused by *Clostridium difficile. Clin Infect Dis* 2002;34:1585.
142. Savola KL et al. Fecal leukocyte stain has diagnostic value for outpatients but not inpatients. *J Clin Microbiol* 2001;39:266.
143. Johnson S et al. *Clostridium difficile*-associated diarrhea. *Clin Infect Dis* 1998;26:1027.
144. Peled N et al. Predicting Clostridium difficile toxin in hospitalized patients with antibiotic-associated diarrhea. *Infect Control Hosp Epidemiol* 2007;28:377.
145. Nelson R. Antibiotic treatment for *Clostridium difficile*-associated diarrhea in adults. *Cochrane Database Syst Rev* 2007:CD004610.
146. Pepin J et al. Emergence of fluoroquinolones as the predominant risk factor for *Clostridium difficile*-associated diarrhea: a cohort study during an

epidemic in Quebec. *Clin Infect Dis* 2005;41:1254.

147. Teasly DG et al. Prospective randomized study of metronidazole versus vancomycin for clostridium-associated diarrhea and colitis. *Lancet* 1983;2:1043.
148. Tedesco F et al. Oral vancomycin for antibiotic-associated pseudomembranous colitis. *Lancet* 1978;2:226.
149. Pelaez T et al. Reassessment of *Clostridium difficile* susceptibility to metronidazole and vancomycin. *Antimicrob Agents Chemother* 2002;46:1647.
150. Edwards DL et al. Disulfiram-like reaction associated with intravenous trimethoprim-sulfamethoxazole and metronidazole. *Clin Pharm* 1986;5:999.
151. Fekety R et al. Treatment of antibiotic-associated *Clostridium difficile* colitis with oral vancomycin: comparison of two-dosage regimens. *Am J Med* 1989;86:15.
152. Keighley MRD et al. Randomized controlled trial of vancomycin for pseudomembranous colitis and post-operative diarrhea. *BMJ* 1978;2:1667.
153. Aradhyula S et al. Significant absorption of oral vancomycin in a patient with *Clostridium difficile* colitis and normal renal function. *South Med J* 2006;99:518.
154. Dudley NM et al. Absorption of vancomycin. *Ann Intern Med* 1984;101:144.
155. Spizter PG et al. Systemic absorption of vancomycin in a patient with pseudomembranous colitis. *Ann Intern Med* 1984;100:523.
156. Zar FA et al. A comparison of vancomycin and metronidazole for the treatment of *Clostridium difficile*-associated diarrhea, stratified by disease severity. *Clin Infect Dis* 2007;45:302.
157. Reinke CM et al. ASHP therapeutic position statement on the preferential use of metronidazole for the treatment of *Clostridium difficile*-associated disease. *Am J Health-Syst Pharm* 1998;55:1407.
158. Dudley MN et al. Oral bacitracin versus vancomycin therapy for *Clostridium difficile*-induced diarrhea. *Arch Intern Med* 1986;146:1101.
159. Young GP et al. Antibiotic-associated colitis due to *Clostridium difficile:* double-blind comparison of vancomycin with bacitracin. *Gastroenterology* 1985;89:1038.
160. Musher DM et al. Nitazoxanide for the treatment of *Clostridium difficile* colitis. *Clin Infect Dis* 2006;43:421.
161. Farver DK et al. Ramoplanin: a lipoglycodepsipeptide antibiotic. *Ann Pharmacother* 2005;39:863.
162. Freeman J et al. Comparison of the efficacy of ramoplanin and vancomycin in both in vitro and in vivo models of clindamycin-induced *Clostridium difficile* infection. *J Antimicrob Chemother* 2005;56:717.
163. Ariano RE et al. The role of anion-exchange resins in the treatment of antibiotic-associated pseudomembranous colitis. *Can Med Assoc J* 1990;142:1049.
164. Louie TJ et al. Tolevamer, a novel nonantibiotic polymer, compared with vancomycin in the treatment of mild to moderately severe *Clostridium difficile*-associated diarrhea. *Clin Infect Dis* 2006;43:411.
165. Munoz P et al. Saccharomyces cerevisiae fungemia: an emerging infectious disease. *Clin Infect Dis* 2005;40:1625.
166. Novak E et al. Unfavorable effect of atropine-diphenoxylate (Lomotil) therapy in lincomycin-caused diarrhea. *JAMA* 1976;235:1451.
167. Climo MW et al. Hospital-wide restriction of clindamycin: effect on the incidence of *Clostridium difficile*-associated diarrhea and cost. *Ann Intern Med* 1998;128:989.
168. Kyne L et al. Underlying disease severity as a major risk factor for nosocomial *Clostridium difficile* diarrhea. *Infect Control Hosp Epidemiol* 2002;23:653.
169. Chang VT, Nelson K. The role of physical proximity in nosocomial diarrhea. *Clin Infect Dis* 2000;31:717.
170. Karlstrom O et al. A prospective nationwide study of *Clostridium difficile*-associated diarrhea in Sweden. *Clin Infect Dis* 1998;26:141.
171. Beaugerie L et al. Antibiotic-associated diarrhoea and *Clostridium difficile* in the community. *Aliment Pharmacol Ther* 2003;17:905.
172. McDonald LC et al. An epidemic, toxin gene-variant strain of *Clostridium difficile. N Engl J Med* 2005;353:2433.
173. Johnson SJ et al. Treatment of asymptomatic *Clostridium difficile* carriers (fecal excretors) with vancomycin or metronidazole. *Ann Intern Med* 1992;117:297.
174. Kazakova SV et al. A hospital outbreak of diarrhea due to an emerging epidemic strain of *Clostridium difficile. Arch Intern Med* 2006;166:2518.
175. Kyne L et al. Health care costs and mortality associated with nosocomial diarrhea due to *Clostridium difficile. Clin Infect Dis* 2002;34:346.
176. Dallal RM et al. Fulminant *Clostridium difficile:* an underappreciated and increasing cause of death and complications. *Ann Surg* 2002;235:363.
177. Lamp KC et al. Pharmacokinetics and pharmacodynamics of the nitroimidazole antimicrobials. *Clin Pharmacokinet* 1999;36:353.
178. Friedenberg F et al. Intravenous metronidazole for the treatment of *Clostridium difficile* colitis. *Dis Colon Rectum* 2001;44:1176.
179. Kleinfeld DI et al. Parenteral therapy for antibiotic-associated pseudomembranous colitis [Letter]. *J Infect Dis* 1988;157:389.
180. Bolton RP et al. Faecal metronidazole concentrations during oral and intravenous therapy for antibiotic-associated colitis due to *Clostridium difficile. Gut* 1986;27:1169.
181. Guzman R et al. Failure of parenteral metronidazole in the treatment of pseudomembranous colitis [Letter]. *J Infect Dis* 1988;158:1146.
182. Apisarnthanarak A et al. Adjunctive intracolonic vancomycin for severe *Clostridium difficile* colitis: case series and review of the literature. *Clin Infect Dis* 2002;35:690.
183. McFarland LV et al. Recurrent *Clostridium difficile* disease: epidemiology and clinical characteristics. *Infect Control Hosp Epidemiol* 1999;20:43.
184. Barbut F et al. Epidemiology of recurrences or reinfections of *Clostridium difficile*-associated diarrhea. *J Clin Microbiol* 2000;38:2386.
185. Hecht J et al. *Clostridium difficile* colitis secondary to intravenous vancomycin. *Dig Dis Sci* 1989;34:148.
186. Saginur R et al. Colitis associated with metronidazole therapy. *J Infect Dis* 1980;141:772.
187. Fekety R et al. Recurrent *Clostridium difficile* diarrhea: characteristics of and risk factors for patients enrolled in a prospective, randomized, double-blinded trial. *Clin Infect Dis* 1997;24:324.
188. McFarland LV et al. A randomized placebo-controlled trial of *Saccharomyces boulardii* in combination with standard antibiotics for *Clostridium difficile* disease. *JAMA* 1994;271:1913.
189. Kyne L et al. Association between antibody response to toxin A and protection against recurrent *Clostridium difficile* diarrhoea. *Lancet* 2001;357:189.
190. McPherson S et al. Intravenous immunoglobulin for the treatment of severe, refractory, and recurrent *Clostridium difficile* diarrhea. *Dis Colon Rectum* 2006;49:640.
191. Juang P et al. Clinical outcomes of intravenous immune globulin in severe *Clostridium difficile*-associated diarrhea. *Am J Infect Control* 2007; 35:131.
192. Pepin J et al. Management and outcomes of a first recurrence of *Clostridium difficile*-associated disease in Quebec, Canada. *Clin Infect Dis* 2006;42:758.
193. McFarland LV et al. Breaking the cycle: treatment strategies for 163 cases of recurrent *Clostridium difficile* disease. *Am J Gastroenterol* 2002;97:1769.
194. Tedesco F et al. Approach to patients with multiple relapses of antibiotic-associated pseudomembranous colitis. *Am J Gastroenterol* 1985;80:867.
195. Pruksananonda P et al. Multiple relapses of *Clostridium difficile*-associated diarrhea responding to an extended course of cholestyramine. *Pediatr Infect Dis J* 1989;8:175.
196. Buggy BP et al. Therapy of relapsing *Clostridium difficile*-associated diarrhea and colitis with the combination of vancomycin and rifampin. *Clin Gastroenterol* 1987;9:155.
197. Surawicz CM et al. The search for a better treatment for recurrent *Clostridium difficile* disease: use of high-dose vancomycin combined with *Saccharomyces boulardii. Clin Infect Dis* 2000;31:1012.
198. Musher DM et al. *Clostridium difficile* colitis that fails conventional metronidazole therapy: response to nitazoxanide. *J Antimicrob Chemother* 2007;59:705.
199. Johnson S et al. Interruption of recurrent *Clostridium difficile*-associated diarrhea episodes by serial therapy with vancomycin and rifaximin. *Clin Infect Dis* 2007;44:846.
200. Chen XM et al. Cryptosporidiosis. *N Engl J Med* 2002;346:1723.
201. Abubakar I et al. Treatment of cryptosporidiosis in immunocompromised individuals: systematic review and meta-analysis. *Br J Clin Pharmacol* 2007;63:387.
202. Alinia. [package insert]. Tampa, FL: Romark Pharmaceuticals; 2005.
203. Rossignol JA et al. Treatment of diarrhea caused by cryptosporidium parvum: a prospective randomized, double-blind, placebo-controlled study of nitazoxanide. *J Infect Dis* 2001;184:103.
204. Amadi B et al. Effect of nitazoxanide on morbidity and mortality in Zambian children with cryptosporidiosis: a randomized controlled trial. *Lancet* 2002;360:1375.

CHAPTER 63

Intra-Abdominal Infections

Kendra M. Damer and Carrie A. Sincak

INTRODUCTION

Despite the introduction of new antimicrobial agents and improvements in diagnostic and surgical techniques, the treatment of intra-abdominal infections remains a therapeutic challenge. Improvements in radiographic techniques with improved localization of abscesses and early drainage, improved nutritional management, and the selection of appropriate antimicrobial agents all have contributed to a decrease in mortality associated with intra-abdominal infections.

Intra-abdominal infections are those contained within the peritoneal cavity, which extends from the undersurface of the diaphragm to the floor of the pelvis or the retroperitoneal space. Intra-abdominal infections can present as localized infections, a diffuse inflammation throughout the peritoneum, or infections in visceral organs such as the liver, biliary tract, spleen, pancreas, or female pelvic organs. Abscesses can form anywhere within the abdomen, between bowel loops, or in solid organs. If adequate source control is delayed, subsequent bacteremia and multiple organ failure are more likely to occur.

Although antimicrobial therapy should be selected on the basis of the suspected pathogens, judicious use of antimicrobial agents is warranted owing to increasing rates of resistant pathogens.

Normal Gastrointestinal Flora

The stomach of fasting individuals contains very few bacteria (i.e., <100 colony-forming units [CFU]/mL) because of the combined effects of gastric motility and the bactericidal activity of normal gastric fluid, which has a pH of 1 to 2.[1] The bacterial population of the stomach can be altered by drugs or diseases that increase gastric pH or decrease gastric motility. Thus, patients with bleeding or obstructing duodenal ulcers, gastric ulcers, or gastric carcinomas have an increased number of oral anaerobes and facultative gram-negative bacteria colonizing the stomach.

The upper small intestine (duodenum and jejunum) usually contains relatively few bacteria and harbors mainly oral flora. The lower small intestine serves as a transitional zone between the sparsely populated stomach and the abundant microbial flora of the colon.[2] The biliary tree is generally sterile, although colonization with aerobic gram-negative bacilli (particularly *Escherichia coli* and *Klebsiella* spp) is more likely in patients with biliary tract stones, surgical biliary interventions, and in the elderly patient population.[3]

In the ileum, facultative gram-negative and gram-positive species, as well as obligate anaerobes, are encountered. As the distal ileum is approached, the quantity and variety of bacteria increase. Substantial numbers of anaerobic bacteria are present, including *Bacteroides* spp., *E. coli*, and *Enterococcus* are the most commonly encountered gram-negative and gram-positive organisms, respectively.[1,2]

In the large bowel, anaerobic bacteria, particularly *Bacteroides* species, predominate. In the distal colon, bacterial counts average 10^{10} CFU/mL of feces, with anaerobes outnumbering other organisms by a ratio of 1,000 to 10,000:1.[2] Although large numbers of *Clostridia* spp., anaerobic gram-positive cocci, and non–spore-forming anaerobic rods are present, the most prevalent anaerobes are *Bacteroides* species. Among the facultative aerobes, *E. coli* is the most frequently isolated species.[1,2] Given these differences in regional microflora populations, it is not surprising that trauma to the colon carries a much higher risk of intra-abdominal infection than it does to the stomach or jejunum[4] (Fig. 63-1).

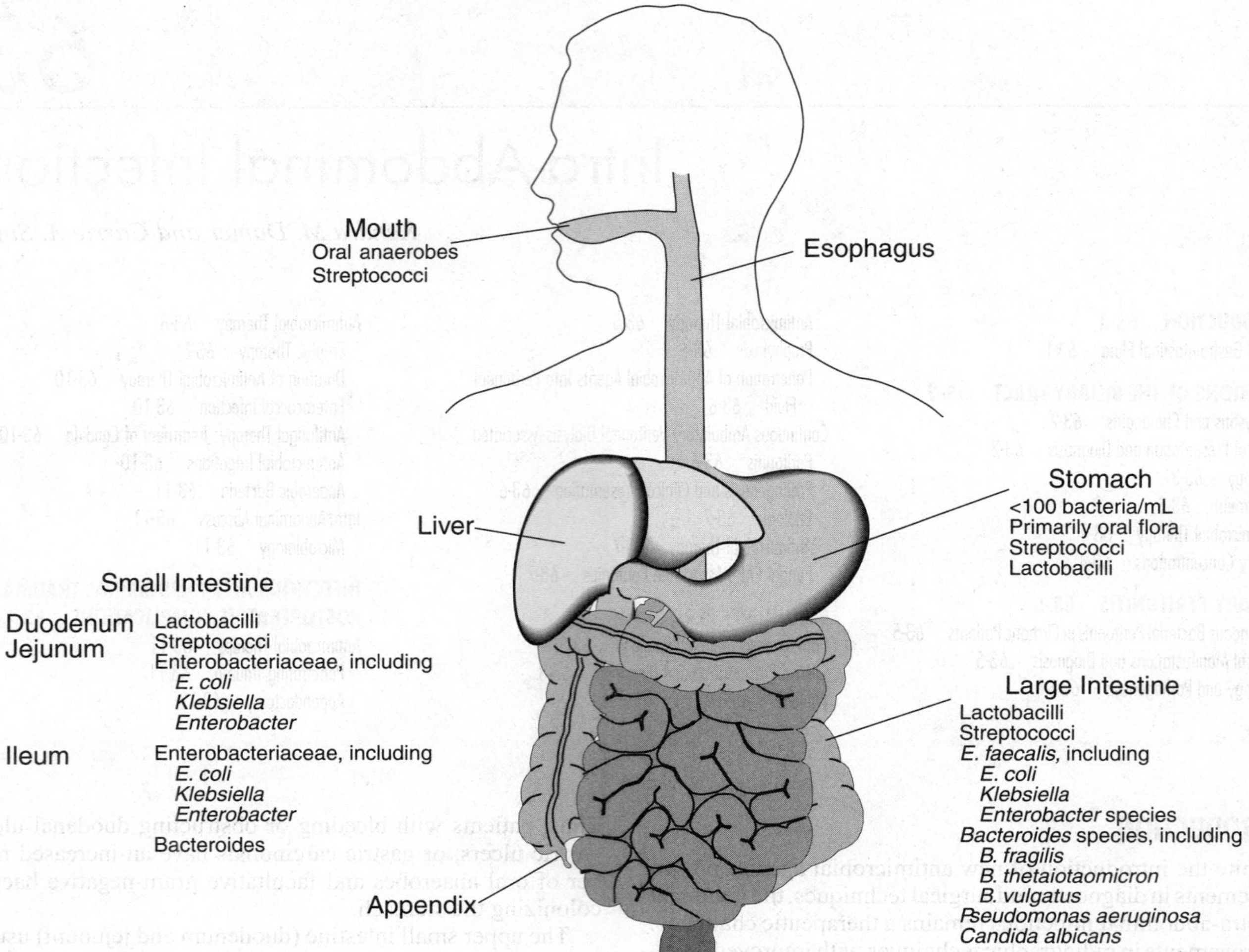

FIGURE 63-1 Microflora of the gastrointestinal tract.

INFECTIONS OF THE BILIARY TRACT

Cholecystitis and Cholangitis

Cholecystitis and cholangitis are intra-abdominal infections that originate as inflammatory conditions of the biliary tract, most commonly as a result of obstruction in the gallbladder or common bile duct. The obstruction is typically caused by the presence of cholelithiasis. The biliary tract is sterile under normal conditions and the flow of bile, along with its bacteriostatic properties, function to maintain the sterility. Infection typically occurs as a secondary event to obstruction.[3,4]

Acute cholecystitis is the acute inflammation of the gallbladder. The presence of gallstones in >90% of cases prevents the outflow of gallbladder drainage by obstructing the neck of the gallbladder, Hartmann's pouch, or the cystic duct.[3] The obstruction causes an increase in intraluminal pressure, gallbladder distention, and edema, which triggers an acute inflammatory response. The potential consequences of this obstruction and inflammation include infection, ischemia, perforation, and necrosis.[3,5] The reduction in gallbladder outflow leads to biliary stasis, which provides an ideal environment for bacterial proliferation and subsequent infection (Fig. 63-2).

Acute cholangitis is an acute inflammation of the common bile duct. The most common cause of cholangitis in the United States is common bile duct obstruction as a consequence of cholelithiasis. Less common causes include neoplastic obstruction, postoperative obstruction following biliary intervention, benign strictures, and primary sclerosing cholangitis.[3] Acute cholangitis characteristically involves the presence of organisms and increased biliary pressure. The decrease in biliary outflow results in biliary stasis and bacterial proliferation. The obstruction of the biliary tree results in increased biliary pressure, which facilitates the spread of bacteria into lymphatics and potentially the bloodstream via alterations in membrane permeability.[3,6]

Clinical Presentation and Diagnosis

1. D.S, a 42-year-old man, presents to the hospital with a 2-day history of abdominal pain and tenderness, localized to the right upper quadrant, fever to 38.9°C, and chills. He complains of nausea, with three episodes of emesis occurring in the past 24 hours. D.S. appears jaundiced and reports dark-colored urine. His laboratory values are white blood cell (WBC) count, 15 × 10^3/mm^3

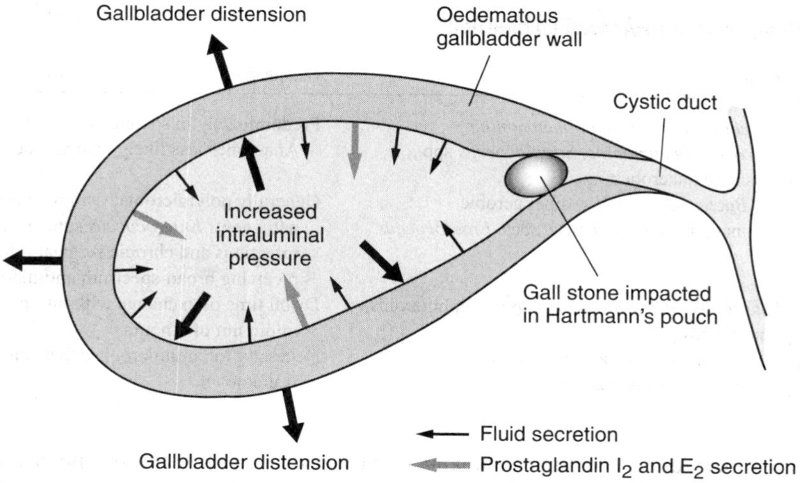

FIGURE 63-2 Pathogenesis of acute cholecystitis.

(normal, 3.2–9.8); serum creatinine (SrCr), 1.2 mg/dL (normal, 0.6–1.2); total bilirubin, 4 mg/dL (normal, 0.1–1); and alkaline phosphatase, 220 U/L (normal, 30–120). What evidence of cholangitis exists in D.S.? How does the presentation of cholecystitis differ from cholangitis?

[SI units: WBC count, 15 × 10^9 /L (normal, 3.2–9.8); SrCr, 106.08 μmol/L (normal, 50–110); total bilirubin, 68.4 μmol/L (normal, 2–18)]

The clinical manifestations of acute cholangitis vary, but the classic presentation involves Charcot's triad, which consists of fever, jaundice, and right upper quadrant abdominal pain. Fever is present in 90% of cases, and jaundice and abdominal pain occur in 60% to 70% of cases.[3] A smaller percentage of patients may present with changes in mental status and hypotension.[3] Laboratory findings of acute cholangitis include leukocytosis, elevated bilirubin and alkaline phosphatase, and mildly elevated liver transaminases.[3,6] The clinical signs and symptoms of cholangitis, as exemplified by D.S., include high fevers (38.9°C), chills, jaundice, and right upper quadrant abdominal pain. Laboratory evidence supportive of cholangitis includes leukocytosis with WBC of 15 × 10^3/mm^3, increased bilirubin of 4 mg/dL, and elevated alkaline phosphatase of 220 U/L.

The clinical presentation of acute cholecystitis involves fever, nausea, vomiting, and a prolonged constant abdominal pain that is typically localized to the right upper quadrant. On physical examination, patients with cholecystitis often have tenderness in the right upper quadrant, which is evident by Murphy's sign (inspiration is inhibited by pain on palpitation).[3,5] Laboratory findings include leukocytosis with increased neutrophils (left shift) and mild elevations in transaminases. Patients with cholecystitis may also present with mild jaundice (bilirubin <60 mmol/L) in comparison to cholangitis.[3,5]

Diagnostic imaging for cholecystitis typically involves ultrasonography, which may reveal pericholecystic fluid, distention of the gallbladder, edema of the gallbladder wall, stones, and a sonographic Murphy's sign.[3] Ultrasound is less sensitive for choledocholithiasis, but may depict the presence of biliary dilation with cholelithiasis to infer cholangitis. Computed tomography (CT) imaging is also commonly utilized for the diagnosis of cholangitis and may be superior in determining the extent of biliary obstruction.[3] Biliary scintigraphy and endoscopic retrograde cholangiopancreatography (ERCP) are alternative modes of imaging for cholecystitis and cholangitis, respectively.[3,6]

Etiology

2. What are the most likely organisms causing infection in D.S.? What clinical specimens are helpful to identify the causative pathogen(s)?

The most common pathogens associated with cholangitis include *E. coli*, *Klebsiella* spp., *Enterococcus* spp., and *Enterobacter* spp. However, *Pseudomonas aeruginosa*, skin flora (*Staphylococcus* spp., *Streptococcus* spp.), and oropharynx bacteria may be cultured. Anaerobic organisms are associated with ~15% of infections, particularly in elderly patients undergoing biliary tract surgery.[3,7] The etiology of cholecystitis typically involves *E. coli, Klebsiella* spp., and *Enterococcus* spp. Anaerobes are less commonly isolated[3,5] (Table 63-1).

As described above, the stasis of bile flow allows bacteria to proliferate within the gallbladder or common bile duct. Acute cholangitis results in increased pressure within the common bile duct with dissemination of bacteria from the biliary tree to the bloodstream. Blood cultures may be positive in up to 40% of patients with symptomatic acute cholangitis.[3] Acute cholecystitis may reveal positive bile cultures in 20% to 75% of patients with symptomatic disease, but the utility of bile cultures has yet to be determined.[2] In contrast to cholangitis, bacteremia is unlikely with cholecystitis. The choice of antibacterial agents is largely empiric covering the aforementioned common causative pathogens.

Treatment

Definitive therapy for both cholangitis and cholecystitis must involve the removal of the obstruction and infected contents, using surgery, percutaneous drainage, or endoscopic intervention. Empiric antibacterial therapy should be added owing to the likelihood of secondary infection and to prevent complications. Supportive measures include fluid and electrolyte supplementation and analgesia.[3–6]

Table 63-1 Common Pathogens in Intra-Abdominal Infection

Disease	*Pathogens*	*Comments*
Primary peritonitis	*Escherichia coli, Klebsiella pneumoniae, Streptococcus pneumoniae, Streptococcus* spp., occasional anaerobes	Predominately in spontaneous bacterial peritonitis in cirrhotics. Anaerobes less likely than aerobes.
Secondary peritonitis	*E. coli, Bacteroides fragilis,* other aerobic gram-negative rods and anaerobes, *Enterococcus*	Generally polymicrobial with both aerobic and anaerobic pathogens. *Enterococcus* spp. are associated with nosocomial infections and chronic surgical infections, particularly in patients receiving broad-spectrum antimicrobials.
Chronic ambulatory peritoneal dialysis	*S. epidermidis, Staphylococcus aureus,* diphtheroids, gram-negative rods	Dwell time of exchange with intraperitoneal antibiotics must be a minimum of 6 hours.
Cholecystitis, cholangitis	*E. coli, K. pneumoniae,* anaerobes, other gram-negative rods, *Enterococcus*	Necessity for antimicrobials that achieve high biliary concentrations is unknown.

To decompress or drain the biliary ductal system in cholangitis ERCP is used, with a success rate of >90% in the treatment of cholangitis.[3] Alternatively, percutaneous transhepatic biliary drainage (PTBD) or endoscopic sphincterotomy (ES) can be utilized to drain the contents. Open surgery is a less favored option to decompress the biliary tree, owing to increased mortality.[3] Acute symptomatic cholecystitis requires removal of the gallbladder (cholecystectomy). The procedure of choice is laparoscopic cholecystectomy within 48 to 72 hours of onset of symptoms. Early intervention is associated with decreased morbidity and length of hospital stay compared with delayed surgical intervention.[3,5] In high-risk patients, where the risks outweigh the benefits of early surgery, percutaneous cholecystostomy can be performed to drain the contents of the gallbladder. The procedure improves the clinical symptoms in 75% to 90% of patients who cannot undergo surgery. Cholecystectomy, however, should take place once the patient is stable for surgery.[3]

Antimicrobial Therapy

3. Based on the most likely causative pathogen(s), what empiric antimicrobial therapy is recommended for D.S., given a diagnosis of cholangitis?

Empiric antimicrobial therapy for cholangitis and cholecystitis should be initiated after blood cultures have been collected. The empiric choice of therapy should cover enteric gram-negative pathogens, particularly *E. coli*. The addition of anaerobic coverage is generally recommended, particularly for patients with cholangitis and elderly patients with previous biliary tract interventions.[3] *Enterococcus* spp. are less commonly encountered pathogens and empiric coverage is typically not necessary in community-acquired intra-abdominal infections.

Antimicrobial therapy must be guided by drug pharmacokinetics and pharmacodynamics, local resistance patterns, and patient factors, such as drug allergies, renal or hepatic dysfunction, and cost. Examples of appropriate empiric regimens include combination therapy with an extended spectrum cephalosporin (ceftriaxone, cefotaxime, or cefepime) or an aminoglycoside, plus metronidazole, or a fluoroquinolone (ciprofloxacin or levofloxacin) plus metronidazole.[8] Utilization of aminoglycosides in uncomplicated, community-acquired infections is not routinely recommended because of the need for therapeutic drug monitoring and potential nephrotoxicity and ototoxicity.[8] Furthermore, the risk of renal toxicity has been suggested to be greater in patients with obstructive jaundice.[9] Therapy with ciprofloxacin or levofloxacin is appropriate in combination with metronidazole owing to the relatively poor anaerobic activity of the fluoroquinolones. Other fluoroquinolones, such as moxifloxacin and garenoxacin, with increased anaerobic activity may represent a potential monotherapy option in the future.[10] Monotherapy with a β-lactam–β-lactamase inhibitor combination (ampicillin–sulbactam, ticarcillin–clavulanate, and piperacillin–tazobactam) or a carbapenem (imipenem–cilastatin, meropenem, and ertapenem) would also be appropriate therapy given the broad spectrum of gram-positive, gram-negative, and anaerobic activity.[8,11] Considering their activity versus multidrug-resistant gram-negative bacilli, the carbapenems generally should be reserved for infection caused by these pathogens.

An appropriate regimen for D.S. is ampicillin–sulbactam 3 g IVPB every 6 hours as monotherapy. Aminoglycoside therapy can be considered in D.S., but given the recent onset of signs and symptoms and the likelihood of community-acquired organisms, other treatment options are available. The presence of hyperbilirubinemia may also place D.S. at higher for the development of aminoglycoside-induced nephrotoxicity.

Biliary Concentrations

4. The physician caring for D.S. questions the need for an antibiotic that concentrates in the bile. Is there a benefit to using an antibiotic that is extensively excreted into bile?

Common bile duct obstruction is a factor that can prevent the entry of antibiotics into the bile, but the need for high biliary concentrations of antibiotics in the treatment of cholangitis has often been questioned.[12] Nagar et al.[13] reviewed the biliary excretion of several antibiotics and concluded that a number of antibiotics with excellent in vitro susceptibility are poorly excreted into bile but are still clinically effective. Biliary antibacterial concentrations have not been correlated with an improved outcome.[3] Highly biliary excreted versus moderately biliary excreted antibiotics have been compared.[12] The investigators concluded that serum concentrations were more important than biliary levels in reducing the septic complications of biliary tract surgery. These authors concluded that biliary excretion of any antibiotic is minimal in the presence of obstruction.[12]

The treatment of D.S.'s biliary tract infection must include biliary drainage. Ampicillin–sulbactam should be continued for 5 to 7 days.

PRIMARY PERITONITIS

Peritonitis is inflammation of the peritoneum as a result of infectious or chemical inflammation within the peritoneal cavity.[2,14] Infectious peritonitis can be classified as primary, secondary, or tertiary. Primary peritonitis involves the development of infection in the peritoneal cavity in the absence of intra-abdominal abnormality.[14,15] Secondary peritonitis classically results from contamination of the peritoneum with gastrointestinal (GI) or genitourinary microorganisms as a result of loss of mucosal barrier integrity. Tertiary peritonitis describes clinical peritonitis along with signs of sepsis and multiorgan dysfunction that persist or recur following the treatment of secondary peritonitis.[2,14]

Primary peritonitis is also known as *spontaneous bacterial peritonitis* (SBP) and is most frequently identified in adults with cirrhosis and ascites. Nearly 10% to 30% of hospitalized patients with cirrhosis and ascites have SBP.[2,15,16] Primary peritonitis can also be associated with postnecrotic cirrhosis, chronic acute hepatitis, acute viral hepatitis, congestive heart failure, metastatic malignancy, or systemic lupus erythematosus.[2,14]

Spontaneous Bacterial Peritonitis in Cirrhotic Patients

Clinical Manifestations and Diagnosis

Patients with SBP may present with fever, signs of peritoneal irritation with abdominal pain, changes in GI motility, nausea, vomiting, diarrhea, or ileus.[16] Fever is the most common sign, occurring in 50% to 80% of patients with SBP.[2] Patients may potentially have an atypical presentation or even lack symptoms.[16] The diagnosis of SBP is made on clinical presentation and examination of the peritoneal fluid via paracentesis. The ascitic fluid is tested for cell counts with WBC differential and the presence of microorganisms based on Gram stain and culture. Ascitic fluid with an elevated polymorphonuclear (PMN) count ($\geq 250/mm^3$) is diagnostic of SBP.[16]

Etiology and Pathogenesis

5. M.W., a 51-year-old man with alcoholic cirrhosis and significant abdominal ascites, presents with a 4-day history of fever to 38.4°C and abdominal pain. Ascitic fluid obtained by paracentesis was cloudy. Culture of the ascitic fluid is pending. Laboratory values are ascitic fluid PMN count, 450/mm^3, serum WBC count, 12.2 × 10^3/mm^3 (normal, 3.2–9.8), and total bilirubin, 4.4 mg/dL (normal, 0.1–1). What organisms are likely to be cultured from M.W.'s ascitic fluid?

[SI units: WBC count, 12.2 × 10^9/L (normal, 3.2–9.8); total bilirubin, 75.2 μmol/L (normal, 2–18)]

An estimated 70% of cases of SBP are caused by aerobic enteric organisms considered normal flora of the GI tract.[16] *E. coli* is the most commonly cultured organism, followed by *Klebsiella pneumoniae*.[2] Other common causes of SBP include *Streptococcus pneumoniae* and other *Streptococcus* spp., accounting for 20% of cases. *Enterococcus* spp. are isolated in ~5% of cases.[16] *Staphylococcus* spp., anaerobes, and microaerophilic organisms are rarely reported in community-acquired SBP. SBP is largely a monomicrobial infection.

One of the main mechanisms of pathogenesis associated with the development of SBP is bacterial translocation, which is the migration of microorganisms through the GI wall to mesenteric lymph nodes and other structures outside the intestine, including the bloodstream. Bacteria will then infect the ascitic fluid by hematogenous or lymphogenous spread.[16,17] Certain characteristics of cirrhotic patients may facilitate the pathogenesis of SBP, including bacterial overgrowth, decreased motility, structural intestinal damage, and decreased host defense mechanisms that function to eliminate microorganisms. Bacterial overgrowth in the face of decreased motility and increased gut wall permeability, secondary to structural damage, facilitates subsequent systemic infection. Reduced opsonic activity and phagocytosis allows the microorganisms to escape the hosts' defenses and subsequently infect the ascitic fluid.[17]

Spontaneous bacterial peritonitis with underlying cirrhosis was previously associated with a >90% mortality rate, but with the advances in antibacterial therapy, the rate has reduced to ~20% to 40%.[2,16] Patient characteristics associated with increased mortality include renal insufficiency, hypothermia, hyperbilirubinemia, and hypoalbuminemia. Gram-negative infections are also associated with a high mortality rate in SBP compared with gram-positive infections.[2] Early diagnosis and effective antibacterial treatment of SBP have been associated with reduced rates of mortality.[18]

Antimicrobial Therapy

6. What empiric antimicrobial therapy is recommended for M.W. pending ascitic fluid culture results? What is an appropriate duration of therapy, and how should the response to therapy be monitored?

Although a positive Gram stain and culture will provide guidance for antibacterial therapy, nearly 60% of patients with signs and symptoms of SBP have negative cultures.[19] Initial antibacterial therapy for patients with a diagnosis of SBP is typically empiric and targeted toward the most likely pathogens as described above. Ampicillin plus an aminoglycoside traditionally was used as empiric therapy; however, third-generation cephalosporins (cefotaxime and ceftriaxone) or β-lactam–β-lactamase inhibitor combinations (ampicillin–sulbactam) as monotherapy represent safer, possibly more effective options.[19,20] An oral fluoroquinolone (ofloxacin or ciprofloxacin) has been recommended in uncomplicated SBP in the absence of renal dysfunction or encephalopathy.[16] The lack of streptococcal activity of these agents suggests, however, they should not be used first line. The treatment of choice for community-acquired SBP is typically a third-generation cephalosporin. As described, aminoglycosides are not recommended in cirrhotic SBP therapy because of the risk of nephrotoxicity.[16] As with all infections, antibacterial therapy should be adjusted on the availability of culture and sensitivity data.

Antibiotic therapy is recommended until the PMN count from the ascitic fluid falls below 250 cells/mm^3, which normally occurs within 5 days.[18] Franca et al.[21] concluded that a 5-day course of cefotaxime for the treatment of SBP was as effective as a 10-day course.

M.W. should receive empiric therapy with an antimicrobial agent effective against *E. coli* and other common pathogens such as *Klebsiella* spp. and *S. pneumoniae*. Any of the abovementioned options would be reasonable empirical choices.

Prophylaxis

7. After treatment is completed, should prophylactic antimicrobial therapy be initiated in M.W.?

Recurrence rates for primary peritonitis are high. Cirrhotic patients who survive an episode of SBP have a 1-year recurrence rate of nearly 70%. Two other types of cirrhotic patients are also considered high risk for the development of SBP: patients with low ascitic protein (<1.0 g/dL) or elevated serum bilirubin (>2.5 mg/dL) and patients presenting with GI hemorrhage.[16] Prophylactic antimicrobial therapy has been shown to be of some benefit in cirrhotic patients at risk for the development of SBP (primary prophylaxis) and those with a high risk for the recurrence (secondary prophylaxis) of SBP: the risks and benefits must be carefully evaluated, however.

Secondary prophylaxis in cirrhotic patients is typically initiated with an antibacterial agent to provide selective decontamination of the GI tract. The goal of this therapy is to reduce the burden of bacteria and subsequently prevent bacterial translocation and therefore infection.[16] Prospective, randomized studies in cirrhotic subjects with ascites provide support for the use of oral antibacterial agents to reduce the rate of recurrence. The agents studied include oral norfloxacin,[22] ciprofloxacin,[23] and trimethoprim–sulfamethoxazole.[24] Long-term secondary prophylaxis is recommended based on the significant reduction in rates of recurrence in clinical trials.

Long-term primary prophylaxis in patients with low ascitic proteins, elevated bilirubin, or both may also be beneficial but is not associated with decreased overall infection or mortality and, therefore, not uniformly recommended.[16,17,22–24] Primary prophylaxis is recommended, however, in all cirrhotic patients presenting with a GI hemorrhage.[16] Clinical trials have provided evidence to support the use of short course therapy (7 days) of norfloxacin or ceftriaxone in patients presenting with GI hemorrhage.[17,25] Prophylactic therapy prevents bacterial infection and reduces the risk of rebleeding.[17] Several cost analyses have been performed demonstrating that prophylactic therapy in high risk groups of cirrhotic patients is cost-effective.[17]

Concerns have been raised regarding the rapid emergence of bacterial resistance in cirrhotic patients receiving norfloxacin prophylaxis. In one study evaluating the influence of prophylactic norfloxacin (400 mg/day) on fecal flora, fluoroquinolone-resistant isolates developed during treatment. Rates of fluoroquinolone-resistant and trimethoprim–sulfamethoxazole-resistant gram-negative bacilli have become more prevalent in patients who receive long-term prophylactic therapy.[26] Because of an increase both in resistance and in gram-positive causative organisms, the utilization of long-term prophylaxis must be considered when initiating antibacterial therapy for the treatment of new infections in this patient population.[27]

M.W. has cirrhosis, a previous episode of SBP, and a high total bilirubin; thus, he is at high risk for recurrence. Prophylactic antimicrobial therapy should be considered and may be a cost-effective measure. Any of the aforementioned prophylactic regimens would be appropriate for M.W. A specific choice for prophylactic therapy for M.W. would depend on institutional resistance patterns.

Penetration of Antimicrobial Agents Into Peritoneal Fluid

8. The physician asks if the agents chosen for treatment and prophylaxis of peritonitis in M.W. will penetrate across the peritoneum. What properties determine the penetration of antibiotics into the peritoneal fluid?

The penetration of antimicrobial agents into tissues or abscess cavities depends on the serum-to-tissue fluid concentration gradient; the binding of the antimicrobial to serum and tissue proteins; the diffusibility of the drug, based on its molecular size and acid dissociation constant (pKa); and lipid solubility.[28] In general, the β-lactam antimicrobials have been shown to achieve peritoneal fluid concentrations that exceed typical minimum inhibitory concentrations (MIC) for most commonly encountered facultative gram-negative and anaerobic bacteria.[28,29]

Continuous Ambulatory Peritoneal Dialysis-Associated Peritonitis

9. H.M., a 43-year-old woman with diabetes mellitus and end-stage renal disease, has undergone continuous ambulatory peritoneal dialysis (CAPD) daily for the past year. She presents with abdominal pain and a cloudy dialysate fluid. H.M. has negligible residual urine output. What are the most common causative organisms related to CAPD-associated peritonitis? What empiric antimicrobial therapy should be initiated? How should antimicrobial agents be administered?

Pathogenesis and Clinical Presentation

Peritonitis continues to remain a major complication of peritoneal dialysis. An estimated 45% of patients undergoing continuous ambulatory peritoneal dialysis will experience at least one episode of peritonitis in the first 6 months of dialysis. Approximately 60% to 70% of patients develop peritonitis during the first year of dialysis, and recurrent infection occurs in 20% to 30% of patients.[2] CAPD-related peritonitis is theorized to originate from contamination of the catheter by organisms of the normal skin flora, contamination of the peritoneum from an exit-site or subcutaneous-tunnel infection, contamination of the dialysate fluid, or bacterial translocation.[2] Alterations in host defenses of the peritoneum may also have a role in the development of CAPD-associated peritonitis.[2]

Clinical manifestations of CAPD-peritonitis include abdominal pain and tenderness, which is observed in 60% to 80% of patients. Nausea and vomiting occur in approximately 30% of patients, whereas 10% will have diarrhea, and 10% to 20% will present with fever. The diagnosis of peritonitis is made based on clinical signs and symptoms along with examination of the dialysate fluid for cell counts, Gram stain, and culture. Characteristically, the dialysate fluid will be cloudy and have a WBC count >100 cells/mm^3 with a neutrophilic predominance (at least 50%).[30] The Gram stain may be negative in 5% to 10% of cases and blood cultures are typically negative.[2] In most cases, peritonitis is commonly caused by a single organism.[31]

Etiology

The most common causative organisms are gram-positive bacteria, accounting for 60% to 80% of isolates. Coagulase-negative *Staphylococcus* spp. (*S. epidermidis*) are the most common causative organisms, followed by *Staphylococcus aureus* and *Streptococcus* spp., Gram-negative bacilli are isolated in approximately 15% to 30% of cases, with *E. coli* being the most common. Other common gram-negative organisms include *Klebsiella* spp., *Enterobacter* spp., *Proteus* spp., and *P. aeruginosa*. Anaerobes, fungi, and mycobacteria constitute the less commonly encountered pathogens.[2]

Antimicrobial Therapy

In general, empiric antibiotic therapy should be directed against the most common causative organisms, both gram-positive and gram-negative, until cultures of peritoneal fluid are available. Intraperitoneal (IP) delivery of antibacterial agents is the preferred route of administration for the treatment of CAPD-associated peritonitis. The IP route provides very high local concentrations of antibacterial agents as well as the ability to avoid a venipuncture and allow the patient to self-administer therapy at home.[30]

Treatment guidelines for CAPD-associated peritonitis provide a systematic approach for antimicrobial selection, dosing guidelines, and duration of therapy. Initial therapy recommendations include vancomycin or a first-generation cephalosporin for gram-positive coverage with an appropriate antibacterial agent for gram-negative coverage.[30] Because of the increasing rates of methicillin resistant *S. aureus* (MRSA) and *S. epidermidis* (MRSE), vancomycin may be the most appropriate initial therapy for gram-positive organisms, although cefazolin remains effective in certain geographical areas.[31–33] Gram-negative therapy options include an aminoglycoside, ceftazidime, cefepime, or a carbapenem.[30,34] Local resistance patterns must govern the decision for initial therapy for both gram-positive and gram-negative causative organisms.[30] Oral treatment with fluoroquinolones represents an option in certain cases of CAPD-peritonitis given the extent of distribution into the peritoneal cavity. An increasing prevalence of fluoroquinolone-resistant gram-negative organisms, particularly *E. coli*, however, exists in many areas and must be considered.[35,36]

When culture and susceptibility results are available, antibacterial therapy should be adjusted as necessary. Antibiotic therapy is recommended for at least 2 weeks and even longer in severe cases. Duration may be determined based on clinical response. When *S. aureus* is isolated from culture, therapy will be determined by susceptibility and may include the removal of the dialysis catheter. Vancomycin plus or minus rifampin is recommended for MRSA, although monotherapy with vancomycin is adequate, particularly if the infected catheter is removed. Conversely, cefazolin alone is adequate for MSSA. Coagulase-negative *Staphylococcus* spp. generally require vancomycin owing to the high rate of methicillin resistance. *Enterococcus* spp. or *Streptococcus* spp. should be treated with ampicillin if susceptible. The addition of synergistic doses of gentamicin may be considered, although clear benefit has not been established in the treatment of enterococcal peritonitis. Furthermore, patients with CAPD do not eliminate gentamicin well and may be at additional risk of aminoglycoside ototoxicity. Vancomycin should be used for ampicillin-resistant enterococcus; however, vancomycin resistant *Enterococcus* spp. (VRE), requires treatment with linezolid, quinupristin–dalfopristin, or daptomycin. In the case of culture-negative peritonitis and clinical improvement after 3 days of empiric coverage, a single agent directed toward gram-positive organisms may be continued for a total of 2 weeks.[30]

When a single gram-negative organism is cultured (e.g., *E. coli, Klebsiella* spp., or *Proteus* spp.), therapy can be narrowed based on susceptibility. Isolation of *P. aeruginosa* most often indicates a severe infection which may also involve the dialysis catheter. Two antibacterial agents can be considered for 2 weeks. Monotherapy, however, appears to be as efficacious. Therapy options include an antipseudomonal β-lactam such as ceftazidime, cefepime, or imipenem–cilastatin with or without an oral fluoroquinolone or an aminoglycoside. Aztreonam can be used in the case of severe IgE-medicated penicillin allergy. Polymicrobial peritonitis is uncommon, and may indicate a more complicated intra-abdominal process. Therapy should include activity for anaerobes with metronidazole, in combination with gram-positive, gram-negative coverage according to culture and susceptibility data. Table 63-2 lists antimicrobial dosing guidelines for the treatment of peritonitis associated with CAPD.[30]

An example of an appropriate regimen for H.M. may include vancomycin plus cefepime or an aminoglycoside given intraperitoneally. The clinician should follow culture and sensitivity results to adjust therapy based on guidelines, local sensitivity patterns, and therapeutic response.

Fungal CAPD-Associated Peritonitis

10. Two years later, H.M. presents with abdominal pain and cloudy dialysate fluid. *Candida albicans* is cultured from the dialysate fluid. No other organisms are present. How should H.M. be treated?

Fungal peritonitis is a rare complication of CAPD that is associated with significant morbidity and mortality. The rate of mortality in fungal peritonitis is approximately 25%.[30] It is recommended to remove the dialysis catheter in patients with evidence of fungal peritonitis because of the high rates of failure associated with maintaining the catheter.[30] Patients who have received prolonged or multiple courses of antibiotics are at increased risk for fungal peritonitis owing to a shift in normal flora.[37] Most cases are caused by *Candida spp.*, most commonly *C. albicans*. An increase in nonalbicans species has emerged in many areas.[37] Antifungal therapy options include amphotericin B and flucytosine, caspofungin, fluconazole, or voriconazole. Amphotericin B may be administered intravenously (IV) or IP, but when given IP it is very irritating to the peritoneum.[30] The azole antifungal agents can be administered orally, IV, or IP. Fluconazole is active against *C. albicans* but has decreased activity against certain types of nonalbicans species, such as *C. glabrata*. In general, fluconazole would be appropriate, safe therapy for *C. albicans*, however, other options, such as a polyene or echinocandin, would be needed for *C. glabrata*. Initial therapy is commonly amphotericin B plus flucytosine until the culture results are obtained. Therapy should continue for a minimum of 2 weeks after catheter removal and total duration may be based on severity and clinical response.[30]

Table 63-2 Intraperitoneal Antibiotic Dosing Recommendations for CAPD Patients. (Dosing of Drugs With Renal Clearance in Patients with Residual Renal Function (Defined as >100 mL/day Urine Output): Dose Should Be Empirically Increased by 25%)

Drug	Intermittent (per exchange, once daily)	Continuous (mg/L, all exchanges)
Aminoglycosides		
Amikacin	2 mg/kg	LD 25, MD 12
Gentamicin	0.6 mg/kg	LD 8, MD 4
Tobramycin	0.6 mg/kg	LD 8, MD 4
Cephalosporins		
Cefazolin	15 mg/kg	LD 500, MD 125
Cefepime	1 g	LD 500, MD 125
Cephalothin	15 mg/kg	LD 500, MD 125
Ceftazidime	1,000–1,500 mg	LD 500, MD 125
Ceftizoxime	1,000 mg	LD 250, MD 125
Penicillins		
Ampicillin	ND	MD 125
Oxacillin	ND	MD 125
Nafcillin	ND	MD 125
Amoxicillin	ND	LD 250–500, MD 50
Penicillin G	ND	LD 50,000 units, MD 25,000 units
Quinolones		
Ciprofloxacin	ND	LD 50, MD 25
Others		
Vancomycin	15–30 mg/kg every 5–7 days	LD 1,000, MD 25
Aztreonam	ND	LD 1,000, MD 250
Antifungals		
Amphotericin	NA	1.5
Combinations		
Ampicillin–sulbactam	2 g every 12 hours	LD 1,000, MD 100
Imipenem–cilastatin	1 g BID	LD 500, MD 200
Quinupristin–dalfopristin	25 mg/L in alternate bags[a]	

[a] Given in conjunction with 500 mg intravenous twice daily.

BID, twice daily; CAPD, continuous ambulatory peritoneal dialysis; LD, loading dose, in mg; MD, maintenance dose, in mg; NA, not applicable; ND, no data.

From reference 30, with permission.

H.M.'s treatment should include temporary catheter removal and administration of antifungal agents. Antifungal therapy with fluconazole 200 mg orally everyday should be continued for at least 14 days.

SECONDARY PERITONITIS

Pathogenesis and Epidemiology

Secondary peritonitis usually occurs after fecal contamination of the peritoneal cavity or its surrounding structures.[1,8] Infections most often occur after perforation of the GI tract (e.g., appendicitis, diverticulitis, perforated ulcer, abdominal trauma, bowel neoplasm). Secondary peritonitis most commonly occurs after penetrating or blunt abdominal trauma.

Localization of infection without eradication of bacteria results in intraperitoneal or visceral abscesses. Intraperitoneal abscesses occur most often in the right lower quadrant in association with appendicitis or a perforated peptic ulcer. Other causes can include diverticulitis, pancreatitis, inflammatory bowel disease, trauma, and abdominal surgery. Visceral abscesses generally are found in the pancreas but also occur in the liver, spleen, or kidney.[2]

11. A.H., a 52-year-old man, presents with severe abdominal pain and nausea. Colonoscopy reveals a perforated colon. Vital signs include temperature of 102°F and tachycardia (pulse, 110 beats/minute). Bowel sounds are absent. Laboratory values are WBC count, 19 × 10^3/mm^3 (normal, 3.2–9.8), and blood urea nitrogen (BUN), 34 mg/dL (normal, 8–18). What signs and symptoms of secondary peritonitis does A.H. display?

[SI units: WBC count, 19 × 10^9/L (normal, 3.2–9.8); BUN, 11 mmol/L (normal, 3–6.5)]

Clinical Presentation and Diagnosis

Making the diagnosis of a localized intra-abdominal infection may be difficult, despite the presence of signs and symptoms typical of severe infection. The patient may experience pain and voluntary guarding of the abdomen. Generalized abdominal pain usually is followed by a rigid, "boardlike" tensing of the abdominal muscles.[2] Inflammation around the intestines and peritoneal cavity results in local paralysis and reflex rigidity of the abdominal wall muscles and the diaphragm, causing rapid and shallow respirations.[2] Bowel sounds may be faint or absent with concomitant abdominal distention, nausea, and vomiting. Fever usually is present with tachycardia and decreased urine output secondary to fluid loss into the peritoneum. These signs usually are accompanied by an elevated WBC count with a predominance of neutrophils (left shift). The hematocrit (Hct) and BUN may be elevated as a result of dehydration. Initially, patients are usually alkalotic as a result of vomiting and hyperventilation, but in the later stages of peritonitis, acidosis usually occurs. Untreated peritonitis can result in generalized sepsis and hypovolemic shock.[1,2]

Gram stain and culture should be performed immediately on infected material before the initiation of antimicrobial therapy. The presence of pleomorphic gram-negative bacilli, a strong odor, or tissue gas is strongly suggestive of infection with anaerobes, particularly *Bacteroides fragilis*.

12. Given these findings, what are the most likely pathogens for A.H.'s secondary peritonitis?

Etiology

Because secondary peritonitis can result from perforation of the intestinal tract, the normal flora consistent with the perforated segment determines the most likely pathogens. Studies consistently document a mixed culture of aerobes and anaerobes. The presence of anaerobic bacteria in the culture is indicative of a polymicrobial infection with a predictable group of pathogens.[1,2]

The most commonly isolated facultative bacterium is *E. coli*, which is found in approximately 60% of cultures. A variety of other gram-negative bacteria also are isolated, including *Klebsiella* spp., *Proteus* spp, *Enterobacter* spp., and *P. aeruginosa* (Table 63-3).[1,38–40] Highly antibiotic-resistant strains of

Table 63-3 Bacteriology of Intra-Abdominal Infections[1,38–40]

Bacteria	Patients (%)
Facultative and Aerobic	
Escherichia coli	42–64
Proteus sp.	4–20
Klebsiella or *Enterobacter* sp.	6–23
Streptococci (including enterococci)	3–27
Staphylococci	3–10
Pseudomonas aeruginosa	4–15
Anaerobes	
Bacteroides fragilis	30–50
Other *Bacteroides* sp.	9–16
Peptostreptococci	10
Clostridium sp.	2–20
Fusobacterium sp.	10

Candida, P. aeruginosa, Serratia, Acinetobacter, Enterobacter spp., and *Enterococcus* often are isolated from patients who develop secondary peritonitis while hospitalized.[2,8] *B. fragilis* is recovered from intra-abdominal sites because of its particular virulence factors and is the most frequently isolated anaerobe following perforation of the colon.[2,41] Anaerobic cocci (*Peptostreptococcus*) and facultative gram-positive cocci, such as *Enterococcus*, are also isolated.[2,8,39,41] *B. fragilis* and *E. coli* are the most common pathogens found in blood culture samples after bacteremia associated with an intra-abdominal infection.[2]

In summary, A.H. is likely to have an intra-abdominal infection caused by mixed flora, containing both aerobic and anaerobic bacteria. His current clinical status, highlighted by an elevated temperature, is probably secondary to the presence of facultative gram-negative bacteria, such as *E. coli, Proteus, Klebsiella*, or *Enterobacter. P. aeruginosa, Candida* spp., or other resistant bacteria are more likely with prolonged hospitalization or receipt of broad-spectrum antimicrobial agents.

Antimicrobial Therapy

Empiric Therapy

13. How should A.H. be treated? Based on clinical studies, what empiric antimicrobial therapy is appropriate for A.H. at this time?

Therapy for secondary peritonitis should include early administration of antimicrobial agents directed at gram-negative bacteria and anaerobes, fluid therapy, and support of vital organ function, as well as source control measures. *Source control* is a term used to involve all physical measures needed to eradicate an infection, such as debridement of necrotic tissue or drainage of an abscess or fluid collections. Surgical debridement and drainage, in conjunction with appropriate antimicrobial therapy, decrease the morbidity and mortality associated with this disease.[1,2,42] Therapy with an agent with activity against *P. aeruginosa* is desirable if the infectious process develops while the patient is hospitalized or has received broad-spectrum antimicrobials. This is not necessary in A.H.

In general, when an intra-abdominal infection is present, antimicrobial agents should be started immediately after appropriate specimens (e.g., blood, peritoneal fluid, abscess drainage) are obtained for culture and sensitivity and before any surgical procedures are performed.[1,2,8,43] The parenteral route should be used to ensure adequate systemic and tissue concentrations, especially in patients in whom shock or poor perfusion of the muscles or GI tract precludes the use of oral or intramuscular (IM) routes of administration. Therefore, antimicrobial therapy is generally empiric, based on the expected pathogens at the site of infection. Table 63-4 outlines dosing recommendations for antibiotics commonly used in the treatment of intra-abdominal infections.

Table 63-4 Treatment of Intra-Abdominal Infections

Regimen	Dosage
Combination Therapy	
1. Metronidazole	500 mg IV every 8 hr
Plus	
Aminoglycoside	5–7 mg/kg/day (normal renal function)
2. Metronidazole	500 mg IV every 8 hr
Plus	
Aztreonam	1–2 g IV every 8 hr
3. Metronidazole	500 mg IV every 8 hr
Plus	
Ceftriaxone	1–2 g IV every 24 hr
Or	
Cefotaxime	1–2 g IV every 8 hr
Or	
Cefepime	1–2 g IV every 8 hr
4. Metronidazole	500 mg IV every 8 hr
Plus	
Ciprofloxacin	400 mg IV every 12 hr
Monotherapy	
Ampicillin–sulbactam	3 g IV every 6 hr
Cefoxitin	1–2 g IV every 6 hr
Ertapenem	1 g IV every 24 hr
Imipenem–cilastatin	500 mg IV every 6 hr
Meropenem	1 g IV every 8 hr
Piperacillin–tazobactam	3.375–4.5 g IV every 6 hr
Ticarcillin–clavulanic acid	3.1 g IV every 6 hr

IV, intravenous.

Early clinical trials of clindamycin combined with gentamicin are efficacious.[2] Increasing resistance rates, the potential for oto- and nephrotoxicity secondary to aminoglycosides, and clindamycin-associated enterocolitis have resulted, however, in many other options.[38,44–49] For mild to moderate community-acquired infections, monotherapy with a β-lactam–β-lactamase inhibitor is recommended. Combination therapy with either a cephalosporin or a fluoroquinolone plus metronidazole is also reasonable.[8,44] A third- or fourth-generation cephalosporin, ciprofloxacin, aztreonam, or an aminoglycoside in combination with metronidazole represent alternative options for severe infections.[9,45] Meropenem, or imipenem–cilastatin[8,44] should be reserved for presumed or documented multidrug-resistant pathogens or in sepsis. Although meropenem and imipenem should be reserved as last-line agents, ertapenem may have a role in mild to moderate intra-abdominal infection. In comparative trials of ertapenem versus piperacillin–tazobactam, the two agents were shown to be similar in efficacy and safety.[45–47] Moxifloxacin with mixed aerobic and anaerobic coverage may be a monotherapy option; however, resistance to *E. coli* and anaerobes may limit its utility.[39] Because monotherapy has been shown to be efficacious in numerous trials, combination therapy is now rarely used.

Meropenem and imipenem–cilastatin, because of their broad spectrum of activity, should be reserved for the treatment of more resistant gram-negative organisms associated with nosocomial infections. Although piperacillin–tazobactam, ticarcillin–clavulanic acid, and ampicillin–sulbactam may have utility in complicated intra-abdominal infections, ampicillin–sulbactam has inferior activity against nosocomial gram-negative organisms and should not be used in patients with long-term hospitalization or extensive antibiotic history.

A.H. should receive antimicrobial therapy with activity against facultative gram-negative bacteria and anaerobes, including *B. fragilis.* IV ertapenem 1 g every 24 hours would be an appropriate treatment for A.H.'s mild to moderate infection.

Duration of Antimicrobial Therapy

14. For how long should A.H. receive antimicrobial therapy?

Recommendations for the duration of therapy for intra-abdominal infection vary from 5 to 7 days and depend primarily on the patient's clinical response to therapy and need for surgical drainage.[8,44] In general, antimicrobial therapy should be continued until resolution of signs of infection takes place, including return of WBC count to normal and elimination of fever.

Enterococcal Infection

15. S.S. is a 66-year-old, nonobese man with a strangulating bowel obstruction. One day after undergoing surgical resection of the duodenum, he develops a fever of 101°F, shaking chills, and abdominal pain. Laboratory values are WBC count, 18.4 × 10^3/mm^3 (normal, 3.2–9.8), and creatinine, 1.2 mg/dL (normal, 0.6–1.2). S.S.'s peritoneal fluid cultures grow *E. coli, B. fragilis, C. albicans,* and *Enterococcus.* Blood cultures are negative. Should he receive additional antimicrobial therapy active against *Enterococcus*?

Although *Enterococcus* is commonly cultured in patients with secondary peritonitis, its pathogenicity has been questioned. *Enterococcus* can cause serious infections (e.g., endocarditis, urinary tract infections), but is less virulent in the setting of polymicrobial infections such as intra-abdominal infections.

An important issue is whether empiric treatment should have included antibiotics directed specifically against *Enterococcus.* Some investigators believe that *Enterococcus* spp. are commensal organisms that need not be treated in most clinical settings. They point to clinical studies in which antibiotic regimens lacking in vitro activity against *Enterococcus* have been successful. The pathogenicity of *Enterococcus* lies in its ability to enhance the formation of abscesses.[1,2]

In general, coverage is warranted if *Enterococcus* is present in blood cultures, is the sole organism on culture, or is the predominant organism on Gram stain.[2,44] Antienterococcal therapy may also be recommended in patients with nosocomial or health care-associated infections.[44] Because S.S.'s blood cultures are negative and ascitic culture has demonstrated mixed pathogens, *Enterococcus* coverage is not necessary. S.S. should be treated with an antimicrobial regimen that has activity against gram-negative pathogens and anaerobes.

Antifungal Therapy: Treatment of Candida

16. Should S.S.'s antimicrobial therapy include an agent with antifungal activity?

The need to treat *Candida* species as a solitary isolate or as part of a polymicrobial infection is controversial. Certainly, *Candida* has the potential to cause peritonitis, IP abscesses, and subsequent candidemia. Parenteral administration of amphotericin B is an option for fungal peritonitis.[14,44] Concern over the toxicity of amphotericin is warranted, however, and the risk-to-benefit ratio must be assessed carefully for each patient. To date, no clinical trials have assessed the efficacy and safety of lipid-based amphotericin B, voriconazole, or caspofungin in the treatment of intra-abdominal fungal infections. The use of antifungal agents, such as fluconazole, may offer decreased toxicity in these patients. The potential risk of the development of resistance must, however, be addressed in clinical trials. Fluconazole is considered an appropriate drug of choice for *C. albicans.*[44] For *Candida glabrata* or other fluconazole-resistant species, an echinocandin or an amphotericin product is an appropriate option.[8]

Therapy with an antifungal agent is not warranted at this time unless positive blood cultures for *Candida* are isolated or S.S. fails to respond to appropriate antimicrobial therapy.

Antimicrobial Irrigations

17. S.S.'s physician wishes to irrigate the peritoneum with aminoglycosides to achieve high local concentrations. Is irrigation with antimicrobial agents rational or effective in the treatment of intra-abdominal infections?

Hypothetic concerns regarding irrigation of the peritoneal cavity include spread of local infection, damage to the mesothelium, dilution of opsonins, or suspension of bacteria in a fluid medium where they are less amenable to phagocytosis. Gravity and the movement of the diaphragm during respiration, however, spread bacteria throughout the peritoneal cavity even in the absence of irrigation. In addition, free circulation of fluids within the peritoneal cavity facilitates lymphatic clearance of microorganisms and toxins.[50]

Although data are limited, systemic antibiotic therapy and antibiotic irrigations appear to be efficacious for both the prevention and treatment of postoperative infections.[51,52] The clinician, however, must recognize the potential for systemic toxicity resulting from systemic absorption of antimicrobial agents from the peritoneal cavity. Most antimicrobials are readily absorbed from mucosal surfaces, especially when they are inflamed. When large volumes of irrigating solution containing antibiotics are used (especially in combination with IV doses), systemic drug concentrations can markedly exceed the therapeutic range. Neuromuscular blockade, renal failure, and ototoxicity have been reported after absorption of aminoglycosides from mucosal surfaces. Although a greater margin of safety exists for many of the penicillins and cephalosporins, the potential for toxicity is still of concern.[53]

Few data support the superiority of antibiotic-containing irrigating solutions over systemic therapy. Given the potential for systemic toxicity secondary to absorption of antimicrobial agents from the peritoneum, the paucity of controlled trials documenting the efficacy of this method of administration, and the proved efficacy of systemic therapy, it seems prudent to use systemic therapy alone for the treatment of intra-abdominal infections.[51,52]

Anaerobic Bacteria

18. The surgical resident initiated S.S. on piperacillin–tazobactam for the treatment of his intra-abdominal infection. Should culture and sensitivity results be used to monitor for anaerobic activity?

With the introduction of broad-spectrum antimicrobial agents with in vitro activity against *B. fragilis* and a significant problem of increasing resistance, the choice of a specific antianaerobic agent has become more complex. Multiple mechanisms of resistance are encountered, and resistance rates differ among various geographic areas of the United States. Although *Bacteroides* resistance to metronidazole is rare,[14,54] resistance to clindamycin has increased.[14] Although the carbapenems and the β-lactamase inhibitor combinations are exquisitely active against *Bacteroides*, resistance has been reported.

The Clinical and Laboratory Standards Institute (CLSI), formerly known as the National Committee for Clinical Laboratory Standards (NCCLS), has suggested that susceptibility testing be performed to determine patterns of anaerobic susceptibility to new antimicrobial agents and to monitor susceptibility patterns periodically on a geographic and local basis.[55]

Because most anaerobes are cultured in the setting of mixed flora, isolation of individual components of a complex mixture can be time-consuming. In addition, most anaerobes are very slow growing, and it may take days to weeks for a definitive culture and sensitivity report. If specimens are not collected and transported in optimal media or in a timely manner, inaccurate or misleading results may be reported. The methods for susceptibility testing of anaerobic bacteria are not well standardized, and many hospital laboratories do not have resources to perform extensive culture and sensitivity testing. It has been argued that routine cultures may be unnecessary because few routine cultures affect the choice of antibiotic regimen, and empiric therapy usually determines outcome.[56] Therefore, empiric therapy must be aimed at the most likely pathogens, and the clinician must be aware of the usual sensitivity patterns at the institution, if anaerobic testing takes place. Routine susceptibility testing for patient-specific cases is not recommended because of the prolonged time needed to achieve results.

Intra-Abdominal Abscess

19. F.S. is a 32-year-old man who has undergone abdominal surgery. Two weeks postoperatively, he develops abdominal pain and purulent material begins to drain from his abdominal wound. An intra-abdominal abscess is visualized by plain films. How did this abscess develop? What considerations should be taken into account in the selection of appropriate antimicrobial agents?

Abscesses are collections of necrotic tissue, bacteria, and WBC that form over a period of days to years. They generally result from chronic inflammation and the body's attempt to localize organisms and toxic substances by formation of an avascular fibrous wall. This isolates bacteria and the liquid core from opsonins and antimicrobial agents.

Microbiology

Although pathogens encountered in abscesses are similar to those encountered in other intra-abdominal infections, abscesses pose a therapeutic challenge because they typically contain large bacterial inocula that are likely to include subpopulations of resistant bacteria.[42] Furthermore, the rate of penetration of antibiotics into abscesses is hindered by the low surface-to-volume ratio, low pH, and decreased permeability.

Although surgical debridement and drainage of F.S.'s abscess is crucial, adjunctive therapy with antimicrobial agents is warranted. The optimal antimicrobial agent should penetrate into the abscess in adequate concentrations with adequate spectrum of activity.[14,42] F.S. should be placed on an antimicrobial regimen that covers gram-negative bacteria and anaerobes, such as piperacillin-tazobactam 3.375 g IV every 6 hours.

INFECTIONS AFTER ABDOMINAL TRAUMA AND POSTOPERATIVE COMPLICATIONS

Risk factors for infection after penetrating abdominal trauma include the number, type, and location of injuries; the presence of hypotension; large transfusion requirements; prolonged operation; advanced age; and the mechanism of injury.[57]

Most investigators stress the importance of instituting antimicrobial therapy as close to the time of trauma as possible. Bozorgzadeh et al.[58] demonstrated a significant reduction in the incidence of postoperative infections when antibiotics were administered before surgical repair of the penetrating abdominal trauma.

Antimicrobial Therapy

Penetrating Trauma

20. M.S., a 23-year-old man, is admitted to the emergency department within 1 hour after sustaining a penetrating knife wound to the stomach and colon. He is to undergo emergency laparotomy. What antimicrobial therapy is appropriate at this time?

As with other types of intra-abdominal infections, antibiotics active against both aerobic and anaerobic pathogens should be used.

Anti-infective therapy has been studied in patients who have sustained penetrating trauma to the abdomen (usually from knife or gunshot wounds). In several comparative trials, single-drug therapy with cefoxitin was as effective as the combination of clindamycin or metronidazole plus an aminoglycoside.[59] In evaluating these studies, however, it is important to note that most patients did not sustain injuries to the colon, where the risk of infection is highest. Although the age of this patient suggests he would tolerate aminoglycoside therapy, monotherapy with cefoxitin or one of the β-lactamase inhibitor combinations would be appropriate.

21. How long should antibiotic therapy be administered to M.S.?

Consensus guidelines regarding the duration of therapy were published by the Eastern Association for the Surgery of Trauma (EAST) Practice Management Group. These investigators reviewed all literature from 1976 to 1997 regarding the duration of antimicrobial use following penetrating abdominal trauma. They concluded that antimicrobial use should not exceed 24 hours in this patient population.[57]

The shortest duration of therapy that has been shown to be effective has been 12 hours with the possibility that a short course (<48 hours) of antimicrobial therapy is as efficacious as 5- to 7-day courses of therapy if antimicrobial therapy is promptly instituted.[44] Several other trials have confirmed no additional benefit exist in providing a longer treatment duration.[44,56,57,60–62]

Because antimicrobial therapy carries a risk of adverse reactions, the development of resistance and unnecessary cost, short-term therapy seems warranted as long as it is instituted soon after the injury.[57,63] If the initial dose of antibiotic is administered >3 to 4 hours after injury, therapy should be continued for 3 to 7 days because the incidence of infection in this circumstance is high.

Antimicrobial therapy was instituted soon after M.S. sustained the colonic injury; therefore, a short course of antimicrobial therapy is appropriate. Therapy should be continued for 24 hours.

Appendectomy

22. B.B. is a 17-year-old girl with a 2-day history of periumbilical pain migrating to the right lower quadrant, abdominal distention, fever of 101.6°F, diarrhea, and decreased bowel sounds. Her WBC count is 16 × 10³/mm³ (normal, 3.2–9.8). A presumptive diagnosis of acute appendicitis is made. What antimicrobial therapy is indicated, and for how long should it be continued?

[SI unit: WBC count, 16.1 × 10⁹/L (normal, 3.2–9.8)]

Clinical manifestations commonly encountered with acute appendicitis include right lower quadrant abdominal pain, rebound tenderness, and low-grade fever complicated by nausea, vomiting, and anorexia.[2]

A variety of antimicrobial agents are effective in the treatment of peritoneal contamination associated with acute appendicitis.[64–68] Most studies, however, have included patients without gangrenous or perforated appendices, which are associated with the highest risk of infection. In several well-designed, randomized, placebo-controlled trials, the combination of clindamycin or metronidazole plus an aminoglycoside has been compared with imipenem–cilastatin, β-lactams, and β-lactamase inhibitor combinations. These single agents were found to be as efficacious as combination therapy.[21,65,67] Patients with gangrenous or perforated appendices who were afebrile for 48 hours have been treated for durations ranging from a single dose[68] to 3 or more days.[66]

Overall, the studies justify the use of single-agent therapy with a β-lactam or β-lactamase inhibitor combination active against both gram-negative aerobes and anaerobes. In patients with uncomplicated appendicitis, single-dose therapy is sufficient; however, patients with gangrenous or perforated appendicitis should be treated for 3 or more days.

B.B. should receive a preoperative dose of any of the aforementioned β-lactam antimicrobials with activity against facultative gram-negative and anaerobic bacteria, such as cefotaxime (1 g IV × 1). Cost, potential side effects, and ease of administration can be used to guide selection of a specific agent. If a gangrenous or perforated appendix is found during surgery, antimicrobial therapy should be continued for a minimum of 3 days or until B.B. has been afebrile for 48 hours.

REFERENCES

1. Marshall JC. Intra-abdominal infections. *Microbes Infect* 2004;6(11):1015.
2. Levison ME et al. Peritonitis and Intraperitoneal Abscesses. In: *Mandell, Bennett, and Dolin: Principles and Practices of Infectious Diseases.* 6th ed. Philadelphia: Churchill Livingstone; 2005: 927.
3. Yusoff IF et al. Diagnosis and management of cholecystitis and cholangitis. *Gastroenterol Clin N Am* 2003;32:1145.
4. Johannsen EC et al. Infections of the liver and biliary system. In: *Mandell, Bennett and Dolin: Principles and Practice of Infectious Diseases.* 6th ed. Philadelphia: Churchill Livingstone; 2005: 951.
5. Indar AA et al. Acute cholecystitis. *BMJ* 2002;325: 639.
6. Carpenter HA. Bacterial and parasitic cholangitis. *Mayo Clin Proc* 1998;73:473.
7. Podnos YD et al. Intra-abdominal sepsis in elderly persons. *Clin Infect Dis* 2002;35:62.
8. Solomkin JS et al. Guidelines for the selection of anti-infective agents for complicated intra-abdominal infections. *Clin Infect Dis* 2003;37(8): 997.
9. Gumaste VV. Antibiotics and cholangitis. *Gastroenterology* 1995;109:323.
10. Goldstein EJ. Intra-abdominal anaerobic infections: bacteriology and therapeutic potential of newer antimicrobial carbapenem, fluoroquinolone, and desfluoroquinolone therapeutic agents. *Clin Infect Dis* 2002;35:S106.
11. Bassotti G et al. Empirical antibiotic treatment with piperacillin-tazobactam in patients with microbiologically-documented biliary tract infections. *World J Gastroenterol* 2004;10(15):2281.
12. Keighley MR et al. Antibiotics in biliary disease: the relative importance of antibiotic concentrations in the bile and serum. *Gut* 1976;17:495.
13. Nagar H et al. The excretion of antibiotics by the biliary tract. *Surg Gynecol Obstet* 1984;158:601.
14. Johnson CC et al. Peritonitis: update on pathophysiology, clinical manifestations, and management. *Clin Infect Dis* 1997;24:1035.
15. Gines P et al. Management of cirrhosis and ascites. *N Engl J Med* 2004;350(16):1646.
16. Garcia-Tsao G. Current management of the complications of cirrhosis and portal hypertension: variceal hemorrhage, ascites, and spontaneous bacterial peritonitis. *Gastroenterology* 2001;120:726.
17. Riordan SM et al. The intestinal flora and bacterial infection in cirrhosis. *J Hepatol* 2006;45:744.
18. Runyon BA et al. Short-course versus long-course antibiotic treatment of spontaneous bacterial peritonitis. A randomized controlled study of 100 patients. *Gastroenterology* 1991;100:1737.
19. Tuncer I et al. Oral ciprofloxacin versus intravenous cefotaxime and ceftriaxone in the treatment of spontaneous bacterial peritonitis. *Hepatogastroenterology* 2003;50:1426.
20. Ricart E et al. Amoxicillin-clavulanic acid versus cefotaxime in the therapy of bacterial infections in cirrhotic patients. *J Hepatol* 2000;32:596.
21. Franca A et al. Five days of ceftriaxone to treat spontaneous bacterial peritonitis in cirrhotic patients. *J Gastroenterol* 2002;37:119.
22. Gines P et al. Norfloxacin prevents spontaneous bacterial peritonitis recurrence in cirrhosis: results of a double-blind, placebo-controlled trial. *Hepatology* 1990;12:716.
23. Rolachon A et al. Ciprofloxacin and long-term prevention of spontaneous bacterial peritonitis: results of a prospective controlled trial. *Hepatology* 1995;22:1171.
24. Alvarez RF et al. Trimethoprim-sulfamethoxazole versus norfloxacin in the prophylaxis of spontaneous bacterial peritonitis in cirrhosis. *Arq Gastroenterol* 2005;42(4):256.
25. Fernandez J et al. Norfloxacin vs. ceftriaxone in the prophylaxis of infections in patients with advanced cirrhosis and hemorrhage. *Gastroenterology* 2006;131(4):1049.
26. Fernandez J et al. Bacterial infections in cirrhosis: epidemiological changes with invasive procedures and norfloxacin prophylaxis. *Hepatology* 2002;35:140.
27. Frazee LA et al. Long-term prophylaxis of spontaneous bacterial peritonitis in patients with cirrhosis. *Ann Pharmacother* 2005;39:908.
28. Gerding DN et al. The penetration of antibiotics into peritoneal fluid. *Bull NY Acad Med* 1975;51: 1016.
29. Wittman DH et al. Penetration of eight beta-lactam antibiotics into the peritoneal fluid. A pharmacokinetic investigation. *Arch Surg* 1983;118:205.
30. Piraino B et al. Peritoneal dialysis-related infec-

tions recommendations: 2005 update. *Perit Dial Int* 2005;25:107.
31. Toussaint N et al. Efficacy of a non-vancomycin-based peritoneal dialysis peritonitis protocol. *Nephrology* 2005;10:142.
32. Salzer W. Antimicrobial-resistant gram-positive bacteria in PD peritonitis and the newer antibiotics used to treat them. *Perit Dial Int* 2005;25:313.
33. Khairullah Q et al. Comparison of vancomycin versus cefazolin as initial therapy for peritonitis in peritoneal dialysis patients. *Perit Dial Int* 2002;22:339.
34. Leung CB et al. Cefazolin plus ceftazidime versus imipenem/cilastatin monotherapy for treatment of CAPD peritonitis-a randomized controlled trial. *Perit Dial Int* 2004;24:440.
35. Passadakis P et al. The case for oral treatment of peritonitis in continuous ambulatory peritoneal dialysis. *Adv Perit Dial* 2001;17:180.
36. Goffin E et al. Vancomycin and ciprofloxacin: systemic antibiotic administration for peritoneal dialysis-associated peritonitis. *Perit Dial Int* 2004;24:433.
37. Prasad N et al. Fungal peritonitis in peritoneal dialysis patients. *Perit Dial Int* 2005;25:207.
38. Dupont H et al. Monotherapy with a broad-spectrum beta-lactam is as effective as its combination with an aminoglycoside in treatment of severe generalized peritonitis: a multicenter randomized controlled trial. The Severe Generalized Peritonitis Study Group. *Antimicrob Agents Chemother* 2000;44:2028.
39. Malangoni MA et al. Randomized controlled trial of moxifloxacin compared with piperacillin-tazobactam and amoxicillin-clavulanate for the treatment of complicated intra-abdominal infections. *Ann Surg* 2006;244:204.
40. Erasmo AA et al. Randomized comparison of piperacillin/tazobactam versus imipenem/cilastatin in the treatment of patients with intra-abdominal infection. *Asian J Surg* 2004;27(3):227.
41. Nathens AB. Relevance and utility of peritoneal cultures in patients with peritonitis. *Surg Infect* 2001;2(2):153.
42. Sirinek KR. Diagnosis and treatment of intra-abdominal abscesses. *Surg Infect (Larchmt)* 2000;1:31.
43. Minton J et al. Intra-abdominal infections. *Clin Med* 2004;4(6):519.
44. Mazuski JE et al. The Surgical Infection Society Guidelines on Antimicrobial Therapy for Intra-Abdominal Infections: An Executive Summary. *Surg Infect (Larchmt)* 2002;3:161.
45. Solomkin J et al. Treatment of polymicrobial infections: post hoc analysis of three trials comparing ertapenem and piperacillin-tazobactam. *J Antimicrob Chemother* 2004;53(S2):ii51.
46. Namias N et al. Randomized, multicenter, double-blind study of efficacy, safety, and tolerability of intravenous ertapenem versus piperacillin/tazobactam in treatment of complicated intra-abdominal infections in hospitalized adults. *Surg Infect (Larchmt)* 2007;8(1):15.
47. Solomkin JS et al. Ertapenem versus piperacillin/tazobactam in the treatment of complicated intraabdominal infections: results of a double-blind, randomized comparative phase III trial. *Ann Surg* 2003;237:235.
48. Cohn SM et al. Comparison of intravenous/oral ciprofloxacin plus metronidazole versus piperacillin/tazobactam in the treatment of complicated intraabdominal infections. *Ann Surg* 2000;232:254.
49. Matthaiou DK et al. Ciprofloxacin/metronidazole versus beta-lactam-based treatment of intra-abdominal infections: a meta-analysis of comparative trials. *Int J Antimicrob Agents* 2006;28:159.
50. Hau T et al. Irrigation of the peritoneal cavity and local antibiotics in the treatment of peritonitis. *Surg Gynecol Obstet* 1983;156:25.
51. Platell C et al. The influence of lavage on peritonitis. *J Am Coll Surg* 2000;191(6):672.
52. Platell C et al. A meta-analysis of peritoneal lavage for acute pancreatitis. *J Gastroenterol Hepatol* 2001;16(6):689.
53. Carver P. Postoperative use of antibiotic irrigations. *Clin Pharm* 1987;6:352.
54. Snydman DR et al. National survey on the susceptibility of group report and analysis of trends in the United States from 1997 to 2004. *Antimicrob Agents Chemother* 2007;51(5):1649.
55. Clinical and Laboratory Standards Institute (CLSI). *Methods for Antimicrobial Susceptibility Testing of Anaerobic Bacteria; Approved Standard.* 7th ed. Approved Standard M11-A7. Wayne, PA: CLSI; 2007.
56. Dougherty SH. Antimicrobial culture and susceptibility testing has little value for routine management of secondary bacterial peritonitis. *Clin Infect Dis* 1997;25(Suppl 2):S258.
57. Luchette FA et al. Practice management guidelines for prophylactic antibiotic use in penetrating abdominal trauma: the EAST Practice Management Guidelines Work Group. *J Trauma* 2000;48:508.
58. Bozorgzadeh A et al. The duration of antibiotic administration in penetrating abdominal trauma. *Am J Surg* 1999;177(2):125.
59. Fabian TC. Infection in penetrating abdominal trauma: risk factors and preventive antibiotics. *Am Surg* 2002;68(1):29.
60. Delgado G Jr. et al. Characteristics of prophylactic antibiotic strategies after penetrating abdominal trauma at a level I urban trauma center: a comparison with the EAST guidelines. *J Trauma* 2002;53:673.
61. Demetriades D et al. Short-course antibiotic prophylaxis in penetrating abdominal injuries: ceftriaxone versus cefoxitin. *Injury* 1991;22:20.
62. Fabian TC et al. Duration of antibiotic therapy for penetrating abdominal trauma: a prospective trial. *Surgery* 1992;112:788.
63. Bratzler DW et al. Antimicrobial prophylaxis for surgery: an advisory statement from the national surgical infection prevention project. *Clin Infect Dis* 2004;38:1706.
64. Berne TV et al. Surgically treated gangrenous or perforated appendicitis. A comparison of aztreonam and clindamycin versus gentamicin and clindamycin. *Ann Surg* 1987;205:133.
65. Lau WY et al. Randomized, prospective, and double-blind trial of new beta-lactams in the treatment of appendicitis. *Antimicrob Agents Chemother* 1985;28:639.
66. Heseltine PN et al. Imipenem therapy for perforated and gangrenous appendicitis. *Surg Gynecol Obstet* 1986;162:43.
67. Lau WY et al. Cefoxitin versus gentamicin and metronidazole in prevention of post-appendectomy sepsis: a randomized, prospective trial. *J Antimicrob Chemother* 1986;18:613.
68. Foster MC et al. A randomized comparative study of sulbactam plus ampicillin vs. metronidazole plus cefotaxime in the management of acute appendicitis in children. *Rev Infect Dis* 1986;8(Suppl 5):S634.

CHAPTER 64

Urinary Tract Infections

Douglas N. Fish

INTRODUCTION

This chapter begins with a brief review of urinary tract infections (UTI), but focuses on the treatment of patients with UTI. For a more detailed discussion of the etiology, pathophysiology, and diagnosis of UTI, the reader is referred to some excellent texts and review articles.[1–9] Additionally, a glossary of associated terms is supplied at the end of this chapter.

Epidemiology

Urinary tract infections occur frequently in both community and hospital environments and are the most common bacterial infections in humans.[1] UTI encompass a spectrum of clinical entities ranging in severity from asymptomatic infection to acute pyelonephritis with sepsis.[1,6] Approximately 7 million cases of acute cystitis and 250,000 cases of acute pyelonephritis occur annually in the United States, resulting in more than 100,000 hospitalizations.[4,10] Direct costs associated with the diagnosis and treatment of UTI have been estimated at more than $2.5 billion annually in the United States.[8,10] After 1 year of age until about age 50, UTI is predominantly a disease of females. From ages 5 through 14, the incidence of bacteriuria is 1.2% among girls and 0.03% among boys. Of women between the ages of 15 and 24 years, 1% to 5% have bacteriuria; the incidence increases 1% to 2% for each decade of life until approximately 10% of women are bacteriuric after age 70.[1,7,11] Approximately 25% to 40% of all women will experience a UTI during their lifetime.[4] Women have more UTI than men, probably because of anatomic and physiologic differences. The female urethra is relatively short and allows bacteria easy access to the bladder. In contrast, males are partly protected because the urethra is longer and antimicrobial substances are secreted by the prostate.[1,7]

The incidence of UTI in neonates is about 1% and is most frequent among male neonates, many of whom prove to have congenital structural abnormalities.[12] The mortality rate among newborns with UTI was earlier reported to be as high as 10%[12]; more recently, this rate has decreased because of an increased awareness of the high frequency of UTI in children, improved diagnostic techniques, and more effective management.[12]

Urinary tract infections again become a problem for males after the age of 50, when prostatic obstruction, urethral instrumentation, and surgery influence the infection rate. Infection in younger men is rare and requires careful evaluation for urinary tract pathology.[13,14]

In general, 5% to 20% of the elderly living at home have bacteriuria. This increases to 20% to 50% in extended care facilities and 30% in hospitals.[11,15,16] The frequency of infection also rises with increasing age for those 65 years or older. Most UTI in these patients are asymptomatic, but are still important because they often result in symptomatic infection.[11,15,16] Whether bacteriuria in old age is associated with decreased survival is controversial[17,18]; however, the presence of asymptomatic bacteriuria is associated with decreased functional ability of institutionalized persons.[11,15] Reasons for higher UTI rates in elderly persons include the high prevalence of prostatic hypertrophy in men, incomplete bladder emptying caused by underlying diseases or medications, dementia, and urinary and fecal incontinence.[7,15,16]

Etiology

Community-Acquired Infections

Most UTI are caused by gram-negative aerobic bacilli from the intestinal tract. *Escherichia coli* cause 75% to 90% of community-acquired, uncomplicated UTI.[1,2,19] Coagulase-negative staphylococci (i.e., *Staphylococcus saprophyticus*) account for another 5% to 20% of UTI in younger women.[1,2,4] Other Enterobacteriaceae (*Proteus mirabilis, Klebsiella*) and *Enterococcus faecalis* also are common pathogens.[1,2,19] Uncomplicated infections are nearly always caused by only a single organism.

Hospital-Acquired Infections

Urinary tract infections occur in up to 10% of hospitalized patients and represent 30% to 40% of all nosocomial infections.[20] *E. coli* remains the most common pathogen in hospital-acquired or other complicated UTI, but it is responsible for only 15% to 20% of these infections. Other gram-negative organisms such as *Pseudomonas aeruginosa, Proteus, Enterobacter, Serratia,* and *Acinetobacter* cause significantly more infections (up to 25%) than in community-acquired infections.[4,21,22] *Enterococcus* is also a common pathogen in hospital-acquired infections and causes approximately 25% of infections.[21,22] UTI caused by *Staphylococcus aureus* are usually the result of hematogenous spread, although this pathogen is also associated with urinary catheterization.[1,23,24] Finally, *Candida albicans* is a common pathogen in hospital-acquired infections and may be involved in 20% to 30% of cases.[20,22] In contrast to uncomplicated infections that are usually monomicrobial, hospital-acquired UTI associated with structural abnormalities or indwelling urinary catheters are often caused by multiple organisms.[1,20,21,23,24]

Pathogenesis

The usual pathway for the spread of bacteria to the urinary tract is the ascending route. A UTI usually begins with heavy and persistent colonization of the introitus (i.e., vaginal vestibule and urethral mucosa) with intestinal bacteria, especially in women with recurrent UTI. Once introital colonization has occurred, colonization of the urethra leads to retrograde infection of the bladder.[3,25]

The bladder has additional defense mechanisms that prevent spread of the infection after urethral colonization occurs. Urination washes bacteria out of the bladder and is effective if urine flows freely and the bladder is emptied completely. Substances in the urine, including organic acids (which contribute to a low pH) and urea (which contributes to a high osmolality), are antibacterial. The bladder mucosa also has antibacterial properties.[1,2] Lastly, other substances, including IgA and glycoproteins (e.g., Tamm-Horsfall protein), are actively secreted into the urine and act to prevent adherence of bacteria to uroendothelial cells.[3,25]

Focal renal involvement may result from the spread of bacteria via the ureters and may be facilitated by vesicoureteral reflux or decreased ureteral peristalsis. Reflux can be produced by cystitis alone or by anatomic defects. Ureteral peristalsis is decreased by pregnancy, ureteral obstruction, or gram-negative bacterial endotoxins.[1,3,25]

Predisposing Factors

Extremes of age, female gender, sexual activity, use of contraception, pregnancy, instrumentation, urinary tract obstruction, neurologic dysfunction, renal disease, previous antimicrobial use, and expression of A, B, and H blood group oligosaccharides on the surface of epithelial cells are among the many predisposing factors for the development of UTI.[1,3,5,26]

The overall likelihood of developing a UTI is approximately 30 times higher in women than in men.[2] The incidence of bacteriuria in pregnant women is 2% to 10%, which is approximately twice that of similarly aged nonpregnant women.[1,11,27] The incidence of acute symptomatic pyelonephritis in pregnant women with untreated bacteriuria also is high. Many factors contribute to the increased susceptibility of the pregnant female to infection; these include hormonal changes, anatomic changes, progressive urinary stasis, and glucose in the urine.[27]

Instrumentation of the urinary tract (i.e., urethral and ureteral catheterization) is an important predisposing factor for hospital-acquired UTI in particular. As many as 67% of nosocomial UTI are preceded by urinary tract instrumentation.[20,24] Other urologic procedures, such as cystoscopy, transurethral surgery, prostate biopsy, and upper urinary tract endoscopy, are much less likely to result in infection unless there is preexisting bacteriuria or other contaminated sites (e.g., prostate, renal stones).

Any obstruction to the free flow of urine (e.g., urethral stenosis, stones, tumor) or mechanical difficulty in evacuating the bladder (e.g., prostatic hypertrophy, urethral stricture) predisposes patients to UTI. Furthermore, infections associated with urethral or renal pelvic obstruction can lead to rapid destruction of the kidney and sepsis.[1]

Renal disease increases the susceptibility of the kidney to infection.[1] The incidence of UTI among renal transplant recipients has been reported to range from 35% to 80%.[28]

Patients with spinal cord injuries, stroke, atherosclerosis, or diabetes may have neurologic dysfunction that can cause UTI. The neurologic dysfunction can cause urinary retention, which may lead to catheterization. Furthermore, prolonged immobilization facilitates hypercalciuria and stone formation in some of these patients.[1,3,4]

Previous antimicrobial use (within the previous 15–28 days) has been shown to increase the relative risk for UTI in women by approximately three- to sixfold.[5] This increased infection risk applies to prior antimicrobial use for treatment of UTI as well as other infections. The proposed mechanism for increased risk is alteration of normal flora of the urogenital tract and predisposition to colonization with pathogenic bacterial strains.[5]

Diabetes mellitus has often been associated with an increased risk for UTI because of glucose in the urine, which both promotes bacterial growth and impairs leukocyte function. Diabetes is also often associated with anatomic, neurologic, and immunologic abnormalities of the urinary tract that increase risk of infection, often because of increased need for urinary tract instrumentation.[29,30] Several studies have documented a two- to threefold increase in UTI in diabetic women compared with nondiabetic women; rates of complications, such as pyelonephritis, are also increased.[29,31] Patients with diabetes who have no neurologic complications resulting in bladder dysfunction and who have not had instrumentation are apparently not at increased risk compared with nondiabetic patients.[3] With autonomic neuropathy affecting the bladder (i.e., cystopathy) or following instrumentation, UTI in diabetic patients are both more frequent and more severe.[3,30]

Studies also have supported an association between sexual intercourse and UTI among otherwise healthy women.[3,26,32] Specific contraceptive practices, particularly the use of spermicides, have also been associated with increased risk for UTI. The use of a diaphragm, cervical cap, or condom in combination with spermicidal jelly has been shown to increase the risk of UTI compared with the use of the barrier method alone.[26,33] Although the greatest risk has been associated with the spermicide nonoxynol-9, the use of other types of spermicidal jellies has also been associated with a significantly higher risk for UTI.[34] Oral contraceptive use has also been associated with increased risk of UTI.[26] The exact mechanisms of infection related to sexual intercourse and contraceptive methods are unclear but appear to be related to alterations in vaginal flora that allow for bacterial overgrowth and subsequent infection.[35,36]

Clinical Presentation

Symptoms commonly associated with lower UTI (e.g., cystitis) include burning on urination (dysuria), frequent urination, suprapubic pain, blood in the urine (hematuria), and back pain. Patients with upper tract infection (e.g., acute pyelonephritis) also may present with loin pain, costovertebral angle (CVA) tenderness, fever, chills, nausea, and vomiting.[1,2,4,6]

Clinical signs and symptoms correlate poorly with either the presence or the extent of the infection. Symptoms common to lower UTI often are the only positive findings in upper UTI (i.e., subclinical pyelonephritis).[1,6] The probability of true infection in women who present with one or more symptoms of UTI is only about 50%.[37] The presence of dysuria, back pain, pyuria, hematuria, bacteriuria, and a history of previous UTI enhance the probability of true infection; the absence of dysuria or back pain and history of vaginal discharge or irritation significantly decrease the likelihood of infection.[37] It has also been determined that the combination of dysuria and frequency in the absence of vaginal discharge or irritation increases the probability of true infection to >90%.[37] Fever, chills, flank pain, nausea and vomiting, or CVA tenderness are highly suggestive of acute pyelonephritis rather than cystitis.[4,6] Many elderly patients with UTI are asymptomatic without pyuria. Additionally, because many patients have frequency and dysuria, it is difficult to distinguish between noninfectious and infectious causes based on symptoms.[1] Nonspecific symptoms, such as failure to thrive and fever, may be the only manifestations of UTI in neonates and children <2 years of age.[1]

Laboratory Diagnosis

The urinalysis (UA) is a series of laboratory tests commonly performed in patients suspected of having a UTI.[38] A technician first performs a macroscopic analysis by describing the color of the urine; measuring its specific gravity; and estimating the pH and glucose, protein, ketone, blood, and bilirubin contents using a rapid "dipstick" method. Then the urine sediment, obtained by centrifugation, is examined under a microscope for the presence and quantity of leukocytes, erythrocytes, epithelial cells, crystals, casts, and bacteria.

Microscopic examination of urine sediment in patients with documented UTI reveals many bacteria (usually >20 per high-power field [HPF]). Gram staining of uncentrifuged ("unspun") urine shows at least one organism per immersion oil field and usually correlates with a positive urine culture. Pyuria (i.e., ≥8 white blood cells [WBC] per mm^3 of unspun urine or 2–5 WBC/HPF of centrifuged urine) frequently is seen in patients with UTI. WBC casts in the urine strongly suggest acute pyelonephritis.[1]

A rapid diagnostic dipstick test for the detection of bacteriuria, the nitrite test, detects nitrite formation from the reduction of nitrates by bacteria. This test is widely available and easily performed; however, at least 10^5 bacteria/mm^3 are necessary to form sufficient nitrite for the reaction to occur. Although a positive nitrite reading is useful, false–negative results do occur. Dipstick testing can also be used to perform the leukocyte esterase test, which detects the esterase activity of leukocytes in the urine. A positive test correlates well with significant pyuria[39]; however, both false–negative and false–positive findings can occur with the leukocyte esterase panel. Nitrite and lekocyte esterase tests are useful in ruling out the presence of infection if results of both tests are negative, whereas positive results of both tests in combination are highly suggestive of the presence of infection. Confirmatory tests (e.g. urine culture) should be performed, however, if one or both dipstick test finding is positive owing to the possibility of false–positive test results.[39]

The major criterion for the diagnosis of UTI is the urine culture. Proper interpretation of these cultures depends on appropriate urine collection techniques. Urinating into a sterile collection cup using the midstream clean-catch technique is the most practical method of urine collection. This method of urine specimen collection is especially useful for male patients, but is less useful in female patients because contamination is extremely difficult to avoid.[1] The external urethral area must first be thoroughly cleaned and rinsed, then the urine specimen collected after initiation of the urine stream (hence "midstream").

Suprapubic bladder aspiration, although unpleasant from a patient's point of view, generally is not painful and is quite reliable. It is not practical for routine office or clinic practice, but may be useful when voided urine samples repeatedly yield questionable results or when patients have voiding problems. Because contamination is negligible, any number of bacteria found by this method reflects infection.[1]

Urinary catheterization for a urine culture sample yields fairly reliable results if performed carefully. Infections can result from the procedure itself because organisms might be introduced into the bladder at the time of catheterization.

Urine must be plated on culture media within 20 minutes of collection to avoid erroneously high colony counts from bacterial growth in urine at room temperature. Otherwise, urine should be promptly refrigerated until it can be cultured. Colony counts are also affected by the concentration of bladder urine; bacterial counts are higher in first-voided morning urines compared with those obtained from the same patient later in the day.

Urine cultures in the bacteriology laboratory usually are evaluated by the pour-plate or streak-plate method. Greater than 10^5 colonies of bacteria/mm^3 cultured from a midstream urine specimen confirms a UTI. A single, carefully collected urine specimen provides 80% reliability, and two consecutive cultures of the same organism are virtually diagnostic.[1,2]

It is important to understand that the classic definition of UTI as $\geq 10^5$ bacteria/mm^3 is fairly insensitive in accurately diagnosing patients with UTI. Approximately 30% to 50% of actual cases of acute cystitis have $<10^5$ bacteria/mm^3.[4,11] Particularly in a symptomatic patient, using a definition of $\geq 10^2$ bacteria/mm^3 is much more sensitive and avoids failure to diagnose infection in many patients.[4]

Diagnosis of UTI in men also requires different interpretation of laboratory data. Contamination of urinary specimens is much less likely to occur in men compared with women, and numbers of bacterial colonies in specimens are therefore much lower. Greater than 10^3 bacteria/mm^3 is thus highly suggestive of UTI in men.[13,14,40] In addition, although a positive nitrite test in a symptomatic man is highly indicative of the presence of an acute UTI, a negative nitrite test does not necessarily exclude infection and should be confirmed with a urine culture.[41]

Diagnosis of UTI in children is particularly problematic because of the difficulties and high contamination rates associated with commonly used methods of urine specimen collection. Suprapubic aspiration is the most accurate method in children, followed by urinary bladder catheterization.[9] Although clean-catch and bag methods (i.e., collecting urine into a bag placed around the urogenital area) are most susceptible to contamination and inaccurate results, they are also the most preferred methods for parents and health care personnel because they are simple and noninvasive. The choice of diagnostic tests for children will therefore be based on the experience, skill, and preferences of those involved with the child, and no one technique will be ideal in every setting.[9]

Simplified culture methods such as the filter-paper method (e.g., Testuria-R), dip-slide method (e.g., Uricult), and pad-culture method (Microstix) are as reliable as traditional laboratory methods for bacterial identification and quantification. The filter-paper method is relatively inexpensive but does not differentiate between gram-positive and gram-negative organisms. The dip-slide and pad-culture methods are accurate, differentiate between gram-positive and gram-negative organisms, and are similar in cost. The dip-slide method has the added advantages of ease of storage and a nitrite indicator pad.

LOWER URINARY TRACT INFECTION

Initiation of Therapy

1. V.Q., a 20-year-old woman (married, no children) with no previous history of UTI, complains of burning on urination, frequent urination of a small amount, and bladder pain. She has no fever or CVA tenderness. A clean-catch midstream urine sample shows gram-negative rods on Gram stain. A culture and sensitivity (C&S) test is ordered, and the results of a STAT UA are as follows: appearance, straw-colored (normal, straw); specific gravity, 1.015 (normal, 1.001–1.035); pH, 8.0 (normal, 4.5–7.5); and protein, glucose, ketones, bilirubin, and blood are all negative (normal, all negative); WBC, 10 to 15 cells/mm^3 (normal, 0–2 cells/mm^3); red blood cells (RBC), 0 to 1 cells/mm^3 (normal, 0–2 cells/mm^3); bacteria, many (normal, 0 to rare); epithelial cells, 3 to 5 cells/mm^3 (normal, 0 to few cells/mm^3). Based on these findings, V.Q. is presumed to have a lower UTI. What should be the goals of therapy and treatment plan at this time?

Drug treatment of a lower UTI often is started before C&S results are known because the most probable infecting organism and its sensitivity to antibiotics can be predicted (Table 64-1). Approximately 75% to 90% of community-acquired infections are caused by Enterobacteriaceae (especially *E. coli*). Although these organisms may be sensitive to ampicillin, amoxicillin, and the sulfonamides such as trimethoprim-sulfamethoxazole (TMP-SMX), resistance to these agents is common.[42,43] Ampicillin resistance has been reported in as many as 25% to 70% of community-acquired isolates; resistance nationwide is currently about 30% to 40%.[1,4,19,42,44] TMP-SMX has been a traditional agent of choice for many years; however, TMP-SMX resistance has significantly increased in recent years and may be as high as 20% to 30% among community-acquired *E. coli* isolates.[19,42,45] Although traditionally associated with hospital-acquired infections, resistance among *E. coli* and *Klebsiella* caused by production of extended-spectrum β-lactamase (ESBL) enzymes which confer resistance to penicillins and cephalosporins has also been increasing among community-acquired pathogens.[46] Another relatively common organism is *S. saprophyticus*. Most strains are susceptible to sulfonamides, TMP-SMX, penicillins, and cephalosporins. Alternative medications and doses are shown in Table 64-2.

The goals of therapy for treatment of acute cystitis are to effectively eradicate the infection and prevent associated complications, while minimizing adverse effects and costs associated with drug therapy. To accomplish these goals, selection of a specific antimicrobial agent should be made after considering several factors: (a) pathogens likely to be causing the infection, (b) resistance rates to various antimicrobials within the specific geographic area, (c) desired duration of therapy, (d) clinical efficacy and toxicity profiles of various agents, and (e) costs of specific agents. Because resistance rates among various pathogens vary considerably among geographic areas, clinicians involved in the treatment of patients with UTI must be familiar with resistance rates prevalent within the specific area within which they practice.[19,42,43]

Table 64-1 Urinary Tract Infections

Organisms Commonly Found	Antibacterial of Choice
Uncomplicated UTI	
Escherichia coli	TMP-SMX[c]
Proteus mirabilis	TMP-SMX[c]
Klebsiella pneumoniae	TMP-SMX[c]
Enterococcus faecalis	Amoxicillin
Staphylococcus saprophyticus	First-generation cephalosporin or TMP-SMX
Complicated UTI[a,b]	
Escherichia coli	First-, second-, or third-generation cephalosporin; TMP-SMX[c]
Proteus mirabilis	First-, second-, or third-generation cephalosporin
Klebsiella pneumoniae	First-generation cephalosporin; fluoroquinolone
Enterococcus faecalis	Ampicillin or vancomycin ± aminoglycoside
Pseudomonas aeruginosa	Antipseudomonal penicillin ± aminoglycoside; ceftazidime; cefepime; fluoroquinolone; carbapenem
Enterobacter	Fluoroquinolone; TMP-SMX; carbapenem
Indole-positive *Proteus*	Third-generation cephalosporin; fluoroquinolone
Serratia	Third-generation cephalosporin; fluoroquinolone
Acinetobacter	Carbapenem; TMP-SMX
Staphylococcus aureus	Penicillinase-resistant penicillin; vancomycin

TMP-SMX, trimethoprim-sulfamethoxazole; UTI, urinary tract infection.
[a] Oral therapy when appropriate.
[b] Drug selection based on culture and susceptibility testing when possible.
[c] Caution in communities with increased resistance (>10%–20%). Fluoroquinolone, nitrofurantoin, or cephalosporins should be used in areas with increased TMP-SMX resistance.

Duration of Therapy

2. What treatment duration options are available for V.Q.?

Outpatients with acute, uncomplicated UTI can be treated successfully with a 7- to 14-day course of oral medications, a 3-day course of therapy, or by single-dose therapy.[1,4,47] A urine C&S may be obtained before antibacterial therapy and repeated 2 to 3 weeks after the completion of therapy,[1,2,4] although this practice is seldom necessary in young adult females with a lower UTI.[1,4]

The duration of therapy for UTI has been extensively studied and progressively shortened. The traditional 7- to 14-day course of antibiotic therapy now is considered excessive for most patients with uncomplicated infections.[1,2,4,43,47,48] A 3-day antibiotic treatment regimen is just as effective as a 10-day regimen in achieving clinical cures and eradicating urinary tract organisms, although this is somewhat antibiotic class-specific.[1,2,4,43,47,48] TMP-SMX and the fluoroquinolones are recommended as the preferred agents for 3-day treatment regimens. β-Lactam antibiotics and nitrofurantoin are more appropriately reserved for longer treatment courses of 7 to 14 days[4,49]; however, a recent study has shown that a 5-day course of nitrofurantoin is as effective as a 3-day course of TMP-SMX.[50] Longer treatment courses are also used in cases of treatment failure following regimens of shorter duration. Because of the relatively high incidence of *E. coli* resistance to ampicillin and amoxicillin, some experts do not recommend these agents for initial, empiric use.[2,4,42–44,48,49] Although TMP-SMX is still recommended as the preferred agent for acute, uncomplicated UTI, this agent also may not be a suitable choice for empiric therapy in certain geographic areas because of increasing resistance. Use of trimethoprim or TMP-SMX has been discouraged in geographic areas where the incidence of *E. coli* resistance exceeds 15% to 20%.[42,43,45,48,51,52] The fluoroquinolones have become favored agents in many geographic areas with high rates of resistance to ampicillin, TMP-SMX, and trimethoprim because of excellent activity against common urinary pathogens and the ability to use short 3-day courses of therapy. The choice of a specific agent should be based on geographic susceptibilities as well as any patient allergies and the relative cost of the drugs.

Even a single dose of an antibiotic may be effective. Bacteria disappear from the urine within hours after antibacterial therapy has been initiated.[48] This, coupled with the urinary bladder's ability to defend itself through micturition, acidification, and inherent antibacterial activity, gives theoretic support to the clinical evidence that a large single dose of an antibiotic can eradicate a UTI.

Single-Dose Therapy

3. Would a 3-day course of therapy or single-dose therapy be preferred for V.Q.?

A single antibiotic dose is reasonably effective in treating acute, lower UTI in young adult females.[4,7,48] Commonly used regimens are TMP-SMX (two or three double-strength tablets), trimethoprim 400 mg, amoxicillin-clavulanate 500 mg, amoxicillin 3 g, ampicillin 3.5 g, nitrofurantoin 200 mg, ciprofloxacin 500 mg, and norfloxacin 400 mg.[1,48,49] Again, choice of a specific agent should be based on local susceptibility patterns, patient allergies, and relative drug costs. Female patients with history or clinical presentation suggestive of complicated infection (e.g., systemic manifestations of infection, renal disease, anatomic abnormalities of the urinary tract, diabetes mellitus, pregnancy), a history of antibiotic resistance, or a history of relapse after single-dose therapy should not receive single-dose regimens. Single-dose therapy is also not appropriate for male patients with UTI. Because V.Q. does not have any of these contraindications, she could potentially receive single-dose therapy with an appropriate agent.

The advantages of single-dose treatment of UTI include improved compliance, cost savings, proved efficacy in a defined population of patients (i.e., young women with acute, uncomplicated lower UTI), minimal side effects, and a potentially decreased incidence of bacterial resistance associated with antibiotic overuse. Furthermore, failure to eradicate the organism with a single dose of an antibiotic may help identify patients who have subclinical pyelonephritis and require more intensive evaluation of their urinary tract.

Some concerns also exist about single-dose therapy.[4,7,48,49] First, sample sizes in most of the comparative studies to date have been relatively small. Consequently, it is difficult to determine whether differences in effectiveness or incidence of side effects between single-dose and multiple-dose therapy are clinically significant. Meta-analysis of studies comparing

Table 64-2 Commonly Used Oral Antimicrobial Agents for Acute Urinary Tract Infections[1,2,4,27,48,49,96]

	Usual Dose				
Drug	***Adult***	***Pediatric***	***Pregnancy[a]***	***Breast Milk[a]***	***Comments[b]***
Amoxicillin	250 mg Q 8 hr or 3 g single dose	20–40 mg/kg/day in three doses	Crosses placenta (*cord*) = 30% (maternal)[c]	Small amount present	Watch for resistant organisms.
Amoxicillin + potassium clavulanate	500 + 125 mg Q 12 hr	20 mg/kg/day (amoxicillin content) in three doses	Unknown	Unknown	
Ampicillin	250–500 mg Q 6 hr	50–100 mg/kg/day in four doses	Crosses placenta	Variable amount (*milk*) = 1%–30% (serum)[c]	Watch for resistant organisms. Should be taken on an empty stomach.
Cefadroxil	0.5–1 g Q 12 hr	15–30 mg/kg/day in four doses	Crosses placenta	Enters breast milk (*milk*) = 20% (serum)[c]	Alternate choices for patients allergic to penicillins, although cross-hypersensitivity can occur. May be associated with high failure rates.
Cephalexin	250–500 mg Q 6 hr	15–30 mg/kg/day in four doses	Crosses placenta		
Cephradine	250–500 mg Q 6 hr	15–30 mg/kg/day in four doses	Crosses placenta (*cord*) = 10% (maternal)[c]		
Norfloxacin[d]	400 mg Q 12 hr	Avoid	Arthropathy in immature animals	Unknown	Useful for pseudomonal infection. *Avoid antacids and ditrivalent cations and sucral-fate. May cause dizziness.*
Ciprofloxacin[d]	250–500 mg Q 12 hr	Avoid	Arthropathy in immature animals	Unknown	Alternate choices for patients allergic to β-lactams
Levofloxacin	250 mg Q 24 hr	Avoid	Arthropathy in immature animals	(milk) = 100% (serum)[c]	
Nitrofurantoin	50–100 mg Q 6 hr	5–7 mg/kg/day in four doses	Hemolytic anemia in newborn	Variable amounts; not detectable to 30%; may cause hemolysis in G6PD-deficient baby	Alternate choice. *To be taken with food or milk. May cause brown or rust-yellow discoloration of urine.* See Questions 47–49.
Sulfisoxazole Sulfamethoxazole (SMX)	0.5–1 g Q 6 hr 1 g Q 12 hr	50–100 mg/kg/day in four doses 60 mg/kg/day in two doses	Crosses placenta; hemolysis in newborn with G6PD deficiency; displacement of bilirubin may lead to hyperbilirubinemia and kernicterus; teratogenic in some animal studies	Enters breast milk; displacement of bilirubin may lead to neonatal jaundice; may cause hemolysis in G6PD deficient baby	Alters bowel flora to favor resistant organisms. *To be taken on an empty stomach with a full glass of water. Photosensitivity may occur.*
Trimethoprim (TMP)	100 mg Q 12 hr		Crosses placenta (cord) = 60%; (maternal) folate antagonism; teratogenic in rats	(*milk*) >1 (serum)[c]	Alternate choice.
TMP-SMX	160 + 800 mg Q 12 hr or 0.48 + 2.4 g single dose	10 mg/kg/day (TMP component in two doses)	Crosses placenta (cord) = 60%; (maternal) folate antagonism; teratogenic in rats	(*milk*) >1 (serum)[c]	*To be taken on an empty stomach with a full glass of water. Photosensitivity may occur.* Monitor HIV-infected patients closely for development tof adverse hematologic reactions First-line agent for prostatitis

[a] Also see Chapter 46, Obstetric Drug Therapy.
[b] Includes unique patient consultation information in italics.
[c] Denotes drug concentration.
[d] May increase theophylline concentrations when given concurrently. Carefully monitor theophylline serum concentrations during quinolone use.
TMP = SMX, trimethoprim-sulfamethoxazole.

either single-dose or 3-day regimens with multiple-dose TMP-SMX therapy has demonstrated that single-dose therapy is significantly less effective in eradicating bacteriuria than regimens of either $\geq$5 days (83% vs. 93%, respectively, $p < 0.001$) or $\geq$7 days in duration (87% vs. 94%, respectively; $p = 0.014$).[47,48] Although side effects were more common with longer courses of therapy (11%–13% with single-dose versus 19%–28% with longer regimens), they were mild and well tolerated.[47,48] Although fewer studies have directly compared single-dose versus 3-day therapies, numerous studies have shown that 3-day courses are as effective as courses of longer duration.[47,48] A 3-day course of therapy is therefore currently recommended for uncomplicated cystitis.

A second area of concern relates to recurrences in patients treated with single-dose therapy. Recurrent infections may represent either a relapse caused by incomplete eradication of more deep-seated kidney infection or a true reinfection in a high-risk patient. If it is assumed that patients who receive single-dose therapy are selected properly, then reinfection is a more likely explanation. It has also has been suggested, however, that relapse following single-dose therapy actually suggests subclinical upper urinary tract infection.[4] In either case, single-dose therapies have been associated with higher rates of recurrence compared with therapies of longer duration. Finally, the safety of single-dose therapy in patients with subclinical pyelonephritis needs further evaluation, and these regimens are not currently recommended in this setting.

Based on the preceding information, a 3-day antibiotic course is reasonable in V.Q. and would be the recommended treatment for her infection. Although single-dose regimens are considered appropriate for some carefully selected patients with acute, uncomplicated lower tract infection, 3-day courses are generally preferred for most patients.[4]

When using short-course (i.e., 1- or 3-day) regimens, it is important to counsel the patient that the clinical signs and symptoms of infection may often not be completely resolved for 2 to 3 days following initiation of therapy. Therefore, symptoms that persist after beginning therapy (or actually completing therapy, in the case of single-dose regimens) are not necessarily indicative of treatment failure.

Trimethoprim-Sulfamethoxazole

4. TMP-SMX, one double-strength tablet twice daily (BID) for 3 days is prescribed for V.Q. Is this appropriate therapy?

Yes. TMP-SMX (Co-trimoxazole, Bactrim, Septra) has been shown to be effective for single- and multiple-dose therapy of uncomplicated cystitis.[1,2,48] Gram-positive and gram-negative organisms, with the notable exceptions of *P. aeruginosa, Enterococcus,* and anaerobes, generally are susceptible to TMP-SMX.[53] Although TMP-SMX may appear active against enterococci in vitro, clinical efficacy against this pathogen is variable and does not always correlate well with in vitro susceptibilities. The efficacy of TMP-SMX largely depends on the sensitivity of the organism to trimethoprim, although *Neisseria gonorrhoeae* is relatively more susceptible to the sulfonamide component. Individually, trimethoprim and sulfamethoxazole are bacteriostatic, but in combination they are bactericidal against most urinary pathogens.[53] Furthermore, this combination is almost uniformly successful in the treatment of uncomplicated UTI, even against organisms that originally were resistant to either agent alone. Although rates of trimethoprim resistance have increased over the past several years,[19,45,45,54] resistance rates remain relatively low in many geographic areas and trimethoprim alone would be effective in managing many simple UTI.

The ratio of trimethoprim to sulfamethoxazole in the available tablet products is 1:5 (e.g., 80 mg trimethoprim and 400 mg sulfamethoxazole). This combination has been chosen to achieve peak serum concentrations of the two drugs that approximate a 1:20 ratio. This ratio is optimal for synergistic activity against most microorganisms, although the drugs remain synergistic and bactericidal in ratios ranging from 1:5 to 1:40 in vitro.[53,55] Urinary concentrations of trimethoprim and sulfamethoxazole far exceed the minimum inhibitory concentrations (MIC) for most susceptible urinary pathogens. Therefore, good in vitro activity, excellent clinical success, relatively low resistance rates among common pathogens in many geographic areas, and low cost make TMP-SMX a reasonable choice in V.Q. Many consider TMP-SMX the initial agent of choice in the treatment of acute, uncomplicated lower UTI in geographic areas where the incidence of TMP-SMX resistance among *E. coli* is <20%.[4,42,43,48,51,52]

Interpretation of Culture and Sensitivity

5. C&S studies in V.Q. show a few *Klebsiella* and >10^5 bacteria per milliliter of *P. mirabilis,* which are sensitive to ampicillin, amoxicillin-clavulanate, cephalosporins, TMP-SMX, and gentamicin. The *Proteus* is intermediately sensitive to nitrofurnatoin, and is resistant to ciprofloxacin. Based on V.Q.'s clinical presentation and recent culture reports, did she have a true UTI?

Yes. Most women with either lower or upper UTI have >100,000 bacterial colonies/mm^3 of urine. As previously mentioned, a major revision in the diagnostic criteria for symptomatic UTI has been the abandonment of the absolute requirement for growth of at least 10^5 bacterial colonies/mm^3 of urine. The criterion of $\geq$100 bacteria/mm^3 appears to provide excellent sensitivity and specificity for the purpose of correctly diagnosing and treating women with symptomatic infection.[11] This same criterion should also be applied to lower UTI when *S. saprophyticus* is isolated, because UTI caused by this pathogen often are associated with low urine bacterial colony counts, suboptimal growth on commonly used media, and negative findings on nitrite screening.

Mixed flora (more than two organisms) is rare except in severely debilitated persons and other complicated infections. Thus, mixed flora in the setting of uncomplicated infection frequently suggests contamination, and a repeat specimen should be obtained.

6. What is the correlation between sensitivity of the organism to a particular drug and treatment outcome in acute cystitis?

Bacterial susceptibility to different antimicrobial drugs usually is tested by placing discs impregnated with antibacterial agents on an agar surface that has been seeded with the infecting organism. Bacterial susceptibility is indicated by a zone of inhibited growth around the disc containing the drug. Most discs are impregnated with a quantity of drug that correlates with achievable serum concentrations. Drugs useful in the treatment of UTI are excreted primarily by the kidney, however, and urine concentrations of these drugs may be 20 to 100 times greater than serum concentrations. Therefore, an organism that is only intermediately sensitive, or even "resistant" to the concentration of antibacterial drug in the testing disc, might be sensitive to the high concentration of drug present in the urine.

Although in vitro susceptibility testing is not always predictive of patient response to therapy, studies clearly show that patients infected with a resistant pathogen are at increased risk of treatment failure.[52,56–58] Several studies reported clinical response to infection in only 24% to 61% of patients with organisms resistant to TMP-SMX compared with 83% to 92% of patients infected with susceptible organisms.[52,56,57,59] Another study found that patients infected with TMP-SMX-resistant pathogens were 17 times more likely to fail therapy compared with patients with susceptible strains.[60] Patients treated with TMP-SMX who were infected with drug-resistant organisms were also found to have longer median times to symptom resolution (14 vs. 7 days, $p = 0.0002$), more frequent return clinic visits within 1 week (36% vs. 6%, $p < 0.0001$), more frequent need for subsequent antibiotic therapy (36% vs. 4%, $p < 0.0001$), and higher rates of significant bacteriuria after 1 month (42% vs. 20%, $p = 0.04$).[57] Although 50% to 60% of patients with resistant organisms may experience failure of TMP-SMX therapy, antimicrobial therapy is usually chosen empirically without the benefit of C&S testing results. Appropriateness of antibiotic therapy is thus usually judged according to subsequent clinical response. If the infecting organism is sensitive, the urine will usually be sterile in 24 to 48 hours. If a urine specimen collected 48 hours after initiation of therapy is not sterile and the patient has been taking the medication properly, the antibiotic may be inappropriate or the focus of infection may be deeper (e.g., pyelonephritis, abscess, obstruction). If the urine specimen is sterile and the patient is symptomatically improved, the appropriate antimicrobial is being used (regardless of sensitivity studies) and the full course of therapy should be completed.

7. Was it necessary to order a pretreatment urine C&S for V.Q.?

Some investigators question the value of pretreatment urine cultures.[1,4] Women with lower UTI usually have pyuria on urinalysis and respond rapidly to antimicrobial treatment. Pyuria appears to be a better predictor of treatable infection than the colony count obtained on urine culture. Furthermore, the urine culture accounts for a large portion of the cost of treating a patient with a UTI. Consequently, in patients with uncomplicated, acute, lower UTI, it is more cost-effective to order a urinalysis and, if pyuria is present, to forego a urine culture. Instead, the patient should be empirically treated with a conventional 3- to 7-day course of antibiotic therapy. If V.Q. remains symptomatic 48 hours later, a C&S test can be ordered.

Fluoroquinolone Therapy

8. I.B., a 48-year-old woman, presents with a community-acquired UTI. She has experienced a rash with TMP-SMX and has a type I hypersensitivity reaction to penicillins. What is the role of fluoroquinolones in the treatment of I.B.'s community-acquired UTI?

Several fluoroquinolones are indicated for the treatment of uncomplicated or complicated UTI; these include norfloxacin, ciprofloxacin, and levofloxacin. The fluoroquinolones are usually administered orally in the treatment of UTI and have excellent in vitro activity against most gram-negative organisms, including *P. aeruginosa*.[61] They are also active in vitro against many gram-positive organisms including *S. saprophyticus*.[61] Resistance to fluoroquinolones among organisms causing acute uncomplicated UTI is usually $<1\%$ to 2%.[19] Fluoroquinolone resistance may, however, be more frequent in some geographic areas (5%–10%) and in complicated infections[44,54]; these quinolone-resistant strains also tend to be resistant to multiple other antimicrobials.[62] The activity of many fluoroquinolones in vitro is antagonized by urine (acidic pH, divalent cations); however, this is unlikely to be clinically significant because urine concentrations are several hundred-fold greater than serum levels.[61]

Although the fluoroquinolones are as effective as TMP-SMX in the treatment of uncomplicated UTI, they are not recommended as first-line therapy because they are more expensive and provide no additional treatment benefits.[4,7,42,43,48,61] Concerns also exist regarding the overuse of fluoroquinolones and the promotion of drug resistance among community-acquired pathogens. These agents are appropriate alternatives for patients with allergies to first-line agents or for patients infected with organisms resistant to multiple antibiotics, such as *P. aeruginosa*. Fluoroquinolones are also recommended as first-line agents in geographic areas with $>20\%$ resistance of *E. coli* to TMP-SMX.[42,43,48,51] Finally, the fluoroquinolones are effective in treating patients with structural or functional abnormalities of the urinary tract and other types of complicated infections.[61,63,64]

A fluoroquinolone is appropriate for I.B. because it will be effective and because she has experienced previous adverse reactions to penicillins and sulfas. The fluoroquinolones are considered similar in efficacy in this setting[63,64]; choice of a specific agent should be based on comparative costs and compliance considerations. The duration of fluoroquinolone therapy in I.B. would be 3 days.

Drug Interactions

9. I.B. also is taking Maalox for a duodenal ulcer. What is the likelihood that this antacid will affect the action of the fluoroquinolones?

It is imperative that clinicians question patients such as I.B. regarding other medications (both prescription and nonprescription) that they may be taking. Products containing divalent and trivalent cations (Mg^{2+}, Ca^{2+}, Zn^{2+}, Al^{2+}, Fe^{2+}) invariably cause significantly decreased fluoroquinolone absorption (20%–70% decrease in area under the concentration curve [AUC]), and this may result in therapeutic failures. Although this interaction can be avoided by taking the antacids or other products at least 2 hours before or 4 to 6 hours after the fluoroquinolone dose, this is complicated and inconvenient for the patient.[65] Patients simply should avoid these products while taking fluoroquinolones. Interactions of the fluoroquinolones with H_2-receptor antagonists and proton pump inhibitors are usually not clinically significant, and these agents can be used for patients with gastrointestinal (GI) ulcers.[65]

Some older fluoroquinolones also interfere with theophylline metabolism, especially ciprofloxacin (20%–90% increase in AUC). Norfloxacin increases the theophylline AUC by approximately 15%.[66] Therefore, theophylline levels should be monitored closely in patients receiving these quinolones and theophylline together. Levofloxacin does not significantly alter methylxanthine metabolism.[65] Whereas ciprofloxacin interferes with the metabolism of caffeine, levofloxacin does not.[65] Although the clinical significance of the interaction between caffeine and most fluoroquinolones is minimal, patients should be monitored carefully for signs and symptoms of caffeine toxicity. This is especially important for patients ingesting large quantities of caffeine and in older patients.

There have been isolated reports of a clinical interaction between certain quinolones (e.g., ciprofloxacin) and warfarin. Although there seems to be no truly relevant pharmacokinetic or pharmacodynamic interactions, patients receiving both warfarin and quinolone therapy should nevertheless be carefully monitored for changes in their anticoagulation.[65] Isolated cases have also been reported of increased toxicity with coadministration of quinolones and nonsteroidal anti-inflammatory drugs (NSAID), phenytoin, and cyclosporine; whether these interactions truly exist is unknown.[65]

HOSPITAL-ACQUIRED ACUTE URINARY TRACT INFECTION

10. P.M., an alert, 70-year-old woman with chest pain, was hospitalized to rule out acute myocardial infarction. This is her third hospitalization for chest pain in the past 6 months. A urinary catheter was temporarily placed as part of her routine medical care. Two days after admission, she complained of burning on urination and bladder pain. TMP-SMX double strength, one tablet BID was ordered after microscopic examination of the urine indicated a UTI. Why was this empiric therapy appropriate?

Hospital-acquired (or nosocomial) UTI occur in about one-half million patients per year and most are associated with the use of indwelling bladder catheters. Approximately 10% to 30% of catheterized patients develop infection.[24] Complications of catheter-associated UTI are significant. Nosocomial UTI are the source of up to 15% of all nosocomial bloodstream infections, occurring in about 4% of all catheterized patients[67]; the associated mortality rate is approximately 15%.[24] Nosocomial UTI also prolong hospitalization by an average of 2.5 days and cost an additional $600 to $700.[21,24,67] Prevention is the best way to manage nosocomial UTI, but antibiotic treatment is usually initiated in hospitalized patients who develop UTI symptoms.

The susceptibility of hospital-acquired pathogens to antimicrobial agents differs from community-acquired bacteria, and these susceptibilities frequently vary from one hospital to another. Therefore, the microbiology department of a particular hospital should be consulted to determine current trends in the antibiotic susceptibility of bacteria acquired in that setting. In general, *E. coli* is still the predominant urinary tract pathogen. An increased proportion of infections is caused, however, by other gram-negative bacteria such as *Proteus* and *Pseudomonas,* gram-positive pathogens such as *Staphylococcus* and *Enterococcus,* and yeast (e.g., *Candida*).[20,22,24]

Repeated courses of antibiotic therapy, anatomic defects of the urinary tract, old age, increased hospital length of stay, and repeated hospital admissions are associated with a higher incidence of infection with antibiotic-resistant organisms.[20,24,68,69] *Pseudomonas, Proteus, Providencia, Morganella, Klebsiella, Enterobacter, Citrobacter,* and *Serratia* are particularly difficult to eradicate because they usually are less susceptible to commonly used antimicrobial agents.

P.M. is elderly, hospitalized, and has been repeatedly exposed to potentially resistant organisms during her previous hospitalizations. Because prompt treatment is deemed necessary, oral TMP-SMX is a reasonable first choice because *E. coli* still is the most likely causative agent, and P.M. is only mildly ill with signs and symptoms of lower UTI. Oral fluoroquinolones are more commonly used in this setting, however, because of the high potential for infection with resistant pathogens.[20,70,71] Cultures of P.M.'s urine should be performed and, once C&S test results are known, therapy promptly changed according to susceptibility reports. To achieve the most cost-effective therapy, oral agents should be administered to all patients capable of taking medications by mouth unless the isolated pathogens are resistant to oral medications or underlying GI dysfunction makes adequate absorption of oral antibiotics questionable.[70,71]

11. If P.M. had additional symptoms of fever, chills, flank pain, and vomiting, how would her treatment differ?

In seriously ill patients with possible sepsis, broad-spectrum parenteral antibiotics with activity against *P. aeruginosa* are usually preferred as initial therapy (Table 64-3). Suitable antibiotic choices include antipseudomonal cephalosporins (e.g., ceftazidime, cefepime), extended-spectrum penicillins (e.g., piperacillin-tazobactam, ticarcillin-clavulanate), carbapenems (imipenem-cilastatin, meropenem), intravenous (IV) fluoroquinolones (ciprofloxacin), and aztreonam. These antibiotics appear to be at least as effective as the aminoglycosides and lack the ototoxic and nephrotoxic potential. These newer agents are more costly, however, and may be associated with the emergence of resistant organisms and superinfection with organisms such as *Enterococcus* and *Candida.*

In general, antipseudomonal β-lactam antibiotics remain the drugs of choice for nosocomial urologic sepsis.[71] The combination of a β-lactam plus an aminoglycoside may be advantageous in neutropenic patients. Once the susceptibility pattern of the infecting organism is known, therapy should be altered to single-agent therapy whenever possible to decrease both the risks of drug toxicity and the drug costs.[71]

ACUTE PYELONEPHRITIS

Signs and Symptoms

12. L.B., a 45-year-old woman with diabetes, comes to the emergency department (ED) complaining of frequent urination, fever, shaking chills, and flank pain. She takes 20 U of NPH insulin subcutaneously (SC) every morning. Positive physical findings include a temperature of 103°F, a pulse of 110 beats/minute, blood pressure (BP) of 90/60 mmHg, and CVA tenderness. A Gram stain

Table 64-3 Parenteral Antimicrobial Agents Commonly Used in the Treatment of Urinary Tract Infections

		Average Adult Daily Dose			
Class	Drug	UTI	Sepsis	Usual Dosage Interval[a]	Comments
Penicillins	Ampicillin	2–4 g	8 g	Q 4–6 hr	Use should be based on local susceptibility patterns.
	Ampicillin-sulbactam	6 g	12 g	Q 6 hr	
Extended-spectrum penicillin	Ticarcillin-clavulanate	9–12 g	18 g	Q 4–6 hr	
	Piperacillin-tazobactam	9 g	18 g	Q 4–6 hr	
First-generation cephalosporins	Cefazolin	1.5–3 g	6 g	Q 8–12 hr	More effective than second- or third-generation cephalosporins against gram-positive organisms.
Second-generation cephalosporins	Cefoxitin	3–4 g	8 g	Q 4–8 hr	Intermediate between first- and third-generation cephalosporins against gram-negative organisms.
	Cefuroxime	2.25 g	4.5 g	Q 8 hr	
	Cefotetan	1–4 g	6 g	Q 12 hr	
Third-generation cephalosporins	Cefotaxime	3–4 g	8 g	Q 6–8 hr	Better coverage than first- and second-generation cephalosporins against gram-negative organisms.
	Ceftizoxime	2–3 g	8 g	Q 8–12 hr	
	Ceftriaxone	1 g	2 g	Q 12–24 hr	Ceftazidime and cefepime are most effective against *Pseudomonas*. All generations of cephalosporins are ineffective against *Enterococcus faecalis* and methicillin-resistant staphylococci.
	Ceftazidime	1.5–3 g	6 g	Q 8–12 hr	
Fourth-generation cephalosporins	Cefepime	1–2 g	4 g	Q 12 hr	
Carbapenems	Imipenem-cilastatin	1 g	2 g	Q 6 hr	The most broad-spectrum coverage of any antibiotics listed. Ertapenem not active against *Pseudomonas*. Resistance may develop especially with *Pseudomonas*. Toxic in some pregnant animals
	Meropenem	1.5–3 g	3 g	Q 8 hr	
	Doripenem	0.5 g	0.5g	Q 8 hr	
	Ertapenem	0.5–1 g	1 g	Q 24 hr	
Monobactam	Aztreonam	1–2 g	6–8 g	Q 8–12 hr	Active against gram-negative aerobic pathogens, including *Pseudomonas* sp.
Aminoglycosides	Gentamicin	3 mg/kg	5 mg/kg	Q 8 hr	Potent against gram-negative bacteria including *Pseudomonas*. Associated with possible eighth nerve toxicity in the fetus. Amikacin should be reserved for multiresistant bacteria.
	Tobramycin	3 mg/kg	5 mg/kg	Q 8 hr	
	Amikacin	7.5 mg/kg	15 mg/kg	Q 12 hr	
Quinolones	Ciprofloxacin	400–800 mg	800 mg	Q 12 hr	Use for resistant organisms. Change to oral therapy when indicated
	Levofloxacin	250–500 mg	500–750 mg	Q 24 hr	

[a]Assuming normal renal function.

of L.B.'s urine reveals gram-negative rods, and a STAT UA demonstrates glucosuria, macroscopic hematuria, 20 to 25 WBC/mm³, numerous bacteria, and WBC casts. She also has a blood sugar level of 400 mg/dL (normal, 70–105 mg/dL). L.B. is admitted to the hospital with a diagnosis of acute bacterial pyelonephritis, and routine laboratory tests including a blood chemistry profile, complete blood count (CBC) with differential, and specimens of urine and blood for C&S are ordered. L.B. is started on IV normal saline, ampicillin 1 g IV every 6 hours, and a sliding-scale schedule of regular insulin based on every 6-hour blood sugars. Which signs and symptoms in L.B. are consistent with a kidney infection?

[SI units: blood sugar, 22.20 mmol/L (normal, 3.88–5.82)]

It is not always possible to differentiate clinically between upper and lower urinary tract infections. Symptoms common in lower UTI often are the only positive findings in upper UTI (i.e., subclinical pyelonephritis).[1,4,6,72] L.B., however, does manifest signs and symptoms of systemic infection consistent with acute bacterial pyelonephritis, including tachycardia, hypotension, fever, shaking chills, flank pain, CVA tenderness, hematuria, and WBC casts. In addition, her diabetes may predispose her to various renal infections, including pyelonephritis, possibly because diabetic patients have altered antibacterial defense mechanisms.[6,72,73]

Treatment

Triage for Hospitalization

13. Why was L.B. hospitalized?

Most patients with clinical pyelonephritis have relatively mild infection and usually can be treated as outpatients. The need for hospitalization often is determined by the patient's social situation and ability to maintain an adequate fluid intake and tolerate oral medications.[6,7,72] Patients such as L.B. with evidence of bacteremia (e.g., fever, shaking chills) or sepsis (e.g., hypotension) should be hospitalized and treated with parenteral antibiotics.[6,7,72] L.B. should be hospitalized because her acute pyelonephritis may predispose her to diabetic ketoacidosis.

Although blood cultures are usually obtained in patients with moderate-to-severe pyelonephritis, one study found that blood cultures were of low yield in the setting of acute uncomplicated pyelonephritis; they rarely provided any additional information not already obtained from the urine culture and were not helpful in the clinical management of such cases.[74] Blood cultures may be positive in up to 25% of patients with severe or complicated pyelonephritis, however, and they are still recommended for patients such as L.B.[6,72]

Antimicrobial Choice

14. Was ampicillin appropriate treatment for L.B.?

Ampicillin is not an appropriate choice for L.B. because diabetic patients (and patients treated with corticosteroids) are susceptible to colonization with unusual or more resistant organisms. As with lower tract UTI, pyelonephritis is often classified as uncomplicated or complicated. L.B.'s infection would be classified as a complicated infection because of her underlying diabetes.[6,72] *E. coli* remains the predominant pathogen in complicated pyelonephritis, but other gram-negative organisms (e.g., *Klebsiella, Proteus, Pseudomonas*) are found relatively more frequently.[6,72] Because L.B. is acutely ill and has gram-negative organisms in her urine, she should be treated with an antibiotic that has a better spectrum of activity against gram-negative organisms. Broad-spectrum antibiotics appropriate for initial therapy would include parenteral third-generation cephalosporins (e.g., ceftriaxone), IV fluoroquinolones (e.g., ciprofloxacin, levofloxacin), and piperacillin-tazobactam; aminoglycosides are also sometimes recommended as monotherapy.[6,7,75] Aztreonam may also be considered for treatment of patients with severe β-lactam allergies. It is not always necessary to initially treat patients with antipseudomonal therapy; thus, agents such as ceftriaxone with relatively less activity against *Pseudomonas* are often appropriate as initial therapy in patients such as L.B.[6,7,72,75] Because most hospital laboratories can report C&S results within 48 hours, these antibiotics can be replaced with more specific ones if appropriate.

Serum versus Urine Concentrations

15. Is it necessary to achieve bactericidal concentrations of antimicrobials in the serum, or are high urinary concentrations adequate for L.B.? How long should she be treated? How should therapeutic success be determined?

In patients with pyelonephritis and infection of the renal parenchyma, adequate tissue concentrations of antimicrobial agents are needed. Therefore, antibiotics that achieve bactericidal concentrations in serum and kidney tissues should be selected.[70] Patients requiring hospitalization should be treated with parenteral antibiotics until fluids can be taken orally and the patient is symptomatically improved and afebrile for 24 to 48 hours. This should be followed with a course of oral antibiotics for a total duration of antimicrobial therapy of 14 to 21 days; less severe infections not requiring hospitalization are usually treated with 7- to 14-day courses. Although it is customary to observe the patient in the hospital for 24 hours after switching from parenteral to oral antibiotics before discharge, this is probably of limited benefit.[6,7,72,75] Specimens for C&S should be obtained on the second day of therapy (to rule out treatment failure), 2 to 3 weeks after the completion of therapy, and again at 3 months.[1,6]

For patients who have relapsed after 14 days, retreatment for 6 weeks usually is curative. There have been reports of successful therapy with 5 days of treatment[74]; however, longer courses are recommended.[7,72,75]

Oral Therapy

16. When should oral therapy be recommended for the initial treatment of acute pyelonephritis?

Patients with mild, acute pyelonephritis (no nausea, vomiting, or signs of sepsis) can be treated with oral antibiotics such as TMP-SMX for 14 days.[6,72,75] This regimen is as effective as 6 weeks of TMP-SMX and significantly better than 6 weeks of ampicillin. The fluoroquinolones may be useful for patients infected with resistant organisms because of their excellent in vitro activity against gram-negative organisms and high kidney tissue concentrations (two- to tenfold greater than serum).[61] Agents, such as amoxicillin-clavulanate, cefixime, or cefuroxime, also can be used in this setting.

SYMPTOMATIC ABACTERIURIA

Clinical Presentation

17. R.D., a 22-year-old woman, complains of urinary frequency and painful urination, which have developed over the past 4 to 5 days. UA reveals 10 to 15 WBC/mm³ (normal, 0–2 WBC/mm³), but no bacteria are seen on a Gram stain of the urine. Phenazopyridine 200 mg three times daily (TID) is prescribed. What is a reasonable assessment of R.D.'s clinical presentation?

Acute urethral syndrome is defined as symptoms consistent with lower UTI but with no organisms evident on Gram stain or culture. The lack of detectable pathogens may mean that the urine specimen is sterile or that the concentration of the organism in the urine sample is small. Patients with these findings still may have a UTI even though the voided urine is sterile or contains $<10^5$ microorganisms per milliliter.[76] The causative organisms and the pathogenesis of infection in these cases are the same as for lower UTI. Other organisms that can cause urethritis in this setting are *Chlamydia trachomatis, N. gonorrhoeae,* and *Trichomonas vaginalis*.[76]

Most cases of UTI with low bacterial counts are associated with bacteriuria or *C. trachomatis* and also demonstrate pyuria (>8 WBC/mm³).[76] Conversely, pathogens are seldom present in patients with the acute urethral syndrome when pyuria is absent. Because R.D. is symptomatic, has 10 to 15 WBC/mm³ in her urine, and no bacteria on Gram stain, infection with *C. trachomatis* or some other more atypical pathogen is likely.

Interstitial cystitis is a chronic clinical syndrome characterized by bladder or pelvic pain and urinary frequency or urgency.[77] Although the exact cause of interstitial cystitis is not known, it is not an infection-related disorder and does not respond to antibiotic therapy. The clinical presentation of interstitial cystitis is very similar to that of symptomatic abacteriuria, but absence of pyuria is a key difference. Interstitial cystitis should be suspected in patients with clinical findings suggestive of lower UTI but who do not manifest pyuria and who have not responded to previous empiric antibiotic therapy; no antibiotics should be administered without further diagnostic evaluation.[77]

Antibiotic Treatment

18. Should R.D. be treated with antibiotics?

Yes. A double-blind, placebo-controlled study evaluated the use of doxycycline 100 mg BID in patients with UTI and low bacterial counts. Clinical cure of bacteriuria and pyuria was significantly greater in the doxycycline-treated group, but doxycycline did not alter symptoms in patients without pyuria.[76] Because *E. coli,* other gram-negative bacteria, and *C. trachomatis* are the usual causes of acute urethral syndrome, an antibiotic such as doxycycline with activity against *Chlamydia* is reasonable initial treatment for patients such as R.D. presenting with urinary tract symptoms (without bacteriuria) if pyuria also is present. All tetracyclines and sulfonamides, with or without trimethoprim, also are likely to be effective in such patients, but doxycycline has been best studied to date. Of the fluoroquinolones, newer agents, such as levofloxacin, offer promise as alternatives to doxycycline but have not been well studied in this setting.[76] Azithromycin as a single dose also has a major role in treating chlamydial infections (see Chapter 65, Sexually Transmitted Diseases).

Prolonged therapy of 2 to 4 weeks in duration and treatment of sexual partners may be required to prevent reinfection through intercourse. Prolonged therapy is appropriate if the patient has a history consistent with *Chlamydia* urethritis; a sexual partner with recent urethritis; a recent new sexual partner; a gradual, rather than abrupt, onset of symptoms that has occurred over a period of days (as in R.D.); and no hematuria. Patients without such a history can be treated with a short course of antibiotics as any other patient with a lower UTI.

Phenazopyridine

19. Was phenazopyridine appropriate for R.D.?

Phenazopyridine, a urinary tract analgesic, often is prescribed alone or along with an antibacterial agent for the symptomatic relief of dysuria. Although 200 mg orally TID may relieve dysuria, it is ineffective in the actual eradication of true UTI. Phenazopyridine plus an antibiotic is not any better than an antibiotic alone; therefore, the drug is not likely to be of significant value in R.D. and should seldom be prescribed for such patients.

Although most patients have resolution of symptoms within 24 to 48 hours after beginning therapy, some patients with severe dysuria or delayed response to antibiotic therapy may benefit symptomatically from a short trial (1–2 days) of phenazopyridine.[4] The need for, and duration of, analgesic therapy must be individualized.

Side Effects

20. What side effects have been associated with phenazopyridine?

Phenazopyridine is an azo dye and may discolor the urine to an orange-red, orange-brown, or red color that can stain clothes. Other adverse effects of phenazopyridine occur following acute overdose, or as a result of accumulation in older patients or in patients with decreased renal function who take the drug chronically. In vivo, about 50% of phenazopyridine is metabolized to aniline, which can cause methemoglobinemia and hemolytic anemia. The hemolytic anemia associated with phenazopyridine occurs primarily in patients with glucose-6-phosphate dehydrogenase (G6PD) deficiency.[78] Cases of reversible acute renal failure and allergic hepatitis have also been rarely reported following brief exposure to phenazopyridine.[78]

ASYMPTOMATIC BACTERIURIA

Antibiotic Treatment

21. A.K., an asymptomatic 6-year-old girl, is found to have significant bacteriuria on routine screening. Should she be treated with an antimicrobial agent?

The treatment of patients with asymptomatic bacteriuria depends on the clinical setting in which it is found. Asymptomatic bacteriuria occurs in a heterogeneous group of patients with different prognoses and risks. Therefore, recommendations for treatment of asymptomatic patients with significant bacteriuria (two consecutive voided urine specimens showing $\geq 10^5$ bacteria per milliliter of urine in women, or a single clean-catch voided specimen in men) are based on specific age, sex, and clinical characteristics.[1,11,12,79] These recommendations are based on the risk for development of acute UTI and subsequent long-term complications. Generally, patients who appear to benefit most from antibiotic treatment are those with complicating factors such as urinary tract structural abnormalities, immunosuppressive therapy, and procedures requiring urinary tract instrumentation or manipulation.[1,2,11] Short-course regimens (i.e., single-dose or 3-day) are usually recommended when treatment is desired,[2] although longer regimens have also been recommended.[11]

Urinary tract infections in infants and preschool children (predominantly girls) occasionally are associated with renal tissue damage.[80] Asymptomatic bacteriuria of childhood also is important because it may be a manifestation of an anatomic or mechanical defect in the urinary tract. Therefore, it should be evaluated fully. Because most cases of renal scarring as a result of bacteriuria occur within the first 5 years of life, it is controversial whether treatment should be limited to infants and preschool children or whether all children should be treated regardless of age. Screening for bacteriuria in children and treating those with positive cultures, regardless of their clinical presentation, seems reasonable and is frequently recommended.[80] Treatment of A.K., although still controversial, seems prudent because renal damage resulting from asymptomatic bacteriuria generally occurs during childhood. Should the decision be made to treat, principles of therapy are similar to those for symptomatic infections.

Pregnant Patients, the Elderly, and Other Adult Populations

22. The decision to treat the asymptomatic bacteriuria of A.K. was based primarily on the increased probability of renal damage during childhood. What other population groups should be treated for asymptomatic bacteriuria?

Without urinary tract obstruction, UTI in adults rarely lead to progressive renal damage.[2,4] Therefore, asymptomatic bacteriuria does not require treatment in most adult patients who have no evidence of mechanical obstruction or renal insufficiency. Aggressive antimicrobial therapy is appropriate during pregnancy, however, because as many as 40% of pregnant women with asymptomatic bacteriuria later develop symptomatic UTI, particularly pyelonephritis.[11] In addition, studies have confirmed associations between acute pyelonephritis during pregnancy with increased rates of preterm labor, premature delivery, and lower birth-weight infants.[26] The treatment of asymptomatic bacteriuria in pregnancy is therefore justified to decrease the risk of associated complications.[11]

Treatment should be based on in vitro susceptibility testing or by selecting the least expensive, least toxic agent. Sulfonamides should be avoided in late pregnancy because they can contribute to kernicterus in the neonate. Fluoroquinolones should be avoided during pregnancy because of the risk of arthropathies (see Question 37).

Bacteriuria in the elderly is common.[15,16] Although bacteriuria in this population often leads to symptomatic infection, clinical studies, however, have consistently documented no beneficial outcomes in treated patients compared with untreated patients.[11,15] Consequently, therapy is not recommended for the asymptomatic older patient because the expense, side effects, and potential complications of drug therapy appear to outweigh the benefits.[11,15] Patients experiencing symptomatic infections should be treated as usual.

The treatment of asymptomatic bacteriuria in women with diabetes has recently been shown not to reduce complications and is not currently recommended.[11,79] Similarly, because asymptomatic bacteriuria in patients with urinary catheters is very common (~25% with short-term catheterization and virtually 100% long-term) but is associated with few complications, antibiotic therapy is not recommended as long as the catheter remains in place. Antibiotic treatment may be considered in asymptomatic women who still have bacteruria ≥48 hours after removal of the catheter.[11]

RECURRENT URINARY TRACT INFECTIONS

Relapse versus Reinfection

23. T.W., a 28-year-old woman with a history of recurrent infections, recently was treated for an *E. coli* UTI with TMP-SMX for 10 days. A repeat UA was scheduled, but she canceled her appointment because she "felt fine." Eight weeks later, she returned to the clinic with signs and symptoms of another UTI. The only other medication she has taken is an oral contraceptive. Why would C&S testing of a urine sample be especially useful at this time?

Recurrent infections develop in approximately 20% to 30% of women with acute cystitis.[2,4,81,82] Repeat C&S data should help determine whether this infection represents a relapse or a reinfection. *Relapse* refers to a recurrence of bacteriuria caused by the same microorganism that was present before therapy initiation. Most relapses occur within 1 to 2 weeks after the completion of therapy and are caused by persistence of the organism in the urinary tract. Relapses often are associated with an inadequately treated upper UTI, structural abnormalities of the urinary tract, or chronic bacterial prostatitis.[1,81,83]

Reinfection implies recurrence of bacteriuria with a different organism than was present before therapy. Reinfections can occur at any time during or after the completion of treatment, but most appear several weeks to several months later. Approximately 80% of recurrences are caused by reinfection.[1] Reinfection is generally caused by introital colonization with *Enterobacteriaceae* from the lower intestinal tract[1]; of these, *E. coli* is the most common. Certain *E. coli* strains have been shown to adhere to vaginal epithelial cells and, in women with recurrent UTI, adherence of these organisms to epithelial cells is increased.[25] That T.W. was symptom free for 8 weeks suggests that this is a reinfection.

Oral Contraceptives as a Risk Factor

24. Is there an association between T.W.'s use of oral contraceptives and her risk of contracting a UTI?

Information regarding the association between oral contraceptive use and UTI is controversial. The two most recent studies to examine this association disagree in their conclusions. A well-designed, prospective study examined 796 women and found the incidence of UTI to be exactly the same between oral contraceptive users and nonusers.[33] A subsequent case-control study in 229 women with recurrent UTI and 253 control subjects, however, found that oral contraceptive users were at significantly higher risk for recurrent infection.[26] The association between oral contraceptive use and risk of UTI remains unclear.

The association between diaphragm use and UTI is much stronger. Diaphragm users are approximately three times more likely to develop a UTI than women using other contraceptive methods, especially when the diaphragm is used in conjunction with spermicidal jelly.[26,33] Possible explanations include urethral obstruction by the diaphragm together with increased vaginal colonization by coliform organisms caused by the spermicide. Use of a spermicide-coated condom also has been shown to increase the risk of UTI.[26,84]

Treatment for Reinfection

25. Pending the C&S results, what therapy should be instituted in T.W.?

T.W. has a history of recurrent infections and now probably has a reinfection. Because reinfection is not caused by failure of previous therapy, TMP-SMX may be a reasonable choice once again. The probability that a resistant organism will be responsible for the infection increases when the interval between infectious episodes is short. If several months elapse between each episode of antimicrobial therapy, normal fecal bacterial flora become re-established and the risk of infection with resistant pathogens is reduced.

The alteration of fecal flora caused by the sulfonamides makes these drugs poor choices for repeated use in cases of frequent reinfection, especially when C&S results are unknown. The development of bacterial resistance also may limit the usefulness of these agents for chronic antimicrobial therapy.[19,44,81,82]

26. If T.W. developed an adverse reaction to TMP-SMX, what are some other therapeutic alternatives?

Nitrofurantoin is effective against 80% to 90% of *E. coli* strains. It does not significantly alter the fecal or introital flora, and the development of resistance in previously sensitive strains does not often occur.[19,44,85] Therefore, it generally is a useful agent for the treatment of recurrent *E. coli, S. saprophyticus,* and *Enterococcus* infections. On the other hand, *Proteus, Enterobacter,* and *Klebsiella* tend to be somewhat resistant to this drug (susceptibility <60%).[19]

Nitrofurantoin is absorbed orally. Food substantially decreases the rate of absorption, but increases the total bioavailability of nitrofurantoin from both the macrocrystalline capsules and the microcrystalline tablets by about 40%. This effect lengthens the duration of therapeutic urine concentrations by about 2 hours.[86] Nitrofurantoin barely reaches detectable levels in the plasma because it is eliminated rapidly (half-life, 20 minutes) into the urine and bile; urine levels are 50 to 250 mg/L.[86] Thus, nitrofurantoin is used only for UTI. The Kirby-Bauer disc sensitivity test measures the sensitivity of an organism to the expected serum levels of most antibiotics, whereas in the case of nitrofurantoin, the test measures sensitivity to urinary levels.

The fluoroquinolones also are useful in this setting. Their widespread use should not be encouraged for reinfections as in T.W. in light of their high cost and selection of resistant organisms.[49] Cephalexin and trimethoprim also have been recommended as alternative agents in this setting.[2,81,82]

Evaluation Procedures (Localization)

27. Greater than 10^5 bacteria per milliliter of *P. mirabilis*, sensitive to ampicillin and TMP-SMX, are cultured in T.W.'s urine. One week after completing her second course of TMP-SMX therapy, signs and symptoms of a UTI again appear. How should T.W. be assessed at this time?

First, attempt to rule out common causes for relapse. Inadequate therapy resulting from patient noncompliance with the prescribed treatment, inappropriate antibiotic selection, or bacterial resistance to the prescribed agent should be considered if significant bacteriuria persists despite treatment. Next, consider renal infections (e.g., subclinical pyelonephritis), which cause many relapsing UTI.[1,2,81,82] Finally, if these common causes are not present, radiologic tests should be performed to rule out surgically correctable structural abnormalities of the urinary tract (e.g., IV pyelogram). Infected kidney stones and unilateral atrophic kidneys are common but correctable abnormalities in females.

Radiologic tests are indicated when UTI start to recur in children, in men <50 years of age, and in patients with UTI associated with bacteremia, ureteral colic, or passage of stones. These populations are most likely to have surgically correctable lesions. In contrast, these procedures rarely are necessary in adult women and elderly men until the common causes of relapse in these populations have been eliminated.[4,23,83] Chronic bacterial prostatitis should be considered as a frequent cause of recurrent infections in male patients.

Treatment of Relapse

Trimethoprim-Sulfamethoxazole

28. Pending C&S results, TMP-SMX is again prescribed. Is this still a reasonable medication for T.W. at this time?

Because the *P. mirabilis* cultured during the last recurrence was still susceptible to TMP-SMX, this agent would again be a reasonable choice until C&S results are obtained. Alternatively, use of a different agent (e.g., fluoroquinolone) could be considered because the relapse occurred within 1 week of completing the previous treatment and resistance may have developed.[4]

29. How long should this therapy be continued?

The duration of therapy for relapsing infections usually is 14 days. In patients who relapse after a second 2-week course of therapy, treatment for 6 weeks should be instituted.[1,2,83] If relapse occurs after a 6-week course, some experts recommend longer courses of 6 months to 1 year.[1,2] These prolonged courses should be reserved for children, adults who have continuous symptoms, or adults who are at high risk for developing progressive renal damage. Asymptomatic adults without evidence of obstruction should not receive these longer courses. T.W. should be treated for at least 2 weeks and perhaps as long as 6 weeks.

Trimethoprim

30. T.W. was previously treated with TMP-SMX and experienced nausea and vomiting after taking the medication. Why would trimethoprim alone be an appropriate substitute?

Trimethoprim alone and in combination with sulfamethoxazole is active in vitro against many of the *Enterobacteriaceae* associated with UTI and is an effective alternative to TMP-SMX in the management of both chronic and acute UTI.[1,2,4,83] It would be especially appropriate for T.W. because GI intolerance to TMP-SMX is most commonly attributed to the sulfamethoxazole component, and trimethoprim is associated with a lower incidence of side effects. Some concern exists for the potential development of resistant organisms, but studies using trimethoprim alone have failed to demonstrate a significant increase in bacterial resistance.[81] Trimethoprim is used for the treatment of acute, uncomplicated UTI in a dosage of 200 mg/day.

Chronic Prophylaxis

31. T.W. was treated successfully with trimethoprim for 6 weeks. Is prophylactic antimicrobial therapy indicated? If so, how long should it be continued?

Cases if chronic UTI in adult patients may be managed by treating each recurrent infection with an appropriate antibacterial. A single dose or longer course may be used. Chronic UTI may also be managed by administering chronic, low-dose prophylactic therapy. The frequency of urinary infections probably is the main determinant of whether chronic suppressive therapy should be used, because data suggest that repeated treatment of recurrent infections eventually will result in a decreased incidence of subsequent infections.[1,82,87] Long-term prophylactic therapy clearly reduces the frequency of symptomatic infections in nearly all patients.[15,87]

From a cost-effectiveness standpoint, women having more than one episode of cystitis per year may benefit from antimicrobial prophylaxis.[81,83] For women with three or more episodes of cystitis per year, prophylaxis clearly is more cost-effective than treating individual infections. Therefore, chronic antimicrobial prophylaxis should be considered in any adult patient with two or more episodes of UTI per year.[82,83]

The duration of prophylactic therapy also is determined by the frequency of infection. Women with three or more UTI in the 12 months before a 6-month course of antimicrobial prophylaxis have a significantly higher recurrence rate (75%) in the 6 months following prophylaxis than women who have had only two infections in the 12 months before prophylaxis (26% recurrence rate).[87] Therefore, prophylaxis should be continued for 6 months in patients with fewer than three UTI per year and for at least 12 months in adult patients with three or more UTI per year.

Before chronic antimicrobial suppressive therapy is initiated, active infections must be completely eradicated with a full course of appropriate antibiotic therapy. The low doses of antimicrobials used for chronic prophylaxis suppress bacterial growth but do not eliminate active infection. Furthermore, surgically correctable anatomic abnormalities that predispose the patient to recurrent infections (e.g., obstruction, stones) should be ruled out. Patients with urologic abnormalities respond poorly to prophylactic therapy.[81,83] Age also should be considered when contemplating chronic antimicrobial therapy. An asymptomatic, elderly patient taking many other medications is usually not an ideal candidate for chronic prophylactic treatment because of problems of noncompliance, cost, and potential drug interactions or toxicities.[81,83] Younger patients, however, are good candidates for long-term suppressive therapy.[82,83]

Because T.W., a 28-year-old woman, has had at least three UTI in the past few months, has undergone extensive evaluation, and has just been successfully treated with a standard course of trimethoprim, a 12-month course of antimicrobial prophylaxis would seem reasonable. She also should be evaluated at regular intervals for recurrent UTI and for the development of resistant organisms.

Although the foregoing discussion applies to antimicrobial prophylaxis in adults, relatively few data are available concerning long-term prophylaxis of recurrent UTI in children. One recent study examined risk factors for recurrent UTI and associations with antimicrobial prophylaxis in a prospective cohort study involving nearly 75,000 children 6 years of age or younger.[88] Among the children in this study, antimicrobial prophylaxis was not associated with decreased risk of recurrent UTI; however, prophylaxis was associated with a 7.5 times increased risk of infection caused by resistant bacteria. Long-term antimicrobial prophylaxis, therefore, should not be routinely recommended for prevention of recurrent UTI in children until such time as more favorable data become available.[1,2,81,82]

32. What drugs can be used for long-term suppressive therapy?

Although numerous drugs are used for prophylaxis, TMP-SMX may be the drug of choice for chronic antimicrobial therapy owing to extensive experience, proved efficacy, infrequent toxicities, and low cost.[82,83] TMP-SMX also has the effect of decreasing vaginal colonization with uropathogens.[82] TMP-SMX one-half tablet daily is commonly prescribed for chronic UTI prophylaxis; TMP-SMX TID is also an effective, well-tolerated and convenient prophylactic regimen.[82,83]

Successful prophylaxis, however, is significantly decreased in patients with urologic abnormalities or renal dysfunction. Also, infections that are not eradicated by a short-term therapeutic trial of TMP-SMX are not likely to respond to a long-term regimen.[81] Finally, enterococci may colonize introitally in patients taking chronic TMP-SMX.[87]

Fluoroquinolones are effective for chronic suppressive therapy but should be used only when antimicrobial resistance exists among cultured organisms or if the patient is intolerant to other recommended drugs. Cephalosporins also have been recommended as being appropriate for long-term prophylactic therapy, but are perhaps best reserved for patients intolerant to or failing prophylaxis with other agents.[81,83]

When selecting a drug for chronic antimicrobial therapy, it is important to consider efficacy, the likelihood that resistant organisms will develop, long-term toxicity, convenience, and cost to the patient. The most commonly used agents are listed in Table 64-4.

Based on the available information, it appears that T.W. could be switched to TMP-SMX. Although she has a history of GI distress because of this drug, this may not be a problem with the lower doses used for prophylaxis. If it is, trimethoprim alone, nitrofurantoin, or a fluoroquinolone also should be effective.

Cranberries and probiotics have long been of interest for their potentially beneficial effects in preventing UTI. Cranberries contain two known compounds that prevent *E. coli* from adhering to uroepithelial cells in the urinary tract.[89] A number of clinical trials have examined the efficacy of cranberries in the prophylaxis of UTI, but the results are inconclusive

Table 64-4 Antimicrobial Agents Commonly Used for Chronic Prophylaxis Against Recurrent UTIs[1,2,4,81–83,87]

Agent	Adult Dose	Comments[a]
Nitrofurantoin	50–100 mg nightly	Contraindicated in infant <1 month of age. *To be taken with food or milk. May cause brown or rust-yellow discoloration of urine.*
Trimethoprim	100 mg nightly	Not recommended in children <12 years of age.
Trimethoprim 80 mg + Sulfamethoxazole 400 mg	0.5–1 tablet nightly or 3/week	Not recommended for use in infants <2 months. *To be taken on an empty stomach with a full glass of water. Photosensitivity may occur.*
Norfloxacin	200 mg/day	Avoid antacids; monitor theophylline levels.
Cephalexin	125–250 mg/day	
Cefaclor	250 mg/day	
Cephradine	250 mg/day	
Sulfamethoxazole	500 mg/day	

[a] Includes unique patient consultation information in italics.

overall.[89,90] Importantly, studies have used a wide variety of cranberry products (e.g., juice concentrate, juice cocktail, capsules, tablets) as well as different dosing regimens.[89,90] Although two trials found that cranberry juice may decrease the number of symptomatic UTI over a 12-month period in younger women, it is not known whether it is effective for other groups such as children and elderly men and women.[89,90] Probiotics (particularly *Lactobacillus* strains) have also been examined as a means of supplementing or re-establishing normal rectal or vaginal flora and thereby preventing colonization with pathogenic strains associated with UTI.[91] Studies of probiotics for prophylaxis, however, are inconclusive at this time. Further research is required to clarify unanswered questions regarding the role of cranberries or probiotics in the prevention of UTI.[89,91]

SPECIAL CASES

Prostatitis

Prostatitis is a common but poorly understood entity. The most prevalent forms include acute and chronic bacterial prostatitis, chronic calculus prostatitis, nonbacterial prostatitis, and prostatodynia.[13,14]

Acute Bacterial Prostatitis

Acute bacterial prostatitis is characterized by the sudden onset of chills and fever; perineal and low back pain; urinary urgency and frequency; nocturia, dysuria, and generalized malaise; and prostration. Patients also may complain of myalgias, arthralgias, and symptoms of bladder outlet obstruction. Rectal examination usually discloses an exquisitely tender, swollen prostate that is firm and warm to the touch. The pathogens generally can be identified by culture of the voided urine and usually are similar to those causing UTI in women (Table 64-1). In patients with acute bacterial prostatitis, prostatic massage should be avoided because of patient discomfort and the risk of bacteremia.[13,14]

Chronic Bacterial Prostatitis

Chronic bacterial prostatitis is one of the most common causes of recurrent UTI in men. Except in male patients with spinal cord injuries, infectious stones, or obstructive abnormalities of the urinary tract, recurrent infections are almost always relapses caused by persistence of bacteria in the prostate. Normally, men secrete a prostatic antibacterial factor; however, this substance is absent in men with chronic prostatitis. Simple UTI will often eventually involve the prostate gland, where bacteria are difficult to eradicate.

The clinical manifestations of chronic bacterial prostatitis are highly variable and, in many patients, are asymptomatic. The disease usually is suspected when a male patient treated for UTI relapses, and the diagnosis is confirmed by examination of expressed prostatic secretions.[13,14] To ensure accurate localization (i.e., to distinguish prostatic from urethral bacteria), segmented urine samples are taken. The first 10 mL of voided urine represents the urethral sample, the midstream urine collected represents the bladder sample, and the first 10 mL voided immediately after prostatic massage represents the prostate sample. When the bladder sample is sterile or nearly so, bacterial prostatitis is diagnosed if the bacterial count in the prostate sample is at least one logarithm greater than that in the urethral sample. The bacterial pathogens responsible for chronic prostatitis often are similar to those of acute prostatitis and UTI in general (Table 64-1).[13,14]

Treatment

33. D.G., a 60-year-old man, experienced his first UTI at age 40, with symptoms of frequency, dysuria, nocturia, perineal pain, chills, and fever, but no flank pain. Acute prostatitis was diagnosed. *E. coli* was cultured from the urine, and treatment with a sulfonamide was successful. After 12 asymptomatic years, acute prostatitis caused by *E. coli* recurred and again responded to sulfonamide therapy. Two more *E. coli* infections that responded to sulfonamide therapy occurred over the next 8 years. Why were sulfonamides appropriate treatment for D.G.'s acute episodes of bacterial prostatitis?

Most antibacterial drugs appropriate for UTI, including sulfonamides, can be used to treat acute bacterial prostatitis because the diffuse, intense inflammation of the prostate gland allows many drugs to readily penetrate into the prostatic fluid and tissues. Antimicrobial therapy should be continued for at least 1 month to prevent the development of chronic prostatitis.[13,14,92]

In addition to antibiotics, other supportive measures may provide symptomatic relief to patients with acute bacterial prostatitis. These measures include liberal hydration, NSAID for pain relief, sitz baths, and stool softeners.

In retrospect, sulfonamides were appropriate for D.G. because they effectively treated his infections.

34. Taking into account the pathophysiology of prostatitis, what would be a reasonable choice of therapy for D.G. should he have future recurrences of prostatitis?

Because inflammation is minimal in patients with chronic prostatitis, most antibiotics that are acidic do not readily cross the prostatic epithelium into the alkaline prostatic fluid. Theoretically, the high alkalinity of prostatic fluids should impair the diffusion of trimethoprim and enhance the diffusion of the tetracyclines, certain sulfonamides, and the macrolide antibiotics, such as erythromycin. Nevertheless, TMP-SMX historically has the best documented cure rates in the treatment of acute and chronic bacterial prostatitis. Long-term therapy of chronic bacterial prostatitis with TMP-SMX for 4 to 16 weeks is associated with a cure rate of 32% to 71%, which significantly exceeds the cure rate associated with short-term therapy of 2 or fewer weeks.[13,14]

The fluoroquinolones have become well-accepted alternatives to TMP-SMX and are even considered by many to be the agents of choice for the treatment of prostatitis.[92] A number of studies have documented bacteriologic cure in 80% to 90% of patients treated with norfloxacin, ciprofloxacin, or levofloxacin for 4 to 12 weeks, rates comparable to or substantially higher than those achieved with agents such as TMP-SMX.[13,14] The fluoroquinolones have assumed an important role in the treatment of prostatitis owing to their bactericidal activity against common pathogens and excellent penetration into prostatic tissues and fluid. The fluoroquinolones are often used as initial empiric therapy of prostatitis and are also excellent alternatives to other agents in patients who are unresponsive or intolerant to conventional therapy, or in those infected with resistant organisms.[13,14,92] Fluoroquinolones also have been used for chronic suppressive therapy (one-half normal doses) in patients who relapse after conventional treatment.[1]

D.G. should be treated with TMP-SMX for a minimum of 6 weeks; some authorities recommend a 2- to 3-month total course of therapy. If an adequate trial of TMP-SMX is unsuccessful, fluoroquinolone therapy can be used. Alternatively, a fluoroquinolone could be used as initial therapy.[92]

If D.G. continues to develop recurrent infections following a trial of fluoroquinolone therapy, chronic low-dose treatment with TMP-SMX, fluoroquinolones, or nitrofurantoin can alleviate the symptoms of episodic bladder infection associated with chronic bacterial prostatitis. Infections eventually recur with greater frequency in most of these patients, although some become asymptomatic, even with chronic bacteriuria. Chronic, low-dose antibacterial therapy sterilizes the bladder, alleviates symptoms, confines bacteria to the prostate, and prevents infection of and damage to the rest of the urinary tract. Chronic bacterial prostatitis is one of the few indications for continuous antibiotic therapy.

Urinary Tract Infection and Sexual Intercourse

35. On routine screening, asymptomatic bacteriuria is noted in W.W., a 30-year-old pregnant woman in her first trimester. Five years ago, during her first pregnancy, she developed acute bacterial pyelonephritis, which required hospitalization and treatment with parenteral antibiotics. Since that time, she has had recurrent UTI, apparently related to sexual intercourse. These subsided when she began taking a single dose of nitrofurantoin after coitus, but she discontinued the practice before this pregnancy because she was afraid of the potential effects of this drug on the fetus. What is the association between sexual intercourse and the occurrence of UTI?

Studies strongly support an association between sexual intercourse and UTI.[1,2,26,33,83] A direct relationship seems to exist between the number of days with intercourse within the previous week and the risk of developing a UTI.[33] One study found the relative risk of infection in women with 1, 4, and 7 days of intercourse within the previous week to be 1.4, 3.5, and 9.0, respectively, compared with women who were sexually inactive within the previous week. Another study found that the risk of UTI was doubled in women having intercourse more than four times per month compared with those women who did not.[26] Studies also indicate that introital colonization by fecal bacteria has a definite role in recurrent infections related to intercourse. The migration of these colonizing bacteria into the bladder appears to be facilitated during intercourse, but the exact mechanism remains unclear.[1,2,33,83] Because UTI are uncommon in men, transmission of an infection from the man is unlikely. Occasionally, bacteria harbored under the foreskin of an uncircumcised man may be transmitted to his partner through intercourse.[3]

36. Was it rational to treat these infections with a single dose of an antibiotic after intercourse?

Postcoital antibiotic prophylaxis often is recommended when recurrent UTI are thought to result from sexual intercourse. Theoretically, a single dose of an antimicrobial agent produces bactericidal activity in the urine before bacteria have a chance to multiply, and the infection is averted. Patients should be instructed to empty their bladder just after intercourse and before taking the medication to minimize the number of bacteria present in the bladder and to eliminate unnecessary dilution of the drug in the urine. Because most drugs effective for UTI are rapidly excreted by the kidney and reach high urinary concentrations, this regimen appears reasonable and does lower the incidence of postcoital infections.[87,93] It has the same drawbacks as does any other type of antibiotic prophylaxis, however, and is not recommended in patients with structural abnormalities of the urinary tract or decreased renal function. It also is important to treat symptomatic infection before beginning prophylaxis.

Depending on the frequency of intercourse, postcoital prophylaxis may result in less antibiotic use compared with continuous prophylaxis. TMP-SMX or nitrofurantoin is the most commonly recommended agent; however, other agents such as fluoroquinolones and cephalexin may be used.[81,83,93,94]

Urinary Tract Infection and Pregnancy

37. Because W.W.'s UTI is asymptomatic at this time, should treatment be withheld because of her pregnancy?

W.W. should be treated because acute symptomatic pyelonephritis may develop in pregnant women with untreated bacteriuria. In addition, evidence suggests that maternal UTI during pregnancy are associated with increased rates of preterm labor, premature delivery, and lower birth-weight infants.[26] Although a cause-and-effect relationship has not been definitely established, treatment with an appropriate antimicrobial agent is currently recommended for all pregnant patients with significant bacteriuria.[11,27]

Nitrofurantoin is often recommended during pregnancy because teratogenic effects have not been observed clinically. In vitro investigations, however, suggest a slight mutagenic potential. Nitrofurantoin also could cause hemolytic anemia in a G6PD-deficient nursing infant; however, only small amounts have been detected in breast milk.[95,96] The fluoroquinolones are contraindicated in pregnancy because of the arthropathy observed in immature animals.[68]

The penicillins, cephalosporins, and aminoglycosides appear to be relatively safe for use during pregnancy, although caution with the aminoglycosides is warranted because of possible eighth nerve toxicity in the fetus. These drugs, along with the others listed in Tables 64-2 and 64-3, cross the placental barrier; thus, the risk of toxicity or teratogenicity to the fetus always must be considered before deciding to treat a pregnant patient with a UTI.[95,96]

In this case, a cephalosporin or sulfisoxazole could be safely prescribed for treatment of W.W.'s UTI. Ampicillin or amoxicillin would also be reasonable choices if W.W. resided in a geographic area where rates of resistance to these agents were known to be low. W.W. was correct in discontinuing her nitrofurantoin before pregnancy because of the risk to the fetus, although small, tends to offset the advantage of antimicrobial prophylaxis. W.W. must receive proper follow-up care.

38. How long should W.W. be treated?

Few studies have compared single-dose and 3-day therapy with conventional 7-day therapy in pregnant patients. Initial trials demonstrated, however, that cure rates of single-dose therapy were lower than 7- to 10-day therapy.[26] Although more recent trials have shown that single-dose therapy effectively eradicates bacteriuria in pregnancy, these studies were conducted in a small number of patients. Therefore, it is recommended that pregnant patients receive either a 3-day regimen or a 7- to 10-day regimen rather than single-dose therapy.[11,26]

Irrespective of the duration of therapy, appropriate follow-up of patients is crucial. Clinicians must document elimination of pathogens 1 to 2 weeks after therapy and follow the patient monthly for the remainder of gestation. If bacteriuria recurs, therapy should be given for relapse or reinfection and the patient evaluated radiologically for structural abnormalities.[1,26]

Urinary Catheters

Catheter-associated UTI, the most common type of hospital-acquired infection, occur in up to 30% of catheterized patients.[24] Catheterization and other forms of urologic instrumentation are involved in 65% to 95% of all hospital-acquired UTI.[20] These UTI also are a major cause of nosocomial gram-negative bacteremia.

Catheter infection can occur by bacterial entry from several routes. The urethral meatus and the distal third of the urethra normally are colonized by bacteria; therefore, initial catheter insertion can introduce bacteria into the bladder. Bacteria contaminating catheter junctions and the urine collection bag can migrate through the catheter lumen to the bladder, initiating infection.[24] The extraluminal space in the urethra also has been considered a potential route of contamination. The risk of infection is directly related to catheter insertion technique, care of the catheter, duration of catheterization, and the susceptibility of the patient. A diagnostic or single, short-term catheterization is associated with a much lower risk of infection than indwelling, long-term catheterization. Despite careful technique, the risk of contaminating a sterile bladder with urethral bacteria is always present. The incidence of infection following a single catheterization is 1% in healthy young women and 20% in debilitated patients. Each reinsertion of the catheter introduces a risk of infection.[24]

Infections have been reduced dramatically by the closed, sterile drainage system, the most common type of catheter currently in use. With this system, the drainage tube leads from the catheter directly to a closed plastic collection bag. The overall incidence of infection from the closed system with careful insertion and maintenance is about 20%; the risk increases to 50% after 14 days of catheterization. If the system is disconnected or contaminated accidentally, the infection rate is similar to that of an open system.[24]

Condom catheters appear to be associated with a lower incidence of bacteriuria than indwelling urethral catheters. These catheters avoid problems associated with insertion of a tube directly into the urinary tract; nevertheless, urine within the catheters may have high concentrations of organisms so that colonization of the urethra and subsequent cystitis may develop.[24]

To prevent bacterial contamination of the bladder when the catheter is inserted, the periurethral area should be cleansed carefully with soap and water followed by some type of antiseptic solution. An iodophor solution often is recommended. Once the catheter is in place, proper maintenance and strict adherence to good catheter care are imperative to minimize the incidence of infections. Thus, caregivers must be trained in the techniques of obtaining urine samples from closed systems. Application of antibacterial substances to the collection bag and the catheter–urethral interface do not appear to decrease the incidence of bacteriuria.[24,97,98] The use of antimicrobial-coated catheters (e.g., silver, rifampin plus minocycline) have been shown in some studies to decreased rates of bacteriuria and UTI.[97,98] The overall effects of these catheters on infection rates, patient outcomes, and antibiotic resistance are not known, however. The routine use of antibiotic-coated catheters is not currently recommended.[95,97]

39. J.W., an 18-year-old man, was hospitalized following a diving accident that resulted in a spinal cord injury with paralysis. Included among several initial interventions was insertion of an indwelling catheter with a closed drainage system because of bladder incontinence. Two weeks after admission to the hospital, J.W. has developed asymptomatic bacteriuria. Should this be treated?

A systemic antibiotic selected specifically for the infecting organism will temporarily result in sterile urine. Reinfection, often by a resistant organism, occurs in 30% to 50% of these cases if closed drainage catheterization is continued during therapy.[1,24] For this reason, it generally is recommended that systemic antimicrobial therapy be initiated after or just before catheter removal.[1,24] Because long-term catheterization is necessary in many patients and because bacteriuria is an inevitable consequence, it is often recommended that asymptomatic patients (such as J.W.) be left untreated to avoid the complications of recolonization and potential infection with resistant organisms.[1,11,24] Therapy must be started, however, if fever, flank pain, or other symptoms indicative of UTI develop.[1,24]

40. Is systemic antimicrobial prophylaxis useful for J.W.?

The benefits of systemic antibiotics in preventing catheter-induced UTI are not clear. Studies using closed drainage systems with diligent catheter care indicate that systemic antibiotics decrease the daily and overall incidence of infection in patients with sterile urines before catheterization.[97,98] The preventive effect of antimicrobials is greatest for short-term catheterizations or during the first 4 to 7 days of long-term catheterization.[97,98] Thereafter, the rate of infection increases. Although the overall infection rate remains lower than in untreated patients, the emergence of resistant organisms is significant. Therefore, in deciding to use systemic antimicrobials, it is important to consider the patient's underlying diseases, risk factors, probable duration of catheterization, and potential complications of drug toxicity or resistant organisms that can result from the chronic use of antimicrobials. Because long-term catheterization is anticipated for J.W., antimicrobial prophylaxis for J.W. is not recommended.

41. C.A., a 60-year-old woman admitted for coronary bypass, is catheterized for urinary incontinence. Two days after removal of the catheter, she still has asymptomatic bacteriuria. How should she be treated?

Catheter-acquired bacteriuria that persists 48 hours after catheter removal may be treated with either a single large dose or a 3-day regimen of TMP-SMX, even if the patient is asymptomatic.[11,24,92] Older women (>65 years) probably should be treated with a 10-day course; however, the optimal duration in this age group is unknown. Whether these treatment regimens can be used in male patients requires further study.

Renal Failure

42. K.M., a 55-year-old man with a history of hypertension and chronic renal failure, develops a UTI. His creatinine clearance (ClCr), determined from a recent 24-hour urine collection, is 20 mL/minute. What antimicrobial agent should be prescribed?

[SI unit: SrCr, 0.33 mL/sec]

The major problem in treating UTI in patients with renal failure is how to achieve adequate urine concentrations of the drug without causing systemic toxicity. The ideal drug would be (a) inherently nontoxic, even at high serum concentrations, making dosage adjustments unnecessary; (b) excreted unchanged in the urine (i.e., not metabolized); and (c) eliminated by renal tubular secretion rather than glomerular filtration. Because renal tubular secretion remains active in all but the most severe cases of renal failure, antibiotics eliminated by this mechanism would reach adequate urinary levels; however, no such ideal drug exists.

Nitrofurantoin, doxycycline, and many sulfonamides are substantially metabolized by the liver and generally produce low urine levels in uremic patients. The aminoglycosides are eliminated almost exclusively by the kidneys, but uremic patients are at high risk of drug-induced toxicities and alternative agents are usually recommended. Penicillins, cephalosporins, and trimethoprim are partially metabolized by the liver but are also eliminated by the kidney to a significant extent. These agents are suitable for use in renal failure according to the criteria described above. Certain fluoroquinolones, specifically ciprofloxacin and levofloxacin, are highly excreted in the urine through a combination of filtration and tubular secretion and reach extremely high urinary concentrations. These agents are also considered safe and effective in the treatment of UTI in patients with renal failure.

ADVERSE DRUG REACTIONS AND DRUG INTERACTIONS

Trimethoprim-Sulfamethoxazole

Hemolytic Anemia

43. G.R., a 45-year-old black man with an 8-year history of congestive heart failure, was admitted to the hospital with increasing shortness of breath. His hematocrit (Hct) was stable at around 42% (normal in men, 40%–49%) and his total serum bilirubin was 0.8 mg/dL (normal, 0.2– 1.1 mg/dL). Sixteen days after admission, an *E. coli* UTI was diagnosed and G.R. was treated with TMP-SMX 160 mg/800 mg twice daily. Four days after beginning TMP-SMX, the Hct suddenly dropped to 25% and the hemoglobin (Hgb) to 8.4 g/dL (normal in men, 14–18 g/dL). There were no signs of bleeding, but his sclerae became icteric. After 7 days of TMP-SMX therapy, the Hct was still 25%, but the reticulocyte count had risen to 6.6% (normal, 0.5%–1.5%) and the total serum bilirubin was 3.0 mg/dL. The TMP-SMX was discontinued, and over a period of 2 weeks the Hct steadily rose to 40%. What mechanism might explain G.R.'s sulfonamide-induced hemolytic anemia? Is his presentation typical? Are there any other drugs used to treat UTI that can cause a similar reaction?

[SI units: Hct, 0.39 to 0.43, 0.25, and 0.40, respectively (normal, 0.40–0.49); bilirubin, 13.7 and 51.3 μmol/L, respectively (normal, 3.4–18.8); Hgb, 84 g/L (normal, 140–180 g/L); reticulocyte count, 0.066 (normal, 0.005–0.015)]

Hemolytic anemia is associated with sulfonamide administration and may be mediated by several mechanisms, including abnormally high blood levels, acquired hypersensitivity as reflected by the development of a positive Coombs' test, genetically determined abnormalities of red blood cell metabolism (e.g., G6PD deficiency), or an "unstable" hemoglobin in RBC (e.g., Hgb Zurich, Hgb Towns, Hgb H).[91,92] Although the defect appears to be most common in Mediterranean male patients, one variant affects as many as 11% of American black men.[92]

Acute hemolytic anemia induced by sulfonamides in G6PD-deficient patients does not appear to be dose related. It usually is abrupt in onset and occurs within the first week of therapy. Typical symptoms include nausea, fever, vertigo, jaundice, hepatosplenomegaly, and occasionally, hypotension. Hematocrit and hemoglobin values may fall precipitously and may be reduced to 30% to 50% of the normal values, as illustrated by G.R., Leukocytosis and reticulocytosis are common, and acute renal failure may result from the hypotension and hemoglobinuria. A mild hemolytic episode is characterized by reticulocytosis without a significant fall in hemoglobin or hematocrit. Nitrofurantoin has also been reported to induce G6PD-deficiency hemolysis.[99]

Clinical illness, as well as drug administration, can precipitate hemolysis in patients with G6PD deficiency. Patients with chronic bacterial infections of the urinary or upper respiratory tract who receive chronic or repetitive courses of certain drugs are particularly predisposed to hemolysis.[99]

Patients with enzyme deficiencies, especially those enzymes associated with the pentose-phosphate shunt (as is G6PD), can develop hemolytic reactions when taking drugs commonly used to treat UTI. Future use of sulfonamides or nitrofurantoin should be avoided in G.R.

Rash and Drug Fever

44. J.P., a 63-year-old diabetic woman taking glipizide 10 mg/day, developed an acute UTI for which TMP-SMX 160 mg/800 mg BID for 10 days was prescribed. Seven days later she presented to the ED with a pruritic maculopapular rash and fever. Are the rash and fever in J.P. typical of that caused by the sulfonamides?

Yes. Rash is one of the more common side effects associated with sulfonamide use and occurs in approximately 1% to 2% of patients treated with TMP-SMX. Various hypersensitivity skin and mucous membrane reactions have been reported, including morbilliform, scarlatinal, urticarial, erysipeloid, pemphigoid, purpuric, and petechial rashes. Erythema nodosum, exfoliative dermatitis, photosensitivity reactions, and the Stevens-Johnson syndrome also are associated with sulfonamides. Skin eruptions usually appear after 1 week of treatment, although more rapid onset may occur in a sensitized person.[53] The hypersensitivity reactions that occurred in J.P. signify that an alternate drug should be used to treat future UTI.

Folate Deficiency

45. D.M., a 50-year-old epileptic woman, has been taking prophylactic TMP-SMX nightly for 3 months for chronic recurrent

UTI. She also takes phenytoin 300 mg/day, which effectively controls her seizures, and diazepam 2 mg TID. She smokes one pack of cigarettes/day and drinks 1 pint of gin/day. Routine CBC after a clinic visit shows a Hgb of 9 g/dL (normal in females, 13.5–16.7 g/dL), a Hct of 30% (normal in females, 40%–49%), a mean corpuscular volume (MCV) of 105 mm^3 (normal, 80–100 mm^3), and a mean corpuscular hemoglobin concentration (MCHC) of 32% (normal, 32%–36%). Could TMP-SMX account for D.M.'s megaloblastic anemia?

[SI units: Hgb, 90 g/L (normal, 135–167); Hct, 0.30 (normal, 0.40–0.49); MCV, 105 fL (normal, 80–100); MCHC, 0.32 (normal, 0.32–0.36)]

Megaloblastic anemia secondary to folate deficiency has been rarely associated with the use of TMP-SMX.[53] Sulfonamides inhibit folic acid synthesis in bacterial and protozoal cells but do not affect the human cell to a significant degree, except when given in high doses. It is especially a problem in patients with known or potentially deficient folic acid stores, such as pregnant women, older persons, patients with malabsorption or malnutrition, alcoholics, patients receiving anticonvulsants, or those with chronic hemolysis (e.g., sickle cell disease). Concomitant administration of folic acid reverses these effects without interfering with antimicrobial activity.[53] It is doubtful that significant folate deficiency occurs following short-term TMP-SMX therapy or in patients without the above risk factors.

In D.M., both phenytoin and alcohol undoubtedly contributed to folate deficiency anemia. Whether or not TMP-SMX was a significant factor may be questioned, but an alternate antibacterial may be preferable in a patient already at risk for folate deficiency.

Nitrofurantoin

Gastrointestinal Disturbance

46. J.R., a 45-year-old, 110-pound woman, is given nitrofurantoin 100 mg four times daily (QID) for 14 days for an acute UTI. She complains of nausea and GI upset after the ingestion of each dose of nitrofurantoin. How can this effect be minimized?

Nausea is a fairly common complication of nitrofurantoin therapy, and the patient's compliance with the prescribed regimen may be severely affected by this common side effect. It is not known whether the mechanism by which nitrofurantoin produces nausea is central or local. The following approaches can be used to decrease nitrofurantoin-induced nausea:

- *Take Each Dose With Food.* Nitrofurantoin should be taken with food or milk. If the nausea is a locally mediated effect, the food may serve as a buffer; if the nausea is centrally mediated, then food may slow the rate of absorption and lower the peak serum concentration of the drug. Food, however, may also increase the bioavailability of nitrofurantoin. Slowing of absorption is particularly beneficial in decreasing the incidence of nausea and vomiting associated with the microcrystalline product.[94]
- *Change to a Macrocrystalline Product.* Use of the macrocrystalline preparation results in significantly fewer adverse effects without affecting clinical cure rates. The larger particle size of the macrocrystalline preparation results in slower rates of dissolution and absorption, and lower serum levels. This may decrease the nausea and vomiting associated with the microcrystalline product.[94] A disadvantage of the macrocrystalline form is the cost, which may be 2 to 10 times that of the microcrystalline form, depending on the product source.
- *Lower the Dose.* Nausea and vomiting appear to be dose related and occur more frequently in small persons.[94] The minimal effective dose of nitrofurantoin generally is stated to be 5 mg/kg/day and the average dose is usually 7 mg/kg/day. At daily doses >7 mg/kg, the incidence of nausea appears to increase significantly, so the dose in this 110-pound (50 kg) patient could be decreased.

Pneumonitis

47. J.R. tolerated the macrocrystalline form taken with meals and continued her regimen. However, 10 days later she presented with dyspnea, tachypnea, coughing, and wheezing. Examination revealed a temperature of 38.4°C, pulse of 115 beats/minute, and soft inspiratory and expiratory rhonchi with a few bibasilar rales. Nitrofurantoin was stopped, and inhaled β_2-agonists and steroids were administered. Symptoms gradually disappeared after a few days; however, rechallenge with a single 50-mg dose of nitrofurantoin caused a recurrence of the respiratory distress. What is the nature of the apparent nitrofurantoin-induced respiratory reaction that occurred in J.R.?

Several hundred cases of nitrofurantoin-induced pulmonary reactions have been reported.[100] Acute, subacute, and chronic reactions have been described. The acute form, illustrated by J.R., often manifests within several days of initiating the drug with a sudden flulike syndrome consisting of fever, dyspnea, and cough. The subacute form tends to occur after at least a month of exposure; symptoms include fever and dyspnea. The chronic form tends to be more insidious with milder dyspnea and low-grade fever. In all forms, rales are commonly heard and pulmonary infiltrates can be demonstrated on chest radiograph. Although eosinophilia frequently occurs with the acute form, it may be absent with the subacute and chronic forms. Antinuclear antibodies are elevated in the latter two forms. Discontinuation of nitrofurantoin results in complete symptomatic recovery after several weeks; however, permanent fibrotic changes may persist with the chronic pulmonary reaction. Although steroids are frequently administered when the adverse reaction is diagnosed, their efficacy has not been demonstrated. Rechallenge with oral nitrofurantoin results in rapid reappearance of pulmonary symptoms in those who have had an acute reaction.[100]

Neurotoxicity

48. G.T., a 55-year-old woman, has been taking nitrofurantoin 100 mg QID for an acute UTI. Pertinent history includes hypertension and moderate renal failure. Medications include lisinopril, hydrochlorothiazide, and allopurinol. On the tenth day of therapy, she complains that both her hands and feet feel numb and weak. Physical examination shows significant sensory loss to the hands and feet as well as no ankle reflexes, although knee and arm reflexes are present. What are the characteristics of neuropathy associated with nitrofurantoin therapy?

Peripheral neuropathy usually is characterized by symmetric dysesthesia and paresthesia in the distal extremities, which progresses in a central and ascending fashion. It usually occurs within the first 60 days of treatment, although neuropathy can be recognized up to 6 weeks after discontinuation of therapy in 16% of patients. Symptom severity is not dose related and is generally reversible, although more severe cases may require up to several months to resolve completely; a few patients may develop permanent neuropathy. Renal failure is a risk factor for toxicity, but neuropathy has also been reported in patients with normal renal function.[86,94]

Nitrofurantoin excretion is impaired in renal failure; however, serum levels do not rise proportionately, suggesting that the drug might be sequestered in an extravascular space. It has been postulated that neurotoxicity is caused by accumulation of nitrofurantoin in neural tissue, or that toxic metabolites are involved.[86,94] In view of the inability to achieve adequate urinary concentrations of nitrofurantoin, even in mild renal failure, G.T. should not be given this drug.

Fluoroquinolone Use in Pediatric Infections

49. C.S. is a 2-year old girl with a history of multiple recurrent UTI caused by congenital urinary tract abnormalities that have not been corrected. She has had at least nine UTI since birth and has received multiple courses of antibiotics, including ampicillin, amoxicillin, amoxicillin-clavulanate, and TMP-SMX. She has also been on chronic low-dose antibiotic prophylaxis with TMP-SMX. C.S. was brought to her pediatrician 48 hours ago with signs and symptoms consistent with a new UTI. Suprapubital aspiration was performed and urine samples sent for C&S testing at that time, and C.S. was empirically begun on amoxicillin-clavulanate pending laboratory test results. C&S results, however, are now available and show $>10^5$ colonies/mm^3 of *P. mirabilis.* The organism is susceptible to ciprofloxacin, gentamicin, and ertapenem; and resistant to ampicillin, trimethoprim, TMP-SMX, cephalexin, cefaclor, cefpodoxime, tetracycline, nitrofurantoin, and erythromycin. C.S. has not clinically improved while receiving empiric amoxicillin-clavulanate. What antibiotic therapy would be most appropriate for continued management of this acute infection in C.S.?

This case illustrates the serious dilemmas caused by antibiotic resistance among uropathogens. The pathogen isolated from C.S. is resistant to all commonly used, orally administered antibiotics that have been proved effective in the treatment of UTI in pediatric patients. Although penicillins, cephalosporins, nitrofurantoin, and sulfonamides are frequently recommended for treatment of pediatric UTI, multiple past treatment regimens and chronic antibiotic prophylaxis have led to these agents being unsuitable for treatment of this new infection. Although in vitro susceptibility testing does not accurately predict clinical response to therapy in all cases, the risk of treatment failure and poor patient outcome is significantly increased when agents to which isolates are resistant are administered.[42,43,51,52,56,57] Alternative treatment is required; however, few desirable options exist for C.S.

The recommended duration of antibiotic therapy in C.S. would be at least 2 weeks for the treatment of this complicated and recurrent infection. Although the organism isolated from C.S. is susceptible to gentamicin and this drug would be effective, parenteral (intramuscular or intravenous) administration would be required and the lengthy required treatment duration makes this far from ideal. Use of aminoglycosides would also be less desirable because of toxicity concerns. Although ertapenem would also likely be effective, there is relatively little clinical experience with this agent in the pediatric population and ertapenem would also require parenteral administration for the duration of the treatment regimen.

Fluoroquinolones are contraindicated in children and adolescents <18 years of age because of concerns regarding potential musculoskeletal toxicities in juvenile populations. Although not approved for pediatric use, fluoroquinolones have been formally studied for febrile neutropenia, infectious gastroenteritis, otitis media, bacterial meningitis, and other uses.[101–103] In addition, the use of fluoroquinolones has been noted to be dramatically increasing in children and adolescents, most likely owing to resistance to other antimicrobials; approximately 520,000 prescriptions were written for patients <18 years of age during 2002, of which nearly 3,000 prescriptions were for children <2 years.[101] Several recent reviews have summarized data related to the safety of fluoroquinolones in children; while tendinopathy or other musculoskeletal toxicities have been recorded, they were usually mild in severity, reversible, and occurred at rates comparable to that seen in adults.[101–103] Based on currently available information and in consideration of problems related to antimicrobial resistance, the American Academy of Pediatrics has published recommendations regarding the use of fluoroquinolones in children and adolescents.[101] According to these recommendations, fluoroquinolones may be considered in special circumstances including (a) infections caused by multidrug-resistant pathogens for which there are no other safe and effective alternatives; and (b) parenteral therapy is not feasible and no other effective oral agent is available. Treatment of UTI caused by multidrug-resistant, gram-negative pathogens are specifically mentioned as a potentially appropriate use for fluoroquinolones in pediatric patients.[101]

Selection of a specific agent for the treatment of UTI in C.S. should be based on careful consideration of potential risks and benefits of available antibiotic options. The feasibility, risks, expenses, and inconvenience associated with prolonged ($\geq$2 weeks) parenteral administration of an aminoglycoside or carbapenem may pose a difficult problem; however, the ease of oral fluoroquinolone administration must be carefully balanced against the possible risks of using these agents in this population. Clearly, no antibiotic of choice exists for treatment of C.S. and both the providers and the child's parents must be involved in development of an acceptable and well-informed treatment plan.

GLOSSARY

Acute pyelonephritis: Inflammation of the kidney, with flank pain and tenderness, bacteriuria (often bacteremia), pyuria, and fever.

Bacteriuria: Bacteria cultured from urine when it is obtained by either suprapubic aspiration, catheterization, or from a freshly voided specimen. Asymptomatic bacteriuria exists if colony counts exceed 10^5/mL in a patient without UTI symptoms. Clinically significant bacteriuria probably exists if colony counts are $\geq 10^2$/mL in patients with UTI symptoms.

Chronic pyelonephritis: A chronic, inflammatory condition of the kidney with associated calyceal dilation and overlying cortical scarring. A nonspecific pathologic appearance of the kidney seen with many disease entities, only one of which is bacterial infection of the kidney.

Complicated urinary tract infection: Infections associated with conditions that increase the risk for acquiring infection, the potential for serious outcomes, or the risk for therapy failure. Such conditions are often associated with abnormalities that may interfere with normal urine flow or the voiding mechanism. Infections in men, children, and pregnant women are considered complicated. Other examples of complicated infections include those associated with structural and neurologic abnormalities of the urinary tract, metabolic or hormonal abnormalities, impaired host responses, and those caused by unusual pathogens (e.g., yeasts, *Mycoplasma*).

Cystitis: An inflammation of the bladder and urethra with dysuria, frequency, urgency, pyuria, clinically significant bacteriuria, and suprapubic tenderness on examination.

Prostatitis: An inflammatory condition affecting the prostate. It can be acute or chronic. Frequently, specific bacterial organisms cannot be detected.

Pyuria: White blood cells in the urine. A WBC count of $\geq$8/mm^3 of uncentrifuged urine or 2 to 5 per HPF in centrifuged urine sediment is consistent with a UTI.

Subclinical pyelonephritis: A kidney infection, but with lower UTI signs and symptoms only. Uncomplicated urinary tract infection: Infections occurring in otherwise healthy persons, usually women, who have none of the underlying risk factors known to increase the risk for treatment complications or failure (see Complicated UTI above).

Urethritis: An inflammation of the urethra with dysuria. The etiologic organisms most commonly implicated are *Neisseria gonorrhoeae, Ureaplasma urealyticum, Chlamydia trachomatis,* and herpes simplex virus.

Urinary tract infection: Microorganisms (bacteria, fungi, viruses) in the urinary tract, including the bladder, prostate, kidneys, and collecting duct. Although fungi and viruses are occasional etiologic agents, UTI are predominantly caused by bacteria.

Vaginitis: Inflammation of the vagina with dysuria, vaginal discharge, and vaginal odor. Common etiologic agents include *Candida albicans, Gardnerella vaginalis,* and trichomonads.

REFERENCES

1. Sobel JD et al. Urinary tract infections. In: Mandell GL et al., eds. *Principles and Practice of Infectious Diseases.* 6th ed. New York: Churchill Livingstone; 2006:875.
2. McLaughlin SP et al. Urinary tract infections in women. *Med Clin North Am* 2004;88:417.
3. Finer G et al. Pathogenesis of urinary tract infections with normal female anatomy. *Lancet Infect Dis* 2004;4:631.
4. Mehnert-Kay SA. Diagnosis and management of uncomplicated urinary tract infections. *Am Fam Physician* 2005;72:451.
5. Smith HS et al. Antecedent antimicrobial use increases the risk of uncomplicated cystitis in young women. *Clin Infect Dis* 1997;25:63.
6. Ramakrishnan K et al. Diagnosis and management of acute pyelonephritis in adults. *Am Fam Physician* 2005;71:933.
7. Kucheria R et al. Urinary tract infections: new insights into a common problem. *Postgrad Med J* 2005;81:83.
8. Foxman B et al. Urinary tract infection: self-reported incidence and associated costs. *Ann Epidemiol* 2000;10:509.
9. Craig JC. Urinary tract infection: new perspectives on a common disease. *Curr Opin Infect Dis* 2001;14:309.
10. Brown P et al. Acute pyelonephritis among adults: cost of illness and considerations for the economic evaluation of therapy. *Pharmacoeconomics* 2005;23:1123.
11. Nicolle LE et al. Infectious Diseases Society of America guidelines for the diagnosis and treatment of asymptomatic bateriuria in adults. *Clin Infect Dis* 2005;40:643.
12. Hansson S et al. The natural history of bacteriurua in childhood. *Med Clin North Am* 1997;11:499.
13. Hua VN et al. Acute and chronic prostatitis. *Med Clin North Am* 2004;88:483.
14. Lummus WE et al. Prostatitis. *Emerg Med Clin North Am* 2001;19:691.
15. Wagenlehner FM et al. Asymptomatic bacteriuria in elderly patients: significance and implications for treatment. *Drugs Aging* 2005;22:801.
16. Nicolle LE. Urinary tract infection in long-term-care facility residents. *Clin Infect Dis* 2000;31:757.
17. Richards CL. Urinary tract infections in the frail elderly: issues for diagnosis, treatment and prevention. *Int Urol Nephrol* 2004;36:457.
18. Matsumoto T. Urinary tract infections in the elderly. *Curr Urol Rep* 2001;2:330.
19. Gupta K et al. Antimicrobial resistance among uropathogens that cause community-acquired urinary tract infections in women: a nationwide analysis. *Clin Infect Dis* 2001;33:89.
20. Bagshaw SM et al. Epidemiology of intensive care unit-acquired urinary tract infections. *Curr Opin Infect Dis* 2006;19:67.
21. Tambyah PA et al. The direct costs of nosocomial catheter-associated urinary tract infection in the era of managed care. *Infect Control Hosp Epidemiol* 2002;23:27.
22. Laupland KB et al. Incidence and risk factors for acquiring nosocomial urinary tract infection in the critically ill. *J Crit Care* 2002;17:50.
23. Wagenlehner FM et al. Current challenges in the treatment of complicated urinary tract infections and prostatitis. *Clin Microbiol Infect* 2006;12(Suppl 3):67.
24. Tambyah PA. Catheter-associated urinary tract infections: diagnosis and prophylaxis. *Int J Antimicrob Agents* 2004;24(Suppl 1):S44.
25. Kim BY et al. Invasion processes of pathogenic *Escherichia coli. Int J Med Microbiol* 2005;295:463.
26. Scholes D et al. Risk factors for recurrent urinary tract infection in young women. *J Infect Dis* 2000;182:1177.
27. Le J et al. Urinary tract infections during pregnancy. *Ann Pharmacother* 2004;38:1692.
28. Tolkoff-Rubin NE et al. Urinary tract infection in the immunocompromised host. *Infect Dis Clin North Am* 1997;11:707.
29. Stapleton A. Urinary tract infections in patients with diabetes. *Am J Med* 2002;113(Suppl 1A):80S.
30. Nicolle LE. Urinary tract infection in diabetes. *Curr Opin Infect Dis* 2005;18:49.
31. Boyko EJ et al. Diabetes and the risk of acute urinary tract infection among postmenopausal women. *Diabetes Care* 2002;25:1778.
32. Foxman B et al. First time urinary tract infection and sexual behavior. *Epidemiology* 1995;6:162.
33. Hooton TM et al. A prospective study of risk factors for symptomatic urinary tract infection in young women. *N Engl J Med* 1996;335:468.
34. Handley MA et al. Incidence of acute urinary tract infection in young women and use of male condoms with and without nonoxynol-9 spermicides. *Epidemiology* 2002;13:431.
35. Eschenbach DA et al. Effects of vaginal intercourse with and without a condom on vaginal flora and vaginal epithelium. *J Infect Dis* 2001;183:913.
36. Gupta K et al. Effects of contraceptive method on the vaginal microbial flora: a prospective evaluation. *J Infect Dis* 2000;181:595.
37. Bent S et al. Does this woman have an acute uncomplicated urinary tract infection? *JAMA* 2002;287:2701.
38. Simerville JA et al. Urinalysis: a comprehensive review. *Am Fam Physician* 71:1153.
39. Deville WL et al. The urine dipstick test useful to rule out infections. A meta-analysis of the accuracy. *BMC Urol* 2004;4:4.
40. Dimitrakov J et al. Recent developments in diagnosis and therapy of the prostatitis syndromes. *Curr Opin Urol* 2001;11:87.
41. Koeijers JJ et al. Evaluation of the nitrite and leukocyte esterase activity tests for the diagnosis of acute symptomatic urinary tract infection in men. *Clin Infect Dis* 2007;45:894.
42. Miller LG et al. Treatment of uncomplicated urinary tract infections in an era of increasing antimicrobial resistance. *Mayo Clin Proc* 2004;79:1048.
43. David RD et al. Rational antibiotic treatment of outpatient genitourinary infections in a changing environment. *Am J Med* 2005;118(Suppl 7A):7S.
44. Mazzulli T. Resistance trends in urinary tract pathogens and impact on management. *J Urol* 2002;168(Suppl):1720.
45. Gupta K et al. Increasing prevalence of antimicrobial resistance among uropathogens causing acute uncomplicated cystitis in women. *JAMA* 1999;281:736.
46. Pitout JD et al. Emergence of Enterobacteriaceae producing extended-spectrum beta-lactamases (ESBLs) in the community. *J Antimicrob Chemother* 2005;56:52.
47. Milo G et al. Duration of antibacterial treatment for uncomplicated urinary tract infection in women. *Cochrane Database Syst Rev* 2005;2:CD004682.
48. Warren JW et al. Guidelines for antimicrobial treatment of uncomplicated acute bacterial cystitis and

acute pyelonephritis in women. *Clin Infect Dis* 1999;29:745.
49. Nicolle LE. Urinary tract infection: traditional pharmacological therapies. *Dis Mon* 2003;49:111.
50. Gupta K et al. Short-course nitrofurantoin for the treatment of acute uncomplicated cystitis in women. *Arch Intern Med* 2007;167:2207.
51. Le TP et al. Empirical therapy for uncomplicated urinary tract infections in an era of increasing antimicrobial resistance: a decision and cost analysis. *Clin Infect Dis* 2001;33:615.
52. Raz R et al. Empiric use of trimethoprim-sulfamethoxazole (TMP-SMX) in the treatment of women with uncomplicated urinary tract infections, in a geographical area with a high prevalence of TMP-SMX-resistant uropathogens. *Clin Infect Dis* 2002;34:1165.
53. Masters PA et al. Trimethoprim-sulfamethoxazole revisited. *Arch Intern Med* 2003;163:402.
54. Muratani T et al. Bacterial resistance to antimicrobials in urinary isolates. *Int J Antimicrob Agents* 2004;24(Suppl):S28.
55. Zinner SH et al. Sulfonamides and trimethoprim. In: Mardell GL et al., eds. *Principles and Practice of Infectious Diseases*. 6th ed. New York: Churchill Livingstone; 2006:440.
56. Talan D et al. Comparison of ciprofloxacin (7 days) and trimethoprim-sulfamethoxazole (14 days) for acute uncomplicated pyelonephritis in women: a randomized trial. *JAMA* 2000;283:1583.
57. McNulty CAM et al. Clinical relevance of laboratory–reported antibiotic resistance in acute uncomplicated urinary tract infection in primary care. *J Antimicrob Chemother* 2006;58:1000.
58. Gupta K et al. Outcomes associated with trimethoprim/sulfamethoxazole (TMP/SMX) therapy in TMP/SMX resistant community-acquired UTI. *Int J Antimicrob Agent* 2002;19:554.
59. Noskin GA et al. Disappearance of the uncomplicated urinary tract infection: the impact of emerging resistance. *Clin Drug Invest* 2001;21(Suppl):13.
60. Brown PD et al. Prevalence and predictors of trimethoprim-sulfamethoxazole resistance among uropathogenic *Escherichia coli* isolates in Michigan. *Clin Infect Dis* 2002;34:1061.
61. Hooper DC. Quinolones. In: Mandell GL et al., eds. *Principles and Practice of Infectious Diseases*. 6th ed. New York: Churchill Livingstone; 2006:451.
62. Karlowsky JA et al. Fluoroquinolone-resistant urinary isolates of Escherichia coli from outpatients are frequently multidrug resistant: results from the North American Urinary tract Infection Collaborative Alliance-Quinolone Resistance Study. *Antimicrob Agents Chemother* 2006;50:2251.
63. Richard GA et al. Levofloxacin versus ciprofloxacin versus lomefloxacin in acute pyelonephritis. *Urology* 1998;52:51.
64. Pisani E et al. Lomefloxacin versus ciprofloxacin in the treatment of complicated urinary tract infections: a multicenter study. *J Chemother* 1996;8:210.
65. Fish DN. Fluoroquinolone adverse effects and drug interactions. *Pharmacotherapy* 2001;21(Suppl):253S.
66. Ho G et al. Evaluation of the effect of norfloxacin on the pharmacokinetics of theophylline. *Clin Pharmacol Ther* 1988;44:35.
67. Saint S. Clinical and economic consequences of nosocomial catheter-associated bacteriuria. *Am J Infect Control* 2000;28:68.
68. Nguyen-Van-Tam SE et al. Risk factors for hospital-acquired urinary tract infection in a large English teaching hospital: a case-control study. *Infection.* 1999;27:192.
69. Wagenlehner FM et al. Spectrum and antibiotic resistance or uropathogens from hospitalized patients with urinary tract infections: 1994–2000. *Int J Antimicrob Agents* 2002;19:557.
70. Wagenlehner FM et al. Emergence of antibiotic resistance amongst hospital-acquired urinary tract infections and pharmacokinetic/pharmacodynamic considerations. *J Hosp Infect* 2005;60:191.
71. Liu H et al. Appropriate antibiotic treatment of genitourinary infections in hospitalized patients. *Am J Med* 2005;118(Suppl 7A):14S.
72. Miller O et al. Urinary tract infection and pyelonephritis. *Emerg Med Clin North Am* 2001;19:655.
73. Scholes D et al. Risk factors associated with acute pyelonephritis in healthy women. *Ann Intern Med* 2005;142:20.
74. McMurray BR et al. Usefulness of blood cultures in pyelonephritis. *Am J Emerg Med* 1997;15:137.
75. Roberts JA. Management of pyelonephritis and upper urinary tract infections. *Urol Clin North Am* 1999;26:753.
76. Hamilton-Miller JM. The urethral syndrome and its management. *J Antimicrob Chemother* 1994;33(Suppl A):63.
77. Nickel JC. Interstitial cystitis: a chronic pelvic pain syndrome. *Med Clin North Am* 2004;88:467.
78. Phenazopyridine Hydrochloride. In: *American Hospital Formulary Service.* Bethesda, MD: American Society of Hospital Pharmacists; 2003:3468.
79. Harding GK et al. Antimicrobial treatment in diabetic women with asymptomatic bacteriuria. *N Engl J Med* 2002;347:1576.
80. Zore JJ et al. Diagnosis and management of pediatric urinary tract infections. *Clin Microbiol Rev* 2005;18:417.
81. Franco AV. Recurrent urinary tract infections. *Best Pract Res Clin Obstetr Gynaecol* 2005;19:861.
82. Hooton TM. Recurrent urinary tract infection in women. *Int J Antimicrob Agents* 2001;17:259.
83. Stapleton A et al. Prevention of urinary tract infection. *Infect Dis Clin North Am* 1997;11:719.
84. Fihn SD et al. Use of spermicide-coated condoms and other risk factors for urinary tract infection caused by *Staphylococcus saprophyticus*. *Arch Intern Med* 1998;158:281.
85. McOsker CC et al. Nitrofurantoin: mechanism of action and implications for resistance development in common uropathogens. *J Antimicrob Chemother* 1994;33(Suppl A):23.
86. Hooper DC. Urinary tract agents: nitrofurantoin and methenamine. In: Mardell GL et al., eds. *Principles and Practice of Infectious Diseases*. 6th ed. New York: Churchill Livingstone; 2006:473.
87. Albert X et al. Antibiotics for preventing recurrent urinary tract infection in non-pregnant women. *Cochrane Database Syst Rev* 2004;3:CD001209.
88. Conway PH et al. Recurrent urinary tract infections in children. Risk factors and association with prophylactic antimicrobials. *JAMA* 2007;298:179.
89. Raz R et al. Cranberry juice and urinary tract infection. *Clin Infect Dis* 2004;38:1413.
90. Jepson RG et al. Cranberries for preventing urinary tract infections. *Cochrane Database Syst Rev* 2004;2:CD001321.
91. Reid G et al. Probiotics to prevent urinary tract infections: the rationale and evidence. *World J Urol* 2006;24:28.
92. Wagenlehner FM et al. Current challenges in the treatment of complicated urinary tract infections and prostatitis. *Clin Microbiol Infect* 2006;12(Suppl 3):67.
93. Stapleton A et al. Post-coital antimicrobial prophylaxis for recurrent urinary tract infection. *JAMA* 1990;264:703.
94. Guay DR. An update on the role of nitrofurans in the management of urinary tract infections. *Drugs* 2001;61:353.
95. Christensen B. Which antibiotics are appropriate for treating bacteriuria in pregnancy? *J Antimicrob Chemother* 2000;46(Suppl 1):29.
96. Briggs GG et al. Drugs in Pregnancy and Lactation. 7th ed. Baltimore: Williams & Wilkins; 2005.
97. Johnson JR et al. Systematic review: antimicrobial urinary catheters to prevent catheter-associated urinary tract infection in hospitalized patients. *Ann Intern Med* 2006;144:116.
98. Trautner BW et al. Prevention of catheter-associated urinary tract infection. *Curr Opin Infect Dis* 2005;18:37.
99. Frank JE. Diagnosis and management of G6PD deficiency. *Am Fam Physician* 2005;72:1277.
100. Ben-Noun L. Drug-induced respiratory disorders: incidence, prevention and management. *Drug Saf* 2000;23:143.
101. Committee on Infectious Diseases. The use of systemic fluoroquinolones. *Pediatrics* 2006;118:1287.
102. Sabharwal V et al. Fluoroquinolone use in children. *Pediatr Infect Dis J* 2006;25:257.
103. Velissariou IM. The use of fluoroquinolones in children: recent advances. *Expert Rev Anti Infect Ther* 2006;4:853.

CHAPTER 65

Sexually Transmitted Diseases

Jeffery A. Goad and Karl M. Hess

Although descriptions of sexually transmitted diseases (STDs) can be discerned in the earliest written records, only recently have the common STDs been differentiated from each other; unique STD syndromes continue to be described today. For example, of the common STDs, bacterial vaginosis (BV) was not described clearly as a syndrome (initially called *Haemophilus vaginalis* vaginitis) until the 1950s; herpes simplex virus (HSV) type 2 (the cause of genital herpes) was not differentiated from HSV type 1 until the 1960s; the spectrum of genital chlamydial infections was not well worked out until the 1970s; and the human immunodeficiency virus (HIV) as an STD, was not recognized until the 1980s. Since 1980, eight additional sexually transmitted pathogens have been identified. They include the human papillomaviruses (HPV), human

T-lymphotropic virus (HTLV-I and II), *Mycoplasma genitalium, Mobiluncus* species, HIV-1 and -2, and the human herpes virus type 8 (associated with Kaposi sarcoma).[1]

GONORRHEA

Gonorrhea is caused by *Neisseria gonorrhoeae,* a Gram-negative diplococcus. In 130 AD, Galen coined the term gonorrhea (Greek for "flow of seed") for the syndrome associated with this infection because he believed the urethral exudate was semen. Although the role of the gonococcus in causing urethral discharge in men has been known for years, the manifestations of gonorrhea in women were determined later. In the 1930s, sulfonamides became the first form of effective antimicrobial therapy for gonorrhea until penicillins and tetracyclines became the mainstays of therapy. Considering the high levels of resistance to these two antimicrobial agents, neither are recommended in the treatment of this disease state.

In the United States, the incidence of gonorrhea rose steadily (15% per year) from the early 1960s through 1975, then fell 74% between 1975 and 1997. Since 1998, the rate has been stable, however, greater than the Centers for Disease Control and Prevention (CDC) goal of <100 cases per 100,000 people (Fig. 65-1).[2] Notably, the incidence of gonorrhea in heterosexuals rose sharply in 1985 for the first time in a decade. Since this time, the rate has declined, although only in whites and Asians. In contrast, the rate among African Americans was approximately 18 times higher than the rate among whites in 2005. The highest incidence of gonorrhea is in men aged 20 to 24 years and in females aged 15 to 19 years and aged 20 to 24 years.[3] Additional risk factors for gonorrhea include low socioeconomic status, urban residence, unmarried marital status, illicit drug use, inconsistent condom use, new or multiple sex partners, prostitution, and a history of gonorrhea or other sexually transmitted infections.[4–6] Although the risk of gonorrhea was greater in homosexual men than in heterosexual men in the past, the incidence dropped in homosexual men during the 1980s AIDS epidemic, in large part due to a reduction in sexual risk behaviors. Since 1988, the rate of gonococcal isolates from homosexual men has increased from 4% to a high of 17% in 2001, then fell to 11% in 2005.[3,7]

Uncomplicated Gonorrhea

Transmission

1. D.S., a 23-year-old male naval officer recently stationed in the Philippines, complains of dysuria, meatal pain, and a profuse yellow urethral discharge for 2 days. He admits to extramarital sex with a prostitute over the past week. He is accompanied by his pregnant wife, C.S., who is asymptomatic. D.S. engages in vaginal sex but there is no history of oral or anal sex with either partner. Assuming the prostitute has gonorrhea, what is the likelihood that D.S. and C.S. have been infected?

After one or two episodes of unprotected vaginal intercourse with an infected prostitute, a man has approximately a 50% risk of acquiring a urethral infection; the risk increases with repeated exposures and high prevalence among commercial sex workers.[8] The prevalence of infection in women who are secondary sex contacts of infected men is as high as 80% to 90%.[9] Therefore, the likelihood that D.S. and C.S. are infected is high. Because D.S. had sex with a prostitute, both D.S. and C.S. should also be tested for HIV infection.

Signs and Symptoms: Males

2. What signs and symptoms in D.S. are consistent with the diagnosis of gonorrhea? Describe D.S.'s anticipated clinical course if he remains untreated.

In males, gonorrhea usually becomes clinically apparent 1 to 7 days after contact with an infected source. A purulent discharge associated with dysuria is the first sign of infection; D.S. exhibits both. The discharge, which is presumably caused by chemotactic factors such as C5a released when antigonococcal antibody binds complement, may become more profuse and blood tinged as the infection progresses. Some strains of gonorrhea have a propensity to cause asymptomatic or minimally symptomatic infection with negative Gram stain, probably owing to different auxotypes.[10]

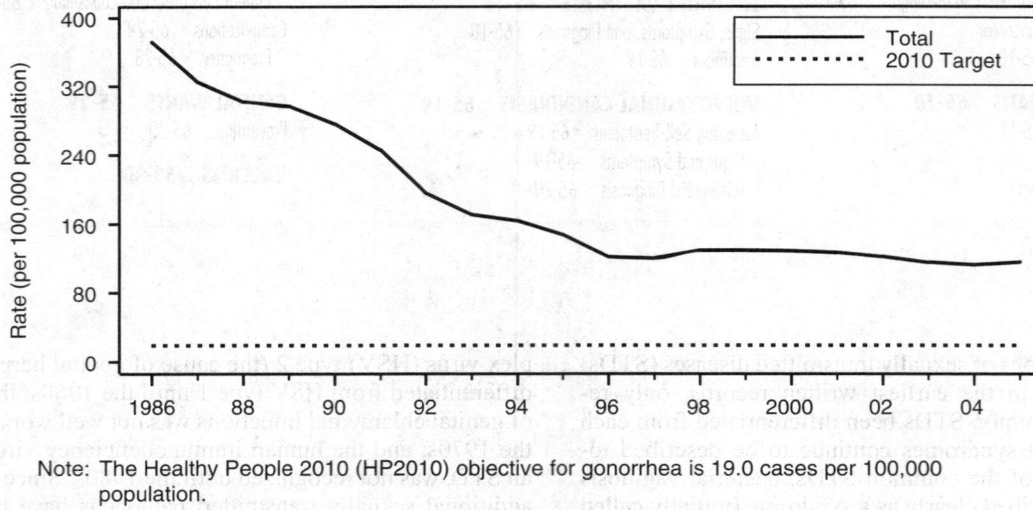

FIGURE 65-1 Gonorrhea: reported rates in the United States, 1986 to 2005 and the *Healthy People 2010* Target. Gonococcal Isolate Surveillance Project (GISP). (From reference 2.)

Patients with asymptomatic or minimally symptomatic disease may serve as reservoirs for the infection, evading treatment for prolonged periods of time.[11] At one time, only females were thought to have asymptomatic gonorrhea, but now it is known that men may be asymptomatic carriers as well.[12]

In the pre-antimicrobial era, gonococci occasionally spread to the epididymis, causing unilateral epididymitis; the prevalence was 5% or more in patients in some studies. Now epididymitis occurs in <1% of men with gonorrhea. Urethral stricture after repeated attacks and sterility after epididymitis are rare complications of gonococcal infection owing to the effectiveness of antibiotics.

Diagnosis: Males

3. Intracellular Gram-negative diplococci were seen on the Gram stain of D.S.'s urethral exudate. Is any further diagnostic testing required?

Demonstration of intracellular Gram-negative diplococci in the Gram-stained exudate confirms the diagnosis in symptomatic men. Until recently, some experts recommended that cultures be reserved for individuals with negative Gram stain of urethral exudate. However, today cultures are recommended for all patients to permit isolation and testing of the bacteria for antibiotic susceptibility. Cultures usually are performed on Thayer–Martin medium, an enriched chocolate agar to which vancomycin, colistimethate, and nystatin have been added. Cultures from the throat should be obtained if D.S. was exposed by cunnilingus to the prostitute. In D.S.'s case, a urethral culture is indicated.

Signs and Symptoms: Females

4. C.S., D.S.'s wife, is asymptomatic. What symptoms would be consistent with gonorrhea in C.S.? Do the symptoms differ because she is pregnant? What is the natural course of gonorrhea in women if left untreated?

Because the endocervical canal is the primary site of urogenital gonococcal infection in women, the most common symptom is vaginal discharge. Many women infected with gonorrhea have abnormalities of the cervix, including purulent or mucopurulent endocervical discharge, erythema, friability, and edema of the zone of ectopy.[9] The incubation period for urogenital gonorrhea in women is variable.[13] Pelvic inflammatory disease (PID) is a serious complication in 10% to 20% of women with acute gonococcal infection and can lead to infertility and chronic pelvic pain.[9] The assessment of signs and symptoms in women with gonorrhea often is confounded by nonspecific signs and symptoms and a high prevalence of coexisting infection, especially with *Chlamydia trachomatis* or *Trichomonas vaginalis.*

Although lower genital tract symptoms in women may disappear, they remain carriers of *N. gonorrhoeae* and should be treated. Complications of urogenital gonorrhea in pregnancy include spontaneous abortion, premature rupture of the fetal membranes, premature delivery, and acute chorioamnionitis.[14,15] Other complications include gonococcal arthritis (see Question 16) conjunctivitis, and ophthalmia neonatorum in the newborn.[16] For these reasons, it is critical that C.S. be worked up thoroughly for gonorrhea.

Diagnosis: Females

5. How should gonorrhea be ruled out in C.S.?

C.S. should undergo an endocervical culture, which is positive in 80% of women with gonorrhea and is still considered the "gold standard."[17] This test should be a part of every pelvic examination of sexually active women. Nucleic acid amplification tests (NAATs), such as polymerase chain reaction (PCR), may yield sensitivities and specificities in the 90% to 100% range, but results must be confirmed with endocervical culture in low-prevalence communities (i.e., <4%).[18] In C.S., anal cultures also could be performed because the rectum can serve as a reservoir for gonococci.

Treatment

6. Compare the various drug regimens used for uncomplicated gonorrhea.

The CDC recommendations are summarized in Table 65-1. Many strains of *N. gonorrhoeae* exhibit plasmid-mediated resistance to penicillin and tetracycline (penicillinase-producing *N. gonorrhoeae* [PPNG] and/or tetracycline-resistant *N. gonorrhoeae* [TRNG]; Fig. 65-2). In addition, significant levels of chromosomally mediated resistance to penicillin, tetracycline, and cefoxitin have been reported.[2] In 2005, all isolates in the Gonococcal Isolate Surveillance Project (GISP) were susceptible to ceftriaxone; therefore, a single dose of intramuscular (IM) ceftriaxone is preferred for the treatment of gonorrhea. Cefixime 400 mg orally as a single dose is also recommended by the CDC; however, tablets are currently unavailable from the manufacturer. Recently, the CDC withdrew recommendations for use of fluroquinolones such as ciprofloxacin and ofloxacin because of unacceptably high levels of quinolone-resistant *N. gonorrhoeae* (QRNG).[19]

Table 65-1 CDC Recommendations for Treatment of Uncomplicated Gonorrhea

Presentation	Drugs of Choice (% Cured)	Dosage	Alternative Regimens
Urethritis, cervicitis,[a] rectal	Ceftriaxone (98.9)	125 mg IM once	Cephalosporin single dose regimens[c]
	Cefixime (97.4)[b]	400 mg PO once	
Pharyngeal	Ceftriaxone	125 mg IM once	

[a]Because a high percentage of patients with gonorrhea have coexisting *Chlamydia trachomatis* infections, many clinicians recommend treating all patients with gonorrhea with a 7-day course of doxycycline or single-dose azithromycin for treatment of Chlamydia.
[b]In July of 2002, Wyeth discontinued oral cefixime (Suprax); currently, only an oral suspension is available.
[c]Additional cephalosporin regimens include ceftizoxime 500 mg IM, cefoxitin 2 g IM (administered with probenecid 1 g PO), and cefotaxime 500 mg IM. Limited evidence suggests that cefpodoxime 200 mg and cefuroxime axetil 1 g might be oral alternatives.
Adapted from reference 6.

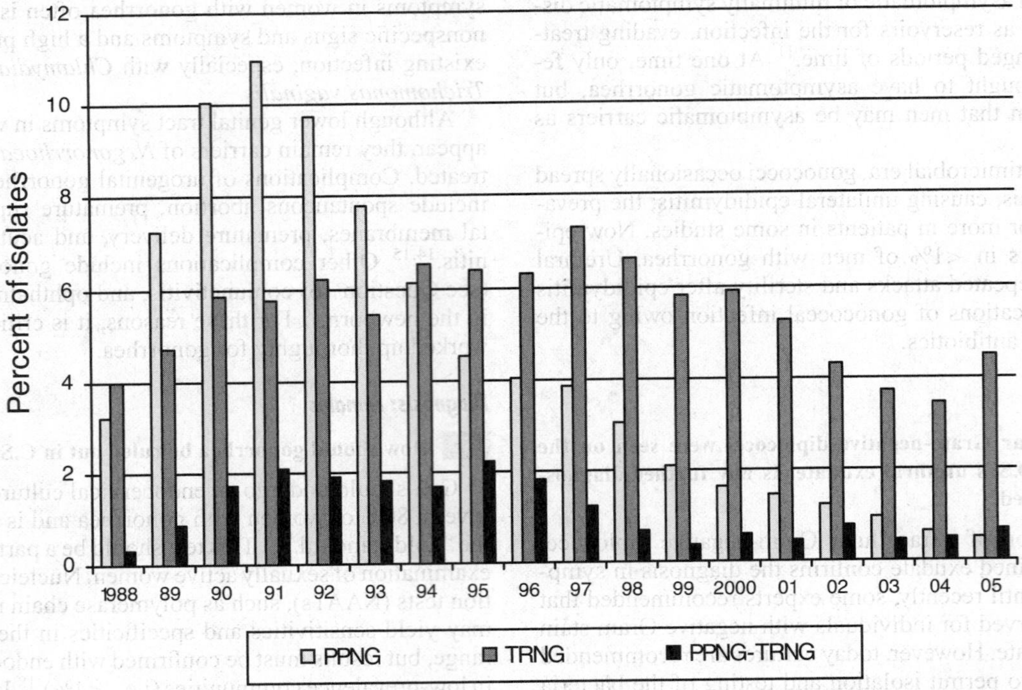

FIGURE 65-2 Plasmid-mediated resistance to penicillin and tetracycline among GISP isolates, 1988 to 2005: Gonococcal Isolate Surveillance Project (GISP). PPNG, penicillinase-producing *N. gonorrhoeae*; TRNG, tetracycline-resistant *N. gonorrhoeae*; PPNG–TRNG, resistant to both penicillin and tetracycline. (From reference 2.)

Because a high percentage of patients with gonorrhea are also coinfected with *C. trachomatis*, a single dose of azithromycin or a 7-day course of doxycycline is recommended to be taken concurrently for a presumed infection (see Question 22).

IM spectinomycin, which traditionally had been used in individuals who could not tolerate either fluoroquinolones or cephalosporins, is also unavailable from the manufacturer. Spectinomycin was the recommended treatment option for gonorrhea in those with either penicillin or cephalosporin allergies.[20] Individuals who have either penicillin or cephalosporin allergies can be desensitized to cephalosporins before treatment begins.[21]

CEFTRIAXONE

Ceftriaxone, a third-generation cephalosporin, is given as a single, small-volume IM injection (e.g., 125 mg diluted with normal saline or 1% lidocaine solution). Ceftriaxone eradicates anal and pharyngeal gonorrhea and is also safe in pregnancy (U.S. Food and Drug Administration [FDA] pregnancy category B). Other injectable cephalosporins (notably ceftizoxime, cefoxitin, and cefotaxime) have been found to be safe and highly effective, although efficacy in pharyngeal infections is not as well-established. Considering the limited availability of cefixime tablets, other oral cephalosporins have been studied. Although not meeting the strict CDC definition of success, evidence suggests that the oral cephalosporins cefpodoxime and cefuroxime axetil are effective in the treatment of uncomplicated urogenital gonorrhea.[6]

Ceftriaxone is ineffective against *C. trachomatis* and in the prevention of postgonococcal urethritis, whereas ofloxacin and levofloxacin for 7 days have similar efficacy to doxycycline.[6]

FLUOROQUINOLONES

Fluoroquinolones have been routinely used since the 1990s for the treatment of gonorrhea; however, since 2002, the GISP has documented increasing rates of fluoroquinolone resistance in *N. gonorrhoeae* isolates (Fig. 65-3), which has necessitated changes in the CDC's Sexually Transmitted Treatment guidelines for 2006. Because of this increased resistance, the CDC no longer recommends ciprofloxacin, levofloxacin, ofloxacin, and other fluoroquinolones for the treatment of gonorrhea. This recommendation also extends to the treatment of gonorrhea-associated conditions such as PID.[19]

PRESCRIBING PATTERNS

The CDC's 2005 Sexually Transmitted Disease Surveillance Program observed that ceftriaxone 125 mg, followed by the fluoroquinolones ciprofloxacin and ofloxacin, were the most commonly prescribed agents (Fig. 65-4).[2] Cefixime is currently only available in a generic suspension (100 or 200 mg/5 mL) form.[22] Cefixime 400 mg tablets were unavailable since 2002, but in 2008, they were re-introduced onto the market. Their use should increase as they are the CDC preferred agent for uncomplicated gonorrhea.

7. How should D.S.'s urethritis be treated? Because C.S. is totally asymptomatic and the results of her cultures are pending, should she be treated empirically? If so, what drug(s) would you recommend?

Because D.S. has gonococcal infection limited to the urethra (uncomplicated), a few treatment regimens are possible, as outlined in question 6. Either ceftriaxone or cefixime is the preferred treatment. With the current unavailability of cefixime

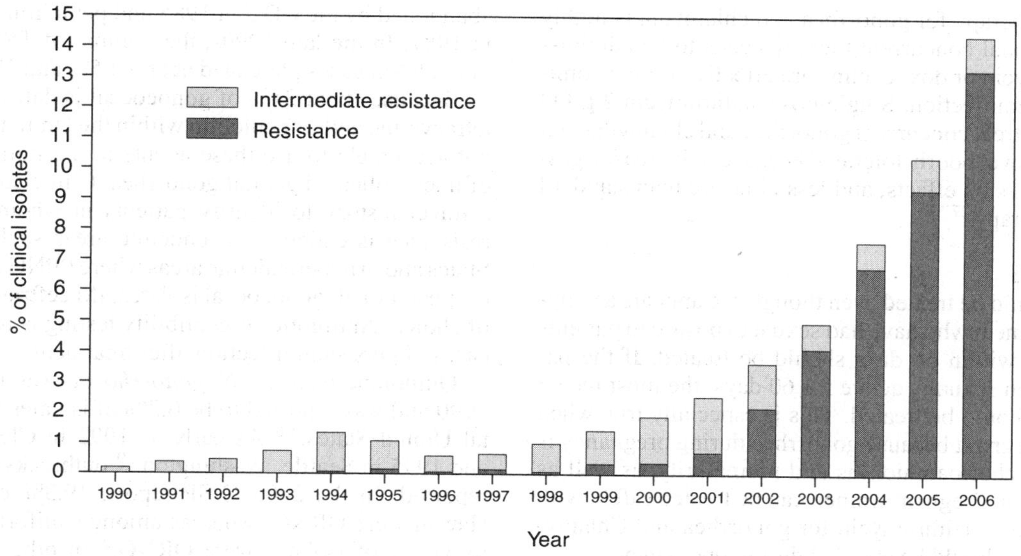

FIGURE 65-3 Percentage of *N. gonorrhoeae* isolates with intermediate resistance or resistance to ciprofloxacin, 1990 to 2006: Gonococcal Isolate Surveillance Project (GISP). *Note:* Resistant Isolates have ciprofloxacin MICs 1 mcg/ml or higher. Isolates with intermediate resistance have ciprofloxacin MICs of 0.125 to 0.5 mcg/ml. Susceptibility to ciprofloxacin was first measured in GISP in 1990. (From reference 2.)

tablets, alternative oral agents may need to be considered if ceftriaxone is not appropriate. Quinolones should be avoided because of increased resistance in *N. gonorrhoeae* and because D.S.'s infection was likely obtained in the Philippines, where quinolone resistance occurs in over half of all isolates.[19,23] Cefpodoxime 200 mg PO and cefuroxime axetil 1 g PO are active in vitro against PPNG, chromosomally mediated resistant *N. gonorrhoeae* (CMRNG), and TRNG, but have limited clinical evidence to support their use. They are, however, FDA approved to treat uncomplicated *N. gonorrhoea.*[24–26] Because

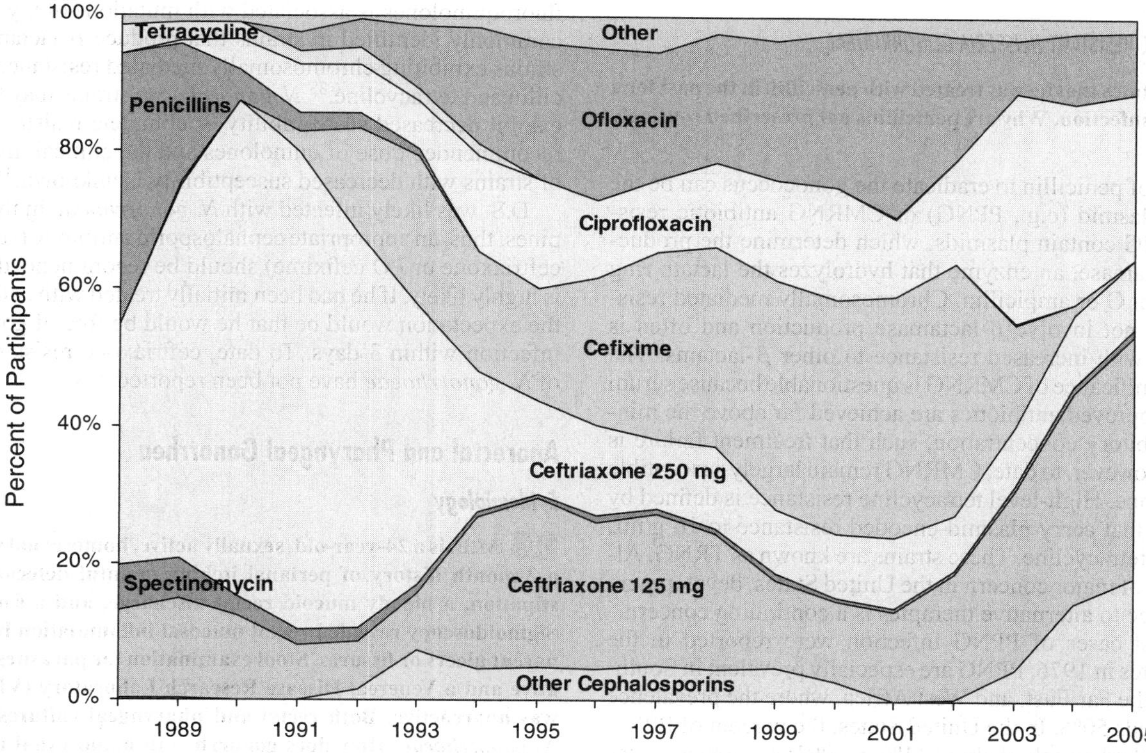

Note: For 2005, "Other" includes no therapy (1.4%), azithromycin 2 g (0.1%), levofloxacin (0.4%), and other less frequently used drugs.

FIGURE 65-4 Drugs used to treat gonorrhea in GISP participants, 1988 to 2005. (From reference 2.)

no single-dose therapy for gonorrhea and chlamydia is highly effective, additional concurrent therapy needs to be administered. Azithromycin or doxycycline are effective for concomitant chlamydia coinfection. Single-dose azithromycin 2 g PO has been used to treat concurrent gonorrhea and chlamydia, but it is more expensive, poorly tolerated because of increased gastrointestinal (GI) side effects, and less effective than standard combination therapy.[27]

SEXUAL PARTNERS

C.S. also should be treated even though she appears asymptomatic. All partners who have had sexual exposure to patients with gonorrhea within 60 days should be treated. If the patient has not been sexually active for 60 days, the most recent sexual partner should be treated. This is especially true when the partner is pregnant because gonorrhea during pregnancy is associated with chorioamnionitis and prematurity, as well as neonatal infection. Pregnant women can be treated safely with cephalosporins and azithromycin for gonorrhea and Chlamydia. Doxycycline should be avoided during pregnancy.

FOLLOW-UP

8. How does one determine whether the drug therapy of gonorrhea has been effective in D.S. and C.S.?

If recommended therapies are used for treatment of uncomplicated gonorrhea (see Table 65-1), a test of cure is not necessary for either C.S. or D.S. because cure rates are close to 100%.[6,9] If symptoms persist in D.S., who was treated with ceftriaxone, cultures should be done to rule out other causes of urethritis.

ANTIBIOTIC-RESISTANT *NEISSERIA GONORRHOEAE*

9. D.S. states that he was treated with penicillin in the past for a gonococcal infection. Why are penicillins not prescribed routinely today?

Failure of penicillin to eradicate the gonococcus can be the result of plasmid (e.g., PPNG) or CMRNG antibiotic resistance. PPNG contain plasmids, which determine the production of lactamase, an enzyme that hydrolyzes the lactam ring of penicillin G or ampicillin. Chromosomally mediated resistance does not involve β-lactamase production and often is associated with increased resistance to other β-lactams. The clinical significance of CMRNG is questionable because serum levels of approved antibiotics are achieved far above the minimum inhibitory concentration, such that treatment failure is unlikely. However, to date, CMRNG remain largely susceptible to ceftriaxone. High-level tetracycline resistance is defined by gonococci that carry plasmid-encoded resistance to 16 g/mL or more of tetracycline. These strains are known as TRNG. Although not of major concern in the United States, development of resistance to alternative therapies is a continuing concern.

The first cases of PPNG infection were reported in the United States in 1976. PPNG are especially prevalent in Southeast Asia, the Far East, and West Africa, where the prevalence often exceeds 50%. In the United States, the percent of PPNG strains reached a peak of about 11% in 1991; since then, cases have steadily declined to 0.5% in 2005, according to the CDC's GISP[2] (Fig. 65-3). Strains of TRNG were first identified in 1985, but fortunately most TRNG isolates still are sensitive to β-lactam antibiotics. The use of tetracycline was officially abandoned by the CDC in 1985 and penicillin was abandoned in 1987. In the late 1990s, the number of TRNG and PPNG plus TRNG cases plateaued at about 5% and 1%, respectively.

Because about 21% of gonococcal isolates are resistant to tetracycline and/or penicillin within the United States, it is still not acceptable to use these agents in the initial management of uncomplicated genital gonorrhea. Clinicians should obtain a travel history to identify patients in whom multiple drug resistance is endemic. In endemic areas such as the United States and in hyperendemic areas where PPNG accounts for 3% or greater of all gonococcal isolates, IM ceftriaxone is the drug of choice. Antibiotic susceptibility testing is recommended in cases of persistent infection after treatment.

Quinolone-resistant *N. gonorrhoeae* was first reported in 1990 and was reported to be 0.2% of isolates in the continental United States.[2,6] As early as 1992 in Cleveland, Ohio,[28] and 1995 in Seattle, Washington,[29] outbreaks of QRNG were reported. In the 2005 GISP report, 19.3% of isolates from Hawaii were QRNG, whereas among California sites, 14.5% to 31.3% of isolates were QRNG.[2] In other geographic regions, strains exhibiting resistance to ciprofloxacin are as high as 63% in the Philippines and 48.8% in Hong Kong, with slightly lower rates reported in the rest of Asia.[30,31] For this reason, quinolones have not been recommended for gonorrhea acquired in Hawaii, California, or Asia.[32] However, more recently, *N. gonorrhoeae* resistance to quinolones has increased and has become widespread in the United States, resulting in the CDC recommending against using quinolones for the treatment of gonococcal or related conditions (e.g., PID) acquired in the United States. In 2006, 13.3% of all isolates collected by the GISP demonstrated resistance to ciprofloxacin.[19] Resistance to fluoroquinolones is associated with mutations of GyrA and is commonly identified in strains that produce β-lactamase and strains exhibiting chromosomally mediated resistance to penicillin and tetracycline.[33] *N. gonorrhoeae* strains may therefore exhibit decreased susceptibility or complete resistance to the recommended dose of quinolones and the clinical importance of strains with decreased susceptibility is unknown.[34]

D.S. was likely infected with *N. gonorrhoeae* in the Philippines; thus, an appropriate cephalosporin antibiotic (such as IM ceftriaxone or PO cefixime) should be recommended; QRNG is highly likely. If he had been initially treated with ceftriaxone, the expectation would be that he would be free of gonococcal infection within 3 days. To date, ceftriaxone-resistant strains of *N. gonorrhoeae* have not been reported.

Anorectal and Pharyngeal Gonorrhea

Epidemiology

10. M.B. is a 24-year-old, sexually active, homosexual male with a 2-month history of perianal itching, painful defecation, constipation, a bloody mucoid rectal discharge, and a sore throat. Sigmoidoscopy revealed rectal mucosal inflammation but no apparent ulcers or fissures. Stool examination for parasites was negative and a Venereal Disease Research Laboratory (VDRL) test was nonreactive. Both rectal and pharyngeal cultures revealed *N. gonorrhoeae*. How does gonorrhea in homosexual men compare with gonorrhea in heterosexual men?

The most prevalent bacterial STD among the homosexual male population is gonorrhea.[35] Rectal infection occurs rarely in strictly heterosexual men, whereas in the male homosexual population, anorectal (25%) and pharyngeal (10%–25%) gonococcal infections occur more often.[9,36] Because pharyngeal[36,37] and anorectal gonococcal infections are often asymptomatic, a large reservoir of carriers in the homosexual male population may exist, diagnosed only with more sensitive DNA amplification techniques.[38] By comparison, very few urethral gonococcal infections are asymptomatic. In addition, recent data indicate that pharyngeal infections may be an important source of urethral gonorrhea in homosexual men, spread by fellatio.[36]

Signs and Symptoms

11. Are M.B.'s signs and symptoms consistent with gonorrhea?

Rectal gonorrhea produces the syndrome of proctitis with anorectal pain, mucopurulent anorectal discharge, constipation, tenesmus, and anorectal bleeding. The differential diagnosis of proctitis in the homosexual male includes rectal infection with *N. gonorrhoeae, C. trachomatis,* HSV, and syphilis. Proctitis, limited to the distal rectum, should be differentiated from proctocolitis, which is often caused by *Shigella* species, *Campylobacter* species, or *Entamoeba histolytica* in homosexual men. The incidence of rectal gonorrhea and Chlamydia has dramatically risen since 1996.[39] Rectal Chlamydia is often asymptomatic and observed more often than gonorrhea, necessitating testing for both pathogens.[40]

Treatment

12. How should M.B.'s diagnosis be managed?

The treatment of choice for patients such as M.B. with anorectal and/or pharyngeal gonorrhea is ceftriaxone 125 mg IM as a single dose (see Table 65-1). Azithromycin or doxycycline should be given to those with rectal gonorrhea to treat possible coexisting rectal chlamydial infection. Patients such as M.B. with either anorectal or pharyngeal gonorrhea should be advised to avoid further unprotected sexual activity and should be counseled and tested for infection with HIV.

13. What are alternative regimens for patients with isolated anal or pharyngeal gonorrhea?

Women with anorectal gonorrhea alone can be treated with either ceftriaxone or cefixime. Alternative regimens for isolated anorectal infection include a single-dose cephalosporin regimen such as with ceftizoxime. Because spectinomycin is unavailable, patients with anorectal gonorrhea who are allergic to penicillin or cephalosporins can be desensitized before treatment is initiated. Patients with gonococcal infections of the pharynx should be treated with ceftriaxone; however, infections of this nature are more difficult to eradicate than infections at anorectal sites. Chlamydial coinfection is uncommon in pharyngeal gonorrhea, but should be treated with either doxycycline or azithromycin.[6]

Prevention

14. What measures have been used to prevent the sexual transmission of infection?

Condoms, when used properly, seem to provide a high degree of protection against the acquisition and transmission of STDs.[41] Previous studies indicated that the use of the spermicide nonoxynol-9 had activity against gonorrhea and Chlamydia, although more recent studies show no effect.[42,43] In light of recent evidence that suggests nonoxynol-9 might actually increase the chance of acquiring HIV, the CDC recommends that it should not be used for the prevention of any sexually transmitted infection.[6,44] Thus, widespread use of this agent for the purpose of decreasing the risk of STDs cannot be recommended at this time. Topical antibacterial agents, urinating, and washing after intercourse are of little value in preventing the transmission of STDs. Douching may increase the risk other STDs such as trichomoniasis.[45]

The prophylactic administration of antibiotics immediately before or soon after sexual intercourse is not recommended owing to increased costs and antimicrobial resistance. Use of rapid, specific tests and empiric syndromatic management should be used to enhance detection and treatment of gonorrhea.

PELVIC INFLAMMATORY DISEASE

The term *pelvic inflammatory disease* (*PID*) commonly refers to a variety of inflammatory disorders of the upper female reproductive tract. This term does not denote the primary infection site (the fallopian tubes) nor the causative micro-organisms. PID also has been used to connote an infection that occurs acutely when either vaginal or cervical micro-organisms traverse the sterile endometrium and ascend to the fallopian tubes. Acute salpingitis also may be used to describe an acute infection of the fallopian tubes. Therefore, the terms PID and salpingitis are used interchangeably in this discussion to denote an acute infection involving the fallopian tubes.

PID affects 1 million women annually in the United States.[46] However, since 1985, the rate of hospitalization owing to PID has decreased 68%.[47] Many cases of acute PID occur by sexual transmission, especially in young women 16 to 24 years who are more likely to have multiple sexual partners.[47] Not all PID is caused by Chlamydia or gonorrhea. Up to 70% of cases may be polymicrobial and include *M. genitalium* and BV.[48] Other risk markers and factors include unprotected sexual intercourse before age 15, douching, BV, sex while menstruating, and smoking.[49] It is unclear whether an intrauterine device (IUD) increases the risk of PID, but it may be prudent to avoid placement when the patient has chlamydial or gonococcal cervicitis.[50] Two-thirds of PID cases resulting in infertility are asymptomatic, and up to one-third are incorrectly diagnosed owing to low specificity of diagnostic techniques. In the United States, infertility occurs in about 12.1% of women after the first episode of PID.[51] The estimated cost of direct medical expenditures for PID and its sequelae was estimated to be $1.88 billion in 1998 with most of this cost associated with treatment of acute PID.[52]

Etiology

Most cases of PID are caused by *C. trachomatis* and *N. gonorrhoeae.*[6] Some micro-organisms that comprise the vaginal flora are also associated with PID, including *Gardnerella vaginalis, H. influenzae*, and *Streptococcus agalactiae.*[6] *Mycoplasma hominis, Ureaplasma urealyticum,* and *M. genitalium* have been associated with PID, but a causative role is unclear.[51] Facultative enteric Gram-negative bacilli and a variety of anaerobic bacteria have also been isolated from the upper genital tract of up to 70% of women with acute PID.[48] Women diagnosed with acute PID should be tested for *C. trachomatis* and *N. gonorrhoeae* and screened for HIV.[6]

Signs and Symptoms

The onset of symptoms of abdominal pain attributable to PID caused by either gonococci or chlamydia often occurs soon after the menstrual period. Symptoms of PID, if present, are often nonspecific, which can create a delay in or failure of diagnosis. Vaginal discharge, menorrhagia, dysuria, and dyspareunia are commonly associated with PID. Signs include cervical motion tenderness, uterine tenderness, or adnexal tenderness. Temperatures above 101°F, abnormal cervical or vaginal mucopurulent discharge, white blood cells (WBC) on saline microscopy of vaginal secretions, elevated erythrocyte sedimentation rate, or an elevated C-reactive protein support a diagnosis of PID.[6] Clinical diagnosis has sensitivity for PID of about 65% to 90%, whereas laparoscopy and a newer technique, transvaginal Doppler ultrasound, are about 100% specific, resulting in the combination of laparoscopy and clinical impression serving as the gold standard.[6,53,54] Unfortunately, laparoscopy and Doppler ultrasound are costly and often not readily available for acute cases nor is it diagnostic for endometritis; thus, clinical impression is critical. A key to reducing the incidence of PID may be through active screening of *chlamydia* in young, sexually active women.[55,56]

Clinical Sequelae

An abscess may form in the pelvic or abdominal cavity and in one or both fallopian tubes. Chronic abdominal pain develops in 18% of women with PID and may be the result of pelvic adhesions surrounding the tubes and ovaries. After a single episode of PID, tubal occlusion and fibrosis secondary to fallopian tube inflammation (salpingitis) result in 12% infertility, 25% infertility after two episodes, and 50% infertility after three or more episodes.[51] Other sequelae include ectopic pregnancy (9%) and chronic pelvic pain (18%).[57] The risk of ectopic pregnancy is increased approximately eightfold after one or more episodes of PID.

Diagnosis and Treatment

15. H.C., a 19-year-old, sexually active woman, complains of mild dysuria, a purulent vaginal discharge, fever, and moderately severe, bilateral, lower abdominal pain of 3 days' duration. Examination confirms uterine and adnexal tenderness, a purulent cervical exudate, and a temperature of 39°C. Laboratory examinations show a nonreactive VDRL and negative urinalysis. A pregnancy test performed at this time was negative. The peripheral WBC count was mildly elevated (11,000/mm^3) with 70% polymorphonuclear leukocytes. Does H.C. have PID? How should she be treated?

Although fever and leukocytosis are often absent in mild or subacute PID, these findings in a woman with uterine and adnexal tenderness with cervical exudate increases the likelihood of acute PID. Treatment should be initiated immediately after diagnosis of PID to prevent clinical sequelae; confirmation of the actual pathogen rarely takes place (Table 65-2). Patients such as H.C. with mild to moderate PID can be hospitalized and treated with parenteral antibiotics; however, clinical efficacy and overall outcomes are equal between parental and oral therapy, and H.C. could also be treated on an outpatient basis. For inpatient treatment, the 2006 CDC guidelines recommend either intravenous (IV) cefotetan 2 g every 12 hours or IV cefoxitin 2 g every 6 hours for at least 24 hours beyond the first signs of clinical improvement. Once clinical improvement is noted, parenteral therapy may be discontinued and PO doxycycline 100 mg every 12 hours can continue to complete 14 days of therapy. For outpatient treatment, the CDC guidelines recommend either IM ceftriaxone 250 mg as a single dose or IM cefoxitin 2 g as single dose (with probenecid 1 g PO × 1) plus PO doxycycline 100 mg twice a day for 14 days with or without PO metronidazole 500 mg twice daily for 14 days. A tetracycline derivative or an alternative agent that is active against *C. trachomatis* should be included in the treatment of PID; however, monotherapy with a tetracycline is not recommended because of the lack of activity against Gram-negative aerobic and anaerobic organisms and *N. gonorrhoeae.* The addition of metronidazole, which covers anaerobic bacteria, should also be considered; anaerobes have been isolated from the upper reproductive tract of women with PID and may cause tubal and epithelial destruction.[6] Metronidazole is widely used by clinicians, although its application is theoretical because the role of anaerobes in PID is not well understood. Quinolones (e.g., levofloxacin, ofloxacin) are no longer recommended for the treatment of PID because of the increase in prevalence of QRNG in the United States.[19]

Both oral and IV doxycycline have similar bioavailability; therefore, doxycycline should be given PO whenever possible because IV administration may be painful.[6] Substantial clinical improvement is usually seen within 3 days after initiation of therapy. Clindamycin plus gentamicin can be used alternatively in penicillin-allergic and pregnant females.[6] Because H.C. is sexually active, any sexual partners within the previous 60 days (or if >60 days, then the most recent sexual partner) should be empirically treated because of the risk of gonococcal or chlamydial urethritis as well as to reduce the risk of reinfection.[6]

COMPLICATED GONORRHEA

Disseminated Gonococcal Infection

Signs and Symptoms

16. S.P., a 28-year-old, sexually active woman, was seen for stiffness and pain of the right wrist and left ankle and fever (38°C). On physical examination, the knee and wrist joints were found to be hot, red, and swollen; papules and pustular lesions were observed on S.P.'s legs and forearms. A latex fixation test for rheumatoid factor was negative. A tap of the right knee yielded an effusion with a WBC count of 34,000/ mm^3 (80% polymorphonuclear leukocytes). Cultures of the skin lesions were negative, but *N. gonorrhoeae* was isolated from the throat, cervix, blood, and synovial fluid. A chest radiograph, echocardiogram, and electrocardiogram all were normal, and no murmur could be appreciated. Assess S.P.'s clinical presentation.

S.P.'s signs, symptoms, and laboratory findings are consistent with gonococcal bacteremia, which today occurs in less than 1% of women and men with gonorrhea. The most common manifestation of gonococcemia is the gonococcal arthritis–dermatitis syndrome or disseminated gonococcal infection (DGI) exhibited by S.P. Symptoms include fever, occasional chills, a mild tenosynovitis of the small joints,

Table 65-2 Antimicrobial Regimens Recommended by the CDC for Treatment of Acute Pelvic Inflammatory Disease

Treatment Setting, Drugs, Schedule	*Advantage*	*Disadvantage*	*Clinical Considerations*
Inpatient			
Regimen A Cefotetan 2 g IV Q 12 hr or cefoxitin 2 g IV Q 6 hr plus doxycycline 100 mg IV or PO[a] Q 12 hr Continue doxycycline (100 mg PO BID) after discharge to complete 14 days of therapy	Optimal coverage of *N. gonorrhoeae* (including resistant strains) and *C. trachomatis*	Possible suboptimal anaerobic coverage	Penicillin-allergic patients also may be allergic to cephalosporins; doxycycline use in pregnant patients may cause reversible inhibition of skeletal growth in the fetus and discoloration of teeth in young children
Regimen B Clindamycin 900 mg IV Q 8 hr plus gentamicin loading dose IV or IM (2 mg/kg) followed by a maintenance dose of 1.5 mg/kg Q 8 hr[b] Continue clindamycin 450 mg PO QID or doxycycline 100 mg PO BID after discharge to complete 14 days of therapy	Optimal coverage of anaerobes and Gram-negative enteric rods	Possible suboptimal coverage of *N. gonorrhoeae* and *C. trachomatis*	Patients with decreased renal function may not be good candidates for aminoglycoside treatment or may need a dosage adjustment
Alternative regimen Ampicillins/sulbactam 3 g IV Q 6 hr plus doxycycline 100 mg PO or IV Q 12 hr	Optimal coverage of *N. gonorrhoeae* and *C. trachomatis*	Inadequate coverage of anaerobes necessitates use of metronidazole or ampicillin/sulbactam	Not appropriate in pregnancy or in young children
Outpatient			
Regimen A Ceftriaxone 250 mg IM in a single dose plus doxycycline 100 mg PO BID for 14 days with or without metronidazole 500 mg PO BID for 14 days or cefoxitin 2 g IM in a single dose and probenecid, 1 g PO administered concurrently in a single dose plus doxycycline 100 mg PO BID for 14 days with or without metronidazole 500 mg PO BID for 14 days or other parenteral third-generation cephalosporins (e.g., ceftizoxime or cefotaxime) plus doxycycline 100 mg PO BID for 14 days with or without metronidazole 500 mg PO BID for 14 days	Good to excellent coverage of *N. gonorrhoeae* and optimal coverage of *C. trachomatis*	Possible suboptimal anaerobic coverage necessitating the addition of metronidazole	Optimal cephalosporin is unclear; more complicated regimen requiring combination of parenteral and oral therapies

[a]Because of the pain involved with doxycycline infusions and the comparable PO/IV bioavailability, IV therapy should be replaced with PO as soon as possible.
[b]Single daily dosing may be substituted.
Adapted from reference 6.

and skin lesions; the latter primarily involving the distal extremities are petechial, papular, pustular, and hemorrhagic in appearance.[58]

Diagnosis of DGI is made by Gram stain and culture. However, blood cultures are positive in only 33% of DGI cases, even when patients are cultured early in the course of the infection.[59] The low positive yield from blood cultures may be due to the low inoculum and/or intermittent bacteremic period. Routine culture of the urethra, cervix, pharynx, and rectum should be performed in any patient suspected of having DGI.

Treatment

17. How should S.P. be managed? How quickly will she respond to therapy?

Patients like S.P. with gonococcal arthritis and bacteremia should be hospitalized for treatment with ceftriaxone 1 g IV daily until clinical improvement, such as decreased fever and pain, is sustained for 24 to 48 hours, at which time therapy may be switched to an appropriate oral agent. Unfortunately, owing to the increased incidence of QRNG in the United States, only oral cefixime 400 mg daily for 7 days is currently recommended (Table 65-3).[6,19] Symptoms and signs of tenosynovitis should be improved markedly within 48 hours. Septic gonococcal arthritis with purulent synovial fluid may require repeated aspiration and resolves more slowly.

Treatment of Gonococcal Endocarditis and Meningitis

18. How should gonococcal endocarditis and meningitis be treated?

Gonococcal endocarditis and meningitis, occurring in only 1% to 3% of DGIs, require high-dose IV therapy such as ceftriaxone (1–2 g IV every 12 hours) for 10 days or more in the case of meningitis and for 4 weeks in the case of endocarditis.[6,9]

Table 65-3 Treatment of Disseminated Gonococcal Infection[a]

No Penicillin Allergy
Parenteral
Ceftriaxone 1 g IV or IM Q 24 hr or cefotaxime 1 g IV Q 8 hr or ceftizoxime 1 g IV Q 8 hr and doxycycline 100 mg PO BID[b] or erythromycin base 500 mg PO QID[b] (if pregnant)
Oral
Cefixime 400 mg PO BID
Penicillin Allergy
Parenteral
Spectinomycin 2 g IM Q 12 hr and doxycycline 100 mg PO BID[b] or erythromycin base 500 mg PO QID[b] (if pregnant)

[a] Duration of treatment is 7 days.
[b] For possible concomitant chlamydial infection, treat for 7 days.
Adapted from reference 6.

Neonatal Disseminated Gonococcal Infection: Treatment

19. How should neonatal DGI and meningitis be managed?

Neonatal DGI and meningitis can be treated with either ceftriaxone or cefotaxime for 7 days; however, if meningitis is documented, 10 to 14 days of treatment is required. Ceftriaxone is given at 25 to 50 mg/kg (IV or IM) Q 24 hr and cefotaxime is given at 25 mg/kg (IV or IM) Q 12 hr.

CHLAMYDIA TRACHOMATIS

C. trachomatis was first isolated from patients with lymphogranuloma venereum (LGV). However, laboratory diagnoses for this pathogen were not developed until the 1960s and 1970s.[60] From 1986 to 2005, the rate of reported Chlamydia infections in the United States rose from 35.2 to 332.5 cases per 100,000 individuals and was largely attributable to the increased development and use of more sensitive screening tests and improved national reporting efforts. Women are three times more likely than men to be infected with Chlamydia—496.5 cases versus 161.1 cases per 100,000 individuals, respectively, in 2005; however, from 2001 to 2005, the infection rate among men increased by 43.5% compared with 15.6% in women over.[61] In U.S. family planning clinics, the chlamydial test positivity, a proxy for prevalence, is 6.3% in 15- to 24-year-old women and probably much lower for men, although men are less frequently screened.[62] If left untreated, chlamydial infection in women can lead to serious sequelae such as PID, ectopic pregnancy, and infertility. Asymptomatic infection is also observed in both men and women; however, routine screening is only recommended for sexually active women at least 25 years old and women with risk factors for infection (e.g., multiple sexual partners, new sexual partners). Screening sexually active men for *C. trachomatis* can be considered in settings with a high prevalence of the infection.[6]

C. trachomatis, an intracellular obligate organism, can be diagnosed either by culture, direct immunofluorescence assay (DFA), enzyme immunoassay (EIA), or NAATs of endocervical or male urethral swabs.[6] However, *C. trachomatis* is a difficult organism to demonstrate in clinical specimens because cell culture techniques are not readily available to the practitioner. Because few practitioners have access to facilities for isolation of *C. trachomatis,* most chlamydial infections are diagnosed and treated based on clinical impression and laboratory techniques. Diagnostic tests, such as NAATs, DFA, and EIA, are generally sensitive methods for detecting *C. trachomatis.* Ligase chain reaction and PCR are two NAATs with wide commercial availability, are relatively simple to use, can be performed using urine or genital swab specimens, and are more sensitive than non-NAATs.[16] A test of cure is not necessary unless patient compliance is questionable, symptoms persist, or reinfection is suspected. Repeat testing fewer than 3 weeks after initiation of treatment is not recommended because false-negative results may occur as a result of undetectable *C. trachomatis* organisms. Moreover, false positives may occur with repeat NAATs as the result of the continued excretion of dead organisms.[6]

The variety of clinical syndromes that are now known to be caused by *C. trachomatis* are cervicitis, urethritis, bartholinitis, endometritis, salpingititis, and perihepatitis in women, and urethritis, epididymitis, prostatitis, proctitis, and Reiter syndrome in men.[63] It is interesting to note that the spectrum of chlamydial infections closely resembles those caused by the gonococcus, which is why many patients presenting with these syndromes are treated with drugs effective against both organisms (Table 65-4).

Table 65-4 Clinical Parallels Between Genital Infections Caused by *N. gonorrhoeae* and *C. trachomatis*: Resulting Clinical Syndromes

Gender	Site of Infection	*N. gonorrhoeae*	*C. trachomatis*
Male	Urethra	Urethritis	NGU, postgonococcal urethritis
	Epididymis	Epididymitis	Epididymitis
	Rectum	Proctitis	Proctitis
	Conjunctiva	Conjunctivitis	Conjunctivitis
	Systemic	DGI	Reiter syndrome
Female	Urethra	Acute urethral syndrome	Acute urethral syndrome
	Bartholin gland	Bartholinitis	Bartholinitis
	Cervix	Cervicitis	Cervicitis
	Fallopian tube	Salpingitis	Salpingitis
	Conjunctiva	Conjunctivitis	Conjunctivitis
	Systemic	DGI	Arthritis-dermatitis (Reiter syndrome)

Adapted from Schachter J. Chlamydial infections. *N Engl J Med* 1978;298:428, 490, 540. Copyright 2008 Massachusetts Medical Society.

There is controversy in how *C. trachomatis* is cultured and what the in vitro results mean clinically, especially in the 10% to 15% of cases that fail treatment.[64] The CDC thus uses cure rates instead of microbial susceptibilities to make treatment recommendations. Only azithromycin and doxycycline have 97% and 98%, respectively, cure rates.[65] Agents mentioned as alternatives include erythromycin, ofloxacin, and levofloxacin, but not the penicillins, cephalosporins, aminoglycosides, clarithromycin, ciprofloxacin, or metronidazole.[6,66,67]

Nongonococcal Urethritis

Etiology

20. T.K., a 26-year-old, sexually active man, complains of mild dysuria and a mucoidlike urethral discharge that started about 15 days after his last intercourse. He had no fever, lymphadenopathy, penile lesions, or hematuria. A Gram stain smear of an anterior urethral specimen showed 20 polymorphonuclear neutrophilic leukocytes (PMNs) per oil immersion (1,000) field and no Gram-negative diplococci. What pathogens are associated with nongonococcal urethritis (NGU)?

In the United States, NGU is the most common STD in men.[63,68] Depending on the study design and diagnostic technique, causative organisms identified include *C. trachomatis* in 35% to 50%,[63] *U. urealyticum* in 9% to 42%,[69] *M. genitalium* in 15% to 25%,[70] *T. vaginalis* in 5% to 15%,[71] and no identifiable cause in up to 20%.[69] The variety of pathogens and disparity among identification techniques require sound clinical judgment and an algorithmic laboratory testing approach to accurately identify and treat the cause. A NAAT, if available, should be performed to rule out the presence of *C. trachomatis*.

Signs and Symptoms

21. Describe the clinical presentation of a person with NGU. Is T.K.'s presentation consistent with NGU? How does one differentiate between NGU and gonococcal urethritis?

T.K.'s presentation is typical. Compared with gonococcal urethritis, NGU typically produces less severe and less frequent dysuria and less penile discharge. Chlamydial urethral infection is completely asymptomatic more often than gonococcal urethral infection. The incubation period for gonococcal urethritis is 2 to 7 days, whereas the incubation period for NGU is typically 2 to 3 weeks.

Nonetheless, NGU and gonococcal urethritis cannot be reliably differentiated solely on the basis of symptoms and signs. If there is objective evidence of a urethral discharge (expressed by milking the urethra), a Gram stain with fewer than 5 WBCs per oil immersion field in the urethral secretion, positive leukocyte esterase test demonstrating 10 WBCs per high-power field, the diagnosis of NGU is made by excluding the presence of *N. gonorrhoeae* by Gram stain and/or culture.

Treatment

22. How should T.K. be treated?

If *C. trachomatis* cannot be ruled out, therapy with azithromycin should be initiated to cover for both *M. genitalium* and Chlamydia.[6] Doxycycline does not effectively eradicate *M. genitalium*.[72] For NGU, doxycycline 100 mg PO BID for 7 days may also be prescribed. Both azithromycin and doxycycline are considered equally effective against NGU.[6,73–75] Doxycycline is less expensive and has been used more extensively than azithromycin. Erythromycin base 500 mg PO QID or erythromycin ethylsuccinate 800 mg PO QID for 7 days are alternative CDC-approved regimens. Additionally, ofloxacin 300 mg PO BID or levofloxacin 500 mg PO QD for 7 days are other alternatives, but they offer no significant advantages over the previously mentioned agents, may not treat *U. urealyticum* adequately, and are significantly more expensive.[76] Ciprofloxacin should be avoided because treatment failures have been reported.[77] Patient counseling should emphasize the need for abstinence from sexual intercourse at least until the prescribed course of therapy has been completed (or 7 days after single-dose therapy) by the patient and their sexual partner(s).[63] There is some indication that the proportion of NGU caused by *C. trachomatis* is declining, potentially being replaced by an increased proportion of *U. urealyticum,* which is variably cured at 2 weeks by azithromycin (73%) and doxycycline (65%).[73]

RECURRENT INFECTION

23. T.K. was treated with doxycycline 100 mg BID for 7 days. He remained asymptomatic for 14 days after completion of his therapy, when he again noticed similar symptoms of dysuria and a mucoidlike urethral discharge. How should T.K.'s recurrent infection be treated?

The major problem encountered in the treatment of NGU is the high rate of recurrent infections. Approximately 20% to 60% of patients experience recurrent or persistent urethritis within 1 to 2 weeks after treatment.[70] The rate of recurrence is highest in patients with idiopathic urethritis, that is, those not infected with *C. trachomatis* or *U. urealyticum.* Recurrence suggests re-exposure to an untreated partner, whereas persistent urethritis (without improvement during therapy) suggests the presence of other organisms including *M. genitalium, U. urealyticum,* or *T. vaginalis.*[69] NGU that persists or recurs should be retreated with the initial regimen if the patient was not compliant or the sexual partner was not treated.[6] For patients with persistent symptoms who were compliant with the initial regimen and were not re-exposed, the CDC recommends using either metronidazole or tinidazole 2 g PO as a single dose plus a single 1 g dose of azithromycin if not used for the initial episode.[6]

Men with acute epididymitis often have chlamydial or gonococcal infection, particularly if they are younger than 35 years of age or have a urethral discharge. Older men with epididymitis more often are infected with *Escherichia coli* or other urinary pathogens. If testicular tenderness is present with urethritis, and the clinical impression is consistent with epididymitis caused by chlamydia or gonorrhea, some experts recommend a single dose of ceftriaxone 250 mg IM plus doxycycline 100 mg PO twice for 10 days. For a nonsexually transmitted etiology of epididymitis, ofloxacin 300 mg PO BID or levofloxacin 500 mg PO once daily for 10 days may be used.[6]

Sexual Partners

24. A.C., T.K.'s girlfriend, comes into the clinic 3 weeks after T.K.'s last visit. She is worried that she may have a similar infection, although she has no signs or symptoms. What clinical

manifestations of chlamydial infections are seen in women? Should A.C. be treated for suspected chlamydial infection?

In the absence of cultures for Chlamydia, empirical treatment of women who are sexual partners of men with NGU is recommended. Routine partner referral for presumptive therapy is not indicated for nonchlamydial NGU.[69] Many partners are asymptomatic, but from 30% to 70% are culture positive if tested. A.C. should be examined carefully for mucopurulent cervicitis and salpingitis. Although many women with chlamydial infection of the cervix are asymptomatic, up to one-quarter have evidence of mucopurulent discharge.[78] A Gram stain of appropriately collected mucopurulent endocervical discharge from these patients shows many PMNs and an absence of gonococci.

Regardless of findings, treatment should be initiated with the same doxycycline regimen used for NGU. However, if A.C. is pregnant, tetracyclines and fluoroquinolones should be avoided. Azithromycin 1 g PO as a single dose or amoxicillin 500 mg PO TID for 7 days could be used instead. Alternatively, either erythromycin base 500 mg QID for 7 days, erythromycin base 250 mg PO for 14 days, erythromycin ethylsuccinate 800 mg PO QID for 7 days, or erythromycin ethylsuccinate 400 mg PO for 14 days can be used.[6] Erythromycin estolate should be avoided in pregnancy because of the increased risk of hepatotoxicity. Azithromycin seems to be safe and effective during pregnancy.[79,80] High rates of GI complaints limit the use of erythromycin. In pregnant women, a repeat NAAT is recommended 3 weeks after completion of therapy to ensure therapeutic cure.[6] Coinfection with Chlamydia is common in heterosexual men and women with gonorrhea. Therefore, drug regimens effective against both organisms are recommended in patients with gonorrhea to prevent postgonococcal chlamydial morbidity (epididymitis, mucopurulent cervicitis, salpingitis) and to reduce the genital reservoir of *C. trachomatis*.

Lymphogranuloma Venereum

Etiology and Signs and Symptoms

25. S.F., a 32-year-old male student who recently arrived from Uganda, presents to the STD clinic with a chief complaint of pain and swelling in the groin. He reports the appearance of a small ulcer on his penis about 2 weeks ago, which resolved rapidly. Upon examination, he has a bubo (inflammatory swelling of one or more lymph nodes in the groin) with surrounding erythema on his right side. S.F. also has a fever (39°C). Laboratory findings are remarkable for a mild leukocytosis (WBC count, 12,000 cells/mm³). What organisms are responsible for LGV? Describe its clinical course. What subjective and objective manifestations in S.F. are consistent with LGV?

Lymphogranuloma venereum is rare in the United States, occurring mainly in Africa, India, Southeastern Asia, South America, and the Caribbean, but it may be on the rise in Europe and North America.[81,82] The cause of LGV is usually *C. trachomatis* serovars L1, L2, or L3, which is different from those serovars responsible for chlamydia urethritis. Three stages of LGV infection are recognized in heterosexual men.[83] During stage I, a small genital papule or vesicle appears between 3 and 30 days after exposure. The patient usually is asymptomatic; the ulcer heals rapidly and leaves no scar. This primary lesion is consistent with the penile ulcer reported by S.F. Many patients with LGV recall no primary lesion.

Stage II is characterized by acute, painful lymphadenitis with bubo formation (the inguinal syndrome); it often is accompanied by pain and fever, as illustrated by S.F. Without treatment, the buboes may rupture, forming numerous sinus tracts that drain chronically. Adenopathy above and below the inguinal ligament results in the "groove sign." Healing occurs slowly, and most patients suffer no serious sequelae. Patients in this stage also may present with an anogenitorectal syndrome, which is accompanied by proctocolitis and hyperplasia of intestinal and perirectal lymphatic tissue. Late or tertiary manifestations include perirectal abscesses, rectovaginal fistulae (in women), rectal strictures, and genital elephantiasis.[83] Appropriate treatment of stage II LGV usually prevents these late complications.

An acute anorectal syndrome of LGV occurs in homosexual men who acquire the infection through rectal receptive intercourse. In these cases, a primary anal ulcer may be noted with associated inguinal adenopathy (anal lymphatics drain to inguinal nodes). Subsequently, acute hemorrhagic proctocolitis occurs with tenesmus, rectal pain, constipation, and a mucopurulent, bloody rectal discharge. Rectal biopsy may show granulomatous colitis, mimicking Crohn disease. Perirectal pelvic adenopathy also occurs.

Treatment

26. How should S.F. be treated?

Current CDC recommendations for LGV include doxycycline 100 mg PO BID or erythromycin base 500 mg PO QID for 21 days.[6] Surgical intervention may be needed for later forms of the disease. Azithromycin 1 g weekly for 3 weeks may be effective, but clinical data on its use are lacking.[6]

SYPHILIS

Epidemiology

Syphilis is caused by the spirochete, *Treponema pallidum*. The rates of primary and secondary syphilis in the United States are thought to have increased in the late 1980s secondary to crack cocaine use (and associated unsafe sex practices), but from 1990 to 2000, rates have decreased to those reported in 1941 (when reporting began), representing a >86% decrease since 1990.[84,85] However, the number of cases have steadily risen since 2000, reaching a high of 8,724 cases in 2005, primarily in men who have sex with men.[86] Another concern is that syphilis facilitates the transmission of HIV, and recent outbreaks of syphilis have been associated with HIV-positive men who have sex with men.[86,87] From 1996 to 2005, rates of congenital syphilis decreased on average by 14.1% per year (Fig. 65-5). From 2004 to 2005, the overall rate of congenital syphilis decreased by 12.1% from 9.1 to 8 cases per 100,000 births.[86] The *Healthy People 2010* (*HP*) goal (0.2 cases per 100,000 people) is significantly lower than the *HP 2000* goal (4 cases per 100,000). Although we have met the *HP 2000* goal, we still have far to go to surpass the *HP 2010* goal (Fig. 65-6).

The clinical manifestations of syphilis have not changed appreciably since their first description. However, early diagnosis,

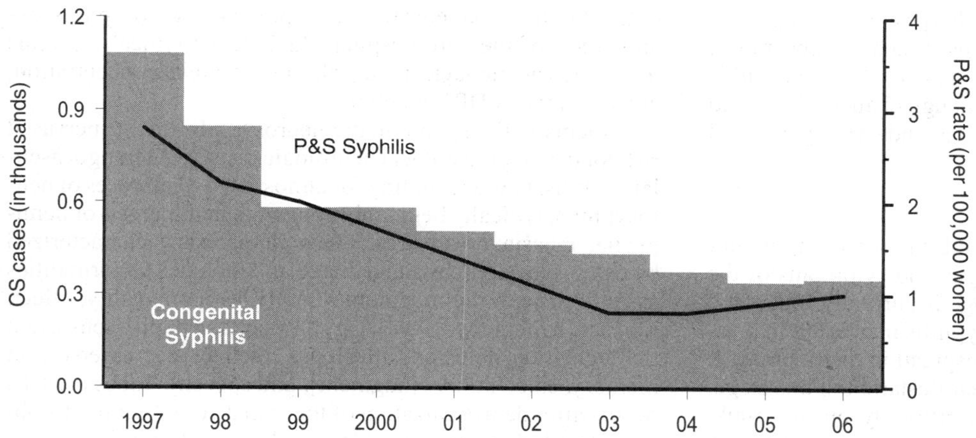

FIGURE 65-5 Congenital syphilis (CS). Reported cases for infants younger than 1 year of age and rates of primary and secondary syphilis among women, 1997 to 2006. (From reference 86.)

treatment, and greater physician/patient awareness of the disease have reduced the incidence of its severe forms. Penicillin continues to be the mainstay of therapy. Vaccine development, although premature, hopefully will advance as more is learned about the biology of *T. pallidum*.

Clinical Stages

27. D.M., a 27-year-old homosexual man, presents to the STD clinic with complaints of malaise, headache, and fever of 4 days' duration. He also reveals that he had a sore on his penis about 8 weeks ago, but it has since resolved. Upon examination, he is afebrile and has a widespread maculopapular skin rash that also involves the soles of his feet; general lymphadenopathy also is appreciated. Medical history is unremarkable except for one episode of gonorrhea 2 years ago that was treated with procaine penicillin. Laboratory findings include a normal peripheral WBC count, a negative serology for HIV antigen, and a positive rapid plasma reagin (RPR) test and fluorescent treponemal antibody absorption (FTA-Abs) test. Describe the clinical course of syphilis. Are D.M.'s symptoms consistent with this infection?

Primary Stage

The average incubation period for syphilis is 3 weeks and ranges from 10 to 90 days.[88] During this incubation period, *T. pallidum* can be demonstrated in the lymph and blood. The primary chancre develops at the site of inoculation as a painless papule that becomes ulcerated and indurated. The ulcer is nontender and filled with spirochetes. The chancre usually involves the penis in the heterosexual male; the penis or anus in the homosexual male; and the vulva, perineum, or cervix in the female. Occasionally, the lip or tongue is involved. Regional lymph nodes are enlarged, firm, and nontender. Unfortunately, the typical chancre described earlier often is missed, particularly in women or homosexual men.[89] Without treatment, the primary chancre resolves spontaneously, usually in 2 to 6 weeks. The differential diagnosis of genital ulcers also includes chancroid and genital herpes. Like chancroid, genital herpes produces painful, superficial, nonindurated ulcers with tender inguinal adenopathy. However, unlike chancroid, lesions of genital herpes characteristically proceed through a vesicular state and often are associated with urethritis, cervicitis, and constitutional symptoms, such as fever and chills.

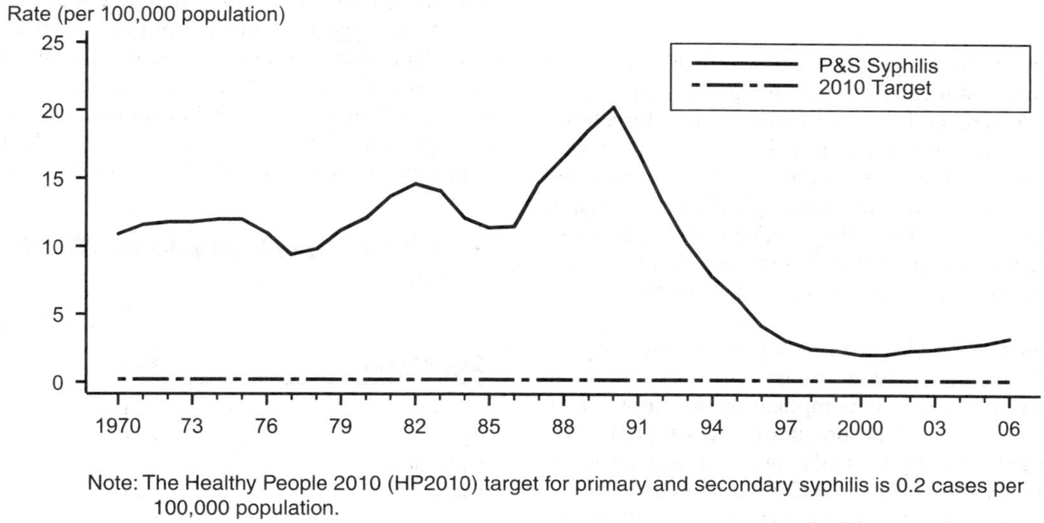

FIGURE 65-6 Primary and secondary syphilis, reported rates, 1970 to 2006 and the *Healthy People 2010* objective (0.2 CASES PER 100,000). (From reference 86.)

Syphilis can be differentiated from herpes by a nonpainful versus painful lesion, a papular versus vesicular appearance, and single versus multiple lesions. Chancroid is more difficult to differentiate from syphilis, although chancroid tends to have a more tender lesion, jagged border, and striking inguinal lymphadenopathy.[90]

Secondary Stage

Approximately 6 weeks after a chancre first appears, the untreated patient begins to manifest signs and symptoms of the secondary stage of syphilis. This stage is currently illustrated by D.M. Skin lesions of secondary syphilis may erupt in a variety of patterns and are usually widespread in distribution. A macular lesion often is the earliest manifestation in this stage. The lesion is round or oval, occurs primarily on the trunk, and is rose or pink in color. As lesions mature, they become papular or nodular with scaling (the so-called papulosquamous rash). The differential diagnosis of diffuse papulosquamous rashes includes psoriasis, pityriasis rosea, and lichen planus. In syphilis, the palms and soles are characteristically involved, and oral lesions (mucous patches) may occur. Generalized lymphadenopathy usually is present, and patching alopecia may be seen. The most infectious lesion of secondary syphilis is condyloma latum. Condylomata lata are characteristically wet, indurated lesions occurring primarily in the perineum or around the anus as a result of direct spread from the primary lesion. Laboratory studies sometimes reveal anemia, leukocytosis, or an increased erythrocyte sedimentation rate. Other manifestations of secondary syphilis include mild hepatitis, aseptic meningitis, uveitis, neuropathies, and glomerulonephritis.[91]

Latent Stage

By definition, untreated, asymptomatic persons with serologic evidence for syphilis have latent syphilis. The latent stage is divided into two phases: the early latent (<1 year's duration) and late latent (>1 year's duration). In the Oslo study of patients with untreated syphilis, 25% experienced secondary relapses, usually within the first year.[92] Patients who relapse to the secondary stage are infectious; those in the late latent stage are not infectious and are immune to reinfection with *T. pallidum.*

Tertiary Stage

Morbidity and mortality of syphilis in adults are due primarily to a variety of late manifestations involving the skin, bones, central nervous system, and cardiovascular system. Infectious granulomas (gummas), the characteristic lesions of tertiary syphilis, now are observed infrequently. Most gummas respond quickly to specific therapy, although if critical organs are involved (heart, brain, liver), they can be fatal.[93] The most common manifestations of syphilitic cardiovascular disease are aortic insufficiency and aortitis, with aneurysm of the ascending aorta.

Neurosyphilis may be classified as asymptomatic early or late, meningeal, parenchymatous, or gummatous. Although neurosyphilis has been a rare complication for more than 40 years because of the widespread of use of penicillin, syphilitic meningitis, an early form of neurosyphilis, may be increasing among HIV-positive patients.[94,95] Late neurosyphilis may be asymptomatic or accompanied by a variety of manifestations; the most common syndromes are meningovascular syphilis, general paresis, tabes dorsalis (locomotor ataxia), and optic atrophy. In patients with asymptomatic neurosyphilis, examination of the cerebrospinal fluid (CSF) typically reveals mononuclear pleocytosis, an elevated protein concentration, and a positive VDRL reaction.

Patients with asymptomatic neurosyphilis are at increased risk for developing clinical neurologic disease. Meningovascular syphilis, now accounting for almost 38% of all cases of neurosyphilis, typically begins abruptly with hemiparesis or hemiplegia, aphasia, or seizures.[96] General paresis is characterized by extensive parenchymal damage and includes abnormalities associated with the mnemonic PARESIS (personality, affect, reflexes [hyperactive], eye [Argyll Robertson pupil], sensorium [hallucination, delusions, illusions], intellect [decreased recent memory, calculations, judgment], and speech). Tabes dorsalis occurs after demyelinization of the spinal cord. Symptoms observed include an ataxic, wide-based gait and foot slap; paresthesias; bladder irregularities; impotence; areflexia; and loss of position, deep pain, and temperature sensation. The Argyll Robertson pupil, seen in both paresis and tabes dorsalis, is a small, irregular pupil that reacts to accommodation but not to light.

Laboratory Tests

28. Evaluate D.M.'s laboratory findings.

Dark-Field Examination

Exudate expressed from the chancre or from condyloma latum is examined with a dark-field microscope. The diagnosis of syphilis is made if spirochetes with characteristic corkscrew morphology and mobility are present. Dark-field examination is the most specific and sensitive method, but only when the microscopist is experienced in the diagnosis of syphilis.[97] Three dark-field examinations on consecutive days should be performed before considering the test negative in suspected primary syphilis.

Serologic Tests

Serologic tests become reactive during the primary stage, but as shown in Table 65-5, they may be negative at the time of presentation with primary syphilis. When the history or examination suggests primary syphilis, a VDRL should be sent to the laboratory, or an RPR test should be performed in the clinic (see discussion on nontreponemal tests, following). If initial serology and dark-field examinations are negative, the serology should be repeated in 1 to 4 weeks to exclude primary syphilis. If the dark-field examination is positive, an RPR

Table 65-5 False-Negative Results With VDRL and FTA-Abs Tests

	Percentage	
Stage of Syphilis	VDRL	FTA-Abs
Primary	24	14
Secondary	<0.1	<0.1
Early latent	5	1
Late latent	28	5

FTA-Abs, fluorescent treponemal antibody absorption; VDRL, Venereal Disease Research Laboratory.

Table 65-6 Causes of False-Positive VDRL and FTA-Abs Test Results

VDRL	FTA-Abs
Technical error	Technical error
Other spirochetal diseases (yaws, bejel, pinta)	Genital herpes
Heroin addiction	
Lupus erythematosus	Leprosy
Hashimoto thyroiditis	Mononucleosis
Malaria	Collagen vascular disease
Mononucleosis	Pregnancy
Pregnancy	
Immunizations	
IV narcotic abuse	

FTA-Abs, fluorescent treponemal antibody absorption; IV, intravenous; VDRL, Venereal Disease Research Laboratory.

may still be ordered to establish a baseline for follow-up after treatment.

Serologic tests are essentially always positive during secondary syphilis.[90] Two types of tests are used for the serodiagnosis of syphilis: nontreponemal tests, which measure serum concentrations of reagin (antibody to cardiolipin), and treponemal tests, which detect the presence of antibodies specific for *T. pallidum.*

NONTREPONEMAL TESTS

Nontreponemal tests are not specific for *T. pallidum*, but can be quantified. They are inexpensive and useful for screening large numbers of people. The most widely used nontreponemal tests are the VDRL test and the RPR Card Test. The RPR test is the most widely used because it is simpler to perform than the VDRL. Results of the VDRL and RPR are not interchangeable; thus, the same test should be used throughout the post-treatment monitoring period.[98]

The result reported in the quantitative VDRL test is the most dilute serum concentration with a positive reaction. This test may be used to follow the decline in VDRL titer after effective therapy (see Question 31). In some individuals, a serofast reaction occurs in which nontreponemal antibodies may remain at a low titer for a long time and even their entire lives. When false-positive tests occur (Table 65-6), the titer usually is low (e.g., VDRL or RPR titer = 1:8).[99] In secondary syphilis, sensitivity of the RPR and VDRL approach 100% owing to the high antibody concentrations.[100]

TREPONEMAL TESTS

Specific treponemal tests are most useful to confirm a positive nontreponemal test. The FTA-Abs test is the most commonly used treponemal test. Because the FTA-Abs test requires fluorescence microscopy, it is relatively difficult and expensive to perform and not appropriate for screening.

The *T. pallidum* immobilization (TPI) test, the microhemagglutination (MHA-TP) test, and the hemagglutination test for syphilis (HATTS) are three other treponemal tests. The TPI test is used rarely because of its cost and complexity. The MHA-TP and HATTS tests are both easier to perform and less expensive than the FTA-Abs test, but they are less sensitive in primary syphilis. Treponemal tests should not be used to assess treatment response because antibody titers correlate poorly with disease progression. A newer test is the *T. pallidum* latex agglutination test, which, in one study, was 100% sensitive and specific for nearly all stages of syphilis and took only 10 minutes to complete.[98,101] This test, however, is not in widespread use.

Treatment

29. How should D.M. be treated?

Penicillin G is the drug of choice for the treatment for all stages of syphilis (Table 65-7).[6] Every effort should be made to rule out penicillin allergy before choosing other antimicrobials that have been studied much less extensively than penicillin in the treatment of syphilis. Considering that penicillin-resistant *T. pallidum* has never been observed, treatment regimens for syphilis have changed relatively little over the years.

As shown in Table 65-7, recommended therapy for primary, secondary, or latent syphilis (with negative findings in the CSF) of <1 year's duration is a single, IM 2.4 MU dose of benzathine penicillin G. If penicillin is contraindicated, tetracycline (500 mg PO QID) or doxycycline (100 mg PO BID) for 2 weeks are the main alternatives.[6] If the patient is allergic to penicillin, not pregnant, and is contraindicated or cannot tolerate tetracycline or doxycycline, a 14-day regimen of azithromycin (500 mg PO QD) or ceftriaxone (500 mg IM QD) may be used (Table 65-7).[102] The CDC lists an alternative regimen of azithromycin 2 g in one dose or ceftriaxone 1 g IM or IV for 8 to 10 days.[6] The use of erythromycin as an alternative is no longer recommended by the CDC because of its poor efficacy. The optimal dose, duration, and efficacy of these alternative regimens are not well-defined, necessitating close follow-up of patients. Skin testing should be performed for individuals who claim allergy to penicillin. If the patient is truly allergic, he or she should be desensitized with oral penicillin in incrementally greater doses over a 4-hour period, after which a full course of penicillin may be given.[6] Latent syphilis (>1 year's duration) and cardiovascular syphilis are treated with IM benzathine penicillin G weekly (2.4 MU) for a total of 3 weeks. The alternative regimen is doxycycline (100 mg PO BID) or tetracycline (500 mg PO QID) for 28 days with close serologic and clinical follow-up. CSF examination is recommended if alternatives to penicillin are being considered.

Neurosyphilis

30. Would D.M.'s treatment differ if his CSF had tested positive for syphilis?

Neurosyphilis can present at any stage of syphilis. When conventional IM doses of benzathine penicillin G are administered, measurable levels of penicillin are not obtainable in the CSF. However, this does not mean that penicillin does not concentrate in meningeal tissue.[102] Treatment failures, as well as late clinical progression to neurosyphilis, can occur after treatment with the recommended IM regimen. After one dose, benzathene penicillin reaches peak plasma concentration slower (13–24 hours) but with more prolonged treponemicidal plasma concentrations (7–10 days) than procaine penicillin (1–4 hours to peak; 12- to 24-hour treponemicidal plasma concentrations).[102] Because of reports of benzathine penicillin

Table 65-7 Treatment Guidelines for Syphilis

Stage	Recommended Regimen	Alternative Regimen
Early (primary, secondary, or early latent)[a]	Benzathine penicillin G 2.4 MU single dose IM	Doxycycline 100 mg PO BID for 14 days *or* Tetracycline 500 mg PO QID for 14 days *or* Ceftriaxone 1 g IM/IV QD for 8 to 10 days *or* Azithromycin 2 g PO ×1 dose
Late latent or latent syphilis of unknown duration	Lumbar puncture	Lumbar puncture
	If CSF normal: Benzathine penicillin G 2.4 MU/wk ×3 wk IM	If CSF normal: Doxycycline 100 mg PO BID for 28 days *or* Tetracycline 500 mg PO QID for 28 days
	If CSF abnormal: Treat as neurosyphilis	If CSF abnormal: Treat as neurosyphilis
Neurosyphilis[b] (asymptomatic or symptomatic)	Aqueous penicillin G 18–24 MU IV QD ×10–14 days[c]	Procaine penicillin 2.4 MU IM QD plus probenecid 500 mg PO QID, both for 10–14 days
Congenital	Aqueous penicillin G 100,000–150,000 U/kg/d, administered as 50,000 U/kg/dose IV Q 12 hr during the first 7 days of life, and Q 8 hr thereafter for a total of 10 days[d] *or* Procaine penicillin G 50,000 U/kg/dose IM a day in a single dose for 10 days	If CSF normal: benzathine penicillin G 50,000 U/kg/dose IM in a single dose
Syphilis in pregnancy	According to stage	According to stage

[a] Some experts recommend repeating this regimen after 7 days for HIV-infected patients.
[b] Because of the shorter duration of therapy as compared with latent syphilis, some experts recommend giving benzathine penicillin G, 2.4 MU/wk for up to 3 weeks, after the completion of these neurosyphilis regimens to provide a comparable total duration of therapy.
[c] Administered as 3–4 MU IV every 4 hours or continuous infusion.
[d] All infants born to women treated during pregnancy with erythromycin must be treated with penicillin at birth.
Adapted from reference 6.

failures in the 1970s, the CDC guideline recommends treatment of neurosyphilis with aqueous penicillin G, 3 to 4 MU IV every 4 hours, or 18 to 24 MU/d continuous infusion, for 10 to 14 days.[6] Alternatively, neurosyphilis can be treated with procaine penicillin (2.4 MU IM/d) plus probenecid (500 mg PO every 6 hours) for 10 to 14 days. Some experts add benzathine penicillin G (2.4 MU IM once a week for up to 3 weeks) after the completion of aqueous penicillin G or procaine penicillin in the hope of providing persistent treponemicidal blood/tissue/CSF levels; the duration of therapy is the same as that for late-stage syphilis. Penicillin-allergic patients should be skin tested to confirm allergy and, if confirmed, the patient should be desensitized and treated with an appropriate penicillin regimen. The World Health Organization also recommends penicillin-allergic nonpregnant patients receive either doxycycline 200 mg PO BID or tetracycline 500 mg PO QID for 30 days.[103]

Follow-Up

31. D.M. was treated with a single IM dose of benzathine penicillin (2.4 MU). How should his response to therapy be monitored?

Physical examination and a quantitative VDRL or RPR test for primary and secondary syphilis should be repeated at least 6 and 12 months after therapy.[6] Retreatment should be considered when the RPR or VDRL titer does not decline by fourfold in 6 months. Patients who also are infected with HIV should have serologic testing every 3 months for 1 year and then a follow-up at 2 years.[90] Patients with latent syphilis should be retested 6, 12, and 24 months after treatment. Close nontreponemal serologic test monitoring is necessary if antibiotics other than penicillin are used; CSF examination should be performed in these patients at their last follow-up visit. Patients with neurosyphilis should be monitored serologically every 6 months; CSF examinations should be repeated at 6-month intervals until normal. If still abnormal at 2 years, retreatment should be considered. Return of lesions, a fourfold increase in titer, or a titer of 1:8 that does not fall at least fourfold within 12 months indicates the need for retreatment because of relapse or reinfection. Suspected treatment failures, especially if there is an abnormal CSF, should be treated as described for neurosyphilis. However, false-positive serologic results should be ruled out (Table 65-6).

Within 2 years, most patients with early syphilis become seronegative. However, if the disease is treated during the late stages, complete seroreversal may not occur. Patients treated with oral doxycycline or erythromycin are less likely to become seronegative.[104] Therapy is considered adequate in patients who never become seronegative if the titer decreases fourfold. Although the disease process may be halted in patients with tertiary syphilis, existing damage to the cardiovascular or nervous systems cannot be reversed.

Pregnancy

32. N.W., a 27-year-old woman in her 19th week of gestation, has a positive VDRL and FTA-Abs. How should N.W. be managed? How would management be altered in the face of penicillin allergy?

Although pregnancy has been a reported cause of false-positive nontreponemal tests,[91] the presence of both a positive treponemal test and a nontreponemal test virtually excludes a false-positive reaction.[97] The next step is to determine whether

N.W. already has been treated adequately. If she has previously received adequate treatment and follow-up and shows no evidence of persistence or recurrence of syphilis, then she requires no further therapy. Pregnancy has no known effect on the clinical course of syphilis.[105] However, her infant should be observed carefully. If N.W. has not been treated previously for syphilis, then she should be treated with penicillin in the same doses recommended for nonpregnant women; some experts recommend a second dose 1 week later of 2.4 MU of benzathine penicillin.[6]

The goal of therapy should be to treat the mother with syphilis as soon as possible. Syphilis transmission can occur transplacentally as early as 9 to 10 weeks' gestation and by direct contact with lesions in the birth canal.[105,106] If the mother is left untreated, 70% to 100% of fetuses born to mothers with primary or 40% with secondary syphilis may be aborted, stillborn, or born with congenital syphilis (see Question 34).[107,108]

There is no completely satisfactory alternative for the pregnant woman allergic to penicillin. Tetracycline, as well as doxycycline, should be avoided during pregnancy, especially during the second or third trimester, because of tetracycline's known effects on the fetus (tooth staining and inhibition of bone growth).[109]

Erythromycin has been used to treat pregnant patients with syphilis. However, the mean transplacental transfer rate (ratio of the concentration between maternal and fetal blood levels) of erythromycin is only 3%.[110] This may explain why some patients treated with erythromycin aborted or had stillborn infants. Therefore, erythromycin is no longer recommended as therapy for syphilis in the pregnant patient.[6] A woman with a history of allergy to penicillin should be skin tested; if allergy is confirmed, she should be desensitized and treated with penicillin.[6] It is possible that the newer cephalosporins and azithromycin may ultimately prove to be more acceptable alternatives to penicillin G in the pregnant woman with syphilis who is allergic to penicillin, but data are insufficient at this time to recommend their use. Even with adequate detection and treatment, fetal infection may still occur; however, more recent evidence suggests that adequate treatment with the appropriate penicillin dose can prevent up to 98% of fetal infections.[111,112] During pregnancy, the patient should be followed up with monthly quantitative VDRL titers to evaluate the effectiveness of therapy; thereafter, she should be followed up as any other patient with syphilis.

Jarisch-Herxheimer Reaction

33. N.W. was treated with an IM injection of 2.4 MU of benzathine penicillin G. Six hours later, she complained of diffuse myalgias, chills, headache, and an exacerbation of her rash. She was tachypneic, but normotensive. What has happened? How should N.W. be managed?

N.W. has developed the Jarisch-Herxheimer reaction (JHR), a benign, self-limited complication of antitreponemal antibiotic therapy that develops in a high proportion of patients within a few hours after treatment of secondary syphilis and less often after primary. The cause of JHR is not well understood, but is probably related to release of cytokines.[113] Clinical manifestations include fever, chills, myalgias, headache, tachycardia, and hypotension. The pathogenesis of the syndrome is uncertain, but the reaction is not an allergic reaction to penicillin. It typically begins 1 to 2 hours after antibiotic administration and normally subsides spontaneously even while antibiotics are continued.[114] Notably, JHR can occur after administration of many antimicrobials and is not exclusive to penicillins, nor is it exclusive to syphilis treatment, occurring in other spirochetal diseases such as Lyme disease and relapsing fever.[115] Usually self-limiting in nonpregnant patients, the primary risk of this reaction in pregnant women is miscarriage, premature labor, or fetal distress.[116] Pregnant women should seek medical attention if contractions or a change in fetal movements are noted. Close monitoring of JHR should be observed for patients with ophthalmic or neurologic syphilis. For these patients, prednisolone 10 to 20 mg three times a day for 3 days given 24 hours before syphilis treatment may prevent fever, but will not control local inflammation.[102] Tumor necrosis factor-α has been demonstrated to have some success in the prevention of JHR in spirochete disease.[117] Although there is no proven effective preventive therapy, some experts still recommend antipyretics, hydration, and patient education; antibiotic therapy should not be discontinued.

Neonatal Syphilis

34. How should N.W.'s baby be treated if a diagnosis of congenital syphilis is confirmed?

Infants born to mothers who have been treated for syphilis during pregnancy should be carefully examined at birth, at 1 month, every 2 to 3 months for 15 months, and then every 6 months until the VDRL is negative or stable at a low titer. Newborn serology is difficult to interpret because of transplacental transfer of nontreponemal and treponemal immunoglobulin G to the infant. Treatment decisions are largely based on evidence of syphilis in the mother, adequacy of maternal treatment, comparison of maternal and neonate nontreponemal serology, and/or presence of clinical or laboratory evidence of syphilis in the neonate. Aqueous penicillin G 50,000 U/kg per dose IV every 12 hours should be used during the first 7 days of life and every 8 hours thereafter for a total of 10 days. Procaine penicillin G 50,000 U/kg per dose IM daily for at least 10 days is an alternative regimen.[6] If more than 1 day of therapy is missed, the CDC recommends restarting the entire course. In addition, infants should be treated at birth, even if they are asymptomatic, when maternal treatment is unknown or inadequate, or when infant follow-up cannot be guaranteed. In most cases, a CSF examination should be performed before treatment is begun to rule out neurosyphilis. Although benzathine penicillin (50,000 U/kg IM) as a single dose is recommended by some clinicians to treat infants who may not be followed up on, data on the efficacy of this treatment regimen are lacking and any abnormalities in the infant's examination (e.g., abnormal or uninterpretable CSF, long-bone radiographs, complete blood count, and platelets) should preclude its use.[6]

CHANCROID

Chancroid or soft chancre is a painful genital ulcer disease that often is associated with tender inguinal adenopathy. It is caused by *Haemophilus ducreyi,* a Gram-negative bacillus. Chancroid is endemic in developing countries and some areas of the United States, but its incidence in the United States has steadily declined from nearly 5,000 cases in 1987 to 17 cases in

2005.[3] Chancroid and other genital ulcers have been implicated in the transmission of HIV. In the United States, up to 18% of people with genital ulcers were also HIV seropositive.[118]

Signs and Symptoms

35. T.G., a 31-year-old uncircumcised man, presents to the STD clinic with complaints of tender lesions on the penis and inguinal regions. He noticed the penile lesions on the external surface of the prepuce (foreskin) 2 days before his visit. The lesions were sharply demarcated, but were not indurated; the base of the penile ulcer was covered by a yellow-gray purulent exudate. Right inguinal adenitis was present and extremely painful on palpation. A dark-field examination of the purulent exudate was negative. Gram stain revealed a mixture of Gram-positive and Gram-negative flora. T.G. claims to have no drug allergies. What is the natural course of chancroid? Does T.G. have signs or symptoms consistent with chancroid? What diagnostic procedures are necessary?

Uncircumcised males may have an increased risk of chancroid infection and may not respond to therapy as well as circumcised males.[6,119] A painful genital ulcer appears 3 to 10 days after exposure and begins as a tender, red papule that becomes pustular and ulcerates within 2 days. As illustrated by T.G., the ulcer may be covered by a grayish or yellow exudate. Multiple ulcers and tender inguinal lymph nodes, which may become fluctuant, are seen in about 50% of cases.[120] Aspiration of fluctuant nodes may be necessary to prevent rupture. A Gram stain can be misleading because of the polymicrobic nature of the ulcer and culture and because isolation of *H. ducreyi* is difficult, requiring specialized specimen collection and growth media.[6,121]

Treatment

36. How should T.G.'s chancroid be treated?

Most strains of *H. ducreyi* produce a TEM-type β-lactamase, and many strains are resistant to the antimicrobials that traditionally were used to treat chancroid, such as sulfonamides and tetracycline.[122,123] Currently recommended treatment regimens include azithromycin 1 g PO for 1 dose, ceftriaxone 250 mg IM once, ciprofloxacin 500 mg PO BID for 3 days, or erythromycin base 500 mg PO TID for 7 days.[6] Ciprofloxacin is contraindicated in pregnant and lactating women and children 17 years of age or younger. Because T.G. does not have a history of penicillin hypersensitivity, ceftriaxone as a single dose is the preferred treatment regimen. Treatment may not be as effective for patients who are coinfected with HIV or who are uncircumcised.[6,119] Follow-up should occur 3 to 7 days after treatment is initiated. Depending on the size of the ulcer, the time required until complete recovery will vary; larger ulcers may require longer than 2 weeks.[6]

VAGINITIS

Vaginitis is one of the most common reasons why women seek gynecologic care. Approximately 10 million physician office visits are made annually in the United States for women seeking evaluation and treatment of their symptoms.[124] The term *vaginitis* refers to such nonspecific vaginal symptoms as itching, burning, irritation, and abnormal discharge that may be caused by infection or other medical conditions. The most common vaginal infections are BV (22%–50% of cases), vulvovaginal candidiasis (VVC; 17%–39% of cases), and trichomoniasis (4%–35% of cases). However, between 7% and 72% of cases of vaginitis may remain undiagnosed.[125]

BACTERIAL VAGINOSIS

Bacterial vaginosis (formerly called nonspecific vaginitis, leukorrhea, *G. vaginalis,* or *H. vaginalis*) is associated with an increased, malodorous vaginal discharge. The normal vaginal lactobacillus flora is replaced by *Mobiluncus* species, *Prevotella* species, *M. hominis,* and increased numbers of *G. vaginalis.*

The prevalence of BV varies widely owing to differing diagnostic criteria, demographics, and lack of a national reporting system, but it probably represents the most common cause of vaginal disharge.[126] Many sexually active women are infected with *G. vaginalis* at any one time, yet fewer than 50% are symptomatic or have signs of abnormal vaginal discharge.[127] The evidence for definitive risk factors in BV is inconclusive. Multiple sexual partners,[6] a new sexual partner,[6] IUDs,[128] and douching[129] have been associated with BV, whereas smoking, abnormal Pap smears, and timing in relation to menstrual cycle have not.[129] There is conflicting information on the role of heterosexual transmission; some nonsexually active postpubertal women had BV,[130] whereas longitudinal cohort studies showed increased incidence of BV after single and multiple sexual experiences.[131,132] A study among sexually active lesbians showed strong evidence for sexual transmission.[133] The routine treatment of sexual partners is not recommended because clinical trials have shown that a women's response to therapy or her likelihood of relapse or recurrence is not affected by the treatment of her sexual partner(s).[6]

Signs, Symptoms, and Diagnosis

37. H.H. is a 24-year-old, sexually active woman with a 1-week history of moderate vaginal discharge that has a "fishy" odor, most notable after coitus. She has no complaints of vaginal pruritus or burning. On examination, the discharge appears thin, white, homogeneous, and notably malodorous. A wet mount of the vaginal secretion revealed few leukocytes and numerous "clue cells." The vaginal pH was 4.8, and a characteristic fishy odor was noted when the discharge was mixed with 10% potassium hydroxide (KOH). Does H.H. have signs and symptoms consistent with BV? What diagnostic tests are required?

H.H.'s signs and symptoms are typical of BV. The clinical diagnosis can be confirmed by a vaginal Gram stain that shows overgrowth of the vagina with *G. vaginalis* and other organisms as noted earlier.

A 10% KOH solution mixed with the vaginal secretions yields a transient "fishy" odor because of the increased production of biogenic diamines (positive amine test). A wet preparation of the specimen reveals "clue cells" (exfoliated vaginal epithelial cells with adherent coccobacillary pathogens), pH >4.5, and the characteristic KOH "whiff" test.[134] If there are many white cells, other infections (e.g., *T. vaginalis*) should be suspected. Self-diagnosis is correct only about 3% to 4% of the time because most women attribute symptoms to poor hygiene.[135]

Treatment

38. How should H.H. be treated?

Nonpregnant women with symptomatic disease require treatment. Oral metronidazole 500 mg twice a day for 7 days is the most effective treatment of BV. Initially, up to 95% of women respond to this regimen, although only 82% still report cure after 4 weeks, indicating the need for follow-up if symptoms persist or recur.[126,136] The FDA has approved metronidazole extended release 750 mg once daily for 7 days and a single dose of clindamycin intravaginal cream for the treatment of BV; however, the CDC reports that limited data have been published evaluating these regimens to other established therapies.[6] Metronidazole 2 g as single-dose therapy is no longer recommended for treatment because this regimen has the lowest efficacy against BV.[6] Ampicillin is no longer considered an alternative treatment because approximately 50% of women develop recurrent symptoms within 6 weeks.[126,137] Clindamycin cream 2%, one full applicator (5 g) intravaginally at bedtime for 7 days or metronidazole 0.75% gel, one full applicator (5 g) intravaginally, once daily for 5 days are CDC-approved topical recommendations.[6,138] Patients should be instructed to avoid consuming alcohol during treatment with metronidazole and for 24 hours afterward. Additionally, clindamycin cream is oil based and may weaken latex condoms or diaphragms. Alternatively, the CDC recommends clindamycin 300 mg PO two times a day for 7 days or clindamycin ovules 100 mg intravaginally once daily at bedtime for 3 days.

BV has been associated with pregnancy complications such as preterm labor and premature delivery. If the decision is made to treat BV during pregnancy, the CDC recommends metronidazole 250 mg PO three times daily for 7 days or 500 mg PO twice a day for 7 days or clindamycin 300 mg PO twice daily for 7 days. Recent teratogenic data suggest that metronidazole is not harmful to the fetus but the use of intravaginal clindamycin cream has been associated with preterm delivery.[6,139]

VULVOVAGINAL CANDIDIASIS

Candida albicans is the causative organism of VVC in 80% to 92% of cases, with *C. glabrata* and *C. tropicalis* accounting for most of the remaining cases.[140,141] The latter organisms have been identified increasingly as the causative agents of VVC over the past two decades. Approximately 75% of women will experience at least one episode of VVC, and 40% to 45% will have two or more episodes within their lifetime.[6] Approximately 5% of women who have VVC have recurrent candidal episodes (defined as four or more episodes of VVC in 1 year).[6] Vulvovaginal candidiasis is not usually described as an STD because celibate women can develop VVC; however, the incidence of VVC increases when women become sexually active.[141] Because of this, VVC is often diagnosed during evaluation for a suspected STD when women present with vaginal symptoms.[6]

Assessing Self-Treatment

39. L.L., a 23-year-old woman, purchases an over-the-counter (OTC) antifungal agent to relieve vaginal symptoms that she believes are caused by a vaginal yeast infection. L.L. asks the pharmacist for assistance in the selection of an antifungal agent. What information should be obtained from L.L. before a medication is recommended?

Table 65-8 Questions to Gain Information About Possible *Candida* Vulvovaginitis[a]

What symptoms are you experiencing currently?
Have you previously been diagnosed by a physician as having a vaginal yeast infection?
What symptoms did you experience with that previous yeast infection? Are the symptoms you are experiencing now the same or similar to those you had with that previous infection?
If you were treated previously for a vaginal infection, what antifungal agent did you use? For how long did you use it? Was it effective?
Did you experience any adverse effects associated with use of the antifungal agent?
Are you pregnant?
Do you have any medical problems?
Are you taking any medications?
Do you have allergies?
Do you use any vaginal preparations (e.g., feminine hygiene sprays or douches)?
If you have sexual intercourse, what contraceptive method do you use? Does your sexual partner use a condom?
You could also ask questions about tight-fitting clothes, nylon undergarments, swimming, etc.

[a] A questionnaire form might also be helpful in collecting information from the patient.

The pharmacist should ask L.L. if this is her first episode of vaginitis or whether she has experienced similar symptoms previously that have been diagnosed as a vaginal yeast infection and treated by a physician. The nonprescription antifungal agents are indicated for the treatment of VVC in women who previously were diagnosed and treated by their physician. She should be referred to her physician if (a) this is her first episode of VVC; (b) she has had two episodes of VVC within the past 6 months; (c) she is pregnant; (d) she is younger than 16 or older than 60 years of age; (e) she currently has abnormal vaginal bleeding or lower abdominal pain; (f) she has been exposed to a STD; or (g) she has a malodorous vaginal discharge (Table 65-8).

Signs and Symptoms

40. L.L. has experienced two episodes of vaginal yeast infections, with the most recent case occurring approximately 1 year ago. On both occasions she was diagnosed as having VVC by her physician and responded to antifungal therapy. L.L. currently describes vaginal and vulvar itching, vaginal soreness, and vulvar burning accompanied by a thick, white vaginal discharge that has the consistency of cottage cheese. She has been unable to have sexual intercourse because of pain. These symptoms are similar to those she experienced with her previous vaginal yeast infections. L.L. has no underlying major health problems. Her current medications include oral tetracycline for acne and Ortho Tri-Cyclen for birth control. She has regular menstrual cycles and her last menstrual period ended 4 days ago. What clinical manifestations does L.L. exhibit that are consistent with VVC? What are other common manifestations?

L.L. exhibits signs and symptoms associated with VVC (i.e., vulvar and vaginal pruritus, vaginal soreness, vulvar burning, dyspareunia, and a thick, white vaginal discharge that appears to be "curdlike").[6] Although vulvar pruritus occurs in most symptomatic patients, many affected women have little or no vaginal discharge.[140] Typically, the vaginal discharge associated with VVC is a nonodorous, highly viscous, white discharge that may vary in consistency from curdlike to watery.[140] Symptoms may be worse before menses and may diminish with the onset of menses.[140]

Differential Diagnosis

41. How can VVC be differentiated from other vaginal infections?

VVC should be differentiated from other vaginal infections (e.g., BV) because a nonprescription antifungal agent could delay the appropriate treatment of other vaginal infections. The physical appearance of the vaginal discharge may be useful in predicting VVC if it is a viscous, nonodorous, white, curdlike discharge and the patient has a normal vaginal pH (pH < 4.5).[6] The quantity of the discharge may be scanty to profuse. Some women with VVC exhibit only vaginal erythema with minimal discharge or an increased amount of normal vaginal secretion. Table 65-9 characterizes the vaginal discharges associated with VVC, BV, and vaginal trichomoniasis. The vaginal discharge from a woman with signs and symptoms of VVC should be examined for the microscopic presence of *Candida* using a wet mount preparation with 10% KOH or a Gram stain of the vaginal discharge. The use of KOH improves the visualization of yeast or pseudohyphae that are seen in approximately 70% of women diagnosed with VVC.[6] If the wet mount is negative, the patient's vaginal discharge should be cultured for *Candida* in an appropriate growth medium. The identification of *Candida* in the absence of signs and symptoms is not diagnostic for VVC and therefore treatment should not be initiated because *Candida* and other species of yeast represent part of the normal flora in approximately 10% to 20% of women.[6] It is the proliferation of *C. albicans* or other yeasts that lead to vulvovaginitis symptoms.

PHYSIOLOGICAL VAGINAL DISCHARGE AND SYMPTOMATIC NORMAL pH VULVOVAGINITIS

42. Do women such as L.L., who have an increased vaginal discharge and symptoms consistent with VVC, necessarily have a vaginal infection?

Although the possibility of vaginal infection must be addressed when a woman presents with an increased vaginal discharge with or without symptoms, other conditions are associated with an increased discharge. First, a physiological vaginal discharge must be distinguished from a pathological discharge. Physiological discharges (Table 65-9) characteristically are nonodorous, white or clear, highly viscous or flocular, and acidic (pH ~4.5). Physiological discharges may become more profuse at midcycle secondary to increased cervical mucus or vaginal epithelial cells. Other conditions resulting in excessive vaginal discharge with or without VVC-like symptoms include retention of foreign bodies (e.g., tampons) and allergic reactions or contact dermatitis secondary to the use of vaginal spermicidal agents, soaps, deodorants, douches, vaginal lubricants, and condoms. Episodes of vulvovaginitis-like symptoms can be secondary to the frequent use of hot tubs, Jacuzzis, or swimming pools that contain chemically treated water (e.g., high levels of chlorine).[142]

Table 65-10 Modified Amsel's Criteria for the Diagnosis of Bacterial Vaginosis

At least three of the following signs must be present for diagnosis:
Homogeneous discharge
Fishy amine odor when 10% KOH is added (sniff test)
Clue cells (i.e., >20% on wet mount)
Vaginal pH > 4.5
No lactobacilli on wet mount
KOH, potassium hydroxide.

From reference 236.

Susceptibility to Vulvovaginal Candidiasis

43. What specific groups of women are most susceptible to VVC? Does L.L. fit into any group at high risk for VVC?

Women are most susceptible to VVC during their childbearing years. Approximately 50% of U.S. college women report having an episode of VVC between menarche and age 25.[141] *Candida albicans* colonization and symptomatic VVC increase during pregnancy and when high estrogen-containing oral contraceptives are used. This increase has been attributed to estrogen enhancement of the binding affinity of vaginal epithelial cells to *C. albicans*.[143] Women with high glycogen concentrations (e.g., uncontrolled or poorly controlled diabetes mellitus); women with depressed cell-mediated immunity secondary to disease (e.g., cancer, HIV infection); and women taking broad-spectrum antibiotics or immunosuppressive drugs (e.g., cytotoxic agents, corticosteroids) may have increased susceptibility to VVC.[141,143] Individual cases of VVC,

Table 65-9 Characteristics of Vaginal Discharge

Characteristics	*Normal*	*Candidiasis*	*Trichomoniasis*	*Bacterial Vaginosis*
Color	White or clear	White	Yellow-green	White to gray
Odor	Nonodorous	Nonodorous	Malodorous	Fishy smell
Consistency	Floccular	Floccular	Homogeneous	Homogeneous
Viscosity	High	High	Low	Low
pH	~4.5	4–4.5	5–6.0	>4.5
Other characteristics		Thick, curdlike	Frothy	Thin

From references 140, 141, and 143.

although not related to intercourse, may be related to orogenital sex.

L.L. is taking tetracycline, which may heighten her risk of developing VVC. Antibacterials (e.g., tetracycline, ampicillin, cephalosporins) increase the risk for *C. albicans* overgrowth by suppressing the normal vaginal flora (e.g., lactobacilli), which normally protect against *C. albicans.* L.L. is also taking a low-estrogen–containing oral contraceptive; however, low-dose oral contraceptives have not been consistently associated with an increased risk of VVC.[144,145] The use of diaphragms, vaginal sponges, and IUDs also may be risk factors for VVC.[146]

Stress-induced VVC and an increased incidence of VVC before menstruation have been described.[143] The cause of both is currently unknown. Although various dietary factors have been postulated as a cause of vaginal yeast overgrowth, the role of diet in the development of VVC remains inconclusive.[143]

Treatment of Vulvovaginal Candidiasis

VAGINALLY ADMINISTERED AZOLES

44. What vaginally administered therapy might be effective for L.L.'s VVC?

L.L. is an appropriate candidate for OTC therapy (Table 65-11) because she had previous vaginal yeast infections with symptoms similar to those she currently is experiencing, and her VVC is uncomplicated (defined as sporadic disease with mild to moderate symptoms in a immunocompetent host).[6] When a patient's VVC appears complicated (defined as recurrent infections, severe symptoms, non-*albicans* candidiasis, presence of uncontrolled diabetes, debilitation, immunosuppression, or pregnancy), she should be referred to her medical practitioner.[6] L.L. should respond to short-term topical azole therapy. In addition, L.L. should ask her physician whether she

Table 65-11 Products Available for the Treatment of *Candida* Vulvovaginitis

Drug	*Availability*	*Trade Names*	*Dosing Regimens*
OTC Products			
Butoconazole	2% vaginal cream[a]	Femstat 3	*Nonpregnant women:* Administer 1 applicatorful intravaginally QHS for 3 consecutive days *Pregnant women during second and third trimesters:* Administer 1 applicatorful intravaginally QHS for 7 consecutive days
Clotrimazole	1% vaginal cream[a]	Gyne-Lotrimin 7; Mycelex-7; Sweet'n Fresh Clotrimazole 7; various generics	Administer 1 applicatorful intravaginally QHS for 7 consecutive days
Miconazole	2% cream[a]	Monistat 7; Femizol-M; various generics	Administer 1 applicatorful intravaginally QHS for 7 consecutive days
	100-mg vaginal suppositories[a]	Monistat 7	Insert 1 suppository intravaginally QHS for 7 consecutive days
	200-mg vaginal suppositories[a]	Monistat 3	Insert 1 suppository intravaginally QHS for 3 consecutive days
	1200-mg vaginal suppositories[a]	Monistat 1 Daytime Ovule	Insert 1 suppository intravaginally HS for 1 dose only
Tioconazole	6.5% vaginal ointment	Vagistat-1, generics	Administer 1 applicatorful intravaginally at HS for 1 dose only
Prescription Products			
Butoconazole (sustained release)	2% vaginal cream[a]	Gynazole 1	*Nonpregnant women:* Administer 1 applicatorful HS for 1 dose only
Clotrimazole	100-mg vaginal tablets	Gyne-Lotrimin; Mycelex-7; Sweet'n Fresh Clotrimazole 7; various generics	Insert 1 tablet intravaginally QHS for 7 consecutive days
	100-mg vaginal tablets	Gyne-Lotrimin; Mycelex-7; Sweet'n Fresh Clotrimazole 7; various generics	Insert 2 tablets intravaginally QHS for 3 consecutive days
Fluconazole	150-mg oral tablet	Diflucan tablet	Take 1 tablet PO for 1 dose only
Nystatin	100,000 U vaginal tablet	Mycostatin; Nystatin; various generics	Insert 1 tablet intravaginally QHS for 14 consecutive days
Terconazole	0.4% vaginal cream[a]	Terazol 7	Administer 1 applicatorful intravaginally QHS for 7 consecutive days
	0.8% vaginal cream[a]	Terazol 3	Administer 1 applicatorful intravaginally QHS for 3 consecutive days
	80-mg vaginal suppositories[a]	Terazol 3	Insert 1 suppository intravaginally QHS for 3 consecutive days

[a] The CDC states that the use of vaginally administered oil-based preparations may weaken latex products such as condoms and diaphragms.
OTC, over-the-counter; QHS, at bed time.
From reference 6.

should continue with oral tetracycline or be prescribed another oral antibiotic instead. If L.L. had been evaluated by her physician, single-dose oral fluconazole or 3-day intravaginal therapy might have been prescribed.

The available azole antifungals are equally effective in treating VVC with cure rates between 80% and 90% when a full course of therapy is completed.[6,147] All the azole antifungal products listed in Table 65-11 are superior to nystatin. The medication used to treat L.L.'s VVC should be selected based on response or failure to previous therapy, convenience, ease of use, length of therapy, dosage form, and cost. L.L. should select a non–oil-based product if a latex condom or a diaphragm is used for contraception (Table 65-11).

OTHER TREATMENTS FOR ACUTE VULVOVAGINAL CANDIDIASIS

Oral lactobacillus and lactobacillus-containing yogurt have long been advocated for the treatment of VVC; however, evidence in support of this treatment is inconclusive.[148] Boric acid (600-mg capsules) inserted high in the vagina at bedtime for 14 days is effective for the treatment of VVC, but vaginal burning and irritation occur in approximately 4% of women and boric acid is poisonous if inadvertently ingested.[148] The primary indication for these extemporaneously prepared boric acid capsules primarily has been in the treatment of fluconazole-resistant *Candida* infection, especially that due to *C. glabrata*. Gentian violet preparations also have limited use in the treatment of candidiasis because they stain clothing and bed linens and cause local irritation and edema. It is important to note that these alternative regimens for the treatment of acute VVC are not currently recommended by the CDC.

ORAL AZOLES

45. How effective are orally administered azoles in the treatment of an acute VVC infection such as the one L.L. is experiencing?

Fluconazole (Diflucan), administered as a single 150-mg oral dose, is the only oral antifungal agent currently recommended by the CDC for the treatment of acute VVC (Table 65-11).[6] In two clinical studies, a single 150-mg oral dose of fluconazole was as effective as 3- to 6-day regimens of intravaginal clotrimazole.[149,150] Although some women may prefer an orally administered drug to one that is administered intravaginally, their use for mild to moderate VVC is of some concern because of the possibility for systemic adverse effects.

Adverse Effects Associated With Azoles

46. What adverse effects might L.L. experience from intravaginally or orally administered azoles?

When used intravaginally, azoles are associated with minimal adverse reactions, many of which are similar to the symptoms women report from candidiasis infections. Thus, it can be difficult to differentiate disease symptoms from adverse drug reactions. If the vaginal symptoms seem to worsen after therapy is started, the patient should contact her health care provider. In addition, if symptoms have not improved within 3 days after initiation of therapy, the patient should contact her physician to rule out more severe disease, treatment of the wrong disease, or drug-related adverse effects. Vulvovaginal irritation, itching, burning, and pelvic cramps are commonly associated with vaginal administration of azoles (3%–4%).[151] Miconazole has also been associated with headaches, allergic contact dermatitis, and skin rashes; clotrimazole with vulvovaginal pruritus, dyspareunia, and bloating; butaconazole with vulvovaginal pruritus (0.9%), burning (2.3%), soreness, discharge, and swelling; terconazole with headaches (21%–30%), dysmenorrhea (6%), genital pain (4.2%), and pruritus (2.3%–5%); and tioconazole with burning (6%) and itching (5%). Oral fluconazole has been associated with headache (13%), nausea (7%), abdominal pain (6%), diarrhea, dyspepsia, dizziness, taste perversion, angioedema, and rare cases of anaphylactic reactions.[151]

Patient Counseling

47. How should L.L. be counseled about the use of a nonprescription (OTC) vaginal antifungal product?

The details of intravaginal administration should be reviewed with L.L., including instructions on how to clean the applicator (if one is used for drug administration) after each use. To minimize leakage and annoyance, L.L. should apply the product at bedtime to increase retention in the vagina. She should be advised that the OTC vaginal antifungal creams and suppositories are oil based and thus may weaken condoms or diaphragms, thereby reducing their effectiveness.

L.L. should be informed about the importance of completing a full course of therapy even if her symptoms subside beforehand and to continue her antifungal treatment through her menstrual period should it occur. In addition, L.L. should be instructed to see her physician if her symptoms persist, if she experiences symptoms that signal a more serious problem (e.g., abdominal pain, fever, a foul-smelling or bloody vaginal discharge), or if another yeast infection occurs within 2 months.

L.L. also should be advised to avoid wearing tight-fitting, unventilated underwear (e.g., nylon panties or panty hose) and tight-fitting jeans because a warm, moist environment can facilitate fungal growth. However, a study addressing risk factors for VVC found no relation between type of underwear and the incidence of VVC.[146] L.L. also could be alerted to the possible relation between candidiasis and swimming in a heavily chlorinated pool or frequent use of a Jacuzzi or hot tub.

Complicated Vulvovaginal Candidiasis

48. How would management of L.L.'s VVC differ if she had poorly controlled diabetes?

VVC in a woman with uncontrolled diabetes is usually considered to be complicated VVC. A diagnosis of complicated VVC is also warranted when the VVC is severe, recurrent (as defined), caused by non-*albicans* species of *Candida,* or when VVC occurs in an immunosuppressed, debilitated, or pregnant woman. Approximately 10% to 20% of VVC cases can be classified as complicated.[6] The treatment of complicated VVC varies depending on the underlying cause of complication. Severe VVC (extensive vulvar erythema, edema, excoriation, and fissures) should be treated with a 7- to 14-day course of topical azoles or two oral doses of fluconazole 150 mg given 72 hours apart.[6] Infection with non-*albicans Candida* should be treated with a 7- to 14-day course of an oral or intravaginal azole.[6] Oral fluconazole has poor activity against non-*albicans Candida* and should not be used; however, a 7-day regimen of terconazole 0.4% cream has been shown to eradicate non-*albicans Candida* in 56% of affected patients.[6,152] Boric acid 600-mg capsules administered intravaginally once daily for 14 days can be used if this regimen is not effective in eradicating the infection.[6]

Recurrent Vulvovaginal Candidiasis

49. L.L. develops another case of VVC 1 month later. Does she have recurrent VVC? How should she be treated?

Most women have only occasional episodes of VVC, but approximately 5% experience recurrent VVC infections defined as four or more episodes per year.[6] To determine whether L.L. has recurrent VVC, a diagnosis of *Candida* needs to be confirmed by vaginal cultures. Then, underlying risk factors for VVC, such as uncontrolled diabetes mellitus, consumption of excess sugars, IUD placement, and use of antibiotics, must be ruled out.[153] Based on the timing of L.L.'s episodes and the absence of risk factors, L.L. does not meet the definition for recurrent VVC. If a patient meets the criteria for recurrent VVC, an underlying cause of the problem may not be determined. In addition, the role of sexual transmission is not currently well understood.[141] In most patients, the pathogenesis of recurrent VVC cannot be determined.

Treatment of recurrent *C. albicans* vulvovaginitis should focus on a prolonged (7- to 14-day) course of topical therapy or a three dose regimen of oral fluconazole (100, 150, or 200 mg) administered every 3 days to eliminate symptoms and induce remission.[6] A 6-month maintenance regimen should be initiated after remission has been achieved. See Table 65-12 for a list of maintenance regimens. Despite the efficacy of these regimens, discontinuation of therapy after 6 months can result in relapse in up to 50% of women.[6,153] Azole-resistant strains of *C. albicans* are rare; therefore, culture and sensitivity testing is not usually performed to help guide treatment before initiation.

Vulvovaginal Candidiasis During Pregnancy

50. What teratogenic risks are associated with the use of azole preparations?

Vaginal colonization with *Candida* and symptomatic VVC are common during pregnancy.[154] Asymptomatic colonization is not associated with increased maternal or fetal risks and need not be treated.[155] However, symptomatic VVC should be treated. Although doses of oral fluconazole used to treat VVC have not been associated with increased fetal defects, higher doses may be teratogenic. Therefore, topical antifungal agents are preferred for treatment of VVC in pregnant women. The CDC currently recommends a 7-day course of topical antifungal therapy for VVC during pregnancy; however, a 3-day regimen with appropriate follow-up to assess efficacy has been shown to be effective in mild to moderate cases.[6,155] Although nystatin is classified as a category B drug during pregnancy, it is not commonly used bits inferior efficacy rate. Clotrimazole is also classified as a category B drug for fetal risk, and the remaining vaginally administered azoles are designated as category C.[155]

Table 65-12 Maintenance Regimens for Recurrent Vulvovaginal Candidiasis

	Dose	Frequency
Topical agents		
Clotrimazole	200 mg	Twice weekly
Clotrimazole vaginal suppositories	500 mg	Weekly
Oral agents		
Fluconazole tablets	100, 150, or 200 mg	Weekly

From reference 6.

TRICHOMONIASIS

Signs and Symptoms

51. N.B. is a 31-year-old woman with a recent history of diffuse vaginal discharge with vaginal irritation. A wet-mount examination of vaginal secretions revealed numerous trichomonads. Examination confirms the presence of an increased, yellow-green vaginal discharge. What subjective and objective clinical data support a diagnosis of trichomoniasis?

Trichomoniasis is an STD caused by the protozoan *T. vaginalis*. The prevalence in women ranges from 5% to 10% and up to 60% in commercial sex workers.[156] Trichomoniasis in women is asymptomatic about 20% to 50% of the time.[157] In men, *T. vaginalis* presumably infects the urethra, although the site of infection (urethra versus prostate) is uncertain. Men with *T. vaginalis* infection usually are asymptomatic. Classic symptoms of trichomoniasis in women include a diffuse, yellow-green discharge with pruritus, dysuria, and a "strawberry" cervix (cervical microhemorrhages). The latter are typically only seen in 2% to 25% of cases.[158] In almost all cases of trichomoniasis, a vaginal pH higher than 5 or 6 is observed.[159] The Pap smear was reported to have a 48.4% error in diagnosis when used alone.[158] Direct microscopic observation of trichomoniasis using a wet mount suffers from low sensitivity, but is up to 99% specific.[160] Broth culture is considered to be the gold standard for identification of trichomoniasis, but it requires up to a 7-day incubation period and the culture system is not widely available.[158] The best approach to diagnosis requires clinical and laboratory confirmation.

Treatment

Metronidazole and Tinidazole

52. How should N.B.'s trichomoniasis be treated?

The only class of drugs that are effective for the treatment of trichomoniasis are the nitroimidazoles. In the United States, metronidazole and tinidazole are the only available nitroimidazoles. Both are CDC-recommended first-line treatments given as a single 2-g oral dose.[6] In addition, sexual partners should be simultaneously treated. Metronidazole cure rates are reported to be 90% to 95%, whereas tinidazole cure rates are reported to be 86% to 100%; concurrently treating sexual partners might increase these rates.[6,161] Clinical trials seem to suggest that tinidazole is equivalent or superior to metronidazole in achieving cure and resolution of symptoms.[162] Approximately 2% to 5% of *T. vaginalis* isolates exhibit resistance to metronidazole therapy, necessitating a dose increase or a change in therapy to tinidazole.[6] If the 2-g metronidazole dose fails and reinfection is excluded, either metronidazole 500 mg PO twice daily for 7 days or tinidazole 2 g PO as a single dose can be used. If either of these regimens fail, either metronidazole or tinidazole 2 g PO daily for 5 days may be used. In the case of allergy to nitroimidazole compounds, patients can be desensitized and subsequently treated with metronidazole.[144]

ADVERSE EFFECTS

53. N.B. was treated with metronidazole 500 mg twice a day for 7 days. On the fourth day of therapy while attending a party, N.B. developed a severe headache, followed by nausea, sweating, and dizziness. Could N.B.'s symptoms be caused by metronidazole?

Minor side effects associated with metronidazole therapy include nausea, vomiting (especially with single-dose therapy), headache, skin rashes, and alcohol intolerance. The alcohol intolerance may be due to a metronidazole-induced inhibition of aldehyde dehydrogenase, which results in the buildup of high serum acetaldehyde levels, although this mechanism is questionable.[163] Severe "antabuse reactions" are uncommon, but according to the manufacturer, patients still should be warned about the possibility of nausea, vomiting, flushing, and respiratory distress after alcohol consumption, although reliable evidence is lacking.[146] As a general rule, patients should avoid alcohol ingestion during treatment and for 24 hours after metronidazole therapy and for 72 hours after tinidazole therapy.[6]

Pregnancy

54. S.G., a 31-year-old woman, is in her first trimester of pregnancy and has a history of recurrent trichomoniasis. She now complains of a diffuse, yellow vaginal discharge. The preliminary diagnosis of trichomoniasis is confirmed by a wet-mount examination of vaginal secretions that revealed numerous trichomonads. S.G. has read much of the lay press on metronidazole and is concerned about her own safety as well as that of her fetus. Can metronidazole be used for S.G.?

During pregnancy, trichomoniasis is associated with premature rupture of the membranes, preterm delivery, and low birth weight.[6] In a recent meta-analysis, an association between metronidazole use and teratogenicity or mutagenicity in infants could not be shown.[164] However, caution should still be exercised if metronidazole must be administered within the first trimester. Metronidazole is mutagenic in facultative bacteria and contains a nitro-reductase enzyme. Long-term, high-dose metronidazole in laboratory mice is associated with the development of pulmonary and hepatic tumors. Midline facial defects have been documented in humans, but two literature reviews indicate that metronidazole is not a teratogen.[165,166] In contrast, the use of metronidazole in asymptomatic women has not been shown to decrease rates of preterm labor despite eliminating the organism from its host.[167]

TREATMENT

55. How should S.G. be treated?

All symptomatic women should be treated with metronidazole 2 g PO as a single dose.[6] Metronidazole is classified as pregnancy category B. Tinidazole 2 g PO as a single dose could be suggested as an alternative regimen; however, it is classified as pregnancy category C.

GENITAL HERPES

The word *herpes* is of Greek origin and means "to creep." HSV is a DNA-containing virus that consists of two antigenic distinct serotypes: HSV-1 and HSV-2. The primary cause of herpes labialis (cold sores), herpes keratitis, and herpetic encephalitis is HSV-1. Genital herpes and neonatal herpes primarily are the result of HSV-2 infections. However, up to 50% of all reported cases of primary genital herpes are due to HSV-1 infections acquired through oral sex.[168,169]

Etiology

Most infants are exposed to HSV-1 early in life with over half being positive for HSV-1 antibodies before 18 years and more than 90% of the population positive by 70 years of age.[170] The infection often is asymptomatic and generally is acquired through primary infection of the respiratory tract. The initial, primary disease is a gingivostomatitis characterized by vesicles in the oral cavity and occasionally an elevated temperature; life-threatening encephalitis or keratitis may appear during this interval. Usually after primary exposure, HSV-1 enters cells of the trigeminal ganglion, where it may remain latent for the lifetime of the host.[171]

Initial HSV-2 infections usually follow puberty and coincide with the onset of sexual activity, although transfer to a neonate from an infected mother can occur. After primary infection, the virus enters a state of latency in the sacral dorsal root ganglia in many infected individuals; a high percentage of infected persons may never manifest the disease clinically.[171,172]

In both HSV-1 and HSV-2 infections, the latent virus can reactivate. Recurrent disease may occur even when circulating antibody and sensitized lymphocytes are present. Clinically, the lesions periodically erupt usually at the same location, and the interval between episodes varies widely between individuals.

Epidemiology

Although herpes was recognized several thousand years ago, genital herpes was not described formally until the 18th century. The seroprevalence of genital herpes has increased dramatically in the United States—from 16.4% in the late 1970s to 21.9% in the early 1990s—making it the most common STD with over 45 million people infected in the United States.[173] In 2001, U.S. physicians saw more than 150,000 new patients presenting with herpes simplex.[3]

The prevalence of antibody to genital herpes is greater among women (26%) than men (18%) and among blacks (45.9%) than whites (17.6%).[170,173] Demographic characteristics obtained at the University of Washington indicate that the mean number of lifetime sexual partners before acquisition of the disease was 8.8 in women compared with 32.8 in men, with the overall chance of acquiring HSV-2 of 5 per 1,000 sex contacts.[174] The mean time from the last sexual exposure to the onset of disease was 5.8 days.[172]

Signs and Symptoms

56. B.J., a 28-year-old, sexually active man, complains of painful penile lesions and tender inguinal adenopathy. The lesions are vesicular and limited to the scrotum, glands, and shaft of the

penis. The onset of the lesions was preceded by a 1-week period of fever, malaise, headache, and itching. Viral culture of the lesions was positive for HSV infection. Describe the typical course and clinical presentation of herpes genitalis in men and women. What subjective and objective clinical data in B.J. are compatible with herpes genitalis?

Most initial episodes of genital herpes, especially in the male, are symptomatic. As illustrated by B.J., the symptoms usually start about 1 week after the initial exposure with prodromal signs of tingling, itching, paresthesia, and/or genital burning.[175] The prodromal stage, which can last from a few hours to several days, is followed by the appearance of numerous vesicles. The vesicles eventually erupt, resulting in painful genital ulcers. The pain and edema associated with genital herpetic lesions, especially if they are infected secondarily, can be severe enough to result in dysuria and urinary retention. Bilaterally distributed lesions of the external genitalia are characteristic. The lesions usually are limited to the glands, corona prepuce, and shaft of the penis in males and to the vulva and vagina in females. However, lesions can occur on the buttocks, thighs, and urethra.[172] Asymptomatic or mucopurulent cervicitis occurs in about 15% to 20% of women with primary HSV-2 infections.[176] Rectal and perianal HSV-2 infections increasingly are being recognized. Herpes simplex virus proctitis usually is seen in homosexual men and heterosexual men who engage in anorectal intercourse. Symptoms include anorectal pain and discharge, tenesmus, and constipation.

Prior infection with HSV-1 seems to ameliorate the severity of the first episode of genital herpes, but does not appear to affect the rate of recurrence.[177] In primary infections, the local symptoms of pain, itching, and urethral or vaginal discharge last from 11 to 14 days, with a complete disappearance of lesions in 3 to 6 weeks.[172,177] The clinical course of primary herpes is presented in Figure 65-7. Most patients, however, have minor symptoms or are asymptomatic and unaware of their disease; they are most infectious within the first year of acquisition of the virus.[178]

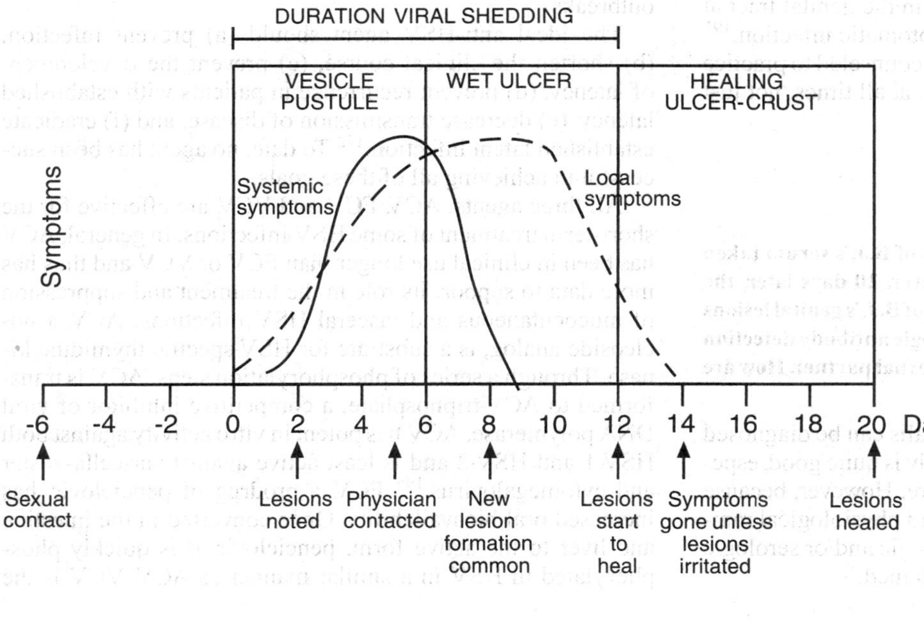

FIGURE 65-7 The clinical time course of primary genital herpes infections. (Reprinted with permission from reference 172.)

Recurrence

57. Is B.J.'s infection likely to recur?

Most patients experience a recurrence of their initial infection. The rate of recurrent infections varies among individual patients. In one study, 38% experienced at least six episodes, and 20% had more than ten recurrences.[177] Natural infection with HSV-2 induces type-specific immunity against exogenous reinfection, but does not affect recurrences.[179] The severity of the primary episode as well as the host's immune response to the disease seem to influence the subsequent recurrence rate.[177] Recurrent infections usually appear at or near the site of the initial infection, and prodromal symptoms are reported by about 50% of persons with recurrent infection. Men seem to have slightly more frequent recurrences. In contrast with primary infections, there are fewer lesions and they are often unilateral.[172] Constitutional symptoms such as lymphadenopathy, fever, and malaise generally are milder. Recurrent infections are shorter in duration (average, 1 week); local symptoms such as pain and itching last 4 to 5 days and the lesions themselves last 7 to 10 days.[172] By about 5 years after the initial infection, recurrence rates tend to decrease.[180] Genital infections with HSV-1, however, recur infrequently and decrease by 50% between 1 and 2 years after infection.[181]

Transmission

58. B.J. states that this is the first time he has had such lesions and that he has had only one sexual partner for the last 14 months. His sexually active female partner has no history of herpes genitalis or any other STD. The couple is very curious as to how B.J. acquired his infection. How is HSV transmitted?

Transmission of HSV occurs by direct contact with active lesions or from a symptomatic or asymptomatic person shedding virus at a peripheral site, mucosal surface, or secretion.[182] Genital HSV-2 infections usually are acquired through sexual (vaginal or anorectal) intercourse, whereas genital HSV-1 infections are acquired via oral–genital sexual practices. Because

HSV is inactivated readily by drying and exposure to room temperature, aerosol and fomite spread are unusual means of transmission.[183] Condoms may act as an effective barrier to viral transmission in women, but this method does not offer complete protection for men.[184,185] Recent evidence suggests that the frequency of condom use is directly proportional to protection against acquisition of HSV-2.[186]

A patient with genital herpes is contagious only when he or she is shedding the virus. The patient begins to shed virus during the prodromal phase, which may be several hours to days before the actual lesions first appear. Subclinical or asymptomatic viral shedding is the most common means of sexual transmission and important from a public health standpoint.[187,188] Lesions are most contagious during the ulcerative phase. The median duration of viral shedding as defined from onset to the last positive culture is about 12 days.[172] The mean time from the onset of vesicles to the appearance of the crust stage (~10.5 days) correlates well with the duration of viral shedding. However, there is considerable overlap between the duration of viral shedding and the duration of crusting. Therefore, patients should be advised to refrain from sexual activity until the lesions have completely healed. Women seem to require a longer total lesion healing time than men, 19.5 and 16.5 days, respectively.[172] The mean duration of viral shedding from the cervix is 11.4 days.

A genital herpes infection may be acquired from an individual who has never had symptomatic genital lesions. States of asymptomatic or subclinical viral shedding occur in the majority of women with recurrent genital herpes as a result of reactivation of latent infection. These recurrent infections can have a primary disease presentation, causing the patient to blame the most proximate sexual partner when in actuality, the exposure could have occurred in the distant past.[189] Serologic and virologic typing can be used to determine whether this is a true primary infection. Using sensitive detection techniques such as PCR, women with recurrent HSV infections demonstrated viral shedding up to 28% of the time, but the relationship between a PCR-positive HSV test and true communicability has yet to be determined.[190] A recent study of men and women seropositive for HSV-2, but with no previous history of symptomatic genital herpes, demonstrated viral shedding in the genital tract at a rate similar to those who reported symptomatic infection.[191] Seropositive HSV patients also should be counseled to practice safer sex, using male or female condoms, at all times, not just during symptomatic episodes.

Diagnostic Tests

59. An HSV antibody test (Western blot) of B.J.'s serum taken on day 1 of the illness was negative. However, 20 days later, the HSV-2 antibody was positive. Viral cultures of B.J.'s genital lesions grew HSV-2. A genital Pap smear and serologic antibody detection tests were negative in B.J.'s asymptomatic sexual partner. How are these laboratory tests to be interpreted?

The accuracy with which herpes genitalis can be diagnosed without the aid of laboratory tests generally is quite good, especially if the infection is recurrent in nature. However, because of the potentially severe psychological and physiological ramifications of such a diagnosis, either virologic and/or serologic confirmation of the diagnosis may be obtained.

The laboratory diagnosis of HSV-1 or HSV-2 infection depends on isolation of virus from tissue culture; detection of viral particles by electron microscopy; visibility of giant cells or intranuclear inclusions by Papanicolaou or Giemsa staining (which are insensitive and nonspecific); direct detection of HSV nucleic acid in cells, blood, or CSF by PCR; or serologic methods using Western blot or EIA.[175] Tissue culture currently is the most sensitive method for detecting mucocutaneous herpes simplex infection. Tests that measure serologic response (as in B.J.'s partner) are valuable in documenting primary infection, but they are not very usefully in recurrent infections. It is possible to differentiate between antibody to HSV-1 and HSV-2 by means of the Western blot assay. Point-of-care devices using HSV-1– and HSV-2–specific antibody testing kits offer ease, reduced time, differentiation between HSV-1 and HSV-2, and high sensitivities and specificities.[6,192,193]

Primary HSV infections are characterized by a fourfold or greater rise in the HSV antibody titer as seen in B.J.'s case. Fewer than 10% of patients with recurrent episodes of disease experience a serologic rise in antibody titer between acute and convalescent sera.[194]

B.J.'s partner's results need to be interpreted cautiously. The negative Pap smear is not completely diagnostic. A nonreactive serology (absence of HSV antibodies) implies the absence of a primary infection, although false-negative reactions have occurred. Absence of antibody to HSV-2 by Western blot would be good evidence against asymptomatic carriage.

Treatment

60. How should B.J.'s lesions be managed? Because the likelihood of recurrence of genital herpes is high, what treatment and prevention measures are recommended currently?

The great anxiety commonly associated with the diagnosis of genital herpes is because there is presently no cure available for the condition. Therapies ranging from antiviral agents and photoinactivation to investigational vaccines have been tried. Currently, only acyclovir (ACV), famciclovir (FCV), and valacyclovir (VCV) are used to treat and prevent genital herpes outbreaks.

The ideal anti-HSV agent should (a) prevent infection, (b) shorten the clinical course, (c) prevent the development of latency, (d) prevent recurrence in patients with established latency, (e) decrease transmission of disease, and (f) eradicate established latent infection.[172] To date, no agent has been successful in achieving all of these goals.

All three agents, ACV, FCV, and VCV, are effective for the short-term treatment of some HSV infections. In general, ACV has been in clinical use longer than FCV or VCV and thus has more data to support its role in the treatment and suppression of mucocutaneous and visceral HSV infections. ACV, a nucleoside analog, is a substrate for HSV-specific thymidine kinase. Through a series of phosphorylation steps, ACV is transformed to ACV-triphosphate, a competitive inhibitor of viral DNA polymerase. ACV has potent in vitro activity against both HSV-1 and HSV-2 and is least active against varicella-zoster and cytomegalovirus.[195] FCV, a prodrug of penciclovir, has increased oral bioavailability. Once converted in the intestine and liver to the active form, penciclovir, it is quickly phosphorylated in HSV in a similar manner as ACV. VCV is the

L-valyl ester prodrug of ACV. The oral bioavailability of VCV is significantly better than ACV, producing plasma levels of ACV comparable to those attained with IV administered ACV, often eliminating the need for parenteral therapy with ACV.[196] All three antiviral drugs seem to have good clinical benefit for genital herpes infections.

In studies of severe, primary genital herpes, IV ACV (5 mg/kg Q 8 hr) significantly reduced the duration of viral shedding, decreased the duration of signs and symptoms of disease by a mean of 5 days, and hastened the time to healing of lesions by a mean of 6 to 12 days over placebo-treated patients.[6,197] Similar findings have been shown in the immunocompromised patient population.[198] IV and oral ACV or VCV also prevent HSV reactivation in seropositive immunocompromised patients who are undergoing bone marrow transplantation.[199] For patients with HIV, ACV 400 mg PO three times daily, FCV 500 mg twice daily, or VCV 500 mg twice daily for 5 to 10 days have been used for recurrent episodes.[6] Currently, IV therapy is recommended only for patients with severe genital or disseminated infections who cannot take oral medication.

Topical therapy with ACV ointment (5% in polyethylene glycol) has minimal effect on the duration of viral shedding, symptoms, and lesion healing in first-episode primary genital herpes and has no effect on the recurrence rate.[197] Currently, topical ACV is not recommended for primary genital herpes. Penciclovir 1% cream is applied every 2 hours while awake and has been shown to be effective for treatment of herpes simplex labialis,[200] but insufficient data exist to recommend its use for genital herpes infections.

The introduction of oral agents (Table 65-13) has replaced the use of topical ACV and thus are indicated for B.J. Oral antivirals speed the healing and resolution of symptoms of first and recurrent episodes of genital HSV-2 infections.[201] Treatment of primary infection after the first week of infection does not seem to change the natural history of recurrent outbreaks; thus, patients should be educated about risk of sexual transmission and prompt recognition of signs and symptoms and the early use of antivirals.[202] The frequency of recurrence decreases with time in most patients. Recurrent episodes of genital HSV-2 infection can be treated with any of the three available oral antivirals (Table 65-13). Rather than having to go into clinic, patients with recurrent infection should have a supply of their antiviral drug with them to allow early initiation of therapy, which may abort or reduce symptoms by 1 to 2 days.[203,204]

Daily suppressive therapy with ACV, FCV, or VCV reduces the frequency of recurrent episodes up to 70% among patients with frequent (more than six episodes per year) genital herpes.[6,205–207] Recurrent outbreaks diminish over time; thus, after each year of continuous suppressive therapy, an effort should be made to discuss discontinuing therapy with the patient.[6] The use of suppressive therapy does not completely eliminate viral transmission. However, a recent randomized, controlled clinical trial of serodiscordant HSV-2–positive couples demonstrated a statistically significant decrease in the rate of transmission to uninfected partners when infected partners took 500 mg/day of VCV.[208] This 8-month study was restricted to heterosexual partners with fewer than ten recurrences per year. The CDC recommends various dosing regimens for VCV, but the 500-mg once-daily dose appears to be less effective than the 1-g once-daily dose in patients with frequent recurrent episodes (i.e., >10 episodes per year).[6] Immunocompromised patients may require higher doses or more frequent intervals for suppression.[209] An increased frequency of resistant strains has been reported in immunocompromised hosts who

Table 65-13 Antiviral Chemotherapy of Genital HSV-2 Infections

	Acyclovir	*Valacyclovir*	*Famciclovir*	*Duration*	*Comments*
First clinical episode	400 mg PO TID *or* 200 mg PO 5 per day	1 g PO BID	250 mg PO TID	7–10 days	May extend treatment duration if healing is incomplete
Episodic recurrent infection	400 mg PO TID *or* 200 mg PO 5 per day *or* 800 mg PO BID	500 mg PO BID *or* 1 g QD	125 mg PO BID	5 days	Most effective if initiated within the first 24 hr of onset of lesions or during the prodrome
Daily suppressive therapy	400 mg PO BID[a]	500 mg PO QD[b] *or* 1 g PO QD	250 mg PO BID	Daily	Reduces the frequency of genital herpes recurrences by ≥75% among patients who have frequent recurrences (i.e., ≥6 recurrences per year); use should be reevaluated at 1 yr
Severe disseminated	5–10 mg/kg IV Q 8 hr	Not indicated	Not indicated	Variable	Hospitalize and treat until clinical resolution of symptoms Follow-up IV therapy with PO ACV to complete 10 days
HIV-infected: episodic	400 mg PO TID *or* 200 mg 5 per day	1 g PO BID[c]	500 mg PO BID	5–10 days	Treat until clinical resolution of lesions
HIV-infected: suppressive	400–800 mg PO BID or TID	500 mg PO BID[d]	500 mg PO BID		

Note: Regimen recommendations derived from 2002 CDC Recommendations.[6]
[a] Safety and efficacy up to 6 years have been documented with the use of acyclovir.
[b] Valacyclovir 500 mg QD seems less effective in patients with >10 episodes per year. Thus, 1 g QD should be used in these patients.
[c] Dosages up to 8 g/day have been used, but an association with a syndrome resembling either hemolytic uremic syndrome or thrombotic thrombocytopenic purpura was observed.
[d] Effective in decreasing both the rate of recurrences and the rate of subclinical shedding among HIV-infected patients.

have used long-term therapy.[210] All ACV-resistant strains are also resistant to VCV, and most are resistant to FCV as well. Foscarnet 40 mg/kg IV every 8 hours may be used for severe ACV-resistant genital HSV infections.[6] Cidofovir 1% gel (not commercially available in the United States, but has been compounded by pharmacists) applied once daily for 5 days may be an alternative to IV foscarnet, but more studies are needed.[6,211]

B.J. is not yet a candidate for daily suppressive ACV therapy. A summary of the indications for ACV, FCV, and VCV is outlined in Table 65-13.

ADVERSE EFFECTS

61. What adverse effects secondary to ACV, FCV, or VCV should be anticipated?

Overall, all forms of ACV, including VCV and FCV, are associated with relatively few adverse reactions largely because of the drugs' affinity for viral thymidine kinase over cellular kinase.

Hematuria and an increase in blood urea nitrogen and serum creatinine may occur, primarily in patients with underlying renal disease or those receiving concomitant nephrotoxic agents. Transient elevations in serum creatinine are associated more frequently with IV than with oral administration. In addition, severe local reactions are possible with IV administration. In immunocompromised patients, VCV at a dosage of 8 g/day was associated with symptoms resembling a hemolytic uremic syndrome or thrombotic thrombocytopenic purpura, but in normal therapeutic doses, this has not occurred according to the manufacturer. When given intravenously in high doses or when significant dehydration exists, ACV has been shown to crystallize in the renal collecting tubules of animals, leading to renal insufficiency.[212] ACV should not be rapidly infused or administered at concentrations >10 mg/mL. If oral ACV or VCV is administered to produce plasma levels equivalent to IV doses, similar changes in renal function may be observed. Dose adjustment is necessary for all three antiviral agents in patients with decreased renal function.

Although neurotoxicity is a rare side effect, case reports of coma and delirium have been reported in patients with renal failure and renally adjusted ACV dosages.[213,214]

Intravenous ACV occasionally has been associated with cutaneous irritation and phlebitis, reversible leukopenia,[215] and transient elevations of liver transaminases. Oral ACV and VCV are relatively safe and do not produce any serious side effects at normal doses. Patients receiving oral ACV, VCV, or FCV may complain of nausea, dizziness, diarrhea, and headaches.

Patient Education and Counseling

62. What are the roles for education and counseling in patients with genital herpes? Are other forms of local or symptomatic care useful?

Most genital herpes infections are benign, and lesions heal spontaneously unless the patient is immunocompromised or the lesions have become infected secondarily. The patient should be instructed to keep the involved areas clean and dry. To prevent autoinoculation, the patient should be told not to touch the lesions and to wash his hands immediately afterward if he comes in contact inadvertently. Local anesthetics provide relief from the pain of genital lesions, but they should be avoided if possible because they counteract efforts to keep the lesions dry. Local corticosteroid therapy is contraindicated because it may predispose the patient to secondary bacterial infections.

Patient counseling is an important facet in the therapy of genital herpes and should include the source contact and any future partner. Health care practitioners should attempt to relieve patients' feelings of guilt and anxiety; discussion of long-term consequences should take place after the acute symptoms of the infection have resolved.

For individuals with frequent recurrences, efforts should be made to identify and avoid stimulatory factors such as sunlight, trauma, or emotional stress. The limitations of therapy and the decreased severity and frequency of recurrences with time should be explained to the patient. The periods of infectivity and the need to avoid sexual activity during these times also should be emphasized, although subclinical or asymptomatic shedding does occur, indicating the need for continuous barrier protection. Women with herpes genitalis should be scheduled for routine Pap smears and should be instructed to discuss the problem with their physicians if they become pregnant.

Currently, there is no completely effective way to prevent the transmission of HSV-2 infection. Barrier forms of contraception, in particular condoms, may reduce the transmission of HSV, but this may be limited only to male-to-female transmission owing to the large area that herpes lesions may occupy on the female.[184] However, recent evidence suggests that a higher frequency of use by males of condoms can increase protection and thus condoms should be recommended routinely to prevent HSV infections in males and females.[186] Nonoxynol-9, a spermicide that has in vitro anti-HSV activity, is ineffective in the treatment of established genital HSV infection and may actually increase the risk of transmission of HSV by causing genital ulceration.[216]

Complications

63. M.F. is a 23-year-old, sexually active female student with a history of frequent and severe recurrences of genital herpes since her initial infection 3 years ago. M.F. has tried numerous therapies, including suppressive and episodic antivirals. None of these therapies has provided M.F. with any relief of her symptoms, nor have they decreased the frequency of her recurrences. M.F. has read much in the lay press about herpes and is concerned about the possible complications of the disease, especially cervical cancer. What are the potential complications of herpes genitalis?

Previous research suggested that HSV-2 might be an oncogenic agent responsible for carcinoma of the cervix. The theoretical association between HSV-2 and carcinoma of the cervix was most likely biased by cross-sectionally designed studies, misclassification, confounding with HPV, now known to cause cervical cancer, and lack of power. A large longitudinal nested case-control study using nearly 20 years of seroepidemiologic and epidemiologic data combined with a meta-analysis concluded that it is very unlikely that HSV-2 is associated with the development of invasive cervical carcinoma.[217]

Pregnancy

64. A.P., a 26-year-old woman in her 32nd week of gestation, was hospitalized with complaints of painful genital lesions, headache, fever, increased vaginal discharge, and dysuria of 1 week's

duration. Multiple ulcerative lesions consistent with genital herpes were present on the cervix, vulva, labia minora, and thighs. How should A.P. be treated?

Herpes genitalis seropositivity in pregnant women occurs more frequently than in nonpregnant women, with 30% to 60% of all pregnant women having serologic evidence of HSV-2 infection.[172] Unfortunately, a large proportion of those infections occurring during pregnancy are limited to the cervix and are totally asymptomatic, often eluding diagnosis.

Pregnant patients with a history of recurrent genital herpes should be examined carefully when they present in labor for evidence of active disease. The safety of systemic ACV and VCV in pregnant women has not been established in controlled trials and therefore is not clearly indicated for A.P. Some small studies suggest ACV administered for several weeks before delivery may decrease recurrent outbreaks and lessen the need for herpes-related cesarean section,[218] whereas a larger randomized clinical trial did not show a benefit on reducing the need for a cesarean delivery with primary infection.[219] In general, it does seem that patients with symptomatic genital herpes benefit from caesarian section.[220] The manufacturer of Zovirax (ACV) maintains an extensive database of fetal complications related to ACV use. To date, no link between ACV and birth defects has been established.[221] The decision to treat HSV with ACV during pregnancy should depend on the clinical severity of infection. Fetal exposure data to FCV or VCV are limited. If the mother has an active herpes genitalis infection at the time of delivery (either active genital lesions or asymptomatic HSV-2 cervicitis), the baby should be delivered by cesarean section within 4 hours after the membranes have ruptured to prevent exposure of the neonate to the virus.[172] However, if no genital lesions are present at the time of labor, vaginal delivery may be recommended.[6] There is evidence that up to 70% of neonatal herpes cases occur in asymptomatic women and the use of ACV or VCV after 36 weeks gestation may decrease clinical disease and viral shedding to the fetus.[222]

Neonatal herpes is a devastating systemic infection of the newborn, associated with high morbidity and mortality. In 1994, assuming an average incidence of 265 cases of neonatal HSV per year, the estimated annual cost to the health care system was $10.5 million.[1] HSV-2 usually is transmitted to the newborn during passage through an infected birth canal, although ascending infections in newborns delivered by cesarean section 6 hours after the membranes have ruptured have been known to occur.[223] The risk of transmission to the newborn is greatest in mothers who acquire an initial infection late in the third trimester and lower in mothers with recurrent infection or those who acquire herpes in the first trimester.[6] A primary episode of clinically apparent HSV-2 results in neonatal HSV-2 infection 50% of the time; 33% of the time in asymptomatic primary infection; 4% if lesions are due to recurrent infection; and 0.04% in nonprimary asymptomatic infection.[224]

GENITAL WARTS

65. S.L., a 19-year-old woman, presents to the women's health clinic for her annual pelvic examination. One week later, her Pap smear is read as showing koilocytosis. A colposcopy is subsequently performed, revealing changes consistent with cervical flat warts. What is the cause of S.L.'s infection? How should she be managed?

HPV, primarily types 6 and 11, are the cause of genital warts, or condylomata acuminata. In the United States, the overall prevalence of HPV infection in women 14 to 59 years is 26.8%, with most occurring among 14- to 24-year-olds.[225] Other types of HPV, including 16 and 18, are strongly associated with cervical cancer.[226] These cause Pap smear changes, including koilocytosis and cervical dysplasia. A common cervical cancer grading system, cervical intraepithelial neoplasia (CIN), uses histologic changes to classify specimens in three categories, CIN1, -2, and -3. The higher the CIN, the greater the chance of progressing to invasive cervical cancer. Most new cases of HPV infection spontaneously regress, but with progressive histologic changes, the chance of spontaneously regressing diminishes (CIN1, 60%; CIN2, 30%; CIN3, 10%).[227] Types of HPV are also classified as high risk, or those likely to cause cancer, and low risk, those less likely to cause cancer. HPV types 16 and 18 are considered high risk and types 6 and 11 are low risk, mostly resulting genital warts. In women, visible warts occur on the labia, introitus, and vagina. Subclinical lesions also commonly occur on these sites and on the cervix, as in S.L.'s case. They are visible only by colposcopy after applying acetic acid. Men can sexually transmit HPV infections to women as well as develop genital warts, and anal and penile cancer associated with oncogenic HPV types, especially type 16.[228]

The goal of HPV therapy is the removal of symptomatic warts. Several therapeutic options are available and include patient-administered treatments to visible warts such as podofilox 0.5% solution or gel and imiquimod 5% cream and provider-administered products such as topical treatments (podophyllin 10%–25%, trichloroacetic acid 80%–90%, and cryotherapy), surgery (laser or scalpel), and intralesional interferon.[6] None of these treatments has been shown to eradicate HPV infection or alter the natural history of HPV. It is important to individualize therapy, considering location and number of warts, patient preference, cost, and convenience.

Podophyllin, compounded as a 10% to 25% solution in tincture of benzoin, is applied by the health care provider to visible warts. After application, it is washed off 3 to 4 hours later and then reapplied once or twice a week until the warts have disappeared. Podofilox 0.5% solution or gel, the active component of podophyllin resin, may be applied by the patient with a cotton swab, or podofilox gel with a finger, to visible genital warts twice a day for 3 days, followed by 4 days of no therapy. A total of four cycles, 0.5 mL/day, or application of an area larger than 10 cm^2 should not be exceeded. Podofilox solution is not suitable for use with perianal warts; the gel is more practical for this region. Podophyllin is potentially neurotoxic if absorbed in large amounts. Podofilox has the advantage over podophyllin resin in that it has a longer shelf life, does not need to be washed off, and has less systemic toxicity.[229] Therefore, it should be applied in limited doses and should also be avoided in pregnancy. The rate of wart recurrence after podophyllin therapy is extremely high, probably 50%. With the high cost of clinic care and the high recurrence rate, home treatment of HPV with podofilox solution may be more cost effective and equally efficacious.[230]

Imiquimod induces cytokines and activates the cell-mediated immune system. In initial trials, complete clearance of warts took place in 37% to 50% of immunocompetent patients, but up to 20% experienced recurrence.[231] A 5% cream may be applied with a finger at bedtime three times per week for up to 16 weeks. It is usually left on for 6 to 10 hours before it is washed off with soap and water. Imiquimod may take as long as 8 weeks before warts are cleared. Mild to moderate local irritation occurs in more than half of the patients who use it, especially when used daily instead of three times weekly.[232]

Cryotherapy by application of liquid nitrogen can be more effective than podophyllin, but requires special equipment and highly trained personnel to avoid over- or undertreating warts. Pain and skin blistering after treatment is not unusual. Cryotherapy is associated with little systemic toxicity and is useful against oral, anal, urethral, and vaginal warts.

Trichloroacetic acid (80%–90%) is used topically in the treatment of some genital warts, but its efficacy is uncertain. To date, interferons are not recommended because of expense, frequent occurrence of toxicity when given systemically, and limited efficacy for intralesional administration. Cases refractory to topical drug therapy should be considered for surgical treatment.

Prevention

In 2006, the first vaccine to prevent HPV types 6, 11, 16, and 18 was approved in the United States. This quadrivalent vaccine was tested in women from 15 to 26 years of age with 98% to 100% protection against HPV types contained in the vaccine.[233,234] This three-dose series can be given as early as 9 years of age, but is CDC recommended at 11 to 12 years as part of a routine adolescent health care visit and ideally before commencement of sexual activity.[235] Because there are more than 30 types of HPV associated with anogenital disease, a previous HPV infection is not a contraindication to vaccination. It is also important to note that receipt of the HPV vaccine does not change the recommendation for Pap smears. It is also not a therapeutic vaccine; it has no effect on clearing a current HPV infection.[236]

VACCINES

Prevention and control of STDs have largely revolved around education and antimicrobials. Immunization, however, holds the promise of protecting large numbers of people before they are at risk for STDs as well as targeting those who already have the infection. Hepatitis B is an example of an STD with a highly effective vaccine that is now mandatory for school-aged children. The quadrivalent HPV vaccine is gaining momentum and a bivalent (HPV 16 and 18) is awaiting review and approval by the FDA. Herpes simplex vaccines have been extensively studied, but no candidate vaccine has been submitted for approval.

REFERENCES

1. Eng T, Butler W, eds. Institute of Medicine: Committee on Prevention and Control of Sexually Transmitted Diseases. *The hidden epidemic: confronting sexually transmitted diseases.* Washington, D.C.: National Academy Press; 1997.
2. U.S. Department of Health and Human Services. Sexually Transmitted Disease Surveillance 2005 Supplement: Gonococcal Isolate Surveillance Project (GISP) Annual Report 2005. 2007. Available at: http://www.cdc.gov/std/GISP2005. Accessed June.
3. Sexually Transmitted Disease Surveillance, 2005 U.S. Department of Health and Human Services, Atlanta, GA. 2006. Available at: http://www.cdc.gov/std/stats/05pdf/Surv2005.pdf. Accessed February 2008.
4. Handsfield HH et al. Localized outbreak of penicillinase-producing *Neisseria gonorrhoeae.* Paradigm for introduction and spread of gonorrhea in a community. *JAMA* 1989;261:2357.
5. Mertz KJ et al. Gonorrhea in male adolescents and young adults in Newark, New Jersey: implications of risk factors and patient preferences for prevention strategies. *Sex Transm Dis* 2000;27:201.
6. CDC. Sexually transmitted diseases treatment guidelines 2006. Centers for Disease Control and Prevention. *MMWR Recomm Rep* 2006;55(RR-11):1.
7. CDC. Resurgent bacterial sexually transmitted disease among men who have sex with men–King County, Washington, 1997–1999. *MMWR Morb Mortal Wkly Rep* 1999;48:773.
8. Holmes KK et al. An estimate of the risk of men acquiring gonorrhea by sexual contact with infected females. *Am J Epidemiol* 1970;91:170.
9. Hook EW et al. Gonococcal infections in the adult. In: Holmes KK, ed. *Sexually Transmitted Diseases.* 3rd ed. New York: McGraw-Hill Health Professions Division; 1999;451.
10. Whittington WL et al. Unique gonococcal phenotype associated with asymptomatic infection in men and with erroneous diagnosis of nongonococcal urethritis. *J Infect Dis* 2000;181:1044.
11. Turner CF et al. Untreated gonococcal and chlamydial infection in a probability sample of adults. [Comment]. *JAMA* 2002;287:726.
12. Mehta SD et al. Unsuspected gonorrhea and chlamydia in patients of an urban adult emergency department: a critical population for STD control intervention. *Sex Transm Dis* 2001;28:33.
13. Emmert DH et al. Sexually transmitted diseases in women. Gonorrhea and syphilis. *Postgrad Med* 2000;107:181.
14. Centers for Disease Control and Prevention (CDC). Control of *Neisseria gonorrhoeae* infection in the United States: report of an external consultants' meeting convened by the division of STD prevention, National Center for HIV, STD, and TB Prevention, Centers for Disease Control and Prevention (CDC). Atlanta: CDC; 2001:19.
15. Watts DH et al. Sexually transmitted diseases, including HIV infection in pregnancy. In: Holmes KK, ed. *Sexually Transmitted Diseases.* 3rd ed. New York: McGraw-Hill Health Professions Division; 1999:1089.
16. Brocklehurst P. Update on the treatment of sexually transmitted infections in pregnancy–2. *Int J STD AIDS* 1999;10:636.
17. Johnson RE et al. Screening tests to detect *Chlamydia trachomatis* and *Neisseria gonorrhoeae* infections–2002. *MMWR Recomm Rep* 2002; 51(RR-15):1.
18. Diemert DJ et al. Confirmation by 16S rRNA PCR of the COBAS AMPLICOR CT/NG test for diagnosis of *Neisseria gonorrhoeae* infection in a low-prevalence population. *J Clin Microbiol* 2002;40:4056.
19. CDC. Update to CDC's sexually transmitted diseases treatment guidelines, 2006: fluoroquinolones no longer recommended for treatment of gonococcal infections. *MMWR Morb Mortal Wkly Rep* 2007;56:332.
20. CDC. Discontinuation of spectinomycin. *MMWR Morb Mortal Wkly Rep* 2006;55(RR-13):370.
21. Park MA, Li JTC. Diagnosis and management of penicillin allergy. *Mayo Clin Proc* 2005;80:405.
22. CDC. Discontinuation of cefixime tablets—United States. *MMWR Morb Mortal Wkly Rep* 2002;51:1052.
23. Aplasca De Los, Reyes MR et al. A randomized trial of ciprofloxacin versus cefixime for treatment of gonorrhea after rapid emergence of gonococcal ciprofloxacin resistance in the Philippines. *Clin Infect Dis* 2001;32:1313.
24. Thorpe EM et al. Comparison of single-dose cefuroxime axetil with ciprofloxacin in treatment of uncomplicated gonorrhea caused by penicillinase-producing and non-penicillinase-producing *Neisseria gonorrhoeae* strains. *Antimicrob Agents Chemother* 1996;40:2775.
25. Thompson EM et al. Oral cephalosporins: newer agents and their place in therapy. *Am Family Phys* 1994;50:401.
26. Tapsall JW et al. The sensitivity of 173 Sydney isolates of *Neisseria gonorrhoeae* to cefpodoxime and other antibiotics used to treat gonorrhea. *Pathology* 1995;27:64.
27. Handsfield HH et al. Multicenter trial of single-dose azithromycin vs. ceftriaxone in the treatment of uncomplicated gonorrhea. Azithromycin Gonorrhea Study Group. *Sex Transm Dis* 1994;21:107.
28. CDC. Decreased susceptibility of *Neisseria gonorrhoeae* to fluoroquinolones—Ohio and Hawaii, 1992–1994. *MMWR Morb Mortal Wkly Rep* 1994; 43:325.
29. CDC. Fluoroquinolone resistance in *Neisseria gonorrhoeae*—Colorado and Washington, 1995. *MMWR Morb Mortal Wkly Rep* 1995;44:761.
30. World Health Organization. Antimicrobial resistance in Neisseria gonorrhoeae. 2001; pg. 65. Available at: http://www.who.int/emc/amrpdfs/Antimicrobial_resistance_in_Neisseria_gonorrhoeae.pdf. Accessed February 2008.
31. Kam KM et al. Ofloxacin susceptibilities of 5,667 *Neisseria gonorrhoeae* strains isolated in Hong Kong. *Antimicrob Agents Chemother* 1993;37: 2007.
32. CDC. Increases in fluoroquinolone-resistant *Neisseria gonorrhoeae*—Hawaii and California, 2001. *MMWR Morb Mortal Wkly Rep* 2002;51:1041.
33. Knapp JS et al. Molecular epidemiology, in 1994, of *Neisseria gonorrhoeae* in Manila and Cebu City, Republic of the Philippines. *Sex Transm Dis* 1997;24:2.
34. Fox KK et al. Antimicrobial resistance in *Neisseria gonorrhoeae* in the United States, 1988–1994: the

emergence of decreased susceptibility to the fluoroquinolones. *J Infect Dis* 1997;175:1396.
35. Tracking the hidden epidemics: trends in STDs in the United States, 2000:36. Available at: http://www.cdc.gov/nchstp/dstd/Stats_Trends/Trends2000.pdf. Accessed 2000.
36. Lafferty WE et al. Sexually transmitted diseases in men who have sex with men. Acquisition of gonorrhea and nongonococcal urethritis by fellatio and implications for STD/HIV prevention. *Sex Transm Dis* 1997;24:272.
37. Jebakumar SP et al. Value of screening for oro-pharyngeal *Chlamydia trachomatis* infection. *J Clin Pathol* 1995;48:658.
38. Page-Shafer K et al. Increased sensitivity of DNA amplification testing for the detection of pharyngeal gonorrhea in men who have sex with men. *Clin Infect Dis* 2002;34:173.
39. Geisler WM et al. Epidemiology of anorectal chlamydial and gonococcal infections among men having sex with men in Seattle: utilizing serovar and auxotype strain typing. *Sex Transm Dis* 2002;29:189.
40. Kent C et al. Prevalence of rectal, urethral, and pharyngeal Chlamydia and gonorrhea detected in 2 clinical settings among men who have sex with men: San Francisco, California, 2003. *Clin Infect Dis* 2005;41:67.
41. Feldblum PJ et al. The effectiveness of barrier methods of contraception in preventing the spread of HIV. *AIDS* 1995;9(Suppl A):S85.
42. Roddy RE et al. Effect of nonoxynol-9 gel on urogenital gonorrhea and chlamydial infection: a randomized controlled trial. *JAMA* 2002;287:1117.
43. Cook RL et al. Do spermicides containing nonoxynol-9 prevent sexually transmitted infections? A meta-analysis. *Sex Transm Dis* 1998;25:144.
44. Centers for Disease Control and Prevention. Nonoxynol-9 spermicide contraception use—United States, 1999. *MMWR Morb Mortal Wkly Rep* 2002;51:389.
45. Sutton M et al. The prevalence of trichomonas vaginalis infection among reproductive age women in the United States, 2001–2004. *Clin Infect Dis* 2007;45:1319.
46. Wiesenfeld HC et al. Lower genital tract infection and endometritis: insight into subclinical pelvic inflammatory disease. *Obstet Gynecol* 2002;100:456.
47. Sutton MY et al. Trends in pelvic inflammatory disease hospital discharges and ambulatory visits, United States, 1985–2001. *Sex Transm Dis* 2005;32:778.
48. Haggerty C, Ness R. Newest approaches to treatment of pelvic inflammatory disease: a review of recent randomized clinical trials. *Clin Infect Dis* 2007;44:953.
49. Barrett S, Taylor C: A review on pelvic inflammatory disease. *Int J STD AIDS* 2005;16:715.
50. Mohllajee AP et al. Does insertion and use of an intrauterine device increase the risk of pelvic inflammatory disease among women with sexually transmitted infection? A systematic review. *Contraception* 2006;73:145.
51. Westrom L et al. Pelvic inflammatory disease. In: Holmes KK, ed. *Sexually Transmitted Diseases.* 3rd ed. New York: McGraw-Hill Health Professions Division; 1999:783.
52. Rein DB et al. Direct medical cost of pelvic inflammatory disease and its sequelae: decreasing, but still substantial. *Obstet Gynecol* 2000;95:397.
53. Ross JDC: An update on pelvic inflammatory disease. *Sex Transm Infect* 2002;78:18.
54. Gaitan H et al. Accuracy of five different diagnostic techniques in mild-to-moderate pelvic inflammatory disease. *Infect Dis Obstet Gynecol* 2002;10:171.
55. Scholes D et al. Prevention of pelvic inflammatory disease by screening for cervical chlamydial infection. *N Engl J Med* 1996;334:1362.
56. Addiss DG et al. Decreased prevalence of *Chlamydia trachomatis* infection associated with a selective screening program in family planning clinics in Wisconsin. *Sex Transm Dis* 1993;20:28.
57. Westrom L et al. Pelvic inflammatory disease and fertility. A cohort study of 1,844 women with laparoscopically verified disease and 657 control women with normal laparoscopic results. *Sex Transm Dis* 1992;19:185.
58. Mehrany K et al. Disseminated gonococcemia. *Int J Dermatol* 2003;42:208.
59. Ross JD. Systemic gonococcal infection. *Genitourin Med* 1996;72:404.
60. Schachter J. Biology of *Chlamydia trachomatis.* In: Holmes KK, ed. *Sexually Transmitted Diseases.* 3rd ed. New York: McGraw-Hill Health Professions Division; 1999:391.
61. U.S. Department of Health and Human Services. Sexually Transmitted Disease Surveillance, 2005. Available at: http://www.cdc.gov/std/stats/05pdf/2005-national-profile.pdf. Accessed September 2007.
62. Centers for Disease Control and Prevention. Sexually transmitted disease surveillance 2005 supplement, Chlamydia Prevalence Monitoring Project Annual Report 2005. Atlanta: U.S. Department of Health and Human Services, Centers for Disease Control and Prevention. December 2006. Available at: http://www.cdc.gov/std/Chlamydia2005/CTSurvSupp2005Short.pdf. Accessed September 2007.
63. Stamm WE: *Chlamydia trachomatis* infections of the adult. In: Holmes KK, ed. *Sexually Transmitted Diseases.* 3rd ed. New York: McGraw-Hill Health Professions Division; 1999:407.
64. Wang S et al. Evaluation of antimicrobial resistance and treatment failures for *Chlamydia trachomatis*: a meeting report. *J Infect Dis* 2005;191:917.
65. Lau C-Y, Qureshi AK. Azithromycin versus doxycycline for genital chlamydial infections: a meta-analysis of randomized clinical trials. *Sex Transm Dis* 2002;29:497.
66. Ridgway GL. Treatment of chlamydial genital infection. *J Antimicrob Chemother* 1997;40:311.
67. Rice RJ et al. Susceptibilities of *Chlamydia trachomatis* isolates causing uncomplicated female genital tract infections and pelvic inflammatory disease. *Antimicrob Agents Chemother* 1995;39:760.
68. Hughes G et al. New cases seen at genitourinary medicine clinics: England 1997. *Commun Dis Rep CDR Suppl* 1998;8:S1.
69. Burstein GR et al. Nongonococcal urethritis—a new paradigm. *Clin Infect Dis* 1999;28(Suppl 1):S66.
70. Horner P et al. Role of *Mycoplasma genitalium* and *Ureaplasma urealyticum* in acute and chronic nongonococcal urethritis. *Clin Infect Dis* 2001;32:995.
71. Krieger JN. Trichomoniasis in men: old issues and new data. *Sex Transm Dis* 1995;22:83.
72. Falk L et al. Tetracycline treatment does not eradicate Mycoplasma genitalium. *Sex Transm Infect* 2003;79:318.
73. Stamm WE et al. Azithromycin for empirical treatment of the nongonococcal urethritis syndrome in men. A randomized double-blind study. *JAMA* 1995;274:545.
74. Steingrimsson O et al. Single dose azithromycin treatment of gonorrhea and infections caused by *C. trachomatis* and *U. urealyticum* in men. *Sex Transm Dis* 1994;21:43.
75. Martin DH et al. A controlled trial of a single dose of azithromycin for the treatment of chlamydial urethritis and cervicitis. The Azithromycin for Chlamydial Infections Study Group. *N Engl J Med* 1992;327:921.
76. Tartaglione TA et al. The role of fluoroquinolones in sexually transmitted diseases. *Pharmacotherapy* 1993;13:189.
77. Hooton TM et al. Ciprofloxacin compared with doxycycline for nongonococcal urethritis. Ineffectiveness against *Chlamydia trachomatis* due to relapsing infection. *JAMA* 1990;264:1418.
78. Meyers DS et al. Screening for chlamydial infection: an evidence update for the U.S. Preventive Services Task Force. *Ann Intern Med* 2007;147:135.
79. Wehbeh HA et al. Single-dose azithromycin for Chlamydia in pregnant women. *J Reprod Med* 1998;43:509.
80. Adair CD et al. *Chlamydia* in pregnancy: a randomized trial of azithromycin and erythromycin. *Obstet Gynecol* 1998;91:165.
81. Perine PL et al. *Lymphogranuloma venereum.* In: Holmes KK, ed. *Sexually Transmitted Diseases.* 3rd ed. New York: McGraw-Hill Health Professions Division; 1999:23.
82. van Hal SJ et al. Lymphogranuloma venereum: an emerging anorectal disease in Australia. *Med J Aust* 2007;187:309.
83. Mabey D et al. Lymphogranuloma venereum. *Sex Transm Infect* 2002;78:90.
84. Centers for Disease Control and Prevention. Primary and secondary syphilis—United States, 1998. *MMWR Morb Mortal Wkly Rep* 1999;48:873.
85. Centers for Disease Control and Prevention. Primary and secondary syphilis—United States, 2000–2001. *MMWR Morb Mortal Wkly Rep* 2002;51:971.
86. Centers for Disease Control and Prevention. Sexually transmitted disease surveillance 2006 supplement: Syphilis Surveillance Report. Atlanta: U.S. Department of Health and Human Services, Centers for Disease Control and Prevention. December 2007. Available at: http://www.cdc.gov/std/Syphilis2006/Syphilis2006Short.pdf. Accessed February 2008.
87. Centers for Disease Control and Prevention. Outbreak of syphilis among men who have sex with men—Southern California, 2000. *MMWR Morb Mortal Wkly Rep* 2001;50:117.
88. Sparling P. Natural history of syphilis. In: Holmes KK, ed. *Sexually Transmitted Diseases.* 3rd ed. New York: McGraw-Hill Health Professions Division; 1999:473.
89. Chapel TA. The variability of syphilitic chancres. *Sex Transm Dis* 1978;5:68.
90. Musher D. Early syphilis. In: Holmes KK, ed. *Sexually Transmitted Diseases.* 3rd ed. New York: McGraw-Hill Health Professions Division; 1999:479.
91. Birnbaum NR et al. Resolving the common clinical dilemmas of syphilis. *Am Fam Physician* 1999;59:2233.
92. Gjestland T. The Oslo study of untreated syphilis: an epidemiologic investigation of the natural course of syphilitic infection based on a restudy of the Boeck-Bruusgaard material. *Acta Derm Venereol* 1955;35(Suppl 34):I.
93. Garnett GP et al. The natural history of syphilis. Implications for the transmission dynamics and control of infection. *Sex Transm Dis* 1997;24:185.
94. Swartz M et al. Late syphilis. In: Holmes KK, ed. *Sexually Transmitted Diseases.* 3rd ed. New York: McGraw-Hill Health Professions Division; 1999;487.
95. Flood JM et al. Neurosyphilis during the AIDS epidemic, San Francisco, 1985–1992. *J Infect Dis* 1998;177:931.
96. Pezzini A et al. Meningovascular syphilis: a vascular syndrome with typical features? *Cerebrovasc Dis* 2001;11:352.
97. Larsen SA et al. Laboratory diagnosis and interpretation of tests for syphilis. *Clin Microbiol Rev* 1995;8:1.
98. Clyne B et al. Syphilis testing. *J Emerg Med* 2000;18:361.
99. Farnes SW et al. Serologic tests for syphilis. *Postgrad Med* 1990;87:37.
100. Hook EW 3rd et al. Acquired syphilis in adults. *N Engl J Med* 1992;326:1060.
101. Matsumoto M et al. Latex agglutination test for detecting antibodies to *Treponema pallidum. Clin Chem* 1993;39:1700.
102. Pao D et al. Management issues in syphilis. *Drugs* 2002;62:1447.
103. World Health Organization (WHO). *Guidelines for the Management of Sexually Transmitted Infections.* Vol 2003. Geneva: WHO Department of HIV/AIDS; 2001:1.

104. Felman YM et al. Syphilis serology today. *Arch Dermatol* 1980;116:84.
105. Genc M et al. Syphilis in pregnancy. *Sex Transm Infect* 2000;76:73.
106. Nathan L et al. In utero infection with *Treponema pallidum* in early pregnancy. *Prenat Diagn* 1997;17:119.
107. Doroshenko A et al. Syphilis in pregnancy and the neonatal period. *Int J STD AIDS* 2006;17:221.
108. Larkin JA et al. Recognizing and treating syphilis in pregnancy. *Medscape Womens Health* 1998;3:5.
109. Niebyl JR. Teratology and Drugs in Pregnancy. In: Danforth DN, Scott JR, eds. *Danforth's Obstetrics and Gynecology.* 8th ed. Philadelphia: Lippincott Williams & Wilkins; 1999.
110. Heikkinen T et al. The transplacental transfer of the macrolide antibiotics erythromycin, roxithromycin and azithromycin. *BJOG* 2000;107:770.
111. Mascola L et al. Congenital syphilis. Why is it still occurring? *JAMA* 1984;252:1719.
112. Alexander JM et al. Efficacy of treatment for syphilis in pregnancy. *Obstet Gynecol* 1999; 93:5.
113. Radolf JD et al. *Treponema pallidum* and *Borrelia burgdorferi* lipoproteins and synthetic lipopeptides activate monocytes/macrophages. *J Immunol* 1995;154:2866.
114. Silberstein P et al. A case of neurosyphilis with a florid Jarisch-Herxheimer reaction. *J Clin Neurosci* 2002;9:689.
115. Negussie Y et al. Detection of plasma tumor necrosis factor, interleukins 6, and 8 during the Jarisch-Herxheimer reaction of relapsing fever. *J Exp Med* 1992;175:1207.
116. Klein VR et al. The Jarisch-Herxheimer reaction complicating syphilotherapy in pregnancy. *Obstet Gynecol* 1990;75:375.
117. Fekade D et al. Prevention of Jarisch-Herxheimer reactions by treatment with antibodies against tumor necrosis factor alpha. *N Engl J Med* 1996; 335:311.
118. Mertz KJ et al. Etiology of genital ulcers and prevalence of human immunodeficiency virus coinfection in 10 U.S. cities. The Genital Ulcer Disease Surveillance Group. *J Infect Dis* 1998;178:1795.
119. Schmid GP. Treatment of chancroid, 1997. *Clin Infect Dis* 1999;28(Suppl 1):S14.
120. Hammond GW et al. Epidemiologic, clinical, laboratory, and therapeutic features of an urban outbreak of chancroid in North America. *Rev Infect Dis* 1980;2:867.
121. Allan RR et al. Chancroid and *Haemophilus ducreyi*. In: Holmes KK, ed. *Sexually Transmitted Diseases.* 3rd ed. New York: McGraw-Hill Health Professions Division; 1999:515.
122. Knapp JS et al. In vitro susceptibilities of isolates of Haemophilus ducreyi from Thailand and the United States to currently recommended and newer agents for treatment of chancroid. *Antimicrob Agents Chemother* 1993;37:1552.
123. National guideline for the management of chancroid. Clinical Effectiveness Group (Association of Genitourinary Medicine and the Medical Society for the Study of Venereal Diseases). *Sex Transm Infect* 1999;75(Suppl 1):S43.
124. Lipsky MS et al. Impact of vaginal antifungal products on utilization of health care services: evidence from patient visits. *J Am Board Fam Pract* 1999;13:178.
125. Anderson MR et al. Evaluation of vaginal complaints. *JAMA* 2004;291:1368.
126. Hillier SL et al. Bacterial vaginosis. In: Holmes KK, ed. *Sexually Transmitted Diseases.* 3rd ed. New York: McGraw-Hill Health Professions Division; 1999:563.
127. West RR et al. Prevalence of *Gardnerella vaginalis:* an estimate. *Br Med J (Clin Res Ed)* 1988;296: 1163.
128. Avonts D et al. Incidence of uncomplicated genital infections in women using oral contraception or an intrauterine device: a prospective study. *Sex Transm Dis* 1990;17:23.
129. Ness RB et al. Douching in relation to bacterial vaginosis, lactobacilli, and facultative bacteria in the vagina. *Obstet Gynecol* 2002;100:765.
130. Amsel R. et al. Nonspecific vaginitis. Diagnostic criteria and microbial and epidemiologic associations. *Am J Med* 1983;74;14.
131. Barbone F et al. A follow-up study of methods of contraception, sexual activity, and rates of trichomoniasis, candidiasis, and bacterial vaginosis. *Am J Obstet Gynecol* 1990;163:510.
132. Hawes SE et al. Hydrogen peroxide-producing lactobacilli and acquisition of vaginal infections. *J Infect Dis* 1996;174:1058.
133. Berger BJ et al. Bacterial vaginosis in lesbians: a sexually transmitted disease. *Clin Infect Dis* 1995; 21:1402.
134. Hay P et al. Evaluation of a novel diagnostic test for bacterial vaginosis: 'the electronic nose.' *Int J STD AIDS* 2003;14:114.
135. Ferris DG et al. Women's use of over-the-counter antifungal medications for gynecologic symptoms. *J Fam Pract* 1996;42:595.
136. Lugo-Miro VI et al. Comparison of different metronidazole therapeutic regimens for bacterial vaginosis. A meta-analysis. *JAMA* 1992;268:92.
137. Spiegel CA et al. Anaerobic bacteria in nonspecific vaginitis. *N Engl J Med* 1980;303:601.
138. Livengood CH 3rd et al. Comparison of once-daily and twice-daily dosing of 0.75% metronidazole gel in the treatment of bacterial vaginosis. *Sex Transm Dis* 1999;26:137.
139. Joesoef MR et al. Intravaginal clindamycin treatment for bacterial vaginosis: effects on preterm delivery and low birth weight. *Am J Obstet Gynecol* 1995;173:1527.
140. Ries AJ. Treatment of vaginal infections: candidiasis, bacterial vaginosis, and trichomoniasis. *JAPhA* 1997;37:563.
141. Sobel JD. Vaginitis. *N Engl J Med* 1997;337:1896.
142. Sobel JD. Vulvovaginitis: when *Candida* becomes a problem. *Dermatol Clin* 1998;16:763.
143. Carr PL et al. Evaluation and management of vaginitis. *J Gen Intern Med* 1998;13:335.
144. Eckert LO et al. Vulvovaginal candidiasis: clinical manifestations, risk factors, management algorithm. *Obstet Gynecol* 1998;92:757.
145. Gieger AM et al. The epidemiology of vulvovaginal candidiasis among university students. *Am J Public Health* 1996;85:1146.
146. Otero L et al. Vulvovaginal candidiasis in female sex workers. *Int J STD AIDS* 1998;9:526.
147. ACOG Committee on Practice Bulletins. ACOG practice bulletin no. 72. *Obstet Gynecol* 2006; 107:1195.
148. Van Kessel K et al. Common complementary and alternative therapies for yeast vaginitis and bacterial vaginosis: a systematic review. *Obstet Gynecol Surv* 2003;58:351.
149. O-Prasertsawat P, Bourlert A. Comparative study of fluconazole and clotrimazole for the treatment of vulvovaginal candidiasis. *Sex Transm Dis* 1995;22:228.
150. Mikamo H et al. Comparative study on the effectiveness of antifungal agents in different regimens against vaginal candidiasis. *Chemotherapy* 1998;44:364.
151. Drug Facts and Comparison. St. Louis: Facts and Comparison; 2002.
152. Sood G et al. Terconazole cream for non *Candida albicans* fungal vaginitis: results of a retrospective analysis. *Infect Dis Obstet Gynecol* 2000;8:240.
153. Sobel JD. Management of patients with recurrent vulvovaginal candidiasis. *Drugs* 2003;63: 1059.
154. Cotch MF et al. Epidemiology and outcomes associated with moderate to heavy *Candida* colonization during pregnancy. *Am J Obstet Gynecol* 1998;178:374.
155. Sobel JD. Use of antifungal drugs in pregnancy: a focus on safety. *Drug Saf* 2000;23:77.
156. Krieger JN et al. *Trichomonas vaginalis* and trichomoniasis. In: Holmes KK, ed. *Sexually Transmitted Diseases.* 3rd ed. New York: McGraw-Hill Health Professions Division; 1999;587.
157. Pabst KM et al. Disease prevalence among women attending a sexually transmitted disease clinic varies with reason for visit. *Sex Transm Dis* 1992;19:88.
158. Petrin D et al. Clinical and microbiological aspects of *Trichomonas vaginalis. Clin Microbiol Rev* 1998;11:300.
159. Haefner HK. Current evaluation and management of vulvovaginitis. *Clin Obstet Gynecol* 1999;42: 184.
160. Egan ME et al. Diagnosis of vaginitis. *Am Fam Physician* 2000;62:1095.
161. Heine P et al. *Trichomonas vaginalis:* a reemerging pathogen. *Clin Obstet Gynecol* 1993;36:137.
162. Forna F, Gulmezoglu AM. Interventions for treating trichomoniasis in women. *Cochrane Database Syst Rev* 2003;2:CD000218.
163. Visapaa JP et al. Lack of disulfiram-like reaction with metronidazole and ethanol. *Ann Pharmacother* 2002;36:971.
164. Caro-Paton T et al. Is metronidazole teratogenic? A meta-analysis. *Br J Clin Pharmacol* 1997;44:179.
165. Burtin P et al. Safety of metronidazole in pregnancy: a meta-analysis. *Am J Obstet Gynecol* 1995; 172:525.
166. Friedman GD. Cancer after metronidazole. *N Engl J Med* 1980;302:519.
167. Klebanoff MA et al. Failure of metronidazole to prevent preterm delivery among pregnant women with asymptomatic trichomonas vaginalis infection. *N Engl J Med* 2001;345:487.
168. Roberts CM et al. Increasing proportion of herpes simplex virus type 1 as a cause of genital herpes infection in college students. [see comment]. *Sex Transm Dis* 2003;30:797.
169. Langenberg AG et al. A prospective study of new infections with herpes simplex virus type 1 and type 2. Chiron HSV Vaccine Study Group. *N Engl J Med* 1999;341:1432.
170. Smith JS et al. Age-specific prevalence of infection with herpes simplex virus types 2 and 1: a global review. *J Infect Dis* 2002;186(Suppl 1):S3.
171. Whitley RJ et al. Immunologic approach to herpes simplex virus. *Viral Immunol* 2001;14:111.
172. Corey L. Genital herpes. In: Holmes KK, ed. *Sexually Transmitted Diseases.* 3rd ed. New York: McGraw-Hill Health Professions Division; 1999: 285.
173. Fleming DT et al. Herpes simplex virus type 2 in the United States, 1976 to 1994. *N Engl J Med* 1997;337:1105.
174. Corey L. Challenges in genital herpes simplex virus management. *J Infect Dis* 2002;186(Suppl 1):S29.
175. Hirsch M. Herpes simplex virus. In: Mandell GL et al., eds. *Principles and Practice of Infectious Diseases.* 4th ed. New York: Churchill Livingstone; 1995:1336.
176. Marrazzo JM, Martin DH. Management of women with cervicitis. *Clin Infect Dis* 2007; 44(Suppl 3): S102.
177. Benedetti J et al. Recurrence rates in genital herpes after symptomatic first-episode infection. *Ann Intern Med* 1994;121:847.
178. Sen P, Barton SE. Genital herpes and its management. *BMJ* 2007;334:1048.
179. Koelle DM et al. Antigen-specific T cells localize to the uterine cervix in women with genital herpes simplex virus type 2 infection. *J Infect Dis* 2000;182:662.
180. Benedetti JK et al. Clinical reactivation of genital herpes simplex virus infection decreases in frequency over time. *Ann Intern Med* 1999;131:14.
181. Engelberg R et al. Natural history of genital herpes simplex virus type 1 infection. *Sex Transm Dis* 2003;30:174.
182. Wald A et al. Virologic characteristics of subclinical and symptomatic genital herpes infections. *N Engl J Med* 1995;333:770.
183. Langenberg A et al. Development of clinically recognizable genital lesions among women previously identified as having "asymptomatic" herpes simplex virus type 2 infection. *Ann Intern Med* 1989;110:882.

184. Wald A et al. Effect of condoms on reducing the transmission of herpes simplex virus type 2 from men to women. *JAMA* 2001;285:3100.
185. Dobbins JG et al. Herpes in the time of AIDS: a comparison of the epidemiology of HIV-1 and HSV-2 in young men in northern Thailand. *Sex Transm Dis* 1999;26:67.
186. Wald A et al. The relationship between condom use and herpes simplex virus acquisition. *JAMA* 2005;143:707.
187. Kimberlin DW, Rouse DJ. Genital herpes. *N Engl J Med* 2004;350:1970.
188. Mertz GJ et al. Risk factors for the sexual transmission of genital herpes. *Ann Intern Med* 1992; 116:197.
189. Diamond C et al. Clinical course of patients with serologic evidence of recurrent genital herpes presenting with signs and symptoms of first episode disease. *Sex Transm Dis* 1999;26:221.
190. Wald A. Herpes. Transmission and viral shedding. *Dermatol Clin* 1998;16:795.
191. Wald A et al. Reactivation of genital herpes simplex virus type 2 infection in asymptomatic seropositive persons. *N Engl J Med* 2000;342: 844.
192. Ashley-Morrow R et al. Time course of seroconversion by HerpeSelect ELISA after acquisition of genital herpes simplex virus type 1 (HSV-1) or HSV-2. *Sex Transm Dis* 2003;30:310.
193. Wald A et al. Serological testing for herpes simplex virus (HSV)-1 and HSV-2 infection. *Clin Infect Dis* 2002;35(Suppl 2):S173.
194. Reeves WC et al. Risk of recurrence after first episode of genital herpes. Relation to HSV type and antibody response. *N Engl J Med* 1981;305:315.
195. Balfour HH Jr. Antiviral drugs. *N Engl J Med* 1999;340:1255.
196. MacDougall C, Guglielmo BJ. Pharmacokinetics of valaciclovir. *J Antimicrob Chemother* 2004;53: 899.
197. Leung DT et al. Current recommendations for the treatment of genital herpes. *Drugs* 2000;60: 1329.
198. Ioannidis JP et al. Clinical efficacy of high-dose acyclovir in patients with human immunodeficiency virus infection: a meta-analysis of randomized individual patient data. *J Infect Dis* 1998;178: 349.
199. Eisen D et al. Clinical utility of oral valacyclovir compared with oral acyclovir for the prevention of herpes simplex virus mucositis following autologous bone marrow transplantation or stem cell rescue therapy. [See comment]. *Bone Marrow Transplant* 2003;31:51.
200. Spruance SL et al. Penciclovir cream for the treatment of herpes simplex labialis. A randomized, multicenter, double-blind, placebo-controlled trial. Topical Penciclovir Collaborative Study Group. *JAMA* 1997;277:1374.
201. Au E et al. Antivirals in the prevention of genital herpes. *Herpes* 2002;9:74.
202. Nadelman CM et al. Herpes simplex virus infections. New treatment approaches make early diagnosis even more important. *Postgrad Med* 2000; 107:189.
203. Drake S et al. Improving the care of patients with genital herpes. *BMJ* 2000;321:619.
204. Strand A et al. Aborted genital herpes simplex virus lesions: findings from a randomised controlled trial with valaciclovir. *Sex Transm Infect* 2002;78:435.
205. Patel R et al. Valaciclovir for the suppression of recurrent genital HSV infection: a placebo controlled study of once daily therapy. International Valaciclovir HSV Study Group. *Genitourin Med* 1997;73:105.
206. Diaz-Mitoma F et al. Oral famciclovir for the suppression of recurrent genital herpes: a randomized controlled trial. Collaborative Famciclovir Genital Herpes Research Group. *JAMA* 1998;280: 887.
207. Gold D et al. Acyclovir prophylaxis for herpes simplex virus infection. *Antimicrob Agents Chemother* 1987;31:361.
208. Corey L et al. Once-daily valacyclovir to reduce the risk of transmission of genital herpes. *N Engl J Med* 2004;350:11.
209. Conant MA et al. Valaciclovir versus aciclovir for herpes simplex virus infection in HIV-infected individuals: two randomized trials. *Int J STD AIDS* 2002;13:12.
210. Chatis PA et al. Resistance of herpesviruses to antiviral drugs. *Antimicrob Agents Chemother* 1992; 36:1589.
211. Lalezari J et al. A randomized, double-blind, placebo-controlled trial of cidofovir gel for the treatment of acyclovir-unresponsive mucocutaneous herpes simplex virus infection in patients with AIDS. *J Infect Dis* 1997;176:892.
212. Perazella MA. Crystal-induced acute renal failure. *Am J Med* 1999;106:459.
213. Revankar SG et al. Delirium associated with acyclovir treatment in a patient with renal failure. *Clin Infect Dis* 1995;21:435.
214. Kitching AR et al. Neurotoxicity associated with acyclovir in end stage renal failure. *N Z Med J* 1997;110:167.
215. Straus SE et al. Acyclovir for chronic mucocutaneous herpes simplex virus infection in immunosuppressed patients. *Ann Intern Med* 1982;96: 270.
216. Wilkinson D et al. Nonoxynol-9 for preventing vaginal acquisition of sexually transmitted infections by women from men. *Cochrane Database Syst Rev* 2002;4:CD003939.
217. Lehtinen M et al. Herpes simplex virus and risk of cervical cancer: a longitudinal, nested case-control study in the Nordic countries. *Am J Epidemiol* 2002;156:687.
218. Tyring SK et al. Valacyclovir for herpes simplex virus infection: long-term safety and sustained efficacy after 20 years' experience with acyclovir. *J Infect Dis* 2002;186(Suppl 1):S40.
219. Watts DH et al. A double-blind, randomized, placebo-controlled trial of acyclovir in late pregnancy for the reduction of herpes simplex virus shedding and cesarean delivery. *Am J Obstet Gynecol* 2003;188:836.
220. Brown ZA et al. Effect of serologic status and cesarean delivery on transmission rates of herpes simplex virus from mother to infant. *JAMA* 2003;289:203.
221. Reiff-Eldridge R et al. Monitoring pregnancy outcomes after prenatal drug exposure through prospective pregnancy registries: a pharmaceutical company commitment. *Am J Obstet Gynecol* 2000;182:159.
222. Sheffield JS et al. Valacyclovir prophylaxis to prevent recurrent herpes at delivery: a randomized clinical trial. *Obstet Gynecol* 2006;108:141.
223. Kibrick S. Herpes simplex infection at term. What to do with mother, newborn, and nursery personnel. *JAMA* 1980;243:157.
224. Scott LL. Prevention of prenatal herpes: prophylactic antiviral therapy? *Clin Obstet Gynecol* 1999;42:134.
225. Dunne EF et al. Prevalence of HPV infection among females in the United States. *JAMA* 2007;297: 813.
226. Munoz N et al. Epidemiologic classification of human papillomavirus types associated with cervical cancer. *N Engl J Med* 2003;348:518.
227. Ostor AG. Natural history of cervical intraepithelial neoplasia: a critical review. *Int J Gynecol Pathol* 1993;12:186.
228. Melbye M, Frisch M. The role of human papillomaviruses in anogenital cancers. *Semin Cancer Biol* 1998;8:307.
229. Longstaff E et al. Condyloma eradication: self-therapy with 0.15%–0.5% podophyllotoxin versus 20%–25% podophyllin preparations — an integrated safety assessment. *Regul Toxicol Pharmacol* 2001;33:117.
230. Lacey CJ et al. Randomised controlled trial and economic evaluation of podophyllotoxin solution, podophyllotoxin cream, and podophyllin in the treatment of genital warts. *Sex Transm Infect* 2003;79:270.
231. Perry CM et al. Topical imiquimod: a review of its use in genital warts. *Drugs* 1999;58:375.
232. Future II Study Group. Quadrivalent vaccine against human papillomavirus to prevent high-grade cervical lesions. *N Engl J Med* 2007;356: 1915.
233. Garland SM et al. Quadrivalent vaccine against human papillomavirus to prevent anogenital diseases. *N Engl J Med* 2007;356:1928.
234. Markowitz LE et al. Quadrivalent human papillomavirus vaccine: recommendations of the Advisory Committee on Immunization Practices (ACIP). *MMWR Recomm Rep* 2007;56:1.
235. Hildesheim A et al. Effect of human papillomavirus 16/18 L1 viruslike particle vaccine among young women with preexisting infection: a randomized trial. *JAMA* 2007;298:743.
236. Sobel JD. Bacterial vaginosis. *Annu Rev Med* 2000; 51:349.

CHAPTER 66

Osteomyelitis and Septic Arthritis

Ralph H. Raasch

Osteomyelitis is an inflammation of the bone marrow and surrounding bone caused by an infecting organism. Any bone can be involved. Serious morbidity often occurs even with early diagnosis and treatment. Despite the continued refinement of diagnostic procedures (e.g., radionuclide imaging, magnetic resonance imaging), advances in antimicrobial therapy, and the use of prophylactic antibiotics before orthopedic procedures, osteomyelitis continues to be a serious problem because the infection is not always cured.

Previously, osteomyelitis was more common in children and the elderly, and the causative microorganisms were usually Gram-positive cocci such as streptococci and staphylococci. Although *Staphylococcus aureus* remains the most common causative organism, the prevalence of infection caused by Gram-negative and anaerobic bacilli is increasing. Osteomyelitis can affect all age groups.[1]

Bone can be infected by three routes: hematogenous spread of bacteria from a distant infection site, direct infection of bone from an adjacent or contiguous source of infection, and infection of bone because of vascular insufficiency. Table 66-1 summarizes important characteristics of these types of osteomyelitis.[1,2] Patients with recurrent osteomyelitis are considered to have chronic osteomyelitis.

BONE ANATOMY AND PHYSIOLOGY

Understanding the pathophysiology of osteomyelitis requires a basic understanding of bone anatomy and physiology. Figure 66-1 is a graphic representation of a long bone. The bone is divided into three sections: the epiphysis, located at the end of the bone; the metaphysis; and the diaphysis. The epiphysis and metaphysis are separated by the epiphyseal growth plate. This is the rapidly growing area of the bone, supported by many blood vessels. Surrounding most of the bone is a fibrous and cellular envelope. The external portion of this envelope is called the *periosteum*, and the internal portion is referred to as the *endosteum*.

The blood vessels that supply bone tissue are located predominantly in the bone's epiphysis and metaphysis. The nutrient arteries enter the bone at the metaphyseal side of the epiphyseal growth plate and lead to capillaries that form sharp loops within the growth plate. These capillaries lead to large sinusoidal veins that eventually exit the metaphysis of the bone through a nutrient vein. Within the sinusoidal veins, blood flow is slowed considerably, and infection can begin if bacteria settle here.

Variations exist in the vasculature of bone in different age groups, leading to different forms of osteomyelitis. In neonates and adults, vascular communications are present between the epiphysis and metaphysis, which can allow infection to spread from bone to the adjacent joint. During childhood, however, this area often is protected from infection because the epiphyseal plate separates the vascular supply for these two regions.

HEMATOGENOUS OSTEOMYELITIS

Hematogenous osteomyelitis classically has been a disease of children, although the number of cases reported in adults is increasing. Osteomyelitis in children tends to be acute and hematogenous and is often responsive to antibiotic therapy

Table 66-1 Features of Osteomyelitis

Feature	*Hematogenous*	*Adjacent Site of Infection*	*Vascular Insufficiency*
Usual age of onset (yr)	<20; >50	>40	>40
Sites of infection	Long bones, vertebrae	Femur, tibia, skull, mandible	Feet
Risk factors	Bacteremia	Surgery, trauma, cellulitis; joint prosthesis	Diabetes, peripheral vascular disease
Common bacteria	*Staphylococcus aureus,* Gram-negative bacilli; usually one organism	*S. aureus,* Gram-negative bacilli; anaerobic organisms; often mixed infection	*S. aureus,* coagulase-negative staphylococci, streptococci, Gram-negative and anaerobic organisms; usually mixed infection
Clinical findings			
Initial episode	Fever, chills, local tenderness, swelling; limitation of motion	Fever, warmth, swelling; unstable joint	Pain, swelling, drainage, ulcer formation
Recurrent episode	Drainage	Drainage, sinus tract	As above

alone. In comparison, osteomyelitis in adults tends to be subacute or chronic and commonly results from trauma, prosthetic devices, or other insult. As a result, surgical débridement often is needed in addition to antibiotics when treating osteomyelitis in adults.

Infection in children develops primarily in the metaphysis of the rapidly growing long bones of the body, probably because the slow blood flow in these areas allows bacteria to settle and multiply. The acute infectious process (e.g., edema, inflammation, small vessel thrombosis) causes a rise in pressure within the bone that compromises blood flow and eventually leads to necrosis. Released cytokines alter bone integrity by promoting osteoclast activity. Eventually, the elevated pressure and necrosis might cause devitalized bone to fragment from healthy bone (sequestra). With continued spread of the infection into the outer layers of the bone and soft tissue, abscess and draining sinus tracts form.[1,2]

In children, hematogenous infection most commonly occurs in the long bones, as a single focus in the femur and tibia.[1] In adults, the vertebrae are more commonly involved,

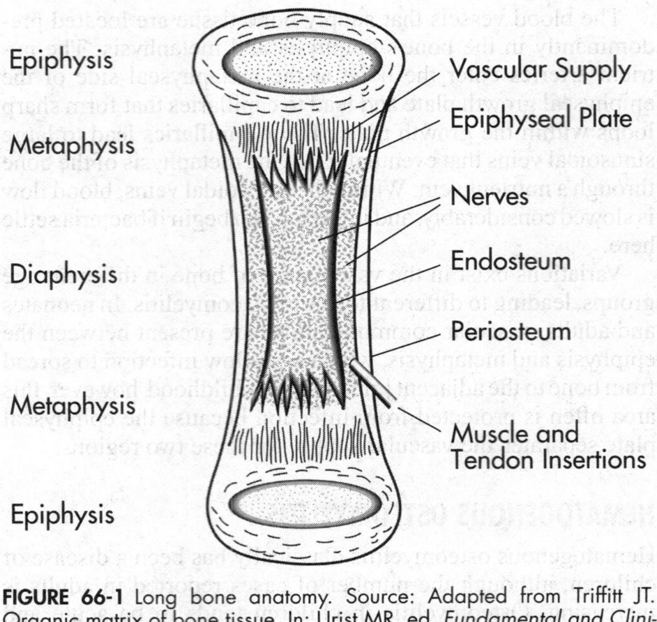

FIGURE 66-1 Long bone anatomy. Source: Adapted from Triffitt JT. Organic matrix of bone tissue. In: Urist MR, ed. *Fundamental and Clinical Bone Physiology*. Philadelphia, Pa.: JB Lippincott; 1980:46.

and infection usually occurs in the fifth and sixth decades of life.[3] In neonates, hematogenous osteomyelitis is an especially serious disease that often involves multiple bones, especially the long bones. Rapid spread across the epiphyseal plate can involve the adjacent joint, making immediate, aggressive treatment crucial.

The most common organism causing hematogenous osteomyelitis in children is *S. aureus*, which is caused partly by the proclivity of this bacterial species to settle and adhere to bone and cartilage. In adults, S. *aureus* is also the most common causative pathogen. Gram-negative bacilli (*Escherichia coli, Klebsiella, Proteus, Salmonella,* and *Pseudomonas*), however, are responsible for an increasing number of cases of osteomyelitis. Intravenous (IV) drug abuse often leads to infection with *Pseudomonas aeruginosa,* whereas *Salmonella* species is a common cause in patients with sickle cell anemia.[1,2]

The clinical features of hematogenous osteomyelitis vary, depending on the patient's age and the infection site. In children, infection usually is characterized by an abrupt onset of high fever and chills, localized pain, tenderness, and swelling. Systemic symptoms often are absent in neonates, delaying the diagnosis. A diagnosis, therefore, must be made on the basis of localized symptoms such as edema and restricted limb movement. Systemic symptoms are also less common in adults. Patients with vertebral osteomyelitis can present with the insidious onset of localized back pain and tenderness.[1,3]

ACUTE OSTEOMYELITIS

Usual Clinical Presentation

1. T.S., a 9-year-old boy, is unable to go to school today because of fever and increasing leg pain. Three to four days ago, he says his upper left leg started to hurt and he began limping last night. There is no history of trauma to the area. His only past medical history is two episodes of otitis media at ages 4 and 6. In the pediatrician's office today, maximal tenderness is focally localized over the left distal femur without knee joint effusion. No visible signs of swelling, warmth, or trauma are seen. His white blood cell (WBC) count is 7,000 cells/mm^3 (normal, 5,000–10,000), with a normal WBC differential. Plain radiographic studies of the left leg are normal, but the erythrocyte sedimentation rate (ESR) is 62 mm/hour (normal, 0–15). Two blood cultures are obtained, and T.S. is sent home with directions for bed rest and use of

acetaminophen as needed for fever. However, 2 days later, he is admitted to the hospital because of severe pain and tenderness in his left leg and a fever of 38.8°C. The blood cultures obtained 2 days ago are positive for *S. aureus,* sensitive to oxacillin (OSSA), and the C-reactive protein (CRP) is 14 mg/dL (normal, <2.0). Another x-ray study is again normal, but a magnetic resonance imaging (MRI) scan is positive for inflammation in the left distal femur. What findings in T.S. are consistent with hematogenous osteomyelitis?

[SI units: WBC, 7, 000 × 10^9/L (normal, 5,000–10,000); ESR, 62 mm/hour (normal, 0–15); CRP, 14 mg/dL (normal, <2.0)]

T.S. displays the usual signs and symptoms of acute hematogenous osteomyelitis in children. He is a previously healthy child who developed acute localized pain and tenderness of the left distal femur, abrupt onset of high fever, and an elevated ESR. The plain radiographic study was normal on two occasions before hospitalization; however, plain radiographs of bone are usually normal during the first 2 weeks of infection. MRI scans usually can detect bone changes earlier in the course of disease, and T.S.'s MRI scan on hospitalization detected inflammation in the left distal femur.[2] Although T.S. did not have a bone biopsy sent for culture, his clinical picture, a positive MRI scan, and blood cultures positive for *S. aureus* establish the diagnosis of osteomyelitis.[2,4] As in many cases of osteomyelitis, the specific event that caused bacteremia with bacterial dissemination to bone is unknown.

Several laboratory tests should be obtained in every child suspected of having osteomyelitis. Although these tests are not specific for the diagnosis of osteomyelitis, they help confirm the clinical diagnosis. A complete blood count (CBC) and an ESR are routinely obtained. The serum CRP, when elevated, is a measure of systemic inflammation.

An increased WBC count is consistent with osteomyelitis, but significant leukocytosis is absent in many children with osteomyelitis at the initial examination. Thus, T.S.'s WBC count of 7,000/mm^3 is not unusual. In adults, leukocytosis does occur, but it is more commonly associated with an acute infection than with recurrent disease. When leukocytosis is present, the WBC count rarely exceeds 15,000/mm^3.[2,5]

Although the ESR and the CRP are relatively nonspecific, most patients with osteomyelitis have ESR values >20 mm/hour and a CRP >2.0 mg/dL.[2] Therefore, the increased ESR and CRP in T.S. are consistent with osteomyelitis. Destructive changes of bone can be seen in plain radiographs, although these do not appear for at least 10 to 14 days after the onset of infection.[2] MRI scans can detect inflammation of bone more quickly than plain radiographs.[6] Hence, a normal plain film does not rule out acute osteomyelitis if obtained within the first 2 weeks of infection. The MRI scan in T.S. was extremely helpful because acute osteomyelitis was detected before the appearance of osteomyelitis on plain x-ray film.

Predisposing factors for hematogenous osteomyelitis include any risk factors that promote bacteremia (e.g., indwelling catheters, hemodialysis shunts, central venous catheters used for chemotherapy or parenteral nutrition). A distant focus in the gastrointestinal or urinary tract can lead to bacteremia and predispose a patient to the development of osteomyelitis. Intravenous (IV) drug abuse leading to bacteremia can be a predisposing factor for osteomyelitis. None of these factors seem to have predisposed T.S. to the development of osteomyelitis. In children such as T.S. who have no history of fractures or penetrating injury, the most common cause for acute hematogenous osteomyelitis is *S. aureus*, including methicillin-resistant strains.[1,2,4,7]

Patient Workup

2. What additional patient and diagnostic information should be obtained before T.S. receives his first dose of antibiotics?

Before T.S. receives antibiotic therapy, he should be assessed for drug allergies, especially penicillin allergy. Patient interviews, discussions with his parents, and a comprehensive review of his medical record are necessary, especially if a history of allergy is reported. Details of an allergic reaction, including symptoms, onset of the reaction, probable causative agent, treatment, and exposure to related compounds, should be sought.

Cultures of blood and bone aspirate material are the best ways to identify the specific bacterial cause for osteomyelitis and are often part of the initial workup. Cultures taken after antibiotics are started often are negative, however, thereby necessitating the use of empiric broad-spectrum antibiotic therapy for several weeks. As a result, both the cost of therapy and the risk of toxicity increase.

In T.S.'s case, the positive blood culture and MRI scan establish the diagnosis of osteomyelitis without the need for a bone culture. If the blood cultures had been negative, however, a bone aspirate for culture to identify the pathogen would be recommended.[1,2] Once material has been obtained for culture, initial empiric therapy should start as soon as possible.

Treatment

Empiric Antibiotic Therapy

3. T.S. has no history of drug allergies; he took amoxicillin for the previous episodes of acute otitis media without incident. What antibiotic treatment should be started? What is the relevance of bone concentrations or protein binding of antibiotics in the selection of therapy for osteomyelitis?

For initial antimicrobial treatment of hematogenous osteomyelitis, the agent chosen should be administered IV at high dosages to achieve adequate levels in the infected bone. It is important to initiate treatment as soon as possible to improve the chances for complete eradication of infection and to avoid the need for surgery. Thus, empiric antibiotic therapy often is instituted before culture and sensitivity results are known.

Based on the epidemiology of T.S.'s infection and the results of the blood culture, he should be treated for *S. aureus* osteomyelitis. In both children and adults, approximately one-third of cases of acute osteomyelitis are currently caused by oxacillin-resistant strains (ORSA).[7–9] Hence, initial, empiric treatment should be with IV vancomycin until susceptibility results indicate the isolate is oxacillin- (or nafcillin-) susceptible. In the absence of susceptibility results or if the isolate is oxacillin-resistant, therapy would continue with vancomycin. Recurrent infection rates with vancomycin therapy are concerning, however; thus, it is crucial that appropriate biopsy and culture results are obtained whenever possible so that patients receive β-lactam–based therapy for

Table 66-2 Empiric Intravenous Antibiotics for Acute Osteomyelitis in Children

Host	Likely Etiologies	Antibiotics	Dosage (mg/kg/day)	Dosage (doses/day)
Neonate	*Staphylococcus aureus*	Oxacillin (or nafcillin) +	100	4
	Group B streptococci	cefotaxime *or*	150	3
	Gram-negative bacilli	Oxacillin (or nafcillin) +	100	4
		gentamicin	5–7.5	3
<3 yr	*S. aureus*	Vancomycin *or*	45	4
	Haemophilus influenzae type b	Cefuroxime *or*	50	2
		Oxacillin (or nafcillin) +	150	4
		cefotaxime	100	4
≥3 yr	*S. aureus*	Vancomycin *or*	45	4
		Oxacillin (or nafcillin) *or*	150	4
		Cefazolin *or*	100	3
		Clindamycin	30–40	3
After puncture wound through shoe	*P. aeruginosa*	Ceftazidime	150	3
Child with sickle cell disease	*Salmonella* sp.	Oxacillin (or nafcillin) +	150	4
	S. aureus	cefotaxime *or*	100	4
		Vancomycin +	45	4
		cefotaxime	100	4

oxacillin-susceptible isolates.[10,11] Because of less experience in treating ORSA osteomyelitis, clindamycin or linezolid should be used only in patients who are vancomycin intolerant. Other organisms that can cause osteomyelitis include *Staphylococcus epidermidis, Streptococcus pyogenes, Streptococcus pneumoniae, Haemophilus influenzae,* and *P. aeruginosa.* In the neonate with osteomyelitis, *S. aureus* and *Streptococcus* species are commonly responsible.[1] T.S.'s blood culture grew OSSA and he is not allergic to penicillin. He is placed on IV oxacillin therapy at 150 mg/kg/day Q 6 hr. He could have been started on IV nafcillin instead of oxacillin because these two drugs are therapeutically equivalent, and are given in similar dosage. His prior exposure to amoxicillin is irrelevant except to establish the absence of a penicillin allergy.

Under circumstances of negative cultures or while blood or bone cultures are pending, the age of the child with acute osteomyelitis is important in the selection of appropriate empiric antibiotics. Table 66-2 summarizes recommended drugs and dosages in children with acute osteomyelitis.[1,4,12]

Antibiotic Bone Penetration and Protein Binding

The importance of selecting an antibiotic that penetrates into bone when treating osteomyelitis is unclear, nor does a clear relationship exist between bone concentrations and outcome of therapy.[1,2,13] Theoretically, drug protein binding could influence clinical efficacy because it is believed that the free drug, rather than the protein-bound drug, diffuses from plasma into bone tissue. Studies evaluating the penetration of highly protein-bound drugs, such as cefazolin (90% protein bound), show high cefazolin bone levels after a single 1-g IV dose, exceeding levels achieved with cephalothin, a drug with only 20% protein binding. In addition, cefazolin and ceftriaxone, two highly protein-bound drugs, usually are effective in treating osteomyelitis, provided high dosages are given for an extended period, and the responsible pathogen is susceptible. In summary, antibiotic bone concentrations and protein binding of antibiotics (when appropriate dosages are used) are not significant factors in the selection of appropriate therapy for osteomyelitis.[1,2]

Duration of Therapy

4. The *S. aureus* grown from T.S.'s blood culture is OSSA. Is oxacillin the best antibiotic choice, or would other antibiotics, given less frequently, also be adequate therapy?

Continuing to treat T.S. with IV oxacillin (or nafcillin) every 6 hours follows treatment recommendations for OSSA osteomyelitis. Antistaphylococcal penicillins achieve high levels in bone and usually provide effective therapy when the treatment regimen is followed with frequent doses for an adequate duration. Changing T.S. to cefazolin would allow slightly less frequent dosing (Q 8 hr), a potential advantage for home treatment. Vancomycin use should be discouraged in T.S.'s case because cultures grew an oxacillin-sensitive organism, and vancomycin is associated with higher rates of treatment failure.[10,11] While the logistics of outpatient therapy in T.S. are being investigated, he should remain on oxacillin while in the hospital.

5. Both of T.S.'s parents are employed, and their work schedules would prevent them from leaving their jobs to transport him to an outpatient antibiotic treatment center. Is T.S. a candidate for outpatient IV antibiotic therapy at home, or could oral antibiotic treatment be considered at this time? Must T.S. remain in the hospital to receive his oxacillin?

Initially, all patients should receive IV antibiotics because early, aggressive therapy offers the best chance to cure the infection. T.S., however, does not necessarily need to stay in the hospital to complete therapy. A peripheral central catheter (PICC) can be inserted for treatment, with antibiotic administered via continuous infusion pump.[1,2,4] Whether T.S. should go home on IV antibiotics must be decided in concert with his parents. If they do not have the resources or are unwilling to oversee IV treatment at home, T.S. should remain hospitalized to assess the first week of treatment. In any case, expecting a 9-year-old boy such as T.S. to complete several weeks of IV therapy at home is overly optimistic. Furthermore, catheter complications (e.g., dislodgment, infection, or occlusion) are concerns. As discussed in Question 6, T.S. may be able to complete most of his course of treatment with oral antibiotics. Oral antibiotics, however, should not be given to T.S. until the effectiveness of the first week of IV therapy can be assessed. The total duration of IV and oral therapy for T.S. should be at least 4 weeks, or until the ESR has returned to the normal range.[1,2,12]

Use of Oral Antibiotics

6. After 1 week of IV oxacillin, T.S. is afebrile and the pain and tenderness in his left leg are significantly reduced. The ESR is 40 mm/hour, and CRP is 6.0 mg/dL. The plan is to switch T.S. to oral antibiotics to complete a 4-week course of treatment at home. What is an appropriate dosing regimen, and how often should he return to the clinic for evaluation?

[SI units: ESR, 40 mm/hour; CRP, 6.0 mg/dL]

Because IV therapy for several weeks is inconvenient and expensive, even at home, patients such as T.S. who have responded to IV antibiotics can be switched to oral therapy. Again, this decision must be made in concert with T.S.'s parents, who must understand the vital importance of frequent antibiotic doses in these circumstances. Oral antibiotics are appropriate only if a clear clinical response to IV therapy has occurred over 7 to 10 days, and the patient can swallow and tolerate oral therapy in adequate dosage.[1,4]

Thus, T.S. is a candidate for oral therapy, assuming his parents agree to supervise treatment once he leaves the hospital. T.S. has responded promptly to the IV therapy: his fever, leg pain, and tenderness have resolved, the ESR and CRP are reduced. The CRP changes more quickly in response to adequate antimicrobial therapy than does the ESR.[14] Oral therapy, however, will be effective only if T.S. is compliant. Therefore, assurances must be in place to guarantee that all doses will be taken. T.S.'s parents have made arrangements with his fourth-grade teacher to help him take his oral antibiotic during the day.

T.S. can complete his 4-week course of antibiotics with oral dosing of cephalexin capsules or suspension, which seems to taste better (and hence is usually better tolerated) than dicloxacillin suspension. Cephalexin dosage should begin at 37.5 mg/kg Q 6 hr. Close follow-up of T.S. (weekly) is required under these circumstances to monitor compliance and clinical response to therapy. Parenteral therapy should be reinitiated promptly if T.S.'s compliance is not perfect, or symptoms (or increased ESR or CRP) recur.[4,12,15] Initial oral therapy with a quinolone is not appropriate for T.S. primarily because staphylococci resistance to ciprofloxacin has emerged, and secondarily because quinolone use is relatively contraindicated in children. Dosages of oral antibiotics for children with osteomyelitis are summarized in Table 66-3.[12]

Table 66-3 Oral Antibiotic Doses for the Treatment of Osteomyelitis in Children

Drug	*Dosage(mg/kg/day)*	*Interval between Doses (hr)*
Penicillin V	125	4
Dicloxacillin	100	6
Amoxicillin	100	6
Cephalexin	150	6
Cefaclor	150	6
Clindamycin	40	8

Duration of Follow-Up for Recurrent Infection

7. T.S. has completed 4 weeks of treatment for his acute staphylococcal osteomyelitis. Clinical evidence shows that the osteomyelitis is completely resolved, and the ESR and CRP are normal. For how long should T.S. be followed for possible recurrence of his infection?

Relapses of osteomyelitis can occur years after the initial acute episode.[1,2] In T.S.'s case of uncomplicated acute osteomyelitis, he should be evaluated for recurrence at least every 3 months for at least 2 years.

SECONDARY OSTEOMYELITIS

Osteomyelitis Secondary to a Contiguous Source Infection

8. R.W., a 56-year-old man, suffered an open right tibial fracture 4 weeks ago in a motorcycle accident. His fracture was set by open reduction and external fixation. Cefazolin, given as surgical prophylaxis, was continued for 24 hours. Antibiotics were then switched to IV ampicillin/sulbactam for 1 week, followed by oral amoxicillin/clavulanic acid, which he is still taking today. The postoperative course was unremarkable until yesterday, when he developed right leg pain and spontaneous drainage from the surgical wound. On presentation, his right shin is tender, warm, swollen, and erythematous, but he is afebrile. Other physical findings are within normal limits. Laboratory data, including WBC count, serum creatinine, and blood urea nitrogen (BUN), are normal, but the ESR is 38 mm/hour, and CRP is 8 mg/dL. Plain bone films and bone MRI show inflammation and nonhealing of the tibial fracture. What findings in R.W. are characteristic of secondary osteomyelitis?

Few of the systemic signs and symptoms usually associated with acute osteomyelitis are seen in secondary osteomyelitis. The objective findings usually present in hematogenous disease, such as fever, leukocytosis, and an elevated ESR, can be absent. The most common subjective complaint in acute contiguous osteomyelitis is pain in the area of infection, which often is accompanied by localized tenderness, swelling, erythema, and drainage. Because several weeks might pass before the patient becomes symptomatic, radiographic studies at the time of diagnosis might reveal abnormalities consistent with bone deterioration.[1,2]

Clinical Presentation

R.W.'s case is consistent with osteomyelitis secondary to a contiguous focus of infection. Probable infection has arisen in his right leg at the site of surgical repair of a fracture of his right tibia. R.W.'s localized symptoms, along with the absence of fever and leukocytosis, are characteristic of secondary osteomyelitis. In these cases, bone becomes infected from an exogenous source, or through spread of an infection from adjacent tissue to bone. Infection can result from any trauma followed by an orthopedic procedure to fix a bone fracture. The bones most commonly involved are the hip, tibia, femur, and fibula.[1,2]

Other associated situations are caused by contiguous spread of an infection. These include any penetrating injury, such as a gunshot wound or a nail puncture, or soft tissue infections, such as pressure sores or those involving the fingers and toes.

Unlike hematogenous osteomyelitis, which occurs mostly in children, acute contiguous infection occurs more often in adults. This is explained by the higher incidence of precipitating factors within this age group, such as hip fractures, orthopedic procedures, oral cancers, sternotomy incisions for cardiac surgery, and craniotomies.[1,2]

Common Pathogens

Whereas hematogenous osteomyelitis usually involves a single pathogen, coinfection with several organisms is common in contiguous-spread osteomyelitis. Thus, although *S. aureus* is the most common pathogen, it is often part of a mixed infection. Other organisms responsible for infection include *Pseudomonas, Proteus, Streptococcus,* and *Klebsiella* species, *E. coli,* and *S. epidermidis.* Most cases of osteomyelitis involving the mandible, pelvis, and small bones (e.g., those of the hands and feet) are caused by Gram-negative organisms. *Pseudomonas* often is isolated from infections after puncture wounds of the foot.[1,2]

Anaerobes also are associated with contiguous-spread osteomyelitis. The anaerobic organisms most commonly isolated are *Bacteroides* species and anaerobic cocci. Possible predisposing factors include previous fractures or injuries resulting from human bites. Adjacent soft tissue infections can also lead to anaerobic bone infections, as in the case of sacral osteomyelitis secondary to severe decubitus ulcers.

To establish the pathogenic organisms, R.W. should have surgical re-evaluation and a biopsy of involved bone at the probable site of infection.[1,2] The bone films and MRI scan will help localize the possible infectious process to direct the surgical biopsy.

Initial Treatment

9. R.W. returns to the operating room for surgical exploration, and bone tissue is obtained for culture. He has no drug allergies. The initial postoperative antibiotic order is for vancomycin, 1 g IV Q 12 hr. Is this adequate antibiotic treatment for R.W.?

R.W. has had surgery to obtain bone material for culture because cultures of adjacent wound or sinus tract material are not predictive of the bacteria actually infecting the bone.[16] Broad antibiotic coverage is necessary now because *S. aureus* and polymicrobial Gram-negative aerobic bacilli most likely are causing this infection.[1] R.W. already has been started on vancomycin to cover for *S. aureus;* however, a third- or fourth-generation cephalosporin (cefotaxime, ceftriaxone, ceftazidime, or cefepime) or a quinolone (ciprofloxacin) should be added for Gram-negative coverage. Cefepime (2 g IV Q 12 hr) or meropenem (1 g IV Q 8 hr) is suggested in cases involving *P. aeruginosa,* although other antipseudomonal drugs (e.g., ceftazidime, aztreonam, imipenem) would also be appropriate.[2] Vancomycin usually is adequate for effective treatment of ORSA infection, although optimal trough concentrations are not defined; some authors suggest trough concentrations should be in the 15 to 20 mcg/mL range.[17,18] Third-generation cephalosporins or quinolones should not be used to treat serious staphylococcal infection; therefore, combined therapy with antistaphylococcal penicillins (if OSSA) or vancomycin is necessary.[1] Oxacillin and vancomycin have activity against Gram-positive anaerobes, but not against an important Gram-negative anaerobe, *Bacteroides fragilis.* If *B. fragilis* is cultured from bone, additional therapy with metronidazole is indicated. Alternatively, combined, broad aerobic (including *Pseudomonas)* and anaerobic Gram-negative coverage could be provided by β-lactam/β-lactamase inhibitor combination therapy with piperacillin/tazobactam. While cultures are pending for R.W., his antibiotic regimen is changed to vancomycin 1.5 g IV Q 12 hr and ciprofloxacin 400 mg IV Q 12 hr.

OSTEOMYELITIS CAUSED BY *PSEUDOMONAS*

10. The bone biopsy from R.W. grows *P. aeruginosa,* which is sensitive to piperacillin, ceftazidime, imipenem, gentamicin, tobramycin, and ciprofloxacin. His leg pain is no worse than it was 2 days ago, and he remains afebrile. How should R.W. now be treated? Is he a candidate for oral therapy?

Traditional aggressive therapy for R.W. would include gentamicin or tobramycin plus a second agent active against *Pseudomonas,* such as piperacillin, ceftazidime, or ciprofloxacin. More recently, anti*pseudomonal* therapy with a β-lactam plus ciprofloxacin combination has been used with increasing frequency to avoid the complications of aminoglycosides. Thus, vancomycin should be discontinued. There is reasonable experience treating *Pseudomonas* osteomyelitis with an antipseudomonal β-lactam, with an aminoglycoside added (both depending on sensitivities), to complete a 4-week course of therapy.[1] R.W. can receive cefipime (2 g IV Q 12 hr) plus gentamicin as initial therapy. To facilitate antibiotic therapy at home, R.W. is a candidate for once-daily dosing of gentamicin.[1] Because his renal function is normal, a single daily dose of 5 to 7 mg/kg can be administered. Although only a few reports exist of extended-dose aminoglycoside use in osteomyelitis, for other Gram-negative infections considerable evidence indicates that once-a-day therapy is as effective and possibly less toxic as multiple daily doses.[19,20] At home, R.W. should have serum creatinine and trough gentamicin concentrations measured weekly. Desired trough levels are $<$1 mcg/mL.

In an effort to avoid aminoglycoside toxicity, some investigators have administered cephalosporins or ciprofloxacin alone for 4 to 6 weeks to treat osteomyelitis caused by *Pseudomonas.* These studies are inadequate, however, because they involved small case series without control groups or their follow-up time was too short (6 months).[21–23] Furthermore, studies do not yet support the use of oral quinolones (ciprofloxacin) alone in these cases.[24] To provide the best chance of cure, R.W. should receive cefipime and gentamicin for the entire 4-week course of therapy. The relative effectiveness of cefipime plus ciprofloxacin is unknown. R.W.'s antibiotic therapy can be reasonably accomplished at home. If gentamicin nephrotoxicity occurs or if he develops an allergic reaction to cefipime, oral ciprofloxacin (750 mg PO Q 12 hr) can be used to complete the full 4-week course of therapy. He should be followed closely thereafter for at least 2 years to detect recurrent infection.

OSTEOMYELITIS ASSOCIATED WITH VASCULAR INSUFFICIENCY

11. P.G, a 60-year-old man, presents to the diabetes clinic with an ulcer on the inferior surface of his left big toe. This lesion began as a red spot about 6 months ago, but is now an ulcer approximately 2 cm wide × 1 cm deep. He has not paid much attention to it because it has not been very painful. The ulcer is not foul smelling. P.G. has had type 2 diabetes mellitus for 20 years and is currently treated with oral glipizide and metformin. Otherwise, he has no other complaints, but notes that his toe sore began after he started using a new pair of shoes about 7 months ago. Laboratory data obtained earlier today show a normal WBC count and differential, and normal electrolytes, BUN, and creatinine. His fasting blood glucose, however, is 240 mg/dL (normal, 65–110), and the ESR is 45 mm/hour (normal, 0–15). What findings in P.G. are consistent with secondary osteomyelitis?

[SI units: fasting plasma glucose, 13.3 mmol/L (normal, 3.6–6.1); ESR, 45 mm/hour (normal, 0–15)]

P.G. has chronic lower extremity vascular insufficiency as a result of type 2 diabetes. Patients such as P.G. with impaired blood flow usually develop osteomyelitis in the toes or small bones of the feet. Infection often first presents as cellulitis, as in P.G.'s case, which commonly progresses to deep ulcers. Finally, the infection spreads to the underlying bone. In many cases of osteomyelitis associated with vascular insufficiency, multiple pathogens can be cultured from surgical specimens or the wound. The most commonly isolated pathogens are *S. aureus;* however, Gram-negative and anaerobic bacteria also are often recovered.

Similar to contiguous-spread osteomyelitis, systemic signs of infection (e.g., fever and leukocytosis) are often absent in patients who develop bone infection secondary to vascular insufficiency. Local symptoms, such as pain, swelling, and erythema, usually dominate the picture.[1,2,25]

P.G. may have a bone infection that underlies a chronic, cutaneous ulcer on the bottom of his left big toe. Because of likely diabetic neuropathy, the skin lesion may not be very painful, and poor blood supply to the site likely contributed to the development of a chronic infection and possibly secondary osteomyelitis. Clinically, osteomyelitis is suggested by his elevated ESR and fasting glucose (consistent with infection). In addition, diabetic foot ulcers that are >2 cm wide and >2 cm deep, or that penetrate to bone, are often predictive for underlying osteomyelitis.[25,26]

Antibiotic Selection

12. P.G.'s wound is débrided, and material obtained from a deep wound swab is sent to the microbiology laboratory for cultures. He is hospitalized to receive wound care and to begin antibiotics. He has no drug allergies, and he is started on vancomycin (1 g IV Q 12 hr) and oral ciprofloxacin (750 mg Q 12 hr). Is this appropriate initial therapy?

The antibiotic treatment selected for P.G. should be active against both Gram-positive and Gram-negative aerobic bacteria. Because anaerobic, Gram-negative bacteria are cultured from bone in diabetic patients with osteomyelitis ≤15% of the time, empiric anaerobic coverage may not be necessary at this stage of treatment.[27,28] Because of the emergence of community-associated ORSA infection, vancomycin plus a third-generation cephalosporin (ceftriaxone, ceftazidime) or a quinolone (ciprofloxacin, levofloxacin) for Gram-negative coverage is a frequently used empiric regimen. If anaerobic bacteria are believed to be clinically involved (e.g., foul-smelling wound), metronidazole (Flagyl) should be added to the regimen. Hence, the initial regimen of vancomycin and ciprofloxacin for P.G. is rational. Further antibiotic refinement should occur after the results of the deep wound swab culture are available. The duration of IV therapy for diabetic foot osteomyelitis is not defined.[26,28] Emerging evidence indicates the effectiveness of oral linezolid (600 mg Q 12 hr) to treat osteomyelitis caused by ORSA in diabetic patients.[29,30] Other useful oral drugs for staphylococcal infections, depending on susceptibilities and patient tolerance, are clindamycin (300 Q 8 hr), trimethoprim-sulfamethoxazole (two DS Q 12 hr), and amoxicillin/clavulanate (Augmentin, 850 mg or Q 12 hr). The overall duration of combination therapy can range from 6 weeks to 10 months or more, depending on the healing rate of the ulcer.[28]

P.G. should also be made aware that osteomyelitis associated with diabetic foot ulcers is difficult to treat because poor circulation can impair antibiotic delivery to the infection site. Despite surgical débridement of the infection followed by appropriate treatment with long-term IV and oral antibiotic therapy, cure rates are low. Even minor amputations (one or two toes) are unsuccessful in eradicating infection. Radical surgical approaches, such as transmetatarsal, below-the-knee, or above-the-knee amputations, often are necessary to cure these infections.[1,2,26,31]

CHRONIC OSTEOMYELITIS

Clinical Presentation

13. F.B., a 48-year-old man, sustained a fracture of the left humerus in an automobile accident 6 years ago. That fracture clinically healed without any immediate consequences. However, 1 year ago, a draining sinus tract developed at the site of the previous fracture without any antecedent events. He has taken various oral antibiotics over this last year, including cephalexin and ciprofloxacin, which he stopped taking 2 months ago. One month ago, he noted increased sinus drainage, pain, swelling, and erythema of his left upper arm, and ciprofloxacin was restarted. A swab culture of the sinus drainage grew *S. epidermidis, E. coli, Peptostreptococcus micros,* and *Bacteroides* species. Two days ago, while off of antibiotics for a week, surgical débridement of bone and tissue was performed because of a further increase in drainage and poor appearance of the wound. Gentamicin-impregnated polymethylmethacrylate (PMMA) beads were placed in the tissue adjacent to the débrided

bone during surgery. Bone cultures grew *Proteus mirabilis, P. micros,* and *B. fragilis.* The *Proteus* was resistant to ampicillin, cefazolin, ticarcillin, and ciprofloxacin, but sensitive to cefotaxime, ceftriaxone, imipenem, gentamicin, and trimethoprim-sulfamethoxazole. Antibiotic sensitivities for the *Bacteroides* were not tested. What aspects of F.B.'s case are characteristic of chronic osteomyelitis?

Inadequate treatment of an acute episode of osteomyelitis can lead to formation of necrotic, infected bone and recurrent symptoms consistent with chronic disease. Even with appropriate initial therapy, osteomyelitis can reactivate, even with different organisms from the initial episode. Some propose that previously infected bone might be a focus of reduced resistance to infection, and then at risk for reinfection.[32] Persistent symptoms or signs lasting longer than 10 days correlate with chronic osteomyelitis and the development of necrotic bone.[1] Draining sinus tracts often develop from the bone to the skin in cases of chronic osteomyelitis.[33]

F.B. probably developed a chronic bone infection after the automobile accident. The reappearance of sinus tract drainage in his left upper arm indicates an indolent infection of bone that was periodically suppressed, but not treated by oral antibiotics. Cultures of sinus drainage now grow multiple organisms, and components of the topical normal bacterial flora are found. These cultures usually do not correlate with the organisms actually causing bone infection.[16] F.B.'s recurrent course of bone involvement with drainage and local symptoms, and lack of any remarkable systemic symptoms, is classic for chronic osteomyelitis.[33]

Surgery and Oral Antibiotics

14. Oral ciprofloxacin (750 mg BID) was restarted 1 month ago when F.B.'s left arm became more painful and drainage increased. Was his poor response to therapy unexpected? How should his case have been managed?

F.B.'s poor response should have been expected for at least two reasons. Antibiotic therapy was started before surgical débridement of avascular tissue, and he was given an antibiotic that is ineffective because of resistance against the cultured organisms from bone.

Surgery plays an important role in the treatment of chronic osteomyelitis. Bone necrosis will progress if decompression and drainage of the infected area is not carried out as soon as possible. Furthermore, without initial surgical removal of necrotic bone and other poorly vascularized, infected material, even IV antibiotics are likely to fail.

After surgery, it is important to achieve high levels of antibiotics that have been selected based on culture results from specimens obtained by deep aspiration or bone biopsy. Antibiotics should not be selected based on culture results from sinus tract drainage because these cultures do not correlate with the actual causative organisms. F.B. should be treated initially with IV antibiotics because of relatively poor blood flow at the infection site. Although the optimal duration of therapy for chronic osteomyelitis is not well studied,[1,2,34] parenteral therapy is generally recommended for 6 to 8 weeks, followed by 3 to 12 months of oral antibiotic therapy, depending on the healing rate.[2]

Finally, F.B. should continue to be evaluated by an orthopedic surgeon because he may require further surgical treatment to eradicate chronically infected bone.

Intravenous Antibiotics

15. What would be reasonable antibiotic therapy for F.B.?

On the basis of the bone culture and sensitivity results, F.B. needs high-dose therapy directed at *P. mirabilis* and *B. fragilis.* For convenience and possible future home therapy, ceftriaxone (2 g IV Q 24 hr) could be started for coverage of *Proteus.* The anaerobic activity of ceftriaxone is inadequate for infections caused by *Bacteroides.* Therefore, metronidazole (500 mg IV Q 8 hr) also should be started. Because of excellent oral bioavailability, the metronidazole can be rapidly converted to oral therapy at the same dose before discharge. Piperacillin/tazobactam (Zosyn) or ertapenem (Invanz) could be an alternative choice for home IV therapy circumstances, assuming it is documented that the *Proteus* isolate is sensitive to either agent. Both of these drugs would also provide excellent activity against anaerobic bacteria. Ertapenem is convenient for home therapy because it can be given once daily (1 g IV Q 24 hr).

After 6 to 8 weeks of parenteral therapy (which can be completed at home), F.B. should be closely evaluated for response. If symptoms have been reduced, then treatment with oral antibiotics (trimethoprim-sulfamethoxazole and metronidazole) should continue for at least 6 to 8 weeks, but treatment can be continued for several additional months based on resolution of the sinus tract drainage, pain, and tenderness in F.B.'s arm. Under these circumstances, F.B. should be monitored closely for possible adverse effects of these drugs given chronically (hepatitis, cytopenias, neuropathy). If the sinus tract does not heal or if F.B.'s arm remains painful, surgical exploration and bone cultures must be repeated.

Local Antibiotics

16. What are the rationale for and effectiveness of local antibiotic administration (the PMMA beads) inserted during F.B.'s orthopedic surgery?

To deliver high concentrations of antibiotics to poorly vascularized bone infection sites, various materials containing antibiotics have been placed at the infection site during surgery. Plaster pellets, fibrin, collagen, hydroxyapatite, and PMMA impregnated with antibiotic, usually an aminoglycoside or vancomycin, have been used. The dosage form is designed for the slow release of antibiotics from the material. The most commonly reported experience with local antibiotic delivery has been with antibiotic-impregnated PMMA cement or beads inserted during joint arthroplasty. Recurrent infection rates have been comparable in patients treated with local antibiotic insertion and those treated with systemic antibiotics. Thus, no evidence suggests that the PMMA beads will improve F.B.'s outcome when added to systemic therapy. Local delivery of antibiotics should never replace systemic antibiotics in the treatment of chronic osteomyelitis.[35]

OSTEOMYELITIS ASSOCIATED WITH PROSTHETIC MATERIAL

Usual Clinical Presentation

17. S.M., a 73-year-old woman, had right hip replacement 8 years ago for chronic osteoarthritis. She is seen today in the orthopedic clinic because of increasing right hip pain for the last 3 months. The hip is painful and warm, but her temperature is 37.5°C. Aspiration of fluid from the hip reveals a total nucleated cell count of 80,000/mm^3 with 90% neutrophils. A Gram stain of this fluid shows 4+ polymorphonuclear leukocytes (PMN) and 1+ Gram-positive cocci. Her peripheral WBC count is 8,800 cells/mm^3. She is started on antibiotic therapy with vancomycin and piperacillin/tazobactam pending culture results, and she is scheduled for operative evaluation and possible removal of her prosthetic joint. Does S.M. have a prosthetic joint infection?

[SI unit: WBC, 8,800 × 10^9 cells/L]

Joint replacement surgery has become a common orthopedic procedure for patients with significant joint destruction as a result of rheumatoid arthritis (RA) and other disabling diseases. Prosthetic knee, shoulder, elbow, or hip devices made of metallic alloys are cemented to adjacent bone to re-establish joint function. Infection of these foreign bodies can occur because of hematogenous dissemination of bacteria or by contiguous spread from a topical wound. *Staphylococcus* species are most commonly involved in prosthetic joint infections, followed by *Streptococcus* species, Gram-negative bacilli, and anaerobes. Bacteria infect bone adjacent to the joint prosthesis, including the bone–cement interface, which results in a loosened and less functional prosthesis.[36]

Chronic pain, swelling, erythema, and tenderness over a prosthetic joint are typical findings associated with prosthetic joint infection. S.M. has a relatively lengthy duration of symptoms associated with her right hip, which also could be caused by joint loosening, but the cell count and differential from the joint aspirate suggest joint infection. Also, the predominance of neutrophils in her joint fluid and Gram-positive cocci on a Gram stain are consistent with an infected prosthesis. As is often the case, she has no obvious source of infection on her skin or other site from which bacteria could disseminate. Occasionally, sources of infection with hematogenous dissemination to the prosthetic joint are identified, such as dental infections, cellulitis, or urinary tract infections. Given the Gram stain result, S.M. should be covered for *Staphylococcus* and *Streptococcus* species with vancomycin, pending the results of cultures and sensitivities. *Staphylococcus* species, including coagulase-negative species such as *S. epidermidis,* are the most commonly isolated bacteria responsible for prosthetic infection. These coagulase-negative *Staphylococci* are especially adherent to prosthetic material and, although coagulase-negative *Staphylococci* are usually considered a contaminant in culture, and when a prosthesis is in place, it should be considered a likely pathogen. Coagulase-negative *Staphylococci* are often resistant to oxacillin, but are susceptible to vancomycin. Because Gram-negative bacteria also can infect these joints, it is reasonable to add Gram-negative coverage to S.M.'s regimen until the results of joint fluid cultures are available.

Surgery

18. Does S.M. need surgery and antibiotics to cure her infection?

Yes. Surgery to remove S.M.'s hip prosthesis and chronic antibiotics for 6 weeks are the current recommendations for optimal eradication of prosthetic joint infection.[1,36] A two-stage orthopedic procedure is involved: removal of the infected prosthesis, placement of an antibiotic-filled spacer or block, joint immobilization, and antibiotics for 6 weeks. If the joint space remains culture negative, a new joint prosthesis is reinserted. Because avascular bone cement and prosthetic material can become seeded with bacteria, complete removal of this material is necessary to have the greatest chance of curing the infection. Six weeks of systemic antibiotic therapy in combination with orthopedic surgery results in restoration of joint function in 85% to 95% of cases. High rates of treatment failure (~70%) occur if the joint prosthesis is not removed and chronic suppressive antibiotics are not given.[36,37]

Antibiotics

19. Because the pelvic portion of S.M.'s hip prosthesis is so firmly attached to bone, the surgeon decides not to remove this portion of the prosthesis because doing so would require a pelvic fracture. Instead, her hip is débrided and the acetabular lining material is replaced. Purulent material is sent for culture. The removed lining material and three swabs of the right hip prosthesis grow OSSA. How should S.M. be treated?

To prevent recurrence of infection, S.M. will need to take antibiotics indefinitely, perhaps for the rest of her life if the original prosthesis remains in place. Lifelong therapy is impractical, expensive, and likely to provoke adverse effects. S.M. should be treated initially with oxacillin (2 g IV Q 4 hr) for at least 2 weeks, although the optimal duration of this initial parenteral therapy is unknown. Thereafter, she should be treated with oral antibiotics. Limited success has been reported with the use of ciprofloxacin plus rifampin, both given orally, in patients with prosthetic joint infections caused by *Staphylococcus* species in which the implant was not removed. In 18 patients with a short duration of symptoms (<21 days), oral ciprofloxacin (750 mg BID daily) and oral rifampin (450 mg BID daily) were given for 3 months. Twelve patients who completed the protocol had no evidence of infection at 24 months of follow-up.[38] S.M.'s symptoms have lasted 3 months, suggesting that her infection may not respond to therapy as well as that reported. Nevertheless, a prolonged course of ciprofloxacin and rifampin could be tried for at least 3 months.[38] Because S.M. grew OSSA (and assuming the isolate is also rifampin-sensitive), she could be treated chronically with dicloxacillin plus rifampin. Rifampin should be used when possible for prosthetic joint infection caused by staphylococci.[36] An important consideration before using rifampin is to make sure the patient is not taking other agents (e.g., warfarin, anticonvulsants) where a detrimental rifampin-induced drug interaction could occur.[39] A third option for oral therapy is linezolid (Zyvox). Limited data exist on the use of linezolid for prosthetic joint infection, however, and chronic use is associated with thrombocytopenia. If linezolid is used for >2 weeks, S.M.'s platelet count should be followed weekly.[29,40]

20. **S.F. is a 48-year-old man with hemophilia A and chronic bilateral knee hemarthroses. He has been human immunodeficiency virus (HIV) seropositive for 12 years; his last CD4 count 1 month ago was 480 cells/mm^3 (normal, >800). One week ago, he had uncomplicated bilateral knee arthroplasty. Cefazolin prophylaxis was administered before surgery and for 24 hours postoperatively. Soon after surgery, he noted intermittent chills and sweats accompanied by documented fevers. Two blood cultures drawn 3 days postoperatively were negative, and he was started on ampicillin/sulbactam (Unasyn) and gentamicin. Two more blood cultures drawn 3 days later are positive for *P. aeruginosa*, sensitive to ceftazidime, piperacillin, imipenem, ciprofloxacin, and gentamicin. The surgical sites are unremarkable. His antiretroviral medications are zidovudine and lamivudine (Combivir) and efavirenz (Sustiva). What is a rational antibiotic therapy plan for S.F.?**

Antibiotic treatment for S.F. should be designed to treat his *Pseudomonas* bacteremia and also to eradicate and then suppress *Pseudomonas* that may have seeded his prosthetic joints. Without symptoms related to his knees (pain, swelling, redness, tenderness), it will be impossible to tell whether the joint has become infected without removing the prosthesis. The conservative approach is to treat S.F. with combined antipseudomonal antibiotics, such as ceftazidime (2 g IV Q 8 hr) and once-daily gentamicin for 6 weeks, followed by chronic suppressive therapy with oral ciprofloxacin for the rest of his life.[36] No evidence indicates that adjunctive rifampin improves outcomes in Gram-negative infections. Also, rifampin would interact significantly with S.F.'s antiretroviral therapy, particularly efavirenz.[39]

SEPTIC ARTHRITIS

Nongonococcal Arthritis

21. **M.T., a 65-year-old man, is referred to the rheumatology clinic for left knee swelling. One week ago, his left knee became painful and swollen and he was unable to flex the joint. He also noted a temperature of 100.5°F to 102°F for at least 5 days. In clinic, a joint effusion is noted, and fluid is aspirated for cell count, a Gram stain, and culture. His medical history is unremarkable except for an episode of hives after receiving cephalexin for cellulitis 2 years ago. M.T.'s WBC count is 14,000 cells/mm^3, and his ESR is 40 mm/hour. The synovial fluid from his right knee contains 50,000 WBCs/mm^3 with 94% neutrophils, and the Gram stain shows Gram-positive cocci in clusters. Culture results are pending. His temperature is 38.5°C. What findings in M.T. are consistent with septic arthritis?**

[SI units: WBC count, 12,000 and 80,000 × 10^9 cells/L, respectively; neutrophils, 0.94; ESR, 40 mm/hour]

Usual Clinical Presentation

Septic arthritis or infectious arthritis usually is acquired hematogenously. The highly vascular synovium of the joint allows easy passage of bacteria from blood into the synovial space. Bacteremia, secondary to *Neisseria gonorrhoeae* or *S. aureus* in particular, often is associated with the development of joint infections. Septic arthritis also can develop secondary to the spread of osteomyelitis into the joint. This is especially a problem in children <1 year of age who still have capillaries perforating the epiphyseal growth plate.[2,4]

Several factors predispose patients to the development of infectious arthritis. Trauma can directly inoculate the synovium or allow infecting organisms to penetrate it more easily. Patients with certain systemic disorders, such as diabetes mellitus, RA, osteoarthritis, chronic granulomatous disease, cancer, or chronic liver disease, are more susceptible to the development of infection. Endocrine factors can predispose pregnant or menstruating women to the development of gonococcal arthritis. In the menstruating patient, this can be explained partially by the increased endocervical shedding of *N. gonorrhoeae*.[41,42]

M.T. has had an acute onset of monoarticular joint pain and swelling, with reduced range of motion and fever. These findings are classic for septic, nongonococcal arthritis. The tap of his joint effusion with a predominance of neutrophils in the joint fluid confirms the diagnosis. In these circumstances, M.T.'s knee has been infected hematogenously from a distant, usually unrecognized, source of infection. The knee is involved most commonly, and *S. aureus* is the usual causative organism. If M.T. had a urinary tract infection, however, Gram-negative bacilli would more commonly be responsible for joint infection. Occasionally, a predisposing factor is present in the involved joint, such as pre-existing arthritis (i.e., RA) or trauma.[41,42]

A single joint is involved in 90% of bacterial arthritis cases. As in M.T.'s case, the joint most commonly involved is the knee. Other potential sites of infectious arthritis in adults include the hip, shoulder, sternoclavicular and sacroiliac joints; the ankle and elbow are common sites of infection in children. The wrist and interphalangeal joints of the hand also may be involved, but in these cases, the infectious pathogens are most often *N. gonorrhoeae* and *Mycobacterium tuberculosis*.[41] The most common systemic indication of infectious arthritis is fever. Localized symptoms include pain, decreased mobility of the involved joint, and swelling.

As illustrated by M.T., most patients also have joint effusion on physical examination. When evaluating a patient who may have a joint infection, any purulent joint effusion should be considered septic until a thorough workup proves otherwise. Alternatively, noninfectious conditions may be present, such as single joint involvement with synovial effusions (e.g., acute RA, gout, chondrocalcinosis).[41]

Aspirated joint fluid should be cultured because isolation of bacteria is the only definitive diagnostic test for bacterial arthritis. M.T.'s joint fluid picture also is typical. The leukocyte count in the synovial fluid usually is significantly elevated, with counts ranging from 50,000 to 200,000 cells/mm^3. Leukocyte counts of <20,000 rarely are seen during infection, except in early cases of bacterial arthritis or in patients with disseminated gonococcal infection (DGI). Synovial fluid from an infected joint also may have a decreased glucose concentration, but this is seen in only about 50% of cases.[41]

Another laboratory finding in M.T. that is consistent with infectious arthritis is the elevated ESR. Although this value is higher in bacterial infection, viral or fungal arthritis also can be associated with this finding. Increased WBC counts in serum are common in younger patients, but rare in adults. Anemia also can be associated with infection, especially in patients with chronic involvement or in cases where predisposing factors such as RA are present.[42]

When attempting to determine the most likely pathogen, the patient's age must be taken into consideration. In adults >30 years of age such as M.T., and in children >2 years of age, *S. aureus* is the most common cause of bacterial arthritis. In adults <30 years of age, *N. gonorrhoeae* is more likely to be the causative agent. *Streptococci,* such as group A β-hemolytic *Streptococci,* can cause infection in children and adults. Other organisms, such as group B *Streptococci,* anaerobic *Streptococci,* and Gram-negative bacteria, can cause infection. Gram-negative bacilli are responsible for approximately 15% of cases and often infect multiple joints. Infections with these organisms usually are associated with predisposing factors, such as RA, osteoarthritis, or heroin use. The organism most commonly isolated from patients with bacterial arthritis who have a history of IV drug abuse is *P. aeruginosa*.[41,42]

Initial Antimicrobial Therapy: Treatment in β-Lactam Allergic Patients

22. M.T. describes his reaction to cephalexin as intense pruritic skin lesions over his trunk and upper extremities that appeared acutely (several hours) after he had received several doses. He did not experience wheezing or shortness of breath, and his reaction was treated symptomatically with diphenhydramine and discontinuation of the cephalexin. He had received several types of oral antibiotics before this episode of pruritus without difficulty, but has not taken antibiotics since then. How should M.T. be treated?

Treatment of nongonococcal arthritis includes drainage of purulent joint fluid (by needle aspiration or surgery) and appropriate antibiotic therapy. Because *S. aureus* is most likely involved, initial empiric therapy with a penicillinase-resistant penicillin, a cephalosporin, or vancomycin should be initiated. M.T.'s reaction to cephalexin is worrisome, however, because readministration of a penicillin or cephalosporin could cause allergic symptoms. An alternative, effective non–β-lactam treatment is available, however. Because M.T.'s septic arthritis is probably caused by *S. aureus* and, perhaps, streptococci, vancomycin (1 g IV Q 12 hr), which covers both organisms, should be started as soon as possible. In patients who are not allergic to penicillin, oxacillin or nafcillin (2 g IV Q 4 hr) is recommended for OSSA infections. β-lactams and vancomycin penetrate joint effusions adequately for Gram-positive infections. If M.T. acquired his infection in the hospital, vancomycin also would be initially indicated because of the possibility that ORSA is involved. In a nonallergic patient, therapy then can be changed on the basis of sensitivity testing to oxacillin if the organism is susceptible.[41,42]

Duration of Therapy

23. How long should M.T. be treated? How should the efficacy of treatment be monitored?

Although few studies have been carried out to determine the optimal duration of therapy for bacterial arthritis, the current recommendation is 2 to 3 weeks; some investigators recommend that treatment be extended to 4 weeks for infectious arthritis caused by *S. aureus* or Gram-negative bacilli.[41,42]

M.T. should be treated for at least 3 weeks.[42,43] His response to therapy should be monitored clinically (resolution of symptoms, fever, and falling ESR, CRP, or both) as well as by periodic evaluation of joint fluid. Frequent aspirations of joint fluid, initially on a daily basis, should be done, with evaluation of cell count and fluid culture. Effective therapy results in a diminishing WBC count in the joint fluid and negative cultures, usually within 3 to 4 days of treatment. A poorer outcome (permanent joint dysfunction) can result if joint fluid cultures are still positive after 6 days of treatment for Gram-positive infection. If fluid cultures are persistently positive, more aggressive surgical management is necessary to preserve joint function.[41,42]

Most joint fluid cultures become negative after 7 days of treatment with IV antibiotics. Joint inflammation and other symptoms also should diminish by this time. The duration of articular symptoms before antibiotic therapy is begun correlates with the subsequent time required to sterilize the synovial fluid. Therefore, delay in initiating antibiotic treatment may necessitate a longer course of therapy.

As in hematogenous osteomyelitis, oral antibiotics have been used in septic arthritis to complete a course of treatment if the initial response to IV therapy is adequate. Oral therapy should not be considered until the patient is afebrile, joint fluid cultures are negative, the ESR or CRP is normal, and there is decreased joint pain and increased joint mobility.[42] There are case series with generally positive results, but adequately controlled, randomized clinical trials comparing IV and oral therapy are not available.[43] Because of M.T.'s allergy to cephalexin, the choice of adequate oral therapy to complete at least 3 weeks of treatment is difficult. Because of the continuing emergence of resistance among Gram-positive organisms to ciprofloxacin, use of this agent is not recommended. Oral clindamycin could be used, but published experience in adults is minimal and there would be concern about the possible development of antibiotic-associated colitis. Use of linezolid (Zyvox) in septic arthritis is also not extensively reported in the literature. If the *S. aureus* isolated from M.T. is sensitive to trimethoprim-sulfamethoxazole, this agent may be an alternative to clindamycin for oral treatment. Published experience with this mode of treatment also is lacking. M.T. should be advised that parenteral treatment with vancomycin, which can be accomplished at home, would be the most effective mode of treatment. Finally, injections of antibiotics into the joint space are of no value. Most antibiotics readily penetrate the joint space and enter the synovial fluid.[41,42]

Gonococcal Arthritis

24. J.E., a 21-year-old woman, presents to the walk-in clinic with right knee and right shoulder pain, nausea, and vomiting. On physical examination, her right knee is swollen and she has decreased range of motion of her right shoulder. Several erythematous, papular skin lesions are noted on both hands. She also has a vaginal discharge. Her temperature is 38.2°C, and her WBC count is 15,000 cells/mm^3. She gives a history of having two recent sexual partners. Cultures of blood, joint fluid, and vaginal discharge are obtained; a joint fluid Gram stain shows 4+ PMNs, but no organisms are seen. Why is J.E. considered to have gonococcal arthritis?

[SI unit: WBC, 15,000 × 10^9 cells/L]

Usual Clinical Presentation

Polyarticular arthritis in a young, sexually active adult, as is the case with J.E., is caused most commonly by *N. gonorrhoeae.* Arthritis in multiple joints is one of the most common features of disseminated gonococcal infection (DGI). Unlike nongonococcal arthritis, which is almost exclusively monoarticular, gonococcal arthritis involves multiple joints in approximately 50% of cases. Clinically, patients present initially with a migratory polyarthralgia and later with fever, dermatitis, and tenosynovitis. Skin lesions are an important clue to the diagnosis of DGI and often begin as tiny erythematous papules and develop into larger vesicles. Other symptoms, such as purulent and swollen joints, are present in only 30% to 40% of patients. As in hematogenously acquired nongonococcal arthritis, the synovial fluid leukocyte count usually is elevated, but to a lesser degree. *N. gonorrhoeae* is recovered in <50% of purulent joint effusions, however, but blood cultures often are positive for this organism and, coupled with the patient's clinical presentation, can be used to make a definitive diagnosis.[41,44]

J.E. has systemic signs of infection, skin lesions, and multiple joint involvement, which are classic for DGI. Her history of recent sexual activity and the presence of a vaginal discharge are consistent with gonococcal infection, although evidence of mucosal infection with *N. gonorrhoeae* is not necessary for disseminated infection to occur.[41,44]

Patient Workup and Treatment in the Clinic

25. What additional workup should be done in J.E.? Can she be treated immediately in the clinic?

J.E. should be evaluated for other sexually transmitted diseases, specifically syphilis and HIV infection. Serologic testing for syphilis (rapid plasma reagent [RPR] or venereal disease research laboratory [VDRL] testing) and for antibody to HIV should be obtained. In addition, she should have a pregnancy test because some of the antibiotics that may be used in J.E. are contraindicated during pregnancy, including doxycycline.

Because of possible penicillinase production by *N. gonorrhoeae,* recommended therapy is with ceftriaxone (1 g intramuscularly or IV Q 24 hr) initially. J.E. should receive her first dose of ceftriaxone in the clinic today. Parenteral treatment should continue for 1 to 2 days after improvement begins; at that point, oral cephalosporin therapy (cefixime 400 mg BID or cefpodoxime 400 mg BID) can be started. Quinolone-resistant *N. gonorrhoeae* are prevalent throughout the United States, so the use of ciprofloxacin or levofloxacin as treatment is no longer recommended by the Centers for Disease Control and Prevention (CDC). The duration of antibiotic treatment is 7 to 14 days.[42,45]

J.E.'s sexual partners should also be evaluated and treated for relevant sexually transmitted diseases.

Full Course of Therapy

26. Results of RPR and pregnancy testing in J.E. are negative. How should she complete her course of therapy?

J.E.'s DGI should be treated for at least 7 days. J.E. also should begin treatment with azithromycin (1 g orally once) or doxycycline (100 mg orally BID for 7 days) for the possibility of concomitant chlamydial infection. J.E. can complete her course of treatment for DGI orally, although parenteral therapy is recommended until signs and symptoms resolve. This usually takes 2 to 4 days.[44] She will have to return to the clinic for daily ceftriaxone administration unless other arrangements for parenteral therapy can be made. Current recommendations from the CDC are that oral treatment should be with either cefixime (400 mg BID) or cefpodoxime (400 mg BID).[45] Treatment guidelines for DGI are included in the gonorrhea section of the chapter on sexually transmitted diseases.

REFERENCES

1. Lew DP, Waldwogel FA. Osteomyelitis. *Lancet* 2004;364:369.
2. Berbari EF et al. Osteomyelitis. In: Mandell GL et al., eds. *Principles and Practice of Infectious Diseases*, 6th ed. Philadelphia, PA: Elsevier Churchill Livingstone; 2005:1322.
3. Priest DH, Peacock Jr JE. Hematogenous vertebral osteomyelitis due to *Staphylococcus aureus* in the adult: clinical features and therapeutic options. *S Med J* 2005;98:854.
4. Kaplan SL. Osteomyelitis in children. *Infect Dis Clin N Am* 2005;19:787.
5. Calhoun JH, Manring MM. Adult osteomyelitis. *Infect Dis Clin N Am* 2005;19:765.
6. Kapoor A et al. Magnetic resonance imaging for diagnosing foot osteomyelitis: a meta-analysis. *Arch Intern Med* 2007;167:125.
7. Arnold SR et al. Changing patterns of acute hematogenous osteomyelitis and septic arthritis. *J Pediatr Orthop* 2006;26:703.
8. Miller LG et al. Clinical and epidemiologic characteristics cannot distinguish community-associated methicillin-resistant *Staphylococcus aureus* infection from methicillin-susceptible *S. aureus* infection: a prospective investigation. *Clin Infect Dis* 2007;44:471.
9. Martinez-Aguilar G et al. Community-acquired, methicillin-resistant and methicillin-susceptible *Staphylococcus aureus* musculoskeletal infections in children. *Pediatr Infect Dis J* 2004;23:701.
10. Tice AD et al. Outcomes of osteomyelitis among patients treated with outpatient parenteral antimicrobial therapy. *Am J Med* 2003;114:723.
11. Gelfand MS, Cleveland KO. Vancomycin therapy and the progression of methicillin-resistant *Staphylococcus aureus* vertebral osteomyelitis. *S Med J* 2004;97:593.
12. Krogstad P. Osteomyelitis and septic arthritis. In: Feigin RD et al., eds. *Textbook of Pediatric Infectious Diseases*, 5th ed. Philadelphia, PA: WB Saunders; 2004:713.
13. Fitzgerald Jr RH et al. Pathophysiology of osteomyelitis and pharmacokinetics of antimicrobial agents in normal and osteomyelitic bone. In: Esterhai JL Jr et al., eds. *Musculoskeletal Infection*. Park Ridge, IL: American Academy of Orthopaedic Surgeons; 1990:387.
14. Roine I et al. Serial serum C-reactive protein to monitor recovery from acute hematogenous osteomyelitis in children. *Pediatr Infect Dis J* 1995;14:40.
15. Jaberi FM et al. Short-term intravenous antibiotic treatment of acute hematogenous bone and joint infection in children: a prospective randomized trial. *J Pediatr Orthop* 2002;22:317.
16. Perry CR et al. Accuracy of cultures of material from swabbing of the superficial aspect of the wound and needle biopsy in the preoperative assessment of osteomyelitis. *J Bone Joint Surg* [*Am*] 1991;73:745.
17. Vuagnat A et al. High-dose vancomycin for osteomyelitis: continuous versus intermittent infusion. *J Clin Pharm Ther* 2004;29:351.
18. El Amari EB et al. High versus standard dose vancomycin for osteomyelitis. *Scand J Infect Dis* 2004;36:712.
19. Bailey TC et al. A meta-analysis of extended-interval dosing versus multiple daily dosing of aminoglycosides. *Clin Infect Dis* 1997;24:786.
20. Ali MZ, Goetz MB. A meta-analysis of the relative efficacy and toxicity of single daily dosing versus multiple daily dosing of aminoglycosides. *Clin Infect Dis* 1997;24:769.
21. Sheftel TG, Mader JT. Randomized evaluation of ceftazidime or ticarcillin and tobramycin for the treatment of osteomyelitis caused by gram-negative bacilli. *Antimicrob Agents Chemother* 1986;29:112.
22. Gentry LO, Rodriguez GG. Oral ciprofloxacin compared with parenteral antibiotics in the treatment of osteomyelitis. *Antimicrob Agents Chemother* 1990;34:40.
23. Stengel D et al. Systematic review and meta-analysis of antibiotic therapy for bone and joint infections. *Lancet Infect Dis* 2001;1:175.
24. Lew DP, Waldwogel FA. Quinolones and osteomyelitis: state-of-the-art. *Drugs* 1995;49(Suppl 2):100.
25. Lavery LA et al. Risk factors for foot infections in individuals with diabetes. *Diabetes Care* 2006;29:1288.
26. Lipsky BA. Osteomyelitis of the foot in diabetic patients. *Clin Infect Dis* 1997;25:1318.
27. Senneville E et al. Culture of percutaneous bone biopsy specimens for diagnosis of diabetic foot osteomyelitis: concordance with ulcer swab cultures. *Clin Infect Dis* 2006;42:57.
28. Embil JM et al. Oral antimicrobial therapy for diabetic foot osteomyelitis. *Foot Ankle Int* 2006;27:771.

29. Rayner CR et al. Linezolid in the treatment of osteomyelitis: results of compassionate use experience. *Infection* 2004;32:8.
30. Lipsky B et al. Treating foot infections in diabetic patients: a randomized, multicenter, open-label trial of linezolid versus ampicillin-sulbactam/amoxicillin-clavulanate. *Clin Infect Dis* 2004;38:17.
31. Lipsky BA, Berendt AR. Principles and practice of antibiotic therapy of diabetic foot infections. *Diab Metab Res Rev* 2000;16(Suppl 1):S42.
32. Uckay I et al. Recurrent osteomyelitis caused by infection with different bacterial strains without obvious source of reinfection. *J Clin Microbiol* 2006;44:1194.
33. Shih H et al. Diagnosis and treatment of subacute osteomyelitis. *J Trauma* 2005;58:83.
34. Lazzarini L et al. Antibiotic treatment of osteomyelitis: what have we learned from 30 years of clinical trials?. *Int J Infect Dis* 2005;9: 127.
35. Zalavras CG et al. Local antibiotic therapy in the treatment of open fractures and osteomyelitis. *Clin Orthop Rel Res* 2004;427:86.
36. Brause BD. Infections with prostheses in bones and joints. In: Mandell GL et al., eds. *Principles and Practice of Infectious Diseases*, 6th ed. Philadelphia, PA: Elsevier Churchill Livingstone; 2005:1332.
37. Brandt CM et al. *Staphylococcus aureus* prosthetic joint infection treated with prosthesis removal and delayed reimplantation arthroplasty. *Mayo Clin Proc* 1999;74:553.
38. Zimmerli W et al. Role of rifampin for treatment of orthopedic implant-related staphylococcal infections. *JAMA* 1998;279:1537.
39. Finch CK et al. Rifampin and rifabutin drug interactions: an update. *Arch Intern Med* 2002;162:985.
40. Bassetti M et al. Linezolid treatment of prosthetic hip infections due to methicillin-resistant *Staphylococcus aureus* (MRSA). *J Infect* 2001;43: 148.
41. Ohl CA. Infectious arthritis of native joints. In: Mandell GL et al., eds. *Principles and Practice of Infectious Diseases*, 6th ed. Philadelphia, PA: Elsevier Churchill Livingstone; 2005:1311.
42. Ross JJ. Septic arthritis. *Infect Dis Clin N Am* 2005;19:799.
43. Syrogiannopoulos GA, Nelson JD. Duration of antimicrobial therapy for acute suppurative osteoarticular infections. *Lancet* 1988;1:37.
44. Rice PA. Gonococcal arthritis (disseminated gonococcal infection). *Infect Dis Clin N Am* 2005;19: 853.
45. http://www.cdc.gov/std/treatment/2006/GonUpdate-April2007. pdf. Accessed July 14, 2007.

CHAPTER 67

Traumatic Skin and Soft Tissue Infections

James P. McCormack and Glen Brown

Skin and soft tissue infections refer to infections involving any or all layers of the skin (epidermis, dermis), subcutaneous fat, fascia, or muscle. Many terms or classifications are used to describe various skin and soft tissue infections, and these often are based on the site of infection and causative organism(s). The terms or classifications, however, add little to the understanding and treatment of these infections. In fact, confusion in terminology may be detrimental if treatment is delayed until a causative organism is identified.

Although mild skin and soft tissue infections often are self-limiting, moderate to severe infections can progress to complicated infections, such as septic arthritis, osteomyelitis, or systemic infections (bacteremia), if not treated appropriately. Soft tissue infections in diabetic patients can lead to gangrene and loss of limb, whereas necrotizing soft tissue infections, even with appropriate treatment, are fatal in 30% to 50% of patients.[1]

This chapter focuses on skin and soft tissue infections that are primarily the result of a break in the skin following an abrasion, skin puncture, ulceration, surgical wound, intentional or unintentional insertion of a foreign body, or blunt soft tissue contusion. Not discussed are superficial skin infections, such as impetigo; infections that originate within the hair follicle (e.g., folliculitis, furuncles, carbuncles) or sweat pores; styes, acne, diaper rash, and skin infestations.

Treatment of traumatic skin and soft tissue infections often is empiric and based on the severity and site of infection, the patient's underlying immunocompetence, and the triggering event (e.g., abrasion, bite, insertion of a foreign object) because attempts to isolate the causative organism often are futile.[2,3]

The organisms that should be considered when empirically treating patients with a traumatic skin or soft tissue infection are outlined in Table 67-1.

CELLULITIS

Definition and Causative Organisms

1. T.E., age 25 years, presents to her family doctor with a 2- to 3-day history of worsening pain, redness, and swelling on her left leg following an abrasion that occurred sliding into second base during a softball tournament. The area is warm to the touch with a defined erythematous border. Over the past 24 to 36 hours, the leg has become increasingly painful and "tight." Mild lymphadenopathy is present, and T.E. has a temperature of 38.2°C. The presumptive diagnosis is a moderate cellulitis, and cloxacillin (Tegopen, Cloxapen) is prescribed. Why is cloxacillin appropriate empiric treatment for T.E.?

Cellulitis (an acute inflammation of the skin and subcutaneous fat) is characterized by local tenderness, pain, swelling, warmth, and erythema with or without a definite entry point. Cellulitis is usually secondary to trauma or an underlying skin lesion that allows bacterial penetration into the skin and underlying tissues. Local treatment (i.e., cleaning or irrigation of the site with soap and water) is all that is required for mild cellulitis in patients with no evidence of a systemic infection. In T.E., however, her elevated temperature, increasing pain, and lymphadenopathy suggest a more serious infection. Antibiotics, in addition to local wound care, should be prescribed

Table 67-1 Potential Organisms Causing Skin and Soft Tissue Infections

	Gram-Positive		*Gram-Negative*			*Anaerobes*		
	Staphylococcal	*Streptococcal*	*Escherichia coli, Klebsiella Species, Proteus Species*	*Pasteurella Multocida*	*Eikenella Corrodens*	*Oral Anaerobes*	*Clostridium Species*	*Bacteroides Fragilis*
Cellulitis	X	X						
Diabetic soft tissue	X	X	X					X
Necrotizing infections	X	X	X			X	X	X
Erysipelas		X						
Animal bites	X	X	X	X		X		
Human bites	X	X	X		X	X		

X, organisms that should be covered empirically with appropriate antibiotic therapy.

for T.E. Cellulitis most often is caused by group A β-hemolytic streptococci (*Streptococcus pyogenes*) and, less often, *Staphylococcus aureus* (Table 67-1).[2,3] In fact, unless there is an abcess or penetrating trauma *S. aureus* rarely causes cellulitis.[4] Wound cultures often are negative, however, and fail to identify the causative organism.[2,3] Other organisms (*Escherichia coli, Pseudomonas aeruginosa, Klebsiella pneumoniae*) also can cause cellulites, but should be suspected only in immunocompromised patients or in patients who fail to respond to antibiotics that have activity limited to gram-positive organisms. Recently the incidence of community acquired methicillin-resistant S. aureus (CA-MRSA) has been increasing.[5]

Empiric Antibiotic Therapy for Moderate Cellulitis

Oral cloxacillin (Tegopen, Cloxapen) is appropriate empiric therapy for cellulitis in an otherwise healthy individual such as T.E. Cloxacillin has good activity against staphylococcal and streptococcal organisms and is better tolerated than erythromycin (E-Mycin) or clindamycin (Cleocin). Dicloxacillin (Dynapen), another antistaphylococcal penicillin, produces slightly higher total serum concentrations than cloxacillin but is more highly protein bound, resulting in slightly lower free-serum concentrations.[6] Flucloxacillin (Floxapen; not available in the United States) provides similar total serum concentrations to dicloxacillin (Dynapen) but is less protein bound and produces higher free concentrations than either cloxacillin or dicloxacillin.[6] These small differences in pharmacokinetics do not affect clinical outcome, and the choice between these agents should be based on cost. If the cellulitis is well demarcated and there are no pockets of pus or evidence of vein thrombosis, penicillin (V-Cillin K, Pen-Vee K) alone can be appropriate because the causative organism is likely to be streptococcal. Many other available antibiotics that have activity against staphylococcal and streptococcal organisms have been evaluated for effectiveness in skin and soft tissue infections. In a surveillance study in the United States, all 405 isolates of *S. pyogenes* isolated from skin and soft tissue infections were sensitive to penicillin. *S. pyogenes* was also 100% susceptible to ceftriaxone, vancomycin, levofloxacin, and moxifloxacin; 6% of the organisms were resistant to azithromycin.[7] Although many antibiotics are effective for the treatment of cellulitis, none is more effective than cloxacillin or dicloxacillin. Cephalexin (Keflex) is probably as effective and as well tolerated as cloxacillin or dicloxacillin and is comparable in cost. Cephalexin has been shown to be just as effective as more expensive agents (ofloxacin).[8] The gram-negative activity of cephalexin (not seen with cloxacillin or dicloxacillin) is not required for most cases of cellulitis in otherwise healthy patients. In many emergency departments (ED), a single dose of a long-acting parenterally administered cephalosporin (e.g., ceftriaxone), followed by oral therapy with one of the agents mentioned above, is often the preferred treatment regimen. This regimen is not more effective than oral therapy alone, and ceftriaxone (Rocephin) adds to the cost of treatment.

In this case, antibiotic treatment is required, and T.E. should receive the least expensive of cloxacillin, dicloxacillin, or cephalexin. Although some of the macrolides and quinolones are effective in treating cellulitis, they do not provide any therapeutic advantage over older and less expensive agents.[4]

However, in areas where the incidence of CA-MRSA has become clinically important (10–15% resistance) and especially if there are additional risk factors (Children, competitive athletes, prisoners, soldiers, selected ethnic populations, Native Americans/Alaska Natives, Pacific Islanders, intravenous drug users, men who have sex with men) empiric treatment should be with antibiotics that have activity against CA-MRSA.[9] At present, most CA-MRSA are still susceptible to trimethoprim-sulfamethoxazole, clindamycin and tetracyclines but clinical trials of these agents for CA-MRSA infections are lacking.[4,10] If these agents are used, a reasonable suggestion would be to re-evaluate (by the patient if they are competent) within 24 to 48 hours to verify that an improvement is occurring. Some clinicians are avoiding the use of clindamycin because of concerns of inducible resistance and in areas with a clinically important incidence of CA-MRSA, laboratories should likely be testing for inducible clindamycin resistance.

In addition to systemic therapy, T.E. should be instructed to keep the area clean with soap and water (if an open wound is present) and to protect the area.

Treatment for the Penicillin-Allergic Patient

2. What agents could be chosen if T.E. were allergic to penicillin?

Oral erythromycin (E-mycin) or clindamycin (Cleocin) could be chosen for patients with a documented history of penicillin or cephalosporin allergy. However, there has been an increase in certain regions of macrolide resistance group A streptococci and if this was the case for TE, then erythromycin may not be a reasonable alternative and oral quinolones such as moxifloxacin or levofloxacin could be considered[4] and local sensitivities should direct the choice. Erythromycin causes nausea, vomiting, diarrhea, and cramps in 30% to 40% of patients, but this can be decreased by taking it with food. Clindamycin causes diarrhea in 20% of patients and can cause serious toxicity secondary to antibiotic-associated colitis. Erythromycin is much less expensive than clindamycin, and unless a patient has documented gastrointestinal (GI) intolerance to erythromycin, it is preferred over clindamycin. Trimethoprim-sulfamethoxazole (Bactrim, Septra) has good activity against *S. aureus*; its activity against *S. pyogenes* is weak, however, and therefore, if a streptococcal organism cannot be ruled out, it should likely not be used as empiric therapy. In addition to the above mentioned agents, moxifloxacin could also be considered as an alternative in the penicillin allergic patient.

Dosages of Antibiotics

3. What dose should be prescribed for T.E.?

The recommended dosages in the literature for cloxacillin (Tegopen, Cloxapen) and dicloxacillin (Dynapen) are 250 to 500 mg orally Q 6 hr and 125 to 250 mg orally Q 6 hr, respectively. Although lower dosages of dicloxacillin can be used, cloxacillin and dicloxacillin produce relatively similar free serum concentrations and should be prescribed at similar dosages. The dosage for mild to moderate infections should be 250 mg orally Q 6 hr; for moderate to severe infections, it should be 500 mg orally Q 6 hr. Dosages up to 1,000 mg orally Q 6 hr have been used, but GI intolerance (usually diarrhea) can occur. These dosages also apply to cephalexin and erythromycin. The dosage for Pen-V is 250 to 500 mg orally Q 6 hr; for oral clindamycin, the dosage is 150 to 450 mg orally Q 6 hr. Because cloxacillin is the drug chosen for T.E., a dosage of 250 mg orally Q 6 hr should be sufficient. If she were more severely ill, however, the higher dosage of 500 mg orally Q 6 hr could be chosen. The dose for doxycycline is 100 mg orally Q 12 hr and the dose for trimethoprim-sulfamethoxazole is one double-strength tablet orally Q12 h. The recommended dose for moxifloxacin is 400 mg orally Q24 hr and 500 mg orally Q24 hr for levofloxacin.

Treatment Duration

4. For how long should T.E. be treated?

While the usual recommended duration of therapy for cellulitis is 10 days, 5 days of antibiotics has been shown to be as good as 10 days for uncomplicated cellulites.[11] An instruction to the patient to continue oral antibiotics for 2 to 3 days after the patient has become afebrile and has improved clinically seems reasonable. T.E. should be counseled to expect a response within 1 to 2 days after therapy begins (although erythema may persist longer). In addition, she should be instructed to return for re-evaluation if the condition does not improve or worsens over the next few days.

Evaluation of Therapy

5. What further diagnostic evaluation should be undertaken for T.E.?

In otherwise healthy individuals, identification of the causative organism in cases of cellulitis is unnecessary. Needle aspiration, fine-needle aspiration biopsy, and punch biopsy have isolated the causative organism in only about 15% to 25% of patients.[2,3] Appropriate empiric treatment is effective in most patients, and an attempt to isolate the organism does not contribute to the success of treatment and adds significantly to the cost of care. Although organisms often are not cultured, attempts to identify the organism are recommended if initial treatment fails and when treating immunocompromised patients, patients with potential joint or tendon damage, and patients with life-threatening infections requiring hospitalization. In these cases, a swab of the primary wound and a needle aspiration or punch biopsy of the leading edge of the cellulitis should be obtained for Gram stain and culture before initiating antimicrobial therapy. Blood for cultures should be drawn in addition to wound cultures in these patients. Anaerobic cultures need to be drawn only when the wound contains necrotic tissue, the wound is foul smelling, or crepitus is present. Even if wound and blood cultures are obtained, many infections will be culture negative (74%).[2] Blood culture results are positive in less than 5% of cases.[12] Culture information, in conjunction with clinical course, can be used to modify subsequent treatment. Because T.E. has only a moderate cellulitis, cultures are not required and therapy can be given empirically.

Role of Topical Antibiotics

6. What role do topical antibiotics play in treating T.E.'s cellulitis?

The value of topical antibiotics in treating skin infections is questionable. Most topical antibiotics have not been evaluated in appropriately designed trials. Although mupirocin produced positive bacteriologic results over placebo in treating some types of wound infections,[13,14] most studies have found no important clinical differences.[14] Mupirocin has been compared favorably with erythromycin and cloxacillin in the treatment of patients with impetigo, minor wound infections, and mild cellulitis; however, most cases of mild cellulitis will improve with only local wound care (e.g., cleansing or irrigation of the area). In patients with moderate to severe infections, mupirocin or any topical antibiotics (neomycin, bacitracin, polymyxin B) should not be used to replace or augment systemic antibiotics. Topical antibiotics likely do little but add to the cost of therapy, and they occasionally cause a contact dermatitis.[14] Therefore, T.E. should not be treated with topical antibiotics because her moderate cellulitis should be managed adequately by her systemic antimicrobial therapy.

Empiric Antibiotic Therapy for Moderate to Severe Cellulitis

7. J.M., age 34 years, presents to the ED with a 3- to 4-day history of increasing pain around his left hip, secondary to an injury he received falling on the sidewalk. In addition, he has a fever and feels weak, lethargic, and nauseated. Examination reveals a swollen, warm, and extremely tender hip. J.M. has a temperature of 39.8°C and appears quite ill. A diagnosis of moderate to severe cellulitis is made, and J.M. is hospitalized because of the severity of the infection. J.M. has no other underlying medical problems. What empiric antibiotic regimen would be reasonable for J.M.?

In moderate to severely ill patients, when hospitalization is required, antibiotics should be administered parenterally. The parenteral agent of choice is nafcillin (Nafcil; cloxacillin in Canada). Some clinicians add penicillin G (2 million units Q 6 hr) to nafcillin to ensure coverage against streptococcal organisms because the minimum inhibitory concentrations for penicillin against streptococci are lower than those with nafcillin. However, this "double coverage" is unnecessary if high-dose nafcillin (2 g intravenously [IV] Q 6 hr) is used. Cefazolin (2 g IV Q 8 hr) would be an appropriate alternative if it is less expensive than nafcillin. Second- and third-generation cephalosporins (cefuroxime [Zinacef], cefoxitin [Mefoxin], ceftriaxone [Rocephin], cefotaxime [Claforan]) and some quinolones may be as effective as nafcillin but provide no clinical advantages and are more expensive. Linezolid is also effective for the treatment of complicated skin and soft tissue infections, but it is no more effective than cloxacillin.[15] In a large study (1,080 subjects) of complicated soft tissue infections linezolid produced similar cure rates to vancomycin overall (92% vs. 89%) but in a subset-analysis of subjects with MRSA, linezolid was associated with a better outcome rate (89% vs. 67%).[16] Newer agents like daptomycin and tigecycline have also been shown to be effective in serious soft tissue infections but at present they don't appear to offer any advantages over other agents unless other agents have been shown to be ineffective or are not tolerated.

Therefore, J.M. should receive either nafcillin or cefazolin, whichever is less expensive. Once J.M. has become afebrile and has clinically improved for 2 days, the parenteral antibiotic should be discontinued and appropriate oral therapy (cloxacillin) initiated to complete at least a 10-day course (2 weeks if the patient responds slowly). In settings where 10% to 15% of community isolates of S. aureus are methicillin resistant or in severe infections (sepsis, necrotizing fasciitis, etc) or if the patient has the risk factors outlined in question 1, empiric treatment with vancomycin, linezolid or daptomycin should be considered until the results of cultures and sensitivities are known.

Penicillin Allergy

8. Two days after starting therapy, J.M. develops a maculopapular skin rash. What alternative therapy should be chosen?

Regardless of when during the course of therapy a drug rash occurs (early or late), the precipitant drug should be discontinued because there is a chance, although small, that the reaction could worsen. In patients who develop a penicillin allergy and who still require parenteral therapy, clindamycin, erythromycin, vancomycin (Vancocin), or linezolid (Zyvox in the United States; Zyvoxam in Canada) moxifloxacin or levofloxacin could be chosen. Because all of these agents are equally effective, the decision on which drug to use in J.M. should be based on cost and dosing convenience (clindamycin 600 mg IV Q 8 hr, erythromycin 500 mg IV Q 6 hr, vancomycin 1,000 mg IV Q 12 hr, and linezolid 600 mg IV Q 12 hr, moxifloxacin 400 mg IV Q24 hr and levofloxacin 500 mg IV Q24 hr). The administration of IV erythromycin is inconvenient because of its significant local irritative properties, and vancomycin, clindamycin, or linezolid, moxifloxacin or levofloxacin is preferred for J.M. The choice between these agents should be based on cost.

Culture and Sensitivity Results

9. After 48 hours of therapy, culture and sensitivity results are available. What changes, if any, should be made in J.M.'s treatment?

If cultures show only streptococcal organisms, in a patient who is not allergic to penicillin, therapy should be switched to penicillin G because it is effective, well tolerated, and less expensive than nafcillin (Nafcil). If cultures show staphylococcal species (*S. aureus*) that are sensitive to methicillin, the initial empiric therapy should be continued. If the organisms are resistant to methicillin, therapy should be switched to vancomycin 15 mg/kg IV Q 12 hr or linezolid 600 mg IV Q 12 hr. The choice between these two agents should be based on oral bioavailability, side effect profile, and cost. Because J.M. has developed a presumed penicillin allergy, he should continue with his existing therapy of either clindamycin or vancomycin.

Switching to Oral Therapy

10. After 72 hours of therapy, J.M. has improved considerably and has been afebrile for 24 hours. Can he be switched to oral therapy?

Once J.M. has been afebrile for at least 24 hours and is virtually asymptomatic, other than some continuing tenderness around the site of the infection, oral therapy can replace IV therapy, assuming J.M. can tolerate oral medications. Although clinicians often switch to an oral version of the drug that was given parenterally, this may not always provide the patient with the most convenient and cost-effective therapy. Clinicians should select the oral agent on the basis of culture results, convenience, and cost.

Intravenous Drug User

11. M.C., age 22 years, presents to the ED with a 3- to 4-day history of pain in her left forearm. On examination, she has a swollen and erythematous area of approximately 8 × 12 cm in the antecubital fossa of the left arm. The area is warm and tender to the touch. M.C. has a temperature of 39.2°C. She admits to injecting heroin daily; track marks are present on both arms. She states that she uses "filtered tap water" as a diluent for her narcotics and that her arm "has only been hurting for the last 3 days." No signs of lymphangitis or thrombophlebitis are seen. What tests are needed to confirm the diagnosis?

M.C. has all the cardinal signs of cellulitis (i.e., induration, edema, erythema, and tenderness to touch). Given her history of an injury (injection), her presentation is compatible with cellulitis. No additional tests are required unless, on clinical examination, there is a suspicion of additional injury beyond the injection site or of a deeper infection (e.g., osteomyelitis). Obtaining a specimen from the infection site (by aspiration) to identify the organism(s) is unnecessary unless the patient has a concurrent condition that could impair her immunologic response.[3] The sensitivity of needle aspiration at the edge of the wound or at the site of greatest inflammation in identifying the infecting organism is only about 10%.[2] Therefore, aspiration of the wound is not warranted. The sensitivity of needle aspiration increases to 25% in patients with underlying immunologic dysfunction (e.g., diabetes, malignancy, poor peripheral circulation) and may be beneficial in identifying the infecting organism(s) in these patients.[3] M.C. possesses risk factor (intravenous drug use) for CA-MRSA.[17] She should be closely examined for any sign of abscess at the infected site, and drained if present. Cultures should be sent of any abscess fluid, but routine cultures for CA-MRSA in cellulitus is not required unless this is a repeat presentation or is part of monitoring for a community outbreak.[17] For patients such as M.C. with signs and symptoms (e.g., fever) where the injury is a significant risk for bacteremia and potentially for endocarditis, blood cultures are warranted. Blood cultures should be drawn before antibiotics are started to assess the presence of bacteria. If the blood cultures return positive, further assessment for potential endocarditis is warranted.

Causative Organisms

12. Are the suspected organisms in this patient population similar to those found in other patients with cellulitis?

A wide range of organisms can cause cellulitis in an IV drug user because of the potential for direct inoculation of any organism with the drug of abuse. Despite the efforts of an IV drug user to make as sterile an IV product as possible, the IV drug user commonly is injecting a contaminated solution. Although almost any organism can be found, the infecting bacteria causing cellulitis in an IV drug user are similar to those found in normal hosts.[18] β-Hemolytic group A streptococci and staphylococci, particularly *S. aureus,* are the most common infecting organisms.[19,20] Intravenous drug use has been identified as a risk factor for infection with CA-MRSA and should be particularly considered if the patient has had recurrent infections or has failed to respond to antibiotic therapy.[17] *Staphylococcus epidermidis* and gram-negative organisms, including *P. aeruginosa,* are rarely the causative organisms unless the IV drug user has taken oral cephalexin concurrent with his or her injections, which is common in IV drug users.[19] In areas with a high prevalence of methicillin-resistant *S. aureus,* a similar resistance pattern may be seen in IV drug users with cellulitis.[21] Some investigators report a high incidence of anaerobic bacteria in cellulitis of IV drug users and hypothesize that these result from the transfer of oral flora.[22]

Empiric Antibiotic Therapy

Antibiotic therapy directed at eradicating all possible infecting organisms is not required. Because streptococci and staphylococci account for >94% of all infecting organisms in IV drug users with soft tissue infections,[19] therapy need cover only the sensitivity patterns of these organisms in the treatment area. Cloxacillin, dicloxacillin, or nafcillin is appropriate therapy (see Question 1). Oral therapy is appropriate for mild cases of cellulitis. Infections that involve a large area or that are associated with lymphangitis should be treated with parenteral antibiotics. Likewise, infections involving the hand should be treated parenterally.[22] Since M.C. may be at risk for CA-MRSA, if this organism is common in her local community, initial therapy of cotrimoxazole (1 double strength tablet bid) or doxycycline (if confirmed not pregnant) would be appropriate. If treatment does not result in some resolution of inflammation within 48 hours, antimicrobial coverage should be expanded to cover gram-negative organisms. The anaerobic organisms found in IV drug users with cellulitis usually respond to treatment with penicillins or cephalosporins.[21]

For patients not responding to initial therapy and for patients with signs or symptoms of a systemic response (e.g., rigors, hypotension), parenteral therapy that covers CA-MRSA is required, such as vancomycin, linezolid, daptomycin or tigecycline.[17] Antibiotic therapy that provides coverage against the other common organisms causing cellulitis (i.e., *E. coli,* and *K. pneumoniae*) in the IVDU population should be added, based on the sensitivity patterns in your local area. This may include the use of a parenteral cephalosporin, quinolone, or aminoglycoside. Although some clinicians suggest that a third-generation cephalosporin or a quinolone be chosen over an aminoglycoside because of concerns about toxicity, an aminoglycoside is effective, safe, and inexpensive when used for a short period (5–7 days).[23] However, in patients with poor renal function (estimated creatinine clearance <60mL/minute) the aminoglycoside should be avoided.

Treatment of cellulitis in an IV drug user should include rest, immobilization and elevation of the infected arm, antibiotics, and surgical drainage or débridement as required. If any sign of pus collection in the wound is noted, the wound must be surgically explored and drained. If no area of pus collection can be seen or palpated, immobilization and elevation, combined with systemic antibiotic therapy, is appropriate treatment. The wound should be assessed daily for local tenderness, pain, erythema, swelling, ulceration, necrosis, and wound drainage until it shows signs of resolution to ensure that subsequent surgical treatment is not required.[22]

SOFT TISSUE INFECTIONS IN DIABETIC PATIENTS

Skin and soft tissue infections are common in patients with diabetes mellitus. Approximately 25% of diabetic patients report a history of skin and soft tissue infections,[24] and 5% to 15% of diabetic patients may undergo limb amputation.[25] In addition to the cost associated with treating skin and soft tissue infections, functional disability can occur, which can significantly decrease the patient's quality of life.

Predisposing Factors

Diabetic patients are at particular risk for foot problems, primarily because of the neuropathies and peripheral vascular diseases associated with longstanding diabetes. The decreased pain sensation allows the patient to continue to bear weight in the presence of skin damage, thereby promoting the formation of an ulcer. In addition, minor trauma (e.g., cuts, foreign body insertion) can go unnoticed and, when left untreated, can become infected and extensive. Although these infections are common, preventive measures can reduce the frequency of amputations.[25]

Causative Organisms

13. P.U., a 67-year-old man with diabetes, presents to his general practitioner for a routine checkup and has no specific complaints. P.U. has a 15-year history of poorly controlled type 2 diabetes and a 3-year history of recurrent foot ulcers. On examination, the physician sees that one ulcer on the underside of the foot, which had

previously healed over, is open and inflamed; purulent fluid can be expressed from the wound. P.U. reports no pain around the area and was unaware that the ulcer had worsened. His temperature is normal, and he shows no other signs of a systemic infection. Does P.U. have an active infection, and is antibiotic therapy required?

All open wounds, in diabetic and nondiabetic patients, will become colonized with bacteria, but only infected wounds should be treated with antibiotic therapy.[26] Often it is difficult to determine whether an open wound is infected, but signs and symptoms (e.g., purulent drainage, erythema, pain, and swelling around the area) are suggestive of infection. Based on his symptoms, P.U. should be considered to have an infection that requires treatment.

Empiric Antibiotic Therapy

14. What treatment should P.U. receive?

Mild infections can be treated empirically as are other soft tissue infections[26] because these are commonly caused by aerobic gram-positive cocci. A penicillinase-resistant penicillin (e.g., cloxacillin, nafcillin) or cephalexin will be effective in most cases. A culture of either the drainage or the infected site should be obtained, however, to help guide future treatment. The choice between these agents should be based on allergy status and cost. If anaerobes are suspected, metronidazole or clindamycin should be added to the regimen. In addition, for all diabetic patients with soft tissue infections, osteomyelitis must be ruled out. In patients with significant vascular compromise, crepitus, or gangrene, a radiograph should be taken to identify any bone involvement.

In moderate to severe infections, antibiotic coverage should be expanded because multiple organisms may be responsible for the infection. An average of two to six organisms are cultured from foot ulcers in patients with diabetes. The following organisms (in no particular order) are found in >20% of wounds in patients with diabetes: *S. aureus, S. epidermidis, Enterococcus faecalis,* other streptococci, *Proteus* species, *E. coli, Klebsiella* species, *Peptococcus* species, *Peptostreptococcus* species, and *Bacteroides* species.[26] These infections are often polymicrobic, but treatment can be effective even if not all cultured pathogens are covered.[26] To determine the pathogens most accurately, a specimen of infected tissue should be obtained that is not directly communicating with an ulcer. If this is not possible, cultures of purulent exudate or curettage should be obtained, versus superficial swab, to determine the true pathogens in the wound.[27] Although antibiotics are important, drainage and surgical débridement to remove all the infected or necrotic tissue are essential and are considered by some to be the mainstay of treatment.[26]

Cultures of the affected areas may not be that useful unless bone involvement is suggested. Although anaerobic organisms often are difficult to culture, anaerobic organisms must be considered if an abscess or devitalized, necrotic, foul-smelling tissue is present or the wound is a result of abdominal surgery. Empiric coverage for *E. faecalis* is required only for severe (necrotizing) infections Even if enterococci are found in the wound, enterococcal coverage probably is needed only if it is the predominant organism.

No "best" regimens exist to treat diabetic soft tissue infections.[28] Clindamycin 600 mg IV Q 8 hr with ciprofloxacin 400 mg or a third-generation cephalosporin is a very effective combination that will provide coverage against most potential pathogens (gram-positive, gram-negative, and anaerobes), with the exception of *E. faecalis.* Clindamycin, however, can cause *Clostridium difficile*-associated diarrhea, and the parenteral formulation is expensive. Aminoglycosides are associated with serious toxicity if used for an extended period and should probably be avoided in diabetic patients with preexisting renal impairment. A β-lactam–β-lactamase inhibitor combination, such as piperacillin and tazobactam (Tazocin), ticarcillin and clavulanic acid, or ampicillin and sulbactam, provides similar coverage but also adds coverage against enterococci and could be chosen over other combinations if it is less expensive.

Other single-agent therapies could include the use of a carbapenem (imipenem or meropenem), but the increased cost and broad spectrum of activity of these agents should limit use to patients unresponsive to other therapies.

In many cases, diabetic foot infections are difficult to treat, but aggressive treatment can prevent extension of the infection, development of osteomyelitis, and on occasion loss of limb. Treatment should be continued for 3 to 4 days after all signs of infection are absent. Oral therapy should be considered once the infection has begun to abate. Because P.U. is an elderly diabetic patient and does not appear to be severely ill, the least expensive of ciprofloxacin–clindamycin or piperacillin–tazobactam, cefoxitin, or ceftizoxime, should be chosen as empiric therapy. In addition, ampicillin and sulbactam (Unasyn) or ticarcillin and clavulanate (Timentin) could be chosen if either is less expensive than the aforementioned agents or if local sensitivity patterns suggest that organisms typically found in these types of infections are routinely resistant to the other less expensive agents. The broad spectrum of carbapenems (e.g., imipenem, meropenem) may appear desirable, but frequent use contributes to isolation in individual patients and patient populations of more resistant pathogens, such as *Stenotrophomonas* organisms. Their use should be limited when possible. In areas where CA-MRSA is an issue, treatment should include antibiotics with activity against this organism. (see Questions 1–3)

Postamputation Antibiotic Treatment

15. Despite aggressive antibiotic therapy and débridement, P.U.'s infection spreads and an amputation is required. How long should antibiotics be prescribed for P.U. following surgery?

The best option for uncontrollable, life-threatening infections often is amputation to remove the infected area. Once the infected area has been removed, antibiotic therapy is no longer required. If it were impossible to remove all of the infected tissue, treatment should be continued as just described.

Prevention

16. What could have been done to prevent this complication in P.U.?

Many of the foot problems associated with diabetes can be prevented with proper foot care (Table 67-2),[25] and these preventive measures must be stressed. Diabetic patients with

Table 67-2 Foot Care for the Diabetic Patient

Inspect feet daily for cuts, blisters, or scratches. Pay particular attention to the area between the toes and use a mirror to examine the bottom of the foot.
Wash feet daily in tepid water and dry thoroughly.
Apply lotion to feet to prevent calluses and cracking.
Ensure that shoes fit properly (not too tight or too loose), and inspect them daily.
Trim nails regularly, making sure to cut straight across the nail.
Do not use chemical agents to remove corns or calluses.

neuropathies or those who are elderly should take care of their feet regularly (every 1–2 days).

NECROTIZING SOFT TISSUE INFECTIONS

Definitions, Terminology, and Causative Organisms

Skin and soft tissue infections are described as *necrotizing* when the inflammation is rapidly progressing and necrosis of the skin or underlying tissue is present. The following clinical signs are associated with necrotizing infections, but not with simple cellulitis: edema beyond the area of erythema, skin blisters or bullae, localized pallor or discoloration, gas in the subcutaneous tissues (crepitus), and the absence of lymphangitis and lymphadenitis. Pain out of proportion to the apparent extent of the infection or the hard wood feel of the infected area may be the only clues of necrotizing infection.[4] Necrotizing soft tissue infections can progress rapidly to cause additional local effects (i.e., necrosis and loss of skin sensation) and severe systemic effects (e.g., hypotension, shock).[29]

Group A β-hemolytic streptococci, *Pseudomonas* species, other gram-negative organisms, *Clostridium perfringens*, peptostreptococci, *B. fragilis*, and *Vibrio* species can cause necrotizing infections.[29]

Necrotizing cellulitis involves the skin and subcutaneous tissues. Necrotizing fasciitis involves both superficial and deep fascia, and necrotizing infections involving the muscle are termed *myonecrosis*. These terms can be used to describe all three of these processes. Gas gangrene is myonecrosis caused by a *Clostridium* subspecies, most commonly *C. perfringens* (70%).[29] Gas in a wound is not necessarily indicative of gas gangrene caused by *C. perfringens*. Gram-negative organisms (e.g., *E. coli, Proteus Species, Klebsiella Species*), or anaerobic streptococci can produce gas in a wound. Air also could have been introduced at the time of the injury. Gas gangrene is characterized by acute onset of worsening pain that is usually out of proportion to the degree of injury.

Clostridial myonecrosis (true gas gangrene), streptococcal gangrene (caused by group A β-hemolytic streptococci), and synergistic bacterial gangrene (caused by anaerobic and aerobic bacteria, usually gram-negative) are other terms used to describe necrotizing skin and soft tissue infections. Fournier's gangrene (a type of synergistic bacterial gangrene of the scrotum), nonclostridial crepitant gangrene (nonclostridial gas gangrene), and necrotizing fasciitis (all necrotizing soft tissue infections other than clostridial myonecrosis, or sometimes just streptococcal gangrene) are other commonly used terms.[29]

Empiric Antibiotic Therapy

17. M.T., a 45-year-old alcoholic man who lives on the streets of the city, presents to the ED with a broken nose and facial lacerations, which he received after a fight outside one of the local taverns. On examination, in addition to the facial wounds, an area of severe inflammation, erythema, and necrosis is found on his left calf. The area is very painful, crepitation is felt over the area, and a purulent discharge is present. M.T. states this is secondary to a knife wound he suffered approximately 1 week ago. What treatment should be provided?

In addition to setting the broken nose and suturing the facial lacerations, the clinician should evaluate the infection on M.T.'s calf. A Gram stain and culture of the purulent discharge should be evaluated before initiating antimicrobial therapy. Because crepitus is present, the area should be incised and a specimen of the infected tissue should be obtained for Gram staining and culture.[1]

The primary treatment for necrotizing soft tissue infections involves extensive débridement of the area to remove all necrotic tissue and drain the area. Thus, a surgical consultation will be required for M.T. In addition, IV antibiotics are required. In this case, gas in the tissues could be caused by many organisms, and empiric antibiotic therapy should be broad spectrum and should include coverage against gram-positive organisms, the Enterobacteriaceae, and *B. fragilis*. Initial therapy should have a broad spectrum until microbiological verification of the pathogen is obtained. Initial therapy with piperacillin/tazobactam plus clindamycin or ampicillin/sulbactam plus clindamycin would be appropriate.[4] If the Enterobacteriaceae in the local community have a high incidence of resistance to these agents, adding ciprofloxacin is recommended.[4] Alternatively, therapy with a carbapenem could be used, with the addition of clindamycin if group A β-hemolytic streptococci is suspected. If the Gram stain of the discharge shows only gram-positive rods (which would likely be clostridial subspecies), the therapy could be streamlined to high-dose penicillin.

Flesh-eating disease is usually a necrotizing fasciitis caused by virulent strains of group A streptococci. High-dose penicillin G (3 million units Q 4 hr) plus clindamycin (900 mg IV Q 8 hr) are the drugs of choice for this condition.[4,30,31] Although only experimental model data exist, the addition of clindamycin to penicillin is more effective in fulminant streptococcal infections than beta-lactam alone, potentially because it inhibits protein synthesis which may reduce toxin expression by the bacteria, and cytokine response by the host.[4] Clindamycin may have adjunctive activities that contribute to reduced morbidity from gram-positive pathogens. In vitro evidence suggests that clindamycin suppresses toxin production by *S. aureus* isolates.[31]

Adjunctive therapy for streptococcal necrotizing skin infections could include IV immunoglobulin G (IVIG) 2 g/kg as a single dose or 0.4 mg/kg daily for 2 days.[32] IVIG is thought to work by binding to the superantigens released by the streptococcal bacteria that are involved in the systemic effects of the infection. The optimal dosage and duration of IVIG therapy are unknown, as is the response to the variability between commercial lots of IVIG products.[4]

Therapy for necrotizing fasciitis should be altered based on the patient's clinical response and culture results.

ERYSIPELAS

Signs, Symptoms, and Causative Organisms

18. D.D., a 70-year-old man, presents to the ED with a red, swollen face. He describes the area as "a swollen red spot" that has appeared over the past 2 days. He also describes feeling unwell for the previous 3 days and having a fever. On examination, D.D. has a bright red, shiny, edematous lesion on his right cheek that is 0.4 cm wide. It is a continuous lesion with a clearly demarcated border. What signs and symptoms support the diagnosis of erysipelas in D.D.?

Erysipelas is a superficial skin infection caused by streptococci, predominantly group A, although groups C or G (and group B in children) also may cause the infection.[33] Erysipelas is diagnosed based on characteristics of the skin lesion and concurrent systemic symptoms.[33] Patients with erysipelas have associated systemic symptoms of high fever, chills, frequent history of rigors, and general malaise. This constellation of systemic symptoms differentiates erysipelas from other local skin disorders. The lesion is a continuous, indurated, edematous area. Early in the course, the lesion is bright red, but it may turn to brown as the lesion ages or grows. The lesion spreads peripherally with no islands of unaffected tissue. The initial lesion results from a small break in the skin that becomes infected, although signs of the initial wound often are not evident.

D.D. has the classic signs and symptoms of erysipelas: a well-demarcated, edematous, red lesion with associated systemic signs. No further diagnostic tests are required because aspiration of the lesion or a superficial swab is not useful in detecting the offending organism.[33]

Empiric Antibiotic Therapy

19. What antibiotic therapy should be initiated for D.D.?

Erysipelas will respond promptly to antibiotics with activity against group A streptococci.[34] Oral penicillin V 250 to 300 mg (depending on available dosage form) Q 6 hr or parenteral penicillin G (1 million units IV Q 6 hr) should reduce the systemic symptoms (e.g., fever, malaise) within 24 to 48 hours.[34] It will take several more days for the skin lesion to resolve. If D.D. does not feel better within 72 hours after initiation of antibiotics, he should be instructed to return for reassessment. If D.D. has an allergy to penicillins, clindamycin or oral quinolone, such as moxifloxacin are alternatives. If your community has increased macrolide resistance to group A streptococci these agents should not be part of empiric therapy.[35] Antibiotic therapy should be continued for 10 days even if signs and symptoms resolve quickly to avoid a relapse, which could lead to chronic infection or scarring.

ACUTE TRAUMATIC WOUNDS

20. J.K., a 25-year-old construction worker, presents to the ED with a deep cut on his left forearm suffered when he accidentally put his hand through a plate glass window. Fourteen stitches are required to close the wound. Is oral antibiotic therapy required for J.K.?

Although almost all traumatic wounds are contaminated with bacteria,[36] routine oral antibiotic therapy is not indicated unless there is evidence of an infection. Contaminated wounds do become infected more often than noncontaminated wounds, but prophylactic antibiotic therapy does not appear to decrease the chance of infection.[36] For all traumatic wounds, aggressive wound care (e.g., irrigation, removal of foreign objects) is required. A meta-analysis of randomized trials of prophylactic antibiotics in patients presenting to an ED for nonbite wounds found no evidence that oral antibiotics would protect against infection.[37] A course of antibiotic therapy should be given only to immunocompromised patients (e.g., those with diabetes mellitus, peripheral vascular disease, human immunodeficiency virus [HIV] or acquired immunodeficiency syndrome [AIDS], chronic corticosteroid use, leukopenia). Other potential candidates for antibiotic therapy include wounds with pus, contamination by feces, and delays in cleansing (>3 hours) of the wound.[38] Antibiotic therapy would be similar to that given for cellulitis (see Question 1). Patients with risk factors for the development of infective endocarditis (i.e., mitral valve prolapse with regurgitation, an indwelling non-native cardiac valve, a previous history of endocarditis, a history of congenital heart malformations, surgically constructed systemic-pulmonary shunts, and cardiomyopathy) should receive prophylactic amoxicillin (Amoxil) 3 g orally followed by 1.5 g in 6 hours or erythromycin 1,000 mg orally followed by 500 mg orally in 6 hours if the patient is penicillin allergic.[39] Because J.K. has no risk factors, all that is required is removal of any glass fragments, irrigation, and suturing of the area.

21. K.M., a 7-year-old boy, presents 30 minutes after falling and scraping his elbow on the pavement. The father requests an antibiotic ointment for the wound. You look at his elbow and notice a mildly abraded, 1-inch square area. What treatment would you recommend?

All minor injuries, such as scratches, cuts, and abrasions, should be thoroughly cleaned with soap and water. The evidence on the use of a topical antibiotic as a preventive measure is contradictory.[34] Placebo was compared with povidone ointment and a topical antibiotic combination (cetrimide–bacitracin–polymyxin) in children with minor dermatologic injuries.[34] The incidence of clinical infection was significantly different in placebo (12.5%) versus the topical antibiotic group (1.6%). No difference was seen in the incidence of clinical infection between povidone and the topical antibiotic group. In addition, no significant difference was noted between any of the preparations in the incidence of microbiologic infections. A randomized, double-blind, prospective trial comparing white petrolatum with bacitracin ointment in wound care following dermatologic surgery showed no difference between the groups in the incidence of wound infection.[40] Some patients can develop skin sensitivities to topical antibiotics. K.M.'s wound should be thoroughly washed and inspected, but a topical antibiotic ointment would not be required.

ANIMAL BITE WOUNDS

Evaluation of Dog and Cat Bites

22. P.J., a 14-year-old boy, presents to the ED 3 hours after being bitten on the leg by a neighbor's dog. He has a laceration, 14 cm long, on his medial calf. Four distinct puncture marks, suggestive of teeth marks, also are present on the calf. There is no suggestion of bone injury. P.J. was healthy before the attack and has no chronic illness. Should P.J. receive any treatment other than suturing of his laceration?

Any wound caused by an animal that results in the skin being cut or punctured should be examined to ensure no underlying tissue damage has occurred. This is especially true in patients with bites of the hand or around other joints. The wound should be washed with clean water as soon as possible after the bite.[42] Irrigation of the wound, including puncture sites, should be extensive to reduce the risk of infection. Obtaining specimens for cultures is not required and wound irrigation should begin as soon as possible.[41]

P.J.'s wound should be evaluated for deep tissue injury, devascularization of any tissue, and bone injury.[42] Loose suturing or closure with adhesive strips is appropriate for lacerations following irrigation.[41] Although the safety of closure of bite wounds has been debated, a good therapeutic response has been obtained following the closure of wounds.[42] P.J. should be instructed to keep his leg elevated and immobilized until signs of any infection have resolved.[43]

The need for antibiotics is controversial and guided by wound characteristics. The patient should receive a course of antibiotics[44] if the wound involves the hand or is near joints[41]; if it involves deep punctures or is difficult to irrigate; if the patient is immunocompromised (e.g., diabetes, splenectomy); or if the wound is not well perfused. Antibiotics are not required for dog bites in which no deep tissue injury is present and the wound can be well irrigated, particularly if the wound is on the lower extremities in healthy adults or children.[45]

Prophylaxis for rabies is required only if the animal is from an area with endemic rabies or if the bite was the result of an unprovoked attack by a wild animal.[46] Contact the local health board to determine the recent rabies risk in the area. If P.J. has not received a tetanus toxoid booster within the past 5 years, a booster should be administered. If P.J. has never been immunized for tetanus, tetanus immune globulin should be administered in addition to the tetanus toxoid (see Question 26).[46]

Causative Organisms and Empiric Antibiotic Therapy

23. Because P.J. has several punctures that are difficult to irrigate, he is a candidate for antibiotic therapy. Which antibiotic(s) should he receive?

The selection of the appropriate antibiotic is based on the most likely pathogens from the specific animal bite. Animals have different oral flora, which alters the potential pathogens associated with bites. The most common pathogens in dog bites are β-hemolytic streptococci, *S. aureus, Pasteurella multocida,* anaerobic bacteria (particularly *Bacteroides* species), and *Fusobacterium* species.[46] Although *P. multocida* often is considered the primary pathogen of dog bites, antibiotic coverage also must address the other common pathogens.[46] Monotherapy with amoxicillin/clavulante 500/875 orally Q12 hr is recommended.[4] If the patient is allergic to penicillin, tetracycline or doxycycline provides adequate coverage. Doxycycline is preferred over tetracycline because it is more convenient to administer (twice daily for doxycycline vs. four times a day for tetracycline); it can be used in patients with decreased renal function, may be taken with food, and is only a little more expensive (in the generic form) than tetracycline.

If the penicillin-allergic patient cannot take doxycycline, a fluoroquinolone, such as moxifloxacin 400mg PO daily, could be used. In all cases, patients should be instructed to watch for a positive response; if the wound does not heal or it worsens within 48 hours, the patient needs to be re-evaluated.

Antibiotic treatment should not extend beyond 5 days unless signs of an infection remain.[41] Appropriate therapy for P.J. would be penicillin V and a penicillinase-resistant penicillin (e.g., dicloxacillin or cloxacillin) orally.

For cat bites, the role of *P. multocida* appears more significant because this organism can be found in the oral flora of up to 75% of cats. Although antibiotic treatment is not required for some dog bites, reports of a >50% incidence of infection after cat bites[43] suggest that all patients with cat bites should receive antibiotics. Because *P. multocida* often is resistant to penicillinase-resistant penicillins and first-generation cephalosporins, use of these agents in cat bites should be avoided. Therapies discussed above for dog bites would be appropriate for treating cat bites.

If the patient presents with an established infection, parenteral therapy is warranted if the infection is over a joint, has lymphatic spread, or involves the hand or head. If the patient has not responded to oral therapy, parenteral second-generation cephalosporins, such as cefoxitin 1 g IV Q 6 hr or ceftizoxime 1 g IV Q 8 hr, have activity against *P. multocida,* streptococci, staphylococci, and anaerobes.[43] The value of parenteral administration of clindamycin or erythromycin is limited by poor activity against *P. multocida*.[2,43] The poor activity of quinolones against anaerobes has limited their use, despite good activity against *P. multocida.*[47] Parenteral therapy should be continued until resolution of the wound is evident, and therapy should then be continued with oral antibiotics. Alternate, but more expensive, therapies would include β-lactam/β-lactamase combinations or carbapenems. There is no evidence that these agents are superior to second or third generation cephalosporins. If anaerobic infection is considered, the addition of metronidazole to the cephalosporin therapy may be warranted.[5] Treatment should continue for at least 7 days or until all clinical signs of the infection have resolved.

HUMAN BITE WOUNDS

Evaluation of Human Bites

24. E.D., a 40-year-old man, presents with a sore arm 24 hours after receiving a bite to his left forearm by his neighbor in a "discussion over property boundaries." E.D. was previously healthy and has no chronic diseases. A 6 $\times$ 8-cm area of his left forearm is swollen and erythematous and includes several distinct puncture marks consistent with a human bite. No joint deformity or bone

abnormality is detected on clinical examination. How should E.D. be treated?

Treating a human bite is similar to any other laceration, including cleansing, irrigating, exploring, débriding, draining, excising, and suturing, as required.[46,48] All human bites should be cleansed as soon as possible, and any lacerations or punctures irrigated copiously. Surgical exploration with débridement, drainage, or excision should be undertaken if deeper tissues may have been injured or if pus collection could have occurred. Exploration for damage to subcutaneous nerves, tendons, joints, or vascularity is particularly important in bites to the hand, especially the knuckles, because subsequent infections could seriously affect hand function. Because E.D. presents 24 hours after the injury, thorough exploration and irrigation of all lacerations or punctures is required. With evidence of pus accumulation in his wound, the area should be explored and drained. E.D. also should receive systemic antibiotic therapy to eradicate potential infecting organisms. Tetanus toxoid booster should be administered if E.D. has not received a booster in the past 10 years.

Empiric Antibiotic Therapy and Causative Organisms

25. Which antibiotic should be prescribed for E.D.?

If E.D. had been seen within 12 hours of the injury, the wound could likely have been treated adequately with simple irrigation. This is especially true if the human bite does not involve the hand.[46] If the hand has been bitten or the patient is immunocompromised, a course of antibiotics using oral agents is appropriate.

If the wound is severe (i.e., involves subcutaneous tissues, a joint, or a large area) or if the patient is unlikely to be compliant with oral antibiotics, parenteral administration of antibiotics is required.[49] The most common pathogens in human bites are β-hemolytic streptococci, *S. aureus, Eikenella corrodens,* and *Corynebacterium* subspecies.[46] Anaerobic bacteria also are commonly involved.[46] Treatment with a combination of penicillin G and a penicillinase-resistant penicillin is appropriate.[46] Therapy with a penicillinase-resistant penicillin or a first-generation cephalosporin alone is not appropriate because *E. corrodens* commonly is resistant to these antibiotics.[43,47] If the anaerobic flora of the patient's community is often resistant to penicillin, alternative anaerobic coverage with amoxicillin–clavulanate may be required.[46] If parenteral therapy is required, a second-generation cephalosporin with antianaerobic activity (e.g., cefoxitin, ceftizoxime) is appropriate.[46] Cefuroxime should not be used as single-agent therapy because it lacks activity against anaerobes and *E. corrodens.*[43] Third-generation cephalosporins and quinolones have good activity against *E. corrodens,* but they cannot be recommended because of their inferior activity against anaerobic organisms.[43] Fluoroquinolones, such as levofloxacin or moxifloxacin, have good activity against the organisms of bite infections, with the exception of poor activity against *Fusobacterium* species.[50] Azithromycin is the macrolide with the best activity against bite organisms.[51] Alternate, but more expensive, parenteral therapy would include β-lactam/β-lactamse inhibitor combinations or carbapenems. Oral regimens for penicillin-allergic patients would include combinations of cotrimoxazole plus metronidazole, or a fluoroquinolone plus clindamycin.[4]

TETANUS PROPHYLAXIS

26. G.T., a 48-year-old woman, presents to the ED 1 hour after receiving a 2-cm laceration to her foot from stepping on a nail while walking around her neighborhood. Examination of the wound found it to be clean, with no subcutaneous extension. The wound was closed with superficial sutures, and no antibiotics, systemic or topical, were prescribed. Should G.T. receive tetanus prophylaxis?

Tetanus is a preventable disease through primary prophylaxis and appropriate wound management. Every child should receive primary prophylaxis of three separate doses of tetanus toxoid. This provides adequate coverage for at least 10 years.[52] Tetanus can develop in patients who have not been immunized or who have not received a booster dose within the past 10 years. If G.T. has received her primary tetanus immunization and had a booster dose within the previous 10 years, no additional tetanus prophylaxis is required for her wound (Table 67-3). If her primary immunization status is unknown or >10 years has elapsed since her last dose, a single 0.5-mL subcutaneous tetanus toxoid dose should be administered. If primary immunization is unknown or incomplete, G.T. should receive the initial 0.5-mL dose immediately and should be scheduled to complete the primary immunization over the next 2 months. For adults, the combination product of tetanus and diphtheria toxoid is the recommended treatment because this will enhance protection against diphtheria.

If G.T. had presented with a dirty wound (contaminated with dirt, feces, soil, or saliva) or if the wound had resulted from a burn, frostbite, missile (bullet), crush, or avulsion, she should receive passive tetanus immunization with tetanus immune globulin in addition to the tetanus toxoid described above. A single 250-U intramuscular dose of tetanus immune globulin will provide passive immunization in addition to the active immunization produced from exposure to the tetanus toxoid (Table 67-3).

Table 67-3 Tetanus Prophylaxis in Routine Wound Management: Adults

History of Adsorbed Tetanus Toxoid	Clean, Minor Wounds		All Other Wounds[a]	
	Td[b]	TIG	Td[b]	TIG
Unknown or <3 doses	Yes	No	Yes	Yes
≥3 doses	No[c]	No	Yes[d]	No

[a] Including, but not limited to, wounds contaminated with dirt, feces, soil, and saliva; puncture wounds, avulsions, and wounds resulting from missiles; crushing, burns, frostbite.

[b] For children <7 years of age, diphtheria-tetanus-pertussis (DTP) is preferred to tetanus toxoid alone. For persons ≥7 years of age, Td is preferred to tetanus toxoid alone.

[c] Yes, if >10 years since last dose.

[d] Yes, if >5 years since last dose. (More frequent boosters are not needed and can accentuate the side effects.)

Td, tetanus and diphtheria toxoid; TIG, tetanus immune globulin.

REFERENCES

1. Sachs MK. Cutaneous cellulitis. *Arch Dermatol* 1991;127:493.
2. Hook EW et al. Microbiologic evaluation of cutaneous cellulitis in adults. *Arch Intern Med* 1986;146:295.
3. Sachs MK. The optimum use of needle aspiration in the bacteriologic diagnosis of cellulitis in adults. *Arch Intern Med* 1990;150:1907.
4. Stevens DL et al. Practice guidelines for the diagnosis and management of skin and soft-tissue infections. *Clin Infect Dis* 2005;41:1373
5. Moellering RC. The growing menace of community-acquired methicillin-mesistant Staphylococcus aureus. *Ann Intern Med*. 2006;144:368
6. Sutherland R et al. Flucloxacillin, a new isoxazolyl penicillin, compared with oxacillin, cloxacillin, and dicloxacillin. *BMJ* 1970;4:455.
7. Critchley IA et al. Antimicrobial susceptibilities of Streptococcus pyogenes isolated from respiratory and skin and soft tissue infections. *Diagnostic Microbiol Infect Dis* 2002;42:129.
8. Powers RD. Soft tissue infections in the emergency department: the case for the use of simple antibiotics. *South Med J* 1991;84:1313.
9. Kowalski TJ et al. Epidemiology, treatment, and prevention of community-acquired methicillin-resistant Staphylococcus aureus infections. *Mayo Clin Proc* 2005;80:1201
10. Sabol KE et al. Community-associated methicillin-resistant Staphylococcus aureus: new bug, old drugs. *Ann Pharmacother*. 2006;40:1125.
11. Hepburn MJ et al. Comparison of short-course (5 days) and standard (10 days) treatment for uncomplicated cellulitis. *Arch Intern Med* 2004;164:1669
12. Perl B et al. Cost-effectiveness of blood cultures for adult patients with cellulitis. *Clin Infect Dis* 1999;29:1483
13. Ward A et al. Mupirocin: a review of its antibacterial activity, pharmacokinetic properties and therapeutic use. *Drugs* 1986;32:425.
14. Hirschmann JV. Topical antibiotics in dermatology. *Arch Dermatol* 1988;124:1691.
15. Stevens DL et al. Randomised comparison of linezolid (PNU-100766) versus oxacillin-dicloxacillin for treatment of complicated skin and soft tissue infections. *Antimicrob Agents Chemother* 2000;44:3408.
16. Weigelt J et al. Linezolid versus Vancomycin in treatment of complicated skin and soft tissue infections. *Antimicrob Agent Chemother,* 2005;49:2260
17. Barton M et al. Guidelines for the prevention and management of community-associated methicillin-resistant *Staphylococcus aurea*: A perspective for Canadian health care providers. *Can J Infect Dis Med Microbiol* 2006;17 (Suppl C):4C.
18. Beaufoy A. Infections in intravenous drug users: a two-year review. *Can J Infect Control* 1993;8:7.
19. Orangio GR et al. Soft tissue infections in parenteral drug abusers. *Ann Surg* 1984;199:97.
20. Sheagren JN. Treatment of skin and skin infections in the patient at risk. *Am J Med* 1984;76(5B):180.
21. Bergstein JM et al. Soft tissue abscesses associated with parenteral drug abuse: presentation, microbiology, and treatment. *Am Surg* 1995;61:1105.
22. Hausman MR et al. Hand infections. *Orthop Clin North Am* 1992;23:171.
23. McCormack JP et al. A critical reevaluation of the therapeutic range of the aminoglycosides. *Clin Infect Dis* 1992;14:320.
24. LeFrock JL et al. Lower extremity infections in diabetics. *Infect Surg* 1986;5:135.
25. Most RS et al. The epidemiology of lower extremity infections in diabetic individuals. *Diabetes Care* 1983;6:87.
26. Cunha BA. Antibiotic selection for diabetic foot infections: a review. *J Ankle Foot Surg* 2000;39:253.
27. Committee of Antimicrobial Agents. Management of diabetic foot infections: a position paper. *Can J Infect Dis* 1996;7:361.
28. Lipsky BA. Medical treatment of diabetic foot infections. *Clinical Infectious Diseases* 2004;39:S104.
29. Kihiczak GG et al. Necrotizing fasciitis: a deadly infection. *J Eur Acad Dermatol Venereol* 2006;20:365.
30. Bisno AL et al. Streptococcal infections of skin and soft tissues. *N Engl J Med* 1996;334:240.
31. Seal DV. Necrotizing fasciitis. *Curr Opin Infect Dis* 2001;14:127.
32. Perez CM et al. Adjunctive treatment of streptococcal toxic shock syndrome using intravenous immunoglobulin: case report and review. *Am J Med* 1997;102:111.
33. Bonnetblanc JM et al. Erysipelas: recognition and management. *Am J Clin Dermatol* 2003;4:157.
34. Langford JH et al. Topical antimicrobial therapy in minor wounds. *Ann Pharmacother* 1997;31:559.
35. Tan K et al. Invasive group A Streptococci reistance to erythromycin and clindamycin at Providence Health Care, Vancouver, 2004–6. *Can J Infect Dis Med Microbiol* 2007;18:77 (Abstract).
36. Rodgers KG. The rational use of antimicrobial agents in simple wounds. *Emerg Med Clin North Am* 1992;10:753.
37. Cummings P et al. Antibiotics to prevent infection of simple wounds: a meta-analysis of randomized studies. *Am J Emerg Med* 1995;13:396.
38. Eron LJ. Targeting lurking pathogens in acute traumatic and chronic wounds. *J Emerg Med* 1999;17:189.
39. Dajani AS et al. Prevention of bacterial endocarditis: recommendations by the American Heart Association. *JAMA* 1990;264:2919.
40. Smack DP et al. Infection and allergy incidence in ambulatory surgery patients using white petrolatum vs bacitracin ointment. *JAMA* 1996;276:972.
41. Anderson CR. Animal bites. Guidelines to current management. *Postgrad Med J* 1992;92:134.
42. Medeiros I et al. Antibiotic prophylaxis for mammalian bites. *Cochrane Database Syst Rev* 2002;4.
43. Goldstein EJ. Bite wounds and infection. *Clin Infect Dis* 1992;14:633.
44. Dire DJ. Emergency management of dog and cat bite wounds. *Emerg Med Clin North Am* 1992;10:719.
45. Higgins MAG et al. Managing animal bite wounds. *J Wound Care* 1997;6:377.
46. Griego RD et al. Dog, cat, and human bites: a review. *J Am Acad Dermatol* 1995;33:1019.
47. Goldstein EJ et al. Comparative susceptibilities of 173 aerobic and anaerobic bite wound isolates to sparfloxacin, temafloxacin, clarithromycin, and older agents. *Antimicrob Agents Chemother* 1993;37:1150.
48. Bunzli WF et al. Current management of human bites. *Pharmacotherapy* 1998;18:227.
49. Smith PF et al. Treating mammalian bite wounds. *J Clin Pharm Ther* 2000;25:85.
50. Goldstein EJC et al. Comparative in vitro activities of azithromycin, Bay y3118, levofloxacin, sparfloxacin, and 11 other oral antimicrobial agents against 194 aerobic and anaerobic bite wound isolates. *Antimicrob Agent Chemother* 1995;39:1097.
51. Goldstein EJC et al. Activities of HMR3004, and HMR3647 compared to those of erythromycin, azithromycin, clarithromycin, roxithromycin and eight other antimicrobial agents against unusual aerobic and anaerobic human and animal bite pathogens isolated from skin and soft tissue infections in humans. *Antimicrob Agent Chemother* 1998;42:1127.
52. Advisory Committee on Immunization Practices, CDC. Diphtheria, tetanus, and pertussis: guidelines for vaccine use and other preventative measures. *MMWR* 1991;40:(RR10).

CHAPTER 68

Prevention and Treatment of Infections in Neutropenic Cancer Patients

Richard H. Drew

Many patients with malignancy have had their lives prolonged through therapeutic advances in chemotherapy, immunotherapy, and bone marrow transplantation. Despite such advances, infectious complications continue to be a major cause of morbidity and mortality in these patients, often replacing the primary disease as the leading cause of death.[1] Although newer broad-spectrum antimicrobial agents and chemotherapeutic agents have altered the frequency and types of infectious complications in patients with both solid and hematologic malignancies, the management of infections in immunocompromised hosts remains a major challenge to health care professionals.

This chapter focuses on the prevention, diagnosis, and management of infectious complications in patients with neutropenia secondary to cancer chemotherapy. The following topics are addressed: principles of prophylactic antimicrobials, empiric antibiotic selection in the febrile patient, modification and duration of therapy, monotherapy versus combination regimens, empiric antifungal and antiviral use, and the use of hematopoietic growth factors.

RISK FACTORS FOR INFECTION

Patients are rendered "immunocompromised" when there is a significant disruption or deficiency of one or more of the host defenses as a result of the underlying disease or chemotherapy. These risk factors include neutropenia, iatrogenic damage to skin and mucosal barriers, and impairment in both humoral (antibody and complement) and cell-mediated immune defenses. Bacteria, fungi, viruses, and protozoa may infect various sites, depending on the specific immunodeficiency (Table 68-1).

Table 68-1 Most Common Pathogens Causing Infections in Neutropenic Cancer Patients

		Pathogen(s)			
Immunologic Defect	*Underlying Condition(s)*	*Bacteria*	*Fungi*	*Parasites*	*Viruses*
Neutropenia	Cancer chemotherapy, acute leukemia	*S. aureus*, coagulase-negative staphylococci, enterococci, *E. coli, K. pneumoniae, P. aeruginosa*	*Candida* spp., *Aspergillus* spp., *Fusarium*	—	—
T-helper lymphocyte (cell-mediated immunity)	Immunosuppressive therapy, Hodgkin disease, transplantation	*Listeria monocytogenes, Nocardia asteroides, Legionella, Salmonella,* mycobacteria	*Cryptococcus, Aspergillus, Candida, H. capsulatum, Mucoraceae*	*Pneumocystis jirovecii, Toxoplasma gondii*	*Herpes simplex,* varicella-zoster, cytomegalovirus
Gamma-globulin (humoral immunity)	Splenectomy, chronic lymphocytic leukemia, hypogammaglobulinemia, bone marrow transplantation	*S. pneumoniae, H. influenzae, N. meningitidis*	—	*Pneumocystis jirovecii, Babesia* spp.	—
Damage to physical barriers	Surgical procedures	*S. aureus;* coagulase-negative staphylococci, *S. pyogenes;* Enterobacteriaceae; *P. aeruginosa, Bacteroides* spp.	*Candida* spp.	—	—
	Indwelling catheters, venipuncture	*S. aureus*, coagulase-negative staphylococci, *Corynebacterium*	*Candida* spp.	—	—
	Chemotherapy, endoscopy, radiation	*S. aureus*, coagulase-negative staphylococci, streptococci, Enterobacteriaceae, *P. aeruginosa, Bacteroides*	*Candida* spp.	—	Herpes simplex
Microbial colonization	Chemotherapy, antibiotics, hospitalization	*S. aureus*, coagulase-negative staphylococci, Enterobacteriaceae, *P. aeruginosa, Legionella*	*Candida* spp., *Aspergillus*	—	—
Transplantation	Bone marrow	—	*Candida* spp.	*Toxoplasma gondii, P. carinii*	Cytomegalovirus, hepatitis B and C, Epstein-Barr virus

Adapted from Armstrong D. History of opportunistic infection in the immunocompromised host. *Clin Infect Dis* 1993;17(Suppl 2):S318.

Neutropenia

Granulocytes, or granular leukocytes, represent an important defense against bacterial and fungal infections. *Neutropenia* (a reduction in the number of circulating granulocytes or neutrophils) predisposes the host to infections. The terms *granulocytopenia* and *neutropenia* are often used interchangeably. The degree of neutropenia is expressed in terms of the absolute neutrophil count (ANC) or the total number of granulocytes (polymorphonuclear leukocytes and band forms) present in the circulating pool of white blood cells (WBCs).

The quantitative relationship between neutropenia and outcome of infections was established more than 40 years ago.[2] It was discovered that the risk of infection in the neutropenic patient is proportional to both the severity and duration of neutropenia. In general, the risk of infection is low when the ANC exceeds 1,000 cells/mm^3, with the frequency and severity of infection inversely proportional to the ANC.[2,3] As the ANC drops to <500 cells/mm^3, the risk of infection rapidly increases. The risk of developing infection is further increased as the ANC drops to <100 cells/mm^3.[2] Conversely, recovery of the ANC is the most important factor determining the outcome of infectious complications in the neutropenic patient. Febrile patients with short durations of neutropenia (<1 week) or in whom neutropenia is not severe (<100 cells/mm^3) generally respond to empiric antibiotics and less frequently develop serious, life-threatening infections.[2] In contrast, patients rendered neutropenic for >1 week (e.g., those receiving more intensive chemotherapy regimens) and/or are severely neutropenic are more vulnerable to serious infection.[2]

Damage to Physical Barriers

The intact skin and mucosal surfaces of the body constitute the host's primary physical defense against microbial invasion. The integrity of this physical barrier may be disrupted by tumor, treatment (e.g., surgery, radiation), or various medical procedures (e.g., insertion of intravenous [IV] or urinary catheters, venipuncture, measurement of rectal temperature).[4] Device-related infections, including those associated with central IV catheters, are commonly caused by migration of skin flora (e.g., staphylococci) through the cutaneous insertion site.[4] Infections secondary to damaged mucosal lining of the gastrointestinal (GI) tract are usually caused by enteric bacteria and fungi such as *Candida* spp.[4]

Alterations in the Immune System

Patients with immunoglobulin deficiencies (e.g., hypogammaglobulinemia, chronic lymphocytic leukemia, or splenectomy) are at increased risk for infections with encapsulated bacteria that must undergo antibody opsonization for efficient phagocytosis. Such bacteria include *Neisseria meningitidis, Haemophilus influenzae,* and *Streptococcus pneumoniae.*[1,4] Hodgkin disease, organ transplantation, and HIV disease can disrupt the cellular immune system, increasing the risk for infections with obligate and facultative intracellular organisms such as mycobacteria, *Listeria, Toxoplasma,* viruses, and fungi.[1,4]

Some chemotherapeutic regimens have profound effects on both cellular and humoral defenses. Corticosteroids exert their immunosuppressive effects on the cellular immune system, particularly at the T-lymphocyte and macrophage level. Therefore, patients receiving corticosteroids have increased susceptibility to infections with viral, bacterial, protozoal, and fungal infections.[5] Infectious complications secondary to glucocorticoid use appear to be dose dependent. The risk of infection increases with daily doses >10 mg or cumulative doses >700 mg of prednisone or its equivalent.[5] Thus, patients receiving corticosteroids in either high doses or for prolonged periods are at increased risk for a wide spectrum of infections caused by bacteria, fungi, and other opportunistic pathogens.[5]

Colonization

Microbial colonization can be a prerequisite to infection in neutropenic patients. *Colonization* may be defined as the recovery of an organism from any particular site (e.g., stool, nasopharynx) without clinical signs of infection. Most infections in neutropenic patients are caused by the host's endogenous microflora or hospital-acquired pathogens that have colonized the alimentary tract, upper respiratory tract, and/or skin.[3,6]

Hematopoietic Stem Cell Transplantation

Transplantation of bone marrow predisposes patients to the development of opportunistic infections secondary to both intensive immunosuppressive therapy and transmission.[7,8] These infections may be acquired from blood products or may represent reactivation of latent host infection.[7,8] The types of infections are detailed in other chapters (see Chapters 35 and 92). The introduction of new therapeutic approaches for treatment of the underlying malignancy (including nucleoside analogs and monoclonal antibodies to CD20 and CD52), along with use of unrelated stem cell donors, has increased the potential for infections in these patients, particularly among allogeneic hematopoietic stem cell transplant (HSCT) recipients.

Radiation Therapy

Side effects associated with the use of radiation therapy for the treatment of malignancy (e.g., mucositis, skin breakdown, or reduction in blood counts) may also predispose a patient with neutropenia to infection.

MOST COMMON PATHOGENS

1. B.C., a 41-year-old woman, was admitted to the cancer center for placement of a central IV catheter for administration of chemotherapy to treat acute nonlymphocytic leukemia in relapse. She was diagnosed 2 years ago and was treated with cytarabine plus daunorubicin, which resulted in a complete remission for 33 months. This admission, she will be treated with high-dose cytarabine plus mitoxantrone for reinduction. What are the most likely pathogens to cause infection in patients like B.C. during periods of chemotherapy-induced neutropenia?

Bacteria are the primary pathogens associated with infection in febrile neutropenic patients, especially those occurring early (Table 68-1).[9] Bacteremia is most often caused by aerobic Gram-negative bacilli (especially *Pseudomonas aeruginosa, Escherichia coli,* and *Klebsiella pneumoniae*) or aerobic Gram-positive cocci (i.e., coagulase-negative staphylococci, *Staphylococcus aureus,* enterococci, viridans streptococci).[10,11] Since the mid-1990s, the proportion of Gram-negative infections has decreased with a proportional increase in Gram-positive infections.[10–14] Gram-positive bacteria now account for approximately 60% to 70% of microbiologically-documented infections in neutropenic cancer patients.[12,13] This is believed to be due (in part) to the frequent use of indwelling intravascular catheters, use of more intensive chemotherapy regimens, and widespread use of broad-spectrum antibiotics for prophylactic and therapeutic use. These factors can contribute to the development of infection in patients such as B.C.

S. aureus (including methicillin-resistant *S. aureus* [MRSA]) and *Staphylococcus epidermidis,* streptococci (including *S. pneumoniae* and viridans streptococci), and *Corynebacterium* species have become important pathogens in some cancer centers.[10–13] Moreover, enterococcal infections (including vancomycin-resistant enterococci [VRE]) are increasing in frequency because of the routine use of broad-spectrum antibiotics.[12] Meningitis caused by the intracellular organism *Listeria monocytogenes* can be observed in patients with defective cellular immunity caused by disease or prolonged corticosteroid use. In general, anaerobic bacteria are an infrequent cause of infection in granulocytopenic patients with hematologic malignancies.[15] However, they may occur more frequently in patients with GI malignancies or with significant disruption of the GI tract secondary to chemotherapy.[15]

Invasive fungal infections are a major cause of morbidity and mortality among neutropenic cancer patients and patients undergoing bone marrow transplantation.[16] They tend to occur later in the illness. Patients with prolonged neutropenia (>7 days), allogeneic HSCT recipients, and those undergoing therapy for graft-versus-host disease (GVHD) are at increased risk of developing systemic fungal infections. In one report, approximately 50% of patients who die during prolonged periods of neutropenia had evidence of deep-seated mycoses at autopsy.[16] Prior to the use fluconazole prophylaxis in selected populations, *Candida* spp. were responsible for most invasive fungal infections. Today, invasive infections due to *Aspergillus* spp. and other moulds are a major cause of invasive fungal infection (IFI)–related death (particularly those with prolonged neutropenia and GVHD).[16]

Viral infections are generally a reactivation of latent infection. These may include herpes simplex virus and varicella-zoster virus.[3,10] Other viruses, such as cytomegalovirus (CMV), can be acquired during hematopoietic stem cell transplantation.[73] Respiratory viruses (e.g., respiratory syncytial virus [RSV], influenza, parainfluenza) and other seasonal viruses may occasionally cause infection in this population.

PROPHYLAXIS AGAINST INFECTION

Infection Control

Exogenous contamination can be prevented by strict protective isolation of patients in specially designed rooms that maintain a sterile environment. These laminar airflow rooms are ventilated with air that is passed through a high-efficiency particulate air (HEPA) filter, which removes >99% of all particles larger than 3 microns. Total protective isolation is accomplished by strict isolation in conjunction with the administration of sterile food and water, local skin care, and intensive microbial surveillance.[8] However, this regimen is burdensome to the patient and health care personnel, difficult to accomplish and maintain, and expensive. Thus, it continues to be used in only a few treatment centers. However, close adherence to adequate handwashing procedures is essential. In addition, contact isolation is advocated in circumstances in which the patient may be colonized or infected with resistant organisms. Finally, isolating the patients from caregivers with potentially contagious respiratory viral illnesses is advocated.

Antimicrobial Prophylaxis

2. What is the role of oral antimicrobial prophylaxis during the neutropenic period?

Studies have demonstrated that the early administration of oral antibiotics (both antibacterials and antifungals) during the afebrile, neutropenic period in select "high-risk" patients can result in a reduction in the number of febrile episodes and subsequent risk of infection.[17] The goals of such prophylactic antibiotic regimens have been aimed at reducing potentially pathogenic endogenous microflora or preventing the acquisition of new micro-organisms in the neutropenic patient.[17] Potential benefits must outweigh the risks of antibiotic-related adverse effects, the development of resistance, and the potential for superinfection. Therefore, prophylaxis is generally considered only in select "high-risk" patients with neutropenia expected to be severe (<100 cells/mm^3) or prolonged (<7 days).[10]

Nonabsorbable Antibacterials

The alimentary tract is recognized as an important reservoir of potential pathogens. Therefore, gut decontamination with and without total protective isolation has been investigated. The rationale behind the use of selective decontamination regimens is based on animal studies that demonstrated that selective elimination of aerobic GI flora, although maintaining anaerobic flora, prevented colonization with potentially pathogenic aerobic Gram-negative bacteria. Early studies focused on the use of nonabsorbable antimicrobials such as gentamicin, polymyxin B, and colistin to eradicate selected bowel flora while reducing the potential for systemic toxicity.

Oral, nonabsorbable antibacterial regimens have not shown consistent efficacy in preventing infection in the neutropenic cancer patient.[17] A major problem with these regimens has been poor patient compliance and tolerance, often because of their unpleasant taste. Of additional concern is the development of aminoglycoside resistance from the nonabsorbable aminoglycoside-containing regimens. Finally, colistin use has recently been identified as a risk factor for staphylococcal infections.[12] Therefore, use of nonabsorbable antibacterial agents have largely been supplanted by oral, absorbable antibiotics.[10,17]

Trimethoprim-Sulfamethoxazole

Several studies have demonstrated the benefit of trimethoprim-sulfamethoxazole (TMP-SMX) in reducing bacterial infections when compared to placebo in febrile neutropenic patients.[18–20] Its benefit in reducing mortality, however, is less clear. In contrast, its role in preventing *Pneumocystis jirovecii* (formerly known as *Pneumocystis carinii* or PCP) pneumonia has been established in many immunocompromised patient populations, independent of the presence of neutropenia.[8,10,19] The potential benefits of TMP-SMX prophylaxis must be carefully balanced against the potential for drug-induced bone marrow suppression, hypersensitivity reactions, the emergence of resistant organisms (e.g., *E. coli*), and the development of superinfections. Patients at high risk for developing *P. jirovecii* pneumonia (i.e., patients with acute lymphocytic leukemia receiving intensive chemotherapy, AIDS, allogeneic HSCT recipients) should be strongly considered for TMP-SMX prophylaxis.[3,10] Recipients of T-cell–depleting agents (e.g., fludarabine or cladribine), cancer patients receiving prolonged corticosteroids (>20 mg prednisone or its equivalent daily), and autologous HSCT recipients should also be considered for prophylaxis with TMP-SMX.[3] In the absence of these risk factors, routine use of TMP-SMX as primary prophylaxis for neutropenia is not currently recommended.[3,10] In patients requiring PCP prophylaxis but unable to tolerate TMP-SMX, patients should be considered for either TMP-SMX desensitization, atovaquone, dapsone, or aerosolized pentamidine as alternate strategies.[3]

Fluoroquinolones

Fluoroquinolones (e.g., ciprofloxacin, norfloxacin, ofloxacin, levofloxacin) are used by some centers as prophylaxis for patients at high risk of infection. Data regarding their use for preventing infection in neutropenic cancer patients have been summarized elsewhere.[21–24] Of concern, however, is the increasing frequency of Gram-positive infections (including viridans streptococci) observed in patients receiving fluoroquinolone prophylaxis,[25,26] combined with the emergence of resistant Gram-negative bacilli (especially *E. coli*)[27] caused by the widespread use of these agents. Recent meta-analyses report reductions in mortality in high-risk patients receiving prophylaxis with fluoroquinolones.[24] Because the benefits of fluoroquinolone prophylaxis may be offset by the emergence of resistant organisms, routine prophylactic use in neutropenic patients should be avoided.[3] However, those at highest risk of bacterial infections (i.e., those patients with an ANC <100 neutrophils/mm^3 for >10 days) should be considered for fluoroquinolone prophylaxis until either the onset of fever or resolution of severe neutropenia (>100 neutrophils/mm^3).[3]

Antifungals

3. What is the role of antifungal prophylaxis in neutropenic patients?

Routine antifungal prophylaxis is not indicated in all patients with neutropenia. However, select patients (i.e., those with acute leukemic patients with prolonged neutropenia [>7 days], allogeneic HSCT recipients, and patients receiving systemic corticosteroids for treatment of GVHD) are at increased risk of developing systemic fungal infections.[16] Because of the frequency with which such infections are encountered, difficulties in establishing a diagnosis, and poor response rates in patients with serious invasive infection who are immunocompromised, effective prophylactic strategies are necessary in these high-risk patients.

NONABSORBABLE ANTIFUNGALS

Various nonabsorbable antifungal agents have been studied for use in fungal prophylaxis in neutropenic patients. Topical agents, such as oral nystatin,[28,29] clotrimazole,[30] and oral amphotericin B,[31] have been studied. Of these agents, only oral amphotericin B and clotrimazole have been successful in reducing the frequency of oropharyngeal candidiasis. None of the antifungals have a role as primary prophylaxis of invasive fungal infections.[3,10]

SYSTEMIC ANTIFUNGALS

The use of systemic antifungals for prophylaxis has been extensively studied. Early trials with the imidazoles miconazole and ketoconazole met with limited success. The toxicities associated with these agents and the availability of newer, less toxic antifungals currently limit their clinical utility in this setting.

In addition to its in vitro activity against many *Candida* spp. (e.g., *C. albicans*), itraconazole is active in vitro against *Aspergillus* species. Randomized, placebo-controlled trials[32,33] as well as comparisons with amphotericin B[34] have demonstrated its efficacy in reducing systemic *Candida* infections in this patient population. A previous limitation to the potential efficacy of itraconazole was the availability of a capsule formulation whose bioavailability following oral administration was significantly dependent on gastric acidity. The oral solution demonstrates improved bioavailability over the capsule. In addition, an IV formulation has also been introduced for use in patients unable to tolerate oral therapy.

Studies have demonstrated that fluconazole prophylaxis has decreased the frequency of both superficial (e.g., oropharyngeal candidiasis) and systemic fungal infections in bone marrow transplant patients[35,36] but not in patients with leukemia.[37,38] When fluconazole 400 mg/day was compared with placebo for fungal prophylaxis in bone marrow transplant recipients, it significantly reduced the incidence of invasive candidiasis and delayed the initiation of empiric amphotericin B from day 17 to day 21.[36] It is unknown, however, if such patients who currently may experience a reduction in the degree and duration of neutropenia due to the administration of colony-stimulating growth factors would also benefit. In contrast, in a study of patients with acute leukemia undergoing chemotherapy, fluconazole prophylaxis was not associated with a reduction in invasive fungal infections or need for empiric amphotericin B.[38] Despite its potential role, concern over its lack of reliable in vitro activity against moulds limits its expanded use in high-risk patients. An increased frequency of isolation of non-albicans *Candida* (e.g., *C. krusei, C. glabrata, C. parapsilosis*) has also been noted in some institutions.[39] Fluconazole may not have a significant impact in reducing mortality in these patients.[40]

Fluconazole is available as both oral and IV formulations, and its oral bioavailability is not significantly influenced by changes in gastric acidity. Like itraconazole, the IV formulation enables fluconazole to be administered to critically ill patients or patients who have difficulty swallowing. However, unlike itraconazole, it is not contraindicated in patients with significant renal impairment. Despite such potential advantages, the efficacy of fluconazole in preventing invasive fungal infections was inferior to that of itraconazole in a randomized, comparative trial performed in 140 patients receiving allogeneic hematopoietic stem cell transplants.[41] In this trial, proven invasive fungal infections occurred in 6 of 71 (9%) itraconazole recipients and 17 of 61 (25%) fluconazole-treated patients. Although overall mortality was not different, fewer fungal deaths were reported in the itraconazole-treated patients (9% vs. 18%), but this difference was not statistically different ($P = 0.13$). In another randomized, comparative trial in allogeneic HSCT patients, fluconazole was compared with itraconazole.[42] Although itraconazole demonstrated superiority during treatment and against mould infections, no differences in invasive fungal infections or mortality were observed between treatments during the entire study period. Treatment-related hepatotoxicity and drug discontinuation because of side effects (predominantly GI intolerance) were more frequent in the group receiving itraconazole (36% vs. 16%, $P < 0.001$).

The prophylactic role of IV amphotericin B has also been investigated.[40,43] In one such evaluation, amphotericin B 0.5 mg/kg given three times weekly was compared with fluconazole 400 mg/day in 90 patients with acute leukemia.[43] Although efficacy against fungal infections was similar in both groups, more side effects (i.e., infusion-related reactions, nephrotoxicity, and electrolyte disturbances) were observed with the amphotericin B regimen. Therefore, the use of amphotericin B deoxycholate for primary prophylaxis is generally discouraged given existing options. There are limited published data on the efficacy of lipid-based formulations of amphotericin B (e.g., amphotericin B lipid complex, liposomal amphotericin B) for prophylaxis. One study compared liposomal amphotericin B versus a combination with fluconazole and itraconazole.[44] No significant differences were detected in terms of efficacy, but toxicity was noted more frequently in the patients receiving liposomal amphotericin B. Lipid-based amphotericin B preparations are generally reserved for patients with underlying renal dysfunction for which alternative strategies would be inappropriate.

The recent introduction of the echinocandin class of antifungals has expanded the number of agents evaluated as a prophylactic strategy in high-risk patients. Micafungin was compared to fluconazole in a randomized, double-blind study conducted in autologous and allogeneic HSCT recipients.[45] Based on a composite endpoint (which included absence of breakthrough fungal infection and absence of empiric modifications to the antifungal regimen due to neutropenic fever), micafungin was found to be superior. Although breakthrough candidemia, survival, and adverse events were similar in both groups, a trend toward a reduction in invasive aspergillosis in the allogeneic HSCT population was noted in the micafungin group. Micafungin is currently U.S. Food and Drug Administration (FDA)–approved for the prevention of *Candida* infections in HSCT patients.

In addition to the echinocandins, extended-spectrum triazoles (posaconazole and voriconazole) have been evaluated. Posaconazole demonstrated improved survival, a reduction in proven or probable IFI, and a reduction in invasive aspergillosis when compared to standard prophylaxis (either itraconazole or fluconazole) for the prevention of fungal infection in patients undergoing chemotherapy for acute myelogenous leukemia or myelodysplastic syndrome.[46] Posaconazole has also proven to be an effective prophylaxis in allogeneic HSCT recipients undergoing therapy for GVHD.[47] Posaconazole is currently available only as an oral formulation, which may limit its use in patients unable to take oral therapy. Although the efficacy of voriconazole in the treatment of invasive aspergillosis has been well documented, published data to support its use as prophylaxis in this patient population is currently lacking. Side effects (most notably hepatotoxicity) and the increased potential (relative to fluconazole and the echinocandins) for drug interactions with voriconazole may limit its use in this setting to patients at highest risk of mould infections. Although use of voriconazole has also been implicated in the emergence of pathogens such as zygomycosis in this patient population, a definitive cause-and-effect relationship is lacking.

Primary antifungal prophylaxis should generally be reserved for high-risk patients with neutropenia (e.g., allogeneic HSCT recipients).[3] Autologous HSCT recipients receiving agents causing significant mucositis, patients undergoing therapy for acute leukemia and those receiving corticosteroids for treatment of GVHD should also be considered for prophylaxis.[3] Although fluconazole has demonstrated efficacy when compared to placebo, select agents (i.e., echinocandins, voriconazole, itraconazole, posaconazole, amphotericin B) might be preferred in patients at increased risk of mold infections. Prophylaxis is generally continued until day 75 after transplant or through induction therapy for patients with leukemia.[3] Patients with a history of documented *Aspergillus* infection undergoing intensive chemotherapy should be considered for voriconazole. Although the addition of a second prophylaxis (e.g., caspofungin) may be considered, the benefits of combination therapy for secondary prophylaxis require further study. Other secondary prophylaxic regimens can be used in patients with a history of IFIs, based on the infection.

Patients receiving cytotoxic chemotherapy for solid tumors have lower rates of invasive fungal infections compared with patients with hematologic malignancies and those receiving allogeneic bone marrow transplantation. This is primarily because of the differences in the duration of neutropenia. In patients receiving cytotoxic chemotherapy for solid tumors, antifungal prophylaxis may not be beneficial and may actually increase the potential for superinfection with resistant fungi. Such patients should be managed with empiric antifungal therapy if they develop persistent fever and neutropenia.

Antivirals

The use of antiviral prophylaxis varies with patient population. High-risk patients (e.g., those receiving allogeneic HSCT, those with acute leukemia undergoing induction or reinduction therapy, those with a past history of infection during neutropenia or patients receiving T-cell–depleting agents such as fludarabine) and those who are seropositive for *herpes simplex* virus (HSV) should be considered for antiviral prophylaxis for the first month after transplant or (for acute leukemics) during periods of neutropenia.[3,8,10] Both acyclovir and valacyclovir may be useful in such settings. Published data for famciclovir for this indication is lacking. Allogeneic HSCT patients who are seropositive for varicella-zoster virus (VZV) should also be considered for acyclovir prophylaxis until the patients have discontinued immunosupression.[3,8,10] In addition, bone marrow transplant recipients at increased risk of CMV infection (e.g., CMV-seropositive patients and CMV-seronegative recipients with a CMV-seropositive donor) should be considered for either ganciclovir prophylaxis or pre-emptive therapy if early evidence of infection is observed.[7,9] The role of valganciclovir as a prophylactic strategy in this population requires further evaluation. Patients experiencing HSV reactivation during treatment should also receive prophylaxis during subsequent periods of neutropenia.[3]

Respiratory tract infections due to RSV, influenza, and parainfluenza are less commonly observed in patients with neutropenia. Although response to influenza virus vaccine may be attenuated, cancer patients should receive annual vaccinations with inactivated influenza vaccine.[3] In contrast, immunocompromised patients should not receive the intranasal live virus vaccine.[3]

Hematopoietic Growth Factors

Updated guidelines have recently been published to readdress the use of granulocyte colony-stimulating factor (G-CSF; filgrastim), granulocyte-macrophage colony-stimulating factor (GM-CSF; sargramostim), or pegylated G-CSF (pegfilgrastim) for use in the prophylaxis of infection in the neutropenic patient.[48,49] These guidelines advocated the use as primary prophylaxis in patients at high risk (>20%) of fever and neutropenia based on risk factors of age (i.e., younger than 65 years), medical history (including prior history of febrile neutropenic episodes, nutritional status, unstable comorbidities, and presence of active infections), disease characteristics (especially those involving bone marrow resulting in cytopenias), and myelotoxicity of the regimen (including both chemotherapy and radiation) used to treat the underlying malignancy. Secondary prophylaxis should be considered for patients who had experienced neutropenic complication from prior cycles of chemotherapy (especially if primary prophylaxis was not administered), or for whom reductions in chemotherapy dose to avoid neutropenia may compromise treatment outcome and disease-free or overall survival.

INFECTIONS IN NEUTROPENIC CANCER PATIENTS

Clinical Signs and Symptoms

4. Seven days after completing chemotherapy, B.C. developed a fever of 102°F (orally). Vital signs are blood pressure (BP), 109/70 mmHg; pulse, 102 beats/minute; and respirations, 25 breaths/minute. Physical examination demonstrates a clear oropharynx without exudates or plaques. Chest and cardiac examination are normal. The exit site for the Hickman catheter is clean and nontender without signs of erythema or induration. The perineum and rectum are nontender, and no masses are noted.

Laboratory data are hematocrit (Hct), 20% (normal, 33%–43%); hemoglobin (Hgb), 7 g/dL (normal, 14–18); WBC count, 1,400 cells/mm^3 (normal, 3,200–9,800), with 3% polymorphonuclear leukocytes (PMNs; normal, 54–62), 1% band forms (normal, 3–5), 70% lymphocytes (normal, 25–33), and 22% monocytes (normal, 3–7); platelet count, 17,000 cells/L (normal, 130,000–400,000); blood glucose, 160 mg/dL (normal, 70–110); serum creatinine (SrCr), 1.1 mg/dL (normal, 0.6–1.2); blood urea nitrogen (BUN), 24 mg/dL (normal, 8–18).

What are the signs and symptoms of infection in B.C.? What are the most common sites and sources of infection in patients such as B.C.?

[SI units: Hct, 0.2 (normal, 0.33–0.43); Hgb, 70 g/L (normal, 140–180); WBC count, 1.4 × 10^{10}/L (normal, 3.2–9.8) with 0.03 PMNs (normal, 0.54–0.62), 0.01 band forms (normal, 0.03–0.05), 0.7 lymphocytes (normal, 0.25–0.33), and 0.22 monocytes (normal, 0.03–0.07); platelets, 17 − 10^{10}/L (normal, 130–400); glucose, 8.88 mmol/L (normal, 3.89–6.11); SrCr, 97.24 mmol/L (normal, 53.04–106.08); BUN, 8.57 mmol/L urea (normal, 2.86–6.43)]

Neutropenia is usually defined as an ANC <500 cells/mm^3, or <1,000 cells/mm^3, and expected to decline to <500 cells/mm^3 within 2 days.[3] B.C. has an ANC of 48 cells/mm^3 (1,400 WBC/mm^3 × [0.03 PMN + 0.01 bands]) and is therefore at high risk for infection. Fever in neutropenic patients is defined as a single oral temperature of ≥38.3°C (101°F) or a temperature of ≥38.0°C (100.4°F) for >1 hour in the absence of an obvious cause.[10,50] As her case illustrates, fever is the earliest (and often the only) sign of infection in neutropenic patients because typical signs can be modified or absent in this patient population.[9,47,48] In contrast, other signs and symptoms consistent with a diagnosis of infection without fever should be considered to be infection in the neutropenic host.

In patients with documented infections, the most common sites are skin, mouth/throat, esophagus, sinuses, abdomen/rectum/liver, vascular access, lungs, and urinary tract.[3] Although the lung is the most common site of serious infection in neutropenic cancer patients, fever and dry cough are often the only presenting signs of pneumonia.[51] The impaired inflammatory response in these patients often makes sputum production scant, and sputum Gram stains often contain few polymorphonuclear cells. Radiologic evidence of a pulmonary infection can be minimal or absent, and the chest examination is frequently nondiagnostic. Pneumonia has a high mortality rate in neutropenic patients, especially if it occurs in conjunction with bacteremia.[10] In the presence of shock, a mortality rate of approximately 80% has been observed in these patients.[52]

Invasive procedures such as venipuncture, central IV catheter placement (e.g., Hickman catheter), and skin biopsies are associated with cellulitis and systemic infections. However, detecting skin and soft tissue infections is also difficult because the typical signs and symptoms of infection (e.g., pain, heat, erythema, swelling) are often absent.[51] This phenomenon exists due to the lack of adequate numbers of granulocytes, as well as the suppression or absence of other components of the inflammatory response.[2] Colonization of these lesions may result in local infection and the potential for systemic dissemination of bacteria and fungi. Bacteremia occurs primarily from entry of bacteria through the skin or through unrecognized ulcerations in the GI and perirectal areas.[10]

Confirmation of Infection

5. How can an infection be confirmed in patients such as B.C.?

Noninfectious sources of fever in the neutropenic cancer patient include inflammation, tumor progression, tumor lysis, adverse drug reactions, and transfusion reactions. Because of the frequent lack of physical signs and symptoms of infection, the clinician must obtain an accurate history (including the cancer type and treatment regimen) and conduct a careful physical examination at the first sign of fever.[51,53] A detailed search for subtle signs and symptoms of inflammation at the most common sites, such as the oropharynx, bone marrow aspiration sites, lung, periodontium, skin, vascular catheter access sites, nail beds, and perineum (including the anus) is necessary. Before antibiotics are initiated, two sets of blood cultures (with each set consisting of two culture bottles) should be obtained.[3] Additional cultures (e.g., stool, urine, IV site, viral) should be obtained if such infections are suspected.[3] Any indwelling urinary or IV catheter should be considered as a potential focus of infection and, if possible, should be removed and cultured.[10] Chest radiographs and oximetry should be obtained if signs and symptoms point to the respiratory tract as a potential infection site.[10] A complete blood count, serum electrolytes, and assessment of organ function (e.g., liver and kidney function) should be obtained to assist in drug dosing and monitoring for treatment-related toxicities.[10]

An infectious cause for fever can be documented either clinically or microbiologically in up to 60% of neutropenic cancer patients.[9] Forty percent of these febrile episodes have a documented microbiological origin; the remaining 20% are attributed to infection based on clinical findings alone.[9]

Significance of Colonization

6. Routine surveillance cultures of swabs taken from B.C.'s axillae, nasopharynx, and rectum grew *C. jeikeium* (axillae), *S. aureus* (axillae and nasopharynx), and *Enterococcus faecium* (rectum). What is the significance of these culture results? Should routine, serial surveillance cultures be performed in patients such as B.C.?

Several factors influence the colonization and subsequent infection by micro-organisms in cancer patients such as B.C. Organisms isolated from infected patients can be found in endogenous flora or acquired during hospitalization.[6] The sources of and factors contributing to colonization are numerous and include staff-to-staff and patient-to-patient transmission (e.g., lack of frequent and adequate hand hygiene), direct transmission from the environment (e.g., inadequately disinfected bathtubs, sinks, toilet bowls), foods (e.g., raw fruits and vegetables), inhalation from contaminated fomites (e.g., respirators, ventilating systems), and IV access devices.

In addition to immunosuppression, the underlying malignancy and chemotherapy diminish the cancer patient's resistance to colonization and infection. For example, chemotherapy induces changes in the microbial binding receptors on epithelial cells in the oropharynx. This allows Gram-negative bacilli to adhere to these surfaces, changing the composition of the oropharyngeal flora from a mixture of Gram-positive aerobes and anaerobes to Gram-negative aerobic bacteria.[54] Colonization with resistant organisms is enhanced by prior antibiotic administration, which may suppress the growth of normal anaerobic flora in the GI tract. This anaerobic suppression may promote the overgrowth of resistant micro-organisms.[54] For example, *P. aeruginosa* and *K. pneumoniae* are not commonly found in the stools of normal healthy adults, but they are recovered from the stools of hospitalized cancer patients.

Organisms that colonize cancer patients differ in their invasiveness and propensity to cause infection.[6,55] Colonization with *P. aeruginosa* is more likely to result in infection than is colonization with less virulent organisms such as *E. coli* or *S. epidermidis*.[56] However, if the host is profoundly impaired, organisms generally considered to be less virulent may become pathogenic.

The acquisition of and subsequent colonization by potentially pathogenic microbes may be detected by serial "surveillance" cultures of specimens obtained from various body sites such as the nasopharynx, axilla, urine, and rectum. Such surveillance cultures can provide information about the dynamic changes in microflora during hospitalization that may be useful for infection control purposes. However, little clinically useful information is gained when infection is absent.[57] Therefore, surveillance cultures are generally restricted to select patients for infection control purposes. In such cases, culture of the anterior nares (for MRSA) or rectal samples (for VRE or multidrug-resistant Gram-negative bacilli) may be performed.

In summary, B.C.'s surveillance culture results indicate that she is colonized with several potential pathogens associated with infection in the immunocompromised host, but these results are probably not useful in selecting empiric antibiotics for her fever.

EMPIRIC ANTIBIOTIC THERAPY

Rationale

7. Should B.C. be started on antibiotic therapy immediately? Is this rational in view of the fact that neither the source of her fever nor the pathogen has been established?

All febrile patients with either an ANC of <500 cells/mm^3 or <1,000 and expected to decline to <500 cells/mm^3 within 2 days should be considered to have a potentially life-threatening infection.[3,10] In addition, afebrile neutropenic patients with signs or symptoms of infection should also receive antibiotic therapy. Once blood cultures and cultures from suspected sources of infection are obtained, these patients should be promptly started on broad-spectrum antibacterials.[3,10] Early studies in the 1950s and 1960s documented the poor prognosis of neutropenic patients whose Gram-negative infections were untreated during the first 24 to 48 hours following the onset of fever. Crude mortality rates secondary to *P. aeruginosa* bacteremia approached 91%.[56] This finding was confirmed in the 1970s when it was demonstrated that withholding antibiotics until a pathogen was isolated resulted in an unacceptably high mortality rate in neutropenic patients. Prompt use of empiric, broad -spectrum antibiotics since the mid-1980s has contributed to significant reductions in infectious mortality rates to <30%, depending on the causative organism.[58] These observations emphasize the need for rapid institution of empiric antibiotic therapy to prevent early morbidity and mortality.

Optimal Antibacterial Spectrum

8. What pathogen- and patient-specific factors should be considered when initiating empiric therapy for B.C.?

Despite advances in the development in antibacterials since the 1960s, the empiric management of febrile neutropenic patients continues to be complicated by the changing spectrum of bacterial pathogens and their antimicrobial susceptibilities. Empiric antibiotic regimens should provide broad-spectrum coverage against the potential Gram-negative bacilli most commonly isolated from neutropenic cancer patients (e.g., *E. coli, K. pneumoniae, P. aeruginosa*), staphylococcal and viridans streptococci.[3,10] Because mortality from untreated bacteremia caused by *P. aeruginosa* was high in early studies,[56] empiric regimens have traditionally included antimicrobials with antipseudomonal activity.

Selecting an initial empiric regimen for a given patient should take into account likely pathogens, their frequency of isolation, infection-specific antibiotic efficacy and institutional susceptibility patterns. Patient-related considerations should include medical stability, allergies, prior and concomitant antimicrobials, and organ dysfunction (e.g., renal or hepatic). Attempts should be made to identify low-risk patients for whom oral antimicrobial therapy may be an option.[3,10] Finally, dosing schedules, acquisition costs, and the potential for significant toxicities should be considered.

In addition to broad-spectrum activity, antibacterial regimens should ideally have bactericidal activity against the infecting pathogen. However, no adequately controlled comparative trials of bacteriostatic versus bactericidal antibiotics have been conducted in humans.

In summary, many organisms, including those recovered from surveillance cultures, may be pathogens in B.C. Those associated with a high mortality rate during the first 48 hours should be empirically treated pending culture and sensitivity results. Therefore, an empiric regimen with optimal activity against commonly isolated Gram-negative bacilli (including *P. aeruginosa*) should be promptly administered to B.C.

Initial Empiric Antibiotic Regimens

9. What would be a reasonable initial empiric antibiotic regimen for B.C.?

Practice guidelines prepared by the National Comprehensive Cancer Network[3] and the Infectious Diseases Society of America (IDSA)[10] identify antimicrobial options for the treatment of fever in the neutropenic cancer patient. The ideal antibiotic regimen for empiric management in this setting remains controversial. Various antibiotics, alone and in combination, have been studied extensively.[10] Monotherapy regimens commonly include a third-generation cephalosporin (e.g., ceftazidime), a fourth-generation cephalosporin (e.g., cefepime), or a carbapenem (e.g., imipenem-cilastatin or meropenem). The combination regimens most frequently recommended (excluding those containing vancomycin) are an aminoglycoside (e.g., gentamicin, tobramycin, or amikacin) plus an antipseudomonal ureidopenicillin with or without a β-lactamase inhibitor (e.g., piperacillin, piperacillin-tazobactam), an aminoglycoside with an antipseudomonal cephalosporin (e.g., ceftazidime, cefepime), or an aminoglycoside in combination with a carbapenem (e.g., imipenem-cilastatin or meropenem).[3,10] Although recommended by some sources,[3] combination β-lactam antibiotics are less frequently used. Comparisons of efficacy rates between studies are complicated by differences in the definitions of neutropenia, the incidence of documented infections, criteria used to assess clinical response, and statistical methodology.[50] Guidelines have been proposed to establish standards for evaluating antimicrobial therapy in this population.[50] Despite such limitations, no striking differences regarding efficacy have been observed between these empiric approaches.[10]

Oral Antibiotics

Carefully selected ("low-risk") adult febrile neutropenic patients may be candidates for oral antibiotic therapy, either as initial therapy or as follow-up to IV antibiotics ("sequential therapy").[10,59,60] This would EXCLUDE patients with any of the following: serious comorbidities, inpatient acquisition of infection, uncontrolled malignancy, pneumonia, recent HSCT, dehydration, hypotension, chronic lung disease, abnormal liver ($>3\times$ upper limits of normal) or renal function (serum creatinine >2 mg/dL), ANC <100 cells/mm^3, or signs/symptoms lasting longer than 7 days.[3] Patients must be without microbiological or clinical evidence of infection (other than fever), clinically stable, and closely observed. An international collaborative study established and validated a risk scoring system in adults that incorporated these principles to identify low-risk patients for whom oral therapy may be an option.[61]

Trials have confirmed the value of oral ciprofloxacin in combination with amoxicillin-clavulanate in low-risk adult patients with febrile neutropenia. Oral ciprofloxacin (30 mg/kg/day in three divided doses) combined with amoxicillin-clavulanate (40 mg/kg/day in three divided doses) has been compared to IV ceftazidime.[62] Treatment was equally successful in both groups, but the ceftazidime group required significantly more modifications in the initial regimen compared with the oral group. Conversely, more patients receiving ciprofloxacin with amoxicillin-clavulanate were unable to tolerate the oral regimen. Similarly, the efficacy of oral ciprofloxacin (750 mg twice daily) in combination with amoxicillin-clavulanate (625 mg three times daily) versus IV ceftazidime and amikacin has been studied.[63] As with the previous trial, the oral regimen was found to be as effective as IV antibiotics. Therefore, ciprofloxacin plus amoxicillin-clavulanate is most frequently used. Clindamycin may be used in place of amoxicillin-clavulanate if the patient is allergic to β-lactam antibiotics.[3,10] Cefixime has been used effectively as an alternative regimen in low-risk pediatric patients initially receiving IV therapy,[64] but there is not adequate experience with cefixime as an initial therapy.[10]

Patients receiving fluoroquinolone prophylaxis would generally be excluded from receiving oral therapy due to the increased risk of infection with resistant organisms. Low-risk patients with adequate home support (e.g., access to emergency facilities, phone access) and the desire for home treatment may be treated as an outpatient (with either IV or oral therapy). Monitoring in the outpatient setting should include either home nursing or office visits daily for 3 days to review progress and to screen for problems (e.g., progression of infection or drug intolerance).[3] Patients who are stable and responding after the initial observation period may continue to receive monitoring by phone contact.[3]

Intravenous Monotherapy

10. Can any of the more potent, extended spectrum β-lactams be used as monotherapy in febrile neutropenic patients?

CEPHALOSPORINS

The antipseudomonal third-generation cephalosporin ceftazidime and the fourth-generation agent cefepime have been extensively studied as monotherapy for empiric therapy in febrile neutropenic patients. In general, these agents are safe and have potent broad-spectrum activity in vitro against many Gram-negative and some Gram-positive pathogens.

Numerous comparative clinical studies in both adults and children have been performed to evaluate the efficacy of ceftazidime as initial empiric monotherapy in febrile neutropenic cancer patients.[65–79] Overall, ceftazidime was as effective as the standard regimen in patients with documented infections and unexplained fever. In some of these trials, the efficacy of ceftazidime in patients with documented staphylococcal infections was suboptimal. Select clinical trials have empirically added antistaphylococcal coverage with a glycopeptide (e.g., vancomycin) and have shown improved outcomes in these patients.[80,81] In addition, pathogens (particularly Gram-negative pathogens) that produce either type 1 β-lactamase or extended spectrum β-lactamase (e.g., *K. pneumoniae*) are not likely to respond to ceftazidime monotherapy.[82,83] These may be seen more frequently in patients with prolonged hospitalization or those who have received prior antimicrobial therapy.[82] Therefore, local in vitro susceptibilities of common Gram-negative pathogens should be examined prior to the routine use of ceftazidime as monotherapy.

Cefepime is a fourth-generation cephalosporin with an FDA-approved indication for monotherapy for empiric management of infection in patients with febrile neutropenia. The potential advantage of this agent over third-generation cephalosporins is its low affinity for major chromosomally mediated β-lactamases.[84,85] Compared with ceftazidime, cefepime has more potent activity in vitro against select Gram-positive bacteria (methicillin-susceptible *Staphylococcus* species, viridans streptococci, and *S. pneumoniae*).[85] Randomized, comparative studies have evaluated the role of cefepime as monotherapy in both adults and children with febrile neutropenia.[66,67,69,71,72,86–93] The improved Gram-positive activity (relative to ceftazidime) may decrease the empiric need for vancomycin in some patients. However, this advantage is less likely in institutions with a high rate of MRSA because cefepime and other cephalosporins are inactive against this pathogen.

CARBAPENEMS

The carbapenems are a unique class of antibiotics with broad-spectrum activity against numerous Gram-positive and Gram-negative bacteria, including anaerobes. Imipenem (in combination with the dehydropeptidase inhibitor cilastatin) and meropenem are two currently available agents in this class. Both imipenem-cilastatin[75,77,79,86,94–103] and meropenem[68,70,74,76,102,104–108] have been studied as monotherapy for febrile, neutropenic patients. The third member of this class available in the United States, ertapenem, possesses microbiological activity similar to that of the other carbapenems, although it lacks in vitro activity against *Acinetobacter* species and *Pseudomonas,* including *P. aeruginosa.*[109] Considering this lack of activity, ertapenem would not be appropriate as empiric therapy for febrile neutropenic patients and has not been evaluated in this setting. Agents with increased anaerobic activity (e.g., carbapenems) might be used as empiric therapy in cases where an intra-abdominal infection is suspected.

Clinical outcomes with imipenem-cilastatin monotherapy have been comparable with those of the β-lactam plus aminoglycoside combinations,[79,94,98,101] as well as combination of two β-lactams.[96] Although proven to be effective, imipenem-cilastatin has generally been associated with a higher incidence of nausea and vomiting compared with ceftazidime or meropenem.[77,110] The GI side effects are generally dose related (3–4 g/day) and associated with the rate of IV administration.[97] Therefore, dosages of 2 g/day (divided Q 6 hr) are generally given to patients with normal renal function.[111]

Meropenem has a broad spectrum of activity (similar to that of imipenem-cilastatin) but is generally associated with fewer GI side effects. Meropenem monotherapy for febrile neutropenia has been evaluated in both adults and children,[68,70,74,76,102,104–108] and the results have supported the value of meropenem as empiric monotherapy for use in febrile neutropenic patients.

In summary, several studies have demonstrated that monotherapy with cefepime, ceftazidime, or a carbapenem (imipenem-cilastatin or meropenem) is appropriate as initial empiric antibiotic therapy in febrile neutropenic patients. There are no convincing data to support one choice over the others as empiric monotherapy. However, routine carbapenem use may be associated with increased drug acquisition cost (relative to cephalosporins) and increased potential for development of carbapenem resistance. Therefore, many institutions have elected to reserve the carbapenems for patients who have failed to respond to prior empiric therapy, have a history of infections with pathogens resistant to third- and fourth-generation cephalosporins, are clinically unstable, or have need for expanded anaerobic coverage.

ALTERNATIVE INTRAVENOUS MONOTHERAPY REGIMENS

Monobactams, fluoroquinolones, and β-lactam/β-lactamase inhibitor combinations have shown efficacy in the management of febrile neutropenic patients. Monobactams and fluoroquinolones have been particularly useful as empiric alternatives in patients with β-lactam allergies.

Monobactams

Aztreonam, the only available monobactam, demonstrates in vitro activity only against Gram-negative aerobic bacilli.[112] Although its in vitro potency against Gram-negative bacteria is comparable to that of ceftazidime, aztreonam lacks activity against Gram-positive bacteria or anaerobes.[112] Considering the lack of Gram-positive activity, aztreonam should not be used as monotherapy in this patient population. Empiric use with aztreonam has been evaluated in combination with either a β-lactam (piperacillin)[113] or vancomycin.[114]

Fluoroquinolones

Select fluoroquinolones offer an approach to the empiric management of febrile neutropenic patients. Most agents in this class are bactericidal against many Gram-negative bacilli. However, they demonstrate variable potency in vitro against certain Gram-positive bacteria, such as *S. pneumoniae, S. aureus,* and *E. faecalis.* Of the currently available fluoroquinolones, ciprofloxacin is generally considered the most active in vitro against *P. aeruginosa.* However, surveys published within the past several years have demonstrated only approximately 60% of *P. aeruginosa* isolates are susceptible to ciprofloxacin.[115,116]

Ciprofloxacin has been studied as both monotherapy[117–121] and as part of combination regimens[122–125] as initial empiric therapy in febrile neutropenic patients. However, monotherapy with ciprofloxacin has met with mixed success. A European Organization for Research and Treatment of Cancer (EORTC) trial comparing ciprofloxacin 400 to 600 mg/day versus piperacillin plus amikacin was terminated prematurely because of significantly poorer response rates in the patients treated with ciprofloxacin (65%) compared with the combination group (91%; $P < 0.002$).[120] This finding may be due in part to the suboptimal ciprofloxacin dosage used and the impact of fluoroquinolone prophylaxis on the institution's nosocomial flora. An additional study demonstrated more favorable results with ciprofloxacin monotherapy.[121] However, the consensus is that the fluoroquinolones should not be used as monotherapy.[3,10]

β-Lactam/β-Lactamase Inhibitor Combinations

Randomized trials have compared piperacillin-tazobactam monotherapy to various antibiotics.[87,100,126–130] Recently published trials have documented that piperacillin-tazobactam is noninferior to cefepime in this patient population.[131,132] Although the results look promising, experience with this agent as monotherapy is limited relative to the carbapenems and antipseudomonal cephalosporins. In addition, piperacillin-tazobactam may interfere with the galactomannan assay used in the diagnosis of select IFIs, including aspergillosis.

Antimicrobial Combinations

11. B.L., a 13-year-old boy, presented with a 3-week history of "always being tired" and a persistent sore throat. Initial evaluation revealed anemia, thrombocytopenia, and a WBC count of 130,000 cells/L (normal, 3,200–9,800 cells/mm^3), with a predominance of immature lymphoblasts. Further evaluation demonstrated that B.L. had "high-risk" acute lymphocytic leukemia. Remission induction treatment was initiated with teniposide plus cytarabine followed by prednisone, vincristine, and L-asparaginase. Seven days after induction chemotherapy, B.L. developed a fever (102°F) and chills. The ANC was 48 cells/mm^3. SrCr and BUN were 1.0 mg/dL (normal, 0.6–1.2 mg/dL) and 15 mg/dL (normal, 8–18 mg/dL), respectively. The physician wants to empirically start B.L. on ceftazidime plus gentamicin combination regimen. What is the role of this combination in the empiric management of febrile

neutropenia? Are there any differences in efficacy between these combinations?

[SI units: SrCr, 88.4 mmol/L (normal, 53.04–106.08); BUN, 5.36 mmol/L urea (2.8–6.43)]

RATIONALE FOR USE

Prior to the introduction of third- and fourth-generation cephalosporins and carbapenems, the empiric use of antibacterial combinations in febrile neutropenic cancer patients was favored because these regimens offered a broader spectrum of activity against bacteria commonly infecting cancer patients. In addition, these combinations offered the potential, in select circumstances, to provide an additive or synergistic effect. Finally, they offered the potential to minimize the development of bacterial resistance. However, infections in neutropenic patients have shifted from Gram-negative to Gram-positive pathogens, against which traditional combination regimens (selected primarily for their activity against Gram-negative pathogens) have limited efficacy. Despite this concern, some clinicians continue to favor antibiotic combinations, especially in patients who are clinically unstable.

Synergy

Antibiotic *synergy* is defined as an interaction between antimicrobial agents in which the effect produced by the combination is greater than the sum of their individual activity. Various in vitro methods may be used to test for synergistic activity between antibacterials, and these methods may result in differing conclusions between similar combinations.

Studies published more than two decades ago reported that the outcome in neutropenic cancer patients with documented Gram-negative bacteremia was significantly improved with the use of antibacterial combinations with the potential for demonstrating synergy in vitro when compared with nonsynergistic combinations.[133,134] Of 18 patients patients with profound persistent neutropenia ($<$100 cells/mm^3) whose regimen demonstrated in vitro synergism or partial synergism against the infecting pathogen, 8 showed clinical improvement.[134] In contrast, none of the 13 patients in the same study receiving nonsynergistic antibiotic regimens responded. This difference was statistically significant ($P < 0.005$). Although these results are of interest, this study was performed using older, less potent Gram-negative agents. It is unknown whether synergistic combinations of newer antimicrobials, such as quinolones with carbapenems or piperacillin, would result in similar findings.

Prevention of Resistant Strains

Another argument in favor of antibiotic combination use is that these combinations may prevent or delay the emergence of resistance during therapy. Although resistant bacterial strains have emerged during therapy with monotherapy, it is not clear whether combination therapy will prevent the emergence of resistance during therapy.

AMINOGLYCOSIDE PLUS β-LACTAM COMBINATIONS

Until the 1980s, most febrile neutropenic patients were treated with two-drug combination regimens that contained an aminoglycoside (gentamicin, tobramycin, or amikacin) plus a β-lactam antibiotic, such as antipseudomonal penicillin or a third-generation cephalosporin. This combination is one of the most established empiric treatment regimens for the management of febrile neutropenia.[10]

Numerous studies have been conducted to evaluate the efficacy of combination therapy of an aminoglycoside with an antipseudomonal cephalosporin. Both ceftazidime[65,79,83,104–106,129,135–146] and cefepime[138,139,147,148] have been evaluated as part of a combination regimen. Cephalosporins without antipseudomonal activity (e.g., ceftriaxone) have also been investigated in combination with aminoglycosides, although this regimen is not routinely recommended.[149] Antipseudomonal penicillins plus β-lactamase inhibitors (in combination with an aminoglycoside) would also be considered.

The duration of combination therapy consisting of an aminoglycoside plus a cephalosporin has also been evaluated. A study conducted by the EORTC evaluated the effectiveness of full-course versus short-course amikacin plus ceftazidime in neutropenic patients with Gram-negative bacteremia.[149] A better outcome was demonstrated with full-course amikacin plus ceftazidime than with a short course (3 days) of amikacin plus a full course of ceftazidime. These data confirm the superiority of combined therapy of ceftazidime plus a full course of an aminoglycoside in profoundly neutropenic patients with Gram-negative bacteremia.

Carbapenem antibiotics are more frequently evaluated as monotherapy in this patient population. Therefore, relative to the numerous trials examining the role of combination therapy with cephalosporins, there are limited studies examining the combination of an aminoglycoside with either imipenem-cilastatin[99,142] or meropenem[104] in this patient population. However, in one such evaluation, the combination of imipenem-cilastatin plus amikacin was found to be superior to imipenem-cilastatin monotherapy.[150] Carbapenems (in combination with aminoglycosides and vancomycin) have been recommended as empiric initial therapy for patients who are clinically unstable.[3]

Aminoglycosides have generally been considered the backbone of combination regimens because of their potential for bactericidal action against various bacteria. However, the addition of an aminoglycoside is associated with increased costs for therapeutic monitoring.[150,151] The benefit of an aminoglycoside for empiric therapy has not been consistently demonstrated.[150,151] In addition, there is an increased potential for the development of nephrotoxicity and ototoxicity.[151] This concern is especially relevant in patients receiving concomitant nephrotoxins such as cisplatin and cyclosporine. Despite these issues, B.L. may benefit from the empiric institution of an aminoglycoside/β-lactam combination because he is profoundly neutropenic (ANC $<$50 cells/mm^3). Serum concentrations of the aminoglycosides should be monitored as needed to achieve optimal outcomes while reducing the risks of toxicity.

12. Seven days into therapy, despite rehydration, B.L.'s SrCr and BUN rose to 2.0 g/dL and 45 mg/dL, respectively. Because B.L. has developed nephrotoxicity (believed to be secondary to the aminoglycoside), what other combination regimens (excluding those containing aminoglycosides) could be used? Are these regimens as effective as aminoglycoside-containing regimens?

[SI units: SrCr, 176.8 mmol/L; BUN, 16.07 mmol/L urea]

DOUBLE β-LACTAM COMBINATIONS

Although numerous β-lactam combinations (usually consisting of either moxalactam or a cephalosporin plus an antipseudomonal penicillin) have been studied, overall response rates have not been significantly different from those of patients treated with aminoglycoside/β-lactam regimens. However, experience is limited with double β-lactam combinations in patients with neutropenia or patients with documented infections caused by *P. aeruginosa,* and the available results are somewhat disturbing. Winston et al. observed a lower response in patients with profound, persistent neutropenia who were treated with moxalactam plus piperacillin (48%) compared with those treated with moxalactam plus amikacin (77%).[152] Because the number of patients studied was small, these differences approached but did not achieve statistical significance ($P < 0.08$). A poorer response in patients with infection caused by *P. aeruginosa* was observed. One of five patients treated with moxalactam plus piperacillin versus seven of nine patients treated with moxalactam plus amikacin responded ($P < 0.06$). Two patients with bacteremia caused by *P. aeruginosa* initially susceptible to the double β-lactam regimen relapsed with isolates resistant to multiple β-lactam antibiotics. These results are compatible with the selection of bacteria producing high amounts of the chromosomally mediated β-lactamase, which is capable of inactivating third-generation cephalosporins and other less stable β-lactams.

OTHER COMBINATIONS

As previously stated, ciprofloxacin has been studied in combination with other antibacterials (either an aminoglycoside or a β-lactam, including an antipseudomonal penicillin) as initial empiric therapy for treatment of suspected infection in febrile neutropenic patients.[122–125] These studies, however, were associated with increased Gram-positive infections in ciprofloxacin-treated patients. In addition, the in vitro activity of ciprofloxacin against *P. aeruginosa* has declined significantly (to <70% in many institutions).[115,116] Therefore, if used as part of combination therapy, ciprofloxacin should be combined with an antimicrobial with favorable in vitro activity against this pathogen.

Summary

Given the limited experience with these regimens in patients with profound persistent neutropenia or infections caused by *P. aeruginosa,* empiric therapy with double β-lactam regimens should not routinely be used as primary therapy. They can be considered, however, in cases where combination therapy is indicated, but the addition of an aminoglycoside may be contraindicated.

Regardless of the empiric regimen selected, patients must be closely monitored for nonresponse, emergence of secondary infections, adverse effects, and the development of drug-resistant organisms.

Empiric Vancomycin

13. B.L. is begun on a three-drug regimen of ceftazidime, tobramycin, and vancomycin. What is the rationale for adding vancomycin to the regimen?

As previously discussed, the number of infections due to Gram-positive pathogens is increasing. Because cephalosporins lack activity against methicillin-resistant staphylococci, vancomycin is often added to empiric regimens. A growing proportion of *S. aureus* infections are methicillin-resistant (as many as 50% in some institutions).[12] However, excessive use of vancomycin has been associated with the rise in vancomycin resistance among Gram-positive organisms, such as VRE. Finally, emergent resistance in *S. aureus* has been seen in the form of vancomycin intermediately resistant *S. aureus* and rare case reports of *S. aureus* fully resistant to vancomycin.

Clinical studies evaluating the need for vancomycin as initial empiric therapy have reached different conclusions, primarily due to differences in the measured end points.[153] For example, febrile neutropenic patients with cancer had more rapid resolution of fever, fewer days of bacteremia, and a lower frequency of treatment failure when vancomycin was added to an initial regimen of antipseudomonal penicillin plus an aminoglycoside.[154,155] Similarly, the addition of vancomycin to ceftazidime showed improved results compared with ceftazidime alone or with a three-drug combination.[156] However, other studies have concluded that mortality was not increased when vancomycin therapy was delayed.[157–159] The mortality from staphylococcal infections is generally considered to be low (<4%) during the first 48 hours after the onset of fever.[153] In contrast, the mortality associated with viridans streptococcal infections may be higher among patients who are not initially treated with vancomycin.[160] Some strains of viridans streptococci are either resistant or tolerant to penicillin, but antibacterials such as piperacillin, cefepime (not ceftazidime), and carbapenems demonstrate excellent activity in vitro against these strains.[160,161]

There has been considerable debate over whether vancomycin should be included in the initial empiric regimen for febrile neutropenic patients. Many clinicians believe that this decision should be based on both patient and institution factors.[10] In general, empiric vancomycin use should be discouraged.[3,10,162] At institutions where these fulminant Gram-positive infections are rare, vancomycin should not be routinely used unless culture results indicate the need. However, for institutions frequently isolating invasive Gram-positive bacterial pathogens (e.g., those caused by viridans streptococci), vancomycin should probably be included in the initial empiric regimen. Other patients in whom empiric vancomycin should be considered in the initial regimen include the following:

- Patients with clinically suspected catheter-related infections[10,163]
- Patients receiving intensive chemotherapy (e.g., high-dose cytarabine) that produces substantial mucosal damage and subsequent increased risk for penicillin-resistant streptococcal infections (i.e., viridans streptococci)[10,163,164]
- Patients receiving prior fluoroquinolone or TMP/SMX prophylaxis[165]
- Patients with a previous history of colonization with β-lactam–resistant pneumococci or MRSA
- Patients with blood cultures positive for Gram-positive bacteria prior to identification and susceptibility testing
- Patients with hypotension or septic shock without an identified pathogen[10,163,164]

Vancomycin has been studied in combination with various antibiotics, including imipenem-cilastatin, meropenem, ceftazidime, cefepime, and various aminoglycosides. The addition of vancomycin to an aminoglycoside-containing regimen should be done with caution because data support an increased risk of aminoglycoside-induced nephrotoxicity in patients receiving these agents concomitantly with vancomycin.[166] Empiric vancomycin should be discontinued after 3 days if a Gram-positive infection is not identified.[3,10]

ALTERNATIVES TO VANCOMYCIN

Options exist for the treatment of invasive Gram-positive infections. Linezolid is an oxazolidinone that can be administered IV or orally.[167] A randomized, double-blind trial comparing the use of linezolid to vancomycin for empiric therapy demonstrated comparable safety and efficacy.[168] It is associated with thrombocytopenia and secondary neutropenia, especially when given for prolonged periods. Considering the reduced marrow reserve in cancer chemotherapy patients, these adverse events are of particular concern. Quinupristin-dalfopristin is available for IV administration only, and concerns regarding potential drug interactions and patient tolerability (including musculoskeletal pain) may limit its use.[167] Daptomycin provides potent in vitro activity against many multidrug-resistant Gram-positive pathogens (including VRE and MRSA), but requires IV therapy and should not be used for the treatment of pneumonia. Further studies are needed with both agents before they could be routinely recommended as an alternative to vancomycin in this patient population.

In the case of B.L., empiric use of vancomycin is not warranted based on the previous discussion, and it should be discontinued unless cultures indicate the need for this antibiotic.

ANTIBIOTIC DOSING, ADMINISTRATION, AND MONITORING CONSIDERATIONS

Intermittent Versus Continuous Infusion of Intravenous Antibiotics

14. Should B.L.'s antibiotics be given intermittently (i.e., divided doses) or as a continuous infusion?

β-lactam antibiotics exhibit time-dependent (i.e., concentration-independent) pharmacodynamic activity.[169] Studies with these agents in both animal and in vitro models of infection suggest that prolonged exposure of bacteria to drug concentrations above the minimum inhibitory concentration (MIC) of the organism for a significant period of time may be linked to improved bacterial killing and survival.[169] Based on these observations and the poor prognosis of neutropenic cancer patients with bacteremia, noncomparative, open-label trials were conducted to evaluate the role of continuous infusions of β-lactams (i.e., ceftazidime) in the empiric treatment of suspected infection in cancer patients.[170–172] These noncomparative trials showed that continuous-infusion ceftazidime was a treatment option and should be evaluated in larger, comparative trials.

In contrast to β-lactam antibiotics, aminoglycosides exhibit concentration-dependent (time-independent) pharmacodynamic activity in both animal and in vitro models of infection.[169] Despite such properties, improved response with continuous rather than intermittent infusion of the aminoglycoside has been reported.[173] Such reports are difficult to evaluate because many of the patients were entered into the studies after "failing" to respond to previous antibiotic regimens. Patients often differed significantly in their immune status (e.g., differences in incidence of neutropenia among study groups, uncontrolled use of granulocyte transfusions), and the total daily dose of the aminoglycoside was often greater in the continuous infusion group. In the only randomized, prospective study conducted to date, no significant difference in efficacy was observed between the two modes of administration.[173] The most convincing argument against the continuous infusion of aminoglycosides relates to the incidence of toxicity. Studies in established animal models of aminoglycoside-induced nephrotoxicity showed that the uptake of aminoglycosides into renal cortical tissue increased, and glomerular function decreased more when the drug was infused continuously rather than given as single or divided doses.[174]

In conclusion, the maintenance of β-lactam antibiotic concentrations above the MIC of the suspected pathogen (as might be provided by continuous infusion) appears rational. However, data demonstrating improved effects with newer, more potent agents in cancer patients are unavailable. Considering the potential for toxicity with this route of administration, B.L. should not receive tobramycin by continuous infusion. Although consideration could be given to administering ceftazidime by continuous infusion, this method of administration would require an IV line dedicated for continuous drug administration. This technique may limit B.L.'s ability to receive intermittent tobramycin infusions unless additional IV ports or lines are available for use. Finally, there are no data showing that this method is superior to intermittent administration.

Consolidated ("Once-Daily") Aminoglycoside Dosing

15. What is the role of consolidated ("once-daily") aminoglycoside dosing in febrile neutropenic patients such as B.L.?

Because of the concentration-dependent pharmacodynamic properties of aminoglycosides and the convenience of administration, studies have been conducted to describe both the pharmacokinetic properties and efficacy of consolidated dosing of aminoglycosides in animals and in neutropenic patients. Pharmacokinetic studies with amikacin[175,176] and gentamicin[177,178] have not revealed pharmacokinetic differences when compared with other populations. Several clinical studies have included consolidated aminoglycoside dosing for amikacin,[104,135,137,139,148,179,180] gentamicin,[147,181–183] and tobramycin.[140] However, most of the studies in this population were not designed to evaluate differences between consolidated aminoglycoside dosing compared to similar regimens using intermittent dosing.[10,184] In general, the various studies suggest that consolidated dosing is as effective and possibly less nephrotoxic than traditional dosing. Therefore, consolidated dosing of aminoglycosides appears reasonable in empiric therapy of neutropenic patients.[184]

Outpatient Administration

Continued administration of antimicrobials in the outpatient setting has been suggested in a subset of low-risk patients.[61,179,185–187] The criteria used to eligibility for outpatient therapy are generally similar to those established and previously discussed for oral therapy. Therefore, outpatient administration of parenteral antibiotics can be considered in a subset of low-risk patients with close medical follow-up.[3]

HOST FACTORS INFLUENCING RESPONSE TO THERAPY

16. What factors may have influenced B.L.'s clinical response to antimicrobial therapy?

The most important prognostic determinants of a favorable outcome in patients with neutropenia and infection are the recovery of the granulocyte count and (for the patient with infection) the selection of agents with appropriate antimicrobial activity against the pathogen.[10] Patients with profound, persistent neutropenia (<100 cells/mm^3 that does not rise during therapy or an initial ANC of 100–500 cells/mm^3 that declines during therapy) tend to respond to antibiotics less favorably than patients whose bone marrow recovers.[10] The initial granulocyte count appears to be less important than the trend toward granulocyte recovery in influencing the patient's overall response to therapy. The site of infection also influences outcome. Septic shock and pneumonia are associated with high mortality in bacteremic neutropenic patients.[10,53]

MODIFYING INITIAL EMPIRIC ANTIBIOTIC THERAPY

17. M.H., a 24-year-old woman with a recent diagnosis of ovarian cancer, developed neutropenia (ANC <150 cells/mm^3) following chemotherapy. Five days after becoming neutropenic, she developed a fever of 101°F and was begun on an empiric antibiotic regimen of ceftazidime 2 g IV Q 8 hr. Although she remained febrile, her initial cultures remained negative at 48 hours. Should M.H. be continued on the same regimen, or should modifications be made? How do the culture results influence this decision? How long should empiric therapy be continued?

Following initiation of empiric antibiotics, a minimum of 3 days (72 hours) of empiric treatment are generally required to determine initial efficacy in the absence of worsening of clinical status. During this time, daily assessments should include history and physical examinations, review of laboratory results, assessment of response, and evaluation of any antibiotic-related toxicities. Modification of the initial empiric treatment is based on whether the fever has resolved or is trending toward normal, whether the patient's condition has improved or deteriorated, ANC, and whether an etiologic pathogen or infection site has been identified.[10] Adjustments to empiric antibiotic therapy should be made prior to 3 days if pneumonia or bacteremia is documented or if the patient's condition deteriorates.

Premature withdrawal of antibiotics may predispose these patients to recrudescence of bacterial infection and increase the risk of infection-related morbidity and mortality. In a clinical study, 142 cancer patients with unexplained fever who became afebrile following empiric antibiotics were randomized to continue or discontinue antibiotic therapy after 7 days.[188] The patients whose neutropenia resolved had no infectious sequelae regardless of whether antibiotics were continued or discontinued. For persistently neutropenic patients randomized to continue or discontinue antibiotic therapy until their ANC was >500 cells/mm^3, the percentages of patients remaining febrile without infections complications were 94% and 41%, respectively.

Responding to Initial Therapy

No Etiology Identified

In general, if the fever improves, and the patient is stable or improves following initiation of empiric antibacterials but no identifiable etiology is identified, empiric therapy should be continued for a minimum of 7 days.[3,10] Patients for whom no infection is identified after 3 days of treatment, who are afebrile for 24 hours or more, and who have an ANC of at least 500 cells/mm^3 for 2 consecutive days can be considered for treatment discontinuation.[3] Although it is most desirable that the patient's ANC be at least 500 cells/mm^3 and increasing, discontinuing antibacterials after 7 to 14 days can be considered for stable patients with prolonged neutropenia in the absence of infection, with no disruption in mucous membranes and integument, and in whom no invasive procedures or ablative chemotherapy is planned. Such patients receiving initial parenteral therapy can be considered for switch to oral therapy. Patients at higher risk of infectious complications (ANC <500 cells/mm^3 at day 7 with initially severe neutropenia [ANC <100 cells/mm^3] or mucositis or who are clinically unstable) should continue antibacterial treatment.[3,10]

M.H.'s slow response to empiric ceftazidime suggests that this regimen may be suboptimal. However, it is prudent to wait at least 72 hours to make that assessment in the absence of clinical worsening. If at 72 hours M.H. becomes afebrile and remains so for 5 to 7 days, it would be reasonable to discontinue ceftazidime after 7 days as long as she appears clinically well and has no apparent evidence of infection. Although it is desirable for M.H.'s ANC to be >500 cells/mm^3 before treatment is stopped, therapy may be discontinued before this time as long as she is closely monitored for recurrent fever and/or evidence of new infection.

Etiology Identified

18. On day 3, M.H.'s temperature is normal (97.6°C). However, two sets of blood cultures drawn 3 days ago have grown *S. aureus* resistant to methicillin and susceptible to vancomycin. Her ANC is 170 cells/mm^3. How should therapy be modified in M.H.? For how long should antibiotics be continued?

Pizzo et al. treated 78 neutropenic cancer patients with documented Gram-positive bacteremias with a single drug (e.g., oxacillin, nafcillin) or a broad-spectrum combination regimen that provided Gram-positive coverage (carbenicillin plus cephalothin plus gentamicin).[189] Of the 15 patients treated with pathogen-directed therapy who remained neutropenic for >7 days, 7 developed a secondary infection. In contrast, none of the 24 patients who continued to receive the broad-spectrum combination regimen developed any secondary infections.

In general, the duration of antibiotic therapy for documented infections in the patient responding to therapy should be based on neutrophil recovery, the rapidity of defervescence, site of infection, and pathogen. For patients such as M.H. for whom an infectious cause of fever is identified but who are afebrile at 3 to 5 days, additional antimicrobials or antibiotic dosage adjustments (based on antimicrobial susceptibility tests and antibiotic serum concentrations) may be required[3,10] (Table 68-2). Despite such modifications, broad-spectrum antibacterial coverage should be maintained in patients who remain persistently neutropenic.[3,10] If M.H.'s neutropenia resolves, broad-spectrum antimicrobials may be discontinued, and narrow-spectrum therapy directed against the infecting pathogen should be continued for duration appropriate for that indication. However, because M.H. remains neutropenic, the ceftazidime should be continued for a minimum of 7 days or until her ANC is >500 cells/mm^3. Vancomycin should be added to treat the MRSA bacteremia and should be continued for an appropriate treatment course of 10 to 14 days (assuming an uncomplicated infection).

Nonresponder to Initial Therapy

No Etiology Identified

19. S.B. is a 55-year-old woman with chronic myelogenous leukemia (CML). She was admitted to the hospital with a 4-day history of fevers and night sweats. On admission, her temperature was 102.3°F, and her WBC count was 100,000 cells/mm^3, with an ANC of 500 cells/mm^3. Blood and urine cultures were obtained, and ceftazidime plus tobramycin was empirically started. Over the next 3 days, S.B. remained persistently febrile and neutropenic. All cultures remained negative. How should she be treated?

One of the most challenging and controversial aspects of empiric antibacterial therapy in the neutropenic host is the management of patients without a microbiologically documented infection who remain persistently febrile on broad-spectrum antibacterial therapy. A persistent fever may be due to tumor lysis, an infection caused by resistant bacteria, slow response to appropriate therapy, drug-related fever, superinfection, infections caused by nonbacterial pathogens (e.g., fungi, viruses), inadequate serum or tissue levels of antibiotics, or avascular infection (e.g., abscess). By day 3 following the initiation of empiric antibiotics, S.B. should be reassessed in an attempt to identify any one or more of these causes.[10] A meticulous physical examination and a thorough review of all culture results should be done. If indicated, additional cultures, diagnostic imaging of suspected areas of infection, and serum drug concentrations should be obtained.

Based on the results and reassessment, options for management are to continue the current empiric regimen, change antimicrobials, or add empiric antifungal therapy with or without changes to antibacterial therapy[10] (Table 68-2). Each treatment option is discussed separately.

Guidelines published in 2002 by IDSA suggest that even if fever persists after 5 days, the initial empiric regimen can be continued without modification as long as the patient remains stable and does not clinically deteriorate.[10] This treatment decision arm works best in patients with neutropenia expected to resolve within the subsequent 5 days.[10] Additional consideration should be given to discontinuing vancomycin (if applicable) in the absence of evidence for a Gram-positive infection. Treatments are generally continued for a minimum of 4 to 5 days after the resolution of neutropenia.[10] The need for further antibiotics can then be reassessed. Patients for whom neutropenia does not resolve generally receive at least 2 weeks of therapy, at which time treatment needs can be reassessed.[10]

Modify Initial Antibiotics

20. S.B., on day 4, continues to feel "lousy" and has started to complain of abdominal pains. What is the significance of this complaint? Should her antibiotic regimen be modified again?

In persistently neutropenic patients with evidence of disease progression or who are clinically unstable, the initial empiric regimen is generally modified (Table 68-2). Such evidence may include catheter site drainage, abdominal pain, or pulmonary infiltrates. In such cases (or in the event of drug-related toxicities), consideration should be given to adding antibiotics or changing to a different antibiotic regimen to broaden coverage against resistant organisms. Because S.B. has developed new abdominal pains suggestive of enterocolitis, her antibiotic regimen should be modified. Although cefepime provides excellent coverage against the common Gram-negative pathogens, it has limited activity against select Gram-positive pathogens (e.g., MRSA or VRE) and anaerobes. A change from cefepime to imipenem-cilastatin or another broad-spectrum regimen with both aerobic and anaerobic activity should be considered.

Antifungal Therapy

21. S.B.'s antibiotic regimen was changed to imipenem-cilastatin plus tobramycin. Despite the change, she continues to have a low-grade fever and does not feel better. What is S.B.'s risk for developing a systemic fungal infection? What is the significance of fungal infections in neutropenic cancer patients?

The incidence of invasive fungal infections in febrile neutropenic patients varies between studies due to differences in definitions, methods of detection, specific patient populations studied, and prior use of antifungal prophylaxis.[190] In one retrospective review, the incidence of documented invasive fungal infections in patients with leukemia was 27% (32 of 119).[191] However, the diagnosis of invasive fungal infection was established before death in only nine of the patients. In general, patients with hematologic malignancies have a higher incidence of fungal infections than those with solid tumors.[190] Early diagnosis and prompt treatment of such systemic fungal diseases are critical to patient survival.[190] However, significant challenges exist in making an accurate and timely diagnosis of invasive fungal infections. Therefore, patients with protracted fever and neutropenia for ≥5 days despite the administration of broad-spectrum antibiotics should be considered for empiric antifungal therapy. Recent studies have also indicated the potential to use newer diagnostic tests (e.g., β-D-glucan tests or galactomannan assays), along with additional diagnostic support, to initiate early pre-emptive therapy prior to the development of severe infection.[192]

Most fungal infections in neutropenic cancer patients are caused by *Candida* and *Aspergillus* species.[193–195] Other less common but important pathogenic fungi are those associated with zygomycosis (e.g., *Mucor* and *Rhizopus* species) and other emerging pathogens (non-albicans *Candida, Trichosporon beigelii, Malassezia* species, *Cryptococcus neoformans,* and *Fusarium* species).[193–195]

Table 68-2 Modifications of Initial Empiric Antibacterials in Patients With Neutropenia and Fever

Clinical Condition	*Type of Modification(s)*
Responding within 3–5 days of treatment	
No etiology identified	Low risk: change to ciprofloxacin + amoxicillin-clavulanate (adults) [alternate clindamycin if penicillin allergic] or cefixime (children).
	High risk: continue antibiotic therapy.
Etiology identified	Adjust antibiotics to most appropriate therapy based on infection.
Unresponsive (3–5 days) without clinical or microbiological evidence of infection	Clinically stable: continue antibiotics.
	Unstable: broaden antibacterial coverage to include anaerobes, resistant Gram-negative rods, and resistant Gram-positive organisms.
	Consider empiric antifungal therapy on days 4 and 5, especially if resolution of neutropenia is not imminent and the patient is at high risk of fungal infection.
	If initial regimen did not include vancomycin: re-evaluate risk factors for Gram-positive infection, consider adding vancomycin.
	Consider addition of G-CSF or GM-CSF.
Positive Gram stain	Gram-positive: add vancomycin, pending further identification (especially in blood culture institutions with high rate of methicillin-resistant *S. aureus*).
	Gram-negative: if monotherapy, consider adding aminoglycoside to carbapenem or β-lactam monotherapy.
Documented infection	
Head, eyes, ears, nose, throat	
Necrotizing ulceration/gingivitis	If initial regimen did not include anaerobic therapy (carbapenem or β-lactam/β-lactamase inhibitor; i.e., piperacillin-tazobactam), consider adding clindamycin or metronidazole or switch to carbapenem (imipenem-cilastatin or meropenem).
	Consider adding antifungal (topical or systemic) and/or antiviral therapy.
Oral vesicular lesions	Add antiviral therapy for *Herpes simplex* virus.
Oral thrush	Add topical (e.g., oral clotrimazole, nystatin) or systemic (e.g., fluconazole) antifungal therapy.
Sinus tenderness, periorbital cellulitis, nasal ulceration	Suspicion of mould infection: add amphotericin B preparation or voriconazole; consider combination antifungal.
	Vancomycin for periorbital cellulitis.
	Reassess antistaphylococcal activity of empiric regimen; consider vancomycin.
Gastrointestinal tract	
Esophagitis	Add antifungal agent (see text); if no response, add acyclovir. Assess CMV risk and (if high) consider ganciclovir or foscarnet.
Acute abdominal pain/perianal	If initial regimen did not include carbapenem or β-lactam/β-lactamase inhibitor (i.e., piperacillin-tazobactam), consider adding clindamycin or metronidazole, or switch to imipenem-cilastatin or meropenem. Assure pseudomonal coverage for perirectal infection.
	Consider enterococcal coverage for infection (not colonization).
	Consider antifungal.
Diarrhea	Add metronidazole if *C. difficile* documented or suspected.
	Contact isolation of rotavirus documented.
Liver abnormalities	Consider anaerobic and enterococcal coverage. Antifungal or antiviral therapy added based on results of diagnostic studies.
Respiratory tract	
Interstitial infiltrates	PCP: institute trial of TMP-SMX or (for sulfa-allergic patients) pentamidine.
	Atypical pathogens *(Mycoplasma, Legionella)*. Add fluoroquinolone, macrolide, or doxycycline.
	CMV: add ganciclovir if high risk.
	Consider influenza. Oseltamivir (preferred) or other directed therapies when indicated.
Focal lesion on chest radiograph	If evidence of mould infection, add voriconazole (preferred) or amphotericin B formulations.
	Consider growth factors (G-CSF, GM-CSF).
	Consider antibiotic coverage for pathogen causing atypical pneumonia.
Skin and skin structure infection	
Vesicular lesions	HSV, VZV treatment: acyclovir, famciclovir, or valacyclovir.
Cellulitis, wound infection	Consider adding vancomycin therapy.
Vascular access device infection, tunnel tract infection	Remove catheter. Consider adding empiric vancomycin therapy initially. Adjust based on culture and susceptibility results.
Central nervous system	β-lactam (cefepime, ceftazidime, meropenem [imipenem if meropenem not available, + vancomycin).
	Add ampicillin if concern for *Listeria*.
	Consider high-dose acyclovir.

CMV, cytomegalovirus; G-CSF, granulocyte colony-stimulating factor; GM-CSF, granulocyte-macrophage colony-stimulating factor; HSV, herpes simplex virus; PCP, *Pneumocystis carinii*; TMP-SMX, trimethoprim-sulfamethoxazole; VZV, varicella-zoster virus.
Adapted from references 3 and 10.

It is difficult to compare clinical trials evaluating empiric antibiotic therapy in neutropenic cancer patients due to clinical trial design elements, such as inclusion of low-risk patients, lack of blinding, changes in concomitant antibacterials obscuring antifungal therapy endpoints, prior antifungal prophylaxis, use of composite endpoints of safety and efficacy, and different endpoint criteria.[190] Although select studies have also demonstrated that empiric antifungal therapy can decrease fungal-related deaths, overall mortality has not been affected.[196,197] This is the case particularly for patients with invasive disease and persistent neutropenia.

Considerations regarding the choice of empiric antifungals should include prior or current antifungal prophylaxis, risks of antifungal-related toxicities, drug interactions, route of administration, and costs. Although prompting evaluation, fever alone does not necessarily indicate the need for intervention with an antifungal in stable patients receiving mould-active prophylaxis.

EMPIRIC AMPHOTERICIN B THERAPY

22. Should amphotericin B therapy be considered in S.B.?

Historically, amphotericin B deoxycholate was most commonly used in this setting because of its reliable activity in vitro against most *Candida* and *Aspergillus* species.[16,198,199] Pizzo et al. demonstrated the impact of empiric amphotericin B deoxycholate in persistently febrile neutropenic patients.[200] After 7 days of empiric broad-spectrum antibiotics, 50 patients with unexplained fever, prolonged granulocytopenia, and evidence of GI colonization with *Candida* species were randomized to one of three groups. Patients in group 1 continued to receive broad-spectrum antibiotics, those in group 2 had their antibiotics discontinued, and those in group 3 had amphotericin B added empirically to their antibiotic regimen. Infectious complications (e.g., bacterial or fungal infection, shock) developed in 9 of 16 patients (56%) in group 2 within 3 days of stopping antibiotics. Of the 16 patients in group 1 who continued to receive antibiotics until neutropenia resolved, an infectious complication developed in 6 (38%), 5 of which were caused by fungal infections. In the 18 patients randomized to receive amphotericin B, only 2 patients developed infectious complications. One of these infections in the latter group was caused by an amphotericin B–resistant organism (*P. boydii*).

Comparative trials have evaluated the role of lipid-based formulations of amphotericin B in the treatment of suspected or documented infections in this population.[201–209] Liposomal amphotericin B,[201–203,205] amphotericin B lipid complex,[203] and amphotericin B colloidal dispersion[204] have demonstrated reductions in nephrotoxicity compared to amphotericin B deoxycholate. In addition, liposomal amphotericin B offers the potential for reducing infusion-related side effects.[202] However, efficacy appears comparable between the preparations, and the lipid formulations are substantially more expensive based on acquisition costs. Therefore, their use is often restricted to patients with underlying renal dysfunction or those with significant risk factors for amphotericin B–induced nephrotoxicity. Although there are limited data to suggest that the continuous infusion of amphotericin B deoxycholate may also reduce nephrotoxicity,[210] efficacy regarding this method of administration has not been established and cannot be recommended at this time.

Because of the alternate treatments options currently available, empiric use of amphotericin B products is generally reserved for patients at highest risk of mould infections. When initiated as empiric therapy, amphotericin B administration is often preceded by attempts to minimize nephrotoxicity (e.g., saline loading) and premedications to minimize infusion-related reactions. Close monitoring of tolerability, renal function, and electrolytes is required during administration. When initiated, amphotericin B is generally continued (in the absence of a documented fungal infection) in a clinically stable patient until the resolution of neutropenia. Clinically stable patients without evidence of fungal infection but with persistent neutropenia often receive a 2-week course of therapy. Patients with documented (invasive) fungal infections are treated with variable durations of treatment, depending on the fungal diagnosis.

ALTERNATIVES TO AMPHOTERICIN B

In stable patients at low risk of mould infections with *Aspergillus* and drug-resistant *Candida* species (e.g., *C. krusei* and some strains of *C. glabrata*), fluconazole may be an acceptable empiric alternative to amphotericin B.[211,212] Patients with suspected mould infections (e.g., aspergillosis) or for whom fluconazole was used as prophylaxis should be excluded. Although itraconazole possesses enhanced activity in vitro against *Aspergillus* spp. and has reduced toxicity relative to amphotericin B, issues regarding oral tolerability, potential for cross-resistance with other azoles, and considerations of alternate treatment options limited its usefulness in this situation. Voriconazole (an azole antifungal agent with increased activity against *Aspergillus* and non-albicans *Candida* relative to fluconazole) has also been tested in this population. When compared with liposomal amphotericin B, it failed to meet the pre-established criteria for noninferiority. However, some believe that voriconazole should be considered as an alternative to amphotericin B preparations for empiric therapy in patients requiring initial empiric antifungal therapy and are at increased risk of mould infections (due to receipt of prior azole prophylaxis). Others continue to support the superiority of liposomal amphotericin B for empiric therapy in this population.[213] Because of the increased potential (relative to fluconazole) for drug interactions (including immunosuppressives and chemotherapy) and adverse events (e.g., phototoxicity, hepatotoxicity), voriconazole therapy should be monitored closely.

The echinocandins (e.g., caspofungin, micafungin, anidulafungin) are a class of antifungals with in vitro activity against *Candida* species (including non-albicans *Candida*) and *Aspergillus* species. Caspofungin was found to be at least as effective and better tolerated than liposomal amphotericin B as empiric therapy in this patient population.[214] Because of its safety profile, caspofungin is often considered for patients requiring initial empiric antifungal therapy and who are at increased risk of mould infections (due to receipt of prior azole prophylaxis); it is currently FDA approved for such use. Published experience with other echinocandins (e.g., micafungin, anidulafungin) as empiric therapy in the febrile neutropenic patient is lacking at present.

Antiviral Therapy

Although necrotizing ulceration in the oropharynx, oral vesicular lesions or esophagitis may be symptoms of a viral infection, empiric use of antiviral agents in the febrile neutropenic patient are not indicated without evidence of such disease.[10] In contrast, clinical evidence of *Herpes simplex* or varicella-zoster virus involving the skin or mucous membranes should be treated with antivirals (e.g., acyclovir, valacyclovir, famciclovir).[10] When oral therapy is used, valacyclovir and famciclovir might be favored due to improved oral bioavailability and need for less frequent dosing. With the exception of patients undergoing bone marrow transplantation,[215] CMV is an uncommon source of infection in the febrile neutropenic patient. However, ganciclovir, valganciclovir, foscarnet, or, less commonly, cidofovir treatment should be initiated in patients with documented CMV infections. Likewise, if influenza or RSV is identified, appropriate antiviral therapy should be initiated.

ANTIMICROBIAL ADJUVANTS

23. S.B. became afebrile 2 days after amphotericin B was initiated, yet she remained neutropenic with an ANC of 480 cells/mm^3. An induction chemotherapy regimen consisting of idarubicin plus cytarabine was initiated for her CML. Because the chemotherapy will further reduce her ANC 7 to 10 days after treatment, is there any way to facilitate marrow recovery and reduce the duration of neutropenia in S.B.?

As previously discussed, the duration of neutropenia is the most important factor affecting outcome in neutropenic cancer patients. Because of this, there has been considerable interest in enhancing the immune system in these patients.

Granulocyte Transfusions

One of the earliest approaches used to boost the patient's defense against infections was the transfusion of WBCs. In the 1970s, granulocyte transfusions were used adjunctively in patients with persistent neutropenia and documented infections who, despite appropriate antibiotics, failed to respond after 24 to 48 hours. This approach had limited value because of the difficulties in obtaining adequate cells for transfusion, as well as the problems with alloimmunization and risk of infection transmission. In addition, the questionable efficacy of WBC transfusions has decreased the use of this strategy.[216] Therefore, granulocyte transfusions are not routinely indicated in this population. However, patients with progressive bacterial or fungal infections unresponsive to appropriate antimicrobial therapy may be considered as candidates.[3]

Hematopoietic Growth Factors

The introduction of hematopoietic colony-stimulating factors (CSFs) such as G-CSF (filgrastim), pegylated G-CSF (pegfilgrastim), or GM-CSF (sargramostim) in clinical practice has raised the hopes of improving survival in cancer patients.[217] CSFs act on various stages of cell proliferation and differentiation in the bone marrow (see Chapter 89). Studies in cancer patients receiving myelosuppressive or myeloablative chemotherapy have demonstrated that concurrent use of the CSFs can reduce the duration of neutropenia.[217] Rash, bone pain, headache, fever, and myalgias have been reported as side effects with both G-CSF and GM-CSF.[217] Bone pain is usually mild to moderate and often responds to nonopiate analgesics (acetaminophen or ibuprofen). The pain usually resolves on discontinuation. A flu-like syndrome consisting of fever, chills, rigors, headache, and GI symptoms has been reported in many patients receiving GM-CSF.[217] The selection of one CSF agent over another is often based on practitioner preference rather than clinical data.

Because these agents have not demonstrated a consistent and significant effect on other infection-related parameters (e.g., duration of fever, use of antibiotics, costs of treatment),[217] routine use of CSFs as adjunctive therapy to antibiotics for febrile neutropenic patients should be avoided. However, patients with high risks for infection-related complications may be considered.[3] Such risks include expected prolonged (>10 days) and profound (<100 cells/mm^3) neutropenia, age older than 65 years, uncontrolled malignancy, pneumonia, hypotension and multiorgan dysfunction (characteristic of sepsis syndrome), and invasive fungal infection.

Immunoglobulins

Data regarding the use of immunoglobulins as adjunctive therapy for the treatment of select infections in the neutropenic cancer patient is primarily limited to case reports. Patients with pneumonia secondary to CMV may benefit from adjunctive immunoglobulin therapy. In addition, IV immunoglobulin G should be considered in those patients with hypogamaglobulinemia.[3]

Summary

G-CSF administration, although likely to reduce the duration of her chemotherapy-induced neutropenia, is not indicated in S.B., who is otherwise stable.

REFERENCES

1. Bow EJ. Management of the febrile neutropenic cancer patient: lessons from 40 years of study. *Clin Microbiol Infect* 2005;11(Suppl 5):24.
2. Bodey G. Quantitative relationships between circulating leukocytes and infection in patients with acute leukemia. *Ann Intern Med* 1966;64:328.
3. National Comprehensive Cancer Network (NCCN). Fever and neutropenia (FEV-1). In: *NCCN Clinical Practice Guidelines in Oncology: Prevention and Treatment of Cancer-Related Infections, V.1.2007*. Available at: www.nccn.org/professionals/physician_gls/PDF/fever.pdf. Accessed August 13, 2007.
4. Viscoli C, Castagnola E. Treatment of febrile neutropenia: what is new? *Curr Opin Infect Dis* 2002;15:377.
5. Stuck AE et al. Risk of infectious complications in patients taking glucocorticosteroids. *Rev Infect Dis* 1989;11:954.
6. Segal BH et al. Antibacterial prophylaxis in patients with neutropenia. *J Natl Comprehensive Cancer Network* 2007;5:235.
7. Neuburger S, Maschmeyer G. Update on management of infections in cancer and stem cell transplant patients. *Ann Hematol* 2006;85:345.
8. Dykewicz CA, Centers for Disease Control and Prevention, Infectious Diseases Society of America, and American Society of Blood and Marrow Transplantation. Summary of the guidelines for preventing opportunistic infections among hematopoietic stem cell transplant recipients. *Clin Infect Dis* 2001;33:139.
9. Barton TD, Schuster MG. The cause of fever following resolution of neutropenia in patients with acute leukemia. *Clin Infect Dis* 1996;22:1064.
10. Hughes WT et al. 2002 Guidelines for the use of antimicrobial agents in neutropenic patients with cancer. *Clin Infect Dis* 2002;34:730.
11. Coullioud D et al. Prospective multicentric study of the etiology of 1051 bacteremic episodes in 782 cancer patients. CEMIC (French-Belgian Study

Club of Infectious Diseases in Cancer). *Support Care Cancer* 1993;1:34.
12. Cordonnier C et al. Epidemiology and risk factors for gram-positive coccal infections in neutropenia: toward a more targeted antibiotic strategy. *Clin Infect Dis* 2003;36:149.
13. Zinner SH. Changing epidemiology of infections in patients with neutropenia and cancer: emphasis on gram-positive and resistant bacteria. *Clin Infect Dis* 1999;29:490.
14. Ramphal R. Changes in the etiology of bacteremia in febrile neutropenic patients and the susceptibilities of the currently isolated pathogens. *Clin Infect Dis* 2004;39:S25.
15. Mathur P et al. A study of bacteremia in febrile neutropenic patients at a tertiary-care hospital with special reference to anaerobes. *Med Oncol* 2002;19:267.
16. Wingard JR. Empirical antifungal therapy in treating febrile neutropenic patients. *Clin Infect Dis* 2004;39:S38.
17. Cruciani M. Antibacterial prophylaxis. *Int J Antimicrob Agents* 2000;16:123.
18. EORTC International Antimicrobial Therapy Project Group. Trimethoprim-sulfamethoxazole in the prevention of infection in neutropenic patients. *J Infect Dis* 1984;150:372.
19. Hughes WT et al. Successful intermittent chemoprophylaxis for *Pneumocystis carinii* pneumonitis. *N Engl J Med* 1987;316:1627.
20. Wade JC et al. A comparison of trimethoprim-sulfamethoxazole plus nystatin with gentamicin plus nystatin in the prevention of infections in acute leukemia. *N Engl J Med* 1981;304:1057.
21. Bow EJ et al. Quinolone-based antibacterial chemoprophylaxis in neutropenic patients: effect of augmented gram-positive activity on infectious morbidity. National Cancer Institute of Canada Clinical Trials Group. *Ann Intern Med* 1996;125:183.
22. Gafter-Gvili A et al. Effect of quinolone prophylaxis in afebrile neutropenic patients on microbial resistance: systematic review and meta-analysis. *J Antimicrob Chemother* 2007;59:5.
23. Engels EA et al. Efficacy of quinolone prophylaxis in neutropenic cancer patients: a meta-analysis. *J Clin Oncol* 1998;16:1179.
24. Gafter-Gvili A, Fraser A, Paul M, Leibovici L. Meta-analysis: antibiotic prophylaxis reduces mortality in neutropenic patients. *Ann Intern Med* 2005; 142:979.
25. Horvathova Z et al. Bacteremia due to methicillin-resistant staphylococci occurs more frequently in neutropenic patients who received antimicrobial prophylaxis and is associated with higher mortality in comparison to methicillin-sensitive bacteremia. *Int J Antimicrob Agents* 1998;10:55.
26. Oppenheim BA et al. Outbreak of coagulase negative staphylococcus highly resistant to ciprofloxacin in a leukaemia unit. *Br Med J* 1989;299:294.
27. Carratala J et al. Emergence of quinolone-resistant *Escherichia coli* bacteremia in neutropenic patients with cancer who have received prophylactic norfloxacin. *Clin Infect Dis* 1995;20:557.
28. Schimpff SC et al. Infection prevention in acute nonlymphocytic leukemia: laminar air flow room reverse isolation with oral, nonabsorbable antibiotic prophylaxis. *Ann Intern Med* 1975;82:351.
29. Young GA et al. A double-blind comparison of fluconazole and nystatin in the prevention of candidiasis in patients with leukaemia. Antifungal Prophylaxis Study Group. *Eur J Cancer* 1999;35:1208.
30. Owens NJ et al. Prophylaxis of oral candidiasis with clotrimazole troches. *Arch Intern Med* 1984; 144:290.
31. Akiyama H et al. Fluconazole versus oral amphotericin B in preventing fungal infection in chemotherapy-induced neutropenic patients with haematological malignancies. *Mycoses* 1993;36: 373.
32. Nucci M et al. A double-blind, randomized, placebo-controlled trial of itraconazole capsules as antifungal prophylaxis for neutropenic patients. *Clin Infect Dis* 2000;30:300.
33. Menichetti F et al. Itraconazole oral solution as prophylaxis for fungal infections in neutropenic patients with hematologic malignancies: a randomized, placebo-controlled, double-blind, multicenter trial. GIMEMA Infection Program. Gruppo Italiano Malattie Ematologiche dell'Adulto. *Clin Infect Dis* 1999;28:250.
34. Harousseau JL et al. Itraconazole oral solution for primary prophylaxis of fungal infections in patients with hematological malignancy and profound neutropenia: a randomized, double-blind, double-placebo, multicenter trial comparing itraconazole and amphotericin B. *Antimicrob Agents Chemother* 2000;44:1887.
35. Chandrasekar PH, Gatny CM. Effect of fluconazole prophylaxis on fever and use of amphotericin in neutropenic cancer patients. Bone Marrow Transplantation Team. *Chemotherapy* 1994;40:136.
36. Goodman JL et al. A controlled trial of fluconazole to prevent fungal infections in patients undergoing bone marrow transplantation. *N Engl J Med* 1992;326:845.
37. Ellis ME et al. Controlled study of fluconazole in the prevention of fungal infections in neutropenic patients with haematological malignancies and bone marrow transplant recipients. *Eur J Clin Microbiol Infect Dis* 1994;13:3.
38. Winston DJ et al. Fluconazole prophylaxis of fungal infections in patients with acute leukemia: results of a randomized placebo-controlled, double-blind, multicenter trial. *Ann Intern Med* 1993;118:495.
39. Safdar A et al. Hematogenous infections due to *Candida parapsilosis:* changing trends in fungemic patients at a comprehensive cancer center during the last four decades. *Eur J Clin Microbiol Infect Dis* 2002;44:11.
40. Gotzsche PC, Johansen HK. Routine versus selective antifungal administration for control of fungal infections in patients with cancer. *Cochrane Database Syst Rev* 2002;CD000026.
41. Winston DJM. Intravenous and oral itraconazole versus intravenous and oral fluconazole for long-term antifungal prophylaxis in allogeneic hematopoietic stem-cell transplant recipients: a multicenter, randomized trial. *Ann Intern Med* 2003;138:705.
42. Marr KA et al. Itraconazole versus fluconazole for prevention of fungal infections in patients receiving allogeneic stem cell transplants. *Blood* 2004;103:1527.
43. Bodey GP et al. Antifungal prophylaxis during remission induction therapy for acute leukemia fluconazole versus intravenous amphotericin B. *Cancer* 1994;73:2099.
44. Mattiuzzi GN et al. Liposomal amphotericin B versus the combination of fluconazole and itraconazole as prophylaxis for invasive fungal infections during induction chemotherapy for patients with acute myelogenous leukemia and myelodysplastic syndrome. *Cancer* 2003;97:450.
45. van Burik JA et al. Micafungin versus fluconazole for prophylaxis against invasive fungal infections during neutropenia in patients undergoing hematopoietic stem cell transplantation. *Clin Infect Dis* 2004;39:1407.
46. Cornely OA et al. Posaconazole vs. fluconazole or itraconazole prophylaxis in patients with neutropenia. *N Engl J Med* 2007;356:348.
47. Ullmann AJ et al. Posaconazole or fluconazole for prophylaxis in severe graft-versus-host disease. *N Engl J Med* 2007;356:335.
48. Smith TJ et al. 2006 Update of recommendations for the use of white blood cell growth factors: an evidence-based clinical practice guideline. *J Clin Oncol* 2006;24:3187.
49. Aapro MS et al. EORTC guidelines for the use of granulocyte-colony stimulating factor to reduce the incidence of chemotherapy-induced febrile neutropenia in adult patients with lymphomas and solid tumours. *Eur J Cancer* 2006;42:2433.
50. Feld R et al. Methodology for clinical trials involving patients with cancer who have febrile neutropenia: updated guidelines of the Immunocompromised Host Society/Multinational Association for Supportive Care in Cancer, with emphasis on outpatient studies. *Clin Infect Dis* 2002;35:1463.
51. Bodey GP. Unusual presentations of infection in neutropenic patients. *Int J Antimicrob Agents* 2000;16:93.
52. Malik I et al. Clinical characteristics and therapeutic outcome of patients with febrile neutropenia who present in shock: need for better strategies. *J Infect* 2001;42:120.
53. Dompeling EC et al. Evolution of the clinical manifestations of infection during the course of febrile neutropenia in patients with malignancy. *Infection* 1998;26:349.
54. Fainstein V et al. Patterns of oropharyngeal and fecal flora in patients with acute leukemia. *J Infect Dis* 1981;144:10.
55. Kurrle E et al. Risk factors for infections of the oropharynx and the respiratory tract in patients with acute leukemia. *J Infect Dis* 1981;144:128.
56. Schimpff SC et al. Significance of *Pseudomonas aeruginosa* in the patient with leukemia or lymphoma. *J Infect Dis* 1974;130(Suppl):S24.
57. de Jong PJ et al. The value of surveillance cultures in neutropenic patients receiving selective intestinal decontamination. *Scand J Infect Dis* 1993;25:107.
58. Hathorn JW, Lyke K. Empirical treatment of febrile neutropenia: evolution of current therapeutic approaches. *Clin Infect Dis* 1997;24(Suppl 2):S256.
59. Castagnola E et al. Clinical and laboratory features predicting a favorable outcome and allowing early discharge in cancer patients with low-risk febrile neutropenia: a literature review. *J Hematother Stem Cell Res* 2000;9:645.
60. Koh A, Pizzo PA. Empirical oral antibiotic therapy for low-risk febrile cancer patients with neutropenia. *Cancer Invest* 2002;20:420.
61. Klastersky J et al. The Multinational Association for Supportive Care in Cancer risk index: a multinational scoring system for identifying low-risk febrile neutropenic cancer patients. *J Clin Oncol* 2000;18:3038.
62. Freifeld A et al. A double-blind comparison of empirical oral and intravenous antibiotic therapy for low-risk febrile patients with neutropenia during cancer chemotherapy. *N Engl J Med* 1999;341:305.
63. Kern WV et al. Oral versus intravenous empirical antimicrobial therapy for fever in patients with granulocytopenia who are receiving cancer chemotherapy. International Antimicrobial Therapy Cooperative Group of the European Organization for Research and Treatment of Cancer. *N Engl J Med* 1999;341:312.
64. Paganini HR et al. Oral administration of cefixime to lower risk febrile neutropenic children with cancer. *Cancer* 2000;88:2848.
65. Jacobs RF et al. Ceftazidime versus ceftazidime plus tobramycin in febrile neutropenic children. *Infection* 1993;21:223.
66. Mustafa MM et al. Comparative study of cefepime versus ceftazidime in the empiric treatment of pediatric cancer patients with fever and neutropenia. *Pediatr Infect Dis J* 2001;20:362.
67. Chuang YY et al. Cefepime versus ceftazidime as empiric monotherapy for fever and neutropenia in children with cancer. *Pediatr Infect Dis J* 2002;21:203.
68. Fleischhack G et al. Meropenem versus ceftazidime as empirical monotherapy in febrile neutropenia of paediatric patients with cancer. *J Antimicrob Chemother* 2001;47:841.
69. Kebudi R et al. Randomized comparison of cefepime versus ceftazidime monotherapy for fever and neutropenia in children with solid tumors. *Med Pediatr Oncol* 2001;36:434.
70. Feld R et al. Meropenem versus ceftazidime in the treatment of cancer patients with febrile neutropenia: a randomized, double-blind trial. *J Clin Oncol* 2000;18:3690.
71. Chandrasekar PH, Arnow PM. Cefepime versus ceftazidime as empiric therapy for fever in neutropenic patients with cancer. *Ann Pharmacother* 2000;34:989.

72. Wang FD et al. A comparative study of cefepime versus ceftazidime as empiric therapy of febrile episodes in neutropenic patients. *Chemotherapy* 1999;45:370.
73. Antabli BA et al. Empiric antimicrobial therapy of febrile neutropenic patients undergoing haematopoietic stem cell transplantation. *Int J Antimicrob Agents* 1999;13:127.
74. Lindblad R et al. Empiric monotherapy for febrile neutropenia: a randomized study comparing meropenem with ceftazidime. *Scand J Infect Dis* 1998;30:237.
75. Aparicio J et al. Randomized comparison of ceftazidime and imipenem as initial monotherapy for febrile episodes in neutropenic cancer patients. *Eur J Cancer* 1996;32A:1739.
76. Equivalent efficacies of meropenem and ceftazidime as empirical monotherapy of febrile neutropenic patients. The Meropenem Study Group of Leuven, London and Nijmegen. *J Antimicrobial Chemother* 1995;36:185.
77. Freifeld AG et al. Monotherapy for fever and neutropenia in cancer patients: a randomized comparison of ceftazidime versus imipenem. *J Clin Oncol* 1995;13:165.
78. De Pauw BE et al. Ceftazidime compared with piperacillin and tobramycin for the empiric treatment of fever in neutropenic patients with cancer: a multicenter randomized trial. The Intercontinental Antimicrobial Study Group. *Ann Intern Med* 1994;120:834.
79. Miller JA et al. Efficacy and tolerability of imipenem-cilastatin versus ceftazidime plus tobramycin as empiric therapy of presumed bacterial infection in neutropenic cancer patients. *Clin Ther* 1993;15:486.
80. Vancomycin added to empirical combination antibiotic therapy for fever in granulocytopenic cancer patients. European Organization for Research and Treatment of Cancer (EORTC) International Antimicrobial Therapy Cooperative Group and the National Cancer Institute of Canada–Clinical Trials Group. *J Infect Dis* 1991;163:951.
81. Rubin M et al. Gram-positive infections and the use of vancomycin in 550 episodes of fever and neutropenia. *Ann Intern Med* 1988;108:30.
82. Ariffin H et al. Ceftazidime-resistant *Klebsiella pneumoniae* bloodstream infection in children with febrile neutropenia. *Int J Infect Dis* 2000;4:21.
83. Fanci R et al. Management of fever in neutropenic patients with acute leukemia: current role of ceftazidime plus amikacin as empiric therapy. *J Chemother* 2000;12:232.
84. Cunha BA, Gill MV. Cefepime. *Med Clin North Am* 1995;79:721.
85. Kennedy HF et al. Antimicrobial susceptibility of blood culture isolates of viridans streptococci: relationship to a change in empirical antibiotic therapy in febrile neutropenia. *J Antimicrob Chemother* 2001;47:693.
86. Biron P et al. Cefepime versus imipenem-cilastatin as empirical monotherapy in 400 febrile patients with short duration neutropenia. CEMIC (Study Group of Infectious Diseases in Cancer). *J Antimicrob Chemother* 1998;42:511.
87. Bohme A et al. Piperacillin/tazobactam versus cefepime as initial empirical antimicrobial therapy in febrile neutropenic patients: a prospective randomized pilot study. *Eur J Med Res* 1998;3:324.
88. Borbolla JR et al. Comparison of cefepime versus ceftriaxone-amikacin as empirical regimens for the treatment of febrile neutropenia in acute leukemia patients. *Chemotherapy* 2001;47:381.
89. Engervall P et al. Cefepime as empirical monotherapy in febrile patients with hematological malignancies and neutropenia: a randomized, single-center phase II trial. *J Chemother* 1999;11:278.
90. Jandula BM et al. Treatment of febrile neutropenia with cefepime monotherapy. *Chemotherapy* 2001;47:226.
91. Montalar JS. Cefepime monotherapy as an empirical initial treatment of patients with febrile neutropenia. *Med Oncol* 2002;19:161.
92. Tamura K et al. Cefepime or carbapenem treatment for febrile neutropenia as a single agent is as effective as a combination of 4th-generation cephalosporin plus aminoglycosides: comparative study. *Am J Hematol* 2002;71:248.
93. Yamamura D et al. Open randomized study of cefepime versus piperacillin-gentamicin for treatment of febrile neutropenic cancer patients. *Antimicrob Agents Chemother* 1997;41:1704.
94. Au E et al. Randomised study comparing imipenem/cilastatin to ceftriaxone plus gentamicin in cancer chemotherapy-induced neutropenic fever. *Ann Acad Med Singapore* 1994;23:819.
95. Bodey G et al. Imipenem or cefoperazone-sulbactam combined with vancomycin for therapy of presumed or proven infection in neutropenic cancer patients. *Eur J Clin Microbiol Infect Dis* 1996;15:625.
96. Bohme A et al. A randomized study of imipenem compared to cefotaxime plus piperacillin as initial therapy of infections in granulocytopenic patients. *Infection* 1995;23:349.
97. Bohme A et al. Prospective randomized study to compare imipenem 1.5 grams per day vs. 3.0 grams per day in infections of granulocytopenic patients. *J Infect* 1998;36:35.
98. Erjavec Z et al. Comparison of imipenem versus cefuroxime plus tobramycin as empirical therapy for febrile granulocytopenic patients and efficacy of vancomycin and aztreonam in case of failure. *Scand J Infect Dis* 1994;26:585.
99. Kojima A et al. A randomized prospective study of imipenem-cilastatin with or without amikacin as an empirical antibiotic treatment for febrile neutropenic patients. *Am J Clin Oncol* 1994;17:400.
100. Marra F et al. Piperacillin/tazobactam versus imipenem: a double-blind, randomized formulary feasibility study at a major teaching hospital. *Eur J Clin Microbiol Infect Dis* 1998;31:355.
101. Ozyilkan O et al. Imipenem-cilastatin versus sulbactam-cefoperazone plus amikacin in the initial treatment of febrile neutropenic cancer patients. *Korean J Intern Med* 1999;14:15.
102. Shah PM et al. Empirical monotherapy with meropenem versus imipenem/cilastatin for febrile episodes in neutropenic patients. *Infection* 1996; 24:480.
103. Rolston KV et al. A comparison of imipenem to ceftazidime with or without amikacin as empiric therapy in febrile neutropenic patients. *Arch Intern Med* 1992;152:283.
104. Akova M et al. Comparison of meropenem with amikacin plus ceftazidime in the empirical treatment of febrile neutropenia: a prospective randomised multicentre trial in patients without previous prophylactic antibiotics. Meropenem Study Group of Turkey. *Int J Antimicrob Agents* 1999; 13:15.
105. Behre G et al. Meropenem monotherapy versus combination therapy with ceftazidime and amikacin for empirical treatment of febrile neutropenic patients. *Ann Hematol* 1998;76:73.
106. Cometta A et al. Monotherapy with meropenem versus combination therapy with ceftazidime plus amikacin as empiric therapy for fever in granulocytopenic patients with cancer. The International Antimicrobial Therapy Cooperative Group of the European Organization for Research and Treatment of Cancer and the Gruppo Italiano Malattie Ematologiche Maligne dell'Adulto Infection Program. *Antimicrob Agents Chemother* 1996;40:1108.
107. Duzova A et al. Monotherapy with meropenem versus combination therapy with piperacillin plus amikacin as empiric therapy for neutropenic fever in children with lymphoma and solid tumors. *Turk J Pediatr* 2001;43:105.
108. Vandercam B et al. Meropenem versus ceftazidime as empirical monotherapy for febrile neutropenic cancer patients. *Ann Hematol* 2000;79:152.
109. Cunha BA. Ertapenem. A review of its microbiologic, pharmacokinetic and clinical aspects. *Drugs Today* 2002;38:195.
110. Raad II et al. How should imipenem-cilastatin be used in the treatment of fever and infection in neutropenic cancer patients? *Cancer* 1998;82:2449.
111. Cometta A, Glauser MP. Empiric antibiotic monotherapy with carbapenems in febrile neutropenia: a review. *J Chemother* 1996;8:375.
112. Asbel LE, Levison ME. Cephalosporins, carbapenems, and monobactams. *Infect Dis Clin North Am* 2000;14:435.
113. Fishman A et al. Aztreonam plus piperacillin: empiric treatment of neutropenic fever in gynecology-oncology patients receiving cisplatin-based chemotherapy. *Eur J Gynaecol Oncol* 1998;19:126.
114. Raad II et al. A comparison of aztreonam plus vancomycin and imipenem plus vancomycin as initial therapy for febrile neutropenic cancer patients. *Cancer* 1996;77:1386.
115. Johnson DM et al. Potency and antimicrobial spectrum update for piperacillin/tazobactam (2000): emphasis on its activity against resistant organism populations and generally untested species causing community-acquired respiratory tract infections. *Eur J Clin Microbiol Infect Dis* 2002;43:49.
116. Livermore DM. Multiple mechanisms of antimicrobial resistance in *Pseudomonas aeruginosa:* our worst nightmare? *Clin Infect Dis* 2002;34:634.
117. Giamarellou H et al. Monotherapy with intravenous followed by oral high-dose ciprofloxacin versus combination therapy with ceftazidime plus amikacin as initial empiric therapy for granulocytopenic patients with fever. *Antimicrob Agents Chemother* 2000;44:3264.
118. Marra CA et al. A new ciprofloxacin stepdown program in the treatment of high-risk febrile neutropenia: a clinical and economic analysis. *Pharmacotherapy* 2000;20:931.
119. Petrilli AS et al. Oral ciprofloxacin vs. intravenous ceftriaxone administered in an outpatient setting for fever and neutropenia in low-risk pediatric oncology patients: randomized prospective trial. *Med Pediatr Oncol* 2000;34:87.
120. Meunier F et al. Prospective randomized evaluation of ciprofloxacin versus piperacillin plus amikacin for empiric antibiotic therapy of febrile granulocytopenic cancer patients with lymphomas and solid tumors. The European Organization for Research on Treatment of Cancer International Antimicrobial Therapy Cooperative Group. *Antimicrob Agents Chemother* 1991;35:873.
121. Johnson PR et al. A randomized trial of high-dose ciprofloxacin versus azlocillin and netilmicin in the empirical therapy of febrile neutropenic patients. *J Antimicrob Chemother* 1992;30:203.
122. Griggs JJ et al. Ciprofloxacin plus piperacillin is an equally effective regimen for empiric therapy in febrile neutropenic patients compared with standard therapy. *Am J Hematol* 1998;58:293.
123. Peacock JE et al. Ciprofloxacin plus piperacillin compared with tobramycin plus piperacillin as empirical therapy in febrile neutropenic patients: a randomized, double-blind trial. *Ann Intern Med* 2002;137:77.
124. Flaherty JP et al. Multicenter, randomized trial of ciprofloxacin plus azlocillin versus ceftazidime plus amikacin for empiric treatment of febrile neutropenic patients. *Am J Med* 1989;87:278S.
125. Chan CC et al. Randomized trial comparing ciprofloxacin plus netilmicin versus piperacillin plus netilmicin for empiric treatment of fever in neutropenic patients. *Antimicrob Agents Chemother* 1989;33:87.
126. Bauduer F et al. A randomized prospective multicentre trial of cefpirome versus piperacillin-tazobactam in febrile neutropenia. *Leuk Lymphoma* 2001;42:379.
127. Del Favero A et al. A multicenter, double-blind, placebo-controlled trial comparing piperacillin-tazobactam with and without amikacin as empiric therapy for febrile neutropenia. *Clin Infect Dis* 2001;33:1295.
128. Hazel DL et al. Piperacillin-tazobactam as empiric monotherapy in febrile neutropenic patients with haematological malignancies. *J Chemother* 1997;9:267.

129. Hess U et al. Monotherapy with piperacillin/tazobactam versus combination therapy with ceftazidime plus amikacin as an empiric therapy for fever in neutropenic cancer patients. *Support Care Cancer* 1998;6:402.
130. Viscoli C et al. Piperacillin-tazobactam monotherapy in high-risk febrile and neutropenic cancer patients. *Clin Microbiol Infect* 2006;12:212.
131. Bow EJ et al. A randomized, open-label, multicenter comparative study of the efficacy and safety of piperacillin-tazobactam and cefepime for the empirical treatment of febrile neutropenic episodes in patients with hematologic malignancies. *Clin Infect Dis* 2006;43:447.
132. Corapcioglu F et al. Monotherapy with piperacillin/tazobactam versus cefepime as empirical therapy for febrile neutropenia in pediatric cancer patients: a randomized comparison. *Pediatr Hematol Oncol* 2006;23:177.
133. Klastersky J et al. Significance of antimicrobial synergism for the outcome of gram negative sepsis. *Am J Med Sci* 1977;273:157.
134. De Jongh CA et al. Antibiotic synergism and response in gram-negative bacteremia in granulocytopenic cancer patients. *Am J Med* 1986;80:96.
135. Ariffin H et al. Single-daily ceftriaxone plus amikacin versus thrice-daily ceftazidime plus amikacin as empirical treatment of febrile neutropenia in children with cancer. *J Pediatr Child Health* 2001;37:38.
136. Bosi A et al. An open evaluation of triple antibiotic therapy including vancomycin for febrile bone marrow transplant recipients with severe neutropenia. *J Chemother* 1999;11:287.
137. Charnas R et al. Once daily ceftriaxone plus amikacin vs. three times daily ceftazidime plus amikacin for treatment of febrile neutropenic children with cancer. Writing Committee for the International Collaboration on Antimicrobial Treatment of Febrile Neutropenia in Children. *Pediatr Infect Dis J* 1997;16:346.
138. Cordonnier C et al. Cefepime/amikacin versus ceftazidime/amikacin as empirical therapy for febrile episodes in neutropenic patients: a comparative study. The French Cefepime Study Group. *Clin Infect Dis* 1997;24:41.
139. Erman M et al. Comparison of cefepime and ceftazidime in combination with amikacin in the empirical treatment of high-risk patients with febrile neutropenia: a prospective, randomized, multicenter study. *Scand J Infect Dis* 2001;33:827.
140. Gibson J et al. A randomised dosage study of ceftazidime with single daily tobramycin for the empirical management of febrile neutropenia in patients with hematological diseases. *Int J Hematol* 1994;60:119.
141. Hoffken G et al. An open, randomized, multicentre study comparing the use of low-dose ceftazidime or cefotaxime, both in combination with netilmicin, in febrile neutropenic patients. German Multicentre Study Group. *J Antimicrob Chemother* 1999;44:367.
142. Laszlo D et al. Randomized trial comparing netilmicin plus imipenem-cilastatin versus netilmicin plus ceftazidime as empiric therapy for febrile neutropenic bone marrow transplant recipients. *J Chemother* 1997;9:95.
143. Marie JP et al. Piperacillin/tazobactam plus tobramycin versus ceftazidime plus tobramycin as empiric therapy for fever in severely neutropenic patients. *Support Care Cancer* 1999;7:89.
144. Nucci M et al. Ceftazidime plus amikacin plus teicoplanin or vancomycin in the empirical antibiotic therapy in febrile neutropenic cancer patients. *Oncol Rep* 1998;5:1205.
145. Pizzo PA et al. A randomized trial comparing ceftazidime alone with combination antibiotic therapy in cancer patients with fever and neutropenia. *N Engl J Med* 1986;315:552.
146. Rossini F et al. Amikacin and ceftazidime as empirical antibiotic therapy in severely neutropenic patients: analysis of prognostic factors. *Support Care Cancer* 1994;2:259.
147. Cornely OA et al. A randomized monocentric trial in febrile neutropenic patients: ceftriaxone and gentamicin vs cefepime and gentamicin. *Ann Hematol* 2002;81:37.
148. Sanz MA et al. Cefepime plus amikacin versus piperacillin-tazobactam plus amikacin for initial antibiotic therapy in haematology patients with febrile neutropenia: results of an open, randomized, multicentre trial. *J Antimicrob Chemother* 2002;50:79.
149. Ceftazidime combined with a short or long course of amikacin for empirical therapy of gram-negative bacteremia in cancer patients with granulocytopenia. The EORTC International Antimicrobial Therapy Cooperative Group. *N Engl J Med* 1987;317:1692.
150. Furno P et al. Monotherapy or aminoglycoside-containing combinations for empirical antibiotic treatment of febrile neutropenic patients: a meta-analysis. *Lancet Infect Dis* 2002;2:231.
151. Paul M et al. Beta-lactam versus beta-lactam-aminoglycoside combination therapy in cancer patients with neutropaenia. *Cochrane Database Syst Rev* 2002;CD003038.
152. Winston DJ et al. Moxalactam plus piperacillin versus moxalactam plus amikacin in febrile granulocytopenic patients. *Am J Med* 1984;77:442.
153. Feld R. Vancomycin as part of initial empirical antibiotic therapy for febrile neutropenia in patients with cancer: pros and cons. *Clin Infect Dis* 1999;29:503.
154. Shenep JL et al. Vancomycin, ticarcillin, and amikacin compared with ticarcillin-clavulanate and amikacin in the empirical treatment of febrile, neutropenic children with cancer. *N Engl J Med* 1988;319:1053.
155. Karp JE et al. Empiric use of vancomycin during prolonged treatment-induced granulocytopenia: randomized, double-blind, placebo-controlled clinical trial in patients with acute leukemia. *Am J Med* 1986;81:237.
156. Kramer BS et al. Randomized comparison between two ceftazidime-containing regimens and cephalothin-gentamicin-carbenicillin in febrile granulocytopenic cancer patients. *Antimicrob Agents Chemother* 1986;30:64.
157. Dompeling EC et al. Early identification of neutropenic patients at risk of gram-positive bacteraemia and the impact of empirical administration of vancomycin. *Eur J Cancer* 1996;32A:1332.
158. Koya R et al. Analysis of the value of empiric vancomycin administration in febrile neutropenia occurring after autologous peripheral blood stem cell transplants. *Bone Marrow Transplant* 1998;21:923.
159. Granowetter L et al. Ceftazidime with or without vancomycin vs. cephalothin, carbenicillin and gentamicin as the initial therapy of the febrile neutropenic pediatric cancer patient. *Pediatr Infect Dis J* 1988;7:165.
160. Shenep JL. Viridans-group streptococcal infections in immunocompromised hosts. *Int J Antimicrob Agents* 2000;14:129.
161. Kennedy HF et al. Antimicrobial susceptibility of blood culture isolates of viridans streptococci: relationship to a change in empirical antibiotic therapy in febrile neutropenia. *J Antimicrob Chemother* 2001;47:693.
162. Paul M et al. Additional anti-gram-positive antibiotic treatment for febrile neutropenic cancer patients. *Cochrane Database Syst Rev* 2005;CD003914.
163. Adcock KG et al. Evaluation of empiric vancomycin therapy in children with fever and neutropenia. *Pharmacotherapy* 1999;19:1315.
164. Blijlevens NM et al. Empirical therapy of febrile neutropenic patients with mucositis: challenge of risk-based therapy. *Clin Microbiol Infect* 2001;7(Suppl 4):47.
165. Razonable RR et al. Bacteremia due to viridans group streptococci with diminished susceptibility to levofloxacin among neutropenic patients receiving levofloxacin prophylaxis. *Clin Infect Dis* 2002;34:1469.
166. Rybak MJ et al. Prospective evaluation of the effect of an aminoglycoside dosing regimen on rates of observed nephrotoxicity and ototoxicity. *Antimicrob Agents Chemother* 1999;43:1549.
167. Eliopoulos GM. Quinupristin-dalfopristin and linezolid: evidence and opinion. *Clin Infect Dis* 2003;36:473.
168. Jaksic B et al. Efficacy and safety of linezolid compared with vancomycin in a randomized, double-blind study of febrile neutropenic patients with cancer. *Clin Infect Dis* 2006;42:597-607.
169. Craig WA. Does the dose matter? *Clin Infect Dis* 2001;33(Suppl 3):S233.
170. Dalle JH et al. Continuous infusion of ceftazidime in the empiric treatment of febrile neutropenic children with cancer. *J Pediatr Hematol Oncol* 2002;24:714.
171. Egerer G et al. Efficacy of continuous infusion of ceftazidime for patients with neutropenic fever after high-dose chemotherapy and peripheral blood stem cell transplantation. *Int J Antimicrob Agents* 2000;15:119.
172. Marshall E et al. Low-dose continuous-infusion ceftazidime monotherapy in low-risk febrile neutropenic patients. *Support Care Cancer* 2000;8:198.
173. Bodey GP et al. The role of schedule of antibiotic therapy on the neutropenic patient. *Infection* 1980;(Suppl 1):75.
174. Powell SH et al. Once-daily vs. continuous aminoglycoside dosing: efficacy and toxicity in animal and clinical studies of gentamicin, netilmicin, and tobramycin. *J Infect Dis* 1983;147:918.
175. Krivoy N et al. Pharmacokinetic analysis of amikacin twice and single daily dosage in immunocompromised pediatric patients. *Infection* 1998; 26:396.
176. Tod M et al. Population pharmacokinetic study of amikacin administered once or twice daily to febrile, severely neutropenic adults. *Antimicrob Agents Chemother* 1998;42:849.
177. MacGowan AP et al. The pharmacokinetics of once daily gentamicin in neutropenic adults with haematological malignancy. *J Antimicrob Chemother* 1994;34:809.
178. Peterson AK, Duffull SB. Population analysis of once-daily dosing of gentamicin in patients with neutropenia. *Austr NZ J Med* 1998;28:311.
179. Paganini HG. Outpatient, sequential, parenteral-oral antibiotic therapy for lower risk febrile neutropenia in children with malignant disease. *Cancer* 2003;97:1775.
180. Suwangool P et al. Empirical antibiotic therapy in febrile neutropenic patients with single-daily dose amikacin plus ceftriaxone. *J Med Assoc Thailand* 1993;76:314.
181. Bakri FE et al. Once-daily versus multiple-daily gentamicin in empirical antibiotic therapy of febrile neutropenia following intensive chemotherapy. *J Antimicrob Chemother* 2000;45:383.
182. Tomlinson RJ et al. Once daily ceftriaxone and gentamicin for the treatment of febrile neutropenia. *Arch Dis Child* 1999;80:125.
183. Warkentin D et al. Toxicity of single daily dose gentamicin in stem cell transplantation. *Bone Marrow Transplant* 1999;24:57.
184. Aiken SK, Wetzstein GA. Once-daily aminoglycosides in patients with neutropenic fever. *Cancer Control* 2002;9:426.
185. Davis DD, Raebel MA. Ambulatory management of chemotherapy-induced fever and neutropenia in adult cancer patients. *Ann Pharmacother* 1998;32:1317.
186. Kern WV. Risk assessment and risk-based therapeutic strategies in febrile neutropenia. *Curr Opinion Infect Dis* 2001;14:415.
187. Rolston KV et al. Early empiric antibiotic therapy for febrile neutropenia patients at low risk. *Infect Dis Clin North Am* 1996;10:223.
188. Pizzo PA et al. Duration of empiric antibiotic therapy in granulocytopenic patients with cancer. *Am J Med* 1979;67:194.
189. Pizzo PA et al. Treatment of gram-positive septicemia in cancer patients. *Cancer* 1980;45:206.

190. Bennett JEP.Forum report: issues in clinical trials of empirical antifungal therapy in treating febrile neutropenic patients. *Clin Infect Dis* 2003;36:S117.
191. DeGregorio MW et al. Fungal infections in patients with acute leukemia. *Am J Med* 1982;73:543.
192. Maertens J et al. Preemptive antifungal therapy: still a way to go. *Curr Opin Infect Dis* 2006;19:551–56.
193. Hagen EA et al. High rate of invasive fungal infections following nonmyeloablative allogeneic transplantation. *Clin Infect Dis* 2003;36:9.
194. Martino R, Subira M. Invasive fungal infections in hematology: new trends. *Ann Hematol* 2002;81:233.
195. Ninin E et al. Longitudinal study of bacterial, viral, and fungal infections in adult recipients of bone marrow transplants. *Clin Infect Dis* 2001;33:41.
196. Gotzsche PC, Johansen HK. Meta-analysis of prophylactic or empirical antifungal treatment versus placebo or no treatment in patients with cancer complicated by neutropenia. *Br Med J* 1997;314:1238.
197. Guiot HF et al. Risk factors for fungal infection in patients with malignant hematologic disorders: implications for empirical therapy and prophylaxis. *Clin Infect Dis* 1994;18:525.
198. Gotzsche PC, Johansen HK. Routine versus selective antifungal administration for control of fungal infections in patients with cancer. *Cochrane Database Syst Rev* 2000;CD000026.
199. Bennett JEP. Forum report: issues in clinical trials of empirical antifungal therapy in treating febrile neutropenic patients. *Clin Infect Dis* 2003;36:S117.
200. Pizzo PA et al. Empiric antibiotic and antifungal therapy for cancer patients with prolonged fever and granulocytopenia. *Am J Med* 1982;72:101.
201. Prentice HG et al. A randomized comparison of liposomal versus conventional amphotericin B for the treatment of pyrexia of unknown origin in neutropenic patients. *Br J Haematol* 1997;98:711.
202. Walsh TJ et al. Liposomal amphotericin B for empirical therapy in patients with persistent fever and neutropenia. National Institute of Allergy and Infectious Diseases Mycoses Study Group. *N Engl J Med* 1999;340:764.
203. Wingard JR et al. A randomized, double-blind comparative trial evaluating the safety of liposomal amphotericin B versus amphotericin B lipid complex in the empirical treatment of febrile neutropenia. L Amph/ABLC Collaborative Study Group. *Clin Infect Dis* 2000;31:1155.
204. White MH et al. Randomized, double-blind clinical trial of amphotericin B colloidal dispersion vs. amphotericin B in the empirical treatment of fever and neutropenia. *Clin Infect Dis* 1998;27:296.
205. Walsh TJ et al. Voriconazole compared with liposomal amphotericin B for empirical antifungal therapy in patients with neutropenia and persistent fever. *N Engl J Med* 2002;346:225.
206. Blau IW, Fauser AA. Review of comparative studies between conventional and liposomal amphotericin B (AmBisome) in neutropenic patients with fever of unknown origin and patients with systemic mycosis. *Mycoses* 2000;43:325.
207. Dupont B. Overview of the lipid formulations of amphotericin B. *J Antimicrob Chemother* 2002;49(Suppl 1):31.
208. Frothingham R. Lipid formulations of amphotericin B for empirical treatment of fever and neutropenia. *Clin Infect Dis* 2002;35:896.
209. Johansen HK, Gotzsche PC. Amphotericin B lipid soluble formulations vs amphotericin B in cancer patients with neutropenia. *Cochrane Database Syst Rev* 2000;CD000969.
210. Eriksson U et al. Comparison of effects of amphotericin B deoxycholate infused over 4 or 24 hours: randomised controlled trial. *Br Med J* 2001; 322:579.
211. Malik IA et al. A randomized comparison of fluconazole with amphotericin B as empiric antifungal agents in cancer patients with prolonged fever and neutropenia. *Am J Med* 1998;105:478.
212. Winston DJ et al. A multicenter, randomized trial of fluconazole versus amphotericin B for empiric antifungal therapy of febrile neutropenic patients with cancer. *Am J Med* 2000;108:282.
213. Jorgensen KJ et al. Voriconazole versus amphotericin B in cancer patients with neutropenia. *Cochrane Database Syst Rev* 2006;CD004707.
214. Walsh TJ et al. Caspofungin versus liposomal amphotericin B for empirical antifungal therapy in patients with persistent fever and neutropenia. *N Engl J Med.* 2004;351:1391.
215. Fassas AB et al. Cytomegalovirus infection and non-neutropenic fever after autologous stem cell transplantation: high rates of reactivation in patients with multiple myeloma and lymphoma. *Br J Haematol* 2001;112:237.
216. Illerhaus G et al. Treatment and prophylaxis of severe infections in neutropenic patients by granulocyte transfusions. *Ann Hematol* 2002;81:273.
217. Dale DC. Colony-stimulating factors for the management of neutropenia in cancer patients. *Drugs* 2002;62(Suppl 1):1.
218. Kojima A et al. A randomized prospective study of imipenem-cilastatin with or without amikacin as an empirical antibiotic treatment for febrile neutropenic patients. *Am J Clin Oncol* 1994;17:400.
219. Murray BE. Vancomycin-resistant enterococci. *Am J Med* 1997;102:284.
220. De Pauw BE. Treatment of documented and suspected neutropenia-associated invasive fungal infections. *J Chemother* 2001;13(Spec No 1):181.
221. Bille J. Laboratory diagnosis of infections in febrile neutropenic or immunocompromised patients. *Int J Antimicrob Agents* 2000;16:87.
222. Newman KA, Schimpff SC. Hospital hotel services as risk factors for infection among immunocompromised patients. *Rev Infect Dis* 1987;9:206.
223. Kern W, Kurrle E. Ofloxacin versus trimethoprim-sulfamethoxazole for prevention of infection in patients with acute leukemia and granulocytopenia. *Infection* 1991;19:73.
224. Lew MA et al. Ciprofloxacin versus trimethoprim/sulfamethoxazole for prophylaxis of bacterial infections in bone marrow transplant recipients: a randomized, controlled trial. *J Clin Oncol* 1995;13:239.
225. Gomez-Martin C et al. Rifampin does not improve the efficacy of quinolone antibacterial prophylaxis in neutropenic cancer patients: results of a randomized clinical trial. *J Clin Oncol* 2000;18:2126.
226. Gurwith MJ et al. Granulocytopenia in hospitalized patients: I. Prognostic factors and etiology of fever. *Am J Med* 1978;64:121.
227. Gill FA et al. The relationship of fever, granulocytopenia and antimicrobial therapy to bacteremia in cancer patients. *Cancer* 1977;39:1704.
228. Schimpff SC et al. Three antibiotic regimens in the treatment of infection in febrile granulocytopenic patients with cancer. The EORTC International Antimicrobial Therapy Project Group. *J Infect Dis* 1978;137:14.
229. Ramphal R. Is monotherapy for febrile neutropenia still a viable alternative? *Clin Infect Dis* 1999;29:508.
230. Furno P et al. Ceftriaxone versus beta-lactams with antipseudomonal activity for empirical, combined antibiotic therapy in febrile neutropenia: a meta-analysis. *Support Care Cancer* 2000;8:293.
231. Shevchuk YM, Conly JM. Antibiotic-associated hypoprothrombinemia: a review of prospective studies, 1966–1988. *Rev Infect Dis* 1990;12:1109.
232. Grasela TH Jr et al. Prospective surveillance of antibiotic-associated coagulopathy in 970 patients. *Pharmacotherapy* 1989;9:158.
233. Boogaerts M et al. Intravenous and oral itraconazole versus intravenous amphotericin B deoxycholate as empirical antifungal therapy for persistent fever in neutropenic patients with cancer who are receiving broad-spectrum antibacterial therapy: a randomized, controlled trial. *Ann Intern Med* 2001;135:412.
234. Groll AH, Walsh TJ. Caspofungin: pharmacology, safety and therapeutic potential in superficial and invasive fungal infections. *Expert Opin Invest Drugs* 2001;10:1545.
235. Ozer H et al. 2000 update of recommendations for the use of hematopoietic colony-stimulating factors: evidence-based, clinical practice guidelines. American Society of Clinical Oncology Growth Factors Expert Panel. *J Clin Oncol* 2000;18:3558.

CHAPTER 69

Pharmacotherapy of Human Immunodeficiency Virus Infection

Julie B. Dumond and Angela D.M. Kashuba

INTRODUCTION

Potent combinations of antiretroviral drugs (also called *highly active antiretroviral therapy* [HAART]) have dramatically altered the natural progression of human immunodeficiency virus (HIV) infection, and significantly improved the quality of life for many patients infected with HIV. As a result, a pronounced decline has occurred in the reported number of new acquired immunodeficiency syndrome (AIDS)-related opportunistic infections and deaths.[1,2] For many, the use of HAART has shifted the outlook of HIV infection from a fatal to a manageable disease. Advances continue to be made for HIV therapy, and most recently include new and more potent antiretroviral agents in existing therapeutic drug classes, new antiretroviral agents in new therapeutic drug classes, and novel, potent combinations of antiretrovirals. Despite these remarkable advances, clinicians working in the area of HIV remain cautious. Although many patients will benefit from these new and more potent regimens, data have shown that up to 25% of patients will fail therapy in the first year,[3] and approximately 25% will have to change regimens within the first year owing to drug-related adverse events.[4] Remaining concerns include the development of resistance and long-term adverse events, suboptimal patient compliance and management of HAART failures, and the rampant spread of HIV throughout developing countries.

This chapter focuses on the antiretroviral treatment of HIV infection. Although many therapeutic options exist, a thorough understanding of viral pathogenesis is essential for clinicians managing patients infected with HIV. By understanding the principles of therapy as they relate to viral pathogenesis, clinicians will be able to rapidly assimilate new data as they become available. Consensus panel recommendations have been published that can be used as a framework for clinical decision making.[5–7] Given the complexity of therapy, this chapter focuses only on treatment of adult HIV infection; the reader is referred to the various Consensus Panel Guidelines on treatment of perinatal transmission, pediatric HIV, and postexposure prophylaxis for both occupational and nonoccupational HIV exposures (located at http://www.hivatis.org).

EPIDEMIOLOGY

Despite a dramatic decline in the number of AIDS-related opportunistic infections and deaths in industrialized countries,[1,2] infection with HIV remains a leading cause of death throughout many regions of the world. Access to newer, more potent antiretroviral regimens and monitoring techniques are often limited, however, by economics and politics. Infected patients residing in countries with a strong economic standing have reasonable access to medications (North America, western Europe, Australia, and New Zealand), whereas patients residing in countries with scarce resources (Africa, south and southeast Asia, the Pacific, Latin America, and the Caribbean) do not. This is extremely alarming given that most infected patients worldwide reside in developing regions of the world.[8]

As of December 2006, the worldwide estimate of persons living with HIV infection is calculated as 39.5 million: 37.2 million adults (17.7 million women) and 2.3 million children

<15 years of age. In 2006, it is estimated that 4.2 million people were newly infected with HIV and 2.9 million people died from AIDS. Two-thirds (63%) of all adults and children infected with HIV live in sub-Saharan Africa, and almost three-quarters (72%) of all adult and child deaths caused by AIDS occurred there in 2006. In the past few years, the number of people living with HIV has increased in every region of the world, but the most striking increases occurred in east Asia, eastern Europe, and central Asia: the number of people living with HIV increased by 21% from 2004 to 2006.[9] Intervention strategies to educate and protect young people have only been effective and sustained in Zimbabwe, where national adult HIV prevalence is declining. Although treatment strategies are difficult to implement in developing countries because of social, political, financial, and resource limitations, expanded provision of antiretroviral treatment has gained an estimated 2 million life years in low- and middle-income countries since 2002.[8]

In the United States, the availability of antiretroviral therapy has resulted in an 80% decline in AIDS death rates between 1990 and 2003. In the past year, approximately 30,000 people died from AIDS, whereas an estimated 1.2 million people are HIV infected. A significant proportion of people (25%) are unaware that they are HIV-positive, and approximately 65,000 acquired HIV infection in the past year. Racial and ethnic minorities continue to be disproportionately affected by HIV: between 2001 and 2004, 50% of AIDS diagnoses were among blacks (who only constitute 12% of the U.S. population) and 20% of AIDS diagnoses were among Hispanics (who constitute 14% of the U.S. population). Compared with white men and women, the rate of new HIV or AIDS diagnoses is 7 times higher in black men and 21 times higher in black women.[8]

Transmission through sexual intercourse remains a predominant route of infection, with unsafe sex between men accounting for approximately 44% of cases, and heterosexual intercourse accounting for approximately 34% of cases. The proportion of women newly diagnosed has increased dramatically (from 15% in 1995 to 27% in 2004). Additionally, patients >50 years of age represent a rapidly expanding group, both from new infections and as a result of effective antiretroviral therapy extending life expectancy.[8]

PATHOPHYSIOLOGY

Infection with HIV can be acquired through unprotected sexual intercourse (both anal and vaginal), injectable drug use, receipt of tainted blood products, and mother-to-infant transmission (both perinatal infection and postpartum through breast feeding).[5] Infection can also be acquired from occupational exposures among health care workers after needle sticks from patients infected with HIV. Rarely, HIV infection has been documented after oral sex.[10,11]

Unprotected sexual intercourse has accounted for approximately 80% of all documented HIV infections to date.[8] Transmission between sexual partners depends on a number of factors, including the HIV viral subtype, stage of infection in the index partner, genetic susceptibility to infection of the potential host, and the fitness (or pathogenicity) of the infecting viral strain. Infectivity via male-to-male receptive anal intercourse represents the greatest sexual risk factor followed by male-to-female vaginal transmission and then female-to-male vaginal transmission.[12]

The HIV attacks and binds to specific cells of the immune system, including monocytes, macrophages, and T-cell lymphocytes (also known as CD4+ T cells, helper T cells, T cells).[13–16] These cells display specific receptor proteins known as CD4 receptors to which HIV binds. Once bound to the CD4 receptor, coreceptor proteins are required for fusion (CCR-5, CXCR-4).[17,18] CCR-5 coreceptors are found on both monocytes and T lymphocytes, and are more abundant in patients newly infected with HIV.[18,19] CXCR-4 coreceptors are predominantly found on T lymphocytes and are more abundant in patients who have been on long-term antiretroviral therapy. The CD4–coreceptor complex causes conformational changes to key HIV proteins (gp41 and gp120) allowing for a more close association between the virus and host cell.[20,21] HIV fuses with the cell and releases its contents into the host cell's cytoplasm: this includes the virus' RNA and specific enzymes necessary for replication (Fig. 69-1). The single-stranded viral RNA is transcribed via reverse transcriptase into a double-stranded proviral DNA that is subsequently incorporated into the host cell's genetic material via the integrase enzyme. HIV then uses the infected cell's machinery to translate, transcribe, and produce immature viral particles that bud and break from the infected cell. For these immature virions to become infectious, the HIV protease enzyme must cleave large precursor polypeptides into functional proteins.[22,23] Once complete, the mature virion is free to infect new host cells and subsequently produce more infectious virus. Over time, HIV-infected host cells can be destroyed by a number of mechanisms: (a) a direct cytolytic effect of the virus (e.g., formation of syncytium induction, cellular dysfunction); (b) the identification and elimination of the infected cell by the host's immune response (e.g., via cytotoxic T-cell lymphocytes); or (c) the cell's natural life cycle coming to completion.[16] In addition, HIV infection can inhibit the production of new CD4 cells.[24]

Once a patient becomes infected, an initial burst of viremia occurs and causes latent infection in various tissues (e.g., lymph nodes) and cells (CD4, macrophages and monocytes).[25,26] Most infectious HIV virions (~99%) reside inside lymph nodes and other immune-cell rich tissues found throughout the body.[15,25,27,28] The immune system reacts by producing antibodies against HIV; however, given the rapid production of new HIV particles and the development of various new viral strains (a result of the error-susceptible HIV reverse transcriptase), the antibody response is inadequate.[29] After this burst of viremia, a transient depletion of CD4 cells occurs (Fig. 69-2). Initially, patients may complain of nonspecific symptoms, such as fever, lymphadenopathy, rash, fatigue, and night sweats.[30,31] This phase of infection is known as the *acute retroviral syndrome.* In most cases, patients are unaware that they are infected. Within 6 months, the host's immune response is able to control the infection to a point where the number of virus particles produced per day equals the number of particles destroyed per day. This steady-state is often referred to as the patient's viral "set point."

The higher a patient's viral set point, the greater the risk for disease progression, because the larger the viral population in a host, the greater the chance for more widespread viral infection and destruction of immune cells and lymphoid tissue. Why some patients establish higher or lower viral set points is currently under investigation, but this may be a consequence of differences in immune responses, cellular receptor populations,

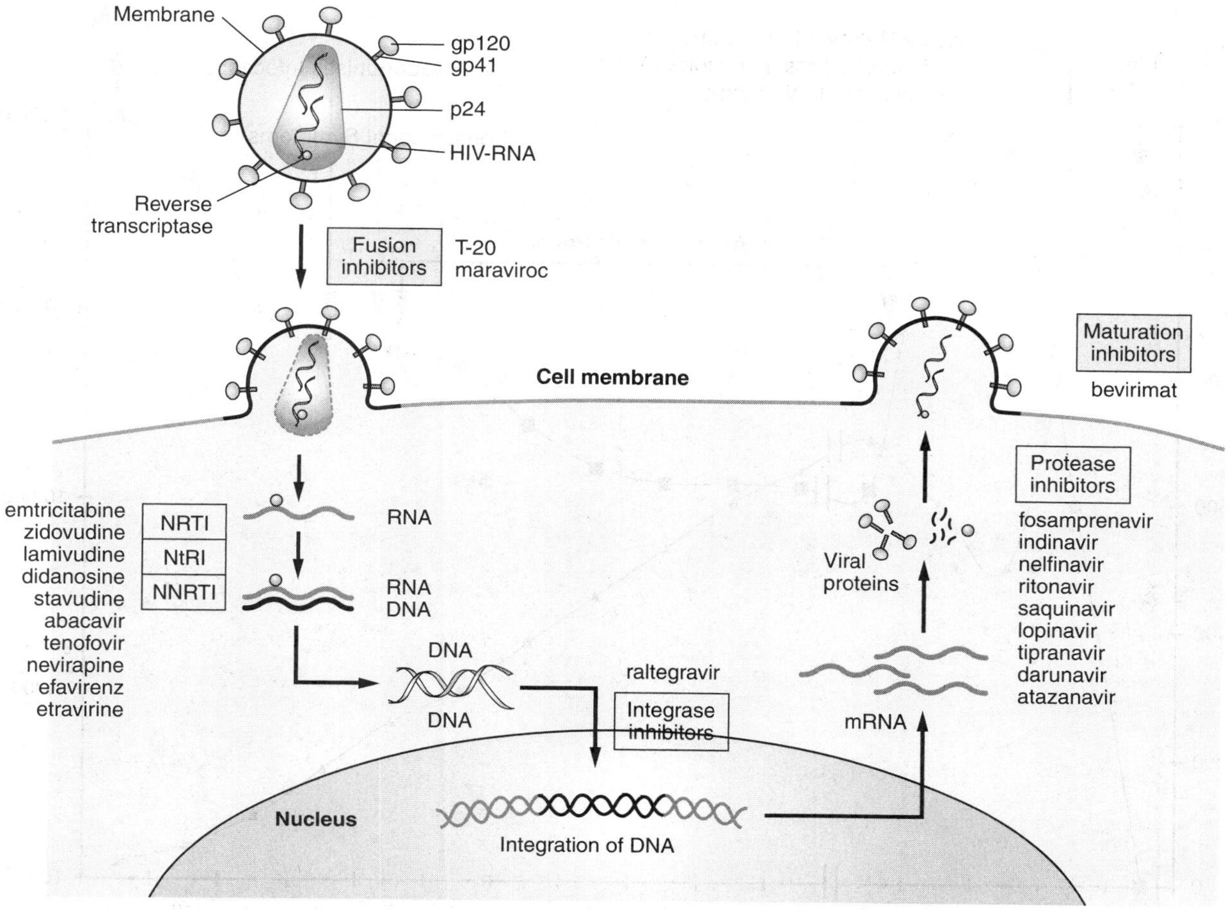

FIGURE 69-1 Schematic Representation of the HIV-1 Life Cycle. Four classes of antiretroviral drugs are available at present. Fusion inhibitors inhibit the entry of virions into a new target cell. The step of reverse transcription can be targeted, using nucleoside/tide analogues or non-nucleoside reverse-transcriptase inhibitors (NRTIs, NTRTI, and NNRTIs, respectively). The class of integrase inhibitors prevent integration of viral DNA into host cell DNA. The class of protease inhibitors interferes with the last state of the life cycle, the proteolytic processing of the viral proteins, which results in the production of non-infectious particles. (Adapted with permission from Simon V, Ho DD. HIV-1 dynamics in vivo: implications for therapy, *Nat Rev Microb* 2003 Dec;1:181.)

viral subtypes, viral fitness, or a combination of these factors. This understanding of viral pathogenesis may lead to a new paradigm of therapy: using antiretrovirals in the acute phase of infection to lower viral set points and potentially reduce the risk of disease progression. A significant challenge, however, remains in identifying patients with acute infection.[32]

Once the initial burst of viremia has been controlled and the viral set point established, infection with HIV results in a constant battle between viral replication and suppression of that replication by the immune system. Mathematical models have calculated the production of HIV at 10 billion particles per day.[15,33–35] To keep the infection controlled, the body must produce an equal immune response. Over time, HIV depletes the body of T cells, which places the host at an increased risk for opportunistic infections (Fig. 69-3). Direct measurements of HIV RNA concentrations in plasma (also called "viral load") can predict disease progression (see below).[36–38] Higher viral load measurements represent an inability of the host to control viral replication, and a greater risk for immune cell destruction. Long-term "nonprogressors" (e.g., patients with asymptomatic HIV infection for >10 years; 5% of all HIV-infected patients) consistently have lower baseline viral loads than patients with rapidly progressive disease (e.g., AIDS within 5 years of infection; 20% of all HIV-infected patients).[39,40]

Without intervention, the natural progression of HIV infection results in depletion of 50 to 100 T cells/mm^3/year.[25,41] The severity of immune dysfunction, as evidenced by T-cell loss, is highly predictive of the potential for developing specific types of opportunistic infections. For example, *Pneumocystis carinii* pneumonia rarely occurs when T-cell counts are >200 cells/mm^3, whereas retinitis from *Cytomegalovirus* (CMV) infection infrequently occurs in patients with CD4 counts >75 cells/mm^3 (Figs. 69-2 and 69-3). The diagnosis of AIDS is made when a significant amount of immune deterioration has occurred, either by direct depletion of CD4 cells or because of the development of new opportunistic infection (Table 69-1 and Table 69-2).[25,42] It is important to recognize that not every patient with HIV has a diagnosis of AIDS. On average, without appropriate drug therapy, death occurs within 10 to 15 years after infection.[25,42]

The interplay between viral load and CD4 T-cell counts is often compared with that of a train heading toward a particular

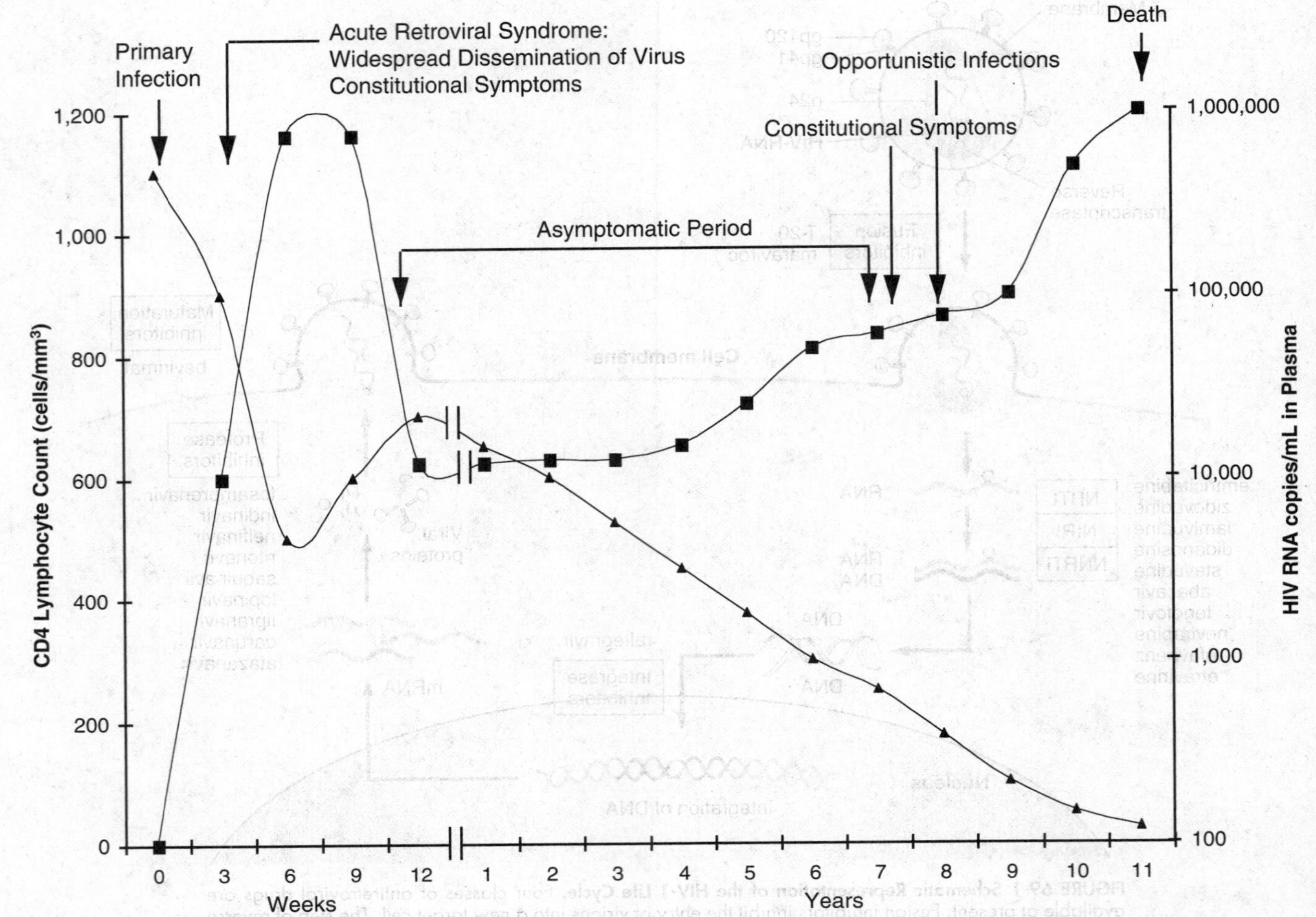

FIGURE 69-2 Sample disease course for an untreated HIV-infected individual showing relationship among immunologic, virologic, and clinical outcomes over time. Constitutional symptoms include fever, night sweats, and weight loss. ■ Viral load values; ▲ CD4 T lymphocytes. (Adapted from References 21 and 25.)

destination. If the destination is immune system destruction (and eventually death), then the T-cell count is the distance of the train from this destination, and the viral load (concentration of HIV RNA in plasma) is the speed of the train. As both higher speeds and shorter distances reach destinations faster, so does a high viral load and low T-cell count result in quicker onset of immune destruction (and death). Potent antiretroviral regimens, by decreasing viral replication, dramatically alter the natural course of infection, and prolong the time to opportunistic infection and death (Fig. 69-4).[43]

PHARMACOTHERAPY

Pharmacotherapy of HIV has been directed at inhibiting key areas of the HIV life cycle (Fig. 69-1; Table 69-3). Much research has been focused on agents that inhibit the reverse transcriptase enzyme. Nucleoside or nucleotide analogue reverse transcriptase inhibitors (NRTIs: zidovudine, didanosine, lamivudine, abacavir, tenofovir, emtricitabine, and stavudine), inhibit this enzyme by incorporating false nucleic acids into the newly forming proviral DNA.[44] This results in a DNA strand that cannot continue elongation. Non-nucleoside reverse transcriptase inhibitors (NNRTIs: nevirapine and efavirenz), inhibit reverse transcriptase by directly binding to the enzyme itself, and prevent DNA transcription from RNA.[45] Protease inhibitors (PI: saquinavir, amprenavir, nelfinavir, indinavir, lopinavir, atazanavir, ritonavir, tipranavir, and darunavir) directly bind to the catalytic site of HIV protease, inactivating the enzyme and preventing maturation of the HIV virion.[46,47] Unlike reverse transcription, which occurs relatively early in the course of the HIV life cycle, protease enzyme activity occurs late in virion development. As a result, inactivation of the protease enzyme inhibits viral replication in any infected cell regardless of the current stage of HIV replication within that cell. In contrast, reverse transcriptase inhibitors can protect newly infected cells only before formation and insertion of proviral DNA into the host cell's genetic material. Subsequently, these agents provide no benefit for those infected cells that are actively producing new strains of virus.

Fusion inhibitors, such as T-20, prevent HIV and CD4+ T cells from being pulled closer together after HIV binds to CD4 and CCR5 or CXCR-4 coreceptors. T-20 prevents

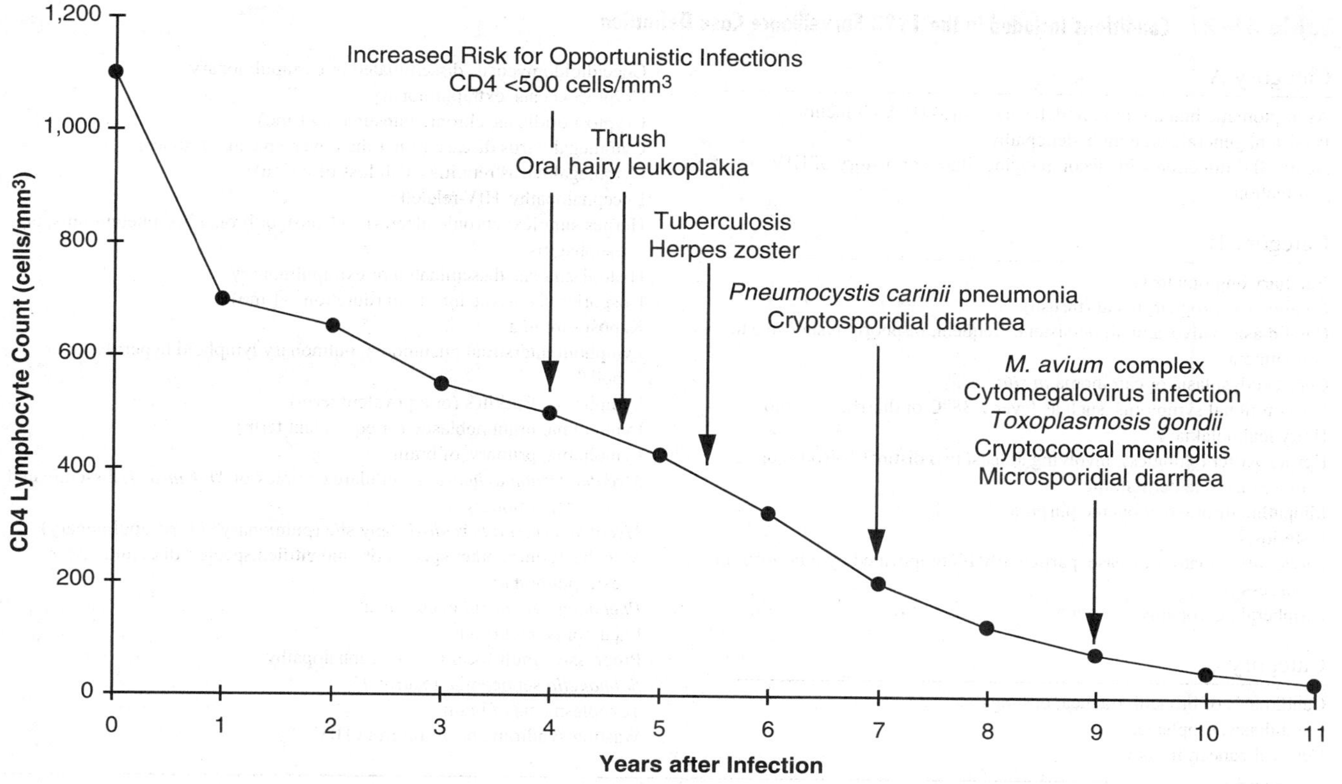

FIGURE 69-3 Relative risk for development of opportunistic infections based on CD4 lymphocyte counts over time.

fusion of the virus with the T-cell by binding to a double coil–coil complex at the gp41–gp120–CD4 receptor area.[21] Two new classes of antiretroviral agents are coreceptor blockers (e.g., via CCR5 and CXCR-4 blockade) and HIV integrase inhibitors.[48,49]

With the development of newer, more potent antiretroviral regimens, researchers have speculated about the possibility of eradicating HIV from an infected patient. This may require complete inhibition of viral replication in all cell lines and body stores where HIV resides (Fig. 69-5).[15] One problem that exists is that some cell lines have shorter half-lives than others (e.g., peripheral T cells, 1–2 days versus macrophages 14 days).[50,51] In addition, long-lived infected T cells with half-lives lasting more than 6 to 44 months have been identified.[52,53] This may require complete HIV suppression for 60 years or more to eradicate infection.[52–54] Another complicating factor is the potential for HIV to reside in sites that achieve low antiretroviral concentrations, thereby serving as sanctuaries for HIV replication (e.g., central nervous system [CNS], testes). Once therapy is discontinued, these sites could theoretically release unaffected virions and repopulate the host. As a result, research has shifted toward immune-based therapies that can identify and destroy HIV-infected cells, in addition to preventing HIV acquisition.

DIAGNOSIS

1. E.J. is a 27-year-old man who presents to your clinic with new complaints of fevers, night sweats, weight loss, and a white

Table 69-1 1993 Revised Classification System for HIV Infection and the Expanded CDC Surveillance Case Definition for AIDS in Adults and Adolescents[a]

	Clinical Categories		
CD4 + T-Cell Categories	*(A) Asymptomatic, Acute (Primary) HIV*	*(B) Symptomatic, Not (A) or (C) Conditions*	*(C) AIDS-Indicator Conditions*
1. >500/mm³	A1	B1	C1
1. 200–499/mm³	A2	B2	C2
1. <200/mm³ (AIDS indicator T-cell count)	A3	B3	C3

[a] The modifications to the prior 1986 Surveillance Case Definition, which have been included in the 1993 revision, include the use of CD4 cell count (<200 cells/mm³) or CD4 cell percent (<14%) and the additional AIDS-indicating conditions of pulmonary tuberculosis, recurrent pneumonia, and invasive cervical cancer (see Table 69-2).
AIDS, acquired immunodeficiency syndrome; CDC, Centers for Disease Control and Prevention; HIV, human immunodeficiency virus.

Table 69-2 Conditions Included in the 1993 Surveillance Case Definition

Category A	Coccidioidomycosis, disseminated or extrapulmonary
Asymptomatic human immunodeficiency virus (HIV) infection	Cryptococcosis, extrapulmonary
Persistent generalized lymphadenopathy	Cryptosporidiosis, chronic intestinal (>1 mo)
Acute HIV infection with accompanying illness or history of HIV infection	Cytomegalovirus disease (other than liver, spleen, or nodes)
Category B	Cytomegalovirus retinitis (with loss of vision)
Bacillary angiomatosis	Encephalopathy, HIV-related
Candidiasis, oropharyngeal (thrush)	Herpes simplex: chronic ulcer(s) (>1 mo); or bronchitis, pneumonitis, or esophagitis
Candidiasis, vulvovaginal; persistent, frequent, or poorly responsive to treatment	Histoplasmosis, disseminated or extrapulmonary
Cervical dysplasia or carcinoma *in situ*	Isosporiasis, chronic intestinal (duration >1 mo)
Constitutional symptoms, such as fever >38°C or diarrhea >1 mo	Kaposi sarcoma
Hairy leukoplakia	Lymphoid interstitial pneumonia, pulmonary lymphoid hyperplasia, or both[a]
Herpes zoster (shingles), involving at least two distinct episodes or more than one dermatome	Lymphoma, Burkitt's (or equivalent term)
Idiopathic thrombocytopenic purpura	Lymphoma, immunoblastic (or equivalent term)
Listeriosis	Lymphoma, primary, of brain
Pelvic inflammatory disease, particularly if complicated by tubo-ovarian abscess	*Mycobacterium avium*-intracellulare complex or *M. kansasii*, disseminated or extrapulmonary
Peripheral neuropathy	*Mycobacterium tuberculosis,* any site (pulmonary[b] or extrapulmonary)
Category C	Mycobacterium, other species or unidentified species, disseminated or extrapulmonary
Candidiasis of bronchi, trachea, or lungs	*Pneumocystis carinii* pneumonia
Candidiasis, esophageal	Pneumonia, recurrent[b]
Cervical cancer, invasive	Progressive multifocal leukoencephalopathy
	Salmonella septicemia, recurrent
	Toxoplasmosis of brain
	Wasting syndrome resulting from HIV

[a]Children <13 years of age.
[b]Added in the 1993 expansions of the acquired immunodeficiency syndrome (AIDS) surveillance case definition for adolescents and adults.

exudate in his mouth. He states that these symptoms have been present for the past 4 to 6 weeks. On physical examination, it is concluded that E.J. has thrush caused by *Candida albicans.* E.J. admits to intravenous drug use in the past; however, he states that he has been "clean" for 3 years. HIV infection is suspected and consent for an HIV test is obtained. Why is HIV suspected and how is it confirmed?

In otherwise healthy, immunocompetent individuals, the appearance of opportunistic infections, such as thrush, is rare. This is because an intact cell-mediated immunity protects against infection. In immunosuppressed individuals, such as those infected with HIV or cancer, the immune system is significantly damaged and places patients at risk for opportunistic infections. Infections such as shingles (*Herpes zoster*), active tuberculosis, oral thrush, and recurrent candidal vaginal infections in an otherwise healthy person warrant further evaluation. More advanced diseases, such as *Pneumocystis jirovecii* pneumonia, *Mycobacterium avium* bacteremia, and *Cytomegalovirus* retinitis infections, among others, generally occur in patients with severely depressed immune systems and strongly suggest HIV infection. This is especially true for those patients with risk factors for HIV infection. Despite E.J.'s discontinuation of intravenous drugs, his prior use places him at risk for HIV infection. Given his social history and current clinical presentation, an HIV test is warranted.

Testing for HIV is based on detection of an antibody to the virus. The most commonly used methods include the enzyme-linked immunosorbent assays (ELISA) and confirmatory Western blot tests.[55,56] ELISA is highly sensitive and specific (>99%) and therefore represents a good screening test. Using this method, the patient's serum is placed in wells coated with HIV antigens. After incubation and washing, an enzyme-labeled antihuman antibody is added, followed by a substrate. If HIV antibodies are present, a color change takes place; this is confirmed with a spectrophotometer. Reactive ELISA are subsequently repeated and, if both tests are positive, a Western blot confirmatory test is performed. The Western blot involves the addition of the host's serum to known HIV antigens that have been separated by gel electrophoresis. After washing and incubation, antihuman immune globulins linked to an enzyme or radioactive probe are added. The spectrum of band patterns on the gel is then interpreted and compared with controls for HIV diagnosis.

Although these tests when used together are highly specific and sensitive, there are situations where both false–negative and false–positive findings can occur.[57] The most troublesome is the situation in which a patient is truly infected but both ELISA and Western blot results are negative, known clinically as *acute HIV infection*. This occurs because, once infected, it takes 1 to 2 months for a person to develop antibodies to HIV.[58] Because both these tests rely on antibody detection, this "window" period of acute infection could result in a false–negative test finding for HIV. If this is suspected, clinicians may wish to order an HIV polymerase chain reaction (PCR) test (viral load measurement; see below); measurements >10,000 copies/mL are present only among patients who are HIV infected. Acute HIV infection is increasingly implicated in sexual transmission

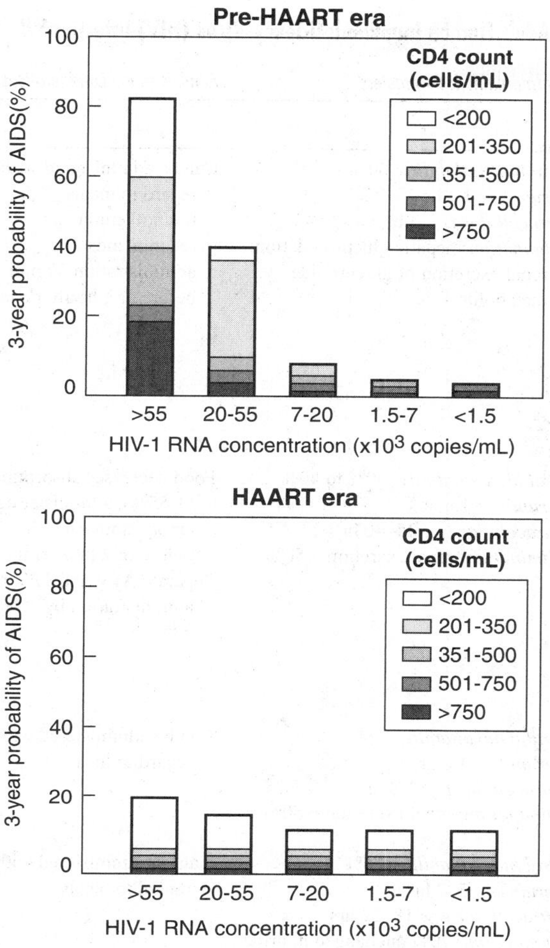

FIGURE 69-4 Prognosis According to CD4 Cell Count and Viral Load in the Pre-HAART and HAART Eras. (Adapted with permission from Elsevier The Lancet, Egger M, et al. ART Cohort Collaboration. Prognosis of HIV-1-infected patients starting highly active antiretroviral therapy: a collaborative analysis of prospective studies, *Lancet* 2002 Jul 13; 360:119.)

of HIV, and cost-efficient methods to detect acute infection using routine viral load measurements have been developed.[59] In all situations, a confirmatory Western blot test should be performed to rule out false–positive findings and mislabeled samples.

Results of the ELISA test take up to 1 to 2 weeks, and this delay means that patients must contact their providers for test results. According to the Centers for Disease Control and Prevention (CDC), in the year 2000 approximately one-third of individuals who tested positive for HIV did not return to the clinic to learn their results. Newer test methods have been developed that allow clinicians to supply definitive negative and preliminary positive results to patients within 20 minutes or less of screening, using whole blood, serum, plasma, or oral fluid.[60] The sensitivity and specificity of these new, rapid screening tests are comparable to those of ELISA. Similar to ELISA, a positive rapid test result should be confirmed by a supplemental test. The use of rapid HIV tests should be strongly considered when expected return rates for test results are low. The CDC has published guidelines on the use and quality assurance of these rapid HIV tests.[61]

SURROGATE MARKER DATA

2. E.J.'s ELISA and Western blot tests both return positive, and he is informed of his HIV status the next week at his follow-up examination. Before making any decisions regarding therapeutic options, what additional laboratory tests should be obtained? What cautions should be used when interpreting these values?

To determine whether therapeutic interventions are necessary, the severity of immune damage and potential for disease progression must be assessed. As stated, HIV predominantly infects and destroys T cells. The larger the viral load, the greater the risk for T-cell destruction and opportunistic infections. Therefore, quantitative measurements of E.J.'s HIV viral load and T-cell counts are necessary to "stage" the severity of infection, assess the risk for disease progression, and provide a reference point (e.g., baseline) for future therapeutic decisions.

Identification and measurement of T-lymphocyte subsets (e.g., CD4, CD8) are based on flow cytometry readings of fluorescent-labeled monoclonal antibodies.[5,42] These values can display wide variability on repeated laboratory evaluations, even in clinically stable patients. Patient samples can display up to 30% intra- and interlaboratory variability.[5] In at least one study, sufficient interlaboratory variability existed to potentially result in conflicting treatment recommendations in 58% of patients (e.g., initiating therapy when T-cell counts fell <500 cells/mm^3).[62] Consequently, it is important to realize that assessment of T-cell measurements should always be interpreted as trends and not as individual values. Variability can also be minimized by using the same laboratory and by sampling patients at a consistent time of day.

The measurement of HIV viral load can be performed by one of three methods: reverse transcriptase-polymerase chain reaction (RT-PCR), branched-chain DNA (bDNA) assay, or nucleic acid sequence-based amplification (NASBA).[63] Measurements using RT-PCR are obtained when viral RNA is amplified and counted. In contrast, bDNA amplifies and enumerates the signal from target probes attached to the viral RNA. NASBA allows real-time, high throughput amplification of viral RNA. All methods report HIV RNA in plasma as the number of copies per milliliter, but have differing lower limits of quantitation.[5] It should be recognized that plasma viral RNA values measure the amount of free virus in the periphery and not the lymph nodes. Because viral concentrations are substantially greater in the lymph node, plasma measurements of HIV indirectly reflect spill over from replication in that compartment.[64,65]

Similar to CD4 counts, viral load measurements (copies/milliliter) can vary by as much as threefold (0.5 log) in either direction.[5] When obtaining a patient's baseline value, a number of issues must be considered. On initial infection with HIV, a burst of viremia occurs until the host's immune responses are able to control the infection. Subsequently, viral load measurements obtained during the first 6 months of infection may not accurately reflect a true baseline value.[5] In addition, factors that activate the immune system, such as the development of a new opportunistic infection or immunizations,[66] can result in transient elevations of viral load measurements. In these situations,

Table 69-3 Characteristics of Antiretroviral Agents for the Treatment of Adult Human Immunodeficiency Virus (HIV) Infection[5,167]

Drug	*Dose*	*Pharmacokinetic Parameters*	*Administration Considerations*
Nucleoside Reverse Transcriptase Inhibitors			
Zidovudine (ZDV; ZDV) **Retrovir (R)** *Preparations* Oral Solution: 10 mg/mL Capsule: 100 mg Tablet: 300 mg IV Solution: 10 mg/mL Combivir (R) with 3TC: ZDV 300 mg + 3TC 150 mg Trizivir (R) with 3TC and ABC: ZDV 300 mg + 3TC 150 mg + ABC 300 mg	300 mg BID or 200 mg TID Combivir(R) or Trizivir(R): one tablet two times per day	*Oral bioavailability:* 60% *Serum* $t_{1/2}$: 1.1 hr *Intracellular* $t_{1/2}$: 3 hr *Elimination:* hepatic glucuronidation; renal excretion of glucuronide metabolite	Can be administered without regard to meals (manufacturer recommends administration 30 min before or 1 hr after a meal)
Didanosine (ddI) **Videx** *Preparations* Videx EC (R): 125 mg, 200 mg, 250 mg, and 400 mg capsule Pediatric powder for oral solution (when reconstituted as solution containing antacid): 10 mg/mL Generic ddI enteric coated capsule also available	>60 kg: 400 mg QD (with TDF, use 250 mg QD) <60 kg: 250 mg QD (with TDF, use 200 mg QD)	*Oral bioavailability:* 30% to 40% *Serum* $t_{1/2}$: 1.6 hr *Intracellular* $t_{1/2}$: 25–40 hr *Elimination:* renal excretion ~50%	Food decreases absorption (↓ 55%); administer ddI on empty stomach (1 hr before or 2 hr after meal) Separate ATV and TPV/r administration by at least 2 hr
Stavudine (d4T) **Zerit** *Preparations* Solution: 1 mg/mL Capsules: 15, 20, 30, 40 mg	>60 kg: 40 mg BID <60 kg: 30 mg BID Sustained release: >60 kg use 100 mg QD; <60 kg use 75 mg QD	*Oral bioavailability:* 86% *Serum* $t_{1/2}$: 1.0 hr *Intracellular* $t_{1/2}$: 3.5 hr *Elimination:* renal excretion ~50%	Can be administered without regard to meals
Lamivudine (3TC) **Epivir** *Preparations* Solution: 10 mg/mL Tablets: 150 mg, 300 mg Combivir: 3TC 150 mg + ZDV 300 mg Epzicom: 3TC 300 mg + ABC 600 mg Trizivir: 3TC 150 mg + ZDV 300 mg + ABC 300 mg	150 mg PO BID or 300 mg PO QD As Combivir: one tablet BID As Epzicom: one tablet BID As Trizivir: one tablet BID	*Oral bioavailability:* 86% *Serum* $t_{1/2}$: 5–7 hrs *Intracellular* $t_{1/2}$: 18–22 hrs *Elimination:* 70% unchanged in urine	Can be administered without regard to meals
Emtricitabine (FTC) **Emtriva** *Preparations* Capsules: 200 mg Oral solution: 10 mg/mL Truvada: FTC 200 mg + TDF 300 mg Atripla: FTC 200 mg + TDF 300 mg + EFV 600 mg	200 mg QD for patients with calculated creatinine clearance (CrCl) >50 mL/min Dose needs to be adjusted for renal dysfunction: CrCl 30–49 mL/min: 200 mg Q 48 hr CrCl 15–29 mL/min: 200 mg Q 72 hr CrCl <15 mL/min: 200 mg Q 96 hr As Truvada: one tablet QD Truvada not for patients with CrCl <30 mL/min As Atripla: one tablet QD Atripla not for patients with CrCl <50 mL/min	*Oral bioavailability:* 93% *Serum* $t_{1/2}$: 10 hr *Intracellular* $t_{1/2}$: >20 hr *Elimination:* 86% recovered in urine	Can be administered without regard to meals
Tenofovir (Viread) *Preparations* Tablets: 300 mg Truvada: TDF 300 mg + FTC 200 mg Atripla: TDF 300 mg + FTC 200 mg + EFV 600 mg	300 mg QD for patients with creatinine clearance >60 mL/min; Truvada: 1 tablet QD Atripla: 1 tablet QD	*Oral bioavailability:* 25% fasting; 39% with high-fat meal *Serum* $t_{1/2}$: 17 hr *Intracellular* $t_{1/2}$: >60 hr *Elimination:* primarily by glomerular filtration and active tubular secretion	Can be administered without regard to meals

Table 69-3 Characteristics of Antiretroviral Agents for the Treatment of Adult Human Immunodeficiency Virus (HIV) Infection[5,167] (*Continued*)

Drug	Dose	Pharmacokinetic Parameters	Administration Considerations
Nucleoside Reverse Transcriptase Inhibitors (*continued*)			
Abacavir **Ziagen** *Preparations* Tablets: 300 mg Oral solution: 20 mg/mL Epzicom: ABC 600 mg + 3TC 300 mg Trizivir: ABC 300 mg + ZDV 300 mg + 3TC 150 mg	300 mg Q 12 hr, or 600 mg QD Epzicom: one tablet QD Trizivir: one tablet BID	*Oral bioavailability:* 83% *Serum* $t_{1/2}$: 1.5 hr *Intracellular* $t_{1/2}$: 12–26 hr *Elimination:* alcohol dehydrogenase and glucuronyltransferase; 82% renal elimination of metabolites	Can be administered without regard to meals Alcohol raises abacavir exposure by 41%
Non-Nucleoside Reverse Transcriptase Inhibitors[a]			
Nevirapine **Viramune** *Preparations* Suspension: 50 mg/5 mL Tablets: 200 mg	200 mg PO QD × 14 days, then 200 mg PO BID	*Oral bioavailability:* >90% *Serum* $t_{1/2}$: 25–30 hr *Intracellular* $t_{1/2}$: Unknown *Elimination:* metabolized by CYP2B6 and CYP3A4 (also a CYP3A4 inducer) with 80% excreted in urine as the glucuronide metabolite	Can be administered without regard to meals
Delavirdine **Rescriptor** *Preparations* Tablets: 100 and 200 mg	400 mg TID (four 100-mg tabs in at least 3 oz water to produce slurry); 200 mg tablets should be taken intact	*Oral bioavailability:* 85% *Serum* $t_{1/2}$: 5.8 hr *Intracellular* $t_{1/2}$: Unknown *Elimination:* metabolized by CYP3A4 (also a CYP3A4 inhibitor) with 51% excreted in urine as metabolites	Can be administered without regard to meals
Efavirenz **Sustiva** *Preparations* Capsules: 50, 100, 200 mg Tablets: 600 mg Atripla: EFV 600 mg + TDF 300 mg + FTC 200 mg	600 mg QHS Atripla one tablet QHS Not for patients with CrCl <50 mL/min	*Oral bioavailability:* ~60%–70% *Serum* $t_{1/2}$: 40–55 hr *Intracellular* $t_{1/2}$: Unknown *Elimination:* hepatically metabolized by CYP2B6 and CYP3A4 (also CYP3A4 mixed inhibitor/inducer)	Avoid taking with high-fat meals, concentrations ↑ 50% (increased risk for CNS toxicity)
Protease Inhibitors			
Indinavir **Crixivan** *Preparations* Capsule: 200, 333, and 400 mg	800 mg Q 8 hrs (BID dosing ineffective when sole protease inhibitor) Indinavir/ritonavir: IDV 800 mg + 100 mg or 200 mg of RTV BID	*Oral bioavailability:* 65% *Serum* $t_{1/2}$: 1.5–2 hr *Intracellular* $t_{1/2}$: Unknown *Elimination:* hepatically metabolized via CYP3A4 (also inhibitor of CYP3A4)	Must be taken on empty stomach (1 hr before or 2 hrs after a meal); may take with skim milk or low-fat meal. Adequate hydration necessary (at least 1.5 L/24 hr of liquid) to minimize risk of nephrolithiasis
Ritonavir **Norvir** *Preparations* Oral solution: 80 mg/mL Capsules: 100 mg	600 mg Q 12 hr (on the rare occasion that RTV is used as the sole PI: day 1–2: 300 mg BID; day 3–5: 400 mg BID; day 6–13: 500 mg BID; day 14: 600 mg BID) Current primary use is as a pharmacokinetic enhancer for other PI, using 100–400 mg/day in one to two divided doses	*Oral bioavailability:* Not determined *Serum* $t_{1/2}$: 3–5 hr *Intracellular* $t_{1/2}$: Unknown *Elimination:* extensive hepatic metabolism via CYP3A4 (also potent CYP3A4 inhibitor and mixed inhibitor/inducer of other isozymes)	Take with food if possible to improve tolerability Dose should be titrated upward to minimize gastrointestinal adverse events Refrigerate capsules but not liquid
Nelfinavir **Viracept** *Preparations* Powder for oral suspension: 50 mg per one level scoop (200 mg per one level teaspoon) Tablets: 250 and 625 mg	750 mg TID or 1,250 mg BID	*Oral bioavailability:* 20%–80% *Serum* $t_{1/2}$: 3.5–5 hr *Intracellular* $t_{1/2}$: Unknown *Elimination:* hepatic metabolism via CYP3A4	Administer with meal or light snack (exposure increased two- to threefold)

(continued)

Table 69-3 Characteristics of Antiretroviral Agents for the Treatment of Adult Human Immunodeficiency Virus (HIV) Infection[5,167] (*Continued*)

Drug	*Dose*	*Pharmacokinetic Parameters*	*Administration Considerations*
Protease Inhibitors (*continued*)			
Saquinavir **Invirase** (hard gel capsules) *Preparations* Hard gel capsule: 200 mg Tablets: 500 mg	Unboosted saquinavir not recommended Saquinavir/ritonavir–1,000/100 BID; 1,600/100 QD under investigation	*Oral bioavailability:* 4% (as the sole PI) *Serum $t_{1/2}$:* 1–2 hr *Intracellular $t_{1/2}$:* Unknown *Elimination:* hepatic metabolism via cytP450 3A4 (inhibitor)	Take within 2 hr of a meal and take with RTV
Amprenavir **Agenerase** *Preparations* Capsules: 50 Solution: 15 mg/mL (capsules and solution NOT interchangeable on mg per mg basis) Fosamprenavir Lexiva Tablet: 700 mg	1,200 mg PO BID capsules, 1,400 mg PIs BID solution Amprenavir/ritonavir–1,200/200 QD (FDA-approved); 600/100–200 BID Do not use APV and RTV solution together owing to competition of the metabolic pathway of the two vehicles In ARV naïve patients: fAPV 1,400 mg BID or fAPV 1,400 mg + RTV 200 mg QD or fAPV 700 mg + RTV 100 mg BID In PI-experienced patients: fAPV 700 mg + RTV 100 mg BID	*Oral bioavailability:* Not determined *Serum $t_{1/2}$:* 7.1–10.6 hr (APV) *Intracellular $t_{1/2}$:* Unknown *Elimination:* hepatic metabolism via CYP3A4 (inhibitor)	Can be taken without regard to meals but should not be taken with high-fat meals
Lopinavir/ritonavir **Kaletra** *Preparations* Tablet: LPV 200 mg + RTV 50 mg Solution: LPV 80 mg+ RTV 20 mg per mL	Two tablets or 5 mL BID or Four tablets or 10 mL QD (recommended for treatment-naïve patients only)	*Oral bioavailability:* Not determined *Serum $t_{1/2}$:* 5–6 hr *Intracellular $t_{1/2}$:* Unknown *Elimination:* hepatic metabolism via CYP3A4 (inhibitor)	Take with food (increases area under the curve by 48%) Tablet stable at room temperature
Atazanavir **Reyataz** *Preparations* Capsules: 100 mg, 150 mg, 200 mg, and 300 mg	400 mg QD Atazanavir/ritonavir: 300/100 QD	*Oral bioavailability:* 60%–70% *Serum $t_{1/2}$:* 6–7 hr *Intracellular $t_{1/2}$:* Unknown *Elimination:* hepatic metabolism via CYP3A4 (modest inhibitor)	Take with food, and avoid acid suppressing agents (which prevent ATV solubility and absorption)
Darunavir **Prezista** *Preparations* Tablet: 300 mg, 600 mg	DRV 600 mg + RTV 100 mg BID	*Oral bioavailability:* 37% alone, 82% with RTV *Serum $t_{1/2}$:* 15 hr *Intracellular $t_{1/2}$:* Unknown *Elimination:* hepatic metabolism via CYP3A4 (inhibitor)	Food ↑ C_{max} and AUC by 30%: administer with food
Tipranavir **Aptivus** Capsules: 250 mg	TPV 500 mg + RTV 200 mg BID DO NOT USE WITHOUT RTV	*Oral bioavailability:* not determined *Serum $t_{1/2}$:* 6 hr *Intracellular $t_{1/2}$:* Unknown *Elimination*: hepatic metabolism via CYP3A4 (inhibitor and inducer)	Administer with food to increase bioavailability
Entry Inhibitors			
Fuzeon (Enfurvitide, T-20)	90 mg SC BID in upper arm, thigh, or abdomen	*Oral bioavailability:* 84.3% compared with IV *Serum $t_{1/2}$:* 3.8 hr *Intracellular $t_{1/2}$:* Not applicable *Elimination:* nonrenal, nonhepatic	Reconstitute with 1.1 mL of sterile water for injection; gently tap vial for 10 sec and then roll gently between hands to avoid foaming and ensure all drug is off vial walls After reconstitution, use immediately or refrigerate for 24 hr. Refrigerated T-20 should be brought to room temperature before injection.

Table 69-3 Characteristics of Antiretroviral Agents for the Treatment of Adult Human Immunodeficiency Virus (HIV) Infection[5,167] (*Continued*)

Drug	*Dose*	*Pharmacokinetic Parameters*	*Administration Considerations*
Chemokine Receptor Antagonists (CCR5)			
Maraviroc **Selzentry** *Preparations* Tablet: 150 mg, 300 mg	300 mg BID (with all NRTIs, NVP, TPV, ENF) 150 mg BID with CYP3A inhibitors (with or without a CYP3A inducer) including: protease inhibitors (except tipranavir/ritonavir), delavirdine, ketoconazole, itraconazole, clarithromycin, and other strong CYP3A inhibitors (e.g., nefazadone, telithromycin) 600 mg BID with CYP3A inducers (without a strong CYP3A inhibitor) including: Efavirenz, etravirine (TMC125), rifampin, carbamazepine, phenobarbital, and phenytoin	*Oral bioavailability:* ~33% *Serum* $t_{1/2}$: 14–18 hr *Elimination:* hepatic metabolism by CYP3A; 20% recovered in urine, 76% recovered in feces	Can be administered without regard to meals (high-fat meal decreases C_{max} and AUC by ~30%)
Integrase Inhibitors			
Raltegravir **Isentress** *Preparations* Tablet: 400 mg	400 mg BID	*Oral bioavailability:* not established *Serum* $t_{1/2}$: 9 hr *Elimination:* hepatic metabolism by UGT1A1 glucuronidation; 32% recovered in urine, 51% recovered in feces	Can be administered without regard to meals (high fat meal decreases C_{max} by ~34% and increases AUC by ~19%)

[a]In clinical trials, the non-nucleoside reverse transcriptase inhibitor (NNRTIs) was discontinued because of rash in 7% of patients taking nevirapine, 4.3% of patients taking delavirdine, and 1.7% of patients taking efavirenz. Rare cases of Stevens-Johnson syndrome have been reported with all three NNRTIs.
APV, amprenavir; ARV, antiviral; BID, twice daily; CNS, central nervous system; DRV, darunavir; ENF, enfuvirtide; fAPV, fosamprenavir; FDA, U.S. Food and Drug Administration; IDV, indinavir; NRTIs, nucleosides; NVP, nevirapine; PI, protein inhibitor; PO, orally; QD, every day; QHS, four times daily; RTV, ritonavir; SC, subcutaneously; TDF, tenofevir disoproxyl fumarate; TID, three times daily; TPV, tipranavir; TPV/r, tipranavir/ritonavir.

concentrations obtained within 4 weeks of the event may not accurately reflect the baseline viral load measurement.[5] Some clinicians would recommend that at least two separate viral load measurements, which are obtained within 1 to 4 weeks of each other, be performed before making decisions regarding therapeutic options.[67] As with T-cell values, viral load measurements should be evaluated as trends.

In addition to quantifying the viral load, baseline resistance testing should be considered, using either genotypic or phenotypic testing,[5] to guide the selection of the initial regimen. Resistance testing is recommended in most clinical situations before beginning treatment, because the rate of transmission of virus resistant to at least one drug is estimated to be between 6% and 16% in European and American cohorts[68–74] (see Resistance, Viral Genotyping, Phenotyping, and Viral Fitness case for further discussion).

E.J. should have a baseline T-cell count, viral load measurement, and viral genotype obtained. A complete blood count, electrolyte panel, and renal and liver function tests should also be performed. These laboratory values help in selecting therapeutic options (see below) and establish baseline values in the event that problems are encountered in the future.

ANTIRETROVIRAL THERAPY

3. E.J.'s T-cell count and viral load measurement (two separate levels obtained within the past 2 weeks) return at 225 cells/mm^3 and 145,000 copies/mL (by RT-PCR assay). Should antiretroviral therapy be initiated?

In deciding to initiate antiretroviral therapy, it is important to consider both the potential benefits of therapy and the potential risk of therapy, including both short-term and long-term side effects and potential for the development of drug resistance (and cross-resistance; see below). Antiretroviral therapy should be offered to any patient who is symptomatic, regardless of T-cell count and viral load measurements. "Symptomatic" refers to any new opportunistic infection or increases in constitutional symptoms (e.g., fevers, night sweats, unexplained weight loss). These events suggest a faltering immune system that necessitates therapy. In patients who are asymptomatic, assessment of the patient's surrogate marker data (T-cell count, viral load measurements), concurrent medical conditions, medication adherence history (if any), and motivation to initiate therapy are necessary. The results of resistance testing should be considered before initiating therapy.

Knowledge of both the T-cell count and the baseline viral load values is necessary to "stage" the severity of infection. In otherwise healthy, immunocompetent persons, T-cell measurements are >1,200 cells/mm^3. In patients who have been chronically infected with HIV, significant T-cell destruction occurs. When T-cell counts fall below 500 cells/mm^3, patients are at increased risk for opportunistic infections (Fig. 69-3). The optimal time to initiate antiretroviral therapy among asymptomatic patients with HIV infection is unknown. Data from

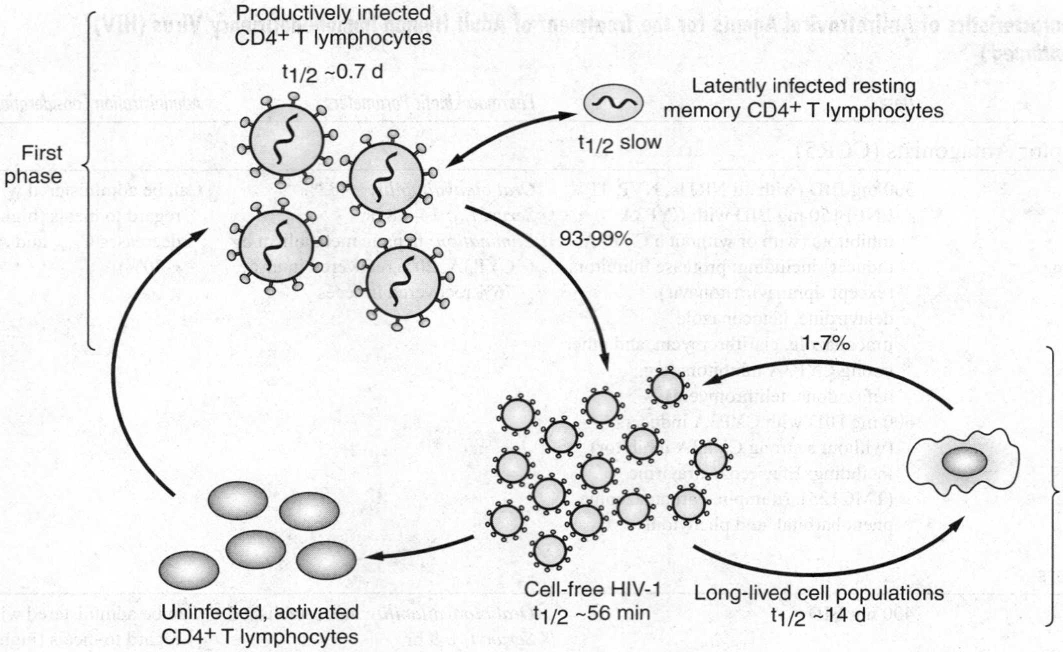

FIGURE 69-5 Schematic summary of the turnover rates of virions and the relative contribution of the different HIV-1-infected cell populations. After initiation of HAART, the viral burden decreases rapidly by several orders of magnitude, which corresponds to the rapid clearance of plasma virions and productively infected T lymphocytes (first phase). Certain cell populations that initially are responsible for only a small proportion of the circulating virions in an untreated HIV-1-infected individual display slower turnovers. Long-lived infected T lymphocytes, latently infected cells that become activated and release of virions from follicular dendritic cells, contribute to the second phase of plasma virus decay. (Adapted with permission from Simon V, Ho DD. HIV-1 dynamics in vivo: implications for therapy, *Nat Rev Microb* 2003 Dec;1:181.)

both clinical trials and observational cohort studies have shown a clear benefit for antiretroviral therapy when CD4 cell counts are <200 cells/mm.[3,5] Currently, the optimal time to initiate antiretroviral therapy in patients with CD4 cell counts between 200 cells/mm^3 and 350 cells/mm^3 is unknown. Information from randomized, controlled trials to guide treatment initiation is lacking, but observational cohorts provide some information on disease progression and initiation of treatment. The risk of disease progression is closely tied to CD4 cell counts, with low CD4 counts (<200 cells/mm^3) predicting both short- and long-term risk of disease progression.[36–38,75,76] High viral load (>100,000 copies/mL), increasing age, acquisition of infection through intravenous drug use, and a previous AIDS diagnosis also increase the risk of disease progression in observational cohorts. Based on these data, the Department of Health and Human Services (DHHS) published guidelines on when to consider antiretroviral therapy in those infected with HIV (Table 69-4). These guidelines provide general principles for when to initiate therapy in an antiretroviral-naïve patient; however, they are not absolute. Most clinicians would prefer to begin therapy before CD4 cell counts become <200 cells/mm^3, and many use <350 cells/mm^3 as a point to begin discussions with the

Table 69-4 Indications for the Initiation of Antiretroviral Therapy in the Chronically HIV-1–Infected Patient[a]

Clinical Category	*CD4+ T-Cell Count*	*Plasma HIV RNA*	*Recommendation[b]*
Symptomatic (AIDS, severe symptoms)	Any value	Any value	Treat
Asymptomatic	CD4+ T cells <200/mm^3	Any value	Treat. The 3-year probability of progressing to AIDS or death is 9%–20%.
Asymptomatic	CD4+ T cells 200–350/mm^3	Any value	Treatment should be offered. The 3-year probability of progressing to AIDS or death is 4.7%–6.1%.
Asymptomatic	CD4+ T cells >350/mm^3	>100,000 copies/mL	Most experienced clinicians defer therapy, but some may consider initiating treatment. The 3-year probability of progressing to AIDS or death is 4.4%
Asymptomatic	CD4+ T cells >350/mm^3	<100,000 copies/mL	Defer therapy. The 3-year probability of progressing to AIDS or death is 3.4%.

[a] The optimal time to initiate therapy in asymptomatic individuals with >200 CD4+ cells is not known. This table provides general guidance rather than absolute recommendations for an individual patient. All decisions to initiate therapy should be based on prognosis as determined by the CD4+ T-cell count and plasma HIV RNA, the potential benefits and risks of therapy shown in Table 69-4, and the willingness of the patient to accept therapy.
[b] Probability of progression to AIDS or death obtained from DHHS Treatment Guidelines, October 2006.
AIDS, acquired immunodeficiency syndrome; HIV, human immunodeficiency virus.
DHHS: Department of Health and Human Services

patient regarding initiating therapy. Increasing data from longitudinal cohort studies suggest that patients who begin HAART therapy at higher CD4 cell counts are more likely to achieve CD4 cell count recovery than patients who begin at counts <200 cells/mm^3,[77–79] although the potential clinical implications of this remain unknown. This evidence plus the ease of dosing and tolerability of new HAART regimens may tip the balance to early treatment. Thus, treatment is offered to patients with CD4 cell counts between 200 cell/mm^3 and 350 cells/mm^3. In the case of CD4 cell counts >350 mm^3, most clinicians would defer treatment, unless viral load is very high (i.e. >100,000 copies/mL), which increases the potential for CD4 cell count decline, and thus the risk of disease progression. In this situation, clinicians may elect to take an approach to early treatment and offer therapy to prevent further immune compromise.

The decision to initiate therapy should not be taken lightly nor should it be based solely on surrogate marker data. Antiretroviral regimens may improve the quality and duration of a patient's life, but they are not without significant risks and adverse effects. Once therapy is initiated, antiretroviral therapy is a lifetime commitment. For some patients, this may be a difficult realization, particularly if the patient is relatively healthy. In addition, the fear of adverse events and toxicities must also be overcome. These guidelines, therefore, should be used as a springboard for discussions with the patient regarding the risks and benefits of therapy. It is critical for practitioners to talk openly with patients about their fears and concerns and make an assessment about their motivation to initiate therapy and ability to take a lifelong regimen. The patient should always make the final decision after careful discussions with the practitioner.

E.J. has a number of significant risk factors for disease progression. He is clinically symptomatic with oral thrush and nonspecific constitutional symptoms (e.g., fevers, night sweats, and weight loss). His surrogate maker data place him at risk for greater disease progression (T-cell count <350 cells/mm^3 and viral load >100,000 copies/mL). Based on these values, E.J. should be counseled on his risk of disease progression, potential adverse events associated with both starting and deferring treatment, and his willingness to adhere to a regimen.

4. After careful discussions, E.J. agrees to initiate therapy. What should be the goals of therapy? What other factors or information needs to be considered in selecting an appropriate regimen?

Before developing a patient-specific regimen, it is important to recognize the benefits and limitations of therapy and identify obtainable and realistic goals.

Goals of Therapy

Goal 1: Maximally and Durably Suppress Viral Load

The ability to measure viral loads has shown that maximal viral suppression often results in significant increases in T-cell counts and improved clinical outcomes.[5] Based on our understanding of viral pathogenesis, this is not surprising. Lower amounts of replicating virus result in decreased risk for T-cell infection and destruction and, subsequently, a more intact immune response. Therefore, therapy should suppress viral replication as much as possible, preferably to nondetectable levels in the plasma, for as long as possible.[5,6] The development of new antiretroviral agents with improved potency and adverse event profiles, in addition to more convenient dosing regimens, makes viral suppression a reasonable goal in most patients, even those who previously have received multiple suboptimal regimens. In the treatment-experienced patient, however, special care must to given to designing a regimen that will suppress viral load, yet not contribute to the development of drug resistance that limits future treatment options. Consultation with an expert in antiretroviral resistance patterns is critical to designing a salvage regimen in such patients.

The development of drug resistance is a consideration in the selection of regimens for patients who are antiretroviral naïve as well. In any given viral population, the potential exists for a spontaneous mutation to occur, which results in a resistant isolate. The larger the population, the greater the risk. HIV replication is a highly error-susceptible process, especially the reverse transcriptase enzyme. Given the high rate of viral replication, the potential exists for the daily production of thousands of replication-competent viral mutants to each and every site on the HIV genome (~10,000 nucleotides in length).[7,35] Under selective pressures from inadequate antiretroviral therapies, isolates with reduced susceptibility to the given regimen eventually flourish and repopulate the host. This is of particular concern given the potential for cross-resistance between antiretroviral agents (see following discussion of resistance). Therefore, the use of a regimen that fully suppresses viral replication reduces the potential for mutations and the development of cross-resistance.

Although >20 U.S. Food and Drug Administration (FDA)-approved antiretroviral agents are currently available to use in combination therapies, many of these agents display similar resistance profiles. As a result, by developing resistance to one or more agents in a given regimen, the loss of activity to other agents with similar resistance profiles can occur (i.e., cross-resistance).[7] Whether drug resistance develops is determined by the genetic barrier associated with the individual agents. Some agents have low genetic barriers; that is, only one or two critical changes in the virus are necessary for resistance to occur. An example of a class of agents with a low genetic barrier is the NNRTIs. One critical point mutation in the viral genome is required for loss of activity among this class of agents.[7] In contrast, the PIs have a wide genetic barrier in that it takes multiple viral changes to incur resistance.[7] It should be recognized, however, that just because an agent has a low genetic barrier does not mean it is virologically inferior or less potent. Potent regimens containing NNRTIs have been shown to be highly effective and provide durable treatment responses.[5] It is also important to realize that the potency of the regimen as a whole is critical to determining whether or not drug resistance develops. If viral replication is suppressed, the development of resistance will be minimal. When viral replication does occur, however, the greater the replication, the greater the risk for development of resistance.[5,6] In situations in which viral replication does occur, having an agent(s) in the antiretroviral regimen with a low genetic barrier may be risky and could result in the loss of activity of the individual agent, the development of cross-resistance to other agents, or both. As a result, it is critical to select an antiretroviral regimen that has a high likelihood of suppressing viral replication and to which the patient will strictly adhere (either through ease of dosing or minimization of adverse drug events).

Given the increased rate of transmission of resistant viruses to patients newly infected with HIV,[68–71,80] current guidelines recommend obtaining a resistance test before initiation of therapy to help in the selection of appropriate agents in the antiretroviral regimen.[5,6] If a regimen is initiated that contains an agent(s) to which the virus has already developed resistance, the potency of the entire regimen may be insufficient for complete viral suppression and further antiretroviral resistance may develop. Because of its more rapid turn-around time, a viral genotype is generally preferred over a viral phenotype.[5]

Goal 2: Preserve and Strengthen the Immune System

Suppression of viral replication usually leads to increased CD4 cell counts and strengthens and preserves the immune system. With increased cell counts, patients are at decreased risk for the development of opportunistic infections and death. With newer and better regimens, strengthening and preserving the immune system may be possible even in treatment-experienced patients, although drug regimens must be designed carefully to prevent development of further resistance. Although full immune reconstitution may not be possible after prolonged time periods with low CD4 cell counts, it is reasonable to attempt to restore immune function as fully as possible. Despite advances in drug therapy, it is important to remember that HIV remains an incurable condition.

Goal 3: Limit Drug Adverse Events, Promote Adherence, and Improve Quality of Life

Treatment with combination therapy has been shown to be highly effective in suppressing HIV replication and improving survival among patients who are HIV infected. Maximal viral suppression, however, should not be obtained at the expense of a patient's overall health and safety. Lifelong adherence to an antiretroviral regimen can be a complex and difficult task,[4,5] although advances in coformulation of drug products and the advent of ritonavir-boosted protease inhibitors have simplified treatment considerably. Several once-daily regimens are recommended as first-line therapy (Tables 69-3 and 69-5). The patient's ability to adhere to therapy may, however, still be the difference between a regimen that fails and one that results in a clinical benefit, and the first regimen generally provides the best chance for treatment success. Adverse events make tolerating these regimens difficult, minimizing drug adherence and subsequent response to therapy. Changes in body composition (known as lipodystrophy), increases in lipids and triglycerides, bone and joint fractures, increased risks for cardiac disease, and the development of lactic acidosis are serious concerns.[81] In addition, both acute and long-term adverse events can be fatal if not properly identified and managed.

Data from studies evaluating nonadherence among those HIV infected shows that at least 10% of patients on PIs miss a dose each day and that at least 20% miss a dose every 2 days.[82] The exact degree of adherence required for clinical success is currently unknown, and patients should be counseled to always take their regimens as prescribed. The four most common reasons for skipping antiretroviral doses among those infected with HIV are simple forgetfulness, a change in daily routine, being too busy with other things, and being away from home.[83,84] Factors associated with poor adherence include (a) the number of medications (the greater the number, the greater the likelihood of poor adherence); (b) the complexity of the regimen (special meal requirements, escalating or de-escalating doses, dose frequency); (c) special storage requirements; (d) interference of medication with lifestyle and daily activities; and (e) poor communication with primary care providers and other health care professionals.[83,84]

Table 69-5 Recommended Antiretroviral Agents for Initial Treatment of Established Human Immunodeficiency Virus (HIV) Infection[a]

	Preferred	*Alternatives*
Dual NRTIs Options	Tenofovir + emtricitabine (coformulated)	Zidovudine + lamivudine (coformulated)
	Abacavir + lamivudine (coformulated)	Didanosine + (lamivudine or emtricitabine)
NNRTIs (one NNRTIs + two NRTIs)	Efavirenz[b]	Nevirapine[c]
PIs (one or two PIs + two NRTIs)	Atazanavir + ritonavir	Atazanavir[d]
	Fosamprenavir + ritonavir twice daily	Fosamprenavir
	Lopinavir/ritonavir (coformulated) twice daily	Fosamprenavir + ritonavir once daily
		Lopinavir/ritonavir (coformulated) once daily
		Saquinaivr + ritonavir
Not recommended: Should not be offered	All monotherapies, dual nucleoside regimens, NRTIs-sparing regimens, triple NRTIs regimens	

[a]This table provides a guide to the use of available treatment regimens for individuals with no prior or limited experience on human immunodeficiency virus (HIV) therapy. In accordance with the established goals of HIV therapy, priority is given to regimens in which clinical trials data suggest the following: sustained suppression of HIV plasma RNA (particularly in patients with high baseline viral load), sustained increase in CD4+ T-cell count (in most cases >48 weeks), and favorable clinical outcome (i.e., delayed progression to acquired immunodeficiency syndrome [AIDS] and death). Additional consideration is given to the regimen's pill burden, dosing frequency, food requirements, convenience, toxicity, and drug interaction profile compared with other regimens. It is important to note that all antiretroviral agents have potentially serious toxic and adverse events associated with their use.

[b]Except during the first trimester of pregnancy or in women with high pregnancy potential (women who are trying to conceive or who are not using effective and consistent contraception).

[c]As an alternative in adult females with CD4+ T-cell counts <250 cells/mm^3 and adult males with CD4+ T-cell counts ≤ 400 cells/mm^3.

[d]When used with tenofovir, atazanavir should be combined with ritonavir 100 mg/day.

NRTIs, nucleotide analogue reverse transcriptase inhibitor; PI, protease inhibitor.

Incorporating these factors into the selection of a patient-specific regimen may improve adherence and, subsequently, the chance for an improved clinical outcome.

Goal 4: Prevent HIV-related Morbidity and Mortality

By successfully treating HIV (i.e., suppressing viral load and restoring immune function), patients are at decreased risk for acquiring HIV-associated opportunistic infections (Fig. 69-3). By achieving goals 1 through 3, goal 4 naturally follows, and truly this is the ultimate goal of the pharmacotherapy of HIV infection. With modern-day HAART therapy, patients infected with HIV are more frequently dying from non–HIV-related conditions that are common in the general population (i.e., cardiovascular disease, hepatic disease, non–HIV-associated malignancies)[85] than in the past. Although this represents a significant achievement in care, it also provides increased complexity in caring for those infected with HIV who are both at risk for HIV-related illness and also receiving treatment for comorbid conditions. This increases the potential for drug–drug and drug–disease interactions that must be considered to optimize patient care and prevent morbidity and mortality.

5. **On questioning, E.J. states that he has had two bouts of alcohol-induced pancreatitis in the past. The last episode was approximately 1 year ago. He admits to occasional binge drinking even though he knows it is not good for him. E.J. has no known drug allergies and is currently taking only temazepam periodically to help him sleep. He is employed as a construction worker and during the day hours is extremely busy. His complete blood count, electrolyte, and liver and renal panel all return within normal limits. E.J. has no particular preference for a specific regimen and appears highly motivated to take control of his disease. What factors should be considered when selecting an appropriate antiretroviral regimen?**

The selection of a patient-specific regimen can be a complex decision. Many potential combinations can be used, but a number of general principles should be followed:

General Rules of Therapy[5,6]

1. Initiate therapy when the potential clinical benefits outweigh the potential risks. Many of the current regimens reduce viral replication to below detectable levels in most patients, and result in durable treatment responses. Reasons for these improved response rates compared with older regimens include the simplification of the regimens (e.g., less pills per day, less frequent dosing per day, use of fixed-dose combination products), improvement in overall potency of the regimens, and minimization of short-term side effects. Consequently, if the correct patient-specific HAART regimen is selected as initial therapy, the patient should be able to adhere to therapy and gain both a virologic and clinical benefit from the regimen.
2. Select the type of antiretroviral regimen. The use of combination HAART therapy is standard medical care and should be considered in all patients. Monotherapy with any agent should be avoided because clinical trials have shown these regimens to be inferior. In addition, the use of dual nucleoside-only–containing regimens should be avoided because initial viral suppression may not be sustained. In general, two types of initial strategies—NNRTIs- or PI-based—are preferred. (Table 69-6). Both types of regimens are potent and can produce sustained virologic response. Currently, no evidence definitively recommends one type over another, and the selection is dependent on patient-specific factors, such as concomitant disease states (i.e., hepatitis, diabetes, cardiovascular disease), and provider preference. In selected patients with compelling reasons to avoid use of a PIs or NNRTIs, triple nucleoside therapy may be considered with lamivudine (3TC), zidovudine (ZDV), and abacavir (ABC), but this regimen should not be routinely used as first-line treatment, particularly in patients with high viral loads (i.e. >100,000 copies/mL).
3. Avoid regimens with overlapping toxicities. In general, the concomitant use of the "D" NRTIs (didanosine [ddI] and stavudine [d4T]) should be avoided owing to an increased risk of pancreatitis and neuropathy. Atazanavir and indinavir can both cause severe hyperbilirubinemia, and concomitant use should be avoided.
4. Avoid regimens that are not virologically additive or synergistic. Zidovudine (ZDV) and d4T should not be used together because both in vitro and in vivo studies have shown these agents to be antagonistic. 3TC and emtricitabine (FTC) should not be used together because they have similar resistance profiles, and concomitant use will not confer any additional virologic benefit. Amprenavir oral solution and fosamprenavir should not be used together, because fosamprenavir is simply the prodrug of amprenavir.

Table 69-6 Advantages and Disadvantages of Antiretroviral Components for Initial Antiretroviral Therapy[a]

ARV Class	*Possible Advantages*	*Possible Disadvantages*
Dual NRTIs	• Established backbone of combination antiretroviral therapy	• Rare but serious cases of lactic acidosis with hepatic steatosis reported (d4T >ddI=ZDV>TDF=ABC=3TC=FTC)
NNRTIs	• Less fat maldistribution and dyslipidemia than PI-based regimens • Save PIs options for future use	• Low genetic barrier to resistance (single mutation confers resistance) • Cross resistance among approved NNRTIs • Skin rash • Potential for cytochrome P450 drug interactions
PI	• Higher genetic barrier to resistance • Save NNRTIs for future use	• Metabolic complications (fat maldistribution, dyslipidemia, insulin resistance) • Cytochrome P450 substrates, inhibitors, and inducers (potential for drug interactions)

[a]Adapted from DHHS treatment guidelines January 2008.
Department of Health and Human Services.
3TC, lamivudine; ABC, abacavir; d4T, stavudine; ddI, didanosine; FTC, emtricitabine; HAART, highly active antiretroviral therapies; NNRTIs, non-nucleoside reverse transcriptase inhibitors; NRTIs, nucleoside reverse transcriptase inhibitor; PI, protease inhibitor; TDF, tenofovir; ZDV, zidovudine.

The use of tenofovir and didanosine as initial therapy is not recommended owing to the potential for virologic failure, suboptimal immunologic response, and the potential for development of drug resistance.

5. If PI-based HAART is desired, consider using a ritonavir-boosted regimen. Various PIs have been evaluated in combination with ritonavir, including saquinavir, lopinavir, indinavir, fosamprenavir, tipranavir, atazanavir, and darunavir. Ritonavir, a potent inhibitor of cytochrome P450 metabolism and p-glycoprotein activity, interacts significantly with a number of agents, including other PIs.[47] This inhibition can be exploited to decrease the metabolism or increase the absorption of the other PIs. In some cases, such as lopinavir, tipranavir, and darunavir, the use of coadministered ritonavir is required for virologically relevant concentrations. The result is a regimen with more potent viral suppression than a regimen using either agent alone. In addition, this combination allows for more convenient once- or twice-daily dosing, often lowers the total daily pill burden, and removes the need for drugfood restrictions. Given that ritonavir can cause significant gastrointestinal side effects in some patients at increased doses and that only small amounts of ritonavir are needed to inhibit metabolism, low doses are sufficient (e.g., 100–200 mg). It should also be remembered that ritonavir interacts with a number of medications and, depending on the severity of the interaction, may require dosage adjustments of other agents or the inability to use ritonavir in the given regimen.[5,6]
6. Avoid regimens shown to be detrimental in specific patient populations. Examples include the use of efavirenz (Pregnancy Class D) in women of child-bearing potential not using reliable methods of birth control or in the first trimester of pregnancy, because this drug has been associated with teratogenic effects; the use of propylene glycol-containing amprenavir solutions in high-risk patients, such as pregnant women, children <4 years of age, patients with renal or liver dysfunction, and those undergoing treatment with metronidazole or disulfiram. Nevirapine has the potential for hepatotoxicity in patients with higher baseline CD4 cell counts (>250 cells/mm^3 for women, >400 cell/mm^3 for men).

6. What initial antiretroviral regimen should E.J. receive?

When selecting a patient-specific regimen, these steps should be followed:

Step 1: Determine Which HAART-Based Regimen Will Be Used

A careful review of the advantages and disadvantages of each interventional strategy should occur (Table 69-6). For example, efavirenz may be avoided for patients with a psychiatric history. Protease inhibitors may be less favored with a familial history or current medical condition consisting of coronary artery disease, hyperlipidemia, or diabetes mellitus.[81]

After discussions with E.J., it appears that he is highly motivated to take control of his disease and is willing to initiate therapy. Subsequently, the use of a combination regimen with either a PI-based or NNRTIs-based regimen is appropriate. Potential treatment options are listed in Table 69-5.

Step 2: Optimize Agents in the Regimen

The next step requires the selection of agents for the regimen. In many situations, absolute contraindications and significant drug–drug interactions limit the agents available for use in the regimen. In this case, ddI is a relative contraindication given a history of alcohol abuse and pancreatitis. The remaining nucleoside or nucleotide reverse transcriptase inhibitors, including ZDV, 3TC, d4T, tenofovir (TDF), FTC, and ABC, are all potential options. With respect to drug interaction issues, any NNRTIs or PIs class can be administered safely with temazepam.

Step 3: Quality-of-Life Considerations

When selecting a regimen, assessment of quality-of-life issues, potential adverse drug events, and patient requests should receive as much consideration as drug–drug interactions and absolute contraindications. In some situations, these issues could mean the difference between a regimen that is effective and one that is not. Considering E.J.'s lifestyle and work requirements, it is best to select a regimen that will minimally interfere with his daily activities. The selection of a regimen with once- or twice-daily dosing is appropriate (Table 69-3), although once-daily dosing might be preferred. The combinations of nucleosides recommended as initial therapy can be given once or twice daily, and are available as coformulated products (Table 69-3). Examples of potential regimens include 3TC plus ABC (dosed once daily) or FTC plus TDF (dosed once daily) with efavirenz, which is the preferred first-line NNRTIs. Using the same nucleoside agents, atazanavir–ritonavir administered once daily, fosamprenavir–ritonavir administered twice daily, or lopinavir–ritonavir administered twice daily are the preferred PI-based regimens.

7. E.J. is starting emtricitabine, tenofovir, and efavirenz (coformulated for once-daily dosing as Atripla). How should therapy be monitored? Are any additional laboratory tests necessary?

Short-Term Assessments

Three important criteria determine whether an antiretroviral regimen is effective: clinical assessment, surrogate marker responses, and regimen tolerability.[5,6] In patients who are clinically symptomatic (e.g., constitutional symptoms such as fatigue, night sweats, and weight loss; new opportunistic infections), the initiation of an appropriate antiretroviral regimen often results in resolution of symptoms, increased strength and energy, and improvement in overall well-being. In some patients, however, the effect may not be as prominent. A careful assessment of clinical symptoms should therefore be regularly performed at all follow-up appointments.

In all patients, repeat viral load and T-cell measurements are necessary. HIV RNA concentrations should be obtained within 2 to 8 weeks of therapy initiation.[5,6] This early value allows clinicians to assess the magnitude of response and ensures declining viral load measurements. Therapy with an effective regimen will result in at least a threefold (0.5 log) and tenfold decrease (1.0 log) in viral load counts by weeks 4 and 8, respectively.[5,6] The viral load should continue to decline over the next 12 to 16 weeks and, in most patients, it will become undetectable.[5,6] Long-term response to therapy correlates with the magnitude of viral suppression on initiation of a regimen. The greater the suppression, the greater the durability of response to that regimen.[86–88] The speed and magnitude of suppression, however, can be affected by a number of factors, including clinical status of the patient (e.g., more advanced disease–low T-cell counts, high viral load value), adherence to therapy, and overall potency of the regimen.[5,6] When the virologic response is less than optimal, evaluation of compliance should be assessed, repeat viral load measurements performed, and drug concentrations of key antiretroviral agents evaluated for subtherapeutic values before considering a change in therapy.

In response to declining viral replication, T-cell destruction decreases and subsequently CD4 counts increase. The magnitude of this rebound can vary significantly, with some patients experiencing large increases and others experiencing little or no change. Given that T-cell changes do not occur rapidly, once therapy is initiated, repeat T-cell counts should be obtained at the 3- to 4-month follow-up visit.[5,6]

Failure either by surrogate marker data or clinical symptomatology can occur when inadequate serum concentrations of antiretrovirals are achieved. The most common reason for this is failure to adhere to the prescribed regimen. It is important to determine the reason for nonadherence so that it can be quickly and adequately addressed (e.g., by education on the management of adverse events, or by switching to a better-tolerated regimen). Drug exposures can also be affected by the addition of new drugs or herbal products to a patient's regimen. Both garlic and St. John's wort have been shown to lower the exposure to non–ritonavir-boosted protease inhibitors.[89,90] In addition, certain medications require specific food requirements to ensure optimal exposure (Table 69-3). Therefore, careful evaluation of new drugs, herbs, and dosing habits should be performed at each follow-up visit. If after discussions with the patient, the clinician does not identify adverse events, adherence issues, and new drug–drug, drug–herb, or drug–food interactions as potential causes of failure, then changing to another viable regimen should be considered. In some cases, therapeutic drug monitoring may assist in identifying physiologic factors such as malabsorption or rapid metabolism.

8. After initiation of therapy, E.J.'s viral load values are 7,000 copies/mL at 4 weeks, and <50 copies/mL (undetectable) at 14 weeks. His T-cell counts have increased from 225 to 525 cells/mm^3. In addition, E.J. states that his night sweats and fevers have disappeared, he "feels great" and that he has had no drug-related problems. Is the therapy effective? How should therapy be monitored?

E.J.'s response to the emtricitabine, tenofovir, and efavirenz does indicate efficacy. Clinically, his symptoms have subsided and his overall health is much improved. His viral load measurements have responded appropriately and are now below the level of assay detection. T-cell counts have increased by 300 cells/mm^3. Finally, E.J. has experienced no drug-related adverse events. Given the response to date, no changes are required and the current regimen should be continued.

Long-Term Assessments

Once the prescribed regimen has been stabilized, the long-term goals of therapy are to maintain maximal viral suppression, sustain clinical and immunologic improvements, and maintain drug tolerability. Periodic assessments should be made of viral load (every 3–4 months) and T-cell counts (every 3–6 months).[5,6] These surrogate marker data allow clinicians to monitor trends in viral activity and immunologic status and assist them in identifying early regimen failure. Clinical assessment of the patient and questioning of tolerability to the prescribed regimen should occur at the 3- to 6-month follow-up visits.

Treatment Failure

9. E.J. has remained on FTC, TDF, and efavirenz for more than a year. To date, his T-cell counts have remained stable at 550 cells/mm^3, and his viral load measurements have remained below the limit of assay detection. He presents with new complaints of fevers and malaise. E.J. reports that he has been compliant with therapy and has not started any new medications. Repeat laboratory tests now show E.J.'s viral load is 3,000 copies/mL and his T-cell count is 375 cells/mm^3 (both repeated and validated). Should E.J.'s regimen be changed?

Up to 25% of patient on HAART fail therapy within the first year.[3] Reasons for failure are not fully known; however, risk factors include a history of low T-cell counts, high viral loads, and extensive use of antiretroviral agents.[3,4] Assessment of regimen failure should be based on data similar to when therapy is initiated: (a) clinical symptoms, (b) surrogate marker data, and (c) regimen tolerability and adherence.[5–7]

In many patients, the first sign of failure is a change in clinical signs and symptoms. These changes can be subtle (e.g., increase in constitutional symptoms, new onset of oral thrush) or more severe (e.g., new opportunistic infections). These situations suggest a failing regimen and necessitate a change in therapy.

Assessment of efficacy should also involve evaluation of surrogate marker data (e.g., T cells and viral load). In many situations, changes to these markers occur before any noticeable clinical signs and symptoms. Therefore, careful evaluation of surrogate marker data may allow clinicians an opportunity to intervene before any significant immune destruction occurs. Virologic failure, defined as new or continued viral replication despite appropriate antiretroviral therapy, suggests a failing regimen. For example, patients with repeated detection of virus in plasma after initial suppression to undetectable levels should be evaluated as potential treatment failures. In patients who do not achieve viral suppression to below detectable levels, a significant increase in viral replication (defined as a threefold increase or greater) should also be viewed as a treatment failure.[5,6]

When assessing viral load, it is important to recognize that these values can increase from vaccinations or other concurrent infections (see Question 2). Therefore, a thorough medical history should be taken to rule out other causes of increasing viral load. In addition, laboratory values should be interpreted as trends over time and not necessarily as individual measurements. A repeat viral load should be performed and evaluated within 4 weeks of the initial viral load increase. In some cases, transient viral "blips" occur (increases in viral load measurements just above the level of assay detection (e.g., 50–1,000 copies/mL), which become undetectable at the next visit.[91–93] The clinical significance of viral blips is unknown and, although they may not directly reflect treatment failure, they may represent the potential for near future viral breakthrough, either because of patient nonadherence or insufficient antiretroviral potency. Careful follow-up of these patients is therefore required, as changes to the current HAART regimen may be necessary.

In response to increasing viral replication, T-cell destruction occurs. A significant decrease in CD4 cells is defined as a decrease of >30% in absolute numbers, or a decrease of 3% in percentage.[5,6] Persistently declining T-cell counts, with or without increasing viral load measurements, represent treatment failure and suggest a change in therapy is warranted.

Other potential causes for failure include nonadherence and drug–drug interactions. When a patient has not taken the prescribed regimen as directed, discussions regarding tolerability, number of doses missed, duration of nonadherence, and lifestyle changes should take place. The decision to reinitiate a prescribed regimen should take into account the future likelihood of adherence and the potential development of resistant strains. In those patients with a history of long-standing nonadherence, the success of reinitiating the prescribed regimen may be limited. The precise effect of the duration and extent of nonadherence on the development of resistance, however, has not been fully evaluated. For the virus to mutate, sufficient drug pressure must be placed on the virus. Some estimate this requires moderate patient adherence of 50%.[94]

Significant drug–drug, drug–food, and drug–herb interactions could also contribute to therapeutic failure. Interactions between a new medication and an herbal product could decrease the bioavailability or increase the metabolism of the HIV medications leading to low serum concentrations.[5,89,90] In addition, many medications require certain food requirements to allow maximal drug absorption. A careful review of all new medications and their potential for clinically significant drug interactions should be evaluated at all visits (Tables 69-7 and 69-8).

Currently, E.J. has a number of signs and symptoms that suggest a failing regimen. E.J. is experiencing new symptoms of fevers and malaise not attributable to any other cause. E.J.'s viral load value has become detectable at 3,000 copies/mL without evidence of concurrent infections or vaccinations in the past 4 weeks. E.J.'s T-cell counts have declined from 550 cells/mm^3 to 375 cells/mm.^{3} Finally, it appears that E.J. has been adhering to his therapy and has not started any new medications that could affect the efficacy of his current regimen. Therefore, a change in therapy is necessary.

10. What potential antiretroviral regimen(s) can be considered for E.J.?

In addition to the general rules of therapy described in Question 5, other issues should be considered when selecting an alternative regimen for a patient failing therapy.

General Rules for Changing Therapies[5,6]

1. If possible, the new regimen should contain all new antiretroviral agents to which the patient has not been exposed. If this is not possible, the new regimen should contain at least two new agents that are not currently contained in the failing regimen. The potential for cross-resistance between antiretroviral drugs should be considered when choosing new regimens, and therefore resistance testing should provide useful information (see Question 12).
2. Given that antiretroviral drug resistance is more likely to occur with increased and prolonged viral replication in the presence of antiretroviral agents, changes to therapy should occur close to the time of treatment failure. Prolonged treatment with a failing regimen is likely to result in the accumulation of resistance mutations (particularly with protease inhibitors), which may limit future treatment options.
3. Resistance testing is recommended to guide the selection of future drug regimens. Optimally, testing via genotype, phenotype, or virtual phenotype should occur while the patient is taking the failing regimen, or within 4 weeks of discontinuation to increase the likelihood of detecting resistant isolates. These tests cannot reliably detect mutations at viral concentrations <1,000 copies/mL, and may have limited usefulness in patients with persistent low-level viremia.
4. To prevent the development of resistance, one new drug should never be added to a failing regimen. An exception to this rule is if the initial response to a first regimen has been inadequate (e.g., nondetectable viral load at 16–20 weeks). In this situation, some clinicians decide to intensify therapy with an additional agent provided that the viral load measurements were trending downward since initiation of therapy.
5. If possible, a regimen that has failed in the past should not be reinitiated; an isolate resistant to the failed regimen could continue to reside within various compartments of the body. If a regimen to which the patient had previously failed were restarted, unimpeded viral replication of the resistant strain would occur, repopulate the host, and eventually result in treatment failure. In some situations (e.g., patients with advanced disease, limited treatment options and prior exposure to most antiretroviral agents), it may be necessary to reinitiate agents or regimens in combination with additional new agents with the goal of suppressing viral replication.
6. When treatment failure is a direct result of drug toxicity (rather than poor drug efficacy), the offending agent should be replaced with an alternative drug from a similar class provided that the potential for cross-resistance is minimal.
7. If an agent in a given regimen must be stopped, it is recommended that all agents in the regimen be stopped and restarted simultaneously to prevent the development of resistance. An exception to this rule is when components of a regimen have differing half-lives, such as NNRTIs and NRTIs. In this situation, if all drugs are discontinued simultaneously, effective NNRTIs monotherapy is likely to result, because detectable concentrations of the NNRTIs will persist for days or weeks longer than detectable NRTIs concentrations. In this situation, many experts would recommend continuing the NRTIs agents for 1 to 2 weeks past NNRTIs discontinuation to provide combination therapy during the NNRTIs elimination "tail."

It should be recognized that many alternative regimens are based on theoretic benefits or limited data. In addition, many potential options could be limited in some patients based on prior antiretroviral use, toxicity, or past intolerances. Therefore, the clinician should carefully discuss these issues with the patient before changing therapy.

Because E.J. is failing to respond to his current regimen, a new antiretroviral regimen must be chosen. In addition to selecting susceptible agents from resistance testing, the new regimen should take into consideration quality-of-life issues. In E.J.'s situation, it is reasonable to switch to a ritonavir-boosted PIs regimen, with two or more nucleoside agents as dictated by the viral resistance profile.

Table 69-7 Drug Effects on Concentration of PI[a]

Drug Affected	Fosamprenavir	Atazanavir	Lopinavir/Ritonavir	Nelfinavir	Ritonavir	Saquinavir*	Tipranavir
Protease Inhibitors							
Darunavir (DRV)	No data.	Levels: ATV concentrations from ATV 300 mg QD when administered with DRV/r were similar to ATV/r 300/100 mg QD DRV was unchanged. Dose: Administer ATV 300 mg QD with DRV/r for exposure similar to ATV/T 300/100 mg QD	Levels: DRV AUC and C_{min} ↓ 53% and 65%, respectively. LPV AUC and C_{min} ↑ 37% and 72%, respectively. Dose: Should not be co-administered, as doses are not established.	No data.	Levels: 14-fold ↑ in DRV exposure in combination with RTV 100 mg bid. Dose: DRV should only be used in combination with RTV 100 mg bid to achieve sufficient DRV exposure	Levels: DRV AUC and C_{min} ↓ 26% and 42%, respectively. SQV exposure similar to when administered with RTV 1000/100 mg bid.‡ Dose: Should not be co-administered, as doses are not established.	No data.
Fosamprenavir (fAPV)	*	Levels: With fAPV/ATV 1,400/400 QD, ATV AUC & C_{min} ↓ 33% and 57%, respectively. fAPV AUC and C_{min} ↑ 78% and 283%, respectively. With fAPV/r 700/100 mg BID + ATV 300 mg QD, ATV AUC and C_{max} ↓ 22% and 24%, respectively; fAPV unchanged. Dose: Insufficient data for dose recommendation.	Levels: With coadministration of fAPV 700 mg BID and LPV/r capsules 400/100 mg BID, fAPV C_{min} 64% and LPV C_{min} ↓ 53%. An increased rate of adverse events was seen with coadministration. Dose: Should not be coadministered, as doses are not established.	*	Levels: fAPV AUC and C_{min} ↑100% and 400% respectively, with 200 mg RTV. Dose: fAPV 1,400 mg + RTV 200 mg QD; or fAPV 700 mg + RTV 100 mg BID.	Levels: APV AUC ↓ 32%. Dose: Insufficient data-for dose recommendation	Levels: APV AUC and C_{min} ↓44% and 55%, respectively, when given as APV/r 600/100 BID with TPV/r. No data with fAPV, but a ↓ in AUC is expected. Dose: Should not be coadministered, as doses are not established.
Indinavir (IDV)	Levels: APV AUC ↑ 33%. Dose: Not established.	Coadministration of these agents is not recommended because of potential for additive hyperbilirubinema.	Levels: IDV AUC and C_{min} ↑. Dose: IDV 600 mg BID.	Levels: IDV ↑ 50%; NFV ↑ 80%. Dose: Limited data for IDV 1,200 mg BID + NFV 1,250 mg BID.	Levels: IDV ↑ 2–5 times. Dose: IDV/RTV 400/400 mg, 800/100 mg, or 800/200 mg BID Caution: Renal events may ↑ with ↑ IDV concentrations.	Levels: IDV-No effect SQV 14-7 tiniest Dose: Insufficient data.	No data. Should not be coadministered, as doses are not established.
Lopinavir/ Ritonavir (LPV/r)	*	Levels: With ATV 300 QD +LPV/r 400/100 BID, ATV C_{min} ↑45%; ATV AUC and C_{max} were unchanged. LPVPK similar to historic data.	*	*	Additional ritonavir is generally not recommended.	*	Levels: LPV AUC and C_{min} ↓ 55% & 70% respectively. Dose: Should not be co-administered, as doses are not established.

(continued)

Table 69-7 Drug Effects on Concentration of PI[a] (*Continued*)

Drug Affected	Fosamprenavir	Atazanavir	Lopinavir/Ritonavir	Nelfinavir	Ritonavir	Saquinavir*	Tipranavir
Nelfinavir (NFV)	Levels: APV AUC ↑ 1.5-fold. Dose: Insufficient data.	No data	Levels: With LPV capsules, LPV ↓ 27%; NFV ↑ 25%. Dose: No data with LPV/r tablets. No dosing recommendation.	No data	No data	No data	No data. Should not be co-administered, as doses are not established.
Ritonavir (RTV)	No data	Levels: ATV AUC ↑ 238%. Dose: ATV 300 mg QD + RTV 100 mg QD.	Lopinavir is co-formulated with ritonavir as Kaletra®. Additional ritonavir is generally not recommended.	Levels: RTV - No effect NFV ↑ 1.5 times. Dose: not established	No data	Levels: RTV no effect SQV ↑20 times.[†‡] Dose: 1,000/100 mg SQV hgc/RTV BID or 400/400 mg BID.	Levels: TPV AUC ↑ 11-fold.
Saquinavir (SQV)	Levels: APV AUC ↓ 32%. Dose: Insufficient data.	Levels: SQV AUC ↑ 60% with SQV/ATV/RTV 1,600/300/100 QD, compared with SQV/RTV 1,600/100 QD. Dose: No dose recommendations can be made.	Levels: SQV[†] AUC and C_{min} ↑ Dose: SQV 1,000 mg BID; LPV/r standard.	Levels: SQV ↑ 3–5 times; NFV ↑ 20%.[†] Dose: NFV standard; Fortovase 800 mg TID or 1,200 mg BID.	No data	No data	Levels: SQV AUC and C_{min} ↓ 76% and 82%, respectively, when given as SQV/r 600/100 BID with TPV/r. Dose: Should not be co-ad ministered, as doses are not established.

*Several drug interaction studies have been completed with saquinavir given as Invirase or Fortovase. Results from studies conducted with Invirase may not be applicable to Fortovase.

[†]Study conducted with Fortovase.

[‡]Study conducted with Invirase.

[a]Reprinted from Guidelines for the Use of Antiretroviral Agents in HIV-1-Infected Adults and Adolescents, January 29, 2008. Developed by the DHHS Panel on Antiretroviral Guidelines for Adults and Adolescents—A Working Group of the Office of AIDS Research Advisory Council (OARAC). Retrieved from http://aidsinfo.nih.gov/contentfiles/AdultandAdolescentGL.pdf, p. 97.

Table 69-8 Drug Effects on Concentration of NNRTIs

Drug Affected	*Delavirdine*	*Efavirenz*	*Nevirapine*
Fosamprenavir (fAPV)	Levels: Presumably, similar PK effects as APV: APV AUC ↑ 130%, and DLV AUC ↓ 61%. Dose: Co-administration not recommended.	Levels: fAPV C_{min} ↓ 36% (when dosed at 1,400 mg QD with 200 mg RTV). Dose: fAPV 1,400 mg + RTV 300 mg QD; or fAPV 700 mg + RTV 100 mg BID.	No data
Atazanavir (ATV)	No data.	Levels: With unboosted ATV, ATV AUC ↓ 74%. EFV no change. Dose: ATV 300 + RTV 100 mg QD with food - ATV concentrations similar to unboosted ATV; if desired ATV concentrations not achieved with ATV/r 300/100 mg, may need to increase the dose of ATV/r - insufficient information for specific recommendation. EFV dose - standard.	No data. A decrease in ATV levels is expected. Co-administration is not recommended. Effect of NVP on ritonavir-boosted ATV combination unknown; if used, consider monitoring ATV level.
Darunavir (DRV)	No data	Levels: DRV AUC and C_{min} ↓ 13% and 31%, respectively. EFV AUC and C_{min} ↑ 21% and 17%, respectively. Dose clinical significance unknown. Use standard doses and monitor closely. Consider monitoring levels.	Levels: NVP AUC and C_{min} ↑ 27% and 47%, respectively. DRV unchanged.† Dose: Standard.
Indinavir (IDV)	Levels: IDV ↑ >40%; DLV-No effect Dose: IDV 600 mg q8h. DLV standard	Levels: IDV ↓ 31%. Dose: IDV 1,000 mg q8h; consider IDV/RTV. EFV standard.	Levels: IDV ↓ 28%; NVP no effect. Dose: IDV 1,000 mg q8h, or consider IDV/RTV. NVP standard.
Lopinavir/Ritonavir (LPV/r)	Levels: LPV levels expected to increase. Dose: Insufficient data	Levels: With LPV/r tablets 600/150 mg BID + EFV 600 mg QD, LPV C_{min} and AUC ↑ 35% and 36%, respectively. No formal study of LPV/r tablets 400/100 mg BID + EFV. EFV no change. Dose: LPV/r tablets 600/150 mg BID, when used with EFV in tx-experienced patients. EFV dose - standard.	Levels: With LPV/r capsules, LPV C_{min} dec. 55%. Dose: LPV/r tablets 600/150 mg BID, when used in combination with NVP in tx-experienced patients. NVP standard.
Nelfinavir (NFV)	Levels: NFV ↑ 2 times. DLV ↓50%. Dose: No data	Levels: NFV ↑ 20%. Dose: Standard.	Levels: NFV ↑ 10%. NVP no effect Dose: Standard.
Nevirapine (NVP)	No data.	Levels: NVP-no effect. EFV AUC ↓ 22%.	*
Ritonavir (RTV)	Levels: RTV ↑ 70%. DLV no effect. Dose: Appropriate doses not established,	Levels: RTV ↑ 18%. EFV ↑ 21%. Dose: Standard.	Levels: RTV ↑ 11%. NVP no effect. Dose: Standard
Saquinavir (SQV)	Levels: SQV‡ ↑ 5 times; DLV no effect. Dose: Fortovase 800 mg TID. DLV standard; monitor transaminase levels.	Levels: SQV‡ ↓ 62%. EFV ↓ 12%. SQV is not recommended as sole PIs when EFV is used. Dose: Consider SQV/RTV 400/400 mg BID.	Levels: SQV ↓ 25%. NVP no effect. Dose: Consider SQV-sgc /RTV 400/400 mg or 1,000/100 mg BID or SQV-hgc/RTV 1,000/100 mg BID.
Tipranavir	No data.	Levels: With TPV/r 500/100 mg BID, TPV AUC and C_{min} ↓ 31% and 42%, respectively. EFV unchanged. With TPV/r 750/200 mg BID, TPV PK unchanged. Dose: No dose adjustments necessary.	Levels: No data on the effect of NVP on TPV/r PK. NVP PK unchanged[a]

‡Study conducted with Invirase.
†Based on between-study comparison.
[a]Study conducted with TPV/r dose(s) other than U.S. Food and Drug Administration (FDA)-approved dose of 500/200 mg BID.
Reprinted from Guidelines for the Use of Antiretroviral Agents in HIV-1-Infected Adults and Adolescents, October 10, 2006. Developed by the DHHS Panel on Antiretroviral Guidelines for Adults and Adolescents—A Working Group of the Office of AIDS Research Advisory Council (OARAC). Retrieved from http://aidsinfo.nih.gov/contentfiles/AdultandAdolescentGL.pdf, p. 88.

Considerations in Antiretroviral-Experienced Patients

11. H.G. is a 46-year-old, HIV-positive man with an extensive history of treatment with a variety of antiretroviral agents. He took ZDV monotherapy in the late 1980s and early 1990s. When 3TC became available, he took the combination of ZDV and 3TC until he failed therapy about 8 years ago. At that time, he began experiencing ZDV-induced myopathies. Since that time, H.G. has been "on and off" various regimens without sustained clinical benefit. He is currently taking 3TC, d4T, TDF, ritonavir, and saquinavir with a CD4 count and viral load measurement of 55 cells/mm^3 and 48,000 copies/mL, respectively. These laboratory values have been stable for the last 9 months. How do patients with extensive antiretroviral histories differ from antiretroviral-naïve patients? Are there any special considerations when selecting therapeutic regimens for patients such as H.G.?

Patients who have been infected for 10 or more years may have been treated with many different regimens, both experimental and FDA approved. As a result, many potential regimens have already been exhausted and therefore may not represent viable choices. Care of such patients is a clinical challenge. Data from clinical trials and clinical experience suggest that many patients previously treated with multiple antiretroviral regimens will exhibit a decreased response and decreased durability to older protease inhibitors such as indinavir and nelfinavir.[5,6] Several newer agents, such as tipranavir, darunavir, etravirine and enfuvirtide, have been developed specifically for highly treatment-experienced patients, and they have the ability to achieve viral suppression in these patients. Maraviroc, the first CCR-5 receptor antagonist approved by the FDA, is also an option for treatment-experienced patients infected with HIV-1 utilizing this coreceptor and failing current treatment. Maraviroc is not recommended for use in patients with dual-trophic viral populations (i.e., able to use CXCR-4 or CCR-5 as coreceptors) or CXCR-4-trophic virus and, thus, patients with extensive treatment histories should undergo trophism testing before maraviroc is initiated. Additional agents in clinical development, including both new drug classes and drugs in existing classes with improved resistance profiles, are expected to further advance the treatment of antiretroviral-experienced patients. Despite these advancements, some highly treatment-experienced individuals will have extensive resistance patterns that limit therapeutic options. In such patients, full suppression of viral load and immune reconstitution may not be possible.

Patients who have experienced several antiretroviral regimens present other unique challenges for clinicians and require consideration of the following factors:

1. *Regimen tolerability*[95–97]: Patients with advanced HIV disease display decreased tolerability to many medications, including antiretroviral agents. Although this is not fully understood, it is probably a result of HIV-induced immune alterations and cytokine dysregulations. Subsequently, clinicians evaluating patients with advanced disease should be alert for possible drug-induced adverse events.
2. *Drug interactions:* Many patients with advanced disease take numerous medications for primary or secondary prophylaxis of various opportunistic infections, as well as other medications for comorbid disease states. Subsequently, the risk for a drug–drug interaction is increased. The addition of any new medication, either prescription or over-the-counter, should be carefully evaluated for potential interactions with the patient's current antiretroviral regimen (see Table 69-7). In addition, any change to the current antiretroviral regimen should also be checked against the patient's current medication list.
3. *Altered bioavailability:* Patients infected with HIV with advanced disease may have unreliable absorption of many medications. Reasons for this finding include episodes of severe diarrhea, anorexia, weight loss, wasting, and gastric achlorhydria. As a result, the bioavailability of some agents, especially certain PIs that require specific dietary requirements, may be affected (Table 69-3). Any changes in dietary habits or bowel function should be carefully assessed as to the potential impact on the patient's antiretroviral regimen.
4. *Antiretroviral drug histories and resistance testing:* The most useful information to guide the choice of alternative regimens is a detailed drug history, in conjunction with appropriate resistance testing. Among patients with extensive prior antiretroviral use, it is critical to identify previously failed regimens and determine the precise cause of the failures. In an experienced patient who has taken many different regimens over a lifetime, the number of remaining viable agents and regimens may be limited. Therefore, it is important to determine whether prior regimens truly failed for virologic reasons or some other cause (e.g., regimen intolerability or an inadequate trial period). In addition, detailed knowledge of regimen intolerabilities and which agent(s) caused the adverse event will help in the selection of a new appropriate regimen. In some situations, the offending agent may be reinitiated if the adverse event was minimal or can be appropriately managed.

RESISTANCE, VIRAL GENOTYPING, PHENOTYPING, AND VIRAL FITNESS

12. Will viral genotyping and phenotyping assist in selecting an appropriate therapeutic regimen for H.G.? What are these tests? What are their limitations and when should they be used? What is viral fitness, and does it have a role in clinical decision-making?

Viral genotyping and phenotyping are tests that assess viral resistance patterns to antiretroviral agents. Genotyping evaluates mutations in the virus' genetic material, whereas phenotyping assesses the ability of the virus to grow in the presence of increasing concentrations of antiretroviral agents. The three potential causes for the development of resistance are

1. Initial infection with a resistant isolate[68–71]
2. Natural selection of a resistant isolate as a consequence of inefficient, error-susceptible viral replication[35,98,99]
3. Generation of resistant isolates via selective pressures from antiretroviral therapies that do not fully suppress viral replication[7,100–109]

Mutations are generated when naturally occurring amino acids in the HIV genome are replaced with alternative amino acids. For example, resistance to 3TC occurs when the amino acid methionine (M) is replaced by valine (V) at the 184th amino acid in the protein chain.[7,110] This mutation is subsequently referred to as an *M184V mutation*. These amino acid substitutions change the proteins that are produced and may alter the shape, size, or charge of the viral enzyme's substrate or primer.[111–113] Subsequently, antiretroviral drug binding to the active site is decreased, affinity for natural substrates is increased, or there is an increased removal of the antiretroviral agent from the enzyme by the virus (known as *pyrophosphorylation*).[114] Whether a mutation results in a clinically resistant, less viable, or indifferent isolate depends on which amino acid(s) is replaced. In addition, certain mutations or combination of mutations have been shown to produce viral isolates that display increased sensitivity to various antiretroviral agents (known as *hypersusceptibility*). Alterations to certain key amino acids can also result in cross-resistance between various antiretrovirals.[7]

Two key enzymes have been extensively studied with regard to their potential for development of resistance: reverse transcriptase (RT) and protease. Replication by the RT enzyme is highly error susceptible. Given that the HIV genome is approximately 10,000 nucleotides in length and that mutations via the RT enzyme occur approximately once in every 10,000 nucleotides copied, it has been estimated that a mutation occurs with every viral replication cycle. With up to 10 billion particles of virus being produced per day, the potential exists for 1,000 to 10,000 mutations occurring at each site in the HIV genome every day.[35] Key mutations to the antiretroviral agents are identified in Figure 69-6 and are updated periodically by expert panels of clinicians.

Over time, countless viral subpopulations known as "quasi-species" develop. In any given host, at any given time, many different quasi-species can exist. In addition, within any compartment of the body (e.g., CNS, testes, lymph nodes), many different quasi-species can also exist. Because these mutant strains represent only a small number of isolates in the total viral population, they must have some replicative disadvantage when compared with the "wild-type" virus.[100,101] Under selective pressures from antiretroviral therapies, however, these mutant isolates can replicate. For example, if wild-type viral replication is inhibited by an antiretroviral regimen, and if any one viral strain of the quasi-species is more fit for growth in the presence of that regimen, then the viral mutant will have

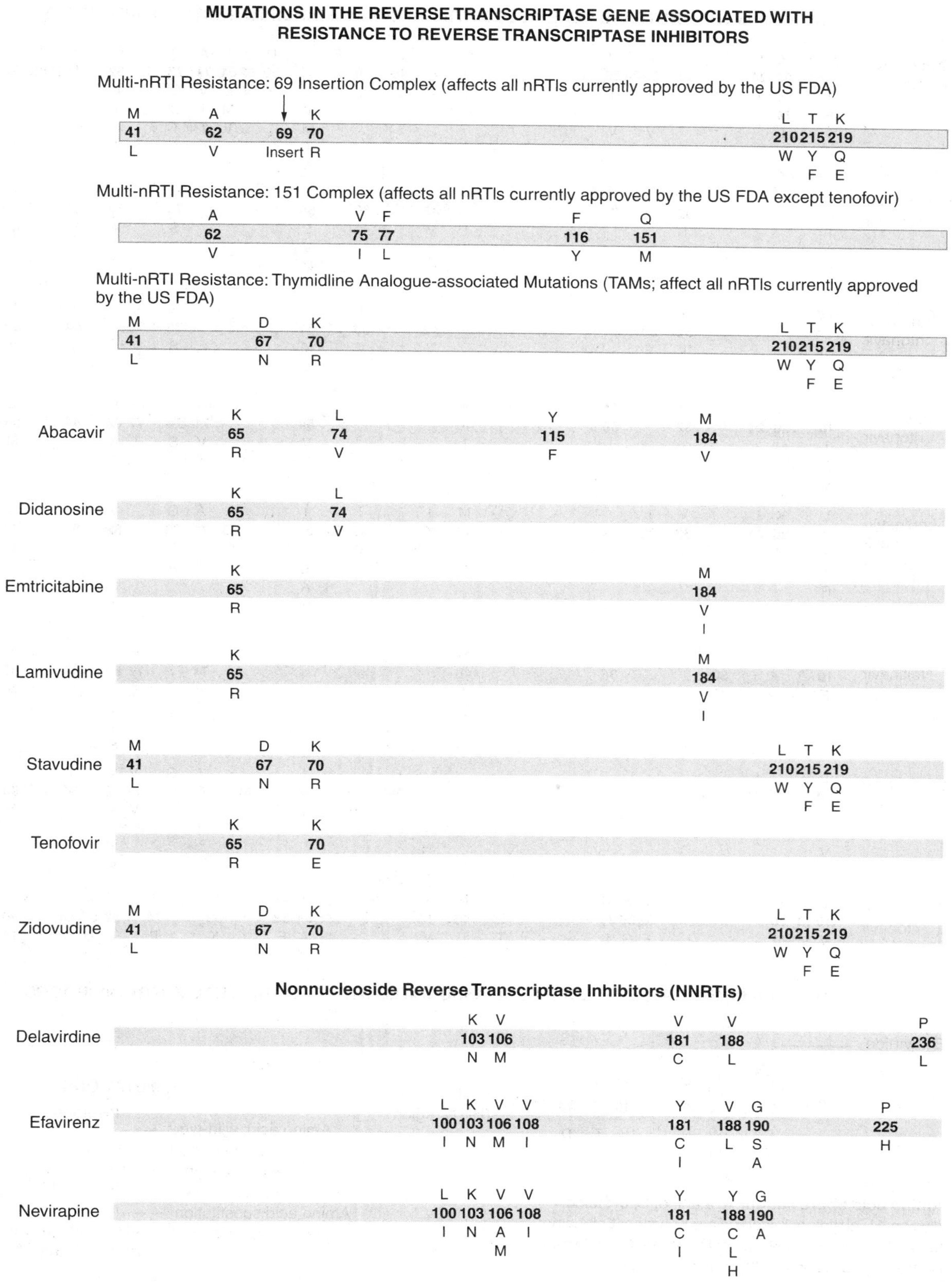

FIGURE 69-6 Mutations associated with resistance to the various classes of antiretroviral agents. Reprinted with permission from the International AIDS Society—USA. Johnson VA, BrunVézinet F, Clotet B, et al. Update of the drug resistance mutations in HIV-1: Spring 2008. *Topics in HIV Medicine.* 2008;16:62. Updated information and thorough explanatory notes are available at www.iasusa.org. (*continued*)

MUTATIONS IN THE PROTEASE GENE ASSOCIATED WITH RESISTANCE TO PROTEASE INHIBITORS

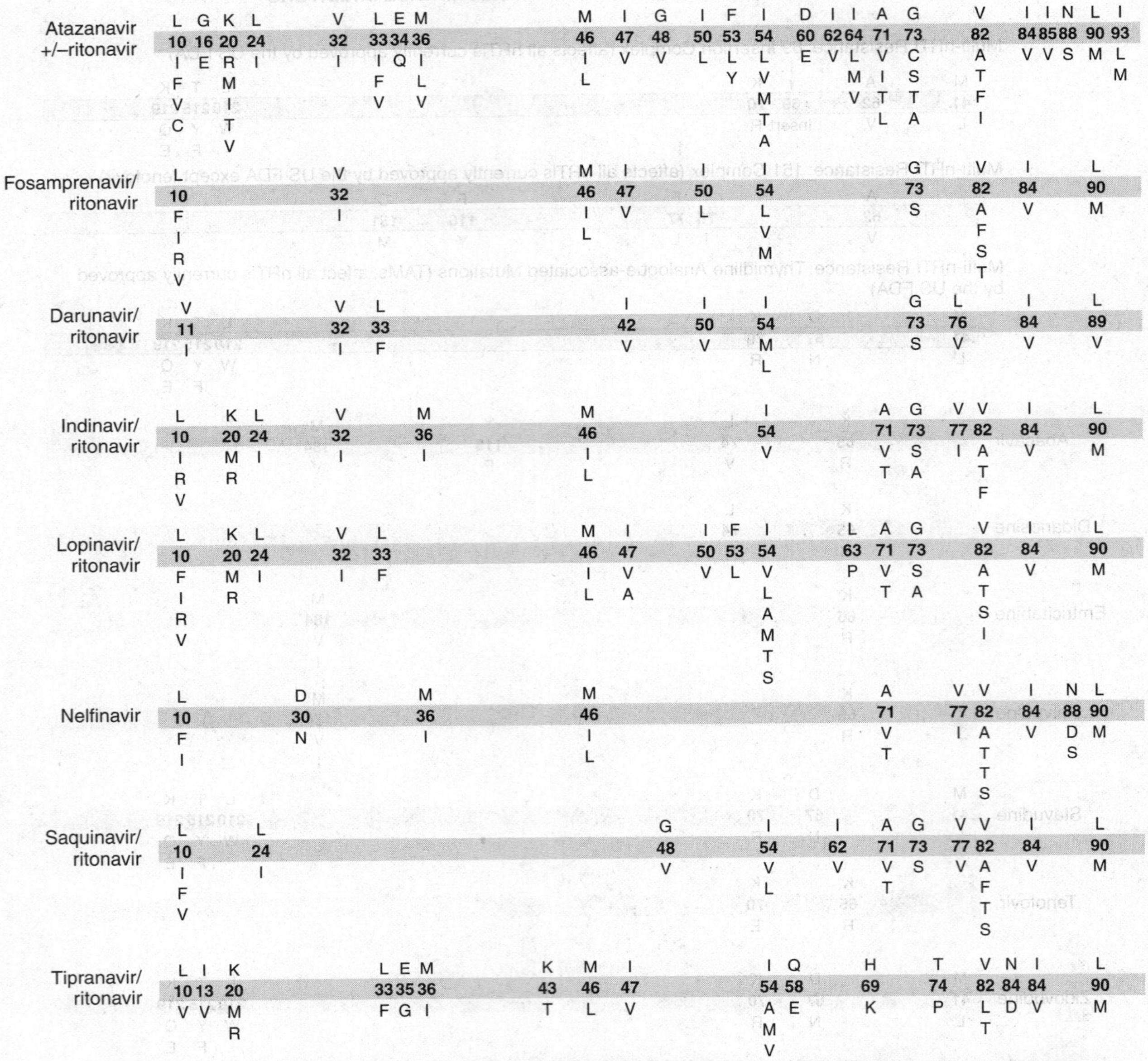

MUTATIONS IN THE GP41 ENVELOPE GENE ASSOCIATED WITH RESISTANCE TO ENTRY INHIBITORS

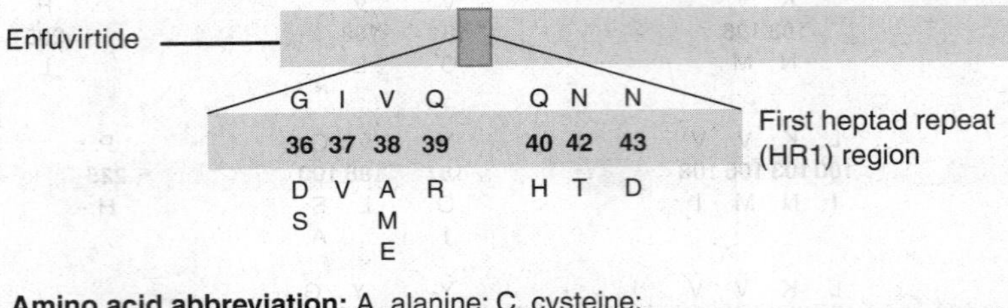

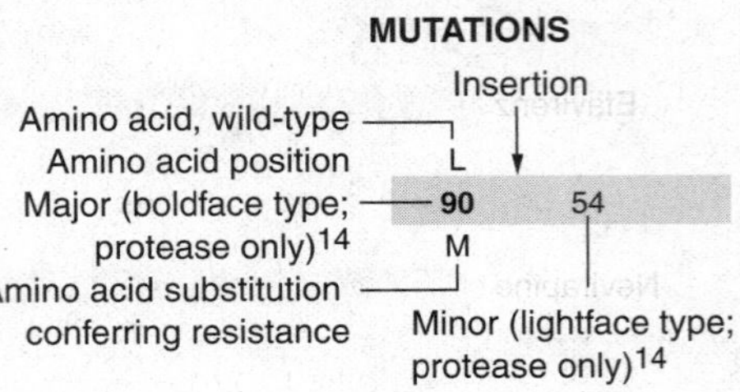

Amino acid abbreviation: A, alanine; C, cysteine; glycine; H, histidine; I, isoleucine; K, lysine; L, leucine; M, methionine; N, asparagine; P, proline; Q, glutamine; R, arginine; S, serine; T, threonine; V, valine; W, tryptophan; Y, tyrosine.

FIGURE 69-6 *(Continued)*

a competitive advantage.[115] It should be recognized that for resistance to develop, viral replication must occur. When viral replication is completely inhibited, the development of resistant isolates is uncommon.

Genotypic analysis involves sequencing the viral genetic material via PCR amplification. Mutations associated with resistance to a given agent are identified by analysis of key sequences of the RT or protease enzymes. These tests can be rapidly processed; however, they detect mutations present only in more than 25% of all HIV isolates in the body, and can only reliably detect resistance patterns in samples with HIV RNA >1,000 copies/mL. Because pressures from antiretroviral therapies select resistant isolates, these tests may not provide information regarding rare, yet potentially clinically significant, isolates.[5]

Phenotypic analysis involves growing virus in the presence of various concentrations of drug and then determining viral susceptibilities (e.g., inhibitory concentrations [IC_{50}]). Phenotyping is limited because it evaluates only one viral isolate at a time and could fail to identify other clinically relevant isolates. In addition, the amount of drug required to inhibit viral growth within a test tube may not represent concentrations required in a given patient, or within various compartments of the body.[5]

An additional methodology, known as the *virtual phenotype*, is also currently available, and compares the genotype information from a sample of interest to a large database of viral isolates where both genotype and phenotype have been performed.[5] This method is only as reliable and robust as the databases from which the virtual phenotype is generated, and may be limited for newer agents with less available genotype-phenotype data.

Genotyping and phenotyping have the potential to provide useful information to clinicians who treat patients with HIV infection. Evidence to date suggests that these tests are effective at predicting which agents will not work, but they are less useful in predicting those that will work.[5,7,116] For example, if testing identifies resistance to an agent, it is highly unlikely this agent will be effective. If testing identifies an agent as susceptible, however, it does not necessarily predict that this agent will be effective. Clinical trials evaluating the use of genotyping and phenotyping for selection of alternative antiretroviral regimens have shown positive treatment responses.[5,6] As with all clinical decisions made for those who are HIV infected, careful assessment of the results in combination with the treatment history are essential for proper clinical decision-making. Consultation with an expert in antiretroviral drug resistance patterns is highly recommended.

One other measure available to clinicians is "viral fitness" or "replication capacity." The genetic changes that occur in a virus to become resistant to antiretroviral therapy often impair the virus' ability to grow.[40,117–119] This measure of growth ability is called "fitness" and is measured by replication capacity during phenotypic evaluation. During amplification of the virus before measuring phenotype, the replication capacity (RC) of the virus is measured and compared with a reference wild-type, drug-sensitive virus. A virus with normal fitness has a RC between 70% and 120% of the reference viral strain; isolates with values <70% are considered to be less fit than wild-type virus. In general, the more mutations that occur to the virus, the more compromised the virus and the lower the fitness (in some situations the interplay between mutations can result in a viral isolate that is relatively fit). Recent data have shown that, despite persistent viral replication, unfit viruses may not cause the same degree of immune destruction as fit viruses.[119] This is important for patients with limited treatment options because they may be able to stay on a HAART regimen that is not completely suppressive, but that produces an unfit virus, with less T-cell depletion. In these situations, it may be best to keep patients on their current therapy despite measurable viral load measurements (provided their CD4 cell counts are stable) until newer treatment options become available.

Given H.G.'s extensive antiretroviral drug history and his current failure, a genotype, phenotype, or virtual phenotype will likely provide some insights into potential therapeutic options.

SPECIAL CIRCUMSTANCES

Immune System Reconstitution

13. Results from H.G.'s genotype analysis suggest that a regimen containing tenofovir, 3TC, ABC, and darunavir–ritonavir may be useful. After thorough discussions with H.G., and careful evaluation of potential drug–drug interactions, this regimen is initiated. Within 2 weeks, H.G.'s T-cell counts increased from 55 to 127 cells/mm^3; however, he now complains of progressive visual loss in his right eye. Physical examination shows macular edema and retinal inflammation consistent with *Cytomegalovirus* infection. Is this a treatment failure? Should H.G.'s antiretroviral regimen be discontinued or changed?

If H.G.'s therapy were evaluated based solely on the rules of therapy (see Questions 7, 8, and 9), this situation would represent a treatment failure. This case, however, is an example of immune reconstitution with disease reactivation after the initiation of potent antiretroviral therapies.[120–122] In patients with advanced HIV disease (e.g., CD4 <100 cells/mm^3), significant immune dysfunction causes an inability to mount an appropriate response to subclinical infections. As a result, these infections replicate unimpeded and often remain undetected by the host (also known as *quiescent disease*). When potent antiretroviral therapies are initiated, immune function is often restored leading to symptoms that can be used to identify and eliminate smoldering infections. During the first 12 weeks of therapy, this increased immune response primarily results from redistribution of memory cells.[123–126] Because of this phenomenon, inflammation at the site of infection often occurs.

The immune reconstitution syndrome can present in any organ system where quiescent disease exists (e.g., CNS, eyes, lymph nodes). Most cases occur within 1 to 4 weeks after the initiation of potent antiretroviral therapies. These cases often occur despite significant increases in T-cell counts to levels well above those generally associated with the detected opportunistic infection.

Although most reports of immune system reconstitution and inflammatory responses have involved infections, one report describes the recurrence of hypersensitivity reactions to trimethoprim-sulfamethoxazole (TMP-SMX) in a small group of subjects ($N = 4$).[127] All had undergone desensitization protocols or dose reductions and were taking TMP-SMX for *Pneumocystis carinii* pneumonia prophylaxis. On initiation of HAART, patients experienced fever (4/4), maculopapular rash

(2/4), and leukocytosis (4/4). The fever did not resolve until TMP-SMX was discontinued. Clinicians should be aware of the possibility of recurrence of hypersensitivity reactions after the initiation of HAART therapies.

In this case, H.G. presents with signs and symptoms of immune reactivation-associated (CMV retinitis, including new onset of visual complaints and inflammation consistent with CMV retinitis on physical examination, in the face of increased T-cell counts (from 55–127 cells/mm^3). Because the new opportunistic infection is a result of immune reconstitution and not clinical failure, the regimen does not need to be discontinued or changed. Appropriate treatment for CMV, however, should be implemented.

Discordant Surrogate Markers

14. H.G. was successfully treated for CMV retinitis and the regimen of tenofovir, 3TC, ABC, and darunavir–ritonavir was continued. Over the following 6 months, H.G.'s T-cell counts increased to 325 cells/mm^3 and his viral load value declined to 5,000 copies/mL. At the last two clinic visits H.G.'s viral load (copies/mL) and CD4 counts (cells/mm^3) were 2,000/275 and <400/225, respectively. H.G. reports no new clinical complaints or adverse drug events. In addition, H.G. states that he has been compliant with therapy. Are changes to therapy necessary?

In most cases, declines in viral load measurements result in increases in CD4 cell counts and increasing viral load measurements result in declining CD4 cell counts. In approximately 20% of cases, however, T cells decline along with viral load decline or T cells increase along with viral load increases.[5,127,128] These situations are referred to as *discordant surrogate marker data*.

In this situation, it may be wise to continue current treatment and monitor the patient closely, because changing or adding an additional drug may not increase CD4 cell counts.[6] When T-cell counts increase despite increasing viral load measurements, decisions regarding therapeutic options are unknown. Although these patients may continue to observe a clinical benefit from the current antiretroviral regimen for a period of time, data suggest that long-term stability of the CD4 count is unlikely.[6] Because this may be an early warning sign of impending CD4 cell destruction, many clinicians would change antiretroviral therapies. Other clinicians, however, might decide to follow patients carefully and change therapies at the first sign of T-cell declines or new clinical signs and symptoms. In these situations, other potential causes of viral load increases (e.g., recent infection, vaccination) should be carefully evaluated to prevent inappropriately changing a nonfailing regimen.

Therapeutic Drug Monitoring

15. P.P. is a 30-year-old HIV-positive man who has failed prior antiretroviral regimens. Based on phenotypic resistance testing, it appears that a regimen including lopinavir–ritonavir may be able to overcome the viral isolate's resistance pattern. Will plasma measurements of P.P.'s antiretroviral drug concentrations be useful? What measurement should be used, which agent(s) should be measured, and how should the samples be collected?

Pharmacokinetic evaluations of various antiretrovirals, including the NNRTIs and PI, have shown wide interpatient variability in drug exposures among cohorts of patients taking the same dose of drug under the same conditions.[46,129,130] Many factors contribute to interpatient variability in drug exposure, such as pharmacogenetics, environment, different physiologic conditions, regimen adherence, and drug–drug, drug–food, and drug–nutraceutical interactions. For most antiretrovirals, a drug exposure–response relationship exists (e.g., the higher the exposure, the faster and more prolonged the viral suppression).[131] In addition, most antiretrovirals also have exposure-toxicity relationships.[130]

Therapeutic drug monitoring (TDM) is currently recommended for selected clinical situations.[131] In patients failing a first regimen, or a regimen that initially was fully suppressive, TDM may identify suboptimal drug concentrations. For patients with uncharacterized drug–drug or drug–food interactions and those with impairments in gastrointestinal, hepatic, or renal function, drug concentrations may help to identify concentrations outside of the recommended range that can be corrected with a dosage adjustment. TDM may also be useful for assuring that a novel antiretroviral combination does not have any unpredictable adverse drug interactions. In treatment-experienced patients, knowledge of drug concentrations and viral susceptibility to the given agent may help to design an optimal dosage regimen in the face of partial viral resistance. Conversely, patients experiencing toxicities thought to be concentration-dependent (e.g., neuropsychiatric effects of efavirenz) may benefit from TDM as well. Monitoring adherence and evaluating pharmacokinetics in special populations, such as pregnant women or pediatric patients, are additional indications for TDM.

Pharmacology experts currently recommend obtaining trough concentrations immediately before the next dose of a PIs or an NNRTIs. For efavirenz, which is usually taken in the evening, samples may be obtained at the 12-hour time point owing to its long half-life.[131] Many factors can affect the trough values of various antiretroviral agents. For proper interpretation of the concentrations, patients should provide a dosing history from the last several days, a list of concomitantly administered drugs to screen for interactions, and the exact time the last dose was taken. The exact time the TDM sample was collected should also be recorded. Another factor that can affect interpretation of drug concentrations over time is intrapatient variability. Although not fully evaluated, it appears that under stringent pharmacokinetic study conditions (e.g., study conditions in which dosing, concomitant food administration, drug–drug interactions, and adherence all are controlled) the day-to-day variability of drug concentrations over time is minimal.[132–134] Outside of a clinical study, however, where patients take their medications under conditions that vary from day to day, the concentrations could be highly variable at clinic visits over time, and a few samples might be required to determine trends in the drug exposure before making a dose adjustment. Finally, to minimize laboratory variability and error in measuring these concentrations, it is also recommended that a laboratory that routinely measures antiretrovirals and participates in both internal and external quality control programs be used. A list of such laboratories can be obtained from www.hivpharmacology.com.

In general, total drug concentration ranges for defining efficacy and toxicity have been developed for PIs and NNRTIs.[131] A limitation of obtaining total drug concentrations is that unbound, active drug fraction is not quantitated. These agents are generally highly protein-bound, and alterations in the bound or unbound fraction can contribute to both reduced efficacy and increased toxicity within accepted total drug concentration ranges. Despite this, total concentrations are generally used owing to technical challenges inherent in determining unbound drug concentrations, and because a reasonable relationship exists between these concentrations and clinical outcomes. The plasma or serum concentrations of NRTIs, however, may or may not be reflective of the active intracellular triphosphate moiety, but may be useful to measure in certain situations. Researchers are evaluating the intracellular triphosphate concentrations of the NRTIs in various cell types, including peripheral blood mononuclear cells (PBMC). Limitations to determining intracellular concentrations include the sophisticated processing of the cellular components before storage, the technical difficulty of the assay itself (generally only found in pharmaceutical companies and academic centers), and the limited availability of instrumentation to measure the low concentrations of these moieties (e.g. femtomoles/10^6 cells).

The interpretation of the drug concentration itself will vary according on the clinical situation. Among treatment-naïve patients with wild-type viral isolates, an assessment should be made whether the concentration lies within a range of the population concentrations: how that range is defined tends to be clinician-specific, but can be the interquartile range, the 90% confidence interval, and so on. If the concentration is below the desired cut-off, and the patient is not responding well to the therapy, the clinician should consider giving more drug or using a pharmacokinetic-enhancing technique (e.g. adding ritonavir). If the concentration is above the cut-off, and the patient is experiencing drug toxicity, a dose reduction should be considered. Clinical trials evaluating TDM among antiretroviral-naïve patients initiating PI-based HAART have shown improved clinical responses compared with patients given standard of care without TDM.[135,136]

Among patients with antiretroviral resistance, the interpretation of the concentration is much more complex and may require the additional assessment of phenotypic resistance data. Higher drug exposure may be needed for patients with drug-resistant viruses to achieve efficacy. Preliminary investigations have evaluated the ratio between drug exposure and viral susceptibility (in a similar fashion to the antimicrobial efficacy ratios of C_{min}: minimal inhibitory concentration [MIC] or area under the curve [AUC]: MIC), also called an inhibitory quotient (IQ).[115] Interpretation of the current IQ data is difficult, however, owing to the various methodologies used for its calculation.[131] Ongoing research is focused on standardizing calculation methods to improve the prediction of appropriate antiretroviral concentrations for maximal efficacy.

In the current case, assuring that P.P.'s lopinavir trough concentration is at least above the IC_{50} value from the phenotype may help improve his chances of optimal antiviral response. If P.P.'s response to treatment is inadequate (e.g., unsatisfactory decline in HIV RNA), then a concentration should be obtained from a trough sample, with a careful concomitant drug and dosing history, and sent to a reliable laboratory for analysis.

Metabolic Complications of Antiretroviral Therapies

16. J.F. is a 37-year-old HIV-positive man who has been taking stavudine, lamivudine, ritonavir, and saquinavir for the past 4 years. Since starting this regimen, J.F.'s T-cell counts have increased from 65 to 475 cells/mm^3, and his viral load has declined from 70,000 to <400 copies/mL (using RT-PCR). J.F. is concerned because he has noticed that his arms and legs have gotten quite thin and the veins in his calves are now very pronounced. In addition, his cheeks have "disappeared," and he cannot seem to get the extra weight off around his belly. Otherwise, he "feels fine." On physical examination, you notice an abnormal accumulation of fat on his posterior neck and upper back. Laboratory tests reveal increased total cholesterol at 8.2 mmol/L (normal, <5.17 mmol/L), triglycerides at 3.8 mmol/L (normal, <2.82 mmol/L), and a fasting blood glucose of 230 mg/dL (normal, <126 mg/dL) with no evidence of ketones or sugar on urine analysis. Before starting this regimen, all laboratory values were within normal limits. J.F. admits to smoking two packs of cigarettes per day, occasional alcohol consumption, poor dietary habits including eating fast foods, and rarely exercising. Are the changes in laboratory values and body shape a result of his current antiretroviral regimen? Is J.F. at increased risk for cardiovascular disease since starting HAART? What interventions, if any, may help?

The discovery and widespread use of HAART in clinical practice has resulted in significant antiviral, clinical, and survival benefit among individuals infected with HIV. These compounds, however, can cause metabolic complications, such as abnormal distribution of body fat, lipid abnormalities (e.g., hypercholesteremia, hypertriglyceridemia, increases in low-density lipoprotein [LDL] and decreases in high-density lipoprotein [HDL]), and new-onset diabetes.[81,137–144] Coronary artery disease, myocardial infarctions, and vascular complications among relatively young patients who are HIV infected taking HAART-containing regimens have also been reported.[145–150] Large observational studies suggest an increased risk for cardiovascular disease among patients taking HAART, particularly among those receiving protease inhibitors. Several theories for the mechanism of these effects have been proposed. One theory is that a sequence of the HIV-1 protease enzyme contains homology to human proteins such as LDL-receptor–related protein, and cytoplasmic retinoic-acid binding protein.[137] By inhibiting these proteins, PIs may inhibit adipocyte growth or promote adipocyte lysis, leading to alterations in serum lipid concentrations, visceral fat accumulation, and impaired insulin signaling. A second theory is that PIs interfere with retinoid signaling within adipocytes (excessive levels of certain retinoids can resemble the lipodystrophy syndrome).[151–153] Additionally, nucleoside analogs can inhibit mitochondrial DNA polymerase and, as a result, have been implicated in lipoatrophy.[154] Finally, metabolic abnormalities have also been reported in patients who are HIV infected before receiving HAART, and may also be a consequence of HIV infection or pre-existing metabolic disorders that are exacerbated by HAART.[155]

Up to 40% of patients on PI-based HAART are reported to experience impaired glucose intolerance owing to significant insulin resistance.[156] Patients with type 2 diabetes mellitus are at increased risk, and PI-based regimens should be avoided if possible in these patients.[81] Fasting glucose measures for all patients are recommended before and during therapy (e.g., every 3–6 months) with PI-based HAART.[81] In many cases, the hyperglycemia will respond to diet and exercise modifications; however, if pharmacologic interventions are necessary, insulin "sensitizers" (thiazolidinediones, metformin) may be most effective.[81,157] For more pronounced hyperglycemia, oral sulfonyureas or insulin may be appropriate, although oral agents may be less efficacious in those who are HIV infected with those who are not HIV infected.[81] Although hyperglycemia is reversible on discontinuation of PIs therapy, the potential benefit of sustained viral suppression with HAART-containing regimens often outweighs the risks for complications in those patients whose hyperglycemia can be controlled.

Elevations in serum levels of triglycerides, total cholesterol, and LDL, with mild decreases in HDL, have also been reported after the initiation of HAART.[81,157,158] These abnormalities may be seen as early as 2 weeks after the initiation of therapy.[81] Although all PIs have been implicated, these laboratory abnormalities appear to occur more frequently in ritonavir-containing regimens, and less frequently in patients receiving atazanavir.[155] The NNRTIs can also cause lipid alterations, although at a lower incidence than the PI. Both efavirenz and nevirapine have been shown to increase HDL concentrations among patients receiving HAART. Generally, nevirapine may have the least detrimental lipid profile (i.e., greater increases in HDL concentrations and less effect on LDL elevations).[159] Of the NRTIs, stavudine appears to affect lipid profiles to the greatest extent: two prospective clinical trials have shown greater increases in triglycerides and total cholesterol among patients receiving stavudine-based HAART compared with zidovudine- or tenofovir-based regimens.[81,155]

The management of HAART-associated hyperlipidemias should involve dietary modifications and regular physical exercise with pharmacologic interventions reserved for those patients who meet criteria for treatment as with the general population. The goals of therapy for patient who are HIV infected are the same for those who are not HIV infected and follow the American Heart Association guidelines.[81,155] When drug therapy is warranted, hydroxymethylglutaryl coacetyl-A reductase inhibitors (HMG-CoA) may be used for hypercholesterolemia and fibric acid derivatives for hypertriglyceridemia.[81,155] Both HMG-CoA reductase inhibitors and PIs are metabolized by the hepatic cytochrome P450 enzyme system, which may result in significant drug–drug interactions (most importantly, decreased clearance of the HMG-CoA reductase inhibitor from the PI, resulting in an increased risk for rhabdomyolysis, myositis, and transaminase elevations). When concomitantly administered with ritonavir, simvastatin concentrations increase significantly, atorvastatin concentrations increase modestly, and pravastatin concentrations decrease significantly.[160] Consequently, simvastatin should not be used in patients receiving ritonavir-based HAART, whereas atorvastatin can be used with caution. Among patients who experience increases in lipids or triglycerides and who are virologically controlled, it may be possible to substitute the current PIs for a different agent that has a lower propensity for raising these laboratory values.[161–170] An NNRTIs, an alternative protease inhibitor, or possibly abacavir may be reasonable options to replace the protease inhibitor. It should be recognized that a detailed history of prior resistance must be known before switching therapies to prevent virologic failure.

Alterations in body composition, both fat loss (arms, legs, face, buttocks) and fat accumulation (dorsocervical fatty deposits or "buffalo humps", increased abdominal girth) are commonly observed among patients taking HAART. Up to 40% to 50% of patients have been reported to experience these changes, although the exact rate is confounded by differences in definition and assessment.[81] Risk factors for this complication include higher baseline body mass index, increased duration of exposure to antiretroviral agents, lower CD4 nadir at time of initiation of HAART and CD4 response to therapy, increasing age, female sex, and prolonged duration of HIV infection. In general, the nucleoside analogs are believed to be responsible for lipoatrophy, and the PIs are believed to be responsible for lipoaccumulation.[81] Because these agents are given in combination, it is difficult to precisely identify which class of agents is responsible for which adverse event.

The causes of lipodystrophy are unknown. For the nucleoside analogs, the greater the ability to inhibit mitochondrial DNA polymerase in vitro (e.g., stavudine), the greater the propensity for lipatrophy. Studies involving the substitution of one NRTIs for another have been done.[166–171] Although the substitution of stavudine with an alternate agent such as zidovudine, tenofovir, or abacavir has shown statistically significant increases in arm and leg fat, and decreases in trunk fat using objective radiographic tests (e.g., dual-energy x-ray absorptiometry, computed tomography scans), these improvements are so modest that they may not be clinically significant. The use of recombinant human growth hormone, an agent with lipolytic effects, has been shown to decrease the size of buffalo humps and abdominal girth; however, once use of the agent is stopped, the growth often returns.[81] Surgical excision or liposuction may be effective; however, recurrences have been reported. In addition, caution should be exercised when using surgical interventions for abdominal girth because of concerns about intestinal perforation and intraperitoneal bleeding. For facial wasting, injection of fat or synthetic polymers into the recessed areas of the cheeks have shown good results but require frequent costly administration, and lack long-term safety data.

Other important long-term complications include nucleoside-associated lactic acidosis, osteonecrosis, and osteopenia.[81] Lactic acidosis has been predominantly associated with the use of stavudine,[5] but it can occur among all nucleoside analogs. This can be managed by discontinuing therapy until lactate levels return to normal and then reinitiating therapy with a nonstavudine or non-nucleoside analog–containing HAART regimen, if possible.

Currently, J.F. has elevated serum levels of cholesterol, lipids, and fasting blood sugars. In addition, he has the classic clinical presentation of body habitus changes with thinning of his arms, legs, and face, as well as accumulation of central fat and a modest buffalo hump on his neck. Although the current antiretroviral regimen has been effective in lowering J.F.'s viral load and increasing his T-cell counts, interventions are necessary to prevent long-term complications such as premature heart disease and other vascular complications. Initially, nonpharmacologic interventions such as diet, exercise, and life-style modifications (e.g., smoking cessation) should be tried. In addition, given the increased reported incidence of these adverse events with ritonavir- and stavudine-containing regimens, modification of J.F.'s current antiretroviral regimen may be reasonable and should be based on treatment history, resistance profiles, and drug intolerances. If these interventions fail, gemfibrozil, atorvastatin, metformin, or a thiazolidinedione (e.g., pioglitazone or rosiglitazone) should be considered.

Limited interventions are currently available for treatment of the buffalo hump. J.F. could consider surgery or recombinant human growth hormone; however, he should be advised that the hump might return. In addition, if the facial lipoatrophy is of significant concern, J.F. should consult a dermatologist who specializes in HIV-associated facial reconstruction.

Structured Treatment Interruptions and Target-Controlled Interventions

17. T.D. is a 32-year-old man infected with HIV whose antiretroviral therapy was initiated with stavudine, lamivudine, and lopinavir–ritonavir 2 years ago when he was first diagnosed with HIV at a routine physical examination. At that time, his CD4 cell count was 125 cells/mm^3 and his viral load was 85,000 copies/mL. T.D. has done well with his current regimen; he has been without any adverse drug events, and his CD4 cell counts have been stable at 575 cells/mm^3 and his viral load measurements have been undetectable (<50 copies/mL). T.D. is concerned about long-term adverse events from HAART and asks if he can stop therapy or at least minimize his exposure to these agents. Can therapy be discontinued once it is stable? If so, how should it be monitored? Are there any interventions that can be implemented to minimize drug exposures and potentially long-term adverse events?

Although HAART-based therapies have been shown to improve survival and minimize the risk for development of opportunistic infections, these agents do have significant adverse effects associated with their use. In addition, given the improved survival rates from HAART, new and more complex long-term adverse events are now recognized. Previously, the goal of antiretroviral therapy was to prolong survival; now, with the use of HAART, the management of HIV has shifted to chronic health maintenance. Consequently, any intervention that can decrease the risk for long-term adverse events or minimize drug exposures over time may represent a key strategy for managing infection with HIV, provided that the intervention does not cause immunologic harm to the patient. Two strategies have been investigated to minimize antiretroviral exposure: structured treatment interruptions (STI) and CD4/viral load–guided discontinuations of therapy.

Structured treatment interruption interventions involve starting and stopping HAART at controlled time points in hopes of minimizing drug exposure, maintaining immunologic control, and minimizing drug resistance. Various dosing schedules have been used (e.g., 7 days on, 7 days off; 3 months on, 2 months off; 5 days on 2 days off) with mixed, although generally unfavorable, results.[172–179] Additionally, this strategy is difficult to adhere to, and short-term adverse drug events may occur when therapy is reinitiated, including the acute retroviral syndrome.[179–181] It appears that antiviral resistance may occur using STI interventions, and should not be undertaken with regimens that contain agents with low genetic barriers or long half-lives.[182,183]

Target-controlled therapy involves patients discontinuing and reinitiating therapy only when certain target values are reached (e.g., CD4 cell counts, viral load, or both).[173,174] This intervention is of particular interest for patients whose therapy was initiated in the past when their CD4 cell counts were >350 cells/mm^3 or for patients whose immune systems have improved to values >350 cells/mm^3 for extended periods of time. Earlier clinical trial data using target values of CD4 cells counts falling <350 cells/mm^3 or a decline of 25% to 30% from baseline demonstrated promising results.[173,174] More recent, larger studies, however, do not support this approach.[184,185] In fact, the most recent studies have been discontinued prematurely because of increases in morbidity and mortality in the treatment interruption arms.

Because of the conflicting evidence and uncertainty surrounding treatment interruption, current guidelines do not recommend these interventions outside of a clinical trial setting.[5,6] As such, if available at the clinical center, T.D. could be referred to a clinical study for close-follow-up and care during treatment interruption. If the patient truly desires cessation of therapy, the clinician should initiate a discussion to explain fully the potential risks, such as disease progression and death, and allow the patient to participate in the decision to stop treatment. The patient should also be counseled that follow-up care and careful monitoring will be required to monitor disease progression and the need to reinstitute antiretrovirals. If treatment is continued, or when it is reinitiated, given the increased risk for side effects with stavudine, it may be reasonable to replace stavudine with ZDV, ABC, or TDF.

KEEPING CURRENT

The management of HIV infection continues to evolve. The overwhelming data presented at scientific meetings and in journals has made staying informed about current issues and new developments a daunting task. As a result, many clinicians, even those actively caring for patient who are HIV infected, remain cautious and often confused as to which therapeutic options to use.

New technologies for the dissemination of medical information are constantly evolving. The internet has allowed clinicians worldwide to exchange ideas, teach new concepts, and obtain access to limited resources. In addition, many research centers, patient advocacy groups, and academic institutions have posted sites on the internet that have resulted in access to large amounts of high-quality medical information. This new technology has also allowed, however, for the dissemination of incomplete, misleading, or inaccurate information. Therefore, clinicians must remain cautious and carefully evaluate the information obtained from various websites.

When evaluating the quality of a website, clinicians should look for a few basic standards:

1. *Author qualifications.* Is the author qualified to write the article or perform the research? Is his or her affiliation or relevant credentials provided?

Table 69-9 HIV Internet Resources

Government Sites	
American Foundation for AIDS Research: http://www.amfar.org	
AIDSinfo from US DHHS: http://www.aidsinfo.nih.gov	
Centers for Disease Control and Prevention: http://www.cdc.gov	
Consensus Panel Guidelines On-line: http://www.hivatis.org	
Government HIV Mutation Charts: http://hiv-web.lanl.gov	
Government HIV Mutation Charts: http://hiv-web.lanl.gov	
National Institute of Allergy and Infectious Diseases: http://www.niaid.nih.gov	
National Prevention Information Network: http://www.cdcnpin.org	
United Nations AIDS WebSite: http://www.unaids.org/	
University Sites	
Johns Hopkins AIDS Service: http://www.hopkins-aids.edu	
University of California, HIV/AIDS Program: http://hivinsite.ucsf.edu	
University of Stanford HIV Drug Resistance Database: http://hivdb.stanford.edu/	
AIDS Treatment/Advocacy Groups	
Project Inform: http://www.projinf.org	
San Francisco AIDS Foundation: http://www.sfaf.org/index.html	
Other Relevant Sites	
The AIDS Map: http://www.aidsmap.com	
AIDS Education Global Information System: http://www.aegis.com	
Clinical Care Options: http://www.clinicalcareoptions.com	
HIV Drug Interactions: http://www.hiv-druginteractions.org	
HIV and Hepatitis: http://hivandhepatitis.com	
HIV Pharmacology: http://www.hivpharmacology.com	
HIV Resistance Web: http://www.hivresistanceweb.com	
HIV Treatment Information: http://www.i-base/info	
Medscape: http://www.medscape.com	
Physician's Research Network: http://www.prn.org	
The Body for Clinicians: http://www.thebodypro.com	
Retroviral Conference: http://www.retroconference.org	

2. *Attribution.* Are references provided to confirm statements? Are all relevant copyrighted information noted?
3. *Currency.* When was the content posted? Is the website updated regularly?
4. *Disclosure.* Who owns the website? Is there a conflict of interest between what is being posted and any commercial interest?

Any internet site that fails to meet these basic competencies should be viewed with caution. In general, the most accurate and informative websites for HIV-specific information come from academic institutions, government organizations, medical societies, and patient advocacy groups. Table 69-9 lists high-quality websites that provide timely and accurate information. A periodic evaluation of these sites often provides sufficient information to stay up-to-date on current issues and controversies.

CONCLUSIONS

Despite significant advances made in the treatment of patients infected with HIV, a cure continues to be out of reach. Pharmacists are in a unique position to assist both clinicians and patients in the general management of HIV infection. In particular, the number of drug–drug interactions in HIV management is unprecedented compared with other therapeutic areas. A basic understanding of drug–drug interactions, absolute contraindications, and adverse event profiles for antiretroviral agents can substantially improve patient compliance, minimize adverse events, and improve clinical outcomes. Although the pharmacologic management of HIV is rapidly evolving, a basic understanding of viral pathogenesis and drug interactions provides a framework that can be used to evaluate new information as it becomes available.

REFERENCES

1. Centers for Disease Control and Prevention. HIV/AIDS Surveillance Report, 2005. Vol. 17. Atlanta: U.S. Department of Health and Human Services, Centers for Disease Control and Prevention; 2006.
2. Murphy EL et al. Viral Activation Transfusion Study Investigators. Highly active antiretroviral therapy decreases mortality and morbidity in patients with advanced HIV disease. *Ann Intern Med* 2001;3;135:17.
3. Lampe FC et al. Changes over time in risk of initial virological failure of combination antiretroviral therapy: a multicohort analysis, 1996 to 2002. *Arch Intern Med* 2006;166:521.
4. O'Brien ME et al. Patterns and correlates of discontinuation of the initial HAART regimen in an urban outpatient cohort. *J Acquir Immune Defic Syndr* 2003;34:407.
5. DHHS. Guidelines for the use of antiretroviral agents in HIV-Infected adults and adolescents Jan 29, 2008; Accessed May 13, 2008. HIV AIDS Treatment Information Service: Online resource: http://www.hivatis.org/trtgdlns.html.
6. Hammer et al. Treatment for Adult HIV Infection; 2006 recommendations of the International AIDS Society–USA Panel. *JAMA* 2006;296:827.
7. Johnson VA et al. Update of the drug resistance mutations in HIV-1: 2006. *Topics in HIV Medicine* 2006;14:125.
8. Orld Health Organization/UNAIDS. AIDS epidemic update. December 2006. Available at http://www.unaids.org. Accessed March 2007.
9. Beyrer C. HIV epidemiology update and transmission factors: risks and risk contexts—16th International AIDS Conference epidemiology plenary. *Clin Infect Dis* 2007;44:981.
10. Lance HC et al. HIV seroconversion and oral intercourse. *Am J Public Health* 1991;81:658.
11. Page-Shafer K et al. Risk of HIV infection attributable to oral sex among men who have sex with men and in the population of men who have sex with men. *AIDS* 2002;16:2350.
12. Royce RA et al. Sexual transmission of HIV. *N Engl J Med* 1997;15:1072.
13. Fauci AS. The human immunodeficiency virus: infectivity and mechanisms of pathogenesis. *Science* 1988;239:617.
14. Fahey JL et al. Quantitative changes in T helper or T suppressor/cytotoxic lymphocyte subsets that distinguish acquired immune deficiency syndrome from other immune disorders. *Am J Med* 1984;76:95.
15. Perelson AS et al. HIV-1 dynamics in vivo: virion clearance rate, infected cell life-span, and viral generation time. *Science* 1996;271:1582.
16. Pantaleo G et al. The immunopathogenesis of human immunodeficiency virus infection. *N Engl J Med* 1993;328:327.
17. Deng HK et al. Identification of a major coreceptor for primary isolates of HIV-1. *Nature* 1996;381:661.
18. Dragic T et al. HIV-1 entry into CD4+ cells is mediated by the chemokine receptor CC-CKR-5. *Nature* 1996;381:667.
19. Berson JF et al. A seven transmembrane domain receptor involved in fusion and entry of T-cell trophic human immunodeficiency virus type 1 strains. *J Virol* 1996;70:6288.
20. Levy J. Infection by human immunodeficiency virus—CD4 is not enough. *N Engl J Med* 1996;335:5280.
21. Wild C et al. A synthetic peptide from HIV-1 gp41 is a potent inhibitor of virus-mediated cell-cell fusion. *AIDS Res Hum Retroviruses* 1993;9:1051.
22. Kohl NE et al. Active human immunodeficiency virus protease is required for viral infectivity. *Proc Natl Acad Sci* 1988;85:4686.
23. Bugelski PJ et al. HIV protease inhibitors: effects on viral maturation and physiologic function in macrophages. *J Leukoc Biol* 1994;56:374.
24. Hellerstein M et al. Directly measured kinetics of circulating T lymphocytes in normal and HIV-1 infected humans. *Nat Med* 1999;5:83.
25. Fauci AS. Immunopathogenic mechanisms of HIV infection. *Ann Intern Med* 1996;124:654.

26. Daar ES et al. Transient high levels of viremia in patients with primary human immunodeficiency virus type 1 infection. *N Engl J Med* 1991;324:954.
27. Fox CH et al. Lymphoid germinal centers are reservoirs of human immunodeficiency virus type 1 RNA. *J Infect Dis* 1991;164:1051.
28. Panteleo G et al. HIV infection is active and progressive in lymphoid tissue during the clinically latent stage of disease. *Nature* 1993;362:355.
29. Richman DD et al. Rapid evolution of the neutralizing antibody response to HIV type 1 infection. *Proc Natl Acad Sci U S A* 2003;100:4144.
30. Schacker T et al. Clinical and epidemiologic features of primary HIV infection. *Ann Intern Med* 1996;125:257.
31. Tindall B et al. Primary HIV infection: host responses and intervention strategies. *AIDS* 1991; 5:1.
32. Pilcher CD et al. Acute HIV revisited: new opportunities for treatment and prevention. *J Clin Invest.* 2004;113:937.
33. Ho DD et al. Rapid turnover of plasma virions and CD4 lymphocytes in HIV-1 infection. *Nature* 1995;373:123.
34. Wei X et al. Viral dynamics in human immunodeficiency virus type 1 infection. *Nature* 1995;373:117.
35. Coffin JM. HIV population dynamics in vivo: implications for genetic variation, pathogenesis, and therapy. *Science* 1995;267:483.
36. Mellors JW et al. Prognosis in HIV-1 infection predicted by the quantity of virus in plasma. *Science* 1996;272:1167.
37. O'Brien WA, et al. Changes in plasma HIV-1 RNA and CD4 lymphocyte counts and the risk of progression to AIDS. *N Engl J Med* 1996;334: 426.
38. Mellors JW et al. Plasma viral load and CD+ lymphocytes as prognostic markers of HIV-1 infection. *Ann Intern Med* 1997;126:946.
39. Pantaleo G et al. Studies in subjects with long-term nonprogressive human immunodeficiency virus infection. *N Engl J Med* 1995;332:209.
40. O'Brien TR et al. Serum HIV-1 RNA levels and time to development of AIDS in the multicenter hemophilia cohort study. *JAMA* 1996;276:105.
41. Moss AR et al. Natural history of HIV infection. *AIDS* 1989;3:55.
42. Stein DS et al. CD4 lymphocyte cell enumeration for prediction of clinical course of human immunodeficiency virus disease: a review. *J Infect Dis* 1992;165:352.
43. Sepkowitz KA. Effect of HAART on natural history of AIDS-related opportunistic disorders. *Lancet* 1998;351:228.
44. Yarchoan R et al. Development of antiretroviral therapy for the acquired immunodeficiency syndrome and related disorder: a progress report. *N Engl J Med* 1987;316:557.
45. Merluzzi VJ et al. Inhibition of HIV-1 replication by a nonnucleoside reverse transcriptase inhibitor. *Science* 1990;250:1411.
46. Deeks SG et al. HIV-1 protease inhibitors: a review for clinicians. *JAMA* 1997;277:145.
47. Acosta E et al. Pharmacodynamics of human immunodeficiency virus type 1 protease inhibitors. *Clin Infect Dis* 2000;30(Suppl 2):S151.
48. Reeves JD et al. Emerging drug targets for antiretroviral therapy. *Drugs* 2005;65:1747.
49. Westby M et al. CCR5 antagonists: host-targeted antivirals for the treatment of HIV infection. *Antivir Chem Chemother.* 2005;16:339.
50. Siliciano R. Latent reservoirs of HIV [Abstract S-36]. Presented at the 37th International Conference on Antimicrobial Agents and Chemotherapy (ICAAC). Toronto, Ontario, Canada. September 28–October 1, 1997.
51. Perelson AS et al. Decay characteristic of HIV-1 infected compartments during combination therapy. *Nature* 1997;387:188.
52. Finzi D et al. Latent infection of CD4+ T cells provides a mechanism for lifelong persistence of HIV-1, even in patients on effective combination therapy. *Nat Med* 1999;5:512.
53. Zhang L et al. Quantifying residual HIV-1 replication in patients receiving combination antiretroviral therapy. *N Engl J Med* 1999;340:1605.
54. Pomerantz RJ. Residual HIV-1 disease in the era of highly active antiretroviral therapy. *N Engl J Med* 1999;340:1672.
55. Steckelberg JM et al. Serologic testing for human immunodeficiency virus antibodies. *Mayo Clin Proc* 1988;63:373.
56. Proffitt MR et al. Laboratory diagnosis of human immunodeficiency virus infection. *Infect Dis Clin North Am* 1993;7:203.
57. Cordes RJ et al. Pitfalls in HIV testing: application and limitations of current tests. *Postgrad Med* 1995;98:177.
58. Gaines H et al. Antibody response in primary human immunodeficiency virus infection. *Lancet* 1987;1249.
59. Pilcher CD et al. Real-time, universal screening for acute HIV infection in a routine HIV counseling and testing population. *JAMA* 2002;288:216.
60. Greenwald JL et al. A rapid review of rapid HIV antibody tests. *Current Infectious Disease Reports* 2006;8:125.
61. CDC. Quality Assurance Guidelines for Testing Using the OraQuick Rapid HIV-1 Antibody Test. http://www.cdc.gov/hiv/rapid_testing/materials/qa-guide.htm. Accessed May 7, 2007.
62. Sax PE et al. Potential clinical implications of interlaboratory variability of CD4 T-lymphocyte counts in patients infected with human immunodeficiency virus. *Clin Infect Dis* 1995;21:1121.
63. Peter JB et al. Molecular-based methods for quantifying HIV viral load. *AIDS Patient Care and STDs* 2004;18:75.
64. Lafeuillade A et al. Human immunodeficiency virus type 1 kinetics in lymph nodes compared with plasma. *J Infect Dis* 1996;174:404.
65. Harris M et al. Correlation of virus load in plasma and lymph node tissue in human immunodeficiency virus infection. *J Infect Dis* 1997;176:1388.
66. Brichacek B et al. Increased plasma human immunodeficiency virus type 1 burden following antigenic challenge with pneumococcal vaccine. *J Infect Dis* 1996;174:1191.
67. Hammer SM. Management of newly diagnosed HIV infection. *N Engl J Med* 2005;353:1702.
68. Hecht FM et al. Sexual transmission of an HIV-1 variant resistant to multiple reverse-transcriptase and protease inhibitors. *N Engl J Med* 1998;339: 307.
69. Yerly S et al. Transmission of antiretroviral-drug-resistant HIV-1 variants. *Lancet* 1999;354: 729.
70. Boden D et al. HIV-1 drug resistance in newly infected individuals. *JAMA* 1999;282:1135.
71. Little SJ et al. Reduced antiretroviral drug susceptibility among patients with primary HIV infection. *JAMA* 1999;282:1142.
72. Weinstock HS et al. The epidemiology of antiretroviral drug resistance among drug-naïve HIV-1-infected person in 10 US cities. *J Infect Dis* 2004;189:2174.
73. Wensing AM et al. Prevalence of drug-resistant HIV-1 variants in untreated individuals in Europe: implications for clinical management. *J Infect Dis* 2005;192:958.
74. Cane P et al. Time trends in primary resistance to HIV drugs in the United Kingdom: multicentre observational study. *BMJ* 2005;331:1368.
75. Egger M et al. Prognosis of HIV-1-infected patients starting highly active antiretroviral therapy: a collaborative analysis of prospective studies. *Lancet* 2002;360:119.
76. Philips A, CASCADE Collaboration. Short-term risk of AIDS according to current CD4 cell count and viral load in antiretroviral drug-naïve individuals and those treated in the monotherapy era. *AIDS* 2004;18:51.
77. Moore RD et al. CD4+ cell count 6 years after commencement of highly active antiretroviral therapy in person with sustained virologic suppression. *Clin Infect Disease* 2007;44:441.
78. Gras L et al. CD4 cell counts of 800 cells/mm^3 or greater after 7 years of highly active antiretroviral therapy are feasible in most patients starting with 350 cell/mm^3 or greater. *J Acquir Immune Defic Syndr* 2007. Epublished ahead of print.
79. Kaufmann GR et al. for the Swiss HIV Cohort Study. Characteristics, determinants, and clinical relevance of CD4 T cell recovery to <500 cells/microL in HIV type-1 infected individuals receiving potent antiretroviral therapy. *Clin Infect Dis* 2005;41:361.
80. Katlama C et al. Safety and efficacy of lamivudine-zidovudine combination therapy in antiretroviral-naïve patients: a randomized controlled comparison with zidovudine monotherapy. *JAMA* 1996;276:118.
81. Schambelan M et al. Management of metabolic complications associated with antiretroviral therapy for HIV-1 infection: recommendations of an international AIDS society–USA Panel. *J AIDS* 2002;31:257.
82. Vanhove GF et al. Patient compliance and drug failure in protease inhibitor monotherapy. *JAMA* 1996;276:1955.
83. Machtinger EL. Adherence to HIV Antiretroviral Therapy. HIV Insite Knowledge Base Chapter. May 2005; content revised Jan 2006. www.hivinsite.ucsf.edu; accessed May 13, 2008.
84. Stone VE. Strategies for optimizing adherence to highly active antiretroviral therapy: lessons from research and clinical practice. *Clin Infect Dis* 2001;33:865.
85. Palella FJ Jr et al. for the HIV Outpatient Study Investigators. Mortality in the highly active antiretroviral therapy era: changing causes of death and disease in the HIV Outpatient Study. *J Acquir Immune Defic Syndr* 2006;43:27.
86. Murphy R et al. Seven-year follow up of a lopinavir/ritonavir (LPV/r)-based regimen in antiretroviral-naïve subjects. Program and abstracts of the 10th European AIDS Conference; November 17–20, 2005; Dublin, Ireland. Abstract PE7.9/3.
87. Gallant JE et al. Efficacy and safety of tenofovir DF vs. stavudine in combination therapy in antiretroviral-naïve patients: a 3-year randomized trial. *JAMA* 2004;292:191.
88. Powderly WG et al. Predictors of optimal virological response to potent antiretroviral therapy. *AIDS* 1999;13:1873.
89. Piscitelli SC. The effect of garlic supplementation on the pharmacokinetics of saquinavir. *Clin Infect Dis* 2002;34:234.
90. Piscitelli SC et al. Indinavir concentrations and St John's wort. *Lancet* 2000;12:547.
91. Lee PK et al. HIV-1 viral load blips are of limited clinical significance. *J Antimicrob Chemother* 2006;57:803.
92. Sungkanuparph S et al. Intermittent episodes of detectable HIV viremia in patients receiving nonnucleoside reverse-transcriptase inhibitor-based or protease inhibitor-based highly active antiretroviral therapy regimens are equivalent in incidence and prognosis. *Clin Infect Dis.* 2005;41:1326.
93. Macias J et al. Transient rebounds of HIV plasma viremia are associated with the emergence of drug resistance mutations in patients on highly active antiretroviral therapy. *J Infect* 2005;51:195.
94. Bangsberg DR et al. Adherence to protease inhibitors, HIV-1 viral load, and development of drug resistance in an indigent population. *AIDS* 2000;14:357.
95. Bayard PJ et al. Drug hypersensitivity reactions and human immunodeficiency virus disease. *J AIDS* 1992;5:1237.
96. Coopman SA et al. Cutaneous disease and drug reactions in HIV infection. *N Engl J Med* 1993;328:1670.
97. Carr A et al. Allergic manifestations of human immunodeficiency virus (HIV) infection. *J Clin Immunol* 1991;11:55.
98. Najera I et al. *pol* gene quasispecies of human immunodeficiency virus: mutations associated with

drug resistance in virus from patients undergoing no drug therapy. *J Virol* 1995;69:23.
99. Mohri H et al. Quantitation of zidovudine-resistant human immunodeficiency virus type 1 in the blood of treated and untreated patients. *Proc Natl Acad Sci* 1993;90:25.
100. Moyle GJ. Current knowledge of HIV-1 reverse transcriptase mutations selected during nucleoside analogue therapy: the potential to use resistance data to guide clinical decisions. *J Antimicrob Chemother* 1997;40:765.
101. Moyle GJ. Use of viral resistance patterns to antiretroviral drugs in optimising selection of drug combinations and sequences. *Drugs* 1998;52:168.
102. Mayers D. Rational approaches to resistance: nucleoside analogues. *AIDS.* 1996;10(Suppl 1):S9.
103. Larder BA et al. HIV with reduced sensitivity to zidovudine (ZDV) isolated during prolonged therapy. *Science* 1989;243:1731.
104. Kozal MJ et al. Didanosine resistance in HIV-infected patients switched from zidovudine to didanosine monotherapy. *Ann Intern Med* 1994;121:263.
105. Schmit J et al. Resistance-related mutations in the HIV-1 protease gene of patients treated for 1 year with the protease inhibitor ritonavir (ABT-538). *AIDS* 1996;10:995.
106. Richman DD et al. Nevirapine resistance mutations of human immunodeficiency virus type 1 selected during therapy. *J Virol* 1994;68:1660.
107. Kellam P et al. Zidovudine treatment results in the selection of human immunodeficiency virus type 1 variants whose genotypes confer increasing levels of drug resistance. *J Gen Virol* 1994;75:341.
108. D'Aquila RT et al. Zidovudine resistance and HIV-1 disease progression during antiretroviral therapy. *Ann Intern Med* 1995;122:401.
109. Frost S et al. Quasispecies dynamics and the emergence of drug resistance during zidovudine therapy of HIV infection. *AIDS* 1994;8:323.
110. Schinazi RF et al. Characterization of human immunodeficiency viruses resistant to oxanthiolanecytosine nucleosides. *Antimicrob Agents Chemother* 1993;37:875.
111. Erickson JW et al. Structural mechanisms of HIV drug resistance. *Annu Rev Pharmacol Toxicol* 1996;36:545.
112. Arts EJ et al. Mechanisms of nucleoside analog antiviral activity and resistance during human immunodeficiency virus reverse transcription. *Antimicrob Agents Chemother* 1996;40:527.
113. Caliendo AM et al. Effects of zidovudine-selected human immunodeficiency type 1 reverse transcriptase amino acid substitutions on processive DNA synthesis and viral replication. *J Virol* 1996; 2146.
114. Mellors J. New Insights into Mechanisms of HIV-1 Resistance to Reverse Transcriptase Inhibitors. Abstract L6. Presented at the 9th Conference on Retroviruses and Opportunistic Infections. February 2002, Seattle, WA.
115. Condra JH et al. Preventing HIV-1 drug resistance. *Science Med* 1997;4:2.
116. Stephenson J. HIV drug resistance testing shows promise. *JAMA* 1999;281:309.
117. Leigh Brown AJ et al. Transmission fitness of drug-resistant human immunodeficiency virus and the prevalence of resistance in the antiretroviral-treated population. *J Infect Dis* 2003;187:683.
118. Baxter JD et al. A randomized study of antiretroviral management based on plasma genotypic antiretroviral resistance testing in patients failing therapy. CPCRA 046 Study Team. *AIDS* 2000;14:F83.
119. Deeks SG et al. Persistence of drug-resistant HIV-1 after a structured treatment interruption and its impact on treatment response. *AIDS* 2003;17:361.
120. Race EM et al. Focal mycobacterial lymphadenitis following initiation of protease-inhibitor therapy in patients with advanced HIV 1 disease. *Lancet* 1998;351:252.
121. Kempen JH et al. for the Studies of Ocular Complications of AIDS Research Group. Risk of immune recovery uveitis in patients with AIDS and cytomegalovirus retinitis. *Ophthalmology* 2006;113:684.
122. Jacobson MA et al. Cytomegalovirus retinitis after initiation of highly active antiretroviral therapy. *Lancet* 1997;349:1443.
123. Lederman MM et al. Immunologic responses associated with 12 weeks of combination antiretroviral therapy consisting of zidovudine, lamivudine, and ritonavir: results of AIDS Clinical Trials Group Protocol 315. *J Infect Dis* 1998;178:70.
124. Parker NG et al. Biphasic kinetics of peripheral blood T cells after triple combination therapy in HIV–1 infection: a composite of redistribution and proliferation. *Nat Med* 1998;4:208.
125. Roederer M. Getting to the HAART of T-cell dynamics. *Nat Med* 1998;4:145.
126. Gray CM et al. Changes in CD4+ and CD8+ T-cell subsets in response to highly active antiretroviral therapy in HIV type-1 infected patients with prior protease inhibitor experience. *AIDS Res Hum Retroviruses* 1998;14:561.
127. Race E et al. Recurrence of trimethoprim-sulfamethoxazole TMP/SMX hypersensitivity following initiation of protease inhibitor (PRI) in patients with advanced HIV-1 [Abstract 535]. Presented at the 4th Conference on Retrovirus and Opportunistic Infections. January 22–26, 1997, Washington, DC.
128. Rabound JM et al. Variation in plasma RNA levels, CD4 cell counts, and p24 antigen levels in clinically stable men with human immunodeficiency virus infection. *J Infect Dis* 1996;174:191.
129. Molto J et al. Variability in non-nucleoside reverse transcriptase and protease inhibitors concentrations among HIV-infected adults in routine clinical practice. *Br J Clin Pharmacol* 2007: Jan. 12. Epub ahead of print.
130. Acosta EP et al. Position paper on therapeutic drug monitoring of antiretroviral agents. *AIDS Res Hum Retroviruses* 2002;18:825.
131. la Porte CJL et al. Updated guideline to perform therapeutic drug monitoring for antiretroviral agents. www.hivpharmacology.com. Accessed May 13, 2007.
132. Burger DM et al. Treatment failure on nelfinavir-containing triple therapy can largely be explained by low nelfinavir plasma concentrations. *AIDS* 2000;14(Suppl 4):P258.
133. Joshi AS et al. Population pharmacokinetic meta-analysis with efavirenz. *Int J Clin Pharmacol Ther* 2002;40:507.
134. Luber AD et al. Serum drug levels of amprenavir display limited inter- and intra-patient variability. *AIDS* 2000;14(Suppl 4):S28.
135. Burger DM et al. Therapeutic drug monitoring of nelfinavir and indinavir in treatment-naïve HIV-1-infected individuals. *AIDS* 2003;17:1157.
136. Fletcher CV et al. Concentration-controlled compared with conventional antiretroviral therapy for HIV infection. *AIDS* 2002;16:551.
137. Dube MP et al. Metabolic complications of antiretroviral therapies. *AIDS Clin Care* 1998; 10:41.
138. Carr A et al. A syndrome of peripheral lipodystrophy, hyperlipidaemia and insulin resistance in patients receiving HIV protease inhibitors. *AIDS* 1998;12:F51.
139. Lumpkin MM. FDA public health advisory: reports of diabetes and hyperglycemia in patients receiving protease inhibitors for the treatment of human immunodeficiency virus (HIV). June 11, 1997.
140. Eastone JA. New-onset diabetes mellitus associated with use of protease inhibitors (Letter). *Ann Intern Med* 1997;11:948.
141. Dube MP et al. Protease inhibitor-associated hyperglycemia. *Lancet* 1997;350:713.
142. Miller KD et al. Visceral abdominal-fat accumulation associated with use of indinavir. *Lancet* 1998;351:871.
143. Lo JC et al. "Buffalo hump" in men with HIV-1 infection. *Lancet* 1998;867.
144. Viraben R et al. Indinavir-associated lipodystrophy. *AIDS* 1998;12:F37.
145. Mary-Krause M et al. Increased risk of myocardial infarction with duration of protease inhibitor therapy in HIV-infected men. *AIDS* 2003;17:2479.
146. Henry K et al. Severe premature coronary artery disease with protease inhibitors. *Lancet* 1998;351:1328.
147. Holmberg SD et al. Protease inhibitors and cardiovascular outcomes in patients with HIV-1. *Lancet* 2002;360:1747.
148. Iloeje UH et al. Protease inhibitor exposure and increased risk of cardiovascular disease in HIV-infected patients. *HIV Med* 2005;6:36.
149. Friis-Møller N et al. for the D:A:D Study Group. Combination antiretroviral therapy and the risk of myocardial infarction. *N Engl J Med* 2003;349:1993.
150. The DAD Study Group. Class of antiretroviral drugs and the risk of myocardial infarction. *N Engl J Med* 2007;356:1723.
151. Lenhard JM et al. HIV protease inhibitors block adipogenesis and increase lipolysis in vitro. *Antiviral Res* 2000;47:121.
152. Mallon PW. Pathogenesis of lipodystrophy and lipid abnormalities in patients taking antiretroviral therapy. *AIDS Rev* 2007;9:3.
153. Cianflone K et al. Protease inhibitor effects on triglyceride synthesis and adipokine secretion in human omental and subcutaneous adipose tissue. *Antivir Ther* 2006;11:681.
154. Brinkman K et al. Mitochondrial toxicity induced by nucleoside-analogue reverse-transcriptase inhibitors is a key factor in the pathogenesis of antiretroviral therapy related lipodystrophy. *Lancet* 1999;354:1112.
155. Dube MP et al. Guidelines for the evaluation and management of dyslipidemia in human immunodeficiency virus (HIV)-infected adults receiving antiretroviral therapy: recommendations of the HIV medicine association of the Infectious Disease Society of America and the Adult AIDS Clinical Trials Group. *Clin Infect Disease* 2003;37:613.
156. Hadigan C et al. Metabolic abnormalities and cardiovascular disease risk factors in adults with HIV and lipodystrophy. *Clin Infect Dis* 2001;32:130.
157. Currier J. Management of metabolic complications of therapy. *AIDS* 2002;16:S171.
158. Distler O et al. Hyperlipidemia and inhibitors of HIV protease. *Curr Opin Clin Nutr Metab Care* 2001;4:99.
159. van Leth F et al. Nevirapine and efavirenz elicit different changes in lipid profiles in antiretroviral-therapy-naïve patients infected with HIV-1. *PLoS Med* 2004;1:e19.
160. Fichtenbaum CJ et al. Pharmacokinetic interactions between protease inhibitors and statins in HIV seronegative volunteers: ACTG study A5047. *AIDS* 2002;16:569.
161. Keiser PH et al. Substituting abacavir for hyperlipidemia-associated protease inhibitors in HAART regimens improves fasting lipid profiles, maintains virologic suppression, and simplifies treatment. *BMC Infect Dis* 2005;5:2.
162. Negredo F et al. Virological, immunological, and clinical impact of switching from protease inhibitors to nevirapine or to efavirenz in patients with human immunodeficiency virus infection and long-lasting viral suppression. *Clin Infect Dis* 2002;34:504.
163. Martinez E et al. Impact of switching from human immunodeficiency virus type 1 protease inhibitors to efavirenz in successfully treated adults with lipodystrophy. *Clin Infect Dis* 2000;31: 1266.
164. Carr A et al. HIV protease inhibitor substitution in patients with lipodystrophy: a randomized, controlled, open-label, multicenter study. *AIDS* 2001;15:1811.
165. Clumeck N et al. Simplification with abacavir-based triple nucleoside therapy versus continued protease inhibitor-based highly active antiretroviral therapy in HIV-1-infected patients with undetectable plasma HIV-1 RNA. *AIDS* 2001;15: 1517.

166. Saag MS et al. Switching antiretroviral drugs for treatment of metabolic complications in HIV-1 infection: summary of selected trials. *Topics in HIV Medicine* 2002;10:47.
167. Carr A et al. Abacavir substitution for nucleoside analogues in patients with HIV lipoatrophy: a randomized trial. *JAMA* 2002;288:207.
168. Dube MP et al. Glucose metabolism, lipid, and body fat changes in antiretroviral-naïve subjects randomized to felfinavir or efavirenz plus dual nucleosides. *AIDS* 2005;19:1807.
169. Moyle GJ et al. for the RAVE Group UK. A randomized comparative trial of tenofovir DF or abacavir as replacement for a thymidine analogue in persons with lipatrophy. *AIDS* 2006;20:1043.
170. Boyd MA et al. Changes in body composition and mitochondrial nucleic acid content in patients switched from failed nucleoside analogue therapy to ritonavir-boosted indinavir and efavirenz. *J Infect Dis* 2006;194:642.
171. Hatano H et al. Metabolic and anthropometric consequences of interruption of highly active antiretroviral therapy. *AIDS* 2000;14:1935.
172. Delaugerre C et al. Virological and pharmacological factors associated with virological response to salvage therapy after an 8-week of treatment interruption in a context of very advanced HIV disease (GIGHAART ANRS 097). *J Med Virol* 2005;77:345.
173. Lawrence J et al. CPCRA 064:Structured treatment interruption in patients with multidrug resistant human immunodeficiency virus. *N Engl J Med* 2003;349:837.
174. Ananworanich J, HIV-NAT 001.4: Highly active antiretroviral therapy (HAART) retreatment in patients on CD4-guided therapy achieved similar virologic suppression compared with patients on continuous HAART. *J Acquir Immune Defic Syndr* 2005;39:523.
175. Ruiz L et al. Antiretroviral therapy interruption guided by CD4 cell counts and plasma HIV-1 RNA levels in chronically infected patients. *AIDS* 2007;21:169.
176. Dybul M et al. A proof-of-concept study of short-cycle intermittent antiretroviral therapy with a once-daily regimen of didanosine, lamivudine, and efavirenz for the treatment of chronic HIV infection. *J Infect Dis* 2004;189:1974.
177. Dybul M et al. Short-cycle structured intermittent treatment of chronic HIV infection with highly active antiretroviral therapy. *AIDS* 2000;14:1935.
178. Cohen CJ et al. Pilot study of a novel short-cycle antiretroviral treatment interruption strategy: 48-week results of the fine-days-on, two-days-off (FOTO) Study. *HIV Clin Trials* 2007;8:19.
179. Deeks S et al. Supervised interruptions of antiretroviral therapy. *AIDS* 2002;16(Suppl 4):S157.
180. Kilby JM et al. Recurrence of the acute HIV syndrome after interruption of antiretroviral therapy in a patient with chronic HIV-1 infection: a case report. *Ann Intern Med* 2000;133:435.
181. Colven R et al. Retroviral rebound syndrome after cessation of suppressive antiretroviral therapy in three patients with chronic HIV infection. *Ann Intern Med* 2000;133:430.
182. Daar ES et al. Acute HIV syndrome after discontinuation of antiretroviral therapy in a patient treated before seroconversion. *Ann Intern Med* 1998;128:827.
183. Jackson JB et al. Identification of the K103N resistance mutation in Ugandan women receiving nevirapine to prevent HIV-1 vertical transmission. *AIDS* 2000;14:F111.
184. Strategies for Management of Antiretroviral Therapy (SMART) Study Group; El-Sadr WM et al. CD4+ count-guided interruption of antiretroviral treatment. *N Engl J Med* 2006;355:2283. *Links Comment in N Engl J Med* 2006;355:2359.
185. Danel C et al. CD4-guided structured antiretroviral treatment interruption strategy in HIV-infected adults in west Africa (Trivacan ANRS 1269 trial): a randomised trial. *Lancet* 2006;9527:1981.

CHAPTER 70

Opportunistic Infections in HIV-Infected Patients

Amanda H. Corbett

The acquired immunodeficiency syndrome (AIDS) is characterized by the gradual erosion of immune competence and the development of opportunistic infections (OIs) and malignancies. Since the era of highly active antiretroviral therapy (HAART) began in 1996, AIDS–related mortality has declined in the United States.[1,2] This decline in mortality more specifically is described by a decline in opportunistic infection associated deaths over the pre-HAART (1992–1995), peri-HAART (1996–1999), and post-HAART (2000–2003) eras with an increase in noninfectious AIDS-related mortality.[3] In 1997, the year after HAART initiation, the U.S. Centers for Disease Control and Prevention (CDC) estimated that approximately 60,000 AIDS-related opportunistic illnesses had occurred in the United States during 1996.[1] This report represents the first calendar year in which the overall incidence of AIDS-associated OIs did not increase in the United States; the 1996 figure represented a decline of 6% compared with 1995. Patients with human immunodeficiency virus (HIV) infection are susceptible to an array of diseases, but most OIs are caused by a few common pathogens, including *Pneumocystis jiroveci*

Table 70-1 Conditions Included in the 1993 Surveillance Case Definition

Category A	Category C *(Continued)*
Asymptomatic HIV infection	Cryptococcosis, extrapulmonary
Persistent generalized lymphadenopathy	Cryptosporidiosis, chronic intestinal (>1 month)
Acute HIV infection with accompanying illness or history of HIV infection	CMV disease (other than liver, spleen, or nodes)
	CMV retinitis (with loss of vision)
Category B	Encephalopathy, HIV related
Bacillary angiomatosis	Herpes simplex: chronic ulcer(s) (>1 month); or bronchitis, pneumonitis, or esophagitis
Candidiasis, oropharyngeal (thrush)	Histoplasmosis, disseminated or extrapulmonary
Candidiasis, vulvovaginal; persistent, frequent, or poorly responsive to treatment	Isosporiasis, chronic intestinal (>1 month's duration)
Cervical dysplasia/carcinoma in situ	Kaposi sarcoma
Constitutional symptoms, such as fever >38°C or diarrhea >1 month	Lymphoid interstitial pneumonia and/or pulmonary lymphoid hyperplasia[a]
Hairy leukoplakia	Lymphoma, Burkitt (or equivalent term)
Herpes zoster (shingles), involving at least two distinct episodes or more than one dermatome	Lymphoma, immunoblastic (or equivalent term)
Idiopathic thrombocytopenia purpura	Lymphoma, primary, of brain
Listeriosis	*Mycobacterium avium-intracellulare* complex or *M. kansasii*, disseminated or extrapulmonary
Pelvic inflammatory disease, particularly if complicated by tubo-ovarian abscess	*Mycobacterium tuberculosis,* any site (pulmonary[b] or extrapulmonary)
Peripheral neuropathy	Mycobacterium, other species or unidentified species, disseminated or extrapulmonary
	Pneumocystis carinii pneumonia
Category C	Pneumonia, recurrent[b]
Candidiasis of bronchi, trachea, or lungs	PML
Candidiasis, esophageal	*Salmonella* septicemia, recurrent
Cervical cancer, invasive	Toxoplasmosis of brain
Coccidioidomycosis, disseminated or extrapulmonary	Wasting syndrome due to HIV

[a] Children <13 years old.
[b] Added in the 1993 expansions of the AIDS surveillance case definition for adolescents and adults.
HIV, human immunodeficiency virus; PML, progressive multifocal leukoencephalopathy.

(carinii), cytomegalovirus (CMV), fungi, and mycobacteria. Persons with AIDS also are susceptible to neoplastic diseases (lymphoma and Kaposi sarcoma [KS]) and other conditions, such as wasting syndrome.[2,4]

The 1993 revised classification system for HIV infection and expanded surveillance case definition for AIDS included stratification for the CD4$^+$ lymphocyte count, as well as subgrouping by clinical categories (Table 70-1). These AIDS-defining OIs or malignancies may also occur in asymptomatic HIV-infected patients (Table 70-1).[4]

The Natural History of Opportunistic Infections

The Decline of the CD4$^+$ Lymphocyte

Within the immune system, the CD4$^+$ lymphocyte functions as a "helper cell" that modulates the actions of the other key cellular components of the immune system. The eventual loss of CD4$^+$ lymphocytes is the underlying pathophysiologic problem that leads to AIDS. (See Chapter 69, Pharmacotherapy of Human Immunodeficiency Virus Infection, and comprehensive immunology texts for a more detailed explanation of immune function and inflammation associated with HIV infection).[5,6] The infected CD4$^+$ lymphocyte can function normally for a period of time, but eventually becomes dysfunctional, as manifested by an abnormal response to soluble mitogens.[7,8] It is this cellular functional deficit, compounded by the eventual decline in the absolute number of CD4$^+$ lymphocytes, that leads to OIs, malignancies, and neurologic dysfunctions. The CD4$^+$ count declines gradually over several years in the untreated HIV-infected person. The average rate of decline of CD4$^+$ lymphocyte cells (CD4 slope) is approximately 40 to 80 cells/mm^3/year in the absence of antiretroviral therapy. An accelerated decline in the CD4$^+$ count occurs at 1.5 to 2 years, just before an AIDS-defining diagnosis.[9,10] Without therapy, the course of infection averages approximately 10 years from the time of initial infection to an AIDS-defining diagnosis. There is individual variation in the decline of the CD4$^+$ count. Some patients have a rapid decline after the acute retroviral presentation, whereas approximately 5% to 15% have a CD4$^+$ count of 500 for longer than 8 years; these patients are considered chronic nonprogressors.[11]

The CD4$^+$ count dictates the need for OI prophylaxis, affects the differential diagnosis of the OI, and is an independent indicator of prognosis. For these reasons, the CD4$^+$ count has become a primary surrogate marker of immune suppression and antiretroviral activity.[12] HIV-1 RNA is the other clinical surrogate marker most predictive of survival and antiretroviral activity.

OIs range from relatively minor events (e.g., oral candidiasis or oral hairy leukoplakia) to sight-threatening episodes of CMV retinitis, or life-threatening *P. jiroveci (carinii)* pneumonia (PCP). The risk for specific OIs varies with the degree of immunosuppression.[13,14,15] Asymptomatic patients with

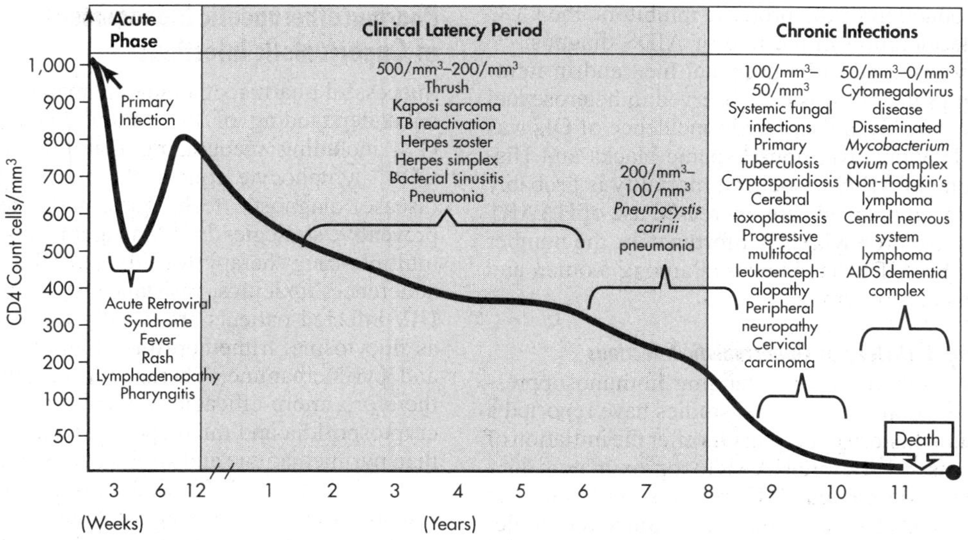

FIGURE 70-1 Natural history of CD4+ cell count in the average HIV patient without antiretroviral therapy from the time of HIV transmissions to death. (Illustration by Mary Van, PharmD.)

moderate immunosuppression (CD4+ counts 200–500) may become infected with herpes viruses and *Candida* species and/or develop pneumonias, enteric infections, and meningitis with common pathogens. Massive destruction of the immune system occurs when the CD4+ count is below 200, which increases the risk for opportunistic pathogens (e.g., PCP), opportunistic tumors, wasting, and neurologic complications. With a CD4+ count of 50 to 100, invasive candidiasis, cerebral toxoplasmosis, cryptococcosis, and various protozoal infections are observed. When the CD4+ count falls below 50, the patient is in an advanced immunosuppressed state, which is associated with non-Hodgkin lymphoma (NHL), CMV, and disseminated *Mycobacterium avium* complex (MAC; Fig. 70-1). Without treatment, the median survival associated with a CD4+ count below 200 is 3.1 years, and the time to an AIDS-defining infection ranges from 18 to 24 months.[9,12,13,15] With the implementation of HAART, the 3-year probability of AIDS (which includes in many cases OIs) has dramatically declined as compared with before HAART; however, much of this may be attributed to the use of prophylactic regimens for OIs.[16]

The Effect of Opportunistic Infections on Viral Load and Survival

Acute OIs upregulate HIV replication, resulting in higher HIV-1 RNA concentrations in the plasma and lymphoid tissues of HIV-infected patients.[17–20] This enhanced replication is presumably caused by antigen-mediated activation of HIV-1 replication in latently infected cells. To assess the impact of OIs on survival, data from a cohort of 2,081 HIV-infected patients followed (in the preprotease inhibitor era) for a mean of 30 months were analyzed.[21] CD4+ counts and incidence of opportunistic disease were used as independent variables. These investigators found that PCP, CMV, MAC, esophageal candidiasis, KS, NHL, progressive multifocal leukoencephalopathy (PML), dementia, wasting syndrome, toxoplasmosis, and cryptosporidiosis were independently associated with death.[21] Additionally, data from a prospective longitudinal study of HIV infection in homosexual men initiated in 1984 (Multicenter AIDS Cohort Study) demonstrated that plasma HIV-1 RNA concentrations strongly predict the rate of decline of the absolute CD4+ count as well as clinical progression to AIDS and death.[22] More recent investigations in the era of HAART have demonstrated that CD4 count is the strongest prognostic factor in patients starting therapy.[16]

Impact of Antiretroviral Agents on the Natural History of Opportunistic Infections

REDUCTION IN THE INCIDENCE OF OPPORTUNISTIC INFECTIONS AND DEATH

The introduction of protease inhibitors, combination therapy, prophylaxis therapy, and improved medical care has reduced the incidence of OIs and death resulting from AIDS in HIV-positive patients. HAART usually consists of two nucleoside reverse transcriptase inhibitors, in addition to one or more protease inhibitors or one non-nucleoside reverse transcriptase inhibitor. HAART generally refers to an antiretroviral regimen that can be expected to reduce the viral load in antiretroviral-naive patients to fewer than 50 copies/mL. A panel of experts convened by the U.S. Department of Health and Human Services and the Henry J. Kaiser Family Foundation recommended HAART as the standard of care for all HIV-infected patients.[23] These potent antiretroviral agents and effective management of OIs have led to an improved quality of life and prolonged duration of survival among HIV-infected patients in the United States.[24–26] A significant decrease in the incidence of OIs and death was first reported in February 1996, when preliminary data from a pivotal study became available. The data demonstrated that the addition of ritonavir to an existing reverse transcriptase regimen in severely immunocompromised patients decreased the incidence of OIs and death.[27] Several studies[16,27,28,29–32] since have shown a decrease in the incidence of OIs in AIDS patients receiving HAART therapy. One such study, a retrospective cohort design of patients in an HIV outpatient clinic observed from January 1994, through June 1997, demonstrated a significant decline in OIs in 1996 and 1997. The most common conditions with reported reduced incidence included KS, HIV wasting, and infections such as PCP, MAC, and CMV.[29]

Since the introduction of the protease inhibitors, the CDC has reported a deceleration in the rate of AIDS diagnosis.[31] This finding was observed in homosexual men and in intravenous (IV) drug users, but was not observed in heterosexual exposure groups. Notably, a decrease in incidence of OIs was not observed in HIV-positive, non-Hispanic blacks and Hispanics. The decline in AIDS-associated mortality is probably the result of improved medical care, increased use of HAART therapy, and effective prophylaxis. Unfortunately, the number of deaths caused by AIDS has increased among women and heterosexual transmission groups.

Changes in the Natural History of Opportunistic Infections

OIs and cancers result from long-standing immunosuppression from HIV infection.[13–15] Several studies have reported a change in the natural history of certain OIs after the initiation of antiretroviral agents.[33,34] Before HAART, approximately 40% of all AIDS patients developed CMV retinitis, with the most cases occurring at CD4+ counts below 100. Since the implementation of HAART, a decrease in the incidence of CMV retinitis and a decline in the rate of retinitis progression have been noted.[33,35]

Ironically, HAART therapy also has been associated with a worsening or an unmasking of occult OIs in patients with advanced AIDS. When antiretroviral therapy strengthens the immune system, inflammatory symptoms in response to infection are more clinically pronounced.[32,36] This syndrome has been referred to as immune reconstitution inflammatory syndrome or IRIS. A subclinical MAC infection syndrome, characterized by severe fever, leukocytosis, and lymphadenitis, was observed in five patients after initiating HAART.[32] CMV retinitis occurred in five patients previously treated with HAART despite a marked improvement in CD4+ counts (195 cell/mm^3) before diagnosis.[35] Elevated liver function tests (LFTs) and hepatitis C viremia have been documented after the initiation of HAART.[37]

The initiation of HAART typically results in an increase in CD4+ lymphocytes and a decrease in HIV-1 RNA to undetectable levels. It is unclear whether the CD4+ lymphocytes associated with HAART therapy are as functional as the cells previously lost over the course of the HIV infection. It is also unknown whether this increase in total CD4+ lymphocytes reflects an increase in memory subtypes, and whether these subtypes mediate a subclinical inflammatory response.[36]

Improvement or Resolution of Opportunistic Infections

With the initiation of HAART, reports of improvement or resolution of some OIs were published.[38–42] These OIs included KS,[38] PML,[39] CMV,[33,35] microsporidiosis, cryptosporidiosis,[40] and molluscum contagiosum,[41] a viral infection caused by a member of the *Poxviridae* family. Furthermore, there are reports of restored immunity and clinical improvement in patients with chronic hepatitis B infection (not classified as a CDC-defined AIDS indicator condition) upon the initiation of HAART.[42] These infections were not eradicated, and in some cases improvement was only transient. Clinical resolution most likely results from immunologic improvement, and the protective immunity against OI is sustained only as long as HAART remains effective.

Pharmacotherapeutic Management of Opportunistic Infections

Successful pharmacotherapeutic management of OIs requires an understanding of the natural history of HIV-associated OIs, including recognizing that OIs occur with declining CD4+ lymphocyte counts, the clinical presentation of each disease, diagnostic techniques, and effective treatment and preventive strategies.[43,44] Management issues, complicated by multiple-drug therapy for OIs and HIV suppression, include adherence, toxicities, resistance, drug interactions, and cost. HIV-infected patients are usually less tolerant to drugs such as flucytosine, trimethoprim-sulfamethoxazole (TMP-SMX), and pyrimethamine. Therapeutic options are often limited; therefore, more efficacious agents (e.g., for the treatment of cryptosporidia and microsporidia) and less toxic agents (e.g., than pyrimethamine and sulfadiazine) need to be developed.[45]

In 1995, the U.S. Public Health Service (USPHS) and the Infectious Diseases Society of America (IDSA) issued guidelines for the prevention of OIs in HIV-infected patients; these were revised in 1997,[46] 1999,[47] and 2002.[48] Nineteen OIs, or groups of OIs, are addressed, and recommendations are included for preventing exposure to opportunistic pathogens, preventing first episodes of disease by chemoprophylaxis or vaccination (primary prophylaxis), and preventing disease recurrence (secondary prophylaxis). Additionally, in 2004 the CDC published the first edition guidelines for treatment of OIs.[49]

Primary Prophylaxis

Primary prophylaxis is defined as therapy that is initiated before the appearance of an OI in high-risk asymptomatic persons. It is used to prevent the initial occurrence of an infection. Primary prevention of OIs is important, considering the inevitable immune depletion associated with chronic HIV infection.[44,50,51] PCP and MAC prophylaxis have significantly prolonged survival and delayed the onset of illness (see sections about PCP and MAC prophylaxis).[50,51]

The guidelines strongly recommend primary prophylaxis against PCP, toxoplasmosis, *Mycobacterium tuberculosis,* MAC, and varicella-zoster virus (VZV). Vaccinations to prevent *Streptococcus pneumoniae,* hepatitis B virus, hepatitis A virus, and influenza virus infection generally are recommended for all HIV-infected patients. Primary prophylaxis for fungal infections (*Cryptococcus neoformans* and *Histoplasma capsulatum*), CMV, and bacterial infections are not routinely recommended for most patients, except in unusual circumstances (Table 70-2).

DISCONTINUATION OF PRIMARY PROPHYLAXIS THERAPY

HAART has diminished the incidence of several OIs.[33,34,38,40] Therefore, it may be possible to discontinue prophylactic OI therapy when CD4+ counts rise above the threshold associated with risk for infection. These data have been particularly encouraging in patients who had PCP prophylaxis discontinued with an increase in CD4+ counts.[48,52–54] In one observational PCP prophylaxis study, no episodes of PCP were observed after discontinuation of primary and secondary PCP prophylaxis.[52] These studies suggest that patients who respond to HAART therapy with a sustained increase in CD4+ count

Table 70-2 Primary Prophylaxis of Opportunistic Infections in HIV-Infected Adults and Adolescents

Pathogen	Indication	Preventive Regimens: First Choice	Preventive Regimens: Alternatives	D/C Prophylaxis
Strongly Recommended as Standard of Care				
Pneumocystis jiroveci (carinii)	$CD4^+$ count <200 or oropharyngeal candidiasis	TMP-SMX, 1 DS PO QD or TMP-SMX 1 SS PO QD	Dapsone 50 mg BID or 100 mg/day; dapsone 50 mg QD + pyrimethamine 50 mg QW + leucovorin, 25 mg PO QW; dapsone, 200 mg PO + pyrimethamine 75 mg PO + leucovorin, 25 mg PO QW; aerosolized pentamadine, 300 mg QM via Respirgard II nebulizer, atovaquone, 1,500 mg PO QD; TMP-SMX 1 DS 3×/wk	Patients on HAART with sustained CD4 >200 cells for ≥3 months may discontinue PCP prophylaxis. Reintroduce if $CD4^+$ <200.
M. tuberculosis				
Isoniazid sensitive	TST reaction ≥5 mm or prior positive result without treatment or contact with case of active tuberculosis regardless of TST result	Isoniazid 300 mg PO + pyridoxine 50 mg PO QD ×9 months or isoniazid 900 mg PO + pyridoxine, 100 mg PO BIW ×9 months	Rifampin 600 mg PO QD ×4 months or rifabutin 300 mg PO QD ×4 months: PZA 1,520 mg/kg PO QD ×2 months + rifampin 600 mg PO QD ×2 months or rifabutin 300 mg PO QD ×2 months	
Isoniazid resistant	Same; high probability of exposure to multidrug resistant tuberculosis	Rifampin 600 mg PO QD or rifabutin 300 mg PO QD ×4 months	Pyrazinamide 15–20 mg/kg PO QD ×2 months; + either rifampin 600 mg PO QD ×2 months or rifabutin 300 mg PO QD ×2 months	
Multidrug resistant (INH and RIF)	Same; high probability of exposure to isoniazid-resistant tuberculosis	Choice of drugs requires consultation with public health authorities	None	
T. gondii	IgG antibody to *Toxoplasma* and $CD4^+$ count <100	TMP-SMX, 1 DS PO QD	TMP-SMZ, 1 SS PO QD: dapsone, 50 mg PO QD + pyrimethamine, 50 mg PO QW + leucovorin, 25 mg PO QW; dapsone 200 mg PO QW + pyrimethymine 75 mg PO QW + leucovorin 25 mg PO QW: atovaquone, 1,500 mg PO QD with or without pyrimethamine 25 mg PO QD + leucovorin, 10 mg PO QD	Patients on HAART with sustained CD4 >200 for ≥3 months may discontinue toxoplasmosis prophylaxis. Restart if CD4 <200.
MAC	$CD4^+$ count <50	Azithromycin, 1,200 mg PO QW or clarithromycin 500 mg PO BID	Rifabutin, 300 mg PO QD; azithromycin, 1,200 mg PO QW + rifabutin, 300 mg PO QD	Patient on HAART with sustained CD4 >100 for ≥3 months may discontinue MAC prophylaxis. Restart if CD4 <50,100.
VZV	Significant exposure to chicken pox or shingles for patients who have no history of either condition or, if available, negative antibody to VZV	VZIG 5 vials (1.25 mL each) IM administered 96 hr after exposure, ideally within 48 hr		
Usually Recommended				
S. pneumoniae	$CD4^+$ >1,200	23 valent polysaccharide Pneumococcal vaccine 0.5 mL IM	None	

(Continued)

Table 70-2 Primary Prophylaxis of Opportunistic Infections in HIV-Infected Adults and Adolescents *(continued)*

		Preventive Regimens		
Pathogen	*Indication*	*First Choice*	*Alternatives*	*D/C Prophylaxis*
Usually Recommended *(continued)*				
HBV	All susceptible (anti-HBc-negative) patients	Hepatitis B vaccine 3 doses	None	
Influenza virus	All patients (annually before influenza season)	Inactivated trivalent influenza virus vaccine 0.5 mL/yr IM	Oseltamivir 75 mg QD (influenza A or B); Rimantadine, 100 mg PO BID, or amantadine, 100 mg PO BID (influenza A only)	
HAV	All susceptible (anti-HAV-negative) patient at increased risk for HAV or patients with chronic liver disease (including HBV or HCV)	Hepatitis A vaccine; 2 doses	None	
Not Recommended for Most Patients; Indicated for Use Only in Unusual Circumstances				
Bacteria	Neutropenia	G-CSF 510 mg/kg SC QD ×24 wk or GM-CSF 250 mg/m² SC ×24 wk	None	
C. neoformans	CD4+ count <50	Fluconazole 100–200 mg PO QD	Itraconazole 200 mg PO QD	
H. capsulatum	CD4+ count <100, endemic geographic areas	Itraconazole 200 mg PO QD	None	
CMV	CD4+ count <50 and CMV antibody positive	Oral ganciclovir 1 g PO TID or valganciclovir 900 mg PO QD	None	

BID, twice a day; CMV, cytomegalovirus; DS, double strength; G-CSF, granulocyte colony-stimulating factor; GM-CSF, granulocyte-macrophage colony-stimulating factor; HAART, highly active antiretroviral therapy; HAV, hepatitis A virus; HBc, hepatitis B core; IM, intramuscularly; INH, isoniazid; MAC, *Mycobacterium avium* complex; PO, orally; QD, daily; QW, weekly; RIF, rifampin; SC, subcutaneously; SS, single strength; TMP-SMX, trimethoprim-sulfamethoxazole; TST, tuberculin skin test; VZIG, varicella-zoster immune globulin; VZV, varicella-zoster virus.

Adapted from USPHS/IDSA Guidelines. *MMWR Morbid Mortal Wkly Rep* 2002;51(RR-8):152.

can have their primary prophylaxis safely discontinued. The OI prophylaxis guidelines suggest that primary PCP prophylaxis may be discontinued for patients on HAART when the CD4+ count is above 200 for at least 3 months. Primary prophylaxis for MAC may also be discontinued when the CD4+ count increases to above 100.[48,55] In addition, the guidelines suggest discontinuing primary prophylaxis for toxoplasmosis when the CD4+ count increases to higher than 200 for at least 3 months.

Acute Therapy

Prompt diagnosis and immediate initiation of therapy are essential to the management of acute infections. Most common OIs can be classified into one of two groups. The first group consists of infections that can be treated by conventional or investigational agents. These include PCP, tuberculosis (TB), cryptococcosis, CMV, MAC, and histoplasmosis. Treatment may result in either effective or moderately effective resolution. These infections may recur if chronic suppressive or secondary prophylaxis is discontinued without an accompanying elevation in the CD4+ count and viral load suppression. The second group includes pathogens for which no therapeutic regimen is currently effective (Table 70-3). These include cryptosporidiosis, microsporidiosis, and PML.[43]

Secondary Prophylaxis or Chronic Suppressive Therapy

Secondary prophylaxis is used to prevent recurrence of an OI once the patient has developed signs and symptoms of active infection. In some cases, secondary prophylaxis regimens can be discontinued after patients achieve a certain CD4+ level. The USPHS and IDSA strongly recommend secondary prophylaxis for PCP, toxoplasmosis (reduced dosage), MAC, CMV, *Salmonella* species, and infections caused by endemic fungi and *C. neoformans.*[48]

DISCONTINUATION OF SECONDARY PROPHYLAXIS OR CHRONIC SUPPRESSIVE THERAPY

In 1999, the USPHS/IDSA guidelines first reported that stopping primary or secondary prophylaxis for certain pathogens was safe if HAART led to an increase in the CD4+ count to above specified threshold levels. The 2002 USPHS/IDSA guidelines incorporated more data to support these initial recommendations and expanded recommendations to other pathogens. Criteria for discontinuing chemoprophylaxis are

Table 70-3 Acute Management of Opportunistic Infections

Group I[a]		Group II
A	B	
Infections effectively treated	Moderate chance of effective treatment	No currently effective therapeutic regimen
• *Pneumocystis jiroveci* pneumonia • Tuberculosis • Cryptococcosis • Histoplasmosis	• CMV • MAC	• Cryptosporidiosis • Microsporidiosis • PML

[a] A and B may recur if secondary prophylaxis is discontinued.
CMV, cytomegalovirus; MAC, *Mycobacterium avium* complex; PML, progressive multifocal leukoencephalopathy.
Adapted from reference 43.

based on specific clinical studies and vary by duration of CD4+ count increase and duration of treatment of the initial episode of disease (in the case of secondary prophylaxis).

Multiple case series have reported that maintenance therapy for CMV can be discontinued safely in patients who have maintained a CD4+ count of >100 to 150 for >6 months on HAART.[33,34,56–60] Whereas CMV retinitis typically reactivated <6 to 8 weeks after stopping CMV therapy in the pre-HAART era, these patients have remained disease free for >30 to 95 weeks. Plasma HIV RNA levels varied among these patients, demonstrating that the CD4+ count is the primary determinant of immune recovery to CMV. The decision to stop CMV prophylaxis should be made in consultation with an ophthalmologist and is influenced by factors such as the magnitude and duration of CD4+ increases and viral load suppression, anatomical location of retinal lesions, and vision in the contralateral eye. Regular ophthalmic examination is critical.[33,34,48,59–61] Secondary PCP prophylaxis may be discontinued among patients whose CD4+ counts have increased to >200 for >3 months while on HAART. Secondary prophylaxis for disseminated MAC may be discontinued among patients who have completed 12 months of MAC therapy, have no signs or symptoms of MAC, and have had a CD4+ count of >100 for >6 months in response to HAART. Similarly, secondary prophylaxis for toxoplasmosis may be discontinued in patients who have completed initial therapy, have no signs or symptoms of infection, and have had CD4+ counts of >200 for >6 months. Using the same criteria, patients with cryptococcosis can discontinue secondary prophylaxis if they have had CD4+ counts of >100 to 200 for >6 months.

Although there are considerable data concerning the discontinuation of primary and secondary prophylaxis, there are no data regarding restarting prophylaxis if the CD4+ count decreases again to levels at which the patient is likely to again be at risk for OIs. For primary prophylaxis, it is unknown whether the same threshold at which prophylaxis can be stopped should be used or whether the threshold below which initial prophylaxis is recommended should be used. For prophylaxis against PCP, the 2002 guidelines use a CD4+ count of 200 as the threshold for restarting both primary and secondary prophylaxis.

PNEUMOCYSTIS JIROVECI PNEUMONIA

As an indication of the relative obscurity of this organism, no comprehensive text on PCP was available until 1983.[62] Since that time, this organism has been reclassified from a protozoan to a fungus on the basis of ribosomal RNA sequence comparisons.[63] The morphologic resemblance of *P. carinii* to a protozoan has led to its life cycle being described as a cyst form, with up to eight sporozoites per cyst. The trophozoite or extracystic form has different staining characteristics (i.e., it does not stain with toluidine-blue O or Grocott-Gomori stains) compared with the cyst or sporozoites. In addition, current literature refers to PCP as *Pneumocystis jiroveci* as opposed to the original terminology of *Pneumocystis carinii*. The former species is the one responsible for infectivity in humans.

Clinical Presentation

1. J.R. is a 38-year-old, HIV-seropositive man who was diagnosed 5 years ago when he had an outbreak of herpes zoster. He refused antiretroviral therapy and was determined to treat himself using natural teas and herbs. J.R. developed a mild, nonproductive cough that has persisted for the last 4 weeks. He has also had a low-grade fever but denies any chills or pleuritic chest pain. His chest radiograph demonstrates a diffuse, symmetric, interstitial infiltrate. Arterial Pa_{O_2} is 80 mmHg (normal, 80–105). His last CD4+ count approximately 3 months ago was 180 cells/mm^3 (normal, approximately 1,000 cells/mm^3) and his viral load was 60,000 copies/mL. He refused primary PCP prophylaxis. After hypertonic saline nebulization for sputum induction and subsequent bronchoalveolar lavage, examination of the specimens with the modified Giemsa stain revealed both intracystic bodies and extracystic trophozoites. How is the clinical presentation of J.R. consistent with PCP?

The clinical features of PCP in AIDS patients differ from non-AIDS patients in that a more subtle onset, with mild fever, a cough, tachypnea, and dyspnea, is typically seen in HIV-infected patients.[64] J.R.'s low-grade fever and mild, nonproductive cough of 4 weeks' duration are consistent with this description of PCP. His history of HIV infection and the finding of trophozoites on Giemsa stain further support a diagnosis of PCP. The characteristic diffuse interstitial pulmonary infiltrates on J.R.'s chest radiograph are consistent with PCP. Limited data exist with regard to the latent state of *P. carinii* after host infection. Some investigators hypothesize that most persons are asymptomatic unless the host immune system becomes impaired. Others believe that the infection is caused by reinfection as opposed to reactivation.[65]

Antimicrobial Selection

2. A diagnosis of PCP is made and J.R. agrees to be treated. What patient factors are important to consider when selecting an antimicrobial? What would be a reasonable drug for J.R., and how might his course of PCP be monitored?

The treatment of acute PCP is determined by the degree of clinical severity on presentation. The arterial oxygen status on presentation is an important indicator of overall outcome. In one study, surviving patients had a mean Po_2 of 70 mmHg, whereas the mean Po_2 of the nonsurvivors was 55 mmHg.[65] Key factors to consider when initiating therapy for PCP include arterial blood gas findings, whether it is an initial or repeat episode of PCP, the need for parenteral therapy, and a prior history of adverse drug reactions or hypersensitivity. Concomitant therapy must also be considered.

Patients with PCP often can be classified as having mild, moderate, or severe disease, based on their oxygenation. Patients with mild PCP often have a room air alveolar-arterial (A-a) oxygen gradient of <35 or $[Po_2]$ >70 mmHg, patients with moderate or severe disease have a gradient >35 mmHg or $[Po_2]$ >70 mmHg. With the advent of corticosteroid use for moderate to severe cases of PCP (discussed later), it is useful to calculate the (A-a) gradient and/or $[Po_2]$. The A-a gradient (normal range, 5–15 mmHg) can be calculated as $Pio_2 - (1.25 \times Pco_2) - Po_2$, where Pio_2 is the partial pressure of oxygen (150 mmHg in room air), and Pco_2 and Po_2 are arterial levels of CO_2 and O_2, respectively, expressed in mmHg.[66]

Several other clinical tests have been used to identify and monitor PCP. The lactate dehydrogenase (LDH) concentration in serum or bronchoalveolar lavage fluid has been used to diagnose and monitor therapy and to predict outcome of PCP. However, many patients have overlapping diseases, preventing LDH from being used alone. Chest radiographs also are variable. The most common picture is one of bilateral diffuse interstitial pneumonitis, but atypical patterns, such as pleural effusion, cavities, pneumatoceles, and nodules, may occur as well. A normal chest radiograph is associated with a better clinical outcome.

The natural course of PCP among untreated HIV-infected patients is progressive dyspnea and hypoxemia. The increased experience with treatment of PCP in AIDS patients (compared with non–HIV-infected patients) indicates that a longer duration of therapy is needed.[62] Despite the greater appreciation of PCP in AIDS patients, some patients may not respond to therapy; many experience worsening hypoxemia during the first 3 to 5 days after treatment is initiated. This period of clinical worsening is least tolerated by those patients with moderate to severe PCP (Po_2 <70 mmHg). In sicker patients, this period may lead to respiratory failure and the need for intubation with continued critical care. Although many would associate the need for intensive care unit admission as a poor prognostic factor, many patients do well despite the need for mechanical ventilation and IV antibiotics. In light of the role of corticosteroids, patients with PCP and respiratory failure may be viewed as manageable if treated aggressively (Table 70-4).

Trimethoprim-Sulfamethoxazole

The decision to hospitalize a patient is based on the severity of his or her illness. Patients who present with mild PCP with reasonable oxygenation and without evidence of clinical deterioration can be managed as outpatients. Patients with reasonably good gas exchange (i.e., Po_2 >70 mmHg), but with signs of clinical deterioration, most often are admitted to the hospital and given oxygen by nasal cannula and are usually started on IV TMP-SMX (15–20 mg/kg/day TMP, 75–100 mg/kg/day SMX) for 21 days. The dosing of IV TMP-SMX must be modified in patients with renal dysfunction. TMP reversibly inhibits dihydrofolate reductase, and sulfamethoxazole competes with para-aminobenzoic acid in the production of dihydrofolate, synergistically blocking thymidine biosynthesis. TMP-SMX is always the first choice for the treatment of PCP unless the patient has a history of life-threatening intolerance. In the treatment of PCP, TMP-SMX is either as effective as, or superior to, all alternative agents. A good response may be expected in >70% of patients receiving TMP-SMX.

TMP-SMX is often prescribed because of its availability as an oral formulation. Tablets are >90% bioavailable. The usual dose is 15 mg/kg (dosed by the TMP component) Q 8 hours for 21 days. Because one double-strength tablet of TMP-SMX contains 160 mg TMP plus 800 mg SMX, a standard regimen is two double-strength tablets three times per day (or Q 8 hours). Taking two double-strength tablets Q 6 hours (eight double-strength tablets per day) does not improve efficacy and causes increased toxicity (gastrointestinal [GI] intolerance, nausea, vomiting, anorexia, and abdominal pain).

Although the TMP-SMX regimen is very efficacious, 25% to 50% of patients may be intolerant. Adverse effects include an erythematous, maculopapular, morbilliform rash and, less commonly, severe urticaria, exfoliative dermatitis, and Stevens-Johnson syndrome. GI intolerance (nausea, vomiting, abdominal pain) is common. Hematologic side effects may include leukopenia, anemia, and/or thrombocytopenia. Neurologic toxicities and hepatitis also may occur. The role of excessive doses, plasma concentration monitoring, and metabolic capability (i.e., rapid or slow acetylation of SMX) in the development of hypersensitivity reactions remains unclear and is under investigation.[67,68] Most patients who develop a mild hypersensitivity (skin rash) reaction can be managed with antipruritics or antihistamines without discontinuation of TMP-SMX. In some patients with mild hypersensitivity reactions, the agent can be restarted after the rash has resolved, using gradual dosage escalation or rapid oral desensitization to reduce adverse effects (Table 70-5).[69] Patients with severe adverse reactions should be switched to another agent rather than being rechallenged with this drug.

Because J.R. seems to have a mild to moderate case of PCP (Po_2, 80 mmHg), has not previously experienced an episode of PCP, and has no history of adverse effects to TMP-SMX, an outpatient course of TMP-SMX would be reasonable.

Alternatives to Trimethoprim-Sulfamethoxazole

3. J.R. experienced exfoliative dermatitis on day 7 of TMP-SMX treatment. What other drugs could be prescribed to treat his PCP?

Because J.R. presents with a significant adverse effect to TMP-SMX, it should be discontinued and he should not be rechallenged or desensitized. Instead, he should be treated with an alternative regimen (Table 70-4).[70]

Table 70-4 Treatment of *Pneumocystis jiroveci* Pneumonia

Regimen	Dose	Route	Adverse Effects/Comments
Approved			
TMP-SMX	15–20 mg/kg TMP (75–100 mg/kg SMX) daily administered IV or PO Q 6–8 hr or 2 DS tabs BID	IV, PO	Hypersensitivity, rash, fever, neutropenia ↑LFTs, nephrotoxicity (15 mg/kg/day preferred to 20 mg/kg/day because of reduced toxicity)
Pentamidine isethionate	4 mg/kg IV daily over 60–90 min ×21 days	IV	Pancreatitis, hypotension, hypoglycemia, hyperglycemia, nephrotoxicity
Trimetrexate + leucovorin	45 mg/m² IV/day ×21 days 20 mg/m² PO or IV Q 6 hr ×24 days	IV PO/IV	Hematologic, GI, CNS, rash
Atovaquone[a]	750 mg BID with meals ×21 days (suspension)	PO	Headache, nausea, diarrhea, rash, fever, ↑LFTs
TMP[a] + dapsone	15 mg/kg/day	PO	Pruritus, GI intolerance, bone marrow suppression
	100 mg/day ×21 days	PO	Methemoglobinemia, hemolytic anemia (contraindicated in G6PD deficiency)
Clindamycin + primaquine	600 mg IV Q 8 hr or 300–450 mg PO Q 6 hr	PO or IV	Rash, diarrhea
	15–30 mg (base) daily ×21 days	PO	Methemoglobinemia, hemolytic anemia (contraindicated in G6PD deficiency)
Prednisone	Within 72 hr of anti-*Pneumocystis* therapy 40 mg Q 12 hr ×5 days, then 40 mg QD ×5 days then 20 mg/day ×11 days	PO	Initiation in patients with moderately severe or severe disease Po_2 <70 mmHg or A-a gradient >35 mmHg

[a]Used only in mild to moderate PCP.
A-a, alveolar-arterial; BID, twice a day; CNS, central nervous system; DS, double strength; GI, gastrointestinal; G6PD, glucose-6 phosphate dehydrogenase; IV, intravenous; PCP, *Pneumocystis jiroveci* pneumonia; PO, oral; QD, daily; LFTs, liver function tests; TMP-SMX, trimethoprim-sulfamethoxazole.

IV pentamidine isethionate can be used to treat acute PCP. The mechanism of action against the organism is unknown, but may be related to interference with oxidative phosphorylation, inhibition of nucleic acid biosynthesis, or interference with dihydrofolate reductase. Pentamidine generally is more toxic than TMP-SMX.[70,71] In a 5-year review of 106 courses of IV pentamidine, 76 (72%) had adverse reactions (nephrotoxicity, dysglycemia, hepatotoxicity, hyperkalemia, and hyperamylasemia). Drug discontinuation occurred in 31 (18%) of the severe cases. Nephrotoxicity and hypoglycemia were the most common causes of drug discontinuation. Nephrotoxicity occurred in 25% to 50% of the patients and was associated with dehydration and concurrent use of nephrotoxic drugs. Hypoglycemia was noted in 5% to 10% of patients after 5 to 7 days of treatment, or several days after discontinuation of treatment. Hyperglycemia is a consequence of decreased β-cells and results in diabetes mellitus in 2% to 9% of patients. Other less common adverse effects and toxicities include thrombocytopenia, orthostatic hypotension, ventricular tachycardia, leukopenia, nausea, vomiting, abdominal pain, and anorexia.[71]

Patients receiving IV pentamidine should be monitored closely, and serum concentrations of glucose, potassium, blood urea nitrogen (BUN), and creatinine should be obtained daily or every other day during treatment. Other tests for periodic monitoring include a complete blood count (CBC), LFTs, amylase, lipase, and calcium.[71] Renal toxicity often responds to a reduction in the dosage of pentamidine to 3 mg/kg/day or 4 mg/kg Q 48 hours (creatinine clearance <10 mL/min); however, the drug should be discontinued in patients who develop signs and symptoms of pancreatitis. Risk factors for pentamidine-induced pancreatitis include prior episodes of pancreatitis and concurrent therapy with other drugs known to cause pancreatitis. The prior use of didanosine or stavudine may be a risk factor for pancreatitis during pentamidine therapy.[72]

The daily pentamidine dose of 4 mg/kg is based on clinical tolerance rather than target plasma concentrations. The exact mechanisms for elimination of pentamidine are not well understood. The drug is not excreted by renal mechanisms, and no metabolites have been identified.[73] The half-life of pentamidine is prolonged with multiple dosing and may increase up to 12 days after the last dose.[73] Nebulized pentamidine should not be considered as an alternative to IV pentamidine.

Trimetrexate (Neutrexin), a lipid-soluble derivative of methotrexate, is a highly potent inhibitor of dihydrofolate reductase. It was first studied as salvage therapy in patients failing to respond to available drugs. The ability of trimetrexate to enhance survival in these often-fatal situations gave hope to the future of this treatment. However, results of subsequent studies have not been as promising. Nonetheless, trimetrexate has been approved for patients with moderately severe and severe cases of PCP who are intolerant or unresponsive to

Table 70-5 TMP-SMX Desensitization Schedule

Time		
Hours: Rapid TMP-SMX Desensitization Schedule[a]		
0	0.004/0.02 mg	1:100,000 (5 mL)
1	0.04/0.2 mg	1:1,000 (5 mL)
2	0.4/2.0 mg	1:100 (5 mL)
3	4/20 mg	1:10 (5 mL)
4	40/200 mg	5 mL
5	160/800 mg	Tablet
Days: Eight-day TMP-SMX Desensitization Schedule (QID)[b,c]		
1		1:1,000,000
2		1:100,000
3		1:10,000
4		1:1,000
5		1:100
6		1:10
7		1:1
8		Standard suspension 1 mL
9		1 DS tablet/day

[a] Serial 10-fold dilutions were given hourly over a 4-hour period.
[b] TMP-SMX given four times daily for 7 days in doses of 1, 2, 4, and 8 mL in accordance with dilution schedule.
[c] 40 mg/TMP, 200 mg SMX/5 mL.
DS, double strength; QID, four times a day; SMX, sulfamethoxazole; TMP, trimethoprim.
Adapted from references 69 and 250.

TMP-SMX.[74] Most clinicians reserve trimetrexate for hospitalized patients intolerant of both TMP-SMX and IV pentamidine. Recently, however, trimetrexate is no longer readily available for routine use in patients. Serious complications associated with trimetrexate administration include bone marrow suppression, oral or GI ulcerations, renal dysfunction, and hepatotoxicity. Patients receiving trimetrexate should be monitored for myelosuppression with daily CBCs and platelet counts. They should also be given leucovorin (80 mg/m^2 daily) to counteract trimetrexate-associated leukopenias. Leucovorin should be continued for 3 to 5 days after completion of trimetrexate therapy (45 mg/m^2 IV once daily over 60–90 minutes for 21 days).[74] Comparative studies with TMP-SMX demonstrate faster resolution of the A-a oxygen gradient and overall superiority of TMP-SMX.[74,75]

Atovaquone (Mepron) suspension, 750 mg BID, is available for treatment of mild to moderate PCP.[75–80] Atovaquone interrupts protozoan pyrimidine synthesis and demonstrates activity against *P. carinii* and *Toxoplasma gondii* in animal models. Thus, this compound may benefit patients with more than one OI. Atovaquone is approved by the U.S. Food and Drug Administration (FDA) for the treatment of mild to moderate PCP in patients intolerant of TMP-SMX. Atovaquone is also an alternative for primary and secondary prophylaxis for both PCP and toxoplasmosis.[48] Atovaquone is well tolerated compared with other PCP therapies. Adverse effects include rash, fever, elevated LFTs, and emesis. A comparative study with oral TMP-SMX in patients with mild to moderate PCP demonstrated fewer side effects with atovaquone but greater efficacy with TMP-SMX.[78] When compared with IV pentamidine in the treatment of mild to moderate PCP, atovaquone and pentamidine were equally efficacious, but significantly more toxicities occurred with pentamidine.[79] Most atovaquone studies were performed using the moderately absorbed oral tablets; reformulation of this drug as a suspension has improved bioavailability by at least 30%. Concomitant administration of fatty foods with atovaquone doubles the absorption.

An oral regimen of dapsone plus TMP is another alternative to TMP-SMX. Dapsone- TMP can be used to treat mild to moderate PCP in patients intolerant of TMP-SMX. Dapsone is a sulfone antimicrobial that is used for leprosy. Although monotherapy (200 mg/day) with dapsone is ineffective for the treatment (not prophylaxis) of PCP, the addition of TMP (20 mg/kg/day) to dapsone (100 mg/day) is an effective alternative regimen.[75,81,82] In a small comparative trial of TMP-dapsone versus TMP-SMX, response rates of 93% and 90% were observed, respectively.[83] When dapsone is coadministered with TMP, the resulting plasma concentrations for both drugs are higher than when either drug is taken alone. In combination with TMP, a pyrimidine, synergistic inhibition of folic acid synthesis occurs.[84] Dapsone-TMP should not be used in sulfonamide-allergic patients with a history of type I hypersensitivity reaction, toxic epidermal necrolysis, or Stevens-Johnson syndrome. Dapsone is associated with hematologic toxicities, including hemolytic anemia, methemoglobinemia, neutropenia, and thrombocytopenia. Patients with glucose-6-phosphate dehydrogenase (G6PD) deficiency cannot detoxify hydrogen peroxide[85] and are at an increased risk for hematologic toxicity from dapsone.

Clindamycin-primaquine has activity in animal models against *P. carinii.* A few trials with small sample sizes have reported success rates of 70% to 100% with clindamycin (600 mg IV Q 6 hours or 600 mg orally TID) given in conjunction with 30 mg/day of primaquine base. Although skin rashes are common with this combination, they often subside with continued therapy. Some patients experience toxicities (fever, rash, granulocytopenia, and methemoglobinemia) requiring discontinuation.[75,83,85] As with dapsone, before starting primaquine, patients should be screened for G6PD deficiency. Patients who test positive for G6PD deficiency are at risk for developing hemolytic anemia.[85]

A double-blind efficacy and toxicity study of 181 patients with mild to moderate PCP compared three oral drug regimens: TMP-SMX versus dapsone-TMP versus clindamycin-primaquine. The doses of TMP-SMX and dapsone-TMP were weight based, and the dosage of clindamycin-primaquine was 600 mg clindamycin TID and primaquine 30 mg/day. All patients with moderately severe PCP (A-a oxygen gradient >45) were treated with prednisone (40 mg BID for 5 days, then once daily for 3 weeks). The three groups differed in toxicities. Rash was the most frequent dose-limiting toxicity: TMP-SMX, 19%; dapsone-TMP, 10%; clindamycin-primaquine, 21% ($p = 0.2$). Hematologic toxicities were observed more frequently in the clindamycin-primaquine arm. Elevated LFTs (five times above baseline) were more frequent in the TMP-SMX arm ($p = 0.003$). The clindamycin-primaquine group demonstrated better quality of life scores at day 7, but by day 21 these differences became less significant.[82] TMP-SMX, dapsone-TMP, and clindamycin-primaquine demonstrated equal efficacy in patients with mild to moderate PCP.

J.R. should be hospitalized to better manage his severe adverse reaction and to complete his treatment of PCP. Because of his severe reaction to TMP-SMX, dapsone-TMP will not be administered because dapsone is a sulfone with a high risk of cross-reaction in patients who present with severe sulfa allergies. IV pentamidine is an option for J.R., but is associated with an extensive adverse effect profile and should be reserved for patients with a more severe PCP presentation. Trimetrexate is used as a parenteral alternative to treat severe PCP in patients who are intolerant of or not responsive to TMP-SMX and IV pentamidine. Although it may be better tolerated, it is not as potent as TMP-SMX or IV pentamidine and is not readily available. Atovaquone is a reasonable option for patients with mild PCP who are intolerant to TMP-SMX and have no evidence of GI dysfunction, but it is not as effective as TMP-SMX or IV pentamidine. Clindamycin-primaquine is as efficacious as TMP-SMX for the treatment of mild to moderate PCP and can be administered orally. Consequently, it is the drug of choice in this patient.

The decision was made to start J.R. on oral clindamycin-primaquine for his mild to moderate PCP. J.R. tested negative for G6PD deficiency and was treated with clindamycin-primaquine for 14 days, completing a 21-day course of PCP therapy (Table 70-4).

Initiation of Corticosteroids

4. Should J.R. receive corticosteroid therapy with PCP treatment? When should corticosteroids be initiated, and what would be a reasonable regimen for patients with PCP?

Corticosteroids have an important role in the management of patients with acute PCP who are clinically ill and have a low Po_2 (<70 mmHg) or an A-a oxygen gradient >35.[86–89] Many patients who are started on PCP therapy have an acute period of clinical deterioration, which may be associated with an acute inflammatory reaction to the rapid killing of *Pneumocystis* organisms. Particularly among patients with moderate to severe PCP (A-a oxygen gradient >35 mmHg or Po_2 <70 mmHg on room air), the use of prednisone during the first 72 hours of treatment may prevent fatal acute deterioration.[90] Data suggest that corticosteroids may also have some benefit in patients exhibiting acute respiratory failure after 72 hours of conventional PCP therapy.[91] The recommended dosing of prednisone is 40 mg given orally twice daily for 5 days, then 40 mg/day for 5 days, and then 20 mg/day for 11 days, for a total of 21 days. Patients requiring IV corticosteroids may receive methylprednisolone at 75% of the prednisone dose. The impact of this therapy on further immunosuppression has not been clearly defined. The major concern is activation of latent infections (such as TB) or exacerbation of an active undiagnosed condition (especially fungal infections). However, the beneficial role of corticosteroids as adjunctive therapy outweighs the relative risk of short-term steroid use in this population.[92] More common side effects of short-term corticosteroids include ulcerative esophagitis, increased appetite, weight gain, sodium and fluid retention, headache, and elevated LFTs. While corticosteroids are being given, it may be prudent for patients with a history of candidiasis to receive suppressive fluconazole therapy; those with a positive TB skin test should receive suppressive TB therapy. Corticosteroids should be used with caution in the presence of uncontrolled diabetes, active GI bleeding, and uncontrolled hypertension.[93]

Considering his mild hypoxemia (Po_2 >70 mmHg), J.R. is not a candidate for corticosteroid therapy.

Prophylaxis

5. J.R. was hospitalized and responded well to treatment. He now is a candidate for secondary prophylaxis. What secondary prophylaxis would be a good choice for J.R. when he is discharged from the hospital?

The early recognized efficacy of TMP-SMX prophylaxis[50] led to the eventual widespread application of prophylaxis and the development of guidelines for PCP prophylaxis (Tables 70-2 and 70-6).[48,94,95] A clear relationship between the $CD4^+$ count and the occurrence of PCP led researchers to conclude that most of the initial episodes of PCP could be prevented or delayed by instituting primary prophylaxis. Studies that examined HIV-infected patients who were not receiving antiretroviral agents or antimicrobial prophylaxis observed a PCP prevalence of 8.4%, 18.4%, and 33.3% at 6, 12, and 36 months, respectively, in patients with a $CD4^+$ count of <200.[95] These

Table 70-6 Antibiotic Regimens for Prophylaxis of *Pneumocystis jirovecii* Pneumonia

Regimen	Dose	Route
Approved		
TMP-SMX	160 mg TMP + 800 mg SMX daily or 3×/wk (1 DS/day or 1 DS 3×/wk) or 80 mg TMP + 400 mg/day SMX (1 SS/day)	PO
Dapsone	50 mg BID or 100 mg QD	PO
Dapsone plus pyrimethamine plus leucovorin	50 mg/day 50 mg/wk 25 mg/wk	PO PO
Dapsone plus pyrimethamine plus leucovorin	200 mg/wk 75 mg/wk 25 mg/wk	
Aerosolized pentamadine isethionate	300 mg every month	Via Respirgard II nebulizer
Atovaquone	1,500 mg QD	PO

BID, twice a day; DS, double strength; IM, intramuscularly; IV, intravenously; PO, orally; QD, daily; SMX, sulfamethazole; SS, single strength; TMP, trimethoprim.

data have formed the basis on which patients receive PCP prophylaxis. In addition to patients with $CD4^+$ counts of <200, other patients at risk for PCP include those with a $CD4^+$ count of <14%, a history of an AIDS-defining illness, a history of oropharyngeal candidiasis, and possibly those with $CD4^+$ counts of 200 to 250.[48] J.R. refused primary prophylaxis and developed PCP. Because the expected relapse rate without prophylaxis among patients (before the use of protease inhibitors) has been documented to be 66% at 12 months' follow-up, secondary prophylaxis is necessary for J.R. to prevent recurrence.

The same agents and dosing schedules are recommended for primary (before an acute event) and secondary (after an acute event) prophylaxis of PCP.[48,96,97] TMP-SMX, one double-strength tablet daily, is the most efficacious prophylactic regimen; a single-strength tablet daily is less toxic and nearly as efficacious.[98] Anti-*Pneumocystis* prophylaxis (TMP-SMX or dapsone) increases survival by 9 to 12 months, improves quality of life, and decreases hospitalization.[27,31,45,48] Patients with a history of non–life-threatening rash or fever owing to TMP-SMX, such as J.R., may benefit from rechallenge with the original (or half) dose, or a dose-escalation technique (desensitization regimen). Desensitization is preferred over switching to an alternative agent and seems to be more successful than the direct rechallenge method.[99,100] Desensitization involves initiating very low doses of TMP-SMX and gradually increasing to the maximum dose over days to weeks (Table 70-5). In addition, patients who develop PCP while receiving prophylactic doses of TMP-SMX usually respond to full therapeutic doses for acute therapy.

The alternative agents used for prophylaxis include dapsone alone, dapsone plus pyrimethamine (with leucovorin), atovaquone suspension, and aerosolized pentamidine administered by the Respirgard II nebulizer (Tables 70-2 and 70-6). TMP-SMX confers additional protection against toxoplasmosis and certain bacterial infections. Regimens containing dapsone plus pyrimethamine or atovaquone with or without pyrimethamine also protect against toxoplasmosis.[48,70,86,96,97] Investigational prophylaxis agents with unproven efficacy include oral clindamycin-primaquine, intermittently administered IV pentamidine, oral pyrimethamine-sulfadiazine, IV trimetrexate, and aerosolized pentamidine administered by other nebulizing devices.[48] TMP-SMX is more efficacious than dapsone or aerosolized pentamidine in the prevention of PCP.[101]

Extrapulmonary (e.g., lymph nodes, spleen, liver, bone marrow, adrenal gland, GI tract) *P. carinii* has been noted in patients receiving inhaled pentamidine prophylaxis,[102,103] a finding rarely observed with IV administration. In addition, aerosolized pentamidine alters the usual chest radiograph findings associated with PCP, complicating the diagnosis of this disease. Upper lobe infiltrates, cystic lesions, pneumothoraces, cavitary lesions with nodular infiltrates, and pleural effusions have been associated with aerosolized pentamidine prophylaxis. Pentamidine prophylaxis is more expensive than TMP-SMX or dapsone but less expensive than atovaquone suspension.

The guidelines for primary prophylaxis indicate that it may be possible to discontinue prophylactic antimicrobial therapy when $CD4^+$ counts rise above the threshold associated with risk for infection (i.e., <200 for PCP).[48,49,52,56–58,104] Reports from three observational studies, one randomized trial, and a combined analysis of eight prospectively followed European cohorts support discontinuing secondary PCP prophylaxis in patients whose $CD4^+$ counts have increased to >200 for ≥3 months.[104–108] The guidelines recommend that prophylaxis be reintroduced if the $CD4^+$ count decreases to <200, or if PCP recurs at a $CD4^+$ count of >200.[49]

J.R. responded well to his PCP treatment with clindamycin-primaquine in the hospital. However, because this regimen is unproven for secondary prophylaxis, it cannot be recommended. Considering his intolerance to TMP-SMX, the best selections would be dapsone (with or without pyrimethamine) or atovaquone suspension.

Children

The prophylaxis of PCP in children needs further clinical research. The $CD4^+$ threshold of 200 is unreliable in infants because they have higher normal values for lymphocyte counts. The current guidelines recommend administering primary PCP prophylaxis to (a) HIV-infected or HIV-indeterminate children born to HIV-infected mothers aged 1 to 12 months (prophylaxis should be discontinued for children subsequently determined not to be infected with HIV); (b) HIV-infected children ages 1 to 5 years with a $CD4^+$ count <500 or $CD4^+$ percentage <15%; and (c) HIV-infected children ages 6 to 12 years old with a $CD4^+$ count <200 or $CD4^+$ percentage <15%. One study of HIV-infected children in Zambia demonstrated a beneficial effect of cotrimoxazole on mortality and hospitalizations.[109,110] The recommended regimen is oral TMP-SMX (150/750 mg/m^2/day) twice daily three times a week on consecutive days. Acceptable alternative dosing strategies include a single oral dose given three times a week on consecutive days, or two divided doses daily, or two divided doses three times per week on alternate days. HIV-infected children with a history of PCP should be administered lifelong secondary prophylaxis to prevent recurrence, because the safety of discontinuing secondary prophylaxis among HIV-infected children has not been studied extensively.[48]

Pregnancy

Primary and secondary PCP prophylaxis is recommended for all HIV-infected women who are pregnant. TMP-SMX is the recommended agent, and dapsone is an alternative. Because of the theoretical risk of teratogenicity from drug exposure during the first trimester, withholding prophylaxis until the second trimester may be considered. As an alternative during this time, aerosolized pentamidine is not systemically absorbed and may be administered during the first trimester.[48]

TOXOPLASMA GONDII ENCEPHALITIS

Clinical Presentation

6. W.O. is a 40-year-old man discovered to be HIV positive during admission to a detoxification program for alcohol and heroin dependency. W.O. presented to the AIDS clinic with esophageal candidiasis, a $CD4^+$ count of 60 cells/mm^3 (normal, approximately 1,000 cells/mm^3), a viral load of 150,000 copies/mL, and a *Toxoplasma* immunoglobulin G (IgG) titer of 1:256. W.O. was started on HAART therapy. He remained well until 2 years later, when he presented to the emergency department reporting two seizures in the past 24 hours. His medications at that time included

daily zidovudine (AZT), lamivudine, lopinavir/ritonavir, and inhaled pentamidine 300 mg monthly. His temperature was 100.1°F, and he was observed to have difficulty walking. His CD4+ count is 90 cells/mm^3 (previously 230 cells/mm^3), viral load is 70,000 copies/mL (previously 4,000), and white blood cell (WBC) count is 4,200 cells/L (normal, 3,800–9,800). A magnetic resonance image (MRI) of the head reveals several ring-shaped lesions in the brain stem. *Toxoplasma* encephalitis is presumptively diagnosed. Should W.O. be isolated from other patients and health care workers to prevent the spread of this organism?

T. gondii is a parasitic protozoan that can infect people and is spread by environmental factors, such as the consumption of raw or undercooked meats and contact with cats. Immunocompetent persons infected with *T. gondii* may develop mild symptoms resembling infectious mononucleosis. However, these symptoms are generally transient and associated with minimal problems (except in pregnant women). Recrudescent disease from *T. gondii* is problematic in patients with a suppressed cellular immune system, including those infected with HIV. Any HIV-positive patient infected with *T. gondii* is at risk for developing clinical disease, particularly at CD4+ counts <100, as illustrated by W.O.[111,112] W.O. presents with encephalitis (an inflammation of the brain or brain stem), the most frequent manifestation of *T. gondii* in HIV-positive patients.

All HIV-infected patients should be tested for IgG antibody to *T. gondii* after HIV diagnosis to detect latent infection. In the United States, as many as 70% of healthy adults are seropositive to *Toxoplasma*. The prevalence of *Toxoplasma* encephalitis among HIV-positive patients varies depending on the geographic region. In the United States, only 3% to 10% of AIDS patients actually develop encephalitis. In countries such as France, El Salvador, and Tahiti, where uncooked meat commonly is ingested, seropositivity is >90% by the fourth decade of life. *Toxoplasma* encephalitis may develop in as many as 25% to 50% of AIDS patients in these countries.[111]

The two major routes of transmission of *Toxoplasma* to humans are oral and congenital. W.O. need not be isolated from other patients and health care workers. HIV-infected patients should be advised not to eat raw and undercooked meat (internal temperature of meat should be at least 165–170°F), especially patients who are IgG negative for *T. gondii*. Patients should wash their hands after touching uncooked meats and soil, and fruits and vegetables must be washed before eating. HIV-infected patients should avoid stray cats, keep their cats inside, and change the litter box daily. If no one else is available to change the litter box, patients should wash their hands thoroughly afterward.[48]

Diagnosis

7. Is there sufficient clinical evidence to establish a presumptive diagnosis of *Toxoplasma* encephalitis in W.O.?

The diagnosis of *Toxoplasma* encephalitis usually is presumptive because demonstration of cysts or trophozoites in brain tissue is required for a definitive diagnosis. The clinical signs and symptoms of *Toxoplasma* encephalitis can be either focal (indicating a specific region of the brain that is infected or inflamed) or generalized (indicating diffuse inflammation of the brain). *Toxoplasma* encephalitis usually occurs in patients with CD4+ counts of <100. Serum titers of antibodies against *T. gondii* typically reflect past infection with the organism and unfortunately do not help delineate whether acute infection is present. In addition, cerebrospinal fluid (CSF) polymerase chain reaction (PCR) for *Toxoplasma* is not always a reliable diagnostic tool. Without prophylaxis, 45% of seropositive HIV-infected patients develop encephalitis as a reactivation of a latent infection. Most patients with encephalitis have single or multiple lesions demonstrated on computed tomography (CT) scan or MRI of the head. Brain biopsy is reserved for patients with symptoms of encephalitis who are seronegative and for those who do not respond to presumptive antitoxoplasmosis therapy.[111–113] Because of the nonspecific diagnosis of *Toxoplasma* encephalitis, a high index of suspicion for other causes of encephalitis (e.g., central nervous system [CNS] lymphoma or TB) should be maintained throughout the treatment period for presumed *Toxoplasma* encephalitis.[112] W.O. has overwhelming clinical evidence suggestive of *Toxoplasma* encephalitis. He is HIV positive, has a CD4+ count of <100, a positive *Toxoplasma* titer of 1:256 IgG, and a ring-shaped lesion in the brain stem on MRI. The development of this infection, in addition to the decline in CD4+ T cells and the increase in plasma HIV RNA concentrations, may signal antiretroviral failure. W.O.'s current antiretroviral therapy should be reassessed, including his adherence to the regimen.

Prophylaxis

8. Should W.O. have been receiving prophylactic therapy for *T. gondii*?

Similar to many other OIs associated with HIV, therapy for toxoplasmosis can be categorized into primary prophylaxis, treatment of acute disease, and secondary prophylaxis. Primary prophylaxis is currently recommended in HIV-infected patients with CD4+ counts of <100 who are also IgG positive for *T. gondii* (Table 70-2). Many of the agents used to prevent PCP have activity against *T. gondii* and afford protection: TMP-SMX, dapsone-pyrimethamine, and atovaquone with or without pyrimethamine are effective as primary prophylaxis for *T. gondii*.[48,115–118] The increased use of PCP prophylaxis with these agents has significantly decreased the incidence of *Toxoplasma* encephalitis.[2,31] The double-strength TMP-SMX tablet daily dose is recommended as first-line prophylaxis. Data do not support the use of macrolides or aerosolized pentamidine for *Toxoplasma* prophylaxis. Similarly, data are conflicting regarding the efficacy of pyrimethamine as monotherapy for primary prophylaxis.[119,120]

Primary prophylaxis may be discontinued in patients who have responded to HAART with an increase in the CD4+ counts to >200 for >3 months. Multiple observational studies[121–123] and two randomized trials[124,125] have reported minimal risk in discontinuing *Toxoplasma* encephalitis prophylaxis in these patients. In these studies, median follow-up ranged from 7 to 22 months. Primary prophylaxis should be reinstituted when CD4+ counts drop below 200.

W.O. is currently receiving inhaled pentamidine for PCP prophylaxis. Because of the localized delivery of inhaled pentamidine, this agent has no antitoxoplasmosis activity, so W.O. was at risk for the development of *Toxoplasma* encephalitis. Considering his CD4+ count and IgG seropositivity, he should have received primary prophylaxis for *T. gondii*.

Treatment

Acute Therapy

9. How should W.O.'s presumptive *Toxoplasma* encephalitis be treated?

Approximately 80% of patients with acute *Toxoplasma* encephalitis can be treated successfully with a combination of sulfadiazine 4 g/day in three or four daily divided doses and pyrimethamine as a single 200-mg loading dose, followed by 50 to 75 mg/day as a single daily dose plus leucovorin 10 to 25 mg orally every day.[111,112] Induction therapy should be continued for 6 weeks after resolution of symptoms (a treatment course of approximately 8 weeks) followed by maintenance therapy (secondary prophylaxis). Sulfadiazine toxicity may limit the completion of a full course of therapy in as many as 40% of patients.[126] However, successful desensitization has been documented.[127] W.O.'s clinical and radiologic response should be monitored closely and other diagnoses considered if there is no improvement.

Alternative therapy includes pyrimethamine plus leucovorin with clindamycin 600 to 900 mg IV Q 6 to 8 hours or 300 to 450 mg orally Q 6 hours for at least 6 weeks. One controlled trial compared the efficacy and tolerability of pyrimethamine plus sulfadiazine versus pyrimethamine plus clindamycin. Although both regimens were effective, pyrimethamine-sulfadiazine was found to be superior to pyrimethamine-clindamycin. The risk of progression of *Toxoplasma* encephalitis was higher for patients who received pyrimethamine-clindamycin therapy. Furthermore, the rate of relapse was twice as high in the pyrimethamine-clindamycin group. The rate of side effects was similar with both regimens; however, pyrimethamine-clindamycin led to fewer discontinuations than pyrimethamine-sulfadiazine (11% versus 30%, respectively).[128] Additionally, anticonvulsants should be given to patients with *toxoplasma* encephalitis and a history of seizures and corticosteroids may be warranted for focal lesions and/or edema, but should be used cautiously.

10. W.O. is treated with sulfadiazine-pyrimethamine. What are the limitations to the use of the sulfadiazine component for the treatment of *Toxoplasma* encephalitis?

As with other sulfonamides in HIV patients, rashes commonly occur with sulfadiazine therapy.[126] Similar to TMP-SMX, various desensitization regimens have been recommended[69,127]; however, it may be simpler to use alternative regimens.

Renal function should be monitored throughout therapy.[129–133] Elevated serum creatinine (SrCr) levels, hematuria, or decreased urine output may occur secondary to sulfadiazine-induced crystalluria. The water solubility of sulfadiazine is less than that of other sulfonamides; therefore, hydration (2–3 L/day) is needed to prevent crystalline nephropathy, and aggressive hydration and alkalinization can be used in cases of crystal formation. Although few manufacturers market sulfadiazine, this drug is available from the CDC and from Eon Labs Manufacturing, Inc.[134,135]

11. What toxicities are associated with the pyrimethamine component?

Pyrimethamine can suppress bone marrow function; thus, concomitant therapy with other medications that suppress marrow function (e.g., AZT or ganciclovir) may not be tolerated. Leucovorin (10–25 mg/day) is always given in conjunction with pyrimethamine to maintain bone marrow function, although it may not always be successful. Folic acid (not folinic acid) should be avoided because it can be used for growth by protozoal organisms, potentially antagonizing pyrimethamine-sulfadiazine activity.[136–138] Vitamin preparations containing large quantities of folic acid should be discontinued during therapy for *T. gondii*.

W.O. is not taking any medications that would make him particularly susceptible to the myelosuppressive effects of pyrimethamine and he is not neutropenic. Consequently, he should be given sulfadiazine and pyrimethamine.

Suppressive Therapy (Secondary Prophylaxis)

12. Once W.O. has completed acute therapy for his *Toxoplasma* encephalitis, should he receive suppressive therapy?

Most antiprotozoal agents do not eradicate the cyst form of *T. gondii*. Therefore, patients should be administered lifelong suppressive therapy unless immune reconstitution occurs as a consequence of HAART. The combination of pyrimethamine plus sulfadiazine plus leucovorin is very effective. Pyrimethamine (25–75 mg/day) plus sulfadiazine (500–1,000 mg PO QID) plus leucovorin is significantly more efficacious than taking this combination twice weekly.[139] A commonly used regimen for patients who cannot tolerate sulfa drugs is pyrimethamine plus clindamycin.[140] However, only the combination of pyrimethamine plus sulfadiazine provides protection against PCP as well. Additionally, one retrospective chart review of 35 patients receiving maintenance therapy for *Toxoplasma* encephalitis suggested that sulfadiazine-pyrimethamine was more effective than clindamycin-pyrimethamine or pyrimethamine alone.[141] Low-dose, intermittent pyrimethamine monotherapy has been associated with an unacceptably high rate of mortality.[142] The use of atovaquone with or without pyrimethamine is also effective as prophylaxis for both *toxoplasma* and PCP.

Patients receiving secondary prophylaxis are at low risk for recurrence of *Toxoplasma* encephalitis when they have completed initial therapy for *Toxoplasma* encephalitis, remain asymptomatic, and have a sustained increase in their $CD4^+$ count to >200 after HAART therapy for >6 months. Clinicians may obtain a brain MRI as part of the evaluation to determine whether to discontinue therapy. There are data to support that discontinuation of primary and secondary prophylaxis for toxoplasmosis is safe if patients are receiving effective antiretroviral therapy and their CD4 count has increased to >200 for ≥3 months.[125] Secondary prophylaxis should be reintroduced if the $CD4^+$ count decreases to <200.

Children aged >12 months who qualify for PCP prophylaxis and who are receiving an agent other than TMP-SMX or atovaquone should have serologic testing for *Toxoplasma* antibody. Severely immunosuppressed children who are not receiving TMP-SMX or atovaquone and are found to be seropositive for *Toxoplasma* should receive prophylaxis for both PCP and toxoplasmosis (i.e., dapsone plus pyrimethamine). Children with a history of toxoplasmosis should be given lifelong prophylaxis to prevent recurrence. The safety of discontinuing primary or secondary prophylaxis among HIV-infected children receiving HAART has not been studied extensively.

In pregnancy, TMP-SMX can be administered for prophylaxis against *Toxoplasma* encephalitis as described for PCP. Because of the possible risk associated with pyrimethamine treatment and the low incidence of *Toxoplasma* encephalitis during pregnancy, chemoprophylaxis with pyrimethamine-containing regimens can reasonably be deferred until after pregnancy. In rare cases, HIV-infected pregnant women who have serologic evidence of toxoplasmic infection have transmitted *Toxoplasma* to the fetus in utero. However, there are no specific guidelines for continuing secondary prophylaxis during pregnancy. Pregnant HIV-infected women who have active toxoplasmosis or evidence of a primary toxoplasmic infection should be evaluated and managed in consultation with appropriate specialists. Infants born to women who have serologic evidence of infections with HIV and *Toxoplasma* should be evaluated for congenital toxoplasmosis.

W.O. will be continued on sulfadiazine-pyrimethamine for suppressive therapy for his *Toxoplasma* encephalitis because his CD4+ count has decreased to <100. W.O. is currently receiving aerosolized pentamidine for PCP prophylaxis, but because sulfadiazine-pyrimethamine is also protective against PCP, the aerosolized pentamidine can be discontinued. Clindamycin-pyrimethamine is an inferior option because it does not protect against PCP.[48,140]

Alternative Therapies

13. What treatment options exist for patients who cannot tolerate sulfadiazine and do not wish to undergo desensitization?

Clindamycin can be substituted for sulfadiazine in the acute treatment of toxoplasmosis (900–1,200 mg IV Q 6 hours or 300–450 mg PO Q 6 hours) plus pyrimethamine and leucovorin at standard doses.[140,143–145,146] Monotherapy with atovaquone,[147–151] trimetrexate, and the tetracyclines, doxycycline and minocycline, has been successful.[49]

Combination therapy with pyrimethamine and folinic acid plus azithromycin (1.2–1.5 g/day), clarithromycin (1 g BID), or atovaquone (750 mg PO QID) was relatively successful in noncomparative trials with limited numbers of patients.[111,151,152]

CYTOMEGALOVIRUS DISEASE

Diagnosis

14. P.Z., a 39-year-old man with AIDS, complains of floating spots, light flashes, and difficulty reading road signs when he drives. His most recent BUN was 17 mg/dL (normal, 8–25) and SrCr was 0.8 mg/dL (normal, 0.5–1.7). His CD4+ count was 40 cells/mm³ (normal, approximately 1,000), and his viral load was 80,000 copies/mL 3 months ago. His current weight is 63 kg. P.Z.'s medications include tenofovir, emtricitabine, atazanavir, ritonavir, dapsone (PCP prophylaxis), and azithromycin (MAC prophylaxis). He has a history of hematologic intolerance to AZT and TMP-SMX. His WBC count is 1,200 cells/L (normal, 3,800–9,800) with 63% polymorphonuclear neutrophil leukocytes. P.Z. is known to have a positive CMV IgG antibody titer. Funduscopic examination reveals alternating areas of hemorrhage and scar tissue (a "cottage cheese and ketchup" appearance) in the proximity of the retina in his left eye. What is the likely cause of P.Z.'s visual problems?

[SI units: BUN, 6.07 mmol/L (normal, 2.9–8.9); SrCr, 70.72 mol/L (normal, 44–150); WBC count, 1.2 × 10^{10}/L (normal, 3.8–9.8) with 0.63 polymorphonuclear neutrophil leukocytes]

P.Z. seems to have an inflammation of the retina (retinitis), most likely because of CMV. Many HIV patients have been previously infected with CMV, and reactivation typically occurs when CD4+ counts are <50. Before HAART, the prevalence of CMV disease in HIV patients with a CD4+ count of <50 was 20% to 40%, and the incidence varied between 15 and 20 per 100 patient-years. Since the introduction of HAART, a more than fivefold decrease in the incidence of CMV disease has been reported by several authors.[154] Although CMV can cause colitis, pneumonitis, esophagitis, hepatitis, and neurologic disease, retinitis is the most common manifestation of active infection. CMV retinitis in HIV patients accounts for 75% to 85% of CMV end-organ disease. A recent investigation describing patients with CMV retinitis in the post-HAART era found a diverse demographic group with infection; most of them had received HAART; and as expected they had very low CD4 counts.[155] In addition, characteristics of the disease in this group were similar to those in the pre-HAART era. A panel of physicians with clinical and virologic expertise was convened by the International AIDS Society to review the available data and develop recommendations for treatment and diagnosis of CMV disease.[44] Diagnosis is usually presumptive because biopsy is difficult given the inaccessibility of the retina. Serology is indicative of previous CMV infection but not active disease. Cultures (serum, urine, and/or saliva) may be useful for monitoring therapy, considering that patients frequently have disseminated CMV disease. Patients with positive cultures for CMV, while receiving therapy, may be at a higher risk for relapse.[156] Typically, the diagnosis of CMV retinitis is based on observations made during a dilated retinal examination and indirect ophthalmoscopy, as was done for P.Z. Lesions appear as fluffy, white retinal patches with retinal hemorrhage.

Once CMV retinitis is diagnosed, the patient should be thoroughly examined for extraocular CMV disease. P.Z. will require regular ophthalmologic examinations, along with retinal photographs, for life. As with HIV therapy, CMV DNA quantification in plasma or blood cells by quantitative branched-chain DNA (b-DNA) or PCR may have a role in evaluating treatment efficacy and predicting symptomatic development of CMV disease.[157–159]

Drug Therapy

15. What are the treatment options for CMV retinitis, and which one would be preferred for P.Z.?

Several treatment options exist for CMV retinitis: oral valganciclovir, IV ganciclovir, IV ganiclovir followed by oral valganciclovir, IV foscarnet, IV cidofovir, and ganciclovir intraocular implants with valganciclovir for induction and maintenance therapy. Alternatives include combined IV ganciclovir plus foscarnet, intraocular injections of ganciclovir, foscarnet, cidofovir, or fomivirsen sodium (Vitravene).[44,160–162] The efficacy of combined parenteral ganciclovir and foscarnet is similar to monotherapy, but it is more toxic. This latter therapy should be reserved for patients with refractory disease (Table 70-7).[163]

Intraocular implants and intraocular injections of ganciclovir have similar efficacy in the treatment of CMV retinitis,

Table 70-7 Treatment of Cytomegalovirus Retinitis[a]

	IV Ganciclovir	Valcanciclovir	IV Foscarnet	Combination IV Ganciclovir and IV Foscarnet Sodium	IV Then Oral Ganciclovir	Intraocular Ganciclovir Implant	IV Cidofovir
Dosing regimens	*Induction*: 5 mg/kg Q 12 hr for 14–21 days	*Induction*: 900 mg Q 12 hr for 14–21 days	*Induction*: 90 mg/kg Q 12 hr for 14–21 days	*Prior ganciclovir induction*: both IV foscarnet 90 mg/kg Q 12 hr and IV ganciclovir 5 mg/kg QD for 14–21 days	*Induction*: same as IV ganciclovir	*Surgical*: intraocular implantation of ganciclovir (4.5 mg) implant releasing 1 mg/hr (duration 68 months; then replacement required every 58 months)	*Induction*: 5 mg/kg every wk for 2 wk
	Maintenance: 5 mg/kg QD	*Maintenance*: 900 mg QD	*Maintenance*: 90–120 mg/kg QD; 750–1,000 mL of 0.9% saline or D_5W solution with each dose	*Maintenance*: both IV foscarnet 90–120 mg/kg and IV ganciclovir 5 mg/kg QD	*Maintenance*: 3,000–6,000 mg/day in 3 divided doses with food	*Maintenance*: 5 mg/kg every 2 wk (*Note*: dose reduction to 3 mg/kg for SrCr by 0.3–0.4 mg/dL above baseline; all doses given with probenecid and IV fluid)	
	Refractory disease induction: 7.5 mg/kg Q 12 hr for 14–21 days *Maintenance*: 10 mg/kg QD (*Note*: dosage should be adjusted for creatinine clearance <70 mL/min; see Table 70-8.)	*Alternative regimen*: with ganciclovir intraocular implant 900 mg QD		*Prior foscarnet sodium induction*: both IV ganciclovir 5 mg/kg Q 12 hr and IV foscarnet 90–120 mg/kg QD *Reinduction*: IV ganciclovir 5 mg/kg and IV foscarnet 90 mg/kg Q 12 hr for 14–21 days			
Select adverse effects	Neutropenia, thrombocytopenia, catheter sepsis	Same as ganciclovir	Nephrotoxicity, electrolyte abnormalities, anemia, catheter sepsis, nausea/irritability, genital ulceration	Same as IV ganciclovir and IV foscarnet	Neutropenia, diarrhea/nausea	*Surgical complications*: transient blurred vision, infection, hemorrhage	Nephrotoxicity, neutropenia, probenecid adverse effects (rash, fever, nausea, fatigue), uveitis, alopecia, hypotonia

Important drug interactions	Neutropenia, with AZT, cancer chemotherapy didanosine levels	Same as ganciclovir	Nephrotoxicity with other nephrotoxic drugs (e.g., amphotericin B, aminoglycosides, IV pentamadine)	Same as IV ganciclovir and IV foscarnet	Same as IV ganciclovir		Nephrotoxicity with other nephrotoxic drugs (e.g., amphotericin B, aminoglycosides, IV pentamadine, NSAIDs) Probenecid: Level of most proximal tubular-excreted drugs
Adjunctive therapy	G-CSF/GM-CSF effective for neutropenia	Same as ganciclovir	IV or oral hydration essential; potassium, calcium/magnesium supplements, antiemetics may be required	Same as both IV ganciclovir and IV foscarnet	Same as IV ganciclovir	Systemic anti-CMV therapy recommended (oral ganciclovir, 4,500 mg/day)	Probenecid and IV hydration essential; antiemetics, antihistamine, acetaminophen premedication commonly used for probenecid toxicity
Advantages	Systemic therapy; anti-HSV activity	Increased bioavailability and decreased pill count compared with PO ganciclovir	Systemic therapy; anti-HSV (acyclovir-resistant) activity; anti-HIV activity	Increased efficacy compared with either IV ganciclovir or IV foscarnet alone; improved response for relapsed disease	Systemic therapy; oral administration; fewer catheter/ sepsis complications	Longest time to retinitis progression in treated eye; no IV dosing or catheter required	Systemic therapy; no indwelling catheter required; infrequent dosing
Disadvantage	Hematologic toxicity; requires daily infusions; indwelling catheter	Must have adequate GI absorption; less clinical data than with ganciclovir	Nephrotoxicity; requires daily infusions/indwelling catheter; supplemental hydration required; prolonged infusion time; requires infusion pump or controlled rate infusion device	Same as IV ganciclovir and IV foscarnet; prolonged daily infusion time and impact on quality of life	Faster time to retinitis progression; high pill count; poor oral bioavailability (6%)	Fellow eye and extraocular disease; requires surgery; postintraocular surgical complications	Requires probenecid and IV hydration; probenecid toxicity; nephrotoxicity (may be prolonged)
Monitoring requirement	*Induction therapy*: (a) CBC with WBC differential, platelet count weekly; (b) SrCr weekly	Same as ganciclovir	*Induction therapy*: (a) SrCr twice weekly; (b) serum Ca^{++}, albumin Mg^{--}, phosphates, and K^{+} twice weekly; (c) Hgb and Hct weekly	Same as both IV ganciclovir and IV foscarnet	*Induction therapy*: IV ganciclovir	No specific laboratory monitoring required for implant; if oral ganciclovir therapy is added, follow monitoring guidelines as outlined	Within 48 hr before each induction and maintenance: (a) SrCr quantitation proteinuria; (b) WBC with differential cell count; monitor intraocular pressure and slit-lamp examination at least monthly

(Continued)

Table 70-7 Treatment of Cytomegalovirus Retinitis[a] *(continued)*

	IV Ganciclovir	Valcanciclovir	IV Foscarnet	Combination IV Ganciclovir and IV Foscarnet Sodium	IV Then Oral Ganciclovir	Intraocular Ganciclovir Implant	IV Cidofovir
	Maintenance therapy: (a) CBC with WBC differential, platelet count weekly; (b) SrCr every 24 wk		*Maintenance therapy*: (a) SrCr weekly; (b) serum Ca^{++}, albumin Mg^{--}, phosphates, and K^{+} weekly; (c) Hgb and Hct every 24 wk		*Maintenance therapy*: oral ganciclovir (a) CBC with WBC differential, platelet count every 2 wk; (b) SrCr every 24 wk		
Precautions and contraindications	Moderate to severe thrombocytopenia (platelet counts <25 × 10^{10}/L)	Same as ganciclovir	Concomitant use with other nephrotoxic drugs (e.g., amphotericin B, aminoglycosides, or IV pentamadine) or in patients with preexisting moderate to severe renal insufficiency (SrCr >168 mmol/L or creatinine clearance <50 mL/min)	Same as both IV ganciclovir and IV foscarnet	Use with caution in patients with immediately sight-threatening (zone 1) retinitis	External ocular or nasolacrimal infection; patients with risk of postoperative intraocular infection	Same as IV foscarnet except parameters are baseline SrCr level (>1.5 mg/dL) or creatinine clearance (<55 mL/min), or 2+ proteinuria (after IV fluid); discontinue therapy for 3+ proteinuria, if SrCr level increases by 0.5 mg/dL above baseline, or intraocular pressure decreases by 50% of baseline value

[a] Fomivirsen intravitreal injection: *Induction therapy*: 330 mg (0.05 mL) every other week for 2 doses (days 1 and 15). *Maintenance dose*: 330 mg (0.05 mL) once every 4 weeks (monthly). *Primary adverse effects*: uveitis (ocular inflammation); increased intraocular pressure.

AZT, zidovudine; CBC, complete blood count; CMV, cytomegalovirus; G-CSF, granulocyte colony-stimulating factor; GI, gastrointestinal; GM-CSF, granulocyte-macrophage colony-stimulating factor; Hct, hematocrit; Hgb, hemoglobin; HIV, human immunodeficiency virus; HSV, herpes simplex virus; IV, intravenously; NSAIDs, nonsteroidal anti-inflammatory drugs; PO, orally; QD, daily; SrCr, serum creatinine; WBS, white blood cells.

Adapted from Consensus Statement: International AIDS Society-USA The Treatment of Cytomegalovirus diseases. *Arch Intern Med* 1998;158:957, and product information.

but their benefit is localized and they may lead to an increased risk of contralateral retinitis and extraocular CMV disease. Concomitant systemic anti-CMV therapy is therefore recommended (e.g., oral valganciclovir or IV ganciclovir). Use of ganciclovir intraocular implants with oral valganciclovir has shown to be more effective at preventing relapse of retinitis than IV ganciclovir and likely oral valganciclovir.[164,165] Therefore, many providers prefer this as first-line therapy, although others chose oral valganciclovir as first line. The choice of agents typically depends on drug efficacy, toxicity, stage of disease, and quality-of-life issues.

Ganciclovir

Ganciclovir is an acyclic nucleoside with CMV activity superior to acyclovir.[166,167] Similar to other nucleosides, ganciclovir must be taken into cells and phosphorylated before it can compete with endogenous nucleotides for binding to viral DNA polymerase.[168] Ganciclovir is poorly absorbed orally (bioavailability, approximately 5%–9%) and its disposition is biexponential after IV administration (terminal half-life, approximately 2.5 hours). The total body clearance is highly dependent on glomerular filtration and tubular secretion.[169]

The induction dose of ganciclovir is 5 mg/kg per dose Q 12 hours IV for 14 to 21 days. It is approximately 80% effective in delaying the progression of CMV retinitis.[44,170–172] The dose-limiting toxicity is bone marrow suppression, with neutropenia occurring in approximately 50% of patients. Thrombocytopenia is also observed. Absolute neutrophil counts (ANCs) and platelets should be monitored weekly during ganciclovir therapy. If the ANC falls to <1,000 cells/mm^3 or the platelet count to <50,000/ mm^3, the monitoring frequency should be increased to twice weekly.[44,173] Ganciclovir is available in two other dosage forms, oral capsules and an intraocular implant (Table 70-7).[44,48] Dosage adjustments must be made in patients with renal dysfunction (Table 70-8).

Patients who develop ganciclovir-induced bone marrow suppression can be given granulocyte colony-stimulating factor (G-CSF). Both G-CSF (filgrastim) and granulocyte-macrophage colony-stimulating factor (GM-CSF [sargramostim])[174,175] have been used successfully. Although neither of these agents is FDA approved for this indication, use of the colony-stimulating factors may result in sight-saving or life-prolonging therapy. Because GM-CSF may stimulate HIV replication in macrophage cell lines,[176,177] patients should receive concomitant antiretroviral therapy.

Valganciclovir

Valganciclovir is an oral monovalyl ester prodrug that is rapidly hydrolyzed to ganciclovir. The absolute bioavailability of ganciclovir from valganciclovir is 60%, and a dose of 900 mg results in ganciclovir blood concentrations similar to those obtained with a dose of 5 mg/kg of IV ganciclovir. The effects of oral valganciclovir to those of IV ganciclovir as induction therapy for newly diagnosed CMV retinitis were compared in patients with AIDS.[165] Seventy-seven percent of patients in the IV ganciclovir group and 72% of patients in the valganciclovir group had a satisfactory response to induction therapy. The median times to progression of retinitis were 125 days in the IV ganciclovir group and 160 days in the oral valganciclovir group. The mean values for the area under the curve (AUC) for the ganciclovir dosage interval were similar at both induction doses and maintenance doses. The frequency and severity of adverse events were similar in the two groups. Based on these data, oral valganciclovir is as effective as IV ganciclovir for induction treatment and is convenient and effective for the long-term management of CMV retinitis in patients with AIDS.

Cidofovir

Cidofovir is a nucleotide analog that is phosphorylated intracellularly to an active diphosphate metabolite. It is the most potent of all the available anti-CMV compounds and is active against herpes simplex virus (HSV) and VZV, including the acyclovir-resistant isolates. Cidofovir does not require viral activation. Because nucleotide analogs do not require virally encoded kinases for their activity, they remain a treatment option for patients who have failed to respond to ganciclovir. Cidofovir is poorly absorbed orally (bioavailability, <5%) and has an intracellular half-life of 17 to 65 hours, resulting in once-weekly induction and every-other-week maintenance therapy. This feature substantially enhances the quality of life relative to foscarnet or ganciclovir, which must be administered much more frequently.

Eighty percent of this poorly soluble agent is excreted unchanged in the urine via filtration and tubular secretion. Cidofovir is nephrotoxic; however, administration of probenecid (2 g administered 3 hours before the start of infusion and two 1-g doses administered at 2 and 8 hours after infusion) blocks tubular secretion and reduces nephrotoxicity. Prehydration with 1 L of normal saline is required 1 hour before each dose and, if tolerated, repeated concomitantly with or after the cidofovir infusion. Because nephrotoxicity is the most significant dose-limiting toxicity, other nephrotoxic agents should be discontinued (e.g., nonsteroidal anti-inflammatory drugs, aminoglycosides), and renal function should be carefully monitored throughout therapy (BUN, SrCr, proteinuria) (Table 70-7). Dosage adjustments must accompany deterioration in renal function (Table 70-8).

The CBC should be checked at baseline because neutropenia has been reported in approximately 20% of patients in clinical trials. Hypotony (reduction in intraocular pressure) and uveitis (inflammation of the uveal tract of the eye) have also been reported. Thus, monthly intraocular pressure checks and slit-lamp examinations of the retina are necessary.[44,178,179]

The role of cidofovir remains unclear. It offers the advantage of weekly and biweekly dosing, but its toxicity greatly limits its utility. Cidofovir appears to be as efficacious as foscarnet and ganciclovir in the treatment of CMV retinitis, but no comparative studies have been performed. Finally, the efficacy of cidofovir in the treatment of extraocular CMV (e.g., GI disease, pneumonitis, encephalitis) remains to be established.[44,178,179]

Foscarnet

Foscarnet is a pyrophosphate analog that acts by selectively inhibiting viral DNA polymerases and reverse transcriptase. At doses currently recommended for induction therapy (60 mg/kg Q 8 hours or 90 mg/kg IV Q 12 hours), peak plasma foscarnet concentrations are attained that should inhibit CMV in vitro (Table 70-7).[180] The dose-limiting toxicity of foscarnet is nephrotoxicity, probably because its poor solubility results in crystallization in nephrons.[173,181]

In one prospective randomized trial, patients receiving foscarnet for CMV retinitis survived approximately 4 months

Table 70-8 Dosage Adjustment for Cytomegalovirus Medications

Drug	Normal Dosage	CrCl (mL/min/1.73 m²)	Adjusted Dosage			
Cidofovir	*Induction dose*: 5 mg/kg IV QW × 2	Increase in SrCr of 0.3–0.4 above baseline	3 mg/kg			
	Maintenance dose: 5 mg/kg IV QOWK	Increase in SrCr of 0.5 above baseline or 3+ proteinuria	Discontinue cidofovir			
		Cidofovir is contraindicated in patients with preexisting renal failure: 1. SrCr concentrations >1.5 mg/dL 2. Calculated CrCl of <55 mL/min 3. Urine protein 100 mg/dL (>2+ proteinuria)				
			Induction Dose		Maintenance Dose	
Foscarnet	Induction dose	CrCl (mL/min/kg)	Low Dose	High Dose	Low Dose	High Dose
	IV Q 8 hr to 90 mg/kg	>1.4	60 mg/kg Q 8 hr	90 mg/kg Q 12 hr	90 mg/kg Q 24 hr	120 mg/kg Q 24 hr
	IV Q 12 hr	1.0–1.4	45 mg/kg Q 8 hr	70 mg/kg Q 12 hr	70 mg/kg Q 24 hr	90 mg/kg Q 24 hr
	Maintenance dose: 90–120 mg/kg	0.8–1.0	50 mg/kg Q 12 hr	50 mg/kg Q 12 hr	50 mg/kg Q 24 hr	65 mg/kg Q 24 hr
	IV QD	0.6–0.8	40 mg/kg Q 12 hr	80 mg/kg Q 24 hr	80 mg/kg Q 48 hr	105 mg/kg Q 48 hr
		0.5–0.6	60 mg/kg Q 24 hr	60 mg/kg Q 24 hr	60 mg/kg Q 48 hr	80 mg/kg Q 48 hr
		0.4–0.5	50 mg/kg Q 24 hr	50 mg/kg Q 24 hr	50 mg/kg Q 48 hr	65 mg/kg Q 48 hr
		<0.4	Not recommended		Not recommended	
Ganciclovir	*Oral (maintenance only)*: 1,000 mg PO TID	CrCl (mL/min)	Maintenance dose			
		70	1,000 mg TID			
		50–69	1,500 mg QD or 500 mg TID			
		25–49	1,000 mg QD or 500 mg BID			
		10–24	500 mg QD			
		<10	500 mg TIW after dialysis			
	IV					
	Induction dose: 5 mg/kg Q 12 hr	CrCl (mL/min)	Induction dose		Maintenance dose	
		>70	5 mg/kg Q 12 hr		5 mg/kg Q 24 hr	
	Maintenance dose: 5 mg/kg QD or 6 mg/kg QD × 5 days/wk	50–69	2.5 mg/kg Q 12 hr		2.5 mg/kg Q 24 hr	
		25–49	2.5 mg/kg Q 24 hr		1.25 mg/kg Q 24 hr	
		10–24	1.25 mg/kg Q 24 hr		0.625 mg/kg Q 24 hr	
		<10	1.25 mg/kg 3 × Q wk after hemodialysis		0.625 mg/kg 3 × Q wk after hemodialysis	
Valganciclovir	*Induction dose*: 900 mg PO BID	CrCl (mL/min)	Induction dose		Maintenance dose	
	Maintenance dose: 900 mg PO QD	40–59	450 mg BID		450 mg QDD	
		10–25	450 mg QOD		450 mg BIW	
		Hemodialysis	Not recommended		Not recommended	

BID, twice a day; BIW, twice a week; IV, intravenously; QD, daily; QOW, every other week; QW, weekly; SrCr, serum creatinine; TID, three times a day; TIW, three times a week.
Modified from references 46, 48, and product information.

longer than those receiving ganciclovir.[182] However, foscarnet-treated patients with reduced creatinine clearance (<1.2 mL/min/kg) had a poor survival rate. Whether the improvement was because of the anti-HIV activity of foscarnet or the ability of foscarnet-treated patients to continue receiving AZT (which was not the case with ganciclovir) is unknown and remains controversial.[183,184]

Because P.Z. has a low ANC, the bone marrow suppressive effects of ganciclovir and valganciclovir are of concern. Adjunctive therapy with G-CSF is an option. Because he has good renal function (SrCr of 0.8 mg/dL), foscarnet or cidofovir probably would be preferred.

NEPHROTOXICITY

16. P.Z. will receive foscarnet, 90 mg/kg IV over 2 hours Q 12 hours. How can the risk of nephrotoxicity be minimized?

During foscarnet therapy, adequate hydration is important to prevent nephrotoxicity. To establish diuresis, 750 to 1,000 mL of normal saline or 5% dextrose should be administered before the first infusion of foscarnet. With subsequent infusions, 500 to 1,000 mL should be administered, depending on the foscarnet dose. Careful dosage titration based on P.Z.'s estimated creatinine clearance may also minimize nephrotoxicity (Table 70-8). The SrCr clearance should be measured at least twice weekly and the dosage recalculated if the creatinine clearance changes. CMV infection itself may also cause an acute increase in the SrCr owing to acute interstitial nephritis. Drugs with nephrotoxic potential, such as amphotericin B or aminoglycosides, should be avoided if possible.[181,182]

ADVERSE EFFECTS

17. What toxicities other than nephrotoxicity have been associated with foscarnet therapy?

Hypocalcemia can occur because foscarnet, a pyrophosphate analog, can bind to unbound calcium. Electrolyte complications can be minimized by avoiding high foscarnet plasma concentrations. Therefore, foscarnet should be infused slowly over 1 to 2 hours.[185] Unbound serum calcium and phosphate levels should be monitored twice weekly during induction therapy and weekly during maintenance therapy, ideally when foscarnet is at its highest concentration. Fatal hypocalcemia occurred in an AIDS patient receiving both foscarnet and parenteral pentamidine; thus, coadministration of these drugs should be avoided.[184]

Penile ulceration from foscarnet has been problematic, especially in uncircumcised men. Characterized as a fixed-drug eruption, careful attention to genital hygiene may minimize the potential for penile ulceration. Other adverse events associated with foscarnet include seizures, hypomagnesemia, anemia, nausea, fever, and rash. Twice-weekly albumin, magnesium, and potassium levels are required during induction therapy and then weekly during maintenance therapy. In general, patients tolerate foscarnet more poorly than ganciclovir.[186]

DOSAGE ADJUSTMENTS

18. After 12 days of foscarnet therapy, P.Z.'s SrCr has increased from 0.8 mg/dL to 1.2 mg/dL despite the coadministration of 2 L of normal saline daily. What dosage adjustments should be made for the remainder of the foscarnet treatment?

[SI units: SrCr, 70.72 and 106.08 mol/L, respectively]

Valganciclovir, ganciclovir, foscarnet, and cidofovir are highly dependent on renal elimination, and dosages (or dosing intervals) should be adjusted for even a modest reduction in renal function (Table 70-8). For example, the creatinine clearance threshold for dosage reduction of ganciclovir is 70 mL/1.73 m^2/min; for dosage reduction of foscarnet, it is 1.6 mL/min/kg. In contrast, the renal threshold for acyclovir and many other drugs is a creatinine clearance of <50 mL/min. Therefore, careful monitoring of renal function is important throughout CMV therapy. P.Z.'s estimated creatinine clearance is 1.2 mL/min/kg; therefore, his foscarnet induction dosage should be adjusted to 70 mg/kg IV Q 12 hours (Table 70-8).[44,183]

Ganciclovir-Foscarnet Combination

In a prospective, randomized, controlled trial of patients with persistent or relapsed retinitis, ganciclovir and foscarnet monotherapy were compared with combination low-dose therapy.[163] Mortality and adverse effects were similar in all three groups. However, combination therapy was associated with significantly delayed time to retinitis progression (median 1.3 and 2 months with foscarnet and ganciclovir monotherapy, respectively, versus 4.3 months in the combination arm). However, the overall prolonged daily infusion time (up to 4 hr/day) and adverse effects detracted from quality of life.[163] Consequently, combination therapy should be reserved for more refractory cases of CMV retinitis[187,188] (see Relapse or Refractory Retinitis).

Suppression Therapy

19. P.Z. completes 21 days of foscarnet induction therapy. How can his CMV retinitis be suppressed in the future?

The currently available antiviral agents used to treat CMV disease are not curative. After induction therapy, chronic maintenance therapy is indicated for the remainder of P.Z.'s life, unless immune reconstitution occurs as a result of HAART. Regimens that have been shown to be effective in randomized controlled clinical trials include parenteral or oral ganciclovir, parenteral foscarnet, combined parenteral ganciclovir and foscarnet, parenteral cidofovir, and (for retinitis only) ganciclovir administration via intraocular implant or repetitive intravitreous injections of fomivirsen. Oral valganciclovir is approved for both acute induction and maintenance therapy, but the published clinical data are limited. The current guidelines do not include this as a preferred option for maintenance, but this may change in the future. In uncontrolled case series, repeated intravitreous injections of ganciclovir, foscarnet, and cidofovir have been shown to be effective for prophylaxis of CMV retinitis. However, because this therapy is effective only locally and does not protect the contralateral eye or other organ systems, it is usually combined with oral ganciclovir.

Foscarnet 90 mg/kg Q 12 hours as IV induction for 14 to 21 days is usually followed by IV foscarnet 90 to 120 mg/kg/day as a single daily maintenance dose. The maintenance dose of 120 mg/kg/day is more efficacious, but may be more toxic than the lower maintenance dose.[189,190] Ganciclovir IV induction (5 mg/kg/dose Q 12 hours) may be followed by IV ganciclovir maintenance (5 mg/kg/day 5–7 times per week). Ganciclovir IV induction may also be followed by oral ganciclovir 3,000 to

6,000 mg daily in three divided doses administered with food. Cidofovir, with induction doses of 5 mg/kg IV each week for 2 weeks followed by a maintenance dose of 5 mg/kg IV every 2 weeks, offers a more convenient dosing schedule and negates the need for an indwelling IV catheter (Table 70-7).

Guidelines suggest that discontinuation of prophylaxis may be considered in patients with CMV retinitis who are taking HAART with a sustained (>6 months) increase in the $CD4^+$ count to >100 to 150. These patients must have remained disease free for >30 weeks. The decision to discontinue suppression should be based on the magnitude and duration of the $CD4^+$ increase and viral load suppression, the anatomical location of the retinal lesions, and the degree of vision loss. An ophthalmology consultation is recommended.[48] All patients who have had anti-CMV maintenance therapy discontinued should continue to undergo regular ophthalmologic monitoring for early detection of CMV relapse as well as for immune reconstitution uveitis.

Relapse or Refractory Cytomegalovirus Retinitis

20. After 5 months of maintenance therapy with foscarnet, a routine funduscopic examination reveals retinal CMV disease progression. How should P.Z.'s retinitis be managed at this time?

Most patients with CMV disease eventually relapse.[44,190] For the first relapse, repeat induction therapy followed by maintenance therapy with the same drug is beneficial in most patients. Because P.Z. has tolerated foscarnet therapy thus far, he should receive another course of induction therapy. After reinduction, P.Z. should receive a higher maintenance dosage (120 g/kg/day).[48]

It is important to distinguish between relapse and refractory disease. Relapse, as in the case of P.Z., is defined as recurrence of clinically apparent viral activity and is usually caused by a decline in immune function, insufficient delivery of drug into the eye, or resistant CMV strains. Relapse can be effectively managed by repeat induction therapy of the same drug.[44] If the relapse is due to a resistant virus, the patient may benefit from a change in therapy. Ganciclovir-resistant CMV strains occur by two mechanisms. DNA polymerase mutation at the UL54 gene is observed in approximately 20% of ganciclovir-resistant strains. This mutation usually confers resistance to cidofovir and, to a lesser extent, foscarnet.[44,191,192] Most ganciclovir-resistant CMV strains have UL97 mutations. UL97 mutations are incapable of monophosphorylating ganciclovir. Cidofovir and foscarnet are appropriate alternatives to treat strains with UL97 mutations. Patients who receive extensive ganciclovir treatment (>6–9 months) may present with highly ganciclovir-resistant strains containing UL54 and UL97 mutations.[193] Cidofovir may be considered in most patients who relapse while receiving ganciclovir or foscarnet. Although ganciclovir- and foscarnet-resistant strains of CMV have been reported, their precise role in the clinical failure of these regimens is not known.[194] Because of the different mechanisms of action of ganciclovir and foscarnet, strains resistant to one drug may retain sensitivity to the other.[191,195] Resistant or relapsing CMV retinitis may be treated by administration of local ocular therapy via intravitreal injection of ganciclovir, foscarnet, or fomivirsen. Fomivirsen is a phosphorothioate oligonucleotide that inhibits the replication of the human CMV through an antisense mechanism. Fomivirsen has potent activity against CMV, including strains resistant to ganciclovir, foscarnet, and cidofovir. Fomivirsen demonstrates a 30-fold greater local activity than ganciclovir.[194,196,197] Ganciclovir intraocular implants are also a potential option (see Local Treatment).

Refractory CMV retinitis is defined by disease progression because of ineffective therapy. This phenomenon is observed in two clinical situations: when the disease persists with minimal or no response during induction therapy, and when long-term control is inadequate with maintenance therapy. Refractory CMV disease has been defined in clinical trials as two relapses occurring within 10 weeks despite repeat induction and maintenance therapy. Treatment options for refractory CMV retinitis include reinduction with ganciclovir at higher dosages (7.5 mg/kg/dose Q 12 hours, followed by maintenance doses of 10 mg/kg/day) or reinduction using combination therapy (IV ganciclovir plus foscarnet).[44] Refractory CMV retinitis can be treated with local ocular therapy via intravitreal injection of ganciclovir, foscarnet, or fomivirsen as well as intraocular implants.[194,196,197]

Local Treatment

Intravitreal Injections

21. What is the role of intravitreal injections in CMV retinitis?

Intravitreal administration of ganciclovir or foscarnet through a small-gauge needle is a method of selectively delivering the drug to the site of infection.[44,198–200] Ganciclovir and foscarnet doses of 0.2 to 2 mg and 1.2 to 2 mg, respectively, are administered two or three times per week for active disease, followed by weekly maintenance injections. Intravitreal fomivirsen induction 330 g (0.05 mL) once a week for 2 doses (days 1 and 15) followed by maintenance doses once every 4 weeks also has been used.[197] Potential complications of intravitreal injections include bacterial endophthalmitis, vitreous hemorrhage, and retinal detachment. Ocular inflammation, with iritis and vitreitis, is the most frequently observed adverse experience with fomivirsen (25%); this complication usually responds to topical corticosteroids.[197] Intravitreous therapy is relatively uncommon because intraocular implants are available. Importantly, in contrast with systemic therapy, local instillation of a drug is associated with a higher risk of CMV disease developing in the contralateral eye as well as extraocular sites (Table 70-7).

Intraocular Ganciclovir Implants

22. Is P.Z. a candidate for ganciclovir intraocular implants?

The intraocular implant is a surgically implantable delivery device (Vitrasert implant) capable of delivering ganciclovir into the vitreous humor at a constant rate of approximately 1 g/hr over a period of 5 to 8 months.[160,201–203] The implant delivers a much higher concentration into the vitreous cavity than can be achieved with systemic therapy. Implants may be an acceptable initial choice for newly diagnosed patients or patients with imminently sight-threatening disease. Surgical complications, such as retinal detachments, infections, and hemorrhage, can occur during or after the procedure. To reduce the risk of contralateral retinitis or extraocular CMV disease, patients receiving the intraocular implant should also be given oral ganciclovir (1,000 mg TID) (Table 70-7).[204]

P.Z. should be reinduced with foscarnet therapy and maintained on a higher foscarnet dose. Neither alternating regimens nor intravitreal administration of antiviral agents is appropriate at present.

Oral Ganciclovir

23. What is the role of oral ganciclovir in the treatment of CMV retinitis? Would P.Z. be a candidate for oral ganciclovir (Cytovene) therapy?

Oral ganciclovir is available in the United States for the suppressive treatment of CMV retinitis in AIDS patients. When taken with food, oral ganciclovir at a dosage of 1,000 mg three times a day provides daily drug exposure (e.g., AUC) that is approximately 75% that of IV doses (5 mg/kg). Peak concentrations associated with oral dosing are substantially lower, but trough levels are higher than with IV dosing. The bioavailability of oral ganciclovir is increased by 22% when administered with food. Therefore, patients should be counseled to take all doses with food to maximize their drug exposure.[205] Although oral ganciclovir is a viable alternative to IV ganciclovir as maintenance therapy, the time to relapse may be shorter.[205] As with the IV formulations, neutropenia or anemia occurs in 40% to 60% of patients; however, the risk seems to be lower with oral administration.

An esterified ganciclovir, valganciclovir, is available. This agent yields an AUC approximately equivalent to that associated with the IV administration of ganciclovir. The maintenance dosage is two 450-mg tablets of valganciclovir once daily.

The expense of oral versus parenteral ganciclovir is controversial. Cost comparisons must take into consideration catheter-associated costs as well as the additional cost of catheter-associated complications, such as sepsis. Furthermore, quality-of-life issues may weigh in favor of oral ganciclovir. Oral ganciclovir seems to suppress CMV disease effectively and is a maintenance therapy option for patients with stable, non–sight-threatening disease. The limited bioavailability decreases its efficacy; however, larger dosages (e.g., 4,500 or 6,000 mg/day) seem more efficacious.[44,204–206] However, OI treatment guidelines state that ganciclovir is not recommended for routine use as treatment or maintenance of CMV owing to the superiority of IV ganciclovir and the availability of valganciclovir.[49] Considering his previous history of neutropenia, P.Z. should not receive oral ganciclovir. Furthermore, oral ganciclovir is less effective as maintenance therapy in sight-threatening cases of retinitis, which exists in P.Z.

24. What is the role of oral ganciclovir or valganciclovir for initial CMV prevention?

The role of oral ganciclovir for primary prophylaxis of CMV retinitis has been evaluated in two studies.[207,208] Oral ganciclovir decreased the 1-year incidence of disease by approximately 50% in one study,[207] but did not demonstrate appreciable efficacy in the second investigation.[208] These two studies had important differences in study design that likely explain the disparate results. One cost-effectiveness study estimated that oral ganciclovir prophylaxis would cost >$1.7 million per year of anticipated life expectancy.[209] Valganciclovir has demonstrated a trend in higher mortality in patients using it for CMV primary prevention.[48] These issues, in addition to adverse effects such as neutropenia and anemia, the lack of proven survival benefit in HIV-infected patients, and the risk for ganciclovir-resistant CMV, are concerns that should be addressed when deciding whether to institute prophylaxis in individual patients. Prophylaxis with oral ganciclovir or valganciclovir is not "strongly recommended as standard of care" by the guidelines, but rather is "usually recommended" for patients who are seropositive and have a CD4+ count of <50 (Table 70-2).[44,48]

CRYPTOCOCCOSIS

Clinical Presentation and Prognosis

25. A.S., age 28, is infected with HIV. She weighs 48 kg. Her boyfriend was an IV drug user who died of AIDS 2 years ago. She presents with a fever (103°F) and a 2-week history of "splitting headaches." Laboratory test results include hemoglobin (Hgb), 11.2 g/dL (normal, 12.1–15.3 for females); WBC count, 4,100 cells/mm^3 (normal, 3,800–9,800); platelets, 73,000/L (normal, 150,000–450,000); SrCr, 0.9 mg/dL (normal, 0.5–1.7); glucose, 94 mg/dL (normal, 65–115); and CD4+ count, 92 cells/mm^3. She is highly nonadherent and has not been to the clinic in more than a year, at which time she was prescribed AZT, lamivudine, fosamprenavir, and ritonavir. Physical examination reveals no nuchal rigidity. With the exception of moderate lethargy, her neurologic examination is unremarkable. Her chest radiograph and three sets of blood cultures for bacteria and fungi are negative. A CT scan is nondiagnostic. Lumbar puncture reveals the following CSF findings: glucose, 45 mg/dL (normal, 40–80); protein, 90 mg/dL (normal, 15–45); WBC count, 10 cells/mm^3 (normal, <5); and a cryptococcal antigen titer of 1:2,048. Her intracranial pressure (ICP) is 240 mm H_2O (normal, 80–220). How is A.S.'s clinical presentation typical of a patient with AIDS and cryptococcal meningitis? What is her likely prognosis?

[SI units: Hgb, 112 g/L (normal, 121–153); WBC count, 4.1 × 10^{10}/L (normal, 3.8–9.8); platelets, 73 10^{10}/L (normal, 150–450); SrCr, 79.56 mol/L (normal, 44–150); peripheral glucose, 5.2 mmol/L (normal, 3.6–6.3); CSF glucose, 2.5 mmol/L (normal, 60%–70% of peripheral glucose); CSF protein, 0.9 g/L]

In the pre-HAART era, cryptococcosis developed in approximately 6% to 10% of AIDS patients in the United States, with meningitis being the most common clinical presentation.[210] In the era of HAART and azole prophylaxis, a significant decline in the incidence of cryptococcosis has been observed.[31,210] After HIV encephalopathy and toxoplasmosis, cryptococcosis is the most common CNS infection associated with AIDS.[210] The initial portal of entry is the lungs, where the organism is normally contained by an intact immune system. Cryptococcal disease typically develops in patients with profound defects in cell-mediated immunity (i.e., CD4+ counts <100). Unlike bacterial meningitis, cryptococcal CNS infection has a much more insidious onset; the most common symptoms are fever and headache. Less frequent signs and symptoms include nausea and vomiting, meningismus, photophobia, and altered mental status. Focal neurologic deficits and seizures are observed in <10% of patients. CSF glucose is decreased, whereas CSF proteins are usually elevated. CSF cryptococcal antigen titer and CSF culture are frequently positive. These findings, along with the clinical presentation, form the basis for the diagnosis. The overall outcome is poor, with a mean survival of 5 months. Relapse within 6 months occurs in 50% of patients who do not receive suppressive therapy. Altered mental status at baseline, CSF WBC count of <20 cells/mm^3, high CSF cryptococcal antigen titer (>1:1,000), and an elevated initial CSF opening pressure of >200 mm H_2O have all been associated with a poor prognosis.[210]

A.S.'s $CD4^+$ count is 92. She has a temperature of 103°F and has experienced "splitting headaches" for about a week. Her clinical presentation is typical of an AIDS patient with cryptococcal meningitis. The CSF WBC count of 10 cells/mm^3, high cryptococcal antigen titer, and ICP >200 mm H_2O, suggest a poor prognosis.[211] If left untreated, cryptococcal meningitis is fatal.

Treatment

Amphotericin B

26. How should A.S.'s acute cryptococcal meningitis be managed?

The current treatment recommended for cryptococcal meningitis is amphotericin B, 0.7 mg/kg/day IV, plus flucytosine (100 mg/kg/day) given orally in four divided doses as induction therapy for 14 days. Once the patient is stable (e.g., afebrile, with resolution of symptoms), then consolidation therapy with oral fluconazole 400 mg/day for 8 weeks or until CSF cultures are sterile can be initiated. After consolidation therapy, daily suppressive therapy with fluconazole 200 mg should be continued indefinitely unless immune reconstitution occurs with HAART.[211] Lipid-based formulations of amphotericin B (specifically the liposomal amphotericin, AmBisome) dosed as 4 mg/kg/day has shown to be effective.[210]

Although the aforementioned regimen is highly effective, the ability to rapidly reduce A.S.'s ICP will also significantly improve her clinical course. Removal of 10 to 20 mL of spinal fluid by repeat lumbar puncture is recommended for patients with an ICP >200 mm H_2O (A.S.'s ICP is 240 mm H_2O). Additional interventions to consider to reduce A.S.'s elevated ICP include administration of acetazolamide (a carbonic anhydrase inhibitor that decreases CSF production) and the insertion of an intraventricular shunt.[210,211]

27. What is the evidence for adding flucytosine to amphotericin B in the acute treatment of A.S.? What are the disadvantages of this combination?

Amphotericin B binds to sterols in the fungal cell membrane, resulting in leakage of cytoplasmic contents.[212] Flucytosine is an antimetabolite type of antifungal drug that is activated by deamination within the fungal cells to 5-fluorouracil. It inhibits fungal protein synthesis by replacing uracil with 5-flurouracil in fungal RNA, and it also inhibits thymidylate synthetase via 5-fluorodeoxy-uridine monophosphate, interfering with fungal DNA synthesis. Although in vitro data have demonstrated synergy between amphotericin B and flucytosine, the addition of the latter agent remains controversial, particularly in AIDS patients, because of the potential for bone marrow toxicity.[210,213] Flucytosine, a purine analog, is approximately 10% converted to 5-fluorouracil, an antimetabolite.

A classic prospective study conducted in HIV-negative patients favored the use of the combination.[214] The protocol randomized patients to receive either amphotericin B monotherapy (0.4 mg/kg/day IV for 6 weeks followed by 0.8 mg/kg/day IV every other day for 4 weeks) or amphotericin B plus flucytosine (150 mg/kg/day orally divided Q 6 hours) for 6 weeks. Fewer failures or relapses, more rapid CSF sterilization, and less nephrotoxicity occurred in the combination group, although overall mortality was no different. However, approximately one-fourth of the patients in the combination arm developed leukopenia, thrombocytopenia, or both.

The addition of flucytosine to the therapeutic regimen in HIV-positive patients warrants careful monitoring. In a retrospective review of 89 AIDS patients with cryptococcal meningitis confirmed by CSF culture, no survival difference was noted between those who received amphotericin B monotherapy and those who were treated with the combination.[212] Flucytosine-induced bone marrow suppression, possibly exacerbated by amphotericin B-induced renal dysfunction, resulted in discontinuation of flucytosine in more than half of the patients. Neutropenia, thrombocytopenia, and diarrhea are more common with sustained blood levels >100 mg/dL. However, not all patients with high blood concentrations experienced adverse effects, suggesting variable patient responses. If flucytosine is chosen as adjunctive therapy, renal function and CBCs should be monitored closely. Whether prospective evaluation of flucytosine blood levels to maintain peak levels <100 mg/dL reduces the incidence of toxicity remains unknown. A.S. is at increased risk of granulocytopenia because of her HIV disease and her concomitant myelotoxic AZT therapy.

The comparative trial forming the basis for the current recommendations for treatment of acute cryptococcal meningitis in HIV-positive patients evaluated a higher dose of IV amphotericin B (0.7 mg/kg/day) with or without flucytosine given at a lower dose (25 mg/kg/dose PO Q 6 hours) for 2 weeks.[211] The study evaluated 381 patients with an acute first episode of cryptococcal meningitis. The second part of this trial re-randomized stable or improved patients to either a fluconazole or itraconazole treatment arm for an additional 8 weeks as consolidation therapy. Sixty percent and 51% of patients receiving amphotericin B plus flucytosine, and amphotericin B alone, respectively, had sterile CSF cultures at 2 weeks of therapy. No significant differences were noted between groups in the percentage of patients who were culture negative at 2 weeks. Importantly, the addition of flucytosine to amphotericin B was not associated with a significant increase in drug toxicities at 2 weeks. Fluconazole and itraconazole were similar in efficacy. However, multivariate analysis revealed two factors that were independently associated with a higher rate of CSF sterilization: the addition of flucytosine and the randomization to fluconazole. Consequently, amphotericin with flucytosine is the preferred initial regimen.

INTRATHECAL OR INTRAVENTRICULAR AMPHOTERICIN B

28. Should A.S. also receive intrathecal or intraventricular amphotericin B?

Although amphotericin B does not penetrate readily into CSF, IV therapy for cryptococcal meningitis is adequate in most patients. One small retrospective review of 13 patients with a first episode of cryptococcal meningitis and underlying malignancy favored insertion of an Ommaya reservoir (a device inserted into the ventricle of the brain to enable the repeated injection of drugs into the CSF).[216] However, the number of subjects was small, and complications from using the Ommaya reservoir occurred in 30% of these patients (e.g., chemical ventriculitis, bacterial superinfection, headache, fever, and tinnitus). Considering the lack of clear efficacy and documented complications associated with the direct instillation of amphotericin into CSF, this method of administration should be avoided.

Fluconazole

29. Could A.S. be treated with fluconazole instead of amphotericin B for acute cryptococcal meningitis?

Fluconazole, one of the triazole antifungal agents, inhibits a fungal cytochrome P450 enzyme necessary for the conversion of lanosterol to ergosterol. Without ergosterol, the fungal cell membrane becomes defective and loses its selective permeability properties.[217] Unlike itraconazole, fluconazole is well absorbed orally even in the presence of an elevated gastric pH. Fluconazole has excellent CNS penetration and a good safety profile,[217] but is likely a secondary choice in the initial treatment of cryptococcal meningitis. In a prospective, randomized, multicenter trial, the National Institute of Allergy and Infectious Diseases Mycoses Study Group and the AIDS Clinical Trial Group (ACTG) compared amphotericin B with 200 mg/day of oral fluconazole (after a 400-mg loading dose) for 10 weeks in 194 patients.[218] The dose of amphotericin B (mean dose, 0.4–0.5 mg/kg/day) and the possible addition of flucytosine were left to the discretion of the individual investigators. Although the overall mortality was similar (14% for amphotericin B versus 18% for fluconazole), more fluconazole-treated patients died during the first 2 weeks of treatment (15% versus 8%; $p = 0.25$). Furthermore, the median time to the first negative CSF culture in the successfully treated patients was shorter in the amphotericin B group compared with fluconazole (16 versus 30 days). In a small, prospective, randomized trial of 20 male patients with AIDS, oral fluconazole (400 mg/day) for 10 weeks was compared with IV amphotericin B (0.7 mg/kg/day for 1 week, followed by the same dose thrice weekly for 9 weeks) combined with flucytosine (150 mg/kg/day).[219] There were four deaths in the fluconazole group and none in the amphotericin B group ($p = 0.27$). Eight of the 14 patients in the fluconazole group failed to respond to treatment, whereas none of the amphotericin B patients failed to respond. The mean duration of positive CSF cultures was 41 days in the fluconazole group and 16 days in the amphotericin B group ($p = 0.02$). These results, taken together, have led most clinicians to choose amphotericin, with or without flucytosine, as initial treatment for severe cryptococcal meningitis. Although increased doses of fluconazole have been proposed, it is unknown whether these will result in improved outcomes. High doses of fluconazole are being investigated further for patients in the developing world where use of IV amphotericin may not always be feasible. Considering the severity of her meningitis, A.S. should be treated acutely with amphotericin and not fluconazole.

Itraconazole

30. What is the role of itraconazole (Sporanox) in the treatment of cryptococcal meningitis?

Although CSF penetration of itraconazole is poor, it has been efficacious in an animal model of cryptococcal meningitis.[220] In a small, uncontrolled trial, all symptoms resolved and cultures were negative in 10 of 14 AIDS patients with cryptococcal meningitis. The median survival of these patients exceeded 10.5 months. In another small, controlled trial, 42% (5 of 12) of itraconazole-treated patients (200 mg orally twice daily) responded completely, compared with 100% (10 of 10) of patients who received amphotericin B (0.3 mg/kg/day IV) plus flucytosine (150 mg/kg/day) for 6 weeks ($p = 0.009$).[221] The lack of efficacy may be the result of erratic absorption of itraconazole capsules and poor penetration into the CSF. The suspension and IV formulations of itraconazole offer better bioavailability and thus may result in improved outcomes. In both studies, itraconazole generally was well tolerated, but its role as initial therapy for acute cryptococcal meningitis remains to be clarified.

In a comparative study of amphotericin B plus flucytosine versus amphotericin B alone for 2 weeks, patients were randomized to receive either fluconazole or itraconazole for an additional 8 weeks of consolidation therapy. Itraconazole produced a lower rate of CSF sterilization than fluconazole. The researchers concluded that itraconazole could be used in consolidation therapy of cryptococcal meningitis only for patients who could not tolerate fluconazole.[211] Itraconazole seems to have a limited role in the treatment of cryptococcal meningitis in HIV-positive patients.

Duration of Therapy

31. For how long should treatment continue for A.S.'s cryptococcal meningitis?

Once A.S. completes 2 weeks of acute induction therapy with amphotericin B and flucytosine, she should be switched, if stable, to oral fluconazole 400 mg/day for consolidation therapy. However, itraconazole could be used if A.S. is intolerant to fluconazole. Consolidation should be continued for an additional 8 to 10 weeks, followed by lifelong suppressive therapy with fluconazole 200 mg/day[211] (see Maintenance Therapy).

Maintenance Therapy

32. Should A.S. receive maintenance therapy after successful treatment?

After induction and consolidation treatment of cryptococcal meningitis, A.S. and all AIDS patients should receive maintenance therapy indefinitely, unless immune reconstitution occurs as a result of HAART.[48,210,211] A higher relapse rate and a shorter life expectancy have been observed in patients who did not receive chronic secondary prophylaxis.[215] Fluconazole (200 mg once daily) has emerged as the suppressive treatment of choice. In a randomized, placebo-controlled trial of 61 AIDS patients, four recurrent cases of meningitis developed in the placebo group and none in the fluconazole group ($p = 0.03$).[222] One multicenter, comparative trial randomized patients to receive either weekly amphotericin B 1 mg/kg/day IV or 200 mg/day of fluconazole orally.[223] Of 189 patients enrolled, 18% of the patients in the amphotericin B group relapsed, compared with 2% in the fluconazole group. Serious toxicities were more frequent in the amphotericin B group. Although data are limited, four of five patients maintained on itraconazole (200–400 mg/day) for 3 to 12 months had a three- to sixfold decline in CSF cryptococcal antigen titers. The fifth patient refused repeat lumbar punctures (see previous section on itraconazole). Thus, itraconazole should be used only as an alternative to fluconazole.[211,224]

According to the OI guidelines,[49] adult and adolescent patients are at low risk for recurrence of cryptococcosis when they have completed a course of initial therapy, remain asymptomatic, and have a sustained increase (e.g., >6 months) in their CD4$^+$ counts to >100 to 200 after HAART. This has been evaluated in limited numbers of patients. Nonetheless, discontinuing chronic maintenance therapy among such patients is reasonable. Recurrences may happen, and certain specialists may perform a lumbar puncture to determine if the CSF is culture negative before stopping therapy. Maintenance therapy should be reinitiated if the CD4$^+$ count decreases to 100 to 200.

Primary Prophylaxis

33. What is the role of primary prophylaxis in cryptococcal meningitis?

Primary prophylaxis against cryptococcal disease in HIV-infected patients has been studied in a few clinical trials.[225,226] In one open-label study, fluconazole (100 mg/day) was administered to all patients (329 HIV-infected patients) with CD4$^+$ counts <68. These results were compared with 337 historical controls from the pre-HAART era.[226] Sixteen cases of cryptococcal meningitis occurred in the historical controls (4.8%) compared with only one case in the fluconazole group (0.3%). In a prospective, randomized ACTG study, fluconazole 200 mg/day was compared with clotrimazole troches (10 mg five times a day) for the prevention of fungal infections in 428 patients with advanced HIV disease. After a median follow-up of 35 months, 32 cases of invasive fungal infection were confirmed. Of these, the majority (17 of 32) were cryptococcosis: 2 cases in the fluconazole group and 15 cases in the clotrimazole group. The greatest benefit derived from fluconazole was observed in patient with CD4$^+$ counts of <50.[226] However, no effect on survival was noted.

The risk for fluconazole resistance has been a concern with primary prophylaxis because fluconazole resistance has been reported in HIV-infected patients receiving long-term therapy.[227] In addition to the potential for resistance, other concerns include the lack of survival benefits associated with prophylaxis, the possibility of drug interactions, and cost. In light of these concerns, the CDC currently does not recommend primary prophylaxis for this disease (Table 70-2).[56] Fluconazole in a daily dose of 100 to 200 mg is reasonable for patients with a CD4$^+$ count of <50.

Additional Therapies

34. What other acute therapies have been investigated for cryptococcal meningitis?

The combination of fluconazole plus flucytosine appears to be superior to fluconazole alone. High-dose fluconazole alone (800–1,600 mg/day for up to 6 months) was compared with high-dose fluconazole and flucytosine (150 mg/kg/day for 4 weeks) in 36 AIDS patients.[228] Nine of 12 (75%) patients in the combination group survived and became CSF culture negative, whereas only 7 of 24 (29%) patients on fluconazole monotherapy had similar outcomes. In a dose-escalation trial of high-dose fluconazole with or without flucytosine, a significant increase in efficacy was observed as fluconazole doses were increased. Potentially, combination fluconazole and flucytosine are useful because of the excellent oral bioavailability of both agents, which is particularly important in developing countries. A randomized trial of 58 AIDS patients with cryptococcal meningitis compared fluconazole and flucytosine with fluconazole monotherapy. Thirty patients received fluconazole 200 mg once daily for 2 months and flucytosine 150 mg/kg/day for the first 2 weeks versus 28 patients who received only fluconazole 200 mg once daily for 2 months. Those who survived for 2 months received fluconazole maintenance therapy at a dose of 200 mg three times a week for 4 months. Combination therapy significantly increased the survival rate compared with monotherapy. No serious adverse effects were observed in either group. Fluconazole and short-term flucytosine may be a cost-effective and safe regimen in developing countries.[229] Additionally, higher doses of fluconazole in these settings (1,800–2,000 mg/day) may be the best option for patients due to the limitations of obtaining and administering flucytosine. These doses are under investigation.

MYCOBACTERIUM TUBERCULOSIS

Clinical Presentation

35. C.J., a 45-year-old male prison inmate with AIDS, presents with fever, cough, and occasional night sweats. A tuberculin purified protein derivative (PPD) skin test is negative, but C.J. is assumed to be anergic based on his response to other skin test antigens. Two acid-fast bacilli (AFB) sputum smears are also negative. Chest radiograph reveals hilar adenopathy with a questionable right middle lobe localized infiltrate. No cavitary lesions are seen. Why is infection with *M. tuberculosis* a strong possibility in C.J.? His antiretroviral medications include abacavir, lamivudine, and efavirenz. Three months ago his CD4$^+$ count was 320 cells/mm^3 (normal, approximately 1,000 cells/mm^3) and his viral load was 5,200 copies/mL.

One-third of the global population is infected with *M. tuberculosis,* with 7 to 8 million new cases every year. Mortality is 2 to 3 million people annually, making TB the most common infectious cause of death worldwide.[230] In 2005, of the 1.6 million deaths due to TB, 195,000 were HIV among infected individuals.[231] The incidence of TB in the United States from 1985 to 1992 increased by 20%, approximately 40,000 more cases than expected.[232–234] Factors associated with this resurgence include the HIV epidemic, urban homelessness, drug abuse, and the dismantling of public health TB control resources. At that time, HIV disease was believed to be a major factor contributing to the emergence of multidrug-resistant *M. tuberculosis* (MDRTB). The recognized link between HIV and TB, along with an increase in clinical and public health resources, has subsequently resulted in a decline in the incidence of TB in the United States.[235] Fortunately in 2006, incidence in the United States was 4.6 per 100,000 persons, the lowest reported rate since TB surveillance began.[235] Nevertheless, TB is the leading cause of death in HIV-infected persons worldwide, and pulmonary TB is an AIDS-defining illness. Furthermore, *M. tuberculosis* strains resistant to isoniazid and rifampin, with or without resistance to other agents, have become a major public health concern.[231–237] MDRTB is defined by resistance to both isoniazid and rifampin. More recently the emergence of extensively drug-resistant TB is increasingly becoming a global health concern as identified in South Africa from 2000 to 2004.[235] In 1991 in New York City, 33% of *M. tuberculosis* cases were resistant to at least one drug and 19% were resistant to both isoniazid and rifampin.[238] In 2005, the first year with complete drug-susceptibility data, 124 cases of MDRTB were reported in the United States.[235] These drug-resistant strains have been identified primarily in large urban areas (e.g., New York and Miami), in coastal or border communities, and in institutional settings.[234,236] Nine outbreaks of MDRTB in hospital and prison settings in New York and Florida in 1990 were investigated by the CDC. A high prevalence of HIV infection (range, 20%–100%), a high mortality rate (72%–89%), and a short median duration of survival (range, 4–16 weeks) were common to these outbreaks. MDRTB strains have been transmitted to health care workers and prison staff.[234,236]

A Community Programs for Clinical Research on AIDS survey evaluating MDRTB in eight metropolitan regions in the United States observed drug-resistant isolates among 37% of all HIV-positive patients versus 18% of HIV-negative patients in New York City. In areas outside of New York City, resistance rates were approximately 15% in both groups.[239]

C.J. presents with fever, cough, night sweats, and a right middle lobe infiltrate with hilar adenopathy, consistent with TB. Furthermore, his HIV status in combination with his incarceration increases the probability of *M. tuberculosis* infection, including multidrug-resistant isolates. C.J. will be started with the standard four-drug regimen: isoniazid, rifampin (or rifabutin), pyrazinamide, and ethambutol.[240] (See Chapter 61 for a more comprehensive approach to TB treatment.)

36. Sputum cultures from C.J. document *M. tuberculosis* resistant to both isoniazid and rifampin. Why are the negative tuberculin skin test, negative sputum smears for AFB, and lack of cavitary lesions in C.J. still consistent with *M. tuberculosis* infection?

The clinical presentation of TB is often different in patients with HIV infection. As many as one-half to two-thirds of AIDS patients presenting with TB have evidence of extrapulmonary sites of infection.[230] These extrapulmonary sites include lymph nodes, bone marrow, spleen, liver, CSF, and blood. *M. tuberculosis* was rarely cultured from blood before the AIDS era; however, bacteremia is well documented today.[239] HIV-infected patients with TB infection are also at risk for developing tuberculous meningitis.[241] The chest radiograph in HIV-infected patients may reveal hilar or mediastinal adenopathy or localized infiltrates in the middle or lower lung fields.

In HIV-infected patients, it is unusual to see typical apical infiltrates or cavitations. Furthermore, concomitant PCP may confuse interpretation of chest radiographs. In addition, AFB smears of sputum are negative in approximately 40% of HIV-infected patients despite a positive culture, as in this patient.[242] Finally, anergy is extremely common in HIV disease. Only 10% to 40% of HIV-infected patients with TB have a positive tuberculin skin test. Anergy testing is not generally recommended because of lack of standardization of anergy test reagents, poor reproducibility, and a failure to show efficacy of prophylaxis in anergic patients.[48,243] Thus, definitive diagnosis of TB rests on positive cultures from sputum or other tissue and body fluid specimens.

Treatment

37. How should C.J. be treated?

C.J.'s organism is resistant to both isoniazid and rifampin (by definition, MDRTB). These two agents should be discontinued, and at least two more drugs should be added to his regimen. The organism must be known to be susceptible to at least three agents in the regimen.[236,238] Treatment additions for C.J. may include an aminoglycoside (e.g., streptomycin, kanamycin, amikacin), capreomycin, and a fluoroquinolone (e.g., ofloxacin, ciprofloxacin, levofloxacin).[236,238] C.J.'s physician decided to treat him with pyrazinamide, 20 mg/kg/day orally (maximum dose, 2 g), ethambutol 15 mg/kg/day orally (maximum dose, 2.5 g), amikacin 15 mg/kg/day IV or intramuscularly, and levofloxacin 500 mg orally or IV daily.

The optimal duration of treatment for MDRTB has not been established. The National Jewish Center for Immunology and Respiratory Medicine treats MDRTB for 24 months after sputum cultures become negative. Parenteral medication is continued for 4 to 6 months if toxicity remains manageable (e.g., amikacin ototoxicity, nephrotoxicity).[234,237,238] Intermittent therapy (administered two or three times per week) is allowable as long as it is directly observed.[244] All patients infected with organisms resistant to either isoniazid or rifampin should have their ingestion of antitubercular medications directly observed. Although directly observed drug regimens are labor intensive, overall they are cost effective.[244]

Whenever isoniazid- or rifampin-resistant organisms are isolated, a medical expert should be consulted. Because many patients suffer from adverse events related to their antituberculosis regimens (particularly GI effects), the National Jewish Center recommends that initial therapy begin in the hospital to monitor toxicity.[244] To minimize side effects, this center also initiates therapy with small doses of each agent followed by gradual escalation to the target dose over 3 to 10 days.

In patients with organisms resistant only to isoniazid, suggested regimens include rifampin or rifabutin, pyrazinamide, and ethambutol daily for 14 days then twice weekly for 6 to 9 months, or for 4 months after sputum conversion. If the organism is resistant only to rifampin, suggested regimens include isoniazid, pyrazinamide, and ethambutol plus streptomycin daily for 8 weeks, then isoniazid, pyrazinamide, and streptomycin two or three times per week for 30 weeks. An alternative to this regimen for rifampin resistance includes isoniazid, pyrazinamide, and ethambutol plus streptomycin daily for 2 weeks, then the same regimen two or three times a week for 6 weeks, followed by isoniazid, pyrazinamide, and streptomycin two or three times a week for 30 weeks.

If the organism is sensitive to both isoniazid and rifampin, then the preferred regimen consists of isoniazid, rifampin, pyrazinamide, and ethambutol or streptomycin for 2 months. The third and fourth drugs (pyrazinamide and ethambutol or streptomycin) may be discontinued after 2 months. The dosing regimens for HIV-infected patients and for non–HIV-infected patients are the same. Treatment should continue for 9 months for both non–HIV-infected and HIV-infected patients. If HIV-positive patients demonstrate a slow or suboptimal response, therapy should be prolonged on an individual

Table 70-9 Tuberculosis Treatment Recommendations for Patients Coinfected With HIV and Tuberculosis

Induction	*Maintenance*	*Comments*
Rifampin-based Therapy (no concurrent use of PIs or NNRTIs)		
INH/RIF/PZA/EMB (or SM) daily ×2 months	INH/RIF daily or 2–3×/wk × 18 wk	RIF-containing regimens used with caution with protease inhibitors and NNRTIs
INH/RIF/PZA/EMB (or SM) daily ×2 wk, then 2–3×/wk ×6 wk	INH/RIF 2–3×/wk ×18 wk	HIV status should be assessed at 3-month intervals to determine need for antiretroviral therapy
INH/RIF/PZA/EMB (or SM) 3×/wk ×8 wk	INH/RIF/PZA/EMB (or SM) 3×/wk ×4 months	
Rifampin-based Therapy (concurrent use of PIs or NNRTIs)		
INH/RFB/PZA/EMB daily ×8 wk	INH/RFB daily or 2×/wk ×18 wk	Monitor for RFB toxicity, arthralgias, uveitis, leukopenia
INH/RFB/PZA/EMB daily ×2 wk, then 2×/wk ×6 wk	INH/RFB 2×/wk ×18 wk	Dose modifications of RFB and PIs/NNRTIs when given concurrently (Table 70-10)
• Nucleoside analogs and nucleotides: not contraindicated/ no dosage changes recommended		
Streptomycin-based Therapy (concurrent use of PIs or NNRTIs)		
INH/SM/PZA/EMB daily ×8 wk	INH/SM/PZA 2–3×/wk ×30 wk	SM is contraindicated in pregnant women
INH/SM/PZA/EMB daily ×2 wk, then 2–3×/wk ×6 wk	INH/SM/PZA 2–3×/wk ×30 wk	If SM cannot be continued for 9 months, add EMB and treatment should be extended to 12 months

EMB, ethambutol; INH, isoniazid; NNRTI, non-nucleoside reverse transcriptase inhibitor; PI, protease inhibitor; PZA, pyrazinamide; RFB, rifabutin; RIF, rifampin; SM, streptomycin.
Adapted from *MMWR* 2002:51(RR-8):152, and references 47 and 254.

basis.[231,236] All HIV-infected patients receiving isoniazid are at risk for peripheral neuropathy and should receive pyridoxine (Table 70-9).[237,244]

38. How should C.J.'s response to therapy be monitored?

C.J.'s response to therapy should be monitored by drug efficacy and toxicity. Efficacy may be assessed by the resolution of symptoms. Symptoms usually improve within 4 weeks, and sputum cultures become negative within 3 months. C.J. should be monitored for a decrease in the frequency of his fevers and night sweats, as well as improvement in his cough. Sputum smear and culture should be monitored at least monthly until a negative culture is documented. Chest radiography may be the last parameter to improve.[235,236,240] In some patients, recurrence of symptoms may be caused by nontuberculous complications associated with HIV. This paradoxical reaction is associated with the initiation of antiretroviral therapy[245] and is the consequence of immune reconstitution. Recovery of delayed hypersensitivity occurs with increases in CD4$^+$ counts, resulting in increased reactions to mycobacterial antigens. Continuation of antimycobacterial and antiviral treatment is recommended, and a short course of prednisone may be considered for severe symptoms.[245]

The second monitoring parameter is drug toxicity. Recommended baseline tests include LFTs, SrCr, CBC, and platelet count. Baseline uric acid is required for patients receiving pyrazinamide. Patients receiving ethambutol require baseline visual acuity and red–green color perception assessment. Reassessment should be performed at least once monthly. Laboratory monitoring usually is not recommended unless symptoms suggest toxicity. Isoniazid and, secondarily, rifampin and pyrazinamide are the agents most associated with hepatotoxicity (see Chapter 61). C.J. is not receiving isoniazid or rifampin but is receiving pyrazinamide. Therefore, if transaminase levels increase to higher than five times the upper limits of normal, pyrazinamide should be discontinued and an alternative agent given. When his LFTs return to their normal limits, pyrazinamide can be reintroduced.[240]

Prophylaxis

HIV-Infected Persons: Multidrug-Resistant Tuberculosis

39. An HIV-infected nurse inadvertently entered C.J.'s room without taking adequate precautions and suctioned respiratory secretions. Four weeks later, her tuberculin skin test converted to positive. What prophylactic regimen should be initiated for this nurse?

There is no known prophylactic regimen with proven efficacy against MDRTB,[48,236] but several regimens have been recommended: pyrazinamide (25–30 mg/kg/day) combined with ethambutol (15–25 mg/kg/day); pyrazinamide with ofloxacin (400 mg BID); and pyrazinamide combined with ciprofloxacin (750 mg BID).[236,246] Other fluoroquinolones, such as levofloxacin, are associated with good in vitro activity and may prove beneficial. Considering that C.J. is HIV infected, multidrug prophylaxis should continue for 12 months.[48,246] The choice of drugs must be based on susceptibility tests and consultation with public health authorities (Table 70-2).[48]

HIV-Infected Persons: Drug-Susceptible Tuberculosis

40. K.D., a 26-year-old HIV-infected man, comes in for a routine clinic visit. It is discovered that he is a household contact of a

person known to have active, untreated, drug-susceptible TB. His $CD4^+$ count is 350 cells/mm^3. A tuberculin skin test (5 tuberculin units of PPD) and two other skin test antigens are administered, and he is instructed to return to the clinic in 48 hours. His PPD has been negative in the past, and he has demonstrated delayed hypersensitivity responsiveness. How should the results of K.D.'s skin tests be interpreted, and should he receive prophylaxis considering his known exposure to TB?

The CDC and the American Thoracic Society currently recommend 9 months of isoniazid prophylaxis (300 mg/day PO) plus pyridoxine (50 mg/day PO) for all HIV-infected persons who have at least a 5-mm induration reaction to PPD and no evidence of active TB (negative chest radiograph and no clinical symptoms), unless otherwise contraindicated and regardless of Bacillus Calmette-Guerin (BCG) vaccination status. The administration of BCG vaccine to HIV-infected persons is contraindicated because of the potential to cause disseminated disease.[48] A >5-mm reaction in HIV-infected persons contrasts to a >10-mm cutoff for HIV-negative persons.[48,240] Few isoniazid prophylaxis failures have been reported, although this finding has not been systematically studied. Additional preferred regimens in instances of questionable compliance include isoniazid 900 mg twice weekly plus pyridoxine 50 mg twice weekly for 9 months, both administered under direct observed therapy. A short-course preferred regimen includes rifampin (600 mg/day) plus pyrazinamide (20 mg/kg/day) for 2 months (Table 70-2).[48,247]

An inverse relationship exists between anergy and a $CD4^+$ count of <500.[248] If K.D. proves to be anergic, he should still be given isoniazid prophylaxis, considering his exposure history.[48] All HIV-infected persons, irrespective of age, PPD results, or prior course of chemoprophylaxis, should be given chemoprophylaxis if they are in close contact with persons who have active TB. Prophylaxis also should be considered for anergic, HIV-infected persons who are members of groups known to have a prevalence of TB infection of >10%. In the United States, these groups include IV drug users, prison inmates, residents of homeless shelters, and persons born in Latin American, Asian, or African countries with high rates of TB. The efficacy of primary prophylaxis in this group has been demonstrated.[48,240,244] Before any prophylactic regimen is begun, active TB needs to be ruled out. K.D. should undergo chest radiography and clinical evaluation to rule out active disease. HIV-infected patients who are anergic or have a negative reaction when tested do not require prophylaxis if they are not close contacts of TB-infected patients.[48,240,244] The CDC no longer recommends routine anergy testing, because several studies have demonstrated inconsistent results.[48,249]

HIV-Infected Persons: Protease Inhibitors or Non-Nucleoside Reverse Transcriptase Inhibitors

41. F.C., a 36-year-old HIV-infected woman, diagnosed 6 months ago, was found to have active TB (pulmonary infiltrates on chest radiographs, sputum AFB stain and culture positive, culture pansensitive). She is taking AZT, lamivudine, lopinavir/ritonavir, and fluconazole, and $CD4^+$ count is 300 cells/mm^3. What factors must be considered when selecting TB therapy for F.C.?

The use of protease inhibitors in the treatment of HIV patients coinfected with TB increases the potential for drug interactions with rifamycin derivatives (rifampin, rifabutin). Because the rifamycins are potent inducers of the hepatic cytochrome P450 system (e.g., CYP3A4), they can induce metabolism of the protease inhibitors, resulting in subtherapeutic levels. Conversely, the protease inhibitors elevate rifamycin serum levels by inhibiting their metabolism and increasing toxicities, such as uveitis (inflammation of the uveal tract of the eye; see Chapter 61).

According to recent guidelines, rifampin should not be coadministered with any standard protease inhibitors (boosted or not with ritonavir) and delavirdine.[250] Rifampin may be used with efavirenz and nevirapine; however, optimal doses are not known for all populations and additive hepatotoxicity exists when nevirapine and rifampin are coadministered. When using rifampin with maraviroc or raltegravir an increased dose of maraviroc (600 mg BID) may be used and the recommended dose of raltegravir (400 mg BID); however, there is no reported clinic experience for these regimens. Rifabutin may be used in place of rifampin but should not be used with the saquinavir (without ritonavir) or delavirdine. Rifabutin should be given at 50% of the usual dose (i.e., reduce from 300 to 150 mg/day) with indinavir, nelfinavir, amprenavir, and fosamprenavir. Rifabutin should be used at 25% of the usual dose (i.e., 150 mg every other day or three times a week), with atazanavir, lopinavir/ritonavir, or any ritonavir-boosted protease inhibitor. When rifabutin is administered with indinavir as a single protease inhibitor, the dosage of indinavir should be increased from 800 mg Q 8 hours to 1,000 mg Q 8 hr or given as 800 mg twice daily with ritonavir 100 mg twice daily. Rifabutin should be given with efavirenz at dosages of 450 to 600 mg/day. There are no data on using rifabutin in the HAART setting of efavirenz plus a protease inhibitor. In this situation, rifabutin dosing may need to be decreased. Rifabutin can be used in full doses with nevirapine and etravirine.[250]

The CDC has recommended three treatment options for patients receiving protease inhibitors and non-nucleoside reverse transcriptase inhibitors (NNRTI). If the patient has not yet been started on a protease inhibitor or NNRTI, it may be best to delay therapy and start antituberculosis medication immediately. If the patient is receiving a protease inhibitor or NNRTI, some physicians may decide to discontinue this treatment for the duration of the antituberculosis medication. If the decision is made to continue or initiate protease inhibitor or NNRTI therapy, an antituberculosis regimen must be selected that modifies the doses of rifampin or rifabutin (Table 70-9).[240,251]

There are currently five options for concomitant TB and antiretroviral therapy; the first three are CDC-recommended options. These are initiating therapy with regimens that do not contain a protease inhibitor or an NNRTI (e.g., abacavir, lamivudine [3TC], AZT), using a concomitant protease inhibitor or NNRTI with streptomycin-based therapy with no use of rifamycins, and initiating rifabutin-based therapy with dose adjustments of the concomitant protease inhibitor or NNRTI (Table 70-9).[252] The other two options are not recommended by the CDC. They are using isoniazid, ethambutol, and pyrazinamide for 18 to 24 months[253] with concomitant protease inhibitor or NNRTI therapy, and using efavirenz 800 mg/day (plus two NRTIs) plus rifampin 600 mg/day or 600 mg twice weekly.[254]

Discontinuing the protease inhibitor for F.C. is not an option considering the rapid viral replication and the risk of developing resistant isolates, especially considering that she recently was started on protease inhibitor therapy and is clinically responsive. A reduced dose of rifabutin (150 mg every other day or three times per week) is recommended when coadministered with lopinavir/ritonavir. Considering that F.C. is receiving lopinavir/ritonavir, she will be treated with a rifabutin-based regimen. She will receive isoniazid, rifabutin, pyrazinamide, and ethambutol daily for 8 weeks followed by isoniazid and rifabutin daily or twice weekly for 18 weeks. An alternative regimen could be isoniazid, rifabutin, pyrazinamide, and ethambutol daily for 2 weeks, then two times weekly for 6 weeks, followed by isoniazid and rifabutin, twice weekly for 18 weeks. Considering the lopinavir/ritonavir-associated reduction in metabolism, rifabutin should be administered 150 mg every other day or three weekly (Table 70-10).

Drug Interactions

42. What additional non-antiretroviral–related drug interactions are of concern to patients like F.C. who are taking antituberculosis medications?

Rifampin induces hepatic microsomal enzymes and therefore increases the metabolism of many drugs frequently prescribed for HIV-positive patients. For example, serum concentrations of fluconazole and ketoconazole are decreased by 25% and 80%, respectively,[255,256] and dapsone concentrations are lowered by as much as 90% with concomitant administration of rifampin. Rifampin may induce acute withdrawal when given with methadone. The activity of oral contraceptives and warfarin anticoagulants also may be reduced. Rifampin also lowers serum concentrations of theophylline, anticonvulsants, corticosteroids, sulfonylureas, and digoxin.

F.C. is receiving rifabutin rather than rifampin. Rifabutin also induces hepatic microsomal enzymes, but the effect is less pronounced. Rifabutin reduces the activity of several agents, including warfarin, barbiturates, benzodiazepines, β-adrenergic blockers, chloramphenicol, clofibrate, corticosteroids, cyclosporine, diazepam, digitalis, doxycycline, haloperidol, oral hypoglycemics, ketoconazole, phenytoin, theophylline, quinidine, and verapamil. A significant reduction in activity is observed with oral contraceptives, dapsone, and methadone (Tables 70-10 and 70-11).

Cytochrome P450 system inhibitors, such as certain macrolides, quinolones, and antifungal azoles, prolong the half-life of rifabutin. The macrolides erythromycin and clarithromycin result in a fourfold increase in rifabutin.[48,234] F.C. is concomitantly taking fluconazole; thus, rifabutin serum levels might increase when given with fluconazole, leading to possible uveitis.[233] However, F.C. is currently taking half the usual dose of rifabutin, minimizing the risk for rifabutin-induced uveitis.

MYCOBACTERIUM AVIUM COMPLEX DISEASE

Clinical Presentation

43. M.E., an HIV-infected 38-year-old woman with a history of IV drug use, presents with fevers, drenching night sweats, a poor appetite, and a 20-lb weight loss (>15% of baseline) over the past 4 months. M.E. has refused all antiretroviral therapy for the past year because of drug intolerance. She has a past medical history of recurrent herpes zoster, PCP, and cryptococcal meningitis. Her current medications include one TMP-SMX double-strength tablet once daily and an occasional acyclovir dose when she feels the herpes zoster "is beginning to start"; she refuses MAC prophylaxis therapy. Physical examination reveals a cachectic woman with mild hepatosplenomegaly. Pertinent laboratory test results include hematocrit (Hct), 23% (normal, 36%–44.6%); WBC count, 3,500 cells/L (normal, 3,800–9,800) with 68% neutrophils, 2% bands, 22% lymphocytes, and 8% monocytes; absolute CD4$^+$ count, 25 cells/mm^3; viral load, 200,000 copies/mL; aspartate transferase, 135 IU/L (normal, 0–35); alanine aminotransferase, 95 IU/L (normal, 0 to 35); and alkaline phosphatase, 186 IU/L (normal, 30–120). Skin testing reveals anergy. The chest radiograph is unremarkable. Based on these findings, a presumptive diagnosis of MAC infection is made. Why is M.E.'s clinical presentation consistent with MAC infection?

[SI units: Hct, 0.23; WBC count, 3.5 × 10^{10}/L with 0.68 neutrophils, 0.02 bands, 0.22 lymphocytes, 0.08 monocytes; aspartate aminotransferase, 135 U/L (normal, 0–35); alanine aminotransferase, 95 U/L (normal, 0–35); alkaline phosphatase, 186 U/L (normal, 30–120)]

Disseminated MAC infection is common in end-stage AIDS patients. On autopsy, MAC organisms are observed in the lungs, spleen, colon, adrenals, kidneys, brain, and skin.[257,258] MAC reduces survival; increased mortality is observed in AIDS patients with disseminated MAC, compared with AIDS patients without disseminated MAC.[257] The predominant organism in HIV-positive patients is *M. avium* (97% of typeable isolates) followed by *Mycobacterium intracellulare* (3%).[259] The risk of developing disseminated MAC infection is strongly associated with a CD4$^+$ count of <100; the highest risk is in patients with a CD4$^+$ count <50.[13] Age, gender, and race do not influence the risk of disseminated MAC infection.[48,257] The overall prognosis is poor, with a mean survival of 3 to 7 months. Poor prognostic indicators include prior OI, severe anemia, AZT dose interruption, and low total lymphocyte count.[260]

M. avium is a ubiquitous organism found in food, water, soil, and house dust. The most likely portal of entry is either the GI or respiratory tract. Sputum and stool samples frequently are colonized with MAC, although the significance of this finding remains controversial. Common presenting symptoms associated with MAC infection include fever, night sweats, anorexia, malaise, profound weight loss (>10% body weight), anemia, lymphadenopathy, and diarrhea.[261] M.E.'s fevers, drenching night sweats, poor appetite, 20-lb weight loss, and mild hepatosplenomegaly are consistent with MAC infection. In particular, her CD4$^+$ count of 25 puts her at risk for this OI.

Treatment

Initiation

44. Why is it appropriate to initiate M.E.'s drug therapy before blood culture results have documented the presence of MAC?

Disseminated MAC is best diagnosed by peripheral blood cultures. The finding of AFB on a blood smear is diagnostic, but the results are variable.[261,262] Conventional culture methods using solid media may have a turnaround time of as long as 8 weeks; however, radiometric broth systems signaling the release of C^{15}-labeled CO_2 from mycobacteria may detect

Table 70-10 Recommendations for Coadministering Rifampin and Rifabutin With Non-Nucleoside Reverse Transcriptase Inhibitors and Protease Inhibitors

Antiretroviral	*Use in Combination With Rifabutin*	*Use in Combination With Rifampin*	*Comments*
Saquinavir HGC	Possibly,[a] if regimen also includes ritonavir	No	Coadministration of saquinavir HGC or tablet with rifabutin 150 mg QOD or 3×/wk is recommended but only if ritonavir is used. Coadministration of saquinavir with rifampin is not recommended because of the demonstration of marked elevations in transaminases when saquinavir/ritonavir and rifampin were combined.
Ritonavir	Probably	Possibly	If the combination of ritonavir and rifabutin is used, then a substantially reduced-dose rifabutin regimen (150 mg 2–3×/wk) is recommended. Coadministration of ritonavir with usual-dose rifampin (600 mg QD or 2–3×/wk) is possible; pharmacokinetic data and clinical experience are limited.
Indinavir	Yes	No	There is limited, but favorable, clinical experience with coadministration of indinavir[c] with a reduced daily dose of rifabutin (150 mg) or with the usual dose of rifabutin (300 mg 2–3×/wk) Coadministration of indinavir with rifampin is not recommended because rifampin markedly decreases concentrations of indinavir.
Nelfinavir	Yes	No	There is limited, but favorable, clinical experience with coadministration of nelfinavir[d] with a reduced daily dose of rifabutin (150 mg) or with the usual dose of rifabutin (300 mg 2–3×/wk). Coadministration of nelfinavir with rifampin is not recommended because rifampin markedly decreases concentrations of nelfinavir.
Amprenavir and fosamprenavir	Yes	No	Coadministration of amprenavir or fosamprenavir with a reduced daily dose of rifabutin (150 mg) or with the usual dose of rifabutin (300 mg 2–3/wk) is a possibility, but there is no published clinical experience. Coadministration of amprenavir or fosamprenavir with rifampin is not recommended because rifampin markedly decreases concentrations of amprenavir.
Atazanavir	Yes	No	Coadministration of atazanavir with a reduced dose of rifabutin (150 mg every other day or 3×/wk) is a possibility, but there is no published clinical experience. Coadministration of atazanavir with rifampin is not recommended because rifampin markedly decreases concentrations of atazanavir.
Lopinavir/ritonavir	Yes	No	Coadministration of lopinavir/ritonavir with a reduced dose of rifabutin (150 mg every other day or 3×/wk) is a possibility, but there is no published clinical experience. Coadministration of lopinavir/ritonavir with rifampin is not recommended because rifampin markedly decreases concentrations of atazanavir.
Darunavir/ritonavir	Yes	No	Coadministration of darunavir/ritonavir with a reduced daily dose of rifabutin 150 mg every other day is recommended. Coadministration of darunavir/ritonavir with rifampin is not recommended.
Tipranavir/ritonavir	No	Possibly	Coadministration of tipranavir/ritonavir is not recommended. A single dose of rifabutin with tipranavir/ritonavir showed an increase in rifaubtin concentrations; however, no multidose data are available. No data are available with the coadministration of rifampin with tipranavir/ritonavir.
Nevirapine	Yes	Possibly	Coadministration of nevirapine with usual-dose rifabutin (300 mg QD or 2–3×/wk) is possible based on pharmacokinetic study data. However, there is no published clinical experience for this combination. Data are insufficient to assess whether dose adjustments are necessary when rifampin is coadministered with nevirapine. Therefore, rifampin and nevirapine should be used only in combination if clearly indicated and with careful monitoring. Some studies have demonstrated additive hepatotoxicity.
Delavirdine	No	No	Contraindicated because of the marked decrease in concentrations of delavirdine when administered with either rifabutin or rifampin.
Efavirenz	Probably	Probably[e]	Coadministration of efavirenz with increased doses of rifabutin 450–600 mg QD or 600 mg 3×/wk is recommended.

[a]Despite limited data and clinical experience, the use of this combination is potentially successful.
[b]Based on available data and clinical experience, the successful use of this combination is likely.
[c]Recommended to increase the indinavir dose to 1,000 mg Q 8 hr or boost with ritonavir (800/100 mg BID) when used in combination with rifabutin.
[d]Usual recommended dose is 750 mg TID or 1,250 mg BID. Some experts recommend increasing the nelfinavir dose to 1,000 mg if used TID and in combination with rifabutin.
[e]Usual recommended dose is 600 mg QD. Some experts recommend increasing the efavirenz dose to 800 mg QD if efavirenz is used in combination with rifampin.
QD, daily; QOD; every other dat.
Adopted from *MMWR* 2000;49:23 and U.S. Department of Health and Human Services Guidelines for Use of Antiretroviral Agents in Adults and Adolescents, Oct 10, 2007.

Table 70-11 Drug Interactions With Tuberculosis and *Mycobacterium avium* complex Medications

Affected Drug	*Interacting Drug(s)*	*Mechanism*	*Recommendation*
Atovaquone	Rifampin	Induction of metabolism drug concentrations	Concentrations might not be therapeutic; avoid combination or ↑ atovaquone dose
Clarithromycin	Ritonavir, indinavir	Inhibition of metabolism ↑ drug concentrations by 77% (w/ritonavir) and 53% with indinavir	No adjustments needed in normal renal function; adjust if CrCl is <30 mL/min
Clarithromycin	Nevirapine	Induction of metabolism ↓ in clarithromycin AUC by 35%, ↑ in AUC of 14-OH clarithromycin by 27%	Effect on *M. avium* prophylaxis might be decreased; monitor closely
Clarithromycin	Rifabutin, rifampin	Induction of hepatic metabolism ↓ clarithromycin concentration 50% (w/rifabutin) to 120% (w/rifampin)	Clinical significance of ↓ clarithromycin levels unknown
Ketoconazole, rifampin	Isoniazid	↓ Serum concentration of ketoconazole ↑ Hepatotoxicity	Possible antifungal treatment resistance May consider discontinuing one or both agents if >5× baseline
Quinolones	Didanosine, antacids, iron products, calcium products, sucralfate	Chelation that results in marked ↓ in quinolone drug levels	Administer interacting drug ≥2 hr after quinolone
Rifabutin	Fluconazole	Inhibition of metabolism with significant ↑ in rifabutin drug levels	Monitor for rifabutin, toxicity such as uveitis, nausea, neutropenia
Antifungals, dapsone, methadone, theophylline, oral contraceptives, phenytoin, digoxin, warfarin (all drugs metabolized via CYP450)	Rifampin	Induction of metabolism-significant decrease in drug levels	Monitor drug levels (theophylline, phenytoin, digoxin) Monitor prothrombin time with warfarin Use alternative birth control method
Theophylline, warfarin, digoxin	Ciprofloxacin	Inhibition of metabolism theophylline levels, digoxin levels, anticoagulant effects	Monitor theophylline and digoxin levels and prothrombin time

AUC, area under the curve; CrCl, creatinine clearance; CYP450, cytochrome P450 enzyme system.
Modified from *MMWR* 1999;48(RR-10).

bacterial growth in 7 to 10 days.[261,262] Identification of the organism (*M. tuberculosis* versus atypical mycobacteria) by conventional biochemical methods may take weeks to months. Techniques using DNA probes make diagnosis possible within several hours.[262] Quantitative blood cultures have been useful to monitor the effects of drug therapy, but may not be practical on a routine clinical basis. Radiometric broth methods also may provide in vitro drug susceptibility in another 7 to 10 days. Even with the availability of all of these laboratory tests, results generally are not available for 2 to 3 weeks. In view of this lag time, it is in the patient's best interest to initiate empiric therapy as quickly as possible. Although MAC is typically isolated from blood, the organism can also be demonstrated via acid-fast smears of lymph node, liver, or bone marrow biopsies. Because these organs are rich in monocytes, the target cells for MAC infection, the organism load may be high (up to 10^{11} colony-forming units [CFU]/mL). Granuloma formation or inflammation may be absent because of profound suppression of cell-mediated immunity in end-stage AIDS patients.[262,263]

45. What is the relevance of M.E.'s discontinued antiretroviral therapy to her development of MAC infection?

The incidence of disseminated MAC in AIDS patients residing in the United States before HAART was 30% to 40%. Treatment with protease inhibitors and the widespread use of primary MAC prophylaxis since mid-1996 substantially lowered the incidence of disseminated MAC infection.[262–265] HIV also is known to infect monocytes and macrophages. In in vitro macrophage culture studies, the intracellular growth rate of *M. avium* was greatly enhanced in HIV-infected cells.[266] Conversely, if macrophages taken from HIV-infected patients were infected with *M. avium,* latent HIV virus began to replicate in some of these cultures.[266] Consequently, the two organisms may act synergistically, leading to a hastened deterioration of the host.[261] Because M.E. has discontinued antiretroviral therapy, the resultant increase in viral load has contributed to her development of MAC.

Drug Susceptibility as a Basis for Treatment

46. Should M.E.'s therapy be based on in vitro drug susceptibility results?

Correlation between in vitro drug susceptibility results and clinical efficacy has not been clearly established for MAC.

Numerous reasons may account for this finding. First, results are method dependent; MAC isolates are more sensitive to antibiotics if broth is used rather than agar.[262,267] Second, current in vitro methods are cell free, which does not take into account the intracellular nature of MAC infection. Thus, drugs that have excellent intracellular penetration may be useful clinically, even if in vitro minimum inhibitory concentration (MIC) data suggest otherwise. Conversely, drugs that have favorable MIC data may be ineffective clinically if they do not reach the intracellular environment.[266,267] An in vitro drug susceptibility testing system that incorporates murine macrophages is under development[266,267] and eventually may be a better predictor of clinical outcome. Clinical laboratories in the United States widely use the radiometric broth macrodilution utilizing Bactec Technology.[267,268]

Drug susceptibility studies also may not correlate with clinical efficacy because in vitro results for individually tested drugs may show resistance, but combination therapy may be additive or synergistic.[269] Finally, some antimycobacterial agents exhibit large differences between the MIC and maximum bactericidal concentration. This finding may reflect the difficulty in eradicating this organism, particularly in a severely immunocompromised host. Despite these limitations, many clinicians still use in vitro drug susceptibility data as a guide to therapy. In summary, in vitro tests for susceptibility, although used, may not predict clinical efficacy.

Drug Therapy

47. What drug regimens could be selected to treat M.E.?

The CDC recommends a two- or three-drug MAC regimen, and at least one of these drugs must be a macrolide. Clarithromycin (500 mg PO BID) is the preferred agent; azithromycin is an alternative. Ethambutol (15 to 25 mg/kg/day PO) is recommended as the second agent. Several drugs can be used as the third agent, including rifabutin (300 mg/day), ciprofloxacin (500–750 mg/day), and amikacin (15 mg/kg/day). The choice of the third agent depends on the severity of the illness, drug interactions, hepatic and renal function, patient tolerability, patient compliance, and cost. Amikacin (15 mg/kg/day) has been used in acute MAC therapy, but it is toxic and does not seem to have a role in long-term therapy. Long-term therapy may be discontinued in patients who have completed a course of >12 months of treatment for MAC, remain asymptomatic, and have a sustained increase (e.g., >6 months) in their $CD4^+$ count to >100 after HAART.[48]

In the late 1980s, whether patients with disseminated MAC infection should be treated at all was controversial. The results of early, uncontrolled trials were disappointing, with poor microbiologic response rates, little improvement in clinical symptoms, and a high incidence of adverse drug reactions. Additional clinical trials have been associated with improvement or eradication of MAC bacteremia and improvement in clinical symptoms. These improved results probably can be attributed to earlier diagnosis, longer follow-up, more potent antiretroviral therapy, and the use of anti-MAC agents that penetrate intracellular spaces more effectively.[269]

The macrolides have potent antimycobacterial activity. Several studies have shown clarithromycin to be efficacious against MAC.[270,271] In a small placebo-controlled trial, seven of eight patients who received 2 g/day of clarithromycin monotherapy eradicated *M. avium* from their blood cultures after 4 weeks. In contrast, all five placebo patients showed increases in CFU/mL. In an uncontrolled, monotherapy trial of azithromycin (500 mg/day), patients showed a mean decrease from 2,028 to 136 CFU/mL. Fevers and night sweats resolved in most patients.[272] However, bacteriologic relapse occurred after treatment was discontinued and in 10 patients who elected to continue azithromycin therapy (250 mg/day), suggesting the emergence of resistance. In another investigation, all isolates initially were susceptible to clarithromycin, but after 12 weeks of monotherapy (1–4 g/day), in vitro resistance developed in 16 of 72 (22%) patients.[273]

Because monotherapy can lead to breakthrough bacteremia and resistance, MAC infections should be treated with a combination of at least two agents, including a macrolide plus ethambutol. Although clarithromycin and azithromycin have excellent activity against MAC, clarithromycin is preferred because the emergence of resistance is more likely with azithromycin.[270–272] Both macrolides demonstrate excellent intracellular penetration and have prolonged half-lives.[274–276] GI toxicity (nausea, vomiting, diarrhea, abdominal pain, and anorexia) is the most frequent adverse effect with either agent.[271,272] These effects may be dose related. Data show that patients receiving 4 g/day of clarithromycin are more likely to have their therapy discontinued because of GI upset than patients receiving lower doses.[277] The dosage of clarithromycin is 500 mg orally twice daily, and the dosage of azithromycin is 500 mg/day.

Ethambutol (15–25 mg/kg/day orally) is preferred as the second agent.[278] In a monotherapy study, 800 mg of ethambutol was more effective than either clofazimine or rifampin.[277] One or more of the following drugs can be added to the macrolide/ethambutol combination: rifabutin, rifampin, ciprofloxacin, and clofazimine, with or without amikacin. Isoniazid and pyrazinamide are not effective for the treatment of MAC.[249,266,268]

Although four-drug regimens have been used, one study observed that a three-drug macrolide regimen (clarithromycin, ethambutol, rifabutin) was more effective than a four-drug regimen (ciprofloxacin, clofazimine, ethambutol, rifampin).[279] Benefits of the macrolide regimen included more rapid clearing of MAC bacteremia and a longer duration of survival. Rifabutin, at 600 mg/day, induced uveitis in approximately one-third of patients. Subsequently, the rifabutin dosage was lowered to 300 mg/day, and the incidence of uveitis decreased to 5.6%. Although clearance of bacteremia was superior at the higher rifabutin dose, no differences in survival were observed. Several recent studies have demonstrated no bacteriologic or clinical benefit with the addition of clofazimine. Clarithromycin and ethambutol, with and without clofazimine, were investigated for the treatment of MAC bacteremia. Survival was found to be significantly decreased in the clofazimine arm; 61% of the patients died versus 38% in the two-drug arm. Based on this analysis, the FDA no longer recommends the addition of clofazimine to clarithromycin and ethambutol.[280]

M.E. is placed on a regimen of clarithromycin 500 mg twice daily and ethambutol 15 mg/kg/day. The choice to use two drugs rather than three is based on M.E.'s poor adherence profile. Other considerations for the addition of a third-line agent include the severity of the illness, potential drug interactions, tolerability, hepatic and renal function, and cost. M.E. must

Table 70-12 Drugs Commonly Used in the Treatment of *Mycobacterium avium* Complex Infection[a]

Agents	*Dose*	*Toxicities*
Initial Therapy Agents		
Clarithromycin	500 mg PO BID[b]	Nausea, vomiting, diarrhea, abdominal pain, serum transferase elevations, bitter taste
Azithromycin	500 mg/day PO	Nausea, vomiting, diarrhea, abdominal pain, serum transferase elevations
Ethambutol	15–25 mg/kg/day PO	Optic neuritis,[c] nausea and vomiting
Rifabutin[d]	300 mg/day PO	Nausea, vomiting, diarrhea, serum transferase elevations, hepatitis, neutropenia, thrombocytopenia, rash, orange discoloration of body fluids, uveitis Clearance of other drugs owing to hepatic microsomal enzyme induction[e]
Secondary Agents		
Ciprofloxacin	500–750 mg PO BID	Nausea, vomiting, diarrhea, abdominal pain, headache, rare insomnia, hallucinations, seizures
Amikacin	10–15 mg/kg/day IV or IM	Nephrotoxicity, ototoxicity

[a] Macrolide plus ethambutol with or without one or more of the drugs listed above.
[b] Clarithromycin dose >500 mg BID is associated with increased mortality.
[c] Visual testing should be done monthly in patients receiving >15 mg/kg/day.
[d] Rifabutin dose 300–600 mg/day; but should not exceed 300 mg/day if given with clarithromycin or fluconazole.
[e] Common drug interactions include protease inhibitors (see Table 70-10).
BID, twice a day; IM, intramuscularly; IV, intravenously; PO, orally.

be counseled regarding the slow response to treatment. If she improves, therapy should be continued and HAART therapy should be reinstituted.

MONITORING THERAPY

48. How should M.E. be monitored?

The primary goals of MAC therapy are to eradicate or reduce the number of *M. avium* organisms, decrease symptoms, enhance quality of life, and prolong survival. M.E. should be monitored for symptomatic relief (temperature spikes and frequency of night sweats), as well as a microbiologic response (CFU/mL). Clinical improvement may not be observed for 2 to 4 weeks, whereas eradication of bacteremia frequently takes longer (4–12 weeks). If no improvement in clinical manifestations is observed in 4 to 8 weeks, a mycobacterial blood culture should be repeated along with susceptibility testing. If resistance is observed or suspected, two new drugs should be added based on susceptibility testing with or without the macrolide. If the organism is found to be susceptible to macrolides, therapy should be continued and adherence, absorption, tolerance, and drug interactions should be considered.[281,282] If the problem is determined to be drug absorption, IV agents can be considered. M.E. also should be followed for development of toxicities related to drug therapy. Furthermore, because many drugs used to treat MAC infections are associated with drug interactions, this issue must be considered each time a new drug is prescribed. In some cases, drug doses need to be modified or alternative drugs selected to prevent adverse events or therapeutic failures (Table 70-11).[283]

Prophylaxis

49. What drug(s) should be used to provide primary prophylaxis against MAC infection?

The most recent official guidelines recommend oral therapy with clarithromycin (500 mg BID) or azithromycin 1,200 mg every week for persons with a $CD4^+$ count <50. Although the combination of azithromycin and rifabutin is more effective than azithromycin alone, the increased cost, adverse events, potential for drug interactions, and absence of a survival benefit preclude this regimen from being routinely recommended. If neither clarithromycin nor azithromycin is tolerated, rifabutin 300 mg/day may be used[48] (Tables 70-2 and 70-12).

Before the use of macrolides, rifabutin was the agent of choice for primary prophylaxis. However, no survival benefit has been demonstrated with the use of this agent, and the drug is associated with high cost, complex drug interactions, and an increased risk for uveitis.[48,283]

Six hundred eighty-two patients with AIDS, $CD4^+$ counts <100, and negative MAC blood cultures were randomized to receive clarithromycin (500 mg PO BID) or placebo.[51] The clarithromycin arm had a 69% reduction in MAC bacteremia and fewer (16% versus 6%) cases of MAC infection. Significantly more patients in the clarithromycin arm survived during the 10-month follow-up (68% versus 59%), with an accompanying longer median duration of survival. This trial was the first prospective MAC prophylaxis study demonstrating a survival benefit and a reduced risk of disseminated MAC infection.[51]

In a randomized, double-blind, placebo-controlled trial, 182 MAC-negative patients with AIDS and $CD4^+$ counts <100 (median 44) were treated with azithromycin 1,200 mg every week or placebo.[284] Azithromycin reduced MAC bacteremia by 57% and infection (23.3% versus 8.2%). Survival benefit was not evaluated. GI disturbance was observed more commonly in the azithromycin arm.[284]

Azithromycin 1,200 mg every week, rifabutin 300 mg/day, and a combination of both drugs in the same doses were compared in patients with AIDS and $CD4^+$ counts <100. The incidence of MAC bacteremia was 13.9% in the azithromycin monotherapy arm, 23.3% in the rifabutin monotherapy arm, and 8.3% in the azithromycin, rifabutin combination arm. Time to death was not significantly different among the treatments; however, the combination arm had an increased incidence of adverse drug effects. Although combination therapy was superior to azithromycin alone, its use is considered second-line because of the increased cost, toxicity, and lack of survival benefit.[285]

In a similar trial, patients with AIDS and $CD4^+$ counts <100 were randomized to receive clarithromycin 500 mg twice daily, rifabutin 450 mg/day, or both.[286] In the midst of the trial, the rifabutin dosage was reduced to 300 mg/day because of a drug interaction with clarithromycin that resulted in rifabutin-induced uveitis. MAC bacteremia occurred in 9% of patients in the clarithromycin monotherapy arm, 15% of patients in the rifabutin monotherapy arm, and 7% of patients receiving the combination. Time to death was not significantly different among the arms, but the combination was more toxic.

The decision to use clarithromycin or azithromycin (both first-line recommendations for primary prophylaxis) is based on patient compliance and the potential for drug interactions. Azithromycin (1,200 mg once weekly) may be preferable for a patient who has difficulty with compliance. In contrast with clarithromycin, azithromycin does not affect the cytochrome P450 enzyme system and is therefore less likely to interact with other drugs. M.E. would have benefited from MAC prophylaxis when her $CD4^+$ count decreased to <50.

Patients whose $CD4^+$ count increases from 100 for >3 months may discontinue primary prophylaxis (Table 70-2).[48] However, prophylaxis should be reintroduced if the $CD4^+$ count decreases to <50 to 100.

ENTERIC INFECTIONS

50. A.B. is a 38-year-old woman with a 4-year history of HIV infection and a $CD4^+$ count of 160 (normal, approximately 1,000). She reports two or three watery, unformed bowel movements per day for approximately 6 weeks, with accompanying abdominal pain. She has refused antiretroviral therapy and is currently taking only one TMP-SMX double-strength tablet each day. What GI pathogens should be considered in the differential diagnosis in HIV-infected patients who develop diarrhea?

GI complications are common in HIV patients (e.g., enteric infections, gastric achlorhydria, pancreatitis, cholangitis, hepatitis, proctitis, KS, lymphoma, carcinoma, and HIV enteropathy). Enteric infections can be caused by fungal, viral, bacterial, or protozoan pathogens. In general, clinical manifestations caused by GI infections appear with a decline in the $CD4^+$ count. Similar to A.B., most patients present with a change in bowel habits, predominantly diarrhea.[287] When evaluating infectious diarrhea, several factors should be considered. The diarrhea first must be categorized as acute or chronic. Acute diarrhea is defined as "greater than or equal to three loose or watery stools for >10 days with fever, blood in the stool, and/or weight loss."[254] In acute diarrhea in patients with AIDS, all potential etiologies should be evaluated, including medication, dietary, or psychosomatic causes. Acute diarrhea is usually associated with bacterial causes, such as *Salmonella, Shigella, Campylobacter jejunii,* or *Clostridium difficile.*

Chronic diarrhea is defined as "greater than two to three loose or watery stools per day for >30 days."[254] Chronic infectious diarrhea also can be caused by protozoans, such as *Microsporidia, Isospora, Cyclospora, Cryptosporidia, Entamoeba histolytica,* and *Giardia.* Chronic diarrhea may also have a viral etiology (e.g., HSV or CMV). Bacteria can also be associated with chronic diarrhea, primarily *Salmonella, Shigella, C. jejuni, C. difficile,* and MAC (Table 70-13).

Fungal Infections

In acute infectious diarrhea, fungal infections are rare; they tend to be isolated to the oropharynx and esophagus and are predominantly caused by *Candida* species, primarily *C. albicans.* Other fungal infections in AIDS patients do not commonly involve the GI tract. However, patients with disseminated histoplasmosis may develop diarrhea (Table 70-12).

Viral Infections

Viruses that infect the GI tract of AIDS patients are unlike those associated with diarrhea in non–HIV-infected patients (e.g., rotaviruses, enteric adenoviruses, Norwalk agent, coronavirus, and coxsackieviruses). More common among HIV patients are CMV and HSV infections. Disseminated CMV infection is common in HIV-infected patients with advanced disease, and although retinitis is the most common CMV infection (see questions 14–25), as many as 2% of patients have GI involvement.[288] CMV usually involves the colon, and the common presentation is diarrhea. Tissue biopsy is preferred for a definitive diagnosis. CMV infection of the pancreas, liver, gallbladder, and biliary tree also has been described.[289] The IV agents used to treat CMV retinitis may also be used to treat CMV disease in the GI tract. In contrast with the treatment of CMV retinitis, therapy for colitis lasts 3 to 6 weeks. Data support the use of ganciclovir over foscarnet for CMV colitis, whereas the efficacy of cidofovir is unknown. Regular ophthalmologic screening for CMV retinitis is recommended for all patients with CMV GI tract disease.[44]

The other common cause of viral GI disease is herpes simplex. The clinical presentation is similar to that of disseminated CMV, but the site of infection and biopsy findings differentiate the viruses. HSV type 1 primarily is associated with ulcerated esophageal lesions. In contrast, HSV type 2 is often the cause of proctitis. Although not usually associated with diarrhea, proctitis may result in bloody, mucousy stools. HSV also can cause large, painful perianal lesions. Herpes simplex GI lesions usually are treated with acyclovir; if herpes-resistant virus is suspected, foscarnet is used (Table 70-12).[254]

Bacterial Infections

Bacteria such as *Salmonella, Shigella,* and *Campylobacter* cause lower GI disease in HIV patients, but these organisms are generally more virulent in HIV-negative patients. The frequency of acute infectious diarrhea caused by *Salmonella* for patients with AIDS is 5% to 15%. *Salmonella* bacteremia is considered an AIDS-defining diagnosis. The clinical features include fever and watery stools, with variable fecal WBCs. Diagnosis is made based on stool and blood cultures. In contrast with immunocompetent persons, antibiotics are recommended for treatment of *Salmonella* in HIV-infected patients; ciprofloxacin (750 mg BID for 2 weeks) is the preferred regimen. Alternative regimens include ampicillin (8–12 g/day IV for 1–4 weeks), amoxicillin (500 mg PO TID to complete a 2- to 4-week course), TMP-SMX (5–10 mg/kg/day IV or PO for

Table 70-13 Enteric Infections Associated With Infectious Diarrhea

Enteric Infections	Treatment
Fungal	
Candida albicans[a]	Fluconazole 100–400 mg PO QD; ketoconazole 200–400 mg PO QD; caspofungin 50 mg IV QD; amphotericin B 0.3–0.5 mg/kg IV; liposomal or lipid amphotericin 3–5 mg/kg IV QD; voriconazole 200 mg BID; itraconazole solution 200 mg QD; efficacy of fluconazole is 85%
Histoplasmosis	Itraconazole 200 mg PO TID ×3 days, then 200 mg PO BID ×12 wks (liquid formulation has better absorption, limited data available on IV) *Alternative*: amphotericin B 0.8–1.5 mg/kg IV or liposomal amphotericin 4 mg/kg QD then itraconazole 200 mg BID ×12 wks
Viral	
CMV	Ganciclovir 5 mg/kg IV BID ×2–3 wk; foscarnet 40–60 mg/kg Q 8 hr ×3–4 wk (efficacy of antiretroviral treatment is 75%) or oral valganciclovir
HSV[a]	Acyclovir 200–800 mg PO 5×/day or 5 mg/kg IV Q 8 hr ×2–3 wk
Bacterial	
Salmonella spp.	Ciprofloxacin 500–750 mg PO/IV BID ×14 days or TMP-SMX 5–10 mg/kg/day PO/IV BID ×2–4 wk or ampicillin 2 g/day PO or 6 g/day IV ×14 days or third-generation cephalosporin or chloramphenicol; treatment may be extended to 4–6 wk
Shigella spp.	Ciprofloxacin 500 mg PO/IV BID ×3–7 days; TMP-SMX 1 DS PO BID ×3–7 days; azithromycin 500 mg ×1, then 250 mg QD ×4 days; antiperistaltic agents (Lomotil or loperamide) are contraindicated
C. jejuni	Ciprofloxacin 500 mg PO BID ×7 days or azithromycin 500 mg QD ×7 days
C. difficile	Metronidazole 250–500 mg PO QID ×10–14 days or vancomycin 125 mg PO QID 10–14 days; antiperistaltic agents (Lomotil or loperamide) are contraindicated
Protozoa	
Isospora	TMP-SMX 1 DS QID or 2 DS BID *Alternative*: pyrimethamine 50–75 mg with folinic acid 5–10 mg or fluroquinolone
Cyclospora	TMP-SMX 1 DS BID
Microsporidia	Albendazole 400–800 mg PO BID until CD4 >200 *Alternative*: metronidazole, atovaquone, and thalidomide
Cryptosporidia	No effective treatment; paromomycin, nitazoxanide, octreotide, azithromycin (marginal benefits and no cure); best treatment approach is antiretroviral therapy to increase CD4 >100.

[a]Primarily esophagitis.
BID, twice a day; DS, double strength; IV, intravenously; PO, orally; QID, four times a day; QD, daily; TID, three times a day; TMP-SMX, trimethoprim-sulfamethoxazole.
Adapted from references 288 and 295.

2–4 weeks), or a third-generation cephalosporin. Eradication of *Salmonella* has been demonstrated only with ciprofloxacin. Bacteremia may be more frequent compared with non–HIV-infected patients and may recur despite antibiotic therapy. For recurrent therapy, ciprofloxacin (500 mg PO BID) is preferred for several months. TMP-SMX (5–10 mg/kg TMP component daily IV or PO) may be considered as an alternative. Lifelong treatment may be required (Table 70-13).[290,291]

The frequency of *Shigella* is 1% to 3% in acute infectious diarrhea in AIDS patients; *S. sonnei* accounts for approximately 70% of the reported U.S. cases. *S. flexneri* is also reported in young homosexual men. Person-to-person spread is the main route of transmission. *Shigella* causes dysentery, fever, and abdominal cramps, which precede voluminous, watery stools. Bloody mucoid stools with fecal urgency may also develop. Fecal WBCs are common, and diagnosis is made by stool culture. Mild to severe cases of *Shigella* bacteremia have been reported, lasting an average of 7 days if untreated. Because this is a self-limiting illness and resistance is common, treatment is recommended only for severely ill patients. Antibiotic therapy should be selected based on susceptibility patterns. Ciprofloxacin (500 mg PO BID) or TMP-SMX (1 double-strength tablet PO BID for 3 days) both are effective regimens. Antiperistaltic agents are contraindicated. As with *Salmonella, Shigella* infections are associated with an increased frequency of bacteremia in HIV-infected patients who may require prolonged therapy (Table 70-13).[291,292]

C. jejuni accounts for 4% to 8% of cases of acute infectious diarrhea in AIDS patients. *Campylobacter* enteritis is associated with a prodrome of fever, headaches, myalgia, and malaise 12 to 24 hours before diarrhea and abdominal pain. Diarrhea varies from loose bowel movements to voluminous, watery, and grossly bloody stools. Fecal leukocytes are variable, and the diagnosis is made by stool culture. *Campylobacter* enteritis is self-limiting, lasting only several days; however, some HIV-infected persons have symptoms lasting >1 week and may relapse if left untreated. Antibiotics are recommended for patients with high fevers, bloody stools, more than eight stools per day, and symptoms for >1 week without improvement. Erythromycin (500 mg PO QID for 5 days) and ciprofloxacin (500 mg PO BID for 3–5 days) are the preferred agents. Quinolone-resistant isolates are well documented. Alternatives to erythromycin or ciprofloxacin include tetracycline, clindamycin, and ampicillin (Table 70-13).[293]

HIV-positive patients should take preventive measures against potential enteric pathogens. Close attention to hand hygiene is recommended, as is not handling or eating raw or uncooked poultry, fruits, vegetables, and nonpasteurized dairy products. Fortunately, the widespread use of TMP-SMX for PCP prophylaxis has reduced the frequency of these bacterial infections. Disseminated MAC disease, *M. tuberculosis, Helicobacter pylori,* and *C. difficile* also can cause diarrhea in HIV-infected patients.

Protozoal Infections

As a group, protozoal infections are the most common cause of diarrhea among HIV-infected patients. Opportunistic protozoans such as *Cryptosporidium, Isospora belli,* and *Microsporidia* are well-known GI pathogens. Other nonopportunistic protozoans such as *Giardia lamblia, E. histolytica,* and *Cyclospora cayetanensis* also cause disease.[287]

Cryptosporidium, a coccidioidin protozoan with a life cycle that occurs entirely within a single host, can be transmitted from animals to humans by fecal water contamination or person-to-person fecal–oral spread.[294] HIV-infected patients should be advised to wash their hands after contact with fecal material (e.g., changing diapers), exposure to pets, gardening, or contact with soil, and they should avoid oral–anal sexual practices. HIV-infected patients also should avoid drinking water from lakes and swallowing water during recreational activities. Outbreaks of cryptosporidiosis have been linked to municipal water supplies.[295] HIV-infected patients should avoid eating raw oysters because the oocysts can survive in oysters for >2 months.[48] In patients with AIDS, the frequency of chronic infectious diarrhea owing to cryptosporidiosis is 10% to 30%.[294] In contrast to the explosive onset that occurs in non-HIV patients, acute cryptosporidiosis in AIDS patients is more insidious and progresses in severity as the degree of immunosuppression increases. Intestinal cryptosporidiosis may be complicated by concurrent biliary involvement, leading to jaundice and hepatosplenomegaly. Although the diagnosis of cryptosporidiosis formerly depended on intestinal tissue biopsy, newer techniques such as staining oocysts in stool (modified acid-fast methods) and fluorescent antibody assays have been developed.[296] No known prophylaxis exists; however, one MAC prophylaxis study suggested that clarithromycin and rifabutin also may prevent cryptosporidiosis.[297] The treatment of cryptosporidiosis remains investigational and studies have progressed slowly. Supportive care that includes fluid and electrolytes, parenteral hyperalimentation, and antidiarrheal agents often is necessary.

The long-acting somatostatin analog octreotide acetate (50–500 g TID subcutaneously or IV at 1 g/hr) also has been used with limited benefit in some patients. However, it is expensive and the parenteral administration is inconvenient for many patients.[296] Trials of α-difluoromethylornithine and oral spiramycin have yielded inconsistent results. Other drugs, such as IV spiramycin, letrazuril, hyperimmune bovine colostrum, transfer factor (a dialyzable leukocyte extract obtained from cow lymph nodes), and IGX-CP (an oral formulation of chicken egg yolks immunized with *Cryptosporidium* antigen), have been investigated, but results are not encouraging.[296]

Paromomycin (500–750 mg PO QID with food for 21 days, then 500 mg PO BID) is a poorly absorbed aminoglycoside antibiotic commonly used to treat HIV-infected patients with cryptosporidiosis.[295] Paromomycin, 1 g BID plus azithromycin 600 mg/day for 4 weeks followed by paromomycin alone, 1 g BID for 8 weeks, was associated with improvement of symptoms and a significant reduction in oocyst excretion. Azithromycin, an azalide antibiotic, when used alone, is ineffective.[298]

Nitazoxanide is an antimicrobial compound with activity against protozoans, helminths, and bacterial organisms. This drug has been approved for use; the usual dosage is 500 mg orally twice daily for 3 days.[254,296,299] Data have demonstrated a 30% favorable response rate in HIV-negative but not HIV-positive subjects. Higher doses or longer durations of therapy may be needed in HIV-infected patients.

Several reports suggest that treatment with HAART results in improved immune function and subsequent resolution of cryptosporidiosis.[40,300]

I. belli, a coccidioidin protozoan, has a life cycle similar to that of *Cryptosporidium.* The frequency of *I. belli* is 1% to 3% in chronic infectious diarrhea in patients with AIDS. *Isospora* is rarely identified as a cause of diarrhea (<1%) in the United States and Europe, in contrast to Africa, Haiti, and Latin America.[301] Clinically, these patients develop diarrhea, steatorrhea, cramping, and weight loss. In AIDS patients, as well as infants or children without AIDS, this disease may become a protracted illness.[296,301] Similar to *Cryptosporidium,* the diagnosis of isosporiasis is made with acid-fast stains. *Isospora* oocysts are larger and morphologically distinct. Importantly, and in contrast to cryptosporidiosis, isosporiasis can be treated with TMP-SMX (160 mg/day and 800 mg/day, respectively). Chronic suppressive therapy often is needed and can be accomplished with lower doses of TMP-SMX or pyrimethamine-sulfadoxine (Table 70-13).

Microsporidium (a ubiquitous, obligate intracellular protozoan parasite) characterizes the four genera (out of hundreds) of *Microsporidia* known to cause human disease; it is responsible for 15% to 30% of chronic infectious diarrhea in AIDS patients. Among AIDS patients, the cornea, liver, peritoneum, and small intestine have been reported to be infected with *Microsporidium.*[301] The primary species associated with AIDS patients are *Enterocytozoon bieneusi* or *Septata intestinalis.* These can be identified in intestinal biopsy specimens using electron microscopy and hematoxylin-and-eosin stained paraffin-embedded sections. Albendazole (400–800 mg PO BID for >3 weeks) has been found to be efficacious in the treatment of *S. intestinalis.* Some patients have been successfully treated with metronidazole, atovaquone, and thalidomide (Table 70-13).[302] Several reports suggest that infection resolves with HAART therapy.[40,48]

GI manifestations of HIV infection become increasingly common in the advanced stages of HIV infection. A.B. presents with chronic infectious diarrhea (two or three watery stools for >30 days). Review of her current medications (to rule out a medication source for diarrhea) revealed only low-dose TMP-SMX. CMV, MAC, *Microsporidia, Isospora,* and *Cyclospora* are common in patients with a $CD4^+$ count <100. Stool analyses, including ova and parasites, AFB smears, bacterial culture, *C. difficile* toxin assay, and *Microsporidia* assay, were ordered. A fecal WBC examination was also ordered. The AFB smear of stool showed *Cryptosporidia* oocysts. A.B. was empirically treated with paromomycin, 500 mg orally four times a day with food for 21 days, then 500 mg orally twice daily with food for chronic suppressive therapy. Baseline auditory and renal function assessment should be done before initiation of therapy to monitor for ototoxicity and nephrotoxicity. A.B. should be treated symptomatically with nutritional supplements and antidiarrheal agents (Lomotil or loperamide). HAART therapy with immune recovery may reverse the progression of her enteritis and should be recommended.

ESOPHAGEAL DISEASE

51. P.J. is a 45-year-old, HIV-positive man who was started on AZT, 3TC, and lopinavir/ritonavir when he was diagnosed 1 year ago. P.J. is a heroin user and has not been seen in the clinic since his initial presentation. He appears today complaining of difficult, painful swallowing and diffuse pain. Upon examination, localized white plaques are observed in the oral cavity. His CD4$^+$ count is 280 (normal, approximately 1,000). What is the most likely cause of this patient's dysphagia and odynophagia?

Esophagitis in HIV-positive patients generally is caused by *Candida* (50%–75% of cases), CMV (10%–20%), HSV (2%–5%), and aphthous ulcers (10%–20%).[254] Symptoms include dysphagia, odynophagia, and thrush (with *Candida* infections). Oral ulcers are common with HSV, rare with *Candida,* and uncommon with CMV or aphthous ulcers. Pain is usually diffuse in *Candida* infections and more focused with HSV, CMV, and aphthous ulcers. Fever is primarily associated with CMV.

Up to 75% of AIDS patients develop oral candidiasis, a consequence of a failing immune system and fungal colonization of the oropharynx. Patients with localized white plaques in the oral cavity likely have oral candidiasis (thrush) and should be started on antifungal therapy. Initially, patients may be treated with local antifungal therapy (e.g., "swish and swallow" nystatin suspension 3 million units four or five times daily or clotrimazole troches four or five times daily). If no response is noted or symptoms of esophageal involvement develop (e.g., dysphagia or odynophagia), these patients should be treated with a systemic agent; the azoles are preferred. Many patients with thrush without esophagitis do not respond to topical treatment and also require systemic azole therapy.

Esophagitis owing to *C. albicans* increases in frequency as HIV progresses. Not all patients with thrush develop esophagitis; however, patients who experience esophageal symptoms generally have esophagitis. Diagnosis is made using endoscopy and microbiology. Multiple white or gray plaques are observed endoscopically; they may be discrete or appear as continuous exudates.[303] Esophageal candidiasis must be treated as a systemic infection; local antifungal agents should never be used. Therapy should be initiated with oral fluconazole (Diflucan) 200 mg orally, then 100 mg orally daily for 2 to 3 weeks (up to 400 mg/day). Fluconazole is the preferred azole because of fewer toxicities, fewer drug–food interactions, and a reduced potential for drug–drug interactions. Alternative oral therapies include itraconazole oral solution or ketoconazole (Nizoral). If azole-resistant candidiasis or severe disease is diagnosed, parenteral amphotericin B (0.3–0.5 mg/kg/day IV with or without flucytosine 100 mg/kg/day) should be used.[304]

CMV esophagitis should be considered in patients who do not respond to a 1-week course of an antifungal. CMV esophagitis is confirmed via endoscopic biopsy demonstrating erythema and single or multiple discrete erosive lesions, usually located distally.[44,289] Acute treatment consists of ganciclovir 5 mg/kg IV per dose twice daily or foscarnet 40 to 60 mg/kg IV per dose Q 8 hours for 2 to 3 weeks. Maintenance therapy, if used, is usually half the dose used for induction treatment. Patients with CMV esophagitis have a poor prognosis.

Diagnosis of esophageal disease caused by HSV is by endoscopy, which reveals erythema and erosions. These small, shallow ulcers usually coalesce. HSV can be successfully treated with acyclovir or valacyclovir. Aphthous ulcers are similar in appearance and location to CMV, and negative results for *Candida,* HSV, and CMV are suggestive of aphthous ulcers. Acute treatment involves prednisone 40 mg/day for 7 to 10 days, tapered to 10 mg/wk. Thalidomide, 200 mg/day, is a promising regimen; one trial demonstrated a 53% response compared with 7% in the placebo group.[305]

A presumptive diagnosis of *Candida* esophagitis can be made for P.J. because he presents with oral pharyngeal candidiasis, dysphagia, and odynophagia. P.J. should be empirically treated with fluconazole, 200 mg/day for 14 to 21 days. If he is unresponsive to fluconazole, endoscopy with biopsy and culture should be performed to confirm the diagnosis. If candidiasis is confirmed, P.J. should be checked for medication adherence and potential drug interactions. If the patient is adherent and does not have malabsorption, parenteral amphotericin B should be considered. Anecdotally, fluconazole doses have been increased in some patients with refractory candidiasis, with successful clinical outcomes. This may be an option before amphotericin therapy.[306] Relapse is common in patients who do not receive secondary prophylaxis. Chronic suppressive therapy (fluconazole 100–200 mg/day) should be considered in all patients responsive to fluconazole therapy who have frequent or severe recurrent esophagitis. However, this practice has been documented to increase the probability of azole resistance.[48,307]

HIV WASTING SYNDROME

52. J.R. is a 38-year-old woman who has been followed in the HIV clinic for 8 years. She has been treated with antiretroviral therapy for 5 years from the time she developed PCP. She has chronic oral candidiasis managed with intermittent fluconazole. Her last CD4$^+$ count was 90 (normal, approximately 1,000). Over the last two visits, J.R.'s weight has declined from a baseline weight of 140 to 115 lb. She reports two or three loose stools per day, intermittent fevers, loss of appetite, and a generalized weakness for at least 5 weeks. What is the potential cause of J.R.'s weight loss, and how should it be managed?

Rapid disease progression is associated with significant weight loss in HIV-infected patients. Wasting syndrome can be defined as "the unintentional weight loss of >10% of baseline body weight plus chronic diarrhea (more than two loose stools a day for >30 days) or chronic weakness with unexplainable fever that is intermittent or constant for >30 days."[308]

The pathophysiology of HIV wasting syndrome is not clearly understood, but it is characterized by depletion of both adipose and lean body tissue. Because weight loss may also

Table 70-14 HIV Wasting Regimens

Agent	Dose	Side Effects	Comments
Approved			
Megestrol acetate[a]	400–800 mg/day	Impotence, GI disturbances, endocrine effects	Dose must be tapered before discontinuation
Dronabinol[a]	2.5 mg BID (before lunch and dinner)	Euphoria, dizziness, confusion, sedation	Use with caution in patients with a history of drug abuse
Somatropin (rhGH)[b]	0.1 mg/kg/day SC (6 mg/day)	Edema, arthralgias, myalgias, paresthesias, diarrhea	Long-term effect unknown Expensive agent
Oxandrolone[b]	520 mg/day	Elevated LFTs	FDA orphan drug
Unlabeled Use			
Oxymetholone[b]	25–50 mg/day	Irritability and aggression	Monitor glucose tolerance
Testosterone[b]	200–400 mg IM Q 2 wk	Irritability, aggression, gynecomastia, acne	Endogenous testosterone levels must be <400 ng/dL for all anabolic steroid administration
Cypionate or enanthate	4 or 6 mg/day		
Testoderm scrotal patch	5 mg/day		
TTS patch	5 mg/day		
Androderm			
Nandrolone[b] decanoate	100–200 mg IM Q 2 wk	Elevated Hgb and Hct, dysmenorrhea	Anabolic steroid
Thalidomide	300–400 mg/day	Teratogenicity, somnolence, rash, peripheral neuropathy	FDA orphan drug
Cyproheptadine[a]	12–20 mg/day	Sedation	Enhanced sedation with other CNS depressants Antihistamine

[a]Appetite stimulants: weight gain predominantly fat, not lean body mass.
[b]Significant increases in lean body mass.
CNS, central nervous system; FDA, U.S. Food and Drug Administration; GI, gastrointestinal; Hct, hematocrit; Hgb, hemoglobin; IM, intramuscularly; LFTs, liver function tests; rhGH, recombinant human growth hormone; SC, subcutaneously.

signal an opportunistic infection (e.g., enteric infection, PCP, or MAC), these etiologies must be ruled out.[2] Wasting syndrome may be multifactorial, resulting from decreased nutritional intake or absorption, accelerated nutrient metabolism, stress, or a combination of these factors.[309,310] J.R. meets the criteria for wasting with an unintentional 18% weight loss accompanied by chronic diarrhea and weakness.

Three appetite stimulants are routinely used to treat HIV-related wasting (Table 70-14). Megestrol acetate is an oral synthetic progestin related to progesterone. This drug is widely used for the treatment of hormone-responsive malignancies, but it is also approved for HIV-infected patients who have lost at least 10% of their ideal body weight. Megestrol 400 to 800 mg/day has been associated with weight gains of up to 10 kg.[309,311] However, a significant portion of the observed weight gain appears to be fat mass rather than lean tissue. Hypergonadism, diabetes, and adrenal insufficiency are the most serious side effects. Other side effects include impotence, diarrhea, reduced testosterone levels, hyperglycemia, and alopecia.

Dronabinol (delta-9-tetrahydrocannabinol), the psychoactive component of marijuana, 2.5 mg twice daily has been approved for treating AIDS-related weight loss. The dronabinol significantly increases appetite,[312] increases body weight (primarily fat), and improves mood. Besides stimulating appetite, dronabinol also has antiemetic effects, which are useful in patients with nausea and vomiting associated with the wasting syndrome. Euphoria, dizziness, confusion, and somnolence occur in 18% of dronabinol-treated patients. A reduction in the dose of dronabinol to 2.5 mg 1 hour before supper or bedtime may reduce adverse events. Because of its potential for misuse, dronabinol should be used with caution in patients with a history of substance abuse. Patients should be counseled to avoid driving, operating machinery, or other potentially hazardous activity until it is established that they can safely perform these activities. Alcohol or other CNS depressants may result in additive CNS depression.

Cyproheptadine is an antihistamine reported to stimulate appetite in HIV-infected patients. The use of cyproheptadine 12 mg/day has been associated with minimal weight gain as a result of an increase in daily caloric intake. This drug, although used for the treatment of anorexia, is not approved by the FDA for HIV wasting (Table 70-14).

Anabolic steroids and testosterone have been shown to increase muscle mass and strength in people with HIV wasting syndrome. Products include oxandrolone (Oxandrin), nandrolone (Deca-Durabolin), oxymetholone (Anadrol-50), and testosterone.[313,314] Oxandrolone at a dosage of 15 mg/day significantly increases body weight but does not improve body strength. The usual dosage for males is 10 to 20 mg twice daily; for females the range is 5 to 20 mg/day. This drug has a low androgenic effect, so it is particularly useful in women. Most weight gain is lean body mass. Minimal hepatotoxicity has been associated with this agent.[313] Oxandrolone can be administered orally, which may improve adherence.[313,315]

Nandrolone increases body weight, muscle mass, and strength. Nandrolone has a high anabolic effect and a low androgenic effect. The dosage of nandrolone for males is 100 to 200 mg intramuscularly every 1 to 2 weeks and for females 25 mg intramuscularly per week or 50 mg intramuscularly every 2 weeks.[315,316]

Oxymetholone is not recommended for use in women because of its high androgenic potential. Hepatic toxicity is common, so LFTs must be carefully monitored. Doses of 50 mg twice daily are used in HIV-infected male patients.[315] In an open-label study, oxymetholone produced a mean weight gain of 5.7 kg with improvement in the Karnofsky score in HIV-infected patients with wasting syndrome.[317] It has high androgenic and some anabolic effects, so it may be better suited for HIV-infected men.

A decrease in testosterone correlates with a decrease in lean body mass in AIDS patients.[314] Testosterone administration produces a significant increase in lean body mass (mean 1.2 kg) in HIV-positive patients without wasting syndrome. It is available as long-acting intramuscular injections (enanthate and cypionate), short-acting intramuscular injections (propionate), and a transdermal system (2.5, 4, 5, and 6 mg/24 hr). The transdermal systems differ in release rate, surface area, and total testosterone content. Testosterone should be used in patients with low endogenous testosterone levels (<400 ng/dL in men). Testosterone has been associated with improved mood, libido, and energy in clinical trials. It is also associated with acne, gynecomastia, alopecia, and testicular atrophy. Testosterone has been shown to be less effective than oxandrolone or nandrolone for weight gain.[318,319] In clinical practice, testosterone is sometimes combined with megestrol acetate or nandrolone, but this combination has not been studied.

Growth hormones (which directly influence nitrogen balance and muscle protein synthesis) have been used in the treatment of HIV wasting syndrome. These include recombinant human insulinlike growth factor-1 and somatropin (Serostim), a recombinant human growth hormone. Disturbances in growth hormone–insulinlike growth factor-1 axis have been described in HIV-positive subjects. In one placebo-controlled trial, 10 mg/day of recombinant human insulinlike growth factor-1 subcutaneously failed to significantly increase weight or lean body mass.[320] Subcutaneous injections of somatropin (0.1 mg/kg/day) have been associated with increases in lean body mass and functional performance.[321] Adverse events include edema, arthralgia, diabetes, acute pancreatitis, and carpal tunnel syndrome. The questionable long-term benefits and the tremendous expense of growth hormone diminish its appeal (Table 70-14).[316]

Several cytokine modulators are used in the treatment of HIV wasting. These include pentoxifylline (Trental), thalidomide, ketotifen, and omega-3 fatty acids (fish oil). Altered metabolism of cytokines, tumor necrosis factor (TNF), interleukin-1, or interferon-may play a role in the wasting syndrome. As an example, an elevation in serum TNF-α has been noted in HIV patients with advanced disease. Thalidomide and pentoxifylline, which decrease TNF-α levels, have been used in patients with HIV wasting syndrome. Thalidomide has been associated with significant weight gain.[315,322] However, thalidomide is associated with numerous adverse effects, including somnolence, rash, teratogenicity, and peripheral neuropathy (additive with other drugs known to cause peripheral neuropathy). It may also be associated with an elevation in HIV-RNA levels; however, more studies are needed for confirmation. Pentoxifylline, a drug used to prevent intermittent claudication, has also been evaluated as treatment for the HIV wasting syndrome. Unfortunately, because pentoxifylline has failed to stimulate the appetite or increase weight gain, it does not have a role in the treatment of HIV wasting.[315]

Exercise has been considered as a possible intervention for HIV wasting. The preliminary results of one study demonstrated an increase in lean body mass and strength after patients underwent an 8-week course of progressive resistance training.[323]

J.R. must be assessed for possible OIs and treated accordingly. Once the diarrhea has resolved, medications to reverse HIV wasting may be started. The patient's lack of appetite should be addressed first with the use of megestrol acetate (400 mg/day oral suspension). In addition, the patient should be started on oxandrolone (10 mg/day PO). A pregnancy test should be performed because most anabolic agents should not be administered to pregnant women. Because of their high androgenic effects, oxymetholone and testosterone should be avoided in J.R.

HIV-ASSOCIATED MALIGNANCIES

53. Despite an extensive microbiologic workup, no organism was identified, and other causes for J.R.'s change in bowel habits were evaluated. What neoplastic conditions could be contributing to J.R.'s GI status?

In addition to the OIs described under enteric infections, GI malignancy is common in patients with HIV. As the $CD4^+$ count declines, patients may develop KS (see Kaposi Sarcoma section), lymphoma, and invasive cervical cancer. The reason for the increased occurrence of malignancy is unknown, but it may be related to impaired immune function. In addition, effective antiretroviral therapy and prophylactic anti-infective therapy have extended the life span of patients with AIDS, increasing the likelihood that malignancies will be detected.[324,325] J.R. has been on HAART therapy and prophylactic anti-infective therapy for many years; thus, she may be at risk for malignancy.

Kaposi Sarcoma

KS previously was well described in non–HIV-infected patients, and its course was fairly uneventful. Consequently, limited studies of innovative chemotherapy regimens were conducted in the past. In contrast, KS in HIV-infected patients is more invasive and is associated with increased morbidity and mortality.[325] Although KS occurs predominantly in homosexual men, the incidence of KS has increased in IV drug users, recipients of blood products, women, and children. The risk of developing KS is 20,000 times higher for HIV-infected patients than for non–HIV-infected persons. The incidence of KS as a presenting AIDS illness has significantly declined since the early 1990s, and this may be indirectly due to HAART.[326] An infectious etiology has been suggested in recent studies. DNA sequencing in KS tissue has detected a herpes virus. A new human herpes virus 8 (HHV-8) has been observed in biopsies of classic KS, African KS, and HIV-positive KS. This finding suggests that HHV-8 is either a causative agent or a recurrent passenger virus (i.e., an "innocent bystander").[327,328]

Other studies have suggested that the pathogenesis of KS in HIV patients is related to the existence of cells with the potential to become KS lesions. Cytokines released from activated immune cells potentially stimulate the proliferation of KS precursor cells at a time when the immune function for such cells is becoming progressively impaired. Furthermore, some cells may produce a growth factor for KS cells (e.g., angiogenic factors), and the expression of the *tat* gene by HIV may produce growth factors that induce vascular KS-like tumors.[324,329–331]

KS presents with three types of lesions: flat, raised, or nodular. The lesions occur primarily on the skin, oral mucosa, GI tract, and lungs. KS lesions may be asymptomatic or painful; intestinal or pulmonary lesions may be associated with significant clinical symptoms such as dyspnea or diarrhea. Cutaneous disease involves initially small, flat lesions that progress to reddish or purple nodules.[331] They are generally asymptomatic and follow a pattern of cutaneous lymphatic drainage. Progression of KS leads to lesions in the oral cavity in approximately one-third of cases.[328] KS has a multifactorial presentation without a primary lesion; therefore, staging according to a standard tumor-node-metastasis classification is not appropriate. A staging system proposed in 1989 by the ACTG Oncology Committee divides patients into good- or poor-risk groups based on tumor characteristics, the patient's immunity (measured by $CD4^+$ count), and the severity of systemic HIV-associated illness.[329,330] Whether staging and the choice or response to therapy are correlated is unclear.

The growth of KS is stimulated by inflammatory cytokines, which are increased in acute OIs and active HIV replication. Successful management of KS includes optimal antiretroviral therapy, prophylactic therapy, and effective treatment of OIs. Mild disease is not treated; therefore, management of KS can be divided into local and systemic therapy.[330] Local therapy involves the use of topical liquid nitrogen cryotherapy, intralesional injections of vinblastine 0.01 to 0.02 mg/lesion every 2 weeks for 3 doses, and low-dose radiation therapy (e.g., 400 rads every week for 6 weeks). Local therapy is used in slowly progressive KS without life-threatening organ involvement. Systemic therapy involves the use of interferon-α, 18 to 36 million IU daily intramuscularly or subcutaneously for 10 to 12 weeks, followed by 18 million units per day with additional chemotherapeutic agents. These include paclitaxel (Taxol) 100 to 135 mg/m^2 IV every 2 to 3 weeks; doxorubicin (Adriamycin), bleomycin, plus either vincristine or vinblastine or bleomycin plus vincristine; liposomal daunorubicin (DaunoXome) 40 to 60 mg/m^2 IV every 2 weeks; or liposomal doxorubicin (Doxil) 10 to 20 mg/m^2.[330]

The use of interferon-α for KS in patients with AIDS has been well studied alone and in combination with antiretroviral therapy.[332,333] Early studies demonstrated that AIDS patients receiving high doses of interferon developed neutropenia and neurologic toxicity, and that nonresponders had high circulating levels of endogenous interferon.[332–335] Later, in vitro data indicated that interferon-α was synergistic with AZT against HIV. As a result, interferon therapy was investigated in combination with AZT.[333,334] Unfortunately, increasing doses of both interferon-α and AZT caused neutropenia, hepatitis, and neurologic toxicity. However, patients who could tolerate the combination had partial or complete remissions and had increased $CD4^+$ counts. The hematologic toxicity caused by this combination has prompted researchers to evaluate the concurrent use of colony-stimulating factors such as G-CSF and GM-CSF. Preliminary results indicate that colony-stimulating factors can attenuate the hematologic toxicity.[335] Although interferon may be helpful for certain patients with KS, many cannot tolerate this agent. For this reason, drugs that inhibit the effects of angiogenic factors are under study. Patients with progressive disease, widespread skin involvement (>25 lesions), extensive cutaneous KS unresponsive to local treatment, and/or visceral organ involvement (especially lung KS) require chemotherapeutic agents. Newer products such as liposomal anthracyclines demonstrate comparable clinical efficacy with reduced toxicities.[336] Experimental therapies include foscarnet, ganciclovir, and cidofovir because of their in vitro activity against HHV-8.[337] Intralesional β-human chorionic gonadotropin injections also have produced favorable responses.[338]

Non-Hodgkin Lymphoma

NHL is more common than KS in people infected with HIV, particularly those with low $CD4^+$ counts (median, 100 cells/mm^3).[339] Unlike KS, NHL occurs in all risk groups of HIV-infected patients and does not predominantly occur in homosexual men.[340] High-grade NHLs account for approximately 3% of initial AIDS-defining illnesses in adults and adolescents.[341] The reason for the increased incidence is unknown; however, similar to KS, cytokine dysregulation may play a role.[324]

HIV-positive patients often have disseminated disease at the time of diagnosis. In fact, many patients with systemic NHL have extranodal disease (87%–95%). Patients also may present with GI involvement at sites such as the oral cavity, esophagus, small bowel, large bowel, appendix, and anorectum. Involvement of the subcutaneous and soft tissue, epidural space, myocardium, and pericardium has been reported. Patients with CNS lymphomas often present with altered mental status, which may be mistaken for cerebral toxoplasmosis or HIV dementia. Only brain biopsy definitively diagnoses CNS NHL. Poor prognostic risk factors for patients with NHL include a $CD4^+$ count of <100, bone marrow involvement, Karnofsky performance status <70, stage IV disease, and a history of a prior AIDS-defining illness. Patients having none of these prognostic risk factors have a threefold greater survival rate compared with patients with one or more of these risk factors.[341,342]

The treatment of NHL is determined by organ involvement. Patients with evidence of CNS lymphoma often require local radiation or intrathecal chemotherapy. Several systemic chemotherapy regimens have been evaluated,[343] including cyclophosphamide with doxorubicin, vincristine, and prednisone (CHOP); cyclophosphamide with methyl GAG, bleomycin, prednisone, doxorubicin, and vincristine (NHL-7); cyclophosphamide combined with vincristine, intrathecal methotrexate, doxorubicin, and prednisone (L-17); and methotrexate, bleomycin, doxorubicin, cyclophosphamide, and dexamethasone (m-BACOD). Of these regimens, low-dose m-BACOD and low-dose CHOP are considered to be the standard therapies for NHL.[344]

Patients with NHL tend to have more advanced HIV disease accompanied by reduced bone marrow reserves. As a result, patients with poor prognostic factors do not tolerate full doses of chemotherapy and often develop leukopenia. These patients benefit from low-dose treatment. Patients with good prognostic risk factors may benefit from full-dose chemotherapy along with a colony-stimulating factor (e.g., G-CSF, GM-CSF) and may still be able to remain on antiretroviral therapy.[341,342]

Because J.R. presents with pathogen-negative, persistent, large-volume chronic diarrhea, KS and NHL must be ruled out.

J.R. has shown no visible skin or oral KS lesions; endoscopy revealed a small GI tumor. Tissue biopsy ruled out KS and confirmed NHL, which was found to be stage II. The bone marrow aspirate was also positive for NHL. The prognostic risk factors for J.R. include a CD4$^+$ count <100 and a past history of an AIDS-defining illness (PCP). Consequently, low-dose m-BACOD was initiated with GM-CSF as needed. J.R. will be monitored for resolution of diarrhea as well as toxicities (e.g., hematologic). Her HAART therapy also should be reevaluated.

Cervical Intraepithelial Neoplasia

54. L.P., a 38-year-old woman, was heterosexually infected with HIV. She also has a history of human papillomavirus (HPV) infection successfully treated with imiquimod cream 5%. During a routine HIV clinic visit, a "cheesy" vaginal discharge is noted. L.P. states that her vagina has been itching. Physical examination is unremarkable with the exception of her vaginal discharge. A potassium hydroxide stain of vaginal secretions is positive for hyphae, indicating a yeast infection. CBC values include Hgb, 13.3 g/dL (normal, 12.1–15.3); WBC count, 5,500 cells/L (normal, 3,800–9,800); and platelets, 95,000/mm^3 (normal, 150,000–450,000). Notably, for the first time, L.P.'s CD4$^+$ count has declined to 435 cells/mm^3 (normal, approximately 1,000). She has received no prior antiretroviral therapy. Is L.P.'s gynecologic presentation typical of a woman with early HIV disease?

[SI units: Hgb, 130 g/L (normal, 121–153); WBC count, 5.5 × 10^{10}/L (normal, 3.8–9.8); platelets, 95 × 10^{10}/L (normal, 150–450)]

Four gynecologic disorders occur more frequently, with greater severity, and with less responsiveness in HIV-infected women[344–346]: HPV, associated cervical intraepithelial neoplasia, *Candida* vaginitis, and pelvic inflammatory disease. All are considered CDC HIV-associated conditions.[4,348] Cervical neoplasia is a CDC AIDS-defining illness.[4] Consequently, L.P.'s presentation with vaginitis is typical. Her vaginal yeast infection should be treated with an antifungal agent such as fluconazole (100 mg/day PO) for ≥7 days. She should be followed closely to ensure that her infection resolves, because HIV-positive patients may not respond to the standard duration of therapy.

55. L.P. returns to the clinic in a week and her vaginal infection has cleared. A routine Pap smear is performed on this visit, demonstrating cellular changes consistent with a low-grade squamous intraepithelial lesion. What therapeutic intervention should follow this abnormal Pap smear?

Women at increased risk of precancerous cervical cytology include those with HIV infection or HPV infection and cigarette smokers.[349–351] HPV infections, types 16, 18, and 33, are more prevalent among HIV-positive women than HIV-negative women and have been causally implicated in the development of preinvasive and invasive cervical neoplasms.[352] Furthermore, the greater the degree of immunosuppression (CD4$^+$ count <200), the higher the risk for cervical intraepithelial neoplasia.[353] Rapidly progressive cervical malignancy and death have been reported in HIV-infected women.[349,354,355]

All HIV-infected women should have Pap smears every 6 months in the first year of diagnosis.[47] Among HIV-infected women, approximately 15% of low-grade squamous intraepithelial lesions progress to high-grade lesions, including moderate to severe dysplasia or carcinoma in situ.[355,356] Because the risk of progression may be greater among HIV-infected women, many gynecologists recommend colposcopic examination (microscopic inspection of the entire cervical area) with directed biopsy.

If a biopsy confirms precancerous cellular changes, as in L.P., a surgical procedure is indicated to destroy or remove the dysplastic tissue.[357] Options include laser therapy, electrosurgery, and cryotherapy. Postsurgical complications may include prolonged bleeding or infertility because of cervical stenosis.[358,359] After surgery, L.P. should have follow-up Pap smears every 3 months for at least 1 year.[357,360] The risk of recurrence is much higher in HIV-infected women.[352]

Pharmacologic Intervention

56. What pharmacologic intervention has proven to be successful in the treatment of cervical intraepithelial neoplasia? Is L.P. a candidate for this therapy?

Interferon has been suggested for the treatment of cervical intraepithelial neoplasia.[361] Many uncontrolled studies have been performed, but the number of women who have been evaluated is insufficient to recommend use of this agent. The best results were observed in one small study with systemic administration, but most patients experienced adverse effects.[361] In an additional trial, 15 women were treated with interferon-β, 2 million IUs intramuscularly daily for 10 days, and their outcomes were compared with 15 women treated with saline.[362] After >6 months, 14 of 15 (93%) of the treated women had a complete response compared with 6 of 15 (40%) of the controls. In a placebo-controlled trial using the same dosage regimen,[363] women with earlier stage cervical intraepithelial neoplasia disease responded, but women with more advanced disease responded poorly. A flulike syndrome characterized by fever, chills, headache, malaise, arthralgia, and myalgia was the most common adverse effect, although these symptoms were better tolerated with continued treatment.[361]

Topical interferon-α is associated with a lower incidence of adverse effects, but this route of administration seems less efficacious.[364,365] Intralesional interferon injections have been tried, but they are inferior to the systemic route, and expert personnel are required for administration.[366,367] In one trial, women with grade II cervical intraepithelial neoplasia were randomized to receive intramuscular β-interferon, intralesional α-interferon, a combination of both, or conventional therapy. Combination therapy demonstrated the best response with respect to lesion progression.[362] L.P. should not be treated with either local or systemic interferon. Systemic therapy seems somewhat more effective in small-scale trials, but it is not well tolerated. The exact role of interferons in the treatment of cervical intraepithelial neoplasia, particularly in HIV-infected women, remains uncertain.

ACKNOWLEDGMENTS

The authors acknowledge Angela D.M. Kashuba, PharmD, Gene D. Morse, PharmD, Alice M. O'Donnell, PharmD, Marjorie Robinson, PharmD, and Mark J. Shelton, PharmD, for their contributions to this chapter in previous editions.

REFERENCES

1. Centers for Disease Control and Prevention. Update: trends in AIDS incidences, United States, 1996. *MMWR Morbid Mortal Wkly Rep* 1997;46: 861.
2. Centers for Disease Control and Prevention. Surveillance for AIDS-defining opportunistic illnesses, 1992–1997. *MMWR Morbid Mortal Wkly Rep* 1999;48(SS-2).
3. Hooshyar D et al. Trends in perimortal conditions and mortality rates among HIV-infected patients. *AIDS* 2007;21:2093.
4. Centers for Disease Control and Prevention. 1993 revised classification system for HIV infection and expanded surveillance case definition for AIDS among adolescents and adults. *MMWR Morbid Mortal Wkly Rep* 1992;41(RR17):1.
5. Cohen O et al. The immunology of human immunodeficiency virus infection. In: Mandell GL et al., eds. *Principles and Practice of Infectious Diseases.* New York: Churchill Livingstone; 2000:1374.
6. Paul WE. *Fundamental Immunology.* New York: Lippincott Williams & Wilkins; 1998.
7. Lane HC et al. Qualitative analysis of immune function in patients with the acquired immunodeficiency syndrome. *N Engl J Med* 1985;313:79.
8. Clerici M et al. Detection of three distinct patterns of T helper cell dysfunction in asymptomatic, human immunodeficiency virus-seropositive patients independent of CD4+ cell numbers and clinical settings. *J Clin Invest* 1989;84:1892.
9. Pantalew G et al. The immunopathogenesis of human immunodeficiency virus infection. *N Engl J Med* 1993;328:327.
10. Niu MT et al. Primary human immunodeficiency virus type 1 infection: review of pathogenesis and early treatment intervention in humans and animal retrovirus infections. *J Infect Dis* 1993;168: 1490.
11. Munoz A et al. Long-term survivors with HIV-1 infection: incubation period and longitudinal patterns of CD4+ lymphocytes. *J Acquir Immune Defic Syndr Hum Retrovirol* 1995;8:496.
12. Fauci AS et al. Immunopathogenic mechanisms of HIV infection. *Ann Intern Med* 1996;124:654.
13. Crowe SM et al. Predictive value of CD4+ lymphocyte numbers for the development of opportunistic infections and malignancies in HIV-infected persons. *J Acquir Immun Defic Syndr Hum Retrovirol* 1991;4:770.
14. Holmberg SD et al. The spectrum of medical conditions and symptoms before acquired immunodeficiency syndrome in homosexual and bisexual men infected with the human immunodeficiency virus. *Am J Epidemiol* 1996;141:395.
15. Moore RD et al. Natural history of opportunistic disease in an HIV-infected urban clinical cohort. *Ann Intern Med* 1996;124:633.
16. Egger M et al. Prognosis of HIV-1-infected patients starting highly active antiretroviral therapy; a collaborative analysis of prospective studies. *Lancet* 2002;360:119.
17. Welles SL et al. Prognostic value of plasma human immunodeficiency virus type 1 (HIV-1) RNA levels in patients with advanced HIV-1 disease and with little or no prior zidovudine therapy. *J Infect Dis* 1996;174:696.
18. Coombs SL. Association of plasma human immunodeficiency virus type 1 RNA level with risk of clinical progression in patients with advanced infection. *J Infect Dis* 1996;174:704.
19. Donovan RM et al. Changes in virus load markers during AIDS-associated opportunistic diseases in human immunodeficiency virus-infected persons. *J Infect Dis* 1996;174:401.
20. Galetto-Lacour A et al. Prognostic value of viremia in patients with long-standing human immunodeficiency virus infection. *J Infect Dis* 1996;173:1388.
21. Chaisson RE et al. Impact of opportunistic disease on survival in patients with HIV infection. *AIDS* 1998;12:29.
22. Mellors JW et al. Plasma viral load and CD4+ lymphocyte as prognostic markers of HIV-1 infection. *Ann Intern Med* 1997;126:946.
23. Guidelines for the use of antiretroviral agents in HIV-infected adults and adolescents. The Department of Health and Human Services and the Henry J. Kaiser Family Foundation. AIDS Treatment Information Service (ATIS). Available at http://www.aidsinfo.nih.gov/guidelines. Accessed February 28, 2008.
24. Sepkowitz KA. The effect of HAART on the natural history of AIDS-related opportunistic conditions. *Lancet* 1998;351:228.
25. Mourton Y et al. Impact of protease inhibitors on AIDS-defining events and hospitalizations in 10 French AIDS reference centres. *AIDS* 1997;11: 101.
26. Mars ME et al. Protease inhibitors lead to a change of infectious diseases unit activity [Abstract]. In: *Programs and Abstracts of the 4th Conference on Retroviruses and Opportunistic Infections.* Washington, DC: IDSA Foundation for Retrovirology and Human Health; 1997.
27. Micheals S et al. Difference in the incidence rates of opportunistic infections before and after the availability of protease inhibitors [Abstract]. In: *Programs and Abstracts of the 5th Conference on Retroviruses and Opportunistic Infections;* Chicago, IL: 1998.
28. Kaplan JE et al. Epidemiology of human immunodeficiency virus-associated opportunistic infections in the United States in the era of highly active antiretroviral therapy. *CID* 2000;30:S5.
29. Palella F et al. Reducing morbidity and mortality among patients with advanced human immunodeficiency virus infection. *N Engl J Med* 1998;338:853.
30. Hammer SM et al. A controlled trial of two nucleoside analogues plus indinavir in persons with human immunodeficiency virus infection and CD4+ cell counts of 200 per cubic millimeter or less. *N Engl J Med* 1997;337:725.
31. Centers for Disease Control and Prevention. Update: trends in AIDS incidences, death and prevalence, United States, 1996. *MMWR Morbid Mortal Wkly Rep* 1997;46:165.
32. Race EM et al. Focal mycobacterial lymphadenitis following initiation of protease inhibitor therapy in patients with advanced HIV-1 disease. *Lancet* 1998;351:252.
33. Tural C et al. Lack of reactivation of cytomegalovirus retinitis after stopping maintenance therapy in HIV-infected patients. *J Infect Dis* 1998;177:1080.
34. Whitcup SM et al. Therapeutic effect of combination antiretroviral therapy on cytomegalovirus retinitis. *JAMA* 1997;277:1519.
35. Jacobson MA et al. Cytomegalovirus retinitis after initiation of highly active antiretroviral therapy. *Lancet* 1997;349:1443.
36. Autran B et al. Positive effects of combined antiviral therapy on the CD4+ T cell homeostasis and function in advanced HIV disease. *Science* 1997;227:112.
37. Rutschmann OT et al. Impact of treatment with HIV protease inhibitors on hepatitis C viremia in patients co-infected with HIV. *J Infect Dis* 1998;177:783.
38. Murphy M et al. Regression of AIDS-related Kaposi's sarcoma following treatment with an HIV-1 protease inhibitor. *AIDS* 1997;11:26.
39. Elliott B et al. 25 year remission of AIDS-associated progressive multifocal leukoencephalopathy with combined antiretroviral therapy. *Lancet* 1997;349: 850.
40. Carr A et al. Treatment of HIV-1 associated microsporidiosis and cryptosporidiosis with combination antiretroviral therapy. *Lancet* 1998;351:256.
41. Hicks CB et al. Resolution of intractable molluscum contagiosum in a human immunodeficiency virus infected patient after institution of antiretroviral therapy with ritonavir. *Clin Infect Dis* 1997;24:1023.
42. Carr A, Cooper DA. Restoration of immunity to chronic hepatitis B infection in HIV-infected patients on protease inhibitor. *Lancet* 1997;349:996.
43. Masur H. Management of opportunistic infections associated with human immunodeficiency virus infection. In: Mandell GL et al., eds. *Principles and Practice of Infectious Diseases.* 5th ed. New York: Churchill Livingstone; 2000:1500.
44. Whitley RJ et al. Consensus statement. Guidelines for the treatment of cytomegalovirus diseases in patients with AIDS in the era of potent antiretroviral therapy. *Arch Intern Med* 1998;158:957.
45. Sepkowitz KA. Effect of prophylaxis on the clinical manifestations of AIDS-related opportunistic infections. *Clin Infect Dis* 1998;26:806.
46. Centers for Disease Control and Prevention. 1997 USPHS/IDSA guidelines for the prevention of opportunistic infections in persons infected with human immunodeficiency virus. *MMWR Morbid Mortal Wkly Rep* 1997;46:1.
47. Centers for Disease Control and Prevention. 1999 USPHS/IDSA guidelines for the prevention of opportunistic infections in persons infected with human immunodeficiency virus. *MMWR Morbid Mortal Wkly Rep* 1999;48(RR-10):1.
48. Centers for Disease Control and Prevention. 2002 USPHS/IDSA guidelines for the prevention of opportunistic infections in persons infected with human immunodeficiency virus. *MMWR Morbid Mortal Wkly Rep* 2002;51:1.
49. Centers for Disease Control and Prevention. Treating opportunistic infections among HIV-infected adults and adolescents. *MMWR Morbid Mortal Wkly Rep* 2004;53(RR15):1.
50. Fischl MA et al. Safety and efficacy of sulfamethoxazole and trimethoprim chemoprophylaxis for *Pneumocystis carinii* pneumonia in AIDS. *JAMA* 1988;259:1185.
51. Pierce MD et al. A randomized trial of clarithromycin as prophylaxis against disseminated *Mycobacterium avium* complex infection in patients with advanced acquired immunodeficiency syndrome. *N Engl J Med* 1996;335:384.
52. Schneider MME et al. Discontinuation of *Pneumocystis carinii* pneumonia (PCP) prophylaxis in HIV-1 infected patients treated with highly active antiretroviral therapy. *Lancet* 1999;353:201.
53. Furrer H et al. Discontinuation of primary prophylaxis against PCP in HIV-1 infected adults treated with combination ARVT. Swiss HIV cohort study. *N Engl J Med* 1999;340:1301.
54. Weverling GJ et al. Discontinuation of *Pneumocystis carinii* pneumonia prophylaxis after start of highly active antiretroviral therapy in HIV-1 infection. EUROSIDA study group. *Lancet* 1999;353:1293.
55. Dworkin MS et al. Risk for preventable opportunistic infections in persons with AIDS after antiretroviral therapy increases CD4+ T lymphocyte counts above prophylaxis thresholds. *J Infect Dis* 2000;182:611.
56. MacDonald JC et al. Lack of reactivation of cytomegalovirus (CMV) retinitis after stopping CMV maintenance therapy in AIDS patients with sustained elevations in CD4 T cells in response to highly active antiretroviral therapy. *J Infect Dis* 1998;177:1182.
57. Jabs DA et al. Discontinuing anticytomegalovirus therapy in patients with immune reconstitution after combination antiretroviral therapy. *Am J Ophthalmol* 1998;126:817.
58. Jouan M et al. Discontinuation of maintenance therapy for cytomegalovirus retinitis in HIV-infected patients receiving highly active antiretroviral therapy. RESTIMOP Study Team. *AIDS* 2001;15: 23.
59. Vrabec TR et al. Discontinuation of maintenance therapy in patients with quiescent cytomegalovirus retinitis and elevated CD4+ counts. *Ophthalmology* 1998;105:1259.
60. Reed JB et al. Regression of cytomegalovirus retinitis associated with protease inhibitors treatment

in patients with AIDS. *Am J Ophthalmol* 1997;124:199.
61. Torriani FJ et al. Lack of progression after discontinuation of maintenance therapy (MT) for cytomegalovirus retinitis (CMVR) in AIDS patients responding to highly antiretroviral therapy (HAART). *J Infect Dis* 1998;177:1182.
62. Young LS. *Pneumocystis carinii* pneumonia. In: Walzer PD, ed. *Pneumocystis carinii* Pneumonia. Rev. ed. New York: Marcel Dekker; 1993.
63. Edman JC et al. Ribosomal RNA sequence shows *Pneumocystis carinii* to be a member of fungi. *Nature* 1988;334:519.
64. Masur H. Pneumocystosis. In: Dolin R et al., eds. *AIDS Therapy*. Philadelphia: Churchill Livingstone; 1999:299.
65. Montgomery AB. *Pneumocystis carinii* pneumonia in patients with the acquired immunodeficiency syndrome. Pathophysiology and therapy. *AIDS Clin Rev* 1991:127.
66. Rose PD. *Clinical Physiology of Acid–Base and Electrolyte Disorders*. 3rd ed. New York: McGraw-Hill; 1989.
67. Sattler FR, Jelliffe RW. Pharmacokinetic and pharmacodynamic considerations for drug dosing in the treatment of *Pneumocystis carinii* pneumonia. In: Walzer PD, ed. *Pneumocystis carinii* Pneumonia. New York: Marcel Dekker; 1993:467.
68. Lee BL et al. Altered patterns of drug metabolism in patients with acquired immunodeficiency syndrome. *Clin Pharmacol Ther* 1993;53:529.
69. Gluckstein D, Ruskin J. Rapid oral desensitization to trimethoprim-sulfamethoxazole (TMP-SMX): use in prophylaxis for *Pneumocystis carinii* pneumonia in patients with AIDS who were previously intolerant to TMP-SMX. *Clin Infect Dis* 1995;20:849.
70. Warren E et al. Advances in the treatment and prophylaxis of *Pneumocystis carinii* pneumonia. *Pharmacotherapy* 1997;17:900.
71. O'Brien J et al. A 5-year retrospective review of adverse drug reactions and their risk factors in human immunodeficiency virus-infected patients who were receiving intravenous pentamidine therapy for *Pneumocystis carinii*. *Clin Infect Dis* 1997;24:854.
72. Foisey M et al. Pancreatitis during intravenous pentamidine therapy in an AIDS patient with prior exposure to didanosine. *Ann Pharmacother* 1994;28:1025.
73. Conte JE et al. Intravenous or inhaled pentamidine for treating *Pneumocystis carinii* pneumonia in AIDS. A randomized trial. *Ann Intern Med* 1990;113:203.
74. Sattler FR et al. Trimetrexate with leucovorin versus trimethoprim-sulfamethoxazole for moderate to severe episodes of *Pneumocystis carinii* pneumonia in patients with AIDS: a prospective, controlled multicenter investigation of the AIDS Clinical Trials Group Protocol 029/031. *J Infect Dis* 1994;170:165.
75. Fishman JA. Treatment of infection due to *Pneumocystis carinii*. *Antimicrob Agents Chemo* 1998;42:1309.
76. Dohn MN et al. Open-label efficacy and safety trial of 42 days of 566C80 for *Pneumocystis carinii* pneumonia in AIDS patients. *J Protozool* 1991;38:220S.
77. Falloon J et al. A preliminary evaluation of 566C80 for the treatment of *Pneumocystis* pneumonia in patients with the acquired immunodeficiency syndrome. *N Engl J Med* 1991;325:1534.
78. Gutteridge WE. 566C80, an antimalarial hydroxynaphthoquinone with broad spectrum: experimental activity against opportunistic parasitic infections of AIDS patients. *J Protozool* 1991;38:141S.
79. Hughes W et al. Comparison of atovaquone (566C80) with trimethoprim-sulfamethoxazole to treat *Pneumocystis carinii* pneumonia in patients with AIDS. *N Engl J Med* 1993;328:1521.
80. Dohn MN et al. and the Atovaquone Study Group. Oral atovaquone compared with intravenous pentamidine for *Pneumocystis carinii* pneumonia in patients with AIDS. *Ann Intern Med* 1994;121:174.
81. Safrin S et al. Dapsone as a single agent is suboptimal therapy for *Pneumocystis carinii* pneumonia. *J Acquir Immune Defic Syndr* 1991;4:244.
82. Safrin S et al. Comparison of three regimens for treatment of mild to moderate *Pneumocystis carinii* pneumonia in patients with AIDS. A double-blind, randomized, trial of oral trimethoprim-sulfamethoxazole, dapsone-trimethoprim, and clindamycin-primaquine. ACTG 108 Study Group. *Ann Intern Med* 1996;124:792.
83. Medina I et al. Oral therapy for *Pneumocystis carinii* pneumonia in the acquired immunodeficiency syndrome. A controlled trial of trimethoprim-sulfamethoxazole versus trimethoprim-dapsone. *N Engl J Med* 1990;323:776.
84. Lee BL et al. Dapsone, trimethoprim, and sulfamethoxazole plasma levels during treatment of *Pneumocystis* pneumonia in patients with the acquired immunodeficiency syndrome (AIDS). *Ann Intern Med* 1989;110:606.
85. Sin DD, Shafran SD. Dapsone and primaquine induced methemoglobinemia in HIV-infected individuals. *J Acquir Immune Defic Syndr Hum Retrovirol* 1996;12:477.
86. Bozzette SA et al. A controlled trial of early adjunctive treatment with corticosteroids for *Pneumocystis carinii* pneumonia in the acquired immunodeficiency syndrome. California Collaborative Treatment Group. *N Engl J Med* 1990;323:1451.
87. Nielsen TL et al. Adjunctive corticosteroid therapy for *Pneumocystis carinii* pneumonia in AIDS: a randomized European multicenter open label study. *J Acquir Immune Defic Syndr Hum Retrovirol* 1992;5:726.
88. Gagnon S et al. Corticosteroids as adjunctive therapy for severe *Pneumocystis carinii* pneumonia in the acquired immunodeficiency syndrome. A double-blind, placebo-controlled trial. *N Engl J Med* 1990;323:1444.
89. Montaner JS et al. Corticosteroids prevent early deterioration in patients with moderately severe *Pneumocystis carinii* pneumonia and the acquired immunodeficiency syndrome (AIDS). *J Acquir Immune Defic Syndr Hum Retrovirol* 1990;113:14.
90. Sistek CJ et al. Adjuvant corticosteroid therapy for *Pneumocystis carinii* pneumonia in AIDS patients. *Ann Pharmacother* 1992;26:1127.
91. LaRocco A Jr et al. Corticosteroids for *Pneumocystis carinii* pneumonia with acute respiratory failure. Experience with rescue therapy. *Chest* 1992;102:892.
92. Bozzette SA, Morston SC. Reconsidering the use of adjunctive corticosteroids in *Pneumocystis* pneumonia? *J Acquire Immune Defic Syndr Hum Retrovirol* 1995;8:345.
93. Briel M et al. Adjunctive corticosteroids for Pneumocystis jiroveci pneumonia in patients with HIV-infection. *Cochrane Database of Systematic Reviews* 2006;3:CD006150. DOI.10.1002/14651858.CD006150.
94. Kovacs JA et al. Prophylaxis for *Pneumocystis carinii* pneumonia in patients infected with human immunodeficiency virus. *Clin Infect Dis* 1992;14:1005.
95. Loannidis JP et al. A meta-analysis of the relative efficacy and toxicity of *Pneumocystis carinii* prophylaxis regimens. *Arch Intern Med* 1996;156:177.
96. Opravil M et al. Once-weekly administration of dapsone/pyrimethamine versus aerosolized pentamidine as combined prophylaxis for *Pneumocystis carinii* pneumonia and toxoplasmic encephalitis in human immunodeficiency virus-infected patients. *Clin Infect Dis* 1995;20:531.
97. El-Sadr W et al. Atovaquone compared with dapsone for the prevention of *Pneumocystis carinii* pneumonia in patients with HIV infection who cannot tolerate trimethoprim, sulfonamides, or both. *N Engl J Med* 1998;339:1889.
98. Selik MA et al. Trends in infectious diseases and cancers among persons dying of HIV infection in the United States from 1987 to 1992. *Ann Intern Med* 1995;123:933.
99. Leoung GS et al. Trimethoprim-sulfamethoxazole (TMP-SMZ) dose escalation versus direct rechallenge for *Pneumocystis carinii* pneumonia prophylaxis in human immunodeficiency virus-infected patients with previous adverse reaction to TMP-SMZ. *J Infect Dis* 2001;184:992.
100. Para MF et al. for the ACTG 268 Study Team. ACTG 286 Trial: gradual initiation of trimethoprim/sulfamethoxazole (T/S) as primary prophylaxis for *Pneumocystis carinii* pneumonia (PCP). In: *Abstracts of the 4th Conference on Retroviruses and Opportunistic Infections;* Washington, DC: 1997. Abstract No. 2.
101. Bozzette S et al. A randomized trial of three anti-*Pneumocystis* agents in patients with advanced human immunodeficiency virus infection. *N Engl J Med* 1995;332:693.
102. Noskin GA et al. Extrapulmonary infection with *Pneumocystis carinii* in patients receiving aerosolized pentamidine. *Rev Infect Dis* 1991;13:525.
103. Telzak EE, Armstrong D. Extrapulmonary infection and other unusual manifestations of *Pneumocystis carinii*. In: Walzer PD, ed. *Pneumocystis carinii* Pneumonia. New York: Marcel Dekker; 1993:361.
104. Lopez Bernaldo de Quiros JC et al; Grupo de Estudio del SIDA 04/98. A randomized trial of the discontinuation of primary and secondary prophylaxis against *Pneumocystis carinii* pneumonia after highly active antiretroviral therapy in patients with HIV infection. Grupo de Estudio del SIDA 04/98. *N Engl J Med* 2001;344:159.
105. Dworkin M et al. Risk for preventable opportunistic infections in persons with AIDS after antiretroviral therapy increases CD4+ T lymphocyte counts above prophylaxis thresholds. *J Infect Dis* 2000;182:611.
106. Kirk O et al. Can chemoprophylaxis against opportunistic infections be discontinued after an increase in CD4 cells induced by highly active antiretroviral therapy? *AIDS* 1999;13:1647.
107. Soriano V et al. Discontinuation of secondary prophylaxis for opportunistic infections in HIV-infected patients receiving highly active antiretroviral therapy. *AIDS* 2000;14:383.
108. Ledergerber B et al. Discontinuation of secondary prophylaxis against *Pneumocystis carinii* pneumonia in patients with HIV infection who have a response to antiretroviral therapy. Eight European study groups. *N Engl J Med* 2001;344:168.
109. Chintu C et al. Co-trimoxazole as prophylaxis against opportunistic infections in HIV-infected Zambian children (CHAP): a double-blind randomised placebo-controlled trial. *Lancet* 2004;364:1865.
110. Grimwade K, Swingler G. Cotrimoxazole prophylaxis for opportunistic infections in adults with HIV (Cochrane Review). In: *The Cochrane Library,* Issue 2, 2004. Chichester, UK: John Wiley & Sons.
111. Montoya JG, Remington JS. *Toxoplasma gondii*. In: Mandell GL et al., eds. *Principles and Practice of Infectious Diseases*. 5th ed. New York: Churchill Livingstone; 2000:2858.
112. Murray HW. Toxoplasmosis. In: Dolin R et al., eds. *AIDS Therapy*. Philadelphia: Churchill Livingstone; 1999:307.
113. Matthews C et al. Early biopsy versus empiric treatment with delayed biopsy of non-responders in suspected HIV-associated cerebral toxoplasmosis: a decision analysis. *AIDS* 1995;9:1243.
114. Harrison PB et al. Focal brain lesions on computed tomography in patients with acquired immune deficiency syndrome. *Can Assoc Radiol J* 1990;41:83.
115. Girard PM et al. Dapsone-pyrimethamine compared with aerosolized pentamidine as primary prophylaxis against *Pneumocystis carinii* pneumonia and toxoplasmosis in HIV infection. The PRIO Study Group. *N Engl J Med* 1993;328:1514.
116. Hardy WD et al. A controlled trial of trimethoprim-sulfamethoxazole or aerosolized pentamidine for secondary prophylaxis of *Pneumocystis carinii*

pneumonia in patients with the acquired immunodeficiency syndrome. AIDS Clinical Trials Group Protocol 021. *N Engl J Med* 1992;327:1842.
117. Carr A et al. Low-dose trimethoprim-sulfamethoxazole prophylaxis for toxoplasmic encephalitis in patients with AIDS. *Ann Intern Med* 1992;117:106.
118. Podzamezer D et al. Intermittent trimethoprim-sulfamethoxazole compared with dapsone-pyrimethamine for the simultaneous primary prophylaxis of *Pneumocystis* pneumonia and toxoplasmosis in patients infected with HIV. *Ann Intern Med* 1995;122:755.
119. Leport C et al. Pyrimethamine for primary prophylaxis of *Toxoplasma* encephalitis in patients with HIV infection: a double-blind, randomized trial. *J Infect Dis* 1996;173:91.
120. Jacobson M et al. Primary prophylaxis with pyrimethamine for *Toxoplasma* encephalitis in patients with advanced HIV disease. Results of a randomized trial. *J Infect Dis* 1994;169:384.
121. Dworkin M et al. Risk for preventable opportunistic infections in persons with AIDS after antiretroviral therapy increases CD4+ T lymphocyte counts above prophylaxis thresholds. *J Infect Dis* 2000;182:611.
122. Kirk O et al. Can chemoprophylaxis against opportunistic infections be discontinued after an increase in CD4 cells induced by highly active antiretroviral therapy? *AIDS* 1999;13:1647.
123. Furrer H et al. Stopping primary prophylaxis in HIV-1-infected patients at high risk of toxoplasma encephalitis. Swiss HIV Cohort Study. *Lancet* 2000;355:22178.
124. Mussini C et al. Discontinuation of primary prophylaxis for *Pneumocystis carinii* pneumonia and toxoplasmic encephalitis in human immunodeficiency virus type I-infected patients: the changes in opportunistic prophylaxis study. *J Infect Dis* 2000;181:1635.
125. Miro JM et al. Discontinuation of primary and secondary *Toxoplasma gondii* prophylaxis is safe in HIV-1 infected patients after immunological restoration with highly active antiretroviral therapy: results of an open, randomized, multicenter clinical trial. *Clin Infect Dis* 2006;43:79.
126. de la Hoz Caballer B et al. Management of sulfadiazine allergy in patients with acquired immunodeficiency syndrome. *J Allergy Clin Immunol* 1991;88:137.
127. Tenant-Flowers M et al. Sulfadiazine desensitization in patients with AIDS and cerebral toxoplasmosis. *AIDS* 1991;5:311.
128. Katlama C et al. Pyrimethamine-clindamycin versus pyrimethamine-sulfadiazine as acute and long-term therapy for toxoplasmic encephalitis in patients with AIDS. *Clin Infect Dis* 1996;22:268.
129. Molina JM et al. Sulfadiazine-induced crystalluria in AIDS patients with *Toxoplasma* encephalitis. *AIDS* 1991;5:587.
130. Oster S et al. Resolution of acute renal failure in toxoplasmic encephalitis despite continuance of sulfadiazine. *Rev Infect Dis* 1990;12:618.
131. Ventura MG et al. Sulfadiazine revisited. *J Infect Dis* 1989;160:556.
132. Simon DI et al. Sulfadiazine crystalluria revisited. The treatment of *Toxoplasma* encephalitis in patients with acquired immunodeficiency syndrome. *Arch Intern Med* 1990;150:2379.
133. Christin S et al. Acute renal failure due to sulfadiazine in patients with AIDS. *Nephron* 1990;55:233.
134. Remington J. Availability of sulfadiazine, United States. *JAMA* 1993;269:461.
135. EON Labs Manufacturers, Inc. Laurelton, NY. Available at: http://www.EONLABS.COM.
136. Holliman RE. Folate supplements and the treatment of cerebral toxoplasmosis. *Scand J Infect Dis* 1989;21:475.
137. Frenkel JK et al. Relative reversal by vitamins (p-aminobenzoic, folic, and folinic acids) of the effects of sulfadiazine and pyrimethamine on *Toxoplasma*, mouse and man. *Antibiot Chemother* 1957;VII:630.
138. Eyles DE et al. The effect of metabolites on the antitoxoplasmic action of pyrimethamine and sulfadiazine. *Am J Trop Med* 1960;9:277.
139. Podzamczer D et al. Twice weekly maintenance therapy with sulfadiazine-pyrimethamine to prevent recurrent toxoplasmosis encephalitis in patients with AIDS. Spanish Toxoplasmosis Study Group. *Ann Intern Med* 1995;123:175.
140. Katlama C. Evaluation of the efficacy and safety of clindamycin plus pyrimethamine for induction and maintenance therapy of toxoplasmic encephalitis in AIDS. *Eur J Clin Microbiol Infect Dis* 1991;10:189.
141. Leport C et al. Long-term follow-up of patients with AIDS on maintenance therapy for toxoplasmosis. *Eur J Clin Microbiol Infect Dis* 1991;10:191.
142. Bhatti N et al. Low-dose alternate-day pyrimethamine for maintenance therapy in cerebral toxoplasmosis complicating AIDS. *J Infect Dis* 1990;21:119.
143. Ruf B et al. Role of clindamycin in the treatment of acute toxoplasmosis of the central nervous system. *Eur J Clin Microbiol Infect Dis* 1991;10:183.
144. Rolston KV. Treatment of acute toxoplasmosis with oral clindamycin. *Eur J Clin Microbiol Infect Dis* 1991;10:181.
145. Foppa CU et al. A retrospective study of primary and maintenance therapy of toxoplasmic encephalitis with oral clindamycin and pyrimethamine. *Eur J Clin Microbiol Infect Dis* 1991;10:187.
146. Dannemann BR et al. Treatment of acute toxoplasmosis with intravenous clindamycin. The California Collaborative Treatment Group. *Eur J Clin Microbiol Infect Dis* 1991;10:193.
147. Araujo FG et al. *In vitro* and *in vivo* activities of the hydroxynaphthoquinone 566C80 against the cyst form of *Toxoplasma gondii*. *Antimicrob Agents Chemother* 1991;36:326.
148. Araujo FG et al. Remarkable in vitro and in vivo activities of the hydroxynaphthoquinone 566C80 against tachyzoites and tissue cysts of *Toxoplasma gondii*. *Antimicrob Agents Chemother* 1991;35:293.
149. Gianotti N et al. Efficacy and safety of atovaquone (556C80) in the treatment of cerebral toxoplasmosis (CT) and *Pneumocystis carinii* pneumonia (PCP) in HIV-infected patients. Paper presented to the IXth International Conference on AIDS in affiliation with the IVth STD World Congress; Berlin: 1993.
150. White A et al. Comparison to natural history data of survival of toxoplasmic encephalitis patients treated with atovaquone. Paper presented to the IXth International Conference on AIDS in affiliation with the IVth STD World Congress; Berlin: 1993.
151. Torres RA et al. Atovaquone for salvage treatment and suppression of toxoplasmic encephalitis in patients with AIDS. *Clin Infect Dis* 1997;24:422.
152. Chang HR et al. In vitro and in vivo effects of doxycycline on *Toxoplasma gondii*. *Antimicrob Agents Chemother* 1990;34:775.
153. Alder J et al. Treatment of experimental *Toxoplasma gondii* infection by clarithromycin-based combination therapies. *J Acquir Defic Syndr Hum Retrovirol* 1994;7:1141.
154. Salmon-Ceron D. Cytomegalovirus infection. *HIV Med* 2001;2:255.
155. Holland GN, et al. Characteristics of untreated AIDS-related cytomegalovirus retinitis II. Findings in the era of highly active antiretroviral therapy (1997 to 2000). *Am J Ophthalmol* 2008;145:12.
156. Jennens ID et al. Cytomegalovirus cultures during maintenance DHPG therapy for cytomegalovirus (CMV) retinitis in acquired immunodeficiency syndrome (AIDS). *J Med Virol* 1990;30:42.
157. Shinkai M et al. Utility of urine and leukocyte cultures and plasma DNA polymerase chain reaction for identification of AIDS patients at risk for developing human cytomegalovirus disease. *J Infect Dis* 1997;175:302.
158. Dodt KK et al. Development of cytomegalovirus (CMV) disease may be predicted in HIV-infected patients by CMV polymerase chain reaction and the antigenemia test. *AIDS* 1997;11:F21.
159. Bowen EF et al. Cytomegalovirus (CMV) viremia detected by polymerase chain reaction identifies a group of HIV-positive patients at high risk of CMV disease. *AIDS* 1997;11:889.
160. Jacobson MA. Treatment of cytomegalovirus retinitis in patients with the acquired immunodeficiency syndrome. *N Engl J Med* 1997;337:105.
161. Masur H et al. Advances in the management of AIDS-related cytomegalovirus retinitis. *Ann Intern Med* 1996;125:126.
162. Parenteral cidofovir for cytomegalovirus retinitis in patients with AIDS: the HPMPC Peripheral Cytomegalovirus Retinitis Trial. A randomized, controlled trial. Studies of Ocular Complications of AIDS Research Group in collaboration with the AIDS Clinical Trials Group. *Ann Intern Med* 1997;126:264.
163. Combination foscarnet and ganciclovir therapy vs monotherapy for the treatment of relapsed cytomegalovirus retinitis in patients with AIDS. The Cytomegalovirus Retreatment Trial. The Studies of Ocular Complications of AIDS Research Group in collaboration with the AIDS Clinical Trials Group. *Arch Ophthalmol* 1996;114:23.
164. Musch DC et al. Treatment of cytomegalovirus retinitis with a sustained-release ganciclovir implant. *N Engl J Med* 1997;337:83.
165. Martin DF et al. A controlled trial of valganciclovir as induction therapy for cytomegalovirus retinitis. *N Engl J Med* 2002;346:1119.
166. Mar E et al. Effect of 9-(1,3-dihydroxy-2-propoxymethyl)guanine on human cytomegalovirus replication in vitro. *Antimicrob Agents Chemother* 1983;24:518.
167. Smee DF et al. Anti-herpesvirus activity of the acyclic nucleoside 9-(1,3-dihydroxy-2-propoxymethyl)guanine. *Antimicrob Agents Chemother* 1983;23:676.
168. Biron KK et al. A human cytomegalovirus mutant resistant to the nucleoside analog 9-([2-hydroxy-1-(hydroxymethyl)ethoxy]methyl)guanine (BW B759U) induces reduced levels of BW B759U triphosphate. *Proc Natl Acad Sci U S A* 1986;83:8769.
169. Fletcher CV et al. Evaluation of ganciclovir for cytomegalovirus disease. *DICP* 1989;23:5.
170. Weisenthal RW et al. Long-term outpatient treatment of CMV retinitis with ganciclovir in AIDS patients. *Br J Ophthalmol* 1989;73:996.
171. Peters BS et al. Cytomegalovirus infection in AIDS. Patterns of disease, response to therapy and trends in survival. *J Infect Dis* 1991;23:129.
172. Crumpacker CS. Ganciclovir. *N Engl J Med* 1996;335:721.
173. SOCA. Morbidity and toxic effects associated with ganciclovir or foscarnet therapy in a randomized cytomegalovirus retinitis trial. *Arch Intern Med* 1995;155:65.
174. Hardy WD. Combined ganciclovir and recombinant human granulocyte-macrophage colony-stimulating factor in the treatment of cytomegalovirus retinitis in AIDS patients. *J Acquir Immun Defic Syndr Hum Retrovirol* 1991;4:S22.
175. Jacobson MA et al. Ganciclovir with recombinant methionyl human granulocyte colony-stimulating factor for treatment of cytomegalovirus disease in AIDS patients. *AIDS* 1992;6:515.
176. Koyanagi Y et al. Cytokines alter production of HIV-1 from primary mononuclear phagocytes. *Science* 1988;241:1673.
177. Perno CF et al. Effects of bone marrow stimulatory cytokines on human immunodeficiency virus replication and the antiviral activity of dideoxynucleosides in cultures of monocyte/macrophages. *Blood* 1992;80:995.
178. Cundy KC et al. Clinical pharmacokinetics of cidofovir in human immunodeficiency virus-infected patients. *Antimicrob Agents Chem* 1995;39:1247.
179. Lalezari JP et al. Intravenous cidofovir for peripheral cytomegalovirus retinitis in patients with AIDS. *Ann Intern Med* 1997;126:257.
180. Aweeka F et al. Pharmacokinetics of intermittently administered intravenous foscarnet in the treatment of acquired immunodeficiency syndrome patients

with serious cytomegalovirus retinitis. *Antimicrob Agents Chemother* 1989;33:742.
181. Deray G et al. Foscarnet nephrotoxicity: mechanism, incidence and prevention. *Am J Nephrol* 1989;9:316.
182. SOCA. Mortality in patients with the acquired immunodeficiency syndrome treated with either foscarnet or ganciclovir for cytomegalovirus retinitis. Studies of Ocular Complications of AIDS Research Group, in collaboration with the AIDS Clinical Trials Group. *N Engl J Med* 1992;326:213.
183. Jacobson MA et al. Foscarnet treatment of cytomegalovirus retinitis in patients with the acquired immunodeficiency syndrome. *Antimicrob Agents Chemother* 1989;33:736.
184. Youle MS et al. Severe hypocalcaemia in AIDS patients treated with foscarnet and pentamidine. *Lancet* 1988;1:1455.
185. Jacobson MA et al. Foscarnet therapy for ganciclovir-resistant cytomegalovirus retinitis in patients with AIDS. *J Infect Dis* 1991;163:1348.
186. Jayaweera DT. Minimising the dosage-limiting toxicities of foscarnet induction therapy. *Drug Safety* 1997;16:258.
187. Jacobson MA et al. Randomized phase I trial of two different combination foscarnet and ganciclovir chronic maintenance therapy regimens for AIDS patients with cytomegalovirus retinitis: AIDS Clinical Trials Group protocol 151. *J Infect Dis* 1994;170:189.
188. Foscarnet-ganciclovir cytomegalovirus retinitis trial 4. Visual outcomes. Studies of Ocular Complications of AIDS Research Group in collaboration with the AIDS Clinical Trials Group. *Ophthalmology* 1994;101:1250.
189. Holland GN et al. Dose-related difference in progression rates of cytomegalovirus retinopathy during foscarnet maintenance therapy. *Am J Ophthalmol* 1995;199:576.
190. Jacobson MA et al. A dose-ranging study of daily maintenance intravenous foscarnet therapy for cytomegalovirus retinitis in AIDS. *J Infect Dis* 1993;168:444.
191. Jabs DA et al. Cytomegalovirus retinitis and viral resistance: ganciclovir resistance. *J Infect Dis* 1998; 177:770.
192. Chou S et al. Frequency of UL97 phosphotransferase mutations related to ganciclovir resistance in clinical cytomegalovirus isolates. *J Infect Dis* 1995;172:239.
193. Smith IL et al. High-level resistance of cytomegalovirus to ganciclovir is associated with alterations in both UL97 and DNA polymerase genes. *J Infect Dis* 1997;176:69.
194. Azad RF et al. Antiviral activity of a phosphorothioate oligonucleotide complementary to human cytomegalovirus RNA when used in combination with antiviral nucleoside analogs. *Antiviral Res* 1995;28:101.
195. Fausto B et al. Single amino acid changes in the DNA polymerase confer foscarnet resistance and slow-growth phenotype, while mutations in the UL97-encoded phosphotransferase confer ganciclovir resistance in three double-resistant human cytomegalovirus strains recovered from patients with AIDS. *J Virol* 1996;70:1390.
196. Kuppermann BD. Therapeutic options for resistant cytomegalovirus retinitis. *J Acquir Immun Defic Syndr Hum Retrovirol* 1997;14:S13.
197. Perry CM, Balfour JA. Fomivirsen. *Drugs* 1999;57:375.
198. Cochereau-Massin I et al. Efficacy and tolerance of intravitreal ganciclovir in cytomegalovirus retinitis in acquired immune deficiency syndrome. *Ophthalmology* 1991;98:1348.
199. Cantrill HL et al. Treatment of cytomegalovirus retinitis with intravitreal ganciclovir. Long-term results. *Ophthalmology* 1989;96:367.
200. Young SH et al. High dose intravitreal ganciclovir in the treatment of cytomegalovirus retinitis. *Med J Aust* 1992;157:370.
201. Musch DC et al. Treatment of cytomegalovirus retinitis with a sustained-release ganciclovir implant. The Ganciclovir Implant Study Group. *N Engl J Med* 1997;337:83.
202. Martin DF. Treatment of cytomegalovirus retinitis with an intraocular sustained-release ganciclovir implant: a randomized controlled clinical trial. *Arch Ophthalmol* 1994;112:1531.
203. Marx JL et al. Use of the ganciclovir implant in the treatment of recurrent cytomegalovirus retinitis. *Arch Ophthalmol* 1996;114:815.
204. Drew WL et al. Oral ganciclovir as maintenance treatment for cytomegalovirus retinitis in patients with AIDS. *N Engl J Med* 1995;333:615.
205. Syntex. *Cytovene package insert.* Palo Alto, CA: 1996.
206. Anderson RD et al. Ganciclovir absolute bioavailability and steady-state pharmacokinetics after oral administration of two 3000 mg/d dosing regimens in human immunodeficiency virus- and cytomegalovirus-seropositive patients. *Clin Ther* 1995;17:425.
207. Spector SA et al. Oral ganciclovir for the prevention of cytomegalovirus disease in persons with AIDS. *N Engl J Med* 1996;334:1491.
208. Brosgart CL et al. A randomized, placebo-controlled trial of the safety and efficacy of oral ganciclovir for prophylaxis of cytomegalovirus disease in HIV-infected individuals. Terry Beirn Community Programs for Clinical Research on AIDS. *AIDS* 1998;12:269.
209. Rose DN, Sacks HS. Cost-effectiveness of cytomegalovirus (CMV) disease prevention in patients with AIDS: oral ganciclovir and CMV polymerase chain reaction testing. *AIDS* 1997;11:883.
210. Powderly WG. AIDS commentary: cryptococcal meningitis and AIDS. *Clin Infect Dis* 1993;17:837.
211. Van der Horst CM et al. Treatment of cryptococcal meningitis associated with the acquired immunodeficiency syndrome. *N Engl J Med* 1997;337:15.
212. Goodman L, Gilman A, eds. *The Pharmacological Basis of Therapeutics.* New York: Macmillan; 1995:1236.
213. Shadomy S et al. In vitro studies with combination 5-fluorocytosine and amphotericin B. *Antimicrob Agents Chemother* 1975;8:117.
214. Bennett JE et al. A comparison of amphotericin B alone and combined with flucytosine in the treatment of cryptococcal meningitis. *N Engl J Med* 1979;301:126.
215. Chuck SL et al. Infections with cryptococcal meningitis and AIDS. *N Engl J Med* 1989;321:794.
216. Polsky B et al. Intraventricular therapy of cryptococcal meningitis via a subcutaneous reservoir. *Am J Med* 1986;81:24.
217. Grant SM et al. Fluconazole: a review of its pharmacodynamic and pharmacokinetic properties, and therapeutic potential in superficial and systemic mycoses. *Drugs* 1990;39:877.
218. Saag MS et al. Comparison of amphotericin B with fluconazole in the treatment of acute AIDS-associated cryptococcal meningitis. The NIAID Mycoses Study Group and the AIDS Clinical Trials Group. *N Engl J Med* 1992;326:83.
219. Larson RA et al. Fluconazole compared with amphotericin B plus flucytosine for cryptococcal meningitis in AIDS. *Ann Intern Med* 1990;113:183.
220. Perfect JR et al. Penetration of imidazoles and triazoles into cerebrospinal fluid of rabbits. *J Antimicrob Chemother* 1985;16:81.
221. deGans J et al. Itraconazole compared with amphotericin B plus flucytosine in AIDS patients with cryptococcal meningitis. *AIDS* 1992;6:185.
222. Bozzette SA et al. A controlled trial of maintenance therapy with fluconazole after treatment of cryptococcal meningitis in the acquired immunodeficiency syndrome. *N Engl J Med* 1991;324:580.
223. Powderly WG et al. A controlled trial of fluconazole or amphotericin B to prevent relapse of cryptococcal meningitis in patients with the acquired immunodeficiency syndrome. The NIAID AIDS Clinical Trials Group and Mycoses Study Group. *N Engl J Med* 1992;326:793.
224. deGans J et al. Itraconazole as maintenance treatment for cryptococcal meningitis in the acquired immune deficiency syndrome. *Br Med J* 1988;296:339.
225. Nightingale SD et al. Primary prophylaxis with fluconazole against systemic fungal infections in HIV-positive patients. *AIDS* 1992;6:191.
226. Powderly et al. A randomized trial comparing fluconazole with clotrimazole troches for the prevention of fungal infections in patients with advanced human immunodeficiency virus infection. *N Engl J Med* 1995;332:700.
227. Darouiche RO. Oropharyngeal and esophageal candidiasis in immunocompromised patients: treatment issues. *Clin Infect Dis* 1998;26:259.
228. Milefchik E et al. High dose fluconazole with and without flucytosine for AIDS-associated cryptococcal meningitis. Paper presented to the IX International Conference on AIDS; Berlin: 1993.
229. Mayanja-Kizza H et al. Combination therapy with fluconazole and flucytosine for cryptococcal meningitis in Ugandan patients with AIDS. *Clin Infect Dis* 1998;26:1362.
230. Chambers HF. Tuberculosis in the HIV-infected patient. In: Sande MA, Volberding PA, eds. *The Medical Management of AIDS.* Philadelphia: WB Saunders; 1999:353.
231. World Health Organization. *Global tuberculosis control: surveillance, planning, financing.* Geneva: WHO; 2007.
232. American Thoracic Society. Treatment of tuberculosis infection in adults and children. *Clin Infect Dis* 1995;21:9.
233. Centers for Disease Control and Prevention. Tuberculosis morbidity, United States, 1996. *MMWR Morbid Mortal Wkly Rep* 1997:46:695.
234. Centers for Disease Control and Prevention. Initial therapy for tuberculosis in the era of multidrug resistance: recommendations of the advisory council for the elimination of tuberculosis. *MMWR Morbid Mortal Wkly Rep* 1993;42(RR-7):1.
235. Centers for Disease Control and Prevention. Trends in tuberculosis incidence, United States, 2006. *MMWR Morbid Mortal Wkly Rep* 2007;56:245.
236. Iseman MD. Treatment of multidrug-resistant tuberculosis. *N Engl J Med* 1993;329:784.
237. Goble M et al. Treatment of 171 patients with pulmonary tuberculosis resistant to isoniazid and rifampin. *N Engl J Med* 1993;328:527.
238. Frieden TR et al. The emergence of drug-resistant tuberculosis in New York City. *N Engl J Med* 1993;328:521.
239. Gordin FM et al. The impact of human immunodeficiency virus infection of drug-resistant tuberculosis. *Am J Respir Crit Care Med* 1996;154:1478.
240. Centers for Disease Control and Prevention. Prevention and treatment of tuberculosis among patients infected with human immunodeficiency virus: principles of therapy and revised recommendations. *MMWR Morbid Mortal Wkly Rep* 1998;47(RR-20):1.
241. Berenguer J et al. Tuberculous meningitis in patients infected with the human immunodeficiency virus. *N Engl J Med* 1992;326:668.
242. Smith RL et al. Factors affecting the yield of acid-fast sputum smears in patients with HIV and tuberculosis. *Chest* 1994;106:684.
243. Centers for Disease Control and Prevention. Anergy skin testing and preventive therapy for HIV-infected persons: revised recommendations. *MMWR Morbid Mortal Wkly Rep* 1997;46(RR-15):1.
244. American Thoracic Society. Treatment of tuberculosis and tuberculosis infection in adults and children. *Am J Respir Crit Care Med* 1994;149:1359.
245. Narita M et al. Paradoxical worsening of tuberculosis following antiretroviral therapy in patients with AIDS. *Am J Respir Crit Care Med* 1998;158:157.
246. Villarino ME et al. Management of persons exposed to multidrug-resistant tuberculosis. *MMWR Morbid Mortal Wkly Rep* 1992;41(RR-11):1.
247. Gordon F et al. A randomized trial of 2 months of rifampin and pyrazinamide versus 12 months of isoniazid for the prevention of tuberculosis in HIV-positive, PPD positive patients. In Program and Abstracts: 5th Conference on Retroviruses and

Opportunistic Infections; Chicago, IL; 1998. Abstract LB5.
248. Brix D et al. Correlation of in vivo cellular immunity with CD4+ number and disease progression in HIV seropositive patients. Paper presented to the 5th International Conference on AIDS; Montreal; 1989.
249. Chin DP et al. Clinical utility of a commercial test based on the polymerase chain reaction for detecting *Mycobacterium tuberculosis* in respiratory specimens. *Am J Respir Crit Care Med* 1995;151:1872.
250. Centers for Disease Control and Prevention 2007. Managing drug interactions in the treatment of HIV-related tuberculosis. [online]. Available from URL: http://www.cdc.gov/tb/TB_HIV_Drugs/default/htm
251. Centers for Disease Control and Prevention. Clinical update: impact of HIV protease inhibitors on the treatment of HIV-infected tuberculosis patients with rifampin. *MMWR Morbid Mortal Wkly Rep* 1996;45:921.
252. CDC. Updated guidelines for the use of rifabutin or rifampin for the treatment and prevention of tuberculosis among HIV-infected patients taking protease inhibitors or nonnucleoside reverse transcriptase inhibitors. *MMWR* 2000;49:185.
253. Havlir D, Barnes P. Tuberculosis in patients with human immunodeficiency virus infection. *N Engl J Med* 1999;340:367.
254. Bartlett JG. *1999 Medical Management of HIV Infection.* Baltimore, MD: Port City Press; 1999.
255. Englehard D et al. Interaction of ketoconazole with rifampin and isoniazid. *N Engl J Med* 1984;311:1681.
256. Lazar JD et al. Drug interactions with fluconazole. *Rev Infect Dis* 1990;12:327.
257. Chaisson RE et al. Incidence and natural history of *Mycobacterium avium*-complex infections in patients with advanced human immunodeficiency virus disease treated with zidovudine. *Am Rev Respir Dis* 1992;146:285.
258. Von Reyn CF et al. The international epidemiology of disseminated *Mycobacterium avium* complex infection in AIDS. *AIDS* 1996;10:1025.
259. Yakrus MA et al. Geographic distribution, frequency and specimen source of *Mycobacterium avium* complex serotypes isolated from patients with acquired immunodeficiency syndrome. *J Clin Microbiol* 1990;28:926.
260. Sathe SS et al. Severe anemia is an important negative predictor for survival with disseminated *Mycobacterium avium-intracellulare* in acquired immunodeficiency syndrome. *Am Rev Respir Dis* 1990;142:1306.
261. Benson CA. Disease due to the *Mycobacterium avium* complex in patients with AIDS: epidemiology and clinical syndrome. *Clin Infect Dis* 1994;18:S218.
262. Woods GL. Disease due to the *Mycobacterium avium* complex in patients infected with human immunodeficiency virus: diagnosis and susceptibility testing. *Clin Infect Dis* 1994;18(Suppl 3):S227.
263. Currier JS et al. Preliminary ACTG 320 OI data analysis (presentation). 23rd AIDS Clinical Trials Group Meeting; Washington, DC; 1997.
264. Baril L et al. Impact of highly active antiretroviral therapy on onset of *Mycobacterium avium* complex infection and cytomegalovirus disease in patients with AIDS. *AIDS* 2000;14:2593.
265. Hoffner SE et al. Control of disease progress in *Mycobacterium avium*-infected AIDS patients. *Res Microbiol* 1992;143:391.
266. Yajko DM. In vitro activity of antimicrobial agents against the *Mycobacterium avium* complex inside macrophages from HIV-1-infected individuals: the link to clinical response to treatment? *Res Microbiol* 1992;143:411.
267. Inderlied CB. Microbiology and minimum inhibitory concentration testing for *Mycobacterium avium* prophylaxis. *Am J Med* 1997;102:2.
268. Heifets L et al. Radiometric broth macrodilution method for determination of minimal complex isolates: proposed guidelines. Denver: National Jewish Center for Immunology and Respiratory Medicine; 1993.
269. Ellner JJ et al. *Mycobacterium avium* infection and AIDS: a therapeutic dilemma in rapid evolution. *J Infect Dis* 1991;163:1326.
270. Heifets LB et al. Clarithromycin minimal inhibitory and bactericidal concentrations against *Mycobacterium avium. Am Rev Respir Dis* 1992;145:856.
271. Heifets LB et al. Individualized therapy versus standard regimens in the treatment of *Mycobacterium avium* infections. *Am Rev Respir Dis* 1991;144:1.
272. Young LS et al. Azithromycin for treatment of *Mycobacterium avium-intracellulare* complex infection in patients with AIDS. *Lancet* 1991;338:1107.
273. Ishiguro M et al. Penetration of macrolides into human polymorphonuclear leukocytes. *J Antimicrob Chemother* 1989;24:719.
274. Girard AE et al. Pharmacokinetic and in vivo studies with azithromycin (CP-62,993), a new macrolide with an extended half-life and excellent tissue distribution. *Antimicrob Agents Chemother* 1987;31:1948.
275. Barradel LB et al. Clarithromycin: a review of its pharmacological properties and therapeutic use in *Mycobacterium avium-intracellulare* complex infections in patients with acquired immune deficiency syndrome. *Drugs* 1993;46:289.
276. Mor N et al. Accumulation of clarithromycin in macrophages infected with *Mycobacterium avium. Pharmacotherapy* 1994;14:100.
277. Kemper CA et al. The individual microbiologic effect of three antimycobacterial agents, clofazimine, ethambutol, and rifampin, on *Mycobacterium avium* complex bacteremia in patients with AIDS. *J Infect Dis* 1994;170:157.
278. Chaisson RE et al. Clarithromycin therapy for bacteremic *Mycobacterium avium* complex disease. A randomized, double-blind, dose-ranging study in patients with AIDS. AIDS Clinical Trials Group Protocol 157 Study Team. *Ann Intern Med* 1994;15;121:905.
279. Shafran SD et al. A comparison of two regimens for the treatment of MAC bacteremia in AIDS: rifabutin, ethambutol and clarithromycin versus rifampin, ethambutol, clofazimine and ciprofloxacin. *N Engl J Med* 1996;335:377.
280. Chaisson RE et al. Clarithromycin ethambutol with or without clofazimine for the treatment of bacteremic *Mycobacterium avium* complex disease in patients with HIV infection. *AIDS* 1997;11:311.
281. Masur H et al. Recommendations on prophylaxis and therapy for disseminated *Mycobacterium avium* complex for adults and adolescents infected with human immunodeficiency virus. *MMWR Morbid Mortal Wkly Rep* 1993;42:14.
282. Dube MP et al. Successful short-term suppression of clarithromycin-resistant *Mycobacterium avium* complex bacteremia in AIDS. California Collaborative Treatment Group. *Clin Infect Dis* 1999;28:136.
283. Flexner C. HIV-Protease inhibitors. *New Engl J Med* 1998;338:1281.
284. Oldfield EC 3rd et al. Once weekly azithromycin therapy for prevention of *Mycobacterium avium* complex infection in patients with AIDS: a randomized, double-blind, placebo-controlled multicenter trial. *Clin Infect Dis* 1998;26:611.
285. Havlir DV et al. Prophylaxis against disseminated *Mycobacterium avium* complex with weekly azithromycin, daily rifabutin or both. California Collaborative Treatment Group. *N Engl J Med* 1996;335:392.
286. Benson CA et al. Clarithromycin or rifabutin alone or in combination for primary prophylaxis of *Mycobacterium* avium complex disease in patients with AIDS: a randomized, double-blind, placebo-controlled trial. The AIDS Clinical Trials Group 196/Terry Beirn Community Programs for Clinical Research on AIDS 009 Protocol Team. *J Infect Dis* 2000;181:1289.
287. Kotler DP. The gastrointestinal and hepatobiliary systems of HIV infection. In: Wormser GP, ed. *AIDS and Other Manifestations of HIV Infection.* New York: Lippincott-Raven; 1998:505.
288. Jacobson MA et al. Retinal and gastrointestinal disease due to cytomegalovirus in patients with the acquired immune deficiency syndrome: prevalence, natural history, and response to ganciclovir therapy. *Queb J Med* 1988;67:473.
289. Wu GD et al. A comparison of routine light microscopy, immunohistochemistry, and in situ hybridization for the detection of cytomegalovirus in gastrointestinal biopsies. *Am J Gastroenterol* 1989;84:1517.
290. Profeta S et al. *Salmonella* infections in patients with acquired immunodeficiency syndrome. *Arch Intern Med* 1985;145:670.
291. Rompalo A, Quinn TC. Enteric bacterial diseases. In: Dolin R et al., eds. *AIDS Therapy.* Philadelphia: Churchill Livingstone; 1999:350.
292. Blaser MJ et al. Recurrent shigellosis complicating human immunodeficiency virus infection: failure of preexisting antibodies to confer protection. *Am J Med* 1989;86:105.
293. Bernard E et al. Diarrhea and *Campylobacter* infections in patients infected with the human immunodeficiency virus. *J Infect Dis* 1989;159:143.
294. Juranels DD. Cryptosporidiosis: sources of infection and guidelines for prevention. *Clin Infect Dis* 1995;21(Suppl 1):S57.
295. Vakil NB et al. Biliary cryptosporidiosis in HIV-infected people after the waterborne outbreak of cryptosporidiosis in Milwaukee. *N Engl J Med* 1996;34:19.
296. Flanigan TP. *Cryptosporidium, Isospora,* and *Cyclospora* infections. In: Dolin R et al., eds. *AIDS Therapy.* Philadelphia: Churchill Livingstone; 1999:328.
297. Holmberg SD et al. Possible effectiveness of clarithromycin and rifabutin for cryptosporidiosis chemoprophylaxis in HIV Disease. *JAMA* 1998;279:384.
298. Smith NH et al. Combination drug therapy for cryptosporidiosis in AIDS. *J Infect Dis* 1998:178:900.
299. Amadi B et al. Effect of nitazoxanide on morbidity and mortality in Zambian children with cryptosporidiosis: a randomized, controlled trial. *Lancet* 2002;360:1375.
300. Grube H et al. Resolution of AIDS associated cryptosporidiosis after treatment with indinavir. *Am J Gastroenterol* 1997;92:726.
301. Goodgame RW. Understanding intestinal spore-forming protozoa: *Cryptosporidia, Microsporidia, Isospora,* and *Cyclospora. Ann Intern Med* 1996;124:429.
302. Weiss LM. Microsporidiosis. In: Dolin R et al., eds. *AIDS Therapy.* Philadelphia: Churchill Livingstone; 1999:336.
303. Blackstone MO. *Endoscopic Interpretation.* New York: Raven Press; 1984:19.
304. Reef SE et al. Opportunistic *Candida* infections in patients infected with human immunodeficiency virus: prevention issues and priorities. *Clin Infect Dis* 1995;21(Suppl 1):S99.
305. Jacobson JM et al. Thalidomide for the treatment of oral aphthous ulcers in patients with human immunodeficiency virus infection. New Institute of Allergy and Infection Disease AIDS Clinical Trials Group. *N Engl J Med* 1997;336:1489.
306. Duswald KH et al. High-dose therapy with fluconazole 800 mg/day. *Mycoses* 1997;40:267.
307. Maenza JR et al. Risk factors for fluconazole-resistant candidiasis in human immunodeficiency virus-infected patients. *J Infect Dis* 1996;173:219.
308. Revision of the Centers for Disease Control and Prevention surveillance case definition for acquired immunodeficiency syndrome. *MMWR Morbid Mortal Wkly Rep* 1987;36(Suppl 1):3S.
309. Von Roenn JH et al. Megestrol acetate in patients with AIDS-related cachexia. *Ann Intern Med* 1994;121:393.
310. Beisel WR. Malnutrition as a consequence of stress. In: Suskind RM, ed. *Malnutrition and the Immune Response.* New York: Raven Press; 1997.

311. Oster MH et al. Megestrol acetate in patients with AIDS and cachexia. *Ann Intern Med* 1994;121:400.
312. Goster R et al. Dronabinol effects on weight in patients with HIV infection. *AIDS* 1992;6:127.
313. Berger JR et al. Oxandrolone in AIDS-wasting myopathy. *AIDS* 1996;10:1657.
314. Engelson ES et al. Effects of testosterone upon body composition. *Acquir Immun Defic Syndr Hum Retrovirol* 1996;11:510.
315. Balog DL et al. HIV wasting syndrome: treatment update. *Ann Pharmacother* 1998;32:446.
316. Grinspoon SK et al. An etiology and pathogenesis of hormonal and metabolic disorders in HIV infection. *Baillieres Clin Endocrinol Metab* 1994;4:735.
317. Hengge UR et al. Oxymetholone promotes weight gain in patients with advanced human immunodeficiency virus (HIV-1) infection. *Br J Nutr* 1996;75:129.
318. Miller K et al. Transdermal testosterone administration in women with acquired immunodeficiency syndrome wasting: a pilot study. *J Clin Endocrinol Metab* 1998;83:2717.
319. Grinspoon S et al. Effects of androgen administration in men with the AIDS wasting syndrome. A randomized, double-blind, placebo-controlled trial. *Ann Intern Med* 1998;128:18.
320. Waters D et al. Recombinant human growth hormone, insulin-like growth factor, and combination therapy in AIDS-associated wasting: a randomized, double-blind, placebo-controlled trial. *Ann Intern Med* 1996;125:865.
321. Schambelan M et al. Recombinant human growth hormone in patients with HIV-associated wasting. A randomized, placebo-controlled trial. Serostim Study Group. *Ann Intern Med* 1996;125:873.
322. Minor JR, Piscitelli SC. Thalidomide in diseases associated with human immunodeficiency virus infection. *Am J Health-Syst Pharm* 1996;53: 429.
323. Roubenoff R et al. Feasibility of increasing lean body mass in HIV-infected adults using progressive resistance training. *Nutrition* 1997;13:271.
324. Pluda JM et al. Parameters affecting the development of non-Hodgkin's lymphoma in patients with severe human immunodeficiency virus infection receiving antiretroviral therapy. *J Clin Oncol* 1993;11:1099.
325. Kaplan LD, Northfelt DW. Malignancies associated with AIDS. In: Sandle MA, Volberding PA, eds. *The Medical Management of AIDS.* Philadelphia: WB Saunders; 1999:467.
326. Jacobson LP et al. Impact of potent antiretroviral therapy on the incidence of Kaposi's sarcoma and non-Hodgkin's lymphomas among HIV-1-infected individuals. Multicenter AIDS Cohort Study. *J Acquir Immun Defic Syndr Hum Retrovirol* 1999;21(Suppl 1):S34.
327. Chang Y et al. Identification of herpesvirus-like DNA sequences in KS tissue from HIV-1 infected men. *Science* 1994;266:1565.
328. Huang YQ et al. Human herpes virus-like nucleic acid in various forms of Kaposi sarcoma. *Lancet* 1995;345:759.
329. Krown SE et al. Kaposi's sarcoma in the acquired immune deficiency syndrome: a proposal for uniform evaluation, response and staging criteria. *J Clin Oncol* 1989;7:1201.
330. Krown S. Kaposi sarcoma. In: Dolin R et al., eds. *AIDS Therapy.* New York: Churchill Livingstone; 1999:580.
331. Gao SJ et al. Seroconversion to antibodies against Kaposi's sarcoma-associated herpes-virus-related latent nuclear antigens before development of Kaposi's sarcoma. *N Engl J Med* 1996;335:233.
332. Lane HC. The role of alpha-interferon in patients with human immunodeficiency virus infection. *Semin Oncol* 1991;18(Suppl 7):46.
333. Kovacs JA et al. Combined zidovudine and interferon-alpha therapy in patients with Kaposi sarcoma and the acquired immunodeficiency syndrome (AIDS). *Ann Intern Med* 1989;111:280.
334. Fischl MA. Antiretroviral therapy in combination with interferon for AIDS-related Kaposi's sarcoma. *Am J Med* 1991;90:2S.
335. Krown SE et al. Interferon-alpha, zidovudine, and granulocyte-macrophage colony-stimulating factor: a phase I AIDS Clinical Trials Group study in patients with Kaposi's sarcoma associated with AIDS. *J Clin Oncol* 1992;10:1344.
336. Uthyakumar S et al. Randomized cross-over comparison of liposomal daunorubicin versus observation for early Kaposi's sarcoma. *AIDS* 1996;10: 515.
337. Kedes DH et al. Sensitivity of Kaposi's sarcoma-associated herpesvirus replication to antiviral drugs. Implications for potential therapy. *J Clin Invest* 1997;99:2082.
338. Gill PS et al. The effects of preparations of human chorionic gonadotropin on AIDS-related Kaposi's sarcoma. *N Engl J Med* 1997;336:1115.
339. Moore RD et al. Non-Hodgkin's lymphoma in patients with advanced HIV infection treated with zidovudine. *JAMA* 1991;265:2208.
340. Armenian HK et al. Risk factors for non-Hodgkin's lymphoma in acquired immunodeficiency syndrome. *Am J Epidemiol* 1996;143:374.
341. Pluda JM et al. Hematologic effects of AIDS therapies. *Hematol Oncol Clin North Am* 1991;5:229.
342. Krown S. Non-Hodgkin lymphoma. In: Dolin R et al., eds. *AIDS Therapy.* New York: Churchill Livingstone; 1999:592.
343. Tirelli U et al. Prospective study with combined low-dose chemotherapy and zidovudine in 37 patients with poor-prognosis AIDS-related non-Hodgkin's lymphoma. French-Italian Cooperative Study Group. *Ann Oncol* 1992;3:843.
344. Kaplan LD et al. Low-dose chemotherapy with standard-dose m-BACOD chemotherapy for non-Hodgkin's lymphoma associated with human immunodeficiency virus infection. National Institute of Allergy and Infectious Diseases AIDS Clinical Trials Group. *N Engl J Med* 1997;336:1641.
345. Centers for Disease Control and Prevention. AIDS in women, United States. *MMWR Morbid Mortal Wkly Rep* 47:845,1990.
346. Feingold AR et al. Cervical cytological abnormalities and papillomavirus in women infected with human immunodeficiency virus. *J Acquir Immun Defic Syndr Hum Retrovirol* 1990;3:896.
347. Irwin KL et al. Pelvic inflammatory disease in human immunodeficiency virus-infected women. *Obstet Gynecol* 1994;83:480.
348. Watts DH et al. Comparison of gynecologic history and laboratory results in HIV-positive women with CD4+ lymphocyte counts between 200 and 500 cells/microl and below 100 cells/microl. *J Acquir Immune Defic Syndr Hum Retrovirol* 1999;20: 455.
349. Maiman M et al. Human immunodeficiency virus infection and cervical neoplasia. *Gynecol Oncol* 1990;38:377.
350. Schiffman MH. Recent progress in defining the epidemiology of human papillomavirus infection and cervical neoplasia. *J Natl Cancer Inst* 1992;84: 394.
351. Winkelstein W Jr. Smoking and cervical cancer current status: a review. *Am J Epidemiol* 1990;131:945.
352. Newman MD, Wofsy CB. Women and HIV disease. In: Sande MA, Volberding PA, eds. *The Medical Management of AIDS.* Philadelphia: WB Saunders; 1999;537.
353. Vermund SH et al. High risk of human papillomavirus infection and cervical squamous intraepithelial lesions among women with symptomatic human immunodeficiency virus infection. *Am J Obstet Gynecol* 1991;165:392.
354. Rellihan MA et al. Rapidly progressing cervical cancer in a patient with human immunodeficiency virus infection. *Gynecol Oncol* 1990;36:435.
355. Monfardini S et al. Unusual malignant tumors in 49 patients with HIV infection. *AIDS* 1989;3:449.
356. Nasiell K et al. Behavior of mild cervical dysplasia during long-term follow up. *Obstet Gynecol* 1986;67:665.
357. Cervical cytology: evaluation and management of abnormalities. ACOG Technical Bulletin #183. *Int J Gynaecol Obstet* 1993;43:212.
358. Ferenczy A et al. Loop electrosurgical excision procedure for squamous intraepithelial lesions of the cervix: advantages and potential pitfalls. *Obstet Gynecol* 1996;87:332.
359. Wetchler SJ. Treatment of cervical intraepithelial neoplasia with the CO_2 laser: laser versus cryotherapy. A review of effectiveness and cost. *Obstet Gynecol Surv* 1984;39:469.
360. Kurman RJ et al. Interim guidelines for management of abnormal cervical cytology. *JAMA* 1994;271:1866.
361. Bornstein J et al. Treatment of cervical intraepithelial neoplasia and invasive squamous cell carcinoma by interferon. *Obstet Gynecol Surv* 1993;48:251.
362. Rotola A et al. Beta-interferon treatment of cervical intraepithelial neoplasia: a multicenter clinical trial. *Intervirol* 1995;38:325.
363. Costa S et al. Intramuscular alpha-interferon treatment of human papillomavirus lesions in the lower female genital tract. *Cervix LFGT* 1988;6:203.
364. Byrne MA et al. The effect of interferon on human papillomaviruses associated with cervical intraepithelial neoplasia. *Br J Obstet Gynecol* 1986;93:1136.
365. Ylikoski M et al. Topical treatment with human leukocyte interferon of HPV 16 infections associated with cervical and vaginal intraepithelial neoplasias. *Gynecol Oncol* 1990;36:353.
366. Puligheddu P et al. Activity of interferon-alpha in condylomata with dysplastic lesion of the uterine cervix. *Eur J Gynecol Oncol* 1988;9:161.
367. Frost L et al. No effect of intralesional injection of interferon on moderate cervical intraepithelial neoplasia. *Br J Obstet Gynecol* 1990;97:626.

CHAPTER 71

Fungal Infections

John D. Cleary, Stanley W. Chapman, and Margaret Pearson

Mycotic (fungal) infections, once observed only occasionally, are now the fourth most commonly encountered nosocomial infection. This increase can be attributed, in part, to the growing numbers of immunocompromised hosts as a result of organ transplants, cancer chemotherapy, and the acquired immunodeficiency syndrome (AIDS) epidemic. Practitioners must be up to date on current concepts in medical mycology that affect the treatment and monitoring of patients with fungal infections. This chapter reviews the mycology, diagnosis, antimycotics, and therapeutics for common mycotic infections. For a more in-depth presentation of the basic biology of fungi, as well as the epidemiology, pathogenesis, immunology, diagnosis, and monitoring of mycotic infections, see Dismukes' *Clinical Mycology.*[1] In addition, other chapters in this book address specific areas of mycology and antifungal therapy. These topics include the treatment of fungal meningitis; endocarditis; intra-abdominal and hepatosplenic infections; bone and joint infections; and infections in immunocompromised patients with and without human immunodeficiency virus (HIV) infections. Treatment of uncommon fungal infections (e.g., paracoccidioidomycosis, alternariosis or fusariosis, mucormycosis, and pseudallescheriasis) is presented associated with immunocompromised hosts.

MYCOLOGY

Morphology

The pathogenic fungi that infect humans are nonmotile eucaryotes that reproduce by sporulation and they exist in two forms: filamentous molds and unicellular yeasts. These forms are not mutually exclusive and, depending on the growth conditions, a fungus may exist in one or even both of these forms (Table 71-1). The dimorphic fungi (e.g., *Histoplasma capsulatum* and *Blastomyces dermatitidis*) grow as a mold in nature (27°C), but quickly convert to the parasitic yeast form after infecting the host (37°C). This mycelium-to-yeast conversion is an important factor in the pathogenesis of disease caused by these organisms. Other pathogenic fungi, such as *Aspergillus* species, grow only as a mold form, whereas *Cryptococcus neoformans* usually grows as a yeast form. *Candida* species grow with a modified form of budding whereby newly budded cells remain attached to the parent cells and form pseudohyphae. Fungi are aerobic and are easily grown on routine culture media similar to that used to grow bacteria. Most fungi grow best at 25°C to 35°C. Fungi that cause only cutaneous and subcutaneous disease grow poorly at temperatures >37°C. This temperature-selective growth explains, at least in part, why

Table 71-1 Organism Classification

Hyphae (Moulds)
Hyalohyphomycoses
Aspergillus spp., Pseudallescheria boydii
Dermatophytes: Epidermophyton floccosum, Trichophyton spp., Microsporum spp.
Phaeohyphomycoses
Alternaria spp., Anthopsis deltoidea, Bipolaris hawaiiensis, Cladosporium spp., Curvularia geniculata, Exophiala spp., Fonsecaea pedrosoi, Phialophora spp., Fusarium spp.
Zygomycetes
Absidia corymbifera, Mucor indicus, Rhizomucor pusillus
Dimorphic Fungi
Blastomyces spp., Coccidioides spp., Paracoccidioides spp., Histoplasma spp., Sporothrix spp.
Yeasts
Candida spp., Cryptococcus neoformans

these organisms rarely disseminate from a primary focus in the skin or subcutaneous tissues.

Classification

Fungal infections are best classified by the area of the body infected (Table 71-2). Superficial mycoses involve only the outermost keratinized layers of the skin (stratum corneum) and hair. The cutaneous mycoses extend deeper into the epidermis and may also infect the nails. The subcutaneous mycoses infect the dermis and subcutaneous tissues; entry into these sites is by inoculation or implantation of dirt or vegetative matter. The systemic mycoses cause disease of the internal organs of the body. Standard definitions that are useful in daily patient care for invasive fungal infections have been developed for epidemiologic and clinical trials. The guidelines are referenced under each infection. The respiratory tract is the most common primary portal of entry into the patient, and infection in the lungs may be symptomatic or asymptomatic. Systemic infection with *Candida* usually results from a primary focus in the gastrointestinal (GI) tract or skin. In each case, the organism may spread hematogenously from the primary focus throughout the body, resulting in disseminated disease. The opportunistic mycoses occur primarily in the immunocompromised host and require more aggressive treatment. The list of fungi that cause opportunistic infection is rapidly expanding, especially with the AIDS epidemic.[2] The nonopportunistic fungi (primary pathogens) usually cause disease in the immunologically normal host. Some primary pathogens, however, result in unique clinical syndromes when infection occurs in the immunocompromised host, such as histoplasmosis in AIDS.[1]

Table 71-2 Clinical Classification of Mycoses

Classification	*Site Infected*	*Example*
Superficial	Outermost skin and hair	Malasseziasis (Tinea versicolor)
Cutaneous	Deep epidermis and nails	Dermatophytosis
Subcutaneous	Dermis and subcutaneous tissue	Sporotrichosis
Systemic	Disease of more than one internal organ	
Opportunistic		Candidiasis Cryptococcosis Aspergillosis Mucormycosis
Nonopportunistic		Histoplasmosis Blastomycosis Coccidioidomycosis

Pathogenesis of Infection

Endogenous

Fungal infection can be acquired from both exogenous and endogenous sources. The only fungi known to be normal flora (commensals) in humans are *Pityrosporum obiculare,* which causes the noninflammatory superficial condition of tinea versicolor, and *Candida* species. Infections with these yeast organisms primarily develop from the patient's own normal flora (endogenous infection). These endogenous fungal infections of the skin or mucous membranes occur when host resistance is lowered and the organism proliferates in high numbers. Excess heat and humidity, oral contraceptive use, pregnancy, diabetes, malnutrition, and immunosuppression facilitate endogenous local infection by both *Pityrosporum* and *Candida.* Systemic candidal infections occur in the immunocompromised host when the organism colonizing the patient's skin or GI tract is disseminated hematogenously throughout the body.

Exogenous

Exogenous infections occur when the fungus is acquired from an environmental source. In the case of dermatophytes (ringworm fungi), the organism can be acquired from dirt, animals, or another infected individual. The subcutaneous mycoses result from direct inoculation of infected material, often a thorn or other vegetable matter, through the skin. Infections of the skin and subcutaneous tissues by *Aspergillus* and the agents causing mucormycosis (e.g., *Rhizopus, Absidia, Mucor*) have resulted from contaminated wound dressings and cast materials.[3] Exogenous fungi colonized or carried on the hands of health care workers can infect patients; therefore, these health care workers, especially in intensive care units (ICU), must wash their hands to prevent cross-infection between patients.[4] Other than candidial infections, the systemic mycoses are primarily the result of inhalation of dust contaminated by the infectious spores, with a primary focus of infection in the lungs. If local or systemic host defenses are unable to control the primary infection, the organism may be spread hematogenously to other organs. Some of the systemic mycoses have defined geographic (endemic) areas in which the fungus is more commonly encountered in the environment. For example, histoplasmosis and blastomycosis occur most often in the regions of the Red, Mississippi and Ohio River valleys, whereas coccidioidomycosis is endemic to the southwestern United States and the Central Valley of California.

Host Defenses

Host defenses against fungal infection involve both nonimmune (also known as nonspecific or natural resistance) and immune (also known as specific or acquired resistance) mechanisms. Nonimmune resistance plays a primary role in preventing colonization and invasion of a susceptible tissue. The normal bacterial flora of the skin and mucous membranes prevent colonization (colonization resistance) by more pathogenic bacteria and fungi. Patients treated with broad-spectrum antibiotics are at greater risk for colonization and infection by fungi because of the alteration in their bacterial flora. The barrier function of the intact skin and mucous membranes is also an important defense against fungal infection. Skin defects, whether the result of intravenous (IV) catheters, burns, surgery, or trauma, predispose individuals to local invasion and fungemia, especially with *Candida* species. When these physical barriers are breached, the polymorphonuclear leukocyte (neutrophil) and monocytes are the cells involved earliest in host defense against fungi. The antifungal activity of neutrophils involves phagocytosis and intracellular killing, but also can include extracellular killing by secreted lysosomal enzymes. Neutropenia is the most common neutrophil defect predisposing to fungal infection, but functional defects of neutrophils, such as those occurring in patients with chronic granulomatous disease of childhood and myeloperoxidase deficiency, have also been associated with an increased frequency of fungal infections, especially with *Candida* and *Aspergillus.*

Antibody and complement may have some role in resistance to certain fungal infections, but they are not the primary effectors of acquired resistance. Cellular immunity, mediated by antigen-specific T lymphocytes, cytokines, and activated macrophages, is the primary acquired (immune) host defense against fungi. Patients with defective cellular immunity (e.g., immunosuppressed organ transplant recipients, patients with lymphomas and AIDS, and those treated with corticosteroids or cytotoxic agents) are at greatest risk for fungal infection. The immunodeficiency noted in these patients is also the primary reason for the poor therapeutic outcome despite appropriate antifungal therapy. An additional factor associated with an increased risk for fungal infection is the use of total parenteral nutrition (TPN).[1]

Table 71-3 Antifungal Agents Approved for Use

Agent (Brand Name)	Formulation
Systemic Agents	
Amphotericin B (Abelcet, AmBisome, Amphotec)	IV
Amphotericin B (generic)	IV
Caspofungin (Cancidas)	IV
Fluconazole (Diflucan)	IV, tablet, oral suspension
Fluorocytosine [Flucytosine] (Ancobon)	Capsule
Griseofulvin (generic)	Tablet, oral suspension
Itraconazole (Sporanox)	IV, capsule, oral solution
Ketoconazole (Nizoral)	Tablet
Miconazole (Monistat)	IV
Potassium iodide	Solution
Terbinafine (Lamisil)	Tablet
Voriconazole (Vfend)	IV, tablet
Topicals, Class I	
Amphotericin B	Cream, lotion, ointment, oral suspension[a]
Butoconazole (Femstat)	Ointment
Ciclopirox (Loprox)	Cream, lotion
Clioquinol (Vioform)	Cream, ointment
Clotrimazole	Cream, lotion, lozenge, pessary, solution, tablet
Econazole (Spectazole)	Cream
Ketoconazole (Nizoral)	Cream shampoo
Miconazole	Aerosol, cream, lotion, pessary, spray, suppository, vaginal tablet
Naftifine (Naftin)	Cream, gel
Nystatin	Cream, lozenge, ointment, powder, suspension, tablet
Oxiconazole (Oxistat)	Cream, lotion
Povidone iodine	Douche, gel, suppository
Sodium thiosulfate (Exoderm)	Lotion
Sulconazole (Exelderm)	Cream, solution
Terbinafine (Lamisil)	Cream
Terconazole (Terazol 7)	Cream, suppository
Tioconazole (Vagistat)	Ointment
Tolnaftate (generic)	Cream, gel, powder, solution, spray
Undecylenic acid	Cream, foam, ointment, powder, soap

[a] No longer available in United States.
IV, intravenous.
Classification identified in reference 182, with permission.

ANTIMYCOTICS

Mechanisms of Action

Table 71-3 lists the U.S. Food and Drug Administration (FDA)-approved topical and systemic antimycotics for the treatment of fungal infections. Griseofulvin and potassium iodide have limited clinical utility and are not used to treat systemic fungal infections. Griseofulvin inhibits growth by inhibiting fungal cell mitosis caused by polymerization of cell microtubules, thereby disrupting mitotic spindle formation. It has activity only against the dermatophyte fungi. The antifungal mechanism of potassium iodide is unclear. It is effective only in the treatment of lymphocutaneous sporotrichosis.

The eight antifungal drugs used for systemic disease fall into five structural classes that act by four mutually exclusive mechanisms. *Amphotericin B* and *nystatin,* polyene macrolides, act principally by binding to ergosterol in the fungal cell membrane, effectively creating pores in the cell membrane and leading to depolarization of the membrane and cell leakage.[5] Amphotericin B binds with greater affinity to ergosterol than to cholesterol.[6] This phenomenon is believed to be mediated through both hydrophilic hydrogen bonding and hydrophobic, nonspecific van der Waals forces. Investigations using P^{32} nuclear magnetic resonance spectroscopy to study the interactions of polyene macrolides with sterols documented that the presence of the double bond in the side chain of ergosterol (not present in cholesterol) accounts for the greater affinity of amphotericin B for ergosterol.[5] Amphotericin B, however, also binds to sterols of mammalian cells (i.e., cholesterol), a fact that is believed to account for most of the toxic effects of amphotericin B. Alteration in the lipid content of the pathogens membrane may play a role in the development of resistance,[7] although this alone is apparently not sufficient to affect that development.[8] The lethal antifungal effects of amphotericin B are, however, the result of not only cell leakage resulting from ergosterol binding, but also immune stimulation and oxygen-dependent killing.[6,9]

5-Flucytosine (5-FC), a fluorinated cytosine analog, is believed to act principally by inhibiting nucleic acid synthesis. It is actively transported into susceptible cells by the enzyme cytosine permease, where it is deaminated to the toxic metabolite 5-fluorouracil. Fluorouracil, when converted to 5-fluorouridine triphosphate, functions as an antimetabolite. It is incorporated into fungal RNA, where it is substituted for uracil and thereby disrupts protein synthesis.[10] 5-Fluorouracil can also be converted to fluorodeoxyuridine monophosphate, which inhibits thymidylate synthase and thus disrupts DNA synthesis.[10]

The *azole* antifungals and the *allylamines* (naftifine and terbinafine) appear to act by the same principal mechanism: inhibition of sterol biosynthesis by interference with either cytochrome P450–dependent lanosterol C14-demethylase (azoles) or squalene epoxidase (allylamines), critical enzymes in the biosynthesis of ergosterol.[11,12] The superior affinity of the triazoles (fluconazole, itraconazole, voriconazole) for fungal versus mammalian enzyme, as compared with the imidazoles (ketoconazole, miconazole), generally is believed to account for their reduced toxicity and improved efficacy.[11] The consequence of sterol biosynthesis inhibition is a faulty cell membrane with altered permeability. In general, the allylamines and older azoles are viewed as fungistatic in their action. The newer triazoles (voriconazole, posaconazole, and ravuconazole) demonstrate fungicidal activity against some fungal species.[13] The clinical relevance of *in vitro* fungicidal versus fungistatic action is the subject of considerable debate. Nevertheless, it seems logical that fungicidal action, if it can also be achieved in vivo, might be preferable in immunosuppressed hosts.

Lipopeptides, which are potent antifungal agents, include the structural class of *echinocandins* (anidulafungin, micafungin, and caspofungin). All share a common mechanism: they act by interfering with 1,3-*β*-D-glucan, preventing synthesis of essential cell wall polysaccharides that protect the cell from osmotic and structural stresses. The result is inhibition of fungal cell wall biosynthesis. Targeting the cell wall (as opposed to the cell membrane, which is the target of polyene, azole, and allylamine) has been an important step in selective inhibition of fungal versus mammalian cells; the fungal cell wall does not share target-associated toxicity with the mammalian cell wall.[14]

Antifungal Spectrum and Susceptibility Testing

The Clinical and Laboratory Standards Institute (CLSI) recommends standardized broth dilution (M27-A2) and disk diffusion (M44-A)[22] methods for determining in vitro antifungal susceptibilities for yeasts.[15] This method stipulates test medium, inoculum size and preparation, incubation time and temperature, end-point reading and quality control limits for amphotericin B, flucytosine, fluconazole, ketoconazole, and itraconazole. Minimum inhibitory concentration (MIC) values for use in clinical interpretation are specified for fluconazole, itraconazole, and flucytosine against *Candida* species after 48 hours of incubation. For fluconazole and itraconazole, a susceptible-dose dependent (S-DD) breakpoint was developed based on data supporting a trend toward better response with higher drug levels for isolates with higher MIC.[16] The S-DD range includes MIC of 16 and 32 mcg/mL along with >0.125 and <0.5 mcg/mL for fluconazole and itraconazole, respectively. *Candida* isolates with MIC less than these ranges are considered susceptible, and isolates with greater MIC are considered resistant. Owing to rapid development of resistance and limited data on correlation of MIC with outcome for flucytosine monotherapy, proposed interpretive breakpoints for this agent are based on a combination of historical data and results from animal studies. *Candida* isolates with a flucytosine MIC ≤4 mcg/mL are considered susceptible, isolates with MIC >16 mcg/mL are considered resistant. Limitations of the M27-A methodology have precluded development of amphotericin B interpretive breakpoints nor have interpretive criteria been proposed for ketoconazole MIC. An E-Test (AB Biodisk; Piscataway, NJ) is commercially available. Difficulties in endpoint determination using this method result from frequent, nonuniform growth of the fungus on the agar medium; yet, when properly performed, correlation between the E-Test and M27-A methods has been satisfactory for the azole antifungal agents against most *Candida.*[17] Other techniques under development for antifungal susceptibility testing for yeasts include flow cytometry and direct measurement of alterations in ergosterol synthesis.[18]

Recently, the CLSI also approved a standardized broth dilution (M38A) method for determining in vitro antifungal susceptibilities for certain spore-producing moulds, namely *Aspergillus* spp., *Fusarium* spp., *Rhizopus* spp., *Pseudallescheria boydii,* and *Sporothrix schenckii.*[19] An E-Test to evaluate mould susceptibilities to the systemic antimycotics is also being studied. Despite these recent advances, the determination of in vitro susceptibilities or resistance in clinical practice is of limited utility and not readily available.

Susceptibility testing for clinical isolates is not routinely recommended; however, published data on the susceptibility of the identified species of yeast or mould should guide the clinician's therapeutic choice. Clinical isolates from patients failing high-dose therapy (i.e., refractory oral pharyngeal candidiasis) or unusual pathogenic yeasts in patients with AIDS can be sent for testing.[18] Testing should be performed in a laboratory where the staff is trained in mycoses. Despite these limitations, certain generalities should be emphasized. First, amphotericin B has broad in vitro activity and clinical efficacy against the yeasts and filamentous moulds. The echinocandins have cidal activity in vitro versus *Candida* spp. and static activity for *Aspergillus* spp.; they are not active in vitro against *Cryptococcus* spp. and many endemic mycoses.[20] The azole antifungals generally have clinically significant activity against only the yeasts and most dimorphic fungi. Additionally, itraconazole, voriconazole and posaconazole have excellent in vitro activity against *Aspergillus* spp., with clinical efficacy demonstrated for itraconazole, posaconazole, and voriconazole. Unlike other azoles, posaconazole has good in vitro activity and has shown clinical efficacy against zygomycetes, fungal infections for which previously only amphotericin B formulations were therapeutic options.[21,22]

New Frontiers for Antifungal Therapy

Various investigative efforts have been directed toward both enhancing efficacy and reducing the toxicity of older antifungal drugs, including biochemical modifications of the agent, improved delivery systems, and combination therapy. Inhalation of amphotericin B, and in lung transplant recipients, lipid complex amphotericin B, has been investigated in immunocompromised patients as a prophylaxis for invasive aspergillosis. Recently, caspofungin has been studied for suitability for aerosol delivery. Antifungal dose and nebulized system required for effective prophylaxis has yet to be established.[23–26] Even more challenging are the attempts to discover or design new prototype antifungal compounds. Substantial hurdles exist because both mammalian cells and fungal cells are eukaryotes and share many similar biochemical processes, unlike bacterial cells, which are prokaryotes. Traditionally, the drug discovery process depended on the ability to detect compounds (either natural products or synthetic compounds) that selectively inhibit or destroy fungal cells. This process is accomplished by either or both of two approaches: (a) the evaluation of existing compounds (natural or synthetic) for potentially useful antifungal activity and (b) the design and synthesis of new compounds that selectively block fungal targets. Recent advances in genomic sequencing of *C. albicans, C. glabrata, A. fumigatus,* and *C. neoformans* have allowed for use of this information within the search for new targets. Other less conventional drug discovery approaches include targeting known traditional virulence factors (e.g., adhesions, secreted enzymes). This approach is based on the principle that killing of the microbe need not occur for an anti-infective agent to be efficacious in reduction of disease.

Lead compounds that appear promising for antimycotic therapy include nikkomycins, sordarins, lytic peptides, hydroxypyridones, and cathelicidins. Nikkomycins inhibit chitin synthase. Chitin synthase catalyzes the polymerization of β-(1,4) linkages of *N*-acetyl glucosamine, which is critical to yeast cell membrane stabilization. Sordarins interfere with elongation factor-2, which is essential for protein synthesis, whereas lytic peptides and cathelicidins bind to cell membrane sterols, thereby reducing cell membrane stability. It appears that inhibition of cellular uptake of essential compounds and loss of other compounds are secondary effects of an unknown primary mode of action for the hydroxypyridone antimycotics.[27] Sordarins, lytic peptides, hydroxypyridones, cathelicidins and antibody directed therapies (i.e., mycograb: antiheat shock protein 90), a novel approach usually reserved for extracellular pathogens,[28] are still in early development.

SUPERFICIAL AND CUTANEOUS MYCOSES

Tinea Pedis: Treatment

1. C.W., a 28-year-old male construction worker, is evaluated for a chronic case of "athlete's foot." He wears boots all day at work and notes intense itching of both feet throughout the day. He has been using tolnaftate powder (Tinactin) for 1 week with no real therapeutic benefit. On examination, the web spaces between all the toes are white, macerated, and cracked. A few vesicles are also present over the dorsum of the foot at the base of the toes. Scrapings of the lesions examined as a potassium hydroxide preparation reveal branching, filamentous hyphae compatible with a dermatophyte infection. The diagnosis of "athlete's foot" is made. What therapeutic options are available for C.W.?

Selection of antifungal therapy should be based on the extent and type of infection. Superficial or cutaneous infections should initially be approached topically. Any follicular, nail, or widespread (>20% of body surface area [BSA]) infection should be treated systemically under medical supervision owing to poor penetration of topical applications. Topical antifungals have been reviewed as a class by the FDA advisory review panel on over-the-counter (OTC) antimicrobial drug products and on an individual basis as newer products have been released. To receive a class I recommendation, each agent (or combination) must have been tested in well-designed clinical trials that show the drug microbiologically and clinically effective against dermatophytosis or candidiasis with insignificant toxicity (irritation). Class I agents are listed in Table 71-4. Class II agents (camphor, candicidin, coal tar, menthol, phenolates, resorcinol, tannic acid, thymol, tolindate) are considered to have higher risk-to-benefit ratios associated with their pharmacotherapy. Class III agents (benzoic acid, borates, caprylic acid, oxyquinolines, iodines, propionic acid, salicylates, triacetin, gentian violet) lack adequate scientific data to determine efficacy. Topical therapy with any class I agent applied twice daily to the affected area for 2 to 6 weeks should be adequate. Therapy should be titrated to response.

Because C.W. could continue tolnaftate powder for 2 to 6 weeks or switch to an antifungal cream or lotion (e.g., miconazole), these products should be applied to the web spaces between all the affected toes twice daily. C.W. should also be careful to use nonocclusive footwear (e.g., cotton rather

Table 71-4 Antimycotic Prophylaxis Regimens and Costs

Agent	*Dose/Day*	*Formulation*	*Recommended Regimen*	*Cost ($)/day[a]*
Selective GI Decontamination				
Amphotericin B	400 mg	Oral suspension[b]	Swish and swallow QID	4.00[b]
Nystatin	4–12 million units	Oral suspension	Swish and Swallow QID	16.60–40.80
Systemic				
Clotrimazole	30–80 mg	Trouche	TID–QID	11.43–40.64
Ketoconazole	200–400 mg	Oral	QD	2.78–5.56
Itraconazole	200–400 mg	Oral	QD	15.56–31.11
Fluconazole	50–400 mg	Oral	QD	5.15–26.48

[a]From Price, AWP. Red Book: Thomson Healthcare, Durham, NC 27703: 2007.
[b]Made from parenteral formulation, no longer commercially available.
GI, gastrointestinal; QD, every day; QID, four times daily; TID, three times daily.

than synthetic fiber socks, and leather rather than vinyl boots). Application of an absorbent or antifungal powder to his footwear would also be helpful (see Chapter 38, Dermatotherapy and Drug Induced Skin Disorders).

Tinea Unguium (Onychomycosis): Treatment

2. If C.W. also suffered from an infection of the toenail (onychomycosis), what additional therapy could be offered to him?

Onychomycosis is typically caused by a dermatophyte, a hyphal fungi, or *Candida.* Nail scrapings and culture should be performed to help plan initial therapy. Once culture results are known, therapy can be initiated with either terbinafine 250 mg/day or itraconazole 200 mg/day for 6 (fingernail) to 12 (toenail) weeks. In some cases, however, successful therapy of tinea unguium can require 3 to 6 months for fingernails and 6 to 12 months for toenails. Therapy should be considered successful when several millimeters of healthy nail have emerged from the nailfold to the margin of infected nail, or when a 25% reduction in size of the infected site has been achieved.

For dermatophyte nail or paronychial infections, griseofulvin therapy could be used if an azole or allylamine is contraindicated. Griseofulvin (microsized or ultramicrosized) administered orally at 10 mg/kg/day and titrated to response should be effective.[22] Owing to the large doses given for prolonged periods, C.W. should be monitored closely at each prescription refill for signs and symptoms of adverse reactions. Terbinafine or itraconazole most commonly causes symptoms of headache, rash, and GI distress. Griseofulvin is more toxic, often causing hypersensitivity (urticaria, angioedema, type II hypersensitivity reactions), photosensitivity dermatitis, GI distress, and neurologic complications (headache, paresthesias, altered sensorium).[22]

Antimycotic pulse therapy is a novel approach to the treatment of onychomycosis. An FDA-approved alternative to daily therapy can now include a course of itraconazole 200 mg twice daily for 1 week in 2 consecutive months for fingernail infections. Double-blind, placebo-controlled trials revealed that this regimen was associated with a 77% clinical response and 73% mycologic response.[29] Overall responses and toxicity to therapy were more desirable with pulse regimens than with traditional regimens. Comparative studies demonstrate promising results for itraconazole pulse therapy for toenail infections[30] and fluconazole pulse therapy administered as a 150- to 450-mg dose once weekly for up to 12 months for mild disease.[31,32] Relapse rates after pulse (intermittent) terbinafine for 4 months have been frequent and longer courses of therapy are under study to enhance long-term efficacy.[33] Longer courses of therapy are being evaluated.

Removal of the nail as the sole therapy is not recommended because of the high relapse rate without concomitant systemic therapy. Likewise, IV antifungals are not indicated.

3. Describe the role of corticosteroids, antibacterials, or other additives to the antimycotic regimen in C.W.

Many patients with superficial, cutaneous, or nail infections will have additional morbidity associated with local inflammation and secondary bacterial infections. Inflammation is caused primarily by a type IV hypersensitivity reaction. Topical corticosteroids in conjunction with antifungals will often relieve itching and erythema secondary to inflammation. Bacterial (*Proteus* or *Pseudomonas* spp.) superinfection can also occur in these inflamed or macerated areas and may require concomitant topical antibacterial therapy. Pharmaceutical manufacturers of OTC preparations often combine a drying agent or astringent (e.g., alcohol, starch, talc, camphor) to their preparations to increase desquamation of the stratum corneum. Hyperhidrosis also can be relieved by these pharmaceutical additions. Such combination treatments should not be used routinely, however, because they increase the risk of toxicity and have not been proven to increase efficacy. If required for symptomatic relief, they should be used only for the initial days of treatment.

The affected web spaces between C.W.'s toes are macerated and cracked and vesicles are present at the base of his toes. A topical corticosteroid cream will probably facilitate the healing process and make him more comfortable during the first few days of antifungal therapy. The selection of topical corticosteroid formulations is presented in Chapter 38, Dermatotherapy and Drug Induced Skin Disorders.

SUBCUTANEOUS MYCOSES

Sporotrichosis

Treatment Options

4. O.M., a 62-year-old man, has had a painless, slowly enlarging ulcer on his left hand for the past 4 months. He is an avid gardener, but can identify no antecedent local trauma. The primary lesion began as a red papule that slowly enlarged and then ulcerated. At the same time the ulcer developed, O.M. also noted painless, red nodules that spread proximally up his arm. He denies any chills, fever, weight loss, or cough. The ulcer has slowly enlarged despite daily application of a povidone-iodine ointment and 2 weeks of cephalexin treatment. On physical examination, O.M. is afebrile. A 1.5-cm^2 ulcer is present on the dorsum of the left hand. Extending proximally from the ulcer is a palpable cord and multiple nontender, erythematous nodules distributed linearly up the forearm, elbow, arm, and axilla. A culture of this ulcer obtained 4 weeks ago is now growing *Sporothrix schenckii.* What is the recommended therapy for O.M.?

Sporothrix schenckii is the dimorphic fungi found in the soil and on many plants. Infection is usually secondary to inoculation into the skin from a thorn or sharp plant matter. *S. schenckii* infection most commonly causes lymphocutaneous disease (Fig. 71-1) as illustrated by this case. Rarely, extracutaneous disease may occur and usually involves the lungs, bones, or joints.

Heat Treatment

In the 1930s and 1940s, local heat was applied to very mild plaque or lymphocutaneous disease. Germination rates of this dimorphic fungus actually can be decreased by increased temperature, and heat therapy 1 hour/day for 3 months is effective in 90% of patients with plaques (very mild disease).[34] Heat treatment could be particularly useful in pregnant patients when pharmacotherapy may be contraindicated.

Itraconazole

Itraconazole is more active in vitro against *S. schenckii* than other imidazoles or saturated solution of potassium

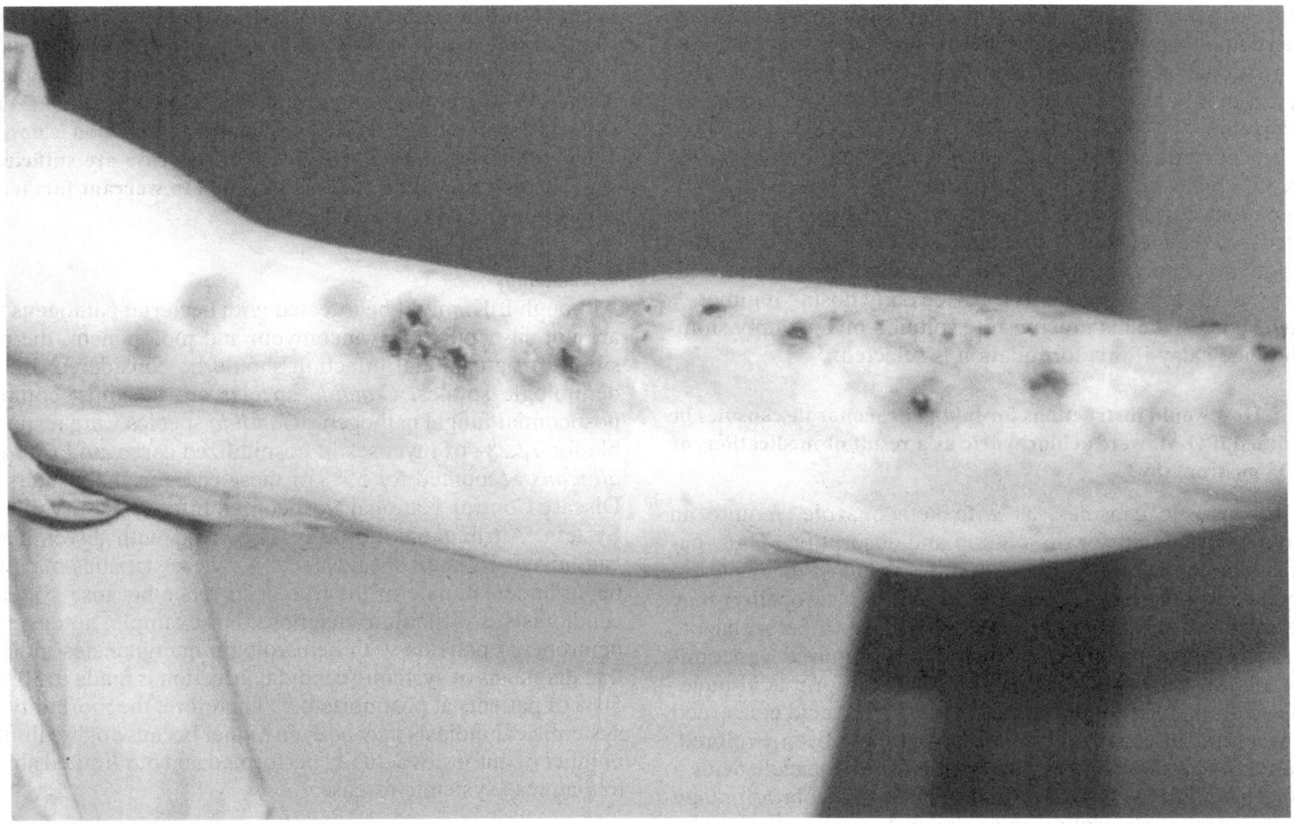

FIGURE 71-1 **Lymphocutaneous sporotrichosis.**

iodide (SSKI) and has dramatically improved the therapy of sporotrichosis. SSKI is seldom used for therapy secondary to treatment-limiting toxicity. Cure rates for sporotrichosis cutaneous and lymphocutaneous disease are >90% with itraconazole 100 to 200 mg/day for 3 to 6 months. For extracutaneous disease, higher dosages of itraconazole (200 mg BID) for 1 to 2 years achieve response rates of 81%, but relapse frequently occurs (27%) after therapy is stopped.[34,35] The toxicity and safety profile for itraconazole also appears favorable in these patients. Patients with extracutaneous disease who are unable to tolerate the higher itraconazole dosages or whose disease continues to progress should be treated with amphotericin B. An amphotericin A total dose of 2.0 to 2.5 g is most often recommended. Although voriconazole, posaconazole and ravuconazole demonstrate amphotericin B in vitro activity against *S. schenckii* (albeit less than itraconazole), their role in the treatment of sporotrichosis has not been defined.[36] Neither ketoconazole or fluconazole is effective in the treatment of sporotrichosis.

Terbinafine

Terbinafine has good in vitro activity against *S. schenckii*. Clinical data, although not abundant, also suggest in vivo efficacy.[37] An unpublished clinical trial comparing 250 mg or 500 mg BID for 3 months for lymphocutaneous disease revealed responses equivalent to itraconazole. Adverse reactions common in this population included GI distress (dysgeusia, dyspepsia, diarrhea), skin rash, and weight gain. Greater clinical experience and peer review of the aforementioned trial will further define the role of terbinafine in the treatment of sporotrichosis.

Therefore, in the case of lymphocutaneous disease; itraconazole 100 mg/day for a minimum of 3 months is the treatment of choice. If significant improvement is not observed in the first 6 weeks, the itraconazole dosage should be increased to 200 mg/day and continued for 6 months or until both the ulcer and lymphangitis have resolved. Most patients will respond to this dosage, but an occasional patient may require dosages of 300 or 400 mg/day.

Itraconazole Dosing

5. What instructions should O.M. receive for taking his itraconazole dose?

The peak serum concentrations of itraconazole capsules are ninefold higher when the drug is taken with food (i.e., 0.18 mcg/mL with food and 0.02 mcg/mL in fasting subjects).[38] The influence of food on absorption appears to be somewhat dependent on the nature of the food. High-carbohydrate meals decrease the absorption of itraconazole, and high-lipid content meals appear to increase itraconazole absorption.[39] Patients who have difficulty eating (e.g., patients with AIDS, those with cancer receiving antineoplastic therapy) may not absorb a sufficient amount from the capsule to achieve therapeutic plasma concentrations following a typical oral dose.[40] Although itraconazole manifests nonlinear serum pharmaco kinetics (i.e., administering the total dose in two divided doses is associated with higher peak serum concentrations than a single larger dose), no clinical benefit of splitting the dose has been demonstrated. Therefore, O.M. could be instructed to take his itraconazole capsule with his highest fat content meal of the day or itraconazole solution could be substituted to improve absorption.

Itraconazole oral solution is a cyclodextrin formulation that has 55% bioavailability in a fed patient; this increases in a fasting patient. Furthermore, bioavailability of this formulation is not affected by level of gastric acidity. Average serum concentration in a cohort of patients with advanced HIV infection was 2.7 mcg/mL following a 28-day twice daily dosing regimen.[41] O.M. should take his itraconazole solution on an empty stomach twice a day if this formulation is selected.

6. How would instructions for taking itraconazole capsules be modified if O.M. were achlorhydric as a result of medications or AIDS gastropathy?

Itraconazole capsules, as with ketoconazole, require an acidic environment for dissolution and absorption. Thus, patients who are achlorhydric, either as a result of medications, surgery, or underlying disease (e.g., AIDS gastropathy) may not absorb itraconazole adequately.[40,42] Use of ketoconazole in achlorhydric patients has historically required concomitant administration of 4 mL, 0.2 N hydrochloric acid aqueous solution.[43] Etching of tooth enamel by the acid concerned many clinicians, and other alternatives have been explored. The administration of ketoconazole and itraconazole with a low pH liquid (e.g., 8 to 16 fluid ounces of a cola or orange juice) improves absorption in 65.2% of healthy patients who are achlorhydric or taking H_2-blockers (Table 71-5).[20,44–59]

Voriconazole does not require an acidic environment for adequate oral absorption, but voriconazole should be administered 1 hour before or after meals as high-fat meals have been shown to reduce voriconazole serum concentrations. Quite the opposite, posaconazole plasma levels are four-fold higher following administration with food or a high fat nutritional supplement.

Because serum ketoconazole or itraconazole concentrations <0.25 mcg/mL have been associated with treatment failures, therapeutic drug monitoring is justified in patients in whom therapy is failing.[60] Serum antimycotic concentrations may be more easily monitored in the future as assays become available and correlations between concentration and efficacy are more clearly established.

SYSTEMIC MYCOSES

Candida Infection

7. L.K., a 21-year-old, 5-foot 8-inch, 170-lb, otherwise healthy man, was admitted to the hospital 16 days ago following a gunshot wound to the abdomen. He has undergone three exploratory laparotomies with repair and resection of damaged small intestine. He was placed on TPN to allow his bowel to rest and Solu-Medrol for stress on admission day 6. Three days ago, he developed a fever of 39.1°C and chills; his blood pressure (BP) of 100/70 mm Hg had dropped >30 mm Hg (systolic). Vancomycin and meropenem were promptly begun after obtaining cultures. Despite 3 days of antibiotics, he remains febrile. His physical examination reveals a Hickman catheter in the right subclavian vein that is functioning normally; no inflammatory changes are evident at the exit site. A single erythematous nodule about 0.5 cm wide is noted near the left wrist. The funduscopic examination of both eyes is normal. A chest radiograph is also normal. The white blood cell (WBC) count is currently 10,950 cells/mm³ and renal function is normal. What subjective and objective data in this case are sufficiently suggestive of a possible *Candida* infection to warrant further diagnostic evaluations in L.K.?

Epidemiology

Although L.K. might be infected with bacterial pathogens that are not susceptible to vancomycin and meropenem, the possibility of a candidal infection should be considered. In epidemiologic studies, *Candida* species are the most common nosocomial fungal pathogens. *Candida* species were responsible for 72.2% of mycoses in hospitalized cases, and *Candida albicans* accounted for 55% of these cases in the Centers for Disease Control, National Nosocomial Infections Surveillance System. Attributable mortality associated with disseminated candidiasis from all species is 38%. These statistics may well be an underestimate of the true occurrence because systemic candidiasis is difficult to diagnose. For example, autopsies in neutropenic patients with hematologic malignancies indicate that diagnosis of systemic candidal infection is made in 30% to 50% of patients at postmortem.[61] Therefore, the morbidity for systemic candidiasis may be even higher because of the limited number of autopsies actually performed and our limited ability to diagnose systemic disease.

Characteristics

The diagnosis and monitoring of therapeutic outcomes for systemic candidal infection are difficult because the characteristics of systemic candidal infection are subtle. Salient clinical features include constitutional symptoms (e.g., fever, chills, hypotension) and evidence of end-organ dissemination, such as nodular skin lesions that are usually erythematous, endophthalmitis, liver abscess, and spleen abscess. In addition, only about 50% of patients or fewer will have a single positive *Candida* blood culture. The Mycoses Study Group has utilized a positive culture from a sterile body site and hypotension (systolic blood pressure [SBP] <100 mm Hg or a SBP decrease >30 mm Hg) or abnormal temperature (<35.5°C or >38.6°C on one occasion or >37.8°C on two separate occasions >4 hours apart), or inflammation at a infected site as diagnostic criteria.

Risk Factors

Risk factors for candidemia include central venous catheters, broad-spectrum antibiotic use, extensive surgical procedures, *Candida* colonization, TPN, neutropenia or neutrophil dysfunction, and immunosuppression (e.g., premature infants, burn patients, mannose-binding lectin deficiency and patients with AIDS).[62]

L.K. has chills, a temperature of 39.1°C and is hypotensive. He is probably immunosuppressed as a result of multiple surgeries and corticosteroids. His Hickman catheter could serve as a possible portal of entry for an infectious agent, and his broad-spectrum antibiotic therapy with vancomycin and meropenem would be expected to be adequate for most of the likely bacterial pathogens. Because L.K. still has manifestations of an

Table 71-5 Pharmacokinetic Properties of Systemically Active Antifungals

Characteristic	Imidazoles			Triazoles			Echinocandins				Other	
	MCZ[a]	*KCZ*[a]	*ICZ*[a]	*FCZ*[a]	*PCZ*[a]	*RCZ*[a]	*VCZ*[a]	*AFG*[a]	*CFG*[a]	*MFG*[a]	*5FC*[a]	*TBF*[a]
Absorption												
Relative bioavailability	<10	75[b]	99.8 (40)[b]	(85–92)[b]		ND	>90[d]	<10	<10	<10	75–90[b]	70
C_{max} (mcg/mL)	1.9	3.29	0.63	1.4	0.851	0.76	2.3–4.7[d]	7.5	12	7.1	70–80	1.34–1.7
T_{max} (hr)	1.0	2.6	4.0	1.0–4.0	3	ND	<2	1	1	1	<2	1.5
AUC[c] (mcg/hr/mL)	ND	12.9 (13.6)	1.9(0.7)	42	8.619	13.84–119.12	9–11 (13)[d]	104.5	97.63–100.5	59.9	ND	4.74–10.48
Distribution												
Protein binding (%)	91–93	99	99.8	11	ND	95	58	80	96.5	99.5	2–4	> 99
CSF or serum concentration (%)	<10	<10	<10	60	ND	ND	~50	ND	ND	ND	60	<10
Excretion												
Beta $t_{1/2}$ (hr)	2.1	8.1[d]	17[d]	23–45	11.9	157	6	25.6	10	13	2.5–6.0	36
Active drug in urine (%)	1	2	<10	60–80	13	ND	<2	<1	2	1	0	80

[a]Above parameters are estimated from the administration of currently recommended doses. Miconazole [MCZ] 7.4–14.2 mg/kg/day (500–1,000 mg) parenterally, ketoconzole [KTZ] 2.8 mg/kg/day orally (200 mg), itraconazole [ITZ] 1.4–2.8 mg/kg/day orally (100–200 mg), fluconazole [FCZ] 0.7–1.4 mg/kg/day orally, voriconazole [VCZ] posaconazole [PCZ] 400 mg bid orally, ravuconazole [RCZ] 400 mg/day orally, anidulofungin [AFG] 200 mg parenterally; caspofungin [CFG] 70(50) mg parenterally on day 1(2–14), micafungin [MFG] 70 mg parenterally, flucytosine [5FC] 150 mg/day parenterally, and terbinafine [TBF] 250 mg/day orally.

[b]With meals (fasting), absorption altered by gastric acidity.

[c]Dose and/or influsion dependent.

[d]Absorption decreased when administered with high-fat meal; C_{max} and AUC reduced by 34% and 24%, respectively.

AUC, area under the concentration-time curve; CSF, cerebrospinal fluid; C_{max}, maximum concentration; CSF, cerebrospinal fluid; ND, no data; T_{max}, time of maximum concentration; $t_{1/2}$, half-life.

infection despite 3 days of antibiotics, additional diagnostic studies appear warranted.

Diagnostic Tests

8. What diagnostic tests could be ordered for L.K. to evaluate a possible fungal infection?

The diagnosis of fungal infection may be made with varying levels of certainty. Sometimes, the diagnosis is absolutely certain, such as when a pathogenic fungus from a clinical specimen is isolated and identified. This is referred to as a definitive or microbiologically confirmed diagnosis. At other times, the physician can determine only that a high probability of infection exists. This is designated as a presumptive diagnosis. To illustrate, a patient with a chest radiograph showing nodular lesions and a high complement fixation antibody against *H. capsulatum* would have a presumptive diagnosis of histoplasmosis. This may be as certain a diagnosis as is possible without performing a more invasive procedure to obtain lung tissue. In this event, a trial of drug therapy can be undertaken on the presumptive diagnosis alone. A diverse spectrum of tests is available for clinicians to diagnose and monitor therapeutic responses.

DIRECT EXAMINATION

Direct examination of the specimen is often useful in diagnosing fungal infection. Traditionally, the specimen is treated with 10% potassium hydroxide (KOH) to digest the cells and debris, resulting in clear visualization of the hyphae or yeast. Treatment of cerebrospinal fluid (CSF) specimens with KOH is not necessary because this fluid is naturally clear. India ink can be added to CSF to increase contrast and outline the organisms. Calcofluor white, a fluorescent fabric brightener that binds to fungi and fluoresces brilliantly when viewed under the ultraviolet microscope, also can be used to assist in recognition of fungal elements.

Histologic examination of biopsy specimens is an important tool for diagnosing and monitoring the presence of fungal infection, but identifying the precise species of fungus involved may be difficult. This is because only the tissue phase can be observed, and the fungal organisms in the specimen may be few. Because recognizing a fungus in hematoxylin- or eosin-stained sections may be difficult, a number of special stains have been developed.[62] Periodic acid–Schiff staining binds linked sugar groups in the fungal cell wall intensely magenta, thus making visualization of the fungal form easier. Likewise, several silver precipitation stains, (Gomori methenamine silver) rely on the presence of a charged fungal surface to reduce oxidized silver to metallic silver. This process coats the fungus with a black layer, again outlining the form.[63] The mucicarmine stain imparts a deep red color to complex polysaccharides, such as mucin. It will also stain the thick capsule of *C. neoformans.* Because no other yeast has a positive mucicarmine stain, the definitive diagnosis of cryptococcosis can be made.[64] The size of the organism, manner of budding, and the presence or absence of septae can all help identify the problem.

Monoclonal antibodies against many fungi are now available. Immunohistochemical procedures using these sera on biopsy specimens will enable the pathologist to detect the presence of a fungus, and determine its identity.[64] Reagents for in situ oligonucleotide probe hybridization to detect fungi in tissue are being developed and will also be extremely helpful.[65]

CULTURE

The most definitive method for diagnosing or monitoring a fungal infection is with culture. Specimens should be inoculated onto several different types of fungal media, some of which contain antibiotics to inhibit bacterial overgrowth. Swab specimens have a very low yield, especially for hyphal fungi and should be avoided in follow-up cultures. Yeast may grow rapidly and be isolated within 24 to 48 hours, but many fungi grow slowly and 4 to 6 weeks of incubation may be necessary to isolate and identify the organism. After growth, yeasts are usually recognized by their patterns of metabolic activity on a variety of substrates, whereas mycelial organisms may produce characteristic spores and fruiting bodies that are used for identification. Occasionally, a mycelial organism will be slow in producing recognizable spores, and immunologic testing for a characteristic isoantigen may be used for identification.

ANTIGEN DETECTION

Fungi synthesize polysaccharides that cannot be broken down by human enzymatic systems. These polysaccharides can accumulate within the body and be excreted in the urine. These fungal antigens can be detected by using antibodies that specifically recognize a particular species of fungus, thereby providing a diagnosis. The most commonly used antigen detection test is a latex agglutination test for cryptococcal antigen. This assay can be performed on serum or CSF. Antigenemia is present in 80% to 100% of patients with culture-proved cryptococcal meningitis. This test can also be used to monitor patient response to therapy by determining the end-point dilution for the positive reaction and following this end-point over time as the patient is treated. If treatment is successful, the titer will decline.[66,67]

Tests (quantitative polymerase chain reaction [PCR], enzyme-linked immunosorbent assay [ELISA], latex agglutination) for other fungal antigens are not as well established. Latex particle agglutination tests to detect candidal antigens are available, but their utility has not been clearly demonstrated. Assays for detecting *H. capsulatum* antigen in serum and urine have been reported.[68] Antigen can be detected in the blood of 50% and in the urine of 80% to 90% of patients with systemic histoplasmosis. Patients with blastomycosis and paracoccidioidomycosis, however, may also have positive cross-reactions. The ELISA for detection of *Aspergillus* galactomannan (GXM) antigen and Candida (1–3)-β-D-glucan has been approved by the FDA. Owing to the reported false–positive and false–negative rates, it is unclear if these assays will improve therapeutic decision-making for patients at risk for this infection.

ANTIBODY DETECTION

Detection of antibody can be useful for some fungal diseases but not for others. Serologic diagnosis of systemic candidiasis is complicated because most people have anti-*Candida* antibodies. A rising titer is not specific for infection and may indicate only colonization. Furthermore, dissemination of *Candida* is most likely in people who are immunocompromised and, therefore, may not respond by producing antibody.[69] On the other hand, seropositivity can be demonstrated in >90% of patients with symptomatic histoplasmosis.[70] The most important serologic tests use the complement fixation, immunodiffusion, and enzyme immunoassay (EIA) techniques. Appropriate evolution of serologic results requires an understanding of the sensitivity, specificity, and predictive value of each methodology. In general, serologic tests allow only a presumptive diagnosis of mycotic infections.

Although any of the aforementioned tests could be ordered for L.K., a direct examination of his blood and urine specimens along with an assessment of signs and symptoms of disseminated candidiasis are reasonable first steps in his evaluation. A blood and urine specimen from L.K. should also be cultured on different fungal media. Because a candidal infection is suspected, the culture could isolate *Candida* within 24 to 48 hours. Cultures and histopathologic examination of a biopsy specimen of skin lesions are often helpful not only in confirming a diagnosis of disseminated candidal infection, but also in monitoring response to therapy. The other fungal tests previously described need not be ordered immediately and should await the results from direct examination and culture.

Necessity of Treatment

9. The clinical laboratory reports that a single blood culture obtained from 2 days ago is growing *Candida* species. In addition, a secondary finding of many budding yeast in the urine was reported on urinalysis (UA). Why is therapy necessary in L.K. with only a single positive blood culture?

Case control studies of candidemia noted an 85.6% mortality rate in the untreated patients compared with a 41.8% mortality rate in patients who were treated early. Isolation of *Candida* from a patient's bloodstream is now viewed seriously, and therapy should be initiated immediately. Delays in therapy of up to 1 week can increase mortality rates by 23%.[71] In fact, delaying therapy 24 hours from the time a blood culture is positive or failure to follow Infectious Disease Society of American (IDSA) treatment guidelines increases mortality nearly 50%.[72,73] Removal of risk factors may improve the clinical outcome of candidemia, and removal of central venous catheters is believed to improve the morbidity and mortality rates.[74,75] Removal of centrally inserted catheters may make pharmacotherapy difficult, however, and L.K.'s other risk factors (e.g., broad-spectrum antibiotics) are perhaps of even greater importance.

Treatment Options and Combination Therapy

10. What therapeutic options are available to treat candidemia? Which option would be best for L.K.?

Therapeutic options are individualized and based on the competence of a patient's host defenses. In immunocompetent patients, amphotericin B, an echinocandin or a triazole, decreases morbidity and mortality associated with this disease.[76–80] Echinocandins have been demonstrated as effective as amphotericin B in neutropenic and non-neutropenic patients; however, amphotericin B clears the bloodstream fastest.[81,82] In the largest, well-controlled comparative trial, 206 non-neutropenic patients were randomized to amphotericin B 0.5 to 0.6 mg/kg/day or fluconazole 400 mg/day for 14 days. Mortality was <9% in both groups with no significant difference in successful outcomes (amphotericin B, 80%; fluconazole, 72%). Less toxicity was noted in the fluconazole group, however.[77] Therefore, fluconazole 400 mg/day is probably equally as effective as amphotericin B for non-neutropenic patients infected with susceptible *Candida.* Candidemic (or other mycotic infections discussed in this chapter) patients who are clinically stable and have no evidence of deep-seated infection should be initiated on a triazole or echinocandin for at least 14 days. Patients who are unstable or have deep-seated (organ involvement) infections should be treated with amphotericin B 0.5 to 0.6 mg/kg/day for at least 14 days; with concomitant septic shock, a minimum daily amphotericin B dose is 1.0 mg/kg. A lipid formulation of amphotericin B should be substituted in intolerant patients or those at high risk of adverse event.

In another trial, higher dosages of fluconazole (12 mg/kg/day) alone or in combination with amphotericin B for a minimum of 3 days, followed by step-down therapy to fluconazole, were given to evaluate the effect of combination therapy on improving clinical efficacy. Outcomes were not different from previously reported success rates. Yet, the fluconazole treatment group experienced higher Acute Physiology and Chronic Health Evaluation (APACHE II) scores, making evaluation of the comparison difficult.[81] In contrast, in another clinical trial the combination of amphotericin B and flucytosine appears more effective than single-agent therapy.[83,84] An amphotericin B-containing regimen does appear more effective in patients with APACHE scores between 10 and 22.

L.K. could be treated with an amphotericin B formulation owing to hemodynamic instablity, with the total dose based on clinical response and resolution of positive cultures (see Question 12). The efficacy of this therapy should be monitored by assessing the previously identified patient-specific signs and symptoms of candidemia. Combination therapy should be tried in patients who are not responding clinically along with a complete examination for focal sites of infection (septic thrombi or intra-abdominal abscess). HSP90 antibody may provide improved outcomes in the future.[28]

11. This fungal species has now been identified as *C. non-albicans.* How does this affect the therapeutic options for L.K.?

Historically, isolation of a non-albicans *Candida* from any patient's blood has been a matter of concern because of decreasing in vitro susceptibilities, clinical resistance observed in animal models, and uncontrolled case reports. Intrinsic resistance (*C. lusitaniae* to amphotericin B, *C. parapsilosis* to echinocandins, and *C. kruseii* to fluconazole) or acquired resistance (*C. tropicalis* or *glabrata* against fluconazole) has been reported.[78,83,84] Acquired in vitro fluconazole drug resistance is probably associated with altered fungal cell membrane permeability, antifungal efflux pumps, and changes in CYP450 enzymes. In observational studies, fluconazole resistance in vitro is up to 9%.[78,83,84] A large, multicenter study of 232 non-neutropenic patients was unable, however, to demonstrate a relationship between a yeast's MIC and patient outcome.[78] An inability to demonstrate a relationship is probably a result of a poor understanding or inadequate management of risk factors for infection. For example, the removal of a colonized IV catheter is probably a more important predictor of outcome than the MIC of the isolated yeast. Also, the therapeutic environment is changing with higher doses, new formulations of older agents, and new agents used in therapeutic regimens.

Therefore, the true rate of acquired clinical resistance to azoles and ultimate failure is unknown. Vigilant monitoring and aggressive therapy of infections caused by *non-albicans Candida* is recommended. In patients in whom susceptibilities are available, fluconazole should be avoided when the MIC are >16 mcg/mL. An antifungal should be avoided if the organism has intrinsic resistance.

Amphotericin

DOSING

12. How should amphotericin B formulation be dosed and administered to L.K.?

The amphotericin B dose and duration of therapy should be individualized based on the severity of infection and immunocompetence of the patient. Once the patient is stable, therapy should be changed to one of the applicable regimens discussed previously. The dose of amphotericin B formulations should be based on lean body mass. Owing to the difficulty in measuring, many clinicians, however, use ideal body weight. Tissues that contain large numbers of macrophages sequester significant amounts of amphotericin B (liver, 17.5%–40.3%; spleen, 0.7%–15.6%; kidney, 0.6%–4.1%; lung, 0.4%–13%), but it does not distribute well into adipose tissue (<1.0%).[79,80] Because L.K. is 5 feet, 8 inches tall and not obese, his ideal body weight should be about 70 kg. Therefore, amphotericin B 35 mg/day (0.5 mg/kg) should be initiated because L.K. is not clinically stable and is likely to need the higher-dose regimen. Half the full dose should be given on the first day of therapy and the full dose given on subsequent days. In more seriously ill patients, the full dose of amphotericin B can be initiated immediately. Although the optimal dosing regimen to initiate amphotericin B is not well established, most clinicians gradually titrate the dose upward to minimize infusion-related reactions. Peak amphotericin B serum concentrations achieved after parenteral administration are a function of dose, frequency of dosing, and rate of infusion. When the amphotericin B total dose is <50 mg, the serum concentration is directly proportional to the dose; doses >50 mg show a plateau in serum concentrations. After administration, amphotericin B undergoes biphasic elimination: peak serum concentrations drop rapidly (initial $t_{1/2}$, 24–48 hours), but low concentrations (0.5–1.0 mcg/mL) are detectable for up to 2 weeks (terminal $t_{1/2}$ 15 days).[85] The long terminal-elimination half-life has been used as a justification for the common practice of every-other-day amphotericin B dosing, in which twice the daily dose is given every other day. Every-other-day regimens have not been carefully evaluated but are rationalized based on the potential for reduced nephrotoxicity. Administration of 0.5 mg/kg/day or 1.0 mg/kg every other day results in trough amphotericin B concentrations with sufficient postdose antifungal effects that inhibit the common pathogenic fungi.[86] Once L.K.'s clinical status has improved, the potential for renal toxicity could outweigh the concerns of potential reduced efficacy, and implementation of amphotericin B every-other-day therapy should be considered.

PREMEDICATION

Premedication to prevent amphotericin B infusion-related reactions and a test dose of amphotericin B are not needed for L.K. Most practices of premedicating are performed out of ritual rather than predicated on scientific study.[87] Test dosing with 1 mg before the first dose is not currently used because of the immeasurably low incidence of anaphylactoid reactions. Until clinical trials clarify the risk-to-benefit ratio of premedications, concomitant therapy should be restricted to acetaminophen for fever or headache and heparin to prevent thrombophlebitis when possible.

INFUSION REACTIONS

13. L.K. has no complaints except for fevers and shaking chills that occur during his 6- to 8-hour amphotericin B infusion for the past 3 days. He has been receiving acetaminophen 650 mg 30 minutes before amphotericin B infusion, but he has refused today's amphotericin B dose. What measures can be taken to minimize these infusion-related reactions?

Adverse reactions, which are common with amphotericin B administration, are best classified as acute infusion-related, dose-related, or idiosyncratic reactions. Infusion-related reactions include an acute symptom complex of fever, chills, nausea, vomiting, headache, hypotension, and thrombophlebitis. Dose-related reactions also can be acute (e.g., cardiac arrhythmias) or chronic (e.g., renal dysfunction with secondary electrolyte imbalances and anemia).

Many infusion-related reactions appear to be mediated by amphotericin B-induced cytokine (interleukin-1β, tumor necrosis factor, prostaglandin E_2) expression by mononuclear cells.[88,89] Hydrocortisone is extremely effective in suppressing cytokine expression[88] and it also blunts the fever and chills associated with amphotericin B administration.[90] Hydrocortisone, however, does not reduce the frequency of chronic dose-related toxicity such as renal insufficiency, and corticosteroid-induced immunosuppression could decrease amphotericin B fungicidal activity.[91] Nonsteroidal anti-inflammatory drugs (NSAID) also prevent fever, most likely by the suppression of prostaglandin E_2 expression.[92] NSAID, however, cannot be recommended for routine use because of their potential for additive nephrotoxicity when used with amphotericin B.

The mild to moderate elevations in temperature and the other infusion-related symptoms usually subside when the infusion is completed, and tolerance to these effects develops over 3 to 5 days. L.K. initially should be counseled that these reactions will abate over the next few days without intervention. If assessment of the reactions suggests the need for more aggressive premedication, a short course of hydrocortisone should be initiated as outlined in Table 71-6. A dose of meperidine 25 to 50 mg by rapid IV infusion reduces amphotericin B-induced rigors and can be repeated every 15 minutes as required while monitoring for signs and symptoms of opiate toxicity. Administration of an average meperidine dose of 45 mg has been found to resolve chills three times faster than placebo.[93]

Faster amphotericin B infusion rates (<4–6 hours) are associated with the earlier onset of infusion-related reactions but not with more severe infusion reactions.[94,95] Many patients prefer rapid infusions (1–2 hours) because the infusion-related reactions abate quickly on completion of the amphotericin B infusion. Electrocardiographic evaluations of 1-hour infusions indicate that this rate of amphotericin infusion is safe at currently recommended doses in patients without renal or heart disease. Rapid infusions are not safe in all patients, however, because cardiac arrhythmias appear to be dose and infusion rate related. If infused too rapidly, high serum concentrations of

Table 71-6 Amphotericin B Desoxycholate Infusion Protocol

1. Administration
   Dilute amphotericin in D_5W; the final concentration should not exceed 0.1 mg/mL. Initial dosing (0.25 mg/kg based on ideal body mass) should not exceed 30 mg. Infuse the dose over 0.75–4 hr immediately after a meal. Record temperature, pulse rate, and blood pressure every 30 min for 4 hours. If patient develops significant chills, fever, respiratory distress, or hypotension, administer adjunctive medication before the next infusion. If initial dose is tolerated, advance to maximal dose by the third to fifth day. Consult an infectious diseases clinician for any questions concerning maximal daily dose, total dose, and duration of therapy.
2. Adjunctive Medications
   1. Heparin 1,000 units may diminish thrombophlebitis for peripheral lines. Observe the contraindications to the use of heparin (e.g., thrombocytopenia, ↑ risk of hemorrhage, concomitant anticoagulation).
   2. Administration of 250 mL of normal saline before amphotericin B may help ↓ renal dysfunction.
   3. Acetaminophen administered 30 min before amphotericin B infusion may ameliorate the fever.
   4. Hydrocortisone 0.7 mg/kg (Solu-Cortef) can be added to the amphotericin infusion. Hydrocortisone is given to ↓ infusion-related reactions. It should be used only for significant fever (>2.0°F elevation from baseline) and chills during infusions and should be discontinued as soon as possible (3–5 days). It is not necessary to add hydrocortisone if the patient is receiving supraphysiologic doses of adrenal corticosteroids.
   5. Meperidine hydrochloride 25–50 mg may be used parenterally in adults to ameliorate chills.
3. Laboratory
   1. At least twice weekly for first 4 wk, then weekly: Hct, reticulocyte count, magnesium, potassium, BUN, creatinine, bicarbonate, and UA. The GFR may fall 40% before stabilizing in these patients. Discontinue for 2–5 days if renal function continues to deteriorate and reinstate after improvement. Hct often falls 22%–35% of the initial level.
   2. Monitor closely for hypokalemia and hypomagnesemia. Supplementation with a nonchloride potassium is preferable for metabolic (renal tubular) acidosis associated with hypokalemia.
4. Caveats
   1. Electrolytes. Addition of an electrolyte to an amphotericin solution causes the colloid to aggregate and probably results in suboptimal therapeutic effect. This includes IV piggyback medications containing electrolytes or preservatives.
   2. Filtering. The colloidal solution is partially retained by 0.22-micron pore membrane filter: do not use filters if possible.
   3. The infusion bottle need not be light-shielded.
5. Patients Needing Closer Monitoring
   1. Addisonian patients tolerate infusion poorly. Treatment with corticosteroids improves patient tolerance.
   2. Patients should receive neither granulocyte transfusion nor indium scanning.
   3. Patients with anuria or previous cardiac history may have an ↑ risk of arrhythmias, and slower infusions are recommended.

BUN, blood urea nitrogen; GFR, glomerular filtration rate; Hct, hematocrit; IV, intravenous; UA, urinalysis. From references 20,21,183,184, with permission.

amphotericin B can precipitate severe cardiac adverse events. Arrhythmias have been reported most often in patients who are anuric or who have previous cardiac disease.[96] Continuous infusion is not recommended based on the pharmacodynamics of this agents and the concentration dependence of activity.

NEPHROTOXICITY

14. On day 4 of therapy with amphotericin B, L.K.'s serum creatinine (SCr) and blood urea nitrogen (BUN) are 2.3 mg/dL and 42 mg/dL, respectively. How could amphotericin B exacerbate L.K.'s renal dysfunction and how could it be prevented from worsening?

[SI units: SCr, 203.32 μmol/L; BUN, 14.99 mmol/L]

Renal dysfunction is the adverse event that most often limits treatment with amphotericin B. The renal toxicity results from amphotericin B-mediated damage to renal tubules, which results in electrolyte wasting and disrupts the tubuloglomerular feedback mechanism. The clinical manifestations of amphotericin B-induced renal damage include azotemia, renal tubular acidosis, hypokalemia, and hypomagnesemia.[87] Generally, amphotericin B-related renal toxicity is reversible within 2 weeks after therapy has been discontinued. Administration of normal saline (250 mL) immediately before amphotericin B administration can decrease amphotericin B-induced nephrotoxicity[97] and should be initiated before L.K.'s next dose. Amphotericin B should not be admixed with normal saline, however, because sodium causes amphotericin B to precipitate into an inactive particulate in IV admixture formulations.[98] The cumulative dose of amphotericin deoxycholate should be kept below 3 g; other nephrotoxins should be avoided (especially diuretics) (Table 71-7), and patients with already compromised renal function should be closely monitored.[98] Hypokalemia and hypomagnesemia also should be monitored closely, and replacement therapy should be initiated as soon as significant declines in potassium or magnesium are detected. These measures to prevent further renal deterioration should be implemented and the amphotericin B therapy continued cautiously in this patient with systemic candidiasis. Anemia, associated with decreased renal production of erythropoietin, should resolve after amphotericin B is discontinued and need not be treated.[99]

15. L.K. has developed significant renal dysfunction resulting from acute tubular necrosis. How should his dose of systemic antifungal drugs be altered?

Renal elimination of the antimycotics varies tremendously. For systemically administered amphotericin B, only 5% to 10% of unchanged drug is eliminated in urine and bile during the first 24 hours,[87] and no evidence indicates it is metabolized to a significant extent. Therefore, no substantial dosage adjustment is required for patients with chronic renal or hepatic failure. Although many clinicians will withhold amphotericin B doses if acute renal dysfunction develops during therapy, concerns

Table 71-7 Significant Drug Interactions

Antifungal	*Interacting agent(s)*	*Class*[a]	*Onset*	*Manifestation*
AmphoB	Acetazolamide	2	R	Severe hyperchloremic acidosis secondary to additive or synergistic renal effects
	Chemotherapeutic agents:			
	Doxorubicin, carmustine, cyclophosphamide, fluorouracil	2	D	Enhanced chemotherapeutic effect secondary to ↑ cellularuptake.
	Cyclosporine	2	D	Enhanced nephrotoxitiy
	Digoxin	2	D	AmphoB-induced hypokalemia leading to ↑ digoxin toxicity
	Leukocyte transfusion	1	R	Severe pulmonary leukostasis with potential for respiratory failure
	NSAID	2	R	Additive or synergistic nephrotoxicity
	Pentamidine	2	D	Additive or synergistic nephrotoxicity
	Potassium-sparing diuretics	2	D	Spironolactone ↓ potassium requirements preventing hypokalemia in neutropenic patients receiving AmphoB
CFG	**Anticonvulsants:**			
	Carbamazepine, phenytoin, mephenytoin	2	D	Carbamazepine and phenytoin to significantly ↓ CFG concentrations through CYP450 induction
	Corticosteroids	2	D	Dexamethasone induces metabolism of CFG, thus ↓ serum concentrations of CFG
	Cyclosporine	2	D	Elevations in transaminases (hepatic toxicity); CFG AUC ↑ by 35%
	Rifampin			Hepatic uptake transporters of CFG might be induced by rifampin; administer CFG 70 mg/day when coadministered with rifampin
Griseofulvin	**Sedative/hypnotics:**			
	Benzodiazepines, ethanol, barbiturates	3	D	↑ Griseofulvin clearance with concomitant barbiturate or ethanol consumption
	Oral contraceptives	1	D	↓ Oral contraceptive efficacy
KI	ACE inhibitors	2	D	Hyperkalemia
	Lithium	2	D	Hypothyroidism
	Potassium-sparing diuretics	2	D	Hyperkalemia

Azole Antifungal Interactions

Effect of other drugs on azole(s)

Azole	*Interacting Agent(s)*	*Class*	*Onset*	*Manifestation*
KCZ	Isoniazid	2	D	↓ Serum antifungal concentration and potential treatment failure
KCZ	Anticholinergics	2	R	↓ Antifungal absorption; antifungal should not be administered concomitantly
KCZ	Sucralfate	2	R	20% ↓ in KCZ concentration
KCZ, ITZ	Didanosine	2	R	Acid neutralizing agents in didanosine prevent ITZ absorption. KCZ extrapolated
ITZ	Dexamethasone	2	D	Dexamethasone hepatically induces metabolism of ITZ
ITZ	Fluoxetine	3	D	Norfluoxetine inhibits CYP3A4, ↑ ITZ concentrations
FCZ	Hydrochlorthiazide	2	D	Significant ↑ in FCZ concentrations; changes attributed to ↓ FCZ renal clearance
KCZ, ITZ, FCZ	Antacids	2	R	Poor dissolution of dosage form, therefore ↓ azole availability Administer KCZ and ITZ 2 hr after antacid dose. Note drug formulations containing antacid buffers.
KCZ, ITZ, FCZ	H_2-blockers	2	R	↓ Antifungal absorption; antifungal should not be administered with H_2-blockers.
FCZ, PCZ, VCZ	Cimetidine	2	R	Alteration of gastric pH ↓ FCZ, and PCZ absorption; VCZ concentrations noted slightly ↑, possibly through nonspecific CYP450 inhibition by cimetidine.
KCZ, ITZ, FCZ, VCZ	Carbamazepine	2	D	↓ ITZ serum concentrations and therapeutic failures have occurred. Carbamazepine likely to significantly↓ VCZ concentration via potent CYP450 induction; coadministration contraindicated.
KCZ, ITZ, FCZ, VCZ	Rifampin	2	D	Rifampin-potent CYP450 inducer. Significant ↓ in serum antifungal concentrations, potentially leading to treatment failure. Doubling VCZ dose does not restore adequate antifungal exposure; coadministration contraindicated.
VCZ	Ritonavir	2	D	Ritonavir-potent CYP450 inducer and both substrate for and inhibitor of CYP3A4. VCZ serum concentrations ↓ by ritonavir in dose-dependent manner; coadministration with low-dose ritonavir should be avoided; high-dose ritonavir contraindicated.
VCZ	Barbiturates	3	D	Long-acting barbiturates likely to significantly ↓ VCZ concentrations.
Azole effects on other drugs				
KCZ, ITZ	Corticosteroids	2	D	Twofold ↑ in serum methylprednisolone observed with concomitant KCZ. Similar reaction with prednisone has been observed. ↑ Systemic effects of inhaled budesonide after ITZ.
ITZ	Fexofenadine	2	R	Significant ↑ fexofenadin AUC not related to dose of ITZ suggesting mechanism related to inhibition of gastrointestinal P-glycoprotein
KCZ, FCZ	Theobromines	2	R	Inhibition of theophylline absorption
FCZ	Oral contraceptives	1	D	↓ Oral contraceptive efficacy

Table 71-7 Significant Drug Interactions (*Continued*)

Azole	*Interacting Agent(s)*	*Class*	*Onset*	*Manifestation*
KCZ, ITZ, FCZ, VCZ	Warfarin	1	D	↓ Warfarin protein binding and hydroxylation by liver (poor documentation) leading to ↑ in prothrombin time response; interaction with VCZ proposed via CYP2C9 inhibition.
KTZ, FCZ, VCZ	Terfenadine Cisapride Astemizole Pimozide Quinidine	1	D	Azoles result in inhibition of metabolism of these drugs. ↑ Plasma concentrations can lead to QT prolongation and rarely *torsade de pointes*. Coadministration of FCZ or VCZ and terfenadine contraindicated.
	Immunologic agents			
KCZ, ITZ, FCZ, PCZ, VCZ	Cyclosporine, Sirolimus, Tacrolimus	2	D	Azole inhibition of CYP3A4 produce significant ↑ in serum immunosuppressant concentration and ↑ toxicity. Monitor cyclosporine and tacrolimus whole blood trough concentrations frequently during and at discontinuation of antifungal therapy. Coadministration of VCZ and sirolimus contraindicated. Data extrapolated for sirolimus and ITZ or PCZ.
KCZ, ITZ, FCZ,	Sulfonylureas	2	D	Significantly ↑ sulfonylurea concentrations. Data extrapolated for VCZ.
PCZ, VCZ, KCZ, ITZ, FCZ, PCZ, VCZ	Benzodiazepines	3	D	20% ↓ in chlordiazepoxide clearance demonstrated with KCZ. Inhibition of CYP3A4 by azole significantly ↑ serum concentrations of benzodiazepines metabolized by this enzyme. Monitor adverse effects frequently and consider dose reduction.
VCZ	Calcium channel blockers	3	D	↑ Plasma concentrations of calcium channel blockers metabolized by CYP3A4.
VCZ	Ergot alkaloids	1	D	Ergotism; coadministration of VCZ with ergot alkaloids contraindicated.
VCZ	Methadone	2	D	R-methadone and S-methadone serum concentrations ↑ via VCZ inhibition of CYP2C9, CYP2C19, and CYP3A4.Monitor for methadone toxicity (QT prolongation).
VCZ	Statins	2	D	VCZ inhibits lovastatin metabolism *in vitro* (CYP3A4 inhibition). Monitor for rhabdomyolysis.
VCZ	Vinca alkaloids	3	D	↑ Plasma concentrations of vinca alkoloids (CYP3A4 substrates) leading to neurotoxicity.
Two-way interactions				
KCZ, ITZ, FCZ, PCZ, VCZ	Phenytoin, mephenytoin	2	D	Phenytoin induction of UDP-G metabolism decreases PCZ concentrations. ↓ VCZ concentrations thought due to phenytoin as CYP2C9 substrate and CYP450 inducer. Avoid concomitant phenytoin and PCZ use; ↑ VCZ maintenance dose. Phenytoin serum concentrations ↑ after FCZ, PCZ, or VCZ administration; postulated mechanism via CYP3A4 inhibition. Monitor plasma phenytoin concentrations.
PCZ, VCZ	Rifabutin	2	D	↓ PCZ concentrations via UDP-G induction. ↓ VCZ concentrations via potent CYP450 induction. ↑ Rifabutin concentrations due to inhibition of CYP3A4 by PCZ and VCZ may ↑ rifabutin adverse effects. Avoid concomitant PCZ or VCZ and rifabutin.
VCZ	Efavirenz	1	D	Efavirenz is a CYP450 inducer, CYP3A4 substrate and inhibitor. Concomitant administration results in ↓ VCZ and ↑ efavirenz concentrations. Coadministration contraindicated. Data extrapolated to other non-nucleoside reverse transcriptase inhibitors; monitor for drug toxicity or antifungal failure.
VCZ	Omeprazole	2	R	↑ Omeprazole and VCZ concentrations via CYP2C19 inhibition. Reduce omeprazole doses of ≥40 mg by one-half. Metabolism of other proton pump inhibitors CYP2C19 substrates may also be inhibited by VCZ.
VCZ	Oral contraceptives	2	D	↑ Oral contraceptive and VCZ concentrations via CYP2C19 inhibition; monitor for oral contraceptive and VCZ adverse events.
VCZ	**HIV protease inhibitors** Saquinavir, amprenavir, nelfinavir	2	D	VCZ and protease inhibitors inhibition of CYP3A4 metabolism (in vitro); monitor patients for toxicity.

[a]Classification: 1, major; 2, moderate; 3, minor
[b]Clinically significant interaction that the authors recommend the reader should focus on.
ACE, angiotensin-converting enzyme; AmphoB, amphotericin B; CYP, cytochrome P; D, delayed; FCZ, fluconazole; HIV, human immunodeficiency virus; ICZ, itraconazole; KCZ, ketoconazole; KI, potassium iodide; NSAID, nonsteroidal anti-inflammatory drugs; PCZ, posaconazole; R, rapid, UDP-G; VCZ, voriconazole.

of drug-induced nephrotoxicity in L.K. must be balanced against the high likelihood of mortality in untreated patients with deep-seated infections.[60,61] Alternative systemic antifungal therapy (i.e., azoles or echinocandins) that is less nephrotoxic should also be considered. Dosing recommendations for echinocandins are unchanged in renal dysfunction or liver dysfunction except for caspofungin. For patients in moderate hepatic insufficiency (Child-Pugh score 7–9), the maintenance caspofungin dose should be decreased to 35 mg/day. No data are available for caspofungin used in severe hepatic impairment and a further dosage reduction should be considered.

Ketoconazole and itraconazole undergo first-pass metabolism and have a biphasic dose-dependent elimination.[38,39] These agents are extensively metabolized and excreted in the bile; small amounts of unchanged drug are excreted in the urine, therefore, no need exists to adjust dosages in patients with renal dysfunction or in patients undergoing dialysis.[100] Fluconazole and voriconazole, unlike ketoconazole and itraconazole, are not extensively metabolized. More than 90% of a fluconazole dose is excreted in urine, of which about 80% is measured as unchanged drug and about 20% as metabolites.[101] Because fluconazole is excreted primarily unchanged in the urine, dosages should be adjusted in patients with renal insufficiency (Table 71-5).[20,21,38–41,87,100–108] Fluconazole or voriconazole may be reasonable alternatives in L.K., but the dosage must be adjusted for renal function based on published nomograms.[102]

16. What is the role of an amphotericin B formulated with a lipid?

Lipid formulations of amphotericin B have been approved by the FDA for patients who are unable to tolerate generic amphotericin B (Table 71-8). In addition, the admixture of amphotericin B in 10% or 20% lipid emulsion has been used for treating systemic mycotic infections. The lipid carriers differ tremendously for each of the amphotericin formulations. The liposomal formulation is a spherical carrier that contains amphotericin both on the inside and outside of the vesicle. Imagine the lipid complex as a snowflake shape, and the colloidal dispersion shaped like a Frisbee with amphotericin bound to the structure. The differences in structure appear to have no effect on therapeutic outcome but confer different protection against amphotericin adverse effects.[109] Amphotericin B admixture with a lipid emulsion cannot be recommended until a stable formulation can be established.[110]

Limited data are available to assist in the management of this case. A single large controlled trial has evaluated amphotericin B lipid complex for the treatment of disseminated candidiases. Amphotericin B 0.6 to 1.0 mg/kg/day for 14 days was slightly, but not significantly, superior to the lipid complex formulation at 5 mg/kg/day for mycologic efficacy (68% vs. 63%) or survival.[111] Renal dysfunction defined as a doubling in serum creatinine, however, was 47% with amphotericin B and 28% with this lipid formulation. Because of the significant cost, lipid formulations of amphotericin B should be reserved for patients who have pre-existing renal dysfunction, and those who have severe adverse reactions to, or are failing, generic amphotericin B. Indications for the lipid formulations are further reviewed in the discussion of sections on aspergillosis and cryptococcosis.

Antimycotic Prophylaxis

17. What measures could have been undertaken to prevent invasive fungal infections in L.K.?

In 2005, the Mycoses Study Group Trial defined patients at high risk patients who could benefit from prophylaxis. Trials are underway to assess efficacy of differing antifungals in those patients who have at least one of the primary risk factors: systemic antibiotics for previous 4 days or presence of a central venous catheter. In addition, each patient would have at least two secondary risk factors: dialysis or use of TPN during previous 4 days; inpatient surgery, pancreatitis, or more than one dose of systemic steroids or immunsuppressive within 7 days before ICU admission. Minimizing these risk factors is instrumental in preventing fungal infections. When such control is not possible, pharmacotherapy should be considered in high risk populations (>10% candidemia incidence).[112]

Selective GI decontamination or systemic antimycotic pharmacotherapy can be used in high-risk, immunocompromised, or surgical patients to prevent the development of fungal infections and could have been used for L.K. In critically ill surgical patients, the risk of invasive infection may be reduced by >50% with systemic fluconazole prophylaxis. No change was seen, however, in patient survival.[113] Alternatively, a nonabsorbable antifungal such as amphotericin B or nystatin could be selected. Oral amphotericin B decreases systemic candidal infections threefold to fivefold in high-risk patients.[114] Yet, the problems of questionable antifungal stool concentrations,[115] decreasing azole cost, and poor compliance have led to preferential azole use. Azoles are more effective in preventing oral pharyngeal candidiasis (OPC) than placebo.[116,117] Only small studies with inadequate sample sizes have compared the clinical efficacy of azoles with polyene antifungals (e.g., amphotericin B) for prevention of either oropharyngeal or systemic candidiasis.

Prophylaxis could be initiated in L.K. and therapy continued until L.K. develops a systemic infection or until immunosuppression ends. If L.K. is discharged from the hospital and treated as an outpatient, a systemic azole (imidazole or triazole) administered once daily is preferable to a polyene to improve adherence. To reemphasize, however, systemic therapy increases the risk of resistance, adverse effects, drug interactions (Table 71-7), and sometimes cost (Table 71-4).

Candiduria

Treatment

18. M.Y., a 24-year-old man, has been hospitalized in the surgical ICU with multiple traumatic injuries resulting from a motor vehicle accident. Shortly after admission, he underwent an exploratory laparotomy for a ruptured spleen and lacerated liver. He subsequently suffered respiratory and renal failure. M.Y. is currently intubated and on mechanical ventilation. Since admission, he has been nutritionally supported with central hyperalimentation and has been receiving broad-spectrum antibiotics (gentamicin, ampicillin, and metronidazole). A Foley catheter is in place. Two recent UA show budding yeast and cultures were positive for >100,000 colony-forming units of *C. albicans*. M.Y. is currently afebrile, his funduscopic examination is normal, and no macronodular skin lesions are present. The WBC count is 8,900 cells/mm^3, and three sets of blood cultures drawn over

Table 71-8 Amphotericin B Formulations

Category	*Amphotericin B (Fungizone)*	*Amphotericin B Lipid Complex (ABLC; Abelcet)*	*Amphotericin B Colloidal Dispersion (Amphotec)*	*Liposomal Amphotericin B (AmBisome)*	*Amphotericin B in Lipid Emulsion (ABLE)*
FDA-approved indication	Life-threatening fungal infections Visceral leishmaniasis	Refractory or intolerant to AmphoB	Invasive Aspergillosis in patients refractory or intolerant to AmphoB	Empirical therapy in neutropenic FUO Refractory or intolerant to AmphoB Visceral leishmaniasis	NA
Formulation					
Sterol	None	None	Cholesterol sulfate	Cholesterol sulfate (5)[a]	
Phospholipid	None	DMPC and DMPG(7:3)[a]	None	EPC and DSPG(10:4)[a]	Safflower and soybean oils 10–20 g/100 mL EPC >2.21 g/100 mL Glycerin >258 g/100 mL
Amphotericin B (Mole%)	34	33	50	10	Variable
Particle size (nm)	<10	1,600–11,000	122(± 48)	80–120	333–500
Manufacturer	Generic	Enzon	Intermune	Fujisawa Pharmaceuticals	Not applicable
Stability	1 wk at 2–8°C or 24 hr at 27°C	15 hr at 2–8°C or 6 hr at 27°C	24 hr at 2–8°C	24 hr at 2–8°C	Unstable
Dosage and rate	0.3 to. 0 mg/kg/day over 1–6 hr	5.0 mg/kg/day at 2.5 mg/kg/hr	3–4 mg/kg/day over 2 hr	3.0–5.0 mg/kg/day over 2 hr	Investigational: 1.0 mg/kg/day over 1–8 hr
Lethal dose 50%	3.3 mg/kg	10–25 mg/kg	68 mg/kg	175 mg/kg	Unknown
Pharmacokinetic Parameters					
Dose	0.5 mg/kg	5.0 mg/kg × 7 days	5.0 mg/kg × 7 days	2.5 mg/kg × 7 days 5 mg/kg × 7 7 days	0.8 mg/kg/day × 13 days
Serum Concentrations					
Peak	1.2 mcg/mL	1.7 mcg/mL	3.1 mcg/mL	31.4 mcg/mL 83.0 mcg/mL	2.13 mcg/mL
Trough	0.5 mcg/mL	0.7 mcg/mL		4.0 mcg/mL	0.42 mcg/mL
Half-life	91.1 hr	173.4 hr	28.5 hr	6.3 hr 6.8 hr	7.75 hr
Volume of Distribution	5.0 L/kg	131.0 L/kg	4.3 L/kg	0.16 L/kg 0.10 L/kg	0.45 L/kg
Clearance	38.0 mL/hr/kg	436.0 mL/hr/kg	0.117 mL/hr/kg	22.0 mL/hr/kg 11.0 mL/hr/kg	37.0 m/hr/kg
Area Under the Curve	14 mcg/mL × hr	17 mcg/mL × hr	43.0 mcg/mL × hr	197 mcg/mL × hr 555 mcg/mL × hr	26.37 mcg/mL × hr

[a] Molar ratio of each component, respectively.
AmphoB, amphotericin B; DMPC, dimyristoyl phosphatidycholine; DMPG, dimyristoyl phosphatidyglycerol; DSPG, distearolyphosphatidyglycerol; EPC, egg phosphatidylcholine; FDA, U.S. Food and Drug Administration; FUO, fever of unknown origin; NA, not applicable.

the past 2 days are negative. How should M.Y.'s candiduria be treated?

[SI unit: WBC count, 8.9 × 10^9/L]

Caution must be used when selecting pharmacotherapy for M.Y. because it is difficult to differentiate among cystitis, urethritis, or systemic infection in the presence of funguria. Similarly, it is difficult to differentiate colonization from infection because candiduric patients are usually asymptomatic. Funguria cannot be used to determine the location or severity of invasion. Signs and symptoms of systemic disease should be monitored diligently until a diagnosis of colonization, cystitis, or urethritis is confirmed and the risk of dissemination is excluded.

Eradication of fungi in the urine (specifically *C. albicans*) should begin with removal of the indwelling urinary catheter and alleviation of risk factors for fungal disease. If catheter removal does not clear the urine within 48 hours, pharmacotherapy should be considered. If M.Y. is scheduled for a genitourinary procedure, he should receive systemic therapy because the rate of candidemia after surgery is high (10.8%). In addition, any patient at high risk for dissemination into the blood should be treated (e.g., patients with diabetes, genitourinary abnormalities, renal insufficiency, or immunosuppression).[118]

Bladder irrigation with amphotericin B has been commonly used and concentrations of 150 mcg/mL effectively kill 5×10^6 *C. albicans* in the urine within 2 hours.[119] Clinical studies evaluating the efficacy of continuous amphotericin B 150 mcg/mL irrigations or intermittent irrigations (15–30 mcg/100 mL) retained for 1 hour × 3 to 7 days are limited, however, and often have had serious design flaws. In two comparative studies, bladder irrigation for 5 days with amphotericin B 50 mcg/mL appeared to be superior to fluconazole 100 mg/day as measured by microbiologic cure rates. Cure rates 2 to 4 weeks days after infection were equal, however, but mortality rates were higher in the amphotericin B-treated groups. Amphotericin B failures may have been associated with dissemination of yeast from the urinary tract.[120,121] Systemic antifungal therapy with flucytosine 100 to 150 mg/kg/day for 7 days[122] and azoles (fluconazole 0.6 to 1.4 mg/kg/day for 7 days)[123,124] also has been used in noncomparative or nonrandomized studies.

Blastomycosis

Etiology

19. C.P., a 17-year-old girl, is admitted to the hospital with a chronic pneumonia that has not responded to antibiotics. Three months ago, she developed a chronic cough that eventually became productive of purulent sputum, which was occasionally streaked with blood. Two months ago, she developed "boils" on her lower extremities and back, which drained spontaneously. She was hospitalized at another hospital but failed to respond to amoxicillin and erythromycin. C.P. denies fever, chills, or night sweats, but has lost 11 pounds. Her temperature is 38.2°C. A 2-cm² subcutaneous, fluctuant, tender mass is seen over the right mandible and a second fluctuant mass about 4 cm wide on the lower back. Also, several 0.5- to 1-cm² ulcers with heaped-up, hyperkeratotic margins are noted on the lower extremities (Fig. 71-2). Rales are heard at the right lung base. C.P.'s leukocyte count is slightly elevated at 13,500 cells/mm³. A chest radiograph shows a masslike infiltrate in the right mid-lung field (Fig. 71-3). A wet preparation of ulcer scrapings and material aspirated from a subcutaneous abscess reveal numerous broad-based, budding yeast forms with refractile cell walls and multiple nuclei typical of *B. dermatitidis*.

Cultures of sputum, skin scrapings, and abscess material eventually confirmed the diagnosis. What was the likely portal of entry for C.P.'s disseminated blastomycosis? Why should it be treated?

[SI unit: WBC count, 13.5×10^9/L]

Typical of the other endemic mycoses, the primary portal of entry for *B. dermatitidis* is the lungs. A pulmonary origin for C.P.'s infection is also supported by her history of cough with purulent, blood-streaked sputum, evident about a month before cutaneous lesions appeared on her legs and back. An acute pulmonary infection is most often asymptomatic and, when symptomatic, usually requires only observation. Chronic pulmonary or extrapulmonary blastomycosis will develop in an unknown number of these patients. C.P.'s rales at the base of her right lung and persistent pneumonia that is unresponsive to antibiotics indicate that she has a chronic pulmonary infection and will require therapy. Chronic pulmonary disease often presents with radiographic studies that can be mistaken

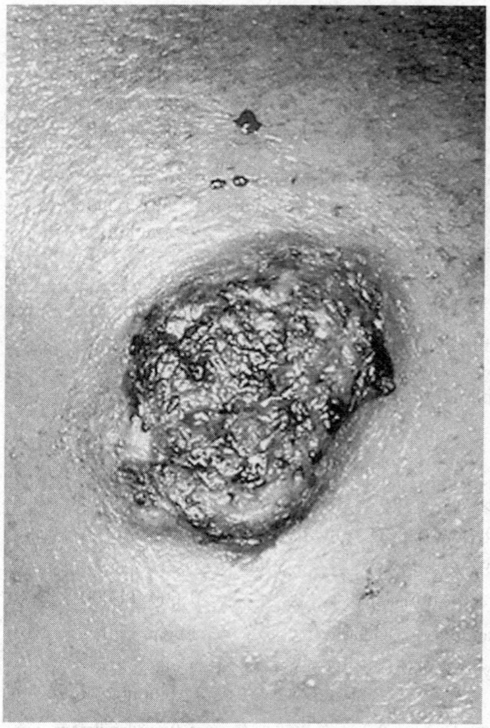

FIGURE 71-2 **Disseminated *Blastomyces dermatitidis* skin ulcers.**

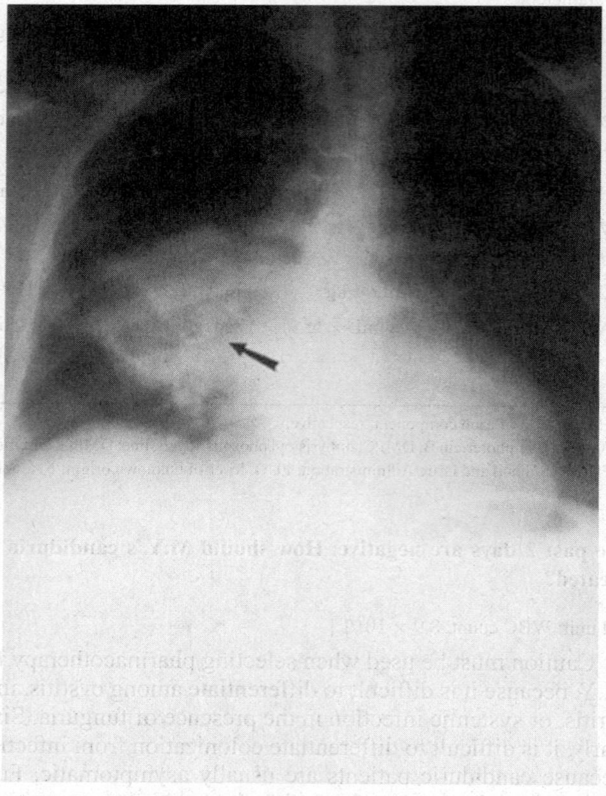

FIGURE 71-3 **Chest radiograph of pulmonary *Blastomyces dermatitidis*.**

for tuberculosis or lung cancer; the masslike infiltrate in her right lung on chest radiograph also is consistent with chronic pulmonary disease. Extrapulmonary infections can involve the skin (verrucous or ulcerative lesions), bone, genitourinary system (prostatitis, epididymo-orchitis), or central nervous system (CNS) (meningitis or brain abscess). If untreated, these chronic pulmonary or extrapulmonary infections will be fatal in at least 21% of patients.[125] Because C.P. presents with pulmonary and cutaneous evidence of blastomycosis, she should be treated.

Treatment

20. What specific therapy should be initiated for C.P.?

Historically, amphotericin B was considered the treatment of choice for blastomycosis and total doses of >2 g were associated with 97% cure rates, low relapse rates, yet 70% toxicity.[125] Ketoconazole and itraconazole currently are advocated as safe and effective alternatives to amphotericin B in patients with non–life-threatening, non-CNS infections. The NIAID -Mycoses Study Group[126] confirmed the effectiveness of azoles for the treatment of chronic pulmonary and extrapulmonary disease caused by the endemic mycoses, blastomycosis, and histoplasmosis. In uncontrolled evaluations of chronic pulmonary and extrapulmonary infections (excluding life-threatening or CNS), ketoconazole at dosages of 400 to 800 mg/day resulted in cure rates of about 89%, failure rates of about 6%, and relapse rates of about 5%.[126] In similar studies, itraconazole capsules 200 to 400 mg/day for a median of 6.2 months resulted in cure rates of 88% to 95%.[127] Fluconazole was ineffective at dosages <400 mg/day. Higher dosages (400–800 mg/day), however, are as effective as ketoconazole in non–life-threatening disease.[128] Although these trials are neither comparative nor controlled, itraconazole appears to be less toxic than ketoconazole and to have the best benefit (efficacy) to risk (toxicity) ratio.

C.P. has mild to moderate disease and can be treated with an initial itraconazole dosage of 200 mg/day. If no clinical improvement is seen within 2 weeks or if the disease progresses despite therapy, the dosage of itraconazole can be titrated upward in 100-mg increments to a maximal dosage of 400 mg/day. Treatment should continue for at least 6 months. If C.P. develops severe or meningeal disease, itraconazole should be discontinued and amphotericin B 0.3 to 0.5 mg/kg/day should be initiated to provide a total dose of 1.5 g. C.P. should be followed up for 12 months because of the possible risk of relapse. Unlike histoplasmosis, skin and serologic testing are not sufficiently sensitive to diagnose blastomycosis or evaluate the effectiveness of treatment.[126,129] Rather, patients should be evaluated closely for resolution of symptoms (constitutional, pulmonary), negative microbiologic samples, and improvement in radiographic studies.

Antifungals in Pregnancy

21. C.P. reports she has not menstruated in 3 months, and a urine pregnancy test is positive. How does this information change the therapeutic options for her?

The data on the safety of antimycotics for treating patients who are pregnant or lactating are limited, but comprehensively reviewed according to FDA categories of the teratogenic risks of drugs (see Chapter 47, Obstetric Drug Therapy).[130,131] The systemic azoles are categorized risk factor C.[132] However, we believe they are contraindicated in pregnant or lactating women who are breast-feeding because of their potential teratogenicity and endocrine toxicity in the fetus or newborn. As with the azoles, griseofulvin and flucytosine have been classified as risk factor C. These agents should not be used in C.P. because the risk clearly outweighs the therapeutic benefit. Few or no data exist on the secretion of these agents in breast milk. Therefore, breast-feeding should be discouraged in women receiving these antifungal agents.

Amphotericin B and terbinafine are classified as risk factor B. Therapeutic agents in this category have no fetal risk based on animal studies or, when risk has been found in animals, controlled human studies have not confirmed the results. No reports apparently exist regarding the use of terbinafine in pregnancy. Therefore, this arbitrary designation is of concern and recommendation is to avoid terbinafine use in pregnancy until published data support a B classification. Furthermore, considerable clinical experience with amphotericin B in pregnant women has documented successful treatment of systemic mycoses with no excess toxicity to either the mother or fetus. Thus, amphotericin B formulations have been the mainstay of antifungal therapy in pregnancy.

Histoplasmosis

Treatment

22. J.N., a 47-year-old man with severe rheumatoid arthritis, has been maintained on daily prednisone for the past 6 years; his current dosage is 20 mg/day. For the past 4 weeks, he has experienced daily fevers to 38.4°C, drenching night sweats, anorexia, and an 8.2-kg weight loss. His prednisone dosage was increased to 40 mg/day with little clinical effect. On admission to the hospital, J.N. appears chronically ill and has many of the stigmata of chronic steroid therapy. His temperature is 37.8°C with an associated rapid heart rate of 105 beats/minute. A shallow mouth ulcer is present on the hard pallet. The liver is enlarged to a total span of 18 cm, and the spleen is palpable 3 cm below the left costal margin. Stool is positive for occult blood. A chest radiograph shows bilateral interstitial infiltrates (Fig. 71-4A). He is pancytopenic, with a hematocrit (Hct) of 29% (normal, 39%–45%), a WBC count of 3,500 cells/mm^3 (normal, 4,000–11,000 cells/mm^3), and platelet count of 78,000 cells/mm^3 (normal, 130 to 400,000 cells/mm^3). The bilirubin is normal but the aminotransferases are elevated to about 1.5 times normal, and serum lactate dehydrogenase is 10 times over normal. A UA reveals 8 to 10 WBC/high-power field. The SrCr is 1.9 mg/dL, and BUN is 42 mg/dL. A bone marrow aspirate and biopsy of the mouth ulcer reveals multiple, small intracellular yeast forms compatible with *H. capsulatum* in macrophages and polymorphonuclear leukocytes (Fig. 71-4B). Cultures of blood and urine, bone marrow aspirate, and mouth ulcer biopsy grew *H. capsulatum*. What should be the primary antifungal therapy in this case of systemic *H. capsulatum*? What clinical parameters should be monitored to assess the efficacy and toxicity of J.N.'s therapy?

[SI units: Hct, 0.29; WBC count, 3.5 × 10^9/L; SrCr, 167.96 μmol/L; BUN, 14.99 mmol/L urea]

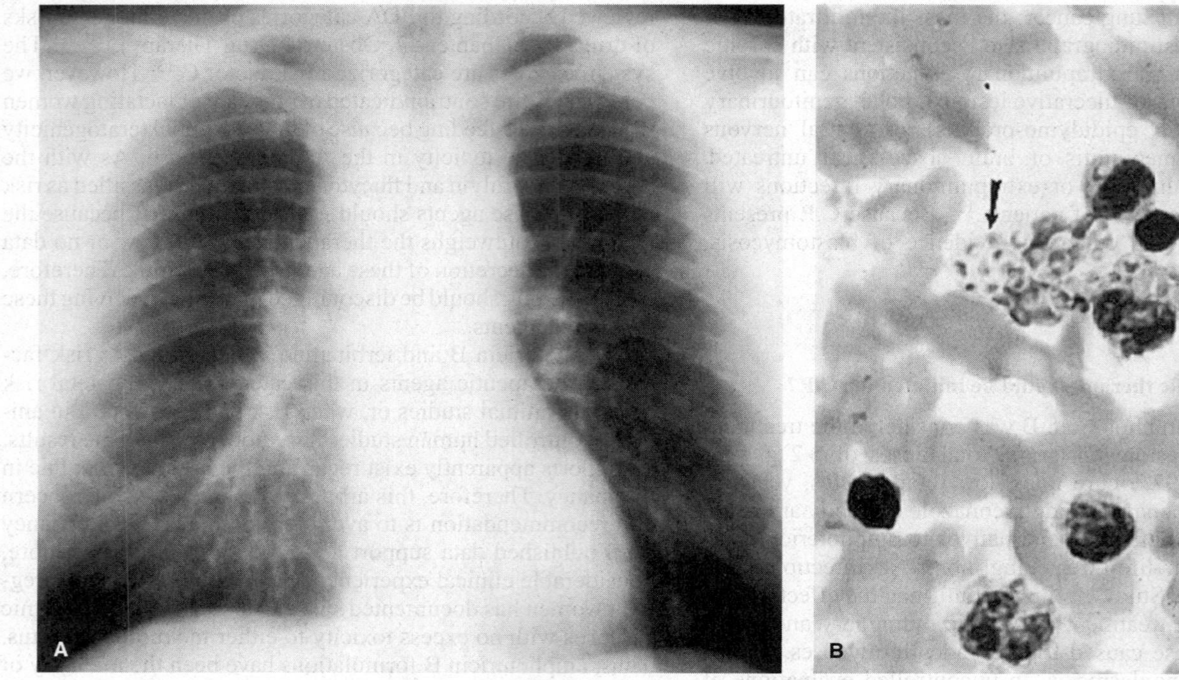

FIGURE 71-4 **Histoplasmosis infection. A:** Chest radiograph showing bilateral interstitial infiltrate. **B:** Gram's stain of peripheral blood showing leukocytes with intracellular organisms.

The treatment benefits of antifungal therapy in systemic histoplasmosis have not been well investigated. Treatment options for histoplasmosis are outlined in Table 71-9.[133] Accordingly, J.N. should be treated with amphotericin B 0.3 to 0.5 mg/kg/day or itraconazole 2.8 mg/kg/day, and his course of therapy should be monitored for both efficacy and toxicity. Amphotericin B was selected for this case.

Blood and urine cultures, pancytopenia (except anemia in amphotericin B-treated patients), constitutional symptoms, serum lactate dehydrogenase (LDH,) and hepatosplenomegaly are excellent measures for evaluating outcome to antifungal therapy of J.N.'s histoplasmosis. Anemia and chest radiographs are poor measures of treatment response. Chest radiographs often reflect calcified granulomas in chronic disease with

Table 71-9 Treatment of Histoplasmosis

Disease	Primary	Secondary
Acute Pulmonary		
Prolonged symptomatology (> 2 wks)	Resolves spontaneously	Not applicable
Immunocompromised [c]	ITZ 50–100 mg/day (3–6 mos)[a]	AmphoB 0.3–0.5 mg/kg/day[a]
Respiratory distress	AmphoB lipid formulation[c]	AmphoB 0.3–0.5 mg/kg/day
(Pao$_2$ <70 mm Hg)	AmphoB 0.5–1.0 mg/kg/day (TD250–500 mg) ± corticosteroids	ITZ 1.5–2.8 mg/kg/day (≥6 mos)[a] ITZ (has not been investigated in life-threatening situations)
Chronic Pulmonary		
Active	ITZ 1.5–2.8 mg/kg/day 9 mos)[a,b]	AmphoB 0.5 mg/kg/day[b]
Inactive		Or KTZ 400 mg/day (≈6 mos)
Histoplasmoma	No treatment	Not applicable
Mediastinal fibrosis	Surgery[d]	Not applicable
Systemic Disease	AmphoB (total dose recommended: 35 mg/kg) or ITZ 2.8 mg/kg/day[a]	Fluconazole 400–800 mg/day[e]

[a] Treatment should be continued until the patient is symptom free and culture negative for 3 mos. The recommendations for duration of therapy or total doses should be used only as guides for initial therapy.
[b] Indicated only for serious symptoms (i.e., hemoptysis).
[c] Lipid formulations of amphotericin B are preferable to generic amphotericin B in HIV-infected patients.[135]
[d] ITZ 200 mg QD or BID for 6–18 mos for most patients.
[e] Fluconazole should only be used in patients who cannot take ITZ.
AmphoB, amphotericin B deoxycholate; ITZ, itraconazole; KTZ, ketoconazole; TD, total dose.

scarring, which rarely resolve even with extensive therapy. Therefore, evaluation of deterioration on radiograph but not of improvement is possible. In addition, amphotericin B-induced renal disease with secondary anemia can confuse evaluation of disease resolution. Anemia must be excluded as a prognostic indicator in patients receiving amphotericin B for durations of 3 weeks regardless of the dose.[99]

Diligent follow-up of patients is required because relapses occur in 5% to 15% of amphotericin B-treated patients within 3 years. Relapses occurred in patients who received <30 mg/kg total dose of amphotericin B, or had concomitant untreated Addison's disease, immunosuppression, vascular infections (endocarditis, grafts, aneurysms), or meningeal infections.[133,134] More than 90% of HIV-positive patients experience a relapse of histoplasmosis subsequent to adequate amphotericin B therapy. A double blind trial in immunocompromised patients (HIV) revealed that liposomal amphotericin B was superior to amphotericin B deoxycholate. It is not known how itraconazole compares with liposomal amphotericin B in those infected with HIV. If this patient was infected with HIV, a lipid based amphotericin may have been preferred.[135] Even the initiation of subsequent immunosuppressive therapy is of particular concern because of the potential for reactivation (relapse) and dissemination of histoplasmosis from dormant foci, especially in patients with residual granulomas.

Potential adverse effects to amphotericin B also should be monitored in J.N. (e.g., infusion-related reactions, nephrotoxicity, anemia, hypokalemia, neurotoxicity, thrombophlebitis). In addition, J.N.'s adrenal status should be monitored closely because of his long-term corticosteroid therapy and his histoplasmosis. Patients who are addisonian secondary to histoplasmosis infections appear to experience more episodes of amphotericin B-induced acute hypotension.

Azole Adverse Effects

23. After treatment with a total amphotericin B dose of 750 mg, clinical improvement of J.N.'s histoplasmosis is subjectively and objectively documented. The clinician selected ketoconazole 400 mg/day as an oral substitute for his amphotericin B regimen because of the patient's economic circumstances. Six weeks later, J.N. complains of impotence and wonders whether this could be caused by his medication. What is the likelihood that ketoconazole is the cause of J.N.'s impotence?

Ketoconazole has been associated with more adverse reactions and greater potential for drug interactions compared with miconazole, itraconazole, and fluconazole. The most common side effects of ketoconazole, however, are nausea and vomiting. GI distress appears to be dose-related because a substantially smaller percentage of patients experience these effects when receiving ketoconazole dosages of 400 mg/day compared with dosages of 800 mg/day.[134] Endocrine and hepatic toxicities are the most significant adverse effects of ketoconazole requiring monitoring. Dose-splitting from daily to twice daily may decrease the nausea and vomiting. Dose-related endocrinologic toxicities (hypoadrenalism, oligospermia, and diminished libido) have been observed during ketoconazole therapy secondary to inhibition of mammalian sterol synthesis,[11,136] and usually resolve with drug discontinuation. Therefore, J.N.'s complaints of impotence might well be attributed to his ketoconazole. Liver enzymes should also be monitored because an approximate 10% risk exists of elevation in transaminases and an occasional case of serious hepatitis and hepatic failure.[11,136]

The triazoles—itraconazole, fluconazole, and voriconazole—are much better tolerated and require less monitoring than ketoconazole therapy. This has been attributed to the greater affinity of the triazoles for fungal cytochrome enzymes and less interference with mammalian enzymes.[137] Neither itraconazole nor fluconazole (6 mg/kg/day) exhibit any substantial hepatotoxicity or antiandrogenic effects, and nausea and vomiting occur in substantially fewer patients (<5%) receiving these agents compared with imidazoles. Abnormal elevations in liver function occurred in 2.7% of patients receiving voriconazole during clinical trials. Abnormalities in liver function tests may be associated with higher azole dosages or serum concentrations, but generally resolve either with continued therapy or dosage modification, including drug discontinuance. Liver function should be determined before and periodically throughout azole therapy because cases of serious hepatic reactions have been reported.[137] A unique adverse event associated with voriconazole is enhanced perception to light, which may be associated with higher plasma concentrations or doses. Generally, drug discontinuance is not required, although monitoring of visual acuity, visual field, and color perception is advised if therapy lasts longer than 28 days. Diarrhea, asthenia, flatulence, and eye pain have been reported with posaconazole therapy.[54] Based on these data, J.N. should be given a trial of itraconazole.

Azole Drug Interactions

24. J.N. chose to continue his ketoconazole therapy. He now returns with Cushnoid signs and symptoms. What potential drug or disease state interaction could be implicated as a cause of this serious problem in J.N.?

Drug interactions with systemic azoles and polyenes can lead to mild inconveniences or life-threatening events (Table 71-7). The interaction between azoles and glucocorticoids is not as serious as the interaction reporting QT prolongation and ventricular arrhythmias with nonsedating H_1-selective antihistamines.[138] The interaction with corticosteroids can be multifaceted, however, and is therapeutically challenging. Although it is clinically possible that corticosteroids could affect outcome, no clinical trial has addressed this important question. Drug interaction trials have measured an increase in corticosteroid serum concentrations leading to recommendations to decrease the steroid dose by 50% when ketoconazole is used concomitantly. The interaction has been suggested between glucocorticoids and other azoles.[139] In addition, dexamethasone has been demonstrated to increase the clearance of caspofungin.

Other significant drug interactions with the azole antifungals revolve around their ability to inhibit the cytochrome (CYP) P450 enzyme system. All five azoles inhibit CYP3A4, but with varying potency: ketoconazole is the most potent inhibitor, followed by itraconazole and voriconazole, then posaconazolze and fluconazole. In addition to the interactions documented in Table 71-7, numerous other agents are substrates to cytochrome CYP3A4, but for which no clinical studies have evaluated an interaction. As azole antifungals could increase serum concentrations and therefore increase activity of these substrates, caution should be exercised during concomitant use. Adding complexity to voriconazole's interactions include its propensity to inhibit CYP2C9 and CYP2C19, two isoenzymes exhibiting polymorphism, thus increasing concentrations of CYP2C9 or CYP2C19 substrates. Conversely, agents that either induce or inhibit the CYP450 system may decrease or increase, respectively, antifungal drug concentrations.

Coccidioidomycosis

Serologic Tests

25. F.W., a 32-year-old Filipino woman and a lifelong resident of the Central Valley in California, is admitted to the hospital with a third recurrence of coccidioidal meningitis. Approximately 4 years ago, she was treated with a total amphotericin B dose of 2.2 g, which resulted in a good clinical response. Nine months later, she relapsed and received a second course of amphotericin B to a total of 1.6 g. She did well over the next 18 months and was able to return to work as a secretary. Over the past 4 months, however, F.W. has had chronic headaches, has been unable to concentrate at work, and is reported by family members to have a very labile personality. A computed tomography (CT) scan of the brain reveals mild hydrocephalus. An opening pressure of 19 mm Hg (normal, 10 mm Hg) was documented at lumbar puncture. Analysis of the CSF showed 110 WBC/mm^3 (normal, 0 WBC/mm^3)); glucose, 18 mg/dL (normal, 60% of serum glucose); and protein, 190 mg/dL (normal, <50 mg/dL). Complement fixation antibodies were positive in the CSF at a titer of 1:32. How should serologic tests for coccidioidomycosis be interpreted?

The most important serologic tests for fungal infections use complement fixation (CF), immunodiffusion, and EIA techniques. Tests for complement fixing antibodies (i.e., CF) to the dimorphic fungi (Table 71-1) are well established and various antigens have been used. Coccidioidin is the mycelial phase antigen for *Coccidioides immitis.* Of patients with coccidioidomycosis, 61% will have coccidioidin CF titers of at least 1:32 and 41% will have titers of 1:64. Rising titers are a bad prognostic sign, and falling titers indicate clinical improvement. Therefore, F.W.'s CSF CF titer of 1:32 is consistent with active coccidioidomycosis. Immunodiffusion testing for coccidioidomycosis using coccidioidin reveals that seropositive results appear 1 to 3 weeks after onset of primary infection in 75% of patients and this positivity usually disappears within 4 months if the infection resolves.[140] IgG- and IgM-specific EIA using a combination of antigens for *C. immitis* have been developed. These tests offer sensitivities of >92% and specificities of 98% for serum and CSF. EIA reactivity appears earlier than CF reactivity.[141,142]

Antifungal Central Nervous System Penetration

26. What is a pharmacokinetic explanation for the treatment failure of F.W.? How might this problem be overcome?

F.W. has received prolonged parenteral amphotericin B administration and the CSF still contains fungal organisms. Treatment failures in this case may partly be owing to the limited penetration of amphotericin B into the CSF.[87] Because amphotericin B is highly bound to lipid (90%–95%), CSF concentrations achieved are only 2% to 4% of the serum concentration[87,137]; peritoneal, synovial, and pleural fluid concentrations are slightly <50% of the serum concentrations (Table 71-5). Flucytosine is not significantly bound to protein and penetrates the CSF, vitreous, and peritoneal fluids; its volume of distribution approximates that of total body water.[143] Flucytosine concentration in the CSF is 74% of the serum concentration, resulting in its extensive use in treatment of CNS mycoses. Flucytosine, however, has no activity in coccidioidomycosis and, therefore, cannot be used in F.W.

The volume of distribution of fluconazole approaches that of total body water,[144] and concentrations of fluconazole in CSF are approximately 60% of simultaneous serum concentrations. Ketoconazole has only about 1% of the dose present as free drug because it is highly bound to plasma proteins (>80%) and to erythrocytes (15%). Therefore, ketoconazole penetrates poorly into the CSF except with dosages of 1,200 mg/day. Itraconazole is similar to ketoconazole in that it is >99% protein bound. Itraconazole concentrates intracellularly in host alveolar macrophages, however, and that may account for its efficacy against fungal CNS infection despite its inability to penetrate into the CSF.[145] Echinocandins also poorly (<5%) penetrate into the CSF.[146] Data on terbinafine and posaconazole penetration are currently unavailable. Therefore, fluconazole might be an alternative to CNS instillation of amphotericin B based only on pharmacokinetic considerations.

Preliminary studies with fluconazole, investigated at dosages of 400 mg/day, are promising for control of disease in patients with coccidioidomycosis meningitis. Relapse rates are high once fluconazole therapy is stopped, however.[140] Ketoconazole, which must be given at very high doses and results in significant toxicity, should be used only if other therapies are contraindicated.[139,147] Oral itraconazole 200 mg twice daily is not superior to fluconazole based on a randomized, double-blind, placebo-controlled trial of nonmeningitis disease; however, it tended toward greater efficency.[148]

Intrathecal Amphotericin

27. What adverse events might be observed with the intrathecal administration of an antifungal in F.W.?

Augmentation of systemic antifungal administration with intraventricular or intrathecal administration may improve the outcome for antifungals with poor penetration into the CSF.[148–153] Intrathecal amphotericin B doses in adults normally range from 0.25 to 0.5 mg diluted in 5 mL of 5% glucose.[140,145] A few studies suggest that doses >0.7 mg improve the cure rate and decrease relapse.[147] Cisternal or intraventricular administration is recommended as the routes of choice because of flow characteristics of CSF from the ventricles to the spinal cord.[148–150] When lumbar administration is necessary, amphotericin B is administered in a hypertonic solution of 10% glucose and the patient is placed in a Trendelenburg position in an attempt to improve distribution of the drug to the basilar meninges and ventricles and reduce local toxicity. Voriconazole, caspofungin, and the lipid amphotericin formulations have not been evaluated.

Cisternal antifungal administration has been associated with headaches, nausea, vomiting, cranial nerve paresis, and cisternal hemorrhage caused by needle trauma.[149,150–152] An Ommaya reservoir often is used to facilitate intraventricular administration of amphotericin B. Common complications of these devices include shunt occlusion, bacterial colonization or bacterial meningitis, parkinsonian symptoms, and seizures.[149–153] Lumbar administration has been used because it is simpler, but it often must be discontinued because of chemical arachnoiditis, headache, transient radiculitis, paresthesia, nerve pulses, difficulty voiding, impaired vision, vertigo, and tinnitus.[153] Acute toxic delirium, demyelinating peripheral neuropathy, and spinal cord injury have also been reported.[154–156] Regardless of the substantial and serious adverse effects, intrathecal administration may be effective in treating patients with meningitis who have severe disease or who are pharmacologic nonresponders.

Aspergillosis

Empiric Therapy (Neutropenic Host)

28. M.Z., an otherwise healthy 29-year-old man, presented for allogeneic bone marrow transplantation (BMT) 12 days ago. He has had no serious complications associated with his chloroquine-induced aplastic anemia during his 7-month wait for BMT. On BMT days −5 to −2, induction therapy was initiated with cyclophosphamide (50 mg/kg) and total body irradiation, and then bone marrow from his HLA antigen-compatible brother was infused on day 0. The onset of neutropenia was noted on day 3 and the WBC count was 50 cells/mm^3. M.Z. has complained only of stomatitis and diarrhea before day 5. On that morning, he was complaining of fever, chest pain, and headache. On physical examination, his temperature is 37°C. Empiric anti-infectives were added, but by day 8 he was not clinically improving. What therapeutic options should be considered for this patient?

Empiric antifungal therapy in a neutropenic host should be initiated when a patient is febrile for >96 hours on appropriate anti-infectives. Routine empiric therapy for a patient without evidence of deep-seated fungal infection historically has been amphotericin B 0.3 to 0.6 mg/kg/day or fluconazole 200 to 400 mg/day until the absolute neutrophil count is >500 cells/mm^3.[157] Therapy results in resolution of signs and symptoms in up to 64% of patients.

Because mould infections are of concern in this neutropenic patient population, drug therapy that is highly active against these organisms should be considered. Assessments of newer antifungals using a composite endpoint for success have failed to show superiority over amphotericcin B. A large, well-controlled, double-blind comparison of amphotericin B 0.6 mg/kg/day versus liposomal amphotericin B 3.0 mg/kg/day can be a guide for this case. Patients who were febrile >96 hours and neutropenic (<500 cells/mm^3) experienced equal survival and clinical success of approximately 50% for both agents.[158] Success rates studies comparing other agents, liposomal amphotericin B (34%) with caspofungin (34%),[159] voriconazole, or itraconazole[160,161] have had similar outcomes. It is important to remember that fever is a late and insensitive measure of infection. Prevention of breakthrough invasive fungal infection may be the most important indicator of an agent's efficacy. Using this measure, voriconazole appears superior when comparing trials, voriconazole versus liposomal amphotericin B (1.9% vs. 5%), amphotericin B versus liposomal amphotericin B (3.2% versus 7.8%).[158,161] Selection of any of these expensive, however less toxic, agents should be weighed against the incidence of invasive fungal disease in institution.

29. What is the role of lipid formulations of amphotericin B in other disease states?

A motivation for developing these formulations was the observation that serum triglycerides and cholesterol decrease adverse drug reactions and may improve efficacy.[112,162] The advantage of the formulations (Table 71-8) is clear in the treatment of diseases such as aspergillosis, which require long-term therapy that can result in patient intolerance to generic amphotericin B.[109] Multiple uncontrolled or retrospective trials have observed that all four lipid formulations of amphotericin B appear to be less nephrotoxic and may be more effective than amphotericin B deoxycholate. A single large randomized, double-blind trial and a historical controlled trial support these observations.[147,163]

Few well-controlled prospective comparative trials exist to guide the decision-making process for fungal infections that require a shorter course of therapy. In addition to the data presented for candidemia (Question 16), liposomal and lipid complex amphotericin B have been evaluated for treatment of cryptococcal meningitis and histoplasmosis in patients infected with HIV.[135,164,165] Each lipid agent appears safer and more effective than amphotericin B deoxycholate. Secondary to the high acquisition cost and relatively low rates of toxicity with short course therapy, generic amphotericin B should be selected over the lipid formulation unless a patient is clearly intolerant, requires extended therapy, or experiences a treatment failure.

Of particular interest are the ongoing studies and case reports in which Intralipid 10% to 20% combined with amphotericin B (1–2 mg/mL) is administered at a dosage of 1 mg/kg/day. This practice cannot be recommended until a prospective, randomized, controlled trial documents efficacy and reduced toxicity of these lipid emulsion–amphotericin B formulations as compared with amphotericin B alone. Current concerns are (a) the inability to formulate a pharmaceutically stable product,[166] (b) difficulty assessing whether inline filtering is required, and (c) the delivery of excessive calories.[167]

Treatment of Aspergillosis

30. Chest auscultation on day 8 reveals right-sided rales with a friction rub. Chest radiograph shows a nodular infiltrate in the right middle lobe. Fiberoptic bronchoscopy identified eroded bronchioles with necrotic tissue, and methenamine silver nitrate stain of a biopsy sample revealed fragmented, closely septated hyphal bodies branched at 45 degree angles. The samples were sent to microbiology for cultures. All previous blood and sputum cultures have been negative, except that *Aspergillus niger* growing from sputum before admission was classified as a "contaminant." The diagnosis at this time is probable aspergillosis. What treatment steps should be taken?

Drug therapy should be approached by first determining whether the infection is likely to be invasive or noninvasive disease (Fig. 71-5). Most patients inhale *Aspergillus* species and never become symptomatic or develop only mild hypersensitivity pneumonitis. Invasive infections are more likely to occur in immunocompromised patients, especially those with prolonged neutropenia associated with bone marrow transplantation. A classic observation reported by radiology is a "halo" sign or a "crescent" sign identified on CT, highly suggestive of this infection. Additionally, an ELISA for a surface protein, galactomannan, has been reported to have high

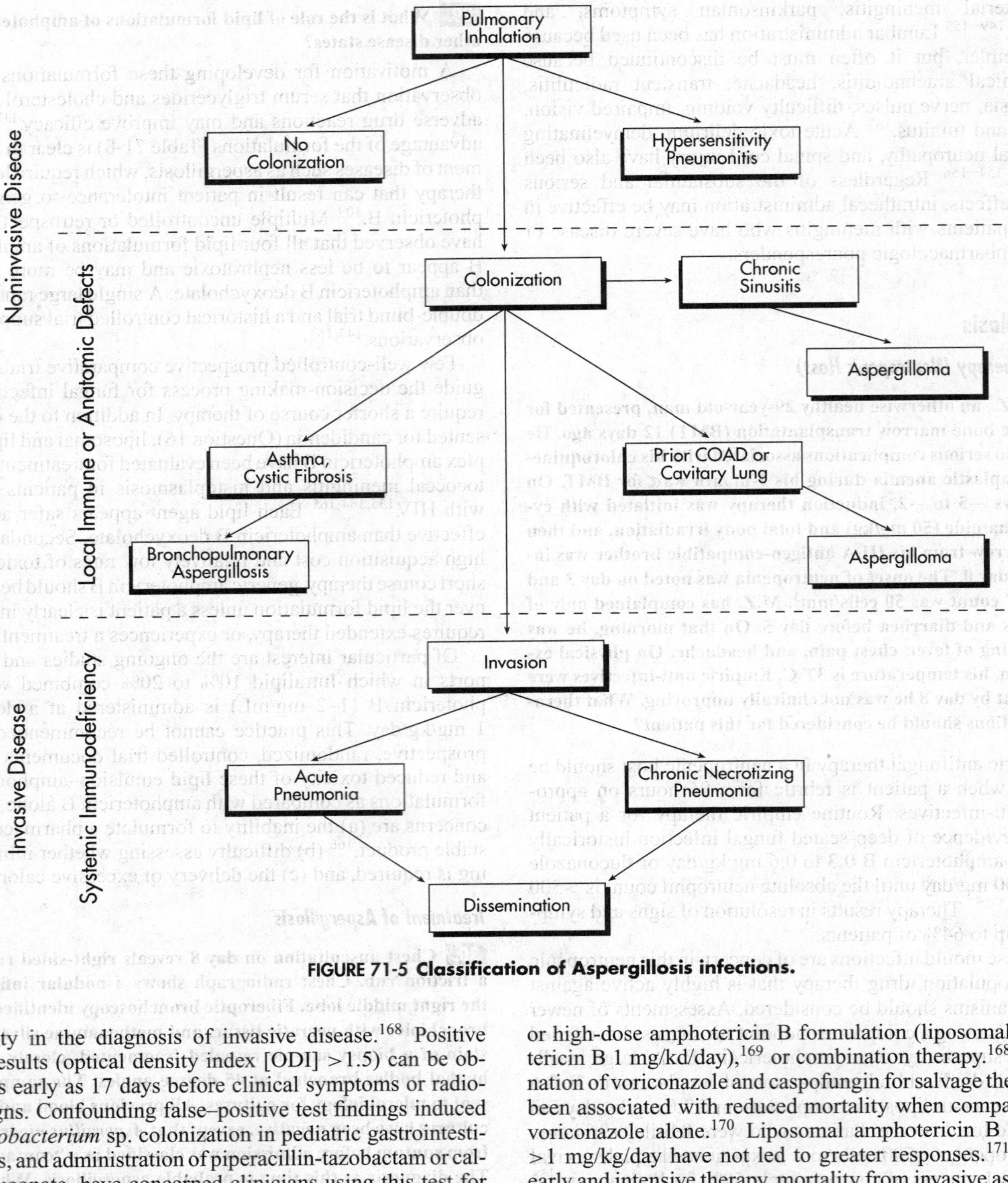

FIGURE 71-5 Classification of Aspergillosis infections.

sensitivity in the diagnosis of invasive disease.[168] Positive serum results (optical density index [ODI] >1.5) can be obtained as early as 17 days before clinical symptoms or radiologic signs. Confounding false–positive test findings induced by *Bifidobacterium* sp. colonization in pediatric gastrointestinal tracts, and administration of piperacillin-tazobactam or calcium gluconate, have concerned clinicians using this test for screening in areas with low case rates. This test should be an excellent prognostic indicator for therapeutic outcome in confirmed cases or screening in areas with high case rates. The subjective and objective data in this case clearly represent invasive symptomatic disease and there is a need for aggressive treatment.

Aspergillosis is a model for invasive mould infections that have a propensity to invade blood vessels and tissue. Antimycotic pharmacotherapy should be initiated rapidly and aggressively (Table 71-10) in conjunction with removal or reversal of immunosuppression if possible. Definite or probable invasive aspergillosis should be treated with voriconazole or high-dose amphotericin B formulation (liposomal amphotericin B 1 mg/kd/day),[169] or combination therapy.[168] Combination of voriconazole and caspofungin for salvage therapy has been associated with reduced mortality when compared with voriconazole alone.[170] Liposomal amphotericin B at doses >1 mg/kg/day have not led to greater responses.[171] Despite early and intensive therapy, mortality from invasive aspergillosis can be >50%.[172] In unresponsive patients, an amphotericin B formulation in combination therapy with an echinocandin, flucytosine, rifampin, or itraconazole; or an echinocandin with voriconazole should be considered.[168,169,173] Flushing, rash, facial swelling, and pruritis can occur with caspofungin administration and is thought to be histamine mediated. Less serious, but more frequent, adverse effects reported in patients receiving caspofungin include fever, elevations in serum transaminases, serum alkaline phosphatase, or both, and headache.[154]

Patients with mild to moderate *Aspergillus* should be treated with voriconazole or itraconazole.[172] Clinical and microbiologic cure rates of 50% to 71% have been reported for

Table 71-10 Therapeutic Options for Treatment of Aspergillosis

Disease	Primary	Secondary
Hyalohyphomycetes		
Aspergillosis		
Allergic bronchopulmonary	Prednisone 1 mg/kg/day followed by 0.5 mg/kg/day or QOD × 3–6 mos; no antifungal therapy	ITZ 200 mg BID × 4 mos[a]
Aspergilloma	Observation	Surgery[b]
Systemic (invasive) Serious	Voriconazole 6 mg/kg/day LD, 4 mg/kg/day divided twice daily	Amphotericin B lipid formulation,[d] or AmphoB 1.0–1.5 mg/kg/day[c]
Mild or moderate	Voriconazole 6 mg/kg/day LD, 4 mg/kg/day divided twice daily	Amphotericin B lipid formulation,[d] or AmphoB 0.5–0.6 mg/kg/day[c] or ITZ 200 mg TID loading dose × 3 days then 200 mg BID with meals (6-mo minimum)

[a]Treatment should be continued until the patient is symptom free and culture negative for 3 months. Noted durations or total doses should be used only as a compass to help guide therapy.
[b]Indicated only for serious symptoms (e.g., hemoptysis).
[c]Lipid formulations of amphotericin B should be utilized preferentially in these patients.
[d]Liposomal amphotericin B at doses up to 15 mg/kg/day appears safe in phase I/II trials.[185]
AmphoB, amphotericin B; BID, twice daily; ITZ, itraconazole; LD, loading dose; QOD, every other day; TID, three times daily.

voriconazole or itraconazole-treated patients with invasive aspergillosis. Further studies are necessary to define the optimal dose, duration, and route of itraconazole in invasive forms of aspergillosis.

Cryptococcosis

31. D.W., a 48-year-old man, was hospitalized with fever and severe headache. His history was significant for Hodgkin's lymphoma, which is in remission. Lumbar puncture revealed an opening pressure of 280 mm Hg (normal, 10 mm Hg), WBC count of 50 leukocytes/mm^3 (normal, 0 leukocytes/mm^3), a positive India ink preparation, and a cryptococcal antigen titer of 1:4,096. Serology for HIV infection was negative. Culture of the CSF eventually grew *C. neoformans*. The presumptive diagnosis is cryptococcal meningitis. What are the treatment options for D.W.?

Currently, only two therapeutic options exist for meningeal cryptococcal disease: amphotericin B formulation with or without flucytosine and fluconazole. Flucytosine cannot be used alone for therapy or prophylaxis because of the rapid development of resistance. This yeast is also resistant to echinocondins. Patients, whether infected with HIV or not, have improved treatment outcomes when the combination of amphotericin B and flucytosine is used.[175,176] Furthermore, when flucytosine (100–150 mg/kg/day divided into four daily doses) is used in combination therapy, the dose of amphotericin B may be reduced to 0.3 to 0.6 mg/kg/day, which decreases the frequency of dose-related amphotericin B toxicity. In patients who cannot be treated with flucytosine, the dosage of amphotericin B must be increased to >0.6 mg/kg/day.

Fluconazole is an alternative to amphotericin B in patients infected with HIV with cryptococcal meningitis. It is important to be mindful of the following caveats, however: sterilization of the CSF occurs more rapidly and mortality is lower during the first 2 weeks of therapy in patients treated with amphotericin B as compared with fluconazole.[162,177] Early mortality was especially high in fluconazole-treated patients who presented with altered mental status.[175,177,178] Thus, initial therapy of cryptococcal meningitis in patients with mental status changes should be initiated with amphotericin B for at least 2 weeks or until the patient has stabilized clinically. At this point, fluconazole may be substituted at an initial dosage of 400 mg/day. The dosage may be titrated upward to a dosage of 800 mg/day depending on clinical response. After a 10-week course of therapy is completed, the dosage of fluconazole is reduced to a maintenance dosage of 200 mg/day for life. Fluconazole 400 mg/day can be used in all other patients. Another alternative may include liposomal amphotericin B 4 mg/kg/day for 21 days.[165] Until larger clinical studies have been completed, however, this regimen cannot be recommended over generic amphotericin B (see Chapter 70, Opportunistic Infections in HIV-Infected Patients).

In D.W., initial treatment should focus on elimination of all factors leading to immunosuppression. Antifungal therapy should then be initiated immediately with amphotericin B 0.3 to 0.6 mg/kg/day plus flucytosine 100 to 150 mg/kg/ for a minimum of 6 weeks to optimize the chance of a cure, especially in transplant recipients.[178] In addition, CSF hypertension, usually presenting as headache, should be resolved through therapeutic spinal tap. Acetazolamide should be avoided in these cases.[179]

32. What parameters should be monitored while D.W. is treated with flucytosine?

The most common side effect of flucytosine is GI distress (e.g., nausea, vomiting, diarrhea). Although flucytosine is not metabolized *per se* by mammalian cells, gut flora may be responsible for metabolism of flucytosine to fluorouracil. This toxic metabolite has been speculated to account, in part, for the GI distress and bone marrow toxicity associated with flucytosine therapy.[180] Other flucytosine adverse effects include leukopenia, thrombocytopenia, and hepatotoxicity.

Dose-dependent bone marrow suppression, which can be fatal, generally is seen in patients whose serum concentration of flucytosine is >100 mcg/mL. Thus, it is important to monitor blood concentrations and maintain concentrations below this level.[176,178] If assays for flucytosine serum concentrations are unavailable, signs and symptoms of bone marrow suppression or worsening renal function should result in a dosage reduction or discontinuation of the drug. Flucytosine is eliminated by glomerular filtration, with 80% to 95% of the dose excreted unchanged in the urine. Renal excretion of flucytosine is directly related to creatinine clearance, and dosages should be adjusted based on creatinine clearance to prevent accumulation to toxic concentrations in patients with renal impairment.[100] Patients with creatinine clearances of 10 to 40 mL/min should have the dosage of flucytosine reduced by 50% (usual dose, 37.5 mg/kg Q 12 hours). For patients with creatinine clearance <10 mL/min, dosing should be initiated at 37.5 mg/kg/day, with frequent monitoring of flucytosine serum concentrations. Dosage adjustment and close monitoring also are required for patients receiving hemodialysis and it is recommended that the dose be given postdialysis.

33. When is combination antifungal therapy indicated?

In vitro results of antifungal combinations against many common mycotic pathogens have been variable. These incomplete and inconsistent findings have been attributed to variable incubation times, variable concentrations of antifungal agents, and the sequence of antifungal addition.[179] As a result, clinical decisions about combination therapy should be based on patient-specific *in vivo* evaluations. Because of the limited clinical data, combination antifungal therapy should be initiated cautiously. Except for the treatment of cryptococcal meningitis and disseminated aspergillosis, combination therapy should be reserved for cases of treatment failure (disseminated candidiasis) with no other established pharmacologic options for therapy or mould infections with high mortality rates.

REFERENCES

1. Dismukes WE ed. *Clinical Mycology.* New York, NY: Oxford University Press; 2003.
2. Rinaldi MG. Systemic fungal infections: diagnosis and treatment. II. Emerging opportunists. *Infect Dis Clin North Am* 1989;3:65.
3. Khardori N et al. Cutaneous Rhizopus and Aspergillus infections in five patients with cancer. *Arch Dermatol* 1989;125:952.
4. Wingard JR. Importance of Candida species other than *C. albicans* as pathogens in oncology patients. *Clin Infect Dis* 1995;20:115.
5. Brajtburg J et al. Amphotericin B: current understanding of mechanisms of action. *Antimicrob Agents Chemother* 1990;34:183.
6. Gruda I et al. Application of different spectra in the UV-visible region to study the formation of amphotericin B complexes. *Biochem Biophys Acta* 1980;602:260.
7. Hitchcock CA et al. The lipid composition and permeability to azole of an azole-and polyene-resistant mutant of *Candida albicans. Journal of Medical and Veterinary Mycology* 1987;25:29.
8. Pierce AM et al. Lipid composition and polyene antibiotic resistance of *Candida albicans. Canadian Journal of Biochemistry* 1978;56:135.
9. Brajtburg J et al. Stimulatory, permeabilizing, and toxic effects of amphotericin B on L cells. *Antimicrob Agents Chemother* 1984;26:892.
10. Chouini-Lalanne N et al. Study of the metabolism of flucytosine in Aspergillus species by ^{13}F nuclear magnetic resonance spectroscopy. *Antimicrob Agents Chemother* 1989;33:1939.
11. Bodey GP. Azole antifungal agents. *Clin Infect Dis* 1992;14(Suppl 1):S161.
12. Petranyi G et al. Allylamine derivative: new class of synthetic antifungal agents inhibiting fungal squalene epoxidase. *Science* 1984;244:1239.
13. Manavathu EK et al. Organism-dependent fungicidal activities of azoles. *Antimicrob Agents Chemother* 1998;42:3018.
14. Walsh TJ et al. New targets and delivery systems for antifungal therapy. *Med Mycol* 2000;38 (Suppl 1):335.
15. Clinical Laboratory Standards Institute. Reference method for broth dilution antifungal susceptibility testing of yeasts. Approved standard CLSI document M27-A. Clinical Laboratory Standards Institute, Wayne, PA; 1997.
16. Rex JH et al. Development of interpretive breakpoints for antifungal susceptibility testing: conceptual framework and analysis of *in vitro-in vivo* correlation data for fluconazole, itraconazole, and *Candida* infections. *Clin Infect Dis* 1997; 24:235.
17. Morace G et al. Multicenter comparative evaluation of six commercial systems and the Clinical Laboratory Standards Institute M27-A. Broth microdilution method for fluconazole susceptibility testing of *Candida* species. *J Clin Microbiol* 2002;40:2953.
18. Rex JH et al. Antifungal susceptibility testing: practical aspects and current challenges. *Clin Microbiol Rev* 2001;14:643.
19. Clinical Laboratory Standards Institute. Reference method for broth dilution antifungal susceptibility testing of yeasts. Approved standard CLSI document M38-A. Clinical Laboratory Standards Institute, Wayne, PA; 2001.
20. Wagner C et al. The echinocandins: comparison of their pharmcokinetics, pharmcodynamics and clinical applications. *Pharmacology* 2006;78:161.
21. Posaconazole (Noxafil) for invasive fungal infections. *Med Lett Drugs Ther* 2006;48:93.
22. Schering-Plough Healthcare Products. *Fulvicin package insert.* Liberty Corner, NJ: January 1994.
23. Drew RH et al. Comparative safety of amphotericin B lipid complex and amphotricin B deoxycholate as aerosolized antifungal prophylaxis in lung-transplant recipients. *Transplantation* 2004;77:232.
24. Wong-Beringer A et al. Suitability of caspofungin for aerosol delivery. Physicochemical profiling and nebulizer choice. *Chest* 2005;128:3711.
25. Mohammad RA et al. Inhaled amphotericin B for prophylaxis against invasive aspergillosis infections. *Ann Pharmacotherapy* 2006;40:2148.
26. Corcoran TE et al. Aerosol deposition of lipid complex amphotericin B (Abelcet) in lung transplant recipients. *Am J Transplant* 2006;6:2765.
27. Sigle HC et al. In vitro investigations on the mode of action of the hydroxypyridone antimycotics rilopirox and piroctone on Candida albicans. *Mycoses* 2006;49:159.
28. Pachl J et al. A randomized, blinded, multicenter trial of opioid-associated amphotericin B alone versus in combination with an antibody-based inhibitor of heat shock protein 90 in patients with invasive candidiasis. *Clin Infect Dis* 2006;42:1404.
29. Odom RB et al. A multicenter, placebo-controlled, double-blind study of intermittent therapy with itraconazole for the treatment of onychomycosis of the fingernail. *J Am Acad Dermatol* 1997;36:231.
30. Havu V et al. A double-blind, randomized study comparing itraconazole pulse therapy with continuous dosing for the treatment of toenail onychomycosis. *Br J Dermatol* 1997;36:230.
31. Scher RK et al. Once-weekly fluconazole (150, 300, or 450 mg) in the treatment of distal subungual onychomycosis of the toenail. *J Am Acad Dermatol* 1998;38:S77.
32. Ling MR et al. Once-weekly fluconazole (450 mg) for 4, 6, or 9 months of treatment for distal subungual onychomycosis of the toenail. *J Am Acad Dermatol* 1998;38:S95.
33. Gupta AK. Single-blinded, randomized, prospective study of sequential itraconazole and terbinafine pulse compared with terbinafine pulse for the treatment of toenail onychomycosis. *J Am Acad Dermatol* 2001;44:485.
34. Kauffman CA. Endemic mycoses: blastomycosis, histoplasmosis, and sporotrichosis. *Infect Dis Clin North Am* 2006;20:645.
35. Breeling JL et al. Pulmonary sporotrichosis treated with itraconazole. *Chest* 1993;103:313.
36. McGinnis MR et al. Sporothrix schenckii sensitivity to voriconazole, itraconazole, and amphotericin B. *Medical Mycology* 2001;39:369.
37. Pappas PG et al. Treatment of lymphocutaneous sporotrichosis with terbinafine: results of randomized double-blind trial. Paper presented to 39th Annual Infectious Diseases Society of America Meeting, San Francisco; 2001:648.
38. Wishart JM. The influence of food on the pharmacokinetics of itraconazole in patients with superficial fungal infection. *J Am Acad Dermatol* 1987;220.
39. Barone JA et al. Food interaction and steady state pharmacokinetics of itraconazole capsules in healthy male volunteers. *Antimicrob Agents Chemother* 1993;37:778.
40. Smith D et al. The pharmacokinetics of oral itraconazole in AIDS patients. *J Pharm Pharmacol* 1992;44:618.
41. Zhao Q et al. Pharmacokinetics of intravenous itraconazole followed by itraconazole oral solution in patients with human immunodeficiency virus infection. *J Clin Pharmacol* 2001;41:1319.
42. Janssen Pharmaceuticals. Sporonox Oral Suspension package insert. Piscataway, NJ: January 1998.
43. Janssen Pharmaceuticals. *Nizoral package insert.* Piscataway, NJ: January 1994.
44. Tatro DS ed. *Drug Interaction Facts.* St. Louis: Facts and Comparisons; 1998.
45. Feron B et al. Interaction of sucralfate with antibiotics used for selective decontamination of the gastrointestinal tract. *Am J Hosp Pharm* 1993;50: 2550.

46. Hoeschst Marion Roussel. *Allegra package insert.* Kansas City, MO: January 1998.
47. Present CA. Amphotericin B induction of sensitivity to Adriamycin, BCNU plus cyclophosphamide in human neoplasia. *Ann Intern Med* 1977;86:47.
48. Kivisto KT et al. Plasma buspirone concentrations are greatly increased by erythromycin and itraconazole. *Clin Pharmacol Ther* 1997;62:348.
49. Cleary JD. Unpublished data, 2002.
50. Antoniskis D et al. Acute, rapidly progressive renal failure with simultaneous use of amphotericin B and pentamidine. *Antimicrob Agents Chemother* 1990;34:470.
51. McNalty RM et al. Transient increase in plasma quinidine concentrations during ketoconazole-quinidine therapy. *Clin Pharm* 1989;8:222.
52. Wright DG et al. Lethal pulmonary reactions associated with the combination use of amphotericin B and leukocyte transfusions. *N Engl J Med* 1981;304:1185.
53. Dutcher JP et al. Granulocyte transfusion therapy and amphotericin B adverse reactions? *Am J Hematol* 1989;31:102.
54. Walsh TJ et al. Treatment of invasive aspergillosis with posaconazole in patients who are refractory to or intolerant of conventional therapy: an externally controlled trial. *Clin Infect Dis* 2007;44:2.
55. Uno T et al. Lack of dose-dependent effects of itraconazole on the pharmacokinetic interaction with fexofenadine. *Drug Metab Dispos* 2006;34:1875.
56. Saad AH et al. Factors influencing the magnitude and clinical significance of drug interactions between azole antifungals and select immunosuppressants. *Pharmacotherapy* 2006;26:1730.
57. Schering Corporation. *Posaconazole package insert.* Kenilworth, NJ: 2006.
58. Roerig Division of Pfizer Inc. VFend package insert. New York, NY: 2004.
59. Roerig Division of Pfizer Inc. *Diflucan package insert.* New York, NY: August 2004.
60. Meunier-Carpentier F et al. Fungemia in the immunocompromised host: changing patterns, antigenemia, high mortality. *Am J Med* 1981;71:363.
61. Rex JH et al. Practice guidelines for the treatment of candidiasis. *Clin Infect Dis* 2000;30:662.
62. Woods GL et al. *Diagnostic Pathology of Infectious Diseases.* Philadelphia: Lea & Febiger; 1993.
63. Arrington JB. Bacteria, fungi, and other microorganisms. In: Prophet EB et al., eds. *Laboratory Methods in Histotechnology. Armed Forces Institute of Pathology.* Washington, DC; American Registry of Pathology: Washington DC; 1992:203.
64. Jensen HE et al. The use of immunohistochemistry to improve sensitivity and specificity in the diagnosis of systemic mycoses in patients with hematologic malignancies. *J Pathol* 1997;181:100.
65. Lischewski A et al. Detection and identification of *Candida* species in experimentally infected tissue and human blood by rRNA-specific fluorescent in-situ hybridization. *J Clin Microbiol* 1997;35: 2943.
66. Coovadia YJ et al. Sensitivity and specificity of a latex agglutination test for detection of cryptococcal antigen in meningitis. *S Afr Med J* 1987;71:510.
67. Loshi G et al. Coagglutination (CoA) test for the rapid diagnosis of cryptococcal meningitis. *J Med Microbiol* 1989;29:189.
68. Wheat LJ et al. Diagnosis of disseminated histoplasmosis by detection of H. capsulatum antigen in serum and urine specimens. *N Engl J Med* 1986;314:83.
69. Crislip MA et al. Candidiasis, in systemic fungal infections: diagnosis and treatment II. *Infect Dis Clin North Am* 1989;2:103.
70. Wheat LJ. Histoplasmosis in systemic fungal infections: diagnosis and treatment I. *Infect Dis Clin North Am* 1988;2:841.
71. Gudiaugsson O et al. Attributable mortality of nosocomial candidemia, revisited. *Clin Infect Dis* 2003;37:1172.
72. Patel M et al. Initial management of candidemia at an academic medical center: evaluation of the IDSA guidelines. *Diagn Microbiol Infect Dis* 2005;52:26.
73. Morrell M et al. Delaying the empiric treatment of candida bloodstream infection until positive blood culture results are obtained: A potential risk factor for hospital mortality. *Antimicrob Agents Chemother* 2005;49:3640.
74. Walsh TH et al. All catheter-related candidemia is not the same: assessment of the balance between risks and benefit of removal of vascular catheters. *Clin Infect Dis* 2002;34:600.
75. Nucci M et al. Should vascular catheters be removed from all patients with candidemia? An evidence-based review. *Clin Infect Dis* 2002;34: 591.
76. Mora-Duarte J et al. Comparison of caspofungin and amphotericin B for invasive candidiasis. *N Engl J Med* 2002;347:2020.
77. Rex JH et al. A randomized trial comparing fluconazole with amphotericin B for the treatment of candidemia in patients without neutropenia. *N Engl J Med* 1994;331:1325.
78. Rex JH et al. Antifungal susceptibility testing of isolates from a randomized, multicenter trial of fluconazole versus amphotericin B as treatment of nonneutropenic patients with candidemia. *Antimicrob Agents Chemother* 1995;39:40.
79. Christiansen KJ et al. Distribution and activity of amphotericin in humans. *J Infect Dis* 1985; 152:1037.
80. Collette N et al. Tissue concentrations and bioactivity of amphotericin B in cancer patients treated with amphotericin B-deoxycholate. *Antimicrob Agents Chemother* 1989;33:362.
81. Rex JH et al. A randomized and blinded multicenter trial of high-dose fluconazole plus placebo vs. fluconazole plus amphotericin B as therapy of candidemia and its consequences in non-neutropenic patients. *Clin Infect Dis* 2003;36:1221.
82. Cappelletty D et al. The echinocandins. *Pharmacotherapy* 2007;27:369.
83. Abele-Horn M. A randomized study comparing fluconazole with amphotericin B/5-flucytosine for the treatment of systemic *Candida* infections in intensive care patients. *Infection* 1996;2496:426.
84. Wingard JR. Infections due to resistant *Candida* species in patients with cancer who are receiving chromotherapy. *Clin Infect Dis* 1994; 19(Suppl.1):S49.
85. Daneshmend TK et al. Clinical pharmacokinetics of systemic antifungal drugs. *Clin Pharmacokinet* 1983;8:17.
86. Ernst EJ et al. Postantifungal effects of echinocandin, azole, and polyene antifungal agents against *Candida albicans* and *Cryptococcus neoformans. Antimicrob Agents Chemother.* 2000;44:1108.
87. Gallis HA et al. Amphotericin B: 30 years of clinical experience. *Rev Infect Dis* 1990;12:308.
88. Cleary JD et al. Inhibition of interleukin 1 release from endotoxin- or amphotericin B-stimulated monocytes. *Antimicrob Agents Chemother* 1992; 36:977.
89. Cleary JD et al. Pharmacologic modulation of prostaglandin $E_2(PGE_2)$ production by bacterial endotoxin (LPS) or amphotericin B (AB) stimulated mononuclear cells (MNCs). Paper presented to 31st Annual Interscience Conference on Antimicrobial Agents and Chemotherapy Meeting, Chicago, September 19, 1991.
90. Tynes BS et al. Reducing amphotericin B reactions. *Am Rev Respir Dis* 1963;87:264.
91. Hoeprich PD. Clinical use of amphotericin B and derivative: lore, mystique, and fact. *Clin Infect Dis* 1992;14:S114.
92. Gigliotti F et al. Induction of prostaglandin synthesis as the mechanism responsible for the chills and fever produced by infusing amphotericin British. *Journal of Infectious Diseases* 1987;156:784.
93. Burks LC et al. Meperidine for the treatment of shaking chills and fever. *Arch Intern Med* 1980;140:483.
94. Cleary JD et al. Effect of infusion rate on amphotericin B-associated febrile reactions. *Drug Intell Clin Pharm* 1988;22:769.
95. Oldfield EC III et al. Randomized, double-blind trial of 1-versus 4-hour amphotericin B infusion durations. *Antimicrob Agents Chemother* 1990;34:1402.
96. Cleary JD et al. Amphotericin B overdose in pediatric patients with associated cardiac arrest. *Ann Pharmacother* 1993;27:715.
97. Branch RA. Prevention of amphotericin B-induced renal impairment: a review on the use of sodium supplementation. *Arch Intern Med* 1988;148:2389.
98. Fisher MA et al. Risk factors for amphotericin B-associated nephrotoxicity. *Am J Med* 1989;87:547.
99. Lin AC et al. Amphotericin B blunts erythropoietin response to anemia. *J Infect Dis* 1990;161:348.
100. Bennett WM et al. Drug prescribing in renal failure: dosing guidelines for adults. *Am J Kidney Dis* 1983;3:155.
101. Grant SM et al. Fluconazole: a review of its pharmacodynamic and pharmacokinetic properties and therapeutic potential in superficial and systemic mycoses. *Drugs* 1990;39:877.
102. Graybill JR. New antifungal agents. *Eur J Clin Microbiol Infect Dis* 1989;8:402.
103. VanCauteren H et al. Itraconazole pharmacologic studies in animals and humans. *Rev Infect Dis* 1987;9(Suppl 1):S43.
104. Hardin TC et al. Pharmacokinetics of itraconazole following oral administration to normal volunteers. *Antimicrob Agents Chemother* 1988;32:1310.
105. Schwartz S et al. Successful treatment of cerebral aspergillosis with a novel triazole (voriconazole) in a patient with acute leukaemia. *Br J Haematol* 1997;97:663.
106. Grasela DM et al. Ravuconazole: multiple ascending oral dose study in healthy subjects. Paper presented to 42nd Interscience Conference on Antimicrobial Agents Chemotherapy. San Diego, September 27, 2002.
107. Ullman AJ et al. Pharmacokinetics, safety, and efficacy of posaconazole in patients with persistent febrile neutropenia or refractory invasive fungal infection. *Antimicrob Agents Chemother* 2006;50:658.
108. Theuretzbacher U et al. Pharmacokinetic/pharmacodynamic profile of voriconazole. *Clin Pharmcokinet* 2006;45:649.
109. Wong-Beringer A et al. Lipid formulations of amphotericin B: clinical efficacy and toxicities. *Clin Infect Dis* 1998;27:603.
110. Cleary JD. Amphotericin B formulated in a lipid emulsion. *Ann Pharmacother* 1996;30:409.
111. Anaissie EJ et al. Amphotericin B lipid complex versus amphotericin B (AMB) for treatment of hematogenous and invasive candidiasis: a prospective, randomized, multicenter trial [abstract LM21]. In: Program and abstracts of the 35th Interscience Conference on Antimicrobial Agents and Chemotherapy.Washington, DC: American Society for Microbiology, 1995:330.
112. Ostrosky-Zeichner L et al. Invasive candidiasis in the intensive care unit. *Crit Care Med.* 2006; 34:857.
113. Pelz RK et al. Double-blind placebo-controlled trial of fluconazole to prevent candidal infections in critically ill surgical patients. *Ann Surg* 2001;233:542.
114. Ezdinli EZ et al. Oral amphotericin for candidiases in patients with hematologic neoplasms. *J Am Med Assoc* 1979;242:258.
115. Degregorio MW et al. *Candida* infections in patients with acute leukemia: ineffectiveness of nystatin prophylaxis and relationship between oropharyngeal and systemic candidiasis. *Cancer* 1982;50:2780.
116. Cuttner J et al. Clotrimazole treatment for prevention of oral candidiasis in patients with acute leukemia undergoing chemotherapy. *Am J Med* 1986;81:771.
117. Yeo E et al. Prophylaxis of oropharyngeal candidiasis with clotrimazole. *J Clin Oncol* 1985;3:1668.
118. Ang BSP et al. Candidemia from a urinary tract source: microbiological aspects and clinical significance. *Clin Infect Dis* 1993;17:662.
119. Fong IW et al. Fungicidal effect of amphotericin B in urine: in vitro study to assess feasibility of bladder washout for localization of site of

candiduria. *Antimicrob Agents Chemother* 1991;35: 1856.
120. Vergis EN et al. A randomized controlled trial of oral fluconazole and local amphotericin B for treatment of Candida funguria in hospitalized patients. Paper presented to Infectious Diseases Society Meeting. San Francisco, September 14, 1997.
121. Jacobs LG et al. Oral fluconazole compared with bladder irrigation with amphotericin B for treatment of fungal urinary tract infections in elderly patients. *Clin Infect Dis* 1996;22:30.
122. Fujihior S et al. Flucytosine in the treatment of urinary fungal infections: clinical efficacy and background factors. *Japanese Journal of Antibiotics* 1991;44:14.
123. Graybill JR et al. Ketoconazole therapy for fungal urinary tract infections. *J Urol* 1983;29:68.
124. Ikemoto H. A clinical study of fluconazole for the treatment of deep mycoses. *Diag Microbiol Infect Dis* 1989;12(Suppl 4):239S.
125. Parker JD et al. A decade of experience with blastomycosis and its treatment with amphotericin B. *Am Rev Respir Dis* 1969;99:895.
126. National Institute of Allergy and Infectious Diseases Mycoses Study Group. Treatment of blastomycosis and histoplasmosis with ketoconazole: results of a prospective, randomized clinical trial. *Ann Intern Med* 1985;103:861.
127. Bradsher RW. Blastomycosis in systemic fungal infections: diagnosis and treatment I. *Infect Dis Clin North Am* 1988;2:877.
128. Pappas PG. Treatment of blastomycosis with higher doses of fluconazole. *Clin Infect Dis* 1997;25: 200.
129. Chapman SW. Blastomyces dermatitidis. In: Mandell GL et al., eds. *Principles and Practice of Infectious Diseases.* New York: Churchill Livingstone; 1990:1999.
130. *Fed Reg* 1980;44:37434.
131. King CT et al. Antifungal therapy during pregnancy. *Clin Infect Dis* 1998;27:115.
132. Pursley TJ. Fluconazole-induced congenital anomalies in three infants. *Clin Infect Dis* 1996; 22:336.
133. Wheat LJ. Histoplasmosis in systemic fungal infections: diagnosis and treatment I. *Infect Dis Clin North Am* 1988;2:841.
134. Sutliff WD et al. Histoplasmosis cooperative study. *Am Rev Respir Dis* 1964;89:641.
135. Johnson PC et al. Safety and efficacy of liposomal amphotericin B compared with conventional amphotericin B for induction therapy of histoplasmosis in patients with AIDS. *Ann Intern Med* 2002;137:105.
136. Pont A et al. Ketoconazole blocks adrenal steroid synthesis. *Ann Intern Med* 1982;97:370.
137. Lyman CA et al. Systemically administered antifungal agents. *Drugs* 1992;44:9.
138. Honig PK et al. Terfenadine-ketoconazole interactions: pharmacokinetic and electrocardiographic consequences. *JAMA* 1993;269:1513.
139. Glynn AM et al. Effects of ketoconazole on methylprednisolone pharmacokinetics and cortisol secretion. *Clin Pharmacol Ther* 1986;39:654.
140. Saubolle MA et al. Epidemiologic, clinical, and diagnostic aspects of coccidioidomycosis. *J Clin Microbiol* 2007;45:26.
141. Peter JB. *Use and Interpretation of Tests in Medical Microbiology.* 3rd Ed. Santa Monica, CA: Specialty Laboratories; 1992.
142. Galgiani JN et al. New serologic tests for early detection of coccidioidomycosis. *J Infect Dis* 1991; 163:671.
143. Vermes A et al. Flucytosine: a review of its pharmacology, clinical indications, pharmacokinetics, toxicity and drug interactions. *J Antimicrob Chemother.* 2000;46:171.
144. Brammer KW et al. Pharmacokinetics and tissue penetration of fluconazole in humans. *Rev Infect Dis* 1990;12(Suppl 3):S318.
145. Phillips P et al. Tolerance to and efficacy of itraconazole in treatment of systemic mycoses: preliminary results. *Rev Infect Dis* 1987;9(Suppl1): S87.
146. Dodds AES, et al. Comparative pharmacokinetics of voriconazole administered orally as either crushed or whole tablets. *Antimicrob Agents Chemother* 2007;51:877.
147. Bowden R et al. A double-blind, randomized, controlled trial of amphotericin B colloidal dispersion versus amphotericin B for treatment of invasive aspergillosis in immunocompromised patients. *Clin Infect Dis* 2002;35:359.
148. Galgiani JN, et al. Comparison of oral fluconazole and itraconazole for progressive, nonmeningeal coccidioidomycosis. A randomized, double-blind trial. Mycoses Study Group. *Ann Intern Med* 2000;133:676.
149. Ratcheson RA et al. Experience with the subcutaneous cerebrospinal fluid reservoir: a preliminary report of 60 cases. *N Engl J Med* 1968;279:1.
150. Witorsch P et al. Intraventricular administration of amphotericin B. *JAMA* 1965;194:109.
151. Sung JP et al. Intravenous and intrathecal miconazole therapy for systemic mycoses. *West J Med* 1977;126:5.
152. Harrison HR et al. Amphotericin B and imidazole therapy for coccidioidal meningitis in children. *Pediatr Infect Dis* 1983;2:216.
153. Fisher JF et al. Parkinsonism associated with intraventricular amphotericin B. *J Antimicrob Chemother* 1983;12:97.
154. Winn RE et al. Acute toxic delirium: neurotoxicity of intrathecal administration of amphotericin B. *Arch Intern Med* 1979;139:706.
155. Haber RW et al. Neurologic manifestations after amphotericin B therapy. *BMJ* 1962;1:230.
156. Carnevale NT et al. Amphotericin-induced myelopathy. *Arch Intern Med* 1980;140:1189.
157. Anaissie EJ et al. Management of invasive candidal infections: results of a prospective, randomized, multicenter study of fluconazole versus amphotericin B and review of the literature. *Clin Infect Dis* 1996;23:964.
158. Prentice HG et al. A randomized comparison of liposomal versus conventional amphotericin B for the treatment of pyrexia of unknown origin in neutropenic patients. *Br J Haematol* 1997;98:711.
159. Walsh TJ et al. Caspofungin versus liposomal amphotericin B for empirical antifungal therapy in patients with persistent fever and neutropenia. *N Engl J Med* 2004;351:1391.
160. Boogaerts M et al. Intravenous and oral itraconazole versus intravenous amphotericin B deoxycholate as empirical antifungal therapy for persistent fever in neutropenic patients with cancer who are receiving broad-spectrum antibacterial therapy. A randomized, controlled trial. *Ann Intern Med* 2001;135:412.
161. Walsh TJ et al. Voriconazole compared with liposomal amphotericin B for empirical antifungal therapy in patients with neutropenia and persistent fever. *N Engl J Med* 2002;346:225.
162. Dismukes WE et al. Treatment of cryptococcal meningitis with combination amphotericin B and flucytosine for 4 as compared with 6 weeks. *N Engl J Med* 1987;317:334.
163. White MH et al. Amphotericin B colloidal dispersion vs. amphotericin B as therapy for invasive aspergillosis. *Clin Infect Dis* 1997;24:635.
164. Leenders ACAP. Liposomal amphotericin B (AmBisome) compared with amphotericin B both followed by oral fluconazole in the treatment of AIDS-associated cryptococcal meningitis. *AIDS* 1997;11:1463.
165. Sharkey PK et al. Amphotericin B lipid complex compared with amphotericin B in the treatment of cryptococcal meningitis in patients with AIDS. *Clin Infect Dis* 1996;22:329.
166. Cleary JD et al. Lipid-associated amphotericin B. *Florida Journal of Hospital Pharmacy* 1994;14:19.
167. Sacks GS et al. Nutritional impact of lipid-associated amphotericin B formulations. *Ann Pharmacotherapy* 1997;31:121.
168. Denning DW et al. Micafungin (FK463), alone or in combination with other systemic antifungal agents, for the treatment of acute invasive aspergillosis. *J Infect.* 2006;53:337.
169. Maertens J et al. Multicenter, noncomparative study of caspofungin in combination with other antifungals as salvage therapy in adults with invasive aspergillosis. *Cancer* 2006;107:2888.
170. Marr KA et al. Combination antifungal therapy for invasive aspergillosis. *Clin Infect Dis* 2004;39:797.
171. Ellis M et al. An EORTC international multicenter randomized trial (EORTC number 19923) comparing two dosages of liposomal amphotericin B for treatment of invasive aspergillosis. *Clin Infect Dis.* 1998;27:1406.
172. Herbrecht R et al. Voriconazole versus amphotericin B for primary therapy of invasive aspergillosis. *N Engl J Med* 2002;347:408.
173. Segal BH et al. Prevention and early treatment of invasive fungal infection in patients with cancer and neutropenia and in stem cell transplant recipients in the era of newer broad-spectrum antifungal agents and diagnostic adjuncts. *Clin Infect Dis.* 2007;44:402.
174. Stevens DA et al. Practice guidelines for diseases caused by Aspergillus. Infectious Diseases Society of America. *Clin Infect Dis* 2000;30:696.
175. Larsen RA et al. Fluconazole compared with amphotericin B plus flucytosine for cryptococcal meningitis in AIDS: a randomized trial. *Ann Intern Med* 1990;113:183.
176. Bennett JE et al. A comparison of amphotericin B alone and combined with flucytosine in the treatment of cryptococcal meningitis. *N Engl J Med* 1979;301:126.
177. Saag MS et al. Comparison of amphotericin B with fluconazole in the treatment of acute AIDS associated cryptococcal meningitis. *N Engl J Med* 1992;326:83.
178. Hibberd PL et al. Clinical aspects of fungal infection in organ transplant recipients. *Clin Infect Dis* 1994;19:S33.
179. Newton PN et al. A randomized, double-blind, placebo-controlled trial of acetazolamide for the treatment of elevated intracranial pressure in cryptococcal meningitis. *Clin Infect Dis* 2002;35: 769.
180. Kauffman CA et al. Bone marrow toxicity associated with 5-fluorocytosine therapy. *Antimicrob Agents Chemother* 1977;11:244.
181. Craven PC et al. Combination of oral flucytosine and ketoconazole as therapy for experimental cryptococcal meningitis. *J Infect Dis* 1984;149: 584.
182. Antimicrobial agents and chemotherapy. *Fed Reg* 1982;47:12480.
183. Ullman AJ et al. Pharmacokinetics, safety, and efficacy of posacnazole in patients with persistent febrile neutropenia or refractory invasive fungal infection. *Antimicrob Agents Chemother* 2006;50:658.
184. Theuretzbacher U et al. Pharmacokinetic pharmacodynamic profile of voriconazole. *Clin Pharmacokinet* 2006;45:649.
185. Walsh TJ et al. Safety, tolerance, and pharmacokinetics of high-dose liposomal amphotericin B (AmBisome) in patients infected with *Aspergillus* species and other filamentous fungi: maximum tolerated dose study. *Antimicrob Agents Chemother* 2001;45:3487.

CHAPTER 72

Viral Infections

Milap C. Nahata, Neeta Bahal O'Mara, and Sandra Benavides

Viral infections are common causes of human disease. An estimated 60% of illnesses in developed countries result from viruses, compared with only 15% from bacteria. These may include the common cold, chickenpox, measles, mumps, influenza, bronchitis, gastroenteritis, hepatitis, poliomyelitis, rabies, and numerous diseases caused by the herpesvirus. Upper respiratory tract infections, such as the common cold or influenza, are one of the most common reasons for visits to a health care professional.[1] Although most of these patients have a self-limiting illness, certain viral infections, such as influenza, can cause significant mortality, particularly in the elderly. For example, in the worldwide Spanish influenza epidemic of 1918 to 1920, between 20 million and 100 million people died.[2] Influenza vaccines can reduce the impact of this illness in susceptible populations, but there are no vaccines against many other potentially severe viral infections, including herpes encephalitis and neonatal herpes. Therefore, the need for safe and effective antiviral agents is obvious.

Substantial progress has been made in antiviral chemotherapy as a result of advances in molecular virology and genetic engineering. Antiviral agents can be designed to inhibit functions specific to viruses; this maximizes their therapeutic benefits while minimizing adverse effects to the host cell.

Current technology also permits rapid diagnosis of viral diseases. It is now possible to make a specific diagnosis of several viral illnesses within hours to a few days; previously, specific diagnosis took days to months. This has made it possible to select an appropriate antiviral drug early for the treatment of acute viral infection.

This chapter describes the etiology, pathogenesis, and treatment of common viral infections. Specific case presentations illustrate the optimal use of antiviral drugs in patients with viral infections.

HERPES SIMPLEX VIRUS INFECTIONS

Herpesvirus is an extremely important pathogen in humans. It causes many illnesses, including herpes encephalitis and neonatal herpes, which are associated with significant mortality and sequelae, and genital herpes, which causes substantial pain and emotional suffering. Fortunately, antiviral drugs can decrease the morbidity, mortality, and duration of symptoms in most cases.[3]

Herpes Encephalitis

Herpes simplex virus (HSV) encephalitis is the most common sporadic viral infection of the central nervous system (CNS). The estimated incidence is approximately 2.3 cases per million population per year, although this may be an underestimate because of the difficulty in diagnosing this disease. It can occur at any age and is characterized by the acute onset of fever, headache, decreased consciousness, and seizures. Any child with fever and altered behavior should be evaluated carefully. This is a devastating infection: without treatment, mortality approaches 70%, and only 2.5% of patients recover enough to lead normal lives.[3]

Herpes simplex virus type 1 (HSV-1) is the etiologic agent in most patients with herpes encephalitis, but herpes simplex virus type 2 (HSV-2) is more common in newborns. The infection may be localized to the brain or involve cutaneous and mucous membranes. Although any area of the brain can be involved, the orbital region of the frontal lobes and portions of the temporal lobes are most often affected.

Herpes encephalitis is often difficult to diagnose and is always a serious disease. A computed tomography (CT) scan is usually indicated to rule out other conditions, including a brain abscess or other space-occupying lesions that may produce similar symptoms. The CT or radionucleotide scans may be unremarkable early in the course of the disease.

Cerebrospinal fluid (CSF) examination usually reveals pleocytosis (predominately lymphocytes) with 50 to 2,000 white blood cells (WBCs)/mm^3. Polymorphonuclear leukocytosis and red blood cells (RBCs) may also be seen. Many patients have an elevated protein level in the CSF (median, 80 mg/dL). The presence of antibody to HSV-1 is useful in making the diagnosis.

The electroencephalogram (EEG) is the most sensitive but least specific test. There are usually CT or brain scan abnormalities, but these may take a day or two longer to appear. The EEG, CT, and brain scan findings compatible with HSV encephalitis can be mimicked by other conditions, and a brain biopsy is required to clearly establish the diagnosis. Rapid diagnosis of herpes encephalitis by a polymerase chain reaction (PCR) assay of HSV DNA in the CSF is available at most medical centers. This is a highly sensitive, specific, and rapid method for diagnosing herpes encephalitis.[4]

Clinical Presentation

1. R.F., a 7-year-old boy weighing 20 kg, was seen in the emergency department (ED) after a seizure. Over the previous 3 days, R.F. had decreased appetite, headache, and fever (101°F–102°F), and was lethargic and disoriented. His leukocyte count was 13,000/mm^3 with a shift to the left. Ceftriaxone (50 mg/kg given intravenously [IV] Q 12 hr) and dexamethasone (0.15 mg/kg IV Q 6 hr) were initiated for presumed bacterial meningitis. Phenobarbital (5 mg/kg IV Q 24 hr) was given for seizure control. The CSF was normal, and no bacteria could be identified. Over the next 2 days, R.F. became increasingly less responsive and lapsed into a coma. A CT scan of the brain revealed decreased density in a localized area of the left temporal lobe. Because of a high suspicion of herpes encephalitis, a brain biopsy was performed. Acyclovir 20 mg/kg IV Q 8 hr was started immediately after the procedure. HSV-1 was isolated from the biopsy specimen 24 hours later. What findings in R.F. are consistent with the diagnosis of herpes encephalitis? Why was a brain biopsy performed?

[SI unit: leukocytes, 13 × 10^6/L]

Fever, headache, lethargy, and disorientation are common features of herpes encephalitis. As illustrated by R.F., the CSF examination can be normal in some patients. The CT scan showing decreased density in the left temporal lobe is suggestive of herpes encephalitis. Finally, a negative CSF culture also suggests the absence of a bacterial infection.[5] However, these findings cannot establish the diagnosis of herpes encephalitis.

Brain biopsy is the most definitive diagnostic procedure for herpes encephalitis. Biopsy is particularly important because some treatable conditions, such as cryptococcosis and aspergillosis, can be missed by other diagnostic procedures. The morbidity (bleeding) caused by brain biopsy is low (1%) in medical centers with extensive experience.

Treatment: Acyclovir

2. As expected, a specific pathogen (HSV-1) was isolated from the biopsy specimen in R.F. What is the treatment of choice for R.F.'s herpes encephalitis?

Two studies comparing acyclovir and vidarabine have demonstrated that IV acyclovir (10 mg/kg Q 8 hr for 10 days) is the treatment of choice in patients with herpes encephalitis.[6,7] The 12-month all-cause mortality was 25% in the acyclovir-treated group and 59% in the vidarabine-treated group. Of great importance was the fact that nearly one-third of the acyclovir-treated patients returned to normal life, compared with only 12% of those treated with vidarabine.[8] In addition, acyclovir is less toxic than vidarabine. Currently, vidarabine is not marketed in the United States.

Acyclovir-resistant herpes is not an important consideration in the management of herpes encephalitis in most patients, but it can be important in AIDS or other immunocompromised patients who receive multiple repeated courses of acyclovir (see Chapter 71). Foscarnet has been successfully used in immunocompromised patients with acyclovir-resistant HSV.[9,10]

Acyclovir is the treatment of choice for R.F. because it has been shown to decrease morbidity in patients with herpes encephalitis.

The role of corticosteroids in the treatment of herpes encephalitis is not well defined. One small, nonrandomized trial found that corticosteroid therapy, in combination with IV acyclovir, was associated with an improved outcome.[11] However, prospective, randomized trials are needed before routine use of corticosteroids can be recommended.[12]

ACYCLOVIR PHARMACOKINETICS

3. Why is the acyclovir dosage regimen appropriate based on the serum concentrations required for the inhibition of viral replication? How should the effect of acyclovir be monitored in R.F.?

In adults receiving single IV doses of acyclovir 2.5 to 5 mg/kg, a peak plasma concentration of 3.4 to 6.8 mcg/mL has been reported.[13,14] The mean peak and trough plasma concentrations were 9.8 and 0.7 mcg/mL, respectively, after multiple doses of 5 mg/kg every 8 hours.[8] At larger IV doses of 10 to 15 mg/kg, the peak plasma concentrations of acyclovir have ranged from 10 to 30 mcg/mL[15] (Tables 72-1 and 72-2).

Limited data are available on acyclovir pharmacokinetics in children, particularly premature infants. Acyclovir pharmacokinetics for children older than 1 year of age are similar to those of adults[16] (Table 72-1). In neonates receiving acyclovir 5 to 15 mg/kg IV Q 8 hr, the peak and trough serum concentrations have ranged from 3.1 to 38 mcg/mL and 0.23 to 30 mcg/mL, respectively.[17,18] Acyclovir distributes into all

Table 72-1 Pharmacokinetic Properties of Antiviral Drugs

Drug	Dose Used in Study	Peak Serum Concentrations (mcg/mL)	% Recovered Unchanged in Urine	Elimination Half-Life (h)
Acyclovir[8,13,16,21]	2.5–10 mg/kg IV	3.4–22.9	69–91	2.5–3.3
	200–800 mg PO	0.83–1.61	NR	2.5–3.3
Amantadine[89]	100–200 mg PO	0.2–0.5	52–88	11–15
Famciclovir[52,159]	125–1,000 mg PO	0.8–6.6	73–94[a]	2.0–3.0[a]
Oseltamivir[87,160]	75 mg PO	0.6–3.5[b]	99[b]	6–10[b]
Ribavirin[117]	0.82 mg/kg INH × 20 h	1–3	NR	6.5–11
Rimantadine[90]	100–200 mg PO	0.2–0.7	20	9–31
Valacyclovir[161,162]	1,000 mg PO	5.7–6.7[c]	46–80[c]	2.5–3.3[c]
Zanamivir[86,163,164]	10 mg INH BID	0.039–0.054	7–17	2.5–5.1

[a] Pharmacokinetic properties of active metabolite, penciclovir.
[b] Active metabolite oseltamivir carboxylate.
[c] Pharmacokinetic properties of active metabolite, acyclovir.
BID, twice a day; INH, inhalation, IV, intravenously; NR, not reported; PO, orally.

tissues, with the highest concentrations occurring in the kidney (10 times the plasma concentration) and the lowest in the CSF (25%–70% of plasma concentration).[8] For R.F., the regimen is appropriate (Table 72-3). Although the pharmacokinetics in children older than 1 year are similar to those in adults, higher dosages are needed in view of its relatively poor distribution into CSF.

HSV-1 clinical isolates have an ID_{50} of 0.02 to 13.5 mcg/mL, with a mean of 0.45 to 1.47 mcg/mL.[8,19] However, antiviral susceptibility testing can be affected by many variables, including the amount of inoculum and the testing method used. The results of antiviral susceptibility tests are usually reported as ID_{50} (the serum concentration necessary to produce 50% inhibition of the viral cytopathic effect). ID_{90} may correlate better than ID_{50} with clinical outcome, but the results are unpredictable.[20] Consequently, the clinical status of patients is monitored for efficacy of acyclovir. Most patients begin to improve within 48 hours after starting treatment.

ADVERSE EFFECTS

4. What type of adverse effects can occur as a result of IV acyclovir therapy in R.F.? How should these be monitored, and how can they be minimized?

Acyclovir is a relatively safe drug, but renal toxicity associated with IV acyclovir should be considered (Table 72-4). Blood urea nitrogen (BUN) and serum creatinine (SrCr) levels can increase in approximately 5% to 10% of patients. These changes are generally reversible. Acyclovir is relatively insoluble: maximum urine solubility at 37°C is 1.3 mg/mL. Therefore, a transient crystal nephropathy may occur at high acyclovir concentrations.[21]

Other common adverse effects include gastrointestinal (GI) complaints such as nausea and vomiting and neurologic disturbances, including lethargy, tremors, confusion, hallucinations, and seizures.[21,22] Neurotoxicity appears to be more common in patients with impaired renal function and tends to be reversible. Transient elevation of liver enzymes may occur. Finally, IV acyclovir can cause phlebitis and pain at the injection site.[21] This can be minimized by administering acyclovir at a concentration of about 5 mg/mL (maximum, 7 mg/mL).[22]

Renal function tests, including BUN, SrCr, and urine output, should be monitored closely. To minimize the risk of acyclovir nephrotoxicity, R.F. should be well hydrated, and each acyclovir dose should be infused over 1 hour. In addition, the IV infusion site should be inspected for inflammation and pain, and R.F. should be asked about pain at the infusion site.

CONVERSION TO ORAL THERAPY

5. After 7 days of IV acyclovir, R.F. is alert, responsive, actively moving about, and eating a normal diet. The intern suggests switching him to oral acyclovir and discontinuing IV therapy. Why is this not appropriate?

Oral therapy is inappropriate for R.F. Based on studies in adults, the absorption of acyclovir after oral administration is variable, slow, and incomplete. The bioavailability of acyclovir is low ($F = 0.15–0.30$) and decreases with increasing doses.[21] The mean peak plasma concentration has ranged from only 0.83 to 1.61 mcg/mL after multiple acyclovir doses of 200 to 800 mg.[21,23] Thus, with only approximately 50% of acyclovir penetrating the blood–brain barrier, the concentrations of acyclovir in the CSF may be inadequate for R.F. Therapy with IV acyclovir should be continued to complete a 10-day course (Table 72-3). The role of long-term oral antiviral agents following IV therapy to further reduce morbidity is currently being studied.[5,24]

Neonatal Herpes

Most neonates acquire herpes from the infected genital secretions of the mother at delivery.[25] The incidence ranges from 1 in 3,000 to 5,000 deliveries per year in the United States. The infection can present in one of three forms: localized to the skin, eye, and mouth (45%); encephalitis (30%); or disseminated disease (25%). The effects of neonatal herpes can be devastating, and severe disabilities persist in many afflicted children.[25] With currently available antivirals, the mortality has ranged from 4% in those with CNS involvement to 29% in those with disseminated disease.[25] Neonatal HSV-1 infections may also be acquired after birth through contact with family members with symptomatic or asymptomatic oral-labial HSV-1 infection or from nosocomial transmission. When the virus is transmitted from the mother, clinical evidence of infection in the neonate usually is present 5 to 17 days after birth. Although skin vesicles are the hallmark of infection, at least one-third

Table 72-2 Clinical Pharmacokinetics of Antiviral Drugs

			Elimination		
Drug	**Type of Patient**	**Total Clearance**	**Volume of Distribution**	**Half-Life (hr)**	**Comments**
Acyclovir[8,14,16,18,21]	Adults	327 mL/min/1.73 m^2	59 L/1.73 m^2	2.5–3.3	Use 100% of recommended dose, but extend dosage interval to 12 and 24 hr if Cl_{Cr} ranges from 25–50 and 10–25 mL/min/1.73 m^2, respectively; use 50% of recommended dose Q 24 hr if Cl_{Cr} ranges from 0–10 mL/min/1.73 m^2.
	Neonates	98–122 mL/min/1.73 m^2	24–30 L/1.73 m^2	3.2–4.1	
Amantadine[89]	Adults	2.5–10.5 L/hr	1.5–6.1 L/kg	11–15	Adjust doses in renal failure: 200 mg on day 1, then 100 mg/d if Cl_{Cr} 30–50; 200 mg on day 1, then 100 mg QOD if Cl_{Cr} 15–29; 200 mg Q 7 days if Cl_{Cr} <15 mL/min/1.73 m^2.
Famciclovir[49,159,165]	Adults	0.37–0.48 L/hr/kg	1.1 L/kg	2.2–3.0	Use 100% of recommended dose, but extend dosage interval to 12 and 24 hr if Cl_{Cr} ranges from 40–59 and 20–39 mL/min, respectively; use 250 mg Q 24 hr if Cl_{Cr} <20 mL/min.
Oseltamivir[87,160,166]	Adults	18.8 L/hr (renal clearance)	NA	6.0–10	Use 75 mg/d in patients if Cl_{Cr} 10–30 mL/min. The effect of hepatic impairment has not been determined.
	Pediatrics (1–12 y)	0.63 L/h/kg	NA	7.8	Dosage recommendations are based on body weight and age. Use 30 mg BID if patient is 15 kg and 1–3 yr, 45 mg if patient is 15–23 kg and 4–7 yr, 60 mg if patient is 23–40 kg and 8–12 yr and normal adult dose if >40 kg and older than 13 yr.
	Adolescents	0.32 L/h/kg	NA	8.1	
Rimantadine[90]	Adults	20–48 L/hr	25 L/kg	9–31	Because it undergoes extensive metabolism, dose may have to be adjusted in patients with severe liver disease. Dose adjustments may also be necessary in elderly and in those with severe renal failure (Cl_{Cr} <10 mL/min). Manufacturer recommends 50% reduction in such cases.
Valacyclovir[23]	See acyclovir (prodrug of acyclovir)				Use 100% of recommended dose, but extend dosage interval to 12 and 24 hr if Cl_{Cr} ranges from 30–49 and 10–29 mL/min, respectively; use 500 mg Q 24 hr if Cl_{Cr} <10 mL/min.
Zanamivir[86]	Adults	2.5–10.9 L/hr	15.9 L	2.5–5.1	4%–17% of inhaled dose systemically absorbed. Although only limited studies with renal or hepatic impairment, dosing adjustment likely unnecessary.
Valganciclovir	See ganciclovir				Use 50% of recommended dose if Cl_{Cr} ranges from 40–59 mL/min; use 450 mg Q 24 hr if Cl_{Cr} ranges from 25–39 mL/min; use 450 mg QOD if Cl_{Cr} <25 mL/min.

BID, twice a day; Cl_{Cr}, creatinine clearance; QD, every day; QOD, every other day.

to one-half of neonates never have skin lesions.[26] In 70% of patients, the disease may progress from isolated skin lesions to involve other organs, including the lungs, liver, spleen, CNS, and eyes.

Diagnosis of this infection can be made by direct fluorescent antibody examination of epithelial cells from the infant or the mother. Examination of the base of a vesicular lesion may show giant cells and intranuclear inclusions, which are characteristic of HSV infections. Serologic test results are also helpful in making a diagnosis of neonatal herpes.

Risk Factors

6. S.P., an 18-year-old woman, was admitted to labor and delivery with premature rupture of the membranes. Four hours later, S.P. vaginally delivered a 2.5-kg baby boy, R.P., who had an estimated gestational age of 33 weeks. Twenty-four hours after

Table 72-3 U.S. Food and Drug Administration (FDA)-Indicated Drugs for Various Viral Infections

Disease	Drug	Dosage (Age Group)	Route	Duration
Herpes encephalitis	Acyclovir (Zovirax)[a]	*>12 yr:* 10 mg/kg Q 8 hr	IV	10 days
		3 mo–12 yr: 20 mg/kg Q 8 hr	IV	10 days
Neonatal herpes	Acyclovir (Zovirax)	*Birth–3 mo:* 10–20 mg/kg Q 8 hr[a]	IV	14–21 days
Oral-facial herpes (for treatment of recurrent infection)	Acyclovir (Zovirax)	*Adults:* 400 mg 5×/days	PO	5 days
	Famciclovir (Famvir)	*Adults:* 1,500 mg	PO	1 dose
	Valacyclovir (Valtrex)	*Adults:* 2,000 mg BID	PO	1 day
Oral-facial herpes[b] (immunocompromised patients)	Acyclovir (Zovirax)	*>12 yr:* 5 mg/kg Q 8 hr	IV	7 days
		<12 yr: 10 mg/kg Q 8 hr	IV	7 days
	Famciclovir (Famvir)	*Adults:* 500 mg BID	PO	7 days
Herpes zoster[b] (immunocompetent patients)	Acyclovir (Zovirax)	*Adults:* 800 mg 5×/days	PO	7–10 days
	Famciclovir (Famvir)	*Adult:* 500 mg Q 8 hr	PO	7 days
	Valacyclovir (Valtrex)	*Adult:* 1,000 mg Q 8 hr	PO	7 days
Herpes zoster[b] (immunocompromised patients)	Acyclovir (Zovirax)	*>12 yr:* 10 mg/kg Q 8 hr	IV	7 days
		<12 yr: 20 mg/kg Q 8 hr	IV	7 days
Varicella (immunocompetent patient)	Acyclovir (Zovirax)	*>40 kg:* 800 mg QID	PO	5 days
		>2 yr and <40 kg: 20 mg/kg (max 800 mg) QID	PO	5–10 days
Varicella (immunocompromised patients)		*>12 yr:* 10 mg/kg Q 8 hr	IV	7–10 days
		< 12 yr: 500 mg/m² Q 8 hr	IV	7–10 days
Cytomegalovirus retinitis (immunocompromised patients)	Ganciclovir (Cytovene)	5 mg/kg Q 12 hr; then 5 mg/kg/days or 6 mg/kg, 5 days a week	IV	14–21 days for induction; maintenance
	Cidofovir (Vistide)	5 mg/kg Q week for 2 wk, then Q 2 wk	IV	Maintenance
	Foscarnet (Foscavir)	90 mg/kg Q 12 hr, then 90 mg/kg QD	IV	Induction for 2 wk; maintenance
	Valganciclovir (Valcyte)	900 mg BID, 900 mg QD	PO	Induction for 21 days; maintenance
Influenza A	Amantadine[c] (Symmetrel)	*> 9 yr:* 100 mg BID	PO	10 days (treatment), 14–28 days (protection with vaccine), 90 days (protection without vaccine)
		1 to 9 yr: 4.4–8.8 mg/kg/days but <150 mg/days	PO	
	Rimantadine[c] (Flumadine)	*>14 yr:* 100 mg BID	PO	7 days (treatment, not approved for treatment in children) up to 6 wk for prophylaxis
		1–13 yr: 100 mg BID	PO	Up to 6 wk for prophylaxis
		1–9 yr: 5 mg/kg div. QD-BID (max 150 mg/days)	PO	
Influenza A and B	Oseltamivir (Tamiflu)	*>13 yr (or >40 kg):* 75 mg BID	PO	5 days (treatment)
		>13 yr (or >40 kg): 75 mg QD	PO	10 days (prophylaxis) Up to 6 wk (community outbreaks)
		23–40 kg: 60 mg BID *15–23 kg:* 45 mg BID *>1 yr–15 kg:* 30 mg BID	PO	5 days (treatment)
		23–40 kg: 60 mg QD *15–23 kg:* 45 mg QD *>1 yr–15 kg:* 30 mg QD	PO	10 days (prophylaxis)
	Zanamivir (Relenza)	*>7 yr:* 10 mg (2 inhalations) BID	Inhalation	5 days (treatment)
		Adolescent and Adult: 10 mg (2 inhalations) QD	Inhalation	10 days (prophylaxis) 28 days (community outbreak)
		>5 yr: 10 mg (2 inhalations) QD	Inhalation	10 days (prophylaxis)
Respiratory syncytial virus	Ribavirin (Virazole)	6 g in 300 mL over 12–18 hr/days	Inhalation	3–7 days

[a]FDA-approved dose is 10 mg/kg. Although doses of 15–20 mg/kg have been used, safety has not been established at these doses.
[b] Foscarnet 40 mg/kg IV Q 8 hr is recommended for acyclovir-resistant herpes simplex virus or varicella-zoster virus.
[c]Amantadine and rimantadine are no longer recommended as drugs of choice for either prophylaxis or treatment of influenza A.
BID, twice a day; IV, intravenously; PO, orally; Q, every; QD, every day; QID, four times a day.

Table 72-4 U.S. Food and Drug Administration-Indicated Drugs for Various Viral Infections

Adverse Effects of Approved Antiviral Drugs

Drug	Adverse Effects
Acyclovir	Local irritation, phlebitis (9%); increased SrCr, BUN (5%–10%); nausea, vomiting (7%); itching, rash (2%); increased liver transaminases (1%–2%); CNS toxicity (1%)
Amantadine	Nausea, dizziness (lightheadedness), insomnia (5%–10%); depression, anxiety, irritability, hallucination, confusion, dry mouth; constipation, ataxia, headache, peripheral edema, orthostatic hypotension (1%–5%); suicide ideation/attempt (<1%)
Cidofovir	Nephrotoxicity (53%); neutropenia (34%); rash (30%); headache (27%); alopecia (25%); anemia (20%); abdominal pain (17%); fever (15%); infection (12%); ocular hypotonia (12%); nausea, vomiting (8%); asthenia (7%); diarrhea (7%)
Famciclovir	Headache (6%–9%); nausea (4%–5%); diarrhea (1%–2%)
Foscarnet	Fever, nausea, vomiting (47%); renal dysfunction (33%); anemia (9%–33%); diarrhea (30%); headache (26%); electrolyte abnormalities (6%–15%); bone marrow suppression (10%); seizure (10%); anorexia (5%); abdominal pain (5%); mental status changes (5%); paresthesia, peripheral neuropathy (5%); cough, dyspnea (5%); rash (5%); first-degree AV block, ECG changes (1%–5%)
Ganciclovir	Increased ScCr (35%–69%); anemia (15%–25%); neutropenia, pancytopenia, thrombocytopenia (5%–8%); abdominal pain, anorexia (15%); diarrhea (44%); nausea, vomiting (13%); retinal detachment, vitreous hemorrhage, cataracts, corneal opacification (6%–15%); neuropathy; rash
Oseltamivir	Nausea, vomiting (9%–15%); diarrhea (3%); abdominal pain (2%); dizziness, vertigo, insomnia (1%); self-injury and psychosis
Ribavirin	Worsening of respiratory status, bacterial pneumonia, pneumothorax, apnea, ventilator dependence; cardiac arrest, hypotension; rash; conjunctivitis
Rimantadine	CNS (insomnia, dizziness, headache, nervousness, fatigue); GI (nausea, vomiting, anorexia, dry mouth, abdominal pain) (1%–3%)
Trifluridine	Burning or stinging on instillation (4.6%); palpebral edema (2.8%); keratopathy; hypersensitivity reaction; stromal edema; hyperemia; increased intraocular pressure
Valacyclovir	Headache (14%); nausea (15%); vomiting (6%); dizziness (3%); abdominal pain (3%)
Valganciclovir	Neutropenia (27%); thrombocytopenia (6%); diarrhea (41%); nausea, vomiting (21%–30%); abdominal pain (15%); increased ScCr (3%); insomnia (16%); peripheral neuropathy (9%); paresthesias (8%); ataxia, dizziness, seizures, psychosis, hallucinations, confusion, drowsiness (<5%); retinal detachment (15% during treatment of CMV retinitis); hypersensitivity
Zanamivir	Bronchospasm; decline in respiratory function, especially if underlying respiratory disease; nasal/throat irritation and/or congestion (2%); headache (2%); cough (2%); diarrhea (3%); nausea, vomiting (1%–3%)

AV, atrioventricular; BUN, blood urea nitrogen; CMV, cytomegalovirus; CNS, central nervous system; ECG, electrocardiogram; GI, gastrointestinal; ScCr, serum creatinine.

delivery, S.P. reported the onset of vesicles in the genital area; she had a history of previous episodes of genital herpes. The last infection was during her first trimester of pregnancy. Is R.P. at risk of developing herpes infection?

R.P. is at risk of acquiring herpes infection because the mother had genital herpes during the first trimester and because he was delivered vaginally rather than by cesarean section.[27] The risk of a newborn acquiring the disease from an infected mother with primary disease is about 35%; that from a mother with reactivation is 3%.

Treatment: Acyclovir

7. Ten days after birth, R.P. developed poor feeding patterns, irritability, and respiratory distress. Three days later, skin lesions appeared. How should R.P. be treated?

R.P. is manifesting signs of HSV infection and should be treated with antiviral therapy (Table 72-3). The drug of choice for neonatal herpes simplex virus infections is IV acyclovir.[25,26] Vidarabine was the first antiviral agent used in the treatment of neonatal HSV. Because of the drastic reduction in morbidity, it became the standard of therapy to which other antiviral agents were compared. In clinical trials comparing vidarabine with acyclovir, acyclovir was shown to be as effective as vidarabine in infants with skin, eye, mouth (SEM) involvement, encephalitis, and disseminated HSV infection.[28] Although both agents were equally effective, acyclovir was safer and easier to administer, making it the standard of care for neonatal HSV.

ACYLOVIR ADMINISTRATION

8. What dosage of acyclovir should R.P. receive?

Although an IV dosage of 30 mg/kg given in three divided doses has been shown to be effective in the treatment of neonatal herpes, the use of 60 mg/kg has been shown to have additional benefits in decreasing morbidity and mortality. The higher dose of acyclovir is associated with a higher frequency of hematologic abnormalities, especially neutropenia.[29,25,30] The minimum duration of therapy should be 14 days, for neonates with only SEM involvement, whereas longer courses (e.g., 21 days) are indicated in infants with CNS involvement or disseminated disease.[25]

The role of prolonged oral suppressive therapy in newborns with SEM involvement has been investigated. Acyclovir, given orally (PO) at 300 mg/m^2 per dose three times a day (TID), resulted in a reduction in the recurrences of lesions. Half of these patients developed neutropenia. One patient had lesions resistant to acyclovir.[31] Because the long-term benefits cannot be fully attributed to the use of suppressive acyclovir, suppressive therapy for patients with SEM involvement is not recommended.[32]

Oral-Facial Herpes

Both primary and recurrent oral-facial HSV-1 infections can be asymptomatic. Gingivostomatitis and pharyngitis are the most common clinical manifestations of a first episode of HSV-1 infection, and recurrent herpes labialis is most commonly caused by reactivated HSV infection. Clinical features include fever, malaise, myalgia, inability to eat, and irritability. Immunocompromised patients with oral-facial herpes have severe pain, extensive lesions, and prolonged viral shedding; thus, they are candidates for antiviral therapy.

Herpes labialis (cold sores) is the most common oral-facial HSV infection. Clinical features include pain or paresthesia and erythematous or papular lesions followed by vesiculation and swelling. These lesions usually crust and heal in the next few days. Viral cultures often are positive within 2 to 3 days. Rapid diagnosis can be made by visualizing viral particles in vesicular fluid with electron microscopy or fluorescent antibody staining of cells from vesicles.

Indications for Antiviral Treatment

9. M.K., a 26-year-old man, developed pain and erythematous skin lesions on his face and around his mouth over a 2-day period after contact with a person with active lesions. Over the next 2 days, significant swelling was noted. M.K. has no previous history of cold sores or any other illnesses. Should he be treated with antiviral drugs?

Most patients with herpes labialis have a self-limiting benign course. Antiviral drugs (e.g., acyclovir, valacyclovir) are indicated only when the patient has a primary infection, an underlying illness, or a compromised immune system that may lead to prolonged illness or dissemination.

Although ice, ether, lysine, silver nitrate, and smallpox vaccine have been used to treat cold sores, no data support their efficacy. Aspirin and acetaminophen are sometimes suggested for symptomatic relief.

10. P.L., a 16-year-old boy diagnosed with acute lymphocytic leukemia 8 months ago, is now admitted for a bone marrow transplant. Admission laboratory tests reveal that he has antibodies against HSV-1 and that 4 months ago, during a course of chemotherapy, he developed an oral-facial herpes infection. What is the significance of these findings for P.L., who is about to undergo a bone marrow transplant?

Immunosuppressed patients have more frequent and severe mucocutaneous HSV infections. Therefore, IV acyclovir should be considered to suppress the reactivation of oral-facial HSV infections.[33,34] Oral therapy with famciclovir is approved for use in HIV-infected patients,[35] but efficacy in other immunocompromised patients is not yet established.

ANTIVIRAL TREATMENT

11. P.L. did not receive antiviral therapy. Two weeks later, he developed oral-mucosal and skin lesions on his face, which were painful and associated with malaise. HSV was identified from the lesion by an immunofluorescence technique. What is the treatment of choice for P.L.?

Acyclovir is administered IV at 5 mg/kg Q 8 hr for 7 days[21] or until the lesions are healed, followed by oral acyclovir 200 mg TID for about 6 months. In patients with marrow transplants and culture-proven recurrent mucocutaneous herpes simplex, oral acyclovir (400 mg five times daily for 10 days) is significantly more effective than placebo in reducing pain, virus shedding, new lesion formation, and lesion healing time.[36] Studies have shown that oral valacyclovir has similar pharmacokinetic parameters as IV acyclovir and may be used as an alternative to IV therapy.[37] However, clinical efficacy of valacyclovir in this population has not been established. The immunocompromised patients in these studies included those receiving corticosteroids, those with leukemia, and recipients of renal allografts.[36,37]

12. N.B., a 43-year-old woman, experiences eight to ten cold sores a year. These are typically preceded by "colds" or sun exposure. She requests a prescription for acyclovir to "prevent" cold sores when she feels one coming on. What is the role of antiviral medications in the acute treatment and prevention in immunocompetent patients with recurrent herpes labialis?

Topical agents which are approved by the U.S. Food and Drug Administration (FDA) for the treatment of recurrent herpes labialis in immunocompetent patients include acyclovir (Zovirax) 5% cream and ointment, docosanol (Abreva) 10% cream, and penciclovir (Denavir) 1% cream. Clinical trials showed that each agent resulted in decreased healing time and decreased pain associated with herpes lesions, when started at the first sign or symptom of a cold sore.[38–44] Penciclovir also decreases viral shedding. Some data have indicated that penciclovir cream may be more effective than acyclovir cream and ointment.[41,42] An advantage of docosanol over the other agents is that it is available without a prescription. The topical agents must be applied within 1 hour of the first sign or symptom of a cold sore and then Q 2 hr for 4 days while awake.

Oral antiviral medications can decrease the duration of pain and healing time in immunocompetent patients. Oral acyclovir 400 mg five times daily for 5 days started within 1 hour of the development of a cold sore was more effective than placebo in reducing mean duration of pain and healing time in immunocompetent patients with a history of one to five episodes of herpes labialis per year.[45] Valacyclovir, 2 g at the first signs of a cold sore followed by 2 g 12 hours later, and famciclovir 1,500 mg as a single dose showed similar clinical efficacy.[46,47] No studies have directly compared the efficacy of the different oral antiviral medications.[48] Frequency of dosing and cost should be considered when choosing a particular agent.[20,23,49]

Daily suppressive therapy may be recommended in patients with six or more recurrences per year or in patients with severe episodes. In immunocompetent patients with six or more episodes of herpes labialis, oral acyclovir 400 mg twice a day (BID) for 4 months was more effective than placebo in decreasing the number of recurrences in patients with herpes labialis.[50] Although not approved by the FDA for suppressive therapy, valacyclovir, 500 mg once daily, also appears to be efficacious in decreasing the number of recurrences.[51]

N.B. should be treated with either a topical antiviral medication or an oral antiviral for the acute episode of herpes labialis. She should be instructed to start treatment as soon as the first sign or symptom of the cold sore appears. If suppressive therapy is desired, N.B. should be treated with continuous oral acyclovir or valacyclovir.

Resistance

13. How should an acyclovir-resistant HSV infection be treated?

The incidence of acyclovir-resistant herpes is higher in immunocompromised patients compared with immunocompetent patients. Current estimates of HSV resistance in the immunocompromised population are about 5%; some populations, such as bone marrow transplant patients, have a resistance rate approaching 30%.[52,53] IV foscarnet 40 mg/kg Q 8 hr was found to be more effective and less toxic than IV vidarabine 15 mg/kg/day in patients with AIDS and mucocutaneous herpetic lesions unresponsive to IV acyclovir.[54] More concerning, however, are the reports of foscarnet-resistant HSV, particularly in the bone marrow transplant population.[55,56] Cidofovir has been used with moderate success in such cases. In patients with recurrent acyclovir-resistant genital herpes, limited evidence suggests that topical imiquimod 5% cream may be effective.[57]

VARICELLA-ZOSTER INFECTIONS

Chickenpox

Chickenpox used to be a common childhood infection, but the incidence has decreased by up to 84% in states with moderate rates of use of the varicella-zoster virus (VZV) vaccine since 1995.[58] This vaccine is now considered a routine childhood vaccine by the American Academy of Pediatrics (see Chapter 96). Before the vaccine was available, approximately 3.5 million cases occurred per year in the United States: 60% of cases occurred in children 5 to 9 years of age, and 80% occurred in those younger than 10 years. Although it is a benign disease in most patients, complications and mortality (7/10,000 cases) can occur in patients younger than 5 years and older than 20 years, and in immunocompromised patients.

This is a highly contagious disease. Children are considered infectious from 2 days before the onset of rash until all vesicles have crusted (usually 4–6 days after the onset of rash). After household exposure, more than 90% of susceptible individuals become infected. Thus, the history can assist in making a diagnosis. A smear of cells scraped from the lesions will show multinucleated giant cells. Viruses also can be identified in vesicular lesions by electron microscopy, or antigen can be detected by countercurrent immunoelectrophoresis. Chickenpox is a primary varicella-zoster infection, whereas herpes zoster (shingles) is caused by reactivation of VZV.

Clinical Presentation

14. A.V., a 10-year-old boy, was admitted to the hospital for evaluation and treatment of possible recurrent chickenpox with progressive lesions. According to his mother and his physician, he had a mild case of chickenpox at age 4 years. At admission, A.V. had a 10-day history of progressive vesicular and pustular lesions that began on his neck and spread to his back, trunk, extremities, and face. Although he had been febrile (up to 40.5°C PO) over the past 3 days, his temperature on admission was 37°C. A.V. had episodes of vomiting during the 4 days before admission. On admission, he was alert, cooperative, and well oriented but had overt ataxia with abnormal cerebellar signs. Lesions consistent with VZV infection were extensive and confluent over the face, neck, chest, and back. Stages of lesions varied from tiny thin-walled vesicles with an erythematous base to umbilicated vesicles. Few crusted lesions were present. Blood analysis revealed a BUN of 9 mg/dL, SrCr of 0.2 mg/dL, and slightly elevated serum transaminase levels (AST 65 IU/L [normal, 0–34] and ALT 122 IU/L [normal, 0–34]). Because of the possibility of cerebellar involvement with VZV infection and possible underlying immunodeficiency, therapy with acyclovir 550 mg IV Q 8 hr (1,500 mg/m²/day) was instituted. Oral diphenhydramine was also prescribed for itching, but A.V. required only two doses on the first hospital day.

New lesions were noted on the second day of acyclovir therapy, but by the third day, no new lesions appeared and previous lesions were healing. The ataxia improved daily. He was discharged on day 7 with no further complaints of nausea and vomiting. Follow-up serologic evaluation demonstrated a fourfold rise in the optical density for the VZV enzyme-linked immunosorbent assay (ELISA) from day 20 to day 60 after the onset of infection. These results suggested primary VZV infection. Why is the use of acyclovir in A.V. appropriate?

[SI units: BUN, 3.213 mmol/L; SrCr, 15.25 mcmol/L; AST, 1.084 mckat/L; ALT, 2.034 mckat/L]

Antiviral Treatment

Neonates, adults, immunocompromised hosts, patients with progressive varicella, and those with extracutaneous complications can benefit from acyclovir therapy. In clinical trials, acyclovir has been shown to be effective in preventing dissemination of VZV infection, accelerating cutaneous healing, and decreasing fever and pain.[59,60] A.V. had a prolonged progressive course of varicella and demonstrated an extracutaneous manifestation of varicella infection (e.g., ataxia with abnormal cerebellar signs). Because of the concern of possible cerebellar involvement, the use of IV acyclovir was appropriate in A.V.

15. C.J., an 8-year-old boy, developed a case of chickenpox and was kept home from school. Four days later, his 15-year-old brother, K.J., began to exhibit similar symptoms. What is the role of acyclovir in immunocompetent patients with chickenpox? Should C.J. or K.J. be treated with acyclovir?

Three studies in children (2–18 years of age) have shown that oral acyclovir 20 mg/kg (when initiated within 24 hours of disease onset) four times a day (QID) for 5 to 10 days was more effective than placebo in accelerating healing and decreasing the formation of new lesions, fever, and itching. However, acyclovir produced only modest benefits (usually healing 1 day sooner than placebo) and was not effective in reducing the complications of varicella.[61] Thus, acyclovir is not indicated for C.J.

Adolescents and adults are more likely to develop complications (e.g., pneumonia, encephalitis) than children. Acyclovir 800 mg PO QID for 5 days in adolescents and 800 mg PO five times daily for 5 days in adults (initiated within 24 hours of disease onset) was more effective than placebo in decreasing the number of lesions, time for healing, fever, and itching. The effect of acyclovir on severe complications could not be assessed.[62–64] Thus, acyclovir therapy should be considered in those at increased risk of severe chickenpox, for example, those like K.J. who are older than 14 years or those with chronic respiratory or skin disease.[65] No data are available to show if famciclovir and valacyclovir are as effective as acyclovir.

Supportive Treatment

16. **What is the role of supportive treatment in A.V. and C.J.?**

Cool baths and application of calamine or other topical antipruritic agents may decrease itching. In severe cases, a systemic antipruritic/antihistamine preparation may be useful because some degree of sedation may be desired. In A.V. and C.J., aspirin should not be used because Reye syndrome has been associated with the use of salicylates in chickenpox or flulike illness (see Chapter 94).

Shingles (Herpes Zoster)

Herpes zoster infections are caused by the reactivation of dormant VZV in the sensory neurons. Reactivation is believed to occur because of waning immunity. The incidence of herpes zoster is higher in immunocompromised patients (e.g., those with HIV or cancer or those receiving immunosuppressive medications), and the incidence of zoster increases with age. It tends to be more severe in the elderly.

Acute herpes zoster infection is characterized by pain, which is described as deep aching or burning. It may be accompanied by excessive sensitivity to touch. Many patients develop a rash that presents initially as erythematous patches and progresses to vesicles that crust in 7 to 10 days. By 1 month, the rash is usually gone, but scarring can occur.

Postherpetic neuralgia (PHN) is pain that continues more than 1 month after the onset of the rash. It is estimated that 10% to 70% of patients experience PHN. PHN is the most common complication of acute herpes zoster, and its prevention is important because PHN pain is difficult to treat.

The goal of pharmacotherapy in acute herpes zoster is to inhibit viral replication to reduce pain and duration of rash. Ultimately, it is hoped that by inhibiting the virus, nerve damage can be prevented, and the incidence and severity of PHN can be decreased. Unfortunately, no therapy can prevent all cases of PHN.

With the approval of the herpes zoster vaccine (Zostavax), it is hoped that the incidence of herpes zoster and the resulting PHN will be reduced (see Chapter 95).

Antiviral Therapy in Immunocompetent Patients

17. **E.O. is a 72-year-old, previously healthy man who complains of a burning pain under his left arm for the last 2 days. The pain radiates across his chest. The pain is worse when the area is touched. This morning, he noticed a rash that starts under his arm and continues to his midline. Pertinent laboratory findings include BUN of 15 mg/dL (normal, 8–18) and SrCr of 2.0 mg/dL (normal, 0.6–1.2). He has not received the herpes zoster vaccine. A diagnosis of herpes zoster is made. What therapy should be initiated?**

[SI units: BUN, 5.4 mmol/L; SrCr, 177 micromolar/L]

Acyclovir is the standard antiviral agent against which new therapies are compared. In immunocompetent patients, oral acyclovir 800 mg five times daily for 7 to 10 days is moderately beneficial in reducing acute pain during the first 28 days. Acyclovir therapy should be initiated within 72 hours of the onset of the rash. The effects of acyclovir in reducing PHN and chronic pain are unclear. Although a number of trials showed no benefit in reducing PHN, a meta-analysis of five placebo-controlled trials of acyclovir treatment in herpes zoster found that the number needed to treat was 6.3 to reduce the incidence of PHN at 6 months.[66]

Famciclovir (Famvir) is approved for the treatment of acute herpes zoster infection. Famciclovir is rapidly absorbed and converted to the active drug penciclovir in the intestine. The bioavailability of famciclovir is higher than acyclovir, resulting in higher concentrations of active drug in the infected cells. In addition, the half-life of famciclovir is considerably longer compared with acyclovir, allowing less frequent administration. In a large clinical trial comparing famciclovir with acyclovir, famciclovir 500 mg TID was as effective as acyclovir 800 mg five times a day in reducing the duration of acute pain and healing of the rash.[67] In another study comparing famciclovir with placebo, famciclovir did not decrease the incidence of PHN but reduced the duration of PHN versus placebo.[68]

A limitation of acyclovir is its poor oral bioavailability (15%–30%). In an attempt to overcome this, valacyclovir (Valtrex), a prodrug of acyclovir, was developed. Valacyclovir is rapidly and extensively absorbed and converted to acyclovir in the body after oral administration. In clinical trials, valacyclovir 1 g TID was equally effective as acyclovir 800 mg five times a day in terms of rash progression and time to rash healing, and valacyclovir was more effective than acyclovir in relieving zoster-associated pain.[69] In comparison to famciclovir, valacyclovir was comparable in duration of acute zoster-associated pain and PHN.[70]

E.O. should be started on acyclovir, famciclovir, or valacyclovir for the treatment of his herpes zoster. Famciclovir or valacyclovir may be preferred because adherence with a three-times-daily regimen will likely be better than with acyclovir, which must be administered five times a day. Therapy should be initiated as soon as possible because most of the clinical trials began therapy within 72 hours of the rash onset. Although therapy may not prevent PHN, it may have an effect on the duration of pain. Because these agents are renally eliminated, the dosage should be adjusted based on E.O.'s creatinine clearance (Table 72-2).

18. **Should E.O. receive a corticosteroid to treat or prevent the pain associated with herpes zoster?**

The use of corticosteroids such as prednisone or prednisolone remains controversial.[71] A number of studies have examined the effect of steroids on pain during acute neuralgia and on the development of PHN. Early studies indicated benefit for both acute pain and PHN, but these studies were small and uncontrolled, lacked statistical analysis, and used various corticosteroid regimens. Studies suggest possible relief of the acute pain but no decrease in PHN.[72–75] Adverse effects of the corticosteroids and the theoretical possibility of dissemination of herpes zoster resulting from their use should be considered when deciding whether to initiate therapy. Based on recent studies demonstrating lack of benefit in preventing PHN, the theoretical concerns of herpes zoster dissemination, and the beneficial effects of antiviral agents such as acyclovir, famciclovir, and valacyclovir for acute pain, corticosteroids should not be used in E.O.

19. **Two months after the onset of the rash, E.O. continues to complain of pain. A diagnosis of PHN is made. What FDA-approved treatments for PHN should be prescribed for E.O.?**

Although many different agents have been studied, the only FDA-approved treatments for PHN are topical capsaicin, topical lidocaine 5% patches (Lidoderm), and pregabalin (Lyrica). Capsaicin depletes substance P, a mediator that transmits pain from the periphery to the CNS. The largest double-blind, placebo-controlled trial of capsaicin evaluated 143 patients with PHN for at least 6 months. After 6 weeks of treatment with capsaicin 0.075% cream, pain scores were reduced in 21% and 6% of the capsaicin and placebo groups, respectively. Following the double-blind phase of the study, a subset of patients continued to use capsaicin cream for up to 2 years, and most patients experienced prolonged pain relief.[76] Lidocaine 5% patches have only been compared with placebo and have been shown to relieve pain for 4 to 12 hours following administration. Either capsaicin cream or lidocaine patches can be considered as a first-line options for E.O. Capsaicin should be applied three or four times per day. A common adverse effect is a burning sensation after application, which is intolerable in up to one-third of patients. The burning sensation usually lessens with continued use.

If lidocaine patches are prescribed, E.O. should be instructed to apply up to three patches to the painful area. Patients should be instructed to wear the patches for a maximum of 12 hours a day, and proper disposal of used patches should be emphasized. Because even a used patch contains a large amount of lidocaine, small children or pets could suffer serious consequences from chewing or swallowing a used patch.[77]

Pregabalin, a newer agent approved for the treatment of PHN, appears to be effective but is associated with a greater risk of adverse effects. Pregabalin binds to a subunit of calcium channels, thereby decreasing calcium influx at nerve terminals and reducing the release of several neurotransmitters, including glutamate, norepinephrine, and substance P.[78] Dizziness and somnolence are common. In clinical trials, dizziness was experienced by 29% of patients treated with pregabalin compared to 9% of placebo-treated patients; somnolence was noted in 22% of patients who received pregabalin compared to 8% of placebo-treated patients. Dizziness and somnolence usually occur soon after the pregabalin is started and appears to be dose dependent.[78]

Other agents that have been used in the treatment of PHN include tricyclic antidepressants (e.g., amitriptyline, desipramine), anticonvulsants (e.g., gabapentin), and opioids.[79]

Antiviral Therapy in Immunocompromised Patients

20. R.F. is a 68-year-old woman seen in the ED with a chief complaint of vesicles on her face associated with severe pain. She has a history of polymyalgia rheumatica and possible temporal arteritis causing headaches that are generally responsive to steroids. She had been having increasing headaches on the right side of her forehead 5 days before admission. Two days before admission, her family physician increased the dosage of prednisone from 30 mg/day to 60 mg/day. Vesicles developed on her face 1 day before admission. She was admitted for pain control and diagnosed with herpes zoster infection. Six hours after admission, R.F. began having visual hallucinations, hearing noises, and talking to herself. A lumbar puncture was performed with the following results: three WBCs (two lymphocytes and one monocyte); three RBCs; protein, 84 mg/dL; and glucose, 86 mg/dL. VZV was isolated from the CSF. IV acyclovir was started at a dosage of 10 mg/kg Q 8 hr. Why is antiviral therapy indicated in R.F.? Should her prednisone be continued or discontinued?

Antiviral therapy is indicated for R.F. Acyclovir may halt the progression of acute herpes zoster infection in immunocompromised hosts such as R.F., who has been taking large doses of corticosteroids.[80]

In clinical trials, IV acyclovir 10 mg/kg Q 8 hr has been shown to be effective in severely immunocompromised patients. Alternatively, in less severely immunocompromised patients, oral therapy with acyclovir 800 mg five times a day, valacyclovir 1,000 mg TID, or famciclovir 500 mg TID, along with close monitoring, can be used.[81] In patients with cutaneous dissemination of disease, there was a more rapid clearance of the herpes zoster virus from vesicles. Pain relief occurred faster in patients who received acyclovir, and fewer acyclovir-treated patients reported PHN, but the differences were not statistically significant.[80] There are no data available regarding the use of famciclovir or valacyclovir in severe herpes zoster infection in an immunocompromised host.

Systemic corticosteroids are of unproven usefulness and may slow the healing of lesions. Therefore, if possible, R.F.'s prednisone should be slowly tapered.

ACYCLOVIR TOXICITY

21. On the fourth day of acyclovir therapy, R.F. developed severe nausea and vomited three times. The laboratory data showed a BUN of 45 mg/dL and SrCr of 3.2 mg/dL (baseline BUN, 10 mg/dL and SrCr, 1.0 mg/dL). Why must R.F.'s acyclovir dosage be altered?

[SI units: BUN, 16.07 and 3.57 mmol/L, respectively; SrCr, 282.88 and 88.40 micromolar/L, respectively]

Nausea and vomiting have been reported with acyclovir therapy in patients with herpes zoster infections.[21] Similarly, elevations of SrCr and BUN can occur in association with acyclovir therapy. This may be secondary to acyclovir crystallization in the renal tubules, particularly when fluid intake is inadequate (Table 72-4). Because R.F.'s creatinine clearance is between 10 and 25 mL/minute per 1.73 m^2, the acyclovir dosage interval should be extended to 24 hours. Every effort should be made to maintain adequate hydration for the duration of acyclovir therapy. (See Table 72-2 and Chapter 2 for creatinine clearance calculation.)

INFLUENZA

Influenza is an acute infection caused by the virus of the *Orthomyxoviridae* family. Epidemics of influenza are usually caused by the type A virus; type B virus is generally associated with sporadic infection. Infection is transmitted by the inhalation of virus-containing droplets ejected from the respiratory tract of a person with influenza. It can be spread by direct contact, large droplets, or articles recently contaminated by nasopharyngeal secretions. The incubation period is typically 2 days (range, 1–4 days).

Influenza A viruses are classified into subtypes of hemagglutinin (H) and neuraminidase (N) surface antigens. Three subtypes of hemagglutinin (H_1, H_2, H_3) and two subtypes of neuraminidase (N_1, N_2) have caused influenza in humans. Infection with a virus of one subtype may confer little or no

Table 72-5 Persons Who Should Receive the Influenza Vaccine[82]

- All healthy children ages 6–59 mo
- All persons 50 years or older
- Nursing home or chronic care facility residents
- Children and adults with chronic pulmonary or cardiovascular disease
- Children and adults who have required medical follow-up because of chronic metabolic diseases (e.g., diabetes mellitus), renal dysfunction, hemoglobinopathies, or immunosuppression (due to medications or diseases such as HIV)
- Children and adults who are at risk for aspiration (e.g., cognitive dysfunction, spinal cord injuries, seizures)
- Children (6 mo–18 yr) receiving long-term aspirin therapy
- Women who will be pregnant during influenza season
- Health care workers
- Household members of person in high-risk groups (including contacts of infants and children 0–59 mo)

protection against viruses of other subtypes. In addition, significant antigenic variation (antigenic drift) within a subtype may occur over time. Thus, infection or vaccination with one strain may not protect against a distantly related strain of the same subtype. This is why major epidemics of influenza continue to occur and influenza vaccines are reformulated each year with likely viral strains to maximize immunity.

Persons at highest risk for influenza infection (Table 72-5) should receive the influenza vaccine each year. Each year's vaccine contains three virus strains (generally two type A and one type B) that are likely to circulate in the community for the upcoming season. The efficacy depends on the similarity of the components of the vaccine to the circulating viruses that year and the immunocompetence of the host. If there is a good match with the circulating viruses, the vaccine can prevent illness in approximately 70% to 90% of healthy adults and children. It appears to be effective in preventing hospitalization and pneumonia in 70% of elderly persons living in the community and in 50% to 60% of elderly persons residing in nursing homes. However, the efficacy of the vaccine in preventing illness is often only 30% to 40% among the frail elderly. Despite the lower efficacy, the illness is less severe, and the risk of complications is reduced in vaccinated individuals.

Individuals who can transmit influenza to persons at high risk include physicians, nurses, and other personnel in both hospital and ambulatory settings; employees of nursing homes and chronic care facilities; providers of home care services; and household members, including children.

Persons at high risk and those who may transmit the virus to those at high risk should be vaccinated annually. Table 72-6 describes the types of vaccines, dosage, number of doses, and route of administration. The optimal time for vaccine administration is between mid-October and mid-November because influenza activity peaks between late December and early March in the United States. Vaccinating an individual too early in the season could result in waning antibody concentrations before the influenza season is over. However, influenza vaccine should be offered throughout the influenza season, even if outbreaks of influenza have already been documented in the community.[82]

Table 72-6 Influenza Vaccines[82]

Age	Dosage	Number of Doses
6–35 mo	0.25 mL IM[a] inactivated vaccine	1 or 2[c]
36–59 mo	0.5 mL IM[a] inactivated vaccine	1 or 2[c]
5–49 yr	0.5 mL IM[a] inactivated vaccine or 0.5 mL IN[b] live vaccine	1 or 2[c]
≥50 yr	0.5 mL IM[a] inactivated vaccine	1

[a] The recommended site is the deltoid muscle for adults and older children and the anterolateral aspect of the thigh in infants and young children.
[b] The live vaccine should not be used in patients with chronic pulmonary or cardiovascular disease and in those with underlying immunodeficiencies.
[c] Two doses given at least 1 mo apart for children younger than 9 years who are receiving the vaccine for the first time.
IM, intramuscularly; IN, intranasally.

Because the parenteral influenza vaccine is an inactivated vaccine and contains no infectious viruses, it cannot cause influenza. The most common adverse effect is soreness at the administration site lasting for up to 2 days.[83] Fever, malaise, myalgia, and other systemic reactions occur infrequently; these may develop within 6 to 12 hours after the vaccine is given and persist for 1 to 3 days.[83,84] Immediate hypersensitivity to egg protein (hives, angioedema, allergic asthma, or systemic anaphylaxis) rarely occurs. Persons with anaphylactic hypersensitivity and those with acute febrile illness should not be given the vaccine. However, minor illnesses with or without fever are not contraindications for the influenza vaccine, particularly in children with a mild upper respiratory tract infection or allergic rhinitis. When the vaccine is contraindicated, a neuraminidase inhibitor (oseltamivir or zanamivir) should be used for prophylaxis.[82] Amantadine and rimantadine are no longer recommended for prophylaxis of influenza because of widespread resistance in the United States.

Clinically, it is impossible to differentiate between influenza A and B. Definitive diagnosis can be made by isolating the virus from throat washings or sputum and by a significant increase in antibody titers during the convalescent period.

Clinical Presentation

22. K.B., a 40-year-old woman, comes into the pharmacy and says she has "the flu." She recently started a new job and is afraid she will lose her job if she misses too many days from work. What questions would you ask her to differentiate the common cold from an influenza infection?

It can be difficult to differentiate the common cold from an influenza infection. Influenza infections typically occur from December through March in the United States. Patients with influenza generally experience more systemic symptoms, such as fever higher than 102°F, headache, myalgia, and cough. Rhinorrhea, nasal congestion, and sneezing are more pronounced in patients with the common cold. Sore throat can occur with both a cold and the flu. Bacterial sore throat (e.g., strep throat) is differentiated from a viral sore throat in that a viral sore throat usually has a slower onset and the throat pain is less severe. Lymph nodes are only slightly enlarged and not tender in a viral sore throat, whereas with a bacterial sore throat, lymph nodes are large and tender.[85]

K.B. should be questioned about her symptoms and exposure to ill contacts, and investigation into whether influenza has been documented in the community should be performed to help differentiate an influenza infection from the common cold.

Treatment

23. K.B. describes symptoms consistent with an influenza infection for the past 24 hours. What treatment options exist for the treatment of influenza? Why is she a candidate for a neuraminidase inhibitor agent such as zanamivir or oseltamivir?

Two agents known as the neuraminidase inhibitors for the treatment of influenza A and B in adults were approved in 1999. Zanamivir (Relenza) and oseltamivir (Tamiflu) work by selectively inhibiting the enzyme neuraminidase, an enzyme necessary for viral replication and spread. Oseltamivir is currently indicated for the prevention and treatment of influenza in patients 1 year of age and older; zanamivir is indicated for the prevention of influenza in patients 7 years of age and older and for the treatment of influenza in patients 5 years of age and older.[86,87]

Zanamivir is available as an oral powder for inhalation. For the treatment of influenza infection in adults, 10 mg (two inhalations) BID for 5 days should be used. Patients should inhale two doses separated by at least 2 hours on the first day and then two doses separated by 12 hours on days 2 through 5.[86] Bronchospasm after use can occur, and if bronchodilators are also prescribed, the bronchodilator should be used before zanamivir.[86] Proper use of the delivery system (Rotadisk Diskhaler) is important, and thus patients should be instructed on proper use, with a demonstration of delivery technique, by the pharmacist.

Oseltamivir is pharmacologically related to zanamivir but has significantly better oral bioavailability, allowing oral dosing. The dosage of oseltamivir for the treatment of influenza in adults is 75 mg BID for 5 days.[87] As with zanamivir, treatment with oseltamivir must be started within 2 days of the onset of symptoms. Common side effects include nausea, vomiting, and headache.[87] In addition, there are reports, predominantly in children, of self-injury and delirium, following the administration of oseltamivir.[88]

Amantadine is approved for patients 1 year of age or older. Rimantadine is only approved for the prevention of influenza A in children.[89,90] However, the incidence of resistance to amantadine and rimantadine has increased dramatically in recent years. In one study, 92% of strains of influenza A demonstrated resistance to influenza A. Consequently, these agents are no longer recommended for the routine prevention or treatment of influenza infections.[82]

When administered within 2 days of onset of illness, zanamivir and oseltamivir reduce influenza symptoms by approximately 1 day.[91–93] Information regarding the effectiveness of the neuraminidase inhibitors in preventing serious complications of influenza, such as pneumonia or worsening of chronic diseases, is limited.[82] Advantages of the neuraminidase inhibitors over amantadine and rimantadine include the efficacy against influenza B or resistant influenza A. Because the causative agent is unknown and symptoms have been present for more than 2 days, K.B. may benefit from a neuraminidase inhibitor. Oral oseltamivir is easier to administer than inhaled zanamivir. Although oseltamivir will not cure influenza, it may reduce the severity and duration of symptoms by about 1 day. Because K.B. is concerned about missing too much time from work, she should be treated with a 5-day course of oseltamivir.

24. J.T., a 74-year-old man, is brought to the ED from a nursing home with chief complaints of fever (103°F), shaking chills, cough, headache, malaise, anorexia, and photophobia. He has been ill for the past 48 hours but suddenly became worse this evening. On physical examination, he appeared flushed, his skin was hot and moist, and he was working hard to breathe. Vital signs were blood pressure, 150/90 mmHg; pulse, 108 beats/minute; respiratory rate, 22 breaths/minute; and temperature, 103°F. Rales were audible on auscultation of both lungs. A chest roentgenogram showed bilateral infiltrates but no consolidation. Blood gas studies showed significant hypoxia, with a PaO_2 of 50 mmHg and a $PaCO_2$ of 50 mmHg. J.T.'s medical history was significant for chronic bronchitis and a stroke 16 months ago. Blood, sputum, and urine cultures were obtained, and J.T. was started on antibiotics (gentamicin 140-mg loading dose, then 90 mg Q 12 hr IV piggyback and clindamycin 900 mg Q 8 hr IV piggyback). Gram stain of the sputum sample showed many WBCs but no bacteria. He was started on oxygen therapy at 4 L/minute via nasal cannula. Twenty-four hours later, his respiratory symptoms worsened, and his arterial blood gases deteriorated slightly (PaO_2, 40 mmHg; $PaCO_2$, 55 mmHg). J.T. was intubated, and a sputum sample was obtained and sent to the virology lab. Three days later, influenza A virus was isolated from the sputum. Blood, urine, and sputum cultures were all negative for bacterial pathogens. Why is this presentation consistent with influenza infection? Is antiviral treatment indicated in J.T.?

[SI units: PaO_2, 6.665 and 5.332 kPa, respectively; $PaCO_2$, 6.665 and 7.332 kPa, respectively]

Although symptoms of influenza may vary depending on age, most patients with influenza A have an abrupt onset of fever, chills, cough, and headache. In elderly patients such as J.T. and those with underlying diseases, the course of influenza can worsen quickly, and patients are more likely to require hospitalization.

Antiviral therapy in J.T. is inappropriate. None of the antiviral agents has been studied in patients presenting with symptoms after 48 hours of onset. In addition, the antiviral agents have shown efficacy only in uncomplicated influenza.[82]

Prevention

25. Over the next 3 weeks, two other nursing home patients develop influenza A infections. What measures should be taken to prevent a further outbreak of influenza among other residents?

Influenza Vaccines

The nursing home residents and staff should receive influenza vaccine plus chemoprophylaxis with oseltamivir, or zanamivir. The Centers for Disease Control and Prevention (CDC) recommends immunization of all high-risk groups[82] (Table 72-5). The top-priority groups include all individuals who are at high risk for influenza-related complications and their household contacts. Second in priority are otherwise healthy adults 50 years of age or older and children with chronic metabolic diseases severe enough to warrant regular follow-up during the preceding year. Any child younger than 9 years in which the vaccine is indicated requires two doses of the vaccine for optimal effectiveness. The first dose should be administered in September, and the second dose is given before influenza infection is present in the community. However, the efficacy of influenza vaccine is incomplete (70%).[94] Therefore, the CDC recommends the use of oseltamivir or zanamivir in high-risk individuals who may not develop an adequate antibody response (e.g., patients with advanced HIV infection) to supplement the protection by vaccine.[82]

A live, attenuated influenza vaccine (FluMist) is an option for healthy, nonpregnant individuals between the ages of 2 and 49 years. In clinical studies with matched influenza strains, live, attenuated influenza vaccine was approximately 87% effective in preventing influenza in children and provided 85% efficacy in adults.[95] Advantages of the intranasal route of administration include ease of administration and patient acceptability of an intranasal preparation compared to an intramuscular (IM) injection. However, because the vaccine is live, viral shedding can occur for 2 or more days after vaccination. Consequently, patients who are immunosuppressed and close contacts of patients who are severely immunocompromised (including health care workers who care for them) should not receive the live vaccine. Others who should not receive the live vaccine include patients with asthma or other chronic disorders of the pulmonary or cardiovascular systems, those with chronic metabolic diseases such as diabetes, renal dysfunction, hemoglobinopathies, and children or adolescents who are receiving aspirin or other salicylates.[82]

Oseltamivir and Zanamivir

Analysis of clinical trials of oseltamivir in the prevention of influenza showed a decreased incidence of laboratory-confirmed influenza: 4.8% in the placebo group and 1.2% in the treatment group.[96] The incidence of influenza in a skilled nursing facility was 4.4% in the placebo group and 0.4% in the oseltamivir group. In addition, oseltamivir lowered the rate of infection in patients exposed to influenza at home from 12% to 1%. Zanamivir also showed decreases in subsequent cases among individuals exposed to influenza in the home setting, although zanamivir is currently not indicated for prophylaxis of influenza.[97,98]

Comparative studies between neuraminidase inhibitors have not been published. Because oseltamivir is available in an oral formulation, it may be easier to administer in nursing home patients compared with zanamivir, which requires proper use of the delivery device and a coordinated inspiratory effort.

AVIAN FLU

Avian flu is an illness caused by an influenza virus that is commonly found in wild poultry. Although many wild birds carry the avian influenza viruses in their intestines, this virus does not commonly cause illness in wild birds. However, the virus is quite contagious and can be deadly in domesticated birds, such as chickens, ducks, and turkeys.

There are two types of avian influenza: the North American H5N1 strain and the Asian H5N1 strain. The low pathogenic or North American strain is common in wild birds and rarely causes symptoms of disease. This strain does not cause disease in humans. Conversely, the high pathogenic or Asian strain spreads rapidly to domesticated poultry and often results in death. This strain is endemic in Asia and has spread to Europe. This strain can infect humans, especially after direct contact with infected birds. There are only rare reports of human-to-human transmission, with none occurring in the United States.

To date, the two H5N1 avian flu strains have not caused widespread disease in humans. For an avian flu pandemic to occur, the virus must be easily spread from human to human. Currently, the transmissibility among humans is poor.

Clinical Presentation

26. **D.D. presents to the urgent care complaining of fever, difficulty breathing, cough, and blood in his sputum. Of note, he works for the poultry industry, and recently, a large number of chickens have died. On physical exam, he is febrile (101.5°F), tachypneic (55 breaths/minute), and has crackles on chest exam. He has a slightly elevated WBC with leukocytosis. Blood, sputum, and respiratory secretions were sent for culture. The PCR for influenza A returns as positive. What signs and symptoms in D.D.'s history support a diagnosis of avian flu?**

The signs and symptoms of infection with avian flu vary widely. Persons infected with the virus can demonstrate signs and symptoms typically seen with human influenza infections, such as fever, cough, sore throat, and muscle aches. Alternatively, infected individuals may have a more fulminant course with pneumonia, severe respiratory distress, and other life-threatening complications. If an avian flu pandemic occurred, those most likely to be seriously affected would be infants, the elderly, and those with chronic medical conditions.[99] Specimens from patients should be sent to the CDC for additional testing if the patient has had a history of contact with poultry or domestic birds and tests positive for influenza A by either PCR or antigen detection testing.[100]

Treatment

27. **How should D.D. be treated?**

For cases of human infection with H5N1, the neuraminidase inhibitors oseltamivir and zanamivir may improve clinical outcome if administered early. Oseltamivir has been used more than zanamivir, but clinical studies are limited. It is believed that the H5N1 virus is susceptible to the neuraminidase inhibitors. Although traditional antibacterial agents are not effective for the H5N1 virus, antibiotics may have a role in secondary bacterial infection such as pneumonia, which often occurs following influenza infections.

In April 2007, the FDA approved the first influenza H5N1 virus vaccine or avian influenza vaccine. The inactivated vaccine is indicated for the immunization of individuals between the ages of 18 and 64 years who are at increased risk of exposure to avian influenza. The vaccine is given as a two-dose series, with the doses separated by 21 to 35 days. In clinical trials, the vaccine has been found to reduce the risk of avian influenza in about 45% of the recipients. In the remaining 55% of recipients, although the antibody concentrations were below the protective threshold concentration, the vaccine may potentially reduce disease severity, influenza-related hospitalizations, and deaths.[101]

RESPIRATORY SYNCYTIAL VIRUS INFECTIONS

Respiratory syncytial virus (RSV) is an important pathogen causing bronchiolitis and bronchopneumonia. RSV infection commonly affects infants younger than 2 years, with more than one-half of the infants becoming infected in the first 2 years of life. Of these infants, approximately 1% to 2% will require hospitalization.[102] Children with underlying congenital heart disease or lung disease may be at increased risk of mortality due to RSV.[103] Patients with RSV infection before 3 years of age appear to be at an increased risk of wheezing and asthma during childhood.[104–106]

RSV infections usually occur in the winter. The chest radiograph and blood gases are often abnormal, and the virus can be isolated in the nasopharyngeal secretions.

Clinical Presentation and Ribavirin Therapy

28. J.R., a 6-month-old infant who is lethargic, tachypneic, and cyanotic, is brought to the ED. J.R.'s medical history is significant for congenital HIV. He has a fever (102°F), his breathing is labored, and wheezing is audible on expiration. The chest roentgenograms show a flattened diaphragm and hyperinflated lung parenchyma. Because of hypoxemia and hypercarbia, J.R. is placed on ambient oxygen to maintain the alveolar oxygen pressure at >60 mmHg. RSV is present in the respiratory secretions. What type of therapy is indicated for J.R., who has an underlying immunodeficiency?

The goal of therapy is to decrease airway resistance in a patient such as like J.R.[107] Treatment of RSV is highly individualized, depending on the presenting signs and symptoms. Oxygen is first-line therapy. Decreases in airway resistance may be achieved with the use of bronchodilators or corticosteroids. However, bronchodilators have led to minimal clinical improvement in only approximately 25% of infants with RSV.[108] The use of corticosteroids in the treatment of RSV is not recommended.[109] Although individual studies differ on the clinical benefits of oral corticosteroids, two meta-analyses found no benefits in decreasing length of stay or disease severity.[110,111]

The use of ribavirin (Virazole), an antiviral agent that possesses unique inhibitory activity against a large number of both DNA and RNA viruses, for the treatment of RSV remains controversial. Early studies with ribavirin showed significant clinical improvement compared to placebo in both healthy children and those with underlying disease.[112] These studies reported clinical recovery and improvement in arterial oxygenation. Subsequent studies found ribavirin to be ineffective in patients with a variety of risk factors.[113,114] Consequently, the routine use in previously healthy infants and children has not been clearly established. Whether ribavirin decreases the long-term sequelae and severity of illness in high-risk groups (including premature infants, patients with bronchopulmonary dysplasia, congenital heart disease, cystic fibrosis, and immunodeficiency) has not been determined.[115] Current recommendations include consideration for use of ribavirin in infants with severe disease or those at risk for severe disease such as infants who may be immunocompromised and/or have hemodynamically significant cardiopulmonary disease.[109] Because J.R. has an underlying immunodeficiency, ribavirin may be considered if J.R.'s condition worsens.

RSV immune globulin (RSV-IGIV, RespiGam) is an IV product made from the blood of donors with high titers of RSV-neutralizing antibodies. The use of RSV-IGIV has been evaluated in children at high risk for severe infections and in previously healthy children. Although administration of RSV-IGIV was safe, studies have shown no efficacy with the use of immune globulins in the treatment of RSV.[116] Thus, this is not recommended for use in the treatment of RSV.

Administration of Ribavirin

29. How is ribavirin administered, and what precautions should be taken during drug administration in J.R.?

Ribavirin is administered as an aerosol through a collision generator that generates particles small enough (1–2 micron wide) to reach the lower respiratory tract. This ensures that high concentrations of ribavirin penetrate the respiratory secretions at the site of viral replication while minimizing systemic absorption. The concentration of the ribavirin solution in the reservoir is 20 mg/mL (6 g in 300 mL of sterile water). The dose is administered over 12 to 18 hours, although in nonventilated patients, 2 g over 2 hours TID (using a 60-mg/mL solution) has been successfully used.[114] Ribavirin therapy is continued for 3 to 7 days.[117]

Ribavirin is approved for use in patients requiring mechanical ventilation. However, ribavirin is hygroscopic, and aerosol particles can deposit in the tubing and around the expiratory valve of a ventilator. The precipitated drug can obstruct the expiratory valve and alter the peak end-expiratory pressure.[117] Ribavirin has been safely used in such patients,[118,119] but close monitoring of respiratory therapy is advised to prevent this problem. In addition to the inspection of tubing, modifications of standard ventilatory circuits have been suggested.[117]

Adverse Effects

30. What are the important adverse effects of ribavirin?

The most common adverse effects of ribavirin are rash, initial mild bronchospasm on drug initiation, and reversible skin irritation.[120] Although long-term follow-up data are limited, a study evaluating the effects of ribavirin in patients 1 year after administration showed a reduction in the incidence and severity of reactive airway disease, as well as in hospitalizations related to respiratory illness. Further long-term evaluation is still necessary.[121]

Ribavirin is contraindicated in women who are or may become pregnant during exposure to the drug. Although there are no human data, ribavirin has been found to be teratogenic and/or embryolethal in nearly all animal species in which it has been tested. Teratogenesis was evident after a single oral dose of 2.5 mg/kg in hamsters and after daily oral doses of 10 mg/kg in rats. Malformation of the skull, palate, eye, jaw, skeleton, and GI tract were noted in animals. Ribavirin has reduced the survival of fetuses and offspring of animals tested. It is lethal to rabbit embryo in daily oral doses as small as 1 mg/kg. There are no studies that address teratogenicity in humans, but hospital personnel who are pregnant or may become pregnant should avoid exposure to this drug.[117]

It is important to consider the environmental effects of ribavirin on the personnel involved with its administration. One study found no detectable plasma or urine concentrations of ribavirin in 19 nurses, whereas another reported its presence in the RBCs of a nurse caring for a patient who received ribavirin via oxygen tent.[122] The ribavirin concentration in the air was highest when it was administered via oxygen tent, followed by mist mask, and was lowest after administration via endotracheal tubes of mechanically ventilated patients. This has led to several recommendations: (a) ribavirin aerosol should be administered solely via endotracheal tube of mechanically ventilated patients in a closed filtered system[102]; (b) children receiving ribavirin should be placed in a containment chamber equipped with a high-efficiency particulate air filter exhaust in an isolation room with negative air pressure[117]; (c) disposable full-body coverings and either a powered air-purifying respirator or disposable particulate respirator should be made available to all health care personnel[117]; and (d) men and women planning to have children should not care for patients receiving ribavirin via oxygen tents.[122] ICN Pharmaceuticals markets an aerosol delivery system for oxygen and ribavirin that decreases the liberation of ribavirin into the environment.[117]

Prevention

31. S.N. is a 7-month-old boy born prematurely at 31 weeks' gestation. He has bronchopulmonary dysplasia (BPD) and uses oxygen at home. RSV season will begin next month. What treatments to prevent RSV infection are available? Why is S.N. a candidate for such treatment?

Two products are available for the prevention of RSV infections. RSV-IGIV may be used to prevent or decrease the severity of lower respiratory tract infections caused by RSV in children younger than 24 months with BPD or a history of premature birth before 35 weeks' gestation. Infants who were born prematurely and who have underlying pulmonary disease (e.g., BPD), cardiovascular disease, or immunodeficiency states are at higher risk for death because of RSV than other infants.

In a large study of infants with BPD and/or prematurity, monthly infusions of RSV-IGIV during RSV season (starting in mid-November and continuing for three to five monthly doses) decreased the number of RSV lower respiratory tract infections, hospital admissions, duration of hospitalizations, and days in the intensive care unit.[123] Other studies have demonstrated similar results.[124]

Palivizumab (Synagis), a humanized monoclonal antibody made from recombinant DNA, is active against RSV and is indicated for children at high risk of RSV respiratory tract infections (e.g., infants with BPD or a history of premature birth prior to 35 weeks' gestation). The efficacy of palivizumab was demonstrated in a randomized, double-blind, placebo-controlled trial involving 1,502 children who had a history of prematurity or BPD.[125] Children received monthly IM injections of placebo or palivizumab for 5 months during RSV season. Palivizumab-treated children had a reduction in RSV hospitalizations and intensive care admissions, and had shorter hospitalizations for RSV disease. Palivizumab is preferred over RSV-IGIV for most high-risk infants because it is easier to administer (IM vs. IV), does not interfere with the response of live vaccines such as measles-mumps-rubella or varicella vaccine, and is not likely to transmit blood-borne diseases because it is a synthetic product rather than one derived from human blood.[126]

Based on S.N.'s age and his underlying immunodeficiency, he is a candidate for palivizumab therapy.[109]

Palivizumab Dosage and Administration

32. How are the doses of RSV-IGIV and palivizumab calculated, and how should they be given?

RSV-IGIV 750 mg/kg is given as an IV infusion. The dose of palivizumab is 15 mg/kg given IM. For both products, the first dose is given before the start of the RSV season, and then monthly doses are given throughout the RSV season. In the Northern Hemisphere, the RSV season is typically November through April.

Because adverse reactions to RSV-IGIV may be related to the infusion rate, infusion titration is important. During the initial 15 minutes, RSV-IGIV should be infused at 1.5 mL/kg/hour (using a 50-mg/mL solution). The infusion rate can then be increased to 3 mL/kg/hour for the next 15 minutes, and, if tolerated, the rate can be increased to a maximum of 6 mL/kg/hours.

HANTAVIRUS INFECTIONS

Rodents are the primary reservoir hosts of Hantavirus, and in the United States, the deer mouse (*Peromyscus maniculatus*) is the main reservoir. These viruses apparently do not cause illness in the reservoir hosts, but infection in humans occurs when infected saliva, urine, and feces are inhaled as aerosols produced by the rodent. Most patients recall exposure to rodents or rodent feces within 6 weeks of the onset of illness.[127] Person-to-person transmission has not been documented.

Four serotypes of Hantavirus have been identified. The case definition used by the CDC includes clinical evidence of (a) febrile illness characterized by unexplained adult respiratory distress syndrome (ARDS) or acute bilateral pulmonary interstitial infiltrates; or (b) an autopsy finding of noncardiogenic pulmonary edema resulting from an unexplained respiratory illness. In addition, laboratory evidence consists of (a) a positive serology (i.e., presence of Hantavirus-specific immunoglobulin M or rising titers of immunoglobulin G), or (b) positive immunohistochemistry for Hantavirus antigen in a tissue specimen, or (c) positive PCR for Hantavirus RNA in a tissue specimen.[128]

Hantavirus infection can cause three different clinical diseases: hemorrhagic fever with renal syndrome, nephropathia epidemica, and Hantavirus pulmonary syndrome (HPS). Hemorrhagic fever with renal syndrome and nephropathia epidemica occur in Asian and European continents. HPS occurs only in the Western Hemisphere, including North America.[129] As of March 2007, there have been 465 cases of HPS in the United States, with 35% of the cases resulting in death.[130] Most have occurred in the southwestern United States during spring and summer.

Clinical Presentation

33. K.C., a previously healthy 55-year-old woman, presented with an abrupt onset of fever, cough, myalgia, and shortness of breath. K.C. lives in western Texas and has not traveled out of state during the past 6 months. Diagnostic evaluation, including a complete blood count with differential and blood and sputum cultures, was negative. On day 3, K.C. remained febrile and had vomiting, hypotension, hypoxemia, and bilateral diffuse infiltrates on the chest radiograph.

Abnormal laboratory findings included a leukocyte count of 22,000/mm^3 with a shift to the left, platelets 70,000/mm^3, and albumin concentration of 2 g/dL. K.C. suddenly developed ARDS. The Hantavirus immunoglobulin M ELISA titer performed from K.C.'s serum specimen at the CDC was elevated. What signs and symptoms are consistent with Hantavirus infection?

The clinical features of patients with HPS include fever, myalgia, headache, and cough. Abdominal pain, nausea, and/or vomiting may also be present. The physical examination has been unreliable. Laboratory abnormalities may include leukocytosis, thrombocytopenia, and hypoalbuminemia. The chest radiograph may initially be normal but can progress rapidly to bilateral infiltrates and ARDS. Other viral pneumonias do not typically progress to ARDS as rapidly as Hantavirus infections. Because of the nonspecific signs and symptoms, some patients may be misdiagnosed as having influenza.

Treatment

34. How should K.C. be treated?

Supportive treatment is important. Oxygen therapy and mechanical ventilation may be necessary. Hypotension can be treated with vasopressor agents and judicious use of IV crystalloids to prevent worsening of pulmonary edema. Universal precautions and respiratory isolation should be instituted.[129]

There is no FDA-approved drug to treat Hantavirus infections. Based on one study in 242 patients, IV ribavirin was more effective than placebo in reducing the mortality and the morbidity (oliguria and hemorrhage) in patients in China. IV ribavirin was given as a loading dose of 33 mg/kg, followed by 16 mg/kg Q 6 hr for 4 days and 8 mg/kg Q 8 hr for the next 3 days. Each dose was infused over 30 minutes. Reversible anemia was the main adverse effect of ribavirin.[131]

Two other clinical trials, however, did not show similar clinical efficacy in the treatment of HPS. One open-label trial conducted by the CDC showed a mortality rate of 47% in patients who received ribavirin compared with 50% to those who did not. Therefore, the trial was inconclusive.[132] In addition, a double-blind, placebo-controlled trial conducted at the National Institutes of Health enrolled 36 patients randomized to either IV ribavirin or placebo.[133] Although the trial was discontinued early and lacked the power to detect statistical differences, ribavirin did not demonstrate trends toward improved clinical outcomes. At this time, the use of ribavirin is controversial and is not recommended.

K.C. should receive supportive treatment, including vasopressors, fluids, oxygen, and mechanical ventilation, if necessary.

WEST NILE VIRUS

West Nile virus (WNV) was first identified in the United States in 1999 in New York City. Since then, the virus has had rapid geographic expansion and has infected individuals in most states in the continental United States.[134] Although WNV normally occurs in tropical climates, the increase in international travel and changes in weather patterns have led to its spread.

WNV is a member of the Flaviviridae family. Culicine mosquitoes (including *Culex pipiens, Culex restuans,* and *Culex quinquefasciatus)* are the vectors, and they infect both birds and humans. Infection with the virus involves direct inoculation by the infecting mosquito. WNV can infect a number of vertebrates, including horses. Transmission requires a mosquito bite, and transmission from person to person or bird to bird is not known to occur. Birds are reservoir hosts. Because of the seasonal variations in the life cycle of the mosquito, cases are most commonly seen during the summer and early fall.

Diagnosis is usually made by high clinical suspicion and laboratory tests. WNV can cause a wide range of illness, from an asymptomatic disease to West Nile fever to encephalitis. Mortality is low except in those with encephalitis. Mortality rates in the elderly, particularly those older than 70 years, can be nine times higher than in the general population.[135] The CDC classification of WNV encephalitis consists of (a) febrile illness with neurologic symptoms plus isolation of the WNV antigen or genomic sequence from a tissue, blood, CSF, or other body fluids; (b) WNV IgM antibody in a CSF sample; (c) a fourfold rise in the antibody titer to WNV; and (d) demonstration of an IgM or rising titers of IgG to WNV in a single serum sample.[136]

Clinical Presentation

35. A.G. is an 84-year-old woman. She is very active and runs the yearly flower festival in the community. She was brought to the ED by her granddaughter, who found her at home, confused and complaining of a headache, fatigue, and increasing muscle weakness. She is found to have a temperature of 103°F. Her Mini-Mental Status Exam score was 21 of 30. She has decreasing muscle strength and an erythematous, macular, papular rash on her arms and legs. The complete blood count and electrolytes were normal, with the exception of slightly decreased sodium. The CSF had increased WBCs, increased protein and normal glucose, and positive IgM antibody to WNV. A CT scan showed no abnormalities. What signs and symptoms are indicative of WNV encephalitis?

Acute signs and symptoms of WNV include sudden onset of fever, anorexia, weakness, nausea, vomiting, eye pain, headache, altered mental status, and stiff neck. A rash may be present on the arms, legs, neck, and trunk. The rash is typically erythematous, macular, and papular with or without morbilliform eruption. Laboratory parameters may show normal or elevated WBC counts. Low serum sodium concentrations may be seen in patients with encephalitis. CSF usually shows pleocytosis, mostly with an elevation of lymphocytes, elevated protein levels, and normal glucose levels. Magnetic resonance imaging (MRI) shows some enhancement of the leptomeninges or the periventricular areas in approximately one-third of patients, but no other abnormalities or evidence of acute disease are present on either CT or MRI examination.

With disease progression, further muscle weakness and hyporeflexia may be seen. Patients may progress to a diffuse, flaccid paralysis similar to Guillain-Barré syndrome. Ataxia, extrapyramidal symptoms, cranial nerve abnormalities, myelitis, optic neuritis, and seizures may be seen.

Treatment

36. What treatment options are available to A.G.?

Currently, treatment of WNV infection is supportive. Patients with febrile infection usually have a self-limiting course. In severe cases, patients with muscle weakness and signs of encephalitis will require admission to an intensive care unit, and many will need mechanical ventilation. The available antiviral medications do not have any activity against WNV in vivo, although ribavirin inhibits replication in vitro.[137] Combination therapy of high-dose ribavirin and interferon-α-2b has been used in patients with severe disease with limited success. Although optimal doses have not been established, the doses needed to inhibit the virus were 2 million units of interferon and 2,400 mg of ribavirin daily.[138] Clinical trials are ongoing to establish the safety and efficacy of intravenous immune globulin, and α-interferon. In addition, a new agent, AVI-4020, is undergoing preclinical trials to determine the pharmacokinetic and safety profile.

SEVERE ACUTE RESPIRATORY DISTRESS SYNDROME

Severe acute respiratory distress syndrome (SARS), a highly infectious disease, was first identified in China in early 2003. Since then, the viral syndrome has been reported in several countries in East Asia, North America (particularly Canada), South America, and Europe. As of April 2004, approximately 8,000 cases have been reported, with a case fatality rate of about 10%.[139,140] Many of the cases reported in Asia and Canada have been traced to a single index case, with outbreaks clustered in apartments, hotels, health care facilities, or biomedical facilities. There is some evidence to suggest that increased age (older than 60 years) may be associated with an increased mortality risk.[141]

The disease is easily spread by airborne microdroplets. Geography and a history of recent travel to affected areas are believed to be important to an individual's likelihood of contracting the disease. In a sample of 100 suspected patients in the United States, 94% traveled within the 10 days before illness onset to an area listed in SARS case definitions.[142] SARS is believed to be transmitted mostly by close contact with an infected person (e.g., sharing eating utensils, <3-feet conversations).

A novel coronavirus, SARS coronavirus (SARS-CoV), was isolated from patients and identified as the causative agent of SARS. Inoculations of a Vero E6 cell line with throat swab specimens from patients with the diagnosis of SARS showed cytopathologic features.[143] Although the natural reservoir of SARS-CoV has not been identified, the virus has been detected in the Himalayan masked palm civet, the Chinese ferret badger, and the raccoon dog.

Clinical Presentation

37. N.Z. is a 48-year-old Asian female who returned 3 days ago from a business trip to Taiwan. Two days after her return, she complained of fatigue, myalgia, chills, and headache. On the third day, she awoke feeling feverish and diaphoretic. Her temperature was 101°F. She complained of a sore throat with cough and shortness of breath when she climbed stairs. She visited her local physician, who noted rales during chest auscultation. As there was concern for SARS, the patient was admitted and placed under quarantine in a local hospital. A chest radiograph revealed bilateral interstitial infiltrates. A routine pneumonia workup was performed with pulse oximetry, blood cultures, and sputum Gram stain and culture. Blood was also collected for antibody analysis. Complete blood count and clinical chemistries were obtained, and the tests were remarkable only for lymphopenia. What signs and symptoms in N.Z. suggest that this is a case of SARS?

The case definition established by the CDC includes clinical, epidemiologic, laboratory, and exclusion criteria.[144] Symptoms of early disease include fever, chills, rigor, myalgia, headache, diarrhea, sore throat, or rhinorrhea. Mild-to-moderate illness includes temperature higher than 100.4°F and clinical findings of lower respiratory illness such as cough or shortness of breath. Severe illness includes the previous criteria plus radiographic evidence of pneumonia or acute respiratory distress syndrome. N.Z. presents to her physician with severe respiratory illness.

Probable or likely exposure to SARS-CoV is a critical component of the SARS case definition. Travel to a location with documented or suspected recent transmission of SARS-CoV or close contact with a person with mild-to-moderate or severe respiratory illness in the 10 days prior to the onset of symptoms are defined as possible exposures to SARS-CoV. Likely exposure is defined as close contact with a person with confirmed disease or symptoms of disease. In N.Z.'s case, travel to Taiwan classifies her as having possible exposure.

For patients suspected of having SARS in the United States, laboratory diagnosis can be confirmed by an enzyme immunoassay detecting serum antibody to SARS-CoV, isolation of SARS-CoV from a clinical specimen, or detection of SARS-CoV RNA by a reverse transcriptase PCR. Both the enzyme immunoassay and the PCR are validated by the CDC. Information regarding the most recent criteria for laboratory diagnosis can be found at the CDC website.

Although the majority of cases of infection are self-limited, initial symptoms may be followed by hypoxemia, which may progress to the need for intubation and mechanical ventilation. Typically, patients do not manifest neurologic or GI symptoms.

Treatment

38. What treatment options are available to N.Z.?

Treatment for SARS during the 2002–2003 outbreak included broad spectrum antibiotics, ribavirin, lopinavir/ritonavir, corticosteroids, interferon, and immunoglobulin.[145] Broad spectrum antibiotics are recommended to cover other potential pathogens until SARS-CoV is isolated. Ribavirin has been used in doses ranging from 400 mg IV every day to 2 g IV followed by 1g IV Q 6 hr.[146] Treatment ranged from 4 to

14 days. Efficacy of ribavirin in the treatment of SARS is unknown due to the self-limiting nature of the disease and the coadministration of other agents. Studies have determined, however, that ribavirin does not inhibit SARS-CoV in vitro, and viral loads remained elevated postmortem despite therapy with ribavirin.[147,148] A high percentage of persons developed adverse drug reactions, including hemolytic anemia (61%), hypocalcemia (58%), and hypomagnesemia (46%). Two of three in vitro studies of lopinavir and ritonavir showed activity against SARS-CoV. Lopinavir 400 mg PO BID with ritonavir 100 mg BID may be effective in reducing mortality in patients with SARS, but data are limited.[145] Treatments with various corticosteroids, interferon, and immunoglobulin remain controversial. No treatment guidelines are available due to the lack of prospective randomized controlled trials.

THE COMMON COLD

The most prevalent viral infection is the common cold. In the United States, approximately 62 million cases of the common cold occur annually.[149] An estimated 20 million and 22 million days of absence from work and school, respectively, occur. The frequency of the occurrence of a cold is greater in younger children and decreases with increasing age. Although the common cold is self-limiting, otitis media occurs in approximately 20% of children following infection.[150]

Many viruses have been isolated from patients with respiratory infections, but rhinovirus is the most common viral pathogen.[151] Rhinovirus accounts for approximately 34% of all respiratory illnesses. More than 100 different serotypes of rhinovirus exist, and the prevalence of each varies with time and geography. Other pathogens include coronavirus, parainfluenza, RSV, adenovirus, and enterovirus. Because of the number of pathogens known to cause the common cold, development of an effective vaccine remains difficult.

Treatment for the common cold is directed at pharmacologic treatment of symptoms. Nonsteroidal anti-inflammatory drugs, oral or intranasal decongestants, antihistamines, and antitussives may be used. However, these products provide minimal relief of symptoms[152] and do not shorten the natural course of infection.[153] In pediatric patients younger than 2 years, the use of cough and cold medications is not recommended by the FDA due to the deaths associated with their use.[154,155] Currently, there are no specific antiviral treatments for the common cold.

Prevention

39. J.C. comes into the pharmacy asking for an herbal product that will help him prevent colds this upcoming cold season. He states that last year he had three colds and his neighbor had none. His neighbor had mentioned an herbal product he had been taking. J.C. cannot remember the name of the product but wonders if there are any products that may be helpful.

Zinc

Zinc, a dietary supplement, has been studied in both the prevention and treatment of the common cold. The proposed mechanism of action is that the rhinovirus 3C protease is inhibited by zinc, and the inhibition of this enzyme prevents viral replication. In vitro, zinc has been shown to have antiviral activity. Several trials conducted in the past several decades have produced conflicting results on the benefits of zinc in decreasing symptom severity or duration. A meta-analysis found no clear evidence to support the use of zinc lozenges in the treatment or prevention of the common cold.[156] Patients who took zinc lozenges for the common cold complained of mouth irritation, unpleasant taste, feeling sick, and diarrhea. Zinc is not currently recommended for treatment or prophylaxis of the common cold.

Echinacea

Echinacea is an herbal product extracted from the *Echinacea* plant, which belongs to the *Compositae* family. Echinacea is believed to stimulate the immune system, specifically phagocytosis. Some clinical trials using echinacea have shown positive results in decreasing the incidence of infection when compared to placebo, but the results remain inconclusive. No benefits were shown in decreasing the severity and duration of the common cold when compared to placebo. In trials evaluating the effectiveness of echinacea in the treatment of the common cold, 9 of 16 trials found a decrease in the severity and duration of symptoms.[157] A recent study showed no benefit of echinacea over placebo but did show an increased incidence of rash in the treatment group.[158] Because the current data are inconclusive and due to the variability of echinacea concentrations in the available products, use of echinacea in the prevention and treatment of the common cold is not recommended.

REFERENCES

1. Hing E, Cherry DK, Woodwell DA. National ambulatory medical care survey: 2004 summary Adv. *Data* 2006;23:1.
2. Murray CJ et al. Estimation of potential global pandemic influenza mortality on the basis of vital registry data from the 1918–1920 pandemic: a quantitative analysis. *Lancet* 2006;368:2211.
3. Whitley RJ et al. Herpes simplex virus. *Clin Infect Dis* 1998;26:541.
4. Aurelius E et al. Rapid diagnosis of herpes simplex encephalitis by nested polymerase chain reaction assay of cerebrospinal fluid. *Lancet* 1991;337:189.
5. Whitley RJ. Herpes simplex encephalitis; adolescents and adults. *Antiviral Res* 2006;71:141.
6. Skoldenberg B et al. Acyclovir versus vidarabine in herpes simplex encephalitis. *Lancet* 1984;2:707.
7. Whitley RJ et al. Vidarabine versus acyclovir therapy in herpes simplex encephalitis. *N Engl J Med* 1986;314:144.
8. Bedford Laboratories. Acyclovir for Injection USP. Product Information. Ben Venue Laboratories, Inc.; 2005.
9. Naik HR et al. Foscarnet therapy for acyclovir-resistant herpes simplex virus 1 infection in allogeneic bone marrow transplant recipients. *Clin Infect Dis* 1995;21:1514.
10. Safrin S et al. A controlled trial comparing foscarnet with vidarabine for acyclovir-resistant mucocutaneous herpes simplex in the acquired immunodeficiency syndrome. *N Engl J Med* 1991;325:551.
11. Kamei S et al. Evaluation of combination therapy using acyclovir and corticosteroid in adult patients with herpes simplex virus encephalitis. *J Neurol Neurosurg Psychiatry* 2005;76:1544.
12. Oppenshaw H, Cantin EM. Corticosteroids in herpes simplex virus encephalitis. *J Neurol Neurosurg Psychiatry* 2005;76:1469.
13. Whitley RJ et al. Pharmacokinetics of acyclovir in humans following intravenous administration. *Am J Med* 1982;73:165.
14. de Miranda P et al. Acyclovir kinetics after intravenous infusion. *Clin Pharmacol Ther* 1979;26:718.
15. Laskin OL et al. Pharmacokinetics and tolerance of acyclovir, a new antiherpes virus agent, in humans. *Antimicrob Agents Chemother* 1982;21:393.
16. Blum MR et al. Overview of acyclovir pharmacokinetic disposition in adults and children. *Am J Med* 1982;73:186.
17. Yeager AS. Use of acyclovir in premature and term neonates. *Am J Med* 1982;73:205.
18. Hintz M et al. Neonatal acyclovir pharmacokinetics in patients with herpes virus infection. *Am J Med* 1982;73:210.

19. Pavia I et al. Flow cytometric analysis of herpes simplex virus type 1 susceptibility of acyclovir, ganciclovir, and foscarnet. *Antimicrob Agents Chemother* 1997;41:2686.
20. Swierkosz EM, Biron KK. Antimicrobial agents and susceptibility testing. In: Murray PR et al, eds. *Manual of Clinical Microbiology*. 6th ed. Washington, DC: ASM Press; 1995:1417.
21. GlaxoSmithKline. *Zovirax (acyclovir). Product Information*. Research Triangle Park, NC; 2005.
22. Wagstaff AJ et al. Acyclovir: a reappraisal of its antiviral activity, pharmacokinetic properties and therapeutic efficacy. *Drugs* 1994;47:153.
23. GlaxoSmithKline Inc. *Valtrex. Product information*. Research Triangle Park, NC; July 2006.
24. Whitley RJ, Kimberlin DW. Herpes simplex: encephalitis children and adolescents. *Semin Pediatr Infect Dis* 2005;16:17.
25. Kimberlin DW. Herpes simplex virus infection in neonates and early childhood. *Semin Pediatr Infect Dis* 2005;16:271.
26. Kohl S. The diagnosis and treatment of neonatal herpes simplex virus infection. *Pediatr Ann* 2002;31:726.
27. American College of Obstetrics and Gynecology (ACOG). ACOG practice bulletin. Management of herpes in pregnancy: clinical management guidelines for obstetricians-gynecologists. *Int J Gynaecol Obstet* 2000;68:165.
28. Whitley R et al. A controlled trial comparing vidarabine with acyclovir in neonatal herpes simplex virus infection. *N Engl J Med* 1991;324:444.
29. Kimberlin DW. Neonatal herpes simplex infection. *Clin Microb Rev* 2004;17:1.
30. Kimberlin DW, Whitley RJ. Neonatal herpes: what have we learned. *Semin Pediatr Infect Dis* 2005;16:7.
31. Kimberlin DW et al. Administration of oral acyclovir suppressive therapy after neonatal herpes simplex virus disease limited to the skin, eyes, and mouth: results of a phase I/II trial. *Pediatr Infect Dis J* 1996;15:247.
32. Gutierrez K, Arvin AM. Long term antiviral suppression after treatment for neonatal herpes infection. *Pediatr Infect Dis J* 2003;22:371.
33. Ljungman P. Prophylaxis against herpesvirus infection in transplant rejection. *Drugs* 2001;61:181.
34. Slifkin M et al. Viral prophylaxis in organ transplant patients. *Drugs* 2004;64:2763–92.
35. Schacker T et al. Famciclovir for the suppression of symptomatic and asymptomatic herpes simplex virus reactivation in HIV-infected persons. *Ann Intern Med* 1998;128:21.
36. Shepp DH et al. Oral acyclovir therapy for mucocutaneous herpes simplex virus infections in immunocompromised marrow transplant patients. *Ann Intern Med* 1985;102:783.
37. Hoglund M et al. Comparable acyclovir exposures produced by oral valacyclovir and intravenous acyclovir in immunocompromised cancer patients. *J Antimicrob Chemother* 2001;47:855.
38. Spruance SL et al. Acyclovir cream for treatment of herpes simplex labialis: results of two randomized, double-blind, vehicle-controlled, multicenter clinical trials. *Antimicrob Agents Chemother* 2002;46:2238.
39. Raborn GW et al. Effective treatment of herpes simplex labialis with penciclovir cream: combined results of two trials. *J Am Dent Assoc* 2002;133:303.
40. Sacks SL et al. Clinical efficacy of topical docosanol 10% cream for herpes simplex labialis: a multicenter, randomized, placebo-controlled trial. *J Am Acad Dermatol* 2001;45:222.
41. Lin L et al. Topical application of penciclovir cream for the treatment of herpes simplex facialis/labialis: a randomized, double-blind, multicentre, acyclovir-controlled trial. *J Dermatol Treat* 2002;13:67.
42. Femiano F et al. Recurrent herpes labialis: efficacy of topical therapy with penciclovir compared with acyclovir (acyclovir). *Oral Dis* 2001;7:31.
43. Spruance SL et al. Penciclovir cream for the treatment of herpes simplex labialis. *JAMA* 1997;277:1374.
44. Raborn GW et al. Penciclovir cream for recurrent herpes simplex labialis: an effective new treatment. *Antimicrob Agents Chemother* 1996;36:178.
45. Spruance SL et al. Treatment of recurrent herpes simplex labialis with oral acyclovir. *J Infect Dis* 1990;161:185.
46. Spruance SL et al. Clinical significance of antiviral therapy for episodic treatment of herpes labialis: exploratory analyses of the combined data from two valacyclovir trials. *J Antimicrob Chemother* 2004;53:703.
47. Spruance SL et al. Single-dose, patient-initiated famciclovir: a randomized, double-blind, placebo-controlled trial for episodic treatment of herpes labialis. *J Am Acad Dermatol* 2006;55:47.
48. Jensen LLA et al. Oral antivirals for the acute treatment of recurrent herpes labialis. *Ann Pharmacother* 2004;38:705.
49. Novartis Pharmaceutical Corp. *Famvir. Product information*. East Hanover, NJ; 2006.
50. Rooney JF et al. Oral acyclovir to suppress frequently recurrent herpes labialis: a double-blind, placebo-controlled trial. *Ann Intern Med* 1993;118:268.
51. Baker D, Eisen D. Valacyclovir for prevention of recurrent herpes labialis: 2 double-blind, placebo-controlled studies. *Cutis* 2003;71:239.
52. Rabella N et al. Antiviral susceptibility of herpes simplex viruses and its clinical correlates: a single center's experience. *Clin Infect Dis* 2002;34:1055.
53. Morfin F et al. Herpes simplex virus resistance to antiviral drugs. *J Clin Virol* 2003;26:29.
54. Safrin S et al. A controlled trial comparing foscarnet with vidarabine for acyclovir-resistant mucocutaneous herpes simplex in the acquired immunodeficiency syndrome. *N Engl J Med* 1991;325:551.
55. Bryant P et al. Successful treatment of foscarnet-resistant herpes simplex stomatitis with intravenous cidofovir in a child. *Pediatr Infect Dis J* 2001;20:1083.
56. Chen Y et al. Resistant herpes simplex virus type 1 infection: an emerging concern after allogenic stem cell transplantation. *Clin Infect Dis* 2000;31:927.
57. Brummitt CF. Imiquimod 5% cream for the treatment of recurrent, acyclovir-resistant genital herpes. *Clin Infect Dis* 2006;42:575.
58. Seward JF et al. Varicella disease after introduction of varicella vaccine in the United States, 1995–2000. *JAMA* 2002;287:606.
59. Carcao MD et al. Sequential use of intravenous and oral acyclovir therapy of varicella in immunocompromised children. *Pediatr Infect Dis J* 1998;17:626.
60. Masaoka T et al. Varicella-zoster virus infection in immunocompromised patients. *J Med Virol* 1993;(Suppl 1):82.
61. Klassen TP et al. Acyclovir for treating otherwise healthy children and adolescents. *Cochrane Database Syst Rev* 2003;(1).
62. Feder HM Jr. Treatment of adult chickenpox with oral acyclovir. *Arch Intern Med* 1990;150:2061.
63. Whitley RJ. Therapeutic approaches to varicella-zoster virus infections. *J Infect Dis* 1992;166(Suppl 1):S51.
64. Wallace MR et al. Treatment of adult varicella with oral acyclovir: a randomized placebo-controlled trial. *Ann Intern Med* 1992;117:358.
65. Committee on Infectious Diseases. The use of acyclovir in otherwise healthy children with varicella. *Pediatrics* 1993;91:674.
66. Jackson JL et al. The effect of treating herpes zoster with oral acyclovir in preventing postherpetic neuralgia: a meta-analysis. *Arch Intern Med* 1997;157:909.
67. deGreef H. Famciclovir, a new oral antiherpes drug; results of the first controlled clinical study demonstrating its efficacy and safety in the treatment of uncomplicated herpes zoster in immunocompetent patients. *Int J Antimicrob Agents* 1995;4:241.
68. Tyring S et al. Famciclovir for the treatment of acute herpes zoster: effects on acute disease and postherpetic neuralgia: a randomized, double-blind placebo-controlled trial. *Ann Intern Med* 1995;123:89.
69. Beutner KR, et al. Valacyclovir compared with acyclovir for improved therapy for herpes zoster in immunocompetent adults. *Antimicrob Agents Chemother* 1995;39:1546.
70. Tyring SK et al. Antiviral therapy for herpes zoster: randomized, controlled trial of valacyclovir and famciclovir therapy in immunocompetent patients 50 years and older. *Arch Fam Med* 2000;9:863.
71. Ernst ME et al. Oral corticosteroids for herpes zoster pain. *Ann Pharmacother* 1998;32:1099.
72. Santee JA. Corticosteroids for herpes zoster: what do they accomplish? *Am J Clin Dermatol* 2002;3:517.
73. Woods MJ et al. A randomized trial of acyclovir for seven days or twenty one days with and without prednisolone for treatment of acute herpes zoster. *N Engl J Med* 1994;330:896.
74. Whitley RJ et al. Acyclovir with and without prednisone for the treatment of herpes zoster. *Ann Intern Med* 1996;125:376.
75. Whitley RJ et al. Acyclovir plus steroids for herpes zoster [letter]. *Ann Intern Med* 1997;126:832.
76. Watson CP et al. A randomized vehicle-controlled trial of topical capsaicin in the treatment of postherpetic neuralgia. *Clin Ther* 1993;15:510.
77. Endo Pharmaceuticals, Inc. *Lidoderm. Product information*. Chadds Ford, PA; 2006.
78. Pfizer, Inc. *Lyrica. Product information*. New York; 2006.
79. Volpi A et al. Current management of herpes zoster. *Am J Clin Dermatol* 2005;6:317.
80. Balfour HH Jr et al. Acyclovir halts progression of herpes zoster in immunocompromised patients. *N Engl J Med* 1983;308:1448.
81. Dworkin RH et al. Recommendations for the management of herpes zoster. *CID* 2007;44:S1.
82. Prevention and control of influenza: recommendations of the Advisory Committee on Immunization Practices (ACIP). *MMWR Morb Mortal Wkly Rep* 2006;55(No. RR-10):1.
83. Margolis KL et al. Frequency of adverse reactions after influenza vaccination. *Am J Med* 1990;88:27.
84. Nichol KL et al. Side effects associated with influenza vaccination in healthy working adults. *Arch Intern Med* 1996;156:1546.
85. Berardi RR et al, eds. *Handbook of Nonprescription Drugs*, 15th ed. Washington, DC: American Pharmaceutical Association; 2006.
86. GlaxoSmithKline. *Zanamivir. Product information*. Research Triangle Park, NC; 2006.
87. Roche Laboratories. *Oseltamivir. Product information*. Nutley, NJ; 2006.
88. Food and Drug Administration, Pediatric Advisory Committee. Dear Healthcare Professional Letter. November 13, 2006. Available at: www.fda.gov/medwatch/safety/2006/Tamiflu_dhcp_letter.pdf. Accessed July 27, 2007.
89. Endo Pharmaceuticals, Inc. *Symmetrel. Product information*. Wilmington, DE, 2003.
90. Forest Pharmaceuticals, Inc. *Flumadine. Product information*. St. Louis, MO; 2006.
91. Hayden FG et al. Use of oral neuraminidase inhibitor oseltamivir in experimental influenza: randomized controlled trials for prevention and treatment. *JAMA* 1999;282:1240.
92. Management of Influenza on the Southern Hemisphere trial (MIST) Study Group. Randomized trial of efficacy and safety of inhaled zanamivir in treatment of influenza A and B virus infections. *Lancet* 1998;352:1877.
93. Jefferson T et al. Neuraminidase inhibitors for preventing and treating influenza in healthy adults. *Cochrane Database Syst Rev* 2003:1.
94. Allison MA et al. Influenza vaccine effectiveness in health 6- to 21-month-old children during the 2003–2004 season. *J Pediatr* 2006;149:755.
95. MedImmune Vaccines, Inc. *FluMist. Product information*. Gaithersburg, MD; 2006.
96. Hayden FG et al. Use of selective oral neuraminidase inhibitor oseltamivir to prevent influenza. *N Engl J Med* 1999;341:1336.

97. Hayden FG et al. Inhaled zanamivir for the prevention of influenza in families. *N Engl J Med* 2000;18:1282.
98. Monto AS et al. Zanamivir in the prevention of influenza in healthy adults: a randomized controlled trial. *JAMA* 1999:282:31.
99. U.S. Department of Agriculture. Avian influenza: low pathogenic H5N1 vs. highly pathogenic H5N1 latest update. September 28, 2006. Available at: http://www.usda.gov/wps/portal/!ut/p/_s.7_Ø_A/7_Ø_10B/.cmd/ad/.ar/sa.retrievecontent/.c/6_2_1UH/.ce/7_2_5JM/.p/5_2_4TQ/_th/J_2_90/_s.7_Ø_A/7_Ø_10B?PC_7_2_5JM_contentid-2006%2FØ8%2FØ296.xml&PC_7_2_5JM_parentnav-LATEST_RELEASES&PC_7_2_5JM_navid-NEWS_RELEASE . Accessed October 11, 2007.
100. Centers for Disease Control and Prevention. Outbreak of avian influenza A (H5N1) in Asia and interim recommendations for evaluation and reporting of suspected cases—United States, 2004. *MMWR Morb Mortal Wkly Rep* 2004;53:97.
101. Sanofi Pasteur, Inc. *Influenza virus vaccine, H5N1. Product information*. Swiftwater, PA; April 2007.
102. Lugo RA, Nahata MC. Pathogenesis and treatment of bronchiolitis. *Clin Pharm* 1993;12:95.
103. Shay DK et al. Bronchiolitis-associated mortality and estimates of respiratory syncytial virus-associated deaths among U.S. children 1979–1997. *J Infect Dis* 2001;183:16.
104. Kotaniemi-Syrjanen A et al. Rhinovirus-induced wheezing in infancy-the first sign of childhood asthma? *J Allergy Clin Immunol* 2003;111:66.
105. Stein RT et al. Respiratory syncytial virus in early life and risk of wheeze and allergy by age 13 years. *Lancet* 1999;354:541.
106. Openshaw PH et al. Links between respiratory syncytial virus bronchiolitis and childhood asthma: clinical and research approaches. *Pediatr Infect Dis J* 2003;22:S58.
107. Panitch HB. Respiratory syncytial virus bronchiolitis: supportive care and therapies designed to overcome airway obstruction. *Pediatr Infect Dis J* 2003;22:S83.
108. Kellner JD et al. Bronchodilators for bronchiolitis. *Cochrane Database Syst Rev* 2000;(2):CD001266.
109. American Academy of Pediatrics, Subcommittee on Diagnosis and Management of Bronchiolitis. Diagnosis and management of bronchiolitis. *Pediatrics* 2006;118:1174.
110. Patel H et al. Glucocorticoids for infant viral bronchiolitis in infants and young children. *Cochrane Database Syst Rev* 2004;(3):CD004878.
111. Garrison MM et al. Systemic corticosteroids in infant bronchiolitis: a meta-analysis. *Pediatrics* 2000;105:E44.
112. American Academy of Pediatrics, Committee on Infectious Diseases. Use of ribavirin in the treatment of respiratory syncytial virus infection. *Pediatrics* 1993;92:501.
113. Wheeler JG et al. Historical cohort evaluation of ribavirin efficacy in respiratory syncytial virus infection. *Pediatr Infect Dis J* 1993;12:209.
114. Englund JA et al. High-dose, short-duration ribavirin aerosol therapy compared with standard ribavirin therapy in children with suspected respiratory syncytial virus infection. *J Pediatr* 1994;125:635.
115. Ventre K et al. Ribavirin for respiratory syncytial virus infection of the lower respiratory tract in infants and young children. *Cochrane Database Syst Rev* 2007;(1):CD000181.
116. Fuller H et al. Immunoglobulin treatment for respiratory syncytial virus infection. *Cochrane Database Syst Rev* 2006;(4):CD004883.
117. ICN Pharmaceuticals. *Product information. Virazole (ribavirin for inhalation solution)*. Costa Mesa, CA; May 1996.
118. Smith DW et al. A controlled trial of aerosolized ribavirin in infants receiving mechanical ventilation for severe respiratory syncytial virus infection. *N Engl J Med* 1991;325:24.
119. Meert KL et al. Aerosolized ribavirin in mechanically ventilated children with respiratory syncytial virus lower respiratory tract disease: a prospective, double-blind, randomized trial. *Crit Care Med* 1994;22:566.
120. Janai HK et al. Ribavirin: adverse drug reactions, 1986 to 1988. *Pediatr Infect Dis J* 1990;9:209.
121. Edell D et al. Early ribavirin treatment of bronchiolitis: effect on long-term respiratory morbidity. *Chest* 2002;122:935.
122. Krilov LR. Safety issues related to the administration of ribavirin. *Pediatr Infect Dis J* 2002;21:479.
123. Groothius JR et al. Prophylactic administration of respiratory syncytial virus immune globulin to high-risk infants and young children. *N Engl J Med* 1993;329:1524.
124. PREVENT Study Group. Reduction of RSV hospitalization among premature infants and children with bronchopulmonary dysplasia using respiratory syncytial virus immune globulin prophylaxis. *Pediatrics* 1997;99:93.
125. The IMpact-RSV Study Group. Palivizumab, a humanized respiratory syncytial virus monoclonal antibody, reduces hospitalizations from respiratory syncytial virus infection in high-risk infants. *Pediatrics* 1998;102:531.
126. Committee on Infectious Diseases. Prevention of respiratory syncytial virus infections: indications for the use of palivizumab and update on the use of RSV-IVIG. *Pediatrics* 1998;102:1211.
127. Khan AS et al. Hantavirus pulmonary syndrome: the first 100 cases. *J Infect Dis* 1996;173:1297.
128. Centers for Disease Control and Prevention. Case definitions for infectious conditions under public health surveillance. *MMWR Morb Mortal Wkly Rep* 1997;46:1.
129. Mertz GJ et al. Hantavirus infection. *Disease-a-Month* 1998;44:89.
130. Center for Disease Control and Prevention. All about Hantavirus. Availabel at: http://www.cdc.gov/ncidod/diseases/hanta/hps/noframes/caseinfo.htm. Accessed September 25, 2007.
131. Huggins JW et al. Prospective, double-blind, concurrent, placebo-controlled clinical trial of intravenous ribavirin therapy of hemorrhagic fever with renal syndrome. *J Infect Dis* 1991;164:119.
132. Mertz GJ et al. Hantavirus infections in the United States: diagnosis and treatment. *Adv Exp Med Biol* 1996;394:153.
133. Mertz GJ et al. Placebo-controlled, double-blind trial of intravenous ribavirin for the treatment of Hantavirus cardiopulmonary syndrome in North America. *Clin Infect Dis* 2004;39:1307.
134. Centers for Disease Control and Prevention. 2007 West Nile Virus Activity in the United States. Available at: http://www.cdc.gov/ncidod/dvbid/westnile/Mapsactivity/surv&control07Maps.htm. Accessed on September 25, 2007.
135. Nash D et al. The outbreak of West Nile Virus infection in the New York City area in 1999. *N Engl J Med* 2001;344:1807.
136. Centers for Disease Control and Prevention. Epidemic/epizootic West Nile virus in the United States: revised guidelines for surveillance, prevention, and control. April 2001.
137. Petersen LR et al. West Nile virus: a primer for the clinician. *Ann Intern Med* 2002;137:173.
138. Anderson JF, Rahal JJ. Efficacy of interferon alpha-2b and ribavirin against West Nile Virus in vitro. *Emerg Infect Dis* 2002;8:107.
139. Centers for Disease Control and Prevention. Current SARS situation. Available at: www.cdc.gov/ncidod/sars/situation.htm. Accessed July 27, 2007.
140. World Health Organization. Summary of probable SARS cases with onset of illness from 1 November 2002 to 31 July 2003. September 26, 2003. Available at: www.who.int/csr/sars/country/table2003_09_23/en/. Accessed July 27, 2007.
141. Donnelly C et al. Epidemiological determinants of spread of causal agent of severe acute respiratory syndrome in Hong Kong. *Lancet* 2003;361:1761.
142. Centers for Disease Control and Prevention. Update: outbreak of severe acute respiratory syndrome, worldwide, 2003. *MMWR Morb Mortal Wkly Rep* 2003;52:269.
143. Ksiazek TG et al. A novel coronavirus associated with severe acute respiratory syndrome. *N Engl J Med* 2003;348:1953.
144. Centers for Disease Control and Prevention. Revised U.S. surveillance case definition for severe acute respiratory syndrome (SARS) and update on SARS cases—United States and worldwide, December 2003. *MMWR Morb Mortal Wkly Rep* 2003;52:1202.
145. Christian MD et al. Severe acute respiratory syndrome. *Clin Infect Dis* 2004;38:1420.
146. Stockman LJ et al. SARS: systemic review of treatment effects. *PLoS Med* 2006;3:1525.
147. Centers for Disease Control and Prevention. Severe acute respiratory syndrome (SARS) and coronavirus testing—United States 2003. *MMWR Morb Mortal Wkly Rep* 2003;52:297.
148. Mazulli T et al. Severe acute respiratory syndrome-associated coronavirus in lung tissue. *Emerg Infect Dis* 2004;10:20.
149. Centers for Disease Control and Prevention. Vital and health statistics: current estimates from the National Health Interview survey, 1996. October 1999.
150. Heikkinen T et al. The common cold. *Lancet* 2003;361:51.
151. Monto AS. Epidemiology of viral respiratory infections. *Am J Med* 2002;112:4S.
152. Arroll B. Non-antibiotic treatments for upper-respiratory tract infections (common cold). *Resp Med* 2005;99:1477.
153. Eccles R. Efficacy and safety of over-the-counter analgesics in the treatment of common cold and flu. *J Clin Pharm Ther* 2006;31:309.
154. Centers for Disease Control and Prevention. Infant deaths associated with cough and cold medications—two states, 2005. *MMWR Morb Mortal Wkly Rep* 2007:56:1.
155. Wingert WE et al. Possible role of pseudoephedrine and other over-the-counter cold medications in the deaths of very young children. *J Forensic Sci* 2007;52:487.
156. Marshall I. Zinc for the common cold. *Cochrane Database Syst Rev* 2000;(2):CD001364.
157. Linde K et al. Echinacea for preventing and treating the common cold. *Cochrane Database Syst Rev* 2006;(1):CD000530.
158. Taylor JA et al. Efficacy and safety of echinacea in treating upper respiratory tract infections in children: a randomized controlled trial. *JAMA* 2003;290:2824.
159. Filer CW et al. Metabolic and pharmacokinetic studies following oral administration of 14C-famciclovir to healthy subjects. *Xenobiotica* 1994;24:357.
160. He G et al. Clinical pharmacokinetics of the prodrug oseltamivir and its active metabolite Ro 64-0802. *Clin Pharmacokinet* 1999;37:471.
161. Glaxo Wellcome, Inc. *Valacyclovir hydrochloride. Product information*. Research Triangle Park, NC, 1997.
162. Soul-Lawton J et al. Absolute bioavailability and metabolic disposition of valacyclovir, the L-valyl ester of acyclovir, following oral administration to humans. *Antimicrob Agents Chemother* 1995;39:2759.
163. Cass LMR et al. Pharmacokinetics of zanamivir after intravenous, oral, inhaled, or intranasal administration to healthy volunteers. *Clin Pharmacokinet* 1999;36(Suppl 1):1.
164. Dunn CJ, Goa KL. Zanamivir: a review of its use in influenza. *Drugs* 1999;58:761.
165. Pue MA et al. Linear pharmacokinetics of penciclovir following administration of single oral doses of famciclovir 125, 250, 500, and 750 mg to healthy volunteers. *J Antimicrob Chemother* 1994;33:119.
166. Bardsley-Elliot A, Noble S. Oseltamivir. *Drugs* 1999;58:851.
167. Skoldenberg B. Herpes simplex encephalitis. *Scand J Infect Dis Suppl* 1996;100:8.

CHAPTER 73

Viral Hepatitis

Curtis D. Holt

One of thefirst references to epidemic jaundice was ascribed to the philosopher Hippocrates. Over the centuries, several epidemics, usually associated with poor hygiene, were observed, especially during wartime. The possibility of a viral etiology was considered as recently as the turn of the 20th century.

Since the 1970s, five distinctly separate hepatitis viruses have been identified with liver disease as their major clinical manifestation, all of which have been characterized and cloned. A sixth virus also has been identified, but has yet to be implicated in liver disease. Five of these viruses are RNA viruses; and one is a DNA virus. The mode of transmission differs, as do the natural history and outcomes. The individual viral types can be distinguished by serologic assays and, in some instances, by genotyping. Although significant progress in the area of disease prevention has occurred, advances in treatment have been limited because of the large amount of virus produced and its rapid mutation. People with chronic hepatitis C produce approximately 1 trillion virus particles daily, compared with 100 billion particles daily for those infected with chronic hepatitis B and 10 billion particles daily for those with HIV infection. This chapter reviews the virology, epidemiology, pathogenesis, clinical manifestations, diagnosis, natural history, prevention, and treatment strategies for viral hepatitis.

CAUSATIVE AGENTS AND CHARACTERISTICS

Viral hepatitis is a major cause of morbidity and mortality in the United States.[1,2] At least six distinct agents are responsible for viral hepatitis. These hepatotrophic viruses are identified by the letters A through G as follows: (a) type A hepatitis caused by hepatitis A virus (HAV), (b) type B hepatitis caused by hepatitis B virus (HBV), (c) type C hepatitis caused by hepatitis C virus (HCV), (d) delta hepatitis caused by the HBV-associated hepatitis D virus (HDV), (e) type E hepatitis caused by the hepatitis E virus (HEV), and (f) type G hepatitis, caused by the hepatitis G virus (HGV) and the GB agents (Table 73-1). Hepatitis A through E viruses primarily affect the liver and have the potential to cause inflammation and hepatocellular necrosis, whereas the clinical manifestations of HGV are unknown.[3] These viruses differ in their immunologic characteristics and epidemiologic patterns (Table 73-2). Fecal-oral transmission is the primary mode of infection for HAV and HEV, whereas percutaneous transmission is characteristic of HBV, HCV, and HDV.[4–7] HGV also appears to be transmitted percutaneously, primarily through volunteer blood donors.[8,9] Several other viruses primarily affect nonhepatic organ systems and may secondarily induce a hepatitis-like syndrome. These include the Epstein-Barr virus (infectious mononucleosis); cytomegalovirus (CMV); herpes simplex viruses; varicella-zoster virus; and rubella, rubeola, and mumps viruses (Table 73-3).

Definitions of Acute and Chronic Hepatitis

Viral hepatitis can present as either an acute or chronic illness. Acute hepatitis is defined as an illness with a discrete date of onset with jaundice or increased serum aminotransferase concentrations >2.5 times the upper limit of normal.[10] Acute viral hepatitis infection is a systemic process and lasts as long as, but not exceeding, 6 months.

Chronic hepatitis is an inflammatory condition of the liver that involves ongoing hepatocellular necrosis for 6 months or more beyond the onset of acute illness.[11] The causes of chronic hepatitis are shown in Table 73-3. The most common cause of chronic hepatitis is chronic viral hepatitis, caused by HBV or HCV.[12,13] Drug-induced and autoimmune chronic hepatitis occur less frequently, whereas metabolic disorders and HDV chronic hepatitis are relatively rare.[14–16] Neither HAV nor HEV infections cause chronic hepatitis. The long-term effects of HGV continue to be investigated, but the virus does not appear to cause liver (or any other) disease, even in immunocompromised patients.[17]

Serologic Evaluation in Presumed Chronic Hepatitis

Because the clinical manifestations and incubation periods are similar among patients with hepatitis, serologies are useful in diagnosing the type of viral infection that is occurring. Appropriate tests include detecting specific antibodies against hepatitis A virus (anti-HAV), hepatitis B surface antigen (HBsAg) and hepatitis C antibody (anti-HCV). A diagnosis of acute hepatitis A virus infection includes the presence of IgM anti-HAV. If HBsAg is present, further testing for hepatitis B envelope antigen (HBeAg) and HBV-DNA is

Table 73-1 Hepatitis Nomenclature

Hepatitis Type	*Antigen*	*Corresponding Antibody*	*Comments*
A	Hepatitis A virus (HAV)	Hepatitis A antibody (anti-HAV)	RNA virus; present in stool and serum early in course of hepatitis A
B	Hepatitis B surface antigen (HBsAg)	Hepatitis B surface antibody (anti-HBs)	DNA virus; found in serum in >90% of patients with acute hepatitis B, anti-HBs appears following infection and confers immunity
	Hepatitis B core antigen (HBcAg)	Hepatitis B core antibody (anti-HBc)	Anti-HBc detected in serum during and after acute infection
	Hepatitis B envelope antigen (HBeAg)	HB envelope antibody (anti-HBe)	HBeAg correlates with infectivity; suggestive of active viral replication
C	Hepatitis C antigen (HCAg)	Hepatitis C antibody (anti-HCV)	RNA virus; previously known as posttransfusion NANB hepatitis
D	Hepatitis D antigen (HDAg)	Hepatitis D antibody (anti-HDV)	Defective RNA virus; requires presence of HBsAg
E	Hepatitis E antigen (HEAg)	Hepatitis E antibody (anti-HEV)	RNA virus present in stool; cause of enteric NANB hepatitis
G	Hepatitis G antigen (HGAg)	Not available	RNA-like virus; named GBV-A, GBV-B, and GBV-C; thought to be of tamarin origin

NANB, non-A, non-B hepatitis.

Table 73-2 Comparison of the Etiologic Forms of Hepatitis A, B, C, D, E, and G Viruses

Virus	HAV	HBV	HCV	HDV	HEV	HGV
Genome	RNA	DNA	RNA	RNA	RNA	RNA
Family	Picornavirus	Hepadnavirus	Flavivirus	Satellite	Calicivirus	Flavivirus
Size (nm)	27	42	30–60	40	32	Unknown
Incubation (days) [mean]	15–50 [30]	45–180 [80]	15–160	21–140 [35]	15–65 [42]	14–35 [NA]
Transmission						
Oral	Common	Rare	Rare	No	Yes, common	Unknown
Percutaneous	Rare	Common	Common	Common	Unknown	Yes
Sexual	No	Common	Common	Common	No	Rare
Perinatal	No	Common	Rare	Common	Rare	Yes, rare
Onset	Sudden	Insidious	Insidious	Insidious	Sudden	Yes, rare
Clinical illness	70%–80% adults 5% children	10%–15%	5%–10%	10%	70%–80% adults	Unknown
Icteric presentation						
Children	<10%	30%	25%	Unknown	Unknown	Unknown
Adults	30%	5%–20%	5%–10%	25%	Common	Unknown
Peak alanine aminotransferase (ALT) (U/L)	800–1,000	1,000–1,500	300–800	1,000–1,500	800–1,000	Unknown
Incidence of acute liver failure (%)	<1	<1	<1	2–7.5	<1; higher in pregnant women	Unknown
Serum diagnosis						
Acute infection	Anti-HAV IgM	HBsAg Anti-HBc IgM	HCV-RNA (anti-HCV)	Anti-HDV IgM	Anti-HEV IgG (seroconversion)	HGV RNA
Chronic infection		HBsAg Anti-HBc IgG	Anti-HCV (ELISA) RIBA	Anti-HDV IgG	NA	HGV RNA
Viral markers	HAV RNA	HBV-DNA DNA polymerase	HCV-RNA	HDV-RNA	Viruslike particles	HGV RNA
Immunity	Anti-HAV IgG	Anti-HBs	NA	NA	Anti-HEV IgG	Unknown
Case-fatality rate	0.1%–2.7% 0.15%–1.7%	1%–3%	1%–2%	<1% coinfect	0.5%–4% 1.5%–21% pregnant women	Unknown
Complete recovery	>97%	85%–97%	50%	90%	99%	Unknown
Incidence of chronic infection	0%	2%–7% >90% neonates	50%	80% superinfect ≤5% coinfection	0%	Unknown
Carrier state	No	Yes	Yes	Yes	No	Unknown
Risk of hepatocellular carcinoma	No	Yes	Yes	Yes	No	No
Drug treatment	None	Interferon, lamivudine adefovir	Interferon, ribavirin + interferon pegylated Interferon pegylated Interferon + ribavirin	Interferon	None	Unknown

ELISA, enzyme-linked immunosorbent assay; NA, not applicable.

indicated to document the presence of active viral replication and assess the viral load. Testing for hepatitis D antibody (anti-HDV) also should be performed in patients with hepatitis B to evaluate the possibility of coexisting delta hepatitis. If the hepatitis serology is negative, rare but treatable causes of chronic active hepatitis should be excluded. These include alcoholic liver disease, Wilson disease, α_1-antitrypsin deficiency, and drug-induced chronic active hepatitis. Drugs associated with reversible chronic active hepatitis syndrome include methyldopa,[18] nitrofurantoin,[19] isoniazid,[20] and rarely, sulfonamides[21] and propylthiouracil.[22]

Following exclusion of these conditions, the patient should be evaluated for the presence of circulating immunologic markers associated with the autoimmune (idiopathic) form of chronic hepatitis. These tests include antismooth-muscle antibody, antimitochondrial antibody, antinuclear antibody titers, and increased serum immunoglobulins.

HEPATITIS A VIRUS

Virology and Epidemiology

Hepatitis A virus is a 27-nm diameter, single-stranded RNA virus that is classified as a picornavirus (Table 73-2).[23] Following attachment to a cell surface receptor, the viral RNA is uncoated. The cell host ribosomes then bind to the viral RNA, and form polysomes. Subsequently, HAV is translated into a polyprotein with three distinct regions: P1, P2, and P3 with the

Table 73-3 Etiologies of Chronic Hepatitis

Viral Infections	
Hepatitis viruses (B, C, D)	
Cytomegalovirus (CMV)	
Epstein-Barr virus (EBV)	
Rubella virus	
Drug-Induced	
Methyldopa	
Nitrofurantoin	
Isoniazid	
Sulfonamides	
Propylthiouracil	
Metabolic Disorders	
Wilson disease	
α_1-Antitrypsin deficiency	
Autoimmune Hepatitis	

P2 and P3 regions encoding for nonstructural proteins associated with viral replication. HAV appears to replicate within the liver; however, enterocytes may also support viral replication.[23] HAV has a single serotype that remains detectable in intact virions and has four different genotypes (I-IV).[23]

Hepatitis A virus has a worldwide distribution.[4,24–26] The prevalence of infection is related to the quality of the water supply, level of sanitation, and age.[26,27] Incidence data are unreliable, however, because the disease is frequently mild and often unrecognized, resulting in underreporting.[24–27] The primary mode of transmission is person-to-person via the fecal-oral route.[24–27] HAV is passed into the stool in high titer. Considering that the virus resists degradation by environmental conditions, gastric acid, and digestive enzymes in the upper gastrointestinal (GI) tract, it is readily spread within a population.[28] Fecally contaminated water or also food is a significant mode of transmission.[24,25,28] Children are considered an important reservoir of infection for others.[29,30]

In the United States, the reported incidence of HAV is 10.8 cases per 100,000, and it is usually associated with outbreaks in lower socioeconomic groups or common-source outbreaks (e.g., day-care centers).[25,27,28,30] Rates in males are greater than those in females by about 20%.[25,28] Children aged 5 to 14 years and Native Americans have the highest incidence of HAV.[25–27] Recent data suggest, however, that with vaccination in children, the incidence of HAV infection is approximately 1.9 cases per 100,000 population, the lowest rate ever recorded.[29] Similar rates of decline have been demonstrated in Native Americans and Hispanics. Additionally, cyclic outbreaks of HAV have been reported among users of injecting and noninjecting drugs and in men who have sex with men.[29] Considering the widespread presence of hepatitis A antibody (anti-HAV), the virus has a high attack rate, with 70% to 90% of those exposed ultimately becoming infected.[24,25]

The most common risk factors for acquiring HAV include close contact with a person positive for HAV (26%), employment or attendance at a day-care center (14%), injection drug use (11%), recent travel (4%), and association with a suspected food- or water-borne outbreak (3%).[4,24,25,27,29] Up to 42% of reported HAV infections have no known source for infection.[26] Exceedingly rare causes of HAV include transfusion of blood or blood products collected from donors during the viremic phase of their infection and from contact with experimentally infected nonhuman primates.[7,25,27,31] Percutaneous transmission is rare because no asymptomatic carrier state for HAV exists, and the incubation period is brief.[1,26,30,32] Occupations at risk for HAV include sewage workers, hospital cleaning personnel, day-care staff, and pediatric nurses.[27,30,31] Furthermore, HAV is the most common preventable (e.g., vaccination) infection in travelers visiting locations with poor hygienic conditions.[30,33] Up to 22% of patients with acute HAV may need to be hospitalized with an associated cost of managing HAV and workdays lost accounting for >$400 million annually.[29]

Pathogenesis

Theoretically, HAV infection results in both a cytopathic and immunologic hepatocyte injury; however, the exact mechanism of injury is unknown.[28,33,34] Viral replication occurs within the liver, based on immunohistochemical analysis in primates. The presence of IgM in sinusoidal cells and hepatitis A viral antigen (HAVAg) in Kupffer cells likely result in the histologic manifestations and functional impairment observed in HAV disease.[30] In addition, circulating T lymphocytes have been isolated from the liver of patients with acute HAV infection.[30]

Nonspecific mechanisms of hepatocyte injury may involve natural killer (NK) cells and lymphokine-activated killer (LAK) cells, which are believed to precede the initiation of damage caused by cytotoxic T lymphocytes (CTL).[30,35] Subsequent hepatocyte death results in viral elimination and eventual resolution of the clinical illness.

Natural History

Hepatitis A virus is typically a benign, self-limited infection, with recovery within 2 months of disease onset. Two atypical courses of acute HAV infection have also been described: prolonged cholestasis and relapsing hepatitis.[30] In patients with prolonged cholestasis, the duration of jaundice exceeds 12 weeks and is associated with pruritus, fatigue, loose stools, and weight loss. Aminotransferase concentrations during this period are <500 U/L.Spontaneous recovery often occurs, yet corticosteroids have been administered to facilitate resolution of the cholestatic phase. Relapsing or polyphasic HAV occurs in 6% to 12% of both adult and pediatric patients and can be characterized by an initial phase of acute infection followed by remission (duration of 4–15 weeks), with subsequent relapse. Aminotransferase concentrations often normalize during the time of remission but increase to >1,000 U/L with relapse. Also, HAV RNA is detectable in the serum, and HAV is usually recovered from the stool during relapse. The pathogenesis of relapsing hepatitis has not been elucidated. Fulminant hepatitis A is rare, occurring in 0.014% to 3.0% of the population infected with HAV, but often fatal.[30,36] Patients >40 years of age or <11 are more susceptible to HAV-induced fulminant hepatic failure (FHF). Chronic HAV does not exist. Typically, the course of HAV includes an incubation phase, an acute hepatitis phase, and a convalescent phase. Complete clinical recovery is usually seen within 2 months in 60% of patients and virtually all patients within 6 months following HAV infection.

Clinical Manifestations

1. E.T., a 34-year-old medical sales representative, presents to the emergency department (ED) with acute onset of jaundice and "dark urine." He was in good health until 2 weeks ago, when he noted feeling fatigued and weak, which he attributed to his demanding work schedule. He also recalled having a mild headache, loss of appetite, muscle pain, diarrhea, and low-grade fevers from 99°F to 101°F. He attributed these symptoms to the flu and took acetaminophen with plenty of fluids. His symptoms persisted until yesterday, when they seemed to resolve unexplainably. He then noted his urine was cola-colored. This morning, he noted jaundice of his eyes and skin and sought medical attention.

E.T.'s medical history includes a recent respiratory tract infection, treated successfully with levofloxacin. His social history is significant for frequenting the local oyster bar, where he regularly ingests raw oysters. He denies smoking and recent travel outside the United States, but admits to occasional alcohol consumption. E.T. has no history of sexual exposure, needle use, or transfusions. His current medications include oral (PO) diazepam 5 mg at bedtime (HS) as needed (PRN) for "muscle spasms," but he has not taken diazepam for "several months." He also has a seizure disorder sustained after a motorcycle accident 2 years before admission, for which he takes phenytoin 400 mg PO HS.

Physical examination is significant for a well-developed, well-nourished man in no acute distress. He is alert and oriented, with a temperature of 99°F. His sclerae and skin are icteric, and his abdomen is positive for a tender, enlarged liver, and right upper quadrant (RUQ) pain. Laboratory tests reveal the following values: hemoglobin (Hgb), 16 g/dL (normal, 12.3–16.3 g/dL); hematocrit (Hct), 44% (normal, 37.4%–47.0%); white blood cell (WBC) count, 5,500 cells/mm^3 (normal, 3.28–9.29 $\times$ 10^3);aspartate transaminase (AST), 120 U/L (normal, 5–40 U/L); alanine aminotransferase (ALT), 240 U/L (normal, 5–40 U/L); alkaline phosphatase, 86 U/L (normal, 21–91 U/L); total bilirubin, 3.2 mg/dL (normal, 0.2–1.0 mg/dL); direct bilirubin, 1.5 mg/dL (normal, 0–0.2 mg/dL); and phenytoin concentration, 12 mg/L (normal, 10–20 mg/L). The albumin, prothrombin time (PT), blood glucose, and electrolytes all are within normal limits. E.T. is negative for anti-HCV, HBeAg, HBsAg, and hepatitis B core antibody (anti-HBc), but is positive for IgM anti-HAV. What clinical features and serologic markers are consistent with viral hepatitis in E.T.?

[SI units: Hgb, 160 g/L (normal, 123–63); Hct, 0.44% (normal, 0.374–0.47%); WBC count, 5,500 $\times$ 10^{9}cells/L (normal, 3,280–9,290 $\times$ 10^9);AST, 120 U/L (normal, 5–40); ALT, 240 U/L (normal, 5–40); alkaline phosphatase, 86 U/L (normal, 21–91); total bilirubin, 54.72 μmol/L(normal, 3.42–17.1); direct bilirubin, 25.65 μmol/L (normal, 0–4)]

The incubation period for HAV is 15 to 50 days (average, 30) following inoculation (Table 73-2). The host is usually asymptomatic during this stage of the infection; thus, E.T. is beyond the inoculation phase of the disease. Because HAV titers are highest in the acute-phase fecal samples, and the period of infectivity is between 14 and 21 days before the onset of jaundice to 7 or 8 days following jaundice, he should be considered infectious at this time. In HAV infections, acute-phase serum and saliva are less infectious than fecal samples, whereas urine and semen samples are not infectious. Family members and persons recently in immediate contact with E.T. should be notified to limit the possibility of disease transmission.

The symptoms of acute viral hepatitis caused by HAV, HBV, HCV, HDV, and HEV are similar. The onset of symptoms in HAV infection, however is less insidious than those seen with HBV and HCV infection.[28–30] Generally, symptoms of HAV present a week or more before the onset of jaundice. The likelihood of having symptoms is related to age. In children age <6 years, 70% of infections are asymptomatic, whereas older children and adults have symptomatic disease with jaundice occurring in >70% of cases. E.T. has signs and symptoms of acute HAV infection, including the nonspecific prodromal symptoms of fatigue, weakness, anorexia, nausea, and vomiting. Abdominal pain and hepatomegaly are common. Less common symptoms include fever, headache, arthralgias, myalgias, and diarrhea. Within 1 to 2 weeks of the onset of prodromal symptoms, patients may enter an icteric phase with symptoms, including clay-colored stools, dark urine, scleral icterus, and frank jaundice. The dark urine is caused by bilirubin, generally occurring shortly before the onset of jaundice. E.T. should be questioned about the presence of pale stools (light gray or yellow), which usually is observed during the icteric phase. His scleral icterus is strongly suggestive of viral hepatitis. Icteric infections usually occur in adults, and are 3.5 times more common than the nonicteric presentation that is seen in children.[37]

The results of E.T.'s liver function tests (LFT) (e.g., elevations in AST, ALT, and bilirubin) also are consistent with viral hepatitis. Serum transaminase concentrations increase during the prodromal phase (usually ALT >AST) of HAV infection, peaking before the onset of jaundice. These concentrations are often >500 U/L, and decline at an initial rate of 75% per week, followed by a slower rate of decline thereafter. Serum bilirubin peaks following aminotransferase activity and rarely exceeds 10 mg/dL. Bilirubin levels decline more slowly than aminotransferases and generally normalize within 3 months. Right upper quadrant tenderness, mild liver enlargement and splenomegaly may also be present in patients with acute HAV infection.

Extrahepatic Manifestations

2. Are there any additional complications that E.T. could develop from his acute HAV infection?

With the appearance of jaundice, prodromal pruritus and extrahepatic manifestations can occur, usually in patients with a more protracted illness. Thus, E.T. should be monitored for additional manifestations of HAV infection, including immune complex-associated rash, leukocytoclastic vasculitis, glomerulonephritis, cryoglobulinemia (less likely than with HCV), and arthritis. Rare extrahepatic manifestations include epidermal necrolysis, fatal myocarditis, renal failure in the presence of hepatic failure (hepatorenal syndrome), optic neuritis, and polyneuritis.[30,38,39] Hematologic abnormalities, although infrequently reported, include autoimmune hemolysis and thrombocytopenic purpura, aplastic anemia, and red cell aplasia.[30,38]

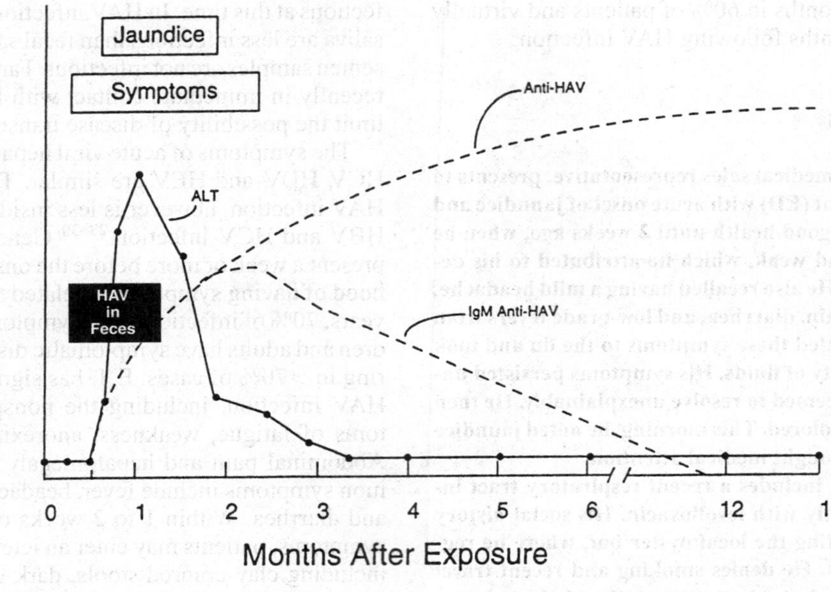

FIGURE 73-1 Typical course of hepatitis A. ALT, alanine aminotransferase; anti-HAV, antibody to HAV; HAV, hepatitis A virus. From reference 40, with permission.

Diagnosis and Serology

Several diagnostic methods are available for detecting HAVAg (antigen) and anti-HAV (antibody). HAV can be detected in stool specimens 1 to 2 weeks preceding clinical illness. Viral RNA can be detected in body fluids and serum using the polymerase chain reaction (PCR), an expensive method usually reserved for research purposes. Because most patients present when the virus is no longer in stool, serum antibody can be detected by radioimmunoassay (RIA) or enzyme-linked immunosorbent assay (ELISA). Two classes of HAV antibodies are detectable: IgM and IgG (Fig. 73-1). Detection of IgM to HAV in a patient who presents with clinical characteristics of hepatitis or in an asymptomatic patient with elevated transaminases is consistent with acute HAV infection. HAV IgG appears following IgM and is indicative of previous exposure and immunity to HAV, whereas a rising IgG is consistent with recent exposure.[28,30,40] Anti-HAV IgM is commonly present throughout the disease course (16–40 weeks), usually peaking early and declining to undetectable levels 3 to 4 months after the initial infection.[30,41] One-quarter of patients infected with HAV have IgM present for up to 6 months, and occasionally longer. HAV IgG appears early in the convalescent phase and is detectable for decades after the acute infection resolves, with a slowly declining titer.[30] Both ELISA and RIA methods of antibody detection are sensitive, specific, and reliable to diagnose acute HAV infection. E.T. has a positive IgM anti-HAV, consistent with acute HAV infection. E.T. has a negative IgM anti-HBc test, ruling out acute HBV infection.[30]

Treatment

General Measures

Hepatitis A virus infection is usually a self-limited disease that does not require a specific therapy. Many treatments have been recommended for acute viral hepatitis, but none significantly alter the course of the disease. The patient with acute viral hepatitis may be treated as an outpatient if symptoms are mild to moderate and regular medical evaluation occurs. Patients infected with hepatitis A usually do not require hospitalization, unless they develop complications of hepatic insufficiency, such as encephalopathy or hemorrhage secondary to hypoprothrombinemia. Patients should continue their normal activities as much as possible while avoiding physical exhaustion. Intravenous (IV) fluid and electrolyte replacement is necessary in some patients with severe nausea and vomiting. Patients should abstain from alcohol during the acute phase of the disease. Following resolution of symptoms and serum biochemical abnormalities, moderate alcohol intake is no longer contraindicated. Ultimately, any patient with fulminant hepatic failure caused by HAV infection should be evaluated for liver transplantation.

Adjustment of Medication Doses

3. Should E.T.'s medications be adjusted during the acute phase of hepatitis A infection?

Dosage adjustments for hepatically eliminated drugs in the setting of liver disease are difficult to predict. This is because hepatic metabolism is complex, involving numerous oxidative and conjugative pathways that are variably affected in hepatic disease. In renal disease, creatinine serves as an endogenous marker to predict the clearance of renally eliminated drugs. In hepatic disease, however, no reliable endogenous markers exist to predict drug hepatic clearance. Laboratory tests that approximate the synthetic function of the liver (albumin, PT) and biliary clearance (bilirubin) are used to estimate the degree of hepatic impairment, but these tests are not dependable in predicting alterations in pharmacokinetic parameters for hepatically metabolized drugs.

Table 73-4 Half-Life Data for Various Agents in Acute Viral Hepatitis Compared With Reference Normal Controls

	Half-life ($t_{1/2}$ hr)	
Drug[7]	Normal Controls	Acute Viral Hepatitis
Acetaminophen[42]	2.1	3.2
Aspirin[43]	0.4	No change[a]
Carbamazepine[43]	12	Increased
Chlordiazepoxide[44]	11.1	91
Chloramphenicol[45]	4.6	11.6
Clofibrate[46]	17.5	No change
Diazepam[47]	37.2	74.5
Lidocaine[48]	3.7	6.4
Lorazepam[49]	21.7	No change
Meperidine[50]	3.4	7
Nitrendipine[51]	2.2	No change
Norfloxacin[52]	4.3	No change
Oxazepam[53]	5.1	No change
Phenobarbital[54]	86	No change
Phenytoin[55]	13.2	No change
Quinine[56]	10	17
Rifampin[57]	2.5	6.5
Theophylline[59]	7.7	19.2
Tolbutamide[59]	5.9	4.0
Warfarin[60]	25	No change

[a]No change indicates that the difference between patients with acute viral hepatitis and normal controls is not statistically significant.

Because of the difficulty in predicting hepatic drug clearance, unnecessary and potentially hepatotoxic medications are best if avoided during the acute phase of the illness. When drug therapy is indicated with agents that undergo hepatic elimination, it is prudent to use the lowest doses possible to achieve the desired therapeutic effect. Data from small pharmacokinetic studies in patients with acute viral hepatitis are shown in Table 73-4.[42–60]

E.T. should be advised to discontinue diazepam (Valium) because this medication undergoes extensive hepatic biotransformation and limited data suggest this agent accumulates in the setting of acute viral hepatitis.[47] If E.T. should require drug therapy for muscle spasms, he should either decrease the diazepam dose or consider using an alternative agent (e.g., lorazepam) that does not accumulate in acute viral hepatitis.[49] Patients with acute viral hepatitis do not require phenytoin dosage adjustments.[55] Because E.T.'s plasma phenytoin concentration is within the desired therapeutic range, no dosage adjustment is needed at this time.

Prevention of Hepatitis A

Prevention of hepatitis A infection can be achieved through immunoprophylactic measures. Immunoprophylaxis may be passive, active, or a combination of both. In passive immunization, temporary protective antibody in the form of immunoglobulin is administered. In active immunization, a vaccine is administered to induce the formation of protective antibody. Prophylaxis can be administered before (pre-exposure prophylaxis) or after exposure (postexposure prophylaxis).

Pre-exposure Prophylaxis

4. M.D., a 22-year-old student, is preparing for a 2-week vacation to Thailand. He plans to travel 3 months from now and wonders if he should receive prophylaxis for HAV.

IMMUNOGLOBULIN

Before hepatitis A vaccine was available, the sole therapy for pre-exposure prophylaxis of hepatitis A infection was immunoglobulin. Immunoglobulin is an injectable solution containing a full complement of antibodies normally present in human serum. Current preparations are manufactured by cold ethanol fractionation of pooled plasma collected from at least 1,000 human donors, providing protective levels of anti-HAV. Although passive immunization with immunoglobulin alone is highly effective in preventing hepatitis A virus infection,[61] the duration of protection is short. When used for pre-exposure prophylaxis (e.g., in travelers who are allergic to a vaccine component or decide against vaccination), a dose of 0.02 mL/kg of immunoglobulin administered intramuscularly (IM) confers protection for <3 months, and an IM dose of 0.06 mL/kg confers protection for ≥5 months.[29,30,61] Patients with continued exposure to hepatitis A require IM administration of immunoglobulin 0.06 mL/kg every 5 months for adequate protection.[29,62]

VACCINE

Active immunization with hepatitis A vaccine has largely supplanted the use of immunoglobulin for pre-exposure prophylaxis of infection caused by HAV. Formulations of inactivated hepatitis A vaccine available in the United States include Havrix and Vaqta. Both vaccines are formalin-inactivated preparations of attenuated HAV strains. The manufacturers use differing units to express antigen content of their respective vaccines. Havrix dosages are expressed in ELISA units (EL.U.), and Vaqta dosages are expressed as units (U) of hepatitis A antigen.

Dosing Regimen

Havrix is available in two formulations that differ according to age: for persons 12 months to 18 years of age, 720 EL.U. (0.5 mL) per dose in a two-dose schedule; and for persons >19 years of age, 1,440 EL.U. (1.0 mL) per dose in a two-dose schedule (Table 73-5).[29,30] This vaccine is usually injected IM into the deltoid muscle using a needle length appropriate for

Table 73-5 Recommended Doses of Hepatitis A Vaccines

Age at Vaccination	Dose (Volume)[a]	Schedule (Months)[b]
Havrix		
Children 12 mos–18 yrs	720 EL.U. (0.5 mL)	0, 6–12
Adults >19 yrs	1,440 EL.U. (1.0 mL)	0, 6–12
Vaqta		
Children 12 mos–18 yrs	25 U (0.5 mL)	0, 6–18
Adults >19 yrs	50 U (1.0 mL)	0, 6

[a]Enzyme-linked immunosorbent assay (ELISA) units.
[b]Zero months represents timing of the initial dose; subsequent numbers represent months after the initial dose.
From references 29,62, with permission.

the person's age and size, with a booster dose administered 6 to 12 months later. Of note, the pediatric Havrix formulation (three-dose schedule) is no longer available. In comparison, Vaqta is available in two formulations, and the formulations differ according to the person's age: for persons 12 months to 18 years of age, 25 U (0.5 mL) in a two-dose schedule; for persons >19 years of age, 50 U (1.0 mL) per dose in a two-dose schedule (Table 73-5).[29,30] Likewise, this vaccine is usually injected IM into the deltoid muscle with a booster dose administered 6 to 18 months later.[29]

The levels of anti-HAV necessary to prevent infection have not been definitively established. The manufacturer-specified protective levels for Havrix and Vaqta are >20 mIU/mL(or >33 mIU/mL in recent studies) and >10 mIU/mL, respectively. The immune response to each preparation has been rapid and complete, with >94% of patients achieving protective antibody levels 1 month after vaccination.[29,62] Following administration of a second dose, 100% of vaccine recipients achieve protective antibody titers.[29,63] Additionally, both vaccines are extensively immunogenic in children (including those with Down syndrome) and adolescents, with 97% to 100% of persons between the age of 2 to 18 years achieving protective antibody levels 1 month after receiving the first dose; 100% achieve protective levels 1 month following the second dose.[29] Additionally, data indicate that inactivated hepatitis A vaccines are immunogenic in children aged <2 years who do not have passively acquired maternal antibody. Vaccination among this group achieves a protective antibody level.[29]

COMBINATION VACCINE

The US Food and Drug Administration (FDA) has also licensed a combined HAV and HBV vaccine (Twinrix, GlaxoSmithKline Biologicals, Rixensart, Belgium) for use in persons aged ≥8 years.[29,64] Twinrix is composed of the same antigenic components used in Havrix and Engerix-B. Each dose of Twinrix contains at least 720 EL.U. of inactivated HAV and 20 mcg of recombinant hepatitis B surface antigen (HBsAg). Trace amounts of thimerosal (<1 mcg) is also present from the manufacturing process.

Primary immunization consists of three doses, given on a 0-, 1-, and 6- month schedule, the same that is used for single antigen hepatitis B vaccine.[29,64] Any person 18 years of age or older having an indication for both hepatitis A and hepatitis B vaccine can be given Twinrix, including patients with chronic liver disease, users of illicit injectable drugs, men who have sex with men, and persons with clotting factor disorders who receive therapeutic blood products.[29,64] For international travel, hepatitis A vaccine is recommended; hepatitis B vaccine is recommended for travelers to areas of high or intermediate hepatitis B endemicity who plan to stay for longer than 6 months and have frequent close contact with the local population.[29,64]

Data from 11 clinical trials in adult patients ages 17 to 70 years indicated, at 1 month after completion of the three-dose series, that seroconversion for anti-HAV (titer >20 mIU/mL) was elicited in 99.9% of vaccines, and protective antibodies against HBsAg (anti-HBs >10 mIU/mL) were elicited in 98.5% of vaccinees.[29,64] Thus, the efficacy of Twinrix likely is comparable with existing single antigen hepatitis vaccines. The persistence of anti-HAV and antibody to hepatitis B surface antigen (anti-HBs) following administration is similar to that following single antigen hepatitis A and B vaccine administration at 4-year follow-up. Observed adverse effects were generally similar in type and frequency to those reported following vaccination with monovalent hepatitis A and B vaccines and no serious vaccine-related adverse events were observed in clinical trials.[29,64]

Efficacy, Safety, and Duration of Response

The efficacy of the hepatitis A vaccine is well established with protective efficacy of 94% to 100%.[64–66] The vaccine is well tolerated with soreness at the injection site, headache, myalgia, and malaise as the most commonly reported adverse effects. A recent postmarketing surveillance study of >6 million doses of vaccine revealed <0.01% of patients reporting adverse events.[67]

The duration of protection has not been studied extensively; however, the little data that exist suggest persistence of protective antibody titers for periods of 6 years with Havrix and 5 to 6 years with Vaqta.[29] Estimates of antibody persistence derived from pharmacokinetic models of antibody decline indicate that protective concentrations of antibody could be present for >20 years.[29,68,69] The US Advisory Committee on Immunization Practices (ACIP) does not have a recommendation regarding the need for booster doses at this time.

Indications

The ACIP continues to recommend administering hepatitis A vaccination for several high-risk groups, including travelers to countries with high endemicity of infection (South and Central America, Africa, South and Southeast Asia, Caribbean, and the Middle East), travelers to countries with intermediate endemicity of infection (Eastern and Southern Europe and the former Soviet Union), children living in communities with high rates of hepatitis A infection and periodic hepatitis A outbreaks (Alaskan Native villages, American Indian reservations), men who have sex with men, IV drug users, researchers or persons who have occupational risk for hepatitis A (health care workers), persons with clotting factor disorders, and persons with chronic liver disease who are at increased risk for fulminant hepatitis A.[29] Because M.D. will not travel for another 3 months, he should receive either Havrix 1,440 EL.U. or Vaqta 50 U as soon as possible and no later than 1 month before travel. This initial injection will provide adequate protection from HAV infection during his travel, and he can receive the booster injection on his return, at least 6 months after the first injection.

Postexposure Prophylaxis

5. L.W., a 26-year-old man, recently was diagnosed with HAV infection. He attends college and works part-time as a retail clerk. He lives with his wife and infant daughter. Which of L.W.'s contacts require postexposure prophylaxis for HAV?

The ACIP recommends using immunoglobulin for people who have been recently exposed to HAV and who have not been previously vaccinated. The recommended dose is 0.02 mL/kg, administered IM as soon as possible but no later than 2 weeks after exposure. Contacts who have received a dose of hepatitis A vaccine at least 1 month before exposure do not need immunoglobulin, because protective antibody titers are achieved in >95% of patients 1 month after vaccination.[29,62]

Administration of immunoglobulin within 2 weeks of exposure to HAV is 80% to 90% effective in preventing acute HAV infection.[29,70] In most cases, when given early, immunoglobulin prevents both clinical and subclinical HAV illness. Protection following immunoglobulin administration is immediate and complete; however, long-lasting immunity to HAV does not develop.

Immunoglobulin is recommended for close personal contacts (household and sexual) of persons with acute hepatitis A infection. L.W.'s wife and infant daughter should receive prophylactic administration of immunoglobulin. Vaccination is not required at this time. Prophylaxis is not recommended for casual contacts at work or school.

Other situations in which immunoglobulin administration may be indicated include hepatitis A infection in day-care centers and in settings with infected persons who prepare and serve food. Immunoglobulin is recommended for all staff and children in day-care settings when a case of hepatitis A virus infection is diagnosed among employees or attendees.[29,62] When a food handler is diagnosed with hepatitis A, immunoglobulin is recommended for other food handlers at the same location. Given the improbability of disease transmission to persons consuming food prepared or served by workers infected with hepatitis A, the routine administration of immunoglobulin in this setting is not recommended.[29,62]

Unvaccinated patients with continued exposure to hepatitis A require IM administration of immunoglobulin 0.06 mL/kg every 5 months for adequate protection.[29] When immunoglobulin is required for infants or pregnant women, preparations that do not contain thimerosal should be used.[29] Additionally, immune globulin does not appear to impede the immune response to inactivated vaccines or to oral poliovirus vaccine or yellow fever vaccine. Immune globulin may, however, interfere with the response to live attenuated vaccines such as measles, mumps, rubella (MMR) vaccine and varicella vaccine when administered as either individual or combination vaccines. Therefore, MMR and varicella vaccine should be delayed for at least 3 months following administration of immune globulin for HAV prophylaxis. Immune globulin should not be given within 2 weeks after the administration of MMR or varicella vaccine. Finally, if immune globulin is administered within 2 weeks of MMR, the person requires revaccination, but not sooner than 3 months after the immune globulin administration for MMR. Serologic tests for varicella vaccination should be performed 3 months after immune globulin administration to determine if revaccination is required.

HEPATITIS B VIRUS

Virology

Hepatitis B virus is a partially double-stranded DNA virus that is a member of the *Hepadnaviridae* family of viruses (Table 73-2).[13,71–74] Unlike HAV, HBV is antigenically complex, and results in an acute illness with or without a chronic disease state. Intact HBV virions are 42 nm wide and contain four major genes (core, X protein, surface X, and polymerase) associated with viral replication.[13,71–76] The core gene encodes the core nucleocapsid protein which aids in viral packaging and production of HBeAg. The surface gene encodes for several proteins (pre-S1, pre-S2, and S). The X gene encodes an X protein that is considered to be associated with hepatic carcinogenesis. Lastly, the polymerase gene encodes a large protein that is responsible for viral packaging and DNA replication. On the surface, coating HBV, is the HBsAg, which is the virus's major envelope protein. This antigen is found in patients with acute or chronic HBV infection and chronic carriers. Two additional proteins, L and M, are also present in the viral envelope. The function of the L protein appears to be viral binding to the hepatocyte surface, whereas the function of the M protein is unknown. Inside the surface envelope of the intact hepatitis B virion is a 27-nm structure called the internal nucleocapsid core, which consists of several copies of the viral core protein or HBcAg surrounding the viral DNA and the virally encoded polymerase. The HBeAg is a secreted product of the nucleocapsid core of HBV, and its presence is also indicative of viral replication.[71–76] In addition to intact virions, several subviral particles (S proteins) are produced that are non-infectious; however, they are severely immunogenic and promote the formation of neutralizing antibodies.[71–76] These particles were used to develop the first HBV vaccines.

Our understanding of HBV replication is based on experiments performed in animals; thus, extrapolation of these results to human disease must be made with caution.[74,76,77] The life cycle of HBV can be summarized as follows: (a) viral attachment and entry; (b) viral uncoating in the cytoplasm through direct membrane fusion; (c) synthesis of complete double-stranded DNA in the nucleus: conversion of relaxed circular HBV-DNA into double-stranded covalently closed circular DNA (ccc-DNA), catalyzed by HBV viral DNA polymerase; (d) synthesis of RNA that forms the template for DNA synthesis by host RNA polymerase; (e) translation of viral transcripts in the cytoplasm, which yields the viral envelop, core, precore, and X proteins, as well as the viral DNA polymerase; (f) encapsidation or packaging of RNA in the cytoplasm with production of viral cores; (g) RNA synthesis of minus strand DNA by reverse transcriptase (RT); and (h) envelopment of viral cores with excretion of infective virions, or transport of viral core back into the nucleus (Fig. 73-2). The final step of replication facilitates horizontal spread of infection throughout the liver.

A basic understanding of the HBV life cycle has provided unique opportunities for drug development. Of special importance, the HBV polymerase functions as both an RT for synthesis of the negative DNA strand from genomic RNA and as an endogenous DNA polymerase. Because the HBV polymerase is remotely related to the RT enzymes of retroviruses (e.g., human immunodeficiency virus [HIV]), it is apparent that some inhibitors of HIV polymerase or RT might have activity against the HBV polymerase. Thus, several RT inhibitors have been evaluated for treating and preventing HBV. Because the proofreading function of the RT is nonexistent, an extremely high mutation rate for HBV occurs resulting in viral resistance to many of these agents.

Epidemiology

Approximately 5% of the world's population is infected with HBV.[1,6,12,73,78] It is estimated that >1.25 million carriers (defined as persons positive for hepatitis B surface antigen for >6 months) occur in the United States, many of whom are immigrants from endemic areas and Alaskan natives (6.4%).[1,6,71,73,78] The incidence of acute HBV has been on the decline in the United States.[1,6,71,73,78] Over the past

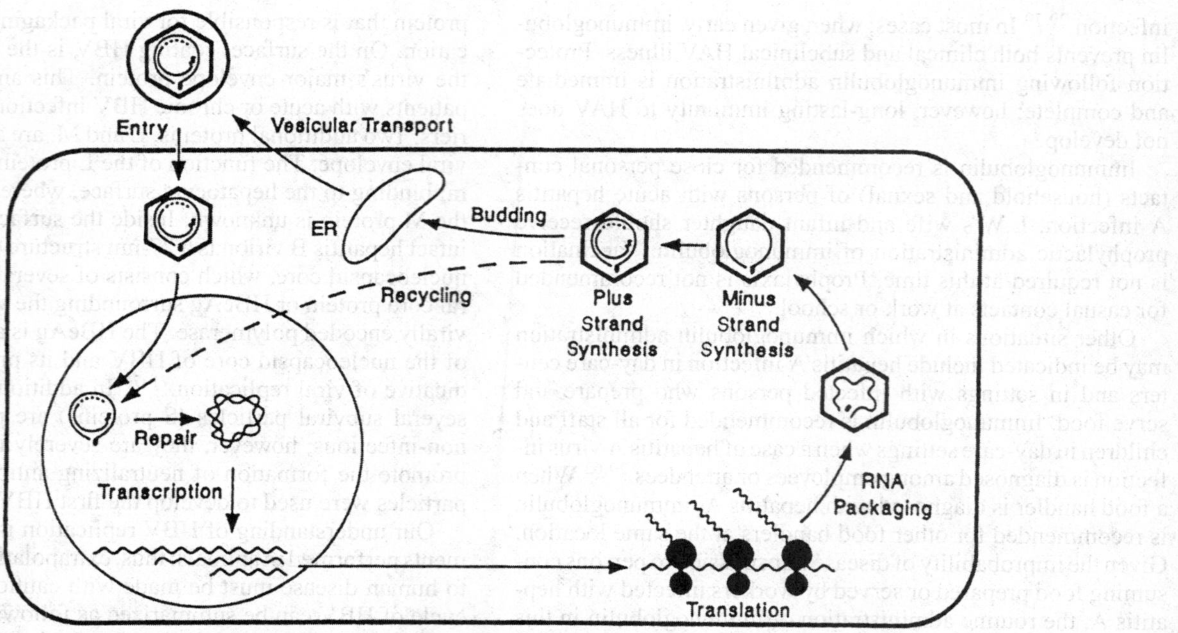

FIGURE 73-2 Life cycle of hepatitis B virus. From Ganem D. Hepadnaviridae: the viruses and their replication. In: Fields BN. Ed. Fundamental Virology. 3rd ed. Philadelphia: Lippincott-Raven; 1996:1199, with permission.

decade, HBV has been reduced from a rate of 438,000 infections per year in the late 1980s to an estimated 185,000 cases in 1997. This reduction has occurred in all age, racial, ethnic, and high-risk groups. The most significant reduction is in children and health care workers, groups with the highest rate of vaccination. The reduced incidence of HBV infection may be attributed to changes in behavior, which has led to decreased transmission of infection. High-risk groups in the United States for acquiring HBV infection include certain ethnic groups (Alaskan natives, Pacific Islanders), first-generation immigrants from regions of high endemicity (Southeast Asia), injection drug users, gay men, black Americans (compared with white Americans), and males (more than females).[1,73,78–80] The most prominent risk factors associated with acute HBV include heterosexual contact (42%), men having sex with men (15%), and injection drug use (21%).[73,78–80] HBV vaccination opportunities include clinics for sexually transmitted disease (and contacts) and in prisons and holding centers for incarceration.

The epidemiology of chronic HBV infection is less well known than that of acute disease. Within the United States, it is estimated that 0.2% of the population is HBsAg positive.[73,78–80] Blacks are more likely to be HBsAg positive than whites, but the highest reported rates of HBsAg symptoms are among Asian Americans, especially those from China and Southeast Asia. In population-based surveys, HBV is responsible for 1% to 14% of chronic liver disease with chronic infection more likely to develop in infants compared with adults.[6]

Transmission

Hepatitis B virus is transmitted by sexual contact, percutaneous or perinatal exposure, and by close person-to-person contact allegedly through open cuts and sores, especially among children in hyperendemic areas. These modes of transmission of HBV are summarized in the following sections.

Sexual Transmission

Sexual activity is the most significant mode of HBV transmission worldwide, including North America, where the prevalence of infection is low.[73,78–81] Heterosexual intercourse accounts for the majority of United States infections (26%). In heterosexuals, factors associated with an enhanced risk of HBV infection include duration of sexual activity, number of sexual partners, and history of sexually transmitted diseases (STD). Sexual partners of injection drug users, prostitutes, and clients of prostitutes are at a very high risk for infection. Sexual partners of infected individuals are at high risk for infection, even in the absence of high-risk behavior. Studies of household of the infected and sexual contacts have reported that 0% to 3% of the spouses or sexual partners and 4% to 9% of the children are HBsAg positive. Because most patients with chronic HBV infection are unaware of their infection and are "silent carriers," sexual transmission is likely to be a significant mode of worldwide transmission. The use of condoms appears to reduce the risk of sexual transmission.[73,78–80]

From 1980 to 1985, a very high rate of HBV infection was observed in homosexual men, accounting for 20% of all reported cases of infection.[73,78–80] Multiple sexual partners, anal-receptive intercourse, and duration of sexual activity were the most common factors associated with HBV acquisition in this population. Current rates of HBV infection in this population have fallen and are estimated to be about 8%, possibly as a result of modifications of sexual behavior in response to HIV. Similar to heterosexuals, the use of condoms in this population may also reduce the risk of sexual transmission.

Blood and Blood Products

Previously, blood was not screened for HBV; by the early 1970s, however, this risk of transmission was significantly reduced through screening of blood (used for transfusions) and blood products before their administration.[73,78–80] Although the risk of transfusion-associated HBV infection has been greatly reduced with the screening of blood (tests for HBsAg and anti-HB core) and the exclusion of donors who engage in high-risk activities, it is estimated that 1 out of 50,000 transfused units transmit HBV infection.[73,78–80]

Perinatal Transmission

Early childhood exposure and perinatal exposure are additional modes of transmission of HBV infection.[73,78–80] High serum concentrations of virus have been linked with increased risk of transmission by vertical routes (and needlestick exposure). Infants born to HBeAg-positive mothers with high viral replication (>80 pg/mL) have a 70% to 90% risk of perinatal HBV acquisition compared with a 10% to 40% risk in infants born to mothers infected with HBV who are HBeAg-negative. Infection generally occurs via inoculation of the infant at the time of birth or soon thereafter and, even with active and passive immunization, 10% to 15% of babies may acquire HBV infection at birth.

In developing countries with high prevalence rates and in regions of the United States with high endemicity, children born to HBsAg-positive mothers with HBV are at risk for acquiring HBV infection in the perinatal period, with infection rates reported to be between 7% and 13%.[73,78–80] In addition, children of HBsAg-positive mothers who are not infected at birth remain at very high risk of early childhood infection, with 60% of those born to HBsAg-positive mothers becoming infected by the age of 5 years. The mechanism of the later infection, which is neither perinatal nor sexual, is not known, however. Furthermore, although HBsAg is detectable in breast milk, breast-feeding is not believed to be a primary mode of HBV transmission.

Injection Drug Use

Recreational drug use in the United States and Europe is an important mode of HBV transmission, accounting for approximately 23% of all patients.[73,78–80] The risk of HBV infection increases with duration of recreational drug use; thus, serologic markers of ongoing or prior HBV infection are usually present after 5 years of drug use.

Other Modes of Transmission

Other risk factors for transmission of HBV include working in a health care setting, transfusion and dialysis, acupuncture, tattooing, traveling abroad, and living in institutions.[73,78–80] Sporadic cases of HBV transmission have been attributed to nonpercutaneous transmission by way of small breaks in the skin, biting, or mucous membranes. Although HBsAg is found in saliva, tears, sweat, semen, vaginal secretions, breast milk, cerebrospinal fluid, ascites, pleural fluid, synovial fluid, gastric juice, urine, and, rarely, feces of HBsAg-positive persons, only semen, saliva, and serum actually contain infectious HBV in experimental transmission studies. Thus, kissing is not considered to be a significant means of HBV transmission, but biting could be.

Pathogenesis

Similar to HAV infection, clinical observations suggest that host immune responses are more important than virologic factors in the pathogenesis of liver injury.[71,73,78,82,83] Host cellular and humoral immune responses are linked to T lymphocytes, which enhance viral clearance from hepatocytes and cause liver injury.[71,73,78,82,83]

Diagnosis

The presence of HBsAg in serum is diagnostic for HBV infection. In 5% to 10% of acute cases in which the HBsAg levels fall below sensitivity thresholds of current assays, the presence of IgM anti-HBc in serum confirms a recent acute hepatitis B infection. Another highly reliable marker of active HBV replication and diagnosis is the presence of HBV DNA in serum through qualitative or quantitative assays, detectable early during the course of acute HBV infection.[71,73,78,84,85] Persisting levels of HBV DNA indicate ongoing infection and a high degree of active viral replication and infectivity.

Diagnostic methods for HBV DNA have expanded in recent years.[71,73,78,86,87] Tests detecting HBV DNA can be classified as (a) dependent on hybridization of labeled probe to the DNA with quantification (Genostics assay; branched-DNA [bDNA]) and (b) PCR-based assays in which viral DNA is amplified with detection through gel electrophoresis. Genostics and bDNA are moderately sensitive in detecting DNA in HBsAg-negative and HBeAg-positive patients and they have high specificity. Values obtained by these assays are not interchangeable and are used primarily as research tools. In general the non–PCR-based assays are available with levels of sensitivity from 10^3 to 10^5 genomic copies/mL of serum. Their results usually correlate with clinical response to antiviral therapy. Because of their many limitations, most clinical laboratories use one of many commercially available PCR assays with enhanced sensitivity (10^2 genomic copies/mL or less).

Serology

Serologic patterns, general definitions, and diagnostic criteria of HBV infection are depicted in Table 73-6. Within the first several weeks after exposure (range, 2–10 weeks), HBsAg appears in the blood and is present for several weeks before serum concentrations of aminotransferases increase and symptoms become apparent (Fig. 73-3A).[41,71,73,78,88,89] Clinical illness usually follows HBV exposure by 1 to 3 months. HBsAg can

Table 73-6 Common Serologic Patterns of Hepatitis B Virus Infection

HbsAg	HbeAg	Anti-HBs	Anti-HBe	Anti-HBc	Interpretation
+	+	−	−	−	Incubation period
+	+	−	−	+ (IgM)	Acute HBV infection (typical case); chronic HBV carrier with high infectivity
−	−	+	−	+ (IgG)	Recovery from HBV infection
+	−	−	−	+ (IgG)	Chronic HBV carrier; chronic hepatitis B
−	−	+	−	−	Successful immunization with HBV vaccine

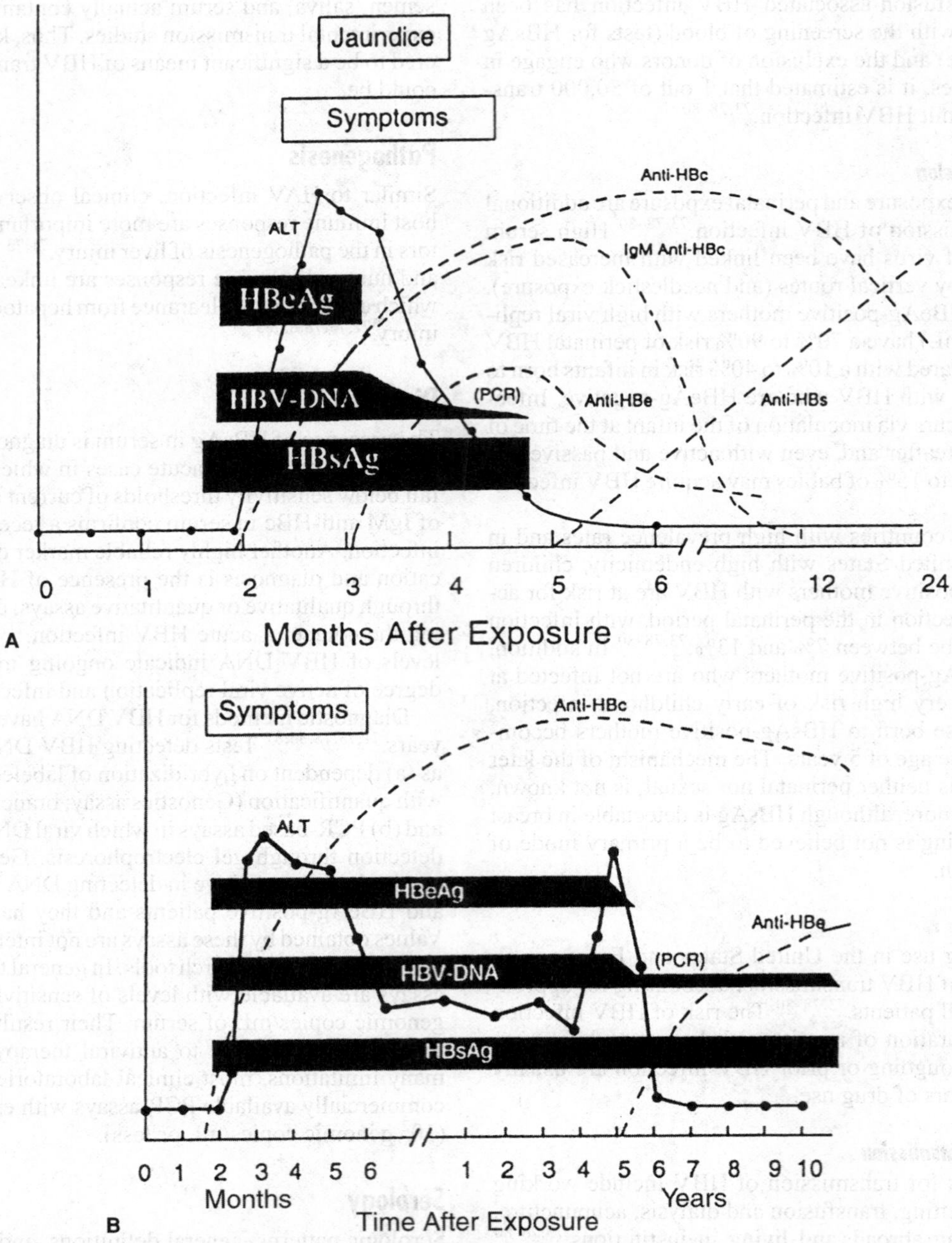

FIGURE 73-3 A: Sequence of events after acute hepatitis B virus infection with resolution. ALT, alanine aminotransferase; anti-HBc, hepatitis B core antibody; anti-HBe, hepatitis B envelope antibody; anti-HBs, hepatitis B surface antibody; HBeAg, hepatitis B e antigen; HBsAg, hepatitis B surface antigen; HBV DNA; hepatitis B virus DNA; IgM anti-HBc, IgM antibody to hepatitis B core virus; PCR, polymerase chain reaction. **B: Sequence of events after acute hepatitis B virus infection converts to chronicity.** ALT, alanine aminotransferase; anti-HBc, hepatitis B core antibody; anti-HBe, hepatitis B envelope antibody; HBeAg; hepatitis B e antigen; HBsAg, hepatitis B surface antigen; HBV DNA, hepatitis B virus DNA; PCR, polymerase chain reaction. (From reference 40, with permission.)

be detected in serum until the clinical illness resolves and usually becomes undetectable after 4 to 6 months. Persistence of HBsAg beyond 6 months implies progression to chronic HBV infection. The antibody to HBsAg (anti-HBs) often appears after a short "window" period during which neither HBsAg nor anti-HBs are detectable. In most patients, anti-HBs persists for years after HBV infection, conferring immunity to reinfection (Fig. 73-3A).

A soluble viral protein, HBeAg is detectable early during the acute phase of the disease and persists in chronic hepatitis B infection. HBeAg is a marker of active HBV replication, and its presence correlates with circulating HBV particles. The presence of both HBeAg and HBsAg indicates a high level of viral replication and infectivity and a need for antiviral therapy. Generally, seroconversion from HBeAg to hepatitis B envelope antibody (anti-HBe) results in a reduction in HBV DNA and suggests resolution of HBV infection. Some patients may, however, continue to have active liver disease and detectable serum HBV DNA levels as a result of the presence of wild-type virus or the presence of precore or promoter mutations that impair HBeAg secretion (HBeAg-negative patients).

Hepatitis B core antigen does not circulate freely in the bloodstream and is not measured. Anti-HBc, the antibody directed against HBcAg, is usually detected 1 to 2 weeks after the appearance of HBsAg and just before the onset of clinical symptoms, and it persists for life. The detection of IgM anti-HBc is the most sensitive diagnostic test for acute HBV infection. During the recovery phase of infection, the predominant form of anti-HBc is in the IgG class. The presence of this antibody suggests prior or ongoing infection with HBV. Furthermore, in areas where HBV is not endemic, isolated detection of anti-HBc in a patient's serum may correlate with low levels of HBV DNA. The presence of HBV DNA may enhance the risk of transmission of HBV and progression to cirrhosis and hepatocellular carcinoma. Patients immunized against HBV do not develop anti-HBc; therefore, the presence of this antibody differentiates successful vaccination from actual HBV infection.

Natural History

Of those patients with acute HBV infection, only 1% develops fulminant hepatic failure (FHF).[35,71,73,90] These patients generally have coagulopathy, encephalopathy, and cerebral edema.[35,90] The cause of fulminant infection is a heightened immune response to the virus, provided that HDV or HCV coinfections are ruled out. Patients with acute liver failure often have early clearance of HBsAg, which may complicate the diagnosis, but a positive IgM antibody to HBcAg generally confirms the diagnosis.

Generally, four phases of HBV infection can be determined: immune tolerance, immune clearance, low level replication or nonreplication phase (inactive carrier), and reactivation phase. Up to 12% (average 5%) of immunocompetent patients acutely infected with HBV remain chronically infected (historically defined as detectable HBsAg in serum for 6 months or longer) (Fig. 73-3B).[71,78,90,91] In these patients, HBsAg generally remains detectable indefinitely and anti-HBs fails to appear. The risk of chronicity following neonatally acquired infection is high (>90%), possibly because neonates have immature immune systems. Of infected neonates, 50% have evidence of active viral replication. Furthermore, patients who have a reduced ability to clear viral infections—including those receiving chronic hemodialysis, immunosuppression following transplantation, chemotherapy, or patients with HIV infection—may have a greater risk for developing chronic HBV infection.[71,92] The outcomes of these patients are mainly determined by the presence or absence of viral replication and by the severity of liver damage.[92,93] Approximately 50% of all chronic carriers have ongoing viral replication, especially with elevated aminotransferases, and 15% to 20% of these develop cirrhosis within 5 years.[71,78,92,93] Spontaneous loss of HBeAg (7% –20%/year) has been reported, possibly as a result of the use of antiviral therapy, whereas loss of HBsAg occurs less frequently (1%–2%/year). In general, chronic carriers remain infected throughout their entire life.[41,88,89] In one study, the 5-year survival rate was 97% in patients with early histologic changes, including chronic persistent hepatitis (in which inflammation is limited to the portal areas), compared with 86% in patients with chronic active hepatitis (in which liver cell necrosis and inflammation are present in the hepatic parenchyma) and 55% in patients with documented cirrhosis.[94] Asymptomatic HBV carriers tend to have mild disease manifestations with few complications, even with a long period of follow-up. Finally, the risk of hepatocellular carcinoma (HCC) is increased up to 300 times in chronic carriers with active viral replication (HBeAg-positive).[95,96]

Clinical Manifestations

6. W.H. is a 35-year-old man who developed nausea, vomiting, anorexia, scleral icterus, and jaundice within the past month. Within the past week he became increasingly lethargic, confused, disoriented, and lapsed into a coma. He is admitted to the ED, intubated, and transferred to the intensive care unit (ICU).

W.H.'s social history is significant for IV drug use for the past 10 years and alcohol abuse (none for the previous 5 years). Physical findings include an older-than-age-appearing, hypertensive (blood pressure [BP], 158/99 mmHg), bradycardic (heart rate (HR), 58 beats/minute) man in respiratory distress (respiratory rate (RR), 26 breaths/minute) with severe jaundice, scleral icterus, and decreased hepatic dullness to percussion (reduced hepatic mass). He shows sluggish pupillary response and increasing muscle tone; neurologic examination reveals him to be stuporous and nonarousable.

The laboratory evaluation shows the following results: Hct, 42%; Hgb, 14 g/dL; platelets, 85,000/mm^3 (normal, 150,000–300,000/mm^3); PT, 25.8 sec (control, 12 sec), international normalized ratio (INR), 3.8; AST, 555 U/L (normal, 5–40 U/L); ALT, 495 U/L (normal, 5–40 U/L); alkaline phosphatase, 101 U/mL (normal, 21–91 U/mL); and total bilirubin, 8.4 mg/dL (normal, 0.1–1.2 mg/dL). Hepatitis serologic tests are positive for HBsAg, HBeAg, IgM anti-HBc, and HBV DNA. IgM anti-HAV, IgM anti-HDV, and anti-HCV are negative. STAT blood gases reveal a metabolic acidosis with a compensatory respiratory alkalosis. W.H.'s serum creatinine is 1.8 mg/dL (normal, 0.5–1.2 mg/dL) with a recent reduction in urine output.

What clinical findings does W.H. have that support the diagnosis of acute hepatitis and acute liver failure?

[SI units: Hct, 0.42; Hgb, 140 g/L; AST, 555 U/L (normal, 5–40); ALT, 495 U/L (normal, 5–40); alkaline phosphatase, 101 U/L (normal, 21–91); total bilirubin, 143.6 μmol/L (normal, 1.7–20.5)]

The clinical features of acute HBV infection are similar to those described for HAV infection. W.H.'s initial symptoms included a recent history of nausea, vomiting, anorexia, scleral icterus, and jaundice. These are consistent with diagnosis of acute hepatitis B. His serologies, notably a positive IgM anti-HBc and HBV DNA, also support this diagnosis.

Acute Liver Failure

The most significant complication of acute HBV infection is acute liver failure (ALF), defined as the onset of hepatic encephalopathy within 8 weeks of the onset of symptoms (Table 73-7).[36,73,78,90] W.H. has several symptoms consistent with ALF. These include recent onset of hepatic encephalopathy, lethargy, confusion, coma, coagulopathy, hemodynamic instability, declining liver function, and acidosis. Patients with ALF often have cerebral edema

Table 73-7 Principal Causes of Acute Liver Failure

Cause	Agents Responsible
Viral hepatitis	Hepatitis A, B, C, D, E virus
Toxins	Carbon tetrachloride
	Amanita phalloides
	Phosphorus
Vascular events	Ischemia
	Veno-occlusive disease
	Heatstroke
	Malignant infiltration
Miscellaneous	Wilson disease
	Acute fatty-liver of pregnancy
	Reyes syndrome
Drug-related injury	Acetaminophen
	Idiosyncratic

(80% mortality rate), a complication of a disrupted blood–brain barrier that allows protein-rich fluid to cross into the extracellular spaces of the brain tissue leading to edema and increased intracranial pressure (ICP) (vasogenic model). Toxins also can induce cerebral damage, edema, and subsequent increases in ICP in patients with an intact blood–brain barrier (cytotoxic model) (Table 73-7). Clinical symptoms (sluggish pupillary response and increasing muscle tone) develop when the ICP >30 mmHg.[36,73,78,90,97–99] Cerebral edema in the confinement of the cranial vault raises the ICP, which may reduce intracerebral perfusion. The edema can result in cerebral ischemia if the cerebral-perfusion pressure (CPP) (systemic blood pressure minus ICP) is not maintained >40 mmHg.

W.H. has symptoms of cerebral edema and may benefit from 100 to 200 mL of a 20% solution of mannitol (0.3–0.4 g/kg) administered by rapid IV infusion to induce an osmotic diuresis with a subsequent decrease in ICP. The dose may be repeated at least once after several hours.[36,73,78,98,99] Because W.H. also has a BP of 158/99 mmHg, a HR of 58 beats/minute, and is at risk for intracranial hemorrhage, an ICP monitoring device should be placed.[36,90,100,101] Although placement of this device is invasive, and bleeding is a potential complication, ICP monitoring devices provide important prognostic information. Patients with a CPP >40 mmHg that is refractory to mannitol therapy are not candidates for liver transplantation.

W.H. also has a coagulopathy typical of ALF. Decreased levels of clotting factors II, V, VII, IX, and X normally synthesized by the liver account for his prolonged PT and elevated INR.[36,90,102] In addition, consumption of clotting factors by low-grade disseminated intravascular coagulation (DIC) is common in ALF. W.H. is also thrombocytopenic and at risk for GI ulceration.[36,90,98] A platelet transfusion should be considered if his counts drop to <50,000/mm^3. Since he is not actively bleeding, fresh frozen plasma is not indicated at this time.[36,90,103]

W.H. also should be monitored for cardiovascular and renal abnormalities as a result of his ALF.[36,90,98] These resemble those associated with cirrhosis and septic shock in certain respects, but differ in others. Although W.H. is hypertensive, most patients with ALF are hypotensive and hypovolemic and present with interstitial edema owing to low levels of oncotic proteins. Functional renal failure, also known as hepatorenal syndrome (HRS) or acute tubular necrosis (ATN), occurs in 43% to 55% of patients with ALF.[36,90] In HRS, renal blood flow is reduced, renin and aldosterone levels are increased, and levels of atrial natriuretic factor are unchanged.[104]

As seen in W.H., patients may develop acid-base disturbances, including respiratory alkalosis as a result of central nervous system (CNS)-mediated hyperventilation or a lactic acid-induced metabolic acidosis.[36,90] Hyponatremia, hypokalemia, hypocalcemia, hypomagnesemia, hypoglycemia, and pancreatitis are additional findings associated with ALF. Thus, sodium, potassium, calcium, magnesium, blood glucose, and amylase should be monitored closely in W.H.[36,90] Finally, pulmonary complications (hypoxemia, aspiration, adult respiratory distress syndrome [ARDS], and pulmonary edema) or sepsis (bacterial, fungal) occur in patients with ALF.[36,90,98]

Prognosis

7. What is W.H.'s prognosis?

Although the incidence of ALF is <1%, the prognosis for these patients is poor once encephalopathy has developed.[36,90,98,105] Survival depends on the etiology and degree of hepatic destruction, the ability of the remaining liver cells to regenerate, and the management of complications that may develop during the course of illness. Survival rates often depend on the etiology of ALF. In one series, patients with non-A, non-B hepatitis and halothane or drug hepatotoxicity had worse survival rates (20% and 12.5%, respectively) compared with those with hepatitis A, hepatitis B, or acetaminophen overdose (66.7%, 38.9%, and 52.9% survival, respectively).[105] Age <14 years, worsening grade of encephalopathy, reduced liver size, and significantly abnormal LFT values (e.g., serum bilirubin, aminotransferases, alkaline phosphatase, PT, and serum albumin) also are poor prognostic indicators in patients with ALF (Table 73-8).[36,105] Because W.H. has evidence of encephalopathy, cerebral edema, and abnormal LFT values, he has a poor prognosis (Table 73-8).

Table 73-8 Criteria for Predicting Death and the Need for Liver Transplantation in Patients With Acute Liver Failure

Cause of Acute Liver Failure	Criteria
Acetaminophen poisoning	pH <7.3 (irrespective of grade of encephalopathy)
	OR
	PT >100 sec *AND*
	Serum creatinine >3.4 mg/dL (300 μmol/L) in patients with grade III or grade IV encephalopathy
All other causes	PT >100 secs
	OR
	Any three of the following variables (irrespective of grade of encephalopathy):
	Age <10 yrs or >40 yrs; liver failure caused by non-A, non-B hepatitis, halothane-induced hepatitis, or idiosyncratic drug reactions; duration of jaundice before encephalopathy >7 days;
	PT >50 secs; serum bilirubin >17.5 mg/dL (300 μmol/L)

PT, prothrombin time.
From reference 105, with permission.

Treatment

8. **Outline an appropriate treatment plan for W.H.'s ALF.**

The primary therapy for ALF is supportive care for the comatose patient. Systemic therapies with heparin, prostaglandin, or insulin and glucagon have shown limited efficacy.[36,90] Blood or plasma exchange, hemodialysis, or other methods implemented to detoxify the blood or improve the coma grade do not result in long-term benefits if liver mass is not reconstituted as well. Thiopental may be useful in lowering ICP, but corticosteroids and prolonged hyperventilation are of no value.[36,90] W.H. could benefit from prophylactic H_2-blockers because they have been shown to reduce the incidence of upper GI hemorrhage.[36,90] Blood products (packed red blood cells, fresh frozen plasma, or platelets) should be given as needed if W.H. develops active bleeding, and pulmonary artery monitoring should be implemented to guide management of intravascular volume and gas exchange. W.H. should be closely monitored for additional complications, especially cardiac abnormalities (arrhythmias), hemodynamic changes, renal failure, acidosis, pulmonary complications, and sepsis.

In cases in which prognostic information indicates <20% chance of survival without transplantation, liver transplantation is indicated (Table 73-8). In patients with acetaminophen poisoning resulting in ALF, a pH <7.3, a PT >100 seconds and a serum creatinine >3.4 mg/dL, with grade III or IV encephalopathy usually require transplantation.[105,106] Other causes of ALF, a PT >50 seconds, or any three of the following variables (irrespective of grade of encephalopathy): age <10 years or >40 years; liver failure caused by non-A, non-B hepatitis, halothane-induced hepatitis, or idiosyncratic drug reactions; duration of jaundice before encephalopathy >7 days or serum bilirubin >17.5 mg/dL indicate a need for transplantation.[105,106] Several strategies to prevent death have been used before liver transplantation with some success. These include hepatic assist devices (e.g., bioartificial liver), auxiliary partial heterotopic transplants, and partial liver graft from living related donors.[36,90]

Extrahepatic Manifestations

9. **What are the extrahepatic manifestations of acute or chronic HBV infection?**

Extrahepatic manifestations, such as arthralgias, rash, angioneurotic edema, and polyarteritis nodosa, have been reported in patients with acute or chronic HBV infection.[71,78] Chronic and, to a lesser extent, acute HBV infection have been associated with immune complex-associated membranoproliferative glomerulonephritis. Neurologic complications of HBV infection include Guillain-Barré syndrome and polyneuropathy. Pericarditis and pancreatitis are infrequent complications of HBV infection. Additional complications of chronic HBV infection include portal hypertension with variceal and esophageal bleeding, encephalopathy, ascites, spontaneous bacterial peritonitis, and hepatorenal syndrome. Although HCC is not considered extrahepatic, many patients with HBV may develop HCC.[71,78,96]

Coinfection with other viruses has been reported in patients with HBV infection. For example, markers of prior or active HBV infection are present in >80% of patients with acquired immunodeficiency syndrome (AIDS), with approximately 10% of these cases seropositive for HBsAg.[107] HIV has also been reported to coexist in up to 13% of patients with chronic HBV infection.[108] Compared with patients with HBV infection alone, patients coinfected with HBV and HIV have significantly higher levels of viral replication, lower ALT levels, and less severe histologic disease. HBV infection does not reduce survival in HIV-positive patients; however, because these patients live longer, hepatic decompensation and manifestations of HBV may occur.

Prevention of Hepatitis B

Comprehensive strategies should be implemented to prevent and maintain protection against HBV infection and should be widely available to eliminate transmission that occurs during infancy and childhood as well as during adolescence and adulthood. Thus, alterations in sexual behavior, screening of high-risk patients or settings (e.g., STD and HIV testing and treatment facilities, drug abuse treatment and prevention settings, heath care settings targeting services to intravenous drug users, heath care settings targeting services to men having sex with men, and correctional facilities) and blood products, developing needle exchange programs, and cultural outreach and education may have an impact on HBV transmission. The goals of preventive therapy should be to identify all persons who require immunoprophylaxis for the prevention of infection and provide long-term protection through vaccination to decrease the risk of chronic HBV infection and its subsequent complications, as well as minimizing adverse effects and cost of therapy.

Pre-exposure Prophylaxis

10. **P.G., a 55-year-old nursing student, is going to start her clinical rotations. She has no history of hepatitis and has not yet been immunized. She is 5 feet 2 inches and weighs 80 kg. What prophylactic regimen should P.G. receive to prevent hepatitis secondary to HBV?**

The available vaccines are manufactured using recombinant DNA technology. Both Recombivax HB (10 mg HBsAg/mL) and Engerix-B (20 mg HBsAg/mL) are yeast-derived HBV vaccines that induce an immunologic response similar to the plasma-derived vaccine (no longer used). Because P.G. will come in contact with potentially infectious bodily secretions during her rotations, she should be immunized against hepatitis B with either Recombivax HB or Engerix-B.

DOSING REGIMEN

The recommended doses of available hepatitis B vaccines are shown in Table 73-9.[109–111] The preferred vaccination schedule uses a three-dose regimen. The first dose is followed 1 month later by a second dose, and the third dose is administered 6 months after the initial dose. The first two doses function as priming doses, inducing antibody to HB surface antigen (anti-HBs) in >85% of healthy persons. The third dose serves as a booster dose, significantly increasing the anti-HBs titer and conferring optimal protection (>90%). The third dose can be administered up to 12 months after the initial dose with comparable efficacy. A four-dose series has been approved for high-risk patients in whom rapid protection is desired. If this schedule is followed, the fourth dose at 12 months is necessary to ensure protective antibody titers.

Table 73-9 Recommended Doses of Currently Licensed Hepatitis B Vaccines[a]

	Recombivax HB		Engerix-B	
Group	Dose (μg)	(mL)	Dose (μg)	(mL)
Birth to 10 yrs	—	—	10	(0.5)
Birth to 19 yrs	5	(0.5)	—	—
Children and adolescents 11–19 yrs	—	—	10	(0.5)
Adolescents 11–15 yrs[b]	10	(1.0)	—	—
Adults >20 yrs	10	(1.0)	20	(1.0)
Dialysis patients and other immunocompromised hosts	40	(1.0)	40[c]	(2.0)

[a] One dose administered three times: at time 0, 1 month, and 6 months.
[b] One dose administered: two times 0 and 4–6 months.
[c] Two 1.0-mL doses administered at one site, in a four-dose schedule at 0, 1, 2, and 6 months.
From references 109–111, with permission.

The recommended doses for the yeast-derived recombinant hepatitis B vaccines were based on dose-response studies that determined the optimal dose necessary to achieve protective antibody titers. Dose-response studies with Recombivax HB in healthy adults using 1.25, 2.5, 5, 10, and 20 mcg of HBsAg all elicited an immune response. Those patients receiving the 10- or 20-mcg dose developed substantially higher antibody titers than those receiving lower doses. No significant difference was observed between the 10- and 20-mcg dose; thus, the 10-mcg dose was selected as the standard adult dose of Recombivax HB. Similar analyses were performed to determine the 5-mcg adolescent and pediatric dosage. Dose-response trials with Engerix-B demonstrated an optimal immune response at higher dosages. The reason for the differing doses necessary to elicit an adequate immune response is unknown. Some have speculated that differences in the manufacturing process (yeast culture, purification methods) may influence the immunogenicity of the final product. For this reason, hepatitis B vaccines produced by different manufacturers may not be equally immunogenic on a microgram-for-microgram basis.[112] Relative potency comparisons are not clinically important because comparative trials using Recombivax HB and Engerix-B in the recommended dosages have demonstrated equivalent immunogenicity and tolerability. P.G. can be immunized with either product, provided she receives the manufacturer's recommended dosage with each injection.

Hepatitis B vaccine should be administered as an IM injection in the deltoid muscle of adults and children or in the anterolateral thigh muscle of neonates and infants. The immunogenicity of hepatitis B vaccine is significantly lower when injections are given in the buttocks, probably because the greater amount of fat tissue in the buttocks inhibits interfacing of vaccine and antigen-recognition leukocytes. The results of a small vaccination series suggest that healthy adults who do not respond to HBV injection to the buttocks have a significantly higher response when vaccinated in the arm. P.G. should be immunized with either Recombivax HB (10 mcg) or Engerix-B (20 mcg) administered as a 1-mL IM injection in the deltoid muscle.

EFFICACY

Recombinant yeast-derived vaccines (e.g., Recombivax HB, Engerix-B) produce similar results.[113] Although a measurable immune response is readily achieved with the current HBV vaccine, a quantitative titer of circulating anti-HBs necessary to prevent infection has not been clearly substantiated. A protective antibody response has been defined as anti-HBs levels ≥10 mIU/mL.[111] This threshold was derived from early HBV vaccine trials in homosexual men, where vaccine recipients with serum antibody levels ≥10 sample ratio units (SRU) were protected from HBV infection.[114–117] A serum antibody level of 10 SRU is roughly equivalent to 10 mIU/mL when the international standard is used. For this reason, an anti-HBs level of ≥10 mIU/mL is considered a protective antibody titer and is the standard used by the US ACIP. Although HBV infections have occurred in vaccine recipients with a detectable immune response, almost all infections have been asymptomatic, identified only through the presence of anti-HBc. These infections have been limited largely to patients with no response or a poor response to vaccination.[116]

NONRESPONDERS

11. P.G. has completed her three-dose vaccination series with Engerix-B. Routine hepatitis serology testing, performed before volunteering for a drug study, reveals that P.G. is anti-HBs negative. Why did P.G. not respond to the hepatitis B vaccine, and how should she be managed?

Two important determinants of vaccine efficacy appear to be the age at vaccination and underlying immune function. In healthy recipients, the immune response to vaccination decreases with advancing age. In one study, 99% of patients age 0 to 19 years, 93% of those age 20 to 49 years, and 73% of those >50 years of age achieved protective anti-HBs levels (>10 SRU) after three doses of the hepatitis B vaccine.[118] Immunocompromised patients, including those receiving hemodialysis,[119] those infected with HIV,[120] or children receiving cytotoxic chemotherapy,[121] respond poorly to the HBV vaccine. Patients who smoke[122–124] or are obese[122,123] also have a reduced response. P.G. has two risk factors for a poor response to the hepatitis B vaccine: she is >50 years of age and she is moderately obese (ideal body weight for her height is 50 kg).

Vaccine recipients who respond poorly to hepatitis B vaccine have been classified either as hyporesponders who can probably be protected by additional doses of vaccine or as true nonresponders. Patients with inadequate initial response to the HBV vaccine series should be revaccinated. Of hyporesponders (anti-HBs levels <10 mIU/mL), 50% to 90% develop a protective level following a single booster injection[125,126] or after repeating the entire three-dose series.[121,129] Of patients not responding to a primary vaccination series with Engerix B, 60% produced an immune response after a three-dose series with HBVax II (Recombivax), suggesting a repeat course with the alternative HBV vaccine may be a reasonable approach in some patients.[127] Revaccination of nonresponders (no detectable anti-HBs) is less successful, and protective levels, if achieved, are not sustained.[128] True nonresponders to HBV vaccination are rare in the immunocompetent population, and these persons may have a genetic predisposition toward nonresponsiveness.[129] P.G. should be revaccinated with a booster dose of hepatitis B vaccine. Her anti-HBs levels can be rechecked 1 month after the injection. If she still has not responded, it is reasonable to administer an additional two injections to complete a second vaccination series.

INTERCHANGEABILITY OF HBV VACCINES

12. T.M., a 32-year-old hospital laboratory technician, received the first two doses of hepatitis B vaccine with Recombivax HB. He has relocated recently and is due for the third injection. The employee health service at his new job uses only Engerix-B for hepatitis B vaccination. Can hepatitis B vaccines produced by different manufacturers be used interchangeably?

Although it is recommended that patients receive the complete vaccination series with the same product, data suggest this is not absolutely necessary to induce a protective antibody titer. In a study to determine whether a hepatitis B vaccination series initiated with Recombivax HB could be completed with Engerix-B, healthy adults received 10 mcg of Recombivax HB at baseline and 1 month. At 6 months, the subjects were randomized to receive either Engerix-B 20 mcg or Recombivax HB 10 mcg. One month after the third dose, 100% of those who had received Engerix-B and 92% of those who had received Recombivax HB had protective anti-HBs levels.[130]

Chan et al.[131] studied the booster response to either recombinant hepatitis B vaccine or plasma-derived vaccine in children who had been vaccinated originally with the plasma-derived product (Heptavax-B). Children were randomized to either 5 mcg of the plasma-derived vaccine or 20 mcg of Engerix-B. One month after the booster injection, all vaccine recipients had significant elevations in their anti-HBs titers, suggesting recombinant hepatitis B vaccines elicit an adequate booster response in persons who originally received the plasma-derived vaccine.[131] According to the ACIP, the immune response from one or two doses of a vaccine produced by one manufacturer, when followed by subsequent doses from a different manufacturer, is comparable with that resulting from a full course of vaccination with a single vaccine.[111]

T.M. may complete the hepatitis B vaccine series with Engerix-B provided he receives the recommended dosage of 20 mcg administered as a 1-mL IM injection to the deltoid region. This dose will significantly increase his circulating anti-HBs titer, thus conferring optimal protection from HBV infection.

DURATION OF RESPONSE

13. Does T.M. require a booster injection for sustained protection from HBV infection?

The duration of vaccine-induced immunity has been evaluated in many long-term studies.[117,132–139] The duration of detectable anti-HBs appears proportional to the peak antibody response achieved after vaccination, and protective anti-HBs levels were sustained in 68% to 85% of patients receiving the plasma-derived HBV vaccine in studies with follow-up ranging from 6 to 12 years.[132–136] Importantly, the protective efficacy of the HBV vaccine in these trials was high, even in patients with anti-HBs levels <10 mIU/mL. HBsAg was only rarely detected and most HBV events consisted of asymptomatic seroconversion to anti-HBc. These studies suggest that successful HBV vaccination is associated with long-lasting protection without the need for additional booster doses for up to 12 years.

The mechanism of sustained protection from HBV, despite low or nondetectable anti-HBs levels, is thought to be related to the phenomenon of immunologic memory in previously sensitized B lymphocytes. This amnestic response, in combination with the long incubation period of HBV, may allow the synthesis of protective antibodies sufficiently quickly to block infection in patients rechallenged with HBV.[140]

In summary, no need exists for routine administration of HBV vaccine booster doses to immunocompetent persons following successful vaccination. Immunocompromised patients may require a persistent minimal level of protective antibody, and the ACIP does recommend annual antibody testing for patients receiving chronic hemodialysis with administration of a booster dose when antibody levels are <10 mIU/mL.[111] Based on available evidence, T.M. does not require a scheduled booster dose of hepatitis B vaccine.

INDICATIONS

14. Why is it appropriate for T.M. to be vaccinated with hepatitis B vaccine, and who else should be vaccinated with this vaccine?

The ACIP has recommended pre-exposure hepatitis B vaccination for the following high-risk groups: health care workers with exposure to blood, staff of institutions for the developmentally disabled, hemodialysis patients, recipients of blood products, household and sexual contacts of HBV carriers, international travelers to HBV-endemic areas, injecting drug users, sexually active homosexual men, bisexual men, and inmates of long-term correctional facilities.[111] Because T.M. is a hospital laboratory technician, he is at high risk for exposure to hepatitis B and should be vaccinated.

UNIVERSAL HEPATITIS B VACCINATION

In addition to the previously listed high-risk groups, all infants should receive hepatitis B vaccination. This recommendation is based on data suggesting the practice of vaccinating only high-risk persons had little impact on decreasing the incidence of HBV disease. Populations at risk for HBV disease (injecting drug users, persons with multiple sexual partners) generally are not vaccinated before they begin engaging in high-risk behaviors. In addition, many persons who become infected have no identifiable risk factors for infection and thus would not be recognized as candidates for vaccination. A program designed to immunize children before they initiate high-risk behaviors is likely to have a greater impact in reducing the incidence of HBV infection. As a means to achieve this goal, the hepatitis B vaccine now is incorporated into the existing pediatric vaccination schedule. The first dose is administered during the newborn period (preferably before the infant is discharged from the hospital) but no later than 2 months of age.[111] The recommended vaccination schedule is shown in Table 73-10.

15. R.M. is a mother of two children aged 11 years and 2 months. Her infant daughter just received a second dose of hepatitis B vaccine as part of her routine well-baby care. R.M. wonders if her son, who did not receive the hepatitis B vaccine during his normal childhood immunizations, should receive the vaccine now.

Table 73-10 Recommended Schedules of Hepatitis B Vaccination for Infants Born to HBsAg (−) Mothers

Hepatitis B Vaccine	*Age of Infant*
Option 1	
Dose 1	Birth (before hospital discharge)
Dose 2	1–2 mos[a]
Dose 3	6–18 mos[a]
Option 2	
Dose 1	1–2 mos[a]
Dose 2	4 mos[a]
Dose 3	6–18 mos[a]

[a]Hepatitis B vaccine can be administered simultaneously with diphtheria-tetanus-pertussis, *Haemophilus influenza* type b conjugate, measles-mumps-rubella, and oral polio vaccines.
From reference 111, with permission.

The Centers for Disease Control and Prevention (CDC) has addressed the issue of immunizing children and adolescents born before 1991 who are potentially at risk for hepatitis B infection. The current recommendations suggest that adolescents who have not received three doses of hepatitis B vaccine should initiate or complete the series at ages 11 to 15 years. A schedule of 0, 1 to 2, and 4 to 6 months is recommended.[141] It is anticipated that universal vaccination of all infants and previously unvaccinated adolescents aged 11 to 12 years, in addition to ongoing immunization of high-risk persons, will reduce the incidence of acute hepatitis B infection, hepatitis B-associated chronic liver disease, and HCC. R.M.'s son should receive either Recombivax HB 5 mcg or Engerix-B 10 mcg as an IM in the deltoid with repeat doses 1 to 2 months and 4 to 6 months from the initial injection.

ADVERSE EFFECTS

Hepatitis B virus vaccination generally has been well-tolerated. The most common side effect is pain at the injection site, observed in 3% to 29% of patients. Transient febrile reactions (defined as temperature >99.9°F) occur in <6% of recipients, and other reactions, including nausea, rash, headache, myalgias, and arthralgias, are observed in <1% of recipients. Ongoing monitoring of vaccine safety by the FDA and CDC is assessed through the Vaccine Safety Datalink (VSD) project and Vaccine Adverse Events Reporting System (VAERS). On the basis of these reporting systems, additional "causal" adverse effects associated with vaccination include anaphylaxis (1 case per 1.1 million vaccine doses), Guillain-Barré syndrome, and multiple sclerosis. Additional rare adverse events that have been reported but remain to be validated are chronic fatigue syndrome, neurologic disorders (leukoencephalitis, optic neuritis, and transverse myelitis), rheumatoid arthritis, type 1 diabetes, and autoimmune disease.

Postexposure Prophylaxis

PERCUTANEOUS EXPOSURE

16. K.N., a 26-year-old medical student, presents to the ED after accidentally sticking herself with a contaminated needle while drawing blood from an HBsAg-positive patient. K.N. was not vaccinated previously and had no known prior episodes of hepatitis or liver disease. Her tetanus status is current. She weighs 56 kg. How should K.N. be treated for percutaneous exposure to hepatitis B?

Table 73-11 Guide to Postexposure Immunoprophylaxis for Exposure to Hepatitis B Virus

Type of Exposure	*Immunoprophylaxis*
Perinatal	Vaccination + HBIG[a]
Sexual	Vaccination + HBIG
Household contact	
Chronic carrier	Vaccination
Acute case	None unless known exposure
Acute case, known exposure	HBIG − vaccination
Infant (<12 months) acute case in primary caregiver	HBIG + vaccination
Inadvertent (percutaneous or permucosal)	Vaccination − HBIG

[a]HBIG, hepatitis B immunoglobulin.
From references 111 and 143, with permission.

Following exposure to HBV, prophylactic treatment with hepatitis B vaccination and possibly passive immunization with hepatitis B immunoglobulin (HBIG) should be considered. The ACIP recommendations for postexposure immunoprophylaxis following hepatitis B exposure are shown in Table 73-11.

K.N.'s percutaneous exposure warrants active immunization with HBV and passive immunization with HBIG. The source of K.N.'s exposure is HBsAg-positive, and K.N. had not been vaccinated previously with the hepatitis B vaccine. She should receive a single dose of HBIG 0.06 mL/kg (3.4 mL) as an IM injection in either the gluteal or deltoid region as soon as possible after exposure, preferably within 24 hours. HBIG is prepared from plasma of persons preselected for high titer anti-HBs. The anti-HBs of HBIG in the United States is 1:100,000 as determined by radioimmunoassay. HBIG is superior to immunoglobulin in the prevention of hepatitis B infection following percutaneous exposure. K.N. also should receive active immunization with IM hepatitis B vaccine (at a separate site) simultaneously with HBIG. The second and third doses should be given 1 month and 6 months later. Passively acquired antibodies against hepatitis B virus from HBIG or immunoglobulin will not interfere with active immunization via hepatitis B vaccine.[142]

If the HBsAg status of the donor source of a percutaneous exposure is unknown, recommendations for prophylaxis of HBV infection depend on whether the donor source is at high risk or at low risk for being HBsAg-positive. High-risk donor sources include homosexual men, IV drug abusers, patients undergoing hemodialysis, residents of mental institutions, immigrants from endemic areas, and household contacts of HBV carriers. Additional ACIP recommendations for hepatitis B prophylaxis following percutaneous exposure are shown in Table 73-12.

SEXUAL EXPOSURE

17. What are the current recommendations for a person who has had sexual contact with an HBsAg-positive person?

Table 73-12 Recommendations for Hepatitis B Prophylaxis Following Percutaneous Exposure[111]

	Treatment When Source Is Found to Be		
Exposed Person	*HBsAg-Positive*	*HBsAg-Negative*	*Unknown or Not Tested*
Unvaccinated	Administer HBIG × 1[a] and initiate hepatitis vaccine	Initiate hepatitis B vaccine[b]	Initiate hepatitis B vaccine[b]
Previously vaccinated			
Known responder	Test exposed person for anti-HBs[c] 1. If inadequate, hepatitis B vaccine booster dose 2. If adequate, no treatment	No treatment	No treatment
Known responder	HBIG × 1[a] as soon as possible, repeat in 1 month *OR* HBIG × 1[a] plus one dose of hepatitis B vaccine	No treatment	If known high-risk source, may treat as if source were HBsAg positive
Response unknown	Test exposed person for anti-HBs[c] 1. If inadequate, HBIG × 1[a] plus hepatitis B vaccine booster dose 2. If adequate, no treatment	No treatment	Test exposed person for anti-HBs[c] 1. If inadequate, hepatitis B vaccine booster dose 2. If adequate, no treatment

[a]HBIG dose 0.06 mL/kg given intramuscular (IM).
[b]For dosing information, see Table 73-9.
[c]Adequate anti-HBs is ≥10 mIU.
HBIG, hepatitis B immunoglobulin.

Sexual transmission of hepatitis B is an important cause of HBV infection, accounting for approximately 30% to 60% of all new cases annually.[143] Passive immunization with a single 5-mL dose of HBIG was found highly effective in preventing hepatitis B infection following sexual exposure when compared with a control globulin (with no anti-HBs activity).[144] The CDC recommends that susceptible persons exposed to HBV through sexual contact with a person who has acute or chronic HBV infection should receive postexposure prophylaxis with 0.06 mL/kg of HBIG as a single IM dose within 14 days of the last exposure. Patients also should receive the standard three-dose immunization series with hepatitis B vaccine beginning at the time of HBIG administration.[143]

PERINATAL EXPOSURE

18. S.L., a 3.2-kg boy, was just born to an HBsAg-positive mother. Is S.L. at risk for acquiring HBV infection, and how should he be treated?

In many Asian and developing countries, perinatal (vertical) transmission accounts for most hepatitis B infections. Infants born to HBV-infected mothers have a >85% risk of acquiring HBV during the perinatal period. Of those who become infected, 80% to 90% become chronic HBsAg carriers.[145–147] Although fulminant cases have been reported, most hepatitis infections in neonates are asymptomatic. Despite the usually innocuous initial disease, significant adverse consequences are associated with chronic HBsAg carriage in neonates. Chronic hepatitis B infection is associated with chronic liver disease and has been clearly implicated as a major risk factor in the development of primary HCC.[148,149]

Mothers who are chronic carriers of hepatitis B, although not acutely infected, pose the risk of transmitting the hepatitis B virus to their infants. The risk is related to the presence of HBsAg and HBeAg (suggesting a high degree of viral replication and infectivity). The likelihood that S.L. will develop HBV infection is high. S.L. requires immediate therapy with HBIG (to provide immediate high titers of circulating anti-HBs) and simultaneous vaccination with hepatitis B vaccine (to induce long-lasting protective immunity). Screening pregnant women for the presence of HBeAg and administration of HBIG and hepatitis B vaccine is 85% to 98% effective in preventing HBV infection and the chronic carrier state.[145,147,150] This compares with a 71% efficacy rate for administration of HBIG alone. Simultaneous administration of HBIG and hepatitis B vaccine does not adversely affect the production of anti-HBs in neonates.[145,147]

Infants born to mothers who are HBsAg positive should receive simultaneous IM injections of the appropriate doses of hepatitis B vaccine (Table 73-9) and HBIG (0.5 mL) within 12 hours of birth. The injections should be administered at separate sites. S.L. should receive HBIG (0.5 mL) as soon as possible after birth, administered as an IM injection. He also should receive 0.5 mL of either Recombivax HB (5 mcg) or Engerix-B (10 mcg) as an IM injection at a separate site.

19. What would the management plan be if the HBsAg status of S.L.'s mother was unknown?

The ACIP has developed recommendations for the prevention of perinatal HBV infection. This includes the routine testing of all pregnant women for HBsAg during an early prenatal visit. HBsAg testing should be repeated late in the pregnancy for women who are HBsAg-negative but who are at high risk of HBV infection or who have had clinically apparent hepatitis. Women admitted for delivery who have not had prenatal HBsAg testing should have blood drawn for testing. While test results are pending, the infant should receive hepatitis B vaccine within 12 hours of birth (Table 73-9). If the mother is found later to be HBsAg-positive, her infant should receive HBIG as soon as possible within 7 days of birth. The second and third doses of vaccine should be administered at 1 and 6 months, respectively. If the mother is found to be HBsAg-negative, her infant should continue to receive hepatitis B vaccine as part of the routine vaccination series.[111]

Evaluation and Management of Patients with Chronic HBV Infection

20. E.A. is a 55-year-old woman who presents to the hepatology clinic with a recent history of mild jaundice. Her previous medical history is unremarkable except for a blood transfusion she received during child birth in 1988. What initial and follow-up tests should be performed to assess the extent of HBV infection in E.A.?

The evaluation of patients infected with chronic HBV is described in Table 73-13. Initially, a thorough history and physical examination should be performed with greater emphasis placed on risk factors for coinfection, alcohol use, and family history of HBV and liver cancer. Laboratory tests should include assessment of liver disease, markers of HBV replication, and screening tests for HCV, HDV, or HIV. Vaccinations for hepatitis A should also be administered as described above. The decision to perform a liver biopsy should be made based on knowledge of a patient's age, the ALT level, HBeAg status, HBV DNA levels, and additional clinical features suggestive of chronic liver disease or portal hypertension. In patients who are not initially considered for treatment (inactive HBV carriers), an algorithm for follow-up based on HBeAg status is described in Table 73-13. Periodic screening for HCC should also be performed in high-risk populations such as Asian men >40 and Asian women >50 years of age, persons with cirrhosis, persons with a family history of HCC, blacks>20 years of age, and any carrier >40 years of age with persistent or intermittent ALT or HBV DNA elevations.

Table 73-13 Evaluation of Patients With Chronic Hepatitis B

Initial evaluation
History and physical examination
Family history of liver disease, hepatocellular carcinoma
Laboratory tests to assess liver disease (CBC, platelets, ALT, AST, bilirubin, prothrombin time/INR) and biopsy
Tests for HBV replication (HBeAg/anti-HBe, HBV DNA)
Tests to rule out coinfection (anti-HCV, anti-HDV, anti-HIV)
Tests to screen for HCC (AFP, and ultrasound for high-risk patients)
Suggested followup for patients not considered for treatment (HBeAg +, HBV DNA >20,000 IU/mL and normal ALT
ALT every 3–6 months, increasing frequency if ALT becomes elevated.
If ALT > 2 × ULN, recheck ALT every 1 to 3 months; consider liver biopsy if age >40, ALT borderline or mildly elevated on serial tests. Consider treatment if biopsy shows moderate or severe inflammation or significant fibrosis.
If ALT >2 × ULN for 3–6 months and HBeAg+, HBV DNA >20,000 IU/mL, consider liver biopsy and treatment.
Consider screening for HCC in relevant population.
Inactive HBsAg carrier
ALT every 3 months for 1 year, if persistently normal, ALT every 6–12 months
If ALT >1 to 2 × ULN, check serum HBV DNA level and exclude other causes of liver disease. Consider liver biopsy if ALT borderline or mildly elevated in serial tests or if HBV DNA persistently >20,000 IU/mL. Consider treatment if biopsy shows moderate or severe inflammation or significant fibrosis.
Consider screening for HCC in relevant population.

ALT, alanine aminotransferase; APF, α-fetoprotein; AST, aspartate aminotransferase; CBC, complete blood count; HCC, hepatocellular carcinoma; INR, international normalized ratio; ULN, upper limit of normal
From references 72, 73, with permission.

21. C.R., a 28-year-old man, presents to the ED with jaundice, complaints of incapacitating fatigue, and vague intermittent abdominal pain for the past month. C.R. was diagnosed with hepatitis B 2 years before admission. His social history includes IV drug abuse (none for 2 years) and alcohol abuse (none for 2 years). Several weeks ago, C.R. noted darkening of his urine and yellowing of his eyes.

Physical examination reveals a thin man in no apparent distress. He is afebrile, and his BP, HR, and RR are within normal limits. Moderate scleral icterus is noted. The abdomen is soft and nondistended. The liver is enlarged, nontender, and smooth with an edge palpable 5 cm below the costal margin and a span of 15 cm. The spleen is palpable. The cardiac, pulmonary, neurologic, and extremity examinations all are within normal limits.

C.R.'s laboratory evaluation is significant for Hct, 44%; Hgb, 15 g/dL; WBC count, 8.8 cells/mm^3; platelets, 225,000/mm^3 (normal, 150,000–300,000/mm^3); PT, 15.4 sec (control, 12 sec), INR, 1.8; AST, 326 U/L (normal, 5–40 U/L); ALT, 382 U/L (normal, 5–U/L); alkaline phosphatase, 142 U/mL (normal, 21–91 U/L); total bilirubin, 4.2 mg/dL (normal, 0.1–1.2 mg/dL); and albumin, 2.8 g/dL (normal, 3.5–4.5 g/dL). Hepatitis serologic tests are positive for HBsAg, HBeAg, and anti-HBc and negative for IgM anti-HBc, IgM anti-HAV, and anti-HCV. HBV DNA is reported as <200 pg/mL. A liver biopsy reveals periportal inflammation as well as piecemeal and bridging necrosis. What clinical findings does C.R. have that support the diagnosis of chronic hepatitis B infection?

[SI units: Hct, 0.44; Hgb, 150 g/L; WBC count, 8.8× 10^3 cells/L; AST, 326 U/L (normal, 5–40); ALT, 382 U/L (normal, 5–40); alkaline phosphatase, 142 U/L (normal, 21–91); total bilirubin, 71.8 μmol/L (normal, 1.7–20.5); albumin, 28 g/L (normal, 35–45)]

The chronic occurrence of jaundice and hepatosplenomegaly with significantly elevated AST and ALT in a young patient such as C.R. is suggestive of chronic hepatitis. Although alcoholic hepatitis secondary to long-term alcohol abuse is consistent with these clinical features, his serologic tests are positive for HBV. Hepatitis serology with positive HBsAg and HBeAg suggest ongoing viral replication and a high degree of infectivity.

Serum concentrations of aminotransferases can range from slightly abnormal to greatly elevated, with ALT concentrations generally greater than AST. Serum bilirubin concentrations >3.0 mg/dL are common, serum concentration of alkaline phosphatase usually is increased, and the PT may be prolonged. Patients such as C.R. with a prolonged PT and low serum albumin concentration generally have a more severe form of chronic hepatitis.

Liver biopsy is important for the diagnosis, treatment, and prognosis of patients with chronic hepatitis. C.R.'s liver biopsy reveals the classic triad of periportal inflammation as well as piecemeal and bridging necrosis. The liver biopsy and hepatitis serologic test results are consistent with a diagnosis of chronic hepatitis B infection.

Treatment of chronic HBV infection requires knowledge of the natural history of the untreated disease and the potential benefits of intervention. Currently six agents are approved by the US Food and Drug Administration (FDA) for treating chronic HBV infection.

22. Does C.R. require treatment for chronic hepatitis secondary to hepatitis B?

The decision to treat C.R. depends on the severity of symptoms, the serum biochemistries, and the liver biopsy results. C.R. has evidence of severe chronic HBV infection. He is symptomatic with jaundice, severe fatigue, and abdominal pain, and the results of his LFT and HBV DNA levels suggest his disease is advanced (decreased albumin, elevated PT). Therefore, he should be treated to reduce the replication of HBV, resolve the hepatocellular damage, and prevent long-term adverse hepatic sequelae.

Goals of Therapy

23. What are the goals of therapy for chronic hepatitis secondary to HBV?

Progression of chronic hepatitis to cirrhosis is thought to be related to continued replication of the hepatitis B virus. Loss of active viral replication usually is associated with a decrease in infectivity, a reduction in inflammatory cells within the liver, and a fall of serum aminotransferase activities into the normal range. The disappearance of detectable HBeAg and HBV DNA is considered an indicator of loss of active viral replication.

The goals of therapy in chronic HBV infection are to achieve sustained suppression of HBV replication and remission of liver disease.[72,73] Ultimately, achieving these goals should lead to resolving ongoing hepatocellular damage and reducing the development of cirrhosis and HCC.[72,73] Clinical trials for chronic HBV infection have used the following markers as endpoints for successful therapy: seroconversion from HBeAg-positive to HBeAg-negative (with appearance of anti-HBe), reductions in serum aminotransferase activity, elimination of circulating HBV DNA, and improvement in liver histology. The elimination of HBsAg (termination of HBV carrier state) has been difficult to achieve in clinical trials. Additionally, the responses to antiviral therapy of chronic HBV can be categorized as biochemical (BR), virologic (VR), or histologic (HR), and as on therapy or sustained off therapy (Table 73-14).

Drug Therapy

24. Would initiating therapy during the acute phase of the HBV infection have benefited C.R.?

Pharmacologic interventions in the management of acute hepatitis B have been disappointing. Early studies demonstrated a transient decrease in serum aminotransferase activity and bilirubin concentration associated with corticosteroids. More recent studies, however, have resulted in a higher incidence of relapse, and mortality[152,153] in patients receiving corticosteroids. Other therapies, including Hepatitis B immunglobulin (HBIG)[154] and α-interferon,[155] have been ineffective in managing acute viral hepatitis secondary to HBV. Nucleoside and nucleotide reverse transcriptase inhibitors reduce HBV DNA levels in patients with chronic disease[71,72,74,156–165]; however, their use in acute HBV infection requires further investigation.[156–158] Thus, administration of antivirals during the acute phase of HBV infection is not recommended in C.R.

Table 73-14 Definition of Response to Antiviral Therapy

Category of Response	*Characteristics*
Biochemical Response (BR)	Decrease in serum ALT to within the normal range
Virologic Relapse (VR)	Decrease in serum HBV DNA to undetectable levels by PCR assays, and loss of HBeAg in HBeAg-positive patients
Primary nonresponse (not applicable to IFN therapy)	Decrease in serum HBV DNA by <2 $\log_{10}$ IU/mL after at least 24 weeks of therapy
Virologic Relapse (VR)	Increase in serum HBV DNA of 1 $\log_{10}$ IU/mL after discontinuation of treatment in at least two determinations more than 4 weeks apart
Histologic response (HR)	Decrease in histology activity index by at least 2 points and no worsening of fibrosis score compared with pretreatment liver biopsy
Complete response (CR)	Fulfill criteria of biochemical and virological response and loss of HBsAg
Time of Assessment	
On therapy	During therapy
Maintained	Persist throughout the course of treatment
End of treatment	At the end of a defined course of therapy
Off therapy	After the discontinuation of therapy
Sustained (SR-6)	6 months after discontinuation of therapy
Sustained (SR-12)	12 months after discontinuation of therapy

ALT, alanine aminotransferase; IFN, interferon; PCR, polymerase chain reaction.
From references 72, 73, with permission.

INTERFERONS

25. What drug therapy should C.R. receive to treat chronic HBV-associated infection?

Previously, the most effective agents for treating chronic hepatitis B have been interferons,[166,167] which appear to activate their target cells by binding to specific cell surface receptors to induce synthesis of effector proteins.[168,169] These intracellular proteins induce the antiviral, antiproliferative, and immunomodulatory actions of the interferons. Gene expression, upregulation of NK cells, cytotoxic T cells, and macrophages are induced by interferons.[168,169] Their antiviral activity possibly arises from their ability to abate viral entry into the host cells and modulate several steps of the viral replication cycle (e.g., viral uncoating, inhibition of messenger RNA [mRNA], and protein synthesis). Several varieties of interferons are commercially available (Table 73-15). Interferon-α2b (Intron-A) and pegylated interferon (PegIFN-α2a), remain the only FDA-approved interferons for the treatment of chronic HBV infection. Pegylated interferons are also used for treatment of HCV infection (see section on Hepatitis C). These agents are known to have increased serum half-life resulting in a prolonged antiviral effect, as well as less immunogenicity.

Table 73-15 Comparison of Interferons Used to Treat Viral Hepatitis

Agent[a]	Trade	Source	Indication	Dose/Route	Comments
Interferon-α					
Interferon-α 2a	Roferon-A	Recombinant	HCV	3 MU TIW IM/SC × 12 months	Most commonly used interferon for HCV
Interferon-α 2b	Intron-A	Recombinant	NANB/HCV	3 MU TIW IM/SC × 6 months	Previous standard of care for HCV
Interferon-α n1	NA	Lymphoblastoid	Not FDA approved for HCV	3 MU TIW IM/SC × 12 months	Originally thought to have higher relapse rate versus recombinant interferon-α (6 months); response rate with 12 months of therapy
Interferon-α-con-1	Infergen	Recombinant	HCV	9 mcg TIW SC × 6 months	Has greater *in vitro* effects versus other interferons; proposed enhanced efficacy against HCV type 1 genotype

[a] Interferons may decrease hepatic cytochrome P450 metabolism of drugs.
NA, not applicable; NANB, non-A, non-B hepatitis; IM, intramuscular; SC, subcutaneously; TIW, three times weekly.

Efficacy

Conventional Interferon

Interferon-α is moderately effective in treating chronic hepatitis B in a small percentage of highly selected patients.[170–174] (Table 73-16 and Table 73-17) HBeAg-positive patients with chronic HBV receiving IFN-α may experience a virologic response based on clearance of HBeAg (27%; range, 15%–41%) or HBV DNA (47%; range, 32%–79%) compared with 9% of untreated controls. Normalization of ALT values is observed in 47% of IFN-α–treated patients versus 13% in untreated controls. Clearance of HBsAg occurs in only 10% to 15% of patients after completion of therapy.[170–174] In one long-term follow-up study of patients responding to IFN-α, delayed clearance of HBsAg was observed in 65% of patients 3 years after completion of therapy.[175] Relapse after successful therapy is rare. In another prospective study, 103 patients with chronic hepatitis B treated with 2 to 5 million units (MU) of IFN-α for 4 to 6 months compared with untreated patients demonstrated greater HBeAg and HBsAg clearance rates (56% versus 28% and 11.6% versus 0%, respectively; $P < 0.001$) at 5 years.[176] All patients with loss of HBeAg also lost HBV DNA and had newly detectable anti-HBeAg antibodies. A trend toward greater survival and fewer clinical complications was also seen in the treatment group.

Pegylated Interferon

In a recent phase III trial, results using PegIFN-α2a 180 mcg weekly plus placebo (n = 271), PegIFN-α2a 180 mcg weekly plus lamivudine 100 mg daily (n = 271), or lamivudine 100 mg daily (n = 272) for 48 weeks were compared. Patients were also followed for an additional 24 weeks after the end of therapy.[177] At the end of the 24-week follow-up, significantly more patients who received PegIFN monotherapy or combination therapy than those who received lamivudine monotherapy had HBeAg conversion (32% versus 19%; $P < 0.001$, and 27% versus 19%; $P = 0.02$, respectively). The use of PegIFN-α2a (alone or in combination) also resulted in HBsAg conversion in 16 patients compared to none in the lamivudine monotherapy group ($P = 0.001$). Additionally, at the end of treatment, viral suppression was most evident in the group that received combination therapy. This trial suggests that use of PegIFN-α2a is superior to lamivudine on the basis of HBeAg conversion, HBV DNA suppression, and HBsAg conversion. Similar results were reported in HBeAg-positive patients receiving PegIFN-α2b.[178] In the only published trial performed in 552 HBeAg-negative patients, PegIFN-α2a 180 mcg weekly (n = 177) was compared with either PegIFN-α2a 180 mcg weekly plus 100 mg lamivudine (n = 179) or 100 mg lamivudine alone (n = 181). Viral suppression was greater in the combination group, but sustained response (HBV DNA and ALT levels at week 72) was comparable in the group that received PegIFN-α2a alone (or in combination), and superior to the lamivudine monotherapy group (15%, 16%, and 6%, respectively). Loss of HBsAg occurred in 12 patients in the pegylated interferon groups as compared with none in the lamivudine group. Ultimately, the addition of lamivudine to PegIFN did not affect post therapy response rates in this patient population.[179]

For these reasons, a trial with IFN (including pegylated IFN) is reasonable for C.R. Long-term follow-up data are sparse in their ability to demonstrate reductions in cirrhosis or hepatocellular cancer in patients receiving IFN-α therapy. Studies comparing the outcome of responders versus nonresponders found that patients who cleared HBeAg had better overall survival and survival free of hepatic decompensation; the benefit was most pronounced in patients with cirrhosis.[72,73]

Predictors of Response

26. Is C.R. likely to respond to IFN-α therapy?

Certain patient variables can predict the response to therapy with standard and pegylated IFN-α (Table 73-18). The most reliable predictor of a positive response to IFN-α in HBeAg-positive patients appears to be pretreatment ALT and HBV DNA levels.[71,73,74] Patients with high pretreatment ALT levels (greater than twice the upper limit of normal) and HBV DNA levels <200 pg/mL (roughly equivalent to 56 million copies/mL on a PCR assay) are more likely to respond to therapy than those with higher levels.[71,73,171] In addition, data suggest that HBeAg seroconversion with IFN treatment is associated with improved survival and reduced complications. Other predictors of a positive response include a short duration of disease, negative HIV status, and a high histologic activity index (HAI) as demonstrated by liver biopsy.[71,73,74,175] Currently, some studies also suggest that persons infected with HBV genotypes A and B respond better than those with genotypes C and D.[72,73,178] No consistent predictor of sustained response

Table 73-16 Responses to Approved Antiviral Therapies Among Treatment-Naïve Patients with HBeAg Positive Chronic Hepatitis B

	Standard IFN-α	*Control*	*Lamivudine*	*Placebo*	*Adefovir*	*Placebo*	*Entecavir*	*Telbivudine*	*PegIFN-α*	*PegIFN-α + lamivudine*
	5 MU QD or 10MU TIW (12–24 weeks)		100 mg QD (48–52 weeks)		10 mg QD (48 weeks)		0.5 mg QD (48 weeks)	600 mg QD (52 weeks)	180 mcg QW (48–72 weeks)	180 mcg QW + 100 mg (48–72 weeks)
Loss HBV DNA	37%	17%	40%–44%	16%	21%	0	67%	60%	25%	69%
Loss HBeAg	33%	12%	17%–32%	6%–11%	24%	11%	22%	26%	30%/34[a]	27%/28%[a]
HBeAg Seroconversion	difference of 18%		16%–21%	4%–6%	12%	6%	21%	22%	27%/32% [a]	24%/27%[a]
Loss HBsAg	7.8%	1.8%	<1%	0	0	0	2%	0%	3%	3%
ALT Normalization	difference of 23%		41%–75%	7%–24%	48%	16%	68%	77%	39%	46%
Histologic Improvement	NA	NA	49%–56%	23%–25%	53%	25%	72%	65%	38%	41%
Durability of Response	80%–90%		50%–80%[b]		90%[b]		69% [b]	80%[b]	NA	

ALT, alanine aminotransferase; NA, not available; QD, every day; QW, every week.
[a]Response at week 48/week 72 (24 weeks after stopping therapy)
[b]Lmivudine and entecavir – no or short duration of consolidation treatment, adefovir and telbivudine – most patients had consolidation treatment.
From references 72, 73, with permission.

Table 73-17 Responses to Approved Antiviral Therapies Among Treatment-Naïve Patients with HBeAg Negative Chronic Hepatitis B

	Standard IFF-α	*Control*	*Lamivudine*	*Placebo*	*Adefovir*	*Placebo*	*Entecavir*	*Telbivudine*	*PegIFN-α*	*PegIFN-α + lamivudine*
	5 MU QD or 10 MU TIW	(6–12 months)	100 mg QD (48–52 weeks)		10 mg QD (48 weeks)		0.5 mg QD (48 weeks)	600 mg QD (52 weeks)	180 mcg QW (48 weeks)	180 mcg QW + 100 mg (48 weeks)
Loss HBV DNA	60%–70%	10%–20%	60%–73%	NA	51%	0	90%	88%	63%	87%
ALT Normalization	60%–70%	10%–20%	60%–79%	NA	72%	29%	78%	74%	38%	49%
Histologic Improvement	NA	NA	60%–66%	NA	64%	33%	70%	67%	48%[a]	38%[a]
Durability of Response	10–22%		< 10%		5%		NA	NA	20%	20%

ALT, alanine aminotransferase NA, not available; QD, every day; QW, every week.

[a]Post treatment biopsies obtained at week 72.

From references 72, 73, with permission.

Table 73-18 Factors Predictive of a Sustained Response to Interferon-Alpha in Patients With Chronic Hepatitis

Chronic hepatitis B
Short duration of disease
High serum, aminotransferase concentrations[a]
Active liver disease with fibrosis[a]
Low HBV DNA concentrations
Wild-type (HBcAg positive) virus
Absence of immunosuppression

[a]One of the most commonly associated factors with a high degree of response to therapy

in patients who are HBeAg negative exist. C.R. is a reasonable candidate for IFN-α therapy. His liver biopsy is consistent with chronic disease, he has high pretreatment aminotransferase levels, his HBV DNA is <200 pg/mL, and his duration of chronic hepatitis is short. Before initiating IFN-α, serologic testing for HIV and genotyping should be performed to assist in the evaluation of C.R.'s response to therapy (Table 73-13).

Adverse Effects

27. What adverse effects to IFN-α should be monitored in C.R.?

Adverse effects associated with standard and PegIFN-α therapy are similar and quite common (Table 73-19). These have been categorized as early side effects that rarely limit the use of IFN, and late side effects that may necessitate dose reduction or discontinuation of therapy altogether.[72,73,167,180] The early side effects of IFN-α therapy generally appear hours after administration and resemble an influenza-like syndrome with fever, chills, anorexia, nausea, myalgias, fatigue, and headache. Virtually all patients receiving IFN-α experience these toxicities, and they tend to resolve after repeated exposure to the drug. Administration of IFN-α at bedtime may decrease the severity of early side effects. Acetaminophen can be used to treat early side effects of IFN-α therapy, but should be limited to 2 g/day to minimize the risk of hepatotoxicity. The late side effects usually are observed after 2 weeks of therapy and are more serious. These toxicities, which limit the use of IFN-α, include worsening of the influenza-like syndrome, alopecia, bone marrow suppression, bacterial infections, thyroid dysfunction (both hypothyroidism and hyperthyroidism), and psychiatric disturbances (emotional lability: irritability, depression, anxiety, delirium, and suicidal ideation). The use of IFN-α can also cause a flare (increase) in ALT levels in 30% to 40% of patients. These flares are considered to be a favorable prognostic indicator, but they have been reported to cause hepatic decompensation, especially in cirrhotic patients. Finally, rare adverse effects, such as development of autoantibodies, retinal changes, and impaired vision, have been reported. C.R. should be questioned at each clinic visit about new or worsening symptoms as well as any changes in mood or the ability to perform daily tasks of living. Additional monitoring parameters should include a complete blood count (CBC) with differential and platelet count after weeks 1 and 2 of therapy and monthly thereafter during treatment. Thyroid function tests and screening tests for autoantibodies should also be performed following initiation of therapy.

Table 73-19 Serious Adverse Events Reported With Interferon-α Therapy

Central Nervous System	Cardiovascular
Psychosis	Cardiac arrhythmias
Depression/suicide	Sudden death
Delirium/confusion	Dilated cardiomyopathy
Extrapyramidal ataxia	Hypotension
Paresthesia	**Other**
Seizures	Retinopathy
Relapse in substance abuse	Hearing loss
Hematologic	Pulmonary interstitial fibrosis
Granulocytopenia	Acute renal failure
Thrombocytopenia	Hyperthyroidism
Anemia	Hypothyroidism
Dermatologic	Systemic lupus erythematosus
Psoriasis	
Erythema multiforme	
Gastrointestinal	
Autoimmune hepatitis	
Primary biliary cirrhosis	
Hepatic decompensation	

From references 167, 179, 180, and 181, with permission.

Dosing

28. What dose of IFN-α should C.R. receive?

Standard interferon doses of 2.5 to 10 MU can be administered subcutaneously (SC) daily or three times weekly for 1 to 12 months. The manufacturer of IFN-α2b recommends 30 to 35 MU/week, administered SC or IM as 5 MU/day or 10 MU three times weekly. For children, the dose should be 6 MU/m^2 SC three times a week with a maximum of 10 MU. The recommended duration of therapy for patients who are HBeAg positive is for 16 to 24 weeks. Current data suggest that patients with HBeAg-negative HBV infection should be treated for at least 12 months and possibly for 24 months to enhance the rate of sustained response.[72,73] The recommended dose of PegIFN-α2a, the only pegylated IFN approved for the treatment of HBV infection in the United States, is 180 mcg SC weekly for 48 weeks. It may be possible, however, to use lower dosages or shorter duration of therapy to achieve a sustained response in HBeAg-positive patients. More trials are needed to support this altered dosing regimen. Whether longer duration of treatment (> 48 weeks) is beneficial in HBeAg-negative patients remains to be determined.

Some authorities believe thrice-weekly administration of IFN-α is associated with more severe flu-like symptoms and headache when compared with daily administration. In contrast, severe bone marrow suppression tends to occur less often with thrice-weekly administration.[180,181] Treatment questions that still need to be adequately assessed are the optimal schedule of IFN administration (daily versus every other day versus three times weekly) and the benefit of combining IFN with other antiviral agents (see below) for the treatment of HBV infection. Because C.R. is HBeAg positive, has normal WBC and platelet counts, he should initially receive either IFN-α2b as a 5-MU SC injection daily for 16 weeks or PegIFN-α2a 180 mcg SC weekly for 48 weeks. The SC route of administration is preferred in C.R. to decrease the possibility of hematoma formation because his PT is prolonged. If conventional doses of IFN lead to liver failure, development of sepsis, or bleeding, low-dose therapy may be of benefit based on results from a trial in patients with decompensated cirrhosis.

The dose should be decreased by 50% if granulocyte or platelet counts decline to <750/mm^3 and 50,000/mm^3, respectively.[182] Profound thrombocytopenia (<30,000/mm^3) or neutropenia (<500/mm^3); serious changes in mood or behavior; and intractable nausea, vomiting, or fatigue warrant the immediate discontinuation of IFN-α.

NUCLEOSIDE ANALOGS

29. If C.R. does not respond to IFN-α, what additional antiviral therapies are available?

Although IFN has been important in the treatment of chronic HBV infection, patients included in most clinical trials represented a highly select group of chronic HBV carriers. Specifically, patients with decompensated liver disease were excluded because they often have leukopenia and thrombocytopenia as a result of hypersplenism, which limits the dose of IFN that can be administered. In addition to IFN-α, the FDA has approved several antiviral agents for treatment of chronic hepatitis B infection (lamivudine, adefovir dipivoxil, entecavir, and telbivudine) with at least three more (emtricitabine, clevudine, and tenofovir disoproxil) that may be approved in the near future.

Lamivudine (Epivir-HBV) was the first nucleoside analog approved by the FDA for use in patients with compensated liver disease who had evidence of active viral replication and liver inflammation caused by chronic hepatitis B infection. Nucleoside analogs represent an alternative approach to treatment.[71,73,74,156–165] Lamivudine, the(–) enantiomer of 3′—thiacytidine is an oral 2′–, 3′—dideoxynucleoside that inhibits DNA synthesis by terminating the nascent proviral DNA chain and interferes with the RT activity of HBV.[183,184] In clinical trials, lamivudine was well tolerated and reduced serum levels of HBV DNA.[71,73,74,162,163,184,185] In a pivotal randomized, placebo-controlled trial patients received 100 mg lamivudine or placebo as initial therapy for chronic hepatitis B for 52 weeks.[186] Patients receiving lamivudine were more likely to have a histologic response, loss of HBeAg in serum, sustained suppression of HBV DNA to undetectable levels, and reduced incidence of hepatic fibrosis. Additional findings were that lamivudine recipients were more likely to experience HBeAg seroconversion (loss of HBeAg), undetectable levels of serum HBV DNA, and the appearance of antibodies against HBeAg. HBeAg responses were maintained in most patients for 16 weeks following discontinuation of therapy. The most commonly reported adverse effects have been headache, fatigue, nausea, and abdominal discomfort. Less common adverse effects include laboratory abnormalities, such as transient asymptomatic elevation in amylase, lipase, and creatinine kinase levels.[71,73,74,78,161–163,184] Although this trial led to widespread use of lamivudine, its major use has been as a continuous long-term therapy in HBV-infected individuals, which can result in resolution of disease and loss of HBsAg.

30. What is the risk of development of resistance in C.R.?

Lamivudine Resistance

Lamivudine, however, has a high rate of antiviral resistance. Considering the high rate of viral turnover and the error susceptible nature of the polymerase (particularly the RT), acquisition of resistance mutations would be predicted. The most common mutation leading to lamivudine resistance is a specific point mutation in the highly conserved methionine motif of the HBV polymerase.[71,73,74,78,96,189] In this mutation, the methionine residue is changed to a valine or isoleucine. These genotypic mutations in the YMDD locus associated with a reduced sensitivity to lamivudine occur following long-term therapy (e.g., 52 weeks). This motif is thought to be representative of the active site of the enzyme, similar to that associated with HIV RT, leading to lamivudine resistance.[71,73,74,78,161–163,184,187,188] Lamivudine-resistant HBV mutants generally are detectable after 6 months or more of continuous therapy. Integrated data from four studies show a 24% (range, 16%–32%) incidence at 1 year, increasing to 47% to 56% at 2 years of therapy and 69% to 75% at 3 years of therapy.[71,73,74,78,96,189] The presence of YMDD mutants results in a loss of the clinical response, a rise in ALT levels, and worsening of hepatic histology.[72,73] Reports of continued improvement despite lamivudine resistance exist, but the long-term consequences of viral resistance (including hepatic decompensation and exacerbation of liver disease) are poor. Thus, lamivudine may have limited benefit in patients similar to C.R. A greater therapeutic benefit in chronic HBV infection would be anticipated with equally or more potent nucleoside analogs with lower rates of resistance.

31. What other drug therapies are available for managing C.R.'s chronic HBV infection?

Adefovir

Adefovir dipivoxil (Hepsera, Gilead) was the second nucleoside analog approved by the FDA for the treatment of chronic hepatitis B in adults with evidence either of active viral replication or of persistent elevations in serum aminotransferases (ALT or AST) or histologically active disease.[190] Adefovir dipivoxil is the oral prodrug of an acyclic nucleotide monophosphate analogue, 9-(2-phosphonylmethoxyethyl)-adenine (PMEA). The active drug is a selective inhibitor of numerous species of viral nucleic acid polymerases and reverse transcriptases. It has broad-spectrum antiviral activity against retroviruses, hepadnaviruses, and herpesviruses. Orally administered adefovir dipivoxil exhibits an inhibitory effect on both the HIV and HBV reverse transcriptases.

Previously, two trials reported the results of adefovir for the treatment of patients who were HBeAg-negative[191] and HBeAg-positive.[192] (Table 73-16 and Table 73-17) The first of these trials, patients with chronic hepatitis B who were negative for hepatitis HBeAg were randomly assigned to receive either 10 mg of adefovir dipivoxil (n = 123) or placebo (n = 61) once daily for 48 weeks.[191] The primary endpoint in this trial was histologic improvement. At week 48, 64% of patients who had baseline liver biopsy specimens available in the adefovir dipivoxil group had improvement in histologic liver abnormalities (77 of 121), as compared with 33% of patients in the placebo group (19 of 57). Additionally, serum HBV DNA levels were reduced to <400 copies/mL in 61 of 123 patients (51%) receiving adefovir and in 0 of 61 patients (0%) receiving placebo. The median decrease in log-transformed HBV DNA levels was also greater with adefovir-treated patients compared with patients taking placebo (3.91 versus 1.35 log copies/mL; $P<0.001$).

Biochemical markers (alanine aminotransferase levels) had normalized at week 48 in 84 of 116 (72%) of patients receiving adefovir compared with 17 of 59 (29%) of those receiving placebo. No HBV polymerase mutations associated with resistance to adefovir were identified within the study period. Adefovir resulted in significant histologic, virologic, and biochemical improvement, with an adverse event profile similar to that of placebo. Emergence of adefovir-resistant HBV polymerase mutations was not observed; however, data suggest rates of resistance to be <1% at 1 year and up to 29% after 5 year.[72,73]

Importantly, it appears that adefovir is capable of inhibiting the enzymatic activity of both wild-type and YMDD mutant variants of both of these viruses. Adefovir resistance may be more common in patients with pre-existing lamivudine resistance, however, and instances of combined resistance have been reported.[189]

In the second clinical trial, adefovir was given to HBeAg-positive patients with chronic hepatitis B.[192] Patients were randomly assigned to receive 10 mg or 30 mg of adefovir dipivoxil or placebo daily for 48 weeks. The primary endpoint was histologic improvement in the 10-mg group as compared with the placebo group. After 48 weeks of treatment, significantly more patients who received 10 mg or 30 mg of daily adefovir had histologic improvement (53% and 59%, respectively) versus 25% in placebo patients. In addition, a significant reduction in serum HBV DNA levels, undetectable levels (<400 copies/mL) of serum HBV DNA, normalization of alanine aminotransferase levels, and HBeAg seroconversion were associated with adefovir. Adefovir-associated resistance mutations were identified in the HBV DNA polymerase gene within the study period. The safety profile of the 10-mg dose of adefovir dipivoxil was similar to that of placebo. More adverse events and renal laboratory abnormalities were observed in the group receiving 30 mg/day of adefovir. In summary, adefovir dipivoxil led to histologic liver improvement, reduced serum HBV DNA and alanine aminotransferase levels, and increased rates of HBeAg seroconversion without adefovir-associated resistance. Again, long-term follow-up is required to validate these findings.

Additional data show that adefovir has been associated with primary nonresponse as shown by only a modest reduction in HBV DNA levels and minimal improvement in ALT in up to one-third of patients with HBeAg-positive HBV infection. Primary nonresponse is associated with high pretreatment HBV DNA levels and may occur owing to the moderate potency of adefovir against HBV. Higher doses could be used; however, they are correlated with renal toxicity. Long-term trials with the drug are ongoing and have shown that high rates of response are possible in patients with HBeAg-negative hepatitis B infection.

Entecavir

Entecavir (Baraclude, Bristol-Myers Squibb) is an acyclic guanosine derivative with potent activity against HBV.[73,74] The drug inhibits HBV replication at three different steps: (a) the priming of HBV DNA polymerase; (b) the RT of the negative strand HBV DNA from the pregenomic RNA; and (c) the synthesis of positive strand HBV DNA. *In vitro* studies have shown that the drug is more potent than lamivudine and adefovir and is highly effective against lamivudine-resistant HBV mutants.

In two published phase III clinical trials, the efficacy of entecavir was reported in patients with HBeAg-positive and HBeAg-negative hepatitis B infection (Table 73-16 and Table 73-17). In the first randomized double-blind trial, 715 patients with compensated liver disease who had not previously received a nucleoside analog were assigned to receive entecavir 0.5 mg (n = 357) or lamivudine 100 mg once daily (n = 358) for a minimum of 52 weeks. By week 48, HBeAg-positive patients receiving entecavir had higher rates of histologic (72% versus 62%; $P = 0.009$), virologic [HBV DNA undetectable by PCR] (67% versus 36%; $P < 0.001$), and biochemical [ALT normalization](68% versus 60%; $P = 0.02$) responses when compared with lamivudine.[193] Of note, the seroconversion rates were similar among the two treatment groups (21% versus 18%; entecavir versus lamivudine, respectively). No viral resistance to entecavir was detected during the study period, but follow-up data suggest a low rate of resistance (3% by week 96 of therapy).[194] The authors concluded that entecavir was as safe and had significantly higher histologic, virologic, and biochemical response rates than HBeAg-positive patients treated with lamivudine. In patients who remained HBeAg positive with low levels of HBV DNA replication, a second year of entecavir and lamivudine therapy resulted in seroconversion in 11% and 13% of patients, respectively.[195]

In another randomized double-blind phase III trial, results were reported in patients with HBeAg-negative hepatitis B infection receiving either entecavir 0.5 mg (n = 331) or 100 mg lamivudine daily (n = 317) for a minimum of 52 weeks. At week 48, patients receiving entecavir had significantly higher rates of histologic (70% versus 61%; $P = 0.01$), virologic (90% versus 72%; $P < 0.001$) and biochemical (78% versus 71%; $P = 0.045$) response rates.[196] Again, no evidence of resistance was seen among patients receiving entecavir. Safety and adverse events were similar in the two groups. The authors concluded that entecavir was as safe and had significantly higher histologic, virologic, and biochemical response rates than HBeAg-negative patients treated with lamivudine. Thus C.R. could receive entecavir 0.5 mg daily. As with all of the nucleoside agents, renal function should be monitored closely and appropriate dosage adjustments should be implemented a when renal function chances (Table 73-20). Furthermore, entecavir may be used for lamivudine-refractory or resistant patients. In these patients, lamivudine should be discontinued to reduce the risk of entecavir resistance. *In vitro* studies showed that entecavir resistant mutations are susceptible to adefovir, but sparse clinical data are available to validate this finding. The dose of entecavir used for lamivudine-resistant patients is 1.0 mg daily.

Telbivudine

Telbivudine (Tyzela, Idenix) is an orally available L-nucleoside analog with potent antiviral activity against HBV.[197–199] In a randomized double-blind phase III trial 1,370 patients with HBeAg-positive (n = 921) or HBeAg-negative (n = 446) chronic hepatitis B infection were randomized to receive 600 mg of telbivudine or 100 mg of lamivudine once daily[197] (Table 73-16 and Table 73-17). The primary efficacy endpoint was noninferiority of telbivudine to lamivudine for therapeutic response (i.e., a reduction in serum HBV DNA levels to <5 log 10 copies/mL, along with a loss of HBeAg, or normalization of aminotransferase levels). Secondary endpoints included

Table 73-20 Adjustment of Adult Dosage of Nucleoside and Nucleotide Analogs in Accordance with Creatinine Clearance

Creatinine Clearance (mL/min)	Recommended Dose	
Lamivudine		
≥50	100 mg QD	
30–49	100 mg first dose then 50 mg QD	
15–29	35 mg first dose, then 25 mg QD	
5–14	35 mg first dose, then 15 mg QD	
<5	35 mg first dose, then 10 mg QD	
Adefovir		
≥50	10 mg daily	
20–49	10 mg every other day	
10–19	10 mg every third day	
Hemodialysis patients	10 mg every other week following dialysis	
Entecavir		
	Nucleoside naïve	Lamivudine refractory/resistant
≥50	0.5 mg QD	1.0 mg QD
30–49	0.25 mg QD	0.5 mg QD
10–29	0.15 mg	0.3 mg QD
<10 or hemodialysis or continuous ambulatory peritoneal dialysis	0.05 mg QD	0.1 mg QD
Telbivudine		
≥50	600 mg daily	
30–49	400 mg daily	
<30	200 mg daily	
Hemodialysis patients	200 mg daily following dialysis	

QD, every day
From references 72, 73, with permission.

histologic response, change in HBV DNA, and HBeAg responses. At week 52, a higher proportion of HBeAg-positive patients receiving telbivudine than lamivudine had a therapeutic response (75.3% versus 67.0%; $P = 0.005$) or a histologic response (64.7% versus 56.3%; $P = 0.01$); telbivudine was also not inferior to lamivudine for these endpoints in HBeAg-negative patients. Elevated creatinine kinase levels were more commonly seen in the patients treated with telbivudine, whereas elevated ALT and AST levels were more common in those treated with lamivudine. Resistance rates were lower among the telbivudine group compared with the lamivudine group during the first year of therapy. The rates of HBeAg loss were similar between the telbivudine and lamivudine treatment groups (26% versus 23%, respectively). With respect to resistance, telbivudine selects for mutations in the YMDD motif. Although resistance rates are lower than those reported with lamivudine, the resistance rate is substantial and increases at a high rate following the first year of therapy.[188] In the phase III trial genotypic resistance after 1 and 2 years of therapy was observed in 4.4% and 21.6% of HBeAg-positive and 2.7% and 8.6% of HBeAg-negative patients who received telbivudine compared with 9.1% and 33% of HBeAg-positive and 9.8% and 21.9% of HBeAg-negative patients who received lamivudine.[74,75] Although telbivudine is more potent with lower rates of resistance than lamivudine, the rates of resistance appear to be higher than for other approved therapies. Thus, telbivudine may not be an optimal choice of nucleoside agent for C.R.

Additional Agents

The safety and efficacy of other antiviral agents for the treatment of chronic HBV infection, including tenofovir (PMPA),[73,74] emtricitabine [Emtriva, FTC (2R,5S)-5-fluoro-1-[2-(hydroxymethyl)-1,3-oxathiolan-5-yl]cytosine],[73,198] and clevudine [L-FMAU (1-(2-fluoro-5-methyl–L-arabinofuranosyl-uracil)][73,74,199] are under investigation. In one study of 248 patients receiving 200 mg daily of emtricitabine(FTC), there were significantly higher rates of histologic (62% versus 25%), virologic (54% versus 2%) and biochemical (65% versus 25%) responses at week 48 compared with placebo. The rates of HBeAg seroconversion were the same in both groups (12%) with FTC resistance rates occurring in 13% of treated patients.[198] Clinical trials with daily clevudine 30 mg for up to 24 weeks demonstrated that the drug is well tolerated and that serum HBV DNA levels were undetectable by PCR assay at the end of treatment in 59% of HBeAg-positive and in 92% of HBeAg-negative patients. A unique characteristic of clevudine is the durability of viral suppression, which persists up to 24 weeks after therapy is discontinued in some patients.[199] Ultimately, this agent has not been shown to increase the rate of HBeAg seroconversion compared with placebo controls and it also may select for mutations in the YMDD motif.

Although several drugs have failed to treat HBV effectively,[200–203] agents such as tenofovir may prove effective against HBV isolates that are resistant to lamivudine.[204–206] Novel agents, such as glycosidase inhibitors, hammerhead ribozymes (short RNA molecules that possess endoribonuclease activity capable of degrading target RNA), and antisense phosphodiester oligodeoxynucleotides (short fragments of DNA that are complementary to HBV-RNA, which result in inhibition of RNA translation) are also under investigation.[207] Pending the results of these trials and the arrival of HBV protease inhibitors and cytokine therapies, combination antiviral therapy as demonstrated in patients with HIV, may enhance response rates, reduce the progression of liver disease, and ultimately enhance survival in patients with chronic HBV infection.[208,209] Because of the relatively high resistance rates for lamivudine and telbivudine, and dosing limitations for adefovir, entecavir 0.5 mg daily should be initiated in C.R. if he fails to respond to IFN or PegIFN. Recommendations for treatment of chronic hepatitis B virus can be found in Table 73-21.

Therapeutic Vaccines

Theradigm-HBV (Cytel, San Diego, CA) is a therapeutic vaccine consisting of the viral protein HBcAg peptide, a T-helper peptide (tetanus toxoid peptide) that enhances immunogenicity, and two palmitic acid molecules. The vaccine appears to be well tolerated, has dose-dependent response rates, and appears to work by inducing HBV-specific major histocompatibility complex (MHC) class I-restricted CTL. Phase I and II studies in patients with chronic HBV are in progress.[210] Another therapeutic vaccine undergoing clinical investigation for chronic HBV is HBV/MF59.[211] This vaccine combines the HBV "Pre

Table 73-21 Recommendations for Treatment of Chronic Hepatitis B

HBeAg	*HBV DNA (PCR)*	*ALT*	*Treatment Strategy*
+	>20,000 IU/mL	≤2 × ULN	Low efficacy with current treatment. Observe, consider treatment when ALT becomes elevated. Consider biopsy in persons >40 years, ALT persistently high normal to 2 × ULN, or family history of HCC Consider treatment if HBV DNA >20,000 IU/mL and biopsy shows moderate to severe inflammation or significant fibrosis
+	>20,000 IU/mL	≥2 × ULN	Observe for 3–6 months and treat if no spontaneous HBeAg loss Consider liver biopsy prior to treatment if compensated Immediate treatment if icteric or clinical decompensation (IFN-α/PegIFN-α, LAM, ADV, ETV, LdT may be used as initial therapy) LAM LdT not preferred due to high rate of resistance
HBeAg to anti-HBe			Endpoint of treatment: seroconversion from Duration of therapy: IFN-α: 16 weeks PegIFN-α: 48 weeks LAM, ADV, ETV, LdT: minimum 1 year, continue for at least 6 months After HBeAg seroconversion IFN-α nonresponders/contraindications to IFN-α → ADV/EDV IFN-α/PegIFN-α, LAM, ADV, ETV, or LdT may be used as initial therapy, LAM and LdT not preferred due to high rate of resistance
	>20,000 IU/mL	≥2 × ULN	High rate of drug resistance; endpoint of therapy not defined Duration of therapy: IFN-α/PegIFN-α: 1 year LAM, ADV, ETV, LdT: >1 year IFN-α nonresponders/contraindications to IFN-α → ADV.EDV
	> 2,000 IU/mL	1–2 × ULN	Consider liver biopsy and treat if liver biopsy shows moderate/severe necroinflammation or significant fibrosis
	<2,000 IU/mL	≤ULN	Observe, treat if HBV DNA or ALT becomes higher
±	Detectable	Cirrhosis	Compensated: HBV DNA >2,000 IU/mL-treat: LAM/ADV/ETV/ LdT may be used as initial therapy; LAM and LdT not preferred due to high rate of resistance HBV DNA <2,000 IU/mL: consider treatment if ALT is elevated Decompensated: Coordinate treatment with transplant center, LAM (or LdT) + ADV or ETV preferred Refer for liver transplant
±	Undetectable	Cirrhosis	Compensated: observe Decompensated: refer for liver transplant

ADV, adefovir; ALT, alanine aminotransferase; ETV, entecavir; IFN-α, interferon alpha; LAM, lamivudine; LdT, telbivudine; PegIFN-α, pegylated interferon alpha; ULN, upper limit of normal.
From references 72, 73, with permission.

S2 and S" antigens with an MF59 adjuvant (enhances immune responses).

32. If C.R. fails therapy with entecavir, is combination therapy appropriate?

Combination Therapies

Combination therapy for HIV and HCV have been proved to be more effective than monotherapy. The potential for additive or synergistic antiviral effects and reduced or delayed rates of viral resistance may also be possible in patients with hepatitis B infection. Several combination therapies have been evaluated in patients infected with hepatitis B (PegIFN and lamivudine, lamivudine and adefovir, lamivudine and telbivudine) but none have been proved to be superior to monotherapy in producing a higher rate of sustained response. Furthermore, combination therapies have shown a reduced rate of resistance in patients treated with lamivudine compared with monotherapy, but no data support the use of combination therapy to reduce mutation rates in agents that have a low risk of drug resistance when used alone.

Liver Transplantation

33. If C.R. fails therapy and continued to decompensate from his chronic HBV infection, what nonpharmacologic interventions are available?

One-year survival rates for patients with cholestatic or alcoholic liver disease are >90% in most transplant centers.[92] Historical data for liver transplants in patients with chronic HBV infection are associated with 1-year survival of 50% compared with non–HBV-infected recipients. In one report, 51 HBsAg-positive patients who received a liver transplant for postnecrotic cirrhosis were compared with 38 transplant recipients with evidence of HBV immunity (HBsAg-negative and anti–HBs-positive).[95] Early post-transplant mortality was similar between the groups but delayed mortality was greater in the HBsAg-positive arm (63% versus 80%, respectively, in patients who survived at least 60 days, or 45.1% and 63.2%, respectively, overall). Recurrent HBV infection was the primary cause of death in HBsAg-positive patients.[92] Patients with active viral replication preceding transplantation as indicated by HBeAg or HBV DNA positivity are less likely to have graft or overall survival compared with those without active viral replication.[212] Reinfection of the allograft takes place in up to 100% of liver transplant recipients, but morbidity is higher in HBeAg-positive patients. HBV DNA levels may be a better predictor of outcome than HBeAg positivity.[212] For this reason, pretransplant HBV DNA status has become the preferred predictor of outcome following transplantation. Because of poor outcomes, several centers have excluded HBsAg-positive patients (in the presence of viral replication) from having liver transplantation. This policy is not universally accepted, however, and with appropriate posttransplant prophylactic strategies, patients who are nonresponders to drug therapy can undergo successful liver transplantation.

34. What are the current recommendations for prevention of recurrent hepatitis B infection following liver transplantation?

The most efficacious approach to preventing HBV recurrence following transplantation has been with high-dose IV hepatitis B immunoglobulin in the anhepatic and postoperative periods.[211,212] Samuel et al. reported that 110 HBsAg-positive patients treated with daily IV HBIG in the early postoperative period to maintain their serum anti-HBs levels $\geq$100 IU/L had an overall survival (84%) that approached that observed in other transplant recipients without HBV infection.[211] These data have been confirmed in a large retrospective analysis of patients (N = 334) undergoing transplantation for HBV infection in Europe. Furthermore, the European trial demonstrated that patients receiving long-term HBIG administration (>6 months) compared with patients receiving short-term HBIG (<6 months) had a lower risk for recurrent HBV infection (35% versus 75%) and longer 3-year actuarial survival (78% versus 48%).[211]

HBIG DOSAGE, ADMINISTRATION, AND ADVERSE EFFECTS

Historically, liver transplant centers routinely administer immunoprophylaxis with IV HBIG 10,000 IU (10 vials, 50 mL in 250 mL of saline) in the anhepatic (recipient liver excised) phase, then 10,000 IU (50 mL infused over 4–6 hours) for the next 6 days postoperatively. HBIG (10,000 IU) is administered on a monthly basis for life, or is discontinued if HBsAg becomes positive, indicating treatment failure. This regimen achieves trough anti-HBs titers of approximately 500 IU/L and up to 2,000 IU/L; however, the link of specific titers and protection from recurrence is controversial at this time. Patients may also experience a serum sickness-like syndrome (fever, myalgias) that is reversible after discontinuation of HBIG therapy. An IV preparation of HBIG is now available for patients undergoing liver transplantation for chronic HBV infection.

Long-term concerns associated with HBIG administration include the potential for HBV reinfection from extrahepatic sites despite adequate anti-HBs titers, emerging mutant viruses that no longer bind to the immunoglobulin, and the prohibitive high cost of therapy (>$60,000/year).[213,214] Current data suggest that pharmacokinetic modeling and use of maintenance therapy with IM administration of HBIG (e.g., 2.5–10 mL every 2–3 weeks) following a reduced induction dose (e.g., 10,000 IU anhepatically, then 2,000 IU IV × 6 doses) may achieve similar outcomes and reduce the cost associated with IV administration of the drug.[215–217]

35. What is the role of oral antiviral agents in liver transplant recipients with HBV?

As previously described, the availability of nucleoside analogs, such as lamivudine, adefovir, and entecavir, are having an impact on the treatment of patients with HBV infection, and they also have a role in patients who undergo transplants for chronic HBV infection.[71,73,184,218–221] Lamivudine monotherapy is effective in converting HBV DNA-positive patients to negative status before and after liver transplantation. Emerging mutations at the YMDD locus in transplant and nontransplant recipients also have been observed, however, rendering lamivudine ineffective.[71,73,184,222,223] Nucleoside analogs are still considered investigational at this time for HBV prophylaxis following transplantation because they have not been FDA approved for this indication in the United States. Several transplant centers, however, have implemented clinical protocols that combine lamivudine with HBIG; ultimately, this combination regimen has emerged as a clinical standard because it has been effective, with low rates of resistance. When lamivudine resistance has occurred following transplant and leads to recurrent hepatitis B, the use of adefovir, entecavir, or tenofovir has been successful in the post-transplant setting. Future considerations for preventing recurrent HBV infection following transplantation include combining nucleoside analogs (lamivudine, adefovir, entecavir), HBIG, or various combinations; however, optimal management strategies continue to be determined. In some patients with low HBV DNA before transplant, the use of RT inhibitors may eliminate the administration of HBIG in the early postoperative course or may allow a "switch" to long-term oral nucleoside- or nucleotide-based therapy. More long-term data are required, however, to validate this approach. Thus, patients who are transplant recipients for chronic HBV infection who fail treatment with HBIG and lamivudine should be treated as part of an investigational protocol.

HEPATITIS D VIRUS

Virology and Epidemiology

Hepatitis D virus is a small, single-stranded RNA animal virus (36 nm) that is similar to defective RNA plant viruses (Table 73-2).[224–226] Discovered in the late 1970s, HDVwas found in the nuclei of infected hepatocytes, and it presents in some, but not all, HBV-infected patients. HDV appears to replicate exclusively in the liver via extensive base-pairing that results in the formation of an unbranched rodlike genome. Although replication of the virus can occur within hepatocytes in the absence of HBV, the latter is required for coating the HDV virions and allowing for their cellular spread. The HDV genome is replicated by an RNA intermediate (antigenome) that depends on the host's RNA-dependent RNA polymerase. During replication, the genomic (positive strand) HDV RNA becomes the template for successive rounds of minus-strand synthesis. The multimeric minus strand then serves as a template for positive strand synthesis. Subsequently, autocleavage and ligation form circular genomes that are produced from this multimeric precursor.

Fifteen million persons are infected with HDV, with the highest incidence reported in Italy, Eastern Europe, the Amazon Basin, Colombia, Venezuela, Western Asia, and the South Pacific.[1,225,226] In the United States, an estimated 7,500 HDV cases occur annually.[1,226] The prevalence of HDV is greatest among persons with percutaneous exposure (e.g., injection drug users) and hemophiliacs (20%–53% and 48%–80%, respectively) and may be affected by additional factors such as age of infection.[1,226] The modes of transmission of HDV are similar to those reported for HBV infection. Thus, HDV clearly represents a potential infectious hazard to patients susceptible to HBV and those who are chronic HBV carriers.[226,227] Because infection by HDV requires the presence of active HBV, preventing HBV infection will prevent HDV infection in a susceptible patient.[1,225,226]

Pathogenesis

Limited data suggest that HDVAg (antigen) and HDV RNA may possess direct cytotoxic effects on hepatocytes, whereas other findings implicate the immune response in pathogenesis.[225,226,228] Furthermore, several autoantibodies associated with chronic HDV infection may play a role in propagating liver disease and could partially explain the differences in disease severity observed in patients with HDV plus HBV compared with those with HBV alone.

Diagnosis and Serology

The ELISA and RIA tests for IgM anti-HDV are available commercially, whereas detection methods for HDV RNA are available only on a research basis to distinguish ongoing from previous HDV infection.[226,229] Measurement of anti-HDV is generally not useful for early diagnosis because detectable antibody levels are usually achieved late in the clinical course of the infection (Fig. 73-4A). Anti-HDV IgM is detectable before anti-HDV IgG in acute HDV coinfection and is diagnostic for acute HDV infection. Anti-HDV IgM levels are not sustained in self-limiting HDV infection but may persist in patients with

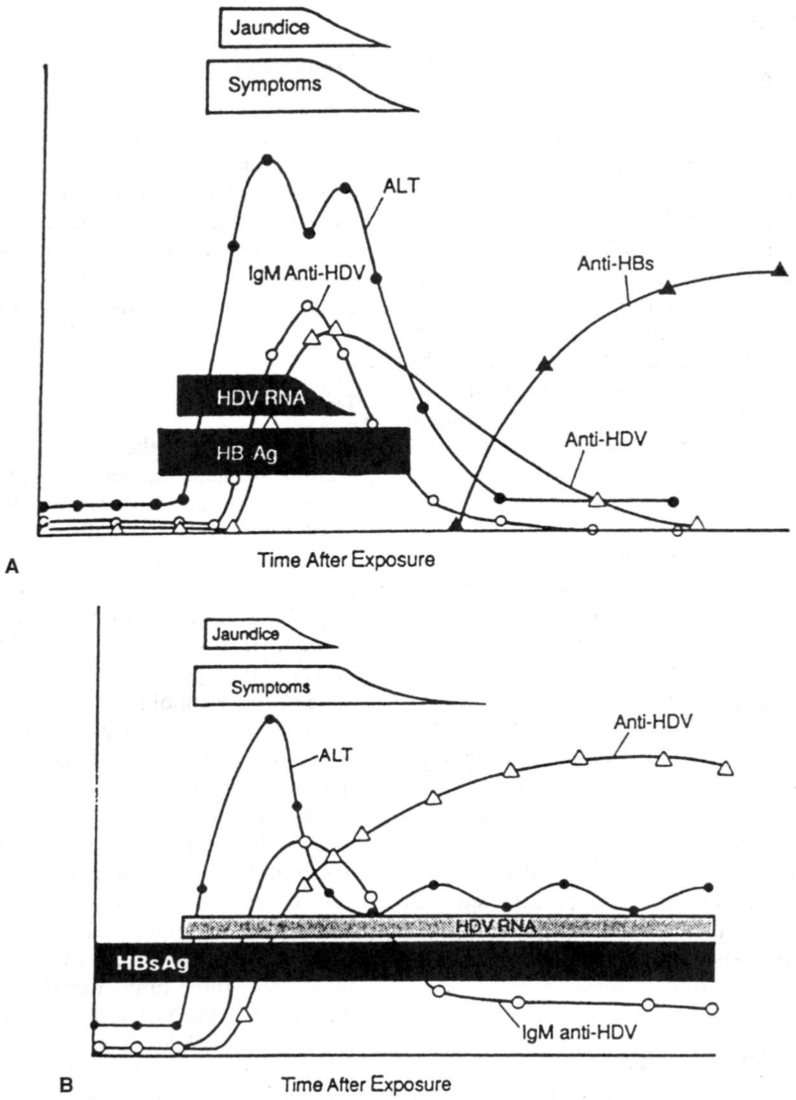

FIGURE 73-4 A: Typical course of acute icteric HBV with HDV coinfection. ALT, alanine aminotransferase; anti-HBs, hepatitis B surface antibody; anti-HDV, antibody to delta hepatitis virus; HBsAg, hepatitis B surface antigen; HDV RNA, delta hepatitis RNA; IgM anti-HDV, IgM antibody to delta hepatitis virus. **B: Typical course of acute icteric HBV with HDV superinfection.** ALT, alanine aminotransferase; anti-HBs, hepatitis B surface antibody; anti-HDV, antibody to delta hepatitis virus; HBsAg, hepatitis B surface antigen; HDV RNA, delta hepatitis RNA; IgM anti-HDV, IgM antibody to delta hepatitis virus.

chronic HDV infection. Also, anti-HDV IgM does not distinguish coinfection (HBV and HDV acquired simultaneously) from superinfection (HDV acquired in chronic HBV carrier) (Fig. 73-4B).

Differentiation between coinfection and superinfection is made by the presence or absence of anti-HBc IgM. In acute coinfection, serum anti-HDV IgM and HDV RNA appear together with anti-HBc IgM, whereas in patients with superinfection, HDV markers are present in the absence of anti-HBc IgM. The presence and titer level of anti-HDV, in the case of persistent infection, also correlate with the severity of disease. Titers of anti-HDV IgG >1:1,000 indicate ongoing viral replication.

Hepatitis D virus antigen is present in the serum in the late incubation period of acute infection and lasts into the symptomatic phase in up to 20% of patients. Because this antigen is transient, repeat testing may be required to detect its presence. The clinical utility of HDVAg detection by ELISA and RIA is limited by the necessity of precise timing of a sample and by its availability only as a research test. In addition, during persistent infection, HDVAg may not be detectable because it is complexed with anti-HDV.

Hepatitis D virus RNA is an early marker of infection in patients with both acute and chronic HDV infection.[226,229,230] HDV RNA is detectable in 90% of patients during the symptomatic phase of HDV infection. HDV RNA levels are nondetectable following symptomatic resolution but remain elevated in chronic infection. A significant correlation exists among HDV RNA detection by hybridization assay, positive results for IgM anti-HDV in serum, and positive immunohistochemistry for HDVAg in liver biopsies. Detection of HDVAg by immunohistochemical analysis of liver tissue is the best diagnostic method for persistent HDV infection; however, antigen staining is only available in research laboratories.[229]

Natural History

Coinfection with HDV and HBV resulting in acute hepatitis is correlated with a higher risk of severe or fulminant liver disease.[226] The rate of chronic disease following coinfection with HDV is similar to that of HBV infection alone, whereas superinfection with HDV is linked to a high rate of chronicity; however, the clinical course may be variable.[226,231] Approximately 15% of patients superinfected with HDV develop rapidly progressive disease with hepatic decompensation (e.g., cirrhosis) within 12 months of the infection. Another 15% of patients have a benign course of illness. Most patients (70%) have a slow progression to cirrhosis, depending on age, IV drug use, and level of viral replication.[225–227] Finally, HBsAg-positive, HBeAg-positive patients who are superinfected with HDV are more likely to develop fulminant disease compared with those who are HBsAg-positive with anti-HBe and who are superinfected and develop chronic disease.[225–227]

Clinical and Extrahepatic Manifestations

Delta infection may be acquired simultaneously in a patient with acute HBV infection (coinfection), or it may occur in a patient with chronic HBV who is a carrier of HBsAg (superinfection). Infection with HDV can lead to both acute and chronic forms of hepatitis. Another pattern of infection, known as latent HDV infection, is documented in liver transplant recipients and is characterized by HDV infection being identified in the liver graft before reinfection of the graft with HBV.[226,232] Acute HDV coinfection is marked by symptoms seen in other acute hepatotrophic viral infections. HDV infection also has a unique biphasic increase in aminotransferase activity, which is rarely observed in HBV infection alone. The clinical features of chronic HDV infection are not specific and are similar to those seen in chronic hepatitis from other causes.

Patients who develop chronic infection are at risk for developing cirrhosis and hepatic decompensation. In contrast to patients with chronic HBV infection, a negative association exists between HDV and HCC.[226,227] Potential reasons for this could be that the delta agent has direct tumor protective effects; delta markers in patients with HCC disappear because the time between infection and cancer detection is longer than in patients with HCC from other causes, or HDV predisposes to early mortality before HCC can develop.[226]

Prevention

Hepatitis D virus replication is dependent on HBV replication; therefore, successful immunization with HBV vaccine also prevents HDV infection.[225–227] No immunoprophylactic therapies are available for patients with chronic HBV infection who are also at risk for superinfection with HDV. Prevention of HDV superinfection is based on behavioral modification, such as the use of condoms to prevent sexual transmission and needle exchange programs to minimize transmission by IV drug use.

Treatment

Supportive care is the general strategy used to treat HDV infection. Because the development of fulminant hepatic failure is more frequent with HDV infection, close monitoring for evidence of encephalopathy, coagulopathy, and other signs of liver failure (e.g., acidosis) is warranted. Liver transplantation is the treatment of choice for patients with fulminant or end-stage liver disease following HDV infection. In patients with chronic HDV infection, antiviral therapy has been attempted; however, therapeutic trials in managing chronic HDV infection have been disappointing (Table 73-22).[226,231] Treatment with either prednisone or azathioprine is ineffective.[233] The use of IFN-α to treat chronic delta hepatitis has been reviewed using meta-analysis of five small, randomized, controlled trials. Patients treated with IFN-α (5 MU/day or 9 MU three times weekly) for 12 months experienced a 30% rate of complete disease remission (normalization of ALT values) compared with 1% observed in untreated controls.[234] In the largest trial published to date, patients with chronic hepatitis D were randomized to either IFN -α2b, 5 MU three times weekly for 4 months then 3 MU three times weekly for an additional 8 months, or placebo. Serum ALT reductions of >50% from baseline were observed in 42% of IFN-α–treated patients at 4 months compared with 7% of untreated controls. The treatment effect was not sustained, however, because only 26% of treated patients maintained reductions in ALT levels at 12 months. Relapses after discontinuation of therapy were common, and histologic improvement was not statistically different from controls.[235] A trial using IFN-α (9 MU three times weekly) demonstrated both

Table 73-22 Efficacy of Interferon in Chronic HDV

Author	N	Interferon	Dosage	Duration (Months)	Response (%) Primary	Response (%) Sustained
Rosina/Rizzetto	12	α2b	5 MU TIW	3	33	8
	12	None	–	–	17	0
Rosina	31	α2b	5 MU TIW then 3 MU TIW	4 then 8	45	25
	30	None	–	–	27	0
Farci	14	α2a	9 MU TIW	12	71	36
	14	α2a	3 MU TIW	12	29	0
	13	None	–	–	8	0
Gaudin	11	α2b	5 MU TIW then 3 MU TIW	4 then 8	66	9
	11	None	–		36	18
Puoti	21	α2b	10 MU TIW and 6 MU TIW	6 and 6	14	9

TIW, three times weekly.
From references 167, 235, 236, with permission.

virologic and histologic improvement after 48 weeks of therapy. As in the previous trials, the treatment effect was not sustained, and relapse was common after drug discontinuation.[236] No clinical, serologic, or virologic factors consistently predict response or lack of response to IFN. In uncontrolled trials involving a small number of patients, the duration of the HDV infection may be significant based on the improved response rates in patients who have had their disease for a relatively short period (i.e., IV drug users) compared with response rates in patients from endemic areas whose infections are acquired early in life. Because of the nature of these reports, verification of this association is needed.

Two small open-label trials evaluated the use of PegIFN-α alone[237] or in combination with ribavirin[238] for the treatment of chronic HDV infection. Castelnua et al.[237] evaluated the efficacy of PegIFN-α2b monotherapy, 1.5 mcg/kg weekly for 12 months in 14 patients with chronic HDV infection. A virologic response, defined as undetectable HDV RNA by PCR, was seen in 57% of patients at the end of therapy and persisted in 43% of patients during the follow-up period. The rate of ALT normalization was higher at the end of follow-up (57%) than at the end of therapy (36%), suggesting that the reduction occurred during the posttreatment phase. A second randomized, controlled trial was performed comparing the efficacy and safety of PegIFN-α alone (1.5 mcg/kg/week) for 72 weeks ($n = 16$) or in combination with ribavirin (800 mg/day) for 48 weeks followed by PegIFN-α monotherapy for 24 additional weeks ($n = 22$).[238] Clearance of HDV RNA at the end of therapy occurred in 19% of patients receiving monotherapy and just 9% of those patients receiving combination therapy. Similarly, the rate of virologic clearance increased to 25% and 19%, respectively, during posttreatment follow-up period. The rates of biochemical response were similar in both groups (25% versus 27% at the end of follow-up) with relapse rates approaching 60%. Although these trials show promise, larger trials with longer follow-up periods are required to confirm the role of PegIFN in HDV infection.

Results from a pilot trial that evaluated the efficacy of 100 mg of oral lamivudine in five patients with HDV (all were positive for HBsAg, antibody to HDV, and HDV RNA) for 12 months demonstrated that serum levels of HBV DNA were reduced in all five patients. All patients remained HBsAg and HDV-RNA positive, however, and serum ALT and liver histology did not improve.[239] Additionally, in patients with chronic HDV infection who received 100 mg of oral lamivudine for 24 weeks followed by a combination of high-dose interferon (9 MU TIW) and 100 mg of oral lamivudine for 16 weeks, biochemical and histologic test findings were not significantly improved compared with baseline characteristics.[240] Nucleoside analogs, such as lamivudine, have not proved to be effective for treating HDV infection because of their inability to cause HBsAg, the only protein required by HDV, to disappear.

In patients with decompensated cirrhosis caused by HDV, liver transplantation is the most appropriate intervention because IFN may precipitate hepatic decompensation.[212,214,236] The presence and amount of HBV DNA before transplantation is the most significant outcome marker, often predicting the posttransplant reinfection rate. Patients who receive a liver transplant for chronic HDV infection have a lower incidence of posttransplant HBV infection than do those with HBV infection alone (67% versus 32%, respectively).[212] This is thought to be related to an inhibitory effect of HDV on HBV replication. Furthermore, 3-year survival is higher for patients with HDV cirrhosis than for patients undergoing transplantation for HBV cirrhosis alone (88% versus 44%, respectively) and is similar to patients having liver transplantation for other indications.[212]

HEPATITIS C VIRUS

Virology

Before the development of methods to identify hepatitis C virus, most post-transfusion hepatitis cases were designated as non-A, non-B (NANB) hepatitis. HCV is recognized now as the most common cause of chronic NANB transfusion-associated hepatitis.[235–238] HCV is a single-stranded, 50-nm RNA virus related to the flaviviruses, a family that includes the yellow fever virus and two animal viruses, bovine viral diarrhea virus, and classic swine fever virus (Table 73-2).[241,245,246]

The genome of HCV contains a single outer reading frame (ORF) capable of encoding a large viral protein precursor that, when cleaved, results in a series of structural (nucleocapsid core and envelops 1 and 2) and nonstructural (NS2, NS3, NS4a, NS4b, NS5a, and NS5b) proteins.[245,247,248] The amino terminal region of NS3 encodes a viral serine protease that cleaves viral peptides, whereas the carboxyl end functions as a helicase, which is essential in unwinding of viral RNA during replication. The NS5b protein functions as an RNA-dependent RNA polymerase; the function of the NS5a protein is unknown, but it may play a role in regulating replication. Furthermore, the positive strand RNA of HCV functions as a template for synthesis of negative strand RNA, as a template for translation of viral proteins, and as genomic RNA to be packaged into new virions. Unlike HBV, HCV has no DNA intermediate and therefore cannot integrate into the host genome.[245,247,248]

The replication process of HCV is poorly understood because there is no *in vitro* or *in vivo* study model system. Available data suggest that viral binding and uptake into the hepatocytes occur through membrane fusion and receptor-mediated endocytosis[245,247,248] (Table 73-2). Following incorporation into the cytoplasm of hepatocytes, the nucleocapsid is uncoated to release RNA. Subsequently, the HCV RNA is translated to several polyproteins that undergo co- and post-translational processing. Subsequently, a complex structure (positive strand RNA) is used as a template for synthesis of negative strand RNA. In primates, HCV RNA is detectable within 3 days of infection, persisting in serum during peak ALT elevation. Detection appears to be associated with the appearance of viral antigens in hepatocytes, the major site of HCV replication. The importance of extrahepatic sites for replication (e.g., mononuclear cells) has not been determined. Kinetic studies in HCV-infected patients have depicted a high viral turnover that may partially explain the rapid emergence of viral diversity in patients with chronic HCV infection and the persistence of the infection, through immune escape, following acute exposure. Mechanisms pertaining to viral packaging and release from the hepatocytes are poorly understood.

Epidemiology

The worldwide seroprevalence based on antibody to HCV (anti-HCV) is approximately 3%, with >170 million people infected chronically. Geographic variations exist, from 0.4% to 1.1% in North America to 9.6% to 13.6% in North Africa.[241,246,249] The prevalence of anti-HCV in the United States has been estimated to be 1.8%, corresponding to an estimated 3.9 million persons infected nationwide. Of these, 2.7 million persons are chronically infected (based on positive HCV RNA), with approximately 230,000 new infections per year.[241,246,249] HCV is the etiologic agent in more than 85% of cases associated with post-transfusional NANB hepatitis.[241,243,244] Following HCV antibody screening of blood donors in the early 1990s, transfusion-related reports of HCV have been dramatically reduced, and non-transfusion-related cases have emerged (e.g., injection drug users).[241,246,250] Sporadic infection with HCV (infection without an identifiable risk factor) accounts for up to 40% of reported HCV infections.[241,243,246] HCV is transmitted through percutaneous (e.g., blood transfusion, needlestick inoculation, high-risk behavior)[241,243,246] and nonpercutaneous (e.g., sexual contact, perinatal exposure) routes.[241,243,246,251,252] The latter appears to occur to a lesser extent than with HBV.

Hepatitis C virus infection occurs among persons of all ages, but the highest incidence is among persons aged 20 to 39 years with a male predominance. Blacks and whites have similar incidence rates of acute disease, whereas persons of Hispanic ethnicity have higher rates. In the general population, the highest prevalence rates of chronic HCV infection are found among persons aged 30 to 49 years and among males.[241,243,246] Unlike the racial or ethnic pattern of acute disease, blacks have a substantially higher prevalence of chronic HCV infection than do whites.

In the United States, the predominant HCV genotype is type 1, with subtypes 1a and 1b accounting for 70% of cases.[241,243,246] Knowledge of the genotype or serotype (genotype-specific antibodies) of HCV is helpful in making recommendations and counseling regarding therapy. Patients with genotypes 2 and 3 are almost three times more likely to respond to therapy with IFN-α or the combination of IFN-α and ribavirin. Furthermore, when using combination therapy, the recommended duration of treatment depends on the genotype. For these reasons, testing for HCV genotype is often clinically helpful. Once the genotype is identified, it need not be tested again; genotypes do not change during the course of infection. Because HCV has a high mutation rate during replication, several so-called quasispecies, a heterogeneous population of HCV isolates that are closely related, may, however, exist in an infected individual.[241,247,248] The number of quasispecies increases over the course of infection, which allows HCV to escape the host's immune system, leading to persistent infection.

Percutaneous Transmission

Before the routine use of blood screening, the incidence of acute HCV infection among transfusion recipients in the 1970s was approximately 5% to 10%. Subsequently, blood donor screening using a first-generation anti-HCV test reduced the risk of transfusion-related hepatitis to 0.6% per patient and 0.03% per unit transfused.[241,250] Following the use of more sensitive second- and third-generation assays for anti-HCV, the risk and incidence of transfusion-related hepatitis approaches that reported in hospitalized patients who have not received a transfusion.

The incidence of HCV infection is 48% to 90% among injection drug users, and the risk of acquiring the infection in these persons is as high as 90%.[241,244,253] Of injection drug users with acute NANB hepatitis, 75% are anti-HCV positive and, unlike transfusion-related hepatitis, the incidence of HCV infection associated with injection drug use has not declined.[241,244,253] Additional risk factors for HCV infection include the presence of HBV or HIV infections.[241,244,253] Other populations at risk for acquiring HCV include patients receiving chronic hemodialysis (up to 45%)[241,244,253] and health care workers (0% to 4% seroconversion following needlestick).[241,244,253,254]

Nonpercutaneous and Sporadic Transmission

Nonpercutaneous transmission includes transmission between sexual partners and from mother to child. This route of transmission is less efficient compared with the percutaneous route, and is supported by data assessing sexual transmission of HCV. Sexual partners of index patients with anti-HCV have an incidence of HCV infection ranging from 0% to 27%, whereas low-risk (anti-HCV negative) index subjects without liver disease or high-risk behavior (injection drug use or promiscuity) have an incidence of anti-HCV of 0% to 7%.[241,244] In contrast, sexual partners of subjects with liver disease or high-risk behavior have an incidence of anti-HCV ranging between 11% and 27%.[241,251] Also, the sexual partners of homosexual men and promiscuous heterosexuals with HCV have shown an increase in anti-HCV positivity.

Compared with the high incidence of perinatal transmission of HBV from mothers to infants, perinatal transmission of HCV infection is relatively low; however, high titers of circulating HCV in the mother may enhance the risk of infection in the infant.[241] Additional concerns and areas for investigation related to mother-to-infant transmission of HCV include the timing of transmission (*in utero*, time of birth), the relative risk associated with breast-feeding, and the natural history of perinatally acquired infection.

In sporadic HCV infection, up to 40% of patients acquire HCV infection without a known or identifiable risk factor.[241] This type of HCV infection may be related to a prevalent nonpercutaneous or percutaneous route that has yet to be identified.

Pathogenesis

The pathogenesis of liver damage as a result of HCV infection most likely results from both direct and indirect, immune-mediated responses instigated by the virus. Direct cellular injury may be caused by the accumulation of intact virus or viral proteins.[248,255] The direct mechanism of injury is supported by the observation that patients with high concentrations of HCV RNA (quantified through branched chain DNA assay) have greater lobular inflammatory activity compared with those with minimal inflammation. Whether specific genotypes (i.e., 1, 1b, 2) are correlated with severe disease continues to be assessed. European data suggest that type 1 genotype is associated with higher viral replication, and infection with the type 1b genotype is associated with more progressive liver disease.[248,256] One reason why HCV genotype 1 may be more difficult to treat than genotypes 2 or 3 is that genotype 1 has a longer half-life (2.9 hours) than that of genotypes 2 or 3 (2.0 hours).[241,257] Viral half-life can be defined as the time for the original amount of virus to be decreased by half, or in this case, die. Other data do not support these findings and have shown that patients with type 2 genotypes have more severe liver disease.[258] Duration of infection is another factor that may be related to disease severity because the expression of genotypes may change over time making the correlation between genotype and severity of disease problematic.

Immune-mediated mechanisms for hepatic injury have been based on the presence of $CD8^+$and $CD4^+$ lymphocytes in portal, periportal, and lobular areas in patients with HCV infection.[248,255] Hepatic $CD8^+$ lymphocytes are activated through an alternative antigen-independent pathway that stimulates CTL, which initiate hepatocellular injury. Helper or inducer T cells ($CD4^+$) have also been implicated in the pathogenesis of chronic HCV infection; however, other data suggest that $CD4^+$ cells may play a protective role against hepatocellular injury. Autoimmune mechanisms of hepatocellular injury (e.g., anti-liver-kidney microsomal antibodies) may play a minor role in the pathogenesis of liver injury.[248,255]

Diagnosis

Serologic Tests

A test for antibodies to HCV is the initial screening test for suspected HCV infection.[241,246,259–261] The two types of antibody tests are (a) the enzyme immunoassay (EIA) and the (b) recombinant immunoblot assay (RIBA). These serologic assays were developed using recombinant antigens derived from cloned HCV transcripts to substantiate a diagnosis of HCV. Predictive values of a positive third-generation EIA test are about 99% (in immunocompetent patients), which obviates the need for a confirmatory RIBA test in the diagnosis of patients with clinical liver disease.[241,246,259–261] A negative EIA test is adequate to exclude a diagnosis of chronic HCV infection in nonimmunocompromised individuals.[241,246,260,261] Occasionally, patients undergoing hemodialysis and those with immune deficiencies may have false-negative findings on EIA. On the other hand, false-positive results can occur in healthy persons without any identifiable risk factors and normal aminotransferases, and in patients with autoimmune disorders.[241,246,259,260,262] In these groups, the results should be confirmed using an assay for HCV RNA to diagnose chronic HCV infection. Anti-HCV antibodies usually are detected in serum late during the course of acute hepatitis C. In many cases, however, seroconversion may take up to a year or longer following exposure to HCV. Anti-HCV is detectable in serum for a variable length of time after acute infection, but it is not protective and its presence does not differentiate between acute, chronic, or resolved infection. The clinical symptoms, changes in HCV RNA, and serologic changes in acute and chronic HCV infection are shown in Figure 73-5A and B. Because of the enhanced specificity and sensitivity rates of the newer EIA tests, RIBA for antibodies to HCV proteins are infrequently used.

Qualitative HCV RNA Assays

Acute or chronic HCV infection in a patients with EIA positivity should be confirmed by a qualitative HCV RNA (PCR) assay with a lower limit of detection of 50 IU/mL or less (~100 viral gene/mL) or with transcription-mediated amplification (TMA), which has a detection limit of 10 IU/mL.[241,246,260,262] Both of these test are highly specific (99%). Qualitative tests detect HCV as early as 1 to 2 weeks after exposure and detect the presence of circulating HCV RNA (viral copies/mL). Results are reported as either "positive" or "negative" and are used to monitor patients receiving antiviral therapy. A single positive qualitative assay for HCV RNA confirms active replication but does not exclude viremia and may only detect a transient decline in viral load below the level of detection of the assay.[241,246,260–262] A follow-up qualitative HCV RNA needs to be obtained to confirm the lack of active HCV replication.[241,246,260–262]

Quantitative HCV RNA Assays

In comparison, quantitative tests are less sensitive than qualitative tests and they are used to determine the concentration of HCV RNA with assays such as semiquantitative PCR-based Amplicor assay (qPCR) or bDNA signal amplification.[241,246,260–262] The lower limit of detection with the second-generation bDNA and Amplicor assays are 250,000 viral equivalents/mL and 200 viral copies/mL, respectively. The qualitative HCV viral load test and third-generation bDNA

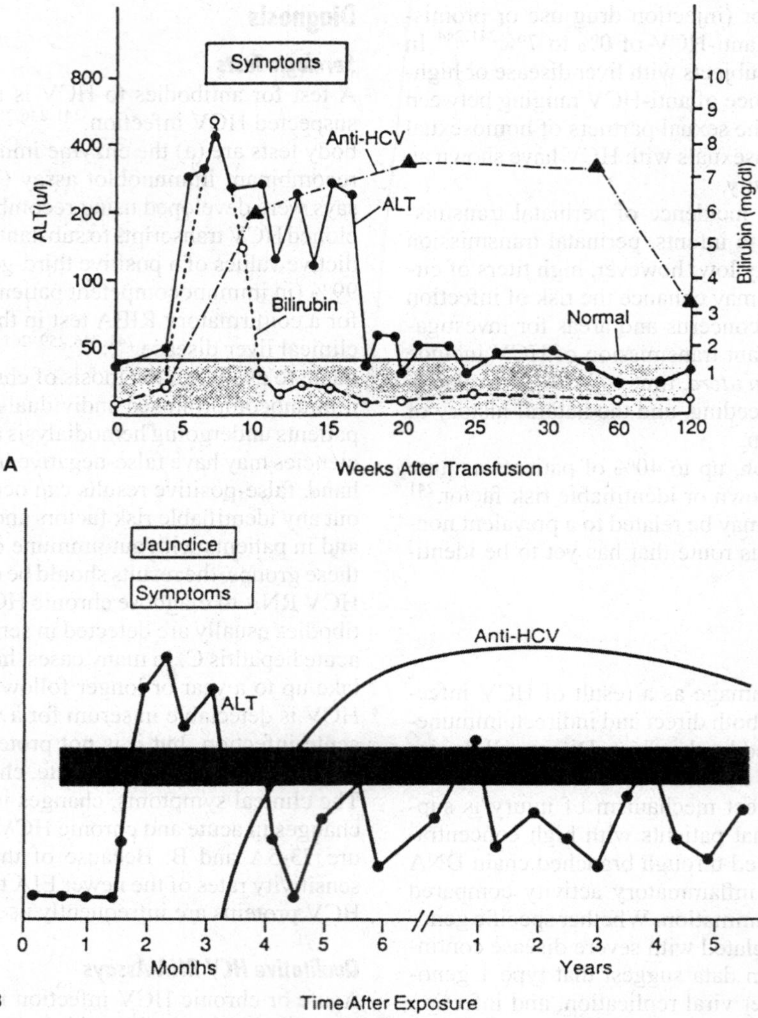

FIGURE 73-5 **A: Typical course of acute hepatitis C virus.** ALT, alanine aminotransferase; anti-HCV, hepatitis C antibody. **B: Typical course of chronic hepatitis C virus.** ALT, alanine aminotransferase; anti-HCV, hepatitis C antibody.

test have a lower limit of detection (sensitivity) of 50 copies/mL and 2,000 to 3,500 copies/mL, respectively. These tests should not be used to exclude the diagnosis of HCV infection or to determine treatment endpoint. An HCV RNA standard has been attempted to allow normalization of reported viral titers in international units. The reported international unit does not correlate with the actual number of viral particles in a preparation and variability does exist. The clinical utility of serial HCV viral concentrations in a patient is based on continued use of the same specific quantitative assay that was used initially.[241,246,260–262] These tests provide significant information with respect to response to treatment in patients receiving antiviral therapy.

Biochemical Markers

Testing for serum ALT concentrations is not a sensitive marker for assessing disease activity and at best has a weak correlation with the histopathologic findings on a liver biopsy.[241,246,260–262] Nevertheless, serial determination of ALT over time appears to be a better indicator of liver injury than is a single ALT test.

Biopsy

Liver biopsy can determine the extent of liver injury caused by HCV.[241,246,260–262] Although some histologic findings are characteristic of HCV infection, such as portal lymphoid aggregates, steatosis, and bile duct injury, these alone are not sufficiently specific to establish a diagnosis of hepatitis C. Currently, no reliable, readily available tests exist to detect HCV antigens in the liver. With respect to liver biopsy in the management HCV, a baseline biopsy (regardless of the extent of aminotransferase elevation) is recommended for the initial assessment of disease. Patients age >40 years or those who wish to defer therapy may benefit most from a liver biopsy.

Selection of Tests

All patients with elevated liver aminotransferases without an obvious source, especially those with known risk factors, should be tested for HCV. A diagnosis of acute hepatitis C can be initiated in a patient with symptoms of acute hepatitis and a positive anti-HCV titer. Confirmation is established by using ELISA tests. If patients are anti-HCV positive by ELISA with an increase in ALT concentration and have a known risk

Table 73-23 Diagnostic Tests for HCV Infection

Test/Type	Application	Comments
Hepatitis C Virus Antibody (Anti-HCV)		
EIA (enzyme immunoassay) Supplemental assay (i.e., recombinant immunoblot strip assay [RIBA])	Indicates past or present infection, but does not differentiate between acute, chronic, or resolved infection. All positive enzyme immunoassay (EIA) results should be verified with a supplemental assay	Sensitivity >97% EIA alone has low positive predictive value in low prevalence populations
Hepatitis C Virus Ribonucleic Acid (HCV RNA)		
Qualitative tests[a] Reverse transcriptase polymerase chain reaction (RT-PCR) amplification of HCV RNA by in-house or commercial assays (e.g., Amplicor HCV)	Detects presence of circulating HCV RNA Monitor patients on antiviral therapy	Detects virus as early as 1–2 weeks after exposure Detection of HCV RNA during course of infection might be intermittent False-positive or false-negative results might occur
Hepatitis C Virus Ribonucleic Acid (HCV RNA)		
Quantitative tests[a] RT-PCR amplification of HCV RNA by in-house or commercial assays (e.g., Amplicor HCV Monitor) Branched chain DNA (bDNA) assays (e.g., Quantiplex HCV RNA Assay)	Determine concentration of HCV RNA Might be useful for assessing the likelihood of response to antiviral therapy	A single negative RT-PCR is not conclusive Should not be used to exclude the diagnosis of HCV infection or to determine treatment endpoint Less sensitive than qualitative RT-PCR

[a]Currently not US Food and Drug Administration approved; lack standardization.

factor for infection exposure (IV drug abuse, blood transfusions, needle stick), confirmatory assays may not be required (Table 73-23).

Tests for HCV RNA may be indicated for diagnosing HCV when HCV antibody tests are unreliable and when indeterminate results are obtained. Thus, direct testing of HCV RNA is preferred to anti-HCV in the early stages of acute HCV infection before HCV antibodies have been produced, when antibody tests are unreliable (e.g., immunocompromised patients), when intermediate results are reported (e.g., RIBA-2 in blood donors), in differentiation between active and past infection, and in the evaluation of patients with chronic liver disease in whom antibody tests are intermediate.

Natural History

Nonimmunocompromised Patients

Once established, infection with HCV persists in most patients.[241,245,246,263] Because disease progression is often asymptomatic, patients are typically diagnosed when they receive routine biochemical testing during a physical examination or before blood donation, for example. Because NANB hepatitis (e.g., hepatitis C) was established in 1974, comprehensive data pertaining to the natural history of the disease are limited. It is known, however, that HCV infection leads to progressive liver disease. Following an asymptomatic period, histologic or clinical cirrhosis can be identified in 8% to 42% of patients as early as 15 months following the infection.[241,245,246,263] Of patients, 10% may also have decompensated liver disease as evidenced by splenomegaly, ascites, coagulopathy, and esophageal varices. In nonimmunocompromised patients, the time between acute infection and manifestations of chronic liver disease is usually 20 to 30 years with rare instances of terminal disease occurring within 3 to 5 years following acute infection. Patients with chronic HCV infection are also at increased risk for HCC.[241,245,246,263]

Patients receiving dialysis have a greater incidence of HCV infection compared with the general population (6% to 22%) because they receive multiple blood transfusions.[264] Kidney transplant recipients also have a high incidence of HCV infection (6%–28%), which may be acquired through dialysis before transplant or from the allograft or blood products following transplantation.[265] Following kidney transplantation, elevation in aminotransferases is more common in anti–HCV-positive compared with anti–HCV-negative patients (48% and 14%, respectively) and cirrhosis has been reported with the former.[266,267] While HCV infection is associated with liver failure, differences in overall patient and graft survival between HCV-positive and HCV-negative patients do not appear to be significant. Long-term studies are needed to confirm these findings.

Immunocompromised Patients

Chronic HCV infection is the most common indication for orthotopic liver transplantation (OLT) in the United States with up to 40% of patients receiving a transplant for the disease.[268–271] Recurrence rates of HCV following transplantation are 100%, possibly because of viremia at the time of transplant.[268–271] In addition, *de novo* acquisition of HCV from the donor liver or from blood products may occur. One-year follow-up studies indicate that 50% of patients with viremia following transplant (HCV RNA) have normal biopsies with no histologic evidence of HCV infection, 40% have mild chronic hepatitis, and 10% have progressive liver damage with chronic active hepatitis and bridging fibrosis or cirrhosis.[268,269] Histologic evidence of disease may also be present even when aminotransferase levels are normal. Reports suggest that high viral loads, as measured by quantitative HCV RNA, have been correlated with early acute hepatitis in the allograft and that genotype 1b may predispose OLT recipients to more severe histologic disease compared with recipients of transplants with other genotypes.[268–270] Controlled trials are needed to further evaluate the relationship between genotype, viral load, amount of immunosuppression, and immunomodulating coinfections (e.g., CMV) and the course of posttransplant HCV infection.

HIV Coinfection

The incidence of HCV infection in HIV-infected patients is variable with up to 100% infection reported in HIV-positive injection drug users.[268] In other populations, such as homosexual men, the incidence is marginally greater than that reported in the general population. Some studies suggest that patients with HCV who are coinfected with HIV may also have more severe hepatic injury and a worse outcome than those infected with HCV alone, whereas other reports contradict these findings.[268,272–274] These conflicting reports may be affected by several factors, including the duration of HCV infection before HIV infection, the route of HCV infection, the genotype associated with infection, and patient selection.

HBV Coinfection

As mentioned above, both HBV and HCV are transmitted parenterally and coinfection is not uncommon, particularly in IV drug users and in countries with a high prevalence of HBV infection.[73,241] Coinfection with chronic HBV and HCV results in more severe liver disease than infection with either virus alone, including increased risk of liver cancer and fulminant hepatitis.[72,241,275,276]

Clinical and Extrahepatic Manifestations

Most patients with acute HCV infection are asymptomatic.[241,246,263,277] In contrast, patients with chronic HCV infection generally complain of fatigue. Nonspecific symptoms are similar to those seen with HBV infection, including nausea, anorexia, abdominal discomfort, and depression. Once patients develop cirrhosis and portal hypertension, they may experience intractable ascites, spontaneous bacterial peritonitis, GI or esophageal bleeding, poor synthetic function (hypoalbuminemia or prolonged PT), or encephalopathy.[241,246,263,277] Jaundice occasionally occurs in acute HCV infection, but it is usually present in chronic infection as a result of decompensated liver disease.

Significant extrahepatic manifestations may also develop as a result of HCV infection.[241,246,263,277] They include membranoproliferative glomerulonephritis, mixed cryoglobulinemia, porphyria cutanea tarda, leukocytoclastic vasculitis, focal lymphocytic sialadenitis, corneal ulcers, idiopathic pulmonary fibrosis, and rheumatoid arthritis.

Prevention of Hepatitis C

Pre-exposure Prophylaxis

No vaccines are effective against HCV, and current measures to prevent hepatitis C infection have largely focused on identifying high-risk uninfected persons and counseling them on risk-reducing strategies to prevent infection.

The CDC and NIH have published recommendations that address these issues.[241,244] Suggested primary preventative measures are that in health care settings, adherence to universal (standard) precautions for the protection of medical personnel and patients be implemented and that HCV-positive individuals should refrain from donating blood, organs, tissues, or semen. In some situations, the use of organs and tissues from HCV-positive individuals may be considered. For example, in emergency situations the use of a donor organ in which the HCV status is either positive or unknown may be considered in an HCV-negative recipient after full disclosure and informed consent. Strategies should be developed to identify prospective blood donors with any history of injection drug use. Such individuals must be deferred from donating blood.

Furthermore, safer sexual practices, including the use of latex condoms, should be strongly encouraged in persons with multiple sexual partners. In monogamous long-term relationships, transmission is rare.[241,244] Although HCV-positive individuals and their partners should be informed of the potential for transmission, insufficient data exist to recommend changes in current sexual practice in persons with a steady partner. It is recommended that sexual partners of infected patients should be tested for antibody to HCV.

In households with an HCV-positive member, sharing razors and toothbrushes should be avoided.[241,243] Covering open wounds is recommended. Injection needles should be carefully disposed of using universal precaution techniques. It is not necessary to avoid close contact with family members or to avoid sharing meals or utensils. No evidence justifies exclusion of HCV-positive children or adults from participation in social, educational, and employment activities.

Additionally, pregnancy is not contraindicated in HCV-infected individuals. Perinatal transmission from mother to baby occurs in <6% of instances.[241,244] No evidence indicates that breast-feeding transmits HCV from mother to baby; therefore, it is considered safe. Babies born to HCV-positive mothers should be tested for anti-HCV at 1 year.

Finally, needle exchange and other safer injection drug use programs may be beneficial in reducing parenterally transmitted diseases.[241,244] Expansion of such programs should be considered in an effort to reduce the rate of transmission of hepatitis C. It is important that clear and evidenced-based information be provided to both patients and physicians regarding the natural history, means of prevention, management, and therapy of hepatitis C.

Postexposure Prophylaxis

Immunoglobulin is no longer recommended for postexposure prophylaxis of hepatitis C infection because it is not effective.[241,244,279]

Treatment of Acute Hepatitis C

36. R.D. is a 37-year-old, 95-kg professional athlete with multiple arm tattoos and a remote history of IV drug use. In 1993, an unscheduled physical examination was performed on R.D. because of the severe fatigue he experienced following inscription of a tattoo. Laboratory tests at that time revealed the following results: ALT, 350 U/L (normal, 5–40 U/L); serum anti-HCV positive (RIBA-2); and an HCV RNA level of 800,000 viral equivalents/mL (bDNA). What were the clinical and serologic features of HCV in R.D. (at that time), and what drug therapy could have been used to treat his acute hepatitis C?

R.D. clearly had a clinical picture consistent with acute HCV infection, including symptoms of fatigue, elevated ALT,

Table 73-24 Comparative Pharmacokinetics of Pegylated Interferons

	Interferon-α	*Peginterferon-α 2b (12 kDa)*	*Peginterferon-α 2a (40 kDa)*
Parameter			
Absorption	Rapid	Rapid	Sustained
Distribution	Wide	Wide	Blood, organs
Clearance	–	10-fold reduction (hepatic/renal)	100-fold reduction (hepatic)
Elimination half-life (hr)	3–5	30–50	50–80
Weight-based dosing	No	Yes	No
Increased concentration with multiple dosing	No	Yes	Yes
Protected from degradation	No	Probable	Yes

and positive anti-HCV RIBA-2 assay and HCV RNA levels. Interferon-α has been studied in patients with acute HCV in an effort to reduce the severity and rate of progression of chronic infection. Limited data suggest that patients with acute HCV infection receiving IFN-α had a lower rate of chronic infection (36%–61%) compared with patients who did not receive therapy (80%–100%).[280,281] These studies, however, have included relatively few patients and used varying dosages and durations (6 months to 1 year). One recent report in Germany evaluated 44 patients with acute hepatitis C.[282] Patients received 5 MU of IFN-α2b SC daily for 4 weeks and then three times per week for another 20 weeks. Serum HCV RNA concentrations were measured before and during therapy and 20 weeks after the end of therapy. At the end of therapy, 43 of 44 patients had undetectable concentrations of HCV RNA in serum and normal serum alanine aminotransferase concentrations. Therapy was well tolerated in all but one patient, who stopped therapy after 12 weeks because of side effects. Thus, if early identification is possible, interferon therapy in the acute phase of the disease appears to be rational. Thus, R.D. could have been started on IFN-α to minimize his risk for developing chronic HCV infection.

Treatment of Chronic Hepatitis C

37. **Initially, R.D.'s hepatologist did not initiate IFN therapy. R.D. now presents to the clinic confused (encephalopathic), with mild ascites and scleral icterus. Significant laboratory findings are as follows: total bilirubin, 4.2 ng/mL (normal, 0.2–1.0 ng/mL); direct bilirubin, 2.2 ng/mL (normal, 0–0.2 ng/mL); ALT, 350 U/L (normal, 5–40 U/L); and AST, 330 U/L (normal, 5–40 U/L). Additionally, genotyping of R.D.'s HCV infection shows that he is genotype 2. What pharmacologic agents are effective in the treatment of patients with chronic hepatitis C?**

R.D. appears to have an atypical accelerated progression of hepatitis C infection based on the current status of his disease. Chronic hepatitis develops in approximately 80% of patients with acute hepatitis C infection. Of patients chronically infected with HCV, approximately 8% to 42% develop histologic or clinical cirrhosis and disability from end-stage liver disease.[241,243,246,263] Up to 10% of cases are associated with decompensated disease with splenomegaly, ascites, coagulopathy, and esophageal varices as early as 15 months after the episode of acute HCV infection. The lack of specific immunoprophylaxis and significant morbidity and mortality associated with chronic HCV infection highlight the need for effective antiviral therapy. Previously, symptomatic patients with chronic hepatitis C infection without decompensated liver disease could be treated with IFN-α[283–298] (Table 73-24) or IFN plus ribavirin[299–301] (Table 73-25) based on controlled studies confirming effectiveness. Furthermore, patients without evidence of fibrosis or significant inflammatory activity are at extremely low risk for the development of cirrhosis or serious hepatic complications; therefore, they can usually defer therapy. Conversely, patients with advanced cirrhosis are poor candidates for current IFN-based treatment regimens because of the increased treatment-associated morbidity seen in these patients and the possible precipitation of decompensation or frank hepatic failure.

GOALS OF THERAPY

The goals of therapy for treating HCV infection are (a) eradicate the virus; (b) decrease morbidity and mortality; (c) normalize biochemical markers; (d) improve clinical symptoms; (e) prevent spread of the disease; (f) prevent progression to cirrhosis and hepatocellular carcinoma; and (g) prevent the development of end-stage liver disease and its manifestations. These goals may be partly achieved through pharmacologic therapy.

Table 73-25 Contraindications to Interferon-α Plus Ribavirin

Interferon	*Ribavirin*
Absolute neutrophil <1.5	Unstable cardiac disease
Platelets <75,000/mm^3	Severe chronic obstructive pulmonary disease (COPD), asthma
Severe depression	Renal dysfunction
Psychiatric instability	Serum creatinine >1.5 mg/dL
Active substance abuse	Creatinine clearance <50 mL/min
Uncontrolled autoimmune disorders	Anemia
Thyroid	Hemoglobin <13 g/dL in males
Diabetes	Hemoglobin <12 g/dL in females
Rheumatoid arthritis	Hemoglobinopathies
Elevated antinuclear antibodies	Thalassemias, sickle cell anemia

Note: Pregnancy risk:
1. Contraindicated in women who are pregnant or by men whose female partners are pregnant.
2. Negative pregnancy test should be obtained before therapy.
3. Women of childbearing potential and men capable of inducing pregnancy must use two reliable forms of birth control during treatment; contraception should be continued for 6 months following discontinuation of treatment.

Interferon

ASSESSMENT OF INTERFERON RESPONSE AND EFFICACY

Several tests are used to assess therapy in HCV infection. These include biochemical markers such as ALT (less reliable), histologic markers (improvement in HAI), clinical progression and mortality, and viral load (HCV RNA). Patterns of response with respect to viral load can be summarized as follows: (a) nonresponder: no reduction in HCV RNA during treatment; (b) partial responder: reduced HCV RNA during treatment, increased HCV RNA following treatment period; (c) relapser: HCV RNA undetectable during treatment followed by high HCV RNA at the end of therapy; and (d) sustained responder: nondetectable HCV RNA throughout the treatment period and beyond the end (usually 6 months) of therapy (Fig 73-6).

In one of the largest trials published to date, patients with chronic hepatitis C were randomly assigned to 3 MU or 1 MU of IFN-α2b three times weekly for 24 weeks or placebo.[283] Response to therapy was assessed by serial measurements of ALT values and liver biopsy results before and after treatment. Of 58 patients treated with 3 MU of IFN-α, approximately one-third had normalized ALT values compared with 16% of patients treated with 1 MU of IFN-α and <5% of untreated controls. Improvement in liver histology was noted in patients receiving IFN-α. The responses to IFN-α were rapid (in general, within 12 weeks). End of treatment response, however, was poor following discontinuation of IFN-α.

Because of the suboptimal response of interferon in early clinical trials, several strategies were attempted to enhance efficacy.[283–298] Explored strategies included longer courses of therapy, higher doses of interferon, and utilization of different formulations of interferon.[302–311] Also, patients developed anemia, thrombocytopenia, neutropenia, and neurologic adverse effects with the prolonged regimens or higher dosing schedules. Ultimately, there did not appear to be a significant difference in efficacy or tolerability between different forms of interferon (e.g., IFN-γ, consensus interferon).[302–310]

38. Are there additional IFN formulations that R.D. could receive that may be more efficacious than IFN-α monotherapy for treating chronic HCV infection?

Additional Treatment Strategies

RIBAVIRIN PLUS INTERFERON

In 1998, reports were published on the results of blinded, placebo-controlled trials of patients infected with hepatitis C with combination therapy utilizing interferon and ribavirin for treatment naïve patients[299–301] (Table 73-25) and in patients with relapsing HCV.[302] In a double-blind, US multicenter trial, patients with chronic HCV infection were randomly assigned to receive recombinant IFN-α2b plus placebo for 24 weeks or 48 weeks, or the combination of IFN-α2b and ribavirin for 24 weeks or 48 weeks.[297] IFN-α2b was administered SC at a dosage of 3 MU three times per week, and oral ribavirin (or matched placebo) was given in daily divided doses of 400 mg (AM) and 600 mg (PM) in patients <75 kg or 600 mg twice daily in patients >75 kg. Efficacy was determined based on sustained virologic response (absence of HCV RNA 24 weeks after treatment was discontinued), biochemical response (reduction in serum aminotransferases), and histologic response (hepatic inflammation and fibrosis based on biopsy).

Greater sustained virologic response took place in patients receiving combination therapy with ribavirin for either 24 weeks (70 of 228 patients; 31%) or 48 weeks (87 of 228 patients; 38%) than in patients who received IFN alone for 24 weeks (13 of 231 patients; 6%) or 48 weeks (29 of 255 patients; 13%). The rate of sustained biochemical response similarly was greater among patients who received IFN and ribavirin for 24 or 48 weeks than among those who received IFN alone. Histologic improvement was observed most often in patients receiving the combination regimen for either 24 weeks (57%) or 48 weeks (61%) compared with IFN alone for either 24 weeks (44%) or 48 weeks (41%). Dose-limiting adverse effects were most commonly associated with combination therapy. Of patients on ribavirin, 8% required dosage reduction for hemoglobin concentrations <10 g/dL. Hemoglobin concentrations remained depressed, yet stable, with the dosage reduction throughout the rest of the trial period and returned to baseline within 4 to 8 weeks after treatment was stopped at 24 or 48 weeks. Dyspnea, pharyngitis, pruritus, rash, nausea, insomnia, and anorexia were also more common with combination therapy than with IFN alone. The most common reason for discontinuation of therapy was depression, which ranged from 2% to 9% in all groups. Despite the favorable outcomes with combination therapy, no difference in overall survival was described between the treatment groups.

Similarly, another placebo-controlled, multicenter, randomized trial was performed in 832 patients with compensated chronic HCV infection.[300] Patients were assigned to one of three regimens: 3 MU IFN-α2b three times per week plus oral ribavirin (400 mg followed by 600 mg daily if <75 kg or 600 mg twice daily if >75 kg) for 48 weeks; 3 MU IFN-α2b three times per week plus oral ribavirin (400 mg followed by 600 mg daily if <75 kg or 600 mg twice daily if >75 kg) for 24 weeks; or 3 MU IFN-α2b three times per week plus placebo for 48 weeks. The primary study endpoint was loss of detectable HCV RNA (serum HCV RNA <100 copies/mL) at week 24 after treatment. A sustained virologic response was observed in 119 (43%) of the 277 patients treated for 48 weeks with the combination regimen, 97 (35%) of the 277 patients treated for 24 weeks with the combination regimen, and 53 (19%) of the 278 patients treated for 48 weeks with IFN alone.

Discontinuation of therapy for adverse events was more frequent with combination therapy (19%) and monotherapy (13%) given for 48 weeks than combination therapy given for 24 weeks (8%).

PREDICTORS OF TREATMENT OUTCOME

These studies have resulted in the identification of several independent factors predicting sustained virologic response to combination therapy.[241,311,312] The most significant of which is HCV genotype. Generally, genotype 1-infected patients have poor response to interferon and ribavirin, irrespective of viral load, and require 48 weeks of therapy. Patients with HCV other than genotype 1 with a viral load <2 million copies/mL, however, have higher response rates and require only 24 weeks of therapy. Additional host factors have been identified and may help predict response to, and duration of, therapy, allowing combination therapy to be tailored more effectively.[241,311,312] In addition to HCV genotype non-1, other factors that predict a good response to interferon and ribavirin include age <40 years, female gender, and little to no portal fibrosis on biopsy.[241,311,312] In addition, black patients with chronic HCV infection have lower response rates than whites to IFN monotherapy and are predominantly infected with genotype 1.[241,311,312]

Based on previous studies, R.D. could have benefited from the combination of ribavirin plus IFN. Other interferon-based therapies exist that are considered to be the standard of care for patients with chronic HCV infection.

Current Treatment Strategies

39. What other IFN-based drug therapy could provide R.D. with therapeutic advantages over IFN alone or IFN plus ribavirin?

Although the advent of combination interferon and ribavirin therapy has led to significant improved clearance of serum HCV RNA and improved both biochemical and histologic evidence of chronic hepatitis, numerous patients with chronic infection are not adequately treated.[241,299–301,311,312] Thus, research in the last few years has examined methodologies for enhancing the effectiveness of interferon-based treatments. The most promising of these explorations has been the development of pegylated interferons.[241,313–316] These compounds are formed through the attachment of polyethylene glycol (PEG) to an interferon molecule, thus changing the pharmacokinetic and pharmacodynamic properties of the drug (Table 73-24).[241,313–316] Of importance, the PEG moiety significantly increases the half-life of IFN, resulting in sustained serum concentrations and permitting once weekly dosing.[241,313–316] The current "standard of care" is PegIFN plus ribavirin for most patients with chronic hepatitis C infection. Subgroups of patients remain in whom standard IFN plus ribavirin combination or pegylated monotherapy may be preferable. Treatment groups are discussed below.

PEGYLATED INTERFERONS

Currently, two forms of PegIFN are FDA approved for treatment of HCV infection. The linear 12 kDa PegIFN, peginterferonα2b (Pegintron; Schering-Plough Corporation), was the first to be FDA approved.[241,313,317,318] The 40-kDa pegylated interferon, peginterferon α2a (Pegsys; Hoffman La Roche), has also received FDA approval (Table 73-24).[241,313,319–321]

Efficacy

In a dose-finding study, PegIFN-α2b (12 kDa) was compared with IFN-α2b for the initial treatment of compensated chronic hepatitis C.[317] Patients received either IFN-α2b 3 MU three-times-weekly or PegIFN-α2b 0.5 mcg/kg, 1.0 mcg/kg, or 1.5 mcg/kg once weekly. Subjects were treated for 48 weeks and then followed for an additional 24 weeks. All three PegIFN-α2b doses significantly improved virologic response rates (loss of detectable serum HCV RNA) compared with IFN-α2b. Unlike the end-of-treatment virologic response, the sustained virologic response rate was not dose related above 1.0 mcg/kg PegIFN-α2b because of a higher relapse rate among patients treated with 1.5 mcg/kg PegIFN-α2b, particularly among patients infected with genotype 1. All three PegIFN-α2b doses decreased liver inflammation to a greater extent than did IFN-α2b, particularly in subjects with sustained responses. Adverse events and changes in laboratory values were mild or moderate.

In another trial using the 40 kDa PegIFN dosage form, PegIFN-α2a was compared with IFN-α2a in the initial treatment of patients with chronic hepatitis C.[319] A total of 531 patients with chronic hepatitis C were randomized to receive either 180 mcg of PegIFN-α2a SC once per week for 48 weeks or 6 MU of IFN-α2a SC three times per week for 12 weeks, followed by 3 MU three times per week for 36 weeks. Patients were assessed at week 72 for a sustained virologic response that was defined as an undetectable level of hepatitis C virus RNA (<100 copies/mL). PegIFN-α2a was associated with a higher rate of virologic response than was IFN-α2a at week 48 (69% versus 28%) and at week 72 (39% versus 19%). Sustained normalization of serum alanine aminotransferase concentrations at week 72 was also more common in the PegIFN group than in the IFN group (45% versus 25%). The two groups were similar with respect to the reported adverse events. Authors concluded that in these patients, a regimen of PegIFN-α2a given once weekly is more effective than a regimen of IFN-α2a given three times per week.

These trials demonstrate that monotherapy with pegylated interferons is superior to conventional interferon alone. Several trials have evaluated the role of combination pegylated interferon plus ribavirin for the treatment of chronic hepatitis C infection.[318,321,322]

Manns et al.[318] compared the combination of PegIFN-α2b (1.5 mcg/kg/week) plus ribavirin 800 mg/day with PegIFN-α2b (1.5 mcg/kg/week with a reduction to 0.5 mcg/kg/week after 4 weeks) plus ribavirin 1,000 to 1,200 mg/day and with IFN-α2b plus ribavirin.[312] No difference in the sustained response was observed between the lower dose of PegIFN-α2b (12 kDa) plus ribavirin and standard IFNα2b plus ribavirin. The difference in the overall treatment response between PegIFN-α2b (12 kDa) (1.5 mcg/kg) plus ribavirin and IFN-α2b plus ribavirin was 6% adjusted for viral genotype and presence of cirrhosis at baseline. As with other IFN-based therapies, patients with genotype 1 infection, regardless of their pretreatment viral load, had a lower response to PegIFN-α2b (12 kDa) plus ribavirin compared with patients infected with other viral genotypes. The superior efficacy of PegIFN plus ribavirin over standard IFN plus ribavirin was only seen in patients with genotype 1 infection. One-third of patients with both genotype 1 infection and a high viral load (>2,000,000 copies/mL, >800,000 IU/mL) responded to therapy in both groups. Similarly, the efficacy of PegIFN plus ribavirin was the same as that observed with standard IFN plus ribavirin in patients with bridging fibrosis or cirrhosis.

Other researchers have compared the efficacy and safety of PegIFN-α2a plus ribavirin, IFN-α2b plus ribavirin, and PegIFN-α2a alone in the initial treatment of chronic hepatitis C.[321] In this trial, patients were randomly assigned to three treatment groups who received at least one dose of study medication consisting of 180 mcg of PegIFN-α2a once weekly plus ribavirin 1,000 or 1,200 mg/day (depending on body weight), weekly PegIFN-α2a plus daily placebo or 3 MU of IFN-α2b three times weekly plus daily ribavirin for 48 weeks. A significantly greater proportion of patients receiving PegIFN-α2a plus ribavirin had a sustained virologic response (defined as the absence of detectable HCV RNA 24 weeks after cessation of therapy) compared with patients who received IFN-α2b plus ribavirin (56% versus 44%; $P<0.001$) or PegIFN-α2a alone (56% versus 29%; $P<0.001$). The proportions of patients with HCV genotype 1 who had sustained virologic responses were 46%, 36%, and 21%, respectively, for the three regimens.

Among patients with HCV genotype 1 and high baseline levels of HCV RNA, the proportions of those with sustained virologic responses were 41%, 33%, and 13%, respectively. The overall safety profiles of the three treatment regimens were similar. Based on these results, it appears that PegIFN-α2a plus ribavirin is superior to IFN-α2b plus ribavirin or PegIFN-α2a alone in the treatment of chronic hepatitis C. Pooled data from these trials suggest that the sustained virologic response (SVR) rates were higher among patients with HCV RNA genotype 2 or 3 (76%–84%) and lower among those patients with genotype 1 (42%–52%).

Predictors of Treatment Outcome for Pegylated Interferons

Independent variables associated with a favorable response to pegylated interferon plus ribavirin include genotype non-1, low pretreatment HCV RNA level, light body weight, young age (40 years), and the absence of bridging fibrosis or cirrhosis.[241,318,321] Ethnicity is also a strong predictor of response to therapy with PegIFN. Based on data from clinical trials, blacks have lower response rates than do whites.[323] Another predictor of SVR has been established by monitoring the rate of HCV RNA reduction following initiation of therapy.[325,326] Assessment of antiviral effects through viral kinetics have been shown to help in predicting the likelihood of a SVR. Because the decline in HCV RNA follows a pattern of biphasic reduction, it enables clinicians to determine whether a rapid virologic response (RVR), defined as undetectable HCV RNA, occurs. If this response is observed, it is a strong predictor of obtaining an SVR. Additionally, if patients with genotype 1 do not have an early virologic response (EVR), defined as $\geq$2 $\log_{10}$ decrease in HCV RNA from baseline or undetectable HCV RNA at 12 weeks, they are unlike to achieve an SVR and therapy may be discontinued.

40. Should weight-based ribavirin dosing be recommended in R. D.?

The most appropriate dose of ribavirin administered in combination with PegIFN-α2b is controversial.[241,246] The FDA-approved ribavirin dose of 800 mg is lower than that approved for standard IFN-α2b. The FDA-approved dose was selected because of concerns regarding additive toxicities associated with peginterferon and ribavirin. Additional data from trials of PegIFN-α2a have suggested that the 800-mg dose is sufficient for treatment of nongenotype 1 infection, but that higher doses (1,000 mg/1,200 mg based on a 75 kg weight) are necessary for effective treatment of genotype 1. Additional data analysis from the pivotal trials has led to patient-specific recommendations for duration and dosing of therapy based on HCV genotype (Fig. 73-6). Patients with genotypes 2 and 3 require only 24 weeks of therapy with 800 mg daily of ribavirin, whereas patients with genotype 1 (and potentially genotype 4), require 48 weeks of therapy and full doses of ribavirin (1,000–1,200 mg daily).

A distinct relationship occurs between successful outcomes (SVR) and exposure to ribavirin. In patients who received <60% of the total ribavirin dose, early virologic response rates and SVR were lower than in patients who had reduced ribavirin exposure (73% versus 79%–84% and 33% versus 57%–67%, respectively).[327] Furthermore subanalysis of the Manns et al.[312] data established that the dose of ribavirin is predictive of achieving SVR. Recent data from an open label, multicenter trial suggest that patients with HCV genotype 1 had improved SVR rates in patients receiving PegIFN-α2b 1.5 mcg/kg/week plus weight-based ribavirin dosing (800–1,400 mg/day) for 48 weeks compared with those receiving PegIFN-α2b 1.5 mcg/kg/week plus 800 mg of ribavirin daily (34% versus 28.9%; $P = 0.005$) for 24 or 48 weeks.[328] In patients with HCV genotype 2 or 3, rates were not significantly different (61.8% versus 59.5%, respectively) regardless of treatment duration. These finding suggest that PegIFN-α2b plus weight-based dosing of ribavirin for 48 weeks may be appropriate for patients with genotype 1, whereas same-dose (800 mg ribavirin) for 24 weeks may be adequate for patients with genotype 2 or 3. Additional data are needed to establish individual dosing recommendation for ribavirin based on HCV genotype. Because R.D. has genotype 2, he should be initiated on PegIFN-α2a in a dose of 180 mcg weekly and oral ribavirin 800 mg daily in two divided doses. At 24 weeks, his aminotransferase and HCV RNA levels should be assessed, and therapy stopped.[329] (Fig. 73-6).

Adverse Effects and Monitoring

41. What adverse effects might be expected if pegylated interferon plus ribavirin are used in R. D., and what are appropriate monitoring parameters?

In the clinical trials with PegIFN and ribavirin, adverse effects resulted in discontinuation of treatment in approximately 10% to 14% of patients.[317–323] Adverse events were similar between those patients receiving PegIFN plus ribavirin and those receiving IFN plus ribavirin, except for a higher frequency of injection site reactions and a higher frequency of neutropenia in the PegIFN plus ribavirin group. Side effects in both groups included influenza-like symptoms, hematologic abnormalities, thyroid dysfunction, and neuropsychiatric symptoms.[317–323] The education of patients, their family members, and caregivers about side effects and their prospective management is an integral aspect of treatment.

Regular monitoring of neuropsychiatric side effects, cytopenias, and adherence to HCV therapy is mandatory (Table 73-25). Psychological conditions, particularly depression, are common among persons with hepatitis C and are frequent side effects of interferon.[314–323] Patients' mental health should be assessed before initiation of antiviral therapy and monitored regularly during therapy, because the ability to comply with the treatment regimen may become compromised. Antidepressants, such as selective serotonin reuptake inhibitors, may be useful in the management of depression associated with antiviral therapy.[314–323]

In certain patients with persistent cytopenias despite dose reductions, treatment with hematopoietic growth factors (i.e., erythropoietin, granulocyte colony-stimulating factor) may be useful to reduce symptoms and maintain adherence to antiviral therapy.[314–323] This therapy is costly, however, and the optimal dosage is not yet clear. Additionally, it is not known if the use of hematopoietic growth factors will enhance the likelihood of an SVR. Thus, the potential benefits of these agents need confirmation in prospectively designed trials before they can be recommended.

Of special importance, severe hemolysis from ribavirin can occur in patients with renal insufficiency.[314–323] In these patients, the ribavirin dose should either be reduced or

1. Make the diagnosis based on aminotransferase elevations, anti-HCV and HCV RNA in serum, and chronic hepatitis shown by liver biopsy.

2. Assess for suitability of therapy and contraindications. Discuss side effects and possible treatment outcomes.

3. Test for HCV genotype

4. Genotype 1: Test for HCV RNA level immediately before starting therapy (baseline level).

   Genotype 1:

   Start therapy with peginterferon alfa-2a in a dose of 180 mg weekly or peginterferon alfa-2b in a dose of 1.5 mg/kg weekly in combination with oral ribavirin in two divided doses of 1,000 mg daily if body weight is < 75 kilograms (165 lbs.) or 1,200 mg daily if body weight is > 75 kilograms.

   Genotype 2 or 3:

   Start therapy with peginterferon alfa-2a in a dose of 180 mcg weekly or with alpha-2b in a dose of 1.5 mcg per kilogram weekly and oral ribavirin 800 mg daily in two divided doses.

   All patients:

   At weeks 1, 2, and 4 and then at intervals of every 4 to 8 weeks thereafter, assess side effects, symptoms, blood counts, and aminotransferases.

   Genotype 1:

   At week 12, retest for HCV RNA level. If HCV RNA is negative or has decreased by at least two log10 units (such as from 2 million IU to 20,000 IU or from 500,000 IU to 5,000 IU or less), continue therapy for a full 48 weeks, monitoring symptoms, blood counts, and ALT at 4- to 8-week intervals. If RNA has not fallen by two log10 units, stop therapy.

   Genotype 2 or 3:

   At 24 weeks, assess aminotransferase levels and HCV RNA and stop therapy.

   All patients:

   After therapy, assess aminotransferases at 2- to 6-month intervals. In responders, repeat HCV RNA testing 6 months after stopping.

FIGURE 73-6 Algorithm for treatment of hepatitis C. Based on reference 241, with permission.

discontinued. Of note, ribavirin is not removed by hemodialysis. Finally, lactic acidosis may be a rare complication of combination therapy in patients undergoing therapy for HIV and HCV. Thus R.D. should be monitored closely to minimize the risk of severe adverse effects in initiated PegIFN plus ribavirin therapy.

Choosing Interferon Formulations

Pegylated interferons offer the convenience of once weekly versus three times weekly dosing, but PegIFN are associated with a greater incidence of cytopenias and injection site reactions compared with standard IFN. Moreover, there are subsets of patients in which treatment response with standard IFN-α2b plus ribavirin is the same with as PegIFN plus ribavirin. These include patients with nongenotype-1 infection and patients with compensated cirrhosis.[241,246] When deciding whether to treat a patient with PegIFN or standard IFN in combination with ribavirin, the patient and provider should weigh the risks and benefits of the two treatment regimens (Fig. 73-6). For example, in the patient with compensated cirrhosis, particularly if he or she has leukopenia before therapy, standard IFN might be the preferred treatment because of a short half-life and reduced likelihood of dose reductions for cytopenias.

Interferon or Pegylated Interferon Monotherapy

For patients with contraindications to the use of ribavirin, such as those with unstable cardiac disease, anemia, renal insufficiency, or those who might conceive while receiving treatment or within 6 months of completing therapy, IFN monotherapy or PegIFN should be considered.[241,246] Pegylated interferons have been shown to be superior to standard IFNα in the treatment of hepatitis C, and PegIFN are the treatment of choice in select patients.[241,246]

As a result of recent trials, combination therapy is the treatment of choice for naïve patients, that is those who have received neither interferon nor ribavirin therapy and who are able to tolerate ribavirin. Pegylated interferons plus ribavirin offer the convenience of once-weekly dosing, but with only a slight increase in efficacy and an increase in adverse events compared with standard IFNα plus ribavirin.[241,246] The FDA-approved dose of ribavirin is 800 mg, but higher doses (1,000/1,200 mg based on a 75 kg weight) may be improve efficacy in patients with genotype 1 infection. A ribavirin dose of 800 mg appears adequate for treatment of genotype non-1 infection. Although the results using PegIFN plus ribavirin are encouraging, the benefits of treatment on important clinical outcomes such as prevention of complications of advanced liver disease and the prevention of hepatocellular carcinoma remain to be demonstrated. Finally, no clinical trials have demonstrated the superiority of one type of PegIFN compared with the other (e.g., PegIFN-α2a versus PegIFN-α2b).

Treatment Options for Relapse of Chronic Hepatitis C

42. What is the role for combination therapy in patients who have relapse of chronic HCV infection?

As noted, HCV relapse rates (based on HCV RNA reappearance) often occur following discontinuation of IFN therapy despite longer courses of treatment. Based on previous trials, the combination of ribavirin plus IFN may reduce HCV relapse. Results from these trials were confirmed in 345 patients with chronic active HCV who relapsed following IFN.[302,323] A total of 173 patients were randomly assigned to receive either standard dose IFN-α2b with ribavirin (400 mg [AM] and 600 mg [PM] in patients $<$75 kg or 600 mg twice daily in patients $>$75 kg) for 6 months or IFN and placebo.[302] The primary endpoints of the study were the disappearance of HCV RNA from the serum and histologic improvement at the end of the 24-week follow-up period. On completion of treatment, serum levels of HCV RNA were undetectable in 141 of 173 patients who received combination therapy compared with IFN alone (82% versus 47%; $P<0.001$). Serum HCV RNA continued to be undetectable in 84 patients (49%) in the combination group and in only 8 patients (5%) in the IFN alone group ($P<0.001$) at 6 months. Patients who achieved a virologic response also had sustained normalization of serum ALT concentrations and histologic improvement. Of note, patients with the greatest response were those with low viral load and genotypes 2 or 3. As in previous trials, patients receiving combined therapy had a significant reduction in their hemoglobin concentrations, but otherwise had a safety profile similar to that of IFN alone. These results appear to be as good or better than those in patients receiving higher doses and longer courses of IFN. Thus, patients with chronic HCV infection without decompensated liver disease who relapse, may benefit from combination therapy.

Adjunctive Therapies

43. In addition to IFN alone, or the combination of IFN plus ribavirin, or PegIFN, are there any other therapeutic options available for R.D.?

Interferon responders have lower serum iron, iron saturation, and hepatic iron levels (which is believed to upregulate cellular immune responses) than do nonresponders to IFN.[324] In pilot trials, iron reduction by phlebotomy has been correlated with an improvement in aminotransferase levels in patients with chronic HCV infection and iron overload. These limited data suggest an enhanced response to IFN may be achieved through iron reduction by phlebotomy.

Other approaches to treating chronic HCV infection include nonsteroidal anti-inflammatory drugs,[330] pentoxifylline,[331] vitamin E,[332] omega-3 fatty acid supplements[333]; herbal remedies, such as glycyrrhizin (licorice root),[334] silymarin (milk thistle),[335] and sho-saiko-to (TJ-9),[336] are unproved for the routine treatment of HCV. These agents are thought to have anti-inflammatory or antifibrotic effects on the liver, which may lead to normalization of biochemical markers (i.e., ALT). Data from patients receiving IL-10 (Tenovil), which inhibits the Th1 T-cell subset, suggest that formation of liver scar tissue may be reduced.[337]

Future therapies for treatment of HCV infection are promising and numerous are in development. Recent studies using hydroxymethylglutaryl-coenzyme A (HMG-CoA) reductase inhibitors (e.g., statins) confirm that cholesterol biosynthesis has an impact on HCV replication and that statins may be useful in interrupting this pathway.[338] In addition to conventional and PegIFN, recombinant human albumin or IFN-α fusion protein (Albuferon), which has a prolonged half-life and excellent antiviral activity, has entered phase II trials.[338–340] Alternatives to ribavirin have also been developed. Viramidine, a ribavirin prodrug, has limited exposure to red blood cells (RBC) and demonstrated significant antiviral activity and erythrocyte-sparing properties.[338–340] In the last few years, the development of *in vitro* replication systems for HCV has led to significant advances in the HCV replication cycle. Specifically targeted antiviral therapy (STAT-C) include those agents that specifically target the viral replication cycle: internal ribosome entry site (IRES) inhibitors, translation (protease, helicase) inhibitors, translation (polymerase) inhibitors, and virus assembly (glycoside) inhibitors.[338–340] Cyclophillin inhibitors and immune mediators (IFN-γ- and IFN-β, thymosin, and levovorin) may also prove useful for treating HCV infection.[338–340] Finally, an experimental vaccine has also been studied in chimpanzees; however, no efficacy or safety data are available with this agent in humans.[341] R.D. should not be initiated on these agents at this time as further investigation is needed.

Summary of HCV in Nonimmunocompromised Patients

Overall, many factors have been identified that are associated with an increased or decreased likelihood of response to IFN therapy in patients infected with HCV. Analyses have generally shown that a decreased pretreatment HCV RNA titer is associated with more favorable response, that genotypes other than type 1b exhibit higher sustained response rates compared with genotype 1b, and that responders have less fibrosis and less inflammatory changes than nonresponders. Furthermore, most trials conducted using IFN or combinations thereof exclude patients with decompensated liver disease (cirrhosis), patients with HCC, patients with cryoglobulinemia or associated membranoproliferative glomerulonephritis, and children infected with HCV. Additional experience is needed in these areas to definitively assess therapy for HCV infection.

Treating Hepatitis C Following Liver Transplantation

44. While discussing treatment options for HCV infection, R.D. experiences a sudden loss of consciousness. He is admitted to the intensive care unit where he will be emergently evaluated for a liver transplant. What are the therapeutic options for preventing or treating HCV-infected patients following liver transplantation?

Uncontrolled trials have reported the efficacy of IFN-α in treating hepatitis C following transplantation.[342–344] In one report, 11 patients were treated with IFN-α (3 MU three times weekly for 6 months).[342] After therapy was stopped, only one patient had normal liver enzyme levels and IFN was not correlated with precipitating allograft rejection. In a similar trial, 4 of 18 patients (22%) had a sustained biochemical response (normal aminotransferase levels) at the end of treatment and in 6-month follow-up.[344] HCV RNA levels were reduced in both responders and nonresponders, but returned to pretreatment levels after discontinuation of IFN. Sustained effects were not observed, nor were improvements in histology. Only one patient had an IFN-associated, biopsy-proved delayed rejection episode. In contrast to these reports, others have identified IFN therapy with precipitating rejection, possibly because of its ability to upregulate the expression of human leukocyte antigen (HLA) class I and II antigens.[345]

Similar to the nontransplant population, the combination of IFN and ribavirin or ribavirin alone has also been assessed in liver transplant recipients for treating recurrent HCV infection following transplantation.[346–348] Data from pilot and randomized, noncomparative trials suggest that combination therapy is effective but poorly tolerated.[346] Furthermore, transplant recipients appear to have a high incidence of hemolysis, thrombocytopenia, and mental status changes with combination therapy. Transplant recipients should also be closely monitored for rejection during and following cessation of IFN plus ribavirin therapy. Finally, the use of PegIFN alone or in combination with ribavirin has also been considered following liver transplantation.[346] Any combination therapy could be considered (based on response criteria for interferon as listed above) in the following areas in liver transplant recipients having transplant because of HCV: (a) as prophylaxis for HCV immediately following liver transplantation (first transplant); (b) as prophylaxis for HCV immediately following liver transplantation (second transplant for recurrent HCV); (c) in patients with HCV recurrence without decompensation with worsening symptoms; and (d) in patients with recurrent HCV with decompensation. These areas are clearly controversial and continue to warrant clinical investigation.

HEPATITIS E VIRUS

Virology, Epidemiology, Transmission, and Pathogenesis

Hepatitis E virus is an icosahedral, nonenveloped virus of the *Caliciviridae* family between 32 and 34 nm wide that was initially identified by immune electromicroscopy in the stool samples of infected persons (Table 73-2).[349,350] The HEV genome is a single-stranded polyadenylated RNA and, unlike HAV, has an RNA genome that encodes for nonstructural proteins through overlapping open ready frames (ORF). Several ORF encode for nonstructural proteins, structural proteins, or proteins of undetermined function. The HEV polyprotein has several sequences, including an RNA-dependent RNA-polymerase, and RNA helicase, and a virally encoded cysteine protease.

Hepatitis E virus occurs in endemic areas such as Africa, Southeast and Central Asia, Mexico, and Central and South America as both epidemic and sporadic infections.[349,351] Sporadic infections also occur in nonendemic areas and are usually associated with travel into areas of endemicity. The attack rate (the percentage of exposed patients who become infected) of HEV is low compared with HAV (1% versus 10%, respectively). In endemic areas, outbreaks usually occur between 5 and 10 years apart and are often associated with times of heavy rainfall, after floods or monsoons, or following the recession of flood waters.[349,351,352] The overall case fatality rate for the general endemic population is 0.5% to 4%, whereas for reasons unknown, pregnant women have a much greater case fatality rate of 20%.[349,353] In particular, the fetal complication rate is increased, especially if the infection occurs in the third trimester of pregnancy.[349,354] The frequency of death *in utero* and immediately following birth is also greater than seen with acute hepatitis of other causes.[349,354]

Transmission of HEV is via the fecal-oral route, and the most common source of transmission is ingestion of fecally contaminated water.[349,351,353] Poor climactic conditions in conjunction with inadequate personal hygiene and sanitation have led to epidemics of HEV infection. Secondary attacks usually are much lower than that observed with HAV, ranging from 0.7% to 2.2% versus 50% to 75%, respectively.[349,351,353] The mechanism for this difference could be related to the instability of HEV to its environment, differences in the quantity of virus needed to propagate infection, or a greater frequency of subclinical disease.

Interference with the production of cellular macromolecules, alteration of cellular membranes, and alteration of lysosomal permeability are some of the proposed mechanisms of hepatic injury.[355,356] In addition, immune-mediated mechanisms are believed to be responsible for lysis of virally infected hepatocytes by direct lymphocyte cytotoxicity or antibody-mediated cytotoxicity.

Diagnosis

Initial assays for detection of anti-HEV used electromicroscopy to detect HEVAg on the surface of HEV particles in stool and serum and immunohistochemistry to detect the antigen in liver tissue.[349,351,353] Fluorescent antibody-blocking assay is currently used to detect anti-HEV reacting to HEVAg in serum and, although highly specific, this assay lacks sensitivity (50%) in acute HEV infection.[349,351] Additional cloning and sequencing of HEV has led to the development of Western blot assays and ELISA that detect anti-HEV by using recombinant expressed proteins from the structural region of the virus. Reverse transcriptase polymerase chain reaction (RT-PCR) has also been used to confirm the diagnosis of HEV by detecting HEV RNA from serum, liver, or stool.[349,351,353] Clinically, HEV is a diagnosis of exclusion.

Clinical Manifestations, Serology, and Natural History

The incubation period following exposure is listed in Table 73-1. Two phases of illness have been described, including a prodromal and preicteric phase as described for HAV infection. Peak serum aminotransferase levels reflect the onset of the icteric phase and generally return to baseline by 6 weeks.[349,354] Stool is often positive for HEV RNA at the onset of the icteric phase and persists for an additional 10 days beyond this period. Viral shedding may also occur for up to 52 days after the onset of icterus. Detection in the serum occurs during the preicteric phase, before detection of virus in the stool, and becomes undetectable following the peak in aminotransferase activity. Because HEV RNA is not detectable in the serum during symptoms, diagnostic tests using HEV RNA have limited utility and a correlation between PCR detection and infectivity has not been observed. Serologically, HEV IgM becomes detectable before the peak rise in ALT, whereas antibody titers peak with peak ALT levels and subsequently decline. In most patients, HEV IgM is present for 5 to 6 months following the onset of illness. HEV IgG appears after HEV IgM and remains detectable for up to 14 years after acute infection; however, the duration of protective immunity has not been fully elucidated.[349,357]

In nonfatal cases, acute HEV hepatitis is followed by complete recovery without any chronic complications. There appears to be protection from reinfection; however, the duration of protection is variable. Fulminant hepatitis has also been associated with HEV infection and has a high association with pregnancy.[349,351,352,354] Maternal mortality was reported to be 1.5% for HEV infection occurring in the first trimester of pregnancy, 8.5% for those in the second trimester, and 21% for those infected in the third trimester.

Prevention and Treatment

No immunoprophylactic measures exist for HEV disease, and effective prevention strategies are dependent on improved sanitation in endemic areas. Travelers going to endemic areas should be educated regarding the risks of drinking water, eating ice, or eating uncooked shellfish or uncooked and peeled fruits and vegetables. Drinking water should be boiled to inactivate HEV. No vaccines or postexposure prophylaxis are available to prevent HEV infection. Results from a phase II randomized trial suggest, however, that in a high-risk population, a recombinant hepatitis E vaccine can be effective in the prevention of HEV infection.[351]

HEPATITIS G VIRUS

Virology

In 1995, the genomes of two previously unidentified RNA viruses were cloned from experimentally inoculated tamarins.[358–360] The original inoculate was obtained from a surgeon (initials G.B.) with NANB hepatitis who was thought to have HCV. The viruses were subsequently named GB virus A (GBV-A) and GB virus B (GBV-B).[358–360] Another unknown RNA virus related to GBV-A and GBV-B was discovered (using representational difference analysis) and was designated GB virus C (GBV-C).[358–360] Similar methods were also implemented in the discovery of one more previously unknown virus, designated TT virus (TTV), obtained from a patient (initials T.T.). In 1996, another independent research group isolated a novel RNA virus (designated HGV) that was associated with hepatitis.[358–360] Sequencing studies comparing GBV-C and HGV have shown these isolates to be two genotypes of the same virus. Apparently, only humans and higher primates can be infected by human GBV-C/HGV.[358–360]

The GBV-C/HGV is a single-stranded enveloped RNA virus that consists of 9,100 to 9,400 nucleotides (Table 73-2).[358–360] GBV-C/HGV belongs to the *Flaviviridae* viruses, and temporarily to the hepacivirus genus together with HCV because the genomic organization of this virus resembles HCV. The biological functions of many GBV-C/HGV proteins have not been entirely defined, although the capsid region of this virus is defective and core proteins are not encoded, unlike with HCV. An envelope region that encodes a surface glycoprotein as well as protease, helicase regions has been identified.[358–360] Additional phylogenetic analysis has depicted four genotypes: genotype 1 (GBV-C; originated from West Africa), genotype 2 (TTV; originated from the United States), and genotype 3 and 4 (originated from Asia).

Epidemiology

Spread worldwide, GBV-C/HGV infection has been observed in healthy persons and in IV drug users, men who have sex with men, patients receiving multiple transfusions, and patients with fulminant hepatic failure.[358,359,361] Viremia has been reported to be between 1% and 4% among healthy populations in Europe and North America and even higher rates (10%–33%) have been documented in residents of South America and Africa.[358–360] The prevalence of resolved GBV-C/HGV infections (using envelope antibodies) appears to be more common than the occurrence of viremic infections. Rates of resolved infections described in blood donors are 3% to 15% in Europe, 3% to 8% in North America, 20% in Africa and South America, and 3% to 6% in Asia.[358–360]

Transmission

Transmission of GBV-C/HGV has been primarily associated with blood transfusions and infections have been observed in the presence of other hepatitis viruses (e.g., HBV, HCV).[358–360] Additional modes of transmission include injection drug use, hemodialysis, sexual contact, and vertical or perinatal transmission.[358] Also, GBV-C/HGV RNA has been isolated in saliva, suggesting that close social contact may be a possible mode of transmission.[358–360]

Pathogenesis and Diagnosis

The pathogenesis and serologic presentation of GBV-C/HGV are poorly described. The natural course of GBV-C/HGV infection appears to vary from an acute self-limited episode to a chronic infection that may persist from years to decades.[358–360,362] GBV-C/HGV can cause mild acute hepatitis, but despite persistent infection, it does not appear to cause clinically significant chronic hepatitis.[358] Diagnosis is usually established through detection of the virus by RT-PCR methodology (HGV RNA).[358,363] Additionally, first generation EIA tests have been utilized to detect specific antibodies to the envelope glycoprotein to diagnose previous infection; however, the specificity and sensitivity of these tests have not been fully elucidated. Reliable serologic assays are needed.

Clinical Manifestations and Treatment

Clinical and extrahepatic manifestations of GBV-C/HGV are unknown, but the virus has been found to be in serum for many years in patients with several types of liver diseases.[358–364,365] No causal relationship has been established between GBV-C/HGV and acute, fulminant, and chronic non B–C-D hepatitis.[358–360,364,365] The role of the GBV-C/HGV in human hepatitis remains unclear. Published studies provide further evidence that GBV-C/HGV may not be a significant cause of acute or chronic liver disease.[358] One report demonstrated that 15% of children with chronic hepatitis C or hepatitis B are infected with GBV-C/HGV; however, GBV-C/HGV coinfection does not appear to cause more severe liver disease. In another report, serum HCV RNA concentrations, liver histology, and response to treatment with IFN-α did not differ between patients with and without GBV-C/HGV coinfection. Loss of serum HGV RNA did not correlate with a biochemical response, whereas loss of serum HCV RNA did. These results show that GBV-C/HGV coinfection frequently occurs in individuals infected with HCV and that GBV-C/HGV does not influence the severity of liver disease or response to treatment with—IFN-α in patients with chronic hepatitis C. Because the significance of GBV-C/HGV is unclear, screening of blood donors for this virus is not presently justified. Currently, no agents are used to treat or prevent GBV-C/HGV infection.[358]

SUMMARY

Viral hepatitis continues to be a significant worldwide infectious disease. To date, prevention strategies through universal vaccination are the most efficient methods for minimizing the incidence of HAV, HBV, and HDV. Patient education with respect to the common ways of spreading these infections may also result in behavioral modifications that reduce the overall incidence of infection. Once HBV and HCV progress to chronic infection, more efficacious and better tolerated antiviral therapies are needed to treat these infections. Similarly, therapeutic modalities that reduce the progression of these diseases are necessary to prevent end-stage liver disease and the development of additional complications (encephalopathy, intractable ascites, coagulation disorders, and HCC). As a better understanding of viral replication is established, as well as appropriate models for study, new agents may become available. Furthermore, more diagnostic tools are needed to better identify new hepatitis viruses and monitor response to drug therapies. The economic impact and quality of life of these patients remains to be fully elucidated.

ACKNOWLEDGMENT

The author would like to acknowledge the contribution of Amy Choi to this chapter.

REFERENCES

1. Alter MJ et al. The epidemiology of viral hepatitis in the United States. *Gastroenterol Clin North Am* 1994;23:437.
2. Hadler SC. Vaccines to prevent hepatitis B and hepatitis A infections. *Infect Dis Clin North Am* 1990;4:29.
3. Berenguer M et al. Hepatitis G virus infection in patients with hepatitis C virus infection undergoing liver transplantation. *Gastroenterology* 1996;111:1569.
4. Melnick J. Proper and classification of hepatitis A virus. *Vaccine* 1992;10 (Supp 1):S24.
5. Purcelli RH. Enterically transmitted non-A, non-B hepatitis. In: Popper H et al., eds. *Progress in Liver Diseases.* New York: Grune and Stratton; 1990;9:371.
6. Margolis H et al. Hepatitis B: evolving epidemiology and implications for control. *Semin Liver Dis* 1991;11:84.
7. Kiyasu PK et al. Diagnosis and treatment of the major hepatotrophic viruses. *Am J Med Sci* 1993; 306:248.
8. Linnen J et al. Molecular cloning and disease association of hepatitis G virus: a transfusion-transmission agent. *Science* 1996;271:505.
9. Matsuko K et al. Infection with hepatitis GB virus C in patients on maintenance hemodialysis. *N Engl J Med* 1996;334:1485.
10. Wrobleski F et al. Serum glutamic oxaloacetate transaminase activity as an index of liver cell injury: a preliminary report. *Ann Intern Med* 1995;43:360.
11. Davis S. Chronic hepatitis. In: Kaplowitz N, ed. *Liver and Biliary Diseases*. 2nd ed. Baltimore, MD: Williams & Wilkins; 1996: 327.
12. Maddrey WC. Chronic hepatitis. *Dis Mon* 1993; 39:53.
13. Lau JYN et al. Molecular virology and pathogenesis of hepatitis B. *Lancet* 1993;342:1335.
14. Dossing M et al. Drug-induced hepatic disorders. *Drug Saf* 1993;9:441.
15. Brewer GJ et al. Wilson's disease. *Medicine* 1992;71:139.
16. Hoofnagle JH et al. Therapy of chronic delta hepatitis: overview. *Prog Clin Biol Res* 1993;382:337.
17. Mphahlele MJ et al. HGV: the identification, biology, and prevalence of an orphan virus. *Liver* 1998; 18:14395.
18. Maddrey WC et al. Severe hepatitis from methyldopa. *Gastroenterology* 1975;68:351.
19. Black M et al. Nitrofurantoin-induced chronic active hepatitis. *Ann Intern Med* 1980;92:62.
20. Maddrey WC et al. Isoniazid hepatitis. *Ann Intern Med* 1973;79:1.
21. Tonder M et al. Sulfonamide-induced chronic liver disease. *Scand J Gastroenterol* 1974;9:93.
22. Weiss M et al. Propylthiouracil-induced hepatic damage. *Arch Intern Med* 1980;140:1184.
23. Lemon S et al. Genetic, antigenic, and biological difference between strains of hepatitis A virus. *Vaccine* 1992;10(Suppl 1):S40.
24. Shapiro C et al. Worldwide epidemiology of hepatitis A infection. *J Hepatol* 1993;18(Suppl 2):S11.
25. Shapiro C et al. Epidemiology of hepatitis A: seroepidemiology and risk groups in the USA. *Vaccine* 1992;10 (Suppl 1):S59.
26. Melnick J. History and epidemiology of hepatitis A virus. *J Infect Dis* 1995;171(Suppl 1):S2.
27. Hoffman F et al. Hepatitis A as an occupational hazard. *Vaccine* 1992;10(Suppl 1):S82.
28. Gust ID et al. Hepatitis A. *Progress in Liver Disease* 1990;306:248.
29. Centers for Disease Control. Prevention of hepatitis A through active or passive immunization: recommendations of the Advisory Committee on Immunization Practices (ACIP). *MMWR* 2006;55: RR-7:1.
30. Cuthbert JA. Hepatitis A: old and new. *Clin Microbiol Rev* 2001;14:38.
31. Shapiro CN. Transmission of hepatitis viruses. *Ann Intern Med* 1994;120:82.
32. Sheretz RJ et al. Transmission of hepatitis A by transfusion of blood products. *Arch Intern Med* 1994;144:1579.
33. Steffen R et al. Epidemiology and prevention of hepatitis A in travelers. *JAMA* 1994;272:885.
34. Margolis H et al. Identification of virus components in circulating immune complexes isolated during hepatitis A virus infection. *Hepatology* 1990; 11:31.
35. Baba H et al. Cytolytic activity of natural killer cells and lymphokine activated killer cells against hepatitis A infected fibroblasts. *J Clin Lab Immunol* 1993;40:47.

36. Lee WM. Acute liver failure. *N Engl J Med* 1993; 329:1862.
37. Romero R et al. Viral hepatitis in children. *Semin Liver Dis* 1994;14:289.
38. Schiff E. Atypical clinical manifestations of hepatitis A. *Vaccine* 1992;10(Supp 1):S18.
39. Scoit R et al. Cholestatic features in hepatitis A. *J Hepatol* 1986;3:172.
40. Hoofnagle JH et al. Serologic diagnosis of acute and chronic hepatitis. *Semin Liver Dis* 1991;11:73.
41. Glikson M et al. Relapsing hepatitis A: a review of 14 cases and literature survey. *Medicine* 1992; 71:14.
42. Jorup-Ronstrom C et al. Reduction of paracetamol and aspirin metabolism during viral hepatitis. *Clin Pharmacokinet* 1986;11:250.
43. Puente M et al. Increase in serum carbamazepine concentrations after acute viral hepatitis. *Ann Pharmacother* 1998;32:1369.
44. Roberts RK et al. Effect of age and parenchymal liver disease on the disposition and elimination of chlordiazepoxide (Librium). *Gastroenterology* 1978;75:479.
45. Narang APS et al. Pharmacokinetic study of chloramphenicol in patients with liver disease. *Eur J Clin Pharmacol* 1981;20:479.
46. Gugler R et al. Clofibrate disposition in renal failure and acute and chronic liver disease. *Eur J Clin Pharmacol* 1979;15:341.
47. Klotz U et al. The effects of age and liver disease on the disposition and elimination of diazepam in adult man. *J Clin Invest* 1975;55:347.
48. Williams RL et al. Influence of viral hepatitis on the disposition of two compounds with high hepatic clearance: lidocaine and indocyanine green. *Clin Pharmacol Ther* 1976;20:290.
49. Kraus JW et al. Effects of aging and liver disease on disposition of lorazepam. *Clin Pharmacol Ther* 1978;24:411.
50. McHorse TS et al. Effect of acute viral hepatitis in man on the disposition and elimination of meperidine. *Gastroenterology* 1975;68:775.
51. Dylewicz P et al. Bioavailability and elimination of nitrendipine in liver disease. *Eur J Clin Pharmacol* 1987;32:563.
52. Eandi M et al. Pharmacokinetics of norfloxacin in healthy volunteers and patients with renal and hepatic damage. *Eur J Clin Microbiol* 1983;2:253.
53. Shull HJ et al. Normal disposition of oxazepam in acute viral hepatitis and cirrhosis. *Ann Intern Med* 1976;84:420.
54. Alvin J et al. The effect of liver disease in man on the disposition of phenobarbital. *J Pharmacol Exp Ther* 1975;192:224.
55. Blaschke TF et al. Influence of acute viral hepatitis on phenytoin kinetics and protein binding. *Clin Pharmacol Ther* 1975;17:685.
56. Karbwang J et al. The pharmacokinetics of quinine in patients with hepatitis. *Br J Clin Pharmacol* 1993;35:444.
57. Holdiness MR. Clinical pharmacokinetics of the antitubercular drugs. *Clin Pharmacokinet* 1984; 9:511.
58. Staib AH et al. Pharmacokinetics and metabolism of theophylline and patients with liver disease. *Int J Clin Pharmacol Ther Toxicol* 1980;18:500.
59. Williams RL et al. Influence of acute viral hepatitis on disposition and plasma binding of tolbutamide. *Clin Pharmacol Ther* 1977;21:301.
60. Williams RL et al. Influence of acute viral hepatitis on disposition and pharmacologic effect of warfarin. *Clin Pharmacol Ther* 1976;20:90.
61. Winokur PL et al. Immunoglobulin prophylaxis for hepatitis A. *Clin Infect Dis* 1992;14:580.
62. Centers for Disease Control. Prevention of hepatitis A through active or passive immunization: recommendations of the Advisory Committee on Immunization Practices (ACIP). *MMWR* 1996;45 (RR-15):1.
63. Westblom TU et al. Safety and immunogenicity of an inactivated hepatitis A vaccine: effect of dose and vaccination schedule. *J Infect Dis* 1994;169: 996.
64. Centers for Disease Control and Prevention. FDA approval for a combined hepatitis A and B vaccine. *MMWR* 2001;50;37:806.
65. Werzberger A et al. A controlled trial of formalin inactivated hepatitis A vaccine in healthy children. *N Engl J Med* 1992;327:453.
66. Innis BL et al. Protection against hepatitis A by an inactivated vaccine. *JAMA* 1994;271:1328.
67. Riedemann S et al. Placebo-controlled efficacy study of hepatitis A vaccine in Valdivia, Chile. *Vaccine* 1992;10(Supp 1):S152.
68. Niu MT et al. Two-year review of hepatitis A vaccine safety: data from the Vaccine Adverse Event Reporting System (VAERS). *Clin Infect Dis* 1998; 26:1475.
69. Totos G et al. Hepatitis A vaccine: persistence of antibodies 5 years after the first vaccination. *Vaccine* 1997;15:1252.
70. Van Damme P et al. Inactivated hepatitis A vaccine; reactogenicity, immunogenicity, and long-term antibody persistence. *J Med Virol* 1994;44:446.
71. Lee WM. Hepatitis B virus infection. *N Engl J Med* 1997;337:1733.
72. Lok AS et al. Chronic hepatitis B. *Hepatology* 2007; 45:507.
73. Hoofnagle JH et al. Management of hepatitis B: summary of a clinical workshop. *Hepatology* 2007; 45:1056.
74. Malik AH et al. Chronic hepatitis B virus infection: treatment strategies for the new millennium. *Ann Intern Med* 2000;132:723.
75. Locarnini S et al. The hepatitis B virus and common mutants. *Semin Liver Dis* 2003;23:5.
76. Kann M et al. Recent studies on replication of the hepatitis B virus. *J Hepatol* 1995;22(Suppl 1):9.
77. Harrison TJ et al. Hepatitis B virus: molecular virology and common mutants. *Semin Liver Dis* 2006: 26:87.
78. Centers for Disease Control. Recommendations of the immunization practices advisory committee (ACIP). Hepatitis B virus: a comprehensive strategy for eliminating transmission in the United States. *MMWR* 2006;55(RR-16):1.
79. Gish RG et al. Chronic hepatitis B: current epidemiology in the Americas and implications for management. *J Viral Hepatitis* 2006;13:787.
80. Alter M. Epidemiology and prevention of hepatitis B. *Semin Liver Dis* 2003;23:39.
81. Perillo RP. Hepatitis B: transmission and natural history. *Gut* 1993;S43.
82. Chang JJ et al. Immunopathogenesis of hepatitis B infection. *Immunol Cell Bio* 2007;85:16.
83. Bertoletti A et al. The immune response during hepatitis B infection. *J Gen Virology* 2006;87: 1439.
84. Zaaijer H et al. Comparison of methods for detection of hepatitis B virus DNA. *J Clin Microbiol* 1994;32:2088.
85. Ke-Qin H et al. Molecular diagnostic techniques for viral hepatitis. *Gastroenterol Clin North Am* 1994;23:479.
86. Zoulim F. New nucleic acid diagnostic tests in viral hepatitis. *Semin Liver Dis* 2006;26:309
87. Bowden S. Serological and molecular diagnosis. *Semin Liver Dis* 2006;26:97.
88. Kumar S et al. Serologic diagnosis of viral hepatitis. *Postgrad Med* 1992;92:55.
89. Sjogren MH. Serologic diagnosis of viral hepatitis. *Gastroenterol Clin North Am* 1994;23:45.
90. Shakil AO et al. Fulminant hepatic failure. *Surg Clin North Am* 1999;79:77.
91. Hyams KC. Risks of chronicity following acute hepatitis B virus infection. *Clin Infect Dis* 1995; 20:992.
92. Hyung JY et al. Natural history of chronic hepatitis B virus infection: what we knew in 1981 and what we know in 2005. *Hepatology* 2006;43:S173.
93. Chia-Ming C et al. Hepatitis B virus-related cirrhosis: natural history and treatment. *Semin Liver Dis* 2006;26:142.
94. Weissberg J et al. Survival in chronic hepatitis B: an analysis of 379 patients. *Ann Intern Med* 1984; 101:613.
95. Chan HL et al. Hepatocellular carcinoma and hepatitis B virus. *Semin Liver Dis* 2006;26:153.
96. Fattovich G. Natural history and prognosis of hepatitis B. *Semin Liver Dis* 2003;23:47.
97. Khan SA et al. Acute liver failure. *Clin Liver Dis* 2006;10:239.
98. Polson J et al. AASLD position paper: the management of acute liver failure. *Hepatology* 2005;41: 1179.
99. Aldersley MA et al. Hepatic disorders. *Drugs* 1995; 49:83.
100. Lidofsky SD et al. Intracranial pressure monitoring and liver transplantation for fulminant hepatic failure. *Hepatology* 1992;16:1.
101. Larsen FS et al. Brain edema in liver failure: basic physiologic principles and management. *Liver Transpl* 2002;8:983.
102. Gazzard BG et al. Early changes in coagulation following a paracetamol overdose and a controlled trial of fresh frozen plasma therapy. *Gut* 1975;16:617.
103. Pereria LMMB et al. Coagulation factor V and VIII/V ratio as predictors to outcome in paracetamol induced fulminant hepatic failure: relation to other prognostic indicators. *Gut* 1992;33:98.
104. Roberts LR et al. Ascites and hepatorenal syndrome: pathophysiology and management. *Mayo Clin Proc* 1996;71:874.
105. O'Grady JG et al. Early indicators of prognosis in fulminant hepatic failure. *Gastroenterology* 1989; 97.
106. Pauwels A et al. Emergency liver transplantation for acute liver failure: evaluation of London and Clichy criteria. *J Hepatol* 1993;17:124.
107. Scharschmidt B et al. Hepatitis B in patients with HIV infection: relationship to AIDS and patient survival. *Ann Intern Med* 1992;117:837.
108. Thio CL. Hepatitis B in the human immunodeficiency virus-infected patient: epidemiology, natural history, and treatment. *Semin Liver Dis* 2003; 23:125.
109. Recombivax HB package insert. West Point, PA: Merck and Company; 1998.
110. Engerix-B package insert. Philadelphia, PA: SmithKline Beecham Pharmaceuticals; 1998.
111. Centers for Disease Control. Recommendations of the immunization practices advisory committee (ACIP). Hepatitis B virus: a comprehensive strategy for eliminating transmission in the United States through universal childhood vaccination. *MMWR* 1991;40;(RR-13):1.
112. Ellis RW et al. Plasma-derived and yeast-derived hepatitis B vaccines. *Am J Infect Control* 1989;17: 181.
113. Dentico P et al. Long-term immunogenicity safety and efficacy of a recombinant hepatitis B vaccine in healthy adults. *Eur J Epidemiol* 1992;8:650.
114. Szmuness W et al. Hepatitis B vaccine: demonstration of efficacy in a controlled clinical trial in a high-risk population in the United States. *N Engl J Med* 1980;303:833.
115. Francis DP et al. The prevention of hepatitis B with vaccine: report of the CDC multi-center efficacy trial among homosexual men. *Ann Intern Med* 1982;97:362.
116. Szmuness W et al. A controlled clinical trial of the efficacy of the hepatitis B vaccine (Heptavax B): a final report. *Hepatology* 1981;1:377.
117. Hadler SC et al. Long-term immunogenicity and efficacy of hepatitis B vaccine in homosexual men. *N Engl J Med* 1986;315:209.
118. Wainwright RB et al. Duration of immunogenicity and efficacy of hepatitis B vaccine in a Yupik Eskimo population. *JAMA* 1989;261:2362.
119. Stevens CE et al. Hepatitis B vaccine in patients receiving hemodialysis: immunogenicity and efficacy. *N Engl J Med* 1984;311:496.
120. Collier AC et al. Antibody to human immunodeficiency virus (HIV) and suboptimal response to hepatitis B vaccination. *Ann Intern Med* 1988;109: 101.
121. Hovi L et al. Impaired response to hepatitis B vaccine in children receiving anticancer chemotherapy. *Pediatr Infect Dis J* 1995;14:931.

122. Wood RC et al. Risk factors for lack of detectable antibody following hepatitis B vaccination of Minnesota health care workers. *JAMA* 1993;270: 2935.
123. Roome AJ et al. Hepatitis B vaccine responsiveness in Connecticut public safety personnel. *JAMA* 1993;270:2931.
124. Winter AP et al. Influence of smoking on immunological responses to hepatitis B vaccine. *Vaccine* 1994;12:771.
125. Goldwater PN. Randomized, comparative trial of 20 μg vs 40 μg Engerix B vaccine in hepatitis B vaccine non-responders. *Vaccine* 1997;15:353.
126. Clemens R et al. Booster immunization of low- and non-responders after a standard three dose hepatitis B vaccine schedule-results of a post-marketing surveillance. *Vaccine* 1997;15:349.
127. Boxall E et al. HBVax II in non-responders to Engerix B. *Vaccine* 1998;16:877.
128. Weissman JY et al. Lack of response to recombinant hepatitis B vaccine in nonresponders to the plasma vaccine. *JAMA* 1988;260:1734.
129. Alper CE et al. Genetic prediction of non-responsiveness to hepatitis B vaccination. *N Engl J Med* 1989;321:708.
130. Bush LM et al. Evaluation of initiating a hepatitis B vaccination schedule with one vaccine and completing it with another. *Vaccine* 1991;9:807.
131. Chan CY et al. Booster response to recombinant yeast-derived hepatitis B vaccine in vaccinees whose anti-HBs response were initially elicited by a plasma-derived vaccine. *Vaccine* 1991;9:765.
132. Tabor E et al. Nine-year follow-up study of a plasma-derived hepatitis B vaccine in a rural African setting. *J Med Virol* 1993;40:204.
133. Milne A et al. Hepatitis B vaccination in children: five year booster study. *NZ Med J* 1992;105:336.
134. Coursaget P et al. Twelve-year follow-up study of hepatitis B immunization of Senegalese infants. *J Hepatol* 1994;21:250.
135. Wainwright RB et al. Protection provided by hepatitis B vaccine in a Yupik Eskimo population: results of a 10-year study. *J Infect Dis* 1997;175:674.
136. Trivello R et al. Persistence of anti-HBs antibodies in health care personnel vaccinated with plasma-derived hepatitis B vaccine and response to recombinant DNA HB booster vaccine. *Vaccine* 1995; 13:139.
137. Resti M et al. Ten-year follow-up study of neonatal hepatitis B immunization: are booster injections indicated? *Vaccine* 1997;15:1338.
138. Yuen MF et al. Twelve-year follow-up of a prospective randomized trial of hepatitis B recombinant DNA yeast vaccine versus plasma-derived vaccine without booster doses in children. *Hepatology* 1999;29:924.
139. Huang LM et al. Long term response to hepatitis B vaccination and response to booster in children born to mothers with hepatitis B antigen. *Hepatology* 1999;29:954.
140. West DJ et al. Vaccine induced immunologic memory for hepatitis B surface antigen: implications for policy on booster vaccination. *Vaccine* 1996;14: 1019.
141. Centers for Disease Control and Prevention. Immunization of adolescents. *MMWR* 1996;45(RR-13):1.
142. Centers for Disease Control and Prevention. 1998 Guidelines for treatment of sexually transmitted diseases. *MMWR* 1998;47(RR-1):1.
143. Seeff LB et al. Type B hepatitis after needle-stick exposure: prevention with hepatitis B immune globulin. *Ann Intern Med* 1978;88:285.
144. Redeker AG et al. Hepatitis B immune globulin as a prophylactic measure for spouses exposed to acute type B hepatitis. *N Engl J Med* 1975;293:1055.
145. Beasley RP et al. Prevention of perinatally transmitted hepatitis B virus infections with hepatitis B immune globulin and hepatitis B vaccine. *Lancet* 1983;2:1099.
146. Beasley RP et al. Efficacy of hepatitis B immune globulin for prevention of perinatal transmission of the hepatitis B virus carrier state: final report of a randomized double-blind, placebo-controlled trial. *Hepatology* 1983;3:135.
147. Wong VCW et al. Prevention of the HBsAg carrier state in newborn infants of mothers who are chronic carriers of HBsAg and HBeAg by administration of hepatitis B vaccine and hepatitis B immunoglobulin: double-blind randomized placebo-controlled study. *Lancet* 1984;1:921.
148. Beasley RP et al. Hepatocellular carcinoma and hepatitis B virus: a prospective study of 22,707 men in Taiwan. *Lancet* 1981;2:1129.
149. Beasley RP. Hepatitis B virus as the etiologic agent in hepatocellular carcinoma: epidemiologic considerations. *Hepatology* 1982;2(Suppl):21.
150. Stevens CE et al. Yeast-recombinant hepatitis B vaccine: efficacy with hepatitis B immune globulin in prevention of perinatal hepatitis B virus transmission. *JAMA* 1987;257:2612.
151. Stevens CE et al. Perinatal hepatitis B virus transmission in the United States: prevention by passive-active immunization. *JAMA* 1985;253:1740.
152. Gregory PB et al. Steroid therapy in severe viral hepatitis: a double blind, randomized trial of methyl-prednisolone versus placebo. *N Engl J Med* 1976;294:681.
153. European Association for the Study of the Liver (EASL). Randomized trial of steroid therapy in acute liver failure. *Gut* 1979;20:620.
154. Sanchez-Tapias JM et al. Recombinant alpha-2c interferon therapy in fulminant viral hepatitis. *J Hepatol* 1987;5:205.
155. Hollinger F et al. Hepatitis B: the pathway to recovery through treatment. *Gastroenterol Clin North Am* 2006;35:425.
156. Farrell GC et al. Management of chronic hepatitis B infection: a new era of disease control. *International Medical Journal* 2006: 36:100.
157. Dienstag JL. Looking to the future: new agents for chronic hepatitis B. *Am J Gastroenterol* 2006; 101:S19
158. Obsborn MK et al. Antiviral options for the treatment of chronic hepatitis B. *J Antimicrob Chemother* 2006;57:1030.
159. Van Thiel DH et al. Lamivudine treatment of advanced and decompensated liver disease due to hepatitis B. *Hepatogastroenterology* 1997;44: 808.
160. Nevens F et al. Lamivudine therapy for chronic hepatitis B: a six month randomized dose ranging study. *Gastroenterology* 1997;113:1258.
161. Dienstag JL et al. A preliminary trial of lamivudine for chronic hepatitis B infection. *N Engl J Med* 1995;25:1657.
162. Ching-lung L et al. A one year trial of lamivudine for chronic hepatitis B. *N Engl J Med* 1998;2:61.
163. Heathcote J. Treatment of HBe Ag-positive chronic hepatitis B. *Semin Liver Dis* 2003;23:69.
164. Hadziyannis SJ. Treatment of HBeAg-negative chronic hepatitis B. *Semin Liver Dis* 2003;23:81.
165. Malaguanrnera M et al. Interferon, cortisone, and antivirals in the treatment of chronic viral hepatitis. *Pharmacotherapy* 1997;17:998.
166. Saracco G et al. A practical guide to the use of interferons in the management of hepatitis virus infections. *Drugs* 1997;53:74.
167. Cirelli R et al. Interferons: an overview of their pharmacology. *Clin Immunother* 1996;5(Suppl 1):22.
168. Farber JM et al. Interferon—in the management of infectious diseases. *Ann Intern Med*. 1995;123:216.
169. Hoofnagle JH et al. Randomized, controlled trial of recombinant human alpha-interferon in patients with chronic hepatitis B. *Gastroenterology* 1988;95:1318.
170. Perrillo RP et al. Prednisone withdrawal followed by recombinant alpha interferon in the treatment of chronic type B hepatitis: a randomized, controlled trial. *Ann Intern Med* 1988;109:95.
171. Perrillo RP et al. A randomized, controlled trial of interferon alfa-2b alone and after prednisone withdrawal for the treatment of chronic hepatitis B. *N Engl J Med* 1990;323:295.
172. Perez V et al. A controlled trial of high dose interferon, alone and after prednisone withdrawal, in the treatment of chronic hepatitis B: long term follow up. *Gut* 1993;33(Suppl):S91.
173. Korenman J et al. Long-term remission of chronic hepatitis B after alpha-interferon therapy. *Ann Intern Med* 1991;114:629.
174. Niederau C et al. Long-term follow-up of the HBeAg-positive patients treated with interferon alfa for chronic hepatitis B. *N Engl J Med* 1996;334: 1422.
175. Perrillo RP et al. Therapy for hepatitis B virus infection. *Gastroenterol Clin North Am* 1994;23:581.
176. Wong DKH et al. Effect of alpha interferon treatment in patients with hepatitis B e antigen-positive chronic hepatitis B: a meta-analysis. *Ann Intern Med* 1993;119:312.
177. Lau GKK et al. Peginterferon alfa 2a, lamivudine, and the combination for HBeAg-positive chronic hepatitis B. *N Engl J Med* 2005;352:2682.
178. Janssen HLA et al. Peglyated interferon alfa 2b alone or in combination with lamivudine for HBeAg positive chronic hepatitis B: a randomized trial. *Lancet* 2005;365:123.
179. Marcellin P et al. Peginterferon alfa 2a alone, lamivudine alone, and the two in combination in patients with HBeAg negative chronic hepatitis B. *N Engl J Med* 2004;351:1206.
180. Perrillo RP et al. Low-dose, titratable interferon alfa in decompensated liver disease caused by chronic infection with hepatitis B virus. *Gastroenterology* 1995;109:908.
181. Intron-A package insert. Kenilworth, NJ: Schering Corporation; 1992.
182. Doong SL et al. Inhibition of the replication of hepatitis B virus *in vitro* by 2', 3'—dideoxy-3' thiacytadine and related analogues. *Proc Natl Acad Sci* USA1991;88:8495.
183. Jarvis B et al. Lamivudine: a review of its therapeutic potential in chronic hepatitis B. *Drugs* 1999; 58:101.
184. Dienstag JL et al. Histological outcome during long-term lamivudine therapy. *Gastroenterology* 2003;124:105.
185. Dienstag JL et al. Lamivudine as initial treatment for chronic hepatitis B in the United States. *N Engl J Med* 1999;341:1256.
186. Honkoop P et al. Lamivudine resistance in immunocompetent chronic hepatitis B: incidence and patterns. *J Hepatol* 1997;26:1393.
187. Chang TT et al. Enhanced HbeAg seroconversion rates in Chinese patients on lamivudine [Abstract]. *Hepatology* 1999;30(Suppl 2):420A.
188. Lai CL et al. Prevalence and clinical correlates of YMDD variants during lamivudine therapy for patients with hepatitis B. *Clin Infect Dis* 2003;36:687.
189. Bartholomeusz A et al. Antiviral drug resistance: clinical consequences and molecular aspects. *Semin Liver Dis* 2006: 26:162.
190. Hadziyannis SJ et al. Adefovir dipivoxil for the treatment of hepatitis Be antigen-negative chronic hepatitis B. *N Engl J Med* 2003;348:800.
191. Marcellin P et al. Adefovir dipivoxil for the treatment of hepatitis Be antigen-positive chronic hepatitis B. *N Engl J Med* 2003;348:808.
192. Sommadossi J-P. Anti-hepatitis B specific beta-L-2'-deoxynucleosides [Abstract]. *Antivir Ther* 1999;4(Suppl 4):8.
193. Chang TT et al. A comparison of entecavir and lamivudine for HBeAg positive chronic hepatitis B. *N Engl J Med* 2006;354:1001.
194. Colonno R et al. Resistance after two years of entecavir treatment in nucleoside naïve patients is rare. *Hepatology* 2006:45:1665.
195. Gish R et al. Entecavir results in substantial virologic and biochemical improvement and HBeAg seroconversion through 96 weeks of treatment in HBeAg (+) chronic hepatitis B patients [Abstract]. *Hepatology* 2005;42(Suppl):267A.
196. Lai CL et al. Entecavir versus lamivudine for patients with HBeAg negative chronic hepatitis B. *N Engl J Med* 2006;354:1011.
197. Lai CL et al. Telbivudine versus lamivudine in patients with chronic hepatitis B. *N Engl J Med* 2007; 357:2576.

198. Lim SG et al. A double blind placebo controlled study of emtricitabine in chronic hepatitis B. *Arch Intern Med* 2006;166:49.
199. Yoo BC et al. Twenty-four week clevudine therapy showed potent and sustained antiviral activity in HBeAg positive chronic hepatitis B. *Hepatology* 2007;45:1172.
200. Hultgren C et al. The antiviral compound ribavirin modulates the T helper (Th) 1/Th 2 subset balance in hepatitis B and C virus-specific immune responses. *J Gen Virol*. 1998;79:2381.
201. Ruiz-Moreno M et al. Levamisole and interferon in children with chronic hepatitis B. *Hepatology* 1993;18:264.
202. Hernandez B et al. Cellular kinases involved in the phosphorylation of beta-L-thymidine and beta-L-2′-deoxycytidine, two specific anti-hepatitis B virus agents [abstract]. *Antiviral Ther* 1999;4(Suppl 4):49.
203. Le Guerhier F et al. 2′3′-Dideoxy-2′3′dideoxyhydro-beta-L-fluorocytidine (beta-L-FD4C) exhibits a more potent antiviral effect than lamivudine in chronically WHV infected woodchucks [abstract]. *Hepatology* 1999;30(Suppl 2):421A.
204. Ying C et al. Inhibition of the replication of the DNA polymerase M550V variant of hepatitis B virus by adefovir, tenofovir, L-FMAU, DAPD, penciclovir and lobucavir [Abstract]. *Antivir Ther* 1999;4(Suppl 4):27.
205. Onbo-Nita SK et al. Screening of new antivirals for wild-type hepatitis B virus and three lamivudine-resistant mutants [Abstract]. *Antivir Ther* 1999;4(Suppl 4):33.
206. Von Weizsacker F et al. Gene therapy for chronic viral hepatitis: ribozymes, antisense oligonucleotides, and dominant negative mutants. *Hepatology* 1997;26:251.
207. Yalcin K et al. Comparison of 12-month courses of interferon-alpha-2b-lamivudine combination therapy and interferon-alpha-2b monotherapy among patients with untreated chronic hepatitis B. *Clin Infect Dis* 2003;36:1516.
208. Barbaro G et al. Long-term efficacy of interferon-alpha-2b and lamivudine in combination compared to lamivudine monotherapy in patients with chronic hepatitis B. *J Hepatol* 2001;35:406.
209. Livingston BD et al. The hepatitis B virus-specific CTL responses induced in humans by lipopeptide vaccination are comparable to those elicited by acute viral infection. *J Immunol* 1997;159:1383.
210. Wright T et al. Phase I study of a potent adjuvant hepatitis B vaccine (HBV/MF59) for therapy of chronic hepatitis B [Abstract]. *Hepatology* 1999;30(Suppl 2):421A.
211. Samuel D et al. Liver transplantation in European patients with the hepatitis B surface antigen. *N Engl J Med* 1993;329:1842.
212. Terrault NA et al. Prophylaxis in liver transplant recipients using a fixed dosing schedule of hepatitis B immunoglobulin. *Hepatology* 1996;24:1327.
213. Waters JA et al. Loss of the common 'A' determinant of hepatitis B surface antigen by a vaccine induced escape mutant. *J Clin Invest* 1992;90:2543.
214. McGory RW et al. Improved outcome of orthotopic liver transplantation for chronic hepatitis B cirrhosis with aggressive passive immunization. *Transplantation* 1996;9:1358.
215. Burbach GJ et al. Intravenous or intramuscular anti-HBs immunoglobulin for the prevention of hepatitis B reinfection after orthotopic liver transplantation. *Transplantation* 1997;63:478.
216. Poterucha JJ. Liver transplantation and hepatitis B. *Ann Intern Med* 1997;126:805.
217. Anselmo DM et al. New era of liver transplantation for hepatitis B: a 17-year single-center experience. *Ann Surg* 2002;235:611.
218. Eisenbach C et al. Prevention of hepatitis B virus recurrence after liver transplantation. *Clin Transplant* 2006;20 Suppl 17:111.
219. Brumage LK et al. Treatment for recurrent viral hepatitis after liver transplantation. *J Hepatol* 1997;26:440.
220. Bain JA et al. Efficacy of lamivudine in chronic hepatitis B patients with acute viral replication and decompensated cirrhosis undergoing liver transplantation. *Transplantation* 1996;10:1456.
221. Grellier L et al. Lamivudine prophylaxis against reinfection in liver transplantation for hepatitis B cirrhosis. *Lancet* 1996;348:1212.
222. Ling R et al. Selection of mutations in the hepatitis B virus polymerase during therapy of transplant recipients with lamivudine. *Hepatology* 1996;24:711.
223. Bartholomew MM et al. Hepatitis-B-virus resistance to lamivudine given for recurrent infection after orthotopic liver transplantation. *Lancet* 1997;349:20.
224. Taylor JM. Hepatitis delta. *Virology* 2005;344:71.
225. Bean P. Latest discoveries on the infection and coinfection with hepatitis D virus. *Am Clin Lab* 2002;21:25.
226. Taylor JM. Hepatitis delta virus. *Intervirology* 1999;42:173.
227. Hoofnagle JH. Type D (delta) hepatitis. *JAMA* 1989;261:1321.
228. Lai M. The molecular biology of hepatitis delta virus. *Ann Rev Biochem* 1995;64:259.
229. Negro F et al. Diagnosis of hepatitis delta virus infection. *J Hepatol* 1995;22 (Suppl 1):136.
230. Smedile A et al. The clinical significance of hepatitis D RNA in serum as detected by a hybridization-based assay. *Hepatology* 1996;6:1297.
231. Rosino F et al. Interferon for HDV infection. *Antivir Res* 1994;24:165.
232. Ottobrelli A et al. Patterns of delta hepatitis reinfection and disease following liver transplantation. *Gastroenterology* 1991;101:1649.
233. Rosina F et al. A randomized controlled trial of a 12-month course of recombinant human interferon—in chronic delta (type D) hepatitis: a multicenter Italian study. *Hepatology* 1991;13:1052.
234. Farci P et al. Treatment of chronic hepatitis D with interferon alfa-2a. *N Engl J Med* 1994;330:88.
235. Rizzetto M et al. Chronic hepatitis in carriers of hepatitis B surface antigen, with intrahepatic expression of the delta antigen. *Ann Intern Med* 1983;98:437.
236. Hadziyannis SJ. Use of alpha-interferon in the treatment of chronic delta hepatitis. *J Hepatol* 1991;13:S21.
237. Castelnau C et al. Efficacy of peginterferon alfa 2b in chronic hepatitis delta: relevance of quantitative RT-PCR for follow up. *Hepatology* 2006;44:728.
238. Niro GA et al. Pegylated interferon alfa 2b as monotherapy or in combination with ribavirin in chronic delta hepatitis. *Hepatology* 2006;44:713.
239. Lau DT et al. Lamivudine for chronic delta hepatitis. *Hepatology* 1999;30:356.
240. Wolters LM et al. Lamivudine-high dose interferon combination therapy for chronic hepatitis B patients co-infected with the hepatitis D virus. *J Viral Hepatitis* 2000;7:428.
241. Strader DB et al. Diagnosis, management, and treatment of hepatitis C. *Hepatology* 2004;39:1147.
242. Stevens CE et al. Epidemiology of hepatitis C virus: a preliminary study in volunteer blood donors. *JAMA* 1990;263:49.
243. Alter MJ et al. Risk factors for acute non-A, non-B hepatitis in the United States and association with hepatitis C virus infection. *JAMA* 1990;264:2231.
244. Centers for Disease Control and Prevention. Recommendations for prevention and control of hepatitis C virus (HCV) infection and HCV-related chronic disease. *MMWR* 1998;47(RR-19):1.
245. Chevaliez S et al. Hepatitis C virus: virology, diagnosis, and management of antiviral therapy. *World J Gastroenterol* 2007: 13:2641.
246. Flamm SL. Chronic hepatitis C infection. *JAMA* 2003;289:2413.
247. Pawlotsky JM et al. The hepatitis c virus life cycle as a target for new antiviral therapies. *Gastroenterology* 2007;132:1979.
248. Kohara M. Hepatitis C virus replication and pathogenesis. *J Dermatol Sci* 2000;22:161.
249. Alter MJ et al. The prevalence of hepatitis C virus infection in the United States. *N Engl J Med* 1999;341:556.
250. Donahue JG et al. The declining risk of post-transfusion hepatitis C virus infection. *N Engl J Med* 1992;327:369.
251. Akahane Y et al. Hepatitis C virus infection in spouses of patients with type C chronic liver disease. *Ann Intern Med* 1994;120:748.
252. Ohto H et al. Transmission of hepatitis C virus from mothers to infants. *N Engl J Med* 1994;330:744.
253. Alter MJ. Epidemiology of community-acquired hepatitis C. In: Hollinger FB et al., eds. *Viral Hepatitis and Liver Disease*. Baltimore: Williams & Wilkins; 1991: 410.
254. Kiyosawa K et al. Hepatitis C in hospital employees with needlestick injuries. *Ann Intern Med* 1991;115:367.
255. Gonzales-Peralta R et al. Pathogenesis of hepatocellular damage in chronic hepatitis C virus infection. *Gastrointestinal Diseases* 1995;6:28.
256. Pol S et al. The changing relative prevalence of hepatitis C virus genotypes: evidence in hemodialyzed patients and kidney recipients. *Gastroenterology* 1995;108:581.
257. Neumann AU et al. Differences in hepatitis C virus (HCV) dynamics between HCV of genotype 1 and genotype 2 [Abstract]. *Hepatology* 1999;30(Suppl 2):191A.
258. Mahaney K et al. Genotypic analysis of hepatitis C virus in American patients. *Hepatology* 1994;20:1405.
259. De Medina M et al. Hepatitis C: diagnostic assays. *Semin Liver Dis* 1995;15:33.
260. Centers for Disease Control and Prevention. Guidelines for laboratory testing and result reporting of antibody to hepatitis C virus. *MMWR* 2003;52(RR-3):1.
261. Wilber JC et al. Serological and virological diagnostic tests for hepatitis C virus infection. *Semin in Gastrointes Dis* 1995;6:13.
262. Gretch DR et al. Assessment of hepatitis C viremia using molecular amplification technologies: correlation and clinical implications. *Ann Intern Med* 1995;123:321.
263. Seef LB. Natural history of hepatitis C. *Hepatology* 1997;26(Suppl 1):21S.
264. Chan T et al. Prevalence of hepatitis C virus infection in hemodialysis patients: a longitudinal study comparing the results of RNA and antibody assays. *Hepatology* 1993;17:5.
265. Chan T et al. Prospective study of hepatitis C virus infection among renal transplant recipients. *Gastroenterology* 1993;104:862.
266. Klauser R et al. Hepatitis C antibody in renal transplant recipients. *Transplant Proc* 1992;24:286.
267. Gane E. Management of chronic viral hepatitis before and after renal transplantation. *Transplantation* 2002;74:427.
268. Garcia G et al. Hepatitis C virus infection in the immunocompromised patient. *Semin Gastrointes Dis* 1995;6:35.
269. Ghobrial RM et al. A 10-year experience of liver transplantation for hepatitis C: analysis of factors determining outcome in over 500 patients. *Ann Surg* 2001;234:384.
270. Charlton M. Hepatitis C infection in liver transplantation. *Am J Transplant* 2001;1:197.
271. Gane EJ et al. Long-term outcome of hepatitis C infection after liver transplantation. *N Engl J Med* 1996;334:815.
272. Eyster ME et al. Natural history of hepatitis C virus infection in multitransfused hemophiliacs: effect of coinfection with human immunodeficiency virus: the multicenter hemophilia cohort study. *J AIDS* 1993;6:602.
273. Sulkowski MS et al. Hepatitis C virus infection as an opportunistic disease in persons infected with human immunodeficiency virus. *Clin Infect Dis* 2000;30:S77.
274. Sulkowski MS et al. Hepatitis C in the HIV-infected person. *Ann Intern Med* 2003;138:197.

275. Liaw YF. Hepatitis C superinfection in patients with chronic hepatitis B virus infection. *J Gastroenterol* 2002;37(Suppl 13):65.
276. El-Serag HB. Hepatocellular carcinoma and hepatitis C in the United States. *Hepatology* 2002;36(5 Suppl 1):S74.
277. Hoofnagle JH. Hepatitis C: the clinical spectrum of disease. *Hepatology* 1997;26(Suppl 1):15S.
278. Koof RS et al. Extrahepatic manifestations of hepatitis C. *Semin Gastrointest Dis* 1995;15:101.
279. Centers for Disease Control and Prevention. Recommendations for follow-up of health-care workers after occupational exposure to hepatitis C virus. *MMWR* 1997;46:603.
280. Viladomiu L et al. Interferon alfa in acute posttransfusion hepatitis C: a randomized controlled trial. *Hepatology* 1992;15:767.
281. Lampertico P et al. A multicenter randomized controlled trial of recombinant interferon alfa 2b in patients with acute transfusion-related hepatitis C. *Hepatology* 1994;19:19.
282. Jaeckel E et al. Treatment of acute hepatitis C with interferon alfa-2b. *N Engl J Med* 2001;245:1452.
283. Davis GL et al. Treatment of chronic hepatitis with recombinant interferon alfa: a multicenter randomized, controlled trial. *N Engl J Med* 1991;321:1501.
284. Di Bisceglie AM et al. Recombinant interferon alfa therapy for chronic hepatitis C: a randomized, double-blind, placebo-controlled trial. *N Engl J Med* 1989;321:1506.
285. Saracco G et al. A randomized controlled trial of interferon alfa-2b as therapy for chronic nonA nonB hepatitis. *J Hepatol* 1990;11:S43.
286. Weiland O et al. Therapy of chronic posttransfusion nonA nonB hepatitis with interferon alfa-2b: Swedish experience. *J Hepatol* 1990;11(Suppl 1):S57.
287. Gomez-Rubio M et al. Prolonged treatment (18 months) of chronic hepatitis C with recombinant alfa-interferon in comparison with a control group. *J Hepatol* 1990;11:S63.
288. Marcellin P et al. Recombinant human alfa-interferon in patients with chronic nonA nonB hepatitis C: a multicenter randomized controlled trial from France. *Hepatology* 1991;13:393.
289. Saez-Royuela F et al. High dose of recombinant alfa-interferon or gamma-interferon for chronic hepatitis C: a randomized controlled trial. *Hepatology* 1991;13:327.
290. Causse X et al. Comparison of 1 or 3 MU of interferon-alfa-2b and placebo in patients with chronic nonA nonB hepatitis. *Gastroenterology* 1991;101:497.
291. Reichen J et al. Fixed versus titrated interferon-alfa 2B in chronic hepatitis C: a randomized controlled multicenter trial. The Swiss Association for the study of the liver. *J Hepatol* 1996;25:275.
292. Poynard T et al. A comparison of three interferon alfa-2b regimens for the long-term treatment of chronic nonA, nonB hepatitis. *N Engl J Med* 1995;332:1457.
293. Diodati G et al. Treatment of chronic hepatitis C with recombinant interferon alfa-2a: results of a randomized controlled clinical trial. *Hepatology* 1994;19:1.
294. Negro F et al. Continuous versus intermittent therapy for chronic hepatitis C with recombinant interferon alfa-2a. *Gastroenterology* 1994;107:479.
295. Chemello L et al. Randomized trial comparing three different regimens of alpha-2a interferon in chronic hepatitis C. *Hepatology* 1995;22:700.
296. Imai Y et al. Recombinant interferon-alpha-2a for treatment of chronic hepatitis C: results of a multicenter randomized controlled dose study. *Liver* 1997;17:88.
297. Rumi et al. A prospective randomized comparing lymphoblastoid interferon to recombinant interferon alfa 2a as therapy for chronic hepatitis C. *Hepatology* 1996;24:1366.
298. Farrell GC et al. Lymphoblastoid interferon alfa-n1 improves the long-term response to a 6-month course of treatment in chronic hepatitis C compared with recombinant interferon alfa-2b: results of an international randomized controlled trial. *Hepatology* 1998;27:1121.
299. McHutchison JG et al. Interferon alfa-2b alone or in combination with ribavirin as initial treatment for chronic hepatitis C. *N Engl J Med* 1998;339:1485.
300. Reichard O et al. Randomised, double-blind, placebo-controlled trial of interferon-alpha-2b with and without ribavirin for chronic hepatitis C. *Lancet* 1998;351:83.
301. Poynard T et al. Randomised trial of interferon-alpha-2b plus ribavirin for 48 weeks or for 24 weeks versus interferon –2b plus placebo for 48 weeks for treatment of chronic infection with hepatitis C virus. *Lancet* 1998;352:1426.
302. Davis GL et al. Interferon alfa-2b alone or in combination with ribavirin for the treatment of relapse of chronic hepatitis C. *N Engl J Med* 1998;339:1493.
303. Iino S et al. Treatment of chronic hepatitis C with high-dose interferon a2b: a multicenter study. *Dig Dis Sci* 1993;38:612.
304. Reichard O et al. High sustained response rate and clearance of viremia after treatment with interferon-alpha-2b for 60 weeks. *Hepatology* 1994;19:280.
305. Picciotto A et al. Interferon therapy in chronic hepatitis C: evaluation of a low dose maintenance schedule in responder patients. *J Hepatol* 1993;17:359.
306. Lee WM. Therapy of hepatitis C: interferon alfa-2a trials. *Hepatology* 1997;26(Suppl 1):89S.
307. Farrell GC. Therapy of hepatitis C: interferon alfa-n1 trials. *Hepatology* 1997;26(Suppl 1):96S.
308. Keefe. Therapy of hepatitis C: consensus interferon trials. *Hepatology* 1997;26(Suppl 1):101S.
309. Tong MJ et al. Treatment of chronic hepatitis C with consensus interferon: a multicenter, randomized, controlled trial. *Hepatology* 1997;26:747.
310. Calleri G et al. Natural beta interferon in acute type-C hepatitis patients: a randomized controlled trial. *Ital J Gastroenterology Hepatology* 1998;30:181.
311. Hoofmagle JH et al. Peginterferon and ribavirin for chronic hepatitis C. *N Engl J Med* 2006;355:2444.
312. McHutchison JG. Hepatitis C advances in antiviral therapy: what is accepted treatment now. *J Gastroenterol Hepatol* 2002;17:431.
313. McHutchison JG. Current therapy for hepatitis C: pegylated interferon and ribavirin. *Clin Liver Dis* 2002;7:149.
314. Baker DE. Pegylated interferons. *Rev Gastroenterol Disord* 2001;2:87.
315. Luxon BA et al. Pegylated interferons for the treatment of chronic hepatitis C infection. *Clin Ther* 2002;24:1363.
316. Perry CM. Peginterferon alfa2a (40kD): a review of its use in the management of chronic hepatitis C. *Drugs* 2001;61:2263.
317. Linsay KL et al. A randomized, double-blind trial comparing pegylated interferon alfa-2b to interferon alfa-2b as initial treatment for chronic hepatitis C. *Hepatology* 2001;34:395.
318. Manns MP et al. Peginterferon alfa-2b plus ribavirin compared with interferon alfa-2b plus ribavirin for initial treatment of chronic hepatitis C: a randomised trial. *Lancet* 2001;358:958.
319. Zeuzem S et al. Peginterferon alfa-2a in patients with chronic hepatitis C. *N Engl J Med* 2000;343:1666.
320. Heathcote EJ et al. Peginterferon alfa-2a in patients with chronic hepatitis C and cirrhosis. *N Engl J Med* 2000;343:1673.
321. Fried MW et al. Peginterferon alfa-2a plus ribavirin for chronic hepatitis C virus infection. *New Engl J Med* 2002;347:975.
322. Mangia A et al. Peginterferon alfa 2a and ribavirin for 12 vs. 24 weeks in HCV genotype 2 or 3. *N Engl J Med* 2005;353:2609.
323. Saracco G et al. A randomized 4-arm multicenter study of interferon alfa-2b plus ribavirin in the treatment of patients with chronic hepatitis C relapsing after interferon monotherapy. *Hepatology* 2002;36:959.
324. McHutchinson JG et al. The impact of interferon plus ribavirin on response to therapy in black patients with chronic hepatitis C. *Gastroenterology* 2000;119:1317.
325. Yu JW et al. Predictive value of rapid virological response and early virological response in HCV patients treated with peglyated interferon alpha 2a and ribavirin. *J Gasteroenterol Hepatol* 2007;22:832.
326. Davis GL et al. Early virologic response to treatment with peginterferon alfa 2b plus ribavirin in patients with chronic hepatitis C. *Hepatology* 2003;38:645.
327. Reddy KR et al. Impact of ribavirin dose reductions in hepatitis C genotype 1 patients completing peginterferon alfa 2a/ribavirin treatment. *Clin Gastroenterol Hepatol* 2007;5:124.
328. Jacobson IM et al. Peginterferon alfa 2b and weight-based or flat-dosed ribavirin in chronic hepatitis C patients: a randomized trial. *Hepatology* 2007;46:971.
329. Shiffman ML et al. Peginterferon alpha-21 and ribavirin for 16 or 24 weeks in HCV genotype 2 or 3. *N Engl J Med* 2007;357:124.
330. Andreone P et al. Interferon alpha increases prostaglandin E2 production by cultured liver biopsy in patients with chronic viral hepatitis: can non-steroidal anti-inflammatory drugs improve the response to interferon? *J Hepatol* 1993;19:228.
331. Lebovics E et al. Pentoxifylline enhances response of chronic hepatitis C to interferon-alpha-2b: a double-blind randomized controlled trial [Abstract]. *Hepatology* 1996;24:402A.
332. Parola M et al. Vitamin E dietary supplementation protects against carbon tetrachloride-induced chronic liver damage and cirrhosis. *Hepatology* 1992;16:1014.
333. Gross JB et al. Vitamin E or omega-3 fatty acid concentrate (Omacor) as suppressive treatment for patients with chronic hepatitis [Abstract]. *Hepatology* 1999;30(Suppl 2):191A.
334. Van Rossim TGJ et al. Review article: glycyrrhizin as a potential treatment for chronic hepatitis C. *Aliment Pharmacol Ther* 1998;12:199.
335. Pares A et al. Effects of silymarin in alcoholic patients with cirrhosis of the liver: results of a controlled, double-blind, randomized and multicenter trial. *J Hepatol* 1998;28:615.
336. Kayano K et al. Inhibitory effects of the herbal medicine Sho-saiko-to (TJ-9) on cell proliferation and pro-collagen gene expression in cultured rat hepatic stellate cells. *J Hepatol* 1998;29:642.
337. Nelson DR et al. A pilot study of recombinant human interleukin 10 (Tenovil) in patients with chronic hepatitis C who failed interferon-based therapy [Abstract]. *Hepatology* 1999;30(Suppl 2):189A.
338. Firpi RJ et al. Current and future hepatitis C therapies. *Arch Med Res* 2007;38:678.
339. Parfieniuk A et al. Specifically targeted antiviral therapy for hepatitis C virus. *World J Gastroenerol* 2007;13:5673.
340. Harrison SA. Small molecule and novel treatments for chronic hepatitis C virus infection. *Am J Gastroenterol* 2007;102:2332.
341. Delpha E et al. Therapeutic vaccination of chronically infected chimpanzees with the hepatitis C virus E1 protein [Abstract]. *Antiviral Ther* 1999;4(Suppl 4):12.
342. Wright HI et al. Preliminary experience with-alpha-2b-interferon therapy in viral hepatitis in allograft recipients. *Transplantation* 1992;53:121.
343. Wright TL et al. Interferon-alpha therapy for hepatitis C virus infection after liver transplantation. *Hepatology* 1994;20:773.

344. Sheiner PA et al. The efficacy of prophylactic interferon alfa-2b in preventing recurrent hepatitis C after liver transplantation. *Hepatology* 1998;28: 831.
345. Arjal RR et al. The treatment of hepatitis c recurrence after liver transplantation. *Aliment Pharmacol Ther* 2007;26:127.
346. Bizollon T et al. Pilot study of the combination of interferon alfa and ribavirin as therapy of recurrent hepatitis C after liver transplantation. *Hepatology* 1997;26:500.
347. Gane E et al. A randomized study comparing ribavirin and interferon alfa monotherapy for hepatitis C recurrence after liver transplantation. *Hepatology* 1998;27:1403.
348. Terrault NA et al. Treating hepatitis C infection in liver transplant recipients. *Liver Transpl* 2006; 12:1192.
349. Mast EE et al. Hepatitis E: an overview. *Annu Rev Med* 1996;47:257.
350. Bradley DW. Hepatitis E virus: a brief review of the biology, molecular virology, and immunology of a novel virus. *J Hepatol* 1995;22(Suppl 1):140.
351. Purdy MA et al. Hepatitis E. *Gastroenterol Clin North Am* 1994;23:537.
352. Khuroo M et al. Spectrum of hepatitis E virus infection in India. *J Med Virol* 1990;43:281.
353. Mast E et al. Hepatitis E: an overview. *Annu Rev Med* 1996;47:257.
354. Tsega E et al. Acute sporadic viral hepatitis in Ethiopia: causes, risk factors, and effects on pregnancy. *Clin Infect Dis* 1992;14:961.
355. Longer C et al. Experimental hepatitis E: pathogenesis in cynomolgus macaques (*Macaca fascicularis*). *J Infect Dis* 1992;168:602.
356. Chauhan A et al. Hepatitis E virus transmission to a volunteer. *Lancet* 1993;1:149.
357. Khuroo M et al. Hepatitis E and long term antibody status. *Lancet* 1993;2:1355.
358. Tucker TJ et al. Review of the epidemiology, molecular characterization and tropism of the hepatitis G virus/GBV-C. *Clin Lab* 2001;47:239.
359. Halasz R et al. GB virus C/hepatitis G virus. *Scand J Infect Dis* 2001;33:572.
360. Tucker TJ et al. GBV/HGV genotypes: proposed nomenclature for genotypes 1–5. *J Med Virol* 2000; 62:82.
361. Frey SE et al. Evidence for probable sexual transmission of the hepatitis G virus. *Clin Infect Dis* 2002;34:1033.
362. Lazdina U et al. Humoral and cellular immune response to the GBV virus C/hepatitis G virus envelope 2 protein. *J Med Virol* 2000;62:334.
363. Schlueter V et al. Reverse transcription PCR detection of hepatitis G virus. *J Clin Microbiol* 1996; 34:2660.
364. Matsumura MM et al. Hepatitis G virus coinfection influences the liver histology of patients with chronic hepatitis C. *Liver* 2000;20:397.
365. Kapoor S et al. Clinical implications of hepatitis G virus (HGV) infection in patients of acute viral hepatitis and fulminant hepatic failure. *Indian Med Res* 2000;112:121.

CHAPTER 74

Parasitic Infections

J.V. Anandan

MALARIA

Distribution and Mortality

Malaria is considered the world's most important parasitic disease, responsible for an estimated 300 to 500 million cases and annual deaths in excess of 1 million.[1–4] Approximately 27 million U.S. travelers visit malaria-endemic areas each year.[5] The distribution of the four *Plasmodium* species of malaria varies worldwide, with *Plasmodium falciparum*, which has the highest mortality, primarily acquired in sub-Saharan Africa, Haiti, the Dominican Republic, the Amazon region in South America, and parts of Asia and Oceania.

Life Cycle

Malarial infection is transmitted by the female mosquito of the genus *Anopheles,* which injects the asexual forms or sporozoites into the human host during a blood meal. After a lapse of about 9 to 16 days and an asexual multiplication stage in the liver called *exoerythrocytic schizogony*, daughter cells, or merozoites, are released into the blood to infect red blood cells (RBC). The merozoites develop into the characteristic ring or trophozoite forms in RBC and then go through another asexual reproductive stage called *erythrocytic schizogony* to produce more merozoites. When the infected RBC rupture, the merozoites invade new blood cells and repeat the erythrocyte cycle. In 1 or 2 weeks, a subpopulation of merozoites differentiates into the sexual forms, resulting in male and female gametocytes. If the gametocytes in the host blood are ingested by a female *Anopheles* mosquito during a blood meal, fertilization and an asexual division in the mosquito midgut will propagate the infective sporozoites to complete the cycle.

The characteristic malarial paroxysms of chills and fever in patients usually coincide with the periodic release of merozoites and other pyrogens in the blood. In *P. falciparum* infections, this periodicity may not always be apparent. However, intervals of 48 hours between paroxysms are reported for *Plasmodium vivax, Plasmodium ovale,* and *P. falciparum* (tertian periodicity), and 72 hours for *Plasmodium malariae* (quartan periodicity). Unlike infections caused by *P. falciparum* and *P. malariae,* infections with *P. vivax* and *P. ovale* have a latent form of the exoerythrocytic phase that can persist in the host liver for months to years. This latent form can produce relapses of the erythrocytic infection (Fig. 74-1).

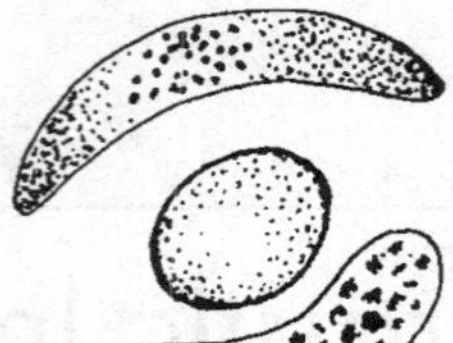

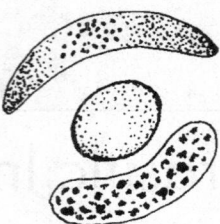

FIGURE 74-1 *P. falciparum gametocytes.*

Epidemiology

Although malaria is endemic to the tropics, approximately 1,324 cases were diagnosed in the United States in 2004.[3,5] Of the 775 U.S. civilians who acquired malaria while abroad, 160 (20.6%) reported that they had been on a chemoprophylaxis regimen recommended by the Centers for Disease Control and Prevention (CDC).[3] Malaria transmission in the United States has occurred from the blood of immigrants and travelers, local transmission, military personnel, and rarely through blood transfusions.[2,3,5,6] In terms of the species of *Plasmodium* identified in the United States, 49% represented *P. falciparum,* and 81% of these infections were acquired in Africa.[3] Transfusion malaria often is the result of *P. malariae,* which can persist in the blood without symptoms for extended periods and has also been reported to cause nephrotic syndrome.[7,8] Malaria can also be transmitted congenitally and through contaminated needles.[3,8,9]

Drug Resistance

Chloroquine-resistant *P. falciparum* (CRPF) is widespread and present in all malaria-endemic areas of the world except Mexico, the Caribbean, Central America (north of the Panama Canal), and parts of the Middle East (except Iran, Yemen, Oman, and Saudi Arabia).[10–14] However, *P. falciparum* malaria, resistant to chloroquine and mefloquine, has been isolated in Thailand, Cambodia, and Myanmar (Burma). Chloroquine-resistant *P. vivax* is an emerging problem in Papua, New Guinea, Irian, Jaya (Indonesia), Myanmar, and Columbia.[10,12,14,15] Most fatal cases of imported malaria in the United States are the result of travelers' failure to comply with appropriate chemosuppressive regimens, delays in seeking treatment, misdiagnosis by physicians or laboratories, and inappropriate antimalarial regimens.[2,13] Prophylactic drug regimens for individuals traveling to endemic areas are problematic (see Question 5).[10,11,15]

Acute Malaria

Signs and Symptoms

1. M.L, a 29-year-old male student, presents to the emergency department (ED) with complaints of malaise, myalgia, headache, and fever of 4 days' duration. A native of Ghana, West Africa, he recently visited his parents and returned to the United States 3 weeks ago. Two days before admission, he had an abrupt onset of coldness and chills, followed 1 hour later by a high fever, headache, nausea, and vomiting. The episode of chills and fever lasted about 24 hours, after which he became asymptomatic. On the afternoon of admission, he again had a bout of chills that preceded a fever of 40°C.

Physical examination reveals a slender black man who is acutely ill and complaining of severe abdominal pain. Abdominal examination reveals a soft, tender spleen that is slightly enlarged. Blood pressure (BP) is 110/70 mmHg; pulse 120 beats/minute, respiration rate 32 breaths/minute, and temperature 40°C. Laboratory findings include hemoglobin (Hgb) 11 g/dL (normal, 12–16); hematocrit (Hct) 34% (normal, 36%–47%); white blood cell (WBC) count 3,300 cells/mm^3 (normal, 4,000–11,000) with 76% neutrophils (normal, 45%–65%), 23% lymphocytes (normal, 15%–35%), and 1% monocytes (normal, 1%–6%); platelets 83 × 10^3/mm^3 (normal, 150–450); and bilirubin 1.0 mg/dL (normal, 0.1–1). Urinalysis reveals trace amounts of albumin and the presence of urobilinogen. Thick and thin films of M.L.'s blood are prepared. A Giemsa stain of the thin film demonstrates *P. falciparum* gametocytes. Why is the presentation of M.L. consistent with *P. falciparum* malaria?

[SI units: Hgb, 110 g/L (normal, 120–160); Hct, 0.34 (0.36–0.47); WBC count, 3.3 × 10^9/L (normal, 4–11) with 0.76 neutrophils (normal, 0.45–0.65), 0.23 lymphocytes (normal, 0.15–0.35), 0.01 monocytes (normal, 0.01–0.06); platelets, 3.3 × 10^9/L (normal, 150–450); bilirubin, 18 mmol/L (normal, 2–18)]

M.L. recently visited Ghana, West Africa, where *P. falciparum* is endemic.[4,9,11] *P. vivax* malaria accounts for about 50% of all cases of malaria reported in the United States. The prevalence of *P. falciparum* malaria has been increasing, however, and it accounts for about 49% of all malarial cases.[3] Infected persons usually experience prodromal symptoms (primarily headache, muscle aches and pains, malaise, nausea, and vomiting) around the second week after exposure.[4,13] This time frame is consistent with M.L.'s onset of symptoms. The incubation period and the onset of primary symptoms for *P. falciparum* malaria can be delayed for months, however.[4,11,16] History of travel to an endemic area, the cyclical paroxysmal episodes of chills and fever, the presence of thrombocytopenia and jaundice, and the identification of *P. falciparum* gametocytes in M.L.'s blood confirm the diagnosis of malaria.

Treatment

2. How should the *P. falciparum* malaria in M.L. be treated? How would M.L.'s treatment differ from that used for other *Plasmodium* species?

P. falciparum malaria, the most severe form of malaria, has the highest mortality rate.[4,5,11,16–25] The fever spikes, unlike those associated with *P. vivax* and *P. ovale* malaria, normally are very high (40°C–41°C), and complications (including confusion, vomiting, diarrhea, severe abdominal pain, hypoglycemia, renal failure, and encephalopathy) are common.[4,13,18–26]

QUINIDINE AND QUININE

M.L. is very ill and may be unable to tolerate oral medications because of nausea and vomiting. He should be admitted to an acute care unit and started on intravenous (IV) quinidine gluconate.[4,9,11,18,27] For doses of IV quinidine, see Table 74-1. If >48 hours of parenteral therapy is required, the dosage of quinidine should be reduced by one-third to one-half.[11,27]

Table 74-1 Drug Therapy of Parasitic Infection [4,7,9,10,11,14,18,27,28,29,32,35,36,39,57,61,64,80,81,90,93,107,111,116,120,124,125,127]

Drug of Choice	*Dosage*	*Adverse Effects*
Amebiasis (Including Cyst Passers)		
Asymptomatic		
Iodoquinol	*Adults:* 650 mg PO TID × 20 days	Rash, acne, thyroid enlargement
or	*Children:* 30–40 mg/kg/days PO TID × 20 days	
Diloxanide furoate	*Adults:* 500 mg PO TID × 10 days	Flatulence, abdominal pain
or	*Children:* 20 mg/kg/day PO TID × 10 days	
Paromomycin	*Adults:* 25–35 mg/kg/day PO TID × 7 days	Nausea, vomiting
	Children: Same as adults	
Mild to Moderate Gastrointestinal Disease		
Metronidazole	*Adults:* 750 mg PO TID × 10 days	Nausea, headache, metallic taste, disulfiram reaction with alcohol, paresthesia
or	*Children:* 35–50 mg/kg/day PO TID × 10 days	
Tinidazole *followed by*	*Adults:* 2 g once daily × 3 days *Children:* 50 mg/kg (max. 2 g) × 3 days	Metallic or bitter taste, anorexia, nausea, vomiting, epigastric discomfort, weakness, seizures, peripheral neuropathy
Iodoquinol	*Adults:* 650 mg PO TID × 20 days	Rash, acne, thyroid enlargement
	Children: 30–40 mg/kg/day PO TID × 20 days	
Severe Gastrointestinal Disease		
Metronidazole	*Adults:* 750 mg PO TID × 10 days	Nausea, headache, metallic taste, disulfiram reaction with alcohol, paresthesia
or	*Children:* 35–50 mg/kg/day PO TID × 10 days	
Tinidazole *followed by*	*Adults* : 2 g once daily × 5 days *Children* : 50 mg/kg/day (max. 2 g) × 5 days	Metallic taste or bitter taste, nausea, vomiting, epigastric discomfort, anorexia and weakness
Iodoquinol	*Adults:* 650 mg PO TID × 20 days	Rash, acne, thyroid enlargement
	Children: 30–40 mg/kg/day PO TID × 20 days	
Alternatives		
Dehydroemetine *followed by*	*Adults:* 1–1.5 mg/kg/day IM × 5 days (max. 90 mg/day)	Arrhythmias, hypotension; ECG: P-R, Q-T, QRS prolongation, S-T depression
	Children: Same as adults	
Iodoquinol	*Adults:* 650 mg PO TID × 20 days	Rash, acne, thyroid enlargement
	Children: 35–40 mg/kg/day PO TID × 20 days	
Amebic Liver Abscess		
Metronidazole	*Adults:* 750 mg PO TID × 10 days	Nausea, headache, metallic taste, disulfiram reaction with alcohol, paresthesia
or	*Children:* 35–50 mg/kg/day PO TID × 10 days	
Tinidazole	*Adults* : 2 g once daily × 5 days	
followed by	*Children* : 50 mg/kg (max. 2 g) × 5 days	
Iodoquinol	*Adults:* 650 mg PO TID × 20 days	Rash, acne, thyroid enlargement
or	*Children:* 30–40 mg/kg/day PO TID × 20 days	
Alternatives		
Dehydroemetine	*Adults:* 1–1.5 mg/kg/d IM × 5 days (max. 90 mg/day)	Arrhythmias, hypotension; ECG: P-R, Q-T, QRS prolongation, S-T depression
followed by	*Children:* Same as adult	
Diloxanide furoate	*Adults:* 500 mg PO TID × 10 days	
or	*Children:* 20 mg/kg/day PO TID × 10 days	
Paromomycin	*Adults:* 25–30 mg/kg/day PO TID × 7 days	Nausea, vomiting
	Children: Same as adults	
Ascariasis (Roundworm)		
Albendazole	Adults/Pediatric: 400 mg once	Nausea and headache
or		
Mebendazole	*Adults and children:* 100 mg BID PO × 3 days	Diarrhea, abdominal pain
Enterobiasis (Pinworm)		
Mebendazole	*Adults and children:* 100 mg once; repeat in 2 wk	Diarrhea, abdominal pain
Pyrantel pamoate	*Adults and children:* 11 mg/kg PO once (max. 1 g), repeat in 2 wk	Nausea, headache, dizziness, rash, fever
or		
Albendazole	*Adult/Pediatric:* 400 mg once; Repeat in 2 wk	Abdominal pain, reversible alopecia, increased transaminases, rarely leukopenia

(continued)

Table 74-1 Drug Therapy of Parasitic Infection [4,7,9,10,11,14,18,27,28,29,32,35,36,39,57,61,64,80,81,90,93,107,111,116,120,124,125,127] ***(Continued)***

Drug of Choice	Dosage	Adverse Effects
Filariasis		
Diethylcarbamazine	*Adults:* Day 1, 50 mg PO; day 2, 50 mg TID; day 3, 100 mg TID; days 4–14, 6 mg/kg/day in 3 doses *Children:* Day 1, 25–50 mg; day 2, 25–50 mg TID; day 3, 50–100 mg TID; days 4–14, 6 mg/kg/day in 3 doses	Severe allergic/febrile reactions, gastrointestinal disturbance, rarely encephalopathy
Flukes (Trematodes)[a]		
Praziquantel	*Adults and children:* 75 mg/kg/day in 3 doses × 1 day (exceptions: *C. sinensis* and *P. westermani*, × 2 days)	Malaise, headache, dizziness, sedation, fever, eosinophilia
Giardiasis		
Metronidazole *or*	*Adults:* 250 mg PO TID with meals × 5 days *Children:* 15 mg/kg/day PO TID × 5 days	Nausea, headache, metallic taste, disulfiram reaction with alcohol, paresthesia
Quinacrine[b]	*Adult:* 100 mg PO TID × 5 days *Pediatric:* 2 mg/kg TID × 5 days (max 300 mg/day)	Gastrointestinal yellow staining of skin and psychosis
Nitazoxanide[c]	*Pediatric:* 12–47 mo 100 mg (5 mL) Q 12 hr × 3 days 4–11 yr 200 mg (10 mL) Q 12 hr × 3 days	Abdominal pain, diarrhea, vomiting and headache
Hookworm		
Mebendazole	*Adults and children:* 100 mg PO BID × 3 days	Diarrhea, abdominal pain
Lice		
1% Permethrin (NIX) *or*	Topical administration	Occasional allergic reaction, mild stinging, erythema
Ivermectin	*Adults and Children* : 200 mcg/kg × 3, day 1, day 2 and day 10	Fever, pruritus, sore lymph nodes, headache, joint pains, rarely hypotension
Leishmaniasis		
Sodium stibogluconate *or*	*Adult:* 20 mg SB/kg IV or IM × 20–28 days *Pediatric:* Same as adult	Gastrointestinal, malaise, headache arthralgias, myalgias, anemia, neutropenia, thrombocytopenia; ECG abnormalities (ST- and T-wave changes)
Liposomal Amphotericin B	*Adult:* 3 mg/kg/day (days 1–5) and 3 mg/kg/days 14 and 21 *Pediatric:* Same as adult	Hypotension, chills, headache, anemia, thrombocytopenia, fever, and elevated serum creatinine
Malaria *All Plasmodia Except Chloroquine-Resistant*		
Parenteral therapy		
Quinidine gluconate	*Adults:* Loading dose 10 mg/kg of salt (6.2 mg base) diluted in 250 mL normal saline and infused IV over 2 hr, followed by a continuous IV infusion of 0.02 mg/kg/min (0.012 mg base) for 72 hr; switch to oral quinine 650 mg Q 8 hr as soon as possible *Pediatric:* Same as adult	ECG: Q-T and QRS prolongation; hypotension, syncope, arrhythmias; cinchonism
Oral therapy		
Chloroquine Phosphate	*Adult:* 1 g (600 mg base), then 500 mg 6 hr later, then 500 mg at 24 and 48 hr later. *Pediatric:* 10 mg base (max. 600 mg base) then 5 mg base/kg 6 hr later, then 5 mg/base at 24 and 48 hr	Gastrointestinal, headache, pruritus, malaise, and cinchonism
Chemoprophylaxis		
Chloroquine phosphate	*Adult:* 500 mg (base) once weekly (beginning 1–2 wk before departure and continuing through stay and up to 4 wk after returning) *Pediatric:* 5 mg/kg base once weekly up to adult dose (300 mg base)	Dose-related: vertigo, nausea, dizziness, light-headedness, headache, visual disturbances, toxic psychosis and seizures
Chloroquine Resistant Therapy (CRF)		
Mefloquine *or*	*Adult:* 750 mg followed by 500 mg 12 hr later *Pediatric:* 15 mg/kg followed 8–12 hr later by 10 mg/kg	Nausea, vomiting, abdominal pain, arthralgias, chills, dizziness, tinnitus and A-V block

(*continued*)

Table 74-1 Drug Therapy of Parasitic Infection [4,7,9,10,11,14,18,27,28,29,32,35,36,39,57,61,64,80,81,90,93,107,111,116,120,124,125,127] ***(Continued)***

Drug of Choice	Dosage	Adverse Effects
Atovaquone/ proguanil	*Adult:* 2 tablets BID × 3 days *Pediatric:* 11–20 kg: 1 adult tablet/d × 3 days 21–30 kg: 2 adult tablets/day × 3 days 31–40 kg: 3 adult tablets/day × 3 days >40 kg: 2 adult tablets BID × 3 days	Rash, nausea, diarrhea, increased aminotransferases, cholestasis
Chemoprophylaxis-CRF		
Mefloquine *or*	*Adult:* 250 mg once weekly beginning 1–2 wk before departure, continuing through stay and for 1–4 wk after return *Pediatric:* <15 kg: 5 mg/kg once weekly 15–19 kg: 1/4 tablet once weekly 20–30 kg: 1/2 tablet once weekly 31–45 kg: 3/4 tablet once weekly >45 kg: 1 tablet once weekly	
Doxycycline	*Adult:* 100 mg daily beginning 1–2 days before departure continuing during stay and 1 wk after return	Nausea, diarrhea and monilial rash
Quinine sulfate *plus*	*Adults:* 650 PO TID × 3 days *Children:* 25 mg/kg/day PO TID × 3 days	Cinchonism
Pyrimethamine-sulfadoxine (Fansidar) *or*	*Adults:* 3 tablets at once (withhold until febrile episode) *Children:* 1/2–2 tablets (depends on age)[c]	Gastrointestinal, erythema multiforme, Stevens-Johnson syndrome, toxic epidermal necrolysis
Mefloquine	*Adults:* 1,250 mg once *Children:* 25 mg/kg once (>45 kg)	Dose-related: vertigo, nausea, dizziness, light-headedness, headache, visual disturbances, toxic psychosis seizures
Prevention of Relapses (P. vivax and P. ovale)		
Primaquine phosphate	*Adults:* 52.6 mg/day (30 mg base) × 14 days; this follows chloroquine or mefloquine regimen	Abdominal cramps, nausea, hemolytic anemia in G6PD
Scabies		
5% Permethrin (Elimite cream)	Topical administration	Rash, edema, erythema
Alternatives		
Ivermectin	*Adults:* 200 mcg/kg PO; repeat in 2 wk	Nausea, diarrhea, dizziness vertigo and pruritus
Lindane (Kwell)	Apply topically once	Not recommended in pregnant women, infants, and patients with massively excoriated skin
Crotamiton 10% (Eurax)	Topically	Local skin irritation
Tapeworm[d]		
Praziquantel	*Adults and children:* 5–10 mg/kg PO × 1 dose	Malaise, headache, dizziness, sedation, eosinophilia, fever
Hydatid Cysts[e]		
Albendazole	*Adults:* 400 mg BID × 8–30 days, repeat if necessary *Children:* 15 mg/kg/day × 28 days, repeat if necessary (surgical resection may precede drug therapy)	Diarrhea, abdominal pain, rarely hepatotoxicity, leukopenia
Trichomoniasis		
Metronidazole	*Adults:* 2 g PO × 1 day or 250 mg PO TID × 7 days *Children:* 15 mg/kg/day PO TID × 7 days	Nausea, headache, metallic taste, disulfiram reaction with alcohol, paresthesia

[a] *Schistosoma haematobium, S. mansoni, S. japonicum, Clonorchis sinensis, Paragonimus westermani.*
[b] Quinacrine is available in the United States: Panorama Compounding Pharmacy, Van Nuys, CA 91406.
[c] Same dose is recommended in children with *Cryptosporidium parvum.*
[d] *Diphyllobothrium latum* (fish), *Taenia solium* (pork), and *Dipylidium caninum* (dog), except for *Hymenolepis nana* where the dose is 25 mg/kg × 1dose.
[e] *Echinococcus granulosus, E. multilocularis.* For neurocysticercosis: 400 mg BID 8–30 days.
BID, twice daily; ECG, electrocardiograph; G6PD, glucose-6-phosphate dehydrogenase; IM, intramuscularly; PO, orally; TID, three times daily.

Because IV quinidine is not routinely used in cardiology care, it may not be available in all hospitals. Because of the serious nature of *P. falciparum* malaria, small stocks of the drug should be kept on hand, or a procedure needs to be established in the hospital to acquire IV quinidine on short notice from an alternative source (Contact Eli Lilly: 800-545-5979).[27] Oral quinine and clindamycin or the combination of atovaquone and proguanil (Malarone) can be used until IV quinidine is available.[4,7,27]

While receiving the IV quinidine, M.L.'s electrocardiogram, BP, and serum glucose should be monitored closely.[4,7,9] Supportive care, including fluid, IV dextrose 5% to 10% and electrolyte management, dialysis, blood transfusion, and mechanically assisted ventilation, are important adjunctive therapies in seriously ill patients. The serum concentration of quinidine should be determined once daily during the continuous infusion. Quinidine levels should remain between 6.1 and 16.5 mcmol/dL. The quinidine infusion should be slowed or stopped if the QRS complex exceeds 25% of baseline, if hypotension is unresponsive to fluid challenge, or if the quinidine serum concentration is >16.5 mcmol/dL.[9,11] When M.L. can be switched to oral therapy, he should receive oral quinine sulfate 650 mg Q 8 hr to complete 3 to 7 days of total therapy.[9,11,18] The quinine is administered for 7 days if *P. falciparum* is acquired in Thailand.[27]

MANAGING CHLOROQUINE-RESISTANT *PLASMODIUM FALCIPARUM*

If M.L. does not respond to the quinidine or quinine regimen within 48 to 72 hours (i.e., failure to reduce parasitemia by 25% of baseline and continued fever over this period), other adjunctive therapies must be considered.[9,27] One of the recommended drug treatments for CRPF infection, which is added to quinine therapy, is doxycycline 100 mg twice daily for 7 days (doxycycline should overlap the quinine for 2 to 3 days before the latter is discontinued) or clindamycin 900 mg three times a day for 5 days.[27] If the patient cannot tolerate oral doxycycline, IV doxycycline 100 mg Q 12 hr can be substituted. An alternative in a patient who can tolerate oral therapy and in whom it is not contraindicated (i.e., history of seizures, or endemic area where *P. falciparum* is not resistant to the agent) mefloquine 750 mg can be initiated, followed by 500 mg 12 hours later.[27] M.L. may also be treated with the combination of atovaquone 250 mg and proguanil 100 mg (Malarone). The dose of Malarone is two tablets twice daily for 3 days.[11,27] Although exchange transfusion has been suggested as an adjunct therapy for serious *P. falciparum* malaria, the role of this intervention remains questionable.[11] The CDC suggests that if patients have parasitemia >10%, or if the patient has altered mental status, nonvolume pulmonary edema, or renal complications, exchange transfusion be considered (www.cdcgov/malaria/pdf/treatmenttable.pdf accessed on 02/26/07).

MANAGING OTHER *PLASMODIA* SPECIES

A patient infected with one of the other species of *Plasmodia* (*P. vivax, P. ovale,* or *P. malariae)* should receive oral chloroquine phosphate (Aralen). The initial dose is 1 g (600 mg base) followed by 500 mg (300 mg base) 6 hours later; subsequently, 500 mg (300 mg base) is administered daily for 2 days.[27] For patients who cannot tolerate the oral doses of chloroquine, parenteral doses of quinidine can be administered (Question 2 lists doses).[27] Patients with *P. ovale* and *P. vivax* also should be given primaquine to prevent relapses from the latent exoerythrocytic stages in the liver. The adult dosage of primaquine is 52.6 mg/day (30 mg base) for 14 days; this should follow the chloroquine regimen.[7,27]

Chemoprophylaxis and Pregnancy

3. T.P., a male medical resident from Indonesia, is planning to visit his seriously ill mother. His wife, T.R., who is 16 weeks pregnant, and their 4-year-old daughter will accompany him. What prophylactic medications for malaria should be administered to each member of the family?

All travelers to endemic areas should receive chemoprophylaxis for malaria. In Indonesia, including Papua, New Guinea, all four types of malaria are present.[7,9,11] T.P. and his family may have to take prophylactic therapy for all malarial species, including a regimen that will protect them against CRPF infections. To verify whether a country is included in the CRPF list or to obtain other relevant information on malaria prophylaxis, T.P. should call the CDC Malaria Hotline, which provides a touch tone-activated, computer-assisted service (770–488-7788).[2,27] Pregnant women are at greater risk for malaria infection and its complications (especially severe hemolytic anemia and splenomegaly) and should be advised not to travel to areas endemic for malaria, if possible.[11,13,28–34] Current publications that provide updated information on parasitic diseases and immunization requirements include *Medical Letter, Morbidity and Mortality Weekly Reports, Health Information for International Travel,* and various Internet sites.[11,13,18]

CHLOROQUINE AND PRIMAQUINE PHOSPHATE

Chloroquine phosphate is an effective chemoprophylactic agent against all species of *Plasmodia* except drug-resistant *P. falciparum.* The adult dosage of chloroquine phosphate is 500 mg (300 mg base) once weekly beginning 1 week before departure and continuing for 4 weeks after last exposure. The pediatric dosage of chloroquine is 5 mg/kg base (8.3 mg chloroquine phosphate) once weekly beginning 1 week before departure and continuing for 4 weeks after exposure. A suspension of chloroquine in chocolate syrup can be prepared for children (5 mg/mL). Chloroquine prophylaxis is safe during pregnancy, and the benefits outweigh the risk of malaria and the drug's possible side effects.[9,11,13,27,29,31] Mefloquine and Malarone may be options for prophylaxis and treatment in pregnancy[29–34]; however, these are not recommended for this particular indication in the United States.[27]

By taking the chloroquine 1 week before travel, the patient can achieve adequate antimalarial chloroquine levels in the blood by the second week. Potential side effects also can be detected early. A weekly dose of 0.5 g of chloroquine phosphate produces average plasma concentrations of chloroquine between 0.47 and 0.78 mcmol/L Most strains of *P. vivax* and *P. falciparum* are susceptible to plasma levels between 0.046 and 0.093 mcmol/L, respectively.[7,18,35] Mefloquine (Lariam) 250 mg (salt) once weekly beginning 1 week before departure and continuing for 4 weeks after leaving a malarious area is an alternative regimen to chloroquine.[7,18,27,36] Mefloquine is not recommended during pregnancy or in children weighing ≤5 kg, however, because the safety of this agent has not been fully established in these populations.[27] Recently, *P. vivax* was reported to be resistant to chloroquine in Indonesia and New Guinea, and despite the lack of data on mefloquine in pregnancy (T.R. is in the second trimester), T.R. may have to be given this agent.[15,18,32,33,37,38] Chloroquine suppresses the asexual erythrocytic forms of the malaria parasite and has no action against the exoerythrocytic phase of *P. vivax* and *P. ovale.*[7,18] However, primaquine phosphate prevents relapses of *P. vivax* and *P. ovale* by inhibiting the exoerythrocytic stage; it also has a significant gametocidal effect against all species.[11,15,18] To prevent an attack after departure from an area where *P. vivax* and *P. ovale* are present, the clinician should also prescribe primaquine phosphate 52.6 mg/day (30 mg base) for 14 days to coincide with the last 2 weeks of the chloroquine regimen. Primaquine should not be administered to pregnant patients.[27] The major toxicity of concern, aside from the teratogenic risk, is hemolytic anemia in patients with RBC glucose-6-phosphate dehydrogenase (G6PD) deficiency[7,18,28,36,39]

PROPHYLAXIS FOR CHLOROQUINE-RESISTANT *PLASMODIUM FALCIPARUM*

Prophylaxis for CRPF also can be achieved by taking mefloquine in the doses indicated above instead of using the chloroquine regimen.[27] An alternative to mefloquine is doxycycline 100 mg/day beginning 1 day before travel and continuing for the duration of the stay and for 4 weeks after leaving the malarial area. Travelers such as T.P. should be advised to take measures to reduce contact with infected mosquitoes by wearing long-sleeved blouses/shirts and pants/trousers, applying insect repellent containing 31% to 35% meta-N, N-diethyl-meta-toluamide (DEET) (e.g., HourGuard-12, Amway Corp.; DEET Plus, Sawyer Products), sleeping in a screened room, or using netting impregnated with permethrin.[30,32,34,37,40] An alternative to the mefloquine chemoprophylaxis regimen in CRPF areas is the combination of atovaquone 250 mg and proguanil 100 mg (Malarone) administered once daily taken 1 to 2 days before departure and continued for 1 week after return.[1,2,27] The pediatric dosage (Malarone Pediatric) contains 62.5 mg of atovaquone and 25 mg of proguanil.[1,27] Instead of doxycycline, T.R. could take Malarone as chemoprophylaxis. The advantage of Malarone is that it can also be used as treatment. The recommended therapeutic dose of Malarone for CRPF is two tablets twice daily for 3 days.[27] Both prophylaxis and treatment of CRPF in nonimmune subjects and pregnant patients continue to pose special problems.[41–47] Pyrimethamine has teratogenic effects and sulfonamides are contraindicated in early pregnancy; however, chloroquine, quinine, and quinidine have been suggested as safe treatments during pregnancy.[2,4,27,29,32,33,39,43] Although not associated with abortions, low birthweight, neurologic retardation, or congenital malformations, mefloquine is associated with an increased risk of stillbirth.[27,34,35,39]

T.P. and T.R. should reconsider their decision to travel together because of the risks of malarial infection during pregnancy. In view of the recent report of *P. vivax* resistance to chloroquine in Indonesia, the family members should consider using mefloquine.[27] The risks and benefits of mefloquine in pregnancy (T.R. is in her second trimester) should be communicated to the family.[15,39] Physical barriers (e.g., clothes, mosquito nets), insect repellent, and a short stay in the endemic area also should be helpful.[29,34,48]

Malaria Vaccine

4. Why could T.R. not be vaccinated as an alternative to prophylaxis with 8-aminoquinolines such as chloroquine?

Currently, no vaccination is available. As a result of successful *in vitro P. falciparum* cultivation and advances in genetic engineering and monoclonal antibody research, some progress has been made, but this vaccine is probably a few years away.[49–54] The malaria plasmodium undergoes many transformations during its development, and each stage expresses a different plasmodial genome that generates a large number of antigens. The development of a malaria vaccine relies on the identification and characterization of these antigens and the subsequent production of monoclonal antibodies.[49,51]

At present, three types of vaccines against *P. falciparum* are under study: a merozoite vaccine that would induce immunity against the erythrocytic forms of plasmodia in the blood, a sporozoite vaccine that would protect against the exoerythrocytic or liver phase, and a gamete vaccine ("transmission blocking") that would prevent transmission of malaria in endemic areas.[49] When a vaccine for malaria is available, it is expected to provide an immune response for at least 1 year. The safety of these vaccines to the fetus and mother during pregnancy will require evaluation.

Multidrug-Resistant Plasmodium Falciparum Malaria

5. F.S., a permanent U.S. resident of Cambodian origin, is planning to travel to the Thai-Kampuchean refugee camp. What antimalarial agents should he use for chemoprophylaxis?

F.S. is traveling to the Thai-Burma border, where *P. falciparum* malaria is epidemic. Chemoprophylaxis against malaria in this region of southeast Asia has become progressively difficult because of the appearance of *P. falciparum* strains resistant to chloroquine, pyrimethamine-sulfadoxine, quinine, and even mefloquine.[7,13,38,41,43,46,47]

F.S. will have to take chemoprophylaxis against both *P. vivax* and multidrug-resistant *P. falciparum*. Mefloquine (Lariam) 250 mg once weekly starting 1 week before travel and continuing weekly for the duration of the stay and for 4 weeks after leaving Thailand is recommended.[27] On return from his visit, primaquine phosphate should be added to F.S.'s regimen to prevent an attack of *P. vivax*, because mefloquine has no effect on the exoerythrocytic phase of *P. vivax* (see Question 3 for doses of primaquine).[27] Another alternative drug for prophylaxis against *P. falciparum* malaria for F.S. would be doxycycline 100 mg taken once daily beginning 1 to 2 days before departure and continuing for 4 weeks after he returns from Thailand.[2,27]

A new chemical entity, ginghaosu, has been undergoing field trials and may prove to be useful for resistant *P. falciparum*. Ginghaosu, a plant extract (artemisinin compounds), has been used for many centuries in China for fever and malaria.[4,7,10,41–45,55–58] Artemisinin and its derivatives (artemether and artesunate) are considered rapidly effective even against CRPF strains and have undergone numerous trials.[7,18,55–58] The antimalarial agent halofantrine (Halfan) may be another alternative to mefloquine, but this agent has been associated with fatal arrhythmias.[27] Clinical trials of fosmidomycin, tefenoquine, lumefantrine, and other new antimalarial agents are ongoing.[1,14,15,47,55–60]

Side Effects of Antimalarials

6. A.K., a 36-year-old Malaysian man, is seen in the ED with a 2-day history of fever, chills, and bouts of diarrhea following his return from west Malaysia, where he was visiting his parents for 3 weeks. A.K. had not taken any prophylaxis for malaria. A blood smear stained with Giemsa solution demonstrated *P. vivax*, and A.K. was given chloroquine 1 g (600 mg base) initially, to be followed by 500 mg (300 mg base) 6 hours later and 500 mg at 24 and 48 hours. On completion of the chloroquine regimen, A.K. was instructed to take primaquine 52.6 mg/day (30 mg base) for 14 days. However, A.K. was seen again in the ED a day later with complaints of abdominal pain, severe headache, vomiting, and a "bitter taste" in the mouth. What subjective evidence does A.K. exhibit that is compatible with the toxicity of antimalarials?

The major side effects of chloroquine (e.g., nausea, abdominal pain, pruritus, vertigo, headache, and visual disturbances)[7,18,39] usually are associated with large doses such as those needed for A.K.'s therapy. The gastrointestinal (GI) complaints and severe headache experienced by A.K. are consistent with chloroquine therapy, and the bitter described is experienced by all patients who are given chloroquine or other 8-aminoquinoline preparations. Because A.K. also will be taking primaquine after the course of chloroquine, he should be told that he probably will experience some GI upset with this drug as well. Abdominal cramps associated with primaquine may be relieved by antacids or by taking the drug after meals. The severe nausea and vomiting may have dehydrated A.K., and he should be encouraged to replenish his fluids. Table 74-1 lists the adverse effects of antimalarials.

Glucose-6-Phosphate Dehydrogenase Deficiency

7. Why is A.K. at risk for primaquine sensitivity?

Primaquine sensitivity, or G6PD deficiency, is an inherited error of metabolism transmitted by a gene of partial dominance located on the X chromosome. Patients with this enzyme deficiency are sensitive to the 8-aminoquinolines, sulfonamides, para-aminosalicylates, nitrofurantoin, sulfone, aspirin, quinine, quinidine, nalidixic acid, and methylene blue.[27,36,39] G6PD in RBC preserves glutathione in the reduced form (Fig. 88-2, Chapter 88, Drug-Induced Blood Disorders) by regenerating nicotinamide adenine dinucleotide phosphate (NADPH). Reduced glutathione protects RBC membranes from increased oxidant stress. Patients with low levels of glutathione and impaired regeneration of NADPH, as seen with G6PD deficiency, are susceptible to the oxidizing effect of drugs.[18,30,61–63] Hemolysis reportedly occurs on the third day of drug ingestion and usually is manifested as abdominal discomfort, anemia, and hemoglobinuria.[61]

The incidence of G6PD deficiency in the southeast Asian refugee population is approximately 5.2%.[63] Because A.K. is a native of Malaysia and may have G6PD deficiency, he may be at risk of hemolysis if primaquine is ingested. Therefore, he should be screened for G6PD deficiency before being treated with this drug.

Although a number of simple and satisfactory screening tests for G6PD deficiency are available, the fluorescent spot test is the simplest, most reliable, and most sensitive. The spot test is based on the addition of a reagent containing NADPH to a hemolysate of the patient's RBC. After an incubation period, the mixture is spotted on filter paper and examined under long-wave ultralight. Fluorescence of the mixture on the filter paper will indicate the presence of NADPH generated by G6PD. In patients who have G6PD deficiency, it will fluoresce only weakly, or no fluorescence will be detected. Large variants exist among those with the mutant gene, and if A.K. has a variant with relatively mild episodic clinical manifestations (variant A, with 10%–60% residual enzyme activity), he may be treated with primaquine at 45 mg/week for 8 weeks.[64]

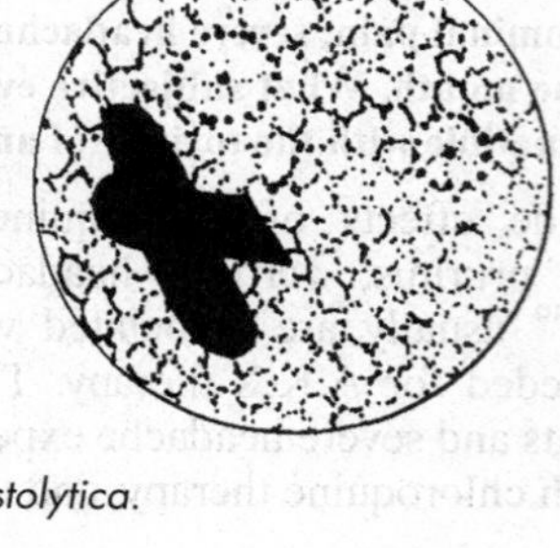

FIGURE 74-2 *E. histolytica.*

AMEBIASIS

Prevalence and Mortality

Amebiasis, caused by the small protozoan parasite *Entamoeba histolytica* (Fig. 74-2), results in amebic dysentery and hepatic abscess.[65–69] Approximately 10% of the world's population (predominately in Latin America, Africa, and Asia) is infected, and about 100,000 die annually from this infection.[64,65] In the United States, amebiasis is considered endemic in 33% of immigrants from Mexico and Central and South America and in 17% from those from Asia and Pacific Islands.[64,66] Most of these individuals are infected with *E. dispar (80%)*, an antigenically different strain from the pathogenic *E. histolytica* (10%) that does not seem to cause symptomatic invasive disease.[66,68] Amebiasis can be asymptomatic, or it can present as colitis or dysentery. Extraintestinal lesions, primarily abscesses in the liver, also can be characteristic.[65–68]

Life Cycle

The amebic parasite or trophozoite lives in the lumen of the colon and the colonic mucosa (Fig. 74-3). Trophozoites do not survive outside the host body and, if ingested, will be destroyed by gastric juice. In contrast, the encysted trophozoites can survive drying and freezing: they are killed only by temperatures in excess of 55°C or by hyperchlorination of water.[66,68] Infection occurs by ingestion of cysts present in contaminated water or food. Once ingested by the host, each cyst dissolves in the alkaline media of the small intestine and undergoes asexual division to produce eight trophozoites.[65–68] The trophozoites, which represent the invasive form of *E. histolytica*, then move to the large bowel, invade the mucosal crypts, and produce ulcerations.[65–68] Ulcerations of the bowel wall can result in amebic dysentery, inflammatory lesions in the bowel (amebomas), amebic appendicitis, and perforation of the colon or intestine[66,68,70–75] The amebae also can enter into the portal vein, which transports them to the liver, where they can initiate multiple abscesses.[66,68,75–78] Cases of genital and cutaneous amebiasis are rare but have been reported.[66,68]

Amebic Dysentery

Diagnosis

8. M.B., a 41-year-old Egyptian immigrant, presented to the ED with a 10-day history of abdominal pain and multiple, loose

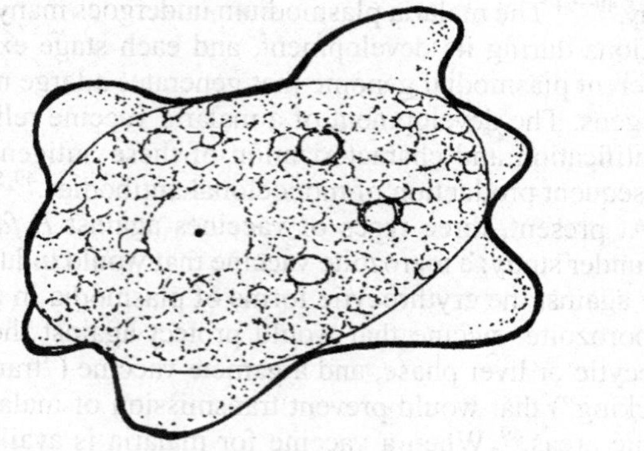

FIGURE 74-3 *E. histolytica trophozoite.*

watery stools with occasional streaks of blood. On physical examination, he is a thin man with abdominal distress. His vital signs are temperature 38°C; pulse 88 beats/minute; and BP 120/80 mmHg. He has no skin lesions, jaundice, or lymphadenopathy. The examination is remarkable for slight abdominal distention with some right lower quadrant tenderness. Rectal examination reveals some tenderness and brown liquid stool positive for occult blood. Proctosigmoidoscopy demonstrates colonic mucosa that is diffusely edematous and friable. A biopsy specimen could not be obtained because M.B. was uncooperative and combative. Initial laboratory findings are Hgb 13.4 g/dL; Hct 40%; leukocyte count, 13,800 cells/mm^3 with 68% neutrophils, 14% bands, 5% lymphocytes, and 13% monocytes; albumin 3.1 g/dL (normal, 3.5–5). A liver scan and liver function tests are normal.

On ultrasound examination, a tender mass palpable in the lower right quadrant proves to be a 3-cm collection of fluid consistent with an abdominal abscess. During an exploratory operation, the clinician drains 100 mL of a brownish-yellow material. Smears of the drained material are positive for *E. histolytica* trophozoites, and culture of the material is negative for bacteria. Fresh stool tested for *E. histolytica* by TechLab's *E. histolytica* II antigen detection test (Blacksburg, VA) is positive.

How was amebic colitis differentiated from ulcerative colitis in M.B.? What is the significance of obtaining serology in M.B.?

[SI units: Hgb, 130.4 g/L; Hct, 0.40; leukocyte count, 13.8 × 10^9/L with 0.68 neutrophils, 0.14 bands, 0.05 lymphocytes, and 0.13 monocytes; albumin, 31 g/L (normal, 35–50)]

M.B.'s abdominal symptoms, elevated temperature, right lower quadrant tenderness, and occult blood in the stool examination, together with the proctosigmoidoscopic findings, strongly suggest either a bacterial or a protozoan infection.[65–69] Stool examination confirms that M.B. has amebiasis; the presence of *E. histolytica* in the abdominal abscess and bloody stools confirm the diagnosis of amebic colitis. Serum antibody tests are useful, especially when the parasite is absent from the stool or abscess material and are considered highly sensitive (>90%).[66,69] The TechLab *E. histolytica* II antigen detection test, which detects specific antibody to the amebae in stool, is helpful in nonendemic areas for the differential diagnosis between ulcerative colitis and amebic colitis.[68,79] Although in M.B. a positive finding of *E. histolytica* in the smear from the abdominal abscess is diagnostic, TechLab's *E. histolytica* II test will document the presence of *E. histolytica.*[69] The test may not differentiate between acute and chronic disease in an area of high endemicity.[69,79] The TechLab test is specific for *E. histolytica* and does not cross-react with the nonpathogenic *E. dispar.*[68] When appropriate stool samples are not available in these cases, endoscopic or colonoscopic specimens may be critical for diagnosis, and positive serology will confirm the diagnosis of acute amebiasis.[65–69] In invasive amebiasis, serum antibodies are found in 90% of individuals by day 7 of illness.[65,68] A positive antibody test of the stool with the TechLab antigen detection test identifies most patients with invasive amebic colitis; the absence of serum antibodies to *E. histolytica* after 7 days of symptoms is evidence against a diagnosis of invasive amebiasis.[68,79] M.B.'s positive antibody test for *E. histolytica* in the stool and identification of *E. histolytica* in the abdominal abscess confirm the diagnosis of amebiasis.[69]

Drugs

9. What are the major drugs that can be used to treat M.B.? What regimen might be preferred?

The two classes of drugs that can be used to treat M.B.'s amebiasis are the luminal-acting drugs, which act only in the bowel lumen, and the tissue amebicides, which have activity in the bowel wall, liver, and other extraintestinal tissues[27,65–68] Luminal-acting drugs achieve high concentrations in the bowel, but only minimal systemic absorption takes place. These drugs include diiodohydroxyquin or iodoquinol (Yodoxin), diloxanide furoate (Furamide), and paromomycin (Humatin).

M.B. needs to be treated with a tissue amebicide in combination with a luminal agent because he has positive serology, which indicates tissue invasion by *E. histolytica.* Tissue amebicides are well absorbed and attain adequate systemic levels to treat extraintestinal amebiasis.[27,65–68] Because the concentrations of the tissue drugs in the bowel may be insufficient to eradicate *E. histolytica,* they must be combined with a luminal-acting agent to treat both serious intestinal amebiasis and extraintestinal amebic lesions.[27,65–68] The tissue amebicides include metronidazole (Flagyl), tinidazole (Tindamax), chloroquine phosphate (Aralen), emetine, and dehydroemetine. Chloroquine is effective only as a liver amebicide.[27] Dehydroemetine is very seldom used but if it is needed, it can be obtained from the CDC.[66] Diloxanide can be obtained from Panorama Compounding Pharmacy, Van Nuys, California (800-247-9767).[27]

M.B.'s acute amebic dysentery should be treated with a combination of metronidazole and a luminal agent, such as iodoquinol or diloxanide furoate. Either tinidazole or nitazoxanide (Alinia) is an alternative to metronidazole.[27] If M.B. is too ill to tolerate the oral tablets, a loading dose of 15 mg/kg of metronidazole can be administered IV over 1 hour, followed by a maintenance dose of 500 mg Q 6 hr.[79] A single oral dose of 2.4 g of metronidazole for 2 to 3 days or tinidazole 2 g once daily for 3 to 5 days is equally effective[27,65,66] (for doses of other agents, see Table 74-1).

M.B. needs to be monitored and his stool should be examined over the ensuing 3 months.

Amebic Cyst Passer

10. P.C., a 47-year-old man whose stool was found to be positive for *E. histolytica* cysts on routine examination, was completely asymptomatic. Would you treat P.C.? What are other drug regimens for amebiasis?

P.C. is an asymptomatic cyst passer and the infection may be chronic. Invasive amebiasis and extraintestinal disease are potential threats to P.C., and he is a source of infection to others.[66,68] For these reasons, he should be treated with a full course of a luminal amebicide (diloxanide or iodoquinol).[65–67] To verify the eradication of the infection, P.C.'s stool should be examined monthly for 3 months. (For other treatment regimens for amebiasis, see Table 74-1 or reference 66.)

11. If P.C. is not treated, what complications might be encountered?

Failure to treat P.C. might lead to significant me-
cal problems. Amebic liver abscess is one of th

common complications of amebiasis, with the right lobe of the liver being involved in 90% of all cases.[65–68,75–78] Patients usually present with fever, tenderness over an enlarged liver, leukocytosis, an elevated sedimentation rate, and anemia.[65–68] Liver scans (using radioactive isotopes with either technetium-99 or gallium), magnetic resonance imaging (MRI), ultrasonography, and serology (enzyme immunoassay or TechLab) usually confirm the presence of an abscess.[65,75–78] Liver abscesses can extend to the lungs through fistulas and can cause empyemas and lung abscesses.[75–79] Amebic peritonitis also can result from liver abscesses.[65–68] Other complications include amebic pericarditis, brain abscess, amebic strictures secondary to dysentery, and cutaneous amebiasis.[65–68] Management of these complications includes exploratory surgery to drain the abscesses, needle aspiration directed by radiologic monitoring, appropriate cultures of aspirate fluid, and drug therapy with metronidazole or tinidazole combined with a luminal agent such as iodoquinol.[27,65–68,79] Most patients respond within 3 days with decreased pain, anorexia, and fever.[66] Lesions may take 4 to 10 months to resolve; healing can be monitored through periodic radiologic studies.[66,75]

TREATMENT DURING PREGNANCY

12. C.R., a 24-year-old woman, presented with a 5-day history of watery stools, bloody mucus, and fever after returning from Thailand. She initially was treated with ampicillin, to which she did not respond. She is 22 weeks pregnant, and her medical history includes rheumatic fever at age 5 and heart murmurs. Her temperature is 38.2°C and her abdomen is soft but nontender; she complains of severe cramps. Fresh stool is positive for occult blood, and the wet mount demonstrates trophozoites with ingested RBC. A trichrome stain shows *E. histolytica* trophozoites. Bacterial culture is negative for pathogenic bacteria. An abdominal computed tomography (CT) scan is negative for abdominal or liver amebiasis, and an antiamebic antibody test is negative. A diagnosis of intestinal amebiasis is made. How would you treat C.R.? If C.R. subsequently develops amebic colitis, how would you treat her, and what are some toxicities of concern with the selected regimens?

C.R. needs to receive a luminal amebicide to treat her intestinal amebiasis. Because she is 22 weeks pregnant and has an underlying cardiovascular problem, the therapeutic options are limited. Metronidazole, iodoquinol, and emetine are not preferred regimens for C.R. because of their potential adverse effects to mother or fetus. A drug with minimal systemic effects would be optimal so as not to jeopardize her fetus. Paromomycin, a nonabsorbable aminoglycoside, is effective and has been used in pregnant patients.[27,66] C.R. should receive paromomycin 25 to 35 mg/kg/day in three divided doses for 7 days.[27,66] The most common side effect of paromomycin is GI upset, manifested as increased frequency of stools.[27,67] At the end of the course of therapy, C.R.'s stools should be tested to verify a cure. A serology for serum amebic antibodies also should be evaluated. If her serology is positive, a full course of metronidazole followed by a luminal agent, either iodoquinol or diloxanide furoate, must be considered.[27,66] Because C.R. would be in the third trimester of pregnancy during this period, her fetus would be less susceptible to the teratogenic effects of the drugs if she develops amebic colitis or hepatic amebiasis.

Used concomitantly with a luminal amebicide, metronidazole or tinidazole remain the drugs of choice for all patients with severe amebic colitis, hepatic abscess, and extraintestinal amebiasis.[27,66,68,79] The most common side effects include metallic taste, nausea, diarrhea, furry tongue, and glossitis.[27,36,66] Metronidazole causes disulfiramlike effects if alcohol is consumed concomitantly.[27,66] Of major concern are the reports of carcinogenicity in rodents and mutagenic activity of metronidazole in bacteria.[66] The clinical significance of carcinogenicity in the human population has not been fully assessed because a cause-and-effect relationship between use of the drug and malignancy has not been documented adequately.[27,66] Although metronidazole is considered safe in C.R., who now is in her third trimester, it should be avoided if possible during the first trimester of pregnancy.[27,66]

If amebic colitis or hepatic amebiasis develops, C.R. needs to receive either iodoquinol or diloxanide furoate to follow her metronidazole or tinidazole regimen. If iodoquinol is selected, the side effects associated with usual dosages include nausea and vomiting, abdominal discomfort, diarrhea, headache, and occasionally enlargement of the thyroid gland.[36,66,67]

If diloxanide furoate is selected instead of iodoquinol, this agent is essentially free of side effects with the exception of some minor GI symptoms such as flatulence (belching and abdominal distention) and stomach cramps.[27,66] This may be preferable to iodoquinol for C.R.

GIARDIASIS

Prevalence and Transmission

Giardiasis, manifested as nausea, abdominal cramping, and diarrhea, is caused by the protozoan *Giardia lamblia*.[80–83] The disease is endemic in many areas of the world, especially where sanitation and sanitary habits are poor.[80,81] Although the prevalence is low in most developed countries, a number of outbreaks of giardiasis have been reported in Sweden, Canada, and the United States.[84–86] *G. lamblia* is the most commonly reported pathogen in infectious diarrhea among Americans.[81] Water-borne outbreaks of giardiasis occur more often than food-borne outbreaks.[80,81,83] Giardiasis seems more prevalent in children, older debilitated individuals, and in those with dysgammaglobulinemias (specifically those with a deficiency of IgA).[80,81,83,87]

Life Cycle

Giardia lamblia exists in two forms: the trophozoite and the cyst (Fig. 74-4). The cyst is excreted in the stool and, if it is ingested in contaminated water or food, it will excyst in the stomach to produce trophozoites.[80,81,83] The trophozoites migrate to the small intestine and produce the GI symptoms characteristic of giardiasis. Symptoms appear 5 to 15 days after ingestion of the cyst.[80]

Diagnosis

Signs and Symptoms

13. J.T., a 23-year-old female student, has just returned from Mexico after spending a month there with a local church group. Two days before returning to the United States, J.T. had a bout

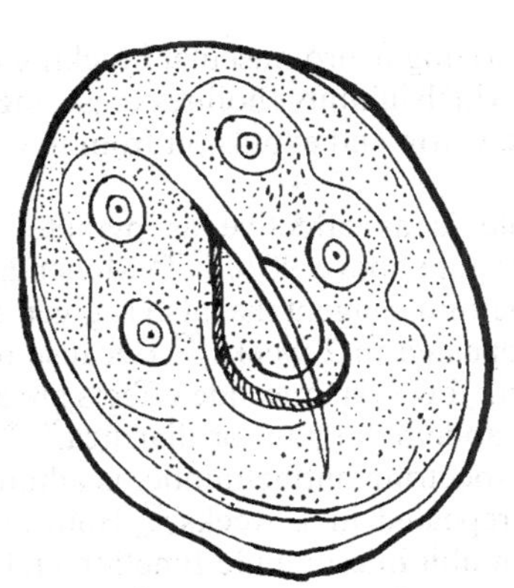

FIGURE 74-4 *G. lamblia* cyst.

of diarrhea with "offensive yellow stools." She now complains of nausea, abdominal discomfort, and occasional foul-smelling diarrhea alternating with constipation. J.T. indicates that she has lost about 10 pounds over the previous 2 weeks. Three stool samples are examined for ova and parasites, and a stool culture is ordered. Two of the three stool samples are positive for *G. lamblia* cysts, and the culture is negative for bacterial pathogens. Why is this a typical presentation of giardiasis?

The symptoms of giardiasis are variable. Some patients present with profuse watery stools, abdominal distention, and cramping for several weeks; others complain only of mild abdominal discomfort, flatulence, and occasional loose stools.[80,81,83] J.T.'s symptoms are typical and consistent with the description of giardiasis. Symptoms usually begin about 2 weeks after transmission of the infection and include anorexia, nausea, and diarrhea with bulky, foul-smelling stools.[80,81,83] The acute phase of giardiasis can be followed by a period of chronic intermittent diarrhea alternating with constipation.[80,81,83] During this period, anorexia and malabsorption will cause weight loss. Malabsorption from severe or chronic giardiasis can result in steatorrhea and deficiencies in vitamins A and B_{12}.[80,81,83,88,89] *G. lamblia* cysts usually are found in the stool, although there may be periods when cysts are difficult to detect because of a low count.[80,81,83] The onset of symptoms, foul-smelling stools, and weight loss are consistent with symptomatic giardiasis in J.T.

14. If the stool examination had been negative for *G. lamblia*, what alternative steps would have been necessary to make a diagnosis in J.T.?

Bacterial infection caused by *Salmonella, Shigella,* or *Campylobacter* was ruled out by a negative stool culture in J.T.[80,83] The next step would be to use the Entero-Test in an attempt to obtain a diagnosis of giardiasis.[81] The Entero-Test consists of a gelatinous capsule attached to a string. The patient swallows the capsule and the other end of the string is secured to the face with tape. After 4 to 6 hours, the string is pulled up and the bile-stained end is examined under a microscope. The Entero-Test sample obtained from the duodenum will demonstrate the trophozoite rather than the cyst and reportedly has a better yield than a stool examination.[80]

Several other tests to detect *Giardia* antigen in the stool have become commercially available.[80,81,83] These tests have a sensitivity of 85% to 98% and a specificity of 90% to 100%.[80,81] However, stool samples are still important to document *G. lamblia.*[82] An immunofluorescence assay using monoclonal antibody against *Giardia* cysts is available (Meridian Diagnostics, Cincinnati, Ohio). Some clinicians may prefer to use these newer tests rather than the Entero-Test. If the Entero-Test finding is negative, however, most clinicians would initiate a therapeutic trial rather than subject a patient to other invasive diagnostic procedures.[80–83] As a last resort, endoscopy with duodenal fluid sampling and biopsy may be performed.[80,81,83]

TREATMENT

15. How should J.T. be treated?

Metronidazole is the drug of choice for giardiasis in J.T.[27] Metronidazole 250 mg three times daily for 7 days is as effective as quinacrine in the treatment of giardiasis.[27,36,80–83] Although metronidazole was reported to be mutagenic in bacteria and carcinogenic at high dosages in animals, no evidence suggests that it currently represents a risk in humans.[80,81,83]

Quinacrine (Atabrine) administered 100 mg three times daily for 5 days, with cure rates of 90% to 95%, was once considered the drug of choice for giardiasis, but is no longer commercially available; it can be obtained from Panorama Compounding Pharmacy (see Question 9).[27,80,81]

Furazolidone (Furoxone), an alternative to metronidazole, is available as a tablet and suspension for the treatment of giardiasis.[27,80–83] Furazolidone has cure rates of 80% to 90%, and the adult dosage is 100 mg four times daily for 7 days.[81]

Furazolidone, which is available as a suspension, is preferred by some clinicians for children. However, metronidazole should be considered the drug of choice for giardiasis in both adults and children.

Tinidazole (Tindamax), an analog of metronidazole, is now available in the United States and is highly effective for giardiasis.[27,90] Other alternatives are paromomycin (25–35 mg/kg/day in three divided doses for 7 days), albendazole (400 mg daily for 5 days), and nitazoxanide (100–500 mg twice daily for 3–7 days).[80,82,91–93]

Following therapy, diarrhea usually subsides within 1 to 2 days and completely resolves in about 10 days.[80–83] Cyst excretion is disrupted 2 days after initiation of therapy. Complete normalization of intestinal functions, especially recovery from malabsorption, may require 4 to 8 weeks.[81] If J.T. does not respond to one course of therapy, she may need a second course of metronidazole.[80–83]

ENTEROBIASIS

Prevalence

Enterobiasis is an intestinal infection caused by the pinworm *Enterobius vermicularis* (Fig. 74-5). Pinworm, the most common helminthic infection in the United States, has an estimated annual incidence of 42 million.[94–98] Enterobiasis is a cosmopolitan disease that usually affects all members of a family when one member is infected. Therefore, all household residents must be treated simultaneously. Institutionalized patients and preschool children in daycare centers may be at greater risk for acquiring enterobiasis.[94,99]

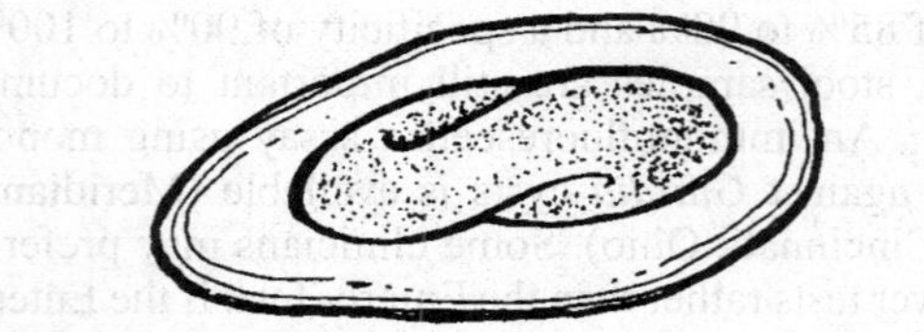

FIGURE 74-5 *E. vermicularis* ovum.

Life Cycle

Infection is initiated with the ingestion of pinworm eggs, which reach the mouth on soiled hands or contaminated food and drink. After ingestion, the eggs hatch in the intestine, releasing the larvae, which attach to the jejunum or upper ileum.[94] After copulation, the female worm migrates to the lower bowel and produces eggs. Under the stimulus of air or change in temperature, the female releases eggs in the perianal skin.[94] Cutaneous irritation in the perianal region produced by migrating females and the presence of eggs can cause severe pruritus.[94,99]

Signs and Symptoms

16. L.C., a 6-year-old boy, is brought in by his mother, K.C., to see the family physician. K.C. states that L.C. was sent home from school because of inattention and disruptive behavior. L.C. has been very irritable and complained of abdominal discomfort and perianal pain on two occasions the previous week. A cellophane tape swab placed over the perianal skin demonstrates the translucent eggs of *E. vermicularis.* Explain the symptoms observed in L.C. What pathologic changes are associated with enterobiasis?

Pinworm infection can be asymptomatic, but the most common symptom is intense pruritus ani caused by the presence of the sticky pinworm eggs in the perianal skin. Pruritus can cause constant scratching and can result in dermatitis and secondary bacterial infections.[94,98,99] A heavy load of worms can cause anorexia, restlessness, and insomnia, resulting in behavioral changes, as illustrated in L.C.[94,99]

Generally, pinworms do not cause any serious intestinal pathology.[94,99] Rarely, *E. vermicularis* ectopic lesions can be caused by a gravid worm that has migrated from the perianal region into the vagina, uterus, or fallopian tubes. The adult worm may travel through the fallopian tubes to the peritoneal cavity.[94–98] The association between cystitis in young females and enterobiasis presumably results when the female worm enters the urethra and makes its way into the bladder carrying enteric bacteria.[96,97]

Treatment

Pyrantel Pamoate, Mebendazole, and Albendazole

17. How should L.C. be treated?

Three different preparations are available to treat pinworm infection in L.C.: pyrantel pamoate (Antiminth), mebendazole (Vermox), and albendazole (Albenza).[27,94,96,99] Either pyrantel pamoate or mebendazole can be considered for this patient. L.C. should receive a single dose of 11 mg/kg (maximum, 1 g) of pyrantel pamoate followed by a second dose in 2 weeks.[27,94,96,99] Some patients experience mild GI upset, headache, and fever from this therapy.[27,97] Pyrantel pamoate acts as a depolarizing neuromuscular blocking agent releasing acetylcholine, which inhibits cholinesterase, thereby leading to paralysis of the worm and expulsion from the host's intestinal tract.[94,100]

Mebendazole is as effective as pyrantel for enterobiasis, with a cure rate above 90%.[97,99] Mebendazole, a broad-spectrum antihelmintic agent that also is given as a single dose (100 mg), is repeated in 2 weeks.[27] Because mebendazole is poorly absorbed, few systemic side effects are associated with its use, except abdominal pain or diarrhea.[94,96] Albendazole, another broad-spectrum antihelmintic, is administered as 400 mg once and repeated in 2 weeks.[27] Both albendazole and mebendazole inhibit microtubule function and deplete glycogen stores in worms, leading to their death.[94,99,100]

Household Contacts

18. What advice should be given to L.C.'s mother?

Pinworm infection can recur as a result of reinfection within families.[99] Therefore, all members of L.C.'s family need to be treated simultaneously. The pinworm's cycle of transmission can be interrupted by encouraging careful handwashing and fingernail scrubbing after using the toilet and before meals.[94,99] Despite meticulous precautions, it still may be difficult to eradicate the infection because of contact with persons outside the home. It may be necessary to repeat treatment for some members of the family at a later date.[94,99] K.C. needs to be reassured that pinworm infection in the home does not represent substandard hygiene.[99]

CESTODIASIS

Description

Cestodiasis (tapeworm infection) is caused by members of the phylum Platyhelminths (flat worms), which include, among others, *Taenia solium* (pork tapeworm), *Taenia saginata* (beef tapeworm), *Diphyllobothrium latum* (broad fish tapeworm), and *Hymenolepis nana* (dwarf tapeworm).[101–104]

The tapeworm's body is made up of an anterior attachment organ called a scolex, accompanied by a chain of segments or proglottids called a strobila. The strobila grows throughout the life of the tapeworm, with the extension taking place just posterior to the scolex.[101,102] At the end of the strobila, mature or gravid segments contain eggs enclosed in the uterus, which, because of its characteristic shape and size, may be used for identifying tapeworm species.[101,102]

Tapeworms remain attached to the mucosal wall of the upper jejunum by the scolex, which contains two to four muscular cup-shaped suckers. The parasite lacks an alimentary canal and obtains nutrients directly from the host's intestine. A protrusible structure called a rostellum is located in the center of the scolex and may contain hooks in some species.[101,102] The scolex, proglottids, and eggs, which are specific for each species, are used for definitive diagnosis.[101]

Tapeworms cause disease in humans in either the adult or larval stage.[101,102] The symptoms in the host primarily are GI when the adult form is present. Larvae or cysticerci become encysted in various visceral organs, causing a disease called cysticercosis.[103,105–107]

Life Cycle

Pork tapeworm (*T. solium*) and beef tapeworm (*T. saginata*) infections are caused by ingestion of poorly cooked meat. The larva or cysticercus is released from the contaminated meat by bile salts and matures in the host jejunum in about 2 months.[101,102] The pork tapeworm has been reported to reach a length of 10 to 20 feet, and adult beef tapeworms can measure up to 30 feet. Gravid proglottids, which contain the eggs, are passed in the host's feces and are the source of infection in animals. When ingested by animals, the embryos are released from the eggs; these migrate through the lymphatics and blood, developing into cysticerci (encysted larvae) in various muscles.[101–103]

Cysticercosis, the systemic infection caused by the larval stage of *T. solium*, is usually acquired by ingestion of the eggs in contaminated food or by autoinfection.[101] The eggs of *T. solium*, when ingested by the host, are digested by gastric juices and develop into the larvae (oncospheres), which penetrate the small bowel and migrate through the bloodstream throughout the body to produce human cysticercosis. Clinical manifestations range over a broad spectrum of symptoms and include both neurogenic and psychiatric: increased intracranial pressure, chronic severe headache, intellectual deterioration, decreased visual acuity, and focal and generalized seizures.[103,105–107]

Epidemiology

The pork tapeworm occurs worldwide and is prevalent in Mexico, Latin America, Slavic countries, Africa, southeast Asia, India, and China.[101,102] The beef tapeworm is cosmopolitan, but is found predominantly in Ethiopia, Europe, Japan, the Philippines, Latin America, and the Middle East.[101,102] Both occur in the United States, although the prevalence is low.[101,102]

Diphyllobothrium latum (broad fish tapeworm) inhabits the ileum in the human host, and infection is acquired by ingesting raw or inadequately cooked freshwater fish.[101,102] *D. latum* also infects other fish-eating animals, including the fox, mink, bear, walrus, and seal. These animals can serve as reservoirs.[101]

Broad tapeworm disease, or diphyllobothriasis, is common in Finland, Scandinavia, Russia, and the lake regions of North Italy, Switzerland, and France.[101] In North America, the highest incidence of infection has been reported in Alaska and Canada.[101]

Hymenolepis nana (dwarf tapeworm) is cosmopolitan in distribution, with a high incidence in children in the tropics and subtropics.[101,102] It is the most common human tapeworm in the United States, particularly in the southeastern section. The infection is passed primarily from person to person by contaminated hands or fomites.

Taenia Saginata and *Taenia Solium*

Signs and Symptoms

19. B.R., a 10-year-old boy from Mexico, has moved to the United States with his parents. The school nurse saw him on several occasions when he complained of vague abdominal discomfort and pain. On questioning, B.R. reports seeing "white noodle-like" objects in his stools. B.R. is seen in the clinic. A cellophane impression of the perianal region and three stool samples over several days demonstrate infection with *T. saginata* (Fig. 74-6). IgE level and eosinophil count are within normal limits. Explain the presenting symptoms in B.R.

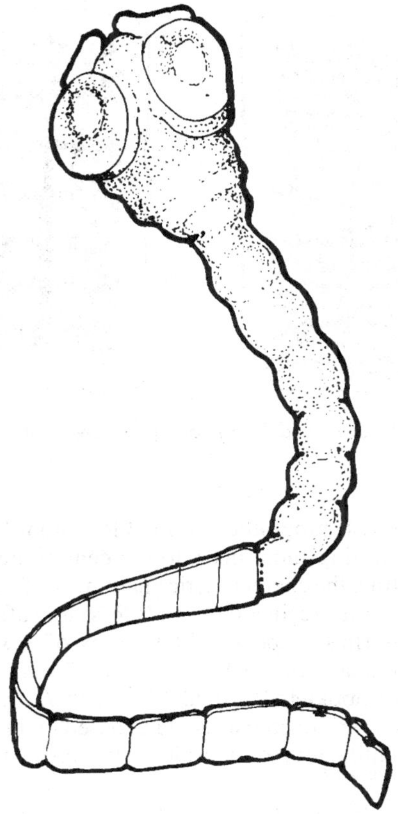

FIGURE 74-6 *T. saginata.*

Patients with tapeworm infections (either *T. saginata*, as in B.R., or *T. solium*) present with symptoms ranging from mild epigastric or abdominal pain to a burning sensation, general weakness, weight loss, headache, constipation, and diarrhea.[101,103] Complications from *T. saginata* include appendicitis, obstruction of pancreatic ducts, and intestinal obstruction.[101,102] Because the adult worm is weakly immunogenic, some patients present with moderate eosinophilia and elevated IgE levels,[101] although B.R. did not. He reported worm segments ("white noodlelike" objects) in the stool. This is commonly how diagnosis is made. Segments are sometimes found in underclothing. An alternative diagnostic method is to use anal swabs (the "Scotch tape" method) as used for pinworm ova.[101]

Diagnosis

20. How can *T. saginata* infection be differentiated from *T. solium* in B.R.?

The eggs of *T. saginata* and *T. solium* are identical and, when found in the stool, will not aid in diagnosis. The presence of gravid proglottids (Fig. 74-7) or a scolex in the stool is necessary to determine the species.[101,102]

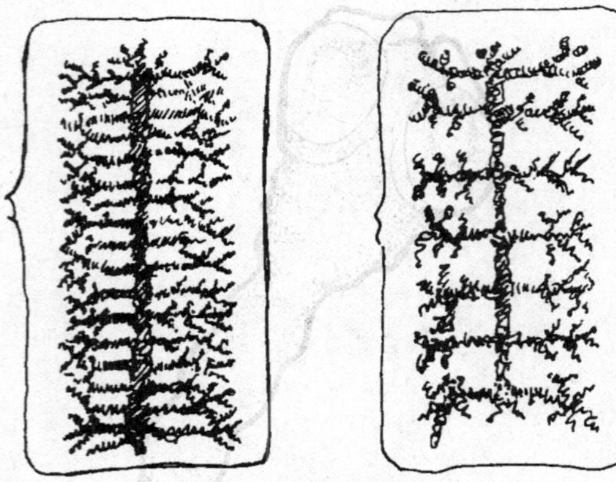

FIGURE 74-7 *T. solium* and *T. saginata* gravid segments.

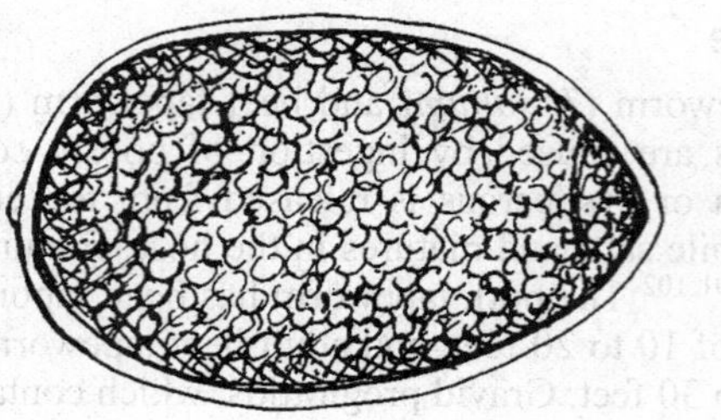

FIGURE 74-8 *D. latus* ovum.

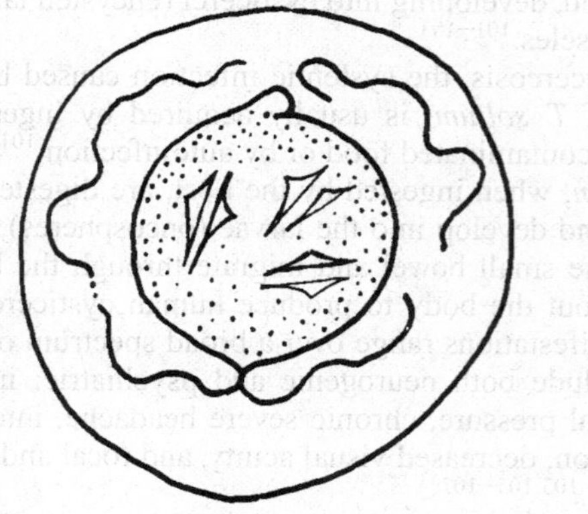

FIGURE 74-9 *H. nana* ovum.

Placing gravid proglottids from B.R.'s stool between two slides and injecting India ink into the central uterine system will demonstrate the characteristic anatomic differences.[101,103]

An intact scolex recovered from B.R.'s stool after treatment also will confirm the species. The scolex of *T. saginata* has no hooklets ("unarmed"), whereas that of *T. solium* contains a double row of hooklets ("armed").[102] With *T. solium*, the diagnosis of neurocysticercosis is made based on history, symptoms, and identification of neurologic lesions by CT scanning and MRI.[103,105–107]

The enzyme-linked immunotransfer blot (CDC-ETIB) assay of cerebrospinal fluid is considered highly sensitive and specific for neurocysticercosis.[106,107]

Treatment

21. How should B.R. be treated, and how should therapy be evaluated?

The drug of choice for both *T. saginata* and *T. solium* intestinal tapeworm infections is praziquantel (Biltricide) 5 to 10 mg/kg as a single dose.[27,101,102] Cure rates for both *T. saginata* and *T. solium* have been reported to be high.[101] The tablets of praziquantel should be swallowed whole with a liquid during meals. In patients who cannot tolerate the single dose because of severe nausea and vomiting, praziquantel can be administered in divided doses; the interval between doses should be 4 to 6 hours.[27,100] Praziquantel kills the adult worm but does not destroy the eggs. The intact or disintegrating segments appear in the stool over a week.[101] Stool specimens should be re-examined to confirm that no regrowth of *T. solium* (5 weeks after treatment) and *T. saginata* (3 months after treatment).[101]

Eggs can be released when gravid segments of *T. solium* disintegrate after treatment, and the release of embryos from the eggs can cause cysticercosis. To minimize this possibility, the clinician should give a purgative (magnesium sulfate 15–30 g) 2 hours after administration of praziquantel when *T. solium* infection is suspected.[102] B.R. should be told that segments of the tapeworm will be passed for several days after treatment.

Diphyllobothrium Latum and Hymenolepis Nana

22. Could B.R. have *D. latum* or *H. nana* infection? How are these treated?

Infection with *D. latum* is highly unlikely in B.R. because diphyllobothriasis is almost exclusively found among raw fish-eating populations of the Baltic countries, Alaska, and Canada,[101,102] and B.R. is from Mexico. In addition, neither the characteristic operculate eggs (Fig. 74-8) nor the distinctive almond-shaped scolex of *D. latum* was found during stool examination.

Hymenolepis nana (dwarf tapeworm) infection is worldwide and is a possibility in B.R. It is unusual to find proglottids of *H. nana* because they usually disintegrate before passage.[101] Instead, identification is made by the presence of the characteristic eggs (Fig. 74-9).

Treatment of *D. latum* is identical to that of *T. saginata*, except that a purgative is not necessary after therapy. *H. nana* infections are treated with praziquantel 25 mg/kg as a single dose.[27]

Cysticercosis and Other Complications

23. V.N. is a 59-year-old native of Guanajuato, Mexico who presented in the E.R at a local hospital with a 3-month history of lethargy, intermittent headaches, and episodes of ataxia. V.N's daughter reports that her father had an episode of seizure the previous evening and he fell off the couch while watching TV. V.N. has been in the United States for about 10 years but has made numerous trips to rural Mexico to see relatives. A lumbar puncture ordered on V.N. showed the following: CSF: WBC 4 cells/mm^3 (93% lymphocytes and 6% polymorphonuclear cells) (normal $<$5 cells), protein 94 mg/dL (normal $<$50 mg/dL), glucose 45 mg/dL (normal $<$60%–70% of serum). India ink capsule stain was negative with no organisms detected. MRI showed multiple intraparenchymal-enhancing lesions with perilesional edema

and some calcified lesions. Enzyme-linked immunoelectrotransfer blot (ETIB) assay was positive for neurocysticercosis.

[S.I Units: CSF glucose: 2.5 mmol/L (normal 60%–70% of serum glucose); protein: 0.92 g/L]

Neurocysticercosis, the deposition of the larval cysts (fluid-filled bladder containing the invaginated scolex) of *T. solium* in the cerebral parenchyma, meninges, spinal cord, and the ventricular system, is considered the most common parasitic disease of the central nervous system.[101,103,105–107] However, debate continues regarding the efficacy of anthelminthic therapy and the optimal dosages of these agents for neurocysticercosis.[103,107,108] If V.N. had subarachnoid or intraventricular cysticercosis, these would normally be treated with surgery. Because of the risk of neurosurgical procedures, others have suggested anthelmintic therapy.[103] Because V.N. has parenchymal disease (cerebral cysticercosis) and multiple cysts, he will receive medical treatment.[27,103,107] Hydrocephalus (blockage of the foramen of Monroe or aqueduct of Sylvius), if present, and elevated intracranial pressure are relieved by a ventriculoperitoneal shunt or temporary ventriculostomy.[101,107] V.N. will need symptomatic therapy (e.g., anticonvulsants) because he presented with seizures and the CT scan and ETIB assay confirmed neurocysticercosis.[105–107] ETIB assay, which uses purified extract of *T. solium* antigen and which detects the specific antibodies, has a sensitivity of 98% and specificity of 100%.[105] Seizures, which occur in 70% to 90% of these cases, are the most common manifestation of neurocysticercosis. For seizures, V.N. will be started on an anticonvulsant with either phenytoin (doses to attain serum levels of 10–20 mcg/mL) or carbamazepine (doses to attain serum levels of 5–12 mcg/mL) before any surgical or medical therapy. Phenobarbital is the preferred anticonvulsant in children.[101] With parenchymal neurocysticercosis, V.N. will receive corticosteroids, which will be used to ameliorate inflammatory reaction from dying parasites. He will be started on this 1 to 2 days before anthelminthic therapy and continued for 4 to 7 days after completion of therapy. However, administration of corticosteroids may not prevent adverse effects in V.N.[105] Dexamethasone 4 to 16 mg/day (or an equivalent dose of prednisone) is the suggested dose for corticosteroid.[101,105,107] Albendazole 400 mg for 8 to 30 days is the preferred agent and may be more cost effective than praziquantel. However, praziquantel 50 to 100 mg/kg/day in three divided doses for 30 days has also been recommended for parenchymal neurocysticercosis.[27,105,107–109] It has been suggested that a better understanding of the pathophysiologic mechanisms, primarily the character of inflammatory response of the host, survival and growth of the organism, and mechanism of anthelmintic activity, may help to identify more definitive therapy for neurocyticercosis in the future.[107,110] On completion of therapy with albendazole (1–3 months), a brain CT scan or MRI and an electroencephalogram should be obtained to monitor the resolution or volume reduction of cysts and seizure activity in V.N.[105,108–110] Some patients may need two or more courses of antiparasitic therapy.[107–110]

24. If V.N. had *D. latum* instead of *T. saginata*, what would be some subjective and objective findings?

If V.N. had been infected with *D. latum* instead of *T. saginata*, he may complain of being tired and possibly sleepy, which may be manifestations of anemia. *D. latum* can cause a megaloblastic anemia because the tapeworm competes with the host for dietary vitamin B_{12}.[101] Although 40% of patients with *D. latum* infection have reduced levels of vitamin B_{12}, less than 2% actually develop anemia from this deficiency.[101] Decreased levels of other nutritional elements have included ascorbic acid, folic acid, and riboflavin.[101] In those who do develop deficiency in vitamin B_{12} from *D. latum* infection, manifestations may include glossitis, tachycardia, and neurologic symptoms such as weakness, paresthesia, and motor coordination disturbances.[101,102]

Praziquantel: Side Effects

25. What are the common side effects of praziquantel?

Praziquantel, which is used for *T. saginata* infections, is associated with headache, dizziness, drowsiness, nausea, abdominal pain, myalgia, and urticaria.[27,102,111] The side effects usually appear about 2 hours after administration and dissipate within 48 hours. The tablets of praziquantel should never be chewed, but should be swallowed whole with fluids, preferably during meals. Chewing the tablets can induce retching and vomiting because of the bitter taste.[27,100]

PEDICULOSIS

Prevalence

Pediculosis (lice infections) can be caused by head lice (*Pediculus humanus capitis*) (Fig. 74-10), body lice (*P. humanus*), or crab lice (*Phthirus pubis*). Lice infections can be present in all socioeconomic groups, but are seen more often among the poor because of crowded living conditions and infrequent washing.[112–116]

Life Cycle

Head and body lice have similar life cycles, but their habitat preferences distinguish the two varieties.[113] The adult fertilized female lays eggs, which remain glued to hair or seams of clothing (Fig. 74-11). The oval-shaped eggs (nits) hatch in 7 to 10 days and produce nymphs, which go through a number of molts to evolve into mature adults.[112,113] Both larvae and adults feed on the host's blood. The lice penetrate the host skin via stylets within their head and attach themselves by a circlet

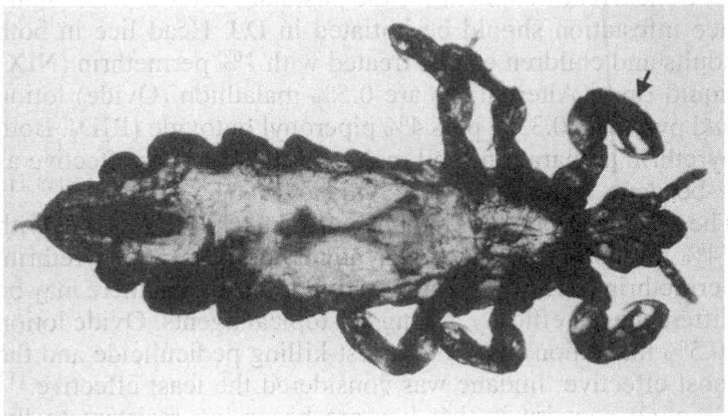

FIGURE 74-10 *Pediculus humanus capitis* (head lice).

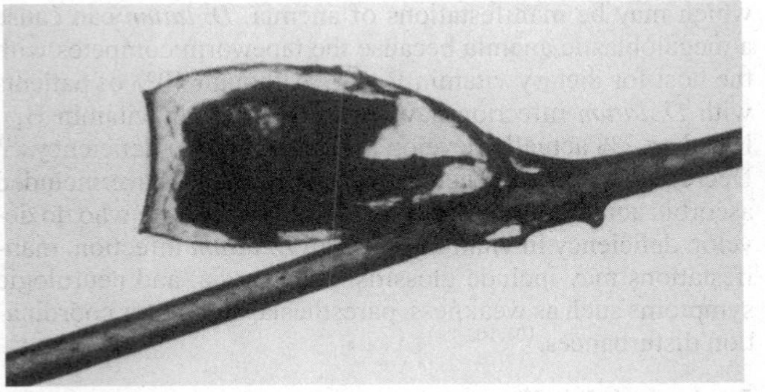

FIGURE 74-11 Nit or egg of lice on hair shaft.

of teeth on their proboscis. Crab lice usually are found in pubic hair, although these organisms can also be found on eyebrows, eyelashes, and axillary hairs.[112,113]

Epidemiology

The highest incidence of head lice is seen among schoolchildren.[113,115,116] The incidence of all types of lice infestation in the United States has been estimated to be 6 to 12 million cases.[116] Head and body lice are transferred between hosts by personal and clothing contact, whereas crab lice are transmitted by sexual contact.[112,113]

Signs and Symptoms

26. D.J., a 54-year-old homeless man who lives in a city shelter, is brought to the clinic by his welfare worker. D.J. has excoriations and numerous pustular lesions all over his body. The welfare worker states that D.J. has "lice all over his body." Why are the symptoms in D.J. consistent with lice infection?

The most common complaint of patients with head and body lice is pruritus of the scalp, ears, neck, and other body parts. With severe infestations, as seen in D.J., intractable itching and scratching can result in folliculitis, hemorrhagic macules or papules, postinflammatory skin thickening, and pigmentation.[112–116] In contrast, schoolchildren who are exposed frequently to head lice may have only minor pruritus affecting the scalp, ears, and neck.[112,116]

Treatment

27. How should D.J. be treated for lice infection of the head, body, and genital areas?

Concurrent treatment for the pustular bacterial lesions and lice infestation should be initiated in D.J. Head lice in both adults and children can be treated with 1% permethrin (NIX) liquid rinse. Alternatives are 0.5% malathion (Ovide) lotion and pyrethrin 0.33% plus 4% piperonyl butoxide (RID). Both pyrethrin preparations and malathion 0.5% are as effective as γ-benzene hexachloride or lindane 1% (Kwell).[27,112,113,116] The eradication rate for lindane is 17% to 61%, compared with 74% to 100% with the new synthetic derivative of pyrethrin, permethrin (NIX).[117] Recent studies indicate that there may be differences in efficacy among the topical agents. Ovide lotion (0.5% malathion) was the fastest-killing pediculicide and the most effective; lindane was considered the least effective.[117] Growing concern is that lice are becoming resistant to the pyrethrin products in the United States.[112,113,116,117]

PYRETHRIN, LINDANE, MALATHION, AND IVERMECTIN

Pyrethrin, which contains extracts of chrysanthemum flowers, acts by blocking the transmission of nerve impulses in lice and kills them in a few minutes.[112,118] Approximately 30 to 50 mL of the pyrethrin lotion should be massaged into D.J.'s scalp, left for about 10 minutes, then rinsed out. The treatment should be followed by a plain shampoo. Nits can be removed from the hair by applying a solution containing equal parts of water and vinegar and using a sturdy fine-tooth comb to remove the nits.[112,113] The whole course of treatment should be repeated within 7 to 10 days to eradicate the organisms hatched after initial therapy.[112,113] Patients who have a history of ragweed allergy occasionally react to pyrethrin preparations.[112] If D.J. has an allergy to pyrethrin, malathion lotion 0.5% may be an alternative. Malathion should be left on for 12 to 24 hours.

For the body and pubic lice in D.J., a pyrethrin combination lotion should be applied. It may be necessary to leave the lotion on for 4 to 6 hours to eradicate crab lice.[113] The applications should be followed by a warm bath. The treatment should be repeated in 7 to 10 days. The pruritus in D.J. can be symptomatically treated with an antihistamine and a low-potency topical steroid.[112]

Alternative treatment for head lice for patients in whom the infestations are not eradicated with either permethrin 1% or lindane are 5% permethrin cream (Elimite) applied to the scalp overnight, or petrolatum (approximately 40 g) applied to the scalp and left overnight while wearing a shower cap.[112] After the application of the petrolatum, a shampoo should be used for 7 to 10 days to remove the residue. Children 2 years or younger should not be treated for lice, and only manual removal should be attempted.[113] Other alternative therapies include two doses of ivermectin 200 mcm/kg administered a week apart or albendazole 400 mg once or for 3 days.[119–121] A recent report advocates use of hot air as a nonpharmacologic treatment for pediculosis.[122]

PETROLATUM

To remove pubic lice from D.J.'s eyelids or eyelashes, plain petrolatum ointment can be used. Petrolatum is applied to the eyelashes and lid margins with cotton swabs three or four times daily. This regimen will either suffocate the lice or physically remove them.

DECONTAMINATION MEASURES

Treatment for pediculosis should include thorough decontamination to avoid reinfection. All personal articles of clothing, including bedding, should be washed (preferably in the hot cycle of the washer at temperature >50°C).[123] Hairbrushes, combs, and other plastic articles can be decontaminated by soaking in rubbing alcohol or pediculicide.[112,113] In institutions and schools where lice infestations are a problem, outer clothing (coats, hats, scarves) of individuals should be isolated in separate plastic bags at the beginning of the day. This measure will reduce reinfection significantly.

Toxicity

28. What are the toxicities of the common pediculicides?

Lindane can cause neurologic symptoms, including tremors, ataxia, insomnia, and seizures in patients who are exposed to it over extended periods.[124,125] It also is reported to cause aplastic anemia.[125] However, when it is applied for 10 minutes to treat head or body lice, it is considered safe and effective in both adults and children. Adverse effects reported with permethrin were local irritative symptoms. Malathion, an organophosphate cholinesterase inhibitor, is degraded rapidly by hepatic enzymes in humans and occasionally can cause some local irritation.[125] These agents are not contraindicated during pregnancy and can be used for treatment.[27,125]

SCABIES

Prevalence

Scabies is caused by *Sarcoptes scabiei var. hominis*.[126–130] The female mite burrows into the skin of the host and lays eggs, which hatch into larvae after 72 to 84 hours. After a number of molts, the adult mites mate and the male dies. The female gravid mite continues to burrow into new areas of skin, primarily in web spaces between the fingers, wrists, elbows, periumbilical skin, and buttocks.[126,127] The hallmark of scabies is intense itching with erythematous papules and excoriations. In infants, scabies may be vesicular or bullous; secondary pyoderma is not uncommon. Transmission is by intimate contact, and institutional epidemics have been reported.[126–128,130]

Treatment

29. A.R., a 4-year-old girl, has a pruritic rash with excoriations in the interdigital areas of both hands. Her mother states that A.R.'s 7-year-old brother, G.R., has a similar rash affecting his hands, groin, and feet. The lesions are scraped and microscopic examination reveals mites and ova of *S. scabiei*. How should A.R. and G.R. be treated? What special instructions and precautions should accompany therapy?

LINDANE, PERMETHRIN, AND CROTAMITON

The agents available for treatment of scabies include lindane 1% (Kwell), crotamiton 10% (Eurax), and permethrin 5% cream (Elimite).[27,125–128,130] The agent that has been used most extensively is lindane, but its safety remains a point of contention.[124,125] When lindane is left on the skin too long (especially excoriated skin), percutaneous absorption can cause neurotoxicity.[124] Crotamiton 10% is presumably safe for infants and pregnant women, but definitive data do not exist. A single application of permethrin 5% cream is more effective than crotamiton or lindane.[121,126,127] Suggestion is that two doses of ivermectin (Stromectol) (200 mcg/kg separated by 1–2 weeks) can be added to the topical therapy if there is no response to permethrin alone. Although ivermectin is not FDA-label approved for scabies, a significant number of studies have used this agent both topically and systemically for scabies.[119,121,126,127] Studies indicate that two doses of ivermectin (200 mcg/kg) separated by a week can be used for scabies epidemics, and the cure rate has been around 100% with this regimen.[119,126]

A.R. and G.R. should have their nails trimmed to minimize further excoriation. They then should be bathed using a soft washcloth to remove loose crusts. Thereafter, permethrin cream should be massaged into the skin from the head (including the scalp) to the soles of the feet.[125–127] The cream should be left on for 8 to 14 hours before they shower again. Permethrin application should be repeated a week later. If crotamiton is selected, it should be applied to the entire body (including the scalp) and left on for 24 hours after the initial bath. A second 24-hour application is recommended before the children are bathed again. When lindane is used, it is applied to the entire body (avoiding the eyes and mucous membranes) and left on the body for approximately 8 hours.[127] After 6 to 8 hours, a cool bath should be taken. Pruritus from scabies can be treated symptomatically with an oral antihistamine such as hydroxyzine (Vistaril) or diphenhydramine (Benadryl), or with a low-potency topical steroid.

Clothes and linens belonging to A.R. and G.R. should be freshly laundered (hot cycle at temperatures >50°C), and they should be re-examined after a week. If evidence remains of active infestation (positive microscopic findings), a second treatment course can be initiated in these patients.[129] They should be informed that pruritus can persist for more than 10 days. Pruritus usually results from retained parts of the mites.

REFERENCES

1. Chen LH, Keystone JS. New Strategies for the prevention of malaria in travelers. *Infect Dis Clin North Am* 2005;19:185.
2. Bledsoe GH. Malaria primer for clinicians in the United States. *South Med J* 2005;98:1197.
3. Skarbinski J et al. Malarial Surveillance—United States, 2004. *MMWR* 2006;55:23.
4. Pasvol G. Management of severe malaria: interventions and controversies. *Infect Dis Clin North Am* 2005;19:211.
5. Newman RD et al. Malaria-related deaths among U.S. travelers, 1963–2001. *Ann Intern Med* 2004;141:547.
6. Local transmission of Plasmodium vivax malaria, Virginia, 2002. *MMWR* 2002;51:922.
7. Hoffman SL, et al. Malaria. In: Guerrant RL et al., eds. *Tropical Infectious Diseases: Principles, Pathogens, & Practice*. Philadelphia, PA: Churchill Livingstone; 2006:1024.
8. Seed CR, et al. The current status and potential role of laboratory testing to prevent transfusion-transmission malaria. *Transfus Med Rev* 2005;19:229.
9. White NJ, Breman JG. Malaria and babesiosis: diseases caused by red blood cell parasites. In: Kasper DL et al., eds. *Harrison's Principles of Internal Medicine*. New York, NY: McGraw-Hill; 2005:1218.
10. Magill AJ. The prevention of malaria. *Prim Care* 2002;29:815.
11. Fairhurst RM, Wellems TE. Plasmodium species (malaria). In: Mandell GL et al., eds. *Principles and Practice of Infectious Diseases*. Philadelphia, PA: Churchill Livingstone; 2005:3121.
12. Chen LH, Wilson ME, Schlagenhauf P. Prevention of malaria in long-term travelers. *JAMA* 2006;296:2234.
13. Franco-Paredes C, Santos-Preciado JI. Problem pathogens: prevention of malaria in travellers. *Lancet Infect Dis* 2006;6:139.
14. Rathore D, et al. Antimalarial drugs: current status and new developments. *Expert Opin Investig Drugs* 2005;14:871.
15. Hill DR et al. The practice of travel medicine: guidelines by the Infectious Diseases Society of America. *Clin Infect Dis* 2006;43:1499.
16. Howden BP, et al. Chronic falciparum malaria causing massive splenomegaly 9 years after leaving an endemic area. *Med J Aust* 2005;182:186.
17. Boirin MJ et al. Cognitive impairment after cerebral malaria in children: a prospective study. *Pediatrics* 2007;119:e360.
18. White NJ. Malaria. In: Cook GC, Zumla A, eds. *Manson's Tropical Diseases*. London: WB Saunders; 2003:1205.
19. Ward DI. A case of fatal Plasmodium falciparum malaria complicated by acute dengue fever in East Timor. *Am J Trop Med Hyg* 2006;75:182.
20. Jarvis JN et al. Lactic acidosis in Gabonese children with severe malaria is unrelated to dehydration. *Clin Infect Dis* 2006;42:1719.
21. Krause G, et al. Chemoprophylaxis and malaria death rates. *Emerg Infect Dis* 2006;12:447.
22. Mohanty S, et al. Adjuvant therapy in cerebral malaria. *Indian J Med Res* 2006;124:245.
23. Elam-Ong S. Malarial nephropathy. *Am J Kid Dis* 2003;23:21.
24. Fraser IP, et al. Case 32–2006: A 3-year old girl with fever after a visit to Africa. *N Engl J Med* 2006;355:1715.
25. Idra R, et al. Pathogenesis, clinical features, and

neurological outcome of cerebral malaria. *Lancet Neurol* 2005;4:827.
26. Ngoungou EB et al. Cerebral malaria and sequelar epilepsy: first-matched case-control study in Gabon. *Epilepsia* 2006;47:2147.
27. Drugs for parasitic infections. In: *Handbook of Antimicrobials Therapy*. The Med Lett (17th Ed.). New Rochelle, NY; 2005:179.
28. Shanks GD, Edstein MD. Modern malaria chemoprophylaxis. *Drugs* 2005;65:2091.
29. Nosten F, McGready R, Matabingwa T. Case management of malaria in pregnancy. *Lancet Infect Dis* 2007;7:118.
30. Desai M et al. Epidemiology and burden of malaria in pregnancy. *Lancet Infect Dis* 2007;7:93.
31. Rogerson S, et al. Malaria in pregnancy: pathogenesis and immunity. *Lancet Infect Dis* 2007;7:105.
32. Ward SA et al. Antimalarial drugs and pregnancy: safety, pharmacokinetics and pharmacovigilance. *Lancet Infect Dis* 2007;7:136.
33. Garner P, Gulmezoglu AM. Drugs for preventing malaria in pregnant women. *Cochrane Database Syst Rev* 2006;Oct18(4):CD000169.
34. Menendez C et al. Reducing the burden of malaria in pregnancy by preventive strategies. *Lancet Infect Dis* 2007;7:126.
35. Krishna S, White NJ. Pharmacokinetics of quinine, chloroquine and amodiaquine. Clinical implications. *Clin Pharmacokinet* 1996;30:263.
36. Rosenthal PJ. Antiprotozoal drugs. In: Katzung BG, ed. *Basic and Clinical Pharmacology*. New York, NY: McGraw-Hill, 2007:845.
37. Lalloo DG et al. Advisory Committee on Malaria Prevention in U.K. travellers. UK Malaria Treatment Guidelines. *J Infect* 2007; 34:111.
38. Maguire JD et al. Mefloquine is highly efficacious against chloroquine-resistant Plasmodium vivax malaria and Plasmodium falciparum malaria in Papua, Indonesia. *Clin Infect Dis* 2006;42:1067.
39. Taylor WRJ, White NJ. Antimalarial drug toxicity. *Drug Saf* 2004;27:25.
40. Toovey S, et al. Special infectious disease risks of expatriates and long-term travelers in tropical countries. Part 1: Malaria. *J Travel Med* 2007;14:42.
41. Ramharter M et al. Artesunate-clindamycin versus quinine-clindamycin in the treatment of Plasmodium falciparum malaria: a randomized controlled trial. *Clin Infect Dis* 2005;40:1777.
42. Ashley EA et al. A randomized, controlled study of a simple, once-daily regimen of dihydroartemisinin-piperaquine for the treatment of uncomplicated, multidrug-resistant Falciparum malaria. *Clin Infect Dis* 2005;41:425.
43. McGready R et al. A randomized comparison of artesunate-atovaquone-proguanil versus quinine in the treatment for uncomplicated Falciparum malaria during pregnancy. *J Infect Dis* 2005;192:846.
44. Sagara I et al. A randomized trial of artesunate-sulfamethoxazole-pyrimethamine versus artemether-lumefantrine for the treatment of uncomplicated Plasmodium falciparum malaria in Mali. *Am J Trop Med Hyg* 2006;75:630.
45. Kuhn S, et al. Emergence of atovaquone-proguanil resistance during treatment of Plasmodium falciparum malaria acquired by non-immune North American traveler to West Africa. *Am J Trop Med Hyg* 2005;72:407.
46. Jennings RM et al. Imported Plasmodium falciparum malaria: are patients, originating from disease-endemic areas less likely to developing severe disease? A prospective, observational study. *Am J Trop Med Hyg* 2006;75:1195.
47. Noedl H et al. Azithromycin combination therapy with artesunate or quinine for the treatment of uncomplicated Plasmodium falciparum malaria in adults: a randomized, phase 2 clinical trial in Thailand. *Clin Infect Dis* 2006;43:1264.
48. Greenwood B et al. Malaria in pregnancy: priorities for research. *Lancet Infect Dis* 2007;7:169.
49. Moore SA, Surgey EGE, Cadwgan AM. Malaria vaccines: where are we and where are we going? *Lancet Infect Dis* 2002;2:737.
50. Ballou WR et al. Update on the clinical development of candidate malaria vaccines. *Am J Trop Med Hyg* 2004;71(Suppl 2):239.
51. Moorthy VS, Good MF, Hill AVS. Malaria vaccine developments. *Lancet* 2004;363:150.
52. Alonso PL et al. Efficacy of RTS, S/ASO2A vaccine against Plasmodium falciparum infection and disease in young African children: randomized controlled trial. *Lancet* 2004;364:1411.
53. Malkin E, Dubovsky F, Moree M. Progress towards the development of malaria vaccines. *Trends Parasitol* 2006;22:292.
54. Makobongo MO, et al. Immunization Aotus monkeys with recombinant cysteine-rich interdomain region 1x protects against severe disease during Plasmodium falciparum reinfection. *J Infect Dis* 2006;193:731.
55. McGready R et al. Pharmacokinetics of dehydroartemisinin following oral artesunate treatment of pregnant women with acute uncomplicated falciparum malaria. *Eur J Clin Pharmacol* 2006;62:367.
56. Davis TME, et al. Artemisinin-based combination therapies for uncomplicated malaria. *Med J Aust* 2005;182:181.
57. Woodrow CJ, et al. Artemisinins. *Postgrad Med J* 2005;81:71.
58. Denis MB et al. Surveillance of the efficacy of artesunate and mefloquine combination for the treatment of uncomplicated falciparum malaria in Cambodia. *Trop Med Int Health* 2006;11:1360.
59. Borrmann S et al. Fosmidomycin plus clindamycin for treatment of pediatric patients aged 1 to 14 years with Plasmodium falciparum malaria. *Antimicrob Agents Chemother* 2006;50:2713.
60. Davis TME, et al. Piperaquine: a resurgent antimalarial drug. *Drugs* 2006;65:75.
61. Luzzatto L. Glucose 6-phosphate deficiency: from genotype to phenotype. *Haematologica* 2006;91: 1303.
62. Tracy JW, Webster Jr LT. Drugs used in the chemotherapy of protozoal infections. Malaria. In: Hardman JG et al., eds. *Goodman and Gilman's The Pharmacological Basis of Therapeutics*. New York, NY: McGraw-Hill; 2001:1069.
63. Chinevere TD et al. Prevalence of glucose-6-phosphate dehydrogenase deficiency in U.S. army personnel. *Mil Med* 2006;171:905.
64. Hill DR et al. Primaquine: report from CDC expert meeting on malaria chemoprophylaxis. 1. *Am J Trop Med Hyg* 2006;75:402.
65. Stanley Jr SL. Amoebiasis. *Lancet* 2003;361:1025.
66. Ravdin JI, Stauffer WM. Entamoeba histolytica (Amebiasis). In: Mandell GL et al., eds. *Principles and Practice of Infectious Diseases*. Philadelphia, PA: Churchill Livingstone; 2005:3097.
67. Haque R, et al. Amebiasis. *N Engl J Med* 2003;348:1565.
68. Petri Jr WA, Singh U. Enteric amebiasis. In: Guerrant RL et al., eds. *Tropical Infectious Diseases: Principles, Pathogens, & Practice*. Philadelphia. PA: Churchill Livingstone; 2006:967.
69. Tanyuksel M, Petri Jr WA. Laboratory diagnosis of amebiasis. *Clin Microbiol Rev* 2003;16:713.
70. Calderaro A et al. Colonic amoebiasis and spirochetosis: morphological ultrastructural and microbiological evaluation. *J Gastroenterol Hepatol* 2006;22:64.
71. Ozdogan M, et al. Amebic perforation of the colon: rare and frequently fatal complication. *World J Surg* 2004;28:926.
72. Hughes MA, Petri WA. Amebic liver abscess. *Infect Dis Clin North Am* 2000;14:565.
73. Lichenstein A et al. Pulmonary amebiasis presenting as superior vena cava syndrome. *Thorax* 2005;60:350.
74. Ng DCK et al. Colonic amoebic abscess mimicking carcinoma of the colon. *Hong Kong Med J* 2006;12:71.
75. Mohan S et al. Liver abscess: a clinicopathological analysis of 82 cases. *Int Surg* 2006;91:228.
76. Nushijima Y et al. Amebic liver abscess rupturing into the lesser omentum space. *J Hepatobiliary Pancreat Surg* 2006;13:252.
77. Khanna S et al. Experience with aspiration in cases of amebic liver abscess in an endemic area. *J Clin Microbiol Infect Dis* 2005;24:428.
78. Blessmann J et al. Ultrasound patterns and frequency of focal liver lesions after successful treatment of amoebic liver abscess. *Trop Med Int Health* 2006;11:504.
79. Farthing MJG, et al. Intestinal protozoa. In: Cook GC, Zumla A, eds. *Manson's Tropical Diseases*. London: WB Saunders; 2003:1373.
80. Hill DR, Nash TE. Intestinal flagellate and ciliate infections. In: Guerrant RL et al., eds. *Tropical Infectious Diseases*. Philadelphia, PA: Churchill Livingstone; 2006:984.
81. Hill DR. Giardia lamblia. In: Mandell GL et al., eds. *Principles and Practice of Infections Diseases*. Philadelphia, PA: Churchill Livingstone; 2005:3198.
82. Petri WA. Treatment of giardiasis. *Current Treatment Options in Gastroenterology* 2005;8:13.
83. Lebwohl B, et al. Giardiasis. *Gastrointestinal Endoscopy* 2003;57:906.
84. Ekdahl K, Anderson Y. Imported giardiasis: impact of international travel, immigration, and adoption. *Am J Trop Med Hyg* 2005;72:825.
85. O'Reilly GE et al. A waterborne outbreak of gastroenteritis with multiple etiologies among resort island visitors and residents: Ohio, 2004. *Clin Infect Dis* 2007;44:506.
86. Hlavsa MC, et al. Giardiasis surveillance—United States 1998–2002. *MMWR* 2005;54:9.
87. Boggild AK et al. Prospective analysis of parasitic infections in Canadian travelers and immigrants. *J Travel Med* 2006;13:138.
88. Walkowiak J, et al. Giardiasis aggravates malabsorption in cystic fibrosis. *Scand J Gastroenterol* 2004;39:607.
89. Girard C et al. Vitamin A deficiency phrynoderma associated with chronic giardiasis. *Pediatr Dermatol* 2006;23:346.
90. Fung HG, Doan T-L. Tinidazole: nitroimidazole antiprotozoal agent. *Clin Ther* 2005;27:1859.
91. Hemphill A, et al. Nitazoxanide, a broad-spectrum thiazolidine antiinfective agent for the treatment of gastrointestinal infections. *Expert Opin Pharmacother* 2006;7:953.
92. Fox LM, Saravolatz LD. Nitazoxanide: a new thiazolidine antiparasitic agent. *Clin Infect Dis* 2005;40:1173.
93. Bailey JM, Erramouspe J. Nitazoxanide treatment for giardiasis and cryptosporidiosis in children. *Ann Pharmacother* 2004;38:634.
94. McCarthy JS, Moore TA. Enterobiasis. In: Guerrant RL et al., eds. *Tropical Infectious Diseases: Principles, Pathogens & Practice*. Philadelphia, PA: Churchill Livingstone; 2006:1248.
95. Arca MJ et al. Clinical manifestations of appendiceal pinworms in children: an institutional experience and review of the literature. *Pediatr Surg Int* 2004;20:372.
96. Thomson JC. Pelvic pain caused by intraperitoneal Enterobius vermicularis (threadworm) ova with associated systemic autoimmune reaction. *J Obstet Gynaecol Res* 2004;30:90.
97. Burkhart CN, Burkhart CG. Assessment of frequency, transmission, and genitourinary complications of enterobiasis (pinworms). *Int J Dermatol* 2005;44:837.
98. Jardine M, et al. Enterobius vermicularis and colitis in children. *J Pediatr Gastroenterol Nutr* 2006;43:610.
99. Maguire JH. Intestinal nematodes (roundworms). In: Mandell GL et al., eds. *Principles and Practice of Infectious Diseases*. Philadelphia, PA: Churchill Livingstone; 2005:3260.
100. Rosenthal PJ. Clinical pharmacology of the anthelmintic drugs. In: Katzung BG, ed. *Basic and Clinical Pharmacology*. New York, NY: McGraw-Hill; 2004:867.
101. King CH. Cestodes (tapeworms). In: Mandell GL et al., eds. *Principles and Practice of Infectious Diseases*. Philadelphia. PA: Churchill Livingstone; 2005:3285.

102. John DT, Petri Jr WA. The cestodes. In: *Markell and Voge's Medical Parasitology*. St. Louis, MO: Saunders Elsevier; 2006:207.
103. Garcia HH et al. RH. Taenia solium cysticercosis. *Lancet* 2003;361:547.
104. Sorvillo FJ, DeGiorgio C, Waterman SH. Deaths from cysticercosis, United States. *Emerg Infect Dis* 2007;13:230.
105. Dua T, Aneja S. Neurocysticercosis: management issues. *Indian Pediatr* 2006;43:227.
106. Prasad S et al. Management of potential neurocysticercosis in patients with HIV infection. *Clin Infect Dis* 2006;42:e30.
107. Nash TE et al. Treatment of neurocysticercosis. Current status and future research needs. *Neurology* 2006;67:1120.
108. Garcia HH et al. New concepts in the diagnosis and management of neurocysticercosis. *Am J Trop Med Hyg* 2005;72:3.
109. Gongora-Rivera F et al. Albendazole trial at 15 or 30 mg/kg/day for subarachnoid and intraventricular cysticercosis. *Neurology* 2006;66:436.
110. Del Brutto OH et al. Meta-analysis: cysticidal drugs for neurocysticercosis: albendazole and praziquantel. *Ann Intern Med* 2006;145:43.
111. Tracy JW, Webster Jr LT. Drugs used in chemotherapy of helminthiasis. In: Hardman JG et al., eds. *Goodman and Gilman's The Pharmacological Basis of Therapeutics*. New York, NY: McGraw-Hill; 2001:1121.
112. Mathieu ME, Wilson BB. Lice (pediculosis). In: Mandell GL et al., eds. *Principles and Practice of Infectious Diseases*. Philadelphia. PA: Churchill Livingstone; 2005:3302.
113. Diaz JH. The epidemiology, diagnosis, management, and prevention of ectoparasitic diseases in travelers. *J Travel Med* 2006;13:100.
114. Mumcuoglu KY et al. Head louse infestation: the "no nit" policy and its consequences. *Int J Dermatol* 2006;45:891.
115. Heukelbach J et al. Epidemiology and morbidity of scabies and pediculosis capitis in resource-poor communities in Brazil. *Br J Dermatol* 2005;153:150.
116. Mumcuoglu KY. Effective treatment of head louse with pediculicides. *J Drugs Dermatol* 2006;5:451.
117. Meinking TL et al. Comparative in vitro pediculicidal efficacy of treatment in a resistant head lice population in the United States. *Arch Dermatol* 2002;138:220.
118. Tomalik-Scharte D et al. Dermal absorption of permethrin following topical administration. *Eur J Clin Pharmacol* 2005;61:399.
119. Fox LM. Ivermectin: uses and impact 20 years on. *Curr Opin Infect Dis* 2006;19:588.
120. Akisu C, et al. Albendazole: single or combination therapy with permethrin against Pediculosis capitis. *Pediatr Dermatol* 2006;23:179.
121. Dourmishev AL, Dourmishev LA, Schwartz RA. Ivermectin: pharmacology and application in dermatology. *Int J Dermatol* 2005;44:981.
122. Goates BM et al. An effective nonchemical treatment for head lice: a lot of hot air. *Pediatrics* 2006;118:1962.
123. Izri A, Chosidow O. Efficacy of machine laundering to eradicate head lice: recommendations to decontaminate washable clothes, linens and fomites. *Clin Infect Dis* 2006;42:e9.
124. Bhalla M, Thami GP. Reversible neurotoxicity after an overdose of topical lindane in an infant. *Pediatr Dermatol* 2004;21:597.
125. Scabicides/Pediculicides. In: *Facts and Comparisons*. St. Louis, MO: Wolters Kluwer; 2007:1699.
126. Chosidow O. Scabies. *N Engl J Med* 2006;354:1718.
127. Mathieu ME, Wilson BB. Scabies. In: Mandell GL et al., eds. *Principles and Practice of Infectious Diseases*. Philadelphia, PA: Churchill Livingstone; 2005:3304.
128. Hengge UR et al. Scabies: a ubiquitous neglected skin disease. *Lancet Infect Dis* 2006;330:1194.
129. Dupuy A et al. Accuracy of standard dermoscopy for diagnosing scabies. *J Am Acad Dermatol* 2007;56:53.
130. Sladden MJ, Johnson GA. More common skin infections in children. *Lancet* 2005;330:1194.

CHAPTER 75

Tick-Borne Diseases

Tom E. Christian

OVERVIEW

Ticks belong to the class Arachnida, which includes scorpions, spiders, and mites. As a vector of human illness worldwide, ticks are second in importance only to mosquitoes. Ticks transmit more infectious agents than any other arthropod. Disease can be spread by ticks, either by transmission of microorganisms or by injection of tick toxin into a host. Bacterial, rickettsial, protozoal, and viral disease pathogens can be transmitted from ticks to humans[1] (Table 75-1).

Tick Genus

Only two of the three families of ticks are of medical significance to humans: the soft-bodied ticks, *Argasidae,* and the hard-bodied ticks, *Ixodidae.*[1] Four of the 13 genera of *Ixodidae* transmit disease in the United States: *Dermacentor, Ixodes, Amblyomma,* and *Rhipicephalus.* Among the five genera of *Argasidae,* only *Ornithodoros* are known to transmit pathogens to humans in the United States. Most hard ticks have a 2-year life cycle, comprising the larval, nymphal, and adult stages. They require one blood meal during each stage before they can mature into the next stage and they usually remain attached to a host for hours or days. In contrast, soft ticks may have multiple nymphal stages, and both nymphal and adult forms can feast on blood multiple times, usually for only 30 minutes. However, *Argasidae* can survive many years without blood sustenance and are long-lived.[1] Humans are the inadvertent hosts for the life cycle of almost all ticks and tick-borne diseases.

LYME DISEASE

Lyme disease, or more accurately Lyme borreliosis, is a multisystem spirochetal disease transmitted by a tick bite.[1–8] Although the responsible spirochete, *Borrelia burgdorferi,* was not identified until 1982,[1] late manifestations of a dermatitis produced by a *Borrelia* species were described in Europe more than a century ago.

Table 75-1 Tick-Borne Diseases

Disease	*Causative Agent*	*Tick Vector*	*Host*	*Region*
Lyme	*Borrelia burgdorferi*	*Ixodes*	Wild rodents	Worldwide
Relapsing fever (endemic)	*Borrelia* species	*Ornithodoros*	Wild rodents	Worldwide
Southern tick-associated rash illness	*Borrelia lonestari?*	*Amblyomma*	?	South-central United States
Tularemia	*Francisella tularensis*	*Dermacentor* *Amblyomma*	Rabbits, ticks	North America
Rocky Mountain spotted fever	*Rickettsia rickettsii*	*Dermacentor* *Rhipicephalus*	Wild rodents, ticks	Western Hemisphere Arizona
Spotted fever group	*Rickettsia parkeri* various rickettsia	*Amblyomma* various species	Horses? ?	United States Worldwide
Boutonneuse fever	*Rickettsia conorii*	*Ixodes*	Wild rodents, dogs	Africa, India, Mediterranean
North Asian tick typhus	*Rickettsia sibirica*	*Ixodes*	Wild rodents	Mongolia, Siberia
Queensland tick typhus	*Rickettsia australis*	*Ixodes*	Wild rodents, marsupials	Australia
Q fever	*Coxiella burnetii*	*Dermacentor* *Amblyomma*	Sheep, goats, cattle, ticks, cats	Worldwide
Babesiosis	*Babesia* species	*Ixodes*	Mice, voles	Europe, North America
Human monocytotropic ehrlichiosis	*Ehrlichia chaffeensis*	*Amblyomma* *Dermacentor*	Deer, dogs Deer	United States, Mexico, Europe, Africa, Middle East
Human granulocytic anaplasmosis	*Anaplasma phagocytophilia*	*Ixodes pacificus* *Ixodes*	Deer, elk, wild rodents	United States, Europe
Human ehrlichial ewingii	*Ehrlichia ewingii*	Amblyomma	Dogs?	United States
Colorado tick fever	*Coltivirus* species	*Dermacentor*	Wild rodents, mammals	North America
Tick-borne encephalitis	*Flavivirus*	*Ixodes*	Rodents	Eurasia
Tick paralysis	Neurotoxin	*Dermacentor*	N/A	North America, Europe, Australia, South Africa

N/A, not applicable.

Spirochete Identification and Pathology

Three genomic subgroups of *B. burgdorferi* worldwide probably account for the clinical variations observed in the disease. The North American strains identified to date belong to the *B. burgdorferi sensu stricto* group. Although all three groups have been found in Europe, most isolates are *Borrelia garinii* or *Borrelia afzelii*. An example of a disease variation is the condition of acrodermatitis chronica atrophicans (Table 75-2), a skin lesion associated predominantly with *B. afzelii* infection.[9]

Lyme disease is a multisystem condition, affecting the skin, joints, and cardiovascular, central, and peripheral nervous systems. The ailment is named for the villages of Lyme and Old Lyme, Connecticut, where arthritic complications of this disease were first recognized. Lyme disease accounts for 96% of cases of vector-borne illness in the United States, with >15,000 cases reported annually.[3,5] Worldwide, it is probably the most commonly reported tick-borne disease.[10]

Tick Vector

Spirochetal Behavior

The tick acquires the *B. burgdorferi* spirochete from feeding on an infected host. The spirochete remains dormant in the tick's midgut until the tick feeds again, at which time the spirochete acquires a mammalian plasminogen, allowing it to penetrate the midgut wall and invade the salivary glands of the tick. In the interim, *B. burgdorferi* activates a tick gene, boosting production of a tick salivary protein, Salp-15, to which it binds. This coating helps camouflage the bacterium from mammalian immune cell detection and destruction.[11] The spirochete then passes through the salivary ducts of the tick and is injected through the skin of the new host with the tick bite. Few spirochetes are transmitted from the tick to its host during the first 24 to 36 hours of attachment. An infected nymphal tick, however, invariably transfers spirochetes when attached to its host for >72 hours.

Tick Identification

Larval and nymphal ticks are small, <3 mm, the size of a freckle or poppy seed. Therefore, the tick often goes unnoticed, and fewer than half of patients with Lyme disease recall having been bitten by a tick. The tick feeds on small, medium, or large mammals; lizards; or birds during its larval and nymphal (immature) stages. Larval ticks are not relevant vectors for Lyme disease, however, because they are rarely infected and become so only after feeding on an infected host.[9] Adult ticks parasitize only medium or large mammals.[1] Humans are inadvertent hosts of any stage of the tick.[1] Although the tick can

Table 75-2 Lyme Disease Clinical Manifestations

Early Localized Infection:
Erythema migrans skin rash
Early Disseminated Disease:
Heart (<4% of untreated patients in United States)
Myocarditis or pericarditis
Conduction defects, varying degrees of atrioventricular or bundle branch block, but permanent pacing not indicated
Nervous System (Neuroborreliosis)
Cranial nerve (Bell's) palsy
Meningitis, lymphocytic
Radiculoneuritis, myelitis
Sensory or motor peripheral neuropathy
Skin
Multiple secondary erythema migrans lesions; lymphocytoma (lymphadenosis benigna cutis) rare in the United States, but 1% in Europe
Late Disease:
Musculoskeletal (less common in Europe)
Persistent (<10% of untreated in United States) or intermittent arthritis of >1 large joint, especially the knee
Skin (10% in Europe; rare in the United States)
Acrodermatitis chronica atrophicans (unique to Lyme disease)
Late Neurologic
Peripheral neuropathy, subacute encephalopathy (memory impairment, sleep disturbance, dementia) and in Europe, progressive encephalomyelitis

feed on many different animals, each tick species has preferred hosts. For example, the immature *Ixodes scapularis* prefers to be hosted by the white-footed mouse, whereas the mature tick prefers white-tailed deer. In the northeastern and midwestern United States, *I. scapularis* (formerly *dammini)* is the primary vector, whereas *I. pacificus* is the primary vector in the western United States. In Europe, *I. ricinus* is the vector, and *I. persulcatus* is the primary vector in Asia. The discovery of organisms such as *B. burgdorferi* from *I. ovatus* in Japan and *Haemaphysalis longicornis* in China, both of which parasitize domestic animals and humans, demonstrates a greater diversity of endemic vectors and cycles in Asia. Therefore, the geographic distribution of Lyme disease matches the geographic range of the specific *Ixodes* species that harbor Lyme *Borrelia.*

Host Identification

The host's ability to harbor and transmit the spirochete to the tick (i.e., reservoir competency) is an important consideration in understanding the epidemiology and prevalence of Lyme disease. The reservoir-competent white-footed mouse and the reservoir-incompetent (i.e., incapable of harboring and transmitting the spirochete) white-tailed deer are the preferred hosts for the immature and adult forms of *I. scapularis* in the northeastern United States, respectively.[1] Subadult *I. pacificus* organisms preferentially feed on the western fence lizard, which is reservoir incompetent. In fact its blood is borreliacidal.[9,12,13] Deer are not important hosts for mature *I. pacificus* organisms. Similarly, in the southern United States, immature *I. scapularis* ticks feed primarily on lizards. The cotton mouse and cotton rat, however, appear to be the predominant reservoir hosts for the spirochete in the southern United States, which the tick may feed upon. In Europe, various reservoir-competent mice and vole species are reported hosts for *I. ricinus.*[1]

How is Lyme borreliosis transmitted to humans in the western United States if the preferred hosts are not reservoir competent? It is suggested that the dusky-footed wood rat and kangaroo rat, which can support *B. burgdorferi,* are the hosts of the spirochete for the few immature *I. pacificus* which incidentally feed on the rats. Thus, an estimated 0% to 14% of *I. pacificus* organisms are infected with spirochetes, contrasting with infection rates for *I. scapularis* in the northeastern United States of 20% to 40%.[9] In Europe, *I. ricinus* infection rates vary from 4% to 40%. In addition, bird parasitism by ticks enables the ticks to be carried long distances, even intercontinentally, during spring and fall migrations. Birds can bring ticks into new areas and also serve as maintenance hosts.[1]

Thus, the complex interplay of spirochete, host, and vector in a particular area influences the risk of Lyme disease after a tick bite. Lyme disease is not transmitted directly between people.[6]

Classification and Laboratory Testing of Lyme Disease

The clinical features of Lyme disease were historically divided into three stages: early localized (stage 1), early disseminated (stage 2), and chronic, persistent, or late disease (stage 3). Many believe that "chronic" Lyme disease is an unproved entity,[9,14] although some disagree.[15,16] Currently, Lyme disease is classified as either "early" or "late" disease with the possible existence of post-Lyme disease syndromes.[9] Although Lyme disease may be debilitating, it is not life threatening.

The most specific marker of Lyme disease is a characteristic skin rash termed *erythema migrans.* This solitary skin lesion occurs in 80% to 90% of patients with the disease.[4,5] No other physical finding of Lyme disease is diagnostic. No laboratory gold standard for diagnosis currently exists. Laboratory diagnosis of Lyme disease is problematic because sufficiently sensitive and specific tests are lacking; deficiencies in laboratory standardization confound the issue. Positive results of blood tests for an antibody response to the spirochete only support a diagnosis of Lyme disease as seropositivity alone does not prove that a given medical condition is caused by Lyme disease.[9] The IgM antibody response develops 4 weeks after infection, peaks at 6 to 8 weeks, and declines to the normal range after 4 to 6 months. In some patients, IgM levels may remain high or reappear. The IgG antibody response begins 6 to 8 weeks after disease onset, peaks at 4 to 6 months, and may remain elevated indefinitely.[17] Overuse of serologic testing and over reliance on the results have resulted in excessive and inaccurate diagnoses of Lyme disease.

Treatment

The clinical manifestations of Lyme disease should govern the treatment strategy used (Table 75-3).[9] To effect a cure, it is not

Table 75-3 Treatment Recommendations for Lyme Disease

Erythema Migrans
Adults: Doxycycline (Vibramycin) 100 mg PO BID × 10 days
Or
Amoxicillin (Polymox) 500 mg PO TID × 14–21 days
Or
Cefuroxime axetil (Ceftin) 500 mg PO BID × 14–21 days
Children (<8 yrs): Amoxicillin 50 mg/kg/day PO in 3 divided doses (maximum, 500 mg/dose) × 14–21 days or cefuroxime 30 mg/kg/day PO in 2 divided doses (maximum, 500 mg/dose) × 14–21 days
Children (>8 yrs): May use doxycycline 1–2 mg/kg PO in 2 divided doses (maximum, 100 mg/dose) × 14–21 days
Cardiac Disease: third-degree heart block
Adults: Ceftriaxone (Rocephin) 2 g IV Daily × 14–21 days
Or
Cefotaxime (Claforan) 2 g IV Q 8 hr × 14–21 days
Or
Penicillin G (Pfizerpen) 3–4 MU IV Q 4 hr × 14–21 days
Or
For first- or second-degree heart block: doxycycline or amoxicillin in doses as noted above × 14–21 days

BID, twice daily; IV, intravenous; MU, million units; PO, by mouth; TID, three times daily.

necessary to continue antibiotic treatment until all symptoms have resolved.[5,9]

1. J.S., age 38 years, visits his local physician with symptoms of low-grade fever and muscle aches 3 days after deer hunting in the state of Washington. After hunting for approximately 6 hours, he noticed a small tick on his thigh and immediately destroyed it. A small, itchy spot that he felt at the site of the tick bite is no longer symptomatic. The temporal relationship of the tick bite with his symptoms of fever and myalgias prompts his physician to collect blood samples for Lyme disease antibody testing. Antibiotic therapy also is initiated. Why is the blood test not likely to be of value? Why is empiric antibiotic therapy not appropriate for J.S.?

In general, the use of serologic testing or antimicrobial prophylaxis after a recognized tick bite is not recommended.[9] The antibody response to *B. burgdorferi* is not detectable for the first 4 weeks after a tick bite.[5] Therefore, the blood tests for antibodies to *B. burgdorferi* are unlikely to be positive, as J.S.'s tick bite occurred only 3 days ago.

The risk of developing Lyme disease can be affected by the rate of transmission of the spirochete from infected ticks to humans; the length of time before the tick is removed during its bite; the degree of blood engorgement of the tick ("scutal index"); the prevalence of spirochete infestation of ticks in an area, which varies with the tick species; and the reservoir competency of host animals in the region.[9]

Although transmission rates of Lyme disease from an infected tick bite are estimated at approximately 10%, the risk is reduced dramatically if the tick is removed within 24 hours of attachment, as in J.S.'s case. The small, itchy spot experienced by J.S. probably represented a hypersensitivity reaction to the bite. These erythematous, noninfectious skin lesions develop within 48 hours of tick detachment or may occur while the tick is still attached. They are usually <5 cm in diameter; they may have an urticarial appearance and usually disappear in 1 or 2 days.[9]

Prophylactic antibiotic preventative therapy with a single dose of 200 mg oral doxycycline, or for children 8 years or older at 4 mg/kg to a maximum 200-mg dose, can be offered if the following criteria are met: (a) there are no contraindications to doxycycline use; (b) administration can start within 72 hours of tick removal; (c) the tick can be reliably identified as a nymphal or adult *I. scapularis* tick with certainty of the duration of attachment of 36 hours or more based on the degree of engorgement or time of exposure; and (d) the local rate of infection of ticks by *B. burgdorferi* in the area of exposure is 20% or greater based on current ecological evidence.[9] Routine testing of ticks themselves for tick-borne infections is not recommended.[9]

Antibiotic prophylaxis after *I. pacificus* tick bites is generally not necessary.[9] The low infection rate of *B. burgdorferi* in *I. pacificus* ticks may be owing to the observation that the western fence lizard's blood can destroy spirochetes in the tick's tissues during feeding.[12] In summary, J.S. would not require prophylactic doxycycline treatment or serologic testing for his tick bite because of the short duration of tick attachment and low prevalence of *B. burgdorferi* infestation of *I. pacificus* ticks.

ERYTHEMA MIGRANS

Signs, Symptoms, and Disease Course

2. K.T., a 34-year-old woman, presents with right knee pain and multiple, large, discrete skin rashes that she has had for the past 10 days. Three months ago, in July, she visited friends in Massachusetts and spent much of her time engaged in outdoor activities (e.g., hiking, biking, swimming). Two months ago, her husband noticed a circular area of intense redness, approximately 9 cm wide, in her left armpit. The rash grew considerably larger over the next 2 weeks and had a red outer border. K.T. attributed the expansion of the rash to having scratched the mildly itchy area. The rash gradually disappeared. In late August, K.T. experienced fatigue, nausea, and headache for a week and thought it was "summer flu." In early September, she experienced right knee pain; ibuprofen produced some relief. On examination, she was afebrile and had mild soft tissue swelling of the right knee. Her white blood cell (WBC) count was normal. Serum samples contained antibody titers to *B. burgdorferi* of 1:60 and 1:400 for IgM and IgG, respectively. A Venereal Disease Research Laboratory (VDRL) test for syphilis and a pregnancy test were negative.

K.T. is started on a 4-week course of oral doxycycline 100 mg twice daily. What characteristics of K.T.'s skin rash are consistent with the erythema migrans of Lyme disease?

The erythema migrans of Lyme disease usually develops within 30 days (median, 7 days) of a usually asymptomatic tick bite at the site of inoculation of the spirochete.[4,10] The rash begins as an erythematous (red) macule or papule typically in the groin, gluteal fold, axilla, torso, popliteal fossa, or thigh.[18] In children, erythema migrans is often found on the head at the hairline, neck, arms, or legs.[18] It expands outwardly at 2 to 3 cm/day to a diameter of 5 to 70 cm (mean, 16 cm), occasionally with some central clearing.[18] The classic annular or ringlike patch may have complex concentric inner erythematous circles, resembling a bull's eye or target, especially in European cases.[18] Some cases of erythema migrans in the United States lack central clearing.[9] The rash may be warm to the touch and is usually painless, but some patients have mild burning or itching.[4] Up to 50% of patients with erythema migrans have multiple secondary lesions that most likely represent blood-borne spread of the spirochete to other skin sites rather than multiple tick bites.[10] If untreated, erythema migrans generally fades within several weeks; if treated, it usually resolves in several days.

Low-grade fever and other nonspecific symptoms, such as fatigue, malaise, lethargy, headache, stiff neck, myalgia, arthralgia, and regional or generalized lymphadenopathy, may accompany erythema migrans. In the United States, 70% to 80% of patients with Lyme disease display erythema migrans.[4,5,19] Some may not have the other early symptoms of the disease. Some clinicians prefer abandoning the term "flu-like illness" in favor of "viral-like syndrome" to describe the nonspecific symptoms of early Lyme disease because cough, rhinitis, sinusitis, and gastrointestinal (GI) symptoms do not usually occur.[16]

Pitfalls in the diagnosis of erythema migrans exist. Lesions commonly misdiagnosed as erythema migrans include streptococcal cellulitis, urticaria, dermal hypersensitivity reaction, *Rhus* contact dermatitis, granuloma annulare, arthropod hypersensitivity reactions, tinea corporis, and serum sickness rashes.[18] K.T.'s skin rash was large (>9 cm), red, and had a red outer border. It gradually faded over a few weeks. These characteristics are consistent with a diagnosis of erythema migrans.

Serologic Testing

3. What might have been the rationale for the laboratory tests that were undertaken in K.T., and what would be reasonable interpretations of laboratory tests in patients with Lyme disease?

An antibody titer measured by enzyme-linked immunosorbent assay (ELISA) is considered positive for IgM when it is >1:100 and positive for IgG when it is >1:130. K.T.'s results (IgM of 1:60 and IgG of 1:400) support a diagnosis of Lyme disease because the IgM can naturally fall by this time, yet IgG levels may remain elevated indefinitely. Syphilis and other known biologic causes (periodontal spirochetes) of false–positive serologic testing should be excluded. Rheumatoid factor or antinuclear antibody tests usually are negative in Lyme disease. These tests help differentiate rheumatoid arthritis or systemic lupus erythematosus from Lyme disease. The WBC count is normal or mildly elevated in Lyme disease. K.T. had a normal WBC. Pregnancy was ruled out before initiating a tetracycline. Most interesting in K.T. is the presence of secondary erythema migrans lesions, which develop in up to 50% of untreated patients in the United States and represent disseminated infection.

The presence of erythema migrans as an early indicator of Lyme disease gives physicians the best opportunity for early diagnosis and treatment. In the United States, the expression of erythema migrans is the *only* manifestation of Lyme disease that is sufficiently distinctive to allow clinical diagnosis in the absence of confirmatory laboratory information.[9] Early treatment can prevent the sequelae of disseminated disease.

LYME DISEASE TREATMENT

Antibiotics

4. Why was doxycycline (Vibramycin) chosen to treat K.T.?

Borrelia burgdorferi is susceptible to amoxicillin, tetracyclines, and some second- and third-generation cephalosporins, based on in vitro data. It is only moderately sensitive to penicillin G (Pfizerpen) and is resistant to first-generation cephalosporins, rifampin (Rimactane), cotrimoxazole (Bactrim), aminoglycosides, chloramphenicol (Chloromycetin), and the fluoroquinolones.[9,19]

Penicillin, tetracycline, and erythromycin historically were the drugs of choice for the treatment of Lyme disease because they are given orally; they are relatively inexpensive and appeared to have good in vitro activity. Disappointing *in vivo* results, however, were found with all these agents except penicillin. Perhaps tetracycline and erythromycin were under dosed, given in too short a duration, or intrinsically have larger time-to-kill ratios than penicillin. In Europe, in particular, penicillin still is used with continued success. Amoxicillin (Polymox) has better absorption and a longer serum half-life than penicillin V (Veetids) and continues to be effective in treating Lyme disease. Amoxicillin is preferred for Lyme disease treatment in pregnant or breastfeeding women and in children <8 years of age.[19]

Compared with the third-generation cephalosporins, the second-generation drug cefuroxime axetil (Ceftin) is available in an oral dosage form and has good in vitro activity as well as in vivo performance. It is more expensive than oral amoxicillin or tetracyclines. Of the third-generation cephalosporins, ceftriaxone (Rocephin) has the strongest in vitro activity. The long half-life of ceftriaxone allows the convenience of once-daily dosing in an outpatient program. Ceftriaxone is expensive, however, and has a higher incidence of diarrhea than other β-lactams, probably because of partial biliary excretion. Risk factors for the development of ceftriaxone-induced biliary disease include age <18 years, daily ceftriaxone dose >40 mg/kg, female gender, and administration of prior courses of the drug. Cefotaxime (Claforan) is an alternative to ceftriaxone that is not associated with biliary complications and comparable in cost, but it must be dosed more frequently.

The macrolides clarithromycin (Biaxin) and azithromycin (Zithromax) may or may not have activity against Lyme spirochetes.[9] As with erythromycin, they have been less effective for the treatment of Lyme disease in controlled clinical trials.[19] The combination of a macrolide with lysosomotropic agents, especially hydroxychloroquine, anecdotally has been suggested to be associated with increased symptom relief probably because of the combined anti-inflammatory activity rather than direct antimicrobial activity.[9] Azithromycin is not considered to be a first-line agent in the treatment of Lyme disease.[9]

Doxycycline is well absorbed orally and is less expensive than third-generation cephalosporins that must be administered parenterally. Doxycycline has a long serum half-life of 18 to 22 hours. In addition, doxycycline penetrates into the cerebrospinal fluid (CSF) at concentrations of at least 10% of serum levels even in the absence of meningeal inflammation. Doxycycline can complex with divalent or trivalent cations in the gut, and absorption may be decreased as a result. On the other hand, administering doxycycline with food, to minimize nausea, is recommended.[9] Compared with other tetracyclines, doxycycline has the least affinity for divalent calcium cations, and oral absorption is reduced by only 20% if given with milk. The major side effect of doxycycline is phototoxicity, which is of concern because Lyme disease usually occurs during sunny times of the year. A less recognized side effect is the risk of doxycycline-induced esophageal ulceration. Patients should be instructed not to take doxycycline or other tetracyclines for 1 to 2 hours before going to bed or lying down and to take the medication while standing up with at least 240 mL of clear fluid, especially with the capsule formulation. Despite less in vitro activity compared with some β-lactam antibiotics, *B. burgdorferi* is sufficiently susceptible to doxycycline, and clinical experience with doxycycline has been very favorable.[20]

In conclusion, doxycycline was a suitable choice for K.T., and the 4-week duration of therapy matches the recommendation for adult arthritis treatment outlined in Table 75-3.

Antibiotic-Refractory Lyme Arthritis

5. K.T. continues to have knee inflammation for 4 months after receiving a second course of antibiotic treatment (ceftriaxone 2 gm daily for 2 weeks) and is now considered to have antibiotic-refractory Lyme arthritis. Why should antibiotic therapy be repeated (or not repeated) for K.T.'s arthritis?

Antibiotic-refractory Lyme arthritis, which in the United States develops in approximately 10% of patients with Lyme arthritis, has been associated with an increased frequency of the class II major histocompatibility complex allele, HLA-DRB1*0401 human leukocyte antigen, and an immune response to outer surface protein A (OspA).[21,22] Patients with these markers may be predestined for the development of chronic arthritis despite antibiotic therapy.[21,22] The HLA-DRB1*0401 allele is associated with lack of response to antibiotic therapy and autoimmunity.[21,22] Destructive changes in the involved joint may occur, with the synovium showing vascular proliferation, villous hypertrophy, and a lymphoplasma cellular infiltrate similar to other inflammatory arthritides. In these patients, persistent arthritis is not the result of the persistence of active infection by the spirochete in a protected site. Such patients often respond well to synovectomy, again suggesting that the presence of synovitis may not be the result of persistence of the infection.

If K.T. is HLA-DRB1*0401 positive and has antibody reactivity to the outer surface protein OspA of *B. burgdorferi,* and a negative polymerase chain reaction (PCR) of synovial fluid for *B. burgdorferi* nucleic acids, she will likely be resistant to further antibiotic treatment. Repeat antibiotics are ineffective in this case. Remittive agents, such as hydroxychloroquine or intra-articular corticosteroid injections, may be helpful. Synovectomy may be offered.[9]

Neuroborreliosis

6. E.C., a 54-year-old man, presents with symptoms of late Lyme encephalopathy, including memory deficits, somnolence, and irritability. CSF analyses confirm the diagnosis. Should E.C. be treated with antibiotics? If so, for how long?

Although very rare, neurologic complications of Lyme disease are the major morbidity of the disease.[10] Lyme encephalopathy is more common in Europe than in the United States.[9] Although the acute neurologic manifestations of Lyme disease can remit spontaneously, IV antibiotic therapy hastens the resolution of symptoms and prevents more chronic sequelae (e.g., mild cognitive dysfunction or low-grade peripheral neuropathies). The development of these other syndromes in E.C. may be evidence of irreversible neurologic damage. Therefore, the approach to diagnosis and treatment should be aggressive. IV antibiotic therapy is indicated according to most clinicians (Table 75-3).[20] Most authorities recommend a minimum of 2 to 4 weeks.[9,19,20] Other candidates for intensive IV regimens of antibiotic therapy include patients with third-degree AV block or acute Lyme meningitis or radiculopathy.[20]

All patients with Lyme disease should be treated with antibiotics because most cases can be managed effectively with appropriately chosen antibiotics. In conclusion, E.C. should be treated aggressively with a parenteral third-generation cephalosporin such as ceftriaxone 2 g IV daily for 2 to 4 weeks.[9] Treatment response, however, is usually slow and possibly incomplete. Unless reliable objective measures indicate relapse, retreatment is not recommended.[9,23]

Laboratory Testing of Lyme Disease

7. P.S., a 35-year-old asymptomatic man with a history of a tick bite from a nonendemic Lyme disease area, just tested positive on ELISA. He was tested because he expressed a fear of Lyme disease. Why is this positive result alone sufficient (or insufficient) to begin treatment for Lyme disease? What other tests could be considered to help confirm the diagnosis?

The *B. burgdorferi* spirochete is long and narrow, with flagella. A flagellar 41-kDa protein is similar to flagellar proteins on other spirochetes, and cross-reactivity can occur. The Osp include two of the major elicitors of antibody response in late Lyme disease, termed OspA and OspB. The OspA antigen was used for vaccine development.

Problems of standardization, sensitivity, and specificity have caused significant interlaboratory and intralaboratory variations in test results in the serodiagnosis of Lyme disease.[24] Serologic testing for an antibody response to the spirochete is incapable of distinguishing between active infection and prior exposure. Demonstration of local CSF antibody production and comparison with serum concentrations, however, are highly useful in the diagnosis of neuro-disease, especially in European cases. Despite these problems, detection of the antibody response to *B. burgdorferi* is the most commonly used laboratory procedure for the diagnosis of Lyme disease.

Immunofluorescent assay (IFA) detection of antibody response was the first tool used in the diagnosis of Lyme disease. This test, however, is labor intensive and interpretation of the results is subjective; it has been replaced by ELISA analysis. Even with ELISA, however, 5% to 7% of test results may be false–positives. The Western blot (immunoblotting) test has been shown to increase the specificity of ELISA results, but it is also insensitive in early Lyme disease.[4] Western blotting supplements ELISA testing but does not confirm it, because they are not independent tests.[25]

Except for research studies, attempting to culture blood or skin for *B. burgdorferi* or PCR testing is not recommended in routine clinical practice in the differential diagnosis of erythema migrans owing to the expense and cumbersome nature of these tests.[9]

In summary, P.S. should not be treated for active Lyme disease based solely on one positive ELISA test. Seropositivity alone does not prove infection by *B. burgdorferi*.[9] Although the Western blot might help to establish a diagnosis, only a careful history and physical examination in combination with the serologic testing will accurately diagnose Lyme disease. The erythema migrans rash is key to early diagnosis.

8. A friend from an area not endemic for Lyme disease calls you to say that she has been recently diagnosed with "chronic Lyme disease." She was never found to have early or late Lyme disease. She'd like more information about it. How should you respond?

Chronic Lyme disease is a confusing term. Most authorities agree that there may be "post-Lyme disease syndromes," but its definition is evolving and not yet well accepted.[9] They agree, however, that objective evidence of a prior *B. burgdorferi* infection must be established before using this terminology. Criteria for diagnosing a post-Lyme disease syndrome include fatigue, widespread musculoskeletal pain, cognitive difficulties, or subjective symptoms of such severity that a substantial reduction in previous levels of activities is encountered. Any of these subjective symptoms must have had onset within 6 months of the initial Lyme disease diagnosis and persisted for at least 6 months after completion of antimicrobial therapy. It is considered clear that if someone has adhered to a recommended treatment regimen for Lyme disease, no convincing biologic evidence establishes the existence of symptomatic, chronic infection by *B. burgdorferi*. The organism has not been shown to develop antibiotic resistance.[9] For these patients with chronic subjective symptoms for >6 months, repeated antibiotic therapy is not useful or recommended.[9,26]

Is post-Lyme disease an autoimmune disease? The usual markers of autoimmune disease, such as increased erythrocyte sedimentation rates (ESR) or C-reactive protein levels, have not been seen. The usual "clustering" of HLA antigen genotypes seen in autoimmune disease has not been shown in case versus control studies in documented Lyme disease in patients. Is it different than fibromyalgia? One can objectively differentiate post-Lyme disease from fibromyalgia because the usual fibromyalgia trigger or pressure points are negative in patients with post-Lyme disease.

Many have attempted to identify useful tools to track Lyme disease response to therapy or supposed disease progression with markers, such as CD57 lymphocyte tests, soluble cd14 levels, anti-C6 antibodies, C6 peptides by ELISA, urinary antigen testing, following Western blot band changes.[27–30] None of these tests have proved to be useful.

What is apparent is that the term "chronic Lyme disease" has been used for patients with vague, undiagnosed complaints who have never had the disease. In fact, most patients regarded as having chronic Lyme disease, when rigorously evaluated at university-based medical centers, have had no evidence of current or prior *B. burgdorferi* infection.[9]

Because of a lack of efficacy, supportive data, or potential harm to the patient, the following are *not* recommended for treatment of any manifestation of Lyme disease: excessive dosing, long-term dosing, pulsed-dosed, or combination antibiotics; IV hydrogen peroxide or immunoglobulins; anti-*Bartonella* treatment with macrolides or other antibiotics (although the DNA of *Bartonella* has been found in some *Ixodes* ticks, no convincing evidence indicates that it can be transmitted to humans by tick bite); hyperbaric oxygen; fever therapy; specific nutritional supplements; ozone; cholestyramine; or magnesium or bismuth (bismacine or chromacine) injections.[9]

Your friend should be encouraged to seek an alternate diagnosis. Even in many patients who have had verified Lyme disease, the aches and pains of daily living they experience appear to be more related to their posttreatment symptoms than Lyme disease itself.[9]

Lyme Disease Prevention

9. P.S. is alarmed that his family members may contract Lyme disease. How do you advise him?

Most vector-borne diseases are prevented through vector control. This has proved difficult for tick-borne diseases because of a lack of efficacy or environmental concerns. Methods tried include habitat destruction by fire, chemical spraying, eradication of host deer, or protection of mice from tick infestation.

The prevention of Lyme disease has been limited thus far to personal protection efforts. Tick repellents may be applied to the skin or clothing. N,N-diethyl-m-toluamide (DEET) skin repellents (Repel Sportsmen) combined with a permethrin (Permanone) clothing repellent offer the best overall protection[9,19]

DEET has been tested against *Ixodid* ticks for repellence and found to be more effective than dibutylphthalate, dimethylphthalate, pyrethrum, and two combination products. Although DEET was considered safe historically, studies suggest that up to 50% of an applied dose may be absorbed through the skin and distributed to fat, liver, and muscle tissue. Half of it is excreted as metabolites in the urine over 5 days. Because DEET is lipid soluble, it can accumulate in fatty tissue and the brain.

Adverse DEET effects reported in adults include tingling, dryness, and some desquamation around the nasal area after repeated application of a 50% DEET solution to the face and arms. Two days after discontinuation of the solution, these side effects usually resolve.

In children, on the other hand, serious reactions after excessive DEET application have been reported.[9] These are rare events, however, and if the products are used according to their labeling, the adverse reaction risk is low, even for children >2 months of age.[4,9] Prolonged or excessive application is not recommended. It may be prudent to use the lowest effective concentration of DEET-containing repellents, such as those containing 20% to 30%. To minimize DEET toxicity apply sparingly, avoid inhalation or introduction into the eyes, wash repellent-treated skin when coming inside, avoid use on children's hands (that are likely to have contact with the eyes or mouth), and apply it only to intact skin or clothing.

A Centers for Disease Control and Prevention (CDC) recommended insect repellent alternative to DEET is picardin

(Cutter Advanced).[31] The effectiveness of picardin against *Ixodes* ticks has not been established, however.[9]

Physical barriers to ticks, such as wearing protective garments, long pants, and long-sleeved shirts, tucking shirts into pants and pants into boots, and wearing closed-toed shoes, should help to prevent infection. Ticks can be easier to spot on light-colored clothing. Checking the body for ticks regularly is recommended; any that are found should be promptly removed. Avoiding tick habitats is the best protection against tick-borne diseases. Human vaccine for Lyme disease has been withdrawn from the market. It may have caused autoimmune arthritis in HLA-DR4 positive patients.[32] Citing low demand, the U.S. manufacturer discontinued production in 2002.

ENDEMIC RELAPSING FEVER

Relapsing fever exists in two forms: epidemic and endemic. The bacterial spirochete *Borrelia recurrentis,* the agent responsible for epidemic relapsing fever, is transmitted between humans by the human body louse. Epidemic relapsing fever prevails in crowded conditions and occurs in the Middle East, Africa, and Asia; it has not been reported in the United States in recent years.[33–35] Mortality rates of up to 40% have been reported in some epidemics. Endemic relapsing fever, which is caused by a variety of *Borrelia* species, occurs worldwide, and is spread by ticks.

Spirochete Identification

In Europe, the identified responsible spirochete is *Borrelia hispanica.* In Africa, they are *Borrelia duttoni,* and *Borrelia crocidurae;* in North America, the species are *Borrelia hermsii, Borrelia turicatae,* and *Borrelia parkeri.*[33,34,36] Other *Borrelia* species may produce Lyme-like diseases or relapsing fevers worldwide. The terms "tick-borne" relapsing fever and "endemic" or "sporadic" relapsing fever are considered interchangeable. In contrast to epidemic relapsing fever, death from tick-borne relapsing fever is rare, and most patients recover.[33]

As the name implies, this disease is characterized by intermittent bouts of fever of variable duration. The *Borrelia* have the genetic ability to alter their outer surface proteins extensively. This capacity of the spirochetes to vary their surface antigens, thus eluding host defenses, is the presumed explanation for the recurrent nature of relapsing fever.[33,34,36]

Tick Vector

Tick Identification

The predominant tick vector for relapsing fever is of the genus *Ornithodoros,* a soft-bodied tick. These ticks feed on wild rodents or domestic animals and, incidentally, on humans. In North America, three tick species carry the agents of endemic relapsing fever with apparent strict specificity. In fact, the names of the responsible *Borrelia* species have been adopted from the three tick species that transmit them: *O. hermsii, O. parkeri,* and *O. turicata.* Although the ticks themselves may serve as reservoir hosts, the *Borrelia* usually circulate between wild rodents and ticks. The assumption that relapsing fever-causing *Borrelia* species are associated only with soft-shelled ticks is challenged by the isolation of *B. miyamotoi* from *I. persulcatus,* the hard-bodied vector tick for Lyme disease in Japan.[37] Similar to Lyme disease, greater worldwide variations of endemic cycles and vectors for tick-borne relapsing fever may exist than in North America.[38]

Tick Geography

In North America, relapsing fever is an uncommon disease largely confined to the geographic distribution of the tick species that harbor the *Borrelia.* These ticks are usually found in the remote natural settings of the mountains and semiarid plains of the far west and Mexico. In the United States, most cases of relapsing fever are caused by *B. hermsii.* It can develop when people visit tick- or rodent-infested cabins or summer homes. *O. hermsii* and *O. parkeri* inhabit forested mountain areas, usually at high altitudes, and have been pinpointed as the common source of relapsing fever outbreaks from human exposure in mountain cabins.[36] *O. turicata* transmits its *Borrelia* in the semiarid plains, from Kansas to central Mexico, creating outbreaks in people visiting caves, especially limestone ones in central Texas.[34,36]

Spirochetal Behavior

Ticks acquire spirochetes from blood feeding on small wild rodents. If high levels of *Borrelia* are present in the animal's blood, large numbers of spirochetes will be ingested by the tick and reside in the tick's midgut. During the next few days, the spirochetes invade the midgut wall, traverse the hemolymph system, and within a few weeks infect the salivary glands as well as other tick tissues and organs. They endure through tick molting and by now are practically absent in the midgut. Females may develop infected ovaries and transmit *Borrelia* to offspring in some *Ornithodoros* species, but this is rare in *O. hermsii.*[34] Having reached the tick's salivary glands, the spirochetes are poised to invade the next host that the tick feeds upon.

Tick Behavior

In contrast to the hard-bodied ticks, these ticks feed rapidly, often detaching after 30 to 90 minutes.[34] They feed at night while people are sleeping, and their bite is usually painless. Therefore, most people are unaware that they have been bitten.[36]

Disease Characterization

The hallmark of endemic relapsing fever is an abrupt onset of high fever (often >39°C) after an incubation period of 4 to 18 days.[34,35] The patient may develop shaking chills, severe headache, tachycardia, abdominal pain, myalgias, arthralgias, nausea, vomiting, and malaise. The fever usually breaks in 3 to 6 days in untreated patients. After a variable afebrile period of 3 to 36 days, (usually 7 days), cyclical periods of fever and constitutional symptoms reappear. Each febrile attack progressively diminishes in severity. Three to five relapses typically occur in untreated patients. A transient skin rash lasting 1 to 2 days appears in 6% to 28% of patients, typically when the primary fever has broken. The rash may be localized or generalized and consist of petechiae, macules, or papules. Neurologic involvement, more common with *B. turicata* infection, may be evident.[33,36]

Routine laboratory testing is of little value. Moderate anemia is common, however, as well as an increased ESR.

Leukocyte counts may be normal, yet thrombocytopenia is regularly encountered but is considered nonspecific.[34,35,36]

The diagnosis of relapsing fever is made by direct observation of the spirochete on a peripheral blood smear while the patient is febrile.[36] The observation of the smear is enhanced with Wright's or Giemsa staining. Further enhancement may be obtained by staining fixed smears with acridine orange. Antibody serology tests, although available, are of little value. Skin biopsy of the rash demonstrating the spirochete is unreliable. Direct culture of the spirochete from the blood into a special culture medium is the most specific diagnostic tool, but this is a slow technique confined to research laboratories.

Treatment

Doxycycline postexposure prophylaxis against a specific species, *B. persica*, of tick-borne relapsing fever has been shown to be successful in an Israeli study.[39] Whether this approach can be translated to other settings for other *Borrelia* species is unknown.

Successful treatment regimens usually include a 7 to 10 day course of antibiotics. Tetracyclines are preferred and doxycycline, 100 mg orally two times a day, is usually used.[36] Tetracycline or erythromycin is also effective at dosages of 500 mg orally four times a day. Hospitalization and administration of IV antibiotics may be required in severely ill patients.

10. O.T. is a 52-year-old man who visits his family practitioner with a sudden onset of high fever, severe headache, malaise, nausea, vomiting, and myalgias. He returned a week ago, at the end of July, from a stay in a rustic cabin on the north rim of the Grand Canyon. The clinician orders a manual complete blood count (CBC) and chemistry panel and asks the laboratory to observe a blood smear with Giemsa stain. What clues does the physician have to suspect endemic relapsing fever as the diagnosis?

The disease occurs more often in males, and the nonspecific constitutional symptoms exhibited by O.T. match the customary features of the ailment. The history is more revealing. The patient visited a location and setting where prior outbreaks of relapsing fever have been documented. In addition, cases of endemic relapsing fever peak in the summer months when ticks are warmer and more active.

11. After confirming the presence of *Borrelia* in the blood smear, the physician prescribes a 10-day course of tetracycline. Two hours after the first dose, O.T.'s wife calls the physician's office with concerns that the disease is worsening. O.T. is experiencing an increased temperature, is feeling faint and chilled, and has a rapid pulse and respiration rate. A skin lesion appears. What is most likely happening? Is this a drug reaction?

Up to 54% of patients with relapsing fever experience a reaction to the first dose of antibiotic, called a *Jarisch-Herxheimer reaction* (see Chapter 65, Sexually Transmitted Diseases).[34–36] It may occur in louse-borne relapsing fever, tick-borne relapsing fever, and in other spirochetal diseases, such as syphilis or Lyme.[9] The dramatic reaction consists of a rise in temperature, chills, myalgias, tachycardia, hypotension, increased respiratory rate, vasodilation, and occasionally exacerbation of skin lesions. Treatment of the reaction consists of supportive care. Severe reactions may require hospitalization for monitoring of vital signs and management of hypovolemia. Although this is a reaction to the administration of an antibiotic drug, it is not an allergic response, and the antibiotic should be continued.

Southern Tick-Associated Rash Illness (STARI)

12. M.G., a 46-year-old man living in southern Missouri, recently developed a rash resembling erythema migrans after a Lone Star tick bite. Because this tick is not known as a vector for Lyme disease, what could be the cause?

Amblyomma americanum (the Lone Star tick) is found through the southeast and south-central United States and along the Atlantic coast as far north as Maine. This tick aggressively bites humans in the southern states, as opposed to *I. scapularis* ticks. Spirochetes detected by microscopy and culture have been found in 1% to 3% of Lone Star ticks and are named *Borrelia lonestari*.[40,41] It is more closely related to the relapsing fever group of *Borrelia* than to Lyme *Borrelia* based on DNA sequencing. *B.* lonestari and *B. burgdorferi,* however, were ruled out as the cause of erythema migranslike skin lesions known as STARI in one investigation in Missouri.[42] Whether antibiotic treatment is even needed for STARI is being investigated.

OTHER BACTERIAL DISEASES: TULAREMIA

Tularemia

Etiology and Epidemiology

In 1911, George W. McCoy and Charles W. Chapin from the U.S. Public Health Service investigated a plaguelike disease in wild ground squirrels harvested in Tulare County, California, and discovered tularemia's cause.[43] The bacterium is a small, nonmotile, aerobic, nonencapsulated, gram-negative coccobacillus now named *Francisella tularensis* in honor of Edward Francis for his fieldwork and contributions to tularemia research.[43] Three tularemia strains, the more virulent biovar A and the less virulent biovars B and C, are recognized.[36] Type A tularemia, formerly thought to exist only in North America was identified as well in Slovakia in 1998.[44] It is fatal in up to 5% of cases.[43,45] The important reservoir hosts for the bacteria are hares, rabbits, and ticks. Before 1950, most human cases of the disease developed from direct contact with infected animals, usually hares or rabbits, and tularemia cases that occur in the fall or winter are usually associated with hunting season exposure. The prime source of serious human infections is the domestic rabbit.[44] Tick bite transmission, however, now accounts for more than half of tularemia cases west of the Mississippi River in the United States. In summer months, tick bites appear to be the main mode of transmission of tularemia to humans.[44] Other modes of transmission include ingestion of, or contact with, infected meat, water, or soil; inhalation of aerosolized bacteria; or bites from infected animals, mosquitoes, or deerflies.[43,46] Direct person-to-person spread of the disease is rare.

Tularemia is found in North America, Europe, Russia, Japan, and the Middle East. Most U.S. cases occur in the south and midwest, primarily in Arkansas, Missouri, Oklahoma, Kansas, and South Dakota.[36,44,47] The North American tick vectors are *Dermacentor variabilis* (dog tick), *Amblyomma americanum* (Lone Star tick), and *Dermacentor andersoni* (wood tick). Tick-borne tularemia occurs most often in the spring and summer, matching the likelihood of exposure. Reported cases of tularemia in the United States have steadily declined since 1950 from a case report high of 2,291 in 1939 to current levels of <200 per year since 1967.

Clinical Presentation

The clinical manifestations of tularemia are related to the mode of transmission. Classically, six types of tularemia presentation are identified: ulceroglandular, glandular, typhoidal, oculoglandular, oropharyngeal, and pneumonic.[43] The last three forms are presumably not tick-borne, reflecting the potential avenues of transmission of the microorganism.

Ulceroglandular is the most common form of tularemia, accounting for 75% to 80% of cases.[36,43] It is characterized by an ulcer that forms at the site of the tick bite, usually on the lower extremities, perineum, buttocks, or trunk. The lesion starts as a firm, erythematous papule that ulcerates and heals over several weeks. It is accompanied by regional, painful lymphadenopathy, usually inguinal or femoral. Glandular tularemia is defined by painful, swollen lymph nodes without an accompanying skin lesion. Typhoidal tularemia is characterized by fever, chills, headache, debilitation, abdominal pain, and prostration. Fever and chills are common with all forms of tularemia.

After exposure to the bacteria and an incubation period of 4 to 5 days, patients become ill with a sudden onset of fever, chills, headache, cough, arthralgias, myalgias, fatigue, and malaise. The severity of symptoms is quite variable, ranging from a mild, limited disease (probably type B tularemia) to rare cases of septic shock (probably type A tularemia). A hallmark manifestation is a high fever without an accompanying increase in pulse, or pulse-temperature disparity.[36] Common complications are mild hepatitis, secondary pneumonia, and pharyngitis. With antibiotic treatment of uncomplicated tularemia, mortality rates are only 1% to 3%. Increased morbidity and mortality are seen in the rare typhoidal forms.

Diagnosis

Laboratory diagnosis of tularemia is limited to the demonstration of an antibody response to the bacteria. Routine laboratory testing is of little help in establishing the diagnosis. Because an antibody response to the illness requires 10 to 14 days for detection, treatment is usually empiric. The diagnosis is based on clinical suspicion from the epidemiologic history and the presence of compatible findings. The customary serologic test demonstrates *F. tularensis* antibody agglutination. Although a single agglutination test with a titer of 1:160 or more in a suspected case is highly suggestive of a tularemia diagnosis, a fourfold or greater rise in titers between the acute and convalescent stages is diagnostic.[43]

Treatment

In adults, streptomycin 7.5 to 10 mg/kg intramuscularly (IM) or IV Q 12 h for 7 to 14 days is the treatment of choice.[43] Pediatric dosing is 20 to 40 mg/kg IM divided twice daily for 7 to 14 days.

13. Streptomycin was historically the drug of choice for tularemia but it is often unavailable commercially. What other antibiotics are alternatives? What are their drawbacks?

Some clinicians believe that gentamicin is the best alternative aminoglycoside for the treatment of nonmeningitic tularemia.[43] Its advantages compared with streptomycin include lower minimal inhibitory concentrations (MIC), less vestibular toxicity, and wider commercial availability. Considered fairly comparable in efficacy to streptomycin treatment, gentamicin therapy has been associated with increased treatment failure and relapse, however.[36] Some of the case reports and studies of gentamicin may have involved inadequate durations of therapy, treatment delays, or sicker patients. Tobramycin (Nebcin) has been associated with lower cure rates and higher failure rates than gentamicin or streptomycin.[36]

Initial cure rates and response to tetracycline are equivalent to those for gentamicin, but therapy with tetracycline has resulted in twice as many relapses. Perhaps bactericidal agents are required for successful tularemia treatment.

Reported cure rates for chloramphenicol therapy of tularemia are significantly lower than those for streptomycin. Chloramphenicol is considered bacteriostaticlike tetracycline. Chloramphenicol does penetrate into the CSF, with or without inflamed meninges, better than aminoglycosides or tetracyclines. Therefore, when tularemic meningitis is suspected, chloramphenicol plus streptomycin should be considered.[36,43]

Cephalosporins, such as ceftriaxone (Rocephin) and ceftazidime (Fortaz), possess favorable MIC data for *F. tularensis;* but inadequate clinical responses and treatment failures were encountered with ceftriaxone. In general, β-lactams and macrolides cannot be recommended for tularemia treatment.[36] Of the fluoroquinolones studied, ciprofloxacin (Cipro) has the optimal minimal bactericidal concentration (MBC) in vitro data. Promising results with ciprofloxacin treatment have been documented.[36,43,48] Because pneumonia is a common complication of tularemia, concern exists about the potential for overwhelming streptococcal meningitis or sepsis during ciprofloxacin therapy. Fluoroquinolones are relatively contraindicated in children.

It is not entirely clear why the in vitro susceptibility of *F. tularensis* to some antibiotics does not correlate with clinical success in treatment of tularemia. It has been suggested that testing pure cell cultures of the organism ("axenic" media) with antibiotics does not correlate well with clinical response. This may be because *F. tularensis* is predominantly an intracellular organism. One study using an in vitro cell system of tularemia antibiotic sensitivity testing found the highest activity with aminoglycosides, tetracyclines, rifampin, and fluoroquinolones, the drugs found to have the most favorable outcomes in treating tularemia today.[49]

In many of the reported studies of antimicrobial therapy for tularemia, short courses of treatment (~7 days) were used. To prevent tularemia from worsening or relapsing, longer regimens (14 days) should be used. Jarisch-Herxheimer reactions can occur with antibiotic treatment of tularemia. Antibiotic prophylaxis for people exposed to those with tularemia is not recommended, but prophylactic antibiotics might be used for suspected bioterrorism attacks of tularemia. Concern for the use of biological warfare agents, such as anthrax, botulinum toxin, plague, or hemorrhagic fever exists as well for Tularemia. Acute febrile illness with pneumonia and other signs of infection would result 3 to 5 days after exposure to aerosolized or airborne Tularemia organisms from an intentionally set weapon.[50] No tularemia vaccines are available in the United States.[43]

THE RICKETTSIA: ROCKY MOUNTAIN SPOTTED FEVER, *RICKETTSIA PARKERI* INFECTION, EHRLICHIOSIS, AND ANAPLASMOSIS

Rocky Mountain Spotted Fever (RMSF)

Rocky Mountain spotted fever is the most prevalent and virulent rickettsial disease in the United States. As early as 1872, RMSF infected white settlers of the Northwest and it may have been prevalent in Native Americans of the region before that time. It was first described in residents of the Bitterroot, Snake, and Boise River valleys of Montana and Idaho in the late 1800s. Howard Ricketts discovered the causative agent, *Rickettsia rickettsii,* in 1906. The rickettsiae is a small (0.3 by 1.5 μm), pleomorphic, gram negative, obligate intracellular coccobacillus that can survive only briefly outside of a host.[36]

Epidemiology

Today, RMSF is reported in every U.S. state except Vermont, Maine, and Hawaii; and in Canada, Mexico, and Central and South America.[51] It has not been documented outside of the Western Hemisphere. The term "Rocky Mountain spotted fever" is actually a misnomer today because the disease has shifted eastward from the Rocky Mountain states, and the greatest incidence of RMSF now occurs in North Carolina, Oklahoma, Arkansas, South Carolina, and Tennessee.[52] Most RMSF infections arise from tick exposure in rural or suburban locations, yet rare outbreaks in urban environments have occurred.

The prevalence of RMSF is highest in children 5 to 9 years of age.[36,53] Another peak prevalence is seen in men >60 years of age. Risk factors are male gender, residence in wooded areas, and exposure to dogs that may bring ticks into households and yards.

Tick Vectors and Hosts

In the east, south, and west coasts of the United States, tick vectors for RMSF have been identified as the dog tick, *Dermacentor variabilis.* In the Rocky Mountains states, the wood tick, *Dermacentor andersoni,* is the vector. In Mexico, they are *Rhipicephalus sanguineus* and *Amblyomma cajennense,* with the latter also being responsible in Central and South America. The brown dog tick, *Rhipicephalus sanguineus*, has been identified as a new tick vector for RMSF in a defined area of Arizona.[36,52,54]

The *Dermacentor* tick feeds on humans only during its adult stage. Larval *Dermacentor* ticks may be infected while feeding on small mammals that develop sufficient rickettsemia for transmission, such as chipmunks, ground squirrels, cotton rats, snowshoe hares, and meadow voles. Dogs are not considered reservoirs for *R. rickettsia* but are susceptible to RMSF and may introduce infected ticks into households.[52] Adult ticks transmit the rickettsia transovarially to their progeny with high efficiency and establish newly infected tick lines. If the rickettsia burden is large in the adult tick, however, it may cause tick death, thereby reducing infected tick lines. Therefore, there must be nontick reservoirs, as mentioned previously, to develop newly infected tick generational lines; otherwise, RMSF would slowly disappear. In summary, ticks are both vectors and hosts for *R. rickettsia.*

Disease Course, Symptoms, and Fatalities

Rickettsia rickettsia is usually transmitted to humans from an infected tick bite.[51] The organism can also gain access to humans through broken skin if an infected tick is being crushed with bare fingers, and such crushing may generate infectious aerosols that might be inhaled. Conjunctival contact with infected tick tissues or feces provides another route for rickettsial entry.

After introduction of the organisms into the body, the rickettsia spread hematogenously with a predilection for the vascular endothelium, especially in capillaries. During an incubation period of 2 to 14 days, induced phagocytosis allows rickettsial entry into endothelial cells, where they replicate by binary fission in the cytoplasm and nuclei of infected cells. This induces a generalized vasculitis leading to activation of clotting factors, capillary leakage, and microinfarctions in various organs.[51] In severe infections, hypotension and intravascular coagulation may coexist and culminate in cell, tissue, or organ destruction.

Dehydration is an early sign of RMSF, followed by increased vascular permeability, edema, decreased plasma volume, hypoproteinemia, reduced serum oncotic pressure, and prerenal azotemia. RMSF is a multisystem disease, but a particular organ may be the major focus of the disease. If the brain or lungs are severely infected, death can ensue. An increased severity of illness is associated with edema, particularly in children, and hypoalbuminemia. Hypotension is present in 17% of patients and hyponatremia in 56%. Extensive infection of the pulmonary microvascular endothelium can cause noncardiogenic pulmonary edema.

A common finding in RMSF is myalgia (72%–83%) or muscular tenderness, which are manifestations of skeletal muscle necrosis. Striking creatinine kinase elevations have been described. Thrombocytopenia resulting from consumption of platelets during intravascular coagulation processes occurs in 35% to 52% of patients. True disseminated intravascular coagulation with attendant hypofibrinogenemia is exceptional, however, even in severe or fatal cases. Blood loss or hemolysis in some may cause anemia, which is seen in 30% of patients and reflects blood vessel damage. Fatalities usually occur 8 to 15 days after illness onset if no treatment is given or if treatment is delayed. Long-term sequelae from severe forms of RMSF can include partial paralysis of the lower extremities, gangrene of extremities requiring amputation, deafness or hearing loss, incontinence, and movement or speech disorders.[52,55]

"Fulminant" RMSF is best defined as a disease with a rapidly fatal course with death occurring in ~5 days. This form of disease is characterized by an early onset of neurologic signs and late or absent skin rash; it is highly associated with glucose-6-phosphate dehydrogenase deficiency, chronic alcohol abuse, advanced age, black race, and male gender.[52] In the preantibiotic era, RMSF mortality rates were as high as 30%, but they have fallen to 5% in antibiotic-treated cases today.[52]

The classically defined triad of RMSF symptoms at initial presentation is fever, rash, and headache, but this is found in only 40% of cases.[36] The RMSF skin rash typically begins, 2 to 4 days after fever onset, as pink, 1- to 5-mm blanchable macules that later become papules.[52] It begins on the ankles, wrists, and forearms and soon thereafter involves the palms or soles. It then spreads to the arms, thighs, and trunk and typically evolves into a petechial exanthem. The utility of these findings in the differential diagnosis is limited because rash may be absent, transient, or late; it may never become petechial or it may have an unusual distribution.

Diagnosis

As for most tick-borne diseases, confirmatory serologic analysis is only retrospective in nature, and antirickettsial treatment should begin immediately to prevent morbidity and mortality.[52] *R. rickettsia* is hard to culture.[36] Immunohistologic demonstration of *R. rickettsii* in biopsy specimens of rash lesions is the only approach that can yield diagnostic results in a timely manner, but this approach is applicable only to those presenting with a skin rash.

The best serologic test for RMSF is the IFA test, but antibodies typically appear only after 10 to 14 days.[51] More striking laboratory abnormalities of RMSF disease include a normal leukocyte count with a shift to the left, hyponatremia, thrombocytopenia, elevated serum transaminases or creatinine kinase, and CSF pleocytosis. These findings are observed late in the disease course, however, and are not helpful in early disease recognition.

Clinical findings and history are key to early diagnosis and successful treatment. In a febrile, tick-exposed person with a rash, RMSF should be considered. RMSF should be strongly considered in febrile children, adolescents, or men >60 years of age, especially if they reside in or have traveled to the southern Atlantic or south-central United States from May through September. A delay in treatment for RMSF beyond 5 days of symptom onset increases the mortality rates from 6% to 22%.[56]

Treatment

In vitro, the MIC for *R. rickettsia* is 0.5 mcg/mL for chloramphenicol, 0.25 mc/mL for tetracycline, and 0.06 mcg/mL for doxycycline. The recommended treatment is doxycycline 100 mg orally or IV two times a day for at least 7 days and for 2 days after the temperature is normal.[57] Chloramphenicol is reserved for use in pregnancy.[51] The erythromycins, penicillins, sulfonamides, aminoglycosides, and cephalosporins are not effective. Although fluoroquinolones have shown activity in other spotted fever rickettsial diseases, no reports are found of their use in human RMSF disease and they cannot be recommended at this time.[36,57]

14. Can tetracyclines be given safely to young children with RMSF?

In 1994, the American Academy of Pediatrics (AAP) Committee on Infectious Diseases revised the RMSF treatment options for young children after considering chloramphenicol's potential toxicity and the dental staining concerns for tetracyclines. The AAP now acknowledges tetracyclines as acceptable treatment in children of any age with RMSF. Doxycycline should be the tetracycline agent of choice in pediatric RMSF because it is dosed less frequently than other tetracyclines, which may improve compliance, and does not bind calcium as strongly as other tetracyclines. The dosage is 4.4 mg/kg orally divided into two doses on day 1 followed by 2.2 mg/kg/day orally each day for 7 to 10 days or 2 to 3 days after the fever abates and clinical improvement occurs.[57]

Prevention

In addition to the same guidelines for prevention of Lyme disease, keeping pets free of ticks should reduce exposure. Ticks must not be crushed in a way that might introduce rickettsia into cutaneous lesions, mucous membranes, or the conjunctiva. No RMSF vaccine is available. Antirickettsial antibiotic prophylaxis after a tick bite is not warranted.

Rickettsia Parkeri and other Spotted Fever Group (SFG) Rickettsia

In the last quarter of the 20th century, a distinct spotted fever group (SFG) rickettsia has been discovered worldwide causing novel rickettsioses.[58] In the United States, SFG rickettsial pathogens other than *R. rickettsia* have recently been recognized, including *R. felis, R. akari,* and *R. parkeri*.[59,60] Three cases of *R. parkeri* human infection transmitted by tick bite have been reported.[58,60,61] *R. parkeri* infection is associated with fever, malaise, and eschar formation (rarely seen in RMSF), especially at the site of the Gulf Coast tick, *Amblyomma maculatum*, bite.[36] *R. parkeri* infection is milder than RMSF and can be diagnosed by PCR testing of an eschar or papule lesion.[60] Doxycycline treatment has resulted in prompt (<1 or 2 days) resolution of symptoms.[58,60]

Ehrlichiosis and Anaplasmosis

Species Identification

Three tick-borne rickettsial human diseases have emerged in recent years: human monocytotropic ehrlichiosis (HME), caused almost exclusively by *Ehrlichia chaffeensis*, human granulocytic anaplasmosis (HGA), caused by *Anaplasma phagocytophilum*, and human *Ehrlichia ewingii* infection (HEE).[9,36,52,62–64] A human mononucleosislike disease first described in Japan in 1954 is caused by *Ehrlichia sennetsu*, a rickettsiallike organism having a fish fluke vector. The disease is termed *Sennetsu fever* and is now indigenous to Japan and Southeast Asia.[64] The agents of HME, HGA, and HEE parasitize white blood cells.

In 1987, the first reported case of human ehrlichial infection in the United States was found in a soldier at Fort Chaffee, Arkansas. It was initially misinterpreted as being the same agent that infects dogs, *Ehrlichia canis*. Subsequent studies revealed that it was a unique species, *E. chaffeensis*. Cases of HME have now been reported in many states, Europe, and Africa.[63] Retrospective analysis revealed that 10% to 20% of unconfirmed, presumptive diagnoses of RMSF were actually HME. The number of HME cases is greater than RMSF in several states today.

Anaplasmosis was first described in 1994. Since HGA's discovery, more cases have been reported than for HME.[52] During 2001–2002, HGA rates were especially high in Rhode Island, Wisconsin, Minnesota, Connecticut, New York, and Maryland.[52]

Tick Vectors and Disease Hosts

The primary tick vector of HME is *A. americanum*, the Lone Star tick, and its geographic distribution matches that of most cases of HME, occurring in the south central and southeastern Unites States.[63] *E. chaffeensis* also has been recovered in *Dermacentor variabilis*, *Ixodes pacificus*, and *Amblyomma cajennense*.[63] Cases of HME that have been diagnosed in the northeastern United States are probably caused by *A. americanum*. HME cases in Europe, Africa, and some U.S. states suggest other vectors. An important reservoir for *E. chaffeensis* is white-tailed deer.[52] Dogs, coyotes, and goats have shown natural infection with *E. chaffeensis*.[52] HME begins with the introduction of *E. chaffeensis* into the skin of a host from the bite of an infected tick. The bacteria spread throughout the body hematogenously. They become established within the cells of monocytic macrophages in the spleen, lymph nodes, liver, bone marrow, lung, and kidney. Characteristic, microscopically visible intracellular inclusion bodies called *morulae* (for their mulberrylike appearance) develop. Each morula is actually a membrane-bound rickettsial colony that grows and divides within the monocyte's cytoplasm. Necrosis in heavily infected cells occurs, and it is believed that cell rupture and the subsequent release of rickettsia allows infection of more monocytes, repeating the cycle.

Tick vectors that harbor the HGA agent include *I. scapularis* and *I. pacificus*, which are also Lyme disease transmitters. In Europe, *Ixodes ricinus* is the vector. The main reservoir for *A. phagocytophilum* is the white-footed mouse. Other hosts include white-tailed deer, elk, and other wild rodents.[52] The events after introduction into a patient's skin of the HGA agent by tick bite are unknown. Rather than directly attacking mature granulocytes, it is suspected that the rickettsia infects a myeloid precursor in the bone marrow and survives or multiplies throughout granulocytic cellular maturation.

Tick removal from the body is less likely to be effective for disease prevention than it is in Lyme disease because of the rapid transmission of *A. phagocytophilum* during the nymphal tick bite.[65] Tick exposure is defined by geography and season. Simply being in an area where ticks can be found, particularly during spring and summer, constitutes exposure.

Clinical and Laboratory Findings

Human ehrlichiosis and anaplasmosis usually present as a nonspecific, febrile, flulike illness resembling RMSF. They begin 5 to 21 days after tick exposure.[9,63,66] Patients may be entirely asymptomatic, but there have been occasional fatalities from the complications of renal failure, respiratory failure, shock, or encephalopathy. HME and HGA share similar clinical features. Both display fever as the major symptom in nearly 100% of cases.[66] The other common symptoms of malaise, myalgia, headaches, and rigors are found in virtually all cases of HGA but somewhat less in HME. Other less common symptoms for both diseases include diaphoresis, nausea, vomiting, cough, diarrhea, abdominal pain, arthralgia, pharyngitis, rash, and confusion. HEE infection has been seen almost exclusively in immunocompromised patients, yet no fatalities have been documented.[52,67]

As with many other tick-borne diseases, serologic findings of antibody response to ehrlichiosis assist only by retrospectively confirming the diagnosis. Currently, indirect IFA serology is the gold standard for both HGA and HME.[63] Blood detection by PCR or culture has been used for HGA. The following signs often are noted, however: hypertransaminemia, leukopenia (often with a shift to the left), thrombocytopenia, and anemia. These findings may increase the suspicion for HME or HGA infection. A peripheral blood smear showing neutrophilic morulae is diagnostic for HGA, but negative results do not rule out the diagnosis.[66] In HME, peripheral blood smears are rarely diagnostic. HME morulae are more likely to be identified in macrophages with biopsy or postmortem specimens of the liver, spleen, or bone marrow anecdotally. A peripheral blood smear examination for morulae should probably be undertaken because this method is the quickest and easiest for making a provisional diagnosis. Confirmatory testing by serology or PCR is still required to establish the diagnosis.[9,52]

15. Because the clinical findings of HME and HGA are similar, how can they be differentiated?

The nonspecific manifestations of HME and HGA are considered indistinguishable. Although considered an uncommon finding, skin rash is consistent with either disease. In HME, skin rashes are seen in almost 60% of children but in <30% of adults.[52] In HGA, skin rashes occur in 10% or less of patients and may actually reflect coinfection with Lyme disease.[36] Therefore, if a skin rash is present, HME is much more likely than HGA (Table 75-4).

Human monocytotropic ehrlichiosis and HGA can be differentiated by serologic evaluation or PCR. Treatment should never be delayed pending the results of testing because the mortality rate is 2% to 3% for HME and 0.5% to 1% for HGA.[52,63] Delays in diagnosis and treatment are related to a substantial proportion of death from the diseases.

HME and HGA as Opportunist/Immunosuppressor

Opportunistic cases of HME have appeared in patients with acquired immunodeficiency syndrome (AIDS), and death from overwhelming HME infection has occurred in other immunocompromised patients. Animal models of *A. phagocytophilum* infection have shown impaired defense responses, such as defects in granulocyte emigration and phagocytosis, suppressed CD4 and CD8 counts, and impaired lymphoproliferation of isolated lymphocytes. HGA fatalities have been associated with concomitant candidiasis, cryptococcal pneumonia, severe herpesvirus infection, and invasive pulmonary aspergillosis. Theoretically, opportunistic infections may be secondary to rickettsial-mediated impairment of the immune response.

Treatment and Prevention

Doxycycline (Vibramycin) 100 mg orally twice daily for 10 to 14 days is the drug of choice for both HME and HGA.[63] For HGA, doxycycline for only 10 days is sufficient.[9] In children <8 years of age, doxycycline is given at a dosage of 4 mg/kg/day PO or IV divided into two daily doses. For those >8 years of age but weighing <45 kg, 4 mg/kg of doxycycline Q 12 h is used; adult doses are used for children weighing >45 kg.[9] (See RMSF for a discussion of the pediatric use of doxycycline.) If tetracyclines are absolutely contraindicated, rifampin 300 mg orally twice daily for 7 to 10 days is an alternative in mild HGA disease.[9] Pediatric rifampin dosing for HGA is 10 mg/kg (to a maximum 300-mg dose) twice daily for 5 to 7 days.[68] Chloramphenicol (Chloromycetin) is ineffective in vitro and should not be used.[63] Although early in vitro data suggested benefit with fluoroquinolones, this finding has not resulted in a clear role for these agents as this time. Ineffective antibiotics for ehrlichiosis or anaplasmosis include gentamicin (Garamycin), ceftriaxone (Rocephin), cotrimoxazole (Bactrim), erythromycin (E-Mycin), metronidazole (Flagyl), clindamycin (Cleocin), sulfonamides, and penicillin.[36] Asymptomatic, seropositive patients with antibodies to *A. phagocytophilum* should not be treated.[9]

Table 75-4 Tick-Borne Disease Findings

	LD	RF	Tularemia	HME	HGA	RMSF	Babesiosis	CTF
Rash	+++	+	+	++	+	+++	–	+/–
Fever	++	++++	+–+++	++++	++++	++++	++	+
Rigors	–	+++	+–+++	+++	++++	+++	++	–
Headache	++	++++	+–+++	+++	++++	++++	+	+
Myalgia	++	+	+–+++	+++	++++	++++	++	+++
Anemia	–	++	–	++	++	+++	+++	+
Nausea/vomiting	+	+++	–	++	++	+++	+	+
Cough	+	++	+	+	++	–	+	–
Confused	+	+	–	+	++	++	–	+
Malaise	++++	++	+–+++	++++	++++	++++	++	–
Arthralgias	+++	++	+	++	+	–	+	–
LFTs	+	++	++	++++	++++	++	+	+
Increased WBCs	+	+	+/–	–	–	+/–	–	–
Decreased WBCs	–	–		++	+++	+/–	–	+++
ESR	–	++	–	–	–	–	+	+
Decreased platelet count	–	+++	–	+++	++++	++	++	+

Caution: Routine laboratory testing is of little value in diagnosing or differentiating tick-borne diseases.

+, ≤25% association; –, not usually associated; CTF, Colorado tick fever; ESR, erythrocyte sedimentation rate; HGA, human granulocytic anaplasmosis; HME, human monocytic ehrlichiosis; LD, Lyme disease; LFTs, liver function tests; RF; relapsing fever; RMSF, Rocky Mountain spotted fever; WBCs, white blood cell counts.

Prevention of ehrlichial disease is preferable to treatment. Tick avoidance and detection strategies, as outlined for Lyme disease, are recommended. No evidence supports the routine administration of prophylactic antibiotics for HME or HGA prevention in patients with known tick bites. Vaccines may be developed.[63]

16. G.K., a 78-year-old man living outside Duluth, Minnesota, presents with an influenzalike illness in late May. He has a 2-day history of fever, shaking chills, headache, myalgias, nausea, and anorexia. On examination, his temperature is 39.4°C, but other physical findings are unremarkable. No skin rashes are found. During questioning, he stated he had multiple tick bites about 2 weeks ago while he was fur trapping. The physician suspects anaplasmosis and prescribes doxycycline 100 mg PO twice daily for 10 days. Blood is drawn for serology, CBC with differential, chemistry profile, C-reactive protein, and a Wright's stain microscopic examination. Immediately available abnormal results include neutrophilic morulae on microscopy, a WBC count of 2.5 × 10^9/L (normal, 4.0–10.7), a platelet count of 80 × 10^9/L (normal, 150–450), C-reactive protein of 136 mg/L (normal, 4–8), aspartate aminotransferase (AST) of 150 U/L (normal, 16–40), and lactate dehydrogenase of 700 U/L (normal, 80–175). Serology is still pending. Two days later, G.K. defervesced and was feeling better. How does this case fulfill a diagnosis of HGA?

G.K.'s history is significant for HGA. He was in the right place, the upper midwestern United States, and was outdoors during the right season; most patients are diagnosed with HGA in May through August.[66] The usual incubation period from tick bite to illness onset ranges from 5 to 21 days.[9]

His symptoms are also important. Nearly 100% of patients with HGA have a fever of >37.6°C. Other symptoms in G.K. consistent with HGA are rigors (shaking chills), headache, myalgias, nausea, and anorexia.[66] Matching laboratory findings include neutrophilic morulae. The observed leukopenia and thrombocytopenia strongly support the diagnosis. Evidence of mild to moderate hepatic injury, as seen by the elevated liver enzyme results, and the elevated C-reactive protein also are helpful in HGA diagnosis.[66] Finally, the good response to doxycycline, with fever resolution in 2 days, is customary. Fever persisting for more than 2 days after doxycycline treatment suggests that the diagnosis of HGA is incorrect.[9]

THE PROTOZOA: BABESIOSIS

Babesiosis

History

Investigating the deaths of 30,000 to 50,000 head of Romanian cattle with febrile hemoglobinuria in 1888, Victor Babes described an intraerythrocytic organism that was thought to be bacterial, and it was named *Haematococcus bovis*.[36,69,70] While investigating a hemolytic cattle fever in Texas in 1893, Smith and Kilborne established that the causative organism was a protozoan, *Babesia bigemina*, and introduced the concept of arthropod-borne transmission of the disease.[36,69,70] The first human case of babesiosis was definitively identified in a 33-year-old Yugoslavian cattle farmer in 1957. His febrile hemoglobinuria and intraerythrocytic organisms were attributed to the bovine pathogen *Babesia divergens*.[69,70] He had undergone a previous splenectomy and died of the disease. Postmortem inquiry revealed that his cattle were infected with a bovine babesial species. Possible tick vectors identified were *Ixodes ricinus* and *Dermacentor sylvarum.* To date, rare, often fatal, human cases of babesiosis in Europe have been caused by *B. divergens* and *B. microti*.[9] Sporadic cases of babesiosis have been reported in Asia, South America, and Africa.[9] European cases present with a fulminant, febrile illness 1 to 3 weeks after a tick bite. In 84% of these cases, the patients have been asplenic. Coma and death has occurred in >50% of cases. Customary findings are hemoglobinuria, hemolysis, jaundice, chills, sweats, myalgia, pulmonary edema, and renal insufficiency.

The first human babesiosis case in a person with an intact spleen was reported in 1969 in a patient from Nantucket

Island, Massachusetts. Since then, "Nantucket fever" has been found to be caused by the babesial rodent agent *B. microti.* In contrast to most European cases and those reported in California, human babesiosis in endemic areas of the Great Lakes regions and the northeastern United States commonly occurs in normosplenic patients.[69,70,71] The presenting complaints are usually nonspecific and consist of malaise, fatigue, low-grade fever or shaking chills, headache, generalized musculoskeletal complaints, emotional lability, nausea, emesis, and weight loss. Fatal cases have been found in distinct areas of Wisconsin, Missouri, Rhode Island, and California. Severe, nonfatal cases have occurred in Minnesota, the state of Washington, and California. Additional cases have been reported in New York, Connecticut, Maryland, Virginia, Georgia, as well as in Mexico. Members of *Babesia* and *Theileria* genusera are called piroplasms because of their pear-shaped appearance of dividing parasites within erythrocytes. A different type of *Babesia*-like piroplasm has emerged in the western United States: designated WA-1, it was originally isolated in a resident in the state of Washington.[69] In Missouri, a pathogen called MO-1 has caused babesiosis.[69,70]

Babesia, Ticks, and Hosts

There are >100 species of *Babesia* having a wide geographic range.[36,69] To date, only four species are known human pathogens: *B. divergens, B. microtti,* WA-1, and MO-1.[36] They are transmitted by *Ixodes, Boophilus, Dermacentor, Haemaphysalis,* and *Rhipicephalus* ticks. *B. microti* is transmitted in the northeastern United States by *I. scapularis,* the deer tick of Lyme disease and HGA, and in the United Kingdom by *I. trianguliceps.* In Europe, bovine babesiosis is transmitted by *I. ricinus.* In the western United States, *I. pacificus* is the probable vector. High infection rates of *B. microti* in field mice (*Microtus pennsylvanicus*) and white-footed mice (*Peromyces leucopus*) have been found on Nantucket Island in Massachusetts during investigations of transmission cycles. Other reservoirs for *B. microti* are chipmunks, meadow voles, shrews, and rats.[69] In the southeastern United States, nymphal stage *I. scapularis* ticks feed on lizards, which are poor reservoirs for *B. microtti,* possibly explaining why babesiosis is rarely reported there. Babesia species also are transmitted from the larval to nymphal stage of the tick (that is, transstadial transmission occurs).[69]

Symptoms and Diagnosis

17. H.W., age 64 years, spent July on Martha's Vineyard. A week later, he felt fatigued and lost his appetite. He presents to his local physician in the middle of August with complaints of fever, headache, drenching sweats, aches and pains, and occasional dark-colored urine. He does not recall a tick bite. On physical examination, he has splenomegaly and hepatomegaly. Laboratory tests show a severe normochromic, normocytic anemia, decreased hemoglobin, hemoglobinuria, thrombocytopenia, and increased liver enzymes. His temperature is 40°C. Examination of a Giemsa-stained thin blood smear reveals the presence of unpigmented ring-shaped intraerythrocytic parasites, some forming tetrads that resemble a Maltese cross, in >10% of his erythrocytes. The physician institutes a clindamycin and quinine regimen. What was the clue to the diagnosis of babesiosis?

The babesiosis diagnosis was confirmed by the direct observation of the protozoan inside the red blood cells. Although the Giemsa-stained test is a commonly used tool, it is subject to false–negative results because the rate of parasitemia is typically low. Usually, multiple blood smears need to be examined because few erythrocytes may be infected early in the course of the disease when most people seek medical help.[9] Because blood smear inspection is often not successful in diagnosing babesiosis or may only detect a few parasites, additional supportive laboratory results are advocated, such as serology using IFA for IgM and IgG antibabesial antibodies or PCR detection of babesial DNA in the blood.[9]

Most patients with *B. microti* babesiosis are asymptomatic. This form of babesiosis can be viewed as a distinct occult, asymptomatic disease with few known sequelae. A number of transfusion-acquired infections have been documented, reflecting the existence of the asymptomatic form of babesiosis in blood donors.

A second form of babesiosis is a potentially life-threatening hemolytic one that occurs in people predisposed to severe infection because of advanced age, immune suppression because of human immunodeficiency virus (HIV) disease or malignancy, or prior splenectomy.[73] Although babesial infection is as prevalent in children as in adults, it is more severe in adults >50 years of age. Complications seen in severe babesiosis include acute respiratory failure, disseminated intravascular coagulation, congestive heart failure, coma, and renal failure, with a 5% to 9% mortality rate.[9,36]

In the northeastern United States, infections commonly occur in patients with spleens, as in H.W. Clinically apparent cases are most common in 50- to 60-year-old patients, many of whom do not recall a tick bite. Most symptoms of babesiosis are caused by hemolysis or the systemic inflammatory responses to parasitemia.[70] The usual incubation period is 1 to 6 weeks after the tick bite.[36] Nonspecific, viral-like symptoms that are gradual in onset appear first, as in H.W.'s case, followed several days later by the other symptoms H.W. displayed. A hallmark of the disease is hemolytic anemia of varying severity. A high index of suspicion for babesiosis should be maintained in any patient with an unexplained febrile illness who lives in or has traveled to a region where the infection is endemic during June through August, as in H.W.'s case, particularly if there is a history of tick bite.[36]

Treatment

18. Why were clindamycin and quinine chosen to treat H.W.? What other drugs have been used?

The discovery of a human babesiosis treatment regimen combining clindamycin (Cleocin) and quinine was a fortuitous one. An 8-week-old infant with presumed transfusion-acquired malaria was initially treated with chloroquine. Because of a lack of response, treatment was switched to quinine plus clindamycin, and the patient defervesced.[70] A correct diagnosis of babesiosis was subsequently confirmed. Although this treatment combination is still used, frequent side effects (e.g., tinnitus, vertigo and diarrhea) occur, often resulting in dose reduction or discontinuation.[9,36] Treatment failures with this regimen have occurred in splenectomized patients, patients with HIV infection, or those receiving concurrent corticosteroids.[9] Dosing recommendations for adults are clindamycin 600 mg orally Q 8 h or 300 to 600 mg IV Q 6 h *plus* quinine 650 mg orally Q 6 to 8 h for 7 to 10 days; children should receive clindamycin 7 to 10 mg/kg (maximum, 600-mg dose) orally or IV Q 6 to 8 hours *plus* quinine 8 mg/kg (maximum, 650 mg dose) orally Q 8 hours for 7 to 10 days.[9,69,70]

Atovaquone (Mepron), the hydroxynaphthoquinone derivative used for opportunistic infections in patients with HIV, has been used with substantial success in patients with *B. microti* infection refractory to conventional therapy. Combination therapy of azithromycin with atovaquone is better tolerated than clindamycin–quinine combinations. This newer regimen is as effective as the clindamycin with quinine combination. The dosing is atovaquone 750 mg orally Q 12 hr *plus* azithromycin 500 mg to 1,000 mg orally on day 1 and 250 mg on subsequent days for 7 to 10 days.[9] Higher azithromycin doses of 600 mg to 1,000 mg/day may be used in immunocompromised patients.[9] Children should receive atovaquone 20 mg/kg (maximum, 750 mg dose) Q 12 hr *plus* azithromycin 10 mg/kg (maximum, 500-mg dose) on day 1 and 5 mg/kg (maximum, 250-mg dose) orally thereafter for 7 to 10 days.[9]

Antimicrobials should be used in all patients with active babesiosis owing to the risk of complications. Antibody seropositive, symptomatic patients without identifiable parasites on blood smear or PCR positivity should not be treated. Similarly, asymptomatic patients should not be treated regardless of serologic results, blood smear examinations, or PCR findings. A course of treatment should be considered in asymptomatic patients, however, if these tests are positive and repeat testing demonstrates persistent parisitemia for >3 months.[9]

Partial or complete red blood cell (RBC) transfusions may be life-saving in severe babesiosis for patients having high-grade parasitemia (10% or more infected erythrocytes), significant hemolysis, or pulmonary, renal, or hepatic compromise.[9] Rapidly increasing parasitemia leading to massive intravascular hemolysis and renal failure mandates immediate treatment for this form of the disease.

Babesiosis prevention is the same as for other tick-borne diseases. Splenectomized patients should avoid areas where babesiosis is endemic. Although developed for use in cattle, babesial vaccines are not available for humans.[69]

THE VIRUSES: COLORADO TICK FEVER AND TICK-BORNE ENCEPHALITIS

Colorado Tick Fever

Disease History

"Mountain fever" has been described since the first immigrants arrived in the Rocky Mountains. It was later renamed Colorado tick fever (CTF) and the Colorado tick fever virus (CTFV) was identified as the cause.

Virus Identification

Colorado tick fever is caused by a double-stranded RNA *Coltivirus*. It is an intraerythrocytic virus. At least 22 strains of CTF virus are known, but the antigenic variation between human strains is low.[72] The virus is an arbovirus because it replicates inside ticks. The primary nidus of infection is thought to be CTFV invasion of hematopoietic progenitor cell lines and it remains sheltered in mature erythrocytes.[72]

Ticks and Host Reservoirs

Colorado tick fever is a viral illness transmitted by the bite of an infected tick.[73,74] Although at least eight tick species have been found to be infected with the virus, *Dermacentor andersoni* is the primary tick vector that transmits the illness to humans.[73,72] *D. andersoni* feeds on numerous mammals, but ground squirrels, porcupines, and chipmunks are primary reservoirs for CTFV.[72–74] Transstadial but not transovarial transmission of CTF virus in the tick has been documented.[72]

Prevalence

The CTF is contracted in forested mountain areas at higher elevations of the Rocky Mountain regions in the United States and Canada, especially on the south-facing brush slopes and dry rocky surfaces of mountains east of the Continental Divide.[73,72] Neutralizing CTFV antibodies are found in up to 15% of perennial campers.[75] Although CTF can develop from March to September, May and June are the peak months for its development.[75]

Symptoms

19. T.M., a previously healthy 28-year-old native of Atlanta, Georgia, returns from a 1-week late spring camping trip in the eastern Colorado Rocky Mountains. Four days later, he experiences fever, chilliness, aching back and leg muscles, photophobia, retro-orbital and abdominal pain, and headache. He recalls no tick bites and has no skin rashes. Suspecting RMSF, his physician prescribes doxycycline. T.M.'s symptoms and fever initially resolve, but 2 days later his symptoms return. Physical examination at this time reveals a temperature of 39°C. Routine laboratory tests are normal, although leukopenia is observed with a WBC count of 2.4 × 10^9/L. Why do T.M.'s symptoms suggest a diagnosis of CTF?

Symptoms of CTF usually start 3 to 6 days after a tick bite, although roughly half of patients do not remember being bitten.[72,74] The most common initial symptoms are fever of rapid onset, headache, and chills without true rigors, and myalgias.[74] A rash, which may be light colored, is occasionally seen.[74,75] A biphasic ("saddle-back") or triphasic pattern of fever and other symptoms lasting 5 to 10 days has been observed.[72,73,74] CTF infection is usually self-limiting and sequelae are rare, although fatigue and malaise may last for months.[74] One- to 3-week periods of convalescence are usual. Children, however, experience complications more frequently than adults.[73] Severe forms of CTF may involve central nervous system (CNS) infection (aseptic meningitis or encephalitis), hemorrhagic fever, myo- or pericarditis.[72,75] A prolonged convalescence does not imply persistent viremia, although viremia can last for 3 to 4 months because of the intraerythrocytic location of the virus avoiding immune clearance.[72,73]

Laboratory Findings

Moderate to significant leukopenia is the most important finding in CTF. Leukocyte counts are usually normal on the first day, but decrease to 2 to 3 × 10^9/L by the fifth or sixth day of illness. In one third of confirmed CTF cases, however, the leukocyte counts remained around 4.5 × 10^9/L. Counts return to normal within a week of fever abatement in most cases. Thrombocytopenia may occur.[72] Occasionally, mildly elevated levels of creatinine phosphokinase and aspartate aminotransferase are reported.

Diagnosis and Treatment

The CTF diagnosis is made serologically, either with IFA staining of erythrocytes, complement fixation, or ELISA.[72] The most sensitive isolation system is intracerebral injection of infected blood into suckling mice.[72] Reverse transcriptase PCR was developed for CTF diagnosis.[72] Treatment is limited to supportive care.[72,73,75] A few deaths have been reported, all with hemorrhagic signs. Long-term immunity is generally conferred by CTFV infection.[72] Experimental CTF vaccines are no longer made.[72]

Tick-Borne Encephalitis (TBE)

Tick-borne encephalitis is divided into three subtypes, European, Siberian, and Far Eastern, and is endemic to central and eastern Europe, Russia, and the Far East, with some overlap in geography.[76,77] The highest incidence of TBE is in Latvia, the Urals, and western Siberia.

The etiologic agent is an RNA virus in the genus *Flavivirus.* The European subtype is transmitted to humans by *I. ricinus* and the Siberian and Far Eastern subtypes by *I. persulcatus,* although the latter tick and subtype were implicated in a Finnish outbreak.[77] Occasional TBE cases have followed the consumption of infected unpasteurized milk or cheese directly without a tick vector.[76] The virus reservoirs are small rodents. Ticks are vectors, and humans are accidental hosts of the virus.[76] Ticks can become infected for life by the virus at larval, nymphal, or adult stages and can transmit it transovarially and transstadially.[76]

As the disease name implies, the ultimate outcome of the infectious process is manifested as CNS involvement, with symptoms of aseptic meningitis, meningoencephalitis, and meningoencephalomyelitis. TBE begins as a febrile headache with progression to CNS manifestations. Treatment is supportive. Human TBE vaccines are available in some countries.[76,78]

THE TOXINS: TICK PARALYSIS

Tick Paralysis

20. **A.M., a 3-year-old girl residing in Spokane, Washington, complains of weakness in both legs. The next day, she begins experiencing flaccid paralysis in both legs and the lower trunk, although she is alert and oriented. Her mother discovers a tick attached to A.M.'s scalp under her hair and removes it. A.M. is back to full health in 2 days. What happened?**

Tick paralysis (tick toxicosis) occurs worldwide in humans and many animals and was first described by the explorer Hovell in Australia in 1824.[79,80] Although 43 tick species worldwide can produce tick paralysis in animals and humans, it is predominantly caused in humans by *Dermacentor andersoni* and *D. variabilis* in North America.[81] The other ticks implicated here are *A. americanum, A. maculatum, I. scapularis,* and *I. pacificus.*[80] In Australia, *I. holocyclus* is the culprit.

Most human cases occur during the spring and summer in Australia and the United States. In the United States, it is most common in the Pacific Northwest and Rocky Mountain states.[79,80] Female ticks are predominantly responsible.[79] In children, girls are more commonly affected, but in adults, more males are affected.[79]

The presumed cause of the disease is the secretion of a neurotoxin present in the saliva of a tick, which must usually be attached for 4 to 7 days before symptoms develop.[79,81] The toxin affects motor neurons and decreases acetylcholine release.[79] Paresthesias and symmetric weakness in the lower extremities with motor difficulties progress to an ascending flaccid paralysis in several hours or days.[82] Cerebral sensorium is usually spared, pain is absent, and the blood and CSF are normal.[80] If the tick is not removed, the toxicosis can progress to respiratory paralysis with death in 10% of cases.[79–81]

In North America, tick removal commonly results in complete recovery within hours to days. In Australia, the disease is more acute and paralysis may continue to progress for 2 days after tick removal. Recovery from the disease in Australia may take several weeks. Treatment is supportive. Antitoxin derived from dogs is the treatment of choice for animals, but not for humans because of the risk of serum sickness or acute reactions.[79]

MIXED INFECTIONS

21. **Because the tick vectors and mammalian hosts are the same for babesiosis, anaplasmosis, and Lyme disease in the northeastern United States, all three diseases, theoretically, could be transmitted to a human from one tick bite. Is there evidence of human coinfection with more than one tick-borne disease?**

Human coinfection by the agents of Lyme disease, babesiosis, or anaplasmosis can occur, especially in endemic areas.[83–85] Some believe that coinfection may alter the natural course for each disease, whereas others have found only an increase in clinical manifestations, especially flulike symptoms, in concurrent Lyme disease with babesiosis or HGA.[83,84]

Dual infection may affect the choice of initial antibiotic therapy. For example, although amoxicillin is sometimes used to treat early Lyme disease, it is not effective for HGA. Doxycycline, however, is useful in both of these diseases. Thus, some cases of Lyme disease that were believed to be treatment failures may actually have been confounded by coinfection. Patients with concurrent Lyme disease and babesiosis have more symptoms and a longer duration of illness compared with patients with single infections.[83,84] When moderate to severe Lyme disease is diagnosed, the possibility of concomitant babesial or anaplasma infection should be considered in regions where both diseases are endemic. Neutropenia and thrombocytopenia are associated with anaplasmosis; anemia and thrombocytopenia are associated with babesiosis and neither is routinely found in Lyme disease. For patients with Lyme disease who experience a prolonged flulike illness that fails to respond to appropriate antiborrelial therapy, clinicians should consider testing for babesiosis and anaplasmosis.[84]

SUMMARY

Most of the research into tick-borne human disease demonstrates a close historical relationship of endemic tick-deer-rodent cycles for various microorganisms. These cycles are almost exclusively identified as having occurred at the geologic sites of the terminal moraines of Ice Age glaciers. Given the recent explosion of deer populations in the United States and Europe, the increase in tick-borne human diseases may reflect the reduction of natural deer predators, the continued expansion of human populations from urban to rural environments, or both. Therefore, it is likely that we will continue to encounter increasing cases of tick-borne human disease of known or unknown origin.

REFERENCES

1. Parola P et al. Ticks and tickborne bacterial diseases in humans: an emerging infectious threat. *Clin Infect Dis* 2001;32:897.
2. Anderson JF. The natural history of ticks. *Med Clin North Am* 2002;86:205.
3. Wilson ME. Prevention of tick-borne diseases. *Med Clin North Am* 2002;86:219.
4. Shapiro ED et al. Lyme disease: fact versus fiction. *Pediatr Ann* 2002;31:170.
5. Steere AC. Lyme disease. *N Engl J Med* 2001;345: 115.
6. Baumgarten JM et al. Lyme disease. Part 1: Epidemiology and etiology. *Cutis* 2002;69:349.
7. Montiel NJ et al. Lyme disease. Part II: Clinical features and treatment. *Cutis* 2002;69:443.
8. Reid MC et al. The consequences of overdiagnosis and overtreatment of Lyme disease: an observational study. *Ann Intern Med* 1998;128:354.
9. Wormser GP et al. The clinical assessment, treatment, and prevention of Lyme disease, human granulocytic anaplasmosis, and babesiosis: clinical practice guidelines by the Infectious Diseases Society of America. *Clin Infect Dis* 2006;43: 1089.
10. Coyle PK et al. Neurologic aspects of Lyme disease. *Med Clin North Am* 2002:86:261.
11. Ramamoorthi N et al. The Lyme disease agent exploits a tick protein to infect the mammalian host. *Nature* 2005;436:573.
12. Lane RS et al. Refractoriness of the western fence lizard (Sceloporus occidentalis) to the Lyme disease group Borrelia bissettii. *J Parasitol* 2006;92: 691.
13. Clark K et al. Molecular identification and analysis of Borrelia burgdorferi sensu lato in lizards in the southeastern United States. *Appl Environ Microbiol* 2005;71:2616.
14. Sigal LH. Misconceptions about Lyme disease: confusions hiding behind ill-chosen terminology. *Ann Intern Med* 2002;136:413.
15. Cameron D et al. Evidence-based guidelines for the management of Lyme disease. *Expert Review Anti-infective Therapeutics* 2004;2:S1.
16. Donta ST. Tick-borne diseases. *Med Clin North Am* 2002;86:341.
17. Kalish RA et al. Persistence of immunoglobulin M or immunoglobulin G antibody responses to *Borrelia burgdorferi* 10 to 20 years after active Lyme disease. *Clin Infect Dis* 2001;33:780.
18. Edlow JA. Erythema migrans. *Med Clin North Am* 2002;86:239.
19. Anon. Treatment of Lyme disease. *Med Lett Drugs Ther* 2005;47:41.
20. Wormser GP et al. Practice guidelines for the treatment of Lyme disease. *Clin Infect Dis* 2000; 31:1.
21. Guerrau-de-Arellano M et al. Development of autoimmunity in Lyme arthritis. *Curr Opin Rheumatol* 2002;14:388.
22. Massarotti EM. Lyme arthritis. *Med Clin North Am* 2002;86:297.
23. Kaplan RF et al. Cognitive function in post-treatment Lyme disease do additional antibiotics help? *Neurology* 2003;60:1916.
24. Marques AR. Lyme disease: an update. *Curr Allergy Asthma Rep* 2001;1:541.
25. Wormser GP et al. A limitation of 2-stage serological testing for Lyme disease: enzyme immunoassay and immunoblot assay are not independent tests. *Clin Infect Dis* 2000;30:545.
26. Krupp LB et al. Study and treatment of post Lyme disease (stop-ld, a randomized double masked clinical trial. *Neurology* 2003;50:1923.
27. Stricker RB et al. Decreased dc57 lymphocyte subset in patients with chronic Lyme disease. *Immunol Lett* 2001;76:43.
28. Lin B et al. Soluble cd14 levels in the serum, synovial fluid, and cerebrospinal fluid of patients with various stages of Lyme disease. *J Infect Dis* 2000; 181:1185.
29. Philipp MT et al. C6 test as an indicator of therapy outcome for patients with localized or disseminated Lyme borreliosis. *J Clin Microbiol* 2003;41: 4955.
30. Peltomaa M et al. Persistence of the antibody response to the vise sixth invariant region (ir6) peptid of Borrelia burgdorferi after successful antibiotic treatment of Lyme disease. *J Infect Dis* 2003;187: 1178.
31. Anon. Picardin–a new insect repellent. *Med Lett Drugs Ther* 2005;47:46.
32. Anon. Lyme disease vaccination lawsuit. *Health-Keepers Magazine Spring* 2000;2:7.
33. Diego D et al. Neuroborreliosis during relapsing fever: review of the clinical manifestations, pathology, and treatment of infections in human and experimental animals. *Clin Infect Dis* 1998;26: 151.
34. Dworkin MS et al. Tick-borne relapsing fever in North America. *Med Clin North Am* 2002;86: 417.
35. Dworkin MS et al. Tick-borne relapsing fever in the northwestern United States and southwestern Canada. *Clin Infect Dis* 1998;26:122.
36. Amsden JR et al. Tick-borne bacterial, rickettsial, spirochetal, and protozoal infectious diseases in the United States: a comprehensive review. *Pharmacotherapy* 2003;25:191.
37. Bunikis J et al. Laboratory testing for suspected Lyme disease. *Med Clin North Am* 2002;86: 311.
38. Richter D et al. Relapsing fever-like spirochetes infecting European vector tick of Lyme disease agent. *Emerg Infect Dis* 2003;9:697.
39. Hasin T et al. Postexposure treatment with doxycycline for the prevention of tick-borne relapsing fever. *N Engl J Med* 2006;355:148.
40. Storch GA. New developments in tick-borne infections. *Pediatr Ann* 2002;31:200.
41. Varela AS et al. First culture isolation of Borrelia lonestari, putative agent of southern tick-associated rash illness. *J Clin Microbiol* 2004;42: 1163.
42. Wormser GP et al. Microbiologic evaluation of patients from Missouri with erythema migrans. *Clin Infect Dis* 2005;40:423.
43. Choi E. Tularemia and Q fever. *Med Clin North Am* 2002;86:393.
44. Hornick R. Tularemia revisited. *N Engl J Med* 2001;345:1637.
45. Bryant KA. Tularemia: lymphadenitis with a twist. *Pediatr Ann* 2002;31:187.
46. Anon. Tularemia transmitted by insect bites—Wyoming 2001–2003. *MMWR* 2005;564:170.
47. Tularemia, United States, 1900–2000. *MMWR* 2002;51:182.
48. Perez-Castrillon JL et al. Tularemia epidemic in northwestern Spain: clinical description and therapeutic response. *Clin Infect Dis* 2001;33: 573.
49. Maurin M et al. Bacterial activities of antibiotics against intracellular Francisella tularensis. *Antimicrob Agents Chemother* 2000;44:3428.
50. Dennis DT et al. Tularemia as a biological weapon: medical and public health management. *JAMA* 2001;285:2763.
51. Sexton DJ et al. Rocky Mountain spotted fever. *Med Clin North Am* 2002;86:351.
52. Centers for Disease Control and Prevention. Diagnosis and management of tickborne rickettsial diseases: Rocky Mountain spotted fever, ehrlichiosis, and anaplasmosis-United States: a practical guide for physicians and other health-care and public health officials. *MMWR* 2006;55(RR-4):1.
53. Marshall GS et al. Antibodies reactive to Rickettsia rickettsii among children living in the southeast and south central regions of the United States. *Arch Pediatr Adolesc Med* 2003;167: 443.
54. Demma LJ et al. Rocky mountain spotted fever from an unexpected tick vector in Arizona. *N Engl J Med* 2005;353:587.
55. Sexton DJ. Acute hearing loss and rickettsial diseases. *Clin Infect Dis* 2006;42:1506
56. Thorner AR et al. Rocky Mountain spotted fever. *Clin Infect Dis* 1998;27:1353.
57. Donovan BJ et al. Treatment of tick-borne diseases. *Ann Pharmacother* 2002;36:1590.
58. Paddock CD et al. Rickettsia parkeri: a newly recognized cause of spotted fever rickettsiosis in the United States. *Clin Infect Dis* 2004;38: 805.
59. Raoult D et al. Rickettsia parkeri infection and other spotted fevers in the United States. *N Engl J Med* 2005;353:6.
60. Whitman TJ et al. Rickettsia parkeri infection after tick bite, Virginia. *Emerg Infect Dis* 2007;13: 334.
61. Raoult D. A new rickettsial disease in the United States. *Clin Infect Dis* 2004;36:812.
62. Zaidi SA et al. Gastrointestinal and hepatic manifestations of tickborne diseases in the United States. *Clin Infect Dis* 2002;34:1206.
63. Olano JP et al. Human ehrlichioses. *Med Clin North Am* 2002;86:375.
64. Buller RS et al. *Ehrlichia ewingii*, a newly recognized agent of human ehrlichiosis. *N Engl J Med* 1999;341:148.
65. des Vinges F et al. Effect of tick removal on transmission of *Borrelia burgdorferi* and *Ehrlichia phagocytophilia* by *Ixodes scapularis* nymphs. *J Infect Dis* 2001;183:773.
66. Bakken JS et al. Human granulocytic ehrlichiosis. *Clin Infect Dis* 2000;31:554.
67. Hongo I et al. Comparison of clinical features among patients infected with Ehrlichial ewingii and Ehrlichial chaffeensis. 44th IDSA abstracts October 2006;133.
68. Krause PJ et al. Successful treatment of human granulocytic ehrlichiosis in children using rifampin. *Pediatrics* 2003;112:e252.
69. Krause PJ. Babesiosis. *Med Clin North Am* 2002;86: 361.
70. Lantos PM et al. Babesiosis: similar to malaria but different. *Pediatr Ann* 2002;31:192.
71. Shulman ST. Ticks! *Pediatr Ann* 2002;31:154.
72. Attoui H et al. Coltiviruses and seadornarviruses in North America, Europe and Asia. *Emerg Infect Dis* 2005;11:1673.
73. Klasco R. Colorado tick fever. *Med Clin North Am* 2002;86:435.
74. Midoneck SR et al. Colorado tick fever in a resident of New York City. *Arch Fam Med* 1994;3:731.
75. Smith DS. Medical encyclopedia: Colorado tick fever. 2006. Available at www.nlm.nih.gov/medlineplus/ency/article/000675.htm. Accessed March 10, 2006.
76. Dumpis U et al. Tick-borne encephalitis. *Clin Infect Dis* 1999;28:882.

77. Jaaskelainen AE et al. Siberian subtype tickborne encephalitis virus, Finland. *Emerg Infect Dis* 2006; 12:1568.
78. Bratu S et al. Active immunization against human tick-borne diseases. *Expert Opin Biol Ther* 2002;2:187.
79. Greenstein P. Tick paralysis. *Med Clin North Am* 2002;86:441.
80. Dworkin MS et al. Tick paralysis: 33 human cases in Washington state, 1946–1996. *Clin Infect Dis* 1999;29:1435.
81. Centers for Disease Control and Prevention. Cluster of tick paralysis cases—Colorado, 2006. *MMWR* 2006;55:933.
82. Lotric-Furlan S et al. Is an isolated initial phase of a tick-borne encephalitis a common event? [letter]. *Clin Infect Dis* 2000;30:987.
83. Thompson C et al. Coinfecting deer-associated zoonoses: Lyme disease babesiosis, and ehrlichiosis. *Clin Infect Dis* 2001;33:676.
84. Krause PJ et al. Disease-specific diagnosis of coinfecting tickborne zoonoses: babesiosis, human granulocytic ehrlichiosis and Lyme disease. *Clin Infect Dis* 2002;34:1184.
85. Steere AC et al. Prospective study of coinfection in patients with erythema migrans. *Clin Infect Dis* 2003;36:1078.

SECTION SIXTEEN

PSYCHIATRIC DISORDERS

Patrick R. Finley and Kelly C. Lee
SECTION EDITOR

CHAPTER 76

Anxiety Disorders

Sally K. Guthrie and Sara Grimsley Augustin

OVERVIEW

Anxiety can be described as an uncomfortable feeling of vague fear or apprehension accompanied by characteristic physical sensations. It is a normal reaction to a perceived threat to one's physical or psychological well-being. The anxiety reaction is normally provoked by stress of some sort and involves activation of neurobiological systems that, when activated, contribute to self-preservation. Anxiety serves the purpose of alerting us to take appropriate measures for dealing with stressful circumstances. Anxiety involves the perturbation of several different neural systems causing two basic components: mental features (e.g., worry, fear, difficulty concentrating) and physical symptoms (e.g., racing heart, shortness of breath, trembling, pacing). An activation of these same systems can also be caused by certain medical illnesses such as pheochromocytoma or hyperthyroidism or medications such as sympathomimetics, resulting in both the physical and psychological manifestations of anxiety. However, when the anxiety is due to an external cause such as a medical illness or a medication, the anxiety abates when the physiological cause is removed.[1]

If the anxiety is not due to an external cause such as a medical illness or a medication, and it is out of proportion to the actual threat or when the anxiety lasts far beyond the presence of the threat, anxiety may impair normal functioning and become an anxiety disorder. The anxiety experienced by a person is excessive for the situation (in intensity or duration) or very distressing, to the point that it interferes with daily functioning. Pathological anxiety can be differentiated according to whether it occurs (a) as a primary anxiety disorder, (b) as a secondary anxiety disorder due to medical causes or substances, (c) in response to acute stress (e.g., loss of a loved one, marital or family problems), or (d) as a symptom associated with other psychiatric disorders. This differentiation can be difficult, but is important in guiding optimal treatment.

Classification and Diagnosis of Anxiety Disorders

The *Diagnostic and Statistical Manual of Mental Disorders, Fourth Edition, Text Revision* (DSM-IV-TR) classifies primary anxiety disorders into six types: generalized anxiety disorder (GAD), panic disorder, phobic disorders (including social anxiety disorder), obsessive-compulsive disorder (OCD), posttraumatic stress disorder (PTSD), and acute stress disorder.[1] The additional category of "Anxiety Disorder Not Otherwise Specified" is used for cases not meeting the diagnostic criteria for any of these six types or for cases in which it cannot be determined whether the anxiety disorder is primary or secondary. Each disorder involves an unhealthy level of anxiety, but the characteristic type and severity of symptoms, as well as course of illness, vary from one disorder to another. Efficacy of drug and nondrug treatments also varies between disorders, indicating underlying biological differences. The DSM-IV-TR secondary anxiety disorders include "anxiety disorder due to a general medical condition" and "substance-induced anxiety disorder."[1] An anxiety disorder may occur in the absence of other psychiatric disorders, but it is often present in addition to other psychiatric disorders, such as mood disorders. Although anxiety disorders and mood disorders are classified separately in the DSM-IV-TR, a perusal of the criteria for both diagnostic categories reveals they have much in common, including fatigue, impaired concentration, restlessness, difficulties with sleep, and somatic symptoms. The main difference is that mood disorders have a prominent mood factor. Both anxiety and mood disorders appear to be associated with dysregulations in the limbic system of the brain, which is involved in emotion, learning, and memory.[2]

Neurobiology of Anxiety

The limbic system is composed of a set of structures that are integral to behavior, including the two key structures, the hippocampus and the amygdala. Hippocampal brain circuits are essential for conversion of short-term to long-term memory and for spatial memory, whereas the amygdala circuits are involved with emotion and its expression. A neurocircuit arising from the output pathways of the central nucleus of the amygdala is believed to mediate fear and anxiety responses in humans.[3] Dysregulated or exaggerated output through various amygdala-related circuits may be a common element underlying the different anxiety disorders, but the specific type of dysfunction probably differs among the various disorders. If it is assumed that a dysregulation of the stress response is the basis of anxiety disorders, then the genesis of anxiety is probably related primarily to interactions between neural pathways in and between the limbic system, the sympathetic nervous system, and the hypothalamic-pituitary-adrenocortical (HPA) axis.[2,4] It is becoming clear that neither anxiety nor depression is solely due to abnormalities of neurotransmitter systems because these systems regulate and are regulated by other neurocircuits. Many neurotransmitter systems interact to modulate the actions of the limbic pathways, including the monoamine neurotransmitters, epinephrine and norepinephrine (NE); corticotrophin-releasing hormone (CRH); the indoleamine, serotonin (5-HT); the inhibitory amino acid, γ-aminobutyric acid (GABA); the excitatory amino acid, glutamate; and the neuropeptides, cholecystokinin (CCK), neuropeptide Y (NPY), and substance P.[3,5]

Interaction of the Hypothalamic-Pituitary-Adrenocortical, Noradrenergic, and Serotonergic Systems

In the event of an acute threat, the fight-or-flight response stimulates both the peripheral and central sympathetic systems. This results in the peripheral reactions such as increased heart rate, heart stroke volume, and vasodilation of blood vessels carrying blood to the muscles. This is accompanied by a release of NE by the locus ceruleus (LC), the main nidus of NE cell bodies in the brain. Central release of NE results in vigilance and arousal, and the ability to focus attention on the threat and its stimulation in response to stress or fear produces arousal and symptoms of anxiety (tachycardia, tremor, sweating). NE innervation of the hippocampus results in an increased state of memory formation, whereas innervation of the amygdala potentiates the formation of aversive memories.[4] Normally, this is important in allowing us to encode emotionally laden memories, but when overactive, it may result in a constant state of arousal and hypervigilance.

During a perceived threat, concomitant with activation of the sympathetic nervous system, the HPA axis is also activated. Initially, both CRH and arginine vasopressin (AVP) are released in the hypothalamus. CRH and AVP activate the anterior pituitary to release adrenocorticotropic hormone (ACTH), which stimulates the release of glucocorticoid steroids from the adrenal cortex. The glucocorticoids act on cells by increasing gene transcription, which can take up to several hours. This explains why the sympathetic response occurs more rapidly than the glucocorticoid response. The glucocorticoids bind to receptors both peripherally and in the brain. Although short-term elevation of glucocorticoids allows the body to adapt to a stressful situation by supporting HPA activation and mobilizing energy stores, prolonged elevation of the same glucocorticoids impairs neural plasticity and may even result in neuronal death. Both the sympathetic system and the HPA axis responses are modulated by limbic brain circuits innervating the amygdala, hippocampus, and orbital/medial prefrontal cortex. CRH is released not only in the hypothalamus, but also in the amygdala as well as in the LC. Its actions involve more than just activation of the HPA axis. CRH binds to at least two specific receptors in the brain, CR_1 and CR_2 receptors. These receptors modulate the actions of a variety of neurotransmitters, including NE, 5-HT, glutamate, and dopamine. When CRH is infused into the LC in rodents, it causes anxiety-like behaviors.[2,4]

Although the inhibitory neurotransmitter, 5-HT, is involved in stress reactions, its role is not entirely clear. 5-HT has roles in sleep, appetite, memory, impulsivity, sexual behavior, and motor function, and seems to decrease aggressive behavior. The site of most 5-HT cell bodies in the brain is the raphe nuclei. There is considerable interconnectivity between the raphe nuclei and the LC, and they tend to mutually inhibit one another. Under normal circumstances, 5-HT connections from the hippocampus decrease activity in the amygdala, which would dampen fear and anxiety responses. However, under conditions of stress, the LC accelerates firing, inhibits the raphe nuclei firing, and increases CRH release—all of which sensitize the limbic system and cause arousal and sensitivity to memory of any stressful or aversive stimuli. This primes the system to a state of arousal to deal with the threat.[2]

One hypothesis is that anxiety states are associated with chronic NE overactivity combined with decreased activity in the 5-HT system.[2] This would maintain the amygdala and hippocampal and cortical pathways associated with the stress reaction in a stable state of hyperarousal. In this state, a minor fear response might be associated with a disproportionately large fear/aversion response. This would result in a chronic activation of the HPA axis. Chronically elevated corticosteroid levels have been shown to contribute to hippocampal and cerebral atrophy. A loss of inhibitory pathways that contribute to a halting of the stress response could lead to a chronic state of arousal and anxiety in the absence of any specific external stimulation of the stress pathways.

Although the specific etiology of anxiety is only hypothesized, the current use of treatments that activate the 5-HT system, or other inhibitory systems such as the GABA system, support the hypothesis.

Epidemiology and Clinical Significance of Anxiety Disorders

As a group, the anxiety disorders are the most common of psychiatric illnesses. Epidemiologic surveys indicate that one in four Americans suffer from an anxiety disorder at some time in their lives and that 18% are affected in any given year.[6,7] Most anxiety disorders are more common in women than in men.[7]

Anxiety disorders are associated with a decrease in quality of life and psychosocial functioning. These factors impact marital, educational, and employment status. Although most anxiety disorders do not require inpatient hospitalization for treatment, their presence is associated with significant impairment in major areas of life functioning.[8]

Today, most anxiety disorders are highly treatable with medications, cognitive or behavioral therapies, or combinations thereof. However, less than one-third of those affected seek help, and many who do are not properly diagnosed.[7] Most medical care for anxiety disorders is rendered in nonpsychiatric settings. Patients commonly present to primary care providers complaining of physical symptoms that cannot be medically explained, while the anxiety continues unrecognized. A large portion of primary care patients with anxiety do not believe in taking medication for emotional problems or are not taking medication to treat their anxiety because their primary care provider did not recommend it.[9]

Because anxiety is a feeling with which everyone is familiar, there is a tendency to trivialize the impact it can have on a sufferer's functioning and quality of life. An increased understanding about pathological anxiety is needed in society in general and health care professionals in particular so that people seek and receive the treatment they need. Widespread public educational campaigns have been initiated to help increase awareness about anxiety disorders and their potential treatments. Practitioners must be knowledgeable about the clinical characteristics and treatment options for various disorders, and must be able to share this information with patients and other health care professionals. A list of consumer and professional resources for information about anxiety disorders and treatment can be found in Table 76-1.

Clinical Assessment and Differential Diagnosis of Anxiety

1. J.K., a 66-year-old man, complains to his physician of having trouble sleeping, feeling nervous, and worrying constantly. J.K.'s wife passed away 1 year ago, and he recently retired from his job as an accountant. Since then, he has become very involved in his hobbies of gardening and writing short stories but claims that he often cannot concentrate well enough to write. J.K. has mild chronic obstructive pulmonary disease (COPD) and suffered a myocardial infarction (MI) 2 years ago. His currently prescribed medications include lisinopril (Zestril), furosemide (Lasix), atorvastatin (Lipitor), niacin, and sucralfate. He also takes over-the-counter (OTC) loratadine and pseudoephedrine for allergies, naproxen for back pain, and docusate sodium as needed (PRN) for constipation. J.K. states that he drinks several cups of coffee each morning and one or two glasses of beer several nights a week to help him calm down when he has had a stressful day. He denies any history of psychiatric illness but states that he has always been a "high-strung" individual. What factors should be considered in the clinical assessment and differential diagnosis of J.K.'s symptoms of anxiety?

A diagnostic decision tree such as that in Figure 76-1 can be used to assist the clinician in differentiating among various causes of anxiety and the different anxiety disorders. According to DSM-IV-TR criteria for primary anxiety disorders, the symptoms should not be secondary to any medical (drug or

Table 76-1 Resource Organizations for Anxiety Disorders

Anxiety Coach 5105 Tollview Drive Rolling Meadows, IL 60008 (847) 481-5251 Website: www.anxietycoach.com
Anxiety Disorders Association of America 8730 Georgia Avenue, Suite 600 Silver Spring, MD 20910 (240) 485-1001 Website: www.adaa.org
Freedom From Fear 308 Seaview Avenue Staten Island, NY 10305 (718) 351-1717 Website: www.freedomfromfear.org
Mental Health America 2000 N. Beauregard Street, 6th Floor Alexandria, VA 22311 (800) 969-6642 Website: www.nmha.org/
MentalHelp.net Website: http://mentalhelp.net
Obsessive Compulsive Foundation 676 State Street New Haven, CT 06511 (203) 401-2070 Website: www.ocfoundation.org
PTSD Gateway (877) 507-PTSD Website: www.ptsdinfo.org
Social Phobia/Social Anxiety Association 2058 E. Topeka Drive Phoenix, AZ 85024 Website: www.socialphobia.org

disease) causes. As illustrated in Table 76-2, the potential "organic" or secondary sources for anxiety symptoms are numerous.

Secondary Causes of Anxiety

A diagnosis *of anxiety disorder due to a general medical condition* is warranted when symptoms are believed to be the direct physiological consequence of a medical condition.[1] In patients such as J.K. who have a number of medical conditions, these illnesses must be considered as possible underlying precipitants of anxiety. A complete physical and laboratory workup, with a thorough medical and psychiatric history, are also needed to exclude other, possibly reversible causes before a primary anxiety disorder diagnosis is considered. In most cases of new-onset anxiety in elderly persons, symptoms can be attributed to some medical or substance-related cause.

Hypoglycemia, hyperthyroidism, electrolyte abnormalities, and angina pectoris are notably associated with anxiety symptoms.[10] Persons with chronic medical conditions such as COPD, Parkinson disease, cardiomyopathy, post-MI, Graves disease, and primary biliary cirrhosis have prevalences of anxiety that are markedly increased compared with healthy controls.[10] Medical illness in general, especially in older patients such as J.K., is associated with higher rates of both anxiety and depression compared with the general population.[10] In some cases, the anxiety is physically induced by the medical condition, but reactional anxiety may also occur in response to being faced with a medical illness, especially a serious illness. In either case, the presence of anxiety may complicate the medical picture and have a negative impact on the course of illness. Successful management of the medical condition often relieves anxiety in such cases, but short-term use of anxiolytic medications or nondrug therapies (biofeedback, psychotherapy) can also be very helpful.

When evaluating for possible causes of anxiety, it is also important to consider all medications a person is taking, including OTC drugs such as cough and cold preparations.[11] A diagnosis of *substance-induced anxiety disorder* is warranted when anxiety symptoms occur in relation to substance intoxication or withdrawal, or when medication use causes the symptoms. Among the medications that J.K. is taking, pseudoephedrine might be contributing to his anxiety. Other medications that can cause anxiety are listed in Table 76-2. Psychoactive substance abuse, withdrawal from CNS depressants (e.g., alcohol, barbiturates, benzodiazepines), excessive caffeine intake, and nicotine withdrawal may go unrecognized as underlying precipitants of anxiety. J.K.'s current pattern of alcohol use, although not excessive, may become problematic if he uses alcohol to self-medicate his anxiety symptoms.

Although anxiety is the hallmark characteristic of anxiety disorders, it is not unique to this diagnostic category. Virtually any psychiatric illness may present with anxiety symptoms. Major depression, schizophrenia, bipolar disorder (both depressive and manic phases), eating disorders, and dysthymia are notably associated with anxiety, and diagnostic differentiation can sometimes be difficult.[1] For example, J.K.'s difficulties with sleeping and concentrating, as well as excessive worry, may be core target symptoms of either anxiety or depression, or possibly both. If anxiety symptoms occur only in relation to another psychiatric disorder, then a separate anxiety disorder diagnosis is precluded. Anxiety in these cases may be alleviated with successful treatment of the primary psychiatric disorder. However, benzodiazepines are often used as adjunctive therapy, especially early in the course of treatment because they have a rapid onset of action.

Individuals with other psychiatric disorders can also have a primary anxiety disorder. In fact, comorbidity with anxiety disorders is the rule rather than the exception.[6] Depression, in particular, is notably associated with anxiety disorders, and there are marked degrees of comorbidity between the two.[12] Concurrent anxiety and depression are associated with greater disability, poorer treatment outcomes, and higher suicide rates than either depression or anxiety alone.

Other factors that should be considered in J.K. are the recent changes in his life (retiring, losing his spouse). Anxiety in response to life stressors may be severe and functionally detrimental, but could be considered appropriate for the

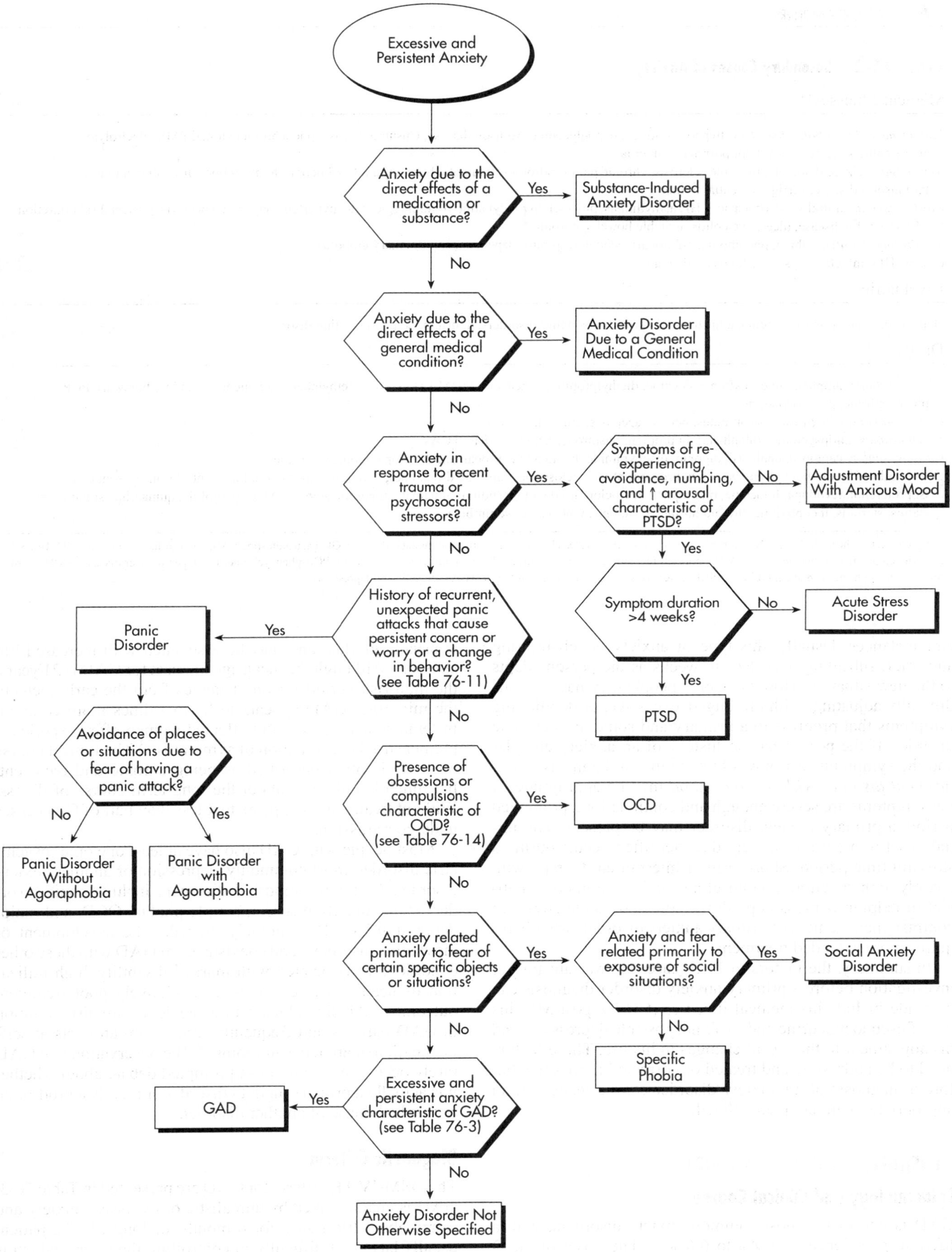

FIGURE 76-1 Diagnostic decision tree for anxiety disorders. GAD, generalized anxiety disorder; OCD, obsessive-compulsive disorder; PTSD, posttraumatic stress disorder.

Table 76-2 Secondary Causes of Anxiety

Medical Illnesses	
Endocrine and metabolic disorders:	hyperthyroidism, hypoglycemia, Addison disease, Cushing disease, pheochromocytoma, PMS, electrolyte abnormalities, acute intermittent porphyria, anemia
Neurologic:	seizure disorders, multiple sclerosis, chronic pain syndromes, traumatic brain injury, CNS neoplasm, migraines, myasthenia gravis, Parkinson's disease, vertigo, essential tremor
Cardiovascular:	mitral valve prolapse, CHF, arrhythmias, post-MI, hyperdynamic β-adrenergic state, hypertension, angina pectoris, postcerebral infarction
GI:	PUD, Crohn disease, ulcerative colitis, irritable bowel syndrome
Respiratory:	COPD, asthma, pneumonia, pulmonary edema, respirator dependence, pulmonary embolus
Others:	HIV infection, systemic lupus erythematosus
Psychiatric	
	Depression, mania, schizophrenia, adjustment disorder, personality disorders, delirium, dementia, eating disorders
Drugs	
CNS stimulants:	amphetamines, caffeine, cocaine, diethylpropion, ephedrine, MDMA (Ecstasy), methylphenidate, nicotine (and withdrawal), PCP, phenylephrine, pseudoephedrine
CNS depressant withdrawal:	barbiturates, benzodiazepines, ethanol, opiates
Psychotropics:	antipsychotics (akathisia), bupropion, buspirone, SNRIs, SSRIs, TCAs
Cardiovascular:	captopril, enalapril, digoxin, disopyramide, hydralazine, procainamide, propafenone, reserpine
Others:	albuterol, aminophylline, baclofen, bromocriptine, cycloserine, dapsone, dronabinol, efavirenz, fluoroquinolones, interferon-α, isoniazid, isoproterenol, levodopa, lidocaine, mefloquine, metoclopramide, monosodium glutamate, nicotinic acid, NSAIDs, pergolide, quinacrine, sibutramine, statins, steroids, theophylline, thyroid hormone, triptans, vinblastine, yohimbine

CHF, congestive heart failure; CNS, central nervous system; COPD, chronic obstructive pulmonary disease; GI, gastrointestinal; MI, myocardial infarction; MDMA, 3,4-methylenedioxymethamphetamine; NSAIDs, nonsteroidal anti-inflammatory drugs; PMS, premenstrual syndrome; PCP, phencyclidine; PUD, peptic ulcer disease; SNRIs, serotonin/norepinephrine reuptake inhibitors; SSRIs, selective serotonin reuptake inhibitors; TCAs, tricyclic antidepressants.

circumstances. Usually, this type of anxiety is self-limiting and brief, subsiding over days to weeks as the person adapts to the new situation. However, some people may have serious difficulty adjusting, with prolonged, excessive, or debilitating symptoms that progress to a primary and sometimes chronic disorder. If the person has no history of an anxiety disorder and the symptoms last only a few months, a diagnosis of *adjustment disorder with anxious mood* may be appropriate. If the symptoms are severe enough and continue for a prolonged period, a primary anxiety disorder may be present. The initial onset of a chronic anxiety disorder often occurs during a stressful time period. Short-term or intermittent therapy with anxiolytic medication or counseling can be extremely beneficial in helping persons cope during times of acute stress. In contrast, management of primary anxiety disorders usually requires more extended treatment.

In summary, the factors in J.K.'s case that warrant further investigation before a primary anxiety disorder diagnosis can be made include his medical illnesses (COPD, post-MI), his use of pseudoephedrine and caffeine, possible depression, and his adjustment to the recent changes in his life. These factors need to be addressed, and treated or corrected if possible, before a diagnosis of an anxiety disorder can be made and an appropriate treatment plan defined.

GENERALIZED ANXIETY DISORDER

Epidemiology and Clinical Course

GAD is one of the most common anxiety disorders, with a lifetime prevalence of 3.9% to 6.6%.[1,7] The onset of GAD is usually gradual and may be associated with increased life stressors. Although the mean age of onset for GAD is 21 years, the high-risk period for onset ranges from the early teens to the mid-50s.[7] GAD appears to be two times more common in females than males, and affected women often experience premenstrual exacerbation of symptoms.[13] The typical course of GAD is often described as being chronic and recurrent, but much is unknown about the long-term course of illness. Without treatment, it appears that less than half of GAD cases undergo remission.

Most people with GAD also have at least one other psychiatric disorder, most commonly, depression or another anxiety disorder. Common comorbid disorders include panic disorder, social anxiety disorder, simple phobia, OCD, and major depression.[6] GAD commonly precedes the development of these other disorders, and coexistence of GAD with these other conditions is associated with marked disability, high utilization of health care resources, and relatively poor treatment outcomes.[7] Alcohol abuse and dependence are also common in GAD patients and frequently result from attempts at self-medication of anxiety symptoms.[14] The observation that GAD rarely occurs in isolation has prompted debate about whether it is actually a primary anxiety disorder or merely a prodromal or residual phase of another disorder.

Diagnostic Criteria

The DSM-IV-TR criteria for GAD are presented in Table 76-3. GAD is characterized by unrealistic or excessive anxiety and worry about life issues for 6 months or longer.[1] The patient usually has great difficulty in controlling the worry, which is

Table 76-3 Diagnostic Criteria for Generalized Anxiety Disorder

1. Unrealistic or excessive anxiety and worry about life circumstances for a period of at least 6 months, during which the person has been bothered more days than not by these concerns
2. Person has difficulty controlling anxiety and worry
3. Anxiety and worry are associated with at least three of the following symptoms:
   a. Restlessness or feeling keyed up or on edge
   b. Easy fatigue
   c. Difficulty concentrating or mind going blank
   d. Irritability
   e. Muscle tension
   f. Sleep disturbances
4. If another psychiatric disorder is present, the focus of the anxiety and worry is unrelated to it
5. Anxiety, worry, or physical symptoms cause significant distress or impairment in social, occupational, or some other important aspect of functioning
6. Disturbance is not due to the direct effects of a substance, medication, or general medical condition and does not occur only during the course of a mood disorder, psychotic disorder, or pervasive developmental disorder

Adapted from reference 1, with permission. Copyright ©2000 American Psychiatric Association.

accompanied by at least three of the associated symptoms listed in Table 76-3. Although some types of physical symptoms are similar between GAD and other anxiety disorders, the course of the symptoms varies between disorders. If the anxiety is related solely to another anxiety disorder (e.g., obsession with germs, fear of being in social situations), a diagnosis of GAD is not warranted.

In children with GAD (also called "overanxious disorder of childhood"), the duration requirement for symptoms is only 1 month.[1] Excessive worry in this younger population typically involves performance in school or sports, punctuality, perfectionism, and the possibility of catastrophic events. Children with GAD commonly seek excessive reassurance and approval from others.

Etiology and Pathophysiology

Genetic factors play a modest, but significant role in the etiology of GAD. The genes involved in the hereditary development of GAD are believed to be the same as those in major depression, with environmental factors determining which disorder is expressed in an individual.[5,15] Biological studies in GAD have found abnormalities in the noradrenergic, serotonergic, and CCK systems, as well as in GABA-A receptor function.[5] Several studies report decreased α_2-adrenergic receptors in GAD patients, and this is believed to represent downregulation of receptors in response to high catecholamine levels. Abnormally low levels of lymphocyte peripheral benzodiazepine receptors (PBRs) have been reported by several investigators. GAD patients have also shown enhanced anxiety in response to CCK-4 administration compared with normal controls, suggesting an increased sensitivity of the CCK system in GAD.

Treatment of Generalized Anxiety Disorder

Nonpharmacologic Treatments

Management of GAD can involve both nonpharmacologic and pharmacologic therapies. Nondrug treatments such as supportive psychotherapy, dynamic psychotherapy, cognitive therapy, relaxation training, and meditation exercises are often helpful in relieving anxiety and improving coping skills.[16] Cognitive therapy is aimed at identifying negative thought patterns that may provoke or worsen anxiety and changing them to be more positive. Combined cognitive-behavioral therapy (CBT) has been associated with significant reductions in anxiety that are maintained over 6 to 12 months, as well as decreased psychiatric comorbidity in GAD.[16] Controlled comparisons of cognitive therapies and benzodiazepine treatment have reported comparable efficacies in GAD.[16] Although psychosocial treatments are commonly recommended as first-line therapy for GAD and other anxiety disorders, they are vastly underused due to cost (many insurance providers offer limited coverage for outpatient psychotherapy) and time requirements, as well as a limited availability of trained therapists. The decline in use of psychosocial therapies for anxiety disorders over the past decade also correlates with the explosion in medication options for treating anxiety disorders.

Benzodiazepines

Benzodiazepines are still widely prescribed anxiolytic agents, and their efficacy in treating GAD and many other anxiety disorders is well established.[14] The benzodiazepines offer distinct clinical advantages over older agents such as barbiturates, meprobamate, paraldehyde, and alcohol. These advantages include more specific anxiolytic effects, lower fatality rates from acute toxicity and overdose (when taken alone), better side effect profiles, lower potential for abuse, and less dangerous interactions with other drugs. Currently, use of these older nonbenzodiazepine agents as anxiolytics is generally considered inappropriate because of the many advantages of benzodiazepines and other newer agents.

MECHANISM OF ACTION

In humans, benzodiazepines have four distinct effects: anxiolytic, anticonvulsant, muscle relaxant, and sedative-hypnotic. These agents are used to treat a wide variety of medical and psychiatric conditions, including muscle spasms, seizures, anxiety disorders, acute agitation, and insomnia. Benzodiazepines with a rapid onset and a short duration of action are commonly used to decrease anxiety and apprehension, as well as induce sedation before surgery and other medical procedures.

The mechanism of action of benzodiazepines involves potentiation of GABA by binding to sites on the central GABA-A receptor. There are four types of GABA-A receptors that are benzodiazepine sensitive; these are distinguished by the type of α subunit they contain (α_1, α_2, α_3, or α_5).[17,18] Benzodiazepine binding sites on α_1-GABA-A and α_2-GABA-A receptors were formerly called BZ-1 and BZ-2 receptors, respectively, but there is a trend away from use of the latter terminology. Receptors with an α_1 subunit are widely distributed throughout most brain areas and are the most abundant type. Benzodiazepine interaction at the α_1-GABA-A receptors produces sedative and amnestic effects, whereas anxiolytic effects are associated with binding to the α_2-GABA-A receptor.[17,19] This latter type of GABA-A receptor is localized mainly in the limbic system, cerebral cortex, and striatum. GABA-A receptors with α_3 subunits are linked with noradrenergic, serotonergic, and cholinergic neurons.

Currently available benzodiazepine anxiolytics do not have selective activity at any of the four GABA-A receptor subtypes. Research is aimed at developing benzodiazepine compounds with specific affinity for the α_2-GABA-A receptor, which would produce anxiolytic effects without sedative and amnestic effects.[20] Agents that are partial agonists at α_2-GABA-A receptors are also being studied as potential anxiolytics; these would be associated with minimal tolerance, dependence, and withdrawal.[20] Zolpidem (Ambien), észopiclone (Lunesta), and zaleplon (Sonata) are examples of selective α_1-GABA-A receptor agonists that have been introduced as selective hypnotic agents.

CLINICAL COMPARISON OF BENZODIAZEPINES

Approximately 35 benzodiazepine compounds are marketed worldwide. Of the 13 benzodiazepines commercially available in the United States, 7 are marketed as antianxiety agents, and 6 as oral sedative-hypnotics. These indications reflect the manufacturers' labeling decisions because the anxiolytics can be effective sedatives and vice versa.

Table 76-4 compares the clinical profiles of marketed oral benzodiazepines. Midazolam (Versed) is not included on Table 76-4. It is a short-acting, water-soluble benzodiazepine, indicated only for induction of sedation before surgery or for short diagnostic or endoscopic procedures. It was previously marketed only in parenteral formulation, but an oral syrup form is now available. Clonazepam (Klonopin) was originally approved only as an anticonvulsant, but is now also indicated for the treatment of panic disorder. Clonazepam and most of the other benzodiazepines also have many unlabeled uses, including treatment of anxiety and agitation associated with various medical or psychiatric illnesses, GAD, and other anxiety disorders; irritable bowel syndrome; premenstrual syndrome; chemotherapy-induced nausea and vomiting; catatonia; tetanus; involuntary movement disorders (restless legs syndrome, periodic limb movements of sleep, akathisia, tardive dyskinesia, essential tremor); and spasticity associated with various neurologic disorders (cerebral palsy, paraplegia).

Antidepressant Agents

Antidepressants have now surpassed benzodiazepines as the recommended first-line treatment for most anxiety disorder patients, even though benzodiazepines are still widely prescribed. One important clinical difference between these two medication classes is that the anxiolytic effects of benzodiazepines occur almost immediately, whereas the effects of antidepressants occur gradually over several weeks. For this reason, it is common practice for short-term benzodiazepine therapy to be prescribed in combination with an antidepressant during initial treatment of many anxiety disorders.

The first indication that antidepressants might be effective in the treatment of anxiety disorders appeared in the late 1970s, when certain tricyclic antidepressants (TCAs) and monoamine oxidase inhibitors (MAOIs) were found to be useful in treating

Table 76-4 Clinical Comparison of Benzodiazepine Agents

Drug (Trade Name, Generic)	*FDA-Approved Indications*	*Usual Dosage Range Through 65 Years of Age*	*Maximum Recommended Dosage Through 65 Years of Age*	*Approximate Dosage Equivalencies*	*Year Introduced*
Chlordiazepoxide (Librium, Limbitrol,[a] Librax,[b] generic)	Anxiety, preoperative anxiety, acute alcohol withdrawal	15–100 mg/day	40 mg/day	50	1960
Diazepam (Valium, generic)	Anxiety, muscle relaxant, acute alcohol withdrawal, preoperative anxiety, anticonvulsant	4–40 mg/day	20 mg/day	10	1963
Oxazepam (Serax, generic)	Anxiety, alcohol withdrawal	30–120 mg/day	60 mg/day	30	1965
Flurazepam (Dalmane, generic)	Sedative-hypnotic	15–30 mg HS	15 mg HS	30	1970
Clorazepate (Tranxene, Tranxene-SD, generic)	Anxiety, alcohol withdrawal, anticonvulsant	15–60 mg/day	30 mg/day	15	1972
Clonazepam (Klonopin, Klonopin wafer, generic)	Anticonvulsant, panic disorder	0.5–12 mg/day	3 mg/day	0.5	1975
Lorazepam (Ativan, generic)	Anxiety, anxiety associated with depression	2–6 mg/day	3 mg/day	1.5–2.0	1977
Alprazolam (Xanax, Xanax XR, Niravam orally disintegrating tablets, generic)	Anxiety, anxiety associated with depression, panic disorder	0.5–6 mg/day (up to 10 mg/day for panic disorder)	2 mg/day	1.0	1981
Temazepam (Restoril, generic)	Sedative-hypnotic	15–30 mg HS	15 mg HS	30	1981
Triazolam (Halcion, generic)	Sedative-hypnotic	0.125–0.25 mg HS	0.125 mg HS	0.25	1983
Quazepam (Doral)	Sedative-hypnotic	7.5–15 mg HS	7.5 mg HS	15	1990
Estazolam (ProSom, generic)	Sedative-hypnotic	1–2 mg HS	1 mg HS	2.0	1991

FDA, U.S. Food and Drug Administration; HS, at bedtime.

[a]Combination product containing amitriptyline.

[b]Combination product containing clidinium bromide (classified as a gastrointestinal antispasmodic agent).

Table 76-5 Summary of Comparative Medication Treatment Options for Anxiety Disorders

Disorder	*First-Line Treatments*[a]	*Second-Line Treatments*	*Possible Alternatives*
Generalized anxiety disorder	Venlafaxine XR Buspirone Benzodiazepines Paroxetine Escitalopram Duloxetine	Sertraline Citalopram	Tricyclic antidepressants[b] Fluoxetine Mirtazapine Nefazodone[b] Hydroxyzine
Panic disorder	Paroxetine Sertraline Fluoxetine Alprazolam Clonazepam	Fluvoxamine Citalopram Clomipramine Lorazepam Escitalopram	Venlafaxine Nefazodone[b] Mirtazapine Imipramine Valproic acid Diazepam
Social anxiety disorder	Paroxetine Sertraline Venlafaxine XR Fluvoxamine CR	Citalopram Clonazepam Alprazolam Escitalopram	Phenelzine[b] Nefazodone Bupropion Buspirone[c] Topiramate Gabapentin
Posttraumatic stress disorder	Sertraline Paroxetine	Fluoxetine Fluvoxamine Venlafaxine Nefazodone Citalopram Escitalopram	Amitriptyline[b] Imipramine[b] Phenelzine[b] Mirtazapine Trazodone[c] Carbamazepine Valproic acid Lamotrigine Topiramate Nefazodone[b] Atypical antipsychotics[c]
Obsessive-compulsive disorder	Paroxetine Fluoxetine Sertraline Fluvoxamine CR Fluvoxamine	Clomipramine[b] Venlafaxine Citalopram Escitalopram	Clonazepam[c] Antipsychotic agents[c] Buspirone[c] Pindolol[c] Nefazodone Lithium[c]

[a]U.S. Food and Drug Administration–approved indications.
[b]Documented efficacy, but not recommended for first-line treatment because of undesirable clinical properties (side effects, potential toxicity, drug interactions).
[c]Adjunctive therapy only.

panic disorder. Clomipramine (Anafranil), a TCA, emerged as an effective treatment for OCD soon thereafter, and as shown in Table 76-5, selective serotonin reuptake inhibitor (SSRIs) have since gained first-line status for treating all five primary anxiety disorders.[21] The distinction between anxiolytics and antidepressants is continually narrowing.

Early controlled studies found trazodone, doxepin, imipramine, and amitriptyline to be comparably effective or even superior to benzodiazepines in treating GAD.[14] Although the benzodiazepines work more quickly, and TCA treatment is often associated with initial increases in anxiety (especially with higher dosages), continued TCA therapy is usually effective if the side effects can be tolerated. However, the TCAs are not widely used for treating anxiety disorders because attention has turned to other much safer and better tolerated antidepressants.

Paroxetine (Paxil) is the best-studied SSRI in GAD and was U.S. Food and Drug Administration (FDA) approved for this indication in 2001. Paroxetine is superior to placebo and as effective as the TCAs in treating GAD, but it is much better tolerated. Results from a large fixed-dose study suggest that a paroxetine dosage of 20 mg/day is effective for most patients with GAD, although some may need 30 to 40 mg/day for optimal benefits.[22] As with TCAs, some patients experience an initial increase in anxiety during SSRI treatment, so that lower-than-normal SSRI starting doses should be used in patients with GAD. A low paroxetine starting dose of 10 mg/day is recommended for the first week in patients with GAD to minimize initial side effects. Paroxetine maintenance therapy significantly decreases the risk of GAD relapse at 6 months.[23] The most common side effects of paroxetine in patients with GAD are sedation, nausea, dry mouth, constipation, asthenia, headache, and sexual dysfunction. With long-term therapy, weight gain may be problematic.

The combination serotonin/norepinephrine reuptake inhibitors (SNRIs), venlafaxine (Effexor XR), and duloxetine (Cymbalta) are efficacious for the treatment of GAD. Several large controlled studies have shown venlafaxine XR to be effective in reducing anxiety associated with depression, as well as in the treatment of pure GAD.[24–26] The recommended venlafaxine starting dose is 37.5 mg/day, and the effective dosage range for GAD is 75 to 225 mg/day.[26] Many patients respond to doses of 75 to 150 mg/day, although some may require up to 225 mg/day. The side effect profile of venlafaxine is similar to the SSRIs, with nausea being the most common complaint. Nausea is dose related, and usually subsides after 1 to 2 weeks of continued therapy. Other common side effects of venlafaxine include dizziness, asthenia, dry mouth, sweating, and either sedation or insomnia. Significant increases in blood pressure are not usually seen within the dosage range used for GAD (75–225 mg/day), but can occur with higher venlafaxine doses. Long-term studies report that GAD response to venlafaxine is maintained during 6 months of continued treatment.[25] Duloxetine recently received FDA approval for the treatment of GAD. Two 10- and one 9-week, randomized, placebo-controlled, double-blind trials in patients suffering from GAD have reported that duloxetine (60–120 mg/day) performed better than placebo.[27–29] In the single trial with a venlafaxine XR comparison arm, both duloxetine and venlafaxine exhibited similar efficacy and tolerability.[27]

SSRIs other than paroxetine can also be beneficial in treating GAD. Escitalopram (Lexapro) received FDA approval for GAD in late 2003, and preliminary reports suggest efficacy for citalopram (Celexa).[21,30] Sertraline (Zoloft), fluvoxamine (Luvox), and fluoxetine (Prozac) are reportedly effective in alleviating anxiety symptoms in patients with depression.[14,31,32] Fluoxetine may be more likely than other SSRIs to cause anxiety as an initial side effect.[21] Fluoxetine use in depressed patients with prominent anxiety or psychomotor agitation has been associated with poor response in some studies, although others report it to be comparably effective and as well tolerated as other SSRIs in this population.[32,33]

Mirtazapine (Remeron) is a non-SSRI antidepressant that appears promising in the treatment of GAD, but controlled studies are few.[34] It causes an especially low incidence of anxiety as a side effect, which is attributed to its serotonin receptor type-2 blocking activity. (See Chapter 79 for more information regarding the clinical use of various antidepressant agents.) Another non-SSRI antidepressant, nefazodone, exhibited anxiolytic effects in patients with GAD but it was associated with several cases of severe hepatotoxicity. In 2004, the trade name brand (Serzone) was voluntarily removed from the market by its manufacturer, although generic nefazodone is still available.[35]

Although decreases in anxiety symptoms during antidepressant treatment may appear within the first 2 weeks, response is gradual and generally continues over 8 to 12 weeks or longer. Therefore, optimal trials of antidepressants in GAD should allow at least 8 weeks of adequate doses before a lack of response is determined. Continued improvements may occur over 4 to 6 months in some GAD patients treated with antidepressants.[23,25]

Overall, advantages of antidepressants over benzodiazepines in treating GAD include their superior efficacy for cognitive symptoms such as excessive worry and their better coverage for common comorbid disorders such as depression and other anxiety disorders. Antidepressants also lack potential for abuse and dependence, although nearly all antidepressants can cause a withdrawal syndrome on abrupt discontinuation.

Other Agents Used to Treat Generalized Anxiety Disorder

Compared with antidepressants and benzodiazepines, buspirone is effective in treating cognitive anxiety symptoms and is not associated with abuse or dependence; however, it has a delayed onset of anxiolytic effects and is not appropriate for as-needed use.

Buspirone (BuSpar) was marketed in the United States in 1986 as the first of a nonbenzodiazepine class of anxiolytics, the azapirones. This class differs pharmacologically and clinically from the benzodiazepines.[14,36] Buspirone does not interact with GABA receptors and works as a partial agonist of the serotonin type 1A (5-hydroxytryptamine [$5HT_{1A}$]) receptor (i.e., it binds to the receptor but exerts a fraction of the effect of a full agonist).[37] This partial agonist activity results in reduced serotonin neurotransmission. In addition, buspirone enhances dopaminergic neurotransmission by blocking presynaptic dopamine receptor-2 auto receptors and also facilitates noradrenergic activity.[36]

β-Adrenergic receptor blocking agents such as propranolol (Inderal) are very effective in reducing certain physical symptoms of anxiety (tremor, flushing, tachycardia) that result from activation of the sympathetic nervous system. These agents are especially effective in preventing performance anxiety or "stage fright" by suppressing peripheral autonomic activity, but they do not modify cognitive symptoms of anxiety. β-Blockers are not as effective as benzodiazepines in the treatment of anxiety disorders and are not recommended as a primary treatment option for GAD.

Histamine-1 (H_1) receptor blocking agents such as hydroxyzine (Vistaril) and diphenhydramine (Benadryl) have been used for years in the treatment of anxiety and insomnia. Because of their potent sedative effects, these antihistamines are generally used on an as-needed basis for insomnia or for their calming effects in a variety of patient types. Although these drugs are considered benign and diphenhydramine is available over the counter, they do possess significant anticholinergic effects, which can produce problems such as confusion, cognitive impairment, nausea, and constipation. Elderly patients, especially those who are medically ill or have dementia, are particularly vulnerable to these side effects, and diphenhydramine is considered inappropriate for use in the elderly.[38] There is no evidence for the efficacy of diphenhydramine in the treatment of primary anxiety disorders.

Several studies have reported hydroxyzine to be beneficial in treating GAD. A large placebo-controlled study in nonelderly patients demonstrated superiority of hydroxyzine (50 mg/day given in three divided doses) over placebo.[39] Hydroxyzine was as effective as benzodiazepine therapy over 3 months of treatment, although it did not work as quickly. No anticholinergic, cognitive impairment, or weight gain adverse effects were reported in hydroxyzine-treated patients, and it was very well tolerated. Minimal sedation was reported with the relatively low daily hydroxyzine dose used in this study. Abrupt discontinuation of hydroxyzine after 3 months was not associated with significant withdrawal symptoms. Hydroxyzine is an inexpensive drug and may be a treatment option for GAD in some patients, but controlled comparisons with antidepressant agents are needed to better define its current role in therapy. It is not a good choice of therapy for elderly persons or patients with GAD and comorbid depression or other anxiety disorders.

Clinical Presentation and Assessment of Generalized Anxiety Disorder

2. N.K., a 25-year-old woman, has been employed as a bank clerk for the past 5 years. She had an excellent work record until 6 months ago, when excessive absences and a tendency to become easily upset at customers and coworkers became noticeable. On clinical assessment, N.K. complains of being tired, irritable, and tense, with frequent stomach upset and diarrhea. She has no history of mental illness; however, she admits to being stressed and worrying too much about "just little things," which she cannot seem to control regardless of how hard she tries. N.K. denies experiencing episodic "attacks" of severe anxiety (which might be indicative of panic disorder) or of having obsessive-compulsive thoughts or behaviors.

N.K.'s physical examination is unremarkable, and she has no history of mental illness in her family, although her mother was a "nervous person." N.K. denies any past or present use of any illicit substances or alcohol. Her mental status examination reveals the following:

- ***Appearance and behavior:* N.K. is neatly groomed and dressed and speaks coherently, but she constantly fidgets and taps her right foot. She states that she often has difficulty falling asleep but generally remains asleep throughout the night.**
- ***Mood:* N.K. is anxious and worried about the clinician's evaluation and admits to occasionally feeling depressed because of her anxiety.**
- ***Sensorium:* N.K. is oriented to person, place, and time.**
- ***Thoughts:* N.K. denies any auditory or visual hallucinations.**

N.K. states that at times she has difficulty speaking, is unable to relax, and startles easily. She realizes that work has been difficult for her lately, and her supervisor has told her that her job is in immediate jeopardy unless she improves her performance. N.K. states that she just wants to be able to perform her job well, relax, and enjoy life. Her insight and judgment are good, and she is motivated to obtain treatment. N.K. denies any suicidal ideation. The physician's provisional diagnosis is GAD (DSM-IV criteria). What clinical features of GAD are present in N.K., and how can her symptoms be assessed objectively?

N.K. exhibits the following target symptoms associated with GAD: excessive worry that is difficult to control, irritability, tension and inability to relax, fatigue, and sleep disturbances. Other typical symptoms of anxiety present in N.K. include gastrointestinal (GI) problems (upset stomach and diarrhea), being startled easily, difficulty speaking, and fidgeting. These target symptoms are not necessarily diagnostic of any particular disorder, but other factors in association with these symptoms are consistent with GAD. The absence of physical or other psychiatric illnesses, as well as use of any illicit substances or alcohol, excludes possible secondary causes of anxiety. The 6-month duration of symptoms is consistent with a diagnosis of GAD, and N.K. is at a common age for onset of GAD. More important, the symptoms are causing significant occupational impairment for N.K. and interfering with her quality of life; therefore, a diagnosis of GAD is appropriate in N.K.

The Hamilton Anxiety Rating Scale (HAM-A) is a useful assessment tool to evaluate clinical anxiety, and it is the standard instrument used in GAD clinical trials. A HAM-A score of >18 is generally correlated with significant anxiety, and a score of 7 to 10 is associated with remission.[40] The HAM-A can be used to assess baseline anxiety symptoms in patients such as N.K. and to monitor response throughout treatment. The Sheehan Disability Scale is a patient-rated instrument, which is commonly used to assess functional impairment due to GAD and other anxiety disorders. A score of 1 reflects mild disability.[40]

Indications for and Selection of Treatment

3. Based on the information presented in N.K.'s case, how can it be determined whether treatment is indicated? What factors should be considered in choosing the most appropriate treatment for N.K.?

N.K. meets the diagnostic criteria for GAD and is suffering significant disability from her anxiety disorder. She also has insight into her illness and desires treatment that will enable her to improve her job performance and quality of life. Appropriate treatment of GAD can help achieve these goals and is therefore indicated for patients such as N.K.

Treatment options for GAD may include both pharmacologic and nondrug therapies. Psychosocial treatments such as CBT can be effective in treating GAD, but use of these therapies alone is generally reserved for patients with mild-to-moderate symptoms. In N.K.'s case, prompt treatment is needed because she feels that her job is in immediate jeopardy owing to impairments associated with her anxiety. Therefore, pharmacotherapy in combination with psychological therapy, if available, is indicated in N.K.

Among potential drug therapies, the benzodiazepines, paroxetine, duloxetine, venlafaxine, and buspirone, are all considered first-line treatments for GAD.[14] A primary consideration when choosing among these options is whether any comorbid psychiatric conditions are present. Venlafaxine, duloxetine, and paroxetine are good initial choices for patients with concurrent depression, which is common in GAD patients. They are also preferred over benzodiazepines in patients with past or present alcohol or substance abuse. Other medical or psychiatric disorders may also be present, which can guide selection toward a treatment that may be dually effective.

Another important consideration when selecting treatment for GAD is how fast therapeutic effects are needed. Benzodiazepines reduce anxiety within a few hours, whereas the antidepressants and buspirone have delayed onsets of anxiolytic effects. Medication cost is another potential factor, and generic benzodiazepines are currently the least expensive anxiolytic medications.

In N.K.'s case, a benzodiazepine may be a good initial choice because of the need for quick symptom relief relating to her problems at work. N.K. is young and healthy with no past or present history of substance or alcohol use that might make benzodiazepines unsuitable for her. GAD is often chronic, and antidepressants or buspirone are usually preferred over benzodiazepines for long-term treatment. Therefore, one of these agents would also be appropriate to use in this case. Combination benzodiazepines-SSRI therapy during initial treatment of anxiety disorders is well tolerated and may result in synergistic anxiolytic effects and quicker response.[41,42]

Benzodiazepine Treatment

Factors Influencing Benzodiazepine Selection

4. The physician decides to treat N.K.'s GAD with venlafaxine XR and also wants to prescribe a benzodiazepine for quick control of her anxiety during the first several weeks until the onset of venlafaxine's anxiolytic effects. What factors are important in the selection of a particular benzodiazepine agent for N.K.?

Of the available benzodiazepines, none has demonstrated clear superior efficacy in the treatment of anxiety. However, certain agents have been used much more extensively than others. Alprazolam (Xanax) is the most commonly used in the United States, lorazepam (Ativan) is the next most popular, followed by clonazepam (Klonopin) and then diazepam (Valium). All four of these benzodiazepines have been successfully used in the treatment of GAD.

Because the overall anxiolytic efficacies of benzodiazepines are similar, other factors must be considered when selecting one agent over another. The one major area of clinically significant differences between benzodiazepines is their pharmacokinetic properties. These are generally the main factors considered in drug selection (Table 76-6).

Benzodiazepines can be differentiated pharmacokinetically according to their elimination half-lives and their metabolism to active or inactive compounds (Fig. 76-2; Table 76-6). Diazepam (Valium) and chlordiazepoxide (Librium) have half-lives between 10 and 40 hours but are metabolized by hepatic oxidative pathways to the active metabolite desmethyldiazepam (DMDZ), which has a half-life of at least 100 hours.[43] Demethylation of diazepam to DMDZ is mediated by several cytochrome P450 (CYP) isozymes, including CYP 2C19, CYP 3A4, and, to a lesser extent, CYP 2B6. CYP 2C19 appears to be the predominate pathway with usual therapeutic diazepam doses, but CYP 3A4 becomes more important with high doses, in overdose cases, and in CYP 2C19 poor metabolizers.[44] The other major active diazepam metabolite, temazepam, is formed through CYP 3A4–mediated hydroxylation.

As shown in Figure 76-2, the prodrugs quazepam (Doral) and clorazepate (Tranxene) are also metabolized to DMDZ.[43] Because of the long half-life of this active metabolite, chronic dosing of benzodiazepines that are converted to DMDZ can lead to drug accumulation and prolonged clinical effects. This can be especially detrimental in the elderly, those with liver disease, or persons taking other drugs that interfere with benzodiazepine metabolism. Although their long durations of action make once-daily dosing possible, small, divided daily doses are often used clinically to minimize side effects.

Clonazepam undergoes various routes of hepatic metabolism, including oxidative hydroxylation, reduction, and acetylation.[43] At least five metabolites have been identified, but their pharmacologic activity is uncertain. The specific enzymes responsible for clonazepam metabolism have not been confirmed, but there is evidence that it is a substrate for CYP 3A4.[45] The elimination half-life of clonazepam ranges from 20 to 50 hours, making once-daily dosing feasible. A new formulation of orally disintegrating clonazepam tablets (Klonopin wafer) has been introduced and is indicated for the treatment of panic disorder. This product dissolves quickly on the tongue and is promoted as being especially convenient because it can be taken without water.

Alprazolam (Xanax, Niravam) and lorazepam (Ativan) have intermediate half-lives of 10 to 20 hours, and oxazepam (Serax) has a short to intermediate half-life of 5 to 14 hours. Alprazolam is a triazolobenzodiazepine that is metabolized by CYP 3A4 to an active metabolite, α-hydroxy alprazolam, which has a short half-life of approximately 2 hours and is considered clinically insignificant. Alprazolam, lorazepam, and

Table 76-6 Pharmacokinetic Comparison of Benzodiazepine Agents

Drug	Elimination Half-Life (hr)[a]	Active Metabolites	Protein Binding	Pathway of Metabolism	Rate of Onset After Oral Administration
Chlordiazepoxide	>100	Desmethyldiazepam	96%	Oxidation	Intermediate
Diazepam	>100	Desmethyldiazepam	98%	Oxidation (CYP 3A4, CYP 2C19)	Very fast
Oxazepam	5–14	None	87%	Conjugation	Slow
Flurazepam	>100	Desalkylflurazepam, hydroxyethylflurazepam	97%	Oxidation	Fast
Clorazepate	>100	Desmethyldiazepam	98%	Oxidation	Fast
Lorazepam	10–20	None	85%–90%	Conjugation	Intermediate
Alprazolam	12–15	Insignificant	80%	Oxidation (CYP 3A4)	Fast
Temazepam	10–20	Insignificant	98%	Conjugation	Intermediate
Triazolam	1.5–5	Insignificant	90%	Oxidation (CYP 3A4)	Intermediate
Quazepam	47–100	2-Oxoquazepam, desalkyloxoquazepam	>95%	Oxidation	Fast
Estazolam	24	Insignificant	93%	Oxidation	Intermediate
Clonazepam	20–50	Insignificant	85%	Oxidation, reduction (CYP 3A4)	Intermediate
Midazolam	1–4	None	97%	Oxidation (CYP 3A4)	NA

NA, not applicable.
[a]Parent drug + active metabolite.

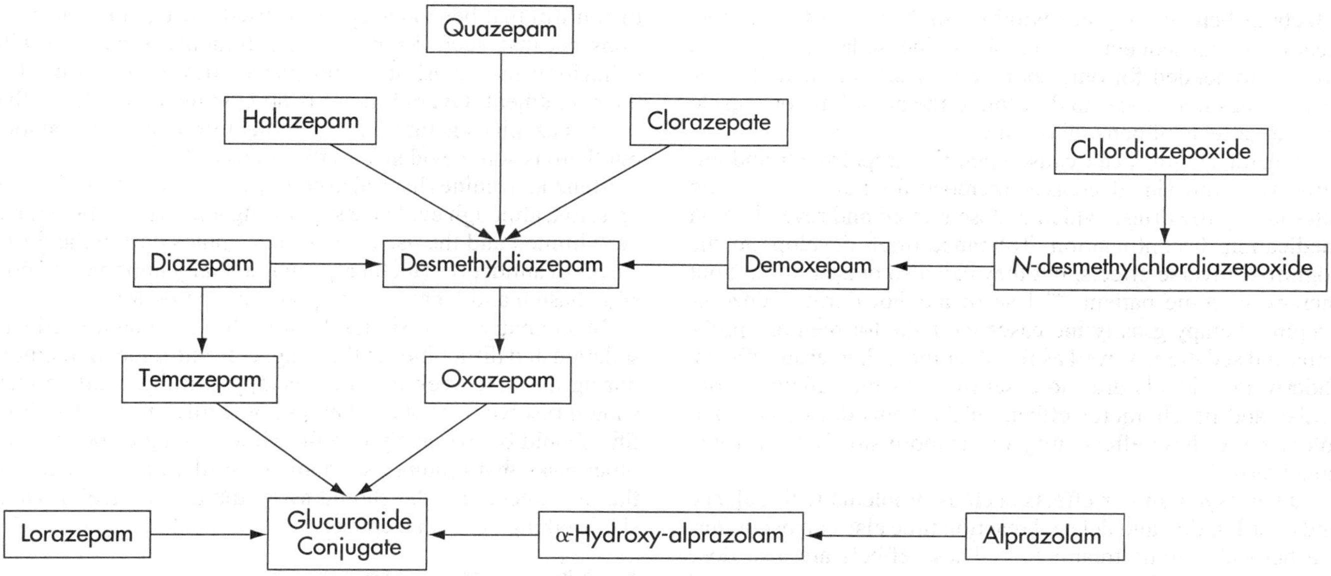

FIGURE 76-2 Metabolic pathways of benzodiazepines.

oxazepam usually need to be taken on a TID to QID dosing schedule for sustained clinical effects, but an extended-release (XR) preparation of alprazolam that allows QD or BID dosing has become available. Alprazolam XR may be associated with less CNS side effects than the immediate-release form because peak alprazolam blood levels are lower.[46] Also, a quickly dissolving tablet of alprazolam (Niravam) has been marketed. Lorazepam, temazepam (Restoril), and oxazepam undergo phase II metabolism by glucuronidation and are believed to be substrates for the uridine diphosphate-glucuronosyltransferase 2B7 isozyme.[47] These agents are free of active metabolites and are unlikely to accumulate with chronic administration; they are preferred over long-acting agents in patients with liver disease and in the elderly. Unlike phase I oxidative metabolism, phase II glucuronidation processes do not appear to decline with age.[47]

Benzodiazepines are readily absorbed within 2 to 3 hours after oral administration.[43] They are widely distributed in the body and accumulate preferentially in lipid-rich areas such as the CNS and fat tissue. Lipid solubility varies among the agents, resulting in differences in rates of absorption and speed of onset, as well as duration of clinical effects (Table 76-6). Diazepam and clorazepate have the highest lipid solubilities and the quickest onsets of action, which can be desirable when rapid anxiolysis is needed; however, both can produce an unpleasant "drugged" or "high" feeling in some patients. Highly lipophilic benzodiazepines are also more quickly redistributed out of the brain, which decreases their duration of action. For example, even though diazepam has a very long half-life, its clinical effects last for a shorter period than lorazepam, which has a relatively short half-life.

Diazepam, lorazepam, chlordiazepoxide, and midazolam are also available for parenteral (intravenous [IV] and intramuscular [IM]) administration.[43] These routes are usually reserved for treatment of severe agitation or seizures or for induction of preoperative sedation and anxiolysis. IM injection of both chlordiazepoxide and diazepam can be very painful. Lorazepam is the preferred agent when parenteral dosing is needed for quick control of anxiety or agitation because it is rapidly and completely absorbed after IM injection. The absorption of sublingual lorazepam, alprazolam, and triazolam (Halcion) is comparable to or slightly faster than oral absorption.[43]

Cost is another important factor in benzodiazepine selection. Brand name benzodiazepines can be relatively expensive, but all are available in less costly generic versions, except the extended-release and quick-dissolving formulations. Potential drug interactions should also be considered in the selection of an agent because they can alter pharmacokinetics and clinical effects (see Question 9).

Because N.K. is young and healthy and is not taking any other medications, the clinician could choose just about any benzodiazepine. Nevertheless, most clinicians still prefer to use shorter-acting high-potency agents such as lorazepam or alprazolam for patients such as N.K. Appropriate starting doses would be lorazepam 0.5 to 1 mg TID or alprazolam 0.25 to 0.5 mg TID. Dosages can be increased every 3 to 4 days, if needed, within the dosage ranges indicated in Table 76-4. N.K. should notice a decrease in her anxiety symptoms within the first few days of treatment. Prescription of a generic formulation is recommended to reduce treatment costs.

Adverse Effects and Patient Counseling

5. Lorazepam 0.5 mg TID is prescribed for N.K. in addition to venlafaxine XR. What side effects may occur with benzodiazepine treatment, and how should N.K. be counseled regarding benzodiazepine therapy?

Overall, benzodiazepines are very safe and well-tolerated medications, and drug discontinuation due to side effects is extremely rare. Sedation and feelings of tiredness are the most common side effects of the benzodiazepines, but sedation can also be beneficial in alleviating the insomnia that often accompanies anxiety. Tolerance usually develops to the sedative effects of benzodiazepines within 1 to 2 weeks of continued treatment; consequently, benzodiazepine sedative-hypnotics are recommended for only short-term use.[48] Fortunately, tolerance does not appear to develop to the anxiolytic or muscle relaxant effects of benzodiazepines.

Benzodiazepines can cause cognitive impairment and anterograde amnesia (decreased memory for new information after taking the drug), which is dose related and reversible on medication discontinuation. Tolerance often develops to the cognitive adverse effects, but they can also persist throughout therapy in some patients.[49] Use of alcohol during benzodiazepine therapy greatly increases the risks for memory problems and sedation, as well as for other more dangerous effects. Elderly individuals are more sensitive to the sedative, cognitive, and psychomotor effects of the benzodiazepines, and tolerance to these effects may occur more slowly than in the nonelderly.[50]

Other psychomotor effects such as problems with balance and coordination and delayed reaction time also can occur during benzodiazepine treatment.[43] These effects are also dose related, but usually subside within a few weeks of continued treatment. However, it is important that patients starting on benzodiazepine therapy be cautioned about possible adverse psychomotor effects. Residual daytime effects after taking a long-acting benzodiazepine the previous night may even pose a hazard while driving the next day.

The link between benzodiazepine use and falls, especially in the elderly, is well documented and may result from a combination of balance impairment, sedation, and muscle relaxant effects.[51] Rapid dosage escalation and use of doses that are too high (of either long-acting or short-acting agents) have been identified as major risk factors, but even use of low doses of short-acting agents greatly increases the fall risk in the elderly.[51,52] Although tolerance can develop to the psychomotor effects of benzodiazepines, elderly individuals may experience persistent impairment. Benzodiazepines should probably be considered second-line therapy in the ambulatory older population.

Respiratory depression is another potential adverse effect of benzodiazepines, but it is usually clinically relevant only in patients with severe respiratory disease, in overdose situations (see Question 11), or when combined with alcohol or substances that depress breathing. It is recommended that benzodiazepines be avoided in patients with sleep apnea. Respiratory complications are encountered most often with IV administration. IV midazolam has been associated with a number of deaths due to cardiorespiratory arrest during its use for conscious sedation, most often in patients premedicated with narcotics or in those with chronic obstructive airways disease. Severe respiratory depression has also occurred with the concurrent use of benzodiazepines and olanzapine (Zyprexa), loxapine (Loxitane), or clozapine (Clozaril).

Paradoxic disinhibition, with increased anxiety, irritability, and agitation, can occur infrequently with benzodiazepines.[43,53] Such effects have been mainly observed in elderly or developmentally disabled patients. Other unusual behaviors, such as increased anger, hostility, and violence, have been attributed to benzodiazepine use in a small number of cases.[43] Most of these reports were anecdotal and involved patients with pre-existing psychiatric disorders such as bipolar disorder, schizophrenia, or personality disorders. It is difficult to confirm that benzodiazepines caused these paradoxic reactions because such disorders are commonly associated with behavioral problems, and benzodiazepines are often used in their treatment. Overall, there is no convincing evidence that benzodiazepines actually cause violent or suicidal behaviors, but there is some evidence to the contrary.[43,53]

Benzodiazepines have also been associated with clinical depression, although evidence supporting a causal relationship is very limited and the use of benzodiazepines during the initial weeks of antidepressant therapy may actually improve and possibly hasten antidepressant response in depression.[12]

In summary, N.K. should be told that she may experience sedation and difficulties in thinking, concentration, or memory during the first week or so of therapy, but these side effects should resolve once she develops some tolerance to the drug. She should be extremely careful while driving or performing other tasks that require psychomotor skills, especially during the first week, and she should avoid the use of alcohol while she is taking benzodiazepines.

Benzodiazepine Abuse and Dependence

6. Two weeks later, N.K. contacts her clinician to discuss a medication concern. She reports that the medication has been extremely effective in relieving her anxiety, and she is currently taking venlafaxine XR, 150 mg Q AM, and lorazepam, 0.5 mg TID, as directed by her physician. However, her mother has told her that she will become addicted to lorazepam, and she wonders if she should stop taking it because of this concern. What potential for abuse and dependence is associated with benzodiazepines? How should N.K. be counseled regarding "becoming addicted" to lorazepam?

Concerns related to abuse and dependence are probably the major drawback to the clinical use of benzodiazepines. These agents are classified as schedule IV controlled substances, reflecting a relatively limited abuse and dependence liability. There may be differences within the class regarding abuse potential. Diazepam, alprazolam, and lorazepam are reported to be more likely to be abused than are oxazepam and chlordiazepoxide.[54] This difference in abuse potential is commonly attributed to the quicker onset of effects for drugs such as diazepam, which may be associated with a subjective euphoric sensation. The XR alprazolam formulation is reported to have a lower abuse potential than immediate-release alprazolam because of its slower onset of effects and lower maximum plasma concentrations.[46]

Abuse is characterized by drug use outside the therapeutic setting and implies recreational use combined with continued use despite negative consequences, dose escalation, and loss of control over use. Patients without a history of substance abuse who take benzodiazepines for therapeutic purposes are unlikely to escalate doses or use them in ways characteristic of abuse.[54]

The potential problems with benzodiazepine abuse and dependence can be avoided or minimized in several ways. First is the identification of patients who have a history of alcohol or substance abuse and using nonbenzodiazepine treatments in such cases.[54] Second, patients should be counseled about the likely duration of benzodiazepine use, the possibility of withdrawal symptoms, and the importance of gradual drug tapering when therapy is to be discontinued. The distinction between "addiction" and appropriate therapeutic use, which may be accompanied by some degree of physical dependence, should be explained.

N.K. should be advised that as long as the medication is helping her anxiety and she is taking it according to her physician's instructions, her use of lorazepam does not constitute addiction. However, her body may develop some physiological dependence to the drug, so if she stops taking lorazepam abruptly, she could experience increased anxiety and other withdrawal symptoms. When lorazepam is to be discontinued, the dose should be decreased gradually over a sufficient period to minimize withdrawal symptoms.

Duration of Treatment

7. Two weeks later at her clinic appointment, N.K. is still doing well and has shown further improvements in her GAD symptoms. She has been taking the prescribed lorazepam and venlafaxine doses for 1 month, and her venlafaxine has been increased to the current dose of 150 mg/day during this time. How long should medication therapy continue?

GAD is a chronic disorder that can fluctuate in severity and often requires long-term treatment. Relapse after discontinuation of benzodiazepine monotherapy is reported to occur in 50% to 80% of GAD patients; however, some of these cases may actually involve benzodiazepine withdrawal.[55] These relapse rates also do not take into account the concurrent use of other medications that may prevent relapse, such as venlafaxine. Although long-term use of benzodiazepines is generally safe and effective, it is desirable to limit treatment to the shortest duration necessary because of the physical dependence potential.[14] When benzodiazepines are used for acute anxiolytic effects during initiation of antidepressant treatment for GAD, they are commonly limited to short-term (2–6 weeks) therapy. N.K. has shown good response after 1 month of combined lorazepam and venlafaxine XR therapy. Because the anxiolytic effects of venlafaxine usually occur between 2 and 4 weeks of therapy and she is taking a therapeutic venlafaxine dose, it is appropriate to start discontinuing lorazepam at this time. N.K. is unlikely to experience significant withdrawal symptoms after only 1 month of treatment, but the dose should still be gradually decreased over several weeks, according to tolerability of the taper.[55]

There is no consensus about the optimal duration of drug therapy for GAD. However, recent recommendations suggest that effective medication treatment be continued for at least 6 to 12 months after response.[14] Continuation treatment with antidepressants significantly reduces the risk of GAD relapse over 6 months.[23,25] Therefore, venlafaxine XR therapy should be continued for another 5 to 11 months in N.K.'s case. After that time period, gradual venlafaxine discontinuation may be considered and reinstitution of treatment is warranted if relapse occurs.

Symptoms and Management of Benzodiazepine Withdrawal

8. G.S., a 43-year-old man, has been taking diazepam 40 mg/day for 6 months for its muscle relaxant effects after sustaining a dislocated shoulder and other injuries in a car accident. Four days ago, G.S. was unable to refill his prescription for financial reasons. A brief mental status examination reveals mild confusion and irritability. Physically, G.S. is trembling and complains of overall body aching and an upset stomach. His medical history indicates no current medical problems or psychiatric illnesses, and G.S. denies the use of tobacco, alcohol, or other drugs of abuse. How should G.S. be treated?

Table 76-7 Symptoms of Benzodiazepine Withdrawal

Common	*Less Common*	*Rare*
Anxiety	Nausea	Confusion
Insomnia	Depression	Delirium
Irritability	Ataxia	Psychosis
Muscle aches/weakness	Hyperreflexia	Seizures
Tremor	Blurred vision	Catatonia
Loss of appetite	Fatigue	

Because G.S. has not taken his prescribed diazepam for 4 days, it is likely that he is experiencing a withdrawal syndrome from long-term benzodiazepine use. His mental and physical symptoms are consistent with benzodiazepine withdrawal. The benzodiazepine withdrawal syndrome implies some degree of physical dependence, and its onset, duration, and severity can vary according to dose, duration of treatment, speed of withdrawal, and elimination half-life of the agent used.[54,55] Withdrawal symptoms that follow discontinuation of agents with short half-lives usually appear within 1 to 2 days and may be more short lived, but more intense, than after discontinuation of long-acting benzodiazepines. Withdrawal symptoms usually appear 4 to 7 days after discontinuation of long-acting agents and may last several weeks. Symptoms of benzodiazepine withdrawal, which are listed in Table 76-7, are generally mild when the drug is tapered gradually during discontinuation.[55] Rarely, serious symptoms such as seizures or psychosis may occur during benzodiazepine withdrawal. Risk factors for seizures include head injury, alcohol dependence, electroencephalogram abnormalities, and use of other drugs that lower the seizure threshold.

Diazepam 10 to 20 mg orally should be administered and repeated within 1 to 2 hours if needed. Resumption of his previous diazepam dosage of 40 mg/day should effectively treat his withdrawal symptoms. However, because his acute injury occurred 6 months ago, it may be desirable to begin discontinuation of the benzodiazepine.

Various dosage reduction regimens have been proposed for benzodiazepine discontinuation. Even when managing withdrawal from low-dose benzodiazepine use, doses should be reduced slowly over 4 to 16 weeks.[55] The rate of the drug taper should be individualized to the patient, but a general recommendation is a 10% to 25% decrease in the dosage every 1 to 2 weeks. The first half of the benzodiazepine taper (down to 50% of the original dose) is generally easier and can proceed more quickly than the last half of the taper.[55] In G.S.'s case, the discontinuation period may take several months.

In general, the same benzodiazepine the patient has been taking should be used to manage withdrawal. However, because withdrawal symptoms are more severe during discontinuation of short-acting compared with long-acting benzodiazepines, a long-acting agent can be substituted at an equivalent dosage and then tapered.[55] In difficult cases, adjunctive medications have been used to ease tolerability of the gradual withdrawal. Carbamazepine (Tegretol) has been effective in attenuating the symptoms of withdrawal from both benzodiazepines and alcohol. Propranolol decreases some physical withdrawal symptoms (tremor, tachycardia), but does not affect the associated anxiety or decrease the seizure risk.[55] CBT, combined with gradual drug taper, has also been effective in facilitating successful benzodiazepine discontinuation.

Benzodiazepine Drug Interactions

9. R.G., a 24-year-old female college student, has been taking alprazolam 1 mg TID for treatment of GAD for almost 1 year. She states that alprazolam has been very helpful for her GAD, but complains to her physician that she is feeling especially stressed lately because she is trying to keep up with extremely difficult schoolwork while making arrangements for her upcoming wedding. She has no medical illnesses, but states that she has suffered from several episodes of vulvovaginal candidiasis since recently beginning oral contraceptives (Ortho-Novum 1/35). R.G. smokes two packs of cigarettes per day and drinks up to 6 cups of coffee per day. Itraconazole, 200 mg QD for 3 days, is prescribed for treatment of recurrent vulvovaginal candidiasis. What potential drug interactions with alprazolam are present in this case?

Reported drug interactions with benzodiazepines are summarized in Table 76-8 and can be divided into two primary

Table 76-8 Drug Interactions With Benzodiazepines

Interacting Drug(s)	*Effect on Object Drug*	*Clinical Significance/Comments*
Hepatic enzyme inducers: carbamazepine, phenobarbital, phenytoin, and rifampin	Decreased Cps and clinical effects of benzodiazepines	Triazolam and midazolam may be ineffective in patients taking rifampin.[163] Carbamazepine greatly decreases the Cps and clinical effects of midazolam, alprazolam, and clonazepam, possibly rendering them ineffective.[164,165]
Hepatic CYP 3A4 inhibitors: ketoconazole, itraconazole, nefazodone, fluvoxamine, fluoxetine, erythromycin, clarithromycin, cimetidine, oral contraceptives, diltiazem, nelfinavir, indinavir, ritonavir, saquinavir, verapamil	Significantly increased Cps of benzodiazepines that undergo oxidative metabolism (alprazolam, triazolam, diazepam, chlordiazepoxide, clonazepam)	Benzodiazepine dosage reductions may be required because of increased clinical effects such as sedation and psychomotor impairment; effects are greatest on alprazolam, triazolam, and midazolam.[166] Ketoconazole and itraconazole should be avoided in patients taking alprazolam or triazolam.[167] Benzodiazepine dosage reductions are recommended when nefazodone, fluoxetine, or fluvoxamine are added to alprazolam, diazepam, or triazolam.[166]
Ritonavir	Initial inhibition of alprazolam and triazolam metabolism, followed by later induction of metabolism	Reduced benzodiazepine dosage is needed initially if ritonavir is added to therapy; a dosage increase may be required later.[168]
Grapefruit juice	Increased Cps of diazepam, alprazolam, and triazolam	Increased benzodiazepine clinical effects (sedation, psychomotor impairment) are possible.[166,169]
Omeprazole	Increased diazepam Cp and prolonged half-life	Increased benzodiazepine clinical effects (sedation, psychomotor impairment) are possible.[56]
Antacids, ranitidine	Decreased rate of benzodiazepine absorption	Possible delayed onset of benzodiazepine clinical effects; separation of administration times is recommended.
Valproic acid, probenecid	Significantly decreased clearance of lorazepam	Lorazepam dosage reductions may be required.[170]
Estrogen-containing oral contraceptives	Decreased Cps of benzodiazepines that undergo glucuronidation (lorazepam, oxazepam, temazepam) and increased Cps of benzodiazepines that undergo oxidative CYP 3A4 metabolism (alprazolam)	Decreased or increased clinical effects of benzodiazepines are possible.[13,47,56]
Central nervous system depressants (alcohol, barbiturates, and opioids)	Increased central nervous system depressant effects of benzodiazepines (sedation, psychomotor impairment)	Avoid use of alcohol with benzodiazepines; exercise caution with use of other depressants.
Alprazolam	Increased digoxin Cp	Digoxin toxicity is possible; monitoring of digoxin level and possible digoxin dosage reduction are recommended.[171]
Benzodiazepines	Respiratory depression and adverse cardiovascular effects reported on addition of benzodiazepines in several patients taking clozapine	Caution with benzodiazepine use in patients taking clozapine.
	Possible decreased efficacy of levodopa in Parkinson disease	Drug interaction is not well established; monitor for possible effect.
	Increased or decreased efficacy of neuromuscular blocking agents	Drug interaction is not well established; monitor for possible effect.

Cp, plasma concentration; CYP, cytochrome P450.

types: pharmacodynamic and pharmacokinetic. The most significant pharmacodynamic drug interactions involve other CNS depressants such as alcohol or barbiturates. These combinations can lead to additive CNS and respiratory depressant effects that can be deadly. Important pharmacokinetic drug interactions mainly involve agents that either inhibit or induce benzodiazepine metabolism.[56] Because the benzodiazepines have a relatively wide margin of safety, elevated plasma levels and/or prolonged elimination half-lives are unlikely to cause serious toxicity. However, they can lead to increased sedative and psychomotor effects, which may be clinically significant in certain cases. Conversely, increased benzodiazepine metabolism by hepatic enzyme inducers may result in medication ineffectiveness. As indicated in Table 76-8, most pharmacokinetic drug interactions with benzodiazepines involve CYP 3A4– or CYP 2C19–mediated mechanisms.

In R.G.'s case, the most important drug interaction is between alprazolam and the newly prescribed antifungal, itraconazole, which is a potent CYP 3A4 inhibitor that can cause a 170% increase in the area under the curve of alprazolam.[57] Therefore, the dosage of alprazolam should be reduced by about one-third, over several days according to tolerability, during the 3 days R.G. is taking itraconazole.

Estrogen-containing oral contraceptives can also inhibit the CYP 3A4 metabolism of benzodiazepines such as alprazolam, potentially resulting in increased side effects.[13] Thus, a reduction in the benzodiazepine dosage may be needed when oral contraceptives are added to ongoing benzodiazepine therapy. The clearance of benzodiazepines that undergo glucuronidation (lorazepam, oxazepam, and temazepam) can be accelerated by oral contraceptives, but this interaction is probably clinically insignificant.[13,47]

Cigarette smoking increases the clearance of some benzodiazepines (clorazepate, lorazepam, oxazepam), but has no effect on others (diazepam, midazolam, chlordiazepoxide).[58] Overall, the effect of smoking is unpredictable and is most likely to be important in patients who either stop or start smoking while taking a benzodiazepine. R.G. should be urged to quit smoking for the sake of her general health and to prevent substantial risks for serious cardiovascular events that occur in smokers taking oral contraceptives. If R.G. does quit, careful monitoring will be needed to determine whether any alprazolam dosage reduction is necessary.

R.G. should also be encouraged to decrease her coffee consumption because caffeine can increase anxiety and possibly decrease the effectiveness of alprazolam. Caffeine has decreased diazepam concentrations by approximately 22%, but studies with other benzodiazepines are lacking.[56]

Benzodiazepine Use in Pregnancy and Lactation

10. At her clinic visit 8 months later, R.G is doing very well. She has graduated from college, is happily married, and states that she and her husband have decided to start a family. R.G.'s candida infection did not recur after a single course of itraconazole, and she has successfully quit smoking. She also has discontinued her oral contraceptive and plans to become pregnant soon. R.G. continues to take alprazolam 0.5 mg BID to TID and wonders whether she should also stop taking this drug before she becomes pregnant. What is the teratogenic potential of alprazolam? What alternative treatments are available for the management of R.G.'s anxiety?

Early reports implicated diazepam in causing several birth deformities, including cleft lip and/or cleft palate and limb and digit malformations, but later studies failed to support this association.[59] Most benzodiazepine anxiolytics are classified as pregnancy category D, indicating that there is some evidence of fetal risk but that the benefits of the medication may outweigh these risks in certain patients.[59] Available evidence suggests that benzodiazepine use during the first trimester increases the risk for oral clefts by approximately 2.4-fold, but the absolute risk is <1%. Alprazolam and lorazepam have not exhibited teratogenic effects, but it is always advisable to avoid drug use during pregnancy when possible, especially in the first trimester.[59] In patients such as R.G., the benzodiazepine should be tapered and discontinued before she becomes pregnant. Nondrug treatments for her GAD such as relaxation therapy, meditation, and biofeedback or cognitive therapy may be helpful. If necessary, single or repeated small doses of benzodiazepines during the second and third trimesters are unlikely to have important adverse effects on the baby. Alprazolam and lorazepam are the preferred agents.[59] Chronic or large doses, especially of long-acting agents, should be avoided because they may accumulate in the fetus. Perinatal sequelae reported in newborns whose mothers took benzodiazepines during pregnancy include withdrawal symptoms, sedation, muscle weakness, hypotonia, apnea, poor feeding, and impaired temperature regulation.[59]

Pregnancies are sometimes unplanned, and the clinical situation of unexpected pregnancy in a woman maintained on benzodiazepines can also arise. The general course of action in such cases is often to discontinue all medications immediately. However, it is unwise to abruptly stop benzodiazepine treatment in someone who has been receiving chronic therapy because the resultant withdrawal syndromes can be detrimental to both mother and child. Benzodiazepine dosages should be tapered as quickly as possible to the lowest dosage necessary and discontinued if possible. The postpartum period is a time of heightened risk for recurrence of anxiety disorders, and new mothers should be monitored carefully for signs of relapse.[60] Benzodiazepines are excreted readily in breast milk, and it is generally recommended that they be avoided by nursing mothers.[61] (Also see Chapter 46.)

Benzodiazepine Overdose and Use of Flumazenil

11. S.P. is a 17-year-old boy who is brought to the hospital by his mother. S.P. is barely conscious, and his breathing is slow and shallow. His mother states that he "took a whole bottle of diazepam" (5 mg, #30) sometime during the previous night. S.P.'s medical history is significant for a severe head injury sustained from a car accident 8 months ago. He currently takes carbamazepine (Tegretol) 200 mg TID for seizure prophylaxis. S.P.'s mother believes that diazepam is the only drug that he ingested because no other medications are missing. What signs and symptoms are consistent with benzodiazepine overdose? Why is it inappropriate to administer the benzodiazepine antagonist, flumazenil, in this case?

Benzodiazepine overdose is characterized by respiratory and CNS depression, both of which are evident in this case (S.P. is almost unconscious, with slow and shallow breathing). Overdose with benzodiazepines as the sole ingested agent is rarely life threatening, and full recovery is the usual outcome.[62]

Flumazenil is a benzodiazepine receptor antagonist that is effective in reversing the sedation associated with benzodiazepine intoxication. Its effects on respiratory depression are inconsistent, but improved breathing may occur secondarily to increased consciousness.[62]

The primary use of flumazenil is in reversing benzodiazepine-induced conscious sedation (primarily with midazolam) in patients who have been sedated for minor surgical or diagnostic procedures. Its use for this purpose is generally safe and effective, and facilitates patient recovery and discharge by decreasing the postprocedural monitoring period.[63] Flumazenil is also approved for treating benzodiazepine overdose, but this use is controversial because of potentially serious complications and questions about its cost effectiveness.[63] Flumazenil administration does not appear to decrease mortality or length of hospital stay in cases of benzodiazepine overdose; therefore, its use for this purpose has become limited.[63]

There are several reports of seizures or cardiac arrhythmias (including fatalities) following the administration of flumazenil in comatose patients who had ingested multiple drugs.[62] These overdoses often included TCAs and carbamazepine. The anticonvulsant effects of benzodiazepines may protect against TCA-induced seizures, and the rapid reversal of their effects with flumazenil removes this protection. Flumazenil is contraindicated in cases of overdose involving TCAs or carbamazepine or overdoses of any agent that decreases the seizure threshold. Toxicology screening and an electrocardiogram (ECG) should be performed before flumazenil is administered. Physical symptoms suggestive of TCA overdose include dry mucous membranes, mydriasis, and motor twitching or rigidity. Flumazenil should also be avoided in patients with increased intracranial pressure or a known history of seizures or head injury, in those who have been receiving chronic benzodiazepine therapy, and in patients with a history of recent illicit drug abuse (cocaine, heroin) because flumazenil can precipitate seizures in these situations. Administration of flumazenil should occur only when acute seizure management measures are available.

Flumazenil reverses benzodiazepine-induced sedation or coma within 1 to 2 minutes after IV administration. The most common side effects include agitation, dizziness, nausea, general discomfort, tearfulness, anxiety, and a sensation of coldness.[62] Rapid or excessive infusion has been associated with tachycardia and hypertension. The elimination half-life of flumazenil is 41 to 79 minutes, and sedation may recur after 1 to 2 hours, especially when large doses of long-acting benzodiazepines are involved. Repeated flumazenil doses or an IV infusion may be indicated in these cases. Full recovery should be verified (3–4 hours of stable alertness) before patients are discharged after flumazenil administration, and they should be advised to avoid driving or performing other potentially hazardous activities for 24 hours. Flumazenil undergoes extensive hepatic metabolism to inactive metabolites.[62] Dosage reductions are recommended in patients with liver dysfunction, but flumazenil pharmacokinetics are not altered significantly by gender, age, or renal impairment.

Flumazenil administration is not appropriate in S.P.'s case because of his history of head injury and seizures. Instead, management should involve general supportive measures and mechanical ventilation, if indicated. It is probably too late for use of activated charcoal or gastric lavage in this case because the ingestion occurred the previous night. These interventions can often be beneficial in managing benzodiazepine overdose, although gastric lavage may provide no extra benefit over administration of activated charcoal alone. A psychiatric evaluation is also indicated in this case to identify and address the reasons for S.P.'s overdose.

Physiological Variables Influencing Benzodiazepines

12. B.G., a 68-year-old man, is brought to the emergency department (ED) by his wife after being involved as the driver in a minor car accident. He has no physical injuries except for several small abrasions caused by the car airbag deployment. However, B.G. appears drowsy, is mildly confused, and has an unsteady gait. A toxicology screen reveals no alcohol or other substances, except for diazepam, which his physician prescribed several months ago. B.G.'s wife states that he has been taking 1 tablet (5 mg) BID or TID and that it has been remarkably effective in improving his mood and anxiety. B.G., who is 5 feet 8 inch tall and weighs 250 lb, is a recovering alcoholic with moderate liver disease caused by years of heavy drinking. He has successfully maintained his sobriety for nearly 2 years. In addition to diazepam, B.G. also occasionally takes OTC omeprazole (Prilosec) and cimetidine (Tagamet) for heartburn. It is determined that B.G. is suffering from adverse effects of diazepam, probably caused by drug accumulation. What factors could be influencing disposition of diazepam in this patient?

Benzodiazepine pharmacokinetics can be affected by various physiological factors, including age, gender, obesity, hepatic and renal disease, and ethnicity (Table 76-9). Several of these factors are present in this case and may have contributed to the accumulation of diazepam with resulting adverse consequences.

B.G.'s age may influence diazepam disposition. Reductions in both CYP 3A4 and CYP 2C19 activity have been reported to occur with aging. The glucuronidation metabolic pathways are minimally affected with age, so no such effect is seen with lorazepam or oxazepam.[47] Although some studies indicate reduced clearance of various benzodiazepines in the elderly (especially males), others have found comparable rates of benzodiazepine clearance between young and elderly groups. Other factors that may contribute to longer benzodiazepine half-lives in the elderly include decreased hepatic blood flow and increased volumes of distribution of lipid-soluble compounds (due to decreased muscle mass and increased fat); the latter effect can increase a drug's half-life in the absence of any clearance changes. As described in Question 5, older patients are more sensitive to the sedative and psychomotor effects of benzodiazepines. For these reasons, the recommended benzodiazepine dosages for patients older than 65 years are generally one-third to one-half of those used in healthy adults (Table 76-4).

Gender also may influence benzodiazepine clearance.[13,64] Studies examining gender effects have yielded mixed results, probably because of wide interindividual differences. In elderly patients, some investigators have found lower clearances of clorazepate, diazepam, and alprazolam in men compared with those in women.[64] Women have been reported to have higher CYP 3A4 and CYP 2C19 activities, which may partially explain these findings. The increased CYP 3A4 activity in women disappears after menopause, which may necessitate the use

Table 76-9 Physiological Factors Influencing Benzodiazepine Pharmacokinetics

Factor	Physiological and Pharmacokinetic Effects	Clinical Significance/Comments
Aging	Increased elimination half-life due to increased Vd of all benzodiazepines[172]	Lower benzodiazepine dosages, and possibly less frequent dosing intervals, recommended in the elderly
	Decreased clearance of benzodiazepines that undergo oxidative hepatic metabolism (Table 76-6)[173]	Benzodiazepines that undergo glucuronidation (lorazepam, oxazepam) preferred in the elderly
	Decreased plasma proteins may lead to increased free fraction of highly protein-bound benzodiazepines (Table 76-6)	Possible increased clinical effects
	Decreased gastric acidity may lead to increased rate of benzodiazepine absorption	Possible faster onset of clinical effects
Gender	Age-related decrease in hepatic oxidative metabolism of benzodiazepines more pronounced in males	Elderly males may require especially low benzodiazepine dosages
	Increased CYP 3A4 and CYP 2C19 activity in premenopausal women may result in higher clearance of drugs that undergo oxidative metabolism[13]	Possible decreased plasma benzodiazepine concentrations and shorter duration of clinical effects of oxidatively metabolized agents in premenopausal women
	Decreased glucuronidation in women may result in slower clearance of benzodiazepines metabolized by conjugation[13]	Women may have longer elimination half-lives of lorazepam and temazepam and may require less frequent dosing
	Increased Vd in women due to lower lean body mass and increased adipose tissue[13]	Possible longer elimination half-lives in women, especially the elderly, and greater drug accumulation
	Lower plasma protein binding in women[13]	Clinical significance unknown
Obesity	Increased benzodiazepine elimination half-lives due to increased Vd	Increased chance of drug accumulation in obese patients; dosage reductions may be indicated
Liver disease	Decreased clearance and increased elimination half-lives of long-acting benzodiazepines and alprazolam in cirrhosis and hepatitis; no changes with oxazepam or triazolam[47]	Avoid long-acting benzodiazepines, or use significantly lower doses to avoid drug accumulation
	Increased elimination half-life of lorazepam in cirrhosis but not acute hepatitis	Decreased lorazepam dose or increased dosing interval recommended in cirrhosis
Kidney disease	Decreased plasma protein binding may lead to increased free fraction of highly protein-bound benzodiazepines (Table 76-6)[174]	Dosage reductions may be necessary
Ethnicity	Decreased oxidative metabolism (via CYP 2C19) of diazepam and alprazolam in Asians[65]	Asians may require lower doses of diazepam, alprazolam, and possibly other benzodiazepines

CYP, cytochrome P450; Vd, volume of distribution.

of lower benzodiazepine dosages during the postmenopausal period. Women have slower glucuronidation metabolic processes than men, resulting in lower clearance of agents such as temazepam and oxazepam.[13,47]

Obesity and liver impairment are other physiological factors that are relevant to B.G.'s case. Obesity increases the volume of distribution of benzodiazepines and the extent of accumulation of long-acting agents. Significant changes in the elimination half-lives of lorazepam and oxazepam are not observed in obese patients. Liver dysfunction can reduce benzodiazepine elimination rates and prolong their half-lives, resulting in recommendations for decreased dosages. The pharmacokinetics of oxazepam or triazolam are unaffected by liver disease.

Decreased protein binding of benzodiazepines can occur in patients with renal insufficiency, and this may lead to increased free fractions of highly protein-bound agents. However, no significant changes in clearance or volume of distribution of free drug have been noted. Regarding ethnicity, up to 20% of Asians are CYP 2C19 poor metabolizers. Decreased clearance of a variety of CYP 2C19 substrates, including diazepam, has been reported in Asian subjects.[65]

In summary, the physiological factors that can alter benzodiazepine disposition in B.G. are his age, obesity, male gender, and liver disease. Accumulation of diazepam due to these combined effects probably led to his mental status changes. In addition to these factors, cimetidine and omeprazole can both significantly impair the metabolism of diazepam, resulting in decreased clearance and increased side effects (Table 76-8).[56]

If continued benzodiazepine therapy is deemed necessary for B.G., lorazepam or oxazepam would be preferred agents because they would be least affected by aging, obesity, liver disease, or drug interactions. Benzodiazepine dosage equivalencies, which are based on relative potencies, can be used to determine an equivalent dose for the selected agent (Table 76-4). However, these equivalencies are inexact, and dosing conversions should take patient variables and usual dosage ranges into consideration. For example, B.G. had been taking 10 to 15 mg/day of diazepam, so the calculated equivalent lorazepam dosage is 2 to 3 mg/day. Because of his age, a somewhat lower initial dose of 0.5 to 1.0 mg BID would be indicated, accompanied by careful monitoring for adverse effects or withdrawal symptoms. However, switching to a nonbenzodiazepine agent should be considered because this may be a better treatment option for B.G.

Buspirone Therapy

13. Several days after recovery from diazepam intoxication, B.G. expresses a desire to discontinue benzodiazepine use. He is being criticized by his fellow Alcoholics Anonymous program members for taking a drug associated with dependency. The

decision is made to switch B.G. from diazepam to buspirone. How does the clinical profile of buspirone compare with that of the benzodiazepines?

Buspirone was the first agent marketed as an anxiolytic that lacks CNS depressant effects. In contrast to the benzodiazepines, it produces no significant sedation, cognitive or psychomotor impairment, or respiratory depression, and it lacks muscle relaxant and anticonvulsant effects.[37] Buspirone is generally well tolerated, and side effects, when they occur, include mild nausea, dizziness, headache, and initial nervousness.[66] Some patients may experience mild drowsiness or fatigue on initiation of therapy. Low sedation potential and lack of cognitive and respiratory depressant effects make buspirone useful in older patients who may have a variety of chronic medical conditions. Unlike many antidepressants, buspirone does not adversely affect sexual functioning and has actually improved sexual functioning in some patients with GAD.[36] Buspirone has minimal potential for abuse and is not classified as a controlled substance. It does not produce physical dependence or withdrawal syndromes on discontinuation, even after long-term therapy."[37,67] It also does not interact with alcohol or other CNS depressants and is relatively safe in overdose.[37]

Buspirone is as effective as benzodiazepines such as alprazolam, oxazepam, lorazepam, diazepam, and clorazepate in the treatment of GAD.[66] Its superiority over placebo has been reported in many, but not all, trials. For example, in a controlled comparison with extended-release venlafaxine, buspirone was no more effective than placebo in treating GAD.[68] Like antidepressants, buspirone is more effective than benzodiazepines in treating the cognitive symptoms of anxiety. However, the anxiolytic effects of buspirone have a more gradual onset than that of benzodiazepines. Initial effects are observed within the first 7 to 10 days, but 3 to 4 weeks may be needed for optimal results. Buspirone must be taken on an ongoing basis if it is effective and the drug should not be taken intermittently or "as needed."

Switching From Benzodiazepine to Buspirone Therapy

14. How should B.G. be switched from benzodiazepine to buspirone therapy?

Because buspirone has no CNS depressant effects and is not cross-tolerant with the benzodiazepines, it is not effective in preventing or treating benzodiazepine withdrawal. Thus, when patients are being converted from benzodiazepine to buspirone therapy, the benzodiazepine must be discontinued gradually. Because it takes several weeks for full therapeutic effects of buspirone to occur, it can be initiated before the benzodiazepine taper begins. This may indirectly ease benzodiazepine withdrawal by providing extra anxiolytic coverage during the benzodiazepine taper period.[69]

Buspirone is completely absorbed, but it undergoes extensive first-pass metabolism, which reduces its absolute bioavailability to approximately 5%.[37] Administration with food may significantly increase bioavailability by decreasing the first-pass effect. Buspirone has an active metabolite, 1-pyrimidinylpiperazine (1-PP), which is present in much higher concentrations than buspirone at therapeutic doses. 1-PP acts on the noradrenergic system rather than serotonin and functions as an α_2-adrenergic antagonist. Some of the side effects of buspirone, such as nervousness, are attributed to this active metabolite.[37,70] The mean elimination half-life of buspirone is short, approximately 2 to 3 hours, but 1-PP is longer acting.

Table 76-10 Buspirone Drug Interactions

Interacting Drug(s)	*Clinical Significance/Comments*
CYP 3A4 inhibitors: nefazodone, fluoxetine, fluvoxamine, erythromycin, itraconazole, ketoconazole, diltiazem, verapamil, grapefruit juice, and ritonavir	Significant increases in buspirone Cp have been reported with these agents, but adverse clinical effects are not always apparent.
	Buspirone dosage reductions are recommended when coadministered with erythromycin, fluvoxamine, nefazodone, fluoxetine, or itraconazole.
Rifampin	Highly significant decreases in buspirone Cp; avoid concurrent use.
Haloperidol	Buspirone may increase haloperidol Cp, but one study found no interaction.
Monoamine oxidase inhibitors	Possible serotonin syndrome; avoid concurrent use.

Cp, plasma concentration; CYP, cytochrome P450.

The clearance of buspirone is significantly reduced in patients with kidney or liver disease, but there is little change in side effects or tolerability.[37] Nevertheless, it is recommended that lower buspirone dosages be used in patients with compromised renal or hepatic function and that it be avoided in cases of severe impairment. Buspirone pharmacokinetics are not significantly affected by age or gender; therefore, no dosage adjustments are needed in the elderly.[37]

Important drug interactions with buspirone are summarized in Table 76-10.[37] Buspirone is metabolized by CYP 3A4, and coadministration of CYP 3A4 inhibitors, including grapefruit juice, can result in significant increases in buspirone levels. In many cases, the half-life of buspirone remained unchanged, suggesting that these interactions are mainly due to inhibition of CYP 3A4–mediated first-pass metabolism in the gut. Because of buspirone's extremely wide margin of safety and tolerability, even very large increases in its plasma levels may be clinically insignificant. Some hepatic enzyme inducers can render buspirone ineffective due to large increases in buspirone clearance. Buspirone should be avoided in patients taking MAOIs due to the risk of serotonin syndrome. Buspirone does not appear to enhance the CNS depressant effects of alcohol.

It was previously believed that patients who had been treated with benzodiazepines in the past did not respond as well to buspirone as benzodiazepine-naive patients. It is now evident that buspirone can provide benefit in this population as long as the benzodiazepine is tapered slowly enough to prevent withdrawal.[14] B.G. has been taking diazepam for several months and needs to be withdrawn gradually over a period of at least several weeks. B.G. can be started on buspirone at this time. The usual recommended starting dosage of buspirone is 15 mg/day given in two to three divided doses, but a lower dosage (10 mg/day) is indicated in B.G. because of his liver disease. Twice-daily dosing is preferred to facilitate compliance and is comparable in efficacy and tolerability to three-times-daily dosing.[71] The daily dosage may be increased in 5-mg/day increments every 3 to 4 days. Optimal anxiolytic doses generally range from 20 to 30 mg/day, with 60 mg/day being the manufacturer's recommended maximum. There are no specific guidelines for adjusting dosages in patients with liver impairment; therefore, dosage titrations in B.G. should be made slowly, according to his response and side effects. "Dividose" 15-mg tablets are available; these tablets are scored and notched, so they may be broken into 5-, 7.5-, or 10-mg doses. A 30-mg "Dividose" tablet is also available, as well as generic buspirone products.

PANIC DISORDER

Diagnostic Criteria

The DSM-IV-TR criteria for panic disorder are presented in Table 76-11.[1] The hallmark characteristic of panic disorder is the occurrence of sudden and distinct panic attacks, which are marked by a tremendous wave of symptoms and feelings listed in Table 76-11. At least four of these symptoms are required to fulfill criteria for a panic attack, and the term "limited symptom attack" refers to those events involving less than four symptoms. Three types of panic attacks have been defined with regard to the context in which they occur: unexpected or uncued panic attacks (the attack is not associated with a situational trigger); situationally bound panic attacks (the attacks invariably occur on exposure to a situational trigger); and situationally predisposed panic attacks (the attacks are more likely to, but do not invariably, occur on exposure to a situational trigger).[1]

The DSM-IV-TR criteria for panic disorder require the occurrence of at least two unexpected or uncued panic attacks that are followed by persistent worry or concern about having another panic attack or a significant change in behavior related to the attacks. Although panic attacks are the hallmark symptom of panic disorder, their occurrence does not always indicate panic disorder.[1] Depressive disorders and other anxiety disorders can also be associated with occasional panic attacks. Situationally bound panic attacks are more characteristic of specific phobias or social anxiety disorder than panic disorder, and situationally predisposed panic attacks may occur in either panic or phobic disorders. Nocturnal panic attacks, which awaken a person from sleep, are almost always indicative of panic disorder. Because panic attacks occur unpredictably, they often lead to generalized anxiety or constant fear of sudden attacks. Two subtypes of panic disorder have been identified: without agoraphobia or with agoraphobia.[1] *Agoraphobia* refers to a fear of being in situations from which escape might be difficult or embarrassing in the event of a panic attack. Mild-to-moderate agoraphobia involves selective avoidance of certain places or situations such as shopping malls, theaters, grocery stores, elevators, and driving alone. Some people may be unable to go anywhere unless accompanied by a companion. In severe cases of agoraphobia, the sufferer may become completely housebound.

Table 76-11 Diagnostic Criteria for Panic Disorder

1. Presence of at least two unexpected panic attacks, characterized by at least four of the following symptoms, which develop abruptly and reach a peak within 10 minutes:
   a. Palpitations, pounding heart, or accelerated heart rate
   b. Sweating
   c. Trembling or shaking
   d. Sensations of shortness of breath or smothering
   e. Feeling of choking
   f. Chest pain or discomfort
   g. Nausea or abdominal distress
   h. Feeling dizzy, unsteady, lightheaded, or faint
   i. Derealization or depersonalization
   j. Fear of losing control or going crazy
   k. Fear of dying
   l. Numbness or tingling sensations
   m. Chills or hot flushes
2. At least one of the attacks has been followed by at least one of the following symptoms for a duration of at least 1 month:
   a. Persistent concern about having another attack
   b. Worry about the implications or consequences of the attack
   c. Significant change in behavior because of the attack
3. Symptoms are not due to the direct effects of a medication, substance, or general medical condition
4. Panic attacks are not better accounted for by another psychiatric or anxiety disorder (e.g., phobias, obsessive-compulsive disorder)
5. May occur with or without agoraphobia (see text)

Adapted from reference 1, with permission. Copyright © 2000 American Psychiatric Association.

Epidemiology and Clinical Course

Approximately 28% of the general population experiences a single isolated panic attack at some time in their lives.[72] Approximately 10% to 12% of persons experience recurrent panic attacks that do not fulfill the diagnostic criteria for panic disorder; however, these persons can still be significantly affected. True panic disorder is estimated to affect 1% to 2% of Americans at some time in their lives.[7,72] Women are affected two to three times more often than men and are more likely to develop agoraphobia.[13] The onset of panic disorder usually occurs in the late teens to mid-30s, and it is rarely seen in the elderly.[7] Most persons report onset of the disorder at some particularly stressful time in their life; in women, this often includes the prenatal and postpartum periods.[13,60]

Panic disorder is accompanied by marked degrees of psychiatric comorbidity; 50% to 60% of patients suffer a major depressive episode at some point. Other common comorbid conditions include social anxiety disorder, GAD, OCD, PTSD, personality disorders, alcohol abuse, and bipolar disorder.[1,72,73] Patients with comorbid disorders have more severe symptoms, show slower and poorer response to treatments, are less likely to experience full remission, and have a greater suicide risk (particularly when depression or substance abuse are present) than those with panic disorder alone.[74,75] Panic disorder causes significant functional disability in areas of work, family relationships, and overall quality of life.[7,76]

Panic disorder is associated with very high rates of health care service utilization.[75] Because of the physical manifestations of panic attacks, repeated ED visits and costly diagnostic tests are common.[77] About 25% to 32% of patients making ED visits related to chest pain actually have panic disorder. The poor recognition of panic disorder in primary care settings further increases use of medical services. Panic disorder is the underlying cause of symptoms in an estimated 10% to 30% of patients referred to specialty vestibular, respiratory, or neurology clinics, and up to 60% of those referred for cardiology consultation.[1] The vast majority of patients with panic disorder do not complain of feeling anxious and report only physical symptoms, such as chest pain, GI problems, headache, dizziness, and shortness of breath, which contributes to misdiagnosis.[77] It is not uncommon for patients to have been in the health care system for up to 10 years before they are correctly diagnosed.

The long-term course of panic disorder is highly variable.[1] Some patients experience episodic periods of remission and relapse, whereas others suffer almost continuously. Follow-up studies conducted several years after treatment reveal that approximately one-third of patients are still well and in remission, 40% to 50% of patients are improved but experience persistent symptoms, and another 20% to 30% are unchanged or worse.[1,78]

Etiology and Pathophysiology

There is substantial evidence that panic disorder is biologically based. A neuroanatomical model for panic disorder has been proposed in which the anxiety and fear response to threatening stimuli are mediated through the amygdala.[5,79] Various projections from the amygdala, including the hypothalamus and the LC, trigger autonomic and neuroendocrine responses that result in anxiety and panic attacks. Patients with panic disorder have a heightened anxiety sensitivity (fear of anxiety-related sensations), and a variety of substances and situations are capable of triggering the neural fear network that activates the anxiety and panic response.[79] Acute panic attacks are believed to be caused by dysregulated firing in the LC as described previously (see Neurobiology of Anxiety section), and hyperresponsiveness of the NE system may be an underlying cause for panic disorder.[80]

Experimental provocation of panic attacks is an important component of panic disorder research. Administration of certain substances induces panic attacks rather consistently in persons with panic disorder, but not in normal healthy subjects.[5,79] These substances include caffeine, noradrenaline, sodium lactate, hypertonic sodium chloride, high concentration carbon dioxide (CO_2), yohimbine, flumazenil, and CCK-B agonists. Administration of effective medication treatments for panic disorder blocks the effects of these panic-inducing substances. Challenge studies such as these provide evidence for possible abnormalities in GABA-A receptor, NE, 5-HT, and CCK functioning that underlie panic disorders. Decreased GABA-A benzodiazepine binding sites, abnormal regulation of neuroactive steroids that modulate GABA-A receptors, hyperactivation of the HPA axis, and CCK-B receptor gene polymorphism are among the findings associated with panic disorder.[73,81]

Hypersensitivity to 35% CO_2 inhalation, as evidenced by precipitation of panic attacks, robustly identifies patients with panic disorder as well as those with other anxiety disorders such as OCD and GAD.[79] This association is specific enough that CO_2 hypersensitivity is considered a biological trait marker, at least for a subset of panic disorder patients. Effective treatment of panic disorder with medication significantly decreases the sensitivity to CO_2 inhalation.[82] Brain imaging studies also have demonstrated abnormal patterns of cerebral glucose metabolism in certain brain areas in patients with panic disorder.[79]

A familial occurrence of panic disorder has been noted; first-degree relatives of individuals with panic disorder have an 8- to 21-fold greater risk of panic disorder than relatives of unaffected persons.[1,15] Genetic and environmental influences both contribute to this familial pattern. The inherited component is believed to involve heightened anxiety sensitivity, which confers increased vulnerability for panic disorder. Heightened anxiety sensitivity in panic disorder has been associated with "catastrophic cognitions," in which harmless normal physical sensations are misinterpreted as being dangerous and cause fear.[78] These negative cognitive patterns are often unconscious and may be integral in potentiating recurrent panic attacks in a biologically predisposed individual.

Developmental experiences may also be important in the etiology of panic disorder. Several studies have shown that distressing childhood events such as separation from parents and abuse are associated with markedly increased risks of developing panic disorder later in life.[79] Behavioral inhibition during childhood, characterized by excessive fear and avoidance of novel stimuli, is also extremely common in panic disorder patients. Obviously, no one biological abnormality can explain panic disorder, and further research is needed to define the complex interplay of the various pathophysiological, genetic, and cognitive findings in this illness.

Treatment of Panic Disorder

Approximately 70% to 90% of patients with panic disorder can experience substantial relief with currently available treatments, which include both pharmacologic therapies and CBTs.[1,73] Medications are most beneficial for reducing panic attacks initially, and their effects on phobic avoidance generally occur later. Nonpharmacologic therapies are especially effective in reducing avoidance behaviors. The two classes of first-line medication treatments for panic disorder are the SSRIs and the benzodiazepines, and these agents are often used in combination.[73] Several TCA and MAOI antidepressants are also effective in treating panic disorder, but are reserved as second- or third-line options because of their clinical disadvantages compared with SSRIs. The heightened anxiety sensitivity common in panic disorder makes patients especially vulnerable to certain initial antidepressant side effects, such as anxiety and agitation. This is seen with most antidepressants, including SSRIs and TCAs, and is the reason why lower than usual starting doses of antidepressants are recommended in patients with panic disorder.

Selective Serotonin Reuptake Inhibitors

The SSRIs, paroxetine, sertraline, and fluoxetine, as well as the SNRI, venlafaxine, are FDA approved for treating panic disorder. There is strong evidence that other SSRIs (fluvoxamine, citalopram, escitalopram) are also effective.[21,30] Several large controlled trials have demonstrated the superiority of paroxetine, sertraline, and fluoxetine over placebo in reducing the frequency of panic attacks, anticipatory anxiety, and associated depression.[83,84] Although low starting dosages are recommended (10 mg/day for paroxetine, 25 mg/day for sertraline, 5–10 mg/day for fluoxetine) to minimize side effects, higher doses are usually required for response. The recommended target dosage range of paroxetine for panic disorder is 20 to 40 mg/day.[85] Fixed-dose sertraline studies showed that the efficacy of 50, 100, and 200 mg/day doses was comparable; there was no consistent dose–response effect.[86] Therefore, 50 mg/day should be targeted as the minimum dose of sertraline that will be needed when treating panic disorder; higher doses may sometimes be required. The target dose of fluoxetine in panic disorder is 20 mg/day, and most patients are unlikely to require higher doses.[83] For citalopram, a 20- to 30-mg/day dosage range has been associated with better efficacy than 40 to 60 mg/day, whereas doses of 10 to 15 mg/day were ineffective.[24] The initial dose of venlafaxine XR should be 37.5 mg/day.

Response to SSRIs and other antidepressants in panic disorder occurs gradually, over the course of several weeks. Reduced frequency of panic attacks usually begins within 4 to 6 weeks. A trial period of 10 to 12 weeks should be allowed to fully assess response, and continued improvements may be seen over a treatment period of 6 months or longer.[73,78] Overall, the SSRIs are as effective as the TCAs in treating panic disorder, but they are better tolerated and may have a slightly faster onset of therapeutic effects.[78,87]

Benzodiazepines

The benzodiazepines, alprazolam and clonazepam, are FDA approved for treating panic disorder and are the most extensively studied agents of this class.[77,78,88] As previously described, new formulations of these agents (Xanax XR, Klonopin wafer) have been introduced specifically for use in panic disorder. Lorazepam is another high-potency agent that appears to be as effective as alprazolam and clonazepam.[78] Other benzodiazepines such as diazepam were previously believed to be ineffective in treating panic disorder, but they can be effective if sufficiently high doses are used.[78]

Optimal benzodiazepine dosing is an important issue in panic disorder because these individuals often need higher doses for response than patients with other anxiety disorders.[89] This may be related to reduced sensitivity of benzodiazepine binding sites in panic disorder.[18] An alprazolam dosage range of 4 to 6 mg/day is effective for most panic disorder patients, but others may require up to 10 mg/day for optimal response. When clonazepam is used, the minimum effective dosage appears to be 1 mg/day, and most panic disorder patients do well in the range of 1 to 3 mg/day.

One problem with alprazolam use in panic disorder is that many patients experience breakthrough anxiety or panic attacks 3 to 5 hours after taking a dose because of its relatively short duration of action.[78] The total daily alprazolam dose usually needs to be taken in three or four, and sometimes five, divided doses to minimize this effect. The extended-release alprazolam formulation (Xanax XR) was developed to address this problem.[46] Xanax XR can be dosed once or twice daily and is associated with minimal interdose anxiety. It may have a lower abuse liability than immediate-release alprazolam, but it is more expensive than generic alprazolam. Clonazepam is longer acting than standard-release alprazolam, and a twice-daily dosing schedule is usually sufficient. A switch to either clonazepam or extended-release alprazolam can be beneficial when breakthrough anxiety is a problem with immediate-release alprazolam. Extended-release alprazolam is more expensive than generic alprazolam or clonazepam and probably offers no clinical advantage in most cases. Panic disorder patients are especially sensitive to benzodiazepine withdrawal effects. For this reason, clonazepam may be preferred over alprazolam in many panic disorder patients.[89]

Tricyclic Antidepressants, Monoamine Oxidase Inhibitors, and Other Antidepressants

TCAs were the first medications widely used in the treatment of panic disorder. Imipramine (Tofranil) and clomipramine (Anafranil) are as effective as alprazolam, but are less well tolerated.[74,85] One trial with desipramine (Norpramin) found that it did not significantly differ from placebo.[78] Well-conducted studies involving other TCAs are lacking. As indicated, especially low starting dosages of TCAs (10 mg/day) are needed to minimize initial anxiety-like side effects. Even so, many patients discontinue therapy because of poor tolerability. Imipramine should be slowly titrated up to the recommended target dosage of 100 mg/day.

Clomipramine appears to be more effective than other TCAs for panic disorder, perhaps because of its greater serotonergic effects.[90] The possibility of a therapeutic dosage window for clomipramine in panic disorder has been suggested, with dosages >80 mg/day being associated with a reduced likelihood of response.[90,91] Clomipramine seems to be most effective within the dosage range of 60 to 80 mg/day, which is relatively low but reasonably well tolerated. Patients who do not respond to clomipramine doses in this range are unlikely to benefit from further dose increases.

Among the MAOIs, phenelzine (Nardil) is often heralded as being remarkably effective in the treatment of panic disorder, but this claim is based on studies that were conducted more than two decades ago in patients who might not meet the current diagnostic criteria for panic disorder.[78] No recent MAOI studies are available to assess phenelzine's efficacy within the context of current diagnostic and treatment standards. Phenelzine may be extremely effective, but it is generally an option of last resort for treatment-refractory cases because of the many clinical disadvantages of MAOIs relative to other antidepressants (see Chapter 79). Preliminary reports suggest that other newer antidepressants, including venlafaxine, nefazodone, mirtazapine, and escitalopram, may also be beneficial in treating panic disorder.[30,78,89] These agents may be useful in patients who do not respond to SSRI therapy.

Miscellaneous Agents

Bupropion (Wellbutrin), buspirone, and trazodone are generally ineffective for panic disorder.[78] Trials of propranolol and clonidine have yielded mixed, but largely negative results.[78] None of these agents are considered appropriate treatment options in panic disorder, although buspirone and pindolol have been effective in augmenting response to SSRI therapy.[89,92] Other medications that are reportedly effective in treating panic disorder include the anticonvulsants carbamazepine, oxcarbazepine, tiagabine, and valproate; the calcium channel blocker verapamil; the antipsychotic agent olanzapine; the antihistamine chlorpheniramine; the serotonin-3 receptor antagonist, ondansetron; and inositol.[78,89] More information is needed before any of these can be recommended for the treatment of panic disorder.

Nonpharmacologic Treatments

CBTs, including exposure treatment and relaxation training, are also established as being effective in panic disorder.[73,78] The cognitive theory of panic disorder is based on the observed heightened anxiety sensitivity in these patients and asserts that physical anxiety sensations are misinterpreted as being serious or life threatening and that these fears trigger a cycle of further worsening anxiety symptoms that finally progress to a panic attack. Reversing the cognitive component of this vicious cycle is an integral part of cognitive therapy and is important in producing lasting therapeutic effects of treatment.[78] Breathing retraining and exposure to fear cues are key components of behavioral therapy.

Some studies have found medications to be superior to CBTs in the treatment of panic disorder, whereas others report opposite results.[73,78] CBTs reportedly result in benefits that are maintained longer after therapy is stopped and have also been effective in easing benzodiazepine discontinuation. Combining medication with CBTs can be useful, especially in patients with severe agoraphobia or those who only partially respond to either treatment modality used alone.[89,93]

Clinical Presentation and Differential Diagnosis of Panic Disorder

15. S.K., a 24-year-old female graduate student, presents to the ED complaining of chest pain, difficulty breathing, dizziness, and nausea. She describes feeling "as if my head is going off in space and I am outside my body." She states that she has been under extreme stress lately with examinations, working too much, and constantly fighting with her roommate. S.K. fears that she has had a heart attack or stroke brought on by her stressful life. S.K. recently visited her family physician for the same symptoms; however, a complete physical examination and laboratory workup yielded no abnormalities, and she was advised to try to relax. She states that her first "attack" occurred out of the blue about 5 months ago while she was studying in the library and that she can never predict when they will occur. Since then, her symptoms have become more severe and frequent, and she has started skipping classes for fear they will return. S.K. denies any drug or alcohol use but states that she has suffered from depression in the past and was hospitalized for one severe episode 2 years ago. An ECG is performed and found to be normal. The physician's diagnosis is panic disorder with mild agoraphobia. What clinical features of panic disorder does S.K. display, and what are the important factors in the differential diagnosis of panic disorder?

S.K. exhibits many typical characteristics of panic disorder. As illustrated in this case, the first panic attack typically occurs without warning while the person is involved in a normal everyday activity and lasts 10 to 30 minutes. Panic attacks are extremely terrifying and usually leave the sufferer feeling anxious and convinced that something is medically wrong. As with S.K., it is not uncommon for persons to make ED visits following or during panic attacks, believing they have had a heart attack or other serious event. Unfortunately, panic disorder is often not recognized in primary care settings, and no medical cause for the symptoms can be identified. Faced with findings that they are apparently healthy, persons may make repeated ED visits and consult different doctors and specialists in an attempt to uncover a physical explanation for their frightening symptoms.

S.K. exhibits the following target symptoms of panic disorder: chest pain, shortness of breath, dizziness, abdominal distress, and depersonalization ("my head is going off in space and I am outside my body"). Mild agoraphobia is present because she has started limiting class attendance because of her panic attacks. Other factors consistent with a diagnosis of panic disorder include her young age, female gender, lack of abnormal physical findings, and absence of possible precipitating substances. This case also illustrates the association between onset of panic disorder and stressful life events, its common association with depression, and the frequent lack of recognition of panic disorder in primary care settings.

Because different substances or medical conditions can cause severe anxiety and panic, it is necessary to rule out these potential causes for panic disorder symptoms.[77] Notable triggers of panic attacks include caffeine, alcohol, nicotine, nonprescription cold preparations, cannabis, amphetamines, and cocaine.[77] Any medication that causes anxiety as a side effect can potentially precipitate panic attacks in predisposed individuals (Table 76-2). Medical illnesses that can cause panic attacks include hyperthyroidism, hyperparathyroidism, pheochromocytoma, seizure disorders, and cardiac arrhythmias. Panic disorder is also associated with higher-than-expected comorbidities with hypertension, mitral valve prolapse, asthma, coronary artery disease, peptic ulcer disease, Parkinson disease, chronic pain syndromes, primary biliary cirrhosis, and irritable bowel syndrome.[78] In patients with comorbid medical conditions, panic disorder can worsen the physical illness.

Panic attacks can also occur in other anxiety disorders. However, in these cases, the panic attacks usually occur on exposure to a feared object or situation (in phobic disorders), an object of obsession (in OCD), or a stimulus associated with a traumatic stressor (in PTSD). S.K. reports that her panic attacks occur unexpectedly, and situationally bound or predisposed attacks are not evident; therefore, the features are consistent with panic disorder.

Treatment Selection for Panic Disorder, SSRI Dosing Issues, and Combination SSRI-Benzodiazepine Therapy

16. S.K. is referred to a psychiatrist who decides to initiate treatment with fluoxetine 20 mg Q AM. Three days later, S.K. calls the doctor complaining that her anxiety and panic attacks have greatly increased since she started taking fluoxetine. The psychiatrist prescribes alprazolam 0.5 mg (tablets) and instructs S.K. to take 1 tablet as needed for the anxiety. What factors should be considered in the selection of an initial medication treatment for panic disorder? Why is the prescribed treatment for S.K. inappropriate?

An SSRI, with or without concurrent benzodiazepine therapy, is appropriate first-line treatment for most panic disorder patients.[88,89] In patients such as S.K. who have a history of depression, SSRIs may also help prevent depressive relapse. Patients with severe or distressing symptoms usually require concurrent benzodiazepine therapy, which provides quick relief from anxiety and panic attacks until the therapeutic effects of SSRI occur. At that time, usually after several weeks, the benzodiazepine can be gradually discontinued. An SSRI-benzodiazepine combination is currently the most commonly prescribed initial treatment for panic disorder and is superior in efficacy to initial monotherapy.[42] Although benzodiazepines are generally avoided in patients with a history of substance abuse, use of low doses for a limited time period may be appropriate for some such patients with disabling symptoms, as long as there is no current substance (especially alcohol) abuse.[54,89] Because of the levels of distress and impairment caused by S.K.'s panic disorder, combined SSRI-benzodiazepine therapy would have been the preferred initial treatment. Scheduled benzodiazepine dosing is preferred over as-needed dosing schedule during initial therapy, so that panic attacks are prevented.[89] Because panic attacks generally last less than 30 minutes, they have usually passed by the time an as-needed benzodiazepine dose can take effect.

In choosing among SSRIs for the treatment of panic disorder, fluoxetine may be more likely to be anxiety provoking in some patients, and there is less published evidence to support its use than for sertraline or paroxetine.[21] If fluoxetine is used, very low initial doses (5–10 mg/day) should be used; in S.K.'s case, the prescribed 20-mg/day starting dose was much too high. Also, scheduled versus as-needed benzodiazepine dosing would have been preferred. After 2 to 4 weeks, the benzodiazepine can be gradually discontinued while the SSRI therapy is continued and gradually titrated to the target effective dose. The potential for drug interactions must also be kept in mind when SSRI-benzodiazepine combinations are used because certain SSRIs can inhibit benzodiazepine metabolism, leading to increased benzodiazepine side effects (see Benzodiazepine Drug Interactions section and Table 76-8).

Patient Counseling Information

Patients such as S.K. who are beginning SSRI therapy for the treatment of panic disorder should be counseled about possible increased anxiety during the first 1 or 2 weeks of treatment, as well as other common SSRI side effects, including nausea, headache, and either insomnia or sedation. Because these are dose-related effects, patients should inform their clinician of any problems, and a dosage reduction may be indicated. These adverse effects usually subside after 1 to 3 weeks of continued treatment. It is also important to inform patients that it may take several weeks before beneficial effects of antidepressant treatment are seen, and 6 to 12 weeks or longer may be required for full response. Patients receiving initial benzodiazepine therapy should be counseled about their relatively quick onset of effects to provide anxiolytic coverage during the initial weeks of SSRI therapy, as well as the likely limited duration of benzodiazepine therapy. Other pertinent counseling information for benzodiazepine treatment should also be included (see Question 5). The desired goals of therapy and likely duration of treatment should also be explained (see Question 18). Providing information about the nature of panic disorder, including reassurance that panic attacks are not life threatening, is also important. Many clinicians recommend that patients keep a "panic diary" in which they record frequency of panic attacks, along with symptoms experienced during attacks.

Clinical Assessment and Goals of Therapy

17. S.K. refuses to continue taking fluoxetine, so paroxetine is prescribed instead. After 1 week of paroxetine therapy at the initial dosage of 10 mg/day, S.K. is tolerating the medication well. The plan is to gradually increase the paroxetine to 40 mg/day over the next several weeks. S.K. is also taking alprazolam, 0.5 mg BID to TID. What are the desired goals of treatment in this case, and how can S.K.'s response to treatment be assessed?

Five domains in panic disorder have been identified in which treatment outcomes should be assessed: frequency and severity of panic attacks, anticipatory anxiety, phobic avoidance behaviors, overall well-being, and illness-related disability in various areas (work, school, family).[78] The treatment goals in this case are first to stop S.K.'s panic attacks, then to reduce her anticipatory anxiety, followed by reversal of phobic avoidance.[40] These outcomes should enable her to attend class regularly and, secondarily, improve her overall functioning and quality of life.

Several different instruments have been used to assess outcomes of treatment in panic disorder.[40] In addition to the panic diary, others include the Fear Questionnaire, the Panic Appraisal Inventory, and the Panic Disorder Severity Scale. The latter is currently considered by many experts to be the most useful because it evaluates outcomes in all five identified target domains of panic disorder.[40,78]

Course and Duration of Therapy

18. After 3 months of paroxetine therapy, S.K. reports that she has had no panic attacks in the past month and that functioning has improved dramatically. She is currently taking 40 mg/day of paroxetine (two 20-mg tablets) and gradually stopped taking the alprazolam 3 to 4 weeks ago. S.K. reveals that she is going to class, making good grades, getting along with her roommate, and dating. S.K. is experiencing no significant side effects from paroxetine but complains that it is expensive. She wonders how long she should continue taking it since she is doing so well. What is the recommended duration of treatment for panic disorder?

Long-term medication trials in panic disorder support the recommendation that treatment should continue for at least 6 to 12 months after acute response.[78,94] The benefits of maintenance pharmacotherapy in preventing relapse are well documented. Maintenance treatment gives patients time to resume normal lifestyles and to re-establish daily activities following acute cessation of panic attacks.

In this case, S.K.'s current paroxetine dosage of 40 mg/day is appropriate because this is within the effective dosage range for panic disorder. Paroxetine therapy should be continued at the current dosage for 3 to 6 more months. Paroxetine is available as a generic and the use of a 40-mg paroxetine tablet instead of two 20-mg tablets each day can decrease the drug expense. After a successful period of full remission, a trial of medication discontinuation may be attempted to determine whether continued treatment is necessary. Medication should not be stopped in patients who are experiencing stressful life events or substantial residual problems in any of the five domains. When medication is discontinued, it should be withdrawn gradually over several months, regardless of which medication class is involved. Because of the devastating impact that panic disorder can have, reinstitution of drug treatment is indicated if relapse occurs. Long-term treatment with antidepressants, and benzodiazepines if necessary, is generally successful in maintaining treatment benefits without detrimental effects or dosage escalations. Panic disorder is accepted as an appropriate indication for long-term benzodiazepine therapy if necessary.[88]

SOCIAL ANXIETY DISORDER AND SPECIFIC PHOBIAS

Classification and Diagnosis of Phobic Disorders

The DSM-IV-TR category of phobic disorders includes two primary types: specific phobia (formerly called *simple phobia*) and social phobia (also called *social anxiety disorder*).[1] The term *social anxiety disorder* is more commonly used and is the term used in this text. These disorders involve fears that are excessive or unreasonable and lead to avoidance behavior to minimize anxiety. The DSM-IV-TR criteria for phobic disorders are presented in Table 76-12.[1] The main difference between specific phobias and social anxiety disorder is that the former involves fear and avoidance of specific objects or situations, whereas the latter involves social situations.

Social Anxiety Disorder

In social anxiety disorder, there is an intense irrational fear of scrutiny or evaluation by others because of concerns about humiliation or being made to appear ridiculous.[1] The *generalized* type of social anxiety disorder refers to cases in which fears relate to most social situations (e.g., fear of general social interactions, speaking to people, attending social gatherings, dating), whereas the *nongeneralized* type involves more specific phobias.[1] Public speaking is by far the most common

Table 76-12 Diagnostic Criteria for Phobic Disorders

Social Anxiety Disorder (Social Phobia)

1. Marked and constant fear of one or more social situations in which the person is exposed to unfamiliar people or possible scrutiny by others and the person fears humiliation or embarrassment
2. Exposure to the situation provokes an immediate anxiety response
3. Person realizes the fear is excessive or unreasonable (not required in children)
4. Feared situation is avoided or endured with intense anxiety or distress
5. Fear or avoidance significantly interferes with the person's normal routine or activities or causes marked distress
6. In individuals younger than 18 years of age, the duration of the fear is at least 6 months
7. Anxiety or phobic avoidance are not better accounted for by another psychiatric disorder (e.g., fear of having a panic attack, obsessions that accompany OCD, trauma related to PTSD)

Specific Phobia

1. Marked and persistent fear of a specific object or situation that is excessive or unreasonable
2. Other criteria (2–7) listed previously for social anxiety disorder

OCD, obsessive-compulsive disorder; PTSD, posttraumatic stress disorder.
Adapted from reference 1, with permission. Copyright © 2000 American Psychiatric Association.

nongeneralized type; others include speaking to strangers, eating in public, and using public restrooms. A defining feature of either type is that the fears and anxiety are confined to social situations, and patients are usually symptom free when alone. The most common symptoms seen in social anxiety disorder include blushing, muscle twitching, and stuttering, in addition to other typical symptoms of anxiety. Panic attacks may also occur in either specific phobia or social anxiety disorder on exposure to the feared object or situation. However, social anxiety disorder is differentiated from panic disorder and agoraphobia in that it involves the fear of humiliation and social scrutiny, rather than the fear of having a panic attack.

The DSM-IV-TR excludes a diagnosis of social anxiety disorder if the person fears public embarrassment due to some physical or medical condition. However, this criterion is controversial because it excludes social anxiety disorder that is due to certain socially stigmatizing conditions, such as Parkinson's disease, stuttering, obesity, and physical disfigurement or deformity.[1] These cases are sometimes referred to as *secondary social anxiety disorder.*

Specific Phobias

Specific phobias are classified into five subtypes: animal type (snakes, dogs, spiders), natural environment type (heights, water, storms), blood-injection type (blood, injury, medical procedures), situational type (flying, bridges, elevators), and others.[1] Exposure to the feared circumstance produces intense anxiety, sometimes to the degree of panic attacks, and avoidance of the stimuli is common. Significant impairment of functioning or marked distress must be present for a diagnosis of specific phobia to be warranted. For example, fear of flying might constitute specific phobia in a person whose job requires airplane travel, but it would not impair functioning in someone who never has occasion to fly.

Management of specific phobias has traditionally involved mere avoidance of the stimuli. Medications generally are not considered beneficial, but CBTs involving repeated exposure to the feared situation and systemic desensitization are very effective. Computer-generated, virtual environment desensitization (virtual reality) therapy has been used successfully to reduce fears associated with flying and heights. Benzodiazepines can not only effectively reduce anxiety associated with a phobic trigger, but they can also interfere with the efficacy of exposure therapies.

Social Anxiety Disorder

Epidemiology and Clinical Course

The lifetime prevalence of social anxiety disorder is approximately 7%, which is lower than previous estimates of 13% to 14%.[7] The male:female prevalence ratio is approximately 2:3. Social anxiety disorder usually begins early in life, with a mean onset between ages 14 and 16 years.[95] More than 50% of patients are affected before adolescence, and a history of shyness and behavioral inhibition throughout childhood is common.[95] Unless effectively treated, the clinical course is often that of a chronic, unremitting, and lifelong disorder. Only 35% of patients recovered over the 10-year follow-up in one recent study.[96]

Comorbidity and Clinical Significance

Because social anxiety disorder usually begins during the teenage years, it can seriously interfere with development of normal social skills and abilities to form interpersonal relationships.[97] This can lead to functional disabilities that may persist for a lifetime. Social anxiety disorder can interfere with achievement of full academic and career potentials and is associated with unemployment, lower levels of education, and dependence on public financial support systems.[7] Persons with social anxiety disorder are less likely to marry, and more than half report moderate-to-severe impairments in their abilities to carry out ordinary daily activities.[97]

Comorbidity in social anxiety disorder is high, with an estimated 70% to 80% of individuals having at least one other psychiatric disorder in their lifetime.[1,95,96] Common comorbid conditions include simple phobia, major depression, GAD, panic disorder, body dysmorphic disorder, and alcohol abuse. Because of its early onset, social anxiety disorder usually precedes the development of comorbid disorders. Alcohol is commonly used to decrease anxiety in social situations. The risk of suicide attempts is very high, especially in those with both social anxiety disorder and another comorbid psychiatric illness.[7]

Etiology and Pathophysiology

Social anxiety disorder is known to be a familial disease, but the relative contributions of genetic versus environmental influences have not been differentiated.[15] Early factors that may predispose to its development include anxious behavior modeling in parents and parental overprotection.[1] Shyness in children, which is associated with later development of social anxiety disorder, has been linked to a specific genetic polymorphism of the serotonin transporter promoter region.[98]

Biological studies suggest that the generalized and nongeneralized types of social anxiety disorder may have different underlying pathophysiologies. Nongeneralized social anxiety disorder may mainly involve disturbances in noradrenergic system functioning, whereas there is substantial evidence for dopaminergic and serotonergic dysfunction in the generalized form.[99,100] Abnormally low dopamine neurotransmission in generalized social anxiety disorder is supported by findings of significantly decreased dopamine-2 receptor binding; markedly reduced dopamine transporter densities; low levels of the dopamine metabolite, homovanillic acid; high rates of social anxiety disorder in persons who later develop Parkinson disease; and several reports of emergence of social anxiety disorder during antipsychotic treatment.[99,100] Social anxiety disorder appears to be unique among the anxiety disorders in its association with dopamine system abnormalities. Pharmacologic challenge studies suggest that serotonin type-2 receptors are hypersensitive in patients with social anxiety disorder, and neuroimaging studies have found specific neural circuits to be activated in this illness.[99]

Treatment of Social Anxiety Disorder

Early detection and treatment of social anxiety disorder are vital in reducing its lifelong functional consequences and may prevent development of comorbid disorders. Because of the very nature of the disorder, some sufferers are reluctant to seek treatment. Those who do seek help, even in psychiatric settings, are rarely diagnosed and treated appropriately.[95] In the past few years, pharmacotherapy has become first-line therapy for social anxiety disorder. Nonpharmacologic treatments also can be very beneficial, and use of the two modalities may be complementary.

SELECTIVE SEROTONIN REUPTAKE INHIBITORS

As with many other anxiety disorders, SSRIs are considered the primary treatment option for most patients with social anxiety disorder.[95] Paroxetine, sertraline, and the SNRI, venlafaxine XR, have received FDA approval for this treatment indication.[101] Fluoxetine, fluvoxamine CR, citalopram, and escitalopram have also demonstrated efficacy in controlled clinical trials.[101–103]

Unlike patients with GAD and panic disorder, those with social anxiety disorder can usually tolerate standard antidepressant starting doses. Target effective SSRI doses for social anxiety disorder are within the normal antidepressant dosage ranges. The one fixed-dose study of paroxetine in social anxiety disorder found no overall difference in efficacy between 20, 40, and 60 mg/day.[104] Although some individuals may respond better to higher dosages, adequate time should be allowed at 20 mg/day before the dosage is increased. Response to SSRI treatment occurs gradually, and an adequate medication trial to assess response should last at least 8 to 10 weeks. Many who experience minimal response at week 8 may show good response at week 12, and improvements have been found to continue throughout 16 weeks of treatment.[105]

OTHER ANTIDEPRESSANTS

The MAOIs phenelzine and tranylcypromine have also demonstrated marked efficacy for social anxiety disorder but are reserved for SSRI nonresponders.[95,101] Before the advent of SSRIs, phenelzine was considered the mainstay of pharmacotherapy for social anxiety disorder. The typically effective dosage ranges are 60 to 90 mg/day for phenelzine and 30 to 60 mg/day for tranylcypromine.

The reversible monoamine oxidase-A inhibitors, moclobemide and brofaromine, which are currently unavailable in the United States, have shown mixed efficacy results in controlled studies.[95] Case reports and/or open studies suggest that other antidepressants, including nefazodone and bupropion, may be useful in treating social anxiety disorder, but controlled trials are needed to define their roles.[95] Imipramine is ineffective for social anxiety disorder, and TCAs are not among the recommended treatment options.[95,101]

BENZODIAZEPINES

The high-potency benzodiazepines, clonazepam and alprazolam, may also be useful in some patients with social anxiety disorder. Clonazepam was markedly efficacious in one controlled study, whereas alprazolam showed only modest efficacy over placebo.[95,101] The usual effective dosage ranges are 1 to 3 mg/day for clonazepam and 1 to 6 mg/day for alprazolam. In contrast to the antidepressants, benzodiazepines have a quicker onset of therapeutic effects and can also be used on an as-needed basis prior to participation in stressful social situations. However, benzodiazepines can reduce the therapeutic effects of exposure therapy. Other disadvantages of the benzodiazepines include their lack of efficacy for many common comorbid psychiatric disorders, potential for abuse and dependence, and a potentially dangerous interaction with alcohol.

Benzodiazepines are generally considered second-line therapy for social anxiety disorder, but in clinical practice they are commonly used on an as-needed basis in combination with SSRI therapy.[101]

β-BLOCKERS AND OTHER MISCELLANEOUS AGENTS

β-Adrenergic receptor blockers reduce peripheral autonomic symptoms of anxiety, but they are not effective in treating generalized social anxiety disorder.[95] However, they are useful for nongeneralized social phobia involving performance-related situations. Propranolol and atenolol are the two recommended agents and can be used on an as-needed basis to reduce performance anxiety. Small doses (10–80 mg of propranolol or 25–50 mg of atenolol) of either agent may be administered 1 to 2 hours before the performance to decrease symptoms such as tremors, palpitations, and blushing. A test dose should be tried before the actual occasion to assess medication tolerability. β-Blockers are not recommended as monotherapy for the treatment of generalized social anxiety disorder.[101] Various other medications, including pregabalin, gabapentin, tiagabine, and levetiracetam have also been reported to be effective in the treatment of social anxiety disorder, but they are considered second-line treatment.[101]

NONPHARMACOLOGIC TREATMENTS

Several studies have demonstrated CBTs to be comparable to medications in the treatment of social anxiety disorder.[106] The cognitive therapy component is aimed at changing the negative thought patterns, such as expectations of performing poorly and overconcern about negative evaluation by others.[106] These negative expectations lead to increased apprehension and anxiety, which further impair performance abilities. The behavioral therapy component, as in other anxiety disorders, involves repeated exposure to the feared social situations and practice at performing in those situations. Cognitive-behavioral group therapies are especially beneficial in social anxiety disorder because group members can practice social interactions with one another. Although medications may work faster, CBTs are believed to result in longer-lasting treatment gains.[106] Social skills training can also be beneficial in improving interpersonal communication skills.

Clinical Presentation of Social Anxiety Disorder

19. S.H., an 18-year-old man, is brought for psychiatric consultation by his mother who complains that her son is extremely shy. S.H. was referred to the psychiatrist by his primary care physician, who reports that S.H. is physically healthy. S.H.'s mother states that he is a very bright young man who made straight As in high school despite frequent absenteeism, but he has no friends and has never been on a date. S.H.'s mother says that during high school, S.H. never attended any school social functions and spent all of his time in his room working on his computer. On graduation from high school, he received a full scholarship to a community college but refused to go. When questioned by the psychiatrist, S.H.'s face turns bright red, and his voice shakes when he speaks. S.H. admits that his behavior is not normal but says that he is afraid that he might "do something stupid" when he is around people and becomes extremely embarrassed when he has to talk to anyone. He has wanted to ask a certain girl for a date for 3 years but experienced severe anxiety attacks on the few occasions he has tried to approach her. S.H. is afraid of being turned down and believes that no girl would ever want to date someone like himself. The psychiatrist's diagnosis is social anxiety disorder. What clinical features of social anxiety disorder are present in S.H.?

S.H. exhibits many characteristic features of the generalized type of social anxiety disorder. S.H. admits that he does not like being around people for fear of embarrassment, and he generally avoids social situations, which are classic traits of social anxiety disorder. His symptoms of blushing and shaking voice are also common in social anxiety disorder, as well as other typical anxiety symptoms such as palpitations, trembling, sweating, tense muscles, dry throat, hot/cold sensations, and a sinking feeling in the stomach. S.H. also displays hypersensitivity to rejection and low self-esteem, and he realizes that his behavior and fears are unreasonable. These symptoms and S.H.'s young age are consistent with a diagnosis of social anxiety disorder.

S.H.'s case illustrates the substantial disability that can result from this illness. S.H.'s anxiety disorder has deprived him of normal social development, making friends, dating, participating in social functions, and pursuit of higher education. Future impairments throughout S.H.'s life are likely to be significant unless his anxiety is treated successfully.

Treatment Selection for Social Anxiety Disorder

20. The physician decides to treat S.H. with medication and prescribes sertraline, 50 mg Q AM. Is the prescribed pharmacotherapy appropriate in this case?

Because S.H.'s generalized social anxiety disorder is severely impacting his life, medication treatment is indicated. The SSRIs are first-line therapy for treating social anxiety disorder, and sertraline is a good choice because it is FDA approved for this indication. Although not applicable in this case, sertraline is also effective for many of the other psychiatric disorders that are commonly seen in patients with social anxiety disorder. The sertraline starting dose of 50 mg/day is appropriate for S.H., and 50-mg increment dosage increases can be made every 4 weeks according to response, up to a maximum of 200 mg/day. Signs of response may be seen within 2 to 4 weeks, but 8 to 12 weeks is usually required for optimal results. If available, CBT may also be combined with pharmacotherapy for S.H.

Goals and Duration of Treatment

21. What are the goals of treatment in this case, and how can S.H.'s response to treatment be objectively assessed? How long should effective therapy be continued?

Three principle domains of treatment outcomes have been defined for social anxiety disorder: symptoms, functionality, and overall well-being.[40] It is recommended that efficacy assessments examine all three of these areas because even if all anxiety symptoms disappear, treatment is not really clinically significant unless functioning also improves. The clinician-rated Liebowitz Social Anxiety Scale (LSAS) and the patient-rated Sheehan Disability Scale can be used for measuring improvements in the symptom and functional ability domains, respectively.[40] In S.H.'s case, the desired outcomes of treatment include reducing his fear and avoidance of social situations, enabling him to comfortably interact socially and attend college, and improving his overall quality of life.

Several studies have examined relapse rates after double-blind discontinuation of effective treatment in social anxiety disorder.[101,105,106] Based on their results, relapse appears to be very common. Long-term studies have shown that sertraline, paroxetine, escitalopram, and clonazepam prevent relapse of social anxiety disorder during continuation treatment. Therefore, pharmacotherapy should be continued for at least 1 year after response.[95,101] After that time, a trial of gradual medication discontinuation may be attempted, accompanied by close monitoring for signs of relapse.

POSTTRAUMATIC STRESS DISORDER AND ACUTE STRESS DISORDER

Diagnostic Criteria

PTSD and acute stress disorder occur in people who have experienced a severely distressing traumatic event. These disorders are characterized by symptoms of intrusive re-experiencing, avoidance features, emotional numbing, and symptoms of autonomic hyperarousal.[1] PTSD has been recognized most commonly in war veterans and was referred to as "shell shock" after World War I. However, PTSD also occurs in persons exposed to events such as natural disasters, serious accidents, criminal assault, rape, physical or sexual abuse, and political victimization (refugees, concentration camp survivors, hostages). The trauma does not have to involve physical injury to the PTSD victim. Witnessing someone else being injured or killed, being diagnosed with a life-threatening illness, and experiencing the unexpected death of a loved one are common types of trauma that may lead to PTSD.[1]

The DSM-IV-TR criteria for PTSD are presented in Table 76-13. PTSD is classified as having either an acute or delayed (after 6 months) onset in relation to the trauma; the latter is extremely rare.[1] Symptoms must persist for at least 1 month to meet the criteria for PTSD. *Acute stress disorder* is a separate diagnostic category in the DSM-IV-TR and refers to cases in which symptoms last <1 month (but at least 2 days).[1] It involves many of the same clinical features as PTSD, but there is an additional requirement of peritraumatic dissociative symptoms (numbing, derealization, depersonalization, amnesia, feeling dazed). In both PTSD and acute stress disorder, the symptoms must be severe enough to interfere with some aspect of functioning.

Table 76-13 Diagnostic Criteria for Posttraumatic Stress Disorder

1. Person has experienced a traumatic event in which the individual witnessed, experienced, or was confronted with actual or threatened death, or serious injury to self or others, and to which the person responded with intense fear, helplessness, or horror
2. Traumatic event is re-experienced persistently in some way (e.g., dreams, nightmares, flashbacks, recurrent thoughts or images), or intense distress is experienced on exposure to stimuli associated with the traumatic event
3. Persistent avoidance of stimuli associated with the event and numbing of general responsiveness involving at least three of the following:
   a. Efforts to avoid thoughts, feelings, or conversations related to the trauma
   b. Efforts to avoid people, places, or activities that are reminders of the trauma
   c. Impaired recall of the traumatic event
   d. Decreased interest or participation in activities
   e. Feelings of detachment
   f. Restricted range of affect
   g. Sense of foreshortened future
4. Persistent symptoms of increased arousal (not present before the event) that include at last two of the following:
   a. Sleep disturbances
   b. Irritability or anger outbursts
   c. Difficulty concentrating
   d. Hypervigilance
   e. Exaggerated startle response
5. Duration of the disturbance (2–4) of at least 1 month
6. Disturbance causes significant impairment in some aspect of daily functioning

Adapted from reference 1, with permission.

Epidemiology and Clinical Course

PTSD was previously believed to affect approximately 1% of the general population, but recent studies reveal a much higher lifetime prevalence of approximately 7% to 8%.[107] PTSD is twice as common in women than in men, although overall men are exposed to trauma more often than women.[107] Rates of PTSD are expected to rise as the frequency of traumatic events throughout the world continues to increase. An estimated 80% to 90% of individuals in the United States today will experience at least one event during their lifetime that is traumatic enough to lead to PTSD.[107]

Most people who are exposed to a traumatic event do not develop PTSD; approximately 90% of individuals experience a normal acute stress response to trauma and fully recover.[107] Risk factors for the development of PTSD include experiencing assaultive violence, more severe and chronic traumas, a history of depressive or anxiety disorders, and experiencing dissociative or other intense symptoms during or soon after the trauma.[107,108] Previous exposure to trauma also increases the risk of developing PTSD after later traumas, and survivors of childhood sexual or physical abuse have been found to be especially vulnerable.[108,109] Among people exposed to various traumatic events, the overall conditional risks for PTSD are reported to be 6% for males and 13% for females.[107] In general, traumas involving personal assault (e.g., rape, combat) are associated with much higher conditional risks of developing PTSD than other types of trauma.

Most PTSD patients also suffer from other disorders at some point in their lifetime, including major depression, GAD, panic disorder, phobic disorders, and alcohol or other substance abuse.[107] Overall, 79% to 88% of those with PTSD have another lifetime psychiatric disorder, most commonly depression or substance abuse.[109–111] High rates of substance abuse and dependence in patients with PTSD are related to attempts to self-medicate PTSD symptoms.[111] The suicide risk in PTSD is high and comparable to that seen in major depression.[112] PTSD causes significant functional disability and has been associated with school failure, teenage pregnancy, unemployment, marital instability, legal problems, and impaired performance in the workplace.[112]

The course of PTSD is highly variable. Most patients who meet criteria for PTSD 1 month after trauma show spontaneous recovery within 6 to 9 months.[110] PTSD continues for years in a significant minority, estimated at 10% to 25%, and some sufferers experience a lifelong course of illness. The overall median duration of PTSD is reported to be approximately 2 years, but has been found to be four times longer in women (4 years) than in men (1 year).[110]

Etiology and Pathophysiology

The effects of stress on the brain have been a topic of intensive research. Apparently, psychological trauma, especially that which occurs early in life or is chronic in duration, can cause persistent changes in various aspects of brain functioning and in neurobiological responses to stress.[113] Evidence of altered NE, 5-HT, glutaminergic, GABA system, neuroendocrine, substance P, and opioid system functioning has been found in PTSD.[114–116] Stress-induced hyperactivity of central noradrenergic systems is believed to lead to the generalized anxiety and autonomic hyperarousal associated with PTSD.[115] These symptoms may also be related to a supersensitivity of the HPA axis system in PTSD because affected patients have a blunted ACTH response to CRH and decreased basal cortisol levels, as well as increased numbers of glucocorticoid receptors.[114] A subset of PTSD patients appear to have an abnormally sensitized 5-HT system, and these patients may represent a neurobiologically distinct subgroup.[116]

Numerous studies have found reduced hippocampal volumes in PTSD, which is a brain area involved in learning and memory that appears to be particularly vulnerable to the damaging effects of stress.[113] Neuropsychological tests show that reduced hippocampal volume is associated with cognitive and memory impairments in PTSD patients.[112] Functional neuroimaging studies in PTSD have found excessive activation of the amygdala and certain other brain areas in response to trauma-related stimuli.[113,117] Thus, the neurobiological consequences of stress and trauma result in both structural and functional changes in the brain. Genetic factors may also play a role in influencing vulnerability to the damaging effects of stress.[117]

Treatment of Posttraumatic Stress Disorder

Both medications and CBTs are useful in treating PTSD. Nonpharmacologic therapies alone may be appropriate for initial treatment of mild PTSD cases, but pharmacotherapy, either alone or in combination with psychological therapies, is usually recommended for patients with moderate or severe illness.[108,109,112] When assessing various treatment options for PTSD, it is important to consider effects on all three core symptom clusters (re-experiencing/intrusive symptoms, avoidance/emotional numbing, hyperarousal symptoms). Not all PTSD treatments are effective for these major symptom domains.

The preferred first-line medications in PTSD are the SSRIs, but various other antidepressants may also be useful. Response to pharmacotherapy occurs very gradually, over 8 to 12 weeks or longer. Partial response at 12 weeks of treatment may be followed by full remission after several more months of therapy; therefore, an adequate time period should be allowed to fully determine response to a particular medication. However, lack of improvement after 4 weeks of therapy is unlikely to be effective with medication continuation, so alternate treatment strategies should be tried in these cases.[118] Early treatment during the first 3 months that follow a trauma may prevent the development of chronic PTSD.[109]

Selective Serotonin Reuptake Inhibitors

Sertraline and paroxetine are currently the only FDA-approved medications for treating PTSD. Large controlled studies have demonstrated that both agents are very effective and superior to placebo in reducing all three PTSD symptom clusters (re-experiencing, avoidance/numbing, and autonomic hyperarousal).[118] They also have beneficial effects on depression and general anxiety symptoms and have been associated with improvements in overall functioning as well as quality of life.[118] Fluoxetine also appears to be effective in treating PTSD in some patients, although study results have been mixed and a lack of significant effects on avoidance/numbing symptoms has been noted.[118] Male war veterans with long-standing combat-related PTSD have been noted to respond poorly to fluoxetine, compared with females and civilians, but this observation may apply to treatment of PTSD in general.[119,120] Citalopram, fluvoxamine, and the SNRI venlafaxine have shown efficacy in the treatment of PTSD in open trials but randomized, double-blind, placebo-controlled studies have yielded negative results, possibly due to the small numbers of subjects studied.[118]

Other Antidepressants

Several open studies and case reports suggest that nefazodone, mirtazapine, and bupropion are also effective in treating the core symptoms of PTSD.[121] Although supporting evidence for these antidepressants is not as strong as for sertraline and paroxetine, they may be considered appropriate alternatives to the SSRIs in certain patients. The TCAs amitriptyline and imipramine and the MAOI phenelzine have also been found to be effective for PTSD in controlled trials, but these agents are generally not recommended because of their poor tolerability and safety profiles.[109] Because of the relatively high risk of suicide in PTSD, TCAs can be especially dangerous in this population.

Miscellaneous Agents

Various other medications have been used successfully in limited numbers of PTSD cases. The anticonvulsants carbamazepine, valproate, topiramate, tiagabine, gabapentin, and lamotrigine have been markedly effective in certain patients and can be particularly useful for reducing irritability, impulsivity, and angry or violent outbursts.[121,122] Anticonvulsant therapy can also be effective for intrusive, re-experiencing, and hyperarousal symptoms. Atypical antipsychotic agents have been used effectively to treat PTSD-related psychotic symptoms (risperidone, clozapine, olanzapine) and sleep disturbances, but they do not appear to be useful for treating core PTSD symptoms.[121] The α_1-adrenergic antagonist, prazosin, and the α_2-adrenergic agonist, clonidine, were reported to decrease nightmares and other core symptoms in patients with PTSD.[123] Benzodiazepines are generally ineffective in treating PTSD, although they may be useful in managing sleep disturbances during the early weeks following trauma. Their use in PTSD should be limited to short-term therapy because chronic use may have detrimental effects.[124]

Nonpharmacologic Treatments

Various types of psychosocial therapies have been used in the treatment of PTSD, including anxiety management training to help patients cope with stress.[124] Cognitive therapies seem to be most effective for symptoms of demoralization, guilt, and shame, whereas exposure therapies are better for reducing intrusive thoughts, flashbacks, and avoidance behaviors. Both cognitive and exposure therapies have been shown to be markedly and comparably effective in controlled PTSD trials, but exposure is probably more critical for optimal results.[109,112]

Clinical Presentation of Posttraumatic Stress Disorder

22. D.D. is a 42-year-old woman who was attacked and raped in the driveway of her home as she was getting out of her car 1 month ago. She did not seek medical treatment at the time and waited several days before reporting the incident to anyone, including her family. She presents to her physician complaining that she cannot sleep and that she is irritable, anxious, and depressed. When asked about any recent stressors in her life, she finally tells her doctor about the rape. D.D. has no history of psychiatric illness, admits that her symptoms have appeared since the attack, and says that she has never had any psychiatric problems until now. She states that she has nightly nightmares and becomes extremely anxious every time she comes home and gets out of her car at night (which she avoids doing when possible). She is startled when the phone rings or when someone approaches her unexpectedly, and she literally freezes if she sees a man who bears any physical resemblance to her attacker. D.D. also states that memories of the rape often flash through her mind for no reason, although she tries hard not to think about it. The assailant has not been caught, and D.D. feels extremely guilty for not promptly reporting the crime. Her symptoms are interfering significantly with her ability to work at her job and have put a strain on her marriage. What clinical features of PTSD does D.D. display?

Persons with PTSD often present with nonspecific complaints indicative of a generalized anxiety, depression, or substance use disorder. They may not realize or want to reveal an association between their symptoms and the trauma they have experienced. Careful evaluation by the clinician is required to elicit a pattern suggestive of PTSD. D.D. displays many target symptoms of PTSD, including re-experiencing (nightmares, recurrent memories), avoidance of the activity that reminds her of the trauma, and symptoms of increased arousal (sleep difficulties, irritability, exaggerated startle response). In addition, she is experiencing feelings of depression, distress, marital problems, and impairment in occupational functioning as a result of her symptoms. The lack of any previous psychiatric illness combined with the temporal relationship between the attack and her symptoms support the presence of PTSD as opposed to another anxiety or depressive disorder. Because her trauma occurred 1 month ago, her condition would be classified as acute-onset PTSD.

Treatment Selection and SSRI Dosing

23. What factors are important in the selection of an initial treatment for D.D.?

Because D.D. is exhibiting moderate-to-severe PTSD symptoms, pharmacotherapy is indicated. Medication treatment can also be combined with CBTs if they are available, but nonpharmacologic therapies alone are generally reserved for patients with mild symptoms. An SSRI is the preferred initial medication treatment for most patients.[118] Sertraline is an appropriate choice of treatment in this case and is FDA approved for PTSD. Low initial SSRI doses are recommended in PTSD, so sertraline can be started at 25 mg/day and gradually increased to the target dosage range of 100 to 150 mg/day, according to response and tolerability.[121] Regarding other SSRIs, studies suggest that a paroxetine dose of 20 to 40 mg/day is sufficient for most PTSD patients; higher doses have not been associated with better response.[121] Persistent sleep complaints during the first month after a traumatic experience may predispose the patient to chronic PTSD, so management of sleep disturbances is an important component of initial PTSD treatment.[123] Low-dose adjunctive trazodone (25–50 mg at bedtime) would be a good choice in this case because it is a safe, effective, and an inexpensive sedative agent.

Even in the absence of formal CBTs, certain aspects of patient and family education are vital to the successful treatment of PTSD.[108,109] Providing information about the nature and prognosis of PTSD are important. The patient should be encouraged to talk with family and friends about the trauma because repeated retelling of the traumatic event is therapeutic and can help facilitate recovery. Significant others need to understand the importance of listening and of being tolerant of the patient's emotional reaction and persistent preoccupation with his or her experience. Peer support groups are widely available and can be very beneficial in the recovery of trauma victims. Patients should be advised to try not to avoid things that remind them of the trauma, but rather to expose themselves to these situations as often as possible.

Clinical Assessment and Goals of Therapy

24. What are the goals of treatment in this case, and how can D.D.'s symptoms be objectively assessed?

The first goal of treatment of PTSD is to reduce the core symptoms of re-experiencing, avoidance, numbing, and hyperarousal. In D.D.'s case, these target symptoms include nightmares, intrusive memories, avoidance behaviors, irritability, startling easily, and sleep difficulties. Improvements should begin within the first 2 weeks and gradually continue over the course of 2 to 3 months. Secondary goals in this case include improving D.D.'s stress resilience, decreasing her work- and marriage-related disability, and improving her overall quality of life. Other general treatment goals in PTSD include decreasing detrimental behaviors (use of alcohol or substances, risky activities, violence) and treating any comorbid psychiatric conditions that may be present.

Several different rating scales have been developed to assess response to treatments in PTSD.[40] The most commonly used clinician-rated scales are the Clinician Administered PTSD Scale (CAPS) and the Treatment Outcome PTSD Scale (TOPS-8). CAPS is most often used in clinical PTSD trials, whereas TOPS-8 is shorter and easier to use in clinical practice. Patient-rated scales for evaluating PTSD symptoms include the Davidson Trauma Scale and the Impact of Events Scale. The Sheehan

Disability Scale is often used to assess functional impairment due to PTSD.

Course and Duration of Treatment

Good treatment response in PTSD is more likely to occur when treatment is begun within 3 months of the trauma.[109,112] There is no well-established definition of response in PTSD, but a decrease in symptoms by 30% to 50%, along with substantial functional improvement, is commonly used in clinical trials. Full recovery during treatment of PTSD is fairly uncommon, and partial responders to either medication or psychosocial therapies may benefit from adding another treatment modality. When an initial SSRI trial is ineffective, the patient may be switched to another SSRI or one of the other antidepressants that have been effectively used in PTSD.[121] Partial responders may benefit from the addition of a second medication, depending on which core symptoms predominate (see Pharmacotherapy of Posttraumatic Stress Disorder section).

For patients who respond, treatment should be continued for an additional 6 to 12 months for acute cases (when symptoms were present <3 months before treatment) and 12 to 24 months for chronic cases (when symptoms lasted >3 months before treatment).[109] Long-term SSRI treatment can prevent relapse of PTSD, especially in those who show good response during the first 3 months of therapy.[124] When pharmacotherapy is discontinued, it should be withdrawn gradually over 1 to 3 months.

OBSESSIVE-COMPULSIVE DISORDER

Diagnostic Criteria

The DSM-IV-TR criteria for OCD are presented in Table 76-14.[1] OCD is characterized by recurrent obsessions or compulsions, which are severe enough to be distressing, consume at least 1 hour a day, or significantly interfere with some aspect of functioning. An *obsession* is an intrusive or recurrent thought, image, or impulse that incites anxiety in the person and that cannot be ignored or suppressed voluntarily. The most common obsessions include germs and contamination; pathological doubt; somatic concerns; need for order and symmetry; and religious, aggressive, or sexual thoughts.[125,126] A *compulsion* is a behavior or ritual that is performed in a repetitive or stereotypic way that is designed to reduce anxiety associated with obsessions or to prevent some future event or situation. However, the compulsions are not actually connected to the obsessions in any realistic way. Frequent compulsions include checking, cleaning, arranging symmetrically, ordering, hoarding, counting, and needing to ask questions or confess.[126] The obsessions and compulsions are unpleasant and disturbing to the sufferer and are not associated with pleasure or gratification. This feature distinguishes OCD from certain other detrimental behaviors (excessive gambling or shopping), which are often described as being "compulsive." Adults with OCD usually realize that their rituals are senseless and excessive at some point, but children may not make this distinction.[1]

OCD is a clinically heterogeneous disorder involving a wide range of symptoms. Five separate OCD symptom dimensions have been defined: symmetry obsessions and repeating, counting, and ordering compulsions; contamination obsessions and cleaning compulsions; hoarding obsessions and compulsions; aggressive obsessions and checking compulsions; and sexual/religious obsessions and related compulsions. Although specific symptoms in an individual may change over time, they usually remain within the same dimension.[126]

Table 76-14 Diagnostic Criteria for Obsessive-Compulsive Disorder

1. Presence of either obsessions or compulsions:
   Obsessions:
   (a) Recurrent and persistent ideas or thoughts are experienced, at some time during the disturbance, as intrusive and senseless
   (b) Thoughts, impulses, or images are not simply excessive worries about real life problems
   (c) Person attempts to ignore or neutralize the ideas or thoughts with some other thought or action
   (d) Person realizes the obsessions are the product of his or her own mind
   Compulsions:
   (a) Repetitive and intentional behaviors or mental acts are performed in response to the obsession or according to rigid rules
   (b) Behavior is designed to prevent or reduce distress or to prevent some dreaded event; however, the activity is clearly excessive and unrealistic to neutralize the situation
2. At some point during the disturbance, the person realizes that the obsessions and compulsions are excessive or unreasonable (not necessary in children)
3. Obsessions or compulsions cause marked distress, are time consuming (>1 hr/day), or significantly interfere with some aspect of daily functioning
4. Content of the symptoms is not related to another psychiatric disorder, and the disturbance is not due to the direct effects of a substance, medication, or general medical illness

Adapted from reference 1, with permission. Copyright © 2000 American Psychiatric Association.

Epidemiology and Clinical Course

OCD once was believed to be a rare disorder, but epidemiologic studies reveal that it affects between 2% and 3% of the worldwide population.[1,127] The overall lifetime prevalence is slightly higher in women, but men tend to have an earlier onset of illness (between ages 6 and 15 years) than women (between ages 20 and 29 years).[1,13,127] Many patients report having mild symptoms for years before full OCD emerges, and an estimated one-third to one-half of patients have onset during childhood or adolescence. Prepubertal OCD is three times more common in boys than in girls.[13] Women with OCD often have worsening of symptoms during the premenstrual and postpartum periods, and onset or worsening of OCD during pregnancy appears to be fairly common.[60] Regardless of gender, the severity of illness usually worsens during stressful life periods.

The course and severity of OCD are highly variable and unpredictable, with some persons only mildly or intermittently affected and others suffering severely and constantly throughout their lifetime. The natural course of untreated OCD was followed for a 40-year period in a group of 144 patients.[126] Although 83% of patients were improved at the end of the follow-up period, only 20% experienced full remission. Two-thirds of patients continued to have some OCD symptoms, and a progressive deterioration was observed in 10%. Observational studies suggest that the long-term course of OCD may be improved substantially with appropriate treatment.[128,129] However, a portion of sufferers still experience a chronic and lifelong course.

It is no surprise that OCD can have seriously detrimental effects on functional abilities and quality of life. In large-scale surveys, OCD patients report that their symptoms significantly interfere with their abilities to socialize, study, work, make friends, and maintain good relationships with family and friends.[130] It is estimated that each person with OCD loses an average of 3 years' wages over his or her lifetime.[130] Quality-of-life ratings in OCD patients indicate marked impairments and are similar to those observed in patients with depression. Fortunately, treatment of OCD can be accompanied by significant improvements in quality of life and functional abilities.

Although several effective treatments are currently available for OCD, most patients do not seek treatment until the disorder is seriously affecting their lives. One study found that OCD patients waited an average of 7.5 years after the onset of OCD before seeking medical evaluation for their disorder.[130] This may be because most OCD patients realize that their symptoms are senseless, so they attempt to hide their disorder due to embarrassment. People with OCD often carry out their rituals privately and may be very successful at concealing their symptoms from others. Initial treatment for OCD is commonly sought outside psychiatric settings, and the obsessive-compulsive symptoms are often missed.

Increased recognition that OCD is a biological disorder for which effective treatments are available is needed among the general public and health care professionals. Four simple questions are recommended for screening for potential OCD.[125] Do you have to wash your hands over and over? Do you have to check things repeatedly? Do you have recurrent distressing thoughts that you cannot get rid of? Do you have to complete actions again and again or in a certain way? Clinicians in a variety of health care settings can incorporate these screening questions into their practice to use when possible signs of OCD are present. Health care providers should be prepared to provide education about the nature and treatability of OCD to suspected sufferers and to make appropriate treatment referrals in these cases.

Psychiatric Comorbidity and Obsessive-Compulsive Spectrum Disorders

As with other anxiety disorders, OCD often is accompanied by psychiatric comorbidity. Two-thirds of those with OCD develop major depression during their lifetime.[1,126] There is a higher-than-expected overlap of OCD with disorders such as specific and social phobias, GAD, panic disorder, schizophrenia, schizoaffective disorder, bipolar disorder, and eating disorders. Identification of comorbid conditions with OCD is important because it can influence choice of treatments. Obsessive-compulsive personality disorder, which is classified as an Axis II disorder, occurs in a small percentage of OCD patients. Despite their name similarities, obsessive-compulsive personality disorder does not involve true obsessions and compulsions (which are senseless and distressing to the sufferer). Rather, it is a personality pattern characterized by rigid and inflexible preoccupation with rules, lists, order, and perfectionism.[1] Although these personality traits cause problems, the person with the personality disorder does not view his or her behavior as abnormal or unreasonable.

The relation between tic disorders and OCD is particularly striking. Tics occur in 20% to 30% of OCD patients, and 5% to 7% have full Tourette syndrome, whereas 35% to 50% of Tourette syndrome patients exhibit OCD symptoms.[126] Individuals with OCD plus Tourette syndrome are believed to represent a genetically and pathophysiologically distinct subtype of illness.[126] These patients are more likely to be male and tend to have an earlier age at OCD onset (before age 10 years), more severe symptoms, and poorer response to SSRIs than those with OCD alone.[131]

Another childhood neurologic disorder commonly associated with OCD is Sydenham chorea. This is the neurologic variant of rheumatic fever, which is an autoimmune disease triggered by infection with group A β-hemolytic streptococcal pharyngitis. Recent reports describe children who developed sudden and severe tics and obsessive-compulsive symptoms after strep throat infections.[132,133] This condition is designated in the medical literature by the acronym PANDAS (pediatric autoimmune neuropsychiatric disorders associated with streptococcal infection), and it has been rapidly reversed by antibiotic or IV immunoglobulin treatment. The possibility of a PANDAS correlation should be considered in any child who develops abrupt onset of obsessive-compulsive symptoms, particularly those who have had pharyngitis within the past 6 months.

The term "obsessive-compulsive spectrum disorder" refers to a diverse collection of psychiatric conditions from various DSM-IV-TR categories that have overlapping characteristics with OCD and involve recurrent or distressing thoughts and/or irresistible or repetitive behaviors.[134] These include somatoform disorders (body dysmorphic disorder [preoccupation with an imagined or slight defect in appearance], hypochondriasis), eating disorders (anorexia nervosa, bulimia nervosa, binge eating disorder), and impulse control disorders (trichotillomania [recurrent impulses to pull out one's hair], pathological gambling, compulsive nail biting, kleptomania, compulsive buying). Tourette syndrome and autism are also often included in this spectrum of disorders. Some of these disorders, such as body dysmorphic disorder, have much higher comorbidities with OCD than others. Like OCD, many patients with these conditions have shown good response to treatment with serotonergic antidepressants such as clomipramine and SSRIs, sometimes preferentially over agents with mainly noradrenergic activity.[134] Examples include body dysmorphic disorder, compulsive buying, pathological gambling, trichotillomania, binge eating disorder, and bulimia nervosa.[134]

Etiology and Pathophysiology

A wealth of research has attempted to identify a specific biological explanation for OCD. Because OCD displays such clinical heterogeneity, there may be several distinct etiologies for different subtypes of illness. One leading hypothesis has focused on the role of 5-HT dysfunction, which is supported by the finding that the only effective medication treatments for OCD mainly influence 5-HT transmission.[135] However, the multitude of studies involving 5-HT challenges and other methods for assessing central 5-HT function in OCD have resulted in no conclusive answers, and the exact role of 5-HT underlying OCD still has not been determined. It is interesting that naturally occurring animal models of OCD have been observed in dogs (canine acral lick) and birds (feather picking disorder), and these conditions have been treated successfully with SSRIs.

More promising areas of OCD research involve functional brain imaging studies.[135] These techniques are used to assess regional metabolic activity in different areas of the brain. Studies in OCD patients have identified abnormal hyperactivity (when compared with normal controls) in certain frontal lobe and basal ganglia regions, specifically the orbital frontal cortex, cingulate cortex, and head of the caudate nucleus.[135,136] Interestingly, these regional brain metabolic abnormalities normalize after successful treatment of OCD, and certain brain metabolism patterns may be associated with preferential response to SSRI versus CBTs.[135,137] These findings have led to one current hypothesis that OCD is a neurologic disorder characterized by a hyperfunctioning circuit involving the aforementioned brain regions. In support of this hypothesis, neurosurgical techniques that interrupt this circuit are often effective in the treatment of OCD. The mechanism of efficacy of the SSRIs may be related to desensitization of terminal serotonin auto receptors in the orbitofrontal cortex, which enhances 5-HT neurotransmission in this brain region.[135,136] Structural abnormalities have also been identified in OCD, including increased brain cortex and opercular volumes, decreased total white matter volume, and smaller pituitary gland size.[125,135] Specific types of cognitive dysfunction have also been found, including problems with nonverbal memory, visuospatial skills, and visual attention.[135] Impairments in memory functioning have been correlated with the aforementioned structural abnormalities in OCD.

In addition to biological factors, twin and family studies support an effect of genetics on risk for OCD.[15] Heredity appears to be most important in early-onset OCD cases (before age 18 years) because familial aggregation has not been observed in OCD cases with a later age at onset.[138] Several studies suggest an association between OCD and specific polymorphisms in the serotonin transporter, $5HT_{1D\beta}$ and $5HT_{2A}$ receptor genes, but others have failed to replicate these findings.[139,140] Other candidate gene studies have linked OCD with functional polymorphisms in the catechol *O*-methyltransferase, dopamine D_4-receptor genes, and a high-affinity neuronal/epithelial excitatory amino acid transporter gene.[140,141]

Treatment of Obsessive-Compulsive Disorder

Both medications and behavioral therapies are effective in the treatment of OCD. Behavioral therapy is vitally important for OCD, and the combination of drugs plus behavioral therapy provides optimal treatment. All medications consistently effective in the treatment of OCD are potent inhibitors of serotonin reuptake. These include clomipramine, and the SSRIs: fluvoxamine, fluoxetine, paroxetine, and sertraline. All five of these medications are FDA approved for the treatment of OCD in adults, and all except paroxetine are indicated for use in children with OCD.

Clomipramine

Clomipramine was the first drug with proven efficacy in treating OCD, and it was considered the standard first-line treatment for several years until the SSRIs gained popularity. Many large well-controlled studies have documented that clomipramine is far superior to placebo and significantly improves OCD symptoms in approximately 60% to 70% of patients.[126,142] Clomipramine is unique among TCAs in its effectiveness for OCD. This distinct property is attributed to its more potent effects on 5-HT reuptake inhibition compared with other TCAs. Clomipramine is often referred to as an SRI (serotonin reuptake inhibitor), not an SSRI, because its major active metabolite, desmethylclomipramine, is a potent inhibitor of norepinephrine reuptake. Clomipramine also blocks adrenergic, histaminergic, and cholinergic receptors similarly to other TCAs, resulting in an adverse effect profile similar to that of imipramine (see Chapter 79).

Although direct comparison studies have shown clomipramine to be similar in efficacy to various SSRIs in treating OCD, several meta-analyses have concluded that clomipramine is superior to SSRIs overall.[142,143] However, clomipramine is less well tolerated than SSRIs, and patients are more likely to discontinue clomipramine treatment because of side effects. Therefore, clomipramine is currently reserved as a second-line treatment option for patients who do not respond adequately to SSRI therapy.[142] Details about the clinical use of clomipramine are discussed in Questions 32 through 34.

Selective Serotonin Reuptake Inhibitors

SSRIs are the only first-line medication treatments for OCD. Double-blind, placebo-controlled studies have documented the efficacies of fluvoxamine, fluoxetine, paroxetine, and sertraline in the treatment of OCD.[144] Citalopram and escitalopram also are effective but there is less evidence to support their use. There is no strong evidence that any one SSRI is more effective than the others in treating OCD, but some patients may respond to or tolerate one agent better than another.[144] Usual SSRI starting dosages can be used in OCD, but at least 4 weeks should be allowed before exceeding the targeted minimally effective dosages (fluvoxamine 200 mg/day, fluoxetine 40 mg/day, paroxetine 40 mg/day, and sertraline 100 mg/day).[144] Details about the clinical use of SSRIs in OCD are discussed in Questions 28 through 31.

Augmentation Strategies

Other than venlafaxine, none of the other miscellaneous agents studied in OCD have demonstrated impressive efficacy as monotherapy. However, several agents appear to be useful as augmentation therapy to boost response to SSRIs or clomipramine in partial responders to these agents.[145] The combination of an SSRI plus clomipramine is one such option for patients who show partial response, although attention must be paid to potential drug interactions, which may lead to clomipramine toxicity (see Question 34).

Antipsychotic agents are useful for augmentation therapy. They may be particularly effective in patients with comorbid tic disorders, although recent reports suggest they are equally effective in patients without tics. Older first-generation antipsychotics, such as haloperidol and pimozide, are effective in augmenting response to fluvoxamine in controlled trials (conducted before the dangerous interaction between pimozide and CYP 3A4 inhibitors, such as fluvoxamine, was identified). Recent reports have focused on newer second-generation antipsychotics because these agents are generally preferred over first-generation antipsychotics and are better tolerated.[145,146] Risperidone (2–4 mg/day), olanzapine (10–20 mg/day), and quetiapine (200 mg/day) have all been used successfully in treatment-resistant OCD to augment response to SSRIs.[145,147,148] It is interesting to note that second-generation antipsychotics (risperidone, clozapine, olanzapine) have been reported to cause or worsen obsessive-compulsive symptoms in schizophrenic patients in a number of cases.[145] This effect is believed to be due to the 5-HT_2-receptor antagonistic activity of antipsychotics. Certain SSRI-antipsychotic combinations can increase antipsychotic plasma levels and side effects, particularly extrapyramidal symptoms. Pimozide should not be used in combination with clomipramine, fluoxetine, sertraline, or fluvoxamine because of the potential for cardiac QT interval prolongation.

Pindolol is another augmenting agent that has been shown to be effective in a placebo-controlled study.[149] This trial involved treatment-resistant OCD patients and found pindolol (2.5 mg TID) to be most beneficial in patients who had shown partial response to SSRI therapy.

Miscellaneous Agents

A wide variety of other medications have been tried in the treatment of OCD, with varying degrees of success. Several controlled studies support the efficacy of venlafaxine in the treatment of OCD.[142] A recent trial comparing venlafaxine with clomipramine in OCD found these agents to be comparably effective, but venlafaxine was better tolerated.[150]

Benzodiazepines are generally not beneficial in treating OCD, although there are several reports of clonazepam being effective as adjunctive therapy or monotherapy.[126] Clonazepam appears to have serotonergic effects, which may explain its potential usefulness in OCD. This agent may be helpful in patients with prominent anxiety symptoms, but it can also interfere with the effectiveness of CBT and should not be used concurrently. As discussed, fluvoxamine and fluoxetine can significantly increase serum levels of clonazepam.

The MAOI, phenelzine, was one of the first medications studied for OCD. Early case reports of its use were favorable, but more recent findings suggest that phenelzine is largely ineffective for OCD.[126]

Nonpharmacologic Treatments

COGNITIVE-BEHAVIORAL THERAPIES

CBT is an extremely important component of treatment for OCD and should be incorporated into the initial treatment plan whenever possible. CBT alone may be appropriate for mild OCD or in cases in which it is desirable to avoid medication (e.g., pregnancy, medical conditions). The combination of CBT and medication is generally superior to either treatment approach used alone.[125,126] Treatment gains achieved with CBT often are maintained long after its discontinuation, which is an advantage over pharmacotherapy.[125]

The cognitive therapy component of CBT is aimed toward changing the detrimental thought patterns in OCD and is most helpful for obsessions such as scrupulosity, moral guilt, and pathological doubt. The behavioral therapy aspect, called exposure plus response prevention, involves exposure to feared objects or situations followed by prevention of the usual compulsive response. This type of therapy is most beneficial for patients with contamination fears, hoarding, and rituals involving symmetry, counting, or repeating. Because exposure plus response prevention is anxiety provoking and can be very distressing, many patients refuse to participate in it.

NEUROSURGERY

Neurosurgical treatment of OCD has been practiced since the 1950s and is considered an option of last resort in treatment-refractory patients. Cingulotomy and capsulotomy are the most commonly used procedures. Indications for neurosurgery include severe disability from obsessive-compulsive symptoms and failed treatments (drugs and behavioral therapies) that have been tried systematically for at least 5 years.[151] Reported success rates of neurosurgery in OCD range from 40% to 60% and complications, including potential infections, personality changes, cognitive impairment, and epilepsy, appear to be rare. A recent, long-term, follow-up study of patients who underwent neurosurgery during the 1970s found that therapeutic effects were maintained but that patients exhibited mild-to-moderate impairments in neuropsychological performance.[151] Permanent cognitive sequelae from neurosurgery may be more common than previously realized. A new neurosurgical procedure using an instrument called the gamma knife (anterior gamma capsulotomy) is being used for treatment-refractory OCD. Results suggest good efficacy with improved short- and long-term safety compared with traditional neurosurgical techniques.[152]

Defining Response to Therapy

Response to medication treatment in OCD is gradual and often delayed. Initial improvements usually begin to appear within the first month, but maximal response may take as long as 5 to 6 months. An adequate period to assess response at lower medication dosages should be allowed before increasing to possibly unnecessary higher dosages. Patients who show unsatisfactory response to lower SSRI dosages by weeks 4 to 9 should have their dosages gradually increased to the manufacturer's recommended maximum (see Question 28). A trial of 8 to 12 weeks at maximum medication dosages is recommended before determining response to a particular medication.

The primary goal of treatment in OCD is to decrease obsessions and compulsions to a level at which the person is able to function normally. Complete elimination of symptoms is rare with current treatments.[153] Most clinical trials in OCD define clinical response as a 25% to 35% reduction in Yale-Brown Obsessive-Compulsive Symptom Checklist (Y-BOCS) scores (see Question 27). Therefore, even those classified as responders may be left with 65% to 75% of their original symptoms, and this may or may not result in significant improvements in functioning or quality of life.

Strategies for Managing Partial Response and Nonresponse

Current estimates are that approximately 40% to 60% of patients show clinically meaningful improvements in obsessive-compulsive symptoms during an initial (SSRI or clomipramine) medication trial, but only a small percentage exhibit marked response.[142] Unfortunately, a fairly large percentage of patients derive minimal or no benefit from an initial trial and require further tactics. Approximately 20% of those who fail a first SSRI trial subsequently respond to another agent in this class; therefore, switching to a second SSRI is usually recommended as the next step before initiating a trial of clomipramine.[125,142] However, clomipramine can be extremely effective in SSRI nonresponders, and it remains a useful treatment option despite its clinical disadvantages.

Partial responders to an initial SSRI trial may be better served by addition of one of the augmentation agents discussed in the previous section than by switching to a new medication. Also, inclusion of CBTs is important for optimizing treatment with any medication. Neurosurgery is an option for severe treatment-refractory cases. Predictors of poor response to treatment in OCD include poor insight; hoarding or sexual/religious dimension symptoms; prepubertal onset of illness; and presence of comorbid personality, mood, or eating disorders.

Clinical Presentation and Assessment

25. R.G. is a 25-year-old woman whose husband complains that she spends 1.5 hours a day cleaning the stove and takes four showers each day. The unusual behavior began about 1 year ago after the birth of their son but has continued to worsen, and R.G.'s husband states that he cannot deal with her "odd habits" any longer. R.G. recently lost her job as a secretary because of tardiness (it took her 3 hours to get ready for work) and spending too much time away from her desk in the ladies' room. R.G. admits that it is silly, but she has irresistible urges to make sure that both she and her surroundings are completely free of germs so that her child will not get sick. She also confines herself to one floor of their three-level house because she is afraid that she will fall down the stairs while carrying her son. R.G. also states that she constantly has "what if" thoughts about horrible things happening to her family, which are very disturbing. The physician's diagnosis is OCD. What clinical features of OCD does R.G. display, and how can her symptoms be objectively evaluated?

R.G. displays many characteristic symptoms of OCD. The most commonly encountered clinical presentation of OCD involves patients with excessive fear of contamination with dirt, germs, or toxins, who repeatedly wash their hands or clean objects or their surroundings. These persons also typically avoid touching possibly dirty objects (e.g., doorknobs, money) or shaking hands with people. Another common clinical presentation is the OCD patient with pathological doubt who constantly worries that something bad will happen because of his or her negligence. These people can be afraid that they have failed to lock the door, turn off the stove, shut the refrigerator door, or secure the medicine cabinet from children. As a result, they continuously check and recheck their actions.

R.G. displays obsessions of contamination and pathological doubt, and compulsions of excessive cleaning and washing. These symptoms are time consuming, cause significant distress, and have led to her unemployment and marital difficulties. As seen in this case, most persons present with a mixture of various obsessions and compulsions. R.G. also realizes that her thoughts and behaviors are "silly," which most often is the case in OCD. This case also illustrates the onset of OCD during times of stressful or significant life events. Pregnancy, death of a relative, and marital discord have been identified as precipitating factors in the onset of OCD.[127,153]

The aforementioned Y-BOCS is a useful tool in the initial evaluation of those who present with symptoms of OCD and may be used in the objective assessment of R.G.'s symptoms. The Y-BOCS is a 10-item scale with a maximum possible score of 40; a score of >15 is generally considered to represent clinically significant obsessive-compulsive symptoms.[154] This scale is a standard tool for evaluating drug efficacy in OCD clinical trials and is often used in clinical practice to assess response to treatments. Other OCD assessment instruments include the National Institute of Mental Health Obsessive-Compulsive Scale, the Leyton Obsessional Inventory, and the self-rated Maudsley Obsessional-Compulsive Inventory. Special versions for use in children have been developed for the Y-BOCS and the Leyton Obsessional Inventory.

SSRI Treatment of Obsessive-Compulsive Disorder

SSRI Selection and Dosing

26. On assessment, R.G.'s Y-BOCS score is found to be 33. Her physician prescribes fluvoxamine and instructs R.G. to take 100 mg Q am for 1 week and then 200 mg Q am thereafter. He also refers R.G. to a psychologist to receive CBT. Is this initial choice of therapy appropriate?

SSRIs such as fluvoxamine are considered the best choice of initial pharmacotherapy for OCD. The primary differences between SSRIs involve pharmacokinetic properties and potential for drug interactions (see Chapter 79). Because there are no overall differences in efficacy among the four SSRIs approved for OCD, fluvoxamine is a suitable selection for R.G. However, the prescribed dosing instructions for R.G. are not appropriate. The initial recommended dosage for fluvoxamine in adults is 50 mg/day (25 mg in children), and it is best taken in the evening because it tends to be sedating. Using higher-than-necessary dosages can increase both adverse effects and medication costs, and these factors can lead to early termination of therapy. The dosage can be increased by 50-mg increments every 3 to 4 days according to patient tolerability, up to the initial targeted dose of 200 mg/day and a maximum of 300 mg/day.[144] Daily doses exceeding 100 mg should be given in two divided doses, based on fluvoxamine's elimination half-life of approximately 15 hours. A controlled-release fluvoxamine formulation can be dosed once daily.[155] This product is reported to be better tolerated than standard-release fluvoxamine and may be associated with a faster onset of therapeutic effects.

Adjunctive Cognitive-Behavioral Therapy

The decision to include CBT in R.G.'s treatment plan is appropriate. The overall efficacy of these nonpharmacologic treatments is estimated to be 50% to 70% when used alone, and their use to complement pharmacotherapy is considered vital.[125] R.G.'s Y-BOCS score of 33 indicates a moderate-to-severe symptom severity, which provides further support for using a combined treatment approach. For R.G., exposure plus response prevention therapy might involve covering her hands with dirt and not allowing her to wash them for a certain time period. These behavioral techniques cause extreme anxiety and discomfort, which often lead to dropout from therapy or noncompliance with "homework assignments" (which involve continuation of the therapy principles outside the clinical setting), but are highly effective if the patient can adhere to treatment.

SSRI Adverse Effects and Patient Counseling

27. What patient counseling information should be provided to R.G. in conjunction with the prescribed treatments?

All OCD patients beginning treatment should be counseled that the medication response occurs gradually and that several weeks may elapse before beneficial effects become noticeable. It is important to emphasize that maximum response may take 3 months or longer and that complete elimination of all symptoms is unlikely. It also is helpful to point out that a variety of other medication treatment options exist for those who do not respond adequately to an initial trial.

R.G. should be educated about possible fluvoxamine side effects, including nausea, sedation or insomnia, and headache. Medication should be taken with food to decrease these effects. Side effects are most common during the initial weeks of therapy, are usually dose related, and often subside with continued treatment. Other aspects of SSRI therapy, including additional adverse effects and their management and drug–drug interactions, are discussed in Chapter 79. Patients should be encouraged to report any problems to their treatment provider. The importance of adhering to prescribed therapies, both pharmacologic and behavioral, should also be stressed.

28. After 4 weeks, R.G. is taking fluvoxamine 200 mg daily and tolerating the medication well. She complains that she has not noticed much improvement, and her Y-BOCS score is slightly decreased at 30. R.G. has been to the cognitive-behavioral therapist twice but is reluctant to return because the therapy was so stressful. R.G. requests to be switched to a more effective medication, and she also asks to be given some Xanax to help calm her anxiety during behavioral therapy sessions. What is the best course of action for R.G. at this point?

Switching to another medication is not recommended at this point because not enough time has elapsed to assess fluvoxamine's efficacy. R.G. is tolerating fluvoxamine well and has shown a mild improvement, so this medication should be continued for at least another 4 weeks. Additional counseling information should be provided to R.G. to emphasize the gradual response to treatment in OCD. An increase in fluvoxamine dosage, up to 250 or 300 mg/day, may be considered after several more weeks because some patients may respond better to higher dosages. If R.G.'s symptoms continue to cause significant functional impairment after 10 to 12 weeks of higher-dose fluvoxamine therapy, a change in treatment (e.g., switching to another SSRI or augmentation therapy) will be indicated.

R.G. should be encouraged to continue CBT to optimize the chance for successful treatment. An anxiety response is integral to the therapeutic benefits of behavioral therapies; because benzodiazepines can blunt this response, they may reduce their efficacy. Therefore, alprazolam should be avoided, and a temporary reduction in the intensity of behavioral therapy may be indicated instead. Fluvoxamine can also inhibit the CYP 3A4–mediated metabolism of alprazolam, resulting in more pronounced effects from a given dose.

Course and Duration of Therapy

29. After 5 months of treatment, R.G. is happy to report that her OCD is much improved (Y-BOCS score of 11). She still has intermittent obsessions related to contamination and doubting, but they are less intense than before. She is usually able to resist urges to clean and wash excessively and is using the stairs in their home with only mild discomfort. Her previous employer has agreed to let her return to her secretarial position when she is ready, and she plans to do so soon. R.G.'s husband is extremely pleased with her progress. Their primary question at this visit is whether treatment can be discontinued now because R.G. is doing so well. What recommendations should be provided regarding the long-term course of therapy for R.G.?

This case illustrates a common outcome of OCD treatment, in which some symptoms persist (as evidenced by a Y-BOCS score of 11), but significant improvements in functioning occur. It is currently recommended that effective treatment for OCD be continued for at least 1 year after response to reduce the risk of relapse. The effectiveness of maintenance pharmacotherapy in preventing relapse of OCD is well documented.[128,154] Therefore, continued drug treatment for at least 7 more months is indicated for R.G. Results from several studies suggest that decreased medication doses (with SSRIs and clomipramine) during maintenance therapy are comparably effective as full doses in preventing relapse.[154] If R.G. were experiencing any fluvoxamine-related problems, a decrease to the minimally effective dose (150 mg/day) during maintenance therapy might be recommended.

After a 1-year maintenance period, discontinuation of medication may be considered by carefully weighing the possible risks and benefits. When medication therapy for OCD is withdrawn, the dosage should be gradually decreased by approximately 25% every 1 to 2 months. Continuous monitoring for signs of relapse is required during this period. Gradual discontinuation also lessens the chance of the withdrawal syndrome that often occurs following abrupt discontinuation of SSRI or TCA therapy (see Chapter 79). Long-term or even lifelong maintenance pharmacotherapy is usually recommended after two to four severe relapses or three to four less severe relapses.

Clomipramine Treatment

Dosing Guidelines

30. K.T. is an 18-year-old Asian man who was diagnosed with OCD 2 years ago and also suffers from mild depression. His physician plans to start him on clomipramine therapy because he has failed previous trials with paroxetine and fluvoxamine. Is clomipramine an appropriate choice of therapy for this patient? What recommendations can be made regarding initiation of clomipramine treatment?

Current guidelines recommend that clomipramine be reserved for OCD patients who fail at least two SSRI trials; therefore, its choice for this patient is appropriate.[126] One precaution relevant to this case is that clomipramine, like other TCAs, is highly dangerous in overdose situations. Because K.T. is depressed, he should be evaluated carefully for any suicidal thoughts before starting clomipramine. If suicidal ideation is detected, it would be preferable to try another SSRI. This case also illustrates the common comorbidity of depression with OCD. Fortunately, most effective treatments for OCD fall into the antidepressant category, and drug treatment can be beneficial for both conditions. Nevertheless, the responses of depression and OCD to treatment are independent of one another so that depression may respond completely to a certain medication while OCD symptoms persist.[154]

Clomipramine should be initiated at a low dosage of 25 to 50 mg/day administered with meals. Divided daily doses are sometimes used initially to minimize side effects, but the total daily dose can be given at bedtime after dose titration. The pharmacokinetic parameters of clomipramine are comparable to other TCAs. Its average elimination half-life of approximately 24 hours makes once-daily dosing appropriate.[144,156]

The clomipramine dosage should be increased to an initial target range of 150 to 200 mg/day over 2 to 4 weeks, guided by patient tolerability. The maximum recommended daily dosage of clomipramine is 250 mg/day because of the sharply increased risk of seizures (2.1%–3.4%) with higher dosages as compared with the risk with dosages <250 mg/day (0.24%–0.48%).[157] Longer duration of clomipramine therapy may also increase the risk of seizures. Clomipramine should be used with caution in persons with a history of seizures, head injury, or any other factors that might lower the seizure threshold.

Clomipramine Side Effects and Monitoring Guidelines

31. What guidelines should be recommended for monitoring the outcomes (both therapeutic and adverse) of clomipramine therapy?

Clomipramine is less well tolerated than the SSRIs and can cause a number of significant adverse effects, especially during the first few weeks of therapy. The most common side effects, reported in more than half of those taking clomipramine, include sedation, dry mouth, dizziness, and tremor.[157] Constipation, nausea, blurred vision, insomnia, and headache also occur frequently. K.T. should be advised that these are not serious effects and usually subside with continued treatment.

Many patients receiving long-term clomipramine (and other TCA) therapy gain substantial amounts of weight. As with the SSRIs, sexual dysfunction can be a problem in both men and women. In men, clomipramine can cause ejaculation abnormalities, which can impair fertility. Patients taking clomipramine should also be counseled about the additive CNS depressant effects with alcohol and to be cautious about the possible sedative effects while driving or performing other potentially hazardous activities.

As with other TCAs, an ECG should be performed before starting clomipramine in individuals at risk for heart disease and in pediatric patients. Elevations in liver enzymes have been observed frequently during the first 3 months of clomipramine treatment, and baseline liver function tests should also be obtained before initiating treatment. The liver enzyme changes are reversible on discontinuation of clomipramine therapy.

No therapeutic range for plasma drug concentrations has been firmly established for clomipramine in OCD, but monitoring plasma levels may be clinically useful in certain patients to guide dosing and/or minimize drug toxicity. Clomipramine metabolism is highly variable from one person to the next, and it is difficult to accurately predict the resulting clomipramine level from any given dose. The initial hepatic metabolism of tertiary TCAs such as clomipramine involves demethylation through various isozymes, including CYP 1A2, CYP 2C19, and CYP 3A4.[156,158] Both the parent drug (clomipramine) and the primary active metabolite (*N*-desmethylclomipramine) then undergo CYP 2D6–mediated hydroxylation. Therefore, the metabolism of clomipramine will be affected by combination with any agent that inhibits CYP 1A2, CYP 2C19, CYP 3A4, or CYP 2D6. Clinically significant drug interactions are possible with several of the SSRIs, including fluoxetine, fluvoxamine, and sertraline (see Chapter 79 Mood Disorders).

Although various studies have failed to find a correlation between clomipramine plasma level and clinical response, the ratio of clomipramine to *N*-desmethylclomipramine may be important.[159] Clomipramine is primarily serotonergic, whereas *N*-desmethylclomipramine is more noradrenergic; higher levels of *N*-desmethylclomipramine relative to clomipramine have been associated with poorer clinical response. Factors that impair the CYP 2D6–mediated elimination of *N*-desmethylclomipramine (concurrent medications that are potent CYP 2D6 inhibitors, CYP 2D6 poor metabolizers) may possibly decrease the efficacy of clomipramine by shifting the metabolic ratio in an undesired direction.

Asian patients such as K.T. have been found to have significantly decreased clearance of clomipramine and higher clomipramine: *N*-desmethylclomipramine ratios compared with whites, which may necessitate use of lower doses.[160] This is probably due to genetic polymorphism of either CYP 2C19 or CYP 2D6, which results in decreased metabolic capacity through these routes in the Asian population. Careful monitoring for possible signs of toxicity should accompany dose increases, and the clomipramine plasma level should be checked in those patients (Asian or otherwise) who show unexpected effects with usual doses. An opposite effect has been described in ultra-rapid CYP 2D6 metabolizers, in which unusually high clomipramine dosages may be required for therapeutic efficacy.

Clomipramine Augmentation

32. After 10 weeks of taking clomipramine 100 mg HS, K.T. has shown partial response. He continues to experience mild-to-moderate anticholinergic side effects and frequent daytime fatigue. His plasma clomipramine level is relatively high for the given dose at 450 ng/mL (clomipramine plus desmethylclomipramine). The physician decides to add another drug to augment treatment. Considering K.T.'s current medication regimen and the evidence supporting the different augmentation strategies, which drug would be the best choice for K.T.?

Many different agents have been used to augment response to either an SSRI or clomipramine. An SSRI could be added to clomipramine. Of the SSRIs, fluvoxamine, fluoxetine, paroxetine, and sertraline are all approved as monotherapy for OCD, and any of these would be likely to augment therapy. However, when adding an SSRI to a TCA, the potential for drug interactions should always be considered. Clomipramine is metabolized by CYP 1A2, CYP 3A4, CYP 2C19, and CYP2D6.[156,158,161,162] The 2D6 pathway is particularly important because it is the rate-limiting metabolic pathway for elimination of both clomipramine and desmethylclomipramine. Fluvoxamine, paroxetine, and fluoxetine are all important inhibitors of clomipramine metabolism. Sertraline also has the potential to cause a clinically significant interaction with clomipramine. Alternatively, escitalopram and citalopram would not be likely to cause a significant drug interaction, but evidence for their efficacy as augmenting agents in combination with clomipramine is lacking. A combination less likely to be associated with a drug interaction is the combination of clomipramine and a second-generation antipsychotic. Up to 2006, ten trials comparing the effectiveness of antipsychotic augmentation had been published. Three trials have been conducted using risperidone, two using olanzapine and four using quetiapine. Unfortunately, most studies are small (<30 patients). However, a meta-analysis of the available data suggested that risperidone was most effective (at a dose near 2 mg/day), and haloperidol was the next most effective agent.[146] Even though it might be efficacious, haloperidol would not be the optimal choice in K.T. because it inhibits clomipramine metabolism, and as a first-generation antipsychotic, it is associated with numerous side effects.

REFERENCES

1. American Psychiatric Association. Diagnostic and Statistical Manual of Mental Disorders. 4th ed., text revision. Washington, DC: American Psychiatric Association; 2000.
2. Ressler KJ, Nemeroff CB. Role of serotonergic and noradrenergic systems in the pathophysiology of depression and anxiety disorders. *Depress Anxiety* 2000;12(Suppl 1):2.
3. Ninan PT. The functional anatomy, neurochemistry, and pharmacology of anxiety. *J Clin Psychiatry* 1999;60(Suppl 2):12.
4. Gunnar M, Quevedo K. The neurobiology of stress and development. *Annu Rev Psychol* 2007;58:145.
5. Jetty PV et al. Neurobiology of generalized anxiety disorder. *Psychiatr Clin North Am* 2001;24:75.
6. Kessler RC et al. Prevalence, severity, and comorbidity of 12-month DSM-IV disorders in the National Comorbidity Survey Replication. *Arch Gen Psychiatry* 2005;62:617.
7. Lepine JP. The epidemiology of anxiety disorders: prevalence and societal costs. *J Clin Psychiatry* 2002;63(Suppl 14):4.
8. Mendlowicz MV, Stein MB. Quality of life in individuals with anxiety disorders. *Am J Psychiatry* 2000;157:669.
9. Weisberg RB et al. Psychiatric treatment in primary care patients with anxiety disorders: a comparison of care received from primary care providers and psychiatrists. *Am J Psychiatry* 2007;164: 276.
10. Wise MG, Griffies WS. A combined treatment approach to anxiety in the medically ill. *J Clin Psychiatry* 1995;56(Suppl 2):14.
11. Anon. Drugs that may cause psychiatric symptoms. *Med Lett Drugs Ther* 2002;44:59.
12. Moller HJ. Anxiety associated with comorbid depression. *J Clin Psychiatry* 2002;63(Suppl 14):22.
13. Pigott TA. Gender differences in the epidemiology and treatment of anxiety disorders. *J Clin Psychiatry* 1999;60(Suppl 18):4.
14. Brawman-Mintzer O. Pharmacologic treatment of generalized anxiety disorder. *Psychiatr Clin North Am* 2001;24:119.
15. Hettema JM et al. A review and meta-analysis of the genetic epidemiology of anxiety disorders. *Am J Psychiatry* 2001;158:1568.
16. Borkovec TD. Psychotherapy for generalized anxiety disorder. *J Clin Psychiatry* 2001;62(Suppl 11):37.
17. Mohler H et al. A new benzodiazepines pharmacology. *J Pharmacol Exp Ther* 2002;300:2.
18. Lydiard RB. The role of GABA in anxiety disorders. *J Clin Psychiatry* 2003;64(Suppl 3):21.
19. Low K et al. Molecular and neuronal substrate for the selective attenuation of anxiety. *Science* 2000;290:131.
20. Gorman JM. New molecular targets for antianxiety interventions. *J Clin Psychiatry* 2003;64(Suppl 3):28.
21. Lee KC et al. Beyond depression: evaluation of newer indications and off-label uses for SSRIs. *Formulary* 2002;37:240.
22. Rickels K et al. Paroxetine treatment of generalized anxiety disorder: a double-blind, placebo-controlled study. *Am J Psychiatry* 2003;160:749.
23. Stocchi F et al. Efficacy and tolerability of paroxetine for the long-term treatment of generalized anxiety disorder. *J Clin Psychiatry* 2003;64:250.
24. Silverstone PH, Salinas E. Efficacy of venlafaxine extended release in patients with major depressive disorder and comorbid generalized anxiety disorder. *J Clin Psychiatry* 2001;62:523.
25. Montgomery SA et al. Effectiveness of venlafaxine, extended release formulation, in the short-term and long-term treatment of generalized anxiety disorder: results of a survival analysis. *J Clin Psychopharmacol* 2002;22:561.
26. Rickels K et al. Efficacy of extended-release venlafaxine in nondepressed outpatients with generalized anxiety disorder. *Am J Psychiatry* 2000;157: 968.
27. Hartford J et al. Duloxetine as an SNRI treatment for generalized anxiety disorder: results from a placebo and active-controlled trial. *Int Clin Psychopharmacol* 2007;22:167.
28. Kaponen H et al. Efficacy of duloxetine for the treatment of generalized anxiety disorder: implications for primary care physicians. *Prim Care Companion J Clin Psychiatry* 2007;9:100.
29. Rynn M et al. Efficacy and safety of duloxetine in the treatment of generalized anxiety disorder: a flexible-dose, progressive-titration, placebo-controlled trial. Depress Anxiety 2007. Available at: www.interscience.wiley.com. Accessed April 27, 2008.
30. Waugh J, Goa KL. Escitalopram: a review of its use in the management of major depressive and anxiety disorders. *CNS Drugs* 2003;17:343.
31. Russell JM et al. Effect of concurrent anxiety on response to sertraline and imipramine in patients with chronic depression. *Depress Anxiety* 2001;13:18.
32. Fava M et al. Fluoxetine versus sertraline and paroxetine in major depression: tolerability and efficacy in anxious depression. *J Affect Disord* 2000;59:119.
33. Flament MF, Lane R. Acute antidepressant response to fluoxetine and sertraline in psychiatric outpatients with psychomotor agitation. *Int J Psych Clin Pract* 2001;5:103.
34. Fawcett J, Barkin RL. A meta-analysis of eight randomized, double-blind, controlled clinical trials of mirtazapine for the treatment of patients with major depression and symptoms of anxiety. *J Clin Psychiatry* 1998;59:123.
35. Spigset O et al. Hepatic injury and pancreatitis during treatment with serotonin reuptake inhibitors: data from the World Health Organization (WHO) database of adverse drug reactions. *Int Clin Psychopharmacol* 2003;18:157.
36. Apter JT, Allen LA. Buspirone: future directions. *J Clin Psychopharmacol* 1999;19:86.
37. Mahmood I, Sahajwalla C. Clinical pharmacokinetics and pharmacodynamics of buspirone, an anxiolytic drug. *Clin Pharmacokinet* 1999;36:277.
38. Beers MH. Explicit criteria for determining inappropriate medication use by the elderly. *Arch Intern Med* 1997;157:1531.
39. Llorca PM et al. Efficacy and safety of hydroxyzine in the treatment of generalized anxiety disorder: a 3-month double-blind study. *J Clin Psychiatry* 2002;63:1020.
40. Ballenger JC. Treatment of anxiety disorders to remission. *J Clin Psychiatry* 2001;62(Suppl 12):5.
41. Stahl SM. Independent actions on fear circuits may lead to therapeutic synergy for anxiety when combining serotonergic and GABAergic agents. *J Clin Psychiatry* 2002;63:854.
42. Goddard AW et al. Early coadministration of clonazepam with sertraline for panic disorder. *Arch Gen Psychiatry* 2001;58:681.
43. Charney DS et al. Hypnotics and sedatives. In: Hardman JG et al., eds. *Goodman & Gilman's The Pharmacological Basis of Therapeutics*. 10th ed. New York: McGraw-Hill; 2001:399.
44. Schmider J et al. Relationship of in vitro data on drug metabolism to *in vivo* pharmacokinetics and drug interactions: implications for diazepam disposition in humans [editorial]. *J Clin Psychopharmacol* 1996;16:267.
45. Bonate et al. Clonazepam and sertraline: absence of drug interaction in a multiple-dose study. *J Clin Psychopharmacol* 2000;20:19.
46. Klein E. The role of extended-release benzodiazepines in the treatment of anxiety: a risk-benefit evaluation with a focus on extended-release alprazolam. *J Clin Psychiatry* 2002;63(Suppl 14):27.
47. Liston HL et al. Drug glucuronidation in clinical psychopharmacology. *J Clin Psychopharmacol* 2001;21:500.
48. Fujita M et al. Changes of benzodiazepine receptors during chronic benzodiazepine administration in humans. *Eur J Pharmacol* 1999;368:161.
49. Gladsjo JA et al. Absence of neuropsychologic deficits in patients receiving long-term treatment with alprazolam-XR for panic disorder. *J Clin Psychopharmacol* 2001;21:131.
50. Lauderdale SA, Sheikh JI. Anxiety disorders in older adults. *Clin Geriatr Med* 2003;19:721.
51. Ensrud KE et al. Central nervous system-active medications and risk for falls in older women. *J Am Geriatr Soc* 2002;50:1629.
52. Wang PS et al. Hazardous benzodiazepines regimens in the elderly: effects of half-life, dosage, and duration on risk of hip fracture. *Am J Psychiatry* 2001;158:892.
53. Rothschild AJ et al. Comparison of the frequency of behavioral disinhibition on alprazolam, clonazepam, or no benzodiazepine in hospitalized psychiatric patients. *J Clin Psychopharmacol* 2000;20:7.
54. Posternak MA, Mueller TI. Assessing the risks and benefits of benzodiazepines for anxiety disorders in patients with a history of substance abuse or dependence. *Am J Addict* 2001;10:48.
55. Rickels K et al. Pharmacologic strategies for discontinuing benzodiazepine treatment. *J Clin Psychopharmacol* 1999;19(Suppl 2):12S.
56. Tanaka E. Clinically significant pharmacokinetic drug interactions with benzodiazepines. *J Clin Pharm Ther* 1999;24:347.

57. Yasui N et al. Effect of itraconazole on the single oral dose pharmacokinetics and pharmacodynamics of alprazolam. *Psychopharmacology* 1998;139:269.
58. Zevin S, Benowitz NL. Drug interactions with tobacco smoking: an update. *Clin Pharmacokinet* 1999;36:425.
59. American Academy of Pediatrics Committee on Drugs. Use of psychoactive medication during pregnancy and possible effects on the fetus and newborn. *Pediatrics* 2000;105:880.
60. Altshuler LL et al. Course of mood and anxiety disorders during pregnancy and the postpartum period. *J Clin Psychiatry* 1998;59(Suppl 2):29.
61. The American Academy of Pediatrics Committee on Drugs. Transfer of drugs and other chemicals into human milk. *Pediatrics* 2002;110:1030.
62. Weinbroun AA et al. A risk-benefit assessment of flumazenil in the management of benzodiazepines overdose. *Drug Saf* 1997;3:181.
63. Mathieu-Nolf M et al. Flumazenil use in an emergency department: a survey. *Clin Toxicol* 2001;39:15.
64. Yonkers KA et al. Gender differences in pharmacokinetics and pharmacodynamics of psychotropic medication. *Am J Psychiatry* 1992;149:587.
65. Wan J et al. The elimination of diazepam in Chinese subjects is dependent on the mephenytoin oxidation phenotype. *Br J Clin Pharmacol* 1996;42:471.
66. Pecknold JC. A risk–benefit assessment of buspirone in the treatment of anxiety disorders. *Drug Saf* 1997;16:118.
67. Dimitriou EC et al. Buspirone vs. alprazolam: a double-blind comparative study of their efficacy, adverse effects and withdrawal symptoms. *Drug Invest* 1992;4:316.
68. Davidson JRT et al. Efficacy, safety, and tolerability of venlafaxine extended release and buspirone in outpatients with generalized anxiety disorder. *J Clin Psychiatry* 1999;60:528.
69. Chiaie RD et al. Assessment of the efficacy of buspirone in patients affected by generalized anxiety disorder, shifting to buspirone from prior treatment with lorazepam: a placebo-controlled, double-blind study. *J Clin Psychopharmacol* 1995;15:12.
70. Uhlenhuth EH et al. International study of expert judgment on therapeutic use of benzodiazepines and other psychotherapeutic medications: IV. Therapeutic dose dependence and abuse liability of benzodiazepines in the long-term treatment of anxiety disorders. *J Clin Psychopharmacol* 1999;19(Suppl 2):23S.
71. Sramek JJ et al. Meta-analysis of the safety and tolerability of two dose regimens of buspirone in patients with persistent anxiety. *Depress Anxiety* 1999;9:131.
72. Kessler RC et al. The epidemiology of panic attacks, panic disorder, and agoraphobia in the National Comorbidity Study Replication. *Arch Gen Psychiatry* 2006;63:415.
73. Roy-Burne PP et al. Panic disorder. *Lancet* 2006; 368:1023.
74. Lepola U et al. Sertraline versus imipramine treatment of comorbid panic disorder and major depressive disorder. *J Clin Psychiatry* 2003;64:654.
75. Roy-Byrne PP et al. Panic disorder in the primary care setting: comorbidity, disability, service utilization, and treatment. *J Clin Psychiatry* 1999;60:492.
76. Hettema JM et al. The structure of genetic and environmental risk factors for anxiety disorders in men and women. *Arch Gen Psychiatry* 2005;62:182.
77. Katon WJ. Panic disorder. *N Engl J Med* 2006;354: 2360.
78. American Psychiatric Association Practice Guidelines. Practice guideline for the treatment of patients with panic disorder. *Am J Psychiatry* 1998;155:1.
79. Cousins MS et al. GABA(B) receptor agonists for the treatment of drug addiction: a review of recent findings. *Drug Alcohol Depend* 2002;65:209.
80. Gorman JM et al. Neuroanatomical hypothesis of panic disorder, revised. *Am J Psychiatry* 2000;157: 493.
81. Strohle A et al. Induced panic attacks shift gamma-aminobutyric acid type A receptor modulatory neuroactive steroid composition in patients with panic disorder. *Arch Gen Psychiatry* 2003;60:161.
82. Perna G et al. Antipanic drug modulation of 35% CO_2 hyperreactivity and short-term treatment outcome. *J Clin Psychopharmacol* 2002;22:300.
83. Michelson D et al. Efficacy of usual antidepressant dosing regimens of fluoxetine in panic disorder. *Br J Psychiatry* 2001;179:514.
84. Pollack MH et al. A double-blind study of the efficacy of venlafaxine extended-release, paroxetine, and placebo in the treatment of panic disorder. *Depress Anxiety* 2007;24:1.
85. Perugi G et al. Diagnosis and treatment of agoraphobia with panic disorder. *CNS Drugs* 2007;21:741.
86. Sheikh JI et al. The efficacy of sertraline in panic disorder: combined results from two fixed-dose studies. *Int Clin Psychopharmacol* 2000;15:335.
87. Bakker A et al. SSRIs vs. TCAs in the treatment of panic disorder: a meta-analysis. *Acta Psychiatr Scand* 2002;106:163.
88. Pollack MH. The pharmacotherapy of panic disorder. *J Clin Psychiatry* 2005;66(Suppl 4):23.
89. Zamorski MA, Albucher RC. What to do when SSRIs fail: eight strategies for optimizing treatment of panic disorder. *Am Fam Physician* 2002;66:1477.
90. Caillard V et al. Comparative effects of low and high doses of clomipramine and placebo in panic disorder: a double-blind controlled study. *Acta Psychiatr Scand* 1999;99:51.
91. Marcourakis T et al. Serum levels of clomipramine and desmethylclomipramine and clinical improvement in panic disorder. *J Psychopharmacol* 1999; 13:40.
92. Hirschmann S et al. Pindolol augmentation in patients with treatment-resistant panic disorder: a double-blind, placebo-controlled trial. *J Clin Psychopharmacol* 2000;20:556.
93. Kampman M et al. A randomized, double-blind, placebo-controlled study of the effects of adjunctive paroxetine in panic disorder patients unsuccessfully treated with cognitive-behavioral therapy alone. *J Clin Psychiatry* 2002;63:772.
94. Mavissakalian MR, Perel JM. Duration of imipramine therapy and relapse in panic disorder with agoraphobia. *J Clin Psychopharmacol* 2002; 22:294.
95. Pollack MH. Comorbidity, neurobiology, and pharmacotherapy of social anxiety disorder. *J Clin Psychiatry* 2001;62(Suppl 12):24.
96. Keller MB. Social anxiety disorder clinical course and outcome: review of Harvard/Brown anxiety research project (HARP) findings. *J Clin Psychiatry* 2006;67(Suppl 12):14.
97. Stein MB. Disability and quality of life in social phobia: epidemiologic findings. *Am J Psychiatry* 2000;157:1606.
98. Arbelle S et al. Relation of shyness in grade school children to the genotype for the long form of the serotonin transporter promoter region polymorphism. *Am J Psychiatry* 2003;160:671.
99. Mathew SJ et al. Neurobiological mechanisms of social anxiety disorder. *Am J Psychiatry* 2001;158:1558.
100. Schneier FR et al. Low dopamine D_2 receptor binding potential in social phobia. *Am J Psychiatry* 2000;157:457.
101. Davidson JRT. Pharmacotherapy of social anxiety disorder: what does the evidence tell us? *J Clin Psychiatry* 2006; 67(Suppl 12):20.
102. Davidson JRT et al. Fluoxetine, comprehensive behavioral therapy, and placebo in generalized social phobia. *Arch Gen Psychiatry* 2004;61:1005.
103. Lader M et al. Efficacy and tolerability of escitalopram in 12- and 24-week treatment of social anxiety disorder: randomised, double-blind, placebo-controlled, fixed-dose study. *Depress Anxiety* 2004;19:241.
104. Liebowitz MR et al. A randomized, double-blind, fixed-dose comparison of paroxetine and placebo in the treatment of generalized social anxiety disorder. *J Clin Psychiatry* 2002;63:66.
105. Stein DJ et al. Predictors of response to pharmacotherapy in social anxiety disorder: an analysis of 3 placebo-controlled paroxetine trials. *J Clin Psychiatry* 2002;63:152.
106. Fedoroff IC, Taylor S. Psychological and pharmacological treatments of social phobia: a meta-analysis. *J Clin Psychopharmacol* 2001;21:311.
107. Breslau N. The epidemiology of posttraumatic stress disorder: what is the extent of the problem? *J Clin Psychiatry* 2001;62(Suppl 17):16.
108. Ballenger JC et al. Consensus statement on posttraumatic stress disorder from the International Consensus Group on Depression and Anxiety. *J Clin Psychiatry* 2000;61(Suppl 5):60.
109. American Psychiatric Association. Practice guideline for the treatment of patients with acute stress disorder and posttraumatic stress disorder. Arlington, VA: American Psychiatric Association; 2004.
110. Breslau N. Outcomes of posttraumatic stress disorder. *J Clin Psychiatry* 2001;62(Suppl 17):55.
111. Jacobsen et al. Substance use disorders in patients with posttraumatic stress disorder: a review of the literature. *Am J Psychiatry* 2001;158:1184.
112. Davidson JRT. Recognition and treatment of posttraumatic stress disorder. *JAMA* 2001;286:584.
113. Nutt DJ, Malizia AL. Structural and functional brain changes in posttraumatic stress disorder. *J Clin Psychiatry* 2004;65(Suppl 1):11.
114. Koob GF. Corticotrophin-releasing factor, norepinephrine, and stress. *Biol Psychiatry* 1999;46: 1167.
115. Southwick SM et al. Role of norepinephrine in the pathophysiology and treatment of posttraumatic stress disorder. *Biol Psychiatry* 1999;46:1192.
116. Friedman MJ. Future pharmacotherapy for posttraumatic stress disorder: prevention and treatment. *Psychiatr Clin North Am* 2002;25:427.
117. Shear MK. Building a model of posttraumatic stress disorder [editorial]. *Am J Psychiatry* 2002;159:1631.
118. Stein DJ et al.Pharmacotherapy for post traumatic stress disorder (PTSD). *Cochrane Database Syst Rev* 2006, Issue 1. Art. No.: CD002795. DOI:10.1002/14651858.CD002795.pub2.
119. Martenyi F et al. Fluoxetine versus placebo in posttraumatic stress disorder. *J Clin Psychiatry* 2002;63:199.
120. Hertzberg MA et al. Lack of efficacy of fluoxetine in PTSD: a placebo controlled trial in combat veterans. *Ann Clin Psychiatry* 2000;12:101.
121. Asnis GM et al. SSRIs versus non-SSRIs in posttraumatic stress disorder. *Drugs* 2004;64:383.
122. Davidson JRT et al. The efficacy and tolerability of tiagabine in adult patients with post-traumatic stress disorder. *J Clin Psychopharmacol* 2007;27:85.
123. Boehnlein JK, Kinzie JD. Pharmacologic reduction of CNS noradrenergic activity in PTSD: the case for clonidine and prazosin. *J Psychiatr Pract* 2007;13:72.
124. Davidson JRT. Long-term treatment and prevention of posttraumatic stress disorder. *J Clin Psychiatry* 2004;65(Suppl 1):44.
125. Stein DJ. Obsessive-compulsive disorder. *Lancet* 2002;360:397.
126. American Psychiatric Association. Practice guideline for the treatment of patients with obsessive-compulsive disorder. Arlington, VA: American Psychiatric Association; 2007.
127. Horwath E, Weissman MM. The epidemiology and cross-national presentation of obsessive-compulsive disorder. *Psychiatr Clin North Am* 2000;23:493.
128. Koran LM et al. Efficacy of sertraline in the long-term treatment of obsessive-compulsive disorder. *Am J Psychiatry* 2002;159:88.
129. Mains G et al. Relapses after discontinuation of drug associated with increased resistance to treatment in obsessive-compulsive disorder. *Int Clin Psychopharmacol* 2001;16:33.
130. Hollander E. Obsessive-compulsive disorder: the hidden epidemic. *J Clin Psychiatry* 1997;58(Suppl 12):3.
131. Rosario-Campos MC et al. Adults with early-onset

obsessive-compulsive disorder. *Am J Psychiatry* 2001;158:1899.
132. Arnold P, Richter MA. Is obsessive-compulsive disorder an autoimmune disease? *Can Med Assoc J* 2001;165:1353.
133. Swedo SE et al. Pediatric autoimmune neuropsychiatric disorders associated with streptococcal infections: clinical description of the first 50 cases. *Am J Psychiatry* 1998;155:264.
134. Phillips KA. The obsessive-compulsive spectrums. *Psychiatr Clin North Am* 2002;25:791.
135. Stein DJ.Advances in the neurobiology of obsessive-compulsive disorder. *Psychiatr Clin North Am* 2000;23:545.
136. Saxena S, Rauch SL. Functional neuroimaging and the neuroanatomy of obsessive-compulsive disorder. *Psychiatr Clin North Am* 2000;23:563.
137. Saxena S et al. Differential brain metabolic predictors of paroxetine in obsessive-compulsive disorder versus major depression. *Am J Psychiatry* 2003;160:522.
138. Nestadt G et al. A family study of obsessive-compulsive disorder. *Arch Gen Psychiatry* 2000;57:358.
139. Melke J. Serotonin transporter gene polymorphisms and mental health. *Curr Opin Psychiatry* 2003;16:215.
140. Pato MT et al. Recent findings in the genetics of OCD. *J Clin Psychiatry* 2002;63(Suppl 6):30.
141. Leckman JF, Kim Y-S. A primary candidate gene for obsessive-compulsive disorder. *Arch Gen Psychiatry* 2006;63:717.
142. Dell'Osso B et al. Diagnosis and treatment of obsessive-compulsive disorder and related disorders. *Int J Clin Pract* 2007;61:98.
143. Ackerman DL, Greenland S. Multivariate meta-analysis of controlled drug studies for obsessive-compulsive disorder. *J Clin Psychopharmacol* 2002;22:309.
144. Blier P et al. Pharmacotherapies in the management of obsessive-compulsive disorder. *Can J Psychiatry* 2006;51:417.
145. Hollander E et al. Refractory obsessive-compulsive disorder: state-of-the-art treatment. *J Clin Psychiatry* 2002;63(Suppl 6):20.
146. Skapinakis P et al. Antipsychotic augmentation of serotonergic antidepressants in treatment-resistant obsessive-compulsive disorder: a meta-analysis of the randomized controlled trials. *Eur Neuropsychopharmacol* 2007;17:79.
147. McDougle C et al. A double-blind, placebo-controlled study of risperidone addition in serotonin reuptake inhibitor-refractory obsessive-compulsive disorder. *Arch Gen Psychiatry* 2000;57:794.
148. Denys D et al. Quetiapine addition to serotonin reuptake inhibitor treatment in patients with treatment-refractory obsessive-compulsive disorder: an open-label study. *J Clin Psychiatry* 2002;63:700.
149. Dannon PN et al. Pindolol augmentation in treatment-resistant obsessive compulsive disorder: a double-blind placebo controlled trial. *Eur Neuropsychopharmacol* 2000;10:165.
150. Albert U et al. Venlafaxine versus clomipramine in the treatment of obsessive-compulsive disorder: a preliminary single-blind, 12-week, controlled study. *J Clin Psychiatry* 2002;63:1004.
151. Dougherty DD et al. Prospective long-term follow-up of 44 patients who received cingulotomy for treatment-refractory obsessive-compulsive disorder. *Am J Psychiatry* 2002;159:269.
152. Greenberg BD et al. Neurosurgery for intractable obsessive-compulsive disorder and depression: critical issues. *Neurosurg Clin N Am* 2003;143:199.
153. Attiullah N et al. Clinical features of obsessive-compulsive disorder. *Psychiatr Clin North Am* 2000;23:469.
154. Hollander E et al. Pharmacotherapy for obsessive-compulsive disorder. *Psychiatr Clin North Am* 2000;23:643.
155. Hollander E et al. A double-blind, placebo-controlled study of the efficacy and safety of controlled-release fluvoxamine in patients with obsessive-compulsive disorder. *J Clin Psychiatry* 2003;64:640.
156. Nielsen KK et al. Single-dose kinetics of clomipramine: relationship to the sparteine and S-mephenytoin oxidation polymorphisms. *Clin Pharmacol Ther* 1994;55:518.
157. Nissen D et al. *Mosby's Drug Consult.* 13th ed. St. Louis, MO: Mosby; 2003.
158. Nielson K et al. The biotransformation of clomipramine in vitro, identification of the cytochrome P450s responsible for the separate metabolic pathways. *J Pharmacol Exp Ther* 1996;277:1659.
159. Oesterheld J, Kallepalli BI. Grapefruit juice and clomipramine: shifting metabolic ratios. *J Clin Psychopharmacol* 1997;17:62.
160. Shimoda K et al. Pronounced differences in the disposition of clomipramine between Japanese and Swedish patients. *J Clin Psychopharmacol* 1999;19:393.
161. Nemeroff CB et al. Newer antidepressants and the cytochrome P450 system. *Am J Psychiatry* 1996;153:311.
162. Michalets EL. Update: clinically significant cytochrome P-450 drug interactions. *Pharmacotherapy* 1998;18:84.
163. Villikka K et al. Triazolam is ineffective in patients taking rifampin. *Clin Pharmacol Ther* 1997;61:8.
164. Backman JT et al. Concentrations and effects of oral midazolam are greatly reduced in patients treated with carbamazepine or phenytoin. *Epilepsia* 1996;37:253.
165. Furukori H et al. Effect of carbamazepine on the single oral dose pharmacokinetics of alprazolam. *Neuropsychopharmacology* 1998;18:364.
166. Dresser GK et al. Pharmacokinetic-pharmacodynamic consequences and clinical relevance of cytochrome P450 3A4 inhibition. *Clin Pharmacokinet* 2000;38:41.
167. Greenblatt DJ et al. Ketoconazole inhibition of triazolam and alprazolam clearance: differential kinetic and dynamic consequences. *Clin Pharmacol Ther* 1998;64:237.
168. Greenblatt DJ et al. Extensive impairment of triazolam and alprazolam clearance by short-term low-dose ritonavir: the clinical dilemma of concurrent inhibition and induction [editorial]. *J Clin Psychopharmacol* 1999;19:293.
169. Ozdemir M et al. Interaction between grapefruit juice and diazepam in humans. *Eur J Drug Metab Pharmacokinet* 1998;23:55.
170. Samara EE et al. Effect of valproate on the pharmacokinetics and pharmacodynamics of lorazepam. *J Clin Pharmacol* 1997;37:442.
171. Guven H et al. Age-related digoxin-alprazolam interaction. *Clin Pharmacol Ther* 1993;54:42.
172. Herman RJ, Wilkinson GR. Disposition of diazepam in young and elderly subjects after acute and chronic dosing. *Br J Clin Pharmacol* 1996;42:147.
173. Kaplan GB et al. Single-dose pharmacokinetics and pharmacodynamics of alprazolam in elderly and young subjects. *J Clin Pharmacol* 1998;38:14.
174. Matzke GR, Frye RF. Drug administration in patients with renal insufficiency: minimizing renal and extrarenal toxicity. *Drug Saf* 1997;16:205.

CHAPTER 77

Sleep Disorders

Julie A. Dopheide and Glen L. Stimmel

"I wake to sleep, and take my waking slow. I learn by going where I have to go."

Theodore Roethke, *The Waking*

The human drive to sleep is strong and enduring. Most healthy people spend one-third of their lives asleep. Such a major part of life deserves full exploration and study. This chapter reviews the impact, epidemiology, and classification of disorders of the sleep–wake cycle. An overview of normal sleep physiology and neurochemistry precedes case discussions.

SOCIETAL IMPACT

The impact of sleep disorders on overall health, productivity, and quality of life has been increasingly appreciated. Untreated sleep disorders, including chronic insomnia, sleep apnea, periodic limb movements during sleep (PLMS), and narcolepsy, are all associated with diminished mental and physical functioning and poor quality of life.[1–4] Sleep research shows that chronic insomnia, for example, can predict untreated illness or may contribute to injury and illness.[2,5,6]

Chronic insomnia is associated with immune system dysregulation and the release of proinflammatory cytokines (IL-6 and tumor necrosis factor alpha [TNF-α]), a disruption of the hypothalamic-pituitary-adrenal (HPA) axis and a depletion of brain serotonin and other neurotransmitters.[6] Persons with insomnia are 10 times more likely to suffer from depression and 17 times more likely to have anxiety compared with people without insomnia.[6] Chronic insomnia is two to three times greater in individuals with high blood pressure, breathing difficulty, gastrointestinal (GI) disorders, cancer, and chronic pain, among other conditions.[7] Insomnia and excessive daytime sleepiness in the elderly are leading predictors of institutionalization.[2]

In 2005, a National Institutes of Health (NIH) panel of sleep experts recommended a major shift regarding insomnia. The panel stated that insomnia is not just a symptom of a medical or psychiatric illness but a condition that contributes to the severity of that disease or disorder. Indeed, when insomnia is effectively treated, co-occurring medical and psychiatric conditions, such as chronic pain or depression, are relieved along with improvement in functioning and quality of life. The relationship between insomnia and medical or psychiatric illness is bidirectional.[2,6] Instead of categorizing insomnia as either primary (with no other co-occurring disorder) or secondary, it should be categorized as either primary or "comorbid" (insomnia that co-occurs with medical or psychiatric illness).[5]

Excessive sleepiness caused by a sleep disorder or sleep deprivation constitutes a serious public health hazard in health care workers, firefighters, policemen, and truck drivers.[8] An alert mind is crucial for maximal productivity in all occupations, particularly when driving is involved. Of all drivers, 20% reportedly have fallen asleep at least once while driving.[8] Motor vehicle accidents also tend to peak during the early morning (1 AM to 6 AM) and mid afternoon (2 PM to 4 PM) hours—times when the circadian cycle for sleepiness is maximal.[8] College students with short sleep times (≤6 hrs/night) had lower grade point averages (GPA) than long sleepers (≥9 hours). Mid range sleepers (7–8 hours) were not significantly different than long sleepers.[9] Medical interns made 35.9% more errors in the Medical Intensive Care Units and Cardiac Care Units when working a 24-hour shift compared with working 16 hours.[10] Medical resident shifts are now limited to 12–16 hours to improve patient safety.[10]

EPIDEMIOLOGY

Sleep Disorders

One in seven Americans has a longstanding sleep–wake disorder.[3–5,11,12] During the course of a year, approximately 30% of the population will experience insomnia, and approximately one-third of this group will consider the problem severe.[2,5] Insomnia is defined as requiring >30 minutes to fall asleep, when individuals awaken throughout the night and cannot immediately return to sleep, when individuals experience early-morning awakening, or when total sleep time is decreased to <6 hours.[2,5,13] Insomnia is the most common sleep complaint, but the resulting daytime sleepiness and fatigue are troubling after-effects. Insomnia is categorized into three general types: transient (lasting a few days), short-term (lasting <4 weeks), or chronic (persisting for ≥1 month). The resulting level of daytime impairment should be assessed to determine insomnia severity.[5,6,13,14]

Major sleep disorders in order of decreasing prevalence are listed in Table 77-1.[2,4] Nightmares, nocturnal leg cramps, and snoring are more benign sleep disorders. Nightmares occur often in 5% to 30% of children 3 to 6 years of age, and approximately 2% to 6% of adults have weekly nightmares.[15] Sleep walking occurs in 1% to 2% of the population. Complex sleep behavior disorders, such as driving or eating while still half-asleep, are uncommon to rare. These behaviors are more common in people taking hypnotic medications, and therefore, counseling is needed.[15,16] In 2007, the U.S. Food and Drug Administration (FDA) issued a black-box warning that applies to all medications marketed for insomnia. It warns of the risk of angioedema (facial swelling), an allergic reaction, as well as complex sleep behaviors as described above.[16]

Table 77-1 Incidence of Major Sleep Disorders[5,13–15,34]

Sleep Disorder	*Incidence (%)*
Insomnia	30–35
Transient (few days)	
Short-term (up to 1 month)	
Chronic (>1 month)	
Sleep apnea	5–15
PLMS (nocturnal myoclonus)	5–15
RLS	5–15
Narcolepsy	0.06

PLMS, periodic limb movements during sleep; RLS, restless legs syndrome.

Hypnotic Use

Cognitive-behavioral therapy (CBT) is the preferred treatment for insomnia because of well-established efficacy, absence of drug side effects, and sustained benefit over time.[5,14,17–20] Hypnotic medications are recommended when nondrug interventions fail, cannot be implemented, or when rapid results are essential.[5,14,20]

Prescribing trends have shifted away from older benzodiazepine hypnotics toward sedating antidepressants, namely trazodone, sedating antipsychotics such as quetiapine, and newer benzodiazepine receptor active "Z-hypnotics" (zaleplon, zolpidem, eszopiclone).[21] Age, gender, and socioeconomic status influence hypnotic prescribing. One study of 2,966 outpatient visits for insomnia or sleep complaint over 1996 to 2001 showed that 48% received a prescription for medication only—with no CBT. Z-hypnotics were prescribed at 25% of these visits. Factors that increased the likelihood of receiving a Z-hypnotic included female gender, co-occurring psychiatric illness, and upper socioeconomic status.

An analysis of 147,945 patient visits for sleep difficulty between 1997 and 2002 in the United States showed women were 1.5 times more likely to have insomnia-related visits. In all ages, the most frequently prescribed or recommended medications were either zaleplon or zolpidem (28.5%), and trazodone (32%). Z-hypnotics were prescribed or recommended significantly more often in patients <65 years of age compared with older patients (54.6% vs. 29.8%, respectively). Temazepam was prescribed to 18.3% of those >65 years of age compared to 15.7% of those <65 years of age. Triazolam or flurazepam was prescribed in 4.9 to 7.9% of patients from all age groups.[22]

With aging, sleep typically changes in quality, partially because of sleep disruption related to chronic illnesses.[23,24] Elderly persons consume more sleep-promoting medications than younger adults. The 2003 National Sleep Foundation's "Sleep in America" poll found 11% of older adults take prescription medications to promote sleep compared with 6% of younger adults.[23]

THE SLEEP STAGES

Normal Sleep

Each sleep stage serves a physiologic function and can be monitored in sleep laboratories by polysomnography. Polysomnography is the term used to describe three electrophysiologic measures: the electroencephalogram (EEG), the electromyogram (EMG), and the electro-oculogram (EOG). The pattern of brain waves, muscle tone, and eye movements can be used to categorize sleep as rapid eye movement (REM) sleep or nonrapid eye movement (NREM) sleep.[25,26]

Nonrapid Eye Movement Sleep

Nonrapid eye movement sleep is divided further into four stages, with different quantities of time spent in each stage. Stage 1 is a transition between sleep and wakefulness known as *relaxed wakefulness*, which generally comprises approximately 2% to 5% of sleep. Approximately 50% of total sleep time is spent in stage 2, which is rapid-wave (alpha) or lighter sleep. Stages 3 and 4 are slow-wave (delta) or deep sleep. Stage 3 occupies an average of 5% of sleep time, whereas stage 4 comprises 10% to 15% of sleep time in young, healthy adults. At sleep onset, the brain quickly passes through stage 1 and moves to stage 2. Muscle activity shuts down and brain waves become less active. After a brief REM period, the brain moves into slow-wave sleep (NREM stages 3 and 4) approximately 1 to 3 hours after a person falls asleep. The body continually moves through all of the sleep stages over the course of the night (Fig. 77-1). REM periods become longer and deep sleep lessens over the last half of the night.[25–27]

Nonrapid eye movement sleep stages differ qualitatively as well as quantitatively. The function of stage 1 is to initiate sleep. Stage 2 provides rest for the muscles and brain through muscle atonia and low-voltage brain wave activity. Arousability from sleep is highest during stages 1 and 2. In contrast, it is difficult to awaken someone during stages 3 and 4, or delta sleep. Delta sleep, also known as *restorative sleep*, is enhanced by serotonin, adenosine, cholecystokinin, and IL-1. The ability of IL-1 to promote slow-wave sleep supports a widely held theory linking deep sleep to the augmentation of immune function. Some hormones (e.g., somatostatin, growth hormone) are released mainly during slow-wave sleep. Deep sleep is most abundant in infants and children and tends to level off at approximately 4 hours a night during adolescence.[24,25] At age 65, deep sleep accounts for only 10% of sleep and at age 75, it often is nonexistent.[23,25] Age-related increased awakenings, decreased deep sleep, and daytime sleepiness have been associated with increases in cortisol and the proinflammatory cytokine, IL-6.[6,24,26]

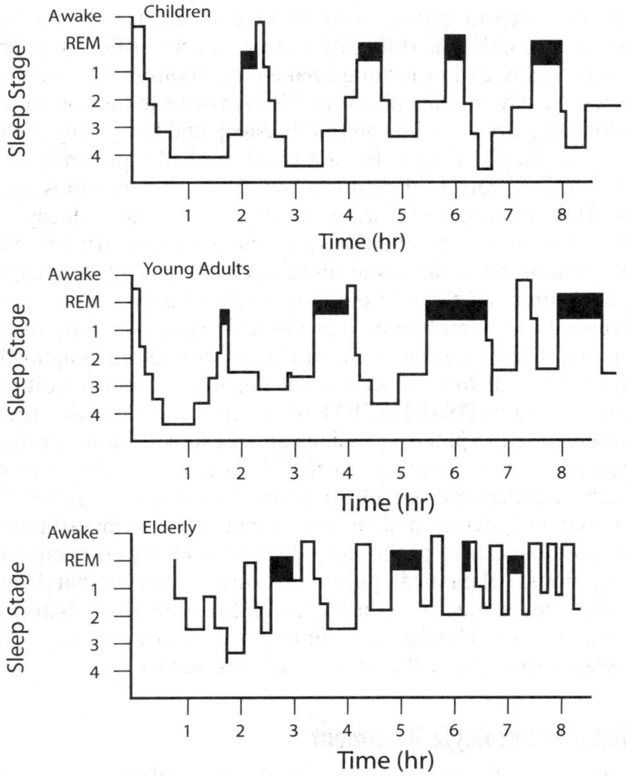

FIGURE 77-1 Normal sleep cycles.

Rapid Eye Movement Sleep

Whereas NREM sleep is necessary for rest and rejuvenation, the purpose of REM sleep remains a mystery. REM sleep also is called *paradoxical sleep* because it has aspects of both deep sleep and light sleep. Body and brainstem functions appear to be in a deep sleep state as muscle and sympathetic tone drop dramatically. In contrast, neurochemical processes and higher cortical brain function appear active. Dreaming is associated closely with REM sleep, and when a person is awakened from REM, alertness returns relatively quickly.

Numerous physiologic functions are altered during REM sleep. Breathing is irregular, consisting of sudden changes in respiratory amplitude and frequency corresponding to bursts of REM. Temperature control is lost and the body temperature typically lowers. REM sleep brings on variability in heart rate, blood pressure (BP), cerebral blood flow, and metabolism. Cardiac output and urine volume decrease. Blood may become thicker as a result of autonomic instability and temperature changes.[26,28]

Rapid eye movement periods cycle approximately every 90 minutes throughout the night. Duration of REM increases in the last half of the night, becoming longer and more intense just after the time when body temperature is at its lowest, around 5 AM. Although the reason for the importance of REM sleep is unknown, it is clear that the human body needs REM sleep. When deprived of REM sleep, whether through poor sleep, drugs, or disease states, the brain and body try to catch up. REM rebound occurs, which may result in vivid dreams or an overall less restful sleep.[25–27]

Abnormal Sleep

Primary insomnia (difficulty sleeping not attributable to a drug, psychiatric disorder, or medical condition) can resemble a normal sleep pattern, but may be associated with an increased time to fall asleep, multiple awakenings, or decreased total sleep time. Polysomnographic readings evaluating insomnia secondary to psychiatric disorders can be markedly different. In depressive disorders, decreased REM latency (i.e., the time from sleep onset to the appearance of REM) is a classic finding. Acute psychotic disorders feature prolonged global sleeplessness, with sleep onset latency, fragmented sleep, and decreased slow-wave sleep. Medical disorders (e.g., arthritis, cancer, infections) can be associated with significantly altered sleep-stage pattern. Uncontrolled pain can result in frequent awakenings and decreased total sleep time. Oxygen saturation is at its lowest during REM sleep; therefore, less time in REM may be advantageous for patients with cystic fibrosis and other breathing disorders.[25,26,28]

Primary sleep disorders, including PLMS, can cause intermittent partial arousals out of stage 2 sleep and can impair the progress to slow-wave sleep. This may disrupt the quality of sleep and contribute to daytime impairment. Sleep apnea syndrome signals the brain to initiate multiple miniarousals in response to breathing cessation during sleep and, therefore, decreases the quality of sleep. Patients with narcolepsy may have the most unique pattern of sleep disruption because they fall almost immediately into REM sleep (instead of the usual 90-minute latency) and may experience an increased number of REM episodes.[4]

Although polysomnographic readings from sleep laboratories are interesting and can be useful diagnostic and assessment tools, they are neither routinely available nor are the costs routinely reimbursable by insurance companies. A thorough history of sleep problems obtained through patient interviews, along with both physical and psychiatric evaluations, are the most widely used methods of patient assessment. Although acknowledging the usefulness of clinical assessment, certain patients with more serious sleep problems, such as sleep apnea, narcolepsy, or excessive daytime impairment, should have sleep laboratory evaluations.

NEUROCHEMISTRY OF SLEEP–WAKE CYCLE

Wakefulness-and Sleep-Promoting Neurochemicals

A basic understanding of brain neurochemistry is essential in understanding sleep disorders and the clinical use of hypnotics. Hypnotics exert their effects by modulating brain neurotransmitters and neuropeptides (e.g., serotonin, norepinephrine, acetylcholine, histamine, adenosine, and γ-aminobutyric acid [GABA]). The neuronal systems where neurotransmitters and neuropeptides act to control the sleep–wake cycle lie in the brainstem, hypothalamus, and basal forebrain, with connections in the thalamus and cortex. Noradrenergic, histaminergic, and acetylcholine-containing neurons promote wakefulness as they modulate cortical and subcortical neurons. Excitatory amino acids, such as glutamate, and stimulating neuropeptides (e.g., substance P, thyrotropin-releasing factor, corticotropin-releasing factor) also promote wakefulness.[27] Hypocretin 1 and 2, also known as orexin a and b, are neuropeptides that modulate the sleep–wake cycle. Hypocretin 1 and 2 are deficient in people with narcolepsy and primary hypersomnia.[29,30]

Wakefulness and sleep are antagonistic states competing for control of brain activity. Sleep takes over as the wakefulness-maintaining neuronal systems weaken and sleep-promoting neurons become active. Serotonin-containing neurons of the brainstem raphe dampen sensory input and inhibit motor activity, promoting the emergence of slow-wave sleep.[6,25,27,31] Opiate peptides (e.g., enkephalin, endorphin) and GABA, an inhibitory neurotransmitter, also promote sleep.[27,31–33]

Drug-Induced Effects on Neurochemicals

The neurochemistry of sleep also can be understood by considering the effect of hypnotic drugs on specific neurotransmitters. GABA is facilitated when a benzodiazepine compound attaches to the benzodiazepine-chloride-ionophore complex and causes chloride channels to open and inhibit the overexcited areas of the brain. GABA-facilitating hypnotics, such as benzodiazepines, induce sleep and decrease arousals between stages, providing more continuous stage 2 sleep. Benzodiazepines, however, also may decrease stage 4 slow-wave sleep and suppress REM, leading to REM rebound on abrupt discontinuation.[27,31,34] Some antihistamines promote sleep by blocking histamine-containing neurons involved in maintaining wakefulness. The excitatory effects of caffeine and other methylxanthines are attributed to their antagonism of adenosine receptors. Adenosine is a sleep-promoting neurotransmitter or neuromodulator.[27,30]

Neurotransmitter alteration may or may not affect REM sleep. Drug-induced noradrenergic and serotonergic modulation usually decreases REM sleep. An increase in dopaminergic neurotransmission can increase wakefulness but has no direct effect on REM sleep.[27,32] In contrast, increased cholinergic neurotransmission triggers REM sleep.[27,32] Cortisol decreases REM sleep in young and old with unpredictable effects on slow-wave sleep and increased wakefulness in the elderly.[6,25,35,37] It is useful to think of the brain centers, neurochemicals, and neuropeptides involved as an interactive network regulating our sleep–wake cycle. Certainly, drugs or disease states that alter neurotransmission can have significant impact on the sleep–wake cycle. Sensory input (visual and acoustic) works with the internal network and signals brain centers to either wake or sleep. Thus, darkness is a visual cue that prepares the brain for sleep. Similarly, bright light serves to prepare the brain for wakefulness.[25,38]

DYSSOMNIAS

Patient Assessment

Questions to Ask Patients

The first step in patient assessment is to determine whether the sleep problem is difficulty falling asleep, difficulty maintaining sleep, early-morning awakening, poor quality sleep, or excessive daytime sleepiness (EDS). Answers to the questions, "How long does it take you to fall asleep and how many hours do you sleep?" should be compared with the patient's normal sleep pattern to determine how it varies. Questions such as "How do you feel during the day: well rested, sleepy, or something else?" can help assess functional impairment. Not all patients need the same amount of sleep. Approximately 7 to 9 hours of sleep is optimal for most people: too much sleep can be as problematic as too little sleep.[13,25] The International Classification of Sleep Disorders and the Diagnostic and Statistical Manual of Mental Disorders, Fourth Edition, Text Revision (DSM-IV-TR) have categorized sleep disorders largely based on pathophysiology and presumed etiology rather than numbers of hours of sleep.[39,40] Four main categories of sleep disorders are useful for clinical assessment (Table 77-2). The next step in patient assessment involves investigating the possible causes of the sleep disorder and any co-occurring conditions. All medical, psychiatric, drug, environmental, and social causes must be considered and treated along with the sleep disorder. The degree of functional impairment should be assessed to evaluate the severity of the disorder.

Nonpharmacologic Treatment

Cognitive-behavioral therapies are the most effective interventions for insomnia according to the American Academy of

Table 77-2 Classification of Sleep Disorders

Dyssomnias[a]	
	Intrinsic: idiopathic insomnia, narcolepsy, sleep apnea, periodic limb movements during sleep
	Extrinsic: inadequate sleep hygiene, substance-induced sleep disorder
	Circadian rhythm sleep disorders: jet lag, shift work, delayed sleep phase syndrome
Parasomnias[b]	
	Arousal: confusional arousals, sleep walking, sleep terrors
	Sleep–wake transition disorders: sleep talking, nocturnal leg cramps
	Associated with REM: nightmares, sleep paralysis, impaired sleep-related penile erections
	Other: Primary snoring, sudden infant death syndrome, sleep bruxism
Medical, Psychiatric, and Substance-Induced Sleep Disorders	
	Associated with mental disorders: mood disorders, anxiety disorders, psychotic disorders
	Associated with neurologic disorders: Parkinson disease, Huntington disease, dementia
	Associated with other medical disorders: heart disease, renal insufficiency, pulmonary disease
	Associated with a substance: medication/substance abuse (e.g., phenylpropanolamine, cocaine)
Proposed Sleep Disorders	
	Menstrual-associated sleep disorder, pregnancy-associated sleep disorder, short or long sleeper

[a] Any sleep pattern that is abnormal (e.g., insomnia or excessive sleepiness).
[b] Any unusual behavior that emerges during sleep.
From references 6, 13, 15, with permission.

Table 77-3 Nonpharmacologic Treatments for Insomnia

1. Cognitive-behavioral therapy: most effective; can be from any trained provider.
   Cognitive: identify and stop thought patterns that interfere with sleep (e.g., "I'm never going to sleep" or allowing 15 minutes to review a worry list, then putting worries aside).
   Behavioral: stimulus control, sleep restriction, relaxation, paradoxical intention.
   (a) Stimulus control: train the brain to reassociate the bed and bedroom with sleep and re-establish a consistent sleep–wake schedule.
   (b) Sleep restriction: create "sleep-debt" by curtailing amount of time in bed, then increasing time in bed as sleep efficiency improves.
   (c) Relaxation therapy: progressive tensing and relaxing of muscles, yoga, stretching.
   (d) Paradoxical intention: encourage patient to engage in most feared behavior, "staying awake" to reduce performance anxiety associated with trying to sleep.
2. Sleep hygiene: not considered effective on its own; useful adjunctive treatment.
   Avoid caffeine, stimulants, heavy meals and etoh at bedtime; exercise early in the day before dinner to relieve stress and prime brain for sleep. Turn the face of the clock away from view; establish a pre-bedtime ritual, make sure bedroom is dark, quiet, comfortable

From references 14, 20, with permission.

Sleep Medicine and the NIH. These interventions can take 2 to 10 weeks to successfully implement based on the individual and the severity and chronicity of that person's insomnia, however, results are long-lasting. Table 77-3 lists established cognitive and behavioral interventions with brief descriptions in addition to some sleep-hygiene tips to include in patient counseling. Sleep hygiene techniques have not been demonstrated as effective without adjunctive CBT.[5,14]

The sleep environment should be dark and comfortable, free from noise or distractions, and not too warm or too cold. Along with creating a sleep-friendly setting, establishing regular sleep hours, particularly a regular wake time, is necessary to condition the body to sleep. Even after a poor night's sleep, it is important for healthy sleepers to avoid daytime naps and stay awake until the regular sleep time. In some cases, brief (e.g., 20-minute) naps may be refreshing without disrupting nocturnal sleep. Phototherapy, bright light exposure for 30 minutes to 1 hour on awakening in the morning, is an additional tool that can help set the circadian rhythm for regular sleep–wake cycles.[14,21,38] Healthy sleep often can be facilitated by avoiding problem-solving activities (e.g., finances, crossword puzzles), strenuous physical exercise, or exciting movies while in bed. Exercise early in the day can improve sleep. Exercise should be completed before dinner time so that the body has a few hours to relax before it is time to sleep. Relaxation is the key to healthy sleep. If a sleeper finds himself or herself tossing, turning, or worrying, it is time to get out of bed and stretch, read, or listen to soft music to relax. Health care practitioners should remind patients to avoid large meals at bedtime because the digestion of heavy meals can impair sleep. Last, chemicals that can disrupt sleep (e.g., alcohol, caffeine, other stimulants) should be eliminated when possible.[14,20,21]

Pharmacologic Treatment

When rapid relief of transient or short-term insomnia is needed or when chronic insomnia persists despite nondrug therapeutic interventions, hypnotic medication is indicated. Benzodiazepine hypnotics or newer, benzodiazepine omega-1 selective hypnotics, sometimes called "Z-hypnotics," are first-line therapies because they offer significantly greater efficacy than over-the-counter (OTC) products; they are safer than barbiturates and are more effective compared with sedating antidepressants.[5,21,41]

Some patients need pharmacologic treatment for insomnia but do not seek treatment from their health care providers.[5,41] Alcohol and OTC sleep aids containing antihistamines are widely used to self-medicate insomnia, although the results are less than ideal.[5,21]

The ideal hypnotic has a rapid onset of effect (within 20 minutes, the natural time to fall asleep), helps the patient sleep throughout the night, does not cause daytime impairment, and has no abuse potential. Currently, there are no ideal hypnotics. Hypnotics that act at benzodiazepine receptors come closest to the ideal.[42] Available agents vary in onset, duration, and potential for daytime impairment, mostly because of their individual pharmacokinetic profiles.[41,42] The selection of the appropriate hypnotic should consider the type of insomnia to be treated and the physiologic characteristics of the patient. For example, if someone cannot fall asleep but has no trouble staying asleep and wants no carry-over effect into the next day, a rapid-acting hypnotic with a short half-life and no active metabolites is desirable.[21,41,42]

Less common sleep disorders are treated with a variety of medications as well as some nondrug therapies. PLMS and restless legs syndrome (RLS) can be relieved with dopamine agonists, opioids, gabapentin, or clonazepam.[4] Narcolepsy is best treated with planned naps, modafinil, stimulants, sodium oxybate, or some antidepressants.[4] Both sleep apnea and primary snoring can be worsened with central nervous system (CNS) depressants but usually improve with nondrug therapies such as continuous positive airway pressure (CPAP).[43] Sleep disturbances associated with medical and psychiatric diagnoses require special attention because a hypnotic can either improve or worsen the problem.[6,13]

In a Normally Healthy Patient

1. E.P., a 31-year-old woman, is requesting a medication for treatment of her insomnia. She just returned to California from Hong Kong 2 days ago and is now having difficulty getting to sleep. When she arrived in Hong Kong, she went to sleep immediately at 4 PM and awoke at 3 AM. Her sleep pattern adjusted during her 6-week visit in Hong Kong, but on returning to California, it now takes her 2 to 3 hours to fall asleep. She has difficulty awakening in the morning and, as a result, sleeps past noon. She needs to be alert during the day to fulfill her obligations as a school teacher. What information provided by E.P. is important in the assessment of her insomnia? What additional information should be obtained from E.P. to assist in the assessment of her sleep disturbance?

E.P. describes a time-zone shift or disruption in circadian rhythm, which is a common cause of transient insomnia. Her major complaint is difficulty falling asleep, because she reports no trouble staying asleep or awakening too early. It is important for E.P. not to be sedated during the day because she is a teacher. Additional information needed from E.P. includes the duration of insomnia, methods already tried to relieve insomnia and their efficacy, concurrent medications, coexisting medical or psychiatric problems, alcohol use, caffeine use, and current life stresses. E.P. should be advised that assessing all of the aforementioned information is necessary in treating her sleep problem.

2. In response to your additional questions, you learn that E.P. has no medical problems and takes no prescription medications. She has been taking pseudoephedrine at night for nasal stuffiness since returning from Hong Kong. She denies drinking alcoholic beverages and coffee but admits to recently increasing her tea intake to try to stay awake during the day. She denies a long history of insomnia, but adds, "I have not been able to sleep as well in my new apartment; I don't know why." What factors could be contributing to E.P.'s?

Several factors are contributing to E.P.'s type of insomnia, which can be classified as circadian rhythm sleep disorder related to jet lag. Her circadian rhythm has been disrupted because of travel, but she also takes a stimulating decongestant (i.e., pseudoephedrine) and drinks a caffeine-containing beverage (i.e., tea). In addition, she sleeps in new surroundings that may require time for adjustment. All these factors can contribute to her difficulty in falling asleep. Circadian rhythm sleep disorder results from a mismatch between the sleep–wake schedule required by a person's environment and the circadian sleep–wake pattern.

Nonprescription Sleep Aids

3. E.P. would like to purchase a nonprescription sleep medication. What would you recommend?

An individual risk-versus-benefit assessment is essential before recommending any medication, even OTC products. Most nonprescription sleep aids contain antihistamines such as diphenhydramine (Benadryl). Antihistamines can cause drowsiness and can help patients fall asleep. The ability to cause sedation does not necessarily lead to hypnotic efficacy. Some patients do not feel well rested the next day after taking an antihistamine, but instead feel slow, lethargic, and not mentally sharp. This "hangover effect" can be significant and may be related to the lipid solubility and central histaminic (H_1) and muscarinic blocking effects of the antihistamine.[21,41] Antihistamines with low lipid solubility (e.g., fexofenadine, loratadine) do not cross the blood–brain barrier readily and do not cause sedation. Although diphenhydramine is the most common antihistamine found in nonprescription sleep medications, some preparations contain the antihistamines doxylamine or hydroxyzine. Tolerance can develop to the sedative effects of antihistamines after 3 to 7 days of continued use.[21,41] Because of a high incidence of daytime sedation and risk of cognitive impairment,[44] antihistamines are a poor choice for E.P., a teacher who must stay alert and functional throughout the day. Therefore, E.P.'s insomnia should be managed with nonpharmacologic interventions before initiating any drug therapy.

Time-Zone Shift: Nonpharmacologic Treatment versus Triazolam or Z-hypnotic

4. Why is E.P. especially susceptible to the effects of time-zone shift (i.e., "jet lag"), and what counseling is needed?

Time-zone shift disrupts the natural circadian rhythm, which helps regulate sleep. E.P. traveled west, then east through multiple time zones. Symptoms and severity of jet lag are related to the direction traveled and the number of time zones crossed.[38] Individuals >50 years of age and those traveling eastward have more difficulty in adjusting their circadian rhythm to time-zone changes. Eastward travelers have difficulty falling asleep and westward travelers complain of difficulty staying asleep and early morning awakening.[38] Travelers should be made aware of the problem and should take steps to help their systems adjust. On arrival in the new time zone, travelers such as E.P. should reset their watches and participate in activities corresponding to the new time. Staying active until the new time-zone bedtime and avoiding naps and stimulants can be helpful.[38]

E.P. should be informed about the likely causes of her insomnia (i.e., jet lag, tea, pseudoephedrine, new surroundings). She also should understand that it may take 1 to 3 weeks for her system to readjust after traveling.[38] The importance of nonpharmacologic interventions to improve sleep (Table 77-3) should be emphasized. For E.P., it is necessary to pay particular attention to regulating her sleep cycle by awakening at the same time each day and resisting daytime naps even after a poor night of sleep. This process, called *chronotherapy*,

Table 77-4 Pharmacokinetic Properties of Hypnotics Acting at Benzodiazepine Receptors[22,41,54–76,111]

Active Substance	Lipid Solubility	T_{max} (hr)	Onset (min)	Half-Life (hr)	Duration (hr)[a]
Zaleplon	Moderate	1.1	30	1.1	1–2
Zolpidem	Low	1–2	30	2.5	2–4
Zolpidem ER	Low	2	45	2.8	3–5
Eszopiclone	Low	1–1.6	30–45	6	5–8
Triazolam	Moderate	1	15–30	2–5	2–4
Temazepam	Moderate	1.5–2.0	60–120	10–20	8–12
Flurazepam[b]					
Hydroxyethyl-[b]	Low	1		2–3	
Aldehyde-[b]	Low	1		1	
N-desalkyl-[b]	Moderate	10	30–60	50–100	10–30

[a]Time the patient feels the effects after a single dose; usually approximates half-life with multiple doses; individual variability exists; and tolerance may develop with continued use, lessening the duration. T_{max}, time of maximum concentration.
[b]Flurazepam metabolite.

regulates the internal time clock. In addition, an hour of bright light in the morning can serve as an environmental stimulus, normalizing the circadian rhythm.[38] If E.P.'s insomnia persists despite adhering to cognitive-behavioral interventions, a prescription hypnotic may be necessary.

5. E.P. asks if she can try one of her husband's triazolam tablets. She notes, "He is immediately out like a light when he takes it, and I worry it may be too strong for me."

Short-acting hypnotics (Table 77-4) like triazolam are effective to induce and regulate sleep if the stay will be relatively short (<5 days) and if critical activities must be accomplished during the first 48 hours after arrival at the destination.[38] Advantages of triazolam for E.P. include well-established efficacy, an onset of 15 to 30 minutes and no next-day impairment at recommended doses (0.25 mg, 0.125 mg for elderly). Women may be more affected from hypnotics than men, possibly because of greater oral bioavailability.[21,41] E.P. could ask her physician to prescribe triazolam 0.125 mg in case it is needed. Triazolam is less optimal than zaleplon or zolpidem for E.P. because it can cause impairment in new learning or anterograde amnesia. These effects can be sufficiently severe to result in inability to remember new information learned on the trip. Triazolam is also associated with rebound insomnia (i.e., daytime nervousness, jitteriness, and insomnia worse than before) if abruptly stopped after >7 to 10 days of continuous use. Of the benzodiazepine hypnotics, triazolam is most commonly associated with rebound insomnia and withdrawal problems likely related to its high binding affinity to the benzodiazepine GABA-chloride–ionophore receptor complex.[41,45] Also, triazolam's short half-life (2–5 hours), and rapid decrease in blood levels create the potential for withdrawal symptoms including anxiety and insomnia. Anterograde amnesia is not a problem with "Z"-hypnotics at recommended doses because they are selective for the Ω-1 receptor and do not have significant anxiolytic effects.[41] Triazolam is highly effective in inducing sleep when used on an as-needed basis. Long-acting hypnotics, such as flurazepam (Dalmane), may prevent the traveler from awakening in the morning and should be avoided.

Melatonin

6. E.P. states she would like to try melatonin for improved sleep but wonders whether it is safe and effective. What information is available on the safety and efficacy of melatonin for jet lag or other types of insomnia?

Melatonin is a naturally occurring hormone secreted by the pineal gland, located in the center of the brain. The pineal gland is connected to the retina via a nerve pathway that runs through the suprachiasmatic nucleus of the hypothalamus, the body's circadian clock. The pineal gland produces melatonin (a byproduct of serotonin metabolism) only during the nocturnal phase of the circadian cycle and only in relative darkness.[41]

Several studies show melatonin has at least mild sleep-promoting properties when administered before the period of natural increase in endogenous melatonin (~10 PM to midnight). Studies in adults show melatonin causes significantly more sleepiness when taken at 8 PM compared with 11:30 PM, theoretically because the brain's receptors are already saturated with melatonin late at night.[41]

Eight of ten clinical trials for jet lag found that melatonin, between 0.5 and 5 mg taken close to the target bedtime in the new time zone decreased jet lag. A systematic review of 10 clinical trials showed melatonin was more effective for travel eastward crossing multiple time zones.[46] Melatonin 0.5 to 10 mg has been found effective for entraining the circadian rhythms in blind people, for alleviating insomnia in developmentally disabled or handicapped children and adults, and treating short-term, initial insomnia in children with attention deficit hyperactivity disorder (ADHD).[41,47] It has no established effectiveness for chronic insomnia.[5] Consumers selecting melatonin should be advised that the safety and effectiveness of melatonin for long-term use have not been clearly established and the purity of melatonin is not regulated by the FDA. Melatonin side effects include sleepiness, headache, and nausea, although usual doses of melatonin 0.5 to 5 mg are well tolerated.[41,48] Melatonin use has been associated with reports of depression, liver disease, and vasoconstrictive, immunologic, and contraceptive effects.[38,41,46]

Ramelteon

7. E.P. is concerned about using melatonin because it is not regulated by FDA and the purity and product integrity cannot be guaranteed. Her doctor gave her a prescription for ramelteon (Rozerem) 8 mg at bedtime, how does ramelteon compare with melatonin?

Ramelteon is a highly selective agonist for melatonin receptors 1 and 2 (MT 1, MT 2). Melatonin receptor 1 regulates sleepiness and MT 2 regulates phase shifts from day to night. The clinical significance of ramelteon's selectivity for MT 1 and MT 2 is not well-described.[49] Ramelteon is approved by the FDA for insomnia characterized by difficulty falling asleep. Clinical studies in primary insomnia show it decreases the time to fall asleep by 10 to 19 minutes and it increases total sleep time by 8 to 22 minutes. Its half-life ranges from 1 to 2.6 hours. Half-life of its active metabolite, M II, is 2 to 5 hours. Ramelteon undergoes hepatic metabolism by CYP1A2. Increases in serum concentration occur even with mild liver disease, so caution is recommended for patients who have at least moderate liver disease. Fluvoxamine inhibits CYP1A2, dramatically increasing the serum concentration of ramelteon, and coadministration with all potent CYP1A2 inhibitors should be avoided. The most common adverse events observed with ramelteon include headache (7%), dizziness (5%), somnolence (5%), fatigue (4%), and nausea (3%).

No evidence of cognitive impairment, rebound insomnia, withdrawal effects, or abuse potential was noted in clinical trials. Adults with a history of sedative abuse took triazolam 0.25, 0.5, 0.75 mg, and ramelteon 16, 80, 160 mg, versus placebo over 18 days. Ramelteon demonstrated no potential for abuse or motor and cognitive impairment up to 20 times the recommended therapeutic dose, whereas triazolam demonstrated potential for abuse at all doses.[50]

Ramelteon is a reasonable option for initial insomnia with no abuse potential and little to no risk of next-day impairment. In the absence of published trials comparing ramelteon with other sedative-hypnotic agents, its place in therapy is unclear.

"Z-hypnotics" (Zolpidem and Zaleplon and Eszopiclone)

8. It has been a month and E.P. continues to have difficulty falling asleep. What alternative medications (aside from triazolam and ramelteon) offer rapid onset, have low risk of daytime sedation, and can be administered safely over weeks to months if necessary?

Considering their rapid onset of action, Z-hypnotics (zaleplon, zolpidem, and eszopiclone) are all potential alternatives for E.P. They have varying degrees of selectivity for Ω-1 receptor on the benzodiazepine receptor complex. This selectivity imparts hypnotic efficacy with no significant anxiolytic, muscle relaxant, or anticonvulsant effects. Consequently, Z-hypnotics have a lower risk of abuse, withdrawal, and tolerance compared with older nonselective benzodiazepines such as triazolam and temazepam. These attributes makes Z-hypnotics more desirable for the treatment of chronic insomnia. Both zolpidem controlled-release and eszopiclone are FDA approved for chronic insomnia and are effective for up to 3 to 6 months of therapy.[51] Although the abuse potential of Z-hypnotics is less than for nonselective benzodiazepines, they are problematic in active substance abuse disorders, however. Z-hypnotics are C-IV controlled substances with more potential for abuse than ramelteon. Tolerance and withdrawal have been reported with abrupt discontinuation of zolpidem, particularly with self-escalation of dose, thus monitoring and counseling are needed.

Another potential advantage of Z-hypnotic's Ω-1 selectivity is little to no change in sleep architecture or sleep stages. Temazepam and flurazepam increase the percentage of stage 2 sleep but can suppress REM and stage 3 and 4 deep restorative sleep. In contrast, Z-hypnotics do not interfere with these sleep stages and have lower rates of uncomfortable REM rebound (vivid dreams, increased autonomic instability) on discontinuation.[51]

The Z-hypnotics differ with respect to pharmacokinetics and adverse events. Zolpidem (Ambien), the first Z-hypnotic, marketed in the United States in 1991 is absorbed rapidly, reaches peak serum levels in 1.5 hours and is eliminated rapidly with an average half-life of approximately 2.5 hours.[41] Zolpidem is metabolized by the oxidative cytochrome P450 isoenzyme CYP3A4; therefore, drug interactions should be considered when zolpidem is coadministered with CYP3A4 inhibitors such as diltiazem or fluoxetine. Zolpidem has no active metabolites and it has a low risk of residual daytime sedation in recommended doses.[51,52] It should be taken on an empty stomach for faster absorption. The usual adult dose of zolpidem is 10 mg at bedtime; elderly or patients such as E.P., who expresses concern that a medicine may be too strong, should begin with 5 mg at bedtime. Zolpidem controlled release (CR) has no clear advantage over zolpidem, except that it may provide a slightly longer duration of sleep. Serum concentrations peak in 2 hours compared with 1.5 hours for immediate release zolpidem with an associated longer latency to effect.[42]

Zaleplon (Sonata) offers a shorter elimination half-life (1.1 hour) and duration of effect than zolpidem. It is least likely of all hypnotic agents to cause residual daytime sedation and has the least effect on memory and psychomotor performance. An assessment of psychomotor performance, arousal, memory, and cognitive functioning with zaleplon revealed no cognitive impairment.[51] The most common adverse effects with zaleplon include dizziness, headache, and somnolence. In dose escalation studies using up to 60 mg, symptoms appear at approximately 30 minutes after dosing, peak at 1 to 2 hours, and are no longer evident after 4 hours. It can be taken in the middle of the night as long as the individual has 4 hours left in bed (Table 77-4).[41] Zaleplon is metabolized primarily via aldehyde oxidase, and CYP3A4 is a secondary route of metabolism, and there are no active metabolites; it has less potential for drug or food interactions compared with zolpidem or eszopiclone.[41]

Eszopiclone (Lunesta) maintains efficacy with no evidence of tolerance after 6 months of continuous use, resulting in an FDA approval for long-term use.[53] Hypnotic efficacy has been demonstrated for up to 6 months in younger patients taking 2 to 3 mg nightly, and in elderly patients taking 1 to 2 mg nightly, although only the higher range of doses significantly improved sleep maintenance. As with zolpidem and zaleplon, eszopiclone has a rapid onset of effect, but differs in that it has a longer duration of effect (Table 77-4). Time of maximum concentration (T_{max}) is delayed up to 1 hour when eszopiclone is administered after a high-fat meal, potentially delaying the onset of sleep.[54]

Eszopiclone has less receptor selectivity than either zaleplon or zolpidem, potentially resulting in some anxiolytic, amnestic, and anticonvulsant activity.[52] Among the three Z-drugs, eszopiclone has a dose-related unpleasant bitter taste in 16% to 33% of patients.[54] Headache and dizziness were reported more commonly with eszopiclone than placebo, and at higher doses, next day confusion and memory impairment have been reported in up to 3% of patients.[51,54] Eszopiclone is primarily metabolized by CYP3A4, so drugs that induce or inhibit this isoenzyme can have an impact on metabolism and a clinical effect.[54]

E.P. needs a medication that will hasten sleep onset, but does not need continued drug effect later in the night. Both zolpidem and zaleplon are useful alternatives for E.P. because of their efficacy for her sleep onset difficulty. Among the Z-hypnotics, eszopiclone has the longest half-life and the greatest risk for next-day impairment.

9. **As an alternative to ramelteon, zolpidem immediate-release, 5 mg is prescribed. E.P. expresses concern over possible adverse effects owing to its labeling as a CIV controlled substance and the recent FDA warning of complex sleep behaviors such as night eating and night driving. How should E.P.'s concerns be addressed?**

Patient counseling is most effective when it is interactive with both patient and practitioner actively listening to each other while exchanging information. It is best to begin by emphasizing the benefits of zolpidem to improve her sleep and daytime functioning. Next, E.P. should be reassured that zolpidem is generally well-tolerated and she will be prescribed the lowest dose to minimize the likelihood of adverse effects. Counseling should include a discussion of common and potentially serious adverse effects along with management strategies. Common possible adverse effects include headache (28.4%), drowsiness (26.2%), fatigue (16.6%), and dizziness (14.0%).[51] Gastrointestinal side effects occurred in 1.7% of patients; this side effect is more common with Z-hypnotics compared with nonselective benzodiazepines. Confusion, disorientation, obsessive ideas, delirium, and psychosis occurred at a rate of 1% in postmarketing surveillance studies. Hallucinations, mostly visual, are more common in elderly patients, or in those taking high doses or patients with impaired metabolism of zolpidem.[21] E.P. should be encouraged to report both effectiveness and all adverse effects to her clinician. Alcohol may be ingested 3 to 4 hours before taking zolpidem but they should not be taken together because it may cause excessive side effects and interfere with E.P.'s sleep.

To address E.P.'s concern about the FDA's hypnotic warning, a reasonable response would be, "rarely, individuals taking sleeping medication have been reported to be making phone calls, eating, having sex, or driving while half asleep. The risk for these potentially dangerous reactions increases if consumers take a higher than recommended dose, or drink alcohol or mix hypnotics with other sedating medications."[16] Another rare allergic reaction is facial swelling (angioedema). All manufacturers of hypnotic medication are required to include this information in their package inserts.[16]

IN A MEDICALLY ILL PATIENT

Insomnia and Effect on Sleep Stages

10. **A.T., a 42-year-old woman with a 5-year history of hypothyroidism and a 2-year history of hypertension and chronic lower back pain, was just transferred from the intensive care unit (ICU) into a medical unit. Her cardiac status is considered "stable" 2 days after a myocardial infarction (MI). She is 5 feet 9 inches tall and weighs 72 kg. She is receiving aspirin (enteric-coated), levothyroxine, and felodipine. Her main complaint is insomnia, including difficulty falling asleep, difficulty maintaining sleep, and early-morning awakenings. A.T. reports insomnia for 6 weeks before admission, which only worsened during the hospitalization. What type of insomnia does A.T. have and how might the insomnia affect her?**

A.T.'s insomnia is considered chronic because she experienced it for 6 weeks before hospital admission. It is severe because it involves difficulty falling asleep, maintaining sleep, and early-morning awakening. Careful monitoring and effective treatment of A.T.'s sleep disturbance is crucial; studies show disrupted sleep can increase the risk of another adverse cardiac event owing to worsening autonomic instability and poor perfusion to the myocardium.[2]

Because normal sleep moves through all the stages of NREM and REM in a continuous cycle, a patient deprived of continuous sleep may not receive sufficient time in each sleep stage. When stage 2 is diminished, muscles have insufficient opportunity to rest and rejuvenate. If NREM stages 3 and 4 are eliminated, immune function and the healing process can be disrupted. If REM sleep is deprived or excessive, neurotransmitter function may be altered and physiologic homeostatic processes can be disrupted.[6,13,25]

Drug or Disease Etiologies

11. **What individual drug or disease state factors should be assessed in A.T. before developing a treatment plan?**

Numerous medical disorders and primary sleep disorders are associated with difficulty falling asleep and maintaining sleep (Table 77-5 and Table 77-6).[2,6] First, A.T.'s pain management should be assessed for optimal efficacy. Acute post-MI pain adds to A.T.'s chronic lower back pain. Of patients with lower back pain, 50% experience chronic poor sleep patterns.[27,38] Second, A.T. was just transferred out of the ICU. Sleep deprivation in an ICU is common and is attributed to the continuous lighting, noise, and constant interventions. Sleep deprivation may prolong or worsen a disease process through diminished natural killer cell activity and decreased stages 3 and 4 of NREM sleep (when healing occurs).[6,13,41] Medications also may be contributing to A.T.'s insomnia (Table 77-5). Levothyroxine can overstimulate the CNS if given in excessive doses.[55] A.T.'s thyroid status should be re-evaluated to ensure appropriateness of the thyroid dose, especially considering her post-MI status. Calcium channel blockers have been associated with occasional sleep disturbances; therefore, felodipine should be evaluated as a potential contributing factor.[55]

Another clue to a possible cause of A.T.'s sleep problem is her description of early-morning awakening, which could be related to hospital activity during these hours or to the presence of a major depressive disorder. A.T. requires psychiatric evaluation to rule out depression, which occurs in 33% to 88% of patients after an MI.[28] In general, patients with chronic illnesses are at increased risk of developing major depression, which typically presents with insomnia or hypersomnia. Interestingly, medical outcome studies of other chronic illnesses (cardiovascular, pulmonary, renal, neurologic disease) show a high prevalence of sleep disturbance even in those not suffering from depression.[2,7] Chronic insomnia related to multiple causes can be resistant to treatment; however, treatment of underlying causes increases the likelihood of insomnia resolution.

Table 77-5 Potential Causes and Contributing Factors for Each Chronic Sleep Complaint

Difficulty Falling Asleep
Learned or conditioned activation (primary insomnia); restless legs syndrome (RLS)
Medications: methylphenidate, modafinil, fluoxetine, bupropion, steroid, β-blocker
Substances: caffeine, guarana, alcohol
Psychiatric disorders: schizophrenia, depression, anxiety disorder, bipolar disorder
Medical disorder: chronic pain, neuropathy, gastrointestinal disorder, cardiopulmonary disorders (particularly if in recumbent position).
Difficulty Maintaining Sleep
Excessive time in bed
Psychiatric disorder: major depression, anxiety or bipolar disorder, substance abuse
Sleep disordered breathing: sleep apnea, acute respiratory distress syndrome
Cardiac disease: atrial fibrillation, heart failure, angina
Neurologic disorder: dementia, Parkinson disease, multiple sclerosis
Early Morning Awakening
Major depression
Advanced sleep phase syndrome; learned or conditioned activation (primary insomnia)
Forced to get up because of family or work obligations
Excessive Daytime Sleepiness
Medications: clonidine, antihistamines, antipsychotic, antidepressant, benzodiazepine, chloral hydrate, opioid, anticonvulsant, α_1-adrenergic blockers
Obstructive sleep apnea, central sleep apnea, narcolepsy
Chronic sleep deprivation

Based on Table 1 from reference 13.

Comparing Available Hypnotics

12. A.T.'s pain is now under control, her levothyroxine dose is appropriate, and felodipine-induced sleep disturbance, sleep-disordered breathing, RLS, and PLMS have all been ruled out. A psychiatric evaluation finds that A.T. does not have major depression, but she is anxious about "life after a heart attack." She meets criteria for primary insomnia and adjustment disorder with anxiety. She continues to have trouble falling asleep and staying asleep. She will be discharged in 2 days. The pain management team suggests an adjunctive medication with anxiolytic properties that may also help with sleep. Which hypnotic is best for A.T., considering her individual clinical characteristics?

The ideal hypnotic for A.T. should act quickly and continue working throughout the night to provide her with uninterrupted sleep. A hypnotic that is not metabolized in the liver would have a lower potential for drug interactions and lessen the opportunity for systemic accumulation. If daytime drug concentrations are needed to calm anxiety, however, a hypnotic with slowly eliminated active metabolites may be desirable. The comparable doses of the hypnotic medications are listed in Table 77-7. When considering available hypnotic medications, differences

Table 77-6 Potential Causes of Chronic Sleep Disorders[25–69,70]

Psychiatric Disorders	
Anxiety disorders	Depressive disorders
Bipolar disorder	Psychotic disorders
Personality disorders	Somatoform disorders
Organic mental disorders	Substance abuse
Medical and Neurologic Disorders	
Angina pectoris	Dementia
Bronchitis	Peptic ulcer disease
Chronic fatigue	Hyperthyroidism and hypothyroidism
Cystic fibrosis	Asthma
Huntington disease	COAD
Parkinson disease	Epilepsy
Hypertension	Gastroesophageal reflux
Arthritis	Renal insufficiency
Cardiac disease	Connective tissue disease
Chronic pain	
Cancer	
Sleep Disorders	
RLS	Sleep apnea (obstructive or central)
PLMS (nocturnal myoclonus)	Primary snoring
Circadian rhythm sleep disorder (jet lag, shift work, delayed sleep phase)	Narcolepsy
Drugs Associated with Sleep Disturbance	
Insomnia	Hypersomnia
Alcohol	Alcohol
Bupropion	Benzodiazepines
Fluoxetine	Antihypertensives
Sertraline	Clonidine
MAO inhibitors	α-Adrenergic blockers
TCA	ACE inhibitors
Thyroid supplements	β-Blockers
Calcium channel blockers	Anticonvulsants
Decongestants	Analgesics
Appetite suppressants	Chloral hydrate
Theophylline	Antipsychotics
Corticosteroids	Antihistamines
Dopamine agonists	Opioids

ACE, angiotensin-converting enzyme; COAD, chronic obstructive airway disease; MAO, monoamine oxidase; PLMS, periodic limb movements during sleep; RLS, restless legs syndrome; TCA, tricyclic antidepressants.

Table 77-7 Hypnotic Dosing Comparison

Drug	Dose (mg)	Range (mg)
Midazolam (Versed)	15	10–30
Zaleplon (Sonata)	10	5–10
Zolpidem (Ambien)	10	5–10
Zolpidem ER (Ambien CR)	12.5	6.25–12.5
Triazolam (Halcion)	0.25	0.125–0.25
Temazepam (Restoril)	15	7.5–30
Flurazepam (Dalmane)	15	15–30

in pharmacodynamic and pharmacokinetic properties should be considered (Table 77-4).

A nonselective benzodiazepine hypnotic is preferable in A.T. because of the need for anxiolytic properties in addition to hypnotic efficacy. Z-hypnotics are not effective anxiolytic agents. Onset of effect is related to lipophilicity, receptor binding affinity, and T_{max}.[41,42]

The pharmacodynamic and pharmacokinetic properties of triazolam (Halcion) have already been presented. Its rapid onset is an advantage for A.T.; however, the duration of action would not be sufficient to help A.T. stay asleep. In addition, it should not be used for >7 to 10 days because of the greater potential for adverse effects with prolonged use and the possibility of significant rebound insomnia on withdrawal.[41] A.T. may require a hypnotic for >7 to 10 days, which is the maximal duration for triazolam use.

Flurazepam (Dalmane) induces sleep within 15 to 45 minutes during chronic dosing. On the first night of use, however, flurazepam does not induce sleep as well as triazolam. It has intermediate fat solubility but depends on plasma concentrations of its metabolite, desalkylflurazepam, for most of its activity.[41] Desalkylflurazepam concentrations take approximately 24 hours to accumulate and induce sleep. Studies show flurazepam maintains efficacy in sleep induction for at least 30 days; desalkylflurazepam has weak receptor binding affinity and a long half-life, resulting in gradual elimination and little chance for rebound insomnia.[41] Desalkylflurazepam can accumulate during chronic dosing and affect daytime cognition in some patients or compete for hepatic metabolism, resulting in altered levels of other hepatically metabolized medications.[41,56] Accumulation and daytime sedation can be therapeutic for some patients with daytime anxiety. A.T. has difficulty moving around during the day because of her chronic lower back pain, and oversedation from accumulation may impair her daytime functioning. Although flurazepam is a viable alternative, it is useful to explore other options.

Temazepam (Restoril) takes 1 to 2 hours to induce sleep. It has moderate fat solubility, similar to desalkylflurazepam, but it has a longer dissolution time. Temazepam takes 1.5 to 2 hours to reach peak plasma concentrations. Temazepam's longer dissolution time is caused by its large drug particle size in a gelatin capsule. The European product formulation, consisting of a solution in a wax matrix, induces sleep in 30 minutes.[41,56] A potential advantage for using temazepam in A.T.'s case is its lack of hepatic oxidative metabolism and intermediate duration of action of 8 to 12 hours. It does not interfere with the metabolism of other hepatically metabolized drugs and it does not accumulate, minimizing the potential for daytime impairment.[35,41] The long onset of action may be of concern, although A.T. could take the drug an hour before bedtime to optimize timing for sleep.

For A.T., the most appropriate choice is temazepam. Temazepam's advantages are intermediate duration of activity that would keep her asleep throughout the night, and low risk of daytime impairment owing to no known active metabolites.[35,41]

Dependence and Tolerance

13. On further discussion with A.T., who prefers to try cognitive-behavioral interventions for anxiety reduction and sleep induction, temazepam 15 mg at bedtime is prescribed on an as-needed basis. A.T. will be monitored regularly as an outpatient for efficacy and tolerability. As A.T. is preparing to leave the hospital, her daughter, B.T., expresses concerns about the potential for physical dependence on temazepam and the risk of A.T. becoming an addict. How would you respond to her concerns?

Fear of dependence and addiction to medications is a concern among the general public. Television station "medical experts" and popular magazine "health sections," while providing information, may increase the potential for confusion, erroneous impressions, and misinformation. For health care practitioners, it becomes even more crucial to provide sound drug information in common, easy-to-understand terms.

An example of the practitioner's response may be, "I'm glad you have expressed a concern; it gives us a chance to discuss temazepam therapy before your mother leaves the hospital. Temazepam has been prescribed for a medical reason, to improve your mother's sleep and to aid in her healing process. One therapeutic benefit of temazepam is an 8-hour duration of effect. Your mother will be able to sleep throughout the night so that she is well rested during the day. It also may decrease her anxiety over not sleeping, and that puts less stress on her heart.

"The possible side effects of temazepam include sedation, unsteadiness, and dizziness. She should let her doctor know if she experiences any adverse effects. Right now, it is unclear how long your mother will be taking temazepam. Duration of therapy needs to be assessed on an ongoing basis. If your mother takes temazepam every night for more than 4 weeks, two things could happen: (a) she may develop a tolerance and it may not help her sleep anymore, or (b) her system may develop a dependence in which she may have worse insomnia if she does not take it. These two scenarios do not always occur and are not likely because your mother will be taking it on an as-needed basis. If one or the other does happen, some other intervention may be tried to help with her sleep, or the temazepam dose can be gradually decreased to prevent withdrawal problems. It is important to advise your mother to take the medication only as directed (no more or less), avoid alcohol, and report any decrease in effectiveness or any adverse effects to her health care practitioner. Your mother, without a history of substance abuse, is not likely to become an addict. Although dependence is something to pay attention to, it is not the same as addiction and what matters is the functional ability of your mother while on and off the medication."

Epidemiologic data indicate that benzodiazepines are widely used primarily for brief periods of time, but less commonly used on a long-term basis. Dependence can occur after continued use over 2 to 4 months.[36] Daily users for >1 year tend to be older, medically ill, and chronically dysphoric and have panic disorder or chronic insomnia. Most chronic use appears to be medically appropriate and does not lead to dose escalation or abuse. Among chronic dysphoric patients, the indications are less clear, and dose escalation is noted sometimes without notable therapeutic benefit. Benzodiazepine hypnotics rarely are taken alone for pleasure, and generally are not likely to be abused. Among substance abusers, however, they frequently are taken as part of a polysubstance abuse pattern by alcoholics and narcotic, methadone, and cocaine users. In these groups, abuse is highly prevalent. Benzodiazepines are used to augment euphoria (narcotics and methadone users), to decrease anxiety and withdrawal symptoms (alcoholics), and to ease the "crash" from stimulant-induced euphoria (cocaine users).[37]

Physiologic dependence on benzodiazepines, resulting in a withdrawal and abstinence syndrome, develops usually after 2 to 4 months of daily use of the longer half-life benzodiazepines. Shorter half-life benzodiazepine use can result in physiologic dependence earlier (days to weeks) and may be associated with more withdrawal problems.[41,45] See Table 77-4 for a comparison of pharmacokinetic properties of hypnotics.

IN PSYCHIATRIC DISORDERS

Stepwise Approach to Selecting a Hypnotic

14. P.H., a 35-year-old man, is hospitalized after a suicide attempt with an amphetamine and alcohol overdose 1 week ago. Before the overdose attempt, P.H. had been clean (i.e., abstinent) and sober for 2 years. He is diagnosed with major depression and organic mood disorder secondary to psychoactive substance abuse. His target symptoms include a 20-pound weight loss, low energy, social withdrawal, depressed mood, hopelessness, inability to experience pleasure, trouble falling asleep, and early-morning awakening. His medications include fluoxetine (Prozac), 20 mg daily; lansoprazole (Prevacid), 30 mg daily; and a multivitamin daily—all started 5 days ago. After completing an interview with P.H., you learn that he was doing well until 2 months ago when his significant other left him and he became increasingly depressed. He began to attend Alcoholics Anonymous groups more regularly, but his depression worsened. Two weeks before admission, he went on a drinking binge that led to the suicide attempt. P.H. reports feeling restless and sleeping only 3 to 4 hours a night. Use Table 77-8 to compare the clinically significant differences between available hypnotics and to demonstrate how such information can be used to develop patient-specific treatment plans. What is the best approach to solving P.H.'s sleep problem?

The stepwise approach for selecting a hypnotic outlined in Table 77-8 serves as a useful guide for applying the information to an individual patient. Once the type of insomnia is known (difficulty falling asleep, difficulty maintaining sleep, early-morning awakening), possible causes or contributing factors must be identified and treated. Cognitive-behavioral interventions can be implemented if P.H. is willing and able to participate. At step 3, if significant insomnia persists and CBT is not feasible, a medication can be considered.

Step 4 lists factors to consider in the drug selection process. For example, agents with long-acting metabolites (e.g., flurazepam,) may accumulate or cause daytime hangover. Therefore, it is best to avoid flurazepam in the elderly. If the hypnotic has no hepatic metabolism, it will not be subject to drug interactions with other agents that are hepatically metabolized. If insomnia is chronic and resistant to hypnotic treatment, or if a low abuse potential agent is desired (e.g., person with existing addictive disorder), trazodone or another sedating antidepressant may be selected.

Sleep Disturbance of Depression

15. What type of insomnia does P.H. have and how is it different from other types of insomnia?

P.H. has trouble falling asleep and early-morning awakening, and sleep time has decreased to 3 or 4 hours a night. He is diagnosed with major depression, and sleep difficulty is part of the disorder. Generally, initial insomnia and early-morning wakening are associated with depression, although difficulty maintaining sleep and next-day fatigue are common as well. P.H. is most bothered by trouble falling asleep, early-morning awakening and next-day fatigue.

The insomnia of depression probably is related to a dysregulation of neurotransmitters, such as serotonin, norepinephrine and dopamine, in addition to dysregulation of the hypothalamic-pituitary axis. All are involved in regulating mood and the sleep–wake cycle.[6,13] Neurotransmitter activity is modified by the effects of antidepressants on REM sleep. Most effective antidepressants (excluding trazodone, and bupropion) suppress REM, causing increased REM latency and decreased total REM time.[32,57] Indeed, REM sleep deprivation can elevate mood.[57,58] Depressed patients deliberately deprived of REM sleep have had a reduction in depressive symptoms. In addition to effects on REM, antidepressants redistribute slow-wave sleep to more physiologically natural patterns, with increased intensity in the first half of the night.[58] Sedating antidepressants with serotonin 2 (5HT-2) antagonist properties, such as trazodone and mirtazapine, alleviate insomnia and improve sleep architecture.[32]

Causes: Psychiatric and Substance Abuse

16. What other factors may be contributing to insomnia in P.H.? How can his sleep problem be solved?

P.H. has been prescribed fluoxetine to treat his depression. Fluoxetine can cause insomnia in 10% to 40% of patients and thus should be dosed in the morning. P.H. also was using alcohol and stimulants before admission. Drug withdrawal and the lingering "abstinence syndromes" often are associated with insomnia, although sometimes hypersomnia is the predominant symptom.[36,59]

Treatment

The treatment for P.H.'s insomnia should begin with patient education. P.H. should be informed that >90% of depressed patients have some sleep disturbance, either too little or too much, and his sleep should improve as depressive symptoms improve (over 2–8 weeks). Counseling on cognitive-behavioral interventions to improve sleep may be appropriate when P.H.'s depression begins to clear and he is more motivated to improve his sleep hygiene. In the meantime, the potential contribution of fluoxetine to his restlessness or insomnia should be assessed by confirming that the drug is being dosed in the early morning to minimize this effect. An alternate, less activating selective serotonin reuptake inhibitors (SSRI) such as sertraline, citalopram, paroxetine, or a sedating antidepressant such as mirtazapine may be preferred unless P.H.'s history includes a positive response with fluoxetine that would justify ongoing treatment.

Hypnotics

All antidepressants, including SSRI, such as fluoxetine, can improve sleep as the depression lifts; however, fluoxetine, bupropion, and monoamine oxidase inhibitors can all cause

Table 77-8 Stepwise Approach to Selecting a Hypnotic for Insomnia

Step 1. Determine type of insomnia: DFA, DMS, EMA; duration.
Step 2. Consider possible causes: medical, psychiatric, drug; treat causes.
Step 3. CBT and sleep hygiene ineffective or only partially effective; significant insomnia persists.
Step 4. Assess type of patient: age, size, diagnosis, organ function, drug interactions, abuse potential.

	Type of Insomnia		
Treatment Options	**DFA**	**DMS**	**EMA**
Antidepressants	Duration of therapy: Chronic use in depressive diagnosis Onset and duration of effects: Intermediate to long onset Pharmacokinetic considerations: See individual antidepressant Clinical considerations: Substance abuse; treatment-resistant insomnia		Duration of therapy: Chronic use in depressive diagnosis Onset and duration of effects: Intermediate to long onset Pharmacokinetic considerations: See individual antidepressant Clinical considerations: Substance abuse; treatment-resistant insomnia
Chloral hydrate	Duration of therapy: Short-term use, 2–7 days Onset and duration of effects: Rapid onset; intermediate duration Pharmacokinetic considerations: Major metabolite, trichloroethanol, is active Clinical considerations: GI side effects; rapid tolerance; no EEG effects; drug interactions		
		Duration of therapy: Short term and chronic Onset and duration of effects: Long onset; moderate duration Clinical considerations: Hepatic metabolism	
Flurazepam or quazpam	Duration of therapy: Short term and chronic Onset and duration of effects: Rapid onset; long duration Pharmacokinetic considerations: Active metabolite Clinical considerations: Efficacy long term	Duration of therapy: Short term and chronic Onset and duration of effects: Rapid onset; long duration Pharmacokinetic considerations: Active metabolite Clinical considerations: Efficacy long term	
Temazepam		Duration of therapy: Short term and chronic Onset and duration of effects: Long onset; moderate duration Pharmacokinetic considerations: No hepatic metabolism	
Zolpidem, zaleplon, or triazolam	Duration of therapy: Short-term use, 7–10 days for triazolam, 2–4 weeks for zaleplon and several months for zolpidem Onset and duration of effects: Rapid onset; short duration Pharmacokinetic considerations: Short half-life Clinical considerations: Rebound insomnia; CNS side effects		

CNS, central nervous system; DFA, difficulty falling asleep; DMS, difficulty maintaining sleep; EEG, electroencephalogram; EMA, early-morning awakening; GI, gastrointestinal.

insomnia as well.[55,60] Prescribing a hypnotic short term or a sedating antidepressant is recommended for depressed patients with insomnia because a good night's sleep can improve treatment adherence and daytime functioning until antidepressant effects become apparent.[2,6] A study of 545 patients with major depression and insomnia taking fluoxetine in the morning were randomized to receive either eszopiclone 3 mg or placebo for 8 weeks. Eszopiclone cotherapy resulted in improved sleep quality, faster antidepressant response, and significantly more responders and remitters at week 8 compared with placebo.[61] Unpleasant taste was the only adverse effect reported significantly more in the eszopiclone group versus the placebo group (22.7 vs. 0.7%). In separate studies, zolpidem and trazodone have demonstrated efficacy for residual insomnia in depressed patients with partial antidepressant response.[6]

Hypnotics that act at benzodiazepine receptors are not recommended for P.H. because of his drug use history. Nonselective benzodiazepines can have a euphoric effect, are cross-tolerant with alcohol, and are likely to be abused by patients with substance-abuse problems.[36,41] Abuse, dependence, and withdrawal reactions have been reported with Ω_1 selective agents Z-hypnotics (zolpidem, zaleplon, eszopiclone); therefore, neither class of drugs is appropriate for P.H.[51]

If the clinician determines that fluoxetine treatment is preferred over an alternate SSRI or mirtazapine, then trazodone may be added to alleviate insomnia.[62] The addition of trazodone to fluoxetine, bupropion, or monoamine oxidase inhibitors decreased time to sleep and increased duration of sleep but caused intolerable sedation in a few patients who received fluoxetine. Tolerance did not develop to the sedative effects of trazodone in short-term studies (<6 weeks) used adjunctively for depression; however, decreased benefit over time has been reported.[62] The 5HT-2 antagonist properties of trazodone at low dosages and its α-adrenergic blocking effects provide the rationale for its efficacy as a sedating agent.

Antidepressants

17. What is the evidence for trazodone's use in managing insomnia? What other antidepressants are used in the treatment of insomnia? Discuss the advantages and disadvantages of using sedating antidepressants for the treatment of insomnia in P.H.

Trazodone is not thought to be a highly effective antidepressant because most people cannot tolerate an effective dose (300–600 mg/day). Because of its sedating properties, trazodone has become a commonly prescribed adjunctive medication (50–200 mg/day) to induce sleep while awaiting the onset of the primary antidepressant's effect. Trazodone's half-life is approximately 6.4 hours in younger adults and 11.6 hours in the elderly. It undergoes hepatic metabolism via CYP 2D6 and 3A4, so inhibitors can increase blood levels and worsen side effects. The most common side effects of trazodone include drowsiness (29.1%), dizziness (21.9%), and dry mouth (17.7%). Cardiac arrhythmias are possible at doses >200 mg/day as is priapism, a painful prolonged erection that occurs in 1 of 1,000 to 10,000 males. Although priapism is considered, rare, it can lead to impotence if untreated, therefore P.H. should be counseled about priapism.[60,62]

In the only placebo-controlled trial of trazodone conducted in primary insomnia, investigators compared the hypnotic efficacy of trazodone and zolpidem with placebo in 306 adults (aged 21–65 years). Subjects were randomly assigned to receive trazodone 50 mg, zolpidem 10 mg, or placebo nightly for 2 weeks. Sleep parameters were assessed using a subjective sleep questionnaire that patients completed each morning and at weekly office visits. Trazodone was found as effective as zolpidem for the first week of treatment, but during the second week, only zolpidem was more effective than placebo.[62]

Tricyclic antidepressants (TCA) (e.g., amitriptyline, doxepin) were used to treat primary insomnia for years based on case reports describing efficacy in doses of 10 to 75 mg/night.[41] TCAs, however, increase the risk of cardiovascular problems and anticholinergic side effects (see Chapter 79, Mood Disorders I: Major Depressive Disorders). TCA have not been proven to be as effective and safe as benzodiazepine hypnotics or trazodone.

For P.H., TCAs raise additional safety concerns. P.H. has a history of substance abuse and prior suicide attempts. Both are risk factors for future suicide attempts. TCAs are more toxic in overdose when compared with trazodone, and there are multiple reports of TCA plasma levels increasing to toxic levels when administered in combination with fluoxetine (see Chapter 79).

Switching to mirtazapine as an antidepressant that offers more sedation is a reasonable consideration for P.H. Mirtazapine has 5HT-2 antagonist effects, which imparts sedation, and they are safer than TCAs in overdose.[32] Mirtazapine is not associated with priapism but it can cause weight gain. Paroxetine (Paxil) is another option for treating both depression and insomnia in P.H. Paroxetine relieved insomnia for 15 primary insomnia patients in a 6-week, open, flexible-dose study.[33]

IN THE ELDERLY

Patient Assessment

18. S.B., a 78-year-old woman, just moved to a skilled nursing facility from her daughter's home because her family could not take care of her. She was unable to sleep at night and paced the house. Six weeks ago, she fell and broke a hip. She had a total hip replacement and uses a walker now. S.B. takes the following medications: salsalate 750 mg BID, lorazepam 0.25 mg TID, lisinopril 10 mg daily, hydroxyzine 50 mg in the morning, and Senokot one tablet in the morning and at bedtime. Zaleplon 10 mg at bedtime has just been prescribed to treat insomnia, with the first dose to start tonight. What additional information is needed to evaluate S.B.'s sleep problem?

Thus far, it is unclear what type of insomnia S.B. has: difficulty falling asleep, difficulty staying asleep, early-morning awakening, or just overall less restful sleep. Identifying the type of insomnia helps to guide proper treatment. As discussed in previous cases, many factors can contribute to sleep problems (e.g., disease states, medications, psychosocial factors, poor sleeping habits). The usual thorough evaluation is needed to understand the etiology of S.B.'s sleep disorder, after which her medication regimen can be optimized.

19. S.B. typifies the nursing home patient, struggling with medical problems and adjusting psychologically to new life situations. On review of the progress notes in the medical record, the consultant discovers S.B.'s type of insomnia is described as difficulty falling asleep and maintaining sleep. S.B. is charted as "stable" medically, with satisfactory pain control and no dementia or major psychiatric diagnosis. The progress notes mention situational anxiety secondary to her move to the nursing home. Lorazepam (Ativan) was prescribed 3 days ago to treat the anxiety. No side

effects had been documented in the medical record, but the nursing notes describe S.B. taking 2-hour naps two to three times a day and awakening two to three times nightly to urinate. What considerations are important for the assessment and treatment of insomnia in an elderly patient such as S.B.?

Age-Related Effects on Sleep

S.B.'s age is an important consideration because sleep is qualitatively different in the elderly, despite the continued need for the same quantity of sleep. A circadian shift advance may occur in which older individuals go to bed earlier and awaken earlier.[38] Fewer cycles into slow-wave sleep and more frequent awakenings occur, which results in the experience of "lighter sleep."[63] The proportion of sleep time spent in REM does not change significantly with aging.[64] Chronic disease, depressed mood, poor perception of health, and the use of sedatives, but not age, were all associated with insomnia in one large, epidemiologic study of 6,800 individuals >65 years. Of these, 28% had insomnia at baseline, but nearly half (48%) did not report symptoms at follow-up 3 years later,[65] demonstrating that insomnia is not always persistent in the elderly. Persistent chronic medical illness (arthritis, cardiovascular disease, prostate problems) predicts persistent sleep disturbance.[2,7] Sleep-related respiratory disturbances and periodic leg movements are more common in the elderly,[1,3,12] and they contribute to insomnia and excessive daytime sedation. EDS occurs in 7% to 30% of those >65 years of age; cardiovascular disease, dementia, excessive night-time awakenings, and sedating medications are factors associated with EDS.[63,64,66] All of these causes should be ruled out as contributors to poor sleep patterns in S.B.

Elderly individuals with chronic illness or social isolation report significantly more problems with sleep than those who are actively involved (e.g., club membership, religion, work) or have a close friend.[23,64] Anxiety and depression often are associated with insomnia, and the elderly tend to be more susceptible to anxiety and depression coping with bereavement, retirement, financial security, and social and functional losses. All of the aforementioned factors contribute to poor sleep patterns.[23,64] An often overlooked problem in the elderly is an alarmingly high rate of alcohol and drug use. Alcohol ingestion is associated with more fragmented, poor-quality sleep.[59] The observation that S.B. has several chronic medical conditions and functional impairment, and has recently changed living environments all have an impact on treatment decisions.

For S.B., several studies document success with nonpharmacologic interventions to improve sleep in the elderly.[14,20,67] A controlled clinical trial in 78 older adults demonstrated that CBT emphasizing good sleep habits was more effective than temazepam in improving sleep as measured by sleep diaries. Polysomnography showed comparable efficacy between CBT and temazepam in improving sleep.[67] Of note is the observation that more than half of the patients screened and deemed eligible for the study (85/163) were excluded because of sleep apnea (40/163), medical or psychiatric conditions (17/163), or an inability to stop taking sedative-hypnotic agents (22/163). These exclusions exemplify the complex etiology of insomnia, the need for careful screening to rule out sleep apnea, and the reality of sedative-hypnotic dependence in a significant percentage of older adults.

Another study in 175 consecutive hospitalized elderly described how a nonpharmacologic sleep protocol (warm drink, massage, relaxation tapes) administered by nurses was effective for improving sleep and decreasing sedative-hypnotic use from 54% to 31% ($p < 0.002$). Back massage was useful in promoting sleep in a group of 24 critically ill men.[67,68] Light therapy administered in the evening by a visor for 30 minutes at 2,000 lux to 10 elderly women in the community improved sleep efficiency and decreased fatigue.[69] These nonpharmacologic interventions should be tried for S.B. to avoid the risk of unsteady gait and excessive daytime cognitive impairment associated with any sedating medication.

AGE-RELATED EFFECTS ON HYPNOTIC DISPOSITION

Pharmacokinetic and Pharmacodynamic Differences

Small doses elicit pronounced pharmacologic effects in the elderly, and pharmacokinetic differences greatly affect the amount of drug available at the receptor site.[35] Absorption of benzodiazepines can be decreased by diminished gastric acidity and decreased GI motility. The volume of distribution of a hypnotic drug can be affected because the elderly may have increased or decreased plasma proteins, depending on whether they have inflammatory disease or poor nutrition. Excessive fat stores can increase the volume of tissue into which lipophilic drugs redistribute.[35] Bioavailability of zolpidem and eszopiclone is increased in the elderly requiring dosage reduction.[52] Oxidative metabolism might be compromised in the elderly.[63] A significantly diminished metabolism is seen in individuals >75 years compared with those 65 to 75 years of age. In young elderly, hypnotic drugs that undergo oxidative biotransformation (e.g., flurazepam) may accumulate more as a result of competition for hepatic metabolism and a decline in renal function than to inherent changes in oxidative metabolism. Elderly patients typically are on multiple drugs competing for metabolism in the liver. Excretion of more hydrophilic active metabolites can be slowed in the elderly secondary to a well-documented, age-related decline in renal function.[52,63]

Other Drugs Used as Hypnotics

20. **What are the potential problems with S.B.'s current medication regimen, and what changes are needed to improve her sleep?**

S.B. is receiving lorazepam three times daily and hydroxyzine every morning. The hydroxyzine can exert intense, long-lasting sedation in the elderly and cause frequent daytime naps when combined with multiple daily doses of lorazepam.[48,70] One short nap during the day often is normal for elderly people and usually does not impair nocturnal sleep; however, in S.B., multiple naps during the day could prevent a restful sleep throughout the night.[23,64] Although lorazepam is not marketed as a hypnotic, it possesses sedative effects as do all benzodiazepine compounds. The elderly are particularly sensitive to cognitive impairment from benzodiazepine medications so the risk versus benefit of continued lorazepam use must be considered carefully.[23,64]

Lorazepam does not undergo oxidative hepatic metabolism and interacts only with a few drugs. It has an intermediate elimination half-life of 10 to 20 hours, which could help S.B. maintain sleep, and it has no active metabolites.[35] Because S.B. currently is taking lorazepam for anxiety, a change in her dosing schedule from 0.25 mg three times daily to 0.25 mg every morning and 0.5 mg at bedtime may be useful in shifting daytime sedation more toward bedtime to help S.B. initiate and then maintain sleep throughout the night. Zaleplon can be discontinued because no need exists for it to be combined with lorazepam. In addition, the starting dose of 10 mg is too high for an elderly individual; a 5-mg dose is more appropriate (Table 77-4). Neither zaleplon nor lorazepam may be needed at bedtime if behavioral interventions are successful. The risks of hydroxyzine (i.e., cognitive impairment caused by central anticholinergic effects and excessive daytime sedation) outweigh its potential benefits for S.B. and it should be discontinued.

Rebound Insomnia and Withdrawal Symptoms

21. An attendant at a skilled nursing facility seeks assistance for one of his patients by presenting the following problem: "L.R. really has been complaining since his sleeping medication was changed. He is agitated, irritable, sweaty, and tosses and turns all night, barely sleeping. I have even noticed some BP and pulse fluctuations. He was taking flurazepam 15 mg at bedtime for many years and approximately a week ago his new doctor replaced flurazepam with zolpidem 5 mg at bedtime. Do you think this problem could be caused by the medication change?" What is causing L.R.'s symptoms?

L.R. is experiencing symptoms of benzodiazepine withdrawal. He took flurazepam every night for years and apparently developed a physical dependence. Withdrawal reactions are more common with short half-life benzodiazepines, such as triazolam, but long half-life drugs, such as flurazepam, also can elicit withdrawal responses.[41,71] With long half-life drugs, the withdrawal symptoms typically occur 1 to 2 weeks after drug discontinuation. The lag time is caused by the slow elimination of flurazepam. Zolpidem displays cross-tolerance with benzodiazepines, including flurazepam; it could not, however, prevent the withdrawal reaction because it was given in a significantly lower relative dose. In addition, zolpidem is metabolized and eliminated rapidly.

22. What therapeutic interventions should be initiated to manage L.R.'s withdrawal symptoms and rebound insomnia?

A slow, gradual dosage reduction is tolerated better by patients than immediate benzodiazepine discontinuation. Because L.R. is experiencing withdrawal symptoms, his nightly flurazepam should be restarted. Once the withdrawal symptoms (e.g., agitation, irritability, autonomic fluctuations, insomnia) subside and L.R. is comfortable, his physician can discuss the gradual dosage reduction process with him. The gradual discontinuation of flurazepam in L.R. should begin by administering the flurazepam every other night. Subsequently, flurazepam should be administered every few nights until L.R. no longer needs the medication. The withdrawal process may require several weeks. The physical withdrawal he experienced may, however, contribute to his becoming psychologically dependent on the flurazepam. L.R. needs reassurance, and nonpharmacologic treatment approaches, such as stimulus control, sleep restriction, and CBT.[36,67]

SLEEP APNEA

Clinical Presentation

23. O.R., a 56-year-old man, presents to an ambulatory care clinic complaining of chronic fatigue, low energy, excessive snoring, and overall less restful sleep. He describes his sleep: "It feels like I'm just skimming the surface of sleep. I'm tired all day and my wife says my loud snoring and gasping to breathe keeps her awake." His symptoms have worsened over the past year and a half since early retirement. He has gained weight (5 feet 10 inches, 202 pounds, body mass index [BMI] 29) and has developed hypertension. O.R.'s current BP reading is 140/90 mm Hg. Medications include hydrochlorothiazide 25 mg in the morning and aspirin 81 mg in the morning. What are the possible causes of O.R.'s sleep disorder, and why is it important for O.R. to have his problem evaluated in a sleep laboratory?

O.R. reports diminished sleep quality, excessive snoring, gasping for air, and weight gain. Although a number of causes could be responsible for O.R.'s symptoms, one of the most serious is sleep apnea. Sleep apnea is a neurologic disorder characterized by mini-episodes of cessation of breathing, which can occur 10 to 200 times an hour. If there is a reduction in airflow but no cessation of breathing, it is called *hypopnea*. The brain responds to episodes of apnea and hypopnea with "mini-arousals," waking the individual to stimulate breathing.[4,72,73] These frequent mini-arousals prevent the individual from obtaining quality sleep by not allowing sufficient time in deep, slow-wave sleep, or REM. Obstructive sleep apnea (OSA), the most common type, may be induced when extra body weight (note O.R.'s weight gain) places pressure on the throat and uvula, narrowing the space into which air must travel; this results in the difficulty in breathing and excessive snoring. Biochemically, proinflammatory cytokines such as C-reactive protein, TNF-α, and IL-6 have been associated with the pathogenesis of EDS and sleep apnea.[11,12,74]

Hypertension may be contributing to O.R.'s sleep difficulty. Several studies show an increased risk of sleep apnea in patients with hypertension, coronary artery disease, and cerebrovascular disease.[66,75] Although sleep apnea occurs in approximately 5% of women and 15% of men in the general population, it occurs in up to 40% of patients with hypertension.[75] Treatment of OSA can improve BP control and lead to more restful sleep. Of note, OSA occurs in nonobese individuals and in all ages, including infants.[11,43,66] Sleep-disordered breathing, including snoring, is a significant risk factor for hypertension even in young individuals of normal weight.[76]

Overnight evaluation by polysomnography (i.e., EEG, EOG, EMG) in a sleep laboratory would confirm or rule out sleep apnea and allow distinction between OSA and the less common, central sleep apnea.[43,72] Patients with central sleep apnea lack respiratory effort (i.e., the diaphragm does not move in attempts to take in air); they frequently gasp for air during the night.[72] Treatment of central sleep apnea requires continuous positive airway pressure (CPAP) as opposed to being alleviated through weight loss or anatomic manipulations. Central sleep apnea frequently occurs along with OSA.

Drug Treatment Considerations

24. Results from the sleep laboratory study clearly document O.R.'s sleep problem as OSA. He experiences an average of 56 apneic episodes per hour. O.R.'s weight gain and inactivity probably contribute to the problem. Both are serious, potentially life-threatening conditions. Why should O.R.'s sleeping difficulties not be treated with a hypnotic medication?

Hypnotics, alcohol, or any CNS depressant can be lethal for patients with sleep apnea and should not be prescribed for O.R. CNS depressants interfere with the mini-arousals required to stimulate breathing once it has stopped. In this case, the sleep laboratory study may have saved O.R. from a potential life-threatening breathing disorder that could have been exacerbated by a hypnotic with CNS depressant activity.

Obstructive sleep apnea can be treated by tracheostomy, nasal surgery, tonsillectomy, uvulopalatoplasty, and either nasal or orally administered CPAP.[12,43,77] Weight loss and CPAP therapy are the most effective treatments and must be maintained for continued therapeutic efficacy.[11,72] In CPAP, the patient wears a lightweight mask to bed each night and a constant flow of air is provided mechanically to prevent breathing cessation and to allow for more restful sleep. Although CPAP is effective for both obstructive and central sleep apnea, the results are short lived and apneic episodes typically reappear when CPAP therapy is stopped. Preliminary studies in individuals with nocturnal bradycardia and sleep apnea show that insertion of a permanent cardiac pacemaker significantly improved bradycardia and sleep apnea.[78] More studies are needed. At this time, the best treatment for O.R.'s hypertension and sleep apnea is weight loss and CPAP.

25. If weight loss, surgery, and CPAP are all ineffective or impractical, what drug treatments are potentially effective for O.R.'s sleep apnea?

Modafinil, an agent approved for narcolepsy, is also FDA approved to treat excessive daytime sleepiness caused by OSA or shift work sleep disorder. For O.R., it is best used as an adjunct to CPAP at doses of 200 to 400 mg in the morning.[79,80] Protriptyline, medroxyprogesterone, theophylline, and acetazolamide have been used successfully in small numbers of patients with sleep apnea.[80] A decrease in apneic episodes is statistically significant, but not, however, clinically significant for most patients.[80] Fluoxetine and paroxetine show promise in treating sleep apnea by increasing upper-airway patency during sleep.[80,81] To date, no clinically significant improvement has been documented with either agent.

NARCOLEPSY

Narcolepsy is an incurable neurologic disorder characterized by two main features: irrepressible sleep attacks and cataplexy. Sleep attacks can intrude at any time during the individual's waking state. Cataplexy is the loss of muscle tone in the face or limb muscles and often is induced by emotions or laughter. Cataplexy can be subtle, where the patient is limp and not moving, or dramatic, whereas persons with narcolepsy collapse to the floor.[82] Hypnagogic hallucinations and sleep paralysis are other secondary symptoms not present in all persons with narcolepsy. Hypnagogic hallucinations are perceptual disturbances (i.e., auditory, visual, tactile) that occur while experiencing a sleep attack. The patient may see imaginary objects, hear sounds, or feel sensations. Sleep paralysis is a terrifying experience that can occur when falling asleep or when awakening. Patients are unable to move their limbs, to speak, or even to breathe deeply. Narcoleptics learn, however, that sleep paralysis episodes are benign and brief (lasting <10 minutes). Except for daytime sleepiness, these symptoms are thought to be expressions or partial expressions of REM sleep.[4,15]

Symptoms of narcolepsy often begin at puberty, but patients usually are not diagnosed until years later, in their late teens or early 20s. Early symptoms consist of excessive daytime sedation and poor sleep quality. The sleep cycle becomes progressively more erratic with frequent bursts of REM and decreased regularity of deep or slow-wave sleep. Polysomnography in a sleep laboratory is necessary to confirm narcolepsy. Sleep architecture is notably different. Instead of the 90-minute delay before REM, individuals with narcolepsy progress directly into REM sleep.[4]

In the 1970s, genetic research in narcoleptic dogs (Doberman pinchers) and humans, revealed narcolepsy is associated with deficits in the hypocretin receptor-2 gene (Hcrtr2).[4,29] An autoimmune response of unknown origin is thought to damage hypocretin or orexin secreting cells in the hypothalamus. Without functional hypocretin and orexin cells, the sleep-wake cycle is disrupted. Hypocretin and orexin are also involved in body weight, control of water balance and temperature.[4]

Comparing Treatments

Optimal treatment of narcolepsy involves treating both sleep attacks and cataplexy. Schedule II controlled substances, methylphenidate (Ritalin) and dextroamphetamine (Dexedrine), were the first drugs used to treat narcolepsy, with 65% to 85% of patients deriving significant improvements in wakefulness. Mixed amphetamine salts are also FDA approved for narcolepsy.[4] The mechanism of action of methylphenidate and amphetamines is related to increasing neurotransmission of dopamine and norepinephrine. Modafinil (Provigil), a schedule IV controlled substance, is an effective treatment with less abuse potential. Its exact mode of action is not fully understood, but it is thought to increase wakefulness through noradrenergic, adrenergic, histaminergic, GABA-modulating, glutamatergic, and hypocretin or orexin stimulating mechanisms.[4,79] In summary, these stimulating drugs decrease the number of sleep attacks, improve task performance, and increase the time to fall asleep, but cannot eliminate sleep attacks altogether. Research is under way exploring the possible use of immunosuppression at the time of narcolepsy onset. One hypothesis suggests that immunosuppression therapy during a period of pathologic immune response could prevent or reduce damage to the hypocretin system that otherwise would lead to the development of narcolepsy.[4,83]

Cataplexy does not respond to psychostimulants or modafinil but may be lessened with low doses of antidepressants. Tricyclic antidepressants (imipramine and clomipramine) were the first antidepressants used, but protriptyline, desipramine, and SSRI (fluoxetine, sertraline, and paroxetine) are also used.[4] SSRI and protriptyline offer the advantage of less daytime sedation, compared with tertiary TCA. The effectiveness of antidepressants for the treatment of cataplexy is thought to be related to REM-suppressant effects. A Cochrane database review concluded insufficient evidence exists to recommend antidepressants as effective treatments for cataplexy, given that most studies are small and uncontrolled. It should be recognized, however, that large-scale studies on such a rare disorder are difficult to conduct.[84] Antidepressants are not considered effective in decreasing sleep attacks.[4,83,84]

Sodium oxybate (Xyrem), a salt form of the CNS depressant-γ-hydroxybutyrate, is the only FDA-approved treatment for cataplexy. Its therapeutic effects are related to decreased REM, improved sleep consolidation, and increased stage 3 and 4, slow-wave sleep.[4,82] In two randomized, double-blind, placebo-controlled trials, sodium oxybate 9 g/night (i.e., 450 mg at bedtime, then 450 mg 2 to 4 hours later), but not 3 or 6 g/night, significantly reduced the median frequency of cataplexy attacks by 69% in patients with narcolepsy, whereas 4.5 to 9 g over 8 weeks significantly reduced the median frequency of cataplexy attacks by 57% to 85% in a dose-related manner. Both trials showed 6% to 30% reduction in excessive daytime sleepiness as measured on the Epworth Sleepiness Scale and 20% to 43% reduction in daytime sleep attacks.[82]

Improved daytime wakefulness is an advantage of sodium oxybate compared with antidepressants. Adverse effects include nausea, headache, dizziness, and enuresis. Sodium oxybate can be administered safely with stimulants; however, coadministration with other CNS depressants, including hypnotic medication, is contraindicated because of the risk of respiratory depression.[82] Individuals taking sodium oxybate should take it on an empty stomach for maximal efficacy, and it should not be given to those with sleep-disordered breathing, sleep apnea, or an alcohol or substance abuse disorder.[82] Because of a significant abuse potential, sodium oxybate is available only through restricted distribution, the Xyrem Success Program, by calling 1-866-997-3688 Orphan Medical. It is a schedule III controlled substance.[82]

Methylphenidate and Imipramine

26. G.B., a 23-year-old man with narcolepsy, is receiving methylphenidate long-acting (Ritalin LA) 60 mg every AM and imipramine 75 mg at bedtime to treat his narcolepsy and cataplexy. What are the potential risks of using both methylphenidate and imipramine to treat G.B.?

Anorexia, stomach pain, nervousness, irritability, insomnia, and headaches are common side effects of stimulant drugs.[4] Psychotic reactions can occur in narcoleptic patients taking stimulants at any dose; however, these symptoms resolve when the stimulant is discontinued. Hypertension and abnormal liver function are more serious complications of long-term stimulant use. Stimulants, even at high dosages (e.g., 80 mg methylphenidate), usually do not bring a patient to a normal level of alertness, and sometimes nocturnal sleep is disrupted. To prevent stimulant-induced insomnia, doses should be taken before 3 PM. Tolerance to the therapeutic effects of stimulants may, however, develop in some patients with narcolepsy.[4,83] Drug holidays sometimes can allow the patient to recapture therapeutic benefit; however, many patients opt for an increased stimulant dose instead. Exceeding maximal recommended doses of stimulant significantly increases the risk of psychosis, substance abuse, psychiatric hospitalization, tachyarrhythmia and anorexia according to a case-control study in 116 patients with narcolepsy taking stimulants.[85]

Imipramine, as with all TCAs, can cause orthostatic hypotension, anticholinergic side effects, sedation, cardiac conduction changes, and periodic limb movements. In addition, G.B.'s imipramine therapy will be more complex because methylphenidate can inhibit the metabolism of imipramine, resulting in higher levels of imipramine.[86] G.B. should be monitored closely during the initiation of imipramine therapy and imipramine plasma levels should be assessed to minimize side effects and prevent toxicity. The optimal therapeutic plasma concentration of imipramine for treatment of cataplexy has not been established, but low doses may be effective and the risk of toxicity from imipramine increases when serum imipramine concentrations are >300 ng/mL.

Modafinil

27. G.B. develops intolerable nervousness, irritability, and nocturnal insomnia on methylphenidate as the dose is increased to 80 mg/day in an attempt to further decrease sleep attacks. He asks about switching to modafinil (Provigil). Does modafinil offer any advantage for G.B.?

Modafinil's efficacy relative to other CNS stimulants has not been adequately assessed in controlled clinical trials; however, it has less potential for insomnia and adverse CNS reactions at recommended dosages between 200 and 400 mg/day administered in the morning.[4] It also has less abuse potential compared with stimulants and is a schedule IV controlled substance. Headache was the only adverse experience rated significantly higher than placebo in 283 patients taking the recommended dose of either 200 or 400 mg/day of modafinil. Anorexia, nervousness, restlessness, and pulse and BP changes are dose-related side effects to discuss during counseling. The maximal tolerable single daily dose may be 600 mg/day, because 800 mg/day produced increased BP and pulse in one tolerability study.[87] Gradual dosage titration improves tolerability. Armodafinil, an active stereoisomer of modafinil has a similar adverse effect profile as modafinil and is being studied for narcolepsy.[4]

28. What counseling should G.B. receive as he changes from methylphenidate to modafinil?

People taking modafinil should receive counseling regarding the potential for drug interactions. Modafinil induces CYP 3A4 metabolism primarily in the gut; decreased levels of triazolam and ethinyl estradiol have been associated with modafinil coadministration.[88] Enzyme inhibition may also occur. Modafinil's inhibition of CYP 2C19 is the proposed mechanism behind modafinil-associated clozapine toxicity.[89] Monitoring for drug interactions is more crucial because modafinil is increasingly used for other indications, including daytime sleepiness associated with Parkinson disease, fibromyalgia, sleep apnea, fatigue associated with multiple sclerosis, and ADHD.[90,91,92]

Naps and Other Behavioral Interventions

29. The benefits, possible risks, and importance of regular physician assessment have been explained to G.B., and he agrees

to report efficacy and adverse effects to his primary care provider regularly. G.B.'s last imipramine level 2 weeks ago on the lower methylphenidate dose was 115 ng/mL, and G.B. is reminded to take the medicine at regular intervals along with daytime naps. Why are naps helpful in the treatment of G.B. and what other behavioral interventions are useful in treating narcolepsy?

Strategically timed 15- to 20-minute naps taken at lunch and then again at 5:30 PM can be refreshing for narcoleptics and increase their time between sleep attacks. Narcolepsy support groups are available and may help G.B. better cope with such a life-changing chronic illness. It also is important for G.B. to avoid alcohol and to regulate his bedtime and wake-up time in the attempt to normalize his sleep habits.[4,83]

RESTLESS LEGS SYNDROME AND PERIODIC LIMB MOVEMENTS DURING SLEEP

Restless legs syndrome is a condition characterized by unpleasant leg sensations occurring at rest, worsening at night, with an irresistible urge to move. Patients use descriptors such as painful, aching, creeping, crawling, pulling, grabbing, tingling sensations relieved by movement. For some patients, RLS may also involve the arms.[3,4] Up to 15% of the population suffers from RLS while awake, and up to 85% of these also have PLMS.[3] PLMS, also known as nocturnal myoclonus, is best described as involuntary clonic-type movements of the lower extremities while sleeping that usually involve bilateral ankle dorsiflexion, knee flexion, and hip flexion. They typically last 0.5 to 5 seconds and occur every 20 to 40 seconds. Five or more movements per hour of sleep as recorded by EMG during polysomnography is considered pathologic. Depending on the severity, both RLS and PLMS contribute to insomnia and prevent restful sleep, and patients with RLS report impaired daytime functioning. Akathisia is different from RLS in that akathisia is more of a generalized urge to move which occurs throughout the day without the characteristic worsening symptoms in the evening associated with RLS.[3,4]

Restless legs syndrome and PLMS can occur at any age, but may be most common in the elderly. Sudden remissions, which may last for months or even years, are as difficult to explain as relapses, which appear without any apparent reason. Parkinson disease, hypothyroidism, uremia, chronic bronchitis, iron deficiency, folate, B_{12} deficiency, and pregnancy are all associated with symptomatic RLS. The pathophysiology of both conditions involves dopaminergic neurotransmission because decreased D_2 receptor binding in the striatum of patients with RLS and PLMS has been documented.[4]

Treatment

Nonpharmacologic management includes reduction in caffeine and alcohol intake, regular exercise, and cessation of smoking.[4] Dopaminergic agents, benzodiazepines, opioids, and selected anticonvulsants have all demonstrated efficacy for RLS and PLMS. Drug selection is based on severity of symptoms, co-occurring conditions, and tolerability.[4]

L-dopa with carbidopa was the first dopaminergic agent to demonstrate efficacy for RLS. It is seldom recommended, however, because with chronic use, L-dopa treatment was associated with RLS earlier in the night (augmentation) and rebound RLS in the middle of the night. L-dopa may be useful on an as needed basis (i.e., when going to the movies, for example). Bromocriptine 7.5 mg/night is effective but causes excessive nausea, and CNS adverse events. Pramipexole (Mirapex) and ropinirole (Requip) both stimulate D_2 and D_3 receptors; they are FDA approved for RLS and are considered first-line therapy. Studies show they are effective in alleviating RLS and increasing total sleep time for 70% to 90% of patients.[4] Ergot-derived dopaminergic agonists (pergolide and cabergoline) should be avoided for safety reasons. Pergolide was recently removed from the market because of the risk of cardiac valve regurgitation. A comparative study in patients with Parkinson showed pramipexole and ropinirole were not associated with clinically significant valvulopathies and are much safer than pergolide.[93]

Pramipexole should be initiated at 0.125 mg given 2 to 3 hours before bedtime every night. The dose can be increased every 4 to 7 days based on symptoms. The usual effective dosing range is (0.375–1.5 mg/night) Ropinirole should be initiated at 0.25 mg given 1 to 3 hours before bedtime with a dosing range between 1 and 4 mg/day. Dizziness, hypotension, nausea, daytime fatigue, and somnolence can occur with both agents; therefore, careful monitoring and counseling are needed. Pramipexole is eliminated renally; ropinirole is eliminated by hepatic metabolism via the CYP 1A2 isoenzyme. Careful dosage adjustment to control symptoms with tolerable side effects is important with dopamine agonists. Insomnia is a potential problem with all dopaminergic agents and benzodiazepines are sometimes necessary in combination to alleviate this symptom.[4]

Benzodiazepines, particularly clonazepam 0.5 to 2 mg and temazepam 7.5 to 30 mg, may be effective in relieving mild to moderate RLS. Most studies, however, have shown reduction in arousals from PLMS rather than elimination of movements. These agents should not be used if sleep apnea coexists because of respiratory depressant effects. The most common adverse effect with clonazepam is excessive daytime somnolence.[4] Agents with intermediate to long half-lives are preferred because agents with short half-lives (<5 hours) may contribute to confusional states and nocturnal wandering in patients with RLS.[94]

Opioids have been demonstrated effective; however, their use is limited because of side effects (constipation, sedation, nausea), dependence, and concern over addiction. Propoxyphene (65–130 mg) or codeine 30 mg may be useful in mild cases of RLS or PLMS for intermittent symptoms. Higher-potency agents, such as oxycodone 4.5 to 5 mg or methadone 5 to 10 mg, should be reserved for severe or resistant symptoms.[94] Opioids must be used with caution in those who have sleep apnea.[94]

Anticonvulsants are another potential treatment for RLS and PLMS without the insomnia of dopamine agonists or addiction potential of benzodiazepines or opioids. Carbamazepine 200 to 400 mg/day was found to be superior to placebo in one double-blind study and in small open trials.[4,95] Several open trials and one double-blind, placebo-controlled study found gabapentin in divided doses of 900 to 3,000 mg/day to be effective, particularly when RLS occurred with pain.[4,95]

Tramadol, a central analgesic with less abuse potential than opioids, was found effective and well tolerated in 10 of 12 patients when given over 15 to 24 months in doses of 50 to

150 mg/day.[96] Magnesium supplementation of 12.4 mmol over 4 to 6 weeks was effective in significantly improving symptoms in 7 of 10 patients with RLS or PLMS in one open trial.[97] Iron supplementation is recommended for RLS associated with iron deficiency.[4]

PEDIATRIC INSOMNIA

Typical sleep need in children varies from 12 to 14 hours in children 1 to 3 years of age to between 8.5 and 9.5 hours in adolescents.[98] All major sleep disorders can occur in youth and therefore evaluation for insomnia, RLS, PLMS, sleep apnea, and narcolepsy are needed whenever symptoms warrant. Trouble initiating and maintaining sleep are more common in children with ADHD (25%–50%) and autism spectrum disorders (44%–83%). Of infants and toddlers, 10% to 30% have bedtime sleep resistance that can be managed behaviorally with parental education. Inconsistent bedtime, falling asleep away from bed, fears, and psychiatric and medical conditions can all contribute to poor sleep in children.[98]

At least 5% to 10% of high school students have delayed sleep phase syndrome, a physiologic condition where they do not fall asleep until between 1 and 3 AM and they awaken between 9 AM and noon. School schedules dictate earlier awakening resulting in chronic sleep deprivation. Recent poll data indicate that 28% of high school students fall asleep in school at least once a week and 14% are late or miss school because of oversleeping.[98]

Behavioral interventions to promote good sleep habits (e.g., consistent bedtime and wake-time, prebedtime ritual) should be initiated during childhood and continued throughout adolescence to promote a lifetime of healthy sleep. No hypnotics are FDA approved for insomnia in children and adolescents and significant data are lacking to guide clinicians on medications to improve sleep in youth. Diphenhydramine, clonidine, melatonin, and chloral hydrate are commonly used in children and some adolescents; however, the use of Z-hypnotics is also increasing, although this class has not been well-studied in this population.[99]

30. What is the evidence for the safety and efficacy of diphenhydramine, melatonin, clonidine, chloral hydrate, and benzodiazepine-active hypnotics in children and adolescents?

Diphenhydramine is the most commonly used sedative in children according to a survey of 800 pediatricians in four states.[99] It has been shown to decrease both time to fall asleep and awakenings in children and adults. The lowest effective dose should be given to minimize anticholinergic side effects and impaired cognition.

Melatonin at an average dose of 2 mg/night administered 1 hour before bedtime was effective and well-tolerated for 29 of 32 children age 9.6 (±4.5 years) with chronic sleep initiation and sleep maintenance problems over an average of 2.1 months.[100] Melatonin 0.3 to 5 mg given 1 to 2 hours before bedtime has been effective for delayed sleep phase syndrome in adolescents.[101]

After diphenhydramine, clonidine, an α_2-adrenergic agonist, is the most prescribed medication to improve sleep in youth despite the lack of data to support its safety and effectiveness for insomnia. Mostly, it is prescribed to treat difficulty initiating sleep. Dosing is 50 to 100 mcg at bedtime.[99] Common side effects include sedation, dry mouth, constipation, dizziness, and bradycardia.[102] Rebound hypertension is possible on abrupt discontinuation of regular use of clonidine.

Chloral hydrate is the most extensively studied sedative agent in youth,[103] and several reasons exist for its widespread use: rapid onset, moderate duration, and lack of significant effects on the EEG. Chloral hydrate induces sedation and allows brain-wave assessment without drug interference.[104] The most common adverse effects of chloral hydrate are nausea, vomiting, or diarrhea, which can be minimized by giving the drug diluted or with food. Tolerance to the sedative effects develops rapidly over a 5- to 14-day period of continued use.[104] Chloral hydrate generally is void of cardiac and respiratory toxicity at its usual dose of 50 mg/kg, but it has been linked to arrhythmias and even respiratory failure in children with compromised cardiac or respiratory systems. Therefore, it should not be used (or used only with extreme caution) in patients with severe cardiac or respiratory disorders.[103,105] The tolerability of preprocedure chloral hydrate was evaluated in children with significant cardiac disease (<1 month to 5 years of age) undergoing echocardiograms. The drug was well-tolerated with only 10.8% of patients experiencing adverse effects; decreases in heart rate and blood pressure occurred but were not significant.[106]

Therapeutic effects and known potential toxicities from chloral hydrate are associated with its two active metabolites: trichloroethanol and trichloroacetic acid. A single dose of trichloroethanol, the metabolite responsible for sedation, induces sedation within 30 minutes and has a usual duration of action of 4 to 8 hours, similar to its half-life of 8 to 12 hours in adults. The half-life can be longer (9–40 hours) in children, depending on the age and maturity of the patient. Trichloroacetic acid is a minor metabolite that does not achieve significant levels in most patients after a single dose. On multiple dosing, trichloroacetic acid can displace bilirubin or warfarin from albumin binding sites, potentially resulting in hyperbilirubinemia or hypoprothrombinemia.[101,105,107] The half-life of trichloroacetic acid is much longer (2–6 days), and this metabolite can accumulate under multiple dosing conditions.

Midazolam oral syrup (0.6 mg/kg dose of a 2 mg/mL solution) is used as a premedication for children undergoing brief procedures (e.g., dental). Premedication dosing of midazolam in children is generally recommended at 0.25 to 0.5 mg/kg. Metabolism occurs via CYP3A4 isoenzyme with a half-life of 2.9 to 4.5 hours. Although more studies are needed, midazolam represents an alternative to chloral hydrate with fewer GI side effects, less potential for accumulation, and lower risk of cardiotoxicity.[56,108] Temazepam has also been used as a premedicant in children, but the long onset of effect requires dosing 1 to 2 hours before procedures.[109] Clonazepam 0.25 to 0.5 mg at bedtime has a long half-life of 30 to 40 hours and has been used to prevent sleep terrors or sleep walking in children.[101]

Z-hypnotics are increasingly prescribed in youth despite a lack of data. Both zaleplon and zolpidem have been used to treat initial insomnia in older children and adolescents and delayed sleep phase syndrome in adolescents. Studies show zolpidem clearance is three times greater in children compared with young adults; therefore, usual dosing of 10 mg is recommended in children who are able to swallow tablets or capsules. Using lower doses may result in lack of effectiveness or parasomnias including hypnagogic hallucinations.[101]

When considering the best sedative for a child, it is useful to compare the advantages and disadvantages of available agents. Barbiturates (e.g., phenobarbital, pentobarbital) are sedating, but can have a higher incidence of cardiac, respiratory, and CNS depression than chloral hydrate or benzodiazepine-active agents.[103] Benzodiazepines have not been studied systematically in children, but there are some reports of paradoxic excitatory reactions, psychomotor impairment, and excessive sedation in young age groups.[109] Respiratory depression and altered EEG patterns can occur secondary to benzodiazepine therapy. An analysis of adverse sedation events in pediatric patients found that 60 of 95 cases resulted in death or permanent neurologic injury. Negative outcomes were associated with drug overdose, the use of multiple sedating medications, drug interactions, prescription or transcription errors, or inadequate monitoring and resuscitation of children undergoing sedation. Among chloral hydrate, barbiturates, ketamine, or benzodiazepines, no evidence indicates that one drug or route of administration was associated with greater toxicity.[103] Any sedative should be used for the shortest period of time possible, with careful monitoring of respiratory, cardiac, and CNS functions, particularly in very young children.

FORMULARY MANAGEMENT OF HYPNOTICS

31. Balancing high-quality care with economic common sense is the responsibility of formulary managers in all health care organizations. The Pharmacy and Therapeutics Committee has decided that four hypnotics should be designated as first-line agents to promote the safe and effective treatment of insomnia. Other agents will require special permission for use. What factors should be involved in the selection of four first-line hypnotics?

Therapeutic efficacy, versatility, and patient tolerability should be foremost in identifying priority hypnotics for a health care system's core formulary. Adverse-effect profiles should be known and manageable. Another important factor is cost, which should be measured both directly (drug cost, frequency of health care utilization) and indirectly (functional ability, productivity and quality of life).[110] When balancing the clinical therapeutics against the economic realities of the available hypnotics, five factors should be considered: onset, duration of effect, metabolism, tolerability, and cost (see Table 77-4 to review pharmacokinetic profiles).

A hypnotic with a rapid onset and short duration with no accumulation of active metabolites is best for patients who only have difficulty falling asleep and who want no risk of next-day impairment. Zaleplon (Sonata), triazolam (Halcion), and ramelteon (Rozerem) best fit this clinical profile. Compared with triazolam, zaleplon has fewer adverse reactions on discontinuation, does not affect sleep stages, and may be used for several weeks if needed. In contrast, triazolam is limited to 7 to 10 days of continuous use. Zaleplon's advantages warrant formulary status whereas triazolam does not.

Ramelteon is the only FDA-approved hypnotic without abuse potential owing to its lack of activity at the benzodiazepine receptor complex. It acts by stimulating melatonin receptors. It is rapid acting with a short duration of action and no risk of next-day impairment in its recommended 8-mg dose. Although ramelteon has not been established as effective as benzodiazepine hypnotics, it should be included on the formulary because it has the clear advantage of no abuse potential. It is more effective at initiating sleep compared with placebo, and it is well-tolerated over 4 to 5 weeks; long-term studies are underway. It is a good option for those with trouble falling asleep who request a medication with no abuse potential.

Zolpidem and eszopiclone both have a rapid onset but there is a risk of next-day impairment. A 10-mg dose of zaleplon is free of residual hypnotic or sedative effects when administered as little as 2 hours before waking in normal subjects, whereas residual effects are still present up to 5 hours after a 10-mg zolpidem dose.[19] Residual effects with eszopiclone would likely be longer than zolpidem because of its longer half-life.[41] Eszopiclone offers a little longer duration of effect compared with zolpidem, but it causes more unpleasant taste, limiting patient acceptability. Zolpidem controlled release may allow for somewhat longer sleep duration compared with immediate release zolpidem, but no comparative trials have shown a distinct clinical advantage. Availability of zolpidem immediate-release generic lowers drug cost as well. For these reasons, immediate release zolpidem merits formulary status over zolpidem extended release and eszopiclone.

Temazepam (Restoril) has a long onset of action (1–2 hours) and intermediate duration (8–10 hours) of action. Temazepam offers several advantages with regard to liver metabolism. It is not oxidized in the liver and does not compete for metabolism with other hepatically metabolized drugs nor accumulate with chronic use. In addition, temazepam has been studied in both young age groups as a premedication and in older age groups as a hypnotic. Unlike Z-hypnotics, it has anxiolytic activity as well. When dosed 1 to 2 hours before bedtime, it is useful in initiating and maintaining sleep. It is an inexpensive and versatile hypnotic meriting formulary status.

Flurazepam (Dalmane) is hepatically metabolized with long-acting active metabolites. It is able to keep the patient asleep throughout the night and provide residual daytime sedation if needed for agitation or anxiety. It maintains hypnotic efficacy over at least 30 days of continuous use. Flurazepam's disadvantage includes the highest risk of next-day cognitive impairment. It does not deserve formulary status.

Chloral hydrate has a rapid onset and short-to-intermediate duration of action with no daytime hangover in patients with good hepatic function. Chloral hydrate has clinical usefulness in all age groups and, unlike other hypnotics, it is available in liquid, capsule, and suppository form, and is inexpensive. Chloral hydrate has been studied in all age groups. Disadvantages, including GI irritation, protein-binding interactions, and lack of usefulness for short-term or chronic insomnia, make it a poor choice for formulary status.

In consideration of the available clinical and cost data, zaleplon, zolpidem, temazepam, and ramelteon should be considered priority hypnotics. Zaleplon initiates sleep with the least risk of daytime hangover and can even be dosed during the night. Zolpidem initiates sleep effectively and maintains sleep longer than zaleplon for those with midnocturnal awakenings. Temazepam has a sufficient duration of action to benefit those with intolerable midnocturnal awakenings and it has an anxiolytic effect that is beneficial for many patients. Ramelteon has a rapid onset, no next-day impairment and no abuse potential.

All have been demonstrated effective and safe in the elderly. If insomnia is effectively treated with proper use of medications and nonpharmacologic interventions, costs may be decreased through decreased health care utilization, reduced work absenteeism, and improved quality of life.[5,41,110] A review of any formulary decision should be conducted every 6 months to determine whether these selections need to be changed based on therapeutic outcome data.

REFERENCES

1. Gooneratne NS et al. Consequences of comorbid insomnia symptoms and sleep disordered breathing disorder in elderly subjects. *Arch Intern Med* 2006;166:1732.
2. Ancoli-Israel S. The impact and prevalence of chronic insomnia and other sleep disturbances associated with chronic illness. *Am J Managed Care* 2006;12:S221.
3. Kushida CA. Clinical presentation, diagnosis and quality of life issues in RLS. *Am J Med* 2007;120:S4.
4. Erman MK. Selected sleep disorders: RLS, PLMD, sleep apnea, narcolepsy. *Psychiatr Clin North Am* 2006;947.
5. NIH State-of-the-Science Conference Statement on Manifestations and Management of Chronic Insomnia in Adults. *NIH Consens Sci Statements* 2005;22:130.
6. Krystal AD. Sleep and psychiatric disorders: future directions. *Psychiatr Clin North Am* 2006; 1115.
7. Taylor DJ et al. Comorbidity of chronic insomnia with medical problems. *Sleep* 2007;30:213.
8. Engleman HM et al. Sleep, driving and the workplace. *Clin Med* 2005;5:113.
9. Millman RP. Excessive sleepiness in adolescents and young adults: causes, consequences, and treatment strategies. *Pediatrics* 2005;115:1774.
10. Lockley SW. When policy meets physiology: the challenge of reducing resident work hours. *Clin Orthop* 2006;449:116.
11. George CFP. Screening and case finding. In: Kushida CA, ed. *Obstructive Sleep Apnea: Diagnosis and Treatment.* New York: Informa Healthcare USA; 2007:21.
12. Fiorentino L et al. Obstructive sleep apnea in the elderly. In: Kushida CA, ed. *Obstructive Sleep Apnea: Diagnosis and Treatment.* New York: Informa Healthcare USA; 2007:281.
13. Becker PM. Insomnia: prevalence, impact, pathogenesis, differential diagnosis and evaluation. *Psychiatr Clin North Am* 2006;29:855.
14. Morgenthaler T et al. Practice parameter for the psychological and behavioral treatment of insomnia: an update. *Sleep* 2006;29:1415.
15. Mason TBA et al. Pediatric Parasomnias. *Sleep* 2007;30:141.
16. FDA strengthens hypnotic warning. www.cder.fda.gov. Accessed, June 1, 2007.
17. Walsh JK et al. Lack of residual sedation following middle-of the night zaleplon administration in sleep maintenance insomnia. *Clin Neuropharmacol* 2000;23:17.
18. Allen D et al. The effects of single doses of CL284,846, lorazepam, and placebo on psychomotor and memory function in normal male volunteers. *Eur J Clin Pharmacol* 1993;45:313.
19. Danjou P et al. A comparison of the residual effects of zaleplon and zolpidem following administration 5 to 2 h before awakening. *Br J Clin Pharmacol* 1999;48:367.
20. Espie C et al. Randomized clinical effectiveness trial of nurse-administered small group CBT for persistent insomnia in general practice. *Sleep* 2007;30(5):574.
21. Benca RM. Diagnosis and treatment of chronic insomnia: a review. *Psychiatr Serv* 2005;56:332.
22. Morlock RJ et al. Patient characteristics and patterns of drug use for sleep complaints in the U.S. *Clin Ther* 2006;28:1044.
23. Benca RM et al. Special considerations in insomnia diagnosis and management: depressed, elderly, and chronic pain populations. *J Clin Psych* 2004;65(Suppl 8):26.
24. Zisapel N. Sleep and sleep disturbances, biological basis and clinical implications. *Cell Mol Life Sci* 2007;63:1174.
25. Carskadon MA et al. Normal human sleep: an overview. In: Kryger MH et al., eds. *Principles of Sleep Medicine.* 3rd ed. Philadelphia: WB Saunders; 2000:15.
26. Zeman A. The Science of Sleep. *Clin Med* 2005;97.
27. Jones B. Basic mechanisms of sleep-wake states. In: Kryger MH et al., eds. *Principles of Sleep Medicine.* 3rd ed. Philadelphia: WB Saunders; 2000:134.
28. Verrier RL et al. Cardiovascular physiology: central and autonomic regulation. In: Kryger MH et al., eds. *Principles of Sleep Medicine.* 3rd ed. Philadelphia: WB Saunders; 2000:179.
29. Ebrahim IO et al. Hypocretin(orexin) deficiency in narcolepsy and primary hypersomnia. *J Neurol Neurosurg Psychiatry* 2003;74:127.
30. Taber KH et al. Functional neuroanatomy of sleep and sleep deprivation. *J Neuropsychiatry Clin Neurosci* 2006;18:1.
31. Lancel M. Role of $GABA_A$ receptors in the regulation of sleep: initial sleep responses to peripherally administered modulators and agonists. *Sleep* 1999;22:33.
32. Thase ME. Antidepressant treatment of the depressed patient with insomnia. *J Clin Psychiatry* 1999;60(Suppl 17):28.
33. Nowell PD et al. Paroxetine in the treatment of primary insomnia: preliminary clinical and electroencephalogram sleep data. *J Clin Psychiatry* 1999;60:89.
34. Greenblatt DJ et al. Neurochemical and pharmacokinetic correlates of the clinical action of benzodiazepine hypnotics. *Am J Med* 1990;88(Suppl 3A):18S.
35. Greenblatt DJ et al. Clinical pharmacokinetics of anxiolytics and hypnotics in the elderly. *Clin Pharmacokinet* 1991;21:165.
36. Salzman C. Benzodiazepine dependency: summary of the APA task force on benzodiazepines. *Psychopharmacol Bull* 1990;26:61.
37. Dement WC. Overview of the efficacy and safety of benzodiazepine hypnotics using objective methods. *J Clin Psychiatry* 1991;52(Suppl):27.
38. Fahey CD et al. Circadian rhythm sleep disorders and phototherapy. *Psychiatr Clin North Am* 2006;(29):989.
39. Thorpy MJ. Classification of sleep disorders. In: Kryger MH et al; eds. *Principles of Sleep Medicine.* 3rd ed. Philadelphia: WB Saunders; 2000:547.
40. *The Diagnostic and Statistical Manual of Mental Disorders.* 4th ed. Text Revised (DSMIV-TR) Washington, DC: American Psychiatric Association; 2000.
41. Curry DT et al. Pharmacologic management of insomnia: past, present and future. *Psychiatr Clin North Am.* 2006:871.
42. Erman MK. Influence of PK profiles on safety and efficacy of hypnotic medication. *J Clin Psychiatry* 2006;67(Suppl 13):9.
43. Kushida CA et al. Practice parameter for the use of continuous and bilevel airway pressure devices to treat adult patients with sleep-related breathing disorders. *Sleep* 2006;29:375.
44. Basu R et al. Sedative-hypnotic use of diphenhydramine in a rural, older adult, community-based cohort: effects on cognition. *Am J Geriatr Psychiatry* 2003;11:205.
45. Bunney WE et al. Report of the institute of medicine committee on the efficacy and safety of Halcion. *Arch Gen Psychiatry* 1999;56:349.
46. Herxheimer A et al. Melatonin for the prevention and treatment of jet lag. *Cochrane Database Syst Rev* 2005;4:1.
47. Sajith SG et al. Melatonin and sleep disorders associated with intellectual disability. *J Intellect Disabil Res* 2007;51:2.
48. Van der Heijden KB et al. Effect of melatonin on sleep, behavior and cognition in ADHD and chronic sleep-onset insomnia. *J Am Acad Child Adolesc Psychiatry* 2007;46:233.
49. Borja NL et al. Ramelteon for the treatment of insomnia. *Clin Ther* 2006;28:1540.
50. Johnson MW. Ramelteon: a novel hypnotic lacking abuse liability and sedative adverse effects. *Arch Gen Psychiatry* 2006;63:1149.
51. Morin AK et al. Therapeutic options for sleep-maintenance and sleep-onset insomnia. *Pharmacotherapy* 2007;27:89.
52. Drover DR. Comparative pharmacokinetics and pharmacodynamics of short-acting hypnosedatives. *Clin Pharmacokin* 2004;43:227.
53. Krystal AD et al. Sustained efficacy of eszopiclone over 6 months of nightly treatment: results of a randomized, double-blind, placebo-controlled study in adults with chronic insomnia. *Sleep* 2003;26:793.
54. Najib J. Eszopiclone, a nonbenzodiazepine sedative-hypnotic agent for the treatment of transient and chronic insomnia. *Clin Ther* 2006;28:491.
55. The Medical Letter, Inc. Drugs that cause psychiatric symptoms. *Med Lett Drugs Ther* 2002; 44:1134.
56. Greenblatt DJ et al. Pharmacokinetic determinants of dynamic differences among three benzodiazepine hypnotics. *Arch Gen Psychiatry* 1989;46:326.
57. Vogel GW et al. Drug effects on REM sleep and on endogenous depression. In: *Neuroscience and Biobehavioral Review.* New York: Pergamon Press; 1990;14:49.
58. Winokur A. Comparative effects of mirtazapine and fluoxetine on sleep physiology measures in patients with major depression and insomnia. *J Clin Psychiatry* 2003;64:1224.
59. Christian-Gillin J et al. Medication and substance abuse. In: Kryger MH et al., eds. *Principles of Sleep Medicine.* 3rd ed. Philadelphia: WB Saunders; 2000:1176.
60. Kaynak H et al. The effect of trazodone on sleep in patients treated with stimulant antidepressants. *Sleep Med* 2004;5:15.
61. Fave M et al. Eszopiclone co-administered with fluoxetine in patients with insomnia coexisting with major depressive disorder. *Biol Psychiatry* 2006;59:1052.
62. Mendelson WB. A review of the evidence for the efficacy and safety of trazodone in insomnia. *J Clin Psychiatry* 2005;66:469.
63. Dolder C. The use of non-benzodiazepine hypnotics in the elderly. *CNS Drugs* 2007;21:389.
64. Kamel NS et al. Insomnia in the elderly: cause, approach and treatment. *Am J Med* 2006;119:463.
65. Foley DJ et al. Incidence and remission of insomnia among elderly adults: an epidemiologic study of 6,800 persons over three years. *Sleep* 1999;22(Suppl 2):S366.
66. Shamsuzzaman AM et al. Obstructive sleep apnea: implications for cardiac and cardiovascular disease. *JAMA* 2003;290:1906.
67. Morin CM et al. Psychological and behavioral treatment of insomnia. *Sleep* 2006;29:1398.

68. Richards KC. Effect of back massage and relaxation intervention on sleep in critically ill patients. *Am J Crit Care* 1998;7:288.
69. Cooke KM et al. The effects of evening light exposure on the sleep of elderly women expressing sleep complaints. *J Behav Med* 1998;21:103.
70. Simons KJ et al. Pharmacokinetic and pharmacodynamic studies of the H_1-receptor antagonist hydroxyzine in the elderly. *Clin Pharmacol Ther* 1989;45:9.
71. Rickels K et al. Pharmacologic strategies for discontinuing benzodiazepine treatment. *J Clin Psychopharm* 1999;19(Suppl 2):12.
72. Flemons WW. Obstructive sleep apnea. *N Engl J Med* 2002;347:498.
73. Littner MR. Polysomnography and cardiorespiratory monitoring. In: Kushida CA, ed. *Obstructive Sleep Apnea: Diagnosis and Treatment.* New York: Informa Healtcare USA; 2007:35.
74. Yokoe T et al. Elevated levels of c-reactive protein and interleukin-6 in patients with obstructive sleep apnea syndrome are decreased by nasal continuous positive airway pressure. *Circulation* 2003;107:1129.
75. Borgel J et al. Obstructive sleep apnea and blood pressure. *Am J Hypertens* 2004;17:1081.
76. Bixler EO et al. Association of hypertension and sleep-disordered breathing. *Arch Intern Med* 2000;160:2289.
77. Smith PL et al. A physiologic comparison of nasal and oral positive airway pressure. *Chest* 2003;123:689.
78. Garrigue S et al. Benefit of atrial pacing in sleep apnea syndrome. *N Engl J Med* 2002;346:404.
79. Keating GM et al. Modafinil: A review of its use in excessive sleepiness associated with obstructive sleep apnea/hypopnea syndrome and shift work sleep disorder. *CNS Drugs* 2005;19:1785.
80. Dopheide JD. Medication Effects. In: Kushida CA, ed. *Obstructive Sleep Apnea: Diagnosis and Treatment.* New York: Informa Healtcare USA; 2007:295.
81. Kraiczi H et al. Effect of serotonin uptake inhibition on breathing during sleep and daytime symptoms in obstructive sleep apnea. *Sleep* 1999;22:61.
82. Robinson DM et al. Sodium oxybate: a review of its use in the management of narcolepsy. *CNS Drugs* 2007;21:337.
83. Green P et al. Narcolepsy: signs, symptoms, differential diagnosis, and management. *Archives of Family Medicine* 1998;7:472.
84. Vignatelli L et al. Antidepressant drugs for narcolepsy. *Cochrane Database Syst Rev* 2005;3.
85. Auger RR et al. Risk of high-dose stimulants in the treatment of disorders of excessive somnolence. *Sleep* 2005;28(6):667.
86. Ritalin LA *Insert.* East Hanover, NJ: Novartis; 2006.
87. Wong YN et al. A double-blind, placebo-controlled, ascending-dose evaluation of the pharmacokinetics and tolerability of modafinil tablets in healthy male volunteers. *J Clin Pharmacol* 1999;39:30.
88. Robertson P et al. Effect of modafinil on the pharmacokinetics of ethinyl estradiol and triazolam in healthy volunteers. *Clin Pharmacol Ther* 2002;71:46.
89. Dequardo JR. Modafinil-associated clozapine toxicity. *Am J Psychiatry* 2002;159:1243.
90. Hogl B et al. Modafinil for the treatment of daytime sleepiness in Parkinson disease: a double-blind, randomized, crossover, placebo-controlled polygraphic trial. *Sleep* 2002;25:905.
91. Rammohan KW et al. Efficacy and safety of modafinil for the treatment of fatigue in multiple sclerosis: a two centre phase 2 study. *J Neurol Neurosurg Psychiatry* 2002;72:179.
92. Biederman J et al. A comparison of once-daily and divided doses of modafinil for ADHD: a randomized, double-blind, placebo-controlled study. *J Clin Psychiatry* 2006;67:727.
93. Dewey RB et al. Cardiac valve regurgitation with pergolide compared to non-ergot agonists in Parkinson disease. *Arch Neurol* 2007;64:377.
94. Lauerma H. Nocturnal wandering caused by restless legs and short-acting benzodiazepines. *Acta Psychiatr Scand* 1991;83:492.
95. Garcia-Borreguero D et al. Treatment of restless legs syndrome with gabapentin: a double-blind, cross-over study. *Neurology* 2002;59:1573.
96. Lauerma H et al. Treatment of restless legs syndrome with tramadol. *J Clin Psychiatry* 1999; 60:241.
97. Hornyak M et al. Magnesium therapy for periodic leg movements-related insomnia and restless legs syndrome: an open pilot study. *Sleep* 1998;21:501.
98. Meltzer LJ et al. Sleep and sleep disorders in children and adolescents. *Psych Clin of North Am* 2006;29:1059.
99. Schnoes CJ. Pediatric prescribing practices for clonidine and other pharmacologic agents used for children with sleep disturbance. *Clin Pediatrics* 2006;45:229.
100. Ivaneko A et al. Melatonin in children and adolescents with insomnia: a retrospective study. *Clin Pediatr* 2003;42:51.
101. Pelayo R et al. So you want to give my child sleeping pills? *Pediatr Clin North Am* 2004;51:117.
102. Glaze DG. Childhood Insomnia. Why Chris can't sleep. *Pediatr Clin North Am* 2004;51:33.
103. Cote CJ et al. Adverse sedation events in pediatrics: analysis of medications used for sedation. *Pediatrics* 2000;106:633.
104. Pershad J. Chloral hydrate: the good and the bad. *Pediatric Emergency Care* 1999;15:432.
105. Mace SE. Clinical policy: critical issues in the sedation of pediatric patients in the emergency department. *Annals of Emergency Medicine* 2008;51: 378.
106. Heistein LC et al. Chloral hydrate sedation for pediatric echocardiography: physiologic responses, adverse effects and risk factors. *Pediatrics* 2006;117:e434.
107. Onks DL et al. The effect of chloral hydrate and its metabolites, trichloroethanol and trichloroacetic acid, on bilirubin-albumin binding. *Pharmacol Toxicol* 1992;71:196.
108. Haas DA et al. A pilot study of the efficacy of oral midazolam for sedation in pediatric dental patients. *Anesth Prog* 1996;43:1.
109. Coffey B. Review and update: benzodiazepines in childhood and adolescence. *Psychiatr Ann* 1993;23:332.
110. Botteman MF et al. Cost-effectiveness of long-term treatment with eszopiclone for primary insomnia in adults. *CNS Drugs* 2007;21:319.
111. McNamara F et al. Obstructive sleep apnea in infants and its management with nasal continuous positive airway pressure. *Chest* 1999;116:10.

CHAPTER 78

Schizophrenia

Rene A. Endow-Eyer, Melissa M. Mitchell, and Jonathan P. Lacro

Schizophrenia is a debilitating and emotionally devastating illness with long-term impact on patients' lives. Many experts consider schizophrenia to be the most severe expression of psychopathology, encompassing significant disruptions of thinking, perception, emotion, and behavior. Schizophrenia is usually a lifelong psychiatric disability. Family relationships, social functioning, and employment are frequently affected, and periodic hospitalizations are common. The management of schizophrenia involves multiple strategies to optimize the patient's functional capacity, reduce the frequency and severity of symptom exacerbations, and reduce the overall morbidity and mortality from this disorder. Many patients require comprehensive and continuous care over the course of their lives.

The aim of this chapter is to provide a framework for the clinician to develop skills in schizophrenia management by considering the pathophysiology, assessment, clinical course, and treatment of schizophrenia.

EPIDEMIOLOGY

In the United States, approximately 1% of the population develops schizophrenia during their lifetime. Although schizophrenia affects men and women with equal frequency, there are differences in the age of onset and course of illness. The onset of schizophrenia usually occurs during late adolescence or early adulthood. Studies have shown women have, on average, an onset of schizophrenia 3 to 5 years after men.[1] Women also have their first admission due to psychiatric illness 3 to 6 years after men on average.[1] Prevalence rates are similar throughout the world, but pockets of high prevalence have been reported in some areas. After adjusting for differences in diagnostic criteria for schizophrenia, similar prevalence rates across cultures have been observed.

ECONOMIC BURDEN

Mental disorders constitute a large part of the global burden of disease, with schizophrenia being among the greatest causes of disability in the United States and the world.[2] Unlike other chronic diseases such as diabetes and hypertension, which occur late in life, schizophrenia usually affects people when they are young followed by a chronic course persisting throughout the patient's lifetime. Most people with schizophrenia experience multiple hospitalizations and generally require social assistance. Even during relatively stable phases of their illness, most people with schizophrenia require support that ranges from a family member to daytime hospitalization. As of 2002, total costs for schizophrenic patients in the United States averaged $62.7 billion annually, taking into account direct and indirect costs, as well as unemployment costs. Direct costs include hospitalization, rehabilitation, professional services, medication, and office visits. Indirect costs include loss of productivity caused by illness, disability, premature death, and economic burden to families.[3] Schizophrenia accounts for approximately 2.5% of total annual health care costs in the United States. Persons afflicted by schizophrenia represent approximately 10% of this country's permanently disabled population and consume 20% of Social Security benefit days.[4,5] In 2004, it was estimated that 70% of patients with schizophrenia receive medications through Medicaid. Because of the advent of newer atypical antipsychotics over the past 20 years, the cost of psychotropic medications now exceeds $10 billion annually.[6]

ETIOLOGY (NEUROBIOLOGY)

Schizophrenia is a complex disorder with multiple causes. Considering the lack of consistent neuropathology or biomarkers, current theories of the disorder have moved away from the view that it is a single entity, toward a conceptualization of schizophrenia as a collection of etiologically disparate disorders with common clinical features.[7,8] In this section, the genetic and environmental factors, neuroanatomical, and neurochemical features of schizophrenia are considered.

Genetic and Environmental Risk Factors

First-degree biologic relatives of persons with schizophrenia have a tenfold higher risk of developing the disease than the general population.[9] The risk is highest (40%–50%) in a monozygotic (identical) twin of a person with schizophrenia.[10,11] There is also higher concordance for schizophrenia in monozygotic twins compared with dizygotic twins, with respective rates being approximately 50% and 15%.[12] Because the concordance rate is not 100% in monozygotic twins or 50% in dizygotic twins, other nongenetic factors must contribute to the development of the disorder. Environmental factors such as prenatal difficulties (e.g., malnutrition in the first trimester of pregnancy or influenza in the second trimester), perinatal complications, and various nonspecific stressors may also influence the development of schizophrenia. Despite the overwhelming evidence that schizophrenia is an inherited illness, a single "schizophrenia gene" has not been found. Risk for schizophrenia is, to some extent, genetically transmitted and is probably determined by multiple genes. A review of the molecular genetics of schizophrenia cited linkage studies implicating chromosomes 6, 8, 10, 13, and 22.[13]

Neuroanatomy

Studies comparing the brains of individuals with schizophrenia with the brains of normal controls have uncovered a number of important differences. Although these studies suggest that anatomical and functional abnormalities are associated with schizophrenia, no single pathognomonic abnormality consistently has been found. In addition, localization of the site(s) responsible for the pathophysiology of schizophrenia remains elusive.

The most consistent structural finding seen with computed tomography and magnetic resonance imaging in patients with schizophrenia has been enlarged ventricles, particularly the lateral and third ventricles. In addition, there seems to be a relationship between brain asymmetry and the disease process.[14] When unilateral abnormalities have been reported, they have typically involved the left hemisphere.[14] As imaging technology has advanced, magnetic resonance imaging studies in schizophrenia frequently have shown morphologic abnormalities involving the temporal, frontal, and parietal lobes, and the subcortical structures.[15–19] Findings include decreased neuronal volume and density, decreased synaptic connections, decreases in synaptophysin (a membrane protein of synaptic vesicles), and loss of microtubule associated protein and synaptosomal protein in certain regions of the cortex.[20,21] The lack of gliosis in association with the neuroantomical abnormalities in the brains of schizophrenia patients suggests that these changes occur neurodevelopmentally.[22] Functional imaging studies, such as positron emission tomography, single photon emission computed tomography, and functional magnetic resonance imaging have demonstrated alterations in either cerebral perfusion or glucose metabolism in frontal, temporal, and basal ganglia areas of the brain.[23–26] Additional attention has been directed toward the correlation of regional brain abnormalities with specific symptoms or subtypes of schizophrenia. Thus far, the most robust findings have been found in the relation between negative symptoms and the prefrontal cortex, positive symptoms and temporal lobes, and thought disorder and the planum temporale.[27]

In summary, neuroimaging studies have identified anatomical and functional abnormalities that affect different areas of the brain, particularly the prefrontal and temporal areas, corresponding with the impairments observed in schizophrenia.[28] Medial temporal structures are important for the processing of sensory information, and abnormalities in this area may explain distortions in the interpretation of external reality that are characteristic of schizophrenia. The prefrontal cortex is responsible for some of the complex and highly evolved human functions, including the integration of information from other cortical areas. The prefrontal cortex is largely responsible for the regulation of working memory, which involves maintaining information in temporary memory while that information is used for executive functions. Hence, these abnormalities in prefrontal areas could explain the deficits in working memory and attention that are often present in schizophrenia. New theories of schizophrenia that have been proposed include the "cognitive dysmetria" theory (implicating the thalamus and its cortical and cerebellar connections), the "disconnection model" (implicating temporolimbic and prefrontal disconnections), and the "asynchronous neural firing" model.[29–31]

Neurochemistry

The discovery of the antipsychotic properties of chlorpromazine led to a fundamental understanding of the neurochemistry of schizophrenia. The finding that chlorpromazine and other antipsychotic drugs decrease dopamine activity by blocking specific postsynaptic receptors served as the foundation for the dopaminergic hypothesis of schizophrenia. Nearly all drugs that decrease dopamine activity decrease the positive symptoms of schizophrenia. Furthermore, the clinical efficacy of antipsychotic agents is roughly proportional to their affinity for a particular subtype of dopamine receptors, the D_2 receptor.[32,33] Although other classes of dopamine receptors have been identified (e.g., D_1, D_3, D_4), this close relationship to clinical potency exists only for the D_2 receptor subtype.[34] Indirect evidence supporting the dopamine hypothesis is found in the observation that dopamine agonists such as amphetamine, levodopa, methylphenidate, and other aminergic agents can worsen schizophrenia symptoms in some patients.[35–37] Although these observations indicate that manipulating the dopaminergic system can regulate the positive symptoms of schizophrenia, they do not directly implicate a central excess of dopamine as the sole cause of schizophrenia symptoms. This simplistic theory does not explain, for instance, cases of schizophrenia in which residual or negative symptoms predominate. The "hypofrontality theory" suggests that reduced or dysfunctional dopaminergic neurotransmission within the prefrontal cortex or mesocortical area of schizophrenic patients may be responsible for negative symptoms.[38,39] In addition to negative symptomatology, prefrontal dopaminergic dysfunction has been correlated with cognitive dysfunction, particularly in the area of working memory. It has also been proposed that a chronically low level of striatal dopamine release causes negative symptoms (caused by low levels of dopamine in the prefrontal cortex). The diminished dopamine release leads to an upregulation of dopamine receptors, resulting in supersensitivity to phasic dopamine release in the context of environmental stressors (exhibited behaviorally as positive symptoms).[40] This theory explains why dopamine-blocking drugs improve positive symptoms, but not negative symptoms.

Serotonin also seems to play a role in schizophrenia. Alteration in monoamine activity in the limbic circuit has been proposed as a possible link to the dopamine hypothesis of schizophrenia.[41] Serotonin receptors are abundant in mesocortical areas, and agonism at these receptor sites may have an inhibitory effect on dopaminergic receptors or dopamine release, possibly contributing to negative schizophrenia symptoms.

Another area of focus is the involvement of excitatory amino acids and the glutamate transmitter system in the pathogenesis of schizophrenia.[42] Decreased activation of *N*-methyl-D-aspartic acid (NMDA) or glutamate receptors may increase cortical dopamine release and produce a syndrome resembling schizophrenia. This hypofunctional NMDA receptor theory was supported by findings of low glutamate levels in the cerebrospinal fluid of persons with schizophrenia and by the observation that phencyclidine (PCP), an NMDA antagonist, could produce florid psychosis.[43] In utero exposure to excitotoxins or viruses has been proposed as a possible mechanism for destruction of NMDA receptors within the brain. The clinical effect of neuronal destruction may not be expressed until late adolescence or early adulthood (when symptoms of schizophrenia usually arise). γ-Aminobutyric acid (GABA), a major inhibitory amino acid, may act as a third link between the neuromodulation of glutamate and dopamine receptors. It has been suggested that GABA receptor function may be impaired within the prefrontal region, resulting in abnormal NMDA receptor concentrations.[44] It has also been proposed that an imbalance between NMDA, GABA, and dopamine receptors may cause the symptoms of schizophrenia. Studies examining the clinical effects of direct glycinergic agonists or inhibitors of glutamate uptake in persons with schizophrenia are needed to clarify the role of excitatory amino acid neurotransmission in this disorder.

Substantial progress has been made in neuropathological and neuroanatomical studies of schizophrenia. Insights from physiological imaging studies in living patients, studies of brain development and its genetic control, and pharmacologic studies using newer atypical antipsychotics are promising stepping stones that may lead to a better understanding of the pathogenesis of schizophrenia.

CLINICAL PRESENTATION

Historical Concept of Schizophrenia

Kraepelin[45] provided the first thorough description of the constellation of symptoms that make up schizophrenia, which he called "dementia praecox" (a syndrome of cognitive and behavioral deficits that tend to appear early in life). Kraepelin emphasized that dementia praecox generally followed a chronic course with no return to the premorbid level of functioning. Kraepelin also noted that no single pathognomonic symptom or cluster of symptoms served to characterize dementia praecox, an illness he considered so mysterious that he referred to it as a disorder whose causes were shrouded in "impenetrable darkness." Bleuler[46] concurred with Kraepelin's initial description of schizophrenia, although he suggested that some patients did recover and subsequently could lead productive lives. For Bleuler, the most important and fundamental feature was a fragmentation in the formulation and expression of thought, referring to it as "loosening of associations." Bleuler described the "4 *A*s" of schizophrenia, which include autism (preoccupation with internal stimuli), inappropriate affect (external manifestations of mood), loose associations (illogical or fragmented thought processes), and ambivalence (simultaneous, contradictory thinking). Thus, Bleuler focused on negative symptoms and thought disorganization rather than on the positive symptoms of schizophrenia, such as delusions and hallucinations. Another important contribution to the defining features of schizophrenia was Schneider's "first-rank" symptoms[47] of schizophrenia that assisted the clinician in diagnosing schizophrenia. First-rank symptoms include delusions, auditory hallucinations, thought withdrawal, thought insertion, thought broadcasting, and experiencing feelings or actions that are under someone else's control. Schneider's first-rank symptoms provided the framework for the systematic diagnostic criteria used today in psychiatry.

Diagnosis and Differential Diagnosis

The *Diagnostic and Statistical Manual of the American Psychiatric Association,* text revision (DSM-IV-TR), is the latest edition of the guide for diagnosing and classifying schizophrenia and other psychiatric disorders. Compared with previous DSM editions, the DSM-IV-TR places a greater emphasis on negative symptoms and the social and occupational dysfunction associated with schizophrenia.[11] Psychosis has many causes, and all must be excluded before the diagnosis of schizophrenia is made. In addition, a diagnosis can be made only if the DSM-IV-TR criteria are met (Table 78-1). Clinicians can misdiagnose psychotic patients when the diagnosis is based on presenting symptoms alone without regard to the longitudinal clinical course. An accurate diagnosis is important because treatments vary for psychoses with different origins. Schizophreniform disorder is similar to schizophrenia except that it lasts for >1 month but for <6 months. Brief psychotic disorder is diagnosed when positive symptoms present suddenly and are present for ≥1 day but <1 month. After the episode subsides, premorbid functioning usually returns. Various personality disorders, including schizotypal, schizoid, and paranoid types also can resemble schizophrenia; however, these disorders lack the chronic thought disturbances seen in schizophrenia. Bipolar disorder, manic or depressive phase, and major depression can have psychotic features that usually are mood congruent. Negative symptoms of schizophrenia such as akinesia, anergy, apathy, and social withdrawal may resemble depression, but do not respond to antidepressant therapy. It is also important to differentiate extrapyramidal side effects of drugs, particularly akinesia seen with antipsychotic-induced parkinsonism, from the negative symptoms of schizophrenia. Common differential diagnoses are listed in Table 78-2.

Drug-induced psychosis is an important differential diagnosis when evaluating patients with schizophrenia-like symptoms. Illicit drugs may cause psychotic symptoms in any individual, but do not cause the illness of schizophrenia in persons without a predisposition to mental illness or an underlying psychiatric disorder. Drugs causing acute psychotic symptoms include amphetamines, cocaine, cannabis, phencyclidine ("angel dust"), lysergic acid diethylamide, and ketamine. In addition, anticholinergic delirium can occur if excessive doses or combinations of therapeutic agents with anticholinergic properties are prescribed. A urine toxicology screen can help to evaluate the contribution of substance abuse to psychosis, but because of the risk of false-negative results, the quality and progression of the presenting symptoms and physical findings also must be considered to make an accurate diagnosis. A particularly difficult problem is evaluating the cause of psychosis in a patient with schizophrenia and concurrent drug or alcohol abuse.

Table 78-1 DSM-IV-TR Criteria for Schizophrenia

A. Characteristic Symptoms

At least two of the following, each present for a significant portion of time during a 1-month period (or less if successfully treated):

1. Delusions
2. Hallucinations
3. Disorganized speech (e.g., frequent derailment or incoherence)
4. Grossly disorganized or catatonic behavior
5. Negative symptoms (i.e., affective flattening, alogia, or avolition)

Note: Only one "A symptom" is required if delusions are bizarre or hallucinations consist of a voice keeping up a running commentary on the person's behavior or thought, two or more conversations with each other.

B. Social/Occupational Dysfunction

For a significant portion of the time since the onset of the disturbance, one or more major areas of functioning such as work, interpersonal relationships, or self-care is markedly below the level achieved before the onset.

C. Duration

Continuous signs of the disturbance persist for at least 6 months. This 6-month period must include at least 1 month of symptoms (or less if successfully treated) that meet criterion A (i.e., active-phase symptoms) and may include prodromal and/or residual periods when the "A criterion" is not fully met. During these periods, signs of the disturbance may be manifested by negative symptoms or by two or more symptoms listed in "criterion A" present in an attenuated form (e.g., blunted affect, unusual perceptual disturbances).

D. Schizoaffective Disorder and Mood Disorder Exclusion

Schizoaffective disorder and mood disorder with psychotic features have been ruled out because either (a) no major depressive, manic, or mixed manic episodes have occurred concurrently with the active phase symptoms or (b) if mood episodes have occurred during active phase symptoms, their total duration has been brief relative to the duration of the active and residual periods.

E. Substance/General Medical Condition Exclusion

The disturbance is not due to direct physiological effects of a substance (drug of abuse or medication) or a general medical condition.

F. Relationship to a Pervasive Development Disorder

If there is a history of autistic disorder or another pervasive development disorder, the additional diagnosis of schizophrenia is made only if prominent delusions or hallucinations also are present for at least a month (or less if successfully treated).

From reference 11.

Table 78-2 Differential Diagnosis for Schizophrenia (DSM-IV-TR)

Drug-induced Psychoses

Amphetamine
Cocaine
Cannabis (marijuana)
Phencyclidine (PCP)
Lysergic acid diethylamide (LSD)
Anticholinergics

Primary Psychiatric Disorders

Brief psychotic disorder
Schizophreniform disorder
Bipolar affective disorder, manic type
Mood disorder with psychotic features

Personality Disorders

Schizotypal
Schizoid
Paranoid

Distinguishing between the two may not be possible until the patient becomes drug free and residual symptoms are assessed. There are some differences in the presentation of drug-induced psychosis and schizophrenia. For example, chronic stimulant use usually does not present with a formal thought disorder. Cannabis psychosis may be differentiated from acute paranoid schizophrenia because patients with the former usually experience a subjective feeling of panic and retain insight into their problem.[48] Acute PCP ingestion can cause psychotic symptoms such as paranoia and acute catatonia, but other concomitant symptoms such as ataxia, hyperreflexia, nystagmus, and hypertension are not found in schizophrenia.

Target Symptoms

Schizophrenia is a complex disorder comprising different clusters of signs and symptoms. The characteristic symptoms of schizophrenia have often been conceptualized as falling into two broad categories: positive and negative (or deficit) symptoms. Positive symptoms can be further divided into two distinct groups, positive symptoms and disorganized symptoms. Positive symptoms include hallucinations (auditory, visual) and delusions (persecution, guilt, religion, mind control). Disorganized symptoms include disorganized speech, thought disorder (tangentiality, derailment, circumstantiality) and disorganized behavior (clothing, appearance, aggression, repetitive actions). Negative symptoms include affective flattening, decreased thought and speech productivity (alogia), loss of ability to experience pleasure (anhedonia), and decreased initiation of goal-directed behavior (avolition). Most patients with schizophrenia exhibit both positive and negative symptoms, although the dominance of one type over the other usually varies throughout the course of the illness. Younger patients tend to exhibit more positive symptoms, whereas in older patients negative symptoms predominate. Table 78-3 provides a glossary of commonly used terms in schizophrenia, and Table 78-4 lists positive and negative symptoms of schizophrenia.

Cognitive deficits, including problems with attention, memory, and concentration, are another frequently cited problem for people with schizophrenia. These impairments are common, affecting as many as 70% of individuals with schizophrenia.[49] The most consistently replicated deficits are observed on tasks measuring attention, information processing speed, working memory, learning, and executive (frontal systems) functions.[50] These domains are not only commonly impaired in schizophrenia, but they are also strongly associated with functional outcomes (social and community functioning).[50] Although it is likely that the overall dysfunction observed in schizophrenia encompasses factors such as psychopathology, drug treatment, and social isolation, evidence suggests that cognitive impairments have a stronger relationship to the long-term functional outcome than positive symptoms.[50]

Table 78-3 Glossary of Commonly Used Terms in Schizophrenia

Affect: behavior (usually an expression of an emotion) observed by the interviewer. Common types of disturbances in affect include: *restricted*—mild decrease in range and intensity of the expression of emotion; *blunted*—significant decrease in intensity of the expression of emotion; *flat*—absence of expression of emotion; *inappropriate*—incongruency between patient's affect and mood or behavior; and *labile*—abrupt shifts in expression of emotion.

Akathisia: syndrome consisting of subjective feelings of anxiety and restlessness, and objective signs of pacing, rocking, and an inability to sit or stand still for extended periods of time.

Akinesia: absence or decrease in voluntary movement; may be antipsychotic induced (extrapyramidal side effects) or a manifestation of negative symptoms of schizophrenia.

Alogia: impoverished thinking usually manifested through speech and language deficits. Speech is brief and lacks spontaneity; replies to questions are very concrete (*poverty of speech*). *Poverty of content* refers to speech that is adequate in amount, but is of little substance (overly abstract), repetitive, or stereotyped.

Anergy: lack of energy.

Anhedonia: loss of interest or pleasure.

Avolition: an inability to initiate and sustain goal-directed activities. The patient may sit for extended periods of time and show minimal interest in participating in social or work-related activities.

Circumstantiality: a form of disorganized speech characterized by "talking in circles" or taking an unusually long length of time in answering a question or expressing one's point of view.

Delusions: a false belief that is firmly held despite evidence to refute the belief. The belief does not qualify as a delusion if it is a cultural or religious belief accepted by a group of individuals. Types of delusions include grandiose, persecutory, and somatic type.

Executive function: the ability to design and carry out a solution to a plan when the solution is not obvious. Loss of executive function presents as failure to learn from past experience and failure to plan or organize life events.

Hallucination: a sensory perception (e.g., auditory, visual, somatic, tactile) experienced in the absence of external stimuli. Hallucinations may be recognized as false sensory perceptions in some, whereas others may believe that the experiences are reality based.

Loose associations: a form of disorganized, illogical speech characterized by unrelated words, phrases, and sentences used in a fashion that makes comprehension very difficult, if not impossible.

Mood: a pervasive and sustained emotion that is experienced by the patient. Examples include depressed, anxious, angry, or irritable mood.

Mood-congruent delusions or hallucinations: delusions or hallucinations that are consistent with a mood or behavior (e.g., delusions/hallucinations of death, guilt, or punishment in the presence of a depressed mood).

Mood-incongruent delusions or hallucinations: delusions or hallucinations that are not consistent with a mood or behavior (e.g., delusions/hallucinations of death, guilt, or punishment in the presence of mania).

Tangentiality: a form of disorganized speech in which answers are remotely or completely unrelated to questions, and patients' thoughts frequently shift in an unconnected fashion.

Thought broadcasting: a delusion that one's thoughts are being broadcast to others (e.g., a patient feels that others can read his or her mind).

Thought disorder: a general term often used to describe any type of abnormal thought process (e.g., delusion, loose association, conceptual disorganization).

Thought insertion: a delusion that one's thoughts are being inserted into one's mind by others.

Table 78-4 Positive and Negative Symptoms of Schizophrenia

Positive	Negative
Combativeness, agitation, and hostility	Psychomotor retardation
Tension	Affective flattening
Hyperactivity	Avolition
Hallucinations	Lack of socialization
Delusions	Alogia
Disorganized speech (loose associations, tangential, blocking)	Loss of emotional connectedness
Unusual behavior	Loss of executive functions

Case Presentation

J.C., a 22-year-old, single, unemployed man, was brought into the emergency department (ED) of a mental health hospital by the police after he was found running barefoot downtown dodging cars in subzero weather. In the ED, J.C. was extremely frightened, and stated, "They won't let me go."

History of Present Illness: J.C. is not a poor historian. He is agitated easily and threatens the interviewer when asked questions regarding his illness. J.C. said he came to this city 5 years ago "to be the king of jazz music." He did not complete high school, has lost touch with his family and has been living at the Salvation Army for the past 3 years. He has no close friends, and does not trust most people. He hears voices of "dead people" who tell him he is worthless and "will be killed." He says, "The newscasters on the television are reading my mind and telling everyone my personal secrets." These problems and insomnia have been disturbing him for the past year.

Medical History: J.C. has no history of a previous psychiatric illness and has never been hospitalized. The administrator at the Salvation Army confirms that J.C. has been living at the facility for 3 years. His behavior has always been rather "odd and unusual"; he has recently become more agitated. He does not get along with other tenants and staff and he has been unable to care for himself for the past year or so.

Psychosocial History: The hospital social worker reveals that J.C.'s mother was frequently hospitalized for unspecified psychotic episodes and his father was "never around." J.C. admits that he was somewhat of a "rebel" as a child; he has never held steady employment and relies on Social Security income and money from strangers to survive.

Physical Examination/Laboratory Tests: J.C. was given a complete physical examination, which was noncontributory. His laboratory tests, including complete blood count (CBC) with differential, SMA-28 laboratory panel, and thyroid and liver function tests (LFTs) were within normal limits. The urine drug screen was negative, his neurologic examination was unremarkable, and no further tests were ordered.

Mental Status Examination: *Appearance and Behavior*: J.C. is a thin, disheveled-looking man with very poor hygiene, who appears much older than his stated age. He is extremely suspicious of the interviewer and his surroundings and continually asks, "Where am I, who are you, and what do you want?" He also is agitated easily. *Mood*: J.C. is very anxious and worried, concerned that the "dead people" are going to track him down and "bury me alive." His affect is blunted, with a minimal range of reactivity to his emotions. *Memory*: Remote memory seems to be intact, although his immediate and short-term memory are difficult to assess because he is uncooperative. *Sensorium*: He is oriented to person, place, time, and situation. *Thought Content*: He hears dead people talking to him. He seems to be responding to internal stimuli, mumbling to himself and answering his own questions. *Thought Process*: J.C. is very suspicious and exhibits loose associations such as "What are you doing to me? Don't you like my hat? Jazz musicians will save us all. You are with the FBI!" *Insight and Judgment*: Both are poor as evidenced by J.C.'s denial of his illness and need for treatment, and his behavior, which precipitated this admission.

Provisional Diagnosis: Schizophrenia, Paranoid Type

1. What target symptoms of schizophrenia are present in J.C.? How are target symptoms used to monitor treatment?

J.C. exhibits many of the classic Schneider's first-rank symptoms of schizophrenia, including auditory hallucinations (hearing voices from "dead people" telling him that he will be killed), delusions ("Jazz musicians will save us all. You are with the FBI. They will bury me alive."), and thought broadcasting ("The newscasters on the television are reading my mind."). Other target symptoms include agitation, suspiciousness, loose associations, poor grooming and hygiene, impaired sleep, decreased social skills, and impaired insight and judgment. These target symptoms are the basis of assessing a change in clinical status and monitoring J.C.'s response to medications.

Typical Course and Outcome

Onset of Illness

The onset of schizophrenia starts with the prodromal phase that begins with the first changes in behavior and lasts until the onset of psychosis.[51–53] It is characterized by a slow and gradual onset of signs and symptoms that can last weeks to years, but typically persists for at least a year.[51] Common prodromal signs and symptoms include anxiety, blunted affect, depression or dysphoric mood, irritability, loss of initiative, low energy, poor concentration, sleep disturbance, social isolation and withdrawal, and suspiciousness. Subthreshold or attenuated positive symptoms, and mild disorganization (digressive, vague, overly abstract, or concrete thinking) may begin during the prodrome. Gradual deterioration in functioning commonly occurs. The prodrome is difficult to recognize; however, family members may interpret the earliest subtle changes as normal adolescence, a phase, relational problems, depression, or drug use. Some researchers have viewed the prodromal phase as the optimal point to begin pharmacologic intervention. Research has shown that many patients are ill for months or even years before seeking treatment; this delay in treatment is related to outcome and level of remission. Early recognition of the prodrome could lead to interventions that delay or prevent the emergence of psychosis. Eventually, a symptom characteristic of the active phase appears (Table 78-1, criterion A), marking the disturbance as schizophrenia.

Course of Illness

In contrast with the notion of an inevitable progressive deterioration in schizophrenia as proposed by Kraepelin, longitudinal studies of schizophrenia suggest that the course of illness is highly variable. The majority suffers from episodic exacerbations and remissions with some degree of residual symptoms.[45,54–56] Complete remission (i.e., a return to full premorbid functioning) is not common in this disorder. Of the patients who remain ill, some seem to have a relatively stable course, whereas others show a progressive worsening associated with severe disability. Reported remission rates range from 10% to 60%, and a reasonable estimate is that 20% to 30% of all schizophrenic patients are able to lead somewhat normal lives. About 20% to 30% of patients continue to experience moderate symptoms, and 40% to 60% of patients remain significantly impaired by their disorder for their entire lives. Early in the illness, negative symptoms may manifest as prodromal features. Subsequently, positive symptoms appear. Because these positive symptoms are particularly responsive to treatment, they typically diminish, but in many individuals negative symptoms persist between episodes of positive symptoms. As patients with schizophrenia age, the frequency and severity of acute episodes may decrease; however, negative symptoms may become more prominent in some individuals, a state often referred to as burn-out.[54,56,57]

Prognosis

Predictors of an improved long-term outcome in patients with schizophrenia include female gender, a positive family history of an affective disorder, a negative family history of schizophrenia, good premorbid functioning, higher IQ, married marital status, acute onset with precipitating stress, fewer prior episodes (both number and length), a phasic pattern of episodes and remissions (i.e., fewer residual symptoms), advancing age at onset, minimal comorbidity, paranoid subtype, and symptoms that are predominantly positive (delusions, hallucinations) and not disorganized (thought disorder, disorganized behavior).[58] Despite modern treatment advancements, schizophrenia remains a severe disease with a relatively poor outcome. Many patients experience repeated hospitalizations and exacerbations of symptoms, and suicide attempts are relatively common. Individuals with schizophrenia have a 20% shorter life expectancy than the general population.[59] This is due in part, to an increased incidence of general medical illness (such as diabetes or cardiovascular disease) and suicide.[58] Patients with schizophrenia have approximately a 50% lifetime risk for a suicide attempt and as many as 9% to 13% complete suicide.[60]

2. What other factors in J.C.'s history are consistent with the diagnosis of schizophrenia, and what is his prognosis?

Other factors that are consistent with schizophrenia in J.C. include onset of illness in early adulthood (typical age of onset is late adolescence to early 30s), a positive family history of psychiatric illness, inability to maintain steady employment and establish interpersonal relationships with others, and the apparent chronicity of the illness over the past year. His acute exacerbations of psychosis are also characteristic of schizophrenia. Because of J.C.'s young age at the time of his initial psychotic episodes, a positive family history for thought disorder, an unstable home environment, and a low premorbid level of functioning, his long-term prognosis is not good.

TREATMENT

Schizophrenia is a chronic disease for which there is no cure. Pharmacotherapy can reduce symptoms to improve social and cognitive functions; however, patients have multiple relapses and experience residual symptoms throughout their lives. Treatment can decrease acute symptoms, decrease the frequency and severity of psychotic episodes, and optimize psychosocial functioning between episodes. However, many patients require comprehensive care and life-long treatment. Comprehensive care consists of pharmacologic, psychosocial, and rehabilitative treatment.

Goals of Treatment

The American Psychiatric Association Practice Guideline for the Treatment of Schizophrenia describes three phases of illness for the purpose of integrating treatment.[58] Treatment is divided into three phases—acute, stabilization, and stable—with each phase using different drug and nondrug strategies to achieve the desired therapeutic outcome. These phases are not always distinct or separate, but instead tend to overlap.

Acute Phase

During the acute phase of illness, patients suffer from floridly psychotic symptoms such as delusions and/or hallucinations, are severely disorganized, and usually require hospitalization or are placed in a supervised outpatient setting. Negative symptoms become more severe during this phase as well. The initial treatment goal is to calm agitated patients who may be physical threats to themselves or others. Medication is usually required to achieve this outcome, although nondrug interventions such as emotional support from the staff and use of quiet areas can also be helpful. An antipsychotic should be initiated as soon as feasible because prolonged psychotic episodes may be associated with a worsening of their course of illness.[61]

Stabilization Phase

During the stabilization phase, acute symptoms gradually decrease in severity as the patient begins to stabilize. The goals of treatment during the stabilization phase of the illness are to reduce the likelihood of symptom exacerbation and develop a plan for long-term treatment.[58] The hope is that a patient will return to his or her premorbid level of functioning, although this is unlikely. Treatment should consist of a combination of pharmacologic and nonpharmacologic strategies. Treatment guidelines recommend that patients continue the same medication and dosage from which they received benefit from during the acute phase of illness. Treatment should be continued for at least 6 months.[58] During this phase, the individual is most vulnerable to relapse. Another concern during the stabilization phase is that clinicians, patients, and families may wrongly conclude that the antipsychotic stopped working if psychotic symptoms persist during this phase. For example, a patient may have suffered from hallucinations that were loud and derogatory before initiation of treatment; after 8 weeks of treatment, the voices might remain but become quieter and less demeaning. Because antipsychotics have been shown to provide gradual improvement over a period of months after the initial episode was treated, the current regimen should be continued.[62]

Stable Phase

During the stable phase, a level of functioning considered optimal for that individual patient is attained. Although complete resolution of symptoms is desired, many patients never achieve this goal. Negative symptoms may persist and patients may experience nonspecific symptoms such as tension, anxiety, or mood instability during the stable phase. Treatment during the stable or maintenance phase is designed to optimize functioning and minimize the risk and consequences of relapse. Antipsychotics are highly effective in preventing relapse. There are no reliable predictors of relapse for an individual patient. When developing a long-term strategy to prevent relapse and rehospitalization, the dose and type of antipsychotic, and the duration of therapy should be considered. Long-term pharmacotherapy reduces the risk of relapse in schizophrenic patients and also may reduce the risk of environment- and stress-induced relapse relative to untreated patients.[63,64] The effectiveness of antipsychotics in remission prevention was demonstrated in studies in which stable patients were either continued on an antipsychotic or changed to placebo. In these studies, relapse rates were higher in patients who did not remain on an antipsychotic. Although results vary, approximately 70% of the patients who were switched to placebo experienced a relapse within 12 months. In contrast, only about 30% of drug-maintained patients had a relapse of their condition.[65] This supports the need for continuing antipsychotic treatment in patients after they have recovered from a psychotic episode. All patients with schizophrenia should receive maintenance therapy for at least 1 year, unless antipsychotic agents are not tolerated or the diagnosis is uncertain. If a patient has only a single episode with predominately positive symptoms and is symptom free for 1 year after the acute episode, then discontinuation of the medication with careful follow-up can be considered.[58] Patients with a history of multiple episodes may be candidates for medication discontinuation after stability has been demonstrated for 5 years.[58] Lifelong treatment is indicated in patients who present a significant risk to themselves or others when unmedicated.[58]

3. What are the specific treatment goals for J.C.?

The immediate treatment goal for J.C. is to reduce his agitation because he may be a physical threat to himself and others. Intermediate goals during the stabilization phase are to attenuate, or to eliminate, if possible, symptoms of psychoses and the thought disorder. Long-term goals during the stable phase should include assisting J.C. in developing a psychosocial support system (e.g., caretakers, mental health workers, peer groups) to promote enhanced medication adherence, enable him to live semi-independently, and possibly obtain part-time employment.

Nonpharmacologic Interventions

Nonpharmacologic interventions are often combined with drug treatment and can provide additional benefits in such areas as relapse prevention, improved coping skills, better social and vocational functioning, and ability to function more independently. Interventions should be started as early as possible, even during the management of an acute episode. As a patient begins to stabilize during an acute episode, nonpharmacologic strategies can be implemented.[58] Individual therapy (e.g., supportive, insight oriented, reality oriented) can improve insight into the illness, improve medication adherence, teach ways to cope with medication side effects and stress, and help the patient to identify early warning signs of relapse. Group therapy can enhance socialization skills. In patients who are less stable and who continue to exhibit negative symptoms, supportive therapy is generally more effective than group or other more complex, insight-oriented therapies. Family therapy is also important because family members need to learn ways to cope with such a devastating illness and how to be supportive of their loved one, while not being overly controlling. Vocational training can benefit patients who will likely need a significant amount of assistance in finding and maintaining long-term employment.[66] Evidence-based practice guidelines for psychosocial treatment of schizophrenia now include interventions such as social skills training, cognitive/cognitive–behavioral therapy, family psychoeducation, and vocational rehabilitation.[67–71]

4. Is nonpharmacologic therapy indicated for treatment of J.C.?

J.C. should be placed in an area of the hospital ward with low amounts of noise and stimulation until his agitation subsides. He needs careful observation by staff until he is fully assessed for the cause of his symptoms and his level of dangerousness. If the treatment team determines that he is very dangerous, he may need one-to-one supervision by an individual staff member. As his behavior calms, J.C. can receive more ward privileges and should begin to attend group therapy. Initial therapy focuses on issues such as "what is schizophrenia?" and "what are the ways to treat it?" Basic issues related to medication education are also discussed. These include symptoms that are improved with medication and recognition of common acute adverse effects. Socialization with other patients and staff should also be encouraged. As J.C. improves further, therapy and education can shift toward coping skills, stress management, recognition of prodromal symptoms of relapse, long-term adverse effects, and ways to enhance adherence to treatment. Family therapy should also be considered if J.C. allows contact to occur. Family therapy focuses on decreasing family stress surrounding the illness, family problem solving, and communication. If J.C. enters a stable phase after discharge from the hospital, other strategies such as psychosocial clubhouses to improve socialization, social skills training, and vocational rehabilitation can increase his quality of life and productivity.[58]

5. How should the staff and family members communicate most effectively with J.C., considering his paranoid state?

Communication should be calm and nonjudgmental in any acutely psychotic and agitated patient. Open-ended questions should be used, with a switch to closed-ended questions if J.C. is unwilling to respond. His paranoid delusions should not be challenged directly because he may feel attacked and become angry and more agitated. Instead of challenging the delusional thoughts, the clinicians should acknowledge that J.C. believes the "dead people" are real and that he is "the king of jazz," but that they do not share his belief. Direct eye contact should also be intermittent to avoid making the patient feel threatened. If the patient is violent, they should be interviewed in the presence of another health care provider. The clinician must not react to the provocation of a threatening patient and should avoid using a loud voice or aggressive words. When interviewing a violent patient, questions should be focused on issues that need immediate attention, such as medication adherence before admission to the hospital, presence of medical conditions, and recent consumption of drugs and alcohol.[72,73] As J.C. calms, he will likely be more cooperative with questions and assessments.

Assessment

Because a diagnosis of schizophrenia cannot be made or monitored by laboratory or physical tests, the clinician must use target symptoms gathered from a patient interview and historic records to assess treatment response. A complete medical, psychiatric, and medication history, physical examination, laboratory panel (electrolytes; glucose; liver, renal, and thyroid function tests; CBC with differential; urinalysis; urine toxicology screen), and electrocardiogram (ECG) should be obtained as soon as possible during the acute phase of illness or once the patient is cooperative (e.g., stable phase). A complete evaluation is needed to rule out other causes of psychosis, to identify comorbid conditions requiring treatment, and to give guidance for selecting an antipsychotic and for determining the length of treatment.

Given the lack of insight that characterizes schizophrenia patients, collateral information should be gathered from the patient's relatives, friends, and significant others. Target symptoms for schizophrenia are specific for an individual patient, and they must be clearly identified and documented before and during the course of treatment to determine response to an intervention. Both specific treatment goals and the patient's previous baseline level of functioning should be clearly established at the onset of drug therapy. These data are used to give a direction for treatment and as a way of determining whether the outcome has been achieved.

Pharmacologic Interventions

Non-Antipsychotic Agents

BENZODIAZEPINES

Benzodiazepines are commonly added to antipsychotics and have been found to be useful in some studies for anxiety, agitation, global impairment, and psychosis.[74] Adjunctive use of benzodiazepines can spare the need for higher dosages of antipsychotics. However, some studies found that the benefits of benzodiazepines were sometimes not sustained.[58] Unfortunately, it is not possible to predict who will respond to adjunctive benzodiazepine treatment, and any potential benefit must be balanced against the risks of benzodiazepines. Common side effects of benzodiazepines include sedation, ataxia, cognitive impairment, and behavioral disinhibition. This latter effect can be a serious problem in those patients who are being treated for agitation. Withdrawal reactions, including psychosis and seizures, can significantly complicate management if a patient suddenly becomes noncompliant with benzodiazepine treatment. In addition, patients with schizophrenia are vulnerable to both abuse and addiction to benzodiazepines. For these reasons, the use of benzodiazepines should be limited to short trials (2–4 weeks in duration) for the management of severe agitation and anxiety.

LITHIUM

The use of lithium in schizophrenia has been investigated as monotherapy as well as an adjunctive treatment with antipsychotics. Studies evaluating the antipsychotic properties of lithium monotherapy indicate that it has limited effectiveness in schizophrenia and may be harmful for some patients.[58] In combination with antipsychotics, lithium has been observed to improve psychosis, depression, excitement, and irritability.[58,75,76] In general, adjunctive lithium therapy may be considered in patients who have a partial or poor response to an antipsychotic agent. The dose of lithium should be sufficient to obtain a blood level in the range of 0.8 to 1.2 mEq/L. Patients should be monitored for adverse effects that are commonly associated with lithium (e.g., polyuria, tremor). Reports of increased neurotoxicity from combined use of lithium and antipsychotic agents are inconclusive, and the risk seems to be no different with either medication used alone.[77]

ANTICONVULSANTS

Anticonvulsants such as carbamazepine and valproate are often prescribed in patients with schizophrenia as adjunctive treatment of psychosis, agitation, aggression, impulsivity, and mood lability.[78,79] However, as with lithium, there is little support for the efficacy of these agents as monotherapy. In general, the evidence to support the use of carbamazepine for schizophrenia is inconsistent. Neppe[80] reviewed the literature and concluded that patients with nonresponsive psychosis and agitation, aggression, or "interpersonal difficulties" may benefit from the addition of carbamazepine. In a recent meta-analysis, Leucht et al. described a nonsignificant trend for a benefit from carbamazepine as an adjunct to antipsychotics.[78] An important consideration with carbamazepine is that the drug alters the metabolism of most antipsychotic agents, and dosage adjustment is often required. Carbamazepine should never be used concurrently with clozapine because of the additive risk of agranulocytosis.

Recent evidence indicates that valproate is being prescribed more frequently for schizophrenia and that the use of lithium and carbamazepine is declining.[81] This shift in utilization may reflect a more favorable side effect profile of valproate. In a recent investigation of hospitalized patients treated with risperidone and olanzapine for an acute exacerbation of schizophrenia, concurrent administration of divalproex resulted in earlier improvements in a range of psychotic symptoms.[82] Additional research is needed to confirm this finding. Dosages and target serum levels of carbamazepine and valproate are similar to those useful in the treatment of bipolar disorder (see Chapter 80 Mood Disorders II: Bipolar Disorders).

PROPRANOLOL

Propranolol, in combination with antipsychotic drugs, has been evaluated in nonresponders, with variable results. Potential explanations for the enhanced efficacy include a drug interaction leading to higher antipsychotic drug serum concentrations, relief of akathisia, or a primary improvement in psychosis. In addition, propranolol has improved chronic aggression in individuals with schizophrenia.[83] When used to treat aggression or to enhance the response to antipsychotic agents, high doses are needed. Propranolol is started at 40 to 80 mg twice a day and is increased every other day until intolerable adverse effects occur (systolic blood pressure [BP] of $<$90 mm Hg or a heart rate $<$50 beats/minute). Dosages as low as 160 mg and as high as 1,920 mg have been effective; however, a reasonable trial usually is considered to be 240 mg/day for 2 months.[83,84]

Antipsychotics

CLASSIFICATION AND NOMENCLATURE OF THE ANTIPSYCHOTICS

Antipsychotics have been broadly classified into two groups. The older agents (i.e., those introduced in the United States before 1990) are referred to as *typical* or *conventional* antipsychotics or dopamine receptor antagonists, with pharmacologic activity attributed to the blockade of central dopamine receptors, particularly the D_2 receptor subtype. These agents have also been referred to as *major tranquilizers* and *neuroleptics*. The term major tranquilizer is inaccurate, because these agents, particularly the high-potency agents, can improve psychosis without associated sedation. *Neuroleptic* refers to the tendency of these drugs to cause neurologic side effects, particularly extrapyramidal symptoms (EPS). Typical antipsychotics are further classified as high- or low-potency agents, based on their relative ability to block dopamine receptors. They can also be classed by chemical structure (phenothiazine and nonphenothiazine) and potential for common adverse effects (EPS, sedation, anticholinergic, and cardiovascular effects).[66,85] Examples of typical agents include haloperidol, fluphenazine, thiothixene, chlorpromazine and thioridazine.

Newer agents, *atypical* or *serotonin-dopamine antagonists*, consist of clozapine, risperidone, olanzapine, quetiapine, ziprasidone, aripiprazole, and paliperidone. These agents demonstrate postsynaptic effects at 5-HT_{2A} and D_2 receptors. Some of the general characteristics that may be considered as features of atypical antipsychotic include an absence or decreased incidence of EPS and tardive dyskinesia (TD), lack of effect on serum prolactin, greater efficacy for refractory schizophrenia, and greater activity against negative symptoms.[86] However, currently there are no widely accepted characteristics that define an "atypical" antipsychotic, and clozapine is actually the only atypical agent which fulfills *all* of the criteria stated above. Recently, the term *second-generation antipsychotic* has also been proposed to describe this class of medications, although there is no consensus on the nomenclature at the present time.[87]

MECHANISM OF DRUG ACTION

Although the specific mechanism of action of antipsychotics has not been elucidated, the focus is postsynaptic blockade at dopamine D_2 and serotonin 5-HT_{2A} receptor sites. It is generally accepted that D_2 receptor antagonism plays a key role in the treatment of positive symptoms of schizophrenia as well as in the production of EPS and hyperprolactinemia-related side effects. Knowledge of the central dopamine pathways in the brain can be used as a model to understand the therapeutic and side effects of the antipsychotics. The central dopamine system is composed of four tracts: mesolimbic, mesocortical, nigrostriatal, and tuberoinfundibular (Fig. 78-1). Drug action can be predicted if a clinician understands the function of each tract, along with the binding affinity of an agent for receptors located in the tract (Tables 78-5 and 78-6). Blockade of dopamine receptors in the mesolimbic tract is likely responsible for the reduction of positive symptoms of schizophrenia. Blockade of the other dopamine tracts is largely responsible for the adverse effects of antipsychotic treatment. The mesocortical tract is responsible for higher-order thinking and executive functions. Dopamine hypofunctioning in this area, either from the schizophrenia itself or by antipsychotic action, may be responsible for negative symptoms. The nigrostriatal tract modulates body movement. Antipsychotic-induced blockade in this area causes EPS. Lastly, antipsychotic-induced blockade of the dopamine tract in the tuberoinfundibular area of the anterior pituitary leads to hyperprolactinemia.[39] Ideally, selective dopaminergic blockade of the mesolimbic tract would be preferred. Unfortunately, typical antipsychotics block all four of these dopaminergic pathways. Studies have demonstrated that antipsychotic effects require a striatal D_2 receptor occupancy of 65% to 70%; D_2 receptor occupancy greater than 80% significantly increases the risk of EPS.[88,89] During chronic treatment with typical antipsychotic agents, between 70% and 90% of D_2 receptors in the striatum are usually occupied.[90] Not surprisingly, all the typical antipsychotic agents have been observed to be effective in reducing positive symptoms of schizophrenia and they all can cause EPS and TD.

In contrast with typical antipsychotic agents that affect all four dopamine tracts, atypical antipsychotics primarily affect dopamine tracts in the limbic system and have been termed *limbic specific*.[39] For example, therapeutic doses of risperidone, olanzapine, and ziprasidone produce >70% occupancy at D_2 receptors.[91,92] However, attributing antipsychotic efficacy solely to D_2 receptor effects is an oversimplification because many patients do not respond to medication despite adequate D_2 occupancy.[88] Furthermore, low levels of D_2 striatal receptor occupancy (<70%) have been observed with therapeutic doses of clozapine and quetiapine. This may explain the low propensity of these agents to produce EPS, but also calls into question the minimum receptor occupancy necessary for antipsychotic efficacy as proposed for typical agents.[92,93]

Blockade of the 5-HT_{2A} receptors, a shared property of the atypical agents, has been investigated with regard to its significance in mediating antipsychotic effects.[94] At therapeutic doses, most atypical agents occupy more than 80% of cortical 5-HT_{2A} receptors.[92,95,96] Blockade of 5-HT_{2A} receptors, independent of D_2 antagonism, has not been demonstrated to produce antipsychotic effects. However, it is postulated that a high 5-HT_{2A} to D_2 receptor affinity ratio may underlie the enhanced therapeutic efficacy and low propensity for EPS observed with atypical antipsychotics.[39] Serotonin is known to exert a regulatory effect on dopaminergic receptors or dopamine release, but the degree of control may vary depending on the pathway. Specifically, serotonin tonically inhibits dopamine release. Therefore, 5-HT_{2A} antagonism should enhance dopaminergic transmission. It has been proposed that the atypical properties of antipsychotics (efficacy against negative symptoms and low propensity to produce EPS) are due in part to augmentation of dopaminergic function via 5-HT_{2A} blockade in the mesocortical and nigrostriatal pathways and limbic specificity.[39,97] Aripiprazole is an antipsychotic agent with unique effects at D_2 and 5-HT receptors. Specifically, this agent has partial agonist activity at D_2 and 5-HT_{1A} receptors and antagonist activity at serotonin 5-HT_{2A} receptors. Aripiprazole is a functional antagonist at D_2 receptors under hyperdopaminergic conditions but exhibits functional agonist properties under hypodopaminergic conditions.[98] Paliperidone (Invega) is the newest atypical agent approved by the U.S. Food and Drug Administration (FDA). Because paliperidone is the primary active metabolite of risperidone, 9-hydroxyrisperidone, we should expect the mechanism of action of paliperidone to be similar to that of risperidone.[99,100]

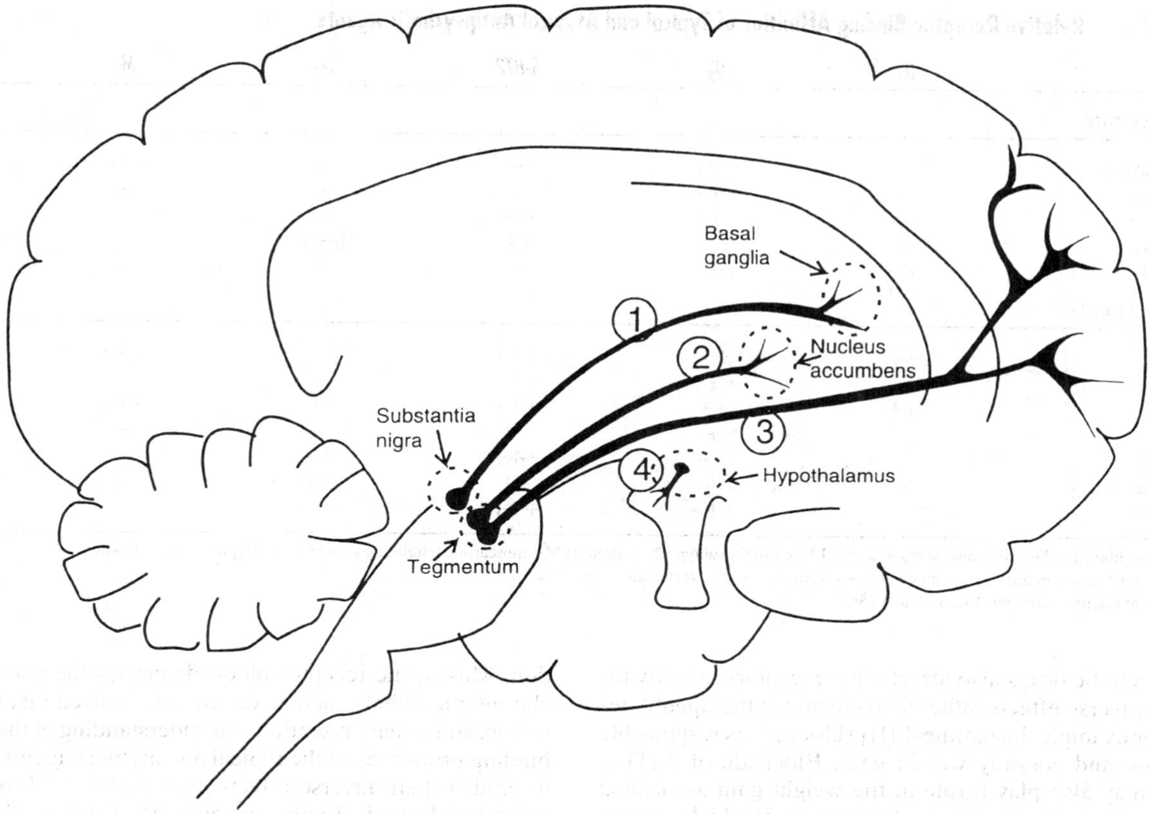

FIGURE 78-1 Four dopamine pathways in the brain. The neuroanatomy of dopamine neuronal pathways in the brain can explain both the therapeutic effects and the side effects of the known antipsychotic agents. (1) The nigrostriatal dopamine pathway projects from the substantia nigra to the basal ganglia, and is thought to control movements. (2) The mesolimbic dopamine pathway projects from the midbrain ventral tegmental area to the nucleus accumbens, a part of the limbic system of the brain thought to be involved in many behaviors, such as pleasurable sensations, the powerful euphoria of drugs of abuse, as well as delusions and hallucinations of psychosis. (3) A pathway related to the mesolimbic dopamine pathway is the mesocortical dopamine pathway. It also projects from the midbrain ventral tegmental area, but sends its axons to the limbic cortex, where it may have a role in mediating positive and negative psychotic symptoms or cognitive side effects of neuroleptic antipsychotic medications. (4) The fourth dopamine pathway of interest is the one that controls prolactin secretion, called the tuberoinfundibular dopamine pathway. It projects from the hypothalamus to the anterior pituitary gland.

Table 78-5 Neurotransmitter Tract Function and Effect of Typical Versus Atypical Antipsychotics

Neurotransmitter Tract	*Clinical Function*	*Typical Agent Effects*	*Atypical Agent Effects*
Dopamine-nigrostriatal	Modulates EPS	Potent D_2 blockade causes EPS	Minimal EPS owing to greater specificity for mesolimbic system
Dopamine-mesolimbic	Modulates arousal, memory, behavior	Effectively treats positive symptoms	Effectively treats positive symptoms
Dopamine-mesocortical	Modulates cognition, socialization, and other negative symptoms	Less effective for negative symptoms	Clozapine (possibly others) greater efficacy for negative symptoms; clozapine, risperidone (others?) may improve cognition
Dopamine-tuberoinfundibular	Regulates prolactin release	Increases prolactin release (dose related)	No increase in prolactin with clozapine, dose-related with risperidone, no significant increase with others
Serotonergic (5-HT2)	5-HT2 blockade reduces EPS, improves negative symptoms	Minimal affinity for 5-HT2 receptors	Greater affinity for 5-HT2 receptors

EPS, extrapyramidal side effects.
Adapted from references 39, 86, and 97.

Table 78-6 Relative Receptor-Binding Affinities of Typical and Atypical Antipsychotic Agents

Receptor	D_1	D_2	5-HT2	α_1	M_1	H_1
Typical Agents						
Chlorpromazine	−	+++	++	+++	+++	++
Fluphenazine	−	+++	+	+	−	−
Perphenazine	−	+++	++	++	−	++
Thioridazine	+	+++	++	+++	+++	+
Haloperidol	++	+++	+	+	−	−
Atypical Agents						
Clozapine	++	++	+++	+++	+++	+
Risperidone	−	+++	+++	+++	−	+
Olanzapine	++	++	+++	++	+++	++
Quetiapine	−	+	++	+++	+	+
Ziprasidone	±	++	+++	++	−	+
Aripiprazole	+	+++	++	++	−	+
Paliperidone	−	+++	+++	+++	−	+

D_1, dopamine subtype 1; D_2, dopamine subtype 2; 5-HT2, serotonin subtype 2; 1, alpha 1; M_1, muscarinic (cholinergic) subtype 1; H_1, histamine subtype 1.
−, none; ±, unclear; +, minimal; ++, moderate; +++, high; ++++, very high.
Compiled from references 90, 99, 100, 143, and 266.

Antipsychotic drugs also affect other receptors, usually resulting in adverse effects rather than enhanced therapeutic response. For example, histamine-1 (H_1) blockade is responsible for sedation and possibly weight gain. Blockade of 5-HT_{2C} receptors may also play a role in the weight gain associated with some atypical agents. α_1-Adrenergic blockade causes orthostatic hypotension and plays a role in sexual dysfunction. Muscarinic receptor blockade causes the classical anticholinergic effects such as dry mouth, blurred vision, constipation, and urinary retention. An understanding of the receptor-binding properties of the typical and atypical agents is helpful to predict their adverse effects profiles.[66,85,101] Properties of typical and atypical antipsychotics are listed in Tables 78-6 and 78-7.

Table 78-7 Relative Incidence of Antipsychotic Drug Adverse Effects

	Sedation	EPS	Anticholinergic	Orthostasis	Seizures	Prolactin Elevation	Weight Gain
Typical—Low Potency							
Chlorpromazine	++++	+++	+++	++++	+++	+++	++
Thioridazine	++++	++	++++	++++	++	+++	+++
Typical—High Potency							
Trifluoperazine	++	++++	++	++	+++	+++	++
Fluphenazine	++	+++++	++	++	++	+++	++
Thiothixene	++	++++	++	++	++	+++	++
Haloperidol	+	+++++	+	+	++	+++	++
Loxapine	+++	++++	++	+++	++	+++	+
Molindone	+	++++	++	++	++	+++	+
Atypicals							
Clozapine	++++	+	++++	++++	++++[c]	0	++++
Risperidone	+++	+[a]	++	+++	++	0 to +++[c]	++
Olanzapine	+++	+[b]	+++	++	++	+[c]	+++
Quetiapine	+++	+	++	++	++	0	++
Ziprasidone	++	+	++	++	++	0	+
Aripiprazole	++	+	++	++	++	0	+
Paliperidone	+++	+[a]	++	+++	++	0 to +++[c]	++

[a] Very low at dosages <8 mg/day.
[b] With dosages <20 mg/day.
[c] Dose related.
0, no effect; +, very low; ++, low; +++, moderate; ++++, high; +++++, very high; EPS, extrapyramidal side effects.
Compiled from references 58, 99, 100, 182, 143, 166, and 266.

Selection of an Antipsychotic

In all patients, the selection of a specific antipsychotic agent should be individualized. The choice of a specific medication is usually based on a number of factors and is frequently more art than science. Important factors include prior experience (efficacy and side effects), the ease of attaining a therapeutic dose, available dosage forms, and formulary or cost considerations. One of the best predictors of response is the patient's previous response to a specific antipsychotic, or a positive response in a first-degree relative. If a patient responded poorly to an antipsychotic in the past, an agent from a different chemical class should be prescribed. Also, if a patient has a particular aversion to an antipsychotic side effect, an appreciation for differences among the available antipsychotics in this regard would be helpful. Drugs with a similar side effect profile should be avoided. Although all the antipsychotic agents have been shown to be efficacious during the acute phase of schizophrenia, atypical antipsychotics (with the exception of clozapine) have become the agents of first choice for the treatment of schizophrenia. The rationale for this practice is based on the lower risk of EPS and TD with the atypical agents.

Efficacy

Typical antipsychotics are effective in reducing positive symptoms of schizophrenia during acute psychotic episodes and in preventing recurrence in many patients.[102] These agents are less effective for treating negative symptoms. In fact, there is concern that typical agents may exacerbate negative symptoms by causing drug-induced akinesia. In general, all typical antipsychotic agents are believed to be equally effective when used in equivalent doses.

Clinical trials demonstrate that the atypical agents—clozapine, risperidone, olanzapine, quetiapine, ziprasidone, aripiprazole, and paliperidone—are superior to placebo, and are at least as effective as typical antipsychotics for treatment of the positive and negative symptoms of schizophrenia.[98,103–113] In a meta-analysis of 52 randomized clinical trials comparing atypical agents (including clozapine, risperidone, quetiapine) with typical agents (haloperidol or chlorpromazine), Geddes et al.[114] found no difference in efficacy between these two drug classes if the dose of the typical agent was considered. The apparent superiority of atypical antipsychotics (in terms of efficacy and drop-out rates) could be attributed to the use of excessive doses of typical agents (>12 mg/day haloperidol or equivalent). In contrast, two other meta-analyses concluded that the atypical agents have efficacy and tolerability advantages over typical agents independent of haloperidol dosage.[115,116] Davis et al.[116] concluded that available evidence demonstrates an efficacy advantage for some (clozapine, risperidone, olanzapine) but not all atypicals (quetiapine, ziprasidone, and aripiprazole) when compared with typical agents. These authors suggest that the atypical agents are at least as efficacious as typical agents for positive symptoms, and that atypical agents are likely more efficacious with negative and cognitive symptoms. This potential advantage of the atypical agents continues to be a source of much debate. On one hand, there are some who believe that atypical agents have a unique therapeutic effect on the primary negative symptoms, whereas others contend that this finding is actually a secondary impact upon other related symptoms and disease manifestations.[117] Data on risperidone and olanzapine suggest a direct effect on primary negative symptoms independent of their effect on psychotic, depressive, or EPS.[118,119]

The National Institute of Mental Health Clinical Antipsychotic Trials of Intervention Effectiveness trial (CATIE) was a real-world trial evaluating schizophrenic patients. The trial compared the effectiveness of atypical antipsychotics (quetiapine, risperidone, clozapine, olanzapine, and, later, ziprasidone) to that of perphenazine, a midpotency typical antipsychotic.[120] Perphenazine was chosen owing to a lower incidence of EPS compared with high and other midpotency typical antipsychotics, as well as decreased sedation when compared with low-potency typical antipsychotics. In this study, 1,460 patients were included from 57 sites in 24 states. The results indicated olanzapine was least likely to be discontinued; however, it (and clozapine) had the most metabolic side effects. Perphenazine was as effective as the atypical agents, however, it had the highest incidence of EPS, even after patients with TD were excluded from receiving the medication.[121,122]

Dosage Forms

ORAL DISINTEGRATING TABLET

Pharmacotherapy during the acute phase is administered orally (as tablets or liquid concentrate) or intramuscularly (IM), depending on the patient's willingness to take medication, the risk of imminent harm, and dosage form availability. Usually, antipsychotic therapy is administered orally. The newest technology available is the oral disintegrating tablet (ODT). ODT can be in the form of a compressed tablet, compression molded tablets, and freeze-dried (lyophilized) wafers that dissolve or disintegrate within a matter of seconds when placed on the tongue. Of the atypical agents, risperidone, olanzapine, and aripiprazole are available as ODT.

SHORT-ACTING INJECTABLES

Although all of the antipsychotics are available in oral formulations, only a few are available as injectables. Short-acting IM preparations of an antipsychotic may be preferred over oral medication if a patient is agitated and not likely to be cooperative. IM preparations bypass the gastrointestinal tract and first-pass metabolism and have a faster onset of action. For example, most IM antipsychotics reach a maximum plasma level within 30 to 60 minutes and patients usually experience substantial calming within 15 minutes.[123] Of the short-acting agents available for IM use, most clinical experience has been with high-potency typical antipsychotic medications such as haloperidol or fluphenazine. Haloperidol and fluphenazine have the advantage of being calming without being sedating, but they can cause severe EPS. Some clinicians prefer low-potency agents such as chlorpromazine, because they are more sedating. Low-potency agents can also cause severe hypotension. High-potency agents can be given in larger doses because they have a lower risk of anticholinergic and cardiovascular complications than low-potency agents. In general, the use of oral typical agents has declined because of the neurologic risks. Studies have shown that the FDA-approved IM formulations of the atypical agents (olanzapine, aripiprazole, and ziprasidone) seem to be better tolerated than typical agents and are equally effective as haloperidol in the acute treatment of psychoses in patients with schizophrenia.[124,125]

Agitation is a problem that many mental health providers face. It can affect whether or not a patient can be treated at any point in time. A patient who is acutely agitated may behave in a way that may result in harm of self, others, or property. In these cases, medication is needed to calm the patient. In the past, sleep was thought to be essential in the treatment of acute agitation. This is no longer true, though, some facilities may still use this as an endpoint or goal.[126] If rapid tranquilization is required for a patient who is acutely agitated and exhibiting dangerous behavior, the combination of IM haloperidol and IM lorazepam appears more effective than either alone.[127] However, rapid tranquilization is not necessarily more effective than traditional dosing methods, and is associated with a greater incidence of acute side effects such as dystonic reactions.[128,129] Rapid tranquilization can be achieved when repeated IM injections of high-potency antipsychotics or benzodiazepines are given until the patient is either adequately calmed, a maximum recommended daily dose is reached, or dose-limiting adverse effects such as acute dystonia (antipsychotics), ataxia, or slurred speech (benzodiazepines) occur. The most commonly used regimen is haloperidol 2 to 5 mg combined with lorazepam 2 mg injected IM every 30 to 60 minutes to a maximum of three doses.[130] Patients should be monitored for severe adverse events, particularly those patients with underlying medical or neurologic problems. Vital signs should be monitored and the dose should be held if clinically significant adverse effects occur.[129,131] The concept of rapid tranquilization should not be confused with rapid neuroleptization, which implies the use of very high loading dosages of antipsychotics (e.g., administering a series of closely spaced IM doses over a period of hours) to produce a more rapid remission of psychotic symptoms.[130] The practice of rapid neuroleptization leads to a higher incidence of EPS without advantages of efficacy when compared with the administration of lower doses of the same drugs. Rapid neuroleptization is no longer recommended.[128] Most recently, with the advent of IM and fast-acting oral formulations of atypical antipsychotics, the combination has changed to decrease the incidence of EPS. Clinical trials have shown that risperidone, ziprasidone, aripiprazole, and olanzapine are at least as effective as haloperidol and lorazepam (Table 78-8).[125,126,132–139]

6. How should pharmacotherapy be used to treat the acute phase of schizophrenia in J.C., and what should be done first to manage his acute symptoms?

Aripiprazole 9.75 mg IM injection can be given to J.C. so further assessment can be completed. Aripiprazole for any a typical IM agent is a good choice because it has efficacy in calming rather than sedating the patient, it has a lower propensity for EPS and TD, and is available in a short-acting IM formulation. These are important features because J.C. is likely to refuse oral medications because of his paranoid symptoms. Also, aripiprazole IM has limited cardiovascular problems such as hypotension, bradycardia with or without hypotension, tachycardia, and syncope as compared with olanzapine IM.[132,139] Lorazepam 0.5 to 1 mg PO or IM every 4 to 6 hours as needed may be given to J.C. to control ongoing agitation, however, greater sedation and orthostatic hypotension have been observed with the combination of lorazepam and aripiprazole as compared to aripiprazole alone.[132] Subsequent doses of aripiprazole IM can be given every 2 hours if needed for agitation, up to a maximum of 30 mg/day.

7. J.C. was given a single dose of aripiprazole 9.75 mg IM. His agitation resolved after the first injection but you are later informed that this medication is not covered by J.C.'s healthplan. What is the next medication you would recommended for J.C., and what factors should be considered when selecting an antipsychotic for the acute and stabilization phases?

An antipsychotic prescribed at a dose reflective of the needs during the stabilization phase should be started now. Olanzapine, 10 mg at bedtime, is an appropriate choice for pharmacologic treatment of schizophrenia in the acute phase. With the exception of clozapine, any of the other atypical agents would also be appropriate choices.

Past experience with antipsychotics predicts therapeutic success in the selection of a regimen. J.C. does not have a past psychotropic medication history to guide drug selection. He also does not have a history of nonadherence, which would direct the choice toward a depot product. A common starting dose for olanzapine is 10 mg/day.

Table 78-8 Agents to Treat Acute Agitation

Medication	Dosage Form	Dose	Onset	Half-life	Duration of Action
Lorazepam	PO (tablet), IM, IV	1–2 mg	60–90 min	12–15 hr	8–10 hr
Typical Antipsychotics					
Haloperidol	PO (tablet), IM, IV	5–10 mg	30–60 min	12–36 hr	up to 24 hr
Droperidol	IM, IV	5–10 mg	15–30 min	2–4 hr	6–8 hr
Atypical Antipsychotics					
Olanzapine	PO (tablet), IM, ODT	10 mg	15–45 min	30 hr	24 hr
Risperidone	PO (tablet, liquid), ODT	2 mg	60 min	20 hr	Not available
Ziprasidone	PO (tablet), IM	20 mg	30–60 min	2–5 hr	4 hr
Aripiprazole	PO (tablet, liquid), IM	9.75 mg	1–3 hr	75–94 hr	Not available

IM, intramuscularly; IV, intravenously; ODT, oral disintegrating tablet; PO, orally.
Compiled from references 125, 126, and 132–139.

8. When should J.C.'s target symptoms start to respond to olanzapine?

During the first week, often known as the medicated cooperation stage, J.C. should respond to the calming properties of the antipsychotic, and his symptoms of hostility, agitation, and insomnia should improve. During the next 2 to 6 weeks, the improved socialization stage, J.C. should begin to obey hospital rules, attend ward meetings, and generally become more sociable. Severely ill schizophrenic patients with chronic disease may never reach this stage. The elimination of the thought disorder stage can occur within any time frame, but usually takes at least 2 to 3 weeks and up to several months to occur. During this stage, the core symptoms of schizophrenia such as delusions, hallucinations, and thought disturbance improve. If no improvement of J.C.'s core symptoms is observed after 3 weeks of olanzapine 10 mg/day, then the dose should be increased slowly to 15 or 20 mg/day and the patient should be observed for another 3 to 4 weeks.

9. It is 6 months later. Most of J.C.'s symptoms have improved, he is residing in assisted living housing and working part-time at Goodwill Industries. Although he is not troubled by any side effects, he sees no point in continuing his medication. Should olanzapine be discontinued? What are the current practice guidelines regarding long-term treatment?

J.C. clearly is responding well to olanzapine and has no side effects. To minimize risk of relapse, he should continue his current regimen for at least another 6 months. If his symptoms remain stable and he maintains good psychosocial functioning (e.g., continues work, keeps close contact with social workers, attends medication groups), discontinuation of therapy can be considered.

When J.C. has been stabilized for a total of approximately 1 year on olanzapine 10 mg/day, then the dose can be reduced by 20% every 3 to 6 months until it is discontinued or relapse occurs. If he exhibits recurrent target symptoms of schizophrenia or decompensation, then the dose should be increased to the previous effective dose (or medication restarted if it was discontinued). Because it is likely that J.C. will require lifelong antipsychotics, it is important to determine the minimal effective dose to prevent recurrence, while minimizing the risk of adverse effects. J.C. is not a candidate for intermittent therapy during the stable phase. He is not a decanoate candidate because he is compliant with treatment.

LONG-ACTING DEPOT INJECTABLES

Long-acting depot medications are not recommended for acute psychotic episodes because these medications take months to reach a steady-state concentration and are eliminated very slowly.[58] Hence, it is difficult to correlate clinical effect with dosage, and it is extremely difficult to make dosage adjustments to manage side effects. However, long-acting depot medications can be useful for maintenance therapy in patients with a history of nonadherence to their oral medication and in those who prefer the convenience of long-acting or depot injections. In these situations, the oral form of available depot medications should be initiated first. If the oral form has been shown to be safe and effective, the patient can be converted to the depot form. Fluphenazine, haloperidol, and risperidone are available as long-acting decanoate injections. Long-acting injectable risperidone appears to combine the most valuable features of an atypical antipsychotic (broadly efficacious and well tolerated) with those of injectable long-acting antipsychotics (improved bioavailability and assured medication delivery).[141,142]

Pharmacokinetics and Drug Interactions

Dosing considerations also have a major influence on safe and effective antipsychotic selections. Specific factors include the number of times a day a medication needs to be administered, the difference between a starting dose and a "target" therapeutic dose (i.e., titration required), and the risk for drug–drug interactions. The long half-life (12–24 hours) and active metabolites of most oral antipsychotic drugs allow for once- to twice-daily dosing.[143] Most antipsychotics, with the exception of clozapine and ziprasidone, can be safely given once a day. Most antipsychotics achieve a steady-state concentration in 4 to 7 days, but it is important to understand that the onset of antipsychotic effect is not related to achieving steady state. Pharmacologic effects often persist for longer than pharmacokinetics would imply. In some instances, treatment is initiated at a subtherapeutic dose and gradually titrated upward to an effective dose. This approach is taken to allow the patient to develop tolerance to adverse events such as sedation or orthostatic hypotension. In the case of acute agitation, antipsychotic doses are also often divided, despite the long half-lives of these drugs, such that the sedative effects are maintained over the day. Once a patient has been stabilized or has become tolerant to the adverse effects, the goal is to give medication once a day, usually at bedtime. Bedtime dosing enhances medication adherence and concentrates ongoing adverse effects such as sedation at night.

Both pharmacokinetic and pharmacodynamic drug interactions can occur with antipsychotic agents. Cytochrome P450 enzymes, especially the 1A2, 2D6, and 3A4 isoenzymes, are responsible for the metabolism of many antipsychotics.[144] Induction or inhibition of these enzymes by other drugs may result in clinically important drug interactions. Table 78-9 summarizes the metabolic pathways for commonly used antipsychotic drugs. In the case of clozapine, serious complications such as seizures can occur when drug interactions cause serum concentrations of clozapine to rise significantly. Examples of drugs that have the potential to cause serious interactions with antipsychotics include fluvoxamine (CYP 1A2 inhibitor), erythromycin, ketoconazole, and ritonavir (CYP 3A4 inhibitors), quinidine, risperidone, fluoxetine, and paroxetine (CYP 2D6 inhibitors), and cimetidine (multiple enzyme inhibition).[145] Conversely, inducers of drug metabolism such as carbamazepine (induces multiple enzymes) or cigarette smoking (induces CYP 1A2) can reduce the plasma concentrations of antipsychotic drugs. For example, carbamazepine has been shown to reduce plasma concentrations of haloperidol by 50%.[146] Cigarette smoking has been shown to increase the metabolism of clozapine and olanzapine.[144] Pharmacodynamic interactions may occur when medications with similar unwanted properties are concurrently prescribed. For example, concomitant use of low-potency typical agents or clozapine along with diphenhydramine or hydroxyzine may cause augmentation of anticholinergic effects. Pharmacodynamic drug interactions of greatest concern are those that can cause

Table 78-9 Pharmacokinetic Comparisons of Antipsychotics

Antipsychotic Agent	Mean Half-Life (hr)	Major Cytochrome P450 Pathway	Plasma Concentration Range
Chlorpromazine	8–35	2D6	Not well defined
Thioridazine	9–30	2D6	Not well defined
Perphenazine	8–21	2D6	Not well defined
Fluphenazine	14–24	2D6	0.2–2.8 mg/mL
Fluphenazine decanoate	8 days	2D6	0.2–2.8 mg/mL
Thiothixene	34	2D6	2–15 mg/mL
Haloperidol	12–36	2D6	4–12 ng/mL
Haloperidol decanoate	21 days	2D6	4–12 ng/mL
Loxapine	5–15	None	Not well defined
Molindone	10–20	None	Not well defined
Clozapine	16	1A2, 3A4	350–420 μg/mL suggested
Risperidone	22	2D6	Not well defined
Olanzapine	30	1A2	>23.2 ng/mL @ 12 hours post dose
Quetiapine	7	3A4	Not well defined
Ziprasidone	4–5	3A4	Not well defined
Aripiprazole	75–94	2D6, 3A4	Not well defined
Paliperidone	23	Limited 2D6, 3A4	Not well defined

Compiled from references 99, 132, 143, 144, 248, and 266.

significant orthostatic hypotensive, anticholinergic effects, and sedation. Pharmacokinetic and dosing information for the antipsychotics are provided in Tables 78-9 and 78-10.

Pharmacoeconomic Considerations

Although medication expenditures represent only a small portion of total resource utilization associated with the management of schizophrenia, concern exists about the cost of atypical antipsychotics and whether their relative advantages over typical agents are worth their increased cost.[147] Drug acquisition costs for atypical antipsychotics can be 100-fold higher than typical antipsychotics. Most pharmacoeconomic studies with atypical antipsychotics show that these agents are at least cost neutral and may offer cost advantages compared with traditional agents when total mental health costs are considered.[148] Depending on the individual study, the higher costs associated with atypical antipsychotics are offset by decreased number of hospital admissions, length of inpatient stay, and number of outpatient visits. Hence, drug costs should not be the sole factor considered when selecting an antipsychotic. The selection of a medication should be individualized and factors such as efficacy, side effects, patient acceptance, and total health care costs should be considered.

Adverse Effects

An important factor in the selection of an antipsychotic is the potential risk for adverse events. Key adverse effects that differentiate the antipsychotics include EPS, anticholinergic side effects, cardiac effects, hyperprolactinemia, metabolic effects and sedation. Table 78-7 compares antipsychotic agents with regard to the risk of these adverse effects.

EXTRAPYRAMIDAL SIDE EFFECTS AND TARDIVE SYNDROMES

EPS is a broad term that describes several types of acute and chronic drug-induced movement disorders. Acute dystonia, parkinsonism, and akathisia all occur early in treatment, whereas TD, tardive dystonia, and tardive akathisia have a late onset, usually after years of treatment. The acute forms of EPS usually develop soon after the initiation of antipsychotics, are dose dependent, and are generally reversible soon after discontinuation of the offending agent.[149] It has been estimated that 60% of patients who receive typical antipsychotics develop some form of EPS acutely.[58] In general, typical agents are more likely to cause EPS than atypical agents when these medications are used at usual therapeutic doses. Among the seven currently available atypical agents, clozapine and quetiapine are associated with the lowest risk for EPS. The rising prescription rate of atypical antipsychotics (and decrease in use of the typical agents) have substantially reduced the problem of EPS. Similarly, the risk of antipsychotic-induced TD is suggested to be lower with atypical agents compared with typical agents. Most of the evidence documenting a decreased incidence of TD with atypical agents is derived from data and clinical experience with clozapine, risperidone, olanzapine, and quetiapine.[150–153]

Acute Dystonia

Acute dystonia has the earliest onset of all the EPS symptoms. Most cases occur within the first few hours or days after initiation or dose increase of antipsychotic medication. Dystonia is characterized by sustained muscle contractions. Common presentations of antipsychotic-induced dystonia include a sudden onset of brief or sustained abnormal postures, including tongue protrusion, oculogyric crisis (eyes rolling back into head), trismus (spasm of the jaw), torticollis (torsion of the neck); opisthotonos (arching of back), and unusual positions in the trunk, limbs, and toes. Laryngeal dystonias are the most serious dystonias and are potentially fatal. Risk factors for acute dystonia include younger age, male gender, high dosage of high-potency typical antipsychotics, and previous history of dystonia.[58]

The exact pathophysiology of acute dystonia is uncertain. Conflicting theories describe either a hypodopaminergic or hyperdopaminergic state after an antipsychotic-induced blockade of postsynaptic dopamine receptors. Acute dystonia likely is caused by dysregulation of the dopamine system and

Table 78-10 Antipsychotic Relative Potency and Adult Dosing

Drug and Chemical Class	Dose Equivalence	Usual Starting Dose (mg/day)	Acute Phase Dosage (mg/day)	Maintenance/Stable Phase Dosage (mg/day)
Typical Agents–Phenothiazines				
Aliphatic type				
Chlorpromazine (Thorazine)	100	50–200	300–1,500[a]	150–800
Piperidine type				
Thioridazine (Mellaril)	100	50–200	300–800	150–600
Piperazine type				
Perphenazine (Trilafon)	10	4–16	32–64[a]	8–48
Trifluoperazine (Stelazine)	5	2–10	10–80	5–30
Fluphenazine (Prolixin)	2	2–10	5–80	2–20
Typical Agents–Nonphenothiazines				
Thioxanthene				
Thiothixene (Navane)	4	2–10	5–60[a]	5–30
Butyrophenone				
Haloperidol (Haldol)	2	2–10	5–100	2–20
Dibenzoxazepine				
Loxapine (Loxitane)	10	10–20	50–250[c]	25–100
Dihydroindolone				
Molindone (Moban)	10	25–75	25–225	25–100
Diphenylbutylpiperidone				
Pimozide (Orap)	1	1–2	10–30	2–6
Atypical Agents				
Risperidone (Risperdal)	2	1–2	2–16	2–8
Clozapine (Clozaril)	50	12.5–25	150–900	150–600
Olanzapine (Zyprexa)	5	5–10	10–20	10–20
Quetiapine (Seroquel)	75	50–100	300–750	400–600
Ziprasidone (Geodon)	60	40–80	80–200	80–160
Aripiprazole (Abilify)	7.5	10–15	10–30	15–30
Paliperidone (Invega)	3	6	6–12	6–12

[a]Dosages can be exceeded with caution, but high-dose therapy is rarely needed.
Compiled from references 57, 66, 80, 144, 151, 239, 241, and 256.

imbalance between neurotransmitter systems after acute antipsychotic administration.[154]

10. J.P., a 19-year-old man, was brought to the psychiatric ED because of assaultive behavior toward his mother. J.P. states he struck her because the devil told him to do it. Trifluoperazine 5 mg IM Q 4 to 6 hr PRN was started to control his assaultive behavior. He received four IM injections over 24 hours and was converted to 15 mg PO HS. On day 2 of the admission he complained of a stiff neck and protruding tongue. J.P. became very upset and wanted to leave the hospital and never take these medications again. No other medical conditions were noted. What evidence suggests that J.P. is experiencing an acute dystonia reaction?

The sudden appearance of a stiff neck and a protruding tongue in J.P. is consistent with acute dystonia. In addition, J.P.'s young age, male gender, and use of a high-potency typical antipsychotic agent also place him at high risk for experiencing a dystonic reaction.

11. How should acute dystonia be treated in J.P.?

Acute dystonic reactions are sudden in onset, dramatic in appearance, and can cause patients great distress. It requires immediate treatment. The initial goal of treatment is to relieve symptoms as soon as possible with either benztropine 1 to 2 mg or diphenhydramine 25 to 50 mg by IM injection. Although the IV route has a faster onset of action, it is not needed in J.P. because his reaction is not severe. If symptoms do not resolve within 15 to 30 minutes, then the dose should be repeated. If there are contraindications to the use of anticholinergic drugs, lorazepam 1 to 2 mg IM can be used. J.P. must be reassured that this is a temporary condition that can be prevented and treated. To prevent another reaction, J.P. should be given oral anticholinergic drugs in doses commonly used for pseudoparkinsonism for 2 weeks after this dystonic reaction.[154]

Parkinsonism

The clinical presentation of antipsychotic-induced parkinsonism includes bradykinesia or akinesia, which may be associated with decreased arm swinging, a masklike face, drooling, decreased eye blinking, and soft, monotonous speech, tremor, which is most commonly a rhythmic, resting tremor, and rigidity of the extremities, neck or trunk (most identifiable in the limbs as a "cogwheel" rigidity during passive motion).[154] Antipsychotic-induced parkinsonism occurs in approximately 20% of patients treated with antipsychotic agents.[58] Symptoms can occur at any time, but usually develop within 4 weeks after antipsychotic initiation or a dose increase. Advanced age,

Table 78-11 Common Rating Instruments for Schizophrenia and Antipsychotics

Psychosis
Brief Psychiatric Rating Scale (BPRS)
Positive and Negative Symptom Scale for Schizophrenia (PANSS)
Scale for Assessment of Positive Symptoms (SAPS)
Scale for Assessment of Negative Symptoms (SANS)
Movement Disorders—Tardive Dyskinesia
Abnormal Involuntary Movement Scale (AIMS)
Dyskinesia Identification System Condensed User Scale (DISCUS)
Movement Disorders—Parkinsonism
Simpson Angus Scale for Extrapyramidal Symptoms
Movement Disorders—Akathisia
Barnes Akathisia Scale

Table 78-12 Agents to Treat Antipsychotic-Induced Parkinsonism and Akathisia

Medication	*Equivalent Dose (mg)*	*Dose/Day (mg)*
Anticholinergic		
Benztropine (Cogentin)[a]	0.5	2–8
Biperiden (Akineton)[a]	0.5	2–8
Diphenhydramine (Benadryl)[a]	25	50–250
Procyclidine (Kemadrin)	1.5	10–20
Trihexyphenidyl (Artane)	1	2–15
Dopaminergic		
Amantadine	–	100–300
GABAminergic		
Diazepam (Valium)	10	5–40
Clonazepam (Klonopin)	2	1–3
Lorazepam (Ativan)[a]	2	1–3
Noradrenergic Blockers		
Propranolol (Inderal)	–	30–120

[a]Oral dose or IM injection can be used.

antipsychotic dose and potency, and preexisting EPS are the major risk factors for antipsychotic-induced parkinsonism.[155] The Simpson Angus Rating Scale is used commonly to assess the presence and severity of EPS (Table 78-11).[156]

Antipsychotic-induced parkinsonism (as well as idiopathic Parkinson's disease) is thought to be due to postsynaptic dopamine receptor blockade in the nigrostriatal system, leading to an imbalance between the dopaminergic and cholinergic systems. Reasons for the delay in onset between receptor blockade, which occurs within hours after initiating an antipsychotic, and development of symptoms are not well understood.[154]

Atypical antipsychotics are the mainstay of the pharmacologic management of psychosis in patients vulnerable to developing antipsychotic-induced parkinsonism. The reduced parkinsonian liability of atypical antipsychotics has been associated with their limbic specificity, 5-HT_{2A} blocking effects and in some cases less D_2 receptor blockade.[89,92,97]

12. S.B., a 46-year-old man, has a diagnosis of chronic undifferentiated schizophrenia and was treated with loxapine 50 mg TID with inadequate response. The dose cannot be increased due to oversedation. Because of the incomplete response, S.B. was switched to haloperidol 5 mg Q AM and 10 mg QHS. One week after the switch, S.B. returns to the clinic complaining of feeling "real slow." He has a bilateral hand tremor that improves when he picks up his coffee cup. Physical examination detected cogwheel rigidity in both arms, although it was worse on the right side. S.B. wants to be taken off this "bad" medication. What evidence suggests that S.B. has antipsychotic-induced parkinsonism?

The onset of symptoms within 1 week of starting a new, high-potency typical antipsychotic is the first clue to the presence of EPS. The "slow feeling" possibly is indicative of akinesia, and S.B.'s bilateral tremor and cogwheel rigidity also are features of antipsychotic-induced parkinsonism.

13. What antiparkinsonian drug could be selected for S.B., if any?

In mild cases of antipsychotic-induced parkinsonism, immediate intervention may not be required if the movement disorder is not bothersome to the patient. For troublesome cases, as experienced by S.B., the simplest intervention is to reduce the antipsychotic (haloperidol) dose to the lowest effective level. If dose reduction is not possible, then an antiparkinsonian agent can be added (Table 78-12).[154]

All anticholinergic antiparkinsonian agents are equally effective for antipsychotic-induced parkinsonism, although there are differences in adverse effects and duration of action. Trihexyphenidyl is the least sedating but more prone to abuse, whereas diphenhydramine is the most sedating. Benztropine has the longest duration and can be used once or twice a day if needed, whereas the others have to be used three to four times a day. Benztropine 1 mg twice a day orally could be initiated for S.B. because he is likely too psychiatrically unstable to tolerate a reduction in the haloperidol dose. The tremor, rigidity, and akinesia should begin to resolve within the first few days of treatment. Alternatively, a switch to an atypical antipsychotic may negate the need for an antiparkinsonian drug in S.B.

14. Benztropine 1 mg BID is started one week later, all of S.B.'s acute symptoms of parkinsonism have disappeared. How long should benztropine be continued in S.B. now that his EPS are resolved?

The long-term treatment of antipsychotic-induced parkinsonism with antiparkinsonian medication is controversial.[154] The World Health Organization published a consensus statement recommending that the prophylactic use of anticholinergic medication in patients receiving antipsychotics should be avoided or used only in cases where alternative strategies have failed.[157] For S.B., an attempt to taper and discontinue the antiparkinsonian treatment should be initiated 6 weeks to 3 months after symptoms resolve. Unfortunately, as many as 30% of patients chronically treated with typical antipsychotics continue to experience parkinsonian symptoms.[90] If that should occur with S.B., he should be switched to an atypical agent.

15. What risks are associated with long-term anticholinergic treatment?

The risks of anticholinergics include constipation, dry mouth leading to dental caries, and blurred vision. They can also impair memory, especially in older patients. Some patients develop tolerance to these adverse effects, but others do not, even with chronic use. Patients sometimes abuse anticholinergic medications for their mood-elevating and hallucinogenic effects. Abuse may be confused with reluctance to discontinue antiparkinsonian medication because of the fear of recurrent EPS or ongoing symptoms.

16. One week after the benztropine was started, S.B.'s psychiatric symptoms began to respond to the haloperidol, but he developed acute urinary retention. Reduction of the benztropine dose to 1 mg/day did not improve his urinary retention. What alternative treatments without anticholinergic effects are available to manage S.B.'s pseudo-parkinsonian symptoms?

S.B. is just beginning to gain benefit from his haloperidol; therefore, the haloperidol dose should not be reduced. Amantadine, an antiparkinsonian medication that directly stimulates postsynaptic dopamine receptors and restores the cholinergic and dopaminergic balance in the nigrostriatum, would be a reasonable alternative to benztropine in S.B. Amantadine is an option for patients who cannot tolerate or who respond poorly to anticholinergic drugs. It often is preferred in the elderly because of the lower incidence of cognitive impairment. The parkinsonian symptoms usually respond within 24 hours.

S.B. should be started on amantadine 100 mg twice a day and benztropine should be discontinued. He should be monitored to determine whether EPS reappear and his urinary retention problem is corrected. S.B. also should be monitored for the appearance of amantadine-associated, dose-related adverse effects such as tremor, slurred speech, ataxia, depression, hallucinations, rash, orthostatic hypotension, and insomnia. If he cannot tolerate amantadine, or if amantadine does not control his EPS, an atypical antipsychotic agent can be considered.

Akathisia

Akathisia is a syndrome consisting of subjective feelings of restlessness or the urge to move and an objective motor component expressed as a semipurposeful movement most often involving the lower extremities (pacing, rocking, and an inability to sit or stand in one place for extended periods of time). Akathisia is observed in up to 50% of patients treated with typical antipsychotics and ranges from 5% to 15% of patients treated with atypical agents.[58,158] Akathisia is often extremely distressing to patients, is a common cause of medication nonadherence and, if allowed to persist, can produce dysphoria and possibly aggressive or suicidal behavior.[58] It is often difficult to distinguish from psychomotor agitation and worsening psychosis. Hence, the clinician must take care not to misdiagnose akathisia because an increase in antipsychotic dose could worsen this adverse event. It usually develops within days to weeks after initiating antipsychotic therapy.

The pathophysiology of akathisia is unclear, but much attention has focused on two theories.[154] One theory states that the mesocortical postsynaptic dopamine blockade leads to increased locomotor activity. An alternate theory claims that akathisia is caused by dopamine antagonist-induced dysregulation of noradrenergic tracts that project from the locus ceruleus to the limbic system.

17. J.P. was diagnosed with paranoid schizophrenia. His acute episode improved with trifluoperazine 15 mg HS, and he had no other dystonic reactions. Two weeks later he became increasingly agitated, began pacing the floor, was unable to sit or lie down for longer than 10 minutes at a time, and subjectively had a feeling that he described as "I have ants in my pants." J.P. is observed rocking back and forth from one foot to the other while standing in line for his dinner. He has no symptoms of antipsychotic-induced parkinsonism. Should the dose of trifluoperazine be increased?

J.P.'s symptoms of rocking, pacing, agitation, and the inability to sit still are consistent with akathisia. Because his psychiatric symptoms have improved and the new symptoms developed within 2 weeks after the initiation of trifluoperazine, a diagnosis of akathisia is more probable than unresponsiveness to the antipsychotic medication. Therefore, the trifluoperazine dose should not be increased because it can worsen the akathisia.

18. How should J.P.'s akathisia be managed?

Akathisia is less responsive to treatment than are antipsychotic-induced parkinsonism and dystonia.[58] As an initial approach to manage his akathisia, a small reduction (5 mg/day) in his trifluoperazine dosage should be attempted. If symptoms of his psychosis return or if the akathisia persists, the addition of a β-blocking agent, an anticholinergic drug, or a benzodiazepine can be considered.[58,154] Propranolol would be a recommended agent because there is a suggestion that its efficacy and safety profile may be preferable compared with other agents.[159] Anticholinergic drugs are appropriate alternatives if antipsychotic-induced parkinsonism is present. If his symptoms do not improve in response to a dosage reduction of his trifluoperazine within 1 week, J.P. should be started on propranolol 20 mg three times a day, and the dose should be increased by 20 mg every other day to a maximum of 120 mg, if necessary.[159] He has no contraindications to β-blocker therapy and does not have antipsychotic-induced parkinsonism; therefore, antiparkinsonian agents (Table 78-12) are not preferred over propranolol. If the akathisia persists after a trial of propranolol 120 mg/day therapy for 1 week, benzodiazepines should be tried or he should be switched to an atypical antipsychotic.

Tardive Dyskinesia (TD)

TD is a syndrome characterized by involuntary choreoathetoid movements that occurs in individuals taking long-term antipsychotics. The face (tics, blinking, grimacing), tongue (chewing, protrusion, tremor, writhing), lips (smacking, pursing, puckering), neck and trunk (torsion and torticollis), and limbs (toe tapping, pill rolling, and writhing) are commonly involved. The movements may be choreiform (rapid, jerky, nonrepetitive), athetoid (slow, sinuous, continual), or rhythmic (stereotypic) in nature.

TD occurs in approximately 20% of patients who receive long-term treatment with typical agents.[149] The cumulative annual incidence is approximately 5% through the first 4 years of treatment in an adult who receives typical antipsychotic treatment.[160] Advancing age is the most consistently observed risk factor for the development of TD.[161] The annual incidence rates of developing TD are three- to fivefold higher in older patients compared with younger adults.[162,163] Other risk factors include higher mean daily and cumulative antipsychotic doses, and presence of extrapyramidal signs early in treatment.[162,163] Although there is some indication that the risk of TD may be higher in women, nonwhites, patients with affective psychiatric disorders, and patients taking concomitant anticholinergic agents, these findings have not been consistently observed.[161]

For most patients, TD does not seem to be progressive or irreversible; it can be reversed with discontinuation of the antipsychotic agent. The onset of symptoms tends to be subtle with a fluctuating course.[161] Most TD cases are relatively mild. However, a portion of patients (5%–10%) may develop a form of TD that is severe enough to impair functioning.[164] Severe oral dyskinesia may result in dental and denture problems that can progress to ulceration and infection of the mouth as well as muffled or unintelligible speech. Severe orofacial TD can impair eating and swallowing, which in turn could produce significant health problems. Gait disturbances owing to limb dyskinesia may leave patients vulnerable to falls and injuries.

Although the exact cause of TD is unknown, dopaminergic hypersensitivity, disturbed balance between dopamine and cholinergic systems, dysfunction of GABAergic and noradrenergic systems and neurotoxicity via free radicals have been proposed.[149]

19. C.M., a 31-year-old woman, was diagnosed with chronic paranoid schizophrenia 9 years ago. She responds to antipsychotic drugs, but has been hospitalized six times because of nonadherence to her medications. She has taken loxapine, haloperidol, and fluphenazine in the past and currently is being treated with trifluoperazine 25 mg HS (decreased from 30 mg 1 month ago). C.M. also has been taking trihexyphenidyl 2 mg TID for the past 5 years. Involuntary movements (including tongue protrusion, frequent blinking, and writhing movements of her legs) were noted during a recent evaluation. What data in C.M.'s history are consistent with TD?

The 9 years of antipsychotic treatment and the symptoms of tongue protrusion, blinking, and writhing leg movements are consistent with TD. Long-term anticholinergic treatment (trihexyphenidyl) also may contribute to the development of C.M.'s abnormal movements.

20. C.M. has no history of abnormal movements and currently has no EPS. What disorders or medications can produce symptoms similar to those of TD?

Tourette syndrome, dental problems, Huntington's or Sydenham's chorea, chorea of pregnancy, and systemic lupus erythematosus are among the disorders that have been associated with dyskinetic movements. Medications such as metoclopramide, amoxapine, bromocriptine, levodopa/carbidopa, and pramipexole[165] also can cause TD. Spontaneous dyskinesia resembles TD but can occur in patients without previous exposure to antipsychotic medications.[161] This form of abnormal movement is noticeably more common in elderly patients. A baseline dyskinesia rating is essential before treating elderly patients with antipsychotic medications to avoid the potential diagnostic dilemma of differentiating spontaneous dyskinesia from antipsychotic-induced TD.

TD varies in severity and presentation and is reversible in many cases; therefore, rating scales are needed to standardize assessments (Table 78-11). A temporal relationship between an antipsychotic dose change and movement severity should be evaluated when performing assessments. An increase in the antipsychotic dose can clinically suppress the symptoms, whereas a decrease in dose can transiently unmask the movements often called "withdrawal dyskinesia."[165] For example, the movements C.M. is exhibiting may have worsened as a result of the recent dose reduction in trifluoperazine. On the other hand, a dose increase may produce a temporary lessening of movement severity. Patients taking long-term antipsychotics should be evaluated for TD every 3 to 6 months using a standardized rating scale (Table 78-11). Findings always should be documented in patient records to ensure continuity of care.

21. C.M. is diagnosed with antipsychotic-induced TD. How should C.M.'s TD be managed?

Management of TD should focus first on prevention. That is, antipsychotic drugs must be reserved to treat conditions known to respond (e.g., psychotic disorders such as schizophrenia, major depression with psychotic features, schizoaffective disorder), and the total dose and duration of treatment should be minimized. Because C.M.'s long-term exposure to antipsychotics is the likely cause of her TD, discontinuation of her trifluoperazine would be the ideal treatment. Unfortunately, she has experienced multiple recurrent psychotic episodes and requires lifetime treatment with antipsychotics. Because of the reduced TD liability with atypicals, C.M. should be switched to an atypical agent.[150–153] It has been recommended that an atypical antipsychotic be used for mild TD symptoms, and that clozapine be considered when TD is severe or distressing to the patient.[150,166] Rapid reduction in the dose of trifluoperazine must be avoided to prevent severe withdrawal dyskinesias, but her dose should be slowly reduced as an atypical antipsychotic is titrated to the lowest effective dose. This minimizes both her exposure to antipsychotic medications and her corresponding dyskinesia risk. Trihexyphenidyl should also be discontinued because of its possible contribution to TD. Because C.M. has already been diagnosed with TD, an evaluation of the risks and benefits of continued antipsychotic treatment must be discussed with her and documented in the chart.

22. Are there other medications for treating T.D.?

A number of other agents have been studied for their potential therapeutic effects on TD. Drugs that augment GABA neurotransmission (e.g., diazepam, clonazepam, valproic acid), adrenergic drugs (propranolol, clonidine) and free-radical scavengers (vitamin E) have all been used, with limited or inconsistent results.[160,167,168] These agents may be useful as adjunctive treatments when TD persists despite the use of atypical agents.

ANTICHOLINERGIC EFFECTS

Anticholinergic effects are more significant with low-potency typical antipsychotics, and with the atypical agents, clozapine and olanzapine. Clinically, patients complain of constipation, urinary retention, and dry eyes, mouth, and throat. Dry mouth and throat can cause several additional problems, including dental caries and weight gain if thirst is satisfied with high-sugar drinks. Oral fungal infections can also occur if gum or liquids with high sugar content are regularly consumed. The most serious complications from medications with anticholinergic properties are delirium and adynamic ileus.[169,170] Interestingly, clozapine causes significant hypersalivation despite its anticholinergic effects. The mechanism is unknown, but it may be caused by clozapine's augmentation of the adrenergic receptors that control salivation.[171] Drug therapy with benztropine, amitriptyline, and clonidine may alleviate hypersalivation; however, these agents are not effective in all patients and when they are beneficial tolerance may develop. Although anticholinergic effects are a minor problem with high-potency typical agents, some patients may still have problems when anticholinergic antiparkinsonian agents are added to treat EPS.

CARDIOVASCULAR EFFECTS

Orthostatic Hypotension

Antipsychotic drugs can cause a variety of cardiovascular complications, but the most common problem is orthostasis from α_1-adrenergic blockade. Low-potency typical agents and atypical antipsychotics pose the greatest risk for producing orthostatic hypotension. Orthostasis is most likely to occur during the first few days of treatment or when increasing the dose of medication. Although tolerance usually occurs within 2 to 3 weeks, orthostasis necessitates slow dose titration early in treatment for patients who are particularly prone to this side effect (e.g., the elderly).

Tachycardia

Tachycardia may occur as a result of the anticholinergic effects of antipsychotic medications on vagal inhibition, or secondary to orthostatic hypotension.[58] Clozapine produces the most pronounced tachycardia. If tachycardia is sustained or becomes symptomatic, low doses of a β-blocker such as atenolol or propranolol can be useful once an ECG has ruled out other medical causes.

Electrocardiographic Changes

ECG changes such as prolongation of the QT and PR intervals, ST-segment depression and T-wave flattening have been observed with antipsychotics.[172] The most clinically important of these potential changes is prolongation of the QTc interval (which is the QT interval adjusted for heart rate) and has drawn the attention of the FDA. QTc prolongation may lead to the development of ventricular tachyarrhythmias such as torsades de pointes and ventricular fibrillation, which can cause syncope, cardiac arrest, or sudden cardiac death. All antipsychotics have the potential to prolong the QTc interval to varying degrees. In 2000, Pfizer in consultation with the FDA, completed a study in which the QTc intervals of patients taking several antipsychotics, at usual therapeutic dosages and in the presence of a metabolic inhibitor, was compared (Fig. 78-2).[173] Thioridazine was shown to prolong the QTc interval at least 20 msec longer than haloperidol, risperidone, olanzapine, or quetiapine. This led to a boxed warning on the FDA-approved product labeling stating that thioridazine has been shown to prolong the QTc interval in a dose-related manner and its use should be limited to patients who cannot be managed on other antipsychotics. In the same study, ziprasidone prolonged the QTc interval 5 to 15 msec longer than did haloperidol, risperidone, olanzapine, or quetiapine. Unlike thioridazine, the ziprasidone effects were not dose related. The exact point at which QTc prolongation becomes clinically dangerous is unclear. Because most reported cases of torsades de pointes have appeared in individuals with a QT interval >500 msec, discontinuation of the suspected offending agent has been recommended if the interval consistently exceeds 500 msec. It is important to note that no patients in this study had QTc intervals exceeding 500 msec or arrhythmias. Despite the fact that no increased risk of arrhythmia or sudden death has been demonstrated with ziprasidone, caution is warranted in patients with some types

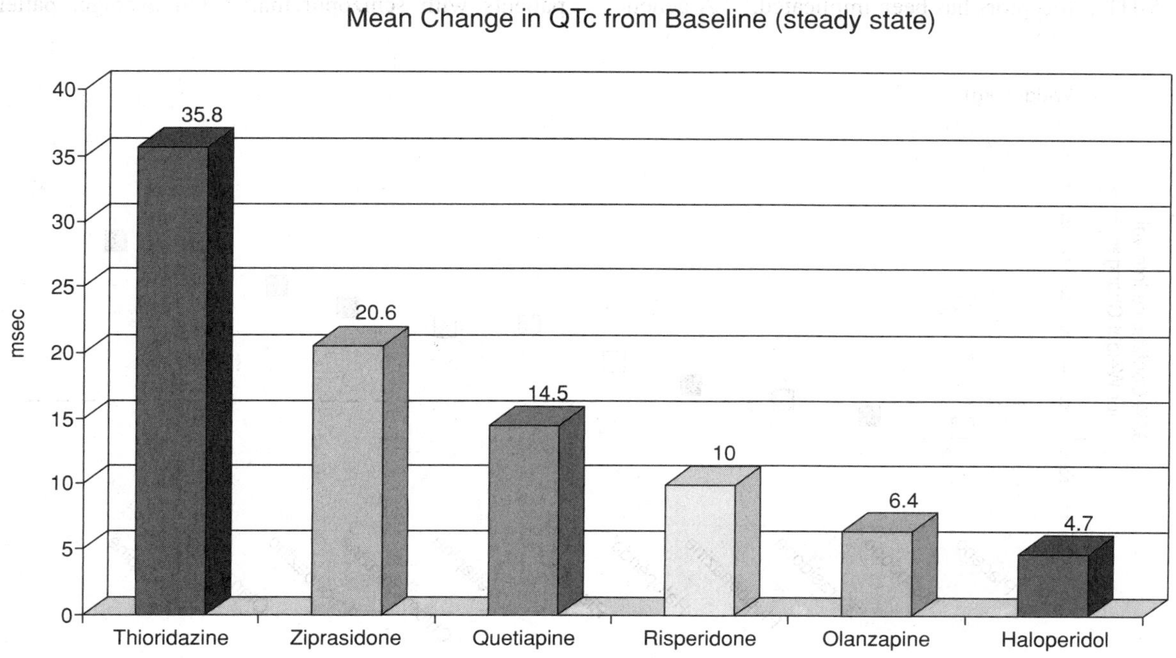

FIGURE 78-2 Comparison of QTc changes with antipsychotics. (Adapted from reference 173.)

of cardiac disease and with an uncontrolled electrolyte disturbance. The coprescription of ziprasidone with other drugs that prolong the QT interval should be avoided. Under most clinical circumstances, however, ziprasidone may be safely used without ECG monitoring or other special precautions.

METABOLIC EFFECTS

Hyperprolactinemia

Antipsychotic-induced hyperprolactinemia has come to the forefront because of differences found among the atypical agents. Before the introduction of the atypical agents, prolactin elevation was unavoidable because all typical antipsychotics elevate serum prolactin by blocking the tonic inhibitory actions of dopamine in the tuberoinfundibular tract.[174] Among the atypical agents, risperidone and, to a lesser extent, olanzapine produce a dose-related increase in prolactin levels that is equal to or greater than that seen with typical antipsychotics.[175,176] The remaining atypical agents have little impact on serum prolactin levels.[175] Hyperprolactinemia is of clinical importance because it may lead to galactorrhea, gynecomastia, amenorrhea, anovulation, impaired spermatogenesis, decreased libido and sexual arousal, and anorgasmia.[177] Interestingly the hyperprolactinemia is not always associated with clinical symptoms. For example, Kleinberg et al.[176] failed to find an association between sexual dysfunction and risperidone-associated hyperprolactinemia. This may be a product of the multifactorial nature of sexual dysfunction or methodologic limitations in data collection. Patients often do not spontaneously report symptoms of sexual dysfunction and clinicians must remember to ask about these potential side effects.[175]

Weight Gain

Weight gain is emerging as one of the most significant concerns associated with the use of antipsychotics, particularly among the atypical agents. The mechanism of antipsychotic-induced weight gain is unclear, but antagonism of histamine H_1 and serotonin 5-HT_{2C} receptors has been implicated.[178] A genetic predisposition exists for weight gain; a mutation in the 5-HT_{2c} receptor gene may increase risk for weight gain from atypical antipsychotics. No genetic tests exist to predict which patients will gain weight from the atypical antipsychotics.[179,180] Another theory is the potential decreased signaling of two serotonin receptors, 2A and 2C, increased calorie intake and appetite, and/or decreased metabolic rate.[180,181] The higher the binding affinity to the histaminergic receptor, the more that agent is likely to be associated weight gain.[180] Among the atypical agents, weight gain is most common with clozapine and olanzapine, lowest with ziprasidone and aripiprazole, and intermediate with risperidone and quetiapine.[182] In a meta-analysis, Allison et al.[183] found that the estimated weight gain at 10 weeks of therapy was greater with clozapine (4.45 kg) and olanzapine (4.15 kg) relative to risperidone (2.1 kg) and ziprasidone (0.04 kg), as illustrated in Figure 78-3. Moderate short-term weight gain has been demonstrated with quetiapine and is minimal with aripiprazole.[98,184] Similarly, clozapine and olanzapine have the largest associated weight gain with long-term treatment.[184] The weight gain observed with clozapine and olanzapine is not dose dependent and plateaus 6 to 12 months after treatment initiation.[185,186] However, other authors suggest that antipsychotic-associated weight gain plateaus within the first several months of treatment with risperidone, quetiapine, and ziprasidone can continue over several years for clozapine and olanzapine.[175] The issue of weight gain has important clinical implications in light of the link with impaired glucose tolerance and type II diabetes, hyperlipidemia, and increased mortality.[58,187–190] Patients who had no weight gain due to atypical antipsychotics can still develop diabetes mellitus. In a case review of 45 patients who developed or had worsening of their diabetes, nearly 50% had no weight gain. Atypical antipsychotics may impair insulin sensitivity or glucose regulation independent of weight gain, although the true reason for diabetes is still unknown.[179,181]

Cardiovascular disease is the leading cause of death among patients with schizophrenia.[191] On average, patients with

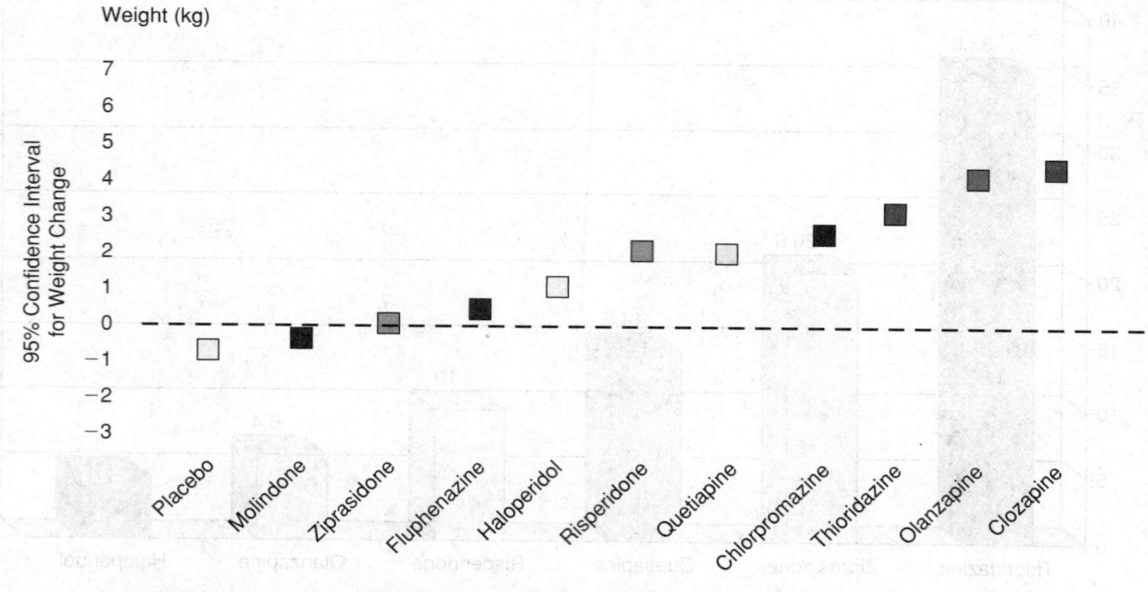

FIGURE 78-3 Comparison of weight change among antipsychotics. (Adapted from reference 183.)

Table 78-13 Monitoring Protocol for Atypical Antipsychotics[a]

	Baseline	Week 4	Week 8	Week 12	Quarterly	Annually	Every 5 years
Personal/Family history	X					X	
Weight (BMI)	X	X	X	X	X		
Waist circumference	X					X	
Blood pressure	X			X		X	
Fasting plasma glucose	X			X		X	
Fasting lipids profile	X			X			X

[a]More frequent assessments may be warranted based on clinical status.
Compiled from references 219 and 220.

schizophrenia live 20% shorter than the general population. They commit suicide up to 20 times more than the general population; and patients with schizophrenia specifically aged 25 to 44 years old, are three times more likely to die compared with the general population. This number has continued to increase as patients are no longer institutionalized.[179]

23. L.A., a 45-year-old woman with chronic paranoid schizophrenia, had been managed successfully with haloperidol for many years. She subsequently developed TD and was switched to olanzapine 20 mg HS. Before initiation of olanzapine 4 months ago, L.A. was 54 and weighed 132 lb. She has responded well to the olanzapine; however, she now weighs 148 lb. Can L.A.'s weight gain be attributed to olanzapine?

Weight gain has been reported with typical antipsychotics, but even greater weight gain has been seen with atypical agents such as clozapine and olanzapine, and to a lesser extent, risperidone and quetiapine.[182–184] The cause of antipsychotic-induced weight gain is multifactorial and may include a change in food preferences, increased food or fluid intake, carbohydrate craving, or a lack of activity. Blockade of the histamine and 5-HT_{2C} receptors are also contributory. H_1 blockade causes sedation that may produce inactivity. H_1 blockade may also increase weight by interfering with normal satiety signals from the gut, resulting in overeating. Evidence for a role of 5-HT_{2C} antagonism is derived indirectly from appetite-suppressing drugs, such as fenfluramine, which are thought to act via 5-HT agonism.[192]

L.A.'s weight gain should be taken seriously because it may contribute to medical conditions such as diabetes, hyperlipidemia, coronary artery disease, gastrointestinal disorders, cancer, and hypertension.[193,194] A significant weight gain may cause her to have a poor self-image, which may lead to treatment nonadherence. Obese patients with schizophrenia are 2.5 times more likely to discontinue their medication than nonobese patients.[194] She should be enrolled in a weight management program. If a patient gains 5% or more of their pretreatment body weight, switching to another antipsychotic should be considered.[195] For L.A., switching to another antipsychotic with lower weight gain liability may be considered; however, this decision must be balanced against her current positive response to olanzapine.

24. How should the potential metabolic complications associated with antipsychotics be monitored?

Although the risk of TD seems to be significantly reduced with the use of atypical antipsychotics, there is concern regarding other long-term side effects with these agents including impaired glucose tolerance, type 2 diabetes, and hyperlipidemia.[175,187]

L.A. should be informed about these potential complications. The routine monitoring of weight, fasting glucose levels, and lipid panels have been recommended and appropriate therapeutic options should be initiated if abnormalities are observed.[175,187] Guidelines have been created for the monitoring of metabolic issues associated with atypical antipsychotic use (Table 78-13). At baseline, a personal and family medical history should be obtained, as well as height and weight (to determine body mass index), waist circumference, BP, fasting plasma glucose, and a fasting lipid panel.[195,196] Fasting blood glucose and lipid levels, as well as BP measurements, should be completed 3 months after drug initiation, then every year if the patient is within normal limits.[195,196] Weight should be reassessed at weeks 4, 8, and 12, then quarterly, after drug initiation.[195,196] L.A. should be encouraged to self-monitor her weight and report any significant weight fluctuations. Subjective evidence of a weight change may include a change in clothes or belt size. In addition, she should be routinely monitored for the presence of diabetic symptoms (e.g., polyuria, polydipsia) at every clinic visit.

NEUROLEPTIC MALIGNANT SYNDROME

25. C.B., a 25 year-old man, was hospitalized with the diagnosis of schizophrenia, paranoid type, and was started on loxapine 25 mg HS. After 2 days of therapy, C.B. became rigid, seemed confused at times, and had a fever of 41°C. A diagnosis of neuroleptic malignant syndrome (NMS) was made. What features of this syndrome does C.B. have and how should it be treated?

NMS is a rare but potentially lethal adverse effect of antipsychotic therapy. The risk of NMS seems to be lower for atypical agents than for typical agents.[143] However, cases of NMS have been linked to treatment with clozapine, risperidone, olanzapine, quetiapine, ziprasidone, and aripiprazole.[197–203]

NMS can occur hours to months after the initial drug exposure, and the mortality rate is reported to be as high as 20%.[58] The incidence is estimated at between 0.02% and 3.23% of patients taking typical antipsychotic drugs.[204] The cardinal features include muscular rigidity, hyperthermia, autonomic dysfunction, and altered consciousness. Extrapyramidal dysfunction (e.g., rigidity) and akinesia usually develop initially or concomitantly with a temperature elevation as high as 41°C. Autonomic dysfunction includes tachycardia, labile BP, profuse diaphoresis, dyspnea, and urinary incontinence. The patient's level of consciousness may vary from alert to mutism, stupor, and coma. Other neurologic findings include sialorrhea, dyskinesia, and dysphagia. Symptoms usually develop rapidly over 24 to 72 hours. Creatine kinase, CBC, and LFTs are usually increased.

C.B.'s fever of 41°C, rigidity, and confusion are consistent with NMS. C.B.'s loxapine should be discontinued and supportive measures initiated to treat hyperthermia and prevent dehydration (e.g., antipyretics, a cooling blanket, and IV fluids).[205] Secondary complications such as pneumonia and renal failure should be managed as they develop.

If C.B.'s condition does not show a trend toward improvement or worsens after 1 to 3 days of observation and supportive therapy, a number of additional pharmacologic interventions should be considered.[205] NMS has been attributed to dopamine depletion caused by neuroleptic drug blockade of dopamine pathways in the basal ganglia and hypothalamus. For that reason, dopamine agonists such as amantadine or bromocriptine sometimes are beneficial. Dantrolene relaxes skeletal muscle and is specifically recommended for severe hyperthermia. C.B. should be started on dantrolene 50 mg four times daily and either bromocriptine 2.5 mg three times daily or amantadine 100 mg three times daily to accelerate reversal of his condition.[206] If he is unable to take oral medications, 1.25 to 1.5 mg/kg IV dantrolene should be used.

NMS is self-limiting and usually lasts 2 to 14 days after the oral antipsychotic is discontinued, or longer after discontinuation of depot medications. C.B.'s response to therapy can be assessed by frequently monitoring his vital signs and by measuring creatine kinase daily. After several weeks of recovery, treatment may be cautiously resumed with another atypical antipsychotic.[205,207]

SEDATION

Sedation can occur with any antipsychotic agent; however, it is most pronounced with the low-potency typical agents and with clozapine and quetiapine. Sedation at the beginning of treatment may be desirable for anxious or aggressive patients. However, persistent sedation during long-term treatment may adversely affect daily functioning and quality of life. Most patients develop some tolerance to these sedating effects over time, but it can be minimized by reducing the dose or shifting administration to bedtime.

HEPATIC DYSFUNCTION

26. **A.S., a 24-year-old woman, is brought to the hospital because of unusual behavior and violence toward her mother. A.S. is diagnosed with schizophrenia, paranoid type, acute exacerbation. Quetiapine 25 mg BID was prescribed initially and the dose gradually increased until 200 mg TID was achieved. Her baseline laboratory tests (CBC with differential, a chemistry profile that included LFTs, and serum electrolytes) were within normal limits. The same tests were repeated 10 days after her psychosis was under evaluation. The aspartate aminotransferase and alanine aminotransferase are now 2.5 times normal, but she has no GI complaints or medical problems. Should quetiapine be discontinued at this time?**

Benign elevations in LFTs (i.e., increases in aspartate aminotransferase or alanine aminotransferase less than two to three times normal) have long been reported early in the course of therapy with most antipsychotic drugs.[34,66,85] Such increases are rarely problematic; thus, no routine assessment of liver function in mandated by the FDA.

A more specific hepatic complication, cholestatic jaundice, has been associated with certain antipsychotic agents. The phenothiazines, especially chlorpromazine, have been implicated. Most cases develop within the first month of therapy and usually are preceded by prodromal symptoms of fever, chills, nausea, upper gastric pain, malaise, and pruritus. Discontinuation of the phenothiazine and symptomatic care are the primary modes of treatment because the cholestatic jaundice generally is self-limiting and usually resolves within 2 to 8 weeks. Occasionally, a more chronic course may develop. Once the signs and symptoms have resolved, an alternate class of antipsychotic, preferably a nonphenothiazine, should be prescribed.

The LFTs in A.S. are only modestly abnormal, and she is not experiencing symptoms of hepatotoxicity or cholestatic jaundice. Therefore, quetiapine should be continued. Routine laboratory monitoring of LFTs does not prevent drug-induced cholestatic jaundice; thus, no follow-up laboratory tests are required unless symptoms of hepatic dysfunction develop. Awareness and evaluation of A.S. for prodromal symptoms is the most appropriate action at this time.

OCULAR EFFECTS

27. **Are there any additional baseline tests that should have been performed on A.S. before starting quetiapine?**

The ocular effects of antipsychotic agents are well recognized and are generally of minor clinical consequence. Corneal and lens changes have been reported with several phenothiazines and thiothixene. Chlorpromazine is the most commonly implicated, with the risk being greatest with long-term, high-dose exposure (1–3 kg lifetime dose).[208]

If A.S. has not yet had a slit-lamp evaluation, an ophthalmologist should evaluate her as soon as possible. A 6-month follow-up examination is also indicated. Quetiapine should probably be discontinued if lens changes were noted on any of the examinations.

TEMPERATURE DYSREGULATION AND DERMATOLOGIC EFFECTS

28. **N.M., a 27-year-old man, recently was diagnosed with undifferentiated schizophrenia and was stabilized with chlorpromazine 400 mg HS during a 3-month stay in an inpatient unit. N.M. has continued chlorpromazine 400 mg HS as an outpatient and has done so well that he is ready to return to work as a laborer at a construction site. What precautions should he take when working outside?**

N.M. should be advised to wear a hat when working outside, drink fluids, stay in the shade as much as possible, and seek a cooler environment if he feels hot. Antipsychotics can cause temperature dysregulation, likely by inhibiting hypothalamic temperature regulation. The net result is poikilothermia (the normal body temperature cannot respond to heat or cold, and patients become hypothermic or hyperthermic, depending on the surrounding temperature).[209] The strong anticholinergic effects of N.M.'s chlorpromazine can impair cutaneous heat elimination and further exacerbate the problem. Olanzapine and clozapine also have strong anticholinergic properties, necessitating caution for patients exposed to excessive heat.

N.M. should also be advised to use a sunscreen with maximum sun protection factor, along with protective clothing because chlorpromazine-induced photosensitivity can predispose him to severe sunburns. The tricyclic structure of some antipsychotic drugs absorbs ultraviolet rays, producing free radicals that damage skin. Chlorpromazine is the most common cause of photosensitivity, but it can occur with all phenothiazines and with thiothixene.[209]

Other dermatologic reactions can occur with antipsychotics, and N.M. should be advised to report any skin abnormalities to his physician. Dermatitis, presenting with a maculopapular rash on the face, neck, and upper chest, occurs in approximately 5% of patients shortly after starting chlorpromazine. Localized or generalized urticaria also can develop. Antihistamines usually provide adequate relief, but the antipsychotic agent may have to be discontinued in severe cases. The rash rarely reappears after resumption of treatment.

SEIZURES

29. R.A., a 26-year-old woman recently diagnosed with chronic paranoid schizophrenia, is brought to the hospital after assaulting a neighbor. She presents in an acute psychotic state and has not calmed down since entering the hospital. She has struck two staff members on the psychiatric unit. R.A. has had generalized tonic–clonic seizures since age 14 and currently is taking carbamazepine 300 mg TID (serum concentration on admission is 8.2 mg/mL). R.A. has not been taking any antipsychotic medications and has been seizure free for 1 year. She needs acute treatment with an antipsychotic because of her dangerous behavior. How should an antipsychotic be initiated to treat her schizophrenia in light of her seizure disorder?

Antipsychotic drugs can lower the seizure threshold, producing seizures in patients who previously were seizure free. Seizures are most common with low-potency typical antipsychotics and clozapine.[58] Clozapine-induced seizures are dose related. The seizure rate is approximately 1% at doses below 300 mg/day, 2.7% at doses between 300 and 600 mg/day, and 4.4% at doses above 600 mg/day.[210] Because R.A. is currently a danger to herself and to others, the benefits of antipsychotic treatment outweigh the risks. Strategies to minimize the risk of seizures should be employed and include slow dose titration, use of lowest effective doses, and possible concurrent administration of an antiepileptic drug (e.g. carbamazepine).[211]

Haloperidol, an agent with a low risk for causing seizures, is a good selection. An initial dose of 5 mg PO or 2.5 mg IM should be given immediately, and additional dosages should be carefully administered until the psychosis resolves or she is no longer dangerous. The decision to use scheduled or as-needed medications should be based on whether she remains dangerous after a few immediate doses and the underlying cause of the psychosis. Supplemental benzodiazepines may be used to avoid high doses of haloperidol. If necessary, R.A.'s carbamazepine dose should be adjusted to maintain good seizure control and serum concentrations should be monitored. Carbamazepine (and other enzyme-inducing antiepileptic drugs) can influence the hepatic metabolism of antipsychotic agents. R.A. should be monitored for recurrent symptoms of schizophrenia if her carbamazepine dosage is increased.

SEXUAL DYSFUNCTION

30. K.J., a 24-year-old man with chronic paranoid schizophrenia, was rehospitalized for an acute exacerbation secondary to nonadherence with thioridazine 400 mg HS. During the medication history, it is discovered that he stopped taking thioridazine because he lost his interest in sex. When he tries to have intercourse, he experiences delayed ejaculation. About a week after stopping the thioridazine he is able to have a normal ejaculation. How does thioridazine contribute to K.J.'s sexual dysfunction?

Thioridazine is recognized as the most common cause of antipsychotic-induced sexual dysfunction.[212] Sexual side effects such as diminished libido, impaired arousal, and erectile and orgasmic dysfunction, however, have also been reported with both other typical agents and atypical agents.[175] The causes of antipsychotic-induced sexual dysfunction are related to a number of factors including hyperprolactinemia via dopamine blockade, α-adrenergic blockade, and anticholinergic and sedative effects.[213] Impaired sexual function has also been observed in untreated patients with schizophrenia, making the distinction between drug-induced and disease-induced symptoms difficult.[214] K.J.'s sexual dysfunction likely is related to the thioridazine because the symptoms resolved after he stopped the medication. Lowering the dose of thioridazine or converting him to another antipsychotic with less influence on sexual function may be helpful, although no reliable evidence is available to indicate which drugs are least likely to cause sexual dysfunction.

Predictors of Medication Response

As a general rule, antipsychotic agents should be initiated and titrated over the first few days to an average effective "target" therapeutic dose unless the patient's physiological status or history indicates that this dose may result in unacceptable adverse events.[215] After 1 week on the "target" dose, a modest dosage increase (within the recognized therapeutic range) may be considered if minimal or no improvement has been observed. In instances in which symptoms improve after the dose is increased, it may be difficult to know whether the response resulted from the dose change or from additional days on the drug. The duration of a therapeutic trial is 3 to 8 weeks in patients with little to no response, and 5 to 12 weeks in patients with a partial response.[166,215] Dosing recommendations for the antipsychotics are provided in Table 78-10.

Factors to Consider When Evaluating a Poor Response

A large proportion of patients with schizophrenia do not have an adequate response to antipsychotic therapy. Inadequate response may be caused by inadequate dosing, poor adherence, or true resistance to antipsychotic treatment.[216] Some of these factors can be addressed. In some patients, the therapeutic antipsychotic dose cannot be reached because of intolerable side effects. As mentioned, a therapeutic trial of 3 to 12 weeks at an optimal dosage may be necessary to determine the full benefit from an antipsychotic agent. Nonadherence with medications is a common obstacle in the management of schizophrenia, even in supervised settings. Blood level monitoring may be helpful to identify nonadherent patients as well as those in whom a pharmacokinetic factor may account for a poor response (e.g., poor drug bioavailability, rapid metabolizer, concomitant use of a metabolism-inducing agent). Therapeutic ranges of some antipsychotics are provided in Table 78-9.

A single definition of treatment resistance does not exist, but factors to consider in this definition include chronic or repeated hospitalizations, persistent positive symptoms, lack of improvement in negative symptoms, and breakthrough symptoms despite adherence to treatment.[216] Guidelines for determining treatment resistance have been proposed and include at least two prior drug trials of 4 to 6 weeks duration at 400 to 600 mg chlorpromazine (or equivalent, i.e., 8–12 mg of risperidone) with no clinical improvement, >5 years without a sustained period of good social or occupational functioning, and persistent psychotic symptoms.[216,217]

Several strategies have been proposed if a change in antipsychotic medication is necessitated by side effects or insufficient efficacy.[140] These include an abrupt switch (abrupt cessation of the current drug, with abrupt introduction of the new one at the expected therapeutic dose), a gradual switch (slow downward adjustment of the dosage of the current medication, with slow upward adjustment of the dosage of the new drug) or an overlapping switch (abrupt introduction of the new medication overlapping with the current medication, followed by downward adjustment of the dosage of the previous medication). None of these strategies has been demonstrated to be superior to another in terms of efficacy or safety, and the switch strategy depends on the clinical presentation.

31. M.S., a 24-year-old man, was brought to the ED by the police because voices told him to strike his mother. His medical workup and urine drug screen were negative. M.S. has a diagnosis of schizophrenia, undifferentiated type, and has been hospitalized four times in the last 2 years secondary to poor adherence to his prescribed medication. He has had the same presentation on all previous hospitalizations. During his last hospitalization, M.S. was stabilized on thiothixene (Navane) 20 mg orally at bedtime without any signs of adverse effects. How can IM depot therapy decrease readmissions, and how do we determine if M.S. is a good candidate for IM depot therapy?

M.S.'s history suggests that he is a good candidate for depot therapy. He responds to typical antipsychotics, but relapses owing to nonadherence. He should be able to tolerate higher potency antipsychotics because he has tolerated moderate doses of thiothixene. The patient should also be asked whether he is willing to take injections before proceeding with this strategy.

Conversion From Oral to Depot Therapy

32. How could M.S. be converted from oral therapy to depot therapy?

For patients such as M.S. who have never taken risperidone, haloperidol, or fluphenazine (the currently available long-acting depot forms of antipsychotics), an oral trial lasting several days to weeks is needed before conversion. The trial is necessary to ensure tolerability, evaluate response, and, when possible, determine the minimum effective dose.

Various formulas to convert from oral formulations to the decanoates have been proposed, but no method has been proved clinically superior. Clinicians should strive to use the longest dosing interval between injections and minimize the duration of combination oral and depot therapy. Careful evaluation of both tolerance and response is required for several months after initiating depot therapy.

FLUPHENAZINE DECANOATE CONVERSION

After stabilizing the patient on oral fluphenazine, multiply the total daily fluphenazine oral dose by 1.2 and administer as fluphenazine decanoate IM every 1 to 2 weeks.[218] Alternatively, 12.5 mg of fluphenazine decanoate can be administered IM every 1 to 2 weeks for every 10 mg (rounding to the nearest 10-mg increment) of oral fluphenazine per day (e.g., 25 mg/day PO rounded to 30 mg/day and given as 37.5 mg of decanoate).[219] The decanoate dosing interval may be increased to every 3 weeks after 4 to 6 weeks of therapy because of fluphenazine accumulation. There are no specific guidelines for the continuation of oral therapy after initiating the depot formulation; however, combination oral and IM therapy should be limited to the initiation period (1–4 weeks) or during times of decompensation.

HALOPERIDOL DECANOATE CONVERSION

Elderly patients or those stabilized on <10 mg of oral haloperidol per day should receive haloperidol decanoate in an IM dose that is 10 to 15 times the oral daily dose every 4 weeks. If higher oral doses are needed for stabilization, then the first decanoate dose should be 15 to 20 times the oral daily dose to a maximum of 450 mg.[220] The first injection of haloperidol decanoate should not exceed 100 mg. If more is required, the balance of the dose can be given in an additional one to two injections (provided that there are no EPS) over 3 to 7 days. Because haloperidol accumulates, the monthly decanoate dose should be decreased every 3 to 4 months by 25% until a minimum effective dose is achieved. Most patients can be effectively managed with a maintenance dose of 50 to 200 mg every 4 weeks.[166] Guidelines for concomitant oral therapy remain unclear and should be based on response and adverse effects, with the goal of depot alone after the first month of treatment if the aforementioned strategy is used.[218]

Using these guidelines, M.S. should be converted from thiothixene 20 to 10 mg of oral haloperidol per day (Table 78-10). Oral haloperidol should be continued alone for at least 1 week, until M.S. is stabilized. Once stabilization with oral haloperidol has occurred, haloperidol decanoate 100 mg IM can be administered. This can be followed with 50 mg IM 3 days later if no adverse effects are noted after the first injection. The total initial dose is 150 mg every 4 weeks (15 times the oral dose). A 200-mg total dose is also acceptable if the clinician believes the patient needs more drug. No oral medication is needed after the second injection and should only be given if M.S. shows signs of decompensation. M.S. should be monitored carefully for extrapyramidal side effects and response. M.S. should receive haloperidol decanoate 150 mg IM every 4 weeks with the dose adjusted according to response and tolerance; the dose can be decreased after 3 to 4 months because of drug accumulation.

LONG-ACTING RISPERIDONE FORMULATION

It is recommended that patients establish tolerability with oral risperidone prior to initiating treatment with Risperdone CONSTA. In published clinical trials, IM doses of 25, 50, or 75 mg have been administered at 2-week intervals.[141,142] The recommended dose is 25 mg IM every 2 weeks. Oral therapy of risperidone should be continued for 2 to 3 weeks after the first IM injection and then discontinued.

Inadequate Response

33. J.H., a 33-year-old man, was diagnosed with chronic paranoid schizophrenia at age 21 and has been hospitalized 15 times because of his illness. He repeatedly presents in a paranoid and hostile state complaining of auditory hallucinations and paranoid delusions in which the police and the people in his apartment building are trying to kill him. His symptoms have prevented him from obtaining employment, and he has no close friends. He has been treated with fluphenazine 20 mg HS and perphenazine 48 mg HS, but has had only a partial response to each medication. After each discharge, J.H. stays out of the hospital for approximately 6 months, then relapses, even with good adherence. He currently is taking haloperidol 15 mg HS with only minimal improvement after 2 months of treatment. What can be done to improve his response?

J.H. meets criteria for treatment-resistant schizophrenia, and clozapine is the "gold standard" for the treatment of this type of patient.[216] However, considering the risk of agranulocytosis, the burden of side effects, and the requirement of white blood cell (WBC) monitoring associated with clozapine therapy, one of the other atypicals should be tried before proceeding to clozapine.[166,216]

Clozapine

INDICATIONS

34. J.H. did not respond to an adequate trial of quetiapine 400 mg BID and was just admitted to the hospital again. He is becoming increasingly isolated and paranoid. He has no other medical conditions and is taking only lorazepam 1 to 2 mg Q 4 to 6 hr PRN. His last dose of quetiapine was 2 days ago. Because of his refractory illness, J.H. is being considered for clozapine therapy. What are the advantages and disadvantages of clozapine therapy? What makes him a good candidate for clozapine?

Clozapine is approved by the FDA for treatment of resistant schizophrenia or when adverse effects such as TD and EPS preclude use of other antipsychotics. Clozapine is contraindicated in patients with a history of a myeloproliferative disorder, uncontrolled epilepsy, paralytic ileus, clozapine-induced agranulocytosis or granulocytopenia a current WBC count below 3,500 mm^3 or ANC count below 2,000/mm^3. Clozapine also should be used with caution in patients who cannot tolerate anticholinergic effects, in those at risk for drug-induced orthostasis, or in patients with significant renal or hepatic disease.[221] Because of J.H.'s progressive decline in social functioning and inadequate response to haloperidol, fluphenazine, perphenazine, and quetiapine, clozapine should be considered.

Clozapine has clearly demonstrated superiority to typical agents in treating refractory schizophrenia. In the pivotal study by Kane et al.,[222] 30% of clozapine-treated subjects versus 4% of chlorpromazine-treated subjects met criteria for response at 6 weeks. A review and meta-analysis of seven controlled trials compared clozapine with typical antipsychotics in treatment-resistant schizophrenia and found that clozapine was superior in terms of overall therapeutic response, EPS, and adherence rate.[223] However, similarly favorable response rates have not yet been seen with other atypical agents in treatment resistant schizophrenia. Risperidone and olanzapine have been most often studied in this regard. In a double-blind trial comparing risperidone with haloperidol in treatment-refractory schizophrenia, a significantly higher response rate favoring risperidone was observed at week 4 but not at week 8.[224] In a 6-week clinical trial, only 7% of patients prospectively determined to be resistant to haloperidol responded to olanzapine, a rate that did not differ from chlorpromazine.[225] In general, atypical agents other than clozapine have not been consistently found to be as effective in treatment-resistant schizophrenia.[226] Nevertheless, given the problems associated with clozapine (risk of agranulocytosis, burden of other side effects, and the requirement for hematologic monitoring), atypical agents should be tried before proceeding to clozapine in most patients.[216] However, some patients do not respond to clozapine after an adequate trial of at least 6 months at a therapeutic dose. In such situations, it is reasonable to prescribe the antipsychotic to which they had the historic best response. Augmentation strategies, such as the addition of mood stabilizers (lithium and valproate), benzodiazepines, propranolol, antidepressants, or another antipsychotic agent, may be attempted. However, evidence for this approach is lacking.[226] Treatment guidelines recommend reserving augmentation strategies for patients who fail or cannot tolerate clozapine, although in practice these strategies are often tried before a trial of clozapine.[58,227]

INITIATION OF THERAPY

35. How should clozapine be initiated in J.H.? What are its side effects and how should he be monitored?

Whenever possible, clozapine should be initiated when a patient is medication free. However, if the patient is too ill to be taken off all antipsychotic drugs before adding clozapine, the current medication can be discontinued after a therapeutic clozapine dose has been achieved. Alternatively, clozapine can be titrated upward while the first antipsychotic is slowly tapered downward. Whenever possible, high-potency antipsychotics should be the concurrent agent used during the clozapine titration to minimize additive adverse effects such as sedation, anticholinergic effects, and orthostasis. Benzodiazepines should not be used for early behavioral and anxiety control, because their combined use with clozapine can lead to respiratory or cardiac arrest.[58]

Clozapine can be started in an outpatient setting if patients are carefully monitored for tolerability, especially orthostasis. The starting dose is 12.5 to 25 mg once or twice a day with increases of 25 to 50 mg/day until a target dose is reached. Clozapine is given in divided doses. The optimal dose has not been specifically delineated although an initial target of 300 to 450 mg/day is reasonable based on clinical experience. The maximum daily dose is 900 mg, but titration should proceed slowly to such high doses, and only after adequate trials at lower doses. Response is based on improvement of individual target symptoms and can be monitored by psychometric rating scales (Table 78-11). In addition, the overall ability of a patient to function and care for oneself during clozapine therapy also should be considered.[228] Most patients improve significantly during the first 6 weeks, but some take longer. Although the exact length of an appropriate trial is unclear, 12 weeks is adequate for most clients; however, improvement may continue for 6 to 12 months after initiating therapy.[58,229,230]

Clozapine has been issued five blackbox warnings from the FDA. These included agranulocytosis, seizures, myocarditis, increased mortality in elderly patients with dementia-related psychosis, and other adverse cardiovascular and respiratory effects.[231] The risk of seizures is dose dependent. The risk of fatal myocarditis is most frequent in the first month of treatment with clozapine. Other adverse cardiovascular and respiratory effects indicates orthostatic hypotension that may or may not be accompanied by syncope. Rarely, collapse with respiratory or cardiac arrest may occur. This is why it is essential to start patients on 12.5 mg once or twice daily, whether it is initiation of treatment, or the patient has been off of clozapine for 2 or more days.[231]

Clozapine causes agranulocytosis in approximately 1% of patients; therefore, baseline and weekly CBCs are required during treatment. Clozapine is automatically discontinued if a patient is noncompliant with the blood work. After 6 months of continuous, stable treatment, patients can be changed to biweekly WBC monitoring if their WBC counts are acceptable (≥3,500 mm³ and the absolute neutrophil count [ANC] is ≥2,000 mm³). After an additional 6 months on a continuous, stable regimen, the patient may be changed to WBC monitoring every 4 weeks.[231] If a patient takes clozapine for <6 months with no problems, but stops the drug for <1 month, WBC monitoring can restart where it was left off for a total of 6 months. If the break is >1 month, then an additional 6 months of weekly testing are needed.

If baseline laboratory work is within normal limits and an informed consent is obtained, J.H. can start on clozapine 25 mg at bedtime. His clozapine dose should be increased by 25 to 50 mg every day until the dose is 300 mg/day, the minimum dose at which most patients respond. The doses should be split and given as 150 mg twice a day. Subsequently, clozapine should be increased incrementally according to the guidelines described. If J.H. has no response to 300 mg after 4 to 8 weeks (based on a reduction in Brief Psychiatric Rating Scale scores and global improvement), then the dose can be increased to 450 mg (150 mg TID). If response still is inadequate, then the dose can be increased slowly to a maximum of 900 mg/day. Careful monitoring for orthostasis, hyperthermia, and oversedation is needed, especially during early titration. Serum concentration monitoring can also help to guide dose increases.

Clozapine may also cause sialorrhea, or hypersalivation. This is most often worst at night, and may lead to social withdrawal, choking, or aspiration pneumonia.[232] The incidence ranges from 31% of patients (premarket studies) to up to 80% in several clinical trials.[233] Several case reports have indicated that the scopolamine patch (1.5 mg/72 hour), ipratropium sublingual spray (0.03% or 0.06% given 2 sprays up to three times daily), atropine 1% ophthalmic solution (2 drops swish and swallow twice daily), botulinum toxin (150 IU injected into each parotid gland), and guanfacine (1 mg every morning) are effective in reducing, if not eliminating, sialorrhea.[232–236] Other medications commonly used are clonidine, anticholinergics (biperiden, benztropine, and diphenhydramine), amitriptyline, terazosin, and propranolol.[235,237]

36. Four weeks after starting clozapine, J.H.'s WBC count drops to 4,000/mm³ from a baseline of 6,800/mm³. Two weeks later, he has a WBC count of 2,100/mm³ and an ANC of 980/mm³. What action, if any, should be taken?

[SI unit: WBC count, 4.0 and 2.1 × 10^9/L, respectively]

The hematologic adverse effect profile for clozapine is very different from that of other antipsychotic agents. The incidence of clozapine-induced agranulocytosis is at least 10 to 20 times greater than the incidence with typical antipsychotic medications.[221] The incidence increases with age and is higher among women.[238] Analysis of data from 150,409 patients followed by the Clozaril National Registry found agranulocytosis in 585 patients resulting in 19 deaths.[238] The risk of agranulocytosis is greatest early in treatment with most cases appearing during the first 3 months of treatment. After 6 months, the risk for agranulocytosis decreases substantially but may occur in rare instances up to 5 years into treatment.[228,231] Trends in the weekly tests showing a continual decline in WBC count, even if it remains >3,000/mm³, require careful attention. Guidelines for responding to reduction in WBC are described in Table 78-14.

Clozapine should be discontinued immediately, J.H. should be hospitalized, and hematology and infectious disease

Table 78-14 Guidelines for Response to Clozapine-Induced White Blood Cell Abnormalities

Do Not Initiate Clozapine
Initial WBC count <3,500/mm³ Initial ANC <2,000/mm³ History of myeloproliferative disorder History of agranulocytosis or granulocytopenia related to clozapine
WBC <2,000/mm³ and/or ANC <1,000/mm³
Discontinue clozapine immediately Do not rechallenge patient Monitor WBC and differential: until normal and for at least 4 weeks: —Daily until WBC > 3,000/mm³ and ANC > 1,500/mm³ —Twice weekly until WBC > 3,500/mm³ and ANC > 2,000/mm³ —Weekly after WBC > 3,500/mm³ Consider bone marrow aspiration Protective isolation initiated if deficient granulopoiesis
WBC 2,000–3,000/mm³ or ANC 1,000–1,500/mm³
Discontinue clozapine Monitor WBC and differential: —Daily until WBC > 3,000/mm³ and ANC > 1,500/mm³ —Twice weekly until WBC > 3,500/mm³ and ANC > 2,000/mm³ May restart clozapine when: —if no symptoms of infection present —WBC > 3,500/mm³ and ANC > 2,000/mm³
WBC Drops to 3,000–3,500/mm³; >3,000/mm³ Over 1–3 Weeks; Immature WBCs Present
Repeat WBC with differential If repeated WBC between 3,000 and 3,500/mm³ and ANC <2,000/mm³ —repeat WBC with differential until WBC > 3,500/mm³ and ANC >2,000/mm³

ANC, absolute neutrophil count; WBC, white blood cell.
Compiled from references 58 and 231.

specialists should manage his care. Granulocyte colony-stimulating factor has been used successfully to manage clozapine-induced agranulocytosis.[239] Clozapine should not be reinstituted in J.H. because he has a very low ANC. However, it should be noted that agranulocytosis can be reversible upon discontinuation of clozapine, in most cases, with no persisting hematologic sequelae.[238]

37. What pharmacotherapy options could be tried to improve J.H.'s response now that clozapine is contraindicated?

Sequential monotherapy trials with other atypical agents that he had not been previously exposed to may be initiated. Alternatively, strategies such as the combination of an antipsychotic and a mood stabilizer or another antipsychotic have been attempted. Because J.H. has no precautions or contraindications to an adjunctive trial of lithium, he is a candidate for a 1-month lithium trial along with an antipsychotic medication other than clozapine. The antipsychotic is selected after reviewing his medication history and choosing the agent to which he had the best previous response. Lithium should be given at doses to achieve a target level of 0.8 to 1.2 mEq/L and continued for 1 month to allow the best chance for response. If the patient is unchanged at the end of 1 month, the lithium should be discontinued and another adjunctive agent tried for a 1-month trial.

Serum Concentration Monitoring

38. E.H., a 68-year-old woman who was diagnosed with chronic undifferentiated schizophrenia >30 years ago. She requires maintenance therapy with antipsychotic drugs because she relapsed when her haloperidol dose was decreased to 10 mg/day. Currently, she is responding poorly to haloperidol 15 mg HS for 6 weeks despite good adherence to her therapy. She has moderate pseudoparkinsonism controlled by benztropine 1 mg BID. Why should a serum concentration of haloperidol be obtained before increasing E.H.'s dose of this drug?

Antipsychotic drug serum concentrations are not part of routine clinical care, but can be considered under the following circumstances[240]:

- Poor response to moderate doses after an adequate trial (dose and duration)
- Serious or unexpected adverse effects at moderate dosages
- Deterioration in a compliant and previously stable patient
- Use of higher than usual dosages
- Evaluating whether the lowest effective dose is used in maintenance therapy
- Children, elderly, and medically compromised patients with potentially altered pharmacokinetics

It is unnecessary and not cost effective to obtain serum concentrations for antipsychotic drugs that do not have defined therapeutic ranges. Most studies describe haloperidol's therapeutic range to be between 4 and 12 ng/mL.[241,242] The recommended ranges for fluphenazine and thiothixene are 0.2 to 2.8 ng/mL and 2 to 15 ng/mL, respectively.[243–245] Evaluation of clozapine trials suggest an optimal range of 350 to 420 ng/mL.[246,247] Greater response rates were observed in olanzapine-treated patients whose plasma concentrations were >23.2 ng/mL in blood samples collected 12 hours after the dose.[248] Samples should be collected 5 to 7 days after a fixed dose and 10 to 12 hours after the last dose for oral preparations. Two to three months should elapse before samples are collected in patients taking depot preparations.[240]

E.H. has received an adequate trial of haloperidol and has moderate antipsychotic-induced parkinsonism. To prevent exposure to higher than necessary doses, a serum haloperidol concentration is warranted before increasing the dose. The target serum concentration should be between 4 and 12 ng/mL.

Treatment Adherence

Poor adherence with prescribed antipsychotic therapy is a significant problem in the long-term management of schizophrenia. Comprehensive reviews suggest that deviation (primarily underuse) from prescribed regimens occurs in about 50% of patients with schizophrenia.[249,250] Recent advances in medication treatments with atypical agents have produced fewer side effects, which some studies have shown has increased adherence.[251,252] During any phase of illness, nonadherence with maintenance antipsychotic therapy places patients at risk for exacerbation of psychosis, increased clinic and emergency room visits, and rehospitalization.[253,254] Nonadherence to prescribed regimens can also compromise patients' daily functioning and quality of life. Long-acting depot antipsychotics should be strongly considered for patients who have a history of nonadherence. In addition to assured medication delivery, another benefit of depot preparations is avoidance of potential bioavailability problems. Clinicians should suspect poor absorption if serum concentrations are much lower than expected for a given oral dose; however, factors such as nonadherence or drug–drug interactions must also be ruled out. Disadvantages of long-acting depot formulations include the time required to reach optimal dosing and the inability to immediately withdraw the drug if unpleasant side effects develop.[58,255] Because of this, patients should be converted to a depot form after confirmation that the oral dosage form is safe and effective.

CONSIDERATIONS IN SPECIFIC POPULATIONS

Pregnancy

39. D.M., a 26-year-old woman, has a 6-year history of chronic undifferentiated schizophrenia that has been treated with chlorpromazine 400 mg HS. She is psychiatrically stable and was last hospitalized 2 years ago. When D.M. decompensates, she isolates herself, is unable to care for herself, does not eat properly, and does not maintain her grooming and hygiene. She just found out that she is 8 weeks pregnant. Should her chlorpromazine be continued and what are the risks if the medication is continued?

Most of the available evidence regarding the use of antipsychotics during pregnancy has focused on typical antipsychotics. Among the typical antipsychotics, pooled results of large retrospective and small prospective controlled studies suggest an increased risk of congenital anomalies in patients treated with low-potency phenothiazines, particularly when treated during the first trimester.[256] Guidelines have recommended that the use of antipsychotic medication during the first trimester should be minimized or avoided if possible, especially between weeks 6 and 10.[58] If an antipsychotic is necessary during this period, high-potency typical antipsychotics may be safer.[58] In addition to their teratogenic effects, there are other reasons to avoid low-potency antipsychotics. Low-potency agents can worsen constipation and cause orthostatic hypotension and uteroplacental insufficiency. Guidelines have also recommended that medications should be tapered 1 week before delivery to minimize neonatal complications such as dystonia, withdrawal dyskinesias, temperature dysregulation, and irritability.[58]

Medication management should balance the needs of D.M. against those of her unborn child. D.M.'s schizophrenia has been stable for 2 years. Chlorpromazine should be discontinued because it is a low-potency phenothiazine and D.M. is currently in her first trimester. Because she is a danger to herself when ill, it is critical that treatment be initiated at the first evidence of decompensation. D.M. should be monitored by her clinician, family members, and caseworker at frequent intervals for reemergence of psychotic symptoms. If D.M. decompensates, treatment should be restarted with a nonphenothiazine, high-potency agent at the lowest possible dose (e.g., haloperidol or fluphenazine 2–5 mg at night). If D.M. does not respond to low-dose haloperidol or fluphenazine, or if she develops intolerable extrapyramidal side effects, then a lower potency antipsychotic drug or an atypical agent can be selected. D.M.'s chart should include the following documentation: specific behaviors that necessitate treatment (danger to self, fetus, or others), goals of therapy (acute control of dangerous behavior or remission), dose, route of administration, schedule, and projected duration of treatment, obstetric history and other medications used during pregnancy, alcohol or illegal drug use; regular progress notes on response and need for continued treatment; and informed consent from the patient or guardian.

Children

40. M.J. is the 5-year-old son of a close friend of the family who was diagnosed with autism. His mother, R.J., knows you are a psychiatric pharmacist and asks your opinion about the use of atypical antipsychotics in children with autism. What can you tell her?

Risperidone is the only atypical antipsychotic agent that is approved by the FDA for the symptomatic treatment of irritability in autistic children and adolescents.[99] In a study of 5- to 17-year-old children with autism accompanied by severe tantrums, aggression, or self-injurious behavior, the children were randomly assigned to flexible doses of either placebo or risperidone treatment (dose range, 0.5–3.5 mg/day) for 8 weeks.[257] A significantly greater percentage of children receiving risperidone responded to treatment than those receiving placebo (56.9% vs. 14.1% respectively, $p < 0.001$); 69% of the risperidone group had at least a 25% improvement on the irritability subscale of the Aberrant Behavioral Checklist as rated by a parent or primary caretaker and confirmed by a clinician and a rating of much or very much improved on a global improvement scale compared with only 12% in the placebo group ($p < 0.001$). The benefit from risperidone treatment was maintained for six months in two-thirds of the risperidone responders. The overall reduction in the level of irritability was 57% at 8 weeks of risperidone in comparison with a reduction of only 14% with placebo ($p < 0.001$). Troost et al.[258] evaluated the long-term effects of risperidone for an additional 24 weeks after the initial 8-week open-label trial. Risperidone was effective in reducing disruptive behavior in about one-half of the children, although considerable weight gain was observed.

Data with other atypical antipsychotics for the treatment of autism are limited. Olanzapine has the most data to date with open-label trials suggesting efficacy; quetiapine, ziprasidone, and anpiprazole may also be effective.[259–265] Hollander et al.[120] found olanzapine to be a potential alternative to risperidone for improving global functioning of pervasive developmental disorders but the risk of significant weight gain may limit its use in children/adolescents. In contrast, ziprasidone was not associated with significant weight gain.[264]

REFERENCES

1. Piccinelli M, Gomez Homen F. Gender Differences in the Epidemiology of Affective Disorders and Schizophrenia. Geneva: World Health Organization; 1997:61.
2. Murray CJL, Lopez AD, eds. *Global Burden of Disease.* Cambridge, MA: Harvard University Press; 1996.
3. Wu EQ et al. The economic burden of schizophrenia in the United States 2002. *J Clin Psych* 2005;66:1122.
4. Rupp A, Keith SJ. The costs of schizophrenia. Assessing the burden. *Psychiatr Clin North Am* 1993; 16:413.
5. National Advisory Mental Health Council. Health care reform for Americans with severe mental illnesses: report of the National Advisory Mental Health Council. *Am J Psychiatry* 1993;150:1447.
6. Rosenheck RA. Outcomes, Costs, and Policy Caution: A Commentary on the Cost Utility of the Latest Antipsychotic Drugs in Schizophrenia Study (CUtLASS 1). *Arch Gen Psych* 2006;63:1074.
7. Andreasen NC, Carpenter WT. Diagnosis and classification of schizophrenia. *Schizophr Bull* 1993;19:199.
8. Seaton BE et al. Sources of heterogeneity in schizophrenia: the role of neuropsychological functioning. *Neuropsychol Rev* 2001;11:45.
9. Kendler KS, Diehl SR. The genetics of schizophrenia: a current genetic-epidemiologic perspective. *Schizophr Bull* 1998;19:261.
10. Kendler KS, Robinett CD. Schizophrenia in the National Academy of Sciences-National Research Council Twin Registry: a 16-year update. *Am J Psychiatry* 1983;140:1551.
11. American Psychiatric Association. *Diagnostic and Statistical Manual of Mental Disorders Text Revision,* 4th ed. (DSM-IV-TR). Washington, DC: American Psychiatric Press; 2000.
12. Pearlson GD. Neurobiology of schizophrenia. *Ann Neurol* 2000;48:556.
13. Pulver AE. Search for schizophrenia susceptibility genes. *Biol Psychiatry* 2000;47:221.
14. Crow T et al. Schizophrenia as an anomaly of development of cerebral asymmetry: a postmortem study and a proposal concerning the genetic basis of the disease. *Arch Gen Psychiatry* 1989;46:1145.
15. Andreasen NC et al. Magnetic resonance imaging of the brain in schizophrenia. *Arch Gen Psychiatry* 1990;47:35.
16. Gur R et al. Magnetic resonance imaging in schizophrenia: I. Volumetric analysis of brain and cerebrospinal fluid. *Arch Gen Psychiatry* 1991; 48:407.
17. Kelsoe JR et al. Quantitative neuroanatomy in schizophrenia: a controlled magnetic resonance imaging study. *Arch Gen Psychiatry* 1988;45:533.
18. Suddath RL et al. Temporal lobe pathology in schizophrenia: a quantitative magnetic resonance imaging study. *Am J Psychiatry* 1989;146:464.
19. Suddath RL et al. Anatomical abnormalities in the brains of monozygotic twins discordant for schizophrenia. *N Engl J Med* 1990;322:789.
20. Harrison PJ. On the neuropathology of schizophrenia and its dementia: Neurodevelopmental, neurodegenerative, or both? *Neurodegeneration* 1995; 4:1.
21. Bogrest B et al. Hippocampus-amygdala volumes and psychopathology in chronic schizophrenia. *Biol Psychiatry* 1991;33:239.
22. Roberts G. Is there gliosis in schizophrenia? Investigation of the temporal lobe. *Biol Psychiatry* 1987;22:1459.
23. Kindermann SS et al. Review of functional magnetic resonance imaging in schizophrenia. *Schizophr Res* 1997;27:143.
24. Weinberger DR et al. Physiological dysfunction of dorsolateral prefrontal cortex in schizophrenia, I: Regional cerebral blood flow evidence. *Arch Gen Psychiatry* 1986;43:114.
25. Stevens AA et al. Cortical dysfunction in schizophrenia during auditory word and tone working

memory demonstrated by functional magnetic resonance imaging. *Arch Gen Psychiatry* 1998;55:1097.
26. Mubrin Z et al. Regional cerebral blood flow patterns in schizophrenic patients. *Cerebral Blood Flow Bull* 1982;3:43.
27. Andreasen NC et al. "Cognitive dysmetria" as an integrative theory of schizophrenia: a dysfunction in cortical-subcortical-cerebellar circuitry? *Schizophr Bull* 1998;24:203.
28. Herz MI, Marder SR. Neurobiology. In: *Schizophrenia: Comprehensive Treatment and Management*. Philadelphia: Lippincott Williams & Wilkins; 2002:3.
29. Andreasen NC et al. Defining the phenotype of schizophrenia: cognitive dysmetria and its neural mechanisms. *Biol Psychiatry* 1999;46:908.
30. Weinberger DR. Neurodevelopmental perspectives on schizophrenia. In: Bloom FE, Kupfer DJ, eds. *Psychopharmacology: The Fourth Generation of Progress*. New York: Raven Press; 1995.
31. Green MF, Neuchterlein KH. Should schizophrenia be treated as a neurocognitive disorder? *Schizophr Bull* 1999;25:309.
32. Creese I et al. Dopamine receptor binding predicts clinical and pharmacological potencies of antischizophrenic drugs. *Science* 1976;192:481.
33. Seeman P et al. Antipsychotic drug doses and neuroleptic/dopamine receptors. *Nature* 1976;261:717.
34. Marder SR, van Kammen DP. Dopamine receptor antagonists. In: Kaplan H, Saddock B, eds. *Comprehensive Textbook of Psychiatry VII*. New York: Lippincott Williams & Wilkins; 1999:2356.
35. Davidson M et al. L-Dopa challenge and relapse in schizophrenia. *Am J Psychiatry* 1987;144:934.
36. Lieberman J et al. Methylphenidate challenge as a predictor of relapse in schizophrenia. *Am J Psychiatry* 1984;141:633.
37. Snyder S. Catecholamines in the brain as mediators of amphetamine psychosis. *Arch Gen Psychiatry* 1972;27:169.
38. Littrel RA et al. The neurobiology of schizophrenia. *Pharmacotherapy* 1996;16:143S.
39. Risch SC. Pathophysiology of schizophrenia and the role of newer antipsychotics. *Pharmacotherapy* 1996;116(Suppl 1 Pt 2):11S.
40. Davis KL et al. Dopamine in schizophrenia: A review and reconceptualization. *Am J Psychiatry* 1991;148:1474.
41. Joyce JN. The dopamine hypothesis of schizophrenia: Limbic interactions with serotonin and norepinephrine. *Psychopharmacology* 1993;112:S16.
42. Olney JW et al. Glutamate receptor dysfunction and schizophrenia. *Arch Gen Psychiatry* 1995;52:998.
43. Kim JS et al. Low cerebrospinal fluid glutamate in schizophrenia patients and new hypothesis on schizophrenia. *Neurosci Lett* 1980;20:379.
44. Akbarian S et al. Gene expression for glutamic acid decarboxylase is reduced without loss of neurons in prefrontal cortex of schizophrenics. *Arch Gen Psychiatry* 1995;52:528.
45. Kraepelin E. Dementia praecox and paraphrenia. *Trans. RM Barclay*. Chicago: Chicago Medical Book; 1919.
46. Bleuler E. Dementia Praecox or the Group of Schizophrenias (1911). *Trans. J Zinkin*. New York: International Press; 1950.
47. Schneider K. *Clinical Psychopathology*. New York: Grune & Stratton; 1959.
48. Thacore VR, Shukla SRP. Cannabis psychosis and paranoid schizophrenia. *Arch Gen Psychiatry* 1976;33:383.
49. Palmer BW et al. Is it possible to be schizophrenic and neuropsychologically impaired? *Neuropsychology* 1997;11:3437.
50. Green MF et al. Neurocognitive deficits and functional outcome in schizophrenia: are we measuring the "right stuff"? *Schizophr Bull* 2000;26:119.
51. Beiser M et al. Establishing the onset of psychotic illness. *Am J Psychiatry* 1993;150:1349–1354.
52. McGorry PD et al. The prevalence of prodromal features of schizophrenia in adolescence: a preliminary study. *Acta Psychiatr Scand* 1995:92:241–249.
53. Duzyurek S, Wienerm JM. Early recognition in schizophrenia: the prodromal stages. *J Pract Psychiatr Behav Health* 1999;5:187–196.
54. Bleuler M. The Schizophrenic Disorders: Long-Term Patient and Family Studies. New Haven, CT: Yale University Press; 1978.
55. Ciompi L. Catamnestic long-term study on the course of life and aging of schizophrenics. *Schizophr Bull* 1980;6:608.
56. Huber G et al. Longitudinal studies of schizophrenic patients. *Schizophr Bull* 1980;6:592.
57. McGlashan TH, Fenton WS. Subtype progression and pathophysiologic deterioration in early schizophrenia. *Schizophr Bull* 1993;19:71.
58. American Psychiatric Association. Practice guideline for the treatment of patients with schizophrenia. 2nd ed. 2004. Available at http://www.psychiatryonline.com/pracGuideTopic_6.aspx.
59. Newman SC, Bland RC. Mortality in a cohort of patients with schizophrenia: a record linkage study. *Can J Psychiatry* 1991;36:239.
60. Caldwell CB, Gottesman II. Schizophrenics kill themselves too: a review of risk factors for suicide. *Schizophr Bull* 1990;16:571.
61. Wyatt RJ. Neuroleptics and the natural course of schizophrenia. *Schizophr Bull* 1992;17:325.
62. Robinson DG et al. Predictors of treatment response from a first episode of schizophrenia or schizoaffective disorder. *Am J Psychiatry* 1999;156:544.
63. Rifkin A. Pharmacologic strategies in the treatment of schizophrenia. *Psychiatr Clin North Am* 1993;16:351.
64. Kane JM. Treatment programme and long term outcome in chronic schizophrenia. *Acta Psychiatr Scand* 1990;358(Suppl):151.
65. Davis JM. Overview: maintenance therapy in psychiatry. I: schizophrenia. *Am J Psychiatry* 1975;132:1237.
66. Janicak PG et al. Principles and Practice of Psychopharmacotherapy. Baltimore, MD: Williams & Wilkins; 1997:97.
67. Heinssen RK et al. Psychosocial skills training for schizophrenia: Lessons from the laboratory. *Schizophr Bull* 2000;26:21.
68. Beck AT, Rector NA. Cognitive therapy for schizophrenia patients. *Harvard Ment Health Lett* 1998;15:4.
69. Dixon L et al. Update on family psychoeducation for schizophrenia. *Schizophr Bull* 2000;26:5.
70. Cook JA, Razzano L. Vocational rehabilitation for persons with schizophrenia: Recent research and implications for practice. *Schizophr Bull* 2000;26:87.
71. Garety PA et al. Cognitive-behavioral therapy for medication-resistant symptoms. *Schizophr Bull* 2000; 26:73.
72. Saddock BJ, Saddock VA. The doctor-patient relationship and interviewing techniques. In: *Kaplan & Sadock's Synopsis of Psychiatry: Behavioral Sciences, Clinical Psychiatry*. Philadelphia: Lippincott Williams & Wilkins; 2003:1.
73. Saddock BJ, Saddock VA. Psychiatric history and mental status examination. In: *Kaplan & Sadock's Synopsis of Psychiatry: Behavioral Sciences, Clinical Psychiatry*. Philadelphia: Lippincott Williams & Wilkins; 2003:229.
74. Wolkowitz OM, Pickar D. Benzodiazepines in the treatment of schizophrenia: a review and reappraisal. *Am J Psychiatry* 1991;148:714.
75. Growe GA et al. Lithium in chronic schizophrenia. *Am J Psychiatry* 1979;136:454.
76. Small JG et al. A placebo-controlled study of lithium combined with neuroleptics in chronic schizophrenic patients. *Am J Psychiatry* 1975;132:1315.
77. Goldney RD, Spence ND. Safety of the combination of lithium and neuroleptic drugs. *Am J Psychiatry* 1986;143:882.
78. Leucht S et al. Carbamazepine augmentation for schizophrenia: how good is the evidence? *J Clin Psychiatry*. 2002;63:218.
79. McElroy SL et al. Sodium valproate: its use in primary psychiatric disorders. *J Clin Psychopharmacol* 1987;7:16.
80. Neppe VM. Carbamazepine in nonresponsive psychosis. *J Clin Psychiatry* 1988;49(Suppl 4):22.
81. Citrome L et al. Changes in use of valproate and other mood stabilizers for patients with schizophrenia from 1994 to 1998. *Psychiatr Serv* 2000;51:634.
82. Casey DE et al. Effect of divalproex combined with olanzapine or risperidone in patients with an acute exacerbation of schizophrenia. *Neuropsychopharmacology*. 2003;28:182.
83. Sorgi PJ et al. Beta-adrenergic blockers for the control of aggressive behaviors in patients with chronic schizophrenia. *Am J Psychiatry* 1986;143:775.
84. Lindstrom L, Persson E. Propranolol in chronic schizophrenia: a controlled study in neuroleptic treated patients. *Br J Psychiatry* 1980;137:126.
85. Perry PJ et al. Psychotropic Drug Handbook. Washington, DC: American Psychiatric Press; 1997.
86. Ames D et al. Advances in antipsychotic pharmacotherapy: clozapine, risperidone, and beyond. *Essent Psychopharmacol* 1996;1:5.
87. Lohr JB, Braff DL. The value of referring to recently introduced antipsychotics as "second generation." *Am J Psychiatry* 2003;160:1371.
88. Nordstrom AL et al. Central D2-dopamine receptor occupancy in relation to antipsychotic drug effects: a double-blind PET study of schizophrenic patients. *Biol Psychiatr* 1993;33:227.
89. Kapur S et al. Relationship between dopamine D2 receptor occupancy, clinical response, and side effects: a double-blind PET study. *Am J Psychiatry* 2000;157:514.
90. Marder SR, Van Putten T. Antipsychotic medications. In: Schatzberg AF, Nemeroff CB, eds. *The American Psychiatric Press Textbook of Psychopharmacology*. Washington, DC: American Psychiatric Press; 1995:247.
91. Bench CJ et al. The time course of binding to striatal dopamine D2 receptors by the neuroleptic ziprasidone (CP-88,059-01) determined by positron emission tomography. *Psychopharmacology (Berl)* 1996;124:141.
92. Kapur S et al. Clinical and theoretical implications of 5-HT2 and D2 receptor occupancy of clozapine, risperidone and olanzapine in schizophrenia. *Am J Psychiatry* 1999;156:286.
93. Kapur S et al. A positron emission tomography study of quetiapine in schizophrenia: A preliminary finding of an antipsychotic effect with only transiently high dopamine D_2 receptor occupancy. *Arch Gen Psychiatry* 2000;57:553.
94. Meltzer HY. The role of serotonin in antipsychotic drug action. *Neuropsychopharmacology* 1999;21(2 Suppl):106S.
95. Nordstrom AL et al. D1, D2, and 5-HT2 receptor occupancy in relation to clozapine serum concentration: a PET study of schizophrenic patients. *Am J Psychiatry* 1995;152:1444.
96. Fischman AJ et al. Positron emission tomographic analysis of central 5-hydroxytryptamine2 receptor occupancy in healthy volunteers treated with the novel antipsychotic agent, ziprasidone. *J Pharmacol Exp Ther* 1996;279:939.
97. Stahl SM. Antipsychotic agents. In: *Essential Psychopharmacology: Neuroscientific Basis and Practical Applications*. New York: Cambridge University Press; 2000;401.
98. Kane JM et al. Efficacy and safety of aripiprazole and haloperidol versus placebo in patients with schizophrenia and schizoaffective disorder. *J Clin Psychiatry*. 2002;63:763.
99. Janssen LP. Paliperidone package insert. Titusville, NJ; February 2008.
100. Paliperidone (Invega) for schizophrenia. *Med Lett Drugs Ther*. 2007;49:21.
101. Casey DE. Side effect profiles of new antipsychotic agents. *J Clin Psychiatry* 1996;57(Suppl 11):40.
102. Lehman AF, Steinwachs DM. Translating research into practice: the Schizophrenia Patient Outcomes Research Team (PORT) treatment recommendations. *Schizophr Bull* 1998;24:1.
103. Marder SR et al. The effects of risperidone on the

five dimensions of schizophrenia derived by factor analysis: combined results of the North American trials. *J Clin Psychiatry* 1997;58:538.
104. Hoyberg OJ et al. Risperidone versus perphenazine in the treatment of chronic schizophrenic patients with acute exacerbations. *Acta Psychiatr Scand* 1993;88:395.
105. Tollefson GD et al. Olanzapine versus haloperidol in the treatment of schizophrenia and schizoaffective disorder and schizophreniform disorders: results of an international collaborative trial. *Am J Psychiatry* 1997;154:457.
106. Beasley CM Jr et al. Olanzapine versus placebo and haloperidol: acute phase results of the North American double-blind olanzapine trial. *Neuropsychopharmacology* 1996;14:111.
107. Arvanitis LA et al. Multiple fixed doses of "Seroquel" (quetiapine) in patients with acute exacerbation of schizophrenia: a comparison with haloperidol and placebo. *Biol Psychiatr* 1997;42:233.
108. Peuskens J, Link CG. A comparison of quetiapine and chlorpromazine in the treatment of schizophrenia. *Acta Psychiatr Scand* 1997;96:265.
109. Goff DC et al. An exploratory haloperidol-controlled dose-finding study of ziprasidone in hospitalized patients with schizophrenia or schizoaffective disorder. *J Clin Psychopharmacol* 1998; 18:296.
110. Daniel DG et al. Ziprasidone 80 mg/day and 160 mg/day in the acute exacerbation of schizophrenia and schizoaffective disorder: a 6-week placebo-controlled trial. *Neuropsychopharmacology* 1999;20:491.
111. Kane J et al. Treatment of schizophrenia with paliperidone extended-release tablets: a 6-week placebo-controlled trial. *Schizophr Res* 2007;90: 147.
112. Davidson M et al. Efficacy, safety and early response of paliperidone extended release tablets (paliperidone ER): results of a 6-week, randomized, placebo-controlled study. *Schizophr Res* 2007;93: 117.
113. Marder SR et al., in press. Efficacy and safety of paliperidone extended-release tablets: results of a 6-week, randomized, placebo-controlled study. *Biol Psychiatry.*
114. Geddes J et al. Atypical antipsychotics in the treatment of schizophrenia: systematic overview and meta-regression analysis. *Br Med J* 2000;321: 1371.
115. Leucht S. Efficacy and extrapyramidal side-effects of the new antipsychotics olanzapine, quetiapine, risperidone, and sertindole compared to conventional antipsychotics and placebo: a meta-analysis of randomized controlled trials. *Schizopr Res* 1999;35:51.
116. Davis JM et al. A meta-analysis of the efficacy of second-generation antipsychotics. *Arch Gen Psychiatry* 2003;60:553.
117. Marder SR, Meibach RC. Risperidone in the treatment of schizophrenia *Am J Psychiatry* 1994;151: 825.
118. Moller HJ. Neuroleptic treatment of negative symptoms in schizophrenic patients. Efficacy problems and methodological difficulties. *Eur Neuropsychopharmacol* 1993;3:1.
119. Tollefson GD, Sanger TM. Negative symptoms: a path analytic approach to a double-blind, placebo- and haloperidol-controlled clinical trial with olanzapine. *Am J Psychiatry* 1997;154:466.
120. Hollander E et al. A double-blind placebo-controlled pilot study of olanzapine in childhood/ adolescent pervasive developmental disorder. *J Child Adolesc Psychopharmacol* 2006;16:541.
121. Nasrallah HA. The Roles of Efficacy, Safety, and Tolerability in Antipsychotic Effectiveness: Practical Implications of the CATIE Schizophrenia Trial. *J Clin Psych* 2007;68(Suppl 1):5.
122. Stroup TS, et al. Effectiveness of olanzapine, quetiapine and risperidone in patients with chronic schizophrenia after discontinuation of perphenazine: a CATIE Study. *Am J Psych* 2007;164: 415.
123. Milton GV, Jann MW. Emergency treatment of psychotic symptoms: pharmacokinetic considerations for antipsychotic drugs. *Clin Pharmacokinet* 1995;28:494.
124. Brook S et al. Intramuscular ziprasidone compared with intramuscular haloperidol in the treatment of acute psychosis. *J Clin Psychiatry* 2000;61:933.
125. Daniel DG et al. Intramuscular ziprasidone 20 mg is effective in reducing agitation associated with psychosis: a double-blind, randomized trial. *Psychopharmacology* 2001;155:128.
126. Battaglia J. Pharmacological management of acute agitation. *Drugs* 2005;65:1207.
127. Garza-Trevino ES et al. Efficacy of combinations of intramuscular antipsychotics and sedative-hypnotics for control of psychotic agitation. *Am J Psychiatry* 1989;146:1598.
128. Baldessarini R et al. Significance of neuroleptic dose and plasma level in pharmacological treatment of psychoses. *Arch Gen Psychiatry* 1988; 45:79.
129. Hillard JR. Emergency treatment of acute psychosis. *J Clin Psychiatry* 1998;59(Suppl):57.
130. Altamura AC et al. Intramuscular preparations of antipsychotics: uses and relevance in clinical practice. *Drugs* 2003;63:493.
131. Dubin WR. Rapid tranquilization: antipsychotics or benzodiazepines? *J Clin Psychiatry* 1988; 49(Suppl):5.
132. Bristol Myers Squibb. Aripiprazole package insert. Princeton, NJ: May 2008.
133. Andrienza R et al. Intramuscular aripiprazole for the treatment of acute agitation in patients with schizophrenia or schizoaffective disorder: a double-blind, placebo-controlled comparison with intramuscular haloperidol. *Psychopharmacology* 2006; 188:281.
134. Janssen LP. Risperidone package insert. Titusville, NJ: February 2008.
135. Currier GW et al. Acute treatment of psychotic agitation: a randomized comparison of oral treatment with risperidone and lorazepam vs. intramuscular treatment with haloperidol and lorazepam. *J Clin Psychiatry* 2004;65:386.
136. Lesem MD et al. Intramuscular ziprasidone, 2 mg versus 10 mg, in the short-term management of agitated patients. *J Clin Psychiatry* 2001;62:12.
137. Breier A et al. A double-blind, placebo-controlled dose-response comparison of intramuscular olanzapine and haloperidol in the treatment of acute agitation in schizophrenia. *Arch Gen Psychiatry* 2002;59:441.
138. Pfizer. Ziprasidone package insert. New York: March 2007.
139. Eli Lilly and Company. Olanzapine package insert. Indianapolis, IN: March 2008.
140. Ganguli R. Rationale and strategies for switching antipsychotics. *Am J Health-Syst Pharm* 2002;59:S22.
141. Kane JM et al. Long-acting injectable risperidone: efficacy and safety of the first long-acting atypical antipsychotic. *Am J Psychiatry* 2003160: 1125.
142. Martin SD et al. Clinical experience with the long-acting injectable formulation of the atypical antipsychotic, risperidone. *Curr Med Res Opin* 2003;19:298.
143. Burns MJ. The pharmacology and toxicology of atypical agents. *J Clin Toxicol* 2001;39:1.
144. Ereshefsky L. Pharmacokinetics and drug interactions: update for new antipsychotics. *J Clin Psychiatry* 1996;57(Suppl 11):12.
145. Michalets EL. Update: clinically significant cytochrome P450 drug interactions. *Pharmacotherapy* 1998;18:84.
146. Jann MW et al. Effects of carbamazepine on plasma haloperidol levels. *J Clin Psychopharmacol* 1985;5:106.
147. Rice DP. The economic impact of schizophrenia. *J Clin Psychiatry* 1999;60(Suppl 1):4.
148. Hudson TJ et al. Economic evaluations of novel antipsychotic medications: a literature review. *Schizophr Res* 2003;60:199.
149. Casey DE. Neuroleptic-induced extrapyramidal syndromes and tardive dyskinesia. In: Hirsch SR, Weinberger DR, eds. *Schizophrenia.* Oxford, UK: Blackwell; 1995:546.
150. Casey DE. Tardive dyskinesia and atypical antipsychotic drugs. *Schizophr Res* 1999;35(Suppl): 55–62.
151. Dolder CR, Jeste DV. Incidence of tardive dyskinesia with typical versus atypical antipsychotics in very high risk patients. *Biol Psychiatry* 2003;53:1142.
152. Beasley CM et al. Randomized double-blind comparison of the incidence of tardive dyskinesia in patients with schizophrenia during long-term treatment with olanzapine or haloperidol. *Br J Psychiatry* 1999;174:23.
153. Jeste DV et al. Lower incidence of tardive dyskinesia with risperidone compared with haloperidol in older patients. *J Am Geriatr Soc* 1999;47:716.
154. Holloman LC, Marder SR. Management of acute extrapyramidal effects induced by antipsychotic drugs. *Am J Health-Syst Pharm* 1997;54:2461.
155. Jeste DV, Naimark D. Medication-induced movement disorders. In: Tasman A, Kay J, Lieberman J, eds. *Psychiatry.* Philadelphia: WB Saunders; 1996: 1304.
156. Simpson G, Angus JWS. A rating scale for extrapyramidal side effects. *Acta Psychiatr Scand* 1970;46(Suppl 221):11.
157. World Health Organization. Prophylactic use of anticholinergics in patients on long-term neuroleptic treatment: a consensus statement. World Health Organization heads of centres collaborating on WHO co-ordinated studies on biological aspects of mental illness. *Br J Psychiatry* 1990;156:412.
158. Shirzadi AA and Ghaemi SN. Side effects of atypical antipsychotics: extrapyramidal symptoms and the metabolic syndrome. *Harv Rev Psych* 2006;14:152.
159. Fleischhacker WW et al. The pharmacological treatment of neuroleptic-induced akathisia. *J Clin Psychopharmacol* 1990;10:12.
160. Kane JM et al. Tardive dyskinesia: prevalence, incidence, and risk factors. *J Clin Psychopharmacol* 1988;8(4 Suppl):52S.
161. Kane JM et al. Tardive Dyskinesia: A Task Force Report to the American Psychiatric Association. Washington, DC: American Psychiatric Association; 1992.
162. Jeste DV et al. Risk of tardive dyskinesia in older patients. A prospective longitudinal study of 266 outpatients. *Arch Gen Psychiatry* 1995;52:756.
163. Woerner MG et al. Prospective study of tardive dyskinesia in the elderly: rates and risk factors. *Am J Psychiatry* 1998;155:1521.
164. Yassa R. Functional impairment in tardive dyskinesia: medical and psychosocial dimensions. *Acta Psychiatr Scand* 1989;80:64.
165. Lantz MS. Tardive dyskinesia: an antipsychotic side effect that has not gone away. *Clin Geriatr* 2005;13:18.
166. McEvoy JP et al. The expert consensus guideline series. Treatment of Schizophrenia, 1999. *J Clin Psychiatry* 1999;60(Suppl 11):1.
167. Boomershine KH et al. Vitamin E in the treatment of tardive dyskinesia. *Ann Pharmacother* 1999;33:1195.
168. Adler LA et al. Vitamin E treatment for tardive dyskinesia. *Arch Gen Psychiatry* 1999;56: 836.
169. Kane JM et al. Does clozapine cause tardive dyskinesia? *J Clin Psychiatry* 1993;54:327.
170. Janicak PG et al. Principles and Practice of Psychopharmacotherapy. Baltimore, MD: Williams & Wilkins; 1997:188.
171. Rogers DP, Shramko JK. Therapeutic options in the treatment of clozapine-induced sialorrhea. *Pharmacotherapy.* 2000;20:1092.
172. Buckley NA, Sanders P. Cardiovascular adverse effects of antipsychotic drugs. *Drug Saf* 2000;23: 215.
173. FDA Psychopharmacological Drugs Advisory Committee. 19 July 2000 Briefing Document for

Ziprasidone HCl. Available at http://www.fda.gov/ohrms/dockets/ac/00/backgrd/3619b1a.pdf.
174. Petty R. Prolactin and antipsychotic medications: mechanism of action. *Schizophr Res* 1999;35:S67.
175. Wirshing DA et al. Understanding the new and evolving profile of adverse drug effects in schizophrenia. *Psychiatr Clin North Am* 2003;26:165.
176. Kleinberg DR et al. Prolactin levels and adverse events in patients treated with risperidone *J Clin Psychopharmacol* 1999;19:57.
177. Dickson RA, Glazer WM. Neuroleptic-induced hyperprolactinemia. *Schizophren Res* 1999;35:S75.
178. McIntyre RS et al. Mechanisms of antipsychotic-induced weight gain. *J Clin Psychiatry* 2001; 62(Suppl 23):23.
179. Goff DC et al. Medical Morbidity and Mortality in Schizophrenia: Guidelines for Psychiatrists. *J Clin Psych* 2005;66:183.
180. Nasrallah HA. Atypical antipsychotic-induced metabolic side effects: insights from receptor-binding profiles. *Mol Psych* 2008;13:27.
181. Nasrallah HA, Newcomer JW. Atypical antipsychotics and metabolic dysregulation: evaluating the risk/benefit equation and improving the standard of care. *J Clin Psychopharm* 2004;24:S7.
182. Tandon R. Safety and tolerability: how do newer generation "atypical" antipsychotics compare? *Psychiatr Q* 2002;73:297.
183. Allison DB et al. Antipsychotic-induced weight gain: a comprehensive research synthesis. *Am J Psychiatry* 1999;156:1686.
184. Sussman N. Review of atypical antipsychotics and weight gain. *J Clin Psychiatry* 2001;62(Suppl 23):5.
185. Henderson D et al. Clozapine: Diabetes mellitus, weight gain and lipid abnormalities: a five year naturalistic study. *Am J Psychiatry* 2000;157:975.
186. Kinon BJ et al. Long-term olanzapine treatment: weight change and weight-related health factors in schizophrenia *J Clin Psychiatry* 2001;62:92.
187. McIntyre RS et al. Antipsychotic metabolic effects: Weight gain, diabetes mellitus, and lipid abnormalities. *Can J Psychiatry* 2001;46:273.
188. Fontaine KR et al. Estimating the consequences of antipsychotic induced weight gain on health and mortality rate. *Psychiatry Res* 2001;101:277.
189. Goldstein LE, Henderson DC. Atypical antipsychotics agents and diabetes mellitus. *Prim Psychiatry* 2000;7:65.
190. Melkersson KI et al. Elevated levels of insulin, leptin, and blood lipids in olanzapine-treated patients with schizophrenia or related psychoses. *J Clin Psychiatry* 2000;61:742.
191. Newcomer JW. Metabolic considerations in the use of antipsychotic medications: a review of recent evidence. *J Clin Psych* 2007;68(Suppl 1):20.
192. Garattini S et al. Reduction of food intake by manipulation of central serotonin: current experimental results. *Br J Psychiatry* 1989;155:41.
193. Must A et al. The disease burden associated with overweight and obesity. *JAMA* 1999;282:1523.
194. Meyer JM. Strategies for the long-term treatment of schizophrenia: real world lessons from the CATIE trial. *J Clin Psych* 2007;68:28.
195. Consensus Development Conference on Antipsychotic Drugs and Obesity and Diabetes. *Diabetes Care* 2004;27:596.
196. Treating Schizophrenia: A Quick Reference Guide. American Psychiatric Association Website. Available at: http://www.psych.org.
197. Farver DK. Neuroleptic malignant syndrome induced by atypical antipsychotics. *Expert Opin Drug Saf* 2003;2:21.
198. Ozen ME et al. Neuroleptic malignant syndrome induced by ziprasidone on the second day of treatment. *World J Biol Psychiatry* 2007;8:42.
199. Evcimen H et al. Neuroleptic malignant syndrome induced by low dose aripiprazole in first episode of psychosis. *J Psychiatr Pract* 2007;13:117.
200. Liebold J et al. Neuroleptic malignant syndrome associated with ziprasidone in an adolescent. *Clin Ther* 2004;26:1105.
201. Molina D et al. Aripiprazole as the causative agent of neuroleptic malignant syndrome: a case report. *Prime Care Companion J Clin Psychiatry* 2007;9:148.
202. Borovicka MC et al. Ziprasidone and lithium-induced neuroleptic malignant syndrome. *Ann Pharmacother* 2006;40:139.
203. Kang SG et al. Atypical neuroleptic malignant syndrome associated with aripiprazole. *J Clin Psychopharmacol* 2006; 26:534.
204. Caroff SN et al. Neuroleptic malignant syndrome. *Med Clin North Am* 1993;77:185.
205. Pelonero AL et al. Neuroleptic malignant syndrome: a review. *Psychiatr Serv* 1998;49:1163.
206. Lazarus A. Therapy of neuroleptic malignant syndrome. *Psychiatr Dev* 1986;4:19.
207. Rosebush PI et al. Twenty neuroleptic rechallenges after neuroleptic malignant syndrome in 15 patients. *J Clin Psychiatry* 1989;50:295.
208. AstraZeneca Pharmaceuticals. Quetiapine Package Insert. Wilmington, DE: May 2008.
209. Simpson CM et al. Adverse effects of antipsychotic drugs. *Drugs* 1981;21:138.
210. Devinsky O et al. Clozapine-related seizures. *Neurology* 1991;41:369.
211. Hummer M, Fleichhacker WW. Nonmotor side effects of novel antipsychotics. *Curr Opin CPNS Invest Drugs* 2000;2:45.
212. Kotin J et al. Thioridazine and sexual dysfunction. *Am J Psychiatry* 1976;133:82.
213. Meston CM, Frohlich PF. The neurobiology of sexual function. *Arch Gen Psychiatry* 2000;57:1012.
214. Aizenberg D et al. Sexual dysfunction in male schizophrenic patients. *J Clin Psychiatry* 1995;56:137.
215. Mossum D. A decision analysis approach to neuroleptic dosing: insights from a mathematical model. *J Clin Psychiatry* 1997;58:66.
216. Conley RR, Kelly DL. Management of treatment resistance in schizophrenia. *Biol Psychiatry* 2001;50:898.
217. Woods SW. Chlorpromazine equivalent doses for the newer atypical antipsychotics. *J Clin Psychiatry* 2003;64:663.
218. Ereshefsky L et al. Future of depot neuroleptic therapy: pharmacokinetic and pharmacodynamic approaches. *J Clin Psychiatry* 1984;45:50.
219. McEvoy GK, ed. *American Hospital Formulary System Drug Information*. Bethesda, MD: American Society of Hospital Pharmacists; 1998:1864.
220. McNeil Pharmaceutical. Haldol decanoate package insert. Raritan, NJ: September 2001.
221. Meltzer HY. New drugs for the treatment of schizophrenia. *Psychiatry Clin North Am* 1993;16:365.
222. Kane J et al. Clozapine for treatment resistant schizophrenia. A double blind comparison with chlorpromazine. *Arch Gen Psychiatry* 1988;45:789.
223. Chakos M et al. Effectiveness of second-generation antipsychotics in patients with treatment-resistant schizophrenia: a review and meta-analysis of randomized trials. *Am J Psychiatry* 2001;158:518.
224. Wirshing DA et al. Risperidone in treatment-refractory schizophrenia. *Am J Psychiatry* 1999;156:1374.
225. Conley RR et al. Olanzapine compared with chlorpromazine in treatment-resistant schizophrenia. *Am J Psychiatry* 1998;155:914.
226. Pantelis C, Barnes TR. Drug strategies and treatment-resistant schizophrenia. *Aust N Z J Psychiatry* 1996;30:20.
227. Miller AL et al. The TMAP schizophrenia algorithms. *J Clin Psychiatry* 1999;60:649.
228. Breier A et al. Clozapine treatment of outpatients: outcome and long-term response patterns. *Hosp Comm Psychiatry* 1993;44:1145.
229. Meltzer HY. Duration of a clozapine trial in neuroleptic-resistant schizophrenia. *Arch Gen Psychiatry* 1989;46:672.
230. Meltzer HY. Treatment of the neuroleptic-nonresponsive schizophrenic patient. *Schizophr Bull* 1992;18:515.
231. Novartis Pharmaceuticals. Clozapine package insert. East Hanover, NJ: May 2008.
232. Freudenreich O et al. Clozapine-induced sialorrhea treated with sublingual ipratropium spray: a case series. *J Clin Psychopharmacol* 2004;24:98.
233. Gaftanyuk O, Trestman RL. Scopolamine patch for clozapine-induced sialorrhea. *Psych Serv* 2004;55:318.
234. Webber MA, et al. Guanfacine treatment of clozapine-induced sialorrhea. *J Clin Psychopharmacol* 2004;24:675.
235. Kahl KG et al. Botulinum toxin as an effective treatment of clozapine-induced sialorrhea treatment. *Psychopharmacology* 2004;173:229.
236. Sharma A et al. Intraoral application of atropine sulfate ophthalmic solution of clozapine-induced sialorrhea. *Ann Pharmacother* 2004;38:1538.
237. Praharaj SK et al. Clozapine-induced sialorrhea: pathophysiology and management strategies. *Psychopharmacology* 2006;185:265.
238. Alvir JMJ et al. Clozapine-induced agranulocytosis: incidence and risk factors in the United States. *N Engl J Med* 1993;329:162.
239. Gerson SL. G-CSF and the management of clozapine-induced agranulocytosis. *J Clin Psychiatry* 1994;55(Suppl 9B):139.
240. Preskorn SH et al. Therapeutic drug monitoring: principles and practice. *Psychiatr Clin North Am* 1993;16:611.
241. Volavka J et al. Plasma haloperidol levels and clinical effects in schizophrenia and schizoaffective disorder. *Arch Gen Psychiatry* 1995;52:837.
242. Van Putten T et al. Haloperidol plasma levels and clinical response: a therapeutic window relationship. *Am J Psychiatry* 1992;149:500.
243. Levison DF et al. Fluphenazine plasma levels, dosage, efficacy, and side effects. *Am J Psychiatry* 1995;152:765.
244. Mavroides M et al. Clinical relevance of thiothixene plasma levels. *J Clin Psychopharmacol* 1984;4:155.
245. Yesavage J et al. Correlation of initial thiothixene serum levels and clinical response. *Arch Gen Psychiatry* 1983;40:301.
246. Perry PJ et al. Clozapine and norclozapine plasma concentration and clinical response of treatment-refractory schizophrenic patients. *Am J Psychiatry* 1991;148:231.
247. Freeman DJ et al. Will routine therapeutic drug monitoring have a place in clozapine therapy? *Clin Pharmacokinet* 1997;32:93.
248. Perry PJ et al. Olanzapine plasma concentrations and clinical response: acute phase results of the North American Olanzapine Trial. *J Clin Psychopharmacol* 2001;21:14.
249. Fenton WS et al. Determinants of medication compliance in schizophrenia: empirical and clinical findings. *Schizophr Bull* 1997;23:637.
250. Lacro JP et al. Prevalence of and risk factors for medication nonadherence in patients with schizophrenia: a comprehensive review of recent literature. *J Clin Psychiatry* 2002;63:892.
251. Dolder CR et al. Antipsychotic medication adherence: is there a difference between typical and atypical agents? *Am J Psychiatry* 2002;159:103.
252. Rosenheck R et al. Medication continuation and compliance: a comparison of patients treated with clozapine and haloperidol. *J Clin Psychiatry* 2000;61:382.
253. Weiden PJ, Olfson M. Cost of relapse in schizophrenia. *Schizophr Bull* 1995;21:419.
254. Terkelsen KG, Menikoff A. Measuring the costs of schizophrenia: implications for the post-institutional era in the U.S. Pharmacoeconomics 1995;52:173.
255. Barnes TR, Curson DA. Long-term depot antipsychotics. A risk-benefit assessment. *Drug Saf* 1994;10:464.
256. Altshuler LL et al. Pharmacologic management of psychiatric illness during pregnancy: dilemmas and guidelines. *Am J Psychiatry* 1996;153:592.
257. McCracken JT et al for Research Units on

Pediatric Psychopharmacology (RUPP) Autism Network. Risperidone in children with autism and serious behavioral problems. *N Engl J Med* 2002;347:314.

258. Troost PW et al. Long-term effects of risperidone in children with autism spectrum disorders: a placebo discontinuation study. *J Am Acad Child Adolesc Psychiatry* 2005;44:1137.
259. Kemner C et al. Open-label study of olanzapine in children with pervasive developmental disorder. *J Clin Psychopharmacol* 2002;22:455.
260. Malone RP et al. Olanzapine versus haloperidol in children with autistic disorder: an open-pilot study. *J Am Acad Child Adolesc Psychiatry* 2001;40:887.
261. Roychoudhury K, Demb HB. Use of olanzapine in children with developmental disabilities and challenging behaviors. *J Investig Med* 1999;47:65a.
262. Potenza MN et al. Olanzapine treatment of children, adolescents, and adults with pervasive developmental disorders: an open-label pilot study. *J Clin Psychopharmacol* 1999;19:37.
263. Martin A et al. Open-label quetiapine in the treatment of children and adolescents with autistic disorder. *J Child Adolesc Psychopharmacol* 1999;9:99.
264. McDougle CJ et al. Case series: use of ziprasidone for maladaptive symptoms in youths with autism. *J Am Acad Child Adolesc Psychiatry* 2002;41:921.
265. Valicenti-McDermott MR, Demb H. Clinical effects and adverse reactions to off-label use of aripiprazole in children and adolescents with developmental disabilities. *J Child Adolesc Psychopharmacol* 2006;16:549.
266. Marken PA, Stanislav SW. Schizophrenia. In: Koda-Kimble MA, Young LY, eds. *Applied Therapeutics: The Clinical Use of Drugs.* Baltimore, MD: Lippincott Williams & Wilkins; 2001;76.

CHAPTER 79

Mood Disorders I: Major Depressive Disorders

Patrick R. Finley

We who squander our sorrows
How we look beyond them
into the mournful passage of time
To see whether they might end

—*Rainer Marie Rilke*

INTRODUCTION

Depression is a common, chronic, and potentially debilitating illness that has tempered the human condition since the beginning of recorded history. The ancient Egyptians, for instance, wrote about depression more than 3,000 years ago. In the First Book of Samuel (dated about 700 BC), Saul, the King of Israel, is overcome by an "evil spirit" that causes him to feel "incapacitated, guilt-ridden and hopeless," leading ultimately to his suicide.[1]

Cultures throughout history have speculated on the origin of depression. The ancient Greeks believed that depression was caused by an excess of bile. Hippocrates thoroughly described the condition as a somatic illness and is believed to have coined the term "melancholia," which literally translates to "black bile." During the Middle Ages, depression and other psychiatric illnesses were considered to be punishment or afflictions from a vengeful God rather than actual illness. At that time, the church and society believed depression to be the result of being weak minded or sinful. Even today, many people suffering from a depressive episode carry the stigma of "having a nervous breakdown," and medications are viewed as a "crutch" to help cope with daily life. Throughout history, depression has affected the lives of many famous people, including Ludwig Van Beethoven, Meriwhether Lewis, Abraham Lincoln, Charles Dickens, Winston Churchill, Ernest Hemingway, and Marilyn Monroe.[1]

Although many people experience "the blues" on occasion, the term "depression" is reserved in psychiatry to define a specific medical condition with distinctive biological and pharmacologic implications. Similarly, the term "clinical depression" is liberally applied in popular culture to a condition that approximates the psychiatric diagnosis of major depression. In general, depressive disorders are enormous health concerns that are often misdiagnosed or undertreated. The physical and social dysfunction associated with depression is profound and is believed to outweigh many other chronic medical conditions, including hypertension, diabetes, and arthritis.[2] The Medical Outcomes Study, for instance, determined that the degree of impairment in depressed individuals is comparable to that seen in patients with chronic heart disease.[3] The financial ramifications of depression are tremendous and place an overwhelming burden on our society. In 2000, the estimated cost of depression in the United States was $83.1 billion annually, with most of these costs ($51.5 billion) attributed to lost productivity and absenteeism in the workplace.[4]

Epidemiology

Since World War II, the lifetime incidence of depression has been rising steadily in studied populations. A recent investigation concluded that the annual incidence of mood disorders is approximately 10% in the adult population, and 1 in 15 adults (6.7%) will suffer from an episode of major depression during any 12-month period.[5] Various studies from Europe and the United States have estimated the lifetime prevalence to be 5% to 12% in adult males and 9% to 26% in females.[6] Although the incidence of depression is remarkably similar across various races and ethnic groups, the illness may be slightly more common in lower socioeconomic classes.[7]

The onset of depression occurs most commonly in the late 20s, but there is a wide range, and the first episode may actually present at any age. One prevailing misconception is that depression is more common among elderly individuals.[8] Epidemiologic evidence suggests that the incidence is slightly lower in older persons than in the general population, but certain subtypes may be more common (e.g., melancholia, depression with psychotic features), and new-onset depression that initially presents during geriatric years may carry a worse prognosis.

Genetic factors appear to play a major role in the cause of depression. The offspring of depressed individuals are 2.7 times more likely to have depression if one parent is afflicted, and 3.0 times more likely if both parents suffer from depression.[9] Concordance rates for monozygotic (identical) twins range from 54% to 65%, whereas dizygotic (fraternal) twins range from 14% to 24%.[10] Genetic factors may also predispose individuals to an earlier onset of depression (younger than 30 years of age).[11]

Alternatively, there is clear evidence that depression may occur as a result of stressful events (i.e., environmental factors) in one's life. These factors include a difficult childhood, physical or verbal abuse, pervasive low self-esteem, death of a loved one, loss of a job, and the end of a serious relationship. Acute depressive episodes are often attributed to a combination or diatheses of environmental or genetic factors. For instance, individuals carrying a genetic predisposition to mood disorders may undergo a traumatic experience that ultimately triggers the manifestation of depressive symptomatology. Depression may also occur spontaneously, however, among people who appear to lack any obvious genetic or environmental factors.

Diagnosis and Classification

Both the diagnosis and the classification of depression have undergone many transformations since Emil Kraepelin's biological model of the late 19th century. Kraepelin separated the functional psychoses into two groups: manic-depressive insanity and dementia praecox. Kraepelin's detailed descriptions of these two mental illnesses laid the foundation for modern psychiatry.[12] In 2000, the American Psychiatric Association (APA) published refined, standardized criteria for diagnosing depressive disorders in the *Diagnostic and Statistical Manual of Mental Disorders,* Fourth Edition, Text Revision (DSM-IV-TR).[13] Depressive disorders are classified under Mood Disorders in DSM-IV-TR and include major depressive disorder; single-episode or recurrent, dysthymic disorder; and depressive disorder, not otherwise specified. See Table 79-1 for the classification of mood disorders.

As previously stated, a major depressive disorder may occur as a single episode, but it is more commonly a recurrent event and looked on, therefore, as a chronic illness.[6] The frequency of recurrent episodes is highly variable, with some people experiencing discrete episodes separated by many years of relatively normal mood (i.e., euthymia), and others experiencing residual symptoms between episodes that may never completely remit. The risk of future episodes appears to increase disproportionately with the chronicity of the illness. For instance, after the first episode there is a 50% likelihood of a second. After the second, there is a 70% chance of a third, and with the third episode comes nearly a 90% incidence of a fourth.

Table 79-1 Classification of Mood Disorders

I. Mood Disorders
- A. Depressive Disorders
  1. Major Depressive Disorder, Single Episode
  2. Major Depressive Disorder, Recurrent
  3. Dysthymic Disorder
  4. Depressive Disorder Not Otherwise Specified
- B. Bipolar Disorders
  1. Bipolar Disorder, Single Episode
  2. Bipolar Disorder, Recurrent
  3. Cyclothymic Disorder
  4. Bipolar Disorder Not Otherwise Specified
- C. Secondary Mood Disorder due to Nonpsychiatric Medical Condition
- D. Substance-Induced Mood Disorder
- E. Mood Disorder Not Otherwise Specified

From reference 13.

Depressive disorders may be subclassified using cross-sectional symptom features, or specifiers, according to DSM-IV-TR.[13] For example, the phrase "with melancholic features" is used when patients possess primary neurovegetative symptoms, early morning awakening, marked psychomotor agitation or retardation, and significant anorexia or weight loss. Melancholia is often a more severe form of depression, and the cause is rather autonomous (i.e., lacking apparent environmental triggers).[14] It may also be less likely than other forms of depression to remit spontaneously. The phrase "with atypical features" is used when depressive symptoms include weight gain, hypersomnia, leaden paralysis, or rejection sensitivity. When hallucinations or delusions occur in patients who are primarily depressed, the phrase "with psychotic features" is applicable to the mood disorder. Other diagnostic specifiers used in DSM-IV-TR include "chronic," "with catatonic features," and "with postpartum onset."

Dysthymic disorder is a type of depressive illness characterized by fewer symptoms than major depression, but the course is much more chronic with symptoms being present most of the time for at least 2 years. In practice, the distinction of major depression from dysthymia may be difficult to make and requires a detailed psychiatric history. Some patients may experience an episode of major depression superimposed on a history of dysthymia, a condition commonly known as *double depression.* The treatment for dysthymia has traditionally focused on psychotherapy, but recent evidence suggests that antidepressant medications may also be effective.[15]

Differential Diagnosis

Symptoms of depression may be induced or exacerbated by numerous medical illnesses or medications (Tables 79-2 and 79-3). Consequently, DSM-IV-TR specifies that whenever an "organic cause" is temporally related to the onset of depressive symptoms, the patient does not fit the criteria for major depression, even if all other criteria are met.[13] The rationale for this

Table 79-2 Selected Medical Conditions That May Mimic Depression

Central Nervous System	Women's Health
Alzheimer disease	Premenstrual dysphoric disorder
Cerebrovascular accident	Antepartum/postpartum
Epilepsy	Perimenopause
Multiple sclerosis	
Parkinson disease	
Cardiovascular	**Other**
Cerebral arteriosclerosis	Chronic fatigue syndrome
Congestive heart failure	Chronic pain syndrome(s)
Myocardial infarction	Fibromyalgia
Endocrine	Irritable bowel syndrome
Addison disease	Malignancies (various)
Diabetes mellitus (types I and II)	Migraine headaches
Hypothyroidism	Rheumatoid arthritis
	Systemic lupus erythematosus

stipulation is that if the medical illness is successfully treated or the offending agent is discontinued, the depressive illness will spontaneously resolve, eliminating the need for somatic intervention. Although lists of medical illnesses or medications are helpful, the clinician should be aware that the actual evidence demonstrating an association between depression and specific organic causes is often very limited and anecdotal. If a medication or condition is suspected of causing depression, the chronologic association should be investigated rigorously before other action is taken.

Clinical Presentation

For a diagnosis of major depressive disorder to be made, symptoms must be present for at least 2 weeks and must not be precipitated or influenced by a medical illness or medication (according to DSM-IV-TR criteria). Individuals must possess at least five symptoms, one of which is either depressed mood *OR* anhedonia (diminished interest or pleasure in activities). The other seven symptoms are as follows:

Table 79-3 Selected Medications That May Induce Depression

Cardiovascular Agents	Hormonal Agents
β-blockers (?)	Anabolic steroids
Clonidine	Corticosteroids
Methyldopa	Gonadotropin-releasing hormone
Reserpine	Progestins
	Tamoxifen
Central Nervous System Agents	**Others**
Barbiturates	Efavirenz
Benzodiazepines (?)	Interferon
Chloral hydrate	Isotretinoin
Ecstasy (MDMA)	Mefloquine
Ethanol	Levetiracetam

1. Change in appetite
2. Change in sleep
3. Low energy
4. Poor concentration (or difficulty making decisions)
5. Feelings of worthlessness or inappropriate guilt
6. Psychomotor agitation or retardation
7. Recurrent thoughts of suicide

The diagnostic criteria also stipulate that the mood disturbance must cause marked distress or result in clinically significant impairment of social or occupational functioning. To distinguish depression from grief reactions or bereavement, it is also stipulated that the symptoms of major depression must persist for at least 2 months after the precipitating event. Table 79-4 lists the specific criteria for a diagnosis of major depressive disorder.

Although low energy and changes in sleep or appetite are present in most depressed patients, the clinical presentation of depression can be highly variable. Many patients, for example, will readily express profound sadness or hopelessness, but others can project a more anxious or irritable appearance. Psychomotor agitation may be apparent, featuring wringing of the hands, grimacing, pacing, or cursing. Conversely, psychomotor retardation can be evident, with slowed speech or thinking, soft monotone voice, or minimal facial expression. On occasion, psychotic symptoms (e.g., auditory hallucinations, persecutory delusions, somatic delusions of serious medical illness) may also occur.

Although the criteria for detecting major depression are exactly the same in the elderly population as in the general population, the presentation may be slightly different than in younger individuals. Elderly patients may be less likely to acknowledge sadness or melancholy and choose to dwell instead on somatic complaints such as headache, insomnia, joint pain, dizziness, or constipation.[16] As a result, clinicians are advised to consider the possibility of depression whenever a person presents with vague, chronic symptoms of physical illness and unclear etiology.

Table 79-4 Diagnostic Criteria for Major Depressive Disorder

- At least five of the following symptoms have been present during the same 2-week period and represent a change from previous functioning. One of the symptoms must be either depressed mood or loss of interest/pleasure.
  - Depressed mood most of the day, nearly every day
  - Loss of interest in pleasurable activities most of the day, nearly every day
  - Change in weight or appetite (increase or decrease) when not dieting
  - Insomnia or hypersomnia nearly every day
  - Fatigue or loss of energy nearly every day
  - Diminished ability to think or concentrate, or indecisiveness
  - Feelings of worthlessness or excessive or inappropriate guilt nearly every day
  - Psychomotor agitation or retardation nearly every day
  - Recurrent thoughts of death or suicidal ideation
- Symptoms cause clinically significant distress or impairment in social, occupational, or other important areas of functioning.
- Symptoms are not caused by an underlying medical condition or substance (e.g., medications or recreational drugs).

Pathophysiology

Our understanding of the biological basis for depressive disorders has come a long way since Hippocrates first identified bile as a possible cause. Several modern theories addressing the origin of depression have evolved over the past three decades, focusing on neurotransmitter systems, including norepinephrine, serotonin, and dopamine. As unique antidepressant medications are developed and our understanding of the mechanisms of pharmacologic action improve, other cogent theories of depression will undoubtedly evolve.

In the past, the *monoamine hypothesis* proposed that decreased synaptic concentrations of norepinephrine and/or serotonin caused depression. The norepinephrine depletion theory was originally based on the observation that reserpine, which depleted catecholamine stores in the central nervous system (CNS), was capable of causing depression.[17,18] This theory evolved into the *permissive hypothesis*, which emphasized a greater role for serotonin in promoting or "permitting" a decline in norepinephrine function. Specifically, this hypothesis suggests that low concentrations of serotonin or norepinephrine in the CNS precipitated depressive symptoms, while low levels of serotonin and increased activity of norepinephrine resulted in manic symptoms. Antidepressants were believed to relieve depression by inhibiting the reuptake of norepinephrine and/or serotonin from the synapse back up into the neuron, and effectively increasing neurotransmitter concentrations in the synaptic cleft.[19]

Although these theories were initially helpful in enhancing our understanding of how antidepressants worked, there were multiple reasons to suspect that other mechanisms and systems were involved. First, antidepressants were capable of blocking the reuptake of neurotransmitters almost immediately after administration, yet several weeks lapsed before therapeutic effects were evident (i.e., delayed onset).[20] Second, synaptic concentrations of biogenic amines are not always decreased in depressed individuals and can actually be higher than those seen in normal controls.[21] Last, antidepressants in development can work via other mechanisms, which do not involve relative increases in synaptic neurotransmitter concentrations (e.g., can block substance P, or can antagonize corticotropin-releasing factor or corticosteroid receptors).[22–24]

The *dysregulation hypothesis* has evolved more recently and suggests that depression, as well as other psychiatric disorders, is the result of a dysregulated neurotransmitter system. Specific criteria for dysregulation have been proposed as follows: (a) an impairment in the regulatory or homeostatic mechanisms, (b) an erratic basal output of the neurotransmitter system, (c) a disruption in normal periodicities (circadian rhythm), (d) a less selective response to environmental stimuli, (e) perturbation of the system resulting in a delayed return to baseline, and (f) restoration to efficient regulation through the use of pharmacologic agents.[25]

Regardless of the antidepressant mechanism of action, changes in the presynaptic and postsynaptic receptor densities (or sensitivities) have been described as being "downregulated."[26] Changes include a decrease in postsynaptic alpha-adrenergic receptor sensitivity, along with alterations in the sensitivities of the alpha-adrenergic, dopaminergic (D2) and serotonin receptor subtypes (5-HT_{1A} and 5HT_{2A}). For example, selective serotonin reuptake inhibitors (SSRIs) can increase the efficiency of serotonergic neurotransmission acutely (through reuptake blockade), but their therapeutic effects are linked temporally with increased release of serotonin through downregulation of presynaptic autoreceptors (5-HT_{1A}).[27]

Today, emphasis continues to be placed on serotonin, norepinephrine, and dopamine neurotransmitters, and additional attention is also being paid to their differential effects on specific depressive symptoms. For instance, appetite, sleep, libido, motor function, anxiety, and aggression all appear to be strongly influenced by serotonin transmission. Research evidence for serotonergic influence has demonstrated that the concentration of serotonin's primary metabolite (5-hydroxyindoleacetic acid [5-HIAA]) is decreased in the cerebrospinal fluid (CSF) of depressed patients.[27] Low 5-HIAA concentrations have also been found in the CSF of patients attempting suicide and may have a role in triggering other violent activities.[28] Dietary depletion of L-tryptophan, a serotonin precursor, has induced relapse in depressed patients previously responsive to SSRIs, and symptoms such as irritability and disrupted sleep/appetite appear to return preferentially[29] (Fig. 79-1).

Alternatively, deficiencies in norepinephrine (and dopamine to some extent) are believed to mediate depressive symptoms such as anhedonia, decreased energy, memory impairments, and executive dysfunction.[30] Administration of α-methyl paratyrosine (which inhibits the synthesis of norepinephrine) has resulted in the return of these depressive symptoms among patients previously treated successfully with noradrenergic antidepressants.[31] The role of dopamine in mediating this constellation of symptoms has been implied through postmortem studies, neuroimaging results, and the demonstrated effectiveness of pure dopamine agonists (e.g., amantadine, pramipexole) in relieving depression.[32] Ultimately, it is still believed that a common circuitry is influenced by the different neurotransmitters, resulting in the clinical manifestation of depression.[31]

Neuroendocrine Findings

Along with dysregulated neurotransmitter systems, neuroendocrine abnormalities may contribute to the development of depression. Depressed patients often have abnormal thyroid function tests (including low triiodothyronine [T_3] and/or thyroxine [T_4] levels).[33] They also may exhibit an abnormal response to challenge with thyroid-releasing hormone (TRH), consisting of a blunted or exaggerated thyroid-stimulating hormone (TSH) response.[34] Clinical hypothyroidism can also induce depressive symptoms, and thyroid supplementation can reverse this pathology, suggesting an indirect association between mood disorders and thyroid homeostasis.[35]

The hypothalamic-pituitary-adrenal (HPA) axis may also influence the manifestation of depression, with a relative hyperactivity of this system commonly reported in depressed individuals. Pituitary and adrenal glands are often enlarged in depressed patients, and concentrations of corticotropin-releasing factor (CRF) are often elevated during depressive episodes and decline with the administration of antidepressant medications or electroconvulsive therapy (ECT).[24,36] Exogenous administration of CRF has elicited classic symptoms of depression in laboratory animals (including decreased appetite, anxiety, insomnia, and decreased libido).[37] In humans, medications that block postsynaptic corticosteroid receptors have also displayed antidepressant properties, as demonstrated with

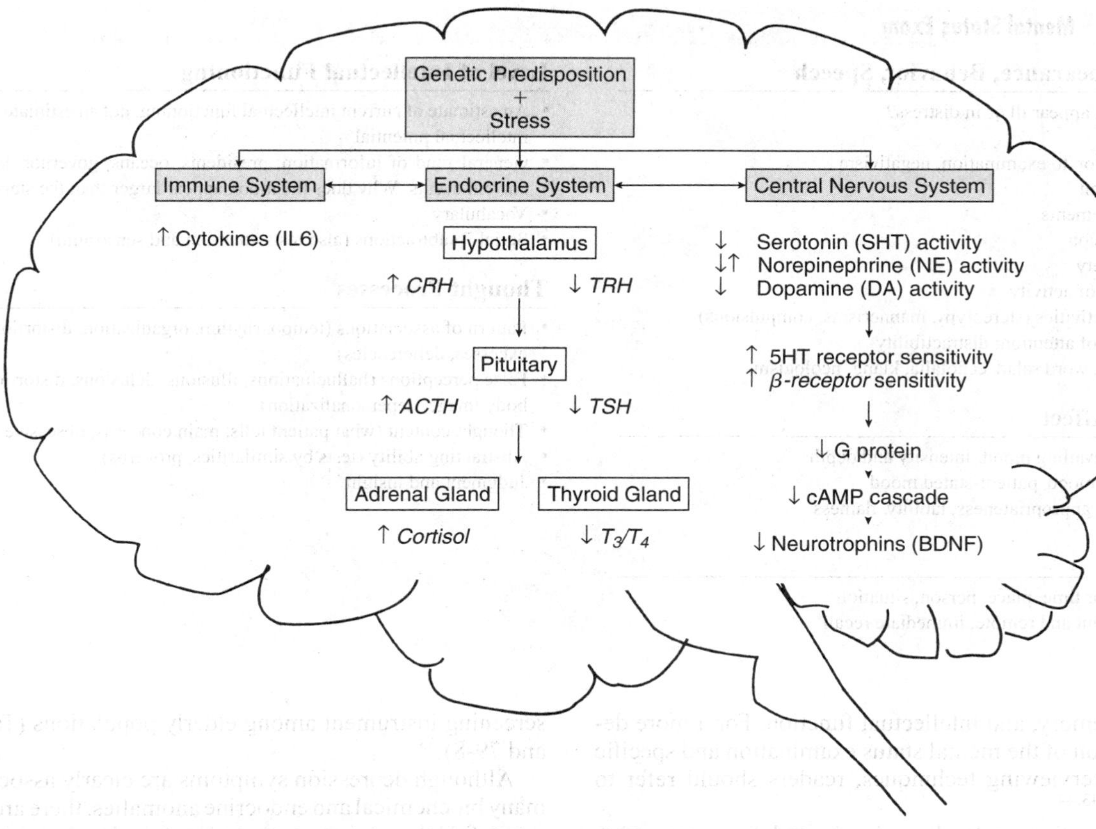

FIGURE 79-1 Influence of genetic and environmental factors on the immune system, endocrine system, and central nervous system. CRH, corticotropin-releasing hormone (also known as corticotropin-releasing factor [CRF]); TRH, thyrotrophin-releasing hormone; ACTH, adrenocorticotropic hormone; TSH, thyroid-stimulating hormone; T_3/T_4, thyroxine/triiodothyronine. (Copyright JL Corbitt, PR Finley 2003.)

ketoconazole and mifepristone.[38,39] Interestingly, serotonin exerts a strong influence on the HPA axis (and vice versa). Activation of the postsynaptic serotonin receptors (5-HT2) along the hypothalamic paraventricular nucleus can stimulate corticotropin-releasing hormone–secreting neurons. Corticosteroids can also modulate serotonin synthesis, metabolism, and reuptake.[24]

Not all of the evidence, however, supports a causative role of HPA overactivity in the manifestation of depression. The acute administration of high-dose corticosteroids, for instance, is more commonly associated with mood elevation (e.g., euphoria or hypomania), leading some to suggest that the exaggerated HPA response seen with depression is actually the body's attempt to overcome this mood disorder. Furthermore, HPA overactivity has not been observed in certain populations of depressed patients, such as adolescents and young adults. Given the strong association of depression with chronic inflammatory conditions, further exploration of the relationship of the HPA axis to depressive symptoms is imperative.

Imaging Studies

Imaging studies (including computed tomography, magnetic resonance imaging, positron emission tomography [PET], and single-photon emission computed tomography) suggest that patients with depression have regional brain dysfunction, most often affecting the limbic structures and prefrontal cortex. Alterations in cerebral blood flow and/or metabolism in the frontal-temporal cortex and caudate nucleus are associated with common depressive symptoms such as dysphoria, anhedonia, hopelessness, and flat affect.[40] Increased firing of the amygdala in the left hemisphere has been linked in PET studies with the future development of depression.[41] Because subtypes of depression have been linked to different regional dysfunctions, a network hypothesis has begun to emerge that may lead to improvements in depression diagnosis and targeted treatments.[42]

Patient Assessment Tools

Pharmaceutical care in the depressed patient requires specialized knowledge of the illness and treatments, as well as refined interviewing skills. To obtain specific information about the target symptoms of depression and to assess the therapeutic impact of psychotropic medications, effective and productive interpersonal communication is vital. The structured mental status examination is an established systematic way of assessing a patient's mental health (Table 79-5). Many functional domains are assessed in a mental status examination. Through this structured interview, the clinician has an observational basis for evaluating a patient's appearance, behavior, speech, mood, affect (i.e., outer manifestation of inner emotional states),

Table 79-5 Mental Status Exam

General Appearance, Behavior, Speech

- Apparent age; appear ill or in distress?
- Dress
- General reaction to examination, negativism
- Posture and gait
- Unusual movements
- Facial expression
- Signs of anxiety
- General level of activity
- Repetitious activities (stereotypy, mannerisms, compulsions)
- Disturbances of attention: distractibility
- Speech: mute, word salad, echolalia, klang, neologisms

Mood and Affect

- Quality of prevailing mood; intensity and depth
- Constancy of mood, patient-stated mood
- Affect: range, appropriateness, lability, flatness

Sensorium

- Orientation for time, place, person, situation
- Memory: recent and remote, immediate recall

Level of Intellectual Functioning

- An estimate of current intellectual functioning, not an estimate of original intellectual potential
- General fund of information: presidents, oceans, governor, large cities, current events. Why does the moon appear larger than the stars?
- Vocabulary
- Serial 7 subtractions (also tests attention and sensorium)

Thought Processes

- Pattern of associations (tempo, rhythm, organization, distortions, excesses, deficiencies)
- False perceptions (hallucinations, illusions, delusions, distortions of body image, depersonalization)
- Thought content (what patient tells, main concerns, obsessive ideation)
- Abstracting ability (tests by similarities, proverbs)
- Judgment and insight

sensorium, memory, and intellectual function. For a more detailed discussion of the mental status examination and specific psychiatric interviewing techniques, readers should refer to other sources.[43,44]

Behavioral rating scales have been used for many years in drug efficacy studies and are being used routinely in the clinical arena today. Rating scales can be helpful in assessing the severity of mental illness, quantifying changes in target symptoms, and determining treatment efficacy, but they are not necessarily diagnostic. Rating scales can vary in length, content, and format, and can be completed by providers, patients, researchers, family members, or conservators. Numerous depression scales have been developed over the years, including the Hamilton Rating Scale for Depression (HAM-D), the Beck Depression Inventory, the Zung Depression Scale, the Hopkins Symptom Checklist, the Montgomery Asberg Depression Rating Scale, the Center for Epidemiological Studies Depression (CES-D) Scale, the Patient Health Questionnaire, and the Quick Inventory of Depressive Symptoms (QIDS).[45–52] The HAM-D was initially designed to measure the efficacy of antidepressant medications given to severely depressed individuals in controlled clinical trials (Table 79-6).[45] Over the years, this instrument emerged as the gold standard of depression rating scales, although many clinicians are unaware of its limitations. For instance, the HAM-D was never designed for routine use in the general ambulatory care patient population and fails to address a number of target symptoms required for a DSM-IV-TR diagnosis of major depression (e.g., low energy, poor concentration, reverse neurovegetative symptoms). The QIDS has emerged recently as a more valuable instrument in the hands of primary care providers. It contains a total of 16 items, can be completed within 10 to 15 minutes, and is available at no cost to clinicians. It has been validated and used extensively in clinical and research settings and is available in a clinician-rated or patient-rated format. The CES-D is also available in an abbreviated format and has served as a useful screening instrument among elderly populations (Tables 79-7 and 79-8).[53]

Although depression symptoms are clearly associated with many biochemical and endocrine anomalies, there are currently no useful laboratory tests that are routinely administered to aid the clinician in establishing a diagnosis of depression. For many years, the dexamethasone suppression test (DST) was used to confirm the diagnosis of depression, but now it is rarely indicated. The rationale for this test lies in the apparent inability of depressed patients to suppress cortisol concentrations after dexamethasone administration. The standard protocol consists of administering a 1-mg dose of dexamethasone at 11 PM and obtaining blood samples at 4 PM and 11 PM on the following day for the purpose of measuring subsequent cortisol concentrations. The results are considered abnormal (positive) if either of the two samples are >5 mcg/dL. Studies have demonstrated that the DST is often more abnormal in older depressed subjects, and a meta-analysis concluded that a positive baseline DST was predictive of worse treatment outcomes.[54] Unfortunately, many medical conditions and medications may augment the cortisol response, resulting in a greater likelihood of false-positive findings. Furthermore, as many as half of depressed subjects may have a normal DST (i.e., manifesting in false-negative findings). The APA Task Force on Laboratory Tests in Psychiatry has outlined some of the potential indications for the DST, and it may, in fact, be useful in certain clinical situations to confirm a diagnosis of depression.[55] However, in general, the DST is not recommended as a routine screening instrument at present.

Nondrug Therapies for Depression

The successful treatment of depression provides a most formidable challenge to modern medicine. In addition to the emotional turmoil and social disability that a depressed individual endures, the illness can have an affect on other disease

Table 79-6 Hamilton Depression Scale (HAM-D 17)

For Each Item, Check the Box Next to the Response That Best Characterizes the Patient

1. Depressed mood (sadness, hopeless, helpless, worthless)	0 ☐	Absent
	1 ☐	These feeling states indicated only on questioning
	2 ☐	These feeling states spontaneously reported verbally
	3 ☐	Communicates feeling states nonverbally (i.e., through facial expression, posture, voice, and tendency to weep)
	4 ☐	Patient reports VIRTUALLY ONLY these feeling states in his or her spontaneous verbal and nonverbal communication
2. Feelings of guilt	0 ☐	Absent
	1 ☐	Self-reproach, feels he or she has let people down
	2 ☐	Ideas of guilt or rumination over past errors or sinful deeds
	3 ☐	Presents illness as a punishment; delusions of guilt
	4 ☐	Hears accusatory or denunciatory voices and/or experiences threatening visual hallucinations
3. Suicide	0 ☐	Absent
	1 ☐	Feels life is not worth living
	2 ☐	Wishes he or she were dead or any thoughts of possible death to self
	3 ☐	Suicide ideas or gesture
	4 ☐	Attempts at suicide (only serious attempt rates 4)
4. Insomnia early	0 ☐	No difficulty
	1 ☐	Complains of occasional difficulty falling asleep (i.e., more than one-half hour)
	2 ☐	Complains of nightly difficulty falling asleep
5. Insomnia middle	0 ☐	No difficulty
	1 ☐	Patient complains of being restless and disturbed during the night
	2 ☐	Waking during the night—any getting out of bed rates 2 *(except for purposes of voiding)*
6. Insomnia late	0 ☐	No difficulty
	1 ☐	Waking in early hours of the morning but goes back to sleep
	2 ☐	Unable to fall asleep again if gets out of bed
7. Work and activities	0 ☐	No difficulty
	1 ☐	Thoughts and feeling of incapacity, fatigue, or weakness related to activities, work, or hobbies
	2 ☐	Loss of interest in activities, work, or hobbies—either directly reported by patients, or indirect in listlessness, indecision, and vacillation (feels he or she has to push self)
	3 ☐	Decrease in actual time spent in activities or decrease in productivity, in hospital, rate 3 if patient does not spend at least 3 hours a day in activities or decrease in productivity, in hospital, rate 3 if patient does not spend at least 3 hours a day in activities (hospital job or hobbies), exclusive of ward chores
	4 ☐	Stopped working because of present illness, in hospital, rate 4 if patient engages in no activities except ward chores, or if patients fails to perform ward chores unassisted
8. Retardation (slowness of thought and speech, impaired ability to concentrate, decreased motor activity)	0 ☐	Normal speech and thought
	1 ☐	Slight retardation at interview
	2 ☐	Obvious retardation at interview
	3 ☐	Interview difficult
	4 ☐	Complete stupor
9. Agitation	0 ☐	None
	1 ☐	"Playing with" hands, hair, etc.
	2 ☐	Hand wringing, nail biting, hair pulling, biting of lips
10. Anxiety psychic	0 ☐	No difficulty
	1 ☐	Slight retardation at interview
	2 ☐	Obvious retardation at interview
	3 ☐	Interview difficult
	4 ☐	Complete stupor
11. Anxiety somatic	0 ☐	Absent — Physiological concomitants of anxiety, such as
	1 ☐	Mild — Gastrointestinal (GI)—dry mouth, wind, indigestion, diarrhea, cramps, belching
	2 ☐	Moderate — Cardiovascular—palpitations, headaches
	3 ☐	Severe — Respiratory—hyperventilation, sighing
	4 ☐	Incapacitating — Sweating
12. Somatic symptoms—GI	0 ☐	None
	1 ☐	Loss of appetite but eating without staff encouragement; heavy feelings in abdomen
	2 ☐	Difficulty eating without staff urging; requests or requires laxatives or medication for bowels or medication for GI symptoms
13. Somatic symptoms—general	0 ☐	None
	1 ☐	Heaviness in limbs, back, or head; backaches, headache, muscle aches; loss of energy or fatigability
	2 ☐	Any clear-cut symptoms rates 2

(continued)

Table 79-6 Hamilton Depression Scale (HAM-D 17) (Continued)

14. Genital symptoms	0 ❑	Absent Symptoms such as Loss of libido
	1 ❑	Mild Menstrual disturbances
	2 ❑	Severe
15. Hypochondriasis	0 ❑	Not present
	1 ❑	Self-absorption (bodily)
	2 ❑	Preoccupation with health
	3 ❑	Frequent complaints, requests for help, etc.
	4 ❑	Hypochondriacal delusions
16. Loss of weight (answer only A or B)		A. When rating by history:
	0 ❑	No weight loss
	1 ❑	Probably weight loss associated with present illness
	2 ❑	Definite (according to patient) weight loss
		B. On weekly ratings by ward psychiatrist, when actual weight changes are measured:
	0 ❑	<1-lb weight loss in week
	1 ❑	>1-lb weight loss in week
	2 ❑	>2-lb weight loss in week
17. Insight	0 ❑	Acknowledges being depressed and ill
	1 ❑	Acknowledges illness but attributes cause to bad food, climate, overwork, virus, need for rest, etc.
	2 ❑	Denies being ill at all
Investigator's Signature:		

From Hamilton M. Development of a rating scale of primary depressive illness. *Br J Soc Clin Psychol* 1967;2:278.

states, slow the recovery process, or even promote complications. Furthermore, the likelihood of future depressive episodes increases with each recurrence, dampening the patient's prognosis over time.

Although pharmacologic intervention has become the primary treatment modality for relieving depressive symptoms, the efficacy and suitability of other therapeutic options should not be overlooked. Most experts now advocate a three-pronged approach to relieving and preventing depressive symptoms, involving (a) psychotherapy, (b) somatic interventions, and (c) lifestyle adjustments. Because these interventions address different aspects of the illness at different stages in the recovery process, they work synergistically together, and a brief summary of these approaches can be found later in this chapter. (*Note:* Because discussion of medications comprises the bulk of this chapter; readers are advised to refer to the "Drug Management" section for information specific to pharmacotherapy.)

Psychotherapy

For the treatment of mild to moderate depression, psychotherapy has proved to be comparable to pharmacologic intervention and may actually be preferred by some patients. For the acute treatment of severe depression, antidepressants appear to be more effective than psychotherapy alone and have a more rapid onset of therapeutic action.[56] The beneficial effects of psychotherapy, however, may persist longer than medication-related benefits after the interventions have been formally discontinued. In addition, psychotherapy may be particularly beneficial for preventing relapse among patients who previously demonstrated a therapeutic response to antidepressants.[57] Overall, the combination of treatments is superior to either intervention alone, although the routine use of both modalities is often not feasible in today's health care environment.[56]

Several forms of psychotherapy are available, including cognitive-behavioral therapy (CBT), interpersonal therapy, and psychoanalytic and psychodynamic therapies. CBT, in particular, often focuses on identifying and reversing negative thought patterns that perpetuate depressed emotions. It has been studied extensively in the depression field and is now available in a manual-driven, evidence-based format. A more precise explanation and description of psychotherapeutic alternatives is beyond the scope of this textbook. However, clinicians in the field are strongly encouraged to develop familiarity with these approaches, as well as general supportive counseling techniques, which can serve to promote the recovery process and decrease the likelihood of future episodes.[58]

Somatic Interventions

ECT is a safe, rapid-acting, and highly effective therapeutic intervention that continues to suffer, ostensibly, from a poor public image. ECT was enormously popular during the 1940s and 1950s and was used without discretion to treat a wide variety of psychiatric conditions. This practice waned with the advent of effective psychotropic medications, and with the accumulation of case reports describing fractures and severe cognitive impairment in treated patients. Since the 1950s, the ECT procedure has undergone considerable transformation and refinement.[59] Adjunctive medications are now routinely administered to prevent adverse effects and reduce morbidity (e.g., a short-acting barbiturate for general anesthesia, an anticholinergic agent to prevent bradycardia and dry excessive airway secretions, succinylcholine to prevent fractures from tonic-clonic contractions). The electric stimulus itself is no longer applied in one steady current but now consists of a series of brief pulses that have been shown to decrease the severity of postictal headaches and memory impairment.

Fundamentally, ECT features the induction of generalized seizures through an electric current delivered by bilateral or

Table 79-7 Quick Inventory for Depressive Symptomatology (Clinician-Rated) (QIDS-C16)

NAME:________________ TODAY'S DATE:________

Please circle the one response to each item that best describes the patient for the past 7 days.

1. Sleep Onset Insomnia:
   a. Never takes longer than 30 minutes to fall asleep.
   b. Takes at least 30 minutes to fall asleep, less than half the time.
   c. Takes at least 30 minutes to fall asleep, more than half the time.
   d. Takes more than 60 minutes to fall asleep, more than half the time.
2. Midnocturnal Insomnia:
   a. Does not wake up at night.
   b. Restless, light sleep with few awakenings
   c. Wakes up at least once at night
   d. Awakens more than once at night and stays awake for 20 minutes or more, more than half the time.
3. Feeling Anxious or Tense:
   a. I do not feel anxious or tense.
   b. I feel anxious (tense) less than half the time.
   c. I feel anxious (tense) more than half the time.
   d. I feel extremely anxious (tense) nearly all of the time.
4. The Quality of Your Mood:
   a. The mood (internal feelings) that I experience is very much a normal mood.
   b. My mood is sad, but this sadness is pretty much like the sad mood I would feel if someone close to me died or left.
   c. My mood is sad, but this sadness has a rather different quality to it than the sadness I would feel if someone close to me died or left.
   d. My mood is sad, but this sadness is different from the type of sadness associated with grief or loss.
5. Sleep During the Night:
   a. I do not wake up at night.
   b. I have a restless, light sleep with a few brief awakenings each night.
   c. I wake up at least once a night, but I go back to sleep easily.
   d. I awaken more than once a night and stay awake for 20 minutes or more, more than half the time.

   Please complete *either* 6 *or* 7 (not both)
6. Decreased Appetite:
   a. There is no change in my usual appetite.
   b. I eat somewhat less often or lesser amounts of food than usual.
   c. I eat much less than usual and only with personal effort.
   d. I rarely eat within a 24-hour period, and only with extreme personal effort or when others persuade me to eat.
7. Increased Appetite:
   a. There is no change from my usual appetite.
   b. I feel a need to eat more frequently than usual.
   c. I regularly eat more often and/or greater amounts of food than usual.
   d. I feel driven to overeat both at mealtime and between meals.
8. Aches and Pains:
   a. I don't have any feeling of heaviness in my arms or legs or any aches or pains.
   b. Sometimes I get headaches or pains in my stomach, back, or joints, but these pains are only sometime present and don't stop me from doing what I need to do.
   c. I have these sorts of pains most of the time.
   d. These pains are so bad they force me to stop what I am doing.
9. Concentration/Decision Making:
   a. There is no change in my usual capacity to concentrate or make decisions.
   b. I occasionally feel indecisive or find that my attention wanders.
   c. Most of the time, I struggle to focus my attention or to make decisions.
   d. I cannot concentrate well enough to read and cannot make even minor decisions.
10. Energy Level:
    a. There is no change in my usual level of energy.
    b. I get tired more easily than usual.
    c. I have to make a big effort to start or finish my usual daily activities (e.g., shopping, homework, cooking, or going to work).
    d. I really cannot carry out most of my usual daily activities because I just don't have the energy.
11. General Interest:
    a. There is no change from usual in how interested I am in other people or activities.
    b. I notice that I am less interested in people or activities.
    c. I find I have interest in only one or two of my formerly pursued activities.
    d. I have virtually no interest in formerly pursued activities.
12. Capacity for Pleasure or Enjoyment (excluding sex):
    a. I enjoy pleasurable activities just as much as usual.
    b. I do not feel my usual sense of enjoyment from pleasurable activities.
    c. I rarely get a feeling of pleasure from any activity.
    d. I am unable to get any pleasure or enjoyment from anything.
13. View of Myself:
    a. I see myself as equally worthwhile and deserving as other people.
    b. I am more self-blaming than usual.
    c. I largely believe that I cause problems for others.
    d. I think almost constantly about major and minor defects in myself.
14. View of My Future:
    a. I have an optimistic view of my future.
    b. I am occasionally pessimistic about my future, but for the most part I believe things will get better.
    c. I'm pretty certain that my immediate future (1–2 months) does not hold much promise of good things for me.
    d. I see no hope of anything good happening to me anytime in the future.
15. Thoughts of Death or Suicide:
    a. I do not think of suicide or death.
    b. I feel that life is empty or wonder if it's worth living.
    c. I think of suicide or death several times a week for several minutes.
    d. I think of suicide or death several times a day in some detail, or I have made specific plans for suicide or have actually tried to take my life.

Please review this test and write in this space ____the numbers of the three items that were the most difficult to understand.

Which three items (questions) were the easiest to understand?____

Thank you.

Range 0–42 Score:________

Table 79-8 Comparison of Selected Depression Rating Scales

Instrument	*Minimal*	*Mild*	*Moderate*	*Severe*
Hamilton (HAM-D)—17-item Clinician-rated	<8	8–15	16–27	>27
Beck Depression Inventory (BDI) Clinician-rated	<10	10–16	17–29	>29
BDI Patient-rated	<10	10–15	16–23	>23
Quick Inventory for Depressive Symptoms (QIDS-C) Clinician-rated	<6	6–10	11–15	>15
QIDS-SR Patient-rated	<6	6–10	11–15	>15
Montgomery-Asberg Depression Rating Scale (MADRS) Clinician-rated	<7	7–19	20–34	>34

unilateral electrode placement. Certain medications may raise seizure thresholds (benzodiazepines) or promote cognitive impairment (lithium) and should be discontinued before the procedure. Adverse effects are generally minimal and consist mainly of transient anterograde amnesia (i.e., difficulty remembering events around the time of the procedure), retrograde amnesia, confusion, headaches, and muscle aches. Cardiovascular effects (e.g., ventricular arrhythmias, myocardial infarction [MI]) are the most ominous sequelae, but these events are actually quite rare.

Many years of clinical experience have enabled clinicians to identify patient populations most likely to benefit from this intervention. Today, ECT is recommended for patients with treatment-resistant depression, severe vegetative depression, psychotic depression, and depression in pregnancy. Overall response rates are rather impressive, ranging from 70% to 90%, and ECT has the distinct advantage of inducing a therapeutic response within the first week or two of treatments.[60] The recommended frequency of ECT treatments is variable. Most institutions have used three sessions weekly to induce a therapeutic response acutely, although evidence suggests that twice-weekly sessions are better tolerated and more cost effective.[61] The frequency of treatments thereafter (i.e., maintenance therapy) is unknown, although recent evidence suggests that ECT administered weekly for 1 month and less frequently thereafter may be as effective as aggressive pharmacotherapy in preventing relapse.[62]

Other somatic interventions have also been used successfully to treat depression. Transcranial magnetic stimulation (TMS) is a noninvasive procedure involving the application of an electrical stimulus across the scalp, which ultimately generates an electrical field in the cerebral cortex.[63] Unlike ECT, TMS does not generate an actual seizure and is very well tolerated. Evidence of efficacy has been demonstrated in several investigations using repetitive high-frequency techniques, and imaging studies have shown functional improvements consistent with antidepressant properties. However, it is not currently U.S. Food and Drug Administration (FDA) approved for the treatment of depression. Vagal nerve stimulation (VNS) involves the surgical implantation of an electrical device in the subcutaneous tissue below the clavicle, which sends an impulse along the left vagal nerve into the cerebral cortex.[64] This intervention has proven to be effective for intractable seizures. It is currently FDA approved for the management of treatment-resistant depression as well, although the safety and cost effectiveness of this expensive procedure have not been extensively studied.

Light therapy or phototherapy is particularly effective for relieving the irritability and malaise associated with seasonal affective disorder, a milder form of depression that has been attributed to decreases in natural sunlight found with seasonal variation.[65] Phototherapy is administered in the form of a light box delivering 1,500 to 10,000 lux over a period of 1 to 2 hours daily. It is generally very well tolerated, although case reports of mania have surfaced as with any other somatic intervention used for depression. Sleep deprivation may be an effective adjuvant to antidepressants and has also been studied as a remedy for premenstrual dysphoric disorder. The goal of sleep deprivation is to gradually advance sleep cycles by altering wake schedules, ultimately minimizing the duration of rapid eye movement (REM) sleep.[66]

Lifestyle Adjustments

Any therapeutic approach to mood disorders should seek to reverse unhealthy or destructive lifestyle habits and consider other activities that may relieve stress and facilitate well-being. Alcohol, recreational drug use, and excessive caffeine consumption should be minimized (if not prohibited) in patients suffering from depression or anxiety disorders. Sleep habits should be evaluated and improved to ensure optimal rest. This also promotes the restoration of normal physiological and immunologic processes that can ward off chronic illness. Dietary factors should be modified to promote diverse, balanced, and nutritional eating habits.

Increased physical activity and sustained cardiovascular exertion can impart a variety of health benefits, as well as relief from mood disorders. Although investigations examining the effectiveness of exercise for clinical depression have met with mixed results, exercise can certainly regulate appetite, improve sleep patterns, increase energy, enhance self-esteem, and indicate a return to euthymic status.[67] Exercise has been shown to increase circulating concentrations of serotonin in the periphery and enhance neurogenesis in the hippocampus.[68] Other activities may also serve to relieve stress and help patients develop insights into their emotional well-being. These pursuits can range from daily journal writing (or "journaling"), to prayer or meditation, to yoga and tai chi. Classes in mindfulness-based meditation, in particular, are now being offered at many medical centers, and the health benefits of this approach have been demonstrated in a wide range of medical conditions (e.g., cancer, chronic pain syndromes, HIV illness).[69] Certain herbal remedies may also be effective and are discussed in Chapter 3.

MAJOR DEPRESSIVE DISORDER

Diagnosis

1. A.R. is a 25-year-old woman who presents to the student health clinic for a routine physical examination. During her visit, A.R. states, "I've been feeling pretty down lately and just want to give up." Her physical examination is unremarkable, and all laboratory tests (complete blood count with differential, chemistry panel, and thyroid function tests) are within normal limits. A human chorionic gonadotropin test is negative. Her medical history is noncontributory, the only prescription medication she has received is an oral contraceptive (which she has taken faithfully for the past 6 months), and she denies drinking alcohol or using other recreational substances.

When asked, A.R. states that she has had increasing periods of depressed mood over the past few months and often finds herself crying in the morning for no particular reason. She reports that she has no interest in her old hobbies (playing the piano, mountain biking, gardening). She is engaged to be married in 3 months but feels that she does not deserve to be a wife. Over the past 2 months, her appetite has decreased, and she has lost 15 lb. She feels overwhelmed about all of the plans that she needs to make for her wedding ("I don't even deserve a wedding this nice") and has difficulty sleeping, often waking in the middle of the night and being unable to fall back asleep. She has no energy during the day and finds it difficult to concentrate or make decisions. This is a major concern because she is a graduate student at the local university.

The mental status examination reveals an appropriately dressed female who appears sad but who is alert, coherent, and logical. Her affect is constricted, apprehensive, and sad. Mood is depressed, and she admits having suicidal ideation but no specific plans. She is oriented to person, place, and time but shows some recent memory deficits. Her intelligence is estimated to be above average. Concentration and abstractions (e.g., "don't cry over spilled milk," "a rolling stone gathers no moss") are satisfactory. She denies hearing voices or other hallucinations. She has good insight and judgment into her illness. What signs and symptoms does A.R. have that support the diagnosis of major depressive disorder?

The target symptoms of depression are listed in Table 79-9 and can be recalled by the pneumonic D-SIG-E-CAPS or DIG-SPACES. Based on A.R.'s history, she describes a dysphoric or depressed mood as well as anhedonia (lack of interest in hobbies or pleasurable activities). In addition, she demonstrates frequent episodes of crying, decreased appetite (with an unintentional 15-lb weight loss), poor concentration, low energy, suicidal ideation, worthlessness, and inappropriate guilt. Her mental status examination is consistent with these target symptoms, revealing a constricted, sad affect (physical manifestation of inner emotional states) and frequent crying episodes during the interview.

Based on the DSM-IV-TR criteria, A.R. has major depressive disorder. Over the past 2 weeks, she has consistently exhibited at least five of the associated symptoms, one of which is depression or anhedonia. It does not appear that her symptoms are the result of any medical condition, medication, thought disorder, or uncomplicated bereavement. The anhedonia and vegetative symptoms (e.g., midnocturnal insomnia, decreased appetite, weight loss) are consistent with the depressive subtype of melancholia.

Suicide Assessment

2. What is the risk of A.R. hurting herself? How should suicidal ideation be assessed?

Patients with major depression should always be assessed for the presence of suicidal thoughts (e.g., "Do you ever feel like giving up?", "Are you thinking about hurting yourself?"). Suicide is viewed by the depressed patient as a remedy to insurmountable problems when all other options appear hopeless. Comments made by the patients alluding to suicide (e.g., "Life is not worth living anymore," "I am leaving and may never see you again") should be taken seriously. Misunderstandings about suicidal ideation abound in the general public. Common myths include the ideas that people are more likely to commit suicide if asked about it, that people who attempt suicide are just looking for attention, or that suicide is usually attempted after a sudden traumatic event.

Several factors may place a person at greater risk for a suicide attempt. A detailed plan, for instance, suggests a serious intent and a higher risk for successful suicide. The clinician should be concerned if a change takes place in A.R.'s personality (e.g., giving away possessions, making a will, purchasing a firearm, asking about the lethal dose of medications). Other risks for suicide include living alone, having a physical illness, being unemployed, being 15 to 24 years of age or older than 65 years of age, having a history of alcohol/drug abuse, or having a family history of suicide.[70] Gender plays a role as well, with women much more likely to attempt suicide, while men are more often successful.

The management of patients who are potentially suicidal depends on the attendant risk, incorporating many of the

Table 79-9 Depressive Disorder Target Symptom Mnemonic

D	SIG	E	CAPS
Depressed mood	Sleep (insomnia or hypersomnia)	Energy loss	Concentration (loss)
	Interest (loss of, including libido)		Appetite (loss or gain)
	Guilt		Psychomotor (agitation or retardation)
			Suicide (ideation)

From ref. 67.

factors just cited. For patients who are actively suicidal, hospitalization is often necessary and may even be facilitated against the patient's will in high-risk settings. Other life-saving interventions include establishing close contact with the patient's family and health care provider, convincing the patient to contract for his or her safety, ensuring that firearms and other lethal means are removed from the home, and avoiding antidepressants with a narrow therapeutic index (e.g., tricyclic antidepressants [TCAs]) or limiting the dispensed quantity to <10 days. Depressed patients surface in any health care environment, so all clinicians should have an emergency hotline or crisis telephone number at their disposal.

A.R. is at some risk for suicide, although she does not have a detailed plan at present. She should be monitored closely during the first few weeks of therapy by friends or family members. If her suicidal ideation becomes severe, A.R. should be admitted to a facility for her own safety. Unfortunately, it is not always possible to predict whether A.R. (or any depressed patient) will attempt to commit suicide. Even with the most conservative precautions, a small percentage of patients succeed in their suicide attempts.

DRUG MANAGEMENT

Drug Selection: General Considerations

3. A.R. is diagnosed as follows: Axis I—major depressive disorder, single episode, with melancholic features; Axis II—none; and Axis III—none. What drug options are available for A.R.'s depressive symptoms? What considerations should be made when selecting antidepressant therapy?

At present, 23 medications have received FDA approval in the United States for the treatment of depression. They can be conveniently grouped into six categories:

1. SSRIs
2. Serotonin norepinephrine reuptake inhibitors (SNRIs)
3. Norepinephrine reuptake inhibitors (NRIs)
4. TCAs
5. Monoamine oxidase inhibitors (MAOIs)
6. Miscellaneous (e.g., trazodone, mirtazapine)

All available antidepressants are equally effective in the general depressed patient population, and all appear to have the same delayed onset of therapeutic effects. Historically, it has been reported that 65% to 70% of patients given a therapeutic trial of an antidepressant will have a positive response (therapeutic response traditionally defined as a ≥50% drop in depression rating scores), and 35% to 40% achieving remission (i.e., virtual absence of symptoms).[71] These treatment effects, however, were usually measured in randomized controlled trials (RCTs) among patients with minimal comorbidity who were exhibiting moderate-to-severe psychopathology. Recent efforts have been made to examine these response patterns under less rigidly controlled conditions (i.e., more naturalistic studies). Most notably, a series of investigations that came to be known as the STAR*D (Sequenced Treatment Alternatives to Relieve Depression) trials enrolled nearly 3,000 patients from primary care clinics and mental health centers across the United States in an effort to determine the effectiveness of first-line treatments, as well as second-line agents and augmentation strategies.[72] All eligible patients received a relatively rigorous course of citalopram (average dose = 41.8 mg daily), and the results suggested that response rates are closer to 50% and remission is achieved in 30% of patients treated under "real world" conditions.

Table 79-10 Factors to Consider in Selecting an Antidepressant

- History of prior response (personal or family member)
- Safety in overdose
- Adverse effect profiles
- Patient age
- Concurrent medical/psychiatric conditions
- Concurrent medications (e.g., potential for drug interactions)
- Convenience (e.g., minimal titration, once-daily dosing)
- Cost
- Patient preference

Because the response rates for all currently available antidepressants are comparable, other important considerations should influence decision making (Tables 79-10–79-13). The first factor to consider is the patient's history of previous response. If this history is unavailable (or the patient has never received an antidepressant before), the clinician should inquire about family history. If a first-degree relative had a successful course of antidepressant treatment with minimal adverse effects, that specific medication (or another from the same antidepressant class) would be a prudent choice for initiating therapy.

The potential impact of an antidepressant on concurrent medical conditions or disease states is often considered next. For example, certain antidepressants (e.g., TCA, paroxetine, mirtazapine) are associated with significant weight gain and would not be desirable choices for obese patients. Similarly, bupropion should be avoided in patients with a history of seizures, and venlafaxine may not be ideal for patients with hypertension.

Many clinicians select an antidepressant by matching the patient's presenting symptoms to the side effect profile of antidepressant medications. For example, if a depressed patient is sleeping and eating excessively, and possesses little energy or motivation, the clinician may choose an agent that will address these baseline symptoms, perhaps through the enhancement of noradrenergic transmission (e.g., bupropion). Patients with substantial anxiety or irritability may benefit preferentially from antidepressants that facilitate serotonergic transmission (e.g., SSRI) because nearly 50% of patients with major depression are believed to be suffering from a concurrent anxiety disorder. Conversely, some clinicians argue that if an antidepressant is clinically effective, it will relieve all target symptoms eventually, regardless of the adverse effect profile. Nonetheless, tailoring antidepressant medications to a patient's presentation is a common practice that may minimize the initial side effect burden and promote adherence.

Other important patient-specific factors to consider in the selection of an agent include safety in overdose, potential for drug interactions, ease of administration (once daily vs. divided doses), necessity of titration practices, cost (to the patient/institution), and patient preference.

Because A.R. is a student, the clinician may want to select an antidepressant that has minimal effects on alertness or cognitive function, such as an SSRI or bupropion. Of these

Table 79-11 Pharmacology of Antidepressant Medications

Medication	*Serotonin*	*Norepinephrine*	*Dopamine*	*Bioavailability (Oral)*	*Protein Binding*	*Half-Life (in hours) (Active Metabolite)*
Selective Serotonin Reuptake Inhibitors						
Fluoxetine (Prozac)	+ + + +	0/+	0	80%	95%	24–72 (146)
Sertraline (Zoloft)	+ + + +	0/+	+	>44%	95%	26 (66)
Paroxetine (Paxil)	+ + + +	+	0	64%	99%	24
Citalopram (Celexa)	+ + + +	0	0	80%	<80%	33
Escitalopram (Lexapro)	+ + + +	0	0	80%	56%	27–32
Serotonin Norepinephrine Reuptake Inhibitors						
Venlafaxine (Effexor)	+ + + +	+ + +	0	92%	25–29%	4 (10)
Duloxetine (Cymbalta)	+ + ++	++++	0	50%	>90%	12 (8–17)
Norepinephrine Reuptake Inhibitors						
Bupropion (Wellbutrin)	0/+	+	+	>90%	85%	10–21
Tricyclic Antidepressants						
Desipramine (Norpramin)	+	+ + + +	0/+	51%	90%	12–28
Nortriptyline (Pamelor)	+ +	+ + +	0	46%–56%	92%	18–56
Amitriptyline (Elavil)	+ + + +	+ + + +	0	37%–49%	95%	9–46 (18–56)
Imipramine (Tofranil)	+ + +	+ +	0/+	19%–35%	95%	6–28 (12–28)
Doxepin (Sinequan)	+ + +	+	0	17%–37%	68%–85%	11–23
Others						
Mirtazapine (Remeron)	+ + +	+ + + +	0	50%	85%	20–40

0, negligible; +, very low; + +, low; + + +, moderate; + + + +, high.

two options, an SSRI may be preferred for A.R. because she is experiencing a significant decrease in appetite and insomnia, which may be exacerbated with bupropion.

Response Rates of Target Symptoms

4. **A.R. is given a prescription for sertraline 50-mg tablets. She is instructed to take a half tablet (25 mg) for the first week and increase to a whole tablet daily thereafter. She is also asked to return to the clinic in 4 weeks for follow-up. How soon should A.R.'s target symptoms begin to resolve?**

A similar delayed pattern of therapeutic response has been observed with all antidepressant medications. Traditionally, patients have been informed that approximately 4 to 6 weeks must elapse before they will experience any therapeutic benefit from medication. However, researchers in the field consider this a conservative estimate, gleaned from standard drug efficacy studies ill suited to answer this question.[73] In such studies, patients will begin to show signs of clinical response during the first 1 or 2 weeks of active treatment, but because the difference from placebo is assessed every 7 days and will not ordinarily achieve statistical significance until the third or fourth week, these early response patterns are misinterpreted to suggest that it may take a month or more for patients to improve. Some experts have contended, in fact, that trials uniquely designed to investigate the onset of therapeutic effect will conclusively show that patients exhibit substantial improvement during the first 2 weeks of treatment, and *maximum* improvement may not be evident for 4 weeks or more.[74]

The *pattern* of patient response can also be generalized, with neurovegetative symptoms often the first to subside (e.g., altered sleep or appetite, decreased energy, excessive worrying and irritability). The cognitive symptoms are slower to respond, and 3 to 4 weeks or more may elapse before improvements are evident. These symptoms include excessive guilt or pessimism, poor concentration, hopelessness or sadness, and decreased libido.

A.R. should be counseled concerning this anticipated delay in therapeutic response and advised that optimal improvement may take at least 4 weeks. If she is not aware of this time frame, she may stop the medication prematurely, prolonging her distress and further delaying the recovery process.

Selective Serotonin Reuptake Inhibitors

Adverse Effects

5. **What are the most common side effects reported with SSRIs, and how should they be managed?**

Although it is not accurate to say that SSRIs (or SNRIs) cause fewer side effects than TCAs, the adverse effects associated with these newer antidepressant classes are generally milder and less likely to lead to discontinuation.[75] There are

Table 79-12 Adverse Effects of Antidepressant Medications

Medication	Sedation	Agitation/Insomnia	Anticholinergic Effects	Orthostasis	GI Effects (Nausea/Diarrhea)	Sexual Dysfunction	Weight Gain
Selective Serotonin Reuptake Inhibitors							
Fluoxetine (Prozac)	+	++++	0/+	0/+	++++	++++	+
Sertraline (Zoloft)	+	+++	0/+	0	+++	+++	+
Paroxetine (Paxil)	+++	++	++	0	+++	++++	++
Citalopram (Celexa)	++	++	0/+	0	+++	+++	+
Escitalopram (Lexapro)	+	++	0/+	0	+++	+++	+
Serotonin Norepinephrine Reuptake Inhibitors							
Venlafaxine (Effexor)	++	++	+	0	+++	+++	+
Duloxetine (Cymbalta)	++	++	+	0	+++	++	0/+
Norepinephrine Reuptake Inhibitors							
Bupropion (Wellbutrin)	0	+++	+	0	+	0/+	0
Tricyclic Antidepressants							
Desipramine (Norpramin)	++	+	++	+++	0/+	+	++
Nortriptyline (Pamelor)	++	+	++	++	0/+	+	++
Amitriptyline (Elavil)	++++	0/+	++++	++++	0/+	++	+++
Imipramine (Tofranil)	+++	0/+	+++	++++	0/+	++	++
Doxepin (Sinequan)	++++	0/+	++++	++++	0/+	++	++
Others							
Mirtazapine (Remeron)	++++	0	++	0/+	+	0/+	++

0, negligible; +, very low; + +, low; + + +, moderate; + + + +, high.

also generally fewer concerns with SSRI (or SNRI) and comorbid illnesses than one encounters with TCAs, suggesting that SSRIs may often be a better choice in medically complex patients.

As clinical experience accumulates with the SSRI (and SNRI) agents, a distinct side effect profile has emerged, consisting of gastrointestinal (GI) complaints, CNS disturbances, and sexual dysfunction. All these medications may induce nausea, but this tends to be a transient effect that diminishes after the first week of treatment. Typically, the SSRI can cause some local GI irritation 1 to 2 hours after oral administration. For this reason, patients should always be advised to take the medication after a meal or snack, particularly during the first week of therapy. Nausea with SSRIs may also be mediated centrally through the stimulation of certain serotonin receptors (5-HT_{3C}) that activate the chemoreceptor trigger zone.[76] Nausea triggered by this mechanism has a more delayed onset, corresponding to the accumulation of medication until steady-state dynamics are reached, and often persists throughout the dosing interval. Patients who experience nausea mediated by CNS stimulation may be unable to tolerate this effect and often require dosage reduction or drug discontinuation.

SSRIs may also have transient and bothersome effects on bowel function. Unlike nausea, there does appear to be clinically relevant differences among SSRIs in this regard. Sertraline, fluoxetine, and citalopram have been associated with a 15% to 20% incidence of diarrhea.[77] Fortunately, the diarrhea often remits after 1 week or so of continued therapy and rarely requires an interruption of treatment. In contrast, paroxetine possesses a mild affinity for blocking muscarinic receptors that can manifest as anticholinergic side effects, such as constipation, dry mouth, or urinary hesitancy. This may discourage the use of paroxetine in patients with pre-existing constipation or those receiving other medications with anticholinergic potential.

SSRIs can have myriad effects on the CNS, with disturbances in sleep or disposition being a primary concern. Overall, the SSRIs appear to have significant but highly variable effects on sleep architecture. For example, in sleep studies, SSRIs have been shown to increase sleep latency and decrease sleep efficiency, often resulting in morning sleepiness or malaise. Many patients also notice that their dreams become more vivid and memorable, which is not always a desirable experience, and may prolong the REM stage, resulting in less fitful sleep.[78] It should be emphasized, however, that sleep may actually improve once the antidepressant properties of the medications are apparent and baseline depressive symptoms are relieved (e.g., midnocturnal insomnia).

Compared with older antidepressants, SSRIs are generally considered activating compounds, and there does appear to be a hierarchy among the individual agents. Fluoxetine, for example, is widely regarded as the most activating of the SSRIs, a property that may be desirable in anergic patients or undesirable in those who are agitated or have difficulty falling asleep.[79]

Table 79-13 Dosage Ranges and Costs of Antidepressant Medications

Medication	Brand Name	Starting Dose (mg/day)	Maximum Dosage (mg/day)	Usual Dosage (mg/day)	Relative Cost[a]
Selective Serotonin Reuptake Inhibitors					
Fluoxetine	Prozac	10	80	10–20 mg QD	$[b]
Sertraline	Zoloft	25	200	50 mg QD	$$[b]
Paroxetine	Paxil	10	50	10–20 mg QD	$[b]
Citalopram	Celexa	10	60	20 mg QD	$$[b]
Escitalopram	Lexapro	5	20	10 mg QD	$$$$
Serotonin Norepinephrine Reuptake Inhibitors					
Venlafaxine	Effexor	25	375	50 mg BID	$$$$
Venlafaxine	Effexor XR	37.5	225	150 mg QD	$$$$
Duloxetine	Cymbalta	30	120	60 mg QD	$$$$
Norepinephrine Reuptake Inhibitors					
Bupropion	Wellbutrin	200	450	100 mg TID	$$[b]
Bupropion	Wellbutrin SR	150	400	150 mg BID	$$[b]
Bupropion	Wellbutrin XL	150	450	300 QD	$$$$[b]
Tricyclic Antidepressants					
Desipramine	Norpramin	25	300	200 mg HS	$
Nortriptyline	Pamelor	10–25	150	100 mg HS	$
Others					
Mirtazapine	Remeron	15	45	15–30 mg HS	$$[b]

[a] Based on average wholesale prices for usual therapeutic doses (July 2007).
[b] Price reflects cost of generic formulation.
$ = $0–25/month; $$ = $25–50/month; $$$ = $50–70/month; $$$$ = >$70/month.

For this reason, fluoxetine is usually administered in the morning after breakfast. However, it should be noted that fluoxetine is not necessarily activating for all patients. In fact, some find it to be slightly sedating or numbing. Daytime drowsiness can be experienced with fluoxetine, perhaps as a result of light, restless sleep. Sertraline, escitalopram, and citalopram have also been associated with comparatively more insomnia than sedation, but they are generally considered to be less activating than fluoxetine in this regard. The effects of paroxetine appear to be somewhat mixed, with approximately equal proportions of patients complaining of sedation and insomnia, respectively.

Another type of CNS side effect reported with SSRIs involves the extrapyramidal system. SSRIs have been associated with extrapyramidal side effects (EPS), consisting of akathisia, dystonias, and parkinsonian symptoms that are qualitatively identical to those commonly seen with high-potency antipsychotics. Fortunately, the reported incidence of EPS effects is much lower than with antipsychotic agents.[80] Although EPS reactions have been documented with all SSRIs, most case reports have featured paroxetine. Because paroxetine has the highest affinity for serotonin receptors, this may lend support to the theory that these EPS effects are mediated through the indirect influence of serotonergic neurons on dopaminergic activity. In certain areas of the brain, serotonin and dopamine appear to have an inverse relationship, whereby central stimulation of serotonin receptors results in a net decline in dopaminergic transmission. Therefore, management of EPS effects induced by SSRI is identical with that of those precipitated by antipsychotics. Dystonias and parkinsonian side effects can be treated with anticholinergic agents and subsequent dosage reduction. Akathisia usually responds to a dosage decrease and/or administration of low-dose β-blockers.

The deleterious effects of SSRI on sexual function were overlooked in early clinical trials, but it is now widely recognized that these adverse effects are very common and potentially profound consequences of SSRI treatment that can often lead to medication nonadherence.[81] In the medical literature, the reported incidence of sexual dysfunction ranges from 1.9% to 75%, reflecting the diversity of research methods (or lack thereof) used to detect this occurrence.[82,83] The actual incidence of SSRI-induced sexual dysfunction is approximately 30% to 50%, and it appears to be slightly more common in men, but the severity may be worse in women. Delayed orgasm is the most common sexual complaint attributed to SSRIs or SNRIs, and should be distinguished from decreases in desire or libido, which are considered to be an aspect of the psychopathology of depression itself. This iatrogenic effect on orgasms has actually been used to clinical advantage in men reporting premature ejaculation, but most patients find it undesirable.[84] All SSRIs are commonly implicated with sexual dysfunction, but there are several indirect lines of evidence suggesting that paroxetine and fluoxetine are the worst in this regard.[85,86] It also appears that this is a dose-dependent phenomenon, which may respond favorably to a decrease in daily dosage. Unlike the GI and CNS side effects reported with SSRIs, sexual dysfunction is not usually a transient adverse effect and must be addressed by clinicians if patients are to complete a full course of therapy.

6. Are there any other adverse effects of SSRIs about which A.R. should be aware?

In addition to GI, CNS, and sexual side effects, a variety of other, less common, adverse sequelae may jeopardize treatment. Dry mouth and headache occur with many antidepressants, and, although these somatic complaints are prevalent in the general population, placebo-adjusted rates suggest that SSRIs may induce this phenomenon.[77] Increased sweating has also been reported with SSRIs and can be particularly uncomfortable or embarrassing.[87] Dosage reduction may help relieve this adverse effect, and alpha-blockers (e.g., terazosin, prazosin) and anticholinergic antidotes have been used as well (e.g., benztropine or low-dose TCA at bedtime).[88,89] Bruxism, or teeth grinding, can also be an unfortunate consequence of SSRI treatment, leading to chipped or cracked teeth and generally poor dentition.[90] Often, patients may not be aware of this nocturnal effect and complain merely of a dull, persistent headache during the morning hours. This, too, may be a dose-dependent side effect of all SSRIs, and several antidotes have been prescribed (e.g., buspirone, benzodiazepines, gabapentin).[91,92] In small retrospective studies and several case reports, SSRIs have been linked to dilutional hyponatremia or syndrome of inappropriate antidiuretic hormone.[93,94] All SSRIs (and venlafaxine) have been associated with this phenomenon, and elderly patients appear to be uniquely at risk.

The long-term effects of SSRIs on body weight are more variable and difficult to predict. It is worthwhile to recall that decreased appetite is one of the most common depressive symptoms and that a small weight gain after an antidepressant course may actually be viewed as a therapeutic effect of successful treatment. Early reports of weight loss with fluoxetine generated much optimism for the use of SSRI in obesity, but longitudinal studies found this to be a brief, transient phenomenon.[95] All SSRIs have been implicated with significant weight gain after long-term use, but it is relatively rare phenomenon believed to be mediated by genetic markers that have not been conclusively identified. The exception is with paroxetine, which has been implicated much more often than other SSRIs. One long-term RCT compared the effects of fluoxetine, sertraline, and paroxetine on total body weight.[96] After 7 months of SSRI use, 25% of the patients receiving paroxetine gained a clinically significant amount of weight (defined as a >7% increase in total body weight) compared with 7% with fluoxetine and 4% with sertraline. Long-term studies with citalopram and escitalopram suggest that 3% to 5% of patients will experience a significant weight gain. Because weight gain may occur with any SSRI, it is best to monitor weight changes closely during long-term treatment and respond accordingly.

Retrospective studies have also linked SSRI with an increased risk for severe GI bleeds.[97] This has been attributed to the SSRI effects on decreasing platelet activation and aggregation. Interestingly, these pharmacologic properties may also confer a therapeutic advantage, as longitudinal studies have suggested that SSRI may be cardioprotective and prevent future MI. Because the bulk of evidence addressing SSRI effects on GI bleeds and MI has been inferred from nonrandomized retrospective studies that may be strongly influenced by other confounding factors (e.g., lifestyle habits, depression itself), future prospective trials are clearly indicated.

Dosage Titration

7. A.R. calls the clinic 2 weeks later requesting a dosage increase. She reports that she has been taking 50 mg of sertraline every morning for the past week and has noticed considerable improvement in her sleep, appetite, and outlook ("Little things don't bother me so much anymore"), but believes she could be doing better. She still feels as though her mood and concentration could improve, and admits that she has yet to resume her exercise regimen ("I still don't have the energy"). She asks you if she could increase her dosage. What changes would you make to her antidepressant regimen at this time?

It is very important to establish realistic expectations for treatment with antidepressants from the very beginning of therapy. Patients need to be informed of the anticipated course of antidepressant treatment and should be advised, for instance, that the onset of side effects usually precedes that of therapeutic effects. Also, patients should be advised that, although antidepressants may relieve their acute symptoms and prevent relapse, they do not abolish environmental stressors, increase self-esteem, or reverse negative perceptions and emotions.

Dosing and prescribing patterns with SSRI have changed since the first SSRI (fluoxetine) was introduced in the United States in 1988. In general, clinicians have come to realize that "one size fits all" prescribing philosophies and early aggressive dosing practices were largely unnecessary and often compromised medication adherence. Providers have found, in fact, that lower dosages of SSRIs may actually suffice (e.g., 10 mg/day of fluoxetine, paroxetine, or citalopram) if patients are informed of the delayed onset of therapeutic effects and are closely monitored for tolerance and response. Because preclinical fixed-dose studies were rarely conducted with these lower dosages, it is difficult to endorse this practice empirically. However, there is experimental evidence demonstrating that daily doses as small as 5 mg of fluoxetine are more effective than placebo and comparable to 20 mg in a significant segment of the depressed populace.[98]

For A.R., many factors must be considered before increasing her dosage. She has been receiving the medication for only 2 weeks (25 mg daily for 1 week, 50 mg daily thereafter), and the improvement she is exhibiting in neurovegetative symptoms may suggest that the resolution of cognitive symptoms is soon to follow. She should be reminded that the optimal effects of antidepressants may not be evident for 4 to 6 weeks. Furthermore, it is possible that the lack of improvement in her concentration and energy may be largely situational as the day of her wedding approaches. An increase in medication at this time would not necessarily address these environmental factors and would serve only to increase the side effect burden. Therefore, a reasonable recommendation would be to continue with the current daily dose of 50 mg and to re-evaluate the medication's effects when she returns to clinic in 2 weeks.

8. At the end of 4 weeks of treatment, A.R. is seen in the clinic and asked about side effects she has experienced. She recalls some mild nausea during the first week of treatment but continued to take the medication after breakfast (as directed) and noticed that

Table 79-14 Management of SSRI-Induced Sexual Dysfunction

- Patience (may improve after 2–4 weeks)
- Reduced dosage (if possible)
- Drug holidays (sertraline, paroxetine, citalopram, escitalopram *only*)
- Antidotes
  - Bupropion SR 150 mg QD–BID
  - Sildenafil 50–100 mg QD PRN
  - Mirtazapine 7.5–15 mg HS
  - Cyproheptadine 4–12 mg PRN (1 hour prior)
  - Methylphenidate 2.5–5.0 mg QD
  - Others: yohimbine, amantadine, buspirone, gingko
- Change of antidepressants (e.g., bupropion, mirtazapine)

this effect went away after approximately 3 or 4 days of therapy. She denies diarrhea, insomnia, or headache. Before leaving, she reluctantly admits that the only side effect she is experiencing is sexual. ("I love my fiancee, but sex isn't as enjoyable anymore.") How should this side effect be managed at this time?

From a clinician's standpoint, the detection and proper management of SSRI-induced sexual dysfunction can be one of the most important factors in ensuring medication adherence (Table 79-14). Clinicians may be uncomfortable asking patients about their sexual activities and satisfaction, but the high incidence of this side effect (and low likelihood of patients volunteering information) necessitates a thoughtful and direct approach. Some patients acknowledge sexual dysfunction but decide that the improvement in their mood and overall health outweighs limitations in sexual performance; however, many others simply stop the medication if the side effect is never addressed.

It may be wise to advise patients that sexual function may change over time, depending on the type and etiology of sexual dysfunction experienced. Depression itself is associated with a decreased libido in 70% to 90% of untreated patients.[99] This symptom will most likely subside with a successful course of antidepressant treatment. Delayed ejaculation or anorgasmia, however, is usually an iatrogenic phenomenon with SSRIs and SNRIs, often persisting and jeopardizing treatment. Because A.R. has been taking the medication faithfully for the first 4 weeks and the time course is consistent with the SSRI effects, it is unlikely that the condition will spontaneously remit now, and some action must be taken.

Ordinarily, one of the first options in managing sexual dysfunction is to reduce the dosage, but this may precipitate a recrudescence of the original depressive symptoms in some patients. In A.R.'s case, she is taking a relatively low therapeutic dosage of sertraline, and a further decrease may be a risky proposition. An alternative solution for A.R.'s problem may be to recommend drug holidays. Small open-label studies with short-acting SSRIs (e.g., sertraline, paroxetine) suggested that if patients skipped their doses on Friday and Saturday, sexual function would return to normal on the weekends.[100,101] Although this method was reported to be successful, it may also promote nonadherence with medication and lead to increased risk of relapse or withdrawal symptoms.

If the patient has had a therapeutic response to the antidepressant, the next option in this setting is to consider antidotes to SSRI-induced sexual dysfunction, and the most popular treatment at present is bupropion. Clinical reports and controlled investigations suggest that the addition of this antidepressant can be helpful for restoring sexual desire and may relieve delayed orgasm or anorgasmia in approximately 50% of patients.[102–104] This therapeutic effect has been demonstrated in depressed and nondepressed patients alike. A common dosing technique is to start with 150 mg of bupropion daily. If unsuccessful, the dose can be increased to 150 mg SR twice daily after several days (or 300 mg of the XL preparation).

From a mechanistic standpoint, sexual arousal and orgasm constitute a complex physiological process, and it is not well understood how SSRIs induce adverse effects or how bupropion may provide relief. Some researchers have theorized that delayed ejaculation or orgasm is mediated by a stimulation of postsynaptic 5-HT_2 or 5-HT_3 receptors, whereas others suggest that the indirect effects of SSRIs on dopamine may be involved.[105] Additional theories point to the inhibitory effects of SSRIs on prolactin or nitric oxide synthetase.[105]

Other remedies have been prescribed for SSRI-induced sexual dysfunction. A large randomized, controlled trial examined the impact of sildenafil on male patients suffering from this side effect.[106] Overall, 54% of patients randomized to sildenafil found it be effective compared with a 4% response rate with placebo. Open-label trials of sildenafil in women experiencing SSRI-induced anorgasmia have also reported improvements, suggesting that controlled trials in this population are warranted.

Cyproheptadine is an obscure antihistamine with potent antiserotonergic properties, which has also received some attention as a potential antidote. It has been used successfully for the treatment of SSRI-induced sexual dysfunction in doses of 4 to 12 mg just before intercourse.[107] Unfortunately, cyproheptadine is sedating and appears to have a limited role in this capacity. If it is used, one should never administer the medication on a routine or daily basis because reports of relapse in depressed patients have surfaced. Amantadine, buspirone, and yohimbine have also been used successfully to reverse delayed ejaculation or decreased libido, but the evidence for efficacy is rather limited.[108–110] One small double-blind study compared the effects of amantadine with buspirone or placebo among depressed patients developing sexual dysfunction on antidepressants.[111] All three treatments improved sexual dysfunction to a comparable extent, and the only statistically significant finding was related to an increase in energy reported among patients receiving amantadine (vs. placebo). An open-label trial of *Ginkgo biloba* in men and women with sexual dysfunction reported very high success rates, but mixed results have been experienced in actual practice.[112] Mirtazapine is capable of blocking postsynaptic 5-HT_2 receptors and theoretically may relieve ejaculatory difficulties, but controlled trials have not been conducted. Finally, stimulants such as methylphenidate or dextroamphetamine may increase libido in SSRI-treated patients, but the potential for dependence and abuse discourages their routine administration.[113]

The onset of A.R.'s sexual dysfunction is consistent with the introduction of sertraline, and it appears, at this time, that her situation will not improve if she continues to take the SSRI. Because she is exhibiting some evidence of a therapeutic response, one would prefer to continue sertraline and discuss possible antidotes for sexual dysfunction with her. A.R. states that she would prefer to not to start another prescription medication to treat her problem, but she will "think about it."

Table 79-15 Duration of Antidepressant Treatment

Acute treatment phase:	3 mo
Continuation treatment phase:	4–9 mo
Maintenance treatment phase:	Variable

- Acute *and* continuation treatment recommended for all patients with major depressive disorder (i.e., minimal duration of treatment = 7 mo)
- Decision to prescribe maintenance treatment is based on the following.
  - Number of previous episodes
  - Severity of previous episodes
  - Family history of depression
  - Patient age (worse prognosis if elderly)
  - Response to antidepressant
  - Persistence of environmental stressors
- Indefinite maintenance treatment is recommended if any one of the following criteria are met.
  1. Three or more previous episodes (regardless of age)
  2. Two or more previous episodes and age older than 50 yr
  3. One or more and age older than 60 yr

Table 79-16 Discontinuation of Antidepressants

Withdrawal syndrome
- Worse with paroxetine, venlafaxine
- Symptoms: dizziness, nausea, paresthesias, anxiety/insomnia, flulike symptoms
- Onset: 36–72 hr
- Duration: 3–7 days

Taper schedule (for patients receiving long-term treatment)
- Fluoxetine: generally unnecessary
- Sertraline: decrease by 25–50 mg every 1–2 wk
- Paroxetine: decrease by 5–10 mg every 1–2 wk
- Citalopram: decrease by 5–10 mg every 1–2 wk
- Escitalopram: decrease by 5 mg every 1–2 wk
- Venlafaxine: decrease by 25–50 mg every 1–2 wk
- Nefazodone: decrease by 50–100 mg every 1–2 wk
- Bupropion: generally unnecessary
- Tricyclics: decrease by 10%–25% every 1–2 wk

Note: Risk of relapse greatest 1 to 6 months after discontinuation.

Duration of Treatment

9. At 6 weeks, A.R. reports that her depressive symptoms are effectively in remission ("I feel like I have my old life back!"). Her energy has improved, and she is doing well in her studies and looks forward, once again, to her wedding day. How long should A.R. continue taking the antidepressant?

According to the guidelines issued by the Agency for Health Research and Quality (formerly known as the Agency for Heath Care Policy and Research), antidepressant treatment can be broken down into three stages (Table 79-15).[114] The first stage, *acute treatment,* lasts approximately 12 weeks; during this time, the clinician attempts to resolve the presenting symptoms and induce remission. The second stage is commonly called *continuation treatment* because the patient continues to receive the same antidepressant regimen that induced the initial treatment response, and the clinician attempts to keep the acute symptoms in remission. The duration of continuation treatment is variable (4–9 months after initial treatment or response), but it is recommended that all patients suffering from major depression complete these first two stages. Therefore, the minimum duration of treatment is 7 months. Alternatively, others have advocated that the minimum duration of treatment should be for 6 months after the complete resolution of symptoms.

The third stage of treatment, *maintenance treatment* or prophylaxis, is not indicated for all patients, and the necessity of continuing medication beyond the first 6 to 7 months depends on many patient-specific factors. One must consider the number of previous episodes, family history of depression, patient's age, severity of presenting symptoms, response to therapy, and persistence or anticipation of environmental stressors. There are specific populations for whom indefinite pharmacologic treatment is advocated: (a) individuals with three or more previous episodes of major depression, (b) individuals older than 50 years with two or more previous episodes, and (c) individuals older than 60 years with one or more previous episodes.[114] Many experts believe that pharmacotherapy should also be continued indefinitely in all elderly people (older than 65 years) suffering from major depression, but research evidence to conclusively support this recommendation is currently lacking.[115]

Because A.R. is exhibiting a full therapeutic response to sertraline, the recommendation would be for her to continue with the effective dosage (50 mg/day) for at least 7 consecutive months. At the end of this time frame, the clinician should sit down with the patient and review the considerations that enter into the decision to continue treatment. Ultimately, the decision to continue antidepressant medications is left to the patient's judgment, and he or she should be well informed of the potential consequences of stopping treatment.

In the future, if A.R. decides to discontinue her antidepressant, she should be advised of potential withdrawal symptoms (Table 79-16). Abrupt discontinuation of chronic SSRI treatment (e.g., treatment >2 months) has been associated with dizziness, headache, anxiety, flulike symptoms, and paresthesias.[116] The onset of these symptoms is generally within 48 to 72 hours of stopping treatment, and effects may persist for at least 1 week. Withdrawal symptoms generally are mild and self-limiting but can be uncomfortable and alarming. Because of their relatively short half-life (and absence of long-acting metabolites), paroxetine, fluvoxamine, and venlafaxine have been associated with a more profound withdrawal presentation than other SSRIs and SNRIs. Due to its long-half life (and that of its active metabolite), fluoxetine has not been commonly associated with withdrawal symptoms. Nonetheless, one is best advised to taper slowly off all antidepressant medications after an extended treatment course.

After A.R. has completed a full course of pharmacotherapy, it is advisable to taper her sertraline over several weeks to minimize the risk of withdrawal, as well as to monitor for signs and symptoms of relapse (e.g., decrease to 25 mg daily for 2–4 weeks, then discontinue). The risk of relapse is relatively low during the first month off medication, and depressive symptoms often return during the second or third months. The risk of relapse is highest during the first 6 months overall.[117]

Antidepressants in Pregnancy and Lactation

10. Eight months after starting her antidepressant, A.R. reports that she has continued to be symptom free and is now living

happily with her husband. She has taken the sertraline faithfully each morning and is willing to do so for as long as it is prescribed ("I don't ever want to go through that again!"). She also reveals that she and her husband are thinking of stopping her birth control pills for the purpose of starting a family. She asks if it is necessary to continue the antidepressant through her pregnancy. How should A.R. and her husband be counseled at this time?

The risk for depression is substantial during pregnancy and during the postpartum period.[118] Historically, patients have been informed that pregnancy is relatively protective in regard to depression, but more recent evidence does not support this perception.[119] A recent prospective investigation reported that women who discontinued their antidepressant on learning they were pregnant were much more likely to relapse prior to delivery (68% relapse rate vs. 26% who continued treatment; hazard ratio = 5.0).[120]

Before deciding to treat with an antidepressant during pregnancy, one should make a careful inventory of the benefits and risks. The consequences of maternal depression on the mother and fetus must be compared with the potential risks of in utero medication exposure (i.e., teratogenicity, growth impairment, other adverse birth outcomes). From the mother's perspective, untreated depression carries with it a great deal of distress during an emotional time. Sleep and appetite may be compromised at a time when these functions are most important for the baby's development. Mothers may also be tempted to drink alcohol or abuse substances, and studies have also shown that depressed mothers are much less likely to attend prenatal clinic visits. Depression during pregnancy is a very strong risk factor for postpartum depression as well. Neonatal studies have shown that infants of mothers who became depressed during pregnancy were smaller at birth, had lower Apgar scores, and experienced more irritability and emotional problems.[121] Abnormal activation along the HPA axis has also been demonstrated among infants born to mothers who were depressed during pregnancy, and other factors suggesting enhanced susceptibility to depression later in life may be engendered as well.

The attendant effects of antidepressants on the developing fetus have been difficult to predict or quantify. For obvious reasons, RCTs of potential teratogens are seldom conducted in expectant mothers, so study methods to assess fetal risk are less than ideal, and recommendations may change in coming years with subsequent investigations.

At the present time, it is believed that most of the SSRIs and newer antidepressants pose little risk for the development of serious fetal malformations, and they have been subsequently categorized as Class C by the FDA (suggesting that the risk to the fetus is not definitively known). Their relative safety has been corroborated recently by two large case-control studies published in the *New England Journal of Medicine,* where a very small increase in risks was reported.[122,123] One notable exception to the SSRI safety profile can be found with paroxetine, which was recently reclassified as Class D by the FDA following the demonstration of a sixfold increase in the risk of persistent pulmonary hypertension in newborns.[124] Interestingly, the FDA also speculated that the benefits of paroxetine to the mother may still outweigh the risks to the developing fetus.

An additional concern with SSRIs and SNRIs in pregnancy can be found in the risk for neonatal withdrawal symptoms immediately after delivery. This has been reported with TCA in the distant past as well. A small controlled investigation (n = 40) examined the effects of fluoxetine and citalopram on CNS effects in newborns and found a significant increase in restlessness, tremor, shivering, and hyperreflexia during the first 4 days of life (vs. controls) that spontaneously remitted shortly thereafter.[125] Although some clinicians have interpreted these findings to suggest that antidepressants should be tapered and discontinued prior to delivery, others have argued that delivery and the postpartum period constitute major stressors for the new mother and the risk of relapse during this time would be unacceptably high if the medication is withdrawn. This same study did not find any substantial difference in birthweight or preterm deliveries, but there was a significant decline in Apgar scores on average. Other studies have also reported a small but significant decrease in birthweight among babies exposed in utero to SSRI (vs. TCA).

The safety of bupropion in pregnancy has also not been extensively studied. A recent review of animal studies uncovered an increased risk of congenital abnormalities, but retrospective reviews in humans have failed to identify an enhanced risk of fetal malformation or spontaneous abortions. Due to these findings in animal trials, however, the FDA recently changed bupropion to a Class C rating. Data are even more sparse with mirtazapine, venlafaxine, or duloxetine, but again no cause for alarm has been identified among infants exposed to these antidepressants in utero. Similarly, fetal malformations have been rarely reported with TCA and they are generally regarded as safe in pregnant women. MAOIs, however, should be avoided due to increased risks for hypertensive crises.

For A.R., it is important to assess her risk for depression if she stops taking her antidepressant. This was her first episode of depression (which occurred under stressful circumstances), and she does not have a strong genetic predisposition to mood disorders. If she is committed to starting a family, she may want to consider being tapered off the sertraline over several weeks just before conception. If she becomes pregnant and her depression returns, the risk to the fetus appears to be quite low with most SSRIs, including sertraline. Theoretically, this risk can be reduced further if the antidepressant is started after the first trimester (when most major fetal development occurs), and lower doses would be prudent as well to minimize fetal exposure.

11. What are the risks of continuing antidepressant medications during breast-feeding?

Approximately 70% of mothers report sadness or anxiety during the first few days after delivery ("baby blues"), but these feelings will usually resolve within 1 to 2 weeks. Approximately 10% of women will develop unremitting symptoms that ultimately satisfy criteria for major depressive disorder. Although psychotherapy may be appealing and obviate the need for medication exposure via breast milk, it is often inconvenient and impractical for new mothers to leave the house on a weekly basis without their infants. Antidepressant medications, therefore, are frequently prescribed to manage postpartum mood disorders.

Because breast-feeding is widely advocated in contemporary medical circles, the passive transfer of medication from mother to infant must be considered. Studies with TCAs and

SSRIs suggest that concentrations of antidepressants in breast milk are *not* negligible. However, subsequent concentrations in the infant's bloodstream are relatively low, and the sequelae from this exposure have been limited to scattered case reports of increased infant irritability. Among the available agents, doxepin and fluoxetine have been associated with the highest concentrations in infants, and although the clinical or developmental consequences of this finding have not been elucidated, it has been recommended that these medications be avoided.[126] Recent studies with SSRIs suggest that the concentrations achieved in breast milk are lowest with sertraline and that paroxetine, citalopram, and escitalopram are somewhere between the extremes of fluoxetine and sertraline.[126,127] If an antidepressant is to be continued in a mother who is breast-feeding, the lowest dosage should be prescribed, and the mother may want to take the medication just before the infant's longest sleep period. It may also be useful to note that the concentration of SSRI in breast milk will generally peak approximately 4 to 8 hours after oral administration. If a new mother is particularly concerned about breast milk exposure, she can be advised to pump and save breast milk immediately prior to taking their antidepressant, and pump and dump breast milk (if possible) between the 4- and 8-hour postadministration period.

Drug Interactions

12. A.R. was recently diagnosed with an uncomplicated urinary tract infection and given a prescription for a short course of oral antibiotics. She is not yet pregnant, but has called to ask if there are any drug interactions to be concerned with in regard to her antidepressant (sertraline). What can you tell her?

There is a growing awareness of the potential for certain antidepressants (e.g., certain SSRIs, duloxetine) to inhibit the metabolism of other medications that are cleared through the cytochrome P450 system of isoenzymes (Table 79-17). In general, these drug interactions are concentration dependent and most clinically relevant when the affected medication has a narrow therapeutic index, requires conversion to an active metabolite, or cannot be eliminated through other metabolic routes.[128] Important examples of affected medications include TCAs, calcium channel blockers, estrogen, theophylline, phenytoin, warfarin, triazolobenzodiazepines, and cisapride.

The SSRIs are potent inhibitors of the cytochrome P450 isoenzymes, but important differences exist among the individual agents in their affinity for the isoenzymes and for the specific metabolic pathways involved (Table 79-17). For instance, the cytochrome P450 1A2 isoenzyme (or CYP 1A2) is most sensitive to the inhibitory effects of fluvoxamine, whereas fluoxetine and paroxetine have the highest affinity for CYP 2D6.[128] Fluoxetine's active metabolite has moderate inhibitory effects on the CYP 3A4 isoenzyme. In comparison, sertraline citalopram and escitalopram have a lower potential for drug interactions but may still inhibit the metabolism of various medications based on the individual circumstances (e.g., high dose, genetic predisposition).[128–130]

Although in vitro affinities of antidepressants for the respective isoenzymes can be very helpful for predicting potentially dangerous drug combinations, there is wide interpatient variability in the susceptibility for these interactions. Much of this variability can be attributed to genetic polymorphism. With CYP 2D6, for example, approximately 5% to 10% of whites and 1% to 2% of Asians are considered poor metabolizers via this isoenzyme (i.e., possess a nonfunctional variant of the enzyme); and the rest of these respective populations are regarded as extensive metabolizers.[131] However, genetic variation does not explain the unpredictable nature of the situation entirely.

One of the best examples of this variability can be found with desipramine, a secondary amine of the TCAs, which is metabolized almost exclusively through the CYP 2D6 pathway. In vitro affinities suggest that paroxetine would have the greatest impact on metabolism occurring via this route, but controlled investigations discovered that fluoxetine increased the plasma desipramine concentrations of adult volunteers by 350%, paroxetine by 125%, and sertraline by 20%.[132–134] One plausible explanation for this unexpected finding may be that therapeutic doses of fluoxetine are associated with much higher plasma concentrations than other SSRIs because of a smaller first-pass effect. Levels may also be higher at steady state because of the longer plasma half-life of fluoxetine and norfluoxetine compared with other SSRIs. It is also worth mentioning that even though sertraline had less of an impact on desipramine concentrations, two patients experienced a doubling of steady-state desipramine levels, emphasizing the wide variability in patient response.[134] Other investigations have reported that bupropion increased the area under the curve for desipramine by 500%, duloxetine by 300%, and escitalopram by 100%, respectively.

The CYP 3A4 isoenzyme is actually the most abundant CYP enzyme found in the human body, and it has been estimated that nearly half of all medications prescribed will ultimately undergo metabolic degradation via this isoenzyme. Fortunately, the only two antidepressants that can have significant inhibitory effects on this enzyme are norfluoxetine and fluvoxamine. Serious drug interactions have been mediated through this pathway, the most notable involving cardiotoxicity and malignant ventricular arrhythmias precipitated by elevated concentrations of several medications that have subsequently been withdrawn from the market (terfenadine, astemizole, and cisapride). Another clinically significant interaction may occur when fluoxetine is coadministered with the triazolobenzodiazepines (triazolam, alprazolam, and midazolam). Because these psychotropic medications are occasionally combined to manage anxiety disorders or depression, clinicians are advised to empirically reduce the initial dosage of the triazolobenzodiazepines (75% with triazolam, 50% with alprazolam) in patients currently receiving these SSRIs.

Serotonin Syndrome

13. What is serotonin syndrome, and is A.R. at risk for this interaction?

Serotonin syndrome is a rare but potentially fatal interaction that has been precipitated by the combination of two or more drugs that enhance serotonin transmission.[135] The syndrome consists of a constellation of associated symptoms, including anxiety, shivering, diaphoresis, tremor, hyperreflexia, and autonomic instability (increased/decreased blood pressure and pulse rate).[136] Fatalities have been attributed to malignant hyperthermia.

Table 79-17 Drug Interactions of the Cytochrome P450 System

Relative Rank	*CYP1A2*	*CYP2C9/19*	*CYP2D6*	*CYP3A4*
Offending Agent (inhibits enzyme)				
High	Fluvoxamine	*Cyp2C9* Fluoxetine Fluvoxamine *Cyp2C19* Fluvoxamine	Paroxetine Fluoxetine Duloxetine Bupropion	Fluoxetine (norfluoxetine) Fluvoxamine
Moderate	Fluoxetine Paroxetine	*Cyp2C19* Fluoxetine Sertraline	Citalopram Escitalopram Sertraline	
Low	Citalopram Escitalopram Sertraline Venlafaxine Duloxetine Bupropion	*Cyp2C9/19* Citalopram Escitalopram Paroxetine Sertraline Venlafaxine	Venlafaxine Mirtazapine	Citalopram Escitalopram Paroxetine Sertraline Venlafaxine Duloxetine
Other Inhibitors				
	Quinolones (ciprofloxacin, enoxacin, etc.) Macrolides (erythromycin, clarithromycin) Grapefruit juice	Modafinil (2C9, 2C19) Cimetidine (2C19) Omeprazole (2C19) Imidazoles (2C9, 2C19) (ketoconazole, fluconazole)	Fenfluramine Yohimbine Methadone Quinidine Celecoxib	Macrolides (Erythro, Clarith) Cimetidine CCB (verapamil, diltiazem) Imidazoles (ketoconazole, fluconazole) Protease inhibitors Grapefruit juice
Other Inducers				
	Cigarettes Caffeine St. John's wort	St. John's wort	Modafinil Phenytoin and phenobarbital Carbamazepine Rifampin Prednisone Testosterone	St. John's wort
Affected Agent (increased concentration)				
	TCA-tertiary amines (imipramine, amitriptyline) Phenothiazines (chlorpromazine) Thiothixene Haloperidol Clozapine Olanzapine Caffeine Theophylline Propranolol Tacrine	*Cyp2C9* Phenytoin Tolbutamide Warfarin NSAIDs *Cyp2C19* TCA-tertiary amines (imipramine, amitriptyline) Citalopram Barbiturates Propranolol Omeprazole	TCA-secondary amines (desipramine, nortriptyline) Fluoxetine Paroxetine Venlafaxine Duloxetine Amphetamines Atomoxetine Risperidone Donepezil Codeine Hydrocodone Tramadol Dextromethorphan Chlorpheniramine Beta-Blockers (propranolol, metoprolol)	Fluoxetine Sertraline Venlafaxine Modafinil Quetiapine Ziprasidone Aripiprazole Buspirone Benzodiazepines (triazolam, alprazolam) Zolpidem Carbamazepine Donepezil CCB (verapamil, diltiazem, nifedipine) Sex hormones (estrogen) Corticosteroids Statins (lovastatin, simvastatin) Protease inhibitors Sildenafil

mcpp, 1-(m-chlorophenyl) piperazine; NSAIDs, nonsteroidal anti-inflammatory drugs; TCA, tricyclic antidepressant; CCB, calcium channel blockers.

With mild cases of serotonin syndrome, the symptoms ordinarily resolve 24 to 48 hours after the serotonergic agents have been discontinued. Supportive treatment is usually not necessary. For more severe reactions, various serotonergic antagonists, such as cyproheptadine, methysergide, and propranolol, have been used.[137–139] Dantrolene has been administered successfully to manage hyperthermia.[140]

Most case reports of serotonin syndrome (and most fatalities) have occurred with a combination of an MAOI and an SSRI, which is now considered an absolute contraindication. Other case reports involve the combination of an MAOI (or SSRI) and tryptophan, meperidine, SNRI, tricyclics, dextromethorphan, linezolid, and tramodol.[135] One case of serotonin syndrome was reportedly induced by the combination of clomipramine with S-adenosylmethionine.[141] Serotonin syndrome has also been reported with concurrent administration of multiple SSRIs. Theoretically, the combination of an SSRI with St. John's Wort may also precipitate this pharmacodynamic interaction, but more recent evidence has suggested that the MAOI properties of the herbal preparation are minimal with therapeutic doses. Nonetheless, a case series of five older patients who developed symptoms reminiscent of serotonin syndrome has appeared in the literature, and, given the degree of uncertainty that persists, this combination of antidepressant agents is best avoided.[142] The safety of combining an SSRI with certain migraine medications (e.g., sumatriptan) has not been elucidated, and clinicians are advised to avoid this combination if possible as well.

The combination of a phenylpiperazine (e.g., trazodone) with an SSRI may pose some concern because both classes of antidepressants augment serotonin activity in the CNS. Trazodone has been associated with serotonin syndrome in two incidences, one involving the coadministration of buspirone and the other associated with a concomitant MAOI.[136] However, in practice, trazodone has been commonly prescribed to patients receiving an SSRI for the treatment of insomnia, and no confirmed cases of serotonin syndrome have surfaced in the medical literature.[143]

Refractory Depression

14. F.H. is a 55-year-old postmenopausal woman presenting to the women's health clinic who has suffered from multiple depressive episodes since the age of 30 years. She reports that she has been hospitalized on three different occasions. Although F.H. is unable to recall details of any specific antidepressant trials, her prescription record reveals treatment with imipramine (100 mg/day), nortriptyline (75 mg/day), diazepam (10 mg/day), and fluoxetine (20 mg/day for the past 8 weeks). Eventually, she recalls that imipramine made her "dizzy and left a strange taste in my mouth" and that diazepam made her "even more depressed." She says that the fluoxetine may be "helping a little bit but I feel so jumpy and irritable that no one can stand me." F.H. has grown rather despondent over her situation ("I almost feel like giving up"). What would be the next reasonable step for managing F.H.'s depressive illness?

Pooled results of clinical trials suggest that the majority of patients with major depression receiving an adequate trial of any antidepressant will have a therapeutic response, traditionally defined as at least a 50% reduction in depressive symptoms. However, for a patient who is severely depressed, a 50% reduction in symptoms still leaves him or her with significant psychopathology and associated disability. Consequently, there has been a strong movement in recent years to consider full remission as the preferred therapeutic end point.[71] Scientific support for this ideologic shift comes from long-term studies demonstrating that patients achieving remission are much less likely to suffer relapse. One longitudinal investigation found that patients with residual symptoms were three times more likely to suffer relapse during the 12 months after treatment than those who had remitted.[144] Although remission can be generally defined as the virtual absence of residual depressive symptoms, it can also be quantified with a corresponding threshold value on a depression rating scale (e.g., QIDS <6; 17-item HAM-D <7).[71] As more clinical trials use these rigorous standards, it has become evident that approximately only 30% to 40% of patients receiving an adequate trial of an antidepressant actually achieve remission. Therefore, strident efforts are being made to make patients feel well and not merely better, and providers must undertake a thorough, rational, and perhaps aggressive approach to optimize treatment and achieve this goal.

For F.H., the first step would be to confirm her diagnosis and rule out potential medical explanations for her distress. Iatrogenic causes should also be explored, such as recent changes in her hormone replacement therapy. Persistent stressors or substance abuse patterns may be hindering her sustained recovery and should be addressed.

An assessment of F.H.'s attitude toward medication adherence is also vital, and her complete medical records should be obtained to verify the dose, duration, and results of previous antidepressant trials. It is critical to confirm that she received full therapeutic trials of the antidepressants that she was prescribed before seeking other therapeutic options. A full therapeutic trial for the treatment of depression is considered to be a minimum of 4 weeks receiving a clinically effective dosage of medication. Although some improvement may be noted during the first 1 or 2 weeks of treatment, maximal response is rarely evident until 4 weeks of medication have been received. An open-label study with fluoxetine, for instance, randomized patients who were not fully responsive after 3 weeks of treatment (20 mg/day) to either continue with the original regimen or receive an increased dosage (60 mg/day) for 5 additional weeks.[145] At the end of the study period, 49% of the patients receiving 20 mg converted to full responders, suggesting that 3 weeks is an inadequate period to confidently assess patient response. Because 50% of the patients receiving 60 mg/day converted to full responders, it may also be inferred that dosage increases are not necessary in many patients.

Drug Selection

Serotonin Norepinephrine Reuptake Inhibitors

15. After a careful interview and workup, it was determined that F.H. is suffering from an acute episode of major depression with a probable history of dysthymia as well (i.e., double depression). She denies substance abuse, which is supported by a subsequent toxicology screen. From her medical chart and interview, it is confirmed that she received a therapeutic trial of nortriptyline and fluoxetine with inadequate clinical benefit. She is not interested in psychotherapy. Her provider decides to start

venlafaxine (37.5 mg SR preparation daily). Is this a reasonable choice?

Because 30% to 40% of patients will effectively achieve remission and about 20% to 25% of patients will stop an antidepressant because of side effects, it is safe to say that *most* patients started on a given antidepressant ultimately need a significant adjustment or change to their original regimen.[146] Clinicians, therefore, are obligated to have a thorough understanding of several antidepressant medications and classes if they are to facilitate successful outcomes.

In F.H.'s case, she has previously failed a therapeutic trial of nortriptyline and is currently expressing vague suicidality, so an additional TCA would not be a reasonable choice (see full discussion of TCAs in the text that follows). Although she has also failed a fluoxetine trial, open-label studies and large controlled investigations suggest that 50% to 70% of patients who are unresponsive or intolerant of one SSRI will experience a therapeutic response to a different SSRI.[145,147,148] For example, in the STAR*D trials patients failing an initial course of citalopram were just as likely to respond if they were randomized to a subsequent trial of a different SSRI (sertraline) as they were to other antidepressant classes (venlafaxine and bupropion, specifically).[149] If a different SSRI is to be initiated, it may be wise to opt for one with less activating properties than fluoxetine (e.g., sertraline, paroxetine, citalopram, escitalopram). Alternatively, a medication from a different antidepressant class would possess the hypothetical benefit of a unique mechanism of action (e.g., venlafaxine, bupropion). Because F.H. is evidently experiencing much torment and despair, a sense of urgency may be perceived, justifying a different pharmacologic approach altogether.

Venlafaxine is the first member of a relatively new class of antidepressants known as SNRIs. Duloxetine (Cymbalta), which possesses a very similar mechanism of action, is the only other SNRI that is approved in the United States for the treatment of depression at the present time.[150] Studies in severe melancholic depression and treatment-resistant depression suggest that venlafaxine is at least as effective as other antidepressants in these populations, and it has emerged as a valuable alternative agent.[151–153] At dosages <150 mg/day, venlafaxine's therapeutic effects are mediated exclusively from the blockade of serotonin reuptake. Therefore, associated adverse effects at low dosages are qualitatively and quantitatively very similar to those found with SSRIs: GI distress, sleep disturbances, and sexual dysfunction. At higher dosages, effects on norepinephrine are observed, which distinguish venlafaxine from an SSRI in terms of adverse effects (e.g., causes hypertension) but may also confer additional therapeutic benefit. Duloxetine does not appear to exhibit a dose-dependent differential effect on neurotransmitters.

Venlafaxine has a relatively brief plasma half-life (5–8 hours) and is demethylated to an active metabolite (*O*-desmethyl-venlafaxine) that has a short half-life as well (11 hours). This metabolite was recently approved by the FDA for the treatment of depression. Duloxetine also has a relatively short half-life (12 hours) and, as with the SSRI, withdrawal reactions may occur when the SNRI are abruptly discontinued after chronic administration. Venlafaxine is not a potent inhibitor of cytochrome P450 isoenzymes, so drug interactions are less of a concern than with certain SSRIs, but duloxetine is a moderate inhibitor of the CYP 2D6 isoenzyme. Both SNRIs have been associated with serotonin syndrome, so clinicians should be aware of the potentially dangerous drug combinations that can occur with these antidepressants.[154]

For F.H., the choice of venlafaxine seems to be prudent. It is fairly safe in overdose, possesses a unique mechanism of action, and is generally less activating than fluoxetine (which had provoked some irritability in her). In comparison to SSRIs, venlafaxine possesses a wide therapeutic range and ordinarily requires more dosage titration (which can increase resource utilization). A starting dose of 37.5 mg (XR) is reasonable, but baseline vitals should be recorded for F.H. with every dosage change in order to monitor the effect of this SNRI on her blood pressure and heart rate. Most patients respond to daily doses between 150 and 225 mg. Because F.H. is suffering from a relatively severe depression, it may be wise to increase her daily dose to 75 mg once she has exhibited good tolerance (i.e., after 4–7 days). In the event that F.H. has not exhibited a satisfactory response to 75 mg/day after 4 weeks, the dosage may be increased in increments of 37.5 to 75 mg every few weeks to a daily maximum of 225 mg. Although daily doses of the XL preparation above 225 mg are not recommended by the manufacturer, anecdotal success and relative safety have been reported for doses as high as 300 mg daily.[155]

Other Agents: Bupropion and Mirtazapine

16. Are there any other antidepressants to consider if F.H. fails her venlafaxine trial?

Bupropion is an aminoketone with a mechanism of action that is clearly different from that of any other antidepressant that has received FDA approval. The direct effects of bupropion on serotonin transmission are negligible, but it may act by enhancing dopamine and/or norepinephrine activity.[156] At therapeutic dosages, bupropion has an attractive adverse effect profile, limited to occasional nausea and insomnia or jitteriness. Seizures, which were reported shortly after it was released in 1985, appear to be very unlikely with therapeutic dosing of bupropion, provided that patients are not predisposed (e.g., history of epilepsy, bulimia, or recent history of heavy drinking). Bupropion is one of the few antidepressants that may actually decrease appetite. A recent randomized, placebo-controlled investigation of bupropion in depressed obese patients observing caloric restriction found that bupropion was much more likely to induce significant weight loss than placebo.[157] After 26 weeks of treatment, 40% of the bupropion-treated patients lost $>5\%$ of their total body weight versus 16% with placebo. This weight loss was positively correlated with an improvement in depressive symptoms.

Bupropion is converted via the cytochrome P450 2B6 isoenzyme to an active metabolite (9 hydroxy-bupropion). Bupropion (or its metabolite) appears to have a moderate affinity for inhibiting the CYP 2D6 isoenzyme, and significant elevations of venlafaxine and metoprolol have been demonstrated to occur with concurrent administration. Because of its short half-life (approximately 8 hours for the parent compound and 12 hours for the active metabolite), bupropion has historically been administered in divided doses, although a once-daily preparation is now available (Wellbutrin XL, or generic). For the regular-release product, the recommended starting dose is 100 mg BID, increasing to 100 mg TID after at least 3 days. Individual doses must not exceed 150 mg and should be given at least 6 hours apart. With the SR formulation, initial daily doses are 150 mg QD, increased to 150 mg BID by the fourth day at the earliest. Individual doses of bupropion SR can be as large as 200 mg, and divided doses should be given at least 8 hours apart. For the XL formulation, the package insert recommends initiating at 150 mg QD and increasing to 300 mg QD as early as the fourth day. Maximum daily doses are 450 mg for regular and XL products and 400 mg for SR products.

Mirtazapine is a novel antidepressant capable of modulating serotonin and norepinephrine activity through a complex mechanism of action. In vitro studies reveal that mirtazapine is an antagonist at presynaptic alpha$_2$-autoreceptors and postsynaptic 5-HT$_2$ and 5-HT$_3$ receptors.[158] In addition, it appears to possess some mild inhibitory properties at serotonin reuptake transporters. Therefore, the net effect of mirtazapine is to enhance serotonin and norepinephrine in a manner that is clearly distinct from any other antidepressants. In a comparative randomized trial with fluoxetine for moderate to severe depression, mirtazapine appeared to be much more effective than the SSRI after 4 weeks of treatment (58% responders vs. 30% with the SSRI; $p < 0.05$), but the differences were no longer significant at 6 weeks (63% vs. 54%; $p = 0.67$).[159]

The most common adverse effects experienced with mirtazapine are sedation and weight gain. Because mirtazapine has potent antihistaminergic effects, it is considered to be quite sedating. Anecdotally, it has been reported that higher daily doses of mirtazapine (>30 mg) are less sedating than lower doses owing to an increase in noradrenergic effects. In addition to the substantial risk of increasing appetite and total body weight, mirtazapine has also been associated with significant increases in total cholesterol and triglycerides.[160] The recommended starting dosage is 15 mg at bedtime, and the therapeutic dosage ranges from 15 to 45 mg/day.[160] Data from controlled trials have demonstrated safety and efficacy in doses up to 60 mg daily.[159,161]

Irreversible MAOIs (e.g., phenelzine, tranylepromine) may also be an alternative for patients who have failed multiple antidepressant trials. Like venlafaxine, TCAs, and mirtazapine, MAOIs are believed to relieve depressive symptoms by enhancing the activity of multiple neurotransmitters, which may be desirable for refractory cases. Because serious drug and dietary interactions are encountered with MAOIs, candidates for treatment should be chosen carefully; a full discussion of the clinical usefulness of MAOIs can be found in the "Depression With Atypical Features" section at the end of this chapter.

Antidepressant Augmentation

17. Three months later, F.H. reports that she feels less hopeless on venlafaxine XL (150 mg/day) and that her appetite has improved as well. However, she is still somewhat depressed and lethargic and attempts to increase her dosage have been limited by nausea and recurring insomnia. What pharmacologic options remain to help manage her refractory depression?

Because F.H. has obtained considerable relief from her venlafaxine trial but is experiencing dose-limiting side effects, one would prefer to add a second medication (i.e., augmentation therapy) rather than changing antidepressants at this time (Table 79-18). A reasonable next step would be to augment her current venlafaxine regimen with another medication such as lithium, thyroid hormone, or bupropion. Lithium's antidepressant properties appear to apply to both unipolar and bipolar patients. Seven of nine antidepressant augmentation trials with lithium have reported positive therapeutic effects, usually within 1 week of achieving steady-state dynamics (i.e., 3–7 days of daily dosing).[162] Effective lithium blood levels are generally within the range used to treat bipolar disorder (0.5–1.2 mEq/L). As with the use of lithium therapy in bipolar disorder, all appropriate clinical monitoring parameters should be followed carefully (see Chapter 80).

Table 79-18 Partial Response to Antidepressant Treatment Augmentation Strategies (With SSRIs)

Ensure completion of full therapeutic trial (4–6 wk).
Ensure optimal dose of antidepressant.
Consider augmentation therapies:

- Bupropion
- Lithium
- Thyroid supplements
- Pindolol (?)
- Buspirone
- Atypical antipsychotics
- Modafinil
- Lamotrigine

T$_3$ also has a long history of use in psychiatric circles for patients exhibiting partial or suboptimal responses to antidepressant monotherapy. Five of six RCTs support the use of T$_3$ supplementation for antidepressant augmentation, with an average effect size of 0.58 reported.[163] Triiodothyronine (Cytomel), at a dosage of 25 mg/day can accelerate as well as augment antidepressant response, and superior effects have been reported in female patients, in particular. The response to the thyroid supplementation should be noticeable within 1 to 2 weeks, much like that found when lithium is used to augment therapy. Thyroxine (T$_4$) has also been administered successfully in a dose of 0.1 mcg daily. Whether T$_3$ is superior to T$_4$ has not been resolved, although one study seemed to indicate that more patients respond to the former (T$_3$) than to the latter (T$_4$).[163] In the recently concluded STAR*D trials, T$_3$ was compared to lithium for antidepressant augmentation in patients with two previous treatment failures.[164] Remission rates were modest for both agents in this challenging population (24.7% with T$_3$ vs. 15.9% with lithium, NS).

Bupropion has also been used successfully as an augmenting agent for many years in several open-label trials and one RCT.[165,166] Patients receiving SSRI or SNRI who continue to complain of fatigue, hypersomnia, or executive dysfunction are excellent candidates, and the combination treatment is usually well tolerated. With F.H., one should be mindful that bupropion may increase her venlafaxine levels and hasten the return of GI and CNS effects.[104] Although the stimulating properties of bupropion may help relieve her lethargy, it may also exacerbate her insomnia.

Lamotrigine is FDA approved for the treatment of bipolar depression. Like lithium, its clinical utility has also extended to the treatment of unipolar disorder, but the evidence supporting lamotrigine in this capacity is currently preliminary. If indicated, lamotrigine should be initiated at a low dose of 25 mg at bedtime and slowly advanced to a target of 150 mg daily over a period of 6 to 8 weeks to minimize the potential for serious life-threatening rashes (e.g., 25 mg daily × 2 weeks, 50 mg daily × 2 weeks, 100 mg daily × 2weeks, 150 mg daily thereafter). CNS side effects such as sedation, dizziness, and ataxia have also been commonly repted.

Buspirone augmentation has be supported by multiple open-label studies and one large R Unfortunately, an additional RCT failed to find a statistic significant benefit from buspirone augmentation due, prir ly, to an inexplicably high placebo response rate. Theoretic buspirone may be of benefit to patients with residual syn ms of anxiety, in particular, and titration up to daily doses 0 to 45 mg daily are often required.

Among other options, p ol is a unique alpha-blocker with intrinsic sympathomi properties that has received some attention as an aug g agent.[167] Early open-label studies and one double- controlled trial suggested that pindolol may enhance erate the therapeutic effects of other antidepressants. These benefits were attributed, in part, to the inhibi cts that pindolol has on the 5-HT1A autoreceptor. e recent double-blind placebo-controlled investig lled 86 depressed patients, and, after 6 weeks of t here was no statistical advantage to pindolol aug terms of the onset or extent of antidepressant e -week, single-blind, crossover followed the initi e, and again no benefits from the alpha-blocker Given the obvious discrepancies in study results, ch appears warranted to adequately assess whet hances response to SSRIs or other antidepress s.

Modaf oved for the treatment of narcolepsy, but it ha nsively to increase energy and alertness, p depressed patients. A large placebo-contro ducted among 311 subjects exhibiting a par n SSRI.[171] Significant improvements were s and fatigue scales, as well as overall ong patients randomized to a fixed dose

r p older y in o n, and pa ded that classes RI were o side than d are

depal or second-generation antipsychotics ofigement of treatment-resistant depression y common among mental health providers controlled trials are currently lacking. Al- riety of anecdotal evidence suggests that ctive for unipolar, bipolar, or psychotic de- vestigations have featured an open-label de- d number of subjects. One common finding in , however, has been a very rapid therapeutic re- latively low doses (e.g., 1–2 mg of risperidone, of olanzapine). Given the high acquisition costs of edications, and the significant metabolic effects that een demonstrated, it is hoped that additional trials will onducted to examine the wisdom of this practice in the ar future.

The Elderly

18. **R.M., a 71-year-old man, is brought in to see a primary care provider by his daughter with whom he has been living since the death of his wife 6 months ago. His daughter reports that R.M. had been in good health until his wife's death and that since then he has been keeping to himself, showing little interest in social activities. She reports that he used to be a happy, outgoing person but is now very irritable and becomes agitated over insignificant things. Over the past 4 months, he has lost approximately 12 lb and has trouble falling asleep. He used to be a voracious reader but seems uninterested in current events now. He appears to be confused or preoccupied at times and is incapable of understanding new concepts. His only documented medical problem is benign prostatic hypertrophy (BPH), and current medications consist of a stool softener and bulk laxative. Today's physical examination is normal, and the laboratory examination is significant only for a mildly elevated prostate-specific antigen (PSA) of 10.0 ng/mL.**

On mental status examination, R.M. is perceived to be a thin, nervous, sad-appearing elderly man. He is oriented × 3. His response to questions is slow, and his volume of speech is reduced. Affect is sad. Mood is dysthymic. He shows mild impairments in his ability to think through problems and perform simple mathematical exercises. There is no evidence of delusions, hallucinations, or paranoia. He denies suicidal thoughts but feels hopeless at present and admits "there's no reason to live anymore." How does a depressive episode in late life, such as that in R.M., differ from an episode earlier in life?

Depression in late life is typically more difficult to recognize than depression in younger adults. Clinicians and patients may inappropriately attribute depressive symptoms to the "aging process" and minimize their significance. In addition, functional expectations are often lowered after retirement, making the degree of impairment difficult to evaluate. Because medical comorbidities are also more common in the elderly, depressive symptoms may be overlooked or misinterpreted in the workup as well.[172]

In general, the elderly present with the same depressive target symptoms as younger adults, which is reflected in the fact that DSM-IV-TR diagnosis for major depression in adults is not specific for age. However, qualitatively, the presentation of depression among the elderly may be quite different.[173] For instance, older patients are more likely to present with psychomotor retardation and are less likely to acknowledge "depression" per se, preferring instead to dwell on somatic concerns (e.g., poor sleep, low energy, changes in bowel function, bodily aches and pains). They are also much less likely to share or admit suicidal thoughts, and because elderly men have the highest suicide success rate, an accurate assessment of depression and attendant risks is critical (see "Drug Selection" section).[174]

19. **What is R.M.'s differential diagnosis? Should he receive antidepressant therapy?**

In assessing nonspecific behavioral and cognitive symptoms in the elderly, a careful differential diagnosis between medical and other psychiatric disorders is essential because numerous medical illnesses can mimic depressive symptoms. Anemia, malignancies, congestive heart failure (CHF), and endocrine abnormalities may all present in a manner similar to that in depressive illness and can be ruled out only with a careful line of questioning and systematic physical workup.

One of the more difficult differential diagnoses in this setting involves the distinction of depression from dementia.[175,176] Like depression, patients with dementia may present with apathy, poor memory or concentration, reduced facial expression, and lack of spontaneous interaction. The illnesses are often comorbid, as 30% to 70% of patients with dementia also suffer from major depression.[176] Some experts have suggested, in fact, that new-onset depression in elderly patients may actually be part of a prodrome toward the manifestation of Alzheimer Dementia (AD).[176,177] A longitudinal cohort study found that, among elderly patients suffering from an acute episode of major depression, 57% were ultimately diagnosed with AD within the next 3 years.[175] Diagnostically, there are three notable differences between dementia and depression: (a) the symptoms (slow and subtle changes with dementia, rapid with depression), (b) orientation (markedly impaired with dementia, intact with depression), and (c) principal CNS impairment (short-term memory with dementia, concentration with depression).

Drug Selection

A therapeutic trial of an antidepressant in a depressed individual with cognitive impairment may reverse the symptoms of the affective illness and restore functional capacity. Cognitive function may also improve to some degree. Moreover, because primary degenerative dementia is largely a diagnosis of exclusion, a successful trial of an antidepressant may help clarify the underlying pathological condition and is strongly recommended in patients with a positive personal or family history of mood disorders. Patients with dementia, in fact, may benefit from antidepressant therapy, even if they do not present with a major mood disorder.[178] Overlapping pathophysiology and neuroanatomical dysfunction in these two disorders might explain the efficacy of antidepressants for selected symptoms of degenerative dementia. Although R.M.'s physical examination and laboratory workup were normal, a therapeutic trial of an antidepressant is warranted based on his current depressive target symptoms.

The overall efficacy of antidepressants in elderly patients is believed to be comparable to that observed in younger subjects, although the response to treatment is somewhat slower (i.e., 6-week therapeutic trial usually warranted). Similarly, the comparative therapeutic effects of individual antidepressants do not appear to differ qualitatively between elderly patients and the general population. The selection of antidepressants for geriatric depression, therefore, is quite similar to the process recommended for younger patients, although the presence of medical comorbidities and current medications will often have a greater influence on treatment plans due to the higher overall disease burden found in older patients. For example, the anticholinergic effects of certain antidepressants (TCA, paroxetine) may discourage their use in elderly patients suffering from narrow angle glaucoma, chronic constipation, or urinary hesitancy. The cognitive effects of antidepressants may also be more pronounced in elderly people due to differences in pharmacokinetic disposition (prolonged half-life) and pharmacodynamic properties (compromised integrity of blood–brain barrier). Although sedating antidepressants such as mirtazapine may serve to promote sleep in depressed patients suffering from insomnia, other geriatric clients may be candidates for more activating medications that can increase energy or enhance alertness (e.g., bupropion).

In the case of *R.H., mirtazapine might* be a judicious choice due to the fact that his appetite and sleep have diminished considerably over the past several months. A conservative starting dose of 7.5 mg at bedtime might be considered to ensure his tolerability of a new medication, although it is quite possible that eventual dosage increases might be required to achieve a therapeutic response.

Tricyclic Antidepressants

20. B.H. is an obese 52-y[ear]-old man suffering from his first episode of major depressive d[iso]rder, melancholic subtype. He has an 8-year history of CHF (Ne[w Yo]rk Heart Association functional class II) with an ejection frac[tion] of 35% and atrial fibrillation. He is currently taking digoxin [illegible] mg PO QD and enalapril 10 mg PO BID. His CHF has been controlled on this regimen, and he remains asymptomatic w[ith reg]ard to the CHF. His atrial fibrillation occurs about once ev[ery] [illegible] months. All other laboratory parameters are within normal [illegible] His cardiologist believes that TCA are the most effective an[tidepres]sants for melancholic depression. Are they any safety con[cerns for s]tarting a TCA in this patient?

For many years, the TCAs were [illegible] popular class of medications used to treat depression[illegible]uisition cost for TCAs was quite low, we had severa[illegible] of experience using them, and there continue to b[illegible] who prefer antidepressant medications that enhan[illegible]n *and* nor-epinephrine for the treatment of severe [illegible]ic depression (i.e., dual-action antidepressants).[17?] [illegible]ue to be prescribed for other indications that are c[illegible] depression as well (e.g., migraine prophylaxis, c[illegible] Unfortunately, TCAs possess a variety of adve[illegible]ging from bothersome (dry mouth, sedation, co[illegible]ous (cardiovascular effects), which often pre[illegible] receiving therapeutic doses of medication.[1?] [illegible]rience with prescribed medication may also b[illegible] with TCAs.[181]

The SSRIs are widely regarded as a major [illegible] in the pharmacologic management of depressi[illegible] and have largely supplanted the TCA in their role [illegible] agents for the treatment of mood disorders. The[illegible] can be attributed to numerous advantages over [illegible] pounds, including a lower side effect burden, safe[illegible] dose, less dosage titration, once-daily administratio[illegible] tient preference. Results of a meta-analysis conclu[illegible] although the overall efficacy of the two antidepressan[illegible] was comparable, primary care patients receiving an SS[illegible] much less likely to discontinue therapy prematurely due [illegible] effects.[182] Although SSRIs were once more expensive [illegible] TCAs, most are now available in generic formulations an[illegible] relatively inexpensive.

Side Effects

21. B.H.'s cardiologist is concerned about the effect of a TC[A] on his cardiac status. What are the major adverse effects and toxicities of the TCAs, and how should these be managed?

The most common adverse effects of the TCAs are listed in Table 79-12. Anticholinergic effects are commonly encountered with the TCAs and may adversely affect adherence.[183] These side effects include dry mouth, blurred vision, constipation, and urinary retention. Although patients may develop tolerance to these effects, they may never disappear completely. Clinicians should be prepared to counsel patients about the daily over a period of 6 to 8 weeks to minimize the potential for serious life-threatening rashes (e.g., 25 mg daily × 2 weeks, 50 mg daily × 2 weeks, 100 mg daily × 2 weeks, 150 mg daily thereafter). CNS side effects such as sedation, dizziness, and ataxia have also been commonly reported.

Buspirone augmentation has been supported by multiple open-label studies and one large RCT. Unfortunately, an additional RCT failed to find a statistically significant benefit from buspirone augmentation due, primarily, to an inexplicably high placebo response rate. Theoretically, buspirone may be of benefit to patients with residual symptoms of anxiety, in particular, and titration up to daily doses of 30 to 45 mg daily are often required.

Among other options, pindolol is a unique alpha-blocker with intrinsic sympathomimetic properties that has received some attention as an augmenting agent.[167] Early open-label studies and one double-blind, controlled trial suggested that pindolol may enhance or accelerate the therapeutic effects of other antidepressants.[167–169] These benefits were attributed, in part, to the inhibitory effects that pindolol has on the 5-HT_{1A} autoreceptor.[170] A more recent double-blind placebo-controlled investigation enrolled 86 depressed patients, and, after 6 weeks of treatment, there was no statistical advantage to pindolol augmentation in terms of the onset or extent of antidepressant effect.[169] A 3-week, single-blind, crossover followed the initial study phase, and again no benefits from the alpha-blocker were evident. Given the obvious discrepancies in study results, further research appears warranted to adequately assess whether pindolol enhances response to SSRIs or other antidepressant medications.

Modafinil is FDA approved for the treatment of narcolepsy, but it has been used extensively to increase energy and alertness, particularly among depressed patients. A large placebo-controlled RCT was conducted among 311 subjects exhibiting a partial response to an SSRI.[171] Significant improvements were seen on sleepiness and fatigue scales, as well as overall depression scores, among patients randomized to a fixed dose of 200 mg daily.

The use of atypical or second-generation antipsychotics (SGAs) for the management of treatment-resistant depression has become relatively common among mental health providers but definitive well-controlled trials are currently lacking. Although a wide variety of anecdotal evidence suggests that SGAs may be effective for unipolar, bipolar, or psychotic depression, most investigations have featured an open-label design or a limited number of subjects. One common finding in these reports, however, has been a very rapid therapeutic response to relatively low doses (e.g., 1–2 mg of risperidone, 5–10 mg of olanzapine). Given the high acquisition costs of these medications, and the significant metabolic effects that have been demonstrated, it is hoped that additional trials will be conducted to examine the wisdom of this practice in the near future.

The Elderly

18. **R.M., a 71-year-old man, is brought in to see a primary care provider by his daughter with whom he has been living since the death of his wife 6 months ago. His daughter reports that R.M. had been in good health until his wife's death and that since then he has been keeping to himself, showing little interest in social activities. She reports that he used to be a happy, outgoing person but is now very irritable and becomes agitated over insignificant things. Over the past 4 months, he has lost approximately 12 lb and has trouble falling asleep. He used to be a voracious reader but seems uninterested in current events now. He appears to be confused or preoccupied at times and is incapable of understanding new concepts. His only documented medical problem is benign prostatic hypertrophy (BPH), and current medications consist of a stool softener and bulk laxative. Today's physical examination is normal, and the laboratory examination is significant only for a mildly elevated prostate-specific antigen (PSA) of 10.0 ng/mL.**

On mental status examination, R.M. is perceived to be a thin, nervous, sad-appearing elderly man. He is oriented × 3. His response to questions is slow, and his volume of speech is reduced. Affect is sad. Mood is dysthymic. He shows mild impairments in his ability to think through problems and perform simple mathematical exercises. There is no evidence of delusions, hallucinations, or paranoia. He denies suicidal thoughts but feels hopeless at present and admits "there's no reason to live anymore." How does a depressive episode in late life, such as that in R.M., differ from an episode earlier in life?

Depression in late life is typically more difficult to recognize than depression in younger adults. Clinicians and patients may inappropriately attribute depressive symptoms to the "aging process" and minimize their significance. In addition, functional expectations are often lowered after retirement, making the degree of impairment difficult to evaluate. Because medical comorbidities are also more common in the elderly, depressive symptoms may be overlooked or misinterpreted in the workup as well.[172]

In general, the elderly present with the same depressive target symptoms as younger adults, which is reflected in the fact that DSM-IV-TR diagnosis for major depression in adults is not specific for age. However, qualitatively, the presentation of depression among the elderly may be quite different.[173] For instance, older patients are more likely to present with psychomotor retardation and are less likely to acknowledge "depression" per se, preferring instead to dwell on somatic concerns (e.g., poor sleep, low energy, changes in bowel function, bodily aches and pains). They are also much less likely to share or admit suicidal thoughts, and because elderly men have the highest suicide success rate, an accurate assessment of depression and attendant risks is critical (see "Drug Selection" section).[174]

19. **What is R.M.'s differential diagnosis? Should he receive antidepressant therapy?**

In assessing nonspecific behavioral and cognitive symptoms in the elderly, a careful differential diagnosis between medical and other psychiatric disorders is essential because numerous medical illnesses can mimic depressive symptoms. Anemia, malignancies, congestive heart failure (CHF), and endocrine abnormalities may all present in a manner similar to that in depressive illness and can be ruled out only with a careful line of questioning and systematic physical workup.

One of the more difficult differential diagnoses in this setting involves the distinction of depression from dementia.[175,176] Like depression, patients with dementia may present with apathy, poor memory or concentration, reduced facial expression, and lack of spontaneous interaction. The illnesses are often comorbid, as 30% to 70% of patients with dementia also suffer from major depression.[176] Some experts have suggested, in fact, that new-onset depression in elderly patients may actually be part of a prodrome toward the manifestation of Alzheimer Dementia (AD).[176,177] A longitudinal cohort study found that, among elderly patients suffering from an acute episode of major depression, 57% were ultimately diagnosed with AD within the next 3 years.[175] Diagnostically, there are three notable differences between dementia and depression: (a) the symptoms (slow and subtle changes with dementia, rapid with depression), (b) orientation (markedly impaired with dementia, intact with depression), and (c) principal CNS impairment (short-term memory with dementia, concentration with depression).

Drug Selection

A therapeutic trial of an antidepressant in a depressed individual with cognitive impairment may reverse the symptoms of the affective illness and restore functional capacity. Cognitive function may also improve to some degree. Moreover, because primary degenerative dementia is largely a diagnosis of exclusion, a successful trial of an antidepressant may help clarify the underlying pathological condition and is strongly recommended in patients with a positive personal or family history of mood disorders. Patients with dementia, in fact, may benefit from antidepressant therapy, even if they do not present with a major mood disorder.[178] Overlapping pathophysiology and neuroanatomical dysfunction in these two disorders might explain the efficacy of antidepressants for selected symptoms of degenerative dementia. Although R.M.'s physical examination and laboratory workup were normal, a therapeutic trial of an antidepressant is warranted based on his current depressive target symptoms.

The overall efficacy of antidepressants in elderly patients is believed to be comparable to that observed in younger subjects, although the response to treatment is somewhat slower (i.e., 6-week therapeutic trial usually warranted). Similarly, the comparative therapeutic effects of individual antidepressants do not appear to differ qualitatively between elderly patients and the general population. The selection of antidepressants for geriatric depression, therefore, is quite similar to the process recommended for younger patients, although the presence of medical comorbidities and current medications will often have a greater influence on treatment plans due to the higher overall disease burden found in older patients. For example, the anticholinergic effects of certain antidepressants (TCA, paroxetine) may discourage their use in elderly patients suffering from narrow angle glaucoma, chronic constipation, or urinary hesitancy. The cognitive effects of antidepressants may also be more pronounced in elderly people due to differences in pharmacokinetic disposition (prolonged half-life) and pharmacodynamic properties (compromised integrity of blood–brain barrier). Although sedating antidepressants such as mirtazapine may serve to promote sleep in depressed patients suffering from insomnia, other geriatric clients may be candidates for more activating medications that can increase energy or enhance alertness (e.g., bupropion).

In the case of R.H., mirtazapine might be a judicious choice due to the fact that his appetite and sleep have diminished considerably over the past several months. A conservative starting dose of 7.5 mg at bedtime might be considered to ensure his tolerability of a new medication, although it is quite possible that eventual dosage increases might be required to achieve a therapeutic response.

Tricyclic Antidepressants

20. B.H. is an obese 52-year-old man suffering from his first episode of major depressive disorder, melancholic subtype. He has an 8-year history of CHF (New York Heart Association functional class II) with an ejection fraction of 35% and atrial fibrillation. He is currently taking digoxin 0.25 mg PO QD and enalapril 10 mg PO BID. His CHF has been well controlled on this regimen, and he remains asymptomatic with regard to the CHF. His atrial fibrillation occurs about once every 6 months. All other laboratory parameters are within normal limits. His cardiologist believes that TCA are the most effective antidepressants for melancholic depression. Are they any safety concerns in starting a TCA in this patient?

For many years, the TCAs were the most popular class of medications used to treat depression. The acquisition cost for TCAs was quite low, we had several decades of experience using them, and there continue to be providers who prefer antidepressant medications that enhance serotonin *and* norepinephrine for the treatment of severe or melancholic depression (i.e., dual-action antidepressants).[179] TCAs continue to be prescribed for other indications that are comorbid with depression as well (e.g., migraine prophylaxis, chronic pain). Unfortunately, TCAs possess a variety of adverse effects, ranging from bothersome (dry mouth, sedation, constipation) to serious (cardiovascular effects), which often prevent patients from receiving therapeutic doses of medication.[180] Patient adherence with prescribed medication may also be compromised with TCAs.[181]

The SSRIs are widely regarded as a major breakthrough in the pharmacologic management of depressive symptoms and have largely supplanted the TCA in their role as preferred agents for the treatment of mood disorders. Their popularity can be attributed to numerous advantages over older compounds, including a lower side effect burden, safety in overdose, less dosage titration, once-daily administration, and patient preference. Results of a meta-analysis concluded that, although the overall efficacy of the two antidepressant classes was comparable, primary care patients receiving an SSRI were much less likely to discontinue therapy prematurely due to side effects.[182] Although SSRIs were once more expensive than TCAs, most are now available in generic formulations and are relatively inexpensive.

Side Effects

21. B.H.'s cardiologist is concerned about the effect of a TCA on his cardiac status. What are the major adverse effects and toxicities of the TCAs, and how should these be managed?

The most common adverse effects of the TCAs are listed in Table 79-12. Anticholinergic effects are commonly encountered with the TCAs and may adversely affect adherence.[183] These side effects include dry mouth, blurred vision, constipation, and urinary retention. Although patients may develop tolerance to these effects, they may never disappear completely. Clinicians should be prepared to counsel patients about the appropriate way to manage these problems. Patients with dry mouth, for instance, may tend to drink excessive fluids to relieve discomfort. To minimize the inherent potential for weight gain with TCAs, patients should be advised to avoid caloric beverages and drink water or dietetic fluids instead. Sugarless gum or hard candy is often recommended as well.

TCAs also can be very sedating and are usually administered at bedtime to minimize functional impairments. Confusion or memory deficits may also occur with TCAs and can be particularly onerous in elderly patients. The secondary amines may be more tolerable in this regard, but all TCAs can impair concentration or alertness to some extent.

The impact of TCAs on cardiovascular function is a legitimate and serious concern. The most potentially dangerous adverse effect of the TCAs is their quinidinelike properties (type IA) on prolonging cardiac conduction through the His-Purkinje system. This, in conjunction with positive chronotropic and adrenergic-blocking properties of the TCAs, can lead to re-entry arrhythmias (e.g., torsades de pointes and other ventricular arrhythmias). In patients with pre-existing conduction defects and in overdose, there is a greater risk for cardiac arrhythmias.[184] Therefore, B.H. should receive a baseline electrocardiogram (ECG) before therapy.

Orthostatic hypotension is the most common and troublesome cardiovascular effect of the TCAs and MAOIs because it can result in significant morbidity and mortality.[185,186] Major clinical consequences of orthostatic hypotension include falls leading to bone fractures, lacerations, and even MI. Patients with CHF, such as B.H., are at greatest risk for developing orthostatic hypotension.

Imipramine and nortriptyline have been best studied with respect to their association with orthostatic hypotension. Amitriptyline, desipramine, doxepin, and clomipramine are also capable of producing it to varying degrees. Although systematic comparisons of the propensity of the TCAs to cause orthostatic hypotension are generally lacking, the tertiary amines (e.g., imipramine) may cause more severe orthostatic hypotension than the secondary amines (e.g., nortriptyline), and research evidence supports the contention that nortriptyline has the lowest risk for causing orthostatic hypotension among TCAs.[184,187]

Antidepressants and Cardiac Disease

22. Will the choice of antidepressant affect B.H.'s arrhythmia?

There are substantial differences among antidepressants (and antidepressant classes) in regard to overall cardiac safety and arrhythmogenic effects in particular. The SSRIs, in general, appear to be relatively safe in patients with a history of arrhythmias or recent MI.[188] In a placebo-controlled investigation, hospitalized patients with unstable cardiac disease were randomized to either sertraline or placebo.[189] Overall, both treatment arms were very well tolerated, and there was actually a lower risk of severe cardiac events reported in the sertraline group (vs. placebo). Retrospective data suggest that SSRIs may be somewhat cardioprotective in depressed patients with heart disease, a benefit that might be explained by their ability to decrease platelet activation.[190,191]

TCAs increase heart rate, probably via intrinsic anticholinergic properties that increase sinus node activity. Clinically, this effect is generally not significant, especially in medically healthy, depressed patients.[192] However, it may be important in those with underlying conduction disease, coronary artery disease, or CHF. TCAs, when used at therapeutic dosages for the treatment of depression, decrease premature atrial and ventricular contractions in both depressed and nondepressed patients.[193,194] Antidepressants with class 1A antiarrhythmic activity (e.g., TCAs) may also have arrhythmogenic activity and thus increase the chances of ventricular arrhythmias and sometimes of sudden death. This effect on rhythm and conduction is believed to be related to the inhibitory effects of TCAs on the fast sodium channels and a decrease in Purkinje fiber action potential amplitude, membrane responsiveness, and slowed conduction.[194] Even nortriptyline, which is believed to be one of the safer TCAs in patients with heart disease, was associated with a greater risk for adverse cardiac events than paroxetine in an RCT.[195]

Bupropion and mirtazapine appear unlikely to affect cardiac rhythm or induce arrhythmias in susceptible patients.[188] Bupropion, however, should be used with caution in patients with pre-existing hypertension because of potential increases in BP.[196] Its safety has not been well studied in patients with heart disease. Similarly, venlafaxine does not appear to be arrhythmogenic, but increases in BP may be seen with higher dosages (>150 mg daily) limiting its usefulness in certain patient populations.[155] The nonselective MAOIs do not seem to affect rhythm significantly, although they generally do slow heart rate and can cause or worsen orthostatic hypotension.[197] Trazodone was associated with ventricular aggravation in the past, but this risk has not been further elucidated, and its widespread use as a sedative hypnotic in institutional settings has generally been well tolerated.[188]

Plasma Concentration Monitoring

23. Are plasma concentrations clinically useful in monitoring antidepressant therapy? When should plasma antidepressant concentrations be obtained?

Attempts to demonstrate an association between plasma concentrations and therapeutic response for SSRIs, venlafaxine, and bupropion have been largely unsuccessful. In contrast to the newer agents, the serum concentration of some TCAs correlates well with clinical response. Nortriptyline exhibits a curvilinear effect, whereas imipramine demonstrates a sigmoidal relationship between serum levels and clinical response.[198,199] Maximum benefit of imipramine is usually associated with serum levels of imipramine plus its demethylated metabolite, desipramine, in excess of 250 ng/mL. The relationship between plasma concentration of desipramine and clinical response is less clear, but it appears that a linear relationship is likely.[200] The most controversy surrounds amitriptyline; studies have shown a linear relationship, a curvilinear relationship, and no relationship between serum concentration and outcome.[201–203]

The APA Task Force on the Use of Laboratory Tests in Psychiatry recommends plasma concentration monitoring of TCA when patients are elderly, not responding to therapy, nonadherent, experiencing adverse effects, or on multiple medications that may result in a possible drug interaction.[204] Plasma concentrations of imipramine, nortriptyline, and desipramine should be obtained after at least 1 week of a constant dosage when steady state has been achieved. Samples should be drawn 12 hours after the last dose has been administered. Routine therapeutic blood monitoring of other antidepressants is not recommended because information concerning their usefulness is limited; however, serum levels may be useful for evaluating adherence in some patients or ruling out serious toxicities.[205]

Other Medical Comorbidities

Diabetes

24. B.L. is a 43-year-old woman who has become increasingly depressed over the past 4 months after the unexpected death of her father. She mentions that she was very upset immediately following his death, unable to sleep at night, and frequently crying at work. These symptoms have not abated over the past few months. She is slightly obese and has always been "borderline diabetic," but her blood sugar control has worsened since her father's death, and she has subsequently gained 30 lb (HbA_{1c} = 8.2 last week, up from 6.1, 4 months ago). She is very upset that she has recently been diagnosed with type 2 diabetes and does not believe that she is capable of following the lifestyle modifications recommended. How strong is the association between depression and diabetes? Would an antidepressant be an appropriate treatment for her symptoms at this time, and, if so, which agent(s) would be recommended?

The potential association of depression with diabetes has been discussed in the medical literature for more than 300 years.[206] Results of a meta-analysis confirmed that diabetic patients are twice as likely to be suffering from depression than the general population, an association that appears to hold true for type 1 and type 2 diabetic illness.[207] Theories abound as to why diabetic patients become depressed, citing complex physiological, psychological, and social factors, and a precise explanation has not been elucidated. Conversely, longitudinal studies have shown that depressed patients are twice as likely to develop type 2 diabetes with time, and in 80% to 90% of cases, the mood disorder preceded the metabolic condition.[208] It has also been established that depressed diabetic patients are much more likely to suffer long-term complications with this metabolic disorder, and successful treatment of depression has been demonstrated to improve glycemic indices.[209–211]

Successful treatment of mood disorders in patients with diabetes is important for several reasons. Patients with depression or diabetes are at risk for cardiovascular illness, and successful antidepressant treatment, therefore, may substantially decrease morbidity and mortality. Depressed patients are also much less likely to comply with treatment recommendations in general because of their hopelessness, cognitive impairment, and social isolation. As a result, they are three times more likely to stop taking their medications, leading to a worsening of diabetes and other medical conditions.[212] Most depressed patients also report a change in their appetite at baseline, which may lead to a compromise in blood sugar control. Moreover, decreases in energy and motivation may also sabotage diabetes treatment plans.

Although the number of clinical studies conducted with depressed diabetic patients is limited, antidepressants appear to possess the same efficacy rates for this particular comorbidity as previously found in the general population.[211] Currently, there is no evidence to suggest that one class of antidepressant is more efficacious than another. Selection of an antidepressant in the diabetic population, therefore, rests largely on differences in adverse effect profiles, potential impact on diabetes complications, and potential for drug interactions.

One important consideration in selecting an antidepressant is the potential impact of the agent on appetite, blood sugar control, and total body weight. Although research on the effects of antidepressants on glycemic control is limited primarily to rat populations, important differences appear to exist among antidepressants in regard to weight gain potential.[213] As discussed previously, the risk of clinically significant weight gain appears to be highest with mirtazapine, TCAs, and MAOIs, and these medications should be avoided. Although SSRI and SNRI may occasionally induce weight gain in susceptible patients (estimated incidence of 3%–5%), this adverse effect appears to be of greatest concern with paroxetine (25% incidence). Bupropion may cause appetite suppression in some patients, which may be beneficial for the obese but may also pose a theoretical concern about hypoglycemia in diabetic patients.

Because one of the long-term complications of diabetes is sexual dysfunction, this potential side effect of antidepressants may also be worth considering. It should be emphasized, however, that erectile dysfunction and impotence are the sexual side effects most commonly encountered by male diabetics. Thus, although the SSRI may impair sexual performance by delaying or preventing orgasm, this impairment occurs at a different stage of the sexual process and would not necessarily discourage use of SSRIs. Diabetic neuropathies may also influence antidepressant selection. SNRIs have proven quite effective for the management of neuropathic pain, but clinicians should also be aware that venlafaxine and duloxetine may increase blood pressure and heart rate as well.

Pharmacokinetic drug interactions may also be a concern for certain antidepressants in diabetic patients. For instance, many of the oral antidiabetic agents are substrates for metabolism by the cytochrome P450 isoenzyme system. Inhibition of this metabolic step may precipitate a serious drug interaction by increasing plasma concentrations of the antidiabetic agents and enhancing hypoglycemic effects. Several of these agents are metabolized via the CYP 2C9 isoenzyme (e.g., tolbutamide, glyburide, glipizide, rosiglitazone), and the administration of certain SSRIs (e.g., fluoxetine or fluvoxamine) may potentiate their effects. Repaglinide and some of the sulfonylureas are metabolized via the CYP 3A4 isoenzyme, which may also be inhibited by fluoxetine or fluvoxamine.

For B.L., the depressive symptoms she experienced after her father's death may be considered a natural response to this serious loss. Because her symptoms have persisted for longer than 2 months, her psychiatric illness would no longer be categorized as a grief reaction (or bereavement) and should be managed medically as an acute episode of major depression. Thus, it is advisable that her depression receive serious attention (i.e., thorough assessment of psychiatric condition) and necessary treatment. Medical history, previous antidepressant trials, and concurrent use of other prescription medications should also be investigated. If B.L. is amenable to an antidepressant, an SSRI that is unlikely to induce weight gain or potentiate drug interactions may be a prudent choice. Such agents would include sertraline, citalopram, or escitalopram.

Epilepsy

25. C.B., a 20-year-old woman, was recently diagnosed with major depressive disorder, single episode. Since the age of 8, she has also experienced complex partial seizures. Her seizures have been difficult to control in the past (at least six seizures per month), but her condition has improved recently (none for 8 months) on a combination of carbamazepine and gabapentin. Are there any special considerations with regard to antidepressant selection in this patient?

Although seizures are a relatively uncommon effect of antidepressant medications, they are frightening and serious when they occur. The overall risk of seizures with most antidepressants is quite low at therapeutic dosages, and, as a result, the precise risk is difficult to quantify with any statistical certainty.[214] Furthermore, the risk of new-onset seizures in the general population (i.e., not necessarily receiving antidepressants) is approximately 0.073% to 0.086% annually, suggesting the likelihood of occasional coincidental case reports.[215] Among the antidepressants marketed in the United States, imipramine may be the best studied, and the frequency of seizures was reported to be 0.1% among patients prescribed therapeutic dosages (–200 mg/day).[216]

Generally, it is believed that iatrogenic seizures are a dose-related phenomenon, so it is not surprising that most case reports of antidepressant seizures have involved overdose ingestions, most commonly with the TCAs. Seizures have been correlated to peak plasma concentrations of tricyclics (e.g., levels >1,000 ng/mL) and typically occur within 6 hours after the overdose.[217]

The specific antidepressant may also be of some importance, but one may want to recall the methodologic difficulties inherent in estimating accurate figures. An older review cited amoxapine with the highest risk of seizures in overdose, followed by maprotiline and the TCAs (collectively).[218] Bupropion was withdrawn from the market in 1986 after the appearance of new-onset seizures in bulimic patients receiving the antidepressant as part of a placebo-controlled trial (4 of 69 subjects).[219] After a re-examination of the original dosing recommendations, bupropion was released again in 1989, and a new SR preparation appeared in 1998. Among the 3,100 patients to receive the new preparation for up to 1 year, the cumulative seizure risk was 0.15%.[220] Although SSRIs have been associated with seizures in acute overdose, the comparative risk encountered with dosages in the therapeutic range has not been determined.

Because of C.B.'s seizure history, choosing a medication with a low risk of seizures is prudent. Bupropion, for instance, is contraindicated in patients with a pre-existing seizure disorder. Because carbamazepine has a narrow therapeutic index and is metabolized by multiple isoenzymes within the cytochrome P450 system, antidepressants that may inhibit its clearance and raise plasma levels, such as duloxetine (CYP 2D6), fluoxetine (CYP 2D6 and 3A4), and paroxetine (CYP 2D6), should be avoided. Similarly, carbamazepine may induce the metabolism of certain TCAs, and it also possesses some of the cardiotoxic effects of these antidepressants (e.g., slowed conduction) further discouraging its use. Among the remaining alternatives, one may opt for an SSRI less likely to inhibit metabolic pathways (e.g., sertraline, citalopram) or venlafaxine.

AIDS

26. K.H., a 33-year-old HIV-positive woman, has been reasonably healthy over the past 2 years but recently developed AIDS after an episode of oral candidiasis. During the past few months, she has noticed a loss of interest in life, accompanied by decreased energy, easy fatigability, and difficulty concentrating (she has to read a sentence several times before she can comprehend its meaning). She also reports a depressed mood but denies suicidal ideation. Her current medications are zidovudine (Retrovir), lamivudine (Epivir), ritonavir (Norvir), and oral clotrimazole troche (Mycelex). After a thorough medical workup, other opportunistic infections have been ruled out. What precipitating factors may be contributing to K.H.'s current symptoms of depression?

Patients with serious illnesses such as HIV/AIDS or certain cancers are faced with an extreme psychosocial stressor that can precipitate a depressive episode. Research evaluating the severity of emotional distress in persons with HIV has shown elevated anxiety, depression, social isolation, and suicidal ideation.[221] Chronic depression in AIDS patients has, in fact, been associated with an acceleration of the disease progression, as well as a significant reduction in the perceived quality of life (vs. nondepressed HIV-infected controls).[222,223] K.H. currently is, or will be, confronted with a number of psychological issues, including fear of developing an opportunistic infection, chronic somatic preoccupations, debilitation, anger, possible death at a young age, and reactive depression.[224,225]

Although K.H.'s target symptoms (fatigue, decreased concentration, and depressed mood) may represent a depressive episode secondary to psychosocial stressors, her differential diagnosis also includes HIV-1–associated cognitive/motor complex or dementia resulting from HIV disease (formally known as *AIDS dementia complex*).[226] HIV-associated dementia closely resembles the symptoms of a depressive disorder and is part of the Centers for Disease Control and Prevention classification system for HIV infection (category C).[227] Neoplasms and opportunistic infections of the CNS secondary to AIDS can also alter mental status. However, a thorough medical workup ruled out opportunistic infection in K.H.

27. Based on K.H.'s target symptoms, is she a candidate for antidepressant therapy? What considerations should be made when selecting antidepressant therapy for K.H.?

K.H. would benefit from antidepressant therapy to help ameliorate her target symptoms of decreased energy, lack of concentration, and depressed mood, regardless of whether it is a major depressive episode or direct HIV involvement within the CNS. Although antidepressant trials in the general HIV population are lacking (and particularly scarce among populations of women or underrepresented minorities), several factors should be taken into account when selecting antidepressant medication in an HIV/AIDS patient.[228,229] In general, comparative trials with conventional agents have been associated with high dropout rates because of adverse effects, suggesting that HIV/AIDS patients may be more vulnerable to toxic effects, or that lower doses of antidepressant medications should be considered.[230,231]

Drug interactions can be a primary concern because several of the protease inhibitors undergo metabolic transformation via the cytochrome P450 system, primarily through the

CYP 3A4 and CYP 2B6 isoenzymes. Therefore, fluoxetine and fluvoxamine are best avoided. Among the alternatives, SSRIs and TCAs have demonstrated comparable efficacy in the depressed HIV/AIDS population, but the side effect burden of SSRIs may be more tolerable to these patients. Bupropion has become increasingly popular in depressed HIV/AIDS patients, and the activating properties may be attractive in this particular patient.[232] Inhibition of bupropion metabolism has been demonstrated with concurrent administration of ritonavir, efavirenz, and nelfinavir, however, which may complicate its use under certain circumstances.[233] Low-dose psychostimulants (e.g., methylphenidate, dextroamphetamine) or modafinil may also be helpful because some limited evidence has demonstrated improved cognition and mood in AIDS patients.[234] For appetite stimulation, mirtazapine would be a reasonable option in some AIDS patients, although the sedating potential should be carefully considered. An additional option may be ECT, which has been administered safely and effectively to the depressed AIDS population as well.[235]

Depression With Atypical Features (Atypical Depression)

Monoamine Oxidase Inhibitors

28. **G.R., a 38-year-old, 73-kg woman, presents at the university outpatient psychiatric clinic with a chief complaint of extreme lethargy and depressed mood more days than not for the past 6 weeks. During this period, she has also been sleeping too much and overeating (she says she has gained at least 10 lb in this time frame). On interview, she also reports an intense fear of heights and consequently does not travel if it involves driving over a bridge or flying in an airplane. She reports that this episode seems to have started around the time of the break-up with her boyfriend, and she becomes extremely anxious and tearful in revealing this piece of her history. Her psychiatric history is consistent with at least two other similar depressive episodes, the first when she was 18 years old and the second occurring around age 25 years. She currently weighs 73 kg, and her physical examination and laboratory assessments are within normal limits. In the past, she has exhibited a poor response to trials of fluoxetine and nortriptyline. During her last episode, she is noted to have responded to phenelzine 60 mg/day.**

G.R.'s depressive illness manifests differently from that expected in most cases of depression. How is this depression of G.R. different from melancholic depression?

G.R. suffers from hysteroid dysphoria, more commonly known as atypical depression (Table 79-19). DSM-IV-TR now refers to it as depression with atypical features.[13] Clinically, atypical depression has generally been regarded as a fairly heterogenous group of depressive symptoms that represent a specific form of depressive illness. Traditionally, atypical depression has been regarded as a more persistent, debilitating, and treatment-resistant mood disorder. Patients with this disorder tend to respond better to MAOIs than other antidepressant classes.[236]

The term "atypical depression" was first used to describe patients with symptoms of depression, such as a worsening of mood in the evening, lethargy, phobic and somatic anxiety, and emotional overreactivity to environmental events. In studying atypical depression, one group of investigators has identified a set of explicit operational criteria for atypical depression (the "Columbia" criteria) based on the literature and their own clinical experience.[237] Briefly, the requirements are as follows: patients must meet criteria for DSM depressive disorder; however, they are excluded if they have pervasive anhedonia (i.e., they have a mood reactivity or enjoy some activities or daily experiences). Furthermore, they must have at least two of the following: (a) hypersomnia, (b) leaden paralysis (profound lethargy), (c) hyperphagia, or (d) pathological sensitivity to interpersonal rejection (rejection sensitivity). The features of atypical depression and melancholia are compared in Table 79-19.

Table 79-19 A Comparison of Atypical Depression and Melancholia

Feature	*Atypical Depression*	*Melancholia*
Onset	Teens (or younger)	Thirties (avg)
Gender	Females > males	Females > males
Course	Chronic	Episodic
Phenomenology		
Appetite/weight	Increased	Decreased
Sleep	Increased	Decreased
Energy	Low with leaden paralysis	Low
Reaction to rejection	Very sensitive	Indifferent
Treatment response	MAOI = SSRI = TCA	MAOI = TCA = SSRI

MAOI, monoamine oxidase inhibitor; SSRI, selective serotonin reuptake inhibitor; TCA, tricyclic antidepressant.

G.R. reports a depressed mood, extreme lethargy, phobic avoidance of bridges or high places, and a recent problem with hypersomnia and hyperphagia with subsequent weight gain. She also seems to have a prominent rejection sensitivity regarding the relationship with her boyfriend.

INITIATION

29. **What role do MAOIs have in the management of depression today? Would this class of antidepressant be appropriate for G.R.? Outline a dosage titration and treatment plan.**

For the treatment of depression, the modern pharmacologic era was ushered in by the discovery of iproniazid, an antitubercular medication and potent inhibitor of MAO.[238] Subsequent research with this MAOI ultimately led to the formulation of the biogenic amine hypothesis of depression, and it influenced antidepressant drug development for the next 20 years.

Although the MAOIs, most notably phenelzine and tranylcypromine, were commonly prescribed for the treatment of depression in the 1970s and 1980s, their popularity has waned in recent years primarily because of the risks of serious drug–drug and drug–food interactions.[239] However, for the treatment of atypical depression, the MAOIs are among the most effective pharmacologic agents available and are still prescribed for patients with this depressive subtype usually after failing an SSRI. Double-blind trials featuring MAOIs versus TCAs have consistently demonstrated a superior response to the MAOIs, and a controlled trial comparing moclobemide with fluoxetine reported that the MAOI was superior as well.[240–242] Limited data comparing TCAs with SSRIs for atypical depression suggest that the two classes are comparable in efficacy, and both were superior to placebo.[243]

Because of G.R.'s positive response to phenelzine in the past, this choice of an antidepressant would be reasonable, but one should ask about the patient's previous experience with this medication (therapeutic effects, side effects, adherence, duration of treatment, and reason for discontinuation). If the dietary restrictions were difficult for G.R. to follow, she may be a good candidate for an MAOI transdermal patch (selegiline, Emsam). This transdermal agent is available in 6, 9, and 12 mg strengths, but only the 6 mg patch was approved by the FDA as safe without the need for dietary restrictions. She should remain wary, however, of the variety of drug interactions that may occur with concurrent MAOI use.

ADVERSE EFFECTS

30. G.R.'s insurance company is not willing to approve the nonformulary use of the MAOI patch, and she is unable to afford its monthly cost. Phenelzine is restarted at a dose of 30 mg daily (15 mg in the morning and at lunchtime). G.R. is being monitored closely for suicidal ideation, especially because the MAOIs are potentially lethal when taken in overdose. What other adverse effects of the nonselective MAOIs should be looked for in G.R. while she is being treated with phenelzine?

Orthostatic hypotension, weight gain, edema, and sexual dysfunction are common during MAOI therapy.[244] As is the case with the TCAs, the nonselective MAOIs can cause clinically significant postural decreases in BP. However, with the MAOIs, the mechanism is believed to be a direct sympatholytic effect because both the lying and the standing systolic BP readings are decreased.[245,246] Phenelzine seems to cause orthostatic hypotension more commonly than does tranylcypromine.[247] Because the orthostatic hypotension appears to be dose related, a reduction in dosage may be helpful.[248] For more difficult cases, orthostatic hypotension has been managed pharmacologically by the addition of 25 mg/day of triiodothyronine or initiation of fludrocortisone 0.025 to 0.05 mg once to twice a day.[249] Monitoring for BP changes, as well as edema and serum electrolyte changes (e.g., hypokalemia), is paramount if these pharmacologic interventions are used. MAOI-induced weight gain may be managed by monitoring carbohydrate and fat intake. Edema can be treated by elevating the affected limbs and/or using a thiazide diuretic (e.g., hydrochlorothiazide 25–50 mg BID), with careful monitoring of other medications (e.g., serum lithium levels) for potential drug interactions.[249] Sexual dysfunction occurs in up to 20% of patients taking MAOIs but may diminish and disappear spontaneously over time.[250,251] If necessary, it can be managed with bethanechol (Urecholine) at dosages up to 50 mg/day in both men and women.[244]

A switch into mania has been reported in up to 10% of patients with a history of bipolar disorder. Therefore, MAOIs should be avoided in this population.[244] Although MAOIs are not known as antimuscarinic medications, some patients complain of anticholinergiclike side effects, including blurred near vision and urinary retention. Dosage reduction may be helpful, but these effects may also diminish over time. Paresthesias have also been reported with the MAOIs and can be treated with pyridoxine 50 to 150 mg/day.[252] The nonselective MAOIs are not associated with proarrhythmic, antiarrhythmic, or contractility effects when used in therapeutic dosages. Rash is by far the most common side effect reported with the selegiline patch, with an approximate incidence of 30% to 40%. Like other MAOI, selegiline can be quite activating, and insomnia is frequently reported.

DRUG–FOOD INTERACTIONS

31. G.R. states that what she most fears is the "cheese reaction." What steps can be taken to avoid it?

The "cheese reaction," which can manifest as a hypertensive crisis, is so named because it occurred in patients who were taking nonselective MAOIs and ingested foods high in tyramine, a byproduct of tyrosine metabolism that is found in certain foods and beverages, such as aged cheese or Chianti wine (Table 79-20). When tyramine is ingested in the absence of an MAOI, it is rapidly metabolized by MAO in the GI tract before systemic absorption. In the presence of an MAOI, more tyramine is absorbed and relatively high concentrations of tyramine may be achieved in circulation, resulting in the displacement of norepinephrine (and other catecholamines) from presynaptic storage granules. Norepinephrine surges out into the synapse, and as metabolic degradation is inhibited by the MAOI, a profound pressor response is triggered.[253] The transdermal application of low-dose selegiline (i.e., 6 mg patch) does not cause appreciable MAOI activity in the GI tract, so normal tyramine degradation continues to occur locally, and dietary restrictions are unnecessary with this strength.

Hypertensive crisis can occur at any time after ingesting the tyramine-containing food and is probably not related to the duration of MAOI therapy.[244] Reports of hypertensive crisis are sporadic and difficult to quantify. About 8% of phenelzine

Table 79-20 Foods Containing Tyramine

High Amounts of Tyramine[a]
Smoked, aged, or pickled meat or fish
Sauerkraut
Aged cheeses (e.g., Stilton, blue cheese)
Yeast extracts (e.g., Marmite)
Fava beans
Moderate Amounts of Tyramine[b]
Beer (microbrewed > commercial)
Avocados
Meat extracts
Red wines such as Chianti
Low Amounts of Tyramine[c]
Caffeine-containing beverages
Distilled spirits
Chocolate
Soy sauce
Cottage and cream cheese
Yogurt and sour cream

[a]May not consume.
[b]May consume in moderation.
[c]May consume.
Adapted from Shulman KI et al. Dietary restriction, tyramine, and the use of monoamine oxidase inhibitors. *J Clin Psychopharmacol* 1989;9:397.

patients and 2% of tranylcypromine patients reported hypertensive reactions based on a chart review of 198 patients taking MAOIs.[244] However, it is a relatively rare event and is certainly found less often than MAOI-induced orthostatic hypotension.

Patients who are to receive nonselective MAOIs should be reliable and willing to comply with food and medication restrictions. This adverse event can be minimized with a low-tyramine diet that begins several days before starting the MAOI and continues for 3 to 4 weeks after stopping the MAOI. The severity of the cheese reaction is related to the amount of tyramine in any given food (i.e., 20 mg of tyramine can produce a severe hypertensive reaction), and the amount of tyramine can vary greatly in "high-tyramine food items."[254,255] Foods that absolutely should not be consumed with nonselective MAOIs include aged cheeses, concentrated yeast extracts, fava beans, and sauerkraut.[256] Microbrewed beers have much higher tyramine content than large, commercially produced varieties and are best avoided. Likewise, consumption of any food that has spoiled, is overripe, or has fermented, even if it is not found in the restricted list, should be avoided. Foods that typically contain tyramine and therefore should be avoided or consumed with caution when taking an MAOI are listed in Table 79-20.

32. How should an MAOI-induced hypertensive crisis be managed in G.R.?

A hypertensive crisis should be considered a medical emergency. In a hospital setting, general supportive measures are used, with attention to respiratory, metabolic, and cardiovascular systems. The urine should be acidified (e.g., with vitamin C), and IV beta-blockers are often given (e.g., phentolamine [Regitine] 5 mg IV followed by 0.25–0.50 mg IV every 4–6 hours). On occasion, patients have also received prescriptions for nifedipine with instructions to carry the medication with them and administer a 10-mg sublingual dose (if necessary).[257]

DRUG–DRUG INTERACTIONS

33. What common drug–drug interactions are associated with the nonselective MAOIs?

Several potentially fatal drug–drug interactions occur with this group of antidepressants. Like the reaction with tyramine, indirect sympathomimetics such as phenylpropanolamine and pseudoephedrine (common ingredients in over-the-counter cold preparations and diet pills) can cause a precipitous rise in BP that can result in cerebrovascular accident.

The potential for inducing serotonin syndrome with the combination of SSRIs and MAOIs has been well chronicled. A washout period of at least 14 days should separate the use of an SSRI and an MAOI. Because fluoxetine (and its primary active metabolite norfluoxetine) has a much longer half-life, the recommended washout period is at least 5 weeks after discontinuing this particular SSRI. Caution is advised when other serotonergic mediations are prescribed (see "Serotonin Syndrome" section). In addition, patients should avoid medications such as carbamazepine and cyclobenzaprine, which are structurally related to the TCAs.[258] Meperidine (Demerol) can cause a life-threatening interaction with MAOIs that is somewhat reminiscent of serotonin syndrome. This reaction is a result, in part, of the MAOI interfering with the degradation of the meperidine and is manifested by agitation, hyperthermia, and circulatory collapse.[259] Other narcotic analgesics such as meperidine, methadone, and tramadol may also trigger this reaction. Codeine and hydrocodone do not appear to have this effect when combined with MAOIs.

Depression With Psychotic Features (Psychotic Depression)

34. R.S., a 41-year-old man, is brought to the crisis stabilization unit (CSU) by the police because of extremely agitated behavior. His wife had called the police because R.S. was on the roof of their home with a gun shooting into the shingles. R.S. had worried for some time that the mortgage balance on the house was too large; now he was yelling that the house was "killing his spirit" and that he could not handle it any longer. He had told his wife that he was "inadequate as a provider" for her and their two children. In your interview with him at the CSU, he tells you that for the past week he has been hearing the voice of his deceased father telling him to kill himself after destroying the house. This has distressed him greatly. Of note, he was fired from his job as a computer analyst 6 weeks ago. His sleep is reported by his wife to be poor over the past month, with difficulties in falling asleep as well as waking up during the night and being unable to resume sleeping. His mood is depressed, and he has lost 15 lb in the past 2 weeks as a result of decreased appetite. His psychiatric history is positive for two past episodes of depression, one at age 22 and the other at age 35. Both episodes resolved after 8-week courses of imipramine 250 mg/day. He is diagnosed with major depressive disorder, recurrent, with psychotic features, and is admitted to the adjacent hospital for treatment. What features of psychotic depression are evident with R.S.?

Psychotic depression, also known as *delusional depression* or *depression with psychotic features,* is a type of affective illness in which the individual manifests with primary mood symptoms found in major depression and also demonstrates secondary psychotic features, such as delusions (fixed, false beliefs) and/or hallucinations (generally auditory). This disorder may be regarded as an extreme form of depression in which the individual's mood is so disturbed that perception is significantly impaired or distorted. Endocrine abnormalities and imaging studies strongly suggest that depression with psychotic features is distinct from unipolar depression, and there is evidence that it more closely resembles bipolar illness. Psychotic depression has been estimated to occur in at least 5% of the depression admissions to acute care hospitals in the United States, and it may be comparatively more common in the geriatric population.[260]

The delusions and hallucinations encountered with psychotic depression can be classified as either mood congruent or mood incongruent. Mood-congruent psychotic features imply that the psychosis is consistent with the depressive illness. In depression, mood-congruent delusions might include self-deprecatory thoughts as well as extreme feelings of guilt, sinfulness, or nihilistic ideation. Mood-incongruent psychotic features imply that the psychotic content is not consistent with the overall mood but, rather, is bizarre, much like that seen in schizophrenia. An example of mood-incongruent features may be a giggle or grin as a patient describes his or her misery and desire to commit suicide.

R.S. described mood-congruent hallucinations when he spoke of his dead father commanding him to kill himself. His ideas of being inadequate and not a good provider are also consistent with a mood-congruent delusion.

35. Why is it critical to resolve R.S.'s psychotic depression promptly? What treatment options are available for R.S.?

Psychotic depression is associated with much greater morbidity and mortality than other forms of major depression and also carries a higher risk of suicide than other types of depressive illness. This factor is currently a major concern in R.S.'s case because he has reported suicidal ideation.

Psychotic depression is often refractory to antidepressant monotherapy.[261,262] If pharmacotherapy is used in R.S., the historical approach has been to prescribe an antipsychotic medication in addition to an antidepressant medication. The combination of an antipsychotic and an antidepressant has proved to be superior to either component alone in psychotic depression. Several combination products are available that contain both an antipsychotic and an antidepressant (e.g., Symbyax contains fluoxetine and olanzapine). Although these combination products may appear to be convenient, they are fixed-dose combinations, and it is impossible to titrate the dosages of the individual agents independently. In psychotic depression, as the psychosis lifts, it is often prudent to taper and discontinue the antipsychotic agent while maintaining the antidepressant medication for a full course of treatment. If the antipsychotic drug is continued after the psychosis has lifted, the patient may be at greater risk for the neurotoxic effects of the antipsychotic (e.g., pseudoparkinsonism, tardive dyskinesia) as well as an increased side effect burden overall.

Atypical or second-generation antipsychotics, such as risperidone and olanzapine, are believed to possess some antidepressant properties, leading researchers to consider their usefulness as monotherapy for this disorder.[263] There is still some controversy as to whether the atypical agents are relieving depressive symptoms or the negative symptoms of schizophrenia; however, their ability to block postsynaptic 5-HT_2 receptors and facilitate dopamine transmission in certain areas of the brain suggests genuine antidepressant properties. Furthermore, their proven efficacy in treating bipolar disorder (both mania and depression) may suggest some clinical benefit in managing refractory depression or depression with psychotic features. At present, evidence supporting their use in psychotic depression is preliminary. The most rigorous trial compared the effects of risperidone with combination therapy with haloperidol and amitriptyline.[264] Although combination treatment did appear to be more efficacious, risperidone produced substantial declines in depression and general psychopathology. Several other case reports suggest that the atypical antipsychotics are worthy of additional study.

If pharmacotherapy is unsuccessful, ECT has proven to be a particularly effective remedy for this psychotic depression. ECT has a reported success rate of 80% to 85% in this population, and the onset of effect is quite rapid. The ideal frequency of maintenance treatments, however, has not been established.

In summary, Table 79-21 offers seven points that everyone should know about depression.

Table 79-21 Seven Things That Everyone Should Know About Depression

- **Depression is NOT a personality flaw or a weakness of character.**
  Depression has been associated with a chemical imbalance in the nervous system, which can be easily corrected with antidepressant medications and associated counseling.
- **All antidepressants are equally effective.**
  Approximately 65% of patients receiving a therapeutic trial of any antidepressant medication will have a beneficial response.
- **Most patients receiving antidepressants will experience some side effect(s) initially.**
  Identify an accessible health professional who can answer your questions.
- **Antidepressants should be taken at the same time daily.**
  This will make it easier for you to remember to take the medication and may also minimize side effects.
- **The response to antidepressants is delayed.**
  Several weeks may pass before you begin to feel better, and it may take 4 to 6 weeks before maximal benefits are evident.
- **Antidepressants must be taken for at least 6 to 9 months.**
  Even if you are feeling completely better, studies have shown that people who stop their medication during the first 6 months are much more likely to become depressed again.
- **Antidepressants are NOT addictive substances.**
  Antidepressants may elevate the moods of depressed individuals, but they do not act as stimulants and are not associated with craving or other abuse patterns. However, if certain antidepressants are discontinued abruptly, mild withdrawal reactions may occur.

REFERENCES

1. Andreasen NC. *The Broken Brain: The Biological Revolution in Psychiatry.* New York: Harper & Row; 1984.
2. Ustun TB, Sartorius N, eds. *Mental Illness in General Healthcare: An International Study.* London: John Wiley & Sons; 1995.
3. Wells KB et al. The functioning and well-being of depressed patients. *JAMA* 1989;262:914.
4. Greenberg PE et al. The economic burden of depression in the United States: how did it change between 1990 and 2000? *J Clin Psychiatry* 2003;64:1465.
5. Kessler RC et al. Prevalence, severity and comorbidity of 12-month DSM-IV disorders in the national comorbidity survey. *Arch Gen Psychiatry* 2005;62:617.
6. Hirschfeld RMA, Cross CK. Epidemiology of affective disorders. *Arch Gen Psychiatry* 1982;29:35.
7. Hollingshead AB, Redlich FC. *Social Class and Mental Illness.* New York: Wiley; 1958.
8. Kanowski S. Age-dependent epidemiology of depression. *Gerontology* 1994;40(Suppl 1):1.
9. Lieb R et al. Parental major depression and the risk of depression and other mental disorders in offspring: a prospective-longitudinal community study. *Arch Gen Psychiatry* 2002;59:365.
10. McGuffin P, Katz R. The genetics of depression and manic-depressive disorder. *Br J Psychiatry* 1989;155:294.
11. Blehar MC et al. Family and genetic studies of affective disorders. *Arch Gen Psychiatry* 1988;45:289.
12. Kraepelin E. *Manic Depressive Insanity and Paranoia.* Edinburgh: ES Livingstone; 1921.
13. American Psychiatric Association. *Diagnostic and Statistical Manual of Mental Disorders.* 4th Ed. Text Revision (DSM-IV-TR). Washington, DC: American Psychiatric Association; 2000.
14. Thase ME, Friedman ES. Is psychotherapy an effective treatment for melancholia and other severe depressive states? *J Affect Disord* 1999;54:1.
15. Silva de Lima M, Hotopf M. A comparison of active drugs for the treatment of dysthymia. *Cochrane Database Syst Rev* 2003;3:CD004047
16. Blazer D. Depression in the elderly. *N Engl J Med* 1989;320:164.
17. Schildkraut JJ. Neuropsychopharmacology and the affective disorders. *N Engl J Med* 1969;281:302.
18. Maas JW. Biogenic amines and depression. *Arch Gen Psychiatry* 1975;32:1357.
19. Prange A. L-tryptophan in mania: contribution to a permissive hypothesis of affective disorders. *Arch Gen Psychiatry* 1974;30:56.
20. Stahl SM. Basic psychopharmacology of antidepressants, part 1: antidepressants have seven distinct mechanisms of action. *J Clin Psychiatry* 1998;59(Suppl 4):5.
21. Schatzberg A, Rosenbaum A. Studies on MHPG levels as predictors of antidepressant response. *McLean Hosp J* 1980;6:138.
22. Kramer MS et al. Distinct mechanism for

antidepressant activity by blockade of central substance p receptors. *Science* 1998;281:1640.
23. Gold PW, Drevets WC, Charney DS. New insights into the role of cortisol and the glucocorticoid receptor in severe depression. *Biol Psychiatry* 2002;52:381.
24. Nemeroff CB. New directions in the development of antidepressants: the interface of neurobiology and psychiatry. *Hum Psychopharmacol* 2002;17(Suppl 1):13.
25. Siever LJ, Davis KL. Overview: toward a dysregulation hypothesis of depression. *Am J Psychiatry* 1985;142:1017.
26. Charney DS et al. Receptor sensitivity and the mechanisms of action of antidepressant treatment. *Arch Gen Psychiatry* 1981;381:1160.
27. Risch SC, Nemeroff CB. Neurochemical alterations of serotonergic neuronal systems in depression. *J Clin Psychiatry* 1992;53(Suppl 10):3.
28. Mann JJ et al. Serotonin and suicidal behavior. *Ann NY Acad Sci* 1990;600:476.
29. Delgado PL et al. Serotonin function and the mechanism of antidepressant action. *Arch Gen Psychiatry* 1990;47:411.
30. Miller HL et al. Noradrenergic function and clinical outcome in antidepressant pharmacotherapy. *Neuropsychopharmacology* 2001;24:617.
31. Bremner JD et al. Regional brain metabolic correlates of alpha-methylparatyrosine-induced depressive symptoms: implications for the neural circuitry of depression. *JAMA* 2003;289:3125.
32. Dunlop BW, Nemeroff CB. The role of dopamine in the pathophysiology of depression. *Arch Gen Psychiatry* 2007;64:327.
33. Morely JE, Shafer RB. Thyroid function screening in new psychiatric admissions. *Arch Intern Med* 1982;42:591.
34. Nemeroff CB, Evans DL. Thyrotropin-releasing hormone (TRH), the thyroid axis, and affective disorder. *Ann NY Acad Sci* 1989;553:304.
35. Fauci AS et al., eds. *Principles of Internal Medicine.* 14th ed. New York: McGraw-Hill; 1998.
36. Banki CM et al. Cerebrospinal fluid corticotropin-releasing factor-like immunoreactivity in depression and schizophrenia. *Am J Psychiatry* 1987;144:873.
37. Gold PN et al. Neuropeptide function in affective illness: corticotropin-releasing hormone and somatostatin as model systems. In: Meltzer HY, ed. Psychopharmacology The Third Generation of Progress. New York: Raven; 1987:617.
38. Wolkowitz OM, Reus VI. Treatment of depression with antiglucocorticoid drugs. *Psychsom Med* 1999;5:698.
39. Belanoff JK et al. An open label trial of C-1073 (mifepristone) for psychotic major depression. *Biol Psychiatry* 2002;5:386.
40. George MS et al. SPECT and PET imaging in mood disorders. *J Clin Psychiatry* 1993;54:6.
41. Nemeroff CB. The neurobiology of depression. *Sci Am* 1998;278:42.
42. Mayberg HS. Modulating dysfunctional limbic-cortical circuits in depression: towards development of brain-based algorithms for diagnosis and optimised treatment. *Br Med Bull* 2003;65:193.
43. Shea SC. *Psychiatric Interviewing: The Art of Understanding.* 2nd ed. Philadelphia: WB Saunders; 1998.
44. Carlat DJ. *The Psychiatric Interview.* 2nd ed. Baltimore: Lippincott Williams & Wilkins; 2005.
45. Hamilton M. A rating scale for depression. *J Neurol Neurosurg Psychiatry* 1960;23:56.
46. Beck AT et al. An inventory for measuring depression. *Arch Gen Psychiatry* 1961;4:561.
47. Zung WK. A self-rating depression scale. *Arch Gen Psychiatry* 1965;12:63.
48. Derogatis LR et al. The Hopkins Symptom Checklist (HSCL): a self-report symptom inventory. *Behav Sci* 1974;19:1.
49. Montgomery SA, Asberg M. New depression scale designed to be sensitive to change. *Br J Psychiatry* 1979;134:382.
50. Radloff LS. The CES-D scale: a self-report depression scale for research in the general population. *Appl Psychol Measure* 1977;1:385.
51. Kroenke K et al. The PHQ-9: validity of a brief depression severity measure. *J Gen Intern Med* 2001;16:606.
52. Rush AJ et al. The 16-item Quick Inventory Of Depressive Symptomatology (QIDS), Clinician Rating (QIDS-C), and Self-Report (QIDS-SR): a psychometric evaluation in patients with chronic major depression. *Biol Psychiatry* 2003;54:573.
53. Irwin M et al. Screening for depression in older adults. *Arch Intern Med* 1999;159:1701.
54. Ribeiro SC et al. The DST as a predictor of outcome in depression: a meta analysis. *Am J Psychiatry* 1993;150(11):1618.
55. American Psychiatric Association (APA) Task Force on the Use of Laboratory Tests in Psychiatry. The dexamethasone suppression test: an overview of its current status in psychiatry. *Am J Psychiatry* 1987;144:1253.
56. Keller MB et al. A comparison of nefazodone, the cognitive behavioral-analysis system of psychotherapy, and their combination for the treatment of chronic depression. *N Engl J Med* 2000;342:1462.
57. Arnow BA, Constantino MJ. Effectiveness of psychotherapy and combination treatment for chronic depression. *J Clin Psychol* 2003;59:893.
58. Brody DS et al. Strategies for counseling depressed patients by primary care physicians. *J Gen Intern Med* 1994;9:569.
59. Sadock BJ, Sadock VA. *Synopsis of Psychiatry.* 9th ed. Baltimore: Lippincott Williams & Wilkins; 2003.
60. Devanand DP et al. Electroconvulsive therapy in the treatment-resistant patient. *Psychiatr Clin North Am* 1991;14:905.
61. Shapira B et al. Cost and benefit in the choice of ECT schedule. *Br J Psychiatry* 1998;172:44.
62. Kellner CH et al. Continuation electroconvulsive therapy vs. pharmacotherapy for relapse prevention in major depression: a multisite study from the consortium for research in electroconvulsive therapy (CORE). *Arch Gen Psychiatry* 2006;63:1337.
63. Gershon AA et al. Transcranial magnetic stimulation in the treatment of depression. *Am J Psychiatry* 2003;160:835.
64. Groves DA, Brown VJ. Vagal nerve stimulation: a review of its applications and potential mechanisms that mediate its clinical effects. *Neurosci Biobehav Rev* 2005;29:493.
65. Gross F, Gysin F. Phototherapy in psychiatry: clinical update and review of indications. *Encephale* 1996;22:143.
66. Wehr TA. Manipulations of sleep and phototherapy: nonpharmacological alternatives in the treatment of depression. *Clin Neuropharmacol* 1990;13:S54.
67. Lawlor DA, Hopker SW. The effectiveness of exercise as an intervention in the management of depression: systematic review and meta-regression analysis of randomized controlled trials. *Br Med J* 2001;322:763.
68. Brene S et al. Running is rewarding and antidepressive. *Physiol Behav* 2007;92(1–2):136.
69. Carlson LE et al. Mindfulness-based stress reduction in relation to quality of life in breast, mood, symptoms of stress and levels of cortisol, dehydroepiandrosterone and melatonin in breast cancer and prostate cancer outpatients. *Psychoneuroendocrinology* 2004;29:448.
70. Kaplan HI, Saddock BJ, eds. *Synopsis of Psychiatry.* 9th ed. Baltimore: Lippincott Williams & Wilkins; 2003.
71. Nierenberg AA, Wright EC. Evolution of remission as the new standard in the treatment of depression. *J Clin Psychiatry* 1999;60(Suppl 22):7.
72. Trivedi MH et al. Evaluation of outcomes with citalopram for depression using measurement-based care in STAR*D: implications for clinical practice. *Am J Psychiatry* 2006;163:28.
73. Katz MM et al. Can the effects of antidepressants be observed in the first two weeks of treatment? *Neuropsychopharmacology* 1997;17:110.
74. Montgomery S. Are two week trials sufficient to indicate efficacy? *Psychopharmacol Bull* 1995;31:41.
75. Hotopf M et al. Discontinuation rates of SSRIs and tricyclic antidepressants: a meta-analysis and investigation of heterogeneity. *Br J Psychiatry* 1997;170:120.
76. Dubovsky SL. Beyond the serotonin reuptake inhibitors: rationale for the development of new serotonergic agents. *J Clin Psychiatry* 1994;55(Suppl 2):34.
77. Preskorn SH. Comparison of the tolerability of bupropion, fluoxetine, imipramine, nefazodone, paroxetine, sertraline and venlafaxine. *J Clin Psychiatry* 1995;56(Suppl 6):12.
78. Vogel GW et al. Drug effects on REM sleep and on endogenous depression. *Neurosci Biobehav Rev* 1990;14:49.
79. Finley PR. Selective serotonin reuptake inhibitors: pharmacologic profiles and potential therapeutic distinctions. *Ann Pharmacother* 1994;28:1359.
80. Leo RJ. Movement disorders associated with selective serotonin reuptake inhibitors. *J Clin Psychiatry* 1996;57:449.
81. Gregorian RS et al. Antidepressant-induced sexual dysfunction. *Ann Pharmacother* 2002;36:1577.
82. *Physicians' Desk Reference.* 48th ed. Montvale, NJ: Medical Economics Data; 1994.
83. Patterson WM. Fluoxetine-induced sexual dysfunction. *J Clin Psychiatry* 1993;54:71.
84. Lee HS et al. An open-label trial of fluoxetine in the treatment of premature ejaculation. *J Clin Psychopharmacol* 1996;16:379.
85. Modell JG et al. Comparative sexual side effects of bupropion, fluoxetine, paroxetine and sertraline. *Clin Pharmacol Ther* 1997;61:476.
86. Waldinger MD et al. Effect of SSRI antidepressants on ejaculation: a double-blind, randomized, placebo-controlled study with fluoxetine, fluvoxamine, paroxetine and sertraline. *J Clin Psychopharmacol* 1998;18:274.
87. Vida S, Looper K. Precision and comparability of adverse event rates of newer antidepressants. *J Clin Psychopharmacol* 1999;19:416.
88. Schatzberg AF, Cole JO, DeBattista C. *Manual of Clinical Psychopharmacology.* 4th ed. Washington, DC: American Psychiatric Publishing; 2003.
89. Mercadante S. Hyoscine in opioid-induced sweating. *J Pain Symp Manage* 1998;15:214.
90. Romanelli F et al. Possible paroxetine-induced bruxism. *Ann Pharmacother* 1996;30:1246.
91. Ellison JM, Stanziani P. SSRI-induced nocturnal bruxism in four patients. *J Clin Psychiatry* 1993;54:432.
92. Rugh JD, Harlan J. Nocturnal bruxism and temporomandibular disorders. *Adv Neurol* 1988;49:329.
93. Kirby D, Ames D. Hyponatremia and selective serotonin re-uptake inhibitors in elderly patients. *Int J Geriatr Psychiatry* 2001;16:484.
94. Arinzon ZH et al. Delayed recurrent SIADH associated with SSRIs. *Ann Pharmacother* 2002;36:1175.
95. Levine LR et al. Use of a serotonin re-uptake inhibitor, fluoxetine, in the treatment of obesity. *Int J Obes* 1987;11(Suppl 3):185.
96. Fava M et al. Fluoxetine versus sertraline and paroxetine in major depressive disorder: changes in weight with long-term treatment. *J Clin Psychiatry* 2000;61:863.
97. Paton C et al. SSRIs and gastrointestinal bleeding. *BMJ* 2005;331:529.
98. Wernicke JF et al. Low dose fluoxetine therapy for depression. *Psychopharmacol Bull* 1988;24:180.
99. Casper RC et al. Somatic symptoms in primary affective disorder: presence and relationship to the classification of depression. *Arch Gen Psychiatry* 1985;42:1098.
100. Shen WW, Hsu JH. Female sexual side effects associated with selective serotonin reuptake inhibitors: a descriptive clinical study of 33 patients. *Int J Psychiatry Med* 1995;25:239.

101. Rothschild AJ. Selective serotonin reuptake inhibitor-induced sexual dysfunction: efficacy of a drug holiday. *Am J Psychiatry* 1995;152:1514.
102. Labbate LA, Pollack MH. Treatment of fluoxetine-induced sexual dysfunction with bupropion: a case report. *Ann Clin Psychiatry* 1994;6:13.
103. Ashton AK, Rosen RC. Bupropion as an antidote for serotonin reuptake inhibitor-induced sexual dysfunction. *J Clin Psychiatry* 1998;59:112.
104. Kennedy SH et al. Combining bupropion SR with venlafaxine, paroxetine or fluoxetine: preliminary report on pharmacokinetic, therapeutic, and sexual dysfunction effects. *J Clin Psychiatry* 2002;63:181.
105. Rosen RC et al. Effects of SSRI on sexual function: a critical review. *J Clin Psychopharmacol* 1999;19:67.
106. Nurnberg HG et al. Treatment of antidepressant-associated sexual dysfunction with sildenafil. *JAMA* 2003;289:56.
107. Aizenberg D et al. Cyproheptadine treatment of sexual dysfunction induced by serotonin reuptake inhibitors. *Clin Neuropharmacol* 1995;18:320.
108. Shrivastava RK et al. Amantadine in the treatment of sexual dysfunction associated with selective serotonin reuptake inhibitors. *J Clin Psychopharmacol* 1995;15:83.
109. Norden MJ. Buspirone treatment of sexual dysfunction associated with selective serotonin re-uptake inhibitors. *Depression* 1994;2:109.
110. Jacobsen FM. Fluoxetine-induced sexual dysfunction and an open-label trial of yohimbine. *J Clin Psychiatry* 1992;53:119.
111. Michelson D et al. Female sexual dysfunction associated with antidepressant administration: a randomized, placebo-controlled study of pharmacologic intervention. *Am J Psychiatry* 2000;157:239.
112. Cohen AJ, Bartlik B. Ginkgo biloba for antidepressant-induced sexual dysfunction. *J Sex Marital Ther* 1998;24:139.
113. Delgado PL et al. Treatment strategies for depression and sexual dysfunction. *J Clin Psychiatry* 1999;17:15 [Monograph 1].
114. Depression Guideline Panel. Clinical Practice Guideline Number 5: Depression in Primary Care. Volume 2: Treatment of Depression. Rockville, MD: U.S. Department of Health and Human Services, Agency for Health Policy and Research; 1993. AHCPR Publication No. 93-0550.
115. Alexopoulos GS et al. Recovery in geriatric depression. *Arch Gen Psychiatry* 1996;53:305.
116. Zajecka J et al. Discontinuation symptoms after treatment with serotonin reuptake inhibitors: a literature review. *J Clin Psychiatry* 1997;58:291.
117. Judd LL. The clinical course of unipolar major depressive disorders. *Arch Gen Psychiatry* 1997;54:989.
118. Nonacs R, Cohen LS. Depression during pregnancy: diagnosis and treatment options. *J Clin Psychiatry* 2002;63(Suppl 7):24.
119. Altschuler LL et al. Course of mood and anxiety disorders during pregnancy and the postpartum period. *J Clin Psychiatry* 1998;59(Suppl 2):29.
120. Cohen LS et al. Relapse of major depression during pregnancy in women who maintain or discontinue antidepressant treatment. *JAMA* 2006;295:499.
121. Orr ST, Miller CA. Maternal depressive symptoms and the risk of poor pregnancy outcome: review of the literature and preliminary findings. *Epidemiol Rev* 1995;17:165.
122. Louik C et al. First-trimester use of selective serotonin reuptake inhibitors and the risk of birth defects. *N Engl J Med* 2007;356:2675.
123. Alwan S et al. Use of serotonin-reuptake inhibitors in pregnancy and the risk of birth defects. *N Engl J Med* 2007;356:2684.
124. Chambers CH et al. Selective serotonin-reuptake inhibitors and persistent pulmonary hypertension of the newborn. *N Engl J Med* 2006;354:579.
125. Laine K et al. Effects of exposure to selective serotonin reuptake inhibitors during pregnancy on serotonergic symptoms in newborns and cord blood monoamine and prolactin concentrations. *Arch Gen Psychiatry* 2003;60:720.
126. Spigstet O, Hagg S. Excretion of psychotropic drugs into breast milk: pharmacokinetic overview and therapeutic implications. *CNS Drugs* 1998;9:111.
127. Wisner KL et al. Serum sertraline and n-desmethylsertraline levels in breast-feeding mother-infant pairs. *Am J Psychiatry* 1998;155:690.
128. Greenblatt DJ et al. Human cytochromes and some new antidepressants: kinetics, metabolism and some drug interactions. *J Clin Psychopharmacol* 1999;19(Suppl 1):23.
129. Gram LF et al. Citalopram: interaction studies with levomepromazine, imipramine and lithium. *Ther Drug Monit* 1993;15:18.
130. von Moltke LL et al. Escitalopram (s-citalopram) and its metabolites in vitro: cytochromes mediating the biotransformation, inhibitory effects, and comparison to r-citalopram. *Drug Metab Dispos* 2001;29:1102.
131. Jefferson JW, Griest JH. Brussel sprouts and psychopharmacology: understanding the cytochrome P450 system. *Psychiatr Clin North Am* 1996;3:205.
132. Crewe HK et al. The effect of selective serotonin re-uptake inhibitors on cytochrome P4502D6 (CYP2D6) activity in human liver microsomes. *Br J Clin Pharmacol* 1992;34:262.
133. Preskorn SH et al. Pharmacokinetics of desipramine coadministered with sertraline or fluoxetine. *J Clin Psychopharmacol* 1994;14:90.
134. Brosen K et al. Inhibition by paroxetine of desipramine metabolism in extensive but not in poor metabolizers of sparteine. *Eur J Clin Pharmacol* 1993;44:349.
135. Sporer KA. The serotonin syndrome—implicated drugs, pathophysiology and management. *Drug Saf* 1995;13:94.
136. Sternbach H. The serotonin syndrome. *Am J Psychiatry* 1991;148:705.
137. Lappin RI, Auchincloss EL. Treatment of serotonin syndrome with cyproheptadine. *N Engl J Med* 1994;331:1021.
138. Sandyk R. L-dopa induced "serotonin syndrome" in a parkinsonian patient on bromocriptine. *J Clin Psychopharmacol* 1986;6:194.
139. Guze BH, Baxter LR. The serotonin syndrome: case responsive to propranolol. *J Clin Psychopharmacol* 1986;6:119.
140. Graber MA et al. Sertraline-phenelzine drug interaction: a serotonin syndrome reaction. *Ann Pharmacother* 1994;28:732.
141. Iruela LM et al. Toxic interaction of S-adenosylmethionine and clomipramine. *Am J Psychiatry* 1993;150:522.
142. Lantz MS et al. St. John's wort and antidepressant drug interactions in the elderly. *J Geriatr Psychiatry Neurol* 1999;12:7.
143. Nirenberg AA et al. Trazodone for antidepressant-induced insomnia. *Am J Psychiatry* 1994;151:1069.
144. Paykel ES et al. Residual symptoms after partial remission: an important outcome in depression. *Psychol Med* 1995;25:1171.
145. Brown WA, Harrison W. Are patients who are intolerant to one serotonin selective reuptake inhibitor intolerant to another? *J Clin Psychiatry* 1995;56:30.
146. Bull SA et al. Discontinuing or switching selective serotonin-reuptake inhibitors. *Ann Pharmacother* 2002;36:578.
147. Thase ME, Ferguson J, Wilcox C. Citalopram treatment of paroxetine intolerant patients. *Depress Anxiety* 2002;16:128.
148. Calabrese JR et al. Citalopram treatment of fluoxetine-intolerant depressed patients. *J Clin Psychiatry* 2003;64:562.
149. Rush AJ et al. Bupropion-SR, sertraline or venlafaxine-XR after failure of SSRIs for depression. *N Engl J Med* 2006;354:1231.
150. Kirwin JL, Goren JL. Duloxetine: an antidepressant that inhibits both norepinephrine and serotonin uptake. *Formulary* 2003;38:29.
151. Poirier MF, Boyer P. Venlafaxine and paroxetine in treatment resistant depression. *Br J Psychiatry* 1999;175:12.
152. Clerc GE et al. A double-blind comparison of venlafaxine and fluoxetine in patients hospitalized for major depression and melancholia. *Int Clin Psychopharmacol* 1994;9:139.
153. Thase ME et al. Remission rates during treatment with venlafaxine or selective serotonin reuptake inhibitors. *Br J Psychiatry* 2001;178:234.
154. Diamond S et al. Serotonin syndrome induced by transitioning from phenelzine to venlafaxine: four patient reports. *Neurology* 1998;51:274.
155. Anon. *Effexor product labeling information.* Philadelphia: Wyeth-Ayerst; 2003.
156. Ascher JA et al. Bupropion: a review of its mechanism of antidepressant activity. *J Clin Psychiatry* 1995;56:395.
157. Jain AK et al. Bupropion SR vs. placebo for weight loss in obese patients with depressive symptoms. *Obes Res* 2002;10:1049.
158. De Boer T. The effects of mirtazapine on central noradrenergic and serotonergic neurotransmission. *Int Clin Psychopharmacol* 1995;10(Suppl 4):19.
159. Wheatley DP et al. Mirtazapine: efficacy and tolerability in comparison with fluoxetine in patients with moderate to severe major depressive disorder. *J Clin Psychiatry* 1998;59:306.
160. Anon. *Remeron product labeling information.* West Orange, NJ: Organon; 1996.
161. Guelfi JD et al. Mirtazapine versus venlafaxine in hospitalized severely depressed patients with melancholic features. *J Clin Psychopharmacol* 2001;21:425.
162. Bauer M et al. Lithium augmentation in treatment-resistant depression: meta-analysis of placebo-controlled trials. *J Clin Psychopharmacol* 1999;119:427.
163. Altshuler LL et al. Does thyroid supplementation accelerate tricyclic antidepressant response? A review and meta-analysis of the literature. *Am J Psychiatry* 2001;158:1617.
164. Nierenberg AJ et al. A comparison of lithium and T3 augmentation following two failed medication treatments for depression: a STAR*D report. *Am J Psychiatry* 2006;163:1484.
165. Bodkin JA et al. Combining serotonin reuptake inhibitors and bupropion in partial responders to antidepressant monotherapy. *J Clin Psychiatry* 1997;58:137.
166. DeBattista C et al. A prospective trial of bupropion SR augmentation of partial responders and non-responders to serotonergic antidepressants. *J Clin Psychopharmacol* 2003;23:27.
167. Artigas F et al. Pindolol induces a rapid improvement of depressed patients treated with serotonin reuptake inhibitors. *Arch Gen Psychiatry* 1994;51:248.
168. Blier P, Bergeron R. Effectiveness of pindolol with selected antidepressant drugs in the treatment of depression. *J Clin Psychopharmacol* 1995;15:217.
169. Berman RM et al. Effect of pindolol in hastening response to fluoxetine in the treatment of major depression: a double-blind, placebo-controlled trial. *Am J Psychiatry* 1997;154:37.
170. Hoyer D. 5-HT receptors: subtypes and second messengers. *J Recept Res* 1991;11:197.
171. Fava M et al. A multi-center, placebo-controlled study of modafinil augmentation in patients with partial response to selective serotonin reuptake inhibitors with persistent fatigue and sadness. *J Clin Psychiatry* 2005;66:85.
172. Diagnosis and treatment of depression in late life: the NIH consensus development conference statement. *Psychopharmacol Bull* 1993;29:87.
173. Rothschild AJ. The diagnosis and treatment of late-life depression. *J Clin Psychiatry* 1996;57(Suppl 5):5.
174. Duberstein PR et al. Suicide in widowed persons. *Am J Geriatr Psychiatry* 1998;6:328.
175. Reding M et al. Depression in patients referred to a dementia clinic: a three year prospective study. *Arch Neurol* 1985;42:894.
176. Meyers BS. The depression-dementia conundrum. *Arch Gen Psychiatry* 1998;55:102.

177. Green RC et al. Depression as a risk factor for Alzheimer disease. *Arch Neurol* 2003;60:753.
178. Cummings JL. Dementia and depression: an evolving enigma. *J Neuropsychol* 1989;1:236.
179. Perry PJ. Pharmacotherapy for major depression with melancholic features: relative efficacy of tricyclic versus selective serotonin reuptake inhibitor antidepressants. *J Affect Disord* 1996;39:1.
180. Katon W et al. Adequacy and duration of antidepressant treatment in primary care. *Med Care* 1992;30:67.
181. Sclar D et al. Antidepressant pharmacotherapy: economic outcomes in a health maintenance organization. *Clin Ther* 1994;16:715.
182. MacGillivray S et al. Efficacy and tolerability of selective serotonin reuptake inhibitors compared with tricyclic antidepressants in depression treated in primary care: systematic review and meta-analysis. *Br Med J* 2003;326:1014.
183. Snyder SH. Antidepressants and the muscarinic acetylcholine receptor. *Arch Gen Psychiatry* 1977;34:236.
184. Cassem N. Cardiovascular effects of antidepressants. *J Clin Psychiatry* 1982;43:22.
185. Rabkin JG et al. Adverse reactions to monoamine oxidase inhibitors: II. Treatment correlates and clinical management. *J Clin Psychopharmacol* 1985;5:2.
186. Glassman AH. Cardiovascular effects of tricyclic antidepressants. *Ann Rev Med* 1984;35:503.
187. Freyschuss U et al. Circulatory effects in man of nortriptyline, a tricyclic antidepressant drug. *Pharmacologia Clin* 1970;2:68.
188. Alvarez W, Pickworth KK. Safety of antidepressant drugs in the patient with cardiac disease: a review of the literature. *Pharmacotherapy* 2003;23:754.
189. Glassman AH et al. Sertraline treatment of major depression in patients with acute MI or unstable angina. *JAMA* 2002;288:701.
190. Sauer WH et al. Selective serotonin reuptake inhibitors and myocardial infarction. *Circulation* 2001;104:1894.
191. Serebrauny VL et al. Effect of selective serotonin reuptake inhibitors on platelets in patients with coronary artery disease. *Am J Cardiol* 2001;87:1398.
192. Bigger JT Jr et al. Cardiac antiarrhythmic effect of imipramine hydrochloride. *N Engl J Med* 1977;296:206.
193. Giardina EGV, Bigger JT Jr. Antiarrhythmic effect of imipramine hydrochloride inpatients with ventricular premature complexes with psychological depression. *Am J Cardiol* 1982;50:172.
194. Muir WW et al. Effects of tricyclic antidepressant drugs on the electrophysiological properties of dog Purkinje fibers. *J Cardiovasc Pharmacol* 1982;4:82.
195. Roose SP et al. Comparison of paroxetine and nortriptyline in depressed patients with ischemic heart disease. *JAMA* 1998;279:287.
196. Roose SP et al. Cardiovascular effects of bupropion in depressed patients with heart disease. *Am J Psychiatry* 1991;148:512.
197. Davidson J, Turnbull CD. The effects of isocarboxazid on blood pressure and pulse. *J Clin Psychopharmacol* 1986;6:139.
198. Asberg M et al. Relationship between plasma level and therapeutic effect of nortriptyline. *Br Med J* 1971;3:331.
199. Glassman AH et al. Clinical implications of imipramine plasma levels for depressive illness. *Arch Gen Psychiatry* 1977;34:197.
200. Nelson JC et al. Desipramine plasma concentrations and antidepressant response. *Arch Gen Psychiatry* 1982;39:1419.
201. Ziegler VE et al. Amitriptyline plasma levels and therapeutic response. *Clin Pharmacol Ther* 1976;19:795.
202. Moyes ICA et al. Plasma levels and clinical improvement—a comparative study of clomipramine and amitriptyline in depression. *Postgrad Med J* 1980;56:127.
203. Robinson DS et al. Plasma tricyclic drug levels in amitriptyline-treated depressed patients. *Psychopharmacology* 1979;63:223.
204. American Psychiatric Association (APA) Task Force. The use of laboratory tests in psychiatry: tricyclic antidepressants—blood level measurements and clinical outcome. An APA Task Force Report. *Am J Psychiatry* 1985;142:155.
205. Linder MW, Keck PE. Standards of laboratory practice: antidepressant drug monitoring. *Clin Chem* 1998;44:1073.
206. Willis T. *Diabetes: A Medical Odyssey*. New York: Tuckahoe; 1971.
207. Anderson RJ et al. The prevalence of comorbid depression in adults with diabetes: a meta-analysis. *Diabetes Care* 2001;24:1069.
208. de Groot M et al. Association of depression and diabetes complications: a meta-analysis. *Psychosom Med* 2001;63:619.
209. Lustman PJ et al. Effects of nortriptyline on depression and glucose regulation in diabetes: results of a double-blind, placebo-controlled trial. *Psychosom Med* 1997;59:241.
210. Lustman PJ et al. Fluoxetine for depression in diabetics: a randomized double-blind placebo-controlled trial. *Diabetes Care* 2000;23:618.
211. Lustman PJ, Clouse RE. Treatment of depression in diabetes: impact on mood and medical outcome. *J Psychsom Res* 2002;53:917.
212. DiMatteo MR et al. Depression is a risk factor for noncompliance with medical treatment: meta-analysis of the effects of anxiety and depression on patient adherence. *Arch Intern Med* 2000;160:2101.
213. Gomez R et al. Acute effect of different antidepressants on glycemia in diabetic and non-diabetic rats. *Braz J Med Biol Res* 2001;34:57.
214. Lee KC et al. Risk of seizures associated with psychotropic medications: emphasis on new drugs and new findings. *Expert Opin Drug Saf* 2003;2:233.
215. Hauser WA, Kurland LT. The epidemiology of epilepsy in Rochester, Minnesota, 1935 through 1967. *Epilepsia* 1975;16:1.
216. Alldridge BK. Drug-induced seizures: controversies in their identification and management. *Pharmacotherapy* 1997;17:857.
217. Bigger JT Jr et al. Tricyclic antidepressant overdose: incidence of symptoms. *JAMA* 1977;238:135.
218. Wedin GP et al. Relative toxicity of cyclic antidepressants. *Ann Emerg Med* 1986;15:7.
219. Horne RL et al. Treatment of bulimia with bupropion: a multicenter controlled trial. *J Clin Psychiatry* 1988;49:262.
220. Dunner DL et al. A prospective safety surveillance study of bupropion sustained-release in the treatment of depression. *J Clin Psychiatry* 1998;59:366.
221. Atkinson JH Jr et al. Prevalence of psychiatric disorders among men infected with human immunodeficiency virus infection: a controlled study. *Arch Gen Psychiatry* 1988;45:859.
222. Leserman J et al. Progression to AIDS: the effects of stress, depressive symptoms and social support. *Psychosom Med* 1999;61:397.
223. Sherbourne CD et al. Impact of psychiatric conditions on health-related quality of life in persons with HIV infection. *Am J Psychiatry* 2000;157:248.
224. Beckett A, Rutan JS. Treating persons with ARCH and AIDS in group psychotherapy. *Int J Group Psychother* 1990;40:19.
225. Faulstich ME. Psychiatric aspects of AIDS. *Am J Psychiatry* 1987;144:551.
226. Perry AW. Organic mental disorders caused by HIV: update on early diagnosis and treatment. *Am J Psychiatry* 1990;147:696.
227. Revised Classification System for HIV infection. *Morb Mortal Wkly Rep MMWR* 1992;41:1.
228. Olatunji BO et al. A review of treatment studies of depression in HIV. *Int AIDS Society* 2006;14:112.
229. Himmelhoch S, Medoff DR. Efficacy of antidepressant medication among HIV-positive individuals with depression: a systematic review and meta-analysis. *AIDS Patient Care* 2005;19:813.
230. Elliott AJ et al. Randomized, placebo-controlled trial of paroxetine versus imipramine in depressed HIV-positive outpatients. *Am J Psychiatry* 1998;155:367.
231. Rabkin JG et al. Fluoxetine treatment for depression in patients with HIV and AIDS: a randomized, placebo-controlled trial. *Am J Psychiatry* 1999;156:101.
232. Currier MB et al. A prospective trial of sustained-release bupropion for depression in HIV-seropositive and AIDS patients. *Psychosomatics* 2003;44:120.
233. Hesse LM et al. Ritonavir, efavirenz and nelfinavir inhibit CYP2B6 activity in vitro: potential drug interactions with bupropion. *Drug Metab Dispos* 2001;29:100.
234. Fernandez F et al. Response of HIV-related depression to psychostimulants: case reports. *Hosp Commun Psychiatry* 1988;39:628.
235. Schaerf FW et al. ECT for major depression in four patients infected with human immunodeficiency virus. *Am J Psychiatry* 1989;146:782.
236. Paykel ES et al. Response to phenelzine and amitriptyline in sub-types of outpatient depression. *Arch Gen Psychiatry* 1982;39:1041.
237. Stewart JW et al. Atypical depression: a valid clinical entity? *Psychiatr Clin North Am* 1993;16:479.
238. West ED et al. Effect of iproniazid in depressive symptoms. *Br Med J* 1959;1:1491.
239. Zisook S. A clinical overview of monoamine oxidase inhibitors. *Psychosomatics* 1985;26:240.
240. Ravaris CL et al. Phenelzine and amitriptyline in the treatment of depression. *Arch Gen Psychiatry* 1980;37:1075.
241. Davidson J et al. A comparison of phenelzine and imipramine in depressed inpatients. *J Clin Psychiatry* 1981;42:395.
242. Lonnquist J et al. Moclobemide and fluoxetine in atypical depression: a double-blind trial. *J Affect Disord* 1994;32:169.
243. McGrath PJ et al. A placebo-controlled study of fluoxetine versus imipramine in the acute treatment of atypical depression. *Am J Psychiatry* 2000;157:344.
244. Rabkin JG et al. Adverse reactions to monoamine oxidase inhibitors. Part II: treatment correlates and clinical management. *J Clin Psychopharmacol* 1985;5:2.
245. Murphy DL et al. Monoamine oxidase-inhibiting antidepressants: a clinical update. *Psychiatr Clin North Am* 1984;7:549.
246. Kronig MH et al. Blood pressure effects of phenelzine. *J Clin Psychopharmacol* 1983;3:307.
247. Salzman C. Clinical guidelines for the use of antidepressant drugs in geriatric patients. *J Clin Psychiatry* 1985;46:38.
248. Mallinger AG et al. Pharmacokinetics of tranylcypromine in patients who are depressed: relationship to cardiovascular effects. *Clin Pharmacol Ther* 1986;40:444.
249. Pollack MH, Rosenbaum JF. Management of antidepressant-induced side effects: a practical guide for the clinician. *J Clin Psychiatry* 1987;48:3.
250. Robinson DS et al. Phenelzine and amitriptyline in the treatment of depression. *Arch Gen Psychiatry* 1978;35:629.
251. Mitchell JE, Popkin MK. Antidepressant drug therapy and sexual dysfunction in men: a review. *J Clin Psychopharmacol* 1983;3:76.
252. Stewart JW et al. Phenelzine-induced pyridoxine deficiency. *J Clin Psychopharmacol* 1984;4:225.
253. Haefely W et al. Biochemistry and pharmacology of moclobemide, a prototype RIMA. *Psychopharmacology* 1992;106:S6.
254. Sheehan DV et al. Monoamine oxidase inhibitors: prescription and patient management. *Int J Psychiatry Med* 1980;10:99.
255. Blackwell B et al. Hypertensive interactions between monoamine oxidase inhibitors and foodstuffs. *Br J Psychiatry* 1967;113:349.
256. Shulman KI et al. Dietary restriction, tyramine, and the use of monoamine oxidase inhibitors. *J Clin Psychopharmacol* 1989;9:397.

257. Clary C, Schweizer E. Treatment of MAOI hypertensive crisis with sublingual nifedipine. *J Clin Psychiatry* 1987;48:249.
258. Anon. *Emsam product labeling information.* Princeton, NJ: Bristol-Myers Squibb; 2006.
259. Hansten PD, Horn JR. *Drug Interaction Analysis and Management.* Vancouver, WA: Applied Therapeutics; 1998.
260. Spiker DG et al. The pharmacological treatment of delusional depression. *Am J Psychiatry* 1985;142:430.
261. Glassman AH, Roose SP. Delusional depression. *Arch Gen Psychiatry* 1981;38:424.
262. Chan CH et al. Response of psychotic and nonpsychotic depressed patients to tricyclic antidepressants. *J Clin Psychiatry* 1987;48:197.
263. Blier P et al. Potential mechanisms of action of atypical antipsychotic medications in treatment-resistant depression and anxiety. *J Clin Psychiatry* 2005;66(Suppl 8):30.
264. Muller-Siecheneder F et al. Risperidone versus haloperidol and amitriptyline in the treatment of patients with combined psychotic and depressive symptoms. *J Clin Psychopharmacol* 1998;18:111.

CHAPTER 80

Mood Disorders II: Bipolar Disorders

James J. Gasper, Mary C. Borovicka, and Raymond C. Love

Manic-depression distorts moods and thoughts, incites dreadful behaviors, destroys the basis of rational thought, and too often erodes the desire and will to live. It is an illness that is biological in its origins, yet one feels psychological in the experience of it; an illness that is unique in conferring advantage and pleasure, yet one that brings in its wake almost unendurable suffering and, not infrequently suicide.

Kay Redfield Jamison[1]

INTRODUCTION

Bipolar disorder (formerly known as *manic-depression)* is a chronic and progressive illness that disrupts and disables the lives of those afflicted. Impairment in day-to-day functioning continues even when mood symptoms have dissipated.[2] Based upon a report from the National Institute of Mental Health patients typically spend one-fourth of their adult lives in the hospital and half of their lives disabled.[3] In fact, the burden of bipolar disorder exceeds many severe illnesses such as human immunodeficiency virus, diabetes mellitus, and asthma.[4]

Diagnosis and Classification

Mood disorders are diagnosed using the criteria established in the *Diagnostic and Statistical Manual of Mental Disorders,* Fourth edition, Text Revision (DSM-IV-TR).[5] Discrete periods of mood disturbance are defined as *major depressive episodes, manic episodes, hypomanic episodes,* or *mixed episodes.*

Manic or hypomanic episodes (Table 80-1) are periods of abnormally and persistently elevated, expansive, or irritable mood.[5] Hypomanic episodes are less intense than manic episodes, which are severe enough to impair functioning (self-care, occupational, social), complicate a medical condition, result in psychotic features, or require hospitalization.[5] Although manic and hypomanic episodes are characteristic symptoms of bipolar disorder, it is depressive episodes that predominate. Depressed mood is ordinarily the initial presenting symptom.[6,7] Bipolar disorder and major depressive disorder share the same criteria with major depressive episodes (Table 79-4).[5] A mixed episode is diagnosed when a patient meets criteria for both a major depressive episode and a manic episode concurrently for at least a 1-week period.[5] Associated symptoms with mixed episodes include agitation, insomnia, changes in appetite, psychosis, and suicidality.

A person who has experienced one or more manic or mixed episodes with or without a depressive episode is diagnosed as having *bipolar I disorder.* An individual who has experienced one or more episodes of both hypomania and depression (without a history of manic or mixed episodes) is diagnosed as having *bipolar II disorder.*[5]

The diagnosis of a *cyclothymic disorder* is used for a person who has experienced at least 2 years of mood cycling characterized by numerous periods with hypomanic symptoms and separate periods with depressive symptoms that do not meet the criteria for a major depressive episode. *Bipolar disorder, not otherwise specified* (NOS), refers to disorders with features of mania or hypomania that do not meet the criteria for a specific bipolar disorder.[5]

The DSM-IV-TR also uses a series of descriptors called *specifiers* to further characterize the course of illness and the

Table 80-1 DSM-IV-TR Criteria for a Manic Episode[a]

1. A distinct period of abnormally and persistently elevated, expansive, or irritable mood, lasting ≥1 week (or of any duration if hospitalization is necessary).
2. During the period of mood disturbance, ≥3 of the following symptoms have persisted (4 if the mood is only irritable) and have been present to a significant degree:
   - Inflated self-esteem or grandiosity
   - Decreased need for sleep (e.g., feels rested after only 3 hours of sleep)
   - More talkative than usual or pressure to keep talking
   - Flight of ideas or subjective experience that thoughts are racing
   - Distractibility (i.e., attention too easily drawn to unimportant or irrelevant external stimuli)
   - Increase in goal-directed activity (either social, at work, at school, or sexually) or psychomotor agitation
   - Excessive involvement in pleasurable activities that have a high potential for painful consequences (e.g., the person engages in unrestrained buying sprees, sexual indiscretions, or foolish business investing)
3. The symptoms do not meet the criteria for a Mixed Episode.
4. The mood disturbance is sufficiently severe to cause marked impairment in occupational functioning or in usual social activities or relationships with others, or to necessitate hospitalization to prevent harm to self or others, or there are psychotic features.
5. The symptoms are not due to the direct physiologic effects of a substance (e.g., a drug of abuse, a medication, or other treatment) or a general medical condition (e.g., hyperthyroidism).

[a]Criteria for a hypomanic episode are identical to a manic episode however the symptoms need only be present for 4 days and are not severe enough to cause marked impairment in occupational functioning or in usual social activities or relationships with others, or to necessitate hospitalization to prevent harm to self or others, or for psychotic features to be present. Manic-like episodes that are clearly caused by somatic antidepressant treatment (e.g., medication, electroconvulsive therapy, light therapy) should not count toward a diagnosis of bipolar I disorder.

Reprinted with permission from American Psychiatric Association. Mood Disorders. In: Diagnostic and Statistical Manual of Mental Disorders. Fourth Ed. Text Revision. Washington, DC: American Psychiatric Association; 2000;362:368.

most recent type of episode experienced by the individual. Recent episodes are first classified as hypomanic, manic, mixed, or depressed. They may be described further in terms of severity (mild, moderate, severe), the presence of psychotic features (in partial or full remission), with or without catatonic features, or with onset during the postpartum period. Other specifiers convey information regarding the pattern of illness. For example, some individuals experience major depressive episodes at a characteristic time of the year (usually the winter) or switch from depression to mania during a particular season. The specifier "with seasonal pattern" applies only to the pattern of major depressive episodes. Other specifiers describe whether full recovery between episodes (i.e., with or without full interepisode recovery) occurs and whether individuals experience rapid cycling (four or more mood episodes/year).[5]

Epidemiology and Cost Burden

Using DSM-IV criteria, the lifetime prevalence of bipolar I disorder is estimated to be 1.0%; bipolar II disorder is slightly more common at 1.1%.[8] The prevalence rate for the bipolar spectrum of illnesses which includes bipolar I, bipolar II, and subthreshold bipolar disorder (mood symptoms present but not meeting full diagnostic criteria) is 4.4%.[8] Bipolar I and II are more common in females than in males, whereas subthreshold illness predominates in males.[8] The familial nature of bipolar disorder has been well established. The estimated relative risk of bipolar disorder in first-degree relatives of probands has been estimated to be 10.7.[9] Twin studies add further support to the genetic linkage of bipolar disorder. Goodwin and Jamison report a 63% concordance rate (rate of illness in co-twin of affected proband) for monozygotic twins compared with 13% for dizygotic twins.[9] The cost of bipolar illness in 1991 was reported to be $45 billion.[10] Direct costs accounted for 17% of the total, whereas the remaining 83% was owing to indirect costs such as lost wages, suicide, institutional care, and caregiver burden.

Clinical Signs and Symptoms

A manic episode usually begins with a change in sleep patterns along with mood elevation. Target symptoms typically include increased talkativeness, staying awake all night, and bursts of energy during which projects are begun but rarely completed. Mania often is characterized by thought disturbances. Patients may exhibit "flight of ideas" (rapid speech that switches among multiple ideas or topics) and delusions of grandeur (false beliefs of special powers, knowledge, abilities, importance, or identity). The behavior of manic patients is characterized as being intrusive, loud, intense, irritable, suspicious, and challenging. They often exercise poor judgment. For example, they may spend large sums of money in business deals that ultimately fail, become sexually promiscuous, take excessive risks, or fail to obey laws.

These symptoms usually develop gradually over several days to more than a week in three stages. *Stage I* is characterized by euphoria, irritability, labile affect, grandiosity, overconfidence, racing thoughts, increased psychomotor activity, and an increase in the rate and amount of speech. This stage corresponds to an episode of hypomania. *Stage II* features increased dysphoria (a feeling of extreme discomfort and unrest), hostility, anger, delusions, and cognitive disorganization without apparent cause. This stage corresponds to acute mania. Many patients progress no further than this stage. Others may proceed to *stage III*, in which the manic episode progresses to an undifferentiated psychotic state. Individuals in stage III experience terror and panic. Their behavior is bizarre and psychomotor activity is frenzied. They may experience hallucinations. They progress from disorganized thought patterns to incoherence and disorientation. Just as the manic episode gradually builds, it often declines in a gradual manner. Psychotic symptoms usually resolve first, whereas irritability, paranoia, and excessive behavior continue. Slowly, remaining symptoms such as hyperverbosity, seductiveness, and dysphoria decrease.[11]

Course of Illness

The mean age of onset for the bipolar spectrum of illnesses is 21 years.[8] Bipolar I is the earliest in onset at 18 years, compared with bipolar II at 20 years and subthreshold bipolar disorder at 22 years.[8] Approximately 20% to 30% of new cases occur in children between 10 and 15 years old.[12,13] Patients may present initially with mania, hypomania, depression, or a mixed episode. However, 75% of patients report having had multiple episodes of depression before the development of a manic episode.[12] Misdiagnosis is common early in the illness with a startling 69% of patients reporting being misdiagnosed.[12] Furthermore, up to 26% reported visiting as many as five physicians before an accurate diagnosis was made. Interestingly, although 70% of patients reported having at least one symptom of mania before, only about 40% reported these symptoms to a physician.[12] After 60 years of age, there is a significant decrease in the new onset of bipolar disorder.[14] Therefore, a presentation of mania later in life should alert the clinician to an underlying medical problem as the possible cause.

Bipolar disorder is a recurrent illness; single episodes of mania occur in fewer than 10%.[5] Most suffer multiple episodes of mania, hypomania, or depression separated by periods of euthymia (normal mood) throughout the course of their lives. In the majority, mania occurs just before or immediately after a depressive episode.[5] There may be a 5- to 10-year period from the onset of illness until the first hospitalization or diagnosis.[14]

The course of illness is characterized by episode, length duration of euthymic intervals, frequency of relapse, severity of episodes, and predominant syndrome (mania, hypomania, or depression). These factors do not remain fixed throughout an individual's illness. For instance, individuals may experience episodes of dysphoria and depression before ever experiencing hypomania or mania. Often, the euthymic interval and cycle length decrease with additional episodes. Over time, a course of alternating manic and depressive episodes without intervening euthymic periods can develop.

People diagnosed with either bipolar I or II disorder who experience shorter cycle lengths and who suffer from four or more episodes of depression, hypomania, mania, or a mixed episode in a year are identified as "rapid cyclers." Rapid cycling occurs in 20% of cases; women are more often affected than men.[15] Individuals with rapid cycling bipolar disorder often are refractory to conventional treatment and suffer significant morbidity and mortality because of their rapid changes in mood. They may have little or no euthymic period between manic and depressive episodes. This can have drastic family, social, and occupational consequences.

Unfortunately, despite adequate treatment, 73% of individuals with bipolar disorder relapse within 5 years. Furthermore, nearly half continue to experience significant mood symptoms between episodes, and fewer than 20% are euthymic or have minimal symptoms.[16]

Complications of Bipolar Illness

Patients with bipolar illness have higher rates of mortality from both natural and unnatural causes. Higher rates of natural mortality largely result from cardiovascular disease.[17] Suicide (primarily in depressive and mixed episodes) and excessive risk-taking behaviors (primarily during manic or hypomanic episodes) also contribute to the high mortality rate. Significant risk factors for suicide in bipolar patients include drug abuse, hospitalization for depression, age younger than 35 years, a recent (within 2 years) hospitalization, previous suicide attempts, and a family history of affective disorders.[18,19] Overall mortality as well as deaths owing to suicide or cardiovascular causes are significantly reduced in bipolar patients who are adequately treated.[16]

Bipolar patients are especially prone to substance abuse. Approximately 42% have comorbid substance use disorders.[8] Rapid cyclers and those with dysphoric mania have the highest rates of concomitant substance abuse.[19] Individuals in a manic phase may engage in sexual indiscretions or risky sexual practices that expose them to sexually transmitted diseases.

The World Health Organization recently identified the top ten causes of disability-adjusted life-years in the world; bipolar disorder ranked sixth.[20] Individuals with bipolar disorder are likely to experience stress and upheaval in many areas of their lives, including relationships, employment, and finances. Of bipolar patients, 88% have been hospitalized once and 66% at least two times.[20] Patients with manic and depressive episodes have divorce rates that are two- to threefold higher than those found in nonaffected populations. Patients often report having poor relationships with family members, and nearly 75% report that their family members have a limited understanding of bipolar disorder.[12] Employment problems may result from bizarre, inappropriate, or unreliable behavior. In one study, 60% of patients reported being unemployed, 88% felt the disease affected how well they performed at work, and 63% felt that they were treated differently from their peers.[12] Financial and legal problems may result from excessive spending, involvement in schemes, substance abuse, and risk-taking behavior. Caregivers and family members may also suffer significant distress in caring for a relative with bipolar illness.[20]

Treatment Overview

Several North American guidelines for the treatment of bipolar disorder exist.[14,21–24] The most recent guidelines to be updated are from the Texas Implementation of Medication Algorithms and the Canadian Network for Mood and Anxiety Treatments.[21,23] The goals of treatment across the phases of illness include the control of acute symptoms, symptom remission, return to normal level of functioning, prevention of relapses, and reduction of suicide.[14] Both the acute treatment of manic and depressive episodes and maintenance treatment for prevention of future episodes require individualization of therapy; treatment decisions should take into account presenting symptoms, history of response, patient preference, and comorbid medical or substance use conditions.

Initial treatment strategies for hypomanic/manic episodes includes the preferred and well established antimanic agents lithium, valproate, or an atypical antipsychotic (AAP). Mixed episodes are more likely to respond to valproate or an AAP than lithium. Carbamazepine (CBZ) and the AAP olanzapine are effective in manic or mixed episodes; however, safety concerns preclude their use as first-line agents.[21,25] Short-term use of benzodiazepines may be needed, particularly for severely ill or agitated patients.[14] In the case of severe manic symptoms or in those only partially responsive to an adequate trial (generally 1–2 weeks) of monotherapy, a two-drug combination of lithium, valproate, or an AAP is recommended.[21] CBZ, oxcarbazepine, or a typical antipsychotic alone or in combination with a preferred antimanic drug are potential alternatives. For treatment-resistant cases, electroconvulsive therapy (ECT), clozapine, or a three-drug combination of lithium plus an anticonvulsant (CBZ, oxcarbazepine, valproate) plus an AAP are recommended. When drug combinations are used, the individual agents should employ different mechanisms of action.

The treatment of acute depressive episodes emphasizes the use of drugs that target the depressed phase without inducing mania or cycle acceleration. Lithium or lamotrigine are preferred treatments for bipolar depression.[14,21,23,24] For patients with a history of severe, recent, or recurrent mania, lamotrigine should only be used in combination with an antimanic agent.[21] Despite being the only U.S. Food and Drug Administration (FDA)-approved treatments for bipolar depression, quetiapine and the olanzapine/fluoxetine combination (OFC), should be reserved for second-line use because of the risk of side effects such as metabolic complications.[25] After failure of these second-line options, a two-drug combination of lithium, lamotrigine, quetiapine, or OFC is appropriate.[21] Subsequent medication trials can include antidepressants, such as selective serotonin reuptake inhibitors (SSRIs), bupropion, or serotonin and norepinephrine reuptake inhibitors (SNRIs), but only when used in combination with an antimanic agent.[21] The use of antidepressants at this stage in treatment has been hotly debated.[21,26] Because of concerns of undertreated depression, some authors have suggested earlier use of antidepressants; however, others advocate for an "antidepressant-sparing" strategy because of the risks of inducing mania and cycle acceleration. Owing to an increased risk of switching into mania and side effects, the use of monoamine oxidase inhibitors and tricyclic antidepressants (TCA) should be reserved for refractory cases.

Maintenance treatment of bipolar disorder should include continuing the acute phase treatment while periodically simplifying and moving toward monotherapy with lithium, valproate, or lamotrigine. Although several AAPs are effective in preventing relapse, they are considered alternative treatments owing to safety concerns.[21] Patient and family education to improve medication adherence are vital to promote long term recovery. Causes of nonadherence that should be considered include ambivalence, side effects, lack of insight, and a reluctance to surrender the "high" of the manic episode.[14] Patients should also be advised to maintain regular patterns of daily activities, a consistent sleep–wake cycle, meals, exercise routines, and other schedules.

CLINICAL ASSESSMENT

Clinical Presentation and Diagnosis

1. H.M., is a 23-year-old man, accompanied to the clinic by his wife, A.M. She called the clinic before bringing H.M. in and reported much of the following information. A.M. says that he was doing well until about 3 weeks ago, when his niece was killed in an automobile accident. At the funeral, he borrowed some "nerve pills" from his cousin. Since then, H.M. has been acting increasingly "wild." He has been staying up later and later at night and often bursts into the bedroom at 2 or 3 A.M. and loudly awakens A.M. Sometimes, he presents her with expensive gifts, which they cannot afford. He often jumps on the bed and starts singing her love songs in a loud voice. A.M. notes that H.M. then almost always demands sex, after which he sleeps for a few hours and then loudly gets up and leaves the house.

H.M. recently has experienced problems at work, where he is a snack delivery truck driver. Over the last several weeks, he was noted to be loading his truck in a rapid and reckless manner. His boss received several reports that H.M. was driving unsafe and at high speeds. Store owners called to complain that he was giving away free cases of snacks to customers. He often did not complete deliveries to the stores at the end of his route.

Last week, when his boss called to express concern over his behavior, H.M. said he was quitting his job. He wrote an illegible resignation note, which was at least 10 pages long, called an overnight air delivery service to deliver the note to his employer (who is located only 3 miles from his home), and then left the house before the driver arrived to pick it up. H.M. returned several hours later driving a brand new foreign car and wearing an expensive new suit, red cowboy boots, and a bright green hat with a large feather. He told A.M. that he had a new job, which was going to make him a millionaire.

Last night, she found a large sum of money in his pants pocket when emptying the clothes hamper. He did not come home at all, but he called her at 4 A.M. to tell her to pack for Dallas, where he was going to become the new head coach of the professional football team.

Upon arriving at the clinic, H.M. insists, "I don't need no doc. I am supercalifragilistic!" He then bursts into song. He is dressed flamboyantly but needs a shave and shower. He gives the examiner (a stranger) a bear hug and has trouble sitting still, listening, or allowing others to talk. His speech is pressured and loud; he often fails to complete sentences or communicate entire ideas, and he is rhyming and punning. His mood obviously is elevated, but he becomes increasingly irritable throughout the examination. He insists he must get to Texas to sing the national anthem at a football game before the CIA can stop him; he then breaks down in tears. Within moments, he is again smiling and talking of money-making schemes. He is oriented to person and place, but thinks it is tomorrow. Intelligence seems average. When asked to interpret a proverb, H.M. becomes angry, throws a chair across the room, and yells, "Enough of this! Air Force One is waiting for me!" He then storms out of the office. How is H.M.'s presentation consistent with the diagnosis of a manic episode?

The hallmark of a manic episode is changes in mood, behavior, cognition, and perception (Table 80-1).[11] H.M. first demonstrates an elevated mood. He is exuberant and notes how great he feels. However, manic patients often demonstrate lability in their mood, and they may become irritable and easily frustrated, especially when challenged. In this case, H.M. becomes irritable and resentful when questioned by the examiner. His quick displays of sadness and anger further demonstrate the volatility of his mood.

H.M. displays behavior and speech typical of acute mania. He has a reduced need for sleep, behaves recklessly, and is overactive. His speech is pressured, loud, and full of rhymes and puns, and he sings to express his emotion. As illustrated by H.M., speech may skip from topic to topic in a "flight of ideas." Behavior often is characterized as being excessive and expansive. H.M. dresses flamboyantly, hugs his examiner, writes an unnecessarily lengthy letter of resignation, seeks an overnight courier service for local delivery, presents his wife with lavish gifts, and distributes merchandise to strangers.

Delusions are often present in acute mania and are grandiose in nature and deal with inflated abilities, self-importance, wealth, or special missions in life. H.M. makes unrealistic comments about his money-making schemes, his singing ability, his position as the coach of a professional football team, and his intended use of the presidential plane. Persecutory delusions may also be present such as H.M.'s fear that the CIA is going to stop him.

Patients with acute mania are often disorganized and do not complete tasks. They tend to skip from idea to idea and scheme to scheme. In this case, H.M. neglects his hygiene, fails to complete his deliveries, and neglects sending out his resignation letter.

Precipitating Factors

2. What factors make H.M. vulnerable to the occurrence of a manic episode at this time?

The mean age of onset for bipolar disorder is 21 years of age.[8] Thus, H.M. is at the age in which his disorder would be likely to first manifest itself. In addition, manic episodes are often precipitated by psychosocial stressors.[27] The death of H.M.'s niece may have served as a predisposing factor for the development of a manic episode.

A variety of medications and clinical states can induce or precipitate manic episodes (Table 80-2). The most common drug causes of mania involve medications that affect monoamine neurotransmitters,[28] such as antidepressants and stimulants. Corticosteroids, anabolic steroids, isoniazid, levodopa, caffeine, and over-the-counter stimulants can induce or aggravate mania. Sleep loss also can be a significant cause of mania.[27] A reduction in sleep after the death of his niece could have contributed to the development of H.M.'s manic episode.

3. If the "nerve pills" borrowed by H.M. were antidepressants, could they have contributed to the development of his manic episode?

All major classes of antidepressants including monoamine oxidase inhibitors, TCAs, SSRIs, and SNRIs may precipitate mania in an estimated 20% to 40% of patients with bipolar disorder.[29] Despite the purported risk, up to 78% of patients with bipolar disorder are treated with antidepressants, but only 56% receive mood stabilizers.[26] There are numerous case reports of induction of mania or hypomania with antidepressant treatment, but few controlled studies making it difficult to make comparisons across antidepressant classes. A comparison of the monoamine oxidase inhibitor, tranylcypromine, and the TCA, imipramine, found a similar rate of treatment emergent mania between groups (21% and 25%, respectively).[30] A meta-analysis found a higher switch rate for TCAs (11.2%) than for SSRIs (3.7%), which approximated placebo (4.2%).[31] A controlled trial with bupropion, sertraline, and venlafaxine (in combination with a mood stabilizer) found an overall switch rate of 19% during acute treatment and 37% during the continuation phase of the study with no significant difference between agents.[32] Antidepressants may also cause cycle acceleration in bipolar disorder, which effectively decreases the time between mood episodes. The risk for cycle acceleration may be heightened for patients who develop manic or hypomanic symptoms on antidepressants despite receiving antimanic treatment concurrently.[33] In the case of H.M., an antidepressant may have precipitated the manic episode or shortened his cycle, moving him into an episode of mania from a preexisting state of depression or euthymic mood.[34]

Table 80-2 Selected Drugs Reported to Induce Mania

Anticonvulsants	Gabapentin, lamotrigine, topiramate
Antidepressants	Monoamine oxidase inhibitors, TCAs, SSRIs, SNRIs, bupropion, nefazodone, trazodone, mirtazapine
Antimicrobials	Clarithromycin, ofloxacin, cotrimoxazole, erythromycin, isoniazid, metronidazole, zidovudine, efavirenz
Anti-Parkinsonian Drugs	Levodopa, amantadine, bromocriptine
Anxiolytics/hypnotics	Buspirone, alprazolam, triazolam
AAPs	Aripiprazole, olanzapine, quetiapine, risperidone, ziprasidone
CNS stimulants	Caffeine, cocaine, methylphenidate, amphetamine,
Drugs of abuse	Marijuana, PCP, LSD
Endocrine	Corticosteroids, thyroid supplements, androgens
Herbals	St. John's wort, SAMe, Ma-huang, omega-3 fatty acids, tryptophan
Sympathomimetics	Ephedrine, phenylpropanolamine, pseudoephedrine, phenylephrine
Miscellaneous	Cimetidine, tramadol, sibutramine

AAPs, atypical antipsychotics; CNS, central nervous system; LSD, lysergic acid diethylamide; PCP, phencyclidine; SAMe, *s*-adenosyl-L-methionine; SSRI, selective serotonin reuptake inhibitor; SNRI, serotonin and norepinephrine reuptake inhibitors; TCA, tricyclic antidepressant.

Compiled from references 28, 29, 132, 134, 135, and 139–155.

TREATMENT OF ACUTE MANIA

4. Why does H.M. require treatment?

Manic episodes have a number of severe complications. Left untreated, severe mania can result in confusion, fever, exhaustion, and even death. The impairment in judgment, the excesses, and the risk-taking that occur during manic episodes may devastate relationships, careers, and finances, and lead to physical harm and loss of life. Manic individuals may engage in illegal activities or behave in a manner that results in a violation of the law. H.M. drives recklessly, may have lost his job, spends excessive amounts of money on gifts, clothing, and automobiles; and plans to participate in a variety of money-making schemes. He has acquired a great deal of cash suddenly, perhaps from withdrawing all of his family's savings or from some type of illegal enterprise. Manic patients also may engage in risky sexual encounters, leading to infection with sexually transmitted diseases or human immunodeficiency virus. Alcohol and drug abuse are common. Irritability, such as that demonstrated by H.M., can lead to episodes of violence, resulting in potential harm to the patient or to others. The goals of treatment are to reduce the severity and duration of the current mood episode as well as to prevent recurrence of future episodes.

Valproate (Divalproex, Valproic Acid)

5. What is the appropriate treatment for H.M.'s acute manic episode?

Depending on the type and severity of mania, first-line treatment includes lithium, valproate, AAPs (aripiprazole, quetiapine, risperidone, ziprasidone), or a combination of these agents.[14,21–24] Table 80-3 lists the treatment recommendations as summarized by North American Treatment Guidelines. Considering H.M.'s presentation, monotherapy with a first-line agent is appropriate.[14,21–24] In the past, lithium was the preferred first-line agent for mania, but its use is limited by a

Table 80-3 Initial Choice of Treatment for Manic and Mixed Episodes

	APA	TIMA	Expert Consensus[c]	CANMAT
Euphoric	Li, VPA, AAP	Li, VPA, ARP, QTP, RIS, ZIP	Li[a], VPA, Li or VPA + AAP[b]	Li, VPA, AAP, Li or VPA + AAP[b]
Mixed	VPA	VPA, ARP, RIS, ZIP	VPA[a], VPA + AAP[b]	

[a] Drug of choice.
[b] Olanzapine, risperidone, quetiapine.
[c] Initial and preferred treatment only.
AAP, atypical antipsychotic; ARP, aripiprazole; Li, lithium; OLZ, olanzapine; QTP, quetiapine; RIS, risperidone; VPA, valproate; ZIP, ziprasidone.
Adapted from American Psychiatric Association (APA). Practice guideline for the treatment of patients with bipolar disorder (revision) *Am J Psychiatry* 2002;159(Suppl 4):1; Texas Implementation of Medication Algorithms (TIMA). Update to the algorithms for treatment of bipolar I disorder. *J Clin Psychiatry* 2005;66:870; Expert Consensus. Expert consensus guideline series: treatment of bipolar disorder. Postgraduate Medicine: A special report. December 2004:1. Canadian Network for Mood and Anxiety (CANMAT). Treatments guidelines for the management of patients with bipolar disorder: update 2007. *Bipolar Disord* 2006;8:721.

narrow therapeutic index, drug interactions, and bothersome side effects. However, some experts indicate that lithium remains the preferred mood stabilizer in euphoric mania. The efficacy of valproate in acute mania has been shown to be comparable with lithium; approximately one-half of patients will demonstrate at least a 50% reduction on the Mania Rating Scale derived from the Schedule for Affective Disorders and Schizophrenia.[35] Valproate may also be preferred in patients who have characteristics that predict a poor response to lithium, such as substance abuse, rapid cycling, mixed states, or multiple prior episodes.[22]

Dosing and Monitoring

6. Valproate was chosen for the management of H.M.'s mania because of comparable efficacy to lithium as well as the more rapid onset of effect.[14] How should valproate therapy be initiated, and what baseline tests are necessary? How will H.M.'s response to therapy be monitored?

The initial dose of valproate for H.M. should be 250 mg three times per day.[14] The dosage should then be increased by 250 to 500 mg every 2 to 3 days to obtain steady-state serum valproate levels between 45 and 125 mcg/mL or a maximum dosage of 60 mg/kg/day.[36] An alternative strategy is to use an oral loading regimen of 20 to 30 mg/kg/day given on a TID schedule during an acute episode of mania. This approach has been used during inpatient management, and may result in a more rapid onset of effect.[37] The correlation between serum concentration and efficacy is not well established with valproate levels of 45 mcg/mL being a minimum threshold and higher concentrations offering greater benefit. In fact, those achieving a serum concentration of 80 mcg/mL by day 3 had greater symptom improvement at days 3 and 5 of treatment.[37] A pooled analysis demonstrated a linear relationship between serum concentration and efficacy with the greatest improvement found in patients with valproate levels >94 mcg/mL.[38] Above valproate levels of 125mcg/mL, the risk of side effects increases.[39]

Before valproate is initiated, baseline laboratory tests, including a complete blood count (CBC) with differential and platelets, and liver function tests should be obtained. H.M.'s baseline weight and neurologic status should be recorded. In premenopausal women who have not undergone surgical sterilization, a baseline pregnancy test is warranted. Attention should be given to any medications that might be administered concurrently with valproate because interactions with aspirin, phenytoin, phenobarbital, lamotrigine, rifampin, warfarin, felbamate and carbamazepine are cited frequently (also see Chapter 54).

Valproate should decrease the severity and duration of H.M.'s current manic episode, decrease the frequency of subsequent episodes, and increase the euthymic period between episodes. Once treatment has started, H.M. should be monitored for response of his initial target symptoms, including grandiosity, decreased need for sleep, pressured speech, distractibility, and impulsivity. Symptom improvement with valproate can be expected in approximately 5 days.[40]

SIDE EFFECTS

7. What are the potential side effects of valproate therapy? How should H.M. be monitored for these possible effects?

H.M. should be monitored for potential dose-related adverse reactions of valproate including various gastrointestinal (GI) complaints (nausea, diarrhea, dyspepsia, anorexia), sedation, ataxia, tremor, benign hepatic transaminase elevations, and thrombocytopenia. GI complaints may be mitigated by reducing the dosage, changing to an extended-release preparation, or administering an antacid or H_2-antagonist. Central nervous system (CNS) effects such as ataxia and sedation may respond to dosage reduction, although sedation may resolve with continued treatment. If tremor is bothersome or interferes with the patient's functioning, dosage reduction or change to the extended-release preparation may provide relief.[41] Alopecia occurs in 0.5% to 12% of patients and may improve with dose reduction.[42] Small elevations in transaminases are considered benign; however, valproate should be discontinued if elevations are more than two to three times the upper limit of normal.

Weight gain occurs in up to 20% of patients receiving valproate.[39] The increase in body weight is particularly distressing to some patients and may contribute to medication nonadherence. Weight gain has been associated with valproate serum concentrations >125 mcg/mL; therefore, dosage reduction may be helpful.[39] Valproate also has been associated with the development of polycystic ovary syndrome in women.[43] Core features of polycystic ovary syndrome include oligomenorrhea and hyperandrogenism, which develop concurrently in about 10% of women with bipolar disorder after taking valproate. The clinical features associated with polycystic ovary syndrome include menstrual irregularities, infertility, hirsutism, alopecia, insulin resistance, hyperlipidemia, and obesity.

There are several reports of valproate-induced hyperammonemic encephalopathy in psychiatric patients.[44,45] Patients presenting with coma or mental status changes should have serum ammonia and liver functions tests ordered. If valproate-induced hyperammonemic encephalopathy is suspected, then valproate should be discontinued. Other serious adverse events with valproate include fulminant hepatic failure, agranulocytosis, and pancreatitis, all of which require discontinuation of therapy as well.

Once valproate therapy is initiated, liver function tests, valproate serum levels, and CBCs with differential and platelets should be monitored at least monthly for the first 3 months and every 3 to 6 months thereafter.[14] Body weight should also be determined at baseline and monitored monthly during therapy.

8. H.M. was titrated to a total daily valproate dosage of 2,500 mg/day and a steady-state plasma concentration of 95 mcg/mL was reported after 1 month of treatment. A routine CBC with differential and platelet count was ordered at this time and the following data were reported: white blood cell (WBC) count, 8.5 × 10^3/mm^3; hemoglobin, 14.5 g/dL; hematocrit, 43%; red blood cells, 5.2 × 10^6/mm^3; neutrophils, 59%; lymphocytes, 27%; monocytes, 6%; eosinophils, 2%; basophils, 0.5%; and platelets, 75 × 10^3/mcL. How should H.M.'s valproate-induced thrombocytopenia be managed?

[SI units: WBC count, 8.5 × 10^9/L (normal, 3.2–9.8); hemoglobin, 145 g/L (normal [male], 115–155); hematocrit, 0.43 L (normal [male], 0.39–0.49); red blood cells, 5.2 × 10^{12}/L (normal [male], 4.3–5.9); neutrophils, 0.59 L (normal, 0.54–0.62); lymphocytes 0.27 L (normal, 0.25–0.33); monocytes, 0.06 L (normal, 0.03–0.07); eosinophils, 0.02 L (normal, 0.01–0.03); basophils, 0.005 L (normal, 0–0.0075); platelets, 75 × 10^9/L (normal, 130–400)]

Valproate-induced thrombocytopenia occurs rarely and is associated with higher serum levels.[39] Nevertheless, clinicians should educate patients to look for signs such as easy bruising or bleeding. In most patients, thrombocytopenia is asymptomatic and responds to a lowering of the valproate dosage; complete discontinuation of the drug is often unnecessary.[46] H.M.'s dosage should be reduced, and his platelet count should be monitored closely. In addition, he should be observed for reemerging symptoms of mania.

Lithium

PRELITHIUM WORKUP

9. C.N., a 21-year-old woman, was diagnosed with her first episode of mania 3 weeks ago. At that time, she was hospitalized and treated with lithium at a dose of 1,200 mg/day (serum level, 0.8 mEq/L). C.N.'s manic episode was stabilized, and after 10 days she was discharged from the hospital. She was scheduled to see her outpatient psychiatrist for follow-up 1 week later, but failed to keep the appointment. Today, C.N. arrives at the emergency department at the request of her mother. C.N. is pulling her mom's hair and kicking wildly as she is pulled from the car. She can be heard screaming "The FBI is after me, Mom! You want them to find me, don't you? I would have made it out of the country if you hadn't gotten in the way! I was going to marry Prince Charles and become the new queen of England." Upon evaluation, C.N.'s mood is irritable, and she is pacing around the interviewer. She is dressed in a short skirt and high heels and is wearing an excessive amount of makeup and costume jewelry. During the interview, she interrupts the examiner, smiles, and says in a loud, provocative voice "Let's you and me get out of here!" Her mother states that after C.N. was discharged from the hospital, she lost her prescription and within several days, stopped attending her classes at the local community college. She began staying out late, playing her radio loudly, and driving recklessly, finally hitting the side of the garage while parking early this morning. What laboratory tests are required before initiating lithium therapy for C.N.?

Because lithium can affect many organ systems, baseline laboratory values must be evaluated before therapy is initiated. These values will serve to determine whether future abnormal values are lithium related. Furthermore, various physiologic states may affect lithium's excretion or predispose one to lithium toxicity. In these cases, baseline laboratory tests are useful in determining the presence of factors that contraindicate the use of lithium or require an adjustment in dosage. As a young, healthy female, C.N.'s prescreening laboratory battery should include electrolytes, blood urea nitrogen, creatinine, urine-specific gravity, thyroid-stimulating hormone (TSH), thyroxine (T_4), and a CBC (Table 80-4). Also, a pregnancy test should be obtained before starting therapy.

Table 80-4 Lithium Monitoring

	Baseline	*Weekly × 4 Weeks*	*Monthly × 3 Months*	*Quarterly*	*Yearly*	*If Symptoms Arise*
Pregnacy[a]	x					x
CBC	x					x
Electrolytes	x				x	x
Kidney (BUN/SCr)[b]	x				x	x
ECG[c]	x				x	x
Urine	x					x
Thyroid function	x				x	
Lithium level		x	x	x		x
Weight/BMI/waist size	x				x	

[a]Women of childbearing potential.
[b]More frequent monitoring for patients with preexisting kidney disease.
[c]Patients ≥45 years or with preexisting cardiac disease.
BMI, body mass index; CBC, complete blood count; ECG, electrocardiogram; SCr, serum creatinine
Reprinted with permission from: Gelenberg AJ. A concise guide to psychotropic medications: laboratory testing, patient warnings, and drug interactions, part I of II. *Biological Therapies in Psychiatry* 2006;29:37.

DOSING

10. C.N.'s baseline laboratory parameters were normal. How should lithium treatment for C.N. be initiated?

Because C.N. has previously responded to lithium and does not have rapid cycling or mixed bipolar disorder, she is likely to respond to lithium again. Although there are many strategies for calculating lithium dosage requirements, it is simplest to begin C.N. at a dosage of 300 mg two times a day. This is a common starting dose for a healthy adult patient.

Patients experiencing an acute manic episode require higher lithium levels than are required during maintenance therapy. The goal for the acute management of C.N. is a serum level between 0.5 and 1.2 mEq/L.[14] Because lithium is not immediately effective, C.N.'s lithium dosage can be adjusted based on the results of lithium serum levels checked twice weekly until the manic episode resolves. As she recovers and enters the maintenance phase of treatment, both C.N.'s lithium dosage and her lithium levels will require reevaluation (see Question 25).

11. How long will it take to get the full effect of lithium?

The half-life of lithium is approximately 24 hours; therefore, steady-state concentrations are achieved in approximately 5 days. The onset of action is slow taking as long as 1 to 2 weeks to fully exert its therapeutic effects.[14] Because of the delay in onset, it is appropriate to use an adjunctive medication to help reduce C.N.'s acute symptoms. Both benzodiazepines and antipsychotics have been used in this manner.[14] AAPs (see Chapter 78) are preferred over typical antipsychotics and have been demonstrated to enhance efficacy and accelerate time to response when used in combination with lithium.[21] Benzodiazepines reduce agitation, anxiety, and insomnia.[47]

SIDE EFFECTS

12. After 3 weeks of therapy, C.N. is demonstrating significant improvement in her sleep, impulsivity, delusions, and activity level. She has achieved her previous lithium carbonate dose of 1,200 mg/day and her lithium level is 0.8 mEq/L. However, today she is complaining to the nursing staff that she has developed a hand tremor. Soon after her physician arrives to evaluate her, she asks to be excused so that she can go to the bathroom. How might C.N.'s presentation be related to her medication?

[SI unit, lithium, 0.8 mmol/L]

When considering side effect management early in lithium therapy, it becomes important to monitor lithium levels closely. When patients start to recover from acute mania, the rate of lithium clearance may decrease and patients may demonstrate an increase in lithium levels and worsening side effects (Table 80-5). This does not seem to be the case with C.N. because her lithium level is within the accepted range for the management of acute mania.

C.N. is complaining of a hand tremor. She should be interviewed and examined to determine its origin. In this case, the likely medication-related cause for the tremor would be lithium. Lithium-induced tremor occurs in 10% to 65% of patients treated and is characteristically rapid, regular, and fine in amplitude (8–12 cycles/sec).[47,48] Often, this tremor occurs early in therapy and improves over time. Caffeine, personal or

Table 80-5 Lithium Adverse Effects

Organ System	Clinical Presentation	Comments
Cardiovascular	ECG changes	T-wave suppression, delayed or irregular rhythm, increase in PVCs; SSNS; myocarditis
	Edema	Primarily ankles and feet; transient or intermittent; secondary to effects on sodium/carbohydrate metabolism; caution about diuretics and sodium restriction to avoid lithium toxicity
Dermatologic	Acne	Worsens
	Psoriasis	Treatment-refractory worsening
	Rashes	Maculopapular and follicular
Endocrine	Hypothyroidism	About 5% goiter; about 30% clinically significant hypothyroidism; may diminish sex drive
	Hyperparathyroidism	Clinically nonsignificant
Fetus (teratogenic)	Tricuspid valve malformation, atrial septal defect	Ebstein anomaly
Gastrointestinal	Anorexia, nausea (10%–30%)	Usually early in treatment and usually transient; may be early sign of toxicity
	Diarrhea (5%–20%)	Slow-release preparations may help
Hematologic	Leukocytosis	May be useful in disorders such as Felty syndrome, iatrogenic neutropenia. May counter CBZ-induced leukopenia
Neurologic	Tremor (10%–65%)	Dose-related; men > women; worse with antidepressants/antipsychotics; reduce dose or use β-blocker
	Cognitive disruption (10%)	Worsens compliance; perceived as "mental dulling"
	Poor concentration/memory; fatigue/weakness	May be early toxicity; may mimic depression
Renal	Polyuria-polydipsia (nephrogenic diabetes insipidus)	May be an indication of morphological changes; requires adequate hydration

CBZ, carbamazepine; ECG, electrocardiogram; PVC, premature ventricular contraction; SSNS, sick sinus node syndrome.

Reprinted with permission from: Janicak PG et al. Treatment with Mood Stabilizers. In: Principles and Practice of Psychopharmacotherapy, 2nd ed. Philadelphia: Lippincott Williams & Wilkins; 2006:426.

family history of tremor, alcoholism, anxiety, antidepressants, antipsychotics, and possibly increased age enhance the risk of lithium-induced tremor.[48] The tremor is more common in patients with higher serum concentrations and may be worse at times of peak serum levels.[14] If C.N. is not bothered by the tremor and suffers no impairment, treatment is not necessary. If the tremor becomes problematic, her lithium dosage may be reduced or a β-adrenergic blocking agent can be added. Switching to a sustained-release lithium preparation may reduce peak serum levels and ameliorate tremors associated with the peak of absorption.[14] Because it is fairly early in treatment and C.N. has only a moderate lithium level, it is more reasonable to add propranolol 10 mg three times a day rather than to reduce the lithium dosage if an intervention is required. Propranolol usually is effective at dosages <160 mg/day.[48] C.N. also should be educated about her tremor and instructed to reduce her caffeine consumption.

In addition, C.N. should be asked about her trip to the bathroom during this clinic visit, because lithium may cause both diarrhea and polyuria. Polyuria and polydipsia are common, occurring in up to 60% of patients.[49] Nephrogenic diabetes insipidus is present in 12% of patients on long-term treatment.[50] With the lower serum levels of lithium commonly used today, the actual increase in urine volume may be as low as 20%; thus, a decrease in C.N.'s lithium dosage may help to reduce polyuria if this is a problem. Urine output also has been correlated with trough lithium levels.[51] Although the advantages of once-daily administration of lithium are not universally accepted, switching a stabilized patient to this schedule with its lower trough levels may help to reduce urine volume.[14] If C.N. were to fail to respond to either of these interventions, amiloride could be prescribed concurrently.[14] Amiloride seems to antagonize the effect of lithium on free water clearance by reducing the ion entry into renal epithelial cells.

If C.N.'s trip to the bathroom was because of diarrhea, lithium should be evaluated as a possible cause; up to 20% of patients started on lithium experience diarrhea, epigastric bloating, and sometimes pain early in therapy.[51] Diarrhea from lithium is associated with high serum levels, once-daily dosing, and rapidly absorbed preparations; therefore, divided doses may help to alleviate the problem. Use of lower doses and switching to sustained-release preparations are alternative strategies that could be used. Sustained-release preparations can potentially lead to lower lithium levels in patients with rapid GI motility because the product must be present in the small intestine for several hours to achieve maximal absorption. If C.N. has diarrhea or polyuria, her fluid status and lithium levels should be monitored carefully. Dehydration leads to increased lithium reabsorption in the proximal tubule and could result in accumulation to toxic levels.

13. Should C.N. be switched to a sustained-release preparation of lithium?

Sustained-release dosage forms have often been used to aid in medication adherence and reduce side effects. Although standard lithium preparations are often administered three or four times per day, many clinicians prescribe them for once- or twice-daily administration. Sustained-release lithium is usually administered once or twice daily, results in lower peak levels, and may decrease side effects associated with high peak concentrations. Both lithium-induced tremor and gastric symptoms may respond to a change to sustained-release preparations.[14] If C.N. is no longer experiencing problems with tremor or GI side effects, she should be maintained on a standard preparation of lithium carbonate.

14. What should C.N. be told regarding potential renal damage from lithium?

C.N. should be informed that lithium can cause renal side effects; however, cases of irreversible kidney damage are relatively rare and have occurred mainly when patients have preexisting renal disease, have experienced episodes of lithium intoxication, or have been poorly monitored with regard to lithium levels.[52] Communication with her physician regarding situations that increase the risk of lithium toxicity (see Question 16) and cooperation with regular lithium and renal function monitoring can vastly reduce the risk of renal disease secondary to lithium therapy. Finally, C.N. must be informed that polyuria is not related to any of the more serious renal side effects.

PATIENT EDUCATION

15. What does C.N. need to know about lithium before she is discharged?

As with all drugs, C.N. should be instructed to disclose the medications she is taking to all of her health care providers. She should be informed that dehydration, fever, vomiting, or sodium-restricted diets could lead to increases in her lithium level. Therefore, she needs to drink plenty of fluids and eat a diet consistent in the amount of sodium. C.N. should be instructed to contact her physician if she starts to experience any symptoms of lithium toxicity, including worsening tremor, slurred speech, muscle weakness or twitches, or difficulty walking.

C.N. also should be told to use caution in selecting over-the-counter medications. Specifically, she should be warned to avoid the use of preparations containing any of the nonsteroidal anti-inflammatory drugs, which can increase lithium levels.[53] C.N. should know that caffeine can sometimes be troublesome in patients taking lithium. On a short-term basis, caffeine can worsen lithium tremor; on a longer term basis, it may lower lithium levels.[53] With regard to serum lithium level monitoring, C.N. needs to know that lithium levels usually are drawn approximately 12 hours after a dose of lithium. If she is taking lithium in the evening and the morning, she should take her evening dose and then report for a blood sample to be drawn in the morning before taking her morning dose.

TOXICITY

16. One day, C.N.'s mother calls, concerned that C.N. has been complaining of nausea, vomiting, and diarrhea for several days. Over the past few hours, C.N. has become confused and has developed a coarse tremor and slurred speech. It has been 4 months since C.N.'s lithium level has been checked. The only change is that C.N. started taking ibuprofen recently for headaches. What action should be taken?

There is a strong possibility that C.N. is suffering from lithium toxicity, which can occur acutely from an overdose or insidiously if lithium excretion is reduced. *Mild toxicity* at levels <1.5 mEq/L usually includes feelings of apathy, lethargy, and muscle weakness accompanied by nausea and irritability. *Moderate toxicity* occurs between 1.5 and 2.5 mEq/L with symptoms progressing to coarse tremor, slurred speech, unsteady gait, drowsiness, confusion, muscle twitches, and blurred vision. *Severe toxicity* at levels >2.5 mEq/L can result in seizures, stupor, coma, renal failure, and cardiovascular collapse. C.N. seems to be experiencing moderate lithium toxicity. She should be taken to the emergency department immediately, where stat laboratory tests, including a lithium level, electrolytes, and renal function tests, should be ordered. Intravenous solutions should be started to ensure that C.N. is hydrated adequately, and electrolyte abnormalities should be corrected promptly. Depending on the results of physical examination and laboratory tests, cardiac monitoring should be instituted. Her ibuprofen should be discontinued.

Lithium levels must be interpreted with caution if they were drawn within 12 hours of lithium ingestion, because levels drawn sooner than 12 hours may be falsely elevated. In contrast, levels that are drawn too soon may be falsely low in individuals who have ingested large quantities of a sustained-release lithium formulation. Twelve-hour serum lithium levels >2.5 mEq/L, coma, shock, further deterioration, and failure to improve with conservative management are indications for dialysis. Although peritoneal dialysis has been instituted in cases of lithium intoxication, hemodialysis is preferred.[14]

HYPOTHYROIDISM

17. After receiving lithium at 1,200 mg/day for 1 year, C.N. returns complaining that the lithium is slowing her down. She is tired and has gained weight in recent weeks and thinks that she is becoming depressed. In the examining room, C.N. complains that the temperature is too cold. What is the most likely cause of C.N.'s complaints? What treatment should be instituted?

C.N.'s symptoms are consistent with those of hypothyroidism. Lithium affects the incorporation of iodine into thyroid hormone, interferes with secretion of thyroid hormones, and may interfere with the peripheral degradation of T_4 to T_3 (tri-iodothyronine).[54] Using laboratory indices, the incidence of hypothyroidism in lithium-free bipolar patients ranges from 6% to 11% as compared with 28% to 32% in lithium-treated patients.[55] Subclinical hypothyroidism with elevated levels of TSH may be present in an even larger number of patients taking lithium. Risk factors for developing lithium-induced hypothyroidism include female gender, family history of hypothyroidism or thyroid illness in first-degree relatives, weight gain, elevated baseline TSH, preexisting autoantibodies, an iodine-deficient diet, rapid cycling, and elevated lithium levels.[56] For women, the first 2 years of treatment may be a period of heightened risk as well for any patient starting lithium in middle age.[56]

Thyroid function tests should be ordered to evaluate C.N.'s current symptoms. If she is found to be hypothyroid, discontinuation of therapy is *not* necessary. She should receive levothyroxine in doses that normalize her thyroid function tests. Even if she has an elevated TSH with normal levels of T_3 and T_4, low-dose thyroid supplementation may help to resolve her symptoms, and prevent breakthrough depressive symptoms.[54]

DRUG AND DIETARY INTERACTIONS

18. T.J., a 35-year-old man, is hospitalized and treated with lithium for a severe manic episode. He had a stable lithium level of around 0.80 mEq/L for several weeks, but his last two levels have dropped to 0.65 and 0.61 mEq/L without any change in his drug therapy. T.J. insists that he is taking the medication as prescribed. The nursing staff believes that he is compliant with his medication but notes that he is spending more time off the ward and in the cafeteria. What factors could contribute to a decrease in T.J.'s lithium levels?

[SI units: lithium, 0.80, 0.65, and 0.61 mmol/L]

Drug interactions are a common cause of changes in lithium levels, but there have been no changes in T.J.'s regimen (Table 80-6 provides a list of clinically significant drug interactions). Changes in formulation or brand may sometimes have an impact on lithium levels. However, lithium is relatively well absorbed and has a long elimination half-life, so this usually does not result in large changes in the 12-hour postdose lithium level. Occasionally, patients switched from lithium citrate to solid dosage forms experience small changes in lithium levels.

T.J. should be questioned regarding his visits to the cafeteria because diet can have a major influence on lithium excretion. If T.J. is consuming large amounts of caffeinated beverages or salty snacks, a reduction in lithium levels could occur. Increases in dietary sodium intake and the ingestion of methylxanthines (e.g., caffeine, theophylline) can increase lithium clearance.[53]

Finally, acute mania can increase lithium clearance.[57] If T.J. was showing signs of a relapse, his decrease in lithium levels might be attributable to his return to a manic state.

LITHIUM IN PREGNANCY

19. A.J., a 36-year-old woman, has been maintained successfully on lithium therapy for 5 years for bipolar disorder. She asks whether she should stay on lithium because she plans to become pregnant in the near future.

Lithium has been associated with a variety of congenital malformations, including the rare cardiac malformation, Ebstein anomaly.[58] There is considerable disagreement about the importance of lithium as a teratogen. Lithium was originally thought to increase the risk of the Ebstein anomaly 400 times; however, the risk is more likely 20 to 40 times higher than in the general population.[59] The estimated overall risk for congenital malformations is approximately 4% to 12% compared with 2% to 4% in controls.[60] Still, lithium is a pregnancy category D drug because of evidence of the risk to the human fetus. Because malformations of this type are most likely to occur in the first trimester of pregnancy, it is advisable for patients to discontinue lithium therapy, when possible, during the first trimester.

In addition to cardiac malformations, infants exposed to lithium have been reported to develop hypotonia, nephrogenic diabetes insipidus, and thyroid abnormalities.[58] Lithium administration during pregnancy increases the risk of premature delivery by a factor of two to three.[61] Unfortunately, the relative safety of other psychotropics commonly used in bipolar disorder is either not ideal or is unknown. Valproate and CBZ are categorized as FDA category D during pregnancy and the general consensus is that these medications are genuine teratogens and should be avoided.[62] Lamotrigine has not been

Table 80-6 Lithium Drug Interactions of Clinical Significance

Drug	Interaction
Drugs That May Increase Lithium Levels	
NSAIDs	Many NSAIDs have been reported to increase lithium levels as much as 50%–60%. This probably is due to an enhanced reabsorption of sodium and lithium secondary to inhibition of prostaglandin synthesis.
Diuretics	All diuretics can contribute to sodium depletion. Sodium depletion can result in an increased proximal tubular reabsorption of sodium and lithium. Thiazidelike diuretics cause the greatest increase in lithium levels, whereas loop diuretics and potassium-sparing diuretics seem to be somewhat safer.
ACE inhibitors	ACE inhibitors and lithium both result in volume depletion and a reduction in glomerular filtration rate. This results in reduced lithium excretion.
Drugs That May Decrease Lithium Levels	
Theophylline, caffeine	Theophylline and caffeine may increase renal clearance of lithium and result in a decrease in levels in the range of 20%.
Acetazolamide	Acetazolamide may impair proximal tubular reabsorption of lithium ions.
Sodium	High dietary sodium intake promotes the renal clearance of lithium.
Drugs That Increase Lithium Toxicity	
Methyldopa	Cases of sedation, dysphoria, and confusion owing to the combined use of lithium and methyldopa have been reported.
Carbamazepine	Cases of neurotoxicity involving the combined use of lithium and carbamazepine have been reported in patients with normal lithium levels.
Calcium channel antagonists	Cases of neurotoxicity involving the combined use of lithium and the calcium channel blockers verapamil and diltiazem have been reported. Lithium does interfere with calcium transport across cells.
Antipsychotics	Cases of neurotoxicity (encephalopathic syndrome, extrapyramidal effects, cerebellar effect, EEG abnormalities) have been reported due to the combined use of lithium and various antipsychotics. The interaction may be related to increase in phenothiazine levels, changes in tissue uptake of lithium, and/or dopamine-blocking effects of lithium. Studies attempting to demonstrate this effect have yielded differing results.
Serotonin-selective reuptake inhibitors	Fluvoxamine and fluoxetine have been reported to result in toxicity when added to lithium. Sertraline has been reported to cause nausea and tremor in lithium recipients.

ACE, angiotensin-converting enzyme; EEG, electroencephalogram; NSAIDs, nonsteroidal anti-inflammatory drugs.

associated with fetal anomalies thus far in available surveys but the data is best regarded as preliminary at the present time. Typical antipsychotics are classified as pregnancy category C, suggesting that adverse morphologic outcomes are less likely to occur (in comparison with mood stabilizers), although this is not necessarily predictive. Data on AAPs are also preliminary, but it is worth noting that, in a recent comparison of placental passage, olanzapine was associated with the highest exposure (72% ratio of umbilical cord-to-maternal plasma concentrations), followed by haloperidol (65%), risperidone (49%), and quetiapine (24%).[63] Olanzapine was also associated with the highest rates of low birth weight and neonatal intensive care unit admissions. For additional information on the safety of psychotropic medications see Chapters 54, 76, 78, and 79.

A.J. and her physician should discuss her individual risks related to lithium treatment. In addition to the risks of teratogenicity, they must consider the harm that could result from the possible recurrence of episodes of mania or depression and the risks inherent in discontinuing lithium or switching to another antimanic agent. Also, A.J. should be actively involved in the decision-making process.

If A.J. and her physician decide that she is to remain on lithium, her levels must be monitored closely during pregnancy and her dosage adjusted periodically. Lithium clearance increases during the third trimester by 30% to 50%, resulting in a reduction in lithium levels and a need for dosage adjustment.[59] Approximately 16 to 18 weeks after conception, screening tests, high-resolution ultrasound, and fetal echocardiography can be used to determine whether cardiac defects have developed.[59] If possible, A.J.'s physician should consider decreasing the lithium dose before delivery to minimize lithium levels in the newborn and to offset the reduction in lithium excretion that occurs after delivery.[59]

If A.J. and her physician decide that she is to discontinue lithium, they must be prepared to deal with the risks of lithium discontinuation. Several cases of what are thought to be rebound manic episodes have resulted from the abrupt cessation of lithium therapy. If lithium is to be discontinued in A.J., it should be gradually reduced over 4 weeks.

20. A.J. did not use lithium throughout her pregnancy. After delivery, A.J. and her physician decide to restart lithium. How soon can this take place?

Lithium can be restarted as soon as A.J.'s urine output is established and she is fully hydrated. However, this decision also may be affected by whether or not A.J. chooses to breastfeed her child because lithium passes into breast milk and is present in concentrations up to 72% of that found in the maternal blood.[58] Risks to the newborn include hypothyroidism, cyanosis, hypotonia, lethargy, and cardiac dysrhythmias. Hydration status must be closely monitored because lithium toxicity may develop during infantile illnesses. Thus, A.J. and her physician must discuss the advantages of breast-feeding versus the risks of exposing the newborn to lithium or withholding lithium during the postpartum period. A.J. should be informed that approximately 40% to 70% of bipolar women experience affective episodes after delivery.[58]

If A.J. chooses to breast-feed while taking lithium, she should consider using infant formula when the child becomes ill because febrile illness, vomiting, and diarrhea can increase the risk of lithium toxicity. She also should be instructed to contact her pediatrician if the infant experiences diarrhea, vomiting, hypotonia, poor sucking, muscle twitches, restlessness, or other unexplained changes in behavior or status.

Atypical Antipsychotics

21. D.W., a 34-year-old female singer and musician, recently experienced her fourth hospital admission for a manic episode. She also suffers from psoriasis and asthma. A trial of lithium led to worsening of her psoriasis and unacceptable tremor, which interfered with her guitar playing. Use of β-blockers was not considered because of her asthma. She was subsequently switched to valproate monotherapy. However, tremor has again become problematic. Furthermore, she is concerned about her appearance because she has begun to experience weight gain and hair loss from the valproate. What other drugs are available for the treatment of acute mania?

AAPs are acceptable first-line choices for the treatment of acute mania (Table 80-3) and aripiprazole, olanzapine, quetiapine, risperidone, and ziprasidone are FDA approved for this indication (Table 80-7). Three recent systematic reviews and meta-analyses support the efficacy of AAPs as a class.[64–66] Perlis et al.[64] reviewed data from 12 randomized, placebo-controlled, monotherapy studies and 6 adjunctive studies finding a collective response rate of 53% for AAPs compared with 30% for placebo. There was no difference in response between the individual AAPs. In adjunctive studies, the mean odds ratio was 2.4 for a 50% improvement with the addition of an AAP to a mood stabilizer (primarily lithium or valproate). Scherk et al.[65] conducted a meta-analysis of 24 randomized controlled trials and found superiority of AAPs for acute mania in comparison to placebo and equal efficacy to lithium, valproate, and the typical antipsychotic haloperidol. In this analysis, the addition of an AAP to lithium, valproate, or CBZ was found to be more effective in reducing manic symptoms and lead to less treatment discontinuation than lithium or the anticonvulsant alone. The results of a different meta-analysis specifically designed to evaluate combination treatment of AAPs with lithium or an anticonvulsant also found greater efficacy for the combined regimen.[66] In most combination therapy studies, AAPs were limited to patients having no response or only a partial response to lithium or an anticonvulsant. Thus, the utility of drug combinations as initial therapy cannot be addressed.

Table 80-7 FDA-Approved Medications for Bipolar Disorder

Drug	*Mania*	*Mixed*	*Depression*	*Maintenance*
Carbamazepine (extended-release capsule)	X	X		
Lamotrigine				X
Lithium	X			X
Valproate (divalproex sodium)	X	X		
Aripiprazole	X	X		X
Olanzapine	X	X		X
Olanzapine/fluoxetine			X	
Quetiapine	X		X	
Risperidone	X	X		
Ziprasidone	X	X		

Although the AAPs seem to be equally effective for the treatment of acute mania, these agents differ in their adverse effect profiles. A significant concern regarding the use of AAPs is the risk of metabolic complications, including weight gain, glucose dysregulation, and dyslipidemia. Clozapine and olanzapine have the highest risk for metabolic complications, quetiapine and risperidone are associated with an intermediate risk, and ziprasidone and aripiprazole seem to have the lowest risk.[25,21] Clozapine is also associated with significant safety concerns, including agranulocytosis, seizures, sialorrhea, anticholinergic side effects, and orthostasis. The requirement for frequent monitoring of WBC count is also a deterrent to its use. Efficacy data with clozapine are limited compared with the other AAPs, but clozapine seems to be effective in treatment-resistant mania and in long-term mood stabilization.[67–69]

Sedation is common with clozapine, olanzapine, and quetiapine and this effect may be beneficial in the treatment of acute mania. However, sedation can also lead to nonadherence with long-term use.[70] Aripiprazole and ziprasidone are less sedating, and the adjunctive use of a benzodiazepine is often necessary in the acute management of mania. The use of adjunctive benzodiazepines may also benefit treatment emergent akathisia, which occurs in 11% to 18% of patients treated with aripiprazole.[71,72] Ziprasidone may cause activation; however, this effect is attenuated at doses of 120 mg/day or more. Results of the Clinical Antipsychotic Trials of Intervention Effectiveness study in schizophrenia suggest that risperidone may overall be the best tolerated of the AAPs; however, this drug carries a higher risk for serum prolactin elevation and extrapyramidal symptoms.[73]

D.W.'s concern over her weight gain makes aripiprazole or ziprasidone rational choices for her manic episode. Aripiprazole should be started at 30 mg/day with the option to decrease the dose to 15 mg/day. If ziprasidone is selected, it should be started at 40 mg BID with food and increased to 60 to 80 mg BID with food on the second day of therapy. In addition to symptom response, D.W. should be monitored for metabolic complications of AAP therapy. If D.W. fails to respond to the initially selected AAP, a switch to a different AAP may prove beneficial given the variability in individual response.[21] Table 80-8 provides dosing information for AAPs in acute mania.

22. What alternative agents are available for acute mania if lithium, valproate, or an AAP fail?

Alternative and Adjunctive Therapies

ANTICONVULSANTS

CBZ represents an alternative treatment for the management of acute mania when lithium, valproate and AAPs fail.[14,21,23,24]

Table 80-8 Atypical Antipsychotic Dosing in Acute Mania

Atypical Antipsychotic	Initial Dose	Titration	Effective Dose Range
Aripiprazole	30 mg/day	Not required	15–30 mg/day
Olanzapine	10–15 mg/day	5 mg/day	5–20 mg/day
Quetiapine	50 mg BID	50 mg BID	200–400 mg BID
Risperidone	2–3 mg/day	1 mg/day	1–6 mg/day
Ziprasidone	40 mg BID	20–40 mg BID	40–80 mg BID

Adapted from: Bristol Myers Squib. Abilify package insert. Princeton, NJ: 2006 Nov. Eli Lilly and Company. Zyprexa package insert. Indianapolis, IN: 2006 Nov. Astra Zeneca Pharmaceuticals. Seroquel package insert. Wilmington, DE: 2007 May. Janssen, L.P. Risperdal package insert. Titusville, NJ: 2007 Feb. Pfizer. Geodon package insert. NY, NY: 2007 March.

Initial interest with CBZ in affective disorders dates back to the early 1970s with expanding clinical use in the 1980s.[74] In 2005, the FDA approved the extended-release CBZ capsule for the treatment of acute manic and mixed episodes based on the results of two double-blind, randomized, placebo-controlled trials.[74] To enhance power, a pooled analysis of these two studies has been conducted.[75] The primary endpoint, reduction in manic symptoms, was superior to placebo at days 7, 14, and 21 with a mean decrease in the Young Mania Rating Scale (YMRS) of 12 points compared with a 6-point reduction with placebo. The response rates at study endpoint were 52% for CBZ-treated patients and 26% for placebo-treated patients. Significant reductions in the YMRS were achieved in both manic and mixed episodes. The mean final dose of extended release CBZ was 707 mg/day.

CBZ should be started at 100 to 200 mg twice daily. The dose should be increased by 200 mg every 3 to 4 days until adequate serum levels have been reached.[14] Although no correlation between CBZ serum levels and response in bipolar disorder has been established, serum levels >12 mcg/mL are associated with sedation and ataxia. The recommended target serum level is from 4 to 12 mcg/mL.[14] Average daily doses for maintenance therapy range from 200 to 1,600 mg/day.

Adverse effects occur in up to 50% of patients receiving CBZ.[14] Neurologic adverse effects, including ataxia, blurred vision, diplopia, and fatigue, are most frequently reported. CBZ can cause adverse hematologic effects, including transient leukopenia, and more rarely, agranulocytosis, thrombocytopenia, and aplastic anemia. CBZ therapy may also cause hyponatremia, skin rashes, elevation of liver enzymes, weight gain, and GI complaints. Women of child-bearing potential should be tested for pregnancy because CBZ is classified as pregnancy category D and has the potential to cause teratogenic effects, especially neural tube defects.

Before receiving CBZ, patients should undergo baseline laboratory testing, including a CBC with differential and platelets, and liver function tests. Subsequent hematologic and liver function monitoring should be occur every 2 weeks during the first 2 months of treatment and every 3 months thereafter (see Chapter 54).[14] During therapy, patients should be monitored for abnormal bleeding or petechiae, skin rashes, signs and symptoms of infection, and signs of hyponatremia such as mental status changes.

CBZ can induce the metabolism and, thereby, reduce the effect of a number of drugs, including oral contraceptives, warfarin, theophylline, haloperidol, lamotrigine, and TCAs. The concurrent use of erythromycin, cimetidine, fluoxetine, or calcium channel blockers may lead to increased levels of CBZ and unanticipated toxicity (see Chapter 54). CBZ has a complex pharmacokinetic interaction with valproate. CBZ can increase the metabolism of valproate, resulting in reduced serum concentrations and efficacy. Conversely, valproate may inhibit the metabolism of CBZ, leading to increased serum concentrations and adverse effects. The combination of CBZ and lithium may increase the risk of neurotoxicity, particularly in patients with preexisting neurologic diseases. Therefore, the combination should be avoided in these patients. CBZ also has the ability to induce its own metabolism. This autoinduction effect may cause CBZ levels to decrease for up to 1 month after a dose adjustment is made; thus, dose increases may be needed to maintain a therapeutic effect.

Oxcarbazepine, a structural analog of CBZ, may be an option for the treatment of bipolar disorder. Oxcarbazepine has some advantages over CBZ, including improved tolerability and fewer drug interactions. However, there is a paucity of well-designed clinical trials of oxcarbazepine in bipolar disorder.[76] Case reports, retrospective chart reviews, open-label trials, and small double-blind studies have found oxcarbazepine monotherapy or adjunctive treatment to be effective in acute mania.[76] The only study of oxcarbazepine in bipolar disorder with adequate statistical power to detect an effect did not report a significant difference between placebo and oxcarbazepine for the primary endpoint (mean reduction in YMRS). This study included 116 children and adolescents (the majority of patients were between ages 7 and 12 years old) with a manic or mixed episode.[77]

Other anticonvulsants studied in mania include lamotrigine, gabapentin, topiramate, tiagabine, zonisamide, and levetiracetam. Initial open-label studies of lamotrigine in mania were promising, and there is one published double-blind trial to date that showed a similar response between lamotrigine, lithium, and olanzapine.[78,79] However, there are two unpublished trials of lamotrigine in mania, both of which are negative.[78] Currently, experts doubt that lamotrigine has any significant effect in acute bipolar mania.

Another anticonvulsant, gabapentin, has been studied in bipolar disorder. Open trials and case reports suggested that adjunctive treatment with gabapentin was effective in manic, hypomanic, and depressive states of bipolar disorder.[80–82] A more recent controlled trial found no benefit of gabapentin.[83] In this double-blind, placebo-controlled trial, gabapentin dosed flexibly between 900 and 3,600 mg/day was administered as an adjunct to lithium, valproate, or lithium plus valproate in patients with bipolar I disorder whose current episode was manic, hypomanic, or mixed. At 12 weeks, gabapentin failed to show any significant benefit over placebo. In fact, the placebo group did significantly better than the gabapentin-treated patients.

Topiramate was also originally suspected to have antimanic effects based largely on open add-on studies.[84] However, in four double-blind, placebo-controlled trials, topiramate did not separate from placebo and was less effective than lithium in the treatment of acute mania.[85] Tiagabine has not been evaluated in randomized, controlled trials in the treatment of bipolar disorder. In the two open trials conducted, no benefit on manic or hypomanic symptoms was demonstrated and some patients experienced serious side effects such as seizures.[86,87] Two separate, open-label adjunctive trials with levetiracetam and zonisamide in treatment-resistant bipolar patients have shown reductions in manic symptoms; however, these studies included patients in a variety of bipolar mood states (depression, mania, cycling, euthymia), not just acute mania.[88,89] Caution is warranted; zonisamide was discontinued in 32% of patients for worsening mood symptoms. Also, 7 out of 16 levetiracetam-treated patients with manic symptoms dropped out and 6 of the remaining patients developed an exacerbation of manic symptoms.

Despite the array of treatments available for the management of acute mania, large numbers of patients fail to respond to monotherapy, and combination therapy is becoming increasingly common.[90] Potentially useful combinations include lithium plus AAPs, valproate plus AAPs, and lithium plus valproate.[22,23] A combination to be avoided is CBZ and clozapine owing to the increased risk of hematologic adverse effects.

Benzodiazepines and Antipsychotics for Acute Agitation

23. M.B. is a 39-year-old man hospitalized for an acute manic episode but refusing all medications, reporting "I will be robbed of my superpowers." He is found pacing around the inpatient unit shouting orders for his release. When asked to return to his room by the nursing staff, he becomes agitated, picks up a chair, and begins swinging it wildly at anyone who approaches him. In the past M.B. developed an acute dystonic reaction to haloperidol. M.B. has a medical history of diabetes mellitus and hypertension. What is an appropriate pharmacologic intervention for M.B.?

Benzodiazepines and antipsychotics are useful in treating agitation, irritability, and hyperactivity associated with acute manic episodes. Oral formulations are preferred and are favored by patients in psychiatric emergencies.[91] Oral dose delivery can be facilitated with liquid concentrates and orally disintegrating tablets. Uncooperative patients may require intramuscular (IM) injections of benzodiazepines or antipsychotics.[92] Traditionally, the combination of IM haloperidol and IM lorazepam has been used; however, the rapid-acting IM AAPs are becoming increasingly popular with improved tolerability over typical antipsychotics. Currently, ziprasidone, aripiprazole, and olanzapine are available in rapid-acting IM dosage forms. IM ziprasidone at doses of 10 and 20 mg is effective in psychotic agitation.[93,94] IM aripiprazole is effective at doses of 9.75 and 15 mg for manic or mixed-state agitation (however, oversedation is more common with a 15-mg dose).[95] Olanzapine 10 mg IM is effective for manic or mixed-state agitation.[96] Repeat doses of IM ziprasidone, aripiprazole, and olanzapine can be administered 2 to 4 hours after the first dose, if needed. The concurrent use of a benzodiazepine with an antipsychotic is generally safe and potentially more effective than either agent alone; however, IM olanzapine should not be used with benzodiazepines owing to concern regarding excessive sedation and cardiorespiratory depression.[97,98]

Lorazepam is the preferred benzodiazepine for acute manic agitation. Benefits of lorazepam include availability of both IM and oral formulations (tablet and concentrate), lack of active metabolites, and safety in hepatic and renal impairment. The Expert Consensus Guideline recommends dosing lorazepam at 1 to 3 mg orally or 0.5 mg to 3 mg IM, with repeated doses at least 60 minutes apart and a maximum dose of 10 to 12 mg in the first 24 hours.[99] The primary concerns regarding the use of benzodiazepines for agitated mania are sedation and potential for abuse and addiction. Because adjunctive therapy with benzodiazepines is usually administered on an inpatient basis for a short time period, abuse and addiction are unlikely to be important considerations.

M.B. is uncooperative and an immediate danger to others, thus warranting IM administration. Because of M.B.'s history of acute dystonia to haloperidol, an IM AAP (such as olanzapine, ziprasdone, or aripiprazole) should be used. The combination of ziprasidone 10 mg IM and lorazepam 2 mg IM is an appropriate intervention. IM administration of aripiprazole and lorazepam may also be used. As M.B. becomes calmer and more receptive to treatment, he should be transitioned to oral therapy. Adjunctive benzodiazepine treatment may be necessary during M.B.'s hospitalization to control his manic symptoms.

TREATMENT OF ACUTE BIPOLAR DEPRESSION

24. H.C., a 31-year-old woman, was hospitalized for treatment of an acute manic episode 3 months ago. She was discharged on valproate 1,750 mg/day with a favorable response. Recently, her parents have become concerned because H.C. has been in bed most of the day for the last 2 weeks. When out of bed, H.C. sits on the couch without moving for hours. She only nibbles at the food her parents offer her. She has no other signs or symptoms of physical illness and has not taken any additional medications, alcohol, or drugs of abuse to her parents' knowledge. On further questioning, they admit that she is intermittently tearful and expresses remorse for her behavior when she was manic. They also quote her as saying that she is "as low as I can go and I just want to die." They suspect she is suicidal. H.C.'s parents report that she is taking valproate as prescribed and that the last time she was this depressed lithium did not seem to help even in combination with valproate. Her valproate level on discharge was 80 mcg/mL. What change in H.C.'s treatment should be instituted at this time?

Lithium

Acute bipolar depression is a recurring and chronic problem for many patients. The depression is often difficult to control and puts patients at significant risk for suicide. Until recently, little attention was paid to bipolar depression and few data are available regarding the best treatment options for these patients. Remission of depressive symptoms should be the primary goal for bipolar depression. Ideal treatment for bipolar depression should target acute depressive symptoms, decrease suicide risk, prevent future mood episodes (both manic and depressive), and not precipitate mania or mood cycling.[100] A logical first step in the management of bipolar depression is to optimize the dose of the current mood stabilizer.[21] Although most studies of lithium for acute bipolar depression are nearly two decades old, this agent remains one of the drugs of choice.[14] Seven of eight placebo-controlled cross-over studies demonstrated the benefit of lithium in bipolar depression with a mean response rate of 76%.[100] Higher serum lithium concentrations ($\geq$0.8 mEq/L) may be required and are associated with antidepressant activity in bipolar depression.[101]

Lamotrigine

Lamotrigine is considered a first-line agent for bipolar depression by all North American guidelines.[14,21–24] A double-blind, placebo-controlled trial of lamotrigine monotherapy in bipolar depression found that 51% of patients receiving lamotrigine 200 mg/day met criteria for response on the Hamilton Rating Scale for Depression (HAM-D), compared with 45% of those treated with lamotrigine 50 mg/day, and 37% of placebo-treated patients.[102] The difference in response rates among the three groups did not reach statistical significance. However, a significant difference between both treatment groups and placebo was noted on the Montgomery-Asberg Depression Rating Scale (MADRS). A cross-over study of lamotrigine, gabapentin, and placebo reported response rates of 45%, 26%, and 19%, respectively.[103] Lamotrogine was recently compared with OFC in a large 7-week trial of bipolar I depression.[104] Improvement from baseline on the Clinical Global Impressions-Severity of Illness Scale was significantly greater with OFC (−1.85) than for lamotrigine (−1.62), the response and remission rates did not differ between groups. Also, patients receiving lamotrigine did not achieve the 200 mg/day target dose until week 5 (leaving only 2 weeks of study treatment at the target dose). Patients treated with OFC experienced more adverse effects than those treated with lamotrigine.

Because H.C. did not respond to lithium in combination with valproate during her past depressive episode, lamotrigine is a reasonable alternative treatment for the current episode. Lamotrigine metabolism is affected by the concomitant use of enzyme-inducing (e.g., CBZ) and enzyme-inhibiting drugs (e.g., valproate). Thus, the initial dose and titration schedule for lamotrigine must be adjusted for patients taking these and other interacting drugs. For patients receiving no enzyme inducers or inhibitors, the initial dose is 25 mg/day for weeks 1 and 2, followed by 50 mg/day for weeks 3 and 4, 100 mg/day for week 5, and then increased to 200 mg/day at the beginning of week 6. Patients receiving enzyme inducers should begin lamotrigine treatment with 50 mg/day for weeks 1 and 2, then 100 mg/day in divided doses for weeks 3 and 4. Thereafter, the dose can be increased by 100 mg/day each week to a target dose of 400 mg/day in divided doses (usually BID). In this case H.C. is taking valproate, which is known to inhibit the metabolism of lamotrigine. Therefore, the initial dose for H.C. is 25 mg every other day for weeks 1 and 2 followed by an increase to 25 mg/day for weeks 3 and 4. The dose can be increased to 50 mg/day for week 5, and then increased to the maximum recommended dose of 100 mg/day beginning at week 6. For some patients, doses higher than the target dose may be useful. Dizziness, headache, ataxia, sedation, blurred vision, and GI disturbances are the most common side effects. Lamotrigine may cause a skin rash, especially when dosages are increased quickly and in patients receiving concomitant valproate. Lamotrigine-induced rash may progress to the life-threatening Stevens-Johnson syndrome. H.C. should be instructed to contact her physician immediately at the first sign of a skin rash.

Atypical Antipsychotics

AAPs offer another option for the treatment of bipolar depression. Quetiapine has been studied in two identical, double-blind, placebo-controlled studies for patients with bipolar I or II depression. In both studies, patient were randomized to quetiapine 300 or 600 mg/day, or placebo for 8 weeks. The primary efficacy outcome was mean reduction in MADRS from baseline to week 8. The first study (BOLDER I) randomized 542 patients.[105] The mean change in MADRS from baseline to study endpoint was similar in the 300 and 600 mg/day treatment groups and both were superior to placebo. Discontinuation due to adverse effects was most common in the 600 mg/day group. The second study (BOLDER II) randomized 509 patients.[106] In both active treatment groups, the reduction in MADRS was again superior to placebo. Discontinuation owing to adverse effects (most commonly dry mouth, sedation, somnolence, dizziness) was most common in the 600 mg/day group. Based on these two studies, the target dose of quetiapine for bipolar depression should be 300 mg/day.

Olanzapine and olanzapine–fluoxetine combination have been studied in patients with bipolar I depression. In the first published study, patients were randomized to olanzapine ($n = 370$), placebo ($n = 377$), or olanzapine–fluoxetine combination ($n = 86$).[107] The 4:4:1 ratio of treatment allocation was explained by the authors: "the primary objective of this 8-week, randomized, double-blind, parallel study was to compare the efficacy and safety of olanzapine monotherapy and placebo in the treatment of bipolar I disorder, depressed. An olanzapine–fluoxetine combination treatment arm was also included concurrently for exploratory purposes." Thus, the primary objective was to compare olanzapine with placebo in bipolar depression. Both the olanzapine and the olanzapine–fluoxetine combination groups had greater improvement in MADRS than placebo throughout the study. This benefit was evident as early as week 1 of the study. Additionally, the olanzapine–fluoxetine combination was superior to treatment with olanzapine alone from weeks 4 through 8. As mentioned, olanzapine–fluoxetine combination therapy was statistically superior to lamotrigine in bipolar depression; however, the clinical significance of this difference remains to be established.[104] A prominent concern with the use of olanzapine–fluoxetine combination or quetiapine is the substantial risk of metabolic complications. Because of these risks, quetiapine and olanzapine–fluoxetine combination are reserved for second-line use in bipolar depression, despite being the only FDA-approved drugs for this indication.[21]

Antidepressants

Antidepressant use in bipolar depression is controversial and current guidelines suggest that they should be used only when other preferred treatments such as lithium, lamotrigine, quetiapine, or olanzapine–fluoxetine combination have failed (either alone or in combination).[21] Antidepressant monotherapy should be avoided in bipolar disorder at all times.[14,21] However, there is conflicting evidence regarding the protective role of antimanic agents against the development of mania triggered by antidepressants.[26,108–110] The largest controlled trial of antidepressant augmentation in bipolar depression was conducted as part of the Systematic Treatment Enhancement Program for Bipolar Disorder (STEP-BD) study. This study was a 26-week, double-blind, placebo-controlled trial comparing antidepressants (bupropion or paroxetine) with placebo as adjunctive treatment to a mood stabilizer (any FDA-approved antimanic agent).[111] The primary endpoint of durable recovery (euthymia for 8 weeks) was achieved in 24% of antidepressant treated subjects compared with 27% of subjects receiving placebo. There was no significant difference between groups in treatment emergent mood switch. These findings suggest that there is no advantage of adjunctive treatment with an antidepressant in patients with bipolar depression receiving a FDA-approved antimanic agent.

MAINTENANCE THERAPY OF BIPOLAR DISORDER

25. R.L., a 33-year-old man, has been treated for an episode of acute mania with lithium 600 mg BID for 3 weeks. He is no longer overtly manic. However, because R.L. may have had past episodes of depression and mania, his physician decides to institute prophylactic (maintenance) lithium therapy. What are the goals of maintenance lithium therapy for R.L.? How should he be monitored during this maintenance phase? How long should R.L. be maintained on lithium?

Lithium

Appropriate goals for maintenance therapy include an increase in the interval between episodes, a decrease in the frequency of episodes, and a reduction in the duration and severity of single episodes. Maintenance therapy with lithium clearly reduces the frequency and severity of mood episodes in patients with bipolar disorder. Goodwin and Jamison[112] have shown that in patients receiving maintenance lithium, only 34% relapsed, compared with 81% of patients receiving placebo. However, some studies indicate that lithium's effectiveness may be much lower. Naturalistic studies that followed patients on maintenance lithium indicate an episodic recurrence rate of 43% to 55%.[113,114] It is possible that these studies failed to identify patients with rapid cycling disorder who may have done poorly on lithium. Beyond preventing mood relapses, lithium therapy may have the added benefit of reducing mortality from suicide.[115] Conflicting results have been published recently regarding lithium's effectiveness for prevention of any mood episode in patients with bipolar I disorder.[116,117]

Target levels for maintenance therapy with lithium should be in the range of 0.5 to 0.8 mEq/L.[14] However, one study found that patients with lithium levels ranging from 0.4 to 0.6 mEq/L had relapse rates 2.6 times higher than patients with levels ranging from 0.8 to 1.0 mEq/L. Although these higher levels reduced the number of relapses, they also resulted in a higher incidence of side effects.[118]

In addition to determining appropriate maintenance lithium levels for R.L., it is appropriate to consider whether once-daily administration of lithium can improve adherence or side effects. During periods of dosage readjustment, R.L. will require monitoring of his lithium serum level more frequently. Once stabilized, the monitoring frequency can be reduced to quarterly. See Table 80-4 for recommended lithium monitoring parameters.

The decision to institute maintenance lithium therapy usually is made because of the severity of affective episodes and the belief that they will recur in the future. A period of successful maintenance therapy means that the individual is controlled, not cured, because most patients who are withdrawn from lithium eventually relapse. With each recurrent manic episode, the risk of experiencing subsequent and more frequent manic episodes increases. Furthermore, as individuals experience successive episodes, they tend to recover less completely and function at a diminished level between occurrences.[112] Because the goal is to prevent the trauma of repeated episodes and the deterioration that may accompany them, R.L. may require lithium for the remainder of his life.

Lithium Refractoriness

26. P.B. is a 42-year-old woman with five previous hospitalizations for manic and/or depressive episodes. She has experienced approximately six severe mood swings in the past year, including episodes of depression and hypomania. Despite adequate plasma levels, she has not responded to a regimen that includes lithium and paroxetine. She now presents as depressed, with expressions of suicidal hopelessness about her condition, sleep disturbances, and poor appetite. Why is P.B. failing to respond to lithium?

There are several potential reasons for P.B.'s poor response. Poor adherence always must be considered as a potential reason for lithium failure; however, P.B. has an adequate level of lithium. If P.B. had been intermittently compliant in the past or if her therapy had been stopped, she might have developed a syndrome called *lithium discontinuation–induced refractoriness*. This phenomenon occurs in patients who once responded to lithium and then had their lithium discontinued. When an affective episode recurs, they fail to fully respond to lithium reintroduction. However, there is conflicting evidence regarding lithium refractoriness, and it is unclear how often this phenomenon occurs.[119,120] If P.B. had been having more and more breakthrough affective episodes gradually, she simply could have become tolerant to lithium. Thus, a careful review of P.B.'s history of adherence and the pattern of her affective episodes is necessary.

P.B. has another potential reason for nonresponse. She has had at least six affective episodes in the past year. Therefore, she meets criteria for rapid cycling. Approximately 70% to 80% of rapid cyclers have a poor response to lithium.[14] P.B.'s trough lithium level should be assessed to ensure that it exceeds the lower limit of the usual therapeutic range. Potential causes of rapid cycling such as the paroxetine should be discontinued. Medical etiologies (e.g., hypothyroidism) and substance abuse should also be evaluated. The addition of valproate or lamotrigine may be warranted.[14]

27. What other maintenance treatments for bipolar disorder are available?

Anticonvulsants

Because of the side effects of lithium, many patients become intolerant or unwilling to continue lithium therapy. Valproate and lamotrigine are reasonable alternatives that have shown efficacy in bipolar maintenance therapy. The first controlled trial of valproate in the maintenance treatment of bipolar disorder randomized 372 patients with a recent manic episode to valproate, lithium, or placebo.[117] Patients were followed for 52 weeks. The primary outcome of time to any mood episode did not differ between groups. However a lower percentage of patients discontinued treatment for any reason in the valproate group (62%) than lithium (76%) or placebo (75%) and patients on valproate remained in the study longer (198 days) than patients on lithium (152 days) but not placebo (165 days). The mean valproate serum concentration was 85 mcg/mL.

Lamotrigine has been studied rigorously in the maintenance treatment of bipolar I disorder. A pooled analysis of two placebo-controlled studies involving 638 patients found that lamotrigine and lithium more than doubled the time to intervention (e.g., addition of pharmacotherapy or ECT) for any mood episode compared with placebo.[121] The time to intervention was 197 days for lamotrigine, 187 days for lithium, and 86 days for placebo. Interestingly, lamotrigine was also superior to placebo in delaying the time to an intervention for a depressive episode, making it an attractive agent for patients with frequent depressive relapses.

Limited evidence supports the role of CBZ in the maintenance treatment of bipolar disorder. In a 2-year study of 94 patients randomized to lithium or CBZ, more patients had a mood relapse on CBZ (42%) than lithium (27%).[122] Mean drug blood levels were within the predefined range for both CBZ (6.8 mcg/mL) and lithium (0.75 mmol/L). Another study compared CBZ and lithium as prophylactic therapies for patients with bipolar I disorder ($n = 114$), bipolar II disorder, or bipolar disorder NOS ($n = 57$).[123] For bipolar I patients, CBZ failed more often than lithium with regard to all criteria (hospitalization, recurrence, concomitant medication, side effects, and subclinical recurrence). In contrast, the failure rate for lithium and CBZ in bipolar II or bipolar NOS was dependent on the failure criterion used. The authors summarize that CBZ was equally as effective as lithium in this population. In a separate analysis, patients were stratified into classical (bipolar I disorder without mood incongruent delusions or comorbidity; $n = 67$) and nonclassical (all other patients; $n = 104$) bipolar subtypes. The rate of hospitalization was significantly lower for lithium than for CBZ (26% vs. 62%, respectively) in the subgroup of patients with classical bipolar disorder. No significant difference was found in the subgroup of patients with nonclassical bipolar disorder subtype.

Atypical Antipsychotics

AAPs have become increasingly popular alternatives and adjunctive treatments for maintenance therapy of bipolar disorder. To date aripiprazole and olanzapine have received FDA approval for the maintenance treatment of bipolar disorder; however, the mood-stabilizing properties of the AAPs may be shared among all agents in the class. A 26-week, double-blind, placebo-controlled relapse prevention study of aripiprazole was conducted in 161 patients with a recent manic or mixed episode.[124] After patients met stabilization criteria (YMRS $\leq$10 and MADRS $\leq$13) during an aripiprazole open-label phase they were randomized to aripirazole (mean, 24 mg/day) or placebo. On the primary outcome of time to a mood episode, aripiprazole was superior with a hazard ratio of 0.52 for relapse on aripiprazole relative to placebo. An extension phase of this study found that aripiprazole was superior to placebo in delaying time to mood episode for an additional 74 weeks; however, only 12 patients completed the study.

Olanzapine and lithium were compared in an open-label relapse prevention study of 431 patients with a recent manic or mixed episode who met remission criteria (YMRS $\leq$12 and HAM-D $\leq$8) on a open-label combination therapy of lithium and olanzapine.[125] Patients were then randomized to lithium (mean serum level, 0.7 mEq/L) or olanzapine (mean dose, 13.5 mg/day) monotherapy for 52 weeks of follow-up. Mood relapse occurred in 30% of olanzapine-treated patients and in 39% of lithium-treated patients. This result met the authors predefined criteria for statistical noninferiority of olanzapine relative to lithium. In a more recent study, 361 patients achieving remission (YMRS $\leq$12 and HAM-D $\leq$8) during open-label treatment with olanzapine were randomized to placebo or olanzapine (mean 12.5 mg/day) for 48 weeks of follow-up.[126] Time to any mood episode was significantly longer with olanzapine (174 days) than with placebo (22 days). Despite strong evidence of efficacy for olanzapine, the risk of metabolic complications limits the use of this drug in the long-term treatment of bipolar disorder (see Question 21).

28. What is the role of psychotherapy in bipolar disorder?

Psychotherapy can have a profound effect on the prevention of acute illness, as well as a sustained effect on maintenance treatments. Excessive stress, for example, is often implicated in the onset of affective episodes, particularly early in the lifetime course of bipolar illness.[27] If individuals and their families can learn to avoid these triggers or to develop coping skills, the acute impact can be minimized and future episodes averted.

Therapy may also help the family to cope with the extreme emotions and disruption that are the hallmark of acute manic and depressive episodes. Violent outbursts, infidelity, financial debts, and loss of self-esteem may all be a byproduct of relapse, and family members must come to terms with such calamities, as well as fears surrounding future episodes. Improvements in sleep hygiene may be encouraged in these sessions, because regular sleep–wake cycles seem vital to the maintenance of euthymic states. Last, sustained medication adherence must also be emphasized; individuals with bipolar disorder will often stop their mood stabilizers in an effort to resume the "highs" of mania. Many other patients also find the cumulative side effect burden of complex psychotropic regimens to be prohibitive.

The specific psychotherapeutic approach to bipolar disorder is generally quite similar to interventions offered to individuals with schizophrenia. Family-focused therapy seems to be quite effective, as are cognitive–behavioral, interpersonal, and social rhythm therapy. Collaborative care models have been extensively studied for unipolar depression in primary care settings, but the effectiveness of collaborative care models for bipolar illness is less clear. In the STEP-BD trials, subjects were randomized to one of four therapy approaches and collaborative care was the least effective.[127] Reported response rates were 77% with family-focused therapy, 64% with interpersonal and social rhythm therapy, 60% with cognitive–behavioral therapy, and 54% with collaborative care. However, some authorities contend that the collaborative care intervention was comparatively less intensive than the other three treatment modalities in this report.

29. Are there other treatment options for bipolar disorder?

Although most experts advocate for regular physical activity to prevent bipolar mood swings, the body of literature supporting such an approach is very limited. Lifestyle surveys have demonstrated that people afflicted with bipolar disorder are less likely to exercise and more likely to exhibit poor dietary habits than those without a serious mental illness.[128] Theoretically, exercise may improve dietary habits, regulate sleep, increase energy, and promote euthymic moods. Because all of these factors would be expected to improve the prognosis of bipolar illness, exercise should be encouraged.

A wide variety of herbal preparations and dietary supplements have been studied for the treatment of bipolar disorder. There has been considerable interest in the benefits of omega-3 fatty acid supplementation. A meta-analysis of double-blind, placebo-controlled trials of combined bipolar and unipolar depression found significant benefit of omega-3 fatty acid supplementation over placebo in patients with bipolar and unipolar depression.[129] In most cases, omega-3 fatty acid supplementation was used as adjunctive treatment and included eicosapentaenoic acid (EPA) alone or a combination of EPA and docosahexaenoic acid (DHA). The doses studied ranged from 1 gm/day of EPA all the way up to 9.6 g/day of combined EPA and DHA. Frangou et al.[130] compared 1- and 2-g/day doses of ethyl-EPA with placebo. Although both doses were superior to placebo, there was no difference between the 1- and 2-g/day doses. In a separate dose-ranging study for unipolar depression, results demonstrated a difference in response between the 1-g/day group and the placebo group; however, the 2- and 4-g/day treatment results did not differ from placebo.[131] Both of these studies suggest that 1 g/day of EPA may be adequate; but, the optimal dose of DHA and the optimal ratio of EPA to DHA remains unknown. The value of omega-3 fatty acids in the treatment and prevention of future manic episodes has been less clear. In fact, in one small randomized trial, 3 of 14 subjects treated with omega-3 fatty acids withdrew from the study due to the occurrence of manic or hypomanic symptoms.[132]

Among the other options, inositol was recently compared with lamotrigine and risperidone in an augmentation trial for bipolar depression.[133] The three treatments were equivalent with regard to recovery from depression; however, the study was open label and the sample size was small ($n = 66$). St. John's wort and *S*-adenosyl-L-methionine may be effective for depressive episodes; however, these agents should generally be avoided in bipolar disorder owing to the risk of switching to mania.[134,135] Chromium shows some promise for the treatment of acute depressive episodes. In one study, approximately one-third of bipolar patients with treatment-resistant rapid cycling bipolar disorder had a positive response.[136] The number of affective episodes also decreased for those patients remaining in the study; however, only 23% of patients were available for follow-up evaluation at 1 year. The adjunctive use of intravenous magnesium has been found to be beneficial for treatment resistant acute mania.[137]

ECT has been shown to have benefit in acute mania, mixed states, depression, and as a therapy to prevent relapse.[14] The rapid onset of effect of ECT in acute mania has been well documented. This therapy is also well tolerated, when used with a pretreatment regimen that includes a short-acting barbiturate, a skeletal muscle depolarizing agent, and atropine. The optimal placement of ECT electrodes (unilateral versus bilateral placement of electrodes) and the optimal frequency of ECT treatments to prevent a relapse are still unknown. The influence of concurrent psychotropic medications on ECT treatment success also should be considered.[138] Anticonvulsants and benzodiazepines may raise the seizure threshold and interfere with seizure induction. Lithium may increase confusion and memory impairment after ECT. Antipsychotics agents seem to be relatively safe in patients receiving ECT.

REFERENCES

1. Jamison Kay R. An Unquiet Mind. New York: Vintage Books; 1996.
2. Fagiolini A et al. Functional impairment in the remission phase of bipolar disorder. *Bipolar Disord* 2005;7:281.
3. National Institute of Mental Health. Key facts about mental illness. Rockville, MD: Nation Institutes of Mental Health; 1993.
4. Murray CL, Lopez AD. Global mortality, disability, and the contribution of risk factors: global burden of disease study. *Lancet* 1997;349:1436.
5. American Psychiatric Association. Mood disorders. In: *Diagnostic and Statistical Manual of Mental Disorder*. 4th ed. Text Revision. Washington, DC: American Psychiatric Association; 2000: 382.
6. Lish JD et al. The national depressive and manic-depressive association (DMDA) survey of bipolar members. *J Affect Disord* 1994;31:281.
7. Judd LL et al. The long-term natural history of the weekly symptomatic status of bipolar I disorder. *Arch Gen Psychiatry* 2002;59:530.
8. Merikangas KR et al. Lifetime and 12-month prevalence of bipolar spectrum disorder in the national comorbidity survey replication. *Arch Gen Psychiatry* 2007;64:543.
9. Goodwin FK, Jamison KR. Genetics. In: *Manic-Depressive Illness: Bipolar Disorders and Recurrent Depression*. New York: Oxford University Press; 2007:411.
10. Wyatt RJ, Henter I. An economic evaluation of manic-depressive illness: 1991. *Soc Psychiatry Psychiatr Epidemiol* 1995;30:213.
11. Goodwin FK, Jamison KR. Clinical description. In: *Manic-Depressive Illness: Bipolar Illness and Recurrent Depression*. New York: Oxford University Press; 2007:29.
12. Hirschfeld RM et al. Perceptions and impact of bipolar disorder: how far have we really come? Results of the national depressive and manic-depressive association 2000 survey of individuals with bipolar disorder. *J Clin Psychiatry* 2003;64: 161.
13. Kupfer DJ et al. Demographic and clinical characteristics of individuals in a bipolar disorder case registry. *J Clin Psychiatry* 2002;63:121.
14. American Psychiatric Association. Practice guidelines for the treatment of patients with bipolar disorder (revision). *Am J Psychiatry* 2002;159(4 Suppl):1.
15. Schneck CD et al. Phenomenology of rapid-cycling bipolar disorder: Data from the first 500 participants in the systematic treatment enhancement program. *Am J Psychiatry* 2004;161:1902.
16. Gitlin MJ. Swendsen J. Relapse and impairment in bipolar disorder. *Am J Psychiatry* 1995;152:1635.
17. Angst F et al. Mortality of patients with mood disorders: follow up over 34–38 years. *J Affect Disord* 2002;68:167.
18. Lopez P et al. Suicide attempts in bipolar patients. *J Clin Psychiatry* 2001;62:963.
19. Tsai SY et al. Risk factors for completed suicide in bipolar disorder. *J Clin Psychiatry* 2002;63;469.
20. Woods SW. The economic burden of bipolar disorder. *J Clin Psych* 2000;61(Suppl 13):38.
21. Suppes T et al. The Texas implementation of medication algorithms: update to the algorithms for treatment of bipolar I disorder. *J Clin Psychiatry* 2005; 66:870.
22. Yatham LN et al. Canadian Network for Mood and Anxiety Treatments (CANMAT) guidelines for management of patients with bipolar disorder: consensus and controversies. *Bipolar Disord* 2005; 7(Suppl 3):5.
23. Yatham LN et al. Canadian network for mood and anxiety treatments (CANMAT) guidelines for the management of patients with bipolar disorder: update 2007. *Bipolar Disord* 2006;8:721.
24. Keck PE et al. The expert consensus guideline series: treatment of bipolar disorder 2004. *Postgraduate Medicine Special Report* 2004:1.
25. American Diabetes Association et al. Consensus development conference on antipsychotic drugs and obesity and diabetes. *Diabetes Care* 2004;27: 596.
26. Ghaemi SN et al. Diagnosing bipolar disorder and the effect of antidepressants: a naturalistic study. *J Clin Psychiatry* 2000;61:804.
27. Goodwin FK, Jamison KR. Course and outcome. In: *Manic-Depressive Illness: Bipolar Disorders and Recurrent Depression*. New York: Oxford University Press; 2007:119.
28. Peet M, Peters S. Drug-induced mania. *Drug Saf* 1995;12:146–153.
29. Goldberg JF, Truman CJ. Antidepressant-induced mania: an overview of current controversies. *Bipolar Disord* 2003;5:407.
30. Himmelhoch JM et al. Tranylcypromine versus imipramine in anergic bipolar depression. *Am J Psychiatry* 1991;148:910.
31. Peet M. Induction of mania with selective serotonin re-uptake inhibitors and tricyclic antidepressants. *Br J Psychiatry* 1994;164:549.
32. Leverich GS et al. Risk of switch in mood polarity to hypomania or mania in patients with bipolar depression during acute and continuation trials of venlafaxine, sertraline, and bupropion as adjuncts to mood stabilizers. *Am J Psychiatry* 2006;163:232.
33. Mattes JA. Antidepressant-induced rapid cycling: another perspective. *Ann Clin Psychiatry* 2006;18: 195.

34. Altshuler LL et al. Antidepressant-induced mania and cycle acceleration: a controversy revisited. *Am J Psychiatry* 1995;152:1130.
35. Bowden CL et al. Efficacy of divalproex vs. lithium and placebo in the treatment of mania. *JAMA* 1994;271:918. Erratum In: *JAMA* 1994;271:1830.
36. Bowden CL et al. Relation of serum valproate concentration to response in mania. *Am J Psychiatry* 1996;153:765.
37. Hirschfeld RMA et al. The safety and early efficacy of oral-loaded divalproex versus standard-titration divalproex, lithium, olanzapine, and placebo in the treatment of acute mania associated with bipolar disorder. *J Clin Psychiatry* 2003;64:841.
38. Allen MH et al. Linear response of valproate serum concentration to response and optimal serum levels for acute mania. *Am J Psychiatry* 2006;163:272.
39. Bowden CL. Valproate. *Bipolar Disord* 2003;5:189.
40. Bowden CL et al. A randomized, placebo-controlled, multicenter study of divalproex sodium extended release in the treatment of acute mania. *J Clin Psychiatry* 2006;67:1501.
41. Smith MC et al. Clinical comparison of extended-release divalproex versus delayed-release divalproex: pooled data analyses from nine trials. *Epilepsy Behav* 2004:5;746.
42. Mercke Y et al. Hair loss in psychopharmacology. *Ann Clin Psychiatry* 2000;12:35.
43. Joffe H et al. Valproate is associated with new-onset oligoamenorrhea with hyperandrogenism in women with bipolar disorder. *Biol Psychiatry* 2006;59:1078.
44. Kimmel RJ et al. Valproic acid-associated hyperammonemic encephalopathy: a case report from the psychiatric setting. *Int Clin Psychopharmacol* 2005:20;57.
45. Elgudin L et al. Ammonia induced encephalopathy from valproic acid in a bipolar patient: case report. *Int J Psychiatry Med* 2003;33:91.
46. Acharya S, Bussel J. Hematologic toxicity of sodium valproate. *J Pediatr Hematol Oncol* 2000; 22:62.
47. Janicak PG et al. Treatment with mood stabilizers. In: *Principles and Practice of Psychopharmacotherapy*. 2nd ed. Philadelphia: Lippincott Williams & Wilkins; 2006:369.
48. Gelenberg AJ et al. Lithium tremor. *J Clin Psychiatry* 1995:283.
49. Henry C. Lithium side-effects and predictors of hypothyroidism in patients with bipolar disorder: sex differences. *J Psychiatry Neurosci* 2002;27:104.
50. Bendz H, Aurell M. Drug induced diabetes insipidus: incidence, prevention, and management. *Drug Saf* 1999;21:449.
51. Mellerup ET. The side effects of lithium. *Biol Psychiatry* 1990;28:464.
52. Hetmar O et al. Lithium: long-term effects on the kidney. *A prospective follow-up study ten years after kidney biopsy. Br J Psychiatry* 1991;158:53.
53. Dunner DL. Drug interactions of lithium and other antimanic/mood-stabilizing medications. *J Clin Psychiatry* 2003;64(Suppl 5):38.
54. Kleiner J, Altshuler LL. Lithium-induced subclinical hypothyroidism: review of the literature and guidelines for treatment. *J Clin Psychiatry* 1999;60:249.
55. Zhang ZJ et al. Differences in hypothyroidism between lithium-free and lithium-treated patients with bipolar disorders. *Life sciences* 2006:771.
56. Livingstone C, Rampes H. Lithium: a review of its metabolic adverse effects. *J Psychopharmacol* 2006;20:347.
57. Goodwin FK, Jamison KR. Medical treatment of hypomania, mania, and mixed states. In: *Manic-Depressive Illness: Bipolar Illness and Recurrent Depression*. New York: Oxford University Press; 2007:721.
58. Ernst CL, Goldber JF. The reproductive safety profile of mood stabilizers, atypical antipsychotics, and broad-spectrum psychotropics. *J Clin Psychiatry* 2002;63(Suppl 4):42.
59. Jain AE, Lacy T. Psychotropic drugs in pregnancy and lactation. *J Psychiatr Pract* 2005;11:177.
60. Cohen LS et al. A reevaluation of risk of in utero exposure to lithium. *JAMA* 1994;271:146.
61. Troyer WA et al. Association of maternal lithium exposure and premature delivery. *J Perinatol* 1993; 13:123.
62. Ward S et al. Collaborative management of women with bipolar disorder during pregnancy and postpartum: pharmacologic considerations. *J Midwifery Womens Health* 2007;52:3.
63. Newport DJ et al. Atypical antipsychotic administration during late pregnancy: placental passage and obstetrical outcomes. *Am J Psychiatry* 2007;164: 1214.
64. Perlis RH et al. Atypical antipsychotics in the treatment of mania: a meta-analysis of randomized, placebo-controlled trials. *J Clin Psychiatry* 2006; 67:509.
65. Scherk H et al. Second-generation antipsychotic agents in the treatment of acute mania. *Arch Gen Psychiatry* 2007;64:442.
66. Smith LA et al. Acute bipolar mania: systematic review and meta-analysis of co-therapy vs. *monotherapy. Acta Psychiatr Scand* 2007;115:12.
67. Banov MD et al. Clozapine therapy in refractory affective disorders: polarity predicts response in long-term follow-up. *J Clin Psychiatry* 1994;55:295.
68. Calabrese JR et al. Clozapine for treatment-refractory mania. *Am J Psychiatry* 1996;153:759.
69. Suppes T et al. Clinical outcome in a randomized 1-year trial of clozapine versus treatment as usual for patients with treatment-resistant illness and a history of mania. *Am J Psychiatry* 1999;156:1164.
70. McIntyre RS, Konarski JZ. Tolerability profiles of atypical antipsychotics in the treatment of bipolar disorder. *J Clin Psychiatry* 2005;66(Suppl 3):28.
71. Sachs G et al. Aripiprazole in the treatment of acute manic or mixed episodes in patients with bipolar I disorder: a 3-week placebo-controlled study. *J Psychopharmacol* 2006;20:536.
72. Keck PE et al. A placebo-controlled, double-blind study of the efficacy and safety of aripiprazole in patients with acute bipolar mania. *Am J Psychiatry* 2003;160:1651.
73. Lieberman JA et al; Clinical Antipsychotic Trials of Intervention Effectiveness (CATIE) Investigators. Effectiveness of antipsychotic drugs in patients with chronic schizophrenia. *N Engl J Med* 2005;353:1209.
74. Post RM et al. Thirty years of clinical experience with carbamazepine in the treatment of bipolar illness. *CNS Drugs* 2007;21:47.
75. Weisler R et al. Extended-release carbamazepine capsules as monotherapy in bipolar disorder: pooled results from two randomised, double-blind, placebo-controlled trials. *CNS Drugs* 2006;20:219.
76. Pratoomsri W et al. Oxcarbazepine in the treatment of bipolar disorder: a review. *Can J Psychiatry* 2006;51:540.
77. Wagner KD et al. A double-blind randomized placebo controlled trial of oxcarbazepine in the treatment of bipolar disorder in children and adolescents. *Am J Psychiatry* 2006;163:1179.
78. Yatham LN. Third generation anticonvulsants in bipolar disorder: a review of efficacy and summary of clinical recommendations. *J Clin Psychiatry* 2002:63:275.
79. Berk M et al. Lamotrigine and the treatment of mania in bipolar disorder. *Eur Neuropsychopharmacol* 1999;9(Suppl 4):S119.
80. Young TL et al. Gabapentin as an adjunctive treatment in bipolar disorder. *J Affect Disord* 1999; 55:73.
81. Schaffer CB et al. Gabapentin in the treatment of bipolar disorder. *Am J Psychiatry* 1997;154:291.
82. Ghaemi SN et al. Gabapentin treatment of mood disorders: a preliminary study. *J Clin Psychiatry* 1998;59:426.
83. Pande AC et al; Gabapentin Bipolar Disorder Study Group. Gabapentin in bipolar disorder: a placebo-controlled trial of adjunctive therapy. *Bipolar Disord* 2000;2:249.
84. Chengappa KNR et al. The evolving role of topiramate among other mood stabilizers in the management of bipolar disorder. *Bipolar Disord* 2001; 3:215.
85. Kushner SF et al. Topiramate monotherapy in the management of acute mania: results of four double-blind placebo-controlled trials. *Bipolar Disord* 2006;8:15.
86. Grunze H et al. Tiagabine appears not to be efficacious in the treatment of acute mania. *J Clin Psychiatry* 1999;60:759.
87. Suppes T et al. Tiagabine in treatment refractory bipolar disorder: a clinical case series. *Bipolar Disord* 2002;4:283.
88. McElroy SL et al. Open-label adjunctive zonisamide in the treatment of bipolar disorders: a prospective trial. *J Clin Psychiatry* 2005;66:617.
89. Post RM et al. Preliminary observations on the effectiveness of levetiracetam in the open adjunctive treatment of refractory bipolar disorder. *J Clin Psychiatry* 2005;66:370.
90. Wolfsperger M et al. Pharmacological treatment of acute mania in psychiatric in-patients between 1994 and 2004. *J Affect Disord* 2007;99:9.
91. Allen MH et al. What do consumers say they want and need during a psychiatric emergency? *J Psychiatr Pract* 2003;9:39.
92. Currier GW, Medori R. Orally versus intramuscular administered antipsychotic drugs in psychiatric emergencies. *J Psychiatr Pract* 2006;12:30.
93. Lesem MD et al. Intramuscular ziprasidone, 2 mg versus 10 mg, in the short-term management of agitated psychotic patients. *J Clin Psychiatry* 2001;62: 12. Erratum In: *J Clin Psychiatry* 2001;62:209.
94. Daniel DG et al. Intramuscular (IM) ziprasidone 20mg is effective in reducing acute agitation associated with psychosis: a double-blind, randomized trial. *Psychopharmacol* 2001;155:128.
95. Zimbroff DL et al. Management of acute agitation in patients with bipolar disorder: efficacy and safety of intramuscular aripiprazole. *J Clin Psychopharmacol* 2007;27:171.
96. Meehan K et al. A double-blind, randomized comparison of the efficacy and safety of intramuscular injections of olanzapine, lorazepam, or placebo in treatment acutely agitated patients diagnosed with bipolar mania. *J Clin Psychopharmacol* 2001;21:389.
97. Battaglia J et al. Haloperidol, lorazepam, or both for psychotic agitation? A multicenter, prospective, double-blind, emergency department study. *Am J Emerg Med.* 1997;15:335.
98. Zyprexa package insert. Indianapolis, In: Eli Lilly; 2006.
99. Allen MH et al. Treatment of behavioral emergencies 2005. *J Psychiatr Pract* 2005;11(Suppl 1):1.
100. Yatham LN et al. Bipolar depression: criteria for treatment selection, definition of refractoriness, and treatment options. *Bipolar Disord* 2003;5:85.
101. Keck PE et al. New approaches in managing bipolar depression. *J Clin Psychiatry* 2003;64(Suppl 1):13.
102. Calabrese J et al. A double-bind placebo-controlled study of lamotrigine monotherapy in outpatients with bipolar I depression. *J Clin Psychiatry* 1999; 60:79.
103. Frye MA et al. A placebo-controlled study of lamotrigine and gabapentin monotherapy in refractory mood disorders. *J Clin Psychopharmacol* 2000;20:607.
104. Brown EB et al. A 7-week, randomized, double-blind trial of olanzapine/fluoxetine combination versus lamotrigine in the treatment of bipolar I depression. *J Clin Psychiatry* 2006;67:1025.
105. Calabrese JR et al. A randomized, double-blind, placebo-controlled trial of quetiapine in the treatment of bipolar I or II depression. *Am J Psychiatry* 2005;162:1351.
106. Thase ME et al. Efficacy of quetiapine monotherapy in bipolar I and II depression. *J Clin Psychopharmacol* 2006;26:600. Erratum In: *J Clin Psychopharmacol* 2007;27:51.
107. Tohen M et al. Efficacy of olanzapine and olanzapine-fluoxetine combination in the treatment of bipolar I depression. *Arch Gen Psychiatry* 2003;60:1079.

108. Prien RF et al. Drug therapy in the prevention of recurrences in unipolar and bipolar disorders: report of the NIMH Collaborative Study Group comparing lithium carbonate, imipramine, and a lithium carbonate-imipramine combination. *Arch Gen Psychiatry* 1984;41:1095.
109. Bottlender R et al. Mood stabilizers reduce the risk of developing antidepressant-induced maniform states in acute treatment of bipolar I depressed patients. *J Affect Disord* 2001;63:79.
110. Boerlin HL et al. Bipolar depression and antidepressant-induced mania: a naturalistic study. *J Clin Psychiatry* 1998;59:374.
111. Sachs GS et al. Effectiveness of adjunctive antidepressant treatment for bipolar depression. *N Engl J Med* 2007;356:1711.
112. Goodwin FK, Jamison KR. Maintenance medical treatment. In: *Manic-Depressive Illness*. New York: Oxford University Press; 1990:665.
113. Harrow M et al. Outcome in manic disorders. *Arch Gen Psychiatry* 1990;47:665.
114. O'Connell RA et al. Outcome of bipolar disorder on long-term treatment with lithium. *Br J Psychiatry* 1991;159:123.
115. Tondo L et al. Lithium treatment and risk of suicidal behavior in bipolar disorder patients. *J Clin Psychiatry* 1998;59:405.
116. Bowden CL et al. A placebo controlled 18-month trial of lamotrigine and lithium maintenance treatment in recently manic or hypomanic patients with bipolar I disorder. *Arch Gen Psychiatry* 2003;60:392.
117. Bowden CL et al. A randomized, placebo-controlled 12 month trial of divalproex and lithium in treatment of outpatients with bipolar I disorder. *Arch Gen Psychiatry* 2000;57:481.
118. Gelenberg AJ et al. Comparison of standard and low serum levels of lithium for maintenance treatment of bipolar disorder. *N Engl J Med* 1989;321:1489.
119. Tondo L et al. Effectiveness of restarting lithium treatment after its discontinuation in bipolar I and bipolar II disorders. *Am J Psychiatry* 1997;1543:548.
120. Coryell W et al. Lithium discontinuation and subsequent effectiveness. *Am J Psychiatry* 1998;155:895.
121. Goodwin GM et al. A pooled analysis of 2 placebo-controlled 18 month trials of lamotrigine and lithium maintenance in bipolar I disorder. *J Clin Psychiatry* 2004;65:432.
122. Hartong E et al. Prophylactic efficacy of lithium versus carbamazepine in treatment-naive bipolar patients. *J Clin Psychiatry* 2003;64:144.
123. Kleindienst N et al. Differential efficacy of lithium and carbamazepine in the prophylaxis of bipolar disorder: Results of the MAP study. *Neuropsychobiology* 2000;42(Suppl 1):2.
124. Keck PE et al. A randomized double-blind, placebo controlled 26-week trial of aripiprazole in recently manic patients with bipolar I disorder. *J Clin Psychiatry* 2006;67:626.
125. Tohen M et al. Olanzapine versus lithium in the maintenance treatment of bipolar disorder: a 12-month, randomized, double-blind, controlled clinical trial. *Am J Psychiatry* 2005;162:1281.
126. Tohen M et al. Randomized, placebo-controlled trial of olanzapine as maintenance therapy in patients with bipolar I disorder responding to acute treatment with olanzapine. *Am J Psychiatry* 2006;163:247.
127. Miklowitz DJ et al. Intensive psychosocial intervention enhances functioning in patients with bipolar depression: results from a 9-month randomized controlled trial. *Am J Psychiatry* 2007;164:1340.
128. Kilbourne AM et al. Nutrition and exercise behavior among patients with bipolar disorder. *Bipolar Disord* 2007;9:443.
129. Freeman MP et al. Omega-3 fatty acids: Evidence basis for treatment and future research in psychiatry. *J Clin Psychiatry* 2006;67:1954.
130. Frangou S et al. Efficacy of ethyl-eicosapentaenoic acid in bipolar depression: Randomized double-blind placebo-controlled study. *Br J Psychiatry* 2006;188:46.
131. Peet M, Horribin DF. A dose-ranging study of the effects of ethyl-eicosapentaenoate in patients with ongoing depression despite apparently adequate treatment with standard drugs. *Arch Gen Psychiatry* 2002;59:913.
132. Stoll AL et al. Omega 3 fatty acids in bipolar disorder: a preliminary double-blind, placebo-controlled trial. *Arch Gen Psychiatry* 1999;56:407.
133. Nierenberg AA et al. Treatment-resistant bipolar depression: a STEP-BD equipoise randomized effectiveness trial of antidepressant augmentation with lamotrigine, inositol, or risperidone. *Am J Psychiatry* 2006;163:210.
134. Gören JL et al. Bioavailability and lack of toxicity of S-adenosyl-L-methionine (SAMe) in humans. *Pharmacotherapy* 2004;24:1501.
135. Moses EL et al. St. John's wort: three cases of possible mania induction. *J Clin Psychopharmacol* 2000;20:115.
136. Amann BL et al. A 2-year, open-label pilot study of adjunctive chromium in patients with treatment-resistant rapid-cycling bipolar disorder. *J Clin Psychopharmacol* 2007;27:104.
137. Heiden A et al. Treatment of severe mania with intravenous magnesium sulphate as a supplementary therapy. *Psychiatry Res* 1999;89:239.
138. Naquib M et al. Interactions between psychotropics, anaesthetics and electroconvulsive therapy. Implications for drug choice and patient management. *CNS Drugs* 2002;16:229.
139. Ogawa N, Ueki H. Secondary mania caused by caffeine. *Gen Hosp Psychiatry* 2003;25:138.
140. Sultzer DL, Cummings JL. Drug-induced mania—causative agents, clinical characteristics and management: a retrospective analysis of the literature. *Med Toxicol Adverse Drug Exp* 1989;4:127.
141. Padala PR et al. Manic episode during treatment with aripiprazole. *Am J Psychiatry* 2007;164:172.
142. Rachid F et al. Possible induction of mania or hypomania by atypical antipsychotics: an updated review of reported cases. *J Clin Psychiatry* 2004;65:1537.
143. Abouesh A et al. Antimicrobial-induced mania (antibiomania): a review of spontaneous reports. *J Clin Psychopharmacol* 2002;22:71.
144. Blanc J et al. Manic syndrome associated with efavirenz overdose. *Clin Infect Dis* 2001;33:270.
145. Jochum T et al. Topiramate induced manic episode. *J Neurol Neurosurg Psychiatry* 2002;73:208.
146. Margolese HC et al. Hypomania induced by adjunctive lamotrigine. *Am J Psychiatry* 2003;160:183
147. Short C, Cooke L. Hypomania induced by gabapentin. *Br J Psychiatry* 1995;166:679.
148. Watts BV et al. Tramadol-induced mania. *Am J Psychiatry* 1997;154:1624.
149. Rego MD, Giller EL. Mania secondary to amantadine treatment of neuroleptic-induced hyperprolactinemia. *J Clin Psychiatry* 1989;50:143.
150. Price WA, Prepubertal M. Buspirone-induced mania. *J Clin Psychopharmacol* 1989;9:150.
151. Gupta N. Venlafaxine-induced hypomanic switch in bipolar depression. *Can J Psychiatry* 2001;46:760.
152. Bhanji NH et al. Dysphoric mania induced by high-dose mirtazapine: a case for norepinephrine syndrome? *Int Clin Psychopharmacol* 2002;17:319.
153. Zaphiris HA et al. Probable nefazodone-induced mania in a patient with unreported bipolar disorder. *Ann Clin Psychiatry* 1996;8:207.
154. Benazzi F. Organic hypomania secondary to sibutramine-citalopram interaction. *J Clin Psychiatry* 2002;63:165.
155. El-Mallakh RS. Bupropion manic induction during euthymia, but not during depression. *Bipolar Disord* 2001;3:159.

CHAPTER 81

Attention Deficit Hyperactivity Disorder in Children, Adolescents, and Adults

Paul Perry and Samuel Kuperman

The popular culture book *Ritalin Nation* suggests that modern Western society's high-speed lifestyle and rapid-fire culture have significant consequences for children.[1] Because children are being continuously bombarded with sophisticated sensory stimuli via television and video games, many never learn to concentrate on free-play activities. By the time they reach school age, they have not learned the skills necessary to attend to activities such as reading, writing, and arithmetic. It is hypothesized that children become "addicted to" and "dependent" on continuous sensory stimulation. DeGrandpre hypothesizes that the symptoms of attention deficit hyperactivity disorder (ADHD)—hyperactivity and an inability to attend to low-stimulation activities—reflect an escape behavior used by children to maintain sensory stimulation.[1] In this theory, methylphenidate is effective only because it provides stimulation in this case, pharmacologic stimulation as opposed to auditory or visual stimulation. This minority opinion contends that ADHD is a diagnosis invented by 20th-century psychiatrists and pharmaceutical companies. In the well-known European children's story of Fidgety Phillip written in the 1863 book, *Struwwelpeter*, by Heinrich Hoffmann[2] "Phil stop acting like a worm, the table is no place to squirm. Thus speaks the father to his son severely say it, not in fun. Mother frowns and looks around, although she doesn't make a sound. But Phillip will not take advice, he'll have his way at any price. He turns and churns, he wriggles and jiggles. Here and there on the chair, Phil, these twists I cannot bear." Today, Phil may have been diagnosed with ADHD.

Among the vocal critics of ADHD are included the Church of Scientology, newspaper reporters, talk show hosts, Drug Enforcement Agency officials, conservative legislators, and a small number of physicians and psychologists. Safer categorized the objections of the ADHD faultfinders into seven criticisms: (a) physicians are haphazard in their diagnosis and treatment of ADHD; (b) school alternative programs for treating ADHD are neglected or ignored because of stimulant treatment; (c) ADHD is caused by 20th- and 21st-century social and cultural pressures and is not really a legitimate diagnosis; (d) stimulant treatment has profound limitations; (e) stimulants are harmful and abused by ADHD patients; (f) methylphenidate is overprescribed; and (g) pharmaceutical companies influence the "pro-Ritalin" parent support groups excessively to legitimize the acceptance of Ritalin as the treatment of choice in ADHD.[3] However, the data do not support these assertions. These claims are countered by the following data: (a) on average, a physician requires an hour to make the initial ADHD diagnosis; (b) 25% of ADHD children do not receive a prescription; (c) most pediatricians offer nonmedical treatment alternatives for ADHD; (d) 45% of methylphenidate-treated ADHD diagnosed children are in special education classes because of learning disabilities; (e) genetic determinants are the major causative factor in explaining the etiology of ADHD; (f) stimulants are clearly more effective than behavioral therapy for the treatment of ADHD; (g) stimulants are safe, well tolerated, and rarely abused by ADHD youth; (g) because of diversion, pharmaceutical company production quotas cannot be used to determine or estimate the number of treated ADHD individuals; (h) in reality, stimulants may be underprescribed for ADHD children and adolescents because of the social stigma associated with taking methylphenidate or amphetamines; and (i) parents have the same attitudes toward ADHD, regardless of whether they are members of a pro-Ritalin parent support group.[3]

DIAGNOSTIC CRITERIA

The effectiveness of stimulants in improving academic performance is often misunderstood. On occasion parents may pressure clinicians into writing stimulant prescriptions for a "let's see if it helps" trial. If the drug does help, they may assume that the diagnosis of ADHD is validated. However, stimulant medications improve vigilance performance (attention/concentration) in both normal and hyperactive children.[4] Other commonly used dopamine agonists such as caffeine and nicotine also benefit concentration and the ability to study. Table 81-1 presents the *Diagnostic and Statistical Manual of Mental Disorders*, Fourth Edition, Text Revision (DSM-IV-TR) criteria required to make a diagnosis of ADHD.

Table 81-1 DSM-IV-TR Diagnostic Criteria for Attention Deficit Hyperactivity Disorder

Inattention Factor

(Six or more of the following nine behaviors need to be present for ≥6 months in two or more settings, such as home, school, or physician's office.)

1. Careless mistakes or inattention to detail
2. Reduced attention span
3. Poor listener
4. Cannot follow instructions and does not complete tasks
5. Difficulty organizing tasks and activities
6. Avoids and/or dislikes chores or homework
7. Loses things needed for tasks and activities
8. Easily distracted by extraneous stimuli
9. Forgetful in daily activities

Hyperactivity/Impulsivity Factor

(Six or more of the following nine behaviors need to be present for ≥6 months in two or more settings, such as home, school, or physician's office.)

Hyperactivity

1. Fidgets with hands/feet or squirms in chair
2. Cannot remain seated in the classroom
3. Uncontrollable/inappropriate restlessness
4. Difficulty in engaging in play or leisure activities quietly
5. Often on the go and appearing driven by a motor
6. Excessive talking

Impulsivity

7. Blurts out answer prior to completion of question
8. Difficulty waiting turn
9. Interrupts or intrudes on others

Reprinted with permission from reference 73.

ADHD impacts the child and his or her family, the child's social interactions, and the child's self-esteem. Often children are aware of these difficulties and resist doing their normal day-to-day tasks. Establishing a diagnosis of ADHD in an adult who has never been treated for the disorder during childhood is difficult. Symptoms tend to be more subjective, with less overt hyperactivity. Unlike teachers who are often familiar with the symptoms associated with ADHD in children, spouses, coworkers and employers are often unfamiliar with ADHD as a disorder that can also affect adults. They may attribute the individual's difficulties to being lazy or to "underachievement". Symptoms of ADHD in adulthood often interfere with social relationships and employment.

PREVALENCE

ADHD is classified into three subtypes depending upon the hallmark clinical features: hyperactive-impulsive, inattentive, or combined. The Centers for Disease Control and Prevention analyzed data from the 2003 National Survey of Children's Health.[5] In 2003, approximately 7.8% (4,418,000; 95% confidence interval = 4,234,000–4,602,000) of U.S. children ages 4 to 17 years were diagnosed with ADHD. ADHD diagnosis was reported approximately 2.5 times more frequently among males than females.

COMORBIDITY

There is a high rate of comorbidity between ADHD and other psychiatric conditions including conduct disorder, oppositional defiant disorder, depression, major affective disorder, and anxiety disorders, including obsessive-compulsive disorder and Tourette syndrome (TS). Family histories from first-degree relatives of probands with ADHD reveal increased rates of ADHD (25% concordance rate), polysubstance dependence, antisocial personality disorder, depression, and anxiety disorders.[6] Children with ADHD are at an increased risk of having antisocial behavior, depression, and polysubstance abuse problems as adults. ADHD symptoms persist into adulthood in approximately 10% to 60% of patients.[7] Adults with ADHD are usually self-sufficient, but they have poorer academic performance, poorer job performance, and lower socioeconomic status than do their siblings. They also have more frequent divorces, job changes, changes of residence, and car accidents. Most adults with ADHD report a high level of subjective distress (79%) and interpersonal problems (75%).[8]

DIFFERENTIAL DIAGNOSIS

ADHD should not be diagnosed until head injuries, absence seizures, cerebral infection, substance abuse, hyperthyroidism, anxiety disorders, and mood disorders have been excluded. Of these conditions, anxiety disorders and mood disorders are most commonly misdiagnosed as ADHD. The ADHD workup should include teacher and parent–child ratings using an accepted rating scale such as the Iowa Connors Rating Scale for ADHD; a physical examination; lead screening; a neurological examination; antenatal, perinatal, social, family, school, and medical history; developmental milestones; cognitive testing that includes an IQ test and a reading test; and psychometric tests that quantify errors of omission (inattention) and errors of commission (hyperactivity/impulsivity).

SIGNS AND SYMPTOMS

1. C.B., a 6-year-old boy, was brought into a child psychiatry clinic after his mother attended his first-grade school conference and was told that her son was having difficulty adjusting to first grade. C.B.'s mother reported that C.B. had always been a somewhat difficult child. He showed disruptive behavior and did not respond well to direction to put toys away, and he never seemed to be able to keep track of what was going on around him. As an infant, he was irritable and overactive. At 7 months, when he began crawling, he would disrupt the entire house. He was unable to follow through with parental instructions to keep his feet off the furniture, not walk on the tops of tables, and not walk through the living room carrying melting chocolate popsicles. When he learned to talk, he talked incessantly and continuously. Attempts to ignore his attention-seeking behavior seemed to have little effect on him. He was disruptive and impulsive in preschool, with noisy, attention-seeking behaviors that continued through first grade. He was oblivious to the pleas of teachers and teaching assistants to get him to sit still and pay attention. He would not sit in his seat.

Often he would get up and run around the room. He could not stay on task on assignments for more than 5 minutes without becoming distracted. Before he even started his assignments, looking for his lost pencil would distract him. His partially completed class assignments would be incomplete and filled with careless errors. He would talk to his classmates when they were working, pointing out to them what was going on outside. He was in constant motion, moving his legs and arms and wiggling in his seat. It was difficult for C.B. to participate in school activities/games because he interrupted others or participated out of turn, which made other kids not like him. During the clinic evaluation, C.B. was quite active. He jumped on his chair rather than sitting on it. When he eventually did sit, he remained in his chair for only 2 to 3 minutes. He then began pulling books off the shelves. When he was told to leave them alone, he threw two books onto the floor and then headed toward the doctor's desk to examine the pens, pencils, and paperweights. C.B. had trouble attempting to put a puzzle together (a five-piece puzzle); he would put one piece in place, lose interest, and throw the remaining pieces across the room. He would reverse letters when asked to write the letters of the alphabet, and he reversed the letter *r* when writing his name. His physical exam was otherwise within normal limits. What symptoms of ADHD does C.B. present? For which of the three diagnostic subtypes of ADHD does he meet the criteria?

Based on his history, C.B. exhibits the symptoms of ADHD, combined subtype. C.B. represents a child with ADHD who is more likely to present to a child psychiatry clinic rather than a pediatrician or family doctor. If his medical history was explored, C.B. would likely be a risk taker, having more accidents requiring stitches and involving broken bones then other children his age. It is likely that his parents and perhaps C.B. himself would say that he has trouble making and maintaining friendships or that his friends were more likely to be children who themselves have behavior difficulties. Finally, it appears that C.B. has comorbid oppositional defiant disorder. Although establishing a learning disorder diagnosis at his current age is unlikely, as C.B. ages the probability of this occurring is likely to increase, and he should be monitored and tested for a learning disorder.

NEUROBIOLOGY

Various abnormal neurochemical and genomic abnormalities are associated with ADHD. A decrease in 3-methoxy-4-hydroxyphenylglycol (MHPG), the major metabolite of norepinephrine, supports a norepinephrine deficiency hypothesis, whereas low levels of homovanillic acid, the major metabolite of dopamine, is postulated to support a dopamine deficiency hypothesis.[9] In addition, an excess of platelet monoamine oxidase (MAO) has been observed in children with ADHD. Normally, there is an age-related decrease in MAO in the platelets of children.[10] However, this decrease in MAO activity was not observed in children with ADHD. The computerized electroencephalogram brain mapping of ADHD children show an excess of theta (slow wave) activity in the frontal lobe, which may relate to a decrease in glucose metabolism in this area and suggest dysregulation of arousal and attention.[11] The neurochemical changes are also hypothesized to have a genetic basis. Candidate genes associated with ADHD can be grouped into four categories: (a) genes coding for various neurotransmitter functions (i.e., dopamine-transporter receptor [DAT1], dopamine-4 receptor [DRD4], dopamine-5 receptor [DRD5], synaptosome-associated protein of 25 kDA [SNAP25]); (b) genes coding for enzymes involved in dopamine biosynthesis (i.e., tyrosine hydroxylase [chromosome 11p15.5], dihydroxyphenylalanine [DOPA], decarboxylase [chromosome 7p11], dopamine-beta-hydroxylase [chromosome 9q34]); (c) genes coding for enzymes involved in the metabolism of catecholamines (i.e., catechol-*O*-methyltransferase [COMT], MAO); and (d) other genes (i.e., glutamate receptor inotropic N-methyl-D-aspartate [NMDA] 2A [GRIN2A] [chromosome 16p13], serotonin transporter gene).[12]

PHARMACOTHERAPY

Although central nervous system (CNS) stimulant or psychostimulant medications are currently the drugs of choice, tricyclic antidepressants (TCAs), atomoxetine, bupropion, and clonidine are also useful medications in the treatment of patients with ADHD. Stimulants that are norepinephrine and/or dopamine agonists benefit the symptoms of ADHD. Patients, teachers, and clinicians rate 75% of children with ADHD to be improved on stimulants, compared to 18% of placebo-treated children.[13] Approximately 20% to 25% of those who respond poorly to one medication will respond positively to another.[14]

Central Nervous System Stimulants

The short- and long-term effectiveness and safety of pharmacological and nonpharmacological interventions for ADHD in children and adults was suggested in a meta-analysis based on 77 randomized controlled trials.[15] There were no obvious differences in effectiveness among the stimulants methylphenidate, dextroamphetamine, and pemoline. However, the six randomized controlled trials that compared drugs with nondrug interventions consistently showed that stimulants, particularly methylphenidate, were more effective than nonpharmacologic interventions. The 20 combined therapy (stimulants plus psychotherapy) randomized controlled trials were unable to identify any additional benefit from the nonpharmacologic interventions. The analysis concluded that psychostimulants are first-line drugs in the treatment of ADHD, and the stimulants methylphenidate, dextroamphetamine, mixed amphetamine salts, and pemoline are equivalent in efficacy. ADHD symptoms that should improve with treatment include hyperactivity; attention span; impulsivity and self-control; compliance; physical and verbal aggression; social interactions with peers, teachers, and parents; and academic productivity. ADHD symptoms that may or may not improve include reading skills, social skills, learning (less improvement in this area than behavior), academic achievement, antisocial behavior, and arrest rates.[16] Although stimulants are more effective for improving behavioral symptoms than academic performance, these agents can improve classroom learning. Methylphenidate 0.3 mg/kg per dose improves performance on arithmetical and language tasks.[17] In addition, aggressive behavior, including stealing and vandalism, is improved by standard doses of methylphenidate 0.3 to 0.6 mg/kg. Stimulants decrease friction between siblings and peers and improve maternal–child interactions. Patients most likely to respond are characterized as having low ADHD severity, low anxiety, higher IQs, being younger, and being highly inattentive. The response from a single stimulant dose predicts the home and school behavioral response at 4 weeks.[18] Finally, patient adherence to stimulant medication correlates with greater improvement on teacher-reported symptoms, an effect that is stable for up to 5 years.[19]

2. C.B. and his mother come to the local pharmacy with a prescription for Concerta 18 mg, #30 tablets, one tablet in the morning with zero refills. The mother is upset with the cost of the medication. Her assumption was that methylphenidate was inexpensive. What relevant patient/caregiver counseling points can you make with respect to the cost of the immediate- and extended-release medications presented in Table 81-2? Suggest to the mother a simple quantitative method whereby she can monitor whether C.B. is responding to the medication. She is also concerned about potential side effects of psychostimulants that she has read about, such as drug addiction, tics, growth retardation, and other adverse effects. What counseling points would you make to her regarding these issues?

According to Table 81-2, generic formulations of short- and intermediate-acting psychostimulants are available. The intermediate-acting formulations of methylphenidate are effective for 6 to 8 hours. If the rationale for nonimmediate-release formulations is to spare the child the embarrassment of taking the medication at school, one of these less expensive products would be suitable.

The Iowa Connors Teacher's Scale—Revised is an example of an ADHD monitoring tool that is used by teachers for monitoring of children and adolescents at school. The scale consists of ten items scored as *not at all* (0), *a little bit* (1), *pretty much* (2), or *very much* (3). They are divided into two symptom clusters: the Attention Factor and the Conduct Factor. The five items of the Attention Factor consist of (a) fidgeting, (b) hums and makes other odd noises, (c) excitable (impulsive), (d) inattentive (easily distracted), and (e) fails to finish thing he starts. The five items of the Conduct Factor consist of (a) quarrelsome, (b) acts smart, (c) temper outburst (explosive, unpredictable behavior), (d) defiant, and (e) uncooperative. This scale has been updated such that normative data exist by both gender[20] and ethnicity.[21] Typically, children with untreated ADHD typically score 2 standard deviations above the mean for their comparison group. Following successful treatment, their score should decrease to <1 standard deviation above the mean.

Adverse drug reactions (ADRs) are relatively infrequent with the therapeutic use of psychostimulants for ADHD. According to a parental survey, the only side effect of methylphenidate more severe than at baseline was appetite suppression, whereas dextroamphetamine caused more severe insomnia and appetite suppression. Methylphenidate was better tolerated than dextroamphetamine because of more severe insomnia, appetite suppression, irritability, proneness to crying, anxiety, dysphoria, and nightmares. Only four of 125 subjects (3.2%) discontinued the medication because of side effects.[22] The association between psychostimulant use and growth retardation is controversial. Some authors contend that growth retardation occurs as a function of the disease rather than a result of psychostimulant use.[23] Others suggest that it is indeed possible for stimulants to cause growth retardation, but that this effect is reversible with drug holidays such as on the weekends or during the summer.[24] However, drug holidays have the risk of disruption of the psychosocial development of the child during the medication-free intervals. Stimulants have been alleged to precipitate or exacerbate tics in children in approximately 1.3% to 60% of ADHD patients.[25] Multiple randomized controlled trials have challenged the veracity of this adverse effect. As an example, the Tourette's Syndrome Study Group contrasted the effect of methylphenidate, clonidine, and the combination of the two to placebo in the treatment of 136 children (7–14 years old) diagnosed with ADHD and Tourette's Syndrome. The group concluded that prior recommendations to avoid methylphenidate in these children because of concerns of worsening tics were unsupported.[26]

Table 81-2 Characteristics of Psychostimulants

Product	*Maximum Dose (mg/d)*	*Peak Concentration (hr)*	*Duration of Action (hr)*
Short-acting psychostimulants (IR)			
Methylphenidate (Ritalin, Methylin, generic)	60	1–2	3–4
d-Methylphenidate (Focalin)	20	1–2	4–5
Dextroamphetamine (generic)	40	3	3–5
Intermediate-acting psychostimulants			
Methylphenidate (Ritalin SR, Methylin ER, Metadate ER, generic)	60	4–5	6–8
Dextroamphetamine (Dexedrine Spansules)	40	1st peak, 3; 2nd peak, 8	5–8
Mixed amphetamine salts (Adderall, generic)	30	3	3–7
Long-acting psychostimulants			
Methylphenidate (Metadate CD) 30:70 ratio of IR:ER product	60	1st peak, 1.5–3; 2nd peak, 4–6	6–9
Methylphenidate (Ritalin LA) 50:50 ratio of IR:ER product	60	1st peak, 1–2; 2nd peak, 5–7	8–10
Methylphenidate (Concerta)	54	1st peak, 1–2; 2nd peak, 6–8	12
Mixed amphetamine salts (Adderall XR)	30	1st peak, 3; 2nd peak, 7	10–12

CD, controlled dose; ER, extended release; IR, immediate release; LA, long acting; SR, sustained release; XR, extended release.

C.B.'s mother concerned about stimulant treatment increasing risk of her child becoming a substance abuser. This concern is probably unfounded. A meta-analysis of epidemiologic literature led to the conclusion that stimulant-treated patients with a diagnosis of ADHD were less likely to be diagnosed with substance use disorder than those not treated with stimulants.[27] However, C.B.'s mother's concerns are not completely without merit. In 2005, the U.S. Food and Drug Administration (FDA) added a warning to amphetamine package prescribing inserts to note that misuse of amphetamine may cause sudden death and serious cardiovascular adverse events.[28] Amphetamines should not be used in patients with structural cardiac abnormalities because of the risk of sudden unexplained death. In addition, there are a small number of cases of sudden unexplained death in children without cardiac abnormalities taking Adderall.

Tricyclic Antidepressants

3. Because of economic issues, C.B. has been treated with generic immediate-release methylphenidate for several years. He has two bottles of medication, one he keeps at home, while the other is held by the school nurse. When C.B. started junior high school, his mother noticed his home supply was gone before it needed refilling. It was discovered that C.B. was selling the methylphenidate to his friends at school. At this time, it was decided to treat C.B. with another class of drugs than the psychostimulants. His primary care practitioner asks for your recommendation regarding an alternative agent to treat C.B.'s ADHD. What alternatives would be recommended for C.B.?

TCAs have been used in the treatment of patients diagnosed with ADHD for nearly 30 years. There may be an ADHD subgroup that responds better to the TCAs than to stimulants. Because TCAs may be effective for the treatment of major depression and anxiety disorders in children and adolescents, this class of drugs might best be reserved for patients diagnosed with ADHD accompanied by major depression or any of the anxiety disorders such as obsessive-compulsive disorder. Six randomized controlled trials in ADHD have established the efficacy of amitriptyline,[29] imipramine,[30,31] desipramine,[32,33] and nortriptyline.[34] TCAs are more effective than placebo in treating ADHD, but they are less effective than methylphenidate. TCAs such as imipramine and clomipramine can also cause significant daytime sedation. This sedation is likely to adversely affect cognition in children diagnosed with ADHD. An additional concern that limits the utility of the TCAs in this patient population is their potential adverse effects on cardiac conduction. Six fatalities have been associated with desipramine administration in children; therefore, careful cardiac monitoring is imperative.[35] A baseline electrocardiogram (ECG) should be obtained, and then repeated when dosages reach 1.5 mg/kg/day, 3.0 mg/kg/day (typical maintenance dose), and 5 mg/kg/day (the maximum dose). With respect to the use of TCA in children and adolescents, the American Heart Association recommends a baseline history and physical, a current medication history, and a baseline ECG within the following parameters of PR interval = 200 milliseconds, QRS duration = 120 milliseconds, and QTc = 460 milliseconds.[36] Follow-up ECG and history are indicated after steady state is achieved and at the dosage thresholds listed above. Nortriptyline, because it is twice as potent, is dosed at 1.5 to 2.5 mg/kg/day and requires ECG monitoring at doses that reflect the difference in potency.

Bupropion

Six randomized controlled trials have established the effectiveness of bupropion as an alternative medication to the psychostimulants in the treatment of ADHD among children, adolescents, and adults.[37,38] One of the studies found bupropion at an average dose of approximately 3 mg/kg/day to be as effective as methylphenidate in the treatment of adolescents with ADHD.[39] The two most common adverse effects encountered with bupropion in ADHD studies were dermatologic reactions and seizures. Dermatologic reactions occurred twice as often as the placebo with severe bupropion-induced urticaria requiring discontinuation in 5.5% (4/72) of the patients in one study.[40] In adults, the risk of seizures increases by about fourfold if bupropion doses of >450 mg/day are exceeded.[41] Although there are no case reports of seizures in children receiving therapeutic doses of bupropion, it is recommended to confine the dose range for treating ADHD to less than 6 mg/kg/day.

Atomoxetine

Atomoxetine inhibits the presynaptic norepinephrine transporter and is not classified as a psychostimulant. Clinical trials have shown that atomoxetine is superior to placebo in reducing the symptoms of ADHD in children, adolescents, and adults.[42,43] However, a trial comparing atomoxetine to the mixed amphetamine salt product, Adderall, found atomoxetine to be less effective than the psychostimulant.[44] Atomoxetine requires a 10- to 14-day titration to the therapeutic dose of 1 to 1.5 mg/kg/day. The slow titration is necessitated by the high rates of nausea (12%), vomiting (15%), and asthenia (11%).[45] In addition, atomoxetine can raise blood pressure and heart rate. Two or more episodes of high systolic and diastolic blood pressures occurred in 8.6% and 5.2% of pediatric subjects, respectively. Heart rate increases of >110 beats/minute and more than 25 beats/minute over baseline were observed in 3.6% of patients.[45]

An additional concern regarding the use of TCAs, atomoxetine, and bupropion is the prescribing insert warning regarding an increase in suicidal thinking and behavior. Pooled analyses of short-term (4–16 weeks) placebo-controlled trials of nine antidepressant drugs in children and adolescents with major depressive disorder, obsessive-compulsive disorder, or other psychiatric disorders (a total of 24 trials involving more than 4,400 patients) revealed a greater risk of suicidal thinking or behavior during the first few months of treatment in those receiving antidepressants. The average risk of such events on drug was 4%, twice the placebo risk of 2%.[46] The seriousness of this warning has been questioned because no suicides occurred in these trials, and because the suicide rates for the 15- to 24-year-old age group in the United States decreased from 13.2/100,000 in 1990 to 9.9/100,000 in 2001.[47] The FDA has authored a patient information handout for pharmacists to give to parents whose children are receiving antidepressant prescriptions entitled *Medication Guide—Antidepressant Medicines, Depression, and Other Serious Mental Illnesses and Suicide Thoughts or Actions*.[48] Thus, this information packet should be given to the parents for patients receiving a TCA, bupropion, or atomoxetine prescription, even though they are being treated for ADHD.

Modafinil

Modafinil, at single daily doses ranging from 170 to 425 mg/day, has been found to be effective in the treatment of ADHD-diagnosed prepubescent, adolescent, and adult patients.[49,50] One small preliminary study found it to be as effective as dextroamphetamine in the treatment of adults with ADHD.[51] Common adverse effects include insomnia, headache, and decreased appetite, although discontinuation rates are similar to placebo.[52]

Because C.B. was selling a short-acting methylphenidate, considering a change to a different medication is reasonable. After discussion with C.B. and his parents, the treating physician may believe that C.B. is aware of the seriousness of this act and thus may elect to continue treatment with the stimulant medication. Conversely, a long-acting stimulant medication with less abuse potential could be considered. However, most clinicians would elect to change the patient's medication to a class without known abuse potential. Based on the available literature, both atomoxetine and bupropion would be reasonable alternatives. Both medications have the disadvantage of taking several days to weeks to become effective. Atomoxetine is not available in generic form; bupropion, even though it is available as a generic product, would be more expensive than methylphenidate. However, the safety margin for misuse of atomoxetine is greater than for bupropion and thus atomoxetine would be preferred by some providers as an alternative to C.B.'s use of methylphenidate.

4. A.D., a 6-year-old first grader, has responded well to his methylphenidate (Concerta) treatment during the school year. His mother sends him off to his father and stepmother for his annual summer visit, with explicit directions for the parents regarding how to use the medication. One month later, he returns home with a full bottle of medication. As he bounces around the room, A.D. reports that his father and stepmother said he did not need these "poison pills". A.D.'s mother phones the stepmother to find that they put A.D. on the Feingold diet along with sugar restriction to control his behavior. What are the roles of diet and alternative therapies in the treatment of ADHD?

The Feingold diet is the most widely known dietary intervention associated with the treatment of ADHD.[53] It is based on the theory that many children are sensitive to dietary salicylates and artificially added colors, flavors, and preservatives. The elimination of these substances from the diet has been proposed to improve learning and behavioral problems associated with ADHD. However, most randomized controlled trials do not support this hypothesis. In addition, the prevalence who have food sensitivities consistent with the Feingold diet among children with ADHD is very small.[53] Another dietary intervention hypothesis is that the elimination of all dietary sugars will reverse the hyperactivity associated with ADHD. However, the claims of an association between sugar intake and hyperactivity have not been supported, even in those children who are reportedly sensitive to the effects of sugar.[54] The use of very high doses of vitamins and/or minerals, known as megavitamin therapy, to treat ADHD is another intervention that lacks data to support its claim. All randomized controlled trials conducted to evaluate the effectiveness of megavitamin therapy in ADHD are negative. The American Psychiatric Association and American Academy of Pediatrics concluded that the use of megavitamin therapy to treat behavioral and learning problems is unjustified.[55]

5. G.S. is a 6-year-old boy referred to the Tourette Syndrome clinic by his pediatrician because of worsening motor (blinking, grimacing) and vocal (throat clearing, coprolalia, grunting) tics. He is treated successfully with clonidine 250 mcg/day. However, his behavior and performance in school is still so poor that his teacher refers him to the school psychologist, who diagnoses ADHD, combined type. A trial of stimulant treatment is considered. The parents are concerned about treating his two disorders simultaneously with the clonidine and a stimulant. Can stimulants be used in children with both disorders?

The two commonly prescribed alpha-2-adrenergic agonists in child-adolescent psychiatry, clonidine and guanfacine, are not approved by the FDA for any psychiatric indication. However, a large randomized controlled trial supports the use of clonidine in the treatment of comorbid Tourette Syndrome and ADHD.[56] The Tourette Syndrome Study Group compared the effect of methylphenidate (mean, 26 mg/day), clonidine (mean, 250 mcg/day), and the combination (methylphenidate ~26 mg/day + clonidine mean, 280 mcg/day) to placebo in the treatment of 136 children (7–14 year olds) diagnosed with ADHD and Tourette Syndrome. Teacher ratings showed that both clonidine and methylphenidate used as individual treatments were more effective than placebo. However, the greatest improvement was seen with the combination therapy. Clonidine primarily benefited the symptoms of impulsivity and hyperactivity, while methylphenidate primarily benefited inattention. A meta-analysis of trials evaluating the efficacy of the clonidine for the treatment of children and adolescents with ADHD concluded that the effect size of the drug was modest (0.58) and less than that of the psychostimulants.[57] Despite its widespread use, there is just one randomized controlled trial that documents the effectiveness of guanfacine in the treatment of patients diagnosed with ADHD and/or a tic disorder. Thirty-four medication-free elementary school–age children with ADHD and a tic disorder participated.[58] After 8 weeks of treatment with a modal dose of 1 mg guanfacine TID, the children had a mean improvement of 37% in their total score on the teacher-rated ADHD Rating Scale, compared to 8% improvement for placebo. Continuous Performance Test commission errors decreased by 22% and omission errors by 17% in the treated group, compared with increases of 29% in commission errors and of 31% in omission errors in the placebo group. However, the parent-rated hyperactivity on dextroamphetamine improved by 27% in the guanfacine group and 21% in the placebo group, a nonsignificant difference.

6. G.S.'s mother places a call to the clinic asking to talk to his physician. She tells the physician that the school psychologist recommended a complicated behavioral modification program that the parents were to institute for G.S. The mother instituted the program, but after two weeks, she was exhausted. In her opinion, the behavioral modification provided no benefit after one month. She asks the physician whether behavioral modification benefits the symptoms of ADHD.

The Multimodal Treatment Study of Children with ADHD (MTA) Cooperative Group was designed to compare long-term medication and behavioral treatments with respect to efficacy. A group of 579 children between 7 and 10 years of age with ADHD combined type were recruited and randomized to four different treatment groups.[24] The children were included even if they had comorbid diagnoses, including conduct disorder, oppositional defiant disorder, or a learning disability. The treatment groups included drug treatment regimen, behavioral treatment, drug treatment regimen plus behavioral treatment, or typical community treatment. Behavioral interventions were delivered in a group-based recreational setting and included an 8-week, 5-days-per-week, 9-hours-per-day, intensive program administered by a counselor/aid. Once school started, the subjects in this arm of the study received 60 school days of a part-time, behaviorally trained, paraprofessional aid who worked directly with the child. In addition, the child's teacher received 10 to 16 sessions of biweekly consultation that focused on classroom behavior management strategies. Daily behavior report cards were sent home to parents. At the same time, families were involved in 27 group therapy meetings plus 8 individual family meetings. The goal of this behavioral management treatment was to train the parents to administer appropriate techniques so they could continue the treatment on their own. Of the children receiving medication, 75% received methylphenidate; 10% received dextroamphetamine; and 15% received pemoline, imipramine, clonidine, guanfacine, or bupropion. It was concluded that drug treatment was more effective than behavioral treatment according to parents' and teachers' ratings of inattention, and teachers' ratings of hyperactivity-impulsivity. Combined treatment (drug treatment plus behavioral modification) was equally effective as medication management only and more effective than behavioral treatment and community care according to parent- and teacher-reported ADHD symptoms. A regimented drug treatment protocol for ADHD appears to be both beneficial and cost effective. However, the study did confirm that if comorbid disorders such as conduct, oppositional defiant, anxiety, or affective were present, then behavior management with or without drug treatment was beneficial for these comorbid conditions. The behavioral management techniques used in this study were costly and highly labor-intensive.

7. G.S. returns to clinic 3 months later for a follow-up appointment. He is doing quite well receiving a combination of methylphenidate and clonidine but no behavioral therapy. His mother has been using the Iowa Connors Rating Scale for ADHD which she was taught to use as a way to monitor her son's behavior. Her observational scores show him to have an approximate average score of 8 for the past week. This score is significantly decreased from a score of 24 at his initial workup. The teacher's scores on the rating scale are similar to the mothers' scores. The mother asks the physician if they could talk privately for a few minutes. She relates to the physician that out of curiosity, she has been sporadically scoring the test for her husband, G.S.'s biological father, for several weeks. Although the conduct factor was normal, she reports that he scores about a 12 on the attention factor. She inquires whether her husband would be a candidate for psychostimulant therapy for ADHD. He was treated for 2 years as a child for hyperactivity, but then his parents stopped the treatment when his hyperactive behavior improved. What is the natural course of ADHD through adulthood? Are the effective treatments for adolescents and children diagnosed with ADHD effective in adults as well?

The experience of G.S.'s father is similar to that of many adults who were diagnosed with ADHD as children. Thus, in a series of 128 boys, hyperactivity and impulsivity symptoms were seen to decline at a higher rate than inattention symptoms.[59] Among 18 to 20 years olds with ADHD who were followed up over 4 years, 40% continued to meet the *Diagnostic and Statistical Manual of Mental Disorders*, Third Edition, Revised (DSM-III-R) criteria for ADHD. Importantly more than 90% of the 18 to 20 year olds continued to experience functional problems with inattention.[59] Other researchers have followed children with ADHD to adulthood by comparing the academic records of controls and ADHD adults. The latter had significantly higher rates of repeated grades, tutoring, placement in special classes, and reading disability.[60,61] Adults with ADHD have been found to achieve lower socioeconomic status and experience more work difficulties and more frequent job changes.[62] In a study comparing 172 ADHD adults to 30 non-ADHD adults, the adults with ADHD reported more psychological maladjustment, more speeding violations, and more frequent changes in employment.[63] More adults with ADHD had their driver's licenses suspended, had performed poorer at work, and had quit or been fired from their job. Adults with ADHD also were more likely to have had multiple marriages.

Numerous studies have documented the effectiveness of methylphenidate,[64] desmethylphenidate,[65] mixed amphetamines,[66] desipramine,[67] bupropion,[38] atomoxetine,[68,69] and modafanil[50] in the treatment of adults with ADHD. All of the trials were similar in that the experimental drug was compared with placebo with the exception of modafinil, where an amphetamine comparator was used along with placebo. A notable finding is that the effect sizes for improvement relative to placebo were lower with atomoxetine (0.35 and 0.40 in two studies) than with methylphenidate and amphetamine (effect sizes of 0.8 to 1.0). This indirect evidence suggests that atomoxetine may be less effective than the stimulants for ADHD treatment. Doses for immediate-release methylphenidate are more conservative (0.3 mg/kg per dose in adults) when inattention is the predominate feature. In contrast, doses of up to 0.6 mg/kg immediate-release methylphenidate are often necessary to optimally control the behavioral feature of the disorder.[70] These methylphenidate doses are consistent with 0.5 to 1.0 mg/kg/day doses found to be effective in adults.[64] Mixed amphetamine salts are effective in doses of 20 to 60 mg/day.[66] The effective dose of desipramine is approximately 150 mg/day. Bupropion is generally dosed at 3 mg/kg/day.[41] The two large studies of atomoxetine used doses that ranged from 60 to 120 mg/day.[69] The mean effective dose for modafinil was 207 mg/day.[50]

8. An editorial by a community newspaper criticized the local school district for the widespread prescribing of psychostimulants by school psychologists. The editorial provided the stimulus for a review by the school board of the clinical practices of the psychologist staff. A regional expert on ADHD pharmacotherapy was contacted by the board and asked to present a rational set of medication prescribing guidelines for the treatment of children and adolescents diagnosed with ADHD. The expert decided that the

most straightforward approach to this issue would be to present the Texas Medication Algorithm Project (TMAP) guidelines for the treatment of ADHD in children and adolescents. Describe the TMAP algorithm for the treatment of children and adolescents diagnosed with ADHD.

The goal of the TMAP algorithm is to provide systematic guidance and structure regarding the potential array of therapeutic options for the ADHD population. There are five algorithms for ADHD treatment; one each for the following diagnoses: (a) ADHD, (b) ADHD with major depressive disorder, (c) ADHD with any anxiety disorder, (d) ADHD with a tic disorder such as Tourette Syndrome, and (e) ADHD with aggression.[71] The algorithms and the details of their use can be found on the Texas Department of State Health Services website (http://www.dshs.state.tx.us/mhprograms/ CMAP.shtm).[73] For patients with ADHD only, it is recommended to initiate treatment with either methylphenidate or an amphetamine. Patients who fail the first psychostimulant can then be treated with the alternate psychostimulant. For patients that fail the stimulants, a trial of atomoxetine is warranted. If atomoxetine fails, a TCA or bupropion can be tried. If these drugs both fail, the alpha-adrenergic agonists, clonidine and guanfacine, should be considered. Patients diagnosed with comorbid ADHD and major depressive disorder can be treated according to both the TMAP ADHD and Major Depressive Disorder algorithms. In patients with comorbid ADHD and an anxiety disorder, initial treatment with atomoxetine or a psychostimulant is recommended. If these treatments fail, the combination of atomoxetine with a psychostimulant, or a psychostimulant with a selective serotonin reuptake inhibitor should be considered. Patients with ADHD and a tic disorder can be treated similarly to those with ADHD only. However, if the tics worsen, an alpha-adrenergic agonist, atypical antipsychotic haloperidol, or pimozide can be tried individually until the patient responds. For patients with significant comorbid aggression, the standard ADHD algorithm should be used; behavioral interventions are added if the patient's behavior does not improve. If behavioral modification fails, an atypical antipsychotic, lithium, or valproate should be considered. Clinicians should not follow the algorithm blindly. It should be emphasized that algorithms integrate available research and clinical consenus into user-friendly, hierarchical decision trees of mediation options. The algorithms are not intended to serve as a substitute for clinician judgment.

REFERENCES

1. DeGrandpre R. *Ritalin Nation.* New York: W. W. Norton; 2000.
2. Hoffmann H. Struwwelpeter; 1863. Available at: http://www.fln.vcu.edu/struwwel/struwwel.html. Accessed March 2, 2008.
3. Safer DJ. Are stimulants overprescribed for youths with ADHD? *Ann Clin Psychiatry* 2000;12:55.
4. Sostek AJ et al. Effects of amphetamine on vigilance performance in normal and hyperactive children. *J Abnorm Child Psychol* 1980;8:491.
5. Centers for Disease Control and Prevention (CDC). Mental health in the United States. Prevalence of diagnosis and medication treatment for attention-deficit/hyperactivity disorder–United States, 2003. *MMWR Morb Mortal Wkly Rep* 2005; 54:842.
6. Weiss G, Hechtman LT. *Hyperactive Children Grow Up: Empirical Findings and Theoretical Considerations.* New York: Guilford Press; 1988.
7. Wilens TE et al. Pharmacotherapy of adult attention-deficit hyperactivity disorder: a review. *J Clin Psychopharmacol* 1995;15:270.
8. Fargason RE, Ford CV. Attention deficit hyperactivity disorder in adults: diagnosis, treatment, and prognosis. *South Med J* 1994;87:302.
9. Cohen DJ et al. Dopamine and serotonin metabolism in neuropsychiatrically disturbed children: CSF HVA and 5-HIAA. *Arch Gen Psychiatry* 1977; 34:545.
10. Young JG et al. Platelet monoamine oxidase activity in children and adolescents with psychiatric disorders. *Schizophren Bull* 1980;6:324.
11. Zametkin A et al. Treatment of hyperactive children wit monoamine oxidase inhibitors: I. clinical efficacy. *Arch Gen Psychiatry* 1985;42:962.
12. Voeller KKS. Attention-deficit hyperactivity disorder (ADHD). *J Child Neurol* 2004;19:798.
13. Green W. Pharmacotherapy: stimulants. *Child Adolesc Psychiatr Clin N Am* 1992;1:411.
14. Dulcan MK. Using psychostimulants to treat behavioral disorders of children and adolescents. *J Child Adolesc Psychopharmacol* 1990;1:7.
15. Jadad AR et al. Treatment of attention-hyperactivity disorder. *Evid Rep Technol Assess (Summ)* 1999;11:1.
16. Swanson JM et al. Effects of stimulant medication on learning in children with ADHD. *J Learn Disabil* 1991;24:219.
17. Douglas VI et al. Short-term effects of methylphenidate on the cognitive, learning and academic performance of children with attention deficit disorder in the laboratory and the classroom. *J Child Psychol Psychiatry* 1986;27:191.
18. Buitelarr JK et al. Prediction of clinical response to methylphenidate in children with attention-deficit hyperactivity disorder. *J Am Acad Child Adolesc Psychiatry* 1995;34:1025.
19. Charach A et al. Stimulant treatment over five years: adherence, effectiveness and adverse effects. *J Am Acad Child Adolesc Psychiatry* 2004;43: 559.
20. Pelham WE Jr, et al. Normative data on the IOWA Conners Teacher Rating Scale. *J Clin Child Psychol* 1989;18:259.
21. Reid R et al. Using behavior rating scales for ADHD across ethnic groups: the IOWA Conners. *J Emot Behav Disord* 2001;9:210.
22. Efron D et al. Side effects of methylphenidate and dextroamphetamine in children with attention deficit hyperactivity disorder: a double-blind, crossover trial. *Pediatrics* 1997;100:662.
23. Spencer TJ et al. Growth deficits in ADHD children revisited: evidence for disorder-associated growth delays? *J Am Acad Child Adolesc Psychiatry* 1996;35:1460.
24. MTA (Multimodal Treatment Study of Children with ADHD) Cooperative Group: National Institute of Mental Health Multimodal Treatment Study of ADHD follow-up: changes in effectiveness and growth after the end of treatment. *Pediatrics* 2004;113:762.
25. Lipkin PH, et al. Tics and dyskinesias associated with stimulant treatment in attention-deficit hyperactivity disorder. *Arch Pediatr Adolesc Med* 1994;14:859.
26. The Tourette's Syndrome Study Group. Treatment of ADHD in children with tics: a randomized controlled trial. *Neurology* 2002;58:526.
27. Wilens TE et al. A systematic chart review of the nature of psychiatric adverse events in children and adolescents with selective serotonin reuptake inhibitors. *J Am Acad Child Adolesc Psychiatry* 2003;13:143.
28. U.S. Food and Drug Administration. Patient information sheet. Adderall and Adderall XR extended release capsules, 2005. Available at: http://www.fda.gov/cder/drug/infosheets/patient/adderallPatientSheet.pdf.
29. Krakowski AJ. Amitriptyline in the treatment of hyperkinetic children: a double-blind study. *Psychosomatics* 1965;6:355.
30. Gross MD. Imipramine in the treatment of minimal brain dysfunction in children. *Psychosomatics* 1973;14:283.
31. Rapoport JL et al. Childhood enuresis. II. Psychopathology, tricyclic concentration in plasma, and antineuritic effect. *Arch Gen Psychiatry* 1980; 37:1146.
32. Donnelly M et al. Treatment of childhood hyperactivity with desipramine: plasma drug concentration, cardiovascular effects, plasma and urine catecholamine levels and clinical response. *Clin Pharmacol Ther* 1986;39:72.
33. Biederman J et al. A double-blind placebo controlled study of desipramine in the treatment of ADD: I. efficacy. *J Am Acad Child Adolesc Psychiatry* 1989;28:777.
34. Prince JB et al. A controlled study of nortriptyline in children and adolescents with attention-deficit hyperactivity disorder. *J Child Adolesc Psycholpharmacol* 2000;10:193.
35. Varley CK, McClellan J. Case study: two additional sudden deaths with tricyclic antidepressants. *J Am Acad Child Adolesc Psychiatry* 1997;36: 390.
36. Gutgesell H et al. Cardiovascular monitoring of children and adolescents receiving psychotropic drugs: a statement for healthcare professionals from the Committee on Congenital Cardiac Defects, Council on Cardiovascular Disease in the Young, American Heart Association. *Circulation* 1999;9:979.
37. Simeon JG et al. Bupropion effects in attention deficit and conduct disorders. *Can J Psychiatry* 1986;31:581.

38. Kuperman S et al. Bupropion SR vs methylphenidate vs placebo for attention deficit hyperactivity disorder in adults. *Ann Clin Psychiatry*, 2001; 13:129.
39. Barrickman LL et al. Bupropion versus methylphenidate in the treatment of attention deficit hyperactivity disorder. *J Am Acad Child Adolesc Psychiatry* 1995;34:649.
40. Conners CK et al. Bupropion hydrochloride in attention-deficit disorder with hyperactivity. *J Am Acad Child Adolesc Psychiatry* 1996;35:1314.
41. Davidson J. Seizures and bupropion: a review. *J Clin Psychiatry* 1989;50:256.
42. Michelson D et al. Atomoxetine in the treatment of children and adolescents with attention-deficit hyperactivity disorder: a randomized, placebo-controlled, dose-response study. *Pediatrics* 2001;108:e83.
43. Michelson D et al. Once-daily atomoxetine treatment for children and adolescents with ADHD: a randomized, placebo-controlled study. *Am J Psychiatry* 2002;159:1896.
44. Wigal J et al. A laboratory school comparison of mixed amphetamine salts extended release (Adderall XR) and atomoxetine (Strattera) in school-aged children with attention deficit/hyperactivity disorder. *J Atten Disord* 2005;9:275.
45. Eli Lilly. Strattera [atomoxetine] package insert. Indianapolis, IN; 2004.
46. U.S. Food and Drug Administration. Revisions to product labeling. 2007, May 2. Available at: http://www.fda.gov/cder/drug/antidepressants/antidepressants_MG_2007.pdf. Accessed March 27, 2008.
47. National Center for Health Statistics. Deaths: final report for 2001. Rockville, MD: National Center for Health Statistics; 2003. DHEW Publication No. (HSM) 2003-1120.
48. U.S. Food and Drug Administration. Revisions to product labeling. 2007, May 2. Available at: http://www.fda.gov/cder/drug/antidepressants/antidepressants_label_change_2007.pdf. Accessed March 2, 2008.
49. Biederman J et al. A comparison of once-daily and divided doses of modafinil in children with attention-deficit/hyperactivity disorder: a randomized, double-blind, and placebo-controlled study. *J Clin Psychiatry* 2006;67:727.
50. Taylor FB, Russo J. Efficacy of modafinil compared to dextroamphetamine for the treatment of attention deficit hyperactivity disorder in adults. *J Child Adolesc Psychopharmacol* 2000;10:311.
51. Greenhill LL et al. A randomized, double-blind, placebo-controlled study of modafinil film-coated tablets in children and adolescents with attention-deficit/hyperactivity disorder. *J Am Acad Child Adolesc Psychiatry* 2006;45:503.
52. Biederman J et al. Efficacy and safety of modafinil film-coated tablets in children and adolescents with attention-deficit/hyperactivity disorder: results of a randomized, double-blind, placebo-controlled, flexible-dose study. *Pediatrics* 2005;116:e777.
53. Ekvall SW, Ekvall VK. *Pediatric Nutrition in Chronic Diseases and Developmental Disorders.* 2nd ed. New York: Oxford University Press; 2005.
54. American Dietetic Association. American Dietetic Association position paper: use of nutritive and nonnutritive sweeteners. *J Am Diet Assoc* 2004;104:255.
55. Marcason W. Can dietary intervention play a part in the treatment of attention deficit and hyperactivity disorder? *J Am Diet Assoc* 2005;105:1161.
56. The Tourette's Syndrome Study Group. Treatment of ADHD in children with tics: a randomized controlled trial. *Neurology* 2002;58:526.
57. Connor DF et al. A meta-analysis of clonidine for symptoms of attention-deficit hyperactivity disorder. *J Am Acad Child Adolesc Psychiatry* 1999;38:1551.
58. Scahill L et al. A placebo-controlled study of guanfacine in the treatment of children with tic disorders and attention deficit hyperactivity disorder. *Am J Psychiatry* 2001;158:1067.
59. Biederman J et al. Age-dependent decline of symptoms of attention deficit hyperactivity disorder: impact of remission definition and symptom type. *Am J Psychiatry* 2000;157:816.
60. Biederman J et al. Patterns of psychiatric comorbidity, cognition, and psychosocial functioning in adults with attention deficit hyperactivity disorder. *Am J Psychiatry* 1993;150:1792.
61. Biederman J et al. Gender differences in a sample of adults with attention deficit hyperactivity disorder. *Psychiatry Res* 1994;53:13.
62. Borland BL, Heckman HK. Hyperactive boys and their brothers: a 25-year follow-up study. *Arch Gen Psychiatry* 1976;33:669.
63. Murphy K, Barkley RA. Attention deficit hyperactivity disorder adults: comorbidities and adaptive impairments. *Compr Psychiatry* 1996;37:393.
64. Spencer T et al. A double-blind, crossover comparison of methylphenidate and placebo in adults with childhood-onset attention-deficit hyperactivity disorder. *Arch Gen Psychiatry* 1995;52:434.
65. Spencer TJ et al. Efficacy and safety of dexmethylphenidate extended-release capsules in adults with attention-deficit/hyperactivity disorder. *Biol Psychiatry* 2007;15:1380.
66. Weisler RH et al. Mixed amphetamine salts extended-release in the treatment of adult ADHD: a randomized, controlled trial. *CNS Spectr* 2006; 11:625.
67. Wilens TE et al. Six-week, double-blind, placebo-controlled study of desipramine for adult attention deficit hyperactivity disorder. *Am J Psychiatry* 1996;153:1147.
68. Spencer T et al. Effectiveness and tolerability of tomoxetine in adults with attention deficit hyperactivity disorder. *Am J Psychiatry* 1998;155:693.
69. Michelson et al. Atomoxetine in adults with ADHD: two randomized, placebo-controlled studies. *Biol Psychiatry* 2003;53:112.
70. Sprague RL, Sleator EK. Methylphenidate in hyperkinetic children: differences in dose effects on learning and social behavior. *Science* 1977;198:1274.
71. Plizka SR et al. The Texas Children's Medication Algorithm Project: revision of the algorithm for pharmacotherapy of attention-deficit/hyperactivity disorder. *J Clin Psychiatry* 2006;45:642.
72. Texas Department of Health Services. CMAP: Attention-deficit hyperactivity disorder, May 16, 2006. Available at http://www.dhs.state.tx.us/ mhprograms/Adhdpage.shtm. Accessed March 27, 2008.
73. American Psychiatric Association (APA). *Diagnostic and Statistical Manual of Mental Disorders.* 4th ed. Washington, DC: APA; 2000.

CHAPTER 82

Eating Disorders

Martha P. Fankhauser and Kelly C. Lee

Control of eating and maintenance of normal body weight are common problems in our society. Despite the public and medical pressure to "stay fit," the incidence of obesity has doubled over the past two decades, particularly among children and adolescents.[1] A review of eating disorders and obesity, as well as recommendations for self-help books and websites related to eating disorders, can be found in the *Clinical Manual of Eating Disorders*[2] and the second edition of *Eating Disorders and Obesity: A Comprehensive Handbook*.[1] The third edition of the American Psychiatric Association *Practice Guidelines for the Treatment of Patients with Eating Disorders* provides the most recent diagnostic and treatment guidelines for anorexia nervosa, bulimia nervosa, and binge-eating disorder.[3] Although effective therapies for eating disorders exist, many people do not seek treatment and many cases are not recognized in clinical settings.

DEFINITIONS: EATING AND RELATED DISORDERS

Eating Disorders

Eating disorders should be considered a syndrome characterized by a cluster of symptoms that define the condition.[1–4] Anorexia nervosa, bulimia nervosa, binge-eating, and obesity are examples of eating or metabolic disorders that evolve as a result of weight loss behaviors and/or by a complex interaction of social, developmental, and biological factors. Diagnosis of eating disorders is based on weight, engagement in weight loss behaviors (e.g., restricting or avoiding food, vomiting, laxative and diuretic abuse, use of appetite suppressants, overexercising), binge-eating behaviors, abnormal attitudes and preoccupation with weight, shape, and food, and medical consequences.[4] Preoccupations with body weight and shape, food avoidance, and overeating are relatively "modern" clinical disorders. In Western societies, men have less pressure to be slim and to diet compared with young females (e.g., less media influences on dieting and exposure to abnormally thin body images). It is estimated that up to two-thirds of teenage girls and one in six adult women in the United States diet each year.[1,2,5] Compared with men, women are twice as likely to report current dieting or a history of dieting. Adolescent girls often start dieting around 12 to 13 years and the rates increase between the ages of 12 and 16.[1] Dieting in males is more likely to be associated with participation in sports, gender identity conflicts, past obesity, and fear of medical complications than from any sociocultural pressures for dieting. Many "fad" diets provide inadequate nutrition, are medically dangerous, and result in

Table 82-1 Body Mass Index and Guidelines for Weight Classes

Metric Conversion Formula Using Kilograms and Meters

$$\text{BMI} = \frac{\text{Weight in kilograms}}{\text{Height in meters}^2}$$

Nonmetric Conversion Formula Using Pounds and Inches

$$\text{BMI} = \frac{\text{Weight in pounds}}{\text{Height in inches}^2} \times 703$$

Weight Status	*BMI*	*Obesity Class*
Anorexia nervosa	≤17.5	
Underweight	<18.5	
Normal	18.5–24.9	
Overweight	25.0–29.9	
Obesity	30.0–34.9	I
	35.0–39.9	II
Extreme obesity	≥40	III

Adapted from reference 14.

rebound weight gain after dieting owing to starvation-induced reduction in metabolic rate. Starvation or the lack of regular intake of food produces both physiologic and psychological symptoms (i.e., anxiety, irritability, and distractibility), a preoccupation with food, a drive to eat, and binge-eating behaviors.[1]

People without eating disorders seem to integrate cultural, behavioral, and chemical changes (release of chemicals from the stomach, intestine, and brain) to produce an appropriate perception of hunger or satiation and are more likely to maintain an ideal weight. Ideal body weight can be measured by a number of calculations, but the body mass index (BMI) is most commonly used for assessing weight based on age and gender norms.[6,7] For calculations of BMI and guidelines for weight classes, see Table 82-1. Behaviors associated with each eating disorder are unique, but may overlap and occur throughout the individual's lifetime (Table 82-2 compares eating disorders).

Anorexia Nervosa

The term *anorexia* (the medical term for loss of appetite) was first used in 1873 by an English physician, Sir William Gull, who described a young woman with restrictive dieting and amenorrhea. When the focus on weight and thinness becomes pathological and detrimental to the person's health (e.g., deficiency in essential amino acids, vitamins, minerals, and electrolytes; bone loss; depression; and cardiac changes) it is called *anorexia nervosa.* Criteria from the *Diagnostic and Statistical Manual of Mental Disorders,* Fourth Edition-Text Revision (DSM-IV-TR) are listed in Table 82-3.[4] Anorexia nervosa is defined by a BMI ≤17.5 kg/m^2. Because linear growth may be impaired in people with anorexia nervosa owing to poor nutrition, adjustments to height and weight calculations must be made based on expected values for the age range.[1] Weight loss, a refusal to maintain a minimal normal weight for age and height, and amenorrhea are characteristic features of the disorder. Classic symptoms and attitudes include persistent and irrational fear of becoming overweight, a distorted perception of body image, and denial of the seriousness of the illness.[8]

Anorexia nervosa is divided into two subtypes: restricting and binge-eating/purging.[4] Weight loss is accomplished primarily by the reduction in total food intake (restriction), although most eventually try purging (misuse of laxatives and diuretics or self-induced vomiting) and use of excessive exercise to lose weight. Approximately 50% of women with anorexia nervosa develop bulimic symptoms; some women who initially have bulimic symptoms later develop anorexic symptoms.[3] Patients with anorexia can alternate between restricting and bulimic subtypes throughout their illness. Individuals with the binge-eating/purging type are likely to exhibit more impulse control behaviors such as suicidal and self-harm behaviors, drug and alcohol abuse, mood lability, and increased sexual activity.[3,8]

Bulimia Nervosa

Bulimia, or binge eating (consuming a large amount of food over a short period of time), was first described in 1979 by

Table 82-2 Comparison of Eating Disorders

	Anorexia Nervosa	*Bulimia Nervosa*	*Binge-Eating Disorder*
Lifetime prevalence	0.5%–1% females	1%–4% females	Unknown
Prevalence rates			0.7%–4% (community) 20%–30% (weight control programs)
Female:male	10:1	10:1	1.5:1
Onset	Mid to late adolescence (14–18 years)	Late adolescence or early adulthood	Late adolescence or early 20s
Cross-over from AN to BN or vice versa	15%	~1%	NA
Subthreshold eating disorder	15%	20%	Unknown
Persistent disorder	10%	10%	Unknown
No clinical eating disorder after long-term follow-up (10 yr after referral)	50%	70%	Unknown
Death	<10%	~1%	Unknown

AN, anorexia nervosa; BN, bulimia nervosa; NA, not applicable.
Adapted from references 1, 2, and 4.

Table 82-3 DSM-IV-TR Diagnostic Criteria for Anorexia Nervosa[4]

A. Refusal to maintain body weight at or above a minimally normal weight for age and height (e.g., weight loss leading to maintenance of body weight <85% of that expected; or failure to make expected weight gain during period of growth, leading to body weight <85% of that expected).
B. Intense fear of gaining weight or becoming fat, even though underweight.
C. Disturbances in the way that one's body weight or shape is experienced, undue influence of body weight or shape on self-evaluation, or denial of the seriousness of the current low body weight.
D. In postmenarchal females, amenorrhea (the absence of at least three consecutive menstrual cycles). (A woman is considered to have amenorrhea if her periods occur only following hormone [e.g., estrogen] administration.)

Specify types:

Restricting type: During the current episode of anorexia nervosa, the person has not regularly engaged in binge eating or purging behavior (i.e., self-induced vomiting or the misuse of laxatives, diuretics, or enemas).

Binge eating/purging type: During the current episode of anorexia nervosa, the person has regularly engaged in binge eating or purging behavior (i.e., self-induced vomiting or the misuse of laxatives, diuretics, or enemas).

Table 82-4 DSM-IV-TR Diagnostic Criteria for Bulimia Nervosa[4]

A. Recurrent episodes of binge eating. An episode of binge eating is characterized by both of the following:
   1. Eating, in a discrete period of time (e.g., within any 2-hour period), an amount of food that is definitely larger than most people would eat during a similar period of time and under similar circumstances
   2. A sense of lack of control over eating during the episode (e.g., a feeling that one cannot stop eating or control what or how much one is eating)
B. Recurrent inappropriate compensatory behavior to prevent weight gain, such as self-induced vomiting; misuse of laxatives, diuretics, enemas, or other medications; fasting; or excessive exercise
C. The binge-eating and inappropriate compensatory behaviors both occur, on average, at least twice a week for 3 months
D. Self-evaluation is unduly influenced by body shape and weight
E. The disturbance does not occur exclusively during episodes of anorexia nervosa

Specify types:

Purging type: During the current episode of bulimia nervosa, the person has regularly engaged in self-induced vomiting or the misuse of laxatives, diuretics, or enemas

Nonpurging type: During the current episode of bulimia nervosa, the person has used other inappropriate compensatory behaviors, such as fasting or excessive exercise, but has not regularly engaged in self-induced vomiting or the misuse of laxatives, diuretics, or enemas

Gerald Russell, a London psychiatrist, who observed that several of his anorectic patients went on eating binges. Bulimia was first recognized as a separate disorder from anorexia nervosa in 1980 in the DSM-III. Originally, the criteria emphasized binge-eating behaviors without the associated features of self-induced vomiting, laxative abuse, and preoccupation with shape and weight. Individuals with bulimia have a powerful urge to overeat in combination with a fear of becoming fat; thus, they induce vomiting or abuse purgatives or both to get rid of ingested foods. One essential distinction from anorexia is that patients with bulimia nervosa usually maintain a normal weight, although a few patients are overweight or obese.[2]

The diagnostic criteria for bulimia nervosa have evolved over time to the most current DSM-IV-TR criteria (Table 82-4).[4] The characteristics of bulimia nervosa include binge-eating along with inappropriate compensatory behaviors and methods to prevent weight gain that occur, on average, at least twice weekly for 3 months. Patients must satisfy all five criteria (Table 82-4) to be diagnosed with bulimia nervosa and may be further classified as either the purging or nonpurging type. Individuals with bulimia nervosa may use several methods to compensate for binge-eating. Vomiting after binge-eating (or purging) is the most common technique and is used by 80% to 90% of individuals with bulimia nervosa.[3] In comparison with nonpurging bulimics, those with purging behaviors have more anxiety about eating, a greater disturbance in body image, more self-injurious behaviors, and a higher incidence of comorbid anxiety, depression, and alcohol abuse.[1] Nonpurging forms of bulimia nervosa may include excessive exercise or fasting, taking appetite suppressants or stimulants, and use of insulin for weight control in patients with diabetes mellitus.[1]

Eating Disorder Not Otherwise Specified

A subset of individuals may have characteristics of anorexia nervosa and bulimia nervosa, but do not meet the complete diagnostic criteria of the disorder.[2] In the DSM-IV-TR, these individuals are classified as having an "Eating Disorder Not Otherwise Specified" (ED-NOS), which also has been called an *atypical eating disorder.*[4] Subsyndromal or subclinical eating disorders have been found in 7% to 10% of young women. Up to 50% of individuals presenting to eating disorder programs are given the diagnosis of ED-NOS because they fail to meet one DSM-IV-TR criteria (e.g., <2 eating binges per week for 3 months, <3 months of amenorrhea).[3] Individuals who abuse weight reduction medications, take anabolic steroids, or use excessive exercise to lose weight and those with binge-eating behaviors are diagnosed with ED-NOS. Extreme vegetarians or vegans may be a type of eating disorder due to their obsessive aversion to ingesting meat or animal byproducts and strict avoidance of animal-derived foods. Cases of food refusal and undernutrition secondary to hypochondriasis may be an atypical eating disorder.[1] Individuals with a subsyndromal eating disorder are at risk for developing anorexia nervosa and bulimia nervosa and need professional help to reduce abnormal eating habits, food restriction, body image distortion, and compulsive exercising.[3]

Binge-Eating Disorder

Binge-eating disorder is a proposed diagnostic entity in the DSM-IV-TR and is characterized by recurrent binge-eating episodes unaccompanied by behaviors to prevent the weight gain, such as self-induced vomiting or laxative abuse.[2–4] The diagnostic criteria requires binge-eating episodes that are associated with three (or more) of the following: eating very rapidly; eating until feeling uncomfortable; eating large amounts of food when not physically hungry; eating alone because of embarrassment about how much is eaten; and feeling disgusted, guilty, or depressed about overeating.[2,4] Binge-eating episodes must occur at least 2 days a week for 6 months and cause significant distress about binge-eating. In some individuals, binge-eating may be triggered by dysphoric moods such as anxiety and depression, whereas others may feel "numb" or "spaced out" during the eating episode.[2,4] Binge-eating patients are more likely to overeat in response to negative emotional states, and obese binge-eaters often eat in response to emotional stress.[2] A night eating syndrome characterized by insomnia with evening hyperphagia has been recognized as a type of binge-eating disorder.[1] Nighttime eaters suffer from frequent awakenings and their snack intake is usually high carbohydrate-to-protein foods. During the night, they can consume more than 50% of their normal daily caloric intake.

Approximately 15% to 50% (average, 30%) of people in weight control programs fit the criteria for a binge-eating disorder; approximately one-third of these individuals are male.[3,4] Binge-eating disorder may be a type of nonpurging bulimia nervosa or an overeating disorder, because this pattern of eating is found in both bulimia nervosa and obesity.[9] Chronic, recurrent binge-eating and dieting are associated with obesity, which leads to significant morbidity and mortality.[8] Comorbid psychiatric disorders associated with binge-eating disorder include anxiety, depression, obsessive-compulsive disorder, impulsive behaviors, substance-related disorders, and personality disorders.[4,8]

Obesity

Obesity is not recognized as a psychiatric or eating disorder in the DSM-IV-TR, although individuals often have comorbid anxiety and depression, a history of "yo-yo" dieting (weight loss attempts followed by weight gain), binge-eating behaviors, and obsessions about food and body weight.[9] Obesity is a chronic metabolic disorder that is determined by multiple biological and environmental factors, a sedentary lifestyle, and a genetic predisposition. The current worldwide epidemic of obesity may be secondary to overconsumption of high-fat, energy-rich foods; unhealthy snacking between meals; more food choices at restaurants, snack bars, and grocery stores; readily available inexpensive food 24 hours a day; larger sized portions of food and drinks; increased advertising of high-fat/high-carbohydrate foods and drinks; and the lack of physical activity and sleep. The addition of 20 to 30 kcal/day over a number of years can lead to significant weight gain; thus, energy intake and energy output through physical activity must be balanced for weight control.[1] The increase in the prevalence of obesity and negative health outcomes (diabetes, hyperlipidemia, cardiovascular disease) are major public health problems in industrialized countries. Despite the improvements in treatment for cardiovascular disorders over the last decade, a study has shown that obesity has significant impact on activities of daily living and functional impairment as people age.[10] In addition, obesity has been shown to be associated with a 25% increased risk of mood and anxiety disorder, although a causal relationship has not been established.[11]

Obesity is defined as a BMI $\geq$30 kg/m^2 and obese patients have an estimated 50% to 100% increased mortality rate compared with patients with BMI in the range of 20 to 25 kg/m^2 (Table 82-1).[7,12–15] People with a BMI range of 25 to 29.9 kg/m^2 are considered overweight and those >28 have an increased risk of developing chronic illnesses (e.g., musculoskeletal disorders, cardiovascular disease, diabetes).

EPIDEMIOLOGY

The prevalence of anorexia nervosa, bulimia nervosa, binge-eating, and obesity have increased over the past 50 years.[1,5] An estimated 5 million Americans have an eating disorder (anorexia nervosa, bulimia nervosa, binge-eating disorder, and variations of disturbances in eating). Eating disorders are more common in women (90%–95% of cases are women, and lifetime male:female prevalence ratios range from 1:6–1:10).[3] Overall lifetime prevalence rates of eating disorders (including any binge eating) ranged from 0.6% to 4.5% in adults surveyed in 2003.[8] Homosexual orientation and premorbid obesity are risk factors for eating disorders among males.[1,3]

Anorexia Nervosa

The prevalence of anorexia nervosa has increased in industrialized societies where there is an abundance of food and where being thin is linked with attractiveness and success.[1,3] Patients with anorexia nervosa are predominantly female (90%–95% of cases), typically middle to upper-middle class, and white. Prevalence rates among late adolescent and early adulthood females is 0.5% for narrowly defined and up to 4.1% for more broadly defined anorexia nervosa.[3,4] The incidence and prevalence of childhood-onset anorexia nervosa is not known. It is estimated that 19% to 30% of preadolescent patients with anorexia nervosa are male.[1–3] Common comorbid conditions associated with anorexia nervosa in both men and women include poor self-esteem, mood disorders (major depression, dysthymia, and bipolar), anxiety disorders (especially obsessive-compulsive disorders and social phobia), substance abuse, and personality disorders (cluster C spectrum, particularly avoidant personality disorder and obsessive-compulsive personality disorder).[1–3] Women who have recovered from anorexia nervosa are likely to have perfectionism, inflexible thinking, overly compliant behavior, social introversion, as well as a continued drive for thinness and rigid eating habits.[1,2]

Bulimia Nervosa

The true prevalence of bulimia nervosa is not known because most patients seem to be within the standards of a healthy weight and are secretive about their eating habits. Furthermore, estimates of lifetime prevalence among women vary widely (1%–4%) because most studies have examined selected populations such as high school or college students.[3] Male cases of bulimia nervosa are uncommon, whereas the ratio of binge-eating disorder is more equivalent between genders.[1] Bulimia nervosa is four to six times more common than anorexia nervosa. Comorbid disorders associated with bulimia nervosa and binge-eating include obesity, substance (alcohol, cocaine, nicotine) use disorders, personality disorders (cluster B and C spectrum, particularly borderline personality disorder and avoidant personality disorder, impulsive, and narcissistic personality), anxiety disorders (obsessive-compulsive disorder, panic disorder, and social phobia), mood disorders (major depression, dysthymia, and bipolar disorder), and impulse control disorders (compulsive buying, kleptomania, and self-mutilation).[2,3,8] Individuals who have recovered from bulimia nervosa often continue to have obsessional symptoms, abnormal eating behaviors, overconcern with body image, dysphoric mood, and low self-esteem.[1,16]

Binge-Eating Disorder

The onset of binge-eating usually first occurs in late adolescence or in the early 20s and after significant weight loss from dieting.[4] Binge-eating is more common in women than men (~1.5 times) and its estimated prevalence rate in the United States is between 2% and 5% of adult women.[4,16] The prevalence of binge-eating disorder is between 0.7% and 4.0% in community samples; 20% to 30% in individuals participating in weight loss programs; and up to 50% in patients seeking bariatric surgery.[2,4] Approximately 1.5% of the general population has night eating syndrome, which is characterized by morning anorexia, evening hyperphagia, insomnia, and occurs more often in obese individuals during periods of high stress.[17] The prevalence of night eating disorder ranges from 9% to 14% of patients being treated at obesity clinics and between 8% and 42% among bariatric surgery patients.[17]

Obesity

Obesity is a major public health concern worldwide and is the leading cause of numerous medical conditions (e.g., cardiovascular disease, hypertension, dyslipidemia, diabetes, sleep apnea) and premature death.[7,14,18] Approximately 97 million adults in the United States are overweight or obese.[14] Adult obesity usually results from a steady weight gain from the mid-20s to between ages 50 and 59, when the prevalence of obesity peaks.[19] The increased prevalence of obesity with increasing age may be secondary to continued consumption of calories that are not expended because of reduction in daily exercise, reduction in the amount of energy the body needs for daily functions, and smoking cessation.[19] In 2003 and 2004, 66% of adults were considered overweight or obese and 32% of patients had BMI $\geq$30 kg/m^2.[19] Obesity is more common in women (with higher rates in low socioeconomic status groups) and in those with diabetes mellitus.[3] In the recent National Health and Nutrition Examination Survey (NHANES) report, obesity and overweight were more prevalent among non-Hispanic black women consistent with previous years.[19] The rate of extreme obesity (BMI $\geq$40) was also highest among black women (14.7% versus 6.9% among all U.S. adults).[19] The economic impact of obesity in the United States in 1994 was estimated to be $68 billion for medical expenses and loss of income and more than $30 billion for diet programs and products.[20,21] Future research is needed to assess the impact of obesity and weight loss on direct/indirect costs of medical care and lost productivity outcomes.[22]

In recent years, the incidence of obesity (BMI $\geq$30 kg/m^2) and severe obesity (BMI >40 kg/m^2) has been rising in industrialized countries, particularly among children and adolescents.[23] According to the latest report from the NHANES taken from data collected during 2003 and 2004, 17% of children in the United States were overweight and the prevalence of overweight increased 2.2% and 4.2% in females and males, respectively.[19] From 1999 to 2000 to 2003 to 2004, non-Hispanic black female children/adolescents had the highest prevalence (2.8%) of overweight. Childhood obesity is unfortunate because typical weight reduction methods may not be successful and there is a greater negative psychological impact on the child secondary to comments by his or her peers. It is known that children who are overweight often remain overweight as adults.[24] Although the cause for the increased prevalence of overweight among children is unclear, poor diet, lack of physical activity, and sleep deprivation have been shown to be potential contributors.[25–27] As in adults, type 2 diabetes mellitus is a significant concern in overweight children.[28] The weighted prevalence of type 2 diabetes mellitus in adolescents was recently estimated to be 29% of all adolescents who had diabetes; in addition, 11% of all U.S. adolescents were estimated to have impaired fasting glucose.[28] Furthermore, the prevalence of metabolic syndrome in adolescents was estimated to be 4.5% from the NHANES 1999 to 2004 study.[29] Treatment of childhood obesity should always be initiated as early as possible; most programs recommend a reduction in weight gain rather than weight loss.

ETIOLOGY AND PATHOPHYSIOLOGY

Eating behavior reflects an interaction between the individual's genetic makeup, physiologic state (e.g., balance of neurotransmitters and neuropeptides, metabolic state and rate, sensory receptors for smell and taste, condition of the gastrointestinal [GI] tract), and environmental factors (e.g., sight of the food, accessibility of food, ambient temperature, stress, social gatherings).[1,30,31] Cultural and religious beliefs and traditions about food also affect eating behaviors. Medical conditions, psychiatric disorders, medications, and substances (e.g., nicotine, central nervous system [CNS] stimulants) may influence appetite and eating behaviors as well (see Table 82-5 for a list of medications and medical conditions that may cause weight gain and loss). Normally when a person has eaten an adequate amount of food, neurotransmitters or peptides in the brain signal the satiety centers in the hypothalamus and there is a reduced desire to eat. Because more bulimia patients starve themselves or use strict dieting between binges, their bodies may sense a "food-deprived state" and this changes brain chemistry to stimulate appetite.[31] When the "starving" person begins to eat, the brain neurotransmitters (e.g., serotonin) that normally turn off appetite may fail to work; thus, the person eats excessive amounts of food. Studies in patients with eating disorders have shown that the perceptions of hunger and satiety are abnormal in patients who binge and purge.[31]

The exact etiology and pathogenesis of anorexia nervosa are unknown, but are likely a combination of familial, psychological, sociocultural, and biological factors.[1,30] Fluctuations in serotonin, dopamine, norepinephrine, leptin, neuropeptide Y (NPY), and cortisol levels modulate appetite, satiety, and eating behavior.[1,32] The neuropeptide, neurotransmitter, and

Table 82-5 Medications and Medical Conditions That May Cause Weight Gain and Weight Loss

WEIGHT GAIN	WEIGHT LOSS
Medications	**Medications**
α- and β-blockers (e.g., terazosin, atenolol, propranolol)	Alcohol/sedative-hypnotics
Antidepressants (e.g., mirtazapine, paroxetine, phenelzine, trazodone, tricyclic antidepressants)	Antidepressants/noradrenergic agents (e.g., atomoxetine, bupropion)
Antidiabetics (e.g., insulin, sulfonylureas, thiazolidinediones)	Antidiabetics (e.g., acarbose, exenatide, metformin, pramlintide)
Antiepileptic drugs (e.g., carbamazepine, gabapentin, pregabalin, valproic acid)	Antiepileptic (e.g., felbamate, topiramate, zonisamide)
Antihistamines (e.g., diphenhydramine, cyproheptadine, histamine-2 blockers)	Cardiovascular/antihypertensive agents (e.g., ACE inhibitors, clonidine, digoxin, diuretics)
Antipsychotics (e.g., most typicals, clozapine, olanzapine, risperidone, quetiapine)	Modafinil
Glucocorticoids (e.g., prednisone)	Nicotine
Mood stabilizers (e.g., lithium)	Stimulants (e.g., amphetamine, cocaine, dextroamphetamine, dopaminergic agents, pseudoephedrine, sibutramine)
Progestin-containing hormones (e.g., medroxyprogesterone)	Theophylline
Protease inhibitors (e.g., ritonavir, indinavir)	
Medical Conditions	**Medical Conditions**
Chronic heart failure	Addison's disease
Cushing syndrome	Cancer (e.g., stomach, gallbladder, liver, ovarian, pancreatic)
Depression (e.g., seasonal affective disorder, premenstrual dysphoric disorder)	Diabetes mellitus type 1 and 2
Diabetes mellitus type 2	Digestive conditions (e.g., Crohn disease, inflammatory bowel disease, intestinal motility disorders, malabsorption, ulcerative colitis)
Hypothyroidism	Human immunodeficiency virus/acquired immunodeficiency syndrome
Polycystic ovarian syndrome	Hyperthyroidism
Schizophrenia	Mood disorders (e.g., depression, mania)

ACE, angiotensin-converting enzyme.
Adapted from reference 2.

hormonal disturbances found in anorexia nervosa are secondary to malnutrition and weight loss and seem to normalize after weight normalization and long-term recovery.[30,32]

There are many possible causes for obesity, such as genetic predisposition, disturbances of hunger and satiety centers in the brain, endocrine abnormalities, environmental and cultural influences, socioeconomic status, medical conditions such as hypothyroidism, medications that stimulate appetite, and inactivity.[14,31] Obese individuals tend to have more restrained eating (dieting with chronic caloric restriction) and lower levels of activity compared with persons with normal weight. This behavior can lead to lowered basal metabolic rates, less energy expenditure, and increased weight gain secondary to periodic overeating and binge-eating.[9] Recently, there have been several association studies linking short sleep duration and metabolic changes such as obesity, insulin resistance, and diabetes.[33] One study showed that children aged 30 months and younger who lacked sleep were at risk of developing obesity at 7 years.[34] Alteration of the hypothalamic regulation of appetite and energy expenditure owing to sleep loss has been one explanation. Sleep loss has also been shown to be associated with low leptin levels and high ghrelin levels; both factors contribute to signaling of energy deficit and hunger, which may contribute to overeating and obesity.[35]

Individuals with mental illness are especially prone to developing obesity. Psychotropic medications including chlorpromazine, clozapine, and olanzapine cause significant weight gain.[2] Associated physiological changes may increase the risk of type 2 diabetes mellitus. Of patients with severe chronic mental illness, 40% to 62% are overweight before initiation of medication.[36] Contributing factors may include reduced access to medical care, lifestyle habits (decreased physical activity, poor diet), and economic issues that restrict participation in healthy living regimens.

Psychological, psychodynamic, and cognitive theories have attempted to explain the emotional, perceptual, and phobic fears of eating disorders, but there are few studies evaluating these hypotheses.[1,3] Examples of psychological and familial factors associated with anorexia nervosa include the fear and avoidance of sexuality and growth, failure of parents to encourage independence and self-expression, rigidity and overinvolvement of parents, and premorbid perfectionism and high-achieving characteristics.[3] Childhood sexual abuse or early sexual trauma may be a contributing factor in the etiology of eating disorders.[1]

Genetics

There is a genetic risk for anorexia nervosa, with higher rates among first-degree biological relatives and higher concordance rates for monozygotic twins (~55%) compared with dizygotic twins (~5%).[1–3,37,38] A large epidemiologic twin study found a strong genetic association between anorexia nervosa and bulimia nervosa; thus, these eating disorders share a familial risk.[30,39] Comorbid mood disorders and an increased risk of mood disorders have been found among first-degree biological relatives of individuals with the binge-eating/purging type of eating disorder.[30] Eating disorders and excessive exercising have been linked to obsessive-compulsive personality disorder and to obsessive-compulsive disorder.[30,40] There is an increased frequency of bulimia nervosa, mood disorders, obsessive-compulsive disorders, and substance abuse and dependence among first-degree biological relatives of patients with bulimia nervosa.[39] Genetic studies show that 80% of children with two obese parents are obese compared with 40% of children with one obese parent, and 10% of children with two normal-weight parents.[31] Genetic risks for obesity are associated with a higher "set-point" for appetite and food intake, which causes individuals to eat more before feeling full. Recently, investigators have found a variant in the fat mass and obesity associated gene that may be linked to BMI and obesity.[41]

Hypothalamus Dysregulation

Neurobiological theories of eating disorders have focused on dysregulation of the hypothalamic–pituitary–adrenal, hypothalamic–pituitary–gonadal, and hypothalamic–pituitary–thyroid axes as well as dysregulation of neurotransmitters, neuropeptides, endogenous opioids, growth hormone, insulin, and leptin.[1,30,31,42] Alterations in hypothalamic functioning are associated with appetite changes, mood disorders, and neuroendocrine disturbances.[1,30] The hypothalamus is the major appetite and eating control center in the brain and is sensitive to a variety of facilitatory and inhibitory neurotransmitters and polypeptide neurohormones from the brain and GI tract.[1,31] Disruption of the ventromedial hypothalamus produces hyperphagia and obesity, whereas lesions of the lateral hypothalamus cause hypophagia and weight loss. This suggests that there is a ventromedial "satiety" and lateral "feeding" center in the hypothalamus. The hypothalamus receives input from peripheral satiety sites (e.g., gastric and pancreatic peptides released secondary to food passing through the GI tract), from leptin that is produced by fat cells, and from the catecholamine and indoleamine neurotransmitter system in the brain.[1,30,43]

Neurotransmitter Dysregulation

Serotonin

Serotonin plays an important role in postprandial satiety, anxiety, sleep, mood, obsessive-compulsive, and impulse control disorders.[1,30] Serotonin is synthesized from the essential amino acid, *l*-tryptophan, which must come from the diet.[44] Under the influence of darkness, serotonin is metabolized in the pineal gland to melatonin, a major neuromodulator of sleep and reproductive function. Serotonin activity in the region of the medial hypothalamus has an inhibitory effect on appetite and is responsible for satiety or the feeling of fullness after food intake.[40,44,45] Pharmacologic treatments that increase intrasynaptic serotonin or those that directly activate serotonin receptors cause satiety and reduce food consumption.[40] Serotonin has an inhibitory effect on dopamine activity and its release is increased with motor activity. Excessive exercising and hyperactivity are found in many patients with eating disorders, particularly anorexia nervosa.[46] Physical exertion increases central serotonin synthesis and turnover, which perpetuates reduced food intake and body weight.

Conversely, reduction of serotonergic activity in the CNS is associated with eating disorders, depression, anxiety disorders, and obsessive-compulsive disorder.[30,40,45] Low cerebrospinal (CSF) fluid levels of 5-hydroxyindoleacetic acid, the major metabolite of serotonin, are associated with aggressive, impulsive, and suicidal behavior and have been found in low-weight patients with anorexia nervosa and in patients with more frequent bingeing.[40] Diminished serotonin activity (either by tryptophan depletion or serotonin antagonists) can contribute to increased food intake and carbohydrate craving.[16,45] Dietary restriction of tryptophan has been shown to reduce brain serotonin synthesis, causing a deficiency state. The reduction in serotonin activity may upregulate the appetite or satiety centers in the brain, thereby increasing the amount of food a person wants to eat. Agents that block postsynaptic serotonin activity (e.g., clozapine, olanzapine, risperidone, quetiapine, cyproheptadine, mirtazapine) can stimulate appetite and may cause weight gain.

Dopamine

Disturbances in dopamine activity and feedback regulation at different receptors have been postulated as a cause of anorexia nervosa.[40] Agents that increase dopamine activity (e.g., apomorphine, a dopamine agonist; levodopa, a metabolic precursor of dopamine; and amphetamine, a releaser of dopamine from presynaptic stores) have been shown to have anorexic effects.[47] Dopamine agonists increase dopaminergic transmission and motor activity, which causes loss of appetite and hyperactivity; at higher doses, these agents may cause psychosis (hallucinations and delusions) and repetitive/stereotypical behaviors.[47] The CNS effects of dopaminergic agents occur in the cerebral cortex, in the reticular-activating system, and in the hypothalamic feeding center. The mesolimbic–mesocortical dopaminergic circuits are important for behavior reward and reinforcement, and are involved with "addictive" behaviors.[47] Dopamine-augmenting agents such as amphetamines are used for the treatment of exogenous obesity and may produce tolerance, dependence, and withdrawal reactions. Conversely, dopamine receptor antagonists such as clozapine, pimozide, and chlorpromazine may cause dysphoria and are often associated with weight gain.

Norepinephrine

The hypothalamus is innervated by noradrenergic pathways; thus, norepinephrine is involved in the regulation of eating behavior, the hypothalamic control of thyrotropin-releasing hormone secretion, corticotropin-releasing hormone (CRH) release, and gonadotropin secretion.[47] D-Amphetamine, which inhibits the reuptake of norepinephrine, decreases hunger sensations and food intake. Abnormalities in leptin and β_3-adrenergic activity have been associated with obesity and diabetes.[18,48] The human β_3-adrenoceptor is involved in a feedback loop with leptin to regulate energy balance, lipolysis in adipocytes, serum insulin levels, and food intake.[49] People with hereditary obesity or non–insulin-dependent diabetes mellitus may have abnormalities in the β_3-adrenoceptor or in leptin activity, signaling, or receptors.[48] A genetic variant of the β_3-adrenoceptor in humans has been associated with morbid obesity and non–insulin-dependent diabetes. It is possible that some cases of obesity may be secondary to failure of the β_3-adrenoreceptor on brown adipocytes to respond appropriately to leptin-induced sympathetic activity.[50] β_3-Adrenergic receptor agonists are being studied to induce thermogenic activity and promote weight loss when combined with a calorie-restricted diet.[49]

Neuropeptide and Leptin Dysregulation

Leptin

Leptin is thought to act as an afferent satiety signal in the brain to regulate body fat mass.[1,51,52] Leptin reduces food intake, decreases serum glucose and insulin levels, increases metabolic rate, and reduces body fat mass and weight by reducing NPY activity.[51,53] Leptin serum levels are highly correlated with BMI and body fat,[52] and its secretion has a circadian rhythm and an oscillatory pattern similar to other hormones.[48,54] Leptin is supposed to signal the brain to stop eating, but the signal may not get through properly in some overweight people.[51] It has been postulated that some obese individuals may have partially resistant hypothalamic receptors or that there is a defect in the blood–brain barrier transport system for bringing leptin into the brain.[51,54,55] CSF leptin levels in some obese humans have been found to be much lower than expected compared with serum leptin levels which suggests that the brain uptake of leptin may be defective.[1] Leptin and leptinlike products currently are being investigated for weight reduction in obese patients and in overweight patients with non–insulin-dependent diabetes mellitus.[51]

Malnourished or underweight individuals with anorexia nervosa have reduced plasma and CSF leptin compared with normal weight controls.[52,56,57] In anorexic patients, CSF leptin levels return to normal before full weight restoration and may contribute to difficulties in patients achieving and maintaining a normal weight.[30] In women with bulimia, serum leptin levels are correlated with body weight and are similar to normal controls.[30]

Neuropeptides

NPY and peptide YY are chemically related, 36–amino-acid peptides and are two of the most potent stimulators of appetite.[1,45] Both enhance food intake in animals, possibly by causing hunger.[58] Peptide YY is three times more potent in stimulating food intake than NPY.[30] Injection of NPY into the brain causes all of the features of leptin deficiency (e.g., hyperphagia and obesity).[55] Many of leptin's effects on food intake and energy expenditure are centrally mediated in the hypothalamus by neurotransmitters such as NPY.[51,53] NPY levels are high in the CSF of anorectic patients but are ineffective in overriding the appetite suppressant neurotransmitters and neuropeptides.[31,59] Plasma leptin and CSF levels of NPY and peptide YY return to normal concentrations in women who have recovered from anorexia nervosa or bulimia nervosa.[45] Regardless, a recent study of 497 obese patients showed that NPY Y5 receptor antagonism did not produce increased weight loss when added to 6 months of either orlistat or sibutramine therapy.[60]

Opioid Peptides/Endorphins

Endogenous opiates play a role in food reward. Altered opioid activity may contribute to changes in feeding behavior, reproductive activity, and cortisol release.[30] β-Endorphin, an endogenous opiate peptide, stimulates feeding behavior in animals and humans, and levels are highly correlated with body weight.[58] Underweight anorexic and some bulimic patients have reduced CSF β-endorphin concentrations that may contribute to changes in feeding behavior.[30] Dynorphin, an endogenous opioid receptor ligand, enhances feeding behavior and acts at the paraventricular nucleus in the hypothalamus.[31] Opioid agonists stimulate feeding, whereas opioid antagonists inhibit feeding; however, there have been few data to support a therapeutic role opioid antagonists in weight loss.[61]

Miscellaneous Neurohormones and Peptides

Food intake and gastric emptying are regulated by the peripheral release of GI peptides such as cholecystokinin, glucagon, calcitonin, bombesin, and somatostatin, all of which inhibit feeding.[1,62] Other hormones, neurotransmitters, and peptides involved in the regulation of hunger and satiety (e.g., histamine, oxytocin, vasopressin, galanin, CRH, melanocyte-stimulating hormone, hypocretin, and orexin) and lipotic action (e.g., growth hormone and dehydroepiandrosterone) are being investigated. Histamine is involved in the regulation of appetite, and histamine$_1$-blocking agents (e.g., tricyclic antidepressants [TCAs], antipsychotics, antihistamines) cause sedation and increased appetite in animals and humans.[63] Growth hormone, a lipolytic hormone that acts at adipose tissue, reduces and redistributes body fat by releasing glycerol and free fatty acids into the circulation.[64] Growth hormone secretion is significantly lower in obese individuals and lipolysis is, therefore, reduced. As people age, the secretion of growth hormone declines (it is estimated that 50% of people >65 years have growth hormone deficit).[64] Replacement doses of growth hormone have been suggested to treat obesity and to reverse body changes associated with aging.

Brain Changes

Once malnutrition occurs, the normal mechanisms for regulating eating behavior change and anorexia is perpetuated because of neurochemical dysregulation and, possibly, brain atrophy. Brain imaging studies have found generalized atrophy and/or ventricular dilation in patients with anorexia nervosa that reverse with weight gain.[30] Reduced regional cerebral blood flow in the temporal lobe has been reported in childhood-onset anorexia, indicating a possible functional abnormality of the brain.[65] Electroencephalograms of anorexic patients often show generalized abnormalities secondary to electrolyte, glucose, and fluid changes in the brain.[30] Morphologic brain changes (e.g., sulcal widening, enlarged ventricles) have been found on brain positron emission tomography and computed tomography scans in some bulimic patients. Electroencephalographic changes (e.g., paroxysmal spike pattern) have been reported in some patients with bulimia nervosa, but brain wave changes usually are more disturbed with anorexia nervosa.[30]

INITIAL ASSESSMENT

A comprehensive evaluation of patients with eating disorders is essential in determining the diagnosis and selecting treatment options (Table 82-6).[2–4,66] A psychiatric assessment is

Table 82-6 Assessment and Management of Eating Disorders

Assessment	*Examples*
Develop a therapeutic alliance with the patient	
Collaborate with other clinicians and providers	Other physicians, dieticians, mental health professionals, school personnel
Assess and monitor eating disorder symptoms and behaviors	DSM-IV-TR criteria, structured interviews, rating scales, screening tools
Determine diagnosis and target behaviors	Binge-eating, purging behaviors, laxative abuse, excessive exercise, food restrictions
Assess and monitor medical status	Vital signs, weight and height, BMI, cardiovascular status, dental exam, comorbid medical disorders, laboratory tests (Tables 82-7 and 82-8)
Assess and monitor for psychiatric disorders	Anxiety, obsessions/compulsions, insomnia, depression, suicidal ideation or plan, substance abuse, impulsive behaviors, personality disorders
Assess family issues	History of eating disorders, family dynamics and support, family attitudes toward eating, exercise, appearance
Management	
Provide education about eating disorder, management, and treatment approaches	
Provide appropriate treatment setting	Inpatient hospitalization, residential treatment, partial hospitalization, or intensive outpatient care depending on medical or psychiatric conditions
Provide psychosocial treatments	Individual, group, family and couples therapy, self-help, online resources, 12-step programs
Restore or maintain a healthy weight	Monitor weight, growth, and individual characteristics
Nutritional rehabilitation for anorexia nervosa	Resume eating and weight gain for seriously underweight, normalize eating patterns and normal perceptions of hunger and satiety
Minimize target behaviors	Food restrictions, binge-eating, purging, and excessive exercising
Treat physical and medical complications	
Treat associated psychiatric conditions	
Prevent relapse	

BMI, body mass index; DSM-IV-TR, Diagnostic and Statistical Manual of Mental Disorders, Fourth Edition, Text Revision.
Adapted from references 2 and 3.

required to establish the diagnosis, identify any comorbid psychiatric disorders, determine the risk of suicide, and evaluate psychosocial stressors.[3] Concurrent mood, anxiety, obsessive-compulsive, personality, and substance abuse disorders often accompany anorexia and bulimia nervosa and need to be identified. Medical complications are numerous with eating disorders (Table 82-7) and require a multi-system assessment and laboratory monitoring (Table 82-8). An interdisciplinary treatment team consisting of physicians, nurses, dietitians, and mental health professionals is recommended for the management of children and adolescents with eating disorders.[1–3]

A detailed weight history and growth chart are needed to detect the onset of an eating disorder.[3] Evaluation of eating behaviors, and purging helps to identify patterns and factors that precede binge-eating. Determining the frequency, type, and length of exercising identifies pathological or excessive physical activity. Assessing body image beliefs and distortions, cultural attitudes about size and shape, and family attitudes toward appearance are important in determining perceptions and attitudes about appropriate weight. Menstrual cycle history and duration of amenorrhea identifies women with increased risk of osteopenia and osteoporosis. Males also develop osteopenia and osteoporosis and may have a lower bone density compared with females with anorexia nervosa.[1] Lowered libido and infertility are common owing to diminished sex hormones, cessation of menstruation, and gonadal atrophy.[1] Diagnosis of comorbid psychiatric disorders (e.g., affective, anxiety, substance abuse, and personality disorders) and medical conditions (e.g., diabetes, thyroid abnormalities, inflammatory bowel disease) helps to determine which management strategies should be used to correct an underlying condition.[2,3]

TREATMENT APPROACHES

A multifaceted treatment approach that addresses medical, dental, nutritional, psychiatric, and family needs is recommended for anorectic, bulimic, or obese patients.[1–3,31,67] Guidelines for the medical and psychiatric assessment and management of eating disorders have been published (Tables 82-6 and 82-7).[3,66] Because patients may be resistant or disinterested in treatment, family members or friends may initiate medical attention.[31] Interventions include education about the disorder, exercise, nutritional counseling, modification of eating behavior, psychotherapy, and pharmacotherapy. Obtaining the patient's cooperation in the program to establish healthy eating patterns is vital.[3] Most patients receive weekly outpatient assessments and therapy to monitor progress toward treatment goals over several months. Hospitalization is recommended for patients with severe anorexia nervosa who require life-saving intensive medical management, including refeeding.[3] Caloric intake, weight, urine output, serum electrolytes, heart rate, and blood pressure are monitored daily.[1,2] Indications for inpatient treatment include a 75% or less expected body weight, intractable purging, rapid weight loss, cardiac disturbances, severe electrolyte imbalances, psychosis, or suicidal ideation.[3] Residential eating disorder programs that specialize in the long-term treatment of eating disorders for those individuals who need more intensive therapy are available.[3]

Table 82-7 Medical Complications of Eating Disorders

Organ System	Signs and Symptoms	Associated Laboratory Abnormalities
Cardiac	Acrocyanosis; arrhythmias; bradycardia; chest pain; cold extremities; dizziness or lightheadedness; faintness; orthostatic hypotension; palpitations; peripheral edema; syncope; tachycardia; weakness	Electrocardiogram changes (e.g., QTc prolongation, ST-segment depression, T-wave inversion); mitral valve prolapse; left ventricular changes (e.g., decreased mass and cavity size); cardiomyopathy (emetine toxicity from ipecac)
Central nervous system	Anxiety; apathy; cognitive impairment; decreased attention and concentration; depression; fatigue; headache; irritable mood; lethargy; neuropathies; obsessional thinking; peripheral neuropathy; seizures (large fluid shifts or electrolyte disturbances); weakness	Brain imaging changes (e.g., cortical atrophy, decreased gray and white matter, increased ventricular:brain ratio, ventricular enlargement); electroencephalogram changes (e.g., diffuse abnormalities, metabolic encephalopathy); abnormal cerebral blood flow and metabolism
Dental	Dental caries (from acidic vomitus); dental enamel erosion (from acidic vomitus); gingivitis; swollen cheeks/neck; enlarged salivary glands	Increased serum amylase (benign parotid hyperplasia); erosion of dental enamel
Dermatologic	*Anorexia nervosa*: acne, alopecia, brittle nails, dry skin and hair, hair thinning, lanugo (fine body hair), yellow skin (hypercarotenemia) *Vomiters*: scarring or calluses on dorsum of hand (Russell's sign); petechiae	Increased serum carotene (in anorexia nervosa); vitamin deficiencies
Endocrine/metabolic	Cold intolerance; diuresis; fatigue; low body temperature; pitting edema; poor skin turgor; impaired temperature regulation; weakness	Carbohydrate intolerance; dehydration (e.g., increased urine specific gravity, osmolality); electrolyte abnormalities (e.g., hypokalemia, hypomagnesemia, hypophosphatemia); hyperamylasemia; hypercholesterolemia in anorexia nervosa; hypercortisolism; hypoglycemia; hypothermia; hypothyroidism (e.g., low T_3, elevated TSH); lipid abnormalities; low basal metabolic rate
Fluid/electrolyte/renal	Decreased or increased urinary volume; dehydration; diuresis; peripheral edema (cessation of laxative and diuretic abuse); pitting edema	Decreased glomerular filtration rate; decreased serum creatinine; hypochloremia; hypokalemia; hypomagnesemia; hyponatremia; hypophosphatemia (especially on refeeding); hypozincemia; increased blood urea nitrogen; ketonuria; metabolic acidosis (laxative abuse); metabolic alkalosis (vomiting); renal calculi; renal failure
Gastrointestinal	*Anorexia nervosa*: abdominal pain, abnormal bowel sounds; abnormal taste sensation (zinc deficiency); bloating (abdominal distension with meals); constipation; dehydration; delayed gastric emptying; gastric dilation (rapid feeding); parotitis; vomiting *Laxative abuse*: constipation; decreased intestinal motility; diarrhea *Vomiters*: dental caries; esophagitis; gastroesophageal erosions; gastric tears; gastritis; gastroesophageal reflux; heartburn; parotid hyperplasia	Abnormal liver function tests; increased serum amylase (in purging); gallstones; increased pancreatic amylase; pancreatitis Gastric motility: delayed emptying Endoscopy: Barrett esophagus or inflammation; Mallory-Weiss (esophageal) or gastric tears or perforation Stool guaiac: positive for purging or laxative abuse
Hematologic	Fatigue; cold intolerance; bruising; clotting abnormalities	Anemia (normocytic, microcytic, or macrocytic); leukopenia; neutropenia; thrombocytopenia
Musculoskeletal	Bone pain with exercise; delayed linear growth; fractures (from bone loss); muscle wasting, weakness, and aches; myopathy	Osteopenia or osteoporosis (decreased bone density); short stature (arrested skeletal growth); stress fractures
Nutrition	Low body weight; cachexia; dehydration; hypothermia; weakness; vitamin and mineral deficiencies (stomatitis, glossitis, diarrhea)	Hypoalbuminemia; low weight and BMI; low body fat percentage; anemia; hypercholesterolemia; decreased serum calcium, ferritin, B_{12}, folate, niacin, thiamine, zinc
Reproductive	*Anorexia nervosa*: amenorrhea; arrested sexual development (atrophy of breasts, delayed puberty, ovarian/uterine regression, regression in secondary sexual characteristics); loss of libido; infertility; oligomenorrhea; pregnancy complications and neonatal complications (low weight gain and low-birth-weight infant)	Decreased serum estradiol (women); follicle-stimulating hormone and luteinizing hormone (prepubertal levels); decreased serum testosterone (men)

BMI, body mass index; T_3, tri-iodothyronine; TSH, thyroid-stimulating hormone.
Adapted from references 1–4, 30.

Table 82-8 Laboratory Assessment and Monitoring

Patient Type	*Laboratory Parameter*
All eating disorders	Complete metabolic panel (serum electrolytes, blood urea nitrogen, serum creatinine) Thyroid functioning (T_3, free T_4, TSH) CBC with differential Urinalysis Liver function tests: aspartate aminotransferase, alanine aminotransferase, alkaline phosphatase
Malnourished or severely symptomatic	Serum calcium, magnesium, phosphorus, ferritin Electrocardiogram 24-hour urine for creatinine clearance
Amenorrhea for >6 months	Osteopenia/osteoporosis assessment (DEXA bone density scan) Women: serum estradiol, luteinizing hormone, follicle-stimulating hormone, β-human chorionic gonadotropin, prolactin Men: serum testosterone
Other tests/screens	Urine drug screens for suspected substance abuse; serum amylase for vomiting; brain magnetic resonance imaging and computerized tomography for severe malnutrition

CBC, complete blood count; T_3, tri-iodothyronine; T_4, thyroxine; TSH, thyroid-stimulating hormone; DEXA, dual energy x-ray absorptiometry.
Adapted from reference 3.

Relapse prevention requires long-term outpatient psychotherapy as well as psychopharmacologic agents when appropriate.

Treatment of obesity generally does not involve hospitalization, although the patient's degree of overweight/obesity and its impact on quality of life is an important consideration. Before recommending treatment, assessment of the BMI, waist circumference, presence of obesity-related diseases, risk factors for cardiovascular disease and related conditions, and patient's motivation to lose weight should be assessed.[14] Patients should also be screened for medical conditions and/or medications that can increase the risk for obesity, and these underlying factors should be corrected before recommending treatment.

ANOREXIA NERVOSA

Clinical Features

1. S.B., a 16-year-old girl, is referred to her physician because of a 30-lb weight loss over the past 6 months and amenorrhea for the past 9 months. She had a normal menarche at age 12 years and reached her maximum weight of 140 lb at age 11. S.B. is a star player on her high school tennis team and previously was involved in gymnastics as a child. Her current weight is 98 lb and height is 5 feet 5 inches. S.B. feels that her weight is perfect, because it helps her move better on the tennis court, an opinion she believes is reinforced by her coach. S.B. rarely eats three meals a day and is on an extreme no-fat diet. She runs an average of 8 miles/day and practices tennis 2 to 3 hours/day after school. Despite her parents' concern about her weight, S.B. feels that if she gains weight, she will be fat and unable to play competitive tennis.

Upon further questioning, S.B. admits to a previous weight loss at around age 13 from 140 to 100 lb, which resulted in amenorrhea for 6 months. At that time, she was involved in gymnastics and was told she needed to lose weight to stay on the team. S.B. started exercising to burn off calories and skipping breakfast to lower her caloric intake. At times, she became dehydrated and had episodes of hypotension that resulted in dizzy spells. She also took "diet pills" that a friend gave her, which made her heart beat fast and caused insomnia. At times she had difficulty controlling her diet and would binge on foods that were "bad"; this usually only happened when she was under more stress at school and at home. During this time, S.B. was on the honor roll and involved in competitive gymnastics and tennis at her school. S.B. was referred by her school nurse to the school psychologist because of the noticeable weight loss. The psychologist recommended that she be evaluated by her pediatrician to receive treatment for an eating disorder. What characteristics does S.B. have that are related to anorexia nervosa?

Anorexia nervosa, a condition of self-induced weight loss, is characterized by a BMI ≤17.5, weight loss of at least 15% of ideal body weight, a preoccupation with body weight and food, behaviors directed toward weight loss, intense fear of gaining weight, disturbances of body image, and amenorrhea (Table 82-3).[4] S.B.'s BMI is 16.3 (98 lb ÷ [65 in]^2 × 703), which fits the criteria for anorexia nervosa. The main clinical feature of anorexia nervosa is a morbid fear of becoming fat and losing control over eating.[4] Anorectic behaviors include restrictive dieting (e.g., drastically reducing the amount of food ingested, minimizing foods high in fat and carbohydrates, and vegetarianism), purging behaviors (e.g., self-induced vomiting and excessive use of laxatives or diuretics), and strenuous exercise. The anorectic person often has a starved appearance that is caused by loss of subcutaneous fat tissue.[30] Associated behaviors include looking in mirrors to check for thinness, expressing concern about being fat, and preoccupation with food (e.g., collecting recipes, preparing elaborate meals, hiding or hoarding carbohydrate-rich foods, throwing away food, cutting food into small pieces, eating slowly). Personality traits include low self-esteem, sensitivity to rejection, perfectionism, competitiveness, an extreme sense of responsibility, excessive conformity, guilt, and an intolerance of angry feelings.[2] Sleep disturbances, depression, anxiety, phobias, social isolation, and sexual disinterest are commonly associated with anorexia nervosa. Anorexia nervosa has been considered a type of obsessive-compulsive disorder with obsessive thoughts about food and weight and compulsive acts or rituals to alleviate the thoughts or fears of being "fat."[1,30]

Course and Prognosis

2. How does S.B.'s clinical course resemble others with anorexia nervosa and what is her prognosis?

As illustrated by S.B., anorexia nervosa typically begins in adolescent girls between the ages of 13 and 18 years (mean, 17) and rarely occurs after age 40.[2] However, the incidence of anorexia nervosa has increased in prepubertal children owing to overconcern and obsession about weight and dieting.[1,68] The onset of anorexia nervosa frequently is associated with a major change in life (e.g., leaving home for college) or after a stressful life event. Anorexia usually begins with significant food deprivation (e.g., related to dieting, stress, or severe illness) along with strenuous physical exercising.[3] Most patients with anorexia nervosa are extremely overactive and obsessive about exercise routines to burn off calories and induce weight loss. Exercise is typically solitary and rigid, and patients feel guilty if they do not exercise. Individuals like S.B., who have occupational or athletic pressures to be thin (e.g., gymnasts, figure skaters, long distance runners, ballet dancers, and models) are at increased risk for developing anorexia nervosa.[2,3] Among males, wrestlers, body builders, and runners seem to be at greatest risk for developing an eating disorder and for abusing anabolic steroids.[3]

The course and prognosis for anorexia nervosa is variable and individuals may only have a single episode, recurring cycles of weight loss and weight gain, or a chronic deteriorating course that may result in death.[1,2] Some individuals may be overweight initially, then develop anorexia nervosa when they start dieting, and later develop bulimia nervosa or obesity. Approximately 30% to 50% of patients with anorexia nervosa develop symptoms of bulimia during the course of their illness.[3] Approximately 45% to 50% of people with anorexia nervosa or bulimia nervosa recover completely, approximately 30% achieve a partial recovery, 20% to 25% are plagued with a long-term illness with no substantial change in symptoms, and fewer than 10% of persons with anorexia nervosa die.[1,3,30,69] Patients with anorexia nervosa may have extreme anxiety, restlessness, and insomnia owing to food deprivation. Many patients who have recovered from anorexia nervosa continue to suffer from social phobias and generalized anxiety, obsessional thinking, compulsive behaviors, perfectionism, dysthymia, and depression.[3,30]

In severe weight loss cases, hospitalization is required to restore weight and correct electrolyte and fluid abnormalities. Those who require hospitalization have higher rates of mortality (~6%–10%) secondary to suicide or from the physical effects of starvation.[70] The mortality rate of anorexia nervosa is approximately 0.56%/year, which is 12 times higher than the mortality rate of young women in the general population.[3,71] Recurrent depressive episodes and suicide have been reported in up to 5% of patients with chronic anorexia nervosa.[1] A follow-up study of women with eating disorders reported a 7.4% mortality rate with 4 out of 10 deaths due to suicide in women with anorexia.[72] Mortality rates among women with anorexia are higher in those with low weight at intake, low serum albumin levels, longer duration of illness, bingeing and purging, poor social functioning, and comorbid substance abuse and affective disorders.[73]

Medical Complications

3. The physician treating S.B. is concerned about possible medical complications caused by her anorexia nervosa. What laboratory and other medical tests should be ordered when assessing S.B. for her anorexia nervosa? What are the most common laboratory abnormalities that you would expect to see and why do they occur?

Starvation can affect all major organ systems and result in serious laboratory, cardiac, bone, and brain abnormalities.[1–3] Self-induced vomiting and the use of laxatives, diuretics, and enemas also can cause physiologic changes and abnormal laboratory tests (Tables 82-7 and 82-8). Appropriate laboratory tests for evaluation of patients with anorexia nervosa include the following: complete blood count, urinalysis, electrolytes, lipid profile, serum albumin, amylase, renal function, liver function, thyroid function, electrocardiogram (ECG), and a bone density scan.[3] Follicle-stimulating hormone, luteinizing hormone, prolactin, and estradiol levels should be assessed in females and testosterone levels should be evaluated in males.

In anorectic patients, the metabolic rate declines due to a loss of body mass that causes a reduction of tri-iodothyronine. Other abnormalities include elevated liver enzymes, increased lipid metabolism resulting in increased free fatty acids, hypoalbuminemia, fasting hypoglycemia, and glucose intolerance. Hypokalemia from emesis or chronic diarrhea after laxative abuse can cause skeletal and smooth muscle weakness, cardiac conduction abnormalities, arrhythmias, and possibly, cardiac arrest.[30] Amenorrhea may occur early in the illness before significant weight loss has occurred (i.e., when BMI is between 17 and 19) and can persist after weight gain, leading to infertility and bone loss. The decrease in bone density correlates with the duration of amenorrhea in women with anorexia nervosa.[74] Bone loss and inadequate bone formation (osteopenia and osteoporosis) may be caused by calcium, vitamin, and micronutrient deficiencies; estrogen and testosterone deficiency; hypercortisolemia; insulinlike growth factor-I deficiency; and excessive exercise.[74,75] Bone density is correlated with caloric intake, fat mass, leptin levels, and BMI. Studies have reported that young women with anorexia nervosa may have a bone density similar to menopausal women in their 70s and 80s.[74] Although body density may increase with weight recovery, osteopenia may be a permanent consequence of the disease, resulting in significant morbidity from bone fractures.[74] In males, weight restoration leads to increased testosterone levels, but 10% to 20% of men may have some type of testicular abnormality secondary to prolonged starvation.[1]

Treatment

Medical Management

4. The laboratory tests for S.B. indicate that she has a low tri-iodothyronine level, mild anemia, an elevated blood urea nitrogen (BUN), hypokalemia, and hyponatremia. T-wave inversions and bradycardia are found on the ECG. Low estradiol and luteinizing hormone levels and reduced bone density on the bone scan are reported. S.B. has orthostatic hypotension from dehydration and is severely constipated. Physical examination reveals lanugo (fine body hair), dry skin and hair, and atrophy of the breasts. The physician recommends that S.B. be admitted to an inpatient program that specializes in eating disorders. Based on S.B.'s presentation, does this patient require hospitalization? What is the usual approach for correcting and monitoring these complications from anorexia nervosa?

Patients should be hospitalized for any of the following conditions: rapid weight loss of >15% of body weight, hypotension with a systolic blood pressure <90 mmHg, bradycardia (heart rate, <50 beats/minute), core body temperature <97°F, suicidal ideation, medical complications, and nonresponsiveness to outpatient treatment (after 3–4 months).[3] S.B. should be hospitalized because of her medical complications of anorexia nervosa. Because the majority of medical complications associated with anorexia nervosa improve with nutritional rehabilitation, the first step in most eating disorder programs is to restore weight, rehydrate, and correct serum electrolytes under close medical supervision.[1–3] Vitamin and mineral deficiencies secondary to restricted dieting require supplementation of vitamins, minerals, and electrolytes (potassium, magnesium) along with nutritional refeeding.

The primary treatment for anorexia nervosa is to improve overall nutritional status, restore weight, restore gonadal function, and establish normal eating patterns (Table 82-6).[3] Weight gain reduces the core symptoms of anorexia nervosa and improves dysphoric mood and obsessive-compulsive behaviors.[16] A minimum goal weight is approximately 90% of ideal weight for height using standard tables, but a final "healthy" goal weight is the weight at which normal ovulation and menstruation occur.[3] Inpatient weight restoration programs can increase weight at a rate of 2 to 3 lb/week, whereas outpatient programs usually have lower weight goals of 0.5 to 1 lb/week. Guidelines for calorie intake and monitoring during refeeding can be found in the American Psychiatric Association's Practice Guideline for the Treatment of Patients with Eating Disorders.[3] Parenteral or enteral nutrition is used for patients with severe undernutrition who are refractory to other methods of weight gain.[3] Rapid refeeding and weight gain are not recommended because they increase the risk of a "refeeding syndrome," characterized by gastric bloating, edema, cardiac changes, and congestive heart failure.[71] Initial caloric intake of 30 to 40 kcal/kg/day (1,000–1,600 kcal/day) with progressive increase up to 70 to 100 kcal/kg/day during the weight gain phase are usual standards for nutritional rehabilitation.[3] For the weight maintenance phase, intake of 40 to 60 kcal/kg/day is required to maintain growth in children and adolescents.[3]

Weight gain results in improvement in psychological and medical complications associated with starvation and patients are more likely to participate and benefit from psychosocial treatments. Treatment should continue for at least 3 to 6 months after achieving the goal weight and until menstrual periods resume.[16] Cognitive and physiological abnormalities may persist for months after achieving the goal weight, thus abnormal eating behaviors and body image distortions may return without a comprehensive treatment approach.[16]

Routine monitoring of laboratory tests (e.g., complete blood count and platelets, renal and hepatic function tests, electrolytes, BUN, urinalysis, ECG), weight, and vital signs is required to assess medical status (see Table 82-8).[2,3,76,77] Patients who are emaciated often have cognitive difficulties and psychological changes that can interfere with their participation in behavioral and cognitive therapies.[31] Patients with a history of vomiting must be watched closely to prevent this compensatory behavior during hospitalization. Cardiac monitoring (e.g., blood pressure, pulse, ECG) is indicated to assess cardiac arrhythmias, ventricular tachycardia, or prolonged QT interval.[3]

Bone density studies at baseline and at 6- to 12-month intervals are recommended to assess lumbar spine bone density and to determine the risk of compression fractures.[74] Weight restoration has been shown to be important in reversing menstrual irregularities, pubertal delay, and bone loss that may result in fractures.[78] Prolonged amenorrhea (>6 months) has been associated with irreversible osteopenia (loss of bone density), greater risk of osteoporosis, a higher rate of spine and hip fractures, and infertility.[74]

Cognitive–Behavioral Therapy, Behavioral Therapy, and Family Therapy

5. S.B. and her family meet with a psychologist from the eating disorder's program to receive education about anorexia nervosa and to review treatment goals. At first, S.B. refuses to be admitted, but her parents strongly support a structured program because they argue about her eating behaviors and excessive exercising. Because of the seriousness of her medical status, S.B. finally agrees to participate in therapy. What are the standard therapeutic approaches for patients with anorexia nervosa?

Anorexia responds to a variety of psychotherapeutic approaches that include individual, group, and family therapy.[1,3,31] Behavioral positive reinforcement programs (i.e., operant conditioning) and response–prevention techniques are very helpful in reducing destructive eating behaviors. Positive rewards, such as increasing social activities, visitations, and physical exercise, can be used when preset weight gain goals are met. Those who use self-induced vomiting after eating can be observed for several hours after meals to prevent purging behavior. These techniques can be modified for both inpatient and outpatient programs to monitor progress toward treatment goals.

Cognitive–behavioral therapy (CBT) helps patients to identify false thinking, distortions in processing and interpreting events, and their relationship to mood and behavior.[2] Patients are encouraged to evaluate thoughts and feelings related to eating, fears, anxiety, and control issues. Cognitive techniques are taught to help the person restructure his or her thought process, to improve problem solving skills, and to better cope with life stresses. Cognitive therapy can help the person to better understand his or her overvaluation of being thin and obsession with food.

Family counseling or therapy may be helpful in younger adolescents, particularly if family dynamics or unfair parental expectations are issues that increase stress.[3] Individual and family therapy provide opportunities to help patients understand themselves and their relationships with others.

Pharmacotherapy

6. S.B.'s mother asks the attending psychiatrist in the eating disorders program about medications used for anorexia nervosa. The mother is also worried about S.B.'s depressed mood and hopelessness about the future. The physician explains that psychotropic medications usually are not effective in treating the primary symptoms of anorexia nervosa until the person has gained at least 85% of their expected body weight. Are there any effective medications for anorexia nervosa? Which agent should be recommended for S.B.?

Many pharmacologic agents have been tried in the acute treatment of anorexia nervosa, but none have been shown to be more effective than placebo. Malnourished patients may be prone to side effects of medications, and some antidepressant agents (e.g., TCAs) can increase the risk of dehydration, hypotension, arrhythmias, and seizures.[3] The pharmacokinetics of medications also can be altered in patients with anorexia nervosa owing to changes in body fat and protein. For example, hypoalbuminemia can result in more free (unbound) drug and a decrease in body fat can reduce the volume of distribution of fat-soluble drugs, resulting in increased steady-state plasma levels.[79] Because of the increased risk of drug toxicity, any drug therapy should be started with very low doses that are titrated gradually based on adverse effects. In one systematic review, the literature on the efficacy of medications and behavioral interventions for anorexia nervosa in adults and children was weak or nonexistent.[80]

Serotonin-augmenting agents such as *selective serotonin reuptake inhibitors* (SSRIs) are more effective in the treatment of bulimia nervosa than in underweight patients with anorexia nervosa.[2,3] Patients with reduced dietary tryptophan have low CSF serotonin levels; therefore, SSRIs may not work owing to low serotonin production and release.[2,16] After weight gain and adequate protein intake, SSRIs are more likely to have a therapeutic effect in weight-restored anorexic patients. SSRIs such as fluoxetine may have a potential role in preventing relapse in weight-restored individuals with anorexia.[2] Antidepressants generally are reserved for patients with prominent depressive or obsessive-compulsive symptoms that persist after weight has been regained.[3] SSRIs are considered the safest class of antidepressants and are the drugs of choice for comorbid anxiety, obsessive-compulsive-impulsive behaviors, social phobia, and depression.[2] SSRIs are better tolerated than other classes of antidepressants (e.g., TCAs, monoamine oxidase inhibitors [MAOIs]).[3] Serotonin–norepinephrine reuptake inhibitors such as duloxetine and venlafaxine have not been adequately studied. Bupropion, a norepinephrine–dopamine reuptake inhibitor is contraindicated in patients with anorexia because of an increased risk of seizures.[2]

Antipsychotics, such as chlorpromazine and pimozide, were initially used to treat psychotic-like obsessional thinking, but there is no evidence that they are effective in anorexia nervosa.[2,16] Atypical antipsychotic agents with serotonin antagonist effects (i.e., olanzapine, quetiapine, risperidone) may exacerbate obsessive-compulsive disorder, worsen binge-eating, and cause weight gain due to blockade of serotonin receptors.[16] Cyproheptadine (serotonin antagonist with antihistamine effects that increases appetite and promote weight gain) has been tried in anorexia nervosa with mixed results.[2] There is no evidence that mood stabilizers or anticonvulsants help with the treatment of anorexia. Lithium carbonate has been tried, but has a narrow therapeutic range and may cause neurotoxicity at high plasma levels; it does not seem to be effective in increasing weight gain.[16]

Estrogen replacement is inadequate to increase bone density in patients with anorexia nervosa, particularly without weight restoration and normalization of body fat composition.[74,75] Oral contraceptives may cause weight gain, but have no effect on bone density.[2] Calcium supplementation alone has not been shown to increase bone density in anorexia nervosa.[75] Controlled trials of zinc supplementation have been conducted but results are mixed.[1] Adequate nutrition, weight gain, calcium and vitamin D supplementation, restoration of the regular menstrual cycle, and moderate weight-bearing aerobic exercise are currently the treatments of choice to maintain bone density.[74,75]

Other agents have been used to treat anorexia nervosa. Benzodiazepines (e.g., lorazepam 0.5–1 mg or oxazepam 15–30 mg) have been given before feeding to reduce anxiety symptoms, but these agents may cause CNS depression, dependence, and withdrawal reactions. Clonidine has not been found to increase weight or have therapeutic effects.[16] Metoclopramide and domperidone (dopamine antagonists) have been investigated for increasing gastric emptying and reducing abdominal distension and bloating, but there is concern about extrapyramidal reactions when these agents are used in high doses.[2]

BULIMIA NERVOSA

Clinical Features

7. S.B., now a 21-year-old woman, still struggles to maintain her normal weight despite several relapses of her anorexia nervosa. Since starting college, she has started gaining weight when living in the dorms with a self-serve cafeteria. Over the past year, rather than exercising excessively to keep the weight off, she sometimes binge-eats at fast food restaurants late at night. The binge-eating episodes have become very expensive and S.B. has started shoplifting and stealing money to support her "habit." Currently, S.B. has been binge-eating at least three times a week over several months. She is beginning to gain weight even though she restricts food between bingeing episodes and induces vomiting afterward to help control her weight. S.B. is very secretive about her binge-eating and purging despite living in a sorority house at college. She plans the episodes late at night and often drives into the country to consume the food and to vomit. S.B. is scared of gaining weight, so she often does not eat for several days between the binge-eating episodes and is thinking about using laxatives to lose weight. What characteristics and behaviors of S.B. suggest that she may be suffering from bulimia nervosa?

Many aspects of S.B.'s history are consistent with bulimia nervosa with compensatory mechanisms (Table 82-4). She has a long history of secretive bingeing and purging. Bulimia nervosa is often a chronic disorder with multiple episodes of relapse and remission that begins in late adolescence or in early adult life between the ages of 15 and 24 years.[1,3] Bulimia may occur in normal weight, obese, or anorexic individuals, as is the case with S.B. Binge-eating usually is preceded by emotional factors (e.g., anxiety, depression, boredom, relationship or family problems) or a stressful life event.[3] Younger women tend to have family problems or are seeking independence from parents, whereas women older than age 20 are more likely to have marital or relationship difficulties preceding the onset of bulimia nervosa. Before the onset of the disorder, individuals may be overweight and report periods of severely restricting food intake, fasting, and using "fad" diets to lose weight.[1] Binge-eating occurs when the person loses his or her control over food restriction and becomes "out of control" when consuming food. Before starting to binge-eat, women can become sweaty, tachycardic, anxious, and tense, all of which may be related to starvation from dieting. During the bingeing episode, a sense of freedom and a reduction in anxiety or negative thoughts often is reported. Afterward, the person may feel depressed, guilty, and anxious about gaining weight and try to reduce these negative emotions with the act of vomiting.

Course and Prognosis

8. How does the clinical course of S.B. resemble others with bulimia nervosa and what is her prognosis ?

The course of the disorder may be intermittent, with periods of remission and recurrences of binge-eating, or it may be chronic.[1–3] Between binges, individuals often diet rigorously, try to resist the urge to eat, and are fearful of weight gain. Over time, the frequency and severity of the binge-eating increases and bulimia nervosa develops. Low self-esteem, anxiety, guilt about binge-eating, depression, impulsive behaviors, sexual conflicts, and problems with intimacy are commonly found in women with bulimia nervosa.[3] In one sample of women with eating disorders, 35% of women had relapse of bulimia nervosa at the 9-year follow-up period; in addition, relapse was associated with greater body image disturbances and psychosocial dysfunction.[81] Approximately 5% of those with bulimia nervosa develop anorexia nervosa.[30]

9. In addition to bingeing, S.B. now admits to using laxatives several times a day. She has also recently started smoking cigarettes and occasionally uses cocaine for its euphoric and appetite suppressant effects. How are these common compensatory mechanisms used to prevent weight gain in patients with bulimia nervosa?

Most binge eaters end the episode because they become nauseated, full, or have discomfort.[3,4,31] Several strategies are used to reduce the fear of gaining weight. The most popular is to reduce the amount of calories absorbed from the food they have eaten by inducing vomiting or restricting food between binges.[31] As many as 80% to 90% of bulimic patients have induced vomiting after an episode of binge-eating to decrease abdominal discomfort and to reduce the chance of gaining weight, and approximately 60% of patients regularly use self-induced vomiting. Initially, individuals may use a variety of methods to induce vomiting, such as gagging themselves with their fingers, a toothbrush, or a spoon. Later, individuals may be able to vomit without self-induction techniques.

Between 75% and 90% of binge eaters have abused laxatives during their illness but this method is less effective in controlling body weight. Laxatives act primarily on the large bowel to empty, but this occurs after food already has been absorbed in the small intestine. Excessive laxative intake may lead to electrolyte disturbances, particularly potassium deficiency. Approximately 60% have used over-the-counter (OTC) diet pills that may contain some form of laxative.

Some individuals may restrict food or starve between eating binges, use excessive exercise, and ingest appetite-suppressant products in an attempt to compensate for binge-eating. A number of appetite-suppressing medications with sympathomimetic effects have addictive properties. Approximately 40% of binge eaters have used diuretics to lose weight, but this only loses fluid weight and is ineffective for reducing energy from food. Approximately 10% use prescription anorectic medications and at least 20% of bulimic patients abuse alcohol or drugs.

Misuse of diuretics and enemas, consuming syrup of ipecac to induce vomiting, or taking thyroid hormones are less frequently used methods to reverse binge eating effects. Women with eating disorders, especially in those who binge and purge, seem to be at higher risk of smoking than controls.[82]

Medical Complications

10. S.B. has been experiencing constant headaches, muscle cramps, and fatigue for several days and feels that she has the flu. She makes an appointment at the student health clinic and is evaluated by a nurse practitioner in a walk-in clinic. During the physical examination, the nurse notes abrasions on the top of her hand, hypertrophy of the salivary and parotid glands, and enamel loss on her teeth. S.B. is dehydrated and complains of chronic constipation. What signs and symptoms of bulimia nervosa are present on S.B.'s physical examination? What laboratory screening tests are recommended to rule out a medical diagnosis or medical complications from bulimia nervosa?

Individuals with bulimia nervosa are usually within their normal weight range; thus, medical complications, morbidity, and mortality associated with weight loss or obesity are less of a problem.[3] Common physiologic changes and abnormal laboratory tests associated with purging are listed in Table 82-7. Baseline laboratory tests often include serum electrolytes, a complete blood count, liver and renal function tests, thyroid function tests, and an ECG (Table 82-8).[3]

Purging behavior can produce electrolyte abnormalities (e.g., hypochloremia, hypokalemia, hyponatremia), fluid disturbances, and dehydration.[3,31] Metabolic alkalosis (elevated serum bicarbonate) is associated with loss of stomach acid through vomiting; metabolic acidosis may occur secondary to diarrhea through laxative abuse. Hypokalemia occurs secondary to aldosterone secretion and increased potassium excretion from the kidneys, and through self-induced vomiting.[31] Electrolyte disturbances can cause lethargy, weakness, and, possibly, cardiac arrhythmias.

Permanent loss of dental enamel, especially on the front teeth, and dental cavities are common secondary to the effects of stomach acid.[31] Enlargement or inflammation of salivary glands (sialadenitis), particularly the parotid glands, from recurrent vomiting often is reported. Elevated serum amylase owing to increases in salivary isoenzymes often results. Calluses or scars on the dorsal part of the hand secondary to trauma by the teeth (known as the *Russell sign*) is caused by repeated self-induction of vomiting.[83] Individuals who chronically abuse syrup of ipecac to induce vomiting may develop myopathy (e.g., muscle weakness, aching, hyporeflexia, slurred speech) and/or cardiotoxicity (e.g., atrial premature contractions, supraventricular tachycardia, ventricular tachycardia, flattened or inverted T waves, prolonged QT and P-R intervals, changes in the QRS complex, decreased contractility, and cardiac arrest).[31] Ipecac contains a cardiotoxin that, in high doses, may cause permanent necrosis of heart fibers and interstitial edema.

Laxative abuse initially causes diarrhea, but continued use may result in rebound fluid retention and electrolyte disturbances. A withdrawal syndrome associated with discontinuation of laxatives is characterized by constipation, abdominal bloating and cramping, agitation, and feeling "sick." Diuretics or OTC slimming tablets cause electrolyte disturbances, particularly potassium deficiency. Fluid retention may result when long-term diuretic use is discontinued.

Approximately 40% of women with bulimia nervosa have irregular menstruation and 20% have amenorrhea. Menstrual disturbances usually cease when body weight is stabilized and when dangerous methods of weight control, including excessive exercise and intermittent starvation, are stopped.

Treatment

Medical Management

11. The nurse practitioner feels that S.B. has bulimia nervosa based on the physical examination and laboratory tests (serum potassium, 3.0 mEq/L; BUN:creatinine ratio, >30; volume depletion; scarring on the dorsum of the hand; and severe dental caries and enamel erosion). She confronts S.B. about her eating habits and recommends referral to a therapist and psychiatrist who have experience in eating disorders. S.B. finally confesses about how horrible she feels and asks for help. A plan is established that includes a psychiatrist, therapist, and nutritionist to manage the medical, psychological, and nutritional aspects of treatment. How should physiologic complications be monitored and assessed in SB?

Individuals who seek medical help may not tell their physician about their eating habits; thus, bulimia nervosa may be missed. Most patients with bulimia nervosa do not require hospitalization unless there is a medical or psychiatric indication such as severe depression with suicidal thoughts, severe concurrent drug or alcohol abuse, or a life-endangering medical problem (e.g., severe hypokalemia, metabolic alkalosis/acidosis, severe dehydration, acute pancreatitis, cardiomyopathy, cardiac arrhythmia).[3,16] Common medical complaints include GI problems (irritable bowel syndrome, spastic colon), menstrual irregularities, depression, or panic attacks. Those who seek treatment for bulimia nervosa have usually started inducing vomiting or taking purgatives, or both. Patients with self-induced vomiting should be monitored for esophageal tears, dehydration, metabolic alkalosis (hypochloremia and hypokalemia), elevated serum amylase, weakness and lethargy, cardiac arrhythmias, erosion of dental enamel or dental caries, and vitamin, electrolyte, and mineral deficiencies.[3] Correcting serum electrolyte abnormalities helps to reduce the risk of medical complications such as cardiac arrhythmias. Individuals who abuse ipecac require monitoring of blood pressure (hypotension), heart rate (tachycardia), ECG to assess cardiac failure, and liver enzymes. An echocardiogram may be needed to diagnose cardiomyopathy.

Cognitive–Behavioral Therapy and Interpersonal Therapy

12. S.B. agrees to participate in an intensive outpatient eating disorder treatment program that is coordinated through the student health clinic. Her team feels that she will need help with self-esteem development, coping skills, and adherence with treatment, so they develop biweekly sessions to work on goals. What are the standard nonpharmacologic therapies for patients with bulimia nervosa or binge eating disorder?

Psychoeducational groups, nutritional counseling, self-help manuals, and self-monitoring have all been used as treatments for bulimia nervosa. However, the literature suggests that individuals who receive CBT have higher remission rates; thus, this treatment should be considered the first-line treatment of choice for most patients.[2] Most patients benefit more from structured CBT approaches, requiring an average of 20 sessions over a 4- to 6-month period.[3,16] Beside CBT, interpersonal psychotherapy may be useful in treating bulimia nervosa and binge-eating disorder.[2] Time-limited interpersonal psychotherapy, up to 16 weeks, also has been shown to improve interpersonal problems and role transitions and reduces bulimic behaviors over the long term. Reviews of psychological and pharmacotherapy comparative studies for bulimia nervosa and binge-eating disorders can be found elsewhere.[1]

Behavioral and cognitive techniques help individuals to self-monitor their binge-eating and purging episodes and document changes in mood and circumstances related to the binge–purge behavior.[2] CBT helps the person to examine distortions in his or her thought processing and interpretation of events, and uses cognitive restructuring to change the way he or she thinks and reacts. Several studies have reported that CBT or CBT in combination with antidepressants is more effective in reducing bulimic symptoms than giving antidepressant medications alone.[2,3,16,84] CBT has been reported to be more effective than supportive psychotherapy and the addition of an antidepressant may significantly improve depression and binge-eating behaviors.[85] Psychoeducational approaches along with individual and group therapy are commonly used for CBT. Behavioral therapy is used to stop the binge-eating and purging behaviors by restricting exposure to situations or cues that trigger a binge–purge episode, by finding alternative behaviors that are less destructive, and by delaying the purging response to eating. Response prevention techniques are used to prevent vomiting by placing an individual in a more restrictive environment or situation where it is very difficult to vomit.

Pharmacotherapy

13. The psychiatrist has several individual sessions with S.B. to assess the severity of the eating disorder and to rule out other psychiatric or medical disorders. S.B. has mild symptoms of depression that do not meet the criteria for a major depressive episode. Nicotine and cocaine help her mood, so S.B. wonders if an antidepressant would help her feel less anxious and reduce the urge to binge and purge. The psychiatrist agrees that the comorbid substance abuse, mild depression, anxiety symptoms, and obsessive-compulsive behaviors may respond to an antidepressant. What medications have been used to treat bulimia nervosa? How safe and effective are these agents, and how long should patients be maintained on treatment?

If medications are required, antidepressants are considered the drugs of choice for bulimia nervosa.[1–3,16] Bulimic patients do not need to be clinically depressed to benefit from treatment. Several short-term, double-blind, placebo-controlled studies have demonstrated that antidepressants are effective for reducing binge-eating and vomiting episodes, although some classes such as TCAs and MAOIs have more adverse effects and may not be tolerated.[86,87] Serotonin-augmenting agents are the most commonly prescribed antidepressants for bulimia nervosa and binge-eating disorder and have a more favorable side effect profile in comparison with other classes.[16] Nutritional counseling has been shown to be effective in bulimia nervosa and may have beneficial effects when combined with SSRI treatment.[88] Few long-term controlled studies have been done with antidepressants to evaluate if modifications in eating behaviors and weight are maintained over time. Fluoxetine and fluvoxamine combined with CBT was shown to be more effective than drug therapy alone in the treatment of binge eating disorder at 1-year follow-up based on BMI and eating disorder rating scales.[84] A summary of randomized controlled trials of antidepressants versus placebo for bulimia nervosa can be found elsewhere.[2]

Fluoxetine was approved by the U.S. Food and Drug Administration (FDA) in 1996 for the treatment of bulimia nervosa. Higher daily doses of fluoxetine (60 mg/day) may be superior to the standard antidepressant dose of 20 mg/day.[16] Other serotonin-augmenting agents (e.g., citalopram, escitalopram, fluvoxamine, paroxetine, sertraline, and venlafaxine) are alternative treatments for bulimia nervosa or binge-eating disorder.[2,16] The efficacy and ideal dose of SSRIs other than fluoxetine have not been established.[16] Common side effects reported with SSRIs include diarrhea, nausea, headache, insomnia, and sexual dysfunction. Bradycardia and hyponatremia have been reported with SSRIs; thus, monitoring of heart rate, blood pressure, and serum electrolytes is recommended, particularly for patients who use diuretics or have purging behaviors.

In a review of double- and single-blind, placebo-controlled studies, TCAs, MAOIs, topiramate, ondansetron, and inositol have shown some benefit in bulimia nervosa.[2,89] Bupropion is not recommended for the treatment of eating disorder patients owing due to reported risks of seizures in patients with bulimia nervosa.[2] Topiramate, a novel antiepileptic agent, has been reported to decrease binge-eating episodes and improve quality of life in patients with bulimia nervosa in several double-blind, placebo-controlled studies.[2]

Duration of antidepressant therapy is an important issue because patients treated for at least 6 months have a better long-term outcome than patients who receive shorter antidepressant trials.[86] Only 50% of patients achieve a complete remission after antidepressant treatment and a majority have relapses after the initial intervention has stopped.[16] Approximately one-third of patients may relapse with prophylactic antidepressant treatment.[16] A rapid relapse of binge-eating behaviors has been reported when antidepressants are withdrawn in both bulimia nervosa and binge-eating disorder.[86] In general, antidepressants should be prescribed for at least 6 months, and some patients may require long-term prophylactic antidepressant treatment.[16] Daily recordings of mood and binge-eating behaviors, weekly weighings, and close monitoring may have their own therapeutic benefits as well.

OBESITY

Clinical Features

14. S.B., now 50 years old, is married and has 3 children. She has been treated successfully for her eating disorders that she suffered as a young woman and has lived without any complications for several decades. Unfortunately, after 3 children, she has noticed a slow but progressive increase in her weight over the past few years. She is currently being evaluated at a chronic pain clinic for lower back and knee pain secondary to degenerative joint disease. Her current height is 5 feet 6 inches tall; she weighs 250 lb, has a waist circumference of 40 inches, and is unable to move without significant joint and back pain. In the past 15 years, she has developed diabetes, hypertension, and hyperlipidemia. S.B. is currently being treated for depression and perimenopausal symptoms. S.B.'s current medications include metformin, atenolol, atorvastatin, and paroxetine. How is obesity defined and assessed in a patient like S.B.? What common clinical features of obesity and risk factors are useful for determining the need for treatment in S.B.?

Obesity is an excessive accumulation of body fat secondary to poor appetite regulation and decreased energy metabolism. Appropriate treatment of the overweight/obese patient requires assessment of the degree of overweight and overall risk status. The best method to determine the degree of overweight/obesity is to measure the BMI, which is associated with total body fat content.[14] The waist circumference is an independent predictor of risk factors and morbidity and correlates to abdominal fat content.[7,14] High relative health risks are seen in patients with waist circumference >102 cm (40 inches) in men and >88 cm (35 inches) in women compared with patients with normal weight. Fat deposited around the waist seems to be more likely than fat on the hips or thighs to lead to health risks such as cardiovascular disease, insulin resistance, type 2 diabetes, hyperlipidemia, and increased blood pressure. The waist circumference may not be as predictive or helpful in patients with BMI >35 kg/m^2 and height <5 ft.[14] Waist:hip ratio indicates regional fat distribution and increased health risk is seen in patients with high intra-abdominal fat (waist:hip ratio >1 in men and >0.8 in women).[7] Skin-fold thickness can be used to assess body fat at various sites, but measurements may vary between observers and it does not provide information about intramuscular or abdominal fat.[7] S.B.'s BMI is 40.3 (250 lb ÷ $[66 \text{ in}]^2 \times 703$), which is in obesity class III (extreme obesity). To determine absolute risk and need for treatment of overweight/obesity, clinicians should be familiar with related diseases and other risk factors (Table 82-9).

Patients who are overweight/obese need to be monitored for other cardiovascular risk factors as recommended by the guidelines published by the National Cholesterol Education

Table 82-9 Conditions That Increase the Risk Status in Overweight/Obese Patients

Disease Conditions	*Risk for Disease Complications, Mortality*
Coronary heart disease	Very high
Atherosclerotic disease	
Type 2 diabetes mellitus	
Sleep apnea	
Other obesity-related diseases	
Gynecologic abnormalities	High
Osteoarthritis	
Gallstones and complications	
Stress incontinence	
Cardiovascular risk factors	
Cigarette smoking	Very high if ≥2 risk factors
Hypertension	
Increased LDL cholesterol	
Low HDL cholesterol	
Impaired fasting blood glucose	
Family history of premature CHD	
Age (men >45, women >55 or postmenopausal)	
Physical inactivity	
High serum triglycerides	

CHD, coronary heart disease; HDL, high-density lipoprotein; LDL, low-density lipoprotein.
Adapted from reference 14.

Program and the Joint National Committee on Prevention, Detection, Evaluation and Treatment of High Blood Pressure. The impact of S.B.'s current medications for her various chronic conditions and her limited mobility to participate in exercise regimens should be taken into consideration. Patients' motivation to lose weight is a significant predictor of success or failure in the weight management program. The willingness to participate in a regimen may depend on past history of diets, social support at home and workplace, patient's understanding of the illness, time, and financial burden.[14] Obesity is considered a chronic medical condition because it causes multiple physical complications.[7] The greater the degree of obesity, the harder it is for a person to lose weight permanently without medical and behavioral interventions. Major depressive disorder, anxiety disorders, and low self-esteem are common in obese patients owing to social prejudice and discrimination in the work force.[9]

Course and Prognosis

15. S.B. has steadily gained weight since her early 30s after the birth of her first child. She has always struggled with her weight and has three other siblings who are obese. She has tried more than 15 diets to lose weight, but each time she stops the diet she regains even more weight. S.B. admits to overeating and, at times, uses laxatives and OTC diet pills to help her control her weight and appetite. What is the typical course and prognosis of obesity?

Obesity is a chronic disease that can begin in childhood or adolescence and can be characterized by a slow and steady increase in body weight during adult life. In a retrospective cohort study comparing long-term mortality of people undergoing bariatric surgery with obese patients in the control group, the rate of death from any cause was 40% lower in the surgical group.[90]

Overeating or binge-eating along with restrictive dieting is a common occurrence among Americans and may be a chronic lifelong problem that leads to obesity. Recent studies have shown that 10% to 25% of obese people regularly engage in binge-eating behavior and that the greater their weight, the more likely they are to be binge eaters[16]; at least 25% to 45% of obese individuals have symptoms that meet the criteria for binge-eating disorder.[9,16,83] Unlike individuals with bulimia nervosa, obese binge-eaters usually do not vomit or purge and may or may not restrict food intake between binge-eating episodes. Obese binge-eaters often have a preoccupation with their body shape and weight, but they have poor control of their eating habits. Women tend to be more concerned about their body shape and weight and are more likely to diet than men. More than 80% of people who lose weight gradually regain it; patients who continue on weight maintenance programs consisting of dietary, physical, and behavioral therapy have a better chance of not regaining weight than those who discontinue weight maintenance programs.[14]

Medical Complications

16. The physician in the pain management clinic is very concerned about S.B.'s weight because of her current medical conditions and the likelihood of further complications during her lifetime. What are the most common medical conditions associated with obesity?

Obesity has a tremendous impact on physiologic functioning and medical illnesses. Obese people tend to die young, and the more abdominal body fat, the greater the mortality. Obesity-related medical conditions in the United States result in 300,000 deaths per year and cost approximately $70 billion in health care costs.[91] Obesity is linked with many disabling diseases such as diabetes mellitus (non–insulin-dependent and insulin-resistant), pulmonary impairment (hypoventilation, hypoxia, hypercapnia, and sleep apnea), gallbladder disease (gallstones and cholecystitis), cancers (colorectal, prostate, breast, cervical, endometrial, uterine, and ovarian), osteoarthritis (hips, knees, and back), gout, cardiac disease (hypertension, stroke, congestive heart failure, and coronary heart disease), increased cholesterol and triglycerides (TG) (increased low-density lipoproteins and decreased high-density lipoproteins), dermatologic problems (intertrigo and stretching of skin), and menstrual irregularities.[14,31] The Nurses Health Study showed that the risk of developing diabetes in women with BMI >35 was 60 times higher than the lowest risk group (BMI <22 kg/m^2).[92] It is estimated that >60% of type 2 diabetes mellitus cases are due to obesity.[20] Weight loss helps to control diseases associated with obesity and may even help prevent development of these diseases. Weight loss has been shown to be beneficial in lowering blood pressure, total cholesterol, low-density lipoproteins, TG, blood glucose in patients with diabetes mellitus type 2, and increasing high-density lipoproteins.[14]

Treatment

Medical Management

17. The physician recommends that S.B. reduce her weight over the next 12 months to help improve the quality of her life, reduce the associated morbidity from related medical conditions, and prolong her life. What would be appropriate goals for weight loss with F.W.? What type of nutritional and exercise plan should be recommended?

According to the National Heart, Lung, and Blood Institute guidelines, weight loss treatment should be initiated for patients who are overweight, who have increased waist circumference plus two or more risk factors, or are obese (BMI ≥30).[14] The general goals of weight loss and management are to prevent weight gain, reduce body weight, and maintain weight loss over a long period.[14] Treatment options to facilitate weight loss include moderate caloric restriction, medications (e.g., appetite suppressants, lipase inhibitors), physical activity, and behavior therapy. Obese patients (like S.B.) should strive to lose 10% of baseline weight at a rate of 1 to 2 lb/week with an energy deficit of 500 kcal/day over 6 months. Overweight patients should ideally lose 0.5 lb/week with an energy deficit of 300 to 500 kcal/day over 6 months. A low-calorie diet consistent with National Cholesterol Education Program Step 1 or Step 2 diet has been shown to be most effective. A low-fat diet does not decrease weight unless total caloric intake is decreased. Total fat intake should account for 30% or less of total calories consumed per day.[14] Drastic caloric restriction is difficult to maintain and may lead to reduced metabolism and overeating due to hunger. Severe caloric restriction and rapid weight loss can be harmful and result in rebound binge-eating behavior and weight gain.[93]

Increased physical activity can facilitate weight loss and is essential in preventing weight gain. Overweight children and adults should have at least 30 minutes of moderate-intensity physical exercise daily (with a gradual increment of increasing exercise by several minutes each day up to 30 minutes per day). It has recently been shown that moderate exercise (e.g. 4 kcal/g per week) can improve physiologic variables.[94] Modest weight loss is beneficial, because even a small amount of weight loss, as little as 5%, is associated with significant improvements in health status.

Obese patients should be evaluated for hypothyroidism because it is a potential cause of weight gain. However, use of thyroid hormones to cause weight reduction in patients with normal thyroid function is not recommended.

Nonpharmacologic Therapy

18. S.B. has never participated in a behavior modification weight reduction or maintenance program. The physician recommends that she attend weekly social support meetings and learn more desirable behaviors for self-monitoring her diet and exercise. What types of nonpharmacologic therapies or programs are available for weight reduction and relapse prevention?

Behavioral modification programs using support groups, a balanced diet, and exercise are most effective for mild obesity (20%–40% overweight).[31] Behavioral modification programs (e.g., nutritional education, exercise, cognitive restructuring, self-monitoring) are the most effective for overweight children and help to motivate parents and children to alter their lifestyles.[14] Supportive family therapy is desirable, particularly for obese children. Obesity may be related to cultural attitudes, family eating behaviors, and social events involving food. Relapse prevention should identify high-risk situations or events that may cause weight gain so that the person can learn new coping strategies to avoid overeating.

Because of the high demand by consumers, there are numerous types of weight loss programs, diets, and products that may or may not be effective. Individuals who want to lose weight frequently seek out popular structured programs (e.g., Jenny Craig, Weight Watchers). Other weight loss programs include low-fat, low-sodium, vegetarian, soy, Atkins, and Zone diets. Regardless of which weight loss program is chosen, patients should select a program that emphasizes the following: (a) counseling for lifestyle changes, (b) trained staff, (c) coping strategies for stressful times, (d) weight loss maintenance, and (e) flexible and appropriate food choices.[95]

Overall, a combination of low-calorie diet, behavioral modifications, and increased physical activity are most effective for reducing and maintaining weight loss. These measures must be attempted and maintained for at least 6 months before considering pharmacotherapy.[14]

Pharmacotherapy

19. S.B. asks the physician about medications that can help with weight loss. What is the current status of pharmacologic agents for obesity therapy? What are their mechanisms of action, efficacy, and potential adverse effects?

A comprehensive treatment approach to obesity includes a weight loss diet, exercise, supportive psychotherapy, and behavioral modification techniques. If indicated, medications such as an anorectic agent (to suppress hunger and appetite) or a GI lipase inhibitor (to reduce fat absorption) may be prescribed.[96] Weight loss is possible for most patients, but the main problem is that the vast majority of people regain the weight over time.[2] Obesity is a chronic, lifelong illness that may require long-term medication therapy. Medication should be considered only for patients with a BMI >30 kg/m^2 without risk factors or >27 kg/m^2 with an obesity-related risk factor (Table 82-9).[14] Anorectic medications or lipase inhibitors should not be considered a replacement for diet, behavioral modification, and exercise, but rather as add-on therapy.

Medications used for the treatment of obesity in the United States are found in Table 82-10. Although there are many medications with varying mechanisms of action that have been theorized to be effective for weight loss, currently marketed drugs for weight loss do so by suppressing the appetite or decreasing the absorption of fat.[96] According to recent meta-analyses and critical reviews, sibutramine and orlistat have been shown to have consistent and sustained, albeit modest, weight loss effects over other pharmacologic classes of drugs up to 1 year.[97,98]

AMPHETAMINES AND SYMPATHOMIMETICS

Amphetamines, dextroamphetamine, and sympathomimetics have been used as appetite suppressants and thermogenic agents for several decades.[99] The enhancement of dopaminergic activity is believed to be responsible for amphetamine's rewarding, reinforcing, and addictive properties.[100] Because of their euphoric properties and risks of drug abuse, amphetamines are schedule II controlled agents and are not routinely used for weight loss.[101] Additional concerns with sympathomimetics are the potential for rebound binge-eating, weight gain, lethargy, and depression when the medication is discontinued.[31] Other centrally active appetite suppressants that augment catecholamines (e.g., phentermine, mazindol, phendimetrazine, and diethylpropion) were developed for the treatment of obesity and may have a lower incidence and severity of CNS side effects compared with the amphetamines.[99]

Although amphetamines and sympathomimetics may be quite effective for weight loss, they are not without significant risks. Fenfluramine and dexfenfluramine were voluntarily removed from the United States market in 1997 due to studies linking their usage to valvular heart disease and primary pulmonary hypertension.[102] As of April 2004, the FDA has prohibited the sale of dietary supplements containing ephedrine alkaloids (ephedra) owing to the many reports of serious adverse effects (e.g., stroke, seizures, and death).[103] Ephedrine (found in ephedra and ma huang) was included in several OTC and herbal products that promoted their ability to increase energy expenditure, thus causing weight loss. Phenylpropanolamine (PPA), a popular synthetic catecholamine that was widely found in OTC weight-loss products and decongestants, was also voluntarily withdrawn in 2000.[104] PPA increased satiety by stimulating norepinephrine and dopamine release in the hypothalamic feeding center, but studies found an increased risk of hemorrhagic stroke in women who took appetite suppressants containing more than 32 mg/day PPA.[105] Because of significant adverse effects of sympathomimetics, these agents are no longer recommended for weight loss.

Table 82-10 Medications Marketed or Used for the Treatment of Obesity

Generic Name	Trade Name	Dosage	DEA Schedule or Class
Amphetamine/dextroamphetamine	Adderall	5–30 mg/day	II[a]
	Biphetamine	12.5–20 mg/day	II[a]
Benzphetamine hydrochloride	Didrex	25–50 mg one to three times daily	III
Dextroamphetamine			
Immediate release	Dexedrine	5–10 mg before meals	II[a]
Extended release	Dexedrine	10–30 mg	II[a]
Diethylpropion hydrochloride			
Immediate release	Tenuate	25 mg TID; 75 mg AM	IV
Controlled release	Tenuate Dospan	75 mg AM	IV
Ephedrine	Various products	20–60 mg/day	OTC
Mazindol	Sanorex	1 mg TID; 2 mg AM	IV
Methamphetamine hydrochloride			
Immediate release	Desoxyn	2.5–5 mg before meals	II[a]
Orlistat	Xenical, Alli	120 mg TID, 60 mg TID	Prescription, OTC
Phendimetrazine tartrate	Bontril, Plegine, Prelu-2, X-Trozine	35 mg TID; 105 mg AM	III
Phenmetrazine	Preludin	25 mg BID–TID	II[a]
Phentermine			
Hydrochloride	Adipex-P, Fastin, Oby-Cap, Phentride	8 mg TID; 30–37.5 mg AM	IV
Resin	Ionamin	15–30 mg AM	IV
Sibutramine	Meridia	5–15 mg/day	IV

[a]High abuse potential, not recommended for routine or long-term use.
BID, twice a day; OTC, over the counter; TID, three times a day.
Adapted from references 53 and 125.

ANTIDEPRESSANTS

Serotonin- and/or norepinephrine-augmenting agents (e.g., serotonin or norepinephrine reuptake inhibitors) are the most effective agents for suppressing appetite drive and reducing weight. For obese binge-eating patients, SSRI antidepressants such as fluoxetine have been used successfully to reduce binge-eating behavior, but this is not always associated with weight loss.[65] The reason for the weight regain is unclear, but may relate to the development of tolerance or the lack of frequent follow-up visits.[106] In a recent meta-analysis, high-dose fluoxetine was shown to produce a pooled weight loss of 4.74 kg at 6 months and 3.15 kg at 12 months.[98] Studies with other SSRIs are either lacking, limited by small sample size or have shown nonsignificant results.[98] Bupropion, an antidepressant that inhibits dopamine reuptake, has been shown to have some weight loss (2.77 kg) effects at 6 and 12 months when combined with other weight loss measures (diet, exercise).[98] Antidepressants that have histamine-antagonist effects (i.e., TCAs) or block serotonin receptors (e.g., mirtazapine) cause sedation and increase appetite and weight, and thus should not be used in obese patients.[63]

SEROTONIN/NOREPINEPHRINE REUPTAKE INHIBITORS

Sibutramine (Meridia), a prescription medication marketed for weight loss, is structurally related to amphetamines (β-phenylethylamine) and is classified as a schedule IV controlled agent.[107] Sibutramine and its two active metabolites inhibit the reuptake of serotonin and norepinephrine and, to a lesser extent, dopamine, thereby increasing concentrations of these neurotransmitters in the brain.[107–109] By increasing serotonin and norepinephrine activity, α-adrenergic, β-adrenergic, and serotonin$_{2A/2C}$ receptors are stimulated, which in turn causes a downregulation of α- and β-adrenergic and serotonin receptors.[44,107] This promotes a sense of satiety and thus decreases appetite. A synergistic interaction between norepinephrine and serotonin has been shown to maximize reduction in food intake.[100,110] When a norepinephrine or serotonin reuptake inhibitor is given alone, food intake generally is not altered unless these agents are given in significantly higher dosages. Sibutramine also is thought to cause a sympathetic stimulation of brown adipose tissue (thermogenesis to increase glucose utilization) via the β_3-adrenoceptors.[100,110]

In a recent meta-analysis for long-term administration of sibutramine, including 10 trials and more than 2,600 patients, sibutramine reduced weight by 4.3% over those taking placebo and increased the percentage of patients achieving successful weight maintenance.[97] In addition, cardiovascular risk profiles also improved with sibutramine (increased high-density lipoprotein cholesterol and lower TG concentrations). It should be noted that sibutramine was associated with elevations in diastolic and systolic blood pressure as well as heart rate.

In a 1-year trial, 224 obese patients were randomized to receive sibutramine alone, lifestyle modification counseling alone (in group sessions), sibutramine plus group sessions of lifestyle modification, or sibutramine plus brief lifestyle modification counseling by a primary care provider. All patients were restricted to a 1,200 to 1,500 kcal/day diet and similar exercise regimen.[111] Patients who received the drug and group sessions of lifestyle modification lost the most weight (an average of 12.1 kg) versus those in the other groups, who only lost about half the average weight. It should be stressed that sibutramine should always be combined with lifestyle modifications.

Common adverse effects of sibutramine include headache, decreased appetite, dry mouth, constipation, and insomnia.[108,112] Other less common side effects include sweating, irritability, excitation, dizziness, insomnia, and increases in blood pressure and heart rate (increase in blood pressure by 1–3 mmHg and in heart rate by 4 to 5 beats/minute). Frequent blood pressure and pulse rate monitoring is recommended because these cardiovascular effects are believed to be dose related. Sibutramine must be used cautiously in patients with high blood pressure and its use is not recommended in patients with heart disease, congestive heart failure, conduction disorders (arrhythmias), or stroke. Sibutramine is absolutely contraindicated in patients taking certain CNS medications that increase levels of norepinephrine or serotonin (e.g., MAOIs) and other centrally acting appetite suppressants. Precautions should be taken in patients who are coadministered lithium, antimigraine agents (e.g., sumatriptan, dihydroergotamine), and some opioid analgesics (e.g., tramadol, dextromethorphan). Drugs that inhibit liver enzymes (cytochrome P450 3A4), such as ketoconazole and erythromycin, can increase serum concentrations of sibutramine. Sibutramine is well absorbed and has high first-pass liver metabolism to produce two active metabolites, both with long elimination half-lives of 14 to 16 hours.[108] Initial dosing of sibutramine is 10 mg once daily with or without food (typically in the morning) and the dose can be increased to 15 mg once daily if needed. A 5-mg dose is available for patients who do not tolerate the recommended starting dose.

LIPASE INHIBITORS

Orlistat (Xenical), an FDA-approved weight loss medication, works to reduce dietary fat absorption by inhibiting GI (stomach and pancreas) lipase activity.[113,114] In February 2007, the FDA approved the OTC marketing of orlistat under the trade name, Alli.[115] Orlistat is a hydrogenated derivative of lipstatin (a naturally occurring lipase inhibitor produced by *Streptomyces toxytricini*) that is a potent inhibitor of lipases and weak inhibitor of other intestinal hydrolases.[114] Gastric and pancreatic lipase are enzymes that play a pivotal role in the digestion of dietary fat (TG). Before digestion and absorption of dietary fat is possible, each TG molecule must be hydrolyzed by lipase enzymes into absorbable products—two fatty acid molecules and one 2-monoacylglycerol molecule. Orlistat inhibits lipase by binding to and inactivating the enzyme. Subsequently, TG cannot be absorbed, and approximately 30% of ingested fat is excreted in the feces.[114] The therapeutic activity of orlistat takes place in the stomach and small intestine and effects are seen as soon as 24 to 48 hours after dosing.

Orlistat does not exert appetite suppressant effects, has no CNS effects, and has no systemic absorption.[114] It is most effective if combined with a reduced fat and calorie diet[113] and is indicated to reduce the risk of weight regain after prior weight loss. It also is indicated for obese patients with an initial BMI $\geq$30 kg/m^2 or $\geq$27 kg/m^2 in the presence of other obesity-related risk factors. In a recent meta-analysis, orlistat was shown to produce less weight loss (2.9 kg) than sibutramine; orlistat also improved blood pressure, low-density and high-density lipoprotein concentrations.[97] GI adverse events were common, although there was no report of vitamin deficiencies. Orlistat may also reduce the risk of related diseases; in a 4-year study, orlistat plus lifestyle changes was associated with a 37% risk reduction of diabetes in over 3,300 obese patients.[116]

The most common adverse effects associated with orlistat include GI problems (loose stools, oily spotting, flatus with discharge, fecal urgency, fatty/oily stools, increased defecation, fecal incontinence, bloating, and cramping).[117] The most common adverse events reported are fatty/oily stool, fecal urgency, and oily spotting. The most common non-GI adverse effect was headache (6%). Side effects usually develop early in treatment and persist for 1 to 4 weeks, but occasionally last longer than 6 months. Because GI adverse effects are worse with a high-fat diet, orlistat may enhance dietary compliance with a low-fat diet.

Orlistat may reduce the absorption of fat-soluble vitamins (A, D, E, and K) and patients should take a multivitamin supplement that contains these vitamins.[117] The supplement should be taken once a day at least 2 hours before or after the administration of orlistat, such as at bedtime. Orlistat may interfere with vitamin K absorption and potentiate the bleeding effects of warfarin. Orlistat may also reduce the absorption of amiodarone and cyclosporine. When used in diabetic patients, weight loss may be accompanied by improved control of diabetes, which requires a reduction in doses of diabetic medications, including insulin. Orlistat has additive effects when combined with lipid (cholesterol)-lowering agents such as pravastatin; thus, the dose of statins may be reduced.[114] The dosage of prescription orlistat in adults is 120 mg three times daily (OTC dose is 60 mg three times daily), during (or up to 1 hour after) each main meal containing fat. If a meal occasionally is missed or contains no fat, the dose may be omitted. Dosages exceeding 120 mg three times daily do not provide additional benefit.

MISCELLANEOUS AGENTS

Topiramate is a second-generation antiepileptic agent which acts as an agonist at γ-aminobutyric acid ($GABA_A$) receptors and as an antagonist at non–*N*-methyl-D-aspartic acid glutamate receptors. It has been shown to produce a dose-dependent weight loss between 1 and 8 kg and may also produce weight loss in patients with bipolar affective disorder.[118] In a pooled analysis of 6 studies with wide range of dosages, topiramate produced a 6.5% weight loss compared with placebo at 6 months.[98] Paresthesia, CNS, and GI effects were commonly seen at higher doses. Zonisamide has been recently studied in randomized controlled trials for weight loss in obese patients with and without binge-eating.[119,120] One double-blind, placebo-controlled study showed that the active treatment group lost an average of 6% of baseline body weight compared with the placebo group at the end of 4 months.[119] In the binge-eating population, tolerability was low for zonisamide and resulted in a 20% dropout rate.[120]

20. S.B. is willing to try a pharmacologic interventions along with behavioral modification, but she has heard about the use of surgery to reduce the size of her stomach. When should surgical intervention be used? What are potential complications related to surgery and postsurgical precautions?

Surgery

Surgery should be used only for morbidly obese individuals (BMI $\geq$40 or $\geq$35 kg/m^2 with comorbid conditions) in whom behavioral or pharmacologic treatments have failed.[121] For severely obese patients (>100% over normal weight), the most effective treatment is a surgical procedure to reduce the size of the stomach. Surgical procedures either reduce the absorptive surface of the GI tract resulting in malabsorption, or reduce the stomach volume so that the person feels full after a smaller meal. According to recent guidelines, gastric banding, vertical banded gastroplasty, Roux-en-Y gastric bypass, and biliopancreatic diversion are effective options, although the degree of weight loss and complications may differ.[122] Gastric bypass has been shown to produce a greater weight loss compared with gastroplasty procedures.[123] In addition, laparoscopic (vs. open surgical approaches) may be preferred for reducing postoperative complications and hospital stay.[122] The mortality rate from bariatric surgery is estimated to be 0.3% to 1.9% and literature has shown that centers who perform surgeries at high volume have better outcomes.[96]

Some of the complications of bariatric surgery include nausea, stomach ulceration, stenosis, anemia, and cholelithiasis. Postsurgical precautions include careful evaluation of meal sizes and timing along with meal content, especially immediately after surgery. Patients should be aware that they will not be able to resume their normal eating habits and they should be properly educated on lifestyle modifications for maintenance of weight loss. In addition, medications and adequate intake of necessary nutrients are important considerations after surgery. Medication such as nonsteroidal anti-inflammatory drugs, salicylates, and bisphosphonates may cause ulcerations and medications that are delayed- or extended-release may not be absorbed owing to changes in gastric size.[124] Medications may need to be administered using liquid formulation and other dosage routes. Transdermal formulations need to be carefully dosed to account for changes in body surface area postsurgically.[124]

REFERENCES

1. Fairburn CG, Brownell KD, eds. *Eating Disorders and Obesity: A Comprehensive Handbook*. 2nd ed. New York: The Guildford Press; 2002.
2. Yager J, Powers PS, eds. *Clinical Manual of Eating Disorders*. Washington, DC: American Psychiatric Publishing; 2007.
3. American Psychiatric Association. Practice guideline for the treatment of patients with eating disorders, 3rd ed. *Am J Psychiatry* 2006;163(7 Suppl):4.
4. American Psychiatric Association. *Diagnostic and Statistical Manual of Mental Disorders*. 4th ed. Text Revision. Washington, DC: American Psychiatric Association; 2000.
5. Hoek HW, van Hoeken D. Review of the prevalence and incidence of eating disorders. *Int J Eat Disord* 2003;34:383.
6. Hammer LD et al. Standardized percentile curves of body-mass index for children and adolescents. *Am J Dis Child* 1991;145:259.
7. Willet WC et al. Guidelines for healthy weight. *N Engl J Med* 1999;341:427.
8. Hudson JL et al. The prevalence and correlates of eating disorders in the National Comorbidity Survey Replication. *Biol Psychiatry* 2007;61:348.
9. Kaplan AS, Ciliska D. The relationship between eating disorders and obesity: psychopathologic and treatment considerations. *Psychiatr Ann* 1999;29:197.
10. Alley DE, Chang VW. The changing relationship of obesity and disability, 1988–2004. *JAMA* 2007;298:2020.
11. Simon GE et al. Association between obesity and psychiatric disorders in the U.S. adult population. *Arch Gen Psychiatry* 2006;63:824.
12. World Health Organization. Physical status: the use and interpretation of anthropometry. Report of a WHO Expert Committee. *World Health Organ Tech Rep Ser* 1995;854:1.
13. Freedman DM et al. Body mass index and all-cause mortality. *Int J Obes* 2006;30:822.
14. Expert Panel on the Identification, Evaluation, and Treatment of Overweight in Adults. Clinical guidelines on the identification, evaluation, and treatment of overweight and obesity in adults: executive summary. *Am J Clin Nutr* 1998;68:899.
15. Ogden CL et al. The epidemiology of obesity. *Gastroenterology* 2007;132:2087.
16. Kaye WH, Walsh BT. Psychopharmacology of eating disorders. In: Davis KL et al, eds. *Neuropsychopharmacology: The Fifth Generation of Progress*. Philadelphia: Lippincott Williams & Williams; 2002.
17. Allison KC et al. Binge eating disorder and night eating syndrome: a comparative study of disordered eating. *J Consult Clin Psychol* 2005;73:1107.
18. Kuczmarski RJ et al. Increasing prevalence of overweight among U.S. adults: The National Health and Nutrition Examination Surveys, 1960–1991. *JAMA* 1994;272:205.
19. Ogden CL et al. Prevalence of overweight and obesity in the United States, 1999–2004. *JAMA* 2006;295:1549.
20. Wolf AM, Colditz GA. Current estimates of the economic costs of obesity in the United States. *Obes Res* 1998;6:97.
21. Wolf AM, Colditz GA. The cost of obesity: the U.S. perspective. *Pharmacoeconomics* 1994;5:34.
22. Wolf AM. Economic outcomes of the obese patient. *Obes Res* 2002;10(Suppl 1):58S.
23. Sturm R. Increases in clinically severe obesity in the United States, 1986–2000. *Arch Intern Med* 2003;163:2146.
24. Nader PR et al. Identifying risk for obesity in early childhood. *Pediatrics* 2006;118:594.
25. Physical Activity and Health: A Report of the Surgeon General. Atlanta, GA: U.S. Dept of Health and Human Services, Centers for Disease Control and Prevention, National Center for Chronic Disease Prevention and Health Promotion; 1996.
26. Graunbaum JA et al. Youth risk behavior surveillance—United States, 2001. *MMWR* 2002; 51:1.
27. Goran MI, Treuth MS. Energy expenditure, physical activity and obesity in children. *Pediatr Clin North Am* 2001;48:931.
28. Duncan GE. Prevalence of diabetes and impaired fasting glucose levels among U.S. adolescents. National Health and Nutrition Examination Survey, 1999–2002. *Arch Pediatr Adolesc Med* 2006;160:523.
29. Ford ES et al. Prevalence of the metabolic syndrome among U.S. adolescents using the definition from the International Diabetes Federation. *Diabetes Care* 2008;31:587.
30. Kaye W, Strober M. The neurobiology of eating disorders. In: Charney DS et al, eds. *Neurobiology of Mental Illness*. New York: Oxford Press; 1999.
31. Halmi KA. Eating disorders: anorexia nervosa, bulimia nervosa, and obesity. In: Hales RE et al, eds. *The American Psychiatric Press Textbook of Psychiatry*. 3rd ed. Washington, DC: American Psychiatric Press; 1999.
32. Kaye WH et al. The role of the central nervous system in the psychoneuroendocrine disturbances of anorexia and bulimia nervosa. *Psychiatr Clin North Am* 1998;21:381.
33. Taheri S. The link between short sleep duration and obesity: we should recommend more sleep to prevent obesity. *Arch Dis Child* 2006;91:881.
34. Reilly JJ et al. Early life risk factors for obesity in childhood: cohort study. *BMJ* 2005;330:1357.
35. Taheri S et al. Short sleep duration is associated with reduced leptin, elevated ghrelin, and increased body mass index. *PLoS Med* 2004;1:e62.
36. Homel P et al. Changes in body mass index for individuals with and without schizophrenia, 1987–1996. *Schizoph Res* 2002;55:277.
37. Hinney A et al. Genetic risk factors in eating disorders. *Am J Pharmacogenomics* 2004;4:209.
38. Landt MC S. Eating disorders: from twin studies to candidate genes and beyond. *Twin Res Hum Genet* 2004;8:467.
39. Lilenfeld LR et al. A controlled family study of anorexia and bulimia nervosa: psychiatric disorders in first-degree relatives and effects of proband comorbidity. *Arch Gen Psychiatry* 1998;55:603.
40. Kaye WH. Anorexia nervosa, obsessional behavior, and serotonin. *Psychopharmacol Bull* 1997;33:335.
41. Frayling TM et al. A common variant in the FTO gene is associated with body mass index and predisposes to childhood and adult obesity. *Science* 2007;316:889–94.
42. Licinio J et al. The hypothalamic-pituitary-adrenal axis in anorexia nervosa. *Psychiatry Res* 1996;62:75.
43. Valassi E et al. Neuroendocrine control of food intake. *Nutr Metab Cardiovasc Dis* 2008;18:158.
44. Blundell JE, Halford JCG. Serotonin and appetite regulation: implications for the pharmacological treatment of obesity. *CNS Drugs* 1998;6:473.
45. Jimerson DC, Wolfe BE. Neuropeptides in eating disorders. *CNS Spectr* 2004;9:516.
46. Monteleone P et al. Serotonergic dysfunction across the eating disorders: relationship to eating behaviour, purging behaviour, nutritional status and general psychopathology. *Psychol Med* 2000;30:1099.
47. Gorwood P et al. Genetics and anorexia nervosa: a review of candidate genes. *Psychiatr Genet* 1998;8:1.
48. Sinha MK, Caro JF. Clinical aspects of leptin. *Vitam Horm* 1998;54:1.
49. Sawa M et al. Recent developments in the design of orally bioavailable beta3-adrenergic receptor agonists. *Curr Med Chem* 2006;13:25.
50. Collins S et al. Role of leptin in fat regulation. *Nature* 1996;380:677.
51. Ferron F et al. Serum leptin concentrations in

patients with anorexia nervosa, bulimia nervosa and non-specific eating disorders correlate with body mass index but are independent of the respective disease. *Clin Endocrinol* 1997;46:289.
52. Houseknecht KL et al. The biology of leptin: a review. *J Anim Sci* 1998;76:1405.
53. Campfield LA et al. Strategies and potential molecular targets for obesity treatment. *Science* 1998;290:1383.
54. Considine RV et al. Serum immunoreactive-leptin concentrations in normal-weight and obese humans. *N Engl J Med* 1996;334:292.
55. Flier JS, Maratos-Flier E. Obesity and the hypothalamus: novel peptides for new pathways. *Cell* 1998;92:437.
56. Mantzoros C et al. Cerebrospinal fluid leptin in anorexia nervosa: correlation with nutritional status and potential role in resistance to weight gain. *J Clin Endocrinol Metab* 1997;82:1845.
57. Nakai Y et al. Role of leptin in women with eating disorders. *Int J Eat Disord* 1999;26:29.
58. Ericsson M et al. Common biological pathways in eating disorders and obesity. *Addict Behav* 1996;21:733.
59. Ahima RS et al. Role of leptin in the neuroendocrine response to fasting. *Nature* 1996;382:250.
60. Erondu N et al. NPY5R antagonism does not augment the weight loss efficacy of orlistat or sibutramine. *Obesity* 2007;15:2027.
61. Marrazzi MA et al. Naltrexone use in the treatment of anorexia nervosa and bulimia nervosa. *Int Clin Psychopharmacol* 1995;10:163.
62. Rowland NE, Kalra SP. Potential role of neuropeptide ligands in the treatment of overeating. *CNS Drugs* 1997;6:419.
63. Stahl SM. *Essential Psychopharmacology: Neuroscientific Basis and Practical Applications*. 2nd ed. New York: Cambridge University Press; 2000.
64. Gertner JM. Effects of growth hormone on body fat in adults. *Horm Res* 1993;40:10.
65. Gordon I et al. Childhood onset anorexia nervosa: towards identifying a biological substrate. *Int J Eat Disord* 1997;22:159.
66. Golden NH et al. Eating disorders in adolescents: a position paper of the Society for Adolescent Medicine. *J Adolesc Health* 2003;33:496.
67. Pike KM. Long-term course of anorexia nervosa: response, relapse, remission, and recovery. *Clin Psychol Rev* 1998;18:447.
68. Stice E et al. Risk factors for the emergence of childhood eating disturbances: a five-year prospective study. *Int J Eat Disord* 1999;25:375.
69. Steinhausen HC. The outcome of anorexia nervosa in the 20th century. *Am J Psychiatry* 2002;159:1284.
70. Neumarker KJ. Mortality and sudden death in anorexia nervosa. *Int J Eat Disord* 1997;21:205.
71. Becker AE et al. Eating disorders. *N Engl J Med* 1999;340:1092.
72. Franko DL et al. What predicts suicide attempts in women with eating disorders? *Psychol Med* 2004;34:843.
73. Keel PK et al. Predictors of mortality in eating disorders. *Arch Gen Psychiatry* 2003;60:179.
74. Grinspoon S et al. Mechanisms and treatment options for bone loss in anorexia nervosa. *Psychopharmacol Bull* 1997;33:399.
75. Powers PS. Osteoporosis and eating disorders. *J Pediatr Adolesc Gynecol* 1999;12:51.
76. Beresin E. Anorexia nervosa. *Compr Ther* 1997;23:664.
77. Mitchell JE, Crow S. Medical complications of anorexia nervosa and bulimia nervosa. *Curr Opin Psychiatry* 2006;19:438.
78. Miller KK et al. Determinants of skeletal loss and recovery in anorexia nervosa. *J Clin Endocrinol Metab* 2006;91:2931.
79. Kleifield E et al. Cognitive-behavioral treatment of anorexia nervosa. *Psychiatr Clin North Am* 1996;19:715.
80. Bulik CM et al. Anorexia nervosa treatment: A systematic review of randomized controlled trials. *Int J Eat Disor* 2007;40:310.
81. Keel PK et al. Postremission predictors of relapse in women with eating disorders. *Am J Psychiatry* 2005;162:2263.
82. Anzengruber D et al. Smoking in eating disorders. *Eat Behav* 2006;7:291.
83. Daluiski A et al. Russell's sign: subtle hand changes in patients with bulimia nervosa. *Clin Orthop* 1997;343:107.
84. Ricca V et al. Fluoxetine and fluvoxamine combined with individual cognitive-behavioral therapy in binge eating disorder: a one-year follow-up study. *Psychother Psychosom* 2001;70:298.
85. Walsh BT et al. Medication and psychotherapy in the treatment of bulimia nervosa. *Am J Psychiatry* 1997;154:523.
86. Agras WS. Pharmacotherapy of bulimia nervosa and binge eating disorder: longer-term outcomes. *Psychopharmacol Bull* 1997;33:433.
87. Jimerson DC et al. Medications in the treatment of eating disorders. *Psychiatr Clin North Am* 1996;19:739.
88. Beaumont PJV et al. Intensive nutritional counseling in bulimia nervosa: a role for supplementation with fluoxetine. *Aust N Z J Psychiatry* 1997;31:514.
89. Ramoz N et al. Eating disorders: an overview of treatment responses and the potential impact of vulnerability genes and endophenotypes. *Expert Opin Pharmcother* 2007;8:2029.
90. Adams T et al. Long-term mortality after gastric bypass surgery. *N Engl J Med* 2007;357:753.
91. Colditz GA. Economic costs of obesity and inactivity. *Med Sci Sports Exerc* 1999;31:S663.
92. Colditz GA et al. Weights as a risk factor for clinical diabetes in women. *Am J Epidemiol* 1990;132:501.
93. Wilfley DE, Cohen LR. Psychological treatment of bulimia nervosa and binge eating disorder. *Psychopharmacol Bull* 1997;33:437.
94. Church TS et al. Effects of different doses of physical activity on cardiorespiratory fitness among sedentary, overweight or obese postmenopausal women with elevated blood pressure. A randomized controlled trial. *JAMA* 2007;297:2081.
95. U.S. Department of Health and Human Services, Public Health Service, National Institutes of Health, National Institute of Diabetes & Digestive & Kidney Diseases. Choosing a safe & successful weight-loss program, NIH Publication No. 03-3700. Bethesda, MD: DHHS; May 2003, Revised Feb. 2006.
96. Snow V et al. Pharmacologic and surgical management of obesity in primary care: a clinical practice guideline from the American College of Physicians. *Ann Intern Med* 2005;142:525.
97. Rucker D et al. Long-term pharmacotherapy for obesity and overweight: updated meta-analysis. *BMJ* 2007;335:1194.
98. Li Z et al. Meta-analysis: pharmacologic treatment of obesity. *Ann Intern Med* 2005;142:532.
99. Bray GA. Use and abuse of appetite-suppressant drugs in the treatment of obesity. *Ann Intern Med* 1993;119:707.
100. Heal DJ et al. Sibutramine: a novel anti-obesity drug. A review of the pharmacological evidence to differentiate it from d-amphetamine and d-fenfluramine. *Int J Obes Relat Metab Disord* 1998;22(Suppl 1):S18.
101. Silverstone T. Appetite suppressants: a review. *Drugs* 1992;43:820.
102. McCann UD et al. Brain serotonin neurotoxicity and primary pulmonary hypertension from fenfluramine and dexfenfluramine: a systematic review of the evidence. *JAMA* 1997;278:666.
103. Jequier E et al. Thermogenic effects of various beta-adrenoceptor agonists in humans: their potential usefulness in the treatment of obesity. *Am J Clin Nutr* 1992;55:249S.
104. FDA/Center for Drug Evaluation and Research. Questions and Answers: Safety of Phenylpropanolamine. November 6, 2006. Available at: http://www.fda.gov/cder/drug/infopage/ppa/qa.htm. Accessed August 21, 2002.
105. Morgenstern LB et al. Use of ephedra-containing products and risk for hemorrhagic stroke. *Neurology* 2003;60:132.
106. Mayer LE, Walsh BT. The use of selective serotonin reuptake inhibitors in eating disorders. *J Clin Psychiatry* 1998;59(Suppl 15):28.
107. Luque CA, Rey JA. Sibutramine: a serotonin-norepinephrine reuptake-inhibitor for the treatment of obesity. *Ann Pharmacother* 1999;33:968.
108. Lean JEJ. Sibutramine—a review of clinical efficacy. *Int J Obes Relat Metab Disorder* 1997;21(Suppl 1):S30.
109. Heal DJ et al. A comparison of the effects on central 5-HT function of sibutramine hydrochloride and other weight-modifying agents. *Br J Pharmacol* 1998;125:301.
110. Bray GA et al. Sibutramine produces dose-related weight loss. *Obes Res* 1999;7:189.
111. Wadden TA et al. Randomized trial of lifestyle modification and pharmacotherapy for obesity. *N Engl J Med* 2005;353:2111.
112. Weintraub M et al. Sibutramine in weight control: a dose-ranging, efficacy study. *Clin Pharmacol Ther* 1991;50:330.
113. James W et al. A one-year trial to assess the value of orlistat in the management of obesity. *Int J Obes* 1997;21(Suppl):S24.
114. Guerciolini R. Mode of action of orlistat. *Int J Obes* 1997;21(Suppl):S12.
115. Williams G. Orlistat over the counter. *BMJ* 2007;335:1163.
116. Torgerson JS et al. Xenical in the prevention of diabetes in obese subjects (XENDOS) study: a randomized study of orlistat as an adjunct to lifestyle changes for the prevention of type 2 diabetes in obese patients. *Diabetes Care* 2004;27:155.
117. Padwal RS, Majumdar SR. Drug treatments for obesity: orlistat, sibutramine and rimonabant. *Lancet* 2007;369:71.
118. Werneke U et al. Options for pharmacological management of obesity in patients treated with atypical antipsychotics. *Int Clin Psychopharmacol* 2002;17:145.
119. Gadde KM et al. Zonisamide for weight loss in obese adults: a randomized controlled trial. *JAMA* 2003;289:1820.
120. McElroy SL et al. Zonisamide in the treatment of binge-eating disorder with obesity: a randomized controlled trial. *J Clin Psychiatry* 2006;12:1897.
121. Greenway FL. Surgery for obesity. *Endocrinol Metab Clin North Am* 1996;25:1005.
122. Sauerland S et al. Obesity surgery: evidence-based guidelines of the European Association for Endoscopic Surgery (E.A.E.S.) *Surg Endosc* 2005;19:200.
123. Maggard MA et al. Meta-analysis: surgical treatment of obesity. *Ann Intern Med* 2005;142:547.
124. Miller AD, Smith KM. Medication and nutrient administration considerations after bariatric surgery. *Am J Health-Syst Pharm* 2006;63:1852.
125. DeWald T et al. Pharmacological and surgical treatments for obesity. *Am Heart J* 2006;151:604.

SUBSTANCE ABUSE

CHAPTER 83

Drug Abuse

Wendy O. Zizzo and Paolo V. Zizzo

DEFINITIONS

Physical addiction or dependence occurs when repeated administration of a drug causes an altered physiologic state (neuroadaptation). Following neuroadaptation, a characteristic set of withdrawal symptoms occurs when the drug is abruptly discontinued. Psychological addiction or psychological dependence refers to a "maladaptive pattern of substance use leading to clinically significant impairment or distress."[1] Habituation is a state of either chronic or periodic drug use characterized by a desire (but not a compulsion) to continue using the drug, no tendency to increase the dose, and an absence of physical addiction despite some degree of psychological dependence.

These conditions collectively are now thought of as addictive disease. A different clinical syndrome is associated with each drug, but all involve a chronic process with progressive deterioration of psychological and physiologic activity secondary to the habitual use of a drug. Although the neurochemistry of the addictive process is possibly the same for all drugs, the psychosocial and pharmacokinetic aspects vary from drug to drug. Evidence, consistent with models established for alcoholism, indicates that genetically inherited traits may result in expression of addictive disease when the person is exposed to certain drugs and other habituating psychic stimuli.[2]

The *Diagnostic and Statistical Manual of Mental* Disorders, fourth edition (*DSM-IV*) cites criteria for substance-related disorders and divides them into two groups: the substance use disorders (including criteria for distinguishing between substance dependence and substance abuse) and the substance-induced disorders (intoxication, withdrawal, and others).[1]

DRUG CULTURE

The drug-using population has developed colloquialisms referring to specific drugs as well as many of the aspects of their drug-using lives. Clinicians encountering unfamiliar expressions should simply ask the patient to explain any terms that are not mutually understood. Most patients are surprisingly willing to describe their drug use if they trust the clinician's ability to help them.

It is worthwhile to look at the business aspects of the illicit drug trade to gain some perspective on the accuracy of historical information provided by the patient. The supply of drugs to the illicit marketplace is subject to the demand for such commodities and obeys laws of economics just as other businesses. Nevertheless, some notable differences exist. There is no quality control at illicit drug laboratories such as that mandated by the US Food and Drug Administration (FDA) for legally sanctioned pharmaceutical manufacturers. Premarketing research for efficacy and safety is not of concern to illicit drug laboratories. The chemicals that the underground chemist must use to synthesize the desired products are to some degree controlled and monitored by the "narcs" (law enforcement officers, specifically plainclothes narcotics officers). As a particular drug synthesis process becomes known to law enforcement authorities, the sale of the required chemicals becomes restricted, and the illicit drug chemists will use alternate methods of synthesis, sometimes with unpredictable results. The dealer (drug seller) is generally attempting to maximize profits and may dilute the relatively expensive drug with cheaper sugars, local anesthetics, and other substances. Frequently, a cheaper or more readily available chemical is substituted for the one desired by the customer (e.g., ephedrine sold as amphetamine). Generally, substituted drugs are in the same pharmacologic class; otherwise, the customer would not obtain the desired psychic effect and would not purchase more drug from that dealer. Nor will a dealer wish to put any acutely toxic chemical in the drugs sold because such an action discourages further purchases.

Despite a trend toward drugs of higher purity in the illicit marketplace, clinicians should be aware that the patients often do not really know which drug they have taken. Any history obtained from users concerning drug use should be substantiated by looking for the expected physical symptoms and obtaining appropriate laboratory studies. Any paraphernalia, such as syringes or drug samples, brought to the clinician may provide valuable evidence to explain a pathologic state. Needles should be considered infectious and should never be handled; they should be promptly discarded into appropriate needle disposal boxes.

URINE SCREENING

1. J.R., who is applying for a new job, has been told that his pre-employment physical will include a urine drug screen. He is worried because for the past 6 months he has been smoking one joint (i.e., cigarette) of marijuana per day, using cocaine twice per week, and drinking a half-pint of brandy to sleep on the days when he has been using cocaine. He last used these drugs 1 week ago. Now he wants to know if he can cleanse his urine of drugs in 2 days by drinking lots of water and exercising heavily. What is a reasonable answer to his question?

Drug users try several methods to avoid detection of illicit drugs in their urine. In addition to exercise and hydration, attempts at enhancing excretion include taking diuretics (attempted forced diuresis), drinking vinegar or cranberry juice; taking vitamin C (attempted pH manipulation for ion trapping of drugs in the urine and enhancing excretion); taking saunas (attempted hastening of drug elimination from fat stores); buying clean urine from a drug-free individual (assumes that the urine collection is unobserved so the switching of samples can be accomplished); and adding bleach, isopropanol, or salt (NaCl) to the urine sample (inactivates the enzymes used by the popular immunoassay "urine drug screen" systems). Commercial products specifically created for the purpose of adulterating urine samples ("Urinaid," "Urine Luck," "Klear") are widely available in head shops (commercial establishments that sell drug paraphernalia) and on the internet. These products either destroy the drug or interfere with the assay. Most of these methods are derived from research literature describing the immunoassay techniques. Although each of the above techniques may decrease the urinary concentration of a drug to some small degree, none of these methods will enhance the total body clearance of drug. Dehydration (e.g., from diuretics) may actually increase the effective drug concentration in the urine, allowing easier detection. Forced fluid administration, resulting in a greatly increased output of dilute urine, or adding water to the specimen in an effort to lower the drug concentration below the cutoff level of the assay may result in a false-negative result, but this technique is often detected by the laboratory by measuring the creatine concentration and the specific gravity of the urine.[3]

The immunoassay techniques used for drug detection are not 100% accurate. Several medications (over-the-counter and prescription), foods, and workplace chemicals are cross-reactive and may produce false-positive results for certain intoxicating drugs. For example, diphenhydramine and quetiapine in the urine can cause a false-positive result for methadone, cloxacillin may test positive for benzodiazepines, fluoroquinolones may cross-react with assays for opiates, efavirenz may cause a false-positive result for marijuana, ephedrine may cause a false-positive test result for amphetamines, and tramadol and venlafaxine have caused false-positive test findings for phencyclidine.[3–8] Current product information should be studied for specific test systems, which are constantly being altered to minimize spurious results.

Many factors influence the length of time a drug can be detected in body fluids (e.g., individual metabolism and excretion rates); therefore, drug detection periods are rough estimates. Urine tests for most drugs of abuse are usually negative within a week of the last use. Heavy, chronic use of marijuana or phencyclidine may, however, produce positive urine results for up to several weeks.[9] Drug testing does not pick up sporadic use that falls outside of these ranges, nor does it indicate chronicity of use. A positive test obtained by random screening is as likely to represent first-time use as it is chronic use.[10] Drug test results should be interpreted only by persons familiar with the laboratory technology and the pharmacokinetics of the drugs being tested.

Hair, saliva, and sweat testing for abused drugs is gaining popularity. Abused drugs can be detected for a longer time in hair. A question of racial bias in hair testing has been raised because the coarse hair of some blacks may absorb proportionately more cocaine than the hair of whites.[10] Commercial products to clean the hair and saliva have also become available to beat these drug tests.[11]

Passive exposure to drugs resulting in a positive urine test is possible but highly improbable. It would take exposure to the smoke from 30 marijuana joints in a small, unventilated space to produce a positive urine drug screen.[3] Passive exposure to drugs may be problematic, however, with the hair testing method.[10]

Therefore, J.R.'s urine is likely to be positive only for marijuana when he is tested, assuming he uses no drugs in the meantime. Forced fluids and exercise will not affect his urinary drug tests.

OPIOIDS

Abuse of opioids includes illicit drugs, such as heroin, and the nonmedical use of prescription pain relievers. According to the Drug Enforcement Administration (DEA), prescription pain relievers appear to be increasingly diverted from legitimate and illegitimate sources of supply via the internet.[12] In the 2006 National Survey on Drug Use and Health, the rate of past month and past year use among persons aged 12 years or older reporting nonmedical use of pain relievers was second only to marijuana and far surpassed those of cocaine and heroin. The survey reported 5.2 million Americans had used prescription pain relievers nonmedically in the past month.[13] Diverted oxycodone is generally sold as 20- or 40-mg tablets at $1 per milligram.[14]

Heroin

2. D.J., age 28, has been "fixing" (injecting) two "quarter bags" ($25 worth) of "junk" (heroin sold on the street) daily for about a month. This "run" (daily use) began when he met a new "connection" (drug supplier) at a party. D.J. describes a steady supply of "Mexican tar." He explains he began smoking the heroin but has now progressed to injecting. What is "Mexican tar"?

Over the past 2 decades, a dramatic shift occurred in the heroin market in the United States. Southeast Asia, formerly the dominant supplier, has been replaced by South America, particularly in the East, and in the West, "Mexican tar" or "black tar" heroin from Mexico is the predominant form. The South American heroin (sold as a white powder) is frequently >90% pure, and this has resulted in increased availability of high-purity heroin from all sources. According to the Office of National Drug Control Policy, South American heroin ranges from 40% to 95% pure, and Mexican black tar heroin ranges from 5% to 64% pure.[14] This has led to a new, younger user population, who can smoke or snort this high-purity heroin and avoid the stigma and hazards associated with needle use. As the addiction progresses and the user's "habit" (amount used daily) increases, however, the user will often begin injecting the drug. The DEA estimates there are roughly 800,000 heroin addicts in the United States. The 2006 National Survey on Drug Use and Health, which does not survey institutionalized populations, found the number of current heroin users in the United States had increased from 136,000 in 2005 to 338,000 in 2006.[13]

Heroin is often sold in glassine bags referred to as "dime" ($10) or "quarter" ($25) bags. A dime bag contains 40 to 50 mg of heroin.[15] Mexican tar, which looks and feels like sticky black roofing tar, is sold as a gummy, pasty chunk, the size of a matchhead, which is enough for two to five doses. The cost of a chunk of Mexican tar this size is $20 to $25. The cost of heroin dependence can range from $20 to $200/day, depending on the level of use.

Heroin Addiction

3. D.J. developed a "big habit" (tolerance developed, and his daily requirement of drug to maintain euphoria had increased). He could not "hustle" (obtain by any means) any more cash on a daily basis. When he tried "kicking" (abrupt cessation of drug use) the drug "cold turkey" (without any therapy for withdrawal symptoms), he became "dope sick" (typical heroin withdrawal symptoms), which was extremely unpleasant. He has been "chipping" (using only occasionally) since his withdrawal. Is D.J. "hooked" (addicted)?

Abstinence precipitated a withdrawal syndrome in D.J.; therefore, he is by definition physically addicted to heroin. The powerful ability of the drug to rapidly alleviate withdrawal symptoms results in reinforcement to continue using the drug. D.J.'s ongoing desire to continue using heroin despite his inability to afford it and his all-day hustling constitutes a psychological dependence on heroin.

Noticeable opioid physical dependence is highly variable, but it is assumed that the potential for an abstinence syndrome exists after repeated administration for only a few days.[16]

Opioid Withdrawal

4. D.J. arrives at the detoxification clinic 10 hours after his last dose of heroin. He is sweating and shaking and keeps yawning. Should he be treated for opioid withdrawal?

Six to 12 hours after the last dose of morphine or heroin (diacetylmorphine), patients addicted to heroin will typically develop symptoms of anxiety, hyperactivity, restlessness, and insomnia with yawning, sialorrhea, rhinorrhea, and lacrimation. There may also be profuse diaphoresis with concurrent shaking chills and pilomotor activity resulting in waves of gooseflesh of the skin (thus, the term "cold turkey"). Anorexia, nausea, vomiting, abdominal cramps, and diarrhea may occur. Severe back pain may accompany muscle spasms that cause kicking movements ("kicking the habit"). These symptoms are most severe 48 to 72 hours after the last opioid dose. D.J. is exhibiting typical heroin withdrawal symptoms, and supportive therapy would be appropriate.

During withdrawal, the heart rate and blood pressure may be elevated. Failure to take in food and fluids, combined with vomiting, sweating, and diarrhea, can result in marked weight loss, dehydration, ketosis, and acid-base imbalance. Rarely, cardiovascular collapse has occurred during the peak phase of opiate withdrawal.

The more dramatic symptoms of heroin withdrawal subside after 7 to 14 days of abstinence even without treatment; however, a return to complete physiologic equilibrium may require months or longer.[17]

The character, severity, and time course of withdrawal symptoms that appear when an opioid drug is discontinued depend on many factors, including the particular opioid, total daily dose, interval between doses, duration of use, intent of drug use, and the health and personality of the user. Unlike the withdrawal symptoms from sedative-hypnotic drugs, opioid withdrawal symptoms are seldom life-threatening.

Withdrawal From Different Opioids

5. R.F. a 33-year-old man, says he is addicted to methadone, but hours after his last dose he does not exhibit any signs of opioid withdrawal. Why is this reasonable?

Physiologic withdrawal symptoms from all opioid drugs are qualitatively similar but quantitatively different in onset, duration, and severity. Opioids with shorter durations of action tend to produce brief, intense abstinence syndromes, whereas those eliminated from the body at much slower rates produce prolonged but milder withdrawal syndromes. The abstinence syndrome of methadone is consistent with that expected for a long-acting opioid. Methadone withdrawal symptoms generally do not become apparent until 36 to 48 hours after the last dose.[17] Although the symptoms are qualitatively similar to those of morphine and heroin, they are less severe overall but are most intense around the sixth day of abstinence, and persist for 14 days or more.[15] R.F. could be telling the truth because his methadone withdrawal symptoms should not occur until 2 to 3 days after his last dose.

Iatrogenic Dependence

6. J.B., a 21-year-old man who underwent bowel surgery, required morphine 10 mg intramuscularly Q 4 hr for 10 days. Is J.B. physically dependent on morphine?

Physical dependence occurs in any patient after 2 to 10 days of continuous administration of an opioid.[18] In the setting of the treatment of acute pain, the dependence is generally not clinically significant because the patient will taper the therapeutic dose naturally as the pain condition resolves. If the opioid is abruptly stopped, the patient may experience withdrawal symptoms, however the intensity of those symptoms varies depending on the individual's physiology, as well as the dose and duration of use of the opioid. Higher doses and longer times of administration are likely to produce more severe symptoms of withdrawal on cessation of opioid use.

Therapeutic physical dependence should not be confused with addiction. Physical dependence is defined as a neurobiological adaptation that occurs with chronic exposure, whereas addiction is a set of maladaptive behaviors involving adverse consequences owing to use of drugs, loss of control over drug use, and preoccupation with acquisition of the drug.[1] Physical dependence and tolerance (the need for increasing doses to achieve the initial effects of the drug) can occur in the setting of addiction, but are also expected, nonpathological sequelae of chronic opioid therapy.

Most studies evaluating the occurrence of opioid addiction resulting from the therapeutic treatment of pain have concluded the risk is low.[19] Historically, a much greater problem has been the undertreatment of pain. It has been theorized that pain may actually reduce the risk of addiction by attenuating the euphoric effects of opioids.[18]

Certain pharmacologic properties, such as high potency, rapid onset and shorter duration of action, and water solubility may increase the likelihood of abuse of that medication. Although all opioids have some abuse liability, some are intrinsically more abusable than others. For example, the controlled-release formulations have been promoted as less likely to cause addiction than immediate-release products, because when used as intended, the reinforcing properties of the opioid are reduced. When tablets, such as OxyContin, are crushed, however, the drug's controlled-release properties are compromised, and the result is much higher dosages than what is available in the immediate-release formulation tablets. Mixed agonist–antagonist opioids (pentazocine, nalbuphine, butorphanol) and partial mu agonist opioids (buprenorphine, tramadol) have less potential for abuse and addiction than the pure mu agonists (e.g., morphine, hydromorphone, oxycodone); however, abuse and addiction to all has been observed.[18]

The term "pseudoaddiction" has been coined to describe the inaccurate interpretation of certain "drug-seeking behaviors" in patients who are inadequately treated for pain.[18,19] Their preoccupation actually reflects a need for pain relief, but is erroneously interpreted as addiction.

J.B. may experience a mild withdrawal syndrome on cessation of his morphine treatment, unless the doses are tapered.

Medical Complications

7. C.F., age 30, presented to the emergency department with violent shaking chills. She admitted that she was a heroin addict and was forced into "doing some cottons" because of an acute financial crisis. She now fears that she has "cotton fever." How should "cotton fever" be managed, and what other medical complications of heroin addiction might be suspected?

When heroin is prepared for self-administration, cotton is used as a filter to trap adulterants; thus, some of the drug remains trapped in the cotton. These crude filters are saved, and when money or drug availability is poor, water or other solvents are added to the "old cottons" to extract any remaining drug for intravenous (IV) use. "Cotton fever" is an acute febrile reaction. The onset is within 30 minutes of injection, with shaking chills, diaphoresis, postural hypotension, tachycardia, and low-grade fever. These symptoms are initially suggestive of sepsis, but most of the symptoms resolve without treatment in 2 to 4 hours, with complete recovery in 1 day. In the past, cotton fever was believed to be an allergic reaction to tiny cotton fibers injected with the drug, but a case report suggests that the causal agent is probably *Pantoea (formerly Enterobacter) agglomerans*, via a heat-stable endotoxin.[20] Cotton and cotton plants are heavily colonized with *P. agglomerans*.[21] IV drug users will often use the term "cotton fever" to describe any short-term illness characterized by fever, chills, aches, and pains. C.F. should have blood cultures performed and receive empiric therapy with a broad-spectrum antimicrobial, such as a third-generation cephalosporin.

According to the Drug Abuse Warning Network (DAWN), heroin is consistently among the top three drugs reported in emergency department visits and drug-related deaths.[22,23] Bacterial endocarditis, sepsis, embolism, septic and aseptic abscesses, thrombophlebitis, cellulitis, and necrotizing fasciitis have also resulted from both improper sterilization of injection apparatus and needles and poor injection techniques.

The common practice of sharing "works" (needle and syringe) between friends has resulted in transmission of various infectious diseases. Chief among those is viral hepatitis, specifically the hepatitis C virus (HCV). Approximately 3.2 million Americans are infected with HCV and most of the cases resulted from injection drug use.[24] According to the Centers for Disease Control and Prevention (CDC), in the United States, human immunodeficiency virus (HIV) infection caused by injection drug use had an overall prevalence of 14% in 2005.[25] Other infectious diseases such as syphilis, tetanus, botulism, and malaria can be transmitted in a similar manner and should be considered when evaluating this patient.

Heroin Overdose

8. T.F., age 21, was unconscious after an alleged "OD" (overdose) on "smack" (heroin). He had a decreased respiratory rate of four breaths per minute, cyanosis, symmetrically "pinned" (maximally miotic or pinpoint) pupils, and a slightly decreased blood pressure. He has one "fresh track" (needle puncture wound) and several "old tracks" (healed scars from needle puncture wounds) in the antecubital fossa area. What is the immediate treatment of choice for this patient?

Immediate treatment includes airway management, cardiorespiratory support, and opioid reversal with naloxone. Naloxone is a full opioid competitive antagonist that rapidly reverses the respiratory depression and hypotension associated with overdose. The preferred route of administration is IV; if access cannot be gained, it may be given intramuscularly (IM), subcutaneously (SC), or by endotracheal tube.[26]

Initial IV administration of 0.2 to 0.4 mg naloxone should be slow and should be discontinued if T.F. responds. It is not necessary to precipitate opioid withdrawal symptoms; the endpoint of naloxone therapy is a relative stabilization of the patient's vital signs. A naloxone-precipitated, sudden-onset withdrawal syndrome is more severe than the symptoms produced by abstinence alone. Repetitive doses should be given if the patient remains unresponsive, up to a maximal dose of 10 mg of naloxone.[26] If the patient still has not responded, the diagnosis of opioid overdose should be reconsidered.[26,27]

The duration of action of naloxone ranges from 20 to 60 minutes, depending on the dose and route of administration. Treatment of the methadone-overdosed patient will require serial dosing of naloxone every 20 to 60 minutes because the toxic effects of this long-acting opiate recur.[26] The patient must be carefully observed following the termination of naloxone therapy to detect any reappearance of opioid intoxication. An IV infusion of naloxone may be appropriate if high doses are needed or if the patient has recurrent respiratory depression.

Treatment of Opioid Dependence

9. A.X. age 27, has been addicted to heroin for 3 years but is tired of the street scene and wants to "get clean" (complete abstinence). He can no longer afford his growing daily habit but is not sure he can stop using opioids. He seems willing and determined to receive treatment for his heroin dependence. What therapeutic options are available to him?

The ultimate goal of most detoxification programs is to transform the narcotic addict into a responsible, drug-free, emotionally stable, and productive member of society. Despite many claims, no program to date fulfils all of these goals. Furthermore, all programs either have a high recidivism rate or do not produce a drug-free state in the patient. Heroin addiction, or any other chronic, compulsive form of drug abuse, is a symptom of a wide range of problems in the addictive disease patient. Therefore, no single treatment modality can be universally applied to all patients.

Treatment options can be loosely divided into either *social model programs* or *medical model programs*. Either model may be inpatient or outpatient based. Social model programs use a nonmedical approach to detoxification and ongoing recovery. Detoxification usually involves the "cold turkey" method of abrupt cessation of the opioid without supportive therapy. Medical model programs are based on pharmacotherapeutic treatment managed by medical professionals and additionally offer recovery-oriented counseling. One therapeutic approach involves opioid substitution for detoxification or maintenance. Currently, methadone and buprenorphine are FDA-approved for these indications.[28] Another approach involves symptomatic treatment of withdrawal. The mainstay of this approach is the α_2-agonist clonidine. A third approach uses rapid detoxification precipitated by an opioid antagonist under general anesthesia.

Methadone treatment for opioid dependence is federally regulated and is only available through specially licensed opioid treatment programs. The Drug Addiction Treatment Act of 2000 allows qualified physicians to prescribe Schedule III, IV, and V medications approved for the treatment of opioid dependence in an office-based setting.[29] Currently, only buprenorphine, a schedule III medication, is approved for this indication.

With A.X.'s apparently strong psychological addiction to heroin (he does not know if he can live without opioids) and his desire to be abstinent, it would seem appropriate to attempt gradual detoxification with intensive psychosocial counseling rather than maintenance therapy.

Substitution Pharmacotherapies for Opioid Dependence

Methadone Detoxification

10. A.X. starts a methadone detoxification program at a local methadone clinic. He claims to have a $100/day habit. What is the recommended methadone dose for starting treatment?

Methadone is a synthetic, potentially addictive, orally acting opiate with a prolonged duration of action of 12 to 24 hours. Pharmacologically, it is qualitatively identical to morphine and other opioid analgesics. Pioneered by Dole et al.,[30] methadone substitution was considered the treatment of choice for opioid addiction by many researchers. It continues to be widely used today, but methadone has emerged as a drug of abuse and many deaths have resulted from its excessive use.[26,31] In 2004, there were 3,800 deaths from methadone overdose, compared with 780 in 1999.[15]

Purportedly, methadone (at a dose of 80–150 mg or more) blocks the euphoriant effects of other opioids without producing euphoria itself. This dose allegedly produces a high degree of cross-tolerance to other opioids so that it is extremely difficult to "get off" (obtain euphoria) with IV injection of other opioids. Addicts, however, have been able to obtain euphoria from doses of 60 to 100 mg of methadone. Furthermore, at lower maintenance doses of methadone that do not produce euphoria, addicts have been able to reach euphoric states through the concomitant IV administration of other opioids. The higher purity heroin available today has required even higher doses of methadone to achieve cross-tolerance.[32]

Methadone detoxification involves stabilizing the patient on a daily methadone dose that is determined by the patient's response based on objective symptoms of withdrawal. This may involve the use of standard rating scales for withdrawal, such as the Clinical Institute Narcotic Assessment (CINA).[33] Initially methadone may be given in 5 mg increments up to a total of 10 to 20 mg over the first 24 hours.[31] Larger methadone doses (i.e., 20 mg starting dose) may be required for patients with larger habits. If initial withdrawal symptoms persist 2 to 4 hours after initial dose administration, the dose can be supplemented with another 5 to 10 mg. Federal regulations allow a maximum of 40 mg as initial dose unless a program physician documents that 40 mg was insufficient to suppress opioid withdrawal symptoms.[34] Once a stabilizing dose has been reached (usually, 40–60 mg/day, but may be as high as 120 mg/day), methadone is tapered by 20% a day for inpatients or 5% a day for outpatients.[26,31,34] Studies have suggested that slow tapers are associated with better outcomes. The duration of the taper varies, but a period of 3 to 4 weeks is generally used. The gradual taper may last as long as 6 months. The most common side effects of methadone are constipation, sweating, and sexual difficulties. A Cochrane review of studies comparing methadone tapers with other detoxification methods (adrenergic agonists and other opioid agonists) found that programs vary widely in design, duration, and treatment objectives, but overall the effectiveness of the treatments was similar, with most patients relapsing to heroin use.[35] Persistent drug craving, often lasting months, probably accounts for the high relapse rate. Even temporary reductions in heroin use are seen as a benefit, however, because heroin use is associated with major health (HIV, hepatitis C) and social (crime) issues. Medical management of opioid dependence should be accompanied by psychosocial treatments, such as cognitive-behavioral therapies, behavioral therapies, and self-help groups, such as Narcotics Anonymous (NA).

A reasonable starting dose of methadone for A.X. would be 20 mg orally. An additional 5 to 10 mg could be administered after 2 to 4 hours for persistent withdrawal symptoms. The daily dose should be titrated upward every third day by 10 mg until he is stabilized on a methadone dose of 60 mg/day. The drug can then be tapered slowly (e.g., 3 mg/day) with A.X. on an outpatient over a period of 4 weeks, while attending counseling sessions and NA meetings.

Buprenorphine Detoxification

11. A.X. heard about a medication called buprenorphine that can be used instead of methadone. How might this medication be used for A.X.?

Buprenorphine, a synthetic partial opioid agonist, was approved by the FDA in October 2002 for the treatment of opioid dependence. It is a partial agonist at mu receptors, and in opioid-dependent patients it prevents withdrawal symptoms. Because of its partial effects, it produces maximal "ceiling" analgesia with sublingual doses of 24 to 32 mg, a dosage equivalent to approximately 60 to 70 mg of oral methadone. This limits its use in the management of heroin addiction. Buprenorphine is associated with a milder withdrawal syndrome compared with full opioid agonists.

Buprenorphine has a long half-life owing to its prolonged occupancy on mu receptors and it produces a relatively mild withdrawal when discontinued. It is believed to be a safer alternative to methadone because life-threatening respiratory depression is much less likely to occur than with a pure mu agonist, unless another central nervous system (CNS) depressant is taken concurrently. Most deaths involving buprenorphine have been caused by a combination of the drug with benzodiazepines.[28,36] Naloxone bolus doses often are ineffective in reversing respiratory depression caused by buprenorphine because of its prolonged occupancy on mu receptors. Evidence suggests that continuous infusion of naloxone is necessary to overcome buprenorphine-induced respiratory depression.[37]

Because buprenorphine is a schedule III medication, it can be prescribed in an office-based setting under the Drug Addiction Treatment Act of 2000, as previously discussed. It is available as 2- and 8-mg tablets for sublingual use. The tablets contain buprenorphine hydrochloride alone (Subutex) or in combination with naloxone (Suboxone). The naloxone is poorly absorbed orally, and its presence in the combination tablets is to discourage the IV abuse of buprenorphine. Both tablet forms can be used in an inpatient setting, but Suboxone is preferred in the outpatient setting, to decrease the risk of diversion. When initiating buprenorphine, the first dose should not be given until >4 hours after the last dose of a short-acting opioid, such as heroin, or 24 hours after a long-acting opioid, such as methadone. Evaluation of objective opioid withdrawal signs may involve use of standard rating scales.[33] Induction dosing should begin with 2 or 4 mg on the first day, which can be repeated every 2 to 4 hours if withdrawal symptoms subside and then reappear, up to a maximum of 8 mg. The dose can then be titrated the second day in 2- to 4-mg increments to a dose of 12 to 16 mg.[38] Higher doses during induction may precipitate withdrawal symptoms. In the inpatient setting, the patient may be stabilized on a relatively low daily dose (e.g., 8 mg/day) and then tapered in increments of 2 mg/day over several days.[26] In the outpatient setting, the patient should be initially stabilized on a daily dose (probably 8–32 mg/day) of buprenorphine that suppresses withdrawal. The dose should then be gradually tapered over a period of 10 to 14 days. Buprenorphine is not associated with any significant adverse effects when used to manage opioid withdrawal. Buprenorphine detoxification should be accompanied by psychosocial treatments and support groups as mentioned.

A Cochrane review found that relative to clonidine, buprenorphine is more effective in alleviating opioid withdrawal symptoms; patients treated with buprenorphine stay in treatment longer, and are more likely to complete treatment.[17] The severity of withdrawal appears to be similar for withdrawal managed with buprenorphine or methadone, but withdrawal symptoms may resolve more quickly with buprenorphine. The authors of the meta-analysis concluded that, although there is limited evidence comparing buprenorphine with methadone, both agents have similar effectiveness in the management of opioid withdrawal. Buprenorphine has a higher unit-dose cost compared with methadone. A depot preparation of buprenorphine is being investigated for the management of opioid withdrawal.

Maintenance Therapy

12. A.X.'s friend B.P. also attends the methadone clinic but is on methadone maintenance. How is methadone used in maintenance therapy? Are there any maintenance alternatives?

Methadone maintenance is the most common form of pharmacologic treatment for opioid dependence. During methadone maintenance, heroin-dependent patients are stabilized on a dose of methadone that will be sufficient to suppress withdrawal symptoms for 12 to 24 hours without producing euphoria. Studies have shown that patients maintained on methadone doses of 60 mg or more had better outcomes than those maintained on lower doses.[32] Most patients do well on a dose range of 60 to 120 mg/day, although some patients require more and some require less.[39] Drugs that induce CYP 450 enzymes can precipitate withdrawal in patients maintained on methadone. Drugs that inhibit CYP 450 enzymes extend the duration of methadone's effects. The drug is administered in one daily oral dose to maintain daily contact with the patient. With the aid of daily counseling and rehabilitation, most clinicians attempt to detoxify the patient eventually from methadone as well. Patients who relapse repeatedly despite supportive treatment may require long-term maintenance therapy.

The ultimate goal of methadone maintenance is controversial. By enabling addicts to escape from the illicit drug scene, review their present lifestyles, and reorient their goals, rehabilitation becomes possible. Early enthusiasm for methadone maintenance has now been tarnished by its use in the same abuse patterns as other opioids. Methadone is now a desired substitute for heroin among the addict population, although the "high" it provides is generally considered inferior to that of heroin, codeine, and other opioids.

Whether rehabilitation occurs or is even possible is confused by the lack of clear and widely accepted goals of therapy. The addition of social objectives to the therapeutic medical goal of cessation of heroin self-administration further confuses the issue. Some people believe the patient must remain completely drug-free for life (including methadone) to consider the treatment program a success. Others see opioid addictive disease as a disorder in which some opioid (methadone for example) must always be administered to the addict to correct the underlying biochemical pathology before any social rehabilitation can occur.

Medical staffing problems and disruption of the patient's employment schedules brought about by the necessity for daily doses of methadone stimulated a search for alternative drugs to methadone. "Take home" dosing, allowing patients to obtain more than a single day's dose of methadone for self-administration, has frequently led to drug diversion and heroin recidivism. Another alternative for maintenance therapy is buprenorphine (see Question 11). Most patients can be stabilized on 8 to 32 mg/day of buprenorphine.[26]

Once stabilized, it may be possible to switch to alternate-day or three-times-a-week dosing schedules. As discussed, buprenorphine has the advantage of office-based availability, thus removing the stigma associated with attending a methadone clinic. There has been interest in developing office-based methadone treatment as well.

When levomethadyl acetate (removed from the US market in 2003 following reports of severe cardiac-related adverse events), buprenorphine, and high-dose methadone (60–100 mg) therapies were compared with low-dose methadone (20 mg)[40]; all three therapies were effective in treating opioid dependence and were superior to low-dose methadone. Trials comparing 12 to 16 mg/day of buprenorphine with moderate doses of methadone (50–60 mg/day) have generally shown comparable outcomes, although higher doses of methadone (>80 mg) appear to be superior to buprenorphine. Buprenorphine may be best suited for patients with mild to moderate physical dependence.

Pain Management

13. T.A., a 44-year-old man maintained on 120 mg daily of methadone, is in severe pain owing to a fractured femur. What type of analgesic, and how much, can be used safely in this patient?

Neuroplastic changes in pain perception occur with chronic opioid use and can result in increased pain sensitivity, or hyperalgesia. In addition cross-tolerance to the analgesic effects extends to all opioids. Therefore, patients maintained on opioid agonist treatment for addiction may actually require higher doses of opioid agonist analgesics given at shorter intervals.[41] Addiction relapse because of the use of opioid analgesics is less likely than relapse because of untreated pain. Careful clinical assessment for objective signs of pain will decrease the physician's concerns of being manipulated. For T.A., it would be appropriate to control his pain acutely using patient-controlled analgesia (PCA) with IV morphine. Given his narcotic tolerance, the initial PCA pump settings could include a 2-mg IV bolus dose of morphine with a 6-minute lock-out interval delivering a maximum of 20 mg/hour. T.A.'s pain should be evaluated and the regimen adjusted as needed to achieve adequate control. T.A.'s usual maintenance dose of methadone should be continued while he is receiving morphine for his acute pain. Many clinicians would divide the daily dose (e.g., 30 mg every 6 hours) to avoid excessive peak levels of narcotic. Opioid withdrawal should be strictly avoided in this patient because it is associated with hypersensitivity to painful stimuli, followed by exaggerated catecholamine and anxiety responses. The partial antagonist–agonist narcotics pentazocine (Talwin), butorphanol (Stadol), and nalbuphine (Nubain) should be avoided because their narcotic antagonist properties may precipitate opioid withdrawal symptoms when used in a methadone-maintained patient.

There is less experience in treating acute pain in patients maintained on buprenorphine.[41] Buprenorphine's high affinity for the mu receptor risks competition with, or even displacement of, full opioid agonists. Naloxone should be on hand when opioid analgesics are used in the buprenorphine-maintained patient. Alternatively, the buprenorphine maintenance dose can be converted to methadone for the duration of opioid analgesia treatment.

T.A. should be reassured that his methadone will be continued and his pain aggressively treated. T.A.'s physician should consult with the methadone maintenance program to verify methadone dose and alert them to any controlled substances used in his treatment that may be detected with drug testing.

Methadone in Pregnancy

14. J.R., age 28, has been maintained on 100 mg methadone daily for the past year. She is now 3 months pregnant. What is the teratogenic potential of methadone?

Methadone has been accepted since the late 1970s to treat opioid addiction during pregnancy.[34] Methadone maintenance was determined to be the standard of care for pregnant women with opiate addiction by a 1998 National Institutes of Health (NIH) consensus panel.[42] Currently, methadone is the only opioid medication approved by the FDA for medication-assisted treatment of opioid addiction in pregnant patients. Women maintained on methadone frequently have regular menstrual periods, ovulate, conceive, and have normal pregnancies. Heroin-addicted mothers, however, generally experience more complicated pregnancies because their lifestyles often predispose them to a poor general state of health and precludes adequate prenatal medical care.[43] Infants born to heroin-addicted mothers may also be exposed to other substances (e.g., alcohol, cocaine, tobacco). These infants tend to be smaller, to weigh less at birth, and to be born prematurely compared with the children of women not using opiates.[43]

Withdrawal During Pregnancy

15. Are there alternatives to methadone in the treatment of opioid-dependence in pregnancy? Should methadone be continued in J.R.?

J.R. should continue methadone maintenance to avoid precipitating a withdrawal syndrome. Withdrawal from methadone is not recommended for pregnant women.[34] A structured methadone maintenance program that provides access to counseling and medical care is probably at least as beneficial to the pregnancy as the pharmacologic prevention of withdrawal. Lowering the maternal methadone dosage is associated with decreased incidence and decreased severity of neonatal withdrawal symptoms.[44] Therefore, the dose of methadone should be titrated individually throughout the pregnancy. The neonate can be managed for either opioid-induced CNS depression or methadone withdrawal after delivery, as needed.

Methadone continues to be the standard of care for the management of opioid dependence in pregnancy; however, a growing body of evidence suggests buprenorphine may be a reasonably safe alternative.[26,39] Also some evidence suggests that infants born to buprenorphine-maintained women have a lower incidence of neonatal abstinence syndrome.[45,46]

Neonatal Addiction

16. Because methadone crosses the placental barrier, will J.R.'s infant exhibit opioid withdrawal symptoms after birth and, if so, how should they be managed?

Methadone crosses the placental barrier and can cause CNS and respiratory depression as well as opioid abstinence in the newborn. In one study, 46% of the infants born to methadone-maintained mothers exhibited withdrawal signs and required treatment for neonatal abstinence sydrome (NAS).[44] In general, the most common NAS symptoms include restlessness, tremors, a high-pitched cry, hypertonicity, increased reflexes, regurgitation, tachypnea, diarrhea, and sneezing. Seizures are associated with, but not necessarily caused directly by, opioid withdrawal in the neonate. The withdrawal symptoms in the newborn may be delayed for up to 3 days.

Management of the neonate's opioid withdrawal syndrome entails careful attention to hydration with demand feeding and symptomatic care. Mild withdrawal symptoms need no therapy, but moderate to severe symptoms may require 14 or more days of treatment. Therapy of neonatal withdrawal should begin when symptoms occur. Prophylactic therapy is not recommended.

Symptoms of physiologic addiction are usually apparent within 48 hours of birth. At this time, treatment can be initiated. Currently, NAS is treated with either morphine or phenobarbital. Studies have suggested that morphine is superior to phenobarbital in both decreasing time of treatment and need for higher intensity of care.[45,47] Morphine can be started at a dose of 50 mcg/kg given orally four times daily and titrated to control symptoms. Once the NAS symptoms have stabilized, the dose can be decreased daily by 20% until discontinuation of the drug. Phenobarbital is preferred for the treatment of NAS in cases of combined dependence or benzodiazepine dependence.[45] If used, phenobarbital is instituted in doses of 5 to 10 mg/kg/day in the first 24 hours, then tapered symptomatically, usually about 20% per day. If J.R.'s infant displays opioid withdrawal symptoms (e.g., feeds poorly, becomes tremulous or agitated), morphine at a dosage of 50 mcg/kg orally given four times daily would be an appropriate intervention. This dosage is given until symptoms stabilize and then gradually tapered over the next week.

Breast-Feeding

17. Should J.R. breast-feed her infant?

Methadone is excreted into the breast milk of methadone-maintained mothers. The amount of methadone in the breast milk is unlikely, however, to have adverse effects on the infant.[48] Furthermore, studies have found minimal transfer of methadone into breast milk.[34] Breast milk offers advantages clearly beneficial to infants and J.R. should be encouraged to breast-feed her infant.

Opiate Antagonist Treatments

18. A.J. is a 41-year-old anesthesiologist seeking rehabilitation and reinstatement of his medical license following 5 years of fentanyl abuse. Are there any special considerations in chemical dependency treatment in health care providers? Would opiate antagonist treatment be appropriate for A.J.?

Experts suggest that the lifetime risk for substance abuse is higher among physicians than the general population.[49] The risk is largely based on access to drugs of abuse, and drug dependence is described as an "occupational hazard" for health care providers. Abuse of fentanyl by anesthesiologists and abuse of meperidine by nurses has long been recognized. Fentanyl (injectable as well as transdermal formulations) and meperidine are primarily, but not exclusively, drugs of abuse among health care providers. Hospice workers and veterinarians also have access to high potency opioids. Medical residents in anesthesiology and psychiatry have higher rates of substance abuse than do residents in other specialties, and psychiatrists are more likely to abuse benzodiazepines than physicians in other specialties.[49] Fentanyl is associated with rapid development of dependence, intense tolerance, and drug-seeking behavior in addicted physicians over a period of months rather than years.

A comprehensive assessment of addicted health care providers is necessary to determine if professional impairment is present, and whether issues involving public health and safety or violations of ethical standards, such as professional boundary violations or improprieties, require that the heath care provider be reported to his respective medical board. A physician's registration with the federal DEA may need to be suspended. It generally is accepted that physicians require longer durations of treatment because they are held to a higher standard of recovery owing to concerns of public safety, and they may be clever at concealing their illness.[49] Physicians should have structured posttreatment monitoring for at least 5 years.

If opioid addiction results from a process of classic and instrumental conditioning and is positively reinforced by self-administration and drug-seeking behavior, then narcotic antagonists may break this addiction cycle. The narcotic antagonists naloxone and naltrexone can block the euphoriant effects of heroin and other opiates, prevent the development of physical dependence, and afford protection from opioid overdose deaths. Of these two antagonists, only naltrexone appears to have any practical utility. Naloxone (Narcan) is impractical because of its short duration of action and its variable potency when taken orally. Naltrexone (Trexan) is orally active and provides a dose-related duration of opioid blockade. An oral dose of 100 mg of naltrexone will block opiate effects for 2 days, and 150 mg for 3 days. Thus, dosing on Monday, Wednesday, and Friday is possible and convenient for the patient. Naltrexone is also available in an injectable extended-release formulation for once-monthly use.[50] Patients selected for naltrexone therapy must be opioid free to avoid precipitation of withdrawal. For heroin or morphine dependent patients, a 4- to 7-day wait is recommended, whereas methadone addiction requires a 10- to 14-day wait. Patients who are highly motivated to abstain have been most successfully treated with this drug. A.J. is a good candidate for naltrexone therapy because of his desire to become rehabilitated and his need to remain drug-free despite continued access to opioids at work.

Ultrarapid Opiate Detoxification

19. Before A.J. can start naltrexone therapy, he must undergo fentanyl detoxification. Would rapid detoxification over a few hours be preferable to the more traditional detoxification methods for A.J.?

Ultrarapid opiate detoxification (UROD) has been advocated to shorten the opioid detoxification period by precipitating withdrawal with an opioid antagonist. The opioid antagonist causes rapid stripping of agonist from opioid receptors. UROD is performed under heavy sedation or general anesthesia so the patient does not consciously experience the acute withdrawal symptoms. The protocols for UROD vary in terms of the opioid antagonist (naloxone, nalmefene, or naltrexone), anesthetic agent, adjunctive medications, and duration of anesthesia. UROD has been performed as an outpatient or inpatient procedure, with costs ranging from $7,500 to $15,000.[51]

The UROD procedure includes risks, such as vomiting with aspiration; cardiovascular complications, including cardiac arrest; pulmonary edema; and death.[51] Some patients have reported residual withdrawal symptoms over several days. Little information exists regarding referral to ongoing treatment or relapse rates after UROD.[52] One randomized, controlled trial found no benefit of UROD over safer, less-expensive treatments using buprenorphine and naltrexone or clonidine and naltrexone.[51] UROD has been criticized for being simply a "quick fix" that fails to address the underlying behavior changes necessary for recovery. Additionally, it subjects patients to possible morbidity and mortality when safer, established procedures are available. The high cost of UROD limits its accessibility. More studies are needed to evaluate the risks and benefits of this approach. UROD would probably not be recommended as a first-line detoxification method for A.J.

Symptomatic Therapy of Opioid Withdrawal

20. How can A.J.'s opioid withdrawal be managed symptomatically? He weighs 72 kg and his blood pressure is 130/80 mmHg.

Methadone treatment for addiction has its limitations (prescribing restrictions, protracted withdrawal, drug of dependence), and many patients prefer an alternative. The discovery of the ability of the α_2-adrenergic agonist, clonidine, to ameliorate some of the opioid withdrawal symptoms, has led to its widespread use as a nonopioid alternative, despite that it is not approved for this indication in the United States. Other α_2-adrenergic agonists (lofexidine, guanfacine, guanabenz acetate) have also been investigated.[53] Noradrenergic outflow from the locus ceruleus is increased during opioid withdrawal and is blocked by administration of mu agonist opioids. Symptoms of opioid withdrawal, therefore, are partly owing to excessive sympathetic activity in the locus ceruleus. Central α_2-adrenergic agonists act on presynaptic autoreceptors to inhibit locus ceruleus noradrenergic outflow during mu agonist opioid withdrawal, thereby significantly reducing some of the symptoms.

Clonidine is therefore best used in a multidrug regimen (Table 83-1). The four primary symptoms of opioid withdrawal are musculoskeletal aches and pains, anxiety, insomnia, and gastrointestinal disorders. Contraindications to clonidine use include diastolic blood pressure <70 mmHg, concurrent dependence on sedative-hypnotics, and clonidine hypersensitivity or previous intolerance. The most common adverse effects are sedation and hypotension. A recent Cochrane review examined studies comparing clonidine with methadone taper and found no significant difference in efficacy between the two for the treatment of heroin or methadone withdrawal.[53] A separate Cochrane review did find buprenorphine to be more effective than clonidine in alleviating opioid withdrawal symptoms.[17]

Table 83-1 Symptomatic Therapy of Opiate Withdrawal

Symptom	*Medication*	*Dose*
Bone or joint pain	Ibuprofen	800 mg Q 8 hr with food as needed
Muscle pain or cramps	Methocarbamol	750 mg Q 6 hr as needed
Insomnia	Trazodone	50–150 mg at bedtime
	Chloral hydrate	500–1,500 mg at bedtime
	Flurazepam[a]	30–90 mg at bedtime
	Doxepin	50–100 mg at bedtime
Gastrointestinal hyperactivity	Belladonna alkaloids with phenobarbital[b]	Two tablets Q 8 hr as needed
	Dicyclomine[b]	20 mg Q 6 hr as needed
Nausea	Prochlorperazine[b]	10 mg Q 6 hr as needed
	Trimethobenzamide[b]	300 mg Q 6 hr as needed

[a] Avoid in concurrent benzodiazepine dependence.
[b] Anticholinergic effects also alleviate rhinorrhea, sialorrhea, diaphoresis, and lacrimation.

A sublingual or oral test dose of 0.1 mg (0.2 mg for patients >91 kg) of clonidine is given: if diastolic blood pressure remains >70 mmHg, additional doses may be instituted, usually as transdermal patches. Transdermal absorption of clonidine from patches (Catapres-TTS) avoids most of the problems encountered with oral therapy. The number of patches applied to a hairless area of the body (usually the upper back or scapular area) depends on the patient's lean body weight: <50 kg, clonidine 5 to 7.5 mg (two or three TTS-1 patches); 50 to 91 kg, 10 mg (two TTS-2 patches or one TTS-2 and two TTS-1 patches), and >91 kg, 10 to 15 mg (two or three TTS-2 patches). Patients <73 kg should use two of the TTS-1 patches and one TTS-2 patch so that one TTS-1 patch can be removed in the event of hypotensive complications. Patches are left on for 7 days, replaced with half the dosage during the second week, and then discontinued. Alternatively, oral clonidine can be used at a dose of 0.1 to 0.2 mg/dose two to four times daily to a maximum of around 1 mg/day for 2 to 4 days after cessation of opioids, then tapered and discontinued by 7 to 10 days.[53]

Clonidine is also used in conjunction with naltrexone for rapidly withdrawing patients from opioid dependence. This technique has been shown to be safe and effective.[26] The withdrawal precipitated by naltrexone is avoided by pretreating the patient with clonidine. Limitations to this technique include the need to monitor the patient for the first 8 hours because of the potential severity of the precipitated withdrawal and the need for blood pressure monitoring. An advantage is the easy transition to opioid antagonist treatment.

A.J.'s blood pressure and drug history should be evaluated for clonidine therapy. Provided his diastolic blood pressure is >70 mmHg after the clonidine test dose, he can receive the clonidine patches (one TTS-2 and two TTS-1 patches) with additional medications to treat his withdrawal symptoms, along with daily intensive psychosocial counseling.

SEDATIVE-HYPNOTICS

The sedative-hypnotics are a diverse group of compounds with broad clinical uses, including anesthesia, treatment of anxiety, and treatment of insomnia. Ethanol, also a sedative hypnotic agent, continues to be the most widely abused substance in the United States and is discussed in Chapter 84, Alcohol Use Disorders. Benzodiazepines, which have replaced barbiturates in clinical practice, have become the prototypical sedative-hypnotic drugs of abuse. Other abused sedative-hypnotic drugs include carisoprodol and γ-hydroxybutyric acid (GHB). Carisoprodol, a nonscheduled skeletal muscle relaxant, has an active metabolite meprobamate, a sedative-hypnotic agent with known abuse potential.[54] GHB is a putative neurotransmitter abused for its euphoric and sedative-hypnotic effects.

Abstinence Syndromes Associated With Sedative-Hypnotic Dependence

21. During a year of therapy for anxiety, B.J. increased his dose of alprazolam to two 1-mg tablets five times a day. He has admitted to "doctor shopping" and buying alprazolam on the street to maintain his daily habit. Will he experience withdrawal symptoms if he suddenly discontinues alprazolam?

Patients who have been on long-term courses of therapeutic doses of sedative-hypnotics often experience withdrawal symptoms on abrupt discontinuation of therapy. Withdrawal syndromes seen with sedative-hypnotics are similar to those seen with alcohol withdrawal and can include insomnia, anxiety, tremors of the upper extremities, muscular weakness, anorexia, nausea, vomiting, and postural hypotension.[55] Postural hypotension may be of value in differentiating the abstinence syndrome from ordinary anxiety states. Generalized tonic-clonic seizures can occur as isolated seizures or as status epilepticus. The psychoses that develop resemble the delirium tremens produced by alcohol withdrawal and are usually characterized by disorientation, agitation, delusions, and hallucinations. During the delirium, hyperthermia and agitation can lead to exhaustion, rhabdomyolysis, cardiovascular collapse, or death. Abstinence from short-acting barbiturates and meprobamate produces symptoms that peak within 2 or 3 days. Discontinuation of short-acting benzodiazepines (e.g., lorazepam, oxazepam, alprazolam, temazepam) results in the abrupt onset of withdrawal symptoms, usually within 12 to 24 hours after the last dose. Long-acting agents, and those with active metabolites, have a gradual onset of milder withdrawal symptoms compared with the short-acting agents. Withdrawal symptoms following chronic use of long-acting benzodiazepines typically peak on the fifth to eighth day after the last dose.[55]

B.J. has been abusing alprazolam, taking more than the recommended maximum dose. Likely, he will experience withdrawal, possibly including seizures, if he were to abruptly discontinue the alprazolam. His withdrawal from this medication should be medically managed. He should undergo an initial physical examination and plan to be absent from his place of employment for at least a week to begin detoxification.

Treatment of Sedative Withdrawal

22. How should B.J.'s sedative-hypnotic dependence be treated?

In clinical practice, three general medication strategies are used for withdrawing patients from sedative-hypnotics: decreasing doses of the drug of dependence (tapering); substituting (and gradual taper) of phenobarbital for the drug of dependence; and the substituting (and gradual taper) of a long-acting benzodiazepine for the drug of dependence.[55] Gradual tapering of the drug of dependence is appropriate for patients with therapeutic dose dependence or those taking long-acting sedative-hypnotics, who are not currently abusing alcohol or other substances. A recent meta-analysis suggests that management of benzodiazepine monodependence by gradual taper is preferable to abrupt discontinuation.[56] The authors also noted that a potential value may exist with carbamazepine used as an adjunctive medication for benzodiazepine taper, but larger, controlled studies are needed. The patient who is abusing sedative-hypnotics already has a strong association between the drug of choice and certain desired effects. Therefore, to minimize exacerbating addictive disease, substitution and taper with a long-acting therapeutic agent is preferred. The pharmacologic rationale for phenobarbital substitution is that it is long acting, producing little changes in serum levels between doses, thereby preventing breakthrough withdrawal symptoms. Lethal doses are many times higher than toxic doses; and dysphoria occurs with elevated dose, rendering it undesirable for users. As a result, the abuse potential is low, and there is little to no street value.

The phenobarbital method is the one most generally applicable; it is widely used in drug treatment programs because it is the best choice for patients who have lost control of their benzodiazepine use or who are polydrug users. The method involves calculating a phenobarbital replacement dose for the total daily dose of the sedative-hypnotic being abused. The calculation is based on phenobarbital equivalents (Table 83-2). If multiple sedative-hypnotics are being used, the totals for each drug and alcohol (amount of pure ethanol) are summated. The total phenobarbital substitution dose should be given in divided doses, three or four times daily (to avoid dysphoria). Because the calculated dosage is an estimate based on patient history, which may be inaccurate, it is advisable to administer a test dose if the calculated replacement dose is >180 mg/day. The test dose, generally one-third the total dose, is given to the patient, who is then observed for 1 to 2 hours. The patient is observed for mitigation of withdrawal symptoms as well as signs of overmedication, such as somnolence or incoordination. Once an appropriate dose is determined, the patient is usually stabilized on that dose for 1 to 2 weeks. Following stabilization, an open-ended taper of phenobarbital is instituted, with dosages reduced by 30 mg every 2 to 3 days as tolerated.[57]

B.J. has an addiction to alprazolam and because it is a short-acting benzodiazepine, it is a poor choice for tapering his dosage. Phenobarbital should be substituted for alprazolam. His total dose of alprazolam is 10 mg/day, so he should receive 300 mg of phenobarbital divided three or four times a day.

γ-Hydroxybutyric Acid

23. L.S. has been attending "raves" (all-night dance parties) every weekend for the past few months. She has been taking "liquid ecstasy" at these parties and believes it is a safe drug because she heard it once was sold in health food stores. What drug is she likely taking, and what are the risks with its use?

γ-Hydroxybutyric acid (GHB), commonly referred to as "liquid ecstasy," is a potent "club drug." Once available as an over-the-counter nutritional supplement, primarily used by bodybuilders, the FDA removed it from the retail market in 1990 because of widespread reports of poisoning. In 2000 it was classified as a schedule I drug; however, a GHB-containing product, sodium oxybate, is available as a schedule III prescription drug for the treatment of cataplexy associated with narcolepsy. GHB prodrugs, γ-butyrolactone (GBL) and 1,4-butanediol are still available for purchase on the internet. GHB is found in mammalian brain tissue, where it is derived from conversion of its parent neurotransmitter, γ-aminobutyric acid (GABA).[58] It is believed to be a neurotransmitter. Experimental evidence suggests that the mechanism of action of exogenously administered GHB involves agonist activity at the $GABA_B$ receptor.[58]

γ-Hydroxybutyric acid has CNS depressant effects and is abused for its euphorigenic properties, disinhibition, and enhanced sensuality. Its psychic effects are similar to those of alcohol, and include increased libido, short-term aterograde amnesia, and a dreamy, altered sensorium. It has a steep dose-response curve, and common adverse effects include dizziness, nausea, weakness, agitation, hallucinations, seizures, respiratory depression, and coma. Its effects are synergistic with alcohol. GHB overdose may be fatal, and there is no antidote. Treatment for GHB overdose is primarily supportive.

Table 83-2 Hypnotic Dose Equivalent to 30 mg Phenobarbital[57]

Pure ethanol 30–60 mL	Clonazepam 1–2 mg	Pentobarbital 100 mg
Alprazolam 1 mg	Diazepam 10 mg	Secobarbital 100 mg
Butalbital 100 mg	Flunitrazepam* 1–2 mg	Temazepam 30 mg
Carisoprodol 350 mg	Lorazepam 2 mg	Triazolam 0.5 mg
Chlordiazepoxide 25 mg	Oxazepam 30 mg	Zolpidem 5 mg

*Not approved for use in the United States.

Highly addictive, tolerance and physical dependence can occur with regular use of GHB, and a withdrawal syndrome has been seen in people who have taken high doses of it (~18 g/day or more, although doses are variable in solution form) with frequent dosing (Q 1–3 hr).[58] Withdrawal symptoms can include muscle cramps, nausea, vomiting, tremor, anxiety, insomnia, tachycardia, restlessness, and delirium or frank psychosis. Death caused by pulmonary edema has been reported. Treatment of withdrawal involves supportive care, including use of benzodiazepines (e.g., lorazepam or diazepam) for sedation. Withdrawal can last up to 2 weeks.[58]

Misrepresented sometimes as a natural and safe hypnotic, the low therapeutic index and the unknown purity of illicit supplies, particularly when sold in solution, make GHB a potentially dangerous drug. Physical dependency is a possibility as well. L.S. should be educated about GHB's potential risks. If she chooses to use GHB, she should be encouraged not to drink alcohol or use other drugs, not to drive, and to be cautious about the amount she ingests.

CENTRAL NERVOUS SYSTEM STIMULANTS

Cocaine

Cocaine is a naturally occurring alkaloid derived from the *Erythroxylon coca* plant, found mainly in the Andes Mountains of South America. Cocaine was first isolated in the 1800s and was a common ingredient in tonics and elixirs of the 1900s. The Harrison Narcotic Act of 1914 prohibited nonmedical use, and in 1970 it became a schedule II controlled substance. Today, it is second to marijuana as the most frequently used drug of abuse. According to the 2006 National Survey on Drug Use and Health, an estimated 35 million people in the continental United States have tried cocaine; 6 million people used cocaine within the previous year, and 2.4 million used cocaine at least once within a month before the survey.[13] Cocaine is a CNS stimulant and has vasoconstrictive and local anesthetic properties. Cocaine's stimulant effects are primarily caused by blockade of reuptake of dopamine, norepinephrine, and serotonin. It also facilitates the release of dopamine and norepinephrine. This results in an overall increase in availability of neurotransmitters. Cocaine also has other indirect effects on neurophysiology, including effects on the endogenous opioid systems.[59,60] Cocaine is associated with compulsive use. The powerful reinforcing effects of cocaine have been identified as occurring in brain regions rich in dopaminergic nerve terminals.

Dosage Forms and Routes of Administration

24. C.H. and his friends bought an "eight ball" (one eighth of an ounce) of "blow" (powdered cocaine). C.H. has only snorted cocaine, but one of his friends suggests they cook up some "rocks" to smoke. What are the distinctions between the various dosage forms of cocaine and their respective routes of administration?

In the manufacture of cocaine, organic solvents are used to solubilize the alkaloidal bases from the leaves, which are then precipitated to form a sticky material, called "pasta" or "cocaine paste." The benzoylmethylecgonine (cocaine) in this "pasta" is separated from most of the other plant alkaloids, converted to the hydrochloride or other salts, precipitated, and dried. This product is the white cocaine hydrochloride powder usually seen in the illicit market. The final product is usually "stepped on" or "cut" (diluted) with various adulterants to increase profits for the dealers. According to the DEA, in 2004 the average purity of cocaine was 84%.[12] Cocaine is usually purchased on the illicit market in quantities of gram or ounce increments. The cost varies geographically, but 1 g of powdered cocaine usually sells for $100 in most cities.[14]

Powdered cocaine is generally snorted. Usually 10 to 25 mg of powdered cocaine is placed on a mirror or flat surface, formed into a line, and then insufflated through a straw or rolled dollar bill. A typical low to moderate user may consume 1 to 3 g/week. Cocaine powder can also be used for IV injection. The highly water-soluble powder is usually mixed with water and injected. When cocaine is injected simultaneously with heroin, this is known as a "speedball."

Cocaine hydrochloride melts at a high temperature, destroying much of its psychoactivity in the process. Therefore, it is inefficient to smoke cocaine hydrochloride in this form. The use of "freebase" cocaine became popular during the late 1970s, as this form of cocaine has a lower melting point and can therefore be smoked, producing an intense rush. For freebase, the cocaine hydrochloride is dissolved into ethyl ether. When an alkali, such as bleach (sodium hypochlorite) or sodium bicarbonate, is added to this ethyl ether, the hydrochloride salt is cleaved from the free alkaloidal cocaine base. The sugars, salts, and some of the other water-soluble adulterants are precipitated out of solution, and the free alkaloidal base remains in the ethyl ether solution. When the ether is evaporated, the freebase of cocaine remains in a powder form. The synthesis of freebase is dangerous and the resultant product may contain residual organic solvents, thus making it highly volatile and putting the user at risk of burns.

In the mid-1980s a safer, easier method for extracting the cocaine base supplanted the traditional freebase process. In the manufacture of "crack," cocaine hydrochloride is dissolved in water. When alkali (bleach or sodium bicarbonate) is added to this aqueous solution, the free alkaloidal base ("crack") precipitates out while the salts and some adulterants stay in aqueous solution. The precipitate is commonly referred to as a "rock." The size of the rock varies but generally ranges from one tenth of a gram to a half a gram. Rocks generally sell for $10, but prices range from $2 to $40, depending on the size of the rock.[14] Both manufacturing methods produce cocaine free alkaloidal base of 90% or greater purity. Smoking "crack" has surpassed snorting as the most common way to use cocaine.

Pharmacokinetics and Effects

25. C.H.'s friend gets some baking soda and water from the kitchen and proceeds to convert a few grams of their cocaine into "rock." After smoking a few "hits" (doses), C.H. feels euphoric, energized, and self-confident. Are these typical cocaine effects?

C.H. is describing the typical euphoria associated with cocaine use. Cocaine generally produces a euphoriant action with a rapid onset and short duration. Snorting cocaine generally produces euphoria and stimulation within 2 minutes; smoking produces these effects within 6 to 8 seconds. Cocaine has a short elimination half-life of approximately 30 minutes owing to its rapid metabolism by plasma esterases.[59]

An initial relaxed, euphoric, gregarious, talkative, hyperactive state characterizes the "high" of cocaine. Additionally, the person may report increased interest in sexual matters, diminished short-term memory, periods of intense concentration on one limited subject, diminished hunger, hypervigilance, and a peculiar, slightly out-of-body sense of one's actions. Without additional doses of cocaine, these feelings usually resolve into a state of mild depression, fatigue, hunger, and sleepiness by 1 to 3 hours. Physiologic manifestations include mydriasis, sinus tachycardia, vasoconstriction with hypertension, bruxism, repetitive behavior, hyperthermia, and talkativeness. After a few hours, continuous self-administration of cocaine will begin to progress from euphoria to dysphoria and hallucinosis and then to psychosis. Some users engage in nonstop binges of self-administration until psychological toxicity develops.[61]

Adverse Effects

26. C.H. and his friends continue to smoke crack for the next 10 hours. C.H. decides to go out for a pack of cigarettes and collapses on the sidewalk outside his apartment. A passerby calls 911, and C.H. is rushed to the nearest emergency department in a semiconscious state. What has likely happened to C.H.?

Cocaine is the most frequently mentioned illicit substance in emergency department visits. In 2005, 448,481 cocaine-related visits to an emergency department were reported in the United States.[22] The potential adverse effects associated with both acute and chronic use of cocaine are numerous and involve most organ systems in the body.

The cardiac complications associated with cocaine use include hypertension, arrhythmias, myocardial ischemia and infarction, dilated and hypertrophic cardiomyopathy, myocarditis, aortic dissection, and acceleration of atherosclerosis. These cardiac effects have occurred in individuals with and without underlying heart disease who have taken large or small doses by all routes of administration and may be associated with acute or chronic use. The cardiac events can occur before, during, or after other toxicities, such as seizures, and can be fatal. The mechanism of cocaine-induced myocardial infarction is most likely multifactorial, involving one or more of the following processes: coronary artery vasoconstriction, increased myocardial oxygen demand related to increased blood pressure and increased heart rate, increased platelet aggregation and thrombus formation, coronary vasospasm, and arrhythmia. The risk is greatest within the first hour following use.[62,63] Frequent cocaine users are up to seven times more likely to suffer a heart attack than are nonusers.[59]

The medical management of acute coronary syndromes differs when cocaine is the cause. Specifically, nonselective β-blocker therapy (i.e., propranolol) is contraindicated, thrombolysis should be used with caution, and nitrates and benzodiazepines are part of first-line therapy.[27] In patients with cocaine-associated chest pain, a 12-hour observation period to rule out myocardial infarction or ischemia is probably sufficient before discharge from a medical facility.[64]

Cocaine has also been associated with cerebrovascular catastrophes. Stroke can occur as a result of increased blood pressure, vasoconstriction, or thrombosis. Seizures are another CNS complication. Seizures can occur with first use and are most often single, generalized tonic-clonic seizures. Most occur within 90 minutes of drug use, when drug plasma concentrations are highest. It is estimated that 10% of patients presenting to emergency departments with acute cocaine intoxication have seizures.[65]

The route of cocaine administration also affects the nature of the adverse effects. For example, pulmonary complications, including pneumomediastinum, pneumothorax, pneumopericardium, acute exacerbation of asthma, diffuse alveolar hemorrhage, pulmonary edema, and "crack lung," are associated with smoking crack cocaine. Crack lung is a syndrome of acute pulmonary infiltrates associated with a spectrum of clinical and histologic findings.[66] Snorting cocaine can lead to perforation of the nasal septum because of the drug's local anesthetic and vasoconstrictive effects. IV use of cocaine has been associated with renal infarction, wound botulism, viral hepatitis, HIV infection, bacterial endocarditis, sepsis, and other infectious complications.[67] C.H. could be suffering from cardiovascular, cerebrovascular, or pulmonary complications caused by his crack smoking. His emergency department workup should be thorough and directed by his symptoms.

Cocaine Addiction

27. C.H. is released from the emergency department and returns home to find his friend with more crack. They resume smoking and binge for the next 4 days. They run out of drugs and money, and C.H. begins to "crash." In desperation, he sells his skateboard to his neighbor for $20, buys another rock, smokes it, and feels good again. Is C.H.'s cocaine usage pattern consistent with cocaine dependence?

C.H. continues to use cocaine despite adverse consequences (emergency department visit), uses it compulsively, suffers withdrawal symptoms, and alleviates his symptoms with further use. Per the DSM-IV criteria for substance dependence, C.H. is addicted to cocaine.[1]

Prolonged or heavy use of cocaine has been associated with the development of tolerance to some of its central effects. Tolerance to cocaine's euphoric effects has been shown to occur, but tolerance to its cardiovascular effects may be incomplete.[68] A withdrawal syndrome may follow long-term or binge use. The initial, acute symptoms, referred to as the "crash," consist of depression, fatigue, craving, hypersomnolence, and anxiety. Anhedonia and hyperphagia soon follow. Although most symptoms are mild and resolve within 1 to 2 weeks, the dysphoria and anhedonia can persist for weeks. These symptoms do not produce profound physiologic changes and are generally not life-threatening.[68]

Treatment of Addiction

28. C.H. decides to get clean and seeks help from a detox clinic. What therapeutic options are available to him?

Most cases of simple cocaine withdrawal do not require medical treatment. Multiple pharmacologic therapies to facilitate abstinence from cocaine have been, and continue to be, under investigation, however. Most studies have yielded variable results, and to date no drug exists that is proven effective in treating cocaine dependence.[26] Studies of dopamine agonists (amantadine, selegiline, levo-dopa/carbidopa, pergolide), antidepressants (desipramine, fluoxetine, bupropion), and carbamazepine have yielded inconsistent findings. Methylphenidate (Ritalin) has been investigated as "maintenance treatment" to satisfy the cocaine addict's desire for further enhancement of mood; however, methylphenidate also can stimulate a powerful craving for the more intense euphoria of cocaine and has significant abuse potential. Recent research shows promise for topiramate, baclofen, tiagabine, disulfiram, and modafinil, but these findings require replication. A cocaine vaccine is currently under investigation. Psychosocial treatments focusing on abstinence have been effective in the treatment of cocaine dependence.[26] Cognitive-behavioral therapies and behavioral therapies, such as contingency management, along with 12-step–oriented individual counseling can be useful, although the efficacy of these therapies varies. Participation in a 12-step self-help group (AA, NA), as an adjunct to treatment, seems to predict less cocaine use.

Because currently no drug therapies are effective or approved by the FDA for the treatment of cocaine addiction, C.H. should receive psychosocial treatment, such as cognitive-behavioral therapy and relapse prevention.

Amphetamines

Central nervous system stimulants have been used both with and without social acceptance for thousands of years. The Chinese prepared ephedrine-containing products from a plant called Ma-Huang (*Ephedra vulgaris*).[15] People in East Africa and the Arabian peninsula chew the leaves of the khat bush (*Catha edulis*) for the stimulating effects of the alkaloid cathinone.[59] Caffeine is consumed worldwide in a usually socially acceptable manner in the form of coffee and cola soft drinks. Amphetamine was synthesized in 1887, and methamphetamine in 1919. The legal sanctions against widespread prescribing of amphetamines in the 1970s restricted their supply and fostered a black market thriving on the illicit production of methamphetamine powder ("speed," "meth," "crank," "crystal meth"). During the 1990s, California and the West Coast experienced a dramatic resurgence of methamphetamine-related hospital admissions, poison center calls, and law enforcement actions. Methamphetamine abuse has since become a nationwide problem, prompting government restrictions on retail sales of ephedrine and pseudoephedrine (precursor chemicals used in the manufacture of methamphetamine). A new marketing tool developed by savvy drug dealers aimed at younger, new users involves bright coloring and flavoring (strawberry, cola, cherry, orange) added to crystal methamphetamine to help mask the bitter taste. According to the National Survey on Drug Use and Health for 2006, there were 731,000 current users of methamphetamine in America. The rate of lifetime methamphetamine use in 2006 (5.8%) was higher than in 2005 (5.2%), but lower than in 2002 (6.5%).[13]

Physical and Psychological Effects

29. D.C., a college student, used speed this past weekend when partying with his friends. He has a midterm examination in 2 days and is too tired to study, so one of his friends suggests snorting some more speed and then hitting the books. Will this help overcome his fatigue?

Methamphetamine produces CNS stimulation by enhancing the effects of norepinephrine, serotonin, and dopamine. This is accomplished by both blocking reuptake and stimulating release of these neurotransmitters. These effects are greater for dopamine and norepinephrine than for serotonin. Methamphetamine is metabolized in the liver, and its half-life is 6 to 15 hours.[59]

The powerful stimulating effects of amphetamine and methamphetamine have made their use popular among a wide variety of groups, including students, athletes, the military, dieters, and long-distance truck drivers. Initially, the user may experience alertness, euphoria, increased energy, the illusion of increased productivity, sociability, and decreased appetite. Continuous dosing, however, produces stereotypical grooming and other repetitive motions. Physiologic effects include bruxism, tremor, muscle twitching, mydriasis, hypertension, diaphoresis, elevated body temperature, nausea, dry mouth, weight loss, and malnutrition. Continued use over several days decreases productivity and is associated with disordered thoughts, paranoia, and psychosis. Tolerance develops very rapidly after continued use.[59]

Illicit methamphetamine is commonly insufflated or injected and, less commonly, taken orally. In a pattern similar to that seen with smoking cocaine, users are now freebasing methamphetamine and smoking it. Crystal methamphetamine, known as "crystal meth" or "ice," became popular in Japan, Hawaii, and the US West Coast initially, but use has spread to other parts of the United States. Heating the crystals and smoking the vapor, as with crack, is a common route of administration; however, snorting and IV administration are also used. Absorption is rapid after smoking "ice," and the effects can last as long as 24 hours. Methamphetamine-induced psychosis may occur more frequently with the use of "ice." Acute pulmonary edema has also been reported following inhalation.[69] D.C. will probably be able to stay awake to study if he uses more methamphetamine; however, if he is up for too many days without sleep, his performance on the examination will likely suffer.

Adverse Effects and Toxicities

30. D.C. finds speed very much to his liking and begins to use it daily. He goes many days at a time without sleeping or showering and starts losing weight because he seldom has an appetite. His friends start calling him a "tweaker." He believes his friends are working with the DEA and tapping his phone. What is happening to D.C.?

D.C. is exhibiting classic signs of chronic methamphetamine abuse, which will likely progress if he continues using. A "speed freak" or "tweaker" (chronic methamphetamine user) is generally regarded even by other drug users as mentally unstable, aggressive, and emotionally labile, with unpredictable periods of violent, even homicidal, behavior. Chronic users characteristically develop complex paranoid delusional systems with hallucinations during extended periods of intoxication that may involve several sleepless days and nights of continuous methamphetamine administration. This "speed psychosis" may include tactile hallucinations, such as formication, the sensation of something crawling under the skin. Initial attempts at reassuring, reality-oriented communication ("talking down") may be successful for an acute psychotic episode. An extremely agitated, anxious, psychotic user, however, will often require administration of a benzodiazepine, such as diazepam or lorazepam. If psychosis persists, a high-potency neuroleptic, such as haloperidol, is preferred owing to its minimal anticholinergic activity. Low-potency neuroleptics, such as chlorpromazine, with higher anticholinergic activity, may worsen symptoms of delirium and hyperthermia.[61]

The physiologic toxicity of stimulant drugs includes hypertension, stroke, seizures, hyperthermia, sexual dysfunction, dental caries, rhabdomyolysis, renal failure, cardiac arrhythmias and cardiomyopathies, myocardial infarction, and malnutrition.

The development of neurotoxicities involving dopaminergic and serotonergic neurons has been demonstrated in animals, but it is less clear if such toxicities develop in humans. Although some studies have shown loss of dopamine transporters, resulting in slower motor function and decreased memory, there is evidence of recovery with protracted abstinence.[70]

Withdrawal and Treatment

31. D.C. is arrested for assault following a bar fight. He is held in the county jail and is unable to post bail. What withdrawal symptoms might he experience during incarceration?

D.C. will probably suffer intense cravings for methamphetamine and initial agitation, followed by fatigue and hypersomnolence. A withdrawal state following acute cessation of chronic stimulant use is generally the same as that previously described for cocaine (see Question 27). As with cocaine, the "crash" is notable for marked fatigue, depression, and anhedonia. Most symptoms are mild and will resolve within 1 to 2 weeks, although anhedonia and depression may persist.

Clinical studies investigating treatments for methamphetamine dependence have borrowed from the experience studying cocaine treatments. Currently no effective pharmacologic treatments have been proved effected for methamphetamine dependence. The most effective treatment so far appears to be cognitive-behavioral therapy.[71]

DISSOCIATIVE DRUGS: PHENCYCLIDINE, KETAMINE, AND DEXTROMETHORPHAN

Phencyclidine (phenylcyclohexylpiperidine) and ketamine are arylcycloalkylamine, dissociative, anesthetic agents. Phencyclidine (PCP) at one time was marketed as an IV anesthetic agent under the trade name of Sernyl.[72] Subsequent reports of postanesthetic dysphoric reactions caused the drug to be withdrawn in 1965. It was reintroduced in 1967 as Sernylan and marketed as a veterinary anesthetic until 1978, when the manufacture and sale of the drug became illegal. Ketamine is currently used clinically as an anesthetic in both animals and humans. Ketamine is shorter acting and somewhat less potent than PCP.

Abuse of arylcycloalkylamines occurs primarily in large metropolitan areas. PCP is relatively easy to synthesize and is inexpensive, therefore it is often misrepresented as other street drugs, such as lysergic acid diethylamide (LSD), amphetamine, mescaline, or δ-9-tetrahydrocannabinol (THC). Ketamine ("K," "Special K," "Super K," "cat valium") is commonly used as a "club drug" and is sometimes misrepresented as 3,4-methylenedioxymethamphetamine (MDMA; ecstasy). Ketamine is often diverted from veterinarian supplies. PCP ("angel dust," "dust") in powdered form is often applied to parsley, marijuana ("dusted joint," "superweed"), or tobacco cigarettes and smoked. Oral, intranasal, and parenteral routes of administration are used by some. The combination of cocaine and PCP in a freebase smoking mixture is called "Space-Base." Although ketamine is manufactured as an injectable liquid, it is frequently evaporated to a powder.[73] The powder can be snorted or compressed into tablets.

Dextromethorphan, an antitussive agent commonly found in over-the-counter cough remedies, has emerged as a drug of abuse, especially popular among adolescents. Its appeal may be because it is inexpensive, licit, lacks social disapproval associated with other drugs, available over-the-counter, and is believed to be safe because it is produced by a pharmaceutical company. Street names include "Skittles," "DXM," "Dex," "Robo," "C-C-C," and "Red Devils." Use is referred to as "dexing," "robotripping," and "robodosing." Dextromethorphan is the d-isomer of the codeine analog of levorphanol. The metabolic byproduct of dextromethorphan, dextrophan, has weak *N*-methyl-D-aspartate (NMDA) antagonist properties.[74] When dextromethorphan is ingested in large doses, it produces effects similar to PCP or ketamine. When abused, doses range from 300 to 1,800 mg. The most commonly abused form is Coricidin HBP Cough and Cold (called "C-C-C" on the street) because it contains the highest concentration of dextromethorphan per dosage unit on the market (30 mg). Dextromethorphan is also available for sale on the internet in powdered form, which can be ingested orally or snorted. The dextromethorphan "high" can last 3 to 6 hours and can consist of euphoria, dissociation, hallucinosis, increased perceptual awareness, altered time perception, hyperexcitability, pressure of thought, disorientation; and increased blood pressure, heart rate, and body temperature; and blurry vision.[74,75] Other ingredients found in the over-the-counter preparations, such as acetaminophen, chlorpheniramine, guaifenesin, and alcohol, may be problematic when ingested in large doses. According to the Drug Abuse Warning Network, an estimated 5,581 emergency department visits in 2004 involved nonmedical use of dextromethorphan.[71] PCP is considered the typical dissociative drug, and review of its effects largely applies to ketamine and dextromethorphan as well.[73]

Phencyclidine

Phencyclidine Intoxication

32. J.R., age 18, is brought to the emergency department by police for violent, combative behavior. Friends claim he was smoking a "dusted joint" (PCP applied to a marijuana cigarette). He appears agitated, diaphoretic, and disoriented. His blood pressure is 160/100 mm Hg, pulse 130 beats/minute, and temperature 101°F. He has vertical and horizontal nystagmus. Are these effects consistent with PCP intoxication?

J.R.'s symptoms are consistent with PCP intoxication. PCP and ketamine are noncompetitive antagonists of the NMDA receptor subtype of the major excitatory neurotransmitter, glutamate. The dose, route of administration, and serum concentration of phencyclidine all influence the pharmacologic effects of this drug and, thus, the symptoms of intoxication.[72] PCP in low doses causes inebriation, ataxia, changes in body image, numbness, and a mind-body dissociative feeling. Horizontal, vertical nystagmus, or both are often present, and the anesthetic effect of the drug raises the pain threshold. Amnesia can occur following intoxication.

As the dose of PCP increases, the patient may manifest agitation, combativeness, catatonia (ketamine users refer to this as a "k-hole"), and psychosis. The action of PCP on the autonomic nervous system becomes more prominent and is characterized by a confusing combination of adrenergic, cholinergic, and dopaminergic effects. A hypertensive response is typically encountered. Tachycardia, tachypnea, and hyperthermia may also be noted in the moderately intoxicated patient. The agitated, combative patient often has feelings of great strength. This, combined with the anesthetic effect of PCP, can result in serious injury because there is no pain sensation to stop the physical activity.

With large doses of PCP, marked CNS depression occurs and nystagmus may no longer be present. In addition to the physiologic effects noted earlier, respiratory depression, seizures, acidosis, and rhabdomyolysis may further compromise the patient's condition. Rhabdomyolysis, particularly in the presence of acidemia, can result in acute renal failure.[61] Opisthotonic posturing and muscular rigidity occur frequently in the severely intoxicated patient.

Medical Management of Intoxication

33. How should J.R. be treated?

Diagnosis of PCP intoxication should be confirmed through a blood or urine specimen. Currently, no clinically useful antidote to PCP exists, and treatment should be supportive. Environmental stimuli should be minimized. Even attempts to "talk down" the patient may trigger a combative response, and chemical restraints may be indicated. Physical restraints may increase risk of rhabdomyolysis and should be reserved for patients who pose threat of great danger to themselves or others. Benzodiazepines are useful in the management of the anxious, agitated patient with mild to moderate PCP intoxication. If benzodiazepines are insufficient, haloperidol (5 mg IM) is effective.[57] Low-potency neuroleptics should be avoided because a greater possibility of precipitating a hypotensive response or a seizure exists.

Hypertension may be managed with β-blockers or calcium channel blockers. Diazepam is a useful anticonvulsant for the management of PCP-induced seizures. Because extreme agitation, seizures, and hyperthermia can initiate rhabdomyolysis and secondarily cause myocardial, renal, or hepatic dysfunction, anxiolytics, neuroleptics, anticonvulsants, and cooling measures should be used as needed.

Management may also include attempts to increase elimination of PCP from the body. The urinary excretion of PCP (a basic compound) is enhanced when the urine is acidic; however, the amount excreted usually is not very large compared with the amount ingested.[61] Activated charcoal in a dose of 1 g/kg given every 2 to 4 hours can prevent the intestinal reabsorption of this drug and promote its elimination.

Psychological and Prolonged Effects

34. J.R. is admitted for a 72-hour psychiatric evaluation. His history reveals that he is a chronic PCP abuser. What psychological adverse effects are associated with chronic use?

Chronic PCP use can result in long-term residual psychological symptoms, including anxiety, depression, and psychosis.[61] Pharmacotherapy for these symptoms may be necessary. Prolonged psychiatric sequelae are almost always associated with premorbid psychopathology. Perceptual disorders, including auditory and visual hallucinations, such as after images seen following moving objects ("trails"), may also occur. Flashbacks (discussed in detail in the following section on LSD) have been reported after PCP use.

The DSM-IV does not recognize PCP withdrawal; however about one-fourth of heavy PCP users report symptoms following discontinuation of use.[61] These symptoms include depression, anxiety, irritability, hypersomnolence, diaphoresis, and tremor. Animal studies have described a withdrawal syndrome, but it is unclear if a true withdrawal syndrome occurs in humans.[76] Currently, no pharmacologic treatments for PCP addiction exist. Some animal data indicate neurotoxicity; however, the long-term consequences and significance for humans is unknown and requires further study. Chronic users often complain of feeling "spaced"; they may be irritable and antisocial and feel depersonalized and isolated from people. Memory lapses, speech and visual disturbances, and confusion have been described in long-term users as well.

HALLUCINOGENS

Hallucinogens can be categorized as indole alkylamines (e.g., LSD, psilocybin, and dimethyltryptamine) or phenethylamines (e.g., mescaline; MDMA). LSD is considered the prototype hallucinogen. Although MDMA is classified as a phenethylamine, it has structural similarities to amphetamine and mescaline. It has been labeled an entactogen or empathogen because of its strong empathy-producing effects and mild hallucinogenic effects. The term *entactogen* can be translated as "a touching within." Hallucinogens are commonly referred to as *psychedelics*.

In 2006, >35 million Americans reported using hallucinogens sometime in their lives, 3.9 million had used it in the past year, and >1 million had used it in the past month. The popularity of MDMA (ecstasy, X) has risen dramatically in recent years, partly because of its use as a "club drug." In 2006, 12.2 million Americans reported using MDMA sometime in their lives, 2.1 million had used it in the past year, and 528,000 had used it in the past month.[13]

The usual pattern of use for hallucinogens is occasional self-administration for enhancement of recreational activities, such as dancing, or for "mind expansion." Certain individuals may develop psychological dependence and use hallucinogens in a more chronic and compulsive manner.

LSD

Effects

35. B.T. attended a dinner party with a few close friends and the host suggested they all "trip" (take LSD) after dinner. B.T. had no previous experience with LSD but was very excited to try it. She took a "hit" (dose) and her host told her she should cancel all plans for tomorrow. What can she expect?

Perhaps the most famous of all hallucinogens, LSD-25, was first synthesized by Albert Hofmann of Sandoz Laboratories in 1938.[73] It was developed as an analeptic agent but produced significant uterine stimulation and caused experimental animals to become excited or cataleptic. Five years later, while resynthesizing LSD-25 for further pharmacologic testing, Dr. Hofmann experienced a restlessness that forced him to go home. This was followed by 2 hours of intense visual hallucinations of kaleidoscopic images and colors. Later, he identified LSD-25 as a potent hallucinogen. Clinical experimentation produced hundreds of papers describing LSD as a drug that could facilitate psychotherapy, particularly in the management of addictive behavior. Widespread public self-experimentation with LSD for recreation and self-exploration, coupled with growing attention to adverse psychological consequences, led Sandoz to discontinue production of LSD-25 (as well as psilocybin, psilocin, and related congeners) in August 1965. The United States made LSD a schedule I controlled substance in 1970 after the proliferation of illicit suppliers to meet the huge public demand for this drug.

Although the mechanism of action of classic hallucinogens is not fully understood, they appear to predominately act as agonists or partial agonists at serotonin (5-HT) receptors, specifically the 5-HT_2 receptor.[77] LSD, one of the most potent hallucinogens known, is active at doses of 25 to 250 mcg. Most users take about 100 to 150 mcg of LSD for a significant effect. This dose produces mild to moderate sympathomimetic effects, profound visual hallucinosis, and the sensation of disordered integration of sensory input. For example, sounds and music are perceived as visual imagery, odors are felt, and inanimate objects assume lifelike qualities. In addition to these sensory-perceptual effects, psychic effects occur, such as depersonalization, dreamlike feelings, and rapid alterations of affect. These are accompanied by somatic effects, including dizziness, nausea, weakness, tremor, and tingling skin.[73,77] These combined effects begin within an hour of ingestion of LSD and usually peak in intensity during the first 2 to 3 hours. After taking LSD, most people feel they have returned to a normal psychological state by 8 to 12 hours.

Within an hour after ingestion, B.T. will begin to experience altered sensations of her surroundings, in addition to some psychic and somatic effects.

Adverse Effects

36. After a few hours of "tripping," B.T. begins to think she will never return to a normal state. She fears she has "slipped over the edge" and begins to panic. What is happening to her?

The most frequently encountered adverse reaction associated with the hallucinogenic drugs is a mental state of acute anxiety and fear, typically referred to as a "bad trip." The hallucinogen experience is influenced by set (the user's mental state and expectations of drug effects) and setting (the environment in which drug use takes place, including the social conditions). Users may be able to calm themselves without outside intervention. The initial therapy of people undergoing a bad trip is frequently called "reality therapy" and consists of "talking down" the fear and panic.[61,77] This consists of getting the person to a quiet, relaxed setting and helping him or her focus on explanations for the uncertainties that are causing the panic. This process also tends to reassure the person that he or she is in a safe physical environment and that the drug effects will diminish in a few hours. Most of these bad trips are resolved during the state of intoxication (generally, 6–12 hours), but some last as long as 24 to 48 hours.

If the talk-down approach is not successful in resolving the panic, drug therapy can be considered. Sedation with an oral benzodiazepine (i.e., diazepam 10–30 mg) or a parenteral benzodiazepine (i.e., lorazepam 2 mg IM) will frequently alleviate the panic.[61] Supportive talking down should be continued because the benzodiazepine will not stop the trip; it will simply sedate the patient. Haloperidol 2 mg IM may also be used if benzodiazepines are insufficient. Phenothiazines should not be used for initial management of bad trips because they have been associated with poor outcomes.[61]

With regard to adverse physical effects, classic hallucinogens have a high margin of safety, although patients should be monitored for seizures or elevations in body temperature, which may indicate a potential hyperthermic crisis. Anticonvulsant therapy may not be effective until body temperature has been lowered.[61]

B.T. is experiencing a bad trip. Her friends should try to "talk her down," with reassurance that the effects of the drug will eventually wear off. If this approach is unsuccessful, she should be taken to the emergency room for pharmacologic treatment of her anxiety and panic.

Flashbacks and Long-Term Effects

37. B.T.'s friends "talk her down," but she has heard that people sometimes have flashbacks after LSD use and is worried she will re-experience her bad trip. What are flashbacks? What are the long-term consequences of LSD use?

Use of hallucinogens can trigger a transient psychosis or unmask an underlying psychiatric disorder; however, a true psychotic episode is rare. Psychiatric conditions following hallucinogen use that persist more than a month are likely caused by pre-existing psychopathology.[61] Hallucinogen use does not seem to be associated with any cognitive impairment.[78]

Hallucinogen persisting perceptual disorder (HPPD), commonly referred to as *flashbacks*, is characterized by recurrences of part or all of the hallucinogenic drug experiences following a period of normal consciousness in a person who used the drug previously. The American Psychiatric Association's DSM-IV includes diagnostic criteria for HPPD. The flashbacks may last from minutes to days or months (usually a few hours). The estimated prevalence of flashbacks varies widely in studies and the etiology is still unclear.[79] Flashbacks can occur spontaneously or be triggered by exercise, stress, or another drug (e.g., marijuana).[61] Treatment remains anecdotal; no randomized, controlled trials have evaluated the efficacy of pharmacotherapy for HPPD.

LSD and other classic hallucinogens have low addiction potential. There does not appear to be a clinically important withdrawal syndrome associated with their use. The rapid development of tolerance that occurs with these drugs may explain the intermittent use patterns commonly seen.

MDMA

Effects

38. R.X. and her friend P.B. go to "raves" (all-night dance parties) every weekend and usually take ecstasy (MDMA). R.X. says

it makes her feel like "I love everyone around me," and P.B. likes to be able to "dance all night without getting tired." Are these effects common with MDMA?

Merck Pharmaceuticals patented MDMA in 1914, but it was not until the 1950s that its use was examined in animal studies, when the US Army Intelligence investigated it as a "brainwashing" agent. By the late 1970s, a few therapists and psychiatrists began using the drug with reported success in patients with a wide range of conditions.[80] MDMA produces a very manageable and comfortable entactogenic effect, during which the person has a clear sensorium. The experience can be recalled in detail, and the insights gained during the session can be incorporated into normal life. The public gave several names to this drug, such as ecstasy, XTC, Adam, and M&Ms. The media became aware of the anecdotal reports from both psychiatrists and people self-experimenting with MDMA. In 1985, the DEA made MDMA a schedule I drug. Subsequently, supplies of the drug proliferated in the public illicit marketplace, and its popularity soared. In 2001, following successful lobbying by researchers interested in reinstituting MDMA in clinical practice, the FDA granted approval for a pilot study investigating the therapeutic use of MDMA in the treatment of posttraumatic stress disorder (PTSD).[81] At the time of this writing, the study has nearly completed phase II. The FDA has also approved a phase II dose-response pilot study of MDMA-assisted psychotherapy in subjects with anxiety associated with advanced stages of cancer.

The effects of MDMA are mainly exerted by three neurochemical mechanisms: blockade of serotonin reuptake, stimulation of serotonin release, and stimulation of dopamine release.[82] The common psychological effects of MDMA intoxication include an overall heightened sense of empathy, interpersonal closeness, increased acceptance of others, and a powerful sense of well-being.[83] The experience is influenced by set and setting. The amphetamine-like side effects include mydriasis, tachycardia, sweating, increased energy and alertness, bruxism, nausea, and anorexia.[84] Users generally ingest MDMA in tablet form and the onset of action is usually after 30 to 60 minutes. Some users take a "booster" dose after 2 hours. The usual duration of action of MDMA is 4 to 6 hours and the half-life is approximately 8 hours. MDMA users in the "rave" scene often "stack" multiple doses, and polydrug use is common. The combined use of ecstasy and LSD is referred to as "candy flipping."[82]

R.X.'s feelings of love for everyone are consistent with the empathogenic effects of MDMA, whereas P.B. is enjoying the amphetaminelike effects of increased energy to dance all night.

Adverse Effects

39. Several hours after taking MDMA, P.B. is still dancing. She begins to feel hot and realizes she is profusely sweating. On her way to the bar for a drink, she begins to feel confused and collapses to the floor. Her friends witness her having a seizure and call 911. What is happening to P.B.?

The "rave" scene, with its crowded conditions and often-high ambient temperatures, has contributed to many adverse effects associated with MDMA ingestion. Because of their increased physical activity, the "ravers" may become dehydrated. Additionally, supplies of MDMA have been notoriously unreliable. Many other drugs have been misrepresented as MDMA, including other phenethylamines such as 3,4-methylenedioxyamphetamine (MDA) and paramethoxyamphetamine (PMA); amphetamine; cocaine; opiates; ketamine; and dextromethorphan. The common polydrug use practiced at "raves" compounds the problem. Dextromethorphan taken at high doses for its dissociative properties competes with MDMA for hepatic metabolism and its anticholinergic effects block perspiration, potentially leading to overheating.[80]

The most dangerous adverse physical effect of MDMA is hyperthermia. MDMA has a slight affinity for the 5-HT_2 receptor, and the increased body temperature may be the result of this activation.[82] The hyperthermia has led to rhabdomyolysis, and acute renal and hepatic failure, disseminated intravascular coagulation (DIC), and death.[85] DIC has been the most common cause of death. Treatment of hyperthermia involves cooling measures and IV fluids. Benzodiazepines (e.g., lorazepam 2 mg IM or IV) and dantrolene (1 mg/kg IV) may be helpful. Other adverse physical effects can include hypertension, cardiac arrhythmias, convulsions, cerebrovascular accident, hepatitis, and hyponatremia (from overingestion of water as a harm reduction measure to avoid hyperthermia).[84,85] Although emergency room visits associated with MDMA use continue to be relatively rare, they increased dramatically (>2,000%) from 1994 to 2001, but have remained stable since.[22,86] Adverse psychological effects are also possible, including anxiety, depression, panic attacks, agitation, paranoia, and rarely psychosis. The treatment of these psychological adverse effects is the same as for those associated with the classic hallucinogens, including "talk-down" therapy and benzodiazepine administration. P.B. may be suffering from MDMA-induced hyperthermia and needs urgent medical evaluation.

Long-Term Effects

40. R.X. has read in the newspaper that MDMA is associated with "brain damage" and is worried that she has caused permanent damage to her brain. What are the long-term effects of MDMA?

Animal studies have consistently demonstrated long-term MDMA-induced serotonin depletion. This has been evidenced by lower levels of serotonin, decreased metabolite levels, lowered levels of tryptophan hydroxylase, and loss of serotonin reuptake transporters.[80] MDMA damages serotonin axonal projections; axonal resprouting and regeneration do occur, but it is unclear if these new projections are damaged. Despite this evidence of neurotoxicity, no associated functional changes have been demonstrated.[80,87]

Several retrospective studies in humans have claimed lowered cognitive performance in MDMA users compared with nonusers. These studies have serious methodologic flaws, including their retrospective design and failure to control for important confounding variables, such as other drug use and adulterant exposure and lifestyle factors.[80,87] Well-controlled, prospective clinical trials are required to establish definitively any risk associated with MDMA ingestion.

Use of MDMA does not appear to produce physical dependence, but some users may become psychologically dependent. Tolerance to the empathogenic effects develops rapidly and may last 24 to 36 hours. This may explain in part the more common practice of sporadic dosing of the drug.[83] No distinctive withdrawal syndrome has been described that would require pharmacologic treatment.

MARIJUANA

Marijuana is the most widely used illicit substance in the United States. In 2006, 97.8 million Americans reported using marijuana at some time in their lives, 25.3 million had used in the past year, and 14.8 million had used in the past month.[13] The main psychoactive ingredient in the *Cannabis sativa* plant is THC, although the plant is known to contain more than 70 cannabinoids.[88] In the United States, the dried, chopped leaves and flowers of the *Cannabis* plant (grass, pot, weed, green bud, chronic, mary jane) are rolled into a cigarette paper (marijuana cigarette, known as a joint or blunt; a "roach" is the butt of the marijuana cigarette) or smoked in a pipe or water pipe ("bong"). Each joint usually weighs 0.5 to 1 g, for a THC content of about 5 mg (very weak), 30 mg (average), or 100 mg (highest-quality sinsemilla). The sinsemilla (Spanish for "without seeds") growing technique involves separating the female plants from the males before pollination occurs. This results in female plants with higher amounts of THC, up to 14%.[89]

A dramatic increase in the potency of marijuana has occurred over the past two decades. Marijuana average potency has increased 52.4% (from 5.34% THC to 8.14%) just within the last 5 years.[12] The raw resin of the *Cannabis* plant can be pressed into cakes, balls, or sticks, called hashish ("hash," "temple balls"), which is smoked or eaten. Hashish can contain up to 12% THC. The oils can be extracted from the plant with organic solvents to produce "hash oil," perhaps the most potent *Cannabis* derivative, with THC concentrations of up to 50%.[89] Commercial grade marijuana (marijuana not grown by the sinsemilla technique) sells on average for $100 per ounce, but high-quality marijuana can cost $600 per ounce.[14]

Researchers in cannabinoid neurobiology have discovered two cannabinoid receptors in the CNS: CB_1 and CB_2; however, additional receptors have been proposed. In addition, five endogenous cannabinoids (endocannabinoids) that act at the cannabinoid receptors have been discovered.[90,91] The best-known are arachidonic acid ethanolamide (anandamide) and 2-arachidonoylglycerol (2-AG).[90]

Marijuana's therapeutic potential has been the center of much public controversy. Research on the effects of cannabinoids has led to several potential therapeutic uses, including relief of nausea and vomiting, appetite stimulation; treatment of pain, epilepsy, glaucoma, migraine, anxiety, depression, and movement disorders (Parkinson's disease, Huntington's disease, Tourette's syndrome, multiple sclerosis); and providing neuroprotection after brain injury or cerebral ischemia.[91,92] A synthetic form of THC, dronabinol, is available as prescription tablets, and a synthetic cannabinoid, nabilone, is available as capsules, but advocates of medicinal marijuana use argue that inhalation allows for faster onset and easier titration of the dose. In addition, nauseated patients want to avoid the oral route of administration. Future research may focus on developing a safer delivery system that will be reliable, rapid, and safe.[93] An oromucosal spray, Sativex, derived from botanical material, is under investigation in the United States. The principal active components are THC and cannabidiol. This cannabis extract spray has been approved in Canada, and is also being used in the United Kingdom.

Effects

41. After school one day, P.H. is offered a "joint" by one of his friends. He smokes it and begins to feel light-headed and euphoric. He begins laughing at everything around him. Thirty minutes later he and his friend become very hungry ("the munchies") and eat several candy bars. Are these effects consistent with marijuana use?

Yes. The pharmacologic effects sought by most users of cannabis products are sedation, mental relaxation, euphoria, and mild hallucinogenic effects, and these effects depend on set and setting. Other common effects that are usually perceived as pleasurable include silliness, subjective slowing of time, gregariousness, hunger, and mild perceptual changes of all the senses that engender an absorbing fascination with music, eating, and other sensual and sensory activities. The state of mind generated is referred to as "stoned," "high," "loaded," "wasted," and many other colloquial terms. Smoking marijuana typically causes numbness and tingling of the extremities, light-headedness, loss of concentration, and a floating sensation in the first 3 or 4 minutes. Some of these effects are probably caused by the hyperventilation associated with deep inhalation of the smoke (referred to as a "hit" or "toke") and breath holding to allow maximal absorption from the lungs. Over the first 10 to 30 minutes, the user may experience tachycardia (possibly palpitations), mild diaphoresis, conjunctival injection, drying of the mouth, weakness, postural hypotension, periods of tremulousness, incoordination, and ataxia along with euphoria and the mental effects described above. These effects usually resolve by 1 to 3 hours and are followed by a 30- to 60-minute period of sleepiness before complete clearing and return to normal consciousness. Oral ingestion of cannabis products may delay the onset of effects by 45 to 60 minutes and prolong the duration.[89]

Adverse Effects

42. P.H. smokes more marijuana with his friend. He liked it so much the first time, he decides to take several "hits" this time. He begins to think his friend is laughing at him and notices his heart is beating rapidly. He starts to panic. Is P.H.'s reaction caused by the marijuana?

Consistent with its widespread use, marijuana was the second most frequently mentioned illicit substance in emergency department episodes in the United States in 2005. A total of 242,200 marijuana-related emergency department visits were mentioned in 2005.[22] Despite these numbers, cases have been documented of fatality in humans from marijuana overdose, and adverse effects tend to be self-limiting and often do not require medical treatment.

A syndrome consisting of anxiety, paranoia, depersonalization, disorientation, and confusion that can lead to panic states and incapacitating fear is perhaps the most frequently reported adverse effect of marijuana. Comforting reassurance ("talk down") and reducing stressful stimuli can alleviate this condition. The dysphoria and anxiety usually resolve in a few hours or less with such an approach. More severe incidents that evolve into panic reactions that are not resolved by sympathetic counseling may be relieved with oral benzodiazepine therapy in a dose equivalent to 5 to 10 mg of diazepam.[61] These adverse psychological reactions to cannabis products commonly occur with inexperienced users, high doses, concomitant use of other psychoactive drugs, and overtly stressful situations. Severe reactions requiring pharmacologic therapy are rare.

Currently, there is much debate in the scientific community regarding the association of marijuana and psychosis. A review of the literature found that cannabis use increases the risk of developing psychotic disorders among vulnerable or predisposed individuals and negatively affects the course of pre-existing chronic psychosis.[88] Population statistics argue against a causal relationship.

Adverse physical effects can include slowed psychomotor responses and short-term memory loss. Slowed psychomotor responses have been shown in certain groups of acutely intoxicated subjects and chronic users. Short-term memory loss is a frequently documented acute, reversible effect of marijuana intoxication as well.

The paranoid ideation and panic reaction of P.H. could certainly be caused by the high dose and his inexperience with marijuana.

Long-Term Effects

43. P.H. continues to smoke marijuana daily. His parents discover his marijuana use and confront him, telling him it will make him stupid, unmotivated, and strung out, and may lead to the use of harder drugs. Are P.H.'s parents' concerns valid? What are possible long-term effects of marijuana use?

Chronic use of cannabis has been alleged to produce an "amotivational syndrome" characterized by apathy, lack of long-term goal achievement, inability to manage stress, and generalized laziness, but little scientific evidence supports such a syndrome.[89]

Cognitive impairment can occur after heavy marijuana use, but appears to be reversible with abstinence.[94] The impairment is more pronounced, the longer the drug is used.[89] Other concurrent drug use may also contribute to cognitive impairment associated with marijuana use. Evidence of brain damage associated with marijuana use is equivocal.

The pulmonary complications of chronic heavy marijuana use are potentially significant. Chronic cough, sputum, wheezing, bronchitis, and cellular changes typical of chronic tobacco smokers are reported in chronic cannabis smokers.[89,95] THC has been shown to be a potent bronchodilator. Both oral and smoked THC were shown to produce significant bronchodilation when given to healthy subjects. The bronchodilatory response in asthmatics given THC has been shown to be less vigorous.[66] Tolerance to these effects can develop after some weeks, and chronic marijuana smoking results in increased airway resistance and decreased pulmonary function.[89] Many of the same carcinogens in nicotine cigarettes are also found in marijuana smoke. Epidemiologic studies have suggested an association between marijuana smoking and certain cancers (lung, head and neck); however, controlled studies have not established such a link.[96–98] *Aspergillus*-contaminated marijuana has been reported to cause pulmonary fungal infections in immunocompromised patients, who may be using the drug for its medicinal value.[99] Harm reductionists have recommended that immunocompromised patients microwave their marijuana before use.

Tolerance to the psychoactive effects of marijuana does develop. Chronic users may not experience the full range of effects as new users unless they abstain for several days or weeks to regain initial sensitivity to the cannabis, and chronic users can tolerate large doses that generally are toxic to novices. Tolerance develops rapidly to both physiologic and psychological effects of cannabis. Dependence characterized by a physical withdrawal syndrome occurs after chronic high-dose use of cannabis. The withdrawal syndrome can involve anxiety, depression, irritability, restlessness, decreased appetite, sleep disturbance, sweating, tremor, nausea, vomiting, and diarrhea.[61,89] Dysphoria and malaise similar to that experienced with influenza can also occur. The cumulative dose of cannabis and duration of use necessary to produce dependence have varied significantly. The withdrawal syndrome is generally mild and self-limiting, and pharmacologic treatments usually are not required.

Marijuana has been labeled as a "gateway drug," meaning that it will lead to the use of "harder" drugs, such as cocaine or heroin. Marijuana is the most widely used illicit drug, but use of drugs such as alcohol and tobacco often predates marijuana use. No studies have conclusively demonstrated a causal link between marijuana use and subsequent other drug use.[89]

P.H.'s parents' concerns are understandable, but not entirely accurate. They should attempt to educate P.H. about the true risks involved with marijuana use, such as interference with studies, risk of pulmonary complications, and possible risk of dependence.

INHALANTS

The introduction of anesthetics (nitrous oxide, chloroform, and ether) to medicine in the early 1800s also promoted the widespread and popular recreational use of these inhalants for mind-altering recreational purposes. Today, abused inhalants include a wide variety of chemicals that are found readily in homes, workplaces, or purchased at retail establishments. Inhalants are commonly subdivided into three main categories: the volatile solvents (mostly hydrocarbons); volatile nitrites (amyl, butyl, isobutyl, cyclohexyl); and nitrous oxide ("laughing gas"). The fumes or vapors of these liquids, or paste in the case of glue, are directly inhaled out of their containers ("sniffing"); poured onto a rag which is held to the nose ("huffing"); poured into a plastic bag ("bagging"); or merely cupped in the hands and inhaled. Aerosols and gaseous substances such as nitrous oxide are also used to inflate a balloon and then inhaled out of the balloon by the user. These products can also be ingested orally or sprayed directly into the mouth. Volatile solvents include gasoline, toluene, kerosene, alcohols, airplane glue, lacquer thinner, acetone (nail polish remover), benzene (nail polish remover, model cement), naphtha (lighter fluid), plastic cement, liquid paper (i.e., White Out, usually containing 1,1,1-trichloroethane, also trichloroethylene and perchlorethylene), and many others. The volatile nitrites, once widely available, are prohibited by the Consumer Product Safety Commission but can still be found, sold in small bottles, labeled as "video head cleaner" or "room odorizer." Amyl nitrite is used medically as a vasodilator for treatment of angina and requires a prescription. The volatile nitrites are commonly referred to as "poppers," because of the sound made when an ampule of amyl nitrite is broken open. The most commonly used inhalants are glue, shoe polish, toluene, and gasoline.[100–102] The use of multiple products is common. Silver and gold paints are popular because they contain more toluene than paints of other colors.[103]

In 2006, 22.8 million Americans reported using inhalants at some time in their lives, >2 million had used them in the past year, and 761,000 had used them in the past month.[13] Unlike other drugs of abuse, inhalant use is most common among younger individuals (consistently highest annual prevalence among 8th graders) and tends to decline as youth grow older. The decline likely reflects that other drugs become available and are substituted, and that the inhalants are seen as "kids" drugs. Abuse of inhalants is believed to be popular among children and adolescents because of their low cost, easy availability, rapid onset, and low threat of legal intervention. Additionally, they are easily concealed. The 2006 Monitoring the Future (MTF) study found that 16.1% of 8th graders have abused inhalants.[104] The MTF and other national surveys of adolescents have found that after marijuana, inhalants are the second most widely used class of illicit drugs for 8th graders.[96] Most inhalant users, however, have used alcohol or cigarettes previously.[105] These surveys, most of which are administered in schools, likely underestimate the true prevalence, as a small but high risk group (incarcerated, homeless, and transient adolescents) are not included in the surveys. Historically, use of inhalants in the United States has been highest among native American youth and lowest among black and Asian youth.[100,105]

It was previously believed that inhalant use was more prevalent in rural communities; however, recent surveys indicate use occurs in both urban and rural settings.[103] Inhalant use has been associated with polysubstance use, later IV drug use, delinquency, depression, suicidal behavior, antisocial personality disorder, and impaired family functioning.[100,106,107] Some research has indicated inhalant use is more prevalent in lower socioeconomic groups, but recent studies have failed to show an association between use and family income.[100,105] Inhalant use is not gender-specific; however, sustained abuse is more common in male users.[100,103,107] Friends' influence on drug use (peer pressure) has been shown to be the strongest predictor of drug use in adolescents.[108]

Effects of Inhalants

44. H.K., age 14, has been pouring degreasing solvents, gasoline, and paint thinners onto a rag and "huffing" the fumes to produce intoxication. What clinical presentation might be expected in this young man?

Inhalant abuse includes a broad range of chemicals and they likely have different pharmacologic effects. In fact, the mechanisms of action of the volatile inhalants are poorly understood. Nearly all have CNS depressant effects. Evidence from animal studies suggests the effects and mechanism of action of volatile solvents are similar to those of alcohol and sedative hypnotics.[103,109]

Gases and vapors are rapidly absorbed when inhaled and, because of their high lipophilicity, tend to distribute preferentially to lipid-rich organs such as the brain and liver.[101] Expired air is the major route of elimination, and most are metabolized to some extent.

Inhalation of these products produces a temporary stimulation and reduced inhibitions before the depressive CNS effects occur. Acute intoxication is associated with euphoria, giddiness, dizziness, slurred speech, unsteady gait, and drowsiness.[103] As the CNS becomes more deeply affected, illusions, hallucinations, and delusions develop. The user experiences a euphoric, dreamy high that culminates in a short period of sleep. The intoxicated state lasts a few minutes, but users may continue to inhale repeatedly over several hours.

Nitrous oxide is an antagonist of the NMDA subtype of the glutamate receptor.[72] Its pharmacologic effects are poorly understood. It produces euphoria and symptoms of intoxication similar to those described for the volatile solvents.

The major effect of the volatile nitrites is the relaxation of all smooth muscles in the body, including the blood vessels. This usually allows a greater volume of blood to flow to the brain. The onset of effects takes 7 or 8 seconds and the effects last about 30 seconds. A certain "rush" occurs, which may be followed by a severe headache, dizziness, and giddiness. The volatile nitrites are frequently used in the context of sexual activity, particularly by homosexual males because of the effect of increased tumescence and relaxation of smooth muscle.[110]

Acute Complications of Inhalants

45. What acute complications may H.K. experience from inhalation of these solvents?

In 2005 the Drug Abuse Warning Network reported 4,312 emergency department visits were associated with inhalant use in the United States.[22] Deaths from inhalant use are well documented and may occur from overdose or trauma (falls, drowning, hanging). Death from overdose is often caused by respiratory problems or suffocation after CNS depression.[110] Deaths caused by asphyxiation, convulsions, coma, and aspiration of gastric contents have occurred.[103] Acute cardiotoxicity resulting in cardiac arrest is the most common cause of sudden death.[107] Referred to as "sudden sniffing death," it is likely caused by "sensitization" of the myocardium to catecholamines, exacerbated by physical exercise, resulting in fatal ventricular arrhythmias. Nearly one-third of deaths resulted from first-time use and 90% of deaths are men.[107] A study of cases of inhalant abuse reported to US poison control centers found that three categories of inhalants were disproportionately responsible for most deaths: gasoline, air fresheners, and propane/butane.[111] The author of that study concluded that a potential exists for >200 deaths from volatile solvent abuse per year in the United States.

Toxicities of Inhalants

46. What toxicities are associated with chronic inhalation of solvents?

The wide variety of chemicals inhaled causes a tremendous range of toxicities. Toxicity depends on the chemical, and on the magnitude and duration of exposure. Complications can result from the effects of the solvents or other toxic ingredients, such as lead in gasoline. The lipophilicity of the volatiles enhances their toxicity. Injuries to the brain, liver, kidney, bone marrow, and particularly the lungs can occur and they may result from the effect of heavy exposure or hypersensitivity. Inhalant abusers may develop irritation of the eyes, nose, mouth, including rhinitis, conjunctivitis, and rash.[110] Methemoglobinemia has been associated with volatile nitrite use.[107]

Many of the inhalants produce neurotoxicity, which can range from mild impairment to severe dementia. Studies reveal approximately 10% of chronic inhalant abusers develop evidence of neurotoxicity.[101] Neurologic deficits include cognitive impairment, ataxia, optic neuropathy, deafness, and disorders of equilibrium. Loss of white matter, brain atrophy, and damage to specific neural pathways can result from chronic exposure to some inhalants.

Solvent abusers have been found to have impaired executive functions, including capacity for insight and behavioral self-control.[101] Some damage to the nervous system and other organs may be at least partially reversible when inhalant use is discontinued.[103]

Inhalant Abuse and Dependence

47. Are inhalants addictive?

Compulsive use has been documented with inhalants, although inhalant abuse and dependence is a neglected area of research. Animal studies have shown some of the abused inhalants to have reinforcing properties.[110,112] The DSM-IV sets criteria for inhalant abuse and dependence, but does not provide for physiologic dependence, and it is unclear if a true withdrawal syndrome occurs with chronic use of inhalants. Inhalant use is typically episodic in nature and, thus, users may not be exposed to levels with sufficient frequency necessary to develop physical dependence or tolerance. A review of national surveys of adolescents found 11% of past year users met the criteria for inhalant abuse or dependence.[100] A study of adolescents in drug treatment revealed that inhalant abuse or dependence is relatively uncommon in adolescent treatment programs.[106] Although many adolescents may try inhalants, few meet criteria for DSM-IV–defined inhalant use disorders. Volatile solvent abusers are particularly refractory to drug treatment.[108]

ACKNOWLEDGMENT

The authors acknowledge James F. Buchanan, Howard E. McKinney, Gregory N. Hayner, Darryl S. Inaba, Jeffery N. Baldwin, and Blaine Benson for their authorship of previous editions of this chapter.

REFERENCES

1. American Psychiatric Association. *Diagnostic and Statistical Manual of Mental Disorders.* 4th ed., Text Revision (DSM-IV-TR). Washington, DC: American Psychiatry Press; 2000.
2. Agrawal A et al. Linkage scan for quantitative traits identifies new regions of interest for substance dependence in the Collaborative Study on the Genetics of Alcoholism (COGA) sample. *Drug Alcohol Depend* 2008;93:12.
3. Willette RE. Drug testing in the workplace. In: Graham AW et al., eds. *Principles of Addiction Medicine.* 3rd ed. Chevy Chase: American Society of Addiction Medicine; 2003:993.
4. Hull MJ et al. Postmortem urine immunoassay showing false-positive phencyclidine reactivity in a case of fatal tramadol overdose. *Am J Forensic Med Pathol* 2006;27:359.
5. Santos PM et al. False positive phencyclidine results caused by venlafaxine. *Am J Psychiatry* 2007; 164:349.
6. Widschwendter CG et al. Quetiapine cross reactivity with urine methadone immunoassays. *Am J Psychiatry* 2007:164:172.
7. Straley CM et al. Gatifloxacin interference with opiate drug screen. *Pharmacotherapy.* 2006;26: 435.
8. Gottesman L. Sustiva may cause false positive on marijuana test. *WORLD* 1999;96:7.
9. Dupont RL et al. Drug testing in addiction treatment and criminal justice settings. In: Graham AW et al., eds. *Principles of Addiction Medicine.* 3rd ed. Chevy Chase: American Society of Addiction Medicine; 2003:1001.
10. Hayner G. Drugs of abuse testing. In: Traub S, ed. *Basic Skills in Interpreting Laboratory Data.* 2d ed. Bethesda: American Society of Health Systems Pharmacists; 1996:41.
11. Dasgupta A. Adulteration of drugs-of-abuse specimens. In: Wong RC et al., eds. *Drugs of Abuse: Body Fluid Testing.* Totowa NJ: Humana Press; 2005: 217.
12. United States Department of Justice, National Drug Intelligence Center. National Drug Threat Assessment 2007, Product No. 2006-Q0317-003, October 2006.
13. Substance Abuse and Mental Health Administration. Results from the 2006 National Survey on Drug Use and Health: National findings (Office of Applied Studies, NSDUH Series H-32, DHHS Publication No. SMA 07-4293). Rockville, MD; 2007.
14. Office of National Drug Control Policy. Pulse Check: Trends in Drug Abuse, Drug Markets and Chronic Users in 25 of America's Largest Cities, January 2004. Online. Available at http://www.whitehousedrugpolicy.gov/publications/drugfact/pulsechk/January04/. Accessed October 29, 2007.
15. Inaba DS et al. *Uppers, Downers, All Arounders.* 6th ed. Medford, OR: CNS Productions; 2007:129.
16. Portenoy RK et al. Acute and chronic Pain. In: Lowinson JH et al., eds. *Substance Abuse: A Comprehensive Textbook.* 3rd ed. Baltimore: Williams & Wilkins; 1997:563.
17. Gowing L et al. Buprenorphine for the management of opioid withdrawal. *Cochrane Database Syst Rev* 2006;(Issue 2.) Art.No.:CD002025.DOI: 10.1002/14651858.CD002025.pub3.
18. Savage SR. Opioid medications in the management of pain. In: Graham AW et al., eds. *Principles of Addiction Medicine.* 3rd ed. Chevy Chase: American Society of Addiction Medicine; 2003: 1451.
19. Ling W et al. Abuse of prescription opioids. In: Graham AW et al., eds. *Principles of Addiction Medicine.* 3rd ed. Chevy Chase: American Society of Addiction Medicine; 2003:1483.
20. Ferguson R et al. *Enterobacter agglomerans*-associated cotton fever. *Arch Intern Med* 1993;153: 2381.
21. Rylander R et al. Bacterial contamination of cotton and cotton dust and effects on the lungs. *Br J Ind Med* 1978;35:204.
22. Substance Abuse and Mental Health Services Administration, Office of Applied Studies. Drug Abuse Warning Network, 2005: National Estimates of Drug-Related Emergency Department Visits. DAWN Series: D-29, DHHS Publication No. (SMA) 07-4256. Rockville, MD; 2007.
23. Substance Abuse and Mental Health Services Administration, Office of Applied Studies. Drug Abuse Warning Network, 2003: Area Profiles of Drug-Related Mortality. DAWN Series: D-27, DHHS Publication No. (SMA) 05-4023. Rockville, MD; 2005.
24. Armstrong GL et al. The prevalence of hepatitis C virus infection in the United States: 1999–2002. *Ann Intern Med* 2006;144:705.
25. Centers for Disease Control and Prevention. HIV/AIDS Surveillance Report, 2005. Vol. 17. Atlanta: US Department of Health and Human Services, Centers for Disease Control and Prevention; 2006. Online. Available at: http://www.cdc.gov/hiv/topics/surveillance/resources/reports/. Accessed October 29, 2007.
26. Kleber HD et al. Treatment of patients with substance use disorders, second edition. American Psychiatric Association. *Am J Psychiatry* 2007;164(4 Suppl):5.
27. Albertson TE et al. TOX-ACLS: toxicologic-oriented advanced cardiac life support. *Ann Emerg Med* 2001;37:S78.
28. Abramowicz M, ed. Buprenorphine: an alternative to methadone. *Med Let* 2003;45:13.
29. Substance Abuse and Mental Health Services Administration, Center for Substance Abuse Treatment. Buprenorphine, Summary of Drug Addiction Treatment Act of 2000. Online. Available at: http://buprenorphine.samhsa.gov/titlexxxv.html. Accessed October 26, 2007.
30. Dole VP et al. A medical treatment for diacetylmorphine addiction. *JAMA* 1965;193:646.
31. O'Connor PG et al. Management of opioid intoxication and withdrawal. In: Graham AW et al., eds. *Principles of Addiction Medicine.* 3rd ed. Chevy Chase: American Society of Addiction Medicine; 2003:651.
32. Stine SM et al. Pharmacological interventions for opioid addiction. In: Graham AW et al., eds. *Principles of Addiction Medicine.* 3rd ed. Chevy Chase: American Society of Addiction Medicine; 2003:735.
33. Peachey JE et al. Assessment of opioid dependence with naloxone. *Br J Addict* 1988;83:193–201.
34. Center for Substance Abuse Treatment. Medication-Assisted Treatment for Opioid Addiction in Opioid Treatment Programs. Treatment Improvement Protocol (TIP) Series 43. DHHS Publication No. (SMA) 05-4048. Rockville, MD: Substance

Abuse and Mental Health Services Administration; 2005.
35. Amato L et al. Methadone at tapered doses for the management of opioid withdrawal. *Cochrane Database Syst Rev* 2005(Issue 3). Art. No.: CD003409. DOI:10.1002/14651858.CD003409. pub3.
36. Boatwright DE. Buprenorphine and addiction: challenges for the pharmacist. *J Am Pharm Assoc* 2002;42:432.
37. van Dorp E et al. Naloxone reversal of buprenorphine-induced respiratory depression. *Anesthesiology.* 2006;105:51.
38. Wesson D et al. Buprenorphine in pharmacotherapy of opioid addiction: implementation in office-based medical practice. California Society of Addiction Medicine, 1999.
39. Payte JT et al. Opioid Maintenance Treatment. In: Graham AW et al., eds. *Principles of Addiction Medicine,* 3rd ed. Chevy Chase: American Society of Addiction Medicine; 2003:741.
40. Johnson RE et al. A Comparison of levomethadyl acetate, buprenorphine, and methadone for opioid dependence. *N Engl J Med* 2000;343:1290.
41. Alford DP et al. Acute pain management for patients receiving maintenance methadone or buprenorphine therapy. *Ann Int Med* 2006;144: 127.
42. National Institutes of Health Consensus Development Panel. Effective medical treatment of opiate addiction. *JAMA* 1998;280:1936.
43. Dunlop AJ et al. Clinical Guidelines for the use of Buprenorphine in Pregnancy, 2003. Fitzroy, Turning Point Alcohol and Drug Centre.
44. Dashe JS et al. Relationship between maternal methadone dosage and neonatal withdrawal. *Obstet Gynecol* 2002;100:1244.
45. Ebner N et al. Management of neonatal abstinence syndrome in neonates born to opioid maintained women. *Drug Alcohol Depend* 2007;87:131.
46. Jones HE et al. Buprenorphine versus methadone in the treatment of pregnant opioid-dependent patients: effects on the neonatal abstinence syndrome. *Drug Alcohol Depend* 2005;79:1.
47. Jackson L et al. A randomised controlled trial of morphine versus phenobarbitone for neonatal abstinence syndrome. *Arch Dis Child Fetal Neonatal Ed* 2004;89:300.
48. Jansson LM et al. Methadone maintenance and lactation: a review of the literature and current management guidelines. *J Hum Lact* 2004;20:62.
49. Talbott GD et al. Physician health programs and the addicted physician. In: Graham AW et al., eds. *Principles of Addiction Medicine.* 3rd ed. Chevy Chase: American Society of Addiction Medicine; 2003:1009.
50. Naltrexone (Vivitrol)—a once-monthly injection for alcoholism. *Med Lett Drugs Ther* 2006;48:1240.
51. Collins ED et al. Anesthesia-assisted vs. buprenorphine- or clonidine-assisted heroin detoxification and naltrexone induction. *JAMA* 2005; 294:903.
52. Gowing L et al. Opioid antagonists under heavy sedation or anaesthesia for opioid withdrawal. Cochrane Review. In: *The Cochrane Library,* Oxford: Update Software; 2003;1.
53. Gowing L et al. Alpha2 adrenergic agonists for the management of opioid withdrawal. *Cochrane Database Syst Rev* 2004(Issue 4). Art. No.: CD002024 DOI:10.1002/14651858.CD002024. pub2.
54. Bailey DN et al. Carisoprodol: an unrecognized drug of abuse. *Am J Clin Pathol* 2002;117:396.
55. Substance Abuse and Mental Health Services Administration, National Clearinghouse for Alcohol and Drug Information. Detoxification from Alcohol and Other Drugs Treatment Improvement Protocol (TIPS) Series 19. Online. Available at: http://ncadi.samhsa.gov/govpubs/BKD172/19e. aspx. Accessed September 24, 2007.
56. Fatseas DC et al. Pharmacological interventions for benzodiazepine mono-dependence management in outpatient settings. *Cochrane Database Syst Rev* 2006(Issue 3). Art. No.:CD005194.DOI:10.1002/14651858.CD005194.pub2.
57. Hayner G et al. Haight-Ashbury Free Clinics Drug Detoxification Protocols. Part 3: Benzodiazepines and other sedative-hypnotics. *J Psychoactive Drugs* 1993;25:331.
58. Snead, OC et al. Gamma-hydroxybutyric acid. *N Engl J Med* 2005;352:2721.
59. Gorelick DA et al. The pharmacology of cocaine, amphetamines, and other stimulants. In: Graham AW et al., eds. *Principles of Addiction Medicine.* 3rd ed. Chevy Chase: American Society of Addiction Medicine; 2003:175.
60. Stefano, GB et al. Nicotine, alcohol and cocaine coupling to reward processes via endogenous morphine signaling: the dopamine-morphine hypothesis. *Med Sci Monit* 2007;13:RA91.
61. Wilkins JN et al. Management of stimulant, hallucinogen, marijuana, phencyclidine, and club drug intoxication and withdrawal. In: Graham AW et al., eds. *Principles of Addiction Medicine.* 3rd ed. Chevy Chase: American Society of Addiction Medicine; 2003:673.
62. Kloner RA et al. Cocaine and the heart. *N Engl J Med* 2003;348:487.
63. Lange RA et al. Cardiovascular complications of cocaine use. *N Engl J Med* 2001;345:351.
64. Weber JE et al. Validation of a brief observation period for patients with cocaine-associated chest pain. *N Engl J Med* 2003;348:510.
65. Boghdadi MS et al. Cocaine pathophysiology and clinical toxicology. *Heart Lung* 1997;26:466–483.
66. Tashkin DP. Airway effects of marijuana, cocaine, and other inhaled illicit agents. *Curr Opin Pulm Med* 2001;7:43.
67. Saitz R. Medical and surgical complications of addiction. In: Graham AW et al., eds. *Principles of Addiction Medicine.* 3rd ed. Chevy Chase: American Society of Addiction Medicine; 2003:1027.
68. Gold MS et al. Cocaine (and crack): neurobiology. In: Lowinson JH et al., eds. *Substance Abuse: A Comprehensive Textbook.* 3rd ed. Baltimore: Williams and Wilkins; 1997:166.
69. Nestor TA et al. Crystal methamphetamine-induced acute pulmonary edema: a case report. *Hawaii Med J* 1989;48:457.
70. Volkow ND et al. Loss of dopamine transporters in methamphetamine abusers recovers with protracted abstinence. *J Neurosci* 2001;21:9414.
71. Department of Health and Human Services, National Institutes of Health. National Institute on Drug Abuse, Research Report Series. Methamphetamine Abuse and Addiction. NIH Pub. No. 02-4210. 2002.
72. Domino EF. The pharmacology of NMDA antagonists: psychotomimetics and dissociative anesthetics. In: Graham AW et al., eds. *Principles of Addiction Medicine.* 3rd ed. Chevy Chase: American Society of Addiction Medicine; 2003:287.
73. Department of Health and Human Services, National Institutes of Health. National Institute on Drug Abuse, Research Report Series. Hallucinogens and Dissociative Drugs. NIH Pub. No. 01-4209. 2001.
74. Bobo WC et al. Dextromethorphan as a drug of abuse. In: Graham AW et al., eds. *Principles of Addiction Medicine.* 3rd ed. Chevy Chase: American Society of Addiction Medicine; 2003:154.
75. Substance Abuse and Mental Health Services Administration, Office of Applied Studies. Emergency Department Visits Involving Dextromethorphan. The New DAWN Report. Issue 32, 2006. Rockville, MD, 2006.
76. Department of Health and Human Services. Phencyclidine (PCP) and Related Substances. Drug Abuse and Drug Abuse Research, Third Triennial Report to Congress, 1991.
77. Glennon RA. The pharmacology of serotonergic hallucinogens and "designer drugs." In: Graham AW et al., eds. *Principles of Addiction Medicine.* 3rd ed. Chevy Chase: American Society of Addiction Medicine; 2003:271.
78. Galloway GP. Lysergic acid diethylamide (LSD) and other classical psychedelics. In: Graham et al., eds. *Principles of Addiction Medicine.* 3rd ed. Chevy Chase: American Society of Addiction Medicine; 2003:286.
79. Halpern JH et al. Hallucinogen persisting perception disorder: what do we know after 50 years? *Drug Alcohol Depend* 2003;69:109.
80. Grob CS. Deconstructing ecstasy: the politics of MDMA research. *Addiction Research* 2000;8: 549.
81. Doblin R. A clinical plan for MDMA (ecstasy) in the treatment of post-traumatic stress disorder (PTSD): partnering with the FDA. Multidisciplinary Association for Psychedelic Studies, 2002. Online. Available at: http://www.maps.org/research/mdmaplan.html. Accessed October 29, 2007.
82. Malberg JE et al. How MDMA works in the brain. In: Holland J, ed. *Ecstasy: The Complete Guide.* Rochester: Park Street Press; 2001:29.
83. Bravo GL. What does MDMA feel like? In: Holland J, ed. *Ecstasy: The Complete Guide.* Rochester: Park Street Press; 2001:21.
84. Henry JA et al. Medical risks associated with MDMA use. In: Holland J, ed. *Ecstasy: The Complete Guide.* Rochester: Park Street Press; 2001:71.
85. Hall AP et al. Acute toxic effects of ecstasy (MDMA) and related compounds: overview of pathophysiology and clinical management. *Br J Anaesth* 2006;96:678.
86. Substance Abuse and Mental Health Services Administration, Office of Applied Studies. Club Drugs, 2001 Update. The Drug Abuse Warning Network, The DAWN Report; 2002.
87. Baggott M et al. Does MDMA cause brain damage? In: Holland J, ed. *Ecstasy: The Complete Guide.* Rochester: Park Street Press; 2001:110.
88. Ben Amar M et al. Cannabis and psychosis: What is the link? *J Psychoactive Drugs* 2007;39:131.
89. Welch SP et al. The pharmacology of marijuana. In: Graham AW et al., eds. *Principles of Addiction Medicine.* 3rd ed. Chevy Chase: American Society of Addiction Medicine; 2003:249.
90. Mechoulam R. Plant cannabinoids: a neglected pharmacological treasure trove. *Br J Pharmacology* 2005;146:913.
91. Drysdale AJ et al. Cannabinoids: mechanisms and therapeutic applications in the CNS. *Curr Med Chem* 2003;10:2719.
92. Chong MS et al. Cannabis use in patients with multiple sclerosis. *Multiple Sclerosis* 2006;12: 646.
93. Watson SJ et al. Marijuana and medicine: assessing the science base: a summary of the 1999 Institute of Medicine report. *Arch Gen Psychiatry* 2000;57:547.
94. Pope HG et al. Neuropsychological performance in long-term cannabis users. *Arch Gen Psychiatry* 2001;58:909.
95. Tetrault JM et al. Effects of marijuana smoking on pulmonary function and respiratory complications: a systematic review. *Arch Intern Med* 2007;167:221.
96. Sidney S et al. Marijuana use and cancer incidence California, United States. *Cancer Causes Control* 1997;8:722.
97. Zhang ZF et al. Marijuana use and increased risk of squamous cell carcinoma of the head and neck. *Cancer Epidemiol Biomarkers Prev* 1999;8:1071.
98. Fung M et al. Lung and aerodigestive cancers in young marijuana smokers. *Tumori* 1999;85:140.
99. Szyper-Kravitz M et al. Early invasive pulmonary aspergillosis in a leukemia patient linked to aspergillus contaminated marijuana smoking. *Leukemia Lymphoma* 2001;42:1433.
100. Wu LT et al. Inhalant abuse and dependence among adolescents in the United States. *J Am Acad Child Adoles Psychiatry* 2004;43:1206.
101. Rosenberg NL et al. Neuropsychiatric impairment and MRI abnormalities associated with chronic solvent abuse. *J Toxicol Clin Toxicol* 2002;40:21.
102. Office of Applied Studies. Patterns and Trends in Inhalant Use by Adolescent Males and Females:

2002–2005. The National Survey on Drug Use and Health Report. Rockville, MD. 2007.

103. Department of Health and Human Services, National Institute of Health. National Institute on Drug Abuse, Research Report Series. Inhalant Abuse. NIH Pub. No. 05-3818; 2005.

104. Johnston LD et al. Monitoring the Future National Results on Adolescent Drug Use: Overview of Key Findings, 2006. NIH Pub. No. 07-6202. Bethesda, MD: National Institute on Drug Abuse.

105. Office of Applied Studies. Characteristics of Recent Adolescent Inhalant Initiates. The National Survey on Drug Use and Health Report. 2006. Issue 11. Rockville, MD.

106. Sakai JT et al. Inhalant use, abuse, and dependence among adolescent patients: commonly comorbid problems. *J Am Acad Child Adoles Psychiatry.* 2004;43:1080.

107. Wille SMR et al. Volatile substance abuse-postmortem analysis. *Forensic Science Int* 2004;142:135.

108. Beauvais F et al. Inhalant abuse among American Indian, Mexican American, and non-Latino white adolescents. *Am J Drug Alcohol Abuse* 2002;28:171.

109. Beckstead MJ et al. Glycine and gamma-aminobutyric acid (A) receptor function is enhanced by inhaled drugs of abuse. *Mol Pharmacol* 2000;57:1199.

110. Balster RL. The Pharmacology of Inhalants. In: Graham AW et al., eds. *Principles of Addiction Medicine.* 3rd ed. Chevy Chase: American Society of Addiction Medicine; 2003:295.

111. Spiller HA. Epidemiology of volatile substance abuse (VSA) cases reported to US poison centers. *Am J Drug Alcohol Abuse* 2004;30:155.

112. Riegel AC et al. The abused inhalant toluene increases dopamine release in the nucleus accumbens by directly stimulating ventral tegmental area neurons. *Neuropsychopharmacology.* 2007;32:1558.

CHAPTER 84

Alcohol Use Disorders

George A. Kenna

ALCOHOL CONTENT AND DEFINITIONS

Beverages containing alcohol (ethanol) have a wide range of ethanol content. Alcoholic proof is a measure of how much ethanol is in an alcoholic beverage, and is twice the percentage of alcohol by volume (ABV), the unit that is commonly used as percent. This system dates to the 18th century, and perhaps earlier, when spirits were graded along with gunpowder. A solution of water and alcohol "proved" itself when it could be poured on a pinch of gunpowder and the wet powder could still be ignited. If the gunpowder did not ignite, the solution had too much water in it and the proof was considered insufficient. A "proven" solution was defined as 100 degrees proof (100).[1,2]

In the United States, the proof is twice the percentage of alcohol content measured by volume at a temperature of 60°F. Therefore "80 proof" is 40% alcohol by volume, and pure alcohol (100%) is "200 proof." One hundred percent ethanol does not stay 100%, because it is hygroscopic and absorbs water from the atmosphere.

Alcohol is produced by yeast during the process of fermentation. The amount of alcohol in the finished liquid depends on the amount of sugar initially present for the yeast to convert into alcohol. Low alcohol beer is beer with very low or no alcohol content. Legally, in the United States, beers containing up to 0.5% alcohol by volume can be called nonalcoholic. In some states (e.g., Minnesota, Colorado, and Utah), beer sold in supermarket chains and convenience stores must be <3.2% alcohol by weight (4% alcohol by volume or ABV). Alcohol content is generally listed by volume (e.g., a beer that is 4.0% by volume is about 3.2% by weight). Light beers range from 2% to about 4% ABV; beers range from 4% to 6% ABV; ales, stouts, and specialty brews can be as high as 10% ABV.

Depending on the strain of yeast, wines are produced at about 14% to 16% (28–32 proof), because that is the point in the fermentation process where the alcohol concentration denatures the yeast. Since the 1990s, a few alcohol-tolerant 'super yeast' strains have become commercially available, which can ferment up to 20%. Yeast organisms multiply as long as there is sugar to metabolize, gradually increasing the alcoholic content of the solution and killing off competing microorganisms, and eventually themselves. There are fortified wines with a higher alcohol concentration because stronger alcohol has been mixed with them. As this is usually done before fermentation is complete, these products contain a much higher quantity of sugar and therefore are typically sweet.

Stronger liquors are distilled after fermentation is complete to separate the alcoholic liquid from the remains of the source of sugar (e.g., grain, fruit). The idea of distillation is that a mixture of liquids is heated; the one with the lowest boiling point will evaporate first, followed by the one with the next lowest boiling point, and so on. Water and alcohol form a mixture called an *azeotrope* that has a lower boiling point than either one of them, so what distills off first is the mixture that is 95% alcohol and 5% water. Distilled liquor therefore cannot be stronger than 95% (190 proof). Other techniques can separate liquids that can produce 100% ethanol (called "absolute alcohol"), but they are used only for scientific or industrial purposes. A standard drink in the United States is considered to be 0.5 ounces or contain 15 grams of alcohol. This is equal to 12 ounces (355 mL) of 5% beer, 5 ounces (148 mL) of 12% wine, or 1.5 ounces (44 mL) of 40% spirits.[1,2]

Epidemiology

Slightly more than half (50.9%) of Americans aged 12 or older, reported being current drinkers (at least one drink in the past 30 days) of alcohol in the 2006 National Survey on Drug Use and Health survey.[3] This translates to an estimated 125 million people, which is similar to the 2005 estimate of 126 million people (51.8%). More than 57 million people (23.0%) aged 12 or older participated in binge drinking (five or more drinks on the same occasion; i.e., at the same time or within a couple of hours of each other, on at least 1 day in the past 30 days) in 2006. In 2006, heavy drinking (five or more drinks on the same occasion on each of 5 or more days in the past 30 days) was reported by 6.9% of the population aged 12 or older.[3] In 2003, alcohol use disorders (AUD) in the United States accounted for 12,766 person deaths in alcohol-related traffic crashes, constituting almost 30% of the total traffic crash fatalities.[4] Currently, >700,000 people a day in the United States receive treatment for alcohol dependence.[5]

Approximately 10% of Americans will be affected by alcohol dependence sometime during their lives.[6,7] In 2001–2002, prevalences of *Diagnostic and Statistical Manual of Mental Disorders*, Fourth Edition (DSM-IV) alcohol abuse and dependence were estimated to be 4.7% and 3.8%, respectively.[8] Abuse and dependence were more common among males and among younger respondents. The prevalence of abuse was greater among whites than among blacks, Asians, and Hispanics. The prevalence of dependence was higher in whites, Native Americans, and Hispanics than Asians.[8]

Alcohol dependence is a chronic disorder with genetic, psychosocial and environmental factors influencing its development and manifestations. Although treatment outcomes have improved, still much remains to address unsuccessful treatment of alcohol abuse and dependence for many others.[9] As defined by the DSM-IV,[10] alcohol dependence is characterized by the preoccupation with alcohol use, use despite adverse consequences, as well as tolerance and withdrawal (Table 84-1).

Treatment of alcohol dependence consists mainly of psychological, social, and pharmacotherapy interventions aimed at reducing alcohol-related problems.[11] Treatment usually consists of two phases: detoxification and rehabilitation. Detoxification manages the signs and symptoms of withdrawal. Once detoxified, rehabilitation helps the individual avoid future problems with alcohol. Most rehabilitation treatments are psychosocial, consisting of individual and group therapies, residential treatment in alcohol-free settings, and self-help groups, such as Alcoholics Anonymous. Although psychosocial treatments show effectiveness in reducing alcohol consumption and in maintaining abstinence, reviews of treatment studies report 40% to 70% of patients return to drinking within the year following treatment.[12] An evidence report prepared by the Agency for Health Care Policy and Research[13] concludes that there is both a significant need to improve current alcohol treatments, as well as to develop new strategies.

Interest in using pharmacotherapies to improve treatments for alcohol dependence is growing.[14,15] The rationale for pharmacotherapy is based on several considerations. Advances in neurobiology have identified neurotransmitter systems that initiate and sustain alcohol drinking; pharmacologic modification of these neurotransmitters or their receptors may alter dependence.[16] Promising genetic research confirms that alcoholics are a heterogeneous population and that several gene variations can predispose some to increased alcohol use and other gene variations can confer protection.[16] Animal models have identified pharmacologic agents that reduce alcohol consumption in animals, suggesting similar agents could reduce

Table 84-1 Diagnostic Criteria for Alcohol Abuse and Dependence[10]

DSM-IV defines **abuse** as a maladaptive pattern of substance use leading to clinically significant impairment or distress, as manifested by one (or more) of the following, occurring within a 12-month period:

1. Recurrent substance use resulting in a failure to fulfill major role obligations at work, school, home
2. Recurrent substance use in situations in which it is physically hazardous
3. Recurrent substance-related legal problems
4. Continued substance use despite having persistent or recurrent social or interpersonal problems caused or exacerbated by the effects of the substance

DSM-IV defines **dependence** as a maladaptive pattern of substance use, leading to clinically significant impairment or distress, as manifested by three (or more) of the following, occurring at any time in the same 12-month period:

1. Tolerance, as defined by either of the following:
   - A need for markedly increased amounts of the substance to achieve intoxication or desired effect
   - Markedly diminished effect with continued use of the same amount of substance
2. Withdrawal, as manifested by either of the following:
   - The characteristic withdrawal syndrome for the substance
   - The same (or a closely related) substance is taken to relieve or avoid withdrawal symptoms
3. The substance is often taken in larger amounts or over a longer period than was intended
4. There is a persistent desire or unsuccessful efforts to cut down or control substance use
5. A great deal of time is spent in activities to obtain the substance, use the substance, or recover from its effects
6. Important social, occupational or recreational activities are given up or reduced because of substance use
7. The substance use is continued despite knowledge of having a persistent or recurrent physical or psychological problem that is likely to have been caused or exacerbated by the substance (e.g., continued drinking despite recognition that an ulcer was made worse by alcohol consumption)

alcohol consumption in humans. Finally, medications have improved the treatment of other addictive disorders, such as nicotine and opiate dependence, suggesting better pharmacotherapies may be developed for the treatment of alcoholism.

Risks and Benefits of Alcohol Consumption

The role of alcohol in the development of medical problems such as cardiovascular disease, hepatic cirrhosis, and fetal abnormalities is well documented. Alcohol use and abuse contribute to thousands of injuries, auto collisions, and violence.[17] Alcohol can dramatically affect worker productivity and absenteeism, family interactions, and school performance.[18] Some studies suggest, however, that individuals who abstain from using alcohol may also be at greater risk for a variety of conditions, particularly coronary heart disease (CHD), than people who consume small to moderate amounts of alcohol.[19]

Over the past 20 years, a number of studies have documented an association between moderate alcohol consumption and lower risk for CHD[20] and myocardial infarction (MI).[21] Binge drinking after an MI, however, increases the risk of mortality.[22] U.S. guidelines define moderate drinking as one drink or less daily for women or people aged 65 and older, and two drinks or less per day for men.[23] An association between moderate drinking and lower risk of CHD does not mean that alcohol is the cause of the lower risk. A review of population studies indicates that the higher mortality risk among abstainers may be attributable to socioeconomic and employment status, mental health, and overall health, rather than abstinence from alcohol use.[24] Benefits of moderate drinking on CHD mortality are offset at higher drinking levels by increased risk of death from other types of heart disease, cancer, cirrhosis, and trauma. The risk of a disease outcome from low to moderate drinking is less than the risk from either no drinking at all or heavier drinking. This produces a U-shaped curve when examining the association of alcohol consumption with rates of deaths from all causes.[19]

The exact mechanism by which alcohol use may be protective against morbidity in those with CHD is not clear. Some evidence indicates that different types of alcoholic beverages, such as red wines which are high in tannins, may lower blood lipids and fats by increasing antioxidants. It is also possible however that how a person drinks alcoholic beverages matters as well. For example, wines are ingested more slowly as they are typically consumed in moderate amounts with food. Binge drinking of any type of beverage, however, increases the risk of mortality from CHD in particular.[22]

NEUROSCIENCE AND NEUROBEHAVIOR

Pharmacokinetics and Pharmacology

When consumed in amounts typical of normal social drinking, the absorption of ethanol from the stomach, small intestine, and colon is complete; however, the rate is variable. Peak blood ethanol concentrations after oral doses in fasting subjects generally are reached in 30 to 75 minutes, but several factors can influence the rate and extent of absorption.[25] The most rapidly absorbed formulations are carbonated beverages containing 10% to 30% ethanol. In contrast, high concentrations of alcohol can produce vasoconstriction in the gastrointestinal (GI) mucosa, which results in slowed or even incomplete absorption of ethanol. Absorption of ethanol from the small intestine appears to be more rapid than any other part of the GI tract and does not depend on the presence or absence of food. Factors that control the rate of gastric emptying significantly control the rate of absorption by controlling the rate at which ethanol is delivered to the small intestine.[26,27] For example, food in the stomach slows the absorption of ethanol, probably by slowing gastric emptying.

The level of intoxication achieved is not solely related to the plasma concentration. For any particular plasma concentration, greater cognitive impairment is seen during times when the plasma level is rising compared with when ethanol is primarily being eliminated. The degree of intoxication also appears to be directly related to the rate at which pharmacologically active plasma concentrations are attained. Alcohol negatively affects cognitive performance and has a differential effect on the descending versus ascending limb of the blood alcohol concentration curve. The latter finding may have important ramifications relating to the detrimental consequences of alcohol intoxication.[28]

The blood alcohol level (BAL) or blood alcohol concentration (BAC) is calculated using the weight of ethanol in milligrams and the volume of blood in deciliters. This yields a BAC expressed as a proportion (i.e., 100 mg/dL or 1.0 g/L) or as a percentage (i.e., 0.10% alcohol). Ethanol concentrations are usually converted to equivalent blood alcohol concentrations for standardization purposes when measured in other body fluids. Ethanol in expired air or breath alcohol concentration is usually stated as grams per 210 liters of breath.

Breath alcohol measurement has been used as an estimate of blood ethanol concentrations since the 1970s. Breath measurement relies on the property of ethanol to partition from blood into inspired air. At equilibrium, the concentration of ethanol in the vapor depends on the ethanol concentration in the fluid and the temperature. If air is inhaled deeply into the lungs and the breath is held briefly, ethanol vapor rapidly diffuses out of the pulmonary capillary blood into air in the alveoli and the ethanol vapor in the alveolar air approaches the equilibrium concentration. The concentration of ethanol vapor in alveolar air at body temperature is a small fraction of the ethanol concentration in blood, which generally varies from person to person, depending on pulmonary blood flow and the diffusibility of alcohol. Regardless of variability, a uniform breath to blood ethanol partition coefficient of 1:2,100 has been defined for legal purposes in almost all countries, and is used to calibrate almost all breath alcohol measurement devices.[29]

Specificity of alcohol metabolism affects an individual's sensitivity to alcohol, and vulnerability to specific behavioral and physiologic effects of alcohol. The alcohol dehydrogenase (ADH) pathway is the major enzyme system responsible for alcohol metabolism in humans. The main alcohol metabolism occurs with ADH isoenzymes, in the stomach (ADH6 and ADH7) and in the liver (ADH1, ADH2 and ADH3). The pathway involves conversion of ethanol to acetaldehyde by these ADH isoenzymes, resulting in the reduction of nicotine-adenine-dinucleotide (NAD) to NADH. In the second step, acetaldehyde is converted to acetate via the enzyme aldehyde dehydrogenase, which also reduces NAD to NADH. These are the rate-limiting steps in ethanol metabolism, and this route becomes saturated when large amounts of ethanol deplete NAD.[29]

Acetate ultimately is converted to carbon dioxide and water. An additional pathway that is more involved in alcohol-dependent individuals than those who are not, involves the catalase pathway of peroxisomes and the microsomal ethanol oxidizing system (MEOS), in the smooth endoplasmic reticulum. The main functional component of the MEOS is the cytochrome P250 (CYP) 2E1.

Of a dose of ethanol, 90% to 98% is oxidized in the liver, with the remaining drug excreted unchanged in the alveolar air and urine. Ethanol metabolism formerly was described by zero-order kinetics; however, Michaelis-Menten and other nonlinear, concentration-dependent models are more accurate.[30,31] In some situations, a portion of the absorbed dose of ethanol does not appear to enter the systemic circulation, suggesting first-pass metabolism. The relative contribution of hepatic versus gastric ADH to this response continues to be debated, however.[32,33] Using a two-compartment, Michaelis-Menton pharmacokinetic model as well as experimental data, Levitt et al.[34,35] suggest that gastric metabolism contributes negligibly to first-pass metabolism. In contrast, Lieber et al.[36] believe that gastric metabolism accounts for gender and ethnic differences in first pass metabolism. Estimates of total gastric ADH suggest that the enzyme can metabolize 0.9 to 1.8 g/hour of ethanol, depending on the concentration of ethanol consumed.[37] Although gastric alcohol dehydrogenase has a lower affinity for ethanol compared with hepatic alcohol dehydrogenase, it may be capable of exerting modest metabolic effects at alcohol concentrations found in the stomach after a drink. The extent of first-pass extraction tends to decrease as the dose of alcohol increases. This is likely because of saturation of alcohol dehydrogenase, regardless of the source. When plasma ethanol levels >0.2 g/mL, the alcohol dehydrogenase system becomes saturated. As hepatic alcohol dehydrogenase becomes saturated, there is increased unchanged excretion of alcohol. This results in a more intense odor of alcohol on the breath as the plasma ethanol concentration increases. The metabolism of alcohol also then tends to become nonlinear because of stimulation of CYP2E1, which produces metabolic tolerance to ethanol in chronic users.

Lower first-pass metabolism has been found in alcohol-dependent individuals, women, the elderly, and Japanese subjects.[34,36] Gastric alcohol dehydrogenase may also play a role in the effect of food in reducing ethanol bioavailability. Food, by delaying gastric emptying, allows for more extensive gastric metabolism.[37]

The accepted average rate of ethanol oxidation commonly reported in the medical literature is 0.15 g/mL/hour for men and 0.18 g/mL/hour for women.[38] Although this rate still is widely used for both legal and medical purposes, other data suggest wide variability in ethanol metabolism. For example, wide differences in alcohol dehydrogenase activity have been demonstrated and attributed to heredity and other causes.[39,40] Chronic heavy drinkers frequently oxidize ethanol at twice the normal rates, with their metabolic rates returning to baseline after a period of abstinence.[41] The rate of oxidation in chronic heavy drinkers may also increase with elevated blood ethanol levels.[41] In contrast, patients with end-stage liver disease may progress to the point at which they have almost no metabolic capacity. Thus, serial determinations of plasma ethanol concentrations are needed to evaluate pharmacokinetic parameters in a particular patient.

Chronic alcohol use is associated with characteristic changes in the liver. Hyperlipidemia and fat deposition in the liver occur because of shunting of the excess hydrogen into fatty acid synthesis and direct oxidation of ethanol for energy instead of body fat stores being used for energy. Fatty liver is the first step in a sequence of events that ultimately leads to alcoholic cirrhosis. Accumulated acetaldehyde, which interferes with mitochondrial function by shortening and thickening microtubules, has been implicated as playing a role in the hepatotoxic process. The damaged microtubules then inhibit the secretory functions of the hepatocytes, which results in an increase in size and weight of the liver.[42] Nutritional deficits and impaired hepatic protein metabolism may contribute as mechanisms of hepatotoxicity in chronic ethanol consumers.[43,44] Although beyond the scope of this chapter, various other mechanisms of hepatotoxicity may be involved to various extents in producing damage to the liver.[45]

Acetaldehyde is believed to play a role in most actions of alcohol.[46] Elevated acetaldehyde concentrations during ethanol intoxication cause the commonly seen sensitivity reactions, including vasodilatation and facial flushing, increased skin temperature, increased heart and respiration rates, and lowered blood pressure. Acetaldehyde also contributes to the sensations of dry mouth and throat associated with bronchoconstriction and allergic-type reactions, as well as nausea and headache. These adverse effects mediated by acetaldehyde certainly have the potential to protect drinkers against the excessive ingestion of alcohol, but acetaldehyde also has the potential to produce euphoric effects that may reinforce alcohol consumption. Acetaldehyde also contributes to the increased incidence of GI and upper airway cancers that are seen with increased incidence in heavy consumers of alcohol and which may also play a role in the pathogenesis of liver cirrhosis.

Ethanol ingestion can depress the central nervous system (CNS) through all the different stages of anesthesia. Tolerance to this effect occurs after chronic use such that a blood ethanol level of 0.150 g/mL will not produce apparent behavioral or neurologic dysfunction in persons who drink a pint or more of 80-proof liquor (or its equivalent) daily for several years.

Neurobiological Basis of Alcohol Dependence

Previously, theories of alcohol action suggested that alcohol dissolved in cellular membranes and increased membrane fluidity.[47] This action in turn altered the function of macromolecules in the cell membrane, leading to intoxication. More recent evidence indicates that alcohol binds to hydrophobic pockets of proteins, changing the structures of proteins and altering their function. Proteins that are particularly sensitive to alcohol include ion channels, neurotransmitter receptors, and enzymes involved in signal transduction.[5] Notable neurotransmitters and their receptors include γ-aminobutyric acid (GABA), glutamate, dopamine (DA), serotonin (5-HT), adenosine, neuropeptide-Y (NPY), norepinephrine, cannabinoid receptors, and opioid peptides. These neurotransmitters or their receptors are potential targets for pharmacotherapy.

The key inhibitory neurotransmitter in the CNS is GABA, which is associated with a chloride-ion channel that is affected by low concentrations of alcohol. Normally, when GABA binds to the $GABA_A$ receptor, the chloride channel opens, allowing negatively charged chloride ions to enter the cell and inhibiting neuronal cell activity. In the presence of alcohol, GABA-induced inhibition is inhibited.[48] Receptor compensation for continual inhibition by alcohol is to reduce $GABA_A$ receptor subunits.[49] Other sedative medications, such as benzodiazepines, also bind to the chloride channel at slightly different sites and facilitate GABA inhibition. The existence of a common receptor mechanism for the actions of alcohol and sedative-hypnotics accounts for the cross-tolerance between these substances.

Glutamate is the major excitatory neurotransmitter in the CNS. After concurrent events of α-amino-3-hydroxy-5-methyl-isoxazole-4 propionic acid (AMPA) depolarization and glutamate binding to *N*-methyl-D-aspartate (NMDA) receptors, a Ca^{2+} ion channel opens and makes the depolarization process more likely. Low doses of alcohol strongly inhibit NMDA receptors and inhibit neuronal activity.[50] After continual exposure to high doses of alcohol, NMDA receptors upregulate in an attempt to balance alcohol's inhibitory action. Thus, the combined effect of alcohol on $GABA_A$ and glutamate is to inhibit excitation and facilitate sedation.

Several other ion channels and receptors neurotransmitters are also affected by alcohol. One of the serotonin (5-hydroxytryptamine or 5-HT) receptors, the $5\text{-}HT_3$ receptor, is an ion-channel receptor. This receptor is particularly sensitive to the action of low doses of alcohol, and may result in an activation of serotonin and dopamine. Alcohol also modifies the activity of β-adrenergic and adenosine neurotransmitter receptors linked to adenylate cyclase through membrane-bound G-proteins. Low doses of alcohol can facilitate the activity of norepinephrine, serotonin, dopamine, endocannabinoid signaling system, and other neurotransmitter receptors linked to G-proteins.[47,51,52]

Other lines of research also suggest important roles for NPY and the cannabinoid receptor 1 (CB1). NPY is a peptide neurotransmitter implicated in the control of food intake, cerebrocortical excitability, cardiovascular homeostasis, and integration of emotional behavior.[53] Evidence suggests that a polymorphism in the NPY gene, Leu7Pro, may be associated with alcoholism and that central NPY activity is recruited in response to ethanol consumption. Moreover, activation of NPY may act as a protective feedback mechanism to prevent high ethanol drinking.[53] Recent studies also show that the endocannabinoid signaling system plays a key role in the reinforcing effects of ethanol by mediating actions on the signal transduction coupled to G-proteins.[53] In particular, the cannabinoid receptor (CB1) is activated by delta-9-tetrahydrocannabinol (Δ^9-THC), the major psychoactive component of marijuana, and stimulated by naturally occurring endogenous cannabinoid agonists. Chronic alcohol administration may downregulate CB1 receptors, facilitating a compensatory increase in endocannabinoids, subsequently influencing neurotransmitter release.[52] Endogenous cannabinoid agonists are found to promote alcohol craving in animals and mimic the psychoactive effects of Δ^9-THC.[52] By contrast, an antagonist of the CB1 receptor, rimonabant, decreases food intake in animals as well as humans and decreases alcohol consumption in rodents.[54,55]

On a neurobiological-behavioral level, the mesolimbic dopaminergic pathway from the ventral tegmental area to the nucleus accumbens is activated by most dependence-producing drugs, including alcohol, cocaine, opiates, and nicotine.[56,57] Putatively, activation of this pathway mediates drug reward and is responsible for the dependence-producing properties of all drugs of abuse.[58] Repeated alcohol use sensitizes the system, so that behavioral stimuli associated with alcohol also begin to release dopamine and to facilitate additional alcohol use.[59] Dopamine released by drugs of abuse are two- to tenfold that of natural rewards. This sensitization may account for the craving and preoccupation with alcohol, which are the hallmarks of alcohol dependence.

Cessation of chronic alcohol use results in an abstinence or withdrawal state of nervous system excitation that is dysphoric and negatively reinforcing. It has been suggested that abstinence contributes to alcohol craving and the preoccupation with alcohol use, in that dependent individuals will continue alcohol use to avoid this state.[60] As noted, chronic alcohol use causes $GABA_A$ downregulation and NMDA upregulation, leading to CNS hyperactivity. The locus coeruleus, a nucleus of norepinephrine-containing cells in the pons, becomes hyperactive during withdrawal and is proposed as mediating some of the negative effects of withdrawal. Chronic alcohol and drug use alters gene expression and increases levels of adenylyl cyclase, upregulates cyclic adenosine monophosphate (cAMP)-dependent protein kinases, activates cAMP-response element binding protein (CREB) and several phosphoproteins in this brain region mediating tolerance and dependence.[61]

MANAGEMENT OF ACUTE ETHANOL INTOXICATION

Clinical Presentation

Toxicology

1. S.L. is brought to the emergency department (ED) unresponsive except to noxious stimuli. Her friends report an evening of heavy drinking to celebrate her 21st birthday. Her respirations are 8 breaths/minute and shallow. Blood pressure (BP) is 100/60 mm Hg, pulse is 100 beats/minute, and temperature is 36°C. A stat arterial blood gas determination reveals a pH of 7.29 (normal, 7.36–7.44), P_{CO_2} of 52 mmHg (normal, 35–45), and HCO_3 of 19 mEq/L (normal, 21–27). Why is S.L.'s respiratory status of concern?

Frequently, individuals reaching their 21st birthday consume alcohol in excess (e.g., attempt to have 21 drinks, often as quickly as during the first hour after turning 21). This can lead to lethal blood alcohol levels, particularly in those who are alcohol naive. In the medulla, ethanol can depress respirations by inhibiting the passive neuronal flux of sodium via a mechanism similar to that of general anesthetic agents.[62] The enzyme Na^+/K^+-adenosine triphosphatase (ATPase) is inhibited, cAMP concentrations are reduced, and GABA synthesis is impaired. Ethanol is clearly a CNS depressant, and even the uninhibited behavior associated with its use is caused by preferential suppression of inhibitory neurons. More global neuronal inhibition is seen at high ethanol concentrations.

Treatment of alcohol intoxication is essentially supportive. In highly intoxicated patients, however, the prolonged slowing of the respiratory rate can lead to arrhythmias, cardiac arrest, and death, often accompanied by aspiration of vomit. Respiratory depression is responsible for the acid-base abnormality in S.L., which causes a respiratory acidosis. Even when blood ethanol levels are below those associated with medullary paralysis, a blunted respiratory response to hypercapnia and hypoxia is seen.[63,64] This makes the assessment of respiratory status a primary concern in severely intoxicated patients.

Management of Respiratory Depression

2. What therapy should be initiated to manage S.L.'s respiratory depression?

Highly intoxicated patients with depressed respiration such as S.L require immediate supportive care that may include endotracheal intubation for respiratory support. This should be sufficient to restore her acid-base balance to within normal limits, because her acidosis is primarily of respiratory origin (pH 7.29, Pco_2 52 mmHg). When metabolic acidosis is a significant component of the acid-base disturbance, it may be necessary to administer sodium bicarbonate. This should be done only in conjunction with appropriate respiratory support to prevent the development of hypercapnia.

S.L. was brought to the ED in a comatose state, and it is unknown whether she has ingested other drugs. She should be given 0.4 to 2 mg of naloxone (Narcan) because alcohol intoxication often is complicated by coingestion of other drugs and can rapidly reverse narcotic-induced respiratory depression. This dose can be repeated at 2- to 3-minute intervals for up to 10 mg, depending on the patient's response and the clinician's index of suspicion for ingestion of respiratory depressants other than alcohol. Naloxone has been used to reverse alcohol-induced coma, to reverse clonidine-induced coma, to treat septic or cardiogenic shock, and to treat acute respiratory failure,[65,66] based on its postulated ability to reverse the effects of endogenous opiate-like agonists in the CNS.

Serum Ethanol Concentration

3. Thirty minutes later, the following laboratory results are reported: glucose, 49 mg/dL (normal, 70–110); sodium (Na), 142 mEq/L (normal, 135–147); potassium (K), 3.5 mEq/L (normal, 3.5–5.0); chloride (Cl), 104 mEq/L (normal, 95–105); HCO_3, 20 mEq/L (normal, 20–27); blood urea nitrogen (BUN), 18 mg/dL (normal, 5–22); creatinine, 0.9 mg/dL (normal, 0.6–1.1); and ethanol, 475 mg%. Based on the blood ethanol level, how severe is S.L.'s intoxication?

Chronic use of alcohol can produce significant tolerance, therefore, the blood alcohol level cannot be used as a sole determinant of physiologic status. By contrast, for alcohol naive patients such as new college students, BAC in the 0.30 mg% range can be fatal, although chronic drinkers can be awake and alert at such a level. The blood ethanol concentration generally correlates with the clinical presentation of the patient (Table 84-2), although tolerance varies among individuals. Impairment in motor function may become observable at levels of 0.05 mg%. Moderate motor impairment usually is seen at 80 g/L, which is the legal definition of intoxication in all states when driving. Respiratory depression may occur with ethanol concentrations 0.45 mg%.[67]

The accepted median lethal dose (LD_{50}) for ethanol in humans is a blood concentration of 0.50 mg%, although fatalities have been reported with ethanol concentrations ranging from 0.295 to 0.699 mg%.[68,69] Factors that may be associated with fatalities at lower ethanol concentrations include lack of tolerance to alcohol, ingestion of other drugs, heart disease, and pulmonary aspiration. For example, patients who died of combined ethanol and barbiturate ingestions had a mean ethanol concentration of only 0.359 mg%.[69] Therefore, the clinician should order a toxicologic screening panel of S.L.'s urine to rule out possible concurrent drug ingestion.

Table 84-2 Blood Alcohol Relationship to Clinical Status

Blood Ethanol Concentration	*Clinical Presentation*[a]
50 mg/dL (0.05 mg%)	Motor function impairment observable
80 mg/dL (0.08 mg%)	Moderate impairment; legal definition of intoxication in all states when driving
450 g/L	Respiratory depression
500 g/L	LD_{50} for ethanol

[a] Tolerance to alcohol varies among individuals.

Acute Management

4. After S.L.'s respiratory support needs are attended, what other clinical conditions warrant attention?

In the alert intoxicated patient, general management is supportive and protective. Volume depletion resulting in hypotension often occurs in ethanol-intoxicated patients. Hypothermia also is a complication of severe intoxication and can contribute to hypotension. S.L.'s BP is not severely low and should normalize with fluid replacement and Trendelenburg bed positioning (i.e., foot of the bed is elevated such that the head is lower than the pelvis). Hypoglycemia most often occurs in conjunction with reduced carbohydrate intake. This situation is common in malnourished alcoholics but also might be particularly pronounced in S.L. if she were dieting. If intravenous (IV) fluids are given, thiamine administration should precede that of glucose, to prevent Wernicke's encephalopathy (see Question 10). Because she is hypoglycemic, 50 mL of 50% glucose solution should be administered to her by IV push (after administering 100 mg thiamine intramuscularly [IM]).[70] Additionally, administration of a short-acting benzodiazepine, such as lorazepam, should be considered. Although not appropriate at this time, if S.L. becomes violent or severely agitated, 2 to 5 mg of haloperidol IM or IV can be administered as needed.

5. What medical interventions can facilitate removal of ethanol from S.L.?

Gastrointestinal Decontamination

Gastric lavage may be useful if ingestion of other drugs is expected, or when the large consumption of alcohol is very recent. Activated charcoal absorbs ethanol poorly but should be administered when coingestion of other drugs is suspected. In addition to S.L.'s clinical presentation, information obtained from friends who brought her in to the hospital should be considered to assess concominant drug and alcohol use by S.L.

Hemodialysis

Hemodialysis rapidly removes ethanol from the body,[71] but the role of this treatment modality is unclear. In uncomplicated cases, it has been suggested that dialysis be initiated when

Table 84-3 Acute Alcohol Intoxication: Symptoms and Treatment

Symptom	Course	Treatment
Respiratory acidosis	Alcohol-induced respiratory depression; blunted response to hypercapnia and hypoxia	Endotracheal intubation for respiratory support
Coma	Alcohol-induced CNS depression; ingestion of other drugs	Gastric lavage, naloxone (Narcam) 1 mg, repeat every 2 to 3 minutes up to 10 doses, depending on response and suspicion of ingestion. Dialysis possible
Hypotension	Hypovolemia	IV fluid replacement
Hypoglycemia	Most often occurs in malnourished patients. Pyruvate is converted to lactate, rather than glucose, through gluconeogenesis.	50% glucose (50 mL) by IV push

CNS, central nervous system; IV, intravenous.

the blood ethanol concentration >0.6 mg%.[68] Ventilatory assistance and good supportive care usually are most important because respiratory depression is the primary cause of death in ethanol intoxication. With good supportive care, dialysis is generally unnecessary. Dialysis may be considered if the patient cannot be stabilized or has other complicating factors, such as coexisting disease states or ingestion of other drugs. The management of acute alcohol intoxication is summarized in Table 84-3.

MANAGEMENT OF ALCOHOL WITHDRAWAL

Signs and Symptoms

6. J.M. is a chef at a nursing home where his wife is the administrator. He drinks at work and was found unconscious and brought to the hospital. His wife states that J.M. regularly drinks half a gallon of vodka daily and has suffered an alcohol withdrawal seizure in the past. J.M.'s wife states that she does not believe that he ever abused street or prescription drugs. His blood alcohol concentration (BAC) on admission was 0.52 mg%. J.M has a history of hepatic insufficiency secondary to cirrhosis. What signs and symptoms evident in a clinical diagnosis of alcohol withdrawal need to be monitored in J.M.? The following laboratory results are reported: Total bilirubin 0.4 mg/dL (normal, 0.2–1.2 mg/dL); direct bilirubin 0.2 (normal, 0–0.4 mg/dL); alkaline phosphatase 74 (normal, 35–131 U/L); aspartate aminotransferase (AST), 129 (normal, 11–36 U/L); alanine aminotransferase (ALT) 72 (normal, 6–43 U/L); blood urea nitrogen (BUN) 18 mg/dL (normal, 5–22 mg/dL); creatinine 0.8 mg/dL (normal, 6–1.3 mg/dL); glucose 101 mg/dL (normal, 70–110 mg/dL); uric acid 6.3 mg/dL (normal, 2.5–8.5 mg/dL); calcium 9.9 mg/dL (normal, 8.3–10.6 mg/dL); albumin 4.7 (normal, 3.3–4.9 g/dL); cholesterol 423 mg/dL (normal, <200 mg/dL); creatine kinase, 1,344 U/L (normal, <18–198 U/L); sodium (Na), 143 mEq/L (normal, 132–147); potassium (K), 4.2 mEq/L (normal, 3.4–5.0); bicarbonate (HCO_3), 25.2 (normal, 17.0–30.6 mEq/L); chloride (Cl), 107 mEq/L (normal, 95–105); magnesium (Mg) 0.9 mg/dL, (normal, 1.5–3.1 mg/dL); γ-glutamyl transpeptidase (GGT) 992 U/L (normal 10–61 U/L)

For many alcohol-dependent individuals with significant physical dependence, a cluster of withdrawal symptoms known as "alcohol withdrawal syndrome" (AWS) may occur on cessation or reduction of alcohol consumption. Depending directly on the degree of physical dependence, AWS can range from creating significant discomfort to mild tremor to alcohol withdrawal-related delirium, hallucinosis, seizures, and potentially death.[72–73] A GGT of 992 U/L suggests that J.M is a heavy drinker.

Patients may present with AWS in a variety of settings, because alcohol-dependent patients may be unrecognized and experience withdrawal after inpatient hospital admission for unrelated medical reasons. For example, a sample from a primary care practice indicated that 15% of patients presented with at-risk drinking patterns or identified alcohol-related problems.[74] Also a continual need exists to assess preoperatively surgical patients for possible alcohol dependence, to treat them adequately and prevent AWS-related complications during and after surgery.[75] Institutional protocols for support and treatment of AWS may vary considerably, and confusion often exists regarding standards of care.[76]

The DSM-IV[10] defines the set of criteria necessary for a diagnosis of AWS. Diagnosis requires cessation or reduction in alcohol use that has been heavy and prolonged, and two or more of the following developing within several hours to a few days after the first criterion: autonomic hyperactivity, increased hand tremor, insomnia, nausea or vomiting, transient hallucinations or illusions (tactile, visual, or auditory), psychomotor agitation, anxiety, and grand mal seizures. These symptoms must cause significant distress or impairment of important areas of functioning, and not be caused by a general medical condition or another mental disorder. Withdrawal-related seizure is considered a more severe manifestation of withdrawal, as is alcohol withdrawal delirium (AWD), or delirium tremens as traditionally called. AWD is estimated to have a mortality rate of approximately 5% of patients who go into alcohol withdrawal.[77] Recognized predictors for AWS complications include the duration of alcohol consumption, total number of prior detoxifications from alcohol, and previous withdrawal-related seizures and episodes of AWD.[78]

7. How could the severity of J.M.'s withdrawal symptoms be assessed?

Of currently used instruments available for measuring the degree of withdrawal in an alcohol-dependent patient, the most commonly used is the revised Clinical Institute Withdrawal Assessment (CIWA-Ar).[79] Additionally the Sedation-Agitation Scale (SAS) could also be used to assess agitation.[80] The CIWA-Ar is a validated 10-item scale used for grading severity of alcohol withdrawal symptoms. The CIWA-Ar provides a final AWS score with a maximum of 67 points. A CIWA-Ar

Table 84-4 Comparison of Benzodiazepines Used for Alcohol Withdrawal

Benzodiazepine	*Onset of Action*	*Peak Level Onset*	*Pathway Metabolized*	*Elimination Half-life (hrs)*	*Comparative Dose*
Chlordiazepoxide	Intermediate (PO)	1–4 hrs (PO)	Hepatic	3–29 (parent drug) 28–100 (metabolite)	10 mg
Diazepam	Rapid (IV or PO)	1–2 (PO) 1 hrs (IM) 8 min (IV)	Hepatic	14–70 (parent drug) 30–200 (metabolites)	5 mg
Lorazepam	Intermediate (PO) Rapid (IV)	1–6 hrs (PO) 45–75 min (IM/SL) 5–10 min (IV)	Hepatic; no active metabolites	8–24	1 mg
Oxazepam	Slow (PO)	1–4 hrs (PO)	Hepatic; no active metabolites	3–25	15 mg

Onset of Action: Rapid, within 15 minutes; Intermediate, 15–30 minutes; Slow, 30–60 minutes.
IM, Intramuscular; IV, intravenous; PO, oral; SL, sublingual.

rating of 8 points or less represents mild withdrawal and needs little pharmacologic support. A rating of 9 to 15 is associated with moderate withdrawal and may require some pharmacotherapy. A rating >15 corresponds to severe withdrawal, with an increased risk of seizures and AWD, and requires close monitoring. Treatment of AWS can be initiated based on a particular patient's CIWA-Ar score. Providers should also consider concomitant illnesses and medications when interpreting CIWA-Ar scores. Indeed, individual items in the scale are not specific to AWS, and likewise some manifestations of withdrawal may be blunted. The SAS can be used in combination with the CIWA-Ar to evaluate the level of agitation and consciousness of a patient, and be linked to administer benzodiazepines on a symptom-triggered regimen when a patient becomes agitated (for scores >4 on a 7-point scale).

Therapy

8. What drugs are demonstrated to be the most clinically effective for alcohol withdrawal particularly in a patient such as J.M. with evidence of cirrhosis?

Benzodiazepines

Benzodiazepines modulate anxiolysis by stimulating $GABA_A$ receptors and, in doing so, substitute pharmacologically for alcohol.[81]

Evidence

Considered the drugs of choice for alcohol withdrawal for some time,[75,81,82] long-acting benzodiazepines (e.g., chlordiazepoxide and diazepam) and short-acting agents (e.g., lorazepam and oxazepam) represent the most efficacious pharmacotherapies for the treatment of acute alcohol withdrawal.[83] They are effective in preventing both first seizures and subsequent seizures during alcohol withdrawal.[84] Longer-acting benzodiazepines may provide for easier weaning because they gradually self-taper on metabolism and excretion; this allows for less fluctuation in plasma drug levels.[85] Longer-acting benzodiazepines also cause fewer rebound effects and withdrawal seizures on discontinuation. Shorter-acting agents (e.g., lorazepam or oxazepam), which undergo hepatic metabolism but are oxidized to inactive metabolites, require more frequent dosing but may be more appropriate for alcoholics with liver disease and the elderly.[82,86] Short-acting lorazepam and long-acting diazepam also demonstrate a higher potential for abuse because of a shared rapid onset of action.[76] As all benzodiazepines appear equally effective in ameliorating the signs and symptoms of alcohol withdrawal, however, the choice of a benzodiazepine is dependent on factors such as pharmacokinetic properties, dosage formulation, presence of liver impairment, and ease of dosage titration (Table 84-4).[76]

Benzodiazepines are shown to be more effective than placebo in reducing the signs and symptoms of alcohol withdrawal.[87] The results of a meta-analysis on treatments for alcohol withdrawal indicated a statistically significant decrease of 4.9 cases of delirium for every 100 patients treated with benzodiazepines.[76] Likewise, a significant difference was shown with treatment in regard to withdrawal-related seizures, with a reduction of 7.7 cases per 100 patients treated. In a Canadian meta-analysis, no difference was seen in adverse effects between benzodiazepines and alternative agents.[88] Even in elderly, cognitively impaired patients, benzodiazepines are recommended.[86] Notably, these patients may be at an even greater risk for adverse events related to ethanol withdrawal. (Refer to Table 84-5 for general AWS treatment guidelines.)

Dose

Two strategies for dosing benzodiazepines in AWS include fixed-schedule and symptom-triggered regimens. Fixed-schedule regimens involve a set dose and interval for the agent chosen, which is to be tapered off at specific times, usually starting on the second day of treatment. Symptom-triggered regimens depend on the use of a rating scale of withdrawal severity, such as the CIWA-Ar previously noted, which is repeated at set intervals. Medication is only administered if the scoring from the scale is above a predetermined threshold value for treatment. In this way, the risk of under- or overmedicating patients may be minimized, because dosing is guided by the degree of withdrawal symptoms. Several studies confirm that symptom-triggered regimens compared with fixed-dose regimens appear to result in a shorter duration of necessary therapy and less medication administered in total, an advantage that appears to come without any loss of efficacy.

The treatment challenge associated with individuals who are in alcohol withdrawal with a comorbid medical illness is illustrated by the case of a patient with AWS who has coronary artery disease. Such a patient may be more aggressively treated for withdrawal-related hypertension and thus treated with a β-blocker or clonidine. The result of such adjuvant treatment may be a reduced sensitivity of the CIWA-Ar owing to a masking of the patient's autonomic manifestations of

Table 84-5 Suggested Treatment Strategies for Alcohol Withdrawal Syndrome

Protocol	Special Considerations	Drug	Dose Range	Benefits
Symptom-Triggered Regimen based on CIWA-Ar Score assessed as medically appropriate	Assess patient and administer one of these drugs every hour until CIWA-Ar = 8–10 for 24 hrs.	Chlordiazepoxide Diazepam Lorazepam	50–100 mg 10–20 mg 2–4 mg	Less abuse potential for outpatients, low cost. Long-acting Available in IM and IV form-More appropriate in elderly and hepatic impairment
Fixed-Schedule Regimens (Provide additional medication as needed when symptoms are not controlled (i.e. CIWA-Ar = 8 10)	Consider if: **Mild:** CIWA-Ar 8–10; SBP >150 mmHg or DBP >90 mmHg; HR >100; T >100°F. Titrate dose. **Moderate:** CIWA-Ar 8–15; SBP 150–200 mmHg or DBP 100–140 mmHg; HR 110–140; T = 100°F to 101°F; Tremors, Insomnia and agitation. Titrate dose. **Severe Withdrawal Symptoms:** CIWA-Ar >15; SBP >200 mmHg or DBP >140 mmHg; HR >140; T >101°F; Tremors, Insomnia and agitation. Endpoint is sedation.	Example of fixed dosing schedule using lorazepam.	**Mild:** 1–2 mg PO every 4–6 hours as needed for 1–3 days **Moderate:** on days 1 and 2 give 2–4 mg PO four times a day. On days 3 and 4 give 1–2 mg PO four times a day. On day 5 give 1 mg by mouth twice a day. **Severe:** Give 1–2 mg IV every 1 hour while awake for 3–5 days.	Rapid onset of action; ease of administration.
Alternative Therapies	In patients with benzodiazepine allergy or when use of a benzodiazepine is deemed medically inappropriate.	Carbamazepine Gabapentin	Taper from 600–800 mg on day 1 down to 200 mg over 5 days. 400 mg TID for 3 days then 400 mg BID for 1 day then 400 mg for 1 day.	**For both drugs:** Non-addicting Few drug interactions Cause relatively little cognitive impairment.
Adjunctive Therapies	Adrenergic hyperactivity-	Clonidine	0.1 mg twice daily as needed.	For mild to moderate hyperactivity
	Adrenergic hyperactivity	β-Blockers (e.g. atenolol)	50 mg daily.	Shown to improve vital signs faster than oxazepam alone
	Adrenergic hyperactivity	Carbamazepine	800 mg/day tapered down to 200 mg over 5 days.	Anticonvulsant activity
	Agitation, hallucinations, delirium	Neuroleptics (e.g. haloperidol)	0.5–5 mg every hour; maximal dose 100 mg/day.	Rapid onset of action.

BID, twice daily; CIWA-Ar, Clinical Institute Withdrawal Assessment; DBP, diastolic blood pressure; HR, heart rate; PO, oral; SBP, systolic blood pressure; TID, three times daily.
Reprinted with permission from Guirguis AB and Kenna GA, Treatment Considerations for Alcohol Withdrawal Syndrome, U.S. Pharmacist; 2005.

withdrawal. This could then lead to a higher likelihood of undermedicating the patient for withdrawal and may put the patient at higher risk for severe sequelae from withdrawal. Because of these exclusion criteria, the symptom-triggered approach has not been tested in such populations or those with histories of severe withdrawal including seizures or delirium. Therefore, traditional fixed-dose regimens are recommended in these populations.[76]

An effective approach is most likely to consider combining these two dosing strategies. For example, for a low-risk patient (no history of AWS or AWD, the patient consumes low weekly amounts of alcohol and no signs or symptoms of early AWS) that patient receives a symptom-triggered regimen (e.g., lorazepam 1 mg every hour as needed). Alternatively, a high-risk patient (history of AWS, AWD, or withdrawal seizures, consume large daily amounts of alcohol, signs or symptoms of early AWS) receives fixed-dose lorazepam or diazepam with a tapering dose schedule and as needed benzodiazepine administration for uncontrolled alcohol withdrawal signs or symptoms.

Contraindications, Warnings, Interactions

Elderly patients, those with hepatic or renal insufficiency, and those with medical illnesses require close observation to prevent overmedication. In patients receiving calcium channel blockers, β-blockers, and α_2-adrenergic agonists, some signs of withdrawal such as hypertension, tachycardia, and tremor may not be apparent.

Summary

Patients with a history of severe withdrawal symptoms, withdrawal seizures, or delirium tremens; multiple previous detoxifications; concomitant psychiatric or medical illness; recent high levels of alcohol consumption; pregnancy; and lack of a reliable support networks should be considered for inpatient treatment regardless of the severity of their symptoms.

Many clinicians have adopted lorazepam as the drug of choice to treat AWS because it has no active metabolites and has an intermediate half-life. Therefore, alcoholic patients with liver disease are at less risk for developing toxicity from detoxification with lorazepam than other benzodiazepines. The choice of agent is based on pharmacokinetics. Diazepam and chlordiazepoxide are long-acting agents that have been shown to be excellent in treating AWS. Because of the long half-life of these medications, withdrawal is smoother, and rebound withdrawal symptoms are less likely to occur. Lorazepam and oxazepam are intermediate-acting medications with excellent records of efficacy. Treatment with these agents may be preferable in patients who metabolize medications less effectively, particularly the elderly and those with liver failure. Lorazepam is the only benzodiazepine with predictable intramuscular absorption (if intramuscular administration is necessary). Rarely, it is necessary to use extremely high dosages of benzodiazepines to control the symptoms of alcohol withdrawal. Because clinicians often are reluctant to administer exceptionally high dosages, undertreatment of alcohol withdrawal is a common problem. Ultimately, controlled studies comparing the advantages and disadvantages of the various benzodiazepines in alcohol detoxification have not been performed, and no evidence exists to definitively support the use of lorazepam as the first-line agent in the treatment of AWS.

In most patients with mild to moderate withdrawal symptoms, outpatient detoxification is safe and effective, and costs less than inpatient treatment. If outpatient treatment is chosen, the patient and support person(s) should be instructed on how to take the prescribed medication, its side effects, the expected withdrawal symptoms, and what to do if symptoms worsen. Small quantities of the withdrawal medication, especially benzodiazepines, should be prescribed at each visit. Because close monitoring is not available in outpatient treatment, a fixed-schedule regimen should be used.

Given J.M.'s elevated liver enzymes, a reasonable approach would be to start with lorazepam. Shorter-acting agents, such as lorazepam that do not undergo extensive hepatic metabolism, are more appropriate for patients with evidence of hepatic insufficiency.

9. Is there an advantage to treating J.M. with an anticonvulsant given his history of seizures?

Anticonvulsants Evidence

Certain anticonvulsant agents show promise for a greater role in the treatment of alcohol withdrawal, although a place in treatment is still not definitive.[93,94] Interest for their use include the possibility that anticonvulsants may curb the *kindling* phenomenon suspected in withdrawal and may therefore be neuroprotective.[89] Kindling refers to long-term neuronal changes resulting from repeated detoxifications and may be associated with progressively worse AWS on subsequent detoxifications.[90] Additionally, anticonvulsants have low abuse potential and a minimal effect on cognition.[91] Finally, benzodiazepines may increase the level of alcohol craving and relapse to alcohol use after abstinence.[92]

The anticonvulsant agent, carbamazepine, widely used in Europe for AWS, effectively decreases the severity of withdrawal symptoms; it is comparable to the benzodiazepines in terms of adverse events and is equally effective as lorazepam in decreasing the symptoms of alcohol withdrawal.[92] Although limited information is available on whether carbamazepine can reduce seizures or delirium associated with alcohol withdrawal in humans,[76] carbamazepine was found to be superior to lorazepam in preventing rebound withdrawal symptoms and reducing post-treatment drinking.[91] Also, patients treated with carbamazepine had a better success rate for subsequent rehabilitation than those treated with benzodiazepines. In that study, carbamazepine was dosed on a tapering schedule of 600 to 800 mg divided through day 1, down to 200 mg as a single dose on day 5. It was as equally efficacious as lorazepam in reducing most withdrawal symptoms during detoxification, and was better at reducing anxiety and promoting sleep.[93] It should be noted that this study involved patients with mild-to-moderate AWS who were treated on an outpatient basis. An earlier study among alcohol-dependent inpatients with severe withdrawal symptoms found that carbamazepine was equally safe and effective as oxazepam.[94]

The major concerns with the clinical use of carbamazepine are the risk of agranulocytosis or aplastic anemia, both potentially lethal conditions.[82] Additionally, in a study comparing carbamazepine with lorazepam, pruritus was the most frequent side effect in 18.9% of patients.[92] Strong evidence indicates human fetal risk with carbamazepine use (category D) and should only be considered if no other safer drugs can be used or are ineffective. Carbamazepine is not intended for outpatient use and can potentiate the sedative effects of alcohol.

Valproate sodium has been used in the treatment of AWS for many years, although most studies suggesting efficacy were open label.[95,96] In a small trial of patients with uncomplicated AWS, valproate was equivalent to lorazepam in suppressing alcohol withdrawal symptoms.[96] One well-controlled study compared valproate and carbamazepine with placebo and reported a high rate of side effects and concluded that the initial dosages of these drugs (oral dose of 600 mg every12 hours) were too high.[97] In a randomized, double-blind placebo-controlled trial evaluating the addition of divalproex with standard of care with benzodiazepines, divalproex reduced progression of withdrawal symptoms as measured by the CIWA-Ar, and likewise reduced benzodiazepine requirements.[98] The investigators speculated that a loading dose of divalproex could potentially increase the magnitude of these benefits. Use of valproic acid during pregnancy may cause teratogenic effects, such as spina bifida, or other neural tube defects. Use in women of childbearing potential for AWS is therefore not recommended (category D). Furthermore, no evidence exists for the use of valproic acid outside of a controlled setting such as inpatient detoxification.

Gabapentin is a U.S. Food and Drug Administration (FDA)-approved adjunctive treatment for partial seizures, and has been studied in additional trials for off-label indications including AWS. Gabapentin is not metabolized in humans; it is eliminated via renal mechanisms and, therefore, is safe for use in those with compromised hepatic function. Additionally, because gabapentin does not induce or inhibit hepatic enzymatic function, the impact of potential drug interactions, such as with alcohol, is lessened. Its major side effects leading to discontinuance include somnolence (1.2%) and ataxia (0.8%). Gabapentin was administered to six patients in one trial,[99] and 49 patients in another.[100] The 5-day dosing schedule for both of these trials was 400 mg three times a day for 3 days, 400 mg twice a day for 1 day, and 400 mg for 1 day. The results of these trials suggest that gabapentin may be useful for patients with mild to moderate AWS. For example, in the second larger study,[100] those individuals who reported larger amounts of alcohol use before treatment required more as-needed benzodiazepines, suggesting that those with higher CIWA-Ar scores do not do as well on gabapentin.

If gabapentin is used, avoid abrupt withdrawal, which can precipitate seizures. Also, gabapentin should be used cautiously, and the dose appropriately reduced, in patients with compromised renal function. Because the drug can potentiate the sedative and respiratory depression effects of alcohol, it is important to ensure that the patient is alcohol-free. Although newer anticonvulsants, such as gabapentin, may be useful for some patients with mild or moderate AWS, benzodiazepines are still the drugs of choice for most patients.

Drugs having antiglutamatergic activity have also been studied, but more research is needed before clinicians can recommend their use. A placebo-controlled, randomized, single-blind trial, randomized 127 alcohol-dependent patients undergoing withdrawal, to receive placebo, diazepam 10 mg three times daily, lamotrigine 25 mg four times daily, memantine 10 mg three times daily, or topiramate 25 mg four times daily. Additional diazepam was allowed when the assigned medication failed to suppress withdrawal symptoms adequately. Only diazepam and lamotrigine were significantly superior to placebo in reducing CIWA-AR scores, although diazepam was most frequently associated with side effects.[101]

Summary

Currently, no specific indication exists for using anticonvulsants to treat alcohol withdrawal, yet because these agents are used internationally in the treatment of AWS, clinicians should be aware of this approach. Because gabapentin undergoes renal elimination, there is some advantage over lorazepam; however, support for gabapentin has been demonstrated in patients with mild to moderate AWS. At this time, no clear convincing evidence indicates that an advantage to using an anticonvulsant over lorazepam. Anticonvulsants, particularly carbamazepine and gabapentin, may offer advantages over benzodiazepines in some patients. Specifically, because they have low abuse potential and interact minimally with alcohol, anticonvulsants may eventually be an option for outpatient treatment, particularly for those who are at sufficiently low risk not to require hospitalization. Although gabapentin may be useful for some patients, benzodiazepines are still the drugs of choice for most patients, including J.M.[102]

10. What adjunctive support might be considered for J.M.?

ADJUNCTIVE TREATMENTS

The hydration, electrolyte (especially, potassium and magnesium), and nutritional status of patients should be assessed at presentation. Support with IV fluids may be necessary in those patients with excessive losses through vomiting, sweating, and hyperthermia.[90] Thiamine and multivitamins should be routinely administered to patients in alcohol withdrawal. If IV fluids are given, thiamine administration should precede that of glucose, to prevent precipitation of Wernicke's encephalopathy.[103] Alcohol-dependent patients are deficient of thiamine and have a higher risk for developing Wernicke's encephalopathy.[104] Wernicke's encephalopathy is a disorder caused by thiamine deficiency. In 1881, Dr. Carl Wernicke, a Polish neurologist, described the condition as a triad of acute mental confusion, ataxia, and ophthalmoplegia. Korsakoff amnestic syndrome is a late neuropsychiatric manifestation of Wernicke's encephalopathy with memory loss and confabulation; hence, the condition is referred to as Wernicke-Korsakoff syndrome or psychosis. It is most often seen in alcohol-dependent patients, but it can also be seen in disorders associated with malnutrition such as long-term hemodialysis or patients with acquired immunodeficiency syndrome (AIDS).

Thiamine deficiency results in a diffuse decrease in cerebral glucose utilization. The body usually stores about 3 weeks of thiamine with daily requirements of about 1.5 mg. The body can absorb about 4.5 mg of a 100-mg oral dose of thiamine. Rapid correction of brain thiamine deficiency can occur with high plasma concentrations of thiamine, achieved by parenteral supplementation only because absorption of the oral thiamine by the GI tract is minimal, even with massive oral daily dosing.[104] According to the 2004 Evidence-Based Guidelines of the British Association of Psychopharmacology,[105] to prevent the neuropsychiatric effects of thiamine deficiency, patients should receive at least 100 mg IM on the first day and patients should be taking 100 to 200 mg/day of thiamine for up to 30 days. Because parenteral thiamine supplementation has been associated with anaphylactic reactions, it is only recommended as a slow IV injection in the presence of resuscitation facilities, although some reviews cite lower grade evidence in favor of oral thiamine supplementation during outpatient detoxification.[106]

Several adjunctive medications, aside from the sedative-hypnotics, may serve ancillary roles in the therapy of AWS. Their selection should be based on treating specific symptoms associated with the syndrome. For instance, β-blockers (e.g., propranolol,[107] atenolol[108]) or α_2-adrenergic agonists (e.g., clonidine[109]) can be used for moderate to severe hypertension or other autonomic manifestations. These agents can, however, mask symptoms of severe withdrawal that may herald the onset of a seizure without providing any antiseizure activity. Antipsychotics (e.g., haloperidol) can be used for managing hallucinations and severe agitation, but care must be used because these drugs can reduce the seizure threshold.[81,102]

MANAGEMENT OF ALCOHOL DEPENDENCE

Screening for Alcohol Problems

Patients who are awake and cognitively responsive should be interviewed to assess their alcohol use history.[110] Several instruments are available to screen and delineate the extent of a patient's alcohol use. Ultimately, time and purpose for use are always major factors when deciding which instrument to use. The simplest screen to assess risk of alcohol abuse is to ask: During the past year on how many occasions have you had five or more drinks (for a man) or four or more drinks (for a woman) at one time?[111] An affirmative answer would suggest that further follow-up of the patient's alcohol use history is needed. A second tool called the **C-A-G-E** consists of four questions: (1) Have you ever felt you should Cut down on your drinking?; (2) Have people Annoyed you by criticizing your drinking?; (3) Have you ever felt bad or Guilty about your drinking?; (4) Have you ever felt you needed a drink first thing in the morning to steady your nerves or get rid of a hangover (Eye opener)? Positive responses to two questions suggest an alcohol problem (Table 84-6).[112] The Rapid Alcohol Problems Screen (RAPS4) is a short screen that has demonstrated effectiveness in an emergency setting.[113] The RAPS4 questions assess heavy alcohol consumption. The Alcohol Use Disorders Identification Test (AUDIT), which was developed by the World Health Organization, has also been shown to be effective in screening individuals and distinguishing problem drinkers from others.[114]

Treatment Aims

It is important to keep in mind that unknown numbers of people with alcohol dependence heal themselves. These people have had the ability to just stop drinking. For a good many other patients who need assistance and who meet diagnostic criteria for substance abuse or dependence, psychosocial approaches are the foundation of treatment for these patients (Table 84-7). By contrast, should the patient need pharmacologic support, then consideration of a medication plan is entirely appropriate.

Table 84-6 Useful Screens for Assessing Alcohol Problems

The C-A-G-E Screening Questions (CAGE)
Have you ever felt you should Cut down on your drinking?
Have other people Annoyed you by criticizing your drinking?
Have you ever felt Guilty about drinking?
Have you ever taken a drink in the morning to calm your nerves or get rid of a hangover (Eye opener)?

The Rapid Alcohol Problems Screen (RAPS4)
Remorse: During the last year, have you had a feeling of guilt or remorse after drinking?
Amnesia: During the last year, has a friend or family member ever told you about things that you could not remember you said or did when you were drinking?
Perform: During the last year, have you failed to do what was normally expected of you because of drinking?
Starter: Do you sometimes take a drink when you get up in the morning?

Methods for Determining Recent Alcohol Consumption
Acute Consumption
- Blood alcohol
- Urine (Ethyl glucuronide)
- Saliva
- Breath

Recent Heavy Consumption
- Gamma-glutamyl transferase (GGT)
- Carbohydrate-deficient tranferrin (CDT)
- Mean corpuscular volume (MCV)

Pharmacotherapy

The pharmacologic treatments of alcohol dependence focus on relapse prevention once detoxification is complete. Treatment

Table 84-7 Psychosocial and Behavioral Interventions Used with AUD

Type of Therapy	*Underlying Processes*	*Key Ingredients*
Cognitive Behavioral Therapy (CBT)	The foundation is the belief that by identifying and monitoring maladaptive thinking patterns, patients can reduce or eliminate negative feelings and substance use.	Alter cognitive processes that lead to maladaptive behaviors of SUD Intervene in the behavioral chain that leads to substance use. Help patients deal with acute or chronic substance craving. Promote and reinforce the development of social skills and behaviors compatible with abstinence
Motivational Enhancement Therapy (MET)	Brief treatment is characterized by an empathetic approach in which the therapist helps to motivate the patient by asking about the pros and cons of the target behavior (e.g., substance use).	Develop discrepancy (e.g., comparing given behavior with peer norms) Eliciting self-motivational statements Listen with empathy Avoid argumentation Support self-efficacy
Medical Management (MM)	Brief 20-minute intervention by a health care professional (e.g., nurse, pharmacist, or physician).	Focus on medication adherence Monitor alcohol use Assess side effects Encourage 12-step meeting attendance Set goals Educate
Brief Behavioral Compliance Enhancement Therapy (BBCET)	Brief 10-minute intervention by a health care professional.	Focus on medication adherence Monitor alcohol use Assess side effects Allow patient to set goal
12-Step Facilitation	Any support group that is a self-help group. Commonly called Alcoholics Anonymous, for example.	Find a support group one feels comfortable with Get a sponsor Work the 12 steps to recovery

Table 84-8 Selected Double-Blind, Placebo-Controlled Trials for Alcohol Dependence

Medication (dose)	*Type of Agent*	*Weeks/Study Design*	*Alcoholic Subtype*	*Drinking/ Nondrinking Days*	*Craving*	*Relapse*
Disulfiram[117] (1 mg, 250 mg)	Aversive	52/Double-blind placebo-controlled	AD	+	NR	NR
Naltrexone[164] (50 mg)	Opiate antagonist	12/Double-blind placebo-controlled	AD	+	+/0	+
Naltrexone[170] (50 mg)	Opiate antagonist	12/Double-blind placebo-controlled	AD	+	+	+
Acamprosate[150] (1,998 mg)	NMDA modulator	48/Double-blind placebo-controlled	AD	+	0	+
Acamprosate[201] (1,332 mg or 1,998 mg)	NMDA modulator	24/Double-blind placebo-controlled	AD	+	+	+
Fluoxetine[202] (60 mg)	SSRI	12/Double-blind placebo-controlled	AD/Type A AD/Type B	0 –	NR NR	0 0
Fluoxetine[203] (60 mg)	SSRI	12/Double-blind placebo-controlled	AD/MD	+	NR	NR
Sertraline[204] (200 mg)	SSRI	14/Double-blind placebo-controlled	AD/Type A AD/Type B	+ 0	NR NR	0 0
Ondansetron[205] (4 mcg/kg)	5-HT3 antagonist	12/Double-blind placebo-controlled	Early onset Late onset	+ 0	NR NR	NR NR
Topiramate[181] (up to 300 mg)	Mixed-action	12/Double-blind placebo-controlled	AD	+	+	NR
Naltrexone[144] (100 mg) or/and Acamprosate (3,000 mg)	Opiate antagonist NMDA modulator	16/Double-blind placebo-controlled	AD	–	NR	NR

+, medication significant compared with placebo ($p < 0.05$); –, significant difference favoring placebo; 0, no significant difference; ±, interaction of subgroup or trend favoring medication; AD, alcohol dependent; Early Onset, onset of alcohol problems <25 years; Late Onset, onset of alcohol problems >25 years; GAD, generalized anxiety disorder; MD, major depression; NR, data not reported; +, medication significant compared with placebo ($p < 0.05$); Type A, later onset of alcohol-related problems, severe dependence, fewer childhood risk factors, alcohol-related problems and psychopathological dysfunction; Type B, early onset of alcohol-related problems, increased number of childhood risk factors, family history of alcoholism, greater severity of dependence.

is intended to be an adjunct to psychosocial treatments (Table 84-7) and not used alone.[115] To date, disulfiram, acamprosate, and naltrexone tablet and injection have been FDA approved for the treatment of alcohol dependence. In addition, several other drugs (Table 84-8) have shown varying degrees of success.[115,116] (Table 84-9). Much is still unknown about the long-term rates of abstinence, how long these drugs should be used once patients are in treatment, the optimal doses, and whether the drugs are more effective in men or women or for which specific subpopulations.

11. R.M. is a 55-year-old man, weighing 140 pounds, who used to drink about 60 drinks a week before going through alcohol detoxification. R.M. is married, has a good job, and is now committed to remain alcohol abstinent. R.M. heard about a drug called disulfiram from a friend and is interested in using this medication to help him abstain from drinking. Is disulfiram an appropriate agent to consider for R.M.? Total bilirubin 0.3 mg/dL (normal, 0.2–1.2 mg/dL); direct bilirubin 0.1 (normal, 0–0.4 mg/dL); alkaline phosphatase 53 (normal, 35–131 U/L); AST 30 (normal, 11–36 U/L); ALT 35 (normal, 6–43 U/L); BUN 14 mg/dL (normal, 5–22 mg/dL); creatinine 1.0 mg/dL (normal, 0.6–1.3 mg/dL); glucose 123 mg/dL (normal, 70–110 mg/dL); uric acid 9.1 mg/dL (normal, 2.5–8.5 mg/dL); calcium 8.7 mg/dL (normal 8.3–10.6 mg/dL); albumin 4.0 (normal, 3.3–4.9 g/dL); cholesterol 255 mg/dL (normal, <200 mg/dL); creatine kinase 78 U/L (normal, <18–198 U/L); Na 132 mEq/L (normal, 132–147); K 3.3 mEq/L (normal, 3.4–5.0); HCO_3 22.6 mEq/mL (normal, 17.0–30.6 mEq/L); Cl, 109 mEq/L (normal, 95–105); Mg 1.7 mg/dL (normal, 1.5–3.1 mg/dL), GGT 30 U/L (normal, 10–61 U/L).

DISULFIRAM

Disulfiram is an irreversible acetaldehyde dehydrogenase inhibitor that blocks alcohol metabolism leading to an accumulation of acetaldehyde. Disulfiram reinforces an individual's desire to stop drinking by providing a disincentive associated with increased acetaldehyde levels, resulting in headache, palpitations, hypotension, flushing, nausea, and vomiting when patients consume alcohol. Although results from clinical trials are inconsistent, some consensus has developed that oral disulfiram reduces the number of drinking days.[115] Supervision of disulfiram administration leads to better outcomes, although not always in the order of a statistically significant effect.[116]

The primary predictor of success with disulfiram is the patient's commitment to total abstinence from alcohol. Although anecdotal reports of success are common, clinical evidence suggests disulfiram appears to be most effective for alcoholics who are involved in special high-risk situations (e.g. weddings, graduations) and particularly when administration is supervised.[115]

Evidence

Controlled clinical trials of disulfiram have failed to demonstrate consistently a therapeutic benefit.[115] Double-blind,

Table 84-9 Recently Completed or Major Ongoing Drug Trials for Alcoholism

Drug	*Pros*	*Cons*	*Comments*
Sertraline 200 mg/day	Selectively targeting LOA subtypes	Most likely little treatment benefit for EOA subtype	$N = 160$; 80 EOA and LOA; results not yet reported
Topiramate[183] 300 mg (maximal dose)	Potentially mimics actions of alcohol without the reinforcement	Not tested in recently abstinent alcoholics; optimal dose unknown	$N = 368$; 14 weeks 6-week titration, 8 week maintenance and 7–16-day taper. Compared with placebo, topiramate significantly lowered % heavy drinking days ($p = 0.002$), drinks/drinking days ($p = 0.006$) and % of days abstinent ($p = 0.002$).
Ondansetron 4 mcg/kg twice a day	Treatment matching in EOA based on SERT may result; nominal side effects	Most likely little treatment benefit for LOA subtype	$N = 320$ 160 with LL 5-HTTLPR and 160 with the SS/SL SERT. Results not yet reported.
Ondansetron 4 mcg/kg twice a day and Topiramate 300 mg (maximal dose)	The combination of ondansetron and topiramate may be additive among EOA	Ondansetron dosing by weight does not easily translate to clinical practice	$N = 360$ 12 weeks; project ends 8/31/09
Aripiprazole[206] 30 mg (maximal dose)	Multiple mechanisms of action	No preclinical or clinical data; not tested in actively drinking alcoholics; optimal dose unknown	$N = 266$ 12 weeks; Also received weekly psychotherapy. Discontinuations (40.3% vs. 26.7%) and treatment-related adverse events (82.8% vs. 63.6%) were higher with aripiprazole than placebo. No significant difference compared with placebo in % days abstinent ($p = 0.227$),% subjects without a heavy drinking day or time to first drinking day. The aripiprazole group had fewer drinks per drinking day ($p < 0.001$).
Naltrexone injection[176] 190 mg or 380 mg	Increased adherence	Pain management	6 months; 380 mg of long-acting naltrexone (n = 205) or 190 mg of long-acting naltrexone (n = 210) or a matching volume of placebo (n = 209) each administered monthly and combined with 12 sessions of low-intensity psychosocial intervention. Compared with placebo, 380 mg of long-acting naltrexone resulted in a 25% decrease in the event rate of heavy drinking days ($p = 0.02$) and 190 mg of naltrexone resulted in a 17% decrease ($p = 0.07$). Sex and pretreatment abstinence each showed significant interaction with the medication group on treatment outcome, with men and those with lead-in abstinence both exhibiting greater treatment effects.
Naltrexone and Acamprosate[144] 100 mg and 3 g (maximal doses)	Targeting positive and negative reinforcement	Not tested in actively drinking alcoholics	$N = 1{,}383$ 16 weeks; patients receiving medical management with naltrexone, CBI, or both fared better on drinking outcomes, whereas acamprosate showed no evidence of efficacy, with or without CBI. No combination produced better efficacy than naltrexone or CBI alone in the presence of medical management. Placebo pills and meeting with a health care professional had a positive effect above that of CBI during treatment.
SR141716, Rimonabant	Unique mechanism of action; potentially useful for nicotine cessation and weight loss	Little research on drugs that block the endocannabinoid system (i.e., potential side effects)	$N = 40$ laboratory study of non–treatment-seeking volunteers using cannabinoid-1 antagonist
Naltrexone and Sertraline	Combination may yield better abstinence rates	Both drugs have gastrointestinal side effects	$N = 198$ Alaskan Native Americans; results not yet reported.
Gabapentin as an adjunct to Naltrexone for alcoholism	Practical application to clinical practice.		Examine if alcoholics receiving naltrexone and adjunctive gabapentin will have less relapse than those treated with naltrexone alone. Project ends 8/31/07.

CBI, combined behavioral intervention EOA, early-onset alcoholism; 5-HTTLPR, serotonin transporter polymorphism, LL, long-long 5-HTTLPR alleles; LOA, late-onset alcoholism; SS/SL, short-short 5-HTTLPR alleles/short-long 5-HTTLPR alleles.

placebo-controlled studies using disulfiram are difficult because the psychological deterrent to use is experienced by both treatment groups and those who relapse will be unblinded when they experience the pharmacologic interaction.

In the most rigorous clinical trial conducted in a population of veterans, no significant difference in abstinence rates was demonstrated between patients taking placebo, 1 mg or 250 mg of disulfiram.[117] Patients randomized to receive 250 mg of disulfiram daily drank less frequently (significantly fewer drinking days per year), however. Patients who were middle-aged and had social stability were more likely to benefit from disulfiram. In another trial in which administration was supervised, patients receiving disulfiram drank less alcohol and less frequently; however on randomization, patients were unblinded to their drug.[118]

The efficacy of disulfiram compared with other drugs such as naltrexone is poorly studied.[119] Although no advantage was seen for combining disulfiram with naltrexone in dually diagnosed alcohol-dependent patients,[120] in one study, disulfiram combined with acamprosate resulted in increased days of cumulative abstinence.[121]

Dosing

The recommended starting dose of disulfiram is 250 mg once daily, with a range of 125 to 500 mg/day.[120] If a patient drinks and does not experience a disulfiram-ethanol reaction, the dose can be increased to 500 mg, as a significant proportion of patients may not experience a disulfiram-alcohol reaction at the usual 250 mg daily dose.[122,123] Side effects are increased, however, at doses >250 mg. Dosing starts at least 12 to 24 hours after abstinence initiation (when the blood or breath alcohol concentration is zero). Treatment continues, depending on the particular needs of the individual, but is generally at least 90 days and maintenance therapy may be required for years.

Contraindications, Warnings, and Interactions

Because of the intense cardiovascular and physical changes that occur in the disulfiram–ethanol interaction, disulfiram is contraindicated in patients with cardiac disease, coronary occlusion, cerebrovascular disease, and renal or hepatic failure. At somewhat higher doses, psychotic reactions have occurred. Many clinicians avoid disulfiram use in elderly patients or in those with any significant medical illness (e.g., diabetes). It is not definitive that disulfiram causes fetal abnormalities when administered during pregnancy,[124] but some data are found regarding limb reduction anomalies in infants born to disulfiram-treated mothers taking disulfiram during the first trimester of pregnancy.[125] As a result, disulfiram should only be used during pregnancy if the expected benefit to the mother and fetus is greater than the possible risk to the fetus; however, it should be avoided in the first trimester (category C). No information is available about the safety of this medicine during breastfeeding.

Disulfiram can also be hepatotoxic and should be used cautiously in patients with liver disease. Liver function should be established at baseline and after 14 days of treatment and a complete blood count (CBC) and liver function tests (LFT) should be obtained every 6 months.[126]

R.M. has normal hepatic function; however, LFT should be monitored at baseline and periodically during treatment. Although not all clinicians agree, most would recommend—at minimum—baseline LFT: ALT, AST, GGT and withholding disulfiram when LFT are more than three times upper limits of normal.[126] If elevated, repeat LFT every 1 to 2 weeks until normal, and then every 3 to 6 months if no elevations, with an awareness that increased LFT results may signal return to drinking rather than disulfiram toxicity.[127,128] Persistently elevated LFT may also indicate viral hepatitis (B or C), for which alcoholics have a higher risk, and thus the need to order a hepatitis profile. Currently no specific guidelines exist to determine whether a patient with elevated LFT should or should not receive treatment for alcoholism. Many clinicians anecdotally feel that as long as a patient's hepatic function is closely monitored, a reduction in alcohol use will lead to more normalized LFT. Wide ranges of psychiatric adverse effects include disorientation, agitation, depression, and behavioral changes such as paranoia, withdrawal and bizarre behaviors, and worsening of schizophrenia, especially at doses >250 mg daily.[129–130] Disulfiram should be avoided or used very cautiously in persons with these conditions. Disulfiram can be used relatively safely at a dose of 250 mg daily in alcohol-dependent patients with co-occurring psychiatric disorders, including schizophrenia.[120,131,132]

Disulfiram is a potent inhibitor of the CYP2E1 oxidase, and can interact with anticoagulants (warfarin), antiepileptics (phenytoin, carbamazepine), some benzodiazepines (e.g., diazepam but not lorazepam), and tricyclic antidepressants (amitriptyline, desipramine), potentially increasing the toxicity of these medications. Delirium can result in combination with monoamine oxidase inhibitors. Other important interactions can occur with metronidazole and omeprazole.[133]

Patient Education

To receive optimal results with disulfiram, patients must receive regular counselling and be closely monitored for any changes in hepatic function. Patients should be advised that the involvement of significant others will facilitate their recovery. Having someone participate in helping to validate the administration process is known to lead to better outcomes. Discontinuation of disulfiram should occur only after consultation with the prescriber and counsellor involved. Common side effects of disulfiram include drowsiness, particularly in the first few weeks of treatment, a metallic or garlic taste, and sexual dysfunction. The dose can be taken at bedtime if drowsiness or tiredness occurs.

Patients must stop the medication for at least 3 days (up to 14 days in some) before being exposed to products containing alcohol. What cannot be overlooked is that patients taking disulfiram must be informed about the dangers of consuming even small amounts of alcohol in foods, in over-the-counter medications, in mouthwashes, and in use of topical lotions. Also, it is important to verify that the patients understand the necessary precautions and the consequences of alcohol use. The patient should call the prescriber to report any respiratory difficulty, nausea, vomiting, decreased appetite, dark colored urine, or a change in pigmentation in the skin or eyes (primarily yellowing).

Summary

Generally, given the special circumstances needed for success, disulfiram is generally not the drug of choice for treating alcoholism. The social, medical, and psychiatric status of a candidate is an important consideration in the use of disulfiram. Conditions that R.M. would appear to possess that may enhance the effectiveness of disulfiram include an agreement by R.M. to have his medication administration supervised (in this case by his wife), a steady job, and his high level of motivation to sustain abstinence. R.M. should also receive counselling and support services on a regular basis.

12. T.M. is a 60-year-old woman who weighs 105 pounds, is 63 inches tall, and is actively drinking about 40–50 drinks a week. Her CIWA-Ar score is 8. T.M. wants a medication that will gradually reduce her alcohol use over time so that she can drink socially with friends. T.M. has heard of acamprosate and asked for some samples but she was refused. Why was she not a good candidate? Total bilirubin 0.8 mg/dL (normal, 0.2–1.2 mg/dL); direct bilirubin 0.2 (normal, 0–0.4 mg/dL); alkaline phosphatase 80 (normal, 35–131 U/L); AST 30 (normal, 11–36 U/L); ALT 23 (normal, 6–43 U/L); BUN 20 mg/dL (normal, 5–22 mg/dL); creatinine 1.2 mg/dL (normal, 0.6–1.3 mg/dL); glucose 91 mg/dL (normal, 70–110 mg/dL); uric acid 3.3 mg/dL (normal, 2.5–8.5 mg/dL); calcium 8.9 mg/dL (normal, 8.3–10.6 mg/dL); albumin 4.5 (normal, 3.3–4.9 g/dL); cholesterol 195 mg/dL (normal, <200 mg/dL); creatine kinase 190 U/L (normal <18–198 U/L); Na 143 mEq/L (normal, 132–147); K 4.2 mEq/L (normal, 3.4–5.0); HCO_3 25.2 (normal, 17.0–30.6 mEq/L); Cl 110 mEq/L (normal, 95–105); BUN 14 mg/dL (normal, 5–22); magnesium 1.9 mg/dL, (normal, 1.5–3.1 mg/dL).

ACAMPROSATE

Acamprosate (Campral) has multiple actions, but is principally a glutamate and GABA modulator. In vitro and in vivo studies in animals suggest that acamprosate interacts with GABA and glutamate to restore the imbalance of neuronal excitation[134] and inhibition[135] caused by chronic alcohol use. The key mechanism of action is considered to be as a weak functional antagonist of the glutamate NMDA receptor possibly mediated through indirect modulation of the receptor site via antagonism at the mGluR5 receptor.[136] A series of meta-analyses and systematic reviews demonstrated that when used as an adjunct to psychosocial interventions, acamprosate improves drinking outcomes such as the length and rate of abstinence.[115,137–139] This effect is doubtful if acamprosate is not initiated quickly after a detoxification.[140,141] Evidence indicates that the effect of acamprosate on abstinence rate lasts after the treatment is stopped.[142] The success of acamprosate, however, seems limited to European trials as recent U.S. trials failed to demonstrate significant results on primary outcome measures.[143,144]

Acamprosate appears to be especially useful in a therapeutic regimen targeted at promoting abstinence and can be used in primary care settings as well as specialized addiction treatment programs.[145] Acamprosate has been studied in thousands of patients, primarily in Europe, and few contraindications to treatment exist. Little consistent information is found about patient characteristics that predict improvement while taking acamprosate. In a meta-analysis of all U.S. and European studies, predictors of abstinence were motivation, readiness to change, baseline abstinence, initial first week compliance, and living with a partner or child.[146] A pooled analysis of seven European trials, however, found no significant predictors of the abstinence outcome measures.[147] Candidates for acamprosate should be committed to abstinence and begin the medication after being abstinent from alcohol.[148,149]

Evidence

In a systematic review of the efficacy data related to acamprosate,[148] proof for efficacy of acamprosate was strong. Moreover, several acamprosate studies have reported positive results. For example, in a study of 272 severely dependent alcoholics, patients receiving acamprosate showed a significantly higher continuous abstinence rate within the first 2 months of treatment compared with patients receiving placebo.[150] Of acamprosate treated patients, 40% were continuously abstinent over a 48-week period compared with 17% of those who received placebo.

Acamprosate has also been studied for periods of up to a year. In a long-term follow-up (12 months) after trial completion, acamprosate still maintained an effect on abstinence rates, but not on nondrinking days.[151] Some studies have found limited to no efficacy,[143,144,152–154] although two of the studies may have been underpowered.[153,154] One of these studies also had a short treatment period,[154] and the other had a long delay in initiating treatment.[152] In summary, most studies suggest that acamprosate is a safe and well tolerated drug for the promotion of alcohol abstinence.

Dose

Acamprosate is dispensed in 333 mg tablets and the usual dose is 666 mg/day three times daily.[155] Patients can be started on the full dose without titration. Acamprosate is not well absorbed from the GI tract and it takes several days to achieve desired blood levels of the medication. The medication appears to be safe and effective in alcoholics, with minimal side effects. It does not appear to produce sedation and does not cause drug dependence. Main adverse effects of acamprosate appear to be GI, including nausea, diarrhea, and bloating. Nausea or diarrhea can be usually managed with bismuth compounds, but if symptoms are severe or persistent, the dose should be reduced by one-third to one-half. Acamprosate has been used in trials for a year, but the duration of therapy depends on treatment success and the willingness of the patient to continue therapy indefinitely.

Contraindications, Warnings, and Interactions

Acamprosate should not be used in patients with impaired kidney function (CrCl <30 mL/minute), nor in patients who previously exhibited hypersensitivity to acamprosate. The dose should be 333 mg three times daily in patients with a CrCl between 30 and 50 mL/minute. Acamprosate should only be used during pregnancy when the benefit clearly outweighs the risk as the drug has been shown to be teratogenic (category C) in rats.[155] Tetracyclines may be inactivated by the calcium component in acamprosate during concurrent administration.[156] Naltrexone increases plasma levels of acamprosate, although the clinical significance of this interaction is unknown.[157,158] Suicidal ideation, and attempted and completed suicides have occurred in patients taking acamprosate. Depression or suicidal ideation must be monitored.

Patient Education

Acamprosate must be used in combination with a psychosocial program such as combined behavioral intervention (CBI) or regular Alcoholics Anonymous (AA) meetings. Acamprosate may be taken without regard to meals. The tablets should not be crushed and should be taken whole. Although no interaction with alcohol occurs, abstinence in combination with counseling and social support are required to attain optimal treatment. Patients should report persistent diarrhea, sudden or excessive weight gain, swelling of the extremities, respiratory difficulties, fainting, or thoughts of suicide.

Summary

Acamprosate was approved by the FDA for the maintenance of abstinence in alcohol-dependent individuals who are abstinent at treatment initiation. Despite a strong showing in many European trials, less favorable results compared with naltrexone were seen in recent U.S. studies, perhaps making acamprosate a good choice for heavily dependent patients coming out of detoxification with verifiable abstinence before starting the drug. Given that T.M. is not abstinent, and wishes to continue drinking socially, the evidence would suggest that she is not a good candidate for acamprosate.

13. T.M. is vacillating over whether or not she wants to continue drinking or not. T.M. is willing to attend weekly counseling sessions. T.M. has never taken a medication for alcoholism and now states that she is willing to stop drinking. Her primary care provider is considering naltrexone. Does the evidence support this choice, and what should be considered before choosing between the oral tablets or the monthly injection in this patient?

NALTREXONE

Naltrexone blocks the action of endorphins when alcohol is consumed, and this results in an attenuation of dopamine release at the nucleus accumbens thought to be crucially important to positive reinforcement, reward, and craving.[60] Although naltrexone therapy has been recommended for all alcohol-dependent patients who do not have a medical contraindication to its use, a survey of 1,388 U.S. physicians specializing in addiction reported that they prescribed naltrexone to an average of only 13% of their patients.[159] The main self-reported reasons why physicians did not prescribe naltrexone to more patients were that patients refused to take the medication or comply with prescribing regimens (23%), and that patients could not afford the medication (21%).

Evidence seems to support the use of naltrexone as an adjunct to psychosocial interventions[122,139,145,160] with higher abstinence rates in short-term treatment[161] and as a deterrent to progressing from a lapse to a full-blown relapse.[115] Naltrexone is as efficacious as disulfiram and probably more efficacious than acamprosate.[144,161–162] The addition of acamprosate to naltrexone does not enhance outcome.[144,163]

Several studies indicate that naltrexone is most effective in patients with strong craving,[164,165] poor cognitive status at study entry,[166] and high compliance.[167,168] This observation is consistent with the demonstrated effect of naltrexone in reducing craving. Evidence also indicates that persons with a family history for alcoholism, early age at onset of drinking, and comorbid use of other drugs are more likely to benefit from naltrexone.[169]

Evidence

A comprehensive review of pharmacotherapies for alcoholism concluded that naltrexone oral (ReVia) produced a consistent decrease in relapse rate to heavy drinking and in drinking frequency, although it did not enhance absolute abstinence rates.[149] More specifically, several studies using naltrexone report the opiate antagonist to be more effective than placebo in reducing relapse rates, in increasing a percent of nondrinking days,[164,167,170] and in reducing craving in heavy drinkers.[171] Yet other studies fail to demonstrate a significant difference with placebo.[172,173] Several factors may explain the discrepancies in results of the different clinical trials with naltrexone. Many of the studies included small sample sizes and may lack the statistical power to demonstrate treatment effects.[162] Several large sufficiently powered studies also reported negative results.[172–174] Nonetheless, the COMBINE trial[144] clearly supports the effectiveness of naltrexone in that each of the groups of patients receiving naltrexone in conjunction with medical management had a higher percentage of days abstinent than those receiving placebo plus medical management without naltrexone or CBI. Naltrexone also reduced the risk of heavy drinking.

Naltrexone injection (Vivitrol), was approved by the FDA and released in June 2006. Injectable naltrexone is safe and well tolerated in alcohol-dependent individuals.[175] In two double-blind, randomized, placebo-controlled trials, the efficacy of once monthly long-acting injectable or depot forms of naltrexone was demonstrated,[176,177] which suggests the advantage of increased compliance. Garbutt et al.[176] found men receiving naltrexone injection had significantly better treatment outcomes than women, and women who received nattrexone demonstrated no difference with those who received placebo. Additionally, because a robust effect was seen for natrexone injection compared with placebo for people coming into the study abstinent, the FDA required the manufacturer to place a requirement for abstinence when starting the medication on its product information.

Dose

Naltrexone has been approved for use in the first 90 days of abstinence when the risk of relapse is highest. It has also been shown to be safe and well tolerated by patients for periods of up to a year. Treatment with naltrexone should continue based on the response to the medication. Discontinuation should only be considered in consultation with the health care provider. The usual dose of naltrexone is 50 mg daily, although doses of 25 mg to 100 mg daily have been reported to be effective, particularly in those with lower blood concentrations of the drug.[178] Side effects, such as nausea or headache, are more common in the initial few days of therapy. Starting with a 25-mg dose (half a tablet) for the first two to four daily doses may reduce the incidence of side effects. Anecdotally, some practitioners suggest that because of its long half-life, naltrexone may also be administered three times weekly in doses of 100 mg on Mondays, 100 mg on Wednesdays, and 150 mg on Fridays (or the equivalent of 50 mg daily). This method may facilitate supervised or observed administration of naltrexone, because only three (versus seven) observations are required per week.

The injection (380 mg) should be administered by deep IM injection into a gluteal muscle, alternating buttocks each injection. No dose adjustment is required for mild or moderate renal or hepatic impairment, but naltrexone has not been studied in severe renal or hepatic impairment.

Contraindications, Warnings, Interactions

Naltrexone is contraindicated in patients with a history of sensitivity to naltrexone with acute hepatitis or liver failure; in those who are physically dependent on opiates, receiving opiate analgesics, or in acute opiate withdrawal. The benefit of using naltrexone during pregnancy should clearly outweigh the risk. The concurrent administration of naltrexone and opiate analgesics is contraindicated. To avoid triggering an acute abstinence syndrome, patients must be opiate free for a minimum of 7 to 14 days before initiating treatment with naltrexone, as substantiated with a urine drug test. Although rarely performed, a naloxone challenge test can be utilized before treatment with naltrexone to rule out concurrent use of opiates. Naltrexone is in the FDA pregnancy category C and it is unknown whether naltrexone passes into breast milk.

Naltrexone injection must be mixed and administered immediately. A special diluent is supplied in the carton and must be administered with the needle supplied with it in the carton. If there is a short delay (e.g., a few minutes) after suspension but before transfer into the syringe, the vial should be inverted a few times to resuspend the product and then transferred into the syringe for immediate use. Substitution of any of the supplied components is not recommended. If the milky white suspension clogs the needle during administration, the needle should be withdrawn from the patient, capped with the attached safety device, and replaced with the spare administration needle provided. The plunger should be gently pushed until a bead of the suspension appears at the tip of the needle. The remainder of the suspension can then be administered into an adjacent site, but in the same gluteal region. Should a patient miss a does, the patient should be instructed to return as soon as possible to receive the next dose; however, no data exist regarding restarting treatment in patients who have missed appointments or discontinued their treatment.

A possible clinical concern with naltrexone tablets or long-acting injectable naltrexone is pain management. Any attempt to overcome the opiate blockade produced by naltrexone using exogenous opioids may result in fatal overdose. Should a patient be in pain after receiving an injection, the first drug of choice should be a nonopiate, such as a nonsteroidal anti-inflammatory drug (NSAID). If the patient is still in pain, an opiate can be used but it will most likely have to be administered in a higher dose and more frequently. When reversal of naltrexone blockade is required for pain management, patients should be monitored in a setting equipped and staffed for cardiopulmonary resuscitation and monitored for signs of respiratory depression.

Patient Education

Naltrexone tablets have been demonstrated to be more effective when used in combination with cognitive behavioral therapy (CBT) or psychosocial therapy. Therefore, to obtain the optimal long-term benefit, the patient must plan on meeting with a counselor and enroll in a behavior modification or support group program such as AA that supports their abstinence. Patients should be reminded not to use opiates or any medications not approved by the prescriber during treatment. Patients receiving naltrexone must be opiate free from 7 to 10 days as substantiated with a urine drug test and should be asked to wear some kind of identifier for medical emergencies. Particularly with naltrexone injection, documentation to alert medical personnel of naltrexone treatment is needed in case of trauma necessitating pain management.

Alert patients that naltrexone can cause nausea, headache, drowsiness, dizziness, or blurred vision. In a year-long safety study, the most common side effects were nausea, headache, anxiety, and sedation.[178] Should such side effects occur, reducing the dosage by one-half often reduces the side effects. Large doses of naltrexone can cause liver failure. Patients should report excessive tiredness, unusual bleeding or bruising, loss of appetite, pain in the upper right part of the stomach, any discoloration of the skin or eyes, a change in stool color or urine, thoughts of suicide, or signs of pneumonia.

An important consumer consideration to note is that, as of this writing, naltrexone injection costs about $800 a month compared with <$150 a month for a month supply of 50-mg tablets. Because the injection is new, some insurance plans might not pay for it, or it may be available on formulary but at a higher co-pay rate to the patient. This cost may represent a significant barrier to affordable treatment for many patients.

Summary

Naltrexone, CBT or a support group would appropriate for T.M. Current evidence suggests, however, that tablets rather than injection would be the most appropriate choice for T.M. Primary concerns would be poor hepatic function (which is normal) or previous failure with the medication. The primary consideration in this case is that no significant difference has been seen in drinking outcomes in women who received naltrexone or placebo injections.[176] While this perhaps anomalous result is still being investigated, sufficient support exists to prescribe naltrexone tablets in this patient. On the other hand, although everyone received a 1-hour low-intensity psychosocial intervention every other week, women compared with men in the control group reduced their alcohol use more than did men, suggesting that using a psychosocial approach such as CBT (Table 84-7) would benefit T.M.

14. T.M. reduces her alcohol use substantially, but is still drinking. Is there any advantage to the combination therapy of acamprosate with naltrexone?

The rationale for combining the drugs is that acamprosate reduces negative reinforcement and naltrexone attenuates positive reinforcement.[60] To test this hypothesis, a randomized, controlled study of 160 patients performed in Europe demonstrated that, although combining naltrexone and acamprosate was more effective than either placebo or acamprosate alone, adding acamprosate was not significantly more effective than naltrexone alone.[163] In a much larger study, the COMBINE trial randomized >1,300 individuals in a double-blind fashion to receive placebo, naltrexone, or acamprosate alone or in combination with medical management or combined behavioral therapy.[144] Results from this study suggest that acamprosate has no significant effect on drinking versus placebo, either by itself or with any combination of the other treatments in the study. Furthermore, patients receiving placebo and medical management (MM) from a health care professional (Table 84-7) had better outcomes than patients receiving CBI (a CBT-like therapy that includes 12-step facilitation) alone. Based on the available evidence, it would not be reasonable to combine acamprosate with naltrexone.

OTHER DRUG THERAPY

15. W.W. is a 48-year-old male executive, who weights 230 pounds and is 73 inches tall. He comes for help with his alcohol use, which he recognizes is out of control. He has previously tried disulfiram, naltrexone, and acamprosate and does not want the naltrexone injection. Currently, W.W. is drinking 55 drinks a week. His CIWA score is 9 (although he does not appear to need inpatient detoxification). His laboratory work reveals the following: Total bilirubin 0.4 mg/dL (normal, 0.2–1.2 mg/dL); direct bilirubin <1 (normal, 0–0.4 mg/dL); alkaline phosphatase 74 (normal, 35–131 U/L); AST 70 (normal, 11–36 U/L); ALT 89 (normal, 6–43 U/L); BUN 14 mg/dL (normal, 5–22 mg/dL); creatinine 1.1 mg/dL (normal, 0.6–1.3 mg/dL); glucose 151 mg/dL (normal, 70–110 mg/dL); uric acid 5.8 mg/dL (normal, 2.5–8.5 mg/dL); calcium 10.0 mg/dL (normal, 8.3–10.6 mg/dL); albumin 3.6 (normal, 3.3–4.9 g/dL); cholesterol 189 mg/dL (normal, <200 mg/dL); creatine kinase 90 U/L (normal, <18–198 U/L); Na 134 mEq/L (normal, 132–147); K 4.5 mEq/L (normal, 3.4–5.0); HCO_3 29.2 (normal, 17.0–30.6 mEq/L); Cl 97 mEq/L (normal, 95–105); magnesium 2.3 mg/dL, (normal, 1.5–3.1 mg/dL). What other medications might be considered?

Topiramate

Topiramate is an FDA-approved medication found to have multiple mechanisms of action, including enhanced $GABA_A$ inhibition that results in decreased dopamine facilitation in the midbrain thought to be of potential benefit in the treatment of addiction.[179] Additionally, there is antagonism of kainate to activate the kainate/AMPA glutamate receptor subtypes[180] and inhibition of type II and IV carbonic anhydrase isoenzymes.

Evidence

Topiramate is not FDA-approved for the treatment of alcoholism. Because the drug is coming off patent soon, it is unlikely the manufacturer will pursue an indication for topiramate in the treatment of alcohol dependence. Johnson et al.,[181] in a randomized, double-blind, placebo-controlled trial used an escalating dose from 25 to 300 mg/day of topiramate or matching placebo in 150 men and women non–treatment-seeking alcoholics during the first 8 weeks of a 12-week period. Patients stayed at the same dose over the last 4 weeks of the study. All patients in the study received brief behavioral compliance enhancement therapy (BBCET) that was a 10- to 15-minute meeting with a health care professional (i.e., a pharmacist, nurse, nurse practitioner, physician, or physician assistant) that focused on resolving side effect issues and facilitated adherence (Table 84-7). Participants receiving topiramate reported significantly fewer drinks per day and drinks per drinking day, significantly fewer drinking days, significantly more days of abstinence, and significantly less craving than those on placebo. The evidence suggests that, although abstinence was not a goal at the start of the topiramate study, the medication may be more beneficial during the abstinence initiation phase of treatment.[182] In a recently completed phase II clinical trial, the use of topiramate for alcohol dependence treatment was confirmed by outcomes demonstrating that topiramate recipients showed a significantly greater lowering of percentage of heavy drinking days (mean difference, 8.4% [95% CI, 3.1–13.8], $p = 0.002$), drinks per drinking day (mean difference, 0.9 [95% CI, 0.3–1.5], $p = 0.006$), and a higher percentage of days abstinent (mean difference, −7.7% [95% CI, −12.5–2.9], $p = 0.002$). Using a repeated-measures mixed model, topiramate showed even greater efficacy over placebo ($p<0.001$) for all comparisons.[183]

In the treatment of alcohol dependence, topiramate is titrated from 25 mg/day up to 300 mg/day over 6 weeks (100 mg in the morning; 200 mg in the afternoon) or to the patient's maximal tolerable dose. Abrupt discontinuation of topiramate has been associated with seizures in patients without a history of seizures and, for this reason, gradual withdrawal of the drug (e.g., a 25% decrease in the dosage every 4 days over 16 days) is recommended.

16. W.W. also reports >2 week period of feeling worthless, suicidal ideation, a 29-pound. weight loss over the last 6 weeks, hypersomnia, and lethargy. These symptoms have alternated with short periods (e.g., ~4 days) of feeling exhilarated, expansiveness, compulsive buying sprees, hyposomnia, and arguments with friends and coworkers. He does not report any psychotic episodes. How should patients with underlying psychiatric and alcohol use disorders be approached?

W.W. reports symptoms that appear consistent with bipolar II disorder (ruling out any other diagnosis) that would include a formal differential diagnosis of major depressive disorder and hypomania without psychosis. Clinicians must consider the potential for dual diagnosis disorders (e.g., depression, bipolar disorder, or schizophrenia) combined with substance dependence (e.g., as with alcohol). Tobacco and caffeine dependence are common. A significant number of individuals with mental health disorders also have an alcohol use disorders compared with the general population.[184] Increased comorbid conditions also lead to a poorer treatment prognosis.

Principles for the optimal treatment of patients with a dual diagnosis include the following: (a) Flexibility (e.g., while the goal of treatment may be abstinence, for some patents movement in the right direction is just as important to keep the person engaged in treatment). (b) Repetition (e.g., a constant refocusing of attention for avoiding alcohol and for confronting their psychiatric symptoms is a priority. (c) Counseling (e.g., matching patients to the appropriate intervention). These factors are all fundamental to long-lasting treatment success. Medications, when appropriate (e.g., early and vigorous drug intervention with nonaddictive medications) may also help the patient stay in treatment; however, every effort must be made to use medications that do not induce euphoria, cause dependence, and are effective and safe even during relapse.

Clinicians must distinguish between drug-induced and drug-related psychiatric disorders. Ideally, but often impractical, is to permit 3 to 4 weeks of abstinence to provide adequate information to determine the relationship off the alcohol use disorder with the psychiatric disorder. A complete drug use history, urinalysis, and blood or hair drug tests should be obtained. A comprehensive history, including age of onset of disorders, persistence of psychiatric illness during abstinence, and very importantly, family history, should provide adequate diagnostic information.

Patients with both drug use and psychiatric disorders constitute a substantial and challenging subpopulation. Treating the alcohol use disorder alone predicts a poorer outcome for other disorders including early relapse. Early and aggressive treatment for each condition should be implemented. Furthermore, care must be taken to ensure that the medications prescribed are safe if combined with alcohol.

A few studies have evaluated the effectiveness of mood stabilizers (e.g., lithium, carbamazepine, divalproex, atypical antipsychotics, and topiramate) in the treatment of comorbid bipolar disorder and alcohol dependence.[185,186] Some evidence suggests that topiramate may be helpful during the depressive phase of bipolar disorder[186] perhaps as a result of reducing alcohol use.[187] Clinicians should monitor weight loss,[188] worsening depression, and suicidal ideation in patients using topiramate.[189]

17. Over an 8-week period, W.W. is taking 300 mg of topiramate a day and is only drinking 10 drinks a week. W.W. complains that he is experiencing pins and needles in his arms and hands. Is this related to symptoms of withdrawal or to topiramate?

It is likely that tingling in the extremities, called paresthesias, is a possible result of withdrawal from alcohol, the more probable reason for this occurrence (given the temporal relationship) is as a side effect of topiramate therapy. In addition to paresthesias, other prominent side effects include mental confusion, slowness in thinking, depression, and somnolence, which may be attenuated by titration when initiating therapy, and the development of renal calculi in about 1.5% of patients.[189] Adequate hydration is encouraged, particularly in patients who may be at risk for developing calculi.

Contraindications, Warnings, Interactions

Topiramate is contraindicated in those hypersensitive to the drug. Topiramate should be used with caution in those who have a history of urolithiasis, paresthesias, secondary angle closure glaucoma, renal or hepatic impairment, and conditions or therapies that predispose to acidosis (e.g., renal disease, severe respiratory disorders, status epilepticus, diarrhea, surgery, ketogenic diet, or drugs). Monitoring for hyperchloremic non–ionic-gap metabolic acidosis is essential, and, therefore, baseline chemistry (e.g., HCO_3 and pH) should be assessed and monitored regularly thereafter. Metabolic acidosis can cause symptoms such as tiredness and loss of appetite, or more serious conditions including arrhythmia or coma. Topiramate has been found to be teratogenic in animal studies and is a pregnancy category C medication.[189]

Concomitant use of oral contraceptives, phenytoin, carbamazepine, and valproic acid has been found to interact with topiramate.[190] Coadministration of another carbonic anhydrase inhibitor, such as acetazolamide, may increase the possibility of renal stone formation and should be avoided.

Patient Education

Patients should be advised not to adjust the dose or discontinue the medication without consulting a health care provider. Unless otherwise instructed, to prevent kidney stones and dehydration, patients should maintain adequate hydration and be advised to drink 2 to 3 L/day of fluid. Patients may be at risk for decreased sweating and increased body temperature and should therefore monitor their exercise, particularly in hot weather. Topiramate can cause drowsiness, dizziness, changes in memory, a change in taste (particularly with carbonated beverages), vision changes (particularly associated with increased intraocular pressure), and pressure to the touch, loss of appetite or unplanned weight loss, and sudden changes in mood.

Summary

Evidence for the effectiveness of topiramate is promising, although more clinical research is needed on topiramate in efficacy and effectiveness trials, as well as determining the proper dose. Although W.W. has some liver impairment (AST and ALT twice the normal limit), some evidence supports the use of valproate as a good choice to treat the diagnosis of bipolar disorder and AUD in this particular patient[191]; drug levels must be monitored, however, because valproate is entirely metabolized by the liver. Topiramate, on the other hand, is renally metabolized and might be considered an adjunctive therapy if W.W. does not completely respond to the drug of first choice.

Balcofen

Baclofen promotes a balance between inhibition of release of GABA, mediated by presynaptic $GABA_B$ receptors and inhibition of neuronal excitability mediated by postsynaptic $GABA_B$ receptors.[192] Putatively, agonism of $GABA_B$ receptors also modulates mesolimbic dopamine neurons.[193] Baclofen is approved for use in the United States to reduce cramping, spasms, and muscle tightness.

Efficacy

Baclofen has been promoted for investigation by the National Institute on Alcohol Abuse and Alcoholism (NIAAA) for alcohol dependence.[194] Studies show that baclofen is effective in reducing alcohol self-administration[195] and motivation to consume alcohol in rats.[196] In a double-blind, placebo-controlled trial using baclofen, alcohol-dependent patients reported less craving, drank on fewer days, and had higher rates of total abstinence than those receiving placebo.[197]

Summary

Because baclofen is metabolized by the kidneys, it would be an alternative adjunct to topiramate to treat the AUD diagnosis in W.W. The evidence for baclofen is limited and should only be considered an alternative if other approved drugs failed or W.W. was known to be allergic to topiramate.

DRUG INTERACTIONS

18. T.C. is a 32-year-old man who has been diagnosed with alcohol dependence and depression. He reports recent weight loss (20 pounds in the last month), excessive 'sluggishness,' an increased need for sleep (10–12 hours a day) and feelings of guilt and worthlessness. His depression is likely substance induced, but the importance of his alcohol use is largely ignored. T.C.'s primary care provider plans to start sustained-release bupropion for depression. Laboratory tests were performed at the visit but are not yet available. What should be considered when prescribing bupropion or any other medication to T.C. and what simple information should T.C. be given?

Prescription drug use and interactions with alcohol are fairly common with individuals diagnosed with alcohol abuse or dependence disorders. Alcohol–prescription drug interactions in patients diagnosed with AUD have been found to be as high as 40%, with more than 20% taking medications with moderate to severe alcohol interactions.[198] The interaction of alcohol with the cytochrome P450 enzyme system may be complex, and depends on duration of consumption. Notably, short-term consumption leads to a competitive inhibition of the CYP2E1, whereas chronic use leads to induction of this enzyme. CYP2E1 induction leads to increased clearance of such drugs as alcohol itself, warfarin, diazepam, rifamycin, meprobamate, pentobarbital, and propranolol, with the effect on liver metabolism lasting for days to weeks after discontinuation of alcohol. More importantly, the CYP2E1 enzyme system converts several substances into highly toxic metabolites. These include cocaine, enflurane and methoxyflurane, isoniazid, phenylbutazone, and acetaminophen. Through induction of this alternate pathway of drug metabolism, otherwise safe doses of drugs may become hepatotoxic. Carbamazepine is also known as a cytochrome P450 3A4 inducer, and can cause several problematic interactions on multiple medications.[198] Obviously, clinicians must consider the impact (e.g., on the liver) of prescribing drugs when patients are also abusing or dependent on alcohol.[199] (See Table 84-10 for more alcohol-drug interactions.)

Table 84-10 Ethanol Drug Interactions

Acetaminophen	Chronic excessive alcohol consumption increases susceptibility to acetaminophen-induced hepatotoxicity. Acute intoxication theoretically protects against acetaminophen toxicity because less hepatotoxic metabolite is generated.
Anticoagulants (oral)	Chronic ethanol consumption induces hepatic metabolism of warfarin, decreasing hypoprothrombinemic effect. Very large acute ethanol doses (>3 drinks/day) may impair the metabolism of warfarin and increase hypothrombinemic effect. Vitamin K-dependent clotting factors may be reduced in alcoholics with liver disease, also affecting coagulation.
Antidepressants	Enhanced sedative effects of alcohol and psychomotor impairment are possible. Acute ethanol impairs metabolism. Fluoxetine, paroxetine, fluvoxamine, and probably other serotonin reuptake inhibitors (SSRI) do not interfere with psychomotor or subjective effects of ethanol.
Ascorbic acid	Ascorbic acid increases ethanol clearance and serum triglyceride levels and improves motor coordination and color discrimination after ethanol consumption.
Barbiturates	Phenobarbital decreases blood ethanol concentration; acute intoxication inhibits pentobarbital metabolism; chronic intoxication enhances hepatic pentobarbital metabolism.
Benzodiazepines	Psychomotor impairment increased with the combination.
Bromocriptine	Ethanol increases gastrointestinal side effects of bromocriptine.
Caffeine	Caffeine has no effect on ethanol-induced psychomotor impairment.
Calcium channel blockers	Verapamil inhibits ethanol metabolism and increases intoxication.
Cephalosporin antibiotics	Ethanol produces flushing, nausea, headaches, tachycardia, and hypotension. Cephalosporin antibiotics that have an ethyltetrazolethiol side chain produce this disulfiramlike reaction (e.g., cefoperazone, cefamandole, cefotetan).
Chloral hydrate	Elevation of plasma trichloroethanol (a chloral hydrate metabolite) and blood ethanol. Combined central nervous system (CNS) depression. Vasodilation, tachycardia, headache.
Chloroform	Ethanol increases chloroform hepatotoxicity.
Doxycycline	Chronic consumption of ethanol induces hepatic metabolism of doxycycline and may lower serum concentration of the antibiotic.
Erythromycin	Ethanol may interfere with absorption of the ethylsuccinate salt. Effects on other formulations are unknown.
Furazolidone	When ethanol is ingested, nausea, flushing, lightheadedness, and dyspnea may occur (i.e., a disulfiramlike reaction).
H_2 antagonists	Cimetidine potentiates ethanol effects. Increases peak plasma ethanol concentrations and area under the plasma ethanol concentration time curve. CNS toxicity from increased cimetidine serum concentration. Nizatidine, and ranitidine may also increase blood alcohol levels slightly by inhibiting gastric alcohol dehydrogenase. Famotidine does not affect blood alcohol levels.
Isoniazid	Consumption of ethanol with isoniazid increases risk of hepatotoxicity. Tyramine-containing alcoholic beverages may cause hypertensive reaction.
Ketoconazole and metronidazole	When ethanol is ingested, nausea, flushing, lightheadedness, and dyspnea may occur (i.e., a disulfiramlike reaction may occur with metronidazole). A sunburnlike rash has been reported with ethanol consumption and ketoconazole. A similar reaction may occur with itraconazole, although no reports exist.
Meprobamate	Synergistic CNS depression.
Metoclopramide	Enhances sedative effects of ethanol.
Monoamine oxidase inhibitors	Tyramine-containing alcoholic beverages (e.g., wines, beer) may cause a hypertensive crisis. Pargyline may inhibit aldehyde dehydrogenase and cause a disulfiramlike interaction with ethanol.
Narcotic analgesics	Volume of distribution of intravenous meperidine increases with increasing ethanol consumption. Clinical significance unknown. Potential for enhanced CNS depression.
Oral hypoglycemic agents	Chlorpropamide, tolbutamide, and tolazamide may cause flushing, lightheadedness, nausea, and dyspnea if alcohol is ingested (i.e., a disulfiramlike reaction).
Paraldehyde	Possible metabolic acidosis.
Phenothiazines	Potentiates psychomotor effects of ethanol.
Quinacrine	Possible inhibits acetaldehyde oxidation.
Salicylates	Increases gastric bleeding associated with aspirin; may increase chance of gastrointestinal hemorrhage.
Tetrachloroethylene	Combined CNS depression.
Trichloroethylene	Flushing, lacrimation, blurred vision, tachypnea may occur when patients exposed to trichloroethylene drink alcohol.

Adapted from reference 190, with permission.

Summary

An alternative to bupropion should be considered particularly in light of the unavailability of T.C.'s laboratory test results. In this case, critical issues need to be considered, particularly hepatic function, which may be associated with an increased risk of seizures. Bupropion is extensively metabolized by the liver and should be used with extreme caution in patients with severe hepatic cirrhosis. In these patients, a reduced dose or frequency of administration is required, as peak plasma levels are substantially elevated, thereby increasing the risk of seizures. The dose should not exceed 150 mg every other day in patients with impaired hepatic function.[200] Additionally, patients should be told that the excessive use or abrupt discontinuation of alcohol may alter their seizure threshold and bupropion is therefore contraindicated in patients undergoing abrupt discontinuation of alcohol. Patients have also reported lower alcohol tolerance during treatment with bupropion. Patients, in general, should be advised that the consumption of alcohol should be minimized or avoided.[200] Moreover a recent study demonstrated that one-third of patients with AUD prescribed drugs were never advised not to take their prescribed medication with alcohol.[198] The study also reported that bupropion, serotonin reuptake inhibitors (SSRI) and acetaminophen were the drugs most frequently involved in drug-alcohol interactions.

REFERENCES

1. Heath DB ed. *International Handbook on Alcohol and Culture.* Westport, CT: Greenwood Press; 1995.
2. Bardon S. Brewed in America: A History of Beer and Ale in the United States. Boston: Little Brown; 1962.
3. Substance Abuse and Mental Health Services Administration. Results from the 2006 National Survey on Drug Use and Health: National Findings, Office of Applied Studies, NSDUH Series H-32, DHHS Publication No. SMA 07-4293. Rockville, MD.
4. Yi H et al. Alcohol Epidemiologic Data System. Surveillance Report #71: Trends in Alcohol-Related Fatal Traffic Crashes, United States, 1977–2003. Rockville, MD: National Institute on Alcohol Abuse and Alcoholism, Division of Biometry and Epidemiology; August 2005.
5. National Institute on Alcohol Abuse and Alcoholism. *Tenth Special Report to the U.S. Congress on Alcohol and Health, 2000*, Washington, DC: U.S. Department of Health and Human Services; 2000.
6. Grant BF. Prevalence and correlates of alcohol use and DSM-IV alcohol dependence in the United States. *J Stud Alcohol* 1997;58:464.
7. Regier DA et al. Comorbidity of mental disorders with alcohol and other drug abuse. *JAMA* 1990;264:2511.
8. Grant BF et al. The 12-month prevalence and trends in DSM-IV alcohol abuse and dependence. United States, 1991–1992 and 2001–2001. *Drug and Alcohol Dependence.* 2004;74:223.
9. Miller WR et al. How effective is alcoholism treatment in the United States? *J Stud Alcohol* 2001;62: 211.
10. Diagnostic and Statistical Manual of Mental Disorders. 4th ed, Text Revision (DSM-IV-TR). Washington, DC: American Psychiatric Association; 2003.
11. Swift RM. Drug therapy in alcohol dependence. *N Engl J Med* 1999;340:1482.
12. Finney JW et al. The effectiveness of inpatient and outpatient treatment for alcohol abuse: the need to focus on mediators and moderators of setting effects. *Addiction* 1996;91:1773.
13. West SL et al., Pharmacotherapy for alcohol dependence. Evidence report number 3. Contract 290-97-0011 to Research Triangle Institute, University of North Carolina, Chapel Hill. AHCPR publication no. 99 E004. Rockville, MD: Agency for Health Care Policy and Research; January 1999.
14. Litten RZ et al. Pharmacotherapies for alcohol problems: a review of research with focus on developments since 1991. *Alcohol Clin Exp Res* 1996;20:859.
15. Chick J et al. Conference summary: Consensus Conference on Alcohol Dependence and the Role of Pharmacotherapy in Its Treatment. *Alcohol Clin Exp Res* 1996;20:391.
16. Enoch MA. Pharmacogenomics of alcohol response and addiction. *American Journal of Pharmacogenomics* 2003;3:217.
17. Cherpitel CJ et al. The effect of alcohol consumption on emergency department services use among injured patients: a cross-national emergency room study. *J Stud Alcohol* 2006;67:890.
18. Cox RG et al. Academic performance and substance use: findings from a state survey of public high school students. *J Sch Health* 2007;77:109.
19. Thun MJ et al. Alcohol consumption and mortality among middle-aged and elderly U.S. adults. *N Engl J Med* 1997;337:1705.
20. Zakhari S. Alcohol and the cardiovascular system: molecular mechanisms for beneficial and harmful action. *Alcohol Health & Research World* 1997;21:21.
21. Mukamal KJ et al. Alcohol consumption and risk for coronary heart disease in men with healthy lifestyles. *Arch Intern Med* 2006;166:2145.
22. Mukamal KJ et al. Binge drinking and mortality after acute myocardial infarction. *Circulation* 2005;112:3839.
23. U.S. Department of Health and Human Services. *Healthy People 2010: Understanding and Improving Health.* 2nd ed. Washington, DC: U.S. Government Printing Office; November 2000.
24. Fillmore KM et al. Alcohol consumption and mortality. I. Characteristics of drinking groups. *Addiction* 1998;93:183.
25. David DJ et al. The acute toxicity of ethanol: dosage and kinetic nomograms. *Vet Hum Toxicol* 1979;21:272.
26. Oneta CM et al. First-pass metabolism of ethanol is strikingly influenced by the speed of gastric emptying. *Gut* 1998;43:612.
27. Jones AW et al. Effect of high-fat, high-protein, and high-carbohydrate meals on the pharmacokinetics of a small dose of ethanol. *Br J Clin Pharmacol* 1997:44:521.
28. Pihl RO et al. Alcohol affects executive cognitive functioning differentially on the ascending versus descending limb of the blood alcohol concentration curve. *Alcohol Clin Exp Res* 2003;27:773.
29. Swift, R. Direct measurement of alcohol and its metabolites. *Addiction* 2003;98(Suppl 2):73.
30. Wilkinson PK et al. Blood ethanol concentrations during and following constant-rate intravenous infusion of alcohol. *Clin Pharmacol Ther* 1976;19:213.
31. Hammond KB et al. Blood ethanol: a report of unusually high levels in a living patient. *JAMA* 1973; 226:63.
32. DiPadova C et al. Effects of fasting and chronic alcohol consumption on the first-pass metabolism of ethanol. *Gastroenterology* 1987;92:1169.
33. Ammon E et al. Disposition and first-pass metabolism of ethanol in humans: is it gastric or hepatic and does it depend on gender? *Clin Pharmacol Ther* 1996;59:503.
34. Levitt MD et al. The critical role of the rate of ethanol absorption in the interpretation of studies purporting to demonstrate gastric metabolism of ethanol. *J Pharmacol Exp Ther* 1994;269:297.
35. Levitt MD et al. Use of measurements of ethanol absorption from stomach and intestine to assess human ethanol metabolism. *Am J Physiol* 1997;273:G951.
36. Lieber CS. Ethnic and gender differences in ethanol metabolism. *Alcoho Clin Exp Res* 2000;24:417.
37. Haber PS. Metabolism of alcohol by the human stomach. *Alcohol Clin Exp Res* 2000; 24:407.
38. Lands WE. A review of alcohol clearance in humans. *Alcohol* 1998;15:147.
39. Crabb DW et al. Alcohol sensitivity, alcohol metabolism, risk of alcoholism, and the role of alcohol and aldehyde dehydrogenase. *J Lab Clin Med* 1993;122:234.
40. Kopun M et al. The kinetics of ethanol absorption and elimination in twins and supplementary repetitive experiments in singleton subjects. *Eur J Clin Pharmacol* 1977;11:337.
41. Adachi J et al. Comparative study on ethanol elimination and blood acetaldehyde between alcoholics and control subjects. *Alcohol Clin Exp Res* 1989;13:601.
42. Lieber CS. Alcoholic fatty liver: its pathogenesis and mechanism of progression to inflammation and fibrosis. *Alcohol* 2004;34:9.
43. Lieber CS. Metabolism of alcohol. *Clin Liver Dis* 2005;9:1.
44. DeFeo P et al. Ethanol impairs post-prandial hepatic protein metabolism. *J Clin Invest* 1995;95: 1472.
45. Lieber CS. Hepatic and other medical disorders of alcoholism: from pathogenesis to treatment. *J Stud Alcohol* 1998;59:9.
46. Eriksson CJP. The role of acetaldehyde in the actions of alcohol. *Alcohol Clin Exp Res* 2001;25: 15S.
47. Hoffman PL et al. Ethanol and the NMDA receptor. *Alcohol* 1990;7:229.
48. Suzdak PD et al. Ethanol stimulates gamma-aminobutyric acid receptor-mediated chloride transport in rat brain synaptoneurosomes. *Proc Natl Acad Sci U S A* 1986;83:4071.
49. Mihic SJ et al. GABA and the $GABA_A$ receptor. *Alcohol & Research World* 1997;2:127.
50. Tsai G et al. The glutamatergic basis of human alcoholism. *Am J Psychiatry* 1995;152:332.
51. Nestler EJ et al. Second messenger and protein phosphorylation mechanisms underlying possible genetic vulnerability to alcoholism. *Ann N Y Acad Sci* 1994;708:108.
52. Basavarajappa BS et al. Neuromodulatory role of the endocannabinoid signaling system in alcoholism: an overview. *Prostaglandins Leukot Essent Fatty Acids* 2002;66:287.
53. Thiele TE et al. A role for neuropeptide Y in alcohol intake control: evidence from human and animal research. *Physiol Behav* 2003;79:95.
54. Naassila M et al. Decreased alcohol self-administration and increased alcohol sensitivity and withdrawal in CB1 receptor knockout mice. *Neuropharmacology* 2004;46:243.
55. Wang L et al. Endocannabinoid signaling via cannabinoid receptor 1 is involved in ethanol

preference and its age-dependent decline in mice. *Proc Natl Acad Sci U S A* 2003;100:1393.
56. Koob GF et al. Neuropharmacology of cocaine and ethanol dependence. *Recent Dev Alcohol* 1992;10:201.
57. Samson HH et al. The role of the mesoaccumbens dopamine system in ethanol reinforcement: studies using the techniques of microinjection and voltammetry. *Alcohol Alcohol Suppl* 1993;2:469.
58. Wise RA et al. A psychomotor stimulant theory of addiction. *Psychol Rev* 1987;94:469.
59. Robinson TE et al. The neural basis of drug craving: an incentive-sensitization theory of addiction. *Brain Res Rev* 1993;18:247.
60. Koob GF et al. Drug addiction, dysregulation of reward, and allostasis. *Neuropsychopharmacology* 2001;24:97.
61. Chao J et al. Molecular neurobiology of drug addiction. *Annu Rev Med* 2004;55:113.
62. Melgaard B. The neurotoxicity of ethanol. *Acta Neurol Scand* 1983;67:131.
63. Kupari I et al. Acute effects of alcohol, beta blockade and their combination on left ventricular function and hemodynamics in normal man. *Eur Heart J* 1983;4:463.
64. Michiels TM et al. Naloxone reverses ethanol induced depression of hypercapnic drive. *Am Rev Respir Dis* 1983;128:823.
65. Barros SR et al. Naloxone as an antagonist in alcohol intoxication. *Anesthesiology* 1981;54:174.
66. Tobin MJ et al. Effect of naloxone on breathing pattern in patients with chronic obstructive pulmonary disease with and without hypercapnia. *Respiration* 1983;44:419.
67. ONeill S et al. Survival after high blood alcohol levels. *Arch Intern Med* 1984;144:641.
68. Sellers EM et al. Alcohol intoxication and withdrawal. *N Engl J Med* 1976;294:757.
69. Poikolainen K. Estimated lethal ethanol concentrations in relation to age, aspiration, and drugs. *Alcohol Clin Exp Res* 1984;8:223.
70. Thomson AD. Mechanisms of vitamin deficiency in chronic alcohol misusers and the development of the Wernicke-Korsakoff Syndrome. *Alcohol Alcohol* 2000;35(Suppl 1):2.
71. Jones AW et al. Pharmacokinetics of ethanol in patients with renal failure before and after hemodialysis. *Forensic Sci Int* 1997;90:175.
72. Kozak LJ et al. National Hospital Discharge Survey: 2000 annual summary with detailed diagnosis and procedure data. *Vital health Stat 13* 2000;153:1.
73. Finn DA et al. Exploring alcohol withdrawal syndrome. *Alcohol Health & Research World* 1997;21:149.
74. Kosten TR et al. Management of drug and alcohol withdrawal. *New Engl J Med* 2003;348:1786.
75. Spies CD et al. Alcohol withdrawal in the surgical patient: prevention and treatment. *Anesth Analg* 1999;88:946.
76. Mayo-Smith MF. Pharmacological management of alcohol withdrawal. A meta-analysis and evidence-based practice guideline. American Society of Addiction Medicine Working Group on Pharmacological Management of Alcohol Withdrawal. *JAMA* 1997;278:144.
77. Trevisan LA et al. Complications of alcohol withdrawal pathophysiologic insights. *Alcohol Health & Research World* 1998;22:61.
78. Asplund CA et al. 3 regimens for alcohol withdrawal and detoxification. *J Fam Pract* 2004;53:545.
79. Sullivan JT et al. Assessment of alcohol withdrawal: the revised Clinical Institute Withdrawal Assessment for Alcohol scale (CIWA-Ar). *Br J Addict* 1989;84:1353.
80. Riker RR et al. Prospective evaluation of the Sedation-Agitation Scale for adult critically ill patients. *Crit Care Med* 1999;27:1325.
81. Schatzberg et al. Manual of Clinical Psychopharmacology. 5th ed. American Psychiatric Publishing; 2005.
82. Lejoyeux M et al. Benzodiazepine treatment for alcohol-dependent patients. *Alcohol* 1998;33:563.
83. Kosten TR et al. Management of drug and alcohol withdrawal. *N Engl J Med* 2003;348:1786.
84. Hillbom M et al. Seizures in alcohol-dependent patients: epidemiology, pathophysiology and management. *CNS Drugs* 2003;17:1013.
85. Ritson B et al. Comparison of two benzodiazepines in the treatment of alcohol withdrawal: effects on symptoms and cognitive recovery. *Drug Alcohol Depend* 1986;18:329.
86. Kraemer KL et al. Managing alcohol withdrawal in the elderly. *Drugs Aging* 1999;14:409.
87. Adinoff B. Double-blind study of alprazolam, diazepam, clonidine, and placebo in the alcohol withdrawal syndrome: preliminary findings. *Alcohol Clin Exp Res* 1994;18:873.
88. Holbrook AM et al. Meta-analysis of benzodiazepine use in the treatment of acute alcohol withdrawal. *J Can Med Assoc* 1999;160:649.
89. Zullino DF et al. Anticonvulsant drugs in the treatment of substance withdrawal. *Drugs Today (Barc)* 2004;40:603.
90. Bayard M et al. Alcohol withdrawal syndrome. *Am Fam Physician* 2004;69:1443.
91. Stuppaeck CH et al. Carbamazepine versus oxazepam in the treatment of alcohol withdrawal: a double-blind study. *Alcohol Alcohol* 1992;27:153.
92. Malcolm R et al. Update on anticonvulsants: for the treatment of alcohol withdrawal. *Am J Addict* 2001;10(Supp):16.
93. Book S et al. Novel anticonvulsants with treatment of alcoholism. *Expert Opinion on Investigational Drugs*. 2005;14:371.
94. Malcolm et al. Double-blind controlled trial comparing carbamazepine to oxazepam treatment of alcohol withdrawal. *Am J Psychiatry* 1989;146:617.
95. Longo et al. Divalproex sodium (Depakote) for alcohol withdrawal and relapse prevention. *J Addict Dis* 2002;21:55.
96. Myrick et al. Divalproex in the treatment of alcohol withdrawal. *Am J Drug Alcohol Abuse* 2000;26:155.
97. Hillbom et al. Prevention of alcohol withdrawal seizures with carbamazepine and valproic acid. *Alcohol* 1989;6:223.
98. Reoux JP et al. Divalproex sodium in alcohol withdrawal: a randomized double-blind placebo-controlled clinical trial. *Alcohol Clin Exp Res* 2001;25:1324.
99. Myrick H et al. Gabapentin treatment of alcohol withdrawal. *Am J Psychiatry* 1998;155:1632.
100. Voris J et al. Gabapentin for the treatment of ethanol withdrawal. *Substance Abuse* 2003;24:129.
101. Krupitsky EM et al. Antiglutamatergic strategies for ethanol detoxification: comparison with placebo and diazepam. *Alcohol Clin Exp Res* 2007;31:604.
102. Mayo-Smith MF et al. Management of alcohol withdrawal delirium. An evidence-based practice guideline. *Arch Intern Med* 2004;164:1405.
103. Asplund CA et al. 3 Regimens for alcohol withdrawal and detoxification. *J Fam Pract* 2004;53:545.
104. Cook CCH et al. B-vitamin deficiency and neuropsychiatric syndromes in alcohol misuse. *Alcohol Alcohol* 1998;33:317.
105. Thomson AD et al. Royal College of Physicians, London. The Royal College of Physicians report on alcohol: guidelines for managing Wernicke's encephalopathy in the accident and Emergency Department. *Alcohol Alcohol* 2002;37:513.
106. Lingford-Hughes et al. Evidence-based guidelines for the pharmacological management of substance misuse, addiction and comorbidity: recommendations from the British Association for Psychopharmacology. *J Psychopharmacol* 2004;18:293.
107. Sellers EM et al. Comparative efficacy of propranolol and chlordiazepoxide in alcohol withdrawal. *J Stud Alcohol* 1977;38:2096.
108. Horwitz RI et al. The efficacy of atenolol in the outpatient management of the alcohol withdrawal syndrome. Results of a randomized clinical trial. *Arch Intern Med* 1989;149:1089.
109. Baumgartner GR et al. Clonidine vs. chlordiazepoxide in the management of acute alcohol withdrawal syndrome. *Arch Intern Med* 1987;147:1223.
110. Fiellin DA et al. Screening for alcohol problems in primary care: a systematic review. *Arch Intern Med.* 2000;160:1977.
111. Vinson DC et al. Comfortably engaging: which approach to alcohol screening should we use? *Ann Fam Med* 2004;2:398.
112. Ewing JA. Detecting alcoholism. The CAGE questionnaire. *JAMA* 1984;252:1905.
113. Cherpitel CJ. A brief screening instrument for problem drinking in the emergency room: the RAPS4. Rapid Alcohol Problems Screen. *J Stud Alcohol* 2000;61:447.
114. Saunders et al. Development of the Alcohol Use Disorders Identification Test (AUDIT): WHO collaborative project on early detection of persons with harmful alcohol consumption. II. *Addiction* 1993;88:791.
115. Garbutt JC et al. Pharmacological treatment of alcohol dependence: a review of the evidence. *JAMA* 1999;281:1318.
116. Berglund M. Pharmacotherapy for alcohol dependence. In: Berglund M et al., eds. *Treating Alcohol and Drug Abuse; An Evidence Based Review.* Wiley-VCH GmbH & Co. Weinheim, FRG, 2003.
117. Fuller RK et al. Disulfiram treatment of alcoholism. A Veterans Administration cooperative study. *JAMA* 1986;256:1449.
118. Chick JK et al. Disulfiram treatment of alcoholism. *Br J Psychiatry* 1992;161:84.
119. De Sousa et al. A one-year pragmatic trial of naltrexone vs. disulfiram in the treatment of alcohol dependence. *Alcohol Alcohol* 2004;39:528.
120. Petrakis IL et al. Naltrexone and disulfiram in patients with alcohol dependence and comorbid psychiatric disorders. *Biol Psychiatry* 2005;57:1128.
121. Besson J et al. Combined efficacy of acamprosate and disulfiram in the treatment of alcoholism: a controlled study. *Alcohol Clin Exp Res* 1998;22:573.
122. Fuller RK et al. Does disulfiram have a role in alcoholism treatment today? *Addiction* 2004;99:21.
123. Brewer C. Recent developments in disulfiram treatment. *Alcohol Alcohol* 1993;28:383.
124. Helmbrecht GD et al. First trimester disulfiram exposure: report of two cases. *Am J Perinatol* 1993;10:5.
125. Reitnauer PJ et al. Prenatal exposure to disulfiram implicated in the cause of malformations in discordant monozygotic twins. *Teratology* 1997;56:358.
126. Saxon et al. Disulfiram use in patients with abnormal liver function test results. *J Clin Psychiatry* 1998;59:313.
127. Wright C et al. Screening for disulfiram-induced liver test dysfunction in an inpatient alcoholism program. *Alcohol Clin Exp Res* 1993;17:184.
128. Wright C et al. Disulfiram-induced fulminating hepatitis: guidelines for liver-panel monitoring. *J Clin Psychiatry* 1988;49:430.
129. Daniel DG et al. Capgras delusion and seizures in association with therapeutic dosages of disulfiram. *South Med J* 1987;80:1577.
130. Knee ST et al. Acute organic brain syndrome: a complication of disulfiram therapy. *Am J Psychiatry* 1974;131:1281.
131. Larson EW et al. Disulfiram treatment of patients with both alcohol dependence and other psychiatric disorders: a review. *Alcohol Clin Exp Res* 1992;16:125.
132. Mueser KT et al. Disulfiram treatment for alcoholism in severe mental illness. *Am J Addict* 2003;12:242.
133. Ciraulo DA et al. Drug Interactions in Psychiatry. 3rd ed. Philadelphia: Lippincott Williams & Wilkins; 2006.
134. Zeise ML et al. Acamprosate (calcium acetylhomotaurinate) decreases postsynaptic potentials in the rat neocortex: possible involvement of excitatory amino acid receptors. *Eur J Pharmacol* 1993;26:47.

135. Daoust M et al. Acamprosate modulates synaptosomal GABA transmission in chronically alcoholised rats. *Pharmacol Biochem Behav* 1992;41:669.
136. Littleton J et al. Pharmacological mechanisms of naltrexone and acamprosate in the prevention of relapse in alcohol dependence. *Am J Addict* 2003;12(Suppl 1):S3.
137. Slattery J et al. Prevention of relapse in alcohol dependence. Health Technology Assessment Report 3. Glasgow: Health Technology Board for Scotland; 2003.
138. Miller WR et al. Mesa Grande: a methodological analysis of clinical trials of treatments for alcohol use disorders. *Addiction* 2002;97:265.
139. Mann K et al. The efficacy of acamprosate in the maintenance of abstinence in alcohol depending individuals: results of a meta-analysis. *Alcohol Clin Exp Res* 2003;28:51.
140. Chick J et al. United Kingdom Multicentre Acamprosate Study (UKMAS): a 6-month prospective study of acamprosate versus placebo in preventing relapse after withdrawal from alcohol. *Alcohol Alcohol* 200;35:176.
141. Gual A et al. Acamprosate during and after acute alcohol withdrawal: a double-blind placebo-controlled study in Spain. *Alcohol* 2001;36:413.
142. Poldrugo F. Acamprosate treatment in a long-term community-based alcohol rehabilitation programme. *Addiction* 1997;92:1537.
143. Mason BJ et al. Effect of oral acamprosate on abstinence in patients with alcohol dependence in a double-blind, placebo-controlled trial: the role of patient motivation. *J Psychiatr Res* 2006;40:383.
144. Anton RF et al. Combined pharmacotherapies and behavioral interventions for alcohol dependence. The COMBINE study: a randomized controlled trial. *JAMA* 2006;295:2003.
145. Kiritze-Topor P et al. A pragmatic trial of acamprosate in the treatment of alcohol dependence in primary care. *Alcohol Alcohol* 2004;39:520.
146. Mason B. Individual patient data meta analysis of predictors of outcome including U.S. and European studies in Acamprosate: New preclinical and clinical findings, Research Society on Alcoholism, Santa Barbara, CA; June 26, 2005.
147. Verheul R et al. Predictors of acamprosate efficacy: results from a pooled analysis of seven European trials including 1,485 alcohol-dependent patients. *Psychopharmacology* 2005;178:167.
148. Carmen B et al. Efficacy and safety of naltrexone and acamprosate in the treatment of alcohol dependence: a systematic review. *Addiction* 2004;99:811.
149. Kenna GA et al. Pharmacotherapy, pharmacogenomics and the future of alcohol dependence therapy. *Am J Health Sys Pharm* 2004;61:2380.
150. Sass H et al. Relapse prevention by acamprosate. Results from a placebo controlled study on alcohol dependence. *Arch Gen Psychiatry* 1996;53:673.
151. Whitworth AB et al. Comparison of acamprosate and placebo in long-term treatment of alcohol dependence. *Lancet* 1996;347:1438.
152. Chick J et al. A multicentre, randomized, double-blind, placebo-controlled trial of naltrexone in the treatment of alcohol dependence or abuse. *Alcohol Alcohol* 2000;35:587.
153. Roussaux JP et al. Does acamprosate diminish the appetite for alcohol in weaned alcoholics? *Journal de Pharmacie de Belgique* 1996;51:65.
154. Namkoong K et al. Acamprosate in Korean alcohol-dependent patients: a multi-centre, randomized, double-blind, placebo-controlled study. *Alcohol Alcohol* 2003;38:135.
155. Acamprosate product information. St. Louis MO: Forest Pharmaceuticals; April, 2004.
156. Hotson JR et al. Disulfiram-induced encephalopathy. *Arch Neurol* 1976;33:141.
157. Johnson BA et al. Dose-ranging kinetics and behavioral pharmacology of naltrexone and acamprosate, both alone and combined, in alcohol-dependent subjects. *J Clin Psychopharmacol* 2003;23:281.
158. Mason BJ et al. A pharmacokinetic and pharmacodynamic drug interaction study of acamprosate and naltrexone. *Neuropsychopharmacology* 2002;27:596.
159. Mark TL et al. Physicians' opinions about medications to treat alcoholism. *Addiction* 2003;98:617.
160. Kenna GA et al. Pharmacotherapy, pharmacogenomics and the future of alcohol dependence therapy. *Am J Health Sys Pharm* 2004;61 Part 1:2272.
161. Srisurapanont M et al. Opioid antagonists for alcohol dependence. In: *The Cochrane Library.* Chichester: John Wiley & Sons; 2003.
162. Kranzler HR et al. Efficacy of naltrexone and acamprosate for alcoholism treatment: a meta-analysis. *Alcohol Clin Exp Res* 2001;25:1335.
163. Kiefer F et al. Comparing and combining naltrexone and acamprosate in relapse prevention of alcoholism: a double-blind, placebo-controlled study. *Arch Gen Psychiatry* 2003;60:92.
164. OMalley S et al. Naltrexone and coping skills therapy for alcohol dependence. *Arch Gen Psychiatry* 1992;49:881.
165. McCaul ME et al. Naltrexone alters subjective and psychomotor responses to alcohol in heavy drinking subjects. *Neuropsychopharmacology* 2000;22:480.
166. Jaffe AJ et al. Naltrexone, relapse prevention and supportive therapy with alcoholics: an analysis of patient-treatment matching. *J Consult Clin Psychol* 1996;64:1044.
167. Monti P et al. Naltrexone's effect on cue-elicited craving among alcoholics in treatment. *Alcohol Clin Exp Res* 1999;23:1386.
168. Volpicelli JR et al. Naltrexone and alcohol dependence. Role of subject compliance. *Arch Gen Psychiatry* 1997;54:737.
169. Rubio G et al. Clinical predictors of response to naltrexone in alcoholic patients: who benefits most from treatment with naltrexone? *Alcohol Alcohol* 2005;40:227.
170. Volpicelli JR et al. Naltrexone in the treatment of alcoholism. Results from a multicenter usage study. The Naltrexone Usage Study Group. *Arch Gen Psychiatry* 1992;49:876.
171. Davidson D et al. Effects of naltrexone on alcohol self-administration in heavy drinkers. *Alcohol Clin Exp Res* 1999;23:193.
172. Kranzler HR et al. Naltrexone vs. nefazodone for treatment of alcohol dependence. A placebo-controlled trial. *Neuropsychiatry* 2000;22:493.
173. Krystal JH et al. Veterans Affairs Naltrexone Cooperative Study 425 Group. Naltrexone in the treatment of alcohol dependence. *N Engl J Med* 2001;345:1734.
174. Gastpar M et al. Lack of efficacy of naltrexone in the prevention of alcohol relapse: results from a German multicenter study. *J Clin Psychopharmacol* 2002;22:592.
175. Galloway GP et al. Pharmacokinetics, safety, and tolerability of a depot formulation of naltrexone in alcoholics: an open-label trial. *BioMed Central Psychiatry* 2005;5:18.
176. Garbutt JC et al. Efficacy and tolerability of long-acting injectable naltrexone for alcohol dependence: a randomized controlled trial. *JAMA* 2005;293:1617.
177. Kranzler HR et al. Naltrexone depot for treatment of alcohol dependence: a multicenter, randomized, placebo-controlled clinical trial. *Alcohol Clin Exp Res* 2004;28:1051.
178. Rohsenow DJ. What place does naltrexone have in the treatment of alcoholism? *CNS Drugs* 2004;18:547.
179. Gerasimov MR et al. GABAergic blockade of cocaine-associated cue-induced increases in nucleus accumbens dopamine. *Eur J Pharmacol* 2001;414:205.
180. Gryder DS et al. Selective antagonism of GluR5 kainate-receptor-mediated synaptic currents by topiramate in rat basolateral amygdala neurons. *J Neurosci* 2003;23:7069.
181. Johnson et al. Oral topiramate for treatment of alcohol dependence: a randomised controlled trial. *Lancet* 2003;361:1677.
182. Swift RM. Topiramate for the treatment of alcohol dependence: initiating abstinence. *Lancet* 2003;361:1666.
183. Johnson BA et al. Topiramate for treating alcohol dependence: a randomized controlled trial. *JAMA* 2007;298:1541.
184. Di Sclafani V et al. Psychiatric comorbidity in long-term abstinent alcoholic individuals. *Alcohol Clin Exp Res* 2007;31:795.
185. Frye MA et al. Bipolar disorder and comorbid alcoholism: prevalence rate and treatment considerations. *Bipolar Disorder* 2006;8:677.
186. Arnone D. Review of the use of Topiramate for treatment of psychiatric disorders. *Ann Gen Psychiatry* 2005;4:5.
187. Huguelet P et al. Effect of topiramate augmentation on two patients suffering from schizophrenia or bipolar disorder with comorbid alcohol abuse. *Pharmacol Res* 2005;52:392.
188. Rosenstock J et al. A randomized, double-blind, placebo-controlled, multicenter study to assess the efficacy and safety of Topiramate controlled-release in the treatment of obese, type 2 diabetic patients. *Diabetes Care* 2007. Epub ahead of print.
189. Topamax Package Insert. Raritan, NJ: Ortho-McNeil Pharmaceutical Inc.; Revised June 2005.
190. Ciraulo D et al. Drug Interactions in Psychiatry. 3rd ed. Philadelphia: Lippincott Williams & Wilkins; 2006.
191. Salloum IM et al. Efficacy of valproate maintenance in patients with bipolar disorder and alcoholism: a double-blind placebo-controlled study. *Arch Gen Psychiatry* 2005;62:37.
192. Misgeld U et al. A physiological role for GABAB receptors and the effects of baclofen in the mammalian central nervous system. *Prog Neurobiol* 1995;46:423.
193. Cousins MS et al. GABA(B) receptor agonists for the treatment of drug addiction: a review of recent findings. *Drug Alcohol Depend* 2002;65:209.
194. Litten RZ et al. Development of medications for alcohol use disorders: recent advances and ongoing challenges. *Expert Opin Emerg Drugs* 2005;10:323.
195. Anström KK et al. Effect of baclofen on alcohol and sucrose self-administration in rats. *Alcohol Clin Exp Res* 2003;27:900.
196. Colombo G et al. Baclofen suppresses motivation to consume alcohol in rats. *Psychopharmacology* 2003;167:221.
197. Addolorato G et al. Baclofen efficacy in reducing alcohol craving and intake: a preliminary double-blind randomized controlled study. *Alcohol Alcohol* 2002;37:504.
198. Brown RL et al. Pharmacoepidemiology of potential alcohol-prescription drug interactions among primary care patients with alcohol-use disorders. *J Am Pharma Assoc* 2007;47:135.
199. DeVane CL et al. Psychotropic drug interactions. *Primary Psychiatry* 1999;6:39.
200. Wellbutrin SR Package Insert. Research Triangle Park, NC: Glaxo Smith Kline; August 2007.
201. Pelc I et al. Efficacy and safety of acamprosate in the treatment of detoxified alcohol-dependent patients. A 90-day placebo-controlled dose finding study. *Br J Psychiatry* 1997;171:73.
202. Kranzler HR et al. Placebo-controlled trial of fluoxetine as an adjunct to relapse prevention in alcoholics. *Am J Psychiatry* 1995;152:391.
203. Cornelius JR et al. Fluoxetine in depressed alcoholics. A double-blind placebo controlled trial. *Arch Gen Psychiatry* 1997;23:193.
204. Pettinati H et al. Sertraline treatment for alcohol dependence. Interactive effects of medication and alcoholic subtype. *Alcohol Clin Exp Res* 2000;24:1041.
205. Johnson BA et al. Ondansetron for reduction of drinking among biologically predisposed patients: A randomized controlled trial. *JAMA* 2000;284:963.
206. Anton RF et al. A randomized, multicenter, double-blind, placebo-controlled study of the efficacy and safety of aripiprazole for the treatment of alcohol dependence. *J Clin Psychopharmacol* 2008;28:5.

CHAPTER 85

Tobacco Use and Dependence

Robin L. Corelli and Karen Suchanek Hudmon

Long before Christopher Columbus traveled to the New World, tobacco use was widespread in the Americas—tobacco preparations were part of religious ceremonies for the Native Americans, and tobacco was also used medicinally. At that time, and for several subsequent centuries, little was known or suspected about the dangers of tobacco use. In retrospect, it is not surprising that these dangers were not recognized initially because the more pressing health issues at that time were related to life-threatening, acute diseases as opposed to chronic diseases such as those imposed by tobacco. However, it is now well established that tobacco is a detrimental substance, and its use dramatically increases a person's odds of dependence, disease, disability, and death.

Cigarettes are the only marketed consumable product that when used as intended will contribute to the death of half or more of its users.[1] Tobacco products are carefully engineered formulations that optimize the delivery of nicotine, a chemical that meets the criteria for an addictive substance: (a) nicotine induces psychoactive effects, (b) it is used in a highly controlled or compulsive manner, and (c) behavioral patterns of tobacco use are reinforced by the pharmacologic effects of nicotine.[2] As a major risk factor for a wide range of diseases, including cardiovascular conditions, cancers, and pulmonary disorders, tobacco is the primary known preventable cause of premature death in our society.[3] During the 20th century, 100 million deaths were caused by tobacco, and currently, an estimated

5.4 million deaths occur annually.[3] Unless tobacco control efforts are able to reverse this trend, the number of annual deaths is likely to exceed 8 million by the year 2030.[4] According to Dr. Margaret Chan, Director-General of the World Health Organization, "Reversing this entirely preventable epidemic must now rank as a top priority for public health and for political leaders in every country of the world."[4]

In the United States, smoking is responsible for approximately 438,000 premature deaths each year.[5] In addition to the harm imposed on users of tobacco, exposure to secondhand smoke results in an estimated 50,000 deaths each year.[6] Furthermore, enormous economic burden accompanies tobacco use. Each pack of cigarettes smoked costs society $7.18 for associated medical care ($3.45) and productivity losses ($3.73), for a total of $157 billion in annual health-related economic losses.[5] Because of the health and societal burdens that it imposes, tobacco use and dependence should be addressed during each clinical encounter with all tobacco users.[7]

EPIDEMIOLOGY OF TOBACCO USE AND DEPENDENCE

Nicotine addiction is a form of chronic brain disease resulting from alterations in brain chemistry.[8] Dr. Alan Leshner, former director of the National Institute on Drug Abuse, defines drug addiction as "compulsive use, without medical purpose, in the face of negative consequences."[8] The addictive properties of nicotine are well documented.

In the United States, experimentation with cigarettes and the development of regular smoking typically occur during adolescence, with 88% to 89% of adult smokers having tried their first cigarette by 18 years of age[9,10] and 71% of adult daily smokers having become regular smokers by age 18.[9] Because most teens who smoke at least monthly continue to smoke in adulthood,[9] tobacco use trends among youth are a key indicator of the overall health trends for the nation.[11] According to the Centers for Disease Control and Prevention (CDC), the prevalence of current smoking (defined as having smoked at least one cigarette in the preceding 30 days) among high school students increased throughout the early and mid-1990s,[12] identifying an urgent need for tobacco prevention and cessation programs focused on younger age groups. These have led to subsequent decreases. In 2007, an estimated 21.6% of 12th graders (23.1% of males and 19.6% of females) had smoked one or more cigarettes in the past 30 days.[13]

Among adults, smoking prevalence varies by sociodemographic factors, including sex, race/ethnicity, education level, age, and poverty level. The CDC reported that in 2006, the percentage of current smokers (defined as having smoked 100 or more cigarettes during their lifetime and currently smoking every day or some days) was 20.8% (23.9% of men and 18.0% of women).[14] Table 85-1 summarizes the smoking prevalence estimates for various population subgroups, stratified by sex. In 2006, the highest median prevalence of current smoking was evident in Kentucky (28.6%), and the lowest prevalence was observed in Utah (9.8%).[15] An estimated 44.3% of cigarettes

Table 85-1 Percentage of Current Smokers[a] Ages 18 Years and Older, by Sex and Selected Characteristics—National Health Interview Survey, United States, 2006

Characteristic	*Category*	*Men (n = 10,715)*	*Women (n = 13,560)*	*Total (n = 24,275)*
Race/ethnicity[b]	White, non-Hispanic	24.3	19.7	21.9
	Black, non-Hispanic	27.6	19.2	23.0
	Hispanic	20.1	10.1	15.2
	American Indian/Alaska Native, non-Hispanic	35.6	29.0	32.4
	Asian[c]	16.8	4.6	10.4
Education[d]	0–12 years (no diploma)	30.6	23.0	26.7
	GED[e] diploma	51.3	40.2	46.0
	High school diploma	27.6	20.4	23.8
	Associate degree	25.4	17.8	21.2
	Some college	26.1	20.0	22.7
	Undergraduate degree	10.8	8.4	9.6
	Graduate degree	7.3	5.8	6.6
Age group (years)	18–24	28.5	19.3	23.9
	25–44	26.0	21.0	23.5
	45–64	24.5	19.3	21.8
	65 and older	12.6	8.3	10.2
Poverty status[f]	At or above federal poverty level	22.9	17.8	20.4
	Below federal poverty level	34.0	28.0	30.6
	Unknown	23.3	14.2	18.3
Total		**23.9**	**18.0**	**20.8**

[a]Persons who reported having smoked ≥100 cigarettes during their lifetimes and who, at the time of interview, reported smoking every day or some days. Excludes 315 respondents whose smoking status was unknown.

[b]Excludes 266 respondents of unknown race or multiple races.

[c]Does not include Native Hawaiians and Other Pacific Islanders.

[d]Persons ages 25 years and older, excluding 305 persons whose educational level was unknown.

[e]GED, general educational development.

[f]Based on family income reported by respondents and 2005 poverty thresholds published by the U.S. Census Bureau.

From reference 15.

smoked in the United States are among persons with mental illness.[16]

Factors Contributing to Tobacco Use

Tobacco addiction is maintained by nicotine dependence.[17] Nicotine induces a variety of pharmacologic effects, described as follows, that lead to dependence.[17,18] However, tobacco dependence is not simply a matter of nicotine pharmacology—it is a result of the interplay of complex processes, including the desire for the direct pharmacologic actions of nicotine, the relief of withdrawal, learned associations, and environmental cues (e.g., advertising, the smell of a cigarette, or observing others who are smoking).[17] Physiological factors, such as preexisting medical conditions (e.g., psychiatric comorbidities[16]) and one's genetic profile, also can predispose individuals to tobacco use. Notably, it has been estimated in twin studies that 40% to 60% of smoking is heritable.[19–21] The rapidity with which nicotine, the addictive component of tobacco, is absorbed and passes through the blood-brain barrier contributes to its addictive nature. After inhalation, nicotine reaches the brain within seconds.[17] As such, smokers experience nearly immediate onset of positive effects of nicotine, including pleasure, relief of anxiety, improved task performance, improved memory, mood modulation, and skeletal muscle relaxation.[17] These effects, mediated by alterations in neurotransmitter levels, reinforce continued use of nicotine-containing products.

Nicotine Pharmacology

Nicotine (*Nicotiana tabacum*), which is composed of a pyridine ring and a pyrrolidine ring, is one of the few natural alkaloids that exist in the liquid state. Nicotine is a clear, weak base (pKa = 8.0) that turns brown and acquires the characteristic odor of tobacco after exposure to air.[22,23] In acidic media, nicotine is ionized and poorly absorbed; conversely, in alkaline media, nicotine is nonionized and well absorbed. Under physiological conditions (pH = 7.3–7.5), approximately 31% of nicotine is nonionized and readily crosses cell membranes.[22,24] Given the relation between pH and absorption, the tobacco industry and pharmaceutical companies are able to titrate the pH of their tobacco products and nicotine replacement therapies (NRTs) to maximize the absorption potential of nicotine.[17,25]

Once absorbed, nicotine induces a variety of central nervous system, cardiovascular, and metabolic effects. Nicotine stimulates the release of several neurotransmitters, inducing a range of pharmacologic effects such as pleasure (dopamine), arousal (acetylcholine, norepinephrine), cognitive enhancement (acetylcholine), appetite suppression (dopamine, norepinephrine, serotonin), learning (glutamate), memory enhancement (glutamate), mood modulation (serotonin), and reduction of anxiety and tension (β-endorphin and GABA).[18] The dopamine reward pathway, a network of nervous tissue that elicits feelings of pleasure in response to certain stimuli, is central to drug-induced reward. Key structures of the reward pathway include the ventral tegmental area, nucleus accumbens, and prefrontal cortex (the area of the brain that is responsible for thinking and judgment). The neurons of the ventral tegmental area contain the neurotransmitter dopamine, which is released in the nucleus accumbens and in the prefrontal cortex. Immediately after inhalation, a bolus of nicotine enters the brain, stimulating the release of dopamine, which induces nearly immediate feelings of pleasure, along with relief of the symptoms of nicotine withdrawal. This rapid dose response reinforces repeated administration of the drug and perpetuates the smoking behavior.[18]

Chronic administration of nicotine has been shown to result in an increased number of nicotine receptors in specific regions of the brain,[26] which is believed to represent upregulation in response to nicotine-mediated desensitization of the receptors and may play a role in nicotine tolerance and dependence.[18] Chronic administration also leads to tolerance to the behavioral and cardiovascular effects of nicotine over the course of the day; however, tobacco users regain sensitivity to the effects of nicotine after overnight abstinence from nicotine, as shown in Figure 85-1.[17,22] Notably, after smoking the first cigarette of the day, the smoker experiences marked pharmacologic effects, particularly arousal. No other cigarette throughout the day produces the same degree of pleasure/arousal. For this reason, many smokers describe the first cigarette as the most important one of the day. Shortly after the initial cigarette, tolerance begins to develop. Accordingly, the threshold levels for both pleasure/arousal and abstinence rise progressively throughout the day as the smoker becomes tolerant to the effects of nicotine. With continued smoking, nicotine accumulates, leading to an even greater degree of tolerance. Late in the day, each individual cigarette produces only limited pleasure/arousal; instead, smoking primarily alleviates nicotine withdrawal symptoms. Lack of exposure to nicotine overnight results in resensitization of drug responses (i.e., loss of tolerance). Most dependent smokers tend to smoke a certain number of cigarettes per day and tend to consume sufficient nicotine per day to achieve the desired effects of cigarette smoking and minimize the symptoms of nicotine withdrawal.[22] Withdrawal symptoms include depression, insomnia, irritability, anxiety, difficulty concentrating, restlessness, and increased appetite.[27–29] Tobacco users become adept at titrating their nicotine levels throughout the day to avoid withdrawal symptoms, maintain pleasure and arousal, and modulate mood.

Nicotine is extensively metabolized in the liver and, to a lesser extent, in the kidney and lung. Approximately 70% to 80% of nicotine is metabolized to cotinine, an inactive metabolite.[17,24] The rapid metabolism of nicotine ($t_{1/2} = 2$ hours) to inactive compounds underlies tobacco users' needs for frequent, repeated administration. The half-life of cotinine, however, is much longer ($t_{1/2} = 18$–20 hours), and for this reason, cotinine is commonly used as marker of tobacco use as well as a marker for exposure to secondhand smoke.[17] Cotinine cannot, however, differentiate between the nicotine from tobacco products and the nicotine from NRT products.

Nicotine and other metabolites are excreted in the urine. Urinary excretion is pH dependent; the excretion rate is increased in acidic urine. Nicotine is excreted in breast milk and can be detected in the blood and urine of infants of nursing smokers.[23,24]

Drug Interactions With Smoking

It is widely recognized that polycyclic aromatic hydrocarbons (PAHs), present in appreciably large quantities in tobacco smoke, are responsible for most drug interactions with smoking.[30,31] PAHs, which are the products of incomplete

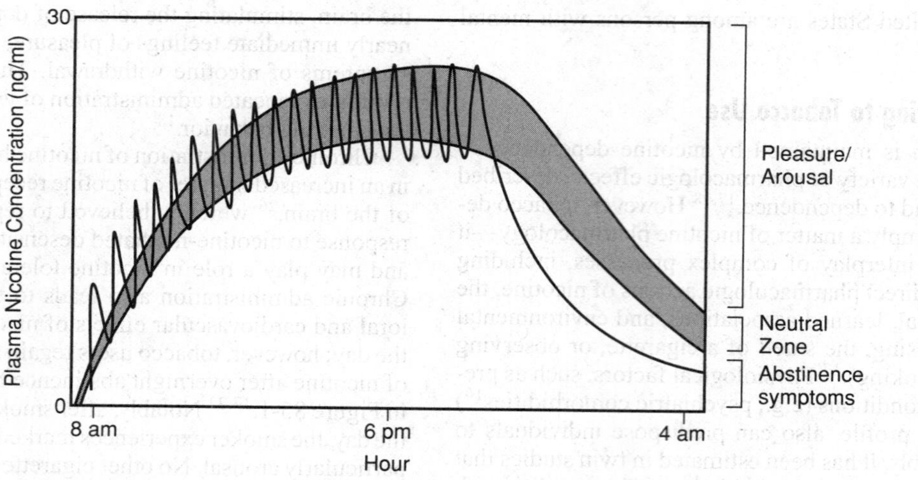

FIGURE 85-1 Nicotine addiction cycle throughout the day.
- The sawtooth line represents venous plasma concentrations of nicotine as a cigarette is smoked every 40 minutes from 8 am to 9 pm.
- The upper solid line indicates the threshold concentration for nicotine to produce pleasure or arousal.
- The lower solid line indicates the concentrations at which symptoms of abstinence (i.e., withdrawal symptoms) from nicotine occur.
- The shaded area represents the zone of nicotine concentrations (neutral zone) in which the smoker is comfortable without experiencing either pleasure/arousal or abstinence symptoms.

Source: Reprinted from reference 22, with permission.

combustion of tobacco, are potent inducers of several hepatic cytochrome P450 microsomal enzymes (CYP1A1, CYP1A2, and possibly CYP2E1). Although other substances in tobacco smoke, including acetone, pyridines, benzene, nicotine, carbon monoxide, and heavy metals (e.g., cadmium), might also interact with hepatic enzymes, their effects appear to be less significant. Most drug interactions with tobacco smoke are pharmacokinetic, resulting from the induction of drug-metabolizing enzymes (especially CYP1A2) by compounds in tobacco smoke. Table 85-2 summarizes key interactions with smoking.[30,32] Patients who begin smoking, or quit smoking, might require dosage adjustments for some medications.

Health Consequences of Tobacco Use

Smoking has a causal or contributory role in the development of a variety of medical conditions (Table 85-3).[3] In the United States, tobacco use accounts for nearly 1 in 5 deaths, and an estimated 8.6 million persons suffer from chronic conditions attributable to smoking.[33] Among current smokers, chronic bronchitis is the most common condition (49%), followed by emphysema (24%). Among former smokers, the most prevalent condition is chronic bronchitis (26%), followed by emphysema (24%) and previous heart attack (24%). Lung cancer, the leading cause of cancer-related mortality for both men and women in the United States and a disease for which the 5-year survival rate is approximately 15%,[34] accounts for an estimated 1% of all smoking-attributable morbidity (i.e., among those who are living) in current smokers and 2% in former smokers.[33]

Secondhand Smoke Exposure

Exposure to secondhand smoke, which includes the smoke emanating from burning tobacco and that exhaled by the smoker, results in an estimated 50,000 deaths annually, in addition to contributing to numerous diseases among nonsmoking children and adults.[6] Major conclusions of the 2006 Surgeon General's Health Effects of Involuntary Exposure to Tobacco Smoke[6] report include (a) Many millions of Americans, both children and adults, are still exposed to secondhand smoke in their homes and workplaces despite substantial progress in tobacco control; (b) Secondhand smoke exposure causes disease and premature death in children and adults who do not smoke; (c) Children exposed to secondhand smoke are at an increased risk for sudden infant death syndrome, acute respiratory infections, ear problems, and more severe asthma. Smoking by parents causes respiratory symptoms and slows lung growth in their children; (d) Exposure of adults to secondhand smoke has immediate adverse events on the cardiovascular system and causes coronary heart disease and lung cancer; (e) The scientific evidence indicates that there is no risk-free level of exposure to secondhand smoke; and (f) Eliminating smoking in indoor spaces fully protects nonsmokers from exposure to secondhand smoke. Separating smokers from nonsmokers, cleaning the air, and ventilating buildings cannot eliminate exposures of nonsmokers to secondhand smoke. Supplementing evidence presented in the Surgeon General's report, in January 2006, the California Environmental Protection Agency designated secondhand smoke as a "toxic air contaminant" and, in addition to the list of diseases described in the Surgeon General's report, specified that exposure is associated with breast cancer in younger, primarily premenopausal women.[35]

Benefits of Quitting

The 1990 Surgeon General's Report on the health benefits of smoking cessation describes numerous and substantial health benefits associated with quitting.[36] Benefits incurred soon after quitting (e.g., within 2 weeks to 3 months) include improvements in pulmonary function, circulation, and ambulation. Within 1 to 9 months of quitting, the ciliary function of

Table 85-2 Drug Interactions[a] With Smoking

Drug/Class	*Mechanism of Interaction and Effects*
Pharmacokinetic Interactions	
Alprazolam (Xanax)	• Conflicting data on significance of a PK interaction. Possible ↓ plasma concentrations (up to 50%); ↓ half-life (35%).
Bendamustine (Treanda)	• Metabolized by CYP1A2. Manufacturer recommends using with caution in smokers due to likely ↓ bendamustine concentrations, with ↑ concentrations of its two active metabolites.
Caffeine	• ↑ Metabolism (induction of CYP1A2); ↑ clearance (56%). • Likely ↑ caffeine levels after cessation.
Chlorpromazine (Thorazine)	• ↓Area under the curve (AUC) (36%) and serum concentrations (24%). • ↓ Sedation and hypotension possible in smokers; smokers may need ↑ dosages.
Clozapine (Clozaril)	• ↑ Metabolism (induction of CYP1A2); ↓ plasma concentrations (18%). • ↑ Levels upon cessation may occur; closely monitor drug levels and reduce dose as required to avoid toxicity.
Erlotinib (Tarceva)	• ↑ Clearance (24%); ↓ trough serum concentrations (2-fold).
Flecainide (Tambocor)	• ↑ Clearance (61%); ↓ trough serum concentrations (25%). • Smokers may need ↑ dosages.
Fluvoxamine (Luvox)	• ↑ Metabolism (induction of CYP1A2); ↑ clearance (24%); ↓ AUC (31%) ↓ plasma concentrations (32%). • Dosage modifications not routinely recommended but smokers may need ↑ dosages.
Haloperidol (Haldol)	• ↑ Clearance (44%); ↓ serum concentrations (70%).
Heparin	• Mechanism unknown but ↑ clearance and ↓ half-life are observed. Smoking has prothrombotic effects. • Smokers may need ↑ dosages due to PK and PD interactions.
Insulin, subcutaneous	• Possible ↓ insulin absorption secondary to peripheral vasoconstriction; smoking may cause release of endogenous substances that cause insulin resistance. • PK & PD interactions likely not clinically significant; smokers may need ↑ dosages.
Irinotecan (Camptosar)	• ↑ Clearance (18%); ↓ serum concentrations of active metabolite SN-38 (~40%; via induction of glucuronidation); ↓ systemic exposure resulting in lower hematologic toxicity and may reduce efficacy. • Smokers may need ↑ dosages.
Mexiletine (Mexitil)	• ↑ Clearance (25%; via oxidation and glucuronidation); ↓ half-life (36%).
Olanzapine (Zyprexa)	• ↑ Metabolism (induction of CYP1A2): ↑ clearance (98%); ↓ serum concentrations (12%). • Dosage modifications not routinely recommended but smokers may require ↑ dosages.
Propranolol (Inderal)	• ↑ Clearance (77%; via side-chain oxidation and glucuronidation)
Ropinirole (Requip)	• ↓ Cmax (38%) and AUC (30%) in study with patients with restless legs syndrome. • Smokers may need ↑ dosages.
Tacrine (Cognex)	• ↑ Metabolism (induction of CYP1A2); ↓ half-life (50%); serum concentrations three-fold lower. • Smokers may need ↑ dosages.
Theophylline (Theo Dur, etc.)	• ↑ Metabolism (induction of CYP1A2); ↑ clearance (58–100%); ↓ half-life (63%). • Levels should be monitored if smoking is initiated, discontinued, or changed. • ↑ Clearance with second-hand smoke exposure. • Maintenance doses are considerably higher in smokers.
Tricyclic antidepressants (e.g., imipramine, nortriptyline)	• Possible interaction with tircyclic antidepressants in the direction of ↓ blood levels, but the clinical importance is not established.
Tizanidine (Zanaflex)	• ↓ AUC (30–40%) and ↓ half-life (10%) observed in male smokers.
Pharmacodynamic Interactions	
Benzodiazepines (diazepam, chlordiazepoxide)	• ↓ Sedation and drowsiness, possibly caused by nicotine stimulation of central nervous system.
Beta-blockers	• Less effective antihypertensive and heart rate control effects; might be caused by nicotine-mediated sympathetic activation. • Smokers may need ↑ dosages.
Corticosteroids, inhaled	• Asthmatic smokers may have less of a response to inhaled corticosteroids.
Hormonal contraceptives	• ↑ Risk of cardiovascular adverse effects (e.g., stroke, myocardial infarction, thromboembolism) in women who smoke and use oral contraceptives. Ortho Evra patch users shown to have 2-fold ↑ risk of venous thromboembolism compared to oral contraceptive users, likely due to ↑ estrogen exposure (60% higher levels). • ↑ Risk with age and with heavy smoking (15 or more cigarettes per day) and is quite marked in women age 35 and older.
Opioids (propoxyphene, pentazocine)	• ↓ Analgesic effect; smoking may ↑ the metabolism of propoxyphene (15–20%) and pentazocine (40%). Mechanism unknown. • Smokers may need ↑ opioid dosages for pain relief.

[a] Shaded rows indicate the most clinically significant interactions.

Adapted from reference 32, with permission.

Table 85-3 Health Consequences of Smoking[3]

Cancer	Acute myeloid leukemia
	Bladder
	Cervical
	Esophageal
	Gastric
	Kidney
	Laryngeal
	Lung
	Oral cavity and pharyngeal
	Pancreatic
Cardiovascular disease	Abdominal aortic aneurysm
	Coronary heart disease (angina pectoris, ischemic heart disease, myocardial infarction)
	Cerebrovascular disease (transient ischemic attacks, stroke)
	Peripheral arterial disease
Pulmonary disease	Acute respiratory illnesses
	Upper respiratory tract (rhinitis, sinusitis, laryngitis, pharyngitis)
	Lower respiratory tract (bronchitis, pneumonia)
	Chronic respiratory illnesses
	Chronic obstructive pulmonary disease
	Respiratory symptoms
	Poor asthma control
	Reduced lung function
Reproductive effects	Reduced fertility in women
	Pregnancy and pregnancy outcomes
	Preterm, premature rupture of membranes
	Placenta previa
	Placental abruption
	Preterm delivery
	Low infant birth weight
	Infant mortality
	Sudden infant death syndrome
Other effects	Cataract
	Osteoporosis (reduced bone density in postmenopausal women, increased risk of hip fracture)
	Periodontitis
	Peptic ulcer disease (in patients who are infected with *Helicobacter pylori*)
	Surgical outcomes
	Poor wound healing
	Respiratory complications

the lung epithelial cells is restored; initially, this might result in increased coughing as the lungs clear excess mucus and tobacco smoke particulates. Smoking cessation results in measurable improvements in lung function[37] (see Chapter 23, Fig. 23-1). Over time, patients experience decreased coughing, sinus congestion, fatigue, shortness of breath, and risk of pulmonary infection. One year after cessation, the excess risk of coronary heart disease is reduced to half that of continuing smokers. After 5 to 15 years, the risk of stroke is reduced to a rate similar to that of people who are lifetime nonsmokers, and 10 years after quitting, the chance of dying of lung cancer is approximately half that of continuing smokers. In addition, the risk of developing mouth, throat, esophagus, bladder, kidney, or pancreatic cancer is decreased. Finally, 15 years after quitting, the risk of coronary heart disease is reduced to a rate that is similar to that of people who have never smoked.[36] Smoking cessation can also lead to a significant reduction in the cumulative risk of death from lung cancer, for both men and women.[38] Quitting at ages 30, 40, 50, and 60 years is associated with 10, 9, 6, and 3 years of life gained, respectively. On average, cigarette smokers die approximately 10 years younger than do nonsmokers, and among those who continue smoking, at least half will die due to a tobacco-related disease. Persons who quit before age 35 add 10 years of life and have a life expectancy similar to those who have never smoked.[1] Reduction in smoking does not equate to a reduction in harm; even low levels of smoking (e.g., 1–4 cigarettes per day) have documented risks,[39,40] and therefore, a reduction in the number of cigarettes smoked per day should be viewed as a positive step toward quitting, but should not be recommended as a targeted end point. For any patient who uses tobacco, the target goal is complete, long-term abstinence from all nicotine-containing products. Thus, it is never too late to quit and to incur subsequent benefits of quitting. But quitting earlier is clearly advantageous.

Tobacco Use and Dependence: Treatment Approaches

Most tobacoo users attempt to quit without assistance, despite the fact that persons who receive assistance are more likely to be successful in quitting.[7,41] Given the complexity of the tobacco-dependence syndrome and the constellation of factors that contribute to tobacco use, treatment requires a multifaceted approach. To assist clinicians and other specialists in providing cessation treatment to patients who use tobacco, the U.S. Public Health Service published the Clinical Practice Guideline for Treating Tobacco Use and Dependence. This document, which represents a distillation of more than 8,700 published articles,[7] specifies that clinicians can have an important impact on their patients' ability to quit. A meta-analysis of 29 studies[7] determined that compared with patients who do not receive an intervention from a clinician, patients who receive a tobacco cessation intervention from a physician clinician or a non-physician clinician are 2.2 and 1.7 times, respectively, more likely to quit (at 5 or more months after cessation). Although even brief advice from a clinician has been shown to lead to increased odds of quitting,[7] more intensive counseling yields more dramatic increases in quit rates.[7]

Numerous effective medications are available for tobacco dependence, and clinicians should encourage their use by all patients attempting to quit smoking—except when medically contraindicated or with specific populations for which there is insufficient evidence of effectiveness (i.e., pregnant women, smokeless tobacco users, light smokers, adolescents).[7] Although both pharmacotherapy and behavioral counseling are effective independently, patients' odds of quitting are substantially increased when the two approaches are used simultaneously. The estimated efficacies of various treatment strategies are shown in Table 85-4. Clinicians can have a significant impact on a patient's likelihood of success by recommending pharmacotherapy agents and by supplementing medication use with behavioral counseling as described later in this chapter.

Assisting Patients With Quitting

Behavioral Counseling Strategies

According to the Clinical Practice Guideline,[7] five key components comprise comprehensive counseling for tobacco cessation: (a) asking patients whether they use tobacco, (b) advising tobacco users to quit, (c) assessing patients' readiness to quit, (d) assisting patients with quitting, and (e) arranging

Table 85-4 Efficacy of Treatment Methods for Tobacco Use and Dependence[7]

Treatment Method	*Estimated Odds Ratio[a] (95% CI)*	*Estimated Abstinence[b] Rate (95% CI)*
Behavioral interventions		
Advice to quit		
No advice to quit	1.0	7.9
Physician advice to quit	1.3 (1.1–1.6)	10.2 (8.5–12.0)
Clinician intervention		
No counseling by a clinician	1.0	10.2
Counseling by a nonphysician clinician	1.7 (1.3–2.1)	15.8 (12.8–18.8)
Counseling by a physician	2.2 (1.5–3.2)	19.9 (13.7–26.2)
Format of smoking cessation counseling		
No format	1.0	10.8
Self-help	1.2 (1.0–1.3)	12.3 (10.9–13.6)
Proactive telephone counseling[c]	1.2 (1.1–1.4)	13.1 (11.4–14.8)
Group counseling	1.3 (1.1–1.6)	13.9 (11.6–16.1)
Individual counseling	1.7 (1.4–2.0)	16.8 (14.7–19.1)
Pharmacotherapy interventions		
Placebo	1.0	13.8
First-line agents		
Bupropion SR	2.0 (1.8–2.2)	24.2 (22.2–26.4)
Nicotine gum (6–14 weeks)	1.5 (1.2–1.7)	19.0 (16.5–21.9)
Nicotine inhaler	2.1 (1.5–2.9)	24.8 (19.1–31.6)
Nicotine lozenge (2 mg)	2.0 (1.4–2.8)	24.2[d]
Nicotine patch (6–14 weeks)	1.9 (1.7–2.2)	23.4 (21.3–25.8)
Nicotine nasal spray	2.3 (1.7–3.0)	26.7 (21.5–32.7)
Varenicline (2 mg/day)	3.1 (2.5–3.8)	33.2 (28.9–37.8)
Second-line agents[e]		
Clonidine	2.1 (1.2–3.7)	25.0 (15.7–37.3)
Nortriptyline	1.8 (1.3–2.6)	22.5 (16.8–29.4)
Combination therapy		
Nicotine patch (> 14 weeks) + *ad lib* NRT (gum or nasal spray)	3.6 (2.5–5.2)	36.5 (28.6–45.3)
Nicotine patch + bupropion SR	2.5 (1.9–3.4)	28.9 (23.5–35.1)
Nicotine patch + nortriptyline	2.3 (1.3–4.2)	27.3 (17.2–40.4)
Nicotine patch + nicotine inhaler	2.2 (1.3–3.6)	25.8 (17.4–36.5)

[a] Estimated relative to referent group.
[b] Abstinence percentages for specified treatment method.
[c] A quitline that responds to incoming calls and makes outbound follow-up calls. Following an initial request by the smoker or via a fax-to-quit program, the clinician initiates telephone contact to counsel the patient.
[d] One qualifying randomized trial; 95% CI not reported in 2008 Clinical Practice Guideline.
[e] Not approved by the U.S. Food and Drug Administration as a smoking cessation aid; recommended by the USPHS Guideline as a second-line agent for treating tobacco use and dependence.
Reprinted from reference 32, with permission.

follow-up care. These steps are referred to as the "5 A's" and are described, in brief, as follows. Figure 85-2 can be used as a guide for structuring counseling interventions.

- ***Ask:*** Screening for tobacco use is essential and should be a routine component of clinical care. The following question can be used to identify tobacco users: *"Do you ever smoke or use any type of tobacco?"* At a minimum, tobacco use status (current, former, never user) and level of use (e.g., number of cigarettes smoked per day) should be assessed and documented in the medical record. Also, consider asking patients about exposure to secondhand smoke.
- ***Advise:*** All tobacco users should be advised to quit; the advice should be clear and compelling, yet delivered with sensitivity and a tone of voice that communicates concern and a willingness to assist with quitting. When possible, messages should be personalized by relating advice to factors such as a patient's health status, medication regimen, personal reasons for wanting to quit, or the impact of tobacco use on others. For example, *"Ms. Crosby, I see that you now are on two different inhalers. It's important that you know that quitting smoking is the single most important treatment for your emphysema. I strongly encourage you to quit, and I would like to help you."*
- ***Assess:*** Key to the provision of appropriate counseling interventions is the assessment of a patient's readiness to quit. Patients should be categorized as being (a) not ready to quit in the next month; (b) ready to quit in the next month; (c) a recent quitter, having quit in the past 6 months; or (d) a former user, having quit more than 6 months ago.[7,42] This classification defines the clinician's next step, which is to provide counseling that is tailored to the patient's level of readiness to quit. As an example for a current smoker: *"Mr. Malkin, are you considering quitting, maybe sometime in the next*

STEP One: ASK about Tobacco Use

➲ Suggested Dialogue

- "Do you ever smoke or use any type of tobacco?"
- "I take time to talk with all of my patients about tobacco use—because it's important."
- "Medication X often is used for conditions linked with or caused by smoking. Do you, or does someone in your household smoke?"
- "Condition X often is caused or worsened by exposure to tobacco smoke. Do you, or does someone in your household smoke?"

STEP Two: Strongly ADVISE to Quit

Advice should be clear, strong, and personalized yet delivered sensitively, with a tone conveying concern for the patient's health and a sincere commitment to help with quitting.

➲ Suggested Dialogue

- "It's important that you quit as soon as possible, and I can help you."
- "I realize that quitting is difficult. It is the most important thing you can do to protect your health now and in the future. I have training to help my patients quit, and when you are ready I will work with you to design a specialized treatment plan."

STEP Three: ASSESS Readiness to Quit

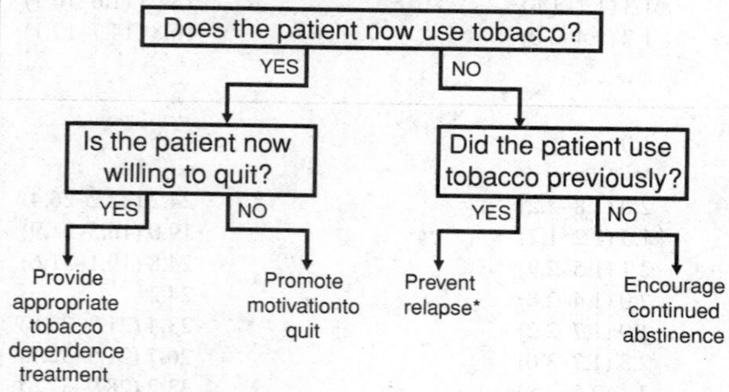

* Relapse prevention interventions not necessary in the case of the adult who has not used to bacco for many years.

Fiore MC, Jaen CR, Baker TB, et al. Treating Tobacco Use and Dependence: 2008 Update. Clinical Practice Guideline. Rockville, MD: U.S. Department of Health and Human Services, Public Health Service. May 2008.

STEP Four: ASSIST with Quitting

✓ **Assess Tobacco Use History**
- Current use: type(s) of tobacco used, brand, amount
- Past use:
  - Duration of tobacco use
  - Changes in levels of use recently
- Past quit attempts:
  - Number of attempts, date of most recent attempt, duration
  - Methods used previously—What did or didn't work? Why or why not?
  - Prior medication administration, dose, compliance, duration of treatment
  - Reasons for relapse

✓ **Discuss Key Issues** (for the upcoming or current quit attempt)
- Reasons/motivation for wanting to quit (or avoid relapse)
- Confidence in ability to quit (or avoid relapse)
- Triggers for tobacco use
- Routines and situations associated with tobacco use
- Stress-related tobacco use
- Social support for quitting
- Concerns about weight gain
- Concerns about withdrawal symptoms

✓ **Facilitate Quitting Process**
- Discuss methods for quitting: pros and cons of the different methods
- Set a quit date: more than 2–3 days away but less than 2 weeks away
- Recommend completion of a Tobacco Use Log
- Discuss coping strategies (cognitive, behavioral) for key issues
- Discuss withdrawal symptoms
- Discuss concept of "slip" versus relapse
- Provide medication counseling: compliance, proper use, with demonstration
- Offer to assist throughout the quit attempt

✓ **Evaluate the Quit Attempt** (at follow-up)
- Status of attempt
- Inquire about "slips" and relapse
- Medication compliance and plans for discontinuation

STEP Five: ARRANGE Follow-up Counseling

✓ Monitor patients' progress throughout the quit attempt. Follow-up contact should occur during the first week after quitting. A second follow-up contact is recommended in the first month. Additional contacts should be scheduled as needed. Counseling contacts can occur face-to-face, by telephone, or by e-mail. Keep patient progress notes.

✓ Address temptations and triggers; discuss relapse prevention strategies.

✓ Congratulate patients for continued success.

FIGURE 85-2 Tobacco Cessation Counseling Guide Sheet. *Source:* Reprinted from reference 32, with permission.

month?" The counseling interventions for patients who are ready to quit will be different from those for patients who are not considering quitting.

- *Assist:* When counseling tobacco users, it is important that clinicians view quitting as a process that might take months or even years to achieve, rather than a "now or never" event. The goal is to promote "forward progress" in the process of change, with the target end point being sustained abstinence.

When counseling patients who are not ready to quit, an important first step is to promote motivation. Some patients who are not ready to quit truly might not believe that they need to quit; however, most will recognize the need to quit but are simply not ready to make the commitment to do so. Often, patients have tried to quit multiple times, and failed, and thus are too discouraged to try again. Strategies for working with patients who are not ready to quit involves promoting motivation to quit, and this can be accomplished by applying the "5 R's"[7] (Table 85-5) and by offering to work closely with the patient in designing a treatment plan. Although it might be useful to educate patients about the pharmacotherapy options, it is inappropriate to prescribe a treatment regimen for patients who are not ready to quit. For patients who are not ready to quit, encourage them to seriously consider quitting by asking the following series of three questions:

1. *Do you ever plan to quit?*
   Most patients will respond "yes," in which case the clinician should continue with question 2. If they respond "no," the clinician should strongly advise the patient to quit and offer to assist, if the patient changes his or her mind.
2. *How would it benefit you to quit later, as opposed to now?*
   Most patients will agree that there is never an ideal time to quit, and procrastinating a quit date has more negative effects than positive.
3. *What is the worst thing that would happen if you were to quit now?*
   This question probes patients' perceptions of quitting, which reveals some of the barriers to quitting that can then be addressed by the clinician.

For patients who are ready to quit (i.e., in the next month), the goal is to work with the patient in designing an individualized treatment plan, addressing the key issues listed under the "Assist" component of Figure 85-2.[32] Except when medically contraindicated or with specific populations for which there is insufficient evidence of effectiveness, patients should be encouraged to use pharmacotherapy (described later in this chapter) in combination with a behavioral intervention.[7] The first steps are to discuss the patient's tobacco use history, inquiring about levels of smoking, number of years smoked, methods

Table 85-5 Enhancing Motivation to Quit: The "5 R's" for Tobacco Cessation Counseling[7]

- **Relevance**—Encourage patients to think about the reasons why quitting is important. Counseling should be framed such that it relates to the patient's risk for disease or exacerbation of disease, family or social situations (e.g., having children with asthma), health concerns, age, or other patient factors, such as prior experience with quitting.
- **Risks**—Ask patients to identify potential negative health consequences of smoking, such as acute risks (shortness of breath, asthma exacerbations, harm to pregnancy, infertility), long-term risks (cancer, cardiac, and pulmonary disease), and environmental risks (promoting smoking among children by being a negative role model; effects of second-hand smoke on others, including children and pets).
- **Rewards**—Ask patients to identify potential benefits that they anticipate from quitting, such as improved health, enhanced physical performance, enhanced taste and smell, reduced expenditures for tobacco, less time wasted or work missed, reduced health risks to others (fetus, children, housemates), and reduced aging of the skin.
- **Roadblocks**—Help patients identify barriers to quitting and assist in developing coping strategies (Table 85-6) for addressing each barrier. Common barriers include nicotine withdrawal symptoms (Table 85-7), fear of failure, a need for social support while quitting, depression, weight gain, and a sense of deprivation or loss.
- **Repetition**—Continue to work with patients who are successful in their quit attempt. Discuss circumstances in which smoking occurred to identify the trigger(s) for relapse; this is part of the learning process and will be useful information for the next quit attempt. Repeat interventions when possible.

used previously for quitting (what worked, what did not work and why), and reasons for previous failed quit attempts. Clinicians should elicit patients' opinions about the different pharmacotherapies for quitting and should work with patients in selecting the quitting methods (e.g., medications, behavioral counseling programs). Although it is important to recognize that pharmaceutical agents might not be appropriate, desirable, or affordable for all patients, clinicians should educate patients that medications, when taken correctly, can substantially increase the likelihood of success by making them more comfortable while quitting.

Patients should be advised to select a quit date that is more than 3 days but less than 2 weeks away. This time frame provides patients with sufficient time to prepare for the quit attempt, including mental preparation, as well as preparation of the environment, such as by removing all tobacco products and ashtrays from the home, car, and workspace and informing their family, friends, and coworkers about their upcoming quit attempt and requesting their support. Additional strategies for coping with quitting are shown in Table 85-6.[32] Patients should be counseled about coping with withdrawal symptoms (Table 85-7)[32] and medication use and compliance, and it is crucial to emphasize the importance of receiving behavioral counseling throughout the quit attempt. Finally, patients should be commended for taking important steps toward improving their health.

- ***Arrange:*** Because patients' ability to quit increases when multiple counseling interactions are provided, arranging follow-up counseling is an important, yet typically neglected, element of treatment for tobacco dependence. Follow-up contact should occur soon after the quit date, preferably during the first week. A second follow-up contact is recommended within the first month after quitting.[7] Periodically, additional follow-up contacts should occur to monitor patient progress, assess compliance with pharmacotherapy regimens, and provide additional support.

Relapse prevention counseling should be part of every follow-up contact with patients who have recently quit smoking. When counseling recent quitters, it is important to address challenges in countering withdrawal symptoms (Table 85-7)[32] and cravings or temptations to use tobacco. A list of strategies for key triggers or temptations for tobacco use is provided in Table 85-6.[32] Importantly, because tobacco use is a habitual behavior, patients should be advised to alter their daily routines; this helps disassociate specific behaviors from the use of tobacco. Patients who slip and smoke a cigarette (or use any form of tobacco) or experience a full relapse back to habitual tobacco use should be encouraged to think through the scenario in which tobacco use first occurred and identify the trigger(s) for relapse. This process provides valuable information for future quit attempts.

TELEPHONE QUITLINES

Clinicians should become aware of local, community-based resources for tobacco cessation, including telephone quitlines. When time or expertise do not afford provision of comprehensive tobacco cessation counseling during a patient visit, clinicians are encouraged to apply a truncated 5 A's model, whereby they *Ask* about tobacco use, *Advise* tobacco users to quit, and *Refer* patients to quit to a telephone quitline. This generally can be accomplished in less than one minute. Telephone services that provide tobacco cessation counseling have proliferated since the late 1990s; these services provide low-cost interventions that can reach patients who might otherwise have limited access to medical treatment because of geographic location or lack of insurance or financial resources. In clinical trials, telephone counseling services for which at least some of the contacts are initiated by the quit line counselor have been shown to be effective in promoting abstinence,[7] and these positive results have been shown to translate into real world effectiveness.[41] The addition of medication to quitline counseling significantly improves abstinence rates compared to medication alone.[7] In addition, preliminary evidence suggests that quitlines are also effective for smokeless tobacco cessation.[43] The telephone number for the tollfree tobacco quitline is 1-800-QUIT NOW. In some states, clinicians can submit a fax referral form, on behalf of a patient, to the quitline. This form initiates a process whereby a quitline counselor then contacts the patient directly.

Pharmacotherapy Options

All smokers who are trying to quit should be encouraged to use one or more U.S. Food and Drug Administration (FDA)-approved pharmacologic aids for cessation; potential exceptions that require special consideration include medical contraindications or use in specific populations for which there is insufficient evidence of effectiveness (i.e., pregnant women, smokeless tobacco users, light smokers, adolescents).[7]

Table 85-6 Cognitive and Behavioral Strategies for Tobacco Cessation

Cognitive strategies	
Focus on *retraining the way a patient thinks*. Often, patients mentally deliberate on the fact that they are thinking about a cigarette, and this leads to relapse. Patients must recognize that thinking about a cigarette does not mean they need to have one.	
Review commitment to quit, focus on downside of tobacco	Reminding oneself that cravings and temptations are temporary and will pass. Have patient announce, either silently or aloud, "I want to be a nonsmoker, and the temptation will pass."
Distractive thinking	Deliberate, immediate refocusing of thinking when cued by thoughts about tobacco use.
Positive self-talks, "pep talks"	Saying "I can do this" and reminding oneself of previous difficult situations in which tobacco use was avoided with success.
Relaxation through imagery	Centering of mind toward positive, relaxing thoughts.
Mental rehearsal, visualization	Preparing for situations that might arise by envisioning how best to handle them. For example, a patient might envision what would happen if he or she were offered a cigarette by a friend—the patient would mentally craft and rehearse a response, and perhaps even practice it by saying it aloud.
Behavioral strategies	
Involve *specific actions to reduce risk for relapse*. For maximal effectiveness, these should be considered prior to quitting, after determining patient-specific triggers for tobacco use. Here, we list some behavioral strategies for several common cues or triggers for relapse.	
Stress	Anticipate upcoming challenges at work, at school, or in personal life. Develop a substitute plan for tobacco use during times of stress (e.g., deep breathing, take a break/leave the situation, call supportive friend or family member, self-massage, use nicotine replacement therapy).
Alcohol	Drinking alcohol can lead to relapse. Patient should consider limiting/abstaining from alcohol during the early stages of quitting.
Other tobacco users	Quitting is more difficult if the patient is around other tobacco users. This is especially difficult if there is another tobacco user in the household. Patients should limit prolonged contact with individuals who are using tobacco during the early stages of quitting. Ask coworkers, friends, and housemates not to smoke or use tobacco in their presence.
Oral gratification needs	Have nontobacco oral substitutes (e.g., gum, sugarless candy, straws, toothpicks, lip balm, toothbrush, nicotine replacement therapy, bottled water) readily available.
Automatic smoking routines	Anticipate routines that are associated with tobacco use and develop an alternative plan. Examples: *Morning coffee with cigarettes:* change morning routine, drink tea instead of coffee, take shower before drinking coffee, take a brisk walk shortly after awakening. *Smoking while driving:* remove all tobacco from car, have car interior detailed, listen to a book on tape or talk radio, use oral substitute. *Smoking while on the phone:* stand while talking, limit call duration, change phone location, keep hands occupied by doodling or sketching. *Smoking after meals:* get up and immediately do dishes or take a brisk walk after eating, call supportive friend.
Postcessation weight gain	The majority of tobacco users gain weight after quitting. Most quitters will gain <10 lb, but there is a broad range of weight gain reported, with up to 10% of quitters gaining as much as 30 lb. Advise patient not to attempt to modify multiple behaviors at one time. If weight gain is a barrier to quitting, advise patient to engage in regular physical activity and adhere to a healthful diet (as opposed to strict dieting). Carefully plan and prepare meals, increase fruit and water intake to create a feeling of fullness, and chew sugarless gum or eat sugarless candies. Consider use of pharmacotherapy shown to delay weight gain (e.g., the 4-mg nicotine gum or lozenge or bupropion SR).
Cravings for tobacco	Cravings for tobacco are temporary and usually pass within 5–10 minutes. Handle cravings through distractive thinking, take a break, change activities/tasks, take deep breaths, or perform self-massage.

Adapted from reference 32, with permission.

Table 85-7 Postcessation Withdrawal Symptoms

Symptoms	*Duration*
Chest tightness	A few days
Constipation, stomach pain, gas	1–2 weeks
Cough, dry throat, nasal drip	A few days
Craving for a cigarette	Frequent for 2–3 days; can persist for months or years
Difficulty concentrating	2–4 weeks
Dizziness	1–2 days
Fatigue	2–4 weeks
Hunger	Up to several weeks
Insomnia	1 week
Irritability	2–4 weeks

Adapted from reference 32, with permission.

Currently, the FDA-approved first-line agents[7] include five NRT dosage forms, sustained-release bupropion (bupropion SR), and varenicline. Pharmacologic agents that have not received FDA approval for smoking cessation but are recommended as second-line agents[7] include clonidine and nortriptyline.

The first approved medication for smoking cessation was the nicotine gum, which was marketed in 1984. This was later followed by the nicotine transdermal patch (prescription-only formulation in 1991 and nonprescription formulations in 1996), bupropion SR and nicotine nasal spray in 1996, the nicotine oral inhaler in 1997, the nicotine lozenge in 2002, and varenicline in 2006. Each product has been shown to be effective in promoting smoking cessation. Dosing information, precautions, and adverse effects for the first-line agents are shown in Table 85-8.

Table 85-8 Pharmacotherapy Options: Products, Precautions/Warnings and Contraindications Dosing, and Adverse Effects

NRT Formulations						
Gum	*Lozenge*	*Transdermal Patch*	*Nasal Spray*	*Oral Inhaler*	*Bupropion SR*	*Varenicline*
Product						
Nicorette,[a] Generic OTC 2 mg, 4 mg Original, cinnamon, fruit, mint (various), orange	**Commit,[a] Generic** OTC 2 mg, 4 mg Cherry, mint	**Nicoderm CQ,[a] Generic[b]** OTC (NicoDerm CQ, generic) Rx (generic) 7 mg, 14 mg, 21 mg (24-hour release)	**Nicotrol NS[c]** Rx Metered spray 0.5 mg nicotine in 50 μL aqueous nicotine solution	**Nicotrol Inhaler[c]** Rx 10 mg cartridge Delivers 4 mg inhaled nicotine vapor	**Zyban,[a] Generic** Rx 150 mg sustained-release tablet	**Chantix[c]** Rx 0.5 mg, 1 mg tablet
Precautions/Warnings and Contraindications						
• Recent (≤2 weeks) myocardial infarction • Serious underlying arrhythmias • Serious or worsening angina pectoris • Temporomandibular joint disease • Pregnancy category: not applicable for OTC formulations	• Recent (≤2 weeks) myocardial infarction • Serious underlying arrhythmias • Serious or worsening angina pectoris • Pregnancy category: not applicable for OTC formulations	• Recent (≤2 weeks) myocardial infarction • Serious underlying arrhythmias • Serious or worsening angina pectoris • Pregnancy category: D for prescription patch, not applicable for OTC formulations	• Recent (≤2 weeks) myocardial infarction • Serious underlying arrhythmias • Serious or worsening angina pectoris • Underlying chronic nasal disorders (rhinitis, nasal polyps, sinusitis) • Severe reactive airway disease • Pregnancy category: D	• Recent (≤2 weeks) myocardial infarction • Serious underlying arrhythmias • Serious or worsening angina pectoris • Bronchospastic disease • Pregnancy category: D	• Concomitant therapy with medications or medical conditions known to lower seizure threshold • Severe hepatic cirrhosis • Pregnancy category: C **Contraindications:** • Seizure disorder • Concomitant bupropion (e.g., Wellbutrin) therapy • Current or prior diagnosis of bulimia or anorexia nervosa • Simultaneous abrupt discontinuation of alcohol or sedatives (including benzodiazepines) • Monoamine oxidase inhibitor therapy in previous 14 days	• Severe renal impairment (dosage adjustment is necessary) • Neuropsychiatric symptoms (behavior changes, agitation, depressed mood, suicidal ideation or behavior) • Safety and efficacy have not been established in patients with serious psychiatric illness • Pregnancy category: C

(continued)

Table 85-8 Pharmacotherapy Options: Products, Precautions, Dosing, and Adverse Effects *(Continued)*

	NRT Formulations					
Gum	*Lozenge*	*Transdermal Patch*	*Nasal Spray*	*Oral Inhaler*	*Bupropion SR*	*Varenicline*
Dosing						
≥25 cigarettes/day: 4 mg *<25 cigarettes/day:* 2 mg Weeks 1–6: 1 piece Q 1–2 hr Weeks 7–9: 1 piece Q 2–4 hr Weeks 10–12: 1 piece Q 4–8 hr • Maximum, 24 pieces/day • Chew each piece slowly • Park between cheek and gum when peppery or tingling sensation appears (~15–30 chews) • Resume chewing when taste or tingle fades • Repeat chew/park steps until most of nicotine is gone (taste or tingle does not return; generally 30 minutes) • Park in different areas of mouth • No food or beverages 15 minutes before or during use • Duration: up to 12 weeks	*First cigarette ≤30 minutes after waking:* 4 mg *First cigarette >30 minutes after waking:* 2 mg Weeks 1–6: 1 lozenge Q 1–2 hr Weeks 7–9: 1 lozenge Q 2–4 hr Weeks 10–12: 1 lozenge Q 4–8 hr • Maximum, 20 lozenges/day • Allow to dissolve slowly (20–30 minutes) • Nicotine release may cause a warm, tingling sensation • Do not chew or swallow • Occasionally rotate to different areas of the mouth • No food or beverages 15 minutes before or during use • Duration: up to 12 weeks	*>10 cigarettes/day:* 21 mg/day × 4 weeks (generic) × 6 weeks (Nicoderm CQ) 14 mg/day × 2 weeks 7 mg/day × 2 weeks *≤10 cigarettes/day:* 14 mg/day × 6 weeks 7 mg/day × 2 weeks • May wear patch for 16 hours if patient experiences sleep disturbances (remove at bedtime) • Duration: 8–10 weeks	1–2 doses/hr (8–40 doses/day) One dose = 2 sprays (one in *each* nostril); each spray delivers 0.5 mg of nicotine to the nasal mucosa • Maximum – 5 doses/hr – 40 doses/day • For best results, initially use at least 8 doses/day • Patients should not sniff, swallow, or inhale through the nose as the spray is being administered • Duration: 3–6 months	6–16 cartridges/day Individualize dosing; initially use 1 cartridge Q 1–2 hr • Best effects with continuous puffing for 20 minutes • Nicotine in cartridge is depleted after 20 minutes of active puffing • Patient should inhale into back of throat or puff in short breaths • Do NOT inhale into the lungs (like a cigarette) but "puff" as if lighting a pipe • Open cartridge retains potency for 24 hours • Duration: up to 6 months	150 mg PO Q am × 3 days, then increase to 150 mg PO BID • Do not exceed 300 mg/day • Treatment should be initiated while patient is still smoking • Set quit date 1–2 weeks *after* initiation of therapy • Allow at least 8 hours between doses • Avoid bedtime dosing to minimize insomnia • Dose tapering is not necessary • Can be used safely with NRT • Duration: 7–12 weeks, with maintenance up to 6 months in selected patients	Days 1–3: 0.5 mg PO Q am Days 4–7: 0.5 mg PO BID Weeks 2–12: 1 mg PO BID • Patients should begin therapy 1 week prior to quit date • Take dose after eating with a full glass of water • Dose tapering is not necessary • Nausea and insomnia are usually temporary side effects • Duration: 12 weeks; an additional 12-week course may be used in selected patients
Adverse Effects						
• Mouth/jaw soreness • Hiccups • Dyspepsia • Hypersalivation • Effects associated with incorrect chewing technique: – Lightheadedness – Nausea/vomiting – Throat and mouth irritation	• Nausea • Hiccups • Cough • Heartburn • Headache • Flatulence • Insomnia	• Local skin reactions (erythema, pruritus, burning) • Headache • Sleep disturbances (insomnia, abnormal/vivid dreams); associated with nocturnal nicotine absorption	• Nasal and/or throat irritation (hot, peppery, or burning sensation) • Rhinitis • Tearing • Sneezing • Cough • Headache	• Mouth and/or throat irritation • Unpleasant taste • Cough • Rhinitis • Dyspepsia • Hiccups • Headache	• Insomnia • Dry mouth • Nervousness/difficulty concentrating • Rash • Constipation • Seizures (risk is 1/1,000 [0.1%])	• Nausea • Sleep disturbances (insomnia, abnormal/vivid dreams) • Constipation • Flatulence • Vomiting • Neuropsychiatric symptoms (rare; see PRECAUTIONS)

[a]Marketed by GlaxoSmithKline.
[b]Transdermal patch formulation previously marketed as Habitrol.
[c]Marketed by Pfizer.
NRT, nicotine replacement therapy; OTC, over the counter (nonprescription); Rx, prescription.
For complete prescribing information, refer to the manufacturers' package inserts.
Adapted from reference 32.

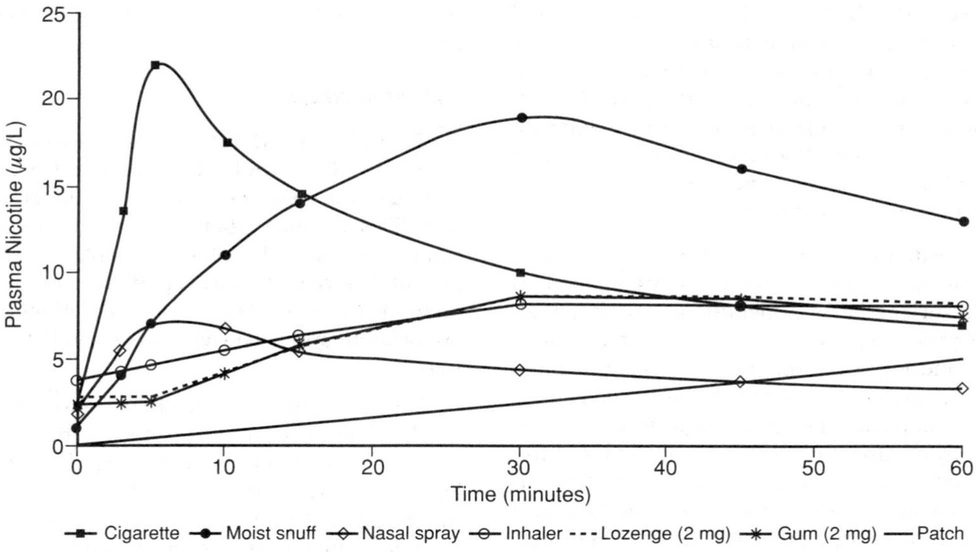

FIGURE 85-3 Plasma nicotine concentrations for various nicotine-containing products. *Source:* Reprinted from reference 32, with permission. Copyright © 1999–2008 The Regents of the University of California, University of Southern California, and Western University of Health Sciences. All rights reserved. Plasma nicotine concentration curves derived from references 52, 66, and 127.

First-Line Agents

NICOTINE REPLACEMENT THERAPY

NRT increases success for quitting by reducing the physical withdrawal symptoms associated with tobacco cessation while the patient focuses on modifying his or her behavior and coping with the psychological aspects of quitting. In addition, because the onset of action for NRT is not as rapid as that of nicotine obtained through smoking, patients become less accustomed to the nearly immediate, reinforcing effects of inhaled tobacco. A meta-analysis of 111 controlled trials, enrolling more than 43,000 participants, found that all NRT formulations (gum, inhaler, lozenge, patch, and nasal spray) result in statistically significant improvements in abstinence rates when compared with placebo. Patients using NRT are 1.6 times as likely to quit smoking than are those receiving placebo.[44] Figure 85-3 depicts the concentration time curves for the various NRT formulations, compared with a cigarette and moist snuff (a form of smokeless tobacco). It can be seen that of the five NRT dosage forms, the nicotine nasal spray reaches its peak concentration most rapidly. The nicotine gum, lozenge, and oral inhaler have similar concentration curves, and the nicotine transdermal patch has the slowest onset, but offers more consistent blood levels of nicotine over a sustained period of time.

BUPROPION SR

Bupropion SR is an atypical antidepressant medication hypothesized to promote smoking cessation by blocking the reuptake of dopamine and norepinephrine in the central nervous system and possibly by acting as a nicotine receptor antagonist. These neurochemical effects are believed to modulate the dopamine reward pathway and reduce cravings for nicotine and symptoms of withdrawal.[7] Use of bupropion SR approximately doubles the long-term abstinence rate when compared with placebo.[7,45]

VARENICLINE

Varenicline is a partial agonist, highly selective for the $\alpha 4\beta 2$ nicotinic acetylcholine receptor.[46] The efficacy of varenicline in smoking cessation is believed to be the result of sustained, low-level agonist activity at the receptor site combined with competitive inhibition of nicotine binding. The partial agonist activity induces modest receptor stimulation leading to increased dopamine levels that attenuate the symptoms of nicotine withdrawal. In addition, by competitively blocking the binding of nicotine to nicotinic acetylcholine receptors in the central nervous system, varenicline inhibits the surges of dopamine release that occur immediately following inhalation of tobacco smoke. The latter mechanism may be effective in preventing relapse by reducing the pleasure associated with smoking.[47] A recent meta-analysis has found that varenicline (2 mg/day) more than triples the likelihood of long-term abstinence from smoking relative to placebo.[7]

Second-Line Agents

Although not FDA-approved specifically for smoking cessation, the prescription medications clonidine and nortriptyline are recommended as second-line agents.[7] Lack of an FDA-approved indication for smoking cessation and side effect profiles currently prohibit these agents from achieving first-line classification.[7]

PHARMACOTHERAPY FOR TREATING TOBACCO USE AND DEPENDENCE

Transdermal Nicotine Patch

1. T.B. is a 32-year-old woman who is enrolled in a worksite smoking cessation program. During the previous group session, the cessation counselor discussed the various medications for

cessation. T.B. has set her quit date for 1 week from today, and she is interested in starting the nicotine transdermal patch. She is currently smoking 1 pack per day (PPD), which is a reduction from the 1.5 PPD she had been smoking for the past 10 years. T.B. reports she smokes several cigarettes in succession immediately after waking in the morning. She takes no medications and has no medical problems. Which nicotine transdermal product should T.B. select, and how should it be used?

Two different transdermal nicotine patch systems are currently marketed. Transdermal nicotine delivery systems consist of an impermeable surface layer, a nicotine reservoir, an adhesive layer, and a removable protective liner. The technology for delivery of nicotine across the skin varies by manufacturer. NicoDerm CQ uses a rate-controlling membrane. The generic patches (previously marketed as Habitrol) use drug-dispersion-type systems whereby release of nicotine is controlled by diffusion of the drug across an adhesive layer.[48] The currently marketed formulations (which continuously release nicotine over 24 hours) deliver nicotine more slowly than the gum, lozenge, nasal spray, and inhaler (Fig. 85-3). Plasma nicotine levels obtained via transdermal delivery are approximately 50% lower than those achieved with cigarette smoking but still alleviate the symptoms of withdrawal.[49]

The efficacy of the transdermal nicotine patch is well documented with significantly improved abstinence rates relative to placebo (Table 85-4).[7,44] A meta-analysis of 25 randomized, controlled trials found treatment with the nicotine patch (6–14 weeks) approximately doubled the likelihood of long-term abstinence compared to placebo.[7]

Dosing

The manufacturers' recommended dosages are listed in Table 85-8. In general, higher levels of smoking necessitate the use of higher-strength formulations and a longer duration of therapy. Ultimately, the starting dose, rate of tapering, and total duration of therapy must be individualized to the patient's baseline smoking levels, development of side effects (e.g., nausea, dyspepsia, nervousness, dizziness, sweating), and the presence or absence of withdrawal symptoms (Table 85-7). T.B. currently smokes 20 cigarettes per day, and thus she should initiate the regimen using the 21-mg/day patch.

Patient Education

Regardless of the product selected, T.B. should be instructed to apply the patch to a clean, dry, hairless area of skin on the upper body or the upper outer part of her arm at approximately the same time each day. To minimize the potential for local skin reactions, the patch application site should be rotated daily, and the same area should not be used again for at least 1 week. After patch application, T.B. should ensure that the patch adheres well to the skin, especially around the edges. The clinician should reassure T.B. that water will not reduce the effectiveness of the nicotine patch if it is applied correctly, and she may bathe, shower, swim, or exercise while wearing the patch. Finally, T.B. should be advised to discontinue use of the nicotine patch and contact a health care provider if skin redness caused by the patch does not resolve after 4 days, if the skin swells or a rash develops; if irregular heartbeat or palpitations occur; or if she experiences symptoms of nicotine overdose such as nausea, vomiting, dizziness, diarrhea, sweating, weakness, or rapid heartbeat.

Adverse Reactions

2. Ten days later, T.B. calls to complain of an itchy rash that she believes is caused by the nicotine patch. She noticed the rash yesterday when she removed the first patch from her left upper arm. This morning, after removing the second patch from her right upper arm, she noticed a similar rash. T.B. describes the skin on her right arm as slightly red but not swollen; the rash on her left arm has only a faint trace of pink discoloration. Her last cigarette was 2 days ago. How should T.B. be managed at this time?

The most common side effects associated with the nicotine patch are local reactions (erythema, burning, and pruritus) at the skin application site. These reactions are generally caused by skin occlusion or sensitivity to the patch adhesives. Rotating the patch application sites on a daily basis minimizes skin irritation; nonetheless, skin reactions to the patch adhesives occur in up to 50% of patch users. Less than 5% of patients discontinue therapy because of a skin reaction.[7] T.B. appears to be experiencing a mild skin reaction and should be reassured that it is normal for the skin to appear erythematous for up to 24 to 48 hours after the patch is removed. T.B. can apply topical hydrocortisone cream (0.5% or 1%) or triamcinolone cream (0.5%), or can take an oral antihistamine for symptomatic treatment.[7] Because the rash on her left arm has nearly resolved, it is reasonable for T.B. to continue using the nicotine transdermal patch provided that the erythema is not too bothersome.

Other less common side effects associated with the transdermal nicotine patch include vivid or abnormal dreams, insomnia, and headache. Sleep disturbances likely result from nocturnal nicotine absorption. Patients experiencing troublesome sleep disturbances should be instructed to remove the patch prior to bedtime and apply a new patch as soon as possible after waking the following morning.[7]

The clinician should also provide behavioral counseling support by asking T.B. about the current quit attempt. Appropriate issues to address include her confidence in remaining tobacco free, situations in which she has been tempted to smoke and potential triggers for relapse, nicotine withdrawal symptoms, her social support system for quitting, and any other questions or concerns she might have. It is reasonable to review potential coping strategies (behavioral and cognitive; Table 85-6) and schedule a future follow-up call. The clinician should commend T.B. for her decision to quit, congratulate her for remaining tobacco free for 48 hours, and reassure her that skin irritation is a common, yet generally manageable, complication with the nicotine patch.

Product Selection Considerations

The primary advantage of the transdermal nicotine patch compared with other NRT formulations is that the patch is easy to use and conceal, releases a continuous dose of nicotine throughout the day, and requires administration only once daily. As a result, patients who have difficulty adhering to regimens that require taking multiple doses of medications throughout the day or those who want a simplified regimen are likely to be more successful with the nicotine patch. Disadvantages of the patch include a high incidence of skin irritation associated with the patch adhesives and the inability to acutely adjust the dose of nicotine to alleviate symptoms of withdrawal. Finally, patients with underlying dermatologic conditions (e.g., psoriasis, eczema, atopic dermatitis) should not use the patch because they are more likely to experience skin irritation.[7]

Nicotine Gum

3. T.B. would like to discontinue the nicotine transdermal patch. She wants to know if the gum is an effective alternative.

Nicotine polacrilex gum is a resin complex of nicotine and polacrilin in a chewing gum base that allows for slow release and absorption of nicotine across the oral mucosa. The product is available as 2- and 4-mg strengths, in multiple flavors (regular, cinnamon, fruit, mint, and orange). The gum has a distinct, tobacco-like, slightly peppery, minty, or fruity taste and contains buffering agents (sodium carbonate and sodium bicarbonate) to increase the salivary pH, which enhances the buccal absorption of nicotine. The amount of nicotine absorbed from each piece is variable, but approximately 1.1 and 2.9 mg of nicotine are extracted from the 2- and 4-mg gum formulations, respectively.[50] Peak plasma concentrations of nicotine are achieved approximately 30 minutes after chewing a single piece of gum and then slowly decline thereafter (Fig. 85-3). Patients using short-term (6–14 weeks) or long-term (>14 weeks) treatment with nicotine gum are significantly more likely to remain abstinent compared to those receiving placebo (Table 85-4).[7]

Dosing

Table 85-8 outlines the manufacturer's recommended dosing schedule for the nicotine gum. Individuals who smoke <25 cigarettes per day should use the 2-mg strength, and those smoking more should use the 4-mg strength. During the initial 6 weeks of therapy, patients should use 1 piece of gum every 1 to 2 hours while awake. In general, this amounts to at least 9 pieces of gum daily. The "chew and park" method described here allows for the slow, consistent release of nicotine from the polacrilin resin. Patients can use additional pieces of gum (to the daily maximum of 24 pieces per day) if cravings occur between scheduled doses. In general, patients who smoke a greater number of cigarettes per day will require more nicotine gum to alleviate their cravings than will patients who smoke fewer cigarettes per day. It is preferable to use the gum on a fixed schedule of administration, tapering over 1 to 3 months rather than using it "as needed" to control cravings.[7]

Patient Education

Proper chewing technique is crucial when using the nicotine gum. Patients should be instructed to chew the gum slowly until a peppery, minty, or fruity taste, or a slight tingling sensation in the mouth is detected; this varies but generally occurs after about 15 chews. When the taste or tingling sensation is noted, the patient should "park" the gum between the cheek and gum to allow absorption of nicotine across the buccal mucosa. When the taste or tingling dissipates (generally after 1–2 minutes), the patient should resume chewing slowly. When the taste or tingle returns, the patient should stop chewing and park the gum in a different area in the mouth. Rotating the gum placement site within the mouth helps decrease the incidence of oral irritation. The chew/park steps should be repeated until most of the nicotine is extracted; this generally occurs after 30 minutes and becomes obvious when chewing no longer elicits the characteristic taste or tingling sensation.

Patients should be warned that the absorption and therefore effectiveness of nicotine gum might be reduced by acidic beverages (e.g., coffee, juices, wine, soft drinks),[51] which transiently reduce the salivary pH. To prevent this interaction, patients should be advised not to eat or drink (except water) for 15 minutes before or while using the nicotine gum.

Product Selection Considerations

Advantages of nicotine gum include the fact that this formulation may be used to satisfy oral cravings and the 4-mg strength might delay weight gain.[7] For these reasons, the gum may be particularly beneficial for patients who have weight gain concerns or for patients who report boredom as a trigger for smoking. The gum might also be advantageous for patients who desire flexibility in dosing and prefer the ability to self-regulate nicotine levels to manage withdrawal symptoms. Some patients may find that the viscous consistency of the gum makes it difficult to use because it sticks to dental work. Others may find it difficult or socially unacceptable to chew the gum so frequently. Nicotine gum should not be used by patients with temporomandibular joint (TMJ) conditions. Finally, to minimize adverse effects and derive maximal therapeutic benefit, it is imperative that patients use enough gum each day and use the correct chewing technique.

Nicotine Lozenge

4. How does the nicotine lozenge differ from the nicotine gum?

The nicotine polacrilex lozenge is a resin complex of nicotine and polacrilin in a sugarfree, light mint, or cherry-flavored lozenge. The product is available in 2- and 4-mg strengths, which are meant to be consumed like hard candy or other medicinal lozenges (e.g., sucked and moved from side to side in the mouth until fully dissolved). Because the nicotine lozenge dissolves completely, it delivers approximately 25% more nicotine than does an equivalent dose of nicotine gum.[52] Like the nicotine gum, the lozenge also contains buffering agents (sodium carbonate and potassium bicarbonate) to increase salivary pH, thereby enhancing buccal absorption of the nicotine. Peak nicotine concentrations of nicotine with the lozenge are achieved after 30 to 60 minutes of use and then slowly decline thereafter (Fig. 85-3). In a trial evaluating the formulation currently available in the United States, the nicotine lozenge approximately doubled the 6-month abstinence rates compared with placebo (23.9% vs. 12.3%).[53] A recent meta-analysis of five studies using either the nicotine lozenge (nicotine polacrilin) or sublingual tablet (not available in the United States) concluded that the odds of abstinence at 6 or more months was 2.0 with the tablet/lozenge relative to placebo (95% CI, 1.6–2.5).[44]

Dosing

Unlike other NRT formulations, which use the number of cigarettes smoked per day as the basis for dosing, the recommended dosage of the nicotine lozenge is based on the time to first cigarette (TTFC). Some experts believe that the best indicator of nicotine dependence is the need to smoke soon after waking.[54] Based on this method, people who smoke their first cigarette of the day within 30 minutes of waking are considered more highly dependent on nicotine than those who smoke their first cigarette more than 30 minutes after waking. Because the nicotine polacrilin lozenge has been studied using the TTFC as a dosage selector, the product is licensed for use in the following manner: Patients who smoke their first cigarette of the day within 30 minutes of waking should use the 4-mg strength lozenge, and patients who smoke their first cigarette of the day more than 30 minutes after waking should use the 2-mg strength lozenge. Patients are more likely to succeed if they use the lozenge on a fixed schedule rather than as needed. During the initial 6 weeks of therapy, patients should use 1 lozenge every 1 to 2 hours while awake. In general, this amounts to at least 9 lozenges daily. Patients can use additional lozenges (up to 5 lozenges in 6 hours or a maximum of 20 lozenges per day) if cravings occur between scheduled doses.

Patient Education

Similar to the gum, the nicotine lozenge is a specially formulated nicotine delivery system that must be used properly for optimal results. The lozenge should be allowed to dissolve slowly in the mouth; when nicotine is released from the polacrilin resin, a warm, tingling sensation may be experienced. The patient should occasionally rotate the lozenge to different areas of the mouth to reduce the potential for mucosal irritation. When used correctly, the lozenge should completely dissolve within 30 minutes. Patients should be counseled not to chew or swallow the lozenge because this increases the incidence of gastrointestinal-related side effects.

Because the nicotine in the lozenge is dissolved in saliva and absorbed through the buccal mucosa, patients should be cautioned that the effectiveness of the nicotine lozenge may be reduced by acidic beverages such as coffee, juices, wine, or soft drinks. As recommended for the nicotine gum, patients should be advised not to eat or drink (except water) for 15 minutes before or while using the nicotine lozenge.

Adverse Reactions

In general, the nicotine lozenge is well tolerated. The most common side effects include nausea, hiccups, cough, dyspepsia, headache, and flatulence. Patients who use more than one lozenge at a time, continuously use one lozenge after another, or chew or swallow the lozenge are more likely to experience dyspepsia or hiccups.

Product Selection Considerations

The nicotine lozenge is similar to the nicotine gum formulation in that it may be used to satisfy oral cravings, the 4-mg strength might delay weight gain,[7,53] and patients can self-titrate therapy to acutely manage withdrawal symptoms. Because the lozenge does not require chewing, many patients find this to be a more discrete nicotine delivery system. The disadvantages of the lozenge are the fact that it requires frequent dosing, and the gastrointestinal side effects (nausea, hiccups, and heartburn) may be bothersome.

Postcessation Weight Gain

5. T.B. is worried about gaining weight after she quits smoking. Is weight gain common after quitting, and if so, how can this be prevented?

Most tobacco users gain weight after quitting, and clinicians should neither deny the likelihood of weight gain nor minimize its significance.[7] For nearly all patients, the health risks associated with postcessation weight gain are negligible compared to the risks of continued smoking.

Studies suggest that most quitters gain less than 10 lb, but there is a broad range of weight gain reported, with up to 10% of quitters gaining as much as 30 lb.[7] In general, women tend to gain more weight than men. In a study of nearly 6,000 smokers who were followed up for 5 years after quitting, the average weight gain during the follow-up period was 19.2 and 16.7 lb among women and men, respectively.[55] For men and women, subgroups that are more likely to gain weight after quitting are African Americans, younger tobacco users (younger than 55 years), and heavier tobacco users (those smoking more than 25 cigarettes per day).

The weight-suppressing effects of tobacco are well known. However, the mechanisms to explain why most successful quitters gain weight are not completely understood. Smokers have been found to have an approximately 10% higher metabolic rate compared with nonsmokers.[56] In some studies, higher caloric intakes were documented after cessation.[57,58] The increased caloric intake may result from an increase in appetite, improved sense of taste, or a change in the hand-to-mouth ritual through the substitution of tobacco with food.

In general, a patient is less likely to be successful if he or she attempts to change multiple behaviors at once. For this reason, strict dieting to prevent weight gain, especially during the early stages of quitting, is generally not recommended.[7] T.B. should be counseled that the average weight gain of less than 10 lb is less detrimental to her overall health than is continued smoking. Because she is concerned about weight gain, it is reasonable for the clinician to recommend that T.B. engage in some form of regular physical activity. Even modest physical activity (e.g., walking 30 minutes daily) has been found to attenuate the weight gain associated with smoking cessation.[58] Although strict dieting is not recommended, T.B. should carefully plan and prepare meals to avoid binge eating, increase her water intake to create a feeling of fullness, chew sugarless gum, and limit alcohol consumption. Furthermore, T.B. may consider pharmacotherapy options that have been shown to delay weight gain—this would include the 4-mg nicotine gum or lozenge or bupropion SR.[7] It is important to note, however, that once the medication is terminated, the quitter gains, on average, an amount of weight that is comparable to that which would have been gained in the absence of medication.[7]

Relapse Back to Smoking

6. During a follow-up contact, the clinician learns that T.B. smoked half a pack of cigarettes at a party over the weekend

and has relapsed to her previous smoking levels after not having smoked for just over a month. How should the clinician respond?

The clinician should thank T.B. for being honest about her smoking and ask her to discuss the circumstances during which the smoking occurred. At the time of her smoking, where was she, who was she with, how did she get access to cigarettes, and how was she feeling at the time? What, specifically, were the triggers for her relapse (e.g., alcohol, depression, friends who were smoking around her)? It is important that the clinician help the patient to use this information as part of the learning process, but it also is important to focus on the "positive," such as T.B.'s ability to have remained tobacco free for more than 1 month. After being smoke free for more than 4 weeks, most physical effects of nicotine withdrawal have completely resolved, and thus, the relapse trigger for T.B. likely was psychological or situational and could be abated through application of effective coping techniques. After an informative discussion about the situation in which the smoking occurred, it is important that the clinician work with the patient in identifying strategies for avoiding relapse in the future (Table 85-6).

Smoking and Cardiovascular Disease

7. P.J. is a 62-year-old man admitted for an elective coronary artery bypass graft (CABG) procedure. His medical history is significant for angina, hypertension, dyslipidemia, peripheral vascular disease (PVD), and allergic rhinitis. He underwent a bilateral carotid endarterectomy procedure 2 years ago and had iliac artery angioplasty with stent placement 5 years ago for PVD. P.J.'s social history is significant for tobacco use (1.5–2 PPD) and alcohol (3–4 drinks/day). He is approximately 10 lb overweight. His preoperative laboratory results are significant for a total cholesterol of 270 mg/dL (desirable, <200), low-density lipoprotein cholesterol count (LDL-C) of 163 mg/dL (optimal, <70), high-density lipoprotein cholesterol count (HDL-C) of 35 mg/dL (low, <40), and triglycerides of 350 mg/dL (normal, <150). His medications before admission include atenolol 50 mg QD, aspirin 81 mg QD, isosorbide dinitrate 20 mg TID, atorvastatin 20 mg QD, fluticasone nasal spray (50 mcg/spray) 1 spray/nostril QD, and nitroglycerin 0.4 mg SL as needed. Which of P.J.'s chronic medical conditions may be caused or exacerbated by his tobacco use?

A wealth of evidence suggests that cigarette smoking is a major cause of cardiovascular disease and is responsible for approximately 138,000 premature cardiovascular-related deaths each year.[5] Smoking is known to accelerate the process of atherosclerosis, leading to chronic cardiovascular disorders, including coronary heart disease, cerebrovascular disease, PVD, aortic aneurysm, and congestive heart failure.[3] In addition, smoking greatly elevates the risk for acute cardiovascular events, including sudden death, myocardial infarction (MI), stroke, and reocclusion of coronary or peripheral vessels after graft surgery or angioplasty.[3,59]

There are numerous plausible pathophysiological mechanisms whereby tobacco smoking contributes to the development of cardiovascular disease. Oxidant gases and other compounds in tobacco smoke are believed to induce a hypercoagulable state characterized by increased platelet aggregation and thrombosis, which greatly increases the risk of MI and sudden death.[59,60] The carbon monoxide in smoke reduces the amount of oxygen available to tissues and organs, including myocardial tissue, and may reduce the ventricular fibrillation threshold.[59] Smoking may accelerate atherosclerosis through effects on serum lipids; smokers tend to have higher levels of total cholesterol, LDL-C, and triglycerides and lower HDL-C than nonsmokers.[3] Smoking increases the levels of inflammatory mediators (C-reactive protein, leukocytes, and fibrinogen), which may contribute to the development and progression of atherosclerosis.[61] Finally, smoking stimulates the release of neurotransmitters (e.g., epinephrine, norepinephrine) that increase myocardial workload and induce coronary vasoconstriction leading to ischemia, arrhythmias, and sudden death.[3,59]

P.J.'s hospital admission for a CABG procedure for coronary heart disease and angina, as well as previous procedures for peripheral vascular disease (angioplasty with stent placement) and cerebrovascular disease (bilateral carotid endarterectomy), are all conditions associated with chronic tobacco use. His elevated total cholesterol, LDL-C, and triglycerides and reduced HDL-C levels are consistent with smoking-induced dyslipidemia. Cigarette smoking in combination with P.J.'s other established cardiovascular risk factors (hypertension, dyslipidemia) have synergistically increased his risk for serious cardiovascular disease.[3,59] Fortunately, the effects of smoking on lipids, coagulation, myocardial workload, and coronary blood flow appear to be reversible, and P.J.'s risk of developing further cardiovascular-related complications will markedly decrease if he is able to quit smoking.[36,62] The clinician should approach this hospitalization as an opportunity to motivate and assist P.J. with quitting smoking.[7] Furthermore, data suggest the initiation of intensive cessation counseling interventions in hospitalized patients is effective in achieving long-term abstinence.[63]

8. The cardiothoracic surgeon has strongly advised P.J. to quit smoking. P.J. is willing to quit completely, but he is worried because he has tried to quit smoking "hundreds of times" and has never been able to quit for longer than 1 week. He expresses a desire for a medication to assist him during this quit attempt. He has tried the nicotine gum and transdermal patch during three previous quit attempts. He did not like the gum because it made his jaw sore. He had temporary success with the nicotine patch but found it to be less flexible than the gum. For example, when he needed extra nicotine during stressful situations, he could not apply a second patch. What treatment alternatives are reasonable for P.J.?

P.J. has failed treatment with the nicotine gum and transdermal patch. First-line treatment options that he has not tried include the nicotine lozenge (see question 4), nicotine nasal spray, nicotine inhaler, bupropion SR, and varenicline. P.J. might also be a candidate for combination therapy (see question 10).

Nicotine Nasal Spray

The nicotine nasal spray is an aqueous solution of nicotine available in a metered-spray pump for administration to the nasal mucosa. Each actuation delivers a metered 50-mcL spray containing 0.5 mg of nicotine. Nicotine in the nasal spray is more rapidly absorbed than other NRT formulations (Fig. 85-3), with peak venous nicotine concentrations achieved within

11 to 18 minutes after administration.[24] Use of the nicotine nasal spray more than doubles long-term (>6 months) abstinence rates when compared to placebo (Table 85-4).[7,44]

Dosing

A dose of nicotine (1 mg) is administered as two sprays, one (0.5-mg spray) in *each* nostril. The recommended initial regimen is one to two doses every hour while awake for 6 to 8 weeks. This may be increased, as needed, to a maximum recommended dosage of five doses per hour or 40 mg/day. For best results, patients should be encouraged to use at least eight doses per day during the initial 6 to 8 weeks of therapy because less frequent administration may be less effective. After 6 to 8 weeks, the dose should be gradually decreased over an additional 4 to 6 weeks.

Patient Education

Before using the nasal spray for the first time, the nicotine nasal spray pump must be primed. This is done by actuating the device into a tissue until a fine spray is visible (about six to eight times). When administering a dose, the patient should tilt the head back slightly and insert the tip of the bottle into the nostril as far as is comfortable. After actuation of the pump, the patient should not sniff, swallow, or inhale through the nose because this increases the irritant effects of the spray. Patients should wait 5 minutes before driving or operating heavy machinery (because of the increased likelihood of tearing, coughing, and sneezing).

Adverse Reactions

Side effects commonly reported with the nicotine nasal spray include nasal and throat irritation (hot peppery sensation), sneezing, coughing, watery eyes, and rhinorrhea. In clinical trials, 94% of patients report moderate-severe nasal irritation during the first 2 days of therapy; 81% of patients still reported mild-moderate nasal irritation after 3 weeks of therapy.[7] Nasal congestion and transient changes in taste and smell have also been reported.[7] Despite the high incidence of local adverse effects, with regular use during the first week, most patients become tolerant to the irritant effects of the spray.[64]

Product Selection Considerations

The primary advantage in using the nicotine nasal spray is the ability to rapidly titrate therapy to manage withdrawal symptoms. However, because nicotine from the spray more rapidly penetrates the central nervous system, there may be higher likelihood of developing dependence during treatment. The nicotine nasal spray has a dependence potential intermediate between tobacco products and other NRT products. About 15% to 20% of patients continue to use the nicotine nasal spray for longer periods than recommended (6–12 months), and 5% use the spray at higher doses than recommended.[7] Individuals with chronic nasal disorders (e.g., rhinitis, polyps, sinusitis) or severe reactive airway disease should not use the nicotine nasal spray because of its irritant effects. Exacerbation of asthma has been reported after use of the nicotine nasal spray.[65]

Nicotine Inhaler

The nicotine inhaler consists of a two-piece plastic device designed to deliver nicotine contained in individual cartridges. Each foil-sealed cartridge contains a porous plug with 10 mg of nicotine and 1 mg of menthol. Menthol is added to reduce the irritant effect of nicotine. Plastic spikes located on the interior of both mouthpiece components pierce the protective foil covering on the cartridge, allowing the release of 4 mg of nicotine vapor following inhalation.

Given that the usual pack-a-day smoker repeats the hand-to-mouth motion up to 200 times per day or 73,000 times each year, it is not surprising that many smokers find they miss the physical manipulation of the cigarette and associated behaviors that accompany smoking. The nicotine inhaler was designed to provide nicotine replacement in a manner similar to smoking while addressing the sensory and ritualistic factors that are important to many patients who smoke.[66]

As a patient puffs on the inhaler, the nicotine vapor is delivered to the mouth and throat, where it is absorbed through the mucosa. Only a small amount (<5% of a dose) of nicotine reaches the lower respiratory tract.[67] With an intensive inhalation regimen (80 puffs over 20 minutes), about 4 mg of nicotine is delivered, and of that, 2 mg is absorbed.[68] Peak plasma nicotine concentrations with the inhaler are achieved after approximal 30 minutes of use[24] and then slowly decline thereafter (Fig. 85-3). Use of the nicotine inhaler approximately doubles long-term (>6 months) abstinence rates when compared to placebo (Table 85-4).[7,44]

Dosing

During the initial 3 to 6 weeks of treatment, the patient should use one cartridge every 1 to 2 hours while awake. This should be increased, as needed, to a maximum of 16 cartridges per day. In clinical trials, most successful quitters used an average of 6 to 16 cartridges per day. The manufacturer recommends that each cartridge be depleted of nicotine by frequent continuous puffing over 20 minutes. The recommended duration of treatment is 3 months, after which patients may be weaned from the inhaler by gradual reduction of the daily dose over the following 6 to 12 weeks.

Patient Education

Patients should be instructed to inhale shallowly (as if puffing a pipe) to minimize the likelihood of throat irritation. When used correctly, 100 shallow puffs from the inhaler mouthpiece over 20 minutes approximates 10 puffs from one cigarette over 5 minutes.[66] The release of delivery of nicotine from the inhaler is temperature dependent and significantly reduced at temperatures below 40°F.[7,66] In cold conditions, patients should store the inhaler and cartridges in a warm place (e.g., inside pocket).[7] Conversely, under warmer conditions, more nicotine is released per puff. However, nicotine plasma concentrations achieved using the inhaler in hot climates at maximal doses will not exceed levels normally achieved with smoking.[66]

As with other forms of NRT that are absorbed across the buccal mucosa, the effectiveness of the nicotine inhaler may be reduced by acidic foods and beverages, such as coffee, juices, wine, or soft drinks. Therefore, patients should be instructed not to eat or drink anything (except water) for 15 minutes before or while using the inhaler.

Adverse Reactions

The most common side effects associated with the nicotine inhaler include mouth/throat irritation (40%) and cough (32%).[7] Most patients rated cough and mouth and throat irritation symptoms as mild, decreasing with continued use. Other less common side effects are rhinitis, dyspepsia, hiccups, and headache. Adverse reactions necessitating discontinuation of treatment occurred in less than 5% of patients using the inhaler.

Product Selection Considerations

Patients who express a preference for therapy that can be easily titrated to manage withdrawal symptoms or one that mimics the hand-to-mouth ritual of smoking may find the nicotine inhaler to be an appealing option. Patients with underlying bronchospastic conditions should use the nicotine inhaler with caution because the nicotine vapor may be irritating and provoke bronchospasm.

Bupropion SR

Bupropion SR was the first non-nicotine medication FDA-approved for smoking cessation. Clinical trials involving enrolling nearly 10,000 patients over the past 16 years have confirmed its effectiveness as an aid for smoking cessation.[45] A recent meta-analysis found that bupropion SR treatment doubles long-term (>6 months) abstinence rates when compared to placebo (Table 85-4).[7]

Pharmacokinetics

Animal data suggest the absolute bioavailability of bupropion ranges from 5% to 20%. It undergoes extensive hepatic metabolism to three active metabolites; one of the metabolites, hydroxybupropion, is formed by the cytochrome P450 isoenzyme CYP2B6. Bupropion and its metabolites are eliminated in urine (87%) and feces (10%), with less than 1% being excreted unchanged in the urine. The half-life for bupropion is 21 hours, and its metabolites have a half-life range of 20 to 27 hours; steady-state plasma concentrations are reached within 5 and 8 days, respectively.[69]

Dosing

Treatment with bupropion SR should be initiated while the patient is still smoking because approximately 1 week of treatment is necessary to achieve steady-state blood levels. Patients should set a target quit date that falls within the first 2 weeks of treatment, generally in the second week. The starting dose of bupropion SR is one 150-mg tablet each morning for the first 3 days. If the initial dose is tolerated, the dosage should be increased on the fourth day to the recommended maximum dosage of 300 mg/day (150 mg BID). Therapy should be continued for 7 to 12 weeks after the quit date; however, some patients might benefit from extended treatment. Whether to continue treatment with bupropion SR for periods longer than 12 weeks for smoking cessation must be determined for individual patients.[69] For patients experiencing side effects with the 300 mg/day regimen, Swan et al suggest that 150 mg/day is better tolerated and exhibits comparable long-term efficacy.[70] Similarly, Hurt and colleagues found no significant difference in long-term (>6 months) abstinence rates between subjects randomized to 150 mg/day or 300 mg/day.[71]

Patient Education

Patients should be instructed to follow the dosing regimen described previously. Advise patients experiencing insomnia to avoid taking the second dose close to bedtime. Inform patients that bupropion might cause dizziness, drowsiness, or reduced alertness, and caution should be exercised when driving or operating machinery. Because alcohol use might increase the likelihood of seizures, patients should avoid or drink alcohol only in moderation while taking bupropion. Patients who consume alcohol regularly should be advised to talk with a health care provider about their alcohol use before initiating bupropion therapy because abrupt cessation of alcohol use while taking bupropion might increase the risk of seizure. Patients should also be advised not to take Zyban and Wellbutrin or generic bupropion formulations concomitantly to avoid dose-related adverse effects, including seizures.

Adverse Reactions

Adverse effects associated with bupropion therapy include insomnia (35%–40%) and dry mouth (10%)[7]; these usually lessen with continued use. Taking the second daily dose in the early evening, but no sooner than 8 hours after the first dose, might reduce insomnia. Less common side effects include headache, nausea, tremors, and rash. Seizures are a dose-related toxicity associated with bupropion therapy. For this reason, bupropion is contraindicated in patients with underlying seizure disorders and those receiving concurrent therapy with other forms of bupropion (Wellbutrin, Wellbutrin SR, and Wellbutrin XL). Bupropion also is contraindicated in patients with anorexia or bulimia nervosa, patients undergoing abrupt discontinuation of alcohol or sedatives (including benzodiazepines), and patients currently taking monoamine oxidase inhibitors due to the increased potential for seizures in these populations. In clinical trials for smoking cessation, the frequency of seizures with bupropion SR is <0.1% (seven seizures among 8,000 bupropion-treated patients),[45] which is comparable to the reported incidence of seizures (0.1%) with the sustained-release formulation (Wellbutrin) when used for the treatment of depression.[72] For this reason, bupropion should be used with extreme caution in patients with a history of seizure, cranial trauma, patients receiving medications known to lower the seizure threshold, and patients with underlying severe hepatic cirrhosis. Animal studies suggest that seizures may be related to the peak plasma concentration of bupropion,[73] and as a precautionary measure, the manufacturer recommends that patients space the doses at least 8 hours apart and limit the total daily dose to no more than 300 mg.

Product Selection Considerations

Bupropion SR may be the drug of choice for patients who prefer to take oral medications (an alternative oral option is varenicline, described as follows). Because bupropion SR is simple to use (twice daily oral dosing), this agent may be preferable for patients with regimen compliance concerns (e.g., those unable to consistently use short-acting NRT formulations that require multiple daily doses). Bupropion SR may be particularly beneficial for use in patients with coexisting depression or in individuals with a history of depressive symptoms during a previous quit attempt. Finally, bupropion SR can be used safely in conjunction with NRT, and data suggest that this combination might be slightly more effective than monotherapy with either agent.[7,74] Disadvantages of bupropion SR include a high prevalence of insomnia and the need to screen patients carefully to prevent the rare complication of seizures.

Varenicline

Varenicline is the most recent agent approved by the FDA for smoking cessation. Data from meta-analyses indicate that varenicline significantly increases long-term abstinence rates relative to placebo and bupropion SR,[7] with a pooled odds ratio of 3.1 for varenicline versus placebo for continuous abstinence at 6 months follow-up (Table 85-4). In clinical trials comparing varenicline with bupropion, varenicline was shown to be significantly superior at 52 weeks with an odds ratio of 1.7 (95% CI, 1.3–2.2).[75]

Pharmacokinetics

Varenicline absorption is virtually complete after oral administration, and oral bioavailability is unaffected by food or time-of-day dosing. Once absorbed, varenicline undergoes minimal metabolism, with 92% excreted unchanged in the urine. Renal elimination is primarily through glomerular filtration, along with active tubular secretion, possibly via the organic cation transporter, OCT2.[76] The half-life is approximately 24 hours, and following administration of multiple oral doses, steady-state conditions are reached within 4 days.[77]

Dosing

Treatment with varenicline should be initiated 1 week before the patient stops smoking. This dosing regimen allows for gradual titration of the dose to minimize treatment-related nausea and insomnia. The recommended dose of varenicline is 1 mg BID (taken as one 1-mg tablet in the morning and one 1-mg tablet in the evening) following a 1-week titration: 0.5 mg daily days 1 to 3, 0.5 mg twice daily days 4 to 7, and 1 mg twice daily weeks 2 to 12. For patients who have successfully quit smoking at the end of 12 weeks, an additional course of 12 weeks may be appropriate to increase the likelihood of long-term abstinence. Varenicline is excreted largely unchanged in the urine, and as such, should be used with caution in patients with severe renal dysfunction (<30 mL/minute). Dosage adjustments may be necessary.

Patient Education

The tablets are to be taken orally, after eating, with a full glass of water. Nausea and insomnia are side effects that are usually temporary. However, if these symptoms persist, patients should notify their provider so dosage reduction can be considered. The typical regimen is a 12-week course of therapy, and patients should be advised to comply with the prescribed dosage for the recommended duration.

Adverse Reactions

Varenicline is generally well tolerated. Common side effects (≥5% and twice the rate observed in placebo-treated patients) include nausea (30%), sleep disturbance (insomnia 18%; abnormal dreams 13%), constipation (8%), flatulence (6%), and vomiting (5%). Per the manufacturer's prescribing information, nausea was the most common adverse event associated with varenicline treatment. Nausea was dose dependent and generally described as mild or moderate and often transient; however, for some patients, it was persistent over several months. Initial dose titration was beneficial in reducing the occurrence of nausea. Approximately 3% of subjects receiving varenicline 1 mg BID discontinued treatment prematurely because of nausea. For patients with intolerable nausea, dose reduction should be considered.[76]

Post marketing, there have been case reports of neuropsychiatric symptoms (behavior changes, agitation, depressed mood, suicidal ideation or behavior) as well as reports of worsening of pre-existing psychiatric illness among patients being treated with varenicline. These reports are rare in comparison to the total number of patients using the medication, but nonetheless warrant ongoing surveillance. In 2008, the FDA alerted heath care providers to advise patients and caregivers that patients should stop taking varenicline and contact their health care provider immediately if agitation, depressed mood, or changes in behavior that are not typical for them are observed, or if the patient develops suicidal ideation or suicidal behavior.[78] Patients with serious psychiatric illness such as schizophrenia, bipolar disorder, and major depressive disorder did not participate in the premarketing studies of varenicline, and as such, the safety and efficacy of the medications in these populations have not been established.[76]

Product Selection Considerations

Varenicline is a first-line agent for the treatment of tobacco use and dependence.[7] It offers a convenient oral dosing regimen and a new mechanism of action that might be particularly appealing for patients who have failed quit attempts with other first-line agents (e.g., NRT or bupropion SR). Its use has not been recommended in combination with other agents and therefore is currently limited to monotherapy. As with any of these medications, varenicline should be combined with behavioral counseling in order to maximize chances for a successful, long-term quit attempt. Given its potential for inducing negative neuropsychiatric effects, varenicline might not be the optimal choice for patients with a current or past history of psychiatric illness.

P.J. has tried the nicotine gum and transdermal patch during previous quit attempts. Because he was intolerant to the nicotine gum (it stuck to his dental work), this form of NRT is not appropriate. P.J.'s experience with the transdermal patch suggests he may benefit from a short-acting NRT formulation that allows for active administration and titration of drug as needed to alleviate symptoms of withdrawal. Other first-line therapies include the nicotine nasal spray, inhaler, and lozenge; bupropion SR; or varenicline. P.J. should not use the nicotine nasal spray because he has allergic rhinitis and may be more susceptible to the irritant effects of the spray. In addition, some data suggest that the bioavailability of nicotine is reduced in patients with rhinitis.[79] Furthermore, the safety and efficacy of the nasal spray in patients with chronic nasal disorders have not been adequately studied. Reasonable choices for P.J. therefore include bupropion SR, nicotine lozenge, nicotine inhaler, or varenicline. Any of these options are reasonable, and the choice of therapy should be dictated by P.J.'s individual preference. Alternatively, it is reasonable to consider combination therapy (see question 10).

Safety of Nicotine Replacement Therapy in Patients With Cardiovascular Disease

9. P.J. would like to try the nicotine inhaler. Is NRT safe for use in patients with cardiovascular disease?

Nicotine activates the sympathetic nervous system leading to an increase in heart rate, blood pressure, and myocardial contractility. Nicotine may also cause coronary artery vasoconstriction.[80] These known hemodynamic effects of nicotine have led to doubts about the safety of using NRT in patients with established cardiovascular disease, particularly those with serious arrhythmias, unstable angina, or MI.

Soon after the nicotine patch was approved, anecdotal case reports in the lay press linked NRT (patch and gum) with adverse cardiovascular events (i.e., arrhythmias, MI, stroke). Since then, several randomized, controlled trials have evaluated the safety of NRT in patients with cardiovascular disease, including angiographically documented coronary artery stenosis, MI, stable angina, and previous coronary artery bypass surgery or angioplasty.[81–83] The results of these trials suggest no significant increase in the incidence of cardiovascular events or mortality among patients receiving the nicotine patch when compared with placebo. However, because these trials specifically excluded patients with unstable angina, serious arrhythmias, and recent MI, the manufacturers of NRT products recommend that these agents be used with caution among patients in the immediate (within 2 weeks) post-MI period, those with serious arrhythmias, and those with unstable angina.[7] It is notable, however, that NRTs (patch, nasal spray) have been shown to have fewer effects on biomarkers of cardiovascular risk than does smoking,[84] and smoking cessation has been shown to improve cardiovascular parameters with no negation of these improvements with use of NRT.[85]

Although one methodologically weak case-control study raised questions regarding NRT use in intensive care settings,[86] NRT use in patients with cardiovascular disease has been the subject of numerous reviews, and it is widely believed by experts in the field that the risks of NRT in this patient population are small in relation to the risks of continued tobacco use.[44,59,80,87,88] The 2008 Clinical Practice Guideline concludes that there is no evidence of increased cardiovascular risk with these medications.[7] Although the use of NRT may pose some theoretical risk in a patient like P.J., cigarette smoking is far more hazardous to his health. Cigarettes, unlike NRT, deliver numerous toxins that induce a hypercoagulable state, reduce the oxygen-carrying capacity of hemoglobin, and adversely affect serum lipids. The amount of nicotine that P.J. would receive using the recommended dose of any NRT product will not exceed the amount he previously obtained from his 1.5–2 PPD smoking habit. The clinician should strongly encourage pharmacotherapy during P.J.'s current quit attempt. P.J. is 10 lb overweight; the additional risk imposed by a modest weight gain after smoking cessation likely will not be of clinical significance, compared with that of continued smoking.

Combination Therapy

10. J.B. is a 60-year-old man referred to the pulmonary clinic for further evaluation and management of his chronic obstructive pulmonary disease (COPD). He complains of decreased exercise tolerance and has noted increasing shortness of breath (SOB) with minimal exertion (e.g., while golfing or climbing stairs). He currently uses an albuterol inhaler (90 mcg/puff), 2 puffs Q 4 hr regularly for SOB. His medical history is otherwise unremarkable except for osteoarthritis controlled with acetaminophen 1 g TID. He has smoked approximately 1.5 to 2 PPD for more than 40 years. J.B. indicates he has made several quit attempts over the past year. On the first attempt (quitting "cold turkey"), J.B. relapsed within 2 days. J.B. was smoke free for nearly 2 weeks on his second quit attempt (using the 4-mg nicotine lozenge), but he found it difficult to adhere to the frequent dosing schedule and relapsed shortly, discontinuing the lozenge. His most recent quit attempt was 6 months ago using varenicline (1 mg BID). After 1 month of abstinence, J.B. self-terminated varenicline ("I thought I didn't need it anymore") and relapsed within 2 weeks. On further questioning, J.B. states that he did not enroll in a behavioral counseling program or seek additional assistance (other than pharmacotherapy) during any of his quit attempts. He expresses an interest in smoking cessation but is discouraged by his inability to quit. On physical examination, coarse breath sounds that clear after coughing are noted. His chest x-ray results are normal. Spirometry reveals a forced expiratory volume in 1 second (FEV_1) of 2.8 L (72% of predicted) and a forced vital capacity (FVC) of 4.1 L (81% of predicted). His FEV_1/FVC ratio is 68%. He weighs 76 kg and is 72 in. tall. J.B. is concerned about his worsening pulmonary function and is committed to making another effort to quit. What treatment options are appropriate for J.B.?

Tobacco smoking is the single most important risk factor for the development of COPD, and most patients diagnosed with COPD are current or former smokers.[89] Medications (e.g., bronchodilators, anti-inflammatory agents) used to treat the symptoms of COPD have not been shown to alter the disease progression.[89] J.B.'s pulmonary function tests indicate he has stage II (moderate) COPD[89]; given his worsening pulmonary symptoms, it is imperative that he stop smoking as soon as possible. J.B. should be advised that medications for COPD offer only limited symptomatic relief; the most important component of his treatment is smoking cessation.[89,90] The clinician should commend J.B. for his interest in quitting and help him devise a patient-specific treatment plan.

In addition to monotherapy with any of the first-line agents, the 2008 Clinical Practice Guideline identified selected combinations of medications that can be considered in the initial treatment of tobacco dependence. Medication combinations that significantly increase long-term (>6 months) cessation rates relative to placebo and are recommended as first-line treatments include combination NRT and the nicotine patch in combination with bupropion SR (Table 85-4).[7]

Combination Nicotine Replacement Therapy

Combination NRT involves the use of a long-acting formulation (patch) in combination with a short-acting formulation (gum, lozenge, inhaler, or nasal spray). The long-acting formulation, which delivers relatively constant levels of drug, is used to prevent the onset of severe withdrawal symptoms, whereas the short-acting formulation, which delivers nicotine at a faster rate, is used as needed to control withdrawal symptoms that may occur during potential relapse situations (e.g., after meals, when stressed, or around other smokers). A recent meta-analysis found that the nicotine patch in combination with a short-acting NRT formulation (gum, inhaler, or nasal spray) was significantly more effective than single-agent NRT. The odds of long-term (>6 months) cessation was 1.4 with combination NRT compared to NRT monotherapy (95% CI, 1.1–1.6).[44]

Nicotine Patch and Bupropion SR in Combination

The combination of bupropion SR and NRT has been evaluated in three long-term controlled trials. Patients receiving combination therapy with bupropion SR and the nicotine patch in standard dosages were significantly more likely to quit than were patients randomized to the nicotine patch alone.[7] The odds of long-term (>6 months) abstinence were 1.3, with the combination compared to nicotine patch monotherapy (95% CI, 1.0–1.8).[7]

TREATMENT SELECTION

Given the severity of J.B.'s condition and his willingness to quit now, the clinician should initiate treatment as soon as possible. His treatment should consist of pharmacotherapy in conjunction with behavioral counseling and appropriate follow-up.

Pharmacotherapy

The clinician should work with J.B. to select the most appropriate pharmacotherapy. As noted previously, appropriate options would include the various NRT formulations, bupropion SR, varenicline, or an effective combination of first-line agents. The choice of therapy is dictated by considerations such as individual patient preference for a given agent, previous experience with cessation medications, current medical conditions, previous levels of smoking, medication adherence issues, and the patient's out-of-pocket cost. For patients reporting a positive experience with a given medication, retreatment with the same agent or a combination of agents might be appropriate, with consideration given to increasing the dose, frequency, or duration of therapy. For patients reporting a negative experience with pharmacotherapy (e.g., poor adherence, side effects, palatability issues, cost), an alternative agent should be considered. Given J.B.'s previous adherence issues with the nicotine lozenge as monotherapy, it might be preferable to use a long-acting cessation medication such as the nicotine patch, bupropion SR, or varenicline. Combination therapy with the nicotine patch and a short-acting NRT formulation (used as needed) or bupropion SR would also be appropriate.

Behavioral Counseling

Although medications are effective alone in helping patients quit smoking, maximizing patients' chances for a long-term, successful quit attempt requires the use of one or more medications in combination with behavioral counseling. J.B's previous 1-month quit attempt highlights the successful impact of varenicline in this patient; however, the relapse is likely attributable to a shortened course of therapy and the absence of a behavioral counseling program. J.B. should be advised that the medications are designed to make patients more comfortable while quitting and that behavioral counseling is needed to address the "habit" of smoking by helping him cope with difficult situations and triggers for relapse. J.B. should be advised to (a) call the tollfree tobacco quitline at 1-800-QUIT NOW, (b) call the tollfree number that accompanies the selected medication (all medications include a free counseling program), (c) enroll in a local group program, (d) join an online quitting program such as Quitnet.com, or (e) request individualized counseling from a health professional with expertise in tobacco cessation. In addition, J.B. should be reminded that compliance with the medication regimen—daily compliance, as well as duration of therapy—will increase his chances of quitting for good. Clinician-delivered counseling might also include a personalized message to further enhance his motivation to quit. For example, the clinician could translate J.B.'s spirometry results into an effective "lung age" (e.g., the age of the average healthy individual with similar spirometry values). Given J.B.'s height (72 in.) and FEV_1 (2.8 L), his estimated "lung age" is almost 80 years.[91] This educational approach has been found to significantly increase long-term (12-month) quit rates in a recent controlled trial.[91]

Complementary Therapies

11. J.B. is worried about "taking more drugs" and asks whether one of the natural herbal products might be better for him than "prescription drugs."

Although many herbal and homeopathic products are available to help people quit smoking, data that support their safety and effectiveness are lacking. Most herbal preparations for smoking cessation contain lobeline, an herbal alkaloid with partial nicotine agonist activity. Although direct-to-consumer advertisements suggest that lobeline-containing preparations are safe and effective, a meta-analysis found no evidence to support the role of lobeline as an effective aid for smoking cessation.[92] Likewise, nicobrevin (an herbal product not available in the United States that contains quinine, menthyl valerate, camphor, and eucalyptus oil),[93] hypnosis,[94] and acupuncture[95] have not been found to be effective treatments for smoking cessation.[7] Furthermore, patients should be cautioned that herbal cigarettes are not safe alternatives because they result in the inhalation of other toxins present in smoke. J.B. should be advised that the efficacy of the herbal therapies are not well established, and use of these agents cannot be recommended at this time.

12. K.M. is a 47-year-old female who has been smoking cigarettes (2 PPD) for almost 30 years. She admits to numerous failed attempts over the past 10 years. K.M. states, "I've tried just about everything to help me quit, but nothing seems to work." K.M. has tried NRT (transdermal patch, lozenge, and inhaler), bupropion SR, varenicline, acupuncture, and hypnotherapy. On questioning, K.M.'s treatment regimens have been appropriate (e.g., correct dosages, duration of therapy). K.M. has enrolled in several worksite cessation classes throughout the years but admits to sporadic attendance due her stressful and unpredictable schedule (she is a paralegal in a busy law firm). Her medical history is significant for TMJ syndrome secondary to nocturnal bruxism (teeth grinding). K.M. is ready to quit now and states, "I want to go to my 30-year high school reunion [4 months from now] as a nonsmoker." What treatment options exist for patients failing first-line therapies?

For most smokers, the quitting process is characterized by a series of quit attempts and subsequent relapses. On average, former smokers report 10.8 quit attempts over a period of 18.6 years before achieving long-term cessation.[96] Most quit attempts are undertaken without assistance, and approximately 95% of attempts end in relapse.[7] As emphasized in the 2008 Clinical Practice Guideline, clinicians should approach the treatment of tobacco dependence in a manner similar to the treatment of other chronic medical conditions such as diabetes, asthma, hyperlipidemia, and hypertension. By acknowledging the chronic nature of tobacco dependence, clinicians will appreciate the need for ongoing care (which includes patient education, behavioral counseling, and pharmacotherapy) rather than episodic care (e.g., a single treatment course or periodic/occasional interventions).[7] K.M. should be congratulated on her renewed interest in quitting, and the clinician should work with her to design an individualized treatment plan.

Second-Line Agents

CLONIDINE

Clonidine is a centrally acting α_2-adrenergic agonist that reduces sympathetic outflow from the central nervous system. Clonidine is approved for use as an antihypertensive agent, but it is also effective in reducing the autonomic symptoms of both opioid and alcohol withdrawal. Studies of clonidine for smoking cessation have been inconsistent, but a recent meta-analysis concluded that clonidine treatment doubles long-term (>6 month) abstinence rates relative compared to placebo (Table 85-4).[7] Dosages for tobacco cessation have ranged from 0.15 to 0.75 mg/day PO and 0.1 to 0.3 mg/day transdermally. The recommended starting dose is 0.1 mg BID or 0.1 mg/day transdermally, increasing by 0.10 mg/day/week as tolerated for up to 10 weeks.[7] The high incidence of side effects, including dry mouth, sedation, dizziness, and constipation, relegate clonidine as a second-line agent reserved for individuals who have failed or are intolerant of first-line agents.

NORTRIPTYLINE

Nortriptyline, a tricyclic antidepressant, has demonstrated efficacy for smoking cessation, approximately doubling long-term (6-month) abstinence rates compared with placebo (Table 85-4).[7] The regimen used for treating tobacco dependence is 25 mg/day, increasing gradually to a target dosage of 75 to 100 mg/day, for approximately 12 weeks.[7] Because the half-life of nortriptyline is prolonged (up to 56 hours), therapy should be initiated at least 10 days before the quit date to allow it to reach steady-state concentrations at the target dose. The side effects most commonly observed with nortriptyline include sedation, dry mouth, blurred vision, urinary retention, lightheadedness, and tremor. This drug should be used with caution in patients with underlying cardiovascular conditions because of the risk of arrhythmias and postural hypotension.

High-Dose Nicotine Replacement Therapy

Plasma levels of nicotine achieved with NRT are generally much lower than those observed during regular smoking.[64,97] Given this incomplete level of nicotine replacement, standard doses of NRT may be insufficient for some individuals, and in particular, for moderate-to-heavy smokers. Studies using transdermal nicotine in doses up to 44 to 63 mg/day suggest that high-dose NRT is safe.[98–102] However, trials evaluating higher doses of NRT have yielded conflicting results. Some studies suggest higher doses of NRT may be more effective in heavy smokers,[100,101,103] whereas others have demonstrated slight but not statistically significant improvements in cessation rates[104,105] or no difference.[106,107] When the results of six studies were pooled, the odds ratio for abstinence was 1.2 for high-dose NRT compared to conventional dose NRT (95% CI, 1.0–1.3), suggesting that high-dose NRT therapy may be advantageous in some patients.[44] This approach should be reserved for patients not able to quit using conventional doses of transdermal NRT.

Extended Use of Medications

In a minority of patients, extended duration medication therapy appears to be safe and effective. Long-term follow-up data from the Lung Health Study have found that approximately 15% of long-term quitters continued nicotine gum therapy with no serious side effects.[108] The 2008 Clinical Practice Guideline states that extended use of medications might be beneficial in individuals who report persistent withdrawal symptoms during treatment, those who have relapsed shortly after medication discontinuation, or those who are interested in long-term therapy.[7] Clinicians should be aware that many of the medications (bupropion SR, varenicline, nicotine nasal spray and inhaler) are FDA approved for long-term (6-month) use.[69,76,109,110] Although the goal should be complete abstinence from all nicotine-containing products, continued use of medicinal nicotine is substantially safer than any level of smoking.[7,111]

K.M. has relapsed following appropriate treatment with several first-line agents, and the clinician should evaluate K.M.'s previous quit attempts, including the dates, methods used (behavioral and pharmacotherapy), and her perceptions of why these methods were ineffective. If K.M. believes a particular medication was more effective than others, it might be reasonable to use the same agent during her next quit attempt.[7] Alternative approaches include the use of a different medication (including second-line agents) or a combination of medications[7] (see question 10). Given that K.M. has TMJ, the nicotine gum formulation should not be used.

Drug Interactions With Smoking

13. M.K. is a new patient presenting to the pharmacy with a new prescription for Ortho Tri-Cyclen (norgestimate/ethinyl estradiol). The new patient history form completed by M.K. reveals that she is 32 years old, weighs 65 kg, and is 70 in. tall. She takes no prescription medications but occasionally uses loratadine 10 mg PRN for allergies and ibuprofen 400 mg PRN for dysmenorrhea. She has no significant medical history. Her father has hypertension and suffered an MI last year. Her mother has type 2 diabetes and dyslipidemia. Her social history is significant for tobacco use (1 PPD for 15 years), alcohol (1 glass of wine per night), and caffeine (5–6 cups of coffee daily). Are there any potential interactions with M.K.'s new prescription?

Smoking and Combined Hormonal Contraceptives

One of the most important, but often unrecognized, precautions to consider with oral contraceptive use is the potential interaction between tobacco smoke and estrogens in combination hormonal contraceptives. Estrogens are known to promote coagulation by altering clotting factor levels and increasing platelet aggregation. As described in question 7, substances present in tobacco smoke, including oxidant gases and other products of combustion, induce a hypercoagulable state increasing the risk of acute cardiovascular events. Exposure to both factors (smoking and high levels of estrogen) greatly increases the risk of thromboembolic and thrombotic disorders. Considerable epidemiologic evidence indicates that cigarette smoking substantially increases the risk of adverse cardiovascular events, including stroke, MI, and thromboembolism in women who use oral combination hormonal contraceptive agents.[112,113] This risk is age related, in that the absolute risk of death from cardiovascular disease in oral contraceptive users who smoke is 3.3 per 100,000 women ages 15 to 34 years compared with 29.4 per 100,000 women ages 35 to 44 years. To put this in perspective, the corresponding risk of death from cardiovascular disease in *nonsmoking* women who use oral contraceptives is much lower, with a death rate of 0.65 per 100,000 women ages 15 to 34 years and 6.21 per 100,000 women ages 35 to 44 years.[114] Because of the increase risk of adverse cardiovascular events, current guidelines from the American College of Obstetricians and Gynecologists (ACOG) and the World Health Organization (WHO) state that combination estrogen-progestin contraceptives should not be used in women who are older than 35 years of age and smoke.[115,116] These organizations recommend the use of progestin-only contraceptives (oral and injectable formulations) and intrauterine devices in this population.[115,116]

M.K. is 32 years of age, and despite her heavy smoking status (20 cigarettes per day), oral contraceptive use is not contraindicated at this time. However, the clinician should strongly advise M.K. to quit smoking and assess her readiness to do so. M.K. should be informed that if she continues to smoke while using oral combined hormonal contraceptives, her risk of developing a blood clot, stroke, or heart attack will continue to increase over time. Her family history (father with recent MI and mother with diabetes and hyperlipidemia) suggests that she may be genetically predisposed to cardiovascular disease, and thus, efforts to minimize preventable risk factors should be encouraged to reduce the likelihood that she will develop cardiovascular-related complications in the future.

14. M.K. is not considering quitting smoking at this time and does not want to discontinue her oral contraceptives because she is sexually active and needs a reliable form of birth control. She wonders if the new low-dose birth control pills or other formulations (e.g., patch, vaginal ring) are safer for smokers.

Combined oral contraceptives available in the United States contain estrogen in doses ranging from 20 to 50 mcg of ethinyl estradiol. The results of in vitro studies have shown that oral contraceptives containing ≥50 mcg of ethinyl estradiol induce greater procoagulatory effects than do preparations containing either 30 mcg or 35 mcg of ethinyl estradiol; formulations containing 20 mcg of ethinyl estradiol appear to have little or no adverse effects on coagulation.[117,118] Early epidemiologic reports linking oral contraceptive use and severe cardiovascular events were largely observed in women using oral contraceptives containing >50 mcg of ethinyl estradiol.[119] Since then, manufacturers have reduced the dose of estrogen in oral contraceptives such that the majority of preparations available in the United States contain 20 to 35 mcg of ethinyl estradiol.[120]

In 2001, the U.S. Surgeon General stated that lower-dose oral contraceptives may be associated with a reduced risk for coronary heart disease (CHD), compared with higher-dose formulations. Despite this conclusion, the report cautioned that heavy smokers who use oral contraceptives still have a greatly elevated risk for CHD.[121] Consistent with the Surgeon General's cautionary statement, a recent study found that women who smoked >25 cigarettes per day had a 20-fold higher risk of MI than nonsmoking women who used oral contraceptives. Interestingly, the elevated risk was independent of the dose of estrogen in the oral contraceptive; women using preparations containing >50 mcg of estrogen were no more likely to experience an MI than were women using preparations containing <50 mcg of estrogen. There was only one case involving the use of a preparation containing 20 mcg of estrogen, and thus, the safety of this dose could not be evaluated.[122]

Serum estrogen levels obtained with the vaginal ring are significantly lower than those achieved with either transdermal or oral combined contraceptive formulations,[123] and theoretically, the contraceptive vaginal ring might be a safer formulation for women who smoke. However, because the contraceptive patch and vaginal ring are relatively new, and their safety has not been established among women who smoke, guidelines issued by the ACOG state that the same precautions for the use of oral combined contraceptions should apply to these newer formulations as well.[116]

M.K.'s prescribed oral contraceptive agent (Ortho Tri-Cyclen) is a triphasic formulation containing 35 mcg of ethinyl estradiol in combination with weekly increasing doses of norgestimate (0.18, 0.215, and 0.25 mg) throughout each monthly cycle. Although some clinicians recommend the use of low-dose (20-mcg) estrogen preparations in smokers, the available evidence suggests that the prescribed regimen poses no additional risk in M.K. However, if M.K. increases her smoking levels to >25 cigarettes per day, some data suggest that her risk for an MI is increased.[122] The clinician should inform M.K. that there are currently no studies demonstrating a reduced risk of adverse cardiovascular events in smokers using oral contraceptives containing low doses (e.g., 20 mcg) of estrogen or the newer transdermal and vaginal ring formulations. In the absence of data, only smoking cessation can be advocated to definitively reduce the risk of stroke, MI, and thromboembolism in women who use combined hormonal contraceptives.

Behavioral Counseling

Although M.K. is not considering quitting at this time, it is appropriate for the clinician to apply the 5 R's (Table 85-5) to promote motivation to quit. This counseling should be *relevant* to M.K.'s situation and should highlight the *risks* of continued tobacco use, such as her elevated risk for thromboembolic and thrombotic disorders (associated with continued use of oral contraceptives). M.K. should be asked to think about the *rewards* of quitting and any potential *roadblocks* to quitting. At subsequent encounters, the clinician should sensitively assess M.K.'s tobacco use status and motivation to quit, and offer assistance with quitting when M.K. is ready. If M.K. decides to quit, it would be important to reassess her caffeine intake because caffeine levels have been reported to increase by 56% in patients who quit smoking.[30]

NONCIGARETTE FORMS OF TOBACCO

Smokeless Tobacco

Classification

15. T.M. is a 29-year-old man who presents to the clinic for evaluation of a painless "white patch" along his lower left gumline, which he noted several weeks ago while flossing his teeth. His social history is significant for the use of smokeless tobacco (consumes

one can of Copenhagen moist snuff every 2–3 days), cigarettes (1 pack per week), and alcohol (one to two beers daily). T.M. reports he has "dipped" for the past 10 years but only recently started smoking "socially" in the evenings when out with friends. He is in otherwise excellent health and takes no medications. What is smokeless tobacco?

Smokeless tobacco is a term used to describe forms of tobacco that are not burned and inhaled but rather held in the mouth to allow absorption of nicotine across the oral (buccal) mucosa. Smokeless tobacco products in the United States are broadly categorized as either chewing tobacco or snuff. Chewing tobacco, which is generally available in loose-leaf, plug, and twist formulations, is chewed or held in the cheek or lower lip. Snuff, which is commonly available as loose particles or sachets resembling mini tea bags, has a much finer consistency and is generally held in the mouth and not chewed. Most snuff formulations in the United States are classified as moist snuff, and users place a small amount (a "pinch") between the cheek and gum (also known as dipping) and suck on the moist mass of tobacco for 30 minutes or longer. Dry snuff, which is generally sniffed or inhaled through the nostrils, is less commonly used. Newer formulations including "spitless" moist snuff (e.g., Snus), and lozenges containing compressed tobacco powder are being marketed as cigarette substitutes for situations where smoking is prohibited.[124]

Epidemiology

According to the U.S. Department of Health and Human Services, in 2006, an estimated 8.2 million Americans ages 12 years and older (3.3%) had used smokeless tobacco in the past month. Males (6.6%) were more likely than females (0.3%) to be current users.[125] The prevalence of smokeless tobacco use is highest among individuals between the ages of 18 and 25 and is substantially higher among American Indians, Alaskan Natives, residents of the southern United States, and persons living in rural areas.[125,126]

Pharmacokinetics

Absorption of nicotine from chewing tobacco and snuff is pH dependent, with more nicotine absorbed across the buccal mucosa under alkaline conditions. Smokeless tobacco manufacturers manipulate the nicotine content and pH of their products by adding alkaline buffering agents and changing the tobacco processing methods to control the delivery of nicotine. For example, a "starter" formulation such as Skoal Bandits has a lower nicotine content and is more acidic (pH = 5.4) to increase tolerability. Once dependence has been established, users generally advance to more alkaline, higher nicotine content products such as Skoal Fine Cut (pH = 7.6) and Copenhagen (pH = 8.6), which are capable of delivering higher levels of nicotine.[126] As depicted in Figure 85-3, the nicotine from smokeless tobacco is absorbed less rapidly than from cigarette smoke, and the peak levels generally occur after 20 to 30 minutes. Plasma levels of nicotine decline slowly even after removal of tobacco from the mouth because of the gradual release of nicotine from mucous membranes and the possible intestinal absorption of nicotine from swallowed tobacco.[127] Although the rate of nicotine absorption from cigarettes exceeds that from smokeless tobacco, the extent of absorption does not. In fact, regular smokeless tobacco users experience comparable exposure to nicotine and are as likely to develop physical dependence as are regular smokers.[126,128]

16. On examination, a superficial whitish lesion with moderate wrinkling of the tissue adjacent to the mandibular left canine and premolars is noted. In addition, there is localized gingival recession and moderate brown staining of the enamel surfaces. T.M. reports that he routinely places snuff between his lower left cheek and gum. He asks if the lesion might be cancerous and wonders if it is related to his snuff use. What are the health consequences of smokeless tobacco use?

Users of smokeless tobacco are often under the mistaken impression that these formulations are a "safe" alternative to smoking cigarettes because it is not inhaled. In addition to the cosmetic concerns (e.g., halitosis, staining of teeth), the use of smokeless tobacco is associated with numerous adverse health effects,[128] including the following:

Soft Tissue Alterations/Leukoplakia

Smokeless tobacco users commonly develop an oral soft tissue condition called leukoplakia or "snuff dipper's lesion." These white-colored patches or plaques, which are observed in approximately 15% of chewing tobacco users and 60% of snuff users, generally develop at mucosal sites in contact with the tobacco.[128,129] Of concern is the fact that a small percentage of these lesions may transform into squamous cell carcinomas.[126,130] Following cessation, the oral leukoplakia appears to regress or completely disappear in the majority of cases.[130,131]

Periodontal Effects

In addition to the soft tissue alterations noted previously, regular users of smokeless tobacco are at significant risk for the development of gingival recession (complete or partial loss of the tissue covering the root of the tooth), caries, and tooth abrasion. The loss of gingival tissue, observed in up to 27% of smokeless tobacco users, generally occurs at sites constantly exposed to tobacco.[129] The high sugar content found in many smokeless tobacco products in contact with exposed tooth root tissue might account for the increased incidence of dental caries in smokeless tobacco users.[126,128,129]

Cancer

The most serious consequence of smokeless tobacco use is an increased risk of developing oral and pharyngeal cancers; the risk appears to be dose related with heavy, long-time users being more likely to develop oral cancer compared with nonusers.[128] Smokeless tobacco contains 28 known carcinogens, including tobacco-specific nitrosamines, polycyclic aromatic hydrocarbons, and radioactive polonium-210, all of which are in direct contact with mucosal tissues for prolonged periods.[132]

Although smokeless tobacco products do not yield many of the risks associated with the inhalation of combusted tobacco (e.g., pulmonary disease, lung cancer), these products impose harm and should not be recommended as aids for smoking cessation, particularly because safer, more effective products (i.e., medications labeled for smoking cessation) are available.[124,128,133]

T.M. is presenting with an oral mucosal lesion commonly observed in smokeless tobacco users. His long-standing history of snuff use and characteristic white, wrinkled lesion appearing at a site where he habitually places snuff are consistent with leukoplakia. T.M. should be informed that the lesion is most likely caused by his chronic snuff use, and he should be strongly advised to quit. With continued exposure to carcinogens present in smokeless tobacco, there is an increased risk that the leukoplakia will undergo malignant transformation. The presence of an identifiable tobacco-induced oral lesion might serve as a powerful motivator for a quit attempt. If he is able to quit snuff use, the gum tissue will likely normalize over a period of 6 weeks.[131] If the lesion persists, he should be referred for biopsy and further diagnostic evaluation. Finally, T.M. already has evidence of localized gingival recession, which increases his risk for serious periodontal disease and further dental-related complications. These periodontal problems will progress as long as he continues to use smokeless tobacco.

Treatment

17. T.M. relates that his new girlfriend is a "militant" nonsmoker who is likely to stop dating him if he does not quit. He is aware that tobacco is "bad for him" and is worried about developing oral cancer. He believes it will not be difficult to quit smoking because he smokes so little. He is more worried about stopping the use of snuff and wants to know if there are any medications to help him quit.

Despite the known health risks and high prevalence of smokeless tobacco use, there are limited evidence-based recommendations to guide clinicians in the treatment use smokeless tobacco use.[7] In a recent meta-analysis, Ebbert et al.[134] reviewed the results of 20 randomized, controlled trials evaluating behavioral counseling and pharmacotherapy interventions for smokeless tobacco use, and their findings are summarized as follows.

BEHAVIORAL THERAPY

Behavioral interventions, including the use of self-help materials (written manuals, pamphlets, videotapes), brief (15- to 20-minute) counseling sessions, telephone support, oral examination with feedback, computerized gradual reduction of tobacco, and use of non-tobacco oral substitutes (herbal and mint snuff, chewing gum), have been shown to significantly increase long-term (>6 month) cessation rates (OR 1.6; 95% CI, 1.4–1.8) compared with control interventions. Interventions that appear to be particularly effective in promoting abstinence among smokeless tobacco users compared to control interventions include telephone support (OR 2.1; 95% CI, 1.7–2.6) or oral examination with clinician-delivered feedback (OR 1.9; 95% CI, 1.1–3.2).[134]

NICOTINE REPLACEMENT THERAPY

To date, the nicotine patch and gum are the only NRT formulations that have been evaluated in randomized controlled trials for smokeless tobacco cessation. A pooled analysis of trials evaluating long-term (>6-month) quit rates did not find a statistically significant improvement with the nicotine patch (OR 1.2; 95% CI, 0.9–1.5) or nicotine gum (OR 1.0; 95% CI, 0.6–1.6) when compared to placebo.[134] Encouraging results from a small open-label trial suggest the nicotine lozenge may be effective for cessation of smokeless tobacco use, but these findings are preliminary.[135] Overall, data from controlled trials suggest NRT is not effective in the treatment of smokeless tobacco use, but further studies are necessary.[7,134]

BUPROPION SR

Bupropion SR for smokeless tobacco cessation has been evaluated in two small randomized, controlled trials with a follow-up duration of at least 6 months. A pooled analysis of these trials failed to find a statistically significant improvement in cessation rates relative to placebo (OR 0.9; 95% CI, 0.5–1.6).[134]

The 2008 Clinical Practice Guideline recommends that smokeless tobacco users receive counseling interventions similar to those recommended for smokers.[7] Based on the available evidence, it appears that behavioral interventions are effective in the treatment of smokeless tobacco use. Limited data suggest that pharmacotherapy with bupropion SR or NRT is ineffective. However, more research is necessary to determine whether combination pharmacotherapy and counseling will provide improved cessation rates in smokeless tobacco users. T.M. should be provided with behavioral counseling tailored to his stage of readiness to quit—if he is ready to quit in the next 30 days, a treatment plan should be devised. If he is not ready to quit in the next 30 days, motivational counseling should be applied using the 5 R's (Table 85-5). Because oral examination with patient feedback appears to promote quitting, T.M. should be referred to a dental provider for additional monitoring and follow-up. T.M. has specifically asked about the use of pharmacotherapy as a cessation aid, and although data do not support the use of bupropion SR or NRT because of insufficient evidence of effectiveness, these agents might be considered. T.M. should also be informed that a non-tobacco oral substitute (herbal and mint snuff) in combination with behavioral counseling is also effective.[134]

Cigars

18. R.N., a 40-year-old man who currently smokes 1 PPD of cigarettes, would like to know whether cutting down to one to two cigars per day is a safe alternative to cigarette smoking.

Cigars are conventionally defined as "any roll of tobacco wrapped in leaf tobacco or in any substance containing tobacco."[136] The types of cigars available in the United States vary and include *little* cigars (shaped like cigarettes and weighing <1.3 g; *small* cigars or cigarillos (some with a plastic mouthpiece and weighing between 1.2 and 2.5 g); *regular* cigars (usually rolled to a tip on one end and banded; generally weighing between 5 and 17 g); and *premium* cigars (expensive, generally hand rolled, and weighing >22 g).[136,137] Cigar tobacco is generally air cured and produces smoke with a more alkaline pH, which allows for buccal absorption of nicotine.[138]

Cigar consumption has significantly increased over the past decade.[139] According to the U.S. Department of Health and Human Services, in 2006, an estimated 13.7 million Americans ages 12 years or older (5.6%) had smoked one or more cigars in the past month. The prevalence of cigar use was highest among individuals ages 18 to 25 years (12.1%); males (9.3%) were more likely than females (2.1%) to be current cigar smokers.[125] Some data suggest that the increased consumption is due to a greater prevalence of occasional cigar smoking by previous nonsmokers, particularly among those of higher socioeconomic status.[136] This trend is likely the result of enhanced marketing and promotional efforts by the tobacco industry; cigar advertisements often depict celebrities or athletes associating cigar smoking with glamour, affluence, and success.[136,140] Increasing numbers of former cigarette smokers switching to cigars and experimentation among adolescents with cigar smoking may also play a role.[136]

Exactly how much nicotine an individual might obtain from a single cigar is difficult to determine or generalize because cigar weight and nicotine content vary widely from brand to brand and from cigar to cigar. Most cigars range in weight from about 1 to 22 g; a typical cigarette weighs less than 1 g. The nicotine content of ten commercially available cigars studied in 1996 ranged from 10 to 444 mg. In comparison, U.S. cigarettes have a relatively narrow total nicotine content range (mean $= 13.5 \pm 0.1$ mg) per cigarette.[141] Relating these data, Henningfield et al. concluded that it is possible for one large cigar to contain as much tobacco as an entire pack of cigarettes and deliver enough nicotine to establish and maintain dependence.[138]

The adverse health effects of cigar smoking have been well described and include an increased risk of cancer of the lung, oral cavity, larynx, esophagus, and pancreas. In addition, cigar smokers who inhale deeply are at increased risk for developing cardiovascular disease and COPD.[136] Cigarette smokers who switch to smoking only cigars decrease their risk of developing lung cancer, but their risk is markedly higher than if they were to quit smoking altogether.[136]

R.N. should be counseled that switching from cigarette smoking to low-level daily cigar smoking will not reduce his risk for developing a tobacco-related disease. The amount of nicotine delivered by one to two cigars per day is capable of sustaining his dependence on nicotine. In addition, former cigarette smokers are more likely to inhale deeply, which further increases the risk of cancer and cardiovascular and pulmonary disease. The clinician should strongly advise R.N. to quit smoking cigarettes and that switching to cigars is not a safe alternative.

Bidis and Clove Cigarettes

19. K.K. is a 16-year-old male who has been suspended from school after his third offense for smoking on campus. K.K. began experimenting with bidis and kreteks a few years ago and then started smoking cigarettes "socially" with his friends. For the past year, he has been smoking about a half-pack of cigarettes per day. What are bidis and kreteks?

Bidis

Bidis are small, hand-rolled cigarettes imported to the United States primarily from India and other Southeast Asian countries. They consist of finely ground tobacco wrapped in a brown tendu or temburni leaf. Bidis, which are similar in appearance to marijuana cigarettes, are readily available in tobacco shops and ethnic stores and via Internet retailers in a variety of flavors (e.g., chocolate, vanilla, strawberry, cherry, mango, orange) and tend to be more popular among younger smokers.[142] In a U.S. survey of nearly 64,000 adults ($\geq$18 years) in 15 states, young adults (18–24 years) reported the highest rates of ever (16.5%) and current (1.4%) bidi use.[143] In 2006, an estimated 2.3% of 12th graders had smoked bidis in the past year.[125] In a previous survey in Massachusetts, reasons cited by urban adolescents for smoking bidis were that they were better tasting, less expensive, safer, and easier to buy than traditional cigarettes.[144]

Although bidis contain less tobacco than standard cigarettes, studies have shown they produce substantial amounts of tar, nicotine, and carbon monoxide.[145,146] A study using standardized smoking machine testing methods found that bidis deliver three times the amount of carbon monoxide and nicotine and nearly five times the amount of tar found in standard cigarettes.[145] Because of the low combustibility of the tendu leaf wrapper, bidis must be puffed constantly to remain lit. As a result, bidi smokers inhale more frequently and more deeply, thereby markedly increasing the delivery of tar and other toxins.[144] Most bidis do not have a traditional filter tip, which further increases exposure to toxic constituents present in smoke. However, a filter does not confer added safety, as evidenced by a study that found that bidi cigarettes containing a filter actually delivered higher levels of tar, nicotine, and carbon monoxide when compared with unfiltered bidi brands. In this study, the filtered bidi cigarettes contained a small wad of cotton instead of the usual cellulose acetate filter found in American cigarettes. The investigators speculated that the inefficient cotton filter and the slightly larger size of the filtered bidi brands led to the observed higher yields of inhaled toxins.[146]

Although by law all packages of bidis sold in the United States must contain the Surgeon General warning about the hazards of smoking, spot-checks in various retail outlets have shown that many of these products are not labeled with health warnings.[147] The absence of federally mandated warning labels may lead to the false impression that these products are safer than other forms of tobacco. However, studies in India have shown that bidi smokers have a comparable or greater risk of developing tobacco-related respiratory, cardiovascular, and neoplastic disease than cigarette smokers. Even low levels of bidi smoking (1–7 bidis/day) are associated with an elevated risk of death (risk ratio estimate, 1.3) compared to nonsmokers. Higher levels of bidi smoking ($\leq$8 bidis/day) incur an even higher risk of death (risk ratio estimate, 2.2).[148]

Clove Cigarettes

Clove cigarettes or "kreteks" are cigarettes imported from Indonesia containing a mixture of approximately 60% to 70% tobacco and 30% to 40% minced cloves.[142] Although usage data in adults are not available, in 2006, an estimated 6.2% of 12th graders had smoked kreteks in the past year.[125] Data from smoking machine tests have found that clove cigarettes deliver twice as much nicotine and carbon monoxide and three times as much tar as conventional cigarettes.[149] In addition to the hazards associated with smoking, clove cigarette use has been implicated in causing rare cases of hemorrhagic pulmonary edema, pneumonia, bronchitis, and hemoptysis.[150–152] It has been speculated that eugenol, a compound possessing local anesthetic properties and present in large quantities in clove cigarette smoke, might be toxic to pulmonary tissue. The anesthetic effects of eugenol might also place users at an increased risk of pulmonary aspiration resulting from an impaired gag reflex.[152]

There is concern among some experts that experimentation with noncigarette tobacco (kreteks, bidis, cigars) provides an alternative form of nicotine exposure to individuals who might not otherwise smoke cigarettes. This concern is heightened by recent data that suggests susceptible youth can become addicted to nicotine shortly (within 1–2 days) after smoking initiation.[153] K.K. began experimenting with bidis and clove cigarettes before he smoked cigarettes socially. It is difficult to know whether K.K.'s previous use of bidis and clove cigarettes led to regular cigarette smoking, but these products can deliver nicotine levels capable of inducing and sustaining dependence.

Water Pipes

20. L.B.C. is a 19-year-old college freshman who resides in an on-campus dormitory. She has been invited by several of her hallmates to "hang-out" at a local hookah bar for the evening. What is hookah, and is this form of tobacco "safe"?

Hookah or water pipe smoking is an ancient method of tobacco use whereby users inhale smoke that is passed through water. Water pipe nomenclature is region specific and includes names such as "hookah" (Africa and Indian subcontinent); "narghile" (Israel, Jordan, Lebanon, Syria); "shisha," "boory," or "goza" (Egypt, Saudi Arabia); and "hubble bubble" (many regions).[154]

A water pipe is a multicomponent apparatus consisting of a mouthpiece, hose, water bowl, body, and head. Maassel (a mixture of tobacco, dried fruit pulp, honey, and molasses in a variety of flavors) is placed in the head and then covered with perforated aluminum foil. Small pieces of burning charcoal are placed on top of the foil. Following inhalation, heat emanating from the burning charcoal is drawn through the tobacco mixture generating smoke. A vacuum created in the water bowl causes the smoke to "bubble" through the water and collect in the air space above the water. The cooled smoke is then transported to the user through the hose and mouthpiece during inhalation.[154]

Hookah bars and cafes, many of which are in close proximity to college campuses, have been emerging throughout the United States,[155] and data suggest this form of tobacco use is becoming increasingly popular among young adults.[156,157] Recent surveys estimate a 13% to 20% prevalence of current water pipe smoking (use within the previous 30 days) among U.S. college students.[156,158] Although many water pipe users assume that the water will filter out toxins and believe this form of smoking is less harmful than cigarette smoking,[156,157,159] data are lacking to substantiate this belief. Indeed, studies have found that water pipe smokers who inhale are exposed to nicotine and other toxins in levels that are comparable to or exceed those found in cigarette smoke,[160–162] suggesting that water pipe smoking is not "safe." Furthermore, preliminary data suggest that water pipe smokers are at risk for developing dependence and other adverse health-related conditions associated with smoking.[154]

REFERENCES

1. Doll R et al. Mortality in relation to smoking: 50 years' observations on male British doctors. *BMJ* 2004;328:1519.
2. U.S. Department of Health and Human Services. The health consequences of smoking: nicotine addiction. A report of the Surgeon General. DHHS Publication No. (PHS) 88-8406. Washington, DC: Government Printing Office; 1988.
3. U.S. Department of Health and Human Services. The health consequences of smoking: a report of the Surgeon General. Washington, DC: U.S. Department of Health and Human Services, Centers for Disease Control and Prevention, National Center for Chronic Disease Prevention and Health Promotion, Office on Smoking and Health; 2004.
4. WHO Report on the Global Tobacco Epidemic, 2008. The MPOWER package. Geneva, Switzerland: World Health Organization; 2008.
5. Centers for Disease Control and Prevention. Annual smoking-attributable mortality, years of potential life lost, and economic costs—United States, 1997–2001. *MMWR Morb Mortal Wkly Rep* 2005;54:625.
6. U.S. Department of Health and Human Services. The health consequences of involuntary exposure to tobacco smoke: a report of the Surgeon General. Atlanta, GA: U.S. Department of Health and Human Services, Centers for Disease Control and Prevention, Coordinating Center for Health Promotion, National Center for Chronic Disease Prevention and Health Promotion, Office on Smoking and Health; 2006.
7. Fiore MC et al. Treating tobacco use and dependence: 2008 update. Clinical practice guideline. Rockville, MD: U.S. Department of Health and Human Services, Public Health Service; May 2008.
8. Leshner AI. Drug abuse and addiction are biomedical problems. *Hosp Pract* 1997:2.
9. U.S. Department of Health and Human Services. Preventing tobacco use among young people: a report of the Surgeon General. Atlanta: U.S. Department of Health and Human Services, Public Health Service, Centers for Disease Control and Prevention, National Center for Chronic Disease Prevention and Health Promotion, Office on Smoking and Health; 1994.
10. Gilpin EA et al. Smoking initiation rates in adults and minors: United States, 1944–1988. *Am J Epidemiol* 1994;140:535.
11. U.S. Department of Health and Human Services. Healthy people 2010. Washington, DC: U.S. Department of Health and Human Services; 2000.
12. Centers for Disease Control and Prevention. Cigarette use among high school students—United States, 1991–2005. *MMWR Morb Mortal Wkly Rep* 2006;55:724.
13. Johnston LD. Teen smoking resumes decline. Press release. Ann Arbor: University of Michigan News Service; December 11, 2007. Available at: www.monitoringthefuture.org. Accessed June 15, 2008.
14. Centers for Disease Control and Prevention. Cigarette smoking among adults—United States, 2006. *MMWR Morb Mortal Wkly Rep* 2007;56:1157.
15. Centers for Disease Control and Prevention. State-specific prevalence of current cigarette smoking among adults and quitting among persons aged 18–35 years—United States, 2006. *MMWR Morb Mortal Wkly Rep* 2007;56:993.
16. Lasser K et al. Smoking and mental illness: a population-based study. *JAMA* 2000;284:2606.
17. Benowitz NL. Clinical pharmacology of nicotine: implications for understanding, preventing, and treating tobacco addiction. *Clin Pharmacol Ther* 2008;83:531.
18. Benowitz NL. Neurobiology of nicotine addiction: implications for smoking cessation treatment. *Am J Med* 2008;121:S3.
19. Li MD et al. A meta-analysis of estimated genetic and environmental effects on smoking behavior in male and female adult twins. *Addiction* 2003;98:23.
20. Sullivan PF, Kendler KS. The genetic epidemiology of smoking. *Nicotine Tob Res* 1999;1(Suppl 2):S51.
21. Xian H et al. The heritability of failed smoking cessation and nicotine withdrawal in twins who smoked and attempted to quit. *Nicotine Tob Res* 2003;5: 245.
22. Benowitz NL. Cigarette smoking and nicotine addiction. *Med Clin North Am* 1992;76:415.
23. Taylor P. Agents acting at the neuromuscular junction and autonomic ganglia. In: Brunton LL, Lazo JS, Parker KL, eds. *Goodman and Gilman's The Pharmacological Basis of Therapeutics.* 11th ed. New York: McGraw-Hill; 2006.
24. Hukkanen J et al. Metabolism and disposition kinetics of nicotine. *Pharmacol Rev* 2005;57:79.
25. Kessler DA. The control and manipulation of nicotine in cigarettes. *Tob Control* 1994;3:362.
26. Perry DC et al. Increased nicotinic receptors in brains from smokers: membrane binding and autoradiography studies. *J Pharmacol Exp Ther* 1999; 289:1545.
27. Hughes JR et al. Symptoms of tobacco withdrawal: a replication and extension. *Arch Gen Psychiatry* 1991;48:52.
28. American Psychiatric Association. *Diagnostic and Statistical Manual of Mental Disorders. 4th ed.* Washington, DC: American Psychiatric Association; 2000.

29. Hughes JR, Hatsukami D. Errors in using tobacco withdrawal scale [letter to the editor]. *Tob Control* 1998;7:92.
30. Zevin S, Benowitz NL. Drug interactions with tobacco smoking: an update. *Clin Pharmacokinet* 1999;36:425.
31. Kroon LA. Drug interactions with smoking. *Am J Health Syst Pharm* 2007;64:1917.
32. Rx for Change: Clinician-Assisted Tobacco Cessation. San Francisco: The Regents of the University of California, University of Southern California, and Western University of Health Sciences; 1999–2008.
33. Centers for Disease Control and Prevention. Cigarette smoking-attributable morbidity—United States, 2000. *MMWR Morb Mortal Wkly Rep* 2003; 52:842.
34. American Cancer Society. Cancer Facts & Figures 2008. Atlanta: American Cancer Society; 2008.
35. California Environmental Protection Agency. Proposed identification of environmental tobacco smoke as a toxic air contaminant: executive summary. January 26, 2006. Available at: www.arb.ca.gov/regact/ets2006/ets2006.htm. Accessed June 6, 2008.
36. U.S. Department of Health and Human Services. The health benefits of smoking cessation: a report of the Surgeon General. DHHS Publication No. (CDC) 90-8416. U.S. Department of Health and Human Services, Public Health Service, Centers for Disease Control and Prevention and Health Promotion, Office on Smoking and Health; 1990.
37. Fletcher C, Peto R. The natural history of chronic airflow obstruction. *Br Med J* 1977;1:1645.
38. Peto R et al. Smoking, smoking cessation, and lung cancer in the UK since 1950: combination of national statistics with two case-control studies. *Br Med J* 2000;321:323.
39. Bjartveit K, Tverdal A. Health consequences of smoking 1–4 cigarettes per day. *Tob Control* 2005; 14:315.
40. Tverdal A, Bjartveit K. Health consequences of reduced daily cigarette consumption. *Tob Control* 2006;15:472.
41. Zhu S et al. Smoking cessation with and without assistance: a population-based analysis. *Am J Prev Med* 2000;18:305.
42. Prochaska JO, DiClemente CC. The Transtheoretical Approach: Crossing Traditional Boundaries of Therapy. Homewood, IL: Dow Jones-Irwin; 1984.
43. Severson HH et al. A self-help cessation program for smokeless tobacco users: comparison of two interventions. *Nicotine Tob Res* 2000;2:363.
44. Stead LF et al. Nicotine replacement therapy for smoking cessation. *Cochrane Database Syst Rev* 2008;CD000146.
45. Hughes JR et al. Antidepressants for smoking cessation. *Cochrane Database Syst Rev* 2007; CD000031.
46. Coe JW et al. Varenicline: an $\alpha 4\beta 2$ nicotinic receptor partial agonist for smoking cessation. *J Med Chem* 2005;48:3474.
47. Foulds J. The neurobiological basis for partial agonist treatment of nicotine dependence: varenicline. *Int J Clin Pract* 2006;60:571.
48. Palmer KJ et al. Transdermal nicotine: a review of its pharmacodynamic and pharmacokinetic properties, and therapeutic efficacy as an aid to smoking cessation. *Drugs* 1992;44:498.
49. Gore AV, Chien YW. The nicotine transdermal system. *Clin Dermatol* 1998;16:599.
50. Benowitz NL et al. Determinants of nicotine intake while chewing nicotine polacrilex gum. *Clin Pharmacol Ther* 1987;41:467.
51. Henningfield JE et al. Drinking coffee and carbonated beverages blocks absorption of nicotine from nicotine polacrilex gum. *JAMA* 1990;264:1560.
52. Choi JH et al. Pharmacokinetics of a nicotine polacrilex lozenge. *Nicotine Tob Res* 2003;5:635.
53. Shiffman S et al. Efficacy of a nicotine lozenge for smoking cessation. *Arch Intern Med* 2002;162: 1267.
54. Heatherton TF et al. Measuring the heaviness of smoking: using self-reported time to the first cigarette of the day and number of cigarettes smoked per day. *Br J Addict* 1989;84:791.
55. O'Hara P et al. Early and late weight gain following smoking cessation in the Lung Health Study. *Am J Epidemiol* 1998;148:821.
56. Perkins KA et al. Acute effects of tobacco smoking on hunger and eating in male and female smokers. *Appetite* 1994;22:149.
57. Hatsukami D et al. Effects of tobacco abstinence on food intake among cigarette smokers. *Health Psychol* 1993;12:499.
58. Kawachi I et al. Can physical activity minimize weight gain in women after smoking cessation?. *Am J Public Health* 1996;86:999.
59. Benowitz NL. Cigarette smoking and cardiovascular disease: pathophysiology and implications for treatment. *Prog Cardiovasc Dis* 2003;46:91.
60. Adamopoulos D et al. New insights into the sympathetic, endothelial and coronary effects of nicotine. *Clin Exp Pharmacol Physiol* 2008;35:458.
61. Bazzano LA et al. Relationship between cigarette smoking and novel risk factors for cardiovascular disease in the United States. *Ann Intern Med* 2003; 138:891.
62. Tonstad S, Johnston JA. Cardiovascular risks associated with smoking: a review for clinicians. *Eur J Cardiovasc Prev Rehabil* 2006;13:507.
63. Rigotti NA et al. Interventions for smoking cessation in hospitalised patients. *Cochrane Database Syst Rev* 2007;CD001837.
64. Benowitz NL et al. Sources of variability in nicotine and cotinine levels with use of nicotine nasal spray, transdermal nicotine, and cigarette smoking. *Br J Clin Pharmacol* 1997;43:259.
65. Roth MT, Westman EC. Asthma exacerbation after administration of nicotine nasal spray for smoking cessation. *Pharmacotherapy* 2002;22:779.
66. Schneider NG et al. The nicotine inhaler: clinical pharmacokinetics and comparison with other nicotine treatments. *Clin Pharmacokinet* 2001;40:661.
67. Bergstrom M et al. Regional deposition of inhaled 11C-nicotine vapor in the human airway as visualized by positron emission tomography. *Clin Pharmacol Ther* 1995;57:309.
68. Molander L et al. Dose released and absolute bioavailability of nicotine from a nicotine vapor inhaler. *Clin Pharmacol Ther* 1996;59:394.
69. GlaxoSmithKline. Zyban package insert. Research Triangle Park, NC; August 2007.
70. Swan GE et al. Effectiveness of bupropion sustained release for smoking cessation in a health care setting: a randomized trial. *Arch Intern Med* 2003;163:2337.
71. Hurt RD et al. A comparison of sustained-release bupropion and placebo for smoking cessation. *N Engl J Med* 1997;337:1195.
72. Dunner DL et al. A prospective safety surveillance study for bupropion sustained-release in the treatment of depression. *J Clin Psychiatry* 1998;59: 366.
73. Johnston AJ et al. Pharmacokinetic optimisation of sustained-release bupropion for smoking cessation. *Drugs* 2002;62(Suppl 2):11.
74. Jorenby DE et al. A controlled trial of sustained-release bupropion, a nicotine patch, or both for smoking cessation. *N Engl J Med* 1999;340:685.
75. Cahill K et al. Nicotine receptor partial agonists for smoking cessation. *Cochrane Database Syst Rev* 2007;CD006103.
76. Pfizer, Inc. Chantix package insert. New York, NY; June 2008.
77. Faessel HM et al. Multiple-dose pharmacokinetics of the selective nicotinic receptor partial agonist, varenicline, in healthy smokers. *J Clin Pharmacol* 2006;46:1439.
78. U.S. Food and Drug Administration, Center for Drug Evaluation and Research. Information for Healthcare Professionals Varenicline (marketed as Chantix). February 1, 2008. Available at: www.fda.gov/cder/drug/InfoSheets/HCP/vareniclineHCP.htm. Accessed June 15, 2008.
79. Lunell E et al. Relative bioavailability of nicotine from a nasal spray in infectious rhinitis and after use of a topical decongestant. *Eur J Clin Pharmacol* 1995;48:71.
80. Benowitz NL, Gourlay SG. Cardiovascular toxicity of nicotine: implications for nicotine replacement therapy. *J Am Coll Cardiol* 1997;29:1422.
81. Joseph AM et al. The safety of transdermal nicotine as an aid to smoking cessation in patients with cardiac disease. *N Engl J Med* 1996;335:1792.
82. Tzivoni D et al. Cardiovascular safety of transdermal nicotine patches in patients with coronary artery disease who try to quit smoking. *Cardiovasc Drugs Ther* 1998;12:239.
83. Nicotine replacement therapy for patients with coronary artery disease. Working Group for the Study of Transdermal Nicotine in Patients With Coronary Artery Disease. *Arch Intern Med* 1994; 154:989.
84. Benowitz NL et al. Cardiovascular effects of nasal and transdermal nicotine and cigarette smoking. *Hypertension* 2002;39:1107.
85. Haustein KO et al. Effects of cigarette smoking or nicotine replacement on cardiovascular risk factors and parameters of haemorheology. *J Intern Med* 2002;252:130.
86. Lee AH, Afessa B. The association of nicotine replacement therapy with mortality in a medical intensive care unit. *Crit Care Med* 2007;35:1517.
87. Joseph AM, Fu SS. Safety issues in pharmacotherapy for smoking in patients with cardiovascular disease. *Prog Cardiovasc Dis* 2003;45:429.
88. McRobbie H, Hajek P. Nicotine replacement therapy in patients with cardiovascular disease: guidelines for health professionals. *Addiction* 2001;96: 1547.
89. Global Strategy for the Diagnosis, Management and Prevention of COPD, Global Initiative for Chronic Obstructive Lung Disease (GOLD) 2007. Available from: www.goldcopd.org. Accessed June 15, 2008.
90. Anthonisen NR. Effects of smoking intervention and the use of an inhaled anticholinergic bronchodilator on the rate of decline of FEV_1. The Lung Health Study. *JAMA* 1994;272:1497.
91. Parkes G et al. Effect on smoking quit rate of telling patients their lung age: the Step2quit randomized controlled trial. *BMJ* 2008;336:598.
92. Stead LF, Hughes JR. Lobeline for smoking cessation. *Cochrane Database Syst Rev* 2000; CD000124.
93. Stead LF, Lancaster T. Nicobrevin for smoking cessation. *Cochrane Database Syst Rev* 2006; CD005990.
94. Abbot NC et al. Hypnotherapy for smoking cessation. *Cochrane Database Syst Rev* 2000; CD001008.
95. White AR et al. Acupuncture for smoking cessation. *Cochrane Database Syst Rev* 2006;CD000009.
96. Hazelden Foundation. Survey on Current and Former Smokers—1998. Available at: www.hazelden.org/web/public/smokers1998.page. Accessed June 6, 2008.
97. Lawson GM et al. Application of serum nicotine and plasma cotinine concentrations to assessment of nicotine replacement in light, moderate, and heavy smokers undergoing transdermal therapy. *J Clin Pharmacol* 1998;38:502.
98. Fredrickson PA et al. High dose transdermal nicotine therapy for heavy smokers: safety, tolerability and measurement of nicotine and cotinine levels. *Psychopharmacology* 1995;122:215.
99. Benowitz NL et al. Suppression of nicotine intake during ad libitum cigarette smoking by high-dose transdermal nicotine. *J Pharmacol Exp Ther* 1998;287:958.
100. Dale LC et al. High-dose nicotine patch therapy: percentage of replacement and smoking cessation. *JAMA* 1995;274:1353.
101. Bars MP et al. "Tobacco free with FDNY": the New York City Fire Department World Trade Center Tobacco Cessation Study. *Chest* 2006;129:979.
102. Hurt RD et al. Nicotine patch therapy based on smoking rate followed by bupropion for prevention of relapse to smoking. *J Clin Oncol* 2003;21:914.

103. Tonnesen P et al. Higher dosage nicotine patches increase one-year smoking cessation rates: results from the European CEASE trial. Collaborative European Anti-Smoking Evaluation. European Respiratory Society. *Eur Respir J* 1999;13:238.
104. Jorenby DE et al. Varying nicotine patch dose and type of smoking cessation counseling. *JAMA* 1995;274:1347.
105. Hughes JR et al. Are higher doses of nicotine replacement more effective for smoking cessation? *Nicotine Tob Res* 1999;1:169.
106. Killen JD et al. Do heavy smokers benefit from higher dose nicotine patch therapy? *Exp Clin Psychopharmacol* 1999;7:226.
107. Paoletti P et al. Importance of baseline cotinine plasma values in smoking cessation: results from a double-blind study with nicotine patch. *Eur Respir J* 1996;9:643.
108. Murray RP et al. Safety of nicotine polacrilex gum used by 3,094 participants in the Lung Health Study. Lung Health Study Research Group. *Chest* 1996;109:438.
109. Pfizer Consumer Healthcare. Nicotrol inhaler prescribing information. Morris Plans, NJ; February 2005.
110. Pfizer Consumer Healthcare. Nicotrol nasal spray prescribing information. Morris Plans, NJ; February 2005.
111. Steinberg MB et al. The case for treating tobacco dependence as a chronic disease. *Ann Intern Med* 2008;148:554.
112. Seibert C et al. Prescribing oral contraceptives for women older than 35 years of age. *Ann Intern Med* 2003;138:54.
113. Burkman R et al. Safety concerns and health benefits associated with oral contraception. *Am J Obstet Gynecol* 2004;190:S5.
114. Schwingl PJ et al. Estimates of the risk of cardiovascular death attributable to low-dose oral contraceptives in the United States. *Am J Obstet Gynecol* 1999;180(1 Pt 1):241.
115. World Heath Organization. Medical Eligibility Criteria for Contraceptive Use. 3rd ed. Geneva, Switzerland: World Health Organization; 2004.
116. ACOG Committee on Practice Bulletins—Gynecology. ACOG practice bulletin no. 73: use of hormonal contraception in women with coexisting medical conditions. *Obstet Gynecol* 2006;107:1453.
117. Fruzzetti F. Hemostatic effects of smoking and oral contraceptive use. *Am J Obstet Gynecol* 1999;180(6 Pt 2):S369.
118. Aldrighi JM et al. Effect of a combined oral contraceptive containing 20 mcg ethinyl estradiol and 75 mcg gestodene on hemostatic parameters. *Gynecol Endocrinol* 2006;22:1.
119. U.S. Department of Health and Human Services. Women and smoking: a report of the Surgeon General. Atlanta: U.S. Department of Health and Human Services, Centers for Disease Control and Prevention, National Center for Chronic Disease Prevention and Health Promotion, Office on Smoking and Health; 2001.
120. Kiley J, Hammond C. Combined oral contraceptives: a comprehensive review. *Clin Obstet Gynecol* 2007;50:868.
121. U.S. Department of Health and Human Services. The health consequences of smoking: cancer. A report of the Surgeon General. DHHS Publication No. (PHS) 82-50179. Rockville, MD: Public Health Service, Office on Smoking and Health; 1982.
122. Rosenberg L et al. Low-dose oral contraceptive use and the risk of myocardial infarction. *Arch Intern Med* 2001;161:1065.
123. van den Heuvel MW et al. Comparison of ethinylestradiol pharmacokinetics in three hormonal contraceptive formulations: the vaginal ring, the transdermal patch and an oral contraceptive. *Contraception* 2005;72:168.
124. Hatsukami DK et al. Changing smokeless tobacco products: new tobacco-delivery systems. *Am J Prev Med* 2007;33:S368.
125. U.S. Department of Health and Human Services, Substance Abuse and Mental Health Services Administration. Results from the 2006 national survey on drug use and health: national findings (Office of Applied Studies, NSDUH Series H-32, DHHS Publication No. SMA 07-4293). Rockville, MD; 2007.
126. Hatsukami DK, Severson HH. Oral spit tobacco: addiction, prevention and treatment. *Nicotine Tob Res* 1999;1:21.
127. Fant RV et al. Pharmacokinetics and pharmacodynamics of moist snuff in humans. *Tob Control* 1999;8:387.
128. Ebbert JO et al. Smokeless tobacco: an emerging addiction. *Med Clin North Am* 2004;88:1593.
129. Taybos G. Oral changes associated with tobacco use. *Am J Med Sci* 2003;326:179.
130. Napier SS, Speight PM. Natural history of potentially malignant oral lesions and conditions: an overview of the literature. *J Oral Pathol Med* 2008;37.1.
131. Martin GC et al. Oral leukoplakia status six weeks after cessation of smokeless tobacco use. *J Am Dent Assoc* 1999;130:945.
132. Hecht SS et al. Similar exposure to a tobacco-specific carcinogen in smokeless tobacco users and cigarette smokers. *Cancer Epidemiol Biomarkers Prev* 2007;16:1567.
133. Henley SJ et al. Tobacco-related disease mortality among men who switched from cigarettes to spit tobacco. *Tob Control* 2007;16:22.
134. Ebbert JO et al. Interventions for smokeless tobacco use cessation. *Cochrane Database Syst Rev* 2007;4:CD004306.
135. Ebbert JO et al. Nicotine lozenges for the treatment of smokeless tobacco use. *Nicotine Tob Res* 2007;9:233.
136. National Cancer Institute. Cigars: health effects and trends. Smoking and Tobacco Control Monograph No. 9. NIH Publication No. 98-4302. Bethesda, MD: U.S. Department of Health and Human Services, National Institutes of Health, National Cancer Institute; 1998.
137. Baker F et al. Health risks associated with cigar smoking. *JAMA* 2000;284:735.
138. Henningfield JE et al. Nicotine concentration, smoke pH and whole tobacco aqueous pH of some cigar brands and types popular in the United States. *Nicotine Tob Res* 1999;1:163.
139. U.S. Department of Agriculture, Economic Research Service. Tobacco outlook. Report TBS-263. October 24, 2007. Available at: http://usda.mannlib.cornell.edu/usda/current/TBS/TBS-10-24-2007.pdf. Accessed June 15, 2008.
140. Wenger LD et al. Cigar magazines: using tobacco to sell a lifestyle. *Tob Control* 2001;10:279.
141. Connolly GN et al. Trends in nicotine yield in smoke and its relationship with design characteristics among popular US cigarette brands, 1997–2005. *Tob Control* 2007;16:e5.
142. Deckers SK et al. Tobacco and its trendy alternatives: implications for pediatric nurses. *Crit Care Nurs Clin North Am* 2006;18:95.
143. Delnevo CD et al. Bidi cigarette use among young adults in 15 states. *Prev Med* 2004;39:207.
144. Centers for Disease Control and Prevention. Bidi use among urban youth—Massachusetts, March-April 1999. *MMWR Morb Mortal Wkly Rep* 1999;48:796.
145. Malson JL et al. Comparison of the nicotine content of tobacco used in bidis and conventional cigarettes. *Tob Control* 2001;10:181.
146. Watson CH et al. Determination of tar, nicotine, and carbon monoxide yields in the smoke of bidi cigarettes. *Nicotine Tob Res* 2003;5:747.
147. Taylor TM, Biener L. Bidi smoking among Massachusetts teenagers. *Prev Med* 2001;32:89.
148. Jha P et al. A nationally representative case-control study of smoking and death in India. *N Engl J Med* 2008;358:1137.
149. Malson JL et al. Clove cigarette smoking: biochemical, physiological, and subjective effects. *Pharmacol Biochem Behav* 2003;74:739.
150. Centers for Disease Control and Prevention. Illnesses possibly associated with smoking clove cigarettes. *MMWR Morb Mortal Wkly Rep* 1985;34:297.
151. American Medical Association. Evaluation of the health hazard of clove cigarettes. Council on Scientific Affairs. *JAMA* 1988;260:3641.
152. Guidotti TL et al. Clove cigarettes: the basis for concern regarding health effects. *West J Med* 1989;151:220.
153. DiFranza JR et al. Symptoms of tobacco dependence after brief intermittent use: the Development and Assessment of Nicotine Dependence in Youth-2 study. *Arch Pediatr Adolesc Med* 2007;161:704.
154. Maziak W et al. Tobacco smoking using a waterpipe: a re-emerging strain in a global epidemic. *Tob Control* 2004;13:327.
155. Lewin T. Collegians smoking hookahs . . . filled with tobacco. New York Times, April 19, 2006. Available at: www.nytimes.com/2006/04/19/education/19hookah.html?ei=5070&en=e29cc03a601b322a&ex=1190001600&pagewanted=print. Accessed June 6, 2008.
156. Eissenberg T et al. Waterpipe tobacco smoking on a U.S. college campus: prevalence and correlates. *J Adolesc Health* 2008;42:526.
157. Ward KD et al. Characteristics of U.S. waterpipe users: a preliminary report. *Nicotine Tob Res* 2007;9:1339.
158. Smith SY et al. Harm perception of nicotine products in college freshmen. *Nicotine Tob Res* 2007;9:977.
159. Smith-Simone S et al. Waterpipe tobacco smoking: knowledge, attitudes, beliefs, and behavior in two U.S. samples. *Nicotine Tob Res* 2008;10:393.
160. Sepetdjian E et al. Measurement of 16 polycyclic aromatic hydrocarbons in narghile waterpipe tobacco smoke. *Food Chem Toxicol* 2008;46:1582.
161. Shihadeh A, Saleh R. Polycyclic aromatic hydrocarbons, carbon monoxide, "tar", and nicotine in the mainstream smoke aerosol of the narghile water pipe. *Food Chem Toxicol* 2005;43:655.
162. Neergaard J et al. Waterpipe smoking and nicotine exposure: a review of the current evidence. *Nicotine Tob Res* 2007;9:987.

SECTION EIGHTEEN

HEMATOPOIETIC DISORDERS

SECTION EDITOR

CHAPTER 86

Anemias

Cindy L. O'Bryant and Kenneth J. Utz

Definition

Anemia is a reduction in red cell mass. It often is described as a decrease in the number of red blood cells (RBC) per cubic millimeter (mm^3) or as a decrease in the hemoglobin concentration in blood to a level below the normal physiologic requirement for adequate tissue oxygenation. The term *anemia* is not a diagnosis, but rather an objective sign of a disease. Diagnostic terminology for anemia requires the inclusion of the pathogenesis (e.g., megaloblastic anemia secondary to folate deficiency, microcytic anemia secondary to iron deficiency). An exact diagnosis is important to the understanding of the problem and to implement specific therapy to correct the anemia.

Pathophysiology

Anemia is a symptom of many pathologic conditions. It is associated with nutritional deficiencies and acute and chronic diseases; it also can be drug induced. Anemia can be caused by decreased red cell production, increased red cell destruction, or increased red cell loss. If the anemia is caused by decreased red cell production, it may be the result of disturbances in stem cell proliferation or differentiation. Anemias caused by increased red cell destruction can be secondary to hemolysis, whereas increased red cell loss may be caused by acute or chronic bleeding. Anemias associated with acute blood loss, those that are iron related, and those caused by chronic disease comprise most of all anemias.[1] Classifications of anemias according to pathophysiologic and morphologic characteristics are shown in Table 86-1.

Normally, RBC mass is maintained by feedback mechanisms that regulate levels of erythropoietin (EPO), a hormone that stimulates proliferation and differentiation of erythroid precursors in the bone marrow. Two types of erythroid precursors reside in the bone marrow: the burst-forming unit,

Table 86-1 Classifications of Anemia

Pathophysiologic (Classifies Anemias Based on Pathophysiologic Presentation)
Blood Loss
Acute: trauma, ulcer, hemorrhoids
Chronic: ulcer, vaginal bleeding, aspirin ingestion
Inadequate Red Blood Cell Production
Nutritional deficiency: B_{12}, folic acid, iron
Erythroblast deficiency: bone marrow failure (aplastic anemia, irradiation, chemotherapy, folic acid antagonists) or bone marrow infiltration (leukemia, lymphoma, myeloma, metastatic solid tumors, myelofibrosis)
Endocrine deficiency: pituitary, adrenal, thyroid, testicular
Chronic disease: renal, liver, infection, granulomatous, collagen vascular
Excessive Red Blood Cell Destruction
Intrinsic factors: hereditary (G6PD), abnormal hemoglobin synthesis
Extrinsic factors: autoimmune reactions, drug reactions, infection (endotoxin)
Morphologic (Classifies Anemias by Red Blood Cell Size [Microcytic, Normocytic, Macrocytic] and Hemoglobin Content [Hypochromic, Normochromic, Hyperchromic])
Macrocytic
Defective maturation with decreased production
Megaloblastic: pernicious (vitamin B_{12} deficiency), folic acid deficiency
Normochromic, normocytic
Recent blood loss
Hemolysis
Chronic disease
Renal failure
Autoimmune
Endocrine
Microcytic, hyperchromic
Iron deficiency
Genetic abnormalities: sickle cell, thalassemia

G6PD, glucose-6-phosphate dehydrogenase.

erythroid (BFUe) and colony-forming unit, erythroid (CFUe). The BFUe is the earliest progenitor, which eventually develops into a CFUe. BFUe is moderately sensitive to EPO and is under the influence of other cytokines (e.g., interleukin [IL]-3, granulocyte-macrophage colony-stimulating factor [GM-CSF]). In contrast, CFUe is highly sensitive to EPO and differentiates into erythroblasts and reticulocytes. Of EPO, 90% is produced in the kidney; liver synthesis accounts for the remaining 10%. Reduced oxygen-carrying capacity is sensed by renal peritubular cells, and this stimulates release of EPO into the bloodstream. Patients with chronic anemia may have a blunted and inadequate response for the degree of anemia present.

Detection

Signs and Symptoms

Signs and symptoms of anemia vary with the degree of RBC reduction as well as with the time interval over which it develops. Onset of anemia can be acute or can develop slowly, resulting in tissue hypoxia caused by the decreased oxygen-carrying capacity of the reduced red cell mass. As a result, perfusion to nonvital tissues (e.g., skin, mucous membranes, extremities) is decreased to sustain tissue perfusion of vital organs (e.g., brain, heart, kidneys). Slowly developing anemias can be asymptomatic initially or include symptoms such as slight exertional dyspnea, increased angina, fatigue, or malaise. Uncorrected tissue hypoxia can lead to a number of complications in quality of life, cognition, and respiratory and gastrointestinal (GI) systems. Changes in the blood hemoglobin concentration also lead to changes in the kidney tissue oxygen tension, as discussed previously.[1,2]

In severe anemia, a hemoglobin (Hgb) <8 mg/dL, heart rate, and stroke volume often increase in an attempt to improve oxygen delivery to tissues. These changes in heart rate and stroke volume can result in systolic murmurs, angina pectoris, high output congestive heart failure, pulmonary congestion, ascites, and edema. Thus, anemia is generally not well tolerated in patients with cardiac disease. Skin and mucous membrane pallor, jaundice, smooth or beefy tongue, cheilosis, and spoon-shaped nails (koilonychia) also may be associated with severe anemia of different causes of anemia.

History

A thorough history and physical examination are essential because of the complexity of the pathologic conditions associated with anemia. A time line, which begins with the onset of symptoms (and surrounding events) and extends to current status, is important. Because longstanding anemias can indicate hereditary disorders, the family history should be noted. Past Hgb or hematocrit (Hct) determinations, transfusion history, as well as occupational, environmental, and social histories may be valuable. Finally, a medication history can help eliminate drug reactions or interactions as the cause of the anemia.

Physical Examination

On physical examination of a patient with anemia, pallor is most easily observed in the conjunctiva, mucous membranes, nail beds, and palmar creases of the hand. In addition, postural hypotension and tachycardia can be seen when hypovolemia (acute blood loss) is the primary cause of anemia. Patients with B_{12} deficiency may exhibit neurologic findings, which include changes in deep tendon reflexes, ataxia, and loss of vibration and position sense; all are consistent with nerve fiber demyelination. Patients with anemia from hemolysis may be slightly jaundiced from bilirubin release. Manifestations of hemorrhage can include petechiae, ecchymoses, hematomas, epistaxis, bleeding gums, and blood in the urine or the stool.

Laboratory Evaluation

Although anemia may be suspected from the history and physical examination, a full laboratory evaluation is necessary to confirm the diagnosis, establish its severity, and determine its cause. A list of the routine laboratory evaluations used in the workup for anemia is found in Table 86-2. The cornerstone of this evaluation is the complete blood count (CBC). Normal hematologic values can be found in Table 86-3. Male patients have higher hematocrit (Hct) values than do female patients. The Hct is increased in individuals living at altitudes above 4,000 feet in response to the diminished oxygen content of the atmosphere and blood.

The morphologic appearance of the RBC provides useful information about the nature of the anemia. Microscopic

Table 86-2 Routine Laboratory Evaluation for Anemia Workup

Complete blood count (CBC): Hgb, Hct, RBC count, red cell indices (MCV, MCH, MCHC), WBC count (and differential)
Platelet count
Red cell morphology
Reticulocyte count
Bilirubin and LDH
Serum iron, TIBC, serum ferritin, transferrin saturation
Peripheral blood smear examination
Stool examination for occult blood
Bone marrow aspiration and biopsy[a]

[a]Performed in patients with abnormal peripheral blood smears.
Hct, hematocrit; Hgb, hemoglobin; LDH, lactic dehydrogenase; MCV, mean corpuscular volume; MCH, mean corpuscular hemoglobin; MCHC, mean corpuscular hemoglobin concentration; RBC, red blood cell; TIBC, total iron-binding capacity; WBC, white blood cell.

evaluation of the peripheral blood smear can detect the presence of macrocytic (large) RBC, which usually are present when anemia results from a vitamin B_{12} or folic acid deficiency; microcytic (small) RBC usually are associated with iron deficiency anemia. Acute blood loss generally is associated with normocytic cells.

Together with the information gained from the history and physical examination, the routine laboratory evaluation can provide sufficient information to distinguish between the most common forms of anemia (Fig. 86-1). If still not identified after routine evaluation, problems such as autoimmune disease, collagen vascular disease, chronic infection, endocrine disorders, or drug-induced destruction may be causing the anemia. When uncertainty exists or an abnormal peripheral blood smear is noted, a bone marrow aspiration with biopsy is indicated.

Table 86-3 Normal Hematology Values

	Pediatric	Adult	
Laboratory Test	*1–15 yr*	*Male*	*Female*
RBC (× 10^6/mm^3)	±4.7–6	5.4–0.7	±4.8–6
Hgb (g/dL)	±13–2	16–2	±14–2
Hct (%)	±40–5	47–5	±42–2
MCV (μm^3)	±80–5	87–7	±90–9
MCH (pg/cell)	±33.5–2	29–2	±34–2
MCHC (g/dL)	±31–36	31–36	±31–36
Erythropoietin (mU/mL)	4–26	4–26	4–26
Reticulocyte count (%)	0.5–1.5	0.5–1.5	0.5–1.5
TIBC (mg/dL)	250–400	250–400	250–400
Fe (mg/dL)	50–120	50–160	40–150
Folate (ng/mL)	7–25	7–25	7–25
RBC folate (ng/mL)	—	140–960	140–960
Fe/TIBC (%)	20–30	20–40	16–38
Vitamin B_{12} (pg/mL)	>200	>200	>200
Ferritin (ng/mL)	7–140	15–200	12–150

Fe, iron; Hgb, hemoglobin; Hct, hematocrit; MCH, mean corpuscular hemoglobin; MCV, mean corpuscular volume; RBC, red blood cell; TIBC, total iron-binding capacity.

There are many causes of anemia. This chapter is limited to the most common anemias managed with drugs. Hemolytic anemias are covered in Chapter 87, Drug-Induced Blood Disorders. Before proceeding, the reader should review the basic hematologic laboratory tests used to evaluate and monitor anemia (see Chapter 2: Interpretation of Clinical Laboratory Tests).

IRON DEFICIENCY ANEMIA

Iron deficiency is a state of negative iron balance in which the daily iron intake and stores are unable to meet the RBC and other body tissue needs. The body contains approximately 3.5 g of iron, of which 2.5 g are found in Hgb. A significant amount of iron is stored as ferritin or aggregated ferritin (hemosiderin) in the reticuloendothelial cells of the liver, spleen, and bone marrow and by hepatocytes. Ferritin circulates at concentrations that reflect total iron body stores. Only a small fraction of iron is found in plasma (100 to 150 mcg/dL), and most is bound to transferrin, the transport protein.

Despite the continuing turnover of RBC, iron stores are well preserved because the iron is recovered and reutilized in new erythrocytes. Only about 0.5 to 1 mg/day of iron is lost from urine, sweat, and the sloughing of intestinal mucosal cells that contain ferritin in men and in non-menstruating women. Menstruating women lose approximately 0.6% to 2.5% more iron per day.[3] Pregnancy and lactation are other common sources of iron loss.

Individuals with normal iron stores absorb roughly 10% of ingested dietary iron. The average American diet contains 6 mg of elemental iron/1,000 Kcal. Thus, the average daily intake ranges between 10 and 12 mg, enough to replace the 1 mg lost daily (based on 10% absorption). For menstruating, pregnant, or lactating women, however, the daily iron intake requirement may be as high as 20 mg.

Iron, which is absorbed from the duodenum and upper jejunum by an active transport mechanism, is enhanced in the presence of an acidic gastric environment. Dietary iron, which is primarily in the ferric state, is converted to the more readily absorbed ferrous form in the acid environment of the stomach. It is the ferrous form that binds to transferrin for its journey to the bone marrow, where it is incorporated into the Hgb of mature erythrocytes.

Gastrointestinal absorption of iron is increased from the usual 10% to as much as three- to fivefold in iron deficiency states or when erythropoiesis occurs at a more rapid rate.[3] Animal sources of iron, heme iron, are better absorbed than plant sources, nonheme iron. A gastrectomy or vagotomy may decrease the conversion of the ferric form of iron to the ferrous state, thereby diminishing iron absorption. In addition, certain foods and drugs can complex with iron, decreasing its absorption.

Anemia caused by iron deficiency is the most common nutritional deficiency worldwide. Although iron deficiency anemia has many causes (Table 86-4), blood loss is considered one of the more common. Each milliliter of whole blood contains 0.5 mg of iron, whereas each milliliter of packed RBC contains 1 mg of iron. Common causes of chronic blood loss include peptic ulcer disease, hemorrhoids, ingestion of GI irritants, menstruation, multiple pregnancies, and multiple blood donations.

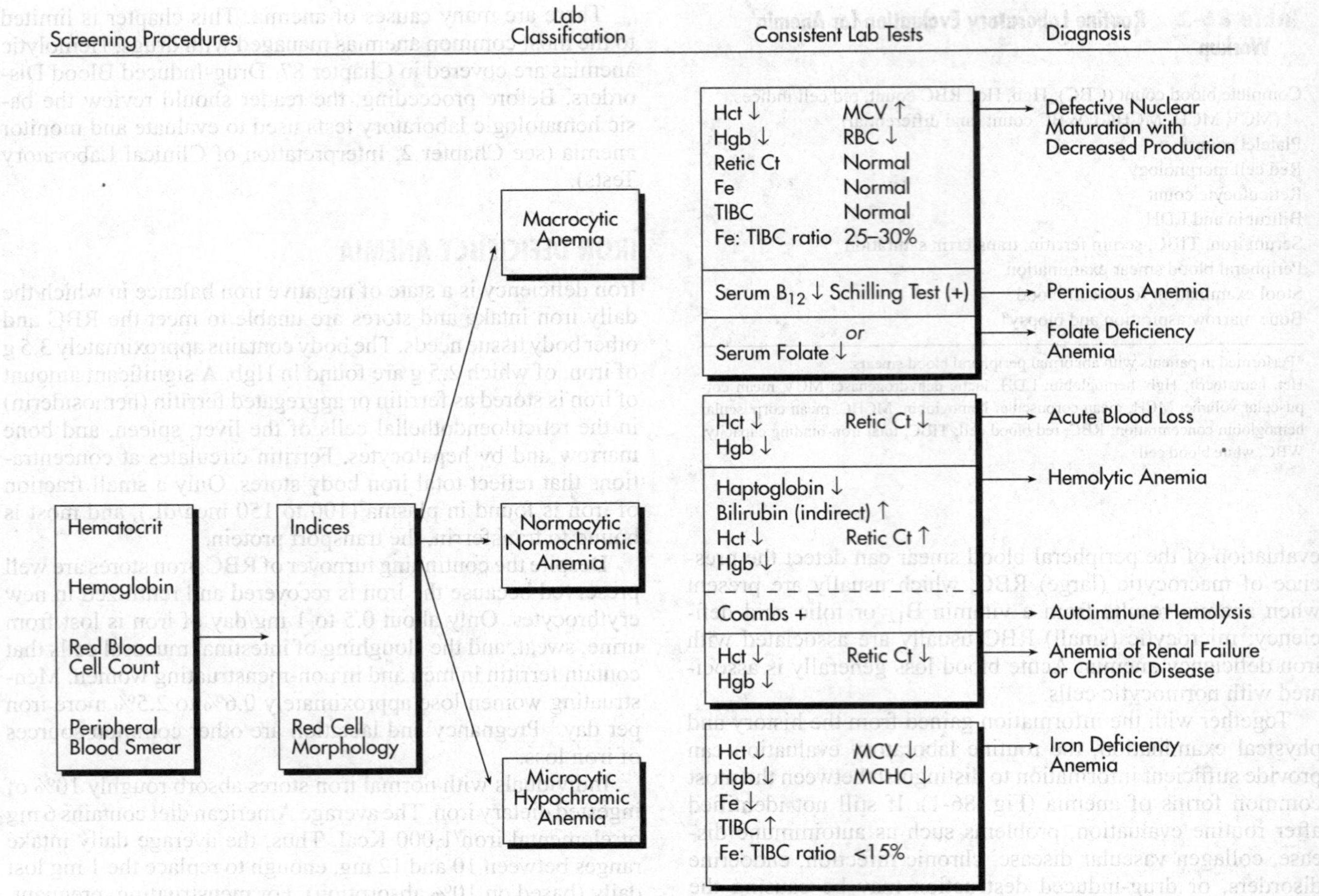

FIGURE 86-1 Laboratory diagnosis of anemia.

Dietary reference intakes (DRI) for iron are listed in Table 86-5. The increased amounts of iron required by pregnant or lactating women are difficult to obtain through diet alone; thus, oral iron supplementation generally is necessary. Although maternal iron usually provides term infants with sufficient stored iron for the first 6 months, infants 6 months to 3 years of age experience rapid growth and a threefold increase in blood volume, which can increase the risk of iron deficiency. Premature infants have reduced iron stores and thus require replacement therapy. Supplementation of 10 to 15 mg/day of iron may be required for up to the first year of life. Maintenance iron therapy for healthy older infants and children is roughly 1 to 2 mg/kg/day (not to exceed 20 mg/day). If iron deficiency develops in the pediatric patient, 3 to 6 mg/kg/day of elemental iron should be administered in two to three divided doses.[4]

Table 86-4 Iron Deficiency Anemia Causes

Blood Loss	Menstruation, gastrointestinal (e.g., peptic ulcer), trauma
Decreased Absorption	Medications, gastrectomy, regional enteritis
Increased Requirement	Infancy, pregnant/lactating women
Impaired Utilization	Hereditary, Iron use

Predisposing Factors

1. D.G., a 35-year-old woman, is seen in the clinic. Her chief complaints include weakness, dizziness, and epigastric pain. She has a 5-year history of peptic ulcer disease, a 10-year history of heavy menstrual bleeding, and a 20-year history of chronic headaches. She has two children who are 1 and 3 years of age. D.G. is currently taking tetracycline (250 mg BID) for acne, ibuprofen

Table 86-5 Dietary Reference Intake for Iron

	mg per day
Healthy, non-menstruating adults	8
Menstruating women	18
Pregnant women	27
Lactating women	9
Vegetarians	16

(400 mg PRN) headaches, and daily esomeprazole (40 mg). A review of her systems is positive for decreased exercise tolerance. Physical examination reveals a pale, lethargic, white woman appearing older than her stated age. Her vital signs are within normal limits; her heart rate is regular at 100 beats/min. Her examination is notable for pale nail beds and splenomegaly.

Significant laboratory results include the following: Hgb, 8 g/dL (normal, 14 to 18); Hct, 27% (normal, 40% to 44%); platelet count, 800,000/mm^3 (normal, 130,000 to 400,000); reticulocyte count, 0.2% (normal, 0.5% to 1.5%); mean corpuscular volume (MCV), 75 μm^3 (normal, 80 to 94); mean corpuscular hemoglobin (MCH), 23 pg (normal, 27 to 31); mean corpuscular hemoglobin concentration (MCHC), 30% (normal, 33% to 37%); serum iron, 40 μg/dL (normal, 50 to 160); serum ferritin, 9 ng/mL (normal, 15 to 200); total iron-binding capacity (TIBC), 450 g/dL (normal, 250 to 400); and 4+ guaiac stools (normal, negative).

Iron deficiency is determined to be the cause of D.G.'s anemia. An upper GI series with a small bowel follow-through are planned to evaluate her persistent epigastric pain. What factors predispose D.G. to iron deficiency anemia?

[SI units: Hgb, 80 g/L; Hct, 0.27; MCV, 75 fL;MCH, 23 pg; MCHC, 0.3; iron, 7.16 mcmol/L; ferritin, 9mcg/L; TIBC, 80.87 mcmol/L; platelets, 800 $\times 10^9$/L;reticulocyte, 0.002]

Several factors predispose D.G. to iron deficiency anemia. Her history of heavy menstrual bleeding and the 4+ stool guaiac indicate menstrual and GI sources of blood loss. The GI blood loss may be secondary to D.G.'s chronic use of nonsteroidal anti-inflammatory drugs, recurrent peptic ulcer disease, or both.

Many women of childbearing age have a borderline iron deficiency that becomes more evident during pregnancy because of the increased iron requirements.[5] D.G. has given birth to two children. Therefore, her iron stores have been repeatedly taxed in recent years. In addition, absorption of dietary iron may be compromised by her use of proton pump inhibitors and tetracycline (see Question 6).

Signs, Symptoms, and Laboratory Tests

2. What subjective or objective signs, symptoms, and laboratory tests are typical of iron deficiency in D.G.?

D.G.'s constitutional symptoms of weakness and dizziness could be a result of her severe anemia. Generally, until the anemia is severe, such symptoms occur with equal frequency in the nonanemic population. The most important signs and symptoms of iron deficiency anemia are related to the cardiovascular system and are a reflection of the imbalance between the ongoing demands for oxygen against a diminishing oxygen supply. D.G.'s increased heart rate, decreased exercise tolerance, and pale appearance are consistent with tissue anoxia and the cardiovascular response that may be seen in iron deficiency anemia.

D.G.'s iron deficiency has advanced to symptomatic anemia. In patients who are not yet symptomatic, however, depletion of iron stores can be detected by measuring ferritin, the iron storage compound. Although ferritin is primarily an intracellular protein, serum concentrations of ferritin correlate closely with iron stores with only a few exceptions.[6,7] Ferritin, an acute-phase reactant, is generally found in higher levels in patients with inflammatory disorders and liver disease.[8] A serum ferritin level <12 ng/mL is consistent with iron deficiency. An increased TIBC also can reflect depletion of storage iron, but it is less sensitive than serum ferritin. Thus, in iron deficiency, the serum ferritin concentration is low, whereas the TIBC is usually high; both of these parameters can be detected before the clinical manifestations of anemia are apparent. These abnormalities persist and worsen as the patient progresses to anemia as illustrated by D.G.'s laboratory values. If the TIBC is low or normal, rather than high, in association with a low serum ferritin, other causes of anemia (e.g., malignancy, infections, or inflammatory disorders) should be considered. In these situations, further documentation (e.g., bone marrow examination) is necessary to determine the cause of the anemia.[9,10]

D.G.'s low serum iron, low serum ferritin, and elevated TIBC are typical of the laboratory findings associated with iron deficiency anemia. Serum transferrin receptor levels, which reflect the amount of RBC precursors available for active proliferation, are increased in iron deficiency.[11]

After the iron in the storage compartment is depleted, heme and hemoglobin synthesis are decreased. In severe iron deficiency, the RBC become hypochromic (low MCHC) and microcytic (low MCV). Usually, the RBC indices do not become abnormal until the Hgb concentration falls to <12 g/dL in male patients or <10 g/dL in female patients. D.G.'s corpuscular indices indicate that her anemia is hypochromic and microcytic.

About 10% of patients who are iron deficient experience neutropenia and either thrombocytopenia or thrombocytosis. Thrombocytosis can occur in 50% to 75% of patients with hypochromic anemia secondary to chronic blood loss. The thrombocytosis (e.g., 800,000 platelets) in D.G. returns to normal after adequate treatment with iron. The reticulocyte count provides an estimate of effective red cell production and is usually normal or low in iron deficiency anemia. D.G. has a reticulocyte count of 0.2% (normal, 0.5 to 1.5%), which also is compatible with iron deficiency anemia.

In the workup of a microcytic, hypochromic anemia, the stool should be examined for occult blood. D.G. has a 4+ stool guaiac, which suggests blood loss via the GI tract. Further diagnostic evaluations (e.g., endoscopy, GI films) are necessary to determine the underlying problem.

In summary, D.G.'s signs, symptoms, and laboratory findings all support the diagnosis of an iron deficiency anemia.

Iron Therapy

Oral Iron Dosing

3. How should D.G.'s iron deficiency be managed? What dose of iron should be given to treat D.G.'s iron deficiency anemia and for how long?

The primary treatment for D.G. should be directed toward control of the underlying causes of anemia, which in this case are many. D.G.'s iron stores are low because of GI blood loss, multiple childbirths, heavy menstrual flow, decreased dietary iron absorption, and perhaps, an inadequate diet. Therefore, the cause of her GI blood loss should be corrected, her dietary intake should be analyzed and modified, and supplemental iron should be prescribed to replenish her stores and correct the anemia.

The usual adult dose of ferrous sulfate is 325 mg (one tablet) administered three times daily, between meals. If no iron is being lost through bleeding, the required daily dose of elemental iron can be calculated using a formula that assumes that 0.25 g/dL/day is the maximal rate of hemoglobin regeneration.

Elemental iron (mg/day) = 0.25 g Hgb/100 mL blood/day (5,000 mL blood)(3.4 mg Fe/1 g Hgb)
= 40 mg Fe/day/20% absorption (approximate absorption rate in iron-deficient states)
= 200 mg Fe/day
= 1,000 mg ferrous sulfate/day (ferrous sulfate contains 20% elemental iron)
= 325 mg TID ferrous sulfate

Product Selection

4. What are the differences between iron products? Which is the product of choice?

The ferrous form of iron is absorbed three times more readily than the ferric form. Although ferrous sulfate, ferrous gluconate, and ferrous fumarate are absorbed almost equally, each contains a different amount of elemental iron.[12] Table 86-6 compares the iron content of several oral iron preparations to assist in making appropriate treatment choices for patients.

PRODUCT FORMULATION

Product formulation is of considerable importance in product selection. Some believe that the more expensive, sustained-release (SR) iron preparations are inherently better. SR preparations fall into three groups: (a) those claimed to increase GI tolerance or decrease side effects, (b) those formulated to increase bioavailability, and (c) those with adjuvants claimed to enhance absorption. Because these products can be given once daily, increased compliance is an additional claim.

Anecdotal claims that SR iron preparations cause fewer GI side effects have not been substantiated by controlled studies. In fact, these products transport iron past the duodenum and proximal jejunum, thereby reducing the absorption of iron.[13] Because poor absorption and poor hematologic responses might occur with ferrous sulfate SR capsules, they should not be used for initial treatment.

Adjuvants are incorporated into many iron preparations in an attempt to enhance absorption or decrease side effects. Several products contain ascorbic acid (vitamin C), which maintains iron in the ferrous state. Doses up to 1 g increase iron absorption by only 10%; however, smaller doses of vitamin C (e.g., 100 mg) do not significantly alter iron absorption.[14]

Table 86-6 Comparisons of Iron Preparations

Preparation	Dose (mg)	Fe^{++} Content (mg)	Fe (%)
Ferrous sulfate	325	65	20
Ferrous fumarate	324	106	33
Ferrous gluconate	300	34	11
Feosol tablets	200	65	33
Slow Fe (time released)	160	50	31

Table 86-7 Combination Iron Products

Drug	DOSS (mg)	Vitamin C (mg)	Fe^{++} Content (mg)
Ferro-Grad 500 (Filmtabs)	0	500	105
Vitron C	0	125	66
Ferro DSS/Ferro-Sequel	100	0	50

DOSS, dioctyl sodium sulfosuccinate; docusate sodium; Fe, iron.

Table 86-7 lists a number of combination products that contain a stool softener or vitamin C.

Stool softeners are added to iron preparations to decrease the side effect of constipation. Generally, these combinations contain suboptimal doses of stool softener and are unwarranted. If constipation does develop, appropriate doses of stool softeners should be taken.

In summary, D.G. should take the least expensive iron preparation containing ferrous sulfate, gluconate, or fumarate. In general, generic preparations of iron salts without adjuvant agents provide the best value.

Goals of Therapy

5. What are the goals of iron therapy? How should D.G. be monitored?

The goals of iron therapy are to normalize the Hgb and Hct concentrations and to replete iron stores. Initially, if the doses of iron are adequate, the reticulocyte count will begin to increase by the third to fourth day and peak by the seventh to tenth day of therapy. By the end of the second week of iron therapy, the reticulocyte count will fall back to normal. The Hgb response is a convenient index to monitor in outpatients. Hematologic response is usually seen in 2 to 3 weeks with a 1 g/dL increase in hemoglobin and a 6% increase in the hematocrit. D.G.'s anemia can be expected to resolve in 1 to 2 months; however, iron therapy should be continued for 3 to 6 months after the hemoglobin is normalized to replete iron stores.[14,15] Therapy duration is related to the absorption pattern of iron. During the first month of therapy, as much as 35 mg of elemental iron is absorbed from the daily dose. With time, the percentage of iron absorbed from the dose decreases, and by the third month of therapy, only 5 to 10 mg of elemental iron is absorbed.

Patient Information

6. What kind of information should be provided to D.G. when dispensing oral iron? What can be done if she experiences intolerable GI symptoms (e.g., nausea, epigastric pain)?

Iron should be dispensed in a childproof container, and D.G. should be told to store it in a safe place away from children. Accidental ingestion of even small amounts (three to four tablets) of oral iron can cause serious consequences in small children[16] (see Chapter 5, Managing Acute Drug Toxicity). D.G. should be told that oral iron therapy produces dark stools. She should try to take her iron on an empty stomach because food, especially dairy products, decreases the absorption by 40% to 50%.[17,18]

Gastric side effects, which occur in 5% to 20% of patients, include nausea, epigastric pain, constipation, abdominal cramps, and diarrhea. Constipation does not appear to be dose related, but side effects (e.g., nausea and epigastric pain) occur more frequently as the quantity of soluble elemental iron in contact with the stomach and duodenum increases.[4] To minimize gastric intolerance, oral iron therapy can be initiated with a single tablet of ferrous sulfate 325 mg/day; the dose is increased by increments of one tablet per day every 2 to 3 days until the full therapeutic dose of ferrous sulfate, 325 mg three times daily, can be administered.[2]

D.G. also should be educated about potential drug interactions that can occur with iron therapy. Currently, she is taking a proton pump inhibitor, which is thought to inhibit serum iron absorption by increasing the pH of the stomach and decreasing the solubility of ferrous salts.[19,20] In addition, antacids can increase stomach pH and certain anions (carbonate and hydroxide) also are thought to form insoluble complexes when combined with iron. Although it is unclear whether this has an impact on therapy, one study showed a therapeutic dose of liquid antacid (containing aluminum hydroxide and magnesium hydroxide) does not significantly alter absorption of iron in adults who are mildly deficient in iron.[21] Although the clinical significance of this is undetermined, D.G. should be advised to take her iron at least 1 hour before or 3 hours after the proton pump inhibitor dose.

D.G. also is taking tetracycline for the treatment of acne. Because the absorptions of both iron and tetracycline are decreased when administered concomitantly, the iron should be taken 3 hours before or 2 hours after the tetracycline dose as well.[22]

Parenteral Iron Therapy

INDICATIONS

7. When would parenteral iron therapy be indicated for D.G.?

Several indications exist for parenteral iron administration. Failure to respond to oral iron therapy would prompt a reevaluation of D.G. Causes of oral therapy failure can include nonadherence, misdiagnosis (e.g., inflammation), malabsorption (e.g., sprue, radiation enteritis, duodenal or upper small intestine resection), and continuing blood loss equal to or greater than the rate of RBC production. Malabsorption can be evaluated by measuring iron levels every 30 minutes for 2 hours after the administration of 50 mg of ferrous sulfate. If her plasma iron levels increase by >50%, absorption is adequate. Besides failure to respond to oral therapy as one indication for parenteral iron administration, other indications include intolerance to oral therapy, required antacid therapy, or significant blood loss in patients refusing transfusion. All can warrant injectable iron therapy.[3] In D.G.'s case, if malabsorption is documented, she would be a candidate for injectable iron.

PREFERRED ROUTE

8. What is the preferred route of parenteral iron administration?

Iron can be given parenterally in the form of ferric gluconate (Ferrlecit), iron dextran (INFeD and Dexferrum), and iron sucrose (Venofer). Iron dextran, the oldest of the parenteral iron agents, is U.S. Food and Drug Administration (FDA)-approved for the treatment of iron deficiency when oral supplementation is impossible or ineffective. In this particular formulation, iron is a complex of ferric hydroxide and dextran. Iron dextran can be administered undiluted intramuscularly or by very slow intravenous (IV) injection. Although not included in the labeling approved by the FDA, iron-dextran injection is commonly diluted in 250 to 1,000 mL 0.9% NaCl and administered by IV infusion. IV administration is preferred to intramuscular (IM) administration when muscle mass available for an IM injection is limited; when absorption from the muscle is impaired (e.g., stasis, edema); when uncontrolled bleeding is a risk (e.g., secondary to hemophilia, thrombocytopenia, anticoagulation therapy); and when large doses are indicated for therapy.

In a few instances, IM iron dextran is the preferred treatment (e.g., patients with limited IV access). In these cases, undiluted drug should be administered using a Z-track technique to avoid staining the skin. (The skin should be pulled laterally before injection; then the drug is injected and the skin is released to avoid leakage of dextran into the subcutaneous tissue.) IM iron dextran is absorbed in two phases. In the first 72 hours, 60% of the dose is absorbed, whereas the remaining drug is absorbed over weeks to months.[23]

Infusion rates of undiluted IV iron dextran should not exceed 50 mg (i.e., 1 mL) per minute. The upper limit of each daily dose is based on the patient's weight and should not be >100 mg/day. Although the data are limited, total dose iron-dextran infusion is given in clinical practice and has proved to be effective and convenient.[24] Infusions generally are given over 1 to 6 hours to minimize local pain and phlebitis.[4] The total dose method of administration can be associated with a higher prevalence of fever, malaise, flushing, and myalgias.

Ferric gluconate and iron sucrose are parenteral iron formulations, which are FDA approved for the treatment of iron deficiency anemia in patients undergoing chronic hemodialysis and receiving supplemental EPO.[4] Ferric gluconate can be administered undiluted as a slow IV injection (rate not to exceed 12.5 mg/minute) or as an IV infusion (125 mg ferric gluconate in 100 mL 0.9% NaCl over 1 hour). Likewise, iron sucrose can be administered undiluted as a slow IV injection (rate not to exceed 20 mg/minute) or as an IV infusion (dilute in a maximum of 100 mL 0.9% NaCl and infuse at a rate of 100 mg over 15 minute). Iron requirements in these patients typically exceed 1 to 2 g and, therefore, multiple doses of ferric gluconate and iron sucrose are needed to achieve the total dose of iron.

DOSAGE CALCULATION

9. How is a total dose of iron dextran for IV infusion that would be needed to achieve a normal hemoglobin value for D.G. and to replenish her iron stores calculated? How quickly should she respond?

The total dose of iron dextran to be administered can be determined using the following equation:

$$\text{Iron (mg)} = [\text{Weight (pounds)} \times 0.3][100 - \{100(\text{Hgb})/14.8\}]$$

where *Hgb* is the patient's measured hemoglobin (g/dL). The equation uses the person's weight (in pounds) and assumes that an Hgb of 14.8 g/dL is 100% of normal. Children weighing <30 lb should be given 80% of the calculated dose because the normal mean Hgb in this population is lower.

For patients with anemia resulting from blood loss (e.g., hemorrhagic diatheses) or patients receiving chronic dialysis, the iron requirement is based on the estimate of iron contained in the blood lost. In this case, the following equation should be used:

Iron (mg) = Blood loss (mL) × Hct (the patient's measured Hct expressed as a decimal fraction)

This formula assumes that 1 mL of normochromic blood contains 1 mg of iron.

After parenteral administration, iron dextran is cleared by the reticuloendothelial cells and processed. The iron is then released back into the plasma and bone marrow. Because the rate of iron incorporation into hemoglobin does not exceed that achieved by oral iron therapy, the response time is similar to that of oral iron therapy, and the Hgb can be expected to increase at a rate of 1.5 to 2.2 g/dL/week during the first 2 weeks and by 0.7 to 1.6 g/dL/week thereafter until normal values are attained.

SIDE EFFECTS

10. What side effects can be expected from parenteral iron therapy?

Anaphylactoid reactions can occur in <1% of patients treated with parenteral iron therapy.[4,25,26] This reaction is more commonly associated with iron dextran than with ferric gluconate and iron sucrose.[25,26] As a result, a 25-mg test dose of iron dextran should be given IM or by IV infusion over 5 to 10 minutes. If headache, chest pain, anxiety, or signs of hypotension are not experienced, the remainder of the dose can be administered parenterally. Nevertheless, delayed reactions (e.g., fever, urticaria, arthralgias, and lymphadenopathy) have occurred 24 to 48 hours after large doses of IV iron dextran and have lasted 3 to 7 days in 1% to 2% of patients.[27] A test dose is not indicated for ferric gluconate and iron sucrose because of the lower incidence of serious anaphylactoid reactions with these agents. Other side effects seen with parenteral iron agents include hypotension, nausea and vomiting, cramps, and diarrhea. Parenteral iron medications should not be mixed with (or added to) other medications or parenteral nutrition solutions for IV infusion.

MEGALOBLASTIC ANEMIAS

Megaloblastic anemia is a common disorder that can have several causes: (*a*) anemia associated with vitamin B_{12} deficiency; (*b*) anemia associated with folic acid deficiency; or (*c*) anemia caused by metabolic or inherited defects associated with decreased ability to utilize vitamin B_{12} or folic acid.[28]

Megaloblastosis results from impaired DNA synthesis in replicating cells, which is signaled by a large immature nucleus. RNA and protein synthesis remain unaffected, and the cytoplasm matures normally. Megaloblastic changes can be observed microscopically in RBC and in proliferating cells (e.g., in the cervix, skin, GI tract).[29]

Although the clinical effects of vitamin B_{12} and folic acid deficiencies can differ in various organ systems, they are similar in their effects on the hematopoietic system. Typically, macrocytic anemia develops slowly and can be identified by large, oval, well-hemoglobinized red cells; anisocytosis; and nuclear remnants. The reticulocyte count is low and the bilirubin level is elevated. Thrombocytopenia is present and the platelets are large. Leukopenia occurs with hypersegmentation of polymorphonuclear leukocyte nuclei. If biopsied, the bone marrow is markedly hypercellular. Nuclear immaturity is present, but the megaloblasts have normal maturation of the cytoplasm. Iron stores in the marrow are increased as a result of the intramedullary hemolysis. Symptoms include fatigue; exaggeration of pre-existing cardiovascular or pulmonary problems; a sore, pale, smooth tongue; diarrhea or constipation; and anorexia. Edema and urticaria also may be present.

Vitamin B_{12} Deficiency Anemia

Vitamin B_{12} Metabolism

Deficiency and poor utilization of vitamin B_{12} are two mechanisms for the development of megaloblastic anemia. Cobalamin (vitamin B_{12}) is naturally synthesized by microorganisms, but because humans are incapable of doing so, vitamin B_{12} must be provided nutritionally. Animal protein, and roots and legumes of plants provide dietary sources of vitamin B_{12}. Meats richest in vitamin B_{12} include oysters, clams, liver, and kidney; moderate amounts of vitamin B_{12} are found in muscle meats, milk products, and egg yolks.

The typical Western diet contains 5 to 15 mcg/day of vitamin B_{12}, an amount sufficient to replace the 1 mcg lost daily. The total body stores of vitamin B_{12} range from 2,000 to 5,000 mcg, 50% to 90% of which is stored in the liver.[30] Because body stores are extensive, 3 to 4 years are required before symptoms of vitamin B_{12} deficiency develop.

In the stomach, the vitamin B_{12} is released from protein complexes and bound to intrinsic factor, which protects it from degradation by GI microorganisms. Intrinsic factor is essential for the absorption of vitamin B_{12}. Specific mucosal receptors in the distal small ileum allow for attachment of the intrinsic factor: B_{12} complex. B_{12} is then transferred to the ileal cell and finally to portal vein blood. The intrinsic factor mechanism is saturated by 1.5 to 3 mcg of B_{12}; however, passive diffusion can occur when B_{12} is present in large quantities.

After vitamin B_{12} is absorbed, it is bound to specific β-globulin transport proteins, transcobalamin I, II, and III. Transcobalamin II is responsible for transporting B_{12} through cell membranes and delivering it to the liver and other organs. All three of the transport proteins prevent loss of B_{12} in the urine, sweat, and other body secretions. In the liver, vitamin B_{12} is converted to coenzyme B_{12}, which is essential for hematopoiesis, maintenance of myelin throughout the entire nervous system, and production of epithelial cells.[31,32]

Pathogenesis and Evaluation of Vitamin B_{12} Deficiency

Vitamin B_{12} deficiency can result from (a) decreased intake, absorption, transport, and utilization; or (b) increased requirements, metabolic consumption, destruction, and excretion. Strict vegetarians most frequently present with signs and symptoms of vitamin B_{12} deficiency. This population also can be iron deficient and the microcytosis of iron deficiency anemia can mask the vitamin B_{12} deficiency–induced macrocytic appearance of RBC. Other causes of vitamin B_{12} deficiency include inadequate proteolytic degradation of vitamin B_{12} from protein, or congenital intrinsic factor deficiency. In addition, the gastric mucosa may be unable to produce intrinsic factor under conditions such as partial gastrectomy, autoimmune destruction (e.g., addisonian or juvenile pernicious anemia), or destruction of the gastric mucosa from caustic agents.

Pernicious anemia can result in vitamin B_{12} deficiency. It can be caused by chronic atrophic gastritis accompanied by reduced intrinsic factor and hydrochloric acid secretion or acquired as a result of gastrectomy, pancreatic disease, or malnutrition. Pernicious anemia occurs commonly in patients with thyrotoxicosis, Hashimoto's thyroiditis, vitiligo, rheumatoid arthritis, or gastric cancer. Anti-intrinsic factor antibodies have been observed in the serum of some patients with pernicious anemia.

The onset of the pernicious anemia is insidious. Patients generally do not feel well for 6 to 12 months and often complain of at least two of the following triad of symptoms: weakness, sore tongue, and symmetric numbness or tingling in the extremities. The neurologic symptoms of vitamin B_{12} deficiency are associated with a defect in myelin synthesis and often are described as stocking-glove peripheral neuropathy or nonspecific complaints (e.g., tinnitus, neuritis, vertigo, headaches). Patients with neurologic symptoms have difficulty determining position and vibration sense and have an increase in deep tendon reflexes. These symptoms may progress to spastic ataxia, motor weakness, and paraparesis. Interestingly, no correlation exists between the extent of neurologic manifestations and the severity of anemia. Anorexia, pallor, and dyspnea on exertion are bothersome symptoms that may overshadow the diagnostic triad.

Laboratory Evaluation

In general, the serum vitamin B_{12} level reliably reflects vitamin B_{12} tissue stores. False low vitamin B_{12} concentrations may be observed in patients with folic acid deficiency, transcobalamin I deficiency, multiple myeloma, pregnancy, or in those who take very large doses of vitamin C. Falsely elevated vitamin B_{12} concentrations may be observed in patients with myeloproliferative diseases, hepatomas, autoimmune diseases, monoblastic leukemias, and histiocytic lymphomas.[33] Measuring serum methylmalonic acid and homocysteine levels may assist in differentiating between folate and vitamin B_{12} deficiency. Once vitamin B_{12} therapy has been instituted, serum levels of these chemicals decrease if true vitamin B_{12} deficiency is present.

The cause of vitamin B_{12} deficiency may be determined by the use of antibody testing (antiparietal cells and anti-intrinsic factor antibodies). Patients with pernicious anemia are not able to absorb vitamin B_{12} because intrinsic factor is not available for binding. Some patients produce intrinsic factor but are still unable to absorb dietary vitamin B_{12}. Malabsorption can be caused by intestinal bacteria that usurp vitamin B_{12}, achlorhydria, pancreatic insufficiency, inadequate disassociation of vitamin B_{12} from proteins, or lack of intrinsic factor receptors secondary to ileal loops, bypass, or surgical resection.[34]

Pernicious Anemia

SIGNS, SYMPTOMS, AND LABORATORY FINDINGS

11. C.L., a 60-year-old Scandinavian man, is seen by a private physician. C.L. has a 1-year history of weakness and emotional instability. He also complains of a painful tongue, alternating constipation and diarrhea, and a tingling sensation in both feet. Pertinent findings on physical examination include pallor, red tongue, vibratory sense loss in the lower extremities, disorientation, muscle weakness, and ataxia.

Significant laboratory findings include the following: Hgb, 9 g/dL (normal, 14 to 18); Hct, 29% (normal, 42% to 52%); MCV, 110 μm^3 (normal, 76 to 100); MCH, 38 pg (normal, 27 to 33); MCHC, 34% (normal, 33% to 37%); reticulocytes, 0.4% (normal, 0.5% to 1.5%); poikilocytosis and anisocytosis on the blood smear; white blood cell (WBC) count, 4,000/mm^3 (normal, 3,200 to 9,800); platelets, 105,000/mm^3 (normal, 130,000 to 400,000); serum iron, 80 μg/dL (normal, 50 to 160); TIBC, 300 g/dL (normal, 200 to 1,000); ferritin, 150 ng/mL (normal, 15 to 200); RBC folate, 300 ng/mL (normal, 140 to 460); serum vitamin B_{12}, 100 pg/mL (normal, 200 to 1,000); and anti-intrinsic factor antibody, positive. What signs, symptoms, and laboratory findings are typical of pernicious anemia in C.L.?

[SI units: Hgb, 90 g/L; Hct, 0.29; MCV, 110 fL; MCH, 38 pg;MCHC, 0.34; reticulocytes, 0.004; WBC count, 4,000/mm^3 × 10^9/L; platelets, 105,000/mm^3 × 10^9/L(normal, 250 to 400); iron, 14.38 μmol/L; TIBC, 53.91 μmol/L; ferritin, 150 μ/L; RBC folate,679.8 nmol/L; vitamin B_{12}, 73.78 pmol/L]

C.L.'s signs and symptoms are classic for pernicious anemia. This disease occurs equally in both sexes (primarily in individuals of northern European descent), with an average onset of 60 years. Pernicious anemia develops from a lack of gastric intrinsic factor production, which causes vitamin B_{12} malabsorption and, ultimately, vitamin B_{12} deficiency. C.L.'s signs and symptoms of vitamin B_{12} deficiency include painful red tongue, loss of lower extremity vibratory sense, vertigo, and emotional instability.

The elevated MCV suggests megaloblastic anemia. Folate and iron are two other factors that can affect the MCV and should be evaluated during the workup of a patient for anemia. In this case, C.L.'s folate and iron levels are normal, but his serum vitamin B_{12} level is low. The presence of poikilocytosis and anisocytosis observed in the blood smear represent ineffective erythropoiesis. Other cell lineages also may be affected in the bone marrow. Erythroid hypercellularity, along with a decrease in the myeloid cells (leukocytes and platelets), increases the erythroid:myeloid ratio in C.L. The patient's low serum vitamin B_{12} levels and the low results obtained from the Schilling test are compatible with the diagnosis of pernicious anemia.

TREATMENT

12. How should C.L.'s pernicious anemia be treated? How soon can a response be expected?

C.L. should receive parenteral vitamin B_{12} in a dose sufficient to provide not only the daily requirement of approximately 2 mcg, but also the amount needed to replenish tissue stores (about 2,000 to 5,000 mcg; average, 4,000 mcg). To replete vitamin B_{12} stores, cyanocobalamin can be given IM in accordance with various regimens. C.L. may receive 100 mcg of cyanocobalamin daily for 1 week, then 100 mcg every other day for 2 weeks, followed by 100 mcg every 3 to 4 days for 2 to 3 weeks. A monthly maintenance dose of cyanocobalamin (100 mcg) would then be required for the remainder of C.L.'s life. Another treatment option may be cyanocobalamin (1,000 mcg) once a week for 4 to 6 weeks followed by 1,000 mcg/mo for lifetime maintenance therapy.[29] IM or deep subcutaneous administration provides sustained release of vitamin B_{12} with better utilization compared with rapid IV infusion. An oral or intranasal cyanocobalamin gel is also available for maintenance therapy, after the patient has achieved hematologic remission.

With adequate vitamin B_{12} therapy, the following response can be expected: Neurologic symptoms should improve within 24 hours. However, with longstanding vitamin B_{12} deficiency, several months may pass before some symptoms are relieved; other symptoms may never resolve. Hematologic parameters should begin to improve within the first few days. The bone marrow becomes normoblastic within 48 hours, the reticulocyte count should peak around day 5 of therapy, and the Hct should return to normal in 1 to 2 months. Because the rapid production of RBC can increase potassium demand, serum potassium should be monitored and potassium supplementation provided as necessary. Peripheral blood counts should be obtained every 3 to 6 months to evaluate the adequacy of therapy. If maintenance therapy is discontinued, pernicious anemia will recur within 5 years.

Oral Vitamin B_{12}

13. What factors affect the oral absorption of vitamin B_{12}? When is oral vitamin B_{12} therapy an effective alternative to parenteral therapy?

The amount of vitamin B_{12} that can be absorbed orally from a single dose or meal ranges from 1 to 5 mcg; approximately 5 mcg of vitamin B_{12} is absorbed daily from the average American diet. The percentage of vitamin B_{12} absorbed decreases with increasing doses. About 50% of a 1 to 2 mcg dose of vitamin B_{12} is absorbed, whereas only about 5% of a 20 mcg dose is absorbed.[35] Doses >100 mcg must be ingested to absorb 5 mcg of vitamin B_{12}. Oral therapy for pernicious anemia using high dosages of oral cyanocobalamin (1,000 to 2,000 mcg) may be indicated in certain patients, especially those who refuse or cannot receive parenteral therapy.[36,37] Overall, oral vitamin B_{12} therapy is considered safe and effective.[38] Patients can be given 1,000 to 2,000 mcg/day for 1 month, followed by 125 to 500 mcg/day as maintenance treatment.[39] Issues of noncompliance or lack of response with oral therapy places the patient at substantial risk for significant neurologic damage. Patients receiving oral vitamin B_{12} therapy should be monitored more frequently to ensure compliance with therapy.

Anemias After Gastrectomy

14. F.M. has just undergone a total gastrectomy for recurrent nonhealing ulcers. What form(s) of anemia would be expected to develop in a patient after gastrectomy? Should F.M. receive prophylactic vitamin B_{12}?

Partial or total gastrectomy often results in anemia, particularly pernicious anemia, because the source of intrinsic factor is lost, and oral vitamin B_{12} absorption will be impaired. The hematologic and neurologic abnormalities associated with B_{12} deficiency do not develop until existing vitamin B_{12} stores are depleted (about 2 to 3 years). Nevertheless, prophylactic vitamin B_{12} should be administered to this patient after total gastrectomy. Because the vitamin B_{12} stores are not currently depleted, maintenance therapy, as discussed in Question 12, should be adequate for F.M.

Malabsorption of Vitamin B_{12}

SIGNS AND SYMPTOMS

15. P.G., a 55-year-old woman, complained of progressive confusion and lethargy 9 months ago. A CBC at that time revealed only mild leukocytosis. Today, she comes to the emergency department with a 4-week history of frequent (three to five per day) stools containing bright red blood. She reports continued lethargy, dizziness, ataxia, and paresthesias in her hands and feet.

Laboratory findings of interest include the following: Hgb, 12.8 g/dL (normal, 12 to 16); MCV, 90 μm^3 (normal, 76 to 100); iron, 150 mcg/dL (normal, 50 to 160); B_{12}, 94 pg/mL (normal, 200 to 1,000); folate, 21 ng/mL (normal, 7 to 25); hypersegmented polymorphonuclear leukocytes (PMN); bilirubin, 3.0 mg/dL (normal, 0.1 to 1.0); and lactate dehydrogenase (LDH), 520 U/L (normal, 50 to 150). A subsequent bone marrow aspirate demonstrates megaloblastic erythropoiesis, giant metamyelocytes, and a low stainable iron. A barium swallow and follow-through show numerous jejunal and duodenal diverticuli. Jejunal and duodenal aspirates reveal aerobic and anaerobic bacterial overgrowth. What signs, symptoms, and laboratory findings are typical for vitamin B_{12} deficiency in P.G.?

[SI units: Hgb, 120 g/L; MCV, 90 fL; iron, 25.87 mcmol/L; B_{12}, 69.35 pmol/L; folate, 47.59 nmol/L; bilirubin, 51.3 mcmol/L; LDH, 520 U/L]

The signs and symptoms in P.G. that are consistent with B_{12} deficiency include confusion, dizziness, ataxia, and paresthesias. Other signs and symptoms may be caused by other underlying conditions. For example, her lethargy may be the result of prolonged blood loss secondary to diverticulitis.

Notably, P.G. initially presented with a mild leukocytosis. Evaluation 9 months later shows a low Hgb, a low serum vitamin B_{12} level, and hypersegmented PMN. The high LDH and bilirubin levels reflect intramedullary hemolysis of megaloblastic RBC consistent with vitamin B_{12} deficiency, even though the MCV is within normal limits. The presence of megaloblastic erythropoiesis and giant metamyelocytes in the bone marrow also is consistent with vitamin B_{12} deficiency.

P.G.'s history of bloody stools and diverticuli suggests substantial long-term blood loss, which increased demand for iron and vitamin B_{12} to replace RBC. Concurrent iron deficiency can mask megaloblastic changes in RBC, which explains the suspiciously normal MCV (dimorphic anemia). The serum folate concentration is also falsely normal. Although the RBC folate level is likely to be low, serum folate concentrations are normal because monoglutamated folates leak from cells into the serum in vitamin B_{12} deficient states.

TREATMENT

16. How should P.G.'s vitamin B_{12} deficiency be treated?

The cause of vitamin B_{12} malabsorption must be corrected before P.G. is given oral vitamin B_{12} therapy. The presence of diverticuli is not the cause of vitamin B_{12} malabsorption because diverticuli typically do not extend into the distal ileum. Instead, given P.G.'s medical history, the most likely cause of vitamin B_{12} malabsorption is bacterial usurpation of luminal vitamin B_{12}. P.G. should first be treated with a broad-spectrum antibiotic (e.g., tetracycline) or a sulfonamide for 7 to 10 days, then begin daily oral vitamin B_{12} supplementation to replenish her body stores. In this case, normal levels of intrinsic factor permit oral therapy. The recommended daily dose of vitamin

B_{12} is 25 to 250 mcg. Following antibiotic therapy, P.G. also should begin to absorb vitamin B_{12} in her diet.

Folic Acid Deficiency Anemia

Folic Acid Metabolism

Folate is abundant in virtually all food sources, especially fresh green vegetables, fruits, yeast, and animal protein. As a result of food fortification, the average American diet provides 50 to 2,000 mcg of folate per day; however, excessive or prolonged cooking (>15 minutes) in large quantities of water destroys a high percentage of the folate that is contained in food.[40] Human requirements for folate vary with age and depend on the rate of metabolism and cell turnover but are generally 3 mcg/kg/day.[40] The minimal daily adult requirement of folate is 50 mcg, but because absorption from food is incomplete, a daily intake of 200 mcg is recommended. Folate requirements are increased in conditions in which the metabolic rate and rate of cellular division are increased (e.g., pregnancy, infancy, infection, malignancies, hemolytic anemia). The following are estimates of daily folate requirements based on age and growth demands: children, 80 mcg; infants, 65 mcg; pregnant or lactating women, 400 to 800 mcg.[37,40,41]

Dietary folic acid is in the polyglutamate form and must be enzymatically deconjugated in the GI tract to the monoglutamate form before it is absorbed. Once absorbed, the inactive dihydrofolate (FH_2) must be converted to active tetrahydrofolate (FH_4, folinic acid) by dihydrofolate reductase (DHFR).

In contrast to the large stores of vitamin B_{12}, the body's folate stores are relatively small (about 5 to 10 mcg). Therefore, deficiency and subsequent megaloblastic anemia can occur within 3 to 4 months of decreased folate intake.

Predisposing Factors

Folate deficiency is most commonly associated with alcoholism, rapid cell turnover, and dietary deficiency. In alcoholics, the daily intake of the folate contained in food may be restricted or absent. In addition, enterohepatic recirculation of folate can become impaired by the toxic effect of alcohol on hepatic cells. Folate deficiency also can develop during the third trimester of pregnancy as a result of a marginal diet and the rapid metabolism of the fetus. Folate coenzymes are required for most metabolic pathways (Fig. 86-2). Therefore, folate deficiency will develop in any condition of rapid cellular turnover (e.g., hemolytic anemias, hemoglobinopathies, sideroblastic

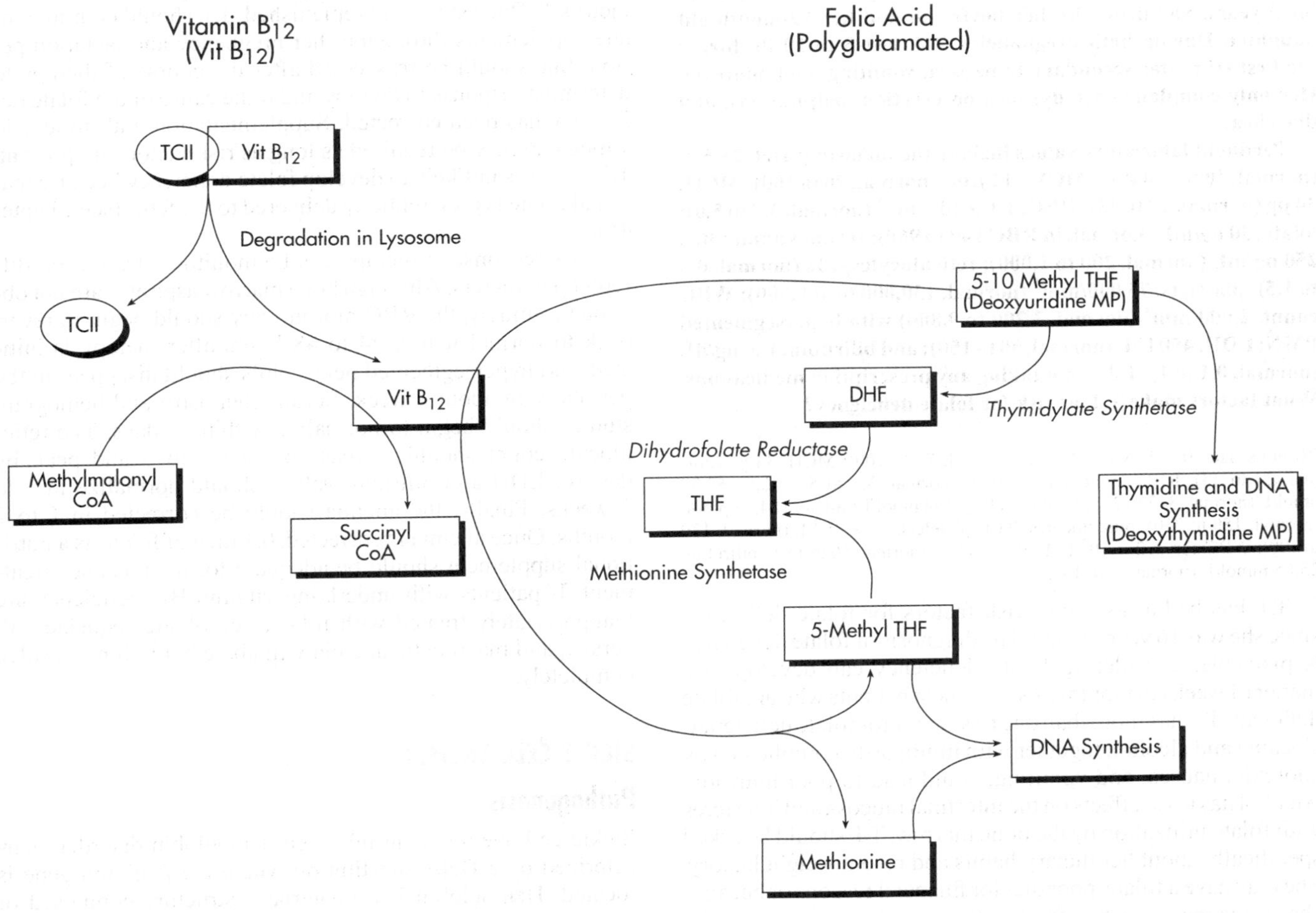

FIGURE 86-2 Intracellular metabolic pathways. Vitamin B_{12} and folic acid are both necessary for nucleic acid precursors used for DNA synthesis. DHF, dihydrofolate; MP, monophosphate; TCII, transcobalamin II; THF, tetrahydrofolate.

anemia, leukemias, lymphomas, multiple myeloma) or a diet lacking in folate (e.g., food faddism or a weight-loss diet). Folate deficiency also can occur with chronic hemodialysis, diseases that impair absorption from the small intestine (e.g., sprue, regional enteritis), extensive jejunal resections, and drugs that alter folate metabolism (e.g., trimethoprim, pyrimethamine, methotrexate, sulfasalazine, oral contraceptives, anticonvulsants).[37,42–44] Few patients have inborn errors of folate metabolism.[45]

The evaluation of megaloblastic anemia must be thorough because indiscriminate use of "shotgun" hematinic therapy can be dangerous. Large doses of folate can partially reverse hematologic abnormalities caused by vitamin B_{12} deficiency; however, folate cannot correct neurologic damage caused by vitamin B_{12} deficiency. Therefore, folate deficiency absolutely must be differentiated from vitamin B_{12} deficiency before folate therapy is initiated. Otherwise, the progression of the neurologic sequelae of vitamin B_{12} deficiency can occur.

17. T.J., a malnourished-appearing woman in her second trimester of pregnancy, presents to the local health clinic for her regular checkup. She is a multiparous, 22-year-old woman who ran away from home when she was 16. T.J. has a 7-year history of excessive alcohol intake and has been using cocaine frequently for 3 years. She lives with her boyfriend and her 19-month-old daughter. During both pregnancies, T.J. lost 8 to 10 lb during the first trimester secondary to nausea, vomiting, and anorexia. Her only complaints are dyspnea on exertion, palpitations, and diarrhea.

Pertinent laboratory values include the following: Hct, 25.5% (normal, 40% to 44%); MCV, 112 μm^3 (normal, 76 to 100); MCH, 34 pg (normal, 27 to 33); RBC, $1.1 \times 10^6/mm^3$ (normal, 3.5 to 5.0); folate, 30 ng/mL (normal, in RBC 140 to 960); serum vitamin B_{12}, 250 pg/mL (normal, 200 to 1,000); reticulocytes, 1% (normal, 0.5 to 1.5); platelets, 75,000/mm^3 (normal, 130,000 to 400,000); WBC count, 2,000/mm^3 (normal, 3,200 to 9,800) with hypersegmented PMN; LDH, 450 U/L (normal, 50 to 150); and bilirubin, 1.5 mg/dL (normal, 0.1 to 1). T.J. is not taking any prescription medications. What factors make T.J. at risk for folate deficiency?

[SI units: Hct, 0.255; MCV, 112 fL (normal, 76 to 100); MCH, 34 pg (normal, 27 to 33); RBC count, 1.1×10^9/L (normal, 3.5 to 5); folate, 67.98 nmol/L (normal, 317 to 2175); vitamin B_{12}, 184 pmol/L; folate, 184.45 pmol/(normal, 150 to 750); reticulocytes, 0.01; platelets, 75×10^9/L (normal, 130 to 400); WBC count, 2×10^9/L; LDH, 450 U/L (normal, 50 to 150); bilirubin, 25.65 mmol/L (normal, 2 to 18)]

T.J. has had a history of risk factors for folate deficiency since she was 16 years of age. The diagnosis of folate deficiency is plausible, considering folate deficiency can develop in a matter of weeks to months. As with most patients who are folate deficient, T.J. has more than one risk factor for folate deficiency. Cocaine and alcohol, together with multiparity complicated by anorexia, nausea, and vomiting, could lead to poor nutrition. Alcohol has toxic effects on the intestinal mucosa and interferes with folate utilization by the bone marrow. T.J. should be asked specifically about her dietary habits and recent weight history. She may have a folate-poor diet for financial reasons or because she is overcooking her food. Alternatively, cocaine may be causing anorexia. The nutritional intake of people who abuse alcohol and drugs is often poor.

Diagnosis and Management

18. Which laboratory values support the diagnosis of folate deficiency? How should T.J. be treated and monitored?

T.J.'s laboratory values reflect macrocytic anemia (Hct, 25.5%; MCV, 112 μm^3) with pancytopenia (reduced number of RBC, WBC, and platelets). Serum vitamin B_{12} concentrations reflect normal vitamin B_{12} stores, but folate stores are inadequate as exemplified by the low RBC folate concentration, pancytopenia, and macrocytic anemia.

Serum folate concentrations generally reflect folate balance over the past 3 weeks, although one balanced meal can raise serum levels and falsely elevate body stores. Tissue folate stores are more accurately reflected by the RBC polyglutamated folate content, which is approximately 10 to 30 times the corresponding serum folate concentrations.[46] Hemolysis or vitamin B_{12} deficiency causes leakage of monoglutamated folates from cells, thereby falsely elevating serum folate levels.[28,29,47]

T.J. should be counseled regarding her nutritional and social habits. Because the estimated total body folate store is only about 5 to 10 mcg, 1 mcg of folic acid given daily for 2 to 3 weeks should be more than adequate to replace her storage pool of folate. Higher dosages (up to 5 mcg) may be needed, however, if absorption is compromised by alcohol or other factors.[48] Once stores are replenished, T.J. should continue folate supplements throughout her pregnancy and lactation period. She should be reassessed after the course of therapy to determine response to therapy and if the cause of the folate deficiency has been corrected. Supplementation with folic acid 1 mcg/day may be required as long as risk factors are present. T.J.'s fetus is unlikely to develop folate deficiency because maternal folate is preferentially delivered to the fetus (see Chapter 46).

T.J.'s response to therapy can be monitored by several different parameters. Although bone marrow aspirates are not obtained routinely, the RBC morphology should begin to revert back to normal within 24 to 48 hours after therapy is initiated, and hypersegmented neutrophils should disappear in the periphery in about 1 week. Serum chemistry and hemogram studies should begin to normalize within 10 days. The reticulocyte count should increase by day 2 to 3 and peak by day 10. LDH and bilirubin values should normalize in 1 to 3 weeks. Finally, the anemia should be corrected in 1 to 2 months. Once anemia is corrected, 0.1 mcg of folate as a nutritional supplement should be adequate for maintenance treatment. If patients with underlying vitamin B_{12} deficiency are inappropriately treated with folate, neurologic sequelae will persist, and macrocytic anemia will abate but will not resolve completely.

SICKLE CELL ANEMIA

Pathogenesis

Sickle cell anemia is an inherited hemoglobin disorder characterized by a DNA substitution where the β-globin gene is located. Hemoglobin is a quaternary structure composed of two α-globin chains and two β-globin chains ($\alpha_2\beta_2$) in adults. The β-globin gene locus encodes several globin gene products during the course of development. These products result from transcription of the embryonic globin gene (ϵ), duplicated fetal genes (γ), and adult genes (β and δ). During fetal development, the γ-globin is the primary β-globin expressed, forming fetal hemoglobin (HbF or $\alpha_2\gamma_2$). Normally, the period from birth to approximately 3 to 6 months of age is marked by the replacement of γ-globin with β-globin, giving rise to the adult form of hemoglobin (HbA, $\alpha_2\beta_2$). Low levels of γ-globin persist throughout life, and HbF, present in F cells, may account for approximately 1% of the total hemoglobin content.[49,50] β^S represents the inheritance of the sickle β-globin gene.[51]

Sickle cell anemia results from a DNA substitution of thymidine for adenine in the glutamic acid codon, forming a B6 valine instead of glutamic acid.[50] The hemoglobin produced from such a substitution has a more negative charge than normal HbA, and the deoxygenated state favors hemoglobin aggregation and polymerization, which forms sickled RBC.[49,50] Sickled RBC are more rigid and may become "lodged" when passing through microvasculature, resulting in vascular occlusions.

In addition, the sickled RBC surface contains rearranged aminophospholipids, which augments the ability of the RBC to initiate coagulation, adhere to vascular endothelium, and activate complement. Abnormal interactions with other cell types produce several complications such as anemia, vaso-occlusive episodes, and multiorgan damage.[49] For these reasons, much effort has been focused on neonatal diagnosis to reduce morbidity and mortality in children <3 years of age.[52]

More than one inheritance pattern results in abnormal hemoglobin polymerization. Patients with sickle cell anemia are homozygous, inheriting a sickle gene from each parent ($\alpha_2\beta^S{}_2$), whereas patients with sickle cell trait are heterozygous and have inherited the sickle cell gene from one parent and the HbA gene from the other parent ($\alpha_2\beta^A\beta^S$). Other inheritance patterns include patients with a sickle cell gene and an HbC gene (where glutamic acid is substituted for lysine B6 [$\alpha_2\beta^S\beta^C$]). Finally, patients may inherit the sickle cell gene and the β-thalassemic gene ($\alpha_2\beta^S\beta^{Sthal}$), in which case the clinical course is less severe than with patients diagnosed with sickle cell anemia.[53] Hematologic abnormalities are more commonly observed in patients with sickle cell anemia and less often in those with sickle cell HbC disease or sickle cell B_O-thalassemia.[49,50]

Laboratory Evaluation

Patients who have inherited the sickle cell gene are diagnosed by electrophoretic procedures that separate different forms of Hgb. Fetal hemoglobin levels vary among patients. The WBC and platelet counts often are elevated, but the WBC differential is normal.[49] The reticulocyte count can range from 5% to 15%, and the MCV may be elevated. If MCV values are within the normal range, iron deficiency or B_O-thalassemia must be considered. Sickled cells may also be visually observed in poorly oxygenated blood of a patient with sickle cell anemia. In contrast, a patient with the sickle cell trait should have normal RBC morphology and WBC, reticulocyte, and platelet counts. Sickled cells are rarely observed. In patients with sickle cell B_O-thalassemia, hematologic abnormalities vary, depending on the amount of HbA present. This form may be difficult to distinguish from sickle cell anemia; RBC microcytosis may be the only differentiating parameter.[49]

Clinical Course and Management

Patients carrying the sickle cell trait experience milder symptoms than those with sickle cell anemia. The kidney is commonly affected by microinfarction, which occurs in the renal medulla and impairs the kidney's ability to concentrate urine. During pregnancy, an increased frequency of urinary tract infections and hematuria are seen. However, vaso-occlusive events are uncommon. If they do occur, they usually are caused by hypoxic conditions resulting from excessive exercise or high altitudes.

Sickle cell HbC disease is usually associated with few clinical complications. These patients may have normal physical examination findings with only splenomegaly. Patients are at risk for bacterial infections and, because of elevated Hgb levels, they may suffer from ocular, orthopedic, and pulmonary vaso-occlusive events.[49,53]

Treatment of sickle cell anemia is largely directed toward prophylaxis against infections and supportive management of vaso-occlusive crises. The clinical course among patients with sickle cell disease is variable and difficult to predict. Some patients suffer from a multitude of health problems. Organs such as the kidneys, retina, spleen, and bones are frequent sites of vaso-occlusive events because these sites have a relatively low pH and oxygen tension. Complications (e.g., pain, anemia, and infections) as well as cardiac, pulmonary, neurologic, hepatobiliary, obstetric/gynecologic, ocular, dermatologic, or orthopedic complications can occur. The management of these complications is organ specific and aimed at supportive interventions.

Hemolytic Anemia

Hemolytic anemia is caused by splenic sequestration of abnormal RBC. Sequestration reduces the RBC life span from 120 days to 15 to 25 days and elevates the reticulocyte count. Erythropoietin response is typically blunted for the degree of anemia, which can be a result of concurrent kidney dysfunction. Some patients may even experience aplastic anemia (bone marrow failure) when extensive hemolysis is accompanied by inadequate bone marrow response. It is usually self-limiting, however. Human parvovirus (HPV) B19 is a common cause of transient red cell aplasia (TRCA) with up to 67% of infections resulting in a hematologic change typical of aplasia.[54] Nearly 70% of all cases of homozygous sickle cell patients are HPV B19 seropositive by 20 years of age.[55] Hemolytic anemia can also present in patients with glucose-6-phosphate dehydrogenase deficiency. Cardiac manifestations include high-output failure secondary to anemia. Management of the underlying anemia may include splenectomy following the first splenic sequestration event. Alternatively, patients can be treated with transfusions and careful observation.[49,56]

Infections

Infections commonly occur in patients with sickle cell anemia because the complement pathway, granulocyte function, and B-cell immunity may be altered. Also, impaired splenic function increases the risk for infection from polysaccharide-encapsulated bacteria such as *Streptococcus pneumoniae, Haemophilus influenzae, Neisseria meningitidis,* and *Salmonella typhimurium.* Pneumonia caused by *S. pneumoniae,* mycoplasma, or viruses can worsen hypoxia, causing progression to vaso-occlusion and acute chest syndrome (chest pain in the presence of a local infiltrate on chest radiograph). Because of such complications, the prophylactic administration of penicillin has significantly reduced morbidity and mortality from pneumonia in children <3 years of age[57], but prophylaxis is recommended to be continued through age 5.[51] Pulmonary complications from pneumonia or vascular occlusion also can lead to right-sided heart failure. Other infectious conditions such as osteomyelitis from *S. aureus* or *S. typhimurium* or urinary tract infections caused by *Escherichia coli* are common complications in patients with sickle cell anemia.[49,51] Because of their susceptibility to infections, antibiotic therapy should be instituted at the earliest sign of infection. Vaccines that are recommended for patients with homozygous sickle cell include all standard pediatric vaccines as well as pneumococcal 23-valent polysaccharide vaccine at 2 and 5 years of age with a booster every 10 years.[51] Because patients with sickle cell typically respond poorly, only 50% of patients will be protected by vaccination.[58]

Vascular Occlusion Episodes

Vascular occlusion episodes, or "sickle cell crises," cause severe pain and organ damage. The pain typically lasts 2 to 6 days and should be managed with narcotic analgesics (morphine or morphine derivatives). Narcotic addiction may occur over time but can be prevented by providing the patient with only a few days supply of analgesics following the crisis.[49,51]

Neurologic Complications

Neurologic complications are age dependent. Stroke most commonly occurs in the first decade of life, whereas intracerebral hemorrhage is a complication associated with adulthood. Primary prevention of stroke with RBC transfusions, targeted to maintain HbS level <30%, reduce the incidence of stroke in high risk patients by 92%.[59] If a stroke occurs, approximately 50% of patients experience recurrent strokes within 3 years unless they are treated by chronic RBC transfusion therapy.[50] Preliminary evidence suggests that transitioning from RBC transfusions to chronic hydroxyurea might be an alternative option to prevent secondary stroke, is being further investigated.[60,61]

Renal and Genital Complications

Renal and genital complications are common in sickle cell disease because the environment (hypoxic, acidotic, and hypertonic) predisposes the renal medulla or corpus cavernosum to infarction. As a result, patients might experience reduced potassium excretion, hyperuricemia, hematuria, hyposthenuria, and renal failure. Patients with renal disease generally have inappropriately low levels of EPO as well. Men experiencing occlusion of the corpus cavernosum can experience acute or chronic priapism. Conservative management includes IV fluid administration and pain control. Refractory cases may require surgery.[49,51]

Microinfarctions

Microinfarctions often produce ophthalmic, hepatic, orthopedic, and obstetric/gynecologic complications as well. Other references address these topics in more detail.[49,56]

Treatment for Frequent Vaso-occlusive Crises

Hemoglobin F (HbF) has a protective effect against hemoglobin polymerization. Investigators have observed that patients with HbF levels >20% experience a relatively mild or benign course with fewer vaso-occlusive crises.[46] Hydroxyurea has been found to increase HbF synthesis, which, in turn, may decrease sickling of RBC and the occurrence of disease-related complications.[48,62,63] Hydroxyurea is used prophylactically in patients with recurrent moderate to severe vaso-occlusive crises, but not in treatment of the crises. The use of hydroxyurea in the sickle cell population should be carefully weighed for risk-versus-benefit, because this drug is a cytotoxic agent associated with bone marrow suppression. Patients taking hydroxyurea should have bone marrow studies performed before therapy and periodically during therapy.[64] Other adverse effects of hydroxyurea include GI effects (nausea, vomiting, diarrhea), dermatologic effects (macular papular rash, pruritus), and potential risk of developing a secondary neoplasm (leukemia) with prolonged use. The treatment dose of hydroxyurea for sickle cell anemia is 15 to 35 mg/kg/day. Following initiation of hydroxyurea therapy, blood counts should be monitored closely and the dose adjusted accordingly. Several clinical trials evaluating hydroxyurea show improvement in the clinical course of patients with sickle cell anemia.[62,65] Other areas of potential promise for the treatment of sickle cell anemia include bone marrow transplantation and gene therapy.[66,67]

Clinical Assessment

19. J.T., an 18-year-old man with sickle cell anemia, presented to the emergency department with the chief complaint of rapid onset of abdominal pain and shortness of breath. Since infancy, J.T. has been severely incapacitated by his disease.

During early childhood, he experienced several episodes of acute pain, swelling of the hands and feet, and jaundice. Three years before this admission, J.T. required a left hip replacement secondary to bony infarctions. Recently, frequent blood transfusions have reduced the frequency of sickling crises.

Physical examination reveals J.T. as a thin black man in acute distress and with scleral icterus. He has a pulse of 110 beats/minute, a respiratory rate of 18 breaths/minute, and a temperature of 98.6°F. His lungs are clear, and cardiac auscultation reveals a hyperdynamic pericardium and a systolic murmur at the left sternal edge. Splenomegaly is noted, and a chest radiograph reveals only cardiomegaly.

A CBC is obtained. Notable results include the following: Hgb, 5.5 g/dL (normal, 14 to 18); Hct, 25% (normal, 42% to 52%); WBC count, 5,000/mm^3 (normal, 3,200 to 9,800); platelets, 325,000/mm^3 (normal, 130,000 to 400,000); reticulocyte count, 1% (normal, 0.5 to 1.5%); bilirubin, 5.8 mg/dL (normal, 0.1 to 1.0); serum creatinine (SrCr), 3.0 mg/dL (normal, 0.6 to 1.2); and blood urea nitrogen (BUN), 52 mg/dL (normal, 1 to 18). The peripheral blood smear shows target cells with an occasional sickled cell. What signs and symptoms are consistent with sickle cell anemia? What is J.T.'s current complication?

[SI units: Hgb, 55 g/L; Hct, 0.25; WBC count, 5 × 10^9/L; platelets, 325 × 10^9/L; bilirubin, 99.18 μmol/L; SrCr,265.2 μmol/L; BUN, 18.56 mmol/L urea]

Based on the presence of splenomegaly and anemia with target and sickled cells, J.T. currently is presenting with an acute splenic sequestration crisis. Splenomegaly rapidly evolves over several hours and is accompanied by progressive anemia. The low reticulocyte count is consistent with acute sequestration because a reticulocyte response would be expected if the anemia had developed in recent days. J.T.'s inadequate reticulocyte response may reflect rapid progression of the anemia, HPV B19 infection, or a blunted EPO response secondary to compromised renal dysfunction. The hyperdynamic pericardium and systolic murmur are consistent with the high cardiac output required to deliver oxygen in an anemic state.

20. How should J.T. be treated?

J.T.'s signs and symptoms are sufficiently serious to justify transfusion therapy. In addition, J.T. should be adequately hydrated, considering his elevated serum creatinine and BUN. Because patients with sickle cell anemia often lose the ability to concentrate urine, they may become dehydrated, which further contributes to cell sickling. Pain control also should be aggressively instituted for J.T.'s comfort and should be continued for a few days after hospital discharge (also see Chapter 8, Pain and its Management). Splenectomy may be indicated in instances of severe splenomegaly, repeated infarction, or pain in adults, and it is indicated when crises occur in children. Those patients with sickle cell anemia who are bedridden should be placed on chronic heparin therapy to prevent vascular occlusions and deep vein thrombosis.

ANEMIA OF CHRONIC DISEASE

Anemia of chronic disease (ACD) refers to a mild to moderate anemia associated with a number of disorders (e.g., rheumatoid arthritis [RA], systemic lupus erythematosus, chronic infections, chronic renal failure, acquired immunodeficiency syndrome [AIDS], neoplastic disease).[68] Because of the common occurrence of such conditions, ACD is encountered frequently and has been estimated to be the second most common anemia behind iron deficiency. Most often, ACD is a normochromic, normocytic anemia, although red cells may be hypochromic and microcytic in some patients. Serum iron and total iron-binding capacity are most often decreased, whereas iron stores (as reflected by serum ferritin) are usually normal or increased. Erythropoietin levels in the serum may be increased, although not to an extent appropriate for the degree of anemia. This implicates bone marrow failure, in the setting of increased EPO, as the primary cause of the anemia associated with chronic diseases.[69]

Although the pathogenesis of ACD is not well understood, inflammatory cytokines are thought to play a major role in its development through multiple mechanisms.[68] Interferon-α (IFN-α), -β (IFN-β), -γ (IFN-γ), tumor necrosis factor-α (TNF-α), and IL-1 inhibit burst BFUe and CFUe proliferation and differentiation. Competition for EPO receptors by IFN-γ and TNF-α may possibly lead to EPO resistance. IL-1 and TNF-α also inhibit hepatic and renal expression of EPO messenger RNA (mRNA), further contributing to the development of ACD. Interleukin-6 (IL-6) promotes expression of hepcidin, a 25-amino acid protein produced in hepatocytes.[70] Hepcidin alters iron hemostasis by decreasing duodenal iron absorption and inhibiting the release of reticuloendothelial iron stores leading to hypoferremia and, therefore, blunted bone morrow erythrocyte production.

Management of mild to moderate ACD usually focuses on the underlying disease process. Anemia of chronic disease is not usually progressive or life-threatening, although it generally affects a patient's quality of life. Patients may require blood transfusions for symptomatic anemia. Unless a concurrent deficiency of vitamin B_{12}, folate, or iron exists, administration of vitamin supplements is not of value. Recombinant human EPO (rhEPO) has been used successfully to treat ACD in patients with RA, AIDS, some neoplastic diseases, and chronic kidney disease[68]; however, medication costs can be significant and may outweigh benefits from the treatment of modest anemia.[71] Patients are less likely to respond to rhEPO if baseline serum EPO and inflammatory cytokine levels are elevated. Although serum iron often is decreased, reticuloendothelial iron stores are usually adequate, and treatment with iron is not warranted.[68]

Human Recombinant Erythropoietin Therapy

Human recombinant erythropoietin therapy is indicated for use in anemia associated with end-stage renal disease, drug-induced anemia (chemotherapy and zidovudine therapy), AIDS; in patients with low endogenous EPO levels; and with autologous blood transfusions for elective surgery. Previously, blood transfusions temporarily deterred symptomatic anemia of chronic disease; however, transfusion therapy is associated with risks such as hepatitis, viral infections, iron overload, treatment-related acute lung injury (TRALI), and immunogenic reactions. Studies with rhEPO show that response is both dose dependent and dependent on the underlying cause of anemia.[72,73] Variables that may predict patient response are both patient specific and disease specific and are not always reliable. For example, response to rhEPO in chronic renal failure is dose related and can vary among patients with chronic renal failure.[74] Repeated dose escalations may occur during therapy until a desirable hemoglobin response is achieved.[75,76] Approximately 75% of patients with cancer respond to rhEPO.[77] Response in this population also is dose related, and therapeutic doses are often higher in those patients than in those with renal failure. Lower rhEPO response rates are seen in patients who have received intensive chemotherapy or radiotherapy.[73] In evaluating response to rhEPO, parameters such as increased serum ferritin, decreased transferrin saturation, increased corrected reticulocyte count, decreased transfusion requirements, and increased Hgb and Hct values have been used. Lack of response to rhEPO therapy in all patient populations is most commonly associated with iron deficiency.[68,78] The ability of rhEPO to stimulate the production of erythrocytes normal in both size and hemoglobin concentration is highly dependent on the availability of functional iron.[78]

Darbepoetin alfa is an erythropoiesis-stimulating protein that differs from rhEPO by the addition of two carbohydrate chains. The significance of the additional carbohydrate chains is an increased sialic acid content that results in decreased clearance, and a serum half-life for darbepoetin alfa that is three times longer than that of rhEPO. These kinetic differences allow darbepoetin alfa to be administered less frequently than rhEPO. Similar to rhEPO, hemoglobin response to darbepoetin is dose related. Most patients with chronic kidney disease[79,80] and cancer achieve the desired hemoglobin response with

Table 86-8 Therapeutic Uses and Regimens for Recombinant Human Erythropoietin (rhEPO)[a]

	Epoetin Alfa[c]		Darbepoetin Alfa[c]			
Anemia Pathogenesis[b]	*Dose (U/kg)*	*Frequency*	*Dose(mcg/kg)*	*Frequency*	*Time to Respond (wk)*	*Overall Response Rate (%)*
Acquired immunodeficiency syndrome (AIDS)	100	3× /wk			8–12	17–35
Chemotherapy-induced malignancy	150 or 40,000 U (total dose)	3× /wk or once a week, respectively	2.25 or 500 mcg (total dose)	Once a week or once every 3 weeks, respectively	2–8	32–61[d] 48–83[e]
Renal insufficiency	50–100	3× /wk	0.45	Once a week	2–8	90–97

[a] Adult dosing: twelve- to sixteen-week course of rhEPO therapy.
[b] Patients with AIDS with endogenous erythropoietin levels ≤500 U/L; zidovudine dose ≤4,200 mg/wk.
[c] Moderate dose escalation is indicated if a partial response is observed after 4 to 8 weeks of therapy.
[d] Epoetin alfa.
[e] Darbepoetin alfa.

darbepoetin treatment.[81] Table 86-8 illustrates current therapeutic uses of rhEPO and darbepoetin alfa.

Renal Insufficiency-Related Anemia

21. K.S., a 35-year-old man with a 25-year history of diabetes mellitus, is diagnosed with renal failure and placed on hemodialysis three times weekly. One year later, K.S. is noted to have become increasingly transfusion dependent for correction of his anemia. Significant laboratory values include the following: Hgb, 7 g/dL (normal, 14 to 18); Hct, 26% (normal, 42% to 52%); ferritin, 360 ng/mL (normal, 15 to 200); and serum iron, 98 μg/dL (normal, 50 to 160). In addition, K.S. complains of constant fatigue, poor appetite, and a low energy level. What treatments are available to correct K.S.'s anemia?

[SI units: Hgb, 70 g/L;Hct, 0.26; ferritin, 1265.4 mmol/day; iron, 17.55 μmol/L]

Unlike the anemia associated with most chronic diseases, the hematocrit of patients with chronic renal failure often is markedly reduced. The cause of the anemia is complex but involves reduced EPO production and a shortened RBC life span. Previously, these patients were treated with transfusions and androgens.[82] Although effective, repeated transfusions cause complications, such as iron overload, infections, reactions to leukocyte antigens, or the development of cytotoxic antibodies.

Because EPO is secreted in the kidney in response to anoxia and is responsible for normal differentiation of RBC from other stem cells, rhEPO is used to treat anemia in patients with renal failure who are undergoing hemodialysis, and K.S. is a candidate for this therapy. A dose-dependent rise in Hct is observed in patients with end-stage renal disease at a usual dosage range of epoetin alfa 50 to 100 U/kg three times weekly or darbepoetin alfa 0.45 mcg/kg. Patients such as K.S. who have renal insufficiency appear to be predisposed to rhEPO-induced hypertension. Adverse effects include functional iron deficiency preceded by an elevated reticulocyte count and a change in the rate of hematocrit rise.[83] Seizures also have been reported in approximately 5% of patients with end-stage renal disease[75] (also see Chapter 32, Chronic Renal Disease). Targeting higher concentrations of Hgb (>12 g/dL) are associated with increased mortality and adverse effects.[84]

Malignancy-Related Anemia

22. T.K. is a 45 year-old woman with non-Hodgkin's lymphoma diagnosed 2 months ago. She is being seen for her third of six cycles of chemotherapy. She complains of shortness of breath and fatigue when she walks up stairs. The only medication T.K. takes is ibuprofen 200 mg PRN for occasional headaches. Her CBC indicates the following: Hgb, 9.7 g/dL (normal, 12 to 16); Hct, 29% (normal, 40% to 44%); MCV, 90 μm³ (normal, 81 to 99); MCHC, 30% (normal, 33% to 37%); serum erythropoietin, 29 U/L (normal, 4 to 26). The peripheral smear shows normochromic and normocytic RBC. What is the most likely cause of T.K.'s anemia? What is the appropriate treatment?

T.K. appears to have malignancy-related anemia, which is often characterized as anemia of chronic disease or is chemotherapy induced. This anemia is generally normocytic and normochromic and develops when a disease has persisted for >1 to 2 months. Generally, the anemia is mild or moderate, with a limited number of distinguishing characteristics. As with T.K., the anemia is often asymptomatic or mildly symptomatic (weakness, decreased exercise tolerance). RBC hypochromia may or may not be present, and RBC size is generally normal unless the patient has an underlying iron deficiency anemia. The reticulocyte count is usually low or within normal limits. Both the serum iron and TIBC are decreased and transferrin saturation is usually less than normal.[85] Serum ferritin is a reliable measurement of iron stores in patients with chronic disease. Serum ferritin usually is increased, but may be normal; if the anemia is caused by iron deficiency, ferritin values will be decreased. A bone marrow aspirate would reveal an elevated hemosiderin content. Factors that can influence the incidence of chronic anemia in patients with cancer are the type of malignancy, the stage and duration of disease; the type, schedule and intensity of treatment; and history of prior myelosuppressive chemotherapy or radiation.[73] Although the prevalence of malignancy-related anemia is difficult to quantify, about 50% to 60% of patients with non-Hodgkin's lymphoma, multiple myeloma, or treatment for ovarian and lung cancer develop anemia that requires blood transfusions. The myelosuppressive and anemia-inducing effects of platinum agents (e.g., cisplatin, carboplatin), are well known.[86] These and other myelosuppressive agents are widely used in the treatment of many malignancies, and patients receiving therapy should be appropriately monitored for the development of anemia. Anemia of chronic disease does not respond to treatment with iron, vitamin B_{12}, or folic acid, unless there is an associated vitamin deficiency. Therapy is directed at treatment of the underlying disease, if possible. Large, randomized, multicenter trials have failed to show a clinical benefit to using erythropoietic stimulating agents (ESA) in anemia which is not chemotherapy-induced.[87] Furthermore, mortality was either increased or trended in that direction in recent trials of anemic patients with head, neck, breast, and lung cancer receiving ESA.[88] Because of these findings, a black-box warning was added to epoetin alfa and darbepoetin alfa product information to advise about increases in serious adverse events or disease progression for these patient populations.[89–91] ESA are not recommended for anemic patients with cancer who are not receiving chemotherapy or radiotherapy.[89–91]

In T.K.'s case, the clinician may choose from a number of anemia management options. For example, the current course of chemotherapy can be delayed to allow for hematologic recovery and resolution of anemia symptoms. Alternatively, an RBC transfusion can be given to relieve her symptoms and allow her to better tolerate chemotherapy. In addition, erythropoietic therapy with epoetin alfa or darbepoetin alfa also should be considered. Treatment with epoetin alfa or darbepoetin alfa increases Hct and Hgb, decreases the need for blood transfusions, and improves quality of life. In clinical studies, response rates are 70% to 80%. Therapy is very well tolerated, with most adverse events being attributable to chemotherapy or the underlying disease. Unlike in the chronic kidney disease population, hypertension is infrequently experienced in patients with cancer.[92–94]

If treatment with epoetin alfa is desired for T.K., therapy can be administered at an initial dose of 150 U/kg subcutaneously three times a week.[95] Alternative dosing regimens, such as 10,000 U three times a week or 40,000 U once a week, have proved to be safe and effective in terms of hematopoietic, quality of life, and transfusion effects.[93,96] Response can be assessed initially by monitoring the reticulocyte count, which should peak by day 10 of treatment. A positive rhEPO response also can be predicted by observation of an increased serum ferritin and decreased transferrin saturation. Epoetin alfa usually is administered for a minimum of 4 weeks, although an increase in Hgb and Hct values should be noted after 2 to 4 weeks. If no hematopoietic response (increase in Hgb by 1 to 2 g/dL) is noted by the fourth to eighth weeks, an additional 4 to 8 weeks of therapy should be considered at an increased dose.[97] Common dose escalation schedules include 300 U/kg three times a week if initially treated with 150 U/kg three times a week dosing[97,98] or 60,000 U once a week if initially on 40,000 U once a week dosing.[99] The most common cause of nonresponse to erythropoietic therapy is iron deficiency. Functional iron deficiency occurs when iron stores are unable to be mobilized at a rate sufficient to satisfy the increased demand brought about by amplified bone marrow activity, which occurs with erythropoietic therapy.[97] Nonresponders should be evaluated for functional iron deficiency and given iron supplement, as appropriate, at any point during erythropoietic therapy. For those who do not respond despite appropriate dose modifications, continuation of therapy for >6 to 8 weeks is not beneficial.[100] Once hemoglobin and hematocrit parameters have increased sufficiently to relieve symptoms, the epoetin alfa dose should be reduced every 2 to 3 weeks until the lowest dose required to maintain these levels has been reached. In addition to laboratory monitoring, patients should be asked about their symptoms, such as fatigue, exercise tolerance, and quality of life at frequent intervals while on therapy.

Darbepoetin alfa is also a treatment option for T.K. Initial dosing of darbepoetin alfa is 2.25 mcg/kg subcutaneously once a week.[81] Also, clinical studies of darbepoetin 200 mcg administered every 2 weeks and 300 mcg or 500 mcg administered every 3 weeks have reported beneficial hematopoietic effects and decreased transfusion requirements.[93,94,101] Therapy response should be monitored in the same manner as epoetin alfa, with dose escalation considered after 6 weeks of therapy for nonresponders.[76]

AIDS-Related Anemia

23. J.M., a 37-year-old man, is currently calling his primary physician with complaints of acute worsening of shortness of breath and pounding in his chest. J.M. has a known history of AIDS and has had recent episodes of *Pneumocystis carinii* pneumonia (PCP) and cytomegalovirus (CMV) esophagitis. J.M. also has complained of frequent diarrhea. Trimethoprim-sulfamethoxazole was given intravenously for treatment of PCP; however, J.M. complained of fever while on maintenance therapy. J.M. is currently taking the following medications: dapsone 100 mg/day PO for PCP prophylaxis, ganciclovir 325 mg IV Monday through Friday for CMV prophylaxis, indinavir 800 mg PO Q 8 hours, lamivudine 150 mg PO BID, zidovudine 300 mg PO BID, fluconazole 100 mg/day PO PRN for thrush, and Imodium liquid 5 mL PRN for diarrhea.

The only remarkable findings on physical examination include a respiratory rate of 24 breaths/min and a heart rate of 120 beats/minute. A chest examination reveals that J.M. is tachypneic and has bilateral dry rales. The Hickman catheter in the left subclavian vein appears dry and clean. Further workup of J.M.'s illness includes an unremarkable chest radiograph and negative cultures of the blood and sputum. The CBC includes normal WBC and platelet counts. Abnormal values include the RBC count of 3,300/mm^3 (normal, 4,500 to 6,200), Hgb of 9.1 mg/dL, Hct of 28% (normal, 42% to 54%), and a CD4 of 387 cells/mm^2 (normal, 440 to 1,600). The morphology of the RBC was moderately anisocytic, normochromic, and normocytic. What factors can contribute to J.M.'s anemia?

[SI units: RBC count, 3.3 × 10^9/L (normal, 4.5to 6.2); Hgb, 91 g/L; Hct, 0.28 (normal, 0.42 to 0.54)]

Anemia occurs in >70% of patients with AIDS and correlates with the severity of the clinical syndrome.[102] In this patient population, anemia is a risk factor for early death.[102] Common symptoms such as fatigue, breathlessness, and difficulties in mental concentration may contribute to this patient population's decreased quality of life.[103] Antibody responses against RBC have been documented in patients with AIDS,[104] although their role in the pathogenesis of AIDS has been challenged (see Chapter 69, Pharmacotherapy of Human Immunodeficiency Virus Infection, and Chapter 70, Opportunistic Infections in HIV-Infected Patients). Anemia occurs more often in patients with opportunistic infections (*Mycobacterium avium intracellulare, Cryptococcus neoformans,* and *Histoplasma capsulatum*), viruses (CMV, herpes simplex viruses type 1 and 2, and parvovirus B-19), or neoplasms.[105] Approximately 1% of all AIDS-related anemias are related to parvovirus and can be treated and reversed with IV gammaglobulin.[106] Enhanced production of cytokines, such as TNF-α, also may be correlated with hematologic abnormalities.[69] Anemia can be a consequence of various human immunodeficiency virus (HIV) drugs (e.g., zidovudine, zalcitabine, didanosine, lamivudine)[107–109] or other drugs often used to treat AIDS-associated illnesses (e.g., bone marrow suppressive chemotherapy, ganciclovir, trimethoprim-sulfamethoxazole, dapsone).[43] Kaposi's sarcoma and lymphoma, which impair normal bone marrow function, also can result in anemia in this population.

Iron stores usually are adequate in patients with AIDS; yet, the characteristics of anemia are similar to those present in anemia of chronic disease: low serum iron and iron-binding capacity or an elevated serum ferritin. Vitamin B_{12} deficiency is a contributing cause to anemia in 15% to 30% of these patients[110–112] and is correlated with progression to AIDS.[113] Vitamin B_{12} malabsorption can result from HIV-infected mononuclear cells within the lamina propia[114] or abnormal binding of vitamin B_{12} to transport proteins. Alterations in the utilization of vitamin B_{12} and folate[110,115] can place a patient at risk for hematologic toxicity of drugs such as zidovudine and trimethoprim. Patients with AIDS generally do not respond to vitamin B_{12} supplementation, however.[116]

As illustrated by J.M., HIV-associated anemia has a characteristic RBC morphology, which is normochromic and normocytic. Mild anisocytosis and poikilocytosis also may be observed. Zidovudine-associated anemia is typically macrocytic.[117]

Erythropoiesis is often defective in patients with AIDS, as reflected by an inappropriately low reticulocyte count and an increased or blunted erythropoietic response for the degree of anemia.[118,119] Treatment with rhEPO therapy increases the quality of life and Hgb in HIV-infected adult patients regardless of zidovudine use, CD4+ count, or viral load.[120]

J.M. has many risk factors for anemia of chronic disease, including AIDS and its accompanying predisposition to malignancy and infection. He is also taking many medications (ganciclovir, zidovudine, and dapsone) that can induce anemia.

24. J.M.'s physician determines that J.M.'s endogenous erythropoietin level is 737 U/L (normal, 4 to 26). Is J.M. a candidate for rhEPO? How can the best response to rhEPO be predicted? What would an appropriate starting dosing regimen be?

Patients taking zidovudine ($\leq$4,200 mg/week) who have baseline EPO levels <500 IU/L experience a significantly higher rate of increase in hematocrit compared with patients with high baseline EPO levels.[121] A patient who develops macrocytic anemia with moderate EPO response (<500 IU/L) may require moderate transfusion support in response to zidovudine. A patient who develops normocytic anemia with a high EPO response (>500 IU/L) may have substantial transfusion requirements.[122] A significant reduction in transfusion requirements has been observed in those patients with macrocytic anemia with moderate EPO response who are given rhEPO 40,000 U subcutaneously once weekly. Therefore, rhEPO may be considered appropriate treatment for patients whose baseline EPO level is <500 IU/L.

J.M.'s anemia is less likely to respond to rhEPO than patients who have endogenous EPO levels <500 U/L. (Note: Although this level far exceeds normal, high values are often seen in anemias of chronic disease.) An rhEPO trial of therapy may be initiated at 40,000 U once weekly. J.M. should be followed by evaluating his RBC indices in another 6 to 8 weeks. If he responds appropriately, the rhEPO dosage may be decreased to the lowest dose necessary to prevent symptoms or RBC transfusions. If J.M. has not responded after 4 weeks of therapy, the dose should be increased to 60,000 U once weekly.[123] If J.M. does not respond to 60,000 U, it is unlikely that he will benefit from further rhEPO therapy.

ACKNOWLEDGMENT

We gratefully acknowledge Ann Bolinger, Jim Koeller, Carla Van Den Berg, and Dan Bestul for their contributions to this chapter.

REFERENCES

1. Bergin JJ. Evaluation of anemia. *Postgrad Med J* 1985;77:253.
2. Dawson AA et al. Evaluation of diagnostic significance of certain symptoms and physical signs in anaemic patients. *BMJ* 1969;4:436.
3. Killip S et al. Iron deficiency anemia. *Am Fam Phys* 2007;75:671.
4. Antianemia drugs. In: McEvoy GK et al. *American Hospital Formulary Service Drug Information 07*. Bethesda, MD: American Society of Health-Systems Pharmacists; 2007.
5. Bentley DP. Iron metabolism and anemia in pregnancy. *Clin Haematol* 1985;14:613.
6. Wheby MS. Effect of iron on serum ferritin levels in iron deficiency anemia. *Blood* 1980;55:138.
7. Harju E, Parkarinen A. The effect of iron treatment on serum ferritin concentrations and bone marrow stainable iron in iron deficient outpatients with gastritis, gastric ulcer and duodenal ulcer. *J Int Med Res* 1984;12:56.
8. Intragumtornchai T et al. The role of serum ferritin in the diagnosis of iron deficiency anemia in patients with liver cirrhosis. *J Intern Med* 1998;243:233.
9. Stojceski T et al. Studies on the serum iron-binding capacity. *J Clin Pathol* 1965;18:446.
10. Beissner RS, Trowbridger AA. Clinical assessment of anemia. *Postgrad Med* 1986;80:83.
11. Cook JD. Newer aspects of the diagnosis and treatment of iron deficiency. *American Society of Hematology Educational Program Book* 2003:40.
12. Ekenved G. Iron absorption studies: studies on oral iron preparations using serum iron and different radioiron isotope techniques. *Scand J Haematol* 1976;28(Suppl):7.
13. Middletown E et al. Studies on the absorption of orally administered iron from sustained-release preparations. *N Engl J Med* 1966;274:136.
14. Harju E, Lindberg H. Ascorbic acid does not augment the restoration effect of iron treatment for empty iron stores in patients after gastrointestinal surgery. *Am Surg* 1986;52:463.
15. Fairbanks VF. Laboratory testing for iron status *Hosp Pract* 1991;26(Suppl 3):17.
16. Saunders JR, Ferguson AW. Ferrous sulfate: Danger to children. *BMJ* 1977;1:57.
17. Grebe G et al. Effect of meals and ascorbic acid on the absorption of a therapeutic dose of iron as ferrous and ferric salts. *Current Therapy Research* 1975;17:382.
18. Norrby A. Iron absorption studies in iron deficiency. *Scandinavian Journal of Haematology* 1974;20(Suppl):5.
19. Ekenved G et al. Influence of a liquid antacid on the absorption of different iron salts. *Scandinavian Journal of Haematology* 1976;28(Suppl):65.
20. Hall G et al. Inhibition of iron absorption by magnesium trisilicate. *Med J Aust* 1969;2:95.
21. Kanazawa S et al. Removal of cobalamin analogue in bile bt enterohepatic circulation of Vit B12. *Lancet* 1983;1:707.
22. Neuvonem P et al. Interference of iron with the absorption of tetracyclines in man. *BMJ* 1970;4:532.
23. Will G. The absorption, distribution and utilization of intramuscularly administered iron-dextran: A radioisotope study. *Br J Haematol* 1968;14:395.

24. Barton JC et al. Intravenous iron dextran therapy in patients with iron deficiency and normal renal function who failed to respond to or did not tolerate oral iron supplementation. *Am J Med* 2000;109:27.
25. Bailie GR et al. Parenteral iron use in the management of anemia in end stage renal disease patients. *Am J Kidney Dis* 2000;35:1.
26. Michael B et al. for the Ferrlecit Publication Committee. Sodium ferric gluconate complex in hemodialysis patients: Adverse reactions compared to placebo and iron dextran. *Kidney Int* 2002;61:1830.
27. Wallerstein RO. Intravenous iron dextran complex. *Blood* 1968;32:690.
28. Beck WS. Diagnosis of megaloblastic anemia. *Annu Rev Med* 1991;42:311.
29. Aslina F et al. Megaloblastic anemia and other causes of macrocytosis. *Clin Med Res* 2006;4:236.
30. Carmel R. Pernicious anemia. *Arch Intern Med* 1988;148:1712.
31. Hagedorn CH, Alpers DH. Distribution of intrinsic factor-vitamin B_{12} receptors in human intestine. *Gastroenterology* 1977;73:1019.
32. Hooper DC et al. Characterization of ileal vitamin B_{12} binding using homogeneous human and hog intrinsic factor. *J Clin Invest* 1973;52:3074.
33. Hsu JM et al. Vitamin B_{12} concentrations in human tissues. *Nature* 1966;210:1264.
34. Murphy MF et al. Megaloblastic anaemia due to vitamin B_{12} deficiency caused by small intestinal bacterial overgrowth: possible role of vitamin B_{12} analogues. *Br J Haematol* 1986;62:7.
35. Nilsson-Ehle H et al. Low serum cobalamin levels in a population study of 70- and 75-year-old subjects. *Dig Dis Sci* 1989;34:716.
36. Lane LA et al. Treatment of vitamin B_{12}-deficiency anemia: Oral versus parenteral therapy. *Ann Pharmacother* 2002;36:1268.
37. Vitamin B complex. In: McEnvoy GK et al., eds. *American Hospital Formulary Service Drug Information ASHP 07.* Bethesda, MD: *American Society of Health-System Pharmacists* 2007.
38. Butler C et al. Oral vitamin B_{12} versus intramuscular vitamin B_{12} for vitamin B_{12} deficiency: A systematic review of randomized controlled trials. *Fam Pract* 2006;23:279.
39. Nyholm E et al. Oral vitamin B_{12} can change our practice. *Postgrad Med J* 2003;79:218.
40. Herbert V. Recommended dietary intakes (RDI) of folate in humans. *Am J Clin Nutr* 1987;45:661.
41. O'Neil-Cutting MA, Crosby WH. The effect of antacids on the absorption of simultaneously ingested iron. *JAMA* 1986;255:1468.
42. Kornberg A et al. Folic acid deficiency, megaloblastic anemia and peripheral polyneuropathy due to oral contraceptives. *Israel Journal of Medical Science* 1989;25:142.
43. McKinsey DS et al. Megaloblastic pancytopenia associated with dapsone and trimethoprim treatment of 0 pneumonia in the acquired immunodeficiency syndrome. *Arch Intern Med* 1989;149:965.
44. Barney-Stallings RA et al. What is the clinical utility of obtaining a folate level in patients with macrocytosis or anemia? *J Fam Pract* 2001;50:544.
45. Anon. Hereditary dihydrofolate reductase deficiency with megaloblastic anemia. *Nutr Rev* 1985; 43:309.
46. Chanarin I. Megaloblastic anaemia, cobalamin, and folate. *J Clin Pathol* 1987:40;978.
47. Snow CF. Laboratory diagnosis of vitamin B_{12} and folate deficiency: a guide for the primary care physician. *Arch Intern Med* 1999;159:1289.
48. Charache S et al. Effect of hydroxyurea on the frequency of painful crises in sickle cell anemia. *N Engl J Med* 1995;332:1317.
49. Embury SH, Vichinsky E. Sickle cell disease. In: Hoffman R et al, eds. *Hematology. Basic Principles and Practice*, 3rd ed. New York: Churchill Livingstone; 1999:510.
50. Frenette PS et al. Sickle cell disease: old discoveries, new concepts, and future promise. *J Clin Invest* 2007;117:850.
51. Redding-Lallinger R, Knoll C. Sickle cell disease pathophysiology and treatment. *Curr Probl Pediatr Adolesc Health Care* 2006;36:346.
52. Karnon J et al. The effects of neonatal screening for sickle cell disorders on lifetime treatment costs and early deaths avoided: A modelling approach. *J Public Health Med* 2000;22:500.
53. Powers DR et al. Outcome in hemoglobin SC disease: A four-decade observational study of clinical, hematologic, and genetic factors. *Am J Hematol* 2002;70:206.
54. Serjeant BE et al. Haematological response to parvovirus B19 infection in homozygous sickle cell disease. *Lancet* 2001;358:1779.
55. Smith-Whitley K et al. Epidemiology of human parvovirus B19 in children with sickle cell disease. *Blood* 2004;103:422.
56. Steinberg MH. Management of sickle cell disease. *N Engl J Med* 1999;340:1021.
57. Gaston MH et al. Prophylaxis with oral penicillin in children with sickle cell anemia. A randomized trial. *N Engl J Med* 1986;314:1593.
58. John AB et al. Prevention of pneumococcal infection in children with homozygous sickle cell disease. *BMJ* 1984;288:1567.
59. Adams RJ et al. Prevention of a first stroke by transfusions in children with sickle cell anemia and abnormal results on transcranial doppler ultrasonography. *N Engl J Med* 1998;339:5.
60. Ware RE et al. Prevention of secondary stroke and resolution of transfusional iron overload in children with sickle cell anemia using hydroxyurea and phlebotomy. *J Pediatr* 2004;145:346
61. Stroke with transfusions changing to hydroxyurea (SWiTCH) (2006). National Heart, Lung, and Blood Institute (NHLBI). http://clinicaltrials.gov/show/nct00122980. Accessed June 18, 2007.
62. Goldberg MA et al. Treatment of sickle cell anemia with hydroxyurea and erythropoietin. *N Engl J Med* 1990;323:366.
63. Ferster A et al. Hydroxyurea for the treatment of severe sickle cell anemia: a pediatric clinical trial. *Blood* 1996;88:1960.
64. Hydroxyurea. In: McEvoy GK et al., eds. *American Hospital Formulary Service Drug Information ASHP 03.* Bethesda, MD: American Society of Health-Systems Pharmacists; 2003:1012.
65. El-Hazmi MAF et al. On the use of hydroxyurea/erythropoietin combination therapy for sickle cell disease. *Acta Haematol* 1995;94:128.
66. Walters MC et al. Impact of bone marrow transplantation for symptomatic sickle cell disease: An interim report. Multicenter investigation of bone marrow transplantation for sickle cell disease. *Blood* 2000;95:1918.
67. Panepinto JA et al. Matched-related donor transplantation for sickle cell disease: Report from the Center for International Blood and Transplant Research. *Br J Haematol* 2007;137:479.
68. Weiss G, Goodnough LT. Anemia of chronic disease. *N Engl J Med* 2005;352:1011.
69. Krantz SB. Pathogenesis and treatment of the anemia of chronic disease. *Am J Med Sci* 1994;307:353.
70. Ganz T. Hepcidin and its role in regulating systemic iron metabolism. *Hematology* 2006;507:29.
71. Bertero MT, Caligaris-Cappio F. Anemia of chronic disorders in systemic autoimmune diseases. *Haematologica* 1997;82:375.
72. Naman A et al. Markers of masked iron deficiency and effectiveness of epo therapy in chronic renal failure. *Am J Kidney Dis* 1997;30:532.
73. Ludwig H. Epoetin in cancer-related anaemia. *Nephrol Dial Transplant* 1999;14(Suppl 2):85.
74. Artune F et al. Serum erythropoietin concentrations and responses to anaemia in patients with or without chronic kidney disease. *Nephrol Dial Transplant* 2007; Epub:doi:10.1093/ndt/gfm316
75. Eschbach JW et al. Recombinant human erythropoietin in anemic patients with end-stage renal disease: results of a phase III multicenter clinical trial. *Ann Intern Med* 1989;111:992.
76. Sabbatini P, Cella D, Chanan-Kahn A et al. NCCN Anemia Panel. *Cancer and Treatment-Related Anemia. National Comprehensive Cancer Network Practice Guidelines* V.3.2007.
77. Vansteenkiste JF. Every 3 weeks dosing with darbepoetin alfa: A new paradigm in anaemia management. *Cancer Treat Rev* 2006;32:S11.
78. Kwack C et al. Managing erythropoietin hyporesponsiveness. *Semin Dial* 2006;19:146.
79. Hertel JE et al. Darbepoetin alfa administration to achieve and maintain target hemoglobin levels for 1 year in patients with chronic kidney disease. *Mayo Clin Proc* 2006;81:1188.
80. Ling B et al. Darbepoetin alfa administered once monthly maintains hemoglobin concentrations in patients with chronic kidney disease. *Clin Nephrol* 2005;63:327.
81. Vansteenkiste J et al. Double-blind, placebo-controlled, randomized phase III trial of darbepoetin alfa in lung cancer patients receiving chemotherapy. *J Natl Cancer Inst* 2002;94:1211.
82. Neff MS et al. A comparison of androgens for anemia in patients on dialysis. *N Engl J Med* 1981;304:871.
83. Eschbach JW et al. Correction of the anemia of end-stage renal disease with recombinant human erythropoietin. *N Engl J Med* 1987;316:73.
84. Phrommintikul A et al. Mortality and target haemoglobin concentrations in anaemic patients with chronic kidney disease treated with erythropoietin: A meta-analysis. *Lancet* 2007;369:381.
85. Dallman PR et al. Prevalence and causes of anemias in the United States, 1976 to 1980. *Am J Clin Nutr* 1984;39:437.
86. Groopman JE, Itri LM. Chemotherapy-induced anemia in adults: incidence and treatment. *J Natl Cancer Inst* 1999;91:1616.
87. http://www.fda.gov/cder/drug/inopage/RHE/default.htm
88. Lappin TR et al. Warning flags for erythropoiesis-stimulating agents and cancer-associated anemia. *Oncologist.* 2007;12:362.
89. Amgen Inc. Aranesp (darbepoetin alfa) prescribing information. Thousand Oaks, CA; April 2007.
90. Amgen, Inc. Epogen (epoetin alfa) prescribing information. Thousand Oaks, CA; March 2007.
91. Ortho Biotech Products, L.P. Procrit (epoetin alfa) prescribing information. Raritan, NJ; March 2007.
92. Hesketh PJ et al. A randomized controlled trial of darbepoetin alfa administered as a fixed or weight-based dose using a front-loading schedule in patients with anemia who have nonmyeloid malignancies. *Cancer* 2004;15;100:859.
93. Schwartzberg LS et al. A randomized comparison of every-2-week darbepoetin alfa and weekly epoetin alfa for the treatment of chemotherapy-induced anemia in patients with breast, lung, or gynecologic cancer. *Oncologist* 2004;9:696.
94. Boccia et al. Darbepoetin alfa administered every three weeks is effective for the treatment of chemotherapy-induced anemia. *Oncologist* 2006; 11:409.
95. Ortho Biotech Division. Procrit (epoetin alfa) prescribing information. Raritan, NJ; February 1997.
96. Demetri GD et al. Quality-of-life benefit in chemotherapy patients treated with epoetin alfa is independent of disease response or tumor type: results from a prospective community oncology study. *J Clin Oncol* 1998;16:3412.
97. Henry DH. Supplemental iron: a key to optimizing the response of cancer-related anemia to rHuEPO? *Oncologist* 1998;3:275.
98. Quirt I et al. Epoetin alfa therapy increases hemoglobin levels and improves quality of life in patients with cancer-related anemia who are not receiving chemotherapy and patients with anemia who are receiving chemotherapy. *J Clin Oncol* 2001;19:4126.
99. Gabrilove JL et al. Clinical evaluation of once-weekly dosing of epoetin alfa in chemotherapy patients: Improvements in hemoglobin and quality of life are similar to three-times-weekly dosing. *J Clin Oncol* 2001;19:2875.
100. Rizzo JD et al. Use of epoetin in patients with cancer: evidence-based clinical practice guidelines

of the American Society of Clinical Oncology and the American Society of Hematology. *Blood* 2002;100:2303.

101. Canon JL et al. Randomized, double-blind, active-controlled trial of every-3-week darbepoetin alfa for the treatment of chemotherapy-induced anemia. *J Natl Cancer Inst* 2006;98:273.
102. Sullivan PS et al. Epidemiology of anemia in human immunodeficiency virus (HIV)-infected persons: Results from the multistate adult and adolescent spectrum of HIV disease surveillance project. *Blood* 1998;91:301.
103. Semba RD et al. The impact of anemia on energy and physical functioning in individuals with AIDS. *Arch Intern Med* 2005;165:2229.
104. Donahue RE et al. Suppression of in vivo haematopoiesis following immunodeficiency virus infection. *Nature* 1987;326:200.
105. Henry DH. Experience with epoetin alfa and acquired immunodeficiency syndrome anemia. *Semin Oncol* 1998;25(Suppl 7):64.
106. Koduri PR et al. Chronic pure red cell aplasia caused by parvovirus B19 in AIDS: use of intravenous immunoglobulin—A report of eight patients. *Am J Hematol* 1999;61:16.
107. Claster S. Biology of anemia, differential diagnosis, and treatment options in human immunodeficiency virus infection. *J Infect Dis* 2002;185:S105.
108. Schacter LP et al. Effects of therapy with didanosine on hematologic parameters in patients with advanced human immunodeficiency virus disease. *Blood* 1992;80:2969.
109. Khawcharoenporn T et al. Lamivudine-associated macrocytosis in HIV-infected patients. *Int J STD AIDS.* 2007;18:39.
110. Beach RS et al. Altered folate metabolism in early HIV infection. *JAMA* 1988;259:519.
111. Harriman GR et al. Vitamin B_{12} malabsorption in patients with acquired immunodeficiency syndrome. *Arch Intern Med* 1989;149:2039.
112. Paltiel O et al. Clinical correlates of subnormal vitamin B_{12} levels in patients with the acquired immunodeficiency virus. *Am J Hematol* 1995;49:318.
113. Tang AM et al. Low serum vitamin B-12 concentrations are associated with faster human immunodeficiency virus type 1 (HIV-1) disease progression. *J Nutr* 1997;127:345.
114. Burkes RL et al. Low serum cobalamin levels occur frequently in acquired immune deficiency syndrome and related disorders. *Eur J Haematol* 1987;38:141.
115. Tilkian SM et al. Altered folate metabolism in early HIV infection. *JAMA* 1988;259:3128.
116. Falguera M et al. Study of the role of vitamin B_{12} and folinic acid supplementation in preventing hematologic toxicity of zidovudine. *Eur J Haematol* 1995;55:97.
117. Richman DD et al. The toxicity of azidothymidine (AZT) in the treatment of patients with AIDS and AIDS-related complex. *N Engl J Med* 1987;317:192.
118. Abels RI. Use of recombinant human erythropoietin in the treatment of anemia in patients who have cancer. *Semin Oncol* 1992;19(Suppl 8):29.
119. Camacho J et al. Serum erythropoietin levels in anaemic patients with advanced human immunodeficiency virus infection. *Br J Haematol* 1992;82:608.
120. Saag MS et al. Once-weekly epoetin alfa improves quality of life and increases hemoglobin in anemic HIV+ patients. *AIDS Res Hum Retroviruses.* 2004;20:1037.
121. Fischl MA et al. A randomized controlled trial of a reduced daily dose of zidovudine in patients with the acquired immunodeficiency syndrome. *N Engl J Med* 1990;323:1009.
122. Fischl M et al. Recombinant human erythropoietin for patients with AIDS treated with zidovudine. *N Engl J Med* 1990;322:1488.
123. Brokering KL, Qaqish RB. Management of anemia of chronic disease in patients with the human immunodeficiency virus. *Pharmacotherapy* 2003;23:1475.

CHAPTER 87

Drug-Induced Blood Disorders

Sana R. Sukkari and Larry D. Sasich

OVERVIEW

Definitions

Drug-induced injuries of the blood are termed *blood dyscrasias*. In this chapter, blood dyscrasias refer to adverse effects that usually are not predictable or are not a direct extension of a drug's pharmacologic action, and they occur in an unknown, although usually small, number of persons exposed to the agent in question. Thus, the decrease in white blood cell (WBC) count that is seen in many patients receiving marrow suppressant cancer chemotherapy would not be considered a blood dyscrasia. The same reaction in someone receiving phenytoin for a seizure disorder would be considered a blood dyscrasia. Exceptions exist and are addressed as necessary. The five major types of drug-induced blood dyscrasias presented are (a) hemolytic anemia, (b) thrombocytopenia, (c) agranulocytosis or neutropenia, (d) aplastic anemia, and (e) pure red cell aplasia. A consensus conference proposed standardized definitions and general criteria for drug-induced blood dyscrasias.[1] These definitions are discussed in specific sections of the chapter. Older reports have used similar, although not necessarily identical definitions and criteria, and not all authors have adopted these standards.

Epidemiology

One study suggests that a substantial proportion of blood dyscrasias could be attributable to drug treatment.[2] Accurate estimates of the incidence of drug-induced injuries, including drug-induced blood dyscrasias, are generally not obtainable. Controlled clinical trials provide incidence estimates of common adverse reactions; however, rare, serious events might not be detected because of the relatively small number of subjects exposed to drugs in clinical trials.

Adverse drug reaction reporting systems such as the U.S. Food and Drug Administration's (FDA) Medwatch program rely on spontaneous reports by health professionals and patients, and do not capture all adverse events. Thus, spontaneous reports cannot provide a reliable numerator for calculating the incidence of adverse reactions. Likewise, prescription sales data used to approximate a denominator in an incidence calculation can only estimate the true number of persons exposed to a drug.

Under-reporting is a widely recognized problem in postmarketing adverse reaction reporting systems. Studies have documented that only 10% to 15% of serious adverse reactions are reported.[3,4]

Spontaneous reporting systems by themselves do not give an accurate insight into the incidence of adverse drug reactions, and often spontaneous adverse event reporting rates are misinterpreted as the incidence of adverse reactions.

The FDA has addressed the misinterpretation of event reporting rates in some drug safety labeling changes. For example, thrombotic thrombocytopenic purpura (TTP) was not seen during clinical trials with the antiplatelet drug ticlopidine (Ticlid), but U.S. physicians reported approximately 100 cases between 1992 and 1997. Based on an estimated patient exposure of 2 to 4 million, and assuming an event reporting rate of 10% (the true rate is not known), the incidence of ticlopidine-associated TTP could be as high as 1 case in every 2,000 to 4,000 patients exposed to the drug.[5]

Spontaneous reporting of suspected drug-induced blood dyscrasias is of greatest value in hypothesis generation and for the detection of new associations. Under specific conditions, spontaneous reports analyzed with prescription sales data can give a fairly accurate estimate of the relative and absolute risk. Calculating the risk using exposure data expressed in patient years might underestimate the risk for long-term treatment. For example, if the risk is highest during the first 3 months of treatment the denominator will include a long period of low risk. On the other hand, risk could be overestimated for short-term treatment when the number of prescriptions is probably a less inaccurate denominator.

In addition to under-reporting, selective reporting is another problem. As a result, spontaneous reports are particularly vulnerable to bias when comparing risks with different drugs within a class or between drug classes. Comparative risk estimates, although vital, are complicated when old drugs are compared with new drugs. In situations when the risk is higher at the beginning of treatment, a population treated with a new drug will always contain a higher proportion of vulnerable patients than those who have tolerated an older drug over time. The best comparison in such cases is to include only first-time users in both groups.[6]

For these reasons, spontaneous reporting data must be interpreted with caution. Spontaneous reporting systems have been developed for signal generation and, thus, must sacrifice specificity for sensitivity. This can lead to possible false associations. Moreover, some well-known associations (e.g., heparin and thrombocytopenia) are not reported because the association already has been established. Voluntary reporting of suspected drug-induced blood dyscrasia and other adverse drug events to the FDA is critical to the prompt identification of drug-induced safety-related problems.

DRUG-INDUCED HEMOLYTIC ANEMIA

Drug-induced hemolysis refers to an increased rate of red cell destruction, caused directly or indirectly by a drug. Destruction can occur within the blood vessels (intravascular hemolysis) or outside the vascular space (extravascular hemolysis). Anemia develops when the rate of hemolysis exceeds the rate that bone marrow is capable of replacing destroyed cells.

Drugs can induce red cell destruction by several mechanisms. The first is by a direct toxic effect on cells as a result of genetically determined enzymopathies or hemoglobinopathies. The red blood cells (RBC) of patients with these inherited abnormalities are predisposed to lysis when exposed to drugs or chemicals that would otherwise not have any predictable toxic effect. Second, several drugs can elicit an immune response that results in destruction of normal RBC. This occurs idiosyncratically (i.e., patients cannot be identified prospectively as being predisposed).[7]

More than 70 drugs are known to cause either positive direct antiglobulin tests (DAT) or immune hemolysis. Second- and third-generation cephalosporins, diclofenac, fludarabine, carboplatin, oxaliplatin, and β-lactamase inhibitors are among the drugs associated with severe or fatal hemolysis.[8,9]

Intravascular Hemolysis

Many drug-induced hemolytic anemias related to genetically determined red cell defects, as well as some classified as immune-mediated, are caused by destruction of RBC within the vessels. Free hemoglobin, a potentially nephrotoxic substance, is released into the bloodstream. The amount of hemoglobin released from erythrocytes during extensive hemolysis overwhelms the mechanisms that usually are capable of efficiently removing hemoglobin (Hgb) from the circulation. Free Hgb initially binds tightly to haptoglobin, a circulating α-globulin. The resulting hemoglobin–haptoglobin complex is too large to be filtered at the glomerulus and is removed from the circulation by the fixed macrophages of the reticuloendothelial system. This occurs primarily in the liver, where the heme portion of the hemoglobin molecule is converted to bilirubin, iron is conserved, and serum levels of haptoglobin fall. Laboratory changes characteristic of hepatic hemoglobin and bilirubin metabolism resulting from extravascular hemolysis (e.g., hyperbilirubinemia, urobilinogenuria) also are observed. If the hemoglobin-binding capacity of haptoglobin is exceeded, either by an acute, severe, or ongoing hemolysis, some hemoglobin will be renally filtered.

The cells of the proximal tubule reabsorb hemoglobin, but as in the case of glucose, there is a threshold concentration beyond which free hemoglobin will spill into the urine. The reabsorbed hemoglobin is degraded to bilirubin and the iron is converted to ferritin and hemosiderin. Bilirubin could appear in the urine and, as the hemoglobin-injured tubular cells slough, so will hemosiderin. Hemoglobin not bound to haptoglobin or filtered at the glomerulus is metabolized to methemoglobin, the hemin moiety of which can then dissociate and bind to the circulating β-globulin, hemopexin. In severe hemolysis, the hemin moiety of methemoglobin binds with circulating albumin to form methemalbumin; serum hemopexin levels will decrease and methemalbumin will be detectable in the serum. Hemin dissociates from albumin and binds to newly synthesized hemopexin as depleted hemopexin supplies are replaced (Fig. 87-1).

Extravascular Hemolysis

Most immune-mediated, drug-induced RBC destruction occurs extravascularly. Reticuloendothelial cells phagocytize the RBC. The heme portion of hemoglobin is metabolized to unconjugated (indirect) bilirubin, which complexes loosely with albumin in the bloodstream and is transported to the liver where it is conjugated with glucuronic acid. When the

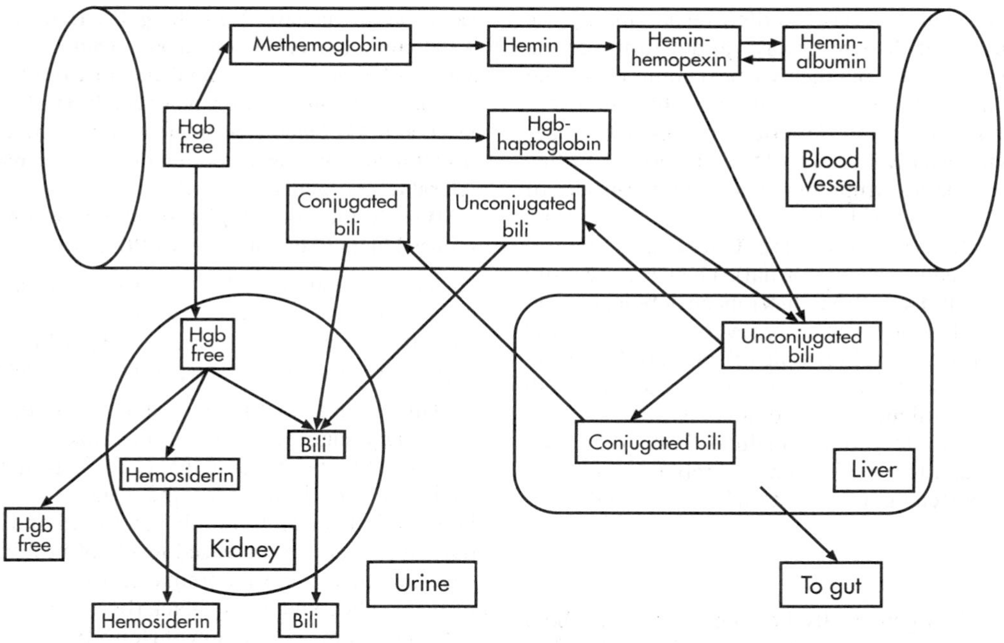

FIGURE 87-1 Intravascular hemolysis. (See Figure 2-1 in Chapter 2, Interpretation of Clinical Laboratory Tests, for bilirubin metabolism after secretion into the gut.)

increased rate of bilirubin formation exceeds the ability of the liver to conjugate it, the serum concentration of indirect bilirubin increases and clinical jaundice can result. The conjugated (direct) bilirubin is passed from the liver to the intestine where it is metabolized to urobilinogen. Most urobilinogen is excreted in the feces, but part is reabsorbed and enterohepatically recycled with some urobilinogen appearing in the urine (also see Fig. 2-1 in Chapter 2, Interpretation of Clinical Laboratory Tests).

Glucose-6-Phosphate Dehydrogenase Deficiency

Etiology

Red blood cells deficient in glucose-6-phosphate dehydrogenase (G6PD) are susceptible to hemolysis when exposed to oxidative stress. The hexose monophosphate shunt in RBC is responsible for maintaining glutathione in the reduced state. Glutathione is an antioxidant that prevents oxidation of hemoglobin to methemoglobin. Nicotinamide adenine dinucleotide phosphate-oxidase (NADPH) is required to keep glutathione in the reduced state and G6PD is needed to reduce NADP to NADPH (Fig. 87-2). When RBC are deficient in G6PD, the amount of NADPH is inadequate to keep glutathione in the reduced state, free radicals accumulate intracellularly, and the oxidation of hemoglobin to methemoglobin cannot be prevented. Heinz bodies (condensations of precipitated, denatured hemoglobin) appear in the RBC. The now fragile cells are removed from the circulation (lysed) prematurely, primarily while passing through the splenic pulp. It is unclear whether methemoglobin contributes to Heinz body formation or is merely a concomitant occurrence. The degree of hemolysis is related both to the oxidant potential of the drug and the dose.[10]

Epidemiology

Deficiency of G6PD is the most common metabolic disorder of RBC and it has been estimated to affect over 400 million individuals worldwide.[11] The disorder is sex linked with transmission from mother to son. Although the defect will be fully expressed in males, female heterozygotes have a mix

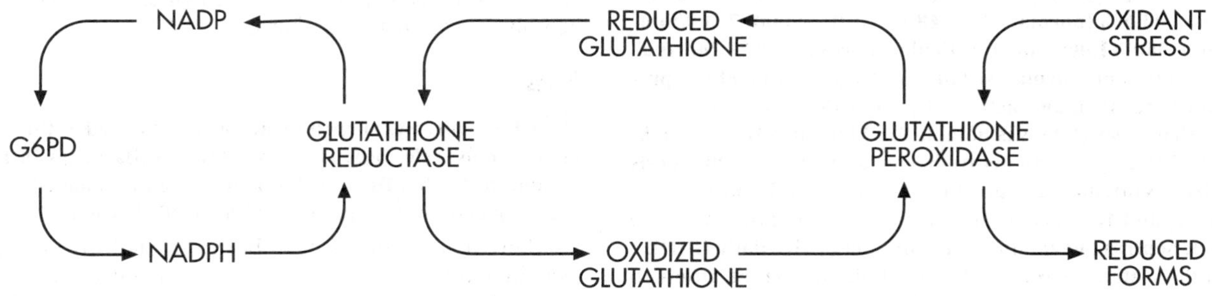

FIGURE 87-2 Nicotinamide adenine dinucleotide phosphate-oxidase (NADPH) is required to keep glutathione in the reduced state, and glucose-6-phosphate dehydrogenase (G6PD) is needed to reduce NADP to NADPH.

of both normal and deficient RBC and correspondingly less severe manifestations of disease. Many variant forms of the enzyme have been identified, but the two most common are the A-type (African) and the Mediterranean type. The less severe A-variant affects about 10% of American blacks. G6PD activity in the A-type usually is 5% to 15% of normal. In this situation, patients remain asymptomatic except for episodes of hemolysis precipitated by oxidant stress. Mediterranean-type deficiency is associated with low levels of G6PD enzyme activity (e.g., in some patients <1% of normal). The RBC are more susceptible to lysis in those with Mediterranean deficiency than those with A-type deficiency. The more severe forms of G6PD deficiency are most prevalent in people of southern European ancestry, particularly Sardinian Italians, Greeks, and Kurdish Jews in whom the prevalence is approximately 50%.[12] Other groups affected by G6PD variants include Sephardic Jews, American Indians, and those of Asian or Arabian ancestry.[13] Cases have been reported rarely in western European and Scandinavian populations.

Classification

Deficiency of G6PD is genetically heterogeneous and about 400 different enzymes mutations have been reported.[12] The World Health Organization (WHO) has established criteria to categorize different variant enzymes into five classes. Class I variants are associated with chronic nonspherocytic hemolytic anemia (CNSHA); class II variants have a G6PD activity of <10% of normal; class III variants have an activity of 10% to 60% of normal; class IV variants have near-normal activity and no clinical manifestations; and class V variants have increased activity.[14] The degree of hemolysis in all classes is related both to the degree of enzyme deficiency and the strength of the precipitating stimulus.

In the case of drugs, both the oxidant potential of the drug and the dose contribute to severity. Even topical administration of 1% silver sulfadiazine in a patient with extensive burns and 10% G6PD activity has resulted in significant RBC destruction.[15] Nondrug inducers of hemolysis include infection, diabetic ketoacidosis, unknown factors during the neonatal period, and ingestion of fava beans. Fava beans (*Vicia faba*), also known as broad beans, are a common dietary staple in some parts of the world and can cause severe hemolysis in some G6PD-deficient patients.

Features

1. F.S., a 55-year-old, Italian-American man, noted suprapubic pain and burning on urination. Laboratory data included the following values: Hgb, 14.0 g/dL (normal, 12–16 g/dL); hematocrit (Hct), 43.6% (normal, 38%–48%); WBC count, 7,500/mm^3 (normal, 4,000–11,000/mm^3); reticulocyte count, 0.5% (normal, 0.2%–2.0%); and normal serum electrolytes, bilirubin, prothrombin time (PT), and activated partial thromboplastin time (aPPT). Urinalysis (UA) was notable for 20 to 50 WBC/per high-power field (HPF) and moderate bacteria. A tentative diagnosis of cystitis was attributed to prostatic hypertrophy. Urine was sent for culture, and F.S. was given a prescription for co-trimoxazole (Bactrim, Septra) one double-strength tablet twice daily (BID).

Four days later, F.S. returned to the clinic noting that, although his original symptoms had resolved, he was experiencing tiredness and that his urine had become dark. Current laboratory values are as follows: Hgb, 9.9 g/dL; Hct, 32.5%; WBC count, 9,100/mm^3; corrected reticulocyte count, 11%; total bilirubin, 3.8 mg/dL (normal, <1.0 mg/dL); and direct bilirubin, 0.7 mg/dL (normal, <1.0 mg/dL). UA now reveals 0 to 5 WBC/HPF, no bacteria, and 4% blood. The urine also is positive for bilirubin and urobilinogen. Physical examination is unremarkable except for scleral icterus and a mild tachycardia.

How is the clinical picture of F.S. compatible with drug-induced hemolysis caused by G6PD deficiency?

[SI units: Hgb, 140 g/dL and 99 g/dL, respectively (normal, 120–160); Hct, 0.436 l and 0.325 l, respectively (normal. 0.36–0.48); WBC, 7.5 × 10^9 L and 9.1 × 10^9 L, respectively (normal, 4.0–11.0); reticulocytes, 0.005 and 0.11, respectively (normal, 0.001–0.024); bilirubin, 65 μmol/L (total), 12 (direct)]

This clinical picture in a man of Mediterranean descent is strongly suggestive for sulfamethoxazole-induced hemolysis caused by G6PD deficiency. F.S.'s asymptomatic hemolysis began 1 to 4 days after the drug was begun. F.S.'s serum hemoglobin concentration began to fall and his urine became dark secondary to increased levels of urobilinogen. In severe cases, weakness and abdominal or back pain may occur and the urine may become nearly black (because of pyrolic substances produced from degradation of Heinz bodies). As F.S.'s levels of indirect bilirubin rise, the presence of scleral icterus is noted. Reticulocytosis is evident and could be attributed to the body's attempt to increase RBC production. In patients with class III deficiency, the hemoglobin will begin to rise toward normal in about 1 week because the younger RBC with greater G6PD activity begin replacing the older, hemolysed RBC. Even with continued drug ingestion, symptoms, if any, resolve and the appearance of the urine becomes normal. With class II deficiency, even the younger RBC are destroyed and significant hemolysis with anemia continues unless the drug is stopped. A G6PD deficiency can be confirmed by assaying G6PD activity. In F.S.'s case, it is too early to determine with certainty the outcome if the drug were to be continued; the prudent course would be to discontinue the co-trimoxazole and substitute an appropriate nonoxidant agent. A cephalosporin or quinolone antibiotic is a possible alternative; at this point, culture results should be available and can be used to guide therapy.

2. Why did F.S.'s urine test positive for blood when no RBC were present?

The urine tests for blood are based on the ability to detect hemoglobin even after some or all of the RBC have disintegrated and are no longer visible microscopically on HPF. Therefore, hemoglobin in the urine will result in a positive urine test for blood. In this case, a positive test for hemoglobin in the absence of RBC helps differentiate hemoglobinuria caused by hemolysis from true hematuria.

Drugs

3. F.S. expresses surprise when he is informed of this reaction to co-trimoxazole, because he has taken sulfa drugs in the past without difficulty. Do all sulfa drugs have the same potential for inducing hemolysis in patients with G6PD deficiency?

Many oxidant drugs have been reported to cause hemolysis in G6PD-deficient patients. In many cases, causality has not been well established. Several drugs, particularly antipyretic and antibiotic agents, have been implicated in causing

Table 87-1 Drugs and Chemicals Associated With Hemolysis in G6PD Deficiency

Acetanilid	Phenazopyridine	Sulfanilamide
Furazolidone	Phenylhydrazine	Thiazolsulfone
Isobutyl nitrate	Primaquine	Toluidine
Methylene blue	Sulfapyridine	Trinitrotoluene
Naphthalene	Sulfacetamide	
Nitrofurantoin	Sulfamethoxazole	

G6PD, glucose 6-phosphate dehydrogenase.
From reference 10, with permission.

hemolysis when, in fact, hemolysis may have been precipitated by the infections for which the drugs were prescribed. Other drugs have been implicated through the use of in vitro enzyme stability tests. The response of RBC in this enzyme stability test does not necessarily correlate with significant in vivo hemolysis, and this test also fails to measure the effect of drug metabolites. The most reliable method of testing for hemolytic potency is to administer the drug in question to normal volunteers who have been infused with Chromium (Cr)-labeled G6PD-deficient RBC.[11]

Drug-induced hemolysis in G6PD-deficient patients can be somewhat confusing. Sulfamethoxazole, alone or in combination as co-trimoxazole, causes hemolysis in class II deficiency, but class III-deficient patients may be at low risk if the daily dose is 3.2 g or less.[16] Sulfisoxazole does not cause significant hemolysis at usually prescribed doses. Therefore, F.S.'s hemolytic response to sulfamethoxazole, but not to sulfisoxazole, is consistent with existing data. Table 87-1 lists other drugs associated with significant hemolysis.

Management

4. How should F.S.'s G6PD deficiency be treated?

Other than discontinuation and avoidance of drugs and substances known to cause hemolysis, no specific therapy exists for G6PD deficiency. If hemolysis is severe, RBC transfusion may be necessary. The patient should be well hydrated to maintain a good urine flow to prevent or attenuate renal toxicity from hemoglobin. Vitamin E and oral selenium have been suggested as possible treatments for G6PD deficiency; however, neither has proved of value.[12] F.S. should be cautioned regarding his G6PD deficiency and the deleterious effects of certain drugs.

Immune Hemolytic Anemia

Drug molecules are potentially antigenic, but they are generally too small to elicit antibody production by themselves. They can, however, serve as haptens and be immunogenic when combined with some larger molecules (e.g., cell membranes, circulating proteins). Likewise, drug metabolites, particularly highly reactive metabolites, can act as haptens (e.g., penicillin and its penicilloyl by-product).[17] Diclofenac has been associated with reports of immune hemolytic anemia and less frequently with immune thrombocytopenia.[18] A metabolite of diclofenac has also been identified as a cause of acute immune hemolytic anemia.[19,20]

Coombs' Test (Antiglobulin Test)

5. R.L., a 53-year-old man, is admitted with gas gangrene of the left leg. His leg was amputated below the knee, and he was given gentamicin 120 mg every 8 hours and penicillin G 4,000,000 units every 4 hours along with aggressive local care. On the ninth hospital day, his Hct was 30%, decreased from 41% 4 days previously. No signs of bleeding were found. Further evaluation revealed a corrected reticulocyte count of 8% (no baseline drawn), elevated indirect bilirubin, and a positive direct Coombs' test. What is the significance of a positive DAT or Coombs' test in R.L.?

[SI units: Hct, 0.3 1 and 0.41 1, respectively; reticulocytes, 0.08 1]

The Coombs', or antiglobulin, test can detect both antibody coating of RBC and circulating immunoglobulins directed against RBC. A DAT is the most important laboratory test in establishing immune hemolysis. The result of this test will direct further investigation. A positive DAT supports, but does not prove, an immune-mediated hemolytic process. The DAT detects IgG class immunoglobulin or complement, or both, on RBC. As few as 100 to 200 molecules of IgG per RBC can be detected by the laboratory. The DAT may be negative even when the patient is hemolyzing, if there are <150 IgG molecules per RBC. Polyspecific antiglobulin serum must be used for the initial DAT to allow detection of both IgG and complement. If the DAT is positive, subsequent testing with monospecific anti-IgG and anti-C3 should be performed. Positive anti-IgG or IgG + C3 indicates warm autoimmune hemolytic anemia. Positive anti-C3 only indicates either drug-induced hemolytic anemia or cold autoimmune hemolytic anemia.[21]

The DAT does not tell whether hemolysis is occurring and, in fact, several drugs, including R.L.'s penicillin, are known to cause a positive test without significant RBC destruction.

Mechanisms

6. How does penicillin cause hemolytic anemia? Why is R.L.'s penicillin a likely cause of his anemia?

The three basic mechanisms by which drugs are thought to cause immunologic hemolytic anemia are (a) a high-affinity hapten-type reaction; (b) a reaction precipitated by low-affinity binding to RBC, either via a low-affinity hapten-type reaction or by circulating immune complex formation, also known as an *innocent bystander reaction*; and (c) an autoimmune reaction (Table 87-2). Because R.L. is receiving 24 million units of penicillin per day, his hemolytic anemia is likely caused by penicillin.

HIGH-AFFINITY HAPTEN-TYPE REACTION: PENICILLIN

Penicillin is the prototype for the high-affinity hapten-type of immunologic drug-induced hemolytic anemia. Penicillin and penicillin metabolites bind strongly to the RBC membrane in a dose-related fashion and are detectable on the cells of nearly all patients receiving >10 million units/day[22] or when penicillin blood levels are high (e.g., presence of diminished renal function). About 3% of patients receiving high-dose penicillin will produce IgG directed against the penicillin-membrane complex as detected by a positive Coombs' test.[23] Antibody-coated RBC in a small number of cases are then recognized and destroyed in significant numbers extravascularly by the macrophages of the reticuloendothelial

Table 87-2 Drug-Induced Immunologic Hemolytic Anemia

Mechanism	*Process*	*Common Drugs*	*Comment*
High-affinity hapten-type reaction	Drug binds tightly to RBC membrane surface; immunoglobulins then form against the drug-membrane complex	Cephalosporins, penicillin, tetracycline	Penicillin is the classic prototype of this dose-related reaction
Low-affinity hapten-type reaction or immune complex formation	Drug binds to either (a) low-affinity specific antigenic loci on the cell membrane or (b) to circulating proteins to form an immune complex that adheres loosely to RBC. Lysis via complement activation ensues	Acetaminophen, ASA, chlorpromazine, chlorpropamide, hydrochlorothiazide, INH, PAS, phenacetin, probenecid, quinidine, quinine, rifampin, sulfonamides	Subsequent to hemolysis, the drug or immune complex dissociates from RBC fragments, adheres to another RBC, and repeats the process. Small doses can cause large-scale hemolysis. Quinidine is the prototype drug
Autoimmune reaction	Drug stimulates production of anti-RBC antibodies. Autoantibodies coat RBC and extravascular lysis occurs	Levodopa, mefenamic acid, methyldopa, procainamide, ceftriaxone, cefotetan	Methyldopa is the prototype drug for autoimmune hemolysis

ASA, acetylsalicylic acid; INH, isoniazid; PAS, para-aminosalicylate sodium; RBC, red blood cell.

system, primarily in the spleen.[24] Other drugs reported to produce high-affinity hapten-type hemolysis, although much less frequently than penicillin, are tetracycline and tolbutamide.

First-generation cephalosporins (e.g., cephalothin) infrequently have been reported to cause immune hemolytic anemia. Severe, sometimes fatal, immune hemolytic anemia has been associated with second- and third-generation cephalosporins,[25] especially cefotetan.[26]

Of 43 cases of drug-induced immune hemolytic anemia that were referred to a single laboratory for investigation over 8 years, 38 were found to be caused by a cephalosporin (35 by cefotetan, 3 by ceftriaxone). Of the 38 cases, 11 (29%) resulted in fatal immune hemolytic anemia; 8 deaths were caused by cefotetan and 3 by ceftriaxone. The fatal cases were sometimes associated with either renal failure or disseminated intravascular coagulation, or both.[26]

The possibility of cefotetan-induced immune hemolytic anemia should be investigated in any patients (particularly healthy young women) who have received prophylactic cefotetan and experienced unexpected anemia after gynecologic or obstetric procedures.

7. Has R.L.'s clinical course been consistent with penicillin-induced hemolytic anemia, and how quickly will the problem resolve once the drug is discontinued?

R.L.'s case is consistent with penicillin-induced hemolytic anemia. Anemia is subacute in onset, usually developing after 7 to 10 days of high-dose therapy. R.L.'s anemia developed after 9 days of treatment. In most cases, no other signs suggest an allergic reaction, and other cell lines rarely are involved. R.L.'s laboratory values are typical of those seen in extravascular hemolysis. The DAT is strongly positive, and the indirect antiglobulin test (IAT) is positive only for penicillin. Hemolysis of decreasing severity can continue for some time after the drug is discontinued, probably because of cell-bound penicillin.

LOW-AFFINITY BINDING: QUINIDINE

Mechanisms

8. H.J. is a 63-year-old woman whose physician prescribed quinidine sulfate 200 mg QID for an "irregular heartbeat." She has taken quinidine for this problem in the past, but stopped taking it 6 months ago. She comes to the emergency department (ED) today with fever, chills, and shakes. H.J. is found to have an Hct of 24%, and her urine tests positive for blood. What drug-induced problem is compatible with this picture?

[SI unit: Hct, 0.24]

The second mechanism by which drugs cause immune hemolysis is through a low-affinity binding process. The classic explanation for this type of hemolysis involves the binding of the offending drug, or drug metabolite, to circulating serum proteins to form a complete antigen. Antibodies, usually IgM, are produced and combine with this antigen to create a circulating immune complex. This immune complex, in turn, is adsorbed onto the surface of an RBC, where it triggers activation of complement. The RBC is lysed and the immune complex, which has a low affinity for the cell membrane, dissociates and goes on to a second RBC to repeat the process. It is this "recycling" of the drug–antibody complex that explains why only small doses of drug are needed to cause large scale hemolysis in previously sensitized patients. Because antibodies are not directed against the cell itself, the RBC is destroyed as an innocent bystander, and thus this immune complex-mediated cell destruction has been termed an innocent bystander reaction. The direct Coombs' test is positive only against complement because washing will remove the immune complexes from the cells.

H.J.'s quinidine is the prototype drug for the immune-complex form of immunologic hemolytic anemia. The innocence of the RBC in this reaction has been questioned, however.[27,28] An alternative explanation for findings in patients such as H.J. is the "low-affinity hapten." According to this hypothesis, the drug or a metabolite binds to a specific antigenic site on the cell membrane. It then forms a complete antigen or causes a conformational change in the membrane that reveals previously protected neoantigenic sites (sites that will not be recognized as "self" by the immune system). Antibodies directed against the new antigen are produced and bind to it, complement is activated, and cell lysis ensues. Because the drug has a relatively low affinity for its binding site, it is free to go on to another cell and repeat the process. Only cells with the particular drug-binding site would be able to form the drug-antigenic site-antibody complex needed to activate complement. The high degree of antigenic specificity inherent in this model applies to the immune destruction of WBC and platelets as well as RBC (see the following discussion) and helps explain why different drugs have a propensity to affect one cell line more frequently than others.[27]

Quinidine is being promoted for use in combination with dextromethorphan for emotional liability and diabetic peripheral neuropathy.[29,30] As a result, practitioners should be aware that patients might be receiving quinidine for off-label uses.

Features

9. Why are H.J.'s symptoms more severe than those of R.L. with high-affinity hapten-type hemolysis?

The symptoms in hemolytic anemia are related to the degree of anemia produced (relative to the baseline blood count) and the severity or rapidity of hemolysis. Immune complex-mediated hemolysis frequently results in more rapid RBC destruction and more acute symptoms. The hemolysis is largely intravascular; therefore, large amounts of free hemoglobin can be released, resulting in hemoglobinuria and possible acute renal failure caused by the renal-toxic effect of hemoglobin.

Management

10. How should H.J.'s case be managed at this point?

The suspected causative agent, quinidine in this case, should be discontinued and an alternative agent selected. A good urine flow should be maintained, with or without urinary alkalinization, to prevent or attenuate renal failure. RBC transfusion might be needed in symptomatic patients or in patients such as H.J. because of a significantly decreased Hct (e.g., H.J.'s hematocrit is 24%). Immune-complex hemolysis resolves soon after the drug is discontinued because the drug must be in the serum to cause hemolysis. An acute, severe RBC destruction can result from even a single dose of drug in a sensitized patient; therefore, this type of hemolysis should not be rechallenged. The patient should be educated about the cause of this reaction and instructed to strictly avoid future use of quinidine or quinine. (See Question 15 and Table 87-2 for other drugs associated with immune complex hemolysis.)

Temafloxacin (Omniflox), a fluoroquinolone, was removed from the U.S. market in 1992 only 6 months after its approval because of frequent reports of serious hemolysis. The hemolysis, with or without organ system dysfunction, became known as the *temafloxacin syndrome*. About 189,000 prescriptions were written for temafloxacin during this brief period.[31]

The core structure of fluoroquinolones resembles that of quinine and quinidine, both of which are known to cause immune hemolytic anemia and thrombocytopenia. Other marketed fluoroquinolones with the same core structure have caused neither a comparable number nor a comparable spectrum of adverse reactions. Interestingly, the structure of temafloxacin most closely resembles that of trovafloxacin (Trovan), a fluoroquinolone that was withdrawn from European markets in June 1999 and whose use was severely restricted in the United States because of hepatotoxicity.[31,32]

In a review of 95 cases of hemolysis associated with temafloxacin, renal dysfunction occurred in 57% of cases, 63% of which required dialysis.[33] The mean onset of symptoms (fever, chills, jaundice) was 6.4 days. Patients who reacted to the first dose of temafloxacin were significantly more likely to have taken quinolone antibiotics in the past, thereby, suggesting a typical anamnestic response and implying cross-reactivity between temafloxacin and other quinolones.

The available data did not permit an accurate estimate of the incidence rate for temafloxacin syndrome. Although an estimate of the number of prescriptions dispensed was available, information about samples given from physicians' offices was not reliable, and thus the denominator (i.e., total number of patients) exposed to temafloxacin could not be determined accurately. More importantly, the actual number of temafloxacin-associated hemolysis cases (i.e., the numerator) was unclear because of probable under reporting.

Autoimmune Reaction: Methyldopa

The third mechanism by which drugs cause immune RBC destruction is by an autoimmune process. Methyldopa (Aldomet) was once the most common cause of hemolysis via this mechanism; however, methyldopa now is seldom prescribed in the United States because of the availability of better antihypertensive agents. Procainamide (Pronestyl),[34] as well as the second- and third-generation cephalosporins, particularly cefotetan (Cefotan) and ceftriaxone (Rocephin), also have been associated with immune-mediated hemolytic anemia.[35] In one report, ceftriaxone was implicated in 19 cases of immune-hemolytic anemia involving 9 children and 10 adults. Six of the children and 3 of the adults died.[36]

Treatment of autoimmune-hemolytic anemia consists of drug discontinuation and RBC transfusion if anemia is severe. Hemolysis resolves gradually over the following several weeks to months, but the antiglobulin test may remain positive for years. Despite the similarity of drug-induced autoimmune-hemolytic anemia with the idiopathic variety, for which the role of corticosteroid therapy is well established, evidence supporting the use of steroids in patients with severe or life-threatening drug-induced autoimmune hemolysis is anecdotal at best.[37,38]

DRUG-INDUCED THROMBOCYTOPENIA

Cases of suspected drug-induced thrombocytopenia are frequently reported to spontaneous adverse drug reaction reporting systems.[39,40] Thrombocytopenia is defined as a decrease in platelet count to $<100,000/mm^3$.[1] Drugs can cause thrombocytopenia by three primary mechanisms: (a) immune-mediated suppression or destruction of platelets; (b) decreased production of platelets through direct suppression of thrombopoiesis; and (c), in the case of heparin, an apparently dose-related, nonimmune direct effect on circulating platelets. It appears that immune platelet destruction occurs through reactions analogous to immunologic RBC destruction.

Most drugs causing thrombocytopenia appear to do so through immune mechanisms, although it has been difficult to distinguish between immune and toxic effects on thrombopoiesis. Well over 100 drugs have been implicated as causes of thrombocytopenia, most in the form of case reports. It is often difficult to determine the cause of a low platelet count, particularly in acutely ill patients undergoing numerous procedures and receiving a large number of potentially platelet-toxic drugs.[41] Diagnostic errors also can result in over- or under reporting of drug-induced thrombocytopenia.[42]

The class of antithrombotic drugs, the glycoprotein IIb/IIIa (GPIIb-IIIa) receptor antagonists (GPRA), has been associated with episodes of thrombocytopenia that are sometimes life threatening. Immune-mediated thrombocytopenia associated with GPRA resembles the classic syndrome of the quinine type with respect to the severity of thrombocytopenia, the risk of bleeding, and anaphylactoid reactions.[43] Severe or profound thrombocytopenia occurs in about 1% of patients treated with abciximab (Reopro), and in about 0.2% to 1% of patients treated with eptifibatide (Integrilin).[44] The incidence appears to be higher with subsequent exposure to the drug, its use with clopidogrel, or in elderly patients. Treatment with intravenous immunoglobulin G (IVIG) after severe thrombocytopenia related to abciximab was of no clinical benefit.[45] Although available data are limited, some reports suggest that the oral ligand-mimetic inhibitors have higher incidents of thrombocytopenia.[46]

Vancomycin-induced immune thrombocytopenia, confirmed by the presence of vancomycin-dependent antiplatelet antibodies, occurred in 29 patients treated with vancomycin based on data in 2007. The mean nadir platelet count in these patients was 13,600/mm^3, and severe bleeding occurred in 10 patients (34%).[47]

Thrombocytopenia and acute onset hemolytic anemia, which were fatal in some cases, have been reported with oxaliplatin (Eloxatin), a new platinum derivative used in colorectal cancer.[9]

In a rigorous 1998 review of 515 case reports of drug-induced thrombocytopenia, a definite or probable causal role for a drug was documented in 247 instances (48%).[48] Among the 98 drugs described in these reports, quinidine was mentioned in 38 reports, gold in 11, and trimethoprim-sulfamethoxazole in 10. Of the 247 patients described, 23 (9%) had major bleeding and 2 (0.8%) died because of the bleeding.

Suppressed Production: Thiazides

Mechanisms

11. J.Y., a 56-year-old man with mild hypertension, started taking hydrochlorothiazide 25 mg/day. Routine blood work at this time showed an adequate platelet estimate (>150,000/mm^3). The platelet estimate after 2 weeks of therapy was likewise normal. At a 1-month follow-up visit, however, J.Y.'s complete blood count (CBC) revealed a decreased platelet estimate, and a subsequent platelet count was 78,000/mm^3. He reported no unusual bleeding, the physical examination was unremarkable, and the CBC was otherwise unchanged. Why should the differential diagnosis include hydrochlorothiazide as a possible cause of J.Y.'s thrombocytopenia?

[SI units: platelet counts, >1.5 × 10^{15}/L and 0.78 × 10^{15}/L, respectively]

Drugs should always be considered in evaluating blood dyscrasias. Thiazide diuretics as well as furosemide are known to be associated with thrombocytopenia. Drug-dependent antiplatelet antibodies have been identified in the serum of some patients with thrombocytopenia who also were taking thiazides,[49,50] suggesting an immune process. In most cases, however, antibodies are not demonstrable and marrow examination typically reveals decreased megakaryocytes, findings more consistent with suppression of platelet production. Thrombocytopenia recurs with rechallenge only after 1 to 4 weeks of drug administration, further supporting a nonimmune process. Although some cases of thiazide-induced thrombocytopenia might have an immunologic basis, the more common mechanism probably is one of direct marrow suppression.

Features

12. A bone marrow examination reveals only decreased megakaryocytes, and the initial workup fails to reveal other reasons for a low platelet count. Why is J.Y.'s clinical picture compatible with thiazide-induced thrombocytopenia?

J.Y.'s course to this point has been typical of thrombocytopenia caused by decreased thrombopoiesis. The onset of thrombocytopenia was delayed and gradual (rather than sudden) and, as usually the case, the thrombocytopenia in J.Y. was not associated with fevers, rash, or other signs of immune reaction. The degree of platelet reduction frequently is mild (J.Y.'s platelets were 78,000/mm^3) and, without other risk factors, bleeding is relatively uncommon unless thrombocytopenia is severe.

Management

13. How should J.Y. be treated and monitored?

With discontinuation of hydrochlorothiazide, the platelet count would be expected to return to normal within about 2 weeks in J.Y. The drug should be discontinued and the platelet count should be monitored to verify resolution of the thrombocytopenia. J.Y. also should be monitored for signs of bleeding until recovery. For treatment of his hypertension, a suitable alternative agent should be prescribed. As always, J.Y. should be advised to avoid this drug in the future and to inform future caregivers of this reaction.

Immune Destruction: Quinine/Quinidine, Sulfamethoxazole/Sulfisoxazole, and Gemcitabine

Mechanisms and Features

15. K.B., a 65-year-old man, began taking quinine sulfate 300 mg at bedtime (HS) for nocturnal leg cramps. He stopped taking the drug after 2 weeks when he read that stretching exercises might help. Three months later, with worsening cramps, he resumed taking the drug. The next morning he noted small, purple splotches on his skin that had not been present the previous evening. This problem became worse throughout the day, particularly on his lower legs, causing him to seek medical attention. When questioned, he recalled experiencing a hot, flushed sensation shortly after taking the quinine dose but thought little of it. Why might quinine be responsible for these events?

Quinine and quinidine are well-studied causes of drug-induced immune thrombocytopenia. When patients have been sensitized through previous exposure to the drug in question, constitutional symptoms (e.g., warmth, flushing, chills, headache) can occur soon after the first dose. The platelet count falls precipitously, often to low levels, with bleeding (should it occur) commencing within hours or days of ingestion. Petechiae, purpura, and hemorrhagic oral bullae are common early signs, but patients can present with overt bleeding as the first indication of a drug reaction. Thrombocytopenia also can occur during initial exposure to the drug, but this normally requires 7 to 10 days of therapy during which time antibodies are formed. Careful questioning of a patient with an acute reaction who denies having previously taken the drug often will reveal previous drug use of which the patient was unaware. Exposure to the small amounts of quinine in tonic beverages is a typical example.

A number of quinine-induced hemolytic uremic syndrome (HUS) have been reported. It is an important cause of acute, often irreversible, renal failure. The clinical manifestations of HUS are inappropriate endothelial cell (EC) activations with secondary activation of both platelets and coagulation cascade that lead to thrombocytopenia, microangiopathic anemia, and leukocytosis.[51]

Quinine is still used, however, for the treatment of nocturnal leg cramps. The FDA ordered firms to stop marketing unapproved quinine products in late 2006 because of serious safety concerns including thrombocytopenia. At least 15 reports of quinine-HUS appear in the medical literature.[52] Gemcitabine (Gemzar), although unrelated to this particular patient, also has been associated with renal toxicity and at least 26 cases of gemcitabine-associated HUS.[53,54]

K.B.'s clinical and laboratory features are compatible with a low-affinity hapten-type reaction (see section on immune hemolytic anemia above). In patients with thrombocytopenia, quinine and quinidine-dependent antiplatelet antibodies react with the GPIIb/IX or GPIIb/IIIa platelet membrane complex[55] and, in some patients, more than one antibody may be present. Similar findings with sulfamethoxazole and sulfisoxazole have been reported.[56] A high degree of antibody specificity is indicated by the low cross-reactivity of quinine/quinidine and sulfamethoxazole/sulfisoxazole antibodies, despite the structural similarities of the drugs.

Management

16. How should K.B.'s acute reaction be treated?

Treatment consists of drug discontinuation and support. The platelet count usually begins to rise within 3 to 4 days and returns to normal in 1 to 2 weeks as the drug and its metabolites are cleared from the body and platelet destruction stops. Platelet transfusions are reserved primarily to control active bleeding because transfused platelets are destroyed rapidly when given during the acute process. Although the use of corticosteroids has not been demonstrated to either reduce bleeding or alter the course of the reaction, some recommend their use.[57] Rechallenge with the suspected drug can result in a potentially fatal reaction and should not be attempted for either diagnostic or therapeutic reasons except under the most extreme conditions. In the case of quinine/quinidine, sensitivity to one does not absolutely preclude use of the other because the antibodies are isomerically specific. Nevertheless, cross-reactivity has been documented;[58] thus, it would be prudent to avoid either substance. The patient should be advised of his serious drug "allergy" and warned to avoid future use of this drug. In this case, K.B. also should be warned against consuming beverages that contain quinine.

Heparin

Mechanisms

17. M.U., a 65-year-old woman with a painful, swollen left leg, was admitted to the hospital to rule out deep vein thrombosis (DVT). A heparin infusion was begun after an appropriate loading dose. The diagnosis of DVT was confirmed by noninvasive venous testing and warfarin was started on the fourth day; the plan was to discontinue heparin after several days of heparin/warfarin overlap. Pain and swelling had resolved by the fourth day with bed rest, leg elevation, and anticoagulation. In the evening of the seventh day, M.U. experienced a recurrence of her symptoms despite an aPPT within the desired range and an international normalized ratio (INR) of 2.2. Her platelet count, which had been 225,000/mm^3 on admission, was now 54,000/mm^3. Why is M.U.'s thrombocytopenia likely to be drug induced?

[SI units: platelet count, 2.25 and 0.54 × 10^{15}/L, respectively]

Heparin is the most common cause of drug-induced thrombocytopenia. Heparin can affect platelet counts by two separate mechanisms. Some patients experience a mild to moderate decrease in platelet count occurring early in therapy, which may resolve despite continued drug administration.[59] This appears to be caused by a direct platelet-aggregating effect of heparin leading to reversible platelet clumping and undercounting by electronic counters, which cannot distinguish between single platelets and platelet aggregates.[60] Counts rarely drop below 50,000/mm^3, the phenomenon is transient, and complications are unlikely. This form of heparin-induced thrombocytopenia (HIT) is classified as HIT type I.

The more threatening form of HIT, which is less common, is classified as HIT type II. Heparin binds relatively weakly to platelets and forms a heparin–platelet factor 4 complex,[61,62] which either serves as a complete hapten or results in a conformational change that exposes membrane neoantigens that normally are concealed.[63,64] IgG directed against this complex causes platelet activation via the platelet Fc receptors. This type of HIT can lead to potentially devastating thromboembolic sequelae. Table 87-3 characterizes the two types of HIT.[65]

Heparin-dependent aggregation of donor platelets exposed to M.U.'s serum would help confirm the diagnosis of HIT. Most widely used is the platelet aggregation test, which measures the aggregation of normal donor platelets by patient serum or plasma with heparin. This test is simple, inexpensive, based on a technique that is in use in most hemostatic laboratories, and can provide a result within 2 to 3 hours. This test, when performed properly (the concentration of heparin and the quality of donor platelets used is important), is reportedly highly specific with a low incidence of false–positive results.[66,67] The test is not highly sensitive, however; that is, a negative test does not

Table 87-3 Characteristics of Type I and II Heparin-Induced Thrombocytopenia

	Type I	Type II
Frequency	10%–20%	2%–30%
Timing of onset	1–4 days	5–10 days
Nadir platelet count	100,000/μL	30,000–55,000/μL
Antibody mediated	No	Yes
Thromboembolic sequelae	None	30%–80%
Hemorrhagic	None	Rarely
Sequelae management	Observe	Cessation of heparin, alternative anticoagulation, additional therapy

From reference 62, with permission.

rule out HIT. A second test to detect heparin-dependent IgG antibodies, the 14C-labeled serotonin-release assay, is more sensitive but may not be as specific. One study used the test in 387 patients treated with unfractionated heparin or enoxaparin (Lovenox) after orthopedic surgery, including 12 patients suspected of having HIT.[68] Of the 20 who tested positive, only 6 actually had thrombocytopenia defined as a platelet count of $<150{,}000/mm^3$ after >5 days of therapy.

Incidence

Although rates of heparin-induced thrombocytopenia as high as 24% to 31% have been reported,[69] reviews of subsequent prospective studies using full doses of heparin and defining thrombocytopenia as a platelet count of $<100{,}000/mm^3$ noted a 2.9% to 5.4% incidence of HIT with bovine source heparin and 1.1% to 2.7% with porcine heparin.[70] The reason for the apparent difference between the two sources of heparin has not been demonstrated clearly, but might be related to differences in charge, degree of sulfation, or average molecular weights.

Heparin-induced thrombocytopenia appears to be more common with full-dose heparin therapy, but it has occurred with various doses. The incidence of thrombocytopenia with prophylactic heparin (5,000 U every 8 to 12 hours subcutaneously) is lower than with full-dose heparin. Thrombocytopenia has even been reported in association with heparin flushes (<500 U/day)[71] and heparin-coated pulmonary artery catheters.[72] Saline flushes, when substituted for heparin flushes whenever possible, minimize the potential for HIT.[73] Female patients might be at greater risk for HIT; therefore, the use of low molecular weight heparin (LMWH) to minimize the potential of HIT, theoretically should be of greatest value in women having surgical thromboprophylaxis.[74]

Although not common, HIT in critically ill patients is one potential etiology to be considered when the platelet count falls to $<150 \times 10^9/L$ or by $>50\%$ from baseline. Thrombocytopenia purportedly occurs in 23% to 41% of patients in critical care units and it is associated with mortality rates of 38% to 54%: the reported mortality rate associated with HIT is 10% and 20%.[75]

The effectiveness of LMWH, when compared with unfractionated heparin for the prevention of postoperative thrombosis, could not be determined in a meta-analysis of studies because of the variable quality of the clinical trials in the analysis.[76] The LMWH are purported to be associated with a lower incidence of HIT compared with unfractionated heparin.[77] Notable differences in the incidence of HIT between the individual LMWH needs further study.

Practitioners involved in selecting a drug for inclusion into a medication formulary should not only conduct a thorough, independent literature search, but also should review FDA drug-approval documents. For example, the FDA safety review for fondaparinux (Arixtra) noted that the prevalence of thrombocytopenia with enoxaparin (3.1%) was similar to that with fondaparinux (2.9%) in preapproval clinical trials.

Features

18. How is the onset of M.U.'s thrombocytopenia typical of thrombocytopenia induced by heparin?

M.U.'s platelet count of $54{,}000/mm^3$ was noted 7 days after the initiation of heparin and consistent with the time frame commonly associated with thrombocytopenia caused by heparin. Heparin-induced thrombocytopenia typically occurs within 6 to 12 days of therapy; however, thrombocytopenia can occur much earlier, particularly in previously sensitized patients.[78] The thrombocytopenia can be profound, but the platelet count can remain above $100{,}000/mm^3$ despite relatively large decreases in total count.[79] Once heparin is discontinued, platelets usually return to normal over the course of 4 to 7 days, although recovery can be delayed.

Thrombotic/Embolic Complications

19. What is the relationship between M.U.'s thrombocytopenia and the recurrence of her symptoms?

Heparin-induced thrombocytopenia can be complicated by the occurrence of embolic and thrombotic episodes.[79] Some patients with heparin-induced thrombocytopenia develop antibodies that deposit on vascular endothelial cells, creating a nidus for thrombus formation.[80] In others, the procoagulant properties of heparin-activated platelets can accelerate coagulation at sites of pre-existing thrombosis, resulting in extension of thrombi in the venous circulation (i.e., "red clots"). Formation of large platelet aggregates (i.e., "white clots") in the arterial circulation can result in stroke or arterial occlusion with or without secondary thrombus formation. The incidence of thromboembolic events, as a complication of HIT, has been reported as high as 75% to 88%.[78] Thromboembolic phenomena associated with heparin-induced thrombocytopenia can be difficult to distinguish from treatment failure and disease recurrence, particularly if the platelet count has not been monitored. Recognition of heparin-associated thrombosis or embolism is important because either is associated with significant morbidity and mortality. In addition, such a high degree of platelet activity can sometimes result in heparin resistance, probably caused by release of platelet factor 4 (antiheparin factor). In M.U.'s case, heparin likely has induced thrombocytopenia and a resultant recurrence of her left leg thrombosis.

Management

20. How should M.U. be treated at this point?

Warfarin therapy should not be postponed once the diagnosis of thrombosis has been established.[81] The prompt initiation of warfarin would permit discontinuation of heparin before the usual onset of heparin-induced thrombocytopenia. Warfarin was delayed in M.U.'s case, but because she is almost fully anticoagulated on warfarin after 4 days of overlap therapy with heparin, the heparin can be discontinued. She should be monitored carefully for signs of pulmonary embolism or further extension of her DVT and observed for signs of bleeding. Surprisingly, bleeding is uncommon in this setting.

Unlike M.U., patients with HIT often are not yet fully stabilized with warfarin, and management decisions are not so easily made. The full benefits of oral anticoagulants are delayed for several days; therefore, they are not immediately effective for treatment of DVT. Antiplatelet agents and dextran-40 have been used in this setting.[78] Although antiplatelet drugs can attenuate or stop further platelet aggregation, they are ineffective in treating either heparin-induced or underlying thrombotic disease and could worsen the risk of bleeding. Corticosteroids are not useful in this situation.

The LMWH preparations to anticoagulate patients with heparin-induced thrombocytopenia have been successful in anecdotal reports; however, routine use of LMWH in patients with heparin-dependent antiplatelet antibodies is potentially hazardous because in vitro cross-reactivity and unfavorable clinical outcomes after substitution have been reported. The low-molecular-weight heparinoid, danaparoid, cross-reacts with standard heparin-dependent antibodies 0% to 19.6% of the time as compared with 25.5% to 94% cross-reactivity of various LMWH (e.g., dalteparin and ardeparin).[82,83]

Ancrod (Viprinex), a defibrinogenating agent that reduces blood coagulability by degrading fibrinogen, has been successful in patients with heparin-induced thrombocytopenia when given in doses sufficient to decrease fibrinogen levels to as low as 50 to 100 mg/dL.[84,85]

Hirudin, a natural anticoagulant from the leech *Hirudo medicinalis,* and its synthetic congeners, bivalirudin (Angiomax) and lepirudin (Refludan), can inhibit coagulation in patients with HIT by binding to sites of circulating and clot-bound thrombin.[86,87] These are approved for use in patients with, or at risk of, HIT or heparin-induced thrombocytopenia and thrombosis syndrome (HITTS) undergoing percutaneous coronary intervention (PCI).[88] Antihirudin antibodies have been observed in about 40% of patients with HITTS treated with lipirudin.[89] The direct thrombin inhibitor, argatroban, also can be utilized for the prophylaxis or treatment of thrombosis in patients with HIT and in patients with, or at risk for, HIT undergoing PCI.[90]

Heparin-induced thrombocytopenia is a life-threatening medical emergency. Awareness of the clinical presentation of this condition and being able to differentiate HIT from other causes of thrombocytopenia are critical in avoiding serious outcomes. The immediate discontinuation of heparin is essential and treatment with therapeutic doses of an alternative nonheparin anticoagulant must be initiated without delay.[91]

Ticlopidine (Ticlid) and Clopidogrel (Plavix)-associated Thrombotic Thrombocytopenic Purpura

Thrombotic thrombocytopenic purpura is a life-threatening, multisystem disease characterized by thrombocytopenia, microangiopathic hemolytic anemia, neurologic changes, progressive renal failure, and fever, with about a 10% to 20% mortality. The cause of TTP is unknown; however, drugs (e.g., penicillin, antineoplastic chemotherapy agents, oral contraceptives, ticlopidine) have been associated with the syndrome.

In a review of 60 cases of ticlopidine-associated TTP, ticlopidine had been prescribed for <1 month in 80% of the cases, and platelet counts had been normal within 2 weeks of the onset of TTP in most patients. Mortality rates were higher among patients who were not treated with plasmapheresis (50% vs. 24%; $p < 0.05$). In these cases, the onset of ticlopidine-associated TTP was difficult to predict, despite close monitoring of platelet counts.[92]

In a retrospective cohort study, 19 cases of ticlopidine-associated TTP occurred in 43,322 patients treated with ticlopidine who had a PCI and received a coronary stent during a 1-year period from 1996 to 1997. The mean time of ticlopidine treatment before the diagnosis of TTP was 22 days (range, 5–60 days). The case fatality rate was 21% (4 of 19), with all 4 deaths occurring in patients not treated with plasmapheresis. No deaths occurred among the 13 patients who received plasmapheresis.[93]

In one postmarketing surveillance, ticlopidine was associated with 259 fatalities, with TTP accounting for 40 of the deaths. Ticlopidine's manufacturer revised the drug's professional product labeling in 1998 to include a black box warning describing an estimated incidence of ticlopidine-associated TTP of 1 in 2,000 to 1 in 4,000 patients.[94]

Clopidogrel (Plavix), as ticlopidine, is a thienopyridine derivative with a chemical structure identical to ticlopidine, except for the addition of a carboxymethyl side group. Active surveillance by blood bank medical directors, hematologists, and the drug's manufacturer has identified cases of clopidogrel-associated TTP.[95]

DRUG-INDUCED NEUTROPENIA

Definitions

Several terms are used to refer to abnormally low numbers of WBC. The broadest description, *leukopenia*, simply denotes a total WBC count of $<3{,}000/mm^3$. *Granulocytopenia* describes a granulocyte count of $<1{,}500$ granulocytes/mm^3 (including eosinophils and basophils), whereas *neutropenia* refers to a neutrophil count (segmented polymorphonucleocytes and band forms) of $<1{,}500/mm^3$. *Agranulocytosis* is defined as a severe form of neutropenia, with total granulocyte counts $<500/mm^3$.[1] Authors, however, use variable definitions when reporting drug-induced WBC dyscrasias. The term agranulocytosis has been used to describe granulocyte counts ranging from <100 to $<1{,}000/mm^3$.

Epidemiology

Agranulocytosis is the most common fatal adverse drug reaction, accounting for 26% of all drug-related deaths and 64% of deaths caused by blood dyscrasias in one series.[97] The mortality rate was about 30% in the 1960s and 1970s,[98] and about 16% at six hospitals from 1970 to 1989 based on data from a diagnosis by exclusion methodology.[99] Mortality rates from more recent reports would be expected to be lower because of advances in medical care. In the elderly, who are over-represented in all published series of agranulocytosis, the estimated mortality rate from idiosyncratic drug-induced agranulocytocis in 2004 was 5% to 10%.[100]

Mechanisms

Drugs cause neutropenia by two basic mechanisms. One is immunologically mediated, either through peripheral destruction of circulating neutrophils or immune suppression of marrow precursors. The second is through a direct, toxic effect on marrow precursors.[101]

Immune Versus Direct Mechanisms: Penicillins

MECHANISMS

21. **S.T., a 54-year-old woman with a WBC count of 12,200/mm^3 (82% neutrophils, 3% band forms, 7% monocytes, 8% lymphocytes) was treated for cellulitis with nafcillin 2 g every 4 hours IV. On the 13th day of therapy, her WBC count was 2,200/mm^3 with 28% neutrophils and 5% bands. At this time, S.T. was**

experiencing no new symptoms and remained afebrile. Why might her neutropenia be attributable to nafcillin?

Administration of penicillins and, to a lesser extent, cephalosporins, in large doses for prolonged periods purportedly results in neutropenia in up to 15% of cases.[102] The problem seems to occur only rarely within the first week of therapy and most often in patients receiving high doses of these β-lactam antibiotics for >2 weeks.[103] S.T. has been receiving high-dose nafcillin (i.e., 12 g/day) for about 2 weeks. Despite this apparent dose relationship, controversy exists whether the neutropenia is immune mediated or caused by toxic suppression of granulocyte development in the marrow. Drug- or metabolite-dependent antigranulocyte antibodies have been noted in patients receiving penicillin[104,105] and cephalosporins.[106] Furthermore, serum from a patient with ceftriaxone-associated agranulocytosis could suppress in vitro proliferation of an early WBC precursor, granulocyte-macrophage colony-forming units (CFU-GM).[107] These findings are consistent with cases of drug-induced agranulocytosis that did not appear to be dose related. In contrast, others have demonstrated dose-dependent inhibition of granulocyte colony growth in vitro, thereby supporting the premise that β-lactam–induced neutropenia is caused by a direct toxic effect on granulopoiesis.[108]

Evidence indicates a potentially important role for reactive metabolites. Reactive metabolites are short lived and produced locally by cells such as neutrophils and neutrophil precursors in the marrow. In predisposed persons, the suggestion is that certain drugs could be converted to reactive metabolites that can then either directly damage precursor cells or cause formation of neoantigens, which would subsequently initiate an immune response directed against the now altered cell.[109] The common finding of apparent maturation arrest of granulocyte precursors on marrow examination is compatible with either toxic suppression or an immune effect on precursors. Fever, rash, and eosinophilia in patients with penicillin-induced neutropenia imply an immune process in many cases despite an apparent dose relationship. Overall, despite significant advances in knowledge, it can be concluded that the mechanisms by which antibiotics cause neutropenia are heterogeneous, and that more study is needed to understand these mechanisms. A few reports implicating >100 drugs as having caused neutropenia provide some insights into mechanisms.

MANAGEMENT

22. How should S.T. have been monitored while receiving high doses of a drug known to be associated with neutropenia?

First, the need for high dosages of drug and long duration of therapy should be reassessed in light of the subjective and objective data (e.g., well-being of the patient, temperature, WBC count, tissue inflammation and pain, culture and sensitivity) that are consistent with cellulitis in this patient. Depending on the situation, some infections do not require maximal antibiotic dosage to achieve bacteriologic and clinical cure, and a shorter course with a lower dose of nafcillin, if appropriate, is considerably less likely to be associated with nafcillin-induced neutropenia. Another consideration might be the selection of a drug dose based on body size, as is the case in pediatric patients, rather than following the common practice of using standardized dosing for all adults.[110] Of course, doses should always be altered appropriately for impaired organ function (e.g., renal insufficiency). The WBC count should be monitored carefully, particularly after the second week of therapy, and the patient should be observed for unexplained fevers and rashes.

23. How should S.T. be treated at this point?

The suspected offending drug, nafcillin in this case, should be discontinued and replaced by an effective antimicrobial with a dissimilar chemical structure (e.g., a fluoroquinolone, vancomycin) if continued therapy is needed for cellulitis. The selection of a substitute antibacterial should be based on culture and sensitivity testing or, if cultures are negative, empirically for likely causative organisms (e.g., *Staphylococcus aureus, S. epidermidis*). Vancomycin also has been implicated as a possible cause of drug-induced neutropenia.[111]

S.T.'s WBC count would be expected to return to normal within several days. Although the neutropenia potentially can resolve after merely decreasing the drug dose, this approach is not without risk and should be considered only if an alternative is unavailable. The patient should be monitored for fever or other signs of new or recurrent infection until the neutropenia has resolved. The precise course of action will be determined by the clinical situation. In S.T.'s case, the nafcillin was discontinued with subsequent hematologic recovery and without recurrence of the original infection.

Idiosyncratic Toxic Effect: Phenothiazines

MECHANISMS

24. J.K., a 34-year-old woman with schizophrenia, was found on routine blood testing to be moderately neutropenic. She started taking chlorpromazine (Thorazine) 8 weeks ago when she began hearing voices warning her that she was being followed by the Central Intelligence Agency (CIA) and that her brain had been bugged. Her chlorpromazine dose was quickly titrated up to 400 mg/day, which she has been taking for 6 weeks with a good clinical response. J.K. has no medical problems and takes no other medications. How likely is it that J.K.'s chlorpromazine is the cause of her neutropenia?

Phenothiazines are one of the most common causes of drug-induced neutropenia, chlorpromazine being the model drug.[112,113] These drugs induce neutropenia through toxic suppression of granulocyte production in the marrow of sensitive patients. In experiments using cultured bone marrow from normal subjects, and from patients who had become neutropenic during chlorpromazine therapy, DNA synthesis resulting in defective granulocyte proliferation occurred in at least half of the patients taking chlorpromazine.[114] The marrow of patients who do not become neutropenic apparently compensate for this interference in DNA synthesis through proliferation of drug-resistant clones of committed stem cells. Patients who go on to develop neutropenia apparently do not have adequate compensatory mechanisms.

FEATURES

25. Why is J.K.'s presentation typical of phenothiazine-induced neutropenia?

As in J.K.'s case, the most common presentation of phenothiazine-induced neutropenia would be that of decreased numbers of neutrophils. Patients usually remain asymptomatic unless they become infected. Phenothiazine-induced neutropenia rarely occurs in <2 weeks or later than 10 weeks into therapy, although latent periods of 3 months have been reported. J.K.'s 6 weeks of chlorpromazine therapy certainly falls within this usual time frame, and her total dose of 10.8 g also is representative of the doses usually associated with chlorpromazine-induced neutropenia. A total cumulative dose of 10 to 20 g of chlorpromazine usually is required; neutropenia occurs only rarely in patients taking less than this amount of the drug. Patients who have developed neutropenia while taking high doses of chlorpromazine have subsequently been treated with reduced dosages uneventfully. Rechallenge with high doses again results in a delayed-onset fall in the neutrophil count. In addition, approximately 10% of patients taking chlorpromazine will experience a transient leukopenia, which resolves despite continuation of the drug.[115] Severe neutropenia is much less common; elderly women appear to be at increased risk. Most other phenothiazine derivatives, with the exception of promethazine (Phenergan), also have been reported to cause neutropenia, although none have been studied as extensively as chlorpromazine.

MANAGEMENT

26. How should J.K. be treated at this point?

No specific therapy is indicated at this time because J.K. is asymptomatic. Although it is possible that the neutropenia might resolve with a simple dose reduction of chlorpromazine, the most prudent course would be to withhold the drug completely until the WBC count returns to normal. Subsequently, the patient could be restarted at a lower dose with close hematologic monitoring, or an alternative neuroleptic agent with less propensity for marrow suppression could be substituted. A more potent phenothiazine or a nonphenothiazine neuroleptic would be preferable because the risk of agranulocytosis appears related to the absolute amount of phenothiazine taken.

27. How quickly should J.K.'s WBC count return to normal once chlorpromazine has been discontinued?

A peripheral hematologic response following the discontinuation of chlorpromazine will be delayed by 4 to 6 days but will then improve rapidly. In some cases, the increase in granulocytes may be preceded or accompanied by a monocyte increase, and myelocytes, metamyelocytes, and band forms may appear in relatively large numbers during the early recovery phase. The neutrophil numbers and total WBC count then rapidly return to normal, sometimes with a WBC count "overshoot" into the 15,000 to 20,000/mm^3 range. Recovery usually is complete within about 2 weeks.

Colony-stimulating Factors

28. How can the rate of WBC recovery be hastened?

Patients with drug-induced agranulocytosis or drug-induced neutropenia have been treated with the granulocyte colony-stimulating factor (G-CSF, filgrastim, Neupogen) and granulocyte-macrophage colony-stimulating factor (GM-CSF, sargramostim, Leukine, Prokine); however, the overall impact of CSF on clinical outcomes is difficult to assess when based on anecdotal case reports. The expectation that granulocyte recovery will be hastened by precursor stimulation cannot be assumed. The time for granulocyte recovery is highly variable and this variability could be sufficiently great to attribute an increase in granulocyte count to either the administration of CSF or to a coincidental increase that would have occurred independent of any additional intervention. Likewise, it is difficult to determine whether patient outcomes would have been different had CSF not been used.

In a review of 70 cases of drug-induced agranulocytosis treated with G-CSF or GM-CSF, peripheral granulocyte recovery time was 1.2 days with mild granulocytopenia, 2.6 days for moderate, and 5.8 days for those with severe granulocytopenia.[116] No difference was noted between G-CSF (mean dose 4 g/kg/day) and GM-CSF (mean dose 7 g/kg/day). The mortality rate was 5%. In a comparison to previous reports in which CSF were not used, recovery time was faster and mortality was lower, but these conclusions are limited by the use of historical controls and the biases inherent in such reviews. Clinicians are much more likely to report cases that are successes rather than failures.

In two randomized, controlled trials, neutrophil recovery time was shortened, but no differences were noted in survival or duration of hospitalization in patients with cancer chemotherapy-induced neutropenia when CSF were administered.[117,118] Although it would not be reasonable to extrapolate these results to the treatment of drug-induced neutropenia, it does appear that hastened white cell recovery does not necessarily result in improved clinical outcomes.

At present, therapeutic trials of CSF are not appropriate as first-line treatment to hasten WBC recovery in drug-induced agranulocytosis or neutropenia. It should also be noted that significant complications related to CSF use for drug-induced agranulocytosis have been reported.[119]

Because J.K. currently is asymptomatic, use of CSF is not indicated.

Idiosyncratic Toxic Effect: Clozapine (Clozaril), Olanzapine (Zyprexa)

29. Why would it be reasonable (or unreasonable) to administer an atypical neuroleptic such as clozapine (Clozaril) to treat J.K.'s schizophrenia subsequent to her recovery from chlorpromazine-induced neutropenia?

Clozapine, a dibenzodiazepine neuroleptic, initially appeared to have a favorable adverse effect profile; however, cases of clozapine-induced neutropenia soon were reported.[120] When discovery of the neutropenia was delayed and clozapine was not promptly discontinued, eight fatalities resulted. As a result, when clozapine was approved for use in the United States for severely ill schizophrenic patients, who were refractory to standard antipsychotic drug treatment, it was available only to patients through a privately contracted drug distribution system, which incorporated mandatory weekly WBC counts and specific criteria for intensified monitoring of patients. Although this drug distribution system was discontinued in 1991, a national registry has continued to collect patient and blood count information; thereby, providing what probably is the most complete postmarketing blood dyscrasia database for any drug available for general use.

In the United States, leukopenia developed in 2.95% of 99,502 patients treated with clozapine through 1994; agranulocytosis occurred in 0.38% of cases, and the death rate was

0.012%.[121] Similarly in the United Kingdom and Ireland, 2.9% of the patients developed neutropenia, 0.8% developed agranulocytosis, and fatal agranulocytosis occurred in 0.03%.[122] The rate of agranulocytosis is lower than the originally estimated 1% to 2%, which could partly be owing to a 97% rate of compliance with the registry protocol for screening for previous blood dyscrasias, monitoring WBC counts weekly, and prompt discontinuation of therapy when neutropenia was noted. The 12 deaths reported represent a fatality rate of 3.2% of agranulocytosis cases, a number that compares favorably with the overall reported population-based rates. In an earlier report of the first 11,555 U.S. patients, the first 6 months of clozapine therapy was the period of greatest risk; only one case of agranulocytosis occurred after a year and a half of clozapine treatment.[123] The risk of agranulocytosis increased with age and was higher in women.

In most, but not all patients, agranulocytosis is preceded by a steady decline in WBC over a period of at least 4 weeks. Nevertheless, leukopenia was not present within 8 days of development of agranulocytosis in 24% of cases. After the discontinuation of clozapine, recovery from agranulocytosis usually occurred within 2 weeks.

A history of clozapine-induced leukopenia might be a risk factor for hematologic reactions to olanzapine (Zyprexa). Eleven reports of olanzapine-induced hematologic reactions (i.e., leukopenia, granulocytopenia, neutropenia, pancytopenia, anemia) were reported to Canadian regulatory authorities through July 2000; in 5 of these cases, the patient had a history of a hematologic reaction with clozapine.[124]

J.K. is not at increased risk for clozapine-induced hematologic toxicity because there does not appear to be cross-reactivity between clozapine and other psychotropic agents, including chlorpromazine.[125,126] Clozapine, however, is not indicated for J.K. because she is not refractory to more typical neuroleptic therapy.

Immune Peripheral Destruction: Metamizole or Dipyrone

30. What drugs have been most commonly associated with acute onset agranulocytosis?

More than two-thirds of the cases of agranulocytosis have been attributable to drugs. The most common drugs associated with agranulocytosis are antithyroid medications and sulfonamides, but almost all classes of drugs have been implicated.[127] According to British reports, neutrophil dyscrasia is the most common life-threatening adverse event with the thionamides, carbimazole and propylthiouracil.[128] The nonsteroidal anti-inflammatory drug (NSAID), metamizole, also known as dipyrone, was withdrawn from the market in the United States in 1979 because of its association with fatal agranulocytosis. Nevertheless, metamizole is still available in other countries, and travelers to these countries are exposed to this drug.[129] Metamizole also is reportedly the most common drug sold to Mexican immigrants by illegal pharmacies in California near the U.S.–Mexican border. This drug also is promoted on the internet by pharmacies specializing in veterinary compounding and it is unknown whether these pharmacies compound metamizole for human use. The risk of developing agranulocytosis from metamizole varies widely and can be partly explained by geographic disparities and differences in use patterns.[130]

DRUG-INDUCED APLASTIC ANEMIA

Aplastic anemia is defined as bicytopenia or pancytopenia, with bone marrow biopsy evidence of decreased cellularity and absence of infiltration and significant fibrosis. The term *pancytopenia* is applied when anemia (Hgb <10 g/dL), neutropenia, and thrombocytopenia are present; and the term *bicytopenia* is applied when two of these three abnormalities are present.[1] Diagnostic criteria also have been established for cases of bicytopenia or pancytopenia with less definitive bone marrow findings. Drugs and chemicals are implicated in 25% to 50% of the cases of aplastic anemia, which is the rarest, most poorly understood, and most serious of the drug-induced blood dyscrasias.

The most serious complication of aplastic anemia is the high risk of infection secondary to the absence of neutrophils. In these patients, overwhelming bacterial sepsis and, especially, fungal infections are the most frequent causes of death.[132] Mortality rates are approximately 10% to 40%; however, patient age, severity of marrow suppression, availability of well-matched marrow transplant donors, and improved treatments influence survival rates.[131] Prognosis is worst for severely affected patients (i.e., severe bone marrow changes and two of the following three criteria: [a] neutrophils $<500/mm^3$, [b] corrected reticulocytes <1%, or [c] platelets $<20/mm^3$).

The underlying pathophysiology of aplastic anemia, including drug-induced mechanisms, remains incomplete despite advances in the understanding of hematopoiesis. An autoimmune process (possibly with genetic predisposition) probably is involved in the pathogenesis of aplastic anemia, even in drug-induced cases.[133,134] Immunosuppressive therapy appears effective for both drug-induced and non–drug-related cases of aplastic anemia. Aplastic anemia caused by direct damage to the pluripotent stem cell (PSC) by toxic insult (e.g., drugs) and true immune-mediated marrow failure might have a common basis in the complex interactions between hematopoiesis and the lymphocyte or monocyte-produced cytokines.

Chloramphenicol

Hundreds of cases of chloramphenicol-induced aplastic anemia have been reported. The aplastic anemia from chloramphenicol is unpredictable; it occurs in about 1:20,000 to 1:30,000 persons and is not related to either dose or duration of use. Chloramphenicol inhibits DNA synthesis and studies from the cells of patients, who have recovered from chloramphenicol-induced aplastic anemia, suggest that some patients might be more sensitive to chloramphenicol's ability to inhibit DNA synthesis.[135,136] A reactive nitrosometabolite of chloramphenicol can affect DNA synthesis irreversibly at low concentrations,[137] and two dehydrometabolites (produced by enterobacteria in the colon) also can be toxic to lymphocytes.[138] Some patients can be predisposed, perhaps genetically, to chloramphenicol-induced aplasia mediated by one or more of these metabolites. The role of enteric bacteria in the pathogenesis of chloramphenicol-induced aplastic anemia might prove to be the most important factor because this adverse effect primarily has been associated with the oral route of administration of this drug.[139] Nevertheless, intravenous[140,141] and ocular[142,143] routes of chloramphenicol administration also have been implicated in aplastic anemia.

Chloramphenicol also can cause an anemia that is dose related, predictable, and reversible. This anemia results from chloramphenicol-induced inhibition of iron utilization and clinically appears with reticulocytopenia, maturation arrest of committed precursors in all cell lines, increased serum concentration of iron, and increased total iron-binding capacity (TIBC). Anemia resulting from inhibited iron utilization with reticulocytopenia and increased serum iron concentrations is common in patients receiving large doses of chloramphenicol. Discontinuation of the drug results in complete recovery.

Importance of a Careful History

31. P.D., a 62-year-old man, notes gradually increasing tiredness and lack of energy over the past month. He seeks medical help after unsuccessful self-medication with stress-formula vitamins. His only other medical problem is osteoarthritis for which he has been taking diclofenac (Voltaren) 50 mg three times daily (TID) for the past 6 months, as well as aspirin 360 mg four to six times daily on an as needed basis. Physical examination is unremarkable except for pallor, several bruises on various parts of the body, and findings typical of osteoarthritis. A blood count, however, reveals an Hgb of 6.2 g/dL, a corrected reticulocyte count of 0.5%, a WBC count of 1,800/mm^3 with 50% neutrophils, and a platelet count of 35,000/mm^3. Diagnostic considerations include drug-induced aplastic anemia. What additional information is needed before P.D.'s anemia might be attributed to a drug-induced etiology?

[SI units: Hgb, 62 g/L; reticulocytes, 0.005 1; WBC 1.8 $\times$ 10^{12}/L; platelets 0.35 $\times$ 10^{15}/L]

Although drug-induced aplastic anemia is a possibility, a more complete medical history is needed. Many drugs and chemicals can cause marrow aplasia, which might not be apparent until long after the last exposure. The family history should be examined for family members who have experienced "blood problems" or sensitivity to drugs or substances. Social history also is important because occupations or military service can provide important information about past or present possible exposure to chemicals. For example, an employee in a paint factory could be exposed to industrial chemicals known to cause aplastic anemia, or a farmer might be exposed to marrow-toxic insecticides. Finally, an exhaustive drug history is mandatory. Use of all drugs past and present, prescription and nonprescription, legal or illegal, regardless of route of administration, should be elicited and documented. This, of course, is true whenever a drug-induced disease is suspected. The relationship between exposure to a causative agent and the onset of aplastic anemia often is not readily apparent and careful scrutiny is needed to uncover a possible association.[144] In one case, a child developed aplastic anemia from use of an herbal remedy 5 weeks before clinical presentation.[145] The product was analyzed with gas chromatography and mass spectrometry and found to contain unlabeled diclofenac and phenylbutazone, two drugs associated with aplastic anemia.

Features

32. A more complete history fails to reveal any additional pertinent information. Which of P.D.'s drugs is most likely to have caused this problem?

A number of commonly used drugs (e.g., NSAID, sulfonamides, antithyroid drugs, antiepileptics, psychotropics, cardiovascular drugs, gold, penicillamine, allopurinol) have been associated with pancytopenia or aplastic anemia.[146]

One year after FDA approval of felbamate (Felbatol) for partial seizures in adults and for Lennox-Gastaut syndrome in children, prescribers were urged to discontinue felbamate use, unless absolutely necessary, because of the potential for aplastic anemia. In all cases, patients had been on the drug for at least 2.5 months. Clinicians were cautioned that even close monitoring cannot protect against the occurrence of aplastic anemia with this drug.[147]

Three cases of dose-dependent, reversible pancytopenia were observed after 2 weeks of linezolid (Zyvox) antibiotic treatment. These cases have features similar to those of the reversible form of chloramphenicol toxicity.[148] Warnings were added to the drug's professional product labeling, cautioning that complete blood counts should be performed weekly in patients who receive linezolid, particularly in those who receive the drug for longer than 2 weeks. Patients with preexisting myelosuppression receiving concomitant drugs that produce bone marrow suppression, or those with a chronic infection who have received previous or concomitant antibiotic therapy also are at higher risk for pancytopenia or aplastic anemia. Discontinuation of linezolid should be considered in patients who develop or have worsening myelosuppression.[149]

The aplastic anemia that has been reported in 57 patients treated with ticlopidine (Ticlid) has been attributed to a direct effect on the PSC. No effective monitoring exists to prevent this adverse effect. Recombinant growth factors do not appear to shorten the neutropenic period.[150]

The professional product labeling for interferon β-1α (Avonex) warns of pancytopenia. Decreased peripheral blood counts in all cell lines, including pancytopenia and thrombocytopenia, have been reported. In some cases, platelets counts were $<$10,000/mm^3, and pancytopenia can reoccur on rechallenge with this drug. Patients using interferon β-1α should be monitored closely for these disorders.[151]

P.D.'s diclofenac has been associated with the development of aplastic anemia. The risk of aplastic anemia with diclofenac has been estimated to occur in about 1 in 150,000. Salicylates have also been linked with aplastic anemia in some,[152] but not all,[146] studies. Diclofenac is the most likely culprit among P.D.'s drugs, but aspirin cannot be ruled out.

33. What subjective and objective data in P.D. are typical of an initial presentation of aplastic anemia?

The symptoms of aplastic anemia at initial presentation usually are nonspecific and are directly related to deficiencies within the suppressed cell lines. P.D.'s pallor, tiredness, and lack of energy likely are caused by anemia. His easy bruisability can be attributable to thrombocytopenia and exacerbated by aspirin. Patients can experience more severe symptoms. For example, when the anemia is severe, high-output congestive heart failure, angina pectoris, and intermittent claudication can occur. When thrombocytopenia is significant, petechiae, purpura, nose bleeds, oozing of blood from the gums, and hemorrhage can be manifested. Symptoms such as oral lesions, fever, and infection can be secondary to leukopenia.

White blood cell counts typically are low at the initial presentation of aplastic anemia, however, the degree of leukopenia varies. The anemia generally is normochromic and either normocytic or macrocytic; and the serum hemoglobin concentration can be as low as 3 g/dL. The serum concentrations of erythropoietin, iron, and transferrin saturation usually are high because erythroid iron-consuming activity is low. Reticulocyte counts generally are low. The WBC count can be low normal or low, but absolute neutropenia almost always is present. P.D.'s WBC count of 1,800/mm^3 with 50% neutrophils (absolute neutrophil count = 1,800 mm^3 × 50% = 900/mm^3) is compatible with this hematologic profile. Total lymphocyte count is affected least and can remain within normal limits until leukopenia becomes severe. Likewise, the platelet count may be near normal or, more commonly, severely depressed. The erythrocyte sedimentation rate (ESR) usually is elevated and bone marrow usually is hypocellular with evidence of fatty replacement.

Management

34. Further evaluation, including bone marrow biopsy, confirms the diagnosis of aplastic anemia. No causes other than drugs are identified. What interventions would facilitate P.D.'s recovery?

First and foremost, as is true in the treatment of most drug-induced diseases, all suspected causative agents should be discontinued. In this case, both diclofenac and aspirin should be stopped. In addition, supportive measures should be initiated as needed.

The approach to treatment is based first on disease severity. Patients with mild aplastic anemia have a relatively benign short-term prognosis and can be treated conservatively. The two basic approaches to treating severe aplastic anemia are bone marrow transplant and immunosuppression.

Bone Marrow Transplantation

Bone marrow transplantation from an HLA antigen-identical sibling donor, if available, achieved about a 72% to 90% long-term survival rate in children and adults <40 to 45 years of age by the mid-1990s.[153–155] Acute and chronic graft-versus-host disease (GVHD) has been a frequent complication of transplant recipients.[156] In one study, GVHD surprisingly was experienced in 4 of 33 transplants from genetically identical twins.[157]

Immunosuppression

Immunosuppression is the treatment of choice for older patients and for young patients without suitable bone marrow donors, and it can appropriate for some patients who would otherwise be transplant candidates.[158] Antithymocyte globulin (ATG) or antilymphocyte globulin (ALG) is administered daily for 8 to 10 days along with a corticosteroid (methylprednisolone 1 mg/kg/day or equivalent) to attenuate the adverse effects of the globulin. Addition of 3 months or more of cyclosporine to the regimen appears to be more effective than ATG or ALG alone.[159] It is postulated that the antilymphocyte activity of these agents results in immunosuppression and inhibits release of PSC-suppressant cytokines responsible for marrow failure. An intradermal skin test of 0.1 mL of a 1:1,000 dilution of ATG along with saline control is recommended before the first infusion.[160]

Androgens

Androgen treatment no longer has a first-line role in the treatment of aplastic anemia and is generally reserved for patients who have failed on immunosuppressants.[161] The use of androgenic steroids as an adjunct to ATG is controversial. Although most trials have failed to demonstrate clear benefit, numerous questions regarding patient selection, timing and duration of therapy, choice of agent, and dosing, any of which can affect results, have been raised.[162,163]

Colony-stimulating Factors

Use of G-CSF and GM-CSF has increased neutrophil counts[164,165] and erythropoietin has increased red cell counts[166] in cases of aplastic anemia. It appears that response, when it occurs, is limited primarily to a subset of patients with nonsevere depression of the cell line in question, and that the response lasts only as long as treatment continues. Interleukin-3 (IL-3) was reported to improve responsiveness to G-CSF in a patient who had not responded to G-CSF alone.[167] The authors speculate this may have been because of an IL-3–induced increase in the number of progenitor cells or an increased responsiveness of those cells to the CSF. One author noted a possible link between G-CSF use and subsequent development of myelodysplasia and leukemia in three children treated with G-CSF for severe aplastic anemia.[168] At this time, therapeutic trials of CSF are not appropriate as first-line treatment of severe aplastic anemia.[169]

Because P.D.'s disease is not severe, discontinuing the drugs and transfusing RBC are the only treatments indicated at this time. It is not possible to predict whether his blood counts will improve once the causative agents are discontinued.

DRUG-INDUCED AUTOIMMUNE PURE RED CELL APLASIA

Definitions

Pure red cell aplasia (PRCA) is a term used for a type of anemia that affects the erythroid cell line. PRCA is a rare condition that has been associated with autoimmune, viral, and neoplastic diseases as well as drug treatment. Other terms (e.g., erythroblastic hypoplasia, erythroplasia, erythroblastopenia, erythroid hypoplasia, red cell agenesis) have been used to describe this particular marrow disorder. PRCA can be classified as an acute, self-limited type; a chronic type; and, either constitutional or acquired. PRCA was first described in 1922.[170,171]

Acquired PRCA might arise in association with thymoma, lymphoid cancer, rheumatoid arthritis, and hepatitis B virus or parvovirus infections. It has also been attributed to drugs, particularly phenytoin, chlorpropamide, and isoniazid. PRCA caused by neutralizing antibodies to erythropoietic proteins also has been described.[172,173]

Exogenous Epoetin and Pure Red Cell Aplasia

Through September 2002, 155 world-wide reports were made of PRCA in patients treated with epoetin alfa (Eprex) confirmed by bone marrow aspirations. Of these, 112 reports had documented the presence of neutralizing antibodies with a high affinity and specificity against the protein moiety of epoetin. All but one of these cases were reported in patients with chronic renal failure.[174]

Eprex, which is marketed outside the United States, accounts for most PRCA cases. Almost all of these cases involved patients with chronic kidney dysfunction who had received epoetin by subcutaneous injection.[175]

When an unexplained progressive drop in hemoglobin levels in the presence of low reticulocyte counts is detected, PRCA is suspected. Treatment with epoetin must be discontinued immediately, and testing for erythropoietin antibodies and bone marrow aspiration should be performed. Patients with suspected PRCA should not be switched to another epoetin treatment. Diagnosis of PRCA is usually confirmed when the bone marrow evaluation shows a virtual absence of red blood cell precursors. Patients diagnosed with epoetin-induced autoimmune PRCA are lifelong transfusion-dependent.[173,176]

Patients who were diagnosed with PRCA before the introduction of epoetin therapy were rarely found to have antibodies against endogenous erythropoietin. One possibility is that a difference in the carbohydrate structure of exogenous epoetin and endogenous erythropoietin creates an epitope on the epoetin polypeptide to which an antibody binds, thereby inactivating both epoetin and the endogenous hormone. The antierythropoietin antibodies are not directed against the carbohydrate moiety on erythropoietin. Removal of the carbohydrate structure by enzymatic digestion had no effect on the antibody affinity for the erythropoietin protein.[173,176]

The precise mechanism of epoetin-induced PRCA is uncertain. Possibilities suggested as the cause of PRCA with epoetin-α are the subcutaneous route of administration and a change in the stabilizer used in the final product formulation or both. Epoetin-α is reported to be sensitive to physical stresses, such as elevated temperature, exposure to light, or extreme shaking.[177] The subcutaneous route is contraindicated for epoetin-α use in patients with chronic renal failure.[174]

The estimated exposure-adjusted incidence of PRCA between 2001 and 2003 is 18 cases per 100,000 patient-years for Eprex formulated with without human serum albumin and 6 cases per 100,000 patient years for a formulation with human serum albumin. The incidence of PRCA peaked in 2001; since then, interventions have resulted in a reduction of more than 80% in the incidence of this dyscrasia caused by Eprex.[175] The increased incidence of PRCA with Eprex, compared with epoetin-α produced in the United States, suggests fundamental differences in the two products.[178]

REFERENCES

1. Benichou C et al. Standardization of definitions and criteria for causality assessment of adverse drug reactions. Drug-induced blood cytopenias: report of an international consensus meeting. *Nouv Rev Fr Hematol* 1991;33:257.
2. Andersohn F et al. Proportion of drug-related serious rare blood dyscrasias: estimates from the Berlin case-control surveillance study. *Am J Hematol* 2004;77:316.
3. Faich GA. Adverse-drug reaction monitoring. *N Engl J Med* 1986;314:1589.
4. Rogers AS et al. Physician knowledge, attitudes, and behavior related to reporting adverse drug events. *Arch Intern Med* 1988;148:1596.
5. Dear Doctor Letter from Russell H. Ellison, MD, Vice President, Medical Affairs, Roche Laboratories, Inc.; August 1998.
6. Wilholm B-E et al. Drug-related blood dyscrasias in a Swedish reporting system, 1994. *Eur J Haematol* 1996;57(Suppl):42.
7. Dhaliwal G et al. Hemolytic anemia. *Am Fam Physician* 2004;69:2599.
8. Wright MS. Drug-induced hemolytic anemias: increasing complications to therapeutic interventions. *Clinical Laboratory Science* 1999;12:115.
9. Koutras AK et al. Oxaliplatin-induced acute-onset thrombocytopenia, hemorrhage and hemolysis. *Oncology* 2004;67:179.
10. Beutler R. G6PD deficiency. *Blood* 1994;84:3613.
11. Glader B. Hereditary hemolytic anemias due to enzyme disorders. In: Greer JP et al., eds. *Wintrobe's Clinical Hematology.* 11th ed. Philadelphia: Lippincott Williams & Wilkins; 2004:1117.
12. Metha AB. Glucose-6-phosphate dehydrogenase deficiency. *Postgrad Med* 1994;70:871.
13. Frank JE. Diagnosis and management of G6PD deficiency. *Am Fam Physician* 2005;72:1277.
14. WHO Working Group. Glucose-6-phosphate dehydrogenase deficiency. *Bull WHO* 1989;67:601.
15. Eldad A et al. Silver sulphadiazine-induced haemolytic anaemia in a glucose-6-phosphate dehydrogenase-deficient burn patient. *Burns* 1991; 17:430.
16. Markowitz N et al. Use of trimethoprim-sulfamethoxazole in a glucose-6-phosphate dehydrogenase-deficient population. *Rev Infect Dis* 1987;9(Suppl 2):S218.
17. Levine BB et al. Studies on the mechanism of the formation of the penicillin antigen: III. The N-(D-alpha-benzylpenicilloyl) group as an antigenic determinant responsible for hypersensitivity to penicillin. *J Exp Med* 1961;114:875.
18. Meyer O et al. Diclofenac-induced antibodies against RBCs and platelets: two case reports and concise review. *Transfusion* 2003;43:345.
19. Salama A et al. Autoantibodies and drug- or metabolite-dependent antibodies in patients with diclofenac-induced immune hemolysis. *Br J Haematol* 1991;77:546.
20. Bougie D et al. Sensitivity to a metabolite of diclofenac as a cause of acute immune hemolytic anemia. *Blood* 1997;90:407.
21. Wright MS et al. Laboratory investigation autoimmune hemolytic anemias. *Clin Lab Sci* 1999; 12:119.
22. Levine BB et al. Immunochemical mechanisms of penicillin induced Coombs positivity and hemolytic anemia in man. *International Archives of Allergy and Applied Immunology* 1967;31:594.
23. Petz LD et al. *Acquired Immune Hemolytic Anemias.* New York, NY: Churchill Livingstone; 1980: 279.
24. Nesmith LW et al. Hemolytic anemia caused by penicillin. *JAMA* 1968;203:27.
25. Garratty G. Immune cytopenia associated with antibiotics. *Trans Med Rev* 1993;7:255.
26. Garratty G et al. Severe immune hemolytic anemia associated with prophylactic use of cefotetan in obstetric and gynecologic procedures. *Am J Obstet Gynecol* 1999;181:103.
27. Packman CH et al. Drug-related immune hemolytic anemia. In: Beutler E et al., eds. *Hematology.* 5th ed. New York: McGraw-Hill; 1995:681.
28. Class FHJ. Immune mechanisms leading to drug-induced blood dyscrasias. *Eur J Haematol* 1996;57(Suppl):64.
29. Smith RA. Dextromethorphan/quinidine: a novel dextromethorphan product for the treatment of emotional lability. *Expert Opin Pharmcother* 2006; 18:2581.
30. Thisted RA et al. Dextromethorphan and quinidine in adult patients with uncontrolled painful diabetic peripheral neuropathy: a 29-day, multicenter, open-label, dose-escalation study. *Clin Ther* 2006;28:1607.
31. Food and Drug Administration. Public Health Advisory-Trovan (trovafloxacin/alatrofloxacin mesylate). June 9, 1999.
32. The European Agency for the Evaluation of Medicinal Products. Public statement on Trovan/Trovan IV/Turvel/Turvel IV (Trovafloxacin/Alatrofloxacin)? Recommendation to suspend the marketing authorization in the European Union. June 15, 1999.
33. Blum MD et al. Temafloxacin syndrome: review of 95 cases. *Clin Infect Dis* 1994;18:946.
34. Kleinman S et al. Positive direct antiglobulin tests and immune hemolytic anemia in patients receiving procainamide. *N Engl J Med* 1984;311:809.
35. Arndt PA et al. The changing spectrum of drug-induced immune hemolytic anemia. *Semin Hematol* 2005;42:137.
36. Anonymous. Hemolysis from ceftriaxone. *Med Lett Drugs Ther* 2002;44:100.
37. Brandt NJ et al. Methyldopa and haemolytic anaemia. *Lancet* 1966;1:771.
38. Surveyor I et al. Autoimmune haemolytic anaemia complicating methyldopa therapy. *Postgrad Med J* 1968;44:438.
39. Pedersen-Bjergaard U et al. Thrombocytopenia induced by noncytotoxic drugs in Denmark 1968–1991. *J Intern Med* 1996;239:509.
40. Wilholm BE et al. Drug-related blood dyscrasias in a Swedish reporting system, 1985–1994. *Eur J Haematol* 1996;57(Suppl):42.
41. Bonfiglio M et al. Thrombocytopenia in intensive care patients: a comprehensive analysis of risk factors in 314 patients. *Ann Pharmacother* 1995;29:835.
42. Burnakis T. Inaccurate assessment of drug-induced thrombocytopenia: reason for concern. *Ann Pharmacother* 1994;28:726.
43. Waekentin TE. Drug-induced immune-mediated thrombocytopenia-from purpura to thrombosis. *N Engl J Med* 2007;356:891.

44. Coons JC. Eptifibatide-associated acute, profound thrombocytopenia. *Ann Pharmacother* 2005; 39:368.
45. Huxtable LM et al. Frequency and management of thrombocytopenia with the glycoprotein IIb/IIIa receptor antagonists. *Am J Cardiol* 2006;97:426.
46. Aster RH et al. Thrombocytopenia resulting from sensitivity to GPIIb-IIIa inhibitors. *Semin Thromb Hemost* 2004;30:569.
47. Von Drygalski A et al. Vancomycin-induced immune thrombocytopenia. *N Engl J Med* 2007;356: 904.
48. George JN et al. Drug-induced thrombocytopenia: a systematic review of published case reports. *Ann Intern Med* 1998;129:886.
49. Nordquist P et al. Thrombocytopenia during chlorothiazide treatment. *Lancet* 1959;1:271.
50. Eisner EV et al. Hydrochlorothiazide-dependent thrombocytopenia due to an IgM antibody. *JAMA* 1971;215:480.
51. Amirlak I et al. Haemolytic uraemic syndrome: an overview. *Nephrology* 2006;11:213.
52. Crum NF et al. Quinine-induced hemolytic-uremic syndrome. *South Med J* 2000;93:726.
53. Saif MW et al. Hemolytic-uremic syndrome associated with gemcitabine: a case report and review of literature. *JOP* 2005;6:369.
54. Walter RB et al. Gemcitabine-associated hemolytic-uremic syndrome. *Am J Kidney Dis* 2002;40: E16.
55. Maguire RB et al. Recurrent pancytopenia, coagulopathy, and renal failure associated with multiple quinine-dependent antibodies. *Ann Intern Med* 1993;119:215.
56. Curtis BR et al. Antibodies in sulfonamide-induced immune thrombocytopenia recognize calcium-dependent epitopes on the glycoprotein Iib/IIIa complex. *Blood* 1994;84:176.
57. George JN et al. Thrombocytopenia due to enhanced platelet destruction by immunologic mechanisms. In: Beutler E et al., eds. *Hematology.* 5th ed. New York: McGraw-Hill; 1995:1315.
58. Christie DJ et al. Structural features of the quinidine and quinine molecules necessary for binding of drug-induced antibodies to human platelets. *J Lab Clin Med* 1984;104:730.
59. Ansell J et al. Heparin induced thrombocytopenia: a prospective study. *Thromb Haemost* 1980;43:61.
60. Bell WR. Heparin-associated thrombocytopenia and thrombosis. *J Lab Clin Med* 1988;11:600.
61. Kelton JG et al. Immunoglobulin G from patients with heparin-induced thrombocytopenia binds to a complex of heparin and platelet factor 4. *Blood* 1994;83:3232.
62. Visentin GP et al. Antibodies from patients with heparin-induced thrombocytopenia/thrombosis are specific for platelet factor 4 complexed with heparin or bound to endothelial cells. *J Clin Invest* 1994;93:81.
63. Warkentin TE et al. Heparin-induced thrombocytopenia. *Prog Hemost Thromb* 1991;10:1.
64. Anderson GM. Insights into heparin-induced thrombocytopenia. *Br J Haematol* 1992;80:504.
65. Brieger DB et al. Heparin-induced thrombocytopenia. *J Am Coll Cardiol* 1998;31:1449.
66. Kelton JG et al. Clinical usefulness of testing for a heparin-dependent platelet aggregating factor in patients with suspected heparin-associated thrombocytopenia. *J Lab Clin Med* 1984;103:606.
67. Chong BH et al. The clinical usefulness of the platelet aggregation test for the diagnosis of heparin-induced thrombocytopenia. *Thromb Haemost* 1993;69:344.
68. Warkentin TE et al. Heparin-induced thrombocytopenia in patients treated with low-molecular-weight heparin or unfractionated heparin. *N Engl J Med* 1995;332:1330.
69. Bell WR et al. Heparin-associated thrombocytopenia: a comparison of three heparin preparations. *N Engl J Med* 1980;303:902.
70. Schmitt BP et al. Heparin-associated thrombocytopenia: a critical review and pooled analysis. *Am J Med Sci* 1993;305:208.
71. Heeger PS et al. Heparin flushes and thrombocytopenia. *Ann Intern Med* 1986;105:143.
72. Laster JL et al. Thrombocytopenia associated with heparin-coated catheters in patients with heparin-associated antiplatelet antibodies. *Arch Intern Med* 1989;149:2285.
73. Garrelts JC. White clot syndrome and thrombocytopenia: reasons to abandon heparin i.v. lock flush solution. *Clin Pharm* 1992;11:797.
74. Warkentin TE et al. Gender imbalance and risk factor interactions in heparin-induced thrombocytopenia. *Blood* 2006;108:2937.
75. Napolitano LM. Heparin-induced thrombocytopenia in the critical care setting: diagnosis and management. *Crit Care Med* 2006;34:2898.
76. Juni P et al. The hazards of scoring the quality of clinical trials for meta-analysis. *JAMA* 1999;282:1054.
77. Martel N et al. Risk for heparin-induced thrombocytopenia with unfractionated and low-molecular-weight heparin thromboprophylaxis: a meta-analysis. *Blood* 2005;106:2710.
78. Laster J et al. Reexposure to heparin of patients with heparin-associated antibodies. *J Vasc Surg* 1989;9:677.
79. Warkentin TE et al. A 14-year study of heparin-induced thrombocytopenia. *Am J Med* 1996;101: 502.
80. Cines DB et al. Immune endothelial-cell injury in heparin-associated thrombocytopenia. *N Engl J Med* 1987;316:581.
81. Hull RD et al. Heparin for 5 days as compared with 10 days in the initial treatment of proximal venous thrombosis. *N Engl J Med* 1990;322:1260.
82. Gouault-Heilmann M et al. Low molecular weight heparin fractions as an alternative therapy in heparin-induced thrombocytopenia. *Haemostasis* 1987;17:134.
83. Vun CM et al. Cross-reactivity study of low molecular weight heparins and heparinoid in heparin-induced thrombocytopenia. *Thromb Res* 1996;81:525.
84. Demers C et al. Rapid anticoagulation using ancrod for heparin-induced thrombocytopenia. *Blood* 1991;78:2194.
85. Yurvati AH et al. Heparinless cardiopulmonary bypass with ancrod. *Ann Thorac Surg* 1994;57: 1656.
86. Chamberlin JR et al. Successful treatment of heparin-associated thrombocytopenia and thrombosis using Hirulog. *Can J Cardiol* 1995;11:511.
87. Harenberg J et al. Anticoagulation in patients with heparin-induced thrombocytopenia type II. *Semin Thromb Hemost* 1997;23:189.
88. Angiomax (bivalirudin) professional product labeling December 2005. The Medicines Company. Parsippany, NJ.
89. Refludan (lepirudin) professional product labeling. October 2004. Berlex Laboratories. Wayne, NJ.
90. Argatroban professional product labeling July 2005. GlaxoSmithKline. Research Triangle Park, NC.
91. Greinacher A et al. Recognition, treatment, and prevention of heparin-induced throbocytopenia: review and update. *Thromb Res* 2006;118:165.
92. Bennett CL et al. Thrombotic thrombocytopenic purpura associated with ticlopidine. *Ann Intern Med* 1998;128:541.
93. Steinhuble SR et al. Incidence and clinical course of thrombotic thrombocytopenic purpura due to ticlopidine following coronary stenting. *JAMA* 1999;281:806.
94. Bennett CL et al. Thrombotic thrombocytopenic purpura associated with ticlopidine in the stetting of coronary artery stents and stroke prevention. *Arch Intern Med* 1999;159:2524.
95. Bennett CL et al. Thrombotic thrombocytopenic purpura associated with clopidogrel. *N Engl J Med* 2000;342:1773.
96. Zakarija A et al. Drug-induced thrombotic microangiopathy. *Semin Thromb Hemost* 2005;31: 681.
97. Kurtz J-E et al. Drug-induced agranulocytosis in older people: a case series of 25 patients [Letter]. *Age Ageing* 1999;28:325.
98. Reizenstein P et al. Mortality in agranulocytosis. *Lancet* 1974;2:293.
99. Julia A et al. Drug-induced agranulocytosis: prognostic factors in a series of 168 episodes. *Br J Haematol* 1991;79:366.
100. Andres E et al. Life-threatening idiosyncratic drug-induced agranulocytosis in elderly patients. *Drugs Aging* 2004:21:427.
101. Bhatt V et al. Review: Drug-induced neutropenia. Pathophysiology, clinical features, and management. *Ann Clin Lab Sci* 2004;34:131.
102. Neftel KA et al. Inhibition of granulopoiesis in vivo and in vitro by beta-lactam antibiotics. *J Infect Dis* 1985;152:90.
103. Houmayouni H et al. Leukopenia due to penicillin and cephalosporin homologues. *Arch Intern Med* 1979;139:827.
104. Murphy MF et al. Demonstration of an immune-mediated mechanism of penicillin-induced neutropenia and thrombocytopenia. *Br J Haematol* 1983;55:155.
105. Salama A et al. Immune-mediated agranulocytosis related to drugs and their metabolites: mode of sensitization and heterogeneity of antibodies. *Br J Haematol* 1989;72:127.
106. Murphy MF et al. Cephalosporin-induced immune neutropenia. *Br J Haematol* 1985;59:9.
107. Rey D et al. Ceftriaxone-induced granulopenia related to a peculiar mechanism of granulopoiesis inhibition. *Am J Med* 1989;87:591.
108. Hauser SP et al. Effects of ceftazidime, a beta-lactam antibiotic, on murine haemopoiesis in vitro. *Br J Haematol* 1994;86:733.
109. Uetrecht JP. Reactive metabolites and agranulocytosis. *Eur J Haematol* 1996;57(Suppl):83.
110. Anonymous. Antibiotic-induced neutropenia [Editorial]. *Lancet* 1985;2:814.
111. Segarra-Newnham M et al. Probable vancomycin induced neutropenia. *Ann Pharmacother* 2004;38:1855.
112. Duggal HS et al. Psychotropic drug-induced neutropenia. *Drugs Today (Barc)* 2005;41:517.
113. Pisciotta AV. Immune and toxic mechanisms in drug-induced agranulocytosis. *Semin Hematol* 1973;10:279.
114. Pisciotta AV. Drug-induced agranulocytosis. *Drugs* 1978;15:132.
115. Pisciotta AV. Agranulocytosis induced by certain phenothiazine derivatives. *JAMA* 1969;208:1862.
116. Sprikkelman A et al. The application of hematopoietic growth factors in drug-induced agranulocytosis: a review of 70 cases. *Leukemia* 1994;12:2031.
117. Anaissie EJ et al. Randomized comparison between antibiotics alone and antibiotics plus granulocyte-macrophage colony-stimulating factor (*Escherichia coli*-derived) in cancer patients with fever and neutropenia. *Am J Med* 1996;100:17.
118. Hartmann LC et al. Granulocyte colony-stimulating factor in severe chemotherapy-induced afebrile neutropenia. *N Engl J Med* 1997;336:1776.
119. Demuynck H et al. Risks of rhG-CSF treatment in drug-induced agranulocytosis. *Ann Hematol* 1995;70:143.
120. Amsler HA et al. Agranulocytosis in patients treated with clozapine: a study of the Finnish epidemic. *Acta Psychiatr Scand* 1977;56:241.
121. Honigfeld G. Effects of the clozapine national registry system on incidence of deaths related to agranulocytosis. *Psychiatr Serv* 1996;47:52.
122. Atkin K et al. Neutropenia and agranulocytosis in patients receiving clozapine in the UK and Ireland. *Br J Psychiatr* 1996;169:483.
123. Alvir JMJ et al. Clozapine-induced agranulocytosis: incidence and risk factors in the United States. *N Engl J Med* 1993;329:162.
124. Olanzapine (Zyprexa): suspected serious reactions. *Can Adv Drug React Newslett* 2000;10:85.
125. Lieberman JA et al. Clozapine-induced agranulocytosis: non-cross-reactivity with other psychotropic drugs. *J Clin Psychiatry* 1988;49:271.
126. Bauer M et al. Clozapine treatment after agranulo-

cytosis induced by classic neuroleptics. *J Clin Psychopharmacol* 1994;14:71.
127. Ibanez L. Population-based drug-induced agranulocytosis. *Arch Intern Med.* 2005;165:869.
128. Pearce SHS. Spontaneous reporting of adverse reactions to carbimazole and propylthiouracil in the UK. *Clin Endocrinol (Oxf)* 2004;61:589.
129. Bonkowsky JL et al. Metamizole use by Latino immigrants: a common and potential harmful home remedy. *Pediatrics* 2002;109:e98.
130. Ibanez L et al. Agranulocytosis associated with dipyrone (metamizol). *Eur J Clin Pharmacol* 2005;60:821.
131. Young NS et al. The treatment of severe acquired aplastic anemia. *Blood* 1995;85:3367.
132. Young NS. Acquired aplastic anemia. *JAMA* 1999;282:271.
133. Young NS. The problem of clonality in aplastic anemia: Dr. Dameshek's riddle, restated. *Blood* 1992;79:1385.
134. Young NS. Autoimmunity and its treatment in aplastic anemia [Editorial]. *Ann Intern Med* 1997; 126:166.8.
135. Yunis AA et al. Chloramphenicol toxicity: pathogenetic mechanisms and the role of the p-NO2 in aplastic anemia. *Clin Toxicol* 1980;17:359.
136. Jimenez JJ et al. Chloramphenicol-induced bone marrow injury: possible role of bacterial metabolites of chloramphenicol. *Blood* 1987;70:1180.
137. Vincent PC. In vitro evidence of drug action in aplastic anemia. *Blood* 1984;49:3.
138. Lafarge-Frayssinet C et al. Cytotoxicity and DNA damaging potency of chloramphenicol and six metabolites: a new evaluation in human lymphocytes and Raji cells. *Mutat Res* 1994;320:207.
139. Yunis AA. Chloramphenicol toxicity: 25 years of research. *Am J Med* 1989;87:44.
140. Plaut ME et al. Aplastic anemia after parenteral chloramphenicol: a warning renewed. *N Engl J Med* 1982;306:1486.
141. West BC et al. Aplastic anemia associated with parenteral chloramphenicol: a review of 10 cases including the second case of possible increased risk with cimetidine. *Rev Infect Dis* 1988;10:1048.
142. Fraunfelder FT et al. Ocular chloramphenicol and aplastic anemia. *N Engl J Med* 1983;308:1536.
143. Doona M et al. Use of chloramphenicol as topical eye medication: time to cry halt. *BMJ* 1995;310:1217.
144. Issaragrisil S. Aplastic anemia-low drug associations. *Current Hematology Reports* 2003;2:1.
145. Nelson L et al. Aplastic anemia induced by an adulterated herbal medication. *Clin Toxicol* 1995;33:467.
146. International Agranulocytosis and Aplastic Anemia Study. Risks of agranulocytosis and aplastic anemia: a first report of their relation to drug use with special reference to analgesics. *JAMA* 1986;256:1749.
147. Food and Drug Administration. Recommendation for the immediate withdrawal of patients from treatment with Felbatol (felbamate). *FDA Medical Bulletin* 1994;24:5.
148. Green SL et al. Linezolid and reversible myelosuppression. *JAMA* 2001;285:1291.
149. Zyvox (linezolid) professional product labeling July 2006. Pfizer, Inc. New York, NY.
150. Symeonidis A et al. Ticlopidine-induced aplastic anemia: two new case reports, review, and meta-analysis of 55 additional cases. *Am J Hematol* 2002;71:24.
151. Avonex (interferon beta-1a) professional product labeling. Revised February 2003. Biogen, Cambridge, Massachusetts.
152. Baurnelou E et al. Epidemiology of aplastic anemia in France: a case-control study. I. Medical history and medication use. *Blood* 1993;81:1471.
153. Young NS. Autoimmunity and its treatment in aplastic anemia [Editorial]. *Ann Intern Med* 1997;126:166.8.
154. Dooney K et al. Primary treatment of acquired aplastic anemia: outcomes with bone marrow transplantation and immunosuppressive therapy. *Ann Intern Med* 1997;126:107.
155. Bacigalupo A et al. Bone marrow transplantation (BMT) versus immunosuppression for the treatment of severe aplastic anemia (SAA): a report of the EBMT SAA working party. *Br J Haematol* 1988;70:177.
156. Young NS et al. The treatment of severe acquired aplastic anemia. *Blood* 1995;85:3367.
157. Hinterberger W et al. Results of transplanting bone marrow from genetically identical twins into patients with aplastic anemia. *Ann Intern Med* 1997;126:115.
158. Paquette RL et al. Long-term outcome of aplastic anemia in adults treated with antithymocyte globulin: comparison with bone marrow transplantation. *Blood* 1995;85:283.
159. Frickhofen N et al. Treatment of aplastic anemia with antilymphocyte globulin and methylprednisolone with or without cyclosporine. *N Engl J Med* 1991;324:1297.
160. Atgam (lymphocyte immune globulin) professional product labeling November 2005. Pfizer, Inc. New York, NY.
161. Guinan EC et al. Acquired and inherited aplastic anemia syndromes. In: Greer JP et al., eds. *Wintrobe's Clinical Hematology.* 11th ed. Philadelphia: Lippincott Williams & Wilkins; 2004:1407.
162. French Cooperative Group for the Study of Aplastic and Refractory Anemias. Androgen therapy in aplastic anemia: a comparative study of high and low-doses and of 4 different androgens. *Scandinavian Journal of Haematology* 1986;36:346.
163. Bacigalupo A et al. Treatment of aplastic anemia (AA) with antilymphocyte globulin (ALG) and methylprednisolone (Mpred) with or without androgens: a randomized trial from the EBMT SAA working party. *Br J Haematol* 1993;83:145.
164. Antin JH et al. Phase I/II study of recombinant human granulocyte-macrophage colony-stimulating factor in aplastic anemia of both acquired and myelodysplastic syndrome. *Blood* 1988;72:705.
165. Kojima S et al. Treatment of aplastic anemia in children with recombinant human granulocyte colony-stimulating factor. *Blood* 1992;77:937.
166. Bessho M et al. Treatment of the anemia of aplastic anemia patients with recombinant human erythropoietin in combination with granulocyte colony-stimulating factor: a multicenter randomized controlled study. *Eur J Haematol* 1997;58:265.
167. Geissler K et al. Effect of interleukin-3 on responsiveness to granulocyte-colony-stimulating factor in severe aplastic anemia. *Ann Intern Med* 1992;117:223.
168. Kojima S et al. Myelodysplasia and leukemia after treatment of aplastic anemia with G-CSF [Letter]. *N Engl J Med* 1992;326:1294.
169. Marsh JCW et al. Haemopoietic growth factors in aplastic anaemia: a cautionary note. *Lancet* 1994;344:172.
170. Erslev AJ. Pure red cell aplasia. In: Beutler E et al.., eds. *Hematology.* 5th ed. New York: McGraw-Hill; 1995:448.
171. Dessypris EN et al. Red cell aplasia. In: Greer JP et al., eds. *Wintrobe's Clinical Hematology.* 11th ed. Philadelphia: Lippincott Williams & Wilkins; 2004:1421.
172. Wooltorton E. Epoetin alfa (Eprex): reports of pure red cell aplasia. *Can Med Assoc J* 2002;166:480.
173. Casadevall N et al. Pure red cell aplasia after treatment with recombinant erythropoietin. *N Engl J Med* 2002;346:469.
174. Committee on Safety of Medicines. Eprex (Epoetin Alfa) and pure red cell aplasia: contraindication of subcutaneous administration to patients with chronic renal disease. December 12, 2002.
175. Bennett CL. Pure red-cell aplasia and epoetin therapy. *N Engl J Med* 2004;351:1403.
176. Bunn F. Drug induced autoimmune red cell aplasia [Editorial]. *N Engl J Med* 2002;346:522.
177. J & J Eprex stability improvements planned in response to aplasia incidence. *The Pink Sheet,* September 16, 2002:24.
178. Schellekens H et al. Eprex-associated pure red cell aplasia and leachates. *Nature Biotechnology* 2006;24:613.

SECTION NINETEEN

NEOPLASTIC DISORDERS

Pamala Jacobson
SECTION EDITOR

CHAPTER 88

Neoplastic Disorders and Their Treatment: General Principles

Mark Kirstein

INTRODUCTION TO NEOPLASTIC DISORDERS

Cancer (neoplasm, tumor, or malignancy) is not a single disease; rather, it is a group of diseases characterized by uncontrolled growth and spread of abnormal cells. Cancer cells do not respond to the normal processes that regulate cell growth, proliferation, and survival, and they cannot carry out the physiologic functions of their normal differentiated (mature) counterparts. Often, cancer cells are described as poorly differentiated or immature. Other characteristics of cancer cells include their ability to invade adjacent normal tissues and break away from the primary tumor (metastasize) and travel through the blood or lymph to establish new tumors (metastases) at a distant site. Their ability to stimulate the formation of new blood vessels (angiogenesis) and their endless replication potential further contribute to their continued growth and survival.[1] Cancers can arise in any tissue in the body and may be classified as benign or malignant. If malignant cancer cells are allowed to grow uncontrollably, they can eventually result in the death of the patient, whereas benign cancer cells cannot spread by tissue invasion or metastasize.

Cancer Statistics

Each year, the American Cancer Society (ACS) publishes the estimated number of new cases and number of cancer-related deaths. The National Cancer Institute (NCI) publishes cancer statistics that also include cancer risk, prevalence, and survival information.[2] The ACS estimates that 1 of 2 American men and 1 of 3 American women will eventually develop cancer

Table 88-1 Leading Sites of New Cancer Cases and Deaths in the United States, 2007, Excluding Basal and Squamous Cell Skin Cancers and In Situ Carcinomas Except Urinary Bladder

New Cancer Cases				*Cancer Deaths*			
Prostate	26%	Breast	26%	Lung and bronchus	31%	Lung and bronchus	26%
Lung and bronchus	15%	Lung and bronchus	15%	Colon and rectum	9%	Breast	15%
Colon and rectum	10%	Uterine corpus	6%	Prostate	9%	Colon and rectum	10%
Urinary bladder	7%	Melanoma of skin	4%	Pancreas	6%	Ovary	6%
Kidney	4%	Non-Hodgkin lymphoma	4%	Esophagus	4%	Pancreas	6%
Non-Hodgkin lymphoma	4%	Thyroid	4%	Leukemia	4%	Leukemia	4%
Oral cavity	3%	Kidney	3%	Liver or intrahepatic bile	4%	Non-Hodgkin lymphoma	3%
Leukemia	3%	Ovary	3%	Kidney	3%	Uterine corpus	3%
Pancreas	2%	Pancreas	2%	Non-Hodgkin lymphoma	3%	Brain or central nervous system	2%
All other sites	19%	All other sites	22%	Urinary bladder	3%	Liver or intrahepatic bile	2%
				All other sites	24%	All other sites	23%
Men 766,860		Women 678,060		Men 289,550		Women 270,100	

From reference 3, with permission.

and that approximately 1,444,920 new cases of cancer will be diagnosed in 2007.[3] The most common cancers and causes of cancer deaths in adult Americans are illustrated in Table 88-1. The incidence of cancer and cancer-related deaths can be affected by both age and ethnic background with the incidence greater in the elderly and black populations.[4] Other factors that can increase an individual's risk for developing a cancer include environmental and lifestyle factors, genetic predisposition, immunosuppression, and exposure to one or more potential carcinogens.[5]

Etiology

Cancers arise from the transformation of a single normal cell. An initial "event" causes damage or mutation to the cell's DNA. These events may include lifestyle, environmental, or occupational factors, as well as some medical therapies (e.g., cytotoxic chemotherapy, immunosuppressive therapy, or radiation therapy) and hereditary factors (Table 88-2). Currently, cigarette smoking is probably the most significant single factor that contributes to the development of cancers. The ACS estimates that tobacco use is responsible for approximately 180,000 cancer deaths per year.[3] In addition, approximately one-third of expected cancer deaths in 2007 are thought to result from preventable causes, such as physical inactivity, obesity, nutrition, and other lifestyle factors.[3,6]

Progress in our understanding about the development of cancer at the molecular level has led to the recognition that cancer is a genetic disease. Two gene classes, oncogenes and tumor-suppressor genes, play a major role in the pathogenesis of cancer. Damage to cellular DNA can result in mutations that lead to the development of oncogenes and loss or inactivation of tumor suppressor genes. Oncogenes are genes whose overactivity or presence in certain forms can lead to the development of cancer. Oncogenes arise from normal genes called *proto-oncogenes* through genetic alterations such as chromosomal translocations, deletions, insertions, and point mutations.

Growth and proliferation of normal cells are influenced by proteins, known as *growth factors*. When growth factors bind to receptors on the cell surface, they activate a series of enzymes within the cell that stimulate cell signaling pathways and gene transcription proteins in the nucleus, which encode for proteins that regulate cell growth and proliferation. The coordination and integration of cellular signaling processes are referred to as *signal transduction*. Proto-oncogenes are responsible for encoding several components of signal transduction pathways, including growth factors, growth factor receptors,

Table 88-2 Carcinogens Associated With an Increased Risk of Cancer

Carcinogenic Risk Factor	*Associated Cancer(s)*
Environmental	
Ionizing radiation (radon gas emitted from soil containing uranium deposits)	Leukemia, breast, thyroid, lung
Ultraviolet radiation	Skin melanoma
Viruses	Leukemia, lymphoma, nasopharyngeal, liver, cervix
Occupational	
Asbestos	Lung, mesothelioma
Chromium, nickel	Lung
Vinyl chloride	Liver
Aniline dye	Bladder
Benzene	Leukemia
Lifestyle	
Alcohol	Esophagus, liver, stomach, oropharynx, larynx
Dietary factors	Colon, breast, gallbladder, gastric
Tobacco	Lung, oropharynx, pharynx, larynx, esophagus, bladder
Medical Drugs	
Diethylstilbestrol	Vaginal in offspring, breast, testes, ovary
Alkylating agents	Leukemia, bladder
Azathioprine	Lymphoma
Phenacetin	Bladder
Estrogens, tamoxifen	Endometrial
Cyclophosphamide	Bladder
Etoposide	Leukemia

signaling enzymes, and DNA transcription factors. Abnormal forms or excessive quantities of these stimulatory proteins disrupt normal cell growth-signaling pathways, leading to excessive growth and proliferation and, ultimately, a malignant transformation. For example, the epidermal growth factor receptor (EGFR) is a member of a family of type I receptor tyrosine kinases, which trigger cell signaling pathways that influence cell growth, proliferation, survival, tissue invasion, and metastases.[7] The family includes four related receptors: EGFR (also referred to as ErbB1 or HER1), ErbB2 (HER2, HER2/neu), ErbB3 (HER3), and ErbB4 (HER4). These receptor proteins are composed of an extracellular binding domain, a transmembrane segment, and an intracellular protein tyrosine kinase domain. In cancer cells, the receptors can become activated through receptor binding to the extracellular ligand, resulting in heterodimerization (different members of the receptor family) or homodimerization (like members of the receptor family).[8]

Ligand-independent receptor dimerization can occur as well and is the principal form of activation of HER2, because HER2 does not bind to any known ligands.[9] The EGFR signaling pathway is depicted in Figure 88-1. Activation of the receptor protein tyrosine kinase leads to autophosphorylation of tyrosine and other intracellular substrates that initiate downstream cellular signaling events.[7] An important signaling route is the Ras-Raf-MAP kinase pathway, which regulates transcription of molecules that are associated with cell proliferation, survival, and malignant transformation.[7] Other important routes for signaling include the phosphatidylinositol 3-kinase (PI3K)-protein-serine/threonine kinase Akt and the stress-activated protein kinase pathways.[7] EGFR is frequently overexpressed in human tumors, including cancers of the lung, head and neck, bladder, breast, ovary, prostate, colon, and glioblastoma.[7] Amplification of the HER2/neu gene or overexpression of the protein is present in 10% to 34% of invasive breast cancers.[10] Increased EGFR or HER2/neu expression in several cancers is associated with a more aggressive cancer growth pattern and poorer clinical outcome.[7]

Tumor-suppressor genes are normal genes that encode for proteins that suppress inappropriate cell division or growth. Gene losses or mutations of these genes can cause these proteins to become inactivated, eliminating the normal inhibition of cell division. Alterations in a third class of genes, DNA repair genes, are also implicated in cancer. DNA repair genes encode for proteins that correct errors that may arise during DNA duplication. Mutations in these genes further contribute to the accumulation of genetic changes that promote cancer progression.

Table 88-3 lists examples of genes frequently associated with human cancers. Multiple genetic mutations, including activation of oncogenes and loss or inactivation of tumor-suppressor genes within a cell, are necessary for malignant transformation.[11] Separate genetic changes are required for tumor invasion of normal tissues and metastases.

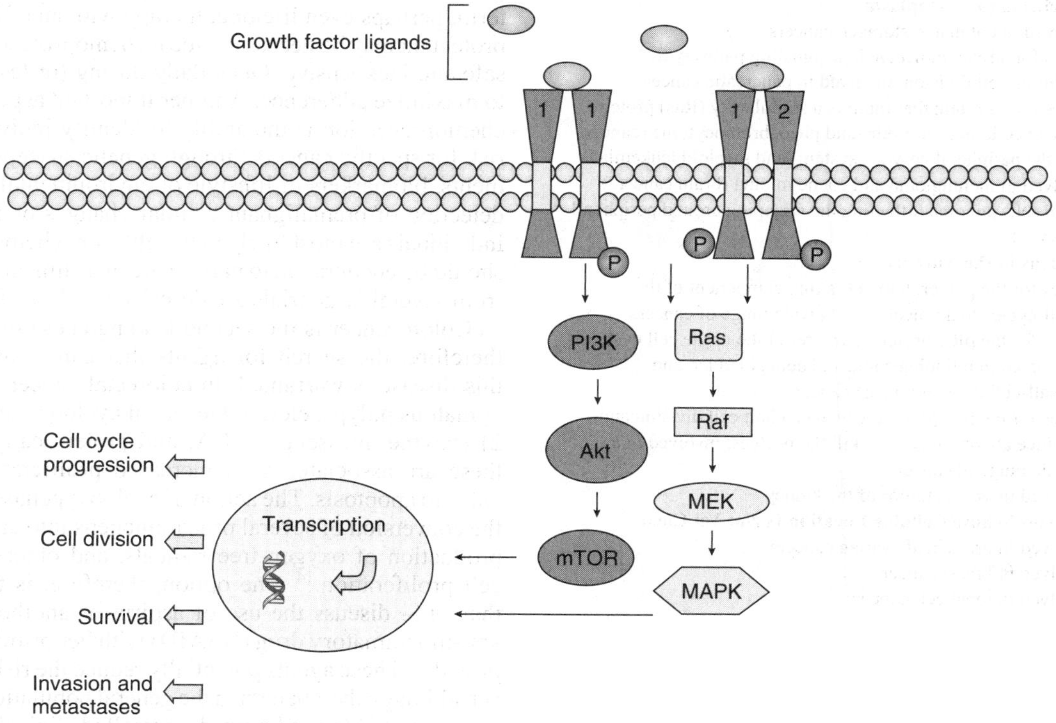

FIGURE 88-1 Epidermal growth factor signaling. Members of the ErbB receptor family become activated by dimerization. Ligand binding to the extracellular domain of epidermal growth factor receptor (EGFR) leads to receptor activation through homodimerization or heterodimerization with other ErbB receptors. Activation of the receptor tyrosine kinase results in tyrosine autophosphorylation and a series of phosphorylations of intracellular substrates that influence cell growth stimulatory signaling and other cellular activities.

Table 88-3 Some Genes Involved in Human Cancers[11]

Oncogenes	
Genes for Growth Factors or Their Receptors	
PDGF	Codes for platelet-derived growth factor; involved in glioma (a brain cancer)
erb-B	Codes for the receptor for epidermal growth factor; involved in glioblastoma (a brain cancer) and breast cancer
erb-B2	Also called *Her-2* or *neu;* codes for a growth factor receptor; involved in breast, salivary gland, and ovarian cancers
RET	Codes for a growth factor receptor; involved in thyroid cancer
Genes for Cytoplasmic Relays in Stimulatory Signaling Pathways	
K-Ras	Involved in lung, ovarian, colon, and pancreatic cancers
N-Ras	Involved in leukemias
Genes for Transcription Factors That Activate Growth-Promoting Genes	
c-Myc	Involved in leukemias and breast, stomach, and lung cancers
N-Myc	Involved in neuroblastoma (a nerve cell cancer) and glioblastoma
L-Myc	Involved in lung cancer
Genes for Other Kinds of Molecules	
Bcl-2	Codes for a protein that normally blocks cell suicide; involved in follicular B-cell lymphoma
Bcl-1	Also called *PRAD1;* codes for cyclin D1, a stimulatory component of the cell-cycle clock; involved in breast, head, and neck cancers
MDM2	Codes for an antagonist of the p53 tumor-suppressor protein; involved in sarcomas (connective tissue cancers) and others cancers
Tumor-Suppressor Genes	
Genes for Proteins in the Cytoplasm	
APC	Involved in colon and stomach cancers
DPC-4	Codes for a relay molecule in a signaling pathway that inhibits cell division; involved in pancreatic cancer
NF-1	Codes for a protein that inhibits a stimulatory (Ras) protein; involved in neurofibroma and pheochromocytoma (cancers of the peripheral nervous system) and myeloid leukemia
NF-2	Involved in meningioma and ependymoma (brain cancers) and schwannoma (affecting the wrapping around peripheral nerves)
Genes for Proteins in the Nucleus	
MTS1	Codes for the p16 protein, a braking component of the cell-cycle clock; involved in a wide range of cancers
RB	Codes for the pRB protein, a master brake of the cell cycle; involved in retinoblastoma and bone, bladder, and small-cell lung and breast cancer
p53	Codes for the p53 protein, which can halt cell division and induce abnormal cells to kill themselves; involved in a wide range of cancers
WT1	Involved in Wilms tumor of the kidney
Genes for Proteins Whose Cellular Location Is Not Yet Clear	
BRCA1	Involved in breast and ovarian cancers
BRCA2	Involved in breast cancer
VHL	Involved in renal cell cancer

Prevention

Chemoprevention

1. M.S., a 37-year-old woman, asks about taking medications to reduce her risk of cancer. Her mother died several years ago of colon cancer, and she fears that she also will develop the disease. Does taking anti-inflammatory medications alter the risk of cancer?

Cancer chemoprevention focuses on suppressing or reversing carcinogenesis in the early phases and preventing the development of invasive cancer. Also, much has been learned about the differences that exist among people and the interindividual variability in their inherited susceptibility to carcinogenic exposures.[12] This type of information will be useful in the design of a chemoprevention program that can be personalized for a specific individual. Chemoprevention strategies can be categorized as primary prevention (i.e., preventing cancer in a healthy individual at high risk), secondary prevention (i.e., preventing cancer in an individual with a premalignant lesion), or tertiary prevention (i.e., preventing a second primary cancer in an individual already cured of a prior malignancy).[13] Chemoprevention may involve treatment with nutrients or natural or synthetic chemicals that exert their protective effects by reversing the abnormal differentiation, inhibiting proliferation, or inducing apoptosis (programmed cell death) of premalignant cells. Other agents can act to block the uptake of carcinogens into cells, inhibit the activation of procarcinogens by various enzymes, or directly detoxify activated carcinogens.[14] Specific phases of carcinogenesis that are current targets for chemoprevention include genes that direct tumorigenesis and metastasis, cell signaling pathways, and genetic (i.e., chromosomal) instability common to malignancies.[14,15]

Chemoprevention studies are designed to detect changes in the incidence of cancer, as well as the rate of regression, progression and recurrence of premalignant lesions. Because long-term, perhaps even lifelong, therapy with an effective chemoprotectant may be necessary, ideal chemoprotectants should be safe and inexpensive. Once-daily dosing (or less) is desirable to maximize adherence. Another important aspect of effective chemoprevention is the ability to identify individuals at high risk for specific cancers through genetic susceptibility assessments, biomarkers of lifestyle or environmental exposures, or detection of premalignant cellular changes or lesions. These individuals are most likely to benefit from chemoprevention or should be encouraged to participate in a clinical trial. Findings from several large trials are described in Table 88-4.

Colon cancer is the second leading cause of cancer death; therefore, the search for agents that can lower the risk for this disease is warranted. In colorectal cancer cells and adenomatous polyps, elevated levels of cyclooxygenase-2 (COX-2) enzyme, messenger RNA, and protein can be found and these are associated with increased proliferation and resistance to apoptosis. The action of cyclooxygenase may enhance the conversion of several procarcinogens into carcinogens, the production of oxygen-free radicals, and otherwise stimulate cell proliferation.[14] One option, therefore, is to recommend that M.S. discuss the use of aspirin or another nonsteroidal anti-inflammatory drug (NSAID) with her primary health care provider. These agents potentially reduce the risk of colon cancer, although their benefit in the general population has not been established.[16] In randomized, controlled clinical trials, aspirin, sulindac, and celecoxib have reduced the development of new or recurrent adenomas in high-risk patients.[16–20] Although aspirin has been shown to prevent adenomatous polyp formation, its use was associated with increased risk for stroke and serious bleeding. For patients with previous colorectal cancer,

Table 88-4 Large, Randomized Chemoprevention Trials

Trial	Agent	Population	Duration of Intervention (yr)	Endpoints	Outcomes
Anti-inflammatory Agents					
Sandler et al.[17]	Aspirin	Patients with history of colorectal cancer (N = 635)	1	Colorectal adenoma recurrence	Positive: lower relative risk for recurrent adenomas and time to detection of first adenoma.
Baron et al.[18]	Aspirin	Patients with a history of colorectal adenomas (N = 1,121)	1	Colorectal adenoma recurrence	Positive: lower relative risk for advanced neoplasms. Nonsignificant increases for stroke and serious bleeding in the aspirin group.
Chan et al.[21]	Aspirin	Patients with colorectal carcinoma (N = 130,274)		Colorectal carcinoma recurrence	Positive: lower incidence for cancers that overexpress cyclooxygenase 2 (COX-2) but not for cancers with weak or absent COX-2 expression.
APC[19]	Celecoxib	Patients with colorectal adenomas (N = 2,035)	3	Colorectal adenoma recurrence	Positive: lower incidence for adenomas. Increased risk for cardiovascular events.
PreSAP[20]	Celecoxib	Patients with colorectal adenomas (N = 1,561)	3	Colorectal adenoma recurrence	Positive: lower incidence for adenomas.
Antiestrogens					
BCPT[22]	Tamoxifen	Women of higher-than-average risk of breast cancer (N = 13,000)	5.7	Newly diagnosed breast cancer	Positive: reduced the risk of invasive and noninvasive cancers and the occurrence of estrogen receptor-positive tumors; tamoxifen received an indication for chemoprevention from the U.S. Food and Drug Administration
MORE[24]	Raloxifene	Postmenopausal women with osteoporosis (N = 7,705)	3	Newly diagnosed breast cancer	Positive: reduced the risk of invasive cancers.
IBIS-I[23]	Tamoxifen	Women of higher risk of breast cancer	5	Newly diagnosed breast cancer	Positive: risk-reducing effect persists for at least 10 yrs; higher risk for deep-vein thrombosis and pulmonary embolism, but not after tamoxifen stopped.
STAR[25]	Tamoxifen versus raloxifene	Postmenopausal women at high risk for breast cancer (N = 19,747)	5	Newly diagnosed breast cancer	Positive: raloxifene as effective as tamoxifen for reducing risk of invasive breast cancer; lower risk of thromboembolic events.

recent studies suggest that aspirin's use for preventing further tumorigenesis will be more beneficial for those with prior tumors that overexpress COX-2 compared with those that do not overexpress it.[21] Celecoxib use also prevents adenomatous polyp formation, but cardiovascular risk is also increased.[19,20]

Finally, M.S. should be encouraged to modify her lifestyle in ways that reduce her overall risk of cancer. These include maintaining a healthy body weight, following a healthy diet, participating in a regular exercise program, avoiding tobacco and other known carcinogens, and avoiding or limiting alcohol consumption.

2. J.M., a 45-year-old woman, tells you that her twin sister was recently treated for breast cancer. She heard on the news that relatives of breast cancer patients are at higher risk for developing the disease and that a drug is now available that can prevent breast cancer. Should J.M. consider taking something to prevent breast cancer?

The Breast Cancer Prevention Trial (BCPT) of the National Surgical Adjuvant Breast Project (NSABP) enrolled 13,000 women who were at higher-than-average risk of developing breast cancer.[22] The trial demonstrated that the risk of invasive breast cancer was reduced by 49% in subjects treated with tamoxifen. During the 69-month follow-up period, 175 of the 6,599 women enrolled in the placebo arm developed invasive breast cancer, compared with 89 of the 6,576 women enrolled in the tamoxifen arm ($p < 0.00001$). Women in this trial received tamoxifen 20 mg/day orally for 5 years. It is important to note that women in the tamoxifen arm had a higher incidence of pulmonary embolism (relative risk [RR], 3.01) and endometrial cancer (RR, 2.53). These risks were greatest in women >50 years of age. The results of this trial led the U.S. Food and Drug Administration (FDA) to approve tamoxifen for the prevention of breast cancer in high-risk women. Longer term, some of the adverse effects associated with tamoxifen therapy (deep vein thrombosis and pulmonary embolism) appear to decrease with time (i.e., 5 years after completion of therapy).[23] Raloxifene, a selective estrogen receptor modulator approved for prevention of osteoporosis, also has been shown to reduce the risk of invasive breast cancer in women with osteoporosis. Patients receiving raloxifene showed an increased risk of thromboembolic disease, but they did not show an increased risk of endometrial cancer in this single trial.[24] Results from a randomized clinical trial comparing tamoxifen and raloxifene (STAR P-2) demonstrated that raloxifene 60 mg/day for 5 years is as effective as tamoxifen 20 mg/day in reducing the risk of invasive breast cancer, and has a lower risk for thromboembolic events.[25] Raloxifene may not be as beneficial as tamoxifen for noninvasive breast cancer because a nonstatistically higher risk for noninvasive breast cancer was found for subjects in the raloxifene group.

Because her sister developed breast cancer before menopause, J.M. may be at a higher-than-average risk for developing breast cancer and she may benefit from preventive therapy. J.M. should discuss the benefits and risks of chemoprevention with her primary health care provider.

Vaccines

3. M.M., a 35-year-old woman, asks you about vaccines to prevent cervical cancer. She heard that a vaccine is now available. Should M.M. consider this vaccine for herself or her daughter? Would this substitute for Pap smear screening?

Human papillomavirus (HPV) is primarily transmitted through sexual contact, and serotypes 16 and 18 (HPV-16, -18) cause approximately 70% of cervical cancers.[26] It is difficult to show that an intervention prevents cancer, because the time between exposure of the virus and tumorigenesis can be protracted. This would require several years and possibly decades to demonstrate efficacy; hence, key surrogate markers, such as cervical intraepithelial neoplasia, are used to assess efficacy. The FUTURE I and FUTURE II trials prospectively randomized 17,622 women between the ages of 15 and 26 years to receive either placebo or GARDASIL (Human Papilloma Virus Quadrivalent Vaccine).[27,28] Subjects received three injections over 6 months and were followed >3 years. The primary endpoint, occurrence of cervical intraepithelial neoplasia was reduced significantly in the vaccine group compared with the placebo group. No effect was observed on previously existing lesions, however, suggesting that the benefit for this vaccine appears to be limited to those with no prior exposure to the virus. The HPV serotypes present in the quadrivalent vaccine include types 6, 11, 16, and 18. At least 15 oncogenic HPV serotypes are not included in the vaccine, thus the vaccine does not prevent the possibility of contracting cervical cancer caused by the less common serotypes. Other vaccines that cover additional serotypes are under evaluation in clinical trials. Efficacy has also not been established in women >26 years of age who might be expected to have had more lifetime sexual partners, nor has it been tested for men. HPV screening should continue for all vaccinated women, because the vaccine does not cover all serotypes of HPV and the duration of vaccine induced anti-HPV immunity is unknown.

Diet

Diet has been linked to the development of colon, prostate, and breast cancers. Worldwide, colon cancer is the third most common cancer in the Western world,[29] but it is relatively uncommon in Africa and Asia, except Japan.[30] Epidemiologic studies show that the incidence of colon cancer in a population increases as individuals migrate from a low-incidence region to a high-incidence region, suggesting that diet or other environmental factors have an important impact on the etiology of colon cancer.[30] Western diets tend to contain more fat and less fiber compared with diets of low-incidence regions. Randomized trials, however, have been unable to show a benefit of high dietary fiber intake in reducing the recurrence of colorectal adenomas in people who have undergone resection of colorectal polyps.[12] Furthermore, the consequences of supplementing fiber in the diet may produce confounding factors, such as decreased fat intake, decreased caloric intake, and even weight loss. Nevertheless, the ACS advocates a healthy diet that consists of vegetables, fruit, whole grains, and fiber and is low in fat and limits red meats.

Similar to the incidence of colon cancer, migrant studies suggest that diet, environmental, or social factors play a role in the cause of prostate cancer, particularly in Asian men.[31] An increasing incidence of prostate cancer has been observed in Japan, which is thought to be associated with a shift toward a more westernized diet.[31] In women, the risk of breast cancer is increased with obesity and physical inactivity, but an association with high-fat diet is less clear.[32] Furthermore, environmental or lifestyle factors influence the risk of breast cancer. For example, even moderate alcohol consumption has been associated with an increased risk of breast cancer.[33]

Sun Exposure

Most risk factors associated with skin cancer are uncontrollable variables, with the exception of sun exposure and other forms of ultraviolet radiation. The interaction between ultraviolet radiation and skin cancers is complex, because nonmelanomas (e.g., basal cell and squamous cell carcinomas) are associated with total cumulative ultraviolet radiation exposure, whereas melanomas are associated with intermittent sun exposure.[34] The risk of melanoma is further increased in people who have a history of five or more severe sunburns in their lifetime, particularly during adolescence.[34] A rising incidence of melanoma skin cancers is thought to be caused by excessive, intermittent sun exposures—particularly among individuals who travel to sunny regions during the winter and to depletion of the ozone layer in the stratosphere.[34] Prevention is simply based on limiting sun exposure. The ACS guidelines recommend avoiding or limiting sun exposure from 10 AM to 4 PM when the ultraviolet rays are the strongest. Protective clothing, including a hat, sunglasses, and long-sleeved shirt and pants, and sunscreens are also advised to minimize exposure. The protective effects of sunscreens alone against melanoma, particularly for intentional sun exposure, is controversial.[35] To reduce the risk of skin cancer, individuals should be cautioned to limit direct sun exposure whenever possible.

Tumors

Growth

CELL CYCLE TRANSITION

Cancer cells, as with normal cells, proceed through a specific and orderly set of events during cellular replication referred to as the cell cycle (Fig. 88-2). The cell cycle contains four phases (S, M, G_1, and G_2) of activity, each responsible for a different task necessary for cell division. During the first activity phase, the M phase, the cell undergoes mitosis, the process of cell division. After mitosis, the cell enters the first gap or resting phase (G_1). During the G_1 phase, the cell makes the enzymes necessary for DNA synthesis. The synthesis of

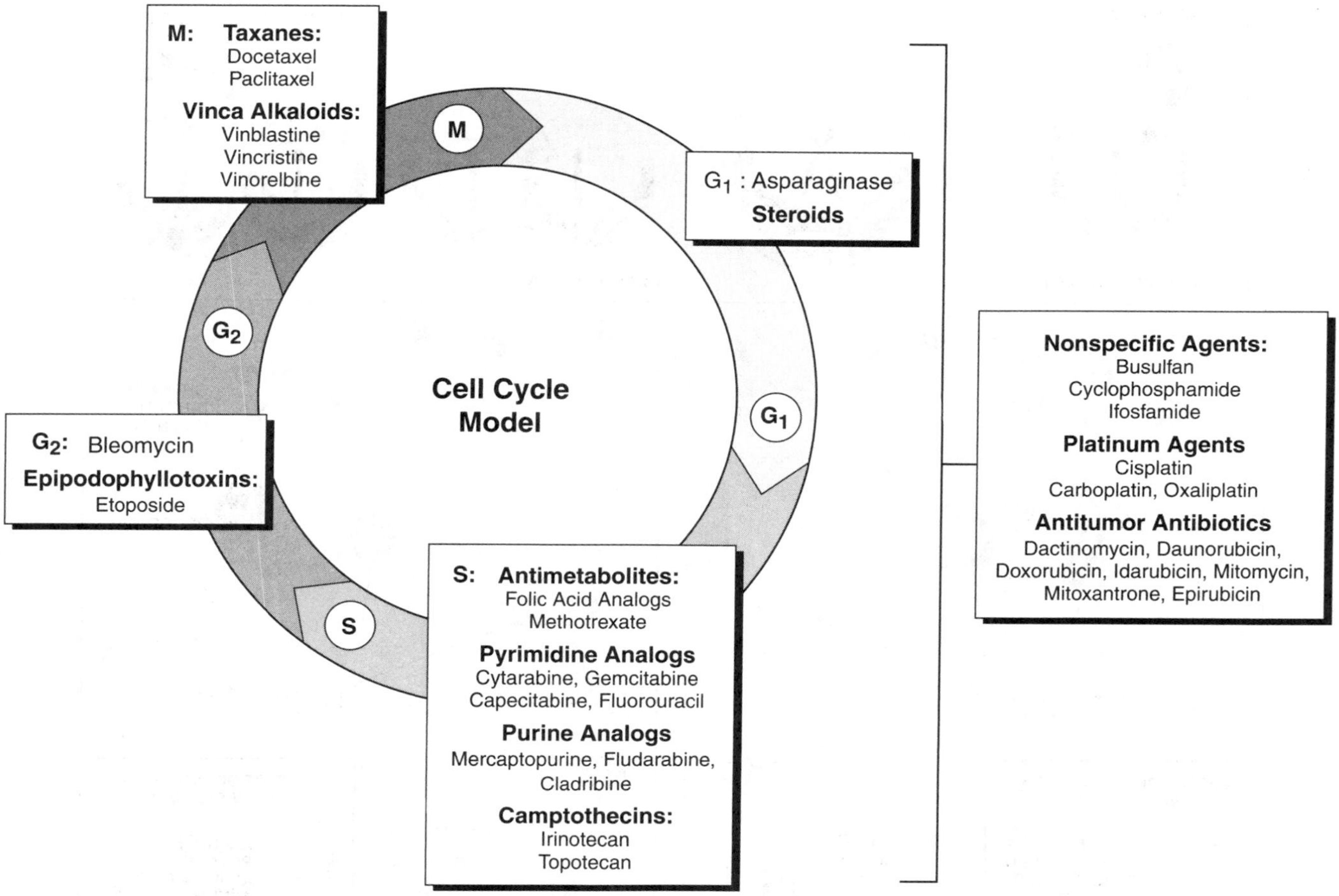

FIGURE 88-2 Cell cycle and effects of cytotoxic drugs on phases of the cell cycle.

DNA occurs during the next activity phase called the S phase. After the S phase, the cell enters a second gap phase (G_2). RNA and other proteins are synthesized during this gap phase to prepare for cell division during the M phase. The cells that complete mitosis may (a) continue to proceed through the cell cycle to divide again, (b) differentiate or mature into specialized cells and eventually die, or (c) enter a third resting phase called G_0.[36]

Proliferation of normal cells (or cell renewal) is under fine control to balance the loss of mature functional cells with the production of new cells. As mentioned, proto-oncogenes and tumor-suppressor genes provide the stimulatory and inhibitory signals, respectively, that regulate the cell cycle. The transition of cells through the cell cycle is an ordered, tightly regulated process, which involves a series of checkpoints that assess these signals and the number and integrity of the cells.[36] *Cyclins,* a group of interacting proteins found in the nucleus, and cyclin-dependent kinases (CDK), make up the molecular machinery that regulates passage of cells through various phases of the cell cycle. The cyclins combine with the CDK to form complexes that act as molecular switches. A molecular switch allows the cell to move through a critical restriction point that occurs late in the G_1 phase to the S phase. If insufficient amounts of cyclins or CDK are present during the G_1 phase, the cell will not enter the S phase to start cell division. Cells that pass through this point are irreversibly committed to the next phase of the cell cycle.[36] A decline in the level of the CDK complex signals the end of the phase.

The levels of cyclins and CDK are influenced by several factors, such as transcription of cyclin genes, degradation of cyclins, activities of CDK inhibitors, and the transfer of phosphate groups to various proteins and enzymes. Cues from the cell's external environment are transmitted to the nucleus via growth factor receptor signaling pathways, which influence formation of cyclins and cyclin–CDK complexes. The complexes generate phosphate groups from molecules of adenosine triphosphate (ATP) and transfer them to a protein called a retinoblastoma protein (pRB). If the pRB acquires enough phosphate groups, it will release the transcription factors the cell needs to make proteins essential for a cell division. Naturally occurring CDK inhibitors block cell cycle progression in response to inhibitory growth signals.

In cancer cells, the regulation and function of cyclins, CDK, and inhibitory proteins may be disrupted by a malignant transformation, or these proteins can undergo changes that cause a malignant transformation. Defects in these processes that are common in human cancers include deletion of the RB gene, a tumor suppressor gene that encodes for pRB, and dysregulation of the CDK through over-activation of CDK or loss of CDK inhibitors.[37] Without appropriate pRB regulation of cell cycle

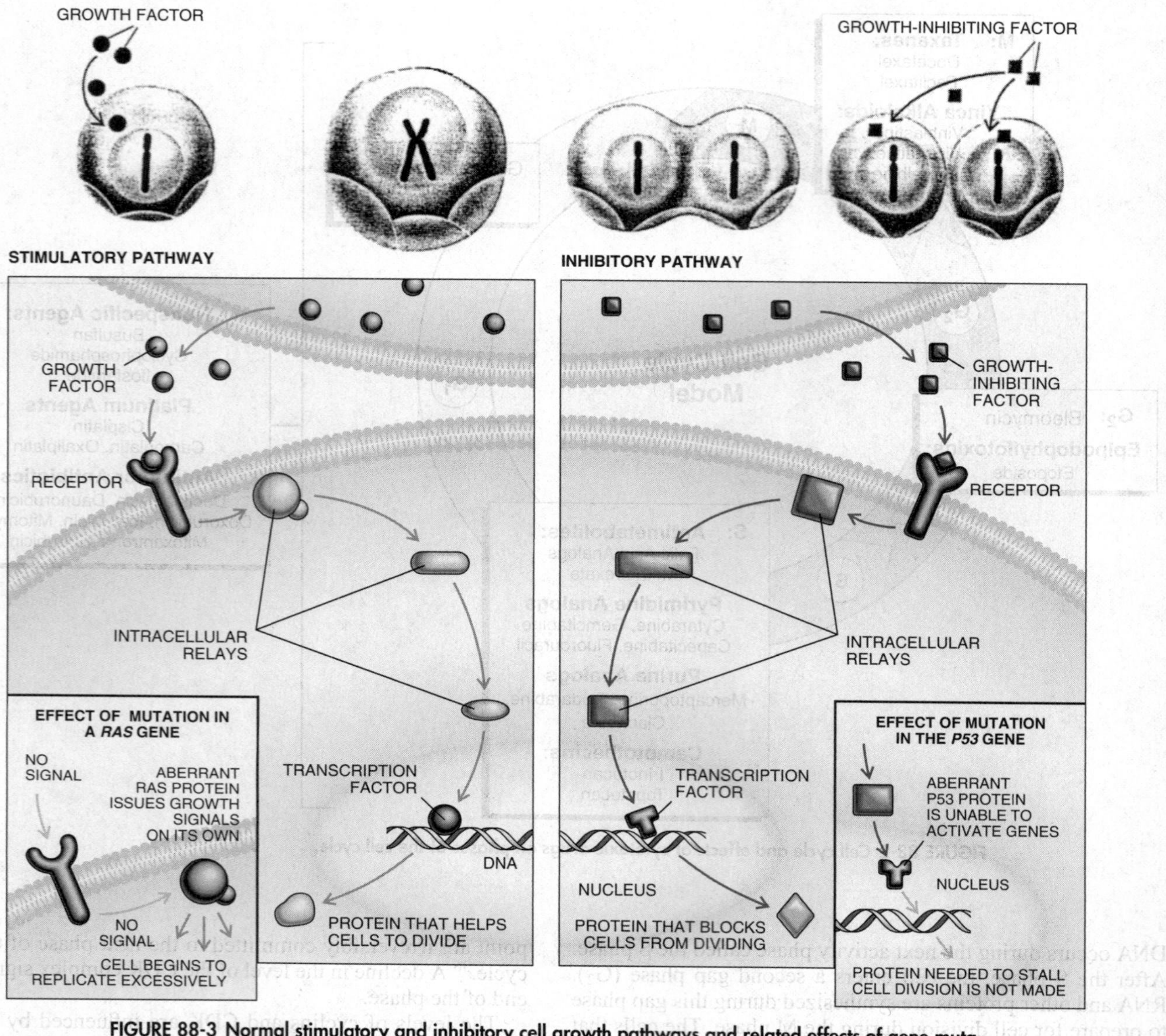

FIGURE 88-3 Normal stimulatory and inhibitory cell growth pathways and related effects of gene mutations on cell proliferation. (From reference 127, with permission.)

transition from the G_1 to the S phase, excessive cell proliferation can occur. Loss or mutation of a second tumor suppressor gene, p53, is also common in human cancers, and is associated with the resistance of cancer cells to undergo cell cycle arrest or apoptosis (e.g., programmed cell death). In normal cells, the *p53* gene is responsible for temporarily arresting cell growth in response to biochemical or molecular damage until the damage can be repaired.[38] If the damage cannot be repaired, apoptosis is a normal cell suicide process that is initiated to prevent genetically damaged cells from growing uncontrollably. Figure 88-3 illustrates the normal stimulatory and inhibitory cell growth pathways and related effects of gene mutations on cell proliferation.

SURVIVAL

If the stimulatory and inhibitory growth signals do not program the cell to stop dividing, mechanisms, such as apoptosis and senescence (aging), can help control excessive cell division. Because abnormalities in the proto-oncogenes and tumor suppressor genes that regulate these processes are present in cancer cells, the balance between cell renewal and loss of mature (senescent) cells is disrupted. Also, cancer cells are less dependent on receiving stimulatory signals from external growth factors.[38] Furthermore, cancer cells possess unlimited replication potential, owing to their ability to activate telomerase.[1,39] Telomerase is an enzyme that synthesizes sequences of telomeres, thereby enabling cells to proliferate endlessly. The expression of telomerase in most normal human cells is suppressed but it is reactivated in most cancer cells.[38,39] Telomeres are repeats of DNA and DNA-binding proteins that form the ends of eukaryotic chromosomes.[39] Telomere loss occurs with each successive cell replication and, after a critical length is reached, the cell undergoes irreversible growth arrest (replicative senescence).[39] Unlike normal cells, in which a finite telomere sequence regulates their life span, cancer cells are capable of immortality through their ability to maintain their telomeres indefinitely. Strategies to inhibit telomerase activity in cancer cells comprise one of many new molecular approaches that are being studied. Efforts are underway to target key genes, proteins, and receptors that facilitate cancer cell growth.

Spread

4. D.J., a 14-year-old boy, presented to the emergency department with a painful, swollen right leg. X-ray examination confirmed a fracture that appeared to be caused by a tumor mass in the bone. Biopsy confirmed osteogenic sarcoma. A routine chest x-ray study showed three nodules that were also believed to be malignant tumors. Does D.J. also have lung cancer? Are the tumors in D.J.'s lungs related to the sarcoma in his leg?

The tumor nodules in D.J.'s lung are most likely metastases from the sarcoma in his leg. The ability of cancer cells to disseminate and form metastases represents their most malignant characteristic. Tumor metastases to distant sites generally have a greater effect than the primary tumor on the frequency of complications and the patient's quality of life (see Complications of Malignancy). Metastases also have a greater effect than the primary tumor on mortality, with metastases associated with most cancer-related deaths. Consequently, individuals diagnosed with metastases face a worse prognosis.

Cancer cells must develop new blood vessels to supply nutrients to the cells and to spread to distant sites (metastasize). In response to low oxygen supply (hypoxia) and other factors, the cancer cells and surrounding tissues secrete growth factors that stimulate the growth of the new blood vessels (or angiogenesis) from existing blood vessels in the surrounding normal host tissue. Although many growth factors secreted by the tumor can be considered angiogenic, vascular endothelial growth factor (VEGF), platelet derived growth factor (PDGF), and basic fibroblast growth factor (bFGF) are considered those most important for sustained endothelial cell growth. Once released by the tumor cells, these growth factors bind to tyrosine kinase receptors on the surface of endothelial cells of existing blood vessels and activate a series of intracellular relay proteins that transmit a signal to genes in the nucleus to produce factors required for new endothelial cell growth.[40] Once the older endothelial cells become activated by the growth factors, they begin making matrix metalloproteinase enzymes (MMP). These enzymes destroy the extracellular matrix of the surrounding cells, allowing the older endothelial cells to invade the extracellular matrix and begin cell division.[40] This process of invasion and proliferation is repeated several times until new blood vessels are formed.

Tumor cells can utilize these newly formed blood vessels to facilitate their spread to distant locations. They must break away from the primary tumor and travel to other sites in the body to form metastases. Normally, cells adhere to both other cells and the extracellular matrix. The cell-to-cell adhesion molecules are called *cadherins,* and the cell-to-extracellular matrix molecules are called *integrins.* In cancer cells, these molecules are often absent, allowing tumor cells to easily move away from the primary tumor mass.

Once a tumor cell breaks off, it can move through the body to form metastatic sites. Two primary pathways, the blood vessels and the lymphatics, play a critical role in determining the location of metastatic sites (Table 88-5). A tumor cell can travel only to a distant site that receives blood or lymph from the primary site. Usually, tumor cells spread to the first capillary bed they encounter after their release from the primary tumor. If the primary site drains its blood supply into the vena cava, the cancer cells will reach the capillary bed in lung. Similarly, if the primary site drains its blood supply into the portal circulation, the cancer cells will reach the capillary bed in the liver. In addition, cancer cells can potentially pass through the first capillary bed they encounter and enter the arterial circulation. If malignant cells reach the arterial circulation, they can distribute to other organs and tissues throughout the body. Growth conditions (e.g., growth factors, physiologic conditions) within a tissue or organ also can determine the location of a metastatic site. After a cancer cell establishes a metastatic site, it must again undergo angiogenesis to ensure continued growth. Together, angiogenesis and hematogenous or lymphatic spread help cancer cells invade healthy tissues and increase morbidity and mortality associated with the disease.

Table 88-5 Common Cancers and Sites of Metastases

Cancer	*Most Common Sites of Metastases*
Bladder	Pelvis, lymph nodes
Breast	
• Premenopausal	Lymph nodes, skin, lung, liver, bone, brain
• Postmenopausal	Lymph nodes, bone, soft tissue
Colon	Lymph nodes, liver, lung, adrenals, ovary, bone
Lung	
• Non–small-cell	Lymph nodes, liver, bone, brain, adrenals
• Small-cell	Lymph nodes, bone, liver, bone marrow, brain
Lymphomas	
• Hodgkin disease lymphoma	Liver, spleen, stomach, bone marrow, lung
• Non-Hodgkin	Gastrointestinal tract, bone marrow, liver, lung, central nervous system
Ovary	Peritoneum, lung
Prostate	Lymph nodes, bone, liver

Screening and Early Detection

Standardized screening tests can help identify disease in asymptomatic individuals (screening) or help diagnose a disease in symptomatic individuals (early detection). Ideally, a screening test should be quick and simple to maximize compliance with screening recommendations. The cancer screening tests recommended by the ACS meet four basic requirements: (a) there must be good evidence that the test is effective in reducing morbidity or mortality (e.g., effective treatment must be available for the screened disease); (b) the benefits of the test should outweigh its risks; (c) the costs of the test should be in balance with its presumed benefits; and (d) the test should be practical and feasible within the existing health care setting. Various professional organizations, including the ACS, regularly publish recommendations for cancer screening[3,41] (Table 88-6).

Recommendations for cancer screening tests have been in existence for decades. As advances are made in screening techniques and the management of certain cancers, recommendations for cancer screening are updated as new information becomes available. Although the concepts of cancer screening and early cancer detection seem intuitively beneficial,

Table 88-6 Guidelines for Screening Cancer

	American Cancer Society[†]	*National Comprehensive Cancer Network*
Self-Examination		
Breast self-examination	20 yr: monthly	20 yr: encouraged
Testicular self-examination	Not recommended	Not recommended
Skin	Not recommended	Not recommended
Clinician Examination		
Clinical breast examination	20–39 yr: every 3 yr 40 yr: annually	20–39 yr: every 1–3 yr 40 yr: annually High risk: begin earlier and more frequently, depending on risk
Digital rectal examination	Colon: not recommended Prostate: if life expectancy 10 yr, 50 yr (normal risk) or 40–45 yr (high risk): annually	Not recommended
Pelvic examination	18 yr: annually	18 yr or within 3 yr of onset of sexual activity: annually
Sigmoidoscopy	Normal risk, 50 yr: every 5 yr, preferably with annual FOBT, as alternative to colonoscopy every 10 yr or double-contrast barium enema every 5 yr High risk: begin earlier than age 50 yr and/or more frequently	Normal risk, 50 yr: every 5 yr with annual FOBT, as alternative to colonoscopy every 10 yr or double-contrast barium enema every 5 yr High risk: begin earlier than age 50 yr and more frequently, depending on risk
Colonoscopy	Normal risk, 50 yr: every 10 yr as alternative to annual FOBT, sigmoidoscopy every 5 yr, or double-contrast barium enema every 5 yr High risk: begin earlier than age 50 yr and more frequently	Normal risk, 50 yr: every 10 yr with annual FOBT, as alternative to sigmoidoscopy every 5 yr, or double-contrast barium enema every 5 yr High risk: begin earlier than age 50 yr and more frequently, depending on risk
Laboratory Tests		
Stool guaiac	50 yr: annually High risk: begin earlier than age 50 yr: annually	50 yr: annually
Prostate specific antigen	If life expectancy 10 yr, 50 yr (normal risk), or 40–45 yr (high risk): annually	Normal risk, life expectancy 10 yr, 50 yr: annually High risk, life expectancy 10 yr, 45 yr: annually
Pap smear	21 yr or within 3 yr of onset of sexually activity if earlier: annually (regular Pap test) or every 2 yr (liquid-based Pap test) 30 yr: every 2–3 yr if three normal prior consecutive Pap test results 70 yr: optional if three or more normal prior consecutive Pap test results and no abnormal Pap test results in the last 10 yr	21 yr or within 3 yr of onset of sexually activity if earlier: annually (regular Pap test) or every 2 yr (liquid-based Pap test) 30 yr: every 2–3 yr if three normal prior consecutive Pap test results 70 yr: optional if three or more normal prior consecutive Pap test results and no abnormal Pap test results in the last 10 yr
Mammogram	40 yr: annually High risk: begin earlier than aged 40 yr and/or have additional tests or more frequent testing	40 yr: annually High risk: begin earlier and more frequently, depending on risk

[†] Listed year is age at which screening begins.
CBE, clinical breast examination; FOBT, fecal occult blood test.

particularly for cancers for which treatments are available, the acceptance of various cancer screening recommendations remains controversial. The question that still needs to be answered is, "Will screening alter the natural history of the disease or simply detect the disease earlier without changing patient morbidity?" The NCI is following up more than 154,000 men and women who enrolled in the Prostate, Lung, Colorectal and Ovary (PLCO) Cancer Screening Trial to determine whether screening affects morbidity or mortality. One-half of participants have specific screening tests; the other half receives routine health care. Because the testing and follow-up occur over 16 years, the results will be unavailable for several years. Interestingly, cancer screening may not alter the mortality or morbidity associated with various cancers. Recent cancer statistics show that patients are still being diagnosed with potentially curable cancers late in the course of the disease, despite the introduction of these recommendations two decades ago.

As new information becomes available, the various professional organizations modestly change their cancer screening recommendations. Only minor changes have been made to the recommendations since the ACS first published its guidelines, because a newly discovered tumor marker or diagnostic procedure must first be validated as a screening test. New tests should fit the four basic requirements the ACS used to develop the current guidelines, including cost:benefit ratio. Because a new screening test could add substantial costs to an already stressed health care system, its costs, benefits, and risks should be evaluated thoroughly before it is recommended for routine use. Screening recommendations also accommodate patients who are at higher than average risk for developing cancer owing to genetic, environmental, and lifestyle factors.

Diagnosis and Staging

The histologic diagnosis of a tumor is the most important determinant of how a malignancy will be treated. This is because a tumor's histologic classification influences its natural history, pattern of progression, and responsiveness to treatment. A surgical biopsy or excision of the primary tumor, followed by a microscopic and a biochemical evaluation by a pathologist, can provide the most accurate histologic diagnosis. Thereafter, staging can begin.

5. J.S. is diagnosed with breast cancer after a large breast mass was biopsied. Chemotherapy, radiation, and surgery all play an important role in the treatment of breast cancer. How does a clinician decide which treatment modalities are most appropriate for J.S.?

The stage of the cancer, as well as the histologic diagnosis, significantly influences both the treatment and prognosis. Staging is the process that determines the extent or spread of the disease. For J.S., staging is crucial to guide therapy. If her disease is limited to her breast, surgery followed by radiation, chemotherapy, or both or hormonal therapy would be recommended. If the cancer has spread beyond the breast, however, surgery may not be recommended. J.S. should immediately consider systemic therapy (chemotherapy or endocrine therapy) if she has advanced disease.

Staging schemas have been developed for all major types of cancers. For solid tumors, the most widely used and accepted staging classification is the TNM system, which incorporates the size of the primary tumor (T), the extent of regional lymph node spread (N), and the presence or absence of metastatic spread to distant organs (M). Within each TNM category, the extent of cancer involvement is related to prognosis. Determining the stage of the cancer often requires tests that can physically or radiographically measure the size of the primary tumor (e.g., radiographs, computed tomography [CT] scans, or magnetic resonance imaging [MRI] scans), dissect and pathologically examine regional lymph nodes, and assess the patient for evidence of tumor spread. In addition, positron emission tomography [PET] scans are being used more frequently to help determine whether tissues contain cancerous cells. To find evidence of a metastatic site, clinicians perform tests that assess the most likely sites of tumor metastases (Table 88-5) and they evaluate symptoms (e.g., pain) or signs (e.g., swelling, abnormal laboratory findings) that may indicate tumor involvement at a distant site.

An example of the TNM classification for solid tumors is shown in Table 88-7. Most solid tumor staging systems also incorporate the TNM classification into broader groups or stages to facilitate comparison among patient populations. Whereas the TNM system adequately stages solid tumors, this staging system does not adequately stage hematologic malignancies, including leukemias, lymphomas, and multiple myelomas. Because hematologic malignancies occur in the blood cells and lymphatic tissues that are widely distributed throughout the body, the TNM staging system cannot sufficiently describe these diseases. To define the extent of disease, guide treatment, and provide prognostic information, specific staging systems have been developed for various hematologic malignancies. Examples of widely accepted staging systems for hematologic malignancies include the Rai system for chronic lymphocytic leukemia and the Ann Arbor system for lymphomas.

Staging systems for some tumors include other characteristics to further determine the stage and prognosis of the disease. These characteristics may include clinical signs or symptoms or biochemical characteristics of the tumor. For example, the staging system used for Hodgkin disease includes a notation for constitutional symptoms (i.e., fever, night sweats, and weight loss). Studies indicate that these symptoms confer a poorer prognosis and could indicate the need for more intensive therapy. A subscript "B" (e.g., stage II_B) next to the stage indicates the patient has experienced these symptoms, whereas the subscript "A" indicates the patient has not experienced these symptoms.

Tumor staging is done at the time of initial diagnosis and periodically during treatment to assess the patient's response to therapy. Staging should also be repeated when (a) evidence shows that the cancer has either progressed during treatment or recurred following therapy to establish the most appropriate second-line therapy and (b) to enable measurement of response to that therapy.

Table 88-7 Staging of Breast Carcinoma

TNM Classification[a]

Primary Tumor (T)	
T1	Tumor 2 cm in greatest dimension
T2	Tumor >2 cm but not >5 cm in greatest dimension
T3	Tumor >5 cm in greatest dimension
T4	Tumor of any size with direct extension to chest wall or skin
Regional Lymph Nodes (N)	
N0	No regional lymph node metastasis
N1	Metastasis to movable ipsilateral axillary lymph node(s)
N2	Metastasis to ipsilateral axillary lymph node(s) fixed to one another or other structures
N3	Metastasis to ipsilateral internal mammary lymph node(s)
Distant Metastasis (M)	
M0	No distant metastasis
M1	Distant metastasis (includes metastasis to ipsilateral supraclavicular lymph nodes)

Stage Grouping

Stage I	T1	N0	M0
Stage II_A	T0	N1	M0
	T1	N1	M0
	T2	N0	M0
Stage II_B	T2	N1	M0
	T3	N0	M0
Stage III_A	T0	N2	M0
	T1	N2	M0
	T2	N2	M0
	T3	N1, N2	M0
Stage III_B	T4	N0, N1, N2	M0
Stage III_C	Any T	N3	M0
Stage IV	Any T	Any N	M1

[a] See text for full explanation of TNM system of classification.
TNM, tumor-node-metastasis.

Table 88-8 Signs and Symptoms Associated With Common Cancers

Cancer	*Local*[a]	*Distant*[b]
Bladder	Hematuria; bladder irritability; urinary hesitancy, frequency or urgency; dysuria; flank or pelvic pain	Edema of lower extremities and genitalia
Breast	Breast lumps; nipple retraction, dimpling, discharge; skin changes; axillary lymphadenopathy	Bone pain; elevated LFT; hypercalcemia
Colorectal	Change in bowel habits; in stool caliber; occult bleeding; constipation	Elevated LFT, CEA, and alkaline phosphatase; obstruction; hepatomegaly; perforation
Lung	New cough; hoarseness hemoptysis, dyspnea; unresolving pneumonias; chest wall pain; pain; dysphagia; effusion; tracheal obstruction	Anorexia; weight loss; elevated LFT; bone pain, hypercalcemia; jaundice; lymphadenopathy; osteoarthropathy; neurologic (brain metastases and neuromuscular disorders); SIADH
Lymphomas	Painless lymphadenopathy	Fever; night sweats; weight loss; bone or retroperitoneal pain; hepatomegaly; splenomegaly; abnormal CBC
Melanoma	Change in size, color, or shape of a pre-existing nevus	Lymphadenopathy; elevated LFT
Ovarian	Abdominal pain, discomfort, or enlargement; postprandial flatulence; vaginal bleeding; abdominal mass; urinary frequency; constipation, nausea; dyspepsia; early satiety	Peripheral neuropathies; pleural effusion; thrombophlebitis; elevated LFT; abdominal distention or pain; Addison or Cushing syndrome
Prostate	Urinary hesitancy; nocturia; poor urine stream; dribbling; terminal hematuria	Bone pain; elevated acid phosphatase, PSA, and alkaline phosphatase
Testicular	Painless enlargement; epididymitis; gynecomastia; back pain; infertility or erectile dysfunction	Elevated βhCG, α-fetoprotein, LD

[a]Local effects include those produced by the primary tumor.
[b]Distant effects include those associated with metastatic spread and paraneoplastic syndromes. Many cancers may not produce symptoms in the early stages, and diagnosis at that time depends on early detection and screening efforts.
CBC, complete blood count; CEA, carcinoembryonic antigen; hCG, beta human chorionic gonadotropin; LD, lactate dehydrogenase; LFT, liver function tests; PSA, prostate-specific antigen; SIADH, syndrome of inappropriate antidiuretic hormone secretion.

Clinical Presentation

The initial signs and symptoms of malignant disease are variable and predominantly depend on the histologic diagnosis, the location (including metastases), and the size of the tumor. Pain secondary to compression, obstruction, and destruction of adjacent tissues and organs is the most common presenting symptom. Other common initial symptoms reported by patients with cancer include anorexia, weight loss, and fatigue. Table 88-8 lists the common signs and symptoms associated with specific cancers. Some symptoms, however, may be obscured by a concomitant illness, such as chronic lung disease in patients with lung cancer. Whereas most tumors cause signs and symptoms early in the course of the disease, some cancers do not cause symptoms until late in the course of the disease and after significant tumor growth. In either of these circumstances, early diagnosis may be difficult. Thus, individuals at a higher-than-average risk should be screened regularly to help detect early disease.

6. P.N., a 59 year-old woman, presents with shortness of breath, fatigue, anorexia, weight loss, and abdominal pain and distention that have worsened significantly over the previous 3 weeks. An evaluation showed a large mass surrounding the head of her pancreas with biopsy results that confirm pancreatic adenocarcinoma. The staging workup confirmed the presence of distant metastases. Her husband states that she was previously an active person, but that she most recently has been unable to dress herself or participate in normal daily activities. He states that she spends most of the day in bed. Will her activity level influence the type of treatment that she can receive?

The description of P.N.'s daily activities indicates that she has a relatively poor performance status. Performance status is a measure of the functional capacity of the patient and reflects a patient's ability to ambulate, care for him- or herself, and carry out normal activities. For several tumors, a poor pretreatment performance status is associated with a decreased ability to tolerate treatment, decreased tumor response to treatment, and a worsened clinical outcome. In these cases, especially if the cancer is not known to respond well to treatment, a less aggressive treatment regimen may be recommended. For this reason, the performance status of a patient is important to assess at the time of staging evaluation and periodically during treatment. Different scales (i.e., Karnofsky score, Eastern Cooperative Oncology Group [ECOG]) can be used to determine performance status. The World Health Organization (WHO) performance scale is depicted in Table 88-9. Because P.N. has a WHO performance status of 3, her oncologist may recommend a less aggressive, less toxic treatment plan. Because other conditions could be responsible for her symptoms, P.N. should undergo a careful evaluation. Depression is a common problem in patients with cancer and, with treatment, can lead to improved patient outcomes.

7. G.D., a 68-year-old man, presents with lethargy, weakness, and nausea. His wife states that he does not take any medications

Table 88-9 World Health Organization (WHO) Performance Status Classification in Cancer

0	Able to carry out all normal activity without restriction
1	Restricted in physically strenuous activity but ambulatory and able to carry out light work
2	Ambulatory and capable of all self-care but unable to carry out work
3	Capable of only limited self-care; confined to bed or chair 50% or more of waking hours
4	Completely disabled; not capable of any self-care; confined to bed or chair

and only occasionally consumes alcohol. He has smoked two packs of cigarettes per day for the past 45 years. Routine laboratory tests reveal a serum sodium (Na) of 129 mEq/L (normal, 135–147). His chest radiograph shows a large mass in his right lung, which is consistent with malignancy. Is the hyponatremia related to G.D.'s lung cancer?

[SI unit: Na, 129 mmol/L (normal, 135–147)]

G.D.'s hyponatremia is likely caused by the syndrome of inappropriate antidiuretic hormone (SIADH) secretion caused by ectopic production of ADH (see Chapter 12, Fluid and Electrolyte Disorders) by his lung carcinoma. Although most signs and symptoms can be associated with the tumor, patients occasionally report symptoms or show clinical signs that are distant to the primary tumor site or metastases. These signs or symptoms, called *paraneoplastic effects*, are produced by substances secreted by the tumor. Table 88-10 lists some of the common paraneoplastic effects.

Complications of Malignancy

Cancer can have a profound effect on the patient's quality of life and his or her ability to tolerate appropriate therapy. For example, patients with malnutrition secondary to anorexia, mechanical obstruction, or pain may not tolerate some therapies because of significant physical debility. Tumor involvement of the liver, kidneys, or lungs also can complicate therapy by causing significant organ dysfunction and metabolic disturbances. In addition, compression or obstruction could produce a "mass effect" by impairing normal organ or tissue function and causing pain or other uncomfortable physical effects. Life-threatening physical effects that require immediate intervention include obstruction of the superior vena cava, spinal cord compression, and brain metastases.

Table 88-10 Paraneoplastic Syndromes Associated With Cancers

Syndrome	*Cancer*
Dermatologic	
Sweet syndrome	Hematologic malignancies and various carcinomas
Endocrine	
Addison syndrome	Adrenal carcinoma, lymphomas, and ovarian cancer
Cushing syndrome	Lung, thyroid, testicular, adrenal, and ovarian cancers
Hypercalcemia (not associated with bone metastases)	Lung cancer
Syndrome of inappropriate antidiuretic hormone secretion	Lung and head and neck cancers
Hematologic or Coagulation	
Anemia	Various cancers
Autoimmune hemolytic anemia	Chronic lymphocytic leukemia, lymphomas, ovarian cancer
Disseminated intravascular coagulation	Acute progranulocytic leukemia, lung and prostate cancers
Thrombophlebitis	Lung, breast, ovarian, prostate, and pancreatic cancers
Neuromuscular	
Dermatomyositis and polymyositis	Lung and breast cancers
Myasthenic syndrome (Eaton-Lambert syndrome)	Small-cell lung, gastric, and ovarian cancers
Sensory neuropathies	Small-cell lung and ovarian cancers

TREATMENT

8. T.J., a 40-year-old man with no significant medical history, presents to his physician with complaints of abdominal pain, nausea and vomiting, weakness, and weight loss. On physical examination, he is noted to be slightly icteric, and the only significant laboratory abnormality is mild anemia (hemoglobin [Hgb], 11 g/dL [normal, 14–18], hematocrit [Hct], 33% [normal, 39%–49%]). A CT scan of the abdomen reveals a mass present in the peripancreatic area that is suggestive of malignancy. T.J. is referred to a surgeon who explains that the first step in evaluating the mass is to obtain a tissue biopsy. T.J. asks the surgeon why he cannot remove all of the mass rather than take only part of it. He also wants to know whether this malignancy will be treated with surgery, radiation, chemotherapy, hormones, or immunotherapy. What is the basis for determining which cancer treatment modality is best suited for T.J.?

[SI units: Hgb, 110 g/L (normal, 140–180); Hct, 0.33 (normal, 0.39–0.49)]

Because a tissue diagnosis of malignancy has not been made, the appropriateness of more extensive surgery for T.J. can not be determined at this time. The choice of specific therapy depends not only on the histology and stage but also on the patient's predicted tolerance of the side effects and complications of the various treatment options. The goal of therapy should always be to cure the patient when possible. No matter what therapeutic options are under consideration, the likelihood of curing the patient is greater when the tumor burden is low. In most cases, either surgery or radiation therapy is the initial choice of therapy for localized tumors.

Surgery

Surgery is the oldest modality available to treat patients with cancer. With the recent advances in surgical techniques and an improved understanding of the patterns of tumor growth and spread, surgeons can now perform successful resections for an increasing number of patients. Surgery can play a significant role in preventing (e.g., removal of colonic polyps or cervical dysplasia), diagnosing, and staging various cancers (e.g., biopsy for histologic evaluation). Surgery can also be used to manage cases of both localized and advanced tumors. When surgery provides definitive (i.e., curative) therapy for a localized tumor, the surgeon removes the tumor plus a margin of normal tissue surrounding the tumor. For extensive, localized tumors that cannot be completely removed, patients may undergo surgery to resect the tumor partially in an attempt to improve the likelihood that subsequent chemotherapy or radiation therapy may successfully kill the tumor. Cytoreductive surgery may be useful only if effective therapies are available to treat the residual disease. Patients with limited metastatic disease (e.g., one or a few metastases at a single site) also may benefit from surgical resection of the metastases if the primary tumor can be controlled with other treatments. Cytoreductive surgery for limited metastatic disease includes resecting pulmonary metastases for sarcomas, hepatic metastases for colorectal cancer, and solitary brain metastases. Patients with metastatic disease also can have surgery to relieve pain or improve functional abnormalities caused by the advanced tumor (e.g., gastrointestinal obstruction). Patients can have palliative surgery to improve their quality of life without prolonging survival. Thus, surgery plays a critical role in cancer treatment.

Radiation Therapy

Radiation therapy can be used to eradicate localized tumor masses. Not all cancers are sensitive to the lethal effects of radiation, so this modality has limited application in the treatment of some cancers (Table 88-11). For others, however, radiation therapy provides potential advantages over surgery. For instance, radiation therapy could encompass a wider area around the tumor and remove the tumor from regions of the body where surgery cannot safely reach. Radiation therapy also can be used when surgery could result in considerable disability or disfigurement. Radiation allows patients to receive treatment to multiple sites simultaneously. The usefulness of radiation therapy can be limited by its toxic effects on normal tissues that surround the tumor, however, and these can be exacerbated if patients receive chemotherapy concomitantly or shortly after radiation therapy. Chemotherapy that follows completion of radiation therapy can produce a "radiation recall" of local toxicity which manifests as skin redness, and swelling and peeling at the radiation site. An established limit exists to the "dose" of radiation that can be delivered, depending on the type of tissue (e.g., bone, liver, brain) that is affected. Two methods are used most often to administer radiation to tumors. External-beam radiotherapy uses a radiation source (typically, a supervoltage electrical machine) that is located a certain distance from the site of intended treatment. Brachytherapy involves placement of radioactive seeds, pellets, or needles within or close to the site of the tumor. Newer radiation therapy techniques, including intraoperative radiation, hyperfractionated radiation, stereotactic radiosurgery, intensity modulated radiation therapy (IMRT), computerized three-dimensional conformal treatment planning, and chemoradiosensitization (e.g., concomitant radiation-sensitizing chemotherapy), may reduce associated toxicities, enhance tumor responsiveness, and improve its clinical usefulness.[42]

Not all cancers can be cured by surgery or radiation therapy. Some patients have tumors that have already metastasized at the time of initial diagnosis, whereas others have tumors that could not be completely eradicated with treatment or have recurred some time after primary therapy with surgery or radiation therapy. In these circumstances, the tumor cells have been released from the primary tumor. Systemic treatments, including chemotherapy, endocrine therapy, signal transduction pathway inhibitors, antiangiogenic agents, and biologic response modifiers, generally offer the only hope of rendering the patient free of disease. Although chemotherapy was developed to treat advanced cancers, these agents are now used to treat many stages of malignant diseases.

Table 88-11 Malignancies Frequently Treated With Radiation Therapy

Acute lymphocytic leukemia (CNS radiation)
Brain tumors
Breast cancer
Head and neck cancers, squamous cell
Lung cancer
• Non–small-cell lung cancer
• Small-cell lung cancer (CNS radiation in limited stage disease)
Lymphomas
Neuroblastoma
Prostate cancer
Rectal cancer
Testicular, seminoma

CNS, central nervous system.

Chemotherapy

Cytotoxic Chemotherapy

The era of cytotoxic chemotherapy can be traced to World War II, when an explosion of mustard gas produced bone marrow and lymphoid hypoplasia in seamen exposed to the gas.[43] This incident led to the use of alkylating agents (derivatives of mustard gas) in the treatment of Hodgkin disease and other lymphomas.[44]

MECHANISM OF ACTION

Classic cytotoxic chemotherapy kills cancer cells by damaging DNA, interfering with DNA synthesis, or otherwise inhibiting cell division. Chemotherapy agents have been classified by their effect on the cell cycle or their mechanism of action. Agents that affect the cell only during a specific phase of the cell cycle often are referred to as *phase-specific agents* or *schedule-dependent agents*. In contrast, agents that affect the cell during any phase of the cell cycle are often referred to as *phase-nonspecific agents* or *dose-dependent agents* (Fig. 88-2). As the understanding of cancer biology continues to grow, other mechanisms of cytotoxicity have been identified for many chemotherapy agents.

The specific mechanisms of action for several chemotherapy agents are described in Table 88-12. Because most agents affect the cell cycle, their lethal effects are not realized until the cells proceed through the cycle. These drugs are most cytotoxic to tumor cells with a high growth fraction (see Tumors: Growth) and least cytotoxic to tumor cells arrested in the G_0 phase.

CELL KILL

Rodent studies done during the 1960s demonstrated that the number of tumor cells killed by the chemotherapy is proportional to the dose when the growth fraction is 100% (i.e., all cells are dividing) and the tumor cells are sensitive to the agent.[45,46] For example, if a dose of chemotherapy reduces the tumor burden from 10^{10} to 10^8 cells, the same dose administered when only 10^7 cells are present should reduce the tumor burden to 10^5 cells. This theory has become known as the cell-kill or log-kill hypothesis (Fig. 88-4).

Table 88-12 Clinical Pharmacology of Commonly Used Chemotherapy Agents

Agents (Trade Name)	*Mechanism of Action*	*Pharmacokinetic Characteristics*	*Major Toxicities*
Alemtuzumab (Campath) Inj: 30 mg/mL	Monoclonal antibody; targets CD52 cell surface antigen; binding leads to lysis of CD52-positive leukemic cells	Half-life ($t_{1/2}$) 12 days; marked interpatient variability	Hypersensitivity and infusion reactions; myelosuppression, pancytopenia, opportunistic infection, nausea, vomiting, dyspnea, hypotension
Bevacizumab (Avastin) Inj: 25 mg/mL	Monoclonal antibody; inhibits development of new blood vessels (angiogenesis) by binding to and inhibiting vascular endothelial growth factor (VEGF) from interacting with receptors	$t_{1/2} = 11–50$ days	Hypertension, diarrhea, constipation; bleeding, thrombosis; gastrointestinal perforation; impaired wound healing; proteinuria; infusion reactions
Busulfan (Myleran, Busulfex) Tab: 2 mg Inj: 60 mg/10 mL	Alkylating agent; forms reactive intermediates that cross-link DNA	Well absorbed orally; metabolized extensively; no intact drug recovered in urine, but metabolites are excreted renally	Myelosuppression, pulmonary fibrosis, hyperpigmentation, hepatic dysfunction, seizures in high dose, suppression of testicular, ovarian, and adrenal function
Capecitabine (Xeloda) Tab: 150, 500 mg	Antimetabolite; prodrug metabolized to fluorouracil; incorporates into RNA and interferes with RNA function; inhibits thymidylate synthase and causes inhibition of DNA synthesis	$t_{1/2} = 0.75$ hr; 35% protein bound; C_{max} and AUC varies >85%.	Nausea, vomiting; stomatitis; hand-foot syndrome; bone marrow suppression; anorexia
Carboplatin (Paraplatin) Inj: 50, 150, 450 mg/vial	Nonclassic alkylating agent; binds to DNA to form interstrand cross-links and adducts	$t_{1/2}\alpha = 12–24$ min; $t_{1/2}\beta = 1.3–1.7$ hr; $t_{1/2}\gamma = 22–40$ hr; >90% excreted in urine	Myelosuppression (especially thrombocytopenia); nausea, vomiting
Cetuximab (Erbitux) Inj: 100 mg/50 mL 200 mg/100 mL	Monoclonal antibody; inhibits cell proliferation by preventing activation of the epidermal growth factor receptor (EGFR)	$t_{1/2} = 41–213$ hr; intrinsic clearance approximately 25% lower in females	Anaphylactic or anaphylactoid reactions; acneiform skin rash; asthenia; nausea, vomiting
Cisplatin (Platinol) Inj: 10, 50 mg/vial	Nonclassic alkylating agents; binds to DNA to form interstrand cross-links and adducts	$t_{1/2} = 20–30$ min; $t_{1/2} = 60$ min; $t_{1/2}\gamma = 24$ hr; >90% excreted in urine	Nephrotoxicity; nausea, vomiting; peripheral neuropathy; ototoxicity; hypomagnesemia; visual disturbances (rare)
Cyclophosphamide (Cytoxan) Inj: 100, 200, 500, 1,000, 2,000 mg/vial Tab: 25, 50 mg	Alkylating agent; metabolite generates reactive intermediates that cross-link DNA	Oral bioavailability 100%; activated in liver by microsomal enzymes to active compounds and toxic metabolites; 22% of parent and 60% of metabolites excreted in urine; $t_{1/2} = 3–10$ hr; 6.5–8 hr (alkylating activity)	Myelosuppression; hemorrhagic cystitis; nausea, vomiting; alopecia; cardiomyopathy (rare); "allergic" interstitial pneumonitis; SIADH
Daunorubicin (Cerubidine) Inj: 20 mg/vial	Antitumor antibiotic, intercalates to DNA double helix; topoisomerase II–mediated DNA damage; produces oxygen-free radicals	Extensive binding to tissues; known routes of elimination account for only 50% to 60% of dose; extensively metabolized by liver; $t_{1/2} =$ 40 min; $t_{1/2} = 45–55$ hr; 20% to 30% biliary excretion; 14%–23% excreted in urine as parent and metabolites	Myelosuppression, mucositis; alopecia cumulative cardiac toxicity; dose-related acute ECG changes; severe tissue damage if extravasated

(*continued*)

Table 88-12 Clinical Pharmacology of Commonly Used Chemotherapy Agents *(Continued)*

Agents (Trade Name)	*Mechanism of Action*	*Pharmacokinetic Characteristics*	*Major Toxicities*
Daunorubicin, liposomal (Daunoxome) Inj: 50 mg/vial	Antitumor antibiotic: intercalates into DNA double helix; topoisomerase II–mediated DNA damage; produces oxygen-free radicals		
Docetaxel (Taxotere) Inj: 40 mg/mL	Taxane; promotes microtubule assembly and arrests cell cycle in G_2 and M phases	$t_{1/2}\alpha = 4$ min; $t_{1/2}\beta = 36$ min; $t_{1/2}\gamma = 11$ hr; Cl 21 L/hr/m^2; Vd = 113 L	Peripheral edema; bone marrow suppression; hypersensitivity reaction
Doxorubicin (Adriamycin, Rubex) Inj: 10, 20, 50, 100, 150, 200 mg/vial	Antitumor antibiotic; intercalates into DNA double helix; topoisomerase II–mediated DNA damage; produces oxygen-free radicals	Extensive binding to tissues; known routes of elimination only account for 50%–60% of dose; extensively metabolized by liver; $t_{1/2}\alpha = 40$ min; $t_{1/2}\beta = 45$–55 hr; 20%–30% biliary excretion; 14%–23% excreted in urine as parent and metabolites	Myelosuppression; mucositis; nausea, vomiting; alopecia; cumulative cardiac toxicity; dose-related acute ECG changes; severe tissue damage if extravasated
Doxorubicin, liposomal (Doxil) Inj: 20 mg	Antitumor antibiotic; intercalates into DNA double helix; topoisomerase II–mediated DNA damage; produces oxygen-free radicals		
Epirubicin (Ellence) Inj: 50 mg/25 mL, 200 mg/100 mL	Anthracycline antitumor antibiotic; intercalates into DNA double helix; topoisomerase II–mediated DNA damage; produces oxygen-free radicals.	$t_{1/2}\alpha = 3$ min, $t_{1/2}\beta = 2.5$ hr, $t_{1/2}\gamma = 33$ hr; protein binding 77%; epirubicin or metabolite excretion in bile (35%) or urine (20%); plasma clearance reduced 35% in patients ≤70 yr	Myelosuppression; nausea, vomiting, diarrhea, mucositis, alopecia; cumulative dose-related cardiomyopathy, acute ECG changes; severe tissue damage (if extravasated);
Erlotinib (Tarceva) Oral tablets: 25, 100, and 150 mg	Small molecule inhibitor; epidermal growth factor receptor (EGFR) tyrosine kinase antagonist.	Oral bioavailability 60%; food increases bioavailability to 100%; protein binding approximately 93%; hepatic metabolism primarily CYP3A4 and also CYP1A1 and CYP1A2; $t_{1/2}$ approximately 36 hr	Diarrhea, acne-form rash, appetite loss, interstitial lung disease
Etoposide (VePesid) Inj: 100 mg/5 mL Cap: 50 mg	Epipodophyllotoxin; produces DNA strand breaks by inhibiting topoisomerase II; arrests cells in late S or early G_2 phase	Oral bioavailability 37%–67% (average 50%); 30%–40% excreted rapidly in the urine (70% of excreted drug is unchanged); terminal $t_{1/2}$ = 6–8 hr; 6%–15% excreted in bile; >2% excreted in feces	Myelosuppression; nausea, vomiting; alopecia; mucositis; hypotension (related to rapid-infusion); hypersensitivity reactions; fever; bronchospasm
Fluorouracil Inj: 500 mg/vial	Antimetabolite; incorporates into RNA, interferes with RNA function; inhibits thymidylate synthase and inhibits DNA synthesis	$t_{1/2} = 6$–20 min; 90% hepatically metabolized.	Mucositis; diarrhea, myelosuppression; dermatologic, nausea, vomiting
Gemcitabine (Gemzar) Inj: 200 mg/vial or 1,000 mg/10 mL	Antimetabolite; inhibits ribonucleotide synthesis reductase and inhibits DNA synthesis	Parameters dependent on infusion; $t_{1/2} = 32$–94 min or 245–638 min; V = 50 L/m^2 or 370 L/m^2	Bone marrow suppression; flulike syndrome; nausea, vomiting; edema
Gemtuzumab ozogamicin (Mylotarg) Inj: 5 mg/20 mL	Monoclonal antibody; linked to a calicheamicin cytotoxic derivative; targets CD33 antigen on leukemic blast cells; binding introduces cytotoxic into cells, causing DNA strand breakage and cell death	$t_{1/2}$ calicheamicin 45 hr (total) and 100 hr (unconjugated); $t_{1/2}$ antibody 72 hr; probably undergoes hepatic metabolism but metabolic studies have not been performed	Myelosuppression (severe); hypersensitivity and infusion reactions; pulmonary events (dyspnea, pleural effusion, pulmonary infiltrates, acute respiratory distress syndrome); hepatotoxicity; nausea, vomiting

Ibritumomab tiuxetan (Zevalin) Inj: 10 mg/10 mL, 50 mg/50 mL	Monoclonal antibody; Yttrium-90 (Y-90)-linked antibody directed against the CD20 antigen on malignant B lymphocytes; binds to antigen and releases radiation (β particles) which induces cell damage and death	Mean effective $t_{1/2}$ for Y-90 = 30 hr; median of 7.2% of injected radioactivity recovered in urine over 7 days; Y-90 particle decay $t_{1/2}$ = 64 hr.	Infusion reactions (hypotension, angioedema, hypoxia, bronchospasm); asthenia, chills, nausea; myelosuppression; see also rituximab
Idarubicin (Idamycin) Inj: 5, 10 mg/vial	Antitumor antibiotic; intercalates into DNA double helix; topoisomerase II–mediated DNA damage; produces oxygen-free radicals.	Terminal $t_{1/2}$ = 15–18 hr	Myelosuppression; muscositis; anorexia; nausea, vomiting; diarrhea; fever; alopecia
Imatinib mesylate (Gleevec) Tab: 100 mg, 500 mg	Tyrosine kinase inhibitor; inhibits kinases for Bcr-Abl, platelet-derived growth factor (PDGF), c-kit, and stem cell factor, thereby inhibiting cell proliferation and inducing apoptosis	Mean bioavailability = 98%; C_{max} 2–4 hr; $t_{1/2}$ of imatinib (18 hr) and major metabolite (40 hr); plasma protein binding 95%; hepatically metabolized via CYP3A4; eliminated as unchanged drug in feces (20%) and urine (5%); interpatient variability in clearance = 40%; susceptible to alterations in clearance with CYP3A4 inducers and inhibitors	Fluid retention, edema; nausea, vomiting, diarrhea; rash, fatigue, muscle cramps, musculoskeletal pain; intratumoral bleeding; myelosuppression, hepatic toxicity
Irinotecan (Camptosar) Inj: 20 mg/mL	Campthothecin; inhibits DNA-strand religation by binding topoisomerase I-DNA complex.	$t_{1/2}$ = 6 hr; 36%–68% protein bound	Diarrhea; cholinergic syndrome; myelosuppression
Isofamide (Ifex) Inj: 1, 3 g/vial	Alkylating agent; metabolites generates reactive intermediates that cross-link DNA	Parameters are dose and schedule dependent; 60%–80% excreted in urine as unchanged drug or metabolite within 72 hr	Myelosuppression; hemorrhagic cystitis (should be administered with MESNA); nephrotoxicity; neurotoxicity; anorexia; nausea, vomiting; alopecia
Mercaptopurine (Purinethol) Tab: 50 mg	Antimetabolite; metabolites incorporated into DNA or RNA and inhibit purine synthesis.	Oral absorption highly variable; $t_{1/2}\gamma$ = 20–60 min; elimination primarily hepatic.	Myelosuppression; anorexia, nausea, vomiting; hepatic toxicity (biliary stasis)
Methotrexate Tab: 2.5 mg Inj: 25, 50, 100, 200, 250, 1,000 mg/vial	Antifolate; inhibits dihydrofolate reductase and depletes reduced folates and inhibits DNA synthesis	Oral absorption appears to be better with smaller doses; exhibits interpatient bioavailability; "third space" collections of fluid may provide a reservoir for drug accumulation; $t_{1/2}$ = 1.5–3.5 hr; $t_{1/2}$ = 8–15 hr; 90% dose excreted in urine within 24 hr	Myelosuppression; nephrotoxicity; hepatotoxicity; mucositis, pulmonary toxicity; neurotoxicity
Oxaliplatin (Eloxatin) Inj: 50 mg/10 mL; 100 mg/20 mL	Nonclassic alkylating agent; binds to DNA to form interstrand cross-links and adducts	$t_{1/2}\,\alpha$ = 0.43 hr, $t_{1/2}\,\beta$ = 16.8 hr, $t_{1/2}$ = 391 hr; Vd ultrafilterable platinum = 440 L; extensive and irreversible plasma protein binding (>90%); nonenzymatically biotransformed; renal primary route of elimination: 54% at 5 days	Anaphylactic or anaphylactoid reactions; peripheral sensory neuropathy, sensitivity to cold, jaw spasm, dysphagia; nausea, vomiting, diarrhea, fatigue; pulmonary fibrosis
Paclitaxel (Taxol) Inj: 30 mg/vial	Taxane; promotes microtubule assembly and arrests cell cycle in G_2 and M phases.	<10% excreted in urine; liver and biliary primary routes of elimination; $t_{1/2}\alpha$ = 0.3 hr; $t_{1/2}\beta$ = 1.3–8.6 hr	Hypersensitivity reactions (premedications recommended); cardiac disturbances; sensory neuropathy; myalgia; arthralgia; myelosuppression

(continued)

Table 88-12 Clinical Pharmacology of Commonly Used Chemotherapy Agents *(Continued)*

Agents (Trade Name)	*Mechanism of Action*	*Pharmacokinetic Characteristics*	*Major Toxicities*
Pemetrexed (Alimta) Inj: 500 mg/20 mL	Multitargeted antifolate; disrupts folate metabolic pathway through inhibition of thymidylate synthase, dihydrofolate reductase, and glycinamide ribonucleotide formyl transferase	Protein binding approximately 81%; 70%–90% excreted unchanged renally; $t_{1/2}$ 2–4 hr	Rash, diarrhea, leukopenia, neutropenia, thrombocytopenia
Rituximab (Rituxan) Inj: 100 mg/10 mL, 500 mg/50 mL	Monoclonal antibody; lyses B cells by recruiting immune effectors	$t_{1/2}$ variable	Tumor lysis; hypersensitivity reactions; mucocutaneous reactions; lymphopenia
Sorafenib (Nexavar) Tabs: 200 mg	Multikinase enzyme inhibitor; raf kinase inhibitor; angiogenesis blockade (VEGFR), PDGFR, Flt3, c-KIT, p-38	Bioavailability 38%–49%; take on empty stomach; protein binding 99.5%; hepatic metabolism primarily CYP3A4 and UGT1A9; $t_{1/2}$ 24–48 hr	Hypertension, rash, hand-foot syndrome, diarrhea, myelosuppression
Sunitinib (Sutent) Cap: 12.5, 25, and 50 mg	Multikinase enzyme inhibitor; angiogenesis inhibitor; VEGFR, PDGFR, bFGF inhibition	Protein binding: 95% for parent molecule and primary metabolite; hepatic metabolism primarily CYP3A4; $t_{1/2}$ 40–60 hr for parent molecule and 80–110 hr for metabolite	Skin discoloration, rash, diarrhea, myelosuppression, prolonged QT interval
Tositumomab (Bexxar) Inj: 35 mg/2.5 mL, 225 mg/16.1 mL	Monoclonal antibody; iodine-131 (I-131)-linked antibody directed against the CD20 antigen on malignant B lymphocytes; binds to antigen and induces apoptosis, complement- or antibody-depended cell cytotoxicity; ionizing radiation induces cell damage and death	Total body clearance influenced by high tumor burden, extent of splenomegaly and bone marrow involvement; I-131 eliminated in urine (98% of administered dose); I-131 and particle decay $t_{1/2} = 8.04$ days	Hypersensitivity reactions; myelosuppression; hypothyroidism; nausea, vomiting, abdominal pain, diarrhea; myelodysplastic syndrome, acute leukemia
Trastuzumab (Herceptin) Inj: 440 mg/30 mL	Monoclonal antibody; inhibits proliferation of human tumor cells that express HER2 proto-oncogene	$t_{1/2} = 5.8$ hr; Vd = 44 mL/kg.	Cardiomyopathy; diarrhea; nausea, vomiting; hypersensitivity reaction
Vincristine (Oncovin) Inj: 1, 2, 5 mg/vial; 2-mg prefilled syringe	Vinca alkaloid; reversibly inhibits of mitosis; binds to microtubule protein, tubulin and ultimately inhibiting formation of mitotic spindles	$t_{1/2}\alpha = <1$ min; $t_{1/2}\beta = 7.4$ min; $t_{1/2}\gamma = 164$ min	Neurotoxicity (primarily distal neuropathy that affects sensory and motor abilities); autonomic neuropathies (high dosages); SIADH; vesicant (if extravasated)
Vinorelbine (Navelbine) Inj: 10 mg/1 mL; 50 mg/5 mL	Vinca alkaloid; reversibly inhibits mitosis; binds to microtubule protein, tubulin and ultimately inhibits formation of mitotic spindles	<20% excreted in urine; $t_{1/2}\alpha = 2$–6 min; $t_{1/2}\beta = 1.9$ hr, $t_{1/2}\gamma = 20$–40 hr	Leukopenia; neurotoxicity; DTR; vesicant (if extravasated)

Cap, capsule; CSF, cerebrospinal fluid; DTR, deep tendon reflexes; GI, gastrointestinal; Inj, injection; PT, prothromboplastin time; PPT, partial thromboplastin time; SIADH, syndrome of inappropriate antidiuretic hormone secretion; $t_{1/2\alpha}$, α-half-life; $t_{1/2\beta}$, β-half-life; $t_{1/2\gamma}$, γ-half-life; Tab, tablet.

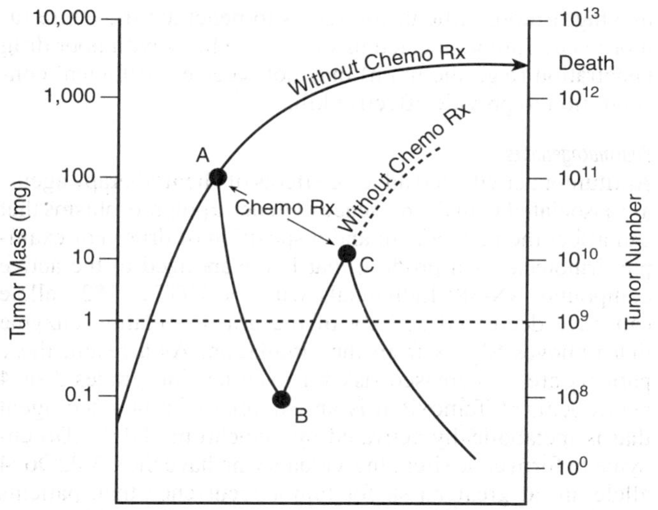

FIGURE 88-4 The growth rate of a tumor is initially very rapid and eventually slows as it approaches 10^{11} cells. Two trillion ($2–10^{12}$) cells or 2 kg of tumor is lethal to humans. An effective chemotherapy treatment given at point A will decrease the tumor number to point B. Regrowth of the tumor will occur during the recovery period until further chemotherapy is given at point C.

FACTORS THAT INFLUENCE RESPONSE TO CHEMOTHERAPY

In the clinical setting, tumor cells do not always decrease predictably with each successive course of chemotherapy. This is because the growth fraction of human tumors is not 100% and because the cell population is heterogeneous and some are resistant to chemotherapy. In patients with large tumors showing a plateaulike growth curve, the fraction of cells killed with each treatment is usually low. The ability of this model to predict cell kill adequately is also limited by the need to administer chemotherapy in cycles (e.g., every 2, 3, or 4 weeks) to allow normal cells to recover from the toxic effects of chemotherapy. During the recovery period, tumor cells can start to replicate again. Therefore, successful treatment requires administration of the next course of therapy before the tumor has grown to its previous size. The objective of successive chemotherapy courses is a further decrease in size of tumor mass. Other factors that influence cell kill include dose intensity, schedule, drug resistance, tumor site, and a patient's performance status.

Dose Intensity

Dose intensity is defined as the chemotherapy dose per unit time over which treatment is given (e.g., mg/m^2/week). Drug resistance might be overcome by escalating the dose intensity of drugs. This can be increased by (a) increasing the dose of chemotherapy per cycle, and (b) shortening the interval between cycles. Unnecessary lengthening of the interval between successive courses of chemotherapy or decreasing the dose can negatively affect treatment outcomes. Evidence suggests that reducing a dose can cause treatment failure in patients with chemotherapy-sensitive tumors who are having their first chemotherapy treatment.[47] Studies with animal models suggest that lower doses may eradicate the bulk of the tumor mass, but residual tumor cells left behind could ultimately be responsible for disease recurrence. A direct relationship between dose intensity and response rate also has been reported in several human tumors, including breast cancer, lymphomas, advanced ovarian cancer, and small-cell lung cancer.[48,49] Dose-dense treatment schedules have been designed to decrease the time period between chemotherapy administration, based on the theory that this would be more effective in reducing the residual tumor burden between treatments than escalating doses.[50] Dose-intensive therapy has not consistently improved the overall cure rate of most solid tumors, however.

The dose intensity for most chemotherapy regimens is limited by the major dose-related toxicity, bone marrow suppression. To minimize this toxicity and administer higher doses, patients have received hematopoietic growth factors, autologous stem cell transplantations, and altered schedules of drug delivery.[51–53]

Schedule Dependency

The schedule of chemotherapy administration is an important determinant of response. It influences dose intensity largely by affecting toxicity.[47] In some circumstances, changing the administration schedule can reduce the toxicity sufficiently to allow patients to receive higher total doses or more frequent courses of therapy, thereby increasing the dose intensity. The optimal schedule is also influenced by the pharmacokinetics of the agent. For example, phase-specific agents can exert their cytotoxic effects only when the cell is in a particular phase of the cell cycle. If a phase-specific agent with a short half-life is administered by intravenous (IV) bolus, a significant number of tumor cells will probably not cycle through the vulnerable phase of the cell cycle during exposure to the agent. Comparatively, the same agent administered by frequent IV bolus or continuous infusion could expose more cells to the agent during the vulnerable phase.[54]

Drug Resistance

9. B.C. is a 39-year-old man with an aggressive non-Hodgkin lymphoma (NHL). At the time of diagnosis, B.C. had enlarged cervical lymph nodes, dyspnea, and a large mediastinal mass noted on chest x-ray examination. Chemotherapy was initiated with the CHOP regimen, which consists of cyclophosphamide, doxorubicin, vincristine, and prednisone. After the first course of chemotherapy, B.C.'s lymphadenopathy was greatly reduced. Chest x-ray examination repeated after the second course of therapy showed marked improvement. When he returned for his fourth cycle of chemotherapy, recurrent lymphadenopathy was noted and the chest radiograph confirmed enlargement of the mediastinal mass. Why is B.C.'s cancer growing despite continued chemotherapy, and how should his treatment be altered?

Most likely B.C.'s cancer is now growing because the tumor has become resistant to the chemotherapy; therefore, it would be wise to discontinue the CHOP regimen. Biochemical resistance to chemotherapy is the major impediment to successful treatment with most cancers.[47] Resistance can occur de novo in cancer cells or develop during cell division as a result of mutation.[47] In 1979, a proposed mathematical model predicted that tumor cells mutate to drug resistance at a rate related to the genetic instability of the tumor.[55] Thus, the probability that a tumor mass will contain resistant clones is related to both the rate of mutation and the size of the tumor. Many specific mechanisms now have been identified by which cancer cells resist the activity of cytotoxic agents (Table 88-13).

Table 88-13 Possible Mechanisms of Anticancer Drug Resistance

Mechanism	*Chemotherapy Agents*
• Proficiency in repair of DNA	Cisplatin, cyclophosphamide, melphalan mitomycin, mechlorethamine
• In drug activation	Cytarabine, doxorubicin, fluorouracil, mercaptopurine, methotrexate, thioguanine
• In drug inactivation	Cytarabine, mercaptopurine
• In cellular uptake of drug	Methotrexate, melphalan
• In efflux of drug (multidrug resistance)	Doxorubicin, daunorubicin, etoposide, vincristine, vinblastine, teniposide, docetaxel, paclitaxel, vinorelbine
• alternative biochemical pathways	Cytarabine, fluorouracil, methotrexate
• alterations in target enzymes (DHFR, topoisomerase II)	Fluorouracil, hydroxyurea, mercaptopurine, methotrexate, thioguanine, etoposide, teniposide, doxorubicin, daunorubicin, idarubicin

Some cell lines that become resistant to a single chemotherapy agent may also be resistant to structurally unrelated cytotoxic compounds. This phenomenon is called *pleiotropic drug resistance* or *multidrug resistance* (MDR).[56] Cell lines that display this type of resistance generally are resistant to natural product cytotoxic agents such as the vinca alkaloids, antitumor antibiotics, epipodophyllotoxins, camptothecins, and taxanes. The primary mechanism believed to be responsible for MDR is an increase in P-glycoprotein in the cell membrane. This protein mediates efflux of the chemotherapy agent, causing a decreased accumulation of drug within the cell (the site of drug activity).[56] Other transport proteins have been implicated in resistance to chemotherapy, as well.[57]

Drugs known to inhibit P-glycoprotein (e.g., verapamil, cyclosporine, quinidine) have been investigated as potential adjunctive therapies to reduce resistance. Dosages of the agents required to inhibit P-glycoprotein have been associated with significant morbidity. Enhanced efficacy is, as of yet, unproved with newer investigational agents that can inhibit P-glycoprotein. A second type of MDR is mediated by altered binding to topoisomerase II, an enzyme that promotes DNA strand breaks in the presence of anthracyclines and epipodophyllotoxins.[58] Because of the likelihood of MDR, B.C. should receive a chemotherapy regimen that does not include chemotherapy agents inactivated by the MDR mechanism. An alternative regimen, such as high-dose methotrexate with leucovorin rescue, would be appropriate because this regimen is effective against NHL and is not affected by the MDR gene.

Tumor Site

The cytotoxic effects of chemotherapy agents are related to the time the tumor is exposed to an effective concentration of the agent (i.e., concentration × time [C × T]). The dosage regimen, including the dose, infusion rate, route of administration, lipophilicity, and protein binding, can influence the concentration-time product. Other factors, such as tumor size and location, can also critically affect an agent's cytotoxicity. As tumors grow larger, their degree of vascularity lessens, making it more difficult for agents to penetrate the entire tumor mass. Tumors located in sites of the body with poor drug penetration (e.g., the brain) may not receive a sufficient concentration to provide effective kill.

Pharmacogenetics

Antitumor activity and adverse effects of chemotherapy agents are associated with the presence of genetic polymorphisms that can affect the metabolism and disposition of drug. For example, irinotecan is a prodrug that is metabolized to the active compound, SN-38. Individuals with the UGT1A1*28 allele can have decreased activity of the glucuronidating enzyme that removes SN-38 from the circulation. As a result, these patients are at increased risk for experiencing grades 3 or 4 neutropenia.[59] Tamoxifen is an example of a targeted agent that is metabolically activated by cytochrome P450 2D6 enzyme to form endoxifen. Individuals who have the CYP2D6*4 allele are at greater risk for tumor recurrence than patients with the common allele, presumably because less of the active molecule is formed.[60] The first example is a polymorphism in an enzyme that affects the ability of the body to remove the active drug and thereby increases unwanted toxicity, whereas the second example is a polymorphism that affects activation to a compound responsible for most of its antitumor activity. A third example relates to the presence of the drug target at the tumor site. Approximately 20% to 30% of patients with early stage breast cancer have tumors that overexpress the HER2/neu growth factor receptor. These patients have more aggressive cancers and shorter survival than those who do not have the overexpressed HER2 receptor. Trastuzumab is a humanized anti-HER2 monoclonal antibody that is effective in treating tumors that overexpress this growth factor receptor. Hence, HER2 amplification status is an important component in the workup of patients with breast cancer, and it represents an example of altered genetic expression of drug target at the tumor site.[61]

Combination Chemotherapy

10. K.K. has advanced Hodgkin disease and is to begin chemotherapy today with the ABVD (doxorubicin [Adriamycin], bleomycin, vinblastine, and dacarbazine) regimen. She is reluctant because of her fear of side effects. She asks if, rather than receiving all four drugs today, she could receive just one and if it does not work then try another one?

CHOICE OF AGENTS

Although single-agent chemotherapy can cause significant early regressions of Hodgkin disease, acute lymphocytic leukemia, and adult NHL, most tumors show only a partial, very short response to single-agent therapy. Recognition that single-agent cytotoxic chemotherapy rarely produced prolonged remission led to the simultaneous use of multiple cytotoxic chemotherapy agents. The optimal activity of adding targeted agents to cytotoxic chemotherapy is less easy to predict. Bevacizumab and trastuzumab are most effective when given in combination with cytotoxic chemotherapy (for colorectal and breast cancers, respectively); agents such as tamoxifen are less effective. Because knowledge about how to combine targeted agents with cytotoxic chemotherapy is limited, this discussion centers around combinations of cytotoxic agents for which there is more long-term experience. In Hodgkin disease, the use of combination cytotoxic chemotherapy results in long-term, disease-free survival for >60% of patients. If K.K. were to receive single-agent therapy, her disease would not be cured. Combination chemotherapy is absolutely recommended to provide her with the best chance for long-term, disease-free survival. She should be reassured that appropriate measures, including prophylactic antiemetic therapy, will be taken to reduce her chances of both acute and chronic toxicities.

Combination chemotherapy provides broader coverage against resistant cell lines within the heterogeneous tumor mass. Table 88-14 lists examples of commonly used chemotherapy regimens. Several principles provide the basis for selecting the agents to be included in a chemotherapy regimen:

- Only agents with demonstrable single-agent activity against the specific type of tumor should be used in combination therapy.
- All agents in the regimen should have different mechanisms of action.
- Agents should not have overlapping toxicities so that the severity and duration of acute and chronic toxicities are minimized.
- All agents in the regimen should be used in their optimal dose and schedule.

APPLICATIONS

Several treatment concepts are noteworthy of discussion. These center around chemotherapy given for recurrent or refractory tumors and the timing of administration, relative to other treatment modalities such as surgery.

Primary Chemotherapy

Primary chemotherapy is defined as first-line treatment and, in the case of leukemia, it is referred to as *induction chemotherapy*. Choice of primary chemotherapy is governed by observations made from clinical trials that demonstrate that a given regimen has the highest known activity against the tumor. Second-line or salvage chemotherapy is administered after the tumor has become refractory to primary therapy or if the patient is unable to tolerate first-line therapy. Chemotherapy is the primary treatment modality used for hematologic malignancies, as well as a number of solid tumors that have metastasized at the time of diagnosis or have recurred at metastatic sites after initial therapy. Chemotherapy is frequently used in different ways during the course of an individual's malignancy (Fig. 88-5). Primary chemotherapy can be either curative or palliative, depending on the specific type of tumor. Following induction therapy for leukemia, patients may receive additional chemotherapy in an attempt to further eradicate residual disease and improve their chances for long-term survival. Postremission therapy (i.e., following induction therapy) can include consolidation, intensification, and maintenance treatment phases.

Adjuvant Chemotherapy

11. F.R., a 36-year-old woman with no other medical problems, recently underwent a lumpectomy and radiation therapy for breast cancer. She has been told that the cancer no longer exists; however, she also is told that she should now receive 6 months of chemotherapy. She knows that chemotherapy will cause her to vomit, lose her hair, gain weight, and place her at risk for life-threatening infections. Why would chemotherapy be recommended now when she is disease free?

Some patients may have unrecognized micrometastases or residual disease after primary treatment. These patients have a high probability of disease recurrence, even though the primary treatment may have successfully removed all visual evidence of the primary tumor. To eradicate any undetectable tumor, the patient could receive systemic therapy after initial curative surgery (or radiation therapy). Systemic chemotherapy administered after primary therapy is referred to as *adjuvant chemotherapy*. Because the tumor burden is relatively low at this time, adjuvant chemotherapy should immediately follow primary therapy. For adjuvant therapy to provide any benefit, the risk of recurrence must be high, and effective agents must be available to eradicate the tumor. Adjuvant therapy is considered standard treatment in the treatment of breast and colorectal cancer, but it also has benefited selected patients with ovarian cancer, Ewing sarcoma, Wilms tumor, and other malignancies.[47] (also see Chapter 91, Solid Tumors.) Because it is impossible to predict which patients have unrecognized disease, it is difficult to determine which patients should receive adjuvant therapy. To help with these decisions, clinicians frequently consider histologic and cytogenetic characteristics of the primary tumor that are associated with high risk of relapse. Some patients who may never relapse will undergo adjuvant chemotherapy, however.

Neoadjuvant Chemotherapy

Neoadjuvant chemotherapy is the therapy given before the primary treatment in patients who present with locally advanced tumors (e.g., large tumors or those that are impinging on surrounding vital structures) that are unlikely to be cured with primary surgery or radiation therapy. The objective is to reduce the tumor mass with neoadjuvant therapy (chemotherapy or hormonal therapy), thereby increasing the likelihood of eradication by subsequent surgery or radiation therapy. Neoadjuvant therapy also can lessen the amount of radical surgery therapy that the patient needs, which can preserve cosmetic appearances and function of the surrounding normal tissues. The tumor can be resistant to the neoadjuvant therapy and continue to grow, however, making surgery or radiation even more difficult. Patients may also experience toxicities with the neoadjuvant therapy that may delay surgery or impair postsurgical healing. Locally advanced tumors in which neoadjuvant chemotherapy has been shown to improve survival rates include stage III_A non–small-cell lung cancer, stage III breast cancer, sarcomas, esophageal cancers, laryngeal cancer, bladder cancer, and osteogenic sarcoma.[47]

Administration

SYSTEMIC

Systemic chemotherapy is most commonly administered by the IV route, either as a bolus injection (generally <15 minutes), a short infusion (15 minutes to several hours), or a continuous infusion (lasting 24 hours to several weeks). Some systemic chemotherapy agents can be administered by the oral route, whereas other agents can be administered by the intramuscular or subcutaneous route. No matter which route of administration is selected for therapy, the individual administering the chemotherapy should be proficient in administering

Table 88-14 Representative Chemotherapy Regimens[a]

Acronym	Agents	Cycle
Breast Cancer		
CMF	Cyclophosphamide[106] Methotrexate Fluorouracil	Every 28 days
Herceptin-tax	Trastuzumab (Herceptin)[107] Paclitaxel	Every 21 days
CAF	Cyclophosphamide[108] Doxorubicin (Adriamycin) Fluorouracil	Every 28 days
AC + T	Doxorubicin (Adriamycin)[109] Cyclophosphamide Paclitaxel	Every 21 days Every 21 days
TAC[137]	Docetaxel Doxorubicin Cyclophosphamide	Every 21 days
FEC[138]	Fluorouracil Epirubicin Cyclophosphamide	Every 28 days
Colorectal Cancer		
FOLFIRI + bevacizumab	Irinotecan[110] Leucovorin Fluorouracil Fluorouracil Bevacizumab	Every 2 wk
FOLFOX4 + bevacizumab	Oxaliplatin[110] Leucovorin Fluorouracil Fluorouracil Bevacizumab	Every 2 wk
CapOx + bevacizumab	Oxaliplatin[110] Capecitabine Bevacizumab	Every 21 days
FU/leucovorin	Flourouracil[111] Leucovorin *Or* Fluorouracil[112] Leucovorin *Or* Fluorouracil[113] Leucovorin	Every 28 days × 2 then every 35 days Every wk × 6 wk Every 4–5 wk
Gastric Cancer		
ECP	Epirubicin[114] Cisplatin Fluorouracil	Every 21 day
FAM	Fluorouracil[115] Doxorubicin (Adriamycin) Mitomycin	Every 8 wk
EAP	Etoposide[116] Doxorubicin (Adriamycin) Cisplatin	Every 21–28 days
Ovarian Cancer		
CP	Cyclophosphamide[117] Cisplatin	Every 21 days
CT	Paclitaxel[117] Cisplatin	Every 21 days
Carbo-tax	Paclitaxel[118] Carboplatin	Every 21 days
Testicular Cancer		
BEP	Bleomycin[119] Etoposide Cisplatin	Every 21 days
EP	Etoposide[120] Cisplatin	Every 21 days
Bladder Cancer		
M-VAC	Methotrexate[121] Vinblastine Adriamycin (Doxorubicin) Cisplatin	Every 28 days
Gemcitabine + CDDP	Gemcitabine[122] Cisplatin	Every 28 days
Small-Cell Lung Cancer		
EP or PE	Cisplatin[123] Etoposide	Every 21–28 days
Non–Small-Cell Lung Cancer		
EP or PE	Cisplatin[124] Etoposide *Or* Cisplatin[125] Etoposide	Every 21 days Every 21–28 days
Carbo-tax	Paclitaxel[126] Carboplatin	Every 21 days
EC	Etoposide[127] Carboplatin	Every 21–28 days
Gemcitabine-Cis	Gemcitabine[126] Cisplatin	Every 28 days
Docetaxel-Cisplatin	Docetaxel[126] Cisplatin	Every 21 days
PC[139]	Paclitaxel Carboplatin	Every 21 days
Head and Neck Cancer		
CF	Cisplatin[128] Fluorouracil	Every 21–28 days
Lymphomas		
Non-Hodgkin Lymphomas		
CHOP	Cyclophosphamide[129] Doxorubicin (Hydroxyl Daunorubicin) Vincristine (Oncovin) Prednisone	Every 21 days

(continued)

Table 88-14 Representative Chemotherapy Regimens[a] *(Continued)*

Acronym	Agents	Cycle
CHOP-Rituximab	Cyclophosphamide[130]	Every 21 days
	Doxorubicin	
	Vincristine (Oncovin)	
	Prednisone	
	Rituximab	
MACOP-B	Methotrexate[131]	Only one cycle
	Leucovorin	
	Doxorubicin (Adriamycin)	
	Cyclophosphamide	
	Vincristine (Oncovin)	
	Prednisone	
	Bleomycin	
ESHAP	Etoposide[132]	Every 21–28 days
	Methylprednisolone	
	Cisplatin	
	Cytarabine	
Hodgkin Disease		
MOPP	Mechlorethamine[133]	Every 28 days
	Vincristine (Oncovin)	
	Prednisone	
	Procarbazine	
ABVD	Doxorubicin (Adriamycin)[134]	Every 28 days
	Bleomycin	
	Vinblastine	
	Dacarbazine	
Multiple Myeloma		
VAD	Vincristine[135]	Every 28 days
	Doxorubicin (Adriamycin)	
	Dexamethasone	
MP	Melphalan[136]	Every 42 days
	Prednisone	

[a] Original citations should be consulted for dosage adjustments owing to toxicity or underlying organ dysfunction.

the agent by the chosen route and be aware of the most common acute and chronic toxicities associated with the chemotherapy. All aspects of drug administration should be discussed with the patient before starting chemotherapy, including any adverse events they may experience during or after the injection and throughout therapy. Printed patient educational materials are recommended to supplement oral instructions.

Currently, most patients receive chemotherapy through a central venous catheter to reduce some of the potential problems associated with recurrent IV administration. Some chemotherapy agents are potent vesicants or irritants if they are extravasated from the vein (see Chapter 89, Adverse Effects of Chemotherapy). Other agents can produce severe irritation and pain to peripheral veins, which can lead to sclerosis and thrombosis. Other potential problems associated with the IV route include unsatisfactory venous access secondary to obesity, prior IV therapy with irritant drugs, or advanced age. Therefore, permanent central venous access devices, such as tunneled central venous catheters (e.g., the Broviac, Hickman, Groshong) or subcutaneous ports (e.g., Port-A-Cath or Infuse-A-Port) are commonly used in patients receiving chemotherapy. A peripherally inserted central catheter (PICC) line is nonpermanent but it can be maintained and used for venous access for extended periods of time.

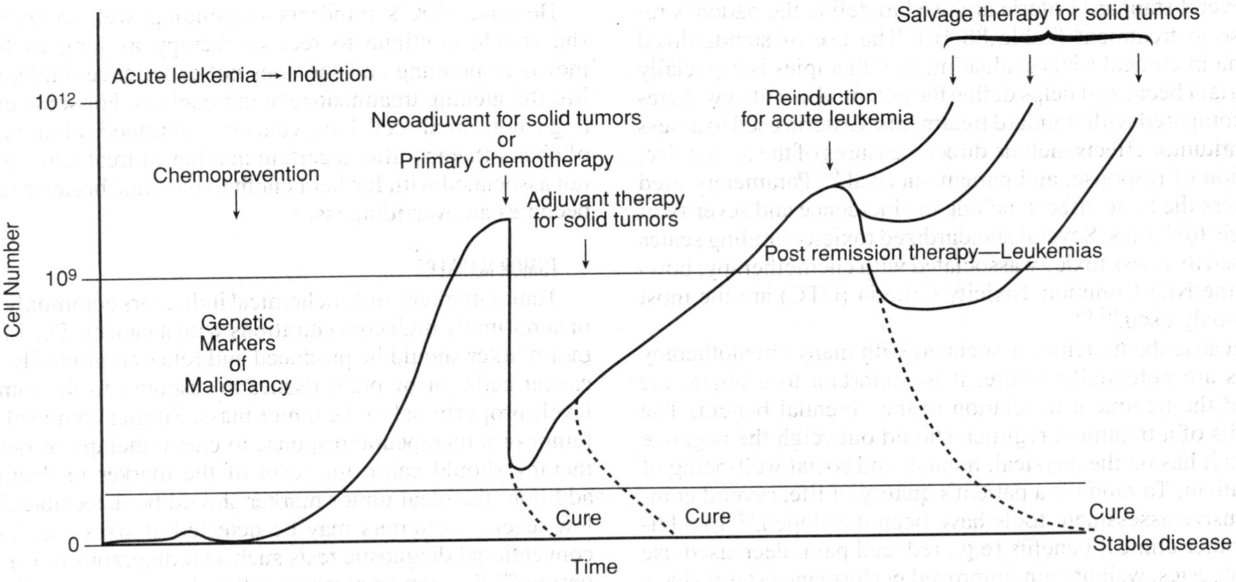

FIGURE 88-5 Chemotherapy during various phases of malignancy. Cell kill hypothesis.

Table 88-15 Local or Regional Routes of Administration of Cancer Chemotherapy

Route of Administration	*Cancer Managed With Alternative Route*
Intrathecal or intraventricular	Leukemia, lymphoma
Intravesicular	Bladder cancer
Intraperitoneal	Ovarian cancer
Intrapleural	Malignant pleural effusions
Intra-arterial	Melanoma, sarcoma
Hepatic artery	Liver metastases
Chemoembolization (intra-arterial or intravenous)	Colon cancer, rectal cancer, carcinoid, liver metastases

Table 88-16 Response Criteria for Evaluating Effects of Chemotherapy of Target Lesion

Complete Response (CR)
Disappearance of all target lesions
Partial Response (PR)
At least a 30% decrease in the sum of the longest diameter (LD) of target lesions, taking as reference the baseline sum LD
Progressive Disease (PD)
At least a 20% increase in the sum of the LD of target lesions, taking as reference the smallest sum LD recorded since the treatment started or the appearance of one or more new lesions
Stable Disease (SD)
Neither sufficient shrinkage to qualify for PR nor sufficient increase to qualify for PD, taking as reference the smallest sum LD since the treatment started
Disease-Free Survival
Time from documentation of complete response until disease relapse or death.
Overall Survival
Time from treatment until time of death.

REGIONAL

Although chemotherapy was initially developed for systemic use, techniques have been developed to locally administer agents to specific sites of the body affected by the tumor (Table 88-15). Regional or local chemotherapy allows high concentrations of agents to be achieved at the site of the tumor while reducing systemic exposure and subsequent toxicity. On the other hand, undetectable metastases at distant sites may not be exposed to the chemotherapy, allowing continued growth of the tumor mass.

Assessing Response to Therapy

A very important step in the process of treating a patient with chemotherapy is to assess his or her response to treatment. The assessment should evaluate the chemotherapy's antitumor and toxic effects, as well as its effect on the patient's overall quality of life and survival. Re-evaluation should occur at regularly scheduled intervals during treatment and should include a physical examination, laboratory tests, and repeat diagnostic tests (radiologic or other tests such as bone marrow biopsy, bronchoscopy) used to stage the cancer. Usually, only tests that previously were positive for the tumor are repeated unless new signs or symptoms suggest additional metastases.

Several standard criteria are used to define the patient's response to treatment (Table 88-16). The use of standardized criteria in clinical trials evaluating new therapies is especially important because it helps define the potential use of new therapies compared with standard treatments. Criteria used to assess the antitumor effects include direct measures of the tumor size, duration of response, and patient survival.[62] Parameters used to assess the toxic effects include the incidence and severity of specific toxicities. Several standardized toxicity grading scales are used to assess toxicity associated with chemotherapy; however, the NCI Common Toxicity Criteria (CTC) are the most commonly used.[63,64]

Because the toxicities associated with many chemotherapy agents are potentially severe, it is important to evaluate the risk of the treatment in relation to the potential benefit. The benefits of a treatment regimen should outweigh the negative effects it has on the physical, mental, and social well-being of the patient. To monitor a patient's quality of life, several comprehensive assessment tools have been developed.[65] In addition, other clinical benefits (e.g., reduced pain, decreased use of analgesics, weight gain, improved performance status) have been recognized by the FDA as acceptable criteria for measuring a patient's quality of life and for approving new chemotherapy agents.

12. G.K. is a 67-year-old woman who was recently diagnosed with metastatic bladder cancer. Her symptoms include widespread pain, anorexia, and fatigue. She began receiving a combination chemotherapy regimen and has received three cycles of treatment. A recent CT scan of her abdomen showed marked shrinkage at several sites of tumor and her pain has decreased. How long should she continue to receive chemotherapy?

Because G.K.'s tumor is responding well to treatment, she should continue to receive therapy as long as her tumor is responding and she does not experience intolerable or life-threatening treatment-related toxicities. For some cancers (e.g., non–small-cell lung cancer), continued administration of chemotherapy after a certain number of treatment cycles is not associated with further benefit to patients, because toxicity becomes an overriding issue.

TUMOR MARKERS

Tumor markers are biochemical indicators commonly found in abnormally high concentrations with a cancer. The ideal tumor marker should be produced and released primarily by the cancer cells (or by other tissues in response to the tumor) at levels proportional to the tumor mass. Surgical removal of the tumor or a therapeutic response to chemotherapy or radiation therapy should cause the level of the marker to decline. In addition, the ideal tumor marker should be detectable at very low levels, so tumors may be detected at sizes smaller than conventional diagnostic tests such as radiographs or CT scans permit.[66] Few tumor markers fulfill these criteria sufficiently to be clinically useful as the sole screening or diagnostic test

Table 88-17 Clinically Useful Tumor Markers

Tumor Marker	Cancers Commonly Associated With Increased Markers
CA-19-9	Pancreatic
CA-15-3	Breast
CA-27-29	Breast
Neuron-specific enolase	Neuroblastoma, small-cell lung cancer
α-Fetoprotein (AFP)	Liver
CA-125	Ovarian, testicular—nonseminoma
Carcinoembryonic antigen (CEA)	Colon, lung
Human chorionic gonadotropin (hCG)	Trophoblastic, testicular
β_2-Microglobulin	Multiple myeloma
Prostate-specific antigen (PSA)	Prostate

(Table 88-17). These markers are also used as confirmatory tests and as part of follow-up care to detect recurrent disease. In most cases, tumor markers lack specificity for the tumor, and they could be elevated owing to other disease states. Patients who have elevated levels of a tumor marker at initial diagnosis should have elevated levels with disease recurrence. Other techniques used to detect very low levels of recurrent cancer in leukemias and lymphomas (e.g., minimal residual disease) include real-time quantitative PCR (RT-PCR) analysis of immunoglobin or gene arrangements or chromosome aberrations in cells.[67] By detecting cancer recurrence at its earliest state, treatments may be more successful.

13. Describe other agents used to treat cancer beyond those that are considered cell-cycle specific or non–cell-cycle specific.

Endocrine Therapy

Endocrine therapy can be used to treat several common cancers, including breast, prostate, and endometrial cancers, which arise from hormone-sensitive tissues (Table 88-18). These tumors grow in response to endogenous hormones that trigger growth signals by binding to specific receptors located on a cell membrane or within the cytoplasm of a cell. Current endocrine therapies inhibit tumor growth by blocking the receptors or by eliminating the endogenous hormone feeding the tumor. (Note: Interruption of hormonal secretion also can be achieved through surgical removal of hormone-producing organs). Not all tumors arising from hormone-sensitive tissues respond to endocrine manipulation. Lack of response could be associated with hormone-resistant tumor cells or inadequate suppression of the endogenous feeding hormones.[68]

Table 88-18 Endocrine Therapy Used for Hormone-Sensitive Tumors

Class	Drug	Dosage	Side Effects	Indication
Antiestrogens	Tamoxifen	10–20 mg PO BID	Disease flare, hot flashes, nausea, vomiting, edema, thromboembolism, endometrial cancer	Breast
	Toremifene	60 mg PO daily		
	Fulvestrant	250 mg IM every month		
Aromatase inhibitors	Anastrozole	1 mg PO daily	Hot flashes, nausea, fatigue, insomnia, increased risk of bone fractures	Breast
	Letrozole	2.5 mg PO daily		
	Exemestane	25 mg PO daily		
	Aminoglutethimide	250 mg PO QID with hydrocortisone 40 mg PO daily	Lethargy, rash, postural dizziness, ataxia, nystagmus, nausea	Breast, prostate
LHRH analogs[a]	Leuprolide	7.5 mg SC every 28 days	Amenorrhea, hot flashes, nausea	Breast, prostate
	Goserelin	3.6 mg SC every 28 days		
	Triptorelin	3.75 mg IM every 28 days		
Antiandrogens	Flutamide	250 mg PO TID	Gynecomastia, hot flashes, breast tenderness, hepatic dysfunction, diarrhea	Prostate
	Bicalutamide	50 mg PO daily		
	Nilutamide	300 mg PO daily for 30 days, then 150 mg PO daily		
Progestins	Medroxyprogesterone acetate	400–1,000 mg IM every week	Weight gain, hot flashes, vaginal bleeding, edema, thromboembolism	Breast, prostate
	Megestrol acetate	10–40 mg PO QID		Anorexia
Estrogens	Ethinylestradiol	1 mg PO TID	Nausea, vomiting, fluid retention, hot flashes, anorexia, thromboembolism, hepatic dysfunction	Breast
	Conjugated estrogens	2.5 mg PO TID		
Androgens	Fluoxymestrone	10 mg PO BID	Deepening voice, alopecia, hirsutism, facial or truncal acne, fluid retention, menstrual irregularities, cholestatic jaundice	Breast

[a]Leuprolide and triptorelin also available in extended release and depot formulations.
BID, twice daily; IM, intramuscular; PO, orally; QID, four times daily; SC, subcutaneously; TID, three times daily.

Signal Transduction Pathway Inhibitors

By understanding the mechanisms by which cancer cells exhibit unregulated growth and immortality, and possess the ability to invade tissues and metastasize,[1] it has been possible to design drugs that inhibit these processes. The EGFR, HER2/neu, and VEGF signaling pathways can be blocked by monoclonal antibodies that inhibit receptor tyrosine kinase activation by binding to the extraceullar domain. Small molecules that directly inhibit tyrosine kinase activation by competing with ATP for binding to the intracellular tyrosine kinase domain have been developed, as well.[7] A potential advantage of targeting the tyrosine kinase activity of the receptor should be the ability to inhibit cells that do not overexpress the receptor on their surface or have mutated forms of the receptor that result in its activation. The first commercially available receptor tyrosine kinase inhibitor was imatinib mesylate, also known as STI-571. Imatinib mesylate specifically inhibits the Abl and c-KIT kinases and platelet-derived growth factor receptors α and β.[69] This agent is active against chronic myelogenous leukemia and gastrointestinal stromal tumors and is under investigation for other malignancies that are dependent on the activity of the Bcr-Abl or c-KIT tyrosine kinases.

Inhibition of the 26S proteosome, which is responsible for the intracellular degradation of ubiquinated proteins, can induce apoptosis in a wide variety of cancer cell lines.[70] VEGF, bFGF, MMP, and receptor tyrosine kinases that are activated in endothelial cells subsequent to endothelial cell activation are also targets for antiangiogenic agents. Unlike most cytotoxic chemotherapeutic agents, bone marrow suppression is not a frequent dose-limiting side effect of signal transduction pathway inhibitors. Because of their mechanism of action, their effects are exerted primarily through inhibition of cell growth rather than through direct cytotoxicity. Occasionally, however, significant tumor regression is observed. Based on current knowledge, treatment regimens that incorporate use of these agents with cytotoxic drugs are most likely to have the greatest impact on patient outcomes in cancer treatments.

Angiogenesis Inhibition

Angiogenesis, the main process for new blood vessel formation postnatally, occurs during wound healing and disease states such as cancer. It occurs through remodeling, migration, and proliferation of pre-existing blood vessels. As discussed in an earlier section, endothelial cells receive stimuli such as VEGF and PDGF from tumor cells.[71,72] These factors trigger cell proliferation and secretion of such factors as MMP, collagenase, and tissue plasminogen activators. These proteases enable the proliferating endothelial cells to invade tissue space and to form new vessels. These tumor vessels often differ phenotypically from normal vessels. Hence, a strategy for inhibiting tumor growth is possible, because agents can be designed to target this process, and thereby starve tumors of nutrients and oxygen. Two classes of molecules have been developed to block angiogenesis: antibody molecules and small molecule inhibitors. Bevacizumab is an example of an antibody molecule that binds to VEGF and inhibits binding to the VEGF receptor. It is approved for use in patients with colorectal cancer and advanced non–small-cell lung carcinoma (NSCLC).[73,74] Sunitinib and sorafenib, which are both small molecule inhibitors, act as antagonists at several locations along the signaling pathways that promote angiogenesis.[75,76] Both of these orally administered agents are approved for use in patients with renal cell carcinoma and are under evaluation for use in treating other solid tumors. Shown in Figure 88-6 is a summary of the angiogenic process and key signaling pathways where anti-angiogenic agents interact.

Biologic Response Modifiers

Biologic response modifiers used to treat cancers include proteins (vaccines), antibodies (monoclonal and polyclonal), and growth factors. These agents can be used to kill cancer cells or to bolster the host's defense mechanisms. An individual's immune system plays a crucial role in developing or eradicating cancer. Normally, an intact immune system can protect the host against malignant cells and infectious pathogens, but current evidence shows that individuals with "weakened" immune systems face an increased risk of developing cancer. For example, individuals with acquired immunodeficiency syndrome (AIDS) face an increased risk of developing lymphomas compared with the normal population. Other individuals with weakened immune systems, including neonates and the elderly, also face an increased risk of developing cancer. Bolstering an individual's immune system could help prevent or treat a malignancy. Some evidence shows that malignancies can undergo spontaneous regression, especially during periods of immune activation (e.g., an acute bacterial infection).[77] Current biologic response modifiers aim to bolster an individual's immune response, as well as provide a direct cytotoxic effect.

Interferon-α

The first recombinant cytokine to become available for the treatment of cancer was interferon-α. This interferon affects tumor cells through several different mechanisms, including (a) a direct antiproliferative effect; (b) an immunomodulatory effect on natural killer cells, T cells, B cells, and macrophages; (c) an induction of tumor cell antigens; and (d) a differentiating effect on tumor cells. Interferons also possess antiangiogeneic effects.[40] Current studies show that interferon-α has antitumor effects against several human malignancies.[78] Interferon-α is sometimes given in combination with radiation therapy, other biologic response modifiers, or chemotherapy agents.

Interleukin-2

Interleukin (IL)-2 is a recombinantly produced lymphokine that has numerous immunoregulatory functions. In normal cells, IL-2 stimulates both T- and B-cell proliferation and differentiation.[79] The idea to use IL-2 to treat cancer arose from the observation that lymphoid cells incubated with IL-2 developed the capacity to lyse tumor cells (lymphokine-activated killer [LAK] cells).[80,81] This observation led to the development of some adoptive immunotherapies. Initial studies showed that patients with advanced tumors, such as renal cell carcinoma and melanoma, experienced tumor regression after receiving IL-2. Subsequent studies using high dosages of IL-2 also reported responses in similar patient populations with advanced disease.[81–83] High-dose IL-2 therapy is accompanied by significant, dose-related toxicity. The most serious

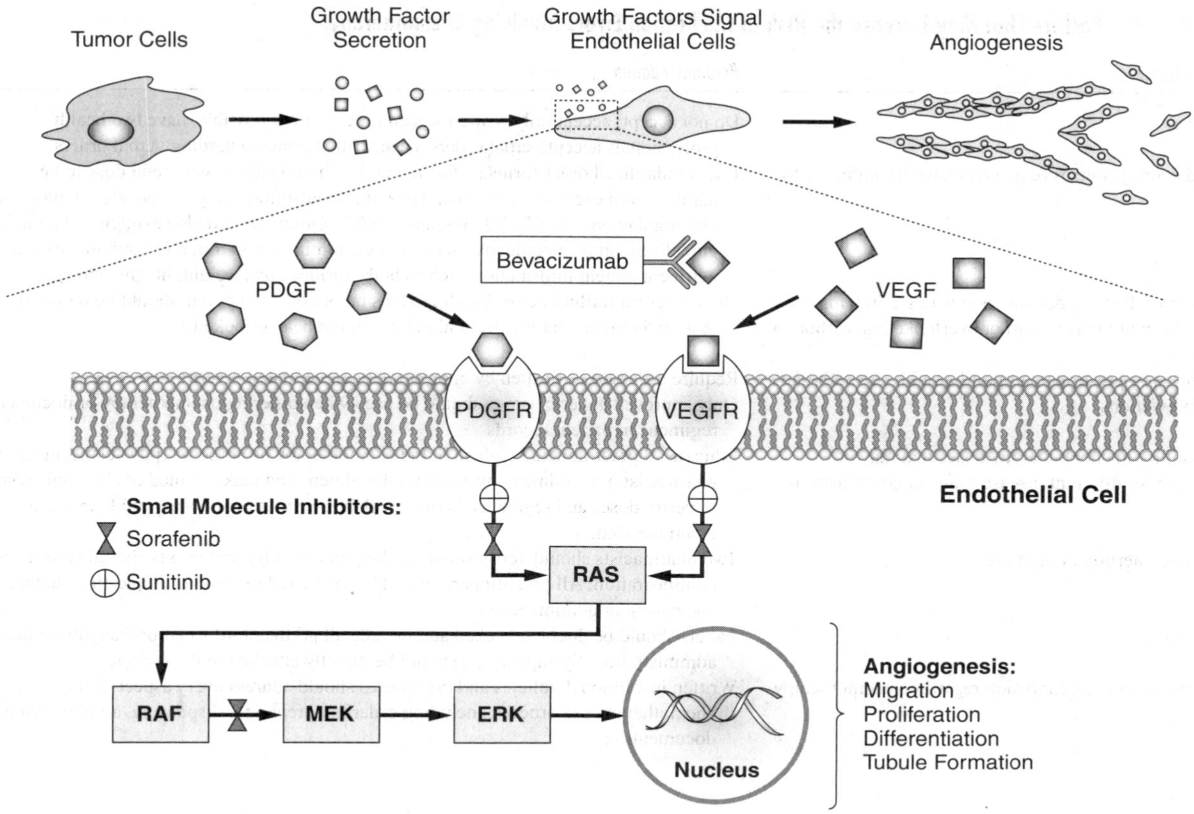

FIGURE 88-6 Angiogenesis and antiangiogenic agents. Tumor cells signal new blood vessel formation through secretion of growth factors such as vascular endothelial growth factor (VEGF) and platelet-derived growth factor (PDGF), which interact and activate receptor tyrosine kinase signaling within the endothelial cells. Subsequent cascade signaling downstream activates the cell nucleus and initiates angiogenesis through endothelial cell proliferation, migration, differentiation, and tubule formation. Agents that block this signaling process are shown as bevacizumab (monoclonal antibody blocks VEGF), and sorafenib and sunitinib (small molecule inhibitors) that block several different targets associated with the angiogenic process. RAF, MEK, ERK-Kinase enzymes.

toxicities (hypotension, pulmonary edema, oliguria, increased bilirubin) occur secondary to a diffuse capillary leak that develops during IL-2 therapy. These signs usually resolve promptly after discontinuing therapy.

HANDLING OF CYTOTOXIC DRUGS

Impact on the Pharmacy

14. The administrator of a health plan recently has announced that two medical oncologists will be joining the professional staff. Previously, patients were referred to outside oncologists, and no cytotoxic drugs were prepared or administered at the clinics. What implications will the addition of these physicians have on the pharmacy department?

New approaches to cancer treatment will affect three areas of the pharmacy department: the budget, the policies and procedures for safe drug handling, and the staff education program. The pharmacy department will need to increase its budget to accommodate the additional personnel and to purchase new equipment, supplies, supportive care medicines, and chemotherapy agents. To estimate the projected increase in the budget, a pharmacist should meet with oncologists to discuss the anticipated volume of chemotherapy orders, the chemotherapy agents they are likely to prescribe, and the supportive care medicines they plan to use. All new chemotherapy agents and supportive care medicines (e.g., antiemetic therapy, analgesics) should be added to the health plan formulary. In addition, the pharmacist should determine the projected use of investigational agents, clinical pharmacy services that will be needed, and any plans to develop an ambulatory infusion program. The department must create new policies and procedures to ensure safe handling of chemotherapy agents by all personnel. These should be conveyed to all personnel through a staff education program, because safe handling of chemotherapy agents can significantly decrease the risk of medication errors and injuries.

Medication Errors

In recent years, several chemotherapy-related medication errors that resulted in death or permanent disability have been highly publicized. These devastating events have brought significant attention to the entire drug use process in oncology and have identified several factors that appear to contribute to the risk (Table 88-19). In particular, the use of abbreviations, verbal orders, multiple-day regimens, poor-quality carbon

Table 88-19 Factors That May Increase the Risk of Medication Errors Involving Chemotherapy

Contributing Factor	*Recommendation*
Verbal orders	Do not accept; accept only written signed orders. If not possible, have two health professionals accept verbal orders, have written policy regarding verbal orders.
Multiple-day drug courses (e.g., etoposide 50 mg/m^2 × 5)	Use standardized order forms or format. Order should clearly state total dose to be administered each day and actual dates of administration (e.g., etoposide 50 mg/m^2/day = 100 mg/day on 3/1, 3/2, 3/3, 3/4, and 3/5/07). Orders should also explicitly state infusion guidelines, other specific instructions (e.g., administer 30 min after antiemetic) and other pertinent patient information such as body surface area, weight, height, and age.
Trailing zeros following decimal points (e.g., 50.0 mg) or the decimal point may be lost or overlooked on carbon or fax copies	Do not permit trailing zeros. Leading zeros before decimal points should be required (e.g., 0.5 mg) so that the decimal point will not be overlooked.
Orders written by prescribers unfamiliar with chemotherapy	Require orders to be written by appropriately credentialed practitioners.
Use of abbreviations	Only approved generic names should be used when ordering chemotherapy or documenting regimens in patient records
Wide variability in chemotherapy doses that may be appropriate for different disease states or combinations	Educate all practitioners involved in the chemotherapy use process (physicians, nurses, pharmacists) regarding commonly used regimens and make printed or electronic resources to verify doses and regimens readily available. Institutional dosing guidelines are recommended.
Inappropriate interpretation of orders	Two pharmacists should verify orders at the point of entry and nurses should reverify before administration. All practitioners should be instructed to resolve all questions before dispensing or administration.
Labeling errors	Labels should be double-checked and include all pertinent information including route of administration. Syringe labels should be directly attached to the syringe.
Poor communication or confusion regarding chemotherapy	Written institutional policies and procedures should address every aspect of the chemotherapy use process, including ordering, preparing, dispensing, administering, and documenting.

orders, poor facsimile medication orders, and incorrect references have contributed to a number of reported medication errors. Several groups have responded to the problem by issuing policy recommendations to minimize such errors.[84–87]

Risks

15. What are the potential risks of handling cytotoxic drugs, and what resources are available to assist the Pharmacy director and the pharmacy staff in the development of policies and procedures?

For almost two decades, the potential hazards of chemotherapy agents have received considerable attention. Many of these agents are carcinogenic, teratogenic, or mutagenic in animal models and in humans at therapeutic doses.[88–91] The danger to health care personnel handling such agents results from both the inherent toxicities of the agents and the extent to which the workers are exposed during drug handling.[92] Various studies have attempted to assess the effect of occupational exposure to hazardous drugs by health care workers. These studies included measurements of urine mutagenicity, chromosomal damage, drug absorption, and, most recently, the level of contamination that occurs in the work areas used for drug preparation and administration.[92–102] Although somewhat controversial, the documentation of urine mutagenicity or chromosomal damage was thought to be a direct result of cytotoxic exposure. Other reports correlate these observations of reproductive and birth defect risks in pregnant workers handling cytotoxic drugs.[101,103] Results of these reports together with the toxicities observed in patients receiving therapeutic doses led the American Society of Hospital Pharmacists to conclude that health care workers both inside and outside the pharmacy exposed to hazardous drugs whenever they are received, stored, prepared, administered, or disposed may be absorbing these drugs and may be at risk for adverse outcomes.[92]

In response to the concerns regarding occupational exposure to hazardous drugs, several groups have published guidelines for the safe handling of these agents in the workplace (i.e., storage, preparation, administration, and disposal).[92,104,105] These documents can be helpful to the pharmacy department when developing policies and procedures.

Policies and Procedures

16. What specific policies and procedures are necessary, and what other departments should be consulted during the development and implementation of the handling guidelines?

Policies must be developed that address the entire scope of potential occupational exposures within the workplace. These policies should include (a) a worker's "right to know" of potential hazards; (b) an education and training program for workers involved with hazardous drug handling; (c) a quality assurance program to monitor adherence to safe handling procedures; and (d) guidelines for workers attempting to conceive a child, who become pregnant, or who are nursing.

Specific procedures that outline the appropriate handling of hazardous agents during all aspects of institutional storage, use, and disposal should be developed. These procedures should include guidelines that outline the appropriate (a) storage in the receiving and storeroom areas, (b) preparation and administration of parenteral formulations, (c) manipulation and dispensing of oral and topical formulations, (d) the clean up of spills, (e) management of acute exposures, and (f) disposal of hazardous agents and supplies used to prepare and dispense chemotherapy. If the oncology program includes ambulatory infusion or home care components, procedures should also be developed for the appropriate handling and disposal of these products in the home.

Other departments that may be affected by these guidelines include the medical staff, nursing, housekeeping (in the clean up of spills and equipment), maintenance (upkeep of equipment), and the receiving area (where cytotoxic drugs may be received from suppliers). The institutional safety office and legal staff also should be consulted to help devise the policies and procedures.

Necessary Equipment and Supplies

17. What equipment and supplies are necessary for handling hazardous drugs?

Various equipment and supplies can minimize occupational exposure in the health care workplace by protecting both the worker and the environment. All handling guidelines recommend that manipulations (e.g., reconstitution, admixing) of hazardous drugs be done in a class II biologic safety cabinet (BSC) to provide maximal protection for the worker and the work environment. Reports of measurable levels of chemotherapy agents found in work areas despite the use of BSC have renewed concerns regarding worker safety.[104] It is not clear how the work areas became contaminated, although the very low vapor pressure of cyclophosphamide at room temperature may result in the release of particles too small to be retained by the high-efficiency particulate air filters within the BSC. Additional research will be required to assess whether other chemotherapy agents vaporize under similar circumstances and subsequently expose individuals in the work area. Workers also should wear gloves (one or two pairs) and a disposable, closed-front gown of lint-free, low-permeability fabric with a solid front, long sleeves, and knit cuffs. In addition, only syringes and IV sets with Luer-Lok fittings should be used. Final products (e.g., syringes, IV bags or bottles) should be placed in sealable containers such as zipper-closure plastic bags and clearly labeled as a hazardous drug. Other supplies that may be necessary for the sterile product preparation area include plastic-back paper liners for the bottom surface of the BSC and 0.2-mm hydrophobic filters.

The disposal of hazardous waste also requires specific receptacles, which should be placed in all areas where workers handle these drugs. Disposal of these agents should follow institutional and state and local regulations. Materials for the clean up of spills (e.g., absorbent material, plastic bags or containers, protective garments) also must be kept in all areas where hazardous drugs are stored, prepared, or administered.

ACKNOWLEDGMENT

The author and editors would like to acknowledge the contribution of Drs. Lisa E. Davis and Celeste Lindley, authors of this topic in the previous edition.

REFERENCES

1. Hanahan D et al. The hallmarks of cancer. *Cell* 2000;100:57.
2. National Cancer Society Surveillance, Epidemiology, and End Results (SEER) Home Page. URL: http://seer.cancer.gov. Accessed May 23, 2007.
3. American Cancer Society. *Cancer Facts & Figures 2007*. Atlanta, GA: American Cancer Society, 2007.
4. Ries LAG et al. *SEER Cancer Statistics Review,* 1975–2004. National Cancer Institute. Bethesda, MD: National Cancer Institute; 2007. URL: http://seer.cancer.gov/csr/1975_2004. Accessed November 15, 2007.
5. Tucker MA. Epidemiology of cancer: epidemiologic methods. In: DeVita VT et al., eds. *Cancer: Principles and Practice of Oncology.* 6th ed. Philadelphia: Lippincott Williams & Wilkins; 2001:219.
6. Calle EE et al. Overweight, obesity, and mortality from cancer in a prospectively studied cohort of U.S. adults. *N Engl J Med* 2003;348:1625.
7. Mendelsohn J et al. Status of epidermal growth factor receptor antagonists in the biology and treatment of cancer. *J Clin Oncol* 2003;21:2787.
8. Ross JS et al. The *Her-2/neu* gene and protein in breast cancer 2003: biomarker and target of therapy. *Oncologist* 2003;8:307.
9. Olayioye MA. Update on HER-2 as a target for cancer therapy: intracellular signaling pathways of ErbB2/HER-2 and family members. *Breast Cancer Res* 2001;3:385.
10. Stern DF et al. p185, a product of the *neu* proto-oncogene, is a receptorlike protein associated with tyrosine kinase activity. *Mol Cell Biol* 1986;6:1729.
11. Weinberg R. How cancer arises: an explosion of research is uncovering the long-hidden molecular underpinnings of cancer-and suggesting new therapies. *Sci Am* 1996;9:62.
12. Sabichi AL et al. Frontiers in cancer prevention research. *Cancer Res* 2003;63:5649.
13. Hong WK et al. Cancer chemoprevention in the 21st century: genetics, risk modeling, and molecular targets. *J Clin Oncol* 2000;18:9S.
14. Steele VE. Current mechanistic approaches to the chemoprevention of cancer. *J Biochem Mol Biol* 2003;36:78.
15. Lippman SM et al. Cancer prevention science and practice. *Cancer Res* 2002;62:5119.
16. Herendeen JM et al. Use of NSAIDs for the chemoprevention of colorectal cancer. *Ann Pharmacother* 2003;37:1664.
17. Sandler RS et al. A randomized trial of aspirin to prevent colorectal adenomas in patients with previous colorectal cancer. *N Engl J Med,* 2003;348:883.
18. Baron JA et al. A randomized trial of aspirin to prevent colorectal adenomas. *N Engl J Med* 2003;348:891.
19. Bertagnolli MM et al. Celecoxib for the prevention of sporadic colorectal adenomas. *N Engl J Med* 2006;355:873.
20. Arber N et al. Celecoxib for the prevention of colorectal adenomatous polyps. *N Engl J Med* 2006;355:885.
21. Chan AT et al. Aspirin and the risk of colorectal cancer in relation to the expression of COX-2. *N Engl J Med* 2007;356:2131.
22. Fisher B et al. Tamoxifen for prevention of breast cancer: report of the National Surgical Adjuvant Breast and Bowel Project P-1 Study. *J Natl Cancer Inst* 1998;90:1371.
23. Cuzick J et al. Long-term results of tamoxifen prophylaxis for breast cancer-96-month follow-up of the randomized IBIS-I trial. *J Natl Cancer Inst* 2007;99:272.
24. Cummings SR et al. The effect of raloxifene on risk of breast cancer in postmenopausal women. Results from the MORE randomized trial. *JAMA* 1999;281:2189.
25. Vogel, VG et al. Effects of tamoxifen vs. raloxifene on the risk of developing invasive breast cancer and other disease outcomes: the NSABP Study of Tamoxifen and Raloxifene (STAR) P-2 trial. *JAMA* 2006;95:2727.
26. Munoz N et al. Epidemiologic classification of human papillomavirus types associated with cervical cancer. *N Engl J Med* 2003;348:518.
27. Future II Study Group. Quadrivalent vaccine against human papillomavirus to prevent high-grade cervical lesions. *N Engl J Med,* 2007;356:1915.
28. Garland SM et al. Quadrivalent vaccine against human papillomavirus to prevent anogenital diseases. *N Engl J Med* 2007;356:1928.
29. Parkin DM et al. Estimates of the worldwide incidence of 25 major cancers in 1990. *Int J Cancer* 1999;80:827.
30. Skibber JM et al. Cancer of the colon. In: DeVita VT et al. eds. *Cancer: Principles and Practice of Oncology.* 7th ed. Philadelphia: Lippincott Williams & Wilkins; 2004:1061.
31. Carroll PR et al. Cancer of the prostate. In: DeVita VT et al., eds. *Cancer: Principles and Practice of Oncology.* 6th ed. Philadelphia: Lippincott Williams & Wilkins; 2001:1418.
32. Chlewboski RT. Reducing the risk of breast cancer. *N Engl J Med* 2000;343:191.
33. Hamajima N et al. Alcohol, tobacco and breast cancer-collaborative reanalysis of individual data from 53 epidemiological studies, including 58,515 women with breast cancer and 95,067 women without the disease. *Br J Cancer* 2002;18:1234.

34. Gilchrest BA. The pathogenesis of melanoma induced by ultraviolet radiation. *N Engl J Med* 1999;340:1341.
35. Christensen D. Data still cloudy on association between sunscreen use and melanoma risk. *J Natl Cancer Inst* 2003;95:932.
36. Park MT et al. Cell cycle and cancer. *J Biochem Mol Biol* 2003;36:60.
37. Sherr CJ. Cancer cell cycles. *Science* 1996;274:1672.
38. Hahn WC et al. Rules for making human tumor cells. *N Engl J Med* 2002;347:1593.
39. Hahn WC. Role of telomeres and telomerase in the pathogenesis of human cancer. *J Clin Oncol* 2003;21:2034.
40. Rundhaug JE. Matrix metalloproteinases, angiogenesis, and cancer. *Clin Cancer Res* 2003;9:551.
41. National Comprehensive Cancer Network Guidelines for Detection, Prevention, and Risk of Cancer National Comprehensive Cancer Network, Inc. 2007. URL: http://www.nccn.org/physician_gls/f_guidelines.html. Accessed November 15, 2007.
42. Heron DE et al. Radiation medicine innovations for the new millennium. *J Natl Med Assoc* 2003;95:55.
43. Hersh SM. *Chemical and Biological Warfare: America's Hidden Arsenal.* New York: Bobbs Merril; 1968.
44. Marshall EK Jr. Historical perspectives in chemotherapy. In: Goldin A et al., eds. *Advances in Chemotherapy.* Vol. 1. New York: Academic Press; 1964:1.
45. Skipper HE et al. Experimental evaluation of potential anticancer agents: XII. On the criteria and kinetics associated with "curability" of experiment leukemia. *Cancer Chemother Rep* 1964;35:1.
46. Skipper HE. Reasons for success and failure in treatment of murine leukemias with the drugs now employed in treating human leukemias. *Cancer Chemotherapy.* Vol 1. Ann Arbor, MI: University Microfilms International; 1978:1.
47. Chu E et al. Principles of cancer management: chemotherapy. In: DeVita VT et al., eds. *Cancer: Principles and Practice of Oncology.* 6th ed. Philadelphia: Lippincott Williams & Wilkins; 2001:289.
48. Wood WC et al. Dose and dose intensity of adjuvant chemotherapy for stage II, node-positive breast carcinoma. *N Engl J Med* 1994;330:1253.
49. Lorigan P et al. Randomized phase III trial of dose-dense chemotherapy supported by whole-blood hematopoietic progenitors in better-prognosis small-cell lung cancer. *J Natl Cancer Inst* 2005;97:666.
50. Citron ML et al. Randomized trial of dose-dense versus conventionally scheduled and sequential versus concurrent combination chemotherapy as post-operative adjuvant treatment of node-positive primary breast cancer: first report of Intergroup Trial C9741/Cancer and Leukemia Group B Trial 9741. *J Clin Oncol* 2003;21:1431.
51. Valley AW. New treatment options for managing chemotherapy-induced neutropenia. *Am J Health Syst Pharm* 2002;59:S11.
52. Richard S et al. Stem cell transplantation and hematopoietic growth factors. *Current Hematology Reports* 2002;1:103.
53. Hawkins TE et al. Blood cell transplantation. *Curr Opin Oncol* 1995;7:122.
54. Mormont MC et al. Cancer chronotherapy: principles, applications, and perspectives. *Cancer* 2003;97:155.
55. Goldie JH et al. A mathematic model for relating the drug sensitivity of tumors to the spontaneous mutation rate. *Cancer Treat Reports* 1979;63:1727.
56. Gottesman MM. Mechanisms of cancer drug resistance. *Annu Rev Med* 2002;53:615.
57. Leonard GD et al. The role of ABC transporters in clinical practice. *Oncologist* 2003;8:411.
58. Pessina A et al. Altered DNA-cleavage activity of topoisomerase from WEHI-3B leukemia cells with specific resistance to ciprofloxacin. *Anticancer Drugs* 2001;12:441.
59. Iyer L et al. UGT1A1*28 polymorphism as a determinant of irinotecan disposition and toxicity. *Pharmacogenomics J* 2002;2:43.
60. Goetz MP et al. The impact of cytochrome P450 2D6 metabolism in women receiving adjuvant tamoxifen. *Breast Cancer Res Treat* 2007;101:113.
61. Slamon DJ et al. Use of chemotherapy plus a monoclonal antibody against HER2 for metastatic breast cancer that overexpresses HER2. *N Engl J Med* 2001;344:783.
62. Therasse P et al. New guidelines to evaluate the response to treatment in solid tumors. *J Natl Cancer Inst* 2000;92:205.
63. Cancer Therapy Evaluation Program, Common Terminology Criteria for Adverse Events (CTCAE) Version 3.0, DCTD, NCI, NIH, NDDS. March 31, 2003 (http://ctep.cancer.gov). Publish date: June 10, 2003.
64. Oken MM et al. Toxicity and response criteria of the Eastern Cooperative Oncology Group. *Am J Clin Oncol* 1982;5:649.
65. Cella D. Advances in quality of life measurements in oncology patients. *Semin Oncol* 2002;29(3 Suppl 8):60.
66. Perkins GL. Serum tumor markers. *Am Fam Physician* 2003;68:1075.
67. van der Velden VH. Detection of minimal residual disease in hematologic malignancies by real-time quantitative PCR: principles, approaches, and laboratory aspects. *Leukemia* 2003;17:1013.
68. Ali S et al. Endocrine-responsive breast cancer and strategies for combating resistance. *Nat Rev Cancer* 2002;2:101.
69. Mauro MJ et al. STI571: a paradigm of new agents for cancer therapeutics. *J Clin Oncol* 2002;20:325.
70. Mitchell BS. The proteasome—an emerging therapeutic target in cancer. *N Engl J Med* 2003;348:2597.
71. Hanahan D et al. Patterns and emerging mechanisms of the angiogenic switch during tumorigenesis. *Cell* 1996;86:353.
72. Jain RK. Normalization of tumor vasculature: an emerging concept in antiangiogenic therapy. *Science* 2005;307:58.
73. Hurwitz H et al. Bevacizumab plus irinotecan, fluorouracil, and leucovorin for metastatic colorectal cancer. *N Engl J Med* 2004;350:2335.
74. Sandler A et al. Paclitaxel-carboplatin alone or with bevacizumab for non-small-cell lung cancer. *N Engl J Med* 2006;355:2542.
75. Escudier B et al. Sorafenib in advanced clear-cell renal-cell carcinoma. *N Engl J Med* 2007;356:125.
76. Motzer RJ et al. Sunitinib versus interferon alfa in metastatic renal-cell carcinoma. *N Engl J Med* 2007;56:115.
77. Mihich E. Historical overview of biologic response modifiers. *Cancer Invest* 2000;18:456.
78. Kirkwood J. Cancer immunotherapy: the interferon-alpha experience. *Semin Oncol* 2002;29(3 Suppl 7):18.
79. Atkins MB. Interleukin-2: clinical applications. *Semin Oncol* 2002;29(3 Suppl 7):12.
80. Lotze MT et al. In vitro growth of cytotoxic human lymphocytes IV: lysis of fresh and cultured autologous tumor by lymphocytes cultured in T cell growth factor (TCGF). *Cancer Res* 1981;41:4420.
81. Rayner AA et al. Lymphokine-activated killer (LAK) cell phenomenon: analysis of factors relevant to the immunotherapy of human cancer. *Cancer* 1985;55:1327.
82. Rosenberg SA et al. A progress report on the treatment of 157 patients with advanced cancer using lymphokine-activated killer cells and interleukin-2 or high-dose interleukin-2 alone. *N Engl J Med* 1987;316:889.
83. Rosenberg SA et al. Treatment of 283 consecutive patients with metastatic melanoma or renal cell cancer using high-dose bolus interleukin 2. *JAMA* 1994;271:907.
84. American Society of Health-System Pharmacists. ASHP guidelines on preventing medication errors with antineoplastic agents. *Am J Health-System Pharm* URL: http://www.ashp.org. Accessed July25, 2007
85. American Society of Clinical Oncology. American Society of Clinical Oncology statement regarding the use of outside services to prepare or administer chemotherapy drugs. *J Clin Oncol* 2003;21:1882.
86. Cohen MR et al. Preventing medication errors in cancer chemotherapy. *Am J Health Syst Pharm* 1996;53:737.
87. Attilio RM. Caring enough to understand: the road to oncology medication error prevention. *Hosp Pharm* 1996;31:17.
88. Berk PD et al. Increased incidence of leukemia in polycythemia vera associated with chlorambucil therapy. *N Engl J Med* 1981;304:441.
89. Stephens JD et al. Multiple congenital abnormalities in a fetus exposed to 5-fluorouracil during the first trimester. *Am J Obstet Gynecol* 1980;137:747.
90. Benedict WF et al. Mutagenicity of cancer chemotherapeutic agents in the Salmonella/microsome test. *Cancer Res* 1977;37:2209.
91. Rieche K. Carcinogenicity of antineoplastic agents in man. *Cancer Treat Rev* 1984;11:39.
92. ASHP technical assistance bulletin on handling hazardous drugs. *Am J Health Syst Pharm* 2006;63:1172.
93. Finley RS et al. Pharmacy practice issues in oncology. In: Finley RS et al., eds. *Concepts in Oncology Therapeutics.* 2nd ed. Bethesda, MD: American Society of Health-System Pharmacists; 1998.
94. Anderson RW et al. Risk of handling injectable antineoplastic agents. *Am J Health Pharm* 1982;39:1881.
95. Falck K et al. Mutagenicity in urine of nurses handling cytostatic drugs. *Lancet* 1979;1:1250.
96. Waksvik H et al. Chromosome analyses of nurses handling cytostatic agents. *Cancer Treat Reports* 1981;65:607.
97. Chrysotomou A et al. Mutation frequency in nurses and pharmacists working with cytotoxic drugs. *Aust N Z Med* 1984;14:831.
98. Hirst M et al. Occupational exposure to cyclophosphamide. *Lancet* 1984;1:186.
99. Venitt S et al. Monitoring exposure of nursing and pharmacy personnel to cytotoxic drugs: urinary mutation assays and urinary platinum as markers of absorption. *Lancet* 1984;1:74.
100. Connor TH et al. Surface contamination with antineoplastic agents in six cancer treatment centers in Canada and the United States. *Am J Health Syst Pharm* 1999;56:1427.
101. Selevan SH et al. A study of occupational exposure to antineoplastic drugs and fetal loss in nurses. *N Engl J Med* 1985;333:1173.
102. Baker ES et al. Monitoring occupational exposure to cancer chemotherapy drugs. *Am J Health Syst Pharm* 1996;53:2713.
103. Hemminki K et al. Spontaneous abortions and malformations in the offspring of nurses exposed to anesthetic gases, cytostatic drugs, and other potential hazards in hospitals, based on registered information outcome. *J Epidemiol Community Health* 1985;39:141.
104. National Institute for Occupational Safety and Health. NIOSH alert: preventing occupational exposures to antineoplastic and other hazardous drugs in health care settings. URL: http://cdc.gov/niosh. Accessed July 25, 2007.
105. AMA Council on Scientific Affairs. Guidelines for handling parenteral antineoplastics. *JAMA* 1985;253:1590.
106. Jonat W et al. Goserelin versus cyclophosphamide, methotrexate, and fluorouracil as adjuvant therapy in premenopausal patients with node-positive breast cancer: the Zoladex Early Breast Cancer Research Association Study. *J Clin Oncol* 2002;20:4628.
107. Slamon DJ et al. Use of chemotherapy plus a monoclonal antibody against HER2 for metastatic breast cancer that overexpresses HER2. *N Engl J Med* 2001;344:783.
108. Bull JM et al. A randomized comparative trial of

Adriamycin versus methotrexate in combination drug therapy. *Cancer* 1978;41:1649.
109. Henderson, IC et al. Improved outcomes from adding sequential Paclitaxel but not from escalating Doxorubicin dose in an adjuvant chemotherapy regimen for patients with node-positive primary breast cancer. *J Clin Oncol* 2003;21:976.
110. National Comprehensive Cancer Network, N.C.C.N., Clinical Practice Guidelines in Oncology. http://www.nccn.org/, 2007. Accessed November 15, 2007.
111. Poon MA et al. Biochemical modulation of fluorouracil: evidence of significant improvement of survival and quality of life in patients with advanced colorectal carcinoma. *J Clin Oncol* 1989;7:1407.
112. Petrelli N et al. The modulation of fluorouracil with leucovorin in metastatic colorectal carcinoma: a prospective randomized phase III trial. *J Clin Oncol* 1989;7:1419.
113. Poon MA et al. Biochemical modulation of fluorouracil with leucovorin: confirmatory evidence of improved therapeutic efficacy in advanced colorectal cancer. *J Clin Oncol* 199;9:1967.
114. Waters JS et al. Long-term survival after epirubicin, cisplatin and fluorouracil for gastric cancer: results of a randomized trial. *Br J Cancer* 1999;80:269.
115. MacDonald JS et al. 5-fluorouracil, doxorubicin, and mitomycin (FAM) combination chemotherapy for advanced gastric cancer. *Ann Intern Med* 1980; 93:533.
116. Preusser P et al. Phase II study with the combination etoposide, doxorubicin, and cisplatin in advanced measurable gastric cancer. *J Clin Oncol* 1989;7:1310.
117. McGuire WP et al. Cyclophosphamide and cisplatin compared with paclitaxel and cisplatin in patients with stage III and stage IV ovarian cancer. *N Engl J Med* 1996;334:1.
118. McGuire WP et al. Chemotherapy of advanced ovarian cancer. *Semin Oncol* 1998;25:340. Erratum in: *Semin Oncol* 1998;25:707.
119. Bokemeyer C et al. First-line high-dose chemotherapy compared with standard-dose PEB/VIP chemotherapy in patients with advanced germ cell tumors: a multivariate and matched-pair analysis. *J Clin Oncol* 1999;17:3450.
120. Motzer RJ et al. Etoposide and cisplatin adjuvant therapy for patients with pathologic stage II germ cell tumors. *J Clin Oncol* 1995;13:2700.
121. Sternberg CN et al. Preliminary results of M-VAC (methotrexate, vinblastine, doxorubicin and cisplatin) for transitional cell carcinoma of the urothelium. *J Urol* 1985;133:403.
122. von der Maase H et al. Gemcitabine and cisplatin versus methotrexate, vinblastine, doxorubicin, and cisplatin in advanced or metastatic bladder cancer: results of a large, randomized, multinational, multicenter, phase III study. *J Clin Oncol* 2000;18: 3068.
123. Evans WK et al. VP-16 and carboplatin in previously untreated patients with extensive stage small cell lung cancer. *Br J Cancer* 1988;58:464.
124. Goldhirsch A et al. Cis-dichlorodiammineplatinum (II) and VP 16-213 combination chemotherapy for non-small cell lung cancer. *Med Pediatr Oncol* 1981;9:205.
125. Dhingra HM et al. Chemotherapy for advanced adenocarcinoma and squamous cell carcinoma of the lung with etoposide and cisplatin. *Cancer Treat Rep* 1984;68:671.
126. Schiller JH et al. A randomized phase III trial of four chemotherapy regimens for advanced non-small-cell lung cancer. *N Engl J Med* 2002;346:92.
127. Pronzato P et al. Carboplatin and etoposide as outpatient treatment of advanced non-small-cell lung cancer. *Chemotherapy* 1994;40:144.
128. Kish JA et al. A randomized trial of cisplatin (CACP) plus; 5-fluorouracil (5-FU) infusion and CACP plus; 5-FU bolus for recurrent and advanced squamous cell carcinoma of the head and neck. *Cancer* 1985;56:2740.
129. Armitage JO et al. Predicting therapeutic outcome in patients with diffuse histiocytic lymphoma treated with cyclophosphamide, Adriamycin, vincristine, and prednisone (CHOP). *Cancer* 1982;50: 1695.
130. Coiffier B et al. CHOP chemotherapy plus rituximab compared with CHOP alone in elderly patients with diffuse large-B-cell lymphoma. *N Engl J Med* 2002;346:235.
131. Klimo P et al. MACOP-B chemotherapy for the treatment of diffuse large cell lymphoma. *Ann Intern Med* 1985;102:596.
132. Velasquez VS et al. ESHAP—an effective chemotherapy regimen in refractory and relapsing lymphoma: a 4-year follow-up study. *J Clin Oncol* 1994;12:1169.
133. DeVita VT Jr et al. Combination chemotherapy in the treatment of advanced Hodgkin disease. *Ann Intern Med* 1970;73:881.
134. Santoro A et al. Alternating drug combinations in the treatment of advanced Hodgkin disease. *N Engl J Med* 1982;306:770.
135. Barlogie B et al. Effective treatment of advanced multiple myeloma refractory to alkylating agents. *N Engl J Med* 1984;310:1353.
136. Alexanian R et al. Combination chemotherapy for multiple myeloma. *Cancer* 1972;30:382.
137. Martin M et al. Adjuvant docetaxel for node-positive breast cancer. *N Engl J Med* 2005; 352:2302.
138. Levine MN et al. Randomized trial comparing cyclophosphamide, epirubicin, and flourouracil with cyclophosphamide, methotrexate, and flourouracil in premenopausal woman with node positive breast cancer: update of the National Cancer Institute of Canada Clinical Trials Group. *J Clin Oncol* 2005; 23:5166.
139. Langer C et al. Randomized phase II trial of paclitaxel plus carboplatin or gemcitabine plus cisplatin in Eastern Cooperative Oncology Group performance status 2 non-small-cell lung cancer patients: ECOG 1599. *J Clin Oncol* 2007;25:418.

CHAPTER 89

Adverse Effects of Chemotherapy and Targeted Agents

Amy Hatfield Seung

Chemotherapy agents are toxic to cancer cells and also to various host tissues and organs. The adverse effects of chemotherapy can be classified as common and acute toxicities, specific organ toxicities, and long-term complications. Common and acute toxicities generally include adverse effects that occur as a result of inhibition of host cell division. Host tissues most susceptible to chemotherapy include tissues with renewal cell populations, such as lymphoid tissues, bone marrow, and epithelium of the gastrointestinal (GI) tract and skin. Some other common and acute toxicities (e.g., nausea and vomiting, hypersensitivity reactions) frequently occur in patients shortly after chemotherapy. Specific organ toxicities often are attributed to a unique uptake of the chemotherapy agent by the organ or a selective toxicity of the agent to the organ. Long-term complications are toxicities that occur months to years after chemotherapy. These long-term toxicities occur secondary to continued immunodeficiencies or from permanent damage to the organ cells from the specific therapy. Acute and chronic toxicities can overlap. For example, many specific organ toxicities are evident within days following treatment, whereas other specific organ toxicities are not evident until months after treatment. Despite the overlapping definitions, this classification system provides some framework to discuss the adverse effects associated with chemotherapy.

The toxicities associated with chemotherapy are the most important factors limiting the use of potentially curative doses. Therefore, all discussions regarding the benefits of chemotherapy agents must include a discussion of toxicities associated with their use. Concerns regarding the toxicities of chemotherapy include the incidence, predictability, severity, and reversibility of the adverse effects. Although the incidence and predictability may be well defined in specific patient populations, the incidence often varies depending on individual susceptibility. In addition, the specific chemotherapy agent, dose intensity, and treatment duration can influence the incidence of several adverse effects. The specific adverse effects that an individual patient will experience can be difficult to predict, however. Because several toxicities do have well-defined characteristics, clinicians treating patients with chemotherapy should be aware of the most common adverse effects.

Clinicians should also be aware of patient-specific factors, such as the stage of disease, concomitant illnesses, and concurrent medications, which could cause signs or symptoms that mimic the adverse effects associated with chemotherapy. Many patients have significant disease involvement and impairment of organ function because of the malignant cells. In addition, most patients with cancer commonly receive many other medications, including antibiotics and analgesics that can cause additional adverse effects or interact with chemotherapy. When the patient reports a new symptom, it may be difficult to determine whether it is secondary to chemotherapy, concurrent medications, or disease progression. Therefore, the clinician needs to be aware of the presentation, management, and prevention of the most common toxicities that could affect patients receiving chemotherapy.

COMMON AND ACUTE TOXICITIES

Hematologic Toxicities

Effects of Chemotherapy on Bone Marrow

The bone marrow contains a population of pluripotent stem cells capable of self-renewal and differentiation into any mature blood cell. At some point, their progeny commit to either the myeloid or the lymphoid cell line. The myeloid stem cell further commits to developing into an erythrocyte, megakaryocyte, granulocyte, or monocyte. After committing to a particular cell line, bone marrow precursor cells undergo a series of divisions (mitosis) to increase the number of cells. The cells then undergo several developmental stages to mature and differentiate into their final forms and leave the bone marrow (postmitotic). The total time required for a cell to pass through the mitotic and postmitotic pool under normal resting conditions is ~10 to 14 days. This process is regulated by several cytokines; although many cytokines have been identified, only a few are now produced through recombinant DNA technology. These growth factors can expand the mitotic pool and accelerate maturation and differentiation. Ultimately, these growth factors decrease the total time spent in these stages ~5 to 7 days.

The development and circulating life span of hematopoietic cell lines determines the severity of the depression of that cell line (nadir) and the time course of peripheral cytopenias. Because red blood cells (RBC) survive approximately 120 days in the peripheral blood, clinically significant anemia is not likely to occur if RBC production is impaired for a short period of time. Instead, anemia usually develops slowly after several courses of chemotherapy. In contrast, platelets survive ~10 days and granulocytes survive approximately 6 to 8 hours. This is why granulocytopenia generally occurs before thrombocytopenia, but both granulocytopenia and thrombocytopenia may be observed after the first or subsequent courses of chemotherapy. The depression of peripheral blood cells following chemotherapy can help determine the dosage and concurrent chemotherapy for subsequent courses. Life-threatening granulocytopenia or thrombocytopenia often necessitates some action to minimize the risk of adverse effects with additional chemotherapy. Previously, clinicians usually reduced the dose of the myelosuppressive agent. The availability of colony-stimulating factors (CSFs) and interleukin-11 (oprelvekin), however, provides an alternative approach to preventing severe neutropenia or thrombocytopenia following myelosuppressive chemotherapy.

MYELOSUPPRESSION

1. J.T., a 45-year-old, 59-kg man with no significant past medical history, presents to the university hospital with complaints of cough and shortness of breath (SOB). Chest radiograph reveals a lesion in the right upper lobe; bronchoscopy washings and cytologic examination are positive for small-cell lung cancer (SCLC). A workup for metastases is negative. J.T. is diagnosed with limited SCLC. His physicians plan to initiate radiation therapy to the right upper lobe with concurrent chemotherapy, to include carboplatin targeted to an area under the concentration-time curve (AUC) of 5 mg/mL/minute on day 1, topotecan 0.5 mg/m^2 daily on days 1 through 3, and etoposide 100 mg/m^2/day orally (PO) on days 4 through 6. Discuss with J.T. the toxicities that might be expected to occur with this regimen. What effects on the bone marrow can be anticipated and how might they clinically appear in J.T.? What factors can influence the incidence and severity of these adverse effects? When can J.T. expect these effects to occur?

Although several toxicities are commonly associated with carboplatin, topotecan, and etoposide, the most predictable and dangerous toxicity associated with this regimen is myelosuppression. This chemotherapy regimen can significantly affect any cell line, including RBC, neutrophils, and platelets, and the cytopenias can cause significant morbidity or mortality. Decreased RBC can cause anemia, and patients usually present with fatigue and decreased exercise tolerance. Having low neutrophil counts significantly increases a patient's risk for bacterial infections. Moreover, reduced platelets can cause thrombocytopenia, which can cause bleeding from the GI and genitourinary tracts.

Both patient- and agent-related factors can significantly influence the degree of cytopenia a patient faces after chemotherapy. Agent-related factors include the chemotherapy agent, dose intensity, and dose density. Because most chemotherapy treatments are not given as a single agent, the effects of concurrent chemotherapy may intensify the myelosuppressive effect of an individual agent. Host factors that specifically may affect the cellularity of the bone marrow compartment also influence the degree of cytopenia. They include the following:

1. Patient age. Younger patients are generally better able to tolerate chemotherapy than elderly patients because they have a more cellular marrow with a decreased percentage of marrow fat.
2. Bone marrow reserve. Certain diseases might present with tumor cells in the bone marrow, such as leukemias and some lymphomas, in which case the bone marrow does not have a healthy reserve of normal hematopoietic cells to help in the recovery process.

3. The degree of compromise from previous chemotherapy, radiation therapy, or both. Prior chemotherapy and radiation therapy to fields involving marrow-producing bone reduce bone marrow reserves.
4. The ability of the liver or kidney to metabolize and excrete the compounds administered. If agents that depend on the liver or the kidney for metabolism to inactive metabolites or for excretion are administered to patients with specific organ insufficiencies, they can cause greater toxicities, including longer cytopenias secondary to lack of clearance.

These factors, along with the kinetics of the stem cells, can help clinicians predict the severity and duration of cytopenia observed following therapy.

With most myelosuppressive agents, the patient's white blood cell (WBC) and platelet counts begin to fall within 5 to 7 days of chemotherapy administration, reach a nadir within 7 to 10 days, and recover within 14 to 26 days. Phase-specific chemotherapy agents, such as the plant alkaloids and antimetabolites, cause a fairly rapid onset of cytopenia that recovers faster than the cytopenias occurring after treatment with phase-nonspecific agents, such as alkylating agents and antitumor antibiotics. For poorly understood reasons, nitrosureas typically produce severe, delayed neutropenia and thrombocytopenia 4 to 6 weeks after therapy. Other agents that exhibit this pattern include mitomycin and mechlorethamine. All of these chemotherapy agents exert their cytotoxic effects during the resting phase of the cell cycle. The nitrosureas as well as mitomycin and mechlorethamine can, however, cause two neutropenic nadirs; the first nadir occurs at the conventional time expected for phase-nonspecific agents and the second nadir occurs approximately 4 to 6 weeks after therapy. Many combination regimens that use these agents recommend 6-week cycles to avoid treatment before the second nadir. Most other myelosuppressive regimens recommend dosing intervals of 3 to 4 weeks to allow the bone marrow time to recover. Many of the targeted therapies do not exhibit bone marrow suppression, because their action is toward a specific molecular event rather than an entire metabolic process. Because these novel agents do not have overlapping myelosuppressive effects, they may be ideal agents to add to regimens that are known to cause cytopenias.

All the agents included in J.T.'s regimen have marked myelosuppressive activity. J.T. should be carefully counseled to contact his physician or report to the emergency department (ED) if he experiences signs or symptoms of an infection (including fever) or bleeding. Typically, these symptoms occur 10 to 14 days after the first day of chemotherapy.

Prevention

2. About 9 days after the first course of chemotherapy, J.T. developed a severe sore throat and fever. He was admitted to the hospital and treated with intravenous (IV) antibiotics. At the time, his WBC count was 300 cells/mm^3. His fever resolved after 3 days, and all cultures were negative for bacterial growth. It is now 3 weeks after chemotherapy, and he is scheduled to receive a second course. Should he receive the same doses he was given initially?

Previously, the chemotherapy doses would have been reduced (usually by 25%) for all subsequent cycles for any patient who experienced febrile neutropenia. Although a dose reduction can clearly cause less neutropenia, it can also compromise the response and survival of patients with chemotherapy-sensitive tumors. Because J.T.'s cancer (i.e., limited-stage small cell lung cancer), is both chemosensitive and potentially curable, a dosage reduction is undesirable. To minimize the risk of neutropenia with future therapy, CSFs can be administered to J.T. to prevent potential complications associated with neutropenia.

The prophylactic administration of CSFs can be used to protect against the myelosuppressive effects of chemotherapy. Three CSFs, granulocyte colony-stimulating factor (G-CSF [filgrastim]) and granulocyte-macrophage colony-stimulating factor (GM-CSF [sargramostim]) and a pegylated long-acting form of filgrastim, pegfilgrastim, are available in the United States. These products were approved by the U.S. Food and Drug Administration (FDA) to enhance neutrophil recovery after chemotherapy. Pegfilgrastim was developed with the aim of providing the same pharmacologic benefit as filgrastim while offering the advantage and convenience of fewer injections. Evidence-based clinical practice guidelines for the use of CSFs have been developed by the American Society of Clinical Oncology (ASCO).[1] These guidelines recommend primary prophylaxis for all patients receiving chemotherapy regimens that have been previously reported to cause an incidence of ~20% of febrile neutropenia. A CSF used in these patients can reduce both the incidence of febrile neutropenia and need for hospitalizations and broad-spectrum antibiotics. Two randomized phase III clinical trials have shown that the risk of neutropenic fever is reduced when primary prophylaxis is used in regimens with a known incidence of ~20% neutropenia. In one trial, 928 patients with breast cancer receiving docetaxel 100 mg/m^2 every 21 days were randomized to receive placebo or pegfilrastim 6 mg subcutaneously (SQ) 24 hours after chemotherapy. Patients who received pegfilgrastim had a lower incidence of febrile neutropenia (1% vs. 17%, respectively) and hospitalizations (1% vs. 14%, respectively).[2] A trial in patients ($N = 171$) with SCLC receiving a dose-intense regimen containing cyclophosphamide 1,000 mg/m^2 day 1, doxorubicin 45 mg/m^2 day 1, and etoposide 100 mg/m^2 days 1 to 3 every 21 days was conducted. Patients were randomized to receive prophylactic antibiotics with or without G-CSF. The rate of febrile neutropenia over all five cycles given was 32% with prophylactic antibiotics alone versus 18% with antibiotics and G-CSF.[3] Because the regimen J.T. received does not typically produce a 20% incidence of febrile neutropenia, a CSF was not recommended for him after his first course of chemotherapy. Because J.T. did experience febrile neutropenia and he has a potentially curable malignancy, a CSF is indicated with subsequent courses of chemotherapy to prevent additional febrile episodes.

3. How are CSFs dosed to prevent chemotherapy-induced neutropenia?

The recommended initial dose of filgrastim (G-CSF) is 5 mcg/kg/day as a single daily subcutaneous (SC) injection, and the recommended initial dose of sargramostim (GM-CSF) is 250 mcg/m^2/day as an SC injection. Pegfilgrastim is given at a dose of 6 mg once per cycle as an SC injection regardless of patient weight. The ASCO guidelines state that rounding the dose of either agent to the nearest vial size may enhance patient convenience and reduce cost without clinical detriment. Because commercially available vials contain either 300 or 480 mcg of G-CSF, adult patients <75 kg should receive 300 mcg daily and adult patients >75 kg should receive 480 mcg daily.[1] Because of differences in commercially available vial sizes, the weight breakpoint for GM-CSF is slightly different; patients who weigh >60 kg should receive 500 mcg daily and patients who weigh <60 kg should receive 250 mcg daily.

The ASCO guidelines also recommend a shorter duration of treatment than does the manufacturer. The manufacturer recommends that therapy with filgrastim or sargramostim continue until the patient's neutrophil count is >10,000 cells/mm^3 after the expected chemotherapy nadir. This is based on the observation that the neutrophil count falls roughly 50% after discontinuing a CSF. The risk of bacterial infection is highest, however, in patients with neutrophil counts of <500 to 1,000 cells/mm^3; patients with neutrophil counts >500 to 1,000 cells/mm^3 are not thought to be at high risk for developing bacterial infections. Thus, many clinicians elect to discontinue CSF when the neutrophil count reaches 2,000 to 4,000 cells/mm^3 following the chemotherapy nadir. This reduces the number of treatment days and the cost associated with therapy without placing the patient at excessive risk for bacterial infections. The ASCO guidelines support this recommendation to discontinue CSF earlier.

To prevent chemotherapy-induced neutropenia, either pegfilgrastim, filgrastim, or sargramostim is used. Many patients find that a single injection of pegfilgrastim is more convenient with fewer injections to receive. Two pivotal, randomized, blinded multicenter phase III trials have evaluated the efficacy of single-dose pegfilgrastim in the prevention of chemotherapy-induced neutropenia in patients with high-risk stage II, stage III, and stage IV breast cancer.[4,5] The patients ($N = 310$)[4] ($N = 157$)[5] received four cycles of doxorubicin 60 mg/m^2 and docetaxel 75 mg/m^2 chemotherapy on day 1 of each cycle and were randomized to either single-dose pegfilgrastim on day 2 or filgrastim 5 mcg/kg/day from day 2 until the absolute neutrophil count (ANC) was >10,000 cells/mm^3 for a maximum of 14 doses. In one study, the pegfilgrastim was a 6-mg fixed dose[5] and in the other study the pegfilgrastim dose was based on weight (100 mcg/kg).[4] The primary endpoint was duration of severe grade IV neutropenia (ANC <500 cells/mm^3 in cycle 1). Secondary endpoints included the degree of ANC nadir, time to recovery, incidence of grade IV neutropenia and incidence of febrile neutropenia. In these phase III breast cancer trials, no significant difference in duration of grade IV neutropenia was seen between the pegfilgrastim and filgrastim groups (1.7 vs. 1.8 days, respectively,[4] and 1.8 vs. 1.6 days, respectively[5]). The incidence of severe neutropenia after chemotherapy was similar in the pegfilgrastim and filgrastim arms. In patients treated with pegfilgrastim, the incidence of febrile neutropenia over four cycles of chemotherapy in the two pivotal phase III trials[4,5] was lower than in the patients treated with filgrastim. In the larger of the trials, this difference was clinically significant ($p = 0.029$). The time to ANC recovery was defined as the time from chemotherapy administration until the ANC increased to >2,000 cells/mm^3. In the larger phase III trial,[4] the mean time to recovery was 9.3 days in the pegfilgrastim group compared with 9.7 days in the filgrastim group. In all studies, pegfilgrastim has been well tolerated. From these data, it appears that a single 6-mg dose of pegfilgrastim is at least equivalent to daily SC injections of filgrastim but offers advantages with respect to convenience and patient comfort.

In summary, J.T. should be given either G-CSF 300 mcg/day or GM-CSF 250 mcg/day SC beginning the day after his last dose of chemotherapy. Treatment should continue until the ANC is >2,000 to 4,000 cells/mm^3. Alternatively, J.T. could receive a single 6-mg injection of pegfilgrastim the day after chemotherapy administration. Patients should not require more than one dose of pegfilgrastim for chemotherapy-induced neutropenia. Self-regulation of pegfilgrastim serum levels, related to its pegylation, is almost entirely dependent on neutrophil receptor-mediated clearance. Serum levels of pegfilgrastim will remain elevated during neutropenia induced by chemotherapy, and decline on recovery of neutrophil counts.[6] Aside from high cost and inconvenience, the only negative effect of G-CSF therapy is mild transient bone pain. Bone pain is most commonly experienced when patients begin to recover peripheral blood cells following their nadir. The proposed mechanism suggests the stimulatory effect of G-CSF on granulopoiesis causes the pain. Most patients commonly report pain in bone marrow-rich areas, such as the sternum and pelvic regions. They should be advised that the bone pain experienced during marrow recovery is normal and usually is relieved with analgesic agents.

Treatment

4. If J.T. was not given G-CSF and presented with febrile neutropenia, would G-CSF therapy be helpful?

Because the duration of neutropenia is the most significant prognostic factor in patients with established febrile neutropenia, the major benefit of CSFs is their ability to reduce the duration of neutropenia. CSFs accelerate hematopoiesis by expanding the mitotic pool of committed progenitor cells and shortening the time spent in the postmitotic pool from 6 days to 1 day. If CSFs reduce the duration of neutropenia in patients who present with febrile neutropenia, then morbidity, mortality, and cost should be significantly reduced.

The ability of CSFs to reduce the duration of neutropenia in patients with established febrile neutropenia has been addressed in numerous randomized, double-blind, placebo-controlled trials,[7] and two meta-analyses of trials have also been completed.[1,8,9] The combined data for G-CSF and GM-CSF reveal minimal to moderate benefit in reducing hospital stays. Additionally, no differences in mortality were reported with the use of CSFs in this setting. Furthermore, questions have been raised as to whether all patients with febrile neutropenia require hospitalization. Several studies have shown equal efficacy and safety with increased cost effectiveness of outpatient treatment of febrile neutropenia.[10–12] Although CSFs do appear to hasten neutrophil recovery, the true cost-to-benefit ratio associated with the use of these products in established febrile neutropenia remains to be determined. The ASCO guidelines currently do not support routine use of CSFs in patients with febrile neutropenia, although they do recognize that certain patients with febrile neutropenia and high risk features predictive of clinical deterioration (e.g., age >65 years, pneumonia, fungal infection, hypotension, sepsis syndrome, uncontrolled primary disease) may benefit from use of CSFs.

5. **Fourteen days after his fourth course of chemotherapy, J.T.'s platelet count is 7,000 cells/mm^3. Although he has no evidence of bleeding, the clinician decides to administer a prophylactic platelet transfusion. Would oprelvekin be helpful in preventing the need for further platelet transfusions?**

Oprelvekin is indicated to prevent severe thrombocytopenia and reduce the need for platelet transfusions following myelosuppressive chemotherapy in patients with nonmyeloid malignancies at high risk for developing severe thrombocytopenia. Because carboplatin has a cumulative myelosuppressive effect on platelet precursors, J.T. is at risk for developing severe thrombocytopenia with future courses of chemotherapy. In a randomized, double-blind clinical trial, oprelvekin reduced the need for platelet transfusions in about 20% of patients who were similar to J.T.[13] The recommended dose is 50 mcg/kg/day SC until the postnadir platelet count is >50,000 cells/mm^3 or up to 21 days following chemotherapy.[14] Side effects can be mild to moderate and include peripheral edema, dyspnea, and pleural effusions. Because only about 20% of patients respond to oprelvekin, J.T. may still require additional platelet transfusions. In addition, the cost:benefit ratio of oprelvekin compared with platelet transfusions has not been demonstrated in clinical trials. Based on current evidence, J.T. should not receive oprelvekin at this time.

Anemia and Erythropoietin

6. **Is erythropoietin useful in cancer patients with anemia?**

Anemia usually is not a dose-limiting toxicity commonly associated with chemotherapy, because RBCs survive ~120 days. Chemotherapy predominantly affects RBCs by causing anisocytosis and macrocytosis. These effects are related to inhibition of DNA synthesis, and they predominantly occur following treatment with antimetabolites, including folic acid analogs, hydroxyurea, purine antagonists, and pyrimidine antagonists. Anemia commonly does not accompany these changes in RBC size. In addition, chemotherapy-induced effects on RBC are rarely the sole factor contributing to the low hemoglobin (Hgb) levels that necessitate an RBC transfusion.

Nevertheless, anemia commonly occurs in cancer patients secondary to the primary disease. The exact mechanism by which this anemia occurs is not well understood. Impaired erythrocyte response to erythropoietin, reduced hematopoietic precursors caused by chemotherapy or radiation therapy, and disrupted marrow architecture caused by invasion of malignant cells may all play a role. Erythropoietin has been shown to ameliorate anemia associated with cancer and chemotherapy, reduce the need for transfusions, and enhance the patient's quality of life.[15–17]

Two erythropoiesis-stimulating agents (ESA) are currently available for patient use. Recombinant human erythropoietin (r-HUEPO, epoietin-α) is approved for use in cancer patients receiving chemotherapy. Multiple dosing strategies have been suggested and evaluated in clinical trials. One recommended starting dose for r-HUEPO is 150 U/kg three times per week rounded to a standard dose of 10,000 U, consistent with the vial size, which is significantly higher than the recommended dose for anemia of renal failure. Alternatively, 40,000 U once weekly has also been shown to be effective and may be more convenient for patients.[18] These initial doses should be given for 4 weeks. If the Hgb increases <1 g/dL, then the dose should be increased to 300 U/kg three times weekly or 60,000 U once weekly. Up to 8 weeks of treatment may be required to decrease transfusion requirements significantly. Only about 50% of patients respond (i.e., reduce their requirement for transfusion or report a significant decrease in symptoms) to erythropoietin, so patients who do not respond positively within 6 to 8 weeks should discontinue therapy. Because pretreatment erythropoietin levels do not consistently correlate with the rate and likelihood of response, clinicians cannot predict which patients will respond to therapy.[19] Adverse effects, such as hypertension, seizures, and angina, that can occur in patients with renal failure following a rapid dose escalation or normalization of hematocrit, have not been observed in patients with cancer; however, reviews of clinical trials in cancer patients have shown an increased risk for thromboembolic events.

Darbepoetin-α (Aranesp) is an ESA closely related to erythropoietin that is produced in Chinese hamster ovary cells by recombinant DNA technology. It stimulates erythropoiesis by the same mechanism as erythropoietin. Darbepoetin, also approved for the treatment of chemotherapy-related anemia, is distinguished from erythropoietin by its approximately threefold longer half-life and greater biologic potency. This allows for an extended dosing interval relative to erythropoietin. Two dose-finding studies in 429 patients found that darbepoetin-α 1.5 mcg/kg, once per week, achieved the same mean hemoglobin change from baseline as that of recombinant human erythropoietin dosed at 150 U/kg, three times a week. At a dose of 3 mg/kg weekly, darbopoetin-α elicited a hematopoietic response after 2 weeks similar to that produced by r-HUEPO 40,000 to 60,000 U once per week.[20,21] Additionally, in a multicenter open-label study of darbepoetin, 500 mcg every 3 weeks was effective in increasing and maintaining hemoglobin levels and was well tolerated.[22] The FDA-approved starting doses of darbepoetin are 2.25 mcg/kg weekly or 500 mcg SC every 3 weeks. Darbepoetin may be increased to 4.5 mcg/kg weekly if no positive response is seen within 6 weeks of the initial dose.[22]

Epoetin-α and darbepoetin-α have been studied in head-to-head prospective comparison trials as well as evaluated in multiple large meta-analyses and systematic literature reviews, and have been shown to be equal in efficacy, including hemoglobin responses and decreases in transfusions.[22–26] ESAs may provide a safe and effective treatment for chemotherapy-associated anemia. ESAs are not recommended in the treatment of anemia in cancer patients caused by underlying diseases when patients are not receiving chemotherapy.

Epoetin-α and darbepoetin-α are indicated only for cancer patients actively receiving chemotherapy to reach and maintain a target hemoglobin level of 11 g/dL. Data have been reviewed by the FDA from four trials in cancer patients receiving ESAs. Collectively they show a higher risk of serious side effects, including thromboembolism, and increased mortality in patients with hemoglobin levels >12 g/dL and in those patients not receiving chemotherapy.[27] The use of erythropoietin agents in patients with cancer is rapidly evolving. Clinical practice guidelines from the American Society of Hematology and American Society of Clinical Oncology have provided updated recommendations and precautions regarding the use of ESA. These guidelines serve as an excellent resource for incorporating the use of ESA into current clinical practice.[22]

Chemotherapy and Coagulation

7. What effect does chemotherapy have on blood coagulation?

Patients with cancer might develop bleeding secondary to chemotherapy-induced thrombocytopenia or thrombosis after chemotherapy. Bleeding can occur after treatment with L-asparaginase or the pegylated formulation PEG-L-asparaginase, which can inhibit the synthesis of fibrinogen and other specific coagulation factors produced by the liver under the influence of vitamin K.[28,29] L-Asparaginase has a widespread effect on protein synthesis, and many plasma protein factors are depressed shortly after treatment with this agent. A patient receiving L-asparaginase can often develop a prolonged prothrombin time (PT) and partial thromboplastin time (PTT). Bleeding or thrombosis occurring as a direct result of changes in coagulation factors has not been frequently reported or conclusively documented, however. Coagulation factors may return to normal levels with continued administration of the agent, which suggests that the impairment of protein synthesis created by L-asparaginase is partially overcome by the liver. Specific treatment of prolonged PT and PTT with coagulation factors, fibrinogen, or vitamin K is not indicated.

THROMBOTIC EVENTS

Thrombotic events have been associated with the administration of chemotherapy.[30] Evidence of intravascular coagulation from plasma fibrinopeptide A, a specific activation peptide of fibrinogen, has been reported after starting chemotherapy.[31] Conversely, a decrease in fibrinolytic activity reflected by a decrease in functional plasminogen activator also has been reported.[31] Other protein abnormalities associated with thrombosis, including a decrease in the anticoagulant proteins C and protein S (free and total),[32,33] have occurred after chemotherapy. Deficiencies of these proteins have been reported to result in spontaneous thrombosis. Although chemotherapy can potentially increase a patient's risk of thrombosis, the underlying disease can also affect risk.

Assessing the risk of thrombosis from administration of chemotherapy is complicated because many cancers are associated with an increased incidence of thrombosis. This is particularly true in tumors of the GI tract and acute promyelocytic leukemia. Trousseau[34] first reported an increased incidence of venous thrombosis in patients with cancer, and many investigators have since confirmed the relationship of multiple or migratory venous thrombosis in up to 15% of patients with cancer.[35] Up to one-third of apparently healthy adults who develop otherwise unexplained deep vein thrombosis eventually are proved to have a malignancy.[36,37] Removal of the tumor often causes thrombotic episodes to disappear. Although warfarin or low-molecular-weight heparin therapy is indicated, thrombosis associated with cancer is often resistant to anticoagulant therapy.

Initiating treatment for acute promyelocytic leukemia commonly is associated (i.e., up to 85%) with disseminated intravascular coagulation.[38] The lysed tumor cells appear to release procoagulant materials following chemotherapy. Use of heparin to minimize risk of coagulation is controversial. Some investigators have reported excellent results in patients treated almost entirely with blood product support (e.g., fibrinogen, antithrombin III) without heparin.[38]

Several chemotherapy agents have been associated with thrombosis risk, including antiangiogenic therapies such as thalidomide, lenalidomide, and bevaciziumab. Thalidomide and lenalidomide in combination with other chemotherapy agents has been associated with venous thromboembolic events when used in the treatment of multiple myeloma and other diseases.[39,40] Prophylaxis may be warranted, although optimal strategies are not defined and have not been studied in randomized trials.

Bevaciziumab is associated with both arterial thrombosis and bleeding events. A retrospective analysis of five trials of patients receiving chemotherapy for colorectal, breast, or non–small-cell lung cancers revealed a 3.8% incidence of arterial thrombosis in patients receiving chemotherapy and bevaciziumb versus 1.7% in chemotherapy alone.[41] Severe major bleeding events have been reported in patients with metastatic colorectal cancer and life-threatening pulmonary hemorrhage and hemoptysis have been described in those with non–small-cell lung cancer; however, most bleeding events associated with bevacizumab use were minor.[42]

Other factors can cause patients to develop thrombosis. Most patients receiving cancer chemotherapy often have other illnesses that may predispose them to developing thrombosis. In addition, surgical procedures and bedrest can increase the risk of thrombosis. Clinicians should maintain a high index of suspicion when a patient with cancer presents with signs or symptoms of thrombosis.

Gastrointestinal Tract Toxicities

The GI tract may be second only to the bone marrow in its susceptibility to toxic effects produced by chemotherapy. GI toxicities include nausea and vomiting, oral complications, esophagitis, and lower bowel disturbances.

Nausea and Vomiting

Nausea and vomiting are common and serious toxicities associated with many chemotherapy agents. Chemotherapy agents, their metabolites, or neurotransmitters may stimulate dopamine or serotonin receptors in the GI tract, the chemoreceptor trigger zone, or the central nervous system (CNS), which ultimately act on the vomiting center. Emesis most commonly occurs on the first day of chemotherapy and often persists for several days thereafter.[43] Most patients who receive traditional chemotherapy agents require antiemetics before and after chemotherapy for several days to control these symptoms. The most appropriate antiemetic regimen is based on patient- and agent-specific factors. Some of the novel targeted therapy agents carry some risk of emetogenicity, although it is generally milder. Guidelines are beginning to incorporate some of these targeted agents into their emetogenic classification schema based on incidence of nausea and vomiting in clinical trials (see Chapter 7, Nausea and Vomiting).

Complications of the Oral Cavity

Complications of the oral cavity include mucositis (or stomatitis), xerostomia (dry mouth), infection, and bleeding. Approximately 40% of patients treated with chemotherapy develop oral complications, and virtually all patients who receive radiation therapy to the head and neck develop oral complications.[44] These toxicities occur because of the nonspecific effects of

Table 89-1 Topical Medications for Oral Complications of Chemotherapy and Radiation Therapy

Problem	*Products*	*Use*
Xerostomia	Pilocarpine 5-mg tablet plus	1–2 tablets TID to QID
	Saliva substitutes and/or	Rinse or spray PRN
	Sugar-free hard candy; sugar-free gum; ice chips	PRN
Mucositis *Generalized*	Dyclonine hydrochloride (HCl) 0.5% or 1% solution	Swish and expectorate 5–15 mL Q 2–3 hr PRN
	or	
	Viscous lidocaine 2% solution	Swish and expectorate 5–15 mL Q 2–3 hr PRN
	or	
	Diphenhydramine capsules (125 mg) plus Dyclonine 1% 30 mL plus Nystatin 1 mL and 120 mL Maalox	Swish and expectorate 5–15 mL Q 2–3 hr PRN
	or	
	Diphenhydramine plus nystatin plus hydrocortisone (various formulations)	Swish and expectorate 5–15 mL Q 2–3 hr PRN
	or	
	Sucralfate suspension (8 tablets in 40 mL sterile water plus 40 mL 70% sorbitol; shake well and add water to 120 mL)	Swish and expectorate 5–15 mL Q 2–3 hr PRN
Localized	Benzocaine in Orabase	Apply to affected dried area Q 2–3 hr; not to be used in the presence of an infection
Local bleeding (gingival)	Topical thrombin solution	Apply to affected area with gauze sponge and hold in place with pressure for 30 min; do not remove formed clots
Mucosal surface bleeding	Aminocaproic acid	Swish and expectorate 250 mg Q 4 hr for up to 12 hr
General infection	Chlorhexidine gluconate 0.12% oral rinse	Rinse BID after breakfast and at HS for 30 sec; do not swallow
Prevention and treatment of oral candidiasis	Nystatin oral suspension	Rinse and swallow (if tolerated) 500,000–1,000,000 units TID to QID
	or	
	Clotrimazole troche 10 mg	Dissolve 1 tablet 5 times/day
Prevention of caries	Acidulated fluoride rinse	Rinse daily for 1 min with 5–10 mL; do not swallow; switch to neutral fluoride if mucositis is present
	or	
	Neutral fluoride rinse	Rinse daily for 1 min with 5 mL; do not swallow; switch back to acidulated fluoride rinse when mucositis resolves
	or	
	Stannous fluoride gel 0.4%	Brush daily at HS; swish for 30 sec; expectorate and rinse
	or	
	Sodium fluoride gel 1.1%	Brush daily at HS; swish for 30 sec; expectorate and rinse

BID, twice daily; HS, at night; PRN, as needed; QID, four times daily; TID, three times daily.

chemotherapy on cells undergoing rapid division, including the cells of the mouth that undergo rapid renewal with a turnover time equal to 7 to 14 days. Chemotherapy reduces the renewal rate of the basal epithelium and can cause mucosal atrophy, as well as glandular and collagen degeneration.[45] Radiation therapy to the head and neck also causes mucosal atrophy by decreasing cell renewal. Radiation can also cause fibrosis of the salivary glands, muscles, ligaments, and blood vessels and damage to the taste buds.[46]

The combined effects of chemotherapy and radiation therapy on the oral mucosa can also cause infection and bleeding in the oral cavity. Infection and bleeding occurs when treatment causes bone marrow suppression, including thrombocytopenia and neutropenia. Because the oral mucosa is highly vascular and frequently traumatized, bleeding occurs commonly with low platelet counts. In addition, chemotherapy and neutropenia can alter the extensive microbial flora harbored in the oral cavity, thus leading to oral infections. Oral complications often compound one another, however. For example, xerostomia can accelerate the development of mucositis as well as the formation of dental caries and local infection. Mucositis can clearly predispose the oral cavity to local bleeding and infection, as well as sepsis. These oral complications can also cause varying degrees of discomfort and adversely affect the patient's ability to eat, which potentially can lead to a compromised nutritional status. Topical treatments of oral complications are summarized in Table 89-1.

XEROSTOMIA

8. J.B. is a 55-year-old man with newly diagnosed, locally advanced head and neck cancer. Neoadjuvant chemotherapy with cisplatin, methotrexate, and fluorouracil, followed by a 2-week course of radiation therapy (200 rads/day for three cycles) and surgical resection of persistent residual disease are planned. A review of systems suggests that J.B. has poor oral hygiene, and a decision is made to consult the dental department of the university hospital before initiating radiation and chemotherapy. Is

J.B. at risk for developing oral complications of chemotherapy? Is there anything that should be done at this point to decrease his risk?

J.B. is at high risk for several of the oral complications previously described. Xerostomia, one of the most frequent side effects of radiation therapy to the head and neck, occurs secondary to radiation-induced changes to the salivary glands. Evidence supports a direct relationship between the dose of radiation to the salivary glands and the extent of glandular changes.[47] In most patients treated with <6,000 rads, radiation-induced changes to the salivary glands are reversible within 6 to 12 months after the end of therapy. J.B., however, also will be receiving chemotherapy agents (i.e., methotrexate, fluorouracil) that can cause xerostomia and enhance the toxicity to the salivary glands. Clinically, xerostomia has been caused by as little as two to three radiation doses of 200 rads.[47]

Damage to the salivary glands causes various effects, including a loss of salivary buffering capacity, lower salivary pH, no mechanical flushing, and decreased salivary IgA. In addition, xerostomia can alter the sense of taste, causing some patients to lose their ability to differentiate between sweet and salty foods and others to report a bitter taste. Xerostomia also commonly causes caries. Caries and decalcification may become sufficiently severe to compromise tooth integrity and cause fracture. Because saliva is no longer available to help clear bacteria from the mouth, xerostomia also predisposes patients to infection secondary to the increases in oral bacteria. Administering a chemoprotectant before chemotherapy or radiation therapy may help reduce these adverse effects.

Amifostine

Amifostine, an organic thiophosphate chemoprotectant agent, is approved to reduce the incidence of moderate to severe xerostomia in patients having postoperative radiation treatment for head and neck cancer when the radiation port includes a substantial portion of the parotid glands. A randomized, clinical trial demonstrated that the incidence of xerostomia was reduced by about 30% in patients receiving 200 mg/m^2 as a 3-minute IV infusion 15 to 30 minutes before each fraction of radiation.[48] Guidelines published by ASCO support the use of amifostine to reduce the incidence of acute and late toxicity in patients receiving fractionated radiation therapy for head and neck cancer.[49] Amifostine cannot, however, prevent xerostomia from occurring in all patients. Amifostine is not used widely for the prevention of radiation-induced xerostomia secondary to its cost and adverse effect profile. Intravenous amifostine can cause nausea and vomiting as well as hypotension. Subcutaneous administration of the agent causes fewer GI effects and less hypotension, but increases the risk of injection site reactions. Because of these toxicities, >20% of patients discontinue amifostine before completing their radiation.[50]

Other Treatments and Prevention

If xerostomia occurs, treatment can stimulate existing salivary flow and replace lost secretions. Relatively low doses of systemically administered pilocarpine (5–10 mg orally three times daily) may stimulate salivary flow and produce clinically significant benefits in patients with postradiation xerostomia.[51] Dose-related adverse effects include cholinergic effects, such as sweating, rhinitis, headache, nausea, and abdominal cramps. Sucrose-free hard candy and sugar-free chewing gum can also stimulate salivation, but these treatments are typically considered oral comfort agents. Saliva substitutes can also provide oral comfort to patients with xerostomia. Commercially available saliva substitutes generally are recommended for use before meals and at bedtime. They are available in several formulations, including sprays, rinses, and chewing gums. Patients who find one product or formulation unacceptable or unsuccessful may benefit from experimenting with other formulations or product lines. Studies have shown that salivary substitutes containing carboxymethylcellulose or hydroxyethylcellulose are more effective in relieving dryness than water- or glycerin-based solutions.[52,53] Other treatment modalities attempt to prevent the complications associated with xerostomia.

Prevention of radiation-induced caries is best accomplished by aggressively using fluorides.[54] Generally, acidulated fluorides are the most effective, although neutral fluorides may be more acceptable to patients with mucositis. Patients are instructed to rinse daily for 1 minute with 5 to 10 mL of a fluoride rinse. Stannous fluoride gels 0.4% or sodium fluoride gel 1.1% tooth brushing agents may be also be used by patients to minimize their risk of caries. Meticulous attention to oral hygiene with regular dental checkups and avoidance of sucrose is essential to minimize the development of caries.

In general, a dentist should see patients who will be receiving radiation therapy to the head and neck or chemotherapy agents with a high risk of oral complications before starting therapy. This includes patients with hematologic malignancies who will most likely experience severe myelosuppression for prolonged periods. Oral evaluation before therapy, intervention to eliminate potential sources of infection or irritation prior to therapy, and preventive measures taken during therapy can dramatically decrease the frequency of oral complications.[55] Given J.B.'s risk factors, a dental examination is indicated before initiating therapy.

MUCOSITIS AND STOMATITIS

9. J.B. successfully completed his first 2-week course of combined chemotherapy and radiation therapy; however, 3 days into his second 2-week cycle, he complains of generalized burning, discomfort, and pain on the ventral surface of his tongue. On clinical observation, both the ventral surface of his tongue and the floor of his mouth appear erythematous, and several discrete lesions are present in both areas. What is the most likely explanation for J.B.'s new onset of symptoms? What treatment is indicated at this time?

J.B.'s symptoms are consistent with therapy-related mucositis. As discussed, this complication occurs as a nonspecific effect of chemotherapy agents and radiation therapy on the basal epithelium of the mouth. Nonkeratinized mucosa is affected most often. Thus, the buccal, labial, and soft palate mucosa; the ventral surface of the tongue; and the floor of the mouth are the most common sites of involvement. Although lesions are usually discrete initially, they often progress to produce large areas of ulceration. The lesions typically do not progress outside the mouth, but they may extend to the esophagus and involve the entire GI tract. Signs and symptoms generally occur about 5 to 7 days after chemotherapy or at almost any point during radiation therapy. The antimetabolites (e.g., methotrexate, fluorouracil, and cytarabine) and the antitumor antibiotics are the chemotherapy agents that most commonly produce direct stomatotoxicity. Lesions generally regress and resolve completely in ~1 to 3 weeks, depending on their severity.

Patients with mucositis can present with various symptoms, but they often complain of pain so severe that parenteral opioid analgesics are required for relief. Other signs or symptoms include decreased ability to eat and speak, and local or systemic infections. Bacterial, fungal, or viral infections can occur. Although different microbial agents can cause a characteristic lesion, the lesion's appearance usually does not always correlate with the infectious agent. This particularly occurs in patients with neutropenia who cannot mount a full inflammatory response. In these individuals, the clinical appearance of an infected lesion may be muted relative to the presence or number of pathogens. Under normal conditions, the mucosa provides a natural barrier to the entry of normal oral flora, but the broken mucosa allows pathogens access to the bloodstream. The patient could develop life-threatening infection or sepsis in addition to a local infection. After assessing the complications associated with mucositis, the patient should be treated to minimize discomfort and morbidity.

Treatment

Treatment of mucositis is palliative. Topical anesthetics, including viscous lidocaine or dyclonine hydrochloride 0.5 or 1%, often are recommended. Equal portions of kaolin, diphenhydramine, and magnesium- or aluminum-containing antacids can be used for their anesthetic and astringent properties. Many institutions may compound mouthwash products containing these ingredients as well as antibiotics, nystatin, or corticosteroids. Corticosteroids provide anti-inflammatory properties, and the antibiotics and antifungals provide antibacterial or antifungal properties. Another topical agent, sucralfate, may provide some benefit by coating the lesion and reducing discomfort. All of these topically applied products are only used for symptom control, and data supporting superior efficacy of one product over another in relieving pain are lacking.

All the topical anesthetic-containing preparations are recommended for use as "swish-and-spit" preparations. Generally, 5 to 10 mL is used three to six times a day. The longer the patient can hold the solution in the mouth, the longer the contact, and, theoretically, the better the symptom relief. Therefore, patients should be advised to hold and swish the solution around the mouth for as long as possible before spitting it out. Other treatment options include topical benzocaine in Orabase and ice chips. For small localized lesions, ointments such as benzocaine in Orabase may be applied after the affected area has been dried with a sponge. Patients may also find ice chips soothing. Most patients, however, require systemic analgesics to alleviate the pain.

Gelclair is a bioadherent oral gel containing polyvinylpyrrolidone and sodium hyaluronate (but no alcohol or anesthetic agent). It provides an adherent barrier over the mucosal surfaces, thereby shielding oral lesions from the effect of food, liquids, and saliva.[56] Controlled clinical data are lacking. In a study of 20 patients with head and neck cancer undergoing radiation therapy presenting with mucositis, Gelclair was compared with standards of care, including sucralfate and lidocaine. No significant difference was found between the two study populations in relieving general pain.[57]

Table 89-2 Guidelines for the Management of Stomatitis

1. Remove dentures to prevent further irritation and tissue damage.
2. Maintain gentle brushing of teeth with a soft toothbrush.
3. Avoid mouthwashes or rinses that contain alcohol because they may be painful and cause drying of the mucosa. Consider normal saline or sodium bicarbonate oral swishes.
4. Lubricants, such as artificial saliva, may loosen mucus and prevent membranes from sticking together. Avoid mineral oil and petroleum jelly because they can be aspirated.
5. Apply local anesthetics for localized pain control, especially before meals (may add an antacid or an antihistamine). Systemic opioid analgesics may be required to control pain associated with severe mucositis.
6. Ensure that adequate hydration and nutrition are maintained:
   - Eat a bland diet, avoiding spiced, acidic, and salted foods.
   - Avoid rough food; process in a blender if necessary.
   - Use sugar-free gum or sugar-free hard candy to stimulate salivation and facilitate mastication.
   - If necessary, provide intravenous nutritional support.
   - Avoid extremely hot or cold foods.
   - Use shakes with nutritional supplements or ice cream.

J.B. appears to have a mild case of stomatitis or mucositis at this time; however, the lesions may progress over the next several days. Appropriate treatment may include the use of any of the topical products listed in Table 89-1. Table 89-2 lists additional guidelines for managing stomatitis.

Prevention

10. Could J.B.'s mucositis have been prevented?

Historically, treatment of chemotherapy- and radiation-induced mucositis has been aimed at reducing symptoms once they occur and avoiding further trauma to the oral mucosa. Cryotherapy has been marginally effective in reducing the severity of chemotherapy-induced mucositis.[58] Ice chips are placed in the mouth 5 minutes before chemotherapy begins and retained for 30 minutes. Theoretically, this will reduce blood flow to the mouth, thereby protecting the dividing cell population from toxins.

Glutamine is an important substrate for rapidly proliferating tissue. In two randomized trials, oral glutamine supplementation was associated with a reduction in the severity and duration of oral pain after chemotherapy. In one trial of bone marrow transplant (BMT) recipients, glutamine significantly reduced the severity and duration of oropharyngeal mucositis in those who had received autologous transplants, but not in those who had received allogeneic transplants.[59] In contrast, glutamine failed to prevent mucositis in two trials of patients receiving standard-dose fluorouracil-based chemotherapy.[60]

Chlorhexidine gluconate 0.12% also may reduce the frequency and severity of mucositis infection,[61,62] although not all studies have shown a benefit. This solution should be used twice daily as a rinse. Side effects include occasional burning (thought to be caused by the product's alcohol content, which can be reduced by diluting it with water) and superficial brown tooth staining, which polishes off easily. Chlorhexidine may reduce the frequency and severity of mucositis by eliminating microorganisms in the oral cavity.

Despite these prophylactic measures, none of these aforementioned methods have a definitive benefit. To date, the only medication with proven efficacy is palifermin, a keratinocyte growth factor, approved for patients with hematologic malignancies having BMT to reduce the incidence and duration of severe oral mucositis. Efficacy was established in a phase III multicenter, randomized, placebo-controlled double-blind trial ($N = 212$) comparing palifermin 60 mcg/kg/day IV starting 3 days before the conditioning regimen and continuing days 0, 1, and 2 of transplant with placebo. Palifermin demonstrated a reduction in severe mucositis of 63% versus 98%, respectively, and duration of mucositis of 6 days versus 9 days, respectively.[63] Palifermin's use is limited thus far and has not shown proven efficacy in other patient populations at risk for mucositis. Other methods for decreasing the incidence and severity of mucositis symptoms include reducing the dose of radiation or chemotherapy, but doing so comes at the risk of compromising treatment outcomes. Stomatitis remains the dose-limiting toxicity for several chemotherapeutic regimens.

Esophagitis

Chemotherapy and radiation therapy can also damage the mucosa lining the esophagus. Although dysphagia is a common symptom reported by patients with esophagitis, other causes of dysphagia should be ruled out. Because patients receiving myelosuppressive chemotherapy may develop infectious esophagitis, bacterial, viral, and fungal cultures should be completed to rule this out before starting treatment for esophagitis. Symptomatic management of esophagitis is similar to the management of mucositis. Other treatment modalities, including behavioral modifications and other medications (e.g., H_2-receptor antagonist, antacids, and proton pump inhibitors) may help reduce esophageal irritation and improve comfort. Patients with severe esophagitis should be carefully monitored to ensure adequate oral hydration and nutritional intake and instructed to avoid acidic or irritating foods. Symptoms should resolve in 1 to 2 weeks as myelosuppression resolves.

Lower GI Tract Complications

Lower GI tract complications associated with chemotherapy include malabsorption, diarrhea, and constipation. These complications may be related to structural changes that occur to the GI tract after chemotherapy or radiation therapy. Several investigators noted villus atrophy and cessation of mitosis within GI crypts in patients and animals treated with combination chemotherapy.[64–66] Other investigators noted swelling and dilation of mitochondria and endoplasmic reticulum and shortening of the microvilli. These or other changes to the small and large bowel can cause decreased absorption of medications that are primarily absorbed in the upper portion of the small intestine. Decreased absorption has been documented with several drugs with narrow therapeutic indexes, including phenytoin, verapamil, and digoxin following chemotherapy.[67–69] Patients receiving medications for concurrent illnesses should be carefully monitored for new signs or symptoms of adverse effects.

Chemotherapy-induced intestinal changes also may be responsible for diarrhea, which frequently occurs with regimens containing irinotecan, high-dose cytarabine, or fluorouracil. Unlike diarrhea, constipation is rare. The vinca alkaloids, which produce colicky abdominal pain, constipation, and adynamic ileus caused by autonomic nerve dysfunction (see Neurotoxicity section), can cause chemotherapy-induced constipation. Additionally, constipation is a problematic side effect of therapy with thalidomide. Constipation should be treated prophylactically with stool softeners and mild stimulants. The true incidence of diarrhea and constipation associated with chemotherapy is difficult to discern, however, because many medications (e.g., opioid analgesics, antiemetics, antacids) and situations (e.g., immobility) commonly associated with cancer and chemotherapy can cause these symptoms as well.

DIARRHEA

11. B.G., a 60-year-old woman with recurrent colorectal cancer refractory to fluorouracil, is beginning her first course of irinotecan 125 mg/m² weekly for 4 weeks followed by a 2-week rest period. What instructions should she receive regarding the management of diarrhea should she experience this complication?

Irinotecan can cause severe diarrhea, both early and late, in the course of chemotherapy. The early- and late-onset diarrhea appears to be mediated by different mechanisms. Early-onset diarrhea (within 24 hours after treatment) may be mediated by parasympathetic stimulation. Patients often report other cholinergic symptoms, such as rhinitis, increased salivation, miosis, lacrimation, diaphoresis, flushing, and abdominal cramping as well. These symptoms can be prevented or managed with atropine IV or SC 0.25 to 1 mg. Late-onset diarrhea (generally occurring >24 hours after treatment) can be prolonged leading to dehydration, electrolyte imbalances, and significant morbidity. Patients should promptly receive loperamide 4 mg with the first episode of diarrhea and repeat doses equal to 2 mg every 2 hours until 12 hours have passed without a bowel movement.[70] For patients who do not respond to initial therapy, some clinicians recommend higher doses equal to 4 mg every 2 hours. Fluid and electrolyte replacement should also be administered, if necessary. With the potential severe complications associated with irinotecan-associated diarrhea, prompt treatment cannot be overemphasized.

If a patient fails to respond to adequate doses of loperamide, the somatostatin analog, octreotide, can be used to manage the diarrhea. Randomized trials comparing loperamide with octreotide in patients with acute leukemia or those undergoing BMT found loperamide to be more effective.[71,72] Nevertheless, some evidence shows that octreotide may be used to successfully manage diarrhea associated with fluorouracil and other high-dose chemotherapy regimens.[73–75] Octreotide produces antisecretory activity in the gut and promotes the absorption of sodium, chloride, and water from luminal content. Patients should receive doses ranging from 100 to 2,000 mcg SC three times daily or 20 to 40 mg of long-acting octreotide.[74,75] Although responses seem to correlate with octreotide dose, more studies are needed to determine the optimal dose. Based on current evidence, octreotide should be limited to second-line therapy for chemotherapy-associated diarrhea.

Dermatologic Toxicities

Dermatologic toxicities associated with chemotherapy include alopecia, hypersensitivity reactions, extravasations, and hyperpigmentation. Toxicities, including alopecia, nail changes, dry skin, and blistering, occur when chemotherapy agents reduce or inhibit mitosis in the epidermis and nail matrix. Other chemotherapy agents can cause various skin reactions when they interact with ultraviolet (UV) light or radiation.

Dermatologic toxicities also can occur when chemotherapy agents with vesicant properties extravasate from the veins into surrounding soft tissue. In addition, some agents produce specific skin eruptions, nonspecific eruptions, or "rashes" by unknown mechanisms. Several reviews serve as excellent references.[76,77]

Alopecia

PATHOGENESIS

12. C.W., is a 45-year-old woman with recently diagnosed breast cancer, who underwent lumpectomy. She will receive 20 fractions or courses of radiation therapy to the affected breast. She will also receive chemotherapy to minimize her risk of recurrence. She is in the clinic today to receive the first of six cycles of cyclophosphamide, doxorubicin, and fluorouracil (CAF regimen). Although C.W. had minimal problems with surgery, she particularly fears receiving combination chemotherapy. You start counseling C.W. about the most common toxicities by reviewing the likelihood and management of myelosuppression, nausea, and vomiting. C.W. is appropriately attentive as you discuss these issues with her; however, her overriding concern is whether or not she will lose her hair. Is C.W.'s concern typical of most cancer patients? How would you respond?

C.W.'s concern regarding hair loss is typical of cancer patients starting chemotherapy. In fact, several investigators have reported that hair loss ranks second only to nausea and vomiting as a patient's greatest fear. Because hair bulb cells replicate every 12 to 24 hours, the cells are susceptible to various chemotherapy agents. Normally, hair follicles independently move cyclically through phases of growth (anagen), involution, or transition (catagen), and rest (telogen). Although most persons normally lose about 100 scalp hairs a day, patients with cancer can lose substantially more. Because ~85% to 90% of hair follicles are in the anagen phase, chemotherapy agents may partially or completely inhibit mitosis or impair metabolic processes in the hair matrix. These effects can cause a thinned or weakened hair shaft or failure to form hair. Even mild trauma, such as normal hair grooming or rubbing the head on a pillow, can fracture the thinned hair shaft and cause hair loss. Hair loss usually begins 7 to 10 days after one treatment, with prominent hair loss noted within 1 or 2 months. Other terminal hairs, such as beards, eyebrows, eyelashes, axillary, and pubic hair can be affected; however, these effects are somewhat variable, depending on the rate of mitosis and the percentage of hairs in the anagen phase.[78]

C.W. should be informed about the expected onset of hair loss, and she should be reassured that alopecia caused by chemotherapy is reversible. She can expect her hair to begin regenerating 1 to 2 months after therapy is completed. The color and texture of her hair may be altered; the new hair may be lighter, darker, or curlier as it regrows. Agents most commonly associated with severe alopecia are listed in Table 89-3.

PREVENTION

Several interventions have been proposed to prevent scalp hair loss during chemotherapy. These procedures attempt to prevent chemotherapy agents from circulating to the hair follicles with either an occlusive scalp tourniquet or an ice cap that produces a localized hypothermia and vasoconstriction. Recognizing that such devices create a refuge for tumor cells, these procedures are contraindicated in patients with hematologic malignancies and in others at risk for scalp metastases. Concerns regarding the efficacy and safety of these devices have prevented them from availability in the U.S. market.[78,79]

Table 89-3 Single Agents Associated With Alopecia, Pigmentation Changes, and Nail Disorders

	Frequent	*Occasional*
Alopecia[a]	Cyclophosphamide	Mechlorethamine
	Ifosfamide	Thiotepa
	Fluorouracil	Methotrexate
	Dactinomycin	Vinblastine
	Daunorubicin	Vincristine
	Doxorubicin	Etoposide
	Bleomycin	Carmustine
	Vindesine	Hydroxyurea
	Paclitaxel	Cytarabine
	Irinotecan	Topotecan
	Epirubicin	Gemcitabine
	Docetaxel	Erlotinib
	Etoposide	Sorafenib
	Mitoxantrone	
Pigmentation	Busulfan	Cyclophosphamide
	Fluorouracil	Methotrexate
	Doxorubicin	Dactinomycin
	Bleomycin	Daunorubicin
	Epirubicin	Hydroxyurea
	Capecitabine	Ifosfamide
		Thiotepa
Nail		Cyclophosphamide
		Fluorouracil
		Daunorubicin
		Doxorubicin
		Bleomycin
		Hydroxyurea
		Epirubicin
		Docetaxel
		Paclitaxel
		Capecitabine
		Erlotinib
		Gefitinib
		Sorafenib
		Sunitinib

[a]Degree and onset of alopecia depend on dose, administration schedule, delivery rate and route, and various agent combinations.

C.W.'s concern is a legitimate one expressed by many patients with cancer, not just patients with breast cancer. C.W. is likely to experience near or complete hair loss, depending on the thickness of her hair and its growth rate. She should be told how to minimize the effect of alopecia on her appearance through the use of hair pieces or stylish head scarves, turbans, or hats. She also should be referred to volunteer groups and organizations that can help her through this difficult time. Hair pieces are tax deductible as a medical expense and are covered by some health insurance policies. If C.W. thinks she will use a hair piece, she should be advised to select a wig before hair loss begins.

Skin and Nail Changes

13. Besides alopecia, what other skin or nail changes should C.W. anticipate?

Several skin and nail changes have been associated with chemotherapy, which C.W. may find disturbing. The major consequences of these toxicities are cosmetic, however, and they usually resolve within 6 to 12 months after discontinuing chemotherapy.

NAIL CHANGES

The growth of fingernails and toenails is arrested in a manner similar to hair growth. A reduction or a cessation of mitotic activity in the nail matrix causes a horizontal depression of the nail plate. Within weeks, these pale horizontal lines ("Beau's lines") begin to appear in the nail beds. They are most commonly seen in patients receiving chemotherapy for >6 months. These growth arrest lines move distally as the nail grows and normally disappear from the fingernails in ~6 months. Nail changes including hemorrhagic onycholysis, discoloration, and acute exudative paronychia are seen in ~40% of patients receiving paclitaxel and docetaxel.[76] Some other nail pigmentation changes that can occur following therapy with cyclophosphamide, fluorouracil, daunorubicin, doxorubicin, and bleomycin are less well understood.[81–83] Brown or blue lines deposit as horizontal or vertical bands in the nails. These lines are seen more commonly in dark-skinned patients. As with Beau's lines, these pigmentation lines generally grow out with the nail.

DERMATOLOGIC PIGMENT CHANGES

Dermatologic pigment changes are among the most common and least well understood side effects of chemotherapy. Hypopigmentation has been reported occasionally in patients receiving chemotherapy, but hyperpigmentation is most frequently reported. Usually, hyperpigmentation is not associated with an identifiable cause or systemic toxicity. It usually occurs following treatment with a wide variety of chemotherapy agents, including antitumor antibiotics, alkylating agents, and antimetabolites. Most agents cause a diffuse, generalized hyperpigmentation, but the pigmentation changes can also be localized, involving only the mucous membrane, hair, or nails. Busulfan, cyclophosphamide, fluorouracil, dactinomycin, and hydroxyurea are examples of specific agents that can cause widespread cutaneous hyperpigmentation.[76,84–87]

Various chemotherapy agents can cause significantly diverse patterns of hyperpigmentation. A peculiar serpiginous hyperpigmentation can occur over veins used to administer fluorouracil and bleomycin.[88,89] Some investigators have attributed this phenomenon to a subclinical phlebitis. Hyperpigmentation has also been noted over pressure points after the use of bleomycin. Bleomycin can also cause peculiar linear or flagellate streaks of hyperpigmentation. Because of their characteristic location and appearance, these streaks may result from scratching during therapy; however, attempts to reproduce these lesions iatrogenically have not been successful. Thiotepa has been reported to cause hyperpigmentation in areas of skin occluded by bandages, which may be caused by secretion of thiotepa in sweat.[90] Interestingly, skin contact with thiotepa has been reported to cause hypopigmentation.[91] Topical contact with mechlorethamine and carmustine also has caused hyperpigmentation.[92,93] Although hyperpigmentation reactions commonly affect the skin, some rare reactions are noted in hair. Methotrexate can cause hyperpigmented banding of light-colored hair. This phenomenon has been described in a patient receiving intermittent high-dose methotrexate and has been referred to by some investigators as the "flag sign" of chemotherapy.[94] To minimize a patient's concern regarding these pigment changes, they should receive counseling before treatment.

As previously stated, pigment changes that occur in patients receiving chemotherapy are basically a cosmetic concern. It is important to anticipate these distressing side effects and educate patients in appropriate cases. At this time, C.W. should receive counseling, explaining that these side effects may occur because she will be receiving several agents that have been implicated in producing both diffuse, as well as localized, cutaneous nail hyperpigmentation. She should be reassured that pigment changes usually resolve with time.

HAND–FOOT SYNDROME

Some patients receiving chemotherapy may develop tender, erythematous skin on the palms of their hands and sometimes on the soles of their feet. Patients may also complain of tingling, burning, or shooting sensations in their hands or feet usually not described as painful. These signs and symptoms may resolve after several days, or they may progress to bullous lesions that can desquamate. This reaction is referred to as *chemotherapy-associated acral erythema* or *the palmar-plantar erythrodysesthesia syndrome*. Agents reported to cause this reaction include cytarabine, fluorouracil, doxorubicin, lipsomal doxorubicin, methotrexate, capecitabine, and hydroxyurea. Additionally, both sunitinib and sorafenib-multiple receptor tyrosine kinase inhibitors- have been associated with hand-foot syndrome.[95,96] No specific therapy exists for hand-foot syndrome. Typically, the offending agent is discontinued at least until recovery occurs.

ACNEIFORM–ERYTHEMATOUS RASH

The most common toxicities reported with the new epidermal growth factor receptor inhibitors are skin related and are probably due to inhibition of the tyrosine kinase pathways in EGFR-dependent tissues, including keratinocytes in the skin. Several EGFR inhibitors currently available include erlotinib and lapatinib, which are small molecule tyrosine kinase inhibitors that target the intracellular domain of the EGFR. Cetuximab and panitumumab are monoclonal antibodies that target the extracellular domain of EGFR. Skin effects occur in >50% of patients who receive these treatments and are reported to be dose dependent. A pustular or maculopapular eruption appears on the upper body, face, and scalp in the first 1 to 2 weeks of treatment. The rashes are predominantly grade 1 or 2 in severity, may be associated with dry skin and itching, and completely resolve without sequelae when the drug is discontinued.[97] Evidence suggests that the severity of the skin rash is associated with increased efficacy of this class of agents. In a retrospective analysis of a phase III trial in patients with NSCLC receiving erlotinib, those who developed a rash had a significantly longer survival time than those who did not. Survival was reported to be 1.5 months in patients with no development of skin rash versus 8.5 months in those with grade 1 rash, and 19.6 months in patients exhibiting a grade 2 or 3 rash.[98] Evidence for correlation between skin rashes and positive response rates has also been seen in patients receiving cetuximab for colorectal cancer.[99] No supportive therapy has, however, been proven to reduce or prevent this bothersome side effect. No randomized, controlled studies have evaluated therapeutic options for relief or treatment of the acneiform rash. Moisturizing creams, steroid creams, sunscreen, antibiotics (e.g., topical clindamycin or systemic tetracyclines), and topical calcineurin inhibitors (e.g., pimecrolimus cream) have been used to manage the effects with varying results. Patients are also advised to minimize sun exposure. All of these agents have demonstrated activity in some patients, but none have worked consistently in all. Therefore, if one agent is not successful, alternative agents may be tried.[97]

DRY SKIN

Many chemotherapy agents (especially bleomycin, hydroxyurea, and fluorouracil) can cause dry skin with fine scaling on the surface. Normally, sebaceous and sweat glands provide lipids, lactates, and other products that contribute to the pliability and moisture retention of the stratum corneum. In patients receiving chemotherapy, the dry skin may be caused by the cytostatic effect of chemotherapy agents on sebaceous and sweat glands. Topical application of emollient creams may provide some symptomatic relief of this dryness.

Interactions With Radiation Therapy

14. C.W. recently completed her course of total breast radiation therapy. She also plans to leave for a 1-week vacation in Florida 3 days after this clinic visit. Are there any interactions between radiation therapy and sunlight exposure with chemotherapy agents? Are there any specific precautions C.W. should take, or signs and symptoms of toxicity that she should know about?

The interactions between chemotherapy and radiation therapy or UV light (from both external beam and natural sources) can be divided into radiation enhancement or sensitization, radiation recall, photosensitivity reactions, and sunburn reactivation (Table 89-4). Several excellent reviews are available that describe each of these interactions in detail. A discussion of the important principles of the interaction between radiation therapy and chemotherapy follows.[100–102]

Table 89-4 Chemotherapy and Radiation Reactions[76,100,103]

Radiation Enhancement Reactions		
Bleomycin	Doxorubicin	Hydroxyurea
Dactinomycin	Fluorouracil	Methotrexate
Etoposide	Gemcitabine	
Radiation Recall Reactions		
All of the above plus		
Vinblastine	Epirubicin	Capecitabine
Etoposide	Paclitaxel	Oxaliplatin
	Docetaxel	
Reactions With Ultraviolet Light		
Phototoxic reactions		
Dacarbazine	Thioguanine	Methotrexate
Fluorouracil	Vinblastine	Mitomycin
Reactivation of sunburn		
Methotrexate		

A synergistic interaction between a small number of chemotherapy agents and radiation therapy results in an enhanced radiation effect. This may be caused by an agent's ability to interfere with radiation repair. Radiation therapy can alter the molecular structure of DNA, but excision repair allows cells to remove small, damaged portions of one strand of DNA and insert new bases using the other strand as a template. This repair mechanism requires several enzymes, including DNA polymerase. Chemotherapy agents can interfere with some of the enzymes and synthetic mechanisms needed to rejuvenate damaged cells. Although the synergistic effects of radiation therapy and chemotherapy are often exploited therapeutically for the treatment of solid tumors, these reactions can inadvertently cause undesirable reactions in non-neoplastic tissues, such as the skin, esophagus, lung, and GI tract. The skin is the most common target of radiation reactions. These reactions can produce severe tissue necrosis, which can compromise organ function and delay or mandate discontinuation of future treatment courses.

These reactions may be further classified as either *radiation sensitization* or *radiation recall* reactions. The primary distinction between radiation sensitization reactions and radiation recall reactions lies in the temporal relationship between radiation therapy and chemotherapy. Generally, sensitization reactions occur when chemotherapy is given concurrently or within 1 week of radiation therapy. In comparison, recall reactions occur several weeks to years after radiation therapy, when a chemotherapy agent causes an inflammatory reaction in tissues previously treated with radiation. Radiation recall is independent of previous, clinically apparent radiation damage. Not surprisingly, the chemotherapy agents that have been associated with radiation recall reactions are the same as those that cause radiation sensitization reactions. Agents most commonly associated with these reactions include the antitumor antibiotics dactinomycin, epirubicin, and doxorubicin; however, other agents, such as bleomycin, fluorouracil, capecitabine, hydroxyurea, methotrexate, etoposide, vinblastine, gemcitabine, oxaliplatin, and paclitaxel, also can cause radiation reactions. Chemotherapy may also interact with UV light to cause similar reactions.[100–103]

Because UV light has sufficient energy to cause photochemical changes in biologic molecules, chemotherapy agents can interact with it. The subsequent reactions are usually less severe than reactions that occur with radiation therapy, and they may be caused by a different mechanism. Photosensitivity reactions, defined as enhanced erythema responses to UV light, have been reported with dacarbazine, fluorouracil, methotrexate, and vinblastine. Methotrexate can also reactivate sunburns, causing a similar, but less severe reaction compared with the radiation recall reactions described previously. The reaction can be more severe than the initial sunburn, resulting in severe blisters, and it usually occurs only in patients who receive large doses of methotrexate. Other agents cited infrequently to cause photoreactivation include paclitaxel, docetaxel, and gemcitabine. Although the precise incidences of photosensitivity reactions caused by chemotherapy agents are unknown, they may be more common than generally believed. For example, photosensitivity may account for many of the erythematous periodic rashes attributed to allergy.

C.W. received doxorubicin and fluorouracil, both of which can interact with radiation therapy. Although not commonly reported, doxorubicin also can cause some increased erythema in the specific area of skin treated with radiation. Because C.W. may have an increased risk for a photosensitivity reaction, she should be advised to avoid direct exposure to the sunlight for several days to a week after chemotherapy. Although no data exist regarding the efficacy of sunscreens in this patient population, C.W. should be advised to use a protective sunscreen with a high sun protective factor (SPF) when she cannot avoid sun exposure. Furthermore, she should periodically assess her skin's reaction to the sun with intermittent periods of rest and observation throughout the day.

15. How will C.W. know if she has a radiation reaction? How should she be treated if such a reaction occurs?

If C.W. has a radiation reaction, she will experience "easy burning" and erythema or redness, followed by dry desquamation. With a more severe reaction, small blisters (vesicles) and oozing can develop. Necrosis with persistent painful ulceration can also occur in more severe cases. Postinflammatory hyperpigmentation or depigmentation may follow. The severity of the reaction can help determine the best treatment option.

Treatment options vary, depending on reaction severity. Milder cases can be treated with topical steroids in an emollient cream base and cool wet compresses. Necrosis and ulcers are notoriously difficult to treat, however, because radiated skin does not heal well. Ulcers are often treated with surgical débridement to keep the ulcer clean. Even when the ulcers are clean, exudation and bacterial contamination can be persistent. Radiation reactions that occur in tissues other than the skin (e.g., the lungs, esophagus, GI tract) often are treated with oral corticosteroids, although data regarding the efficacy of these agents in ameliorating the symptoms or reducing the extent of damage are lacking. If C.W. experiences any of these signs or symptoms, she should immediately seek medical attention.

Irritant and Vesicant Reactions

16. C.W. complained of pain and burning at the injection site immediately following the administration of her third course of IV chemotherapy with cyclophosphamide, doxorubicin, and fluorouracil. She described the sensation as being distinctly different from the mild discomfort she had experienced with previous chemotherapy. Physical examination of the injection site revealed mild erythema and slight induration. What types of local reactions can occur after the administration of chemotherapy?

Several distinct types of local reactions (ranging from transient local irritation to severe tissue necrosis of the skin, surrounding vasculature, and supporting structures) have been reported following chemotherapy[104,105] (Table 89-5). Some of these reactions (particularly those associated with anthracyclines) may be caused by local hypersensitivity reactions. These reactions usually are characterized by immediate local burning, itching, and erythema. Some patients may also experience a "flare" reaction along the length of the vein used for treatment. Hypersensitivity reactions usually are self-limited and subside within a few hours. Administration of the antihistamine, diphenhydramine, before the next course of chemotherapy may reduce the severity or duration of hypersensitivity reactions.[106,107] More severe reactions, including irritation of the vein (or phlebitis) caused by the irritant properties of an agent or a diluent, can occur following chemotherapy.

Table 89-5 Chemotherapeutic Drugs Reported to Produce Local Toxicities[103–105]

Potential Vesicants	
Dactinomycin	Epirubicin
Daunorubicin	Streptozocin
Doxorubicin	Vinblastine
Idarubicin	Vincristine
Mechlorethamine	Paclitaxel
Mitomycin	Oxaliplatin
Potential Irritants	
Carmustine	Etoposide
Cisplatin	Mitoxantrone
Dacarbazine	Melphalan
Vinorelbine	Vindesine
Cyclophosphamide	Teniposide

Extravasation occurs when IV medications are accidentally administered into the surrounding tissue, either by leakage or by a needle puncturing the vein, causing direct exposure to surrounding tissues. Local reactions resulting from the extravasation of agents with vesicant or irritant properties may be more severe. All agents with vesicant properties potentially can produce these devastating reactions. Agents known to bind to DNA (i.e., the anthracyclines) have the propensity to produce the most severe damage. Treatment with a chemotherapy agent with these properties can produce phlebitis and pain, and extravasations can cause local irritation or soft tissue ulcers, depending on the agent, and the amount and concentration of the extravasated drug. In addition, no clear agreement exists regarding the vesicant potential of many chemotherapy agents, and various references may categorize agents differently based on their vesicant or irritant properties. Initially, it may be impossible to distinguish a local irritant reaction from a vesicant extravasation; therefore, if an agent with vesicant or irritant properties has been administered, the reaction should be treated as a potential extravasation.

Patients who experience an extravasation can show a range of different signs or symptoms. Infiltration of a vesicant into tissue often produces a severe burning sensation that may persist for hours. In some cases, however, no immediate symptoms or signs are evident. In the days to weeks that follow, the skin overlying the extravasation site may become reddened and firm. The redness may gradually diminish or progress to ulceration and necrosis.[108,109]

17. What factors increase the risk of extravasation, and what administration techniques and precautions can minimize these risks?

Several factors have been associated with an increased risk of extravasation and subsequent tissue damage following administration of chemotherapy. Risk factors include (a) generalized vascular disease commonly found in elderly and debilitated patients or in patients who have undergone frequent venipuncture and treatment with irritating chemotherapy (the latter causes venous fragility and instability or decreased local blood flow); (b) elevated venous pressure, which typically occurs in patients with an obstructed superior vena cava or venous drainage after axillary dissection; (c) prior radiation therapy to the injection site; (d) recent venipuncture in the same vein; and (e) use of injection sites over joints, which increases the risk of needle dislodgement.[105] In addition, tissue damage may be more severe if extravasation occurs in areas with only a small amount of subcutaneous tissue (e.g., the back of the hand or wrist) because wound healing is more difficult and exposure of deeper structures, such as the tendons, is increased.[107] These risks have led to the increased use of central catheters in patients receiving vesicant chemotherapy.

Extravasations of agents with vesicant properties can produce devastating tissue damage that can potentially cause loss of an extremity or death. To prevent significant morbidity or mortality, major emphasis must be placed on prevention. All caretakers who administer agents with vesicant or irritant properties should be skilled in IV drug administration and receive special instruction before administering these agents. The patient also must be told how agent administration should feel and to report immediately any change in sensation, including pain, burning, or itching. Recommendations to reduce the risk of local complications during cytotoxic agent administration are outlined in Table 89-6.

18. The oncology nurse believes that the doxorubicin may have extravasated during C.W.'s chemotherapy administration. How should this be managed? Do management guidelines differ for other vesicant agents?

Table 89-6 Guidelines for Administration of Cytotoxic Agents[103-105]

Administration of chemotherapy should be performed only by persons familiar with its toxic effects.

The site of infusion is selected with consideration of visualization of the vessel, its size, and potential damage if extravasation occurs in the following order of preference: forearm > dorsum of the hand > wrist > antecubital fossa.

- Limbs with compromised circulation (e.g., invading neoplasm, axillary dissection, severe bruising) should not be used.
- The lower extremities should not be used.
- Pre-existing IV lines should not be used because the site may already have occult vein or tissue irritation or phlebitis.

A 23- or 25-gauge scalp vein ("butterfly") needle is inserted into the vein. Only one venipuncture should be performed on a vein to avoid leakage.

The wings of the needle should be lightly taped in place with care not to obscure the injection site so that it can be visualized during injection.

Test the integrity of the IV line by injecting a small volume of saline solution and withdrawing a small amount of blood. If extravasation of the saline is obvious, select another vein or a site proximal on the same vein to avoid upstream leakage.

Administer the drug at the recommended rate (preferably through the tubing of an IV running by gravity to assess for back pressure).

During the administration, question the patient about discomfort, check for blood return by aspirating the syringe gently, observe the continuous flow of the running IV, and visualize the IV site frequently. If line patency is in doubt at any time, the injection should be stopped and an alternate site selected.

After administration, the IV line should be flushed with at least 10 mL of saline or other IV fluid to flush the needle and tubing of all drug.

If multiple drugs are to be given, the IV should be flushed between each drug.

Apply pressure with sterile gauze for 3–4 minutes after the needle is removed. Inspect the site before applying a bandage.

IV, intravenous.

Table 89-7 Suggested Procedures for Management of Suspected Extravasation of Vesicant Drugs[103-105]

1. Stop the injection immediately, but do not remove the needle. Any drug remaining in the tubing or needle, as well as the infiltrated area, should be aspirated.
2. Contact a physician as soon as possible.
3. If deemed appropriate, instill an antidote in the infiltrated areas (via the extravasated intravenous needle if possible).
4. Remove the needle.
5. Apply ice to the site and elevate the extremity for the first 24–48 hr (if vinca or podophyllotoxin, use warm compresses).
6. Document the drug, suspected volume extravasated, and the treatment in the patient's medical record.
7. Check the site frequently for 5–7 days.
8. Consult a surgeon familiar with extravasations early so that the surgeon can periodically review the site, and if ulceration begins, the surgeon can rapidly assess if surgical débridement or excision is necessary.

Immediate management of a potential vesicant extravasation should include stopping the injection if the entire agent has not been administered. Various other recommended measures may minimize vesicant exposure and subsequent tissue damage (Table 89-7). These include application of cold compresses to the extravasation site and elevation of the extremity. Cold compresses have been shown to cause vasoconstriction, which can help to localize the extravasation and allow time for local vessels to displace the extravasated agent, whereas warm compresses are thought to induce vasodilation, increase drug distribution and absorption, and therefore decrease localized drug concentrations. Warm compresses are recommended for vinca alkaloids and epipodophyllotoxins.[104,105] With the exception of these two classes of agents, cooling has been shown more effective than warm compresses. Specific antidotes thought to inactivate the extravasated agent have been suggested; however, many of these antidotes are based on observations in few patients or animal models, and their effectiveness, in many cases, is unsubstantiated. Antidotes recommended in some guidelines may actually worsen tissue damage (e.g., sodium bicarbonate for doxorubicin). Recommended treatments for suspected extravasation of vesicant agents are outlined in Table 89-8.[104,105]

Because doxorubicin skin damage may be related to the formation of toxic free oxygen radicals, a free radical scavenger may prevent ulceration. Dimethylsulfoxide (DMSO) is a potent free radical scavenger that penetrates all tissue planes. In pig and rat models, topical DMSO has decreased doxorubicin-induced skin ulcers.[110] Several series of case reports and a single-arm clinical study have reported that topical application of DMSO can safely and effectively manage an extravasation with an anthracycline.[111–116] DMSO also has been reported to be beneficial in patients with mitomycin extravasations.[115]

Hypersensitivity Reactions

All cancer chemotherapy agents except altretamine, the nitrosureas, and dactinomycin, have produced at least an isolated instance of a hypersensitivity reaction.[117] All types of hypersensitivity reactions can occur with chemotherapy agents,

Table 89-8 Recommended Extravasation Antidotes[103–105]

Class/Specific Agents	Local Antidote Recommended	Specific Procedure
Alkylating Agents Cisplatin[a] Oxaliplatin Mechlorethamine	1/6 M solution sodium thiosulfate	Mix 4 mL 10% sodium thiosulfate USP with 6 mL of sterile water for injection, USP for a 1/6-M solution. Into site, inject 2 mL for each mg of mechlorethamine or 100 mg of cisplatin extravasated.
Mitomycin-C	Dimethylsulfoxide 99% (w/v)	Apply 1–2 mL to the site Q 6 hr for 14 days. Allow to air dry; do not cover.
Anthracylines	Cold compresses	Apply immediately for 30–60 min for 1 day.
Doxorubicin	Dimethylsulfoxide 99% (w/v)	Apply 1–2 mL to the site Q 6 hr for 14 days. Allow to air dry; do not cover.
Daunorubicin	Dimethylsulfoxide 99% (w/v)	Apply 1–2 mL to the site Q 6 hr for 14 days. Allow to air dry; do not cover.
Vinca alkaloids	Warm compresses	Apply immediately for 30–60 min, then alternate off/on every 15 min for 1 day.
Vinblastine	Hyaluronidase	Inject 150 U into site.
Vincristine	Hyaluronidase	Inject 150 U into site.
Epipodophyllotoxins[a]	Warm compresses	Apply immediately for 30–60 min, then alternate off/on every 15 min for 1 day.
Etoposide	Hyaluronidase	Inject 150 U into site.
Teniposide	Hyaluronidase	Inject 150 U into site.
Taxanes	Cold compresses	Apply immediately for 30–60 min Q 6 hr for 1 day.
Docetaxel	Hyaluronidase	Inject 150 U into site.
Paclitaxel	Hyaluronidase	Inject 150 U into site.

[a] Treatment indicated only for large extravasations (e.g., doses one-half or more of the planned total dose for the course of therapy).
w/v, weight per volume.

although type I is the most common reaction documented following chemotherapy. Type I hypersensitivity reactions are immediate reactions that are most often immunologically mediated, although there are other possible mechanisms for type I hypersensitivities. Anaphylactic or IgE-mediated reactions occur when an antigen interacts with IgE bound to a mast cell membrane, causing degranulation of mast cells. Major signs and symptoms of type I reactions include urticaria, angioedema, rash, bronchospasm, abdominal cramping, and hypotension. Although many reactions associated with chemotherapy agents probably are immunologically mediated, other mechanisms may cause type 1 reactions. Other mechanisms include the degranulation of mast cells and basophils through a direct effect on the cell surface that releases histamine and other vasoactive substances. Activation of the alternative complement pathway also can release vasoactive substances from mast cells. When non–IgE-mediated mechanisms account for the symptoms of a type 1 reaction, it is called an *anaphylactoid reaction.*

Many of the type 1 hypersensitivity reactions produced by chemotherapy agents appear to be mediated by non-IgE mechanisms. Although little research has been conducted on the mechanism of these reactions, two features suggest that they are not mediated by IgE. First, many reactions occur during or immediately after administration of the first dose. This is in contrast to immunologic reactions that require prior exposure (i.e., one must be sensitized before becoming hypersensitized). In addition, certain symptoms or symptom complexes are more diagnostic of immunologically mediated disorders. These symptoms include urticaria, angioedema, bronchospasm, laryngeal spasm, cytopenias, arthritis, mucositis, vasculitic syndromes, and vesicular dermatitis. If not experiencing any of these symptoms after the first dose, the patient most likely did not experience an immunologically mediated hypersensitivity reaction.

Although the spectrum of symptoms and their severity vary widely in the case reports, most hypersensitivity reactions that occur with chemotherapy agents are classified as grade 1 (transient rash, mild) or grade 2 (mild bronchospasm, moderate) by the National Cancer Institute (NCI) Common Terminology Criteria for Adverse Events.[118] Furthermore, a patient who has had a reaction to an agent that is not immunologically mediated safely can receive future courses of chemotherapy if he or she receives appropriate premedication. For example, appropriate premedication allows many (>60%) patients who have previously experienced a hypersensitivity reaction secondary to paclitaxel to continue therapy; this also reduces the incidence of hypersensitivity reactions associated with short duration infusions (i.e., 3 hours). (See Table 89-9 for NCI common toxicity criteria.)[118] Other chemotherapy agents can commonly cause hypersensitivity reactions after the first and subsequent doses of chemotherapy.

The other types of hypersensitivity reactions are less commonly documented with chemotherapy administration. Type II is hemolytic anemia. Type III results from deposition of antigen–antibody complexes that form intravascularly and in tissues that can result in tissue injury. Sensitized T lymphocytes that react with antigens causing a release of lymphokines are responsible for type IV reactions.[117] Chemotherapy agents most frequently reported to produce hypersensitivity reactions and their characteristic reactions are listed in Table 89-10. Most valuable information stems from patient series and case reports. However, they often providing conflicting and contradictory information, particularly with respect to incidence, severity, characteristic symptoms, time course, and the success of rechallenge. If a patient experiences a hypersensitivity reaction and the clinician decides to continue therapy with this regimen, a full review of all of the relevant literature as well as manufacturer's data is advised. Several excellent reviews are available to assist in this effort.[103,117]

MONOCLONAL ANTIBODIES

19. S.R, a 58-year-old man with metastatic colorectal cancer, has progressed through four cycles of FOLFOX (oxaliplatin 85 mg/m² IV on day 1, leucovorin 100 mg/m² IV on days 1, 2, and

Table 89-9 National Cancer Institute Common Terminology Criteria for Adverse Events (CTCAE)[118]

Toxicity[a]	*Grade 1*	*Grade 2*	*Grade 3*	*Grade 4*
Hematologic				
WBC	3.0–3.9	2.0–2.9	1.0–1.9	<1.0
Platelets	75.0–normal	50.0–74.9	25.0–49.9	<25.0
Hgb g/100 mL	10.0–<LLN	8.0–10.0	6.5–7.9	<6.5
Hgb g/L	100–<LLN	80–100	65–79	<65
Hgb mmol/L	6.2–<LLN	4.9–6.2	4.0–4.9	<4.0
Granulocytes/bands cells/mm^3	1.5–<LLN	1.0–1.5	0.5–1.0	<0.5
Lymphocytes	0.8 –<LLN	0.5–0.8	0.2–0.5	<0.2
Hematologic (other)	Mild	Moderate	Severe	Life-threatening
Hemorrhage	Mild without transfusion		transfusion indicated	catastrophic bleeding, requiring nonelective intervention
Gastrointestinal				
Nausea	Loss of appetite without alteration in eating habits	Oral intake decreased without significant weight loss, dehydration, or malnutrition; IV fluids indicated <24 hr	Inadequate oral caloric or fluid intake; IV fluids, tube feedings or TPN indicated >24 hr	Life-threatening consequence
Vomiting	1 episode in 24 hr	2–5 episodes in 24 hr; IV fluids indicated	>6 episodes in 24 hr; IV fluids, or TPN indicated	Life-threatening consequences
Diarrhea	Increase of <4 stools/day over baseline; mild increase in ostomy compared with baseline	Increase of 4–6 stools/day over baseline; IV fluids indicated <24 hr; moderate increase in ostomy output compared with baseline; not interfering with ADL	Increase >7 stools/day over baseline; incontinence; IV fluids >24 hr; hospitalization; severe increase in ostomy output compared with baseline; interfering with ADL	Life-threatening consequences (e.g., hemodynamic collapse)

ADL, activities of daily living; IV, intravenous; LLN, lower limit of normal; PO, orally; TPN, total parenteral nutrition; WBC, white blood cell count.

fluorouracil 400 mg/m^2 IV bolus, followed by 600 mg/m^2 IV over 22 hours on days 1, 2) plus bevacizumab 10 mg/kg. He also progressed through two cycles of FOLFIRI (irinotecan 180 mg/m^2 on day 1, leucovorin 100 mg/m^2 IV on days 1, 2, and fluorouracil 400 mg/m^2 IV bolus, followed by 600 mg/m^2 IV over 22 hours on days 1, 2). S.R. now presents to the clinic for his first weekly dose of cetuximab (400 mg/m^2 IV load, followed by 250 mg/m^2 IV weekly). Discuss the toxicities that S.R may expect and when they might appear. How should these side effects be managed? S.R. asks how these side effects can be prevented.

The most common toxicities observed in patients receiving cetuximab include rash, diarrhea, hypomagnesemia, headache, nausea, and hypersensitivity reactions. Infusion-related reactions occur in 15% to 20% of patients receiving their first infusion with severe hypersensitivity reactions (including allergic and anaphylactic reactions) occurring in 1% to 3% of patients. The reactions are related to the infusion of cetuximab and generally occur during or within 1 hour of completing the first dose. Patients should be premedicated with diphenhydramine before the infusion. The infusion can be stopped or the rate decreased if S.R. begins experiencing these effects. The skin rash and dry skin presenting after cetuximab administration is related to its mechanism of inhibiting EGFR and was the most common side effect seen in clinical trials. The rash occurred in ~80% of patients and appeared in the first 1 to 3 weeks of therapy. Grade 3 or 4 skin rashes occurred in 5% to 10% of patients.[119]

Several of the monoclonal antibodies (e.g., rituximab, trastuzumab, and cetuximab) can cause more hypersensitivity reactions than traditional chemotherapy agents. These agents are genetically engineered humanized monoclonal antibodies containing foreign proteins that can trigger the reaction. During the first infusion with trastuzumab, ~40% of patients experience a symptom complex, mild to moderate in severity, which consists of chills, fever, or both. These symptoms usually do not recur with subsequent injections.[120] In comparison, ~80% of patients receiving rituximab may experience an infusion-related reaction ranging from fever, chills, and rigors to severe reactions (7%) characterized by hypoxia, pulmonary infiltrates, adult respiratory distress syndrome, myocardial infarction, ventricular fibrillation, or cardiogenic shock with the first dose. Approximately 40% of patients receiving rituximab develop infusion-related reactions with subsequent infusions (5%–10% severe).[120] Treatment of these reactions follows the recommendations for treatment of hypersensitivity reactions that occur with more traditional agents.

Treatment

Recommended treatment of hypersensitivity reactions is reviewed in Table 89-11. If a patient develops a severe type I hypersensitivity reaction to any chemotherapy agent, the treatment should be stopped. If a structural analog or another agent in the same chemical class is an effective treatment for the same cancer, subsequent therapy should use the analog or

Table 89-10 Cancer Chemotherapeutic Agents Commonly Causing Hypersensitivity

Drug	Frequency	Risk Factors	Manifestations	Mechanism	Comments
L-Asparaginase[117,282,283]	10%–20%	Increasing doses; interval (weeks to months) between doses; IV administration; history of atopy or allergy; use without prednisone, 6-MP and/or vincristine	Pruritus, dyspnea, agitation, urticaria, angioedema, laryngeal spasm	Type I	Substitute PEG-L-asparaginase, but up to 32% may demonstrate mild hypersensitivity
Paclitaxel[121,284,285]	Up to 10% first or second dose	None known	Rashes, dyspnea, bronchospasm, hypotension	Nonspecific release of mediators; Cremophor	Premedicate with diphenhydramine corticosteroids, and H_2-receptor antagonists Paclitaxel protein-bound particles (Abraxane) may be substituted and better tolerated in some patients
Teniposide[286–291]	6%–40%; can occur with first dose	Increasing doses or number of doses; young age or leukemia	Dyspnea, wheezing, hypotension, rash, facial flushing	Type I versus nonspecific; Cremophor	Etoposide may be substituted in some cases; decrease rate of infusion
Cisplatin[292–297]	Up to 20% intravesicular 5%–10% systemic; case reports of hemolytic anemia	Increasing number of doses Anemia: none known	Rash, urticaria, bronchospasm Anemia: hemolytic anemia	Type I Anemia: type III	Carboplatin may be substituted in some cases but cross-reactivity has been reported
Procarbazine[298–303]	Up to 15%, case reports	None known	Urticaria Pneumonitis	Type I Type III	All patients rechallenged have prompt return of symptoms
Anthracyclines[304–310]	1%–15% depending on anthracycline	None known	Dyspnea, bronchospasm, angioedema	Unknown; nonspecific release	Cross-reactivity documented, but incidence and likelihood unknown
Bleomycin[311–313]	Common	Lymphoma	Fever (up to 42°C), tachypnea	Endogenous pyrogen release	Not technically classified as HSR; premedicate with acetaminophen and diphenhydramine
Rituximab[314]	First treatment 80%; subsequent treatments 40%	Female gender, pulmonary infiltrates, CLL or mantle cell lymphoma	Fevers, chills, occasional nausea, urticaria, fatigue, headache, pain, pruritis, bronchospasm, SOB, angioedema, rhinitis, vomiting, ↓ BP, flushing	Unknown; related to manufacturing process	Stop or ↓ infusion rate by 50%; provide supportive care with IV fluids, acetaminophen, diphenhydramine, vasopressors PRN
Trastuzumab[315]	First treatment 40%; subsequent treatments rare	None known	Chills, fever, occasional nausea or vomiting; pain, rigors, headaches, dizziness, SOB, ↓ BP, rash, asthenia	Unknown, related to manufacturing process	Manage with acetaminophen, diphenhydramine, meperidine
Cetuximab[316]	First treatment 15%–20%; Grade 3–4 3%; subsequent treatmentsuncommon	None known	Airway obstruction (bronchospasm, stridor, hoarseness), urticaria, hypotension, or cardiac arrest		Premedicate with diphenhydramine; stop or decrease infusion rate; provide supportive care with epinephrine, corticosteroids, IV antihistamines, bronchodilators, and oxygen PRN
Alemtuzumab[317]	~90% with IV administration in first week	None known	Hypotension, rigors, fever, shortness of breath, bronchospasm, chills, rash	Unknown	Dose titration over several days; substitute with SC administration rather than IV; premedicate with acetaminophen, diphenhydramine, meperidine
Docetaxel[318]	0.9% with premedication	None known	↓ BP, bronchospasm, rash, flushing, pruritus, SOB, pain, fever, chills	Unknown	Premedicate with acetaminophen, dexamethasone, and diphenhydramine
Doxorubicin[319] liposomal	6.8%	None known	Flushing, SOB, angioedema, HA, chills, ↓ BP	Unknown, related liposomal components	Stop infusion; restart at a lower rate

Type I: antigen interaction with IgE bound to mast cell membrane causes degranulation. Drug binding to mast cell surface causes degranulation. Activation of classic or alternative complement pathways produces anaphylatoxins. Neurogenic release of vasoactive substances. Type III: antigen–antibody complexes form intravascularly and deposit in or on tissues.

BP, blood pressure; CLL, chronic lymphocytic leukemia; HA, headache; HSR, hypersensitivity reaction; IV, intravenous; 6-MP, 6-mercaptopurine; PEG-L-asparaginase, pegaspargase; PRN, as needed; SC, subcutaneous; SOB, shortness of breath.

Table 89-11 Prophylaxis and Treatment of Hypersensitivity Reactions From Antitumor Drugs

Prophylaxis
IV access must be established.
BP monitoring must be available.
Premedication
Dexamethasone 20 mg PO and diphenhydramine 50 mg PO 12 and 6 hr before treatment, then the same dose IV immediately before treatment
Consider addition of H_2-antagonist with similar schedule
Have epinephrine and diphenhydramine readily available for use in case of a reaction.
Observe the patient up to 2 hr after discontinuing treatment.
Treatment
Discontinue the drug (immediately if being administered IV).
Administer epinephrine 0.35–0.5 mL IV Q 15–20 min until reaction subsides or a total of 6 doses are administered.
Administer diphenhydramine 50 mg IV.
If hypotension is present that does not respond to epinephrine, administer IV fluids.
If wheezing is present that does not respond to epinephrine, administer nebulized albuterol solution 0.35 mL.
Although corticosteroids have no effect on the initial reaction, they can block late allergic symptoms. Thus, administer methylprednisolone 125 mg (or its equivalent) IV to prevent recurrent allergic manifestations.

BP, blood pressure; IV, intravenous; PO, orally.

other agent to minimize the risk of future reactions. If the reaction is mild or moderate, the patient may continue with the same chemotherapy if treatment is preceded by methods to prevent or minimize hypersensitivity reactions. General recommendations for preventing anaphylactoid reactions are found in Table 89-10. Pretreatment with prednisone and diphenhydramine significantly decreases the frequency and severity of anaphylactoid reactions; however, the effect of H_2-receptor antagonists and epinephrine remains controversial. Because the success of these preventive measures depends on the cause of the reaction (immunologic or anaphylactoid), the aforementioned characteristics of type I reactions should be used to assess the underlying pathogenesis. In addition, other chemicals present in the formulation or other agents administered concomitantly with the chemotherapy can cause the hypersensitivity reaction. Potential allergens included in the diluent or formulation of chemotherapy agents include Cremophor EL (present in paclitaxel and teniposide), polysorbate 80 (present in docetaxel), and benzyl alcohol (present in the parenteral form of methotrexate and cytarabine). Recognizing potential allergens can significantly affect treatment of the current reaction and minimize the risk of future reactions.

PACLITAXEL PROTEIN-BOUND PARTICLES

To reduce the hypersensitivity reactions observed with paclitaxel, a new formulation has been produced, paclitaxel protein-bound particles (Abraxane), which is an albumin-bound form of paclitaxel. Because paclitaxel protein-bound particles formulation is Cremophor EL-free and less likely to cause hypersensitivity than traditional paclitaxel, it is not necessary to premedicate patients with steroids and antihistamines. The albumin-bound formulation is approved for patients with metastatic breast cancer after failure of a previous regimen containing an anthracycline. Doses between the two agents are not comparable; the recommended dose of paclitaxel protein-bound particles is 260 mg/m^2 every 21 days for six cycles. Although fewer hypersensitivity reactions are associated with this formulation, myelosuppression remains a dose-limiting toxicity.[121]

SPECIFIC ORGAN TOXICITIES

Neurotoxicity

Cytarabine and L-Asparaginase

20. A.L., a 39-year-old woman with acute lymphoblastic leukemia, has been admitted to the hospital for induction chemotherapy. Cytarabine 5 g IV Q 12 hr for eight doses, vincristine 2 mg IV push weekly, prednisone 100 mg/day, L-asparaginase 15,000 U/day for 14 days, and allopurinol 300 mg/day are ordered. Laboratory data obtained on admission include a WBC count of 120,000 cells/mm^3 (normal, 3,200–9,800), with 9% neutrophils (normal, 54%–62%), 11% lymphocytes (normal, 25%–33%), and 80% blasts and a uric acid of 7.5 mg/dL (normal, 2–7). On day 3, A.L. is confused and she has difficulty performing a finger-to-nose neurologic examination. After 3 weeks, she complains of numbness in her hands and feet. In addition, the clinician notes an eyelid lag and ataxia. A.L. also complains of severe constipation. What is the possible cause of A.L.'s mental status? Should chemotherapy be continued?

[SI unit: uric acid, 446 mmol/L]

High dosages of cytarabine (>1 g/m^2 in multiple doses) are associated with CNS toxicity in 15% to 37% of patients.[122,123] These neurotoxicities are dose and schedule related. Doses >18 g/m^2 per course increase the frequency of neurotoxicity. Older patients are more susceptible than younger patients, and the prevalence seems higher in subsequent versus initial courses of therapy. As illustrated by A.L., neurotoxicity may become evident within a few days after treatment with cytarabine and, most commonly, the neurotoxicity is manifested by a generalized encephalopathy with symptoms such as confusion, obtundation, seizures, and coma. Cerebellar dysfunction, presenting as ataxia, gait and coordination difficulties, dysmetria (inability to arrest muscular movement when desired and lack of harmonious action between muscles when executing voluntary movement), also is commonly observed in patients receiving high-dose cytarabine therapy. These neurologic symptoms may partially resolve over days to weeks after discontinuation of therapy. Other neurologic toxicities reported with cytarabine include progressive leukoencephalopathy and chemical meningitis. Leukoencephalopathy typically presents with progressive personality and intellectual decline; dementia; hemiparesis; and, sometimes, seizures. Chemical meningitis can occur with intrathecal administration of cytarabine (see Chapter 90, Hematologic Malignancies). These neurotoxicities also can occur following treatment with other chemotherapy agents, including L-asparaginase.

L-Asparaginase often causes encephalopathy, which presents most commonly as lethargy and confusion.[124] Severe cerebral dysfunction occurs occasionally, and patients may

Table 89-12 Neurotoxicity of Selected Chemotherapeutic Agents[125,126,133,138]

Encephalopathy	Acute Encephalopathy	Chronic Syndrome	Cerebellar Neuropathy	Peripheral Neuropathy	Cranial Neuropathy	Autonomic (IT Dose)	Arachnoiditis Syndrome	Strokelike	SIADH
Alkylating Agents									
Cyclophosphamide									+
Ifosfamide	+		+	+	+				
Thiotepa		+					+		
Cisplatin	+		++	++					
Oxaliplatin				++					
Altretamine	+		+	++					
Procarbazine	++		+	+					
Antimetabolites									
Fluorouracil			++	+	+				
Fludarabine	+		+						
Cytarabine	+	+	++				+		
Nelarabine	++	+		++					
Methotrexate	+	+	+				+	+	
Plant Alkaloids									
Vinca alkaloids									
Vincristine				++		++			+
Vinblastine				++		++			+
Vinorelbine				++		++			+
Taxanes									
Paclitaxel				++					
Docetaxel				++					
Miscellaneous									
Asparaginase	++	+							
Bortezomib				++					
Thalidomide				++					
Lenalidomide				++					

+, reported but appears rare; + +, common in some cases and may present a clinical problem.
IT, intrathecal; SIADH, syndrome of inappropriate secretion of antidiuretic hormone.

present with stupor, coma, excessive somnolence, disorientation, hallucination, or severe depression. Symptoms can occur early (within days of administration of L-asparaginase) or late, depending on the treatment schedule.[125] The acute syndrome usually clears rapidly, but the delayed syndrome can last several weeks.

A.L.'s symptoms most likely are the result of CNS toxicity caused by both cytarabine and L-asparaginase. A decision regarding further treatment with these agents is complicated because decreasing the dose of cytarabine or L-asparaginase could compromise the likelihood of a complete remission. Although L-asparaginase–induced CNS neurotoxicities are usually reversible, high-dose cytarabine cerebellar toxicity may not be. Therefore, the clinician may decide to continue treating A.L. with modified doses.

Other Agents

21. What other chemotherapy agents produce CNS toxicity?

Other agents that produce CNS toxicities include methotrexate, fluorouracil, interferon-α, interleukin-2, fludarabine, altretamine, carmustine, procarbazine, ifosfamide, oxaliplatin, and nelarabine (Table 89-12). Recognition of neurotoxicity resulting from chemotherapy is often difficult because of comorbid conditions such as metastatic disease and other paraneoplastic syndromes, but it is important in assessing the need for potential dose modifications or even discontinuation of the agent. Several reviews provide detailed explanations of signs and symptoms, mechanisms, and potential treatments for chemotherapy-induced neurotoxicities.[125,126]

METHOTREXATE

Methotrexate causes little or no neurotoxicity when administered orally or intravenously in the usual doses; however, high-dose IV methotrexate (usually >1 g/m^2) can occasionally cause acute encephalopathy. Similar to that caused by other agents, the encephalopathy that occurs following therapy with methotrexate is usually transient and reversible. Other patients may develop a progressive leukoencephalopathy following high-dose IV methotrexate. The risk of leukoencephalopathy increases with higher cumulative doses of methotrexate and concomitant cranial radiation therapy.[127–129] As with intrathecal cytarabine, intrathecal methotrexate can cause a chemical meningitis and, less commonly, myelopathy or paraplegia. Patients receiving intrathecal therapy or high-dose methotrexate should be carefully monitored for signs and symptoms associated with neurotoxicity.

FLUOROURACIL

Fluorouracil can cause acute cerebellar dysfunction characterized by the rapid onset of gait ataxia, limb incoordination, dysarthria, and nystagmus.[130,131] Cerebellar dysfunction occurs in approximately 5% to 10% of patients receiving fluorouracil at all treatment schedules in common use and can present weeks to months after beginning therapy. A more diffuse encephalopathy presenting as headache, confusion, disorientation, lethargy, and seizures can also occur. These symptoms can be reversed if fluorouracil is discontinued or the dose is reduced. Other neurotoxicities observed with fluorouracil include rare reports of optic neuropathy and decreased vision. As with methotrexate, patients should be carefully monitored for signs and symptoms associated with neurotoxicity.

INTERFERON-α

Interferon-α can cause a neurologic complex characterized by headache and encephalopathy (weakness, confusion, lethargy). The symptoms occur in one-third of patients receiving interferon and can cause severe reactions in 10%. Severe reactions include coma, obtundation, major depression, and suicidal behavior. Elderly patients receiving high dosages may be more susceptible to these effects. Symptoms typically begin after several weeks of therapy and usually resolve within 3 weeks after dose attenuation or discontinuation of therapy. If further treatment is warranted, lower doses should be used.[132]

FLUDARABINE AND OTHER PURINE ANALOGS

Fludarabine can cause severe neurotoxicity when used at doses >90 mg/m^2 for 5 to 7 days.[133–135] Symptoms include altered mental status, photophobia, amaurosis (blindness that usually is temporary without change in the eye itself), generalized seizures, spastic or flaccid paralysis, quadriparesis, and coma. Some patients die even when therapy is discontinued. This neurotoxicity, however, is not usual with the current recommended dosage of 25 mg/m^2/day for 5 days. Mild neurologic symptoms are typically reported, but severe neurotoxicity[135,136] and optic demyelination can occur occasionally.[137] Patients with signs or symptoms suggestive of significant neurotoxicity should receive a neurologic examination and, if warranted, therapy should be discontinued. Nelarabine has dose-limiting neurotoxicity reported in ~64% of patients treated in phase I and II clinical trials. Clinical presentation includes severe somnolence, convulsions, and peripheral neuropathy ranging from paresthesias to motor weakness. Several cases of ascending peripheral neuropathies and demyelination have been reported. Therapy should be stopped if grade 2 toxicity is present because some cases have been irreversible.[138]

CARMUSTINE AND OTHER AGENTS

Carmustine and other alkylating agents cause little or no neurotoxicity in the usual IV doses, but higher dosages can increase the incidence of these adverse effects. Carmustine produces encephalopathy associated with confusion or seizures with a dose >600 to 800 mg/m^2.[139] Concurrent cranial radiotherapy and intracarotid administration may increase the risk of neurotoxicity.[140,141] Other agents reported to produce CNS toxicity include ifosfamide,[142,143] procarbazine,[144] altretamine,[145] and cisplatin.[146–149] These agents have been associated with encephalopathy that manifests as confusion, lethargy and, in some instances, psychosis and depression. When a patient presents with any signs or symptoms of neurotoxicity, that patient should receive a neurologic examination followed by a dose reduction or discontinuation of therapy. Ifosfamide is associated with an encephalopathy thought to result from one of its metabolites, chloracetaldehyde. The incidence ranges from 10% to 20%; it presents hours to days after initiation of treatment with confusion and disorientation and is generally self-limiting. Methylene blue has been used for both prevention and treatment. Risk factors for this complication include a history of ifosfamide-induced encephalopathy, renal dysfunction, low serum albumin, and abdominal disease.[150,151]

Peripheral Nerve Toxicity

22. What is causing A.L.'s numbness?

Paresthesia (numbness and tingling) involving the feet and hands (or both) is an early subjective symptom of vincristine neurotoxicity, which often appears within the first few weeks of therapy. This peripheral nerve toxicity commonly is bilateral and symmetric and is often referred to as a "stocking-glove" neuropathy. Symptoms initially consist of paresthesias, loss of ankle jerks, and depression of deep tendon reflexes. Areflexia (absent reflexes) typically occurs in about 50% to 70% of patients treated with a cumulative dose >6 to 8 mg. Although older patients appear to be more susceptible to paresthesias than younger ones, almost all complain of paresthesias following combination chemotherapy that incorporates vincristine or vinblastine. Pain and temperature sensory loss is usually more pronounced than vibration and proprioception sensory loss. Patients also may display motor weakness with a foot drop or muscle atrophy. Motor weakness, which can become the most disabling symptom associated with vincristine neurotoxicity, can occasionally cause muscle wasting. Although some patients develop muscle atrophy, true muscle weakness seldom occurs after treatment with vincristine. Stumbling and falling that can occur with this peripheral neuropathy is not usually caused by muscle weakness; instead, it occurs in the dark when patients lose proprioception because they lack visual orientation. These complications are either partially or completely reversible, but recovery often takes several months.[152,153]

23. What other agents may cause similar complaints of numbness?

Other agents that often share the peripheral nerve toxicity of vincristine include vinblastine, vinorelbine, cisplatin, etoposide, oxaliplatin, paclitaxel, docetaxel, bortezomib, thalidomide, and lenalidomide. Other agents causing peripheral nerve toxicity include those commonly associated with CNS toxicity. Unlike the vinca alkaloids, most of these agents cause numbness only and not a loss of reflexes, paresthesias, or weakness. These side effects generally are not dose limiting and are usually reversible. Several reviews provide detailed references for this information.[154,155]

Oxaliplatin causes peripheral neuropathies that differ from those associated with the use of cisplatin. Oxaliplatin-induced neurotoxicity manifests as an acute neurosensory complex as well as a cumulative sensory neuropathy. Hyperexcitability of peripheral nerves causes an 85% to 95% incidence of paresthesia and dysthesias of the hands, feet, and the perioral region. Laryngeal dysthesias have been described as well. These effects are precipitated by exposure to cold. The cumulative dose-limiting chronic neuropathy is described as a sensory neuropathy that is reversible several months after completion of therapy. Dose modifications for patients with persistent neurotoxicities have been developed and include delaying therapy until their condition improves.[156,157] Prevention of these reactions with infusions of magnesium and calcium were evaluated in a retrospective study of patients ($N = 161$) with advanced colorectal cancer receiving regimens of oxaliplatin, fluorouracil, and leucovorin. Calcium gluconate 1 g IV and magnesium sulfate 1 g IV 15 minutes before and immediately after completion of the oxaliplatin administration led to fewer patient withdrawals because of toxicity (4% vs. 31%, respectively). Relative to the control group, fewer treated patients developed distal paresthesias (7% vs. 26%, respectively) and less acute distal and lingual paresthesias. Additionally, no patients in the calcium–magnesium group demonstrated pseudolaryngospasm. Those in the calcium–magnesium group were less likely to develop chronic grade 2 and 3 neuropathy at the end of treatment (20% vs. 45%, respectively). Importantly, calcium and magnesium infusions have not been shown to decrease efficacy.[158] Consequently, calcium and magnesium infusions are given routinely with oxaliplatin administration.

Cranial Nerve Toxicity

24. What is the significance of A.L.'s lid lag?

Cranial nerve toxicity occurs in 1% to 10% of patients receiving vinca alkaloids, and most patients present with ptosis or ophthalmoplegia,[153,159] probably related to damage to the third cranial nerve. Toxicity to other cranial nerves can cause trigeminal neuralgia, facial palsy, depressed corneal reflexes, and vocal cord paralysis.[160] Other nerve toxicities associated with the vinca alkaloids include jaw pain, which can occur after the first or second injection[160]; the pain usually resolves spontaneously and does not recur with subsequent doses. Several of the cranial nerve toxicities, especially with vincristine, may be dose limiting because evidence shows an increased prevalence with increasing doses. A.L.'s eyelid lag probably is caused by vincristine.

25. Do other chemotherapy agents produce cranial nerve toxicity?

Ifosfamide, vinblastine, and cisplatin have been reported to cause cranial neuropathies. Intra-arterial administration of chemotherapy agents such as carmustine may increase the risk of encephalopathy and cranial neuropathies.

Ototoxicity, characterized by a progressive, high-frequency, sensorineural hearing loss, commonly occurs with cisplatin,[161,162] most likely as a result of a direct toxic effect on the cochlea. Ototoxicity occurs more frequently at higher dosages, worsens with concurrent cranial radiation therapy, and appears to be more pronounced in children. The reversibility of cisplatin ototoxicity is questionable. At some centers, routine audiometric tests are performed in patients receiving cisplatin; as a result, these centers have a greater percentage of patients with documented decreases in audio acuity than others. Early cessation of cisplatin may result in greater hearing improvement. Although ototoxicity appears to be a major toxicity associated with cisplatin, it is not commonly caused by other platinum analogs. For example, only 8 of 710 (1.1%) patients who received carboplatin experienced clinical hearing deficits, mainly tinnitus.[163] If ototoxicity is suspected, a hearing test should be performed and therapy discontinued if alternate treatments are available.

Autonomic Neuropathy

26. What is the cause of A.L.'s constipation, and how might this problem have been prevented?

Vincristine, as well as vinblastine, commonly causes an autonomic neuropathy. The earliest symptoms (colicky abdominal pain with or without constipation) are reported by one-third to one-half of patients receiving these agents.[153,159] Because severe constipation can progress to or include adynamic ileus, prophylactic laxatives are recommended on a regular basis for patients receiving vincristine and vinblastine. Stimulant laxatives such as the senna derivatives or bisacodyl are believed to be the most effective agents, and stool softeners also may be used concurrently. No compelling evidence suggests, however, that laxatives prevent constipation. Other less-frequent manifestations of autonomic dysfunction associated with vinca alkaloids include bladder atony with urinary retention, impotence, and orthostatic hypotension.[164,165] Patients should be monitored carefully for these signs or symptoms and receive appropriate management following diagnosis.

Cardiac Toxicities

Doxorubicin

27. D.A., a 35-year-old man with stage IV Hodgkin's disease, is receiving CHOP (cyclophosphamide 750 mg/m^2 IV day 1, doxorubicin 50 mg/m^2 IV day 1, vincristine 2 mg IV day 1, and prednisone 100 mg PO days 1–5) and concurrent radiation therapy to a large mediastinal mass. He comes to the clinic to receive his fifth cycle of CHOP and complains of tachycardia, shortness of breath (SOB), and a nonproductive cough. Physical examination reveals neck vein distention, pulmonary rales, and ankle edema. What is the most likely cause of D.A.'s current symptoms?

D.A. is experiencing symptoms of congestive heart failure (CHF) most likely caused by doxorubicin therapy. Doxorubicin, an anthracycline antibiotic, can cause a dose-dependent cardiomyopathy that generally occurs with repeated administration. Doxorubicin causes myocyte damage by a mechanism that differs from its cytotoxic effect on tumor cells. Because myocytes stop dividing in infancy, they presumably would not be affected by an agent whose cytotoxicity relies on actively cycling cells. Many mechanisms have been proposed to explain the cardiac toxicity associated with doxorubicin.[166,167] The association of anthracycline-induced cardiotoxicity with other agents administered concomitantly, monitoring techniques, and therapies to prevent and treat this condition have been reviewed.[168]

D.A.'s presentation is fairly typical of doxorubicin-induced cardiomyopathy, although he has no significant risk factors usually associated with CHF. The total cumulative dose of doxorubicin is the most clearly established risk factor for the CHF.[166,167,169] Patients, such as D.A., who are receiving bolus doses of doxorubicin at the standard 3-week interval face little risk of CHF until a total dose of 450 mg/m^2 to 550 mg/m^2 has been reached. After a patient has received a total dose >550 mg/m^2, the risk of CHF rises rapidly. Patients receiving <550 mg/m^2 of doxorubicin face a 0.1% to 1.2% risk of developing CHF. Comparatively, patients receiving >550 mg/m^2 face a risk that rises more or less linearly; the probability of CHF in patients receiving a total dose of 1,000/m^2 may be nearly 50%.[169]

Other factors that could increase D.A.'s risk of developing doxorubicin cardiomyopathy include mediastinal radiation therapy, pre-existing cardiac disease, hypertension, and age. Young children, as well as older patients, are likely to experience CHF at a lower cumulative dose. Concurrent chemotherapy agents (e.g., cyclophosphamide, etoposide, mitomycin, melphalan, trastuzumab, paclitaxel, vincristine, bleomycin) may also potentiate doxorubicin cardiac toxicity.[168] When patients receive paclitaxel and doxorubicin, the risk of cardiac toxicity appears to be related to the sequence and proximity of the infusions. In a pharmacokinetic study, paclitaxel increased the AUC of doxorubicin and its active metabolite, doxorubicinol, when paclitaxel administration immediately preceded doxorubicin. Therefore, doxorubicin should be given at least 30 minutes before paclitaxel. The relationship between risk factors and the total cumulative dose of doxorubicin is sufficiently strong to warrant guidelines restricting the total cumulative dose of doxorubicin to 450 mg/m^2 in patients with one or more identified risk factors (high-risk patients) and to 550 mg/m^2 in patients without risk factors (low-risk patients).

It is unusual that D.A., a 35-year-old man who has received a cumulative dose of only 200 mg/m^2 of doxorubicin, would be presenting with symptoms of CHF. Mediastinal radiation therapy, cyclophosphamide, or undiagnosed cardiac disease may, however, have contributed to this event. In addition, Hodgkin's disease involving the myocardium may be responsible for this presentation.

28. Is routine cardiac monitoring recommended in patients receiving doxorubicin?

Prevention of cardiomyopathy is achieved primarily by limiting the total cumulative dose. Limiting the total dose, however, cannot entirely prevent the cardiomyopathy for two reasons. First, individual tolerance to doxorubicin varies such that cardiotoxicity may occur before the arbitrary dose limit; second, some clinical situations warrant exceeding the dose limit to achieve positive chemotherapeutic outcomes.

Early efforts to prevent cardiomyopathy focused on monitoring systolic time intervals, QRS voltage loss, or ST-T segment changes on an electrocardiogram (ECG). These changes were too nonspecific or occurred too late to be useful, however; serial echocardiography has some usefulness in children.[170,171] Other current state-of-the-art monitoring for anthracycline cardiomyopathy includes radionuclide ventriculography (RNV) and endomyocardial biopsy. The use of radionuclide ventriculography (also referred to as radionuclide cardiac angiography; gated blood pool imaging; multiple gated acquisition [MUGA]) for early detection of doxorubicin-induced cardiac dysfunction has been investigated extensively.[172] RNV can accurately detect functional cardiac status, but it is not particularly sensitive in detecting patients who have early myocyte damage. Augmenting the RNV with exercise appears to give a more accurate picture of functional cardiac reserve. Because myocyte damage usually occurs days to weeks after treatment with doxorubicin, the RNV should be obtained just before, rather than just after, a course of the agent. Although guidelines vary, most institutions recommend obtaining an RNV before starting therapy with doxorubicin. Additional RNV should be obtained when a patient shows signs or symptoms of CHF or when low-risk patients receives cumulative doses >450 mg/m^2 or high-risk patients receive >350 mg/m^2, if additional doses are planned. Most guidelines recommend stopping doxorubicin or obtaining an endomyocardial biopsy when there is an absolute decrease in the RNV >10% to 20%, the RNV is <40%, or the RNV fails to increase >5% with exercise. The ASCO currently recommends frequent cardiac monitoring after doses >400 mg/m^2.[49] The study should be repeated after patients receive >500 mg/m^2 and with every additional dose of 50 mg/m^2. The guidelines published by ASCO support the recommendations to discontinue therapy when patients show clinical signs or symptoms of CHF or if the left ventricular ejection fraction decreases below institutional normal limits.[49]

Endomyocardial biopsies, along with a quantitative assessment of morphologic changes, provide the most specific evaluation of myocardial damage induced by anthracyclines. Progressive myocardial pathology is graded on a scale (the Billingham Score) of 0 (no change from normal) to 3 (diffuse cell damage in >35% of total number of cells with marked change in cardiac ultrastructure).[173] The prevalence of abnormal RNV and the appearance of signs and symptoms of CHF correlate with biopsy scores. Usually, a significant change in cardiac function is not seen with scores <2 to 2.5. Several investigators have evaluated the predictive value of this technique. With a score of 2, a patient has less than a 10% chance of developing heart failure if 100 mg more of doxorubicin is given.[174–176] There are occasional false–negative biopsy findings, and fatal CHF has been encountered in at least one patient with a relatively normal (1.0) biopsy score.[177] The most significant risk associated with endomyocardial biopsy is perforation of the right ventricle with associated tamponade; this occurs rarely and depends largely on the experience of the operator.

In summary, RNV and endomyocardial biopsy are complementary procedures that when used together with clinical evaluation can provide a degree of confidence in predicting tolerance to additional doxorubicin dosing. The endomyocardial biopsy provides a distinct advantage by allowing early myocyte damage to be appreciated before the RNV changes or the patient shows signs or symptoms of CHF.

Other Agents

29. How do the other members of the anthracycline class compare with doxorubicin in terms of cardiotoxicity and clinical usefulness?

DAUNORUBICIN

Daunorubicin differs structurally from doxorubicin only by hydroxylation of the fourteenth carbon. Unlike doxorubicin, daunorubicin is primarily used to treat hematologic malignancies, such as acute myeloid leukemia. During its initial clinical evaluations, clinicians lacked a good understanding of this drug's dose-schedule–relationship to toxicity, and it became known on some hospital wards as "the red death." Doxorubicin became favored to treat solid tumors because daunorubicin caused excessive mucositis and myelosuppression when patients received antileukemic dosages to treat these tumors. Since then, clinical trials have given clinicians a better understanding of daunorubicin's side effects and how to provide better supportive care. Daunorubicin safely produces clinical responses in patients with Hodgkin's disease, non-Hodgkin's lymphomas (NHL), melanoma, sarcomas, lung carcinomas, breast carcinomas, and GI tract carcinomas.[178] In randomized trials comparing daunorubicin and doxorubicin, daunorubicin caused less mucositis and a lower incidence of colonic damage and perforation.[179] Cardiac toxicities are similar for both drugs, however, although somewhat higher cumulative doses of daunomycin are typically tolerated.[180] Risk factors for CHF appear to be the same, and similar assessments should be undertaken to monitor for cardiotoxicity.

IDARUBICIN

Idarubicin is an anthracycline that is approved for the treatment of acute leukemias. Although idarubicin appears less cardiotoxic than doxorubicin in animal models[181] and daunorubicin in some early clinical trials,[182–184] other studies show equivalent myelosuppressive doses can cause cardiotoxicity comparable to that of doxorubicin and daunorubicin.[185,186] Until additional studies adequately define the cumulative dose associated with cardiotoxicity, patients receiving idarubicin should be routinely monitored for signs and symptoms of CHF.

EPIRUBICIN

Epirubicin is another anthracycline approved by the FDA for adjuvant therapy of breast cancer after surgical resection. As with the other anthracyclines, epirubicin can cause a dose-dependent, potentially fatal CHF. CHF occurs in 1.6% of patients receiving 700 mg/m^2 and in 3.3% of patients receiving 900 mg/m^2. Risk factors for cardiotoxicity include a history of cardiovascular disease, prior or concomitant radiation therapy to the mediastinum or pericardium, previous therapy with other anthracyclines or mitoxantrone, or concomitant use of other cardiotoxic medications. Cumulative doses should not exceed 900 mg/m^2, which may result in toxicity.[187] Patients receiving epirubicin should receive cardiac monitoring with continued therapy to minimize the risk of severe CHF.

MITOXANTRONE

Mitoxantrone is an anthracenedione that is structurally similar to the anthracyclines. Mitoxantrone is typically one-fifth the dose of doxorubicin or 12 to 14 mg/m^2 every 3 weeks. The important risk factors for mitoxantrone cardiotoxicity include a history of mediastinal radiation, cardiovascular disease, and anthracycline exposure. Predicting mitoxantrone cardiotoxicity is similar to that of doxorubicin and daunorubicin. In patients without risk factors, the risk for cardiotoxicity does not begin to rise significantly until patients receive about 160 mg/m^2. This dose is equivalent to about 800 mg/m^2 of doxorubicin. For patients who previously received doxorubicin (mean cumulative dose, 239 mg/m^2), the risk starts to rise when the cumulative mitoxantrone dose reaches about 100 mg/m^2.[188–190] The guidelines suggested for monitoring doxorubicin-induced cardiotoxicity should be followed with mitoxantrone therapy to minimize the risk for CHF.

Prevention

30. Can CHF be prevented by the use of a different dose or dosing schedule or by agents that protect the myocardium?

Altering the dose schedule of doxorubicin to more frequent, smaller doses while maintaining dose intensity has consistently resulted in reduction of cardiotoxicity without obvious compromise of antitumor effects.[191–196] Several reports suggest that peak plasma levels, as well as cumulative dose, have an important relationship to doxorubicin cardiotoxicity. Low doses of doxorubicin administered weekly or prolonged continuous IV infusions (48–96 hours) can be relatively cardiac sparing, allowing higher cumulative doses to be administered. In a retrospective, uncontrolled study of 1,000 patients receiving weekly doxorubicin, a total dose of 900 to 1,200 mg/m^2 of doxorubicin given in weekly fractions had the equivalent cardiotoxicity of 550 mg/m^2 given in every-3-week fractions.[192] Although well-designed studies comparing cardiac toxicity following bolus doses with fractionated therapy or continuous infusion are lacking, treatment that incorporates these alternative schedules should be considered in patients with pre-existing risk factors or patients who will be receiving total doses of >450 to 550 mg/m^2. The concurrent use of drugs that might minimize the risk of cardiotoxicity without compromising efficacy can be considered as well.

Dexrazoxane is a chemoprotectant that reduces the incidence and severity of cardiomyopathy. It is indicated in women with metastatic breast cancer who have received a cumulative doxorubicin dose of 300 mg/m^2. The recommended dosing ratio of dexrazoxane:doxorubicin is 10:1 slow IV push 30 minutes before starting doxorubicin. Currently, the ASCO guidelines do not support the routine use of dexrazoxane in patients unless a plan exists to continue doxorubicin beyond a total cumulative dose >300 mg/m^2. Clinical trials are evaluating the benefits of dexrazoxane in children and patients receiving other anthracyclines. Some evidence supports the use of dexrazoxane in patients receiving epirubicin.[197]

Another approach to protecting against doxorubicin cardiotoxicity focuses on delivering anthracycline encapsulated in liposomes. A phase III trial of women ($N = 509$) with metastatic breast cancer showed that efficacy with liposomal pegylated doxorubicin may be similar to conventional doxorubicin with decreased cardiotoxicity.[198] More data are needed in adjuvant settings. Additionally, the equivalent dose of liposomal preparations to conventional doxorubicin is not confirmed.

Management

31. How should doxorubicin- or other anthracycline-induced CHF be managed clinically?

Anthracycline-induced CHF presents similarly to other forms of biventricular CHF and occurs between 0 to 231 days after the last dose of doxorubicin (mean, 33 days). Anthracycline-induced CHF should be treated with diuretics, activity restriction, inotropic agents, and vasodilators, but these measures often are ineffective. The clinical course varies, with some patients showing stable disease and others showing improvement. Before cardiotoxicity was a widely recognized toxicity, the course of anthracycline-induced CHF was characterized by a rapid progression that generally led to death in a few weeks. The clinical outcome is better now, perhaps because anthracycline therapy is promptly discontinued after initial presentation and there are better treatments for CHF. These include the use of spironolactone, beta blockers, and angiotensin-converting enzyme (ACE) inhibitors, which have decreased morbidity and mortality in non–anthracycline-induced CHF. Enalapril was evaluated to determine if it would prevent cardiac function decline in a randomized, double-blind, placebo-controlled study of pediatric cancer patients who were at least 2 years out from treatment with anthracyclines and had evidence of CHF. Patients received enalapril at 0.05 mg/kg/day and this dose was progressively escalated to 0.10 mg/kg/day, and finally 0.15 mg/kg/day if there were no side effects. Although enalapril did not increase exercise intolerance, it did increase left ventricular end-systolic wall stress (LVESWS) in the first year of treatment. Side effects included dizziness, hypotension, and fatigue. The follow-up to the study was ~3 years, so the long-term benefits of enalapril are not known.[199]

Other Cardiac Toxicities

32. What other chemotherapy agents have been associated with cardiac toxicities?

Electrocardiographic changes have been observed during or after treatment with doxorubicin, other anthracyclines, cisplatin, etoposide, paclitaxel, cyclophosphamide, mechlorethamine, and arsenic. Most commonly, ECG changes involve ST-T segment changes, decreases in voltage, T-wave flattening, and atrial and ventricular ectopy. Other ECG abnormalities may be seen as well. Most studies suggest that arrhythmias occur in 6% to 40% of patients receiving bolus doxorubicin.[200] Paclitaxel also caused significant arrhythmias and conduction defects in phase I and II trials[201]; most patients developed sinus bradycardia. Arsenic, used in the treatment of relapsed acute promyelocytic leukemia, can cause QT interval prolongation and complete atrioventricular block. QT prolongation can lead to a torsade de pointes-type ventricular arrhythmia. Before initiating therapy, an ECG should be performed and serum electrolytes, including potassium and magnesium, should be assessed and corrected. Additionally, all drugs that are known to prolong the QT interval should be discontinued.[202] All other chemotherapy agents occasionally cause a rhythm disturbance, but these are limited to a few scattered reports and should not be considered clinically significant. Therapy should not be discontinued unless the patient develops a serious cardiac arrhythmia.

FLUOROURACIL

Fluorouracil has been associated with angina pectoris and myocardial infarction. Angina may occur in 1.6% to 18%[203–205] of patients receiving fluorouracil and appears to occur with an increased incidence in patients with a history of ischemic cardiomyopathy or in patients receiving 5-day infusions. Angina has been associated with both initial and subsequent courses. Although ischemia occurs most frequently during continuous infusion, it occasionally is delayed 3 to 18 hours after fluorouracil administration and has been reported after an oral dose. The cause of fluorouracil cardiotoxicity is uncertain. Direct myocyte damage is suggested from animal studies; however, human studies suggest that coronary artery spasm is the most likely cause of angina. Because the chest pain associated with fluorouracil responds to nitrates, this problem, theoretically, could be managed prophylactically or therapeutically with long-acting nitrates or calcium channel blockers.[203] Other agents (including vincristine, vinblastine, etoposide, paclitaxel, and bleomycin) can cause chest pain or infarction based on case reports in the literature.[168]

ALKYLATING AGENTS

Myocardial necrosis rarely has been reported with alkylating agents, including cyclophosphamide, ifosfamide, busulfan, and mechlorethamine. Typically, cardiotoxicity occurs when patients receive high doses, such as the doses used for hematopoietic cell transplantation. Pericarditis and hemorrhagic myocardial necrosis also have been reported in these cases. Risk factors are similar to those associated with doxorubicin and daunorubicin; however, a clear relationship between dose and cardiac dysfunction has not been demonstrated consistently in all case reports.[168]

TRASTUZUMAB

Signs and symptoms of CHF (e.g., dyspnea, increased cough, peripheral edema, S_3 gallop, and reduced ejection fraction) have been reported in 3% to 7% of patients receiving trastuzumab single-agent therapy. Of these patients, 5% had New York Heart Association (NYHA) class III or IV heart failure. The use of trastuzumab in combination with chemotherapy in patients ($N = 469$) with metastatic breast cancer showed a 27% incidence of cardiotoxicity compared with an overall 8% incidence in the anthracycline alone arm. In these same patients, the incidence of NYHA class III or IV heart failure was 16% in the trastuzumab and chemotherapy arm versus 3% in patients receiving anthracyclines alone. Additionally, heart failure occurred in the combination paclitaxel and trastuzumab arm with an overall incidence of 13% and 2%, class III and IV, respectively, versus a 1% incidence in the paclitaxel alone arm.[206] The toxicity seems to be direct and not dependent on cumulative dose or treatment duration. Trastuzumab-associated cardiac toxicity usually responds to standard medical treatment or discontinuation of the drug.[207] Before and periodically during treatment with trastuzumab, patients should undergo cardiac evaluation to assess left ventricular ejection fraction. Therapy should be discontinued if patients develop a clinically significant decrease in left ventricular function.

MULTITARGETED TYROSINE KINASE INHIBITORS AND MONOCLONAL ANTIBODIES

The multitargeted tyrosine kinase inhibitors exhibit a range of cardiovascular toxicities. Because these new agents are dosed chronically, more long-term toxicities may occur with longer follow-up. Imatinib has been associated with the development of CHF. A case series described 10 patients who presented with NYHA class III and IV heart failure, a mean of 7.2 ± 5.4 months (range 1–14 months) from initiation of therapy. The mean ejection fraction was 25% ± 8%. Patients receiving imatinib should be monitored for symptoms and signs of heart failure.[208] Imatinib and dasatinib have also been associated with heart failure, ventricular dysfunction, chest pain, and pericardial effusions.[209] Sunitinib has been associated with a decline in cardiac ejection fraction in 4.7% to 6% of patients in phase II studies in metastatic renal cancer, although most patients were asymptomatic.[210,211] An increased risk of myocardial ischemia and infarction has been observed with the use of sorafenib in patients with metastatic renal cell cancer in a phase III study.[212] Additionally, hypertension has been associated with sorafenib, sunitinib, and bevacizumab. Bevacizumab-related hypertension may be dose-related; it can occur at any time during therapy and is reported to have a 22% to 32% incidence. Hypertension is usually grade 3 or less and can be controlled with standard antihypertensive medications.[213] Patients receiving these agents should be routinely monitored for CHF and hypertension.

Nephrotoxicity

Cisplatin

33. T.J., a 58-year-old man with nonresectable head and neck cancer, is being treated with cisplatin 100 mg/m^2 IV on day 1 and fluorouracil 1 g/m^2/day IV for 5 days. He presents today for the third cycle of this regimen. A 24-hour urine analysis for creatinine collected by T.J. at home revealed a creatinine clearance of 75 mL/minute, down from 110 mL/minute at baseline. Other abnormalities include serum magnesium (Mg) of 1.2 mEq/L (normal, 1.6–2.2 mg/dL); all other electrolyte values are within normal range. Is cisplatin responsible for T.J.'s decreased glomerular filtration rate (GFR) and serum magnesium levels?

[SI units: Cl_{Cr}, 1.25 mL/sec; Mg, 0.6 mmol/L]

Cisplatin, a heavy-metal complex, is widely used clinically because it has activity against various solid tumors. The major dose-limiting toxicity of cisplatin is nephrotoxicity, and various renal and electrolyte disorders, both acute and chronic, have been associated with cisplatin. In the early 1970s, before the need for vigorous hydration was recognized, cisplatin often caused acute renal failure. Today, with the use of vigorous hydration, acute renal failure is uncommon; however, tubular dysfunction and decreased GFR remain problematic.

Morphologic damage is greatest in the straight segment of the proximal renal tubules where the highest concentration of platinum occurs. Acute and cumulative renal tubular damage have been demonstrated by increased urinary excretion of proximal tubular enzymes, such as β_2-microglobulin, alanine aminopeptidase, and *N*-acetyl glucosamine. Increases in proximal tubular enzymes correlate well with urinary excretion of protein and magnesium as well as decreased reabsorption of salt and water in the proximal tubules. T.J. has hypomagnesemia, which is the most common electrolyte abnormality caused by cisplatin. Hypomagnesemia appears to be dose related and may occur after a single treatment. Despite replacement with oral magnesium, renal losses of magnesium and decreased serum magnesium levels can persist for months or even years after completion of cisplatin therapy. Hypocalcemia and hyponatremia occur less frequently. The cause of these electrolyte abnormalities is thought to be similar to that of hypomagnesemia in that a proximal tubular defect occurs that interferes with reabsorption of these electrolytes.[214–216]

Chronic renal toxicity associated with cisplatin presents as a decrease in the GFR. Published reports suggest that the GFR decreases by 12% to 25% in most patients receiving multiple courses.[214,215] The decrease appears to be persistent and only partially reversible. An increase in serum creatinine or a decrease in creatinine clearance does not necessarily reflect the decline in GFR. The renal function of patients receiving cisplatin therapy should be evaluated because dosage reductions may be necessary if the creatinine clearance decreases. Methods that estimate creatinine clearance based on serum creatinine should be avoided, especially in patients with borderline renal function, because poor correlation has been demonstrated in some cancer patient populations. In addition, changes in creatinine clearance are not always reflected by changes in serum creatinine in these patients. Creatinine clearance should be determined using a 12- to 24-hour urine collection for creatinine.

T.J.'s decreased GFR and low serum magnesium likely are caused by cisplatin therapy. Although a dose reduction of cisplatin generally is not recommended for creatinine clearances in this range, the clinician should provide T.J. with adequate and aggressive hydration to prevent cisplatin nephrotoxicity. In addition, T.J. should receive an oral magnesium supplement, although diarrhea usually limits the use of the oral route when large doses are necessary. IV administration should be used if higher magnesium doses are required. Patients should undergo frequent measurements of their electrolytes, including magnesium, to minimize potential complications.

PREVENTION

34. What measures should be taken to prevent cisplatin nephrotoxicity in T.J.?

Several measures have been used to minimize or prevent cisplatin-induced nephrotoxicity, including hydration with saline, mannitol, and prophylactic magnesium. The patient should be vigorously hydrated with 2 to 3 L of normal saline over 8 to 12 hours to maintain a urine output of 100 to 200 mL/hour for at least 6 hours after treatment with cisplatin.[217–219] A loop diuretic (e.g., furosemide) may be required in elderly patients to eliminate excess sodium or in patients with compromised cardiac reserve, but these diuretics should not be used routinely to prevent nephrotoxicity. Mannitol (25–50 g) may be administered just before chemotherapy to prevent cisplatin-induced renal artery vasoconstriction, which can increase the concentration of platinum in the renal tubules.[219,220] Most patients may also benefit from prophylactic magnesium supplementation. Patients who received prophylactic magnesium 16 mEq IV daily during a 5-day course of cisplatin followed by 60 mEq orally (20 mEq three times daily) between courses experienced less nephrotoxicity compared with those who received no supplements in a prospective trial of 16 patients with testicular carcinoma.[221]

Although most of these preventive measures can adequately minimize the risk of nephrotoxicity, amifostine, an organic thiophosphate that is a chemoprotectant, is also available. It is indicated for reducing the cumulative renal toxicity associated with repeated administration of cisplatin in patients with advanced ovarian cancer. Amifostine's mechanism is based on the assumption that oxygen-free radicals generated by cisplatin and radiation therapy are toxic to normal cells. It preferentially enters normal cells where it generates an active thiol metabolite, which scavenges the free radicals. A pivotal clinical trial demonstrated that pretreatment with amifostine significantly reduced grade 4 neutropenia, nephrotoxicity, and neurotoxicity. No evidence indicated that amifostine interfered with the antitumor activity of cisplatin or cyclophosphamide.[222] This trial, along with several others, suggests that amifostine may prevent other toxicities associated with chemotherapy, including neurotoxicity, neutropenia, and ototoxicity. The ASCO guidelines currently support the use of amifostine for the prevention of nephrotoxicity and neutropenia; its use to prevent ototoxicity or neurotoxicity is not supported.[49]

The recommended dosage of amifostine is 910 mg/m^2 administered once daily as a 15-minute IV infusion starting 30 minutes before chemotherapy. Because amifostine can cause significant hypotension, all antihypertensives should be discontinued 24 hours before treatment. In addition, patients should receive IV saline and remain in the Trendelenburg position during the infusion. If a patient experiences significant decreases in systolic blood pressure or signs or symptoms of hypotension during the infusion, treatment with amifostine should be stopped temporarily. In most cases, the systolic blood pressure returns to near normal 5 minutes after interruption of the infusion. Any patient who appears hypotensive or dehydrated should not receive amifostine. Additional adverse reactions include infusion-related flushing, fever or chills, dizziness, hiccups, sneezing, and severe nausea and vomiting.[49] Using amifostine in combination with traditional preventive measures may significantly reduce the incidence of cisplatin-induced nephrotoxicity.

35. At what point would cisplatin therapy be discontinued in a patient with a diminished GFR?

Guidelines to modify the dosage of cisplatin in patients with decreased renal function are available. Most suggest a 50% dosage reduction when the GFR decreases to 30 to 60 mL/minute and discontinuation when the GFR falls to <10 to 30 mL/minute.[214] Percentage dose reductions generally refer to the recommended dose for a specific cancer in a given combination chemotherapy regimen. Because the cisplatin dose ranges from 50 mg/m^2 to 150 mg/m^2, the precise dose for a patient with a GFR of <60 mL/minute must be individualized to the situation. If the tumor responds to carboplatin, substitution should be considered because it does not cause nephrotoxicity. The dose of carboplatin when calculated by the Calvert equation[223] adjusts for with decreased GFR. Carboplatin it is primarily excreted by the kidneys. Other agents requiring dose adjustments or omission are given in Table 89-13.

Table 89-13 Chemotherapeutics and Targeted Agents Requiring Dosage Modifications or Dosage Omissions in Renal Insufficiency[320–322]

Bleomycin	Ifosfamide
Capecitabine	Lomustine
Carboplatin	Melphalan
Carmustine	Methotrexate
Cisplatin	Mitomycin
Cytarabine	Pemetrexed
Dacarbazine	Pentostatin
Fludarabine	Topotecan

Other Nephrotoxic Agents

36. What other chemotherapy agents can cause nephrotoxicity? What are the clinical consequences of nephrotoxicity produced by these agents?

PROXIMAL TUBULE DYSFUNCTION

Other agents reported to cause renal tubular defects include streptozocin, lomustine, carmustine, ifosfamide, and azacytidine.[224] Nephrotoxicity appears to be related to the total cumulative dose for streptozocin, carmustine, and lomustine. Comparatively, a clear relationship between dosage and renal tubular toxicity with ifosfamide has not been established; however, the renal abnormality associated with high doses of bolus ifosfamide did lead to the use of fractionated doses.[224] Most patients show signs and symptoms consistent with proximal tubular dysfunction.

The primary renal lesion associated with each of these agents occurs in the proximal renal tubule, and patients show several electrolyte imbalances, such as loss of protein, glucose, bicarbonate, and potassium. Serum creatinine, bicarbonate, potassium, urinary pH, protein, and glucose should be monitored closely in patients receiving these agents. Because the reversibility of the lesions varies among clinical reports and a significant number of patients who develop renal toxicity with these agents require dialysis,[224] patients should discontinue treatment with these agents if they show any changes in serum creatinine or electrolytes.

METHOTREXATE

37. J.R., a 15-year-old boy with osteogenic sarcoma of the right knee, was treated with amputation of his right leg. His leg is now healed and chemotherapy consisting of high-dose methotrexate, leucovorin rescue, doxorubicin, dactinomycin, bleomycin, cisplatin, and ifosfamide is planned. The dose of methotrexate is 15 g/m^2 administered over 3 hours. What precautions are necessary to prevent the renal and other toxicities associated with high-dose methotrexate therapy in J.R.?

Methotrexate normally is not nephrotoxic, although 90% of the agent is excreted unchanged in the urine; however, acute tubular obstruction can occur with high-dose methotrexate if appropriate precautions are not taken. Acute tubular obstruction is caused by tubular precipitation of methotrexate, which is poorly soluble at a pH <7.0. To prevent this occurrence, preventive measures should be planned for J.R., including hydration and brisk diuresis to produce urine output in the range of 100 to 200 mL/hour for at least 24 hours after the administration of high-dose methotrexate. A urine pH >7.0 usually can be ensured by administration of 25 to 50 mEq/L sodium bicarbonate within the hydration fluid. Acetazolamide, a carbonic anhydrase inhibitor, promotes urinary bicarbonate excretion and is used by some clinicians at doses of 500 mg two to four times daily to assist in maintaining a urinary pH >7.0. J.R.'s urine output and pH must be monitored closely to prevent acute tubular obstruction associated with high-dose methotrexate therapy.[214]

If J.R. has any existing renal insufficiency, methotrexate excretion will be decreased significantly, and he may experience greater bone marrow suppression and GI side effects because of prolonged exposure to high serum methotrexate levels. Leucovorin or folinic acid is a reduced form of folic acid. Leucovorin is given after methotrexate administration to selectively rescue normal cells from the adverse effects of methotrexate caused by inhibiting production of reduced folates. Because leucovorin does not require the action of dihydrofolate reductase for its conversion, it is unaffected by methotrexate's inhibition of this enzyme. Therefore, it is important to ensure that appropriate leucovorin rescue is initiated within 48 hours after the high-dose methotrexate infusion. In addition, intrapatient and interpatient variability in methotrexate clearance is considerable, particularly with high doses of methotrexate therapy. Renal excretion of methotrexate is a complex process involving glomerular filtration, tubular reabsorption, and secretion. Concentrations of methotrexate obtained within 24 hours after the infusion often are not predictive of concentrations at 48 hours. Therefore, methotrexate concentrations between 24 and 48 hours must be monitored in J.R. and in all patients receiving high-dose therapy. Methotrexate levels are necessary to optimize leucovorin rescue (see Chapter 91, Solid Tumors). Leucovorin rescue does not affect the renal toxicity of methotrexate, however. Acute tubular obstruction associated with high-dose methotrexate therapy can be prevented only by appropriate attention to optimal urinary output before and for at least 24 hours after high-dose methotrexate administration and urinary alkalization.[225]

IFOSFAMIDE

38. J.R. also is receiving ifosfamide. What unique bladder toxicity occurs with ifosfamide that requires attention before its administration?

Pathogenesis

Ifosfamide is a structural analog of cyclophosphamide belonging to the oxazaphosphorine class of antitumor alkylating agents, which must be hydroxylated and activated by the cytochrome 3A4/5 and 2B6 in the liver. The 4-hydroxy metabolite spontaneously liberates acrolein, which is excreted in high concentrations in the urine. Acrolein is responsible for urotoxicity causing a direct irritation of the bladder mucosa. Both ifosfamide and cyclophosphamide can produce cystitis, which ranges from mild to severe bladder damage and hemorrhage. Cystitis is characterized by tissue edema and ulceration followed by sloughing of mucosal epithelial cells, necrosis of smooth muscle fibers and arteries, and culminating in focal hemorrhage. Because the metabolic activation of ifosfamide proceeds more slowly than the metabolic activation of cyclophosphamide, the dosages of ifosfamide are three to four times higher than the dosages of cyclophosphamide. This may explain the higher incidence of urotoxicity associated with ifosfamide.

Clinical Presentation

Patients with oxazaphosphorine-induced hemorrhagic cystitis initially go through an asymptomatic stage characterized by complaints of brief episodes of painful urination, frequency, and hematuria. The symptoms may subside over a period of several days or weeks after discontinuing the agent. The course of oxazaphosphorine-induced hemorrhagic cystitis usually is relatively benign, although death from massive refractory hemorrhage has occurred. Factors that may predispose J.R. to hemorrhagic cystitis include IV administration and the high doses he is receiving.

Prevention

Historically, forced hydration was the primary method used to prevent hemorrhagic cystitis in patients treated with cyclophosphamide therapy. Theoretically, hydration flushes the toxic metabolites out of the bladder so that insufficient contact time is available to set up the tissue reaction. The more urotoxic agent ifosfamide was introduced to the market with a uroprotective agent, mesna. Mesna liberates free thiol groups in the bladder, which can neutralize the oxazaphosphorine metabolite. When administered in an appropriate dosing schedule, mesna can prevent the bladder toxicity completely.

The manufacturer and ASCO currently recommend a parenteral mesna dose of 20% of the ifosfamide dose (<2.5 g/m^2) given IV at zero, 4, and 8 hours after ifosfamide (for a total mesna dose of 60% of the ifosfamide dose).[49] The goal is to maintain mesna levels within the urinary tract for some time after treatment with ifosfamide to provide adequate uroprotection. Repeated administration is required because mesna has a short elimination half-life (<1 hour), especially compared with the relatively long half-life of ifosfamide. If patients receive a continuous infusion of ifosfamide, clinicians fear that patients may not receive adequate uroprotection with this divided dose regimen. Therefore, for patients receiving a continuous infusion of ifosfamide, ASCO guidelines recommend an IV bolus mesna dose of 20% of the ifosphamide followed by a 40% mesna dose by continuous infusion given over 12 to 24 hours after the end of the ifosfamide infusion.[49] This regimen ensures that mesna remains in the bladder for an extensive amount of time following the end of the ifosfamide infusion.

Various other mesna dosing schedules are clinically used, but no trials have compared the different regimens. One author suggests that a total mesna dose equivalent to 17% w/w of the ifosfamide dose was just as effective in preventing urotoxicity as the 60% w/w dose.[226] Many investigators use a 1:1 w/w dose of mesna to ifosfamide when administered by continuous infusion. The dosing guidelines become less well defined, however, when patients receive higher dosages of ifosfamide (>2.5 g/m^2).

The lack of data and the unique pharmacokinetic properties of ifosfamide have caused some concerns about the current dosing guidelines. The pharmacokinetics of ifosfamide is dose dependent. The elimination half-life associated with doses of 2.5 g/m^2 is 6 to 8 hours, whereas the elimination half-life associated with doses of 3.5 to 5 g/m^2 is 14 to 16 hours. The current recommendations for mesna administration provide protection for ~12 hours after an IV bolus; thus, with higher dosages of ifosfamide, mesna should be infused beyond the recommended 8 hours after ifosfamide to maintain bladder protection. Based on pharmacokinetics of ifosfamide and mesna and the observation that hematuria can develop 1 to 2 days after combined ifosfamide and mesna infusions have been discontinued, mesna infusions should be continued for some time following discontinuation of ifosfamide.[227] Also, concern exists that the 4-hour dosing interval may be inadequate to maintain sufficient mesna levels within the bladder. Although most of the mesna dose after IV administration is eliminated within 4 to 6 hours, data demonstrate that elimination rates (mg/kg/hour) are highest in the first 2 hours after IV administration.[228,229] To ensure maximal protection against urotoxicity, ASCO currently recommends more frequent or prolonged mesna dosage regimens.[49] Indeed, some centers administer mesna by continuous infusion to avoid the need for frequent bolus dosing. Because ifosfamide and mesna are compatible in solution, combining the ifosfamide and mesna in one IV bag and administering by continuous infusion allows patients to conveniently receive uroprotection.

Another question concerns the influence of urination on the efficacy of mesna uroprotection. Several authors have suggested that the frequency of mesna doses be adjusted based on frequency and amount of urination.[230,231] Although forced hydration has been the mainstay for prevention of cyclophosphamide-induced hemorrhagic cystitis, it is unnecessary and potentially disadvantageous when mesna is used. This is because forced hydration can increase urination and increase the evacuation of mesna from the bladder.

Mesna is often given IV, but an oral formulation is available. The oral bioavailability of mesna is approximately one-half that of IV mesna. Therefore, patients should receive two times the standard IV dose if they receive mesna orally (e.g., oral mesna 40% of the ifosfamide dose) 2 hours before and 4 and 8 hours after ifosfamide.[232] Others have recommended that an oral dose also be given with the ifosfamide dose. Several centers administer the first dose of mesna IV followed by oral doses at 4 and 8 hours, particularly in the outpatient clinic setting.[49] All patients receiving cyclophosphamide should receive saline diuresis or forced saline diuresis to protect urothelial tissue. When patients receive cyclophosphamide for a BMT, they may receive mesna in conjunction with saline diuresis because the higher cyclophosphamide dosages produce more of the urotoxic metabolites than conventional dosing. Other practices to prevent this complication include hyperhydration and the use of continuous bladder irrigation. Data comparing these methods are controversial and report varying rates of hematuria and severe hemorrhagic cystitis. These recommendations are currently supported by the ASCO consensus guidelines[49] (see Chapter 92, Hematopoietic Cell Transplantation).

39. If J.R. develops hemorrhagic cystitis, how should it be treated?

Once hemorrhagic cystitis develops, the chemotherapy agent causing the disorder must be discontinued and vigorous hydration started. If gross hematuria occurs, a large-bore urinary catheter should be inserted to avoid obstruction of the urethra by clots. Some clinicians also use continuous silver nitrate irrigation, local instillation of formalin, or electrocauterization of bladder blood vessels to control bleeding. If these measures fail, surgical intervention may be necessary to divert urine flow away from the bladder.

Pulmonary Toxicities

40. J.A., a 67-year-old man with an 8-year history of chronic lymphocytic leukemia (CLL), was treated intermittently for 7 years with chlorambucil and prednisone. About 1 year ago, increasing lymphadenopathy was noted, and a biopsy revealed that his CLL had transformed to large-cell lymphoreticular lymphoma. (This transformation is called Richter's syndrome.) At that time, he was started on a chemotherapy regimen of cyclophosphamide, doxorubicin, vincristine, prednisone, and bleomycin (CHOP-Bleo), and his disease stabilized. Three weeks after his ninth course, he developed dyspnea, a nonproductive cough, and fever. Chest radiograph showed diffuse bilateral infiltrates; his respiratory rate (RR) was 36 breaths/minute; and his arterial blood gases (ABG) were pH, 7.50 (normal, 7.35–7.45); Po_2, 62 (normal, 80–100 mmHg); Pco_2, 28 (normal, 35–45 mmHg); and an O_2 saturation of 92% (normal, 95%–98%). What are the possible causes of his new pulmonary findings?

J.A. is at risk for several processes that could produce diffuse pulmonary infiltrates and dyspnea. He undoubtedly is immunosuppressed secondary to both his lymphoma and the chemotherapy; therefore, J.A. has an increased risk for infection (e.g., *Pneumocystis carinii* or cytomegalovirus [CMV]). In addition, his lymphoma now may be resistant to the therapy, and the infiltrates may represent progression of the disease. Pulmonary infiltrates also may represent toxicity resulting from one or more of the chemotherapy agents he has received. Further diagnostic workup is necessary to establish the cause.

41. A bronchoscopy with bronchoalveolar lavage and a biopsy with pathologic and microbiologic evaluations were performed. Bacterial, fungal, and viral cultures were negative, and the biopsy revealed inflammation and fibrosis with no evidence of lymphoma. These results are highly suggestive of chemotherapy-induced pulmonary damage. (Note: If the results of the bronchoscopy had not been helpful in establishing a diagnosis, an open-lung biopsy would have been recommended.) Which of the agents that J.A. received are associated with pulmonary toxicity, and what other factors may have increased his risk of pulmonary toxicity?

Many chemotherapy agents have been associated with pulmonary toxicity and the varying types of mechanisms and clinical presentations have been reviewed[233] (Table 89-14). J.A. has received three agents with potential pulmonary toxicity, including chlorambucil, cyclophosphamide, and bleomycin. Because J.A. has received three potentially pulmonary toxic agents and because of his advanced age, he is at increased risk for pulmonary toxicity.

Among the chemotherapy agents, bleomycin most commonly causes pulmonary toxicity. Although several forms have been reported, the most frequent is interstitial pneumonitis followed by pulmonary fibrosis.[233–235] Patients generally present with a nonproductive cough and dyspnea. Clinicians may detect only fine crackling bibasilar rales that often progress to coarse rales. The chest radiograph may be normal in the early stages, but patients can develop bilateral alveolar and interstitial infiltrates. ABG show hypoxia, and pulmonary function tests generally show a progressive fall in the diffusing capacity without a significant decrease in the forced vital capacity.[234] The most significant factor associated with the development of pulmonary toxicity is the cumulative dose of bleomycin. At total doses <400 mg, <10% of patients may develop pulmonary toxicity. When the cumulative dose reaches 450 to 500 mg, the incidence is higher. The incidence may be lower when patients receive bleomycin by a continuous infusion.[236] A rarer, hypersensitivity reaction produces fever, eosinophilia, and diffuse infiltrates, and this pulmonary toxicity is not dose related. The mortality associated with bleomycin pulmonary toxicity

Table 89-14 Chemotherapy-Induced Pulmonary Toxicity

Drug	Histopathology	Clinical Features	Treatment/Outcome
Aldesleukin[323]	Capillary leak, pulmonary edema	*Clinical presentation:* ↓ BP, fever, SOB, anorexia, rash, mucositis	Stop infusion; provide supportive care to cause a quick resolution of symptoms.
Bleomycin[236,237,324,325]	Interstitial edema and hyaline membrane formation; mononuclear cell infiltration pneumonitis with progression to fibrosis; eosinophilic infiltrations seen in patients with suspected hypersensitivity-type reactions	Cumulative dose-related toxicity with risk increasing substantially with total dose >450 mg or 200 mg/m^2; may occur during or after treatment *Clinical presentation:* cough, fever, dyspnea, tachypnea, rales, hypoxemia, bilateral infiltrates, dose-related ↓ in diffusing capacity	Recovery if bleomycin is discontinued while symptoms and radiologic changes still minimal; progressive and usually fatal if symptoms severe. Avoid cumulative doses >200 mg/m^2; monitor serial pulmonary function tests. Discontinue therapy if diffusing capacity ≤40% of baseline, FVC <25% of baseline, or if any signs or symptoms suggestive of pulmonary toxicity occur. Steroids may be helpful if toxicity is result of hypersensitivity.
Busulfan[235]	Pneumocyte dysplasia; mononuclear cell infiltrations; fibrosis	Does not appear to be dose-related, but no cases reported with total doses <500 mg *Clinical presentation:* insidious onset of dyspnea, dry cough, fever, tachypnea, rales, hypoxemia diffuse linear infiltrate, ↓ in diffusing capacity	Fatal in most patients; progressive despite discontinuation of busulfan. High-dose steroids (50–100 mg prednisone daily) have been helpful in a few cases.
Carmustine[326–330]		Dose-related; usually occurs with doses >1,400 mg/m^2 *Clinical presentation:* dyspnea, tachypnea, dry hacking cough, bibasilar rales, hypoxemia, interstitial infiltrates; spontaneous pneumothorax has been reported	May continue to progress after carmustine discontinued. No evidence that steroids improve or alter incidence. High mortality rate if symptoms severe. Serial pulmonary function studies recommended. Total cumulative dose should not exceed 1,400 mg/m^2.
Chlorambucil[234]	Pneumocyte dysplasia; fibrosis	Usually occurs after at least 6 months of treatment with total cumulative doses of >2 g *Clinical presentation:* dyspnea, dry cough, anorexia, fatigue, fever, hypoxemia, bibasilar rales, localized infiltrates progressing to diffusing involvement of both lung fields	Fatal in most cases despite discontinuation of chlorambucil and treatment with high-dose steroids.
Cyclophosphamide[234,329]	Endothelial swelling, pneumocyte dysplasia, lymphocyte infiltration fibrosis	Does not appear to be schedule- or dose-related and may occur after discontinuation *Clinical presentation:* progressive dyspnea, fever, dry cough, tachypnea, fine rales, ↓ diffusing capacity and restrictive ventilatory defect, bilateral interstitial infiltrates	Clinical recovery reported in about 50% of patients within 1–8 wk if therapy stopped. Some of these patients received steroid therapy; however, others have died despite steroid therapy. Occasionally, therapy has been restarted without recurrence.
Cytarabine[331]	Pulmonary edema, capillary leak	*Clinical presentation:* tachypnea, hypoxemia, interstitial or alveolar infiltrates	Not always fatal.
Gemcitabine[332]	Pulmonary edema, rare interstitial pneumonitis	Dyspnea was reported in 23% of patients; severe dyspnea in 3%; dyspnea occasionally accompanied by bronchospasm (<2% of patients); rare reports of parenchymal lung toxicity consistent with drug-induced pneumonitis	Treatment is supportive care measures. Symptoms resolve and are usually not seen with rechallenge.
Fludarabine[333]	Interstitial infiltrates, alveolitis, centrilobular emphysema	*Clinical presentation:* fever, dyspnea, cough, hypoxia; onset 3–28 days after third or fourth course; bilateral infiltrates and effusions	Resolves spontaneously over several weeks with or without corticosteroids.
Melphalan[234]	Pneumocyte dysplasia	Not dose-related *Clinical presentation:* dyspnea, dry cough, fever, tachypnea, rales, pleuritic chest pain, hypoxemia	Most patients die because of progressive pulmonary disease. Most reported cases occurred while patients were receiving concomitant prednisone therapy. Usually progresses rapidly.

Table 89-14 Chemotherapy-Induced Pulmonary Toxicity *(Continued)*

Drug	*Histopathology*	*Clinical Features*	*Treatment/Outcome*
Methotrexate[334–337] *Delayed*	Nonspecific changes; occasional fibrosis	No evidence that dose-related; daily or weekly schedules more likely to cause toxicity than monthly dosing *Clinical presentation:* headache, malaise prodrome, dyspnea, dry cough, fever, hypoxemia, tachypnea, rales, eosinophilia, cyanosis in up to 50% of patients, interstitial infiltrates, ↓ diffusing capacity, restrictive ventilatory defect	Most patients recover within 1–6 wks (some may have persistent infiltrates or ↓ pulmonary function parameters). Steroids may produce more rapid resolution. May resolve despite continuation of methotrexate, but discontinuation may speed resolution. Rarely fatal.
Noncardiac pulmonary edema	Acute pulmonary edema	Occurs very rarely 6–12 hr after PO or IT methotrexate	May be fatal.
Pleuritic chest pain		Not related to other methotrexate toxicities or serum levels; may not occur with each course of therapy *Clinical presentation:* right-sided chest pain, occasional pleural effusion or collapse of lung, thickened pleural densities	Usually resolves within 3–5 days.
Mitomycin[234]	Similar to bleomycin	*Clinical presentation:* dyspnea, dry cough, basilar rales, hypoxemia, bilateral interstitial or finely nodular infiltrates, ↓ diffusing capacity	Fatal in ≈50% of cases. Complete resolution reported in some patients, including some who received steroid therapy.
Procarbazine[338,339]	Hypersensitivity pneumonitis with eosinophilia and interstitial fibrosis	*Clinical presentation:* nausea, fever, dry cough, dyspnea within a few hours of ingestion, bilateral interstitial infiltrates, and pleural effusion	Rapid resolution after discontinuation.
Vinblastine[235]	Hyperplasia, dysplasia, interstitial edema, and fibrosis	Associated with concomitant treatment with mitomycin *Clinical presentation:* acute respiratory distress, bilateral infiltrates	Initial improvement with subsequent progression.

BP, blood pressure; FVC, forced vital capacity; IT, intrathecal; SOB, shortness of breath.

is about 50%.[233–235] If bleomycin is discontinued while symptoms are minimal and before pulmonary function has decompensated significantly, the damage may not progress. In contrast, patients with prominent physical and radiographic findings generally die because of pulmonary complications. Other chemotherapy agents can potentially exacerbate the pulmonary toxicity associated with bleomycin.

Less commonly, chlorambucil and cyclophosphamide induce pulmonary toxicities similar to bleomycin. Chlorambucil-induced lung damage appears to be dose related because most cases have occurred in patients who received a total dose >2 g over >6 months.[234] In most instances, patients died of severe interstitial pulmonary fibrosis. Cyclophosphamide pulmonary toxicity does not appear to be related to the dosage regimen. Approximately 50% to 65% of patients improve clinically after discontinuing cyclophosphamide therapy. If a patient presents with signs or symptoms consistent with pulmonary toxicity, the patient should undergo a diagnostic workup after discontinuing therapy.

42. Why are routine pulmonary evaluations indicated in patients such as J.A. who receive bleomycin or other pulmonary toxic agents?

Because a dose-related decrease in diffusing capacity has been observed in patients receiving bleomycin before the onset of clinical symptoms, routine baseline and serial pulmonary function studies are recommended.[237] Bleomycin therapy should be withheld if the diffusing capacity falls below 40% of the baseline value, if the forced vital capacity falls below 75% of the baseline value, or if patients develop any signs or symptoms of pulmonary damage.[234] Some practitioners also recommend limiting the total cumulative dose to ≤450 mg. Specific screening is not routinely recommended for patients receiving other pulmonary toxic agents; however, if patients develop any symptoms or clinical findings, therapy should be withheld until the cause can be determined.

Management

43. How should J.A.'s agent-induced pulmonary toxicity be managed?

The most effective way to manage pulmonary toxicity is to prevent it. If pulmonary toxicity becomes evident, however, all responsible agents (in J.A.'s case: bleomycin, chlorambucil, and cyclophosphamide) should be discontinued and the patient should receive symptomatic support based on their physical condition (e.g., oxygen). As illustrated by J.A., other treatable causes of pulmonary infiltrates (e.g., infection) also should be ruled out. In many cases, however, pulmonary toxicity is irreversible and progressive, and effective treatments are unavailable. Corticosteroids often are administered but probably are effective only in cases in which hypersensitivity caused the pulmonary damage. Nevertheless, because other effective treatments are lacking, a trial of steroids generally is indicated for all patients; if steroids are discontinued, they must be tapered carefully to avoid clinical deterioration.

Hepatotoxicity

44. J.D. has received two courses of chemotherapy with cytarabine and daunorubicin. Before chemotherapy was started, his liver function tests (LFT) and coagulation studies were within normal limits. His current laboratory values include the following: aspartate aminotransferase (AST), 204 U/L (normal, 8–46); alanine aminotransferase (ALT), 197 U/L (normal, 7–46); lactate dehydrogenase (LDH), 795 U/L (normal, 100–190); alkaline phosphatase, 285 U/L (normal, 25–100); bilirubin, 1.2 mg/dL (normal, <1.5); and PT, 13.1 seconds (normal, 11–16). Why could J.D.'s chemotherapy be responsible for these laboratory abnormalities?

[SI units: AST, 3.4 μkat/L; ALT, 22.98 μkat/L; LDH, 13.25 μkat/L; alkaline phosphatase, 4.75 μkat/L; bilirubin, 20.52 mmol/L]

Elevated LFT occur frequently in cancer patients and their causes are listed in Table 89-15. Other signs and symptoms include jaundice, nausea, vomiting, abdominal pain, and, rarely, encephalopathy. Patients should receive an extensive workup to determine whether they require any immediate attention for tumor involvement of the liver or possible infection. In addition, patients should discontinue any nonessential medications that can potentially cause hepatotoxicity. The clinician may also need to consider discontinuing chemotherapy because some agents may cause the hepatotoxicity observed.

Several chemotherapy agents, including cytarabine given to J.D., have been associated with hepatocellular damage and are reviewed in detail[238] (Table 89-16). The agents most commonly associated with hepatotoxicity include asparaginase, carmustine, cytarabine, mercaptopurine, streptozocin, clofarabine, and gemtuzumab ozogamicin. Methotrexate has caused hepatotoxicity when given on a daily schedule; however, if it is given on an intermittent basis, the incidence of toxicity decreases significantly.[239–240] All of these drugs come in contact with the liver by entering the liver's blood supply; the liver uniquely receives a dual blood supply from the portal and superior mesenteric veins. The liver can detoxify or inactivate noxious substances and metabolizes many chemotherapeutic agents as well. When chemotherapy agents undergo metabolism, they can damage the metabolic processes in the liver. The exact mechanisms by which chemotherapy agents cause hepatotoxicity are unknown, but most agents probably cause hepatic damage by (a) interfering with the mitochondrial function of the hepatocyte, (b) depleting hepatic glutathione stores, (c) eliciting hypersensitivity reactions, (d) decreasing bile flow, or (e) causing phlebitis of the central hepatic vein to produce veno-occlusive disease.[238]

Table 89-15 Common Causes of Elevated LFT in Patients With Cancer

Primary or metastatic tumor involvement of the liver
Hepatotoxic drugs (e.g., cytotoxics, hormones [estrogens, androgens], antimicrobials [trimethoprim-sulfamethoxazole, voriconazole])
Infections (e.g., hepatic candidiasis, viral hepatitis)
Parenteral nutrition
Portal vein thrombosis
Paraneoplastic syndrome
History of liver disease (including hepatitis B and C)

LFT, liver function tests.

Table 89-16 Hepatotoxicity From Select Antineoplastic Drugs

Drug/Schedule	Prevalence	Type
Asparaginase[340–342]		
Daily	Frequent	Hepatocellular fatty metamorphosis
Busulfan[343]		
High dose	Infrequent	Veno-occlusive disease
Carmustine[344,345]		
Weekly bolus	Common	Hepatocellular
Daily × 3	Common	
Bolus	Infrequent	
Clofarabine[346]	Common	Hepatocellular
Cytarabine[347]		
Daily	Common	Cholestatic
Dacarbazine[348,349]		
Daily × 5	Infrequent	Hepatocellular
Bolus		
Etoposide[350]		
High dose	Common with high dose	Hepatocellular
Gemtuzumab ozogamicin[351]	Common	Hepatocellular, veno-occlusive disease
Imatinib[352]	Frequent	Hepatocellular
Lomustine	Infrequent	
Mercaptopurine[353,354]		
Daily	Common	Cholestatic
High dose		Hepatocellular
Methotrexate[239,240]		
Daily	Common	Hepatocellular
Weekly bolus	Rare	Hepatocellular
High dose	Uncommon	Hepatocellular
Mitomycin[355]		
High dose	Infrequent	Veno-occlusive disease
Streptozocin[356]		
Bolus	Common	Hepatocellular
Thioguanine[357]		
Daily	Rare	Veno-occlusive disease
Epirubicin	Infrequent	Hepatocellular

Several laboratory tests can provide markers of liver structure and function. Serum transaminases, alkaline phosphatase, and bilirubin levels should be monitored routinely in patients receiving hepatotoxic chemotherapy. Although these laboratory indices are sensitive indicators of liver injury, they are nonspecific for the type of liver disease and do not necessarily correlate with hepatic function. Serum levels of proteins produced by the liver (e.g., ferritin, albumin, prealbumin, or retinol-binding protein) also may be helpful in assessing liver function. The decision to continue or discontinue chemotherapy in patients with apparent hepatic dysfunction can be difficult. If the chemotherapy is the suspected cause, therapy should be withheld until LFT are within normal ranges. The clinician should also consider alternative (nonhepatotoxic) chemotherapy for future treatment. In addition, agents that are cleared

Table 89-17 Chemotherapeutics Requiring Dose Modification in Hepatic Dysfunction[358,359]

Bilirubin	Aspartate Aminotransferase (AST)	Doxorubicin Epirubicin	Daunorubicin	Vincristine Vinblastine, Etoposide	Methotrexate	Fluorouracil
<1.2	<60	100%	100%	100%	100%	100%
1.2–3.0	60–80	50%	75%	50%	100%	100%
3.1–5.0	>180	25%	50%	Omit	75%	100%
5.0		Omit	Omit	Omit	Omit	Omit

Note: % written as the percentage of the full dose that should be given.

Paclitaxel Dosing in Patients With Liver Dysfunction

AST >2 ULN and Bilirubin ≤1.5	135 mg/m²
Bilirubin = 1.6–3.0	75 mg/m²
Bilirubin ≥3.1	50 mg/m²

Docetaxel Dosing in Patients with Liver Dysfunction

Bilirubin > ULN or	Omit
AST/ALT >1.5 × ULN	Omit

ALT, alanine aminotransferase; AST, aspartate aminotransferase; ULN, upper limit of normal.

predominantly via the liver may require dosage adjustments and should be administered cautiously (Table 89-17).

J.A.'s therapy is likely responsible for his elevated liver enzymes. Therefore, costly workup should be deferred to allow recovery of liver function. Recovery should occur within 2 weeks of chemotherapy. If full recovery does not occur, further therapy (agents, doses, or both) may require modifications.

LONG-TERM COMPLICATIONS OF CHEMOTHERAPY

Second Malignancies After Chemotherapy

Acute Myeloid Leukemia (AML)

45. T.D., a 55-year-old woman, was diagnosed with an early stage breast cancer and successfully treated with radical mastectomy followed by four cycles of adjuvant AC (doxorubicin 60 mg/m² IV on day 1, cyclophosphamide 600 mg/m² IV on day 1). Eighteen months after her breast cancer therapy was completed, T.D. presents to her primary care physician with complaints of fatigue, SOB, easy bruising, and sinusitis. A peripheral blood smear shows a WBC count of 120,000/mm³ with a differential of >90% leukemic blasts and a bone marrow biopsy confirms acute myeloid leukemia (AML). Subsequent cytogenetic analysis revealed abnormalities involving chromosome 11q23. What factors support the diagnosis of chemotherapy-associated acute leukemia in T.D.?

Acute leukemia has been associated with chemotherapy used to treat hematologic malignancies, solid tumors, and nonmalignant diseases.[241] AML also has been reported after combination chemotherapy that involves topoisomerase inhibitors, including teniposide, etoposide, and anthracyclines.[242] These leukemias usually occur 1 to 3 years after the completion of chemotherapy and myelodysplasia does not usually occur before the leukemia. Other characteristics include FAB M4 or M5 classification and chromosomal abnormalities involving chromosome 11q23. This is an important area for research given the widespread use of these agents for many curable diseases.

Acute myeloid leukemia has also been reported in patients who have had previous exposure to alkylating agents. It usually occurs 5 to 7 years after the patient finishes chemotherapy.[243] Myelodysplastic syndrome (preleukemia changes) commonly occurs in 50% of patients before overt acute leukemia.[244,245] Although all alkylating agents can cause acute leukemia, melphalan appears to be the most potent leukemogenic agent in this class; other classes of chemotherapy agents do not appear to carry as significant a risk. Large doses, continuous daily dosing, prolonged treatment periods, age >40 years, and concomitant radiation therapy may increase the risk of developing acute leukemia. Several additional factors may increase a patient's risk of developing acute leukemia.[241,246–248]

Evidence that chemotherapy can cause secondary lymphoid malignancies, particularly non-Hodgkin's lymphoma, is also strong. Immunosuppression from the disease and its treatment rather than the particular chemotherapy agent may be the primary cause of NHL. Other secondary malignancies can occur after chemotherapy as well. Solid tumors have been associated with superficial bladder cancer in patients treated with daily oral cyclophosphamide, and bone sarcoma has occurred after treatment with alkylating agents.[249] The secondary solid tumors in patients treated with other chemotherapy agents are considered coincidental.[249–251]

T.D.'s AML probably occurred secondary to her previous anthracycline therapy. The chemotherapy agent, as well as the time course for her acute leukemia, is consistent with topoisomerase-II agent-induced malignancies. In addition, cytogenetic abnormalities occur in >90% of those patients who have received chemotherapy or radiation therapy and have subsequently developed therapy-related myelodysplastic syndrome or AML.[245] Abnormalities in chromosome 11q23 are involved in many of the cases with cytogenetic abnormalities from topoisomerase inhibitors.[252] The chromosomal abnormalities of 11q23 in T.D. strongly support the diagnosis of chemotherapy-associated acute leukemia rather than *de novo* leukemia.

46. Are the therapy and prognosis of T.D. with treatment-associated AML similar to those of patients with *de novo* AML?

Therapy for patients with treatment-associated AML compares poorly with that of patients with *de novo* leukemia. Complete remissions with standard cytarabine and daunorubicin regimens are obtained in less than half of patients with treatment-associated AML compared with a complete remission rate of 70% to 80% in patients with *de novo* leukemia[253,254] (see Chapter 90 Hematologic Malignancies). High-dose cytarabine produced remissions in 10 of 11 patients with AML secondary to chemotherapy in one series.[255] Most series, however, reported a lower response rate, with responses of short duration and a median survival of only 3 to 4 months. Isolated case reports suggest that BMT may benefit younger patients and those with human leukocyte antigen (HLA) identical donors.[256–258]

The best "treatment" of therapy-associated AML is prevention. In patients such as T.D. receiving adjuvant chemotherapy for curable malignancies, avoiding the use of agents that cause treatment-related AML should be discussed in conjunction with other risks and benefits of therapy.

Fertility and Teratogenicity

Effects on Oogenesis

47. C.L., a 32-year-old woman with recently diagnosed stage II breast cancer, underwent a lumpectomy and external-beam radiation therapy and is scheduled to begin adjuvant chemotherapy with cyclophosphamide, doxorubicin, and fluorouracil (CAF). C.L. was married 12 months before her diagnosis and wishes to have children. What are C.L.'s prospects for fertility following adjuvant chemotherapy?

Chemotherapy is potentially gonadotoxic in humans. Ovarian biopsies taken from women treated for cancer demonstrate loss of ova and follicular elements.[259,260] This injury is evident even in prepubertal female patients treated for cancer.[261] Ova die or become nonfunctional by direct injury to the ova or by indirect injury resulting from loss of supporting follicular cells. If the damage to the follicular elements is extensive and irreversible, fertility is impaired even if the ova are spared.

Agent-induced injury to ova and follicular elements reduces ovarian estrogen and progesterone secretion in menstruating women. This causes the hypothalamus and pituitary to secrete more follicle-stimulating hormone (FSH) and luteinizing hormone (LH), which in turn increase follicular recruitment and the number of follicles vulnerable to chemotherapy agents. If the gonadal toxicity is severe or prolonged, permanent ovarian failure can occur secondary to depletion of ova and follicles. Recovery of some of the affected follicles often occurs, however, and this may be manifested by irregular menses or delayed recovery of menses. If the ova are spared and follicular cells recover sufficiently, ovulation and pregnancy might occur, but premature ovarian failure is inevitable in most women treated with large doses of gonadotoxic agents given over long periods.

Prepubertal girls have a greater reserve of primary follicles and because their ovaries are not producing estrogen and progesterone, increases in FSH and LH with resultant recruitment of follicular elements do not occur. For this reason, prepubertal girls can tolerate large doses without apparent effects even if the pathology previously described occurs. The gonadal effects of chemotherapy in women and girls have been described in several reviews.[261,262]

C.L. is going to receive one of the alkylating agents, which are the most potent gonadotoxic agents. Cyclophosphamide is well known for producing infertility in men and women and gonadal failure even in children. The effect is influenced strongly by the total dose of cyclophosphamide and the patient's age at the onset of chemotherapy. Nearly 100% of women over 20 years of age develop amenorrhea when the mean total dose is 20 to 50 g. The same consequence can be expected in women >35 years of age who receive >6 to 10 g and in women 40 years of age and older who receive more than 5 g.[263] Depending on the exact dose of cyclophosphamide in the CAF regimen planned, C.L. may or may not fall into a dose range that would be expected to produce permanent amenorrhea.

The clinician also must consider that a synergistic gonadotoxic effect has been reported when doxorubicin is combined with cyclophosphamide. The onset of amenorrhea may occur at half the total dose of cyclophosphamide after therapy with doxorubicin and cyclophosphamide than after treatment with cyclophosphamide, methotrexate, and fluorouracil. Fluorouracil is unlikely to play any role in producing ovarian failure. Aside from the alkylating agents, the only chemotherapy agents with strong evidence of gonadal toxicity include vinblastine, etoposide, and cisplatin. Several excellent reviews discuss the doses of chemotherapy agents, used both alone and in combination, and specific incidences of associated gonadotoxicity, as well as the prevalence of temporary and permanent amenorrhea.[264,265]

C.L. most likely will experience amenorrhea along with the signs and symptoms of menopause as both estrogen and progesterone production diminish during chemotherapy. C.L. may recover from chemotherapy-induced amenorrhea months to years after completion of her therapy. Recovery may be manifested as amenorrhea interspersed with normal menstrual periods. Pregnancy is possible during periods of normal menstruation because ovulation does occur in most instances. Premature menopause is inevitable, however. Because the greatest risk of pregnancy exists early in the course of chemotherapy, C.L. should be counseled to practice birth control while receiving chemotherapy. Because oral contraceptives are contraindicated in patients with breast cancer, barrier methods (i.e., diaphragm, condoms, spermicide) should be advised.

Effects on Spermatogenesis

48. J.K., a 25-year-old man with recently diagnosed stage IV Hodgkin's lymphoma, will receive systemic chemotherapy. What effect does systemic chemotherapy have on male gonadal function?

The primary gonadal toxic effect of chemotherapy agents in male patients is a progressive dose-related depletion of the germinal epithelium lining the seminiferous tubule.[266] The clinical manifestations of germinal depletion include a marked reduction in testicular volume and azoospermia. The Leydig cells responsible for testosterone production remain morphologically intact, although mild functional impairment occurs rarely. The major toxicity of chemotherapy in men is loss of reproductive capacity. During treatment, libido and sexual activity may decline, but most men report a return to pretreatment sexual function after chemotherapy.[266]

Of the chemotherapy agents, alkylating agents most commonly are associated with azoospermia. Progressive dose-related oligospermia occurs in men receiving chlorambucil,[267,268] cyclophosphamide,[269,270] nitrogen mustard, busulfan, procarbazine, and nitrosureas; procarbazine appears to be the most gonadotoxic alkylating agent in men. Doxorubicin, vinblastine, cytarabine, and cisplatin also have been associated with azoospermia,[271] and doxorubicin appears to have a synergistic toxic effect in men when given with cyclophosphamide similar to that previously described in women. Phase-specific agents, such as antimetabolites and plant alkaloids, seem unlikely to produce azoospermia when used alone but may play a minor role in combination chemotherapy regimens.

In contrast to oogenesis, in which women are born with a full complement of ova, spermatogenesis occurs in a continuous cycle of regeneration, differentiation, and maturation beginning in the second month of embryogenesis and continuing through old age. Although different chemotherapy agents appear to exert more damage to germ cells in specific phases of spermatogenesis in animal models, in humans, gonadotoxic agents generally are used in sufficiently large doses to affect varying proportions of maturing sperm cells in any stage of development. This has two realistic implications. The first is that because spermatogenesis must start at the beginning after agent-induced azoospermia occurs, the length of recovery is prolonged, usually lasting at least 2 to 3 years. The second is that the relationship of age to the development of azoospermia is far less clear than the relationship of age to ovarian suppression. Although conventional wisdom holds that prepubertal boys are less likely to be affected by chemotherapy agents than adult men, the reserve of primitive sperm cells in male children is far less than it is in adults. Therefore, the spermatogenesis potential in prepubertal testes may make them more vulnerable to cytotoxic damage than those of adults. A review of the literature regarding the effects of chemotherapy administered to male children concluded that agents and regimens known to be toxic in men should be considered toxic in young boys.[264] Short of a testicular biopsy, the damage cannot be detected until puberty.

The two diseases most likely to affect young men who are concerned with their fertility are Hodgkin's disease and testicular cancer. The standard treatment for advanced Hodgkin's disease is doxorubicin, bleomycin, vinblastine, and dacarbazine (ABVD) (see Chapter 88, Neoplastic Disorders and Their Treatment). Azospermia has been observed in 35% of patients receiving ABVD and spermatogenesis nearly always recovered in these patients.[271] A similar scenario exists in patients about to start on chemotherapy for testicular cancer. Evidence to date suggests that chemotherapy-induced azoospermia that follows treatment with vinblastine, bleomycin, and cisplatin for nonseminomatous testicular carcinoma is reversible within 2 to 3 years in approximately 50% of patients treated and that those who recover spermatogenesis are capable of impregnating their partners.[272,273] In this particular patient population, it is important to recognize that retroperitoneal lymph node dissection, which results in retrograde ejaculation, as well as cryptorchidism, which predisposes to infertility, may contribute to the lack of full recovery of fertility potential.

49. Aside from the use of chemotherapy agents with less gonadal toxicity, are there means of circumventing infertility in young patients receiving chemotherapy?

Sperm or gamete cryopreservation should be considered in males. A major limitation of this approach has been the finding of diminished sperm counts, sperm volume, and sperm motility in young men affected with Hodgkin's disease and testicular cancer before combination chemotherapy is initiated.[274,275] Although published studies suggest that the quantity and motility of sperm are important determinants of successful artificial insemination, pregnancies have been reported.[276,277] Thus, sperm banking should be considered even in oligospermic men.

Oocyte and embryo cryopreservation now are feasible options for young women about to undergo cytotoxic chemotherapy. Even in the face of chemotherapy-induced ovarian failure, in vitro fertilization of an ovum, and implantation into the endometrium with proper hormonal support can successfully accommodate a term pregnancy.[278,279] This may be an option for C.L. described in Question 47.

In both genders, it has been hypothesized that gonadal toxicity from chemotherapy could be decreased by inhibiting spermatogenesis or follicular development during chemotherapy. Methods used to suppress gonadal function have included administration of testosterone in men, oral contraceptives in women, and gonadotropin-releasing hormone analogs (LHRH analogs) in both men and women. A review describes approaches in detail[280] and the ASCO provides recommendations on preserving fertility in cancer patients.[281]

Teratogenicity

50. If C.L. or J.K. regain fertility after their planned combination chemotherapy regimens, are they at risk for producing offspring with congenital abnormalities or an excess risk of cancer?

Most of the agents used to treat cancer are designed specifically to interfere with DNA synthesis, cellular metabolism, and cell division. Thus, reason exists to suspect that they may cause mutation of ova or spermatocytes exposed to these effects. The actual outcomes of pregnancies in survivors of cancer are published as case reports, small series, and retrospective case series. Nearly 1,600 children have been born to 1,078 patients previously treated for malignancy in childhood or as adults. A review of the published information suggests no evidence that spontaneous abortion, genetic disease, or congenital anomalies occurs more frequently in the progeny of cancer survivors. Similarly, there does not appear to be an increased risk of malignancy in the offspring of patients treated for cancer.[264] The likely explanation for this is that ova and sperm cells affected by chemotherapy usually are killed. The risk of producing an abnormal offspring thus would be highest at the time of ongoing germ cell exposure. Men and women should be explicitly discouraged from conception during chemotherapy. In general, adults surviving cancer should be advised to wait at least 2 years after completion of therapy before attempting to parent a child; this theoretically allows time for elimination of damaged germ cells. This also provides time to assess the likelihood of the necessity for further treatment that would have grave consequences on the fetus, particularly in the case of female patients.

ACKNOWLEDGMENTS

The authors and editors would like to acknowledge the contribution of Celeste Lindley of this topic in the previous edition.

REFERENCES

1. Smith TJ et al. American Society of Clinical Oncology 2006 update of recommendations for the use of white blood cell growth factors: an evidence-based clinical practice guideline. *J Clin Oncol* 2006;24:3187.
2. Vogel CL et al. First and subsequent cycle use of pegfilgrastim prevents febrile neutropenia in patients with breast cancer: a multicenter, double-blind, placebo-controlled phase III study. *J Clin Oncol* 2005;23:1178.
3. Timmer-Bonte JN et al. Prevention of chemotherapy-induced febrile neutropenia by prophylactic antibiotics plus or minus granulocyte-stimulating factor in small cell lung cancer. A Dutch randomized phase III study. *J Clin Oncol* 2005;23:7974.
4. Holmes FA et al. Blinded, randomized, multicenter study to evaluate single administration pegfilgrastim once per cycle versus daily filgrastim as an adjunct to chemotherapy in patients with high-risk stage II or stage III/IV breast cancer. *J Clin Oncol* 2002;20:727.
5. Green MD et al. A randomized double-blind multicenter phase III study of fixed-dose single-administration pegfilgrastim versus daily filgrastim in patients receiving myelosuppressive chemotherapy. *Ann Oncol* 2003;14:29.
6. Johnston E et al. Randomized, dose-escalation study of SD/01 compared with daily filgrastim in patients receiving chemotherapy. *J Clin Oncol* 2000;18:2522.
7. Garcia-Carbonero et al. Granulocyte colony-stimulating factor in the treatment of high-risk febrile neutropenia: a multicenter randomized trial. *J Natl Cancer Inst* 2001;93:31.
8. Clark OA et al. Colony-stimulating factors for chemotherapy-induced febrile neutropenia: a meta-analysis of randomized controlled trials. *J Clin Oncol* 2005;23:4198.
9. Berghmans T et al. Therapeutic use of granulocyte and granulocyte-macrophage colony-stimulating factors in febrile neutropenic fever patients: a systematic review of the literature with meta-analysis. *Support Care Cancer* 2002;10:181.
10. Hidalgo M et al. Outpatient therapy with oral ofloxacin for patients with low risk neutropenia and fever: a prospective, randomized clinical trial. *Cancer* 1999;85:213.
11. Santolaya ME et al. Early hospital discharge followed by outpatient management versus continued hospitalization of children with cancer, fever, and neutropenia at low risk for bacterial infection. *J Clin Oncol* 2004;22:3784.
12. Innes HE et al. Oral antibiotics with early hospital discharge compared with in-patient intravenous antibiotics for low-risk febrile neutropenia in patients with cancer: a prospective randomised controlled single centre study. *Br J Cancer* 2003;89:43.
13. Isaacs C et al. Randomized placebo-controlled study of recombinant human interleukin-11 to prevent chemotherapy-induced thrombocytopenia in patients with breast cancer receiving dose-intensive cyclophosphamide and doxorubicin. *J Clin Oncol* 1997;15:3368.
14. Neumega package insert. Philadelphia, PA: Wyeth Pharmaceuticals Inc.; September 2006.
15. Abels RI et al. Erythropoietin: evolving clinical applications. *Exp Hematol* 1991;19:842.
16. Oster W et al. Erythropoietin for the treatment of anemia of malignancy associated with neoplastic bone marrow infiltration. *J Clin Oncol* 1990;8:956.
17. Platanias LC et al. Treatment of chemotherapy-induced anemia with recombinant human erythropoietin in cancer patients. *J Clin Oncol* 1991;9:2021.
18. 20030125 Study Group Trial, et al. Randomized comparison of every-2-week darbepoetin alfa and weekly epoetin alfa for the treatment of chemotherapy-induced anemia: the 20030125 Study Group Trial. *J Clin Oncol* 2006;24:2290.
19. Glaspy J et al. Impact of therapy with epoetin alfa on clinical outcomes in patients with nonmyeloid malignancies during cancer chemotherapy in community oncology practice. Procrit Study Group [Abstract]. *J Clin Oncol* 1997;15:1218.
20. Glaspy JA et al. Darbepoetin alfa administered every 1 or 2 weeks (with no loss of dose efficiency) alleviates anemia in patients with solid tumors [Abstract]. *Blood* 2001;98:298a.
21. Glaspy JA et al. Darbepoetin alfa given every one or two weeks alleviates anemia associated with cancer chemotherapy. *Br J Cancer* 2002;87:268.
22. Rizzo JD et al. Use of epoetin and darbepoetin in patients with cancer: 2007 American Society of Hematology/American Society of Clinical Oncology clinical practice guideline update. *Blood* 2008;111:25.
23. Glaspy J et al. Randomized comparison of every-2-week darbepoetin alfa and weekly epoetin alfa for the treatment of chemotherapy-induced anemia: the 20030125 Study Group Trial. *J Clin Oncol* 2006;24:2290.
24. Schwartzberg LS et al. A randomized comparison of every-2-week darbepoetin alfa and weekly epoetin alfa for the treatment of chemotherapy-induced anemia in patients with breast, lung, or gynecologic cancer. *Oncologist* 2004;9:696.
25. Mirtsching M et al. Every two week darbepoetin alfa is comparable to rHuEPO in treating chemotherapy induced anemia. Results of combined analysis. *Oncology* 2002;16(Suppl 11):31.
26. Ross SD et al. Clinical benefits and risks associated with epoetin and darbepoetin in patients with chemotherapy-induced anemia: a systematic review of the literature. *Clin Ther* 2006;28:801.
27. FDA website. U.S. Food and Drug Administration Web page. Available at www.fda.gov/cder/drug/infopage/RHE/default.htm. Accessed May 31, 2007.
28. Whitecare JP Jr et al. L-Asparaginase. *N Engl J Med* 1970;282:732.
29. Ramsay NKC et al. The effect of L-asparaginase on plasma coagulation factors in acute lymphoblastic leukemia. *Cancer* 1977;40:1398.
30. Levine MN et al. The thrombogenic effect of anticancer agent therapy in women with stage II breast cancer. *N Engl J Med* 1988;318:404.
31. Ruiz MA et al. The influence of chemotherapy on plasma coagulation and fibrinolytic systems in lung cancer patients. *Cancer* 1989;63:643.
32. Rogers JS II et al. Chemotherapy for breast cancer decreases plasma protein C and protein S. *J Clin Oncol* 1988;6:276.
33. Kaufman PA et al. Autologous bone marrow transplantation and factor XII, factor VII, and protein C deficiencies: report of a new association and its possible relationship to endothelial cell injury. *Cancer* 1990;66:515.
34. Trousseau A. Phlegmasia alba dolens. *Clinique medicale de L'Hotel-Dieu de Paris*. London: The New Sydenham Society, 1865;3:94.
35. Sack GH Jr. et al. Trousseau's syndrome and other manifestations of chronic disseminated coagulopathy in patients with neoplasms: clinical, pathophysiologic, and therapeutic features. *Medicine* 1977;56:1.
36. Aderka D et al. Idiopathic deep vein thrombosis in an apparently healthy patient as a premonitory sign of occult cancer. *Cancer* 1986;57:1846.
37. Goldberg RJ et al. Occult malignant neoplasm in patients with deep venous thrombosis. *Arch Intern Med* 1987;147:251.
38. Goldberg MA et al. Is heparin administration necessary during induction chemotherapy for patients with acute promyelocytic leukemia? *Blood* 1987;69:187.
39. Zangari M et al. Thrombogenic activity of doxorubicin in myeloma patients receiving thalidomide: implications for therapy. *Blood* 2002;100:1168.
40. Knight R et al. Lenalidomide and venous thrombosis in multiple myeloma. *N Engl J Med* 2006;354:2079.
41. Skillings JR et al. Arterial thromboembolic events in a pooled analysis of 5 randomized, controlled trials of bevacizumab with chemotherapy. *J Clin Oncol* 2005;23:16S (Abstract 3019).
42. Johnson DH et al. Randomized phase II trial comparing bevacizumab plus carboplatin and paclitaxel with carboplatin and paclitaxel alone in previously untreated locally advanced or metastatic non-small-cell lung cancer. *J Clin Oncol* 2004;22:2184.
43. Lindley CM. Incidence and duration of chemotherapy-induced nausea and vomiting in an outpatient cancer population. *J Clin Oncol* 1989;7:1142.
44. Sonis ST et al. Oral complications in patients receiving treatment for malignancies other than of the head and neck. *J Am Dent Assoc* 1978;97:468.
45. Lockhart PB, Sonis ST. Alterations in the oral mucosa caused by chemotherapy agents. *J Dermatol Surg Oncol* 1981;7:1019.
46. Eneroth CM et al. Effects of fractionated radiotherapy on salivary gland function. *Cancer* 1972;30:1147.
47. Dirix P et al. Radiation-induced xerostomia in patients with head and neck cancer: a literature review. *Cancer* 2006;107:2525.
48. Brizel DM et al. Phase III randomized trial of amifostine as a radioprotector in head and neck cancer. *J Clin Oncol* 2000;18:3339.
49. Hensley ML et al. American Society of Clinical Oncology clinical practice guidelines for the use of chemotherapy and radiotherapy protectants. *J Clin Oncol* 1999;17:3333.
50. Brizel DM. Pharmacologic approaches to radiation protection. *J Clin Oncol* 2007;25:4084.
51. LeVeque FG et al. A multicenter, randomized, double-blind, placebo-controlled, dose-titration study of oral pilocarpine for treatment of radiation-induced xerostomia in head and neck cancer patients. *J Clin Oncol* 1993;11:1123.
52. Momm F et al. Different saliva substitutes for treatment of xerostomia following radiotherapy: a prospective crossover study. *Strahlenther Onkol* 2005;181:231.
53. Kam MK et al. Prospective randomized study of intensity-modulated radiotherapy on salivary gland function in early-stage nasopharyngeal carcinoma patients. *J Clin Oncol* 2007;25:4873.
54. Keys HM et al. Techniques and results of a comprehensive dental care program in head and neck cancer patients. *Int J Radiat Oncol Biol Phys* 1976;1:859.
55. Sonis ST et al. Pretreatment oral assessment. *J Natl Cancer Inst* 1990;9:29.
56. Helsinn Healthcare SA. Gelclair drug information. www.gelclair.com. Accessed June, 5 2007.
57. Barber C et al. Comparing pain control and ability to eat and drink with standard therapy versus Gelclair: a preliminary, double centre, randomised controlled trial on patients with radiotherapy-induced oral mucositis. *Support Care Cancer* 2007;15:427.
58. Mahood D et al. Inhibition of fluorouracil-induced stomatitis by oral cryotherapy. *J Clin Oncol* 1991;9:449.
59. Anderson PM et al. Effect of low dose oral glutamine on painful stomatitis during bone marrow transplantation. *Bone Marrow Transplant* 1998;22:339.
60. Okuno SH et al. Phase III controlled evaluation of glutamine for decreasing stomatitis in patients receiving fluorouracil (fluorouracil)-based chemotherapy. *Am J Clin Oncol* 1999;22:258.
61. Ferretti GA et al. Chlorhexidine in prophylaxis against oral infections and associated complications in patients receiving bone marrow transplantation. *J Am Dent Assoc* 1987;114:292.
62. Ferretti GA et al. Chlorhexidine prophylaxis for chemotherapy and radiotherapy-induced stomatitis: a randomized, double-blind trial. *Oral Surg Med Oral Pathol* 1990;69:331.
63. Spielberger R et al. Palifermin for oral mucositis after intensive therapy for hematologic cancers. *N Engl J Med* 2004;351:2590.

64. Shaw MT et al. Effects of cancer, radiotherapy and cytotoxic agents on intestinal structure and function. *Cancer Treat Rev* 1979;6:141.
65. Wurth MA et al. Mechlorethamine effects on intestinal absorption in vitro and on cell proliferation. *Am J Physiol* 1973;225:73.
66. Roche AC et al. Correlation between the histological changes and glucose intestine absorption following a single dose of 5-fluorouracil. *Digestion* 1970;3:195.
67. Kuhlmann J et al. Effects of cytostatic agents on plasma levels and renal excretion of B-acetyldigoxin. *Clin Pharmacol Ther* 1981;30:519.
68. Finchman R et al. Decreased phenytoin levels in chemotherapy therapy. *Ther Agent Monit* 1984;6: 302.
69. Kuhlmann J et al. Verapamil plasma concentrations during treatment with cytostatic agents. *J Cardiovasc Pharmacol* 1985;7:1003.
70. Camptostar package insert. New York, NY: Pfizer Inc.; June 2006.
71. Geller RB et al. Randomized trial of loperamide versus dose escalation of octreotide acetate for chemotherapy-induced diarrhea in bone marrow transplant and leukemia patients. *Am J Hematol* 1995;50:167.
72. Casincu S et al. Octreotide versus loperamide in the treatment of fluorouracil-induced diarrhea: a randomized trial. *J Clin Oncol* 1993;11:148.
73. Petrelli NJ et al. Bowel rest, intravenous hydration, and continuous high-dose infusion of octreotide acetate for the treatment of chemotherapy-induced diarrhea in patients with colorectal carcinoma. *Cancer* 1997;72:1543.
74. Casincu S et al. Control of chemotherapy-induced diarrhoea with octreotide in patients receiving 5-fluorouracil. *Eur J Cancer* 1992;28:482.
75. Rosenoff SH et al. A multicenter, randomized trial of long-acting octreotide for the optimum prevention of chemotherapy-induced diarrhea: results of the STOP trial. *J Support Oncol* 2006;4:289.
76. Payne AS et al. Dermatologic toxicity of chemotherapeutic agents. *Semin Oncol* 2006;33:86.
77. Goolsby TV et al. Extravasation of chemotherapeutic agents: prevention and treatment. *Semin Oncol* 2006;33:139.
78. Seipp C. Alopecia. In: De Vita VT et al., eds. *Cancer: Principles and Practice of Oncology.* 7th ed. Philadelphia: Lippincott Williams & Wilkins; 2005.
79. Grevelman EG et al. Prevention of chemotherapy-induced hair loss by scalp cooling. *Ann Oncol* 2005;16:352.
80. Faulkson G et al. Skin changes in patients treated with 5-fluorouracil. *Br J Dermatol* 1962;74:229.
81. DeMarinis M et al. Nail pigmentation with daunorubicin therapy. *Ann Intern Med* 1978;89:516.
82. Priestman TJ et al. Adriamycin and longitudinal pigmented banding of fingernails. *Lancet* 1975;1: 1337.
83. Shetty MR. Case of pigmented banding of the nail caused by bleomycin. *Cancer Treat Rep* 1977;61: 501.
84. Ma HK et al. Actinomycin D in the treatment of methotrexate-resistant trophoblastic tumours. *J Obstet Gynaecol Br Commonw* 1971;78:166.
85. Kennedy BJ et al. Skin changes secondary to hydroxyurea therapy. *Arch Dermatol* 1975;111:183.
86. Harrold BP. Syndrome resembling Addison's disease following prolonged treatment with busulfan. *BMJ* 1966;1:463.
87. Kyle RA et al. A syndrome resembling adrenal cortical insufficiency associated with long-term busulfan (Myleran) therapy. *Blood* 1961;18:497.
88. Hrushesky WJ. Serpentine supravenous fluorouracil hyperpigmentation. *JAMA* 1976;236:138.
89. Fernandez-Obregon AC et al. Flagellate pigmentation from intrapleural bleomycin. A light microscopy and electron microscopy study. *J Am Acad Dermatol* 1985;13:464.
90. Horn TD et al. Observations and proposed mechanisms of N,N′,N′-triethylenethiophosphoramide (Thio-TEPA)-induced hyperpigmentation. *Arch Dermatol* 1989;125:524.
91. Harben DJ et al. Thiotepa-induced leukoderma. *Arch Dermatol* 1979;115:973.
92. Vonderheid EC. Topical mechlorethamine chemotherapy. *Int J Dermatol* 1984;23:180.
93. DeVita VT et al. Clinical trials with Bis (2-chloroethyl)-1-nitrosourea, NSC-409962. *Cancer Res* 1965;25:1876.
94. Wheeland RG et al. The flag sign of chemotherapy. *Cancer* 1983;51:1356.
95. Tsai KY et al. Hand-foot syndrome and seborrheic dermatitis-like rash induced by sunitinib in a patient with advanced renal cell carcinoma. *J Clin Oncol* 2006;24:5786.
96. Lai SE et al. Hand-foot and stump syndrome to sorafenib. *J Clin Oncol* 2007;25:341.
97. Lynch TJ et al. Epidermal growth factor receptor inhibitor-associated cutaneous toxicities: an evolving paradigm in clinical management. *Oncologist* 2007;12:610.
98. Perez-Soler R. Rash as a surrogate marker for efficacy of epidermal growth factor receptor inhibitors in lung cancer. *Clin Lung Cancer* 2006;8(Suppl 1):S7.
99. Cunningham D et al. Cetuximab monotherapy and cetuximab plus irinotecan in irinotecan-refractory metastatic colorectal cancer. *N Engl J Med* 2004;351:337.
100. Yeo W et al. Radiation-recall skin disorders associated with the use of antineoplastic drugs: pathogenesis, prevalence, and management. *Am J Clin Dermatol* 2000;1:113.
101. Camidge R et al. Characterizing the phenomenon of radiation recall dermatitis. *Radiotherapy and Oncology* 2001;59:237.
102. Kvols LK. Radiation sensitizers: a selective review of molecules targeting DNA and non-DNA targets. *J Nucl Med* 2005;46:187S.
103. Alley E et al. Cutaneous toxicities of cancer therapy. *Curr Opin Oncol* 2002;14:212.
104. Clamon GH. Extravasation. In: Perry MC, ed. *The Chemotherapy Source Book.* 3rd ed. Philadelphia: Lippincott Williams & Wilkins; 2001.
105. Goolsby TV et al. Extravasation of chemotherapeutic agents: prevention and treatment. *Semin Oncol* 2006;33:139.
106. Vogelzang NJ. "Adriamycin flare": a skin reaction resembling extravasation. *Cancer Treat Rep* 1979;63:2067.
107. Souhami L et al. Urticaria following intravenous doxorubicin administration. *JAMA* 1978;240:1624.
108. Luedke DW et al. Histopathogenesis of skin and subcutaneous injury induced by adriamycin. *Plast Reconstr Surg* 1979;63:463.
109. Rudolph R et al. Skin ulcers due to adriamycin. *Cancer* 1976;38:1087.
110. Desao MH et al. Prevention of doxorubicin-induced skin ulcers in the rat and pig with dimethyl sulfoxide (DMSO). *Cancer Treat Rep* 1982;66: 1371.
111. Bertelli G et al. Dimethyl sulfoxide and cooling after extravasation of antitumor agents. *Lancet* 1993;341:1098.
112. Lawrence HJ et al. Dimethyl sulfoxide and extravasation of anthracycline agents [Letter]. *Ann Intern Med* 1983;98:1026.
113. Olver IN et al. A prospective study of topical dimethyl sulfoxide for treating anthracycline extravasation. *J Clin Oncol* 1988;6:1732.
114. Ludwig CU et al. Prevention of cytotoxic agent-induced skin ulcers with dimethyl sulfoxide (DMSO) and alpha-tocopherol. *Eur J Cancer Clin Oncol* 1987;23:327.
115. Alberts DS et al. Case Report: topical DMSO for mitomycin C-induced skin ulceration. *Oncol Nurs Forum* 1991;19:693.
116. Van Slotten-Harwood K et al. Treatment of chemotherapy extravasation: current status. *Cancer Treat Rep* 1984;7–8:939.
117. Weiss RB. Hypersensitivity reactions. In: Perry MC, ed. *The Chemotherapy Source Book.* 3rd ed. Philadelphia: Lippincott Williams & Wilkins; 2001.
118. National Cancer Institute. Common Terminology Criteria for Adverse Events v3.0. (CTCAE) Publish date August 9, 2006. Available at http://ctep.cancer.gov/forms/CTCAEv3.pdf. Accessed June 5, 2007.
119. Saif MW et al. Incidence and management of cutaneous toxicities associated with cetuximab. *Expert Opin Drug Saf* 2007;6:175.
120. Lenz HJ. Management and preparedness for infusion and hypersensitivity reactions. *Oncologist* 2007;12:601.
121. Gradishar WJ et al. Phase III trial of nanoparticle albumin-bound paclitaxel compared with polyethylated castor oil-based paclitaxel in women with breast cancer. *J Clin Oncol* 2005;23:7794.
122. Baker WJ et al. Cytarabine and neurologic toxicity. *J Clin Oncol* 1991;9:679.
123. Graves T et al. Agent-induced toxicities associated with high-dose cytosine arabinoside infusions. *Pharmacotherapy* 1989;9:23.
124. Pratt CB et al. Low dose asparaginase treatment of childhood acute lymphocytic leukemia. *Am J Dis Child* 1971;121:406.
125. Sul JK et al. Neurologic complications of cancer chemotherapy. *Semin Oncol* 2006;33:324.
126. Hildebrand J. Neurological complications of cancer chemotherapy. *Curr Opin Oncol* 2006;18:321.
127. Allen JC, Rosen G. Transient cerebral dysfunction following chemotherapy for osteogenic sarcoma. *Ann Neurol* 1978;3:441.
128. Bleyer WA et al. White matter necrosis mineralizing microangiopathy, and intellectual abilities in survivors of childhood leukemia: associations with central nervous system radiation and methotrexate therapy. In: Gilbert HA et al., eds. *Radiation Damage to the Nervous System.* New York: Raven Press; 1980.
129. Allen JC et al. Leukoencephalopathy following high-dose IV methotrexate chemotherapy with leucovorin rescue. *Cancer Treat Rep* 1980;64:1261.
130. Moertel CG et al. Cerebellar ataxias associated with fluorinated pyrimidine therapy. *Cancer Chemother Rep* 1964;41:15.
131. Lynch HT et al. "Organic brain syndrome" secondary to 5-fluorouracil toxicity. *Dis Colon Rectum* 1981;24:130.
132. Raison CL et al. Neuropsychiatric adverse effects of interferon-alpha: recognition and management. *CNS Drugs* 2005;19:105
133. Meyer M. Neurotoxicity of chemotherapy agents. In: Perry MC, ed. *The Chemotherapy Source Book.* 3rd ed. Philadelphia: Lippincott Williams & Wilkins; 2001.
134. Warrell RP et al. Phase I and II study of fludarabine phosphate in leukemia: therapeutic efficacy with delayed central nervous system toxicity. *J Clin Oncol* 1986;4:74.
135. Chun HG et al. Central nervous system toxicity of fludarabine phosphate. *Cancer Treat Rep* 1986;70:1225.
136. Puccio CA et al. A loading/continuous infusion schedule of fludarabine phosphate in chronic lymphatic leukemia. *J Clin Oncol* 1991;9:1562.
137. Merkel DE et al. Central nervous system toxicity with fludarabine. *Cancer Treat Rep* 1986;70: 1449.
138. Arranon package insert. Research Triangle Park, NC: GlaxoSmithKline; July 2006.
139. Phillips GL et al. Intensive 1, 3-bis (2-chloroethyl)-1-nitrosourea (BCNU) monochemotherapy and autologous marrow transplantation for malignant glioma. *J Clin Oncol* 1986;4:639.
140. Shapiro WR et al. Re-evaluating the efficacy of intra-arterial BCNU. *J Neurosurg* 1987;66:313.
141. Mahaley MS Jr. et al. Central neurotoxicity following intracarotid BCNU chemotherapy for malignant gliomas. *J Neurooncol* 1986;3:297.
142. Watkin SW et al. Ifosfamide encephalopathy: a reappraisal. *Eur J Cancer Clin Oncol* 1989;25: 1303.
143. Merimsky O et al. Ifosfamide-related acute encephalopathy: clinical and radiological aspects. *Eur J Cancer* 1991;27:1188.
144. Brunner KW et al. A methylhydrazine-derivative in Hodgkin's disease and other malignant neoplasms:

therapeutic and toxic effects studied in 51 patients. *Ann Intern Med* 1965;63:69.
145. Weiss RB. The role of hexamethylmelamine in advanced ovarian carcinoma treatment. *Gynecol Oncol* 1981;12:141.
146. Gerritsen van der Hoop R et al. Incidence of neuropathy in 395 patients with ovarian cancer treated with or without cisplatin. *Cancer* 1990;66:1967.
147. Legha SS et al. High dose cisplatin administration without hypertonic saline: observation of disabling neurotoxicity. *J Clin Oncol* 1985;3:1373.
148. Cersosimo RJ. Cisplatin neurotoxicity. *Cancer Treat Rev* 1989;16:195.
149. Thompson SW et al. Cisplatin neuropathy: clinical, electrophysiologic, morphologic, and toxicologic studies. *Cancer* 1984;54:1269.
150. Patel PN. Methylene blue for management of ifosfamide-induced encephalopathy. *Ann Pharmacother* 2006;40:299.
151. David KA et al. Evaluating risk factors for the development of ifosfamide encephalopathy. *Am J Clin Oncol* 2005;28:277.
152. Casey EG et al. Vincristine neuropathy: clinical and electrophysiological observations. *Brain* 1973;96:69.
153. Sandler SG et al. Vincristine-induced neuropathy: a clinical study of fifty leukemic patients. *Neurology (Minn)* 1969;19:367.
154. Hausheer FH et al. Diagnosis, management, and evaluation of chemotherapy-induced peripheral neuropathy. *Semin Oncol* 2006;33:15.
155. Stillman M et al. Management of chemotherapy-induced peripheral neuropathy. *Curr Pain Headache Rep* 2006;10:279.
156. Cassidy J et al. Oxaliplatin-related side effects: characteristic and management. *Semin Oncol* 2002; 29:11.
157. Gamelin E et al. Clinical aspects and molecular basis of oxaliplatin neurotoxicity: current management and development of preventive measures. *Semin Oncol* 2002;29:25.
158. Gamelin L et al. Prevention of oxaliplatin-related neurotoxicity by calcium and magnesium, infusions: a retrospective study of 161 patients receiving oxaliplatin combined with 5-fluorouracil and leucovorin for advanced colorectal cancer. *Clin Cancer Res* 2004;10:4055.
159. Albert DM et al. Ocular complications of vincristine therapy. *Arch Ophthalmol* 1967;78:709.
160. Holland JF et al. Vincristine treatment of advanced cancer: a cooperative study of 392 cases. *Cancer Res* 1973;33:1258.
161. Granowetter L et al. Enhanced cisplatinum neurotoxicity in pediatric patients with brain tumors. *J Neuro Oncol* 1983;1:293.
162. Schaefer SD et al. Ototoxicity of low-and moderate-dose cisplatin. *Cancer* 1985;56:1934.
163. Canetta R et al. Carboplatin, the clinical spectrum to date. *Cancer Treat Rev.* 1985;12:125.
164. Carmichael SM et al. Orthostatic hypotension during vincristine therapy. *Arch Intern Med* 1973;126: 290.
165. Gottlieb RJ et al. Vincristine-induced bladder atony. *Cancer* 1971;28:674.
166. Tan C et al. Adriamycin—an antitumor antibiotic in the treatment of neoplastic diseases. *Cancer* 1973;32:9.
167. Lefrak EA et al. A clinicopathologic analysis of adriamycin cardiotoxicity. *Cancer* 1973;32:302.
168. Ng R et al. Anticancer agents and cardiotoxicity. *Semin Oncol* 2006;33:2.
169. Von Hoff DD et al. Risk factors for doxorubicin induced CHF. *Ann Intern Med* 1977;62:200.
170. Bloom K et al. Echocardiography in adriamycin cardiotoxicity. *Cancer* 1978;41:1265.
171. Biancaniello T et al. Doxorubicin cardiotoxicity in children. *J Pediatr* 1980;97:45.
172. Steinberg JS, Wasserman AG. Radionuclide ventriculography for evaluation and prevention of doxorubicin cardiotoxicity. *Clin Ther* 1985;7:660.
173. Alexander J et al. Serial assessment of doxorubicin cardiotoxicity with quantitative radionuclide angiography. *N Engl J Med* 1979;300:278.
174. Bristow MR. Toxic cardiomyopathy due to doxorubicin. *Hosp Pract (Hospital ed.)* 1982;17:101.
175. Bristow MR et al. Dose-effect and structure-function relationships in doxorubicin cardiomyopathy. *Am Heart J* 1981;102:709.
176. Bristow MR et al. Efficacy and cost of cardiac monitoring in patients receiving doxorubicin. *Cancer* 1982;50:32.
177. Bristow MR et al. Doxorubicin cardiomyopathy: evaluation by phonocardiography, endomyocardial biopsy, and cardiac catheterization. *Ann Intern Med* 1978;88:168.
178. Von Hoff DD. Use of daunorubicin in patients with solid tumors. *Semin Oncol* 1984;11(Suppl 3):23.
179. Yates J et al. Cytosine arabinoside with daunorubicin or adriamycin for therapy of acute myelocytic leukemia. A CALGB study. *Blood* 1982;60:454.
180. Von Hoff DD et al. Daunomycin-induced cardiotoxicity in children and adults. *Am J Med* 1977;62: 200.
181. Cassaza AM. Effects of modifications in position 4 of the chromophore or in position 4′ of the amino sugar on the antitumor activity and toxicity of daunorubicin and doxorubicin. In: Crooke ST, Reich SD, eds. *Anthracyclines: Current Status and New Developments.* New York: Academic Press; 1980:403.
182. Hurteloup P et al. Clinical studies with new anthracyclines: epirubicin, idarubicin, esorubicin. *Agents Exp Clin Res* 1986;12:233.
183. Hurteloup P et al. Phase II trial of idarubicin (4-demethoxydaunorubicin) in advanced breast cancer. *Eur J Cancer Clin Oncol* 1989;25:423.
184. Villani F et al. Evaluation of cardiac toxicity of idarubicin (4-demethoxydaunorubicin). *Eur J Clin Oncol* 1989;25:13.
185. Tan CT et al. Phase I and clinical pharmacological studies with 4-demethoxydaunorubicin (Idarubicin) in children with advanced cancer. *Cancer* 1987;47:2990.
186. Feig SA et al. Determination of the maximum tolerated dose of idarubicin when used in a combination chemotherapy program of reinduction childhood ALL at first marrow relapse and a preliminary assessment of toxicity compared to that of daunorubicin: a report from the Children's Cancer Study Group. *Med Pediatr Oncol* 1992;20:124.
187. Ewer MS et al. Cardiotoxicity of chemotherapeutic agents. In: Perry MC, ed. *The Chemotherapy Source Book.* 3rd ed. Philadelphia: Lippincott Williams & Wilkins; 2001.
188. Crossley RJ. Clinical safety and tolerance of mitoxantrone. *Semin Oncol* 1984;11(Suppl 1):54.
189. Posner LE et al. Mitoxantrone: an overview of safety and toxicity. *Invest New Agents* 1985;3:123.
190. Henderson IC et al. Randomized clinical trial comparing mitoxantrone with doxorubicin in previously treated patients with breast cancer. *J Clin Oncol* 1989;7:560.
191. Weiss AJ et al. Studies on adriamycin using a weekly regimen demonstrating its clinical effectiveness and lack of cardiac toxicity. *Cancer Treat Rep* 1976;60:813.
192. Weiss AJ. Studies on cardiotoxicity and antitumor effect of doxorubicin administered weekly. *Cancer Treat Symp* 1984;3:91.
193. Jain KK et al. A randomized comparison of weekly (Arm I) vs monthly (Arm II) doxorubicin in combination with mitomycin C in advanced breast cancer [Abstract]. *Proc Am Soc Clin Oncol* 1983;2:206.
194. Torti FM et al. Reduced cardiotoxicity of doxorubicin delivered on a weekly schedule. Assessment by endomyocardial biopsy. *Ann Intern Med* 1983;99:745.
195. Valdivieso M et al. Increased therapeutic index of weekly doxorubicin in the treatment of non-small cell lung cancer: a prospective, randomized study. *J Clin Oncol* 1984;2:207.
196. Lum BL et al. Doxorubicin: alteration of dose scheduling as a means of reducing cardiotoxicity. *Agent Intell Clin Pharm* 1985;19:259.
197. Seymour L et al. Use of dexrazoxane as a cardioprotectant in patients receiving doxorubicin or epirubicin chemotherapy for the treatment of cancer. The Provincial Systemic Treatment Disease Site Group. *Cancer Prev Control* 1999;3:145.
198. O'Brien M et al. Reduced cardiotoxicity and comparable efficacy in a phase III trial of pegylated liposomal doxorubicin versus conventional doxorubicin for first-line treatment of metastic breast cancer. *Ann Oncol* 2004;15:440.
199. Silber J et al. Enalapril to prevent cardiac function decline in long-term survivors of pediatric cancer exposed to anthracyclines. *J Clin Oncol* 2004;22:820.
200. Wortman JE et al. Sudden death during doxorubicin administration. *Cancer* 1979;44:1588.
201. Rowinsky EK et al. Cardiac disturbances during the administration of Taxol. *J Clin Oncol* 1991;9:1704.
202. Jones RL et al. Cardiac and cardiovascular toxicity of nonanthracycline anticancer drugs. *Expert Review of Anticancer Therapy* 2006;6:1249.
203. Labianca R et al. Cardiac toxicity of 5-fluorouracil: a study on 1,083 patients. *Tumor* 1982;68:505.
204. Eskilsson J et al. Adverse cardiac effects during induction chemotherapy treatment with cisplatin and 5-fluorouracil. *Radiother Oncol* 1988;13:41.
205. Pottage A et al. Fluorouracil cardiotoxicity. *BMJ* 1978;6112:547.
206. Slamon D et al. Use of chemotherapy plus a monoclonal antibody against HER2 for metastatic breast cancer that overexpresses HER2. *N Engl J Med* 2001;344:783.
207. Keefe DL. Trastuzumab-associated cardiotoxicity. *Cancer* 2002;95:1592.
208. Kerkela R et al. Cardiotoxicity of the cancer therapeutic agent imatinib mesylate. *Nat Med* 2006;12: 908.
209. Sprycel package insert. Princeton, NJ: Bristol-Myers Squibb Company; July 2006.
210. Motzer RJ et al. Sunitinib in patients with metastatic renal cell carcinoma. *JAMA* 2006;295:2516.
211. Motzer RJ et al. Activity of SU11248, a multitargeted inhibitor of vascular endothelial growth factor receptor and platelet-derived growth factor receptor, in patients with metastatic renal cell carcinoma. *J Clin Oncol* 2006;24:16.
212. Escudier B et al. Sorafenib in advanced clear-cell renal-cell carcinoma. *N Engl J Med* 2007;356:125.
213. Gordon MS et al. Managing patients treated with bevacizumab combination therapy. *Oncology* 2005; 69(Suppl 3):25.
214. Patterson WP et al. Renal and electrolyte abnormalities due to chemotherapy. In: Perry MC, ed. *The Chemotherapy Source Book.* 3rd ed. Philadelphia: Lippincott Williams & Wilkins; 2001.
215. Kintzel PE. Anticancer drug-induced kidney disorders. *Drug Saf* 2001;24:19.
216. de Jonge M et al. Renal toxicities of chemotherapy. *Semin Oncol* 2006;33:68.
217. Ries F et al. Nephrotoxicity induced by cancer chemotherapy with special emphasis on cisplatin toxicity. *Am J Kidney Dis* 1986;8:368.
218. Finley RS et al. Cisplatin nephrotoxicity: a summary of preventative interventions. *Agent Intell Clin Pharm* 1985;19:362.
219. Pera MF et al. Effects of mannitol or furosemide diuresis on the nephrotoxicity and physiological disposition of cis-dichlorodiammineplatinum-(II). *Cancer Res* 1979;39:1269.
220. Ries F et al. Nephrotoxicity induced by cancer chemotherapy with special emphasis on cisplatin toxicity. *Am J Kidney Dis* 1986;8:368.
221. Willox JC et al. Effects of magnesium supplementation on testicular cancer patients receiving cisplatin: a randomized trial. *Br J Cancer* 1986;54:12.
222. Kemp G et al. Amifostine pretreatment for protection against cyclophosphamide-induced and cisplatin-induced toxicities: results of a randomized control trial in patients with advanced ovarian cancer. *J Clin Oncol* 1996;14:201.
223. Calvert AH et al. Carboplatin dosage: prospective evaluation of a simple formula based on renal function. *J Clin Oncol* 1989;7:1748.
224. deGeorge M et al. Renal toxicities of chemotherapy. *Semin Oncol* 2006;33:6.

225. Widemann BC et al. Understanding and managing methotrexate nephrotoxicity. *Oncologist* 2006;11:694.
226. Scheef W et al. Controlled clinical studies with an antidote against the urotoxicity of oxazaphosphorines: preliminary results. *Cancer Treat Rep* 1982;18:1377.
227. Klein HO et al. High-dose ifosfamide and mesna as continuous infusion over five days—a phase I/II trial. *Cancer Treat Rev* 1983;10(Suppl A):167.
228. Ormstad K. Pharmacokinetics and metabolism of sodium 2-mercaptoethanesulfonate in the rat. *Cancer Res* 1983;43:333.
229. Brock N et al. Studies of the urotoxicity of oxazaphosphorine cytostatics and its prevention. 2. Comparative study of the uroprotective efficacy of thiols and other sulfur compounds. *Eur J Cancer Clin Oncol* 1981;17:1155.
230. Shaw IC, Graham MI. Mesna—a short review. *Cancer Treat Rev* 1987;14:67.
231. Finn GP et al. Protecting the bladder from cyclophosphamide with mesna [Letter]. *N Engl J Med* 1986;314:61.
232. Goren MP et al. Pharmacokinetics of an intravenous-oral versus intravenous-mesna regimen in lung cancer patients receiving ifosfamide. *J Clin Oncol* 1998;16:616.
233. Meadors M et al. Pulmonary toxicity of chemotherapy. *Semin Oncol* 2006;33:98.
234. Hinson JM et al. Chemotherapy-associated lung injury. In: Perry MC, ed. *The Chemotherapy Source Book.* 3rd ed. Philadelphia: Lippincott Williams & Wilkins; 2001.
235. Stover DE et al. Pulmonary toxicity. In: De Vita VT et al, eds. *Cancer: Principles and Practice of Oncology.* 7th Ed. Philadelphia: Lippincott Williams & Wilkins; 2005.
236. Sikic BI et al. Improved therapeutic index of bleomycin when administered by continuous infusion in mice. *Cancer Treat Rep* 1978;62:2011.
237. Comis RL et al. Role of single breath carbon monoxide diffusing capacity in monitoring the pulmonary effects of bleomycin in germ cell tumor patients. *Cancer Res* 1979;39:5076.
238. Floyd J et al. Hepatotoxicity of chemotherapy. *Semin Oncol* 2006;33:50.
239. Dahl MGC et al. Methotrexate hepatotoxicity in psoriasis—comparison of different dosage regimens. *BMJ* 1972;1:654.
240. Podugiel BJ et al. Liver injury associated with methotrexate therapy for psoriasis. *Mayo Clin Proc* 1973;48:787.
241. Boyce JD. Second malignancies after chemotherapy. In: Perry MC, ed. *The Chemotherapy Source Book.* 3rd ed. Philadelphia: Lippincott Williams & Wilkins; 2001.
242. Pedersen-Bjergaard J et al. Increased risk of myelodysplasia and leukaemia after etoposide, cisplatin, and bleomycin for germ-cell tumors. *Lancet* 1991;338:359.
243. Casciato DA et al. Acute leukemia following prolonged cytotoxic agent therapy. *Medicine (Baltimore)* 1979;58:32.
244. De Gamont A et al. Preleukemic changes in cases of non-lymphocytic leukemia secondary to cytotoxic therapy: analysis of 105 cases. *Cancer* 1986;58:630.
245. Kantarjian HM et al. Therapy-related leukemia and myelodysplastic syndrome: clinical, cytogenic, and prognostic features. *J Clin Oncol* 1986;4:1748.
246. Tucker MA et al. Leukemia after therapy with alkylating agents for childhood cancer. *J Natl Cancer Inst* 1987;78:459.
247. Kaldor JM et al. Leukemia following chemotherapy for ovarian cancer. *N Engl J Med* 1990;332:1.
248. Kaldor JM et al. Leukemia following Hodgkin's disease. *N Engl J Med* 1990;322:7.
249. Tucker MA et al. Bone sarcomas linked to radiotherapy and chemotherapy in children. *N Engl J Med* 1987;317:588.
250. Zarrabi MH. Association of non-Hodgkin's lymphoma (NHL) and second neoplasms. *Semin Oncol* 1980;7:340.
251. Stegman R et al. Solid tumors in multiple myeloma. *Ann Intern Med* 1979;90:780.
252. Smith RE et al. Acute myeloid leukemia and myelodysplastic syndrome after doxorubicin-cyclophosphamide adjuvant therapy for operable breast cancer: the National Surgical Adjuvant Breast and Bowel Project Experience. *J Clin Oncol* 2003;21:1195.
253. Pedersen-Bjergaard J et al. Acute non-lymphocytic leukemia, preleukemia, and acute myeloproliferative syndrome secondary to treatment of other malignant diseases. Clinical and cytogenetic characteristics and results of in vitro culture of bone marrow and HLA typing. *Blood* 1981;57:712.
254. Bloomfield CD et al. Treatment-induced acute non-lymphocytic leukemia (t-ANLL): response to cytarabine-anthracycline therapy [Abstract]. *Blood* 1982;60(Suppl 1):152.
255. Preisler HD et al. Therapy of secondary acute non-lymphocytic leukemia with cytarabine. *N Engl J Med* 1983;308:21.
256. Brusamolino E et al. Treatment-related leukemia in Hodgkin's disease: a multi-institution study of 75 cases. *Hematol Oncol* 1987;5:83.
257. Geller RB et al. Successful marrow transplantation for acute myelocytic leukemia following therapy for Hodgkin's disease. *J Clin Oncol* 1988;6:1558.
258. Larson RA et al. Is secondary leukemia an independent poor prognostic factor in acute myeloid leukemia? *Best Pract Res Clin Haemotol* 2007;20:29.
259. Belohorsky B et al. Comments on the development of amenorrhea caused by Myleran in cases of chronic myelosis. *Neoplasma* 1960;7:397.
260. Sobrinho LG et al. Amenorrhea in patients with Hodgkin's disease treated with chemotherapy agents. *Am J Obstet Gynecol* 1971;109:135.
261. Nicosia SV et al. Gonadal effects of cancer therapy in girls. *Cancer* 1985;55:2364.
262. Maltaris T et al. The effect of cancer treatment on female fertility and strategies for preserving fertility. *Eur J Obstet Gynecol Reprod Biol* 2007;130:148.
263. Meistrich ML et al. Gonadal Dysfunction. In: DeVita VT, ed. *Cancer: Principles and Practice of Oncology.* 7th ed. Philadelphia: Lippincott Williams & Wilkins; 2005.
264. Klein CE. Gonadal complications and teratogenicity of cancer therapy. In: Perry MC, ed. *The Chemotherapy Source Book.* 3rd ed. Philadelphia: Lippincott Williams & Wilkins; 2001.
265. Myers SE et al. Prospects for fertility after cancer. *Semin Oncol* 1992;19:597.
266. Meistrich ML. Critical components of testicular function and sensitivity to disruption. *Biol Reprod* 1986;34:17.
267. Miller DG. Alkylating agents and human spermatogenesis. *JAMA* 1971;217:1662.
268. Cheviakoff S et al. Recovery of spermatogenesis in patients with lymphoma after treatment with chlorambucil. *J Reprod Fertil* 1973;33:155.
269. Fairley KF et al. Sterility and testicular atrophy related to cyclophosphamide therapy. *Lancet* 1972;1:568.
270. Buchanan JD et al. Return of spermatogenesis after stopping cyclophosphamide therapy. *Lancet* 1975;2:156.
271. Vivani S et al. Gonadal toxicity after combination chemotherapy for Hodgkin's disease: comparative results of MOPP vs. ABVD. *Eur J Cancer Clin Oncol* 1985;21:601.
272. Drasga RE et al. Fertility after chemotherapy for testicular cancer. *J Clin Oncol* 1983;1:179.
273. Nijman JM et al. Gonadal function after surgery and chemotherapy in men with stage II and III nonseminomatous testicular tumors. *J Clin Oncol* 1987;5:651.
274. Fossa SD et al. Recovery of impaired pretreatment spermatogenesis in testicular cancer. *Fertil Steril* 1990;54:493.
275. Einhorn LH et al. Cis-diammine-dichloroplatinum, vinblastine and bleomycin combination chemotherapy in disseminated testicular cancer. *Ann Intern Med* 1977;87:293.
276. Lange PH et al. Fertility issues in the therapy of nonseminomatous testicular tumors. *Urol Clin North Am* 1987;14:731.
277. Berthelsen JG et al. Sperm counts and serum follicle-stimulating hormone levels before and after radiotherapy and chemotherapy in men with testicular germ cell cancer. *Fertil Steril* 1984;41:281.
278. Tournage H et al. In vitro fertilization techniques with frozen-thawed sperm: a method for preserving the progenitive potential of Hodgkin's patients. *Fertil Steril* 1991;55:443.
279. Davis OK et al. Pregnancy achieved through in vitro fertilization with cryopreserved semen from a man with Hodgkin's lymphoma. *Fertil Steril* 1990;53:377.
280. Molina JR et al. Chemotherapy-induced ovarian failure. *Drug Saf* 2005; 28:401.
281. Lee, SJ et al. American Society of Clinical Oncology recommendations on fertility preservation in cancer patients. *J Clin Oncol* 2006;24:2917.
282. Evans WE et al. Anaphylactoid reactions to *Escherichia coli* and *Erwinia asparaginase* in children with leukemia and lymphoma. *Cancer* 1982;49:1378.
283. Land VJ et al. Unexpectedly high incidence of allergic reactions with high dose (HD) weekly asparaginase (ASP) consolidation (cons) therapy (Rx) in children with newly diagnosed non-T, non-B acute lymphoblastic leukemia (ALL): a Pediatric Oncology Group (POG) study [Abstract]. *Proc Am Soc Clin Oncol* 1989;8:215.
284. Swenerton K et al. Taxol in relapsed ovarian cancer: high vs. low and short vs. long infusion: a European-Canadian study coordinated by the NCI Canada Clinical Trials Group [Abstract]. *Proc Am Soc Oncology* 1993;12:256.
285. Weiss RB et al. Hypersensitivity reactions from Taxol. *J Clin Oncol* 1990;8:1263.
286. O'Dwyer PJ et al. Hypersensitivity reactions to teniposide (VM-26): an analysis. *J Clin Oncol* 1986;4:1262.
287. Hayes FA et al. Allergic reactions to teniposide in patients with neuroblastoma and lymphoid malignancies. *Cancer Treat Rep* 1985;69:439.
288. Carstensen H et al. Hypersensitivity reactions to teniposide in children. *J Clin Oncol* 1987;5:1491.
289. Canal P et al. Phase I/pharmacokinetic study of intraperitoneal teniposide (VM 26). *Eur J Cancer Clin Oncol* 1989;25:815.
290. O'Dwyer PJ, Weiss RB. Hypersensitivity reactions induced by etoposide. *Cancer Treat Rep* 1984;68:959.
291. Tucci E et al. Etoposide-induced hypersensitivity reactions. Report of two cases. *Chemioterapia* 1985;4:460.
292. Anderson T et al. Chemotherapy for testicular cancer: current status of the National Cancer Institute combined modality trial. *Cancer Treatment Reports* 1979;63:1687.
293. Denis L. Anaphylactic reactions to repeated intravesical instillation with cisplatin. *Lancet* 1983;1:1378.
294. Getaz EP et al. Cisplatin-induced hemolysis. *N Engl J Med* 1980;302:334.
295. Levi JA et al. Haemolytic anemia after cisplatin treatment. *BMJ* 1981;282:2003.
296. Bacha DM et al. Phase I study of carboplatin (CBDCA) in children with cancer. *Cancer Treat Rep* 1986;70:865.
297. Allen JC et al. Carboplatin and recurrent childhood brain tumors. *J Clin Oncol* 1987;5:459.
298. Glovsky MM et al. Hypersensitivity to procarbazine associated with angioedema, urticaria, and low serum complement activity. *J Allergy Clin Immunol* 1976;57:134.
299. Eyre HJ et al. Malignant glioma: a randomized trial of radiotherapy plus BCNU, procarbazine, or DTIC: a SWOG study [Abstract]. *Proc Am Soc Clin Oncol* 1982;1:180.
300. Brunner KW, Young CW. A methylhydrazine derivative in Hodgkin's disease and other malignant neoplasms. *Ann Intern Med* 1965;63:69.

301. Lokich JJ et al. Allergic reaction to procarbazine. *Clin Pharmacol Ther* 1972;13:573.
302. Jones SE et al. Hypersensitivity to procarbazine (Matulane) manifested by fever and pleuropulmonary reaction. *Cancer* 1972;29:498.
303. Ecker MD et al. Procarbazine lung. *AJR Am J Roentgenol* 1987;131:527.
304. Arnold DJ et al. Systemic allergic reaction to adriamycin. *Cancer Treat Rep* 1979;63:150.
305. Solimando DA et al. Doxorubicin-induced hypersensitivity reactions. *Agent Intell Clin Pharm* 1984;18:808.
306. Collins JA. Hypersensitivity reaction to doxorubicin. *Agent Intell Clin Pharm* 1984;18:402.
307. Etcubanas E et al. Uncommon side effects of adriamycin (NSC-123127). *Cancer Chemother Rep (Part 1)* 1974;58:757.
308. Crowther D et al. Management of adult acute myelogenous leukaemia. *BMJ* 1973;1:131.
309. Mathe G et al. Phase II trial of THP-Adriamycin (pirarubicin), the most efficient and least toxic anthracycline in breast cancer. In: Kuemmerle H-P, ed. *Advances in Experimental and Clinical Chemotherapy*. Landsberg, Germany: Ecomed, 1988.
310. Tan CTC et al. Phase I trial of rubidzone (NSC 164011) in children with cancer. *Med Pediatr Oncol* 1981;9:347.
311. Rosenfelt F et al. A fatal hyperpyrexial response to bleomycin following prior therapy: a case report and literature review. *Yale J Biol Med* 1982;55:529.
312. Leung W-H et al. Fulminant hyperpyrexia induced by bleomycin. *Postgrad Med J* 1989;65:417.
313. Bochner BS et al. Anaphylaxis. *N Engl J Med* 1991;324:1785.
314. Rituxan package insert. South San Francisco, CA: Biogen Idec Inc., and Genentech, Inc.; February 2007.
315. Herceptin package insert. South San Francisco, CA: Genentech, Inc.; November 2006.
316. Erbitux package insert. Branchburg, NJ: ImClone Systems Incorporated; March 2006.
317. Campath package insert. Cambridge, MA: Genzyme Corporation; January 2007.
318. Taxotere package insert. Bridegewater, NJ: Sanofi-Aventis; December 2006.
319. Doxil package insert. Raritan, NJ: Ortho Biotech; May 2007.
320. Kintzel PE et al. Anticancer drug renal toxicity and elimination: dosing guidelines for altered renal function. *Cancer Treat Rev* 1995;21:33.
321. Launay-Vacher V et al. Prevalence of renal insufficiency in cancer patients and implications for anticancer drug management: the renal insufficiency and anticancer medications (IRMA) study. *Cancer* 2007;110:1376.
322. Li YF et al. Systemic anticancer therapy in gynecological cancer patients with renal dysfunction. *Int J Gynecol Cancer* 2007;17:739.
323. Yang JC et al. Randomized study of high-dose and low-dose interleukin-2 in patients with metastatic renal cancer. *J Clin Oncol* 2003;21:3127.
324. Goldiner PL et al. Factors influencing postoperative morbidity and mortality in patients treated with bleomycin. *BMJ* 1978;1:1664.
325. Tryka AF et al. Differences in effects of immediate and delayed hyperoxia exposure on bleomycin-induced pulmonary injury. *Cancer Treat Rep* 1984;68:759.
326. Wilson KS et al. Fatal pneumothorax in "BCNU lung." *Med Rad Oncol* 1982;10:195.
327. Durant JR et al. Pulmonary toxicity associated with bischloroethylnitrosurea (BCNU). *Ann Intern Med* 1979;90:191.
328. Schreml W et al. Progressive pulmonary fibrosis during combination chemotherapy with BCNU. *Blut* 1978;36:353.
329. Skarin AT et al. The treatment of advanced non-Hodgkin's lymphoma (NHL) with bleomycin, adriamycin, cyclophosphamide, vincristine and prednisone. *Blood* 1977;49:759.
330. Holoye PY et al. Pulmonary toxicity in long-term administration of BCNU. *Cancer Treat Rep* 1976;60:1691.
331. Haupt HM et al. Ara-C lung: noncardiogenic pulmonary edema complicating cytosine arabinoside therapy of leukemia. *Am J Med* 1981;70:256.
332. Gupta N et al. Gemcitabine-induced pulmonary toxicity case report and review of the literature. *Am J Clin Oncol* 2002;25:97.
333. Hurst PG et al. Pulmonary toxicity associated with fludarabine monophosphate. *Invest New Agents* 1987;5:207.
334. Wall MA et al. Lung function in adolescents receiving high-dose methotrexate. *Pediatrics* 1979;63:741.
335. Zusman J et al. Rapid resolution of "methotrexate lung" with preoperative steroids [Abstract]. *Proc Am Assoc Cancer Res* 1979;20:412.
336. Lascari AD et al. Methotrexate-induced sudden fatal pulmonary reaction. *Cancer* 1977;40:1393.
337. Walden PAM et al. Pleurisy and methotrexate treatment. *BMJ* 1977;2:867.
338. Jones SE et al. Hypersensitivity to procarbazine (Mutalane) manifested by fever and pleuropulmonary reaction. *Cancer* 1972;29:498.
339. Lokich JJ. Allergic reaction to procarbazine. *Clin Pharmacol Ther* 1972;13:573.
340. Pratt CB et al. Duration and severity of fatty metamorphosis of liver following L-asparaginase therapy. *Cancer* 1971;28:361.
341. Ohnuma T et al. Biochemical and pharmacological studies with L-asparaginase in man. *Cancer Res* 1970;30:2297.
342. Oettgen HF et al. Toxicity of *E. coli* L-asparaginase in man. *Cancer* 1969;25:253.
343. Dix SP et al. Association of busulfan area under the curve with veno-occlusive disease following BMT. *Bone Marrow Transplant* 1996;17:225.
344. DeVita VT et al. Clinical trials with 1,3-Bis (2-chloroethyl)-1-nitrosurea, NSC-79037. *Cancer* 1965;25:1876.
345. Takvorian T et al. Single high-dose of BCNU with autologous bone marrow (ABM). *Proc Am Soc Clin Oncol* 1980;21:341.
346. Jeha S et al. Clofarabine, a novel nucleoside analog, is active in pediatric patients with advanced leukemia. *Blood* 2004a;103:784.
347. Slavin RE et al. Cytosine arabinoside-induced gastrointestinal toxic alterations in sequential chemotherapy protocols. *Cancer* 1978;42:1747.
348. Fosch PJ et al. Hepatic failure in a patient treated with DTIC for malignant melanoma. *J Cancer Res Clin Oncol* 1979;95:281.
349. Ceci G et al. Fatal hepatic vascular toxicity of DTIC: is it really a rare event? *Cancer* 1988;61:1988.
350. Johnson D et al. Etoposide-induced hepatic injury: a potential complication of high-dose therapy. *Cancer Treat Reports* 1983;67:1023.
351. Larson RA et al. Final report of the efficacy and safety of gemtuzumab ozogamicin (Mylotarg) in patients with CD33-positive acute myeloid leukemia in first recurrence. *Cancer* 2005;104:1442.
352. Guilhot F et al. Indications for imatinib mesylate therapy and clinical management. *Oncologist* 2004;9:271.
353. Einhorn M et al. Hepatotoxicity of 6-mercaptopurine. *JAMA* 1964;188:802.
354. Clark PA et al. Toxic complications of treatment with 6-mercaptopurine: two cases with hepatic necrosis and intestinal ulceration. *BMJ* 1960;1:393.
355. Lazarus HM et al. Veno-occlusive disease of the liver after high-dose mitomycin C therapy and autologous bone marrow transplantation. *Cancer* 1982;49:1789.
356. Schein PS et al. Clinical antitumor activity and toxicity of streptozotocin (NSC-85998). *Cancer* 1974;34:993.
357. Gill RA et al. Hepatic veno-occlusive disease caused by 6-thioguanine. *Ann Intern Med* 1982;96:58.
358. King PD et al. Hepatotoxicity of chemotherapeutic agents. In: Perry MC, ed: *The Chemotherapy Source Book*. 3rd ed. Philadelphia: Lippincott Williams & Wilkins; 2001.
359. King PD et al. Hepatotoxicity of chemotherapy. *Oncologist* 2001;6:162.

CHAPTER 90

Hematologic Malignancies

John M. Valgus, Maureen Haas, R. Donald Harvey III, and Mark T. Holdsworth

HEMATOLOGIC MALIGNANCIES: ADULT DEFINITIONS AND CLASSIFICATION

Cancers arising from hematopoietic cells and lymphoid tissue are termed "hematologic malignancies," and include leukemias, lymphomas, plasma cell disorders, and myeloproliferative disorders. Compared with other cancers, they are relatively uncommon (<10% of all newly diagnosed cancers) and will account for approximately 52,300 deaths in the United States in 2007.[1] Chemotherapy is the primary treatment for most cases of hematologic malignancies because they are usually disseminated at the time of diagnosis. Focal treatment with surgery and/or radiation therapy is not commonly used to manage these cancers. Compared with solid malignancies, the growth rate of most hematologic malignancies is rapid, and aggressive combination chemotherapy regimens can provide high response rates and cures. Complex supportive care regimens are often needed in conjunction with chemotherapy because of multiple disease symptoms and toxicities associated with chemotherapy. The hematologic malignancies also serve as the most common experimental laboratory models of cancer growth, biology, and treatment effects. In addition, advances in delineating molecular targets and improved disease detection continue to lead to changes in therapeutic approaches.

Leukemias

Leukemias are hematologic malignancies that are derived from cytogenetic alterations in hematopoietic cells. Biologically, they originate in the bone marrow before disseminating to systemic tissues. Leukemias are classified based on the cell of origin (myeloid or nonlymphocytic and lymphocytic) and clinical course. Myeloid leukemias include disorders of granulocytes, monocytes, erythrocytes, and platelets. Lymphocytic leukemias include disorders of B and T lymphocytes. Leukemias are further classified as acute or chronic.

Acute leukemia is characterized by the expansion and differentiation arrest of immature hematopoietic cells. This expansion causes large numbers of early progenitor cells (blasts) to appear in the bone marrow. Leukemic blasts develop a growth advantage that leads to failure of the bone marrow to produce adequate numbers of functional mature blood cells. The immature blast cells generally retain some features that indicate their origin from the hematopoietic lineage. If the blasts have lymphoid features, the leukemia is classified as *acute lymphocytic leukemia* (ALL). If the blasts have myeloid features, the leukemia is classified as *acute myeloid leukemia* (AML). Clinical and laboratory distinction of AML from ALL is illustrated in Table 90-1. AML and ALL can be distinguished based on morphologic examination of the bone marrow and peripheral blood, along with special cytochemical stains, surface membrane phenotyping, and chromosomal analysis. Acute leukemias appear suddenly and progress very rapidly. Death due to infection or bleeding occurs within weeks to months if the patient is not effectively treated.

Chronic leukemias follow a more insidious onset and course than acute leukemias and are associated with proliferation of more mature hematopoietic cells. Chronic lymphocytic leukemia (CLL) is characterized by overproduction of mature lymphocytes. Chronic myeloid (or granulocytic) leukemia (CML or CGL) is associated with overproduction of mature neutrophils or granulocytes. Deposition of these cells in various organs, as well as high numbers in vascular spaces, have profound and unique consequences that are discussed in subsequent cases. Other less common chronic leukemias include hairy cell leukemia and chronic myelomonocytic leukemia. Patients with chronic leukemias also often have decreased production of red blood cells (RBCs) and platelets. Although patients with chronic leukemias may survive for years with suppressive therapies, these disorders are curable in only a fraction of patients who are candidates for immune-based approaches using chemotherapy and progenitor cell replacement (see Chapter 92).

Table 90-1 Distinction of Acute Myeloid Leukemia From Acute Lymphocytic Leukemia

	AML	*ALL*
Clinical Features		
Age	Commonly adults	Commonly children
Lymphadenopathy	Rare	Common
CNS involvement	Unusual	5%
Cytochemical Stains		
Myeloperoxidase	Positive	Negative
Periodic acid (Schiff)	Negative (except M_6)	Positive
Other Studies		
Surface markers	Myeloid	Lymphoid
CALLA	No	In early pre-B lineage ALL
Tdt	Absent	Present
Gene Arrangement Studies		
T-cell receptor	Absent	Present in T-cell ALL
Immunoglobulin	Absent	Present in B-cell ALL
Common Cytogenic Abnormalities		
	t(9;22)	t(9;22)
	t(8;21)	t(4;11) null cell ALL
	t(15;17) in AML-M_3	t(8;14) B-cell Burkitt's type
	5q-, 7q-	t(1;14) B cell
	Inv 16 in AML-M_4Eo	t(1;19) B cell

AML, acute myelogenous leukemia; ALL, acute lymphocytic leukemia; CNS, central nervous system; CALLA, common acute lymphocytic leukemia antigen.

Lymphomas

The lymphomas are a heterogeneous group of hematologic malignancies that originate in lymphoid tissues. A lymphoma may arise within single or multiple lymph nodes or in extranodal sites commonly involving the lymphoid tissue of the gastrointestinal (GI) tract, central nervous system (CNS), or numerous other sites. The two major types of lymphomas are Hodgkin disease (HD) and non–Hodgkin lymphoma (NHL) (Table 90-2). It is estimated that these hematologic malignancies account for >60,000 new cases annually, with seven times as many patients affected by NHL compared with HD.[1] NHLs

Table 90-2 Comparison of Hodgkin Disease and Non-Hodgkin Lymphoma

Characteristic	Hodgkin Disease	Non-Hodgkin Lymphomas: Low Grade	Non-Hodgkin Lymphomas: Intermediate-High Grade
Site(s) of origin	Nodal	Extranodal (10%)	Extranodal (35%)
Nodal distribution	Axial (centripetal)	Centrifugal	Centrifugal
Nodal spread	Contiguous	Noncontiguous	Noncontiguous
Central nervous system involvement	Rare (<1%)	Rare (<1%)	Uncommon (<10%)
Hepatic involvement	Uncommon	Common (>50%)	Uncommon
Bone marrow involvement	Uncommon (<10%)	Common (>50%)	Uncommon (<20%)
Marrow involvement adversely affects prognosis	Yes	No	Yes
Curable by chemotherapy	Yes	No	Yes

represent a spectrum of diseases marked by different pathological features, natural history, response to treatment, and prognosis. NHLs have been divided into categories based on cell of origin (B or T), histology (low, intermediate, or high grade), immunophenotypic characteristics, cytogenetic abnormalities, and natural history. The main classification systems used for NHLs are the Working Formulation (WF) classification and the Revised European-American Lymphoma (REAL) classification. The WF classification is based on the morphology and clinical behavior of the disease; the REAL classification has been advocated because it also incorporates immunophenotypic and molecular characteristics. Further classification of all neoplastic diseases of myeloid and lymphoid tissues by the World Health Organization (WHO) beyond the 1994 REAL system is currently ongoing, with the goal of removing arbitrary clinical groupings of lymphoid neoplasms from clinical practice and relying on more complete information (including morphology, immunophenotype, cytogenetic features, and clinical features) to guide prognosis and therapy.[2] The additional information included with further classification will ideally provide insight into the biological diversity of each type of lymphoma and assist with therapeutic decisions.[3,4]

Plasma Cell Disorders

Plasma cell disorders include a group of neoplasms that arise from antibody-secreting B cells that overproduce excessive amounts of a monoclonal immunoglobulin or part of a monoclonal immunoglobulin (light chains). If the monoclonal protein is in the IgM subclass, the disease is called "Waldenström macroglobulinemia," and the malignant cells are called "plasmacytoid lymphocytes." If the monoclonal protein is in the IgG (70% of cases) or IgA (20% of cases) subclass or if only monoclonal light chains are present in blood, the disease is called "multiple myeloma," and the malignant cells are called "plasma cells."[5] High monoclonal immunoglobulin concentrations can be found in conditions other than multiple myeloma or Waldenström macroglobulinemia, such as monoclonal gammopathy of undetermined significance or amyloidosis. However, the amount of immunoglobulin produced with multiple myeloma or Waldenström macroglobulinemia generally exceeds the amount produced with other conditions. Excessive amounts of protein cause a number of clinical manifestations, including hyperviscosity and renal dysfunction. If plasma cells infiltrate the bone marrow, a decreased production of RBCs and platelets occurs. Multiple myeloma is the most common plasma cell disorder, accounting for 14% of all hematologic malignancies.[1]

ACUTE MYELOID LEUKEMIA

Signs and Symptoms

1. D.M., a 35-year-old woman, presented to the emergency department with increasing fatigue and fever. This past week, a peripheral blood smear (complete blood count [CBC]) revealed a white blood cell (WBC) count of 80,000/mm^3 (normal, 4,000–11,000) with a differential of >90% leukemic blasts (normal, 0%), a hematocrit (Hct) of 31% (normal, 40%–44%), and a platelet count of 46,000/mm^3 (normal, 150,000–400,000). A bone marrow aspirate and biopsy confirmed the diagnosis of AML (FAB-M2, myeloid with maturation; 60% blasts, myeloperoxidase positive; CD13 and CD33 positive). All serum chemistry values were within normal limits, with the exception of potassium (K), 3.2 mEq/L (normal, 3.5–5.5); phosphorus, 5.5 mg/dL (normal, 2.5–4.5); and lactate dehydrogenase (LDH), 3,000 mU/mL (normal, 30–120). Physical examination was unremarkable except for a perirectal cellulitis. Which signs and symptoms exhibited by D.M. are consistent with AML?

[SI units: WBC count, 80 × 10^6/L (normal, 4–11) with differential >0.9 leukemic blasts (normal, 0); Hct, 0.31 (normal, 0.40–0.44); platelets 46 × 10^9/L (normal, >150); K, 3.2 mmol/L (normal, 3.5–5.5); phosphorus, 5.5 mmol/L (normal, 2.5–4.5); LDH, 3,000 (normal, 30–120)]

D.M.'s symptoms of increasing fatigue and fever of 1 week's duration are consistent with a rapid reduction in RBCs leading to anemia (Hct, 31%) and a low neutrophil count leading to infection (perirectal cellulitis). Although her WBC count is high, the differential reveals that >90% are "blasts," which are immature, nonfunctional cells of myeloid or lymphoid origin. Circulating blast cells are typically not present in chronic leukemias or mild-to-moderate infection. However, blasts may also be observed on the peripheral smear in patients with anemia associated with primary bone marrow dysfunction (myelodysplastic syndromes). They are also present in patients with severe infection, stress, or trauma and in those with CML in "transformation" to acute leukemia. D.M.'s platelet count is also low, which may lead to bleeding or bruising. Collectively, these are often the presenting signs and symptoms of acute leukemia.

D.M.'s symptoms are consistent with either AML or ALL. However, patients with ALL also commonly present with

Table 90-3 Classification of Acute Myeloid Leukemia[a]

Designation	Name	Predominant Cell Type	Cytogenetics	Frequency (%)	Morphology
M_0	Undifferentiated myeloblastic				No maturation of myeloblasts
M_1	Undifferentiated myelocytic	Myeloblasts	t(9;22) + 8 del(5), del(7)	2–3	Minimal maturation of myeloblasts
M_2	Myelocytic	Myeloblasts, promyelocytes, myelocytes	t(8;21) + 8 del(5), del(7)	20	Prominent maturation of myeloblasts
M_3	Promyelocytic	Hypergranular promyelocytes	t(15;17)	25–30	Promyelocytic
M_3 variant					Promyelocytic in marrow; atypical monocytes in blood
M_4	Myelomonocytic	Promyelocytes, myelocytes, promonocytes, monocytes	t(4;11), t(9;11) + 8 del(5), del(7)	8–15	Myelomonocytic
M_4Eo			inv(16)		With atypical eosinophils
M_{5a}	Monoblastic	Monoblasts	t(9;11) + 8 del(5), del(7)		Monoblastic
M_{5b}	Differentiated monocytic	Monoblasts, promonocytes, monocytes		20–25	Promonocytic
M_6	Erythroleukemia	Erythroblasts	+ 8 del(5), del(7)	5	Erythroblastic
M_7	Megakaryocytic	Megakaryocytes		1–2	Megakaryoblastic

[a] French-American-British (FAB) classification system.

lymphadenopathy and hepatosplenomegaly. It is important to distinguish between these two disorders because treatment regimens differ significantly. AML is far more common in adults than in children. (For a complete discussion of ALL, see Acute Lymphoblastic Leukemia of Childhood section.)

Classification and Diagnosis

For a definitive diagnosis of AML to be made, the bone marrow aspirate must contain more than 20% leukemic blast cells. A normal bone marrow aspirate would typically contain less than 5% blasts. Eight major variants of AML are defined by the French-American-British (FAB) classification system based on morphologic characteristics (Table 90-3). More recently, the World Health Organization (WHO) has developed a classification system that expands the number of AML subtypes and better incorporates genotypic information, which is important in determining prognosis.[2] Cells of myeloid origin commonly contain myeloperoxidase enzymes and express surface markers CD13, CD33, CD14, and CD15. Specific clonal chromosomal abnormalities are associated with several AML subtypes. These aberrations include gains or losses of whole chromosomes on the long (q) or short (p) arms of chromosomes, as well as a variety of structural rearrangements (e.g., translocations, inversions, insertions). A number of cytogenetic abnormalities in AML have suggested molecular-clinical syndromes, which are now being analyzed at the genetic level. The translocation t(15;17)(q22;q12) is the cytogenetic hallmark of acute promyelocytic leukemia (AML-M3). This translocation splits the retinoic acid receptor gene on chromosome 17 and blocks expression of retinoic acid–controlled genes required for cell differentiation. Treating patients with acute promyelocytic leukemia with all-*trans* retinoic acid (ATRA, tretinoin) has caused complete morphologic responses. This example shows how defining cytogenetic or chromosomal abnormalities in acute leukemia can be critical to understanding its pathophysiology and identifying optimal treatments. Currently, three chromosomal abnormalities are recognized as being associated with a good prognosis[6,7]: t(8;21), t(15;17), and inv 16. In contrast, several chromosomal abnormalities have been associated with a relatively poor prognosis, including inv 3, del 5, del 5q, del 7, and del 7q; trisomy 8; and complex (three or more unrelated cytogenetic abnormalities) cytogenetics. These chromosomal findings are increasingly being used to guide treatment decisions. For example, patients with cytogenetic findings associated with a poor prognosis may be considered for more aggressive postremission therapy such as high-dose chemotherapy with stem cell support (i.e., transplantation). Other poor prognostic signs in AML include age older than 60 years at the time of diagnosis, a pre-existing hematologic disorder (e.g., myelodysplastic syndrome), prior exposure to a chemotherapy agent (e.g., a secondary leukemia), and poor baseline performance status.

D.M. has FAB-M2 (myelomonocytic) AML. Approximately 10% to 20% of patients with FAB-M2 acute leukemia have a translocation of t(8;21)(q22;q22).[6] This translocation is usually seen in young patients such as D.M. and is associated with a favorable response to therapy. D.M.'s bone marrow has been sent for cytogenetic analysis; however, results will not be available for several days. Although the cytogenetic analysis will not alter recommendations for induction therapy for D.M., these findings, in combination with other prognostic features, do influence postremission therapy recommendations.

Treatment

Goal of Therapy

2. What is the goal of treatment, and what type of therapy is indicated for D.M. at this time?

The leukemic cells populating D.M.'s blood are abnormal and incapable of fighting infection. Their rapid proliferation is also suppressing RBC and megakaryocyte production in the bone marrow. D.M. is at substantial risk for both life-threatening infections and bleeding complications. The goal of the initial chemotherapy is to clear the bone marrow and peripheral blood of all blast cells in the hope that normal blood cell components can regenerate.

Induction Therapy

Standard induction chemotherapy for AML includes an anthracycline (either daunorubicin or idarubicin) and cytarabine, an antimetabolite. One commonly used regimen includes idarubicin 12 mg/m^2/day on days 1 to 3 as an intravenous (IV) bolus injection, plus cytarabine 100 mg/m^2/day as a continuous IV infusion on days 1 to 7. This combination (7 + 3) is one of the most successful chemotherapy regimens used to treat AML, with complete response (CR) rates of 60% to 80%.[6] Continuous infusions of cytarabine are preferred because these regimens produce higher response rates than bolus injections during induction therapy.[8,9] Using higher doses of cytarabine by increasing the number of days of therapy to 10, doubling the daily dose to 200 mg/m^2, and using high dose cytarabine (HiDAC) (0.5–6.0 g/m^2/day) has not shown consistent improvement in complete remission rates or survival.[10] Adding etoposide for 7 days may increase the CR rate, response duration, and survival in patients younger than 55 years.[11] However, other investigators have not shown a benefit with the addition of etoposide to the standard 7 + 3 induction regimen.[12]

If a patient presents with a very high WBC count, he or she may experience complications associated with hyperviscosity of the blood (e.g., ringing ears, stroke, blindness, or headache as a result of impaired oxygen delivery to the CNS, pulmonary infarction). Because it may take several days for cytarabine and idarubicin to substantially decrease the WBC count, the patient may receive hydroxyurea 2 to 4 g orally (PO) or undergo leukapheresis to quickly reduce the WBC count.

TRETINOIN AND ARSENIC TRIOXIDE FOR ACUTE PROMYELOCYTIC LEUKEMIA

3. Would induction therapy for other subtypes of AML differ from that described previously?

Induction therapy is standard for all types of AML, with one exception: acute promyelocytic leukemia (APL) or FAB-M3. APL is uniquely characterized by the t(15;17) translocation that fuses the PML gene on chromosome 15 to the retinoic acid receptor-alpha (*RAR-α*) gene on chromosome 17. Severe coagulopathy is also common in patients with APL at the time of diagnosis or during induction therapy. Myeloperoxidase and procoagulant substances released from granules contained within the leukemia cells cause these complications. As discussed previously, tretinoin or ATRA induces promyelocyte differentiation and maturation.[13] In clinical trials, ATRA has induced complete remissions in approximately 90% of patients with APL.[14] Serial bone marrow aspirations after initiation of ATRA therapy demonstrate progressive differentiation without hypoplasia.[14,15] Unfortunately, ATRA typically induces brief remissions. A number of trials have investigated combination treatment with chemotherapy and ATRA.[16,17] Current evidence supports the use of concurrent ATRA plus conventional chemotherapy for induction, with ATRA starting 2 days before chemotherapy. In addition, postremission therapy should include at least two cycles of an anthracycline-based regimen.[17,18] Maintenance therapy with intermittent ATRA has been shown to decrease the relapse rate.[16,19]

ATRA therapy, although avoiding life-threatening myelosuppression, can produce significant toxicities, including the retinoic acid syndrome (RAS), which manifests as fever, weight gain, respiratory distress, lung infiltrates, pleural or pericardial effusion, hypotension, and acute renal failure.[20] If RAS develops, corticosteroid therapy (dexamethasone 10 mg BID for at least 3 days) should be initiated.[21] In patients receiving concurrent ATRA and chemotherapy, ATRA may be stopped if the patient has received ATRA for at least 20 days or if symptoms of RAS are life threatening or not improving with dexamethasone. Patients with leukocytosis seem to be more likely to experience RAS. Concurrent use of chemotherapy and ATRA has been reported to reduce the likelihood of RAS.[21] ATRA also causes dryness of the lining of the mouth, rectum, and skin; hair loss; skin rash; blepharon conjunctivitis; corneal erosions; muscle weakness; nail changes; depression; elevated liver enzymes; and high cholesterol. Despite the risk of serious complications and death during induction therapy, the long-term diseasefree survival (DFS) rate of patients with APL is superior compared with other AML subtypes. Approximately 75% of patients who receive ATRA-based induction and maintenance therapy are alive 3 to 5 years after diagnosis.[19]

Arsenic trioxide (ATO) has also been evaluated in the treatment of patients with APL. Clinical trials have confirmed that ATO is highly effective for the treatment of patients with relapsed APL, with complete remission rates up to 85%.[22] Preliminary results suggest no benefit to adding ATRA to ATO in this setting; however, future studies will determine whether ATO in combination with other strategies will yield superior outcomes.[23] There are several clinically significant adverse effects associated with ATO use. QT interval prolongation and *torsades de pointes* have been reported in a small number of patients, and warrant careful monitoring and management. Signs and symptoms of RAS were also reported, suggesting that this syndrome is not specific to therapy with ATRA and may be more appropriately referred to as APL syndrome. The monitoring and management of APL syndrome with ATO are the same as with ATRA. Coagulopathy, leukocytosis, neuropathy, nausea and vomiting, cough, headache, rash, hypokalemia, and hyperglycemia have also been frequently reported with ATO therapy and should be monitored appropriately.

COMPLICATIONS OF INDUCTION THERAPY

Tumor Lysis Syndrome

4. Twenty-four hours after D.M.'s induction chemotherapy was initiated, the following laboratory values were obtained: WBC count, 28,000/mm^3 (normal, 4–11); K, 5.3 mEq/L (normal, 3.5–5.5); phosphorus, 6.0 mg/dL (normal, 2.5–5.5); uric acid, 9.8 mg/dL (normal, 2.5–8); calcium, 6.0 mg/dL (normal, 9.0–11.5); and creatinine, 1.6 mg/dL (normal, 0.8–1.2). Why have these laboratory values changed so suddenly? Could they have been minimized or prevented? How should these metabolic disturbances be managed?

[SI units: WBC count, 58 × 10^6/L; K, 5.3 mmol/L; phosphorus, 1.94 mmol/L; uric acid, 582.9 mmol/L (normal, 148.7–475.84); calcium, 1.5 mmol/L (normal, 2.25–2.875); creatinine, 141.44 mol/L (normal, 88.4–176.8)]

D.M. presented with a very high number of peripheral blasts. Consequently, chemotherapy resulted in rapid lysis of the blast cells and the release of their cellular contents into the blood. A hypercellular bone marrow with a very high number of blast cells can also lead to rapid lysis of the blast cells and the release of cellular contents. Typical metabolic abnormalities associated with tumor lysis syndrome (TLS) are hyperuricemia, hyperphosphatemia, hypocalcemia, and uremia. These

Table 90-4 Complications Associated With Acute Tumor Lysis Syndrome

Hypocalcemia	Renal failure
Hyperkalemia	Electrocardiogram changes
Hyperphosphatemia	Metabolic acidosis
Hyperuricemia	

disturbances may lead to arrhythmias and acute renal failure (Table 90-4). Patients can present with TLS, but, most commonly, TLS occurs 12 to 24 hours after chemotherapy is initiated. TLS may occur after therapy for other malignancies, particularly in those with a high tumor burden, such as high-grade lymphomas and ALL. TLS rarely occurs after therapy for solid tumors.

Before chemotherapy is initiated, leukapheresis to reduce D.M.'s peripheral WBC count may minimize TLS. Leukapheresis is not routinely done unless the patient is experiencing symptoms of hyperviscosity. Patients should receive IV hydration (2–3 L/day) beginning 24 to 48 hours before chemotherapy to (a) maintain renal perfusion, (b) optimize the solubility of tumor lysis products, and (c) compensate for fluid losses due to fever or vomiting. Alkalinization of the urine may also reduce or prevent uric acid from precipitating in the renal tubules and collection ducts by maintaining the urate in its ionized state. However, increased pH may increase the risk of precipitating calcium phosphate in both soft tissue and kidney tubules, and it may aggravate hypocalcemia.[24]

Allopurinol (a xanthine oxidase inhibitor that blocks the metabolism of uric acid) should be started before chemotherapy to minimize the complications of TLS. The recommended adult dosage is 300 to 600 mg/day. D.M.'s serum uric acid and electrolytes should be monitored at least two to three times a day for 24 to 48 hours after initiating chemotherapy. If severe abnormalities occur, more aggressive measures should be initiated. Allopurinol may be discontinued if the serum uric acid is within normal limits and the WBC count is low. Rasburicase, a recombinant urate oxidase product, can also be used as prophylaxis in patients who are at high risk of developing TLS or for the treatment of patients who present with or develop TLS. Rasburicase acts as a catalyst in the enzymatic oxidation of uric acid to allantoin, which is five to ten times more soluble than uric acid and undergoes rapid renal excretion. The recommended dose of rasburicase for both prevention and treatment of TLS is 0.2 mg/kg/dose. Rasburicase results in a rapid reduction in serum uric acid (within 4 hours of administration) and is generally well tolerated.[25] Most of the clinical data for rasburicase is in the pediatric population; however, data from compassionate use trials suggest that rasburicase is equally effective in adults.[26,27] Although rasburicase has demonstrated excellent efficacy and tolerability, its optimal role in the prevention and management of hyperuricemia in adults remains to be defined because of its high cost and lack of a randomized trial comparing its effect with other interventions.

Although D.M.'s serum potassium was low on admission, it has increased significantly as a result of tumor cell lysis. For this reason, replacement potassium therapy is not recommended before chemotherapy in patients in whom TLS is highly likely. In extreme circumstances, dialysis may be required to correct severe metabolic and electrolyte disturbances associated with TLS.

Myelosuppression

5. D.M. received allopurinol therapy and aggressive hydration throughout her induction chemotherapy. The metabolic abnormalities gradually resolved as her WBC count declined and tumor lysis diminished. What other complications may occur during induction therapy. Can they be treated?

Patients receiving cytarabine and idarubicin induction therapy develop profound anemia, granulocytopenia (e.g., WBC count <100/mm³) and thrombocytopenia (<20,000 platelets/mm³) shortly after therapy is initiated that persists for 21 to 28 days. All infectious complications must be considered life threatening in severely immunocompromised patients such as D.M. (see Chapter 68).

Filgrastim (granulocyte colony-stimulating factor [G-CSF]) and sargramostim (granulocyte-macrophage colony-stimulating factor) stimulate leukemic cells as well as normal granulocyte precursors in vitro; however, several studies have demonstrated that these agents, when used as an adjunct to AML chemotherapy, are safe and do not adversely affect disease outcome.[28,29] Most studies have demonstrated that CSFs can modestly decrease the length of profound neutropenia, and sometimes reduce the incidence of infection-related morbidity, the duration of systemic antibiotic and antifungal therapy, and the number of hospitalization days. Guidelines published by the American Society of Clinical Oncology recommend that patients older than 55 years are most likely to benefit from CSF administration after completion of induction chemotherapy.[30] Despite the reduction in short-term complications, administration of CSFs after induction chemotherapy does not appear to have an impact on the rate of complete remissions or the long-term outcomes of the disease.

Severe thrombocytopenia may result in bleeding episodes that range in severity from oozing gums to massive GI hemorrhage. Serious bleeding complications can usually be avoided if patients receive platelet transfusions when their platelet counts decrease to <10,000/mm³ or when patients experience bleeding. Currently, there are no data to support the use of interleukin (IL)-11 (oprelvekin) or investigational thrombopoietic agents in this setting. Because D.M. is premenopausal, she has a significant risk of excessive vaginal bleeding if she begins menstruating while she is thrombocytopenic. The menstrual cycle can be suppressed with daily, uninterrupted oral contraceptives or progesterone (e.g., medroxyprogesterone 10–20 mg/day PO). If spotting occurs, dosages should be increased until bleeding stops. After D.M.'s platelet count returns to normal, suppressive therapy can be discontinued.

Other common drug-induced complications that may occur during induction therapy include nausea and vomiting, mucositis, fever, and skin rash (see Chapters 7 and 89).

Postremission Therapy

Rationale

6. After completion of her induction chemotherapy, D.M.'s WBC count fell to <100/mm³, and her platelet count fell to 5,000/mm³. She received platelet transfusions approximately

every 2 to 3 days to prevent bleeding complications. On day 9, she developed a fever of 38.8°C. She was started immediately on empiric, broad-spectrum antibiotic therapy, which resolved her fever. On day 29, her WBC count was 5,600/mm^3 with a normal differential, and her platelet count was 168,000/mm^3. She received packed RBC transfusions on two separate occasions when her Hct fell to <30%. A repeat bone marrow aspirate showed no evidence of persistent leukemia, and D.M. was told that her leukemia was in remission. Nevertheless, her oncologist recommended additional chemotherapy, and D.M. questions why this is necessary. Is postremission therapy necessary, and if so, what therapeutic options are available to D.M.?

Although >60% of patients treated for AML achieve complete remission after induction therapy, the median duration of the remission is only about 12 to 18 months, and only 20% to 40% of patients have a DFS exceeding 5 years.[10] Short remissions have been attributed to proliferation of clinically undetectable leukemic cells. Thus, the rationale for administering chemotherapy after remission is to eradicate these residual cells.

In AML, postremission therapy (also referred to as "consolidation therapy") includes two to four cycles of chemotherapy. Clinical trials have shown that high-dose postremission therapy results in a higher percentage (30%–40%) of long-term (>2–5 years) diseasefree survivors than either no or low-dose postremission chemotherapy.[31,32] Postremission therapy regimens usually include HiDAC alone or in combination with one or more agents such as mitoxantrone, idarubicin, or etoposide. Patients 60 years of age and older or those with comorbid disease may not be able to tolerate this intensive postremission therapy. In these circumstances, the risk of life-threatening toxicity may outweigh the potential benefits of postremission chemotherapy. Allogeneic hematopoietic cell transplantation (HCT) has also been studied in the postremission treatment of AML and is addressed in Chapter 92.

Administration of chemotherapy (thioguanine, methotrexate) and biologicals (IL-2) for a prolonged period has been investigated to see if it can prolong survival. This is often referred to as maintenance therapy. With the exception of APL, maintenance chemotherapy has not been shown to improve survival in patients with AML.

High-Dose Cytarabine

7. D.M. does not have any siblings that would be a compatible donor for an allogeneic hematopoietic cell transplant. Consequently, her oncologist recommends three courses of high-dose cytarabine (HiDAC) as postremission therapy while an unrelated compatible donor is sought. One week after she was declared to be in remission, D.M. is readmitted to the hospital to receive cytarabine 3 g/m^2 Q 12 hr, over 3 hours, on days 1, 3, and 5. What are the potential acute and delayed toxicities associated with HiDAC, and how can these effects be prevented?

At conventional dosages of 100 to 200 mg/m^2/day, adverse effects associated with cytarabine include myelosuppression, fever, and skin rashes. Occasionally, liver enzymes rise transiently. The side effect profile for HiDAC (>1 g/m^2/day), however, is very different and can produce major cerebellar, ocular, and skin toxicities.[33,34]

CEREBELLAR TOXICITY

Cerebellar toxicity is a significant problem in patients receiving HiDAC therapy. See Chapter 89 for details regarding cytarabine-induced cerebellar toxicity.

OCULAR TOXICITY

Ocular toxicity results from damage to corneal epithelium, when cytarabine penetrates the epithelium through the anterior chamber of the eye or tears. Symptoms include conjunctivitis, excessive lacrimation, "burning" ocular pain, photophobia, and blurred vision. Artificial tears (two drops every 4–6 hours) administered concurrently with HiDAC generally prevents these symptoms. Corticosteroid eyedrops should be used if symptoms of conjunctivitis occur.[35]

DERMATOLOGIC TOXICITY

Dermatologic toxicity may be manifested as a rash covering most of the body (similar to that seen with conventional doses) or plantar-palmar erythema. Desquamation of the palms and soles can occur with plantar-palmar erythema, causing significant pain and allowing for pathogenic organisms to enter the body.

ACUTE LEUKEMIA IN THE ELDERLY

8. Would recommendations for induction and postremission therapy differ if D.M. were elderly (60 years of age or older)?

The incidence of AML gradually increases with age, with the median age of affected patients between 65 and 70 years. Several clinical trials have shown lower complete remission rates, as well as reduced DFS and overall survival (OS) in patients older than 55 years. The reason for this is most likely multifactorial, including a decreased tolerance to chemotherapy, comorbidities, and compromised organ function, as well as inherent biological differences between AML in the elderly and in younger patients.[36] Poor prognostic factors more common in the elderly include a history of preleukemic syndrome (myelodysplastic syndrome), poor cytogenetic abnormalities, high expression of multidrug-resistant glycoprotein MDR1, and prior radiation therapy or chemotherapy.[37] Whether the elderly should receive aggressive chemotherapy is often debated.[38] Two studies have evaluated a standard induction regimen versus alternatives of low-dose or palliative chemotherapy.[39,40] Both studies demonstrated superior prolonged survival in the standard therapy arms at the cost of increased treatment-related mortality. It must be taken into consideration, though, that these studies were performed approximately 20 years ago and that improvements in supportive care may significantly improve the treatment-related mortality observed in these studies. Nevertheless, many oncologists believe aggressive therapy is warranted in most elderly patients given the rapid progression of the disease and certain death within weeks if the disease is not treated.

The decision of postremission therapy is a difficult decision in elderly patients because they have a higher risk of morbidity and mortality, and, more important, no clinical trials have demonstrated the benefit of postremission therapy specifically in the elderly. The intensity of the regimens must often be attenuated because there is risk of serious toxicities. This is particularly true with HiDAC therapy due to the increased risk of cerebellar toxicity in the elderly. Studies have shown that postremission therapy with low-dose cytarabine (100 mg/m^2 by continuous infusion for 5 days) is as effective as HiDAC and better tolerated in elderly patients.[31]

Refractory or Resistant Acute Myeloid Leukemia

9. A.W., a 65-year-old man, is 30 days post induction therapy with 7 + 3. His neutrophil count has been <200/mm^3 since day 12. Bone marrow biopsy reveals 60% blasts, confirming the diagnosis of refractory AML. What are treatment options for A.W. at this time?

Given the decreased efficacy and tolerability of myelosuppressive chemotherapy in the elderly, novel immunotherapeutic approaches are being developed. Gemtuzumab ozogamicin, a humanized anti-CD33 antibody coupled to calicheamicin, an anthracycline-like toxin, is approved for relapsed or refractory AML in patients 60 years and older who are not considered candidates for further cytotoxic chemotherapy.[41] CD33 is a cluster differentiation antigen present on the majority of blast cells, but not on hematopoietic stem cells. The conjugation of an anthracycline to the anti-CD33 antibody targets the delivery of the toxin to the CD33-positive blast cells. A total of 142 patients participating in open-label trials were treated with gemtuzumab 9 mg/m^2 on days 1 and 15.[41] Gemtuzumab provided an overall response (OR) rate of 30%. Myelosuppression and thrombocytopenia appear to be of longer duration compared to conventional chemotherapy regimens in this setting; however, it is associated with less nonhematologic side effects such as mucositis, nausea and vomiting, and alopecia. Infusion-related adverse events such as rigors, chills, and fever are common and are severe in approximately 30% of patients. This drug may be a reasonable alternative to additional chemotherapy for A.W.

CHRONIC MYELOID LEUKEMIA

Signs and Symptoms

10. S.E., a 66-year-old white female, recently had a routine CBC drawn during her annual checkup. Her CBC showed a WBC count of 60,000/mm^3 with 90% neutrophils, Hct of 32%, and a platelet count of 300,000/mm^3. The only pertinent physical finding was splenomegaly. A bone marrow aspirate revealed a hypercellular marrow with less than 10% blasts. Cytogenetic analysis confirmed a diagnosis of Philadelphia chromosome-positive CML. Explain S.E.'s high WBC counts. What are the possible clinical consequences of these abnormal values?

[SI units: WBC count, 60 × 10^6/L with 0.9 neutrophils; Hct, 0.32, platelets 900 × 10^6/L]

CML is a myeloproliferative disorder characterized by unregulated stem cell proliferation in the bone marrow and an increase in mature granulocytes in the peripheral blood. Common clinical symptoms on presentation include fatigue, fever, anorexia, and weight loss. Approximately 50% to 70% of patients present with a leukocyte count >100,000/mm^3. Symptoms of hyperleukocytosis and hyperviscosity include priapism, headaches, tinnitus, and cerebrovascular accidents. On physical examination, the most common abnormal finding is splenomegaly, which results from increased activity of the reticuloendothelial system to remove increased numbers of WBCs. Although these symptoms are common, approximately 30% to 40% of patients are asymptomatic at presentation, and the initial suspicion for CML is based solely on an abnormal CBC.[42]

Clinical Course and Prognosis

11. What is the expected disease progression for S.E. and others with newly diagnosed CML?

The natural history of CML can be divided into three distinct phases: chronic phase, accelerated phase, and blastic phase. Early in the disease (chronic phase), patients exhibit leukocytosis and associated symptoms as described previously. Bone marrow examination and peripheral blood smear reveal <10% immature blast cells.[43] The duration of the chronic phase may range from a few months to many years. Because symptoms may be nonspecific and relatively minor, CML may remain undiagnosed until patients progress into more advanced stages. The annual transition rate from chronic phase to accelerated phase is 5% to 10% in the first 2 years and 20% in subsequent years. Common signs and symptoms suggestive of this transition include increased leukocytosis, anemia, increased splenomegaly, fever, and bone pain.

During the second phase of the disease, the accelerated phase, leukocytosis progresses (despite therapy), and an increased number of immature leukocytes (blasts) appear in the peripheral blood. Patients often report significant symptoms. The accelerated phase generally lasts <6 weeks. The final phase of the disease (blastic phase or blast crisis) is characterized by a predominance of immature cells. Bone marrow examination of the peripheral blood at this time reveals >20% blasts.[43] During this phase, CML is indistinguishable from AML with the exception of cytogenetics. In blast crisis, patients often experience bone pain, fatigue, worsening anemia, infections, and bleeding complications. The blast phase is often refractory to conventional induction regimens for AML, and median survival is approximately 5 months.[42] Because less than 10% blast cells are present in S.E.'s bone marrow, she is in the chronic phase of the disease.

12. What is the significance of the finding of the Philadelphia chromosome?

The cytogenetic hallmark of CML is the Philadelphia chromosome, which is present in more than 90% of cases. Cytogenetic analysis reveals a translocation of chromosomes 9 and 22 t(9;22)(q34;q11).[44] This translocation creates a new protein (BCR-ABL) that has unregulated tyrosine kinase activity. The three major mechanisms that have been implicated in the malignant transformation by unregulated tyrosine kinase include abnormal cell cycling, inhibition of apoptosis, and increased proliferation of cells.[44] Identifying the Philadelphia chromosome helps confirm the diagnosis of CML and helps with monitoring the efficacy of treatment.

Treatment

13. What therapy is appropriate for S.E.?

In newly diagnosed patients who present with very high leukocyte counts (>100,000/mm^3), the initial goal of therapy is to reduce leukocytosis and its related symptoms.[43] Hydroxyurea is still the most common agent used for initial leukocyte reduction. Treatment is initiated with 2 g/day PO, and the dosage is titrated to a WBC count of <20,000/mm^3. A small dosage decrease often permits a considerable rise in leukocyte count in 1 or 2 days. Hydroxyurea is well tolerated and is relatively free of nonhematologic side effects. Although effective for initial control of high leukocyte counts, hydroxyurea is inferior to other treatments for long-term control of CML.

The ultimate goal of therapy for CML is to cure patients of their disease. The only curative therapy for CML to date is allogeneic HCT. The best results are achieved with HLA-matched related donors; however, HLA-matched unrelated donor transplants in select patients can also yield favorable long-term DFS rates.[45] When patients are transplanted during the blast phase, only 10% to 20% survive >5 years. If patients are transplanted during the chronic phase, 50% to 60% are disease free at 5 years.[46] The highest rate of prolonged DFS occurs in younger patients who undergo transplantation within 1 year of initial diagnosis during the chronic phase.[47]

Because most patients newly diagnosed with CML are not transplant candidates because of their age and lack of a suitable donor, alternative therapies must be considered. When cure is not an option, the primary goals of therapy are to prolong survival, prevent progression of disease, and attain a complete hematologic and/or cytogenetic remission. The definition of a complete hematologic response is a reduction in the leukocyte count to <10,000/mm^3 and the platelet count to <450,000/mm^3. A cytogenetic response is defined by the percentage of cells in metaphase that are positive for the Philadelphia chromosome in the bone marrow (Table 90-5).

Imatinib

In May 2001, the U.S. Food and Drug Administration (FDA) approved imatinib mesylate (Gleevec) for the treatment of patients with CML. Imatinib is a tyrosine kinase inhibitor that occupies the adenosine triphosphate binding site of several tyrosine kinase molecules and prevents phosphorylation of substrates that are involved in regulating the cell cycle. Imatinib was initially tested in patients with chronic phase CML who were refractory to or intolerant of interferon (IFN)-based therapy. Ninety-eight percent of patients receiving 300 mg or more per day of imatinib achieved a complete hematologic response, whereas 31% of patients at the same dose achieved a major cytogenetic response.[48] Imatinib has also shown efficacy in accelerated and blastic phase CML.[49,50] These impressive results set the stage for the pivotal International Randomized Study of Interferon and STI571 (IRIS) trial, which compared imatinib with the combination of IFN-α plus low-dose cytarabine in patients with newly diagnosed CML in the chronic phase. A total of 1,106 patients were randomly assigned to either imatinib (400 mg PO daily) or IFN plus cytarabine.[51] For patients on imatinib, the dose could be escalated to 400 mg BID if no hematologic response was seen within 3 months or if no cytogenetic response was seen within 12 months. All primary and secondary end points of the trial, including rates of complete hematologic remission, major and complete cytogenetic response, and freedom from progression to the accelerated phase or blast crisis, demonstrated superiority of imatinib over IFN plus cytarabine (Table 90-6). Estimated survival rates at 18 months between the two arms were not significantly different (97.2% vs. 95.1% for imatinib and IFN plus cytarabine, respectively; $p = 0.16$). The lack of survival difference is most likely due to a large percentage of patients (89%) in the IFN plus cytarabine arm who crossed over to the imatinib arm due to lack of efficacy or intolerance to therapy. In addition to superior efficacy, imatinib was very well tolerated. The most common toxicities reported with imatinib are superficial edema, nausea, muscle cramps, and rashes. Only 12% of patients in the imatinib arm discontinued therapy due to adverse events compared with 33% in the IFN plus cytarabine arm. More mature data from this trial, with a median follow-up of 60 months, demonstrated an 89% OS of patients who received imatinib as initial therapy.[52] This landmark trial clearly showed the superiority of imatinib over IFN plus cytarabine in the treatment of patients with newly diagnosed CML in chronic phase. Based on these results, imatinib is now considered the front-line standard of care for patients with newly diagnosed CML in chronic phase. Practical management strategies for dosing, treatment and prevention of toxicities, and possible drug interactions have been reviewed extensively elsewhere.[53] The excellent results seen with imatinib challenge the role of allogeneic stem cell transplantation as front-line therapy. Clinicians and patients must carefully evaluate the potential risks and benefits of each treatment modality in order to make the best therapeutic decision for each individual situation.

Table 90-5 Definition of Cytogenetic Response in Chronic Myeloid Leukemia

Cytogenetic Response[a]	*Philadelphia (Ph) Chromosome-Positive Cells (%)*
Complete	0
Partial	1–35
Minor	36–65
Absent	>65

[a] Major response is defined as complete or partial responses.

Table 90-6 Response Rates in International Randomized Study of Interferon and STI571 Trial

Response	*% Imatinib (N = 553)*	*% Interferon Plus Cytarabine (N = 553)*
Complete hematologic	95.3 (93.2–96.9)	55.5 (51.3–59.7)
Major cytogenetic	85.2 (81.9–88.0)	22.1 (18.7–25.8)
Complete cytogenetic	73.8 (69.9–77.4)	8.5 (6.3–11.1)
Partial cytogenetic	11.4 (8.9–14.3)	13.6 (10.8–16.7)

Relapsed and Refractory Disease

14. On routine follow-up, cytogenetics analysis of S.E.'s bone marrow demonstrates a rising percentage of Philadelphia chromosome-positive cells. S.E. has her imatinib dose increased to 400 mg BID. After 3 months at the higher dose, S.E. continues to demonstrate cytogenetic relapse. A bone marrow biopsy results in less than 10% leukemic blast cells, demonstrating chronic phase CML. What available options are there for S.E.?

Based on the most recent update of the IRIS trial, approximately 30% of patients initially treated with imatinib will have to discontinue therapy either due to lack of therapeutic benefit or intolerable side effects. Dasatinib, an orally available, multitargeted kinase inhibitor that is active against BCR-ABL and SRC family kinase, has recently been approved for the treatment of CML patients who are refractory to or intolerant of imatinib. Dasatinib 70 mg BID has demonstrated activity in all phases of CML.[54,55] For patients in chronic phase after failure to imatinib, complete hematologic and cytogenetics responses were seen in 90% and 52% of patients, respectively.[56] Nonhematologic toxicities were mild to moderate, and cytopenias could effectively be managed with dosage reductions.

CHRONIC LYMPHOCYTIC LEUKEMIA

Signs and Symptoms

15. B.R., a 66-year-old male, presents to his physician with a persistent semiproductive cough and increased fatigue. A routine CBC revealed an Hgb of 13.0 g/dL, a WBC count of 34,000 mm³ (80% lymphocytes), and a platelet count of 175 × 10⁶/L. Blood pressure was 120/70 mmHg, heart rate 64 beats/minute, and respiratory rate 23 breaths/minute. He was afebrile. Physical examination was unremarkable. He was prescribed azithromycin for possible community-acquired pneumonia and scheduled for a return visit in 3 weeks. At that time, his CBC results were Hgb 13.2 g/dL, WBC count 32,000 mm³ (82% lymphocytes), and platelets 168 × 10⁶/L. Physical examination was unchanged, the chest radiograph was clear, and his cough had resolved. B.R. was referred to a hematologist for evaluation of his persistent lymphocytosis. What is the most likely cause of persistent lymphocytosis in B.R.?

[SI units: Hgb 130 g/L (normal, 135–175); WBC count, 34 × 10^9/L with 0.8 lymphocytes and 32 × 10^9/L with 0.82 lymphocytes, respectively (normal, WBC 4.5–10 with 0.15–0.5 lymphocytes); platelets, 175 × 10^9/L and 168 × 10^9/L (normal, >150)]

CLL is a chronic lymphoproliferative disorder characterized by an excess of functionally incompetent B-cell lymphocytes derived from a single stem cell clone. CLL should be included in the differential diagnosis of any adult with persistent lymphocytosis (>5,000 lymphocytes/mm³ in peripheral blood). Additional causes of lymphocytosis include transient reactions to acute infections and viruses such as influenza or mononucleosis, as well as other hematologic malignancies, including lymphoma and ALL.

To differentiate between benign and malignant lymphocytosis, examination of the peripheral blood or bone marrow morphology by a hematologist or pathologist may be required. Patients with CLL commonly have lymphocytosis in both the peripheral blood and bone marrow, whereas patients with other disorders have a high percentage of atypical lymphocytes in the peripheral blood alone. The absence of fever or additional signs of infection without significant diagnostic or physical exam findings, together with the presence of mature peripheral blood lymphocytes, make CLL the most likely diagnosis for B.R. Cell surface marker staining (immunophenotyping) is required, and bone marrow biopsy with aspirate may be useful to determine the definitive diagnosis.[57]

Staging and Prognosis

16. Bone marrow examination reveals normal cellularity with >30% of nucleated cells lymphocytes. The immunophenotype indicates that peripheral blood lymphocytes are predominately B cells and are positive for CD5, CD19, and CD20. A diagnosis of CLL is confirmed. What is the usual presentation and prognosis of CLL? What treatment is indicated at this time? B.R.'s cells were sent for routine cytogenetic analysis, which revealed a chromosome abnormality (Deletion 11q-). How does this impact his management?

CLL is the most common type of leukemia in adults, with more than 15,000 estimated new cases annually.[58] CLL is characterized as a disease of the older population. Median age at diagnosis is 65 years with 90% of patients older than age 50 at diagnosis.[59,60] Approximately 40% of patients are asymptomatic at presentation and are diagnosed by routine CBC.[59] Predicting the clinical course of CLL remains a challenge as some patients experience an indolent course with a maintained quality of life, whereas others experience more aggressive disease and debilitation. Therefore, survival is variable and depends on the stage of disease at diagnosis. CLL is staged based on peripheral lymphocyte counts; enlargement of lymph nodes, liver, and spleen; and the presence of anemia and/or thrombocytopenia. The two most commonly used staging systems in clinical practice are included in Tables 90-7 and 90-8. B.R. would be classified as having early stage disease, with a historical median survival of ≥10 years.[59,61]

An accepted treatment modality for early stage disease includes a conservative watchful waiting approach. No clear advantage has been demonstrated in treating asymptomatic patients in early stage disease with alkylator-based chemotherapy

Table 90-7 Binet Classification

	Lymphocytosis[a]	Anemia[b]	Thrombocytopenia[c]	Number of Involved Nodes (Max 5)[d]	Median Survival (Years)
A	+	−	−	<3	12
B	+	−	−	≥3	7
C	+	±	±	Any	2–4

[a]Lymphocytes >5 × 10^9/L in peripheral blood and >30% of total cells in the bone marrow.
[b]Hemoglobin <11 g/dL in men and <10 g/dL in women excluding immune-mediated etiology.
[c]Platelets <100,000 × 10^9/L.
[d]Maximum of five—cervical, axillary, inguinal, spleen, and liver–are counted as one area.
Adapted from reference 61.

Table 90-8 Modified Rai Classification

Risk	*Stage*	*Lymphocytosis*[a]	*Anemia*[b]	*Thrombocytopenia*[c]	*Lymphadenopathy*	*Hepatomegaly or Splenomegaly*	*Median Survival (Years)*
Low	0	+	−	−	−	−	10
Intermediate	I	+	−	−	+	−	7
	II	+	−	−	±	+	
High	III	+	+	−	±	±	1.5–4
	IV	+	±	+	±	±	

[a]Lymphocytes $>5 \times 10^9$/L in peripheral blood and >30% of total cells in the bone marrow.
[b]Hemoglobin <11 g/dL excluding immune-mediated etiology.
[c]Platelets $<100{,}000 \times 10^9$/L.
From reference 409.

as compared to deferred treatment.[62] The survival of patients with smoldering CLL is similar to an age- and gender-matched normal population.[63,64] B.R. decides to delay treatment until he becomes symptomatic.

Biological explanations for the heterogeneity in the clinical course of CLL are under investigation. Recent advances have led to the discovery of chromosomal abnormalities (Deletions 17p-, 11q-), gene mutations (unmutated immunoglobulin variable region and p53), and serum or cell surface markers (increased B_2-microglobulin, zeta-associated protein-70, and CD 38 expression) that may confer poor prognosis and resistance to treatment.[65–68] Because the clinical practice of risk-adapted therapy is still evolving, survival estimation or treatment initiation based on prognostic markers alone cannot be recommended outside a clinical trial.

Treatment

17. B.R. returns to the hematologist every 3 months and does well for about 2 years. At that time, physical examination reveals enlargement of cervical, inguinal, and axillary lymph nodes; hepatomegaly; and splenomegaly. His lymphocyte count has increased from 32,000/mm³ 6 months ago to 68,000/mm³ today. His Hgb is 11.7 g/dL, and his platelet count is 140 × 10⁶/L. Is treatment now indicated?

[SI units: lymphocyte count, 32×10^9/L and 68×10^9/L, respectively; Hgb, 117 g/L; platelets, 140×10^9/L]

Indications for treatment initiation in CLL include significant anemia and/or thrombocytopenia, progressive disease demonstrated by lymphadenopathy, hepatomegaly, splenomegaly, a lymphocyte doubling time <6 months, persistent B symptoms (fever, night sweats, and weight loss), and recurrent infection. Patient performance status, comorbid conditions, pharmacoecomonic variables, and social support should all be taken into consideration when selecting treatment. B.R. should initiate treatment at this time to prevent further deterioration of his hematologic and immune function.

Initial Therapy

CHLORAMBUCIL

Historical therapy for CLL included use of an alkylating agent, most often oral chlorambucil or cyclophosphamide, with or without prednisone. A variety of daily and intermittent dosing schedules have been reported. The OR rate to chlorambucil was approximately 40% to 60%, but only 3% to 5% achieved CR.[59] Chlorambucil therapy requires dose titration and frequent monitoring of blood counts and physical findings to maximize its efficacy and prevent toxicity. Chlorambucil use has diminished, and the use of purine analogs, including fludarabine and cladribine, is more common in clinical practice; however, chlorambucil remains an option for elderly patients or those with contraindications to other therapies.

FLUDARABINE

Fludarabine is now considered the single most active agent in the treatment of CLL. Fludarabine monotherapy at a dose range of 25 to 30 mg/m²/dose IV × 5 days has shown a 70% to 80% OR rate, and CR rates of 20% to 30% with increased progressionfree survival (PFS).[69–71] The impact of fludarabine on OS has yet to be demonstrated. Toxicities associated with fludarabine are typically mild and include fever, myelosuppression, and immunosuppression. Increased incidence of infection and autoimmune hemolytic anemia is also associated with fludarabine therapy. Infectious prophylaxis should be considered in elderly patients and patients with advanced disease or renal dysfunction.

Fludarabine has been combined with chemotherapy and monoclonal antibodies, including cyclophosphamide, epirubicin, and rituximab, in an effort to prevent multidrug resistance (MDR) and increase response. Although combination regimens including fludarabine have demonstrated higher response rates and PFS, no difference in OS has been consistently demonstrated.[72–74] Additional toxicities of the combination regimen include higher rates of leucopenia, thrombocytopenia, nausea, vomiting, and alopecia.

A Cancer and Leukemia Group B trial compared single-agent fludarabine, single-agent chlorambucil, and the combination of fludarabine and chlorambucil.[70] Fludarabine monotherapy achieved higher CR rates than single-agent chlorambucil (20% vs. 4%, $p = 0.001$). Patients in the combination arm experienced more life-threatening toxicities, including infectious complication warranting early termination of this study arm. Patients receiving single-agent fludarabine had a 29% major infection rate versus 17% in patients treated with chlorambucil.[75]

CLADRIBINE

The response to cladribine, a synthetic purine nucleoside, is superior to chlorambucil with OR and CR rates comparable to single-agent fludarabine.[76] A typical dose and schedule is 10 mg/m²/dose PO on days 1 to 5 monthly or on days 1 to 3 at Q 3 weeks. The toxicity profile is similar to fludarabine.

Although cladribine in combination with cyclophosphamide with or without mitoxantrone achieved higher CR rates and less MDR clones, no significant improvement in OR, PFS, or OS has been demonstrated.[77] A higher percentage of grade 3/4 neutropenia was seen with the combination regimens.

RITUXIMAB

Rituximab is a chimeric human-murine anti-CD20 monoclonal antibody. The CD20 surface antigen is expressed on a high percentage of CLL cells. Rituximab monotherapy as initial therapy for untreated patients at a dose of 375 mg/m^2 yielded OR and CR rates lower than those seen with cytotoxic therapy with a disappointing duration of response.[78] Therefore, rituximab therapy is reserved for combination therapy with cytotoxic agents and/or monotherapy maintenance after a CR has been achieved. The optimal dose and schedule for maintenance rituximab therapy is yet to be determined. All patients should be pretreated with acetaminophen and diphenhydramine to prevent a cytokine release reaction associated with rituximab infusion. Rituximab should be omitted from the first cycle of therapy or administered in a split dosing schedule when the absolute lymphocyte count is >25,000.[79] The rate of infusion should be titrated as tolerated to a maximum of 400 mL/hour. In addition, allopurinol may be required to prevent TLS.

A regimen of particular interest for initial treatment is the combination of fludarabine, cyclophosphamide, and rituximab (FCR). In a study of 224 patients with various stage CLL, patients were treated with fludarabine 25 mg/m^2 IV × days 1 to 3, cyclophosphamide 250 mg/m^2 IV × days 1 to 3, and rituximab 375 mg/m^2 IV × day 1 of cycle 1 escalated to 500 mg/m^2 in subsequent cycles. All patients received prophylaxis against *Pneumocystis (carinii) jiroveci* pneumonia (PCP), herpes simplex, and herpes zoster. CR was attained by 70% of patients.[73] Toxicity of this regimen included infusion, related reactions, nausea, vomiting, and myelosuppression. Grade 3/4 neutropenia was noted in 52% of treatment courses, with a major infection rate of 2.6%.

ALEMTUZUMAB

Alemtuzumab is another humanized conjugated anti-CD52 monoclonal antibody that has been used in CLL. Initial doses of 3 mg, titrated to 10 mg, and, ultimately, 30 mg were administered either subcutaneously or intravenously three times weekly. Although the role of alemtuzumab in first-line therapy is still under investigation, CR rates of approximately 20% and OR rates of 80% to 87% have been reported.[80,81] Toxicities associated with alemtuzumab include infusion-related reactions (rigors, fever, dyspnea), neutropenia, and infectious complications.[82,83] The role of alemtuzumab maintenance following cytotoxic therapy is also under investigation.[84]

18. B.R. receives FCR as initial CLL therapy. After the third cycle, he has complete regression of his lymphadenopathy and hepatosplenomegaly, and his lymphocyte count decreases to 8,000/mm^3. B.R. comes to clinic 2 years after completion of therapy. A CBC is obtained that reveals WBC count 55,000 mm^3 with 70% lymphocytes, Hgb of 10 g/dL, and platelet count of 90 × 10^9/L. On physical examination, B.R. is found to have some cervical, inguinal, and axillary lymphadenopathy with no palpable splenomegaly. He complains of excessive fatigue and fever. A 2-month trial of oral chlorambucil is tried with no change in WBC count, lymphadenopathy, or symptoms. What therapies may be helpful to B.R. at this point?

[SI units: WBC count, 55 × 10^9/L; Hgb 100 g/L; platelets, 90 × 10^9/L]

Salvage Therapy

Second-line therapy should be selected based on criteria similar to those used for initial management. Relapsed patients are classified as fludarabine naive, fludarabine sensitive (relapse more than 6 months post treatment), or fludarabine refractory.

Fludarabine Naive and Fludarabine Sensitive

In a follow-up of 91 patients receiving salvage therapy after relapse, approximately 20% of patients achieved CR with either fludarabine monotherapy or a fludarabine combination regimen. Four of the five CRs reported with a fludarabine combination regimen used the combination of fludarabine and cyclophosphamide. In contrast, only 1 of the 28 patients receiving nonfludarabine regimens achieved CR.[69] Patients who failed to respond to initial fludarabine treatment did not respond to salvage treatment with a fludarabine-based regimen. In a subsequent study, the combination of FCR achieved a CR in 25% (45/177) of patients who had received at least one prior regimen. The majority of patients, 82% (145/177), had received prior fludarabine therapy. The estimated median OS was longer than historical data, although this remains to be confirmed.[85]

Fludarabine Refractory

Alemtuzumab has been FDA approved for the treatment of refractory CLL. The OR rate is approximately 30%, with a 0% to 2% CR rate and an OS of 16 to 27.5 months.[86,87] Activity has been demonstrated in patients who relapsed after or were refractory to alkylator or purine analog therapy, including those with the 17p- cytogenetic mutation, which is associated with resistance to most cytotoxic agents.[88] Alemtuzumab is least effective in patients with bulky (>5 cm) disease.[89]

Major toxicities of alemtuzumab include infusion-related events, infections, and cytopenias. The occurrence of opportunistic infections, including PCP and cytomegalovirus (CMV) in as many as 15% to 25% of patients treated with alemtuzumab, warrants the use of prophylactic therapy. An increased risk of infection occurs 3 to 8 weeks post treatment, which corresponds to the T cell nadir. Viral prophylaxis should be continued for at least 2 months after completion of therapy and bacterial prophylaxis until the CD4 count is at least ≥200 cells/μL.[90,91]

Younger patients (age younger than 55 years) with relapsed disease or high-risk features may benefit from autologous or allogeneic HCT. Both clinical and molecular remissions have been reported following autologous HCT, although no plateau in the OS curves has been demonstrated.[92] No prospective randomized trial comparing autologous HCT versus chemotherapy for poor prognosis patients has been conducted. Allogeneic HCT is the only curative treatment for CLL to date. However, the high risk of treatment-related morbidity and mortality must be considered. Patients with relapsed CLL after fludarabine therapy or with high-risk features should be referred for an HCT consultation to determine candidacy.

Infectious Complications

19. Six weeks after the initiation of alemtuzumab, B.R. complains of progressive shortness of breath and fever. On questioning, he reveals that he quit taking his trimethoprim/sulfamethoxazole and valacyclovir because "I felt fine." X-ray of the chest reveals bilateral infiltrates. B.R. is admitted to the hospital for further evaluation and treatment. A CBC reveals a WBC count of 22,000/mm^3 with 80% lymphocytes and an absolute neutrophil count of 800/mm^3, Hgb of 11 g/dL, and platelet count of 70 × 10^9/L. Quantification of serum immunoglobulins reveals profound hypogammaglobulinemia. What are the possible causes of B.R.'s pneumonia, and what treatment is indicated?

[SI units: WBC count, 22 × 10^9/L; Hgb 110 g/L; platelets, 70 × 10^9/L]

Infections contribute significantly to morbidity and mortality in CLL. Immunoglobulin deficiency, abnormal T-cell function, and neutropenia contribute to the increased rate of both common and opportunistic infections.[93] Opportunistic infections (OIs) associated with alemtuzumab therapy include PCP, invasive fungal infections, viral infections, and listeria. The most commonly reported OI associated with alemtuzumab is CMV reactivation. The use of supplemental intravenous immune globulin (IVI_g) is controversial, particularly in the setting of acute infection due, in part, to high cost.[94] However, in patients with low immunoglobulin levels and recurrent infections requiring hospitalization, supplementation can be recommended.[93] Hospitalization for broad-spectrum antimicrobials for neutropenic fever and a thorough workup for opportunistic etiologies is warranted for B.R. Because B.R. has a significant pulmonary infection requiring hospitalization with a documented hypogammaglobulinemia, IVI_g therapy may be considered if his condition worsens.

NON–HODGKIN LYMPHOMA

Clinical Presentation

20. R.G., a 39-year-old female, presents with complaints of swollen lymph nodes and occasional fevers and night sweats over the past month. Physical examination reveals marked cervical, supraclavicular, and inguinal lymphadenopathy >2 cm. Laboratory values are normal with the exception of a mild anemia (Hgb, 11 g/dL) and a slightly elevated LDH. HIV and hepatitis B surface antibody and antigen are negative. Excisional biopsy of a supraclavicular lymph node and immunophenotyping confirms a diagnosis of diffuse large B-cell (DLBC) lymphoma. Flow cytometry is positive for CD20, CD22, CD38, and CD45 surface markers. How does this type of lymphoma differ from other types of NHL?

Lymphomas are a heterogeneous group of disorders that arise from malignant transformation of lymphocytes (B cells, T cells, or natural killer [NK] cells) in the lymphoid system. Approximately 63,000 new cases of NHL are diagnosed annually, making it the fifth most common new cancer in both men and women in the United States.[58] More than 80% of NHL are B-cell neoplasms, with follicular lymphoma and DLBC as the most common subtypes.[3]

Hundreds of lymph nodes designed to process antigens present in the lymphatic fluid can be found throughout the body. Lymph nodes consist of a capsule, cortex, medulla, and

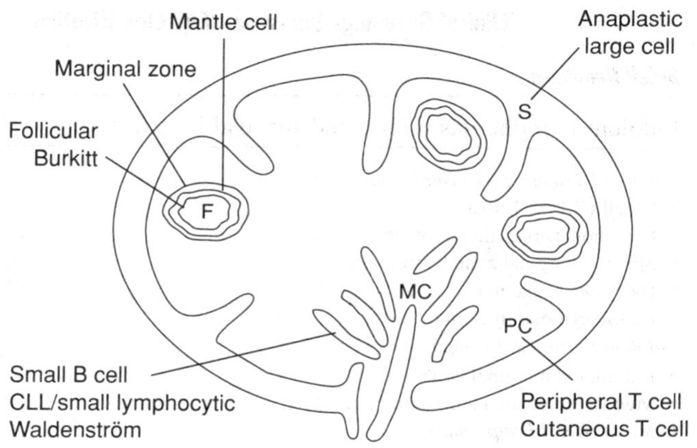

FIGURE 90-1 Sites of origin of malignant lymphomas in a lymph node according to anatomical and functional compartments of the immune system. CLL, chronic lymphocytic leukemia; F, follicles, or germinal centers; MC, medullary cords; PC, paracortex, or interfollicular areas; S, sinuses.

sinuses with anatomical and functional compartments, such as follicular (germinal) centers, follicular mantle, and interfollicular and medullary areas (Fig. 90-1). The growth pattern of lymphoma is described as follicular when malignant B cells take over normal germinal centers of lymph follicles. When the normal architecture of the lymph node is totally replaced by a uniform population of neoplastic lymphocytes, the growth pattern is described as diffuse. Other morphologic features, such as cell type, size, and appearance are determined to establish the specific subtype of NHL and are helpful in determining the best treatment.[95]

Patients with slow-growing indolent lymphomas such as follicular or marginal zone lymphoma typically present with painless generalized lymphadenopathy that can be either transient or persistent. Presentation of fast-growing aggressive lymphomas, such as DLBC, is variable; most patients present with lymphadenopathy and extranodal involvement. The most common extranodal sites include the GI tract, skin, bone marrow, sinus, or central nervous system. Fever (>38°C), night sweats, and weight loss (>10% of body weight over 6 months) are defined as B symptoms and may be associated with more advanced or aggressive disease. Approximately one-third of patients with aggressive lymphomas will report B symptoms.[96]

Numerous classification systems have been used to categorize this diverse group of malignancies. One of the early classification systems was the WF, which classified NHLs into three broad groups (low, intermediate, and high grade) based on their morphology and clinical behavior. The REAL classification includes morphology, immunophenotype, cytogenetics, and clinical information. Clinical groupings—indolent, aggressive, and highly aggressive lymphomas—were added as part of the REAL classification (Table 90-9).[97,98] The WHO updated the REAL classification, including additional disease categories and removing clinical groupings (Table 90-10).[98] For the purpose of this text, the grouping of indolent, aggressive, and highly aggressive will be used. R.G. has DLBC lymphoma, which can be classified as an intermediate-grade lymphoma (WF), aggressive (REAL), and mature B-cell neoplasm (WHO).

Table 90-9 Clinical Groupings Based on REAL Classification

B-Cell Neoplasm	T-Cell and NK Cell Neoplasm
Indolent Lymphomas (Untreated survival is years)	
Indolent Disseminated Lymphomas/Leukemias	
• B-cell CLL/SLL/PLL	• T-cell CLL/PLL
• Lymphoplasmacytic lymphoma	• Large granular lymphocyte leukemia
• Splenic marginal zone lymphoma	
• Hairy cell leukemia	
• Plasmacytoma/myeloma	
Indolent Extranodal Lymphomas	
• Extranodal marginal zone	• Mycosis fungoides
• Mucosa-associated lymphoid tissue (MALT)	
Indolent Nodal Lymphomas	
• Marginal zone	
• Follicular center	
• Mantle cell	
Aggressive Lymphomas (Untreated survival is months)	
• Diffuse large B cell	• Anaplastic large cell • Peripheral T cell
Highly Aggressive Lymphomas/Leukemias (Untreated survival is weeks)	
• Precursor B lymphoblastic • Burkitt lymphoma	• Precursor T lymphoblastic blastic NK cell lymphoma • Adult T-cell lymphoma • Human T-cell leukemia virus type I

CLL, chronic lymphocytic leukemia; SLL, small lymphocytic lymphoma; PLL, prolymphocytic leukemia.
Adapted from reference 97.

Staging and Prognosis

Lymphoma is staged based on its distribution and the number of involved sites; presence or absence of extranodal involvement and constitutional symptoms using the Ann Arbor Staging Classification (Table 90-11).[99] In general, stage I or II is referred to as limited disease, whereas stage III or IV is considered advanced disease. The majority of patients with NHL present with advanced-stage disease. Due to the wide range of outcomes in patients with lymphoma, even within histologic subtypes, factors that predict both response to treatment and outcomes are used to determine overall prognosis and need for aggressive therapy. The International Prognostic Index (IPI) was designed to determine predictors of survival for aggressive lymphomas (Table 90-12). An age-adjusted model for patients younger than 60 years has also been developed (Table 90-13).[100] R.G. has advanced stage III_B disease, an aggressive lymphoma with a high/intermediate IPI; therefore, she will require treatment with systemic chemotherapy. Patients with a high-intermediate IPI have a 50% chance of being cured with standard therapy.[96]

Treatment

Aggressive Lymphomas

21. R.G. had a consultation with a hematologist, and several treatment options were discussed. R.G. elected to receive combination chemotherapy consisting of cyclophosphamide, doxorubicin, vincristine, and prednisone with rituximab (R-CHOP) every 21 days for six to eight cycles. She will then be referred to a radiation oncologist to determine whether she will receive additional benefit from radiation therapy. Is this considered standard therapy? What information should be included in her medication counseling?

Aggressive and highly aggressive lymphomas are potentially curable. Patients with nonbulky (<10 cm) localized stage I/II disease without B symptoms were typically treated with cyclophosphamide, doxorubicin, vincristine, and prednisone (CHOP) for three to eight cycles with or without radiotherapy. For patients with advanced disease; defined as bulky stage II or stage III/IV disease, CHOP for six to eight cycles had been established as the standard of care with a CR rate of 58%.[101] Phase II trials comparing CHOP versus other regimens (m-BACOD, MACOP-B, ProMACE-CytaBOM) appeared promising; however, phase III data showed no difference in CR rate or 3-year survival. Increased toxicities, including fatal toxicity, was described in the non-CHOP arms.[102,103]

The effect of dose intensity (reduction of treatment interval from 3 weeks to 2 weeks) on response was investigated in a study of patients ages 61 to 75 years comparing CHOP every 14 days with traditional CHOP every 21 days. A significant ($p < 0.05$) increase in CR, 5-year eventfree survival (EFS) and 5-year OS was observed in the every 14-day CHOP arm.[104] Growth factor support with G-CSF was required in the every 14-day arm to prevent treatment delay. These results were not reproducible in patients ages 18 to 60 years.[105]

More recently, the Groups d'Étude des Lymphomas de l'Adult compared the 5-year follow-up of CHOP to R-CHOP in

Table 90-10 Proposed World Health Organization Classification of Lymphoid Neoplasms

B-cell neoplasms
- Precursor B-cell neoplasm
  - **Precursor B-lymphoblastic leukemia/lymphoma (precursor B-cell acute lymphoblastic leukemia)**
- Mature (peripheral) B-cell neoplasms[a]
  - **B-cell chronic lymphocytic leukemia/small lymphocytic lymphoma**
  - B-cell prolymphocytic leukemia
  - Lymphoplasmacytic lymphoma
  - Splenic marginal zone B-cell lymphoma (± villous lymphocytes)
  - Hairy cell leukemia
  - **Plasma cell myeloma/plasmacytoma**
  - **Extranodal marginal zone B-cell lymphoma of MALT type**
  - Nodal marginal zone B-cell lymphoma (± monocytoid B cells)
  - **Follicular lymphoma**
  - **Mantle cell lymphoma**
  - **Diffuse large B-cell lymphoma**
    - Mediastinal large B-cell lymphoma
    - Primary effusion lymphoma
  - **Burkitt lymphoma/Burkitt cell leukemia**

T-cell and NK cell neoplasms
- Precursor T-cell neoplasm
  - **Precursor T lymphoblastic lymphoma/leukemia (precursor T-cell acute lymphoblastic leukemia)**
- Mature (peripheral) T-cell neoplasms[a]
  - T-cell prolymphocytic leukemia
  - T-cell granular lymphocytic leukemia
  - Aggressive NK cell leukemia
  - Adult T-cell lymphoma/leukemia (HTLV1+)
  - Extranodal NK/T-cell lymphoma, nasal type
  - Enteropathy-type T-cell lymphoma
  - Hepatosplenic gamma-delta T-cell lymphoma
  - Subcutaneous panniculitislike T-cell/lymphoma
  - **Mycosis fungoides/Sézary syndrome**
  - Anaplastic large cell lymphoma, T-/null cell, primary cutaneous type
  - **Peripheral T-cell lymphoma, not otherwise characterized**
  - **Angioimmunoblastic T-cell lymphoma**
  - **Anaplastic large cell lymphoma, T-/null cell, primary systemic type**

Hodgkin lymphoma (Hodgkin disease)
- Nodular lymphocyte-predominant Hodgkin lymphoma
- Classical Hodgkin lymphoma
  - **Nodular sclerosis Hodgkin lymphoma (grades 1 and 2)**
  - Lymphocyte-rich classical Hodgkin lymphoma
  - **Mixed cellularity Hodgkin lymphoma**
  - Lymphocyte depleted Hodgkin lymphoma

Note. Only major categories are included. Subtypes and variants are discussed in the WHO book.[410] Common entities are shown in **boldface** type.
[a]B- and T-/NK cell neoplasms are grouped according to major clinical presentations (predominantly disseminated/leukemic, primary extranodal, predominantly nodal).
MALT, mucosa-associated lymphoid tissue; NK, natural killer; HTLV1+, human T-cell leukemia virus.
From reference 98.

Table 90-11 Ann Arbor Staging Classification of Lymphoma

Stage	Number of Lymph Nodes	Same Side of Diaphragm	Extranodal Disease
I	Single	N/A	–
II	Multiple	+	–
III	Multiple	–	–
IV	Multiple	±	+
Additional Nomenclature			
A	Absence of B symptoms		
B	Presence B symptoms		
E	Extranodal disease		
X	Bulky disease (>10 cm)		

N/A, not applicable.
From reference 411.

Table 90-12 International Prognostic Index

Risk Factors	Risk Group	Number of Risk Factors	5-Year Survival Rate (%)
All patients Age ≥60 years LDH >normal Performance status ≥2 Ann Arbor stage III/IV Extranodal involvement >1 site	Low	0–1	73
	Low-intermediate	2	51
	High-intermediate	3	43
	High	4–5	26

Adapted from reference 100.

Table 90-13 Age-Adjusted International Prognostic Index

Risk Factors	Risk Group	Number of Risk Factors	5-Year Survival Rate (%)
Age ≤60 years LDH >normal Performance status ≥2 Ann Arbor stage III/IV	Low	0	83
	Low-intermediate	1	69
	High-intermediate	2	46
	High	3	32

From reference 100.

newly diagnosed DLBC patients ages 60 to 80 years. Rituximab is a chimeric human monoclonal antibody to the B-cell surface antigen CD20. Although the exact mechanism is unknown, rituximab is believed to induce lysis through complement-mediated destruction, antibody-dependent cytotoxicity, and induction of apoptosis working in synergy with chemotherapy.[106] EFS, progressionfree survival (PFS), DFS, and OS was higher in the R-CHOP arm. No additional significant long-term toxicity was apparent.[107] Because these results have been confirmed in both young and elderly patients, R-CHOP has become the standard of care in the United States.[108,109]

The standard dose of rituximab is 375 mg/m^2 given intravenously in a variety of dosing schedules. The first infusion should be administered at a rate of 50 mg/hour and can be increased every 30 minutes to a maximum of 400 mg/hour. Subsequent infusions can be initiated at a rate of 100 mg/hour and increased to 400 mg/hour as tolerated. An infusion-related complex consisting of fever, chills, and rigors may occur during rituximab infusion, necessitating premedication. Other less common infusion-related symptoms include nausea, urticaria, pruritus, bronchospasm, angioedema, and hypotension. These reactions generally occur within 30 minutes to 2 hours from the start of the infusion (typically, the first dose) and resolve if the infusion is slowed or interrupted. Another less common side effect associated with rituximab is TLS, which occurs mostly in patients with a high number of circulating CD20-positive cells.[110]

Safety precautions prior to administration of the CHOP regimen include documentation of a normal cardiac ejection fraction (EF) and a baseline peripheral neuropathy assessment. Antiemetics should be given prior to administration to prevent nausea or vomiting, and a bowel regimen should be initiated to prevent constipation. Prophylaxis against febrile neutropenia with G-CSF post chemotherapy should be considered.

22. R.G. has a CR to R-CHOP therapy demonstrated by restaging studies performed after her third and sixth cycle of treatment. Every 3 months, she has a follow-up examination for disease recurrence. At her 15-month follow-up visit, she has radiographic evidence of disease recurrence in her abdomen. What treatment options are available to R.G. at this time?

High-dose chemotherapy immediately followed by autologous HCT should be considered for patients who relapse after conventional chemotherapy. Salvage chemotherapy regimens are administered prior to transplant to assure the disease is sensitive to additional cytotoxic therapy. Regimens use non cross-resistant agents such as ICE (ifosfamide, carboplatin, etoposide) ± rituximab, DHAP (dexamethasone, cytarabine, cisplatin) ± rituximab, and ESHAP (etoposide, methylprednisolone, cytarabine, cisplatin) ± rituximab. Patients who have responded to conventional therapy and demonstrated chemosensitive disease at relapse have the best outcome from HCT. Transplant is not recommended as initial therapy or for those with chemorefractory disease.[111] Allogeneic transplant should be reserved for those who have relapsed after autologous SCT, and the risk–benefit profile should be considered. R.G. received three cycles of R-ICE chemotherapy, and then her stem cells were collected for autologous HCT.

23. How does treatment differ for highly aggressive NHL?

Highly aggressive NHL, such as lymphoblastic or Burkitt lymphoma, progresses very rapidly and commonly metastasizes to the CNS.[95] The majority of adult patients can be cured with aggressive combination therapy. Regimens such as R-CHOP may not be intensive enough to prevent progression between cycles of therapy. Therefore, regimens similar to those for ALL are used because they provide more continuous exposure to more intensive chemotherapy. The hyper-CVAD regimen (hyperfractionated cyclophosphamide, vincristine, doxorubicin, and dexamethasone, alternating with high-dose methotrexate and cytarabine) has a CR rate of 91%.[112] These regimens must include CNS prophylaxis with intrathecal methotrexate or cytarabine.[95] These patients are at increased risk for TLS and should be treated with allopurinol, vigorous IV hydration, and electrolytes.

Indolent Lymphoma

CLINICAL PRESENTATION

24. D.J. is a 64-year-old male who presents to his physician complaining of low-grade fevers and a constant "bloated feeling," despite taking over-the-counter aluminum hydroxide and famotidine. He was otherwise asymptomatic, denying recent weight loss or night sweats. On physical examination, axillary adenopathy was found. An excisional biopsy and pathological examination revealed CD20-positive follicular B-cell lymphoma. CT scans of the chest, abdomen, and pelvis showed axillary and mediastinal lymphadenopathy. What are appropriate treatment options at this time?

The goal of therapy for indolent lymphomas is typically palliative because few patients will be cured of disease. However, the progression of the disease is typically very slow, and median survival is 8 to 12 years after diagnosis.[96] Treatment of localized disease, defined as nonbulky stage I or II, includes radiation with or without systemic therapy. Approximately half of the patients with localized disease will remain lymphoma free at 10 years with radiation therapy alone.[96] The addition of chemotherapy has not been shown to improve OS.[88]

Treatment for advanced disease (bulky stage II, stage III, or IV) is individualized based on age, performance status, comorbid disease states, disease progression, and future transplant possibility. The choice for initial therapy is controversial because observation alone has been associated with a 5-year survival of more than 75%.[113] Most experts advocate treating these patients only after they become symptomatic. Calculation of the Follicular Lymphoma International Prognostic Index (FLIPI) score may also guide treatment decisions (Table 90-14). D.J.'s disease is stage II with a low-intermediate FLIPI score for which he decides to pursue localized radiation therapy and to delay systemic therapy until he becomes symptomatic.

TREATMENT

25. D.J. remains asymptomatic for 3 years. At this time, he develops abdominal and splenic lymphadenopathy, night sweats, and weight loss over a 2-month period. What treatment options are available for D.J.?

Table 90-14 Follicular Lymphoma International Prognostic Index (FLIPI criteria)

Risk Factors	Risk Group	Number of Risk Factors	10-Year Overall Survival (%)
All patients	Low	0–1	70
Age >60 years			
LDH >normal	Low-intermediate	2	50
Hemoglobin <12 g/dL			
Ann Arbor stage III or IV	High	>3	35
Extranodal involvement >5 sites[a]			

[a]Nodal sights include cervical, axillary, mesenteric, inguinal, mediastinal, and para-aortic.
Adapted from references 412 and 413.

Chemotherapy options include single-agent rituximab with a CR rate of 15% and OR rate of 64%, which may be extended by maintenance rituximab.[114] No improvement in OS has been reported. Rituximab, in combination with chemotherapy regimens such as CHOP or cyclophosphamide, vincristine, and prednisone (CVP), achieve higher CR rates and extend the duration of response.[115,116] Other options include purine analogs alone or in combination, such as FND (fludarabine, mitoxantrone, dexamethasone) with or without rituximab, or oral alkylating agents such as chlorambucil or cyclophosphamide.[88,117] The National Comprehensive Cancer Network practice guideline recommends treatment with a rituximab-containing regimen unless contraindicated, although definitive evidence supporting a survival advantage is lacking.[88] A cardiac echocardiogram reports D.J.'s EF as 40%. Therefore, a nonanthracycline-containing regimen (R-CVP) was selected.

26. **D.J. is 6 years out from his initial diagnosis. His disease was stable for 2 years after treatment with R-CVP. However, his most recent CT scan shows progression of his disease. The decision is made to administer single-agent rituximab to D.J. His daughter read on a lymphoma website that rituximab has been combined with radiation (radioimmunotherapy) and transplantation. She asks if these options would be appropriate for D.J.**

Relapsed disease is treated with the same modalities as first-line treatment. Retreatment with rituximab has been found to be efficacious without additional toxicities.[118] Radioimmunoconjugates are monoclonal antibodies (rituximab) linked to radioisotopes that target CD20-positive lymphoma cells, which deliver local radiation therapy. Although radioimmunotherapy may be used first line, it is most often used in the setting of relapsed disease.[119,120] Both iodine-131 (^{131}I) tositumomab and yttrium-90 (^{90}Y) ibritumomab tiuxetan have been developed to treat follicular lymphomas. Both contain anti-CD20 antibodies with β-emitting radioisotopes. ^{131}I tositumomab also emits gamma irradiation.

Patients are candidates if they have <25% bone marrow involvement and $>100 \times 10^9$/L platelets due to the significant hematologic toxicity associated with radioimmunotherapy. Response rates are higher than those seen with rituximab therapy alone. However, due to the complicated administration and high cost, this treatment has not been widely used clinically. ^{131}I tositumomab patients should receive saturated solution of potassium iodide (two drops PO TID) at least 24 hours before the first dose is administered. This should be continued for 14 days after therapy to protect the thyroid gland. Because there are low-level radiation exposure is a concern, patients receiving either agent should be counseled to properly dispose of body fluids, carefully attend to personal hygiene, and limit their social contact for up to 7 days after administration. Hematologic toxicity can occur 7 to 9 weeks after administration, with a median duration of neutropenia and thrombocytopenia of approximately 3 weeks.[119]

High-dose chemotherapy followed by autologous HCT has a higher PFS and OS than standard therapy (RCHOP or other).[121] Patients in second remission should be referred for transplant evaluation. Use of radioimmunoconjugates as part of the preparative regimen prior to autologous HCT has also been explored.[122] Allogeneic or reduced intensity allogeneic HCT are additional options but require careful patient selection due to high risk of morbidity and mortality.[123] D.J. is not a transplant candidate because of his advanced age and EF.

HODGKIN LYMPHOMA

Clinical Presentation and Prognosis

27. **J.R. is a 55-year-old man with complaints of painless swelling around his collarbone, fever, night sweats, cough, and an unintentional 20-lb weight loss over the past 6 months. X-ray of the chest revealed a mediastinal mass, and a CT scan of the neck, chest, abdomen, and pelvis confirmed cervical and mediastinal lymph node enlargement, as well as multiple enlarged lymph nodes in the perisplenic and inguinal areas. A bone marrow biopsy was positive for lymphoma cells. Excisional biopsy of the cervical lymph node revealed nodular sclerosis Hodgkin lymphoma with Reed-Sternberg cells. Is this a typical presentation for Hodgkin lymphoma? What is J.R.'s prognosis?**

Hodgkin lymphoma (or HD) can occur at any age and represents <1% of all cancers in the United States. Presentation can be limited to a single lymph node or to an extralymphatic organ or site, or it can involve multiple lymph nodes and extralymphatic organs. The WHO classification of Hodgkin lymphoma is shown in Table 90-10. Nodular sclerosis Hodgkin lymphoma is the most common subtype and represents about two-thirds of cases. The Ann Arbor staging system for lymphomas is shown in Table 90-11.[99] J.R. has lymphadenopathy above and below the diaphragm and bone marrow involvement; therefore, he has stage IV disease. He has also been experiencing constitutional B symptoms (i.e., fever, night sweats, weight loss), which are designated by the letter B in the staging system. Hodgkin lymphoma is one of the few malignancies that is typically curable, even in the advanced stages. An analysis of patients with up to seven prognostic factors showed 5-year diseasefree progression of 42% to 82%.[124]

Treatment

28. J.R. is scheduled to begin chemotherapy with the ABVD (doxorubicin [Adriamycin], bleomycin, vinblastine, and dacarbazine) regimen. Is this the optimal initial treatment?

Multiple combination chemotherapy regimens have been developed; however, none have demonstrated superiority to ABVD in patients with advanced Hodgkin lymphoma. Other regimens evaluated include MOPP (mechlorethamine, vincristine, procarbazine, and prednisone), BEACOPP (bleomycin, etoposide, doxorubicin, cyclophosphamide, vincristine, procarbazine, and prednisone), and the Stanford V regimen (mechlorethamine, doxorubicin, etoposide, vincristine, vinblastine, bleomycin, and prednisone). In direct comparison with MOPP, ABVD has been shown to have an improved OS and a lower risk of both short- and long-term toxicities, including myelosuppression, infertility, and secondary leukemias.[125–127] Although promising results have been obtained with BEACOPP and Stanford V, they have not been compared with ABVD in well-designed, long-term studies evaluating survival and toxicity.

Hodgkin lymphoma is a chemotherapy-sensitive disease, and administration of full doses given on schedule is critical. Cycles of ABVD are given every 28 days, and all patients should continue treatment for two cycles beyond documentation of complete remission for a total of six to eight cycles. A significant toxicity associated with ABVD use is bleomycin-induced lung injury. Patients should be monitored for pulmonary symptoms and/or abnormal pulmonary function tests or x-rays of the chest. If any of these occur, bleomycin should be discontinued from further treatment. The deletion of bleomycin from ABVD in patients who have pulmonary complications does not appear to reduce long-term survival.[128]

Traditionally, all histologic subtypes of Hodgkin lymphoma have been treated in a similar fashion, and this remains the standard of care. One exception is nodular lymphocyte-predominant Hodgkin lymphoma (LPHL), which overexpresses CD20. Selected patients who are not candidates for standard chemotherapy may benefit from rituximab.[129] The future role of rituximab in combination treatment of LPHL remains to be determined, and these patients should be referred to ongoing clinical trials.

Relapsed Disease

29. J.R. achieved a complete remission and received a total of six courses of full-dose ABVD. Two years after completion of chemotherapy, a routine follow-up x-ray of the chest revealed enlarged lymph nodes, which were subsequently biopsied and found to be recurrent disease. What treatment should J.R. receive?

Patients with relapsed Hodgkin lymphoma have two main treatment options: salvage chemotherapy with or without radiation therapy, or high-dose chemotherapy with autologous stem cell support. Prognostic and patient-specific factors determine which avenue is optimal. Patients whose recurrence occurs in less than 1 year following initial therapy and have stage III or IV disease at relapse need more aggressive therapy if age and performance status permit.[130] Because it has been more than 1 year since he completed initial chemotherapy and he does not have stage III or IV disease, J.R. should be offered salvage chemotherapy. Regimens such as ESHAP, DHAP, or ICE could be considered, along with others. DFS for patients who relapse 1 year or later after initial therapy and are treated with salvage chemotherapy is 45% at 20 years.[131]

MULTIPLE MYELOMA

Clinical Presentation

30. Z.C. is a 59-year-old man who presents with low back pain that has increased over the past month and fatigue. He has been self-medicating his back pain with over-the-counter nonsteroidal anti-inflammatory drugs (NSAIDs), but has achieved little relief. Plain films of the spine show a compression fracture at the L1 level. Further workup reveals hemoglobin (Hgb) of 9 g/dL, serum calcium of 11.5 mg/dL, and serum creatinine of 2.1 mg/dL. Serum and urine protein electrophoreses reveal a monoclonal protein typed as IgG lambda of 8.8 g/dL, IgA of 0.008 g/dL, and IgM of 0.025 g/dL. A 24-hour urine collection showed 5.2 g total protein, with 77% Bence Jones proteins. A serum β-2-microglobulin was 5.7 mg/L. Bone marrow biopsy reveals 47% plasma cells with normal cytogenetics. Skeletal survey shows additional lesions in the skull and ribs. A diagnosis of multiple myeloma (MM) stage III is made. Is this presentation consistent with the diagnosis of MM?

[SI units: Hgb, 90 g/L (normal, 135–165); calcium, 2.5 mmol/L (normal, 2.13–2.55); creatinine, 212.2 μmol/L (normal, 70.7–123.8); IgG, 0.088 g/L (normal, 0.005–0.016); IgA, 0.00008 g/L (normal, 0.0004–0.004); IgM, 0.00025 g/L (normal, 0.0003–0.002); β-2-microglobulin, 0.0045 g/L (normal, 0.0011–0.0025)]

MM is a malignancy of fully differentiated B lymphocytes called "plasma cells." Proliferation and accumulation of plasma cells leads to excessive antibody (immunoglobulin) production, typically IgG or IgA. A variety of clinical manifestations can be seen and are related to excessive immunoglobulin production, plasma cell infiltration, and immune deficiency. Of patients who develop MM, 55% are male, and 98% are 40 years or older.[132,133] The disease occurs twice as often in blacks compared with whites and has increased in each decade since the 1970s.[132] Z.C. presents with a number of the classic features of MM. Bone pain and skeletal disease are common and occur when plasma cells infiltrate the bone marrow and secrete osteoclast-activating factors (e.g., IL-6, tumor necrosis factor, parathyroid hormone–related peptide). Plain radiographic films will reveal osteopenia and/or multiple osteolytic bone lesions (punched-out areas on radiographs). Hypercalcemia and pathological fractures often accompany the osteolytic lesions associated with this disease. When plasma cells infiltrate the bone marrow, they can also lead to a normocytic normochromic anemia in up to 70% of patients. Comparatively, neutropenia and thrombocytopenia are rarely present at the time of diagnosis. Renal dysfunction is generally attributable to deposition of kappa or lambda light chains of immunoglobulin in the distal tubule, and up to 50% of patients have or will develop renal insufficiency with the disease.[134] In most patients with MM, only light chains are found in the urine. Myelomas that overproduce light chains are most commonly associated with renal dysfunction. Renal dysfunction can be further complicated by dehydration secondary to hypercalcemia, the use of NSAIDs for pain relief, and the use of contrast dyes in radiographic evaluation. Z.C. should receive hydration with a sodium chloride–containing solution to restore euvolemia and reduce his calcium; he should avoid NSAIDs and other nephrotoxic therapies. Another feature that may accompany MM is hyperviscosity syndrome, more commonly seen with IgA subtype. Hyperviscosity causes CNS, renal, cardiac, and pulmonary symptoms and complications. Plasmapheresis may be used emergently to alleviate life-threatening cases. Patients may develop recurrent infections as a result of depressed production of other immunoglobulin classes, leading to an inability to opsonize bacteria.

Staging and Prognosis

Plasma cell disorders comprise a spectrum of disorders that range from monoclonal gammopathy of undetermined significance to MM.[135] Differential diagnoses for all plasma cell disorders are shown in Table 90-15. Z.C. clearly meets the criteria for MM. The prognosis for patients diagnosed with MM has traditionally been based on tumor mass and end-organ damage (hypercalcemia, renal dysfunction, anemia, and bone lesions), but recently a large international study demonstrated that staging and prognosis can be predicted reliably from serum β-2-microglobulin (a light chain protein expressed on all nucleated cells) and albumin (Table 90-16).[136] Median survival is 62 months for patients with stage I disease and 29 months for patients with stage III disease.[136] Evaluation of bone marrow cytogenetics also helps determine prognosis. Patients who have deletions of chromosome 13 or 17 and those with a 4;14 or 14;16 translocation have lower responses to initial therapy and shorter times to progression than those without the abnormalities.[137] Based on his serum β-2-microglobulin, Z.C. has stage III disease.

Table 90-15 Diagnostic Criteria for Plasma Cell Disorders[a]

Multiple Myeloma

1. Presence of a serum or urinary monoclonal immunoglobulin protein
2. Presence of clonal plasma cells in the bone marrow or a plasmacytoma
3. Presence of end-organ damage related to plasma cell proliferation, including:
   - Elevated calcium (1 mg/dL above the upper limit of the normal range, or >11 mg/dL)
   - Renal insufficiency (creatinine >1.9 mg/dL)
   - Anemia (2 g/dL below the lower limit of the normal range, or <10 g/dL)
   - Bone lesions (lytic lesions or osteoporosis with compression fractures)

Asymptomatic (Smoldering) Multiple Myeloma

1. Serum monoclonal immunoglobulin >3 g/dL and/or bone marrow plasma cells >10%
2. No end-organ damage related to plasma cell proliferation

Monoclonal Gammopathy of Undetermined Significance

1. Serum monoclonal immunoglobulin <3 g/dL
2. Bone marrow plasma cells <10%
3. No end-organ damage related to plasma cell proliferation

[a] All criteria must be met.
Adapted from reference 135.

Table 90-16 International Staging System for Multiple Myeloma

Stage I—β-2-microglobulin <3.5 mg/L and serum albumin ≥3.5 g/dL
Stage II—neither stage I nor stage III
Stage III—β-2-microglobulin ≥5.5 mg/L

Adapted from reference 136.

Treatment

Initial Therapy

31. The decision is made to begin Z.C. on thalidomide plus dexamethasone. What advantages and disadvantages does this regimen have compared with others?

Patients who meet the diagnostic criteria for MM and who are symptomatic are candidates for systemic chemotherapy (Table 90-17). Prior to treatment initiation, all patients should be evaluated for high-dose chemotherapy with autologous HCT. Those who are eligible for HCT should not be treated with alkylating agents (e.g., melphalan) before the stem cell collection because use of this class of agents may compromise the ability to collect a sufficient number of cells to perform the procedure. Agents such as thalidomide, dexamethasone, doxorubicin, and vincristine have been shown to be effective in induction regimens and do not reduce stem cell yield.

Thalidomide is an immunomodulatory agent with antiangiogenic properties, which are effective in patients with MM. Doses of thalidomide have ranged from 200 to 800 mg daily in the evening. Common adverse effects include sedation, constipation, thrombotic events, and neuropathies. Because of teratogenic effects, thalidomide is available only through a restricted distribution program, and patients must be thoroughly counseled about contraception. Dexamethasone is moderately effective as induction therapy alone and in combination, but has significant adverse effects, including hyperglycemia, insomnia, and increased infection risk.[138] The combination of thalidomide and dexamethasone was compared to dexamethasone alone in 207 previously untreated patients.[139] Response to the combination was 63% compared to 41% with single-agent dexamethasone; however, significant adverse events were also more common with the combination (34% vs. 18%, respectively). Combination therapy with vincristine, doxorubicin, and dexamethasone is another option for patients eligible for autologous HCT. The conventional VAD (vincristine, doxorubicin [Adriamycin], dexamethasone) regimen is a 4-day infusional treatment that was historically preferred over melphalan-based regimens because the response was more rapid and caused less myelosuppression. However, the requirement of a central

Table 90-17 Multiple Myeloma Treatment Regimens

Regimen	*Agents*	*Comments*
Induction Therapy		
Eligible for High-Dose Chemotherapy With Autologous Stem Cell Support		
Thalidomide + dexamethasone	Thalidomide 200 mg PO daily Dexamethasone 40 mg PO daily, days 1–4, 9–12, 17–20 Repeat cycle Q 28 days	Thalidomide should be given in the evening to minimize sedation. Antithrombotic prophylaxis is recommended. Thalidomide ± dexamethasone may also be used as salvage therapy.
DVD	Pegylated liposomal doxorubicin (Doxil) 40 mg/m^2 mg IV once, day 1 Vincristine 1.4 mg/m^2 (max 2 mg) IV once, day 1 Dexamethasone 40 mg PO daily, days 1–4 Repeat cycle Q 28 days	
VAD	Vincristine 0.4 mg/day CIV, days 1–4 Doxorubicin 9 mg/m^2/day CIV, days 1–4 Dexamethasone 40 mg PO daily, days 1–4, 9–12, 17–20 Repeat cycle Q 28 days	Should be administered through an indwelling central venous catheter to reduce extravasation risk. May also be used as salvage therapy.
Dexamethasone	Dexamethasone 40 mg PO daily, days 1–4, 9–12, 17–20 Repeat cycle Q 35 days	
Ineligible for High-Dose Chemotherapy With Autologous Stem Cell Support		
MPT	Melphalan 4 mg/m^2 PO daily, days 1–7 Prednisone 40 mg/m^2 PO daily, days 1–7 Thalidomide 100 mg PO daily Repeat cycle Q 28 days	Melphalan should be given on an empty stomach due to variable absorption when administered with food.
MP	Melphalan 8–10 mg/m^2 PO daily, days 1–4 Prednisone 60 mg/m^2 PO daily, days 1–4 Repeat cycle Q 28–42 days	
Salvage Therapy		
Bortezomib	Bortezomib 1.3 mg/m^2 IV once, days 1, 4, 8, 11 Repeat cycle Q 21 days	Dose reduction to 1 mg/m^2 may be necessary in patients with neuropathy and/or thrombocytopenia. Addition of dexamethasone may be required in patients who do not respond.
Lenalidomide + dexamethasone	Lenalidomide 25 mg PO daily, days 1–21 Dexamethasone 40 mg PO daily, days 1–4, 9–12, 17–20 for the first four cycles, then days 1–4 only in subsequent cycles	Consider prophylactic antithrombotics.
DT-PACE	Dexamethasone 40 mg PO daily, days 1–4 Thalidomide 400 mg PO daily at night Cisplatin 10 mg/m^2/day CIV days 1–4 Doxorubicin 10 mg/m^2/day CIV days 1–4 Cyclophosphamide 400 mg/m^2/day CIV days 1–4 Etoposide 40 mg/m^2/day CIV days 1–4	Thromboembolic events with thalidomide are increased in combination with doxorubicin and require prophylactic antithrombotics.

CIV, continuous intravenous infusion.

venous access device and the length of IV therapy make this a more cumbersome treatment. The substitution of pegylated liposomal doxorubicin (Doxil) for conventional doxorubicin and administration of vincristine on day 1 only with standard dexamethasone (DVD) makes this combination more convenient. A noninferiority comparison of VAD and DVD was conducted in 192 patients with untreated MM. The response was equivalent, and neutropenia, growth factor use, and alopecia were significantly lower in the DVD group, whereas hand-foot syndrome was more common.[140] To date, no comparison of induction with IV therapy and oral therapy has been made in patients eligible for autologous HCT.

In patients ineligible for autologous HCT, melphalan-based regimens are appropriate for induction therapy. Melphalan and prednisone (MP) was the first regimen to show significant activity in myeloma, but it rarely produces a complete remission. The addition of thalidomide to MP (MPT) was compared to MP in patients ages 60 to 85 years.[141] OR and CR rates were significantly improved with MPT (76%, 16%) compared to MP (48%, 2%). In addition, 2-year EFS was superior in patients receiving MPT compared to MP (54% vs. 27%). Thromboembolic events seen in the early part of the trial in patients receiving MPT led to the use of enoxaparin 40 mg SC daily, which reduced thromboembolism from 20% to 3%. Other toxicities seen more commonly with MPT included peripheral neuropathy, constipation, and infection, necessitating discontinuation of thalidomide in 33% of patients prior to completion of 2 months of therapy. Despite these toxicities, MPT is now considered the optimal induction therapy in patients ineligible for HCT.

Because Z.C. is eligible for autologous HCT and oral therapy is more convenient than IV therapy, the combination of thalidomide and dexamethasone is appropriate induction therapy.

Hematopoietic Cell Transplantation

Efforts to improve the outcome of MM treatment have led to the investigation of high-dose chemotherapy (e.g., melphalan 200 mg/m^2) with autologous stem cell support and nonmyeloablative regimens with allogeneic stem cell support. Randomized comparisons of autologous HCT and conventional chemotherapy in previously untreated patients younger than 65 years have been conducted.[142–145] All patients received two to six cycles of conventional chemotherapy before randomization to autologous HCT or standard chemotherapy. Most trials have reported higher response rates and improved survival in patients randomized to receive autologous HCT. Younger age, chemosensitive disease, and fewer pretransplant therapies have emerged as important predictive factors for response to autologous HCT. Despite flaws in study design, autologous HCT is regarded as the current treatment of choice for eligible patients with MM who achieve CRs following induction therapy.[146] The use of allogeneic HCT transplantation in MM is a potentially curative option, but has been associated with excessive mortality. Nonmyeloablative allogeneic regimens are generally associated with fewer regimen-related toxicities than full allogeneic transplants, but allow for a graft-versus-tumor effect that eradicates residual disease (see Chapter 92). Initial trials have been encouraging, particularly in patients who are not heavily pretreated and those with chemotherapy-sensitive disease.[147–149] Z.C. will receive four cycles of thalidomide and dexamethasone and will be evaluated for HCT.

Supportive Care

Bisphosphonates

32. Zoledronic acid 4 mg IV over 15 minutes every 28 days is ordered for Z.C. What is the rationale for bisphosphonate therapy in the presence of normal serum calcium? What benefits and toxicities are associated with bisphosphonate therapy?

The efficacy of IV pamidronate and zoledronic acid for the prevention of skeletal fractures in myeloma patients with osteolytic bone lesions or osteopenia has been established and guidelines for their use developed.[150] Equivalent efficacy with monthly infusion has been shown with pamidronate 90 mg and zoledronic acid 4 mg. Zoledronic acid can be given over 15 minutes, whereas pamidronate is given over 2 hours. Because bisphosphonates can negatively affect kidney function, serum creatinine should be monitored monthly and urine albumin measured every 3 months. Higher doses and shorter infusion times have been associated with renal damage; patients with creatinine clearances between 30 and 60 mL/minute should receive reduced doses of zoledronic acid. In patients with baseline creatinine values of >3 mg/dL, pamidronate 90 mg over 4 to 6 hours is recommended. Bisphosphonate therapy should be held in patients who have creatinine elevations above the normal baseline of 0.5 mg/dL or more until renal function returns to baseline. Osteonecrosis of the jaw (ONJ) is a rare but serious complication of bisphosphonate therapy that appears to increase in likelihood with prolonged treatment. Baseline dental examinations and avoidance of invasive dental procedures during therapy are recommended. The use of zoledronic acid has been associated with a 9.5-fold increased risk of ONJ compared to pamidronate.[151] All patients with responsive or stable disease should be strongly considered for bisphosphonate discontinuation after 2 years of treatment. Z.C. is a candidate for bisphosphonate therapy because he has lytic disease in the skull and ribs.

Relapsed and Refractory Disease

33. Z.C. receives four cycles of thalidomide and dexamethasone, followed by autologous HCT. Three years after HCT, he is found to have relapsed disease. What other therapies may offer benefit for his myeloma?

Treatment options for relapsed and refractory MM (salvage therapy) may include agents and regimens patients were not given in induction or other combinations (Table 90-17). Two newer agents for MM therapy are bortezomib and lenalidomide. Bortezomib acts by inhibiting the proteosome, a multienzyme complex responsible for regulation of proteins that promote cell survival, stimulate growth, and reduce susceptibility to programmed cell death. It is given for 2 weeks every 21 days for up to eight cycles. Dexamethasone 20 mg on the day of and after bortezomib may be added in patients who do not respond after two cycles. Common toxicities include sensory neuropathy, thrombocytopenia, and diarrhea; and dose reductions or omissions may be necessary for neuropathy and thrombocytopenia. In a comparison with dexamethasone, patients receiving bortezomib had a longer time to disease progression (6.2 months vs. 3.5 months) and better OS, leading to a recommendation to halt the dexamethasone arm and allow those patients to receive bortezomib.[152] Lenalidomide is an analog of thalidomide that is more potent with a more favorable toxicity profile. Unlike thalidomide, sedation, constipation, and neuropathy are not seen, but dose-related side effects do include thrombocytopenia and neutropenia. Lenalidomide also causes thromboembolic events and is only available through a restricted access program. The combination of lenalidomide and dexamethasone was compared with dexamethasone alone in 353 patients with relapsed or refractory MM.[153] OR was greater with the combination (61.0% vs. 19.9%); neutropenia was the most common toxicity (41.2% vs. 4.6%).

Results with single-agent thalidomide and few overlapping toxicities led to interest in combination therapy with conventional chemotherapy earlier in the course of disease. A regimen of two cycles of high-dose dexamethasone, thalidomide, and a 4-day continuous infusion of cisplatin, doxorubicin, cyclophosphamide, and etoposide (DT-PACE) given 4 to 6 weeks apart was evaluated in relapsed patients treated with two prior regimens who also remained candidates for HCT.[154] Treatment was delayed or reduced for neutrophil counts <1,000/mm^3 or platelet counts <100,000/mm^3. An OR rate of 48% was seen in patients able to receive full doses of therapy for both cycles. Significant differences were seen in both complete and partial response rates for patients receiving <100% of scheduled doses. Thromboembolic events necessitated anticoagulant prophylaxis during the study and neutropenia, thrombocytopenia, nausea, and sensory neuropathies were seen in 65%, 37%, 21%, and 13% of patients, respectively. DT-PACE represents an effective regimen in patients who can tolerate significant cytopenias and remain eligible for transplantation.

HEMATOLOGIC MALIGNANCIES: PEDIATRIC

ACUTE LYMPHOBLASTIC LEUKEMIA OF CHILDHOOD

The two most common types of childhood leukemia are acute lymphoblastic leukemia (ALL) and acute myelogenous leukemia (AML), with the former accounting for 75% of cases and the latter for approximately 19%. ALL is the most common childhood cancer, accounting for approximately 30% of all malignancies in children.[155] Approximately 2,400 new cases of childhood ALL occur each year in the United States, with an estimated incidence of 34 cases per million in children younger than 15 years.[155]

A distinct peak incidence occurs at ages 2 to 3 years for ALL (>80 cases/million), and then decreases substantially for 8 to 10 year olds (20 cases/million). A higher incidence of ALL is seen in white children than in black children. This racial difference is most apparent in the 2- to 3-year-old age group, with a nearly threefold greater incidence rate for white children. Over the past 20 years, the incidence rate of ALL in U.S. children has increased by approximately 0.9% per year. These incidence figures are derived from the Surveillance, Epidemiology and End Results Program (SEER), which collects data from nine tumor registries throughout the United States.[155] The nine registries account for approximately 13% of the U.S. population. Total U.S. incidence is then estimated by applying the SEER data to the total population size. It is unknown how reflective the SEER data are of the true U.S. incidence and/or if certain unmonitored regions may have significantly different rates of disease.

Before the early 1970s, ALL was a fatal illness; most children did not survive >2 to 3 months after diagnosis. Today, >80% of children will achieve prolonged survival with antileukemic therapy.[155,156] New innovations in therapy for ALL are now focusing on additional refinements in therapy to further improve on survival and to decrease the long-term morbidity associated with the therapeutic components of current treatment regimens.

Etiology

The etiology of ALL is unknown; however, several interesting associations have been discovered. A high incidence of leukemia was found among survivors of the atom bomb explosion in Japan during World War II, and those closest to the epicenter of the blast were at greatest risk.[157,158] Leukemia also occurs in children exposed to radiation in utero.[159] Other unproven factors that have been suggested to cause ALL include exposure to electromagnetic fields, pesticides, maternal use of alcohol, contraceptives, and cigarette smoking.[160–163] Viruses have not been proved to cause childhood ALL.[164] Evidence supporting an association between ALL and electromagnetic field exposure is currently inadequate.[155,165] In particular, the incidence of childhood ALL has not increased markedly over the past 40 years during a time when electricity use has seen a large increase.[166] Clusters of leukemia cases that occur over certain time frames and around certain places may represent merely instances of statistic coincidence.[167] Also of interest, there is a significant correlation between the incidence of childhood ALL and type 1 diabetes around the world. This was found to be related to socioeconomic variables, such as national prosperity, with an apparent relationship to an affluent lifestyle. It is hypothesized that affluence may lower infectious disease prevalence and the childhood exposure pattern to pathogens. This suggests that the prevention of infection in infancy may increase vulnerability to later disease by inappropriate modulation of a naïve infant immune system.[168] Because the incidence of childhood ALL in the United States has increased moderately over the past 20 years and because the SEER program samples data only from a small portion of the U.S. population and excludes several geographic regions, it is unclear whether significant variations in childhood ALL incidences across the nation may be related to certain environmental factors. Recent examination of the relationship between childhood leukemia and environmental benzene exposure demonstrated an association between dwellings close to sources of benzene and the risk of childhood leukemia, particularly for AML.[169]

Pathophysiology

The pathophysiology of ALL involves the replacement of normal bone marrow elements with a clone of immature lymphoid cells. The essential lesion in ALL is a stabilization of a malignant cell in the lymphocyte differentiation process. Many factors are involved in the control of normal cellular proliferation. Leukemia may represent a disruption in one or more of the normal relationships within the cell proliferation pathway, such as an abnormal response to lymphoid cell growth factors.[170]

With the availability of classification systems of lymphoblasts based on morphology, immunology, and cytogenetics, it has become clear that ALL is a heterogeneous disease. This is especially true with regard to cytogenetic abnormalities. The immunologic heterogeneity results from leukemic transformation at various stages of lymphocyte differentiation. In addition, an emerging classification involving gene expression profiling may allow for further classification of ALL cytogenetic subtypes, potentially allowing for prediction of response and adverse events.[171] As discussed later in this section, these classifications have important prognostic value.

Clinical Presentation

The signs and symptoms of ALL are nonspecific, and many are shared with other childhood diseases such as juvenile rheumatoid arthritis (JRA). This occasionally leads to a child with ALL being mistakenly treated with corticosteroids for JRA. As a general rule, children should not be treated with chronic corticosteroids without first performing a CBC and/or a bone marrow aspirate. These signs and symptoms reflect the uncontrolled growth and differentiation of the leukemic clone and the resulting deficiency in normal bone marrow elements, namely, neutrophils, RBCs, and platelets. Frequent clinical findings include fever (61%), bleeding (48%), and bone pain (23%).[172] Bone pain is believed to be the result of hypercellular bone marrow and infiltration of leukemic lymphoblasts into pain-sensitive structures such as the periosteum. Although bone pain may be severe, it quickly resolves once chemotherapy is initiated. On physical examination, many patients have lymphadenopathy (50%), splenomegaly (63%), and/or hepatosplenomegaly (68%).[172]

A CBC will demonstrate that at least 59% of patients have a normal or low WBC count; the remainder have elevated counts.[172] The WBC differential reveals a low percentage of neutrophils and bands and a marked lymphocytosis. Lymphoblasts may be present in the peripheral blood even with a low WBC count (e.g., 2,000–4,000/mm^3), but they are more likely when the WBC count is elevated.[174] A normochromic, normocytic anemia, along with thrombocytopenia, is present in most patients.[172]

A bone marrow aspirate and biopsy are usually necessary to confirm the diagnosis of ALL. Occasionally, in patients with elevated WBC counts, the diagnosis can be confirmed by studies of lymphoblasts in the peripheral blood. The diagnosis of ALL is made when at least 25% of lymphoid cells in the bone marrow are blasts.[173] Most ALL patients have far greater than 25% blasts, and many have complete replacement of bone marrow with lymphoblasts. Once a child is diagnosed with ALL, it is important to determine the various characteristics that influence treatment decisions and the prognosis.

Prognostic Variables

Clinical Variables

Certain clinical and laboratory findings that are present at diagnosis are important to predict a child's prognosis and to classify his or her risk stratification. Children with ALL are classified by their risk of relapse into one of the following categories: low, intermediate, high, or very high risk. It is important to stress that much debate continues over which variables most strongly influence patient outcome. One agreed that the most important risk-defining features of childhood ALL are age and initial WBC count.[174] However, several ongoing investigations are likely to further refine what constitutes different ALL risk populations.

WHITE BLOOD CELL COUNT

The initial WBC count is considered to be among the most important predictors of outcome in childhood ALL. Its importance as a prognostic feature is often retained after the adjustment for other important prognostic criteria.[173] Children with the highest WBC counts at presentation have the shortest duration of complete remissions.[175–177] There appears to be a linear relationship between the duration of remission and the WBC count at presentation (Fig. 90-2). Although exactly where the demarcation line is for predicting a good or a poor prognosis is unknown, an initial WBC count >50,000/mm^3 is generally associated with a poor prognosis.[174]

AGE

Patients younger than 1 year or older than 9.99 years of age at diagnosis tend to have worse prognoses.[174] At least one trial has demonstrated that more intensive therapy may overcome the adverse prognostic factor of adolescent age.[178] These investigators reported that young adults (16–21 years of age) with ALL have an EFS of approximately 60% at 6 years, which is similar to that of patients 10 to 15 years of age and superior to that achieved in most trials of older adults.[178] Age is

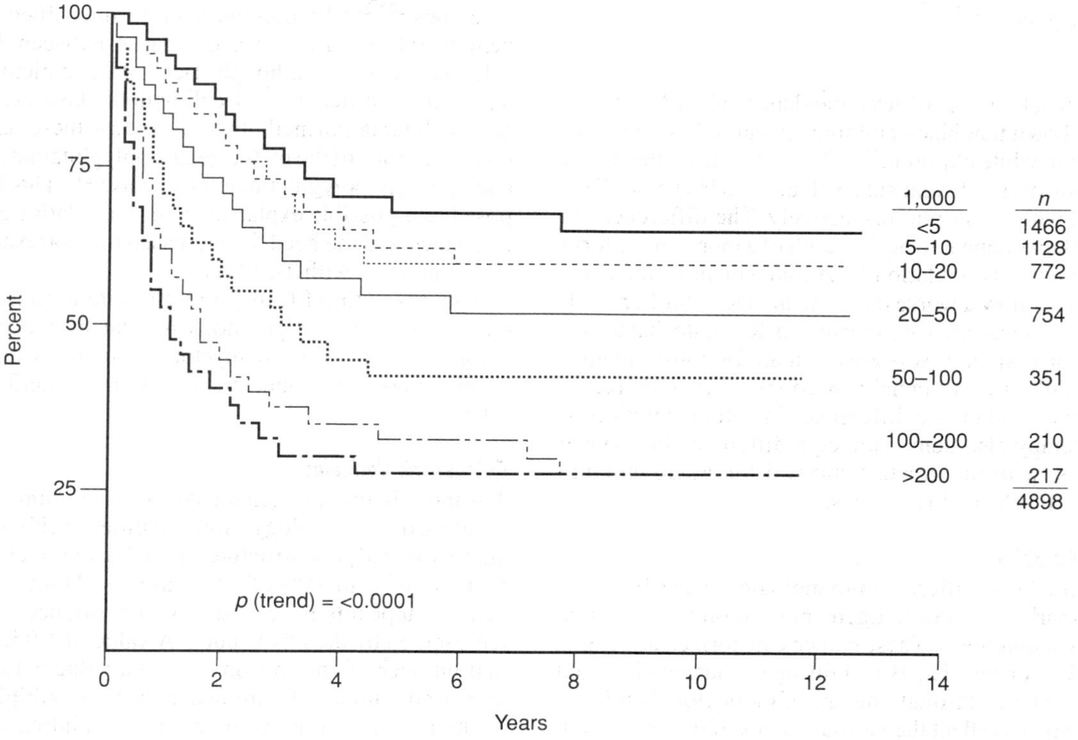

FIGURE 90-2 Percentage of children with acute lymphocytic leukemia in continuous complete remission stratified according to their white blood cell count at the time of diagnosis. *Source:* From reference 185. Reprinted with permission of Wiley-Liss, a subsidiary of John Wiley and Sons, Inc.

the strongest predictor of prognosis with regard to infants, a group in which survival is exceedingly poor compared with other age groups.[179–181] For this group, even with intensified chemotherapy regimens, long-term, DFS is usually <50%, especially when associated with cytogenetic aberrations involving the mixed lineage leukemia (MLL) locus.[182]

GENDER

Patient gender also has been shown to be an important prognostic factor in several studies.[183,184] Testicular relapse is responsible for a somewhat worse prognosis in males, but it is not believed to completely account for the better prognosis of females. However, occult testicular disease is usually not ruled out when males experience relapse. Another factor that may be of importance is the inherent ability of males to tolerate higher doses of chemotherapy.[185] Greater therapy tolerance in males suggests the need to use the maximum tolerated dose intensity to produce the same therapeutic effect achieved in females at lower doses. This finding may be due to a gender difference in the metabolism of certain chemotherapy agents.[186] Whether current improvements in the treatment of childhood ALL have nullified the adverse prognostic association of male gender has recently been re-evaluated. A large series examined the outcome in >2,000 patients treated over >30 years. Females had significantly better outcomes than males in the early era, and although prognosis improved for both genders, an approximate 10% EFS advantage in females remained during the modern era (73.4% vs. 63.5%). After accounting for differences in immunophenotype and DNA index between genders, these differences were no longer present. It was noted that males were significantly more likely to have T-cell ALL, and there was a trend for them to have a less favorable DNA index, indicating that these factors may be responsible for the adverse prognostic factor of male gender.[187]

RACE

Although blacks have a lower incidence of ALL, several studies have shown that black children appear to have a higher relapse rate than white children.[155,188–190] Data from the SEER program demonstrate a 5-year survival rate of 64% versus 78% for black and white children, respectively. The differences in outcome for blacks appear to be the result of a more severe form of ALL in this patient population.[189] A trial with more intensive therapy failed to show a worse outcome in black children.[191] It has also been demonstrated in a recent SEER update that the incidence rate for Hispanics was greater than for non-Hispanics and was the highest of all racial subgroups.[192] A more recent analysis of racial and ethnic differences in outcome with contemporary therapy also demonstrated a difference in survival among groups, with the greatest survival for Asian children and lowest for blacks and Hispanics.[193]

Immunologic Variables

ALL is classified into different immunologic subsets based on cell surface markers and/or antigens present on the leukemic lymphoblasts at diagnosis. These can be categorized as cells of B-cell and T-cell origin. The B-cell lineage is further classified into various subtypes through the use of monoclonal antibodies. These subtypes reflect the various stages of differentiation at which leukemia may develop. Approximately 15% to 20% of children with ALL have leukemia with a T-cell lineage,[194,195] and 1% to 2% of patients have leukemia with a mature B-cell origin.[195,196] Using more sophisticated diagnostic techniques, the majority of patients who were previously classified as non–T-, non–B-cell ALL (null cell ALL) are now known to have leukemia of a more immature B-cell lineage.[197,198,199] Most patients with B-cell lineage ALL (80%) have cells that are positive for the common ALL antigen (CALLA, designated CD10) on their surface[200,201]; this is referred to as common ALL. Additional markers, including CD19 and cytoplasmic immunoglobulin, have been used to further determine the level of differentiation of leukemic cells of the B-cell lineage. Intermediate cells of the B-cell lineage (pre–B cells) possess these markers, but more immature cells (early pre–B cells) do not.[198,202] More than 60% of children with ALL have a leukemia of the early pre–B subtype, and approximately 20% have a leukemia of pre–B cells.

Mature B-cell ALL (or Burkitt ALL) has traditionally been associated with a poor prognosis,[198,203,204] but prognosis has improved greatly with the advent of short-term, very intensive chemotherapy.[205,206] Although differences in outcome have been noted among the B-cell subtypes,[198] when other prognostic factors are considered and when effective therapy is used, these differences may no longer be evident.[183] At present, immunologic features that differentiate B-cell precursor, T-cell, and mature B-cell ALL are believed to be clinically important because different types of chemotherapeutic strategies are employed for these three immunophenotypes.[156,206]

Patients with T-cell ALL have several distinguishing features, including a greater likelihood of being older males with high initial WBC counts and the presence of a mediastinal mass and/or initial leukemic involvement of the CNS.[207,208] Patients with T-cell ALL historically have had a decreased survival, although more intensive treatment is improving their outcomes.[209,210] Studies with more intensified therapy also demonstrate no difference in relapse between T-cell and B-cell lineage ALL, although T-cell ALL patients tend to relapse much earlier.[211,212] T-cell lymphoblasts are less efficient at polyglutamation methotrexate because these cells have lower concentrations of the methotrexate polyglutamate synthesizing enzyme, folylpolyglutamate synthetase.[213] This has been proposed as a possible explanation for the relative chemotherapy resistance and the need for increased methotrexate dose intensity in patients with T-cell ALL.[156]

Patients with ALL may present with a mixed-cell lineage disease, containing lymphoblasts that also express myeloid antigens. Expression of myeloid antigens is not believed to be an important prognostic factor in predicting the risk of relapse.[156]

Cytogenetic Variables

Advances in chromosomal analysis have improved the understanding of ALL biology. Abnormalities in either chromosome number (ploidy) or structure of the leukemic clone have been found in 60% to 75% of ALL cases.[156] Many of these abnormalities appear to have prognostic importance.[156,214] Ploidy is represented by the DNA index. A value of 1.0 indicates a normal number of chromosomes, and a value >1.0 indicates an increased number of chromosomes by a multiplication factor of the normal chromosome number. Children with leukemia blasts containing >52 chromosomes (DNA index >1.16, hyperdiploid) appear to have an increased probability of continuous complete remission versus patients with leukemia blasts containing a diploid chromosome complement or with a DNA index <1.16.[214] Approximately 30% of ALL cases have a DNA index >1.16. Patients whose ALL cells are hyperdiploid also tend to have other favorable prognostic features.[214] For example, children with hyperdiploid ALL may have a more favorable prognosis owing to their increased sensitivity to chemotherapy. An in vitro study of hyperdiploid versus nonhyperdiploid ALL revealed that those cells with a higher DNA index were more sensitive to antimetabolites (e.g., mercaptopurine) and asparaginase.[215] Also, B-precursor hyperdiploid ALL cells contain more reduced folate carriers than diploid B-precursor blasts. Hyperdiploid cells have elevated levels of gene expression for these carriers, which may account for the higher levels of methotrexate polyglutamates noted in these cells as compared to patients with B-precursor diploid ALL.[216,217] In contrast, patients with hypodiploidy (<45 chromosomes and, in particular, those with 24–28 chromosomes) have a significantly worse outcome than nonhypodiploid patients.[218]

Translocations are the most common structural abnormalities occurring in leukemic cells[219] and occur in approximately 75% of childhood ALL cases.[220] Certain translocations are associated with treatment failure and relapse.[156] The translocations most commonly associated with treatment failure are the *MLL* rearrangements—t(4;11), t(11;19), and t(1;11)—and the *BCR-ABL* fusion transcript—t9;22, Philadelphia chromosome. In particular, children with the Philadelphia chromosome appear to represent a population at very high risk of relapse. This translocation occurs in approximately 2% to 5% of childhood ALL cases. A published review compared the outcome of 30 patients with this translocation from a group of 1,322 children enrolled on ALL studies. This study demonstrated a 4-year EFS estimate of only 20% for children with the Philadelphia translocation versus 76% in those without it. This difference remained regardless of patient age, initial WBC count, or rapidity of response to therapy. Most patients with this translocation who were event-free survivors underwent bone marrow transplantation during their first remission.[221] A second case series of 61 children with Philadelphia chromosome-positive ALL identified early treatment response as a strong independent predictor of outcome. In this latter trial, 65% of these patients had a good initial response and a lower risk of treatment failure with either intensive chemotherapy or bone marrow transplantation when compared with the poor initial responders (EFS = 55% vs. 10%, respectively).[222]

Using more sensitive (polymerase chain reaction [PCR]-based) methods than available with classic cytogenetic techniques, the previously unrecognized *TEL/AML1* rearrangement—t(12;21), *ETV6-CBFA2* fusion transcript—has now been identified as the most commonly occurring (approximately 18% of patients) translocation in childhood ALL. This translocation is associated with patients ages 1 to 10 years, and most are precursor B-cell type and nonhyperdiploid. The *TEL/AML1* translocation is an independent predictor of good prognosis; however, relapses tend to occur later in these patients, necessitating a long follow-up to determine the ultimate impact of this translocation.[220] At present, reducing the intensity of chemotherapy for children with this translocation is not recommended.[220] Also, a recent analysis has shown that this fusion transcript was not an independent predictor of outcome in multivariate analysis.[223]

The prognostic value of the main clinical variables can often be explained by cytogenetic abnormalities. For instance, most infants have rearrangements of the *MLL* gene. This abnormality, as well as the Philadelphia chromosome, occurs more often in adolescents and adults.[156] In addition, two cytogenetic abnormalities associated with improved outcome (hyperdiploidy and the *TEL-AML* translocation) are found mainly in the 1- to 9-year age group. In addition to the prognostic significance of the acquired genetic mutations, germ-line mutations may also predict outcomes. There are several polymorphisms that encode for proteins that can affect the pharmacodynamics of certain drugs used to treat ALL. Patients with high-risk ALL who had genotypes expressing greater glutathione S-transferase and thymidylate synthetase activity had a greater risk for relapse. These polymorphisms may be future targets for tailoring antileukemic therapy.[224]

Once a patient achieves complete remission, abnormalities of both ploidy and structure are not evident in the patient's recovered bone marrow by morphologic assessment, although a leukemic cell burden as large as 10^9 may remain.[225] However, new techniques based on PCR assays can detect minimum residual disease (MRD) in many patients.[225] If relapse does occur, the leukemic cell cytogenetic characteristics are usually identical to those observed at diagnosis.[219]

Early Response

An additional factor of prognostic importance in childhood ALL is that of early response to therapy. Several investigations have noted that early response, as measured by either clearance of blasts from the peripheral blood or morphologic bone marrow remission (e.g., <5% bone marrow blasts) on day 7 or 14 of therapy, is predictive of long-term DFS. In a review of 15 trials, early response was an independent prognostic factor in each study.[226] Response was most commonly measured based on morphologic evaluation of day 14 bone marrow results, and it appeared that assessment of early response was more sensitive with bone marrow studies. Children who were slow early responders were 2.7 times more likely to have an adverse event than those with more rapid clearance of blasts. Interestingly, the rapidity of response maintained its prognostic significance within different strata delineated by the initial WBC count, providing further evidence that this variable is an important independent marker of prognosis. The rapidity of response is an intuitive marker of treatment sensitivity. However, the use of morphologic criteria to assign responder status will still include many patients with a significant disease burden. It is important to note that such tests of bone marrow burden may represent a dilute sample or a decrease in marrow cellularity and may not reflect the total leukemia burden in the body. It is estimated that these measures of early response may detect up to 25% of children at risk for early relapse.[226] At present, rapid early response is defined as clearance of bone marrow blasts by day 15 of induction, whereas slow early response refers to the converse. Whether patients are rapid or slow early responders is now being used to determine the type and intensity of further chemotherapy because slow earlier responders benefit from more intensive postinduction chemotherapy.[227] Other groups have examined response to initial treatment with a 7-day course of prednisone (initiated prior to the start of systemic induction chemotherapy) in children with high-risk ALL. Prednisone-poor response, defined as patients with >1,000 blast cells/μL in peripheral blood after 7 days, was a predictor of poor outcome and was used to intensify induction therapy, with a consequent improvement in EFS.[228]

Minimum Residual Disease

Several investigators have examined the prognostic value of detecting MRD in bone marrow samples through the use of sophisticated PCR and flow cytometric–based assays. A variety of lymphoblast characteristics, including gene fusion transcripts, immunophenotype, and antigen receptor gene rearrangements, may be relied on for minimal disease detection in children with ALL. Although specific fusion transcripts can be relied on as PCR targets in only one-third of childhood ALL cases, clonal antigen receptor gene rearrangements occur in virtually all cases.[225] Using various techniques, approximately 50% of children with ALL are MRD positive at the completion of induction therapy, and roughly 45% of these patients will experience a relapse. The association for a negative test for MRD at the completion of induction therapy appears stronger because it has a negative predictive value of 92.5% and a positive predictive value of 44.5% at this time point. In patients positive for MRD, there is a continuous decrease in MRD during the months of chemotherapy treatment. Persistence of MRD beyond 4 to 6 months or re-emergence of MRD is almost always predictive of future relapse.[229] It is now established that the presence of MRD is an important prognostic factor, regardless of the patient's initial WBC count or age at presentation.[225] At the time of this writing, monitoring of MRD has become important in the management of childhood ALL and is being used to risk stratify treatment in current front-line leukemia studies.

Additional Variables

Several additional variables may determine the prognosis of children with ALL. A complete discussion of these factors is beyond the scope of this text, but a few of these deserve brief mention. In addition to having an increased risk for developing ALL, children with Down syndrome are at a slightly greater risk for treatment failure. Their adverse outcome has been ascribed to an excess of therapy-related toxicities, especially associated with high-dose methotrexate.[230] One variable that has not been traditionally listed as a prognostic factor is that of nutritional status. Although this is usually not an important variable in the United States and in developed nations, it may be a significant factor in Third World countries, which are home to the majority of the world's children. In several trials, the outcome in childhood ALL was significantly worse for malnourished patients, and in at least one trial, the most important predictor of relapse was malnutrition.[231] This may be related to a decrease in patient tolerance to chemotherapy. A malnutrition prevalence rate of up to 50% for children with ALL in Third World countries has been reported. When compared with socioeconomic status, malnutrition was more closely related to prognosis than was poverty. It appears that height for age is a more reliable predictor of prognosis than weight for age, suggesting that chronic stunting is more important than acute wasting in malnourished patients.[231]

These prognostic variables can be used to assign patients to various categories based on their risk of relapse. These categories are important in determining the therapy that patients should receive. Although there is considerable agreement regarding the importance of certain variables in assigning patients to a defined risk group (e.g., age, initial WBC, DNA index, translocations), institutions that treat ALL differ in their definitions of what constitutes high-, intermediate-, and low-risk patients. This makes it difficult to compare treatment results from different institutions or treatment groups. Last, newer prognostic variables, especially rapidly evolving cytogenetic prognosticators, complicate the comparisons of treatment regimens over time.

Treatment

Remission Induction Therapy

ALLOPURINOL INTERACTION

34. J.B. is a 4-year-old Hispanic boy presenting with a 2-week history of an upper respiratory tract infection and a 1-week history of otitis media. His symptoms have worsened, and he now presents with a nosebleed and fatigue. Physical examination reveals appreciable pallor and hepatosplenomegaly. A CBC with differential reveals a normochromic, normocytic anemia with Hct of 15.7% (normal, 39%–49%), Hgb of 5.7 g/dL (normal, 14–18), WBC count of 4,300/mm^3 (normal, 3,200–9,800), and platelet count of 13,000/mm^3 (normal, 150,000–400,000). A differential on the WBC count reveals 82% lymphocytes (normal, 30%–40%), 7% neutrophils (normal, 50%–60%), and 11% lymphoblasts (normal, 0%). Based on these findings, a bone marrow biopsy is performed, which reveals 95% lymphoblasts. A diagnosis of ALL is made. The immunologic class is early pre–B cell based on CD10 and CD19 positivity. Analysis of the chromosomes reveals the TEL-AML1 translocation and a DNA index of 1.0. X-ray of the chest does not reveal a mediastinal mass, and a lumbar puncture shows that there are no leukemic lymphoblasts in the cerebrospinal fluid. J.B. is hydrated, alkalinized, and treated with oral allopurinol 200 mg/m^2/day, with a plan to institute induction therapy the next day. (For a discussion of the use of allopurinol in induction chemotherapy for the prevention of TLS, see Complications of Induction Therapy section.) Within a few days, J.B. will be treated with several drugs for his leukemia. Do any of the agents that are likely to be used in J.B. exhibit significant drug interactions with allopurinol?

[SI units: Hct, 0.157 (normal, 0.39–0.49); Hgb, 57 g/L (normal, 140–180); WBC count, 4.3 × 10^6/L (normal, 3.2–9.8) with 0.82 lymphocytes (normal, 0.3–0.4), 0.07 neutrophils (normal, 0.5–0.6), and 0.11 lymphoblasts (normal, 0); and platelets, 13 × 10^6/L (normal, 150–400)]

Xanthine oxidase, the enzyme inhibited by allopurinol, also converts mercaptopurine to 6-thiouric acid.[232] Thus, allopurinol may markedly increase the plasma concentrations of oral mercaptopurine by inhibiting first-pass metabolism, and this may lead to toxicity.[233] This potentially serious drug interaction is usually irrelevant for most patients with ALL because these agents are rarely used together. Allopurinol is usually employed early in the first week of induction therapy, and patients do not receive mercaptopurine until they finish induction therapy in most contemporary childhood ALL protocols.

35. What is the goal of the induction therapy that J.B. will receive? Which agents should be used to achieve this goal?

Table 90-18 Systemic Induction Regimens for Childhood Acute Lymphocytic Leukemia

Agent	Route	Dose/Schedule
Three-Drug Induction Schema		
Prednisone	PO	40 mg/m²/day × 28 days
or		
Dexamethasone[a]	PO	6 mg/m²/day × 28 days
with		
Vincristine	IV	1.5 mg/m²/week (max 2 mg) × 4
and		
Asparaginase	IM	10,000 U/m² 3 times weekly × 9 doses
or		
Pegaspargase	IM	2,500 U/m² × 1 dose
And (if Four-Drug Induction)		
Daunorubicin	IV	25 mg/m² on days 2, 8, 15

[a]Denotes that this agent is only employed in three-drug induction regimens (see text).
PO, orally; IV, intravenously; IM, intramuscularly.
Adapted from references 239–242 and 246–248, 252.

GOAL OF INDUCTION

The goal of induction therapy is complete remission (i.e., the inability to detect leukemic cells in the peripheral blood or the bone marrow by morphologic microscopic evaluation). J.B.'s peripheral blood values must be within the normal range, and the bone marrow must reveal <5% lymphoblasts. This definition also assumes the absence of lymphoblasts in the CSF. Although these findings indicate an adequate response to chemotherapy, they do not indicate a cure. Most patients have a total of 10^{12} cells at diagnosis, and successful induction regimens reduce this cell load by 99% to 10^{9}.[234,235] Therefore, continuation of therapy will be required for J.B. to further reduce the leukemic cell population and to increase his chances of long-term survival. Without continuation of therapy, the majority of patients with ALL will relapse within 1 to 2 months.[236]

INDUCTION COMBINATION CHEMOTHERAPY

The agents most commonly used in remission induction therapy are vincristine (Oncovin), prednisone (Deltasone), dexamethasone (Decadron), asparaginase (Elspar), pegaspargase (Oncaspar), and daunorubicin (Cerubidine) (Table 90-18). The prednisone or dexamethasone dose is not routinely tapered at the end of induction treatment.[237–240] More recently, dexamethasone has begun to supplant prednisone as the corticosteroid employed during induction therapy and/or throughout therapy. This is based on earlier work showing that dexamethasone has greater CSF penetration.[241] In patients with standard-risk ALL, a randomized comparison of dexamethasone to prednisone for induction therapy showed a lower CNS relapse rate in the dexamethasone group.[239] However, the use of a 28-day course of dexamethasone during induction for patients with high-risk ALL was also associated with an increased risk of infectious complications, in particular, sepsis and toxic deaths.[242] This has led to removal or alteration of dexamethasone use during induction therapy in high-risk patients. It is plausible that the addition of dexamethasone to a more intensive chemotherapy backbone that is employed for induction therapy of high-risk ALL may significantly increase the risk of infection in this more myelosuppressive milieu. In addition to the choice of corticosteroids, the efficacy of the long-acting polyethylene glycol (PEG) asparaginase has been compared with the short-acting native *Escherichia coli* asparaginase. One study demonstrated a comparable degree and duration of systemic asparagine depletion with PEG as compared to native asparaginase. However, unlike native asparaginase, PEG did not result in asparagines depletion within the CNS. It is unclear if this could have an impact on CNS relapse in children receiving contemporary chemotherapy regimens.[238] With regard to immunogenicity, PEG asparaginase is less likely to induce high antiasparaginase antibody titers, which are in turn associated with lower asparaginase activity. This resulted in an almost complete avoidance of the silent inactivation noted to occur in approximately 30% of patients receiving native asparaginase.[243]

No chemotherapy drug meets the criteria of an ideal agent (i.e., toxic to leukemic cells only and active in all phases of the cell cycle). Corticosteroids, vincristine, and various asparaginase products come closest to this ideal in terms of activity, primarily against lymphocytic leukemia, because none of these agents is myelosuppressive to normal marrow elements. To improve the success in attaining complete remission, additional agents have been added to vincristine, prednisone, and asparaginase (Table 90-18). The most frequently used additional agent is an anthracycline, such as daunorubicin or doxorubicin. Use of at least a three-drug induction regimen is the current standard of care for children at low or intermediate risk of relapse and results in improvements in both remission rate and duration versus less intensive therapy.[244–246] Currently, a four-drug regimen, or an even more intensive induction regimen consisting of more than four drugs, and often for a duration of >4 weeks, is used for children at high risk of relapse and adult ALL patients.[237,247–250]

If complete remission is not achieved with three agents by the end of induction, patients are treated with additional agents (e.g., an additional 2–4 weeks of daunorubicin and prednisone; initiation of cytarabine with additional asparaginase; vincristine and prednisone for 1–2 weeks). Because this occurs rarely, there is no consensus about the most effective agents or schedules to use in this situation. Most of these patients have a decreased survival and a higher relapse rate.

Intensive induction treatment has benefits for the majority of children with ALL. This treatment strategy supports the hypothesis of Goldie and Coldman,[251] that intensification of early treatment may decrease the chance that drug resistance will develop and may therefore potentially increase the proportion of long-term relapse-free survivors. Although J.B. has a DNA index of 1.0, based on his age, initial WBC count, and translocation, he is a patient with a low to intermediate risk of relapse. A three-drug induction regimen consisting of vincristine, dexamethasone, and pegaspargase is recommended to optimize his chances for long-term DFS.[238,239,243]

Vincristine Toxicity

36. J.B. is discharged from the hospital during the second week of induction chemotherapy. Results of his CBC and differential indicate that he is responding well to his chemotherapy (i.e., WBC count 2,600/mm³, neutrophils 69%, lymphocytes 22%, platelets

229,000/m^3, Hct 28.6%, blasts 0). However, during the third week of induction chemotherapy, J.B. develops severe abdominal pain. It is discovered that he has not had a bowel movement in 6 days. J.B. has also been exhibiting "acting out" behaviors in recent days. How might these symptoms be explained?

[SI units: WBC count, 2.6 × 10^6/L; neutrophils, 0.69; lymphocytes, 0.22; platelets, 229 × 10^6/L; Hct, 0.286; blasts, 0]

The use of vincristine is associated with an autonomic neuropathy, which may substantially reduce GI motility[252]; in severe cases, paralytic ileus may result. Constipation is often accompanied by colicky abdominal pain, which may be quite distressing.[253] These symptoms usually become apparent 3 to 10 days after drug administration and resolve over several days. Prophylactic use of a stool softener (docusate [Colace]) and/or laxative (polyethylene glycol [Miralax]) may lessen the severity of J.B.'s constipation and facilitate defecation. This regimen should have been instituted soon after the first dose of vincristine.

J.B.'s emotional changes are likely the result of the dexamethasone he is receiving. Emotional lability, sleep disturbances, depressed mood, and listlessness have occurred during corticosteroid therapy in children with ALL.[254] These behavioral changes can be quite disruptive, and parents should be prepared for them in advance. Behavioral disturbances typically resolve within 2 weeks after corticosteroid discontinuation.[254]

Central Nervous System Preventive Therapy

37. In addition to the aforementioned drugs, J.B. also receives intrathecal (IT) chemotherapy for CNS prophylaxis with methotrexate at the beginning (week 1) and end (week 4) of induction therapy. What is the purpose of IT chemotherapy? What are the various treatments available for CNS preventive therapy? What determines which one is chosen for J.B.?

PURPOSE

IT or CNS preventive therapy decreases the chance of relapse within the CNS and increase J.B.'s chance of long-term survival. Before CNS preventive therapy was routine, the CNS was the most common site of leukemic relapse and thus predicted bone marrow relapse.[255,256] Patients at greatest risk for CNS relapse include those with very high initial WBC counts, T-cell ALL, and infants.[257,258] However, because all patients with ALL are at risk for CNS relapse, one of the largest incremental improvements in DFS has been the routine use of CNS preventive therapy.[156] Because many antileukemic agents do not distribute well into the CSF, this area becomes a sanctuary site for leukemic lymphoblasts. The aim is to eradicate any CNS leukemic lymphoblasts present at diagnosis and to prevent the emergence of a relapse within the CNS.

CENTRAL NERVOUS SYSTEM PREVENTIVE THERAPY OPTIONS

All treatment protocols for childhood ALL use some form of CNS preventive therapy, although different regimens are used. The first successful CNS prophylaxis treatments were 2,400 cGy of craniospinal radiation with or without IT methotrexate, which markedly reduced the CNS relapse rate.[260] To avoid the myelosuppression and reductions in spinal growth due to craniospinal irradiation, the standard CNS preventive therapy was modified to 2,400 cGy of cranial irradiation, along with IT methotrexate. However, the adverse effects of cranial irradiation remained problematic. These included decreased intellectual function, dysfunctions of the neuroendocrine system, and poorer psychosocial functioning.[261–263] As a result, clinicians sought alternative, potentially safer forms of CNS preventive therapy. For example, lower doses (1,800 cGy) of cranial irradiation were combined with IT methotrexate to reduce the CNS effects, and this has proved to be equivalent to 2,400 cGy in preventing CNS relapse.[258,264] The results of a long-term follow-up study indicate mild, but diffuse deficits in information processing in patients receiving 2,400 cGy of cranial irradiation but not in patients treated with 1,800 cGy, suggesting that the lower radiation dose reduces neuropsychological morbidity. Nevertheless, because concerns regarding the long-term toxicity of cranial radiation remain, especially for younger children, it is currently reserved for patients with detectable CNS disease on presentation, some patients with T-cell ALL and patients with CNS relapse. Currently, CNS preventative therapy includes IT methotrexate alone, triple IT chemotherapy (methotrexate, cytarabine, and hydrocortisone), or IT methotrexate combined with systemic dose–intensified methotrexate.[265–268]

Because patients differ in their risk for developing CNS leukemia, CNS preventive therapy should be tailored accordingly. Children with low- and intermediate-risk ALL have equivalent CNS protection rates with either cranial radiation or IT chemotherapy, as long as adequate intensive systemic therapy is provided.[266,269,270] Patients at low or intermediate risk of relapse may be treated with either triple IT chemotherapy or IT methotrexate, depending on the institutional protocol.[266,269] Some high-risk children who are early responders to chemotherapy and who do not have CNS disease on presentation may also obtain adequate CNS protection with IT methotrexate alone.[271] Currently, most patients with T-cell disease still receive cranial radiation therapy as a component of their CNS preventive therapy, although with current intensive systemic therapy a radiation dose of 1,200 cGy appears to provide adequate CNS protection.[156]

INTRATHECAL CHEMOTHERAPY: CHRONIC ADVERSE EFFECTS

The chronic toxicities of IT chemotherapy are now being determined. When examined for effects on growth, triple IT chemotherapy demonstrated no effect on the final height achieved by children in contrast to a reduced final height in patients receiving cranial irradiation.[272] Limited evidence suggests that IT chemotherapy may be associated with some neuropsychological deficits. At least one study of patients receiving IT chemotherapy without cranial irradiation has demonstrated deficits in higher-order cognitive function tasks and learning disabilities in mathematics.[273] Another study has demonstrated that children who were treated with IT chemotherapy before age 5 years had deficits in the cerebellar-frontal brain subsystem and in neuropsychological performance.[274] It is unclear whether these deficits will translate into significant long-term consequences for these children.

Dosage

38. J.B. is at a low risk for CNS relapse, and the decision is made to treat him with IT methotrexate. What dose of IT methotrexate should J.B. receive?

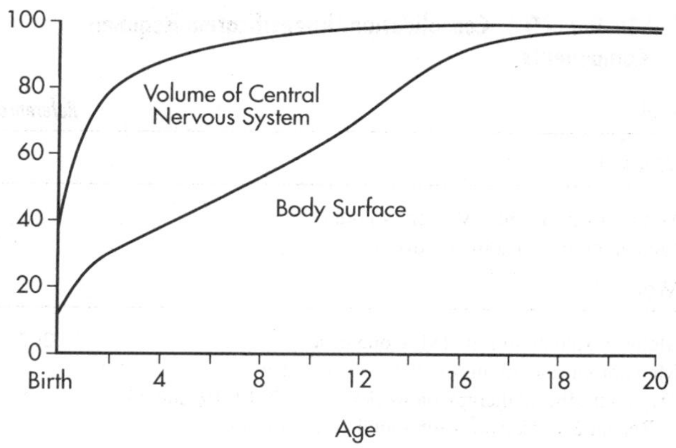

FIGURE 90-3 Relationship between body surface area and central nervous system (CNS) volume as a function of age. CNS volume increases at a more rapid rate than body surface area, reaching adult volume by 3 years of age. From Bleyer WA et al. Reduction in central nervous system leukemia with a pharmacokinetically derived intrathecal methotrexate dosage regimen. *J Clin Oncol* 1:1983:289. Reprinted with permission © 2008 American Society of Clinical Oncology. All rights reserved.

High chemotherapy concentrations can be attained within the CSF with relatively low doses because the CSF volume of distribution is small in contrast to the peripheral plasma volume (140 vs. 3,500 mL).[275,276] Drug exposure is also maximized by the longer half-life of most drugs in the CSF.[277] The approach used for IT dosing differs from systemic administration, the latter of which is based on body weight or body surface area. CSF methotrexate concentrations appear to correlate better with patient age than size.[278] As seen in Figure 90-3, the CSF volume in children approaches that of an adult by the age of 3 years. Because CSF volume does not correlate with body surface area, IT doses based on body size result in subtherapeutic concentrations in young children and potentially toxic concentrations in older children and adults. The age-based dosing regimens shown in Table 90-19 are less neurotoxic and are associated with a lower rate of CNS relapse than doses based on size.[279] Using this dosing regimen, J.B.'s dose of IT methotrexate should be 12 mg. If triple intrathecal therapy were employed, the doses of IT cytarabine and hydrocortisone would be 24 and 12 mg, respectively. These latter doses are also based on age, but no literature exists to support how they were derived. Nevertheless, empiric evidence supports their efficacy.[266]

Table 90-19 Dosage Regimen for Intrathecal Chemotherapy Based on Patient Age

Patient Age (years)	*Methotrexate (mg)*	*Hydrocortisone (mg)*	*Cytarabine (mg)*
<1	6	6	12
1	8	8	16
2	10	10	20
3	12	12	24
≥9	15	15	30

Adapted from reference 280.

PRECAUTIONS

39. J.B.'s triple IT methotrexate is to be administered on the same day as his vincristine dose. Are there any special precautions that should be taken when these medications are administered in close proximity?

Inadvertent IT administration of vincristine is almost uniformly fatal,[280–282] although there is at least one report of a patient in whom death was prevented.[283] Despite widespread educational efforts and numerous precautionary measures used by the pharmaceutical industry in recent years, deaths from the inadvertent IT administration of vincristine continue to be reported.[284] The clinical course in patients mistakenly given IT vincristine has typically progressed from backache and headache on day 1, muscle weakness (generalized) on day 2, apnea on day 5, loss of evidence of electroencephalographic activity by days 7 to 9, and death on day 12.[280] To avoid the tragedy of IT vincristine administration, vincristine should be admixed separately from IT medications, specially labeled, and preferably delivered to the patient area for IV infusion after the administration of IT medications.

Acute Adverse Effects

40. J.B. develops severe nausea and vomiting following his IT methotrexate treatment. Is this common following IT chemotherapy? What can be done to decrease this toxicity for future IT chemotherapy treatments?

Several acute toxicities have been reported following IT chemotherapy. Acute arachnoiditis may occur 12 to 24 hours after injection, resulting in headaches, nausea, vomiting, and various other signs of increased intracranial pressure.[285] Severe symptoms occurred in 4 of 91 children receiving combination IT chemotherapy.[286] IT methotrexate alone produces these side effects in 38% of cases.[287] Fortunately, these reactions are usually self-limiting and can be reduced by use of doses based on patient age.[279]

Nausea and vomiting due to IT chemotherapy is usually mild to moderate in severity.[288] The emetogenic effect of IT chemotherapy is likely the result of direct contact between the chemotherapy and the chemoreceptor trigger zone. IV ondansetron (a 5-HT_3 antagonist) at a dose of 0.15 mg/kg before and 3 to 4 hours after IT chemotherapy or 0.3 mg IV × 1 dose prior to IT chemotherapy can significantly reduce the incidence and severity of nausea and vomiting secondary to triple IT chemotherapy.[288] Without antiemetic protection, only 22% of children receiving IT chemotherapy had no vomiting. With the addition of ondansetron, complete protection from vomiting rose to 69%.[288] The efficacy of ondansetron IV when chemotherapy is administered IT is consistent with animal data demonstrating that 5-HT_3 antagonists administered directly into the brainstem can block the emetic response of systemically administered chemotherapy.[289] (Also see Chapter 7.)

Rarely, a form of methotrexate neurotoxicity resulting in either paraplegia or necrotizing leukoencephalopathy may occur.[290–292] Leukoencephalopathy is associated with cranial irradiation given before or during IT therapy.[292] The preservatives in the chemotherapy diluents (methylhydroxylbenzoate and benzyl alcohol) rather than the chemotherapy agents are believed to be responsible for the paraplegia. This emphasizes the importance of diluting IT chemotherapy with a preservative-free diluent.[290] In addition, acute seizures associated with IT methotrexate have been reported. It also has been shown that methotrexate can increase the CSF concentration of homocysteine, as a consequence of decreased CSF folate. It is known that homocysteine can be metabolized to excitatory neurotransmitters that are agonists of the *N*-methyl-d-aspartate (NMDA) receptor, leading to seizures.[293,294] It is possible that known NMDA receptor antagonists (e.g., dextromethorphan) may decrease the risk of seizures in patients who develop this toxicity.[294]

Consolidation Therapy

41. J.B. had bone marrow aspirations performed at day 8 and at the completion of induction treatment on day 29; both indicated a complete morphologic remission, indicative of a rapid early response. After completion of the induction phase, J.B. was scheduled to receive an intensified phase of chemotherapy known as *consolidation therapy*. What is the purpose of consolidation treatment, and what are some examples of effective regimens for this phase of treatment?

Consolidation or intensification is a period of dose-intensive chemotherapy following induction therapy. This phase of treatment has proved to be an important strategy for the prevention of relapse in children with ALL and has helped produce EFS of greater than 80% in low-risk childhood ALL.[156,295] To date, the optimum consolidation/intensification regimens have yet to be determined. However, a few interesting findings from investigations of consolidation therapy are briefly mentioned. A comparison between methotrexate 1 g/m^2 IV (intermediate-dose methotrexate) and low-dose (180 mg/m^2 divided into six doses) oral methotrexate revealed an approximate 4.4% increase in continuous complete remission with the higher-dose regimen.[295] This study is considered to be one of the pivotal trials demonstrating the superiority of higher-dose methotrexate in childhood ALL.[156] Although this difference was statistically significant, it may not have been clinically significant because leukoencephalopathy also occurred in 4.5% of children treated with the higher-dose regimen, compared with 0.6% of those treated with low-dose methotrexate. Although this study was not designed to examine differences in gender, female patients failed to benefit from the higher-dose regimen. This study has also been criticized for using the same leucovorin dosage with both methotrexate regimens because it is known that a lower-dose oral regimen without leucovorin may produce similar RBC concentrations to that achievable with higher-dose methotrexate with leucovorin.[296]

It is not uncommon for newer consolidation regimens to lead to complications, given the baseline treatment intensity of many contemporary ALL treatments. For example, a trial evaluating the addition of either intensified asparaginase or cytarabine to intermediate-dose methotrexate in standard-risk ALL patients failed to show any incremental benefit in EFS over that achievable with methotrexate alone, although the cytarabine regimen did result in an increase in both infectious morbidity and hospitalizations.[297] Some examples of state-of-the-art consolidation regimens are provided in Table 90-20.[239,247,295,297,298]

Table 90-20 Consolidation/Intensification Regimen Components

Week	Reference
Week 1	
Methotrexate 1 g/m^2 IV over 24 hours	
Mercaptopurine 1 g/m^2 IV over 6 hours	
Week 2	
Methotrexate 20 mg/m^2 IM × one dose	297
Mercaptopurine 50 mg/m^2 PO daily × 7 days	
Triple intrathecal therapy on weeks 1, 2, 3, 7, 12, 19, and 25	
Repeat 2-week cycles for a total of 12 courses	
Cyclophosphamide 1 g/m^2 IV on days 0 and 14	
Cytarabine 75 mg/m^2 SC or IV on days 1–4, 8–11, 15–18, and 22–25	
Mercaptopurine 60 mg/m^2 PO daily × 28 days	300
Methotrexate IT weekly × 4 weeks	
Mercaptopurine 25 mg/m^2 PO daily on days 1–56	249
Methotrexate 5 g/m^2 IV over 24 hours on days 8, 22, 36, and 50	
Methotrexate IT on days 8, 22, 36, and 50	
Methotrexate 1 g/m^2 IV over 24 hours, every 3 weeks × 6 doses	299
Vincristine 1.5 mg/m^2 IV on weeks 8, 9, 17, and 18	
Prednisone 40 mg/m^2 PO daily × 7 days on weeks 8 and 17	
Dexamethasone 10 mg/m^2 PO daily × 21 days + 7-day taper	241
Vincristine 1.5 mg/m^2 IV on days 0, 7, and 14	
L-asparaginase 6,000 U/m^2 IM × 6 doses on days 3–17	
Doxorubicin 25 mg/m^2 IV on days 0, 7, and 14	

IV, intravenously; IM, intramuscularly; PO, orally; SC, subcutaneously; IT, intrathecally.

METHOTREXATE CONCENTRATION MONITORING

42. J.B. receives consolidation therapy with intermediate-dose methotrexate. His methotrexate serum concentrations are monitored after the administration of each dose of methotrexate during this phase of therapy. Why is monitoring of serum concentrations important when giving this dose of methotrexate? Are methotrexate concentrations important in predicting the outcome of ALL therapy?

After dose-intensive methotrexate therapy, concentration monitoring is crucial to establish the dose of leucovorin and the duration of hydration and alkalinization needed to prevent systemic methotrexate toxicity.[299] Before serum methotrexate concentrations were routinely monitored after high-dose methotrexate, severe GI desquamation and myelosuppression led to fatalities in as many as 6% of patients.[300] Methotrexate concentrations are measured approximately 24 hours after completion of the methotrexate infusion and repeated daily until the concentration falls below the toxic threshold of 0.05 μmol/L. Patients who have unexpectedly high concentrations after high-dose methotrexate may require higher doses of leucovorin and prolonged hydration and alkalinization to circumvent methotrexate toxicity.[299] (See Pediatric Tumors:

Osteosarcoma section of Chapter 91 for details on monitoring methotrexate concentrations and dosing leucovorin.)

Investigators have evaluated the influence of serum concentrations of methotrexate on the outcome of ALL patients.[300,301] These studies have determined that children with higher methotrexate clearance values appear to be at higher risk of relapse and suggest that concentration monitoring may also play a role in enhancing the long-term survival of these patients.[301] However, when follow-up was extended, the survival advantage reported in one of these studies was lost.[301,302] A subsequent investigation of individualized chemotherapy versus standard dosing based on body surface area also demonstrated that concentration monitoring and subsequent dose adjustment of methotrexate during consolidation was associated with a significant 10% improvement in continuous complete remission for children with B-cell lineage ALL.[248] It also remains to be seen whether this difference will be lost with further patient follow-up. Given the somewhat conflicting data at present, dose adjustment of methotrexate for efficacy purposes based on serum concentrations should be considered investigational and should not be used for dose adjustments in J.B. Currently, dosage adjustment of intermediate- and high-dose methotrexate should be used only for patients experiencing excess toxicity.

Maintenance Therapy

43. After completion of his induction and consolidation/intensification treatments, J.B. is scheduled to receive maintenance (continuation) treatment for a total therapy duration of 2.5 years from the start of his induction therapy. His parents question why treatment will be of such a long duration and ask whether this is necessary because J.B. is already in remission. What is the purpose of J.B.'s maintenance or continuation treatment for ALL? Which agents should be used in J.B. for this phase of therapy?

PURPOSE

Maintenance or continuation treatment sustains the complete remission achieved from induction chemotherapy. Early trials have shown that without maintenance treatment, the majority of ALL patients will relapse.[236] It must be stressed that patients who have successfully responded to induction and consolidation/intensification therapy may still have a high leukemic cell burden (although undetectable), which must be eradicated by additional treatment. This is supported by the results of bone marrow biopsies from patients who have experienced relapse after several months to years of treatment. The cytogenetic characteristics of the leukemic cells in relapsed patients are identical to those at the time of diagnosis.[303,304] Maintenance therapy is also supported by the results of MRD studies, which demonstrate that some amount of measurable leukemic cells are still present months after the completion of induction therapy.[225]

CHEMOTHERAPY REGIMENS

Drugs that are effective during induction therapy cannot, by themselves, prolong remission during maintenance therapy.[173] However, other agents are effective in sustaining a complete remission. Two of the most effective drugs are mercaptopurine (Purinethol) and methotrexate.[244,305,306] Methotrexate is most effective and least toxic when administered intermittently, usually on a weekly basis in oral doses of 20 mg/m^2/week. Mercaptopurine is effective and well tolerated orally when dosed daily, usually at a dose of 50 to 75 mg/m^2/day.

Other agents have been added to standard maintenance therapy with mercaptopurine and methotrexate to improve remission duration and to increase a patient's chances for long-term survival. There is evidence that monthly pulses of vincristine and prednisone offer advantages (lower bone marrow and testicular relapse rates) in standard-risk patients as well.[307] At present, most contemporary treatment regimens for childhood ALL have intensified induction and consolidation phases, and sometimes include a reinduction and/or a delayed intensification phase within the first 6 months.[247,249,295,297,298] Following this early intensive treatment schema, these newer protocols use a less intensive maintenance therapy consisting of methotrexate and mercaptopurine in combination with periodic IT chemotherapy treatments, either with or without intermittent vincristine/prednisone pulses.[247,249,295,297,298] It is unclear which of these regimens is best because risk criteria used to assign patients to various maintenance treatment arms within these protocols have varied among investigators.

The available evidence suggests that a patient like J.B. with standard-risk ALL will benefit from use of daily mercaptopurine 50 to 75 mg/m^2 PO and weekly methotrexate 20 mg/m^2 PO, IM, or IV, along with periodic pulse therapy with vincristine 1.5 mg/m^2 for 1 day and either prednisone 40 mg/m^2 or dexamethasone 6 mg/m^2 PO for 7 days every 4 weeks. In addition, IT methotrexate should be repeated every 8 to 12 weeks.

Potential Problems

44. After 6 weeks of maintenance therapy with the aforementioned regimen, J.B. has an absolute neutrophil count (ANC) that has ranged between 2,000 and 3,500 cells/mm^3 for >6 weeks. Other CBC findings are also within normal limits. Should any changes in his maintenance therapy be considered at this time? Are there any potential problems with mercaptopurine and methotrexate that could explain his ANC values and that might increase his risk of treatment failure?

Diurnal variation of methotrexate concentration and marked interpatient variability in absorption and metabolism of mercaptopurine have been described, which may explain the varied response among patients to standard doses.[308–310] Most patients are able to tolerate full doses of mercaptopurine, which is inactivated by the enzyme thiopurine methyltransferase (TPMT). It is known that approximately 89% to 94% of patients have high TPMT activity, whereas 6% to 11% have intermediate activity, and 0.3% have deficient activity. Patients with deficient TPMT activity develop severe and even fatal toxicity with standard mercaptopurine doses and require very low doses (approximately 10 mg/m^2 three times per week) for avoidance of profound myelosuppression.[311,312]

Patients receiving half doses of these agents have shorter remission durations[313]; however, those who tolerate maximal protocol dosages may also be at greater risk of relapse.[185] Patients who are able to tolerate maximal doses without significant myelosuppression may require even higher doses than are recommended in some protocols. Investigations, including studies of intracellular concentrations of active metabolites, have not found the pharmacokinetics of mercaptopurine or methotrexate to be predictive of outcome in children with

ALL.[314–316] However, one of these trials did demonstrate that dose intensity of mercaptopurine was a significant predictor of EFS.[314] Because bioavailability is a concern for both agents and because some patients, particularly males, may be able to tolerate high dosages without toxicity, doses are often adjusted upward based on the degree of leukopenia. Some protocols allow for dosage increases of methotrexate or mercaptopurine every 4 to 6 weeks to maintain a target ANC in the range of 300 to 2,000/mm^3.[314,315] This is usually accomplished by alternately increasing the doses of mercaptopurine and methotrexate by 25%.

For J.B., this means an increase in mercaptopurine from 50 mg/day to a daily schedule alternating 50 mg with 75 mg, or an increased methotrexate dose from 20 to 25 mg/week. Although parenteral administration of methotrexate is logical, it does not consistently improve the results of therapy.[316,317] To assess whether J.B. is receiving an adequate dose, weekly WBC counts are essential. This allows one to accurately appraise the adequacy of his dose and to follow his disease status to ensure that remission is continuing. If an inadequate degree of myelosuppression is demonstrated, J.B.'s compliance should be investigated because decreased compliance is a frequent problem in the therapy of childhood ALL.[318–320] At least one investigation has found improved compliance with evening administration of mercaptopurine.[318]

Duration of Therapy

45. How long should J.B.'s maintenance therapy be continued?

Most centers treat children with ALL until a total therapy duration of approximately 2.5 years is reached.[321,322] Extending maintenance treatment to 5 or 6 years adds no benefit.[321,322] Other data suggest that a shorter duration of 18 months may be adequate for girls, but not for boys.[323] Most patients who experience relapse do so during therapy or within the first year of completing therapy. After the second year of therapy and for every year thereafter, relapses become much less common, but are occasionally observed. Some centers are exploring whether more intensive treatment protocols could decrease the duration of maintenance treatment because the optimal duration is based on less aggressive protocols. Until there is more conclusive evidence regarding the duration of ALL maintenance therapy, patients with J.B.'s characteristics should receive chemotherapy for approximately 2.5 years.

High-Risk Acute Lymphoblastic Leukemia

LONG-TERM SEQUELAE

46. N.B. is a 12-year-old Hispanic boy with a 4- to 5-week history of an enlarging right-sided neck mass. On physical examination, he is found to have a 6 × 3-cm right neck mass with extension to the nape of the neck. X-ray of the chest indicates an anterior mediastinal mass. The CBC reveals a WBC count of 62,000/mm^2 (43% lymphoblasts, 27% neutrophils, and 27% lymphocytes), Hct of 41.5%, and platelet count of 83,000/mm^3. Other pertinent laboratory results are urate of 15.1 mg/dL and LDH of 1,636 U/L (normal, 280–540). A bone marrow biopsy confirms the diagnosis of ALL and shows that 85% of the bone marrow is replaced by leukemic lymphoblasts. The leukemic cells are T lymphoblasts, and their DNA index is 1.0. A lumbar puncture reveals a few cells within the CSF that are terminal deoxynucleotidal transferase (TdT) negative, but are rather suspicious.

N.B. is started on rasburicase 0.2 mg/kg/day for 1 to 3 days, instead of allopurinol and hydration and alkalinization. Because N.B. in known to have T-cell ALL, he is begun on an intensive protocol. The induction regimen consists of six drugs, including prednisone 40 mg/m^2/day PO on days 1 to 29; vincristine 1.5 mg/m^2 IV weekly for 5 weeks; cyclophosphamide (Cytoxan) 1 g/m^2 on day 1 and 600 mg/m^2 on day 22; doxorubicin (Adriamycin) 50 mg/m^2 on day 1; cytarabine 100 mg/m^2/day via continuous infusion for 5 days starting on day 22; and asparaginase 10,000 U/m^2 IM on days 27, 29, and 31. Triple IT therapy consists of methotrexate 15 mg, cytarabine 30 mg, and hydrocortisone 15 mg administered weekly for 6 weeks. Why was rasburicase used instead of standard tumor lysis syndrome (TLS) preventive strategies?

Despite the standard prophylactic regimen for TLS, some high-risk patients may develop urate nephropathy. Patients with a significant elevation in uric acid and/or renal dysfunction may not derive significant early benefit from the standard regimen, which is designed to prevent the formation of additional uric acid and to aid in its excretion. Significant elevations in uric acid and/or renal dysfunction may even delay the initiation of chemotherapy. Rasburicase is a recombinant form of urate oxidase, the enzyme that catalyzes the conversion of uric acid to the more water-soluble allantoin. Rasburicase produces a dramatic reduction in uric acid within 4 hours of administration. Uric acid is often reduced below the normal range, and additional daily doses are not necessary if uric acid normalizes and remains within normal limits. Given N.B.'s significantly elevated uric acid, he is at significant risk for TLS and is a good candidate for initial management with rasburicase. Rasburicase obviates the need for allopurinol, hydration, and alkalinization.[324]

47. N.B. achieves a complete remission based on the results of a bone marrow specimen on day 29. His parents are concerned about the doxorubicin because they have heard about heart problems with this drug. His protocol includes significant doses of this agent throughout his treatment plan. They ask about the likelihood for cardiac toxicity, what might be done to screen for it, and whether any preventive strategies exist that might be of value. They also ask about other potential long-term sequelae from his treatment. What are the recommended screening tools and preventive strategies for anthracycline cardiotoxicity in children? What is the evidence for the relationship between osteonecrosis and corticosteroid used in the treatment of childhood ALL?

The relationship between cumulative anthracycline dose and cardiotoxicity is well established; a dramatic increase in congestive heart failure (CHF) is observed at cumulative doses >450 mg/m^2.[156,325] However, because this is a median dose for cardiotoxicity, limiting the total dose to this threshold will not protect all patients. At least one study has demonstrated that both biochemical and echocardiographic abnormalities can be seen in childhood cancer survivors following low cumulative anthracycline doses.[326] Although some early reports suggested reversibility in children, subsequent follow-up data confirm a worsening of CHF over time.[327–330] Late-occurring cardiotoxicity (i.e., years following completion of chemotherapy) has been reported in children.[330,331] One of these studies used a very sensitive echocardiography technique and reported that the majority of patients had either abnormal contractility or afterload.[331] The other study used a less sensitive echocardiography technique and reported a lower prevalence of cardiotoxicity, although the rate of abnormalities was shown to increase substantially with longer patient follow-up.[330] Recent prospective studies of long-term cardiac function following anthracycline therapy in children show a continual decrement in left ventricular function years after chemotherapy.[332] It is currently unclear what the long-term risk of CHF is in children. Close patient follow-up is important for early detection, although currently used screening tools such as echocardiography detect only functional damage and have not demonstrated value in preventing CHF. Newer nuclear medicine probes are showing some promise in the early detection of anthracycline-induced cardiotoxicity and may be used in the future for identifying children before the development of functional deficits.[259] Dexrazoxane (Zinecard), an intracellular iron chelator, has been studied for its effectiveness in preventing anthracycline-induced CHF in adults.[333,334] However, because there was a decreased antitumor response in dexrazoxane-treated patients in one of these trials, it was subsequently studied at a reduced dose. It has been approved for use only in women with breast cancer who have received a cumulative anthracycline dose of 300 mg/m^2. In one small trial in children with sarcoma, dexrazoxane decreased the risk of cardiotoxicity and improved tolerance of higher cumulative anthracycline doses.[335] However, the left ventricular EF declined in both groups receiving higher cumulative anthracycline doses. A more recent study employing serum troponin T elevations as a surrogate marker for cardiac damage demonstrated that children with ALL randomized to receive dexrazoxane with each dose of doxorubicin were less likely to have elevations of troponin T levels, but EFS was not different between the group receiving dexrazoxane versus those receiving doxorubicin alone. Also, it is unclear whether these differences in serum troponin T will translate into differences in cardiotoxicity because the study did not report the results of echocardiography.[336] In summary, whether dexrazoxane circumvents the long-term risk of anthracycline-induced CHF in children is unclear. Some degree of long-term cardiotoxicity or CHF risk in children may be unavoidable when an anthracycline is used, even if it is combined with dexrazoxane. Because anthracyclines are an important component of many ALL treatment protocols and have figured significantly into the improved survival rates achieved in high-risk patients in recent years, the benefits seem to outweigh the risks in these patients at present. Although N.B. will be monitored closely for the occurrence of cardiac deterioration, there is currently no proven way to completely eliminate the risk of cardiotoxicity, although restricting children to a cumulative dose of $<$300 mg/m^2 has resulted in a low frequency of late occurring cardiotoxicity.[337]

Many survivors of childhood ALL therapy are found to have decreased bone mineral density.[338–342] This has been attributed to both corticosteroids and cranial radiation therapy. Studies of osteonecrosis in childhood ALL demonstrate an overall incidence of 1.1% to 1.8%.[339,340] However, patient age at the time of treatment is an important risk factor with an incidence of 0.2% in children younger than 10 years, but 8.9% in patients 10 years and 16.7% in those 15 years. Most patients developed osteonecrosis in two or more joints. There is a fairly clear relationship between the cumulative dose of corticosteroid received and the incidence of osteonecrosis. An increased risk of fractures during chemotherapy has also been reported in children with ALL.[342] These risks of bone pathology in survivors of childhood ALL argue in favor of close monitoring as well as optimization of mineral supplementation.

48. After completing induction therapy, N.B. is scheduled to receive a 25-week consolidation therapy consisting of vincristine/prednisone pulses, along with doxorubicin 30 mg/m^2 Q 3 weeks, in addition to oral mercaptopurine and three IV doses of methotrexate 5 g/m^2 on weeks 7, 10, and 13. Weekly asparaginase at a dose of 25,000 U/m^2 IM will also be given weekly for the first 20 weeks. Is this the usual dose of asparaginase? What is the value of asparaginase in patients with T-cell leukemia?

This dosage of asparaginase is higher than that usually used in the treatment of ALL (6,000–10,000 U/m^2). This is based on a study of T-cell ALL, in which patients were randomized to receive asparaginase 25,000 U/m^2 IM every week or not for 20 doses. There was a significant improvement in continuous complete remission at 4 years for those who had received the additional high-dose asparaginase therapy (68% vs. 55%). This provided evidence that patients with T-cell ALL may achieve long-term remission rates similar to those of other ALL immunologic subtypes.[210] Furthermore, the addition of high-dose methotrexate has increased relapse-free survival rates to approximately 80% in patients with T-cell ALL.

49. Two weeks following his vincristine/doxorubicin/prednisone/mercaptopurine regimen and 5 days following his fifth dose of asparaginase, N.B. develops severe epigastric abdominal pain and hyperglycemia. N.B. has been having normal bowel movements and does not have abdominal distention. The serum amylase is markedly elevated to 450 IU/L (normal, 111–296). Which agent is likely responsible for N.B.'s abdominal pain? What other complications are associated with asparaginase?

Pancreatitis

Pancreatitis has been noted in children following the administration of asparaginase.[343] As illustrated by N.B., this often presents as abdominal pain accompanied by an elevated serum amylase and hyperglycemia. Insulin may be required to control the hyperosmotic, nonketotic hyperglycemia that may result.[344,345] The pancreatitis is occasionally severe, and fatalities have been reported.[346] Unfortunately, the serum amylase may not predict whether patients will develop acute fatal pancreatitis.[346] N.B.'s pancreatitis secondary to asparaginase makes further treatment with this agent inadvisable. Because this reaction is not a hypersensitivity reaction, further therapy with the *Erwinia* form of asparaginase is also not recommended. N.B. may be treated with supportive care and insulin therapy. He should recover fully and be able to receive further chemotherapy.

Hypersensitivity Reactions

Hypersensitivity reactions are common, occurring in 20% to 35% of patients, but they are usually mild, generally presenting as urticarial eruptions.[344] Premedication does not appear to prevent subsequent reactions in most patients.[347] Severe anaphylactoid reactions may occur and can be fatal.[348] Clinical reactions correlate better with asparaginase-specific IgG rather than IgE antibodies, and severe hypersensitivity reactions can be explained in most instances by complement activation.[349,350]

Anaphylactoid reactions appear to be less common when asparaginase is administered intramuscularly.[351,352] This is because the slow absorption of asparaginase after IM administration results in delayed, less severe acute reactions. Because these reactions can be delayed, prolonged monitoring is recommended after IM asparaginase.[353] Most serious hypersensitivity reactions tend to occur after the patient has received several doses.

A significant number of patients receiving asparaginase as a component of ALL treatment test positive for antiasparaginase antibodies, and antibody concentrations are significantly higher in patients who experience a hypersensitivity reaction.[347] Patients who are receiving asparaginase may also develop "silent" immune clearance, resulting in rapid clearance of asparaginase from the plasma (similar to patients with hypersensitivity) but without an allergic reaction.[354–356] These patients may not obtain benefit from asparaginase and may be at greater risk for treatment failure.[357] More recently, the prevalence of antibodies to asparaginase has been investigated. It was demonstrated that asparaginase antibody titers were present in 61% of patients receiving native *E. coli* asparaginase during induction therapy (including 29% with silent hypersensitivity). It was also shown that the majority (73%) of these patients did not have measurable asparaginase activity in their serum. Preliminary analysis from this study also demonstrated a relationship between antibody titers and outcomes, with patients with silent hypersensitivity more likely to have an adverse outcome.[358] Because premedication usually does not prevent future reactions and because of the possibility that patients who exhibit hypersensitivity may derive no benefit from asparaginase, it appears that the best course of action is to switch patients from the *E. coli* preparation to an alternate asparaginase preparation.

Preparations

Asparaginase is available from two natural sources, *E. coli* and *Erwinia*. These two preparations are not 100% cross-reactive, so the *Erwinia* product may be substituted for the *E. coli* product when hypersensitivity reactions occur.[359] However, one should be aware that cross-reactions occur in 17% to 26% of patients.[240,360] Because of the shorter half-life of the *Erwinia* product, a dosage increase of *Erwinia* asparaginase is necessary to mimic the activity of the *E. coli* product.[361] Of note, patients receiving equivalent doses of *Erwinia* asparaginase have a poorer remission rate and survival than those patients receiving the *E. coli* asparaginase.[362] In contemporary protocols, the dose of *Erwinia* asparaginase is typically about 2.5 times greater than the *E. coli* asparaginase dose. The incidences of hypersensitivity reactions are equivalent for these two preparations.[359]

Asparaginase is also available as an altered form known as pegaspargase (Oncaspar). This agent is formed by covalently linking monomethoxy PEG to *E. coli* asparaginase. Pegaspargase has a prolonged half-life of 5.8 days compared with 1.2 days for *E. coli* asparaginase and appears to be safe and effective, even in patients with prior reactions to *E. coli* and *Erwinia* asparaginase.[363] The prolonged half-life allows for less frequent (i.e., every 2 week) dosing of PEG asparaginase than for the natural source asparaginase products (i.e., three times a week).[355] Asparaginase compounds derived from different *E. coli* strains may differ in both enzyme activity and half-life. At least one study has reported an unexpected mortality rate in childhood ALL associated with an assumption of equivalence among different *E. coli* asparaginase preparations.[364]

Asparaginase-Induced Coagulation Disorders

Asparaginase is known to cause decreases in albumin, fibrinogen, and α and β globulins, owing to its effects on general protein synthesis, which can result in inhibition of the synthesis of various clotting factors.[365,366] Asparaginase may also produce abnormalities in the coagulation-inhibiting and fibrinolytic system, along with deficiencies in antithrombin III and plasminogen.[365,366] This complex series of events can result in coagulopathies, occasionally leading to cerebral hemorrhage or infarction.[240,365–367] Some have suggested monitoring markers of the coagulation-inhibiting and fibrinolytic system to identify patients at risk for severe coagulation disturbances,[365] but no prospective studies have documented this practice. A higher risk of thrombotic events has been observed among children with central venous catheters and/or a genetic predisposition.[368,369] There is also a greater risk of thromboembolism in children receiving native asparaginase in combination with prednisone versus dexamethasone, perhaps due to greater inhibition of prostaglandin and thromboxane synthesis by the latter agent.[370]

Relapsed Acute Lymphoblastic Leukemia

50. After 1 year of continuation therapy, N.B. undergoes a routine lumbar puncture. Analysis of the CSF indicates the presence of numerous lymphoblasts. A CBC reveals Hct of 29.5%, platelet count of 120,000/mm^3, and WBC count of 5,300/mm^3, with 45% lymphocytes, 50% neutrophils, and 5% bands. A bone marrow biopsy confirms relapsed ALL, with 53% lymphoblasts. Would routine bone marrow biopsies of N.B. have allowed for early detection of N.B.'s relapse and an increased chance for long-term survival? What are N.B.'s chances of achieving a second remission and long-term survival? Which treatments could be used in N.B. in an attempt to attain a complete remission and improve his chances of long-term survival?

[SI units: Hct, 0.295; platelets, 120 × 10^6/L; WBC count, 5.3 × 10^6/L with 0.45 lymphocytes, 0.50 neutrophils, and 0.05 bands]

N.B. is asymptomatic at the time of relapse, as are most patients experiencing a relapse of ALL. Most of these patients are diagnosed by routine CBCs and/or lumbar punctures.[371] Routine bone marrow biopsies identify some bone marrow relapses before they become evident on a CBC, but it has not been demonstrated that earlier identification of bone marrow relapse by morphologic criteria makes an impact on long-term survival. In the future, recognition of MRD with molecular probes may change the prognostic value of routine bone marrow examination.

N.B.'s chances of achieving a second remission with salvage chemotherapy are good. Approximately 80% to 85% of relapsed patients attain a second complete remission with further chemotherapy.[371–374] Unfortunately, however, bone marrow relapse in childhood ALL is associated with poor long-term survival.[371–377] Only 6% to 29% of patients with bone marrow relapse may be rendered disease free for 2 years after relapse.[375–377] Allogeneic HCT for ALL in relapse results in a 10% to 20% long-term leukemia-free survival.[378] However, better results with HCT are possible after a second remission has been achieved. Studies of children with ALL receiving allogeneic HCT in second remission report 5-year DFS rates of 40% and 64%.[379–381] These results are superior to those of chemotherapy in patients such as N.B.[381–383] However, no randomized trials have established that bone marrow transplantation is superior to chemotherapy for children with ALL in second remission, and some of the reported advantages with transplantation may be due to selection bias.[381] Autologous HCT does not appear to be superior to chemotherapy for children with ALL in second remission.[381,384] N.B.'s family should be offered the option of an HCT if testing determines that he has an acceptable bone marrow donor match.

Agents used in salvage regimens are similar to those used in high-risk ALL regimens. In general, treatment usually consists of an intensive three- or four-agent induction regimen of vincristine, prednisone, and daunorubicin with or without asparaginase. This is accompanied by radiation therapy to sites of local relapse (e.g., testis, CNS) and IT chemotherapy.[374,376,377] After this regimen has been completed, the patient may continue with courses of intensification therapy, continuation therapy, and IT therapy.[376,377] N.B. already has been treated with many different chemotherapeutic agents. Therefore, the regimen selected should include agents to which N.B. has had little or no exposure. This theoretically increases his chances of maintaining a second remission. For example, a regimen that includes doxorubicin, asparaginase, and cyclophosphamide appears most appropriate for N.B. If N.B. fails to respond to the initial reinduction attempt, HiDAC (3 g/m^2 Q 12 hr for four doses) in conjunction with standard-dose asparaginase may be used to induce a remission. This approach has been successful in approximately 40% of patients. However, the median duration of second remission was only 3 months.[385]

PEDIATRIC NON–HODGKIN LYMPHOMA

Lymphomas account for approximately 10% of all childhood malignancies, and they are less common in children than in adults. Children younger than 16 years account for only 3% of all lymphoma cases. The malignancy can occur in any lymphoid cell at any level of differentiation and appears to be a consequence of a genetic alteration. Considerable progress has been made in the treatment of children with NHL, and currently, approximately 80% are cured.[386]

Classification

Numerous classification systems for NHL exist, and there is considerable variation in terminology among these systems.[387–390] Pediatric NHLs are best classified using histopathology, which divides them into three different categories: B-cell lymphomas, lymphoblastic lymphomas, and anaplastic large cell lymphomas.[386] This is a narrower range of histologic types than in adults.

Lymphoblastic lymphomas account for approximately 30% of childhood NHLs, B cell for about 50%, and large cell for the remainder.[386] The lymphoblastic lymphomas are usually immature T cells that are histologically identical to the cells of ALL. The distinction between lymphoblastic lymphoma and ALL is made on the basis of bone marrow involvement, with ALL being diagnosed if there is >25% bone marrow infiltration. This distinction is made by the amount of bone marrow infiltration that is present at the time of diagnosis. B-cell lymphomas may be further divided into Burkitt, Burkitt-like, and large B-cell lymphomas. Anaplastic large cell lymphomas may be T cell or null cell in origin.

Clinical Presentation

Pediatric patients with NHL may present with a number of different symptoms, many of which are related to the cell type of NHL. In general, these symptoms differ from those in adults because of the propensity of pediatric NHLs to be extranodal in origin in contrast to the common nodal presentation of adult NHL.[386] Patients with lymphoblastic lymphoma commonly present with a mediastinal mass or pleural effusions.[386] They also may have pain, dyspnea, or swelling of the face and upper arms if superior vena cava obstruction is present. Lymphoblastic lymphoma also has a predilection for the bone marrow and the CNS.[391,392] Lymphadenopathy in patients with lymphoblastic lymphoma tends to be supradiaphragmatic. Patients with B-cell NHL typically present with an abdominal tumor, abdominal pain, an alteration in bowel function, and possibly nausea and vomiting.[393] In addition, many patients with B-cell NHL present with bone marrow involvement.[378] Lymphadenopathy in these patients typically occurs below the diaphragm in the inguinal or iliac area. Anaplastic large cell lymphomas may involve the gut or unusual sites such as the lung, skin, face, or CNS.[386]

Staging

Several staging systems for pediatric NHLs are used.[393] Today the most commonly used staging system for pediatric NHL is the St. Jude Staging system.[386] This staging system includes four stages, with stage I being a single tumor or a single nodal area, and higher stages including cases with regional involvement or more than one anatomical site involved. The highest stage (stage IV) refers to patients with bone marrow or CNS involvement. The main predictor of outcome in pediatric patients with NHL has historically been determined by tumor burden at presentation.[394] However, with modern chemotherapy regimens that are tailored to the extent of disease, patients with higher-stage disease may achieve a similar EFS to that achieved in patients with lower-stage disease.[386,395] Serum concentrations of several different molecules, particularly serum LDH, help clinicians estimate tumor burden. It has also been demonstrated that serum LDH ≥500 to 1,000 U/L was a significant predictor of adverse outcome.[386]

Treatment

Lymphoblastic (T Cell)

The primary treatment for all stages and histologic types of pediatric NHL is combination chemotherapy because it is a generalized disease at the time of diagnosis.[386] A wide variety of chemotherapy agents have activity in childhood NHL. At present, the best results to date are reported by the BFM group, with an estimated 5-year EFS of approximately 92%[395] (Table 90-21). This regimen employs an intensive scheme of multiagent chemotherapy administered for a treatment duration of

Table 90-21 BFM Group Treatment Protocol for T-Cell Lymphoblastic Lymphoma

Drug	*Dose*	*Days of Administration*
Induction Protocol I (All Stages)		
Prednisone (PO)	60 mg/m^2	1–28, then taper
Vincristine (IV)	1.5 mg/m^2 (max 2 mg)	8, 15, 22, 29
Daunorubicin (IV over 1 hour)	30 mg/m^2	8, 15, 22, 29
L-asparaginase (IV[a] over 1 hour)	10,000 IU/m^2	12, 15, 18, 21, 24, 27, 30, 33
Cyclophosphamide[b] (IV over 1 hour)	1,000 mg/m^2	36, 64
Cytarabine (IV)	75 mg/m^2	38–41, 45–48, 52–55, 59–62
6-Mercaptopurine (PO)	60 mg/m^2	36–63
Methotrexate (IT)	12 mg	1, 15, 29, 45, 59
Protocol M		
Mercaptopurine (PO)	25 mg/m^2	1–56
Methotrexate (IV)	5 g/m^2	8, 22, 36, 50
Methotrexate (IT)	12 mg	8, 22, 36, 50
Reinduction Protocol II (Stages III and IV Only)		
Dexamethasone (PO)	10 mg/m^2	1–21, then taper
Vincristine (IV)	1.5 mg/m^2 (max 2 mg)	8, 15, 22, 29
Doxorubicin (IV over 1 hour)	30 mg/m^2	8, 15, 22, 29
L-asparaginase (IV[a] over 1 hour)	10,000 IU/m^2	8, 11, 15, 18
Cyclophosphamide[b] (IV over 1 hour)	1,000 mg/m^2	36
Cytarabine (IV)	75 mg/m^2	38–41, 45–48
Thioguanine (PO)	60 mg/m^2	36–49
Methotrexate (IT)	12 mg	38, 45
Maintenance (All Stages)		
Mercaptopurine (PO)	50 mg/m^2	Daily until month 24 of therapy
Methotrexate (PO)	20 mg/m^2	Weekly until month 24 of therapy

[a] This agent is typically administered intramuscularly in most treatment protocols in the United States.
[b] With mesna.
Note. Doses were adjusted for children younger than 3 years. Ten percent of the dose was given over 30 minutes, and 90% was given as a 23.5-hour continuous IV infusion.
Leucovorin rescue: 30 mg/m^2 IV at hour 42; 15 mg/m^2 IV at hours 48 and 54.
Additional doses are given on days 8 and 22 for CNS-positive patients.
IV, intravenously; IT, intrathecally.
Adapted from reference 395.

24 months. Patients with lymphoblastic lymphoma require longer treatment duration than patients with B-cell or anaplastic large cell lymphoma. This chemotherapy plan is similar to that employed in the treatment of ALL and is designed to deliver continuous or weekly therapy. All patients with lymphoblastic lymphoma are given CNS preventive therapy, regardless of stage. Few patients with lymphoblastic lymphoma present with limited disease (stages I and II), thus making it difficult to conduct adequate studies in this patient population. Attempts to shorten the duration of therapy for patients with limited-stage disease have been unsuccessful, although less intensive therapy is administered to patients with early-stage disease on some protocols.[386]

B Cell

The main differences between the treatment of lymphoblastic and B-cell lymphoma are the use of more agents and a longer treatment duration in the former. The trend in the treatment of B-cell lymphomas has been toward using short duration, intensive therapy with alkylating agents in conjunction with high-dose antimetabolite therapy (e.g., methotrexate, cytarabine). Chemotherapy is administered in rapid succession with limited recovery from neutropenia (i.e., ANC 500) between cycles. Patients with localized B-cell lymphomas respond as adequately to a four-drug regimen (consisting of cyclophosphamide, vincristine, methotrexate, and prednisone) as they do to more aggressive regimens.[386]

Evidence suggests that a 6-month course is as efficacious as the previously used 18-month course for patients with localized B-cell lymphomas.[386] Studies indicate that even 6 months of chemotherapy may be unnecessary for patients with limited-stage disease because it has been demonstrated that maintenance treatment offered no additional benefit after 9 weeks of combination chemotherapy.[386] Contemporary chemotherapy regimens include varying degrees of treatment intensity from three to seven cycles, depending on whether the tumor is completely resected, and on bone marrow and CNS involvement, and the serum LDH.[396]

With the addition of high-dose methotrexate, ifosfamide, etoposide, and HiDAC to the standard regimen, patients with stage III disease are now achieving survival rates comparable to those of patients with limited-stage disease.[396] Patients with bone marrow disease also benefit from these intensive therapeutic strategies and have achieved impressive survival rates of approximately 80%.[386] Currently, patients with advanced-stage disease are treated with a total of six to eight cycles of chemotherapy, and these treatment protocols achieve superior results to those of a much longer duration (e.g., 1–2 years) used previously.[386,396,397] Although rituximab is now a standard therapy component for B-cell lymphomas in adults, it has yet to be routinely employed in front-line treatment in the pediatric arena. Case reports demonstrate the utility of this agent when added onto a standard chemotherapy backbone for children with relapsed disease.[398,399]

Large Cell

Large cell lymphomas have responded well to both types of regimens.[386,400,401] Thus, the use of shorter, less complicated, B-cell protocols is appropriate. Patients who fail to respond may be treated with additional courses of their prescribed protocol in hopes of eventually inducing a response. Patients who relapse may be reinduced with intensive chemotherapy, but their prognosis for long-term survival is unfavorable.

Lymphoblastic Lymphoma

Treatment

ACUTE TREATMENT

51. D.B., a 16-year-old girl, presents with a history of shortness of breath and chest pain for 3 weeks before admission. A mediastinal mass is found, and a biopsy confirms a lymphoblastic (T-cell) lymphoma. X-ray of the chest reveals a right pleural effusion. Laboratory values show erythrocyte sedimentation rate, 35 (normal, 0–20); WBC count, 22,000/mm^3 (normal, 4,500–11,000); uric acid, 7 mg/dL; and LDH, 1,259 U/L (normal, 280–540). The bone marrow, CNS, and abdomen are negative for lymphoma. How should D.B. be managed acutely? Besides chemotherapy, what types of adjunctive therapies should be initiated to minimize the acute effects of treatment?

Given D.B.'s shortness of breath and chest pain, it is likely that her mediastinal mass may be obstructing the superior vena cava. To alleviate this obstruction, the most appropriate course of action is to decrease the tumor mass by initiating chemotherapy as soon as possible. Radiation therapy offers no additional benefit in patients such as D.B., with a tumor such as NHL, which is highly responsive to chemotherapy.[386,402] Because of the high cell kill that will result from the initial chemotherapy treatment, uric acid nephropathy is also possible. However, the risk of this complication is probably greater in patients with B-cell NHL in whom the fraction of cells in S phase is higher.[403,404]

Alkaline diuresis and allopurinol should be instituted before chemotherapy to prevent this complication (see question 4). Because D.B. has a pleural effusion, fluids may collect in this third space, resulting in weight gain and decreased urine output. Thus, in addition to placement of a chest tube with suction, D.B. should be given diuretics to maintain an adequate urine output. To minimize intravascular volume depletion and maintain electrolyte balances, fluid input and output, body weight, and electrolyte panels should be monitored daily. These values should be used to make appropriate adjustments in D.B.'s electrolyte and fluid balance.

ADVERSE EFFECTS

52. D.B. is treated with the BFM combination chemotherapy regimen. Due to her intrathoracic mass, her disease is characterized as stage III. She is to receive induction therapy for 8 weeks, as outlined in Table 90-21. Which acute adverse effects is D.B. likely to experience with these agents? How can they be monitored, minimized, and treated?

Several toxicities are expected with these chemotherapy agents. For vincristine, both constipation and neuropathy are likely to appear during or following the 4 weeks of therapy.[252] Constipation can be prevented or minimized by use of stool softeners with or without a laxative.[405] Neuropathy may be painful (especially when jaw pain occurs) but can be managed with mild analgesic regimens consisting of NSAIDs and/or acetaminophen with codeine. Both toxicities are self-limiting and are not reasons to discontinue or decrease the dosage of vincristine unless neuromuscular toxicity, as evidenced by motor weakness, develops. As outlined previously, asparaginase can cause several types of toxicities, most of which cannot be prevented.

Prednisone is likely to increase D.B.'s appetite and may cause gastritis, although divided doses will help decrease stomach upset. In addition, prednisone-induced behavioral disturbances are not uncommon.[254]

Unlike prednisone and vincristine, daunorubicin, cyclophosphamide, cytarabine, and mercaptopurine produce significant myelosuppression. Leukopenia is the primary sign, with the nadir occurring in approximately 8 to 14 days and recovery occurring by approximately day 21 after administration. Because the goal of induction therapy is achievement of remission, doses of daunorubicin will not be held for uncomplicated myelosuppression during the first 4 weeks of induction therapy, although during the latter 4 weeks, the combination of cyclophosphamide, cytarabine, and mercaptopurine are typically held until hematologic recovery occurs.

Hemorrhagic cystitis may occur with cyclophosphamide, but it is usually associated with high-dose therapy or with prolonged administration, which D.B. is not receiving. Vigorous IV hydration to maintain urine output of approximately 50 to 100 mL/m^2/hour should reduce the risk of this toxicity at this dose. In addition, this chemotherapy protocol also includes mesna, which will bind to urotoxic metabolites of cyclophosphamide and also reduce the risk of hemorrhagic cystitis. Because most of the induction regimen will be administered on an outpatient basis, patients and/or parents should be instructed to report signs or symptoms of infection (e.g., febrile episodes) immediately so that proper treatment may be instituted as soon as possible. To decrease the risk of hemorrhagic cystitis, parents should be instructed to report whether patients are urinating regularly after cyclophosphamide.

Nausea and vomiting are likely to be induced by both daunorubicin and cyclophosphamide/cytarabine.[406] D.B.'s chemotherapy regimen includes a corticosteroid (prednisone), which may provide some antiemetic activity during the initial 4 weeks.[407] However, to maximize tolerance to her chemotherapy, D.B. should receive a 5-HT_3 serotonin antagonist. Ondansetron may be used in this setting and is more effective than metoclopramide when either is combined with a corticosteroid.[408] D.B. is unlikely to require corticosteroids during the first 4 weeks of induction therapy. However, during the second portion of induction, D.B. will benefit from a few doses of dexamethasone at 10 mg/m^2 PO or IV at the time of cyclophosphamide administration.[406]

Central Nervous System Prophylaxis

53. What is the importance of CNS prophylaxis for D.B., and what type of treatment regimen is typically used?

All pediatric patients with lymphoblastic lymphoma should receive some form of CNS prophylaxis. Although lymphoblastic lymphoma rarely presents with CNS involvement, as illustrated by D.B., it was a common site of relapse before CNS prophylaxis was included as a routine part of the chemotherapy regimen.[391,392] Recurrence of NHL within the CNS is rare when intrathecal methotrexate and/or cytarabine are given.[386] D.B. will be treated with intrathecal methotrexate periodically, as outlined in Table 90-21.

Myelosuppression and Hematopoietic Recovery

54. After completion of initial therapy, the chemotherapy plan for D.B. consists of protocol M and reinduction protocol II, as outlined in Table 90-21. How should D.B.'s hematopoietic recovery be managed, and what guidelines may be used to determine when it is appropriate for her to receive the next sequence of the treatment cycle? Would D.B. benefit from a colony-stimulating factor (CSF) to aid with hematopoietic recovery?

Protocol M will likely not produce significant myelosuppression because leucovorin rescue will tend to minimize the myelosuppression from the high-dose methotrexate. The most challenging problems with this phase of treatment will be to confirm that the methotrexate has been properly eliminated and to continue aggressive hydration, alkalinization, and leucovorin dosing until the methotrexate level is nontoxic. Due to D.B.'s pleural effusion at the time of diagnosis, it should be confirmed that this has resolved prior to administration of high-dose methotrexate in order to avoid significantly delayed clearance because the pleural effusion could allow for third spacing of high doses of methotrexate. Pleural effusions are a relative contraindication to high-dose methotrexate. Methotrexate elimination has high inter- and intrapatient variability, and necessitates close monitoring of methotrexate concentrations and renal function after each dose.

Protocol II will result in significant myelosuppression. However, as with protocol I, dosing of doxorubicin will not be held for uncomplicated myelosuppression. Similarly, during the second phase of this protocol, dosing of cytarabine and thioguanine will also not be held for uncomplicated myelosuppression. However, prior to the start of this second phase on cycle day 36, clinicians will assure adequate hematologic recovery, typically defined as an ANC $>750/\text{mm}^3$ and platelets $>100{,}000/\text{mm}^3$. It is unlikely that D.B. will benefit from a CSF during these phases of therapy. When myelosuppressive chemotherapy is given fairly continuously, as is the case with protocol II, there is little room for inserting doses of CSFs on days where myelosuppressive chemotherapy is not being administered.

REFERENCES

1. American Cancer Society (ACS). Cancer Facts and Figures 2007. Available at: www.cancer.org/downloads/STT/CancerFacts&Figures2007TM.pdf. Accessed April 22, 2008.
2. Harris NL et al. World Health Organization classification of neoplastic diseases of the hematopoietic and lymphoid tissues: report of the Clinical Advisory Committee meeting, Airlie House, Virginia, November 1997. *J Clin Oncol* 1999;17:3835.
3. Armitage JO et al. New approaches to classifying non-Hodgkin's lymphomas: clinical features of the major histologic subtypes. *J Clin Oncol* 1998;16:2780.
4. Koeppen H, Vardiman JW. New entities, issues and controversies in the classification of malignant lymphoma. *Semin Oncol* 1998;25:421.
5. Munshi NC et al. Plasma cell neoplasms. In: De-Vita VT et al., eds. *Cancer: Principles and Practice of Oncology.* 6th ed. Philadelphia: Lippincott Williams & Wilkins; 2001:2465.
6. Lowenberg B et al. Acute myeloid leukemia. *N Engl J Med* 1990;341:1051.
7. Visani G et al. The prognostic value of cytogenetics is reinforced by the kind of induction/consolidation therapy in influencing the outcome of acute myeloid leukemia—analysis of 848 patients. *Leukemia* 2001;15:903.
8. Rai KR et al. Treatment of acute myelocytic leukemia: a study by cancer and leukemia group B. *Blood* 1981;58:1203.
9. Frei E et al. Dose schedule and antitumor studies of arabinosylcytosine. *Cancer Res* 1967;29:1325.
10. Scheinberg DA et al. Acute leukemias. In: De-Vita VT et al., eds. *Cancer: Principles and Practice of Oncology.* 6th ed. Philadelphia: Lippincott Williams & Wilkins; 2001:2404.
11. Bishop JF et al. Etoposide in acute nonlymphocytic leukemia. *Blood* 1990;75:27.
12. Hann IM et al. Randomized comparison of DAT vs. ADE as induction chemotherapy in children and younger adults with acute myeloid leukemia: results of the Medical Research Council's 10th AML Trial. *Blood* 1997;89:2311.
13. Brietman TR et al. Terminal differentiation of human promyelocytic leukemic cells in primary culture in response to retinoic acid. *Blood* 1981;57:1000.
14. Fenaux P et al. Effect of all transretinoic acid in newly diagnosed acute promyelocytic leukemia: results of a multicenter randomized trial. European APL 91 Group. *Blood* 1993;82:3241.
15. Castaigne S et al. All-*trans* retinoic acid as a differentiation therapy for acute promyelocytic leukemia: I. Clinical results. *Blood* 1990;76:1704.
16. Fenaux P et al. A randomized comparison of all transretinoic acid (ATRA) followed by chemotherapy and ATRA plus chemotherapy and the role of maintenance therapy in newly diagnosed acute promyelocytic leukemia. *Blood* 1999;94:1192.
17. Sanz MA et al. High molecular remission rate and low toxicity with modified AIDA protocol omitting cytarabine and etoposide from treatment of newly diagnosed PML-RAR-alpha positive acute promyelocytic leukemia. *Blood* 1999;94:4015.
18. Estey E et al. Treatment of newly diagnosed acute promyelocytic leukemia without cytarabine. *J Clin Oncol* 1997;15:483.
19. Tallman MS et al. All-transretinoic acid in acute promyelocytic leukemia. *N Engl J Med* 1997;337:1021.
20. Tallman MS et al. Clinical description of 44 patients with acute promyelocytic leukemia who developed the retinoic acid syndrome. *Blood* 2000;95:90.
21. DeBotton SD et al. Incidence, clinical features, and outcome of all transretinoic acid syndrome in 413 cases of newly diagnosed acute promyelocytic leukemia. *Blood* 1998;92:2712.
22. Soignet SL et al. United States multicenter study of arsenic trioxide in relapsed acute promyelocytic leukemia. *J Clin Oncol* 2001;19:3852.
23. Raffoux E et al. Combined treatment with arsenic trioxide and all-transretinoic acid in patients with relapsed acute promyelocytic leukemia. *J Clin Oncol* 2003;21:2326.
24. Flombaum CD. Metabolic emergencies in the cancer patient. *Semin Oncol* 2000;27:322.
25. Pui C-H et al. Recombinant urate oxidase for the prophylaxis or treatment of hyperuricemia in patients with leukemia or lymphoma. *J Clin Oncol* 2001;19;697.
26. Pui C-H et al. Recombinant urate oxidase (rasburicase) in the prevention and treatment of malignancy-associated hyperuricemia in pediatric and adult patients: results of a compassionate-use trial. *Leukemia* 2001;10:1505.
27. Bosly A et al. Rasburicase (recombinant urate oxidase) for the management of hyperuricemia in patients with cancer: report of an international compassionate use study. *Cancer* 2003;98:1048.
28. Souza LM et al. Recombinant human granulocyte-colony stimulating factor: effects on normal and leukemic myeloid cells. *Science* 1986;232:61.
29. Rowe JM et al. A randomized placebo-controlled phase III study of granulocyte-macrophage colony-stimulating factor in adult patients (>55 to 70 years of age) with acute myelogenous leukemia: a study of the Eastern Cooperative Oncology Group. *Blood* 1995;86:457.
30. Ozer H et al. 2000 Update of recommendations for the use of hematopoietic colony-stimulating factors: evidence-based, clinical practice guidelines. *J Clin Oncol* 2000;18:3558.
31. Mayer RJ et al. Intensive postremission chemotherapy in adults with acute myeloid leukemia. *N Engl J Med* 1994;331;896.
32. Tallman MS et al. Evaluation of intensive postremission chemotherapy for adults with acute nonlymphocytic leukemia using high-dose cytosine arabinoside with L-asparaginase and amsacrine with etoposide. *J Clin Oncol* 1987;5:918.
33. Graves T, Hooks MA. Drug-induced toxicities associated with high-dose cytosine arabinoside infusions. *Pharmacotherapy* 1989;9:23.

34. Ritch PS et al. Ocular toxicity from high-dose cytosine arabinoside. *Cancer* 1983;51:430.
35. Higa GM et al. The use of prophylactic eye drops during high-dose cytosine arabinoside therapy. *Cancer* 1991;68:1691.
36. Leith CP et al. Acute myeloid leukemia in the elderly: assessment of multidrug resistance (MDR) and cytogenetics distinguishes biologic subgroups with remarkable distinct responses to standard chemotherapy. A Southwest Oncology Group Study. *Blood* 1997;89:3323.
37. Hiddemann W et al. Management of acute myeloid leukemia in elderly patients. *J Clin Oncol* 1999; 17:3569.
38. Stone RM et al. The difficult problem of acute myeloid leukemia in the older adult. *CA Cancer J Clin* 2002;52:363.
39. Tilly H et al. Low-dose cytarabine versus intensive chemotherapy in the treatment of acute nonlymphocytic leukemia in the elderly. *J Clin Oncol* 1990;7:272.
40. Lowenberg B et al. On the value of intensive remission induction chemotherapy in elderly patients of 65-plus years with acute myeloid leukemia: a randomized phase III study of the European Organization for Research and Treatment of Cancer Leukemia Group. *J Clin Oncol* 1989;7:1268.
41. Sievers EL et al. Efficacy and safety of gemtuzumab ozogamicin in patients with CD33-positive acute myeloid leukemia in first relapse. *J Clin Oncol* 2001;19:3244.
42. Garcia-Manero GS et al. Chronic myelogenous leukemia: a review and update of therapeutic strategies. *Cancer* 2003;98:437.
43. National Cancer Institute, U.S. National Institute of Health. Chronic Myelogenous Leukemia Treatment (PDQ). Available at: www.nci.nih.gov/cancerinfo/pdq/treatment/CML/healthprofessional/. Accessed April 22, 2008.
44. Sawyers CL. Chronic myeloid leukemia. *N Engl J Med* 1999;340:1330.
45. McGlave P. Unrelated donor transplant therapy for chronic myelogenous leukemia. *Hematol Oncol Clin N Am* 1998;12:93.
46. Pasweg JR et al. Related donor bone marrow transplantation for chronic myelogenous leukemia. *Hematol Oncol Clin N Am* 1998;12:81.
47. Silver RT et al. An evidence based analysis of the effects of busulfan, hydroxyurea, interferon, and allogeneic bone marrow transplantation in treating the chronic phase of CML: developed by the American Society of Hematology. *Blood* 1999;94:1517.
48. Druker BJ et al. Efficacy and safety of a specific inhibitor of the bcr-abl tyrosine kinase in chronic myeloid leukemia. *N Engl J Med* 2001;344:1031.
49. Talpaz M et al. Imatinib induces durable hematologic and cytogenetics responses in patients with accelerated phase chronic myeloid leukemia: results of a phase 2 study. *Blood* 2002;99:1928.
50. Sawyers CL et al. Imatinib induces hematologic and cytogenetics responses in patients with chronic myelogenous leukemia in myeloid blast crisis: results of a phase II study. *Blood* 2002;99: 3530.
51. O'Brien SG et al. Imatinib compared with interferon and low-dose cytarabine for newly diagnosed chronic-phase chronic myeloid leukemia. *N Engl J Med* 2003;348:994.
52. Druker BJ et al. Five year follow-up of patients receiving imatinib for chronic myeloid leukemia. *N Engl J Med* 2006;355:2408.
53. Deininger MW et al. Practical management of patients with chronic myeloid leukemia receiving imatinib. *J Clin Oncol* 2003;21:1637.
54. Talpaz M et al. Dasatinib in imatinib-resistant Philadelphia chromosome-positive leukemias. *N Engl J Med* 2006;354:2531.
55. Cortes J et al. Dasatinib induced complete hematologic and cytogenetic responses in patients with imatinib-resistant or -intolerant chronic myeloid leukemia in blast crisis. *Blood* 2007;109:3207.
56. Hochhaus A et al. Dasatinib induced notable hematologic and cytogenetic responses in chronic phase chronic myeloid leukemia after failure of imatinib therapy. *Blood* 2007;109:2303.
57. Binet JL et al. Perspectives on the use of new diagnostic tools in the treatment of chronic lymphocytic leukemia. *Blood* 2006;107:859.
58. American Cancer Society (ACS). Cancer Facts and Figures 2007. Available at: www.cancer.org/downloads/STT/CAFF2007PWSecured.pdf. Accessed April 22, 2008.
59. O'Brien S, Keating MJ. *Chronic Lymphoid Leukemias*. Vol. 2, 7th ed. Philadelphia: Lippincott Williams & Wilkins; 2005.
60. Shanafelt TD et al. Narrative review: initial management of newly diagnosed, early-stage chronic lymphocytic leukemia. *Ann Intern Med* 2006;145:435.
61. Binet JL et al. A new prognostic classification of chronic lymphocytic leukemia derived from a multivariate survival analysis. *Cancer* 1981;48:198.
62. Anonymous. Chemotherapeutic options in chronic lymphocytic leukemia: a meta-analysis of the randomized trials. CLL Trialists' Collaborative Group. *J Natl Cancer Inst* 1999;91:861.
63. Oscier D et al. Guidelines on the diagnosis and management of chronic lymphocytic leukaemia. *Br J Haematol* 2004;125:294.
64. French Cooperative Group on Chronic Lymphocytic Leukaemia. Natural history of stage A chronic lymphocytic leukaemia untreated patients. *Br J Haematol* 1990;76:45.
65. Palma M et al. The biology and treatment of chronic lymphocytic leukemia. *Ann Oncol* 2006;17(Suppl 10):144.
66. Byrd JC et al. Select high-risk genetic features predict earlier progression following chemoimmunotherapy with fludarabine and rituximab in chronic lymphocytic leukemia: justification for risk-adapted therapy. *J Clin Oncol* 2006;24:437.
67. Dohner H et al. Genomic aberrations and survival in chronic lymphocytic leukemia. *N Engl J Med* 2000;343:1910.
68. Orchard JA et al. ZAP-70 expression and prognosis in chronic lymphocytic leukaemia. *Lancet* 2004;363:105.
69. Keating MJ et al. Long-term follow-up of patients with chronic lymphocytic leukemia (CLL) receiving fludarabine regimens as initial therapy. *Blood* 1998;92:1165.
70. Rai KR et al. Fludarabine compared with chlorambucil as primary therapy for chronic lymphocytic leukemia. *N Engl J Med* 2000;343:1750.
71. Rummel MJ. Fludarabine versus fludarabine plus epirubicin in the treatment of chronic lymphocytic leukemia—final results of a German randomized phase-III study. *Blood* 2005;106a:2123.
72. Byrd JC et al. Randomized phase 2 study of fludarabine with concurrent versus sequential treatment with rituximab in symptomatic, untreated patients with B-cell chronic lymphocytic leukemia: results from Cancer and Leukemia Group B 9712 (CALGB 9712). *Blood* 2003;101:6.
73. Keating MJ et al. Early results of a chemoimmunotherapy regimen of fludarabine, cyclophosphamide, and rituximab as initial therapy for chronic lymphocytic leukemia. *J Clin Oncol* 2005; 23:4079.
74. Eichhorst BF et al. Fludarabine plus cyclophosphamide versus fludarabine alone in first-line therapy of younger patients with chronic lymphocytic leukemia. *Blood* 2006;107:885.
75. Morrison VA et al. Impact of therapy with chlorambucil, fludarabine, or fludarabine plus chlorambucil on infections in patients with chronic lymphocytic leukemia: Intergroup Study Cancer and Leukemia Group B 9011. *J Clin Oncol* 2001;19:3611.
76. Robak T et al. Cladribine with prednisone versus chlorambucil with prednisone as first-line therapy in chronic lymphocytic leukemia: report of a prospective, randomized, multicenter trial. *Blood* 2000;96:2723.
77. Robak T et al. Cladribine alone and in combination with cyclophosphamide or cyclophosphamide plus mitoxantrone in the treatment of progressive chronic lymphocytic leukemia: report of a prospective, multicenter, randomized trial of the Polish Adult Leukemia Group (PALG CLL2). *Blood* 2006;108:473.
78. O'Brien SM et al. Rituximab dose-escalation trial in chronic lymphocytic leukemia. *J Clin Oncol* 2001;19:2165.
79. Hainsworth JD et al. Single-agent rituximab as first-line and maintenance treatment for patients with chronic lymphocytic leukemia or small lymphocytic lymphoma: a phase II trial of the Minnie Pearl Cancer Research Network. *J Clin Oncol* 2003;21:1746.
80. Lundin J et al. Phase II trial of subcutaneous anti-CD52 monoclonal antibody alemtuzumab (Campath-1H) as first-line treatment for patients with B-cell chronic lymphocytic leukemia (B-CLL). *Blood* 2002;100:768.
81. Hillmen P et al. Preliminary phase III efficacy and safety of alemtuzumab vs chlorambucil as frontline therapy for patients with progressive B-cell chronic lymphocytic leukemia (BCLL). *J Clin Oncol* 2006;24(Suppl).
82. Martin SI et al. Infectious complications associated with alemtuzumab use for lymphoproliferative disorders. *Clin Infect Dis* 2006;43:16.
83. Osterborg A et al. Strategies in the management of alemtuzumab-related side effects. *Semin Oncol* 2006;33:S29.
84. O'Brien SM et al. Alemtuzumab as treatment for residual disease after chemotherapy in patients with chronic lymphocytic leukemia. *Cancer* 2003; 98:2657.
85. Wierda W et al. Chemoimmunotherapy with fludarabine, cyclophosphamide, and rituximab for relapsed and refractory chronic lymphocytic leukemia. *J Clin Oncol* 2005;23:4070.
86. Keating MJ et al. Therapeutic role of alemtuzumab in (Campath-1H) in patients who have failed fludarabine: results of a large international study. *Blood* 2002;99:3554.
87. Rai KR et al. Alemtuzumab in previously treated chronic lymphocytic leukemia patients who also had received fludarabine. *J Clin Oncol* 2002;20: 3891.
88. National Comprehensive Cancer Network (NCCN). *NCCN Clinical Practice Guidelines in Oncology: Non-Hodgkin's Lymphomas*. Vol. 1. Fort Washington, PA: NCCN; 2007.
89. Moreton P et al. Eradication of minimal residual disease in B-cell chronic lymphocytic leukemia after alemtuzumab therapy is associated with prolonged survival. *J Clin Oncol* 2005;23:2971.
90. O'Brien SM et al. Updated guidelines on the management of cytomegalovirus reactivation in patients with chronic lymphocytic leukemia treated with alemtuzumab. *Clin Lymphoma Myeloma* 2006; 7:125.
91. Keating M et al. Management guidelines for use of alemtuzumab in B-cell chronic lymphocytic leukemia. *Clin Lymphoma* 2004;4:220.
92. Gribben JG et al. Autologous and allogeneic stem cell transplantations for poor-risk chronic lymphocytic leukemia. *Blood* 2005;106:4389.
93. Ravandi F, O'Brien S. Infections associated with purine analogs and monoclonal antibodies. *Blood Rev* 2005;19:253.
94. Weeks JC et al. Cost effectiveness of prophylactic intravenous immune globulin in chronic lymphocytic leukemia. *N Engl J Med* 1991;325:81.
95. Fisher R et al. Non-Hodgkin's lymphomas. In: DeVita VT et al., eds. *Cancer: Principles & Practice of Oncology*. 7th ed. Vol. 2. Baltimore: Lippincott Williams & Wilkins; 2005.
96. Ansell SM, Armitage J. Non-Hodgkin lymphoma: diagnosis and treatment. *Mayo Clin Proc* 2005;80:1087.
97. Harris NL et al. A revised European-American classification of lymphoid neoplasms: a proposal from the International Lymphoma Study Group. *Blood* 1994;84:1361.
98. Harris NL et al. World Health Organization classification of neoplastic diseases of the hematopoietic and lymphoid tissues: report of the Clinical

Advisory Committee meeting, Airlie House, Virginia, November 1997. *J Clin Oncol* 1999;17:3835.
99. Carbone PP et al. Report of the committee on Hodgkin's disease staging. *Cancer Res* 1971;31:1860.
100. A predictive model for aggressive non-Hodgkin's lymphoma. The International Non-Hodgkin's Lymphoma Prognostic Factors Project. *N Engl J Med* 1993;329:987.
101. Jones SE et al. Superiority of Adriamycin-containing combination chemotherapy in the treatment of diffuse lymphoma: a Southwest Oncology Group study. *Cancer* 1979;43:417.
102. Gordon LI et al. Comparison of a second-generation combination chemotherapeutic regimen (m-BACOD) with a standard regimen (CHOP) for advanced diffuse non-Hodgkin's lymphoma. *N Engl J Med* 1992;327:1342.
103. Fisher RI et al. Comparison of a standard regimen (CHOP) with three intensive chemotherapy regimens for advanced non-Hodgkin's lymphoma. *N Engl J Med* 1993;328:1002.
104. Pfreundschuh M et al. Two-weekly or 3-weekly CHOP chemotherapy with or without etoposide for the treatment of elderly patients with aggressive lymphomas: results of the NHL-B2 trial of the DSHNHL. *Blood* 2004;104:634.
105. Pfreundschuh M et al. Two-weekly or 3-weekly CHOP chemotherapy with or without etoposide for the treatment of young patients with good-prognosis (normal LDH) aggressive lymphomas: results of the NHL-B1 trial of the DSHNHL. *Blood* 2004;104:626.
106. Cerny T et al. Mechanism of action of rituximab. *Anticancer Drugs* 2002;13:S3.
107. Feugier P et al. Long-term results of the R-CHOP study in the treatment of elderly patients with diffuse large B-cell lymphoma: a study by the Groupe d'ude des Lymphomes de l'Adulte. *J Clin Oncol* 2005;23:4117.
108. Habermann TM et al. Phase III trial of rituximab-CHOP (R-CHOP) vs. CHOP with a second randomization to maintenance rituximab (MR) or observation in patients 60 years of age and older with diffuse large B-cell lymphoma (DLBCL) [abstract]. *Blood* 2003;102:6A.
109. Pfrendschuh M et al. First analysis of the completed mabthera international (MlnT) trial in young patients with low-risk diffuse large B-cell lymphoma (DLBCL): addition of rituximab to a CHOP-like regimen significantly improves outcome of all patients with the identification of a very favorable subgroup with IPI=O and no bulky disease [abstract]. *Blood* 2004;104:48A.
110. Byrd JC et al. Rituximab therapy in hematologic malignancy patients with circulating blood tumor cells: association with increased infusion related side effects and rapid blood tumor clearance. *J Clin Oncol* 1999;17:791.
111. Shipp MA et al. International consensus conference on high-dose therapy with hematopoietic stem cell transplantation in aggressive non-Hodgkin's lymphoma: report of the jury. *J Clin Oncol* 1999;17:423.
112. Kantarjian HM et al. Results of treatment with hyper-CVAD, a dose-intensive regimen, in adult acute lymphocytic leukemia. *J Clin Oncol* 2000;18:547.
113. Young RC et al. The treatment of indolent lymphomas: watchful waiting v aggressive combined modality treatment. *Semin Hematol* 1988;25:11.
114. Ghielmini M et al. Prolonged treatment with rituximab in patients with follicular lymphoma significantly increases event-free survival and response duration compared with the standard weekly × 4 schedule. *Blood* 2004;103:4416.
115. Czuczman MS. CHOP plus rituximab chemoimmunotherapy of indolent B-cell lymphoma. *Semin Oncol* 1999;26:88.
116. Marcus R et al. CVP chemotherapy plus rituximab compared with CVP as first-line treatment for advanced follicular lymphoma. *Blood* 2005;105:1417.
117. McLaughlin P et al. Safety of fludarabine, mitoxantrone, and dexamethasone combined with rituximab in the treatment of stage IV indolent lymphoma. *Semin Oncol* 2000;27:37.
118. Davis TA et al. Rituximab anti-CD20 monoclonal antibody therapy in non-Hodgkin's lymphoma: safety and efficacy of re-treatment. *J Clin Oncol* 2000;18:3135.
119. Witzig TE et al. Treatment with ibritumomab tiuxetan radioimmunotherapy in patients with rituximab-refractory follicular non-Hodgkin's lymphoma. *J Clin Oncol* 2002;20:3262.
120. Witzig TE et al. Randomized controlled trial of yttrium-90-labeled ibritumomab tiuxetan radioimmunotherapy versus rituximab immunotherapy for patients with relapsed or refractory low-grade, follicular, or transformed B-cell non-Hodgkin's lymphoma. *J Clin Oncol* 2002;20:2453.
121. Schouten HC et al. High-dose therapy improves progression-free survival and survival in relapsed follicular non-Hodgkin's lymphoma: results from the randomized European CUP trial. *J Clin Oncol* 2003;21:3918.
122. Gopal AK et al. High-dose [^{131}I]tositumomab (anti-CD20) radioimmunotherapy and autologous hematopoietic stem-cell transplantation for adults $\geq$60 years old with relapsed or refractory B-cell lymphoma. *J Clin Oncol* 2007;25:1396.
123. Branson K et al. Role of nonmyeloablative allogeneic stem-cell transplantation after failure of autologous transplantation in patients with lymphoproliferative malignancies. *J Clin Oncol* 2002;20:4022.
124. Hasenclever D et al. A prognostic score for advanced Hodgkin's disease. International Prognostic Factors Project on Advanced Hodgkin's Disease. *N Engl J Med* 1998;339:1506.
125. Bonfante V et al. ABVD in the treatment of Hodgkin's disease. *Semin Oncol* 1992;19:38.
126. Canellos GP et al. Chemotherapy of advanced Hodgkin's disease with MOPP, ABVD, or MOPP alternating with ABVD. *N Engl J Med* 1992;327:1478.
127. Duggan DB et al. Randomized comparison of ABVD and MOPP/ABV hybrid for the treatment of advanced Hodgkin's disease: report of an Intergroup trial. *J Clin Oncol* 2003;21:607.
128. Canellos GP et al. How important is bleomycin in the Adriamycin + bleomycin + vinblastine + dacarbazine regimen? *J Clin Oncol* 2004;22:1532.
129. Ekstrand BC et al. Rituximab in lymphocyte-predominant Hodgkin disease: results of a phase 2 trial. *Blood* 2003;101:4285.
130. Jostin A et al. New prognostic score based on treatment outcome of patients with relapsed Hodgkin's lymphoma registered in the database of the German Hodgkin's Lymphoma Study Group. *J Clin Oncol* 2002;20:221.
131. Byrne BJ, Gockerman JP. Salvage therapy in Hodgkin's lymphoma. *Oncologist* 2007;12:156.
132. Munshi NC, Anderson KC. Plasma cell neoplasms. In: DeVita VT et al., eds. *Cancer: Principles and Practice of Oncology.* 7th ed. Philadelphia: Lippincott Williams & Wilkins; 2005:2156.
133. Jemal A et al. Cancer statistics 2007. *CA Cancer J Clin* 2007;57:43.
134. Goldschmidt H et al. Multiple myeloma and renal failure. *Nephrol Dial Transplant* 2000;15:301.
135. International Myeloma Working Group. Criteria for the classification of monoclonal gammopathies, multiple myeloma and related disorders: a report of the International Working Group. *Br J Haematol* 2003;121:749.
136. Greipp PR et al. International staging system for multiple myeloma. *J Clin Oncol* 2005;23:3412.
137. Orlowski RZ. Initial therapy of multiple myeloma patients who are not candidates for stem cell transplantation. *Hematology* 2006;338.
138. Alexanian R et al. Primary dexamethasone treatment of multiple myeloma. *Blood* 1992;80:887.
139. Rajkumar SV et al. Phase III clinical trial of thalidomide plus dexamethasone compared with dexamethasone alone in newly diagnosed multiple myeloma: a clinical trial coordinated by the Eastern Cooperative Oncology Group. *J Clin Oncol* 2006;24:341.
140. Rifkin RM et al. Pegylated liposomal doxorubicin, vincristine, and dexamethasone provide significant reduction in toxicity compared with doxorubicin, vincristine, and dexamethasone in patients with newly diagnosed multiple myeloma: a phase III multicenter trial. *Cancer* 2006;106:848.
141. Palumbo A et al. Oral melphalan, prednisone, and thalidomide compared with melphalan and prednisone alone in elderly patients with multiple myeloma: randomised controlled trial. *Lancet* 2006;367:825.
142. Ferman JP et al. High-dose therapy and autologous peripheral blood stem cell transplantation in multiple myeloma: up-front or rescue treatment? Results of a multicenter sequential randomized trial. *Blood* 1998;92:3131.
143. Child JA et al. High-dose chemotherapy with hematopoietic stem-cell rescue for multiple myeloma. *N Engl J Med* 2003;348:1875.
144. Attal M et al. A prospective randomized trial of autologous bone marrow transplantation and chemotherapy in multiple myeloma. *N Engl J Med* 1996;335:91.
145. Lenhoff S et al. Impact on survival of high-dose therapy with autologous stem cell support in patients younger than 60 with newly diagnosed multiple myeloma: a population-based study. *Blood* 2000;95:7.
146. Hahn T et al. The role of cytotoxic therapy with hematopoietic stem cell transplantation in the therapy of multiple myeloma: an evidence-based review. *Biol Blood Marrow Transplant* 2003;9:4.
147. Kroger N et al. Autologous stem cell transplantation followed by a dose-reduced allograft induces high complete remission rate in multiple myeloma. *Blood* 2002;100:755.
148. Badros A et al. Improved outcome of allogeneic transplantation in high-risk multiple myeloma patients after nonmyeloablative conditioning. *J Clin Oncol* 2002;20:1295.
149. Crawley C et al. Outcomes for reduced-intensity allogeneic transplantation for multiple myeloma: an analysis of prognostic factors from the Chronic Leukaemia Working Party of the EBMT. *Blood* 2005;105:4532.
150. Kyle RA et al. American Society of Clinical Oncology 2007 clinical practice guidelines update on the role of bisphosphonates in multiple myeloma. *J Clin Oncol* 2007;25:2464.
151. Zervas K et al. Incidence, risk factors and management of osteonecrosis of the jaw in patients with multiple myeloma: a single-centre experience in 303 patients. *Br J Haematol* 2006;134:620.
152. Richardson PG et al. Bortezomib or high-dose dexamethasone for relapsed multiple myeloma. *N Engl J Med* 2005;352:2487.
153. Weber DM et al. Lenalidomide plus dexamethasone for relapsed multiple myeloma in North America. *N Engl J Med* 2007;357:2133.
154. Lee C-K et al. DTPACE: an effective, novel combination chemotherapy with thalidomide for previously treated patients with myeloma. *J Clin Oncol* 2003;21:2732.
155. Ries LAG et al., eds. Cancer incidence and survival among children and adolescents: United States SEER Program 1975–1995. NIH Publication No. 99–4649. Bethesda, MD: National Cancer Institute, SEER Program; 1999.
156. Pui C-H, Evans WE. Acute lymphoblastic leukemia. *N Engl J Med* 1998;332:605.
157. Bizzozero OJ Jr et al. Radiation-related leukemia in Hiroshima and Nagasaki, 1946–64: I. Distribution, incidence and appearance in time. *N Engl J Med* 1966;274:1095.
158. Folley JH et al. Incidence of leukemia in survivors of the atomic bomb in Hiroshima and Nagasaki, Japan. *Am J Med* 1952;13:311.
159. Morgan KZ. Radiation-induced health effects. *Science* 1977;195:344.

160. Van Steensel-Moll HA et al. Are maternal fertility problems related to childhood leukemia? *Int J Epidemiol* 1985;14:555.
161. Stjernfeldt M et al. Maternal smoking during pregnancy and risk of childhood cancer. *Lancet* 1986;1:1350.
162. London SL et al. Exposure to residential electric and magnetic fields and risk of childhood leukemia. *Am J Epidemiol* 1991;134:923.
163. Greenberg RS, Shuster JL. Epidemiology of cancer in children. *Epidemiol Rev* 1985;7:22.
164. Wyke J. Principles of viral leukemogenesis. *Semin Hematol* 1986;23:189.
165. Michaelson SM. Household magnetic fields and childhood leukemia: a critical analysis. *Pediatrics* 1991;88:630.
166. Pool R. Is there an EMF-cancer connection? *Science* 1990;249:1096.
167. Lewis MS. Spatial clustering in childhood leukemia. *J Chronic Dis* 1980;33:703.
168. Feltbower RG et al. International parallels in leukaemia and diabetes epidemiology. *Arch Dis Child* 2004;89:54.
169. Steffen C et al. Acute childhood leukaemia and environmental exposure to potential sources of benzene and other hydrocarbons: a case-control study. *Occup Environ Med* 2004;61:773.
170. Miller DR. Childhood acute lymphoblastic leukemia: 1. Biological features and their use in predicting outcome of treatment. *Am J Pediatr Hematol Oncol* 1988;10:163.
171. Bhojwani D et al. Potential of gene expression profiling in the management of childhood acute lymphoblastic leukemia. *Paediatr Drugs* 2007;9:149.
172. Miller DR. Acute lymphoblastic leukemia. *Pediatr Clin North Am* 1980;27:269.
173. Margolin JF, Poplack DG. Acute lymphoblastic leukemia. In: Pizzo PA, Poplack DG, eds. *Principles and Practice of Pediatric Oncology.* Philadelphia: Lippincott-Raven; 1997:409.
174. Smith M et al. Uniform approach to risk classification and treatment assignment for children with acute lymphoblastic leukemia. *J Clin Oncol* 1996;14:18.
175. Sather HN. Statistical evaluation of prognostic factors in ALL and treatment results. *Med Pediatr Oncol* 1986;14:158.
176. Mastrangelo R et al. Report and recommendations of the Rome Workshop concerning poor-prognosis acute lymphoblastic leukemia in children: biologic bases for staging, stratification, and treatment. *Med Pediatr Oncol* 1986;14:191.
177. Bleyer WA et al. The staging of childhood acute lymphoblastic leukemia: strategies of the Children's Cancer Study Group and a three-dimensional technique of multivariate analysis. *Med Pediatr Oncol* 1986;14:271.
178. Nachman J et al. Young adults 1621 years of age at diagnosis entered on Children's Cancer Group acute lymphoblastic leukemia and acute myeloblastic leukemia protocols: results of treatment. *Cancer* 1993;71(Suppl):3377.
179. Pui C-H, Evans WE. Acute lymphoblastic leukemia in infants. *J Clin Oncol* 1999;17:438.
180. Lauer SJ et al. Intensive alternating drug pairs after remission induction for treatment of infants with acute lymphoblastic leukemia: a Pediatric Oncology Group pilot study. *J Pediatr Hematol Oncol* 1998;20:229.
181. Reaman GH et al. Treatment outcome and prognostic factors for infants with acute lymphoblastic leukemia treated on two consecutive trials of the Children's Cancer Group. *J Clin Oncol* 1999;17:445.
182. Hilden JM et al. Analysis of prognostic factors of acute lymphoblastic leukemia in infants: report on CCG 1953 from the Children's Oncology Group. *Blood* 2006;108:441.
183. Hammond D et al. Analysis of prognostic factors in acute lymphoblastic leukemia. *Med Pediatr Oncol* 1986;14:124.
184. Lanning M et al. Superior treatment results in females with high-risk acute lymphoblastic leukemia in childhood. *Acta Paediatr* 1992;81:66.
185. Hale JP, Lilleyman JS. Importance of 6-mercaptopurine dose in lymphoblastic leukaemia. *Arch Dis Child* 1991;66:462.
186. Lilleyman JS et al. Childhood lymphoblastic leukemia: sex difference in 6-mercaptopurine utilization. *Br J Cancer* 1984;49:703.
187. Pui C-H et al. Sex differences in prognosis for children with acute lymphoblastic leukemia. *J Clin Oncol* 1999;17:818.
188. Kalwinsky DK et al. Variation by race in presenting clinical and biologic features of childhood acute lymphoblastic leukaemia: implications for treatment outcome. *Leuk Res* 1985;9:817.
189. Walters TR et al. Poor prognosis in Negro children with acute lymphoblastic leukemia. *Cancer* 1972;29:210.
190. Sklo M et al. The changing survivorship of white and black children with leukemia. *Cancer* 1978;42:59.
191. Pui C-H et al. Outcome of treatment for childhood cancer in black as compared with white children: the St. Jude Children's Research Hospital experience, 1962 through 1992. *JAMA* 1995;273:633.
192. McNeil DE et al. SEER update of incidence and trends in pediatric malignancies: acute lymphoblastic leukemia. *Med Pediatr Oncol* 2002;39:554.
193. Bhatia S et al. Racial and ethnic differences in survival of children with acute lymphoblastic leukemia. *Blood* 2002;100:1957.
194. Gupta S, Good RA. Markers of human lymphocyte subpopulations in primary immunodeficiency and lymphoproliferative disorders. *Semin Hematol* 1980;17:1.
195. Brouet JC et al. The use of B and T membrane markers in the classification of human leukemias, with special reference to acute lymphoblastic leukemia. *Blood Cells* 1975;1:81.
196. Brouet JC, Seligmann M. The immunological classification of acute lymphoblastic leukemias. *Cancer* 1978;42:817.
197. Cossman J et al. Induction of differentiation in the primitive B-cells of common, acute lymphoblastic leukemia. *N Engl J Med* 1982;307:1251.
198. Crist WM et al. Immunologic markers in childhood acute lymphocytic leukemia. *Semin Oncol* 1985;12:105.
199. Nadler LM et al. Induction of human B-cell antigens in non-T-cell acute lymphoblastic leukemia. *J Clin Invest* 1982;70:433.
200. Pesando JM et al. Leukemia-associated antigens in ALL. *Blood* 1979;54:1240.
201. Ritz J et al. A monoclonal antibody to human acute lymphoblastic leukemia antigen. *Nature* 1980;283:583.
202. Pullen DJ et al. Southwest Oncology Group experience with immunological phenotyping in acute lymphocytic leukemia of childhood. *Cancer Res* 1981;41:4802.
203. Magrath IT et al. Bone marrow involvement in Burkitt's lymphoma and its relationship to acute B-cell leukemia. *Leuk Res* 1979;4:33.
204. Flandrin G et al. Acute leukemia with Burkitt's tumor cells: a study of six cases with special reference to lymphocyte surface markers. *Blood* 1975;45:183.
205. Reiter A et al. Favorable outcome of B-cell acute lymphoblastic leukemia in childhood: a report of three consecutive studies of the BFM group. *Blood* 1992;80:2471.
206. Patte C. Non-Hodgkin's lymphoma. *Eur J Cancer* 1998;34:359.
207. Bowman WP et al. Cell markers in lymphomas and leukemias. In: Stollerman GH, ed. *Advances in Internal Medicine.* Chicago: Year-Book Medical; 1980:391.
208. Sallan SE et al. Cell surface antigens: prognostic implications in childhood acute lymphoblastic leukemia. *Blood* 1980;55:395.
209. Steinherz PG et al. Improved disease-free survival of children with acute lymphoblastic leukemia at high risk for early relapse with the New York regimen—a new intensive therapy protocol: a report from the Children's Cancer Study Group. *J Clin Oncol* 1986;4:744.
210. Amylon MD et al. Intensive high-dose asparaginase consolidation improves survival for pediatric patients with T cell acute lymphoblastic leukemia and advanced stage lymphoblastic lymphoma: a Pediatric Oncology Group study. *Leukemia* 1999;13:335.
211. Goldberg JM et al. Childhood T-cell acute lymphoblastic leukemia: the Dana-Farber Cancer Institute acute lymphoblastic leukemia consortium experience. *J Clin Oncol* 2003;21:3616.
212. Nachman JB et al. Augmented post-induction therapy for children with high-risk acute lymphoblastic leukemia and a slow response to initial therapy. *N Engl J Med* 1998;338:1663.
213. Rots MG et al. Role of folylpolyglutamate synthetase and folylpolyglutamate hydrolase in methotrexate accumulation and polyglutamylation in childhood leukemia. *Blood* 1999;93:1677.
214. Look AT et al. Prognostic importance of blast cell DNA content in childhood acute lymphoblastic leukemia. *Blood* 1985;65:1079.
215. Kaspers GJL et al. Favorable prognosis of hyperdiploid common acute lymphoblastic leukemia may be explained by sensitivity to antimetabolites and other drugs: results of an in vitro study. *Blood* 1995;85:751.
216. Zhang L et al. Reduced folate carrier gene expression in childhood acute lymphoblastic leukemia: relationship to immunophenotype and ploidy. *Clin Cancer Res* 1998;4:2169.
217. Belkov VM et al. Reduced folate carrier expression in acute lymphoblastic leukemia: a mechanism for ploidy but not lineage differences in methotrexate accumulation. *Blood* 1999;93:1643.
218. Heerema NA et al. Hypodiploidy with less than 45 chromosomes confers adverse risk in childhood acute lymphoblastic leukemia: a report from the Children's Cancer Group. *Blood* 1999;94:4036.
219. Look AT. The cytogenetics of childhood leukemia: clinical and biological implications. *Pediatr Clin North Am* 1988;35:723.
220. Borkhardt A et al. Biology and clinical significance of the TEL/AML1 rearrangement. *Curr Opin Pediatr* 1999;11:33.
221. Uckun FM et al. Clinical significance of Philadelphia chromosome positive pediatric acute lymphoblastic leukemia in the context of contemporary intensive therapies: a report from the Children's Cancer Group. *Cancer* 1998;83:2030.
222. Schrappe M et al. Philadelphia chromosome-positive (Ph^+) childhood acute lymphoblastic leukemia: good initial steroid response allows early prediction of a favorable treatment outcome. *Blood* 1998;92:2730.
223. Loh ML et al. Prospective analysis of TEL/AML1-positive patients treated on Dana-Farber Cancer Institute Consortium Protocol 95-01. *Blood* 2006;107:4508.
224. Rocha JCC et al. Pharmacogenetics of outcome in children with acute lymphoblastic leukemia. *Blood* 2005;105:4752.
225. Foroni L et al. Investigation of minimal residual disease in childhood and adult acute lymphoblastic leukaemia by molecular analysis. *Br J Haematol* 1999;105:7.
226. Gaynon PS et al. Early response to therapy and outcome in childhood acute lymphoblastic leukemia: a review. *Cancer* 1997;80:1717.
227. Nachman JB et al. Augmented post-induction therapy for children with high-risk acute lymphoblastic leukemia and a slow response to initial therapy. *N Engl J Med* 1998;338:1663.
228. Arico M et al. Improved outcome in high-risk childhood acute lymphoblastic leukemia defined by prednisone-poor response treated with double Berlin-Frankfurt-Muenster protocol II. *Blood* 2002;100:420.
229. Willemse MJ et al. Detection of minimal residual disease identifies differences in treatment

response between T-ALL and precursor B-ALL. *Blood* 2002;99:4386.
230. Dordelmann M et al. Down's syndrome in childhood acute lymphoblastic leukemia: clinical characteristics and treatment outcome in four consecutive BFM trials. *Leukemia* 1998;12:645.
231. Gomez-Almaguer D et al. Nutritional status and socio-economic conditions as prognostic factors in the outcome of therapy in childhood acute lymphoblastic leukemia. *Int J Cancer* 1998;11:52.
232. Elion GB et al. Relationship between metabolic rates and antitumor activities of thiopurines. *Cancer Res* 1963;23:1207.
233. Zimm S et al. Inhibition of first pass metabolism in cancer chemotherapy: interaction of 6-mercaptopurine and allopurinol. *Clin Pharmacol Ther* 1983; 34:810.
234. Skipper HE, Perry SE. Kinetics of normal and leukemic leukocyte populations: relevance to chemotherapy. *Cancer Res* 1970;30:1883.
235. Hart JS et al. The mechanism of induction of complete remission in acute myeloblastic leukemia in man. *Cancer Res* 1969;29:2300.
236. Lonsdale D et al. Interrupted vs continued maintenance therapy in childhood leukemia. *Cancer* 1975;336:342.
237. Rivera GK et al. Improved outcome in childhood acute lymphoblastic leukaemia with reinforced early treatment and rotational combination chemotherapy. *Lancet* 1991;337:61.
238. Rizzari C et al. A pharmacological study on pegylated asparaginase used in front-line treatment of children with acute lymphoblastic leukemia. *Haematologica* 2006;91:24.
239. Bostrom BC et al. Dexamethasone versus prednisone and daily oral versus weekly intravenous mercaptopurine for patients with standard-risk acute lymphoblastic leukemia: a report from the Children's Cancer Group. *Blood* 2003;101:3809.
240. Clavell LA et al. Four-agent induction and intensive asparaginase therapy for treatment of childhood acute lymphoblastic leukemia. *N Engl J Med* 1986;315:657.
241. Balis FM et al. Differences in cerebrospinal fluid penetration of corticosteroids: possible relationship to the prevention of meningeal leukemia. *J Clin Oncol* 1987;5:202.
242. Hurwitz CA et al. Substituting dexamethasone for prednisone complicates remission induction in children with acute lymphoblastic leukemia. *Cancer* 2000;88:1964.
243. Avramis VI et al. A randomized comparison of native *Escherichia coli* asparaginase and polyethylene glycol conjugated asparaginase for treatment of children with newly diagnosed standard-risk acute lymphoblastic leukemia: a Children's Cancer Group study. *Blood* 2002;99:1986.
244. Aur RJA et al. Childhood acute lymphocytic leukemia: study VIII. *Cancer* 1978;42:2123.
245. Simone JV. Factors that influence haematological remission duration in acute lymphocytic leukemia. *Br J Haematol* 1976;32:465.
246. Ortega JA et al. L-asparaginase, vincristine, and prednisone for induction of first remission in acute lymphocytic leukemia. *Cancer Res* 1977;37: 535.
247. Reiter A et al. Chemotherapy in 998 unselected childhood acute lymphoblastic leukemia patients: results and conclusions of the multicenter trial ALL-BFM 86. *Blood* 1994;84:3122.
248. Evans WE et al. Conventional compared with individualized chemotherapy for childhood acute lymphoblastic leukemia. *N Engl J Med* 1998;338: 499.
249. Sackmann-Muriel F et al. Treatment results in childhood acute lymphoblastic leukemia with a modified ALL-BFM'90 protocol: lack of improvement in high-risk group. *Leuk Res* 1999;23:331.
250. Gaynon PS et al. Improved therapy for children with acute lymphoblastic leukemia and unfavorable presenting features: a follow-up report of the Children's Cancer Group study CCG-106. *J Clin Oncol* 1993;11:2234.
251. Goldie JH et al. Rationale for the use of alternating non-cross-resistant chemotherapy. *Cancer Treat Rep* 1982;66:439.
252. Kaplan RS, Wiernik PH. Neurotoxicity of antineoplastic drugs. *Semin Oncol* 1982;9:103.
253. Legha SS. Vincristine neurotoxicity: pathophysiology and management. *Med Toxicol* 1986;1:421.
254. Drigan R et al. Behavioral effects of corticosteroids in children with acute lymphoblastic leukemia. *Med Pediatr Oncol* 1992;20:13.
255. Price RA, Johnson WW. The central nervous system in childhood leukemia: I. The arachnoid. *Cancer* 1973;31:520.
256. Evans AE et al. The increasing incidence of central nervous system leukemia in children. *Cancer* 1970; 26:404.
257. Morrison VA. The infectious complication of chronic lymphocytic leukemia. *Semin Oncol* 1998; 25:98.
258. Bleyer WA, Poplack DG. Prophylaxis and treatment of leukemia in the central nervous system and other sanctuaries. *Semin Oncol* 1985;12:131.
259. Carrio I et al. Indium-111-antimyosin and iodine-123-MIBG studies in early assessment of doxorubicin cardiotoxicity. *J Nucl Med* 1995;36:2044.
260. Aur RJA et al. Central nervous system therapy and combination chemotherapy of childhood lymphocytic leukemia. *Blood* 1971;37:272.
261. Hill JM et al. A comparative study of the long term psychosocial functioning of childhood acute lymphoblastic leukemia survivors treated by intrathecal methotrexate with or without cranial radiation. *Cancer* 1998;82:208.
262. Pizzo P et al. Neurotoxicities of current leukemia therapy. *Am J Pediatr Hematol Oncol* 1979;1: 127.
263. Meadows A et al. Declines in IQ scores and cognitive dysfunction in children with acute lymphocytic leukemia treated with cranial irradiation. *Lancet* 1981;1:1015.
264. Nesbit ME Jr et al. Presymptomatic central nervous system therapy in previously untreated childhood acute lymphoblastic leukemia: comparison of 1800 rad and 2400 rad. A report for Children's Cancer Study Group. *Lancet* 1981;1:461.
265. Haghbin M et al. Treatment of acute lymphoblastic leukemia in children with "prophylactic" intrathecal methotrexate and intensive systemic therapy. *Cancer Res* 1975;35:807.
266. Sullivan MP et al. Equivalence of intrathecal chemotherapy and radiotherapy as central nervous system prophylaxis in children with acute lymphatic leukemia: a Pediatric Oncology Group study. *Blood* 1982;60:948.
267. Freeman AT et al. Comparison of intermediate-dose methotrexate with cranial irradiation for postinduction treatment of acute lymphocytic leukemia in children. *N Engl J Med* 1983;308:477.
268. Komp DM et al. CNS prophylaxis in acute lymphoblastic leukemia. *Cancer* 1982;50:1031.
269. Tubergen DG et al. Prevention of CNS disease in intermediate-risk acute lymphoblastic leukemia: comparison of cranial radiation and intrathecal methotrexate and the importance of systemic therapy: a Children's Cancer Group report. *J Clin Oncol* 1993;11:520.
270. Tsurusawa M et al. Improvement in CNS protective treatment in non-high-risk childhood acute lymphoblastic leukemia: report from the Japanese Children's Cancer and Leukemia Study Group. *Med Pediatr Oncol* 1999;32:259.
271. Nachman J et al. Response of children with high-risk acute lymphoblastic leukemia treated with and without cranial irradiation: a report from the Children's Cancer Group. *J Clin Oncol* 1998;16:920.
272. Katz JA et al. Final attained height in patients successfully treated for childhood acute lymphoblastic leukemia. *J Pediatr* 1993;123:546.
273. Brown RT et al. Chemotherapy for acute lymphocytic leukemia: cognitive and academic sequelae. *J Pediatr* 1992;121:885.
274. Lesnik PG et al. Evidence for cerebellar-frontal subsystem changes in children treated with intrathecal chemotherapy for leukemia: enhanced data analysis using an effect size model. *Arch Neurol* 1998;55:1561.
275. Poplack DG et al. Pharmacologic approaches to the treatment of central nervous system malignancy. In: Poplack DG et al., eds. *The Role of Pharmacology in Pediatric Oncology*. Boston: Martinus Nijhoff; 1987:125.
276. Collins JM. Regional therapy: an overview. In: Poplack DG et al., eds. *The Role of Pharmacology in Pediatric Oncology*. Boston: Martinus Nijhoff; 1987:125.
277. Poplack DG et al. Pharmacology of antineoplastic agents in cerebrospinal fluid. In: Wood JH, ed. *Neurobiology of Cerebrospinal Fluid*. New York: Plenum Press; 1980:561.
278. Bleyer WA. Clinical pharmacology of intrathecal methotrexate: II. An improved dosage regimen derived from age-related pharmacokinetics. *Cancer Treat Rep* 1977;61:1419.
279. Bleyer WA et al. Reduction in central nervous system leukemia with a pharmacokinetically derived intrathecal methotrexate dosage regimen. *J Clin Oncol* 1983;1:317.
280. Shepherd DA et al. Accidental intrathecal administration of vincristine. *Med Pediatr Oncol* 1978;5:85.
281. Bain PG et al. Intrathecal vincristine: a fatal chemotherapeutic error with devastating central nervous system effects. *J Neurol* 1991;238:230.
282. Solimando DA, Wilson JP. Prevention of accidental intrathecal administration of vincristine sulfate. *Hosp Pharm* 1982;17:540.
283. Dyke RW. Treatment of inadvertent intrathecal injection of vincristine. *N Engl J Med* 1989;321:1270.
284. Fernandez CV et al. Intrathecal vincristine: an analysis of reasons for recurrent fatal chemotherapeutic error with recommendations for prevention. *J Pediatr Hematol Oncol* 1998;20:587.
285. Geiser CF et al. Adverse effects of intrathecal methotrexate in children with acute leukemia in remission. *Blood* 1975;45:189.
286. Sullivan MP et al. Combination intrathecal therapy for meningeal leukemia: two versus three drugs. *Blood* 1977;50:471.
287. Sullivan MP et al. Remission maintenance for meningeal leukemia: intrathecal methotrexate vs. *intravenous bis-nitrosourea*. *Blood* 1971;38:680.
288. Holdsworth MT et al. Assessment of emetogenic potential of intrathecal chemotherapy and response to prophylactic treatment with ondansetron. *Support Care Cancer* 1998;6:132.
289. Higgins GA et al. 5-HT_3 receptor antagonists injected in the area postrema inhibit cisplatin-induced emesis in the ferret. *Br J Pharmacol* 1989;97:247.
290. Saiki JG et al. Paraplegia following intrathecal chemotherapy. *Cancer* 1972;29:370.
291. Gagliano R, Costani J. Paraplegia following intrathecal methotrexate: report of a case and review of the literature. *Cancer* 1976;37:1663.
292. Rubinstein LJ et al. Disseminated necrotizing leukoencephalopathy: a complication of treating central nervous system leukemia and lymphoma. *Cancer* 1975;35:291.
293. Quinn CT et al. Methotrexate, homocysteine, and seizures [letter]. *J Clin Oncol* 1998;16:393.
294. Quinn CT, Kamen BA. A biochemical perspective of methotrexate neurotoxicity with insight on nonfolate rescue modalities. *J Invest Med* 1996;44:522.
295. Mahoney DH et al. Intermediate-dose intravenous methotrexate with intravenous mercaptopurine is superior to repetitive low-dose oral methotrexate with intravenous mercaptopurine for children with lower-risk B-lineage acute lymphoblastic leukemia: a Pediatric Oncology Group phase III trial. *J Clin Oncol* 1998;16:246.
296. Kamen BA et al. Oral versus intravenous methotrexate: another opinion. *J Clin Oncol* 1998;16: 2283.
297. Tubergen DG et al. Improved outcome with delayed intensification for children with acute lymphoblastic leukemia and intermediate presenting features: a Children's Cancer Group phase III trial. *J Clin Oncol* 1993;11:527.

298. Harris MB et al. Consolidation therapy with antimetabolite-based therapy in standard-risk acute lymphocytic leukemia of childhood: a Pediatric Oncology Group study. *J Clin Oncol* 1998;16:2840.
299. Crom WR, Evans WE. Methotrexate. In: Evans WE et al., eds. *Applied Pharmacokinetics: Principles of Therapeutic Drug Monitoring*. Vancouver, WA: Applied Therapeutics; 1992:29.
300. Borsi JD, Moe PJ. Systemic clearance of methotrexate in the prognosis of acute lymphoblastic leukemia in children. *Cancer* 1987;60:3020.
301. Evans WE et al. Clinical pharmacodynamics of high-dose methotrexate in acute lymphocytic leukemia: identification of a relation between concentration and effect. *N Engl J Med* 1986;314:471.
302. Evans WE et al. Reappraisal of methotrexate clearance as a prognostic factor in childhood acute lymphocytic leukemia [abstract]. *Proc Am Assoc Cancer Res* 1989;30:241.
303. Wright JJ et al. Gene rearrangements as markers of clonal variation and minimal residual disease in acute lymphoblastic leukemia. *J Clin Oncol* 1987;5:735.
304. Secker-Walker LM et al. Bone marrow chromosomes in acute lymphoblastic leukemia: a long-term study. *Med Pediatr Oncol* 1979;7:371.
305. Freireich EJ et al. The effect of 6-mercaptopurine on the duration of steroid induced remission in acute leukemia: a model for evaluation of other potentially useful therapy. *Blood* 1963;21:699.
306. Holland JV, Glidewell OA. Chemotherapy of acute lymphocytic leukemia of childhood. *Cancer* 1972;30:1480.
307. Bleyer WA et al. Monthly pulses of vincristine and prednisone prevent bone marrow and testicular relapse in low-risk childhood acute lymphoblastic leukemia: a report of the CCG-161 study by the Children's Cancer Study Group. *J Clin Oncol* 1991;9:1012.
308. Ferrazzini G et al. Diurnal variation of methotrexate disposition in children with acute leukaemia. *Eur J Clin Pharmacol* 1991;41:425.
309. Lennard L, Lilleyman JS. Variable mercaptopurine metabolism and treatment outcome in childhood lymphoblastic leukemia. *J Clin Oncol* 1989;7: 1816.
310. Kato Y et al. Dose-dependent kinetics of orally administered 6-mercaptopurine in children with leukemia. *J Pediatr* 1991;119:311.
311. Andersen JB et al. Pharmacokinetics, dose adjustments, and 6-mercaptopurine/methotrexate drug interactions in two patients with thiopurine methyltransferase deficiency. *Acta Paediatr* 1998;87: 108.
312. McLeod HL et al. Analysis of thiopurine methyltransferase variant alleles in childhood acute lymphoblastic leukaemia. *Br J Hematol* 1999;105:696.
313. Pinkel D et al. Drug dosage and remission duration in childhood lymphocytic leukemia. *Cancer* 1971;27:247.
314. Relling MV et al. Prognostic importance of 6-mercaptopurine dose intensity in acute lymphoblastic leukemia. *Blood* 1999;93:2817.
315. Balis FM et al. Pharmacokinetics and pharmacodynamics of oral methotrexate and mercaptopurine in children with lower risk acute lymphoblastic leukemia: a joint Children's Cancer Group and Pediatric Oncology Branch study. *Blood* 1998;92:3569.
316. Pearson ADJ et al. The influence of serum methotrexate concentrations and drug dosage on outcome in childhood acute lymphoblastic leukaemia. *Br J Cancer* 1991;64:169.
317. Chessels JM et al. Oral methotrexate is as effective as intramuscular in maintenance therapy of acute lymphoblastic leukemia. *Arch Dis Child* 1987;62:172.
318. Lau RCW et al. Electronic measurement of compliance with mercaptopurine in pediatric patients with acute lymphoblastic leukemia. *Med Pediatr Oncol* 1998;30:85.
319. Festa RS et al. Therapeutic adherence to oral medication regimens by adolescents with cancer. I. Laboratory assessment. *J Pediatr* 1992;120:807.
320. Kamen BA et al. Methotrexate and folate content of erythrocytes in patients receiving oral vs intramuscular therapy with methotrexate. *J Pediatr* 1984;104:131.
321. Land VJ et al. Long term survival in childhood acute leukemia: "late" relapses. *Med Pediatr Oncol* 1979;7:19.
322. Nesbit ME et al. Randomized study of 3-years versus 5-years of chemotherapy in childhood acute lymphoblastic leukemia. *J Clin Oncol* 1983;1: 308.
323. Medical Research Council Working Party on Leukaemia in Childhood. Duration of chemotherapy in childhood acute lymphoblastic leukemia. *Med Pediatr Oncol* 1982;10:511.
324. Pui C-H et al. Recombinant urate oxidase for the prophylaxis or treatment of hyperuricemia in patients with leukemia or lymphoma. *J Clin Oncol* 2001;19:697.
325. Von Hoff DD et al. Risk factors for doxorubicin-induced congestive heart failure. *Ann Intern Med* 1979;91:710.
326. Pinarli FG et al. Late cardiac evaluation of children with solid tumors after anthracycline chemotherapy. *Pediatr Blood Cancer* 2005;44:370.
327. Lewis AB et al. Recovery of left ventricular function following discontinuation of anthracycline chemotherapy in children. *Pediatrics* 1981;68: 67.
328. Goorin AM et al. Congestive heart failure due to Adriamycin cardiotoxicity: its natural history in children. *Cancer* 1981;47:2810.
329. Goorin AM et al. Initial congestive heart failure, six to ten years after doxorubicin chemotherapy for childhood cancer. *J Pediatr* 1990;116:144.
330. Steinherz L et al. Delayed anthracycline cardiac toxicity. In: DeVita VT et al., eds. *Cancer: Principles and Practice of Oncology*. Philadelphia: J.B. Lippincott; 1991:1.
331. Lipshultz SE et al. Late cardiac effects of doxorubicin therapy for acute lymphoblastic leukemia in childhood. *N Engl J Med* 1991;324:808.
332. Poutanen T et al. Long-term prospective follow-up study of cardiac function after cardiotoxic therapy for malignancy in children. *J Clin Oncol* 2003;21:2349.
333. Speyer JL et al. ICRF-187 permits longer treatment with doxorubicin in women with breast cancer. *J Clin Oncol* 1992;10:117.
334. Swain SM et al. Congestive heart failure (CHF) after doxorubicin-containing therapy in advanced breast cancer patients treated with or without dexrazoxane (ICRF-187, ADR-529). *Proc Am Soc Clin Oncol* 1996;15:536.
335. Wexler LH et al. Randomized trial of the cardioprotective agent ICRF-187 in pediatric sarcoma patients treated with doxorubicin. *J Clin Oncol* 1996;14:362.
336. Lipshultz SE et al. The effect of dexrazoxane on myocardial injury in doxorubicin-treated children with acute lymphoblastic leukemia. *N Engl J Med* 2004;351:145.
337. Nysom K et al. Relationship between cumulative anthracycline dose and late cardiotoxicity in childhood acute lymphoblastic leukemia. *J Clin Oncol* 1998;16:545.
338. Arikoski P et al. Reduced bone mineral density in long-term survivors of childhood acute lymphoblastic leukemia. *J Pediatr Hematol Oncol* 1998;20:234.
339. Arico M et al. Osteonecrosis: an emerging complication of intensive chemotherapy for childhood acute lymphoblastic leukemia. *Haematologica* 2003;88:747.
340. Burger B et al. Osteonecrosis: a treatment related toxicity in childhood acute lymphoblastic leukemia (ALL) experiences from trial ALL-BFM 95. *Pediatr Blood Cancer* 2005;44:220.
341. Warner JT et al. Relative osteopenia after treatment for acute lymphoblastic leukemia. *Pediatr Res* 1999;45:544.
342. Atkinson SA et al. Bone and mineral abnormalities in childhood acute lymphoblastic leukemia: influence of disease, drugs and nutrition. *Int J Cancer* 1998;11:35.
343. Haskell CM et al. L-asparaginase: therapeutic and toxic effects in patients with neoplastic disease. *N Engl J Med* 1969;281:1028.
344. Capizzi RL et al. L-asparaginase [abstract]. *Annu Rev Med* 1970;21:2433.
345. Faletta JM et al. Nonketotic hyperglycemia due to prednisone (NSC-10023) following ketotic hyperglycemia due to L-asparaginase (NSC-109229) plus prednisone. *Cancer Chemother Rep* 1972;56:781.
346. Land VJ et al. Toxicity of L-asparaginase in children with advanced leukemia. *Cancer* 1972;30:339.
347. Woo MH et al. Anti-asparaginase antibodies following *E. coli* asparaginase therapy in pediatric acute lymphoblastic leukemia. *Leukemia* 1998;12: 1527.
348. Zubrod CG. The clinical toxicities of L-asparaginase in treatment of leukemia and lymphoma. *Pediatrics* 1970;45:555.
349. Fabry U et al. Anaphylaxis to L-asparaginase during treatment for acute lymphoblastic leukemia in children: evidence of a complement-mediated mechanism. *Pediatr Res* 1985;19:400.
350. Cheung N-KV et al. Antibody response to *Escherichia coli* L-asparaginase: prognostic significance and clinical utility of antibody measurement. *Am J Pediatr Hematol Oncol* 1986;8:99.
351. Nesbit M et al. Evaluation of intramuscular versus intravenous administration of L-asparaginase in childhood leukemia. *Am J Pediatr Hematol Oncol* 1979;1:9.
352. Lobel JS et al. Methotrexate and asparaginase combination chemotherapy in refractory acute lymphoblastic leukemia of childhood. *Cancer* 1979;43: 1089.
353. Spiegel RJ et al. Delayed allergic reactions following intramuscular L-asparaginase. *Med Pediatr Oncol* 1980;8:123.
354. Capizzi RL. Asparaginase revisited. *Leuk Lymphoma* 1993;10(Suppl):147.
355. Capizzi RL, Holcenberg JS. Asparaginase. In: Holland JF, ed. *Cancer Medicine*. 3rd ed. Philadelphia: Lea & Febiger; 1993:796.
356. Ohnuma T et al. Biochemical and pharmacological studies with asparaginase in man. *Cancer Res* 1970;30:2297.
357. Ettinger LJ. Asparaginases: where do we go from here? *J Pediatr Hematol Oncol* 1999;21:3.
358. Panosyan EH et al. Asparaginase antibody and asparaginase activity in children with higher-risk acute lymphoblastic leukemia. *J Pediatr Hematol Oncol* 2004;26:217.
359. Dellinger CT, Miale TD. Comparison of anaphylactic reactions to asparaginase derived from *Escherichia coli* and from *Erwinia* cultures. *Cancer* 1976;38:1843.
360. Evans WE et al. Anaphylactoid reactions to *Escherichia coli* and *Erwinia* asparaginase in children with leukemia and lymphoma. *Cancer* 1982;49:1378.
361. Nowak-Gottl U et al. Changes in coagulation and fibrinolysis in childhood acute lymphoblastic leukaemia re-induction therapy using three different asparaginase preparations. *Eur J Pediatr* 1997;156:848.
362. Duval M et al. Comparison of *Escherichia coli*-asparaginase with *Erwinia*-asparaginase in the treatment of childhood lymphoid malignancies: results of a randomized European Organization for Research and Treatment of Cancer-Children's Leukemia Group phase 3 trial. *Blood* 2002;99:2734.
363. Kurtzberg J et al. The use of polyethylene glycol-conjugated L-asparaginase in pediatric patients with prior hypersensitivity to native L-asparaginase [abstract]. *Proc Am Soc Clin Oncol* 1990;9:219.
364. Liang D-C et al. Unexpected mortality from the use of *E. coli* L-asparaginase during remission induction therapy for childhood acute lymphoblastic leukemia: a report from the Taiwan Pediatric Oncology Group. *Leukemia* 1999;13:155.

365. Urban C, Sager WD. Intracranial bleeding during therapy with L-asparaginase in childhood acute lymphocytic leukemia. *Eur J Pediatr* 1981;137:323.
366. Saito M et al. Changes in hemostatic and fibrinolytic proteins in patients receiving L-asparaginase therapy. *Am J Hematol* 1989;32:20.
367. Cairo MS et al. Intracranial hemorrhage and focal seizures secondary to use of L-asparaginase during induction therapy of acute lymphocytic leukemia. *J Pediatr* 1980;97:829.
368. Rizzari C et al. A pharmacological study on pegylated asparaginase used in front-line treatment of children with acute lymphoblastic leukemia. *Haematologica* 2006;91:24.
369. Nowak-Gottl U et al. Prospective evaluation of the thrombotic risk in children with acute lymphoblastic leukemia carrying the MTHFR TT 677 genotype, the prothrombin G20210 variant, and further prothrombotic risk factors. *Blood* 1999;93:1595.
370. Nowak-Gottl U et al. Thromboembolic events in children with acute lymphoblastic leukemia (BFM protocols): prednisone versus dexamethasone administration. *Blood* 2003;101:2529.
371. Rivera G et al. Recurrent childhood lymphocytic leukemia: clinical and cytokinetic studies of cytosine arabinoside and methotrexate for maintenance of second hematologic remission. *Cancer* 1978;42:2521.
372. Amato KR et al. Combination chemotherapy in relapsed childhood acute lymphoblastic leukemia. *Cancer Treat Rep* 1984;68:411.
373. Ekert H et al. Poor outlook for childhood acute lymphoblastic leukemia with relapse. *Med J Aust* 1979;2:224.
374. Amadori S et al. Combination chemotherapy for marrow relapse in children and adolescents with acute lymphocytic leukemia. *Scand J Haematol* 1981;26:292.
375. Baum E et al. Prolonged second remission in childhood acute lymphocytic leukemia: a report from the Children's Cancer Study Group. *Med Pediatr Oncol* 1983;11:1.
376. Rivera GK et al. Intensive treatment of childhood acute lymphoblastic leukemia in first bone marrow relapse. *N Engl J Med* 1986;315:273.
377. Culbert SJ et al. Remission induction and continuation therapy in children with their first relapse of acute lymphoid leukemia: a Pediatric Oncology Group study. *Cancer* 1991;67:37.
378. Champlin R, Gale RP. Acute lymphoblastic leukemia: recent advances in biology and therapy. *Blood* 1989;73:2051.
379. Brochstein JA et al. Allogeneic marrow transplantation after hyperfractionated total body irradiation and cyclophosphamide in children with acute leukemia. *N Engl J Med* 1987;317:1618.
380. Sanders JE et al. Marrow transplantation for children with acute lymphoblastic leukemia in second remission. *Blood* 1987;70:324.
381. Wheeler K et al. Comparison of bone marrow transplant and chemotherapy for relapsed childhood acute lymphoblastic leukaemia: the MRC UKALL X experience. *Br J Haematol* 1998;101:94.
382. Barrett AJ et al. Bone marrow transplants from HLA-identical siblings as compared with chemotherapy for children with acute lymphoblastic leukemia in a second remission. *N Engl J Med* 1994;331:1253.
383. Butturini A et al. Which treatment for childhood acute lymphoblastic leukemia in second remission? *Lancet* 1987;1:429.
384. Borgmann A et al. Autologous bone-marrow transplants compared with chemotherapy for children with acute lymphoblastic leukaemia in a second remission: a matched-pair analysis. *Lancet* 1995;346:873.
385. Harris RE et al. High-dose cytosine arabinoside and L-asparaginase in refractory acute lymphoblastic leukemia: the Children's Cancer Group experience. *Med Pediatr Oncol* 1998;30:233.
386. Magrath IT. Malignant non-Hodgkin's lymphomas in children. In: Pizzo PA, Poplack DG, eds. *Principles and Practice of Pediatric Oncology*. Philadelphia: Lippincott Williams & Wilkins; 2002:661.
387. Nathwani BW et al. Malignant lymphoma, lymphoblastic. *Cancer* 1976;38:964.
388. Bennett HM et al. Classification of non-Hodgkin's lymphomas. *Lancet* 1974;1:1295.
389. Lukes RJ et al. New approaches to the classification of the lymphomata. *Br J Cancer* 1975;31(Suppl 2):1.
390. National Cancer Institute sponsored study of classifications of non-Hodgkin's lymphomas: summary and description of a working formulation for clinical usage. *Cancer* 1982;49:2112.
391. Wanatabe A et al. Undifferentiated lymphoma, non-Burkitt's type: meningeal and bone marrow involvement in children. *Am J Dis Child* 1973;125:57.
392. Hutter JJ et al. Non-Hodgkin's lymphoma in children: correlation of CNS disease with initial presentation. *Cancer* 1975;36:2132.
393. Magrath IT. Burkitt's lymphoma. In: Mollander D, ed. *Diseases of the Lymphatic System: Diagnosis and Therapy*. Heidelberg, Germany: Springer-Verlag; 1983:103.
394. Magrath IT et al. Prognostic factors in Burkitt's lymphoma: importance of total tumor burden. *Cancer* 1980;45:1507.
395. Reiter A et al. Intensive ALL-type therapy without local radiotherapy provides a 90% event-free survival for children with T-cell lymphoblastic lymphoma: a BFM group report. *Blood* 2000;95:416.
396. Reiter A et al. Improved treatment results in childhood B-cell neoplasms with tailored intensification of therapy: a report of the Berlin-Frankfurt-Munster group trial NHL-BFM 90. *Blood* 1999;94:3294.
397. Patte C et al. The Societe Francaise d'Oncologie Pediatrique LMB89 protocol: highly effective multiagent chemotherapy tailored to the tumor burden and initial response in 561 unselected children with B-cell lymphomas and L3 leukemia. *Blood* 2001;97:3370.
398. Jetsrisuparb A et al. Rituximab combined with CHOP for successful treatment of aggressive, recurrent, pediatric B-cell large cell non-Hodgkin's lymphoma. *J Pediatr Hematol Oncol* 2005;27:223.
399. Claviez A et al. Rituximab plus chemotherapy in children with relapsed or refractory CD20-positive B-cell precursor acute lymphoblastic leukemia. *Haematologica* 2006;91:272.
400. Weinstein HJ et al. APO therapy for malignant lymphoma of large cell "histiocytic" type of childhood: analysis of treatment results for 29 patients. *Blood* 1984;64:422.
401. Murphy SB et al. Non-Hodgkin's lymphomas of childhood: an analysis of the histology, staging, and response to treatment of 338 cases at a single institution. *J Clin Oncol* 1989;7:186.
402. Mott MG et al. Adjuvant low dose radiation in childhood T cell leukaemia/lymphoma (report from the United Kingdom Children's Cancer Study Group—UKCCSG). *Br J Cancer* 1984;50:457.
403. Murphy SB et al. Correlation of tumor cell kinetic studies with surface marker results in childhood non-Hodgkin's lymphoma. *Cancer Res* 1979;39:1534.
404. Hirt A et al. Differentiation and cytokinetic analysis of normal and neoplastic lymphoid cells in B and T cell malignancies of childhood. *Br J Haematol* 1984;58:241.
405. Dorr RT, Von Hoff DD, eds.Vincristine sulfate. In: *Cancer Chemotherapy Handbook*. 2nd ed. Norwalk, CT: Appleton & Lange; 1994:951.
406. Holdsworth MT et al. Acute and delayed nausea and emesis control in pediatric oncology patients. *Cancer* 2006;106:931.
407. Mehta P et al. Methylprednisolone for chemotherapy-induced emesis: a double-blind randomized trial in children. *J Pediatr* 1986;108:774.
408. Roila F. Ondansetron plus dexamethasone compared to the "standard" metoclopramide combination. *Oncology* 1993;50:163.
409. Rai KR et al. Clinical staging of chronic lymphocytic leukemia. *Blood* 1975;46:219.
410. Kay NE et al. Chronic lymphocytic leukemia. *Hematology* 2002;193.
411. Lister TA et al. Report of a committee convened to discuss the evaluation and staging of patients with Hodgkin's disease: Cotswolds meeting. *J Clin Oncol* 1989;7:1630.
412. Solal-Celigny P et al. Follicular lymphoma international prognostic index. *Blood* 2004;104:1258.
413. Montoto S et al. Predictive value of Follicular Lymphoma International Prognostic Index (FLIPI) in patients with follicular lymphoma at first progression. *Ann Oncol* 2004;15:1484.

CHAPTER 91

Solid Tumors

Adult: Susan Goodin; and Pediatric: David W. Henry

Solid tumors include the malignancies that initially present as discrete masses. They arise from malignant transformations of cells within virtually any organ system except the hematopoietic system. Solid tumors are far more common than hematologic malignancies and represent the major causes of cancer-related morbidity and mortality. Depending on the specific type of cancer and its stage, surgery, radiation, chemotherapy, biologic therapy, immunotherapy, and hormonal manipulation all play important roles in patient treatment. The types of solid tumors that occur in adult versus pediatric populations are distinctively different. Specific tumors commonly treated with drug therapy are included in this chapter.

ADULT TUMORS

BREAST CANCER

Risk Factors

1. B.W., a 41-year-old woman, is found to have a 2.2-cm mass in the upper, outer quadrant of her left breast during routine screening mammography. Biopsy of the mass reveals infiltrating ductal carcinoma. Physical examination is unremarkable, and she has no complaints. All laboratory values, including the complete blood count (CBC) and liver function tests (LFT), are within normal limits and a chest radiograph is negative. Her family history is significant in that her mother died of breast cancer at age 42, and her 44-year-old sister had a breast tumor removed about 5 years ago. B.W. reports that she had her first menstrual cycle at age 10 and has had regular periods since that time. She is married but has never been pregnant. What is the incidence of breast cancer in premenopausal women? Did any factors place B.W. at an increased risk of developing breast cancer?

Overall, breast cancer is the most common cancer in women in the United States and accounts for 26% of their cancer occurrences and 15% of their cancer deaths; however, the incidence rates as well as the death rates have been declining since 1990.[1] The lifetime risk of developing breast cancer is approximately one in eight women with the greatest risk occurring after age 65.[1] For women 39 years of age or younger, the chance of developing breast cancer is <1%; however, a strong family history of breast cancer increases the relative risk.[1]

Some cases of familial breast cancer, especially those occurring in premenopausal women, have been linked to specific breast cancer susceptibility genes, BRCA-1 and BRCA-2. Carriers of these genes have an increased risk of breast and ovarian cancer in women, and prostate cancers in men. Women such as B.W. who have a positive family history and who are carriers of the gene have an 85% chance of developing breast cancer and a 60% chance of developing ovarian cancer by age 70.[2] The risk is not as significant in women who are carriers and who do not have a positive family history. Genetic testing is available; however, if a woman chooses to have such testing, appropriate genetic counseling and psychological support should be made available.

Despite the strong relationship with breast cancer development, it is also important to realize that BRCA gene mutations account for only 5% to 10% of all cases. Several additional factors have been associated with an increased risk of developing breast cancer (Table 91-1). Nulliparous women such as B.W. have a higher incidence of breast cancer than women who have had one or more pregnancies, but age at first pregnancy appears to be an even more important determinant. One study indicated that the risk of developing breast cancer was substantially higher in women whose first pregnancy was after age 30, compared with those whose first pregnancy was before age 18. Early menarche also has been associated with an increased risk of breast cancer.[3]

Table 91-1 Risk Factors Associated With Development of Breast Cancer

Strong Risk Factors
History of breast cancer in the contralateral breast
Family history of breast cancer, especially in first-degree relatives
Benign breast "cancer" (i.e., atypical hyperplasia)
Early menarche, late menopause
Late first pregnancy greater than no pregnancy
Advancing age
Possible Risk Factors
Obesity
High-fat diet
Long-term use of exogenous estrogens
Alcohol

Screening

2. Is routine screening mammography recommended for B.W. because of her increased risk of breast cancer? Is it recommended for all women?

Women with a positive family history often are instructed to begin screening at an early age. Several different guidelines for breast cancer screening are available. Although strong evidence of benefit is lacking, it generally is agreed that women should perform monthly breast self-examinations. Annual examination for breast cancer performed by a health care provider is recommended for all women >40 years of age.

Nearly 75% of breast cancers occur in women >50 years of age. Currently, all screening guidelines recommend that women in this age group have annual mammography but disagree over the value of mammography screening in women age 40 to 49 years; therefore, the guidelines differ for this group of patients. Meta-analyses reveal the risk reduction from mammography screening does not differ substantially by age, although absolute benefits are lower in women <50 years compared with women aged 50 years and older.[4] More recently, data have supported the role of magnetic resonance imaging (MRI) in women at higher risk, defined as those with a lifetime risk of approximately 20% to 25%, which includes women with a family history (especially early onset), genetic mutations including BRCA, and certain clinical factors that increase risk. For this reason, the American Cancer Society (ACS) updated their recommendations to include MRI, depending on the presence of risk factors, as an adjunct to annual mammography screening, which should be initiated at age 40.[5]

It is not clear how long screening should be continued. Women >70 years of age are at increased risk for developing breast cancer; however, no randomized trials have evaluated the merits of annual mammography in this group. The ACS states there is no chronologic age at which screening should stop, emphasizing that as long as a woman is in good health she is likely to benefit from annual mammography.

Surgery

3. After receiving the results of the biopsy, B.W. has a partial mastectomy and full axillary lymph node dissection because of a positive sentinel lymph node biopsy. The tumor is estrogen- and progesterone-receptor negative; human epidermal growth factor receptor-2 (erB-2 or HER-2) positive; and 4 of 20 lymph nodes are positive for tumor involvement. Is partial mastectomy as effective as more extensive surgical procedures such as modified radical mastectomy? Is radiation indicated following surgery?

Historically, radical mastectomy (removal of the breast, axillary lymph nodes, and pectoralis muscles) and modified radical mastectomy (radical mastectomy with preservation of the pectoralis muscles) have been the standard surgical procedures used for primary breast cancer. The psychological and cosmetic effects of breast loss can be substantial, however. This has led to the use of more conservative surgical procedures, such as lumpectomy, partial mastectomy, and evaluation of axillary lymph nodes using lymph node mapping with sentinel lymph node biopsy. Lumpectomy consists of gross removal of the tumor without attention to margins; a partial mastectomy includes excision of the tumor with clean surgical margins. It is now standard to evaluate the axilla through the use of the sentinel lymph node by the injection of radioactive colloid or blue dye into the breast to identify the lymph nodes that first receive drainage for the tumor. Use of the sentinel lymph node to assess spread of disease has reduced the number of patients who require axillary lymph node dissection.[6] Early trials evaluating conservative procedures without treatment of the remaining breast tissue or axillary lymph nodes reported high failure rates. Failures presented primarily as cancer recurrences in the remaining breast tissue or axilla.[7] Therefore, postoperative radiation therapy is indicated after conservative breast surgery because it reduces the risk of local recurrence. Additionally, no difference in survival is seen between patients having conservative surgery (e.g., lumpectomy or partial mastectomy) followed by local radiation therapy and those treated with a radical mastectomy.[7,8]

Adjuvant Therapy

4. B.W. recalls that her sister received chemotherapy after her surgery for breast cancer. She now questions whether she should receive any additional therapy and wonders what her chances are that her cancer has been cured. What factors determine the need for adjuvant systemic therapy following surgery, and what are the indications for administering adjuvant chemotherapy, biologic therapy, or hormonal therapy?

A significant portion of women who have early-stage disease experience relapse at distant sites and ultimately die of recurrence-related complications. Distant treatment failures indicate that some women have clinically undetectable micrometastatic disease at the time of diagnosis, therefore locoregional (surgery and radiation) therapy is insufficient. Adjuvant therapy is given to kill any cells that may have spread from the primary site and that are not detectable by radiographic measures. Adjuvant systemic therapy can include chemotherapy, hormonal approaches, biologic therapy, or experimental agents.

Recommendations regarding adjuvant chemotherapy are generally made by estimating the risk of recurrence and the expected benefit of therapy balanced with the anticipated toxicity. The benefit of systemic adjuvant therapy is directly related to the likelihood of disease recurrence. A number of factors determine the likelihood of recurrence and the role of adjuvant therapy for early stage breast cancer. Size of the primary tumor, presence and number of involved axillary lymph nodes, HER-2 oncogene amplification, nuclear or histologic grade of the tumor, and the presence of hormone receptors on the tumor (estrogen, progesterone, or both) appear to be the most important factors that predict prognosis.[9,10] More recently, the enhanced use of molecular markers has improved prognostic profiling to determine risk of recurrence.

Currently, the single most important factor that predicts recurrence of breast cancer in patients such as B.W., whose tumor is initially small and localized, is the presence and extent of lymph nodes positive for cancer. Women with positive lymph nodes (stage II disease) have a 40% to 60% chance of cure with surgery alone. Women with negative lymph nodes (stage I disease) have a 70% to 90% chance of cure with surgery alone. Because B.W., who has four positive nodes, negative hormone receptors, and positive HER-2, is at high risk for recurrence, she should receive adjuvant therapy.

Patients with node-negative, estrogen-receptor positive (ER+) breast cancers have a better prognosis. They may not require adjuvant chemotherapy, and many only need 5 years of hormonal therapy. Genomic tools evaluating the tumor specimen from tissue blocks, utilizing onco*type* DX®[11], and from fresh tissue, utilizing Mammaprint,[12] are being tested in clinical trials to identify patients with node-negative, ER+ tumors at high risk of recurrence that would benefit from adjuvant chemotherapy. The onco*type* DX®, commercially available in the United States, utilizes a 21-gene recurrence score, based on monitoring of messenger RNA (mRNA) levels of 16 cancer-related genes in relation to five reference genes.[11] These recurrence scores have identified patients at low-, intermediate-, or high-risk of recurrence in a retrospective analysis. This analysis revealed that women in the low-risk group (recurrence score <18) need only hormonal therapy, whereas the high-risk group (recurrence score ≥ 31) require both chemotherapy and hormonal therapy.[11] It is not clear from the retrospective analysis which patients in the intermediate-risk group require adjuvant chemotherapy in addition to hormonal therapy. Although onco*type* DX® is not widely used in clinical practice, the prospective study TAILORx (Trial Assigning Individualized Options for Treatment), which is accruing 10,000 women in North America, will further define whether chemotherapy is required in addition to hormonal therapy for the intermediate-risk group defined by the recurrence score of 12 to 25.

Trials of systemic adjuvant therapy in women with breast cancer began in the 1960s. These trials originally focused on patients with stage II disease; however, recognizing the significant rate of disease recurrence in patients with stage I disease, later trials included patients with stage I disease as well. Many trials evaluating the effects of systemic adjuvant chemotherapy, endocrine therapy, and combined chemoendocrine therapy have been conducted over the past 45 years. Because many of the individual trials have included relatively small numbers of patients, multiple patient subsets, or different therapeutic strategies, a series of meta-analyses have been performed by the Early Breast Cancer Trialists' Collaborative Group. The most recent meta-analysis reviewed data from 194 randomized clinical trials conducted worldwide, which included 110,000 women with stages I and II breast cancer. The overview concluded that appropriate use of adjuvant cytotoxic chemotherapy can reduce the rate of death by as much as 10% in women <50 years of age and by 3% for those age 50 to 69 years.[13] Irrespective of age or chemotherapy, for ER+ disease, adjuvant tamoxifen reduces the annual breast cancer death rate by 31%.[13] Anthracycline-containing regimens were associated with a 38% decrease in the annual death rate in women <50 years of age and by 20% in women 50 to 69 years of age.[13] Additionally, the use of anthracycline-based adjuvant regimens led, on average, to improved treatment results compared with non–anthracycline-based regimens in node-positive breast cancer. The proportional reduction in risk of death in stages I and II is approximately equivalent; however, the absolute survival difference is greater in patients with stage II disease who have a higher risk of recurrence. Because B.W.'s risk of recurrence is high and her age is <50 years, systemic adjuvant chemotherapy would be recommended. Common regimens for the adjuvant setting (outlined in Chapter 88, Neoplastic Disorders and Their Treatment) include FAC (fluorouracil, doxorubicin, cyclophosphamide), FEC (fluorouracil, epirubicin, cyclosphosphamide), AC (doxorubicin, cyclophosphamide), EC (epirubicin, cyclophosphamide), TAC (docetaxel, doxorubicin, cyclophosphamide), and CMF (cyclophosphamide, methotrexate, fluorouracil), among others.

Biologic therapy targeting HER-2 has become a standard in the adjuvant setting in patients whose tumors overexpress HER-2. A number of trials evaluating trastuzumab in the adjuvant setting with various combination chemotherapies have shown that adjuvant trastuzumab significantly reduces the risk of recurrence and may prolong overall survival with acceptable toxicity.[14,15] Additionally, concurrent administration of trastuzumab with chemotherapy appears to be superior to sequential administration.

Treatment recommendations for patients with stages I and II breast cancer continue to evolve.[16,17] Early guidelines were based on menopausal status (if unknown, based on age older than or younger than 50 years) and the presence of involved axillary lymph nodes at the time of the initial surgery. The results of these early studies demonstrated conclusively that premenopausal women, particularly those with four or more positive lymph nodes who received chemotherapy, had significant prolongation in disease-free and overall survival compared with untreated controls. These trials also demonstrated that postmenopausal women treated with adjuvant endocrine therapy, such as tamoxifen or an aromatase inhibitor, had significant improvement in disease-free and overall survival compared with untreated controls. Thus, chemotherapy was recommended for premenopausal women and endocrine therapy for postmenopausal women.

The significance of menopausal status for adjuvant therapy is related to hormone receptors in the primary tumor. Whereas most premenopausal women are hormone receptor negative, most postmenopausal women are hormone receptor positive. Endocrine therapy is most likely to benefit women with positive hormone receptors. In early studies, hormone receptor assays were not available and menopausal status served as a surrogate marker of hormone receptor positivity. Although current adjuvant treatment guidelines retain the categories of premenopause and postmenopause, they also incorporate hormone receptor status.

RECOMMENDED REGIMENS

5. Based on current guidelines and the estrogen receptor status of her tumor, B.W.'s physician recommends that she receive adjuvant chemotherapy. What regimens are currently recommended?

B.W. has several poor prognostic characteristics associated with her disease, including the presence of positive lymph nodes, negative hormone receptors, and HER-2 overexpression. The HER-2 oncogene has undergone extensive study as both a prognostic and a predictive factor in early stage breast cancer.[10,18,19] The gene encodes for a growth factor receptor, and its overexpression correlates with a poor prognosis and predicts a stronger likelihood of response to an anthracycline-containing regimen. For this reason, B.W. could receive a doxorubicin-containing regimen with trastuzumab.

It was hypothesized that owing to the importance of doxorubicin in the treatment of breast cancer, increasing the dose would be beneficial. Although trials reveal that increasing the dose of doxorubicin does not appear to influence treatment outcomes, the addition of a taxane results in a significant reduction of the rate of both recurrence and death.[20,21] Dose density has also been shown to be important in the adjuvant setting.[22] Dose density refers to the administration of drugs with a shortened intertreatment interval (e.g., every 2 weeks). Therefore, it is recommend that B.W. receive four cycles of dose-dense doxorubicin and cyclophosphamide followed by 12 weekly doses of paclitaxel with concurrent weekly trastuzumab, which is continued for a total of 52 weeks.

ENDOCRINE THERAPY

6. Should B.W. receive adjuvant endocrine therapy in addition to chemotherapy?

Because B.W.'s tumor was negative for hormone receptors, endocrine therapy is not indicated as it is ineffective against ER– tumors in the adjuvant setting. In premenopausal women with ER+ tumors, however, combined chemoendocrine therapy may be beneficial. Results of the meta-analysis found that ovarian ablation, by surgery or radiation or ovarian suppression by treatment with luteinizing hormone-releasing hormone (LHRH) analogs, in patients <50 years of age was as effective as chemotherapy in reducing recurrence and mortality.[23] This, however, is an indirect comparison of results of trials employing ovarian ablation with those using combination chemotherapy. The report of this meta-analysis has stimulated renewed interest in the value of endocrine therapy (ovarian ablation, tamoxifen, or LHRH analogs) in premenopausal women. Combination chemotherapy often produces permanent ovarian failure in premenopausal women and evidence exists that this is associated with a favorable prognosis.

If B.W.'s tumor had been ER+, both chemotherapy and endocrine therapy would have been indicated. Typically, radiation and adjuvant chemotherapy are completed before the initiation of hormonal therapy. In the meta-analysis, chemoendocrine therapy was associated with the greatest reduction in risk of death in women ages 50 to 69 years.[13] Consequently, chemoendocrine therapy is now recommended for patients with ER+ tumors.

For the last 20 years, interest in adjuvant endocrine therapy for pre- and postmenopausal women with ER+ tumors has concentrated on the optimal use of tamoxifen.[13] Although it is clear from these studies that adjuvant tamoxifen therapy in patients with ER+ tumors for 5 years is superior to 2 years, no evidence indicates that extending tamoxifen beyond 5 years provides any advantage, and benefits are seen independent of age and menopausal status.[24] Whereas adjuvant tamoxifen was considered the classic standard care for the endocrine therapy of ER+ breast cancer, successful trials involving aromatase inhibitors (anastrazole, letrozole, and exemestane) for postmenopausal women in the adjuvant setting have challenged the gold standard, tamoxifen.

Trials of the aromatase inhibitors, used only in postmenopausal women with ER+ tumors, have revealed that both anastrozole and letrozole reduce the recurrence risk when compared with tamoxifen.[24,25] Additionally, use of exemestane for 2 to 3 years following 2 to 3 years of tamoxifen (for a total of 5 years of therapy) was associated with an improvement in relapse-free survival.[24] Although each of the studies involving aromatase inhibitors compared with tamoxifen used different study designs (head-to-head, sequential, extended), aromatase inhibitors are now the standard in the adjuvant setting for postmenopausal women. Finally, letrozole for 5 years after completion of first-line tamoxifen therapy has also been shown to be effective. Currently, no comparative trials exist to document enhanced efficacy of one aromatase inhibitor over another. Concerns with the use of aromatase inhibitors are the reported increased cardiovascular complications versus tamoxifen, which did not reach statistical significance. Increased bone fractures were also observed; a number of studies with new data to be presented over the next few years should clarify this association.

For premenopausal women such as B.W., combining different endocrine modalities such as tamoxifen with ovarian ablation has been investigated. The rationale for these studies is based on data from patients with metastatic disease in whom an improvement in outcomes was noted in those receiving an LHRH agonist in combination with tamoxifen compared with either therapy alone.[24] Ongoing studies evaluating the role of LHRH agonists in combination with tamoxifen or an aromatase inhibitor will better define the role of estrogen suppression in premenopausal women.

Metastatic Disease

Prognosis

7. Approximately 2 years after completing adjuvant chemo- and trastuzumab therapy, B.W. begins experiencing back pain that is partially relieved by ibuprofen 400 mg as needed (PRN). Because the pain was temporally related to moving some furniture in her living room, she did not seek medical attention. Five days after the onset of the back pain, her husband noted that she was mildly confused. He contacted her physician who suggested she come to the clinic immediately. Physical examination was negative for lymphadenopathy or breast masses, and chest and abdominal examinations were unremarkable. Pertinent laboratory values were as follows: calcium (Ca), 15 mg/dL (normal, 9.0–11.5 mg/dL); phosphorus, 4.2 mg/dL (normal, 2.5–4.5 mg/dL); sodium (Na), 138 mEq/L (normal, 136–145 mEq/L); potassium (K), 4.3 mEq/L (normal, 3.5–5.5 mEq/L); albumin, 3.0 g/dL (normal, 3.5–5.5 g/dL); alkaline phosphatase, 580 mU/mL (normal, 15–70 mU/mL); aspartate aminotransferase (AST), 258 mU/mL (normal, 5–20 mU/mL); and alanine aminotransferase (ALT), 96 mU/mL (normal, 5–24 mU/mL). The CBC was within normal limits. Spinal cord radiographs revealed several lytic vertebral lesions consistent with metastatic carcinoma, but a myelogram did not show any evidence of spinal cord compression.

B.W. is admitted to the hospital for acute management of hypercalcemia and restaging of her breast cancer to determine the extent of tumor spread. A bone scan shows positive uptake in the spine and right scapula and a liver scan reveals two small nodules consistent with metastatic disease. A computed tomography (CT) scan of the brain is positive. Is any further assessment of the disease stage necessary at this time? What is the prognosis now that B.W.'s disease has metastasized?

[SI units: Ca, 3.75 mmol/L (normal, 2.25–2.88); phosphorus, 1.36 mmol/L (normal, 0.81–1.45); Na, 138 mmol/L (normal, 136–145); K, 4.3 mmol/L (normal, 3.5–5.5); albumin, 30 g/L (normal, 35–55); alkaline phosphatase, 580 U/L (normal, 15–70); AST, 258 U/L (normal, 5–20); ALT, 96 U/L (normal, 5–24)]

The purpose of documenting all sites of disease involvement is to provide a means by which treatment efficacy can be assessed and to identify any disease sites that may require immediate therapy to avoid life-threatening complications (e.g., brain metastases). B.W. has documented disease in the liver, bones, and brain. Other common sites of disease are the remaining breast tissue, bone marrow, and the lungs. Because her CBC is normal, further examination of the bone marrow is not necessary at this time; however, a chest radiograph should be ordered to rule out involvement of the lungs.

Metastatic breast cancer is rarely curable. After metastatic disease is documented, survival may range from a few months to several years, depending on the site(s) and number of metastases as well as the rate of tumor growth (which may be assessed by the disease-free interval). The median duration of survival after recurrence is approximately 2 years. Multiple sites of metastatic disease, a relatively short disease-free interval (<1 year), liver involvement, negative estrogen and progesterone receptors at the time of diagnosis, and premenopausal status all confer a poor prognosis for B.W.

Chemotherapy and Targeted Therapy

8. What treatment options are available for B.W. at this time?

The goals of therapy for metastatic disease are to prolong survival, alleviate or prevent tumor-related symptoms or complications, and maintain or improve quality of life. Currently, patients such as B.W. with metastatic disease have a 5-year survival rate of 26%.[1] B.W. has tumor in both the liver and bones, and systemic therapy is necessary to treat both disease sites simultaneously. Bone and soft tissue metastases tend to have a better prognosis and are more likely to respond to endocrine therapy. B.W. is unlikely to respond to endocrine manipulations such as hormonal therapy or oophorectomy, however, because her tumor is ER− and she is premenopausal. Liver metastases do not respond well to hormonal therapy. Patients such as B.W. who are symptomatic and unlikely to benefit from hormonal therapy should receive chemotherapy.

Cytotoxic chemotherapy is the mainstay of treatment for advanced breast cancer in patients whose tumors are refractory to endocrine therapy or not sensitive to hormone therapy. With the increased use of adjuvant chemotherapy, however, the choice of first-line treatment for metastatic breast cancer is increasingly complicated and is determined by a complex interaction of tumor, patient tolerability, and oncologist preferences. Many antitumor agents have some degree of activity against breast cancer (Table 91-2).[26] Several combination regimens that have been widely used in advanced breast

Table 91-2 Single-agent Response Rates of Chemotherapy Used as First-line Therapy in the Treatment of Metastatic Breast Cancer[26]

Agent	Dose/Frequency	Response Rates (%)
Doxorubicin	60–75 mg/m^2 every 3 wk	36–41
Pegylated liposomal doxorubicin	40–50 mg/m^2 every 28 days	36–41[a]
Epirubicin	75–90 mg/m^2 every 3 wk	36–41[a]
	20–30 mg/m^2 every wk	
Paclitaxel	135–175 mg/m^2 every 3 wk	22–29[b]
	80–100 mg/m^2 weekly	50–55[c]
Docetaxel	100 mg/m^2 every 3 wk	48
Capecitabine	1,250 mg/m^2 twice a day for 14 days of a 21-day cycle	30–37
Nanoparticle albumin bound paclitaxel	260 mg/m^2 every 3 wk	33
Vinorelbine	25 mg/m^2 every wk	25–40
Gemcitabine	1,200–1,500 mg/m^2 every wk for 3 of 4 wk	15–37

[a] Studies report equivalence to doxorubicin in response rate and time to progression.
[b] Response rates include those patients that were anthracycline pretreated.
[c] Both first- and second-line response rates.

cancer are listed in Chapter 88, Neoplastic Disorders and Their Treatment. Currently, sequential therapy with one agent at a time over concurrent therapy with combination therapy is more common; however, this concept is changing with the targeted therapies. Chemotherapy is commonly continued as long as the patient is achieving a response or has stable disease and is tolerating treatment. Because adjuvant chemotherapy is increasingly common, many patients in the metastatic setting have received many of the active agents utilized in the metastatic setting. Response rates to combination chemotherapy regimens in metastatic disease in patients who have not received prior chemotherapy are high. The response rates to chemotherapy in patients who have had prior exposure to chemotherapy are low, however.

One of the most important factors in determining the choice of first-line metastatic chemotherapy is the type of treatment given in the adjuvant setting. Anthracyclines are considered the most active agents against breast cancer; however, overall response rates in patients who have had prior anthracyclines are only 20% to 30%. In patients who have not received adjuvant anthracyclines, first-line anthracycline therapy should be considered, particularly in patients who have had disease-free intervals >12 months and in whom the maximal lifetime dose of anthracycline has not been achieved; however, data conclusively supporting this approach are lacking. Consideration of a different dose, a different anthracycline, or altered schedule should be given. Taxane-based therapy is considered the standard of care after anthracycline therapy. In patients who have received adjuvant taxane therapy and have had a long disease-free interval, treatment with a different taxane is a reasonable option. Finally, the recent approval of ixabepilone as monotherapy or in combination with capecitabine has been shown to be effective in patients who have previously been treated with an anthracycline and a taxane.

In patients with HER-2 positive tumors, trastuzumab in combination with chemotherapy has been shown to improve response rates and survival. In the largest trial of trastuzumab in patients with HER-2 positive, untreated metastatic breast cancer, trastuzumab plus chemotherapy prolonged the median time to disease progression and median response duration, increased the overall response rate, and improved overall survival time.[27] The greatest improvement was seen in patients receiving the combination of trastuzumab and paclitaxel. Other regimens consisting of other active agents with trastuzumab have been investigated. Weekly trastuzumab and vinorelbine resulted in an 84% response rate in patients receiving this regimen as first-line therapy for metastatic disease.[28] In patients who had previously received paclitaxel, the use of docetaxel in combination with trastuzumab reported a response rate of 20%. As with B.W., however, the use of trastuzumab in a patient who has already been treated with the drug in the adjuvant setting is unclear because the recurrent cancer is likely to be HER-2 positive, further targeting may provide some benefit. B.W.'s cancer recurred 2 years following chemotherapy, so other chemotherapy alternatives should be investigated. Importantly, she has central nervous system (CNS) involvement. Trastuzumab, a large protein, would not be expected to cross the blood–brain barrier to treat the metastases. The oral dual tyrosine kinase inhibitor lapatinib, with specificity for both the epidermal growth factor receptor (EGFR) and HER-2 would be an option for the management of B.W.'s disease at this time. One of the advantages of lapatinib over trastuzumab is that lapatinib does cross the blood–brain barrier. Additionally, lapatinib in combination with capecitabine is active in women with HER-2 positive advanced breast cancer that has progressed after treatment with regimens that include an anthracycline, a taxane, and trastuzumab.[29]

Another novel biologic agent used to treat metastatic breast cancer, bevacizumab, targets tumor angiogenesis through targeting the vascular endothelial growth factor (VEGF). Two randomized phase III trials evaluating single-agent chemotherapy with or without bevacizumab have been reported. The first trial enrolled patients with anthracycline- and taxane-resistant disease who had received one prior therapy for metastatic disease and evaluated bevacizumab in combination with capecitabine. The other trial evaluated bevacizumab with paclitaxel as first-line therapy for locally recurrent or metastatic breast cancer.[30] The bevacizumab and capecitabine therapy in the second-line trial resulted in improved response rates with no significant differences in survival, whereas the first-line treatment resulted in significant improvements in response rates and progression free survival, but no improvement in overall survival. This data, however, are still immature. Recently, bevacizumab was approved for treatment of HER-2 negative metastatic breast cancer as first-line therapy in combination with paclitaxel, but follow-up data from these trials and ongoing studies will better define its role in patients with metastatic breast cancer.

B.W. had received an anthracycline-containing regimen followed by paclitaxel and trastuzumab in the adjuvant setting. In patients treated with anthracyclines, taxanes, or both in the adjuvant setting, first-line treatment options for metastatic disease include re-exposure to the same agent or introduction of a different treatment. Studies evaluating retreatment with anthracyclines and taxanes after prior exposure in the adjuvant setting have yielded conflicting results. B.W.'s oncologist decides to use capecitabine in combination with lapatinib because she now has metastatic disease in multiple locations, including the CNS, and has previously received paclitaxel and trastuzumab.

Hormonal Therapy

ESTROGEN AND PROGESTERONE RECEPTORS

9. M.L., a 68-year-old woman with a history of breast cancer, had a lumpectomy followed by radiation therapy 7 years ago. At the time of initial diagnosis, she had been postmenopausal for approximately 10 years, and her tumor was documented to have high concentrations of both estrogen and progesterone receptors. She received 5 years of tamoxifen, which she completed approximately 2 years ago. She remained disease-free until recently, when she was found to have bone metastases in her left scapula and several ribs. No other sites of disease involvement were identified. Her only symptom is shoulder pain. What would be the appropriate treatment for M.L. at this time?

Breast cancer is one of the few human tumors that can be very sensitive to hormonal manipulations; however, it is also well recognized that only a subset of patients with breast cancer respond to the various endocrine therapies. Patients with tumors that are potentially endocrine-sensitive can be identified by measuring estrogen and progesterone receptors in the tumor tissue. Patients whose tumors are both ER+ and progesterone receptor positive (PR+) have a much higher response rate to endocrine therapy than patients without either receptor (~70% vs. 10%). Patients with ER+, PR− tumors have an intermediate response rate (30%).[31] Patients with endocrine-responsive tumors also are reported to have longer disease-free intervals after initial surgery, such as M.L. experienced.[31,32] In addition, they may have a longer survival after the documentation of metastatic disease. M.L.'s tumor was strongly ER+ and PR+ and she had a long disease-free interval (7 years); therefore, she is likely to respond to endocrine therapy.

Bisphosphonates

10. M.L. starts oral letrozole 2.5 mg every day and intravenous (IV) zoledronic acid 4 mg monthly. Is this a reasonable approach?

Hormonal agents, including antiestrogen (e.g., tamoxifen) and aromatase inhibitors (anastrozole, letrozole, exemestane), are equally effective for the initial treatment of endocrine-responsive breast cancer. As reviewed above, the aromatase inhibitors have dramatically changed the treatment of women with ER+ breast cancer. Because M.L. received adjuvant tamoxifen for 5 years and has ER+ disease, the use of an aromatase inhibitor would be appropriate. Multiple studies with anastrazole, letrozole, and exemestane have shown that they produce equivalent or superior response rates or time to disease progression compared with tamoxifen when used as first-line treatment for advanced disease.[33] Therefore, the use of letrozole is reasonable. Other treatment options for patients with ER+ disease include fulvestrant, an ER antagonist without agonist effects, which has also been shown to be equivalent to tamoxifen with respect to time to disease progression, overall response rate, and median duration of response.

Following the initiation of endocrine therapy, it usually takes 3 months before the therapeutic response can be assessed. In patients such as M.L. with only bone metastases, assessment may be difficult because it may take 4 to 6 months to reossify the involved bones. In such cases, the decision to continue therapy may be based on the lessening of bone pain and disease stabilization (i.e., no new metastatic sites).

Bone metastases occur in approximately 70% of patients with metastatic breast cancer and are associated with a median survival of 24 months with 20% of patients alive at 5 years.[34] Skeletal-related complications caused by the bone metastases are common, including significant bone pain, spinal cord complications, hypercalcemia, and pathologic fractures. An integrated approach to treating these patients includes pain medications, antineoplastic therapy or endocrine therapy (depending on the ER status), radiation therapy for palliation, and bisphosphonates. The bisphosphonates have been shown to decrease the risk for skeletal-related events by approximately one-third.[34] Current guidelines support the use of bisphosphonates in women with radiographic evidence of bony metastases.[35] More recently, zoledronic acid 4 mg was shown to be as effective and as well tolerated as pamidronate 90 mg in the treatment of osteolytic and mixed bony metastases in patients with advanced breast cancer.[36] The advantage of zoledronic acid over pamidronate is that therapy can be administered as a 15-minute infusion versus a 2-hour infusion. Therefore, M.L. should begin zoledronic acid therapy.[35]

11. Over the next 18 months, M.L. continues letrozole therapy and has a complete resolution of her shoulder pain with considerable improvement of the radiographs and no appearance of new lesions. She is now experiencing left hip pain and a bone scan has documented new metastatic disease. What therapy should be considered at this time?

M.L. had a good initial response to letrozole, so she is likely to respond again to another type of endocrine therapy. Exemestane is an irreversible, nonsteroidal aromatase inhibitor that has been shown to be effective as second-line therapy, as has fulvestrant.[33,37] Megestrol also can be considered as a third-line hormonal therapy. Radiation therapy may provide M.L. with palliative relief of pain. If M.L. had rapidly worsening disease involving a visceral organ, such as the liver, or if she had not responded well to prior endocrine therapy, cytotoxic chemotherapy may have been more appropriate.

COLON CANCER

Screening

12. E.R., a 55-year-old man, is having his first physical examination in >10 years because he has noted a change in his bowel habits recently. His father died of colorectal cancer 2 years ago.

E.R. questions whether his risk is increased and if there is anything that he can do to prevent colon cancer or decrease his risk of dying from it.

Colorectal cancer is the third leading cause of cancer deaths in the U.S. adult population.[1] Approximately 70% of these cancers will arise in the colon, whereas 30% will occur in the rectum. Multiple risk factors are well recognized: family history; age >50 years; high-fat, low-fiber diet; obesity; chronic inflammatory bowel disease; and a personal history of colorectal polyps or cancer. Several hereditary syndromes are recognized that place persons at an extremely high risk, such as hereditary nonpolyposis colorectal cancer (HNPCC or Lynch syndrome) and familial adenomatous polyposis (FAP).[38] The American Society of Clinical Oncology currently recommends genetic testing for HNPCC or Lynch syndrome for those at high risk.[39]

Evidence suggests that continuous aspirin or other nonsteroidal anti-inflammatory drug (NSAID) use may prevent the development of colorectal cancer by inhibiting cyclooxygenase (COX-2) expression.[38] Presumably, COX-2 acts as a tumor promoter in the intestine. In fact, celecoxib, a COX-2 inhibitor, is approved as an oral adjunct to usual care in patients with FAP because it was shown to reduce the number and size of colorectal polyps in these patients. Large-scale, prospective clinical trials evaluating aspirin and classic NSAIDs have revealed promising results, and trials with the newer selective COX-2 inhibitors are ongoing.[38] Other potential preventive measures include calcium supplementation and a high-fiber diet.[38] Chemoprevention trials for colorectal cancer are discussed in Chapter 88, Neoplastic Disorders and Their Treatment.

Because E.R. is >50 years of age and has a family history of colorectal cancer, he should undergo screening. He also has symptoms (i.e., change in bowel habits) that heighten suspicion. Current screening recommendations for colorectal cancer include fecal occult blood testing and, depending on age and risk, sigmoidoscopy or total colonic examination.[40]

Fecal Occult Blood Testing (FOBT)

13. What methods to detect FOBT are available, and are there any advantages of one method over another?

A FOBT increases the chance of diagnosing colorectal cancer at an early stage of disease and is associated with a 30% reduction in colorectal cancer mortality.[40] Of the three FOBT methods used, the guaiac test is the most common, simple, and inexpensive, although newer methods may be more sensitive and specific. The guaiac test is a colorimetric test in which guaiac dye is oxidized to a bluish quinone compound in the presence of a peroxidase (e.g., hemoglobin). Foods, other substances, and medical conditions that contain or produce peroxidase activity may yield false–positive readings (Table 91-3). Conversely, large amounts of ascorbic acid can produce false–negative guaiac test results. A second method is a quantitative test based on fluorometry of heme-derived porphyrin. During intestinal transit, hemoglobin is broken down to porphyrin. The third method is an immunochemical test (e.g., HemeSelect) that uses antiserum to human hemoglobin to detect blood in the feces. This test is very sensitive and specific; however, it loses sensitivity if the bleeding is from the proximal colon because bacteria alter the globin. The immunochemical test eliminates the need for dietary restrictions; however, there is a 24-hour delay in reading the results because an extract needs to be prepared from the stool sample. Red meat should be eliminated from the diet for 3 days before occult blood is tested using the guaiac methods and for 4 days before testing using methods based on heme-derived porphyrins.[41] Approximately 2% of persons >50 years of age will have a positive FOBT. Of these, 10% will be diagnosed with cancer, 30% with polyps, and the remaining 60% will have false–positive results.

Table 91-3 Causes of Positive Fecal Guaiac Test

Foods With Peroxidase Activity
Broccoli
Cauliflower
Turnips
Horseradish
Cabbage
Potatoes
Cucumbers
Mushrooms
Artichokes
Medications That Interfere With Fecal Blood Testing
Steroids
Nonsteroidal anti-inflammatory drugs (NSAID)
Reserpine
Common Causes of Blood in the Stool
Colorectal cancer
Colorectal polyps
Diverticulitis
Hemorrhoids
Fissures
Proctitis
Inflammatory bowel disease

Staging and Prognosis

14. E.R.'s fecal occult blood tests are positive on specimens obtained on two consecutive days. Colonoscopy revealed a 2.5-cm mass, and a biopsy of the lesion is interpreted as adenocarcinoma of the colon. Surgical resection of the mass and regional lymph nodes is performed. The tumor is confined to the bowel wall, although four regional lymph nodes show evidence of tumor involvement. Distant metastases of the tumor are not evident at this time, and his colon cancer is stage III. E.R.'s physical examination is otherwise unremarkable and all laboratory values are within normal limits except for an elevated lactate dehydrogenase (LDH) and a carcinoembryonic antigen (CEA) level of 647 ng/mL (normal, <5 ng/mL). What is the prognosis for stage III colon cancer? Could earlier detection have improved the prognosis?

When colorectal cancer is diagnosed in the early stages, it is curable with surgical intervention and >90% of patients survive 5 years. The 5-year survival rate declines to 55% to 60% in patients such as E.R. with stage III disease. Overall 5-year survival rates have increased during the past two decades from 50% to 63%.[42] The tumor node mestasis (TNM) staging system is most commonly used for colon cancer. Stage I indicates penetration into (but not through) the bowel wall. Stage II generally indicates penetration through the bowel wall; stage III indicates lymph node involvement; and stage IV indicates metastatic disease. Optimal node sampling at the time of surgery is critical to staging and should include the evaluation of 12 to 17 lymph nodes. Patients with early-stage colorectal cancer often are asymptomatic; therefore, intensive screening programs as just described are advocated to reduce the mortality of this disease. Of patients with metastatic and recurrent colorectal cancer, 60% to 90% have elevated CEA or CA-19–9 levels. Levels are elevated in relation to the stage and extent of disease, the degree of tumor differentiation, and the site of metastases. If the CEA level is elevated at the time of initial diagnosis, as in E.R., it can be monitored after surgical resection of the tumor for evidence of recurrent disease.[43]

Treatment

Adjuvant Therapy

15. All evidence of tumor is removed, and E.R.'s CEA level declines. Therefore, the surgery may be considered potentially curable. Should E.R. receive any additional therapy at this time?

Tumor recurrence is a significant problem associated with stage III colon and rectal cancers, with up to 60% of all surgically treated patients eventually developing local recurrences. Causes of these relapses may include peritoneal seeding caused by exfoliation of tumor cells in the colonic lumen and spillage during surgery. Most tumor recurrences are secondary to either disease spread to the regional lymph nodes or extension of the tumor into the bowel wall, with subsequent hematogenous dissemination. Metastasis to the liver via hematogenous spread (through the portal circulation) is the most common site of disease spread beyond the regional lymph nodes and occurs in 50% of patients with invasive disease.[44] Lung metastases (without liver metastases) occur rarely and generally are associated with lesions in the lower rectum.

Because of the significant relapse rate in patients with stage III and high-risk stage II colon cancer, adjuvant chemotherapy has been extensively studied. Chemotherapy improves disease-free survival (DFS) and overall survival in patients, such as E.R., who have had "potentially curative surgery."[45] The first definitive adjuvant chemotherapy regimens contained fluorouracil and leucovorin. Currently, agents used in combination chemotherapy for the adjuvant treatment of colorectal cancer (Chapter 88) include fluorouracil, leucovorin, oxaliplatin, and capecitabine in various combinations and doses. Patients such as E.R. who have stage III disease should receive adjuvant therapy consisting of 6 months of FOLFOX (fluorouracil, leucovorin, oxaliplatin). Three clinical trials support the use of FOLFOX or XELOX (capecitabine and oxaliplatin) in the adjuvant setting.[46–48] These trials have shown improved DFS compared with adjuvant fluorouracil and leucovorin, but an overall survival benefit has not been observed.[46,48] The tradeoff for this improved DFS has been increased toxicity caused by the oxaliplatin, including neutropenia and neurotoxicity, which interferes with the activities of daily living. In the X-ACT trial, capecitabine was equivalent to the combination of fluorouracil and leucovorin in the adjuvant setting.[49]

Ongoing trials are evaluating the role of the monoclonal antibodies bevacizumab (targeting VEGF) and cetuximab (targeting EGFR) in combination with FOLFOX in the adjuvant setting. Until the results of these trials are available, the use of monoclonal antibodies in the adjuvant setting is limited to participation in a clinical trial.

Follow-Up Care

16. Within 6 months after surgery, E.R.'s CEA level has fallen to <2.5 ng/mL and he completes the adjuvant therapy without serious sequelae. What follow-up care is recommended at this time?

E.R. continues to be at significant risk for developing recurrent disease. If recurrences are detected early, it is possible to cure them with additional surgery. In most cases, patients with early recurrences are asymptomatic; therefore, an active follow-up program is necessary to detect them, including a medical history, physical examination, and CEA levels every 3 months for the first 3 years, then every 6 months for the next 2 years, and then annually.[43] Colonoscopy is repeated annually for several years and then every 3 to 5 years. He should receive a chest radiograph annually or when prompted by an elevated CEA or symptoms. Additional tests, such as abdominal and pelvic CT scans and liver function chemistries, should be done if routine test findings are abnormal or if symptoms suggest recurrent disease.[43]

Recurrent Disease

Rising Carcinoembryonic Antigen Level

17. Eighteen months after completing adjuvant chemotherapy, E.R. returns for routine follow-up; his CEA levels are elevated. What is the significance of a rising CEA level?

Although widespread serum CEA level monitoring is not an efficient way to screen for colorectal cancer in the general population, a rising CEA level in a patient with a history of colorectal cancer may be the first indication of recurrent disease if the patient had an elevated CEA level at the time of original diagnosis. Generally, the CEA level is measured every 3 months for 3 years and then every 6 months for 2 years.[43] More than 50% of patients who have recurrent disease also have elevated CEA levels.

Chemotherapy for Metastatic Disease

18. On a routine follow-up visit several months later, a CT scan of E.R.'s abdomen shows that the disease in his colon has recurred and the liver CT shows two discrete nodules along with a nodule in the left lung that are consistent with metastatic disease; however, E.R. is feeling well and has no symptoms suggestive of metastases. What is the role of further chemotherapy now that E.R. has recurrent disease?

Of those patients such as E.R. who present initially with localized, resectable disease, 30% will subsequently develop metastatic disease. Among patients with newly diagnosed colorectal cancer, 25% will present with metastatic disease. Significant treatment advances have been made in the last 5 years to manage cases of advanced colorectal cancer such that the median survival is now up to 2 years in treated patients.[50] These include single-agent therapy (irinotecan, oxaliplatin, capecitabine), combination chemotherapy, and the use of monoclonal antibodies (bevacizumab, cetuximab, and panitumumab). Comparisons of irinotecan, fluorouracil, and leucovorin regimens (IFL, FOLFIRI) with oxaliplatin, fluorouracil, and leucovorin (FOLFOX) combinations for the initial treatment of metastatic colorectal cancer have been reported. Patients treated with FOLFOX had a response rate, time to disease progression, and overall survival rate that were superior to those observed with IFL or IROX (irinotecan, oxaliplatin). The overall survival results did not account, however, for second-line therapy, which was not controlled for and could affect survival.[51] Nevertheless, this established FOLFOX as the first-line chemotherapy choice for patients with metastatic disease. Other regimens used first-line therapy for metastatic disease (outlined in Chapter 88) include FOLFIRI (fluorouracil, irinotecan, leucovorin), CAPOX (capecitabine, oxaliplatin), XELOX (capecitabine, oxaliplatin), and XELIRI (capecitabine, irinotecan); however, the optimal sequence of any of these regimens and the effect of sequence on survival are unclear. Often, the decision regarding the choice of combination therapy for first- or second-line therapy is based on prior therapy, quality of life, pre-existing toxicities, and comorbid conditions.

Biologic therapies targeting VEGF (bevacizumab) and EGFR (cetuximab and panitumumab), play a significant role in the metastatic setting. The addition of bevacizumab to IFL significantly improved response and overall survival.[52] As second-line therapy, the combination of FOLFOX and bevacizumab has also demonstrated significant improvement both in response and overall survival.[53] Cetuximab, a chimeric monoclonal antibody against the extracellular domain of EGFR, has shown efficacy, but has not improved survival as a single agent or in combination with irinotecan in patients with irinotecan-refractory malignancies in the metastatic setting.[54] Despite the lack of improvement in survival, cetuximab is approved for second- and subsequent-line therapy in patients with EGFR-positive, irinotecan-refractory metastatic colorectal cancer. A recent trial evaluated the combination of cetuximab plus bevacizumab with or without irinotecan in previously treated patients with advanced colorectal cancer and reported a response rate for the three-drug combination of 37% and a time to disease progression of 7.9 months.[55] These response rates are impressive for an otherwise chemotherapy-refractory population. Finally, panitumumab, a fully human monoclonal antibody also targeting the extracellular domain of EGFR, has shown activity as monotherapy in the treatment of refractory metastatic disease when compared with best supportive care. Ongoing trials are evaluating the efficacy and safety of panitumumab in combination with chemotherapy.

Now that E.R. has metastatic disease in both the liver and the lung, he should receive combination chemotherapy. The choice of regimen depends on prior therapy, and because E.R. has received adjuvant FOLFOX, the use of FOLFIRI in combination with bevacizumab would be a reasonable approach.

Hepatic Metastases

Colorectal-related metastases mainly affect the liver. In one-third of the cases, the metastases are synchronous and in two-thirds, metachronous. Surgical resection, if possible, is the most effective treatment modality for potential long-term survival in colorectal patients with isolated liver metastases. Many patients, however, could potentially benefit from regional therapy. Because liver tumors derive most of their blood supply from the hepatic artery, direct administration of effective anticancer drugs into the artery provides high drug concentrations to the area of tumor involvement.[56] Hepatic intra-arterial administration of fluorouracil, floxuridine, or other chemotherapeutic agents has been extensively studied in patients with metastases confined to the liver. More recently, the intra-arterial use of oxaliplatin- and irinotecan-based chemotherapies has yielded encouraging results. Because E.R. has disease that also involves the lung, he should receive systemic chemotherapy for his disease.

Genomic Markers

19. What is the role of genomic markers in the treatment of colon cancer?

The identification of appropriate patients for treatment could be improved in both the metastatic and adjuvant setting by molecular profiling. This would allow the clinician to individualize therapy based on risk of toxicity and potential for response. Although not standard in today's practice, a number of predictive markers have been identified, including the evaluation of microsatellite instability, protooncogenes such as *K-ras*, and DNA microarray profiling.[57] Microsatellite instability is found in almost two-thirds of colon cancers and these tumors exhibit improved survival from recurrence. Mutations in *K-ras* occur in approximately 30% of colon cancer cases and in early stage disease. These tumors are associated with recurrence and poorer long-term survival, so patients should receive adjuvant chemotherapy. Finally, DNA microarray profiling may allow identification of patients who respond to specific chemotherapies, such as fluorouracil, irinotecan, or oxaliplatin. Although all these markers are currently under investigation in clinical trials, they will allow clinicians to tailor therapy according to an individual patient and tumor profile.

A genetic diagnostic test (Invader UGT1A1 Molecular Assay), which assesses the status of an individual's UGT1A1 enzyme, is available for clinical use. The test allows clinicians to individualize irinotecan therapy by identifying patients at risk for toxicity. Irinotecan is metabolized by enzymes exhibiting polymorphic activity, specifically uridine 5′ diphosphate glucuronosyltransferase (UGT). UGT1A1 is responsible for glucuronidating SN38, an irinotecan metabolite that produces severe toxicity. Individuals with the UGT1A1*28 variant have reduced activity of UGT1A1 and may suffer severe neutropenia. Despite the tremendous advance in using UGT1A1*28 to predict neutropenia risk, more research is needed to identify patients at risk for irinotecan-induced diarrhea. The commercially available test is designed to predict which patients are at risk for enhanced toxicity. In clinical practice, however, genotyping is performed once the patient has severe neutropenia to determine if the patient has reduced enzyme activity.

LUNG CANCER

Clinical Presentation

20. H.H., a 57-year-old, white woman with a 6-month history of weight loss and increasing fatigue, recently noted shortness of breath (SOB) and fever. She also complains of joint pain in her knees and elbows and has noted a change in her fingers and nails over the past several months. Physical examination is significant for swelling and tenderness over her knees and elbows as well as hypertrophy and clubbing of the distal joints of both hands. A chest radiograph and CT scan reveals a central mass causing

obstruction of the middle right lobe as well as mediastinal lymphadenopathy. Bronchoscopy washings and cytology were positive for small-cell lung carcinoma. H.H. denied exposure to any environmental or occupational carcinogens but did admit to a 40-pack/year history of cigarette smoking. Are H.H.'s symptoms typical of those associated with lung cancer?

Signs and symptoms associated with lung cancer depend on the size and location of the tumor and degree of spread outside of the lungs. The most common symptoms at presentation are those associated with the primary tumor and include cough, wheezing, chest pain, hemoptysis, and dyspnea.[58] Because many patients have other medical problems, such as chronic obstructive airway disease related to cigarette smoking, the worsening of these symptoms may go unnoticed for a period or may be attributed to other smoking-related illnesses. A large tumor can result in obstruction, leading to fever and other evidence of pneumonia.

Regional spread to lymph nodes and other structures within the thorax can result in dysphagia, superior vena cava obstruction, pleural effusion, and hoarseness. Patients with distant metastatic spread may have findings associated with the site of disease involvement. For example, if the tumor has spread to the liver, patients are likely to have elevated LFT, or if they have brain metastases, severe headache, neurologic impairment, or seizures may be present.

Almost one-third of patients with lung cancer present with nonspecific symptoms such as anorexia and weight loss.[58] In addition, a few patients will present with paraneoplastic syndromes. Hypertrophic osteoarthropathy, with inflammation of the outer covering of bones and clubbing, can cause pain, tenderness, and swelling over the affected bones such as that experienced by H.H. This often mimics bone metastases (bone scans also may be positive); however, further studies will reveal no evidence of direct tumor involvement of the bones. Other paraneoplastic syndromes commonly seen in patients with lung cancer include ectopic Cushing's syndrome and the syndrome of inappropriate antidiuretic hormone secretion (SIADH). Characteristically, successful treatment of the tumor will reduce the effects of paraneoplastic syndromes.

Prevalence and Risk Factors

21. How common is lung cancer and what factors place H.H. at risk?

Over 160,390 deaths will occur from lung cancer in 2007. Although the World Health Organization recognizes that there are >10 types of primary pleuropulmonary malignancies, four major types of carcinomas account for up to 95% of all lung cancers.[58] The four major types are adenocarcinoma, squamous cell, small-cell, and large-cell carcinoma (Table 91-4).[58] Adenocarcinoma, squamous cell, and large-cell carcinoma are grouped together and referred to as non–small-cell lung cancers (NSCLC) because they are similar in prognosis and response to therapy.

Cigarette smoking is the predominant cause of lung cancer worldwide, and the risk appears to increase with the number of cigarettes smoked each day.[59] Approximately 75% to 80% of lung cancer cases are attributable to smoking.[59] Second-hand smoke exposure is also a risk factor, with approximately 3,000 deaths attributable to this factor. Although the risk of developing any type of lung cancer increases with cigarette smoking, the relative risk of small-cell lung cancer (SCLC) is among the highest. Therefore, patients such as H.H. who have a long history of cigarette smoking have the highest risk of developing lung cancer relative to any other population. Other risk factors for lung cancer include exposure to passive smoke (i.e., nonsmokers who live with smokers); pipe and cigar smoking; and exposure to asbestos, radon, or other occupational carcinogens such as heavy metals, chloromethyl ether, and arsenic.[59]

Table 91-4 Histologic Classification of Lung Cancer[58]

Classification	*Prevalence (%)*
Adenocarcinoma	40
Squamous cell carcinoma	25
Small-cell carcinoma	20
Large-cell carcinoma	10
Adenosquamous carcinoma, carcinoid, bronchial gland carcinoma	<5

Prevention and Screening

22. What are the current recommendations for prevention and screening for early detection of lung cancer in patients like H.H.?

By far, the most important intervention for preventing lung cancer is to avoid or cease smoking and to avoid secondary smoke whenever possible. Antioxidants and β-carotene have no protective effect and, in at least two large trials, an increase in lung cancer was found in persons receiving β-carotene.[60,61] Secondary analysis in a trial of selenium for the prevention of skin cancer revealed a significant reduction in the occurrence of lung cancer,[62] but definitive trials are still in progress.

Lung cancer screening has not affected overall mortality. In the early 1970s, the National Cancer Institute (NCI) launched three studies evaluating sputum cytology and chest radiography as lung cancer screening tests. Although cancers were detected earlier, the overall mortality rates in the two groups did not differ significantly.[63,64] Since the time of these studies, the quality of diagnostic testing has been substantially enhanced and many new tests have become available; therefore, new screening studies, especially for high-risk populations are underway. Presently, no medical or scientific organization recommends testing for early lung cancer detection in asymptomatic individuals. Growing evidence suggests spiral CT may be effective for detecting early lung cancer, but prospective trials confirming a benefit have not been completed.[65] Ongoing trials will better determine its role in the evaluation of patients at high-risk for lung cancer.

Small-Cell Lung Cancer Versus Non–Small-Cell Lung Cancer

23. How do treatment and prognoses for SCLC and NSCLC differ?

The natural history and response to treatment of patients with SCLC and NSCLC differ significantly. Therefore, it is extremely important to establish a histologic diagnosis before contemplating treatment (Table 91-4). In general, the NSCLC are less likely to metastasize early in the course of the disease and are less sensitive to chemotherapy than SCLC. In contrast, SCLC progresses rapidly, but is sensitive to many chemotherapeutic agents.

Surgery is curative only in early stages of NSCLC and is the treatment of choice for patients with stage I through IIIA NSCLC.[58,66] Radiation therapy may be considered an alternative for patients who are poor surgical risks. Radiotherapy also is used as an adjuvant therapy to surgery to treat NSCLC characterized by large tumors or extensive lymph node involvement; however, no survival advantage has been observed with the addition of radiation therapy.[67] In advanced stages of NSCLC, overall response rates to combination chemotherapy are 20% to 40%, with fewer than 5% of patients achieving a complete response.[68,69] The highest response rates for chemotherapy in NSCLC have been achieved with regimens using cisplatin or carboplatin combined with etoposide, paclitaxel, docetaxel, vinorelbine, and gemcitabine. Even with the best therapy, median survival is approximately 12 months.

Small-cell lung cancer is staged as "limited" or "extensive." Limited-stage disease is confined to one hemithorax and the regional lymph nodes and can be encompassed within one radiation port. Extensive disease is that which extends beyond the thorax. Because SCLC disseminates early in the disease, surgery is almost never indicated. The only exception is the rare patient who presents with very early stage disease. Such patients may benefit by resection of the tumor followed by combination chemotherapy. Overall, the use of combination chemotherapy regimens for SCLC has increased median survival by four- to fivefold. In disease limited to the thoracic cavity, optimal chemotherapy regimens produce response rates of 85% to 95%, with 50% to 60% of patients achieving a complete response. Although many patients initially respond to therapy, most eventually relapse and die from their SCLC. The median duration of survival is 12 to 16 months and the 2-year DFS rate is usually 15% to 20% for patients with limited disease. Response rates are somewhat lower for patients with disease outside the thoracic cavity, and the median survival is only 7 to 11 months. The 2-year DFS for these patients is <2%.

Small-Cell Lung Cancer

Staging

24. What information, in addition to the histologic type, is necessary before H.H.'s treatment can be initiated?

Before initiating therapy, the stage of H.H.'s disease should be evaluated. This will help establish a prognosis and identify tumor lesions that can be monitored to evaluate the response to therapy. Staging also will assist in determining if H.H. will benefit from radiation therapy in addition to chemotherapy. Because the TNM staging factors do not appear to correlate with survival, a simple two-stage system is used for SCLC. Staging procedures should include a thorough workup of any areas that are suspicious for tumor involvement, a chest radiograph and CT scans, a CBC, LFT, physical examination of the liver, and a neurologic examination. In addition, H.H.'s physiologic and performance status should be assessed to determine her ability to tolerate the aggressive chemotherapy and possible radiation therapy. This includes evaluation of her nutritional, cardiac, and pulmonary status, as well as her renal and hepatic function.

Combination Chemotherapy

25. H.H. is to start a chemotherapeutic regimen of cisplatin 100 mg/m^2 IV on day 1 and etoposide 100 mg/m^2 IV on days 1 through 3. The chemotherapy is to be repeated every 28 days. She also will receive radiation therapy to the area of tumor involvement. Is H.H. likely to benefit from the addition of prophylactic radiation or other cytotoxic agents to her regimen?

Although combination chemotherapy is clearly superior to single-agent therapy in the treatment of SCLC, no major differences exist between several combination chemotherapy regimens that have been widely studied when compared for response rate or survival. Most current first-line regimens include cisplatin or carboplatin in combination with etoposide. Other active agents for SCLC include topotecan, paclitaxel, docetaxel, ifosfamide, cyclophosphamide, teniposide, doxorubicin, vincristine, and methotrexate.

26. How should H.H. be monitored during therapy?

Approximately 80% of patients respond to initial chemotherapy for SCLC. Because this is a chemosensitive disease, patients typically show evidence of response within days. Follow-up care of a patient receiving chemotherapy should include the following: (a) assessment of chemotherapy-associated toxicities (e.g., mucositis, myelosuppression, renal dysfunction, electrolyte disorders) so that appropriate interventions can be initiated; (b) regular re-evaluation of renal, hepatic, and bone marrow function to assess the patient's ability to tolerate further treatment; and (c) assessment of the antitumor effects of the treatment.

Myelosuppression (i.e., granulocytopenia, thrombocytopenia) is generally only moderate with cisplatin-etoposide regimens; however, the addition of radiation therapy is likely to increase its severity. Therefore, H.H. should have her CBC monitored weekly once therapy begins. Because nephrotoxicity is the usual dose-limiting toxicity of cisplatin, renal function must be evaluated.

Chest radiographs and CT scans should be repeated after every two to three courses of therapy to assess antitumor effects. Therapy should be continued if the tumor is responding to treatment and discontinued or changed with evidence of tumor progression.

Duration of Therapy and Prophylactic Irradiation

27. After six courses of this regimen, repeat chest radiographs and CT scans reveal no evidence of residual tumor in H.H. A repeat bronchoscopy is also negative. Is additional treatment indicated?

Despite the high recurrence rate for patients with SCLC who achieve a complete response, no current evidence supports prolonged administration of chemotherapy after complete response is achieved. Long-term survival rates appear to be similar for patients who receive 4 to 6 months of treatment and those who receive 12 to 24 months. In addition, patients who receive a shorter duration of chemotherapy exposure are less likely to suffer major toxicities. After disease recurrence, however, response rates to second-line therapy are only 20% to

40% with few complete responses; the median survival is only a few months. Today, the topoisomerase inhibitors (topotecan or irinotecan), taxanes, paclitaxel or docetaxel, gemcitabine or vinorelbine are the most widely used second-line agents.

At least 20% to 25% of patients with SCLC eventually develop brain metastases, which produce significant morbidity. Clinical trials have demonstrated that prophylactic cranial irradiation significantly reduces the incidence of symptomatic brain metastases and prolongs disease-free and overall survival.[70] Therefore, prophylactic cranial irradiation is recommended for patients such as H.H. who attain a response to chemotherapy.

Non–Small-Cell Lung Cancer

Metastatic Disease

28. M.D., a 62-year-old man, was recently diagnosed with stage IV adenocarcinoma of the lung. His medical history is not significant, and he is otherwise in good health. What are the current treatment recommendations?

Although NSCLC is less chemosensitive than SCLC, evidence gathered over the past decade substantiates that combination chemotherapy therapy improves median survival from 16 to 26 weeks and enhances 1-year survival rates by 10% over the best supportive care. The American Society of Clinical Oncology now recommends two to eight cycles of platinum-based combination chemotherapy for patients with stage IV disease and good performance status (Eastern Cooperative Oncology Group [ECOG] 0, 1, and possibly, 2).[69] The most widely used first-line regimens include carboplatin or cisplatin plus either paclitaxel, docetaxel, vinorelbine, or gemcitabine. Some newer regimens also incorporate three of these agents. Response is generally re-evaluated after two cycles of chemotherapy and, if a response or stable disease is noted, treatment is continued for up to eight cycles. If disease progression is evident, second-line therapy with agents not previously received or palliative radiation therapy is recommended. One-year survival rates range from 25% to 40% using these newer regimens.

The role of targeted therapies, specifically the antivascular endothelial growth factor agent bevacizumab, has been evaluated in patients with advanced (stage IIIB and IV) NSCLC and it is now U.S. Food and Drug Administration (FDA)-approved for use as first-line treatment of advanced or metastatic NSCLC in combination with standard chemotherapy. The pivotal study utilized paclitaxel 200 mg/m^2 and carboplatin area-under-the-curve (AUC) of 6 (mg/mL × minute) every 3 weeks for six cycles with or without bevacizumab 15 mg/kg continued until disease progression. The regimen containing bevacizumab resulted in significant improvements in median survival (12.5 vs. 10.5 months, respectively) as well as significantly improved response rates and progression-free survival.[71] Women, however, did not experience a survival benefit (13.3 vs. 13.1 months, respectively).

The novel tyrosine kinase inhibitors that act on EGFR, gefitinib and erlotinib, were fast-tracked to the market pending phase III confirmatory trials as single-agent treatment for patients with NSCLC who failed platinum and docetaxel regimens. Use of gefitinib is now limited, however, to those cancer patients who, in the opinion of their treating physician, are currently benefiting, or have previously benefited, from gefitinib treatment because it did not significantly improve overall survival in the randomized phase III setting.[72] The response rates to these agents were highly variable in certain subgroups, with women, those with adenocarcinoma, and nonsmokers having higher response rates. Importantly, clinical trials adding these agents to platinum-based chemotherapy have shown no advantage except in the subset of patients who have never smoked. In them, erlotinib in combination with chemotherapy significantly improved overall survival.[72] Currently, the use of erlotinib is limited to single-agent therapy in the metastatic setting, although ongoing trials are evaluating its use sequentially with chemotherapy.

For patients with unresectable stage III disease, there have now been at least 10 major multi-institutional trials in which patients were randomized to treatment with thoracic radiation with or without platinum-based chemotherapy. A statistically significant survival advantage was seen for the combined modality therapy.[73]

Adjuvant Chemotherapy

29. If M.D. had been diagnosed with stage II disease, what would be the role of chemotherapy after surgical resection?

Surgical resection is the cornerstone of therapy for early stage disease, but relapse is high with 30% to 60% of patients with resected NSCLC still dying of their disease. Until recently, no additional treatment beyond surgery was known to be beneficial. Three randomized trials, however, validated the role of adjuvant chemotherapy for completely resected NSCLC with survival advantages at 5 years ranging from 5% to 15% (Table 91-5).[74–76] The role of surgery in stage IB remains controversial, however, but beneficial trends exist, especially when tumors are large (at least 4 cm in size).[74] Recently, absence of the ERCC1 (excision repair cross-complementation group 1)

Table 91-5 Adjuvant Lung Cancer Trials

			5-yr Survival (%)		
Study/Reference	*Patients (N)*	*Stage*	*Control*	*Chemotherapy Arm*	*p-Value*
IALT/[75]	1,867	I-IIIA	40	45	<0.03
NCICTG/[76]	482	IB-II	54	69	0.03
ANITA/[74]	840	IB-IIIA	43	51	0.013

ANITA, Adjuvant Navelbine International Trialists Association; IALT, International Adjuvant Lung Trial; NCICTG, National Cancer Institute of Canada Trials Group.

protein in operative tumor specimens of patients with NSCLC has been used to identify tumors that appear to benefit most from adjuvant cisplatin-based chemotherapy.[77] Each of the positive adjuvant trials utilized cisplatin-based chemotherapy regimens in combination with etoposide or a vinca alkaloid, with two of the trials utilizing cisplatin and vinorelbine. Therefore, if M.D. was diagnosed with stage II disease, he should receive six cycles of a cisplatin-based regimen.

OVARIAN CANCER

Risk Factors and Clinical Presentation

30. C.R., a 50-year-old woman, presents to her family physician complaining of vague abdominal pain over the last several weeks. A detailed history revealed that she had experienced increasing abdominal girth without significant weight gain and a change in her usual bowel habits. The abdominal and pelvic ultrasound studies reveal a 6- to 10-cm mass, and her serum CA-125 antigen is significantly elevated. C.R. is referred to a gynecologic oncologist who performs a total abdominal hysterectomy and bilateral salpingo-oophorectomy. Pathologic examination of the mass determined it to be epithelial carcinoma of the ovary. The large intra-abdominal mass and numerous peritoneal tumor implants were resected during surgery; however, several small (<0.5 cm) tumor implants were not resectable. What factors are associated with an increased risk of ovarian cancer? Are C.R.'s symptoms consistent with ovarian cancer?

Ovarian cancer is the fifth most common cause of cancer and cancer deaths in women.[1] The three categories of ovarian cancer are named for their cell of origin. Greater than 90% are epithelial cancers, arising from the epithelial layer that covers the surface of the ovaries, whereas the remainder are either germ cell or stromal tumors. Postmenopausal women (median age, 63 years) are most likely to develop epithelial ovarian cancer. Factors that appear to increase the risk of ovarian cancer include positive family history, nulliparity or a low number of pregnancies, first child after age 35, prolonged use of ovulation-inducing drugs, and increasing age.[78] A genetic predisposition may also exist to ovarian cancer, which can be related to hereditary breast cancer. Genetic mutations in the *BRCA1* and *BRCA2* genes may play a role in the development of ovarian cancer.[39]

Ovarian cancer is known as the silent killer because 70% of patients present with advanced disease. As in C.R.'s case, patients with early stages of ovarian cancer may be relatively asymptomatic. The patient's only complaint may be vague abdominal symptoms, and she may not seek medical attention until symptoms become significantly worse. Ovarian carcinoma, however, usually has extended beyond the pelvis at the time of diagnosis. Pain, abdominal distention, and vaginal bleeding are the most common symptoms in patients with advanced disease.[78] Other symptoms may include weight loss, nausea, or a change in bowel or bladder habits if the tumor mass is compressing adjacent structures.

Screening and CA-125

31. C.R. is surprised by the diagnosis and questions why the cancer was not diagnosed earlier. She has always had routine annual physical and gynecologic examinations that included the Papanicolaou (Pap) test.

The diagnosis of ovarian cancer typically does not occur early in the disease. This is because the ovaries are suspended by ligaments in a large spacious pelvic cavity where masses are not easily detectable until they become large. At the time of diagnosis, 75% of women with ovarian cancer have evidence of spread beyond the ovaries and, in 60%, the cancer has spread beyond the pelvis. Although the Pap test is the single most successful screening test used in gynecology, it is not useful for detecting ovarian cancer. The dramatic decrease in invasive cervical cancers along with a 70% reduction in mortality, however, confirms the efficacy of the Pap test as a screening tool for uterine cervical cancer.[79] The pelvic examination is the most common method of screening for ovarian cancer, but it has a low sensitivity; for every 10,000 examinations, approximately one tumor is detected.[80] The presence of a pelvic mass at physical examination is the most important sign of ovarian cancer. Abdominal ultrasounds have been investigated, but produce a high number of false–positive findings, even in high-risk populations.[78] Transvaginal ultrasonography produces clearer images than abdominal scanning and more accurately identifies intrapelvic disease. A CT of the abdominal–pelvic area may aid in the evaluation of a pelvic mass. Currently, none of these tests are recommended for screening women in the general population. The serum CA-125 level has been evaluated as a screening tool for ovarian cancer, but there is a high false-positive rate because a number of gynecologic and nongynecologic conditions can also elevate CA-125 levels. Currently, the primary role of CA-125 is to monitor disease status in patients diagnosed with ovarian cancer. Other candidate biomarkers are under investigation for the early detection of ovarian cancer.[78] Although no data indicate their value as screening tests, annual rectovaginal pelvic examinations, CA-125 levels, and transvaginal ultrasonography are often performed in high-risk women.

Chemotherapy

32. Following surgery, C.R. is advised that she should receive chemotherapy to eradicate the remaining tumor cells. Which antineoplastic drugs are effective in advanced ovarian carcinoma?

The first goal in the treatment of patients with epithelial ovarian cancer is optimal surgical cytoreduction of metastatic disease. Optimal debulking is defined as removal of all disease 1 cm or larger in diameter. The amount of residual disease after primary surgery is generally considered the most important modifiable prognostic factor that influences survival of patients with advanced disease.[81] After surgery, postoperative chemotherapy is administered to patients such as C.R. with a significant risk of recurrence. Single agents that have exhibited activity in the treatment of advanced ovarian cancer include cisplatin, paclitaxel, docetaxel, topotecan, gemcitabine, and altretamine. Several studies have shown that carboplatin and cisplatin have equivalent benefits when used with paclitaxel.[78] Currently, the standard first-line chemotherapy for epithelial ovarian cancer is the combination of carboplatin plus paclitaxel resulting in a 75% complete response rate; however, the relapse rate is 50% within 2 years.

Recurrent Disease

33. After six courses of paclitaxel and carboplatin, C.R. has no remaining evidence of ovarian cancer. Planned follow-up includes repeat serum CA-125 levels and CT scans at 3-month intervals. Six months after completing chemotherapy, the CA-125 level was increased and a CT scan of the abdomen revealed several new masses. Should C.R. receive more paclitaxel and carboplatin therapy at this time?

Although ovarian cancer is initially sensitive to chemotherapy, most women will experience a relapse of their disease. At the time of recurrence, the median survival is 2 years; therefore, the primary goal of therapy is management of symptoms. The relapse-free interval after completion of platinum-based therapy (the platinum-free interval) has been recognized as a predictor of the likelihood of subsequent response to chemotherapy. Patients with disease that recurs within 6 months after treatment are unlikely to benefit from additional therapy with the first-line agents. Therefore, it is most appropriate to treat C.R.'s cancer with a drug that has a different mechanism of action and, it is hoped, a different pattern of resistance. Several agents have shown activity in the second-line setting, including topotecan, liposomal doxorubicin, taxanes, gemcitabine, oral etoposide, altretamine, and ifosfamide. Response rates range from 16% to 30% when these agents are administered as single agents; combination therapy has not been shown to be more effective than any single agent evaluated to date.[78] A number of trials are evaluating the role of novel agents in the setting of recurrent ovarian cancer and, owing to the low response rates from currently available agents, patients should be encouraged to participate in these trials. Bevacizumab has shown promising activity, but its use has been limited by the occurrence of bowel perforation.[82] Ongoing trials will better define the occurrence of this serious adverse effect and the role of bevacizumab in recurrent ovarian cancer.

Intraperitoneal Chemotherapy

34. What is the role of intraperitoneal chemotherapy in ovarian cancer?

Ovarian carcinoma is usually limited to the peritoneal cavity. Commonly, tumor plaques are attached to the underside of the diaphragm as well as to the exterior of other organs within the abdominal cavity. Even following meticulous surgical removal of the tumor, some residual disease nearly always remains. Thus, intraperitoneal (IP) instillation of chemotherapeutic agents allows drug delivery directly to the site of the tumor and produces higher concentrations of drug at the tumor than could be attained by systemic administration. The ideal agent for IP administration is water soluble with a high molecular weight, which will slow its removal from the peritoneal cavity. Although drug delivery to the tumor is primarily by surface diffusion, agents that are then absorbed systemically from the peritoneum also reach the tumor via capillary flow. Intraperitoneal cisplatin has been the most widely studied IP drug in both the adjuvant and metastatic setting. A randomized trial in previously untreated stage III ovarian cancer with minimal disease following surgery compared cisplatin 100 mg/m^2 IV with the same IP dose in conjunction with IP cyclophosphamide 600 mg/m^2.[83] Median survival was significantly longer (41 vs. 49 months) and moderate to severe toxicities were fewer in the IP treatment group. A similar trial compared standard IV cisplatin and paclitaxel with IV carboplatin followed by IV paclitaxel and IP cisplatin; again, the IP arm was associated with significantly improved overall survival.[84] Although these studies were associated with improved outcomes, it was not considered the standard of care until an NCI clinical announcement was made based on results of a recent study.[85] In the most recent study, IV paclitaxel and cisplatin were compared with IV paclitaxel followed by IP cisplatin and IP paclitaxel in patients with stage III disease who had undergone optimal surgical cytoreduction. Although <50% of the patients in the IP arm completed therapy, similar to earlier studies, the progression-free survival and overall survival again favored IP administration.[85] Neutropenia, gastrointestinal (GI) toxicity, fatigue, pain, and metabolic events were more common in the IP group and quality of life was significantly worse. The NCI, however, now recommends a regimen containing IP cisplatin and a taxane administered IV or IV and IP for women with optimally debulked stage III ovarian cancer.[86] Ongoing studies are evaluating the optimal dose and schedule of IP chemotherapy administration.

BLADDER CANCER

Risk Factors and Clinical Presentation

35. B.B., a 65-year-old man, presented with complaints consistent with cystitis, including burning and pain on urination. Urinalysis reveals no white blood cells (WBC) or bacteria and 10 red blood cells (RBC)/high-power field (HPF). B.B. is a textile worker who smokes cigarettes but does not drink alcohol. He is referred to a urologist for cystoscopy, and the biopsy is consistent with multifocal, transitional cell carcinoma of the bladder, grade 3. What factors placed B.B. at risk for bladder cancer?

Risk factors for bladder cancer include age >60 years, male gender, occupational exposure to chemical carcinogens (aryl amines, including organic chemical, aniline dye, rubber, and paint industries), cigarette smoking, drugs (oral cyclophosphamide and phenacetin), and chronic urinary tract infections.[87] Because the whole uroepithelium is chronically exposed to carcinogens excreted in the urine, these cancers tend to recur in multiple sites even after surgical resection. B.B.'s male gender, long career as a textile worker, coupled with his significant history of cigarette smoking, place him at increased risk of bladder cancer.

The only symptom many patients experience before diagnosis is bladder irritation; in women, this may be mistaken for interstitial cystitis. Microscopic or gross hematuria is often the finding that prompts the patient to seek medical intervention. Patients with more extensive tumors may experience flank pain, constipation, or lower extremity edema.

Treatment

Intravesical Therapy

36. Further workup establishes that B.B. has superficial disease. He undergoes transurethral resection (TUR) and

fulguration (tumor is charred and then scraped with a curet). Is further therapy indicated at this time?

Approximately 70% of the newly diagnosed cases of bladder cancer will present with superficial disease. Optimal management of these cases can range from TUR alone to adjuvant intravesical (instillation directly into the urinary bladder) therapy to very aggressive approaches utilizing radical cystectomy. Although resection is highly effective in eradicating existing lesions, 30% to 85% of patients eventually develop new lesions.[88] B.B.'s tumor is grade 3 (poorly differentiated) and multifocal, which further increases his risk for recurrence. Adjuvant intravesical therapy is recommended for high-risk patients to reduce the risk of recurrence. This route places high concentrations of the drug into direct contact with the bladder mucosa and can delay or prevent progression of disease (which could require cystectomy or systemic chemotherapy). The limited systemic absorption of intravesicular therapy also minimizes the risk of serious systemic toxicities.

Drugs that have been used intravesicularly include thiotepa, doxorubicin, valrubicin, mitomycin, and bacillus Calmette-Guerin (BCG).[89] The choice of intravesical therapy is individualized; however, BCG is accepted as the standard therapeutic intervention for carcinoma inside of the bladder and for prophylaxis of tumor recurrence in superficial bladder cancer.[90] Specifically, evidence shows that patients who receive BCG for both the induction and maintenance regimen, have better outcomes than those receiving intravesical chemotherapy. A number of novel agents are currently under investigation, with considerable interest in intravesicular gemcitabine and early trials of intravesicular docetaxel.

Neoadjuvant and Adjuvant Chemotherapy

37. What role does chemotherapy play in the treatment of B.B.'s cancer?

Combining radical cystectomy with chemotherapy is an attractive approach to managing bladder cancer. Whether all patients or only high-risk patients should be treated this way and optimal timing of this approach is an ongoing debate. A small, but significant improvement is seen in survival in patients who receive neoadjuvant MVAC (methotrexate, vinblastine, doxorubicin, cisplatin).[91] The small benefit must be balanced with the potential toxicities associated with this regimen. Alternatively, adjuvant chemotherapy following cystectomy may be offered to patients at high-risk. Currently, no data confirm a survival benefit from adjuvant chemotherapy, although the available trials have had significant flaws in their design.[92] Recent meta-analyses have concluded that adjuvant therapy modestly, but significantly, improved survival over surgery alone.[93,94] An ongoing European trial will better define the impact of adjuvant chemotherapy on overall survival. Because B.B. has high-grade disease, he should receive neoadjuvant chemotherapy with MVAC.

Metastatic Disease

38. Six months after receiving neoadjuvant chemotherapy and surgery, B.B. is found to have recurrent, metastatic disease (stage IV) involving his lungs and liver. What is the incidence of disease dissemination and what type of treatment should B.B. receive?

Approximately 40% of patients with bladder cancer develop metastatic disease during their clinical course. The most common sites of disease spread are the lymph nodes, liver, lung, and bone. Follow-up histories, physical examinations, and assessments should focus on these areas. Once the disease disseminates to a distant site, the prognosis is poor and the objective of treatment is to reduce symptoms and prolong survival. The standard therapy for metastatic disease is systemic chemotherapy with multidrug regimens that contain cisplatin. The classic regimen is MVAC, but more recently the commonly used doublet of gemcitabine and cisplatin has been utilized. In chemotherapy naïve patients, the combination of gemcitabine and cisplatin was associated with a higher response rate and less toxicity, including significantly less neutropenic sepsis and grade III/IV mucositis, compared with MVAC.[95] The taxanes are active agents for bladder cancer, along with pemetrexed in combination with gemcitabine.[92] Because bladder cancer with distant metastases is considered an incurable disease, patients should be encouraged to participate in clinical trials whenever feasible. B.B.'s cancer has recurred within 6 months of treatment with MVAC; therefore, a single-agent taxane could be useful. If he responds, he could be offered treatment with the doublet of gemcitabine and cisplatin, if and when the cancer progresses.

MELANOMA

Risk Factors and Clinical Presentation

39. B.C., a 35-year-old white man, has worked for the past 12 years as a landscaper in south Florida. Two years before this recent admission he had undergone surgical resection of a stage IB malignant melanoma. What risk factors placed B.C. at an increased risk for melanoma?

Melanoma can occur in adults of all age groups and predominantly affects whites. The precise cause of melanoma is unknown; however, epidemiologic studies suggest that sunlight, especially exposure to ultraviolet (UV) rays, is the most important factor in its pathogenesis.[96,97] Individuals with light complexions, an inability to tan, blond or red hair, or blue eyes have a higher risk of melanoma than the general population. Sunburns, especially during childhood, along with sun exposure, and use of tanning beds at an early age have been associated with an increased risk of melanoma.[96,97] Finally, the total number of benign nevi on the body has been directly correlated to the risk of melanoma.[97] For B.C., constant exposure to sun is the most important risk factor for melanoma.

Screening high-risk individuals is extremely important because the initial presentation is often a melanoma lesion. Early recognition involves the ABCD evaluation of lesions (A, asymmetric; B, irregular borders; C, color variegation; D, diameter >6 mm). Commonly, these lesions are located on the back and trunk of men and the lower extremities of women. Cutaneous melanoma can arise on any surface of the skin and is perhaps the most visible of malignancies; therefore, it can be detected in asymptomatic persons. Early detection and recognition of melanoma are essential for possible cure. Occasionally, melanomas develop in noncutaneous tissues (e.g., the retina). The most critical factor in determining the prognosis following surgical removal of a melanoma is the vertical extension of the lesion into the skin and subcutaneous tissue; those that extend into the subcutaneous fat have a high rate of tumor recurrence and a grave prognosis.

Treatment

Adjuvant Therapy

40. At the time of diagnosis, B.C. underwent a wide excision of the area, but because he did not have lymphadenopathy, the regional lymph nodes were not dissected. Should B.C. receive adjuvant therapy?

A number of agents have been evaluated in the adjuvant setting in high-risk patients with cutaneous melanoma. Chemotherapy has been largely unsuccessful, and the significance of adjuvant interferon-alfa-2b treatment is difficult to evaluate because different doses and schedules were utilized. A meta-analysis of high and low dose adjuvant interferon-alfa-2b, however, showed a trend toward a reduction in the risk of melanoma recurrence and melanoma-related deaths.[98] Although no clear differences in high-dose versus low-dose regimens for responses were seen, the high-dose regimen was associated with more severe toxicity. Because of the lack of consistent benefit, the use of interferon-alfa-2b has not been widely adopted. The effectiveness of tumor-specific vaccines in the adjuvant setting is being evaluated for patients with high-risk melanoma.

Accurate staging is necessary to identify patients whose risk of recurrence is high and who may benefit from systemic adjuvant treatment. Staging involves the assessment of lymph node status at the time of surgical removal of the primary lesion. The need to understand lymph node status has led to the emergence of lymph node dissection and sentinel-lymph-node biopsy at the time of surgery. Because B.C. did not have lymph node dissection, information is insufficient to assign an accurate stage to his melanoma.

Metastatic Disease

41. B.C. now presents with complaints of enlarged, painful lymph nodes in his groin; physical examination reveals several enlarged inguinal nodes and hepatomegaly as well. A lymph node biopsy confirms recurrence of malignant melanoma and his LFTs as follows: AST, 190 IU/L (normal, 5–35 IU/L); ALT, 165 IU/L (5–45 IU/L); and bilirubin, 2.2 mg/dL (2–18 mg/dL). Is chemotherapy indicated for B.C., who has metastatic malignant melanoma?

[SI units: AST, 190 U/L; ALT, 165 U/L; bilirubin, 37.62 mmol/L]

To date, the prognosis of patients with stage IV disease is poor because the results of chemotherapy in the treatment of melanoma have been disappointing. Only two agents, dacarbazine and interleukin-2 (IL-2), are FDA approved for the treatment of metastatic melanoma. Other agents that have demonstrated modest activity include carboplatin, carmustine, temozolomide, and cisplatin. Most responses are only partial, however, and the duration of response is generally only 3 to 6 months. Over the past 30 years numerous combination chemotherapy regimens utilizing dacarbazine as the primary active agent have been used but have not consistently demonstrated differences in response or survival. No combination regimen has yet been proved to be superior to dacarbazine alone.[96]

For several reasons, melanoma has been one of the most widely studied tumors in the area of immunotherapy. Commonly, melanoma cells express surface antigens that can be targeted by specific immunotherapy (e.g., monoclonal antibodies) and these surface antigens enhance recognition by the host's own immune system. The latter is supported by the lymphocytic infiltrates commonly observed in tumor biopsies. In addition, melanoma and its normal precursor cells, melanocytes, require growth factors for proliferation. Although melanocytes require exogenous growth factors, melanoma cells (at least sometimes) produce their own. This may explain, in part, the progressive nature of malignant melanomas. The interferons, IL-2, and vaccines are biologic therapies that have been most widely studied in the treatment of melanoma. Other biologic therapies that have been added to IL-2, but have not improved response rates or durable remissions, include monoclonal antibodies, active immunotherapy by vaccination, and adoptive immunotherapy using tumor-infiltrating lymphocytes or lymphokine-activated killer (LAK) cells. Initial studies using high-dose IL-2, either alone or in combination with LAK cells, produced overall response rates of only 10% to 20%. Importantly, about 5% of patients responded completely, most of whom have maintained responses without therapy for many years. Pooled analyses of patients treated with high-dose IL-2 supported the benefit of therapy, with overall objective response rates of 16% and a 6% complete response.[99]

Several different preparations of IL-2 have been used in clinical trials. Variations in dose determination (on a per meter squared or per kilogram of body weight basis) as well as the use of different unit standards has caused dosing confusion. The World Health Organization (WHO) has defined international units (IU).[100] In the case of the commercially available aldesleukin (Proleukin, Chiron Therapeutics, Inc.), a milligram, which had previously been defined as equivalent to 3 million Cetus units, is now defined as equivalent to 18 million IU. Attention to the formulation and units is crucial to ensure the use of appropriate dosages.

Regimens using high doses of IL-2 (e.g., 600,000 IU/kg every 8 hours for 15 days) have been associated with considerable dose-related toxicities.[101] Most of these can be included in a "diffuse capillary leak syndrome" characterized by intravascular volume depletion, oliguria, and edema of all major organs resulting in multiorgan dysfunction. Once therapy is discontinued, the capillary leak and related toxicities resolve quickly. During therapy, fluid balance must be carefully and frequently evaluated and IV hydration administered cautiously. Early administration of vasopressors is usually necessary when patients receive high-dose therapy to maintain systemic perfusion and enhance urinary output. Patients also require H_2-receptor antagonists to prevent gastritis, and premedication with acetaminophen and an NSAID (e.g., indomethacin) to prevent fever and chills associated with IL-2 administration. Meperidine is usually effective in attenuating chills when they occur. Concurrent with resolution of widespread edema, desquamation and intense pruritus often are observed, which can be managed with emollients. Corticosteroids should not be given because they may attenuate the immunomodulatory effects of IL-2. Although patients receiving single-agent IL-2 do not become neutropenic, a high incidence of staphylococcal bacteremia has been observed.

Recent approaches have focused on combining chemotherapy with immunotherapy, a concept labelled "biochemotherapy." Early trials were promising; however, recent phase III studies reveal no survival benefit with biochemotherapy when compared with either chemotherapy or immunotherapy alone.[96]

Active specific immunotherapy (vaccination) uses tumor-associated antigens to induce an immune response against melanoma. Both autologous and allogeneic vaccines have been studied.[99] Therapeutic cancer vaccines, angiogenesis inhibitors, and novel cytotoxic agents are under investigation for the treatment of metastatic melanoma. Because no standard therapy exists, B.C. should be encouraged to participate in a clinical trial.

PROSTATE CANCER

Etiology and Risk Factors

42. J.D., a 65-year-old black man, was diagnosed with prostate carcinoma 18 months ago. At that time, he underwent a radical prostatectomy and was found to have stage II disease (confined to the prostate) with a Gleason score of 7. What are J.D.'s risk factors for prostate cancer?

Although adenocarcinoma of the prostate is the most common malignancy in adult males in the United States, specific risk factors (other than male gender and increasing age) have not been identified. The median age at diagnosis is 66 years and the disease is rare before the age of 40 years. Ethnicity is a well known risk factor, with the highest incidence worldwide in black men. Asian men have the lowest risk.[1] The mortality rate in black men is 2.4 times that of white men. Family history is a risk, most notably if it occurs in a first-degree relative.

The cause of prostate cancer is unknown. Regional variation in incidence worldwide suggests that environmental factors may have a role. Nationalized males have incidence rates that are intermediate between those born in the United States and those who have remained in their native country, which also suggests that environmental factors contribute. Increased risk also has been linked to high-fat diets. High levels of testosterone also have been implicated in prostate cancer development. Support for a hormonal etiology includes the hormone dependence of prostate cancer, the absence of prostate cancer in eunuchs, and the increased incidence in male populations with higher testosterone levels. An increased risk of prostate cancer in patients with benign prostatic hyperplasia has been suggested, although others have not observed this association. Conclusive evidence that widespread screening and early detection of prostate cancer improves survival is lacking. Before the advent of prostate specific antigen (PSA) screening, most prostate cancers were detected by digital rectal examination. Screening leads to earlier diagnosis and most agree that screening for prostate cancer has led to the recent declines in prostate cancer mortality. Because PSA is specific to the prostate and not specific for cancer, it is not a sensitive screening tool when used alone. Furthermore, several situations can falsely elevate PSA. Finasteride reportedly doubles the PSA, and prostate manipulation, biopsy, and the digital rectal examination increase the PSA as well. Nevertheless, the routine evaluation of PSA in men >50 years of age has become the standard of care.

Staging

43. Before surgery, J.D.'s PSA was 25 ng/mL (normal, <4.0 ng/mL). At a regular follow-up examination, his only complaint is mild backache, which he attributes to strain. Now, his PSA is 100 ng/mL and a CT scan of the pelvis shows several enlarged lymph nodes consistent with metastatic prostate cancer. Bone scan reveals blastic lesions in the lumbar region of the spine. J.D. is otherwise asymptomatic. His only other medical problems are a 20-year history of essential hypertension and evidence of early congestive heart failure. Is J.D.'s disease still considered stage II?

Following radical prostatectomy, serum PSA should be undetectable. Lifelong follow-up should occur in these patients. Stage I disease is typically found incidentally when prostate tissue is removed for other reasons, such as benign prostatic hypertrophy. The cells closely resemble normal cells and the gland feels normal to the examining finger. In stage II, which was J.D.'s initial diagnosis, more of the prostate is involved and a lump can be felt within the gland. In stage III, the tumor has spread through the prostatic capsule and the lump can be felt on the surface of the gland. In stage IV disease, the tumor has invaded nearby structures, or has spread to lymph nodes or other organs. Grading is based on cellular content and tissue architecture from biopsies (Gleason), which provides an estimate of the destructive potential and ultimate prognosis of the disease. From the CT scan, J.D. now has obvious spread to the pelvic lymph nodes and bone, indicating stage IV disease. The stage of the disease determines the most appropriate therapy.

Treatment

44. Does J.D.'s disease require therapy at this time? Is there a role for intermittent androgen blockade?

J.D. has advanced disease and is experiencing symptoms that could progress, causing him considerable pain and loss of neurologic function if left untreated. Hormonal manipulation that reduces testosterone to levels consistent with castration is the mainstay of pharmacotherapy for advanced symptomatic prostate cancer. Testosterone deprivation is effective against prostate cancer cells because the growth of both normal and malignant prostate tissue depends on it. Multiple hormonal manipulations can be employed alone or in combination, including (a) ablation of androgen sources, (b) inhibition of testosterone production, and (c) interference of testosterone binding at its receptor site.

Testosterone is produced by the testicles in response to pituitary follicle-stimulating hormone (FSH) and luteinizing hormone (LH) and also by metabolic conversion of androgens produced by the adrenal glands. Testosterone is converted by α-reductase enzymes to dihydrotestosterone, the major intracellular androgen, which then binds to a specific cytoplasmic receptor protein. The receptor–dihydrotestosterone complex is then translocated into the prostatic nucleus where it binds to and activates DNA to induce the production of mRNA. Messenger RNA then codes for proteins essential for the metabolic functions of the prostate cells, including prostate cancer cells.

Therapeutic options for J.D. at this time include (a) orchiectomy; (b) LHRH agonists (e.g., leuprolide, goserelin), which decrease FSH and LH synthesis and production, which in turn decrease testosterone production; (c) a nonsteroidal antiandrogen (e.g., flutamide, bicalutamide, nilutamide), which inhibits dihydrotestosterone binding to its receptor; or (d) combined androgen blockade, using both an LHRH agonist and an antiandrogen.[102]

Bilateral Orchiectomy

Bilateral orchiectomy is considered by many to be the therapy of choice because it permanently removes the primary source of testosterone production (95%) with few surgical complications.[102] Orchiectomy does cause impotence (as do all forms of testosterone ablation) and patients may suffer from hot flashes; however, the need for regular long-term administration of drugs that have potential side effects is avoided.[103] Nevertheless, some patients find this procedure unacceptable.

LHRH Agonists

Medical castration with an LHRH agonist, or bilateral orchiectomy, is recommended as an initial treatment for metastatic prostate cancer.[102] Leuprolide (Lupron) and goserelin (Zoladex) are LHRH agonists. The efficacy of leuprolide and goserelin appears to be similar, although large-scale comparative trials have not been completed. As with LHRH itself, these drugs stimulate the release of FSH and LH by the pituitary, which increases the production of testosterone. Thus, when therapy is initiated, an initial testosterone surge occurs (during the first 10–14 days), which can transiently worsen symptoms such as pain (i.e., flare reactions). Some clinicians choose to initiate short-term antiandrogen therapy before or together with the LHRH agonist and to continue the antiandrogen for about a month. This method is intended to reduce the possibility for the flare reaction. Over several weeks, the LHRH receptors in the pituitary are downregulated by the continuous onslaught of synthetic LHRH, followed by a decline in the release of LH. Ultimately, the levels of FSH, LH, and testosterone become profoundly suppressed.

Long-term use of LHRH agonists is associated with anemia, fatigue, and osteoporosis. Therapy is continued until the disease progresses (i.e., new metastatic sites). Many experts advocate continuing androgen deprivation with these agents for the duration of the patient's life, even after disease progression and the addition of chemotherapy.

Antiandrogens

Monotherapy with antiandrogens such as flutamide, bicalutamide, and nilutamide has been evaluated in previously untreated patients in a small number of trials.[104] The most studied antiandrogen for monotherapy in the metastatic setting is bicalutamide.[104] Although monotherapy with an antiandrogen may be discussed as an alternative, it should not be offered.[102] When compared with castration, bicalutamide was associated with a decreased time to treatment failure, time to objective progression, and increased risk for death, but no statistical difference in survival.[105] The most common antiandrogen-related adverse effects include gynecomastia, hot flashes, GI disturbances, breast tenderness, and liver function abnormalities. Because antiandrogens do not directly reduce testosterone levels, patients often can maintain sexual potency.

Combined Hormonal Blockade

The rationale for combination hormonal therapy is to interfere with multiple hormonal pathways to completely eliminate androgen action. In clinical trials, combination hormonal therapy, sometimes also referred to as *maximal androgen deprivation* or *total androgen blockade*, has been used. The combination of LHRH agonists or orchiectomy with antiandrogens is the most extensively studied combined androgen deprivation approach. Combined hormonal blockade with conventional medical or surgical castration and the addition of a nonsteroidal antiandrogen improves overall survival but increases adverse effects.[102] Combined androgen blockade (e.g., LHRH agonist or orchiectomy plus nonsteroidal antiandrogen) would be an appropriate choice given J.D.'s minimal disease and good performance status.

Intermittent Androgen Blockade

The efficacy of intermittent versus total continuous complete androgen blockade in patients who have never received pharmacologic treatment whose prostate cancer has relapsed has been evaluated in a few studies. This approach involves hormonal therapy (LHRH agonists) for 6 to 9 months until the PSA level is <4 ng/mL followed by a break in therapy until the PSA reaches a predetermined level, such as 10 ng/mL or half of the PSA level when the treatment was initiated.[106] The value of such an approach is to allow periods during which testosterone production resumes and adverse effects are abated. Unknown are the effects on prostate cancer when testosterone levels are allowed to rebound. This approach remains investigational.

Immediate versus Delayed Androgen Ablation

Deferring androgen ablation therapy with active surveillance may be an option in men who have an increasing PSA level, who are asymptomatic or have no clinical or radiographic evidence of metastatic disease after local therapy.[106] Early initiation of androgen ablation for an increasing PSA level only exposes patients to risks of adverse events and provides only temporary benefit. Early therapy is associated with higher costs and greater frequency of treatment-related adverse effects, whereas deferred treatment may increase the risk for the development of hormone independence in the tumor. Patients who opt for active surveillance require close follow-up and ongoing discussions regarding the risks and benefits of deferred therapy. Because J.D. has evidence of metastatic disease, he requires immediate therapy.

Monitoring Therapy

45. J.D. started intramuscular (IM) leuprolide 22.5 mg every 3 months and flutamide 250 mg three times daily (TID). How should his response to therapy be monitored?

Blastic bone lesions heal slowly and have been shown to persist even when biopsy documents absence of disease. Therefore, a repeat bone scan would not be a useful indicator of response; however, it may be used to rule out new lesions or progressive disease. If bony lesions improve, it may take up to

6 months for resolution on the bone scan because of the slow rate of bone remodeling in elderly men.

Measurement of PSA is the most useful tool to follow response to therapy. Because the serum half-life of PSA is only 2 to 4 days, serial measurements provide a rapid indication of tumor status. It also is less expensive and more sensitive than imaging techniques (e.g., CT scans, bone scans). Control of symptoms, such as pain, and maintenance of quality of life are important outcome indicators in this disease and should be monitored frequently.

Androgen-Independent Disease

46. Following initiation of treatment, J.D.'s PSA level fell to 8 ng/mL and remained stable for the next 18 months. During this time, he had no clinical evidence of disease progression. His most recent clinic visit, however, revealed an increase in his PSA level to 75 ng/mL and a repeat bone scan and pelvic CT showed some disease progression. Is a change in therapy warranted at this time?

Various second-line hormonal therapies have been studied. If J.D. had been receiving an LHRH agonist alone, a testosterone level could be checked to ensure castrate levels have been achieved. If castrate testosterone levels (<20 ng/dL) are not achieved, then an orchiectomy or the addition of an antiandrogen is an option.[107] Because J.D. was receiving combined androgen blockade, a trial of antiandrogen withdrawal should be initiated. This approach produces symptomatic improvement and objective signs of tumor regression or a decrease in PSA in up to 35% of patients.[108] This is likely because of a mutation in the androgen receptor and a change in the selectivity or activation of the receptor that allows antagonists to act as agonists. Therefore, J.D.'s flutamide should be discontinued. The addition of an aromatase inhibitor, such as aminoglutethimide, or ketoconazole, is also a reasonable choice. Because J.D. is not experiencing progressive symptoms at this time, the benefits of additional therapy with either aminoglutethimide or ketoconazole probably do not outweigh the potential risks and complications of treatment and its associated costs.

Chemotherapy

47. J.D.'s metastatic disease continues to progress. Would cytotoxic chemotherapy be beneficial at this time?

Almost all patients with metastatic prostate cancer initially treated with androgen deprivation will develop progressive disease within 2 to 3 years. The term *androgen independent prostate cancer* describes the situation in which a patient has a documented castrate testosterone level and progressive disease. These patients typically have a median survival of 6 months.

Chemotherapy is now a standard for men with androgen-independent disease who have metastatic disease. Mitoxantrone with prednisone was the standard of care for a number of years, with approval based on clinically meaningful benefits, such as PSA reduction, pain relief, and a delay in bone scan evidence of disease progression.[106] Docetaxel is now the standard of care for the management of cases of metastatic androgen-independent prostate cancer after a small, but significant, survival benefit was observed in two separate trials when compared with the combination of mitoxantrone and prednisone.[109,110] Therefore, J.D. should receive single agent docetaxel for the management of his disease.

TESTICULAR CANCER

Clinical Presentation

48. M.W., a 26-year-old man, noted painless swelling of his left testicle approximately 2 or 3 weeks before seeing his family physician. Physical examination reveals an indurated mass located in the lower pole of the left testicle. Epididymitis is ruled out because of the location. Laboratory evaluation reveals the following: α-fetoprotein (AFP) is 300 ng/mL (normal, <40), β-human chorionic gonadotropin (β-hCG) (<5 IU/L) is negative, and LDH is 43 U/L. He is referred to a urologist who performs a radical inguinal orchiectomy and a nerve-sparing retroperitoneal lymph node dissection. M.W. has two positive nodes and the pathology report reveals embryonal carcinoma. Following orchiectomy, the AFP declines exponentially; a metastatic workup, including chest radiograph and CT scan of the abdomen and pelvis, reveals no evidence of disease. Is this a typical presentation of testicular cancer?

[SI units: AFP, 300, respectively (normal, <40); LDH, 43 U/L]

Testicular cancer is the most common malignancy in men between ages 15 and 35 years. M.W.'s presentation is typical in that the cancer presents as a painless swelling in one gonad. The cause of testicular cancer is unknown, but approximately 10% of patients have a history of cryptorchidism.[111] Other possible risk factors include race (the incidence is much lower among black male patients) and family history.[112]

Histologic Classification

49. Does histologic classification provide a clinical basis for therapeutic decisions?

Germinal neoplasms are divided into seminomas and various other types known collectively as nonseminomatous germ cell tumors (Table 91-6). Seminomas arise from malignant transformations of spermatocytes, whereas nonseminomas arise from transformation of germ cells of placental origin. Although treatment of advanced disease is similar, seminoma is exquisitely sensitive to radiation and, therefore, early stages of the disease are more frequently treated with radiotherapy.[112]

Table 91-6 Histologic Classification of Primary Tumors of the Testes

Germinal Neoplasms
Seminoma
Embryonal carcinoma
Teratoma
Choriocarcinoma
Yolk sac tumor
Nongerminal Neoplasms
Specialized gonadal stromal neoplasms (e.g., Leydig cell tumor)
Gonadoblastoma
Miscellaneous (e.g., adenocarcinoma, carcinoid, mesenchymal)

Determining the most appropriate therapy depends on both the histology and stage of the disease. Because M.W. has a nonseminoma (i.e., embryonal carcinoma), initial radiation is not indicated.

Staging

50. What is the stage of M.W.'s disease?

Stage I disease is limited to the testes; stage II disease involves the testes and lymph nodes; and stage III disease includes all metastatic tumors. Following orchiectomy, a metastatic workup was completed to rule out spread of the disease. Such a workup should include chest radiograph, CT evaluation of retroperitoneal lymph nodes, and assessment of decline in the tumor markers following orchiectomy. Because M.W. has two positive lymph nodes, his disease is classified as stage II.

Treatment

Adjuvant Chemotherapy

51. M.W. is diagnosed with stage II disease. Following surgery, the AFP declined exponentially. Is adjuvant chemotherapy indicated at this time?

Approximately 30% of patients such as M.W. (less than six positive nodes) whose disease is apparently completely resected (AFP declined following lymph node dissection) ultimately experience relapse, and adjuvant chemotherapy (two cycles of a platinum-based regimen) dramatically reduces this risk.[113] If patients do not receive adjuvant chemotherapy and are monitored closely for early detection of relapse, the chance of cure following aggressive induction of chemotherapy remains high (>80%).[113]

Metastatic Disease

52. The decision is that M.W. will not receive adjuvant therapy at this time. Instead, he will be followed by a monthly history, physical examination, and AFP for the first year, every 2 months during the second year, and every 6 months thereafter. After 4 months, M.W. is lost to follow-up. He returns to his urologist 1 year later with complaints of abdominal discomfort and shortness of breath. A chest radiograph reveals multiple nodules in the lung, and an abdominal CT reveals a 6- to 10-cm mass. His AFP is 360 ng/mL and the β-hCG is 290 ng/mL. Is chemotherapy indicated at this time?

[SI unit: AFP, 360 mg/L]

M.W. now has metastatic testicular cancer and should receive systemic chemotherapy. For many years the combinations of either (a) cisplatin, vinblastine, and bleomycin or (b) cisplatin, etoposide, and bleomycin have produced responses in almost all men and complete responses in 60% to 80% of patients.[114–116] A randomized trial demonstrated a higher long-term survival rate for patients who had received the regimen containing etoposide in a subset of patients at high risk; therefore, this combination is most widely used today.[116]

Before initiating chemotherapy, pulmonary function tests, an audiogram, and a 24-hour urinary creatinine clearance are obtained. M.W. is hydrated with IV D5/0.45% sodium chloride and chemotherapy is initiated with cisplatin 20 mg/m^2/day for 5 days; etoposide 100 mg/m^2 on days 1 to 5; and bleomycin 30 units on days 2, 9, and 16. Courses are repeated every 21 days. Because M.W. disease places him at high risk (i.e., nonseminomatous, extragonadal disease) he should receive a minimum of four courses of chemotherapy.

Monitoring Therapy

53. How should M.W. be monitored for therapeutic and toxic responses to chemotherapy?

Response to chemotherapy would be demonstrated by a reduction in the size of the abdominal mass, a reduction in the size and number of pulmonary nodules, and a steady decrease in the AFP and β-hCG without any other evidence of disease progression. CT scans, chest radiographs, and tumor markers are typically re-evaluated after every second course of therapy.

The most significant toxicities associated with this regimen include myelosuppression and the nephrotoxicity and neurotoxicity associated with cisplatin. A CBC with differential and platelet count should be performed once weekly until the myelosuppression has resolved and just before the next course. Serum creatinine, blood urea nitrogen (BUN), and electrolytes (including potassium and magnesium) should be monitored daily during chemotherapy and weekly thereafter. If evidence of toxicity appears, more intense monitoring may be recommended. Weekly symptom analysis and physical examination should include assessment for cisplatin neurotoxicity and other chemotherapy-associated toxicities. To assess bleomycin lung toxicity, baseline pulmonary function tests should be performed before the first course and after every second or third course.

54. M.W.'s AFP and β-hCG drop dramatically after his first course of chemotherapy and less so after his second course; however, they appear to plateau at an AFP of 170 ng/mL and β-hCG of 200 ng/mL after the third course. No evidence is found of tumor on the abdominal CT scan or chest radiograph. Should the fourth and fifth cycles of chemotherapy be administered?

[SI unit: AFP, 170 mg/L]

The plateau of the tumor markers confirms that M.W.'s disease is not continuing to regress after chemotherapy. First-line, cisplatin-based combination chemotherapy cures 70% of patients with disseminated germ cell tumors.[111] The remaining 30% of patients are candidates for salvage chemotherapy at the time of relapse or disease progression. Additional cycles of chemotherapy with the same regimen are unlikely to produce further tumor regression and normalization of the tumor markers. Because he had an initial good response to cisplatin therapy, it is reasonable to continue cisplatin in this circumstance. M.W. could receive salvage chemotherapy with cisplatin 20 mg/m^2/day for 5 days, vinblastine 0.11 mg/kg on days 1 and 2, and ifosfamide 1.2 g/m^2/day for 5 days. More recently, paclitaxel has replaced the vinblastine in this regimen.[117] As a single agent, ifosfamide produces responses in approximately 22% of patients with refractory germ cell tumors.[118] In patients such as M.W., the combination of ifosfamide with cisplatin and vinblastine has produced a 36% complete response rate with a median duration of remission of 34 months. Mesna should be administered concurrently with ifosfamide to prevent hemorrhagic cystitis.

The response and long-term survival rates reported with both first-line and salvage chemotherapy for testicular cancer are considerably higher than for most solid tumors. Because of the likelihood of long-term survival, efforts are now focused on minimizing the long-term sequelae of chemotherapy (e.g., secondary malignancies, sterility).

Alternatively, at the time it was recognized that M.W.'s AFP and β-hCG plateaued, high-dose chemotherapy and autologous stem cell support could have been considered. Testicular cancer is potentially curable by means of high-dose chemotherapy plus hematopoietic stem-cell rescue, even in the third-line setting.[119]

PEDIATRIC SOLID TUMORS

Statistics

In the United States, more children between 1 and 14 years of age die of cancer than any other disease.[120] Yet, many common pediatric cancers that had low cure rates before the advent of chemotherapy now have 5-year survivals >70%. Acute leukemias are the most common malignancies of childhood (Table 91-7), whereas the solid tumors discussed in this chapter each represent 2.7% to 6.5% of all childhood malignancies.[120] Many common pediatric solid tumors are uncommon in adults. Likewise, many tumors common in adults occur infrequently in children. In general, sarcomas and embryonal tumors are common in children, whereas carcinomas predominate in adults.

Small Round Cell Tumors

Several pediatric malignancies present as small round cell tumors, making morphologic diagnosis by traditional light microscopy more difficult. The most challenging diagnostic problems are the less typical forms of these diseases. The list commonly includes peripheral primitive neuroectodermal tumors, extraosseous Ewing's sarcoma, extranodal lymphoma,

Table 91-7 Relative Incidence of Malignancies in Children 0 to 14 Years of Age

Malignancy	*Relative Incidence (%)*
Acute lymphoblastic leukemia	25.7
Central nervous system	24.8
Neuroblastoma	6.5
Non-Hodgkin's lymphoma	5.6
Wilms' tumor	4.7
Hodgkin's lymphoma	3.5
Acute myeloid leukemia	5.2
Rhabdomyosarcoma	3.5
Retinoblastoma	2.7
Osteosarcoma	2.7
Ewing's sarcoma	1.4
Other histologic types	13.7

Adapted from reference 120, with permission.

rhabdomyosarcoma, metastatic neuroblastoma, and some bone sarcomas.[121] Problems involved with diagnosing these tumors have stimulated the development of newer techniques aimed at detecting tumor-specific antigens or chromosomal aberrations. This information may prove useful in identifying prognostic subgroups as well as tumor types in children and adults with cancer. Identification of the t(11;22) chromosomal translocation in both peripheral primitive neuroectodermal tumors and Ewing's sarcomas has resulted in the classification of both into the Ewing's sarcoma family of tumors.[122]

Genetics

Similar to adult cancers, the association of many pediatric cancers with chromosomal aberrations or genetic defects is well confirmed. Examples include the association of Wilms' tumor with congenital malformations, acute lymphoblastic leukemia with Down syndrome, and the association of some pediatric cancers with loss of the p53 or retinoblastoma tumor suppressor genes[121,123].

Carcinogens

The role of carcinogens in pediatric cancer is probably less prominent than in adults because of the long latency periods required. Carcinogens, however, are implicated in the etiology of some childhood cancers.[124] Postnatal exposure to ionizing radiation is associated with acute leukemias, chronic myelogenous leukemia, and solid tumors, such as brain, thyroid, bone, and other sarcomas.[124] Treatment of pediatric malignancies with alkylators is associated with an increased risk of leukemias.[125] Etoposide and teniposide are associated with an increased risk of secondary acute myelogenous leukemia.[126] Treatment of childhood acute lymphoblastic leukemia, especially in those <5 years of age who received irradiation, results in an increased risk of CNS neoplasms, leukemia, lymphoma, and other neoplasms later in life.[127] The only well-documented prenatal carcinogen is diethylstilbestrol (DES), which is associated with an increased risk of vaginal or cervical cancer in offspring.[128]

Patient Age

Patient age can be a factor in pediatric cancers and their treatment. Neuroblastoma is the most common malignancy in infants; however, an infant's prognosis is typically better than a child's, which is attributed to the biology of the disease in this age group.[129] In contrast, infants with acute lymphoblastic leukemia tend to have a worse prognosis than older children.[130] The biology and location of rhabdomyosarcoma are often different in younger and older children, with younger children having the better overall survival.[131]

Similarly, age may be a consideration with regard to the toxicity of treatments. Children may have increased susceptibility to toxicity from irradiation relative to adults. Normal organ development may be disrupted; the skeletal system and, in children <4 years of age, the brain are particularly susceptible.[124,129] Prepubertal girls may have a decreased risk of fertility problems from chemotherapy, and conversely, children appear to have a greater risk for anthracycline cardiovascular toxicity than adults.[132]

Multi-Institutional Research Groups

With the exception of a few pediatric oncology centers, most treatment centers do not have sufficient patients with specific diagnoses to scientifically establish the efficacy of therapeutic regimens within a reasonable time frame. Thus, most centers join the Children's Oncology Group (COG), the largest pediatric multi-institutional research group in the United States, Canada, Australia, and New Zealand. Through this mechanism, clinical trials often can be finished in 3 to 4 years, allowing for more rapid progress in the treatment of pediatric cancers. With the number of childhood cancer survivors increasing, research is focusing on reducing the long-term risks and complications of treatment modalities. It is important to determine which patients are at greatest risk from their cancer and to stratify treatments such that the minimal treatment needed to produce cure is given when the prognoses are good, and maximal treatment is given when the potential benefits outweigh the risks. Progress is already being made in this direction, and the future holds promise, especially with rapid gains in our understanding of the biology of cancers.

NEUROBLASTOMA

Neuroblastoma develops in immature cells of sympathetic nervous system origin.[133] It is the most common extracranial tumor of childhood, representing 6.5% of all childhood cancers. The median age at diagnosis is 19 months; 36% occur in children <1 year of age, and 89% before 5 years of age.[133] Of neuroblastomas, 65% are abdominal (half of these adrenal) and 20% are thoracic.[133] Neuroblastoma often presents as a fixed, hard, abdominal mass noted on physical examination by the family or physician without any other signs or symptoms, although other findings may be present depending on the location of the primary tumor and metastases. For example, GI fullness, discomfort, or dysfunction can occur. Other less common but characteristic signs include proptosis with periorbital ecchymoses, increased-renin hypertension, secretory diarrhea with increased vasoactive intestinal peptide, respiratory distress, nerve root compression, opsomyoclonus, and unilateral ptosis.[134] The most common sites of metastases are the bone marrow, bone, liver, and skin.[133]

The catecholamine metabolites vanillylmandelic acid (VMA) and homovanillic acid (HVA) are elevated in the urine of 90% of patients with neuroblastoma.[135] Because infants have a better prognosis than older children with neuroblastoma, efforts have been made to screen infants using urinary concentrations of VMA and HVA.[136,137] To date, these efforts have resulted in the diagnosis of more infants with good-risk disease, but have not reduced the number of older children diagnosed with poor-risk disease.

A simplified description of the international staging system is shown in Table 91-8. Twenty percent of infants (<1 yr), and 59% of children have stage IV disease at the time of diagnosis. A large number of prognostic factors have been identified and are discussed elsewhere.[133,138] Patients are stratified for treatment based on age, stage, *N*-myc amplification, histology, and diploidy. The COG guidelines divide patients into three risk levels (Table 91-9).[138] Three-year, DFS for patients at high risk is approximately 30% and for those at low risk it is 90%. Infants have better outcomes for the same stage of disease and stage IVS has a significant incidence of spontaneous regression or regression with minimal treatment.[134,139]

In current U.S. clinical trials, patients with low-risk disease are typically treated with surgery. Progression or recurrence may be treated with surgery again, unless disease is unresectable, in which case chemotherapy is used. Two to four courses of chemotherapy may be used with initial surgery if organ or life-threatening symptoms are present. Intermediate-risk disease is treated with surgery and four or eight courses of chemotherapy (Table 91-10) for favorable or unfavorable histology disease.[139] Chemotherapy for patients with low- or intermediate-risk disease avoids cisplatin to reduce nephrotoxicity and ototoxicity, limits the total doxorubicin dose to avoid cardiac toxicity, limits the total etoposide dose to reduce the risk of secondary acute myelogenous leukemia, and avoids ifosfamide to eliminate Fanconi renal syndrome. Radiation therapy is used only for poor responders.

Table 91-8 International Neuroblastoma Staging System (Abbreviated)

Stage I	Local tumor with complete gross excision
Stage IIA	Unilateral localized tumor with incomplete gross excision
Stage IIB	Unilateral localized tumor, complete or incomplete excision, with ipsilateral nonadherent lymph node spread
Stage III	Involves both sides of the midline
Stage IV	Distant lymph node or organ involvement
Stage IVS	Infants <1 yr of age with localized primary tumor (stage I or II) with dissemination limited to liver, skin, or <10% of bone marrow

Adapted from reference 138, with permission.

Table 91-9 Children's Oncology Group Neuroblastoma Risk Groups

Low Risk
- All stage 1 patients
- Patients >1 year of age with stages IIA or IIB, and *N*-myc not amplified, or amplified but with favorable histology
- Infants <1 year of age with stages IIA, IIB, or IVS with *N*-myc not amplified, favorable histology and hyperdiploidy

Intermediate Risk
- Patients >1 year of age at diagnosis with stage III, *N*-myc not amplified, and favorable histology
- Infants with stages IVS and *N*-myc not amplified, and either diploidy or unfavorable histology
- Infants with stage III or IV and *N*-myc not amplified

High Risk
- Infants with stage III, or stage IV <18 months of age, and *N*-myc amplified
- Patients >1 year of age with stage IIA or IIB, *N*-myc amplified, and unfavorable histology
- Patients >18 months of age with stage IV, or >1 year of age with stage III and *N*-myc amplified, or stage III and *N*-myc not amplified but unfavorable histology

Adapted from reference 138, with permission.

Table 91-10 Typical Cycles of Chemotherapy Used in U.S. Intergroup Low- and Intermediate-Risk Neuroblastoma[a]

Carboplatin, etoposide
Carboplatin, cyclophosphamide, doxorubicin
Cyclophosphamide, etoposide
Carboplatin, doxorubicin, etoposide
Cyclophosphamide, etoposide
Carboplatin, cyclophosphamide, doxorubicin
Carboplatin, etoposide
Cyclophosphamide, doxorubicin

[a] Each line represents a single course of therapy. Generally the first four cycles are used in patients at intermediate risk with favorable histology disease, and all eight for patients with unfavorable histology. Patients at low risk whose disease is potentially organ- or life-threatening may receive the first two to four cycles of these drugs plus their surgery, rather than surgery alone.

Therapy for high-risk disease generally involves a first surgery for biopsy, aggressive chemotherapy (Table 91-11), second-look surgery for residual tumor resection, either additional aggressive chemotherapy or high-dose chemotherapy with autologous progenitor cell rescue, and then radiation to the tumor bed.[138] An alternative regimen of chemotherapy with equivalent short-term results would be four courses of cyclophosphamide, doxorubicin, and vincristine with two courses of cisplatin and etoposide, followed by the transplant.[140] High-dose chemotherapy with progenitor cell rescue has raised 2-year, disease progression-free survival to 49% from historic values of 10% to 20%; however, relapses can occur later, with 7-year disease progression-free survival of only 26%.[141] Evidence suggests that survival can be improved (46% vs. 29% 3-year postchemotherapy disease-free survival) for patients with higher-risk disease if standard-dose or high-dose chemotherapy is followed by six cycles of isotretinoin 80 mg/m^2 given orally twice daily for 14 days of each 28-day cycle.[142] Typical conditioning regimens preceding progenitor cell rescue include carboplatin and etoposide with either cyclophosphamide or melphalan, or thiotepa and cyclophosphamide. Total body irradiation may also be used.

Table 91-11 Typical Cycles of Chemotherapy Used in U.S. Intergroup Trials for High-Risk Neuroblastoma[a]

Cisplatin, etoposide
Vincristine, doxorubicin, cyclophosphamide
Ifosfamide, etoposide
Carboplatin, etoposide
Cisplatin, etoposide
Ifosfamide, etoposide
Vincristine, doxorubicin, cyclophosphamide
Cisplatin, etoposide
Vincristine, doxorubicin, cyclophosphamide
Carboplatin, etoposide

[a] The second five cycles may be skipped if the patient is ready to proceed to high-dose chemotherapy with progenitor cell rescue after the first five combinations. Patients who are not candidates for autologous progenitor cell rescue receive all ten cycles of chemotherapy. Primary tumor removal or debulking is performed before progenitor cell rescue. Radiation to the site of the primary tumor occurs after all chemotherapy and progenitor cell rescue. Patients who are in complete response after this therapy will receive six cycles of isotretinoin (14 of every 28 days).

Clinical Presentation and Diagnosis

55. H.K. is a 2-year-old girl with a 3-month history of constipation and progressive abdominal distention. She has a decreased appetite, 1-week history of vomiting, and is pale and tired. She has a large retroperitoneal mass and multiple bilateral enlarged inguinal lymph nodes. Her hemoglobin is 5.1 g/dL (normal, 11–14 g/dL); the WBC count, differential, and platelets are within normal limits. Serum sodium, potassium, chloride, creatinine, and glucose are within normal limits. LDH is 6,144 U/L (normal, 322–644 U/L), and albumin is 2.3 g/dL (normal, 3.5–5.0 g/dL). Urine HVA is 570 g/mg creatinine (normal, <26 g/mg); VMA, 31 g/mg creatinine (normal, <11 g/mg). Biopsies of the abdominal mass and bone marrow are positive for neuroblastoma. The lymph nodes are negative for neuroblastoma. Scans are negative for other sites of disease. Which of these signs, symptoms, and laboratory results are consistent with a diagnosis of neuroblastoma?

[SI units: hemoglobin (Hgb), 51 g/L (normal, 110–140); LDH, 6,144 U/L (normal, 322–644)]

Virtually all of H.K.'s findings are consistent with neuroblastoma. The low hemoglobin and albumin and high LDH, however, are not specific for this cancer. In addition to the biopsy, the elevated urine VMA and HVA (catecholamine metabolites) are most helpful in confirming the diagnosis of neuroblastoma. Neuroblastomas can contain malignant (neuroblastoma) and benign (ganglioneuroma) cells within the same tumor, which is referred to as *ganglioneuroblastoma*.[133] In H.K., biopsies of the bone marrow, lymph nodes, and primary tumor are necessary to demonstrate the presence or absence of neuroblastoma at more than one site for staging purposes.

Treatment

56. What stage of disease does H.K. have? What treatment will she receive?

H.K.'s abdominal disease with distant bone marrow involvement indicates stage IV disease. Considering her age and disease stage, H.K. has a high risk of dying from her disease. Therefore, she is started on chemotherapy consisting of cisplatin (40 mg/m^2/day on days 1 through 5) and etoposide (100 mg/m^2/dose every 12 hours on days 1 through 3). Subsequent courses will contain vincristine, cyclophosphamide, and doxorubicin; ifosfamide and etoposide; carboplatin and etoposide; and a repeat of the cisplatin and etoposide.

57. H.K. is 81.5 cm tall, weighs 11.65 kg, and has a body surface area of 0.5 m^2. She starts cisplatin and etoposide with hydration fluids of 5% dextrose with 0.45% sodium chloride at 62.5 mL/hour. Urine output is 4 mL/kg/hour. How does monitoring of H.K.'s chemotherapy differ from that of an adult?

Monitoring Vital Signs for Etoposide

Although prevention and monitoring of toxicities from chemotherapy agents in children follow the same basic rules as in adults, there are some differences. When monitoring vital signs for hypotensive reactions to etoposide, normal blood pressure will be lower (90th percentile 104/60 mmHg for a 2-year-old girl) and the pulse higher (mean, 119 beats/minute for a 2-year-old) than in adults.[143] It is important to have baseline vital signs so that hypotension or tachycardia will be recognized.

Monitoring Hydration for Cisplatin

In adults receiving cisplatin, hydration is often standardized with 1 to 2 L of IV fluids given before the drug, 1 to 2 L with the drug, and then continuous hydration for at least 24 hours after the dose.[144] In children, hydration volumes should be calculated based on the child's size. To decrease the risk of cisplatin nephrotoxicity, most pediatric protocols recommend IV fluids at twice maintenance rates to maintain urine outputs of at least 2 mL/kg/hour. The COG calculates maintenance fluids as 1,500 mL/m^2/24 hours, so H.K. should receive 3,000 mL/0.5 m^2 = 1,500 mL over 24 hours (62.5 mL/hour). H.K.'s measured urine output is 4 mL/kg/hour, which should be adequate to prevent nephrotoxicity. Weight should also be monitored throughout cisplatin administration to assure fluid balance. Acute weight gain may require diuretics to prevent overhydration, and weight loss may indicate dehydration with impending reduction of urine output that could lead to acute nephrotoxicity. Increased IV fluids would help prevent the latter.

Adjustment of Creatinine Clearance to Adult Size

58. H.K.'s measured creatinine clearance (ClCr) is 39 mL/minute. Should her cisplatin be withheld or the dose adjusted because of low creatinine clearance?

[SI unit: ClCr, 0.65 mL/second]

Cisplatin is either not administered or administered at a reduced dosage when the creatinine clearance is <50 to 60 mL/minute/1.73 m^2.[145] Although H.K.'s creatinine clearance of 39 mL/minute appears to be low, it is not relative to the patient's size (i.e., 39 mL/minute/0.5 m^2). Guidelines for dosing drugs cleared by glomerular filtration are based on creatinine clearance for normal adult body size, 1.73 m^2. Therefore, it is important to correct H.K.'s creatinine clearance to adult body size.[146] Multiplying by 1.73/0.5, her creatinine clearance is 135 mL/minute/1.73 m^2, so this is not a reason to withhold cisplatin. One precaution is that the accuracy of serum creatinine and creatinine clearance in assessing renal function during cisplatin therapy in children has been questioned.[147]

Partial Response

59. H.K. obtains a partial response to the aforementioned initial chemotherapy regimen with reduction of urine VMA and HVA concentrations and a 50% decrease in the size of the primary tumor in the abdomen. Second-look surgery is performed to debulk the tumor, and pathology results indicate that the residual tumor contains 95% mature (benign) ganglioneuroma cells, but neuroblastoma cells are still present. What further treatment has the most potential benefit for H.K.?

Stem Cell Transplant

The best chance for prolonged DFS for H.K. is dose-intensive chemotherapy combined with autologous peripheral blood progenitor cell rescue. Although improvement in long-term DFS has not been shown in all trials, the 2- to 3-year DFS is better with intensive chemotherapy followed by autologous progenitor cell rescue.[133,138,140–142] The plan for H.K. is to proceed to high-dose chemotherapy with an autologous progenitor cell rescue. If a complete response is achieved, she would then receive 6 months of isotretinoin (cis-retinoic acid) therapy following cell rescue.

Treatments Based on Disease Biology

With rapid advances in neuroblastoma biology being made, future alternatives may include biologic treatments. One agent in clinical trials is iodine-131-metaiodobenzylguanidine (I-MIBG), a compound that delivers radiation directly to catecholamine-secreting cells such as neuroblastoma. Pilot studies have used I-MIBG as part of the conditioning regimen before progenitor cell rescue in patients with neuroblastoma.[148] A published trial has demonstrated improved survival for high-risk patients in complete response who are postchemotherapy and receive isotretinoin.[142]

WILMS' TUMOR

Wilms' tumor, also known as nephroblastoma, is a kidney tumor composed of various kidney cell types at different stages of maturation.[149] Approximately 5% of all childhood cancers are Wilms' tumor, making it the most common intra-abdominal tumor of childhood.[120] The peak incidence occurs at 3 years of age.[150] Wilms' tumor frequently presents as an asymptomatic abdominal mass, although malaise and pain may be reported.[149] Hematuria and high renin hypertension each occur in approximately 25% of patients. Metastases, when present at diagnosis, most commonly involve the lung (80%) or the liver (15%).

The relationship of genetic factors to Wilms' tumor is demonstrated by the approximately 1.5% of patients with Wilms' who have family members with the disease, and the approximately 10% who have aniridia, hemihypertrophy, or genitourinary anomalies.[149] Chromosomal aberrations at 11p13 and 11p15, known respectively as WT1 and WT2, are thought to be losses of tumor suppressor genes that occur in nonfamilial Wilms' tumor. The familial syndrome is probably related to unidentified genes.[149]

Overall, Wilms' tumor has an excellent prognosis. Treatment is based on disease stage following surgical resection or debulking, and favorable histology versus focal or diffuse anaplasia. A simplified description of the staging is as follows: stage I is limited to the kidney and can be completely removed surgically; stage II is extended beyond the kidney but can be completely excised; stage III is characterized by residual tumor confined to the abdomen; stage IV is distant metastases; and stage V is bilateral disease.[151] Metastases are present in only 15% of patients at diagnosis, and even these patients have relatively good prognoses. Four-year, relapse-free survival rates from the fourth National Wilms' Tumor Study (NWTS-4) range from 79% for stage IV with favorable histology to as low as 17% for patients with stage IV and diffuse anaplasia.[151] Survival is approximately 90% for patients with stage I regardless of histology.

Clinical Presentation and Treatment

60. B.N. is a 34-month-old boy who is pale and irritable. He has had abdominal complaints with decreased bowel movements and

reduced oral intake for 2 weeks. He has played less than normal for the last 4 weeks. B.N.'s blood pressure has intermittently been as high as 146/87 mmHg (normal, 90th percentile, 106/69). His Hgb is 7.9 g/dL (normal, 11.5–13.5) and his erythrocyte sedimentation rate is 139 mm/hour (normal, <10). B.N. has a history of hypospadias and left hydronephrosis. Scans show a right kidney mass extending through the capsule plus two distant metastases in the peritoneum. Chest radiography shows one nodule in the lung as well. Pathology from a biopsy sample shows favorable histology Wilms' tumor. What is the current treatment for Wilms' tumor?

The series of five National Wilms' Tumor studies have sought to progressively minimize toxicities from radiation and chemotherapy while maintaining the excellent cure rate. The fourth National Wilms' Tumor Study Group (NWTS-4) study demonstrated that intermittent, higher doses of dactinomycin allowed higher dose intensity with less myelosuppression than lower doses given daily for 5 days. Using greater dose intensity and dose density, 6 months of therapy was shown to be as effective as 15 months of therapy given the traditional way.[152] Also, fewer clinic visits were made and estimated costs were reduced by 50%.[152,153] The fifth NWTS study used surgery followed by 18 to 24 weeks of chemotherapy. The drugs were determined by the stage and histology (Table 91-12). Abdominal radiation therapy is used for stage II disease with unfavorable histology (focal or diffuse anaplasia) or stages III or IV with any histology; pulmonary radiation is used for stage IV disease if the chest radiograph is positive for metastases. For patients with stage V, or those with inoperable tumors, surgery can be delayed until chemotherapy reduces the tumor size.

Table 91-12 National Wilms' Tumor Study V Treatment Regimens by Stage and Histology

Stages I and II, Favorable Histology; Stage I, Focal or Diffuse Unfavorable Histology:
Surgery followed by 18 wk of vincristine and dactinomycin

Stage III, Favorable Histology; Stages II and III, Focal Anaplasia:
Surgery followed by 24 wk of vincristine, dactinomycin, and doxorubicin, with abdominal radiation. *Stage IV, Favorable Histology or Focal Anaplasia:* add pulmonary radiation if chest radiograph shows metastases

Stage II or III, Diffuse Anaplasia; Stages I to III Clear Cell Sarcoma of the Kidney (Unfavorable Histology):
Surgery followed by 24 wk of vincristine, doxorubicin, etoposide, and cyclophosphamide with mesna, abdominal radiation. *Stage IV, Diffuse Anaplasia or Clear Cell Sarcoma of the Kidney:* add pulmonary radiation if chest radiograph is positive for metastases

Stage V:
Biopsy followed by neoadjuvant vincristine, dactinomycin, and doxorubicin, then complete resection or debulking followed by more chemotherapy and, if a poor response, radiation therapy; more aggressive treatment if unfavorable histology (10%)

Stages I–IV, Rhabdoid Tumor (Unfavorable Histology):
Surgery followed by 24 wk of carboplatin, etoposide, and cyclophosphamide with mesna, abdominal radiation

Adapted from reference 151, with permission. http://www.cancer.gov/cancertopics/pdq/treatment/wilms/healthprofessional/.

Dosing Chemotherapy in Infants

61. Are there any special precautions for dosing chemotherapy in B.N.?

The NWTS-2 noted an excessive number of toxic deaths in infants with good prognosis, and this resulted in a dosing change.[154] After chemotherapy doses were decreased by 50%, severe hematologic toxicity, toxic deaths, and pulmonary and hepatic complications were reduced.[155] Importantly, no decrease in therapeutic effect was noted. Reduction of chemotherapy doses in infants may be a consideration for other pediatric cancers as well.[156–158] Reasons for increased toxicity may include altered pharmacokinetics or organ sensitivity as well as the larger body surface area per kilogram relative to older children and adults.[154] In NWTS-5, dosages of chemotherapy agents for children <30 kg were converted from mg/m^2 to mg/kg. By assuming the average 1-m^2 child weighs 30 kg, the dose/m^2 can be divided by 30 to arrive at a dose per kilogram, which can be used in dosing calculations. This adjustment lowers the dose by 20% to 50% in children who weigh <15 kg. In NWTS-5, infants <12 months of age received doses that were further reduced by halving the milligram per kilogram dose.

Interaction of Chemotherapy With Radiation

62. Are there any dosing precautions required because of potential interactions between B.N.'s treatments?

Another drug-related problem that may arise in B.N. is the interaction of dactinomycin and doxorubicin with radiation therapy.[159–163] Two effects have been reported. One is acute enhancement of radiation effects, and the other is recurrence (recall) of radiation effects up to several weeks later, especially to skin and mucous membranes. Because B.N. is to receive abdominal and lung irradiation during his chemotherapy treatment, concurrent doses of dactinomycin and doxorubicin will need to be reduced by 50% or held if wet desquamation of the skin occurs. In many of the Ewing's sarcoma and rhabdomyosarcoma protocols, dactinomycin or doxorubicin is stopped during concurrent radiation treatments.

Doxorubicin Cardiotoxicity in Pediatrics

63. When B.N. receives lung irradiation for his metastases, how will it affect the doxorubicin he is scheduled to receive?

Although it is well known that mediastinal irradiation can increase the risk of anthracycline-induced cardiac toxicity,[164] the only adjustment for B.N. would be temporary reduction of doxorubicin doses as described in Question 62. The total doxorubicin dose should be limited to no more than 5 mg/kg (150 mg/m^2 in larger children). In earlier Wilms' tumor studies, the risk of congestive heart failure was 4.4% at 20 years, or up to 17.4% in patients who relapsed and received more doxorubicin.[165] Thus, cardiovascular toxicity can develop as long as 20 years after therapy is completed, with an apparent decrease in left ventricular wall thickness and increased ventricular afterload, probably related to inadequate numbers of myocytes.[166] These reports emphasize the need to minimize chemotherapy in patients with good prognosis, as the Wilms' tumor studies are doing. New recommendations include better standardization of cardiac monitoring and continuation of monitoring for life in survivors of childhood cancer who receive cardiotoxic agents.

Dactinomycin Hepatotoxicity

64. B.N. is to receive vincristine 0.05 mg/kg weekly for 10 weeks; doxorubicin 1.5 mg/kg on weeks 3 and 9; 1 mg/kg on weeks 15 and 21; and dactinomycin 0.045 mg/kg on weeks 0, 6, 12, 18, and 24. During the third week of treatment, his ALT is elevated to 78 U/dL (normal, 7–56). Is this related to his drug therapy?

Early in the NWTS-4, an increased incidence (14.3%) of severe hepatotoxicity (elevation of AST or ALT 10 times normal with or without ascites) was reported with the pulse-intensive dactinomycin doses (0.060 mg/kg per single dose) in patients receiving no abdominal radiation.[167] Subsequently, dactinomycin doses were reduced. Still, the incidence of hepatotoxicity in patients receiving the newer 0.045-mg/kg pulse doses (3.7%), as well as those receiving the standard 0.015 mg/kg/day for 5 days (2.8%), remained elevated relative to the NWTS-3 results (0.4%), which used 0.015 mg/kg/day for 5 days.[168] The reasons for the increased hepatotoxicity are not known. Liver function usually returns to baseline within 1 to 2 weeks after discontinuation of chemotherapy, although more severe problems with veno-occlusive disease (hepatopathy) have also been reported.[151] Chemotherapy was restarted in some patients, although frequently at lower doses or without dactinomycin. B.N. should be monitored closely in case his liver enzymes continue to rise, especially because he will receive abdominal radiation treatments. If his ALT rises to two to five times normal, or his total bilirubin is 3 to 5 mg/dL, doses of all three of his drugs should be reduced by 50%. If his ALT or bilirubin rises above two to five times normal, the drugs should be withheld until laboratory values return to the aforementioned range.

OSTEOSARCOMA

Osteosarcoma is a malignant bone tumor that occurs most commonly in adolescents or young adults in the second or third decade of life.[169] It occurs most frequently in the metaphyseal ends of the distal femur, proximal tibia, or proximal humerus, but it can occur in the flat bones as well.[170] The age range and bones involved suggest a malignant response associated with the normal childhood growth spurts.[169] The most common manifestation at diagnosis is pain at the site, which can sometimes be present for several weeks to months.[169] Clinically detectable metastases are present in 15% to 20% of patients, usually in the lungs but occasionally in bone.

If surgery alone is used for treatment, 80% of patients will die within 5 years of recurrent metastatic disease, indicating the presence of subclinical micrometastases at the time of diagnosis.[170,171] Although surgery is the main treatment of the primary tumor, chemotherapy is used to prevent development of metastases. Drugs frequently used for osteosarcoma include high-dose methotrexate, cisplatin, doxorubicin, and ifosfamide.[169] Regimens have changed minimally in the last 25 years, with the current standard treatment in the COG being cisplatin and doxorubicin alternating with two courses of high-dose methotrexate. The tumor is relatively resistant to radiation therapy, which is usually reserved for cases in which local control cannot be achieved surgically.[169,172] When chemotherapy is used with surgery, long-term (2–5 years) DFS estimates typically range from 50% to 75%.[169–171,173,174]

65. G.C. is an 18-year-old man with a 2- to 3-month history of left shoulder pain. A tumor is found on radiograph, and biopsy confirms a high-grade conventional osteosarcoma of the left proximal humerus. No apparent metastases are found with CT and bone scans. G.C. begins neoadjuvant chemotherapy consisting of high-dose methotrexate alternating with cisplatin and doxorubicin. Two cycles of this chemotherapy will be given before his surgery, after which he will receive two additional cycles with all three drugs and two more without the cisplatin. What is the goal of chemotherapy? What is the role of presurgical (neoadjuvant) chemotherapy in G.C.?

Because G.C.'s osteosarcoma is in his proximal humerus, the surgeon can remove the primary tumor using one of the various operations that have been described elsewhere.[169] Limb salvages typically work well in the upper extremities, with fewer complications than when they are used for lower extremities. Because patients with osteosarcoma usually die from metastases, the goal of the chemotherapy is to eradicate micrometastases. Neoadjuvant chemotherapy of osteosarcoma was developed to treat micrometastases while waiting for limb salvage surgeries to be arranged, performed, and healed. Neoadjuvant therapy may also facilitate limb-sparing surgery by shrinking the tumor; it also allows histologic grading of the response to initial chemotherapy at surgery, a prognostic factor for risk of relapse. No convincing evidence to date indicates that DFS is better for patients who receive neoadjuvant chemotherapy relative to those who receive only adjuvant therapy.[172,174]

Prognostic Factors

66. At surgery, G.C.'s tumor shows excellent histologic response, with 99% necrosis. At diagnosis, his LDH was 684 U/L (normal, 322–644 U/L). Both of these factors indicate that G.C. is a good-risk patient. How do prognostic factors affect the choice of therapy in osteosarcoma?

Conventional staging systems do not correlate well with prognosis for most bone cancers. Clinically apparent metastases or a location that does not allow complete surgical removal of the primary tumor are associated with a poor prognosis.[172] Newer surgical techniques and treatments have improved the outlook, with 20% to 30% of these patients cured using neoadjuvant chemotherapy and surgery of the primary tumor and metastases.[175] Patients with poor prognostic factors continue to be less likely to benefit from conventional surgery and chemotherapy. Other potential prognostic factors have been identified; however, few of these factors have been used to stratify patients to different treatment regimens.[172] One exception is the histologic grade of the tumor at surgery. In current studies, patients with >90% tumor necrosis after two cycles of neoadjuvant chemotherapy are considered good risk and are treated with standard chemotherapy such as G.C. is receiving. Patients whose tumors have less necrosis at surgery are considered to be standard risk, and efforts are being made to increase their response rates by adding courses of ifosfamide and extending the duration of the standard regimen.

Delayed Clearance After High-Dose Methotrexate

67. After reconstructive surgery using a vascularized fibula graft, G.C. restarts his chemotherapy. During his fourth cycle of chemotherapy, after high-dose methotrexate is given, G.C.'s peak methotrexate concentration is 1,300 micromolar/L and the 72-hour concentration is 0.22 micromolar/L (normal, <0.1 micromolar/L at 72 hours). Recorded urine-specific gravities are <1.015, urine pHs are >6.5, and urine output is >2 mL/kg/hour, all meeting the guidelines to reduce the risk of methotrexate-induced nephrotoxicity. His creatinine has increased from 0.9–1.1 mg/dL (normal, 0.5–1.2 mg/dL), however. Leucovorin rescue (15 mg IV every 6 hours) is continued. What potential problems could be causing his retention of methotrexate?

Accumulations of protein-containing "third-space" fluids, such as pleural effusion and ascites, or GI obstruction, may retain methotrexate and cause slow terminal excretion.[176–178] Slow terminal excretion of methotrexate allows more proliferating cells to be exposed to methotrexate during the S phase of the cell cycle, increasing the cytotoxicity and resulting in more mucositis and myelosuppression. Many drugs interact with methotrexate, which can also slow its terminal excretion. Cisplatin reportedly reduces the excretion of methotrexate, especially at cumulative doses >300 mg/m^2.[179] G.C. has received four doses of 120 mg/m^2 of cisplatin, which may have contributed to the reduced methotrexate excretion. He has not received concomitant nephrotoxins, such as aminoglycosides or amphotericin B. Weak organic acids, such as salicylates, ketoprofen, or trimethoprim-sulfamethoxazole (TMP-SMX), can compete with methotrexate for renal tubular secretion.[180,181]

Although G.C.'s serum creatinine appears to be the same that it was at diagnosis (1.1 mg/dL), serum creatinine is not always a good indicator of renal function, so it is possible that G.C. has had some renal damage that is not apparent from his serum creatinine concentrations.[147] A measured creatinine clearance was 176 mL/minute/1.73 m^2 at diagnosis, and a repeat at this point is 106 mL/minute/1.73 m^2. Even measured creatinine clearance may not always be accurate when compared with Cr-EDTA measurement of glomerular filtration rate.[147] Although the reduced renal clearance may be contributing, it is not clear why G.C. is retaining methotrexate; future courses of methotrexate will need close monitoring.

Leucovorin Rescue

68. How long should leucovorin be administered to G.C.?

Cytotoxic effects of methotrexate depend on concentration and duration of exposure.[182] Many high-dose methotrexate protocols continue leucovorin rescue until serum methotrexate concentrations are 0.1 micromolar/L, which would be expected to occur approximately 72 hours after a 12-g/m^2 dose infused over 4 hours. Because G.C. has delayed clearance with persistence of low methotrexate levels past 72 hours, prevention of GI and bone marrow cytotoxicity may require continuation of leucovorin rescue until methotrexate concentrations are <0.01 to 0.05 micromolar/L.[178] For G.C., methotrexate concentrations did not fall below 0.1 micromolar/L until 108 hours after his dose; thus, leucovorin was continued 24 hours past that time. Other considerations may also be important in patients receiving leucovorin rescue. Because of the competitive nature of leucovorin rescue, higher leucovorin doses may be needed for patients with excessively high methotrexate concentrations.

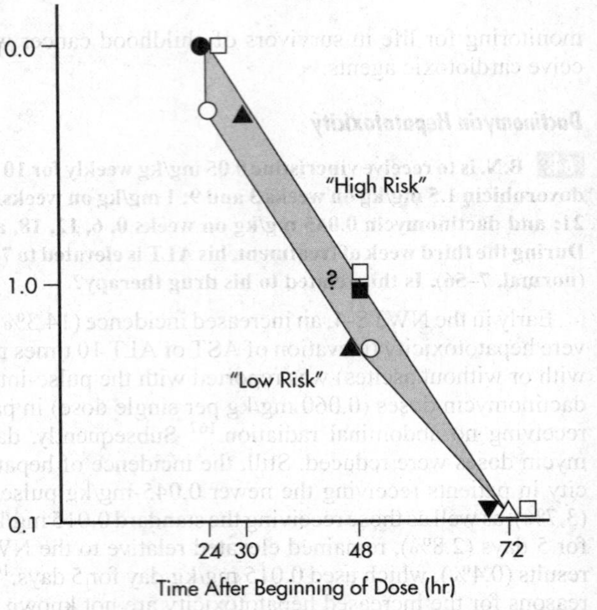

FIGURE 91-1 Composite semilogarithmic plot of serum methotrexate (MTX) concentrations that have been proposed to identify patients at "high risk" to develop toxicity from high-dose MTX if conventional low-dose leucovorin is administered. From Petros WP, Evans WE. Anticancer agents. In: Burton ME, et al., eds. Applied Pharmacokinetics & Pharmacodynamics. 4th ed. Philadelphia: Lippincott Williams & Wilkins; 2006:617.[177] Data for the figure were obtained from reports of: (▲) Evans,[183] (△) Tattersal,[184] (●) Isacoff,[185] (○) Isacoff,[186] (□) Nirenberg,[187] (■) Stoller,[188] and (▼) Rechnitzer.[189]

Petros and Evans[177] have published a figure that helps identify patients who are at high risk for methotrexate toxicity if given the usual low doses of leucovorin rescue [177,183–189] (Fig. 91-1). Using their guidelines, if G.C.'s methotrexate concentrations had remained between 1 and 5 micromolar/L 42 hours after the beginning of the infusion, recommendations would include increasing the dose of the leucovorin to 30 mg/m^2 every 6 hours until methotrexate concentrations fall below 1 micromolar/L. A rough guideline for normal methotrexate concentrations after a 12-g/m^2 dose is infused over 4 hours would be as follows: 1,000 micromolar/L for the peak, 10 micromolar/L at 24 hours, 1 micromolar/L at 48 hours, and 0.1 micromolar/L at 72 hours. If concentrations exceed 1 micromolar/L 42 hours or more after the methotrexate dose, higher doses of leucovorin may be needed. Oral leucovorin administration should not be used when the patient has emesis or requires larger doses (>50 mg), which are often poorly absorbed.[177]

RHABDOMYOSARCOMA

Rhabdomyosarcoma is the most common soft tissue sarcoma of childhood, occurring in 3.5% of all children with cancer.[120] The two most common histologic types are embryonal and alveolar. Embryonal rhabdomyosarcoma cells resemble striated muscle and occur most frequently in young children with involvement in the head and neck or genitourinary tract. Alveolar rhabdomyosarcoma cells resemble lung parenchymal cells and occur more frequently in older children or adolescents with involvement of the trunk or extremities. Generally, patients with alveolar rhabdomyosarcoma have a poorer prognosis than patients with the embryonal type. The clinical presentation of rhabdomyosarcoma varies with its location.

Treatment combines surgery, radiation, and chemotherapy. Complete surgical removal is often difficult, given the locations and infiltrative characteristics of rhabdomyosarcoma. Because good local control improves the prognosis,[131] radiation is generally added to the surgery to achieve this. Combination chemotherapy is necessary because the 5-year survival with local control alone is 10% to 30%. Vincristine, dactinomycin, and cyclophosphamide (VAC regimen) have been used extensively to treat rhabdomyosarcoma.[131] Other agents producing responses include combinations of vincristine, doxorubicin, and cyclophosphamide; ifosfamide and etoposide; and vincristine and irinotecan.[190–192] Results of the fourth Intergroup Rhabdomyosarcoma Study (IRS) indicate a 76% failure-free survival for patients with nonmetastatic disease.[193]

Clinical Presentation and Prognostic Factors

69. F.J. is a 2-year-old girl with a rapidly enlarging mass on the lateral head of the gastrocnemius muscle in the right calf. F.J. has no other complaints. Bone marrow and scans are negative for metastatic disease. The diagnosis is embryonal rhabdomyosarcoma, stage III (unfavorable site and >5 cm mass). Initial expectations were that gross residual tumor would remain after the surgery, making it clinical group III. Chemotherapy consists of 3-week cycles of vincristine 0.05 mg/kg (days 1, 8, and 15 of some cycles, but day 1 only of some cycles); dactinomycin 0.045 mg/kg on day 1 of each cycle; and cyclophosphamide 73 mg/kg on day 1 of each cycle with mesna to reduce the risk of hemorrhagic cystitis. Because of reports of hepatotoxicity during a prior study, especially in patients <3 years of age, the protocol recommends all three drugs be dosed in milligram per kilogram for children <3 years of age. TMP-SMX is begun at 150 mg/m^2/day (TMP) divided twice daily for 3 consecutive days per week. After each course of chemotherapy, F.J. is to receive filgrastim 5 mcg/kg/day subcutaneously for 14 days or until the absolute neutrophil count (ANC) is >1,000. What factors in F.J. are associated with a good prognosis? What are the chemotherapy treatment options for rhabdomyosarcoma?

The embryonal histopathologic classification has a better prognosis than the alveolar one, although evidence indicates that the primary tumor site is more important than the histology.[131,194,195] The primary site affects resectability, route of spread, and how early the diagnosis is made. Additionally, age between 1 and 9 years is associated with a better prognosis. The Intergroup Rhabdomyosarcoma Studies (IRS) have used a clinical grouping system (groups I to IV), which is based on spread of the disease and extent of resection. This system has been useful because of its correlation with prognosis where complete surgical removal and lack of metastases both correlate with good prognosis.[131] The fourth and fifth IRS studies compared the clinical grouping system with a TNM staging system similar to that used in adult cancers. Although the two systems may result in different disease stages for a specific patient, both are considered valuable and current protocols use both systems.

In rhabdomyosarcoma, the tumor site is one important part of the T rating in the staging system. F.J.'s tumor involves an unfavorable site, and is >5 cm, making it stage III. Although her tumor was expected to be clinical group III, after a good response to neoadjuvant chemotherapy, a complete resection was performed, making it clinical group I. This suggests that she has an 80% to 90% chance of 3-year survival based on the IRS-II, IRS-III, and IRS-IV results.[131,193,196] The IRS-V classified patients as having low-, intermediate-, or high-risk disease. Low-risk includes patients with embryonal rhabdomyosarcoma at favorable sites, or at unfavorable sites with no more than microscopic residual tumor.[192] Patients at intermediate risk have the embryonal subtype with gross residual tumor or the alveolar subtype without metastatic disease. Patients at high risk include those with metastatic alveolar or embryonal disease.

Chemotherapy for many patients at low risk is limited to vincristine and dactinomycin.[192] Most at intermediate risk are treated with vincristine, dactinomycin, and cyclophosphamide. New studies are adding courses of vincristine and irinotecan (COG ARST0531). Patients at high risk have not responded well in the past and are candidates for trials with newer drugs added to the vincristine, dactinomycin, and cyclophosphamide. A current study adds courses of vincristine and irinotecan, ifosfamide and etoposide and vincristine, doxorubicin, and cyclophosphamide (COG ARST0431).[192] F.J. would be in the low-risk group; however, her large tumor justifies adding cyclophosphamide to the vincristine and dactinomycin as in the intermediate-risk regimen. Because radiation to her leg would stop bone growth, and her surgical margins were tumor-free, no radiation is being administered.

TMP-SMX Prophylaxis and Filgrastim for Myelosuppression

70. What are the reasons for treating F.J. with TMP-SMX and filgrastim?

F.J.'s VAC regimen (vincristine, dactinomycin, and cyclophosphamide) was associated with a high incidence of neutropenic fevers even during the pilot studies. Because of the frequency of severe myelosuppression, TMP-SMX is used until 6 months after chemotherapy for prophylaxis against *Pneumocystis jiroveci (carinii)*, an opportunistic pathogen. Filgrastim is used to minimize neutropenia so that the chemotherapy dose intensity can be maintained.

Renal Fanconi Syndrome With Ifosfamide

71. F.J.'s mother read on the internet about a patient with rhabdomyosarcoma who had received vincristine, ifosfamide, and etoposide and was cured. She wants to know why that regimen is not being used for her daughter.

The IRS-IV results for local or regional disease (intermediate risk) demonstrated no advantages of vincristine, ifosfamide, and etoposide or vincristine, dactinomycin, and ifosfamide over the standard vincristine, dactinomycin, and cyclophosphamide treatment.[193] Additionally, the ifosfamide-containing regimens caused more toxicity. Ifosfamide has been associated with renal Fanconi syndrome, a proximal tubular defect that is characterized by wasting of electrolytes, glucose, and amino acids, as well as renal tubular acidosis and an increased serum creatinine. Data suggest that the risk of Fanconi syndrome is increased in children <3 years of age; have received total ifosphamide doses >72 to 100 g/m^2; have hydronephrosis, a single kidney, or an elevated serum creatinine; or have received previous platinum therapy.[197–200] During each course of her chemotherapy, F.J. develops ketonuria; however, this is not a toxicity of her chemotherapy. Ketonuria is caused by her mesna therapy, which has been reported to routinely cause false–positive ketone tests.[201]

REFERENCES

1. Jemal A et al. Cancer Statistics, 2007. *CA Cancer J Clin* 2007;57:43.
2. Struewing JP et al. The risk of cancer associated with specific mutations of BRCA1 and BRCA2 among Ashkenazi Jews. *N Engl Med* 1997;336:1401.
3. Armstrong K et al. Assessing the risk of breast cancer. *N Engl J Med* 2000;342:564.
4. Humphrey LL et al. Breast cancer screening: a summary of the evidence for the U.S. Preventive Services Task Force. *Ann Intern med* 2002;137:347.
5. Saslow D et al. American Cancer Society guidelines for breast screening with MRI as an adjunct to mammography. *CA Cancer J Clin* 2007;57:75.
6. Viale G et al. Intraoperative examination of axillary sentinel lymph nodes in breast carcinoma patients. *Cancer* 1999;85:2433.
7. Fisher B et al. Twenty-year follow-up of a randomized trial comparing total mastectomy, lumpectomy, and lumpectomy plus irradiation for the treatment of invasive breast cancer. *N Engl J Med* 2002;347:1233.
8. Clarke M et al. Early Breast Cancer Trialists' Collaborative Group (EBCTCG). Effects of radiotherapy and of differences in the extent of surgery for breast cancer on local recurrence and 15-year survival: an overview of randomised trials. *Lancet* 2005;366:2097.
9. McGuire WL et al. Prognostic factors and treatment decisions in axillary node negative breast cancer. *N Engl J Med* 1992;326:1765.
10. McArthur HL et al. Adjuvant chemotherapy for early-stage breast cancer. *Hematol Oncol Clin North Am* 2007;21:207.
11. Paik S et al. Gene expression and benefit of chemotherapy in women with node-negative, estrogen receptor-positive breast cancer. *J Clin Oncol* 2006;24:3726.
12. van de Vijver MJ et al. A gene-expression signature as a predictor of survival in breast cancer. *N Engl J Med* 2002;347:1999.
13. Early Breast Cancer Trialists' Collaborative Group (EBCTCG). Effects of chemotherapy and hormonal therapy for early breast cancer on recurrences and 15-year survival: an overview of the randomised trials. *Lancet* 2005;365:1687.
14. Smith I et al. 2-year follow-up of trastuzumab after adjuvant chemotherapy in HER2-positive breast cancer: a randomised controlled trial. *Lancet* 2007;369:29.
15. Romond EH et al. Trastuzumab plus adjuvant chemotherapy for operable HER2-positive breast cancer. *N Engl J Med* 2005;353:1673.
16. Khatcheressian JL et al. American Society of Clinical Oncology 2006 update of the breast cancer follow-up and management guidelines in the adjuvant setting. *J Clin Oncol* 2006;24:5091.
17. Goldhirsch A et al. Meeting highlights: international expert consensus on the primary therapy of early breast cancer 2005. *Ann Oncol* 2005;15:1569.
18. Muss HB et al. c-erbB-2 expression and response to adjuvant therapy in women with node-positive early breast cancer. *N Engl J Med* 1994;330:1260.
19. Gusterson BA et al. Prognostic importance of c-erbB-2 expressions in breast cancer. *J Clin Oncol* 1992;10:1049.
20. Henderson IC et al. Improved outcomes from adding sequential paclitaxel but not from escalating doxorubicin dose in an adjuvant chemotherapy regimen for patients with node-positive primary breast cancer. *J Clin Oncol* 2003;21:976.
21. Bria E et al. Benefit of taxanes as adjuvant chemotherapy for early breast cancer. *Cancer* 2006;106:2337.
22. Citron ML et al. Randomized trial of dose-dense versus conventionally scheduled and sequential versus concurrent combination chemotherapy as postoperative adjuvant treatment of node-positive primary breast cancer: first report of intergroup trial C9741/Cancer and Leukemia Group B trial 9741. *J Clin Oncol* 2003;21:1431.
23. Baum M et al. Early Breast Cancer Trialists' Collaborative Group. Ovarian ablation in early breast cancer: overview of the randomized trials. *Lancet* 1998;348:1189.
24. Lonning PE. Adjuvant endocrine treatment of early breast cancer. *Hematol Oncol Clin North Am* 2007;21:223.
25. Goss PE et al. Efficacy of letrozole extended adjuvant therapy according to estrogen receptor and progesterone receptor status of the primary tumor: National Cancer Institute of Canada Clinical Trials Group MA.17. *J Clin Oncol* 2007;25:2006.
26. Mayer EL et al. Chemotherapy for metastatic breast cancer. *Hematol Oncol Clin North Am* 2007;21:257.
27. Slamon DJ et al. Use of chemotherapy plus a monoclonal antibody against HER2 for metastatic breast cancer that over expresses HER2. *N Engl J Med* 2001;344:783.
28. Burstein HJ et al. Clinical activity of trastuzumab and vinorelbine in women with HER2-overexpressing metastatic breast cancer. *J Clin Oncol* 2001;19:2722.
29. Geyer CE et al. Lapatinib plus capecitabine fore HER2-positive advanced breast cancer. *N Engl J Med* 2006;355:2733.
30. Traina TA et al. Bevacizumab for advanced breast cancer. *Hematol Oncol Clin North Am* 2007;21:303.
31. McGuire WL. Hormone receptors: their role in predicting prognosis and response to endocrine therapy. *Semin Oncol* 1978;5:428.
32. Singhakowinta A et al. Estrogen receptor and natural course of breast cancer. *Ann Surg* 1976;183:84.
33. Rugo HS. Hormonal therapy for advanced breast cancer. *Hematol Oncol Clin North Am* 2007;21:273.
34. Layman R et al. Bisphosphonates for breast cancer: questions answered, questions remaining. *Hematol Oncol Clin North Am* 2007;21:341.
35. Hilner BE et al. American Society of Clinical Oncology 2003 update on the role of bisphosphonates and bone health issues in women with breast cancer. *J Clin Oncol* 2003;21:4042.
36. Rosen LS et al. Zoledronic acid versus pamidronate in the treatment of skeletal metastases in patients with breast cancer or osteolytic lesions or multiple myeloma: a phase III, double-blind, comparative trial. *Cancer J* 2001;7:377.
37. Lonning PE et al. Activity of exemestane in metastatic breast cancer after failure of nonsteroidal aromatase inhibitors: a phase II trial. *J Clin Oncol* 2000;18:2234.
38. Tsao AS et al. Chemoprevention of cancer. *CA Cancer J Clin* 2004;54:150.
39. American Society of Clinical Oncology policy statement update: genetic testing for cancer susceptibility. *J Clin Oncol* 2003;21:2397.
40. Smith RA et al. Cancer Screening in the United States, 2007: a review of current guidelines, practices, and prospects. *CA Cancer J Clin* 2007;57:90.
41. Feinberg EJ et al. How long to abstain from eating red meat before fecal occult blood tests. *Ann Intern Med* 1990;113:403.
42. Gill S et al. Colorectal cancer. *Mayo Clin Proc* 2007;82:112.
43. Desch CE et al. Colorectal cancer surveillance: 2005 update of an American Society of Clinical Oncology Practice Guideline. *J Clin Oncol* 2005;23:8512.
44. Weiss L et al. Hematogenous metastatic patterns in colonic carcinoma: an analysis of 1541 necropsies. *J Pathol* 1986;150:195.
45. Wolpin BM et al. Adjuvant treatment of colorectal cancer. *CA Cancer J Clin* 2007;57:168.
46. Andre T et al. Oxaliplatin, fluorouracil, and leucovorin as adjuvant treatment for colon cancer. *N Engl J Med* 2004;350:2343.
47. Schmoll H et al. Early safety findings from a phase III trial of capecitabine plus oxaliplatin (XELOX) vs. bolus 5-FU/LV as adjuvant therapy for patients with stage III colon cancer. *J Clin Oncol* 2005;23(Suppl:16s) (Abstract 3523).
48. Wolmark N et al. A phase III trial comparing FULV, to FULV + oxaliplatin in stage II or III carcinoma of the colon: results of NSABP protocol C-07. *J Clin Oncol* 2005;23(Suppl):16s (Abstract 3500).
49. Twelves C et al. Capecitabine as adjuvant treatment for stage III colon cancer. *N Engl J Med* 2005;352:2696.
50. Grothey A et al. Survival of patients with advanced colorectal cancer improves with the availability of fluorouracil-leucovorin, irinotecan, and oxaliplatin in the course of treatment. *J Clin Oncol* 2004;22:1209.
51. Goldberg RM et al. A randomized controlled trial of fluorouracil plus leucovorin, irrinotecan and oxaliplatin combinations in patients with previously untreated metastatic colorectal cancer. *J Clin Oncol* 2004;22:23.
52. Hurwitz H et al. Bevacizumab plus irinotecan, fluorouracil, and leucovorin for metastatic colorectal cancer. *N Engl J Med* 2004;350:2335.
53. Giantonio BJ et al. High-dose bevacizumab improves survival when combined with FOLFOX4 in previously treated advanced colorectal cancer: results form the Eastern Cooperative Oncology Group (ECOG) study E3200. *Proc Am Soc Clin Oncol* 2005;23;1s (Abstract 2).
54. Cunningham D et al. Cetuximab monotherapy and

cetuximab plus irinotecan in irinotecan-refractory metastatic colorectal cancer. *N Engl J Med* 2004;351:337.
55. Saltz LB et al. Randomized phase II trial of cetuximab/bevacizumab/irinotecan (CBI) versus cetuximab/bevacizumab (CB) in irinotecan-refractory colorectal cancer. *J Clin Oncol* 2005; 23(Suppl):248s (Abstract 3508).
56. Aurora V et al. Adjuvant therapy for resectable liver metastases: can metastatic colorectal cancer be cured? *Current Colorectal Cancer Reports* 2007;3:127.
57. Allen WL et al. Role of genomic markers in colorectal cancer treatment. *J Clin Oncol* 2005;23: 4545.
58. Collins LG et al. Lung cancer: diagnosis and management. *Am Fam Physician* 2007;75:56.
59. Bilello KS et al. Epidemiology, etiology, and prevention of lung cancer. *Clin Chest Med* 2002; 23:1.
60. The Alpha-Tocopherol, Beta Carotene Cancer Prevention Study Group. The effect of vitamin E and beta carotene on the incidence of lung cancer and other cancers in male smokers. *N Engl J Med* 1994;330:1029.
61. Omenn GS et al. Effects of a combination of beta-carotene and vitamin A on lung cancer and cardiovascular disease. *N Engl J Med* 1996;334:1150.
62. Clark LC et al. Effects of selenium supplementation for cancer prevention in patients with carcinoma of the skin. A randomized controlled trial. Nutritional Prevention of Cancer Study Group. *JAMA* 1996;276:1957.
63. Berlin NI et al. The National Cancer Institute Cooperative Early Lung Cancer Detection Program: results of the initial screen (prevalence). Early lung cancer detection: introduction. *Am Rev Respir Dis* 1984;13:545.
64. Maras PM et al. Lung cancer mortality in the Mayo Lung Project: impact of extended follow-up. *J Natl Cancer Inst* 2000;92:1308.
65. International Early Lung Cancer Action Program Investigators et al. Survival of patients with stage I lung cancer detected on CT screening. *N Engl J Med* 2006;355:1763.
66. Beckles MA et al. The physiologic evaluation of patients with lung cancer being considered for resectional surgery. *Chest* 2003;123(1 Suppl): 105S.
67. PORT Meta-analysis Trialists Group. Postoperative radiotherapy in non-small cell lung cancer: systematic review and meta-analysis of individual patient data from randomized controlled trials. *Lancet* 1998;352:257.
68. Non-Small Cell Lung Cancer Collaborative Group. Chemotherapy in non-small cell lung cancer: a meta-analysis using updated data on individual patients from 52 randomized clinical trials. *BMJ* 1995;311:899.
69. American Society of Clinical Oncology treatment of unresectable non-small-cell lung cancer guideline: update 2003. *J Clin Oncol* 2004;22:330.
70. Slotman B et al. Prophylactic cranial irradiation in extensive small-cell lung cancer. *N Engl J Med* 2007;357:664.
71. Sandler A et al. Paclitaxel-carboplatin alone or with bevacizumab for non-small-cell lung cancer. *N Engl J Med* 2006;355:2542.
72. Goodin S. Erlotinib: optimizing therapy with predictors of response? *Clin Cancer Res* 2006;12: 2961.
73. Auperin A et al. Concomitant radio-chemotherapy based on platin compounds in patients with locally advanced non-small cell lung cancer (NSCLC): a meta-analysis of individual data from 1764 patients. *Ann Oncol* 2006;17:473.
74. Douillard JY et al. Adjuvant vinorelbine plus cisplatin versus observation in patients with completely resected stage IB-IIIA non-small-cell lung cancer (Adjuvant Navelbine International Trialist Association [ANITA]): a randomised controlled trial. *Lancet Oncol* 2006;7:719.
75. Arriagada R et al. Cisplatin-based adjuvant chemotherapy in patients with completely resected non-small-cell lung cancer. *N Engl J Med* 2004;350: 351.
76. Winton T et al. Vinorelbine plus cisplatin vs. observation in resected non-small-cell lung cancer. *N Engl J med* 2005;352:2589.
77. Olaussen KA et al. DNA repair by ERCC1 in non-small-cell lung cancer and cisplatin-based adjuvant chemotherapy. *N Engl J Med* 2006;355: 983.
78. Aletti G et al. Current management strategies for ovarian cancer. *Mayo Clin Proc* 2007;82:751.
79. Koss LG. Cervical (PAP) smear. *Cancer* 1993;71: 1406.
80. Creasman WT et al. Screening in ovarian cancer. *Am J Obstet Gynecol* 1991;165:7.
81. Bristow RE et al. Survival effect of maximal cytoreductive surgery for advanced ovarian cancer during the platinum era: a meta-analysis. *J Clin Oncol* 2002;20:1248.
82. Wright JD et al. Bevacizumab combination therapy in recurrent, platinum-refractory, epithelial ovarian carcinoma: a retrospective analysis. *Cancer* 2006;107:83.
83. Alberts DS et al. Intraperitoneal cisplatin plus intravenous cyclophosphamide versus intravenous cisplatin plus intravenous cyclophosphamide for stage III ovarian cancer. *N Engl J Med* 1996;335: 1950.
84. Markman M et al. Phase III trial of standard-dose intravenous cisplatin plus paclitaxel versus moderately high-dose carboplatin followed by intravenous paclitaxel and intraperitoneal cisplatin in small-volume stage III ovarian carcinoma: an Intergroup study of the Gynecologic Oncology Group, Southwestern Oncology Group, and Eastern Cooperative Oncology Group. *J Clin Oncol* 2001;19:1001.
85. Armstrong DK et al. Intraperitoneal cisplatin and paclitaxel in ovarian cancer. *N Engl J Med* 2006; 354:34.
86. National Cancer Institute. Clinical Advisory: NCI issues clinical announcement for the preferred method of treatment for advanced ovarian cancer. www.nlm.nih.gov/databases/alerts/ovarian_ip_chemo.html. Accessed August 1, 2007.
87. Lamm DL et al. Bladder cancer. *CA Cancer J Clin* 1996;46:93.
88. Heney NM et al. TA and T1 bladder cancer: occasion, recurrence and progression. *Br J Urol* 1982; 54:152.
89. Herr HW. Intravesical therapy. *Hematol Oncol Clin North Am* 1992;6:1.
90. Han RF et al. Can intravesical bacillus Calmette-Guerin reduce recurrence in patients with superficial bladder cancer? A meta-analysis of randomized trials. *Urology* 2006;67:1216.
91. Winquist E et al. Neoadjuvant chemotherapy for transitional cell carcinoma of the bladder: a systemic review and meta-analysis. *J Urol* 2004;171: 561.
92. Clark PE. Bladder cancer. *Curr Opin Oncol* 2007; 19:241.
93. Ruggeri EM et al. Adjuvant chemotherapy in muscle-invasive bladder carcinoma: a pooled analysis from phase III studies. *Cancer* 2006;106:783.
94. Adjuvant chemotherapy for invasive bladder cancer (individual patient data). *Cochrane Database System Rev* 2006;CD006018.
95. von der Maase H et al. Long-term survival results of a randomized trial comparing gemcitabine plus cisplatin with methotrexate, vinblastine, doxorubicin, and cisplatin in patients with bladder cancer. *J Clin Oncol* 2005;23:4602.
96. Tsao H et al. Management of cutaneous melanoma. *N Engl J Med* 2004;351:998.
97. Markovic SN et al. Malignant melanoma in the 21st century. Part 1: Epidemiology, risk factors, screening, prevention, and diagnosis. *Mayo Clin Proc* 2007;82:364.
98. Wheatley K et al. Does adjuvant interferon-alpha for high-risk melanoma provide a worthwhile benefit? A meta-analysis of the randomised trials. *Cancer Treat Rev* 2003;29:241.
99. Markovic SN et al. Malignant melanoma in the 21st century. Part 2: Staging, prognosis, and treatment. *May0 Clin Proc* 2007;82:490.
100. Gearing AJH et al. The international standard for human interleukin-2: calibration by international collaborative study. *J Immunol Methods* 1988;114:3.
101. Siegal JP et al. Interleukin-2 toxicity. *J Clin Oncol* 1991;9:694.
102. Loblaw DA et al. Initial hormonal management of androgen-sensitive metastatic, recurrent, or progressive prostate cancer: 2006 update of an American Society of Clinical Oncology Practice Guideline. 2007;25:1596.
103. DiPaola RS et al. State-of-the-art prostate cancer treatment and research. *NJ Med* 2001;98:23.
104. Boccardo F. Hormone therapy of prostate cancer: is there a role for antiandrogen monotherapy? *Crit Rev Oncol Hematol* 2000;35:121.
105. Tyrrell CJ et al. A randomized comparison of 'Casodex' (bicalutamide) 150 mg monotherapy versus castration in the treatment of metastatic and locally advanced prostate cancer. *Eur Urol* 1998;33: 447.
106. Walczak JR et al. Prostate cancer: a practical approach to current management of recurrent disease. *Mayo Clin Proc* 2007;8:243.
107. Oefelein MG et al. Failure to achieve castrate levels of testosterone during luteinizing releasing hormone agonist therapy: the case for monitoring serum testosterone and a treatment decision algorithm. *J Urol* 2000;164:726.
108. Kelly WK et al. Steroid hormone withdrawal syndromes: pathophysiology and clinical significance. *Urol Clin North Am* 1997;24:421.
109. Petrylak DP et al. Docetaxel and estramustine compared with mitoxantrone and prednisone for advanced refractor prostate cancer. *N Engl J Med* 2004;351:1513.
110. Tannock IF et al. Docetaxel plus prednisone or mitoxantrone plus prednisone for advanced prostate cancer. *N Engl J Med* 2004;351:1502.
111. Richie JP. Detection and treatment of testicular cancer. *CA Cancer J Clin* 1993;43:151.
112. Hellerstedt BA et al. Testicular cancer. *Curr Opin Oncol* 2002;12:260.
113. Kondagunta GV et al. Adjuvant chemotherapy for stage II nonseminomatous germ-cell tumors. *Semin Urol Oncol* 2002;20:239.
114. Wozniak AJ et al. A randomized trial of cisplatin, vinblastine, and bleomycin versus vinblastine, cisplatin, and etoposide in the treatment of advanced germ cell tumors of the testis: a Southwest Oncology Group Study. *J Clin Oncol* 1991;9:70.
115. DeWit R et al. Four cycles of BEP versus an alternating regimen of PVB and BEP in patients with poor prognosis metastatic testicular non-seminoma: a randomized trial of the EORTC Genitourinary Tract Center Cooperative Group. *Br J Cancer* 1995;71:1311.
116. Williams SD et al. Treatment of disseminated germ-cell tumors with cisplatin, bleomycin, and either vinblastine or etoposide. *N Engl J Med* 1987; 316:1435.
117. Varuni Kondagunta G et al. Combination of paclitaxel, ifosfamide, and cisplatin in an effective second-line therapy for patients with relapsed testicular germ cell tumors. *J Clin Oncol* 2005;23: 6549.
118. Miller K et al. Salvage chemotherapy with vinblastine, ifosfamide, and cisplatin in recurrent seminoma. *J Clin Oncol* 1997;15:1427.
119. Einhorn LH et al. High-dose chemotherapy and stem-cell rescue for metastatic germ-cell tumors. *N Engl J Med* 2007;357:340.
120. Ries LAG et al., eds. *SEER cancer statistics review.* 1975–2004, National Cancer Institute. Bethesda, MD. http://seer.cancer.gov/csr/1975_2004/, based on November 2006 SEER data submission, posted to the SEER web site, 2007.
121. Triche TJ et al. Diagnostic pathology of pediatric malignancies. In: Pizzo PA et al., eds. *Principles and Practice of Pediatric Oncology.*

5th ed. Philadelphia: Lippincott Williams & Wilkins; 2006:185.
122. Delattre O et al. The Ewing family of tumors—a subgroup of small-round-cell tumors defined by specific chimeric transcripts. *N Engl J Med* 1994; 331:294.
123. Plon SE et al. Childhood cancer and heredity. In: Pizzo PA et al., eds. *Principles and Practice of Pediatric Oncology.* 5th ed. Philadelphia: Lippincott Williams & Wilkins; 2006:14.
124. Malogolowkin M et al. Clinical assessment and differential diagnosis of the child with suspected cancer. In: Pizzo PA et al., eds. *Principles and Practice of Pediatric Oncology.* 5th ed. Philadelphia: Lippincott Williams & Wilkins; 2006:145.
125. Tucker MA et al. Leukemia after therapy with alkylating agents for childhood cancer. *J Natl Cancer Inst* 1987;78:459.
126. Pui CH et al. Acute myeloid leukemia in children treated with epipodophyllotoxins for acute lymphoblastic leukemia. *N Engl J Med* 1991;325: 1682.
127. Neglia JP et al. Second neoplasms after acute lymphoblastic leukemia in childhood. *N Engl J Med* 1991;325:1330.
128. Melnick S et al. Rates and risks of diethylstilbestrol-related clear-cell adenocarcinoma of the vagina and cervix: an update. *N Engl J Med* 1987; 316:514.
129. Reamon GH et al. Infants and adolescents with cancer: special considerations. In: Pizzo PA et al., eds. *Principles and Practice of Pediatric Oncology.* 5th ed. Philadelphia: Lippincott Williams & Wilkins; 2006:452.
130. Crist W et al. Clinical and biologic features predict a poor prognosis in acute lymphoid leukemias in infants: Pediatric Oncology Group study. *Blood* 1986;67:135.
131. Wexler LH et al. Rhabdomyosarcoma and the undifferentiated sarcomas. In: Pizzo PA et al., eds. *Principles and Practice of Pediatric Oncology.* 5th ed. Philadelphia: Lippincott Williams & Wilkins; 2006:971.
132. Bhatia S et al. Late effects of childhood cancer and its treatment. In: Pizzo PA et al., eds. *Principles and Practice of Pediatric Oncology.* 5th ed. Philadelphia: Lippincott Williams & Wilkins; 2006:1490.
133. Brodeur GM et al. Neuroblastoma. In: Pizzo PA et al., eds. *Principles and Practice of Pediatric Oncology.* 5th ed. Philadelphia: Lippincott Williams & Wilkins; 2006:933.
134. Castleberry RP. Biology and treatment of neuroblastoma. *Pediatr Clin North Am* 1997;44:919.
135. LaBrosse EH et al. Urinary excretion of 3methoxy-4-hydroxymandelic acid and 3-methoxy- 4-hydroxy-phenylacetic acid by 288 patients with neuroblastoma and related neural crest tumors. *Cancer Res* 1980;40:1995.
136. Woods WG et al. Screening for neuroblastoma is ineffective in reducing the incidence of unfavorable advanced stage disease in older children. *Eur J Cancer* 1997;33:2106.
137. Yamamoto K et al. Spontaneous regression of localized neuroblastoma detected by mass screening. *J Clin Oncol* 1998;16:1265.
138. Http://www.cancer.gov/cancerinfo/pdq/treatment/neuroblastoma/healthprofessional/. Accessed June 1, 2007.
139. Baker DL et al. A phase III trial of biologically-based therapy reduction for intermediate risk neuroblastoma. *J Clin Oncol* 2007;25:527s (Abstract 9504).
140. Kreissman SG et al. Response and toxicity to a dose-intensive multi-agent chemotherapy induction regimen for high risk neuroblastoma (HR-NB): A Children's Oncology Group (COG A3973) study. *J Clin Oncol* 2007;25:527s (Abstract 9505).
141. Philip T et al. 1070 myeloablative megatherapy procedures followed by stem cell rescue for neuroblastoma: 17 years of European experience and conclusions. *Eur J Cancer* 1997;33:2130.
142. Matthay KK et al. Treatment of high-risk neuroblastoma with intensive chemotherapy, radiotherapy, autologous bone marrow transplantation, and 13-cis-retinoic acid. *N Engl J Med* 1999;341:1165.
143. Taketomo CK et al. *Pediatric Dosage Handbook.* 10th ed. Hudson, Ohio: Lexi-Comp; 2007:222.
144. McEvoy GK et al., eds. *AHFS Drug Information 2007.* Bethesda, MD: American Society of Health-System Pharmacists; 2007:964.
145. Solimando DA. *Drug Information Handbook for Oncology.* 6th ed. Hudson, Ohio: Lexi-Comp; 2007:222.
146. D'Angio R et al. Creatinine clearance: corrected versus uncorrected [Letter]. *Drug Intell Clin Pharm* 1988;22:32.
147. Womer RB et al. Renal toxicity of cisplatin in children. *J Pediatr* 1985;106:659.
148. Yanik GA et al. Pilot study of iodine-131-metaiodobenzylguanidine in combination with myeloablative chemotherapy and autologous stem-cell support for the treatment of neuroblastoma. *J Clin Oncol* 2002;20:2142.
149. Dome JS et al. Renal tumors. In: Pizzo PA et al., eds. *Principles and Practice of Pediatric Oncology.* 5th ed. Philadelphia: Lippincott Williams & Wilkins; 2006:905.
150. Breslow NE et al. Age distribution of Wilms' tumor: report from the National Wilms' Tumor Study. *Cancer Res* 1988;48:1653.
151. http://www.cancer.gov/cancertopics/pdq/treatment/wilms/healthprofessional/. Accessed June 1, 2007.
152. Green DM et al. Comparison between single-dose and divided-dose administration of dactinomycin and doxorubicin for patients with Wilms' tumor: a report from the National Wilms' Tumor Study Group. *J Clin Oncol* 1998;16:237.
153. Green DM et al. Effect of duration of treatment on treatment outcome and cost of treatment for Wilms' tumor: a report from the National Wilms' Tumor Study Group. *J Clin Oncol* 1998;16:3744.
154. Jones B et al. Toxic deaths in the second National Wilms' Tumor Study. *J Clin Oncol* 1984;2:1028.
155. Morgan E et al. Chemotherapy-related toxicity in infants treated according to the second National Wilms' Tumor Study. *J Clin Oncol* 1988;6:51.
156. Woods WG et al. Life-threatening neuropathy and hepatotoxicity in infants during induction therapy for acute lymphoblastic leukemia. *J Pediatr* 1981;98:642.
157. Allen JC. The effects of cancer therapy on the nervous system. *J Pediatr* 1978;93:903.
158. Reaman G et al. Acute lymphoblastic leukemia in infants less than one year of age: a cumulative experience of the Childrens Cancer Study Group. *J Clin Oncol* 1985;3:1513.
159. D'Angio GJ et al. Potentiation of x-ray effects by actinomycin D. *Radiology* 1959;73:175.
160. Tan CTC et al. The effect of actinomycin D on cancer in childhood. *Pediatrics* 1959;24:544.
161. Donaldson SS et al. Adriamycin activating a recall phenomenon after radiation therapy. *Ann Intern Med* 1974;81:407.
162. Greco FA et al. Adriamycin and enhanced radiation reaction in normal esophagus and skin. *Ann Intern Med* 1976;85:294.
163. Phillips TL et al. Acute and late effects of multimodal therapy on normal tissues. *Cancer* 1977;40: 489.
164. Merrill J et al. Adriamycin and radiation-synergistic cardiotoxicity. *Ann Intern Med* 1975;82: 122.
165. Green DM et al. Congestive heart failure after treatment for Wilms' Tumor: a report from the National Wilms' Tumor Study Group. *J Clin Oncol* 2001;19:1926.
166. Lipshultz SE et al. Chronic progressive cardiac dysfunction years after doxorubicin therapy for childhood acute lymphoblastic leukemia. *J Clin Oncol* 2005;23:2629.
167. Green DM et al. Severe hepatic toxicity after treatment with single-dose dactinomycin and vincristine. *Cancer* 1988;62:270.
168. Green DM et al. Severe hepatic toxicity after treatment with vincristine and dactinomycin using single-dose or divided-dose schedules: a report from the National Wilms' Tumor Study. *J Clin Oncol* 1990;8:1525.
169. Link MP et al. Osteosarcoma. In: Pizzo PA et al., eds. *Principles and Practice of Pediatric Oncology.* 5th ed. Philadelphia: Lippincott Williams & Wilkins; 2006:1076.
170. Goorin AM et al. Osteosarcoma: fifteen years later. *N Engl J Med* 1985;313:1637.
171. Link MP et al. The effect of adjuvant chemotherapy on relapse-free survival in patients with osteosarcoma of the extremity. *N Engl J Med* 1986;314: 1600.
172. Jenkin R et al. Osteosarcoma: an assessment of management with particular reference to primary irradiation and selective delayed amputation. *Cancer* 1972;30:393.
173. Meyers PA et al. Chemotherapy for nonmetastatic osteogenic sarcoma: the Memorial Sloan-Kettering experience. *J Clin Oncol* 1992;10:5.
174. Goorin AM et al. Presurgical chemotherapy compared with immediate surgery and adjuvant chemotherapy for nonmetastatic osteosarcoma: Pediatric Oncology Group study POG-8651. *J Clin Oncol* 2003;21:1574.
175. Pastorino U et al. The contribution of salvage surgery to the management of childhood osteosarcoma. *J Clin Oncol* 1991;9:1357.
176. Evans WE et al. Effect of pleural effusion on high-dose methotrexate kinetics. *Clin Pharmacol Ther* 1978;23:68.
177. Petros WP et al. Anticancer agents. In: Burton ME et al., eds. *Applied Pharmacokinetics & Pharmacodynamics.* 4th ed. Philadelphia: Lippincott Williams & Wilkins; 2006:617.
178. Evans WE et al. Pharmacokinetics of sustained serum methotrexate concentrations secondary to gastrointestinal obstruction. *J Pharm Sci* 1981;70:1194.
179. Crom WR et al. The effect of prior cisplatin therapy on the pharmacokinetics of high-dose methotrexate. *J Clin Oncol* 1984;2:655.
180. Tatro DS. *Drug Interaction Facts 2007.* St. Louis: Wolters Kluwer Health; 2007:1017.
181. Gerrazzini G et al. Interaction between trimethoprim-sulfamethoxazole and methotrexate in children with leukemia. *J Pediatr* 1990;117:823.
182. Pinedo HM et al. Role of drug concentration, duration of exposure and endogenous metabolites in determining methotrexate cytotoxicity. *Cancer Treatment Reports* 1977;61:709.
183. Evans WE et al. Pharmacokinetic monitoring of high-dose methotrexate: early recognition of high-risk patients. *Cancer Chemother Pharmacol* 1979; 3:161.
184. Tattersall MHN et al. Clinical pharmacology of high-dose methotrexate (NSC-740). *Cancer Chemotherapy Reports* 1975;6(Pt 3):25.
185. Isacoff WH et al. High-dose methotrexate therapy of solid tumors; observations relating to clinical toxicity. *Med Pediatr Oncol* 1976;2:319.
186. Isacoff WH et al. Pharmacokinetics of high-dose methotrexate with citrovorum factor rescue. *Cancer Treatment Reports* 1977;61:1665.
187. Nirenberg A et al. High dose methotrexate with CF rescue: predictive value of serum methotrexate concentrations and corrective measures to avert toxicity. *Cancer Treatment Reports* 1977;61:779.
188. Stoller RC et al. Use of plasma pharmacokinetics to predict and prevent methotrexate toxicity. *N Engl J Med* 1977;297:630.
189. Rechnitzer C et al. Methotrexate in the plasma and cerebrospinal fluid of children treated with intermediate dose methotrexate. *Acta Paediatr Scand* 1981;70:615.
190. Arndt CA et al. Comparison of results of a pilot study of alternating vincristine/doxorubicin/cyclophosphamide and etoposide/ifosfamide with IRS-IV in intermediate risk rhabdomyosarcoma: a report from the Children's Oncology Group. *Pediatric Blood & Cancer* November 7, 2006. Epub ahead of print.
191. Pappo AS et al. Two consecutive phase II window trials of irinotecan alone or in combination with

vincristine for the treatment of metastatic rhabdomyosarcoma: The Children's Oncology Group. *J Clin Oncol* 2007;25:362.

192. http://www.cancer.gov/cancertopics/pdq/treatment/childrhabdomyosarcoma/healthprofessional. Accessed June 1, 2007.
193. Crist W et al. Intergroup Rhabdomyosarcoma Study-IV: results for patients with nonmetastatic disease. *J Clin Oncol* 2001;19:3091.
194. Crist WM et al. Prognosis in children with rhabdomyosarcoma: a report of the Intergroup Rhabdomyosarcoma Studies I and II. *J Clin Oncol* 1990;8:443.
195. Rodary C et al. Prognostic factors in 281 children with non-metastatic rhabdomyosarcoma (RMS) at diagnosis. *Med Pediatr Oncol* 1988; 16:71.
196. Crist W. et al. The Third Intergroup Rhabdomyosarcoma Study. *J Clin Oncol* 1995;13:610.
197. Raney B et al. Renal toxicity in patients receiving ifosfamide/mesna on intergroup rhabdomyosarcoma study (IRS)-IV Pilot regimens for gross residual sarcoma [Abstract]. *Proceedings of the American Society of Clinical Oncologists* 1993;12: 418.
198. Rossi R et al. Unilateral nephrectomy and cisplatin as risk factors of ifosfamide-induced nephrotoxicity: analysis of 120 patients. *J Clin Oncol* 1994;12:159.
199. Suarez A et al. Long-term follow-up of ifosfamide renal toxicity in children treated for malignant mesenchymal tumors: an International Society of Pediatric Oncology report. *J Clin Oncol* 1991;9: 2177.
200. Skinner R et al. Risk factors for ifosfamide nephrotoxicity in children. *Lancet* 1996;348:578.
201. Yehuda AB et al. False positive reaction for urinary ketones with mesna [Letter]. *Drug Intell Clin Pharm* 1987;21:547.

CHAPTER 92

Hematopoietic Stem Cell Transplantation

Jeannine S. McCune and Douglas J. Black

OVERVIEW

Worldwide, more than 30,000 autologous and 15,000 allogeneic hematopoietic stem cell transplantations (HCTs) are performed annually.[1] HCT is a medical procedure involving the infusion of hematopoietic stem cells into a patient, or the HCT recipient, to treat disease and/or restore normal hematopoiesis and lymphopoiesis. Originally, HCT developed from allogeneic bone marrow transplantation (BMT).[1] These early allogeneic BMTs involved administration of a myeloablative preparative regimen, which was followed by true "transplantation" of bone marrow from one individual to another. Bone marrow contains pluripotent stem cells and postthymic lymphocytes, which are responsible, respectively, for long-term hematopoietic reconstitution, immune recovery, and graft-versus-host disease (GVHD).[1] Subsequently, the "dose intensity" concept for cancer treatment was expanded to using myeloablative preparative regimens followed by autologous HCT. *Autologous HCT,* or infusion of a patient's own hematopoietic stem cells, allows for the administration of higher doses of chemotherapy, radiation, or both to treat cancer.[1,2] In the setting of autologous HCT, the hematopoietic stem cells "rescue" the patient from otherwise dose-limiting hematopoietic toxicity. During the 1990s, there was an improved understanding of the graft-versus-tumor (GVT) effect, where the donor's cytotoxic T lymphocytes suppress the recipient's malignancy. This led to investigations with reduced intensity or nonmyeloablative preparative regimens. These less toxic preparative regimens are used with the hope of expanding the availability of HCT to those patients whose pre-existing medical condition(s) or age prohibits use of myeloablative regimens.[3–5]

HCT is the only treatment available to many patients; however, it is associated with considerable morbidity and mortality with approximately 40% of advanced cancer patients

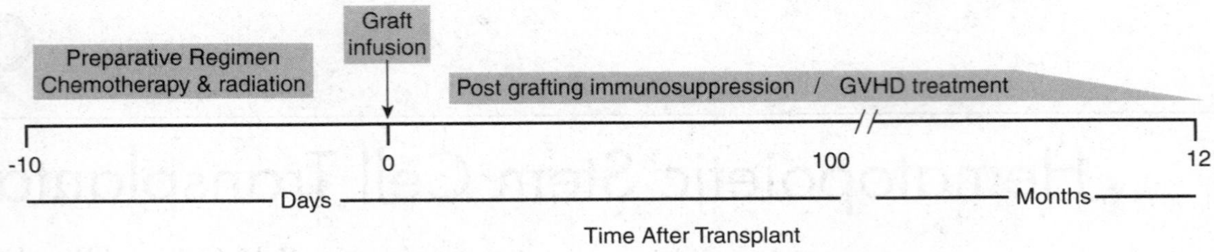

FIGURE 92-1 Basic schema for hematopoietic stem cell transplantation. Day 0 = bone marrow, peripheral blood progenitor cell, or umbilical cord blood infusion. Postgraft immunosuppression or graft-versus-host disease prophylaxis for allogeneic grafts only.

who undergo an HCT dying from complications due to this procedure.[1] The basic schema for HCT is illustrated in Figure 92-1. The combination of chemotherapy and/or radiation administered before infusion of hematopoietic stem cells is referred to as the *preparative* or conditioning regimen.[1] Its purpose is to eradicate the residual malignancy and, in the setting of an allogeneic HCT, to suppress the recipient's immunity.[1] Only myeloablative preparative regimens are used for autologous HCT, whereas myeloablative, reduced intensity, or nonmyeloablative preparative regimen may be used with allogeneic HCT. Myeloablative preparative regimens involve administration of near-lethal doses of chemotherapy and/or radiation, which are generally followed by a 1- to 2-day rest and then infusion of hematopoietic stem cells. Myeloablative preparative regimens have significant regimen-related toxicity and morbidity, and thus, are usually limited to healthy, younger (i.e., usually younger than 55 years) patients.[6] Alternatively, reduced intensity or nonmyeloablative transplantations (Fig. 92-2) are being performed with the hope of curing more cancer patients with less preparative regimen-related toxicity and by using the GVT effect. For most chemotherapy-based preparative regimens, the rest period is necessary to allow for elimination of toxic metabolites from the chemotherapy that could damage infused cells. After chemotherapy and radiation, a period of pancytopenia lasts until the infused hematopoietic stem cells reestablish functional hematopoiesis. This process is called *engraftment* and is commonly defined as the point at which a patient can maintain a sustained absolute neutrophil count (ANC) of >500 cells/mm^3 and a sustained platelet count of at least 20,000/mm^3 lasting 3 consecutive days without transfusions.[7] Graft rejection occurs when the patient cannot maintain functional hematopoiesis. Graft rejection can occur after either autologous or allogeneic HCT.

There are various sources of hematopoietic stem cells that can be used for HCT. The key properties of the hematopoietic stem cells are their ability to engraft, the speed of engraftment, and the durability of engraftment.[8] Peripheral blood progenitor cell transplant (PBPCT) has essentially replaced BMT for autologous HCT and is being increasingly used in the allogeneic setting.[9] Cord blood transplant (CBT) has increased the availability of allogeneic HCT to those in need of an urgent HCT or to those for whom suitable donors are not found.[1] Umbilical

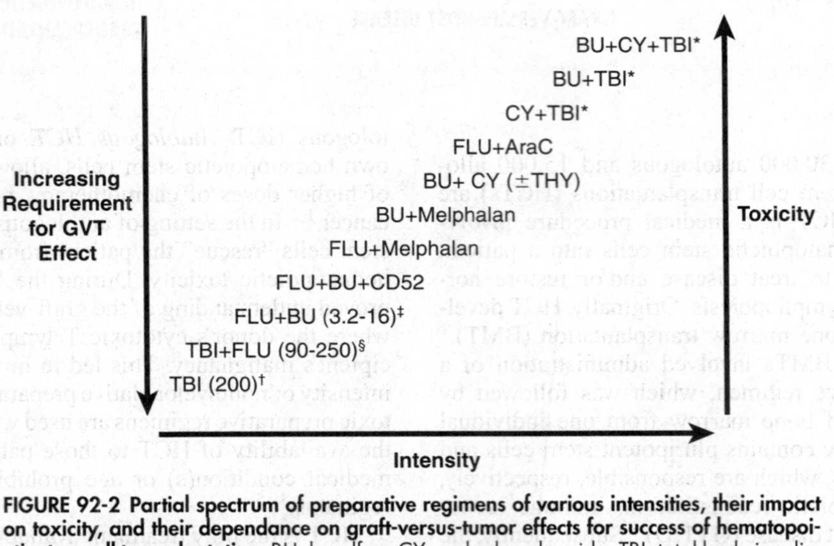

FIGURE 92-2 Partial spectrum of preparative regimens of various intensities, their impact on toxicity, and their dependance on graft-versus-tumor effects for success of hematopoietic stem cell transplantation. BU, busulfan; CY, cyclophosphamide; TBI, total body irradiation, FLU, fludarabine, AraC, cytarabine; THY, Thymoglobulin; CD52, anti-CD52 antibody (alemtuzumab). *TBI >1,200 cGy; †200 cGy; ‡3.2–16 mg/kg; §90–250 mg/m^2. *Source:* Reprinted from reference 70, with permission.

Table 92-1 Comparison of Hematopoietic Stem Cell Transplantation (HCT)

		Myeloablative	Nonmyeloablative
Risk[a]	*Autologous*	*Allogeneic*	*Allogeneic*
Relapse after HCT	+++	+	+
Rejection	–	+	++
Delayed engraftment	++	+	+
Graft-versus-host disease (GVHD)	–	+	++
Infection	+	++ to +++[b]	++ to +++[b]
Transplant-related morbidity	+	+++	++
Transplant-related mortality	+	++	+
Cost of procedure	++	+++	++ to +++

[a]Risk varies depending on underlying disease, patient characteristics, and previous medical history.
[b]Risk of infection increases with prolonged immunosuppression and/or chronic GVHD.

cord blood is rich in hematopoietic stem cells but has a limited volume; thus, both hematologic and immunologic reconstitution is delayed in CBT.[1]

The type of HCT performed depends on a number of factors, including type and status of disease, availability of a compatible donor, patient age, performance status, and organ function. Characteristics of autologous and allogeneic transplantation, with either myeloablative or nonmyeloablative preparative regimens, are compared in Table 92-1.[1] Many diseases are treated with autologous or allogeneic HCT and are listed in Table 92-2.[1] Modifications to the basic schema for HCT are necessary based on the immunologic source (i.e., allogeneic or autologous) and the anatomical source (i.e., bone marrow, peripheral blood progenitor cells [PBPCs], or umbilical cord blood) of the hematopoietic stem cells infused. The number of allogeneic HCTs has plateaued, most likely because of the limited availability of suitable donors, the limited success to date with HLA-disparate donors, and the increasing availability of targeted therapies for diseases that were traditionally treated with HCT (e.g., the replacement of HCT with imatinib as first-line therapy for chronic phase chronic myeloid leukemia [CML]).[10]

AUTOLOGOUS HEMATOPOIETIC STEM CELL TRANSPLANTATION

The defining characteristic of autologous HCT is that the donor and the recipient are the same individual. Consequently, pretransplantation and posttransplantation immunosuppression is unnecessary. Autologous hematopoietic stem cells must be obtained (i.e., harvested) before the myeloablative preparative regimen is administered and subsequently stored for administration after the preparative regimen. Essentially, these hematopoietic stem cells are administered as a rescue intervention to re-establish bone marrow function and avoid long-lasting, life-threatening marrow aplasia that results from the myeloablative preparative regimen.[11]

Indications for Autologous Hematopoietic Stem Cell Transplantation

1. P.J., a 46-year-old man, has diffuse large-cell B-cell non-Hodgkin lymphoma (NHL) in first relapse after a complete remission of 1 year duration. An 80% reduction in measurable disease is noted after two cycles of dexamethasone, high-dose cytarabine, and cisplatin [DHAP] salvage chemotherapy. P.J.'s bone marrow biopsy and lumbar puncture are negative for malignant cells. Is a myeloablative preparative regimen with autologous HCT indicated for P.J.?

Autologous HCT is used to treat a variety of malignancies (Table 92-2). NHL and multiple myeloma are the most common indications for this procedure and represent more than two-thirds of all autologous HCT.[1] Patients with NHL are more frequently treated with an autologous HCT than with

Table 92-2 Diseases Commonly Treated With Hematopoietic Stem Cell Transplantation[a]

Allogeneic	
Nonmalignant	Aplastic anemia
	Thalassemia major
	Severe combined immunodeficiency disease
	Wiskott-Aldrich syndrome
	Fanconi anemia
	Inborn errors of metabolism
Malignant	Acute myelogenous leukemia (AML)
	Acute lymphoblastic leukemia
	Chronic myeloid leukemia
	Myelodysplastic syndrome
	Myeloproliferative disorders
	Non-Hodgkin lymphoma (NHL)
	Hodgkin disease
	Chronic lymphocytic leukemia
	Multiple myeloma
Autologous	
Malignant	NHL
	Multiple myeloma
	AML
	Hodgkin disease
	Neuroblastoma
	Ovarian cancer
	Germ-cell tumors
Other diseases	Autoimmune disorders
	Amyloidosis

[a]Timing relative to diagnosis and other therapies may vary.
From reference 1.

an allogeneic HCT because autologous HCT has equivalent or superior survival to allogeneic HCT.[12,13] The usefulness of reduced intensity preparative regimens with allogeneic HCT is currently being evaluated for the treatment of NHL because of the potential advantages of a graft-versus-lymphoma effect and of using hematopoietic stem cells unexposed to prior cytotoxic chemotherapy.[3–5]

The most appropriate patient population and timing for autologous HCT in the treatment of NHL are being defined. A significant percentage of patients with aggressive NHL are cured with conventional chemotherapy alone. Adding autologous HCT to initial combination chemotherapy does not improve outcomes in patients with aggressive NHL.[14–16] The primary eligibility criterion for autologous HCT is relapsed disease that is chemotherapy sensitive or refractory.[17] In a randomized, controlled trial,[18] autologous BMT, compared with conventional chemotherapy with DHAP, resulted in a 5-year event-free survival of 46% and 12%, respectively ($p = 0.001$). Overall 5-year survival was 53% in the BMT group and 32% in the conventional chemotherapy patients ($p = 0.038$).[18] Prospective studies comparing preparative regimens, stem cell mobilization techniques, and stem cell source (i.e., BMT vs. PBPCT) are not available; however, autologous PBPCT has become the standard of care, most likely owing to the improved outcomes with PBPCT in other disease settings.[14]

P.J. has minimal residual disease that has demonstrated chemotherapy sensitivity (i.e., he had a partial response to chemotherapy). Long-term prognosis will be improved with autologous PBPCT rather than further conventional chemotherapy, as described previously.[18] Thus, autologous PBPCT is indicated.

Harvesting Autologous Hematopoietic Stem Cells

2. What is the best way to harvest and preserve harvested hematopoietic stem cells?

Autologous PBPCs have essentially replaced bone marrow at many HCT centers because PBPCs result in earlier engraftment than bone marrow.[9] Because the harvest occurs before administering the preparative regimen, autologous hematopoietic stem cells must be cryopreserved.[1] Hematopoietic stem cells are usually frozen below –120°C and used within a few weeks, although, when frozen, they are viable for years.[1] Dimethylsulfoxide (DMSO) is the cryopreservative commonly used to protect hematopoietic stem cells from damage during freezing and thawing. Infusion of hematopoietic stem cells stored in DMSO can be associated with toxicities due to the DMSO itself. During infusion, DMSO is associated with skin flushing, nausea, diarrhea, dyspnea, hypotension, arrhythmias, and, rarely, anaphylactic reactions.[19] Although contamination of grafts with tumor cells contributes to relapse of hematologic cancers, purging the grafts of tumor cells does not appear to improve survival.[1]

Relative to a bone marrow graft, a PBPC graft results in a higher number of hematopoietic stem cells that are harvested and thus infused. This results in a PBPC graft having more rapid neutrophil and platelet recovery (i.e., a shorter duration of neutropenia or thrombocytopenia), fewer platelet transfusions, fewer days of intravenous (IV) antibiotics, and a shorter duration of hospitalization compared to a bone marrow graft. Thus, the shift to the use of PBPCs over bone marrow for autologous HCT is primarily because of the more rapid engraftment and less invasive collection methods.[9]

Mobilization and Collection of Autologous Peripheral Blood Progenitor Cells

3. For PBPC mobilization, P.J. received one dose of cyclophosphamide 4 g/m² IV on day 1, followed by filgrastim 10 mcg/kg/day subcutaneously (SC) beginning on day 2 and continuing through completion of pheresis. Twelve days after receiving cyclophosphamide, P.J.'s white blood cell (WBC) count recovered to 3,000/mm³ and pheresis was begun. An adequate number of PBPCs is collected after two pheresis sessions are processed and then stored. What was the rationale for administering filgrastim and cyclophosphamide? What determines the duration of pheresis?

[SI units WBC 3,000 × 10^6 cells/L]

There is a low frequency of PBPCs in the peripheral circulation. Thus, mobilizing PBPC from the marrow compartment and increasing their numbers in the peripheral circulation is necessary to collect sufficient numbers of PBPCs for clinical use. Mobilization will lead to collection of sufficient numbers of autologous PBPCs in most patients, although a significant minority of patients has poor mobilization.[9]

PBPCs are obtained by administering a mobilizing agent(s) followed by leukapheresis, which is an outpatient procedure similar to dialysis.[9] Hematopoietic growth factors (HGFs) alone or in combination with myelosuppressive chemotherapy are used to mobilize of PBPCs.[9] The HGF granulocyte-macrophage colony-stimulating factor (sargramostim, Leukine) and granulocyte colony-stimulating factor (filgrastim, Neupogen) are used as mobilizing agents for PBPC collection.[9,20] Both HGFs reliably mobilize PBPCs, with filgrastim providing a higher PBPC yield.[9] The most frequently used filgrastim doses for autologous PBPC mobilization are in the range of 10 to 24 mcg/kg/day SC.[9,20] PBPC yield is higher when pheresis is started at day 5 (vs. day 6), with the optimal yield being 3 to 7 hours after filgrastim administration.[9]

Myelosuppressive chemotherapy stimulates stem cell and progenitor cell proliferation. The combination of chemotherapy with filgrastim enhances PBPC mobilization relative to filgrastim alone.[9] The chemotherapy also treats the underlying malignancy, but increases the risk of neutropenia.[9] No mobilization chemotherapy regimen is clearly superior, which has led to incorporating PBPC mobilization into a cycle of disease-specific chemotherapy. Examples of PBPC mobilization chemotherapy regimens are single-agent cyclophosphamide or ifosfamide, carboplatin, and etoposide.[9] Stem cell toxic agents, such as melphalan and carmustine, should be avoided because they lower the quantity and quality of PBPCs.[9] The HGF is initiated 24 hours after completion of chemotherapy. Pheresis begins when the peripheral WBC count begins to recover to >1 to 3 × 10^9 cells/L.[9]

Pheresis is continued daily until the target number of PBPCs per kilogram of the recipients' weight is obtained.[9] For adult recipients, the number of cells infused that expresses the CD34 antigen (i.e., $CD34^+$ cells) is the most reliable

Table 92-3 Representative Myeloablative Preparative Regimens Used in Hematopoietic Stem Cell Transplantation (HCT)

Type of HCT	*Disease State*	*Regimen*	*Dose/Schedule*
Allogeneic[102]	Hematologic malignancies[a]	Cyclophosphamide (CY)/total body irradiation (TBI)	CY 60 mg/kg/day IV on 2 consecutive days before TBI 1,000–1,575 rads fractionated over 1–7 days
Allogeneic Autologous[62,81,84]	Acute and chronic leukemias	Busulfan (BU)/CY	BU adult 1 mg/kg/dose PO or 0.8 mg/kg/dose IV Q 6 hr for 16 doses Children <12 kg 1.1 mg/kg/dose IV Q 6 hr for 16 doses CY 50 mg/kg/day IV QD for 4 days after BU or 60 mg/kg/day IV QD for 2 days after BU
Autologous[18]	Non-Hodgkin lymphoma	BEAC (carmustine/etoposide/cytarabine/cyclophosphamide)	Carmustine 300 mg/m^2/day IV, day –6 Etoposide 200 mg/m^2/day BID IV for 4 days, days –5 to –2 Cytarabine 200 mg/m^2/day IV BID for 4 days, days –5 to –2 CY 35 mg/kg/day IV for 4 days, days –5 to –2 Mesna 50 mg/kg/day IV for 4 days, days –5 to –2

[a] Includes acute myelogenous leukemia, acute lymphocytic leukemia, chronic myelogenous leukemia, non-Hodgkin lymphoma, and Hodgkin disease.

indicator of an adequate PBPC population and predictor of durable engraftment.[9] The CD34 antigen is expressed on 1% to 4% of human marrow cells. It is expressed on virtually all unipotent and multipotent colony-forming cells and on precursors of colony-forming cells, but not on mature peripheral blood cells.[21] A variety of different thresholds have been identified regarding the minimal number of $CD34^+$ cells needed for an autologous PBPCT to produce rapid and complete (i.e., WBC, red blood cell [RBC], platelet) engraftment in adults. The threshold range has varied from 1 to 3 $\times$ 10^6 $CD34^+$ cells/kg of recipient weight, with more rapid platelet and neutrophil engraftment occurring with $\geq$5 to 8 $\times$ 10^6 $CD34^+$ cells/kg of recipient weight.

More intensive prior chemotherapy or radiation therapy is associated with a lower yield of $CD34^+$ cells. There is a paucity of information regarding the parameters associated with engraftment in children undergoing an autologous PBPCT.[22] After pheresis, the cells are cryopreserved, stored, thawed, and infused into the patient as described in the "Harvesting Autologous Hematopoietic Stem Cells" section.

Myeloablative Preparative Regimens

4. What are the goals and characteristics of agents used for myeloablative preparative regimens in patients like P.J.?

The primary goal of P.J.'s high-dose, myeloablative preparative regimen is to eradicate residual malignancy. With autologous HCT, there is no need to induce immunosuppression because the donor and recipient are genetically identical.[1] Combination chemotherapy with multiple alkylating agents comprises the most common high-dose regimen before autologous HCT. Alkylating agents are used because they exhibit a steep dose–response curve for various malignancies and are characterized by dose-limiting bone marrow suppression.[2] Ideally, if combinations of antineoplastics are used, they should have nonhematologic toxicities that do not overlap and are not life threatening. Examples of common myeloablative regimens used with hematopoietic stem cell support are illustrated in Table 92-3. The early and late toxicities to myeloablative conditioning are listed in Table 92-4.

Complications of Autologous Hematopoietic Stem Cell Transplantation

5. What complications must be anticipated as a consequence of autologous HCT? How can these be minimized? How can treatment be provided in an outpatient setting?

The most common cause of death after autologous HCT is the primary disease. The more concerning toxicities of the preparative regimen are infection and organ failure, each occurring in less than 5% of the patients. Because autologous HCT is not complicated by profound immunosuppression or GVHD, supportive care strategies vary from allogeneic HCT in the early and later recovery periods. Isolation and use of laminar air flow rooms are unnecessary, although many centers continue to provide care for patients undergoing autologous HCT in high-efficiency particulate air (HEPA)-filtered rooms. The use of autologous PBPCT is associated with shorter periods of neutropenia and less need for clinical resources. Thus, some HCT centers have developed programs that incorporate outpatient care into the initial recovery; these programs also offer cost savings to the payer for health services.[23,24] Successful outpatient care during administration of a myeloablative preparative regimen and the neutropenic period requires careful development and implementation of the necessary supportive care

Table 92-4 Common Toxicities Associated With Myeloablative Allogeneic Hematopoietic Stem Cell Transplantation

Early	*Late*
Febrile neutropenia	Increased susceptibility to infections
Nausea, vomiting, diarrhea	Endocrine disorders (hypothyroidism, hemorrhagic cystitis, infertility, growth retardation)
Mucositis	Neurocognitive changes
Veno-occlusive disease	Secondary malignant neoplasms
Renal dysfunction	Chronic GVHD
Cardiotoxicity	Cataracts
Pneumonitis	
Graft rejection	
Acute graft-versus-host disease (GVHD)	

strategies to prevent or minimize infection, chemotherapy-induced nausea and vomiting (CINV), pain, and bleeding, along with admission criteria for more severe complications. Use of prophylactic oral antibiotics and once-daily IV antibiotics to prevent or treat uncomplicated febrile neutropenia have facilitated outpatient care and prevented many patients from being hospitalized.[25] In addition, outpatient care during autologous HCT demands that HCT centers have appropriate resources, facilities, and staff to provide 24-hour patient care coverage. Patients undergoing outpatient care must meet eligibility criteria, including the availability of caregivers 24 hours a day and housing within close proximity to the HCT center.

Hematopoietic Growth Factors After Autologous Peripheral Blood Progenitor Cell Infusion

6. After 10 days of rest, P.J. is admitted for his autologous BMT. He receives a myeloablative preparative regimen with cyclophosphamide, carmustine, and etoposide with an autologous PBPC graft. An order is written to begin filgrastim 5 mcg/kg/day SC, beginning on day 0 and continuing until the ANC has recovered to 500/mm^3 for 2 consecutive days. What is the rationale for filgrastim in P.J. following the transplant procedure?

[SI units: ANC 500 × 10^6 cells/L]

Autologous HCTs, regardless of the stem cell source, are associated with profound aplasia due to the myeloablative preparative regimen. Aplasia typically lasts 20 to 30 days after an autologous BMT and 7 to 14 days after an autologous PBPCT.[9] During this period of aplasia, patients are at high risk for complications such as bleeding and infection. Filgrastim and sargramostim exert their effects by stimulating the proliferation of committed progenitor cells, and, once engraftment occurs, hematopoietic recovery may be accelerated.

Several factors need to be considered when discussing the role of HGF in accelerating engraftment after HCT. First, the anatomical source of hematopoietic stem cells predicts the degree of benefit. The greatest benefit is enhanced neutrophil recovery and decreased use of associated resources in the setting of autologous BMT. The benefits of the HGF have been shown in several large multicenter, randomized, double-blind, placebo-controlled trials.[26–28] The majority of the trials suggest HGF administration is associated with a shorter time to neutrophil engraftment (by 4–7 days), less infectious complications, and shorter hospitalization after autologous BMT.[26,27,29] Survival is equivalent in those who received an HGF or a placebo.[26,28]

Although some studies in the autologous PBPCT setting note more rapid neutrophil recovery after HGF use, others report no difference in infection rates and minimal decreases in associated resource use such as the duration of hospitalization.[27,29–31] In addition, sargramostim administration had no benefit (i.e., neutrophil and platelet engraftment) over placebo after autologous PBPCT in one trial.[32] Although clinical practice guidelines for HGF support their use after both autologous BMT and PBPCT, pharmacoeconomic analyses are needed to further evaluate the true benefit of HGFs after autologous PBPCT.

Filgrastim is preferred for this indication in clinical practice. The reason most commonly cited, is the desire to avoid febrile reactions associated with sargramostim, which complicate interpretation of febrile neutropenia. Although sargramostim or filgrastim theoretically may stimulate proliferation of leukemia myeloblasts, no evidence to date suggests that the incidence of leukemia relapse is higher in patients who receive these HGFs after autologous or allogeneic HCT.[32,33] This may be due to the fact that patients with leukemia are usually in remission at the time of HCT. Thus, the population of residual leukemia cells is probably minimal.

Although both filgrastim and sargramostim successfully hasten neutrophil recovery, neither agent stimulates platelet production or augments platelet recovery.[26,27] This is an important consideration because thrombocytopenia is often a cause of prolonged hospitalization in the HCT patient. Successful engraftment of all hematopoietic stem cell lines will likely require combinations of growth factors that work in concert to augment hematopoiesis. However, erythropoietin (Epogen, Procrit) and interleukin (IL)-11 (Neumega) have only been used experimentally in the HCT patient. At this time, there is no established role for either agent in the care of these patients.

In summary, P.J. is undergoing autologous PBPCT for the treatment of a lymphoid malignancy. Thus, either sargramostim or filgrastim is an acceptable option for accelerating engraftment. Whether the addition of either agent will reduce infection and improve other clinically relevant outcomes is debatable.[20] A complete blood cell (CBC) count with differential should be obtained daily. Filgrastim should be continued until neutrophil recovery is achieved.

ALLOGENEIC HEMATOPOIETIC STEM CELL TRANSPLANTATION

Allogeneic HCT involves the transplantation of hematopoietic stem cells obtained from a donor's bone marrow, PBPCs, or umbilical cord blood to a patient. Thus, to understand the application of and complications after allogeneic HCT, a working knowledge of immunology and the MHC and HLA in humans is necessary.[34]

Eligibility criteria for allogeneic HCT vary between institutions. Having a matched sibling donor is no longer a requirement for allogeneic HCT, because improved immunosuppressive regimens and the National Marrow Donor Program have allowed an increase in the use of unrelated or related matched or mismatched HCT.[35] Potential donors also include haploidentical donors, who are a parent, sibling, or child of a parent with only one identical HLA haplotype. HCT with a haploidentical donor was initially associated with high rates of graft failure and GVHD, but recent technological advances have improved outcomes. Haploidentical HCT involves another alloreactive mechanism involving NK cells, which may be associated with reduced relapse rates in acute myelogenous leukemia (AML) patients.[1]

Normal renal, hepatic, pulmonary, and cardiac functions are necessary for eligibility at most centers. Historically, patients older than 55 years were excluded from allogeneic HCT because they were more likely to succumb to transplantation-related complications. However, many centers are now considering patients up to 65 years old and basing their selection criteria on physiological rather than biological age.

Indications for Allogeneic Hematopoietic Stem Cell Transplantation

7. B.S., a 22-year-old man, has AML in first remission after induction chemotherapy with standard doses of cytarabine and daunorubicin and consolidation with high-dose cytarabine. B.S. has poor risk cytogenetics, with abnormalities of 11q23 and inversion 3. Thus he will receive an allogeneic HCT as part of postremission therapy. HLA typing performed on family members has identified a fully HLA-matched sibling donor. B.S. returns to clinic today for a pretransplantation workup. At this time, his physical examination is noncontributory. All laboratory values are within normal limits. A bone marrow biopsy reveals <5% blasts. B.S. has a normal electrocardiogram and cardiac wall motion study. His renal and hepatic, and pulmonary function tests are normal. Is an allogeneic HCT indicated for B.S.?

B.S. has a diagnosis of AML, which is one of the most common indications for allogeneic HCT.[1] The primary indications for allogeneic HCT include treatment of otherwise fatal diseases of the bone marrow or immune system (Table 92-2). The optimal role and timing of allogeneic HCT, in contrast to other therapies, remains controversial,[36] especially because treatment options for AML have increased. The National Comprehensive Cancer Network Guidelines for AML patients include the use of allogeneic HCT. A matching sibling or alternative donor (e.g., matched unrelated donor) HCT is recommended as part of postremission therapy in patients with preceding hematologic disease (e.g., myelodysplasia, secondary AML) or poor risk cytogenetics, such as B.S.[37] Current research efforts focus on the use of reduced intensity preparative regimens and the utility of HCT relative to novel targeted agents in the hope of improving the outcome of allogeneic HCT.[37] B.S. is eligible for allogeneic HCT by virtue of his cytogenetics and the availability of a histocompatible donor. In addition, he meets age and organ function eligibility requirements and is in complete remission with minimal residual disease. The decision regarding timing of allogeneic HCT compared with other therapies must be made, weighing the aforementioned risks and benefits. B.S. can either undergo allogeneic HCT now or receive consolidation chemotherapy and delay HCT until early in his first relapse.

Histocompatibility

8. How does histocompatibility influence the risks for graft rejection and graft-versus-host reactions in patients like B.S. who undergo an allogeneic HCT?

Because the tissue transplanted in allogeneic HCT is immunologically active, there is potential for bidirectional graft rejection.[1] In the first scenario, cytotoxic T cells and NK cells belonging to the host (recipient) recognize MHC antigens of the graft (donor hematopoietic stem cells) and elicit a rejection response. In the second scenario, immunologically active cells in the graft recognize host MHC antigens and elicit an immune response. The former is referred to as host-versus-graft disease and the latter as GVHD. Host-versus-graft effects are more common in solid organ transplantation. When host-versus-graft effects occur in allogeneic HCT, they are referred to as graft rejection, which results in ineffective hematopoiesis (i.e., adequate ANC and/or platelet counts were not obtained). Therefore, an essential first step for patients eligible for HCT is finding an HLA-compatible graft with an acceptable risk of rejection and GVHD.

Graft rejection is least likely to occur with a syngeneic donor, meaning that the recipient and host are identical (monozygotic) twins. Identical twins occur spontaneously in nature in approximately 1 in 100 births; thus, it is unlikely that a patient would have a syngeneic donor. In those patients without a syngeneic donor, initial HLA typing is conducted on family members because the likelihood of complete histocompatibility between unrelated individuals is remote. Siblings are the most likely individuals to be histocompatible within a family. However, <30% of potential HCT recipients have an HLA-identical sibling.[1]

Determination of histocompatibility between potential donors and the patient is completed before allogeneic HCT.[34] Initially, HLA typing performed using blood samples and compatibility for class I MHC antigens (HLA-A, HLA-B, and HLA-C) is determined through serologic and DNA-based testing methods.[38] In vitro reactivity between donor and recipient can also be assessed in mixed lymphocyte culture, a test used to measure compatibility of the MHC class II antigens (HLA-DR, HLA-DP, HLA-DQ).[38] Currently, most clinical and research laboratories are also performing molecular DNA typing using polymerase chain reaction (PCR) methodology to determine the HLA allele sequence.[38] A donor–recipient pair with different HLA antigens (i.e., "antigen mismatched") always has different alleles, whereas pairs with the same allele always have the same antigen and are termed "matched." However, some pairs have the same HLA antigen but different alleles and are thus "allele mismatched."[39] (See Chapter 34 for full discussion of histocompatibility.)

Lack of an HLA-matched sibling donor can be a barrier to allogeneic HCT. The use of alternative sources of allogeneic hematopoietic stem cells, such as related donors mismatched at one or more HLA loci, or phenotypically (i.e., serologically) matched unrelated donors has been evaluated.[35] Establishment of the National Marrow Donor Program has helped increase the pool of potential donors for allogeneic HCT.[35] Through this program, an HLA-matched unrelated volunteer donor might be identified. Recipients of an unrelated graft are more likely to experience graft failure and acute GVHD relative to recipients of a matched-sibling donor.[40] Thus, work is ongoing to identify factors that predict graft failure or GVHD to improve the availability and safety of unrelated donor transplants[41] (see "Graft Rejection" section).

The preparative regimen or GVHD prophylaxis may be altered based on the mismatch between the donor and the recipient. The risk of graft failure decreases with better matches, such that those with a class I (i.e., HLA-A, -B, or -C) antigen mismatch have the highest risk of rejection compared with those with just one class I allele mismatch who have a minimal risk. Graft failure does not appear to be associated with mismatch at a single class II antigen or allele.[38] GVHD, both acute and chronic, and survival have also been associated with disparity for class I and II antigens and alleles.[42,43]

Harvesting, Preparing, and Transplanting Allogeneic Hematopoietic Stem Cells

9. What methods can be used to harvest hematopoietic stem cells from B.S.'s histocompatible sibling and prepare them for transplant? Are there any advantages to the use of bone marrow, PBPCs, or umbilical cord blood as a source for hematopoietic stem cells?

The method of harvesting allogeneic hematopoietic stem cells varies according to the site of harvest (i.e., bone marrow, peripheral blood, or umbilical cord blood).

ABO incompatibility increases the complexity of HCT, but is not an obstacle to HCT. The hematopoietic stem cells may need additional processing if the donor and recipient are ABO incompatible, which occurs in 30% to 40% of sibling donor HCTs and is higher in unrelated donor HCT.[44] Various strategies used to manage blood support for ABO-incompatible HCT recipients include removing RBC from the HCT product, as well as transfusing type O RBCs to minimize the risk of immune-mediated hemolytic anemia and thrombotic microangiopathic syndromes.[44]

Bone Marrow

Harvesting bone marrow entails a surgical procedure in which marrow is obtained from the iliac crests. Allogeneic bone marrow is obtained from the donor under local or general anesthesia on day 0 of BMT.[1] Multiple aspirations of marrow are obtained from the posterior iliac crests until a volume with a sufficient number of hematopoietic stem cells is collected (e.g., 600–1,200 mL of bone marrow). The bone marrow is then processed to remove fat or marrow emboli and is usually immediately infused intravenously into the patient like a blood transfusion. Bone marrow is the primary graft source for allogenic transplant in children, accounting for 60% of HCT in this population with PBPCs and cord blood accounting for the remainder.[45]

Peripheral Blood Progenitor Cells

Peripheral blood has replaced marrow for allogeneic HCT in adults.[1,45] Marrow stem cells continuously detach, enter the circulation, and return to the marrow; thus, the peripheral blood is a convenient source of hematopoietic stem cells. The number of PBPCs is estimated by using the cell surface molecule CD34 as a surrogate marker. The number of circulating $CD34^+$ cells in blood is increased by mobilizing them from the marrow. The most commonly used regimen to mobilize allogeneic (healthy) donors is a 4- to 5-day course of filgrastim, 10 to 16 mcg/kg/day SC, followed by leukapheresis on the fourth or fifth day when peripheral blood levels of $CD34^+$ cells peak.[46] An adequate number of hematopoietic stem cells is usually obtained with one to two pheresis collections, with the optimal number of $CD34^+$ collected being 5 to 8 $\times 10^6$ cells/kg of recipient body weight.[47,48] Higher cell doses have been associated with not only more rapid engraftment, but also fewer fungal infections and improved overall survival.[49] Hematopoietic stem cells obtained from the peripheral blood are processed like bone marrow–derived stem cells and may be infused immediately into the recipient or frozen for future use. Allogeneic donation of PBPC has a similar level of physical discomfort to bone marrow donation; however, PBPC donation leads to quicker recovery.[48] The donor may experience musculoskeletal pain, headache, mild increases in hepatic enzyme or lactate dehydrogenase levels due to filgrastim administration, and hypocalcemia due to citrate accumulation, which decreases ionized calcium concentrations during pheresis.[50]

Compared to bone marrow, PBPC infusions are associated with quicker neutrophil and platelet engraftment.[1] In patients with a hematologic malignancy and a matched sibling donor, PBPCT is also associated with lower relapse rates and increased disease-free survival rates.[51] However, PBPC grafts contain more T cells than bone marrow grafts.[1] PBPCT has a similar incidence of acute GVHD, but an approximately 20% higher incidence of extensive stage and overall chronic GVHD.[51]

Umbilical Cord Blood

Blood from the umbilical cord and the placenta is rich in hematopoietic stem cells but limited in volume.[1] Thus, CBT offers an alternative stem cell source to those patients who do not have an acceptable matched related or unrelated donor. After consent is obtained, the cord blood cells are obtained in the delivery room after birth and delivery of the placenta.[52] The cord blood is then processed, and a sample is sent for HLA typing and frozen for future use. At least 2,000 HCTs with cord blood donors have been performed, with more than 70,000 cord blood units banked for future HCT.[52] It is unclear how long cord blood can be viably cryopreserved.[52]

HCT with an unrelated cord blood donor has several potential advantages over unrelated marrow or PBPC donors.[52] Specifically, cord blood is readily available, which leads to a more rapid time to HCT and the ability to tolerate greater degrees of HLA disparity.[52] CBT has less stringent HLA matching requirements than bone marrow or PBPC grafts, because mismatched cord blood cells are less likely to cause GVHD while still maintaining GVT activity.[1] The less stringent HLA requirements increase the likelihood of identifying a suitable allogeneic donor, which is particularly beneficial for minority populations who are underrepresented in adult registries and often lack matched stem cell sources.[1] Outcomes in umbilical cord blood recipients are improved, with fewer HLA mismatches and greater numbers of $CD34^+$ cells.[1] However, the limited number and quality of hematopoietic stem cells in cord blood are potential disadvantages. To improve engraftment, research is ongoing with two cord blood grafts each from different donors, with a cord blood and HLA-matched haploidentical PBPC grafts, and ex vivo expansion of cord blood cells.[1]

Most CBT clinical data are derived from retrospective case series. These data have shown that CBT from a related or unrelated donor is effective in children with cancer and nonmalignant conditions.[52] Platelet and neutrophil engraftment is slower in CBT, with a lower risk of acute and chronic GVHD and similar survival rates relative to a BMT.[52] In children, engraftment is related to the dose of nucleated cells with an optimal dose of approximately 2 $\times 10^7$ nucleated cells per kilogram of recipient body weight.[53] This raises the question as to whether a CBT can provide enough nucleated cells to adequately engraft within an adult. In adults who do not have a related or unrelated donor for bone marrow or PBPC donation, a CBT is feasible when at least 1×10^7 nucleated cells per kilogram of recipient body weight are administered.[54]

In summary, it is most reasonable to harvest PBPCs from B.S.'s sibling to use for his myeloablative HCT.

Graft-versus-Tumor Effect

10. What is the GVT effect? Which tumors are most responsive to this effect?

Initial clinical evidence of a GVT effect came from the observation that patients with GVHD had lower relapse rates compared with those who did not.[55,56] This suggests a GVT effect due to the donor lymphocytes. Further support for a GVT effect is the higher rate of leukemia relapse after T-cell–depleted BMT, in part due to the reduction in GVHD and concomitant loss of GVT effect.[57,58] The effectiveness of donor lymphocyte infusions in patients who experienced relapse after allogeneic HCT also suggests a GVT effect. Lymphocytes are collected from the peripheral blood of the donor and administered to the recipient. Eradication of the recurrent malignancy is due to either specific targeting of the tumor antigens or to GVHD, which may affect cancer cells preferentially. Different illnesses vary in their responsiveness to donor lymphocyte infusions, with CML and acute leukemias being the most and least responsive, respectively.[59] Patients with certain solid tumors (e.g., renal cell carcinoma) also appear to benefit from a GVT effect.[60] These data gave rise to the use of reduced intensity and nonmyeloablative preparative regimens, which rely on the GVT effect.

Preparative Regimens for Allogeneic Hematopoietic Stem Cell Transplantation

Myeloablative Preparative Regimens

11. What is the rationale for using myeloablative preparative regimens for patients like B.S. who are to receive an allogeneic HCT? What types of regimens are used, and what is recommended for B.S.?

The combination of chemotherapy and/or radiation used in allogeneic HCT is referred to as the preparative or conditioning regimen. The rationale for high-dose myeloablative preparative regimens was similar to that discussed in the "Autologous Hematopoietic Stem Cell Transplantation" section of this chapter. Specifically, infusion of hematopoietic stem cells circumvents dose-limiting myelosuppression, maximizing the potential value of the steep dose–response curve to alkylating agents and radiation,[2] and suppressing the host immune system. The preparative regimen is designed to eradicate immunologically active host tissues (lymphoid tissue and macrophages) and to prevent or minimize the development of host-versus-graft reactions. In contrast, a myeloablative preparative regimen may not be necessary if a histocompatible allogeneic HCT is performed on a patient with a poorly functioning immune system (e.g., severe combined immunodeficiency disease).[61] In the absence of a functioning immune system, the likelihood of a host-versus-graft reaction to histocompatible donor hematopoietic stem cells is small. Similarly, patients undergoing syngeneic transplantation do not require immunosuppressive preparative regimens before HCT because the donor and the patient are genetically identical. Thus, the preparative regimen is tailored to the primary disease and to HLA compatibility between the recipient–donor pair.

Examples of common preparative regimens for allogeneic HCT are shown in Table 92-3.[18,62,63] Table 92-4 lists the common toxicities associated with myeloablative allogeneic HCT. Most allogeneic preparative regimens for the treatment of hematologic malignancies contain cyclophosphamide, radiation, or both. The combination of cyclophosphamide and total body irradiation (TBI) was one of the first preparative regimens used, and it is still used widely today. This regimen is immunosuppressive and has inherent activity against hematologic malignancies (e.g., leukemias, lymphomas). TBI is myeloablative and immunosuppressive, does not have cross-resistance to chemotherapy, and also reaches sites not affected by chemotherapy (e.g., the central nervous system).[1] Toxicity to TBI is considerable and although fractionating its dose reduces toxicity, research is ongoing to identify newer methods of selective radiation with increased specificity.[1] The toxicity of TBI and the scarcity of facilities for its delivery have led to the development of radiation-free preparative regimens. Modifications of the cyclophosphamide-TBI preparative regimen include replacing TBI with other agents (e.g., busulfan) and adding other chemotherapeutic or monoclonal agents to the existing regimen. These measures are designed to minimize the long-term toxicities associated with TBI (e.g., growth retardation in children, cataracts) or to provide additional antitumor activity, respectively. In the case of a mismatched allogeneic HCT with a substantially increased chance of graft rejection, antithymocyte globulin (ATG) may also be added to the preparative regimen to further immunosuppress the recipient.

The optimal myeloablative preparative regimen for allogeneic HCT is challenging to study because several indications for HCT (e.g., thalassemia) are rare enough that it is not feasible or is too cost-prohibitive to conduct clinical trials adequately powered to detect clinically relevant differences. However, the long-term outcomes of busulfan/cyclophosphamide (BU/CY) and CY/TBI in patients with AML and CML have been compared in a meta-analysis of four clinical trials.[64] Equivalent rates of long-term complications were present between the two preparative regimens, except for a greater risk of cataracts with CY/TBI and alopecia with BU/CY. Overall and disease-free survival rates were similar in patients with CML, whereas there was a trend for improved disease-free survival with CY/TBI in AML patients. Thus, the preparative regimen can be tailored to the primary disease and HLA compatibility.

Based on these data, the CY/TBI preparative regimen is preferred for B.S. because he has AML in first remission.

Reduced Intensity or Nonmyeloablative Preparative Regimens

12. Describe the rationale for nonmyeloablative preparative regimens. Is B.S. a candidate for such a regimen?

The regimen-related toxicity of a myeloablative preparative regimen (Table 92-4) limits the use of allogeneic HCT to younger patients who have minimal comorbidities. Since most cancer patients are elderly myeloablative HCT cannot be offered to a substantial portion of these patients.[65] An improved understanding of the GVT effect led to the development of a strongly immunosuppressive but not myeloablative (i.e., a reduced intensity) preparative regimens.[1] Now reduced intensity preparative regimens account for 30% of allogeneic transplants.[45] More than 60% of patients receiving reduced intensity preparative regimens are older than 50 years.[45]

There is a wide spectrum of reduced intensity preparative regimens (Fig. 92-2), with the nonmyeloablative regimens causing the least amount of myelosuppression. More intensive myeloablation is required for engraftment in the setting of unrelated donor or HLA-mismatched related HCT.[66] Reduced intensity regimens do not completely eliminate the host's normal and malignant cells and depend on the graft to eradicate remaining cancer. Thus, these preparative regimens may be preferable in those malignancies in which immunologic elimination of the malignant stem cells is possible.[1] The donor cells eradicate residual host hematopoiesis, and the GVT effects generally occur after the development of full donor T-cell chimerism.[60] After engraftment, mixed chimerism should be present as evidenced by the ability to detect both donor- and recipient-derived cells. Thus, if the graft is rejected, autologous recovery should promptly occur. Following a reduced intensity preparative regimen, mixed chimerism (defined as 5%–95% peripheral donor T cells) between the host and recipient develops, which allows for a GVT effect as the primary form of therapy. Chimerism is evaluated to monitor disease response and engraftment at varying time points. Chimerism is assessed within peripheral blood T cells and granulocytes and bone marrow using conventional (e.g., using sex chromosomes for opposite sex donors) and molecular (e.g., variable number of tandem repeats for same sex donors) methods. The methods used to characterize chimerism after HCT are reviewed elsewhere.[67–69] A few months after HCT, donor lymphocytes can be infused (called a "donor lymphocyte infusion") to augment the GVT activity.[1] The challenge is to maximize the GVT effect while minimizing the risk of GVHD. Therefore, GVHD prophylaxis, although different from that used with myeloablative regimens, is still necessary as is follow-up for infectious complications.

The safety and efficacy of these regimens have led to their wider application to nonmalignant conditions.[1] Reduced intensity preparative regimens lead to lower treatment-related mortality rates, but, they may be offset by higher relapse rates.[70] They are most effective in treating slow-growing cancers (e.g., chronic lymphocytic leukemia).[1] Because most of the data for reduced intensity preparative regimens are derived from older patients or those with comorbid conditions, they cannot be compared with data for myeloablative preparative regimens.[70] It is unclear if reduced intensity preparative regimens improve long-term survival of patients with malignant or nonmalignant diseases who are younger or without comorbid conditions. Prospective controlled trials are needed with stratification based on comorbidities, disease characteristics, pretransplant therapy, and hematopoietic stem cell source.[70]

There are a paucity of data regarding the optimal source of hematopoietic stem cells following reduced intensity preparative regimens. Most case series have combined data from PBPC and marrow grafts. But some data suggest that, compared to bone marrow grafts, PBPC is associated with quicker engraftment, earlier T-cell chimerism, longer progression-free survival, and a lower risk of graft rejection.[71,72]

B.S. is young and healthy enough to receive a myeloablative allogeneic HCT. Presently, reduced intensity HCT is not indicated as first-line therapy for any malignant or nonmalignant conditions. It is not an option for B.S.

Posttransplantation Immunosuppressive Therapy

13. What is the rationale for immunosuppressive therapy after an allogeneic HCT? What is recommended for B.S.?

After infusion of hematopoietic stem cells, immunosuppressive therapy is administered to prevent or minimize GVHD. Patients receiving syngeneic transplants or a T-cell–depleted histocompatible allogeneic transplant generally do not receive posttransplantation immunosuppressive therapy. In syngeneic transplantation, the donor and the patient are genetically identical, and GVHD should not be elicited. In T-cell depleted transplantation, the volume of donor T cells infused into the patient is usually insufficient to elicit a significant graft-versus-host reaction.[57,73] Numerous immunosuppressive agents given alone or in combination have been evaluated for the prevention of GVHD. Commonly used regimens after myeloablative HCT include cyclosporine or tacrolimus administered with a short course of low-dose methotrexate.[74] GVHD prophylaxis varies between a myeloablative and reduced intensity HCT (Table 92-5). Corticosteroids may also be used to prevent GVHD, but they are more commonly used to treat GVHD. In allogeneic HCT recipients without GVHD, immunosuppressive therapy is slowly tapered and discontinued over 6 months to 1 year because of immunologic tolerance. Over time, the immunologically active tissue between host and recipient become tolerant of one another and cease recognizing the other as foreign. In contrast, solid organ transplant recipients usually continue immunosuppressive therapy for the duration of the recipient's life.

Thus, B.S. should receive cyclosporine or tacrolimus administered with a short course of methotrexate for posttransplantation immunotherapy. This combination regimen will lower the risk of GVHD after his allogeneic HCT with a myeloablative preparative regimen.

Table 92-5 Common Reduced Intensity Preparative Regimens and Post Grafting Immunosuppresion[230]

Preparative Regimens	*Postgrafting Immunosuppression*
Fludarabine 30 mg/m^2/day IV on 3 consecutive days (–4, –3, –2), TBI 2 Gy as single fraction on day 0	Cyclosporine 6.25 mg/kg PO BID, days –3 to day + 100 with taper from day + 100 to + 180 Mycophenolate mofetil 15 mg/kg PO BID or TID, day + 0 to + 40 with taper from day + 40 to + 90
Fludarabine 25 mg/m^2/day IV for 5 days and melphalan 90 mg/m^2/day IV for 2 days	Tacrolimus to maintain trough blood concentration of 5–10 ng/mL with methotrexate 5 mg/m^2/day IV days + 1, + 3, + 6, + 11
Fludarabine 25–30 mg/m^2/day IV for 3–5 days, busulfan ≤9 mg/kg/total	

COMPARISON OF SUPPORTIVE CARE STRATEGIES BETWEEN AUTOLOGOUS AND ALLOGENEIC MYELOABLATIVE HEMATOPOIETIC STEM CELL TRANSPLANTATION

14. How do supportive care strategies used for myeloablative preparative regimens with an autologous graft differ from those described for an allogeneic graft?

Supportive care strategies common to patients receiving a myeloablative preparative regimen, regardless of whether they have received an autologous or allogeneic HCT, include use of indwelling central venous catheters; blood product support; and pharmacologic management of chemotherapy-induced nausea and vomiting (CINV), mucositis, and pain. These similarities are a function of the side effects of a myeloablative preparative regimen.

Because of the different needs for immunosuppression with an autologous and allogeneic HCT the supportive care differs. Allogeneic HCT patients experience an initial period of pancytopenia followed by a more prolonged period of immunosuppression, which substantially increases the risk of bacterial infections, but more importantly, fungal, viral, and other opportunistic infections.[7] The risk of infection increases as additional immunosuppressive therapy is incorporated to prevent or treat GVHD. Supportive strategies designed to minimize infection during immunosuppression are essential after allogeneic HCT (see "Infectious Complications" section).

COMPARISON OF SUPPORTIVE CARE STRATEGIES BETWEEN ALLOGENEIC MYELOABLATIVE AND NONMYELOABLATIVE HEMATOPOIETIC STEM CELL TRANSPLANTATION

15. How do supportive care strategies used for myeloablative and nonmyeloablative preparative regimens with an allogeneic graft differ?

Nonmyeloablative HCT is the least myelosuppressive reduced intensity regimen (Fig. 92-2). A direct comparison of the toxicities with a myeloablative and nonmyeloablative preparative regimen is difficult because the latter is offered only to patients who are not candidates for myeloablative allogeneic HCT. These preparative regimens differ substantially in terms of the chemotherapy agents used (Tables 92-3 and 92-5) and the degree of myelosuppression. Nonmyeloablative HCT may have a different time pattern for infectious complications but there is a similar incidence and severity of acute GVHD. Nevertheless, comparisons between the preparative regimens are challenging because of the differences in the pre-HCT health of the recipients.[66] Clinical research is focusing on designing optimal preparative regimens with acceptable efficacy and toxicity (i.e., mixed chimerism, disease response). Thus, relative to myeloablative HCT, the preparative regimens and immunosuppression used after graft infusion are more variable for reduced intensity or nonmyeloablative HCT (Table 92-5).

DOSE CALCULATIONS IN OBESITY

16. K.M. is a 36-year-old woman with CML in accelerated phase. After her initial diagnosis, a successful search for an unrelated 6/6 HLA-matched allogeneic donor was conducted. K.M. is being admitted for myeloablative allogeneic PBPCT. Orders for K.M.'s preparative regimen are written as follows: height, 162 cm; actual body weight (ABW), 80 kg; ideal body weight (IBW), 54 kg; body surface area (BSA), 1.85 m^2; body mass index (BMI), 30.5 kg/m^2; and busulfan, 16 mg/kg total dose to be administered over 4 days (1 mg/kg per dose PO Q 6 hr for 16 doses, days –7, –6, –5, and –4). Cyclophosphamide 60 mg/kg/day IV to be administered on days –3 and –2. Day –1 is a "rest" day, followed by infusion of PBPC on day 0. Which weight should be used to calculate doses for K.M.'s preparative regimen?

K.M.'s ABW is 48% over her IBW. She is considered obese because her ABW is 30% greater than her IBW and her BMI is between 27 and 35 kg/m^2. Obesity has numerous effects on the pharmacokinetic disposition of medications; unfortunately, there is a paucity of data regarding the effects of obesity on the clinical outcomes of anticancer agents. The risk associated with inaccurate dosing of the preparative regimen for a myeloablative HCT is particularly challenging, because using a weight that is too high can cause lethal toxicity, while one that is too low could result in inadequate marrow ablation or disease eradication.

Few studies have evaluated the association of body weight and outcome to preparative regimens for myeloablative HCT.[75–77] Routine dosing of oral or IV busulfan based on adjusted IBW or BSA does not require a specific dose adjustment for obesity.[77,78] K.M.'s busulfan dose should not be based on her ABW because it does not accurately correct for her obesity and may predispose her to hepatic veno-occlusive disease (VOD). Her initial busulfan doses should be based on adjusted IBW.

COMPLICATIONS ASSOCIATED WITH HEMATOPOIETIC STEM CELL TRANSPLANTATION

17. What toxicities associated with myeloablative preparative regimen should be anticipated in K.M.? Are they similar to those anticipated after standard-dose chemotherapy?

Myelosuppression is a frequent dose-limiting toxicity for antineoplastics when administered in conventional doses used to treat cancer. However, because myelosuppression is circumvented with hematopoietic rescue in the case of patients receiving HCT, the dose-limiting toxicities of these myeloablative preparative regimens are nonhematologic (i.e., extramedullary) in nature. The toxicities vary with the preparative regimen used. Most patients undergoing HCT experience toxicities commonly associated with chemotherapy, such as alopecia, mucositis, CINV, infertility, and pulmonary toxicity (see Chapter 89). However, these toxicities are magnified in the HCT population.

Table 92-4 depicts a range of toxicities that can occur after myeloablative preparative regimen for HCT, and Figure 92-3 depicts the time course for complications after HCT. Selected toxicities are discussed in the following sections.

Busulfan Seizures

18. In addition to her preparative regimen, the following supportive care agents and monitoring parameters are prescribed

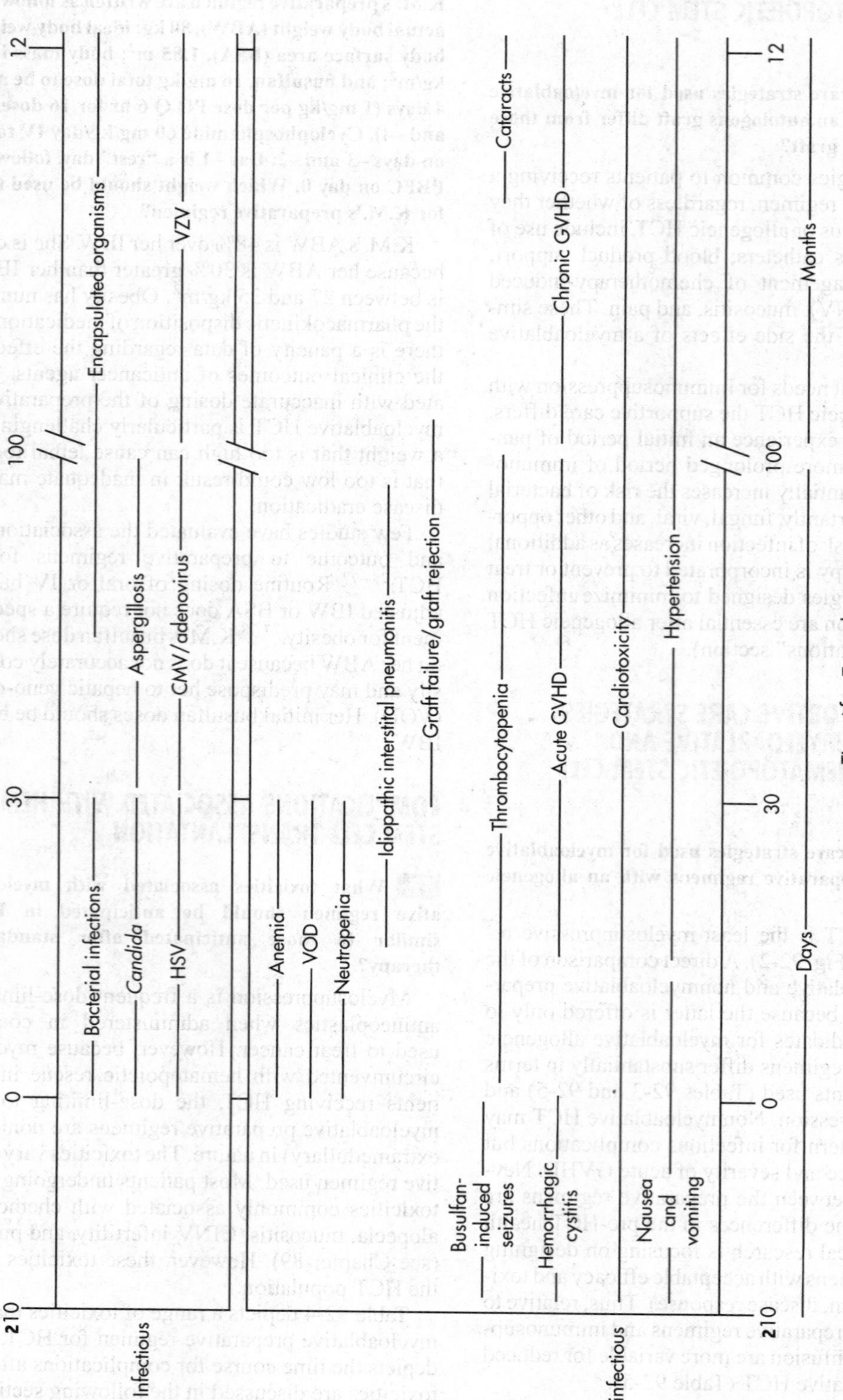

FIGURE 92-3 Complications after hematopoietic stem cell transplantation (HCT) by time for patients undergoing myeloablative allogeneic HCT only. CMV, cytomegalovirus; GVHD, graft-versus-host disease; HSV, herpes simplex virus; VOD, veno-occlusive disease; VZV, varicella-zoster virus.

for K.M.: on the day of admission (day –8), administer a phenytoin loading dose (10–15 mg/kg) orally in divided doses (300, 300, and 400 mg Q 3 hr). Continue 300 mg PO daily from days –8 to –3. Busulfan pharmacokinetic blood sampling is to occur after dose 1 to a target busulfan concentration at steady state (C_{SS}) >900 ng/mL. Begin normal saline hydration 3,000 mL/m^2/day 4 hours before cyclophosphamide and continue for 24 hours after the last cyclophosphamide dose. Mesna is to be given concurrently with cyclophosphamide as 10% of the cyclophosphamide dose administered intravenously 30 minutes before starting the cyclophosphamide dose, then as 100% of cyclophosphamide dose administered as a continuous IV infusion over 24 hours after each dose of cyclophosphamide. Beginning on day –5, weigh patient twice daily, check fluid input and urinary output every 4 hours, and monitor urine for RBCs daily until 24 hours after the last cyclophosphamide dose. If urine output drops below 300 mL over 2 hours, administer an IV bolus of 250 mL normal saline and give furosemide 10 mg/m^2, not to exceed 20 mg IV. What is the rationale for these supportive care therapies and monitoring parameters prescribed for K.M. as they relate to busulfan therapy?

Seizures occur in approximately 10% of patients receiving high-dose busulfan for HCT preparative regimens. Busulfan is highly lipophilic and readily crosses the blood–brain barrier with an average CSF: plasma ratio of 1 or higher. Seizures are probably a direct neurotoxic effect,[79] so, seizure prophylaxis is used. Many HCT centers use phenytoin for seizure prophylaxis, although benzodiazepines (e.g., lorazepam or clonazepam) also have been used.[80] Seizure prophylaxis is started at least 24 hours before the first busulfan dose and is usually discontinued 24 to 48 hours after administering the last busulfan dose. Seizures can occur despite the use of seizure prophylaxis, but they usually do not result in permanent neurologic deficits.

Adaptive Dosing of Busulfan

19. What dosing strategies can be used to minimize busulfan toxicities?

Wide interpatient variability in the clearance of both oral and IV busulfan, along with the identified concentration–effect relationships, has led to adaptive dosing of busulfan. The clearance of Busulfex (IV busulfan) adjusted for weight exhibited interpatient variability with a coefficient of variation (CV, standard deviation/mean) of 25% in 59 patients.[81] Oral busulfan exhibited a similar CV of 21% in 279 adult patients.[77] Weight, disease, and age are factors that may influence the clearance of oral busulfan.[77]

In patients receiving BU/CY, adaptive dosing of busulfan to achieve a target plasma level minimizes veno-occlusive disease (VOD), while improving engraftment and relapse rates.[82–84] The pharmacodynamic relationships are briefly reviewed here; however, more complete reviews of these relationships after oral busulfan administration are available elsewhere.[85,86] When reviewing pharmacodynamic data for busulfan, close attention should be paid to their interpretation because of the potential changes in the concentration–effect relationships between busulfan C_{SS} and outcome in each patient population and for each preparative regimen. Most studies have shown a pharmacodynamic relationship in patients receiving the BU/CY preparative regimens. One must also pay close attention to the units used in these studies. Data are also represented as area under the plasma concentration time curve (AUC) or C_{SS}. AUC data are easily converted to C_{SS} (C_{SS} = AUC/dosing interval). Results are expressed as μM-minute or ng/mL; an AUC of 1,500 μM-minute is roughly equivalent to a C_{SS} of 1,025 ng/mL based on busulfan's molecular weight of 246.

Hepatic VOD was observed more frequently in patients receiving BU/CY with a busulfan C_{SS} >925 to 1,025 ng/mL. In BU/CY regimens, busulfan C_{SS} >600 ng/mL favors engraftment, although contradictory data exist. Higher busulfan concentrations (C_{SS} >900 ng/mL) were associated with lower relapse rates in adult CML patients receiving BU/CY before HLA-matched grafts, with acceptable rates of VOD. Thus, a busulfan C_{SS} >900 ng/mL is targeted for K.M. because she has CML.

IV busulfan (Busulfex) was approved by the U.S. Food and Drug Administration (FDA) for use in combination with cyclophosphamide as a preparative regimen before allogeneic HCT for CML. The FDA-approved dose is 0.8 mg/kg IV Q 6 hr for 16 doses, which is similar to the oral busulfan dose of 1 mg/kg with a mean fraction absorbed (F) of 90%.[87] Busulfex, at 0.8 mg/kg of ABW or 29 mg/m^2 of BSA produces an average AUC of 1,200 μM-minute, within a wide range of 900 to 1,500 μM-minute in 80% of patients.[78] The product labeling states "high busulfan AUC values (>1,500 μM-minute) may be associated with an increased risk of developing hepatic VOD," which has caused many HCT centers to institute adaptive dosing of IV busulfan. See Questions 23–25.

Hemorrhagic Cystitis

20. What is the rationale for these supportive care therapies and monitoring parameters prescribed for K.M. as they relate to cyclophosphamide therapy?

In HCT patients receiving cyclophosphamide, moderate to severe hemorrhagic cystitis occurs in 4% to 20% of patients receiving hydration alone.[88] The putative bladder toxin is acrolein, a metabolite of cyclophosphamide.[89] Mesna donates free thiol groups to bind acrolein. American Society of Clinical Oncology (ASCO) Guidelines for the Use of Chemotherapy and Radiotherapy Protectants recommends the use of mesna plus saline diuresis or forced saline diuresis to lower the incidence of urothelial toxicity with high-dose cyclophosphamide in the setting of HCT.[90] It is important to note that hematuria or hemorrhagic cystitis can occur despite the use of any of these methods.

The optimal mesna dose with high-dose cyclophosphamide in preparation for myeloablative HCT is unknown. A variety of different regimens have been used, including intermittent bolus dosing (mesna dose 20%–40% of cyclophosphamide dose, administered for three or four doses) or continuous infusion regimens (mesna dose 80%–160% of cyclophosphamide dose).[88,91,92] Mesna should be continued for 24 to 48 hours after the last cyclophosphamide dose, such that mesna is present within the bladder to donate free thiol groups at the same time as the urotoxic metabolite acrolein. After IV administration of mesna, most of it (i.e., 60%–100%) is excreted within the urine over 4 hours.[93] Cyclophosphamide has an average half-life of 7 hours after administration of 60 mg/kg,[94] and acrolein may be present within the urine for 24 to 48 hours after cyclophosphamide administration.[95]

Thus, K.M. is receiving hydration with normal saline and mesna, administered as a continuous infusion, to minimize her risk of hemorrhagic cystitis due to cyclophosphamide. K.M. should also be monitored for any RBCs present in the urine, along with her urinary output, to allow for rapid intervention if hemorrhagic cystitis occurs.

Chemotherapy-Induced Gastrointestinal Effects

21. What other end-organ toxicities must be watched for? Should any medications be ordered for K.M. to prevent and treat the gastrointestinal (GI) effects associated with myeloablative therapy?

Preparative regimens for myeloablative HCT result in other end-organ toxicities, such as renal failure[96] and idiopathic pneumonia syndrome.[97] Lung injury post HCT has a mortality rate greater than 60%. Risk factors include total body irradiation (TBI), allogeneic HCT, and acute GVHD, which suggest that donor lymphocytes target the lung.[98] Tumor necrosis factor, induced by GVHD and damage to the intestinal mucosa, contributes to lung injury. Lung injury may be decreased by prompt treatment with etanercept, which inhibits tumor necrosis factor, and corticosteroids.[1]

The preparative regimen causes most patients to be nauseated and anorexic until day +10 to +15. CINV in HCT recipients can be due to highly emetogenic chemotherapy agents, TBI administration, and poor control of CINV prior to HCT. Thus, patients such as K.M. who are undergoing a myeloablative HCT should be treated with a serotonin antagonist plus a corticosteroid.[99] ASCO guidelines state that the use of the neurokinin receptor 1 antagonist, aprepitant, should be considered, although evidence to support its use in HCT patients is lacking.[99] Because aprepitant is a moderate inhibitor of cytochrome P450 3A4, it can theoretically interact with the preparative regimen; thus, well-controlled studies evaluating its efficacy, along with its potential for causing drug interactions, are needed.[99] The serotonin antagonist ondansetron may increase cyclophosphamide clearance in breast cancer patients undergoing a myeloablative HCT[100,101]; however, further work is needed to identify the clinical implications of this finding because, to date, cyclophosphamide concentrations have not been consistently associated with clinical outcomes in patients undergoing a myeloablative HCT.[87,102]

Most patients receiving a myeloablative preparative regimen experience mucositis due to its effects on rapidly dividing cells of the oral epithelium. The use of methotrexate, as GVHD prophylaxis, also contribute to mucositis.[103] Oral mucositis causes nausea and anorexia. In severe cases, parenteral opioid analgesics for pain relief[104] and total parenteral nutrition to prevent the development of nutritional deficits may be needed. Because mucositis can be worsened by superinfection, good oral hygiene should be practiced. Soft toothbrushes should be used and replaced often[105] The FDA recently approved recombinant human keratinocyte growth factor palifermin (Kepivance). The Multinational Association of Supportive Care in Cancer (MASCC) and International Society for Oral Oncology (ISOO) Guidelines recommend palifermin to prevent mucositis for patients with hematologic malignancies receiving myeloablative chemotherapy and TBI with autologous HCT. Palifermin 60 mcg/kg/day should be given for 3 days immediately prior to administering the preparative regimen and for 3 days after infusion of the hematopoietic stem cell graft (i.e., days 0, +1, +2).[105] In these patients, palifermin lowered the incidence and average duration of clinically meaningful oral mucositis. The incidence of bloodborne infections and the use of parenteral opioids also diminished outcomes.[106]

Myelosuppression and Growth Factor Use

22. An order is written to begin filgrastim on day 0 and to continue administration until the ANC has recovered to 500/mm³ for 2 consecutive days. Is this therapy appropriate for K.M.?

[SI units: ANC 500 × 10^6 cells/L]

The use of hematopoietic growth factors (HGFs) after infusion of allogeneic PBPC is controversial and is not recommended by ASCO Guidelines.[20] Administration of HGFs after allogeneic graft infusion decreases the duration of neutropenia, but does not decrease cost, length of hospitalization, or antibiotic use. HGF administration increases the incidence of severe GVHD and lowers survival. K.M. is receiving an allogeneic PBPC graft and, thus, should not receive filgrastim starting on day 0.

Veno-Occlusive Disease of the Liver

23. K.M.'s pretransplantation admission laboratory values are within normal limits. Her weight on admission is 80 kg. During the first 5 days after marrow infusion, K.M.'s weight begins to increase by approximately 0.5 kg/day, her inputs exceed her outputs by about 500 to 1,000 mL/day, and she is mildly febrile with an axillary temperature of 38°C. Blood and urine cultures are all negative. On day +6, her weight is 85 kg. Laboratory values drawn on day +7 are significant for a total bilirubin of 1.5 mg/dL, an aspartate aminotransferase (AST) of 40 U/L (normal, 0–45), and an alkaline phosphatase of 120 U/L (normal, 30–120). By day +10, K.M. is complaining of midepigastric, right upper quadrant pain, and a liver that is tender to palpation. Over the next few days, K.M. begins to look icteric. Her liver function tests continue to rise slowly, until day +18 when they reach the following peak values: total bilirubin 5.0 mg/dL (normal, 0.1–1), AST 150 U/L, and alkaline phosphatase 180 U/L. On day +18, K.M.'s weight is 90 kg. "Rule out VOD of the liver" is included on her problem list in the medical record. What is VOD?

[SI units: total bilirubin 25.6 and 85.5 μmol/L respectively; AST, alkaline phosphatase, same as previously]

Hepatic VOD is a life-threatening complication of HCT.[103] The incidence of VOD varies considerably, ranging from 5.3% to 54%, mainly due to differences in the preparative regimens.[103] Preparative regimens including busulfan, cyclophosphamide, and/or TBI >13.2 Gy have been associated with higher VOD rates.[102,107] Although the pathogenesis is not understood completely, the key event is toxic injury to the sinusoidal endothelial cells. Involvement of the hepatic venules is not essential to developing the clinical signs and symptoms; thus, the term "sinusoidal obstruction syndrome" has been proposed in place of VOD.[108] The endothelial damage initiates the coagulation cascade, induces thrombosis of the hepatic venules, and eventually leads to fibrous obliteration of the affected venules.[103] The cardinal histologic features are marked sinusoidal fibrosis, necrosis of pericentral hepatocytes, and narrowing and eventual fibrosis of central veins.[108] In patients with VOD, early microscopic changes include subendothelial swelling, leading to several physiological changes, including narrowing of hepatic venules and necrosis of centrizonal hepatocytes.[103]

Clinical Presentation

24. What signs and symptoms in K.M. are consistent with a diagnosis of VOD?

The signs and symptoms associated with VOD are hyperbilirubinemia (≥2 mg/dL), weight gain (>5% above baseline), hepatomegaly, azotemia, elevated alkaline phosphatase, ascites, elevated AST, and encephalopathy.[109] Insidious weight gain exceeding 5% of baseline is usually the first manifestation of impending VOD, occurring in more than 90% of patients within 3 to 6 days after marrow infusion.[110] Weight gain is caused by sodium and water retention, as evidenced by decreased renal sodium excretion. This is usually distinguished from cyclophosphamide-induced syndrome of inappropriate secretion of antidiuretic hormone by the time course relative to administration of the preparative regimen. Hyperbilirubinemia, which also occurs in virtually all patients, follows the onset of weight gain and usually appears within 10 days after hematopoietic stem cell infusion. In more than half of the patients, the peak bilirubin concentration is >6 mg/dL. Other liver function test abnormalities usually occur after hyperbilirubinemia and include elevations in AST and alkaline phosphatase. Ascites, right upper quadrant pain, and encephalopathy lag behind changes in liver function tests and develop within 10 to 15 days after infusion of hematopoietic stem cells.[110]

A clinical diagnosis of VOD is made when two of the following features occur within the first 20 days of HCT: (a); hyperbilirubinemia (total serum bilirubin >2 mg/dL), (b) hepatomegaly or right upper quadrant pain, and (c) sudden weight gain.[110] To make a clinical diagnosis of VOD, the features listed previously must occur without other causes of post-HCT liver damage, including GVHD, viral hepatitis, fungal abscesses, and drug reactions. A clinical diagnosis can be confirmed histologically via liver biopsy.

In summary, the signs and symptoms consistent with VOD in K.M. include insidious weight gain, hyperbilirubinemia, and right upper quadrant pain. The onset and timing of these signs and symptoms are consistent with VOD and occurred without other causes of hepatic toxicity.

Prevention and Treatment

25. What is the likelihood that K.M. will recover from her VOD? How should she be treated?

The overall mortality for patients who develop VOD varies considerably (i.e., 0%–67%) due to the variable definitions of VOD and fatal VOD.[103] Patients with greater weight gain and elevations in total bilirubin are more likely to die of VOD when compared to patients with less severe weight gain and elevations in total bilirubin.[103] Severe VOD is usually accompanied by multiorgan system failure, and these patients rarely die from liver failure itself but from renal and cardiopulmonary failure.[103]

Risk factors for severe and/or fatal VOD have been identified in the hope of preventing this condition or its progression through early treatment. Although various risk factors have been identified, their association is variable, and conflicting reports of their association can be found. The most important risk factors are the preparative regimen, TBI dose, the pharmacokinetics of busulfan and/or cyclophosphamide, and liver inflammation and fibrosis pre-HCT.[103] In patients with AML, gemtuzumab ozogamicin (Mylotarg) has been associated with VOD when used prior to and after HCT.[103]

Various pharmacologic methods to prevent VOD have been evaluated. One such method is altering the preparative regimen. The substitution of fludarabine for cyclophosphamide in combination with busulfan (i.e., BU/FLU) and the use of reduced intensity regimens that contain no liver toxins appear to lower VOD risk.[1,103,111,112] When busulfan is dosed based on body weight, VOD rates are lower with IV busulfan compared to oral busulfan.[113,114] Individualizing chemotherapy doses for busulfan or cyclophosphamide may also lower VOD rates. There is interpatient variability in their metabolism and clearance, along with pharmacodynamic relationships, although the relationships vary within the various preparative regimens.[85,115] The association of VOD with busulfan concentrations is discussed in the "Adaptive Dosing of Busulfan" section. Although the data from clinical trials are mixed, some HCT centers routinely use heparin infusions or low-molecular-weight heparin subcutaneously. Single-agent ursodiol (600 mg/day PO) has been associated with a lower incidence of VOD[116,117] or with a lower frequency of total serum bilirubin >3 mg/dL.[118] Ursodiol, which is a bile acid, most likely lowers cholestasis but not toxic liver injury.[103] Prostaglandin E1 and anticytokine strategies, specifically pentoxifylline, have been ineffective in preventing VOD in clinical trials.[103]

Most patients with VOD (70%–85%) spontaneously recover; thus, the mainstay of treatment is managing sodium and water balance and repeated paracentesis for ascites that is associated with pain for pulmonary compromise.[103] Volume expanders such as albumin and colloids may be used to maintain intravascular volume, spironolactone may be used to minimize extravascular fluid accumulation, and protein restriction and lactulose may be used if encephalopathy develops. Unfortunately, improved outcomes with these measures have not been confirmed. In patients with severe VOD and multiorgan failure, available treatment options are limited. Thrombolytic therapy with recombinant human tissue plasminogen activator (rh-TPA) and heparin have had mixed results in terms of efficacy, and can cause fatal intracerebral or pulmonary bleeding.[103] Defibrotide, an investigational new drug, has shown promising results in the treatment of VOD.[119–121] Defibrotide, a ribonucleotide, has antithrombotic, anti-ischemic, and thrombolytic activity without producing significant systemic anticoagulation. In a compassionate use trial of 88 patients with severe VOD and associated organ dysfunction, 36% of patients had complete resolution of VOD and 35% survived past day 100 after HCT.[121]

Because K.M. does not meet the criteria for severe VOD, she should be managed conservatively with fluid restriction and spironolactone. Her signs and symptoms should resolve over the next 2 weeks. Because she has mild VOD, she is likely to recover completely without sequelae.

Graft Rejection

26. E.R. is a 65-year-old woman diagnosed with myelodysplastic syndrome. Past medical history is significant for type I diabetes and renal dysfunction. After her initial diagnosis, a successful search for a completely HLA-matched unrelated donor was conducted. E.R. will receive a nonmyeloablative allogeneic HCT using bone marrow. E.R.'s preparative regimen orders are written as follows: fludarabine, 30 mg/m^2/day on days –4, –3 and –2 and 2 Gy TBI on the day of marrow infusion with postgrafting cyclosporine and mycophenolate mofetil. It now is day +28, and E.R.'s CBC reveals the following: WBC count, 500 cells/mm^3 (normal, 3,200–9,800); no granulocytes or monocytes detected on differential; platelets, 100,000/mm^3 (normal, 130,000–400,000); and hematocrit (Hct), 30% (normal, 33%–43%). Donor T-cell chimerism is <5%. What is E.R. experiencing, and how should she be treated?

[SI units: WBC, <0.1 cells/L platelets, 100 × 10^9 cells/L Hct, 0.22]

Reduced intensity regimens typically consist of fludarabine in combination with an alkylating agent or low-dose TBI (Fig. 92-2). With the nonmyeloablative fludarabine/TBI regimen, there is minimal neutropenia, thrombocytopenia, and nonhematologic toxicity, thus making HCT an outpatient procedure.[1] Engraftment is usually evident within the first 30 days in patients receiving a nonmyeloablative preparative regimen; however, rejection can occur after initial engraftment.[4] Because E.R. has low donor T-cell chimerism on day +28, she is at higher risk of experiencing graft rejection.

In myeloablative allogeneic HCT, graft rejection is less common because the donor PBPC or marrow is unmanipulated and free from the toxic effects of prior chemotherapy. A delicate balance between host and donor effector cells is necessary since residual host-versus-graft effects may lead to graft rejection. The incidence of graft rejection is higher in patients with aplastic anemia and in patients undergoing HCT with histoincompatible marrow or T-cell–depleted marrow. Graft rejection is uncommon in leukemia patients receiving myeloablative preparative regimen with a histocompatible allogeneic donor. After myeloablative HCT, there are limited therapeutic options for the treatment of graft rejection. A second HCT is the most definitive therapy, although the toxicities are formidable.[122] In patients receiving myeloablative allogeneic HCT, graft rejection is best managed with immunosuppressants such as antithymocyte globulin.

E.R. received nonmyeloablative conditioning, and thus, she should have mixed chimerism posttransplant. However, because she is <5% donor she will not benefit from the GVT effect due to the lack of the donor's cytotoxic T lymphocytes that suppress the recipient's malignancy. Current research is focusing on quantitative chimerism monitoring, specifically evaluating the percent donor chimerism, which may be a tool on which to base clinical interventions.[68] Donor chimerism is evaluated in different cell types (e.g., T cells, NK cells, granulocytes). The longitudinal changes in the percent donor chimerism, termed "engraftment kinetics," are influenced by several factors such as, type of HCT conditioning, stem cell source, intensity of postgrafting immunosuppression.[68,123] A balance between the recipient and donor's cells is needed to maximize the GVT effect, which lowers the risk of relapse while minimizing the risk of GVHD. Some HCT centers are evaluating the benefit of clinical interventions to tip this balance.[68,123]

E.R. is at high risk of graft rejection. A trial of discontinuing cyclosporine and mycophenolate mofetil is an option. E.R.'s T-cell chimerism should be monitored periodically, and hematopoietic function should be monitored with daily CBCs and a bone marrow biopsy every 2 weeks.

GRAFT-VERSUS-HOST DISEASE

GVHD is caused by activation of donor lymphocytes leading to immune damage to the recipient. Histocompatibility differences between donor and recipient necessitate posttransplantation immunosuppression after allogeneic HCT because considerable morbidity and mortality are associated with graft rejection and GVHD. Therefore, postgrafting immunosuppression or GVHD prophylaxis is used after allogeneic HCT. However, because allogeneic transplantation offers the potential for a GVT effect in which immune effector cells from the donor recognize and eliminate residual tumor in the recipient, research is focusing on being able to improve GVT effects while lowering the risk of graft rejection and GVHD.[3]

GVHD is the most important complication of allogeneic HCT.[1] GVHD can occur after allogeneic HCT, regardless of the preparative regimen used. The pathophysiology of GVHD is not completely understood, but the current view of its development is described by a three-step process. The pathophysiology for acute GVHD is a multistep phenomenon, including (a) the preparative regimen results in tissue damage and release of inflammatory cytokines into the circulation; (b) both recipient and donor antigen presenting cells and inflammatory cytokines trigger activation of donor-derived T cells; and (c) the activated donor T cells mediate cytotoxicity through a variety of mechanisms, which leads to tissue damage characteristic of acute GVHD.[124]

GVHD is divided into two forms (i.e., acute or chronic) based on clinical manifestations. Acute GVHD damages the skin, GI tract, and liver and usually occurs in the first 100 days after allogeneic HCT.[1] In contrast, chronic GVHD can affect almost any organ system, closely resembles several autoimmune diseases, and usually occurs after day 100.

The vast majority of the data regarding the prevention and treatment of GVHD have been obtained after myeloablative preparative regimens. Therefore, this section refers only to trials conducted in recipients of a myeloablative allogeneic HCT.

Acute Graft-versus-Host Disease

Risk Factors

27. M.P., a 22-year-old, 70-kg man, undergoes a one-antigen mismatched allogeneic HCT from his sister for the diagnosis of Philadelphia chromosome-positive AML. After a preparative regimen of CY/TBI, the following immunosuppressive regimen is ordered: tacrolimus 0.3 mg/kg/day as a continuous infusion from days –1 until tolerating oral medications, then switch to tacrolimus 1.2 mg/kg PO Q 12 hr until day +50. Methotrexate 15 mg/m^2 IV

Table 92-6 Clinical Staging of Acute Graft-versus-Host Disease (GVHD) According to Organ System

Stage	Skin[a]	Liver	Intestinal Tract[b]
+	Maculopapular rash <25% of body surface	Bilirubin 2–3 mg/dL	500–1,000 mL/day diarrhea or persistent nausea[c]
++	Maculopapular rash 25%–50% body surface	Bilirubin 3.1–6 mg/dL	1,000–1,500 mL/day diarrhea
+++	Generalized erythroderma	Bilirubin 6.1–15 mg/dL	>1,500 mL/day diarrhea
++++	Generalized erythroderma with bullous formation and desquamation	Bilirubin >15 mg/dL	Severe abdominal pain with or without ileus

[a] Extent of rash determined by burn chart or "rule of nines."
[b] Diarrhea volume applies to adults.
[c] Persistent nausea requires endoscopic biopsy to show evidence of GVHD histology in stomach or duodenum.
Adapted from Sullivan KM. Graft-versus-host disease. In: Blume KG et al, eds. *Thomas' Hematopoietic Cell Transplantation*. 3rd ed. Malden, MA: Blackwell; 2004:635.

on day +1, then 10 mg/m² day +3, +6, and +11. What factors are associated with an increased risk of acute GVHD?

The single most important factor associated with the development of GVHD is the degree of histocompatibility between donor and recipient.[1] Clinically relevant grade II–IV acute GVHD occurs in 20% to 50% of HLA-matched sibling grafts and 50% to 80% of HLA-mismatched sibling or HLA-identical unrelated donors.[125] The onset of acute GVHD is earlier and severity is increased in mismatched grafts relative to matched grafts, and also in matched unrelated donors relative to matched sibling donors.[40,126] Other factors that increase the risk of developing acute GVHD include increasing recipient (and possibly donor) age, greater intensity of the preparative regimen, use of PBPC rather than bone marrow, and donor/recipient sex mismatch.[124] CBT have a lower risk of acute GVHD.[127–129]

M.P. is receiving allogeneic bone marrow from a female sibling donor that is mismatched at one HLA antigen. These two factors increase his risk of developing acute GVHD.

Clinical Presentation

28. On day +14, the time at which engraftment occurred, M.P. is noted to have a diffuse macular papular rash on his arms, hands, and front trunk. He does not have diarrhea, and his liver function tests are within normal limits. At the onset of his rash, M.P.'s empiric antibiotics are changed from cefepime to imipenem. Despite the change in antibiotics, M.P.'s rash persists. How is M.P.'s presentation consistent with acute GVHD?

The primary targets of immune-mediated destruction of host tissue by donor lymphocytes in acute GVHD are the skin, liver, and GI tract.[125] Acute GVHD of the skin usually manifests as a diffuse maculopapular rash that starts on the palms of the hands or soles of the feet or face. In more severe cases, skin GVHD can progress to a generalized total body erythroderma, bullous formation, and skin desquamation. The earliest symptoms of acute GVHD of the GI tract are usually loss of appetite followed by nausea and vomiting.[103] Abdominal pain and watery or bloody diarrhea also occur, which can result in electrolyte abnormalities, dehydration, or ileus in severe cases. Liver GVHD usually follows skin and/or GI GVHD. Clinical symptoms of liver GVHD include a gradual rise in total bilirubin, alkaline phosphatase, and hepatic transaminases.[103] Acute GVHD is usually not evident until the time of engraftment, when donor lymphoid elements begin to proliferate. The skin is usually the first organ to be involved. The onset of liver or GI GVHD usually lags behind the onset of skin GVHD by approximately 1 week and infrequently occurs without skin GVHD.

Acute GVHD must be distinguished accurately from other causes of skin, liver, or GI toxicity in the HCT patient. For example, a maculopapular rash, which may occur as a manifestation of an allergic reaction to antibiotics, usually begins on the trunk or upper extremities and rarely presents on the palms of the hands or soles of the feet. Diarrhea can be caused by chemotherapy, radiation, infection, or antibiotic therapy.[103] However, diarrhea caused by the preparative regimen is rarely bloody and usually resolves within 3 to 7 days after discontinuation of drugs and radiation. Diarrhea caused by infectious agents such as *Clostridium difficile* or cytomegalovirus (CMV) should be distinguished from GVHD. Liver GVHD must be distinguished primarily from VOD and, to a lesser extent, hepatitis induced by drugs, blood products, or parenteral nutrition.[103] Although liver function test abnormalities between these syndromes are similar, liver GVHD is rarely associated with insidious weight gain or right upper quadrant pain.[103] A tissue biopsy of the affected organ in conjunction with clinical evidence is the only way to definitively diagnose acute GVHD. Acute GVHD is associated with characteristic histologic changes to affected organs. A staging system based on clinical criteria is used to grade acute GVHD. The severity of organ involvement is determined first (Table 92-6), and then an overall grade is established based on number and extent of involved organs (Table 92-7).

Table 92-7 Overall Clinical Grading of Severity of Acute Graft-versus-Host Disease

Grade	Degree of Organ Involvement
I—Mild	+ to ++ skin rash; no liver involvement; no gastrointestinal (GI) involvement; no functional impairment
II—Moderate	+ to +++ skin rash; + liver involvement; + GI involvement; mild functional impairment
III—Severe	++ to +++ skin rash; ++ to +++ liver involvement, ++ to ++++ GI involvement (or both); moderate functional impairment
IV—Life threatening	Any skin involvement, ++ to ++++ liver involvement, ++ to ++++ GI involvement and extreme functional impairment

Adapted from Sullivan KM. Graft-versus-host disease. In: Blume KG et al, eds. *Thomas' Hematopoietic Cell Transplantation*. 3rd ed. Malden, MA: Blackwell; 2004:635.

M.P. developed a rash at the time of engraftment that could have been consistent with either an antibiotic-induced rash or acute GVHD. Although it was appropriate to change antibiotics, the fact that M.P.'s rash did not improve is suggestive of acute GVHD. M.P.'s rash is present on 36% of his body, but because there are no signs of GI or liver involvement at this time, M.P. is likely to have grade I GVHD (Tables 92-6 and Table 92-7).

Immunosuppressive Prophylaxis

29. Why did M.P. receive prophylactic immunosuppressive therapy with tacrolimus and methotrexate?

GVHD is a leading cause of morbidity and mortality after allogeneic HCT. Without post-HCT immunosuppression, serious acute GVHD would occur in almost every allogeneic HCT recipient.[1] The most common method used to minimize GHVD risk is to administer postgrafting immunosuppression. However, these immunosuppressive regimens are associated with significant toxicity and a higher risk of relapse in patients with acute leukemia who are at high risk of relapse.[130] The latter is most likely due to the GVT effect mediated in conjunction with acute GVHD because an inverse relationship between acute GVHD and leukemic relapse has been observed.[3] Patients with acute leukemias at high risk for relapse may receive single-agent prophylaxis for acute GVHD because the development of some acute GVHD may facilitate a GVT effect.

Initially, acute GVHD was prevented with single-drug therapy using ATG, cyclophosphamide, methotrexate, or cyclosporine.[131–133] ATG binds nonspecifically to mononuclear cells and depletes hematopoietic progenitor cells in addition to lymphocytes. Consequently, ATG is rarely used for fear of a high incidence of graft failure.[131] The risk of GVHD is greatly reduced by two-drug combination immunosuppression (Table 92-8). Methotrexate, cyclosporine or tacrolimus, and corticosteroids are the agents most commonly incorporated into combination immunosuppressive regimens. Although the most widely published regimen is short-course methotrexate plus cyclosporine (Seattle regimen),[133] there is no national consensus with regard to the most effective regimen. Methotrexate is administered up to day +11. Several randomized clinical trials have compared tacrolimus and short-course methotrexate with cyclosporine plus short-course methotrexate in patients undergoing allogeneic HCT using HLA-matched siblings[134,135] and unrelated donors.[74] Recipients of matched-sibling grafts treated with tacrolimus had a lower incidence of grade II to IV acute GVHD, but a similar incidence of chronic GVHD.[134] Overall survival was lower in the tacrolimus group as a result of more toxic deaths in patients with advanced stage disease; however, a higher number of advanced stage disease patients in the tacrolimus/methotrexate group make the results of this trial somewhat difficult to determine.[134]

Subsequently, the IBMTR conducted a matched control study, which suggested that the survival difference between the two arms was in fact due to the imbalance in the underlying risk factors.[135] In patients receiving HLA-matched or slightly mismatched unrelated grafts, those given tacrolimus had a lower incidence of grade II to IV acute GVHD, a similar incidence of chronic GVHD and similar disease-free and overall survival rates.[74] Patients with advanced hematologic malignancies were excluded from this study. Both regimens are currently used in allogeneic HCT after myeloablative preparative regimens.

Several studies have compared triple-drug with two-drug immunosuppression. The incidence of acute GVHD has been similar or lower with triple-drug regimens, but infectious complications are higher, and overall survival is similar to two-drug regimens.[136,137] Three-drug immunosuppression regimens are still being evaluated and are used mainly in mismatched or unrelated allogeneic HCT, where the risk of acute GVHD is increased.

M.P. received acute GVHD prophylaxis with a two-drug regimen of short-course methotrexate and tacrolimus.

30. What principles are used in dosing medications used for acute GVHD prophylaxis?

Although the various combination immunosuppressive regimens vary slightly by drug, dose, and combination, several guidelines are consistent throughout all regimens. First, cytotoxic agents used in combination for prophylaxis of acute GVHD (e.g., methotrexate) are withheld or given in reduced doses if mucositis or myelosuppression is severe.[133,136] Methotrexate for GVHD prophylaxis can delay engraftment, increase the incidence and severity of mucositis and cause liver function test elevations. The methotrexate dose is reduced in the setting of renal or liver impairment.[138]

The calcineurin inhibitors (i.e., cyclosporine, tacrolimus) should be initiated before or immediately after donor cell infusion (day –1 or 0) when used for GVHD prophylaxis. This schedule is recommended because of the known mechanism of

Table 92-8 Combination Regimens of Prophylaxis of Acute Graft-versus-Host Disease

Drug	*Dosing Examples*
Cyclosporine/short-term methotrexate[133]	1.5 mg/kg IV or 6.25 mg/kg (Sandimmune) PO Q 12 hr, days –1 to + 50, then taper 5% per week and discontinue by day + 180 Methotrexate 10 mg/m^2 IV, days + 3, + 6, + 11
Tacrolimus/short-term methotrexate[74]	Tacrolimus 0.03 mg/kg/day continuous IV infusion or 0.12 mg/kg/day PO BID Methotrexate 15 mg/m^2 IV day + 1, 10 mg/m^2 IV, days + 3, + 6, + 11
Cyclosporine/methotrexate/ prednisone[136]	Cyclosporine 5 mg/kg/day IV continuous infusion, day –2 to + 3, then 3–3.75 mg/kg IV until day + 35; then 10 mg/kg/day (Sandimmune) PO, dose adjusted to cyclosporine concentrations (via radioimmunoassay) of 200–600 ng/mL. Taper by 20% Q 2 wk; then discontinue by day + 180 Methotrexate 15 mg/m^2 IV day + 1, 10 mg/m^2 IV day + 3, + 6 Methylprednisolone 0.5 mg/kg/day IV, day + 7 until day + 14, then 1 mg/kg/day IV until day + 28, then prednisone 0.8 mg/kg/day PO until day + 42, then taper slowly and discontinue by day + 180

action of cyclosporine, which entails blocking the proliferation of cytotoxic T cells by inhibiting production of helper T-cell–derived IL-2. Administering cyclosporine before the donor cell infusion allows inhibition of IL-2 secretion to occur before a rejection response has been initiated.

Cyclosporine is usually administered intravenously until the GI toxicity from a myeloablative preparative regimen has resolved (e.g., for 7–21 days).[133] This is because GI effects of the preparative regimen (e.g., CINV, diarrhea) and GVHD affect the oral absorption of microemulsion cyclosporine and may result in inconsistent blood concentrations.[139] Most centers use the microemulsion oral formulation (Neoral) or other new generic microemulsion formulations that have improved bioavailability. With the Neoral formulation, a ratio of 1:2 or 1:3 is used. The most common ratio used when converting tacrolimus from IV to oral is 1:4. Different conversion ratios for IV to oral regimens may be used when patients are receiving concomitant medications that affect cytochrome P450 3A or P-glycoprotein, which are involved in the metabolism and transport of the calcineurin inhibitors (e.g., itraconazole). Thus, careful monitoring for drug interactions with the calcineurin inhibitors is warranted.[140]

The dose of cyclosporine or tacrolimus is adjusted based on serum drug levels and the serum creatinine (SrCr) concentration. Doses are usually reduced by 50% if the SrCr concentration doubles above baseline and is withheld for SrCr concentrations >2 mg/dL.[133,141] Although the calcineurin inhibitors do not contribute to myelosuppression, common adverse effects to these agents include neurotoxicity, hypertension, and/or nephrotoxicity (which may lead to an impaired clearance of methotrexate).[79]

When corticosteroids are added to combination immunosuppressive regimens, they are usually withheld until engraftment is expected (7–14 days after marrow infusion). Administering corticosteroids earlier in the posttransplantation period (e.g., day 0) paradoxically increases the incidence of GVHD when used in combination with methotrexate and cyclosporine.[142] Corticosteroids are associated with several adverse effects, including infectious complications, hyperglycemia, and an increased incidence of hypertension when used in combination with a calcineurin inhibitor.

Tapering schedules for cyclosporine or tacrolimus and corticosteroids vary widely among institutions. The general goal is to keep calcineurin inhibitor doses stable to day +50, and then slowly taper with the intent of discontinuing all immunosuppressive agents by 6 months after HCT. By this time, immunologic tolerance has developed, and patients no longer require immunosuppressive therapy.

Adaptive Dosing of Calcineurin Inhibitors

31. On day +18, a tacrolimus level is drawn right before the morning dose and is reported to be 15 ng/mL. Why are tacrolimus levels being obtained for M.P.?

The role of pharmacokinetic monitoring of the calcineurin inhibitors in HCT patients is not well defined but is commonly performed because of the established pharmacodynamic associations within solid organ transplant recipients. In general, desired tacrolimus trough concentrations are 5 to 15 ng/mL. Tacrolimus concentrations >20 ng/mL have been associated with increased risk of toxicity, primarily nephrotoxicity.[143,144] Adjustments in tacrolimus dosing for increased SrCr should be made in a manner similar to that described for cyclosporine.

It is standard practice for HCT centers to adjust cyclosporine or tacrolimus doses based on trough blood concentrations.[144] An association between cyclosporine concentrations and acute GVHD was not found in early studies; however, other studies have suggested that cyclosporine trough concentrations less than 200 ng/mL are associated with an increased risk of acute GVHD.[145,146] Pharmacokinetic monitoring may play a more important role in minimizing the risk of cyclosporine-induced nephrotoxicity. Cyclosporine trough concentrations >400 ng/mL (via radioimmunoassay and high-pressure liquid chromatography assay) are associated with a higher incidence of nephrotoxicity in some series.[147] However, it is important to note that cyclosporine-induced nephrotoxicity can occur despite low or normal concentrations of cyclosporine and may be a consequence of other drug- or disease-related factors known to influence the development of nephrotoxicity (e.g., concurrent use of other nephrotoxic agents, sepsis).

It is reasonable to adjust doses to maintain tacrolimus trough concentrations between 5 to 15 ng/mL in patients undergoing allogeneic HCT with a myeloablative preparative regimen. Recommendations for dose adjustments should be based on tacrolimus concentrations and SrCr concentration. Dosage adjustments should be made for SrCr, regardless of tacrolimus concentration, as recommended previously. No standard dosage adjustment schedule exists, but most centers adopt their own standardized approach. M.P. has a normal SrCr, and his tacrolimus level is 15 ng/mL. Therefore, his tacrolimus dose should be maintained.

Treatment of Established Acute Graft-versus-Host Disease

32. On day +19, the suspicion of acute skin GVHD is confirmed by biopsy. On the same day, M.P. experiences 1,000 mL of diarrhea over the next 24 hours and is noted to have a bilirubin of 2.8 mg/dL. He is started on methylprednisolone 35 mg IV Q 6 hr. What is the rationale for methylprednisolone therapy in M.P.?

[SI units: total bilirubin = 48 μmol/L]

Preventing the development of GVHD is the most effective way to treat this HCT complication. Corticosteroids, often in combination with calcineurin inhibitors, are first-line treatment for GVHD. For this reason GVHD and its treatment cause profound immunodeficiency.[1,148] The combination of GVHD and infectious complications are leading causes of mortality for allogeneic HCT patients.

Corticosteroids are the first-line treatment for established GVHD.[124] A complete response occurs in 25% to 40% of patients, with a lower likelihood of response in more severe cases of acute GVHD.[124] Patients with mild to moderate (grades I–III) acute GVHD who respond to initial therapy have a significantly better survival advantage than patients with severe acute GVHD who do not respond to initial therapy. Patients who do not respond to therapy or have ongoing severe GVHD usually die from a combination of GVHD and infectious complications.[149]

When treating acute GVHD, corticosteroids are generally tapered based on response. There is no consensus on the optimal method for tapering the corticosteroids[148] and the tapering rate depends on the patient. Patients who develop acute GVHD or who experience flares of existing GVHD during a tapering trial will have their dosages increased or tapered more slowly as tolerated.

Because M.P. had objective evidence of established acute GVHD, he was given systemic corticosteroids at the first sign of progressive disease. This was appropriate because single-agent corticosteroids are considered the therapy of choice for established acute GVHD.[150] Corticosteroids indirectly halt the progression of immune-mediated destruction of host tissues by blocking macrophage-derived IL-1 secretion. IL-1 is a primary stimulus for helper T-cell–induced secretion of IL-2, which in turn is responsible for stimulating proliferation of cytotoxic T lymphocytes. The recommended dosage of methylprednisolone for the treatment of established acute GVHD is 1 to 2 mg/kg/day, given intravenously or orally in four divided doses for a minimum of 14 days, followed by a tapering schedule that is determined by response.[149] The dosage of methylprednisolone in M.P., approximately 2 mg/kg/day, is consistent with these recommendations. Trials that compared higher doses of corticosteroids (i.e., 10 mg/kg/day) to 2 mg/kg/day as initial treatment of acute GVHD showed no advantage.[151] Monitoring for acute GHVD response should occur every 3 to 5 days.[124]

A significant portion of patients do not respond to corticosteroids, and they are said to have steroid-refractory GVHD.[124] The timing of treatment response varies among the organs affected by GVHD and patients. If GVHD symptoms worsen over 3 days of treatment and if the skin does not improve by 5 days, it is unlikely that a response will be achieved in a timely manner, and secondary therapy should be considered.[124] Patients with steroid-refractory acute GVHD have a poor prognosis. A variety of medications are being studied for "salvage" or secondary therapy. The salvage therapy depends on the organs affected. For example, phototherapy is used as salvage therapy for skin GVHD and nonabsorbable corticosteroids are used for GI GHVD. Other options for salvage therapy include ATG, denileukin diftitox, TNF-α blockers (e.g., infliximab, etanercept).[124] The most effective dose, timing, or combination of these salvage therapies is still unknown.

M.P. should be evaluated for response to methylprednisolone after 4 to 7 days. If his acute GVHD has improved or stabilized, he should be continued on therapy at this dose for a total of 14 days. If M.P. responds to therapy, his methylprednisolone dose should be tapered slowly over a minimum of 1 month, and he should be monitored for any evidence of recurrent GVHD. If the GVHD flares during his steroid taper as evidenced by worsening skin reactions, increased bilirubin, or increased diarrhea volume, the dose should be increased again until his disease is stable; the subsequent taper should be initiated at a slower rate. If M.P. fails to respond to first-line therapy with methylprednisolone, he should receive salvage therapy.

Chronic Graft-versus-Host Disease

Clinical Presentation

33. M.P. was successfully treated for his acute GVHD, is no longer taking corticosteroids, and is currently tapering his cyclosporine. On day +200, M.P. comes to clinic for follow up after a 2-week vacation in Florida. On examination, M.P. is found to have a mild skin rash on his arms and legs, hyperpigmentation of the tissue surrounding the eyes, and white plaquelike lesions in his mouth. He is also complaining of dry eyes. Laboratory tests reveal an increased alkaline phosphatase and total bilirubin concentration. What is the most likely cause of M.P.'s findings?

Chronic GVHD, the most common late complication of allogeneic HCT, occurs in 20% to 70% of patients surviving more than 100 days.[152] Chronic GVHD is a major cause of nonrelapse morbidity and mortality.[1] Risk factors for chronic GVHD include recipient, donor, and transplant factors. Nonmodifiable recipient risk factors include older age, certain diagnoses (e.g., CML), and lack of an HLA-matched donor. Modifiable factors that may lower the risk of chronic GVHD include selecting a younger donor, avoiding a multiparous female donor, using umbilical cord blood or a bone marrow graft rather than PBPC, and limiting the CD34$^+$ and T-cell dose infused.[152] Development of acute GVHD is a major predictor of chronic GVHD; 70% to 80% of those with grade II to IV acute GVHD develop chronic GVHD.[152]

Chronic GVHD is not a continuation of acute GVHD.[152] Traditionally, the boundary between the two was based on time, but now they are classified based on different clinical symptoms.[152] Signs and symptoms of chronic GVHD in various organ systems are listed in Table 92-9. A consensus guideline for the diagnosis and scoring of chronic GVHD has been published.[153] The diagnosis of chronic GVHD requires (a) being distinct from acute GVHD, (b) having at least one diagnostic clinical sign of chronic GVHD or at least one distinctive manifestation confirmed by pertinent biopsy or other relevant tests, and (c) exclusion of other possible diagnoses. The clinical scoring system uses a numerical value of 0 to 3, with more severe symptoms having a higher, number. A global score is calculated by including the number of organs involved and the severity within each affected organ. The global score reflects the effect of chronic GVHD on the patient's performance status and can be used to evaluate whether treatment with systemic immunosuppression is required.

The signs and symptoms of chronic GVHD in M.P. include a rash in sun-exposed areas of the skin, hyperpigmentation of tissues surrounding his eyes, white plaque-like lesions in the mouth, dry mucous membranes, and increased alkaline phosphatase and total bilirubin levels. These symptoms appeared after a period of complete resolution of acute GVHD. Thus, M.P. has limited involvement, quiescent chronic GVHD.

Pharmacologic Management

34. M.P. is started on prednisone 1 mg/kg PO daily for the treatment of his chronic GVHD. His cyclosporine taper is stopped, and the dosage is raised to therapeutic concentrations. Is this therapy rational? What other agents are available to treat chronic GVHD?

There is no specific prophylactic therapy for chronic GVHD. The mainstay of therapy for chronic GVHD is long-term immunosuppressive therapy. Survival for patients with chronic GVHD is improved by extended corticosteroid therapy, although there are multiple long-term adverse effects associated with the corticosteroids.[152,154] The prednisone dose is 1 mg/kg/day, administered orally in divided doses for 14 days and then converted slowly to alternate-day therapy by increasing the "on-day" and decreasing the "off-day" dose until a total of 1 mg/kg/day on alternate days is administered.[154] Alternate-day therapy is preferred to minimize adrenocortical suppression. Once therapy is initiated, 1 to 2 months may pass before an improvement in clinical symptoms is noted. Therapy is

Table 92-9 Abbreviated Table of Signs and Symptoms of Chronic Graft-versus-Host Disease (GVHD)[a]

Affected Organ	Diagnostic	Distinctive	Other Features[b]	Seen With Both Acute and Chronic GVHD
Eyes		New-onset drug, gritty or painful eyes[c] Cicatricial conjunctivitis Keratoconjunctivitis sicca[c] Confluent areas of punctuate keratopathy, tear formation, dry eyes, burning, photophobia	Photophobia Periorbital hyperpigmentation Erythema of the eyelids with edema	
Gastrointestinal tract	Esophageal web Stricture or stenosis in the upper to mid third of the esophagus[d]		Pancreatic insufficiency	Anorexia Nausea Vomiting Diarrhea Weight loss Failure to thrive (infants and children)
Liver				Total bilirubin, alkaline phosphatase >2 × upper limit of normal[d]
Lung	Bronchiolitis obliterans diagnosis with lung biopsy	Bronchiolitis obliterans diagnosed with pulmonary function tests and radiology[c]		Bronchiolitis obliterans organizing pneumonia
Skin	Poikiloderma Lichen planuslike features Sclerotic features Morphealike features Lichen sclerosuslike features	Depigmentation	Seat impairment ichthyosis Keratosis pilaris Hypopigmentation Hyperpigmentation	Erythema Maculopapular rash Pruritus

[a]Signs and symptoms for nails; scalp and body hair; mouth; genitalia; muscles, fascia, and joints; hematopoietic and immune; and other organs are also described by Filipovich et al.[153]

[b]Can be acknowledged as part of chronic GVHD symptomatology if the diagnosis is confirmed.

[c]Diagnosis of chronic GVHD requires biopsy or radiology confirmation (or Schirmer's test for eyes).

[d]Infection, drug effects, malignancy, or other causes must be excluded.

usually continued for 9 to 12 months and then slowly tapered after signs and symptoms of chronic GVHD have resolved. If chronic GVHD worsens during the tapering or after discontinuation of prednisone, immunosuppressive therapy is restarted. Other potential approaches for patients with refractory chronic GVHD include mycophenolate mofetil, daclizumab, sirolimus, pentostatin, and extracorporeal photochemotherapy.[154]

When immunosuppressive therapy is administered for long periods, the patient must be monitored closely for chronic toxicity. Cushingoid effects, aseptic necrosis of the joints, and diabetes can develop with long-term corticosteroid use. Other severe complications include a high incidence of infection with encapsulated organisms and atypical pathogens such as *Pneumocystis jiroveci* (*P. Jiroveci*) pneumonia, CMV, and herpes zoster.

Thus, it is reasonable to start M.P. on single-agent prednisone for chronic GVHD treatment.

Adjuvant Therapies

35. Suggest some adjuvant therapies that should be instituted in a patient like M.P. with chronic GVHD.

Patients who are being treated for chronic GVHD should receive trimethoprim-sulfamethoxazole for prophylaxis of *P. jiroveci* and encapsulated organisms, such as *Streptococcus pneumoniae* and *Haemophilus influenzae.* Ensuring optimal prophylactic antibiotics in chronic GVHD patients is critical because infection is the primary cause of death during treatment.[155] Artificial tears and saliva may improve lubrication and decrease the occurrence of cracking and fissures in mucous membranes. If nutritional intake is poor, consultation with a clinical nutritionist and use of oral nutritional supplementation may be advisable. Patients should be instructed to apply sunscreens to exposed areas whenever prolonged sun exposure is anticipated. Liver function abnormalities have been improved by up to 30% with the use of ursodiol as bile acid displacement therapy.[116–118] Calcium supplements, estrogen replacement, or other antiosteoporosis agents should be considered in women or other patients at risk for fracture or bone loss while receiving prolonged regimens with immunosuppressant therapy.[156] Patient education regarding the delay in improvement of symptoms, anticipated duration of therapy, and importance of compliance with oral immunosuppressive therapy is essential.

INFECTIOUS COMPLICATIONS

Opportunistic infections are a major cause of morbidity and mortality after myeloablative and nonmyeloablative HCT. There are three general periods of infectious risk (Fig. 92-3). During the early period pre-engraftment, particularly for patients undergoing myeloablative HCT, the primary pathogens are aerobic bacteria, *Candida* spp., and herpes simplex virus (HSV). Chemotherapy-induced mucosal damage creates a portal of entry into the bloodstream for many organisms, such as viridans group *Streptococcus*, *Candida*, and aerobic gram-negative bacteria. *Staphylococcus* is also common because patients undergoing HCT have indwelling IV central catheters.

The routine use of antiviral prophylaxis has decreased the incidence of HSV. Respiratory viruses such as respiratory syncytial virus (RSV), influenza, adenovirus, and parainfluenza are increasingly recognized as pathogens causing pneumonia, particularly during community outbreaks of infection.[157] To reduce potential exposure of HCT recipients to these pathogens, visitors and staff members with signs and symptoms of a viral respiratory illness may not be allowed direct contact with patients.

A potential advantage of reduced intensity or nonmyeloablative preparative regimens is reduced toxicity of the preparative regimen compared to myeloablative HCT. Reduced intensity or nonmyeloablative preparative regimens frequently do not result in true neutropenia,[4] and the incidence of mucositis during the early period is reduced.[158] In a matched controlled study comparing the incidence of infection following nonmyeloablative and myeloablative HCT, the incidence of bacteremia during the first 30 days post-HCT in the nonmyeloablative group was significantly reduced.[158] Moreover, nonmyeloablative HCT recipients experienced significantly fewer infections attributable to mucositis during the early period.

The second or middle period of infectious risk includes the time from engraftment to posttransplantation day +100. Pathogens such as CMV, adenovirus, and *Aspergillus* are common. CMV, adenovirus, *Aspergillus,* and *P. jiroveci* frequently cause interstitial pneumonitis. Patients undergoing reduced intensity or nonmyeloablative preparative regimens that experience acute GVHD and are treated with corticosteroids have a similar risk of infection during this time period as those undergoing myeloablative HCT.[158]

During the late period (after day +100), the predominant pathogens are the encapsulated bacteria (e.g. *S. pneumoniae, H. influenzae, Neisseria meningitidis*), fungi, and varicella-zoster virus (VZV). The encapsulated bacteria commonly cause sinopulmonary infections. The risk of infection during this late period is increased in patients with chronic GVHD as a result of prolonged immunosuppression.

Because of the morbidity associated with opportunistic infection in HCT recipients, optimal pharmacotherapy for prevention and treatment is critical. In 2000, the Centers for Disease Control and Prevention (CDC) published guidelines for prevention of opportunistic infection in HCT recipients.[7] These guidelines were constructed from available data by an expert panel from CDC, the Infectious Disease Society of America (IDSA), and the American Society for Blood and Marrow Transplantation. The following discussion incorporates recommendations from the CDC guidelines and also provides information on the pharmacotherapy of opportunistic infections in all types of HCT.

Prevention and Treatment of Bacterial and Fungal Infections

36. S.D. is a 26-year-old woman with Ph$^+$ acute lymphocytic leukemia (ALL) in first complete remission who is admitted for allogeneic myeloablative HCT. The following orders are written: admit to a room with a positive-pressure HEPA filter. Flush double-lumen Hickman catheter per protocol. Immunosuppressed patient diet as tolerated. Begin fluconazole 400 mg PO Q 24 hr on admission. Begin ceftazidime 2 g IV Q 8 hr with first fever when ANC <500/mm^3. Transfuse 2 units of packed RBCs for hematocrit <25% and 1 unit of single-donor platelets for platelet count <20,000/mm^3. What is the rationale for these supportive measures?

As a result of disease-related immunosuppression, intensive preparative regimens, and posttransplantation immunosuppressive therapy, patients undergoing allogeneic HCT require careful vigilance for regimen-related toxicities and intensive supportive care directed at maintaining adequate blood counts, preventing or treating infection, and providing optimum nutrition.

Placement of a double-lumen or triple-lumen central venous catheter (e.g., Hickman, Groshong, Broviac, Neostar) is mandatory in all patients. The need for prolonged administration of chemotherapy, blood products, antibiotics, parenteral nutrition, and adjunctive medications precludes the use of peripheral access sites. The use of a central venous catheter allows delivery of maximum concentrations of all medications into a high-flow blood vessel. Administration time is reduced and daily fluid infusion is minimized.

After administration of the preparative regimen and before successful engraftment, allogeneic myeloablative HCT patients undergo a period of pancytopenia lasting from 2 to 6 weeks. During this time, patients may require multiple RBC and platelet transfusions. Packed RBCs and platelets are usually given for a hematocrit <25% and a platelet count less than 10,000/mm^3 or 20,000/mm^3. Transfusions with multiple blood products put patients at risk for blood product–derived infection (e.g., CMV, hepatitis). In addition, sensitization to foreign leukocyte HLA antigens (alloimmunization) may cause immune-mediated thrombocytopenia. Thus, blood product support in the myeloablative allogeneic HCT patient must incorporate strategies that reduce the risk of viral infection and alloimmunization. Effective methods include minimizing the number of pretransplant infusions, use of single-donor rather than pooled-donor blood products, irradiating blood products, and filtering blood products with leukocyte reduction filters.

Patients receiving reduced intensity or nonmyeloablative preparative regimens may or may not experience neutropenia and generally have reduced requirements for blood products. In fact, many centers perform reduced intensity or nonmyeloablative HCT in the outpatient setting and admit patients to the hospital only for complications requiring more aggressive management.

Several measures are recommended to minimize the risk of infection in autologous and allogeneic myeloablative HCT patients. Private reverse isolation rooms equipped with positive-pressure HEPA filters and adherence to strict handwashing techniques reduce the incidence of bacterial and fungal infections.[7] To reduce exposure to exogenous sources of bacteria in immunosuppressed patients, low microbial diets are instituted on hospital admission, and visitors are prohibited from bringing plants or flowers into the patient's room. Patients are encouraged to maintain good oral hygiene because the mouth can be a source of bacterial or fungal infection. Frequent (four to six times daily) mouth rinses with sterile water, normal saline, or sodium bicarbonate are effective.[7] Brushing or flossing teeth is avoided during periods of thrombocytopenia and neutropenia.

Aggressive use of antibacterial, antifungal, and antiviral therapy, both prophylactically and for documented infection, is an important aspect of patient management. Antibiotics with a broad gram-negative spectrum may be instituted prophylactically once the patient becomes neutropenic, or empirically after the patient is neutropenic and experiences fever. S.D. will receive ceftazidime empirically. Some transplant centers administer a prophylactic fluoroquinolone such as levofloxacin on admission for HCT and then switch to a broad-spectrum IV antibiotic such as ceftazidime, cefepime, or imipenem when the patient becomes neutropenic and febrile. Fluoroquinolone prophylaxis significantly reduces the incidence of gram-negative bacteremia but generally does not affect mortality.[7] Concerns regarding prophylactic fluoroquinolone use include the emergence of resistant organisms and an increased risk of streptococcal infection.[7,159] The incidence of infection during HCT due primarily to members of the viridans group of streptococci is increasing, and prompt, aggressive treatment is warranted.[7,160] Prophylactic antibiotics (e.g., penicillin, vancomycin) are not recommended due to their lack of proven efficacy in preventing streptococcal infections and the concern about antibiotic-resistant bacteria.[7] At a minimum, broad-spectrum IV antibiotics should be initiated or added at the time of the first neutropenic fever according to treatment guidelines endorsed by the IDSA.[7,161]

S.D. is prescribed fluconazole 400 mg/day because prophylactic use of this agent until day +75 posttransplantation decreases the incidence of systemic fungal infection and fungal death in patients undergoing transplantation.[162,163] The use of prophylactic fluconazole by most HCT centers has been linked to reports of breakthrough infections with resistant fungi such as *C. glabrata* and *Aspergillus*.[164,165] Itraconazole has improved activity *in vitro* against fluconazole-resistant fungi. In a randomized clinical trial, allogeneic HCT patients treated with prophylactic itraconazole (200 mg IV Q 24 hr or oral solution 200 mg BID) developed significantly fewer invasive fungal infections than those treated with fluconazole (400 mg Q 24 hr). Although there was a trend toward fewer fungal deaths in the itraconazole-treated patients, overall mortality was similar. Itraconazole was associated with more frequent GI side effects (e.g., nausea, vomiting).[166]

Published data supporting the use of newer mold-active agents for antifungal prophylaxis are limited. Van Burik et al. compared micafungin (50 mg IV Q 24 hr) to fluconazole (400 mg IV Q 24 hr) in a randomized, double-blind study of patients undergoing HCT. Overall success was defined as the absence of suspected, proven, or probable systemic fungal infection through the end of therapy and as the absence of proven or probable systemic fungal infection through the end of the 4-week posttreatment period. The overall efficacy was greater in the patients who received micafungin (80.0% vs. 73.5% in patients treated with fluconazole, $p = 0.03$). Fewer episodes of aspergillosis occurred in patients treated with micafungin. Patient tolerability of the regimens was similar.[167]

Prevention of Herpes Simplex Virus and Varicella-Zoster Virus

37. On routine screening before transplantation, S.D. is found to be HSV and VZV seropositive. How will this affect her management?

Forty-three to 70% of HSV-seropositive patients undergoing myeloablative allogeneic HCT experience reactivation of HSV.[168,169] Prophylactic acyclovir is commonly used in HSV-seropositive patients undergoing allogeneic or autologous HCT to prevent viral reactivation.[7] Dosing regimens for prophylactic acyclovir vary widely; the dose of IV acyclovir is typically 250 mg/m^2 IV Q 12 hr, whereas oral doses of acyclovir range from 600 mg/day to 1,600 mg/day.[7] The recommended duration of acyclovir prophylaxis for HSV varies from day +30 to day +365 posttransplantation or longer, depending on the specific type of HCT and other factors. Valacyclovir, a prodrug of acyclovir with improved bioavailability, may allow for adequate serum concentrations to prevent HSV in patients with mucositis or GI GVHD.[170] Prophylactic valacyclovir is commonly used at a dose of 500 mg PO Q 12 hr.[171,172]

VZV-seropositive patients are at risk for developing herpes zoster, particularly after day +100 posttransplanation.[170] Prophylactic acyclovir reduces the risk of VZV reactivation.[173] As with prophylaxis for HSV reactivation, the optimum duration of VZV prophylaxis is controversial, often extending to day +365 posttransplantation or longer.

Patients who are HSV or VZV seronegative rarely develop primary HSV or VZV infection and are therefore not administered prophylactic acyclovir. If HSV does occur, lesions usually appear on the oral mucosa, nasolabial mucous membranes, or genital mucocutaneous area and can be managed with acyclovir at appropriate treatment doses.

Because S.D. is HSV and VZV seropositive, she is at risk for viral reactivation and should receive prophylactic acyclovir.

Prevention of Cytomegalovirus Disease

38. S.D. is also CMV seropositive. What is the significance of this finding, and what measures can be taken to prevent reactivation of CMV?

CMV has the ability to establish lifelong latent infection following primary exposure. In immunocompromised patients, the virus may reactivate, resulting in asymptomatic shedding or the development of CMV disease. The incidence of CMV infection (defined as isolation of the virus or detection of viral proteins or nucleic acid in any body fluid) and CMV disease in HCT recipients is 15% to 60% and 20% to 35%, respectively. The most common manifestations of CMV disease after allogeneic HCT are pneumonitis, fever, and GI infection.[174]

In the CMV-seronegative HCT recipient, primary CMV can be prevented by transplanting PBPCs or bone marrow from CMV-seronegative donors and using only blood products from CMV-seronegative donors. In patients who are CMV-seropositive or who have received a CMV-seropositive graft, antiviral drugs are essential to minimize morbidity associated with CMV reactivation or secondary infection. Two general strategies are possible. Universal prophylaxis involves the administration of ganciclovir from the time of engraftment until approximately day +100 posttransplantation. This strategy significantly decreases the incidence of CMV infection and disease compared with placebo.[175] However, prophylactic ganciclovir therapy is associated with neutropenia in 30% of patients, which contributes to an increased risk of invasive bacterial and fungal infections.[175,176] Neutropenia secondary to ganciclovir may lead to interruptions in antiviral therapy or necessitate administration of filgrastim daily or several times per week to maintain adequate neutrophil counts.

Pre-emptive therapy, or risk-adjusted therapy, is the most commonly used strategy for preventing CMV disease after allogeneic HCT.[170,177] This strategy, based on detection of early reactivation of CMV using shell vial cultures, assay of blood for CMV antigens (e.g., pp65), or viral nucleic acid using the PCR results in the selective administration of ganciclovir to those HCT patients at greatest risk for development of CMV disease.[178–180] Antigenemia-based pre-emptive therapy is as effective as universal ganciclovir prophylaxis for prevention of CMV disease and has also been associated with reduced CMV mortality.[176,181–184] The induction dose of ganciclovir is typically 5 mg/kg IV Q 12 hr for 7 to 14 days, followed by a maintenance dose of 5 mg/kg IV daily until 2 to 3 weeks after the last occurrence of antigenemia or until day +100 posttransplantation.[7] Pre-emptive therapy limits patient exposure to the potential toxicity of ganciclovir and thus reduces overall cost.[173] Recent data suggest that oral valganciclovir is a safe and effective alternative to ganciclovir for pre-emptive therapy.[185,186] Foscarnet may be administered in lieu of ganciclovir, but its use is complicated by nephrotoxicity and electrolyte wasting.[184,187]

Autologous HCT recipients who are CMV-seropositive pretransplant should receive antiviral treatment pre-emptively as described previously.[7,188] Because host T cells may persist in the peripheral blood for up to 6 months following reduced intensity or nonmyeloablative preparative regimens, their presence may provide protection against early CMV disease. A matched controlled study comparing the incidence and outcome of CMV infection in myeloablative and nonmyeloablative HCT demonstrated that although the time to onset of CMV antigenemia was similar in the two groups, fewer nonmyeloablative HCT recipients developed CMV disease in the early period.[189] The overall 1-year incidence of CMV disease was also similar, suggesting that nonmyeloablative HCT recipients are at increased risk for developing late CMV disease (>100 days after transplantation) compared to their myeloablative counterparts.[189] It is therefore recommended that nonmyeloablative HCT patients receive pre-emptive antiviral therapy and be monitored for development of CMV antigenemia for 1 year after HCT.[189,190]

S.D.'s absolute neutrophil count recovers to >1,000 cells/μL on day +20, and on day +32, her weekly surveillance blood sample is positive for CMV by PCR. Pre-emptive ganciclovir therapy is initiated at 5 mg/kg IV Q 12 hr. After 3 weeks of therapy, S.D.'s surveillance samples are negative and ganciclovir is discontinued. Weekly surveillance sampling continues until day +100. If surveillance samples again become positive for CMV, ganciclovir therapy should be reinstituted.

Diagnosis and Treatment of *Aspergillus* Infection

Risk Factors

39. A.W., a 60-kg, 165-cm, 15-year-old boy, is day +79 after a matched, unrelated, nonmyeloablative PBPC transplant for ALL in third complete remission. He presents to the clinic for evaluation of a temperature of 102.3°F and a 3-day history of nonproductive cough. Significant medical history includes skin and GI GVHD (stable on his current regimen of cyclosporine, mycophenolate mofetil, and prednisone) and congestive heart failure believed to be secondary to anthracycline exposure. A.W. has chronic low-grade nausea and hypomagnesemia necessitating daily IV hydration with magnesium supplementation. Relevant laboratory values are as follows: Na, 138 mEq/L (normal, 135–147); K, 4.2 mEq/L (normal, 3.5–5.0); Cl, 100 mEq/L (normal, 95–105); CO_2, 23 mEq/L (normal, 22–28); blood urea nitrogen (BUN), 18 mg/dL (normal, 8–18); SrCr, 0.8 mg/dL (normal, 0.6–1.2); total bilirubin, 0.6 mg/dL (normal, 0.1–1); Mg, 1.5 mg/dL (normal, 1.6–2.4); WBC count, 3,500/mm^3 (normal, 3,200–9,800); platelets, 78,000/mm^3 (normal, 130,000–400,000); ANC, 1,810 cells/L (normal, >1,700); and Hgb, 10.8 g/dL (normal, 12–15). He was CMV and HSV seropositive before HCT. Oral medications include cyclosporine 275 mg Q 12 hr, mycophenolate mofetil 900 mg Q 12 hr, prednisone 60 mg Q am and 12.5 mg Q pm (tapering), trimethoprim-sulfamethoxazole (TMP/SMX) 160 mg/800 mg BID on Monday and Tuesday, fluconazole 400 mg Q am, valacyclovir 500 mg BID. digoxin 0.125 mg Q 12 hr, enalapril 10 mg Q 12 hr, and One-a-Day Plus vitamin Q am.

On physical examination, A.W. is a chronically ill–appearing child with moon facies, dry skin with thickened areas, a pleural friction rub, and thinning hair. Blood cultures, urinalysis, and chest x-ray are obtained. Chest x-ray reveals several small cavitary lesions worrisome for fungal disease. A.W. is admitted for further workup and management of presumed *Aspergillus* infection. What risk factors does A.W. have for developing infection with *Aspergillus*?

[SI units: Na, 138 mmol/L; K, 4.2 mmol/L; Cl, 100 mmol/L; CO_2, 23 mmol/L; BUN, 6.43 mmol/L; SrCr, 71 μmol/L; total bilirubin, 10.26 μmol/L; Mg, 0.61 mmol/L; WBC count, 3,500 × 10^6 cells/L; platelets, 78 × 10^9 cells/L; ANC, 1,810 × 10^6 cells/L; Hgb, 108 g/L]

Invasive molds (most commonly *Aspergillus* spp., but also *Fusarium* spp., *Scedosporium*, and *Zygomycetes*) are an increasing cause of morbidity and mortality after allogeneic and autologous HCT.[164] Factors contributing to this trend include (a) more effective prevention of bacterial and viral infection, as described previously; and (b) the use of fluconazole prophylaxis, which has reduced the incidence of candidemia and *Candida*-related mortality.[162–164,191,192] *Aspergillus* infection is reported in up to 26% of HCT recipients, and the mortality rate of invasive aspergillosis (IA) is 74% to 92%.[193]

Several risk factors for development of invasive fungal infection have been identified.[191,192] Given that neutrophils are critical for host defense, prolonged neutropenia is considered the single most important predictor of infection at all time points after HCT.[165,191] GVHD (acute and chronic) and treatment with corticosteroids are also important risk factors, particularly for aspergillosis occurring between day +40 and day +100 posttransplantation, presumably as a result of neutrophil dysfunction.[191,192,194] In addition, the widespread use of fluconazole prophylaxis (400 mg/day) for prevention of invasive candidiasis in transplant patients since the early 1990s has led to a substantial increase in the incidence of IA and also fluconazole-resistant *Candida* species such as *Candida krusei* and *Candida glabrata*.[191,194,195]

A.W. is receiving corticosteroid treatment for GVHD and fluconazole prophylaxis. These therapies increase his risk for developing IA.

Treatment

40. A.W. undergoes bronchoalveolar lavage in an attempt to identify the organism responsible for his infection. Pathological examination of the fluid obtained reveals septate, branching hyphae, and culture results confirm the diagnosis of *Aspergillus fumigatus* infection. CT scans are negative for extrapulmonary involvement. A.W. is started on amphotericin B lipid complex (ABLC) at a dose of 300 mg IV daily. How is aspergillosis usually diagnosed, and what are the acceptable alternatives for treating this infection?

Early diagnosis and treatment of IA, which rely on tissue or fluid obtained from the infected site followed by aggressive antifungal therapy, may improve patient survival.[196] Although the lower respiratory tract is frequently the primary focus of infection, *Aspergillus* may invade blood vessels and spread hematogenously to other organs, including the brain, liver, kidneys, spleen, and skin.[197] Head, chest, abdomen, and pelvic CT scans assist in assessing the extent of disease, treatment options, and overall prognosis. Cultures of respiratory tract secretions lack sensitivity for detecting *Aspergillus*, and the medical condition of the patient may preclude invasive diagnostic procedures altogether. Many clinicians have adopted the European Organization for Research and Treatment of Cancer criteria for diagnosis of proven, probable, and possible IA.[198]

Newer diagnostic tests based on the detection of fungal antigens or metabolites, such as galactomannan, 1,3-β-D-glucan, and fungal DNA detection by PCR, are being developed. Galactomannan is a polysaccharide component of the *Aspergillus* cell wall that is released during fungal cell growth. Galactomannan detection by enzyme-linked immunoassay (GM-EIA) has proved to be a sensitive and specific tool for early detection of *Aspergillus* infection. The test is useful not only for serum samples, but also for bronchoalveolar lavage and cerebrospinal fluid. Concomitant antifungal therapy may cause false-negative GM-EIA results, whereas antibiotics of fungal origin (e.g., piperacillin/tazobactam) have been associated with false positives.[193,199]

Antifungals

Outcomes for patients with IA after HCT are often poor, with approximately 20% of patients alive after 1 year.[191] Treatment success depends not only on the use of intensive antifungal agents, but also on recovery of the host immune system and/or reduction of immunosuppression.[196,200] Conventional amphotericin B (c-AmB) at a dose of at least 1 mg/kg/day has traditionally been the gold standard antifungal therapy for IA. Response rates with c-AmB monotherapy range from 28% to 51%, depending on the severity of the underlying immunosuppression; however, 65% of responders eventually die of their infection.[196] Moreover, toxicity associated with c-AmB frequently limits the dose and duration of therapy. Fortunately, the lipid derivatives of amphotericin B, broad-spectrum triazoles, and echinocandins are available as alternatives to c-AmB.

Three lipid formulations of amphotericin B have been marketed: ABLC (Abelcet), liposomal amphotericin B (L-AmB; AmBisome) and amphotericin B colloidal dispersion (ABCD; Amphotec). Practice guidelines delineating use of these agents for fungal infections in HCT patients have been published.[201] Studies of lipid amphotericin B formulations as monotherapy for patients with IA who have failed or are intolerant to c-AmB therapy demonstrate response rates of 23% to 71%, regardless of which formulation is used. No randomized trials show superiority of lipid amphotericin B products over c-Amb for IA.[200] Doses most commonly used in the studies are 5 mg/kg/day for ABLC and L-AmB and 4 to 6 mg/kg/day for ABCD. The lipid formulations of amphotericin B are clearly less toxic than c-AmB, with L-AmB being the least toxic.[202]

The cost of the amphotericin B lipid formulations, which is 15- to 30-fold higher than c-AmB, is a limiting factor. Drug acquisition cost should be balanced against the potential expense of managing c-AmB nephrotoxicity. A recent pharmacoeconomic evaluation comparing hospital costs for neutropenic patients with persistent fever treated with L-AmB or c-AmB demonstrated significantly higher overall costs for patients receiving L-Amb, principally due to higher acquisition cost.[203] Thus, establishing cost-effective strategies for the appropriate use of the lipid amphotericin b formulations is imperative. Most HCT centers have developed criteria for appropriate use based on risk for nephrotoxicity and severity of the infection being treated.

Three broad-spectrum triazole agents are available for patients who are refractory to or intolerant of amphotericin B therapy. Oral itraconazole capsules (Sporanox) were approved in 1992, followed later by the oral solution and an IV formulation. In an early compassionate use trial of IA unresponsive to amphotericin B, 27% of patients had a complete response to itraconazole, and another 35% experienced improvement in their infection.[204] Patients who had undergone HCT had response rates similar to patients who were less immunocompromised. Unfortunately, oral itraconazole capsules exhibit erratic absorption, and the IV form is complicated by the risk of drug precipitation in the IV line.[200] In addition, itraconazole is a potent inhibitor of common CYP isoforms and also has negative inotropic properties.[205,206]

Voriconazole (Vfend) was approved in 2002. An advantage of voriconazole is excellent (96%) oral bioavailability; however, like itraconazole, the drug is a potent inhibitor of cytochrome P450 enzymes. Voriconazole has been compared to c-AmB in a randomized, unblinded trial as primary therapy for established IA in an immunocompromised host.[207] The primary study objective was to demonstrate the noninferiority of voriconazole compared with c-AmB after 12 weeks of therapy in patients with definite or probable IA. Patients received voriconazole 6 mg/kg IV Q 12 hr × two doses followed by 4 mg/kg IV Q 12 hr for at least 7 days, followed by oral voriconazole 200 mg Q 12 hr or c-AmB at a dose of 1 to 1.5 mg/kg/day. Patients refractory to or intolerant of initial therapy could receive other antifungal drugs. Of 144 evaluable patients who received voriconazole, 76 (52.8%) had a partial or complete response compared to 42 of 133 (31.6%) patients treated with c-Amb. The median duration of therapy for patients treated with voriconazole was 77 days, and 52 of 144 patients switched to an alternative agent. In contrast, the median duration of therapy for patients receiving c-AmB was 10 days, and 107 of 133 patients switched to another agent (most commonly, a lipid formulation of amphotericin B). The survival rate at 12 weeks in the voriconazole group was 70.8% compared to 57.9% in the c-Amb group ($p = 0.02$). These results of initial therapy with voriconazole indicate superior response and improved survival compared to c-AmB in immunocompromised patients, such as allogeneic HCT recipients, with IA. Voriconazole-treated patients also experienced fewer drug-related adverse effects.

Posaconazole (Noxafil) was approved in 2006. This broad-spectrum triazole is available only as a variably absorbed oral suspension, and like itraconazole and voriconazole, it is a cytochrome P4503A4 inhibitor. Posaconazole has the lowest MICs of any available triazole against *Aspergillus* spp., including *Aspergillus terreus*, and it is the only triazole with useful activity against the *Zygomycetes*. Published clinical experience with posaconazole is limited; however, in an open-label externally controlled trial in patients with IA refractory to or intolerant of other therapies, the overall success rate was 42% in posaconazole-treated patients compared to 26% for controls ($p = 0.006$).[208]

Echinocandin antifungal agents (caspofungin, micafungin, and anidulafungin) inhibit the synthesis of β-(1,3)-glucan, an important component of the fungal cell wall. No prospective randomized trials document the efficacy of any echinocandin for primary therapy of IA, and only caspofungin is approved for salvage therapy. An open-label, noncomparative trial evaluated the efficacy of caspofungin in 69 patients with IA who had failed or were intolerant of at least 7 days of standard antifungal therapy.[209] Patients received 70 mg IV of caspofungin on day 1 followed by 50 mg IV daily. Of the 63 evaluable patients, 26 (43%) responded favorably to treatment. Twenty-six of 52 patients (50%) who had received at least 7 days of therapy had a favorable response. In another open-label, noncomparative trial, Denning et al. evaluated the safety and efficacy of micafungin (alone or in combination) in patients with proven or probable IA. Eighty of 225 patients (35.6%) had a favorable response. Most patients received combination therapy; the 34 patients treated with monotherapy had a similar response rate.[210]

In summary, the number of agents available to manage IA has expanded greatly in the past few years. Although some experts believe that voriconazole is the drug of first choice, considerable controversy still exists. Therapy should be tailored to the individual patient based on response, tolerability, and cost.

Antifungal Toxicities

41. Despite premedication with acetaminophen and diphenhydramine, A.W. experiences significant chills and rigors with his ABLC infusions. In addition, he is having daily temperatures exceeding 39°C. On day 5 of therapy, morning laboratory tests reveal a SrCr of 1.4 mg/dL, K of 2.7 mEq/L, and Mg of 1.4 mg/dL. What expected adverse reactions of conventional amphotericin B–based therapy does A.W. demonstrate?

[SI units: SrCr, 123.8 μmol/L; K, 2.7 mmol/L; Mg, 0.57 mmol/L]

The most troublesome side effect of c-AmB therapy is nephrotoxicity. Up to 80% of patients treated with c-AmB will experience an episode of altered renal function.[211] The mechanism of amphotericin B nephrotoxicity is complex and poorly understood. It most likely results from afferent vasoconstriction leading to cortical ischemia and a subsequent decrease in glomerular filtration rate, as well as defective acid secretion by the renal tubule. Risk factors for nephrotoxicity include concomitant administration of other nephrotoxic drugs such as aminoglycosides, cyclosporine, cisplatin, and radiocontrast dye; prolonged duration of therapy; history of chronic renal disease; male gender; and a mean daily dose ≥35 mg.[212]

The lipid derivatives of amphotericin B were developed with the goal of reducing nephrotoxicity, and each is significantly less nephrotoxic compared to c-AmB.[201,213–216] Furthermore, patients treated with c-AmB who experience nephrotoxicity and are then switched to a lipid formulation frequently show improvement in renal function. It is difficult to determine the true incidence of nephrotoxicity associated with the lipid products because most trials evaluate their use in patients who have received prior c-AmB therapy. In addition, many trials do not control for other factors known to reduce the risk of nephrotoxicity, including sodium loading and IV fluid boluses administered before c-AmB infusion. Nonetheless, clinical experience confirms the reduced incidence of nephrotoxicity with these products, and they are recommended as first-line therapy for patients at high risk for nephrotoxicity or in whom baseline renal function is impaired.

Other toxicities of c-AmB include infusion-related reactions (fever, chills, rigors, hypotension, hypoxia), hypokalemia, hypomagnesemia, nausea, and anemia. Premedications such as acetaminophen, diphenhydramine, meperidine, and/or hydrocortisone are typically administered before each dose to lessen or prevent the infusion-related reactions, with mixed results. Patients may also develop tolerance. Fortunately, there appears to be a reduced incidence of infusion-related reactions when the lipid products are used. Significant hypokalemia and hypomagnesemia may persist well beyond discontinuation of c-AmB. Most patients require daily potassium and magnesium supplementation, particularly if they require prolonged antifungal treatment.

Length of Antifungal Therapy and Combination Antifungal Therapy

42. In response to A.W.'s rise in SrCr, his physician elects to discontinue ABLC and begin voriconazole 6 mg/kg IV Q 12 hr × two doses, followed by 4 mg/kg IV Q 12 hr plus caspofungin 70 mg IV on day 1 and 50 mg IV QD thereafter. What is the rationale for combination therapy, and how should the patient be monitored? How long should A.W. receive antifungal therapy for his IA?

Common toxicities reported with voriconazole include reversible visual disturbances (blurred vision, altered color perception, photophobia, visual hallucinations), skin reactions (rash, pruritus, photosensitivity), elevations in hepatic transaminase enzymes and alkaline phosphatase, nausea, and headache.[207,217,218] Caspofungin has fewer adverse effects. Vein irritation and headache are most common; dermatologic reactions related to histamine release (flushing, erythema, wheals) have also been reported. Increased hepatic transaminase enzymes occur in approximately 6% of patients treated with caspofungin.[209] A.W. should be monitored for changes in liver function and counseled regarding the potential visual side effects of voriconazole.

Data supporting improved outcomes with two-drug combinations of triazoles, echinocandins, and polyenes in patients with IA are sparse. However, *in vitro* and animal data suggest that an echinocandin plus voriconazole or a polyene may be synergistic.[219–222] Given the overall poor prognosis of IA in severely immunocompromised patients, many practitioners are choosing to treat patients with two-drug combination therapy. Voriconazole in combination with caspofungin is thus a reasonable alternative for A.W., particularly in view of the ABLC toxicity he is experiencing.

The optimum duration of antifungal therapy for treatment of IA is unestablished.[200] Important considerations include the status of the patient's immune system and the extent of response to treatment. Many clinicians continue aggressive antifungal therapy until the infection has stabilized radiographically and then proceed with less aggressive "maintenance" therapy (e.g., single-agent oral voriconazole) until restoration of the immune system has taken place. It is not uncommon for a patient to require several months of antifungal therapy for effective management of IA.

Prevention of *Pneumocystis jiroveci* pneumonia

43. A.W. is receiving TMP/SMX, one double-strength tablet PO BID on Monday and Tuesday. What is the rationale for its use?

P. jiroveci (formerly *Pneumocystis carinii*) is a common pathogen in patients who have undergone allogeneic HCT. Pneumocystis pneumonia (PCP) is a potentially lethal infection, and therefore, prophylaxis is routinely administered. The optimum prophylactic regimen is unestablished, but most centers administer TMP/SMX for PCP prophylaxis.[7] Dapsone or aerosolized pentamidine are alternatives for patients who are allergic to sulfonamides or do not tolerate TMP/SMX for other reasons.

PCP prophylaxis is usually begun following neutrophil recovery because (a) PCP most commonly occurs after engraftment, and (b) TMP/SMX is potentially myelosuppressing. Patients should be closely monitored for unexplained neutropenia or thrombocytopenia. Rash secondary to the sulfonamide component of TMP/SMX may force its discontinuation. TMP/SMX is usually avoided on days of methotrexate administration because of increased systemic methotrexate exposure resulting from increased methotrexate free fraction and decreased renal clearance of free methotrexate.[223] Prophylaxis is typically continued for 6 to 12 months posttransplantation.

The risk of PCP is lower in autologous HCT patients because posttransplant immunosuppression is not used. However, TMP/SMX prophylaxis may be administered after autologous HCT for non-Hodgkin lymphoma, Hodgkin disease, multiple myeloma, and lymphocytic leukemia because of the immunosuppressive nature of the underlying disease.

ISSUES OF SURVIVORSHIP AFTER HEMATOPOIETIC STEM CELL TRANSPLANTATION

44. H.O. is a 32-year-old woman who received a BU/CY preparative regimen and an HLA-matched sibling BMT for treatment of chronic phase CML at age 21. H.O. received her BMT more than 10 years ago, is disease free, and has not had chronic GVHD for 9 years. Her only medication is one multivitamin tablet PO QD. What issues of cancer survivorship are of concern to H.O.?

A greater proportion of HCT recipients are surviving their cancer diagnosis without evidence of their primary malignancy, but they are at risk for long-term physical and emotional sequelae of their cancer treatments.[1] Since most long-term HCT survivors are no longer under the care of an HCT center, their health care providers may be unfamiliar with the complications of HCT. To facilitate the clinical care of long-term HCT recipients, recommendations for screening and preventative practices have been created for adult and pediatric HCT survivors.[224,225] These guidelines should facilitate the provision of health care to HCT recipients. The following paragraphs describe various concerns associated with the morbidity of long-term HCT survivors.[224–226] Long-term HCT survivors should be regularly screened, or take preventative steps regarding immunity, secondary malignant neoplasm, oral complications, and liver, respiratory, endocrine, ocular, skeletal, nervous system, kidney, vascular, and psychosocial function.

Immune function can take more than 2 years to recover, even without immunosuppressants.[227] Treatment of GVHD exacerbates immune system defects, necessitating prophylaxis and vigilant monitoring for infectious complications. Fevers should be rapidly assessed and treated to prevent a fatal infection. Recipients of HCT also lose protective antibodies to vaccine-preventable diseases. Therefore, HCT survivors need to be revaccinated for selected infectious diseases with due consideration for the risk of vaccination.

HCT survivors have a greater risk of secondary malignant neoplasms.[1] An increased incidence of cancer of the skin, oral mucosa, brain, thyroid, and bone is observed after allogeneic HCT, while an increased incidence of myelodysplasia and acute leukemia can occur after autologous HCT for NHL.[1] HCT survivors should avoid carcinogens (e.g., tobacco) and be screened for secondary malignant neoplasms indefinitely.[1] Long-term impairment of end-organ function may be due to the preparative regimen, infectious complications (either autologous or allogeneic grafts), and posttransplantation immunosuppression (allogeneic grafts only).[224,225] Endocrine dysfunction, specifically of the thyroid, gonads, and growth velocity, is common.[224,225] Adrenal insufficiency can result from long-term corticosteroids therapy used to treat GVHD. Infertility is commonly observed after myeloablative HCT secondary to the high doses of alkylating agents and radiation administered. Frequently, men become azoospermic, and chemically induced menopause develops in women.[1] However, pregnancies have occurred after HCT.[1] Up to 60% of HCT recipients have osteopenia, most likely resulting from gonadal dysfunction and corticosteroid administration; avascular necrosis due to corticosteroids can also occur.[228] A significant portion (15%–40%) of HCT survivors develop pulmonary dysfunction with variable symptoms (e.g., restrictive, chronic obstructive lung disease) from multiple causes.[228] Hepatic infections can occur in HCT recipients, with the prevalence of chronic hepatitis C ranging from 5% to 70% in long-term HCT survivors.[229] Because of this, cirrhosis and its complications may become an important late complication of HCT.[229] Hepatic dysfunction can also result from iron overload, which may occur secondary to multiple PRBC transfusions administered during aplasia after myeloablative preparative regimens and before HCT. Alopecia is a common late effect with BU/CY, as are cataracts with CY/TBI.[64]

H.O. should be routinely monitored for signs of relapse and chronic GVHD. To lower the risk of infectious complications, she should be counseled to obtain prompt medical care for fevers or signs of an infection, and she should be revaccinated if she has not done so since receiving her myeloablative HCT. Thorough evaluation of end-organ function, including renal, hepatic, thyroid, and ovarian function, should be assessed at regular intervals. In addition, her bone mineral density should be determined, and H.O. should be counseled on preventive measures for osteopenia (e.g., calcium supplementation). In addition to standard cancer screening tests, H.O. should be closely monitored for secondary malignant neoplasms.[1]

REFERENCES

1. Copelan EA. Hematopoietic stem-cell transplantation. *N Engl J Med* 2006;354:1813.
2. Eder JP et al. A phase I–II study of cyclophosphamide, thiotepa, and carboplatin with autologous bone marrow transplantation in solid tumor patients. *J Clin Oncol* 1990;8:1239.
3. Appelbaum FR. Haematopoietic cell transplantation as immunotherapy. *Nature* 2001;411:385.
4. McSweeney PA et al. Hematopoietic cell transplantation in older patients with hematologic malignancies: replacing high-dose cytotoxic therapy with graft-versus-tumor effects. *Blood* 2001;97:3390.
5. Khouri IF et al. Transplant-lite: induction of graft-versus-malignancy using fludarabine-based nonablative chemotherapy and allogeneic blood progenitor-cell transplantation as treatment for lymphoid malignancies. *J Clin Oncol* 1998;16:2817.
6. Baron F, Storb R. Allogeneic hematopoietic cell transplantation following nonmyeloablative conditioning as treatment for hematologic malignancies and inherited blood disorders. *Mol Ther* 2006;13:26.
7. Guidelines for preventing opportunistic infections among hematopoietic stem cell transplant recipients. *MMWR Recomm Rep* 2000;49:1.
8. Schmitz N, Barrett J. Optimizing engraftment—source and dose of stem cells. *Semin Hematol* 2002;39:3.
9. Ng Cashin J, Shea T. Mobilization of autologous peripheral blood hematopoietic cells for support of high-dose cancer therapy. In: Blume KG et al., eds. *Thomas' Hematopoietic Cell Transplantation.* 3rd ed. Malden, MA: Blackwell; 2004:576.
10. Hehlmann R et al. Drug treatment is superior to allografting as first-line therapy in chronic myeloid leukemia. *Blood* 2007;109:4686.
11. Anderlini P, Champlin R. Use of filgrastim for stem cell mobilisation and transplantation in high-dose cancer chemotherapy. *Drugs* 2002;62(Suppl 1):79.
12. Rizzo JD, 1998 Summary data from International Bone Marrow Transplant Registry/Autologous Bone Marrow Transplant Registry. *ABMTR Newsl* 1998;5:4.
13. Ratanatharathorn V et al. Prospective comparative trial of autologous versus allogeneic bone marrow transplantation in patients with non-Hodgkin's lymphoma. *Blood* 1994;84:1050.
14. Hahn T et al. The role of cytotoxic therapy with hematopoietic stem cell transplantation in the therapy of diffuse large cell B-cell non-Hodgkin's lymphoma: an evidence-based review. *Biol Blood Marrow Transplant* 2001;7:308.
15. Haioun C et al. Survival benefit of high-dose therapy in poor-risk aggressive non-Hodgkin's lymphoma: final analysis of the prospective LNH87–2 protocol—a groupe d'Etude des lymphomes de l'Adulte study. *J Clin Oncol* 2000;18:3025.
16. Santini G et al. VACOP-B versus VACOP-B plus autologous bone marrow transplantation for advanced diffuse non-Hodgkin's lymphoma: results of a prospective randomized trial by the Non-Hodgkin's Lymphoma Cooperative Study Group. *J Clin Oncol* 1998;16:2796.
17. National Comprehensive Cancer Network (NCCN). NCCN Clinical Practice Guidelines in Oncology: Non-Hodgkin's Lymphoma. Version 2.2008. 2008, February 28. Available at: http://www.nccn.org/professionals/physician_gls/PDF/nhl.pdf. Accessed March 5, 2008.
18. Philip T et al. Autologous bone marrow transplantation as compared with salvage chemotherapy in relapses of chemotherapy-sensitive non-Hodgkin's lymphoma. *N Engl J Med* 1995;333:1540.
19. Rowley SD. Cryopreservation of hematopoietic cells. In: Blume KG et al, eds. *Thomas' Hematopoietic Cell Transplantation.* 3rd ed. Malden, MA: Blackwell; 2004:599.
20. Smith TJ et al. 2006 Update of recommendations for the use of white blood cell growth factors: evidence-based clinical practice guidelines. American Society of Clinical Oncology Growth Factors Expert Panel. *J Clin Oncol* 2006;24:3187.
21. Berenson RJ et al. Engraftment after infusion of CD34+ marrow cells in patients with breast cancer or neuroblastoma. *Blood* 1991;77:1717.
22. Figuerres E et al. Analysis of parameters affecting engraftment in children undergoing autologous peripheral blood stem cell transplants. *Bone Marrow Transplant* 2000;25:583.
23. Meisenberg BR et al. Outpatient high-dose chemotherapy with autologous stem-cell rescue for hematologic and nonhematologic malignancies. *J Clin Oncol* 1997;15:11.
24. Rizzo JD et al. Outpatient-based bone marrow transplantation for hematologic malignancies: cost saving or cost shifting? *J Clin Oncol* 1999;17:2811.
25. Gilbert C et al. Sequential prophylactic oral and empiric once-daily parenteral antibiotics for neutropenia and fever after high-dose chemotherapy and autologous bone marrow support. *J Clin Oncol* 1994;12:1005.
26. Gisselbrecht C et al. Placebo-controlled phase III trial of lenograstim in bone-marrow transplantation. *Lancet* 1994;343:696.
27. Greenberg P et al. GM-CSF accelerates neutrophil recovery after autologous hematopoietic stem cell transplantation. *Bone Marrow Transplant* 1996;18:1057.
28. Rabinowe SN et al. Long-term follow-up of a phase III study of recombinant human granulocyte-macrophage colony-stimulating factor after autologous bone marrow transplantation for lymphoid malignancies. *Blood* 1993;81:1903.
29. Klumpp TR et al. Granulocyte colony-stimulating factor accelerates neutrophil engraftment following peripheral-blood stem-cell transplantation: a prospective, randomized trial. *J Clin Oncol* 1995;13:1323.
30. Spitzer G et al. Randomized study of growth factors post-peripheral-blood stem-cell transplant: neutrophil recovery is improved with modest clinical benefit. *J Clin Oncol* 1994;12:661.
31. Cortelazzo S et al. Granulocyte colony-stimulating factor following peripheral-blood progenitor-cell transplant in non-Hodgkin's lymphoma. *J Clin Oncol* 1995;13:935.
32. Legros M et al. rhGM-CSF vs. placebo following rhGM-CSF-mobilized PBPC transplantation: a phase III double-blind randomized trial. *Bone Marrow Transplant.* 1997;Feb 19:209.
33. Powles R et al. Human recombinant GM-CSF in allogeneic bone-marrow transplantation for leukaemia: double-blind, placebo-controlled trial. *Lancet* 1990;336:1417.
34. Erlich HA et al. HLA DNA typing and transplantation. *Immunity* 2001;14:347.
35. Davies SM et al. Engraftment and survival after unrelated-donor bone marrow transplantation: a report from the national marrow donor program. *Blood* 2000;96:4096.
36. Estey EH. Treatment of acute myelogenous leukemia. *Oncology* 2002;16:343.
37. National Comprehensive Cancer Network (NCCN). NCCN Clinical Practice Guidelines in Oncology: Acute Myeloid Leukemia. Version 1.2008. 2007, December 31. Available at: http://www.nccn.org/professionals/physician_gls/PDF/aml.pdf. Accessed March 5, 2008.
38. Mickelson E, Petersdorf EW. Histocompatibility. In: Blume KG et al, eds. *Thomas' Hematopoietic Cell Transplantation.* 3rd ed. Malden, MA: Blackwell; 2004:31.
39. Petersdorf EW et al. Major-histocompatibility-complex class I alleles and antigens in hematopoietic-cell transplantation. *N Engl J Med* 2001; 345:1794.
40. Weisdorf DJ et al. Allogeneic bone marrow transplantation for chronic myelogenous leukemia: comparative analysis of unrelated versus matched sibling donor transplantation. *Blood* 2002;99:1971.
41. Anasetti C et al. Improving availability and safety of unrelated donor transplants. *Curr Opin Oncol* 2000;12:121.
42. Morishima Y et al. The clinical significance of human leukocyte antigen (HLA) allele compatibility in patients receiving a marrow transplant from serologically HLA-A, HLA-B, and HLA-DR matched unrelated donors. *Blood* 2002;99:4200.
43. Sierra J, Anasetti C. Hematopoietic transplantation from adult unrelated donors. *Curr Opin Organ Transplant* 2003;8:99.
44. O'Donnell MR. Blood Group incompatibilities and hemolytic complications of hematopoietic cell transplantation. In: Blume KG et al., eds. *Thomas' Hematopoietic Cell Transplantation.* 3rd ed. Malden, MA: Blackwell; 2004:824.
45. Report on state of the art in blood and marrow transplantation. *IBMTR/ABMTR Newsl* 2006;12:1.
46. Tjonnfjord GE et al. Characterization of CD34+ peripheral blood cells from healthy adults mobilized by recombinant human granulocyte colony-stimulating factor. *Blood* 1994;84:2795.
47. Brown RA et al. Factors that influence the collection and engraftment of allogeneic peripheral-blood stem cells in patients with hematologic malignancies. *J Clin Oncol* 1997;15:3067.
48. Rowley SD et al. Experiences of donors enrolled in a randomized study of allogeneic bone marrow or peripheral blood stem cell transplantation. *Blood* 2001;97:2541.
49. Bittencourt H et al. Association of CD34 cell dose with hematopoietic recovery, infections, and other outcomes after HLA-identical sibling bone marrow transplantation. *Blood* 2002;99:2726.
50. Bolan CD et al. Controlled study of citrate effects and response to i.v. calcium administration during allogeneic peripheral blood progenitor cell donation. *Transfusion* 2002;42:935.
51. Allogeneic peripheral blood stem-cell compared with bone marrow transplantation in the management of hematologic malignancies: an individual patient data meta-analysis of nine randomized trials. *J Clin Oncol* 2005;23:5074.
52. Broxmeyer HE, Smith FO. Cord blood hematopoietic cell transplantation. In: Blume KG et al, eds. *Thomas' Hematopoietic Cell Transplantation.* 3rd ed. Malden, MA: Blackwell; 2004:550.
53. Gluckman E. Hematopoietic stem-cell transplants using umbilical-cord blood. *N Engl J Med* 2001; 344:1860.
54. Laughlin MJ et al. Hematopoietic engraftment and survival in adult recipients of umbilical-cord blood from unrelated donors. *N Engl J Med* 2001; 344:1815.
55. Weiden PL et al. Antileukemic effect of graft-versus-host disease in human recipients of allogeneic-marrow grafts. *N Engl J Med* 1979;300:1068.

56. Weiden PL et al. Antileukemic effect of chronic graft-versus-host disease: contribution to improved survival after allogeneic marrow transplantation. *N Engl J Med* 1981;304:1529.
57. Ho VT, Soiffer RJ. The history and future of T-cell depletion as graft-versus-host disease prophylaxis for allogeneic hematopoietic stem cell transplantation. *Blood* 2001;98:3192.
58. Marmont AM et al. T-cell depletion of HLA-identical transplants in leukemia. *Blood* 1991;78:2120.
59. MacKinnon S. Who may benefit from donor leucocyte infusions after allogeneic stem cell transplantation? *Br J Haematol* 2000;110:12.
60. Childs RW. Nonmyeloablative allogeneic peripheral blood stem-cell transplantation as immunotherapy for malignant diseases. *Cancer J* 2000;6:179.
61. Pinkel D. Bone marrow transplantation in children. *J Pediatr* 1993;122:331.
62. Clift RA et al. Marrow transplantation for patients in accelerated phase of chronic myeloid leukemia. *Blood* 1994;84:4368.
63. Vassal G et al. Is 600 mg/m^2 the appropriate dosage of busulfan in children undergoing bone marrow transplantation? *Blood* 1992;79:2475.
64. Socie G et al. Busulfan plus cyclophosphamide compared with total-body irradiation plus cyclophosphamide before marrow transplantation for myeloid leukemia: long-term follow-up of 4 randomized studies. *Blood* 2001;98:3569.
65. Balducci L, Extermann M. Cancer and aging. An evolving panorama. *Hematol Oncol Clin North Am* 2000;14:1.
66. Champlin R et al. Nonmyeloablative preparative regimens for allogeneic hematopoietic transplantation: biology and current indications. *Oncology (Huntingt)* 2003;17:94.
67. Bryant E, Martin PJ. Documentation of engraftment and characterization of chimerism following hematopoietic cell transplantation. In: Blume KG et al, eds. *Thomas' Hematopoietic Cell Transplantation.* 3rd ed. Malden, MA: Blackwell; 2004:234.
68. Kristt D et al. Assessing quantitative chimerism longitudinally: technical considerations, clinical applications and routine feasibility. *Bone Marrow Transplant* 2007;39:255.
69. Baron F et al. Kinetics of engraftment in patients with hematologic malignancies given allogeneic hematopoietic cell transplantation after nonmyeloablative conditioning. *Blood* 2004;104:2254.
70. Deeg HJ et al. Optimization of allogeneic transplant conditioning: not the time for dogma. *Leukemia* 2006;20:1701.
71. Michallet M et al. Allogeneic hematopoietic stem-cell transplantation after nonmyeloablative preparative regimens: impact of pretransplantation and posttransplantation factors on outcome. *J Clin Oncol* 2001;19:3340.
72. Maris M et al. Nonmyeloablative hematopoietic stem cell transplants using 10 HLA antigen matched unrelated donors for patients with advanced hematologic malignancies. *Am Soc Hematol* 2002;100:275a.
73. Martin PJ et al. Effects of in vitro depletion of T cells in HLA-identical allogeneic marrow grafts. *Blood* 1985;66:664.
74. Nash RA et al. Phase 3 study comparing methotrexate and tacrolimus with methotrexate and cyclosporine for prophylaxis of acute graft-versus-host disease after marrow transplantation from unrelated donors. *Blood* 2000;96:2062.
75. Kasai M et al. Toxicity of high-dose busulfan and cyclophosphamide as a preparative regimen for bone marrow transplantation. *Transplant Proc* 1992;24:1529.
76. Schuler U et al. Busulfan pharmacokinetics in bone marrow transplant patients: is drug monitoring warranted? *Bone Marrow Transplant* 1994;14:759.
77. Gibbs JP et al. The impact of obesity and disease on busulfan oral clearance in adults. *Blood* 1999;93:4436.
78. Nguyen L et al. Intravenous busulfan in adults prior to haematopoietic stem cell transplantation: a population pharmacokinetic study. *Cancer Chemother Pharmacol* 2006;57:191.
79. Openshaw H. Neurological complications of hematopoietic cell transplantation. In: Blume KG et al., eds. *Thomas' Hematopoietic Cell Transplantation.* 3rd ed. Malden, MA: Blackwell; 2004:811.
80. Tran HT et al. Individualizing high-dose oral busulfan: prospective dose adjustment in a pediatric population undergoing allogeneic stem cell transplantation for advanced hematologic malignancies. *Bone Marrow Transplant* 2000;26;463.
81. Package insert. IV Busulfex (busulfan) injection. Fremont, CA: PDL BioPharma, Inc. 2006, August. Available at: http://www.pdl.com/documents/IV_Busulfex_PI_US.pdf. Accessed March 5, 2008.
82. Dix SP et al. Association of busulfan area under the curve with veno-occlusive disease following BMT. *Bone Marrow Transplant* 1996;17:225.
83. Bolinger AM et al. Target dose adjustment of busulfan using pharmacokinetic parameters in pediatric patients undergoing bone marrow transplantation for malignancy or inborn errors. *Blood* 1997;90:374a.
84. Radich JP et al. HLA-matched related hematopoietic cell transplantation for CML chronic phase using a targeted busulfan and cyclophosphamide preparative regimen. *Blood* 2003;102:31.
85. McCune JS et al. Plasma concentration monitoring of busulfan: does it improve clinical outcome? *Clin Pharmacokinet* 2000;39:155.
86. Slattery JT, Risler LJ. Therapeutic monitoring of busulfan in hematopoietic stem cell transplantation. *Ther Drug Monit* 1998;20:543.
87. McCune JS, Slattery JT. Pharmacological considerations of primary alkylators. In: Andersson B, Murray D, eds. *Clinically Relevant Resistance in Cancer Chemotherapy.* Boston: Kluwer Academic; 2002:323.
88. Shepherd JD et al. Mesna versus hyperhydration for the prevention of cyclophosphamide-induced hemorrhagic cystitis in bone marrow transplantation. *J Clin Oncol* 1991;9:2016.
89. Cox PJ. Cyclophosphamide cystitis—identification of acrolein as the causative agent. *Biochem Pharmacol* 1979;28:2045.
90. Hensley ML et al. American Society of Clinical Oncology clinical practice guidelines for the use of chemotherapy and radiotherapy protectants. *J Clin Oncol* 1999;17:3333.
91. Hows JM et al. Comparison of mesna with forced diuresis to prevent cyclophosphamide induced haemorrhagic cystitis in marrow transplantation: a prospective randomised study. *Br J Cancer* 1984;50:753.
92. Vose JM et al. Mesna compared with continuous bladder irrigation as uroprotection during high-dose chemotherapy and transplantation: a randomized trial. *J Clin Oncol* 1993;11:1306.
93. James CA et al. Pharmacokinetics of intravenous and oral sodium 2-mercaptoethane sulphonate (mesna) in normal subjects. *Br J Clin Pharmacol* 1987;23:561.
94. Ren S et al. Pharmacokinetics of cyclophosphamide and its metabolites in bone marrow transplantation patients. *Clin Pharmacol Ther* 1998;64:289.
95. Fleming RA et al. Urinary elimination of cyclophosphamide alkylating metabolites and free thiols following two administration schedules of high-dose cyclophosphamide and mesna. *Bone Marrow Transplant* 1996;17:497.
96. Cohen EP. Renal failure after bone-marrow transplantation. *Lancet* 2001;357:6.
97. Bilgrami SF et al. Idiopathic pneumonia syndrome following myeloablative chemotherapy and autologous transplantation. *Ann Pharmacother* 2001;35:196.
98. Cooke KR, Yanik G. Acute lung injury after allogeneic stem cell transplantation: is the lung a target of acute graft-versus-host disease? *Bone Marrow Transplant* 2004;34:753.
99. Kris MG et al. American Society of Clinical Oncology guideline for antiemetics in oncology: update 2006. *J Clin Oncol* 2006;24:1.
100. Cagnoni PJ et al. Modification of the pharmacokinetics of high-dose cyclophosphamide and cisplatin by antiemetics. *Bone Marrow Transplant* 1999;24:1.
101. Gilbert CJ et al. Pharmacokinetic interaction between ondansetron and cyclophosphamide during high-dose chemotherapy for breast cancer. *Cancer Chemother Pharmacol* 1998;42:497.
102. McDonald GB et al. Cyclophosphamide metabolism, liver toxicity, and mortality following hematopoietic stem cell transplantation. *Blood* 2003;101:2043.
103. Strasser SI, McDonald GB. Gastrointestinal and hepatic complications. In: Blume KG et al., eds. *Thomas' Hematopoietic Cell Transplantation.* 3rd ed. Malden, MA: Blackwell; 2004:769.
104. Stiff P. Mucositis associated with stem cell transplantation: current status and innovative approaches to management. *Bone Marrow Transplant* 2001;27(Suppl 2):S3.
105. Keefe DM et al. Updated clinical practice guidelines for the prevention and treatment of mucositis. *Cancer* 2007;109:820.
106. Spielberger R et al. Palifermin for oral mucositis after intensive therapy for hematologic cancers. *N Engl J Med* 2004;351:2590.
107. Peters WP et al. Clinical and pharmacologic effects of high dose single agent busulfan with autologous bone marrow support in the treatment of solid tumors. *Cancer Res* 1987;47:6402.
108. DeLeve LD et al. Toxic injury to hepatic sinusoids: sinusoidal obstruction syndrome (veno-occlusive disease). *Semin Liver Dis* 2002;22:27.
109. Jones RJ et al. Venoocclusive disease of the liver following bone marrow transplantation. *Transplantation* 1987;44:778.
110. McDonald GB et al. Veno-occlusive disease of the liver and multiorgan failure after bone marrow transplantation: a cohort study of 355 patients. *Ann Intern Med* 1993;118:255.
111. Russell JA et al. Once-daily intravenous busulfan given with fludarabine as conditioning for allogeneic stem cell transplantation: study of pharmacokinetics and early clinical outcomes. *Biol Blood Marrow Transplant* 2002;8:468.
112. de Lima MD et al. Once-daily intravenous busulfan and fludarabine: clinical and pharmacokinetic results of a myeloablative, reduced-toxicity conditioning regimen for allogeneic stem cell transplantation in AML and MDS. *Blood* 2004;104:857.
113. Kashyap A et al. Intravenous versus oral busulfan as part of a busulfan-cyclophosphamide preparative regimen for allogeneic hematopoietic stem cell transplantation: decreased incidence of hepatic venoocclusive disease (HVOD), HVOD-related mortality, and overall 100-day mortality. *Biol Blood Marrow Transplant* 2002;8:493.
114. Lee JH et al. Decreased incidence of hepatic veno-occlusive disease and fewer hemostatic derangements associated with intravenous busulfan vs oral busulfan in adults conditioned with busulfan + cyclophosphamide for allogeneic bone marrow transplantation. *Ann Hematol* 2005;84:321.
115. McCune JS et al. Cyclophosphamide following targeted oral busulfan as conditioning for hematopoietic cell transplantation: pharmacokinetics, liver toxicity, and mortality. *Biol Blood Marrow Transplant* 2007;13:853.
116. Essell JH et al. Ursodiol prophylaxis against hepatic complications of allogeneic bone marrow transplantation: a randomized, double-blind, placebo-controlled trial. *Ann Intern Med* 1998;128:975.
117. Ohashi K et al. The Japanese multicenter open randomized trial of ursodeoxycholic acid prophylaxis for hepatic veno-occlusive disease after stem cell transplantation. *Am J Hematol* 2000;64:32.
118. Ruutu T et al. Ursodeoxycholic acid for the prevention of hepatic complications in allogeneic stem cell transplantation. *Blood* 2002;100:1977.
119. Richardson PG et al. Treatment of severe veno-occlusive disease with defibrotide: compassionate

use results in response without significant toxicity in a high-risk population. *Blood* 1998;92:737.
120. Chopra R et al. Defibrotide for the treatment of hepatic veno-occlusive disease: results of the European compassionate-use study. *Br J Haematol* 2000;111:1122.
121. Richardson PG et al. Multi-institutional use of defibrotide in 88 patients after stem cell transplantation with severe veno-occlusive disease and multisystem organ failure: response without significant toxicity in a high-risk population and factors predictive of outcome. *Blood* 2002;100:4337.
122. Wolff SN. Second hematopoietic stem cell transplantation for the treatment of graft failure, graft rejection or relapse after allogeneic transplantation. *Bone Marrow Transplant* 2002;29:545.
123. Baron F, Sandmaier BM. Current status of hematopoietic stem cell transplantation after nonmyeloablative conditioning. *Curr Opin Hematol* 2005;12:435.
124. Deeg HJ. How I treat refractory acute GVHD. *Blood* 2007;109:4119.
125. Tabbara IA et al. Allogeneic hematopoietic stem cell transplantation: complications and results. *Arch Intern Med* 2002;162:1558.
126. Beatty PG et al. Marrow transplantation from related donors other than HLA-identical siblings. *N Engl J Med* 1985;313:765.
127. Barker JN et al. Survival after transplantation of unrelated donor umbilical cord blood is comparable to that of human leukocyte antigen-matched unrelated donor bone marrow: results of a matched-pair analysis. *Blood* 2001;97:2957.
128. Rocha V et al. Comparison of outcomes of unrelated bone marrow and umbilical cord blood transplants in children with acute leukemia. *Blood* 2001;97:2962.
129. Rocha V et al. Graft-versus-host disease in children who have received a cord-blood or bone marrow transplant from an HLA-identical sibling. Eurocord and International Bone Marrow Transplant Registry Working Committee on Alternative Donor and Stem Cell Sources. *N Engl J Med* 2000;342:1846.
130. Storb R et al. Methotrexate and cyclosporine versus cyclosporine alone for prophylaxis of graft-versus-host disease in patients given HLA-identical marrow grafts for leukemia: long-term follow-up of a controlled trial. *Blood* 1989;73:1729.
131. Weiden PL et al. Anti-human thymocyte globulin (ATG) for prophylaxis and treatment of graft-versus-host disease in recipients of allogeneic marrow grafts. *Transplant Proc* 1978;10:213.
132. Deeg HJ et al. Cyclosporine as prophylaxis for graft-versus-host disease: a randomized study in patients undergoing marrow transplantation for acute nonlymphoblastic leukemia. *Blood* 1985;65:1325.
133. Storb R et al. Methotrexate and cyclosporine compared with cyclosporine alone for prophylaxis of acute graft versus host disease after marrow transplantation for leukemia. *N Engl J Med* 1986;314:729.
134. Ratanatharathorn V et al. Phase III study comparing methotrexate and tacrolimus (Prograf, FK506) with methotrexate and cyclosporine for graft-versus-host disease prophylaxis after HLA-identical sibling bone marrow transplantation. *Blood* 1998;92:2303.
135. Horowitz MM et al. Tacrolimus vs. cyclosporine immunosuppression: results in advanced-stage disease compared with historical controls treated exclusively with cyclosporine. *Biol Blood Marrow Transplant* 1999;5:180.
136. Chao NJ et al. Cyclosporine, methotrexate, and prednisone compared with cyclosporine and prednisone for prophylaxis of acute graft-versus-host disease. *N Engl J Med* 1993;329:1225.
137. Bacigalupo A et al. Prophylactic antithymocyte globulin reduces the risk of chronic graft-versus-host disease in alternative-donor bone marrow transplants. *Biol Blood Marrow Transplant* 2002;8:656.
138. Goker H et al. Acute graft-versus-host disease: pathobiology and management. *Exp Hematol* 2001;29:259.
139. Schultz KR et al. Effect of gastrointestinal inflammation and age on the pharmacokinetics of oral microemulsion cyclosporin A in the first month after bone marrow transplantation. *Bone Marrow Transplant* 2000;26:545.
140. Leather HL. Drug interactions in the hematopoietic stem cell transplant (HSCT) recipient: what every transplanter needs to know. *Bone Marrow Transplant* 2004;33:137.
141. Storb R et al. Marrow transplantation for chronic myelocytic leukemia: a controlled trial of cyclosporine versus methotrexate for prophylaxis of graft-versus-host disease. *Blood* 1985;66:698.
142. Storb R et al. What role for prednisone in prevention of acute graft-versus-host disease in patients undergoing marrow transplants? *Blood* 1990;76:1037.
143. Wingard JR et al. Relationship of tacrolimus (FK506) whole blood concentrations and efficacy and safety after HLA-identical sibling bone marrow transplantation. *Biol Blood Marrow Transplant* 1998;4:157.
144. Przepiorka D et al. Relationship of tacrolimus whole blood levels to efficacy and safety outcomes after unrelated donor marrow transplantation. *Biol Blood Marrow Transplant* 1999;5:94.
145. Duncan N, Craddock C. Optimizing the use of cyclosporin in allogeneic stem cell transplantation. *Bone Marrow Transplant* 2006;38:169.
146. Schmidt H et al. Correlation between low CSA plasma concentration and severity of acute GvHD in bone marrow transplantation. *Blut* 1988;57:139.
147. Hows JM et al. Use of cyclosporin A in allogeneic bone marrow transplantation for severe aplastic anemia. *Transplantation* 1982;33:382.
148. Couriel D et al. Acute graft-versus-host disease: pathophysiology, clinical manifestations, and management. *Cancer* 2004;101:1936.
149. Deeg HJ et al. Treatment of human acute graft-versus-host disease with antithymocyte globulin and cyclosporine with or without methylprednisolone. *Transplantation* 1985;40:162.
150. Lazarus HM et al. Prevention and treatment of acute graft-versus-host disease: the old and the new. A report from the Eastern Cooperative Oncology Group (ECOG). *Bone Marrow Transplant* 1997;19:577.
151. Van Lint MT et al. Early treatment of acute graft-versus-host disease with high- or low-dose 6-methylprednisolone: a multicenter randomized trial from the Italian Group for Bone Marrow Transplantation. *Blood* 1998;92:2288.
152. Lee SJ. New approaches for preventing and treating chronic graft-versus-host disease. *Blood* 2005;105:4200.
153. Filipovich AH et al. National Institutes of Health consensus development project on criteria for clinical trials in chronic graft-versus-host disease: I. Diagnosis and staging working group report. *Biol Blood Marrow Transplant* 2005;11:945.
154. Perez-Simon JA et al. Chronic graft-versus-host disease: pathogenesis and clinical management. *Drugs* 2006;66:1041.
155. Vogelsang GB. How I treat chronic graft-versus-host disease. *Blood* 2001;97:1196.
156. Stern JM et al. Bone density loss during treatment of chronic GVHD. *Bone Marrow Transplant* 1996;17:395.
157. Bowden RA. Respiratory virus infections after marrow transplant: the Fred Hutchinson Cancer Research Center experience. *Am J Med* 1997;102:27.
158. Junghanss C et al. Incidence and outcome of bacterial and fungal infections following nonmyeloablative compared with myeloablative allogeneic hematopoietic stem cell transplantation: a matched control study. *Biol Blood Marrow Transplant* 2002;8:512.
159. Engels EA et al. Efficacy of quinolone prophylaxis in neutropenic cancer patients: a meta-analysis. *J Clin Oncol* 1998;16:1179.
160. Tunkel AR, Sepkowitz KA. Infections caused by viridans streptococci in patients with neutropenia. *Clin Infect Dis* 2002;34:1524.
161. Hughes WT et al. 2002 guidelines for the use of antimicrobial agents in neutropenic patients with cancer. *Clin Infect Dis* 2002;34:730.
162. Goodman JL et al. A controlled trial of fluconazole to prevent fungal infections in patients undergoing bone marrow transplantation. *N Engl J Med* 1992;326:845.
163. Slavin MA et al. Efficacy and safety of fluconazole prophylaxis for fungal infections after marrow transplantation: a prospective, randomized, double-blind study. *J Infect Dis* 1995;171:1545.
164. Marr KA et al. Epidemiology and outcome of mould infections in hematopoietic stem cell transplant recipients. *Clin Infect Dis* 2002;34:909.
165. Cornely OA et al. Evidence-based assessment of primary antifungal prophylaxis in patients with hematologic malignancies. *Blood* 2003;101:3365.
166. Winston DJ et al. Intravenous and oral itraconazole versus intravenous and oral fluconazole for long-term antifungal prophylaxis in allogeneic hematopoietic stem-cell transplant recipients: a multicenter, randomized trial. *Ann Intern Med* 2003;138:705.
167. Van Burik JA et al. Micafungin versus fluconazole for prophylaxis against invasive fungal infections during neutropenia in patients undergoing hematopoietic stem cell transplantation. *Clin Infect Dis* 2004;39:1407.
168. Saral R et al. Acyclovir prophylaxis of herpes-simplex-virus infections. *N Engl J Med* 1981;305:63.
169. Selby PJ et al. The prophylactic role of intravenous and long-term oral acyclovir after allogeneic bone marrow transplantation. *Br J Cancer* 1989;59:434.
170. Ljungman P. Prevention and treatment of viral infections in stem cell transplant recipients. *Br J Haematol* 2002;118:44.
171. Vusirikala M et al. Valacyclovir for the prevention of cytomegalovirus infection after allogeneic stem cell transplantation: a single institution retrospective cohort analysis. *Bone Marrow Transplant* 2001;28:265.
172. Dignani MC et al. Valacyclovir prophylaxis for the prevention of Herpes simplex virus reactivation in recipients of progenitor cells transplantation. *Bone Marrow Transplant* 2002;29:263.
173. Steer CB et al. Varicella-zoster infection after allogeneic bone marrow transplantation: incidence, risk factors and prevention with low-dose acyclovir and ganciclovir. *Bone Marrow Transplant* 2000;25:657.
174. Razonable RR, Emery VC. Management of CMV infection and disease in transplant patients. *Herpes* 2004;11:77.
175. Goodrich JM et al. Ganciclovir prophylaxis to prevent cytomegalovirus disease after allogeneic marrow transplant. *Ann Intern Med* 1993;118:173.
176. Boeckh M et al. Cytomegalovirus pp65 antigenemia-guided early treatment with ganciclovir versus ganciclovir at engraftment after allogeneic marrow transplantation: a randomized double-blind study. *Blood* 1996;88:4063.
177. Zaia JA. Prevention of cytomegalovirus disease in hematopoietic stem cell transplantation. *Clin Infect Dis* 2002;35:999.
178. Boeckh M et al. Plasma polymerase chain reaction for cytomegalovirus DNA after allogeneic marrow transplantation: comparison with polymerase chain reaction using peripheral blood leukocytes, pp65 antigenemia, and viral culture. *Transplantation* 1997;64:108.
179. St George K et al. A multisite trial comparing two cytomegalovirus (CMV) pp65 antigenemia test kits, biotest CMV Brite and Bartels/Argene CMV antigenemia. *J Clin Microbiol* 2000;38:1430.
180. Nichols WG et al. High risk of death due to bacterial and fungal infection among cytomegalovirus (CMV)-seronegative recipients of stem cell transplants from seropositive donors: evidence for indirect effects of primary CMV infection. *J Infect Dis* 2002;185:273.
181. Boeckh M et al. Successful modification of a pp65 antigenemia-based early treatment strategy for

prevention of cytomegalovirus disease in allogeneic marrow transplant recipients. *Blood* 1999;93:1781.

182. Schmidt GM et al. A randomized, controlled trial of prophylactic ganciclovir for cytomegalovirus pulmonary infection in recipients of allogeneic bone marrow transplants: The City of Hope-Stanford-Syntex CMV Study Group. *N Engl J Med* 1991;324:1005.
183. Goodrich JM et al. Early treatment with ganciclovir to prevent cytomegalovirus disease after allogeneic bone marrow transplantation. *N Engl J Med* 1991;325:1601.
184. Ljungman P et al. Results of different strategies for reducing cytomegalovirus-associated mortality in allogeneic stem cell transplant recipients. *Transplantation* 1998;66:1330.
185. Ayala E et al. Valganciclovir is safe and effective as pre-emptive therapy for CMV infection in allogeneic hematopoietic stem cell transplantation. *Bone Marrow Transplant* 2006;37:851.
186. Diaz-Pedroche C et al. Valganciclovir preemptive therapy for the prevention of cytomegalovirus disease in high-risk seropositive solid-organ transplant recipients. *Transplantation* 2006;82:30.
187. Reusser P et al. Randomized multicenter trial of foscarnet versus ganciclovir for preemptive therapy of cytomegalovirus infection after allogeneic stem cell transplantation. *Blood* 2002;99:1159.
188. Holmberg LA et al. Increased incidence of cytomegalovirus disease after autologous CD34-selected peripheral blood stem cell transplantation. *Blood* 1999;94:4029.
189. Junghanss C et al. Incidence and outcome of cytomegalovirus infections following nonmyeloablative compared with myeloablative allogeneic stem cell transplantation, a matched control study. *Blood* 2002;99:1978.
190. Mohty M et al. High rate of secondary viral and bacterial infections in patients undergoing allogeneic bone marrow mini-transplantation. *Bone Marrow Transplant* 2000;26:251.
191. Marr KA et al. Invasive aspergillosis in allogeneic stem cell transplant recipients: changes in epidemiology and risk factors. *Blood* 2002;100:4358.
192. De La Rosa GR et al. Risk factors for the development of invasive fungal infections in allogeneic blood and marrow transplant recipients. *Transpl Infect Dis* 2002;4:3.
193. Singh N et al. *Aspergillus* infections in transplant recipients. *Clin Microbiol Rev* 2005:1844.
194. Wingard JR et al. Association of *Torulopsis glabrata* infections with fluconazole prophylaxis in neutropenic bone marrow transplant patients. *Antimicrob Agents Chemother* 1993;37:1847.
195. Wingard JR et al. Increase in *Candida krusei* infection among patients with bone marrow transplantation and neutropenia treated prophylactically with fluconazole. *N Engl J Med* 1991;325:1274.
196. Patterson TF et al. Invasive aspergillosis: disease spectrum, treatment practices, and outcomes. I3 Aspergillus Study Group. *Medicine (Baltimore)* 2000;79:250.
197. Soubani AO, Chandrasekar PH. The clinical spectrum of pulmonary aspergillosis. *Chest* 2002;121:1988.
198. Ascioglu S et al. Defining opportunistic invasive fungal infections in immunocompromised patients with cancer and hematopoietic stem cell transplants: an international consensus. *Clin Infect Dis* 2002;34:7.
199. Marr KA et al. Antifungal therapy decreases sensitivity of the Aspergillus galactomannan enzyme immunoassay. *Clin Infect Dis* 2005;40:1762.
200. Marr KA et al. Aspergillosis: pathogenesis, clinical manifestations, and therapy. *Infect Dis Clin North Am* 2002;16:875.
201. Quilitz RE et al. Practice guidelines for lipid-based amphotericin B in stem cell transplant recipients. *Ann Pharmacother* 2001;35:206.
202. Wingard JR et al. A randomized, double-blind comparative trial evaluating the safety of liposomal amphotericin B versus amphotericin B lipid complex in the empirical treatment of febrile neutropenia. *Clin Infect Dis* 2000;31:1155.
203. Cagnoni PJ. Liposomal amphotericin B versus conventional amphotericin B in the empirical treatment of persistently febrile neutropenic patients. *J Antimicrob Chemother* 2002;49(Suppl 1):81.
204. Stevens DA, Lee JY. Analysis of compassionate use itraconazole therapy for invasive aspergillosis by the NIAID Mycoses Study Group criteria. *Arch Intern Med* 1997;157:1857.
205. Ahmad SR et al. Congestive heart failure associated with itraconazole. *Lancet* 2001;357:1766.
206. Terrell CL. Antifungal agents. Part II. The azoles. *Mayo Clin Proc* 1999;74:78.
207. Herbrecht R et al. Voriconazole versus amphotericin B for primary therapy of invasive aspergillosis. *N Engl J Med* 2002;347:408.
208. Walsh TJ et al. Treatment of invasive aspergillosis with posaconazole in patients who are refractory to or intolerant of conventional therapy: an externally controlled trial. *Clin Infect Dis* 2007;44:2.
209. Stone EA et al. Caspofungin: an echinocandin antifungal agent. *Clin Ther* 2002;24:351.
210. Denning DW et al. Micafungin (FK463), alone or in combination with other systemic antifungal agents, for the treatment of acute invasive aspergillosis. *J Infect* 2006;53:337.
211. Luber AD et al. Risk factors for amphotericin B–induced nephrotoxicity. *J Antimicrob Chemother* 1999;43:267.
212. Harbarth S et al. The epidemiology of nephrotoxicity associated with conventional amphotericin B therapy. *Am J Med* 2001;111:528.
213. Prentice HG et al. A randomized comparison of liposomal versus conventional amphotericin B for the treatment of pyrexia of unknown origin in neutropenic patients. *Br J Haematol* 1997;98:711.
214. Walsh TJ et al. Amphotericin B lipid complex for invasive fungal infections: analysis of safety and efficacy in 556 cases. *Clin Infect Dis* 1998;26:1383.
215. White MH et al. Amphotericin B colloidal dispersion vs. amphotericin B as therapy for invasive aspergillosis. *Clin Infect Dis* 1997;24:635.
216. Wingard JR. Efficacy of amphotericin B lipid complex injection (ABLC) in bone marrow transplant recipients with life-threatening systemic mycoses. *Bone Marrow Transplant* 1997;19:343.
217. Walsh TJ et al. Voriconazole compared with liposomal amphotericin B for empirical antifungal therapy in patients with neutropenia and persistent fever. *N Engl J Med* 2002;346:225.
218. Denning DW et al. Efficacy and safety of voriconazole in the treatment of acute invasive aspergillosis. *Clin Infect Dis* 2002;34:563.
219. Petraitis V et al. Combination therapy in treatment of experimental pulmonary aspergillosis: synergistic interaction between an antifungal triazole and an echinocandin. *J Infect Dis* 2003;187:1834.
220. Kirkpatrick WR et al. Efficacy of caspofungin alone and in combination with voriconazole in a Guinea pig model of invasive aspergillosis. *Antimicrob Agents Chemother* 2002;46:2564.
221. Perea S et al. In vitro interaction of caspofungin acetate with voriconazole against clinical isolates of *Aspergillus* spp. *Antimicrob Agents Chemother* 2002;46:3039.
222. Lewis RE, Kontoyiannis DP. Rationale for combination antifungal therapy. *Pharmacotherapy* 2001;21:149S.
223. Ferrazzini G et al. Interaction between trimethoprim-sulfamethoxazole and methotrexate in children with leukemia. *J Pediatr* 1990;117:823.
224. Rizzo JD et al. Recommended screening and preventive practices for long-term survivors after hematopoietic cell transplantation: joint recommendations of the European Group for Blood and Marrow Transplantation, the Center for International Blood and Marrow Transplant Research, and the American Society of Blood and Marrow Transplantation. *Biol Blood Marrow Transplant* 2006;12:138.
225. Children's Oncology Group. Long-term follow-up guidelines for survivors of childhood, adolescent, and young adult cancers. Version 2.0. 2006, March. Available at: http://www.survivorshipguidelines.org/. Accessed March 5, 2008.
226. Goldberg SL et al. Vaccinations against infectious diseases in hematopoietic stem cell transplant recipients. *Oncology (Huntingt)* 2003;17:539.
227. Antin JH. Clinical practice. Long-term care after hematopoietic-cell transplantation in adults. *N Engl J Med* 2002;347:36.
228. Socie G et al. Nonmalignant late effects after allogeneic stem cell transplantation. *Blood* 2003;101:3373.
229. Strasser SI, McDonald GB. Hepatitis viruses and hematopoietic cell transplantation: a guide to patient and donor management. *Blood* 1999;93:1127.
230. Giralt S et al. Reduced-intensity conditioning for unrelated donor progenitor cell transplantation: long-term follow-up of the first 285 reported to the national marrow donor program. *Biol Blood Marrow Transplant.* 2007;13:844.

CHAPTER 93

Pediatric Considerations

Sherry Luedtke, Mark Haase, and Michelle Condren

MEDICATION ADMINISTRATION ISSUES IN CHILDREN

Children represent more than 25% of the population and receive an average of three prescription medications before 5 years of age. The safe and effective use of medications in children, nevertheless, is challenging because of the lack of U.S. Food and Drug Administration (FDA)-approved indications and dosing guidelines for children, limited evidence-based medicine, and paucity of appropriate dosage formulations. About 60% of drugs have not been approved by the FDA for use in children, and even fewer have been approved for use in infants. Most current laws governing FDA approval of drugs are the result of pediatric tragedies (e.g., thalidomide, sulfanilamide), but legislation to encourage research in pediatrics did not occur until the 1990s. The FDA Modernization Act of 1997, Best Pharmaceuticals for Children Act (BPCA), and the Pediatric Research Equity Act are attempts to encourage manufacturers to focus on pediatric indications for medications. As a result, knowledge of pediatric drug therapy has grown significantly; however, information on which to base drug therapy decisions remains inadequate. This chapter focuses on general principles guiding pediatric pharmacotherapy, and reviews the pharmacotherapy of common pediatric disorders by integrating best-evidence medicine and the practical considerations unique to pediatric patients.

Medication Error Prevention

Children are at threefold greater risk for medication errors than adults, and up to 19% of these errors are deemed preventable.[1] The lack of appropriate information or guidelines for use of medications in children, the miscalculation of doses, and the need to either compound oral dosage forms or to dilute commercially available formulations contribute to this disproportionate rate of medication errors in children. In the last decade, efforts have increased to improve medication ordering processes, to standardize medication concentrations, and to educate practitioners about medication error prevention. The Pediatric Pharmacy Advocacy Group and other pediatric organizations have developed guidelines to reduce the potential for medication errors in children and these guidelines and strategies are becoming the focus for many health care systems and health care accrediting organizations.[2]

Drug Administration

Oral Medications

The administration of oral medications to a young child or infant often requires two adults: one to gently restrain the child while the other rapidly and accurately administers the medication. If only one adult is available, one can restrain the arms and legs of the child in a swaddling blanket or large towel as depicted in Figure 93-1.

The administration device (cup, syringe, or dropper) that generally accompanies a liquid medication product provides the most accurate measurement of the desired dose. For infants, liquid medications are most easily administered to the back cheek in 1- to 2-mL amounts with an oral syringe. Household teaspoons should not be used to measure medications because teaspoons are of variable sizes and hold 3 to 8 mL of a liquid. Crushed tablets or capsule contents mixed in small amounts (1–2 teaspoons) of food (e.g., chocolate pudding, applesauce, ice cream, jelly, chocolate syrup) offer an alternative to liquid formulations. The taste of liquid dosage formulations generally is improved by refrigeration and flavoring agents, and "chasers" (i.e., popsicle or flavored drink after a dose) also are helpful. Although medications can be delivered in small amounts (10–15 mL) of liquid in a bottle (juice, milk, formula), doses should not be diluted into an entire scheduled feeding or prepared ahead of time in batches in anticipation of future administration. Limiting the volume more likely facilitates delivery of the entire dose and adding the medication to a feeding bottle immediately before delivery minimizes the potential of drug instability. Drug interactions with foods also should be considered before drugs are added to feeding formulas. Most children are able to swallow tablets at 5 to 8 years of age. Duplicate supplies of medication should be provided to the caregiver when mid-day doses are required for children who attend school or childcare in the event a dose is dropped. Children of all ages should be encouraged and praised for their cooperation in taking their medicine. Rewards, gold stars, or stickers can be useful to gain cooperation in an older child.

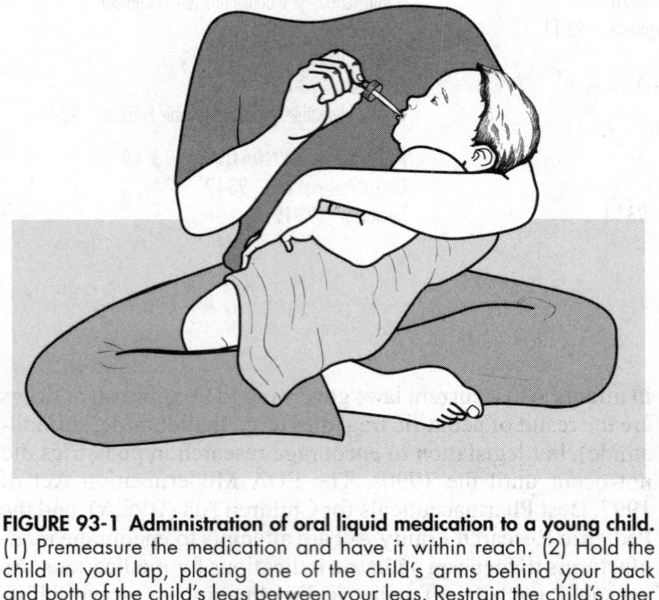

FIGURE 93-1 Administration of oral liquid medication to a young child. (1) Premeasure the medication and have it within reach. (2) Hold the child in your lap, placing one of the child's arms behind your back and both of the child's legs between your legs. Restrain the child's other arm securely with your nondominant arm. (3) Tilt the child's head back slightly, pressing gently on the child's cheeks to open the mouth. Using your dominant hand, aim the dropper or syringe between the rear gum and cheek. Administer small amounts of medication (1–2 mL) at a time, making sure the baby swallows.

Ear, Nose, and Eye Drops

Otic, ophthalmic, and nasal medications usually need to be administered to infants and young children in a different manner than adults. Otic medications should be instilled by pulling the auricle down and out in infants and young children, whereas older children should have the auricle of the ear held up and back to straighten the ear canal. During the instillation of nose and eye drops, position infants and toddlers with their head lower than the rest of the body because gravity assists in dispersing the medication. This can be achieved by laying the infant across a bed with the shoulders projecting over the edge of the bed. Restraining the infant often is required during the administration of ophthalmic formulations. When administering the eye medication (Fig. 93-2), the caregiver must be

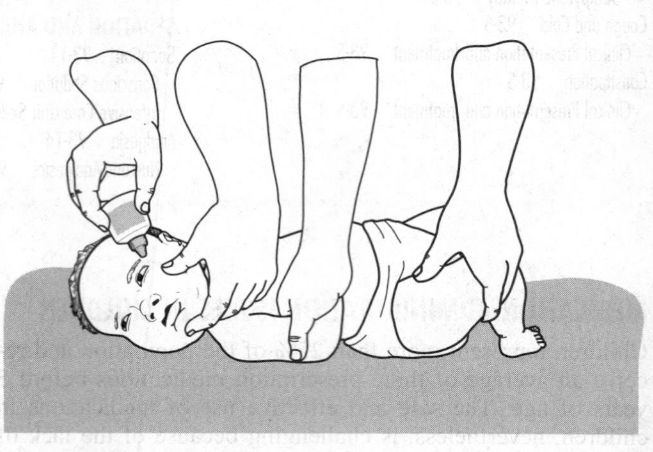

FIGURE 93-2 Administering eye drops to a young child. (1) Place the child on a flat surface. Enlist the help of a second adult to restrain the child or swaddle the child as described in Figure 93-1. (2) Holding the child's head steady, gently pull the eyelids apart. The hand that is holding the medication dropper can rest on the child's head while administering the medication to minimize the potential for injury to the eye if the child's head moves abruptly. Administer the medication as directed.

cautious to avoid injury to the eye caused by sudden movements of the infant. The technique of placing the hand, which holds the eye medication, on the forehead of the infant during administration can help to minimize eye injury because the hand holding the eye dropper will move when the infant's head moves.

To minimize fear and improve cooperation during instillation of eye, nose, or ear drops, the procedure should be explained to the child as simply as possible. It is best to warm the medication in your hand for a few minutes before administration because medications can feel very cold inside the ears or nose even when stored at room temperature.

INFANT CARE

Teething

The growth and development of teeth begin as early as the sixth week of embryonic life. Calcification of the enamel and dentin begins at 4 months of gestation. Normal eruption of primary or deciduous teeth rarely begins before 4 to 5 months of age and usually is completed by 36 months of age.[3] Although premature infants usually experience delayed eruption of their deciduous teeth, their first tooth appears (based on postconceptual age) at about the same time as term infants.[4] In many full-term infants, however, teeth do not erupt until the end of the first year: delayed eruption of all teeth can reflect systemic or nutritional disturbances (e.g., hypothyroidism, hypopituitarism, rickets).[3] Early eruption is less common and also can be associated with medical conditions (e.g., hyperthyroidism, precocious puberty, long-term steroid therapy).

Normal Eruption of Primary Teeth

Signs and Symptoms

1. C.J., a 6-month old, has become increasingly irritable and has been waking up four to five times a night. She is drooling excessively and biting on hard objects constantly. A brief examination of C.J.'s mouth shows red and tender gums. No teeth are present, and C.J. is afebrile. Her mother is concerned that C.J.'s teething has caused a secondary illness. What would be a likely explanation for these symptoms?

C.J.'s regular sleeping pattern has been disturbed by symptomatic teething. As the teeth penetrate the gums, the site can become tender: this process generally is associated with increased salivation. Bacterial invasion through a break in the tissue or under a gingival flap covering the teeth can cause inflammation and edema, but "teething" does not cause systemic disturbances.[5] Restlessness, increased salivation, thumb-sucking, gum-rubbing, and decreased appetite commonly accompany teething.

Treatment

2. What course of treatment can be suggested for C.J.?

GENERAL MANAGEMENT

Gentle irrigation with water often relieves the inflammation around a gum flap. A topical anesthetic can be rubbed gently on the mucous membranes overlying the erupting tooth with a cotton-tipped applicator. Local anesthetics, however, should not be used long-term, and topical products containing lidocaine should not be used for symptomatic relief of teething because absorption of lidocaine can lead to systemic toxicity. Alcohol-free products containing 7.5% benzocaine (e.g., Orajel Baby Gel, Orabase Baby Analgesic Teething Gel) can be used for infants more than 4 months of age.[6] Giving the child a blunt, firm object to chew is helpful; and wrapping cracked ice in a soft cloth also can hasten tooth eruption and relieve pain. Rubber teething rings of various shapes can be beneficial, but trauma from the teething ring might lead to angular cheilitis.[7] Water-containing rings can become contaminated with bacteria and should be avoided.

Ibuprofen and acetaminophen are commonly prescribed for younger children to relieve pain associated with the eruption of primary dentition. Ibuprofen's anti-inflammatory effects last for about 6 to 8 hours and might be especially helpful at bedtime. Pediatric dosage recommendations must be strictly followed. Topical aspirin should never be used because it can cause oral chemical burns. Oral aspirin is not used because of its association with Reye's syndrome, a condition consisting of encephalopathy and fatty degeneration of the liver.

Diaper Rash

Etiology

Diaper dermatitis is commonly encountered in pediatric practice, occurring in up to 35% of infants at any given time. Although the pathogenesis of diaper dermatitis is not well defined, a number of factors (e.g., chemical irritants, friction, bacteria) have been associated with skin inflammation in the diaper area. In particular, skin wetness and pH have been implicated in diaper dermatitis, and wetness appears to have greater influence than that of pH. Overhydration of the skin increases the permeability of low molecular weight compounds and exacerbates the effects of friction.[8] Cloth diapers covered with plastic pants or disposable diapers with plastic outer linings decrease air circulation and increase moisture in the diaper area.[9] Residual chemicals or laundry detergents in the diaper (cloth or disposable), as well as soaps, medications, or lotions that have been applied directly to the infant's skin also have roles in the development of diaper rash. A persistent diaper rash could represent a localized fungal or bacterial infection.[9]

Clinical Presentation

Four clinical presentations of dermatitis are associated with diaper wear:

1. A mild, scaling rash in the perianal area
2. A sharply demarcated confluent erythema
3. Ulceration distributed through the diaper area
4. A beefy red confluent erythema with satellite lesions, vesiculopustular lesions, and diffuse involvement of the genitalia

Treatment

3. K.G., a 3-month-old infant, has had a severe "diaper rash" for the past 4 days. The very inflamed and tender area is confined to the diaper area, and vesicular satellite lesions are present on the periphery of the erythematous area. K.G.'s mother uses only cloth diapers and has not changed soap or her normal pattern of diaper care since K.G. was born. Based on the clinical appearance of the rash and its duration, the clinician prescribed clotrimazole 1% cream and gave K.G.'s mother instructions for treatment. Why

was clotrimazole prescribed? What are some general measures for the prevention and treatment of diaper rash?

K.G.'s rash is consistent with a candidal infection, which typically is beefy red and associated with vesicular satellite lesions. Presence of a rash for >3 days and diffuse involvement of the genitalia and inguinal folds also are characteristic of this form of diaper rash. K.G.'s rash can be treated with clotrimazole or miconazole cream applied to the inflamed area four times daily until it has resolved. Nystatin ointment can be applied, but often is not as effective as the imidazole antifungals because of increasing resistance of candida species to nystatin.

Removal of stool and urine from the diaper area by gentle rinsing with plain water and more frequent diaper changes often help to alleviate diaper rashes. Wiping the baby with diaper wipes that contain alcohol can sting, further irritate the involved area, and should be avoided until the rash has resolved. A good protective agent containing zinc oxide or petrolatum (e.g., Desitin) can be applied with each diaper change to create a barrier to irritants and seal out moisture. Powdered protective agents (e.g., cornstarch, talc) can minimize friction caused by diapers, but should be used cautiously because the infant can aspirate powder particles and develop a chemical pneumonia.[10] When used, powders should be shaken into the diaper or applied close to the body, away from the baby's face. The concern that cornstarch might serve as a culture medium for *Candida albicans* has not been substantiated.[11]

Other prevention and treatment measures should include the following:

1. Change the diaper as soon as it is wet or at least every 2 to 4 hours during the day.
2. Keep the diaper area clean (e.g., nightly baths until resolved).
3. Use super absorbent disposable diapers at night.
4. Expose the diaper area to air as often as possible.
5. Dry the diaper area completely before a new diaper is put on.
6. For cotton diapers, use a bacteriostatic agent in the diaper pail and rinse water or employ a diaper service to ensure that diapers are sterile.
7. Apply a low-potency topical corticosteroid, such as 0.5% to 1% hydrocortisone, twice daily for up to 1 week when severe inflammation is present.[12]

Fever

Normal body temperature varies throughout the day, peaking in late afternoon or early evening. Body temperature can be measured rectally, orally, axillary (under the arm), and tympanically. Rectal temperatures are most reliable in infants <3 months of age. Oral measurements of temperature are not appropriate in children <3 years of age because it is difficult for young children to maintain a tight seal around the thermometer.

Fever is defined as an oral temperature >37.8°C (100°F), an axillary temperature >37.2°C (99.0°F), or in children <5 years of age, a rectal temperature >38°C (100.4°F). (*Fahrenheit temperatures can be converted to or from centigrade temperatures by the formula:* $°F = 1.8°C + 32$.)

Children with fevers might not have other signs or symptoms of an illness. *Any child <2 months of age* who develops a fever (e.g., rectal temperature >100°F) requires a complete evaluation (e.g., blood culture, urinalysis) because clinical manifestations of a serious infection often are subtle, nonspecific, and not predictive of the extent or severity of illness. In this situation, antibiotic therapy usually is initiated while awaiting laboratory results. *Children 6 to 24 months of age* with a temperature >38.9°C (102°F) and white blood cell (WBC) counts <5,000/mm^3 or >15,000/mm^3 are at increased risk for bacteremia. *Children of any age* with fever >41°C should be evaluated not only for bacteremia, but also for possible meningitis. Blood cultures, lumbar puncture, urinalysis, and chest radiograph should be considered on an individual basis to help determine the etiology of infection. *Febrile immunocompromised children* and *febrile children with functional or anatomic asplenia* are at increased risk for sepsis or fulminant infections (e.g., *Streptococcus pneumoniae,* Salmonella species, *Escherichia coli*) and should receive prompt antibiotic therapy.[13]

4. R.B., a 12-month-old, 10-kg baby boy was well yesterday until his mother noticed that he felt warm to her touch later in the afternoon. For the past 24 hours, he has remained warm, is fussy and less active. A rectal temperature 15 minutes ago was 39°C. His mother is concerned R.B.'s temperature will continue to rise. When do fevers progress into febrile seizures? How should R.B.'s febrile illness be treated?

Risk of Febrile Seizures

Febrile seizures occur in approximately 2% to 4% of children 6 months to 5 years of age who have temperature elevations >38°C.[14] The etiology and pathogenesis are unknown, but the temperature and the rate of temperature increase appear to be important factors.[15] Genetic predisposition also appears to be a factor because febrile seizures occur with greater frequency among family members.[14] Febrile seizures are of two types: simple and complex. Simple febrile seizures last <15 minutes and do not have significant focal features. Complex febrile seizures have a longer duration, occur in series, and are associated with focal changes. Typically, febrile seizures occur within the first 24 hours of a febrile episode.[14] Although R.B. is in the age group at greatest risk for having a febrile seizure, he has been febrile for more than 24 hours and a seizure is unlikely during this illness.

Treatment

ANTIPYRETIC THERAPY

Acetaminophen is the most common antipyretic agent used in children. The usual dose, oral or rectal, is 10 to 15 mg/kg/dose administered every 4 to 6 hours as needed to a maximum of 65 mg/kg/day.

Ibuprofen is administered as 5 to 10 mg/kg/dose orally every 6 to 8 hours as needed to a maximum of 40 mg/kg/day. Ibuprofen is as effective as acetaminophen as an antipyretic and is associated with a low incidence of adverse effects.[16,17] Although renal failure has been reported after ibuprofen use in children,[18,19] the risk of renal impairment is small with short-term use and not greater than that with acetaminophen.[17,19]

Acetaminophen or ibuprofen should be effective in lowering R.B.'s fever. Acetaminophen typically is considered to be a first-line drug in children. Dosing errors have occurred when teaspoonful quantities of acetaminophen infant drops (80 mg/0.8 mL) were given instead of the liquid formulation

(160 mg/5 mL) or when regular strength tablets (325 mg) have been substituted for chewable children's tablets (160 mg). Caretakers should be questioned about the dosage form of acetaminophen they have at home, concurrent use of any other products containing acetaminophen, and whether cumulative doses are within the recommended range. Ibuprofen, an alternative to acetaminophen for R.B., is available in two liquid formulations (infant drops, 50 mg/1.25 mL; children's suspension, 100 mg/5 mL) and two chewable tablet dosage formulations (50 mg, 100 mg). Adverse effects are limited when ibuprofen is used in recommended doses for short-term antipyresis. Although some practitioners may alternate acetaminophen and ibuprofen during the day, no data are available to support the efficacy or safety of combination therapy. Aspirin therapy is not recommended for treatment of fever in children or adolescents with chickenpox, gastroenteritis, or respiratory viral infections because of its association with Reye's syndrome.[20]

Cough and Cold

Another common diagnosis in children is viral upper respiratory infection or the common cold.[21] Preschool children have between three and nine colds each year.[21] Children with a cold often present with sore throat, nasal congestion, rhinorrhea, sneezing, cough, and irritability.

Clinical Presentation and Treatment

5. J.K. is a 3-month-old infant who began having nasal congestion, rhinorrhea, and cough yesterday. She has had no fever and is eating well, but did not sleep well last evening. J.K.'s mother called her pediatrician and was told that J.K. most likely has a cold caused by a virus. How can J.K.'s symptoms be treated?

A cool mist humidifier can increase the amount of moisture in room air and decrease irritation in the upper airway when humidity is low. Saline nose drops followed by bulb suctioning can help to clear the nasal passages in J.K. who is <6 months of age.[21] It is especially important to do this before feedings. If a topical nasal decongestant is needed, phenylephrine would be preferred over oxymetazoline and xylometazoline, because of its lesser association with toxicity (e.g., sedation, convulsions, insomnia, coma) in children <6 years of age.[22,23] A decongestant, however, should not be prescribed for J.K. because of her age and the potential for adverse effects.

Several hundred over-the-counter medications for upper respiratory symptoms are available and about 95 million units of these products are sold each year in the United States. Nevertheless, the safety and effectiveness of these cough and cold medications in children have yet to be proved.[24a] The Centers for Disease Control and Prevention (CDC) reported that 1,519 children <2 years of age were admitted to Emergency Departments in 2004 to 2005 because of overdoses and other problems associated with cough and cold medicines. Furthermore, according to the FDA, 54 deaths in children were linked to the use of decongestants (e.g., pseudoephedrine, phenylephrine, ephedrine) and 69 deaths to antihistamines (e.g., diphenhydramine, brompheniramine, chlorpheniramine) from 1969 to September 13, 2006. Most of these deaths occurred in children <2 years of age, and some of the fatalities occurred in children who received overdoses that might have been the result of inadvertent administration of multiple medications containing the same ingredient. Antihistamines are not effective for rhinorrhea caused by the common cold and should not be recommended. Antitussives also should not be used if the child's cough is productive, but might be helpful if a cough is dry and interferes with activities or sleep.[21] Nevertheless, cough suppressant formulations for children, including dextromethorphan or diphenhydramine, have not been proven to be beneficial when compared with placebo. An FDA advisory committee in 2007 voted 13 to 9 to recommend that over-the-counter cold and cough medications not be used in children <6 years of age.[24a] Expectorants, such as guaifenesin, also are not effective and evidence is insufficient to support the use of vitamin C, zinc, or echinacea in children for treatment or prevention of the common cold.

Owing to reports of toxicity and death related to over-the-counter cough and cold products, the CDC has recommended that caregivers avoid giving these products to children <2 years of age unless advised by a clinician.[24] In 2007, pharmaceutical manufacturers already had begun preemptively to stop selling versions of these medications (i.e., over-the-counter decongestants, antihistamines, and cough suppressants) aimed at infants <2 years of age. If deemed necessary by a physician for older children, nonprescription cough and cold medications containing single ingredients should be selected to minimize the potential for adverse effects and administration of multiple products with similar ingredients.

Constipation

Constipation, accounting for approximately 3% of general pediatric office visits,[25] can be defined as a stool frequency of less than 3 per week or occurrence of pain on defecation (signifying hard stools).[25] Beyond the neonatal period, constipation is most commonly idiopathic or functional and may be due to a diet low in fiber, lack of time or routine for toileting, or passage of a painful stool resulting in a fear of defecating. Stool retention over time may result in soiling or encopresis.

Clinical Presentation and Treatment

6. R.J., a 2-year-old boy, has had abdominal pain for several weeks. On average he has one stool weekly and he cries each time because of pain. After obtaining a thorough history and performing a physical examination, the physician determines that R.J. has functional constipation. What treatment measures should be taken to relieve and prevent R.J's constipation?

Before maintenance therapy can be initiated, disimpaction of the patient is necessary first. Although no controlled studies compare efficacy of the oral and rectal routes, oral therapy (mineral oil, polyethylene glycol, bisacodyl) is preferred because it is less invasive and might achieve better adherence than rectal therapy (phosphate soda enemas, mineral oil enemas, glycerin suppositories in infants, bisacodyl suppositories in older children).[26] After disimpaction, a combination of behavioral, dietary, and medication therapies should be initiated to promote regular stool production and prevent reimpaction. Dietary interventions include adequate fluid and fiber intake. Medications (e.g., polyethylene glycol 3350, mineral oil, lactulose, sorbitol) should be titrated to produce one to two soft stools daily; and stimulant laxatives might be needed

Table 93-1 Medications for the Treatment of Constipation[25,26]

Medication	*Initial Dosage*	*Comments*
Osmotic Agents		
Lactulose	1–3 mL/kg/day QD-BID	
Sorbitol	1–3 mL/kg/day QD-BID	Less expensive than lactulose
Barley malt extract	2–10 mL/240 mL of milk or juice daily	Useful for infants drinking from a bottle
Magnesium hydroxide	1–3 mL/kg/day using 400 mg/5 mL	Infants are at risk for hypermagnesemia.
Phosphate enema	≥2 yr of age: 6 mL/kg up to 135 mL	Electrolyte abnormalities more common in children with renal failure or Hirschprung disease. Avoid in children <2 yr.
Lubricant		
Mineral oil	>1 yr of age: Disimpaction: 15–30 mL/yr of age up to 240 mL daily Maintenance: 1–3 mL/kg/day	Better tolerated if chilled. Avoid in children <1 yr. Lipoid pneumonia may occur if aspirated.
Stimulants		
Senna	2–6 yr of age: 2.5–7.5 mL/day 6–12 yr of age: 5–15 mL/day	Not recommended for chronic use
Bisacodyl	≥2 yr old: 0.5–1 suppository or 1–3 tablets per dose	Not recommended for chronic use
Glycerin suppositories	1 suppository per dose	Preferred stimulant for children <2 yr of age

BID, twice daily; QD, every day.

intermittently. The recommended dosing of medications for treatment of constipation is listed in Table 93-1.

Vomiting and Diarrhea

Vomiting and diarrhea, two commonly encountered complaints in pediatric practice, usually are self-limiting, but severe cases can result in serious complications (e.g., dehydration, metabolic disturbances, and even death). Infants and young children are particularly susceptible to more severe complications.

Pathogenesis and Presentation of Vomiting

Vomiting or emesis is defined as forceful expulsion of gastrointestinal (GI) contents through the mouth or nose; nonforceful expulsion of GI contents is considered regurgitation. In newborns, regurgitation of small amounts of breast milk or formula after feeding, especially when burping, is common. In most cases, regurgitation usually resolves by 1 year of age and rarely causes a problem.[27] Extensive evaluation of regurgitation is not needed in a child who is growing well. Other causes of vomiting during the newborn period include pyloric stenosis, gastroesophageal reflux, overfeeding, food intolerance, and GI obstruction. Beyond the neonatal period, the most common cause of vomiting is infection. Vomiting in infants and children also can be caused by central nervous system (CNS) disease (e.g., intracranial tumors), metabolic disease (e.g., urea cycle disorder), inflammatory bowel disease, and ulcers. Conditions causing emesis in older infants and children range from viral gastroenteritis to more severe illnesses, such as bowel obstruction or head injury, that require immediate medical attention (Table 93-2).[27] Acute vomiting also can result from medication or toxic ingestions. In teenagers, migraine, pregnancy, and psychological disorders (e.g., bulimia) have been associated with vomiting.

Pathogenesis and Presentation of Diarrhea

Diarrhea refers to an increase in frequency, volume, or liquidity of stool when compared with normal bowel movements. In developing countries, diarrhea is a common cause of death. In the United States, approximately 38 million cases of diarrhea will occur annually, resulting in approximately 2 to 4 million physician visits, 220,000 hospitalizations, and about 400 deaths.[28]

Acute diarrhea in infants and children generally is abrupt in onset, lasts a few days, and usually is caused by viruses. (See Chapter 62, Infectious Diarrhea for infectious diarrhea of other etiologies.) Diarrhea is considered chronic if it is longer than 2 weeks in duration and can be caused by malabsorption, inflammatory disease, alteration of intestinal flora, milk or protein intolerance, and drugs.[29]

Infants and children are at high risk for morbidity and mortality secondary to diarrhea for several reasons. Dehydration can occur easily as acute net intestinal fluid losses are relatively much greater in young children than in adults. This may result from inefficient transport systems in the developing intestine. In addition, the percent of total body water in children is higher than in adults; thus, they are more susceptible to body fluid shifts. Total body water changes from 80% of total body weight in premature infants to 70% in term infants and 60% in adults. Finally, the renal capacity to compensate for fluid and electrolyte imbalances in the infant is limited compared with an adult's.[30]

VIRAL GASTROENTERITIS

7. J.R., a 15-month-old male infant, had one loose stool and began vomiting this morning but has not had a fever. On questioning, you discover that many children attending day care with J.R. are experiencing vomiting, diarrhea, and low-grade temperatures. How should J.R.'s vomiting be treated?

Table 93-2 Causes of Vomiting in Infants and Children[27]

Causes	Other Signs and Symptoms
Drug Induced	
Cancer chemotherapy	Nausea
Narcotics	
Theophylline/Aminophylline	
Antibiotics	
Alcohol	
Anesthetics	
Metabolic or Endocrine Disorders	Alteration in behavior
Infectious Diseases	Fever
Otitis media	Symptoms of otitis media
Meningitis	Stiff neck, toxic appearance
Appendicitis	Abdominal pain
Urinary tract infection or pyelonephritis	Dysuria, frequency and urgency in older children
Viral or bacterial gastroenteritis	Diarrhea
Mechanical Obstruction	
Bowel obstruction	Abdominal distention, green emesis
Pyloric stenosis	Projectile nonbilious vomiting
	Abdominal pain
Inflammatory	
Pancreatitis	
Inflammatory bowel	Diarrhea
Peptic ulcer disease	Black or red vomitus
Psychologic	
Chemotherapy	
Bulimia	
Miscellaneous	
Gastroesophageal reflux	Usually self-limited; indications for evaluation include recurrent pneumonia, poor growth, gastrointestinal blood loss, dysphagia, or heartburn
Increased intracranial pressure	Mental status alternation
Head injury or trauma	History of trauma, mental status changes
Food or milk intolerance	Irritability, loose stool, blood in stool or allergy

Routine use of antiemetics for acute vomiting in children is not recommended because masking of symptoms may delay diagnosis of a treatable illness. In addition, the safety and efficacy of the antiemetics, metoclopramide, promethazine, trimethobenzamide, and dimenhydrinate have not been demonstrated.[31,32] Ondansetron does decrease vomiting, and it increases oral intake and decreases the need for intravenous rehydration; however, the cost effectiveness of ondansetron for use in gastroenteritis needs consideration because this drug does not significantly decrease hospital admission.[32,33]

Parents should be taught the signs and symptoms of gastroenteritis and vomiting that are sufficiently serious to warrant medical attention. A pediatrician should be contacted if a child is toxic appearing, exhibits unusual behavior or signs of an ear infection, experiences abdominal pain or distention, or has red or black vomitus or stool. In addition, a pediatrician should be called if there is a history or suspicion of toxic ingestion or head trauma. Medical evaluation also is necessary for infants <6 months of age; when persistent vomiting or high volume diarrhea is present; or when chronic medical conditions or prematurity are involved. Because fever can accompany vomiting in viral gastroenteritis, any fever occurring in a neonate warrants medical attention, as well as in older infants and children when fever becomes prolonged or changes in pattern.

When communicating with a health care provider about a vomiting child, it is helpful if the parents have knowledge of the child's fluid intake, and the frequency and volume of vomiting and urination. The amount of vomitus can be estimated by the following rule of thumb: one tablespoon makes a spot four inches wide and a quarter-cup makes a spot approximately 8 inches wide.

Vomiting associated with gastroenteritis usually resolves in 24 to 48 hours. Infants are particularly susceptible to the development of fluid and electrolyte abnormalities; therefore, fluid and electrolyte replacements are critically important (see Question 9).

J.R, who is early in the course of gastroenteritis, must receive sufficient fluids to prevent dehydration. Oral hydration therapy can be successful when given in small volumes, even if J.R. is still vomiting. For example, 5 to 10 mL can be administered every 5–10 minutes, and the volume can be gradually increased as tolerated. Volumes equal to estimated fluid deficit (usually 50–100 mL/kg) should be given over 2 to 4 hours. For each diarrheal stool, an additional 10 mL/kg of oral electrolyte solution should be given. If diarrhea or vomiting recurs, 10 mL/kg and 2 mL/kg of an oral rehydration solution (ORS) can be administered for each stool or emesis, respectively.[31] J.R.'s clinical condition should continue to be monitored by his caregiver. If stool output exceeds 10 mL/kg/hour, ORS might not be sufficient, and the health care provider should again be contacted. ORS should only be abandoned in children with intractable vomiting, loss of consciousness, bowel obstruction, or if the child is in shock. Most infants will tolerate oral hydration when small amounts are given frequently. Using a spoon or oral syringe to administer the fluid may be more effective than using a nipple or cup. As dehydration is corrected, the frequency of vomiting typically decreases. Once rehydration has been achieved, fluids other than ORS and a diet appropriate for age may be started.[31] Breast milk or formula should be given as tolerated.

Assessment of Dehydration

8. On the second day of illness, J.R. develops a mild fever and diarrhea that has increased in frequency and water content. How can the severity of J.R.'s diarrhea be assessed? Should he be hospitalized for intravenous (IV) fluid replacement, or can he be treated on an outpatient basis?

To determine whether IV fluid replacement is needed, consider the following questions:

1. Does the child have any of the following signs and symptoms of severe dehydration? Deeply sunken eyes, parched mucous membranes, significantly prolonged capillary refill; cool, mottled extremities; crying without tears; oliguria or anuria; weak or thready pulses; lethargy; poor oral intake;

deep respirations; history of seizures or convulsions; a fever without perspiration, or thirst?
2. Are a large number of copious stools still being produced (>10 mL/kg/hour)? Is bowel obstruction a possibility?
3. Is there a risk of dehydration from inadequate monitoring, or is the parent unable to care for the child? Specific inquiries should be made about the number and consistency of stools in children with diarrhea.

Estimating the degree of dehydration is particularly valuable in assessing the patient with diarrhea: weight loss is a good criterion. A 3% to 9% weight loss is considered mild to moderate dehydration, whereas >9% is considered severe dehydration.[31] (See Chapter 97, Pediatric Nutrition, for information about IV replacement therapy in children with 10% or more dehydration.)

Oral Replacement Therapy

9. On questioning, J.R. was not considered to be sufficiently dehydrated to warrant hospitalization. How might J.R.'s fluids and electrolytes be managed on an outpatient basis?

The goal of J.R.'s treatment should be focused on the prevention of dehydration and the restoration and maintenance of adequate fluid and electrolyte balance. Mild to moderate diarrhea without dehydration generally is managed at home by continued age-appropriate feeding. Fluid losses in stools can be replaced with a glucose-containing ORS. Glucose provides calories and enhances salt and water absorption in the small intestine through mechanisms that usually are unimpaired in many toxin-induced diarrheas. Parents formerly were instructed to prepare salt and sugar solutions at home; however, frequent errors in the preparation of these solutions resulted in exacerbation of problems with fluid and electrolyte balance. Oral glucose–electrolyte formulations (e.g., Pedialyte), designed to enhance glucose and sodium absorption, are commercially available and should be used in infants and young children. Gatorade is an alternative for older children, but carbonated beverages and fruit juices do not contain sufficient sodium to replace diarrheal losses. Rehydration and maintenance solutions can be made more palatable with sugar-free flavorings (e.g., Kool-Aid, Crystal Lite).

The World Health Organization (WHO) formerly promoted use of an oral replacement solution (WHO formula) containing sodium (90 mEq/L), potassium (20 mEq/L), bicarbonate (30 mEq/L), chloride (80 mEq/L), and 2% glucose for the widespread management of acute diarrhea in third-world countries. The WHO formula, which had a 90% successful rehydration rate for the management of diarrhea, contained a high concentration of sodium because secretory diarrhea (e.g., cholera) is associated with substantial loss of sodium. Malabsorptive diarrheas, such as those associated with rotavirus infections, are associated with much lower loss of sodium (<40 mEq/L). Although commercially available ORS contain less sodium than the WHO formulation, these preparations were equally effective as the WHO formula, even when used to treat the high-sodium losses associated with cholera. Furthermore, these lower sodium-containing formulations were associated with less vomiting, lower stool output, and reduced need for IV infusions in non–cholera-associated gastroenteritis. As a result, the WHO, in 2002, promoted a new formulation that consists of 75 mEq/L sodium and a total osmolarity of 245 mOsm/L.[31] Glucose is added to oral electrolyte solutions to enhance glucose-coupled sodium transport; however, concentrations >3% can impair sodium absorption because the glucose-coupled sodium transport system becomes saturated at this concentration and any additional glucose acts as an osmotically active solute in the bowel lumen. The electrolyte content of commonly used ORS is provided in Table 93-3.

Table 93-3 Oral Electrolyte Solutions[31]

	Compositions			
Solution	Sodium (mmol/L)	Potassium (mmol/L)	Carbohydrate (mmol/L)	Osmolarity
Rehydration				
Rehydralyte	75	20	140	305
WHO formula (1975)	90	20	111	311
WHO formula (2002)	75	20	75	245
Maintenance				
Enfalyte	50	25	167	200
Pedialyte	45	20	139	250
Home Remedies				
Apple juice	0.4	44	667	730
Gatorade	20	3	255	330
Ginger ale	3	1	500	540
Chicken broth	250	8		500
Cola	1.6		622	730

WHO, World Health Organization.

Reinstitution of Oral Feedings

Previously, feeding during an episode of viral gastroenteritis has been delayed because of the malabsorption that typically occurs during and after these bouts. The malabsorption, however, is self-limiting and substantial amounts of carbohydrate, protein, and fat can still be absorbed. The reinstitution of a regular diet, therefore, should not adversely affect mild diarrhea and can be beneficial.[34] Parents are encouraged to continue feeding their children using age-appropriate diet while avoiding simple sugars, which can increase osmotic load and worsen diarrhea. Continuation of oral feeding, despite diarrheal episodes, minimizes the development of protein and energy deficits; facilitates the maintenance and repair of intestinal mucosa; promotes recovery of brush border membrane disaccharidases; decreases the duration of illness; and improves nutritional status.[31,34] Although lactose intolerance can occur with viral gastroenteritis, most children with mild diarrhea can tolerate full-strength animal milk, animal milk-based formula, and breast milk. If the child becomes lactose intolerant during this illness, a lactose-free formula may be substituted for 2 to 6 weeks until GI lactase production returns to normal. Specific diets are often recommended during diarrhea (e.g., BRAT [bananas, rice, applesauce, toast]). Although these diets occasionally can be useful, the nutritional value of these foods is relatively low, and they do not provide optimal nutrition compared with complete diets with fats and proteins.[31]

Drug Therapy

10. What medications can be recommended for the treatment of diarrhea in children?

Medications play a minor role in the treatment of acute infantile diarrhea because most episodes are self-limiting. Antibiotics should be used only when systemic bacteremia is suspected; when immune defenses are compromised; or when a persistent enteric infection is sensitive to antibiotics.[35] In general, antidiarrheal preparations are not recommended for infants or children because they have little effect on acute diarrhea, are associated with side effects, and direct attention away from the use of oral hydration therapy.[31,34] Drugs that alter GI motility should be avoided, especially in children with high fever, toxemia, or bloody mucoid stools, because they may worsen the clinical course of the bacterial infection. Adsorbents, such as Kaopectate, adsorb bacterial toxins and water and lessen the symptoms of diarrhea by producing more formed stools, but they do not decrease the duration of diarrhea or fluid and electrolyte losses. Kaopectate also can adsorb nutrients, enzymes, and antibiotics (especially with prolonged use).[34]

Probiotics, live microbial foods containing species of lactobacillus, bifidobacterium, saccharomyces, and streptococcus, can improve the balance of intestinal flora and diminish the effect of enteric pathogens. These microbes are thought to exert their beneficial effects through various mechanisms (e.g., producing antibacterial chemicals, competing with enteric pathogens, inhibiting the adhesive capabilities of pathogens, altering toxins or toxin receptors).[36] Probiotics are most useful in infectious viral gastroenteritis (but not in bacterial infections) when used early in the course of disease. Lactobacillus GG, in doses of at least 10^6 to 10^9 colony-forming units per day, has been the most consistently beneficial in clinical trials. The manufacture of probiotics is not regulated; therefore, the organism count per dose might be based on the number present at the time of production and not at time of expiration, and the labeling might incorrectly identify the species of organism. As a result, the efficacy of probiotics is difficult to ascertain reliably. Probiotics are not recommended for use in immunocompromised individuals because systemic infections after use have been reported.[31,36] Zinc supplementation hold promise for the treatment and prevention of diarrheal disease; however, its mechanism of action, best method of administration, and its efficacy in different populations are unclear.[31]

GASTROESOPHAGEAL REFLUX

Gastroesophageal reflux (GER) is a common disorder, with 50% to 67% of infants experiencing recurrent vomiting and regurgitation during the first 4 months of life.[37] Most reflux in infants is believed to be caused by transient relaxations of the lower esophageal sphincter (LES). Infants also might be predisposed to reflux because of their body positioning (e.g., slumped over in a car seat or lying supine); their consumption of a liquid feeding that exceeds the volume capacity of the stomach; and in premature infants, a decrease in peristaltic activity.[38] Infants and young children also might have undiagnosed underlying conditions that predisposes them to reflux (e.g., neurologic disorders, hiatal hernia, hypertrophic pyloric stenosis, cow's milk protein allergy).[40] Of cases of reflux in infants, 80% are benign and resolve by 18 months of age,[39] and reflux in older children resolves in a timeframe similar to that of adults. If untreated, GER can result in esophageal strictures; GI hemorrhage; or chronic respiratory disease from the aspiration of GI contents. Children with asthma are noted to have an increased incidence of GER. [41]

Clinical Presentation

In infants, the vomiting and regurgitation of GER occur frequently and other symptoms often are nonspecific (e.g., failure to thrive [FTT], recurrent pneumonia, apnea, dysphagia, reactive airway disease, apparent life-threatening events [ALTE], hematemesis, anemia).[40–42] A thorough diagnostic workup generally is not necessary in a healthy infant with functional GER presenting as recurrent vomiting: empiric drug therapy can be initiated after the diagnosis is made based on clinical findings and after other causes of vomiting have been eliminated.[40,43] Further diagnostic evaluations, however, are indicated for infants and children presenting with additional symptoms (e.g., FTT, irritability, ALTE, respiratory difficulties).[43] Currently, esophageal pH monitoring is considered the standard of practice for diagnosis of GER and endoscopic biopsy when mucosal abnormalities are noted.[41,43] Multichannel intraluminal impedence measurements could replace these techniques.[44] Further evaluations (e.g., barium contrast radiography) might be necessary if anatomic abnormalities (e.g., strictures, pyloric stenosis) are suspected.[43]

Treatment

Because uncomplicated GER usually resolves spontaneously in infants, therapy should focus on providing symptom relief and maintaining normal growth.[43] The goals of therapy are to heal esophagitis and prevent complications in infants and children with pathologic GER so that surgery can be avoided.[43] Infants and young children with underlying neurologic problems (e.g., cerebral palsy) are unlikely to have spontaneous resolutions of GER and frequently require aggressive antireflux therapies and surgical intervention.

Positional and Dietary Measures

11. S.B., a 3-month-old, 6-kg, 60-cm male infant, has a 2-week history of regurgitation after each feeding. The pediatrician noted that S.B. had not gained weight since his last visit 1 month earlier. The presumptive diagnosis is FTT secondary to GER, and S.B. was referred to a pediatric gastroenterologist. The gastroenterologist admitted S.B. to the hospital and confirmed the diagnosis using 24-hour pH monitoring. How should S.B. be treated initially?

S.B. can be treated conservatively because he does not present with life-threatening complications.[43] First, caregiver feedings should be observed to rule out regurgitation caused either by overfeeding or by inappropriate feeding techniques. Sometimes infants with milk protein allergies can have a similar clinical presentation; therefore, a change to a soy protein formula or hypoallergenic formula should be tried.[41] Interventions to modify an infant's body positioning or to modify infant feedings with milk thickeners are not proved to be effective,

Table 93-4 Oral Drugs Used to Treat GER in Infants[42,43,46,49,52–57,60,134,135–137,138,139–141]

Agent	Mode of Action	Oral Dosage
Acid Suppressing Agents		
Antacids (aluminum or magnesium hydroxide)	Neutralizes acid;	0.5–1.0 mL/kg/dose before and after feeding (maximum, 15 mL/dose)
Proton Pump Inhibitors	↓ acid secretion via inhibition of gastric hydrogen-potassium adenosine triphosphatase	
Omeprazole		1 mg/kg/day divided daily–BID
		5–10 mg daily (1–5 yr)
Esomperazole		10–20 mg daily (6–11 yr)
Lansoprazole		15 mg daily (weight <30 kg)
Pantoprazole		30 mg daily (weight > 30 kg)
		20 mg daily (0.5–1 mg/kg/day)
H_2 Receptor Antagonists	Blocks H_2-receptors; ↓ acid secretion	
Cimetidine		40 mg/kg/day divided QID
Famotidine		0.5–1 mg/kg/day div daily-BID
Nizatidine		5–10 mg/kg/day divided BID
Ranitidine		5–10 mg/kg/day divided TID–QID
Prokinetic Agents		
Bethanechol	Cholinergic agent; stimulates peristalsis ↑ LES pressure; ↑ gastric emptying; ↑ colonic motility	0.1–0.2 mg/kg/dose QID given 30–60 min before feeding and HS
	↑ gastric emptying; ↑ LES pressure; augments esophageal clearance	
Cisapride		0.8 mg/kg/day divided QID
Metoclopramide		0.1–0.2 mg/kg/dose QID given 30 min before feeding and HS
Erythromycin	Motilin agonist stimulates smooth muscle contraction	1–3 mg/kg/dose QID
Surface Active Agents		
Sucralfate	Forms paste and adheres to damaged esophageal mucosa	40–80 mg/kg/day divided QID

BID, twice daily; GER, gastroesophageal reflux; HS, at bedtime; LES, lower esophageal sphincter; QID, four times daily; TID, three times daily.

but are reasonable to undertake.[40–45] Maintaining S.B. at a 60-degree angle during the day while sitting and at a 30-degree position at night should be implemented in an effort to promote clearance of acid from the esophagus and to minimize reflux after meals. Milk thickeners (most commonly rice cereal in the United States) and more frequent, smaller feedings also are worthwhile interventions. Mild cases of GER often can be treated successfully by dietary measures alone, as well as by propping infants in an upright position during, and 1 hour after, feedings. Although the placement of infants in a face-down prone position during sleep can reduce reflux, the greater risk of sudden infant death syndrome (SIDS) in infants <12 months of age outweighs the benefits of such positioning.[41] Older children and adolescents should follow the recommended dietary guidelines (i.e., avoidance of caffeine, chocolate, spicy foods) for adults.

Drug Therapy

The efficacy of pharmacologic therapy in altering the course of uncomplicated GER in infants has not been proved[43]; however, a therapeutic trial of a prokinetic agent to manage recurrent vomiting in an infant with uncomplicated GER seems reasonable. In infants or children who present with nonspecific symptoms or complications, such as S.B., acid suppression therapy or prokinetic therapy is warranted even in the absence of documented esophagitis.[43] When esophagitis is present, acid suppression is always recommended to aid in the healing process; however, these agents alone do not rectify the causes of the GER.[43] The various agents to treat infant GER are listed in Table 93-4.

ACID-SUPPRESSANT AGENTS

Antacids

Antacid therapy is not recommended for the treatment of GER in infants and young children because infants treated with aluminum-containing antacids can accumulate sufficient aluminum to cause osteopenia and neurotoxicity.[41–43,46,47] In addition, information on other antacids in infants is limited; nevertheless, antacids can provide short-term relief of symptoms in older children and adults.

Proton-Pump Inhibitors

Proton-pump inhibitors (PPI) are superior to histamine$_2$-receptor antagonists (H_2RA) in relieving symptoms and in promoting healing of significant esophagitis from GER in infants, young children, and adults.[43,48,49] PPI control both basal and meal-stimulated acid secretion, which may in part explain their superior efficacy. The incidence of adverse effects in children from PPI is similar to that reported in adults.[49] Despite concerns about the long-term use of PPI, untoward effects have not been observed from their use for up to 11 years.[50] In children, increased metabolism and decreased bioavailability necessitate larger milligram per kilogram doses to maintain acid suppression than adults; thus, titration of dose to response is necessary, particularly for treatment of esophageal erosions.[44,51] Although most clinicians dose PPI once a day, multiple, divided daily doses can prevent acid breakthrough and better promote healing.[48] Omeprazole and lansoprazole are available in extended-release capsules, which can be separated, opened, and sprinkled on soft foods. Lansoprazole also is available as granules for an oral suspension. Suspension formulations for both omeprazole and lansoprazole have been extemporaneously compounded and evaluated for stability.

Histamine$_2$-Receptor Antagonists

Histamine$_2$-receptor antagonists (H_2RA) reduce histamine-stimulated acid secretion, but have limited effects on acid secretion by other chemical mediators and other stimuli. In randomized, controlled trials, H_2RA in infants and children relieved symptoms and facilitated the healing of esophageal tissue.[52,53] Tolerance to the acid suppressant activity of H_2RA over a relatively short time (<30 days), however,[54,55] can limit their use for long-term treatment of esophagitis. Oral liquid formulations are available for most H_2RA. Ranitidine also is available in an effervescent tablet to facilitate compliance.

PROKINETIC AGENTS

Metoclopramide, a dopamine antagonist with cholinergic and serotonergic effects, accelerates gastric emptying, increases LES pressure, enhances esophageal clearance, and accelerates transit time in the small bowel; however, its effects on vomiting and esophageal pH in children with GER has been equivocal.[56,57] Additionally, metoclopramide has been associated with significant CNS (i.e., restlessness, drowsiness, extrapyramidal) effects and rare reports of gynecomastia and galactorrhea. The prokinetic drug, *cisapride*, is not available in the United States; however, it can be obtained via a limited access protocol for children in whom conventional therapy has failed.[43] *Domperidone*, another prokinetic agent, also has been associated with limited benefits for the treatment of GER in infants.[58] *Erythromycin* increases GI motility by increasing smooth muscle contractions through its motilin agonistic activity, and has been used as a prokinetic agent for GER in children when acid suppression therapy alone was ineffective.[59] Erythromycin-induced development of infantile hypertrophic pyloric stenosis, arrhythmias, and potential changes in bacterial resistance patterns, however, limit its use for GER. The cholinergic agonist, *bethanecol*, reportedly reduces vomiting episodes in infants with GER;[43,60] however, its role in treating GER in infants is limited because of its potential to induce bronchospasm and to stimulate gastric acid secretion. The lack of a suitable commercially available formulation of bethanechol for young infants necessitates its extemporaneous compounding. *Baclofen*, which decreases transient LES relaxations through its γ-aminobutyric acid (GABA) agonist actions, could be a future therapeutic option for GER, pending further study.[61] Generally, prokinetic agents only are marginally effective in the management of GER.

SURFACE ACTIVE AGENTS

Sucralfate (Chapter 26, Upper Gastrointestinal Disorders) was equally effective as cimetidine for use in esophagitis[62]; however, its use for GER is more limiting because of concern about the adverse effects of aluminum-containing products in infants.

12. Four weeks after instituting positional and dietary measures, S.B. continues to vomit and still has not been gaining weight. On physical examination, the gastroenterologist notes bilateral wheezes; endoscopy rules out esophagitis. What would be the next step of therapy?

The treatment of S.B. can include acid suppression therapy and a prokinetic agent. Acid suppression therapy in children who have complications from GER can be implemented by a "step up" approach in which treatment is initiated with a H_2RA followed by a PPI if no improvement is noted, or through a "step down" approach involving a PPI followed by an H_2RA for maintenance therapy.[43] No evidence supports the preferential use of one H_2RA or PPI versus another; however, most pediatric gastroenterologists prefer to use PPI.

The effectiveness of acid suppression for managing symptoms of GER in children is not as well documented as it is for healing esophagitis; however, acid suppression is believed to play a useful role for symptom control, particularly for managing the respiratory symptoms.[43] If additional symptom control is desired, metoclopramide 0.6 mg (0.1 mg/kg/dose) four times daily, 30 minutes before meals and at bedtime can be initiated for S.B. This dose can be adjusted based on his response, with close observation for adverse effects. Treatment should be continued for at least 3 to 4 months, although the optimal duration of therapy is unknown. If S.B. requires additional drug therapy to control symptoms of GER beyond 18 months to 2 years of age, surgery should be considered because GER is unlikely to resolve spontaneously after this age.[39] Surgery might be considered earlier if S.B. fails medical therapy or if he develops an esophageal stricture, apnea, or recurrent respiratory disease.[39,43]

SEDATION AND ANALGESIA

Sedation

Conscious Sedation

Sedation often is needed for children who must undergo diagnostic or therapeutic procedures or when placed in an intensive care setting. Table 93-5 lists characteristics of drugs commonly used to produce conscious sedation. In general, the IV administration of drugs provides the most rapid onset of action. The absorption of intramuscularly (IM), rectally, or orally administered sedatives can be variable, especially in infants and young children.[63]

13. A.J., a 3-year-old, 15-kg girl, is admitted for evaluation of abdominal mass. A computed tomography scan is ordered. What regimen should be used to sedate A.J.?

The ideal sedative should be easy to administer, and have (a) a rapid and predictable onset, (b) minimal adverse effects, and (c) a duration of action that approximates the duration of many common medical procedures. Chloral hydrate, barbiturates (e.g., pentobarbital), narcotic analgesics (e.g., morphine, fentanyl), benzodiazepines (e.g., midazolam, lorazepam), and anesthetic agents (e.g., propofol, ketamine) can be used in pediatric patients for short-duration diagnostic procedures.

Although *chloral hydrate* had been used for sedation for many years without evidence of problems, it has not been tested extensively for toxicity or efficacy.[64] Several years ago, the potential carcinogenicity and genotoxicity of chloral hydrate became of concern because it is a metabolite of trichloroethylene, an industrial solvent and cleaning fluid, which has induced can-

Table 93-5 Drugs Commonly Used for Conscious Sedation[67,71]

Drug	Dosage[a]	Onset of Action	Duration	Comments
Chloral hydrate	25–75 mg/kg (maximum, 1 g/dose to a total of 2 g) *Route:* PO, PR	20–30 min	Unpredictable	Rapidly metabolized to active metabolite trichloroethanol; paradoxical excitation may occur; hyperbilirubinemia has been associated with chloral hydrate (repeated doses) in premature infants and neonates; absorption erratic when given PR
Diazepam (Valium)	*IV:* 0.04–0.3 mg/kg (maximum: 10 mg) *PO:* 0.2–0.3 (maximum: 10 mg)	IV: 2–3 min PO: 30–45 min	2–6 hr	May burn when given IV (lipid soluble); do not use small veins; infuse IV over 3 min and at most 5 mg/min; potentiates the effect of narcotics and barbiturates
Fentanyl (Sublimaze)	*IV:* 1–2 mcg/kg (up to 100 mcg/dose) *PO:* 5–15 mcg/kg (maximum: 400 mcg)	*IV:* 1–1.5 min *IM:* 7–8 min *PO:* 5–15 min	*IV:* 30–60 min *IM:* 1–2 hr *PO:* 1–2 hr	Infuse IV over 3–5 min; effects potentiated by benzodiazepines; Oralet available in 200-, 300-, and 400-mcg doses Maximal dose is 400 mcg. Only about 25% of dose of Actiq is absorbed from the oral mucosa
Lorazepam (Ativan)	*IV:* 0.05 mg/kg *PO:* 0.02–0.1 mg/kg	*IV:* 2–5 min *IM:* 15–30 min *PO:* 30–60 min	6–24 hr	Infuse IV over 2–3 min, not to exceed 2 mg/min; potentiates the effect of narcotics and barbiturates
Meperidine (Demerol)	*IV:* 0.5–1.5 mg/kg *SC/IM:* 1–2 mg/kg (maximum, 100 mg/dose) See combination drugs below for Demerol/Phenergan/Thorazine dosage	*IV:* 1–5 min *SC/IM:* 10 min	*IV:* 1–2 *SC/IM:* 2–4 hr	Metabolite (normeperidine) has neurotoxic effect; accumulation of normeperidine may result in central nervous system manifestation; caution in patients with renal impairment after high or repeated doses; infuse IV dose over 3–5 min
Midazolam (Versed)	*IV:* 0.05–0.1 mg/kg *Intranasal:* 0.2–0.3 mg/kg *PO:* 0.25–0.5 (maximum: 20 mg)	*IV:* 1–3 min *IM:* 10–15 min *Intranasal:* 5 min *PO:* 5–10 min	*IV:* 30–60 min *IM:* 2–6 hr *Intranasal:* 40–75 min *PO:* 30–90 min	3–4 times potency of diazepam; potentiates the effect of narcotics; infuse IV dose over 1–2 min
Morphine	*IV:* 0.05–0.1 mg/kg	*IV:* 1.0–2.5 min	1–2 hr	Maximal respiratory depression occurs within 7 min; effect potentiated by benzodiazepines; infuse IV dose over 3–5 min
Pentobarbital (Nembutal)	*PO/PR/IM:* 2–6 mg/kg (maximum, 100 mg/dose) *IV:* 1–3 mg/kg in increments of 1 mg/kg (maximum: 100 mg/dose)	PO/PR: 15–60 min *IM:* 10–25 min *IV:* 1–2 min	*PO/PR:* 1–4 hr *IM:* 30–60 min *IV:* 15–20 min	IV administration over at least 1 min or not to exceed 50 mg/min
Propofol (Diprivan)	*IV:* ≥2.5 mg/kg × 1 7.5–15 mg/kg/hr	*IV:* 30 sec after bolus	3–10 min, longer with prolonged use	Titrate to desired effect; lower dosages required when used with narcotics; metabolic acidosis with fatal cardiac failure has been reported in children
Combination drugs Demerol/ Phenergan/ Thorazine	*IM:* Demerol: 2 mg/kg (up to 50 mg) Phenergan: 1 mg/kg (up to 12.5 mg) Thorazine: 1 mg/kg (up to 12.5 mg) *IV:* 1/2 of IM dose	*IM:* 10–15 min *IV:* 5–10 min	2–5 hr	Infuse IV dose over 5 min; hypotension can occur with rapid IV infusion; may be mixed in the same syringe
Ketamine	*IV:* 0.5–2 mg/kg *IM:* 3–7 mg/kg *PO:* 6–10 mg/kg	*IV:* 30 sec *IM:* 10–15 min *PO:* 30 min	*IV:* 1–2 hr *IM:* 3–4 hr	Can result in hallucinogenic emergence reactions; less common in younger patients, can be managed in part with benzodiazepines; can cause bronchial secretions
Etomidate	*IV:* 0.1–0.3 mg/kg	*IV:* 30–60 sec	*IV:* 2–10 min; dose dependent	Blocks cortisol production; avoid in critically ill patients and prolonged infusions; myoclonus seen in up to 33% of patients; no analgesic activity, use with opioid
Dexmedetomidine	*IV:* 0.5–1 mcg/kg loading dose, then 0.2–0.7 mcg/kg/hr infusion	*IV:* analgesia, ~30 min	*IV:* 2–3 hr	Sedative and analgesic properties; hypotension common

[a]Use low end of the dose if combined with another agent(s).
IM, intramuscular; IV, intravenous; PO, orally; PR, as needed; SC, subcutaneously.

cer in rodents.[65] Because the extrapolation of animal data to humans is only theoretical, the American Academy of Pediatrics (AAP) continues to support chloral hydrate use because many practitioners are familiar with the use of this drug and because it is associated with a low incidence of toxicity. A sudden switch by practitioners from chloral hydrate to a less familiar agent might pose a greater risk than a theoretic risk of carcinogenesis.[66] Practitioners, nevertheless, should become increasingly familiar with sedating agents other than chloral hydrate, especially for situations when chloral hydrate fails to produce the desired effect. The risks of chloral hydrate in pediatric patients needs further study. Chloral hydrate 25 to 75 mg/kg can be repeated in 30 minutes if needed to a maximal total dose of 120 mg/kg, or 1 g for infants and 2 g for older children.[67] Most children respond to 50 to 75 mg/kg; however, dose requirements can vary.[66,68–70] Repetitive dosing of chloral hydrate to maintain prolonged sedation in infants and children during mechanical ventilation is not recommended because its pharmacologically active metabolites can accumulate and cause excessive CNS depression and other complications.[64,66] Chloral hydrate can be particularly useful for sedating infants and children in preparation for electroencephalogram and pulmonary function tests.[71]

Pentobarbital induces sedation in children more rapidly than chloral hydrate and has shorter duration of action. A lower milligram per kilogram dose of pentobarbital is needed in older patients than younger infants and children. Intravenous pentobarbital should be given in 1 mg/kg increments to minimize risk of respiratory depression. In clinical trials, pentobarbital has compared favorably with chloral hydrate for sedation before imaging studies.[72,73] Paradoxical reactions (e.g., excitation and hyperactivity) can occur with barbiturates; however, the administration of a narcotic (e.g., morphine) to the excited child can convert the reaction to a peaceful sedation.

Morphine and *fentanyl* can provide both sedation and analgesia in patients undergoing painful procedures (e.g., bone marrow biopsy). Narcotics, however, rarely are used alone for sedation because analgesia occurs at lower doses than those required for sedation. Fentanyl oral lozenge (Actiq) is available in 200, 400, 600, 800, 1200, and 1600 mcg strengths for the child to suck on the flavored lozenge until he or she falls asleep. Some clinicians, however, are uncomfortable with the psychological association of candylike preparations with drugs. Comparisons of oral transmucosal fentanyl with oral midazolam as premedication sedatives have shown mixed results.[74,75] Narcotic analgesics can induce respiratory depression (especially when combined with benzodiazepines), however, the respiratory depression can be reversed by naloxone.[76] Fentanyl is usually the preferred agent because of its shorter duration of action, shorter recovery time, and relative lack of tendency to cause histamine-release related side effects.[71]

Benzodiazepines (i.e., lorazepam, diazepam, and midazolam) can induce sedation, hypnosis, muscle relaxation, and amnesia, and can decrease anxiety in patients undergoing procedures.[76] These benzodiazepines usually are administered IV before the procedure, although midazolam also has successfully induced sedation when administered orally, rectally, or intranasally.[71] Flumazenil, a specific benzodiazepine antagonist, can reverse the sedative effects of benzodiazepines.[77]

Propofol, an anesthetic agent, appears safe as a sedative for elective pediatric procedures. It is as effective as other sedatives, and is associated with shorter recovery times and hospital stays.[71,78,80] Transient hypotension and severe respiratory depression can occur, however, and the patient should be closely monitored.[71] Because propofol administration generally requires anesthesiology support and because opioid–benzodiazepine combinations often result in prolonged sedation, the dissociative anesthetic, *ketamine* has been used as an adjunct to benzodiazepines for procedures in children and compares favorably with opioid–benzodiazepine combinations.[79,81,82] Adverse effects associated with ketamine include increased bronchial secretions, hypertension, and increased muscle tone; older children have experienced hallucinations or vivid and disturbing dreams. *Etomidate*, an ultrashort-acting hypnotic is effective for procedural sedation in children, however, it has been associated with respiratory depression, clonus, and adrenal suppression.[71] As a result, propofol remains as the ultrashort-acting agent of choice in most situations.[71] *Dexmedetomidine,* a centrally acting α_2-receptor agonist, has compared favorably with other agents used for conscious sedation in noninvasive procedures, but it might not be as effective as propofol or other agents for invasive procedures.[83] Dexmedetomidine does not affect respiratory or circulatory function to the same extent as propofol,[71] but unlike propofol, a maintenance infusion is needed to supplement the bolus dose.

Any one particular sedative combination has not been shown to be superior to any another. The medication(s) of choice for conscious sedation in children, therefore, usually depend on the type of procedure, degree of sedation required, age of the patient, clinical status of the patient, anatomic location of the procedure, and the expertise of the staff administering the agents. For A.J., any of the above regimens could be appropriate. If anesthesiology support is available, propofol would be a good choice given its safety profile during short-term procedures and the rapid recovery time associated with its use. Nevertheless, chloral hydrate, pentobarbital, an opioid–benzodiazepine combination (e.g., fentanyl–midazolam), ketamine alone or in combination with benzodiazepines, and possibly etomidate and dexmedetomidine, would be appropriate choices as well. Serious adverse events do not appear to be related to medication class or route of administration, although an association exists with adverse outcome when three or more medications are used.[84] Any previous history of successful sedation also can be helpful in the selection of sedation for a patient. The patient should be monitored closely during and after the procedure, and adequate personnel and resuscitation equipment should be readily available.[85]

Intensive Care Unit Sedation

14. M.P., a 5-year-old boy, is admitted to the pediatric intensive care unit (ICU) for sepsis. He currently is intubated and receiving a neuromuscular blocking agent. What are the considerations when sedating critically ill patients such as M.P.?

Children who require mechanical ventilation commonly receive medication to induce sedation to obviate resistance from the patient during ventilator manipulations. Children who receive drugs to induce paralysis also generally need adequate sedation to minimize the fear associated with being aware but unable to move. Critically ill children often require constant sedation; therefore, medication should be administered on a set schedule or as a continuous IV infusion rather than on an as needed (PRN) basis. Intermittent administration results in peak and trough effects, whereas continuous infusions provide a more constant serum concentration and more constant sedation. Incompatibility with other IV medications, however, often can be a problem with continuous IV infusions. IM administration of sedation medications should be avoided because of injection pain and erratic absorption in critically ill patients. The oral administration of medications to induce sedation usually is impractical. Clinicians must be diligent in ensuring that sedation for critically ill children is adequate. In one study, 66% of children receiving morphine and midazolam remembered the pediatric intensive care unit (PICU), many recalled pain, and some stated that they were scared and could not sleep.[86]

Propofol, with its a rapid onset of action and quick recovery from sedation on discontinuation, is commonly utilized in the ICU. This drug does not provide analgesia and should be combined with a narcotic when used after a painful procedure. Adequate sedation is usually achieved with a bolus dose followed by a continuous infusion titrated to effect.[87] Adverse effects of propofol include hypotension, dose-dependent respiratory depression, myoclonus, and seizure activity. Prolonged propofol infusions have been associated with a "propofol-related infusion syndrome" characterized by persistent and worsening metabolic acidosis, cardiovascular instability, arrhythmias often resistant to aggressive management, and fatalities.[88–92] If propofol is to be used as a continuous infusion in the PICU, the acid base and overall clinical status of the patient needs to be carefully monitored. If prolonged mechanical ventilation is required, agents, such as opioids and benzodiazepines, might be more appropriate.

Children who receive repeated doses of agents for sedation may develop tolerance and require larger doses to achieve the desired effect. In addition, pediatric patients who receive narcotics or benzodiazepines for several days to weeks are at risk for developing symptoms of drug withdrawal.[93,94]

15. S.C., a 7-year-old boy, is admitted to the hospital after being hit by a car while riding his bicycle. He sustained multiple fractures and has just returned from surgery after an open reduction and internal fixation of his left femur and left humerus. He is tearful and states that he is in a lot of pain. What classes of pain medication are available for use in children? What problems can be anticipated after the use of analgesics in children?

Analgesia

Inadequate pain control in children usually is the result of inaccurate pain assessment or misconceptions about pain. The pain experienced by infants and children often has been treated less aggressively than pain in adults[95]; however, as the effects of pain on psychological, physiologic, and endocrine systems have become better understood, there has been an increased emphasis on ensuring adequate pain control in pediatric patients.[96]

NARCOTIC ANALGESICS

Morphine is one of the most commonly used agents to treat moderate and severe pain in children and the pharmacokinetic parameters of this drug are well established. The elimination and clearance of morphine in children >5 months of age is similar to that in adults. Neonates demonstrate decreased clearance of morphine and a longer elimination half-life when compared with older infants and children.[96] In neonates, the prolonged half-life may allow for adequate pain control when using intermittent bolus doses. When morphine is administered intermittently, however, older infants and children will require a shorter dosing interval (e.g., every 2–3 hours). This frequent dosing schedule has led to an increased use of continuous IV morphine infusion, patient-controlled analgesia (PCA), and epidural infusion.

Fentanyl, a popular analgesic because of its rapid onset and short duration of action, is most often administered as a continuous or epidural infusion for the management of postoperative pain. It also is administered as an intermittent bolus for short procedures. Fentanyl is highly lipophilic and rapidly penetrates the blood–brain barrier. Because it has a larger volume of distribution in neonates, infants, and toddlers, higher dosages may be needed to achieve a desired effect. Repeated fentanyl dosing or continuous infusion can lead to the accumulation of this drug.[96]

Codeine often is administered orally in combination with acetaminophen to treat mild to moderate pain. It should not, however, be administered parenterally because parenteral administration offers no advantage over the IM administration of morphine or meperidine and is potentially dangerous. Serious adverse events after IV or IM administration of codeine have occurred in both children and adults.

Adverse Effects of Narcotic Analgesics. At equipotent doses, all narcotic analgesic agents cause a similar degree of respiratory depression and constipation. The side effects of nausea and vomiting from these analgesics often occur secondary to stimulation of the chemoreceptor trigger zone in the brain. Fentanyl produces less sedation than meperidine and morphine. Morphine can produce peripheral vasodilation, which can lead to significant hypotension in hypovolemic patients. Meperidine should be avoided in patients with renal failure because accumulation of its metabolite, normeperidine, has been associated with seizures. The most serious adverse effect after administration of opioid analgesics is respiratory depression. Infants <3 months of age are particularly susceptible because of their immature blood–brain barrier and decreased clearance of narcotics.[96] Patients receiving concomitant therapy with benzodiazepines or barbiturates may be at increased risk for cardiorespiratory side effects.

Adverse effects associated with epidural administration of morphine include nausea, pruritus, urinary retention, and late respiratory depression. Although late respiratory depression appears to be less common in children than adults, respiratory status should still be monitored carefully for up to 12 hours after administration of morphine.

NON-NARCOTIC ANALGESICS

Acetaminophen, salicylates, or nonsteroidal anti-inflammatory drugs (NSAID) commonly are used for treatment of mild to moderate pain (Table 93-6.) Salicylates and NSAID can have an opioid-sparing effect and are useful in the management of bone pain and pain associated with inflammation. Aspirin is not used routinely in children because of its association with Reye's syndrome. Ketorolac (Toradol) is the only NSAID available parenterally.[96,97] Side effects associated with

Table 93-6 Analgesic Agents Used in Children[67]

Product	Initial Dose	Comments
Nonopioid		
Acetaminophen	10–15 mg/kg/dose Q 4–6 hr	No anti-inflammatory effect
Salicylates	10–15 mg/kg/dose Q 4–6 hr	Associated with Reye's syndrome; has anti-inflammatory effect
NSAIDs		
Ibuprofen	5–10 mg/kg/dose Q 6–8 hr	Gastritis with prolonged use
Naprosyn	5–7 mg/kg/dose Q 8–12 hr	
Ketorolac	*Adults:* 15–30 mg IM/IV Q 6 hr *Children:* Not well established; 0.4–1 mg/kg IM/IV Q 6 hr; do not exceed adult dose	Increased risk of bleeding if high doses are used for >5 day
Opioids		
Codeine	0.5–1.0 mg/kg/dose Q 4–6 hr (*Adults:* 30–60 mg/dose)	Frequently combined with acetaminophen
Fentanyl	1–2 mcg/kg/dose IV/IM (*Adults:* 50–100 mg/dose) *Infusion:* 3–10 mcg/kg/hr	Chest wall rigidity, especially after rapid IV administration
Meperidine	*IV/IM:* 1.0–1.5 mg/kg Q 2–4 hr *PO:* 1–2 mg/kg Q 3–4 hr (*Adults:* 50–100 mg/dose)	Active metabolite has neurotoxic effect; avoid in renal failure
Morphine	*IV:* 0.05–0.1 mg/kg/dose Q 2–4 hr *IM:* 0.1–0.2 mg/kg Q 2–4 hr *PO:* 0.2–0.5mg/kg Q 4–6 hr *IV infusion:* 0.05–0.1 mg/kg/hr	When changing to sustained release formulation, give daily dose as two to three divided doses

IM, intramuscular; IV, intravenous; NSAID, nonsteroidal anti-inflammatory drug; PO, oral.

salicylates and NSAID are minimal, although gastritis may occur, especially after prolonged use. NSAID also have been associated with renal toxicity.

TOLERANCE AND DRUG WITHDRAWAL

Tolerance can occur in some children receiving several days of narcotic therapy resulting in the need for an increased dose to produce the same pain relief. If the patient continues to have reason for pain, doses should be adjusted accordingly. If narcotics are being used for sedation, an alternative agent should be considered.

Administration Schedules

The choice of drug, dose, frequency, and route of administration must be individualized. As-needed (PRN) dosing schedules are less desirable than scheduled dosing times (around the clock) because patients must endure or complain about pain before receiving analgesia. Generally, less medication is needed to prevent the return of pain than to control it. Continuous IV infusion and scheduled administration of pain medication maintain more constant blood levels and minimizes peak (sedation) and trough (return of pain) effects.

Patient-controlled analgesia (PCA) is an alternative to continuous IV infusion and scheduled administration regimens. PCA allows the patient to administer small bolus doses of analgesia, eliminates the time between pain perception and relief, and gives the patient control over pain therapy. PCA, even in children and adolescents, is safe and effective.[96] Children as young as 6 years of age can be taught to use PCA devices, although the age of children capable of understanding the concept of PCA will vary. In some instances, nurses or parents (especially when providing palliative care) are allowed to activate analgesia for the patients who are too young or unable to activate the pump themselves.[97] If parents are to be allowed to participate, however, education on the appropriate and safe activation of the PCA pump should be provided to them and their actions should be closely supervised by nursing personnel. A low-dose, continuous infusion of a narcotic drug, when combined with PCA, has the benefit of providing baseline pain relief, especially while the patient is sleeping. This combined use, however, can contribute to increased side effects (e.g., hypoxia).[96]

Routes of Administration

Typically, pain medication is administered IV, IM, or orally. The IV route provides the most rapid onset of action. When medication is administered IM, children may deny pain to avoid injections. When changing from parenteral to oral routes of administration, bioavailability and absorption need to be considered. Sustained-release oral formulations may be useful in children with chronic pain, but use of such products often is limited by the ability of the patient to swallow whole tablets and because of "fixed" tablet strengths.

Epidural administration of analgesics can provide pain relief for long periods of time with minimal sedation in children of all ages.[96] The transdermal fentanyl patch also offers a unique approach to pain control, and may be useful in children with severe cancer pain.[96] Patches have limited use in young patients because they cannot be cut to deliver smaller doses. Anesthesia also can be achieved through the administration of local anesthetics (e.g., bupivacaine, lidocaine) or narcotics (e.g., morphine, fentanyl).

16. Z.Z., a 15-month-old, 10-kg boy, has been receiving fentanyl continuous infusion for 3 weeks for pain and sedation during mechanical ventilation. The infusion has been decreased from 10 mcg/kg/hour to 1 mcg/kg/hour over the past 5 days. Because

Z.Z. has been successfully extubated and will be transferred to the ward in the morning, the fentanyl drip must be discontinued. Why is Z.Z. at risk for narcotic withdrawal? If Z.Z. develops signs and symptoms of withdrawal, how should these symptoms be managed?

The risk of fentanyl withdrawal is associated with the total dose and duration of the infusion. When the total fentanyl dose is >1.5 mg/kg or the duration of infusion has >5 days, approximately 50% of patients could experience opioid withdrawal symptoms. When the total fentanyl dose is >2.5 mg/kg or the duration of infusion is >9 days, almost all patients will experience withdrawal.[94] Z.Z. has been receiving fentanyl for 3 weeks; therefore, his risk of withdrawal symptoms is very high.

The fentanyl infusion for Z.Z. should be decreased by 10% every 6 hours, and then converted to an oral narcotic. Once Z.Z. is established on an oral regimen, it can be decreased by 10% to 20% a day. Z.Z. should be monitored for withdrawal symptoms, which usually occur within 24 hours of abrupt discontinuation or dosage reduction. Symptoms of opioid withdrawal include neurologic excitation (irritability, insomnia, tremors, seizures), GI dysfunction (nausea, vomiting, diarrhea), and autonomic dysfunction (sweating, fever, chills, tachypnea, nasal congestion, and rhinitis).[94] If Z.Z. develops withdrawal symptoms, the narcotic agent should be increased to the previously tolerated dose. Clonidine may be a useful adjunct to help prevent symptoms of withdrawal.[95]

UNIQUE PEDIATRIC DISORDERS

Hemolytic Uremic Syndrome

Hemolytic uremic syndrome (HUS) is the most common cause of renal failure in children. It is characterized by microangiopathic hemolytic anemia, thrombocytopenia, and acute renal failure. HUS typically occurs several days to 2 weeks after an episode of gastroenteritis, upper respiratory tract infection, or acute flulike illness. HUS is classified into diarrhea-associated (D+) and non–diarrhea-associated (atypical or D–) illness. Diarrhea-associated HUS is more frequent, has seasonal variation, and occurs primarily between 6 months and 4 years of age. It most often is associated with *E. coli* (usually subtype O157:H7) that produces a vero-cytotoxin similar to the shiga-toxin produced by *Shigella* species. Pathologically, WBC activation and endothelial cell injury in the kidney lead to fibrin deposition and platelet adherence to vessel walls. Glomerular lumens are swollen and occluded resulting in renal insufficiency. Red blood cells (RBC) and platelets are damaged by the fibrin strands as they pass through the narrowed vessels. Abnormalities in coagulation involving prostacyclin-thromboxane axis and von Willebrand factor have been implicated in the pathogenesis of thrombocytopenia.[98,99]

The shiga-toxin–producing *E. coli* (STEC) can be spread by contaminated or undercooked food and through person-to-person contact. In 1993, a single outbreak of STEC (subtype O157:H7) associated with hamburgers from a fast food chain caused over 600 cases of diarrhea, 151 hospitalization, 45 cases of HUS, most in children, and 3 deaths.[100] As a result, all ground beef should be well cooked until juices run clear and are no longer pink. *E. coli O157:H7* outbreaks also have been associated with unpasteurized milk and juices, fresh produce, alfalfa sprouts, home made beer, venison, lettuce, and contaminated swimming and drinking water.[98,101] Although *E. coli O157:H7* is by far the most common etiology, other bacteria and viruses have been implicated in D+ HUS, including *Shigella dysenteriae* type 1, *Salmonella, Campylobacter, Yersinia, Pseudomonas, Bacteroides, Aeromonas, Coxsackie,* influenza, and Epstein-Barr.[101] Atypical HUS can be inherited, caused by drugs (e.g., oral contraceptives, cyclosporine, cancer chemotherapeutic agents), or associated with other conditions (e.g., pneumococcal infections, Kawasaki's disease, postpregnancy, bone-marrow transplant). The estimated prevalence of D+ HUS in the United States ranges from 0.2 to 7 per 100,000 children.[99,102] Children with D– HUS appear to have a worse prognosis.[102]

17. How can STEC infection be prevented?

The risk of STEC infection can be minimized by using the following guidelines.

1. Wash all fresh food thoroughly.
2. Remove the outer leaves of lettuce and greens.
3. Cook chicken and ground meats until all pink is gone and juices run clear.
4. Cook fish until it is opaque and flakes easily.
5. Do not drink unpasteurized milk, milk products, or juices.
6. Do not eat raw eggs.
7. Wash hands with soap and water after using the bathroom, changing diapers, before eating, and after handling raw meat, poultry, or seafood.

Clinical Presentation

18. R.H., a 14-month-old, 9.4-kg girl, has been increasingly irritable and lethargic over the past 24 hours. The sudden appearance of dark urine 24 hours ago and significantly decreased urine output in the past 12 hours caused her mother to bring her in for evaluation. Her recent medical history is significant for 3 days of gastroenteritis with blood, which resolved 2 days before the onset of her present symptoms. R.H.'s diet includes breast milk and table food; her mother states that she fed R.H. hamburger earlier in the week.

On physical examination, R.H. is pale, somnolent, and has small purple bruises over her arms and legs. Significant laboratory results reveal the following: partial thromboplastin time (PTT) 26 seconds (normal, 25–35 seconds); hemoglobin (Hgb) 7.6 g/dL (normal, 11.8 g/dL); hematocrit (Hct) 22.5% (normal, 36%); WBC 15,100 cells/mm^3 (normal, 6,000–17,500 cells/mm^3); platelet count 44,000 cells/mm^3 (normal, 150,000–400,000 cells/mm^3); reticulocytes 4.7% (normal, 0.5%–1.5%); blood urea nitrogen (BUN) 60 mg/dL (normal, 5–18 mg/dL); serum creatinine (SrCr) 3.9 mg/dL (normal, 0.3–0.7 mg/dL); potassium (K) 5.4 mEq/L (normal, 3.5–5.5 mEq/L); urinalysis 3+ protein and 3+ blood; blood smear, schistocytes (fragmented RBC); factor V and VIII within normal limits; fibrinogen within normal limits; and fibrin split within normal limits. R.H. is admitted to the hospital with a diagnosis of HUS. Which signs, symptoms, and laboratory tests are consistent with HUS in R.H.?

[SI units: Hgb 1.178 mmol/L (normal, 1.829); Hct, 0.225 (normal, 0.36); platelet count, 44 × 10^{10}/L (normal, 150–400); WBC, 15.1 × 10^{10}/L (normal, 6–17.5); reticulocytes, 0.047 (normal, 0.005–0.015); BUN, 21.42 mmol/L (normal, 1.8–6.4); SrCr, 344.8, mcgmol/L (normal, 26.5–61.9); K, 5.4 mmol/L (normal, 3.5–5.5)]

R.H. exhibits many signs and symptoms associated with HUS. Her lethargy, irritability, change in mental status, and pale color are symptoms of anemia. The dark color of her urine is indicative of hemolysis and renal damage; other signs of renal damage include anuria and hypertension. The purpura (i.e., bruises) on her arms and legs are evidence for thrombocytopenia.

R.H.'s laboratory abnormalities also help confirm a diagnosis of HUS. The low hemoglobin and hematocrit are consistent with anemia, whereas the high reticulocyte count and presence of schistocytes indicate hemolysis. Nephropathy in R.H. is manifested by proteinuria and elevations in BUN and creatinine. The hyperkalemia is a sign of both nephropathy and hemolysis. Finally, normal coagulation studies, absence of fibrin split products, and normal levels of clotting factors and fibrinogen indicate that R.H., as with many children with HUS, does not have active disseminated intravascular coagulation (DIC) at initial presentation.

Treatment

19. On admission, R.H. is given IV fluids without potassium at half maintenance and oral nifedipine 2 mg (0.2 mg/kg) Q 4 to 6 hr PRN for hypertension. Her urine output decreased significantly and peritoneal dialysis was initiated within 24 hours. How should R.H. be treated? What is the role of antibiotic therapy?

Therapeutic approaches aimed at modifying the acute phase of HUS have been unsuccessful, and supportive care is the only widely accepted form of treatment. Therapy for R.H. should be directed at managing the complications (e.g., fluid and electrolyte imbalance, anemia, thrombocytopenia, renal failure, hypertension, seizures) that are associated with HUS. Antimotility agents should be avoided because, in addition to having little if any clinical benefit, they may increase morbidity.[98] The value of using antibiotics to treat *E. coli* O157:H7 infections is questionable and may increase the rate of progression to HUS. The rate of HUS was increased in children with diarrhea caused by *E. coli* O157:H7 who were treated with either trimethoprim–sulfamethoxazole or β-lactam antibiotics.[103] As a result, until conclusive data indicate otherwise, antibiotics should be avoided.[98]

Correction of Hemostatic and Electrolyte Imbalances

R.H.'s hemostatic and electrolyte imbalances need to be corrected first. Packed RBC are needed when anemia is significant (Hct <15%) or when the patient is symptomatic from the anemia. Infusion of platelets should be limited to those patients with active bleeding and those requiring surgery or central line placement because platelets can exacerbate platelet aggregation and thrombus formation. R.H. should not receive potassium in IV fluids, and her electrolytes should be monitored frequently. If peritoneal dialysis is not initiated, R.H. might require potassium-lowering therapy. Blood pressure elevations should be treated with nifedipine, and seizures should be treated initially with benzodiazepines, followed by phenobarbital or phenytoin if they cannot be controlled.[98,102]

20. What other modes of therapy have been used to treat HUS in children?

Many treatments (e.g., aspirin, dipyridamole, heparin, streptokinase, urokinase, corticosteroids) have been evaluated in cases of HUS, but few have improved outcomes.[98,99] Plasmapheresis and plasma infusion, exchange transfusions, and fresh frozen plasma administration also have been ineffective. Although a vaccine for *E. coli* O157:H7 has been studied, it is not yet approved for clinical use: a toxin binding agent has been clinically evaluated and found ineffective.[104,105]

IDIOPATHIC THROMBOCYTOPENIC PURPURA

Idiopathic thrombocytopenic purpura (ITP) in children generally is an acute, self-limited, benign disease with spontaneous remission occurring in approximately 80% of cases within 6 months of diagnosis whether treated or not.[106] Chronic ITP evolves from the acute form in approximately 25% of cases, although <10% of these are clinically significant.[107,108] Mortality rates are low, and most deaths can be attributed to intracranial hemorrhage, which occurs in <1% of children with platelet counts <10,000/mm^3.[106,109] The social and psychological effects that occur secondarily to restriction of normal childhood physical activity is the primary morbidity.

The etiology of ITP in children is unknown. ITP is thought to primarily be triggered by a viral infection that induces formation of antigen–antibody complexes. These complexes adhere to platelets resulting in increased platelet consumption by the reticuloendothelial system (RES). The chronic form, which is similar to adult ITP, may be caused by production of autoantibodies to platelet antigens.[106,110]

Clinical Presentation

21. J.T., a 3-year-old, 15-kg, previously healthy girl, presents with a 3-week history of increased bruising and repeated nosebleeds after an episode of gastroenteritis. Physical examination is remarkable for generalized petechiae and scattered bruising. Her Hgb, Hct, WBC count and differential, and peripheral smear are within normal limits, but the platelet count is 10,000/mm^3 (normal, 250,000–350,000/mm^3). She is admitted to the hospital with a diagnosis of acute ITP. Which signs, symptoms, and laboratory tests in J.T. are consistent with ITP?

[SI unit: platelet count, 10 × 10^{10}/L (normal, 250–350)]

Diagnosis of ITP is based on clinical presentation, complete blood count (CBC), and examination of peripheral smear.[107] As illustrated by J.T., children with acute ITP classically present with a sudden appearance of purpura or petechiae within 6 weeks of the onset of a viral infection. Approximately 25% of children with acute ITP have epistaxis (nosebleeds), 5% have hematuria, and <4% have massive purpura or retinal hemorrhages. Diagnosis of ITP is confirmed by the presence of thrombocytopenia with no apparent cause. The marked decrease in J.T.'s platelet count to <25,000 cells/mm^3 with a normal CBC is indicative of ITP.

Treatment

22. How should J.T. be treated initially?

Hospitalization is indicated for children with life-threatening bleeding, regardless of the platelet count. J.T. can be treated conservatively because she is not massively hemorrhaging. Medical treatment is indicated in the two groups of children thought to be at highest risk for intracranial hemorrhage: (a) children with platelet counts <20,000 cells/mm^3 who have moderate mucous membrane bleeding and (b) children with platelet counts <10,000 cells/mm^3 with minor purpura.[107] If J.T.'s platelet count were higher, some clinicians would delay treatment because the risk of spontaneous, severe bleeding is low if platelet counts remain >30,000/mm^3. Also, clinicians may not treat children such as J.T. who are not massively hemorrhaging or bleeding internally, regardless of the platelet count, because the incidence of catastrophic hemorrhage is very low.[109]

Splenectomy

The treatment of choice is controversial because the mortality rate is low, the rate of spontaneous remission is high, and data for different therapies are inconsistent.[107] The only therapeutic modality with undisputed efficacy is splenectomy because the major site of platelet phagocytosis and antibody formation is removed. Because splenectomy is a major surgical procedure leaving a child at risk for serious infection and treatment with IV γ-globulin (IVIG) therapy or high-dose steroids is associated with good results, many clinicians reserve splenectomy for children with resistant cases of ITP.[107,108]

23. What treatments are available for acute ITP?

Observation, splenectomy, glucocorticoids, IVIG, and anti-D immune globulin have been used to treat acute ITP. Platelet transfusions are ineffective because infused platelets are removed rapidly by the reticuloendothelial system.

Glucocorticoids

Glucocorticoids have been used as treatment for acute ITP for many years, but their benefits and indications are controversial.[106] Glucocorticoids might decrease the duration of thrombocytopenia by inhibiting platelet phagocytosis and they also might lower the risk of hemorrhage by increasing capillary integrity. Further study is needed to determine whether steroids induce a more rapid rise in platelet levels than would occur spontaneously and whether steroids increase capillary integrity. The indications for the use of steroids vary; however, most clinicians would consider steroids when the patient's platelet count is <50,000/mm^3 in the presence of severe bleeding, <20,000/mm^3 with mucous membrane bleeding, or <10,000/mm^3 with minor purpura.[107]

Prednisone 4 mg/kg for 7 days followed by decreasing tapered doses until day 21, and methylprednisolone 30 to 50 mg/kg/day for 7 days, reportedly facilitate platelet recovery similar to IVIG. A short course of prednisone 4 mg/kg/day for 4 days also was able to increase platelet counts >20,000/mm^3.[110] In a meta-analysis, however, steroids were less likely than IVIG to increase platelet counts to >20,000/mm^3 after 48 hours.[111] Although the optimal steroid regimen for acute ITP has not been determined, the risks of steroids are relatively low because they are used for a short period. Modest adverse effects (e.g., behavioral abnormalities, weight gain, acne, GI upset), however, have been reported in children receiving high-dose glucocorticoid therapy.

Intravenous γ-Globulin and Anti-D Immune Globulin

IVIG has been commonly used for management of acute ITP to induce a rapid rise in platelet counts to minimize the risk of hemorrhaging. IVIG purportedly blocks phagocytosis of antibody-coated platelets by the reticuloendothelial system or eliminates circulating immune complexes and microbial antigens.[106] Adverse reactions (e.g., flushing, chills, fever, headache, dizziness, diaphoresis, nausea) to IVIG usually are mild and related to the rate of administration. These can be minimized by stopping the infusion or decreasing the infusion rate. Anaphylactic reactions have been reported in patients with IgA deficiency, as have other serious adverse effects (e.g., hypotension, dyspnea, myalgias, joint pain, abdominal pain). Another consideration is the relatively high cost of IVIG therapy.

Anti-D immune globulin (anti-D), a polyclonal antiserum against the Rh(D) antigen of RBC that was first licensed to prevent hemolytic disease of newborns caused by Rh isoimmunization, is a treatment option for ITP because it has a lower cost and shorter infusion time (15 minutes) compared with IVIG. It has the greatest efficacy in patients who are D antigen positive and is thought to increase platelet counts in ITP by binding to Rh-positive erythrocytes. This leads to removal of the sensitized RBC by the spleen, allowing the antibody-coated platelets to survive.[110] Most patients experience a mild, transient hemolysis.

Both IVIG and anti-D immune globulin appear to be equally effective, particularly when the anti-D is dosed at 50 mcg/kg.[110] Little exists to guide the clinician in choosing IVIG or anti-D for ITP treatment. Survey data suggest a slight preference for anti-D over IVIG.[110] In a randomized trial in Rh+ children, IVIG at 0.8 g/kg and anti-D at 75 mcg/kg (compared with anti-D at 50 mcg/kg) were equally effective, and adverse effect profiles were acceptable in both groups.[112]

Either IVIG, anti-D, or high-dose glucocorticoids are reasonable treatments for J.T. because she is at high risk for bleeding. On the other hand, some clinicians might elect to withhold therapy and monitor J.T. closely.

Goals of Therapy

24. What are the goals of therapy?

The ultimate goal of therapy for ITP is induction of remission. If remission does not occur, therapy is aimed at maintenance of hemostatic platelet levels and prevention of catastrophic hemorrhage. Severe internal bleeding has occurred in patients, however, despite treatment with steroids or IVIG. Another goal of therapy is to avoid performing a splenectomy, which would put the child at an increased risk for infections.[107]

Prognosis

25. What is J.T.'s prognosis?

J.T.'s prognosis is good, much better than the prognosis of adults with ITP. Only 10% to 20% of children will fail to achieve remission within 6 months of diagnosis.[113] Children with chronic ITP will enter remission slowly over a period of years or after a splenectomy. Although early institution of nonsurgical treatments for acute ITP can decrease morbidity and mortality, they probably cannot prevent the development of chronic ITP.[107]

Chronic Idiopathic Thrombocytopenic Purpura

26. J.T.'s platelet count rose to 260,000/mm³ after she received the IVIG, and her counts have remained within normal limits for the past year. J.T. appears to be in remission. If she had developed chronic ITP, how would she have been treated?

[SI unit: platelet count, 260 × 10^{10}/L]

Chronic ITP is defined as thrombocytopenia lasting >6 months. Different approaches exist for the treatment of chronic ITP, but all agree that splenectomy should be delayed to allow for spontaneous remission as long as hemostatic platelet counts are maintained and the child remains asymptomatic.[107]

To maintain adequate platelet counts or to control symptoms before splenectomy is needed, IVIG, anti-D, or glucocorticoids have been prescribed.[107] IVIG sometimes is cited as the treatment of choice for chronic ITP because it has relatively few side effects. Doses of IVIG (0.8–1 g/kg) or anti-D (50–75 mcg/kg) might need to be repeated to maintain hemostatic platelet counts.[108] Long-term steroid use is discouraged because steroids have not been consistently effective, and because of adverse events (e.g., exacerbation of thrombocytopenia, delayed bone growth). Other modalities (e.g., plasmapheresis, danazol, α-interferon, azathioprine [Imuran], cyclophosphamide [Cytoxan], vincristine [Oncovin], vinblastine [Velban], 6-mercaptopurine) have been attempted for children with steroid or IVIG-resistant chronic ITP, but data are insufficient to support their routine use.[107] Splenectomy is effective in 70% of children with chronic ITP and is indicated in symptomatic children with platelet counts that have remained <30,000/mm³ for 12 months.[107,108] A good response to IVIG could be predictive of good response to splenectomy.[114,115] Steroids or IVIG can be given before splenectomy to obtain platelet counts that will maintain hemostasis during surgery.[107] Children should be immunized with *Haemophilus influenzae* type b (Hib), pneumococcal, and meningococcal vaccines at least 2 weeks before an elective splenectomy. Therefore, if J.T. develops chronic ITP, she could receive a repeat course of IVIG with booster doses to maintain hemostasis; a second line of therapy would be steroids or anti-D. Splenectomy and immunosuppressive drugs would be considered last resorts.

Finally, parents should be educated to avoid medications with antiplatelet effects (e.g., aspirin, dipyridamole, NSAID) in children with ITP. Parents also should be instructed to monitor their child's physical activity in an effort to minimize trauma that could precipitate life-threatening hemorrhage.

NEPHROTIC SYNDROME

Nephrotic syndrome in children typically is characterized by proteinuria, hypoalbuminemia, edema, and hypercholesterolemia.[116,117] Overall, it is a relatively rare pediatric disorder with an incidence of 2 to 7 cases per 100,000 children under 18 years of age.[116,117] This idiopathic nephrotic state can present as minimal change nephrotic syndrome or focal segmental glomerular sclerosis. Minimal change disease is in part characterized by normal glomeruli on microscopic analysis.[118,119] It is by far the more common manifestation in children, with >75% of those <12 years of age having this type of nephritic syndrome.[117,119]

In minimal change disease, a loss occurs in charge selectivity of the glomerular membrane barrier, which allows large plasma proteins such as albumin and immunoglobulins to be filtered into the urine that would otherwise be reabsorbed.[119] The etiology is complex, and has not been fully characterized, but T-lymphocyte dysfunction may play a role in the pathogenesis of nephrotic syndrome.[120]

Clinical Presentation

27. GG, a previously healthy 4-year-old, 21-kg boy, has been noted by his mother to have swelling in his face, (especially of his eyes) the past several mornings. The facial swelling disappears during the day, but at night his feet and lower legs are swollen. Physical examination reveals normal vital signs, mild facial puffiness, 2+ to 3+ pitting edema of the lower extremities. Urinalysis shows 4+ protein (normal, negative or trace) and a specific gravity of 1.029 (normal, 1.002–1.030). His serum albumin is 1.6 g/dL (normal, 3.9–5 g/dL), serum cholesterol is 296 mg/dL (normal, 109–189 mg/dL), and the other chemistry results are within normal limits. What subjective and objective data in this patient are consistent with nephrotic syndrome?

[SI units: albumin, 16 g/L (normal, 39–50), serum cholesterol, 7.7 mmol/L (normal, 2.8–4.8)]

G.G. presents with typical findings of nephrotic syndrome. Edema of the face early in the day, and lower extremities at night is a result of the loss of oncotic pressure caused by hypoalbuminemia. Other manifestations of this complication can include swelling of the scrotum, which can lead to testicular torsion. Decreased oncotic pressure can also result in abdominal pain owing to decreased perfusion to the splanchnic capillary bed.

The main laboratory finding in nephrotic syndrome is proteinuria. Levels of proteinuria associated with nephrotic syndromes generally are >50 mg/kg/24 hours or >3.5 g/1.73 m²/day. Sometimes, the proteinuria merely is described as "heavy proteinuria" or proteinuria that is sufficiently significant to result in the four major clinical findings in nephrotic syndrome.[116,117,119] G.G. has 4+ protein in his "dipstick" urinalysis. If the dipstick protein is persistently elevated (>1+), the first morning urine should be "spot tested" to assess the protein:creatinine ratio (Pr:Cr). If the Pr:Cr is abnormal (normal for children <2 years of age is <0.2 mg Pr/1 mg Cr), a complete workup is warranted.[116]

Serum albumin levels of <2 g/dL will likely result in visible edema. Serum cholesterol and triglyceride concentrations often are increased, perhaps attributable to decreased catabolic capacity of the liver or increased production.[117] Other laboratory abnormalities can include hypocalcemia, hyperkalemia, and hyponatremia. Patients with idiopathic minimal change disease do not usually present with gross hematuria, hypertension, or renal dysfunction.

Treatment

28. G.G. is eventually diagnosed with nephrotic syndrome. How should he be treated initially? What nonpharmacologic interventions can be considered?

Patients with nephrotic syndrome have an increased total body sodium owing to increased retention, even in the presence of low serum levels and decreased intravascular volume.[116,117,119] Therefore, sodium restriction is important. Although it is not practical to set a sodium limit in children, a "no-added salt" diet is usually recommended in which family support and participation is crucial. Many institutions will provide patients with examples of foods that are low in sodium (e.g., fresh beef or chicken, fresh vegetables). Patients may eat the normal recommended daily allowance of protein, because protein restriction does not consistently decrease proteinuria or have an impact on the progression of renal disease.[116,117]

A regimen of prednisone 2 mg/kg/day or 60 mg/m^2/day (80 mg/day maximum) for 4 weeks, followed by 2 mg/kg/day or 40 mg/m^2/day every other day, and subsequently tapered over another 4 weeks generally constitutes the first line of therapy. Single daily dosing is as effective as daily divided dosing. Some data support a longer regimen of 6 weeks of every day therapy followed by 6 weeks of every other day therapy. Longer treatment courses (i.e., 5–7 months, including daily therapy for 4 to 8 weeks followed by every other day therapy) might prove to be more effective in preventing relapse. Adverse effects are not significantly different with the longer regimens.[121]

29. How is G.G.'s response to steroid therapy determined?

Most children with minimal change disease respond within weeks of initiating corticosteroids.[120] Remission is defined as negative or trace protein for at least 3 consecutive days on dipstick urinalysis.[116] Of patients who respond, 60% to 80% will have multiple relapses, defined as 2+ proteinuria for 3 consecutive days or 3+ to 4+ proteinuria with edema. Relapses are treated with high-dose prednisone until the urine is protein free for 3 days. Prednisone is then tapered over 4 to 6 weeks using alternate day therapy.[116]

30. What options are available for patients with frequent relapses or for those who are steroid dependent or resistant?

Many children with nephrotic syndrome will experience frequent relapses (i.e., ≥2 relapses in the first 6 months after initial response or ≥4 relapses in any 1-year period). A patient is deemed to be "steroid dependent" when experiencing two consecutive relapses either during steroid tapering or within 14 days of steroid discontinuation. Steroid resistance is described as a failure to achieve remission after 4 weeks of every day high-dose therapy followed by 4 weeks of alternate day therapy.[116] Several studies have investigated patient characteristics that predict relapses in those with nephrotic syndrome. In one study, patients who responded within 1 week of therapy and did not present with hematuria were less likely to have frequent relapses in the first year.[122] In another, children who relapsed within 1 year or who had short remissions before relapse were more likely to have subsequent relapses.[123] An initial remission time of 9 or more days and concurrent upper respiratory tract infections were predictive of steroid dependency.[124] Age at onset of disease, gender, and race were not associated with risk in any of the studies.

In difficult to manage cases, high-dose alternate day regimens are tapered to monthly IV pulse doses of methylprednisolone at 30 mg/kg (maximum, 1 g).[116,117,120] Such patients should be under the care of a pediatric nephrologist and should be monitored for infusion reactions (e.g., hypertension). Cytotoxics (e.g., cyclophosphamide, chlorambucil), are reserved for patients who do not respond to steroids after multiple courses or for those in whom side effects have become intolerable. Anytime cytotoxic agents are utilized, patients must be monitored for bone marrow suppression. Other potential problems that must be discussed with the family before initiation of these agents include the possibility of malignancy, infertility, alopecia, increased infection risk, and hemorrhagic cystitis with cyclophosphamide. Cyclosporine has become the most popular second-line agent in many institutions.[120]

31. What other complications are possible in children with nephrotic syndrome?

Nephrotic syndrome can lead to a hypercoagulable state, which has been attributable to increased factor V and VIII, increased fibrinogen, decreased coagulation inhibitors (e.g., antithrombin III), and increased platelet activity.[119] This alteration in hemostasis can lead to life-threatening events in children.[125,126] Antiplatelet or anticoagulant agents are recommended for patients who have a history of a thromboembolic event.[116] In addition, diuretics must be used more cautiously in patients with a history of hypercoagulability.

Children with nephrotic syndrome have an increased risk of infection secondary to alterations in circulating immune globulins, cellular immunity, and chemotaxis. Cellulitis and spontaneous bacterial peritonitis occur at higher rates in this population; children with albumin <1.5 g/dL are thought to be at greatest risk.[127] Encapsulated organisms such as *Streptococcus pneumoniae* and gram-negative rods, such as *E. coli,* are the most frequent causes of bacterial infection. Prophylactic antibiotics have been used during active relapse, but no consensus exists among pediatric nephrologists on the management of infection risks in these patients.[116,128] Patients should receive standard vaccination using the childhood immunization schedule. The pneumococcal conjugate vaccine (Prevnar) or the pneumococcal polysaccharide vaccine (Pneumovax) should be administered to children with nephrotic syndrome if they were not immunized as infants.[116,129] Live viral vaccines are appropriate for these patients, but must not be given while receiving high-dose corticosteroids or other immunosuppressive therapy. Varicella vaccine has been studied in cases of nephrotic syndrome and is safe and effective.[116,130]

Hyperlipidemia is a common complication of nephrotic syndrome, but it usually resolves spontaneously in steroid-responsive patients. Lipid levels may remain elevated in steroid-resistant patients and, if diet intervention is insufficient, bile acid sequestrants are FDA approved for use in pediatric patients.[131,132] Therapy with statins appears to significantly reduce total cholesterol and low-density lipoprotein (LDL) and triglycerides, but has no documented impact on disease progression. Statin therapy might have beneficial effects on arterial endothelium.[133]

Renal protein excretion may be decreased by angiotensin-converting enzyme inhibitors (ACE-I). Long-term benefit in children with nephrotic syndrome is not known. ACE-I should be given with caution, especially during initial steroid therapy because of the risk of hypotension, resulting in an increased risk of thrombosis.[116]

32. What is the prognosis of children with nephrotic syndrome?

In minimal change disease, mortality is approximately 2%, mostly caused by peritonitis or thrombotic complications. Most patients will be steroid responsive, but will likely have multiple relapses over several years. Considering all categories of nephrotic syndrome in children, 20% will sustain remission, 50% will have relapses in any 5-year follow-up period, and the remaining 30% will develop nephrosis. Half of this last group can attain remission with combination therapy of prednisone and cytotoxic drugs if they have minimal change disease.[117]

REFERENCES

1. Kaushal R et al. Medication errors and adverse drug events in pediatric inpatients. *JAMA* 2001;285:2114.
2. Levine SR et al. Guidelines for preventing medication errors in pediatrics. *J Pediatr Pharmacol Ther* 2001;6:427.
3. Johnson D et al. Development and developmental anomalies of the teeth. In: Behrman Re et al., eds. *Textbook of Pediatrics*. 16th ed. Philadelphia: WB Saunders; 2000:1108.
4. Golden NL et al. Teething age in prematurely born infants. *Am J Dis Child* 1981;135:903.
5. Wake M et al. Teething and tooth eruption in infants: a cohort study. *Pediatrics* 2000;106:1374.
6. Sims KM et al. Oral pain and discomfort. In: *Handbook of Nonprescription Drugs*. 13th ed. Washington, DC: American Pharmaceutical Association; 2002:654.
7. Skoglund RR. Teething ring cheilitis. *Cutis* 1984;34:362.
8. Berg RW et al. Association of skin wetness and pH with diaper dermatitis. *Pediatric Dermatol* 1994;11:18.
9. Jordon WE. Relationship of diapers to diaper rashes. *J Pediatr* 1980;96:957.
10. Mofenson HC et al. Baby powder—a hazard. *Pediatrics* 1981;68:265.
11. Leyden JJ. Corn starch, Candida albicans and diaper rash. *Pediatr Dermatol* 1984;1:322.
12. Sires UI et al. Diaper dermatitis: how to treat and prevent. *Postgrad Med* 1995;98:79.
13. Jaffe D. Assessment of the child with fever. In: Rudolph AM, ed. *Rudolph's Pediatrics*. 21st ed. New York: McGraw-Hill; 2002:889.
14. Warden CR et al. Evaluation and management of febrile seizures in the out-of-hospital and emergency department settings. *Ann Emerg Med* 2003;41:215.
15. Applegate MS et al. Febrile seizures: current concepts concerning prognosis and clinical management. *J Fam Pract* 1989;29:422.
16. Wilson JT et al. Single dose, placebo-controlled comparative study of ibuprofen and acetaminophen antipyresis in children. *J Pediatr* 1991;119:803.
17. Lesko SM et al. The safety of acetaminophen and ibuprofen among children younger than two years old. *Pediatrics* 1999;104:e39.
18. Lesko SM et al. An assessment of the safety of pediatric ibuprofen: a practitioner-based randomized clinical trial. *JAMA* 1995;273:929.
19. Lesko SM et al. Renal function after short-term ibuprofen use in infants and children. *Pediatrics* 1997;100:954.
20. Delay ED et al. Reye's syndrome in the United States from 1981 through 1997. *N Engl J Med* 1999;340:1377.
21. Katcher ML. Cold, cough, and allergy medications: uses and abuses. *Pediatr Rev* 1996;17:12.
22. Soderman P et al. CNS reactions to nose drops in small children. *Lancet* 1984;1:573.
23. Dunn C et al. Coma in a neonate following single intranasal dose of xylometazoline. *Eur J Pediatr* 1993;152:541.
24. Center for Disease Control and Prevention. Infant deaths associated with cough and cold medications—Two states, 2005. *MMWR* 2007; 56:1.

24a. Dooren JC et al. Cough-medicine dilemma widens. *Wall Street Journal*, October 22, 2007.

25. Felt B et al. Guideline for the management of pediatric idiopathic constipation and soiling. *Arch Pediatr Adolesc Med* 1999;153:380.
26. Baker SS et al. Evaluation and treatment of constipation in infants and children: evaluation and treatment. A medical position statement. Recommendations of the North American Society for Pediatric Gastroenterology, Hepatology and Nutrition. *J Pediatr Gastroenterol Nutr* 1999–2006;2943: 612e1.
27. Ulsher M. Major symptoms and signs of digestive tract disorders. In: Behrman RE, ed. *Nelson Textbook of Pediatrics*. Philadelphia: WB Saunders; 2000:1101.
28. Gastanaduy AS et al. Acute gastroenteritis. *Clin Pediatr* 1999;38:1.
29. Leung AKC et al. Evaluating the child with chronic diarrhea. *Am Fam Physician* 1996;53:635.
30. Blackburn P. Dehydration and fluid replacement. In: Reisdorf EJ et al., eds. *Pediatric Emergency Medicine*. Philadelphia: WB Saunders; 1993:108.
31. Centers for Disease Control and Prevention. Managing acute gastroenteritis among children: oral rehydration, maintenance, and nutritional therapy. *MMWR* 2003;52(RR-16):1.
32. Freedman SB et al. Oral ondansetron for gastroenteritis in a pediatric emergency department. *N Engl J Med* 2006;354:1698.
33. Borowitz SM. Are antiemetics helpful in young children suffering from acute viral gastroenteritis? *Arch Dis Child* 2005;90:646.
34. Armon K et al. An evidence and consensus based guideline for acute diarrhoea management. *Arch Dis Child* 2001;85:132.
35. Phavochitr N et al. Acute gastroenteritis in children: what role for antibiotics? *Pediatr Drugs* 2003;5:279.
36. Szajewska H et al. Use of probiotics in children with acute diarrhea. *Pediatr Drugs* 2005;7:111.
37. Nelson SP et al. Prevalence of symptoms of gastroesophageal reflux during infants: a pediatric practice-based survey. Pediatric Practice Research Group. *Arch Pediatr Adolesc Med* 1997;151:569.
38. DeMeester TR et al. Biology of gastroesophageal reflux disease: pathophysiology relating to medical and surgical treatment. *Ann Rev Med* 1999;50:469.
39. Nelson SP et al. One-year follow-up of symptoms of gastroesophageal reflux during infancy. Pediatric Research Group. *Pediatrics* 1998;102:E67.
40. Vandenplas Y. Gastroesophageal reflux: medical treatment. *J Pediatr Gastroenterol Nutr* 2005;41: S41.
41. Gold BD et al. Gastroesophagel reflux in children: pathogenesis, prevalence, diagnosis, and the role of proton pump inhibitors in treatment. *Pediatr Drugs* 2002;4:673.
42. Wooodard-Knight L et al. Aluminum absorption and antacid therapy in infancy. *J Paediatr Child Health* 1992;28:257.
43. Rudolph CD et al. North American Society for Pediatric Gastroenterology and Nutrition. Guidelines for evaluation and treatment of gastroesophageal reflux in infants and children: recommendations of the North American Society for Pediatric Gastroenterology and Nutrition. *J Pediatr Gastroenterol Nutr* 2001;32(Suppl):S1.
44. Omari T. Gastro-oesophageal reflux disease in infants and children: new insights, developments, and old chestnuts. *J Pediatr Gastroenterol Nutr* 2005;41:S21.
45. Craig WR et al. Metoclopramide, thickened feedings, and positioning for gastro-oesophageal reflux in children under two years.(Cochrane Review). In: *The Cochrane Library, Issue (1), 2007*. Chichester, UK; John Wiley & Sons, LTD.
46. Tsou VM et al. Elevated plasma aluminum levels in normal infants receiving antacids containing aluminum. *Pediatrics* 1991;87:148.
47. Robinson RF et al. Metabolic bone disease after chronic antacid administration in an infant. *Ann Pharmacother* 2004;38:265.
48. Gibbons TE et al. The use of proton pump inhibitors in children: a comprehensive review. *Pediatr Drugs* 2003;6:25.
49. Hassall E et al. and the International Pediatric Omeprazole Study Group. Omeprazole for treatment of chronic erosive esophagitis in children: a multicenter study of efficacy, safety, tolerability and dose requirements. *J Pediatr* 200;137:800.
50. Hassall E et al. Characteristics of children receiving proton pump inhibitors continuously for up to 11 years duration. *J Pediatr* 2007;150:262.
51. Litalien C et al. Pharmacokinetics of proton pump inhibitors in children. *Clin Pharmacokinet* 2005;44:441.
52. Cucchiara S et al. Cimetidine treatment of reflux esophagitis in children: an Italian multicentric study. *J Pediatr Gastroenterol Nutr* 1989;8:150.
53. Simeone D et al Treatment of childhood peptic esophagitis: a double-blind placebo controlled trial of nizatidine. *J Pediatr Gastroenterol Nutr* 1997;25:51.
54. Hyman PE et al. Tolerance to intravenous ranitidine. *J Pediatr* 1987;110:794.
55. Nwokolo CU et al. Tolerance during 29 days of conventional dosing with cimetidine, nizatidine, famotidine, or ranitidine. *Aliment Pharmacol Ther* 1990;4:29.
56. Bellissant E et al. The triangular test to asses the efficacy of metoclopramide in gastroesophageal reflux. *Clin Pharmacol Ther* 1997;61:377.
57. Putnam PE et al. Tardive dyskinesia associated with use of metoclopramide in a child. *J Pediatr* 1992;121:983.
58. Pritchard DS et al. Should domperidone be used for the treatment of gastroesophageal reflux in children? Systematic review of randomized controlled trials in children aged 1 month to 11 years old. *Br J Clin Pharmacol* 2005;59:725.
59. Chicella M et al. Prokinetic drug therapy in children: a review of current options. *Ann Pharmacother* 2005;39:
60. Euler AR. Use of bethanechol for the treatment of gastroesophageal reflux. *J Pediatr* 1980;96:321.
61. Wise J et al. Gastroesophageal reflux disease and baclofen: is there a light at the end of the tunnel? *Curr Gastroenterol Rep* 2004;6:213.
62. Arguelles-Mart F et al. Sucralfate versus cimetidine in the treatment of reflux esophagitis in children. *Am J Med* 1989;86:73.
63. Besunder JB et al. Principles of biodisposition in the neonate: a critical evaluation of the pharmacokinetic-pharmacodynamic interface (part 1). *Clin Pharmacokinet* 1988;l14:189.
64. Steinburg AD. Should chloral hydrate be banned? *Pediatrics* 1993;92:442.
65. Smith MT. Chloral hydrate warning. *Science* 1990;250:359.
66. Committee on Drugs and Committee on Environmental Health, AAP. Use of chloral hydrate for sedation in children. *Pediatrics* 1993;92:471.
67. Taketomo KC et al., eds. *Pediatric Dosage Handbook*. 129th ed. Hudson, OH: LexiComp; 2005.
68. Napoli KL et al. Safety and efficacy of chloral hydrate sedation in children undergoing echocardiography. *J Pediatr* 1996;129:287.

69. McCarver-May DG et al. Comparison of chloral hydrate and midazolam for sedation of neonates for neuroimaging studies. *J Pediatr* 1996;128:573.
70. Hollman GA. Chloral hydrate versus midazolam sedation for neuroimaging studies [Letter]. *J Pediatr* 1996;129.
71. Krauss B et al. Procedural sedation and analgesia in children. *Lancet* 2006;367:766.
72. Chung T et al. The use of oral pentobarbital sodium (Nembutal) versus oral chloral hydrate in infants undergoing CT and MR imaging–a pilot study. *Pediatr Radiol* 2000;30:332.
73. Ziegler MA et al. Is administration of enteric contrast media safe before abdominal CT in children who require sedation? Experience with chloral hydrate and pentobarbital. *AJR Am J Roentgenol* 2003;180:13.
74. Howell TK et al. A comparison of oral transmucosal fentanyl and oral midazolam for premedication in children. *Anaesthesia* 2002;57:778.
75. Klein EJ et al. A randomized, clinical trial of oral midazolam plus placebo versus oral midazolam plus oral transmucosal fentanyl for sedation during laceration repair. *Pediatrics* 2002;109:894.
76. Krauss B et al. Sedation and analgesia for procedures in children. *N Engl J Med* 2000;342:938.
77. Shannon M et al. Safety and efficacy of flumazenil in the reversal of benzodiazepine-induced conscious sedation. *J Pediatr* 1997;131:582.
78. Hertzog JH et al. Prospective evaluation of propofol anesthesia in the pediatric intensive care unit for elective oncology procedures in ambulatory and hospitalized children. *Pediatrics* 2000;106:742.
79. Auden SM et al. Oral ketamine/midazolam is superior to Intramuscular meperidine, promethazine, and chlorpromazine for pediatric cardiac catheterization. *Anesth Analg* 2000;90:299.
80. Havel CJ et al. A clinical trial of propofol vs midazolam for procedural sedation in a pediatric emergency department. *Acad Emerg Med* 1999;6:989.
81. Wathen JE et al. Does midazolam alter the clinical effects of intravenous ketamine sedation in children? A double-blind, randomized, controlled, emergency department trial. *Ann Emerg Med* 2000;36:579.
82. Kennedy RM et al. Comparison of fentanyl/midazolam with ketamine/midazolam for pediatric orthopedic emergencies. *Pediatrics* 1998;102:956.
83. Tobias JD. Dexmedetomidine: applications in pediatric critical care and pediatric anesthesiology. *Pediatr Crit Care Med* 2007;8:115.
84. Cote CJ et al. Adverse sedation events in pediatrics: analysis of medications used for sedation. *Pediatrics* 2000;106:633.
85. Work Group on Sedation, AAP. Guidelines for monitoring and management of pediatric patients during and after sedation for diagnostic and therapeutic procedures: an update. *Pediatrics* 2006;118:2587.
86. Playfor S et al. Recollection of children following intensive care. *Arch Dis Child* 2000;83:445.
87. Reed et al. A pharmacokinetically based propofol dosing strategy for sedation of the critically ill, mechanically ventilated pediatric patient. *Crit Care Med* 1996;24:1473.
88. Hanna JP et al. Rhabdomyolysis and hypoxia associated with prolonged propofol infusion in children. *Neurology* 1998;50:301.
89. Cray SH et al. Lactic academia and bradyarrhythmia in a child sedated with propofol. *Crit Care Med* 1998;26:2087.
90. Strickland RA et al. Fatal metabolic acidosis in a pediatric patient receiving an infusion of propofol in the intensive care unit: Is there a relationship? *Crit Care Med* 1995;23:405.
91. Parke TJ et al. Metabolic acidosis and fatal myocardial failure after propofol infusion in children: five case reports. *BMJ* 1992;305:613.
92. Sulsa GM. Propofol toxicity in critically ill pediatric patients: show us the proof [Editorial]. *Crit Care Med* 1998;26:1959.
93. Fonsmark L et al. Occurrence of withdrawal in critically ill sedated children. *Crit Care Med* 1999;27:196.
94. Katz R et al. Prospective study on the occurrence of withdrawal in critically ill children who receive fentanyl by continuous infusion. *Crit Care Med* 1994;22:763.
95. Tobias JD. Tolerance, withdrawal, and physical dependence after long-term sedation and analgesia of children in the pediatric intensive care unit. *Crit Care Med* 2000;28:2122.
96. Berde CB et al. Analgesics for the treatment of pain in children. *N Engl J Med* 2002;347:1094.
97. Sutters KA et al. Comparison of morphine patient-controlled analgesia with and without ketorolac for postoperative analgesia in pediatric orthopedic surgery. *Am J Orthop* 1999;28:351.
98. Tarr PI et al. Shiga-toxin-producing *Escherichia coli* and haemoltyic uraemic syndrome. *Lancet* 2005;365:1073.
99. Amirlak I et al. Haemolytic uraemic syndrome: an overview. *Nephrology* 2006;11:213.
100. Bell BP et al. A multi-state outbreak of *Escherichia coli* O157:H7-associated bloody diarrhea and hemolytic uremic syndrome from hamburgers. *JAMA* 1994;272:1349.
101. Begue RE et al. *Escherichia coli* and the hemolytic-uremic syndrome. *South Med J* 1998;91:798.
102. Corrigan JJ et al. Hemolytic-uremic syndrome. *Pediatr Rev* 2001;22:365.
103. Wong CS et al. The risk of the hemolytic-uremic syndrome after antibiotic treatment of *Escherichia coli* O157:H7 infections. *N Engl J Med* 2000;342:1930.
104. Konadu EY et al. Investigational vaccine for *Escherichia coli* O157: Phase I study of O157 O-specific polysaccharide—*Pseudomonas aeruginosa* recombinant exoprotein A conjugates in adults. *J Infect Dis* 1998;177:383.
105. Trachtman H et al. Effect of an oral shiga toxin-binding agent on diarrhea-associated hemolytic uremic syndrome: a randomized controlled trial. *JAMA* 2003;290:1337.
106. Di Paola JA et al. Immune thrombocytopenic purpura. *Pediatr Clin North Am* 2002;49:911.
107. George JN et al. Idiopathic thrombocytopenic purpura: a practice guideline developed by explicit methods for the American Society of Hematology. *Blood* 1996;88:3.
108. Blanchette V. Childhood chronic immune thrombocytopenic purpura. *Blood Rev* 2002;16:23.
109. Bolton-Maggs PHB et al. The nontreatment of childhood ITP (or "the art of medicine consists of amusing the patient until nature cures the disease"). *Semin Thromb Hemost* 2001;27:269.
110. Shad AT et al. Treatment of immune thrombocytopenic purpura in children: current concepts. *Pediatr Drugs* 2005;7:325.
111. Beck CE et al. Corticosteroids versus intravenous immune globulin for the treatment of acute immune thrombocytopenic purpura in children: a systematic review and meta-analysis of randomized controlled trials. *J Pediatr* 2005;147:521.
112. Tarantino MD et al. Single dose of anti-D immune globulin at 75 μg/kg is as effective as intravenous immune globulin at rapidly raising the platelet count in newly diagnosed immune thrombocytopenic purpura in children. *J Pediatr* 2006;148:489.
113. Bolton-Maggs PHB. Idiopathic thrombocytopenic purpura. *Arch Dis Child* 2000;83:220.
114. Hemmila MR et al. The response to splenectomy in pediatric patients with idiopathic thrombocytopenic purpura who fail high-dose intravenous immune globulin. *J Pediatr Surg* 2000;35:967.
115. Holt D et al. Response to intravenous immunoglobulin predicts splenectomy response in children with immune thrombocytopenic purpura. *Pediatrics* 2003;111:87.
116. Hogg RJ et al. Evaluation and management of proteinuria and nephrotic syndrome in children: recommendations from a pediatric nephrology panel established at the National Kidney Foundation Conference on Proteinuria, Albuminuria, Risk, Assessment, Detection, and Elimination (PARADE). *Pediatrics* 2000;105:1242.
117. Roth KS et al. Nephrotic syndrome: pathogenesis and management. *Pediatr Rev* 2002;23:237.
118. Schapner HW et al. Nephrotic syndrome: minimal change disease, focal glomerulosclerosis, and related disorders. In: Schrier RW et al., eds. *Diseases of the Kidney*. 6th ed. Boston: Little, Brown, and Company; 1997:64.
119. Orth SR et al. The nephrotic syndrome. *N Engl J Med* 1998;338:1202.
120. Eddy AA et al. Nephrotic syndrome in childhood. *Lancet* 2003;362:629.
121. Hodson EM et al. Evidence-based management of steroid-sensitive nephrotic syndrome. *Pediatr Nephrol* 2005;20:1523.
122. Constantinescu AR et al. Predicting first-year relapses in children with nephrotic syndrome. *Pediatrics* 2000;105:492.
123. Takeda A et al. Prediction of subsequent relapse in children with steroid-sensitive nephrotic syndrome. *Pediatr Nephrol* 2001;16:888.
124. Yap HK et al. Risk factors for steroid dependency in children with idiopathic nephrotic syndrome. *Pediatr Nephrol* 2001;16:1049.
125. Silva JMP et al. Premature acute myocardial infarction in a child with nephrotic syndrome. *Pediatr Nephrol* 2002;17:169.
126. Lin CC et al. Thalamic stroke secondary to straight sinus thrombosis in a nephrotic child. *Pediatr Nephrol* 2002;17:184.
127. Hingorani SR et al. Predictors of peritonitis in children with nephrotic syndrome. *Pediatr Nephrol* 2002;17:678.
128. Shroff A et al. Prevention of serious bacterial infections in new-onset nephrotic syndrome: a survey of current practices. *Clin Pediatr* 2002;41:47.
129. Policy statement: Recommendations for the prevention of pneumococcal infections, including the use of pneumococcal conjugate vaccine (Prevnar), pneumococcal polysaccharide vaccine, and antibiotic prophylaxis (RE9960). *Pediatrics* 2000;106:362.
130. Alpay H et al. Varicella vaccination in children with steroid-sensitive nephrotic syndrome. *Pediatr Nephrol* 2002;17:181.
131. Sanjad SA et al. Management of hyperlipidemia in children with refractory nephrotic syndrome: the effect of statin therapy. *J Pediatr* 1997;130:470.
132. Saland JM et al. Dyslipidemia in pediatric renal disease: epidemiology, pathophysiology, and management. *Curr Opin Pediatr* 2002;14:197.
133. Dogra GK et al. Statin therapy improves brachial artery endothelial function in nephrotic syndrome. *Kidney Int* 2002;62:550.
134. Leung C et al. Use of metoclopramide for the treatment of gastroesophageal reflux in infants and children. *Current Therapy Research* 1984;36:911.
135. Machida HM et al. Metoclopramide in gastroesophageal reflux of infancy. *J Pediatr* 1988;112:483.
136. Chiba N et al. Speed of healing and symptom relief in grade II to IV gastroesophageal reflux disease: a meta-analysis. *Gastroenterology* 1997;112:1798.
137. Grill BB et al. Effects of domperidone therapy on symptoms and upper gastrointestinal motility in infants with gastroesophageal reflux. *J Pediatr* 1985;106:311.
138. Croom KF et al. Lansoprazole in the treatment of gastro-eosophageal reflux disease in children and adolescents. *Drugs* 2005;65:2129.
139. Madrazo de la Garza A et al. Efficacy and safety of oral pantoprazole 20 mg given once daily for reflux esophagitis in children. *Gastroenterology* 2003;36:261.
140. Heyman MB et al. Pharmacokinetics and pharmacodynamics of lansoprazole in children 13 to 24 months old with gastroesophageal reflux disease. *J Pediatr Gastroenter Nutri* 2007;44:35.
141. Zhao J et al. Pharmacokinetic properties of esomeprazole in children aged 1 to 11 years with symptoms of gastroesophageal reflux disease: a randomized, open label study. *Clin Ther* 2006;28:1868.

CHAPTER 94

Neonatal Therapy

Donna M. Kraus and Jennifer Tran Pham

The rational use of medications in neonates depends on an appreciation of both the physiological immaturity and the developmental maturation that influence neonatal drug disposition and pharmacologic effects. Much progress has been made to decrease neonatal mortality and improve survival of more premature and lower-birth-weight newborns. Neonates, particularly those of extremely low birth-weights, pose a pharmacotherapeutic challenge to the clinician. The alterations of body composition, weight, size, as well as physiological and pharmacokinetic parameters that occur with normal growth and maturation during the first few months of life are greater than at any other time. Although the amount of neonatal drug information is increasing, the overall lack of well-designed pharmacokinetic and pharmacodynamic studies still hinders the clinical use of many drugs in this population. This is especially true for newborns of the lowest birth-weights (<750 g).

The term *therapeutic orphans,*[1] which was coined more than 30 years ago to describe the lack of medications labeled for use in children, unfortunately still is applicable today.[2] Although the number of medications under development for children has significantly increased over recent years, 71% of new molecular entities approved by the U.S. Food and Drug Administration (FDA) do not have pediatric drug labeling.[3] In addition, practical issues (e.g., technical problems of drug delivery, a lack of suitable dosage formulations) further complicate neonatal pharmacotherapeutics.

This pediatric dilemma led to the passage of the FDA Modernization Act of 1997.[4] This federal legislation offered incentives (in the form of a 6-month drug patent extension) to pharmaceutical companies to conduct pediatric research. The Best Pharmaceuticals for Children Act of 2002 reauthorizes the use of these incentives and provides a process to increase pediatric studies for medications that are no longer "on patent."[5] In addition, this law specifically includes neonates as a population that should be studied. These and other regulations, plus the establishment of the Pediatric Pharmacology Research Unit Network by the National Institutes of Child Health and Human Development,[3] will increase pediatric drug studies, enhance the neonatal labeling of medications, and lead to more rationale use of medications in neonates. Until that time, the clinical use of drugs in neonates presents unique therapeutic challenges for the clinician.

Terminology

An understanding of common neonatal terminology is important because every newborn is evaluated and classified at birth according to birth-weight, gestational age, and intrauterine growth status. These factors influence patient outcome and long-term prognosis.[6] Common neonatal terminology is listed in Table 94-1. Pharmacokinetic parameters, pharmacodynamics, and dosing recommendations often are specified according to these terms.

Table 94-1 Common Neonatal Terminology[6,8]

Term	Definition
Gestational age	*By dates:* The number of weeks from the onset of the mother's last menstrual period until birth *By examination:* Assessment of gestational maturity by physical and neuromuscular examination; gestational age estimates the time from conception until birth
Postnatal age	Chronologic age after birth
Postconceptional age	Gestational age plus postnatal age
Corrected age	Postconceptional age in weeks minus 40; represents postnatal age if neonate had been born at term (40 weeks' gestational age)
Preterm	<38 weeks' gestational age at birth
Term	38–42 weeks' gestational age at birth
Post-term	≥43 weeks' gestational age at birth
Extremely low-birth-weight	Birth-weight <1 kg
Very low-birth-weight	Birth-weight <1.5 kg
Low birth-weight	Birth-weight <2.5 kg
Small for gestational age	Birth-weight <10th percentile for gestational age
Appropriate for gestational age	Birth-weight between 10th and 90th percentiles for gestational age
Large for gestational age	Birth-weight >90th percentile for gestational age

Neonatal Monitoring Parameters

Many pharmacotherapeutic monitoring parameters used in adults also are used in neonates; however, normal values for neonates may differ from those in adults. The monitoring of pharmacotherapy in neonates must take into account these differences. For example, neonates have higher heart rates (HR) and respiratory rates (RR) and lower blood pressures (BP) compared with adults. Appropriate texts should be consulted for neonatal normal values when providing comprehensive pharmacy care.[7,8]

The physiological transitions from intrauterine to extrauterine life can influence disease states and drug disposition. For example, the change from fetal to adult circulation results in an increase in perfusion of organs that are responsible for the elimination of drugs. The developmental changes in absorption, distribution, metabolism, and excretion affect drug disposition and, ultimately, neonatal drug dosing. This chapter focuses on applied therapeutics for common neonatal disease states and the safe and effective use of drugs in the neonate.

NEONATAL PHARMACOKINETICS

Drug Absorption

Gastrointestinal Absorption

Numerous developmental factors (e.g., gastric acidity, gastric emptying time, intestinal integrity and motility, bacterial colonization) can influence the absorption of enterally administered drugs during the neonatal period. Neonates, especially preterm newborns, have a decreased capacity to secrete gastric acid compared with adults.[9] This relative lack of gastric acid output may be referred to as relative achlorhydria or hypochlorhydria. Although the exact maturational pattern of gastric acid secretion needs more clarity, a biphasic pattern in term infants usually is described. At birth, the pH of gastric contents is neutral owing to the presence of residual amniotic fluid. (Amniotic fluid is swallowed regularly during intrauterine life.) In term infants, acid output begins within minutes after birth and gastric pH decreases to 1.5 to 3 within a few hours. Gastric acidity then decreases (pH increases) over the next 10 days; subsequently, basal acid output gradually rises. The maturational pattern of acid secretion in term infants is different in preterm neonates. Gastric acid rarely is present in the fetal stomach before 32 weeks' gestation, and the early decrease in gastric pH usually is not seen or may be delayed in preterm neonates. Hypochlorhydria with a basal pH above 4.0 is present in approximately 20% of preterm neonates 1 to 2 weeks of age. After 6 weeks of life, gastric pH falls to below 4.[10] Although gastric acid production correlates with postnatal age, extrauterine factors (e.g., initiation of enteral feedings) seem to be responsible for the stimulation of gastric acid output.[10] In general, gastric acidity is lower during the neonatal period, and adult values for maximal acid output are not reached until 2 years of age.[9,11]

Gastric and duodenal pH affect drug ionization and absorption.[11,12] Generally, an acidic environment favors absorption of acidic drugs because these drugs will be un-ionized and, therefore, more lipid soluble. Basic drugs, however, are mostly ionized in an acid environment. As a result, basic drugs in an acidic environment are hydrophilic and less well absorbed. Likewise, an acidic drug in an alkaline environment is also primarily in the ionized form and less well absorbed. Therefore, the hypochlorhydria (relatively alkaline gastric pH) in neonates can result in decreased bioavailability of acidic drugs (e.g., phenobarbital, phenytoin), as well as increased bioavailability of weakly basic drugs or acid-labile drugs (e.g., penicillin, ampicillin, erythromycin) compared with that in adults.[11,13]

Gastric emptying time plays an important role in both the rate and the degree of drug absorption because most drugs are absorbed in the small intestine. During the neonatal period, gastric emptying time can be prolonged by up to 6 to 8 hours and may not attain adult values until 6 to 8 months of age.[11] The rate of gastric emptying is affected by gestational age, disease states, and dietary intake. Prematurity, respiratory distress syndrome (RDS), congenital heart disease, and ingestion of long-chain fatty acids prolong gastric emptying time. The rate of gastric emptying is increased with consumption of human milk and hypocaloric feedings, but is unaffected by osmolality and posture. A prolonged gastric emptying time can delay drug absorption, resulting in a longer time to reach maximal serum drug concentrations and a decrease in the peak concentration.

Small intestine motility is irregular in both neonates and young infants,[13] making it difficult to predict the time for peak absorption or the extent of absorption of enterally administered drugs. In addition, the immature or altered permeability of the intestinal mucosa, which can result in increased drug absorption, actually may be more important than both gastric emptying time and intestinal motility.[14] Osmolality also can influence gastrointestinal (GI) tract integrity and absorption, particularly in preterm infants.[13] Enteral administration of drugs or solutions with high osmolalities can destroy GI tract integrity and increase the risk of necrotizing enterocolitis (NEC) in neonates.

Drug absorption in the neonate also can be affected by other factors. For example, the reduced rate of bile acid synthesis and pancreatic secretions in preterm neonates may decrease the absorption of fat-soluble vitamins D and E.[12,13,15] Absorption of these vitamins may be reduced further by cholestasis, and water-soluble forms of these vitamins may be necessary. Short-bowel syndrome (which may occur as a result of NEC) may decrease the intestinal surface area available for drug absorption and result in decreased drug bioavailability. Changes in bacterial colonization of the GI tract during the neonatal period can influence the fate of conjugated forms of drugs excreted in bile. The high activity of β-glucuronidase in the neonatal intestinal lumen results in hydrolysis of drug glucuronide conjugates and potentially alters the disposition of the parent drug or its metabolite.[11,13]

During the neonatal period, drugs such as phenobarbital, digoxin, and sulfonamides are absorbed at a slower, rate but the total amount absorbed is similar to that of older children.[14] In contrast, the total absorption of drugs such as phenytoin, acetaminophen, carbamazepine, and rifampin is decreased in neonates.[11,13,15]

Rectal Absorption

The routine use of the rectum for administration of drugs (e.g., aminophylline) has been discouraged because of erratic drug absorption and toxicities.[13] With the proper drug and dosage formulation, however, the rectum can be an important alternative route for drug administration, with rapid and efficient absorption.[11,13] For example, rectal administration of diazepam solution for injection produces serum concentrations similar to those from intravenous (IV) administration.[16] This route is therapeutically important in the neonate with seizure activity in whom rapid IV access is not available.

Intramuscular Absorption

Many physiological factors, as well as physicochemical characteristics of drugs, influence intramuscular (IM) absorption.[11–13] During the first few days of life, both the rate and the amount of IM absorption may be reduced owing to the relatively decreased muscle blood flow, higher percentage of water in muscle mass, and diminished strength of muscular contractions.[11] The amount of both muscle and subcutaneous tissue in the newborn is directly proportional to gestational age. The low muscle mass to total body mass ratio in neonates can result in decreased absorption of a drug administered IM because absorption is influenced by the surface area of the muscle that comes into contact with the injected medication. In addition, the degree of muscle activity, which directly affects the rate of drug absorption from both IM and subcutaneous injections, can be greatly decreased in the severely ill, immobile, or paralyzed neonate.[11–13] Adequate perfusion of the injection site also is required for systemic absorption to occur. Blood supply to muscles can be compromised in the critically ill neonate with low cardiac output or hypotensive states such as patent ductus arteriosus (PDA), sepsis, or RDS.[12,17] Drugs that more commonly may be administered IM to neonates include vitamin K, aminoglycosides, phenobarbital, and penicillins.[8,12]

Percutaneous Absorption

Percutaneous absorption is increased in neonates (especially in preterm newborns) because of decreased thickness of the stratum corneum, increased skin hydration, and increased ratio of surface area per kilogram body weight.[11–13] Because the epidermis is barely present before 34 weeks' gestational age, preterm newborns (especially those <2 weeks' postnatal age) are at greatest risk for percutaneous drug absorption. After 2 to

Table 94-2 Pharmacokinetics of Selected Drugs in Neonates and Adults[8,12,21,22]

Drug	Plasma $t_{1/2}$ (hr) Neonates	Plasma $t_{1/2}$ (hr) Adults	Vd (L/kg) Neonates	Vd (L/kg) Adults	% Protein Bound Neonates	% Protein Bound Adults
Caffeine	40–230	3–7	1.0	0.5–0.6	N/A	30–40
Diazepam	25–100	20–30	1.8–2.1	1.6–3.2	84–86	94–98
Digoxin	20–80	25–50	4–10	7	14–26	23–40
Gentamicin	3–12	1.5–3	0.4–0.7	0.2–0.3	<10	< 10
Indomethacin	15–30	4–10	0.35–0.53	0.15–0.26	95–98	90–95
Morphine	5–14	2–4	1.7–4.5	2.4–4.2	18–22	33–37
Phenobarbital	40–400	50–180	1.0	0.6–0.7	28–43	45–50
Phenytoin	15–105	15–30	1.0	0.6–0.7	70–90	89–93
Theophylline	20–60	6–12	1.0	0.45	36–50	50–65
Vancomycin	6–12	5–8	0.48–0.97	0.3–0.7	N/A	30–55

N/A, not available; $t_{1/2}$, half-life; Vd, volume of distribution.

3 weeks' postnatal age, the epidermis of the preterm newborn histologically matures to that seen at term.[18] Although the epidermis of a term neonate is functionally intact, the epidermis continues to develop through 4 months of age. The newborn's ratio of skin surface area to body weight is approximately three times that of an adult. Therefore, for the same percutaneous dose, a neonate absorbs three times more drug per kilogram than an adult. In addition, occlusive dressings or an interruption in the integrity of the skin (e.g., abrasion) increases the amount of drug absorbed percutaneously. Various toxicities have been described in neonates after topical administration of iodine, hexachlorophene, boric acid, salicylic acid, alcohol, epinephrine, corticosteroids, and triple antibiotic (Bacitracin, neomycin, polymyxin B) spray.[18]

The increased percutaneous absorption of drugs in preterm newborns has potential therapeutic implications.[18] For example, transdermal theophylline, administered as a gel with an occlusive dressing, produces therapeutic serum concentrations in preterm newborns who are 30 weeks or less gestational age and 20 days or less postnatal age. Clinical application of transdermal drug delivery in preterm newborns seems promising and may avoid problems associated with other routes of administration. However, transdermal drug delivery is limited by the normal maturation of the epidermis, and drug absorption decreases with increasing postnatal age and in newborns older than 32 weeks' gestational age.[18]

Drug Distribution

Drug distribution—the process of drug partition among various body organs, fluids, and tissues—depends on pH, composition and size of body compartments (e.g., total body water, intracellular and extracellular water, and adipose tissue mass), protein binding, membrane permeability, and hemodynamic factors such as cardiac output and regional blood flow.[19]

Water Compartments

Total body water, as a percentage of body weight, is increased in the newborn (especially the preterm neonate) and decreases with increasing age. The total body water of a preterm, 1-kg newborn is 80% and that of a term newborn is 75%. These values are much higher than those of a 3-month old (60%) or an adult (55%).[20] Newborns also have an increase in extracellular water as a percentage of body weight, and an increase in the extracellular water to intracellular water ratio. Extracellular water decreases from approximately 40% at term to approximately 20% at 3 months of age.[20] The higher total body water and extracellular water in newborns typically result in larger volumes of distribution (Vd) for water-soluble drugs (Table 94-2).[8,12,21,22] In addition, the Vd for water-soluble drugs that distribute to the extracellular water compartment (e.g., gentamicin) roughly parallels extracellular water as a percentage of body weight. Because the Vd in newborns usually is larger for water-soluble drugs, larger mg/kg loading doses of these agents are needed in neonates, particularly preterm newborns, to achieve initial drug concentrations similar to that of an adult. As the neonate grows and matures, total body water and extracellular water decrease, causing the Vd for water-soluble drugs and therefore mg/kg loading doses to decrease with increasing age.

Adipose Tissue

Compared with the adult, the neonate has much less adipose tissue. A preterm newborn is composed of only 1% to 2% fat, whereas a term neonate is approximately 15% fat.[20] Neonatal adipose tissue also contains more water. The decreased amount of adipose tissue and the higher water content in the newborn may decrease the Vd for fat-soluble drugs (e.g., diazepam). Because of the smaller Vd for fat-soluble or lipophilic drugs, smaller mg/kg loading doses should be administered in neonates.

Protein Binding

In general, neonatal protein binding of drugs is decreased compared with adults (Table 94-2). The decrease in plasma protein binding is a result of several factors, including a lower concentration of binding proteins (e.g., albumin, lipoproteins, α_1-acid glycoprotein, and β-globulins); the presence of fetal albumin, which has decreased affinity for drugs; a lower plasma pH, which can decrease protein binding of acidic drugs; and the presence of endogenous substances (e.g., bilirubin and free fatty acids) or transplacentally acquired interfering substances (e.g., hormones and pharmacologic agents) that can compete for protein-binding sites.[11,23] Decreased protein binding (increased free fraction) has been described in neonates for many drugs (e.g., ampicillin, carbamazepine, diazepam, lidocaine, penicillin, phenobarbital, phenytoin, propranolol, salicylic acid, sulfonamides, theophylline).[11,12,23] Total plasma protein concentration, as well as the affinity of albumin for acidic drugs, increases with age and approaches adult values at 10 to 12 months of age.[12] Therefore, as the newborn grows and matures, protein binding also increases.

A decrease in protein binding may result in an increased Vd, increased free (unbound) fraction, or increased free concentration of a drug. Drugs that have an increased Vd may require larger mg/kg loading doses in neonates to attain the same total serum concentration as that of an adult. However, for a given total serum concentration, the increased free fraction results in a higher free concentration. The increased free concentration may result in increased therapeutic or toxic effects. For example, protein binding of theophylline in term newborns (36%) is decreased compared with adults (56%).[24] The commonly accepted total theophylline serum concentration of 10 to 20 mcg/mL in adults produces free theophylline serum concentrations of 4.4 to 8.8 mcg/mL in adults but 6.4 to 12.8 mcg/mL in newborns (i.e., approximately 1.5 times the adult free concentrations). Pharmacologic and toxic effects of drugs are related to the free concentration (i.e., the amount of drug that can pass through membranes and reach the receptor). Therefore, the total theophylline serum concentration range used in adults (10–20 mcg/mL) could result in toxicities if applied to the neonatal population. In neonates, a total theophylline serum concentration of approximately 7 to 14 mcg/mL would produce free concentrations comparable with those seen with total concentrations of 10 to 20 mcg/mL in adults.[24] Likewise, the decreased protein binding of phenytoin in neonates and resultant increased free fraction suggests that total phenytoin therapeutic serum concentrations in newborns should be 8 to 15 mcg/mL rather than the 10 to 20 mcg/mL as accepted in adults.

Decreased protein binding also may be a result of endogenous or exogenous substances displacing highly protein-bound drugs from protein-binding sites. Higher concentrations of free fatty acids in neonates may be responsible for the decreased protein binding of diazepam, propranolol, salicylates, and valproic acid.[23] In addition, bilirubin can displace acidic drugs (e.g., phenytoin) from albumin-binding sites. A positive correlation between total bilirubin concentrations and free fraction of phenytoin has been described. Unbound phenytoin was reported as 11% in normal newborns, but approximately 20% in neonates when bilirubin concentrations were 20 mg/dL.[25]

Some drugs (e.g., sulfonamides) or free fatty acids can displace bilirubin from albumin-binding sites, facilitating the deposition of unconjugated bilirubin in the brain. This condition, known as *kernicterus* or *bilirubin encephalopathy*, may produce neurologic injury and cell death and is frequently fatal. Survivors experience central hearing loss, ataxia, and choreoathetosis.[26] The displacement of bilirubin from albumin-binding sites depends on several factors, including pH, the affinity of albumin for the drug and bilirubin, and the individual molar concentrations of the drug, bilirubin, and albumin. Preterm newborns may be at an increased risk for bilirubin displacement because of lower albumin concentrations, decreased albumin affinity for bilirubin, lower pH, and higher bilirubin concentrations (secondary to overproduction or decreased hepatic glucuronide conjugation). To displace bilirubin, a specific molar concentration of a drug is necessary to occupy a critical portion of the reserve albumin. Generally, if the molar concentration of a drug is much lower than the molar concentration of albumin, displacement of bilirubin from albumin-binding sites is unlikely.[12,27] For example, highly protein-bound drugs such as furosemide, indomethacin, and cardiac glycosides can be administered to neonates without fear of displacing bilirubin from albumin (even though some of them are potent displacers of bilirubin) because they achieve low plasma concentrations.[12] In contrast, ceftriaxone can significantly displace bilirubin off albumin-binding sites and therefore should be avoided in the presence of hyperbilirubinemia.[28,29] Sulfonamides are associated with the development of kernicterus, and therefore generally are avoided in infants younger than 2 months of age. However, not all sulfonamides have the same ability to displace bilirubin. Therapeutic concentrations of trimethoprim-sulfamethoxazole do not alter albumin's capacity to bind bilirubin, and this drug occasionally is used in neonates if no reasonable alternative antibiotic exists.[30]

Other Factors

Decreased skeletal muscle mass and alterations in tissue affinity, membrane permeability, and hemodynamics also can influence drug distribution in neonates. The increased permeability of the central nervous system (CNS) to certain lipophilic drugs, such as phenytoin, may be due to the composition of the immature brain (lower myelin content) and the higher cerebral blood flow as compared with adults.[11] The increased permeability of drugs into neonatal tissues, such as the CNS or red blood cells (e.g., digoxin, theophylline), also may contribute to the increased Vd observed in newborns.[19]

Metabolism

Most drugs are lipophilic and require biotransformation into more water-soluble substances before they can become inactivated and eliminated from the body. Biotransformation (metabolism) of drugs is catalyzed by specific enzymes. Drug-metabolizing enzyme activity is ultimately determined by an individual's underlying genetic makeup (pharmacogenetics); however, it is also greatly influenced by developmental and environmental factors. Thus, the clinically observed rate of enzyme activity and metabolism of a specific drug depends on a patient's genetic constitution, age, development, race, and gender; environmental and nutritional influences; and concomitant drug exposure and disease states.[31] Although biotransformation may take place at various sites (e.g., plasma, skin, GI tract, lungs, and kidney), it typically occurs in the liver with subsequent elimination of metabolites via the kidneys, lungs, or biliary tract. Hepatic biotransformation may include phase I (oxidation, reduction, hydrolysis, and demethylation) and phase II reactions (conjugation with sulfate, glucuronide, glycine, glutathione, and hippurate; acetylation; and methylation).[32] In general, hepatic metabolism is reduced in the neonate because of decreases in hepatic blood flow, cellular uptake of drugs, hepatic enzyme capacity, and biliary excretion. Hepatocellular uptake and intrahepatic transport of drugs may be decreased at birth because of reduced concentrations of the hepatocyte acceptor proteins Y and Z. This may result in decreased hepatic clearance for capacity-limited drugs (i.e., drugs with low extraction ratios and low intrinsic clearance).[11,12] Concentrations of acceptor proteins significantly increase during the first 10 days of life.[12,32]

Phase I Biotransformation Reactions

Phase I biotransformation reactions are significantly reduced in the newborn, but increase with both gestational and postnatal age.[11] Maturation of enzyme activity (phases I and II) occurs at different ages for different metabolic pathways, may be regulated by endogenous hormones (e.g., growth hormone or corticosteroids), and may be substrate specific. The development of isoenzymes, presence of endogenous competitive substrates, and in utero or postnatal induction of hepatic enzymes may alter the maturation of drug metabolism.

The major group of enzymes responsible for phase I biotransformation reactions are the cytochromes P450.[33] Cytochrome P450 enzymes catalyze the biotransformation of many lipophilic drugs and endogenous substances. These enzymes are actually a "superfamily" of heme-containing proteins that exist as many different isoforms (i.e., isoenzymes). Cytochrome P450 isoenzyme nomenclature uses the root symbol CYP, followed in order by (a) an Arabic number to denote the gene family, (b) an upper case letter to designate a subfamily of highly related genes, and (c) another Arabic number to identify the individual isoenzyme within the subfamily. Seventeen human CYP gene families have been described. The most important gene families involved in human drug metabolism include CYP1, CYP2, and CYP3.[34] Table 94-3 lists important drug-metabolizing enzymes, their known developmental pattern, and important neonatal substrates.[33] Isoenzymes can catalyze more than one type of biotransformation reaction, and the metabolism of certain drugs may be catalyzed by more than one isoenzyme. For example, CYP1A2 catalyzes the 3-demethylation and 8-hydroxylation of theophylline. However, theophylline 8-hydroxylation may also be catalyzed by CYP2E1 and CYP3A4. In preterm and newborn infants with low CYP1A2 activity, the contribution to 8-hydroxylation by CYP2E1 and CYP3A4 may become important. However, in general, decreased isoenzyme activity results in decreased drug clearance. Clinical examples of decreased drug metabolism in neonates according to specific phase I biotransformation reactions are described in the following sections.

Oxidation

In term newborns, activity of cytochrome P450 enzymes and NADPH-cytochrome-C-reductase is approximately 50% of the adult value.[35] This decreased oxidative capacity results in a reduced clearance of some drugs (e.g., diazepam, phenobarbital, phenytoin, valproic acid, theophylline, indomethacin, and metronidazole), particularly in the first few weeks of life.[11,32] Compared with other enzyme systems, maturation of oxidative reactions occurs rapidly after birth. For example, in term newborns hydroxylation of phenytoin and phenobarbital matures as early as 2 to 4 weeks' postnatal age.[32] In preterm infants, however, the rapid postnatal maturation of hydroxylation is delayed. Hydroxylation of theophylline is related primarily to postconceptional age (PCA) and approaches adult values by 40 weeks' PCA.[36] In general, oxidative biotransformation pathways have one-third to one-half the adult activity at birth but increase to two to five times that of an adult by 1 year postnatal age.

Hydrolysis

Hepatic and plasma esterase activity is reduced in neonates, especially preterm newborns, and reaches adult values within 10 to 12 months.[11] The decreased esterase activity results in reduced elimination of ester anesthetics such as procaine, tetracaine, and cocaine. This may explain the increased effects and cardiorespiratory depression seen in newborns exposed to local anesthetics.

Demethylation

The dealkylation pathway for some drugs (e.g., diazepam and lidocaine) may be less impaired than the hydroxylation pathway at birth.[11] In contrast, the *N*-demethylation pathways of theophylline are greatly reduced in comparison with

Table 94-3 Important Neonatal Phase I Drug-Metabolizing Enzymes, Substrates, and Known Developmental Patterns

Enzyme	*Neonatal Substrates*	*Known Developmental Pattern*
CYP1A2	Acetaminophen, caffeine, theophylline, warfarin	Not present to an appreciable extent in human fetal liver. Adult levels reached by 4 months of age and may be exceeded in children 1–2 years of age. Activity slowly declines to adult levels, which are attained at the conclusion of puberty. Gender differences in activity are possible during puberty.
CYP2C9 CYP2C19	Phenytoin, S-warfarin; Diazepam, phenytoin, propranolol	Not apparent in fetal liver. Inferential data using phenytoin disposition as a nonspecific pharmacologic probe suggest low activity in first week of life, with adult activity reached by 6 months of age. Peak activity (as reflected by average values for V_{max}, which are 1.5- to 1.8-fold adult values) may be reached at 3–4 years of age and declines to adult values at the conclusion of puberty.
CYP2D6	Captopril, codeine, propranolol	Low to absent in fetal liver but uniformly present at 1 week of postnatal age. Poor activity (approximately 20% of that in adults) at 1 month of postnatal age. Adult competence attained by approximately 3–5 years of age.
CYP3A4	Acetaminophen, alfentanil, carbamazepine, cisapride, diazepam, erythromycin, lidocaine, midazolam, theophylline, verapamil, R-warfarin	Low activity in the first month of life, with approach toward adult levels by 6–12 months of postnatal age. Pharmacokinetic data for CYP3A4 substrates suggest that adult activity may be exceeded between 1 and 4 years of age. Activity then progressively declines, reaching adult levels at the conclusion of puberty.
CYP3A7	Dehydroepiandrosterone sulfate, ethinylestradiol, triazolam	Functional activity in fetus is approximately 30%–75% of adult levels of CYP3A7.

Modified with permission from reference 33.

Table 94-4 Important Neonatal Phase II Drug-Metabolizing Enzymes, Substrates, and Known Developmental Patterns

Enzyme	*Neonatal Substrates*	*Known Developmental Pattern*
N-acetyltransferase-2 (NAT2)	Caffeine, clonazepam, hydralazine, procainamide, sulfamethoxazole	Some fetal activity present by 16 weeks. Virtually 100% of infants between birth and 2 months of age exhibit the slow metabolizer phenotype. Adult phenotype distribution reached by 4–6 months of postnatal age, with adult activity present by approximately 1–3 years of age.
Thiopurine methyltransferase	Azathioprine, mercaptopurine, thioguanine	Levels in fetal liver are approximately 30% of those in adult liver. In newborn infants, activity is approximately 50% higher than in adults, with a phenotype distribution that parallels that in adults. In Korean children, adult activity appears at approximately 7–9 years of age.
Glucuronosyltransferase (UGT)	Acetaminophen, chloramphenicol, morphine, valproic acid	Ontogeny is isoform specific as reflected by pharmacokinetic data for certain pharmacologic substrates (e.g., acetaminophen or chloramphenicol). In general, adult activity as reflected from pharmacokinetic data seems to be achieved by 6–18 months of age.
Sulfotransferase	Acetaminophen, bile acids, chloramphenicol, cholesterol, dopamine, polyethylene glycols	Ontogeny (based on pharmacokinetic studies) seems to be more rapid than that for UGT; however, it is substrate specific. Activity for some isoforms (e.g., that are responsible for acetaminophen metabolism) may exceed adult levels during infancy and early childhood.

Modified with permission from reference 33.

hydroxylation.[36] Maturation of theophylline *N*-demethylation occurs at 55 weeks' PCA and lags behind the maturation of the oxidation pathways seen at 40 weeks' PCA. Despite the earlier maturation of theophylline hydroxylation, theophylline clearance is not increased significantly until the *N*-demethylation pathway matures.[36] Clearances of other drugs such as diazepam, morphine, and meperidine also are affected by low *N*-demethylation activity.

Phase II Reactions

Most phase II reactions are decreased in the newborn (Table 94-4).[33] Sulfation, however, is more developed than other conjugation reactions because sulfotransferase activity may approximate adult values at birth (e.g., estrogen sulfotransferase).[32] Methylation also is functional at birth, as demonstrated by the ability of both term and preterm newborns to methylate theophylline to caffeine. Methyltransferase activity is known to be present even in the fetus because methylation is required for synthesis of pulmonary surfactant. In contrast, acetylation of sulfonamides via *N*-acetyl-transferase 2 is decreased in neonates, especially preterm newborns.[32] Other drugs such as hydralazine that are eliminated via acetylation have decreased hepatic clearance in the neonate. In fact, almost all infants younger than 2 months of age are phenotypically slow acetylators. This is in contrast to 50% of 4- to 7.5-month-old infants and 62% of 7.5- to 11-month-old infants being phenotypically fast acetylators.[33]

Glucuronide Conjugation

Uridine diphosphate–glucuronosyltransferase (UGT) activity is significantly reduced at birth and generally reaches adult levels by 6 to 18 months of age.[33] However, at least ten different UGT isoforms exist, and adult levels of UGT metabolism may be reached at different ages for different substrates (drugs).[37] As a result of the decreased UGT activity, metabolism is significantly decreased in the neonate for compounds that undergo glucuronidation (e.g., chloramphenicol, morphine, lorazepam, corticosteroids, bilirubin, and trichloroethanol [the active metabolite of chloral hydrate]). Toxic effects of these agents may be seen unless doses are decreased appropriately. Reduced glucuronidation with resultant accumulation of chloramphenicol was responsible for the toxic symptoms of the "gray baby syndrome" (cardiovascular collapse and shock).

The effects of decreased glucuronidation may not be as dramatic for drugs that have alternate metabolic pathways because a shift to a more mature pathway may occur. For example, in neonates, the decreased glucuronidation of acetaminophen is partially offset by an increase in acetaminophen-sulfate conjugation. This change to sulfation only partially compensates for decreased glucuronidation because acetaminophen half-life is still prolonged in the newborn.[12]

Glycine Conjugation

Glycine conjugation is decreased in newborns, but increases to adult levels by approximately 8 weeks of age. In adults, benzyl alcohol (a preservative) is converted to benzoic acid (benzoate), which then is detoxified in the liver through conjugation with glycine to form hippuric acid. Because neonates have a decreased capacity to conjugate *p*-amino benzoate and benzoate with glycine, benzoic acid can accumulate in newborns given excess benzyl alcohol or benzoic acid.[38] Accumulation of benzoic acid results in the "gasping syndrome," which consists of multiple organ system failure, severe metabolic acidosis, and gasping respirations. This potentially fatal syndrome is associated with cumulative benzyl alcohol doses of 99 mg/kg or higher in preterm neonates.[39] As recommended by the FDA, drugs containing the preservatives benzyl alcohol or benzoic acid should not be used in neonates.[40] The use of preservative-free IV solutions, diluents, and medications is advised.

Induction of Enzymes

Maturation of hepatic enzymes can be influenced by in utero or postnatal exposure to enzyme-inducing agents.[32] Neonatal enzymes may have a faster and greater response to inducing agents compared with adults. Hydroxylation and glucuronidation pathways are especially affected.[11] For example, the plasma half-life of diazepam is 40 to 100 hours in preterm neonates and 20 to 45 hours in term neonates, but only 11 to

18 hours in neonates briefly exposed to the enzyme-inducing drug, phenobarbital.[41,42] This shortened diazepam half-life is a result of an increase in the hydroxylation and conjugation pathways. Because phenobarbital can induce uridine diphosphate–UGT (and therefore glucuronide conjugation), it sometimes is used to treat neonatal unconjugated hyperbilirubinemia. Antenatal corticosteroid administration, which commonly is used to promote fetal lung maturation, also can induce postnatal metabolism of both theophylline and metronidazole.[11]

Other Effects

Decreased cardiac output, respiratory distress, decreased liver perfusion, or hypoxia may further decrease neonatal hepatic enzymatic activity.[11] Decreased phenobarbital clearance has been demonstrated in asphyxiated neonates.[43]

Renal Elimination

Glomerular filtration, tubular secretion, and tubular reabsorption are decreased in preterm and term newborns compared with adults. Because most drugs and metabolites are eliminated renally, clearance generally is decreased in neonates. As a result, maintenance doses of drugs that are eliminated renally must be decreased. Although overall renal function increases with age, the maturational rates of individual physiological functions vary. For example, glomerular filtration matures several months before tubular secretion, and factors increasing tubular reabsorption mature after tubular secretion. Because renal elimination depends on the balance of filtration, secretion, and reabsorption, predictions of renal clearance of drugs eliminated by more than one of these mechanisms may be difficult in the maturing neonate.

Glomerular Filtration

At birth, the glomerular filtration rate (GFR) is significantly decreased. The GFR for term newborns is 2 to 4 mL/minute, or approximately 10 to 20 mL/minute/1.73 m^2. For preterm newborns, GFR is only 0.7 to 0.8 mL/minute or approximately 0.5% of an adult.[44] In term newborns, GFR increases markedly after birth, doubling by 1 to 2 weeks' postnatal age. Despite the continued increase postnatally, GFR is only 50 mL/minute/1.73 m^2 at 2.5 weeks' postnatal age[45] and does not reach adult values until 3 to 5 months' postnatal age.

In preterm neonates, postnatal development of GFR is delayed and a lower GFR persists beyond the first few months of life, especially in very low-birth-weight (VLBW) newborns ≤30 weeks' gestational age. Even at a corrected postnatal age of 9 months (i.e., 18 months' PCA), GFR is significantly decreased in VLBW infants compared with term infants of the same PCA.[45] Although the exact age at which GFR matures in VLBW infants is not known, a normal GFR should not be assumed in older preterm infants even up to 1 to 2 years postnatal age.

Serum creatinine (SrCr) concentrations in all neonates are elevated at birth, reflecting maternal concentrations. In healthy newborns more than 30 weeks' gestational age, SrCr steadily decreases throughout the first week of life to approximately 0.4 mg/dL. SrCr concentrations in VLBW infants born at 30 weeks' or less gestational age are significantly higher than their term counterparts, even at a corrected postnatal age of 9 months.[45]

Table 94-5 Gentamicin Dosing Guidelines for Neonates and Infants[a8]

Age	Weight	Dosing Regimen
GA <38 wk	<1000 g	3.5 mg/kg/dose Q 24 hr
PNA 0–4 wk	<1200 g	2.5 mg/kg/dose Q 18–24 hr
PNA ≤7 days	≥1200 g	2.5 mg/kg/dose Q 12 hr
PNA >7 days	1200–2000 g	2.5 mg/kg/dose Q 8–12 hr
PNA >7 days	>2000 g	2.5 mg/kg/dose Q 8 hr

[a]Traditional dosing; see Question 33, Dosage and Route of Administration section for discussion of extended-interval aminoglycoside dosing
GA, gestational age; PNA, postnatal age

Clearance of drugs primarily eliminated by glomerular filtration (e.g., digoxin, vancomycin, and the aminoglycosides) is well correlated with GFR. Therefore, maturation of GFR must be considered when developing dosing guidelines for these medications. For example, both vancomycin clearance and gentamicin clearance correlate with postnatal age, weight, and creatinine clearance, as well as PCA.[46–50] Therefore, guidelines that incorporate these patient factors are more likely to result in therapeutic serum concentrations in the developing neonate.[8,51,52] An example of neonatal gentamicin dosing guidelines[8] that are used commonly is given in Table 94-5.

Other conditions such as asphyxia, decreased cardiac output, renal disease, or indomethacin therapy may further decrease GFR and drug clearance during the perinatal period.[53–55] The hypoxia, hypercarbia, hypotension, and decreased cardiac output that occur during asphyxia cause significant decreases in GFR. In addition, compensatory mechanisms such as an increased formation of renovascular constricting prostaglandins may aggravate this condition further.[44] Therefore, dosage regimens of renally eliminated drugs should be empirically decreased in severely asphyxiated neonates. Dosage reduction before the initiation of indomethacin therapy also is necessary because significant elevations of aminoglycoside and digoxin serum concentrations have resulted with concomitant indomethacin therapy.[54,55] For example, a 50% dosage reduction of digoxin is recommended in preterm infants receiving indomethacin.[55]

In contrast, an increase in dosage may be required for drugs (e.g., thiazide and loop diuretics) that depend on GFR for sufficient intraluminal concentrations and pharmacologic effect. A diminished diuretic response may be seen in preterm neonates, particularly during the first month of life. Because furosemide is less dependent on GFR, it is the preferred diuretic in neonates.

Tubular Secretion

Tubular secretion is approximately 20% to 30% of adult values at birth and matures more slowly than GFR. Despite a doubling over the first 7 days of life, tubular secretion does not reach adult values until 30 to 40 weeks' postnatal age. By 1 year of age, tubular secretion is 10 times higher than at birth.[11,12] Therefore, in neonates, a decreased clearance is seen for drugs that are eliminated by proximal tubular secretion (e.g., furosemide, penicillins, thiazides, atropine, and morphine). Tubular secretion, however, can be enhanced in the immature kidney after continued exposure to certain drugs. Substrate stimulation of tubular secretory pathways and subsequent increases in elimination (and therefore dosing requirements) have been reported for penicillin, ampicillin, and dicloxacillin.[12,56]

Tubular Reabsorption

Tubular reabsorption, a passive process that is concentration dependent, is decreased in the neonate owing to the decreased GFR and reduced filtrate load.[11] The low urinary pH seen in neonates results in an increase in reabsorption of weak acids (decreased clearance) and a decrease in reabsorption of weak bases. In addition, the normal diurnal variation in urine pH is not present until 2 years postnatal age.[11]

Clinical Relevance to Dosing

Decreased enzyme activity and renal function in neonates result in a decreased clearance and prolonged half-life for many drugs (Table 94-2). Because drug clearance determines the maintenance dose, mg/kg/day dosages must be reduced in neonates, particularly preterm neonates, to avoid toxicities. As biotransformation reactions and renal function mature, daily dosages subsequently must be increased with age to prevent subtherapeutic concentrations. Because of these dynamic changes, periodic clinical assessment and therapeutic drug monitoring are extremely important in neonates.

RESPIRATORY DISTRESS SYNDROME

RDS is a major cause of morbidity and mortality in preterm neonates, affecting approximately 50,000 infants in the United States each year.[57] This clinical syndrome is characterized by respiratory failure with atelectasis, hypoxemia, decreased lung compliance, small airway epithelial damage, and pulmonary edema. The principle cause of RDS is pulmonary surfactant deficiency. Pulmonary surfactant decreases the surface tension at the air/fluid interface in the alveoli and prevents alveolar collapse. Surfactant also facilitates the clearance of pulmonary fluid, prevents pulmonary edema, and stabilizes alveoli during aeration. At birth, the clearance of residual fetal lung fluid is accompanied by an increase in pulmonary blood flow, which facilitates the transition from fetal to adult circulation.[58,59]

In the fetus, endogenous cortisol stimulates the synthesis and secretion of pulmonary surfactant at 30 to 32 weeks' gestational age.[60] However, sufficient amounts of pulmonary surfactant for normal lung function are not present before 34 to 36 weeks' gestation.[61] Therefore, the incidence and severity of RDS increase as gestational age decreases. RDS occurs in <20% to 30% of neonates born at 30 to 31 weeks' gestational age, but in 50% of neonates born at 26 to 28 weeks' gestational age.[58]

Without adequate amounts of surfactant, the surface tension within the alveoli is so great that the alveoli collapse (atelectasis), resulting in poor gas exchange (e.g., hypoxemia, hypercapnia). Low lung compliance also results and large inspiratory pressures are needed to aerate the lungs. Unfortunately, the extremely compliant neonatal chest wall makes it difficult to create the large negative inspiratory pressures necessary to open the alveoli. This results in an increased work of breathing and alterations of ventilation and perfusion (V/Q mismatch).[58,59]

Aeration of the surfactant-deficient lung also results in the cyclic collapse and distention of bronchioles with resultant bronchiolar epithelial injury and necrosis. This epithelial damage causes pulmonary edema by allowing fluid and proteins to leak from the intravascular space into the air spaces and interstitium of the lung. The necrotic epithelial debris and proteins then form fibrous hyaline membranes.[59] Hyaline membranes and pulmonary edema further impair gas exchange. The term *hyaline membrane disease* has been used to describe the presence of these fibrous membranes. However, because hyaline membrane disease is not specific to surfactant deficiency, the term *respiratory distress syndrome* (RDS) is preferred.

The inadequate oxygenation and ventilation and increased work of breathing caused by RDS may result in the need for assisted positive-pressure ventilation. Complications of RDS may be related to mechanical ventilation and include pulmonary barotrauma (e.g., pneumothorax, pulmonary interstitial emphysema [PIE]), intraventricular hemorrhage (IVH), PDA, retinopathy of prematurity (ROP), and chronic lung disease or bronchopulmonary dysplasia (BPD).[59] (Also see Bronchopulmonary Dysplasia.)

Clinical Presentation

1. L.D., an 800-g male, was precipitously born at 27 weeks' gestational age to a 38-year-old gravida 6 para 5 female. Apgar scores were 5 at 1 minute, and 7 at 5 minutes. One hour after birth, L.D. seems cyanotic and has retracting respirations with grunting and nasal flaring. HR is 160 beats/minute and RR is 65 breaths/minute. An arterial blood gas (ABG) on 100% oxygen by nasal cannula is as follows: pH, 7.26; Pco_2, 50 mmHg; Po_2, 53 mmHg; and base deficit, 7. Arterial to alveolar oxygen tension ratio (a/A) is <0.2. L.D. is intubated immediately and placed on positive-pressure–assisted ventilation. A catheter is inserted in his umbilical artery for frequent ABG monitoring, and an umbilical vein catheter is inserted for central venous access. L.D.'s chest radiographic shows moderate hyaline membrane disease. Ampicillin 50 mg/kg Q 12 hours and gentamicin 3.5 mg/kg Q 24 hours are ordered IV to rule out sepsis. What risk factors does L.D. have for RDS? What signs and laboratory data are consistent with RDS?

[SI units: Pco_2, 6.67 kPa; Po_2, 7.1 kPa]

L.D.'s risk factors for RDS are prematurity and male gender. Other risk factors include gestational diabetes, cesarean section with no labor, second-born twins, perinatal asphyxia, and maternofetal hemorrhage.[58,59,62] Clinical signs and laboratory data consistent with RDS in L.D. include tachypnea (RR, 65 breaths/minute); cyanosis, retracting respirations, grunting, nasal flaring, hypoxemia (PO_2, 53 mmHg); hypercapnia (Pco_2, 50 mmHg); and a mixed respiratory and metabolic acidosis.[58,59,62] Clinical manifestations classically present within the first 6 hours of life.[62]

Tachypnea, the first sign of respiratory distress, is an attempt to compensate for the inadequate ventilation, hypercapnia, and acidosis. L.D.'s retracting respirations (the use of intercostal, subcostal, suprasternal, or sternal accessory muscles) reflect the increased work of breathing necessary to maintain ventilation. His nasal flaring decreases resistance during inspiration and increases oxygenation. Grunting is the result of forceful exhalation against a partially closed glottis in an effort to prolong expiration and maximize oxygenation. Grunting also increases intrathoracic pressure during expiration in an attempt to stabilize the alveoli and prevent atelectasis. L.D.'s cyanosis, hypoxemia, hypercapnia, and mixed respiratory and metabolic acidosis are consequences of inadequate oxygenation and poor ventilation and are consistent with RDS.[58,59]

Prevention

2. What maternal treatment might have prevented RDS in L.D.?

RDS may be prevented if pregnancy can be prolonged long enough for fetal lungs to mature, or if production of pulmonary surfactant can be accelerated in utero. Premature labor can be suppressed pharmacologically with drugs that inhibit uterine contractions (tocolytic agents), such as the β-adrenergic agonists (e.g., ritodrine, terbutaline), prostaglandin inhibitors (e.g., indomethacin), calcium channel blockers (e.g., nifedipine), and magnesium sulfate.[63,64] (See Chapter 46.)

Maternal administration of glucocorticoids can accelerate fetal lung maturation and decrease the incidence and severity of RDS. L.D.'s mother should have been considered a candidate for antenatal corticosteroids, unless immediate delivery was anticipated. In a meta-analysis of 15 antenatal maternal corticosteroid trials with more than 3,400 participants, corticosteroids significantly reduced RDS, NEC, IVH, and neonatal death, regardless of the infant's gender and race. Furthermore, there was no evidence of an increased incidence of fetal, neonatal, or maternal infection, or fetal death associated with the use of antenatal steroids. The incidence of BPD, however, was not affected, and the decrease in RDS was not significant for newborns greater than 34 weeks' gestational age.[65]

A consensus panel formed by the National Institutes of Health (NIH) evaluated the use of antenatal corticosteroids for fetal lung maturation.[64] This panel recommended administration of antenatal steroids in all pregnant women at high risk for premature delivery. Many centers repeated the course of steroids every 7 days until 34 weeks' gestation because the effects of antenatal steroids had not been shown to last beyond 7 days. Although the potential benefits and risks of repeated courses were unknown at the time, multiple-course antenatal steroids became widespread, with usage ranging from 85% to 98%.[66] Subsequently, a decrease in birth-weight and head circumference, and an increase in neonatal sepsis and death have been associated with multiple-course antenatal steroids.[67,68] Investigation by a second NIH consensus panel resulted in a recommendation that a single course of antenatal corticosteroids be considered for all pregnant women between 24 and 34 weeks gestation who are at risk of preterm delivery within 7 days; repeat courses of antenatal steroids are not routinely recommended and should be reserved for patients enrolled in randomized controlled trials.[69]

Since the second NIH consensus panel in 2000, three large randomized controlled trials of single versus repeat courses of antenatal corticosteroids reported conflicting results.[70–72] The issue of repeat courses of antenatal steroids remains controversial. Not all trials found significant decreases in the incidence of RDS and chronic lung disease with repeat courses. A significant decrease in other neonatal morbidities (e.g., PDA, pneumothorax, surfactant use, and the need for oxygen therapy, continuous positive airway pressure, mechanical ventilation, and pressor or volume support) was found in at least one, but not all trials. However, birth-weight and head circumference were significantly decreased and severe IVH was significantly increased with repeat steroid courses in at least one trial. Sepsis and death were not increased with repeat courses.

Despite numerous clinical trials, the appropriate number and timing of repeat courses of antenatal corticosteroids and the risk to benefit ratio are still unknown. Repeat courses might benefit neonates of extreme prematurity because a significant decrease in composite neonatal morbidity was noted in one clinical trial for neonates born less than 28 weeks' gestational age.[70] A randomized clinical trial known as the "Multiple courses of antenatal corticosteroids for preterm birth (MACS)" is currently underway to investigate if a longer interval between repeat courses will maintain efficacy while decreasing composite neonatal morbidity.

Betamethasone injection 12 mg IM Q 24 hours for two doses or dexamethasone injection 6 mg IM Q 12 hours for four doses are the only two NIH-recommended regimens to accelerate lung maturation.[64,69] Fetal lung maturity can be assessed by measuring certain components (e.g., lecithin, sphingomyelin) of lung surfactant in amniotic fluid. A ratio of lecithin to sphingomyelin greater than 2 indicates functionally mature fetal lungs and a decreased risk for RDS.[59] Although both betamethasone and dexamethasone decrease the incidence of RDS, only betamethasone decreases neonatal mortality and the risk for periventricular leukomalacia (PVL).[73,74] Multiple courses of dexamethasone (compared with betamethasone) have been associated with an increased risk for PVL, IVH, ROP, and neurodevelopmental abnormalities.[75] Therefore, betamethasone seems to be the preferred agent.

Maternal administration of glucocorticoids increases the production of fibroblast-pneumocyte factor, which stimulates the biosynthesis of surfactant in type II pneumocytes. This mimics the physiological response of fetal lungs to the increased cortisol production that normally begins at 30 to 32 weeks' gestation.[60] Certain obstetric conditions can stress the fetus and stimulate adrenal activity and corticosteroid release in utero, thereby enhancing fetal lung maturity. For example, an unusually low incidence of RDS occurs in neonates born prematurely to mothers with hypertension, infection, cardiovascular disease, hemoglobinopathies, heroin addiction, premature rupture of membranes >48 hours, and decreased placental function.[59,61] Antenatal steroids also improve postnatal responsiveness to exogenous surfactant administration.[62,64,76] Administration of thyrotropin-releasing hormone (TRH) in combination with antenatal steroids was initially thought to enhance fetal lung maturation, decrease the incidence of RDS, and decrease the incidence of BPD. Unfortunately, in a meta-analysis, prenatal TRH increased neonatal ventilation usage, lowered 5-minute Apgar scores, and was associated with poorer 12-month outcomes.[64,77] Therefore, antenatal use of TRH cannot be recommended.

Treatment

Surfactant Therapy

3. What treatments should be initiated for L.D.?

Before L.D. is treated for RDS, other causes of respiratory distress must be ruled out. For example, infections, (particularly group B streptococcal sepsis or pneumonia), often present with respiratory distress. Because it is difficult to distinguish between RDS and infection, all infants with severe RDS should receive antibiotics. L.D. was started empirically on antibiotics, and a complete evaluation of possible sepsis should be performed.

Exogenous surfactant should be administered intratracheally to L.D. as soon as possible. Until the late 1980s, oxygen supplementation, mechanical ventilation, fluid restriction, and supportive care were the general treatment measures for RDS. Presently, RDS primarily is considered a consequence of surfactant deficiency; therefore, the administration of exogenous surfactant should decrease the severity of RDS and the risk of death.[78]

Human surfactant is synthesized and secreted by type II alveolar epithelial cells of the lung. It contains 80% phospholipids, 8% neutral lipids, and 12% proteins.[79] The major surface-active component is dipalmitoylphosphatidylcholine (DPPC), also known as *colfosceril* or *lecithin*. However, this phospholipid slowly adsorbs to the air/fluid interface in the alveoli. Other phospholipids (e.g., phosphatidylcholine, phosphatidylglycerol), and four surfactant apoproteins (SP-A, SP-B, SP-C, and SP-D) enhance spreadability and surface adsorption.[61,76,80] Adsorption and surface spreading of the surfactant in the alveoli are important determinants of surface-tension activity. SP-A and SP-D both play a role in immune regulation and providing host defense. SP-A may also help to regulate alveolar surfactant reuptake and metabolism.[61] SP-B and SP-C are the two most important apoproteins responsible for promoting adsorption and surface spreading of the surfactant in the alveoli to form a phospholipid monolayer.[79]

Natural surfactants are derived from bovine or porcine lung-lipid or lavage extracts, or from human amniotic fluid. Modified natural surfactants are lung-lipid extracts supplemented with phospholipids or other components.[76] Currently, three surfactant products are commercially available for clinical use in the United States: beractant (Survanta) is a modified natural surfactant, and both calfactant (Infasurf) and poractant alfa (Curosurf) are natural surfactants. Colfosceril palmitate (Exosurf), a synthetic surfactant without a protein analog, is no longer available for clinical use. Beractant and calfactant are FDA-approved for the prevention (i.e., prophylaxis) of RDS, and all three products are approved for the treatment (i.e., rescue therapy) of RDS.[81–83] Lucinactant (Surfaxin), a new synthetic surfactant that contains a protein analogue, is awaiting FDA approval for the treatment and prevention of RDS.[79]

Beractant is prepared by mincing bovine lung, which contains lung surfactant and phospholipids from lung cells. During the extraction process, cholesterol is removed and synthetic DPPC is added to improve surface activity. Surfactant apoprotein B (SP-B), which is thought to be the most critical protein for surfactant activity, is removed with cholesterol. As a result, beractant contains only trace amounts of SP-B (<0.5% of total protein). Ninety-nine percent of the protein in beractant is SP-C.[84,85]

In contrast, calfactant is extracted from washings of newborn calves' lungs; therefore it contains fewer contaminating lung cell components. Forty percent of the protein in calfactant is SP-B and 60% is SP-C. Poractant alfa is extracted from washings of pigs' lungs and is purified by liquid gel chromatography to remove neutralized lipids such as cholesterol. As with calfactant, no synthetic DPPC is added to poractant alfa.[86] It is composed of 99% lipids and 1% apoproteins (SP-B [30%] and SP-C [70%]). Neither beractant, calfactant, nor poractant alfa contain SP-A (refer to Table 94-6 for comparisons).[81–83]

PHARMACOLOGIC AND LONG-TERM EFFECTS

4. What are the effects of exogenously administered surfactant in RDS?

Oxygenation and lung compliance rapidly and markedly improve after the administration of surfactant. Supplemental oxygen and mechanical ventilation can be reduced significantly. The increased lung compliance and decreased need for high inspiratory pressures result in a dramatic decrease in the incidence of pneumothorax and PIE. Survival in treated infants increases by approximately 40% regardless of birth-weight or gestational age, and neonatal mortality from RDS is decreased to approximately 20%.[78] Other complications of RDS such as severe BPD, IVH, and PDA have not been decreased consistently with surfactant therapy. Although the severity of ROP was decreased with the use of exogenous surfactants, overall incidence is unchanged.[78]

NUMBER OF DOSES

5. At 2 hours of age, 4 mL/kg of beractant was administered to L.D. intratracheally. Within 1 hour, oxygenation improved and the FiO_2 was weaned from 100% to 80%. Six hours later, the ABGs revealed the following: pH, 7.36; PCO_2, 45 mmHg; PO_2, 80 mmHg; base deficit, 2; and O_2 saturation of 94% on the following ventilator settings: FiO_2, 0.73; intermittent mechanical ventilation (IMV), 40; peak inspiratory pressure (PIP), 18; and positive end-expiratory pressure (PEEP), +3. The a/A ratio is <0.2. Should another dose of beractant be administered?

[SI units: PCO_2, 6.0 kPa; PO_2, 10.7 kPa]

The response to a single dose of surfactant usually is transient; thus, more than one dose is needed. Response to surfactant therapy can be variable, especially in preterm newborns weighing less than 750 g.[76] Reasons for nonresponse include surfactant inhibition by proteins that have leaked into the alveolar spaces, inactivation of surfactant by inflammatory mediators (free oxygen radicals, proteases), presence of conditions that can decrease surfactant effectiveness (e.g., pulmonary edema), or poor delivery of surfactant to the alveoli (owing to atelectasis). The degree of responsiveness to surfactant also decreases with increasing postnatal age.[76,85]

Although the indications for subsequent doses of surfactant have varied in investigational studies, persistence of respiratory failure is the major clinical indicator for retreatment. A second dose of beractant should be given to L.D. because he still requires mechanical ventilation with relatively high inspiratory pressures and supplemental oxygen ($FiO_2 \geq 0.3$) to maintain an arterial $PO_2 \geq 50$ mmHg and oxygen saturation of 90%. Furthermore, an a/A ratio of <0.2 is an indication for repeat dosing.[78] In meta-analyses, the incidence of neonatal death and pneumothorax is reduced by multiple surfactant doses; however, other large trials have not reported additional benefits with more than two doses of calfactant.[87,88] In practice, despite these conflicting findings, most infants receive an average of two surfactant doses.

PROPHYLACTIC ADMINISTRATION AND TREATMENT OF RESPIRATORY DISTRESS SYNDROME

6. Could prophylactic administration of surfactant have prevented RDS in L.D.?

Prophylactic administration (i.e., at the time of delivery within 30 minutes after birth) of surfactant may reduce the

Table 94-6 Comparison of Currently Marketed Surfactant Products[81–83]

Variable	*Calfactant (Infasurf)*	*Poractant α (Curosurf)*	*Beractant (Survanta)*
Type and source	Natural surfactant, calf lung wash	Natural surfactant, porcine lung mince extract	Modified natural surfactant, bovine lung mince extract
Phospholipids	Natural DPPC with mixed phospholipids	Natural DPPC with mixed phospholipids	Natural and supplemented DPPC with mixed phospholipids
Proteins	Calf proteins SP-B and SP-C	Porcine proteins SP-B and SP-C	Bovine proteins SP-B and SP-C
Dispersing and adsorption agents	Proteins SP-B and SP-C	Proteins SP-B and SP-C	Proteins SP-B and SP-C
Recommended dose	3 mL/kg (phospholipids 105 mg/kg)	*Initial dose*: 2.5 mL/kg (phospholipids 200 mg/kg); *Repeat dose*: 1.25 mL/kg (phospholipids 100 mg/kg)	4 mL/kg (phospholipids 100 mg/kg)
Indications	Prophylaxis and rescue therapy	Rescue therapy	Prophylaxis and rescue therapy
Criteria for prophylaxis	Premature infants <29 weeks' gestational age at high risk for RDS	Not approved	Birth-weight <1,250 g or evidence of surfactant deficiency
Recommended regimen for prophylaxis	Give first dose ASAP after birth, preferably within 30 min; repeat Q 12 hr up to a total of 3 doses if infant remains intubated or repeat as early as 6 hr up to a total of 4 doses if infant remains intubated and requires $FiO_2 \geq 0.3$ with $PaO_2 \leq 80$ mmHg	Not approved	Give first dose ASAP after birth, preferably within 15 min; repeat as early as 6 hours up to a total of 4 doses if infant remains intubated and requires $FiO_2 \geq 0.3$ with $PaO_2 \leq 80$ mmHg
Criterion for rescue therapy	Infants ≤72 hr of age with confirmed RDS who require endotracheal intubation	Infants with confirmed RDS who require endotracheal intubation	Infants with confirmed RDS who require endotracheal intubation
Recommended regimen for rescue therapy	Give first dose ASAP after RDS diagnosed, repeat Q 12 hr up to a total of 3 doses if infant still remains intubated or repeat as early as 6 hours up to a total of 4doses if infant still remains intubated and requires $FiO_2 \geq 0.3$ with $PaO_2 \leq 80$ mmHg	Give first dose ASAP after RDS diagnosed, repeat Q 12 hr up to a total of 3 doses if infant remains intubated and requires mechanical ventilation with supplemental oxygen	Give first dose ASAP after RDS diagnosed, preferably by 8 hours postnatal age; repeat as early as 6 hours up to a total of 4 doses if infant remains intubated and requires $FiO_2 \geq 0.3$ with $PaO_2 \leq 80$ mmHg
Recommended administration technique	Administer through side-port of ETT adapter via ventilator, divide dose into 2 aliquots with position change *or* through disconnect ETT via 5-F catheter, divide dose into 4 aliquots with position change	Administer through disconnected ETT via 5-F catheter, divide dose into 2 aliquots with position change	Administer through disconnected ETT via 5-F catheter, divide dose into 4 aliquots with position change
Formulation	Suspension	Suspension	Suspension
Storage	Refrigerate 2–8°C; protect from light	Refrigerate 2–8°C; protect from light	Refrigerate 2–8°C; protect from light
Volume/vial	3 mL, 6 mL	1.5 mL, 3 mL	4 mL, 8 mL
Special instructions	Gentle swirling of the vial may be necessary for redispersion; warming to room temperature is not necessary; do not shake	Warm to room temperature before use, do not shake	Warm to room temperature before use; do not shake
Stability	If warmed to room temperature for <24 hr, unopened, unused vials may be returned once to refrigerator; single-use vial contains no preservative, discard unused portion	If warmed to room temperature for <24 hr, unopened, unused vials may be returned only once to refrigerator; single-use vial contains no preservative, discard unused portion	If warmed to room temperature for <24 hr, unopened, unused vials may be returned only once to refrigerator; single-use vial contains no preservative, discard unused portion
Cost per vial	\$413.64 (3 mL), \$732.12 (6 mL)[a]	\$340.70 (1.5 mL), \$667 (3 mL)[a]	\$459.60 (4 mL), \$813.46 (8 mL)[a]

[a] Average wholesale price 2007 Red Book.

ASAP, as soon as possible; DPPC, dipalmitoylphosphatidylcholine; ETT, endotracheal tube; F, French; FiO_2, fractional inspired oxygen; PaO_2, partial pressure of oxygen; RDS, respiratory distress syndrome.

incidence and severity of RDS, but does not always prevent the disease.[78] Theoretically, the first dose of surfactant should be given before the newborn's first breath or before positive-pressure ventilation.[78,85] This would avoid the early lung injury in RDS that can interfere with surfactant distribution, bioavailability, and effectiveness.[76] This strategy, however, increases the cost of care because newborns who might never develop RDS would be intubated and treated unnecessarily.[62,76,87] In addition, delivery room treatment may interfere with resuscitation and stabilization of the neonate.[85]

In a Cochrane meta-analysis, prophylactic administration of surfactant to infants at high risk for developing RDS was associated with significant decreases in the risk of pneumothorax, PIE, death and the combined variable of BPD or death, compared to rescue treatment.[89] Although these results are promising, the exact criteria to clinically determine "high-risk" newborns who should receive prophylactic surfactant therapy is still unclear. Additionally, a clinical study has not compared prophylactic use of surfactant to early therapy.

Exogenous surfactant also can be administered "early" (i.e., at 2 hours of age) to treat RDS, or immediately upon diagnosis of RDS as "rescue" therapy. In another Cochrane meta-analysis, mortality, pneumothorax, PIE, and BPD were significantly reduced among neonates receiving early therapy compared with rescue therapy.[90]

In summary, surfactant treatment should be administered as soon as clinical signs of RDS appear.[90] Early therapy avoids progression of the disease and the potential for decreased surfactant effectiveness. Prophylactic administration in the delivery room should be reserved for extremely premature neonates who are at the highest risk for RDS.[78,85]

COMPLICATIONS

7. What complications of surfactant treatment is L.D. at risk of developing?

The most common adverse effects of surfactant therapy are related to the method of administration.[85] Surfactant is administered directly into the lungs via the endotracheal tube (ETT) by using a catheter or a side-port adapter connected to the ETT. During administration, bradycardia and oxygen desaturation may develop secondary to vagal stimulation and airway obstruction.[81–83,85] These adverse events might require temporary discontinuation of surfactant administration and increased ventilator support. Mucous plugging with obstruction, BP changes, and altered electroencephalogram (EEG) tracings also can occur.[85] Airway obstruction can be decreased by delivering surfactant as a continuous intratracheal infusion over 10 to 20 minutes via an infusion pump.[91]

Surfactant therapy may increase the risk of pulmonary hemorrhage. Although the exact mechanism is unknown, surfactant may increase pulmonary blood flow through the ductus arteriosus, increase pulmonary microvascular pressures, and cause hemorrhagic pulmonary edema.[78] The benefits of surfactant therapy, however, far outweigh the increased risk of pulmonary hemorrhage.

Neonates who are given surfactant can be at greater risk for apnea that requires methylxanthine treatment. Surfactant-treated neonates can be weaned from ventilator support sooner and, therefore, might display apnea more easily.[78] Individual trials with natural surfactants have suggested an increased incidence of sepsis and NEC, but most studies have not validated these findings.[78] No difference in the incidence of NEC or apnea treated with methylxanthines was noted between calfactant and beractant.[84]

PRODUCT SELECTION

8. Are there any advantages of one surfactant product over the other?

Not enough data exist to label one commercially available product superior to the other. Although several studies have compared two products, no study has compared all three commercially available surfactant products. Currently, three comparative trials of commercially available natural and modified natural surfactants exist.[84,86,92] In the first randomized, double-blind trial of calfactant and beractant, calfactant-treated infants required significantly less supplemental oxygen and mean airway pressures (MAP) during the acute phase of respiratory distress.[84] However, the duration of mechanical ventilation and the use of supplemental oxygen for the rest of the hospital stay were not significantly different between the two groups. The number of infants requiring four doses of surfactant was significantly less in the calfactant-treated group. In addition, the calfactant group also had a longer dosing interval, indicating that calfactant may have a longer duration of effect. The incidence of death, BPD, and secondary outcomes, including pneumothorax, were not significantly different between the two groups.[84]

The second clinical trial of calfactant versus beractant compared the immediate changes in lung compliance after treatment in infants <37 weeks gestational age with RDS.[92] There was no difference in pulmonary compliance at 1 hour after surfactant administration between the two treated groups. However, calfactant-treated infants had a significant decrease in Fio_2 and MAP at 1 hr after treatment and required fewer doses compared to the beractant-treated infants (2 versus 4, respectively). No significant differences in the incidence of death, BPD, PIE, pneumothorax, PDA, sepsis, or pneumonia were found between the two groups.

In the third randomized trial of poractant alfa and beractant, poractant alfa-treated infants required significantly less supplemental oxygen and mechanical ventilation than infants treated with beractant during the acute phase of RDS.[86] These improvements were significant for up to 24 hours after treatment. Pneumothorax tended to be higher in the beractant-treated infants (5 of 40 versus 2 of 33); however, a significant difference was not detected because of the small sample size. The overall duration of mechanical ventilation and total time of oxygen therapy, mortality, the incidence of BPD, and other secondary outcomes were not significantly different between the two groups.

Based on these three comparative trials, the natural surfactants (calfactant and poractant alfa) seem to have a longer duration of effect and require less supplemental oxygen and MAP than the modified natural surfactant, Survanta, (Beractant). The incidence of BPD, death, and other secondary outcomes are not different between natural and modified natural surfactants. A new synthetic surfactant, lucinactant, contains both phospholipids and a high concentration of recombinant proteins designed to mimic human SP-B and has approvable status from the FDA for the prevention of RDS. A recent Phase III, multicenter, randomized, controlled trial compared the efficacy and safety of poractant alfa and lucinactant in the prevention of RDS in very premature infants at high risk for RDS.[93] There were no significant differences in the incidence of BPD, overall mortality, and the number of doses required per infant. Further comparative trials are needed to better determine if other clinical advantages of surfactant products exist.

Surfactant should be administered by qualified physicians with the presence of nursing and respiratory therapy personnel.[94] Neonates receiving beractant or poractant alfa need to be disconnected from the ventilator before surfactant administration.[81,83] As a result, clinicians transiently increase both Fio_2 and peak inspiratory pressures before disconnecting the ventilator. These higher settings and interruption from the ventilator may be avoided, however, if beractant is given through a neonatal suction valve. This method is equally effective, simpler, and possibly safer than methods with ventilator disconnection.[95] Calfactant, on the other hand, has the advantage of flexible administration techniques. It can be administered intratracheally via a catheter passed through the ETT with brief interruptions in ventilation (as with beractant and poractant alfa) or via a side-port adapter into the ETT without disconnecting the ventilator.[82]

Because beractant, calfactant, and poractant alfa are all derived from natural sources, they contain proteins that are potentially antigenic. Thus, theoretically, they may cause an immunologic response. However, there are no reports of beractant-, calfactant-, or poractant alfa-induced hypersensitivity reactions.[78] Surfactant products are expensive and are commercially available only in single-use vials; two vial sizes are available for each product (Table 94-6). The current availability of a second size vial may make these products more cost effective.[96]

Diuretics

9. What is the role of diuretics in the management of RDS?

The therapeutic role of diuretics in RDS is controversial. In the natural course of RDS, an abrupt diuresis (urine output >80% of fluid intake) occurs within the first 48 to 72 hours of life. This diuresis is followed by an improvement in pulmonary function, which is thought to be due to a decrease of alveolar or interstitial pulmonary fluid. Before surfactant was commercially available, neonates who did not have this diuresis (or had it after 72 hours) were more likely to develop BPD.

ROUTINE USE

Routine early administration of furosemide to pharmacologically mimic the natural course of RDS may facilitate diuresis and weaning from mechanical ventilation. Although diuretics do not decrease the incidence of BPD or mortality, infants receiving early (prophylactic) therapy of furosemide had a greater increase in urine output, decrease in ventilator MAPs, and improvement in oxygenation compared with infants not receiving furosemide.[62] However, infants receiving prophylactic furosemide had hemodynamic instability and a greater postnatal weight loss. Furthermore, long-term use of furosemide can result in hypercalciuria, renal calcifications, and other electrolyte imbalances (e.g., hyponatremia, hypochloremia, and hypokalemia).[62] Finally, treatment with furosemide may promote patency of the ductus arteriosus, which may further worsen pulmonary edema.[97] Therefore, routine administration of diuretics in RDS is not indicated.[62]

SELECTIVE USE

Because pulmonary edema is present in RDS, furosemide occasionally is administered to enhance lung fluid elimination and decrease pulmonary edema. If L.D. had signs of pulmonary edema with compromised pulmonary function (e.g., hypoxemia and hypercapnia), furosemide 1 mg/kg IV push could be given.

BRONCHOPULMONARY DYSPLASIA

Definition and Incidence

10. J.T. is an 80-day-old, 2-kg, female ex-preemie born at 25 weeks' gestation. Her medical history includes RDS, episodes of sepsis and pneumonia, and chronic parenteral hyperalimentation. J.T. has also failed extubation numerous times and is currently requiring mechanical ventilation with an Fio_2 of 0.5. Current vital signs are as follows: RR, 60 breaths/minute; HR, 150 beats/minute; BP, 80/55 mmHg; O_2 saturation, 90%. On physical examination, J.T. has intercostal and subcostal retractions, shallow breathing, and an expiratory wheeze. Bilateral diffuse haziness with lung hyperinflation, focal emphysema (with bleb formation), atelectasis, and irregular fibrous streaks are seen on chest radiograph. J.T. is currently receiving enteral feedings with a standard preterm 20-cal/oz formula at 40 mL Q 3 hr. Based on these findings, the diagnosis of BPD is made. What risk factors for BPD does J.T. have? What is the pathogenesis of BPD? What clinical signs and laboratory evidence of BPD are apparent in J.T?

BPD (also known as chronic lung disease) is the most common form of chronic pulmonary disease in infants. The disease develops in newborns who require supplemental oxygen and positive-pressure ventilation for RDS or other primary lung disorders. A severity-based definition of BPD has been developed by the National Institute of Child Health and Human Development.[98] For infants born <32 weeks' gestational age, assessment of BPD is performed at 36 weeks' PCA or at the time of discharge. Mild BPD is defined as a need for supplemental O_2 >21% for ≥28 days but not at 36 weeks' PCA or discharge; moderate BPD as a need for supplemental O_2 ≥28 days *plus* treatment with <30% O_2 at 36 weeks' PCA or discharge; and severe BPD as a need for supplemental O_2 ≥28 days *plus* treatment with ≥30% O_2 and/or positive pressure at 36 weeks' PCA or discharge. For infants born ≥32 weeks gestational age, the above definitions are different only in that assessments are conducted at 56 days of life rather than 36 weeks' PCA.[98] BPD is a significant cause of infant morbidity and mortality. Approximately 7,500 new cases of BPD occur in the United States each year.[99] The incidence of BPD is inversely related to gestational age and birth-weight. Infants with birth-weights ≤1,000 g have as high as a 77% risk of developing BPD compared with a 7% risk in infants with birth-weights >1,250 g.[100] J.T. has two of the most important risk factors for BPD, low birth-weight and decreased gestational age. She is also at risk for BPD owing to mechanical ventilation, oxygen toxicity, and fluid excess (160 mL/kg/day). Other risk factors include male gender, white ethnicity, and persistent PDA.[101]

Pathogenesis and Clinical Manifestations

The cause of BPD seems to be multifactorial. Lung immaturity, surfactant deficiency, oxygen toxicity, barotrauma/volutrauma, and inflammation all play important roles. Premature infants, especially those <26 weeks' gestation, are at a higher risk for BPD owing to lung immaturity.[102] Surfactant deficiency (which causes severe RDS) and the immature parenchymal structure of the lung and chest wall contribute to the development of BPD. Oxygen therapy, which causes a release of free oxygen radicals, is directly associated with the pathogenesis of BPD. Prolonged exposure to high oxygen concentrations and free oxygen radicals causes tissue damage, alveolar-capillary leaks, and atelectasis with resultant impaired gas exchange and pulmonary edema.[102] This may lead to the chronic pulmonary fibrotic changes seen in infants with BPD. In term infants, the lungs contain antioxidant enzymes that help to protect the lung from damage produced by free oxygen radicals. However, in preterm infants, the concentration of antioxidant enzymes may be low or absent. Therefore, premature infants are more susceptible to develop BPD than term infants.

Barotrauma secondary to positive-pressure ventilation is also a major factor in the pathogenesis of BPD, independent of oxygen toxicity.[102] Barotrauma is caused by repetitive distention of the terminal airways during mechanical ventilation. This results in disruption of the epithelium and an increase in capillary permeability to proteinaceous fluid. The severity of lung injury is related to the amount of positive peak pressure used. Volutrauma is also involved in the pathogenesis of BPD and is caused by high tidal volume ventilation and overdistention. Volutrauma may be due to unusually high peak inflation pressures compared with lung compliance. The combined iatrogenic insults of oxygen toxicity and barotrauma/volutrauma, both inflicted on an immature lung over a period of time, can worsen lung damage.

The inflammatory process in the lung is activated by oxygen toxicity, barotrauma/volutrauma, or other injury. This results in the attraction and activation of leukocytes (e.g., neutrophils, macrophages), which may cause further release of inflammatory mediators, elastase, and collagenase.[99] Elevated levels of elastase and collagenase can destroy the elastin and collagen framework of the lung. α_1-Proteinase inhibitor, a major defense against elastase activity, may be inactivated by free oxygen radicals. Therefore, the combined elevated levels of elastase and the decreased activity of α_1-proteinase inhibitor may enhance lung injury and lead to the development of BPD. Infants who are going to develop BPD also have elevated levels of cytokines such as platelet-activating factor, leukotrienes, tumor necrosis factor, and fibronectin.[102] These agents, combined with the activated leukocytes, cause significant lung damage with breakdown of capillary endothelial integrity and capillary leakage. Furthermore, the increased fibronectin levels found in tracheal aspirate samples of infants with early BPD may predispose them to develop pulmonary fibrosis.[102]

Infection and nutrient deficiency may also play a role in the pathogenesis of BPD. Pathogens such as *Ureaplasma, Chlamydia,* or cytomegalovirus (CMV) may cause chronic infection and contribute to the development of BPD. Studies have shown direct correlations between *Ureaplasma* colonization and the presence of BPD.[102] Deficiencies in nutrients such as vitamin A (retinol) or trace elements such as zinc, copper, and selenium (which are integral components of the antioxidant enzyme structure), may also play a role in the pathogenesis of BPD.

BPD is characterized by tachypnea with shallow breathing, intercostal and subcostal retractions, and expiratory wheezing as demonstrated in J.T. Other signs and symptoms include rales, rhonchi, cough, airflow obstruction, airway hyperreactivity, increased mucus production, hypoxemia, and hypercarbia.[99] J.T.'s chest radiograph shows evidence of BPD, including focal emphysema (with bleb formation), atelectasis, bilateral diffuse haziness (interstitial thickening) with increased expansion of the lungs (hyperinflation), and irregular fibrous streaks. Mucous plugging, sepsis, and pneumonia can also develop in BPD infants on chronic mechanical ventilation. Infants with severe BPD eventually develop cardiovascular complications such as pulmonary hypertension, cor pulmonale, systemic hypertension, and left ventricular hypertrophy. In addition to chronic respiratory and cardiovascular complications, infants with BPD have significant growth, nutritional, and neurodevelopmental problems.

Management

11. What nonpharmacologic and therapeutic agents should be used to manage BPD in J.T.?

The medical management of infants with BPD includes supplemental oxygen therapy, mechanical ventilation, fluid restriction, nutritional management, and various pharmacologic interventions. Supplemental oxygen administered via mechanical ventilation, continuous positive airway pressure, or nasal cannula should be provided to maintain an oxygen saturation of 88% to 92% and prevent hypoxemia.[103] Fluids should be restricted to 120 to 130 mL/kg/day to prevent congestive heart disease and pulmonary edema. Because infants with BPD have a 25% increase in caloric expenditure (owing to the increased work of breathing), hypercaloric formulas (e.g., 24 or 27 cal/oz) may be used to optimize calories while restricting fluid intake.[99] If this increased energy is not provided, infants are at risk for developing a catabolic state that places them at higher risk for developing BPD (inadequate nutrition may potentiate the toxic effects of oxygen toxicity and barotrauma). The goal of nutritional therapy is to produce weight gains of 10 to 30 g/day, which can usually be accomplished by providing 140 to 160 kcal/kg/day.[99,102] If infants do not tolerate enteral feedings, parenteral alimentation should be substituted until the GI tract becomes more functional. Because J.T. is on a 20-cal/oz formula, switching her to a hypercaloric formula (i.e., 24 or 27 cal/oz) would help to optimize her weight gain. Her fluids should be restricted to 240 to 260 mL/day (120–130 mL/kg/day).

Pharmacologic Therapy

The treatment of BPD consists of multiple-drug therapy, which includes diuretics, bronchodilators, and corticosteroids. Despite the advancement of drug therapy, none of these drugs has been shown to reverse pulmonary damage in infants with BPD. Instead, they are used primarily to reduce clinical symptoms and to improve lung function. Pharmacologic therapy and dosage regimens for the management of BPD are shown in Table 94-7.[8,99,101,103–105]

Diuretics

Infants with BPD are particularly prone to pulmonary edema from cardiogenic and noncardiogenic factors. Left ventricular failure may superimpose the already existing right ventricular failure. Pulmonary vascular permeability is increased because of the disruption of the alveolar-capillary unit and causes an increased amount of fluid in the interstitium. Although the precise mechanism in the treatment of BPD is unknown, diuretics help to reduce interstitial lung water. In addition, diuretics lower pulmonary vascular resistance and improve gas exchange, thereby, reducing oxygen requirements. Among the diuretics available, furosemide is the drug of choice because of its potent diuretic effect. It acts by blocking the reabsorption of chloride in the ascending loop of Henle. In addition, it increases lymphatic flow and plasma oncotic pressure and decreases pulmonary interstitial edema. In several studies, the use of furosemide in infants with BPD was associated with short-term improvement in lung compliance and oxygenation, decreased total pulmonary resistance, and facilitation in ventilator weaning.[99,106] However, a more recent meta-analysis did not support all of these findings. The chronic use of furosemide

Table 94-7 Pharmacologic Management of Bronchopulmonary Dysplasia[8,99,101,103–105]

Drug Therapy	*Dosage Regimen*
Diuretics	
Chlorothiazide	*Neonates and infants <6 months:* PO: 20–40 mg/kg/day in two divided doses; maximum dose: 375 mg/day *Infants >6 months:* PO: 20 mg/kg/day in two divided doses; maximum dose: 1 g/day
Furosemide	*PO*: 1–4 mg/kg/dose 1–2 times/day *IV*: 1–2 mg/kg/dose Q 12–24 hr *Nebulized*: 1 mg/kg/dose diluted to a final volume of 2 mL with NS (use IV form)
Hydrochlorothiazide/Spironolactone	*PO*: 1–2 mg/kg/dose Q 12 hr (dose based on hydrochlorothiazide)
Systemic Bronchodilators	
Caffeine citrate	*Loading dose:* 20 mg/kg (10 mg/kg as caffeine base) IV over 30 min *Maintenance dose:* 5 mg/kg/dose (2.5 mg/kg/dose as caffeine base) Q 24 hr; start 24 hr after loading dose; may administer IV (over 10 min) or PO
Theophylline	*Loading dose:* 5 mg/kg IV or PO *Maintenance dose:* 2–3 mg/kg/dose Q 8–12 hr IV or PO
Inhaled Bronchodilators	
Albuterol	0.03–0.06 mL/kg/dose of 0.5% solution (0.15–0.3 mg/kg/dose) diluted to 1–2 mL NS; give via nebulization Q 2–6 hr or PRN; minimum dose: 0.25 mL (1.25 mg); maximum dose: 1 mL (5 mg)
Cromolyn sodium	20 mg (2 mL) via nebulization Q 6–8 hr; may need up to 2–4 weeks for response to occur
Ipratropium bromide	*Neonates*: 0.125 mL/kg/dose of 0.02% solution (25 mcg/kg/dose) diluted to 2–2.5 mL NS; give via nebulization Q 8 hr *Infants*: 0.625–1.25 mL of 0.02% solution (125–250 mcg/dose) diluted to 2–2.5 mL NS; give via nebulization Q 8 hr
Metaproterenol	0.01–0.02 mL/kg/dose of 5% solution (0.5–1 mg/kg) diluted to 1.5–2 mL NS; give via nebulization Q 4–6 hr or PRN; minimum dose: 0.1 mL (5 mg); maximum dose: 0.3 mL (15 mg)

IV, intravenous; NS, normal saline; PO, oral; PRN, as needed.

in infants >3 weeks old with BPD was associated with significant improvements in oxygenation and lung compliance only.[107] The effects of furosemide on the duration of oxygen requirement and mechanical ventilation, length of hospital stay, mortality, and the incidence of BPD could not be assessed owing to limited data. In addition to questionable clinical outcome, furosemide can have significant adverse effects. Chronic furosemide use can result in increased urinary losses of chloride, potassium, and sodium, and may result in hypochloremia, hypokalemia, and hyponatremia. Furthermore, volume depletion, hypercalciuria, nephrocalcinosis, osteopenia, and ototoxicity may also occur.[99] Excessive fluid loss or hypochloremia may result in metabolic alkalosis and worsen respiratory acidosis. Some of these adverse effects may be reduced by using alternate-day furosemide therapy or nebulized furosemide.[106,108] Both of these regimens were not associated with electrolyte imbalances and were shown to significantly increase lung compliance and decrease pulmonary resistance.[106] In summary, because of the limited efficacy data and potential adverse effects, the use of furosemide for the management of BPD cannot be routinely recommended.

Thiazide diuretics (e.g., hydrochlorothiazide) in combination with a potassium-sparing diuretic (e.g., spironolactone) can improve lung function and decrease oxygen requirements with increased diuresis.[99,106] Although less potent than furosemide, the combination of these two diuretics can reduce the incidence of hypokalemia commonly associated with loop or thiazide diuretics. Adverse effects commonly seen with a combination of a thiazide and spironolactone include hyponatremia, hyperkalemia or hypokalemia, hypercalciuria, hyperuricemia, hyperglycemia, azotemia, and hypomagnesia.[99] Various diuretics and dosage regimens are listed in Table 94-7.

Generally, infants with BPD who are treated with diuretics are started on furosemide, but are changed to a combination diuretic (spironolactone/hydrochlorothiazide) if long-term treatment is needed to avoid adverse effects. Suggested indications for initiating furosemide therapy include (a) 1-week-old infants with early BPD and ventilator dependency, (b) infants with stable BPD who significantly worsen owing to fluid overload, (c) infants with chronic BPD who do not improve, and (d) infants requiring an increased fluid intake to provide adequate calories.[102]

Because J.T. has chronic BPD and is not improving (i.e., she has not been able to be weaned off the ventilator), furosemide 1 mg/kg Q 12 hours should be initiated. J.T. should be monitored for electrolyte disturbances while on furosemide. Electrolyte supplements such as potassium chloride or sodium chloride may be required to prevent hypokalemia, hyponatremia, and hypochloremia.

12. J.T. is started on furosemide 2 mg Q 12 hours. One week later, she still requires high ventilatory settings and is unable to be weaned from the ventilator. What other therapeutic agents may be considered to treat J.T.'s BPD?

Systemic Bronchodilators

Methylxanthines (theophylline, caffeine) have been used extensively in infants with BPD because of a direct bronchodilating effect. Methylxanthines can also improve diaphragmatic and skeletal muscle contractility and act as mild diuretics (see the Apnea of Prematurity section). Improvement in skeletal muscle contractility may improve functional residual capacity, which can help to facilitate ventilator weaning. Both theophylline and caffeine reduce pulmonary resistance and increase lung compliance.[99] Unfortunately, most studies in infants with BPD have only evaluated the short-term benefits of methylxanthines in improving lung function; long-term outcome studies are needed. The early use of caffeine to treat apnea of prematurity has recently been shown to decrease the incidence of BPD compared with placebo.[109]

If J.T. is started on theophylline, a loading dose of 5 mg/kg followed by a maintenance dose of 2 mg/kg every 8 hours is recommended (Table 94-7). J.T. should be monitored for adverse effects, including tachycardia, gastroesophageal reflux, vomiting, diarrhea, agitation, and seizures. Caffeine may be preferred because it has fewer side effects and a wider therapeutic index. However, caution should be taken to ensure that the dosing reflects the salt form of the caffeine prescribed (e.g., caffeine base or caffeine citrate).[105] Therapeutic serum concentrations for theophylline and caffeine are not well defined for BPD. However, most clinicians target the upper range cited for apnea of prematurity (see the Apnea of Prematurity section).

Inhaled Bronchodilators

Infants in the early stages of BPD generally have airway hyperactivity and smooth muscle hypertrophy. They are also at higher risk for bronchoconstriction owing to increased airway resistance secondary to hypoxia. Therefore, the use of bronchodilators may be helpful in these infants. β_2-Agonists such as albuterol or metaproterenol have been shown to provide short-term improvements (duration, 4 hours) in lung compliance and pulmonary resistance owing to bronchial smooth muscle relaxation.[99,110] However, inhaled bronchodilators are not effective in all infants with BPD. Infants in the late stages of BPD may have severe pulmonary damage and fibrotic changes. Only half of these infants demonstrate a decrease in pulmonary resistance after albuterol therapy.[111] Although β_2-agonists are more potent bronchodilators than theophylline or caffeine, their adverse effect profile, which includes cardiovascular side effects (e.g., tachycardia, hypertension), limit their use. In addition, tolerance may develop with prolonged administration.[99] Therefore, inhaled bronchodilators should be reserved for infants who clearly demonstrate improvements during therapy. Currently, there are no well-designed studies evaluating the chronic use of inhaled bronchodilators for the treatment of BPD. Further studies evaluating the efficacy and safety of long-term inhaled bronchodilator therapy are needed.

Inhaled anticholinergics such as ipratropium bromide have produced short-term benefits (duration, ~4 hours) in infants with BPD by improving pulmonary function.[112] These drugs work by preventing the action of acetylcholine at the muscarinic cholinergic receptor site, thereby interfering with vagally mediated bronchoconstriction. Anticholinergics relax bronchial smooth muscle and decrease mucus secretion. Inhaled anticholinergics are generally reserved for infants who fail or are intolerant to albuterol, or as an adjunct to albuterol if clinical improvement is not seen.[99] The combined therapy of albuterol and ipratropium may be more effective than either drug alone.[99,112] The adverse effect profile of ipratropium is minimal because the drug is poorly absorbed.

Cromolyn prevents the release of inflammatory mediators from mast cells. In randomized trials, cromolyn has not been shown to prevent BPD or to decrease mortality.[113] Because of the lack of evidence supporting the role of cromolyn for the prevention of BPD, its use is not recommended. Further studies evaluating different dosage regimens and mode of delivery of cromolyn are required.

A major problem with inhaled bronchodilators is their method of administration and drug delivery. Inhaled bronchodilators can be given by jet or ultrasonic nebulization or via a metered-dose inhaler.[106] For ventilator-dependent infants receiving metered-dose inhalers, the metered-dose inhaler is connected to an adapter that is attached to the ventilator circuit and ETT. Metered-dose inhalers can also be given through bag ventilation via the ETT. For nonventilated infants, the metered-dose inhaler can be given using a spacer/AeroChamber and a face mask.

Compared with metered-dose inhalers, nebulization of inhaled bronchodilators has several disadvantages. Loss or inefficient delivery of drug and cooling of the inspired oxygen mixture may occur with nebulization. In several studies in neonates, metered-dose inhalers with a spacer provided more efficient delivery of inhaled bronchodilators and greater improvements in oxygenation and ventilation; smaller doses and a shorter treatment time were also used.[114,115] In addition, metered-dose inhalers are less expensive than nebulization. Therefore, the use of metered-dose inhalers with an appropriate spacing device is preferred for most infants. Various products and dosage regimens can be found in Table 94-7.

Corticosteroids

Corticosteroids, particularly dexamethasone, have been used extensively for the prevention and treatment of BPD. Mechanisms of action of corticosteroids include (a) reduction of polymorphonuclear leukocyte migration to the lung, (b) reduction of lung inflammation, (c) inhibition of prostaglandin, leukotriene, tumor necrosis factor, and interleukin synthesis, (d) reduction of elastase production, (e) stimulation of surfactant synthesis, (f) reduction of vascular permeability and pulmonary edema, (g) enhancement of β-adrenergic receptor activity, (h) reduction of pulmonary fibronectin (which can reduce the risk of interstitial fibrosis), and (i) stimulation of serum retinol concentrations.[99,106,116] Treatment with dexamethasone (initiated ~7 days of life) in infants with documented BPD or with clinical signs and chest radiograph findings consistent with BPD reduces the release of inflammatory mediators, improves pulmonary mechanics and clinical status, facilitates weaning from mechanical ventilation, and decreases the duration of oxygen therapy.[99,102,106,116–118] In most studies, dexamethasone therapy did not significantly reduce the duration of hospitalization or improve survival in infants with BPD.[99,106,116,118,119]

Systemic dexamethasone is associated with many serious short-term adverse effects, including hyperglycemia, increased BP, hypertrophic cardiomyopathy, GI bleeding, intestinal perforation, pituitary-adrenal suppression, bone demineralization, poor weight gain, and increased risk of infection.[99,102,106,116]

Serious long-term adverse effects have also been identified in preterm infants who receive systemic corticosteroids. Two reviews (which assessed infants at ~1 year) reported an increase in the incidence of cerebral palsy, neurodevelopmental delay, and motor dysfunction in preterm infants who received systemic steroids for the prevention and treatment of BPD.[120,121]

The American Academy of Pediatrics does not recommend the use of steroids for the prevention and treatment of BPD in preterm infants because of short- and long-term adverse effects.[122] Systemic corticosteroids should be reserved for preterm neonates enrolled in randomized, double-blind, controlled trials; long-term neurodevelopmental assessment is highly encouraged. In general, the clinical use of systemic steroids should be limited to exceptional circumstances (e.g., an infant on maximal ventilatory and oxygen support) where the benefits may outweigh the risks. The American Academy of Pediatrics advises that parents should be fully informed about the short- and long-term adverse effects of systemic corticosteroids.[122]

Subsequent to the last American Academy of Pediatrics recommendation, several randomized trials have evaluated different corticosteroids and dosing regimens for the prevention and treatment of BPD, in an attempt to minimize adverse effects while maintaining efficacy. A recent placebo-controlled trial of low-dose dexamethasone administered to ventilator-dependent very preterm (gestational age <28 weeks) or extremely low-birth-weight infants (birth-weight <1,000 g) after 1 week of life (median age, 4 weeks) reported a decrease in ventilator settings, improvement in oxygenation, and higher percentage of extubation in the dexamethasone-treated infants.[123] However, the incidence of BPD and mortality were not different between groups. Short-term adverse effects such as hypertension, hyperglycemia, and intestinal perforation were not found. A 2-year follow-up to this study reported no significant differences in the incidence of cerebral palsy, blindness, deafness, developmental delay, and mortality between the two groups.[124] However, the number of patients followed was too small to provide definitive evidence.

Hydrocortisone has also been used for the prevention and treatment of BPD in several clinical trials.[125–128] In a retrospective study, hydrocortisone was as effective as dexamethasone in decreasing supplemental oxygen requirements but produced fewer adverse effects.[125] However, a prospective placebo-controlled trial found no effect of hydrocortisone on survival without BPD or mortality. In addition, an increase in spontaneous GI perforation was found in the hydrocortisone-treated group resulting in an early termination of the study.[126] Long-term adverse effects (e.g., cerebral palsy, neurodevelopmental impairment) have been reported to be similar between hydrocortisone and placebo or nontreated groups.[125,127,128] Based on these clinical findings, a lower dose and a shorter duration of therapy using either dexamethasone or hydrocortisone for the prevention and treatment of BPD may be considered in extremely high-risk ventilated infants. A delay of treatment until >7 days postnatal age may decrease the risk of adverse neurologic outcomes such as cerebral palsy. Some centers have delayed treatment until the infant reaches a postnatal age of >14 days. One currently recommended dosing regimen is dexamethasone 0.2 mg/kg/day in two divided doses for 3 days followed by 0.1 mg/kg/day for 3 days and then 0.05 mg/kg/day for 3 days.[129]

Inhaled steroids such as beclomethasone dipropionate, flunisolide, fluticasone, and budesonide have also been used for the treatment and prevention of BPD.[102,106] Infants receiving inhaled steroids for the treatment of BPD may have reduced oxygen requirements and duration of mechanical ventilation, and improvement in lung mechanics.[102,106,122] However, the onset of clinical improvements may be delayed compared with systemic steroids. In contrast, the preventative use of inhaled steroids has not been shown to decrease the incidence of BPD or the duration of mechanical ventilation and oxygen therapy; however, the use of systemic steroid may be decreased.[110,130] Two meta-analyses assessing comparative trials of inhaled versus systemic steroids found no significant differences in mortality or the incidence of BPD.[131,132] The use of early inhaled steroids (for prevention of BPD) was associated with increased duration of mechanical ventilation and oxygenation. Adverse effects of inhaled steroids reported in BPD infants are less common than with systemic steroids.[129,131,132] These include mild adrenal suppression, bronchospasm, tongue hypertrophy, and oral candidiasis.[133] High-dose inhaled fluticasone (500 mcg Q 12 hours for 2 weeks) has also been associated with moderately severe pituitary-adrenal suppression in VLBW infants.[134] The infant's mouth should be cleaned after each use of inhaled steroid to minimize complications such as oral thrush. As with inhaled bronchodilators, administration is a therapeutic problem with these medications. The amount of drug delivered to the infant can vary from 0.02% (by jet nebulizer) to 14.2% (by metered-dose inhaler with an aerochamber).[116] Further studies evaluating the optimal dose, duration of therapy, route of administration, time of initiation, most appropriate preparation, and long-term adverse effects of corticosteroids are needed before inhaled steroids can be routinely recommended.

Long-Term Sequelae

13. Six months have passed, and J.T. is now 6 months old (corrected age), weighs 5 kg, and ready for discharge. Over the past several months, ventilation requirements slowly decreased and J.T. was eventually extubated. However, she still requires supplemental oxygen at an FiO_2 of 30%, 1/8 L/minute via nasal cannula to maintain an oxygen saturation of 88% to 92%. Discharge medications include multivitamins with iron 0.5 mL Q 12 hours; spironolactone/hydrochlorothiazide suspension, 5 mg Q 12 hours; sodium chloride solution, 2 mEq Q 8 hours; nebulized albuterol (0.5% solution), 0.25 mL Q 6 hours; and fluticasone metered-dose inhaler (44 mcg per actuation), 2 puffs Q 12 hours. What are the long-term complications of BPD that can be expected in J.T.?

Infants with BPD have little pulmonary reserve and, therefore, are at higher risk for developing frequent respiratory exacerbations. BPD places J.T. at risk for recurrent infections of the lower respiratory tract and she may require frequent hospitalizations during the first year for bronchiolitis and pneumonia.[103] Approximately 50% of all children with severe BPD require hospitalization for respiratory exacerbations during the first year of life.[103] Respiratory syncytial virus is a common cause of respiratory distress (airway obstruction, mucus plugging, and airway edema) and recurrent atelectasis. With time, most preterm survivors with BPD have an improvement in pulmonary function owing to lung growth; however, many continue to have airway hyperreactivity. Infants with severe

BPD can also develop pulmonary hypertension, cor pulmonale, systemic hypertension, and left ventricular hypertrophy.

In addition to pulmonary and cardiovascular complications, J.T. may be at risk for developing bone demineralization and rickets. VLBW infants are born with inadequate stores of vitamin D. In general, these premature infants may not receive an adequate intake of vitamin D, either parenterally or through their diet. Most VLBW infants require prolonged parenteral nutrition, which may cause cholestasis or hepatic failure. Prolonged cholestasis or chronic hepatic congestion owing to heart failure may cause malabsorption of calcium and vitamin D. In addition, furosemide may exacerbate calcium deficiencies by causing hypercalciuria. These combined factors may result in bone demineralization and rickets. Infants with BPD usually have a high catabolism and increased oxygen consumption due to an increased work of breathing and chronic hypoxia. Inadequate nutritional support may negatively affect weight gain, growth, and long-term outcome of BPD.

Neurologic and developmental abnormalities such as learning disabilities, speech delays, vision and hearing impairment, and poor attention span can also occur in infants with BPD.[100] BPD itself is not an independent risk factor for neurologic abnormality; related factors include birth-weight, gestational age, and socioeconomic status.[99,102] Long-term follow-up evaluations at 1 to 8 years of age in infants previously treated with dexamethasone revealed an increase in neurodevelopmental abnormalities such as cerebral palsy and decreased school performance.[102,120,125,135] However, it is not known if these abnormalities were due to an adverse effect of dexamethasone on brain development or to an improved survival of infants who may already be at risk for developing these abnormalities. Recent studies assessing the long-term follow-up of infants treated with low-dose or delayed use of dexamethasone (i.e., initiated at >7 days of age), did not find an increase risk of developmental delay or cerebral palsy.[124,129] Hydrocortisone may offer an advantage over dexamethasone, because increases in neurodevelopmental abnormalities were not observed in infants followed up at 2 to 8 years of age.[127,128]

Mortality rates for infants with severe BPD range from 30% to 40%.[104] Approximately 80% of deaths associated with BPD occur during initial hospitalization and are from respiratory failure, sepsis, pneumonia, cor pulmonale, and congestive heart failure.[104]

Prevention

14. What preventive measures could have been used to decrease the incidence of BPD in J.T.?

Prevention of prematurity and other etiologic factors of RDS is the most effective means of preventing BPD. The administration of antenatal steroids to mothers before delivery decreases the incidence of RDS and, potentially, BPD. Exogenous surfactant therapy also reduces the incidence of RDS, but not the incidence of BPD. Early administration of dexamethasone (initiated <96 hours of life) in preterm infants reduces pulmonary inflammation and lung injury, decreases the incidence of BPD and oxygen requirements, improves lung function, and facilitates weaning from the ventilator.[99,116,119] However, early dexamethasone therapy has also been associated with an increased risk of infection, GI bleeding, intestinal perforation, hypertrophic cardiomyopathy, growth failure, and, of greatest concern, neurologic impairment and cerebral palsy.[119] A follow-up study at school age reported significant decreases in motor skills and coordination, lower IQ scores, and clinically significant disabilities in the dexamethasone-treated children.[135] Early dexamethasone therapy is not recommended for routine use because of the inconsistent improvements in outcome and mortality, and the lack of long-term follow-up data.[122] Clinicians should weigh the potential benefits versus the risks of early dexamethasone therapy for the prevention of BPD.

One of the causes of BPD can be vitamin A deficiency, which can predispose infants to BPD owing to impaired lung healing, increased susceptibility to infection and loss of cilia, and decreased number of alveoli.[136,137] Premature infants, especially VLBW infants, are at greatest risk owing to low body stores, inadequate intake during feedings, and decreased enteral absorption of vitamin A. In a meta-analysis evaluating various dosing regimens of IM vitamin A, mortality or oxygen requirement was reduced significantly at 1 month of life.[137] In addition, a significant reduction in oxygen requirements at 36 weeks PCA was observed in infants with a birth-weight <1,000 g. Administration of oral vitamin A 5,000 IU/day did not decrease the incidence of BPD, perhaps because of inadequate dose or poor oral absorption.[138] Vitamin A seems to be a relatively safe drug; the incidence of adverse effects was similar between treated and control groups.[137] Despite the beneficial findings of IM vitamin A, further studies evaluating the efficacy, safety, and optimal dosage regimen of vitamin A for the prevention of BPD are needed before routine use can be recommended.

Optimization of nutritional support may also help to prevent the development of BPD because proper nutrition helps to promote lung maturation, growth, and repair. Excessive fluid administration should be avoided because it may lead to BPD. Fluid restriction decreases both the incidence of BPD and mortality.[106] In addition, the early use of high-frequency ventilation in infants may decrease the severity and incidence of BPD.[99]

PATENT DUCTUS ARTERIOSUS

Pathogenesis

Several major differences between adult and fetal circulation exist. To understand the pathophysiology and clinical manifestations of PDA, fetal circulation and the cardiovascular changes that occur at birth are reviewed.

Fetal Circulatory Anatomy

The fetus has three unique circulatory structures that differ from the adult: (a) the ductus venosus, which permits blood to bypass the liver; (b) the foramen ovale, which allows blood to pass from the right atrium into the left atrium; and (c) the ductus arteriosus, the structure that connects the pulmonary artery to the descending aorta and allows blood to bypass the lungs (Fig. 94-1).[139]

In addition to these structural differences, vascular resistance and pressure play important roles in determining the pathway of fetal circulation. For example, the relative hypoxia that occurs in utero causes pulmonary vasoconstriction. Pulmonary vasoconstriction, along with compression of pulmonary blood

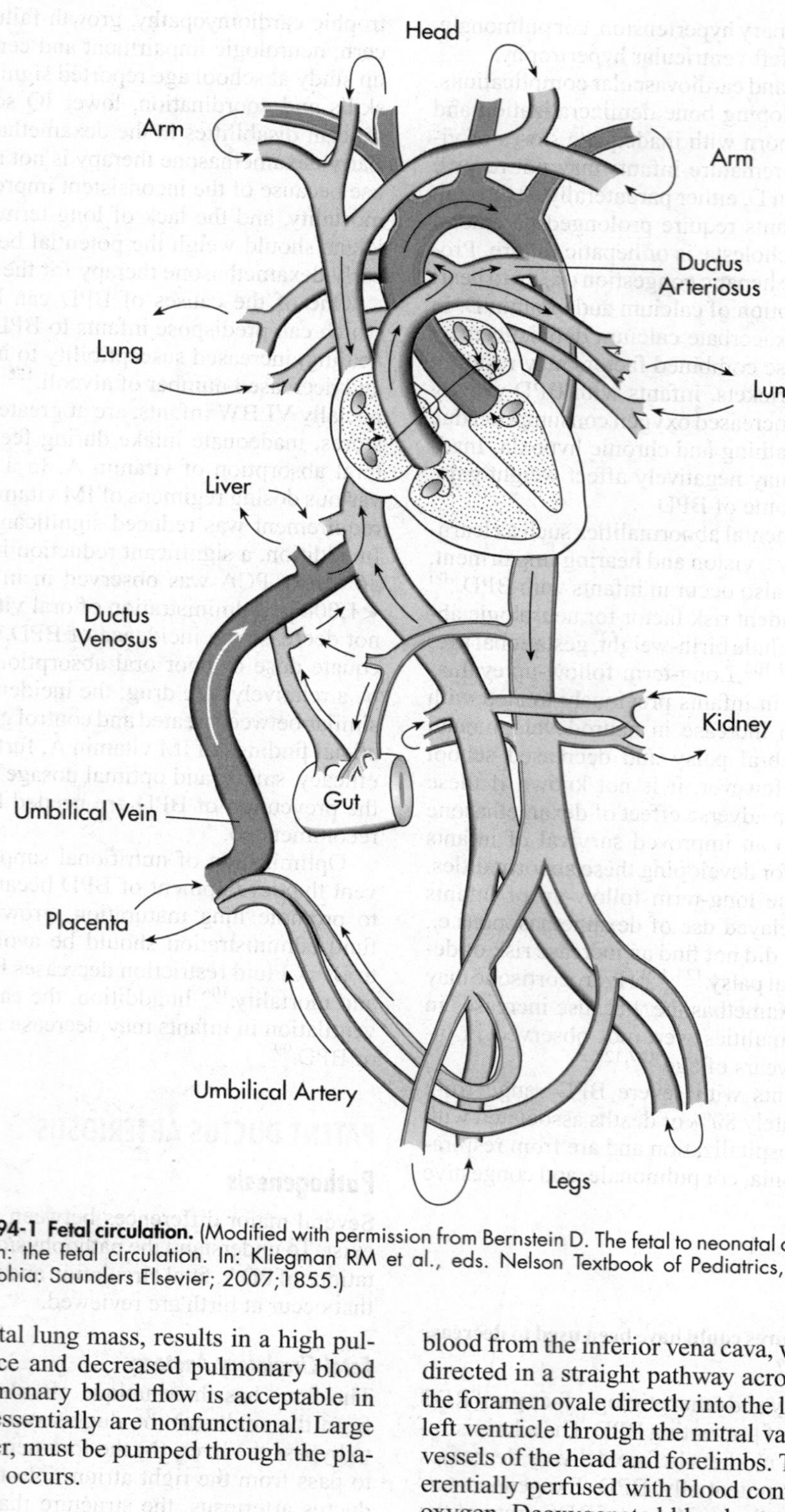

FIGURE 94-1 Fetal circulation. (Modified with permission from Bernstein D. The fetal to neonatal circulatory transition: the fetal circulation. In: Kliegman RM et al., eds. Nelson Textbook of Pediatrics, 18th Ed. Philadelphia: Saunders Elsevier; 2007;1855.)

vessels by unexpanded fetal lung mass, results in a high pulmonary vascular resistance and decreased pulmonary blood flow. This decreased pulmonary blood flow is acceptable in utero because the lungs essentially are nonfunctional. Large amounts of blood, however, must be pumped through the placenta where gas exchange occurs.

Fetal Circulation

Maximally oxygenated blood (Po_2, 30–35 mmHg) flows from the placenta to the fetus through the umbilical vein (Fig. 94-1). Approximately 50% of the umbilical venous blood is shunted away from the liver through the ductus venosus and directed into the inferior vena cava. Blood from the inferior vena cava and superior vena cava then enters the right atrium. Most of the blood from the inferior vena cava, which is well oxygenated, is directed in a straight pathway across the right atrium through the foramen ovale directly into the left atrium. It then enters the left ventricle through the mitral valve and is pumped into the vessels of the head and forelimbs. Thus, the fetal brain is preferentially perfused with blood containing a higher amount of oxygen. Deoxygenated blood returning from the head region via the superior vena cava enters the right atrium and is directed through the tricuspid valve into the right ventricle, where it then is pumped into the pulmonary artery. Most of this blood is diverted through the ductus arteriosus into the descending aorta and then through the two umbilical arteries to the placenta. A small percentage of the blood flows to the lower extremities and then is returned to the heart via the inferior vena cava.[139]

Changes at Birth

At birth, major circulatory changes result from umbilical cord clamping, aeration and expansion of the lungs, and an increase in arterial Po_2. These changes are important in the transition from fetal to adult circulation. When the umbilical cord is clamped, blood flow decreases through the ductus venosus, which closes within 3 to 7 days. Clamping of the umbilical cord also results in a twofold increase in systemic vascular resistance. This increase in systemic vascular resistance increases aortic, left ventricular and atrial pressures and cardiac output. Pulmonary pressures and blood flow also change. After the neonate's first breath, the lungs expand, oxygenation improves, and pulmonary vascular resistance immediately drops. This increases pulmonary blood flow, causing a decrease in pulmonary artery, right ventricle, and right atrium pressures.[139]

If hypoxia occurs after delivery, pulmonary vasoconstriction results and the neonate may develop pulmonary hypertension with a persistence of fetal circulation. This is termed persistent pulmonary hypertension of the newborn or persistent fetal circulation. Oxygenation of these neonates is extremely difficult because of the pulmonary vasoconstriction and resultant decreased pulmonary blood flow. Systemic alkalization (through hyperventilation and the use of sodium bicarbonate) and inotropic support often are necessary.[139] Severe cases may require extracorporeal membrane oxygenation.

Closure of the Foramen Ovale

Because of the decreased right atrium pressure and increased left atrium pressure that occur after birth, blood attempts to flow down the pressure gradient from the left atrium through the foramen ovale into the right atrium. This is in the opposite direction from what occurs in fetal life. The small, valvelike flap that lies over the foramen ovale on the left side of the atrial septum closes over the foramen ovale opening when the pressure in the left atrium exceeds the pressure in the right atrium. Closure of this flap prevents further flow through the foramen ovale. As long as the pressure in the left atrium is higher than the right atrium, the foramen ovale remains functionally closed, until it closes anatomically.

Closure of the Ductus Arteriosus

Closure of the ductus arteriosus is more complex and depends on many factors. In utero, patency of the ductus arteriosus is maintained through the combined vasodilatory effects of a low Po_2 and high concentrations of prostaglandins, particularly prostaglandin E_2 (PGE_2).[140] Prostacyclin also plays a role in maintaining ductal patency.[140,141] After birth, the smooth muscles of the ductus arteriosus constrict as arterial oxygenation increases and concentrations of placentally derived prostaglandins, particularly PGE_2, decrease.[141] In utero, the Po_2 of the ductal blood is 18 to 28 mmHg, whereas after birth in a term neonate, it is approximately 100 mmHg. Normally, the ductus arteriosus of a term neonate functionally closes within the first few days of life (i.e., in 82% of infants within 48 hours of life and in 100% of infants within 96 hours of life).[140] Anatomical closure of the ductus occurs within 2 to 3 weeks of life.[141] When the ductus arteriosus fails to close, it is called *patent ductus arteriosus* (*PDA*). In a term neonate, a PDA beyond the first few days of life generally is permanent. It usually is secondary to an anatomical defect in the wall of the ductus arteriosus and requires surgical ligation. In contrast, a PDA in a preterm neonate may persist for weeks and still close spontaneously.

When a PDA is present, the direction and amount of shunting through this opening are determined by the pressure between the systemic and pulmonary circulation. Usually, blood flows from the aorta into the pulmonary circulation. Because systemic vascular resistance and aortic pressure are increased, and pulmonary vascular resistance and pulmonary artery pressure are decreased after birth, blood pumped from the left ventricle into the aorta flows from the aorta (a high-pressure area) through the PDA and into the pulmonary artery (a lower-pressure area). This flow is called *left-to-right shunting* and is in contrast to the right-to-left shunting that occurs through the PDA during fetal life.

Although the persistence of a PDA is pathological, it is necessary for the survival of patients with cyanotic congenital heart disease while awaiting corrective or palliative cardiac surgery. These patients have congenital cardiac defects that depend on the ductus arteriosus to maintain cardiac output and systemic perfusion (e.g., coarctation of the aorta, aortic stenosis, and hypoplastic left heart syndrome) or to provide pulmonary blood flow and maintain systemic oxygenation (e.g., pulmonary artery atresia or severe stenosis and tricuspid atresia). Patency of the ductus arteriosus can be maintained pharmacologically with a continuous infusion of alprostadil (PGE_1). The initial starting dose of PGE_1 is 0.05 to 0.1 mcg/kg/minute and may be increased every 15 to 30 minutes up to 0.2 mcg/kg/minute until achievement of clinical response. Infusion doses up to 0.4 mcg/kg/minute have also been used by several centers. PGE_1 infusion should be reduced to the lowest effective dose once patency of the ductus arteriosus is achieved.[8,142]

Clinical Presentation

15. **T.S. is a 750-g female who was born at 25 weeks' gestational age to a 22-year-old gravida 2 para 1 female. One hour after birth, T.S. developed symptoms of RDS and two doses of beractant were given within the first 24 hours of life. After the second dose of beractant, T.S.'s respiratory function greatly improved and no further doses of beractant were required. On the third day of life, the nurse noticed that T.S. had tachycardia, a systolic murmur, a hyperactive precordium, and a widened pulse pressure. Her lungs sounded "wet." In addition, the nurse noted that T.S.'s combined IV fluid rates total 160 mL/kg/day instead of the desired fluid intake of 120 mL/kg/day. Current vital signs are as follows: HR, 190 beats/minute; RR, 65 breaths/minute; BP, 55/23 mmHg; and O_2 saturation, 89%. ABGs include pH, 7.22; Pco_2, 55 mmHg; PO_2, 77 mmHg; and base deficit, 10. Ventilator support is increased to compensate for T.S.'s deteriorating respiratory status. Echocardiography is performed and shows a moderate-size PDA with significant left-to-right shunting. The chest radiograph shows pulmonary edema and an enlarged heart. What risk factors for PDA does T.S. have?**

[SI units: Pco_2, 7.33 kPa; Po_2, 10.3 kPa]

T.S. has two major risk factors for developing a symptomatic PDA: prematurity and RDS. The occurrence of a PDA is inversely proportional to gestational age and birth-weight. The incidence of PDA is approximately 45% in premature infants with a birth-weight of <1,750 g but can be as high as 80% in premature infants with a birth-weight of <1,200 g.[141] In contrast, the incidence of PDA in term infants is only 0.04%.[140] Preterm neonates are at a higher risk for PDA than term newborns because the smooth muscle of the immature ductus is more sensitive to the dilatory effects of prostaglandins and less sensitive to the constrictive effects of increased oxygen tension. In addition, circulating concentrations of PGE_2 are often elevated in premature infants owing to the decreased pulmonary metabolism of prostaglandins.[140] These factors contribute to the delayed closure of the ductus arteriosus in premature infants. With advanced gestation, the ductus is less responsive to the relaxant effects of prostaglandins and is more sensitive to the constricting effects of oxygen.[140,143]

RDS also increases the risk for PDA. Exogenous surfactant, especially prophylactic use, also may increase the risk of symptomatic PDA.[143,144] PDA can further complicate the course of RDS.[143,145] T.S.'s course is typical of a preterm neonate with resolving RDS. T.S.'s pulmonary function improved after surfactant administration. Consequently, pulmonary vascular resistance decreased and the degree of left-to-right shunting across the ductus arteriosus increased, causing a deterioration in respiratory status. In addition, the excess fluid that T.S. received is an iatrogenic factor that may have increased the shunting across the PDA, aggravating the degree of pulmonary congestion.[143]

16. How is T.S.'s presentation consistent with that of PDA?

T.S.'s clinical presentation is due to the increased pulmonary blood flow, decreased systemic perfusion, and left ventricular volume overload that resulted from the shunting of left ventricular cardiac output through the PDA into the lungs. To compensate for the inadequate peripheral perfusion, HR increases. This results in an increase in cardiac output and a greater left-to-right shunt through the PDA, creating a vicious cycle. The widened pulse pressure (the difference between systolic and diastolic pressures, 32 mmHg) is a result of diversion of aortic blood flow through the PDA, which is causing the bounding pulses. The systolic murmur, which is not always present, is the result of turbulent blood flow through the ductus arteriosus occurring as the pulmonary vascular resistance decreases. Tachycardia, hyperactive precordium, and a continuous murmur are results of the left-to-right shunting through the ductus arteriosus during systole.[141]

17. What are the potential complications of this hemodynamically significant PDA in T.S.?

The increased pulmonary blood flow and resultant pulmonary edema will worsen T.S.'s respiratory disease and increase the need for ventilatory support. The higher ventilatory settings (increase in MAP and FIO_2) place T.S. at risk for developing BPD. If the PDA is left untreated, T.S. may develop congestive heart failure secondary to an increased left ventricular end-diastolic volume. A hemodynamically significant PDA also places T.S. at risk for IVH and NEC.[143]

Treatment

18. How should PDA be managed in T.S.?

The initial medical management for T.S.'s symptomatic PDA is supportive care, which includes fluid management (e.g., fluid restriction and diuretic therapy), correction of anemia, and treatment of hypoxia and acidosis. Although excessive fluid administration may increase the risk of PDA, fluid restriction alone is unlikely to result in ductal closure. T.S.'s fluid intake should be restricted to 100 to 120 mL/kg/day (approximately 80% of total fluid maintenance requirements) to avoid worsening of her pulmonary edema and to prevent congestive heart failure.[141,143] Furosemide 1 mg/kg IV push should also be given to T.S. immediately to treat her pulmonary edema (see Question 9). In addition to fluid management, correction of anemia is important. Low concentrations of hemoglobin result in an increased cardiac output, which may worsen the infant's cardiac function. Anemia not only increases the demand of left ventricular output to ensure adequate oxygen delivery to the tissues, but may also increase the magnitude of the left-to-right shunt by decreasing the resistance of blood flow through the pulmonary vascular bed.[143] Maintaining a hematocrit level of >40% to 45% is often recommended.[141] Because of T.S.'s gestational age, birth-weight, and size of PDA, it is unlikely that she will respond to these general measures alone. Therefore, T.S. requires treatment with indomethacin. Indomethacin nonspecifically inhibits prostaglandin synthesis, thereby eliminating the vasodilator effects of the PGE series on the ductus arteriosus. Unfortunately, not every infant who is treated with indomethacin responds with constriction of the ductus arteriosus; therefore, surgical ligation of the PDA may be required for T.S. Ligation generally is reserved for neonates who do not respond to indomethacin therapy or those in whom indomethacin therapy is contraindicated (see Question 20).[143]

Indomethacin

19. What is the dose of indomethacin and what route should be used for its administration?

The treatment of choice for T.S. is pharmacologic therapy with IV indomethacin; enteral indomethacin is less effective. This reduced effectiveness may be due to the formulation of the suspension and decreased, erratic, enteral absorption.[146]

A large interpatient variability of indomethacin pharmacokinetics occurs in preterm neonates. Serum concentrations do not correlate consistently with therapeutic or adverse effects.[146] Furthermore, the optimal therapeutic serum concentration is not yet defined. Although many dosage regimens have been reported, dosing guidelines from the National Collaborative Study are commonly used.[145] Three indomethacin doses are given in 12- to 24-hour intervals, with the first dose equal to 0.2 mg/kg IV in all neonates. Because indomethacin clearance is directly proportional to postnatal age, the second and third doses are determined by postnatal age at initiation of indomethacin therapy.[141] If onset of treatment was at less than 2 days postnatal age, neonates receive 0.1 mg/kg/dose; if initiation of therapy occurred at 2 to 7 days postnatal age, neonates receive 0.2 mg/kg/dose; and if therapy began more than 7 days postnatal age, neonates receive 0.25 mg/kg/dose. Second and third doses are administered at 12- to 24-hour intervals. No specific guidelines exist regarding which patients receive every-12-hour versus every-24-hour dosing; however, the individual dosing interval generally is determined by the neonate's urine output.[141] If urine output remains >1 mL/kg/hour after an indomethacin dose, then the next dose may be given in 12 hours.

If urine output is <1 mL/kg/hour but >0.6 mL/kg/hour, then the dosing interval may be extended to 24 hours.

Other indomethacin dosing regimens have been evaluated more recently for the treatment of PDA in preterm infants. An initial dose of 0.2 mg/kg followed by either 0.1 or 0.2 mg/kg for two doses at 12- to 24-hour intervals has been used. In a study measuring serum concentrations, higher doses of indomethacin were required in older neonates (>10 days postnatal age).[147] This may be due to an increased indomethacin clearance in these infants. Because rapid IV administration of indomethacin can vasoconstrict the mesenteric arteries and renal vascular beds, longer infusion rates of 20 to 30 minutes are recommended. Continuous infusion of indomethacin seems to further decrease the adverse effects, but additional studies are needed.[143]

Response to indomethacin therapy can be determined by assessing the clinical signs of PDA such as tachycardia, widened pulse pressure, bounding pulses, heart murmur, and the ability to wean ventilator support. In certain cases, echocardiography may be performed to confirm closure of a PDA.

MONITORING THERAPY

20. What clinical and laboratory data should be monitored during T.S.'s indomethacin therapy?

Before initiating indomethacin therapy, T.S. should receive an echocardiogram to rule out ductal-dependent congenital heart disease and to confirm the presence of a PDA. In addition, a SrCr and blood urea nitrogen (BUN) should be obtained from T.S. before indomethacin therapy because nephrotoxicity is the most common adverse effect. Infants receiving indomethacin can develop transient oliguria with increased SrCr. This occurs as a result of indomethacin-induced decreases in renal blood flow and GFR.[145] Dilutional hyponatremia may occur secondary to either decreased urine output or decreased free water diuresis owing to increased antidiuretic hormone activity.[142] Treatment of hyponatremia should be aimed at decreasing free water intake through fluid restriction rather than by sodium supplementation. Typically, renal function normalizes within 72 hours after the last dose of indomethacin.[142] In general, indomethacin therapy is contraindicated in neonates with renal failure, urine output <0.6 mL/kg/hour, or SrCr $\geq$1.8 mg/dL.[145] Although furosemide has been reported to decrease indomethacin-induced nephrotoxicity without affecting PDA, more studies are needed to confirm these findings.[148] In addition, serum concentrations of aminoglycosides, digoxin, and other renally eliminated drugs should be monitored carefully. Indomethacin therapy may decrease renal drug clearance and cause accumulation of these agents.[149]

A platelet count should also be obtained from T.S. before therapy because indomethacin may decrease platelet aggregation. Thrombocytopenia (platelet count, <50,000/mm^3) is a contraindication to indomethacin therapy.[142,145] In cases of thrombocytopenia, indomethacin may be withheld temporarily until platelets can be transfused. Other potential contraindications to indomethacin therapy include active bleeding and clinical evidence of NEC because GI bleeding, perforation, and NEC have been reported with indomethacin use.[143] These GI effects may be related to decreases in intestinal blood flow usually seen with rapid IV infusions. Grades II to IV IVH also are frequently quoted as contraindications to indomethacin therapy; however, indomethacin treatment probably is not associated with progression of IVH. In fact, prophylactic treatment with indomethacin may be associated with a decrease in the incidence of severe IVH (grades III and IV).[143,144]

Ibuprofen

Because of the adverse effects of indomethacin, other prostaglandin inhibitors such as ibuprofen have been studied for the closure of the ductus arteriosus. Results indicate that ibuprofen is as effective as indomethacin and causes significantly less of a decrease in renal, mesenteric, and cerebral blood flow.[150] In studies comparing ibuprofen to indomethacin, ibuprofen was less likely to cause adverse effects on renal function (e.g., oliguria). The incidence of NEC or IVH were similar for both of these drugs.[151,152] However, one recent meta-analysis found that ibuprofen may increase the risk of developing chronic lung disease (BPD).[153] Thus, until further studies are conducted, many clinicians still consider indomethacin the drug of choice. Ibuprofen may be preferred in select patients who have or are at increased risk for decreased renal function. IV ibuprofen lysine is commercially available in the United States. The initial dose is 10 mg/kg followed by two doses of 5 mg/kg given at 24-hour intervals. If urinary output decreases to <0.6 mL/kg/hour, the second or third doses should be held.[8]

21. When is the best time to initiate indomethacin for symptomatic treatment of PDA?

Conflicting data exist on when to initiate indomethacin therapy for the treatment of symptomatic PDA. Some centers may opt to treat within the first 2 to 3 days of life (early symptomatic PDA) when infants initially present with clinical signs of PDA (i.e., murmur, widened pulse pressures, tachycardia). Others may not treat until clinical signs of congestive heart failure are present (late symptomatic PDA; 7–10 days of life).[144] Both indomethacin treatment strategies (early and late) significantly decrease the incidence of PDA, but both cause significant transient reduction of urine output and SrCr elevation. In some studies, infants receiving early treatment of indomethacin had significant reductions in the incidence of BPD and NEC and the need for surgical ligation.[144] In contrast, one study found that final PDA closure rates and the need for surgical ligation were comparable in early versus late indomethacin-treated neonates. In fact, spontaneous closure was observed in 43% of the late treatment group, which may indicate unnecessary treatment in the early group. In addition, renal adverse effects and ventilatory requirements were higher in the infants treated early.[154] Thus, early administration of indomethacin should not be used routinely.

RECURRENCE

22. T.S. completes a course of indomethacin 0.16 mg IV Q 12 hours × 3 doses. The physicians were able to decrease T.S.'s ventilator support within the first 12 to 24 hours after starting indomethacin treatment. After 3 to 4 days of gradual and consistent ventilator weaning, the ventilator settings could not be decreased further. Over the next 2 to 3 days, T.S.'s respiratory status deteriorates and she requires increased ventilator support. T.S. now has tachycardia, a widened pulse pressure, bounding pulses, and a hyperactive precordium. Repeat echocardiogram shows a small-to-moderate PDA. Current data include the following:

BUN, 10 mg/dL; SrCr, 1.1 mg/dL; sodium (Na), 134 mEq/L; potassium (K), 4.9 mEq/L; chloride (Cl), 97 mEq/L; urine output, 2.3 mL/kg/hour; fluid intake, 130 mL/kg/day; and platelets, 180,000/mm³. Why did PDA recur in T.S.?

[SI units: BUN, 3.6 mmol/L of urea; SrCr, 97.2 mmol/L; Na, 134 mmol/L; K, 4.9 mmol/L; Cl, 97 mmol/L; platelets, 180 × 10^9/L]

Successful closure of the PDA with indomethacin occurs in 70% to 90% of infants; however, ductal reopening or recurrence can occur in 20% to 35% of infants who initially respond to indomethacin.[140,155] Recurrence of PDA occurs especially in lower birth-weight infants.[155] Several reasons might explain T.S.'s transient response to indomethacin. Recurrence of PDA is inversely proportional to gestational age; the incidence of ductal reopening is significantly higher in infants ≤26 weeks' gestational age compared with infants born ≥27 weeks' gestation (37% versus 11%, respectively).[156] The higher recurrence in younger gestational age neonates may be due to resumption of PGE_2 production after indomethacin serum concentrations decline and heightened sensitivity of the immature ductus arteriosus to the dilating effects of PGE.[143,155] This is particularly important in ventilator-dependent patients such as T.S. because mechanical ventilation increases circulating vasodilating prostaglandins.[140] Furthermore, the rate of ductal reopening is independent of indomethacin serum concentrations, but seems to be related to the timing of indomethacin therapy, postnatal age, and the amount of fluid intake 24 hours before indomethacin treatment.[156] The rate of recurrence is lower in infants who were treated with indomethacin within the first 48 hours of life compared with those receiving treatment after 7 days of life.[143] Because anatomical closure of a PDA may be delayed for a couple of weeks, it is not surprising that the ductus arteriosus reopened in T.S. after her initial response to indomethacin.[143]

Although controversial, prolonged indomethacin therapy may prevent recurrences and allow for permanent closure of the ductus arteriosus. Several prolonged treatment regimens have been successful in preventing ductal reopening.[143,155] One such regimen (indomethacin 0.2 mg/kg/dose IV Q 12 hours × 3 doses, followed by 0.2 mg/kg/dose Q 24 hours × 5 doses) was able to significantly decrease the recurrence of PDA in neonates <1,500 g from 47% to 10% without increasing toxicity. The need for surgical ligation also was decreased significantly.[155] However, some studies report an increased mortality in infants receiving prolonged therapy (seven doses) compared with those receiving the short course (three doses).[143] Furthermore, other investigators found a significantly higher PDA closure rate in the short-course group (initial, 0.2 mg/kg then 0.1 mg/kg for two doses, each given at 12-hour intervals). The prolonged course (0.1 mg/kg/dose Q 24 hours × 7 doses) had a higher incidence of NEC and urea retention, and a longer duration of oxygen therapy.[157] Therefore, the optimal duration of indomethacin therapy and dosing regimen need to be identified.

23. Should indomethacin be given to T.S. again? Can future recurrences be prevented?

T.S. remains ventilator dependent and is at increased risk for developing BPD. Because she has no contraindications to indomethacin therapy, a second course should be given. To prevent further recurrences, an additional five doses of indomethacin (0.1–0.2 mg/kg/dose Q 24 hours) may be given to T.S. after she completes the standard three-dose regimen.[155,157] If the PDA fails to respond to this prolonged regimen or if it recurs again after an initial response, and T.S. remains ventilator dependent, surgical ligation most likely will be required to permanently close the PDA.

PROPHYLACTIC ADMINISTRATION

24. Could prophylactic indomethacin have prevented the development of a symptomatic PDA?

Prophylactic indomethacin therapy is defined as the administration of indomethacin to infants who have echocardiographic evidence but no clinical signs of PDA. Only 40% of infants with severe RDS and echocardiographic evidence of PDA during the first day of life go on to develop a hemodynamically significant PDA. Therefore, 60% of infants would be treated unnecessarily if prophylactic indomethacin was given on day 1 of life.[143] Prophylactic use of indomethacin for the prevention of PDA significantly decreases the incidence of PDA and IVH (grades III and IV)[144,158] and the need for surgical ligation.[144] Unfortunately, most studies have not been able to show that prophylactic ductal closure with indomethacin decreases the incidence of death, BPD, or NEC.[144,158] In fact, infants receiving prophylactic therapy had a higher incidence of NEC (when studies were evaluated individually),[158] oliguria, and elevated SrCr.[144,158] Therefore, routine prophylactic administration is not warranted. Preterm neonates, particularly those at high risk for developing a large PDA (e.g., extremely low-birth-weight neonates), should be treated as soon as clinical signs appear.

Prophylactic ibuprofen therapy (administered at <24 hours of life) can significantly increase ductal closure rate without increasing IVH, NEC, or mortality or decreasing renal function.[159,160] However, one study that utilized IV ibuprofen buffered with *tris*-hydroxymethyl-aminomethane (THAM) was terminated early because of three cases of severe hypoxemia and pulmonary hypertension that occurred in ibuprofen-treated infants.[159] Early administration of ibuprofen (i.e., <6 hours of life in this study versus <24 hours of life in other studies) may have prevented the decrease in pulmonary vascular resistance that normally occurs shortly after birth. However, other studies that administered ibuprofen early have not reported this adverse effect.[161] Another explanation is that the THAM–buffered solution allowed the ibuprofen to precipitate, causing microembolization of the lungs with resultant pulmonary hypertension. Although this is a plausible explanation, a case of pulmonary hypertension was reported in Europe after administration of L-lysine ibuprofen.[162] Additional studies are needed before routine use of prophylactic ibuprofen therapy can be recommended.

NECROTIZING ENTEROCOLITIS

Pathogenesis and Classification

25. C.D., an 11-day-old female neonate, was born at 28 weeks' gestational age with a birth-weight of 908 g. Her postnatal course has been complicated by RDS, sepsis, and PDA for which she required intubation and mechanical ventilation, two doses of beractant, a 7-day course of ampicillin and gentamicin, and indomethacin. Enteral feedings with a standard preterm 24-cal/oz formula were started on day 7 of life at 5 mL Q 3 hours (44 mL/kg/

day). Feedings were increased by 5 mL/feed on days 8 through 10 to 20 mL/feed Q 3 hours on day 10 of life (176 mL/kg/day). This morning, C.D. developed a distended abdomen, bloody stools, multiple episodes of apnea that required reintubation and assisted ventilation, and metabolic acidosis. ABG results revealed the following: pH, 7.20; P_{CO_2}, 47 mmHg; and PO_2, 55 mmHg. An abdominal radiograph revealed pneumatosis intestinalis (the presence of gas in the intestinal submucosa). C.D. is to take nothing by mouth (NPO), and gentamicin 3.5 mg/kg IV infusion Q 24 hours and ampicillin 50 mg/kg IV push Q 12 hours are restarted. What clinical signs of NEC does C.D. have? What is the pathogenesis of NEC and what risk factors for NEC does C.D. have?

NEC, a type of acute intestinal necrosis, is the most common life-threatening nonrespiratory condition, affecting 1,200 to 9,600 newborns in the United States each year.[163] The rate of hospitalization associated with NEC is 1.1 per 1,000 live births.[164] Approximately 62% to 94% of NEC occurs in premature infants; however, NEC can infrequently occur in full-term neonates.[163,165] NEC occurs in 3% to 15% of neonatal intensive care unit (ICU) admissions and has a mortality rate of 25% to 30%; approximately 25% of survivors develop long-term complications.[165,166] The age of onset of NEC is inversely related to gestational age and birth-weight; the greater the gestational age of the infant at birth, the sooner the onset of NEC. Although NEC is less common in term infants, it usually develops within 3 to 4 days of age. In contrast, infants born at ~30 weeks' gestation develop NEC at a mean postnatal age of 20 days. Thus, preterm infants are at a risk for NEC for a longer period of time.[163,166] Although C.D. is extremely premature, she developed NEC early (at 11 days of age), most likely due to the aggressive advancement of feedings (see following discussion).

C.D. has several clinical signs of NEC, including abdominal distention, bloody stools, apnea, metabolic acidosis, and pneumatosis intestinalis on abdominal radiograph. Gastric retention of feedings, respiratory distress, occult blood in stools, lethargy, temperature instability, thrombocytopenia, and neutropenia also may occur. NEC may progress to bowel perforation, peritonitis, sepsis, disseminated intravascular coagulopathy (DIC), and shock. On an abdominal radiograph, the presence of gas in the intestinal mucosa or in the portal venous system is diagnostic of NEC, and free air in the abdomen is observed with bowel perforation. Although these radiographic findings confirm the diagnosis of NEC, a lag time may occur between the initial clinical signs of NEC and radiologic confirmation.[165]

NEC can evolve slowly over a period of 24 to 48 hours, from a clinically benign course to an advanced stage of shock, peritonitis, and widespread intestinal necrosis. Although NEC can affect any part of the GI tract, most of the disease is confined to the ileum and colon.[167] A staging system, which categorizes severity according to systemic, intestinal, and radiologic signs, has been developed to permit a more consistent evaluation and treatment of patients.[168] Stages IA and IB NEC include neonates and infants with suspected disease or "rule out" NEC. These patients may have mild GI problems such as emesis and increased gastric residuals, temperature instability, apnea, bright red blood from rectum, or a mild ileus. Infants with stages IIA and IIB have definite NEC and usually present with abdominal distention, bloody stools, and the presence of pneumatosis intestinalis on radiograph. Infants in stage IIB NEC may also develop metabolic acidosis and thrombocytopenia. C.D.'s presentation is most consistent with stage IIB NEC. Infants with stages IIIA and IIIB (advanced disease) are severely ill with clinical signs, including peritonitis, ascites, shock, severe metabolic and respiratory acidosis, and DIC. Those with stage IIIB have intestinal perforation.

The exact pathogenesis of NEC is unknown, but seems to be multifactorial. Most likely, NEC results from the effects of intestinal bacteria and other factors on injured intestinal mucosa (Fig. 94-2). Inflammatory mediators such as platelet-activating factor, tumor necrosis factor-α, interleukin-1β, and interleukin-8 may also contribute to mucosal damage.[169] The neonatal intestinal mucosa is prone to injury for the following reasons: (a) increased permeability to potentially harmful substances, such as bacteria and proteins; (b) decreased immunologic host defenses, including low concentrations of IgA in intestinal mucosa; and (c) decreased nonimmunologic defenses, such as decreased concentrations of proteases and gastric acid. In addition, numerous factors (both prenatal and postnatal) can cause injury to the neonatal intestinal mucosa and increase the risk for NEC.[167] Prenatal maternal factors include eclampsia, prolonged rupture of membranes, fetal distress, maternal cocaine use, and cesarean section. Postnatal factors include prematurity, low birth-weight, ischemia/hypoxemia, asphyxia, hypotension, respiratory distress, apnea, malnutrition, infection, hemodynamically significant PDA, congenital GI anomalies, cyanotic heart disease, toxins, hyperosmolar substances (e.g., feedings, medications), rapid advancement of enteral feedings, exchange transfusions, and the presence of umbilical catheters.[166–168,170] Medications such as corticosteroids, indomethacin, and H_2-blockers significantly increase the incidence of NEC in VLBW infants.[171,172] However, the most significant clinical risk factor for NEC is prematurity.[163,168]

C.D. has several risks for developing NEC, which include prematurity (gestational age of 28 weeks), extremely low birth-weight (908 g), history of infection, and RDS requiring mechanical ventilation. Furthermore, C.D. not only was given a hyperosmolar formula (24 cal/oz instead of 20 cal/oz), but her feedings were advanced aggressively. These two factors may also contribute to the development of NEC. Approximately 90% to 95% of infants with NEC have received enteral feedings, although NEC also occurs in infants who have never been fed.[173] Enteral feedings (breast-milk or formulas) serve as substrates for bacterial proliferation in the gut. As a result, reducing substances, organic acids, and hydrogen gas are produced by bacterial fermentation of these nutrients. Although studies have shown that rapid advancements in the volume of feeds (30 mL/kg/day versus 15–20 mL/kg/day) were associated with an increased risk of NEC, more recent studies report that infants advanced at rate of 30 mL/kg/day reach full enteral intake and regain birth-weight significantly earlier than infants advanced at 15 or 20 mL/kg/day without increasing the risk of NEC.[174,175] Similarly, older studies reported that early initiation of feeds might increase the risk of NEC; however, more recent studies have failed to confirm these findings.[176] Thus, feedings should be increased by 10 to 20 mL/kg/day; however, advancement >20 mL/kg/day (up to 30 mL/kg/day) may enable infants to reach full feeds and regain birth-weight faster without increasing the risk of NEC. C.D. was started at a much higher initial feeding volume (44 mL/kg/day) and aggressively

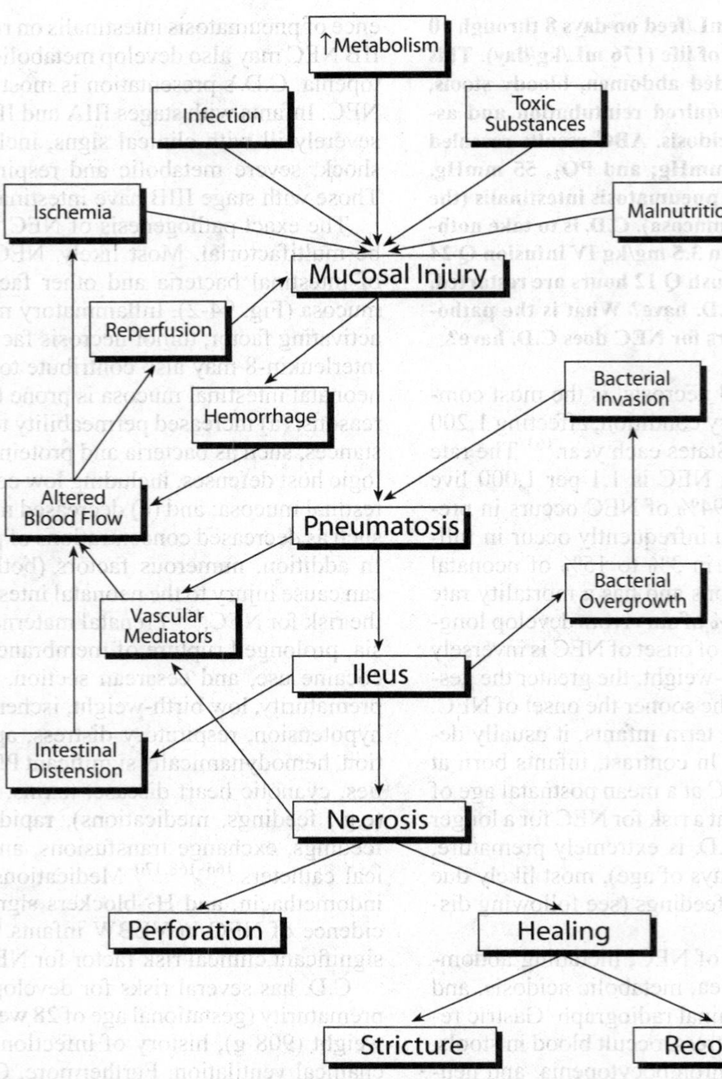

FIGURE 94-2 Necrotizing enterocolitis (NEC). This schematic is a composite of the theories about factors believed to be involved in the pathogenesis of NEC. The progression of this disease is denoted in large type. The factors believed to initiate or propagate the disease process are in smaller type. (Reproduced with permission from Crouse DT. Necrotizing enterocolitis. In: Pomerance JJ, Richardson CJ, eds. Neonatology for the Clinician. Norwalk, CT: Appleton & Lange; 1993:364.)

increased by 44 mL/kg/day. If C.D. were appropriately fed, she would have reached full feedings in 7 to 14 days instead of 4 days. Last, the presence of PDA and the use of indomethacin for the treatment of PDA may also have contributed to NEC in C.D. Her PDA or the use of indomethacin may have decreased mesenteric blood flow with resultant ischemia and intestinal mucosal injury.[166]

Treatment

General Management

26. How should C.D. be managed?

Significant abdominal distention may compromise respiratory function and blood flow to the intestines. Therefore, as soon as NEC is suspected, feedings should be stopped immediately and an orogastric tube with low intermittent suction placed to decompress the abdomen. C.D.'s vital signs and abdominal circumference should be closely monitored for disease progression. A complete blood count (CBC) and platelet count should be obtained frequently to monitor for neutropenia and thrombocytopenia. Blood, urine, and stool cultures should be obtained, and parenteral antibiotics should be started as soon as possible; 20% to 30% of infants with NEC have associated bacteremia. In infants with stage I NEC, antibiotic therapy is usually given for 3 days pending culture results and clinical signs. Once the diagnosis of NEC is ruled out, antibiotics may be discontinued.[168] Enteral feedings can then be initiated slowly. However, if the diagnosis of NEC is made, antibiotics are continued and parenteral nutrition is initiated at that time. Infants require 7 to 14 days of bowel rest (NPO). The length of antibiotic therapy and bowel rest in infants with documented NEC (stages II or III) is determined by the severity of systemic illness (e.g., metabolic acidosis, thrombocytopenia). C.D. has stage

IIB disease and needs to be NPO for at least 10 to 14 days; she requires total parenteral nutrition during that time. Infants with stage III disease may also require fluid resuscitation, administration of inotropic agents such as dopamine and dobutamine, and surgical intervention, especially for those with perforated NEC.[166] In a recent, randomized, controlled trial, significant differences were not noted in survival rate, duration of hospitalization, and dependence on parenteral nutrition (assessed 90 days postoperatively) between primary peritoneal drainage versus laparotomy with bowel resection in preterm infants with perforated NEC.[177]

Antibiotics

27. C.D. just completed a 7-day course of ampicillin and gentamicin. Is it appropriate to restart these antibiotics?

The selection of antibiotics for NEC depends on the common micro-organisms observed in an individual neonatal unit and their sensitivities. Many organisms have been implicated in NEC, including Enterobacteriaceae (e.g., *Escherichia coli, Klebsiella* species), *Pseudomonas, Staphylococcus aureus* (in rare cases, methicillin resistant), *Staphylococcus epidermidis, Clostridium,* enteroviruses, and rotaviruses.[165,168,170] For most cases of NEC, treatment with a broad-spectrum penicillin, such as ampicillin, and an aminoglycoside (e.g., gentamicin) is appropriate.

However, in some nurseries, *S. epidermidis* is the most common cause of neonatal nosocomial infections. Increases in *S. epidermidis*–associated NEC also have been reported. Therefore, vancomycin and an aminoglycoside may be used as routine treatment in some nurseries or in specific patients at risk for *Staphylococcus* infections (e.g., neonates with central catheters or prolonged ICU stays). Vancomycin may be more appropriate than ampicillin because vancomycin has coverage against methicillin-resistant *S. epidermidis,* as well as enterococcal and streptococcal species. Because C.D. has been hospitalized for longer than 1 week, vancomycin and gentamicin may be more appropriate, especially if her neonatal ICU has a high incidence of staphylococcal nosocomial infections. C.D. should be treated with parenteral antibiotics for 10 to 14 days.

Other antibiotic combinations used to treat NEC include cefotaxime and vancomycin, and cefotaxime and ampicillin. The combination of cefotaxime and vancomycin has been shown to prevent severe peritonitis and death in <2,200-g birth-weight neonates with NEC, whereas gentamicin and ampicillin have not. Suppression of aerobic fecal flora by the combination of cefotaxime and vancomycin, but not by ampicillin and gentamicin, may explain these findings.[178]

28. The neonatologist would like to give gentamicin 2.5 mg/kg via the orogastric tube Q 12 hours in addition to parenteral antibiotics. Is there any added benefit to adding enteral gentamicin to the current parenteral antibiotic regimen?

Enteral administration of aminoglycosides does not prevent or change the course of NEC or prevent GI perforation in infants with NEC. In addition, enteral aminoglycosides can be absorbed systemically in neonates with NEC, via the inflamed intestinal mucosa.[168] Systemic absorption may significantly increase the serum concentrations of concomitantly administered parenteral aminoglycosides. Therefore, routine enteral administration of antibiotics such as gentamicin is not warranted for C.D. In select patients and during NEC epidemics, however, prophylactic administration of enteral aminoglycoside antibiotics or vancomycin decreases the incidence of NEC. Unfortunately, prophylactic use of these antibiotics has been associated with the emergence of resistant organisms, which limits their systemic use.[179] Systemic absorption of enterally administered vancomycin also can occur through inflamed intestinal mucosa.

ADDITIONAL ANTIBIOTICS

29. Two days later, C.D. develops peritonitis with ascites, hypotension, metabolic acidosis, neutropenia, and DIC. IV fluids and dopamine are administered for the hypotension, fresh frozen plasma and whole blood are given to treat the coagulopathy, and morphine 0.05 mg/kg IV push Q 4 hours PRN is started for pain control. Free air in the abdomen is observed on abdominal radiograph. Blood and urine cultures have had no growth for 48 hours. What additional antimicrobial coverage should be provided?

Peritonitis secondary to intestinal perforation may be polymicrobial, involving both aerobes and anaerobes. Therefore, an antimicrobial agent with anaerobic activity should be added to C.D.'s current regimen.[166] The two most commonly used agents are clindamycin and metronidazole. Empiric anaerobic coverage in the treatment of NEC without perforation is controversial.[165] Routine use of clindamycin in the treatment of NEC has not decreased the incidence of intestinal gangrene or perforation. In addition, it has been associated with an increased incidence of abdominal strictures.[180]

Complications/Prognosis

30. C.D. is taken urgently to the operating room and 10 cm of necrotic ileum is removed along with the ileocecal valve. What long-term nutritional problems is C.D. likely to develop?

The most common postoperative complications of NEC are intestinal strictures (14%–32%) and short-bowel syndrome (~10%).[181] C.D. is at risk of developing short-bowel syndrome, a condition of malabsorption and malnutrition that results from surgical removal of a significant portion of the small intestine. The most important factors that determine short-bowel syndrome are the length of the remaining small intestine and the presence of the ileocecal valve. Because C.D. has had a majority of her ileum and her ileocecal valve removed, she most likely will suffer from short-bowel syndrome.

Because the terminal ileum is an important site for absorption of vitamins, trace minerals, and nutrients, C.D. will be at risk for decreased absorption of these substances. C.D. also will have a faster GI transit time and diarrhea because her ileocecal valve was removed. (The ileocecal valve plays a major role in controlling intestinal transit time.) Absorption of enterally administered medications also may be decreased in patients with short-bowel syndrome. As C.D. starts to receive most of her nutrition enterally, she should be monitored for fat malabsorption and other nutritional deficiencies (e.g., deficiencies in vitamins A, B_{12}, D, E, and K), and supplemented accordingly.[182]

Owing to advances in earlier diagnosis and aggressive treatment, 56% of VLBW infants and 72% of infants with birth-weight ≥1,000 g with NEC survive.[183] However, infants with NEC are significantly more likely to have neurodevelopmental impairment (e.g., cerebral palsy); those requiring surgical management are at higher risk.[184]

Prevention

31. What could have been done to prevent NEC in C.D.?

Several interventions may decrease the incidence of NEC. Enteral feedings in preterm infants can be withheld for several weeks and parenteral nutrition initiated. Intestinal priming or trophic feeding (i.e., using a small amount of full-strength formula or breast-milk to stimulate GI mucosal development) in addition to parenteral nutrition can improve feeding tolerance and increase GI motility.[185,186] Because breast-milk provides antibodies, growth factors, and cellular immune factors, it may reduce the incidence of NEC. In fact, NEC was six to ten times less common among infants fed human milk exclusively than in those fed formula alone and three times less common in those fed a combination of human milk and formula than in those fed formula alone.[187] In contrast, the use of hyperosmolar formulas or medications can cause osmotic injury to the bowel and may result in NEC. Maternal steroids (commonly used to accelerate fetal lung maturation) can decrease the incidence of NEC due to a maturational effect on the microvillous membranes. Strict infection control measures, such as preventing fecal and oral spread of bacterial pathogens after epidemic outbreaks, also decrease the incidence of NEC.[170]

Probiotics

Probiotics are live, nonpathogenic microbial preparations that colonize the intestine and have a beneficial effect on the health of the host.[188] Probiotic micro-organisms commonly used are strains of lactobacillus and bifidobacterium. Enteral administration of probiotics has been shown to significantly decrease the risk of NEC and death and shorten the time to full feedings in VLBW infants.[189] One major concern is that exposing immunologically immature VLBW infants to probiotics may potentially increase the risk for infections. However, in a recent meta-analysis, no significant risk of sepsis was noted in infants treated with probiotics.[189] Currently, there is no strong evidence to recommend a specific type of probiotic (species, strains, single or combined, live or killed), the timing, dosage, or duration of therapy. In addition, the long-term effects of probiotics for the prevention of NEC in VLBW infants are unknown. Further clinical studies addressing these issues are needed.

NEONATAL SEPSIS AND MENINGITIS

Pathogenesis and Clinical Presentation

32. J.E., a 28-week gestation, 850-g male, was born to a mother with prolonged rupture of membranes (>72 hours). The newborn's mother is febrile with a white blood cell (WBC) count of 20 × 10³/mm³ and differential of 70% segmented neutrophils, 20% bands, 7% lymphocytes, and 3% monocytes. J.E. had Apgar scores of 4 at 1 minute and 3 at 5 minutes after birth. Mechanical ventilation was instituted and J.E. was admitted to the neonatal ICU. Vital signs upon admission were as follows: HR, 190 beats/minute; temperature, 35.8°C; and BP, 56/33 mmHg. Blood and urine cultures are pending. Significant laboratory data include the following: WBC 2,400 cells/mm³ with a differential of 25% segmented neutrophils, 15% bands, 45% lymphocytes, 10% monocytes, 4% eosinophils, and 1% basophils; platelets, 45,000/mm³; and C-reactive protein (CRP), 5 mg/dL. What is the etiology and pathogenesis of neonatal sepsis? What risk factors for sepsis does J.E. have? What clinical signs and laboratory evidence of sepsis are apparent in J.E.?

[SI units: WBC, 2,400 × 10⁶ cells/L with 0.25 neutrophils, 0.15 bands, 0.45 lymphocytes, and 0.1 monocytes; platelets, 45 × 10⁹/L]

Bacterial sepsis significantly contributes to neonatal morbidity and mortality. Neonates, especially preterm newborns, are at increased risk for infections and should be considered immunocompromised. The neonate's decreased immune function (e.g., immature function of neutrophils, lower amounts of immunoglobulin) also results in a reduced ability to localize infections. Once a tissue site becomes infected, bacteria can spread easily, resulting in disseminated disease. In addition, the lack of opsonic antibodies in preterm infants such as J.E. increases the susceptibility to infections caused by bacteria with polysaccharide capsules (e.g., group B streptococcus, *E. coli, Hemophilus influenzae* type B).[190]

The incidence of neonatal sepsis varies from 6 to 9 cases per 1,000 live births, but is higher among low-birth-weight neonates.[191] In VLBW infants with prolonged hospitalization, the incidence increases to 110 to 320 per 1,000.[192] Risk factors (as demonstrated in J.E.) include prematurity, low birth-weight, male gender, and predisposing maternal conditions (e.g., prolonged rupture of membranes, maternal fever, elevated maternal WBC or left shift, chorioamnionitis, and urinary tract infection).[193,194] Despite treatment, mortality rates for neonatal sepsis can be as high as 30% to 50%, with the highest mortality observed in newborns <1,500 g.[195,196] Meningitis occurs as a complication of bacterial sepsis in 10% to 30% of septic neonates[195,196] and has a mortality rate of 20% to 50% depending on the pathogen.[193]

Common Pathogens

The fetal environment within the amniotic membranes is normally sterile until the onset of labor and delivery. Once the membranes are ruptured, the infant may be at risk for colonization of micro-organisms from the maternal genital tract. Many of these organisms do not cause infection in the mother, but may be detrimental to the infant. Early onset neonatal sepsis (sepsis that presents during the first 5–7 days of life) usually is caused by organisms acquired from the maternal genital tract. The most common pathogens found in early-onset neonatal sepsis are group B streptococcus (50%) and *E. coli* (20%). Other primary pathogens include *Listeria monocytogenes, Enterococcus,* and other Gram-negative bacilli (e.g., *H. influenzae, Klebsiella pneumoniae*). Late-onset sepsis (sepsis presenting after 5–7 days postnatal age) usually is caused by these primary organisms or by nosocomial pathogens, such as coagulase-negative staphylococci (CONS), particularly *S. epidermidis, S. aureus, Pseudomonas* species, anaerobes, and *Candida* species.[195,197] The major risk factor for nosocomial septicemia is the presence of IV catheters (umbilical and central).[198] Other risk factors include low birth-weight, prolonged hospital stay, prior antibiotic use, parenteral hyperalimentation, lipid emulsion, invasive procedures, and the presence of other indwelling devices (e.g., ETTs, ventriculoperitoneal shunts).[192,193]

Over the past two decades, CONS such as *S. epidermidis*, have emerged as the most common pathogen for late-onset neonatal nosocomial septicemia, causing 55% to 58% of cases.[198,199] This emergence is most likely due to the increased survival of extremely premature neonates with a resultant prolonged hospital stay and an increase in the associated risks of infection (i.e., placement of umbilical and central venous catheters and arterial lines, use of hyperalimentation and intralipid). More disturbing, however, is the reported persistence of coagulase-negative staphylococcal bacteremia, despite appropriate treatment in low-birth-weight neonates without central venous catheters.[200]

Neonatal sepsis may present with nonspecific or subtle signs, especially in VLBW infants.[193] The most common signs are poor feeding, temperature instability, lethargy, or apnea.[193,196] Other signs of neonatal sepsis include glucose instability (hypoglycemia or hyperglycemia), tachycardia, dyspnea or cyanosis, tachypnea, diarrhea, vomiting, feeding intolerance, abdominal distension, metabolic acidosis, and abnormal WBC.[193] Clinical signs and laboratory evidence of neonatal sepsis observed in J.E. include tachycardia (HR, 190 beats/minute), hypothermia (temperature 35.8°C), leukopenia (WBC, 2.4 × $10^3/mm^3$), neutropenia (absolute neutrophil count of $960/mm^3$), a left shift in the differential (i.e., an immature-to-total neutrophil ratio [I/T] of 0.38), thrombocytopenia (platelets, $45,000/mm^3$), and an elevated CRP (5 mg/dL). Hypothermia is more common than fever in neonatal sepsis, especially in preterm newborns. However, if fever is present, it is strongly associated with bacterial infection. Neutropenia, especially with a left shift (as seen in J.E.) can be a sign of WBC depletion from bone marrow owing to overwhelming sepsis. An elevated WBC also can indicate a neonatal infection, but may be less specific.[194] The I/T ratio, defined as band forms plus any earlier cells divided by the total neutrophil count (including early cells), has been shown to be useful in diagnosing neonatal sepsis. An I/T ratio of <0.3 is normal.[194] CRP, an acute phase reactant protein associated with tissue injury in response to an inflammatory process, may also be included as part of a sepsis workup. A CRP level >1 mg/dL indicates inflammation and possible infection.[194] Late signs of neonatal infection include jaundice, hepatosplenomegaly, and petechiae.[193] A bulging fontanel, posturing, or seizures indicate meningitis, although these CNS signs are not always present when meningitis exists.

Bacterial meningitis should always be considered in infants with neonatal sepsis. The definitive diagnostic method for bacterial meningitis is lumbar puncture. Lumbar puncture should be performed in infants with a positive blood culture, abnormal neurologic signs, an elevated WBC or left shift, or the presence of bacterial antigen in the urine.[201] The cerebrospinal fluid (CSF) should be tested with a Gram stain, cell counts with differential, glucose and protein levels, and bacterial culture. Neonatal CSF cell counts are difficult to interpret because values may overlap with normal neonatal values. The diagnosis of neonatal sepsis is confirmed by isolation of the pathogen from blood, urine, CSF, or other body sites. Latex agglutination tests that detect antigens (e.g., bacterial cell wall fragments) of group B streptococcus, *E. coli, S. pneumonia, N. meningitidis,* and *H. influenzae* type B in body fluids can facilitate a prompt diagnosis, especially in patients who previously were treated with antibiotics.[202]

Treatment of Sepsis

Antibiotic Selection

33. What antibiotic regimen should be prescribed for J.E.?

Empiric treatment with appropriate IV antibiotics must be initiated immediately in J.E. Significant morbidity or fatality would occur if antibiotics were withheld until a diagnosis was confirmed by culture results (in 24–72 hours). This is especially true in patients in whom meningitis is suspected. The initial empiric antibiotic treatment of choice for early onset neonatal sepsis and meningitis is ampicillin plus an aminoglycoside. These antibiotics are used because they (a) are bactericidal against the common neonatal pathogens; (b) penetrate into the CNS; (c) are relatively safe; and (d) have proven clinical efficacy. If group B streptococcus is suspected, antibiotic therapy should be switched to high-dose penicillin G. Penicillin is preferred over ampicillin because of its higher activity against group B streptococcus.[197]

Therefore, ampicillin 45 mg Q 12 hours IV plus an aminoglycoside (e.g., gentamicin 3 mg Q 24 hours IV) should be started in J.E. for suspected neonatal sepsis and possible meningitis. Meningitic doses of ampicillin should be used in J.E. until meningitis can be ruled out. Ampicillin is active against group B streptococci, group D streptococci, *Listeria,* and most strains of *E. coli.* Aminoglycoside antibiotics (e.g., gentamicin or tobramycin) usually are active against gram-negative bacilli. In addition, aminoglycosides may provide synergy with ampicillin against *Listeria* and group B streptococci.[194] Selection of the specific aminoglycoside should be determined by antibiotic resistance patterns within the neonatal ICU. Amikacin should be reserved for gram-negative organisms resistant to gentamicin and tobramycin. Aminoglycoside regimens need to be designed to achieve safe and therapeutic serum concentrations (gentamicin and tobramycin peak 6–8 mcg/mL, trough <2 mcg/mL; amikacin peaks 20–30 mcg/mL, troughs <10 mcg/mL).[8,49]

In some nurseries, a third-generation cephalosporin (e.g., cefotaxime [Claforan] or ceftriaxone [Rocephin]), instead of an aminoglycoside, is added to ampicillin for initial empiric treatment of early-onset neonatal sepsis and meningitis.[197] The spectrum of activity of these third-generation cephalosporins includes many gram-negative organisms and group B streptococci. However, third-generation cephalosporins do not have sufficient activity against *Listeria* or group D streptococci. Therefore, these agents must be used in combination with ampicillin for empiric neonatal therapy. As mentioned, ceftriaxone should be avoided in neonates with hyperbilirubinemia owing to bilirubin displacement from albumin-binding sites. Ceftriaxone has also been associated with sludging in the gallbladder and cholestasis.[8] In addition, calcium-ceftriaxone precipitates have been found in the lungs and kidneys of neonates when ceftriaxone was administered with calcium-containing solutions. Several fatalities have been reported; ceftriaxone should not be administered within 48 hours of calcium-containing solutions or products.[8] Hence, cefotaxime is the preferred cephalosporin for neonatal use.

The third-generation cephalosporins have advantages over the aminoglycosides, including better CNS penetration, the elimination of serum concentration measurements, and less nephrotoxicity. However, these cephalosporins do not significantly improve clinical or microbiological endpoints compared with the standard ampicillin and gentamicin regimen. Furthermore, extensive use of the third-generation cephalosporins in neonatal ICUs may lead to rapid emergence of resistant gram-negative bacilli (e.g., *Enterobacter cloacae, Pseudomonas aeruginosa,* and *Serratia* species) and vancomycin resistance in enterococci. In contrast, gentamicin has not been associated with rapid development of these resistant strains.[197] Thus, combinations such as ampicillin and cefotaxime should be reserved for the following situations: (a) neonatal ICUs where aminoglycoside resistance to Gram-negative enteric bacilli is of concern, (b) neonatal ICUs where serum concentrations of aminoglycosides cannot be measured, and (c) specific neonates in whom aminoglycoside therapy could be of concern (e.g., neonates with known renal failure).[197]

Therapy for late-onset sepsis or meningitis is directed toward nosocomial pathogens plus the primary pathogens of early-onset infection (see Question 32). Selection of initial antibiotic therapy should consider the specific neonatal ICU's nosocomial pathogen and antibiotic resistance patterns, as well as the neonate's risk factors, clinical condition, and previous antibiotic therapy.[203] CONS is now the most common pathogen of late-onset neonatal nosocomial septicemia. Because of the high incidence of methicillin-resistant CONS (as high as 80% in some neonatal ICUs),[203] vancomycin has been used as the drug of choice for empiric therapy for suspected late-onset neonatal sepsis. However, widespread use of vancomycin has led to the emergence of vancomycin-resistant enterococci. Therefore, the routine use of vancomycin as empiric therapy for nosocomial neonatal sepsis should be discouraged. In two retrospective studies, the highly selective use of vancomycin for neonatal CONS septicemia results in low morbidity and mortality, while significantly reducing vancomycin use.[199,204] Guidelines for the selective use of vancomycin should be tailored according to individual neonatal ICU's nosocomial pathogens, susceptibility patterns, and patient risk factors, clinical condition, and antibiotic history. Therefore, if J.E. had a central venous catheter and presented with a late-onset sepsis, initial antibiotic therapy should include an aminoglycoside (for gram-negative coverage) plus either an antistaphylococcal penicillin (e.g., nafcillin, methicillin) or vancomycin (for activity against *S. aureus* and *S. epidermidis*). Vancomycin is used in place of the antistaphylococcal penicillin in neonatal units with methicillin-resistant *S. aureus* and for selective use to cover *S. epidermidis* (a CONS) as outlined.[197,203]

Linezolid, a new oxazolidinone, has activity against staphylococci, streptococci, and enterococci. This drug has been approved by the FDA for treatment of gram-positive infections in neonatal and pediatric patients and is available as IV and oral formulations. A study comparing linezolid with vancomycin for the treatment of resistant gram-positive infections in neonates reported no significant difference in overall clinical cure rate between the linezolid-treated (84%) and the vancomycin-treated groups (77%). About 60% of these infections were due to CONS with similar eradication rates between groups (linezolid 88% versus vancomycin 100%). Linezolid was well-tolerated and had fewer drug-related adverse events than vancomycin.[205] Because of limited studies in term and preterm neonates, linezolid should be reserved for those infants who failed or are intolerant to vancomycin therapy for the treatment of staphylococcal infections. If *Pseudomonas* infection is suspected, an antipseudomonal penicillin (e.g., piperacillin, ticarcillin, mezlocillin) combined with an aminoglycoside should be used for their synergistic bacterial activity.

For systemic fungal infections, amphotericin B (with or without flucytosine) is considered the initial treatment of choice.[196] Because of the high incidence of Candida species colonization (up to 60%) with up to 20% progressing to invasive fungal infections in VLBW infants, prophylactic antifungal agents may be used to prevent candida colonization and infection in these infants. In a multicenter randomized trial, prophylactic fluconazole in preterm neonates significantly decreased the incidence of fungal colonization and invasive fungal disease in the fluconazole-treated infants compared to placebo.[206] Overall mortality, adverse events and emergence of resistant candida species were similar in both groups. Despite these findings, routine use of prophylactic antifungal therapy is not recommended and should be reserved for those units with high incidence of fungal infections. Because uncommon organisms are not suspected in J.E., the regimen of ampicillin 45 mg IV Q 12 hours plus gentamicin 3 mg IV Q 24 hours is appropriate.

Dosage and Route of Administration

Dosage regimens for the antimicrobial agents commonly used in neonates[8,51,52,207,208] are listed in Tables 94-5 and 94-8. Dosing guidelines for tobramycin and netilmicin are the same as gentamicin (Table 94-5). The IV route is preferred for treatment of all septic neonates. If the IV route is not available, the IM route can be used in neonates with sufficient muscle mass, adequate peripheral perfusion, and a normal, stable coagulation status. Oral administration almost never is used in serious neonatal infections because GI drug absorption is extremely variable at this age. Meningitic doses of antibiotics should be used for the treatment of any seriously ill neonate until meningitis is excluded by negative CSF cultures.

Extended-interval aminoglycoside dosing (also known as once-daily dosing or single-daily dosing) has been widely used in the adult population. Aminoglycoside antibiotics display concentration-dependent killing of bacteria. Rationale for the use of extended-interval aminoglycoside dosing include: (a) enhancement of bacterial killing by providing a higher peak serum concentration to minimal inhibitory concentration ratio, (b) provision of a prolonged postantibiotic effect, and (c) minimization of adaptive postexposure microbial resistance.[209] In meta-analyses of clinical studies in adults, extended-interval aminoglycoside dosing seems to have similar efficacy, without increased toxicity, compared with traditional multiple daily dosing.[210] In addition, extended-interval aminoglycoside dosing can reduce costs associated with drug wastage, administration time, and therapeutic monitoring.[211]

Because of these beneficial effects, the use of extended-interval aminoglycoside dosing has been studied in the pediatric population. Most studies have included term or near-term newborns (i.e., gestational age $\geq$34 weeks).[209] As expected, the use of extended-interval aminoglycoside dosing resulted in higher peak and lower trough serum concentrations in

Table 94-8 Antimicrobial Dosage Regimens for Neonates: Dosages and Intervals of Administration

Drug	Weight <1,200 g[52]	Weight 1,200–2,000 g		Weight >2,000 g	
	0–4 Weeks[a] (mg/kg)	0–7 Days[a] (mg/kg)	>7 Days[a] (mg/kg)	0–7 Days[a] (mg/kg)	>7 Days[a] (mg/kg)
Amphotericin B					
Deoxycholate	1 Q 24 hr	1 Q 24 hr	1 Q 24 hr	1 Q 24 hr	1 Q 24 hr
Lipid complex/Liposomal	5 Q 24 hr	5 Q 24 hr	5 Q 24 hr	5 Q 24 hr	5 Q 24 hr
Ampicillin					
Meningitis	50 Q 12 hr	50 Q 12 hr	50 Q 8 hr	50 Q 8 hr	50 Q 6 hr
Other diseases	25 Q 12 hr	25 Q 12 hr	25 Q 8 hr	25 Q 8 hr	25 Q 6 hr
Cefazolin	25 Q 12 hr	25 Q 12 hr	25 Q 12 hr	25 Q 12 hr	25 Q 8 hr
Cefepime	30 Q 12 hr	30 Q 12 hr	30 Q 12 hr[c]	30 Q 12 hr	30 Q 12 hr[c]
Cefotaxime[d]	50 Q 12 hr	50 Q 12 hr	50 Q 8 hr	50 Q 12 hr	50 Q 8 hr
Ceftazidime[d]	50 Q 12 hr	50 Q 12 hr	50 Q 8 hr	50 Q 12 hr	50 Q 8 hr
Ceftriaxone[d]	25 Q 24 hr	25 Q 24 hr	50 Q 24 hr	25 Q 24 hr	50 Q 24 hr
Chloramphenicol	22 Q 24 hr	25 Q 24 hr	25 Q 24 hr	25 Q 24 hr	25 Q 12 hr
Clindamycin	5 Q 12 hr	5 Q 12 hr	5 Q 8 hr	5 Q 8 hr	5 Q 6 hr
Erythromycin	10 Q 12 hr	10 Q 12 hr	10 Q 8 hr	10 Q 12 hr	13.3 Q 8 hr
Fluconazole	6 Q 72 hr	6 Q 72 hr	6 Q 48 hr	6 Q 24 hr	6 Q 24 hr
Linezolid	10 Q 12 hr	10 Q 12 hr	10 Q 8 hr	10 Q 8 hr	10 Q 8 hr
Meropenem[d]	20 Q 12 hr	20 Q 12 hr	20 Q 8 hr	20 Q 12 hr	20 Q 8 hr
Metronidazole	7.5 Q 48 hr	7.5 Q 24 hr	7.5 Q 12 hr	7.5 Q 12 hr	15 Q 12 hr
Oxacillin	25 Q 12 hr	25 Q 12 hr	25 Q 8 hr	25 Q 8 hr	37.5 Q 6 hr
Nafcillin	25 Q 12 hr	25 Q 12 hr	25 Q 8 hr	25 Q 8 hr	37.5 Q 6 hr
Penicillin G					
Meningitis	50,000 U Q 12 hr	50,000 U Q 12 hr	75,000 U Q 8 hr	50,000 U Q 8 hr	50,000 U Q 6 hr
Other diseases	25,000 U Q 12 hr	25,000 U Q 12 hr	25,000 U Q 8 hr	25,000 U Q 8 hr	25,000 U Q 6 hr
Piperacillin/tazobactam	50 Q 12 hr	50 Q 12 hr	100 Q 8 hr	100 Q 12 hr	100 Q 8 hr
Ticarcillin or Ticarcillin/clavulanate	75 Q 12 hr	75 Q 12 hr	75 Q 8 hr	75 Q 8 hr	75 Q 6 hr
Vancomycin	15 Q 24 hr[b]	20 Q 24 hr	15 Q 12 hr	15 Q 12 hr	15 Q 8 hr

[a] Postnatal age.
[b] If weight <750 g and postnatal age <14 days, use 10–12.5 mg/kg Q 24 hr.
[c] Cefepime should be given at 30 mg/kg/dose Q 12 hr for the first 2 weeks of life then increase to 50 mg/kg/dose Q 12 hr (or 50 mg/kg/dose Q 8 hr for *Pseudomonas* infections or meningitis.
[d] Higher dosage may be needed for meningitis.
Adapted with permission from Bradley JS, Nelson JD. Nelson's pocket book of pediatric antimicrobial therapy, 16th ed. Buenos Aires, Argentina: Alliance for World Wide Editing, 2006:23; incorporating references 8, 208.

these neonates compared with traditional multiple-daily dosing. However, neonatal studies have not established optimal regimens to achieve the best peak serum concentration to minimal inhibitory concentration ratio. A meta-analysis in neonates >32 weeks' gestation confirmed these findings and reported no nephrotoxicity or ototoxicity in either group.[212] Several clinical trials have evaluated the use of once-daily dosing of gentamicin in preterm infants <32 weeks' gestation; however, these studies evaluated serum gentamicin concentrations and potential adverse effects and not clinical efficacy or cure rates.[213–215] Furthermore, most studies in neonates used extended-interval aminoglycoside dosing for short periods of time, for example, during the workup to rule out neonatal sepsis (i.e., 72-hour duration). Studies included only a few neonates, who received extended-interval aminoglycoside dosing to actually treat documented neonatal infections. Other neonatal-specific factors, such as the neonate's immature immune function and a potential decreased postantibiotic effect, have not been adequately addressed. Therefore, large, well-designed studies evaluating the clinical efficacy and safety of extended-interval aminoglycoside dosing for the treatment of gram-negative infections in neonates are required before routine use can be recommended.

Once a pathogen is isolated, the antimicrobial susceptibilities should be evaluated and the drug therapy modified appropriately. Blood, CSF, or urine cultures should be repeated to document bacterial sterilization after 24 to 48 hours of appropriate therapy. J.E. should be evaluated carefully for the development of serious bacterial complications such as meningitis, osteomyelitis, abscess formation, or endocarditis.

Duration of Therapy

As long as there is no evidence of meningitis or other focal infection (e.g., abscess formation), the duration of therapy for most systemic bacterial infections is 7 to 10 days (or approximately 5–7 days after significant clinical improvement). Antibiotic therapy may need to be continued for 14 to 21 days if the neonate's clinical response is slow or if multiple organ systems are involved.[196] If cultures are negative at 72 hours and the infant does not have any clinical or laboratory signs of sepsis, antibiotics can be discontinued. In neonates presenting with signs of severe infection followed by improvement after initiation of antibiotics, therapy may be continued despite negative cultures.

Treatment of Meningitis

34. How should J.E. be treated if meningitis is suspected?

Antibiotic Selection

The major pathogens causing neonatal sepsis also are the primary pathogens that cause neonatal meningitis. Seventy-five percent of neonatal meningitis is caused by group B streptococcus and *E. coli; L. monocytogenes* is the third most common organism.[196] Initial empiric antibiotic therapy of choice consists of ampicillin plus an aminoglycoside.[193] Ampicillin plus a third-generation cephalosporin (cefotaxime or ceftriaxone) may be used empirically for early-onset neonatal meningitis in situations as outlined previously for early-onset neonatal sepsis (see Question 33). In addition, because of their greater CSF penetration compared with the aminoglycosides, the combination of a third-generation cephalosporin with ampicillin may be preferred when the CSF Gram's stain indicates a gram-negative infection. Initial empiric antibiotic treatment of late-onset meningitis should follow guidelines similar to those for late-onset sepsis with consideration of nosocomial as well as primary pathogens (see Question 33). As with neonatal sepsis, once an organism is recovered from the CSF, the most appropriate antibiotic is selected based on susceptibility.

Duration of Therapy

If CSF cultures are positive, repeat CSF cultures should be obtained daily or every other day in J.E. to document when the CSF becomes sterilized. The duration of therapy for neonatal meningitis depends on the clinical response and duration of positive CSF cultures after therapy is initiated. Appropriate antibiotics should be continued for a minimum of 14 days after the CSF is sterilized. This is equivalent to a duration of antibiotic therapy for a minimum of 21 days for gram-negative organisms and at least 14 days for gram-positive pathogens.[193,196,216] As a general rule, it takes longer to sterilize the CSF of neonates infected by gram-negative enteric bacilli (72 hours) than those infected by gram-positive bacteria (36–48 hours).[193] Although surgical placement of a ventricular reservoir for intraventricular administration of an antibiotic (usually an aminoglycoside) has been used to treat meningitis not responding to IV antimicrobial therapy, the Neonatal Meningitis Cooperative Study group reported no beneficial effect of this method of administration in infants with gram-negative meningitis. In fact, infants treated with intraventricular gentamicin had a threefold increase in mortality rate compared with infants treated solely on IV antibiotics[196,217] (see Chapter 58).

Intravenous Immune Globulin

35. On day 2 of life, J.E.'s blood culture is reported as positive for group B streptococcus. His current vital signs are as follows: HR, 135 beats/minute; temperature, 37°C; and BP, 59/40 mmHg. Laboratory data include the following: WBC, 7,000 cells/mm^3 with a differential of 53% segmented neutrophils, 15% bands, 25% lymphocytes, and 7% monocytes; platelets, 100,000/mm^3. J.E.'s ventilatory settings are slightly improved. What is the role of IV immune globulin (IVIG) in a patient like J.E.?

[SI units: WBC, 7,000 × 10^6 cells/L with 0.53 neutrophils, 0.15 bands, 0.25 lymphocytes, and 0.07 monocytes; platelets, 100 × 10^9/L]

Rationale

Neonatal humoral immunity is provided primarily by transplacental transport of maternal immunoglobulin (Ig)G to the fetus. Active transfer starts at 17 weeks' gestation and increases with gestational age. By 33 weeks' gestation, fetal IgG levels are equal to maternal IgG.[218] Neonates born before 33 weeks' gestation have very low IgG concentrations. In addition, because of the neonate's poor antibody response to antigenic stimuli, these low concentrations of IgG can decrease further during the first few weeks of life.[219] Low IgG concentrations, as well as a lack of micro-organism–specific antibodies, and opsonic antibody activity against the polysaccharide capsules of certain bacteria (i.e., group B streptococcus, *E. coli,* and *H. influenzae*) significantly contribute to the neonate's increased susceptibility to infections.[219] Exogenous administration of IVIG may correct low IgG serum concentrations and improve neonatal host defenses. Therefore, administration of IVIG has been proposed for the prevention and treatment of neonatal infections.

Efficacy

The efficacy of IVIG as an adjunct to antimicrobial therapy for the prevention and treatment of neonatal sepsis has been assessed in numerous studies. However, comparisons between studies are difficult because of differences in study design, sample size, dosage regimens (dose and duration of therapy), specific product used, pathogen-specific antibodies, lot-to-lot variability, inclusion criteria, and outcome measures. In addition, studies assessing IVIG for treatment of neonatal sepsis differ in the specific infecting organism and the rates and severity of infection.[190] Despite these differences, several meta-analyses have been conducted to try to summarize the data evaluating the effectiveness of IVIG for prophylaxis and treatment of neonatal sepsis.

An early evaluation of published articles assessing prophylaxis of IVIG concluded that its effectiveness depended on the pathogen-specific antibody activity of the individual product used. Other evaluations have found encouraging results or no clear evidence of benefit for preterm infants.[190] In a recent systematic review of 19 studies (representing approximately 5,000 preterm infants) prophylactic IVIG was associated with a significant, but very small reduction in sepsis (3%) and serious infections (4%). However, NEC, IVH, length of hospital stay, and mortality were not significantly affected.[220] Therefore, the use of prophylactic IVIG is of marginal clinical benefit and thus cannot be routinely recommended.

Few studies have evaluated IVIG as adjunctive treatment with antibiotics for treatment of neonatal sepsis. In a Cochrane review of 13 studies of suspected or proven infections in >500 neonates, IVIG treatment was associated with reductions in length of hospitalization (for term infants) and mortality. However, the reduction in mortality for clinically suspected infections was of borderline significance.[221] Owing to the lack of power of this meta-analysis, further studies are needed to determine the effectiveness of IVIG for the treatment of suspected or proven neonatal infections. Clinically, the routine use of IVIG for suspected or proven infections cannot be recommended. IVIG can be considered for select patients with proven infections.

Large, well-designed, prospective studies are required to determine the optimal IVIG dosage regimen, including dose per kilogram, number of doses, and timing of treatment. Studies of the cost-effectiveness of IVIG are also needed. Unlabeled or low concentrations of antibodies against the primary pathogens of neonatal sepsis may limit the use of commercial IVIG preparations. However, the use of preselected lots of IVIG that possess antibodies against specific neonatal pathogens may be of benefit. Other immunologic agents, such as monoclonal antibodies and hyperimmune immunoglobulin preparations, may be more effective and currently are being investigated.

Initiation of Therapy

At this time, routine use of IVIG for all newborns to prevent or treat neonatal sepsis is not indicated.[190,219] However, treatment with IVIG should be considered in septic neonates who are not responding to standard antibiotic treatment and supportive care.[190] Because J.E. has responded to antibiotic therapy, as evidenced by his improvement in vital signs, WBC, differential, platelet count, and ventilatory settings, IVIG would not be indicated.

Dosing, Administration, and Adverse Effects

36. IVIG 500 mg/kg IV push weekly for four doses has been ordered for J.E. because of prescriber preference. How should IVIG be administered and what should be monitored for adverse effects?

The optimal dose of IVIG has not been established. The National Institute of Child Health and Human Development study used prophylactic doses of 900 mg/kg for neonates 501 to 1,000 g and 700 mg/kg for neonates 1,001 to 1,500 g to attain IgG serum concentrations of 700 mg/dL.[222] Doses were repeated every 2 weeks. Trough concentrations after the first dose were ≥700 mg/dL in approximately 50% of the neonates. Only 13% of neonates had all trough concentrations at or above the target concentration during the study period.[222] These findings suggest that the clinical use of these doses or even slightly higher doses would be adequate. However, the optimal total IgG serum concentration for treatment or prophylaxis of neonatal sepsis has not been established. In addition, the amount of specific immunoglobulins directed against the primary neonatal pathogens may be more important. Although many dosing regimens have been studied,[190,219,222] doses of 500 to 1,000 mg/kg are commonly used. Some institutions repeat treatment every 2 weeks.[190] Doses >1,000 mg/kg may not be more effective and may have toxic effects. Suppression of opsonophagocytosis and decreased bacterial clearance have been reported with high-dose IVIG in neonatal animal models.[223]

Although the dose of IVIG prescribed for J.E. is reasonable, IVIG should never be administered via IV push. Rapid IV administration may result in significant adverse effects. Administration rates for IVIG are product specific and most neonatal doses should be infused IV over 2 to 6 hours. Because anaphylaxis can occur, slower initial infusion rates are recommended. In this case, the specific IVIG product used in J.E.'s neonatal ICU should be identified, and an appropriate text[8] or the package insert should be consulted for proper administration rates. Neonates receiving IVIG should be monitored routinely for adverse effects such as tachycardia, dyspnea, hypotension, hypertension, fever, flushing, irritability, tremors, restlessness, and emesis.[222] These reactions may be related to the rate of infusion and generally resolve when the infusion rate is decreased or when the infusion is discontinued temporarily. In the National Institute of Child Health and Human Development study, the overall rate of NEC in the IVIG group (12%) was not statistically higher than in the control group (9.5%). However, a significantly greater number of NEC cases occurred during Phase 2 of the study in the IVIG group (12%) compared with placebo (8.3%).[222] Therefore, because of the potential association with NEC, indiscriminate use of IVIG is not warranted. Other adverse effects may be identified as neonatal investigations continue with IVIG use.

CONGENITAL INFECTIONS

TORCH Titers

37. S.Y., a 2,000-g girl, was born at 34 weeks' gestational age by vaginal delivery. She was born at another institution and transferred to your hospital on day 3 of life. S.Y.'s birth was complicated by prolonged rupture of membranes (>72 hours), a difficult labor and delivery, and fetal distress requiring a fetal scalp monitor. On physical examination, S.Y. is an extremely irritable newborn with RR of 60 breaths/minute. Several vesicular skin lesions located on the scalp and around the eyes are noted. Conjunctivitis also is present. S.Y. is placed on supplemental oxygen and ABGs are obtained. Blood, CSF, and urine were cultured for bacteria and fungus and S.Y. was started on ampicillin 100 mg IV Q 12 hours and gentamicin 5 mg IV Q 12 hours to rule out sepsis. Antimicrobial therapy will not be altered until culture results are available. What other tests and/or information are needed for S.Y. at this time?

Certain bacteria, viruses, and protozoa can cause fetal infections that may result in fetal death, congenital anomalies, serious CNS sequelae, intrauterine growth retardation, or preterm birth.[224] The primary organisms that cause these infections can be remembered by the acronym, TORCH: *t*oxoplasmosis; *o*ther (i.e., syphilis, gonorrhea, hepatitis B, listeria); *r*ubella; *c*ytomegalovirus; *h*erpes simplex. Because of the potential severity of these diseases, newborns who display any signs of infection (e.g., irritability, fever, thrombocytopenia, hepatosplenomegaly) need to be evaluated for these intrauterine and perinatally acquired infections. The diagnosis of each of these infections should be considered separately. A complete infectious disease workup should include specific antibody titer measurements to the suspected organisms rather than sending a single serum sample for TORCH titer measurement.[224]

Primary clinical manifestations and treatment[8,224–228] for selected congenital infections are listed in Table 94-9. The clinical signs of these infections may overlap, and concurrent infection with two or more micro-organisms is possible. The detection of congenital infections often is difficult because many neonates are asymptomatic at birth. Therefore, prenatal maternal screening and accurate evaluation of maternal history for risk factors are very important. Other organisms that can cause congenitally acquired infections include human immunodeficiency virus (HIV), human parvovirus, varicella-zoster virus, and measles virus.[224]

When congenital infections are suspected, appropriate diagnostic tests for each suspected organism should be performed. Viral cultures of the urine, oropharynx, nasopharynx, stool, and conjunctiva and a complete maternal history along with the results of recent maternal vaginal cultures also should be obtained.[224] Measurements of IgM levels specific for each possible organism under consideration are also recommended. S.Y. has signs of a congenital infection (respiratory distress, skin rash, and conjunctivitis). Because of the nature of S.Y.'s skin rash (i.e., vesicular), infection with the herpes simplex virus (HSV) should be highly suspected. Skin vesicles, conjunctiva, oropharynx, nasopharynx, rectum, urine, and CSF

Table 94-9 Selected Congenital and Perinatal Infections in the Neonate[8,224–228]

Organism	*Primary Clinical Manifestations*	*Treatment of Proven or Highly Probable Disease*
Herpes simplex[a,b]	Cutaneous vesicles, keratoconjunctivitis, microcephaly, CNS infection, hepatitis, pneumonitis, prematurity, respiratory distress, sepsis, convulsion, chorioretinitis	*Acyclovir:* 20 mg/kg Q 8 hr IV ×14–21 days *Ocular Involvement:* Acyclovir IV plus topical therapy: 1–2% trifluridine, 1% iododeoxyuridine, or 3% vidarabine
Toxoplasmosis	Chorioretinitis, ventriculomegaly, microcephaly, hydrocephaly, intracranial calcifications, ascites, hepatosplenomegaly, lymphadenopathy, jaundice, anemia, mental retardation	Sulfadiazine 100 mg/kg/day in two divided doses PO for 1 year *and* pyrimethamine 2 mg/kg/day ×2 days then 1 mg/kg/day for 2–6 months then 1 mg/kg QOD to complete 1 year of therapy *and* folinic acid (leucovorin) 5–10 mg 3 times/week ×1 year
Treponema pallidum[a]	*Early:* Osteochondritis, periostitis, hepatosplenomegaly, skin rash (maculopapular or vesiculobullous), rhinitis, meningitis, IUGR, jaundice, hepatitis, anemia, thrombocytopenia, chorioretinitis *Late:* Hutchinson's triad (interstitial keratitis, VIIIth-nerve deafness, Hutchinson's teeth), mental retardation, hydrocephalus, saddle nose, mulberry molars	Aqueous crystalline penicillin G ×10–14 days IV (preferred) or IM: ≤7 days postnatal age: 50,000 U/kg Q 12 hr >7 days postnatal age: 50,000 U/kg Q 8 hr *OR* Procaine penicillin G 50,000 U/kg/day IM Q 24 hr ×10–14 days
Hepatitis B[c]	Prematurity; usually asymptomatic; long-term effects include chronic hepatitis, cirrhosis, liver failure, hepatocellular carcinoma	*Perinatal exposure (maternal HbsAg-positive):* HBIG 0.5 mL IM and hepatitis B vaccine IM (different IM sites) within 12 hours after birth; repeat hepatitis B vaccine at 1 and 6 months
Rubella	*Early:* IUGR, retinopathy, hypotonia, hepatosplenomegaly, thrombocytopenic purpura, bone lesions, cardiac effects *Late:* Hearing loss, mental retardation, diabetes *Rare:* Myocarditis, glaucoma, microcephaly, hepatitis, anemia	Supportive care
Cytomegalovirus	Petechiae, hepatosplenomegaly, jaundice, prematurity, IUGR, increased liver enzymes, hyperbilirubinemia, anemia, thrombocytopenia, interstitial pneumonitis, microcephaly, chorioretinitis, intracranial calcifications *Late:* Hearing loss, mental retardation, learning and motor abnormalities, visual disturbances	IV ganciclovir (optimal dose and duration not established; preliminary data suggests doses of 15 mg/kg/day divided Q 12 hr)
Neisseria gonorrhoeae[a]	Ophthalmia neonatorum, scalp abscess, sepsis, arthritis, meningitis, endocarditis	*Nondisseminated (including ophthalmia neonatorum):* Ceftriaxone 25–50 mg/kg IV or IM ×1 (maximum dose: 125 mg); alternative for ophthalmic neonatorum: cefotaxime 100 mg/kg IM or IV ×1; use saline eye irrigations for ophthalmia neonatorum *Disseminated:* Ceftriaxone 25–50 mg/kg IV or IM Q 24 hr; cefotaxime 25–50 mg/kg IV or IM Q 12 hr Duration of therapy: • Arthritis or septicemia: 7 days • Meningitis: 10–14 days Use cefotaxime if hyperbilirubinemic

[a]See Chapter 65.
[b]See Chapter 72.
[c]See Chapter 73.
CNS, central nervous system; HBIG, hepatitis B immune globulin; HbsAg, hepatitis B surface antigen; IM, intramuscular; IUGR, intrauterine growth retardation; IV, intravenous; QOD, every other day.

should be cultured for HSV and other organisms known to cause congenital infections. Rapid diagnostic testing using tissue scrapings from vesicles and fluorescein-conjugated monoclonal HSV antibody can also be performed. Other appropriate tests for the diagnosis and workup of suspected congenital infections also should be performed (e.g., liver enzymes, prothrombin time, partial thromboplastin time, EEG, computed tomography scan [CT], or magnetic resonance imaging [MRI]).[224]

Congenital Herpes

38. Upon investigation, it is discovered that S.Y.'s mother has genital herpes. This infection is her first known genital HSV episode and was accompanied by fever and headache. S.Y.'s mother had herpes genital lesions present during the vaginal delivery of S.Y. What are risk factors for HSV infection in S.Y.? What interventions could have lowered S.Y.'s risk for HSV?

The incidence of neonatal HSV infection is approximately 1 in 3,200 live births (i.e., ~1,500 estimated new cases each year) in the United States.[229,230] Neonatal HSV may be acquired in utero by either transplacental or ascending vaginal and cervical infections, perinatally via passage through a birth canal with active herpes lesions, or postnatally.[230] Most congenital HSV infections (85%) are acquired during passage through the birth canal in the intrapartum period; 5% are acquired in utero and 10% postnatally through close contact.[230] Ascending infections are more likely to occur with prolonged rupture of membranes. Factors that increased the risk of HSV in S.Y. include primary maternal infection during delivery, prolonged rupture of membranes, presence of active lesions at vaginal birth, and use of a fetal scalp monitor during active herpes infection.[229,231] The most important of these risk factors is primary maternal genital HSV infection at the time of delivery. Neonates born vaginally to these women are ten times more likely to develop HSV infections than neonates born vaginally to women with recurrent HSV infection (33%–50% risk of HSV versus 3%–5%).[228] Identification of newborns at high risk for HSV is difficult, however, because most women who give birth to HSV-infected neonates have asymptomatic or unrecognized HSV infection at the time of delivery. These women also have negative histories for HSV genital infection.

In women with active genital herpes lesions, delivery by cesarean section can reduce the newborn's exposure to HSV lesions by sevenfold and thereby decrease the risk of perinatal transmission.[229] Prolonged rupture of membranes, however, can lessen the protective effect of cesarean delivery by increasing the risk of an ascending HSV infection. Therefore, cesarean section cannot prevent all cases of neonatal HSV. In fact, as many as 33% of infants with congenital HSV infection are delivered by cesarean section.[231] In S.Y.'s case, delivery by cesarean section may have decreased S.Y.'s risk for HSV infection, especially if performed before or shortly (within 4–6 hours) after rupture of the membranes.[231]

Treatment

39. Cultures for HSV and other organisms have been obtained from S.Y. as described in Question 37. Why should therapy be initiated before culture results are available?

Neonatal HSV infections can result in significant morbidity and mortality. Given S.Y.'s signs of infection and risk factors, she should be treated as a case of probable HSV infection until culture results confirm the diagnosis. Three patterns of neonatal HSV infection can occur: (a) disseminated infection (multiple organ involvement) with or without encephalitis; (b) localized CNS infection; and (c) localized infection of the skin, eyes, or mouth (SEM). Approximately 25% to 30% of newborns are symptomatic on the first day of life. Most infants present with SEM disease; however, 60% progress to disseminated disease or CNS infection.[230] S.Y. has several signs of disseminated infection, including irritability, respiratory distress, and skin vesicles. Other signs of disseminated disease include seizures, coagulopathy, jaundice, and shock. Symptoms of CNS infection include temperature instability, irritability, lethargy, poor feeding, bulging fontanel, tremors, and seizures. The onset of illness in neonates with disseminated or SEM disease is at 10 to 12 days of life, whereas those with CNS disease usually present at 16 to 19 days.[230] Morbidity and mortality for neonatal HSV infections are extremely high if left untreated, but can be decreased with appropriate treatment. Even with treatment, disseminated infections have the worst prognosis with a mortality rate of 29%.[230] The mortality rate for CNS disease with treatment is 4% and approximately two-thirds of these infants will have neurologic abnormalities. Mortality from SEM disease is essentially zero; less than 2% have developmental delays. Early treatment also is important because it can halt the progression of less severe SEM infections to more severe forms (i.e., encephalitis and disseminated disease). However, early diagnosis of infection is difficult and treatment is often delayed because the initial symptoms of the disease are often nonspecific.

IV acyclovir, the antiviral of choice for the treatment of neonatal HSV infection, can improve the outcome of neonatal herpes.[228] The recommended acyclovir dose is 60 mg/kg/day in three divided doses, given intravenously for 14 days for those with SEM disease and 21 days for CNS or disseminated HSV disease.[228] Because acyclovir is primarily excreted via the kidneys, the dose must be reduced in neonates with renal dysfunction (e.g., SrCr >0.8 mg/dL). These neonates should receive 20 mg/kg/dose administered every 12 to 24 hours, depending on SrCr.[232] S.Y. should receive acyclovir 40 mg IV Q 8 hours (60 mg/kg/day) for 21 days plus topical antiviral ophthalmic therapy (Table 94-9). Some experts recommend repeating lumbar puncture at the completion of IV acyclovir therapy in all patients with CNS involvement to document virologic clearance from the CSF.[230] Treatment should be continued for those who remain HSV polymerase chain reaction positive (PCR) until their PCR becomes negative. Liver enzymes, SrCr, BUN, and CBC should be monitored for adverse effects of acyclovir. Phlebitis at the injection site also may occur.[8]

Recurrence of mucocutaneous HSV is common and is associated with neurologic sequelae if it occurs more than three times during the first 6 months of life.[228] In a small, Phase I/II trial, oral acyclovir suppressive therapy (300 mg/m^2/dose TID for 6 months), initiated after completion of 10 days of acyclovir treatment for neonatal SEM disease, prevented cutaneous recurrences of HSV.[233] However, approximately 50% of the infants developed neutropenia while receiving suppressive acyclovir therapy. Furthermore, HSV encephalitis has been reported in a preterm infant who was receiving suppressive oral acyclovir therapy.[234] The benefits and risk associated with suppressive therapy are unclear and therefore, routine use of oral acyclovir suppressive therapy is not recommended. A larger study comparing different acyclovir suppressive dosage regimens and the effects on neurologic outcome of infants is needed.

Other Congenital Infections

Toxoplasmosis

Congenital toxoplasmosis, an infection caused by the protozoan organism, *Toxoplasma gondii,* usually results from maternal ingestion of uncooked meat or contact with infected cats. In the United States, 400 to 4,000 cases of congenital toxoplasma infection are reported yearly.[235] The only mode of human-to-human transmission is transplacental. The rate of transmission to the infant is highest (60%) if the disease is acquired during the third trimester of pregnancy. However, if infection occurs earlier in gestation, the infant develops a more severe form of infection. Most newborns infected with *T. gondii* are asymptomatic. The most common manifestation of *T. gondii* infection in neonates is chorioretinitis. These infants may develop permanent visual loss.[235] Other clinical symptoms are listed in Table 94-9. Maternal treatment with spiramycin (currently investigational in the United States) or pyrimethamine with sulfadiazine can be administered to the infected mother to help reduce vertical transmission of *T. gondii.* If the diagnosis of an in utero toxoplasmosis infection is made, treatment of both the mother and the fetus reduces the sequelae in the infant. Because pyrimethamine is teratogenic, it cannot be used during the first trimester. Treatment of neonatal toxoplasmosis includes pyrimethamine, sulfadiazine, and folinic acid (leucovorin). Folinic acid is given to decrease potential hematologic toxic effects of pyrimethamine.[235]

Syphilis

Syphilis is caused by a spirochete, *Treponema pallidum,* and can be acquired by direct contact with ulcerative, denuded lesions of the mucous membranes or skin of the infected person. Vertical transmission of congenital syphilis can either occur transplacentally or during delivery by contact of the newborn with genital lesions. In fact, the rate of transmission can be as high as 100% during the secondary stage of the disease.[228] The incidence of congenital syphilis in the United States has decreased from 107 per 100,000 live births in 1991 to 11.2 cases per 100,000 live births in 2002.[236] Forty percent of pregnancies in women with untreated early syphilis result in spontaneous abortion, stillbirth, nonimmune hydrops, premature delivery, and perinatal death.[228] Clinical manifestations of congenital syphilis are divided into two syndromes, early (occurring before 2 years of life) and late (occurring after 2 years). The most classic presentations of congenital syphilis are bone lesions, hepatosplenomegaly, erythematous maculopapular rash (primarily on the hands and feet), and rhinitis ("snuffles"). Other clinical manifestations are listed in Table 94-9. Parenteral penicillin G is the preferred treatment and is the only drug that has documented efficacy for the treatment of congenital syphilis. IV penicillin G is preferred over IM penicillin G procaine owing to higher CSF concentrations; however, both are considered adequate treatment for congenital syphilis. If more than 1 day of therapy is missed, the entire course must be restarted.[228]

Hepatitis B Virus

Unlike other congenital infections (e.g., toxoplasmosis, syphilis), hepatitis B virus (HBV) infection is rarely transmitted transplacentally, especially if infection occurs during the first or second trimesters. However, the rate of transmission can be as high as 60% if infection occurs in the third trimester.[227] Most infants with HBV are infected around the time of birth as a consequence of exposure to maternal HBV-positive genital tract secretions and blood.[227,237] Newborns with HBV infection are usually asymptomatic initially, but the majority (90%) can become chronic carriers of hepatitis B surface antigen. Many of these infants develop long-term sequelae such as chronic hepatitis, cirrhosis, and hepatocellular carcinoma. Neonatal chronic carrier rates of HBV can be significantly decreased to 0% to 14% with the combined use of hepatitis B vaccination and hepatitis B immune globulin.[227] Owing to these beneficial effects, the Centers for Disease Control and Prevention recommends that all newborn infants should be immunized with hepatitis B vaccination regardless of the mothers' hepatitis status (see Chapter 95).

Rubella

Rubella was a common viral illness affecting humans; however, with the advent of vaccines, the prevalence of rubella has significantly decreased. The virus crosses the placenta and infects the fetus, resulting in spontaneous abortion, stillbirth, or birth defects known as congenital rubella syndrome (CRS). The rate of congenital infection is highest during the first trimester (80%), but transmission can also occur at any time of pregnancy.[225] CRS is characterized by hearing loss, cataracts, and congenital heart disease (primarily PDA and pulmonary artery stenosis); intrauterine growth retardation also commonly occurs. Other clinical findings of CRS are listed in Table 94-9. In a 20-year follow-up study, ocular disease (i.e., cataracts, retinopathy, glaucoma) was found to affect approximately 80% of infants with CRS.[225] Currently, there are no effective antiviral medications for the treatment of CRS; therefore, it is important to provide universal immunization with rubella vaccination to all children.[228]

Cytomegalovirus Infection

CMV is the most common cause of congenital infection, affecting approximately 40,000 infants each year.[238] Transmission of CMV can occur transplacentally at any stage of pregnancy or during delivery. The rate of transmission from the mother to the fetus is much higher in mothers with primary CMV infection (50%) than in those with recurrent infection (0.5%–2%).[239] CMV infection can also be transmitted through breastmilk or close contact.[239] Approximately 10% of infants with CMV infection are symptomatic at birth (i.e., 90% are asymptomatic). The most common manifestations of CMV infection in symptomatic infants <2 weeks of age are petechiae, hepatosplenomegaly, jaundice, and prematurity.[239] Mortality rates in severely affected infants can be as high as 20%, and most infants surviving the infection have permanent damage, such as visual deficits, hearing loss, seizure disorders, and learning and motor disabilities.[238,239] Currently, there is no proven effective antiviral therapy for congenital CMV infection. Ganciclovir has been used to treat infants with symptomatic CMV infection[239]; however, it must be administered intravenously and has been associated with severe adverse effects (e.g., neutropenia, anemia, thrombocytopenia).[8] In addition, the optimal dose and duration of ganciclovir treatment remains unknown. Therefore, routine use of ganciclovir is not recommended.[228] In preliminary findings, oral valganciclovir may be a promising alternative; however, further studies are needed.[240]

APNEA

Pathogenesis

Apnea in neonates is a life-threatening condition that occurs more frequently in premature newborns and newborns of lower birth-weights. Only 7% of infants 34 to 35 weeks' gestational age have apnea.[241] In contrast, the incidence of apnea has been reported to be 78% in infants 26 to 27 weeks' gestational age and 84% in infants with birth-weights <1,000 g.[241] Although several definitions exist,[242,243] clinically significant apnea may be defined as cessation of breathing for ≥15 seconds, or less if accompanied by bradycardia (HR <100 beats/minute), significant hypoxemia, or cyanosis.[244–246] Pallor or hypotonia also may occur.

In neonates, apnea may be caused by a severe underlying illness, drugs, or prematurity itself (Fig. 94-3). Appropriate patient history, physical examination, and laboratory tests must be evaluated to rule out other causes of apnea before the diagnosis of apnea of prematurity can be made.[244,245] It is especially important to rule out sepsis before apnea of prematurity

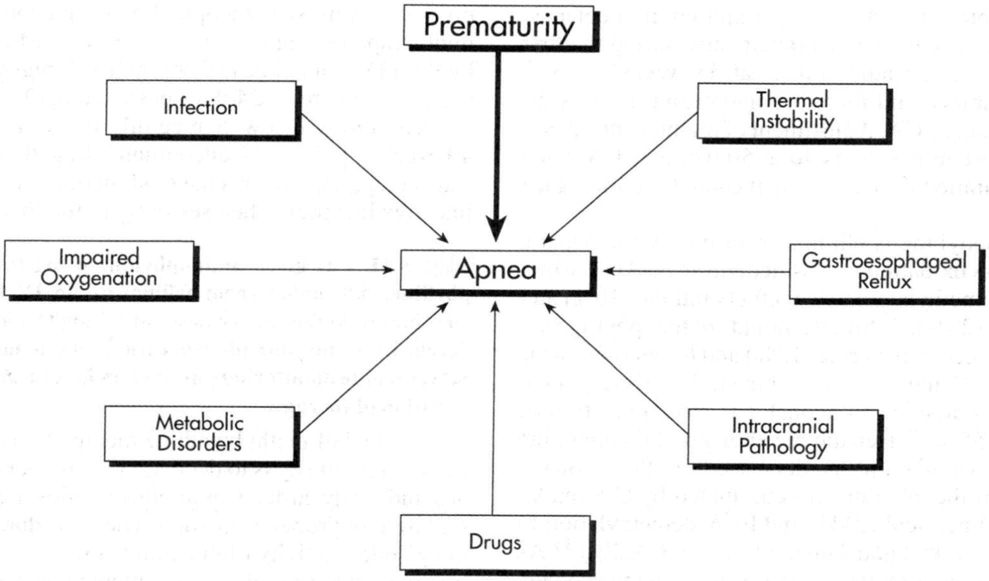

FIGURE 94-3 Causes of apnea in the neonate. (Reproduced with permission from Martin RJ et al. Pathogenesis of apnea in preterm infants. *J Pediatr* 1986;109:738.)

is presumed. If an etiology other than prematurity is identified, therapy would be directed toward that specific cause. For example, antibiotics are used to treat neonatal sepsis with secondary apnea.

Apnea of prematurity is classified into three types: central, obstructive, and mixed. Approximately 40% of apneic episodes are of central origin (i.e., no respiratory effort), 10% are due to obstruction, and 50% are due to both (i.e., mixed events).[247] Although these terms imply separate mechanisms, obstruction/airway closure may be important in all three types (even "central").[241] Treatment of apnea of prematurity includes the use of supplemental oxygen, gentle tactile stimulation, environmental temperature control, oscillation water beds, methylxanthines, nasal continuous positive airway pressure, and positive-pressure ventilation.[244,245]

Treatment

Methylxanthines

40. S.M., a premature male newborn of 29 weeks' gestational age, had a birth-weight of 995 g. On day 2 of life, he develops seven episodes of apnea followed by bradycardia with HR as low as 85 beats/minute. These episodes last 20 to 30 seconds and require administration of oxygen and tactile stimulation. Three prolonged episodes required bag-and-mask ventilation. Between apneic spells, the newborn seems well; physical examination and laboratory tests are normal for gestational age. Appropriate cultures are drawn for a septic workup and ampicillin and gentamicin are initiated. The decision is made to begin aminophylline. What is the rationale for the use of methylxanthines in apnea of prematurity and what dosing considerations must be addressed?

RATIONALE

Methylxanthine therapy generally is initiated for apnea of prematurity when apneic episodes are frequent (e.g., more than three episodes), prolonged (e.g., duration >20–30 seconds), or severe in nature (e.g., accompanied by significant bradycardia or cyanosis) or are not controlled by nonpharmacologic means (e.g., gentle tactile stimulation, environmental temperature control, or oscillation water beds). This infant's apneic episodes are frequent, prolonged, and severe, and therefore require pharmacologic intervention.

Methylxanthines, specifically theophylline and caffeine, are widely accepted as the initial pharmacologic approach for the treatment of idiopathic apnea of prematurity.[245] These agents decrease apneic episodes via both central and peripheral effects. Methylxanthines stimulate the medullary respiratory center and increase receptor responsiveness to carbon dioxide. This results in an increase in respiratory drive and minute ventilation.[245] Central stimulatory effects may be mediated by adenosine receptor blockade. Adenosine is a known inhibitor of respiration, and both theophylline and caffeine competitively inhibit adenosine at the receptor level.[248] Other central effects, such as alteration of sleep–awake patterns, also may be important.[249] Peripherally, methylxanthines increase diaphragmatic contractility, decrease diaphragmatic fatigue, and improve respiratory muscle contraction.[250,251] In addition, methylxanthines increase catecholamine release and metabolic rate. This may improve cardiac output and oxygenation, lessen hypoxic episodes, and decrease apneic spells.

DOSING CONSIDERATIONS

Several developmental pharmacokinetic and pharmacodynamic factors need to be considered when dosing theophylline in neonates. Protein binding of theophylline is decreased in term newborns (36%) compared with adults (65%).[24] The decreased protein binding along with an increased tissue distribution results in a larger Vd of theophylline in neonates (Table 94-2). This larger Vd results in larger loading-dose requirements to attain similar serum concentrations.

Theophylline clearance in preterm newborns (17.6 mL/hour/kg) is much slower than that observed in young children 1 to 4 years of age (100 mL/hour/kg).[24] As a result, smaller theophylline maintenance doses are required in neonates. Theophylline clearance increases dramatically during the first year of life, approaching adult values at 55 weeks' PCA.[36] Theophylline clearance and therefore maintenance doses increase with increasing PCA. Adjustment of maintenance doses is especially important in infants 40 to 50 weeks' PCA when the greatest maturational changes in theophylline clearance occur.[36]

In adults, theophylline is eliminated primarily via hepatic metabolism by C-8 oxidation to 1,3-methyluric acid (39% of a dose) and by *N*-demethylation to 3-methylxanthine (16%) and 1-methyluric acid (20%).[252] Small amounts of theophylline are eliminated unchanged in the urine (13%) and 6% of the dose is *N*-methylated to caffeine.[252,253] In contrast, the primary route of theophylline elimination in neonates is renal excretion of unchanged drug (55%).[36] Hepatic metabolism of theophylline (especially *N*-demethylation) is decreased in the neonate. Lower amounts of theophylline are eliminated by C-8 oxidation to 1,3-methyluric acid (24%) and by *N*-demethylation to 3-methylxanthine (1.4%) and 1-methyluric acid (8.2%).[36] As in adults, theophylline is methylated to caffeine in the neonate. The neonate's decreased demethylation pathway, however, results in a decrease in caffeine elimination and significant serum caffeine accumulation. On average, serum caffeine concentrations can be 40% of the serum theophylline concentration.[36] The theophylline-derived caffeine may contribute to the pharmacologic and toxic effects seen in neonates receiving theophylline. After 50 weeks' PCA, the theophylline-derived serum caffeine concentrations become insignificant.

The generally accepted therapeutic range of theophylline for apnea of prematurity is 6 to 12 mcg/mL. This range is lower than that which is normally accepted for the treatment of asthma (10–20 mcg/mL) for several reasons: (a) the higher free fraction of theophylline found in neonates results in a higher free concentration at any given total concentration; (b) there is a significant accumulation of the unmeasured active metabolite, caffeine; and (c) a different mechanism of action for theophylline is being exploited for apnea (i.e., central stimulation versus bronchodilation for asthma). Although some neonates may respond to theophylline serum concentrations as low as 2.8 mcg/mL,[249] most require concentrations in the generally accepted therapeutic range.[254]

DOSING AND ADMINISTRATION

Although oral aminophylline and theophylline are considered to be well absorbed in the neonate, many neonates initially have feeding problems when apnea and bradycardia are present. Therefore, S.M. should initially receive IV therapy, and an oral nonalcoholic solution can be used when S.M. is stable and tolerating oral feedings. It should be remembered that, depending on the specific product used, aminophylline is 80% to 85% theophylline.

An aminophylline IV loading dose of 6 to 7 mg/kg (4.8–5.6 mg/kg of theophylline) produces theophylline levels of approximately 6.4 to 7.5 mcg/mL. Most centers use initial maintenance doses of aminophylline in the range of 1 to 2 mg/kg/dose given Q 8 to 12 hours, with the lower doses in this range used in younger, more premature infants. For IV administration in neonates, aminophylline should be diluted to 1 mg/mL and infused over 20 to 30 minutes.[8] An aminophylline maintenance dose for S.M. of 1.5 mg/kg/dose Q 8 hours should produce steady-state theophylline serum concentrations in the midtherapeutic range. Lower doses for S.M., as recommended by the FDA guidelines (theophylline 1 mg/kg Q 12 hours for preterm neonates <24 days postnatal age),[255] result in serum concentrations below 5 mcg/mL in most infants less than 40 weeks' PCA.[256] Concomitant drug therapy and disease states (e.g., hepatic or renal dysfunction) also should be taken into consideration when selecting initial theophylline doses.

41. S.M. was given aminophylline 6 mg (6 mg/kg of aminophylline, 4.8 mg/kg theophylline) as an IV loading dose over 20 minutes. Maintenance doses of 1.5 mg Q 8 hours have been ordered. Describe your pharmacotherapeutic monitoring plan for S.M. Include monitoring parameters for efficacy and toxicity and duration of therapy.

The goal of methylxanthine therapy in the treatment of apnea of prematurity is to decrease the number of episodes of apnea and bradycardia. Continuous monitoring of HR and RR is required for proper evaluation. The time, duration, and severity of episodes, activity of the infant, and any necessary intervention performed should be documented. Relationships between the apneic episodes and the feeding schedule and volume of feeds, as well as the dosing schedule of theophylline (e.g., trough), should be examined.

Apnea of prematurity usually resolves by 37 weeks' PCA; however, it may persist in some infants up to or beyond 40 weeks' PCA.[257] In general, the younger the gestational age of the infant at birth, the older the PCA at cessation of apnea. Apnea of prematurity frequently persists beyond 36 weeks' PCA in infants born at 28 weeks' gestational age or less, and persists beyond 40 weeks' PCA in 22% of infants born at 24 weeks' gestational age.[257] Therefore, methylxanthine therapy usually is discontinued at 35 to 37 weeks' PCA provided that the infant has not been having apneic spells.[245] Infants requiring therapy for longer periods of time may be discharged home on methylxanthines with apnea monitors.

Toxicities noted in neonates include tachycardia, agitation, irritability, hyperglycemia, feeding intolerance, gastroesophageal reflux, and emesis or occasional spitting up of food. Tachycardia is the most common toxicity and usually responds to a downward adjustment of the theophylline dose. Tachycardia may persist for 1 to 3 days after dosage reductions owing to the decreased elimination of theophylline-derived caffeine. Seizures also have been reported with accidental overdoses. Methylxanthine toxicity can be minimized with careful dosing and appropriate monitoring of serum concentrations. Serum theophylline concentrations should be monitored 72 hours after initiation of therapy or after a change in dosage. Serum concentrations of theophylline also should be measured if the infant experiences an increase in the number of apneic episodes, signs or symptoms of toxicity, or a significant increase in weight. In asymptomatic neonates, once steady-state levels are obtained, theophylline concentrations may be monitored every 2 weeks.

42. S.M. now is 3 weeks old (32 weeks' PCA) and weighs 1,100 g. His septic workup was negative. Currently, S.M. has several apneic spells per day, which respond to tactile stimulation; his apneic episodes have not required ventilatory assistance. S.M. receives 1 mg aminophylline IV Q 8 hours, and his trough theophylline level this morning was 5.7 mcg/mL. The medical team is considering switching S.M.'s theophylline therapy to caffeine because

of possible improved benefits. How does caffeine compare with theophylline with regard to its pharmacokinetics, efficacy, and toxicity? What treatment should be selected?

PHARMACOKINETICS

The plasma clearance of caffeine is considerably lower and the half-life is extremely prolonged in the premature newborn (Table 94-2). The low clearance is a reflection of the decreased neonatal hepatic metabolism and a resultant dependence of elimination on the slow urinary excretion. In the preterm neonate, the amount of caffeine excreted unchanged in the urine is 85%, compared with <2% in adults. Adult urinary metabolite patterns are seen by 7 to 9 months of age.[258] The half-life of caffeine decreases with increasing PCA[259] and plasma clearance reaches adult levels after 3 to 4.5 months of life.[260] As a result of the maturational changes, doses usually need to be adjusted after 38 weeks' PCA and dosing intervals need to be shortened to 8 hours after 50 weeks' PCA.[259]

EFFICACY, TOXICITY, AND DOSING

Comparative studies have found similar efficacy for theophylline and caffeine in the control of apnea of prematurity.[261] Caffeine, however, may have some advantages over theophylline, including a wider therapeutic index. Adverse effects such as tachycardia, CNS excitation, and feeding intolerance are reported more frequently with theophylline than with caffeine. The prolonged half-life of caffeine in premature neonates results in less fluctuation in plasma concentrations and permits the use of a 24-hour dosing interval. Because the half-life is prolonged and dosing requirements do not change quickly over time, caffeine serum concentrations can be monitored less frequently. Loading doses of 10 mg/kg of caffeine base (20 mg/kg of caffeine citrate), followed 24 hours later by maintenance doses of 2.5 mg/kg (5 mg/kg caffeine citrate) given daily maintain plasma caffeine concentrations in the therapeutic range (5–20 mcg/mL). Loading doses of caffeine citrate are recommended to be given IV over 30 minutes using a syringe infusion pump. Maintenance doses can be administered IV over 10 minutes or given orally.[105] Because of the longer half-life, infants receiving caffeine must be monitored for a longer period of time (e.g., for 7–10 days) for adverse effects if toxicities occur and for efficacy once the medication is discontinued. Another disadvantage of caffeine is its high cost. Although infants who are unresponsive to theophylline may respond to caffeine,[262] S.M.'s theophylline therapy presently is not optimized; his serum concentration is <6 mcg/mL. S.M. seems to have partially responded to theophylline and may benefit from an increase in the dose with resultant therapeutic serum concentrations. S.M.'s aminophylline dose should be increased to 1.5 mg every 8 hours to achieve serum concentrations of approximately 8 mcg/mL. Caffeine may have several advantages over theophylline. Now that a preservative-free caffeine citrate product is available in the United States,[105] its use is increasing. It is important to remember that another IV caffeine product is marketed in the United States as the sodium benzoate salt. Benzoic acid has been associated with the gasping syndrome and also may displace bilirubin from albumin-binding sites.[39,40] Because of these toxicities, the caffeine sodium benzoate product should not be used in neonates.

The short- and long-term safety and efficacy of caffeine to treat apnea of prematurity in VLBW infants was studied in a large, randomized, placebo-controlled trial.[109,263] Caffeine significantly decreased the frequency of BPD.[109] Infants who received caffeine were able to have positive airway pressure discontinued 1 week sooner than those receiving placebo. Although caffeine reduced weight gain, the effect was only temporary (during the first 3 weeks of therapy). No significant short-term effects of caffeine on death rates, ultrasonographic signs of brain injury, or NEC were identified. In a follow-up study at 18 to 21 months' corrected age, caffeine significantly improved the rates of survival without neurodevelopmental disability; no difference in death rates were observed between caffeine and placebo, but the incidence of cerebral palsy and cognitive delay were both decreased in infants receiving caffeine.[263]

Other Agents

43. S.M.'s dose of theophylline has been optimized and theophylline serum concentrations now are 12.4 mcg/mL. S.M. continues to have apneic episodes. What other pharmacologic agents can be used?

Doxapram, an analeptic agent, has been shown to be as effective as theophylline for the treatment of apnea of prematurity.[264,265] Because of the limited number of investigations and uncertain side effects, however, doxapram should be restricted to patients who are refractory to methylxanthine therapy. In addition, the IV preparation commercially available in the United States contains 0.9% benzyl alcohol and should be used with caution. Although doses are not well defined, a loading dose of 2.5 to 3 mg/kg given IV over 15 to 30 minutes followed by a 1 mg/kg/hr continuous infusion has been recommended. Doses may be increased by 0.5 mg/kg/hour increments to a maximum dose of 2.5 mg/kg/hour. Lower doses have been used in infants receiving concomitant methylxanthine therapy with approximately 50% responding to IV doxapram doses of 0.5 mg/kg/hour.[266] A few studies have administered doxapram enterally; however, bioavailability in preterm newborns is not well defined[267] and routine use of oral doxapram cannot be recommended.[268] Side effects associated with doxapram include cardiovascular problems such as increased BP (usually with doses >1.5 mg/kg/hour)[266] and second-degree atrioventricular heart block with prolonged QT interval[269]; GI disturbances such as abdominal distention, regurgitation, increased gastric residuals, and vomiting; and CNS adverse effects such as increased agitation, excessive crying, jitteriness, irritability, disturbed sleep, and seizures. Further studies of doxapram are needed to better delineate its adverse effects and to help define its safety and efficacy for the treatment of apnea of prematurity.

PERIVENTRICULAR–INTRAVENTRICULAR HEMORRHAGE

Pathogenesis

44. M.C., a 3-day-old male infant, was born at 28 weeks' gestation with a birth-weight of 980 g. He was intubated shortly after birth for respiratory distress and last night developed a pneumothorax. This morning, M.C. required a blood transfusion because of a significant drop in hematocrit. Hypotension, hypotonia, and decreased responsiveness now are noted on physical examination. An ultrasound of the infant's head was ordered

to confirm the suspicion of an intraventricular bleed. What factors are associated with an increased risk for the development of periventricular–intraventricular hemorrhage (PV-IVH)?

PV-IVH is a significant cause of death among premature newborns and is one of the most common serious neurologic injuries that occurs during the neonatal period. The incidence and severity of PV-IVH is inversely related to gestational age, with the highest frequency occurring in the most immature neonates.[270] PV-IVH occurs in approximately 3% of healthy, term newborns, in >20% of premature newborns <1,500 g birth-weight, and in >60% of preterm infants <700 g birth-weight.[271,272]

The most common site of origin of the hemorrhage is the periventricular germinal matrix, a highly vascularized cellular region that contains neuronal precursor cells. This vascular network, which is prominent at 26 to 34 weeks' gestational age, contains poorly supported blood vessels that are fragile and vulnerable to injury.[270] Most factors associated with an increased risk of PV-IVH alter cerebral blood flow or arterial BP, which results in damage to these vessels. M.C. has two risk factors that are strongly associated with PV-IVH: prematurity and acute respiratory failure requiring mechanical ventilation.[270] Other associated risk factors include pneumothorax (which M.C. also has), hypotension, hypertension, hypoxia, hypercapnia, asphyxia, acidosis, rapid volume expansion, coagulation defects, infusion of hyperosmolar substances (e.g., sodium bicarbonate), hypernatremia, hyperglycemia, seizures, PDA, heparin use, tracheal suctioning, and inadvertent noxious stimulation.[270–273] The use of low-dose heparin in umbilical catheter infusions (1 unit/mL) may not increase the risk of PV-IVH, but larger studies are required.[274]

Common signs and symptoms of PV-IVH include hypotension, hypotonia, a drop in hematocrit, and a decrease in responsiveness as illustrated by M.C. Apnea, oculomotor disturbances, areflexia, tonic posturing, flaccid quadriparesis, seizures, and death also may occur.[275] Prognosis for normal neurologic development in survivors depends on location and severity of the bleed. Mild hemorrhages (grade I, isolated germinal matrix hemorrhage; grade II, hemorrhage extending into normal-size ventricles) have a better prognosis, but may result in cognitive deficits such as reading disabilities or other learning problems. Approximately 10% of infants with mild hemorrhages develop a major disability, such as spastic diplegia. Infants with moderate (grade III, hemorrhage extending into enlarged ventricles) or severe hemorrhages (grade IV, intraparenchymal hemorrhage) do worse with an increase in major motor (e.g., spastic hemiparesis, quadriplegia) and intellectual deficits. Infants with moderate and severe bleeds also are more likely to develop posthemorrhagic hydrocephalus and seizure activity. Those with severe hemorrhage have a higher mortality rate.[270]

Treatment

45. How is PV-IVH managed and what therapies have been investigated to prevent PV-IVH?

Management and prevention of PV-IVH include the reduction or elimination of known risk factors. Because prematurity is a major risk factor, prevention of premature birth is the most effective way to eliminate PV-IVH. However, antenatal tocolytic agents such as maternal β-sympathomimetics and indomethacin have been shown to increase the incidence of IVH in infants.[272,273] Other antenatal pharmacologic agents (magnesium sulfate, phenobarbital, vitamin K, and corticosteroids) have been investigated to reduce PV-IVH, but only antenatal corticosteroids are currently recommended.[64,270,272,273] Antenatal maternal corticosteroids significantly reduce the incidence and severity of PV-IVH (as well as the incidence of RDS and infant mortality).[64,272] Corticosteroids may prevent PV-IVH by stabilizing or promoting maturation of the endothelium of the fragile blood vessels of the germinal matrix.[270,273] Because even partial courses of maternal corticosteroids are beneficial, M.C may have benefited from prompt treatment of his mother with corticosteroids as soon as the risk for preterm delivery was identified (see Respiratory Distress Syndrome section).[64,271,273]

To prevent PV-IVH after birth, wide variations in BP and cerebral blood flow, abnormalities in serum osmolality and blood gases, and noxious stimulations should be avoided. Several postnatal pharmacologic agents, including phenobarbital, indomethacin, ibuprofen, ethamsylate, vitamin E, and pancuronium have been investigated for the prevention of PV-IVH.[270] At present, none are widely accepted for routine use in newborn infants. Of the agents studied, low-dose indomethacin offers the best potential for PV-IVH prophylaxis.[272,276] A multicenter, randomized, placebo-controlled trial using indomethacin (0.1 mg/kg/dose IV at 6–12 hours after birth and every 24 hours for two additional doses) significantly lowered the incidence and severity of IVH in neonates of weighing 600 to 1,250 g at birth.[276] Postnatal low-dose indomethacin therapy also significantly lowered the incidence of IVH in infants whose mothers received antenatal corticosteroid therapy.[277]

Indomethacin, a cyclo-oxygenase inhibitor, may prevent IVH by reducing the synthesis of vasodilating prostanoids and prostaglandins. This results in a decrease in baseline cerebral blood flow and changes in cerebral blood flow modulation. Inhibition of cyclo-oxygenase also may decrease formation of harmful free radicals. Because indomethacin lowers cerebral blood flow, concerns about increased risks of cerebral ischemic injury and neurodevelopmental handicaps exist. One follow-up study conducted at 36 months of corrected age showed that low-dose indomethacin did not result in any adverse cognitive or motor outcomes.[277] Although this seems promising, further long-term follow-up investigations are needed before the use of low-dose indomethacin in premature infants can be recommended universally.[271,273]

In animal studies, ibuprofen enhances cerebral blood flow autoregulation and may offer neuroprotection after oxidative stress.[152] However, in clinical trials, IV ibuprofen did not prevent IVH. In two placebo-controlled double-blind, randomized studies of early administration of ibuprofen (within 6 hours after birth), ibuprofen did not reduce the frequency of IVH (grades II–IV).[161,278] In addition, comparative trials of ibuprofen and indomethacin for the treatment of PDA did not find significant differences in the incidence IVH.[153] Thus, ibuprofen has no proven effect on IVH risk and cannot be recommended.

NEONATAL SEIZURES

Pathogenesis and Diagnosis

46. F.H., a term female newborn (weight 3.5 kg), has a history of perinatal asphyxia. Apgar scores were 2 and 4 at 1 and 5 minutes,

respectively. Forty-eight hours after birth, F.H. begins to have rhythmic clonic twitching of the right hand, repetitive chewing movements, fluttering of the eyelids, and occasional pendular movements of the extremities that resemble swimming motions. What interventions should be initiated immediately for F.H.?

Seizure activity may be difficult to recognize in the term or premature neonate. Because of the immaturity of the cortex, neonatal seizures rarely are generalized tonic–clonic events, but can be clonic (focal or multifocal), tonic (focal or generalized), myoclonic (focal, multifocal, or generalized), or subtle in nature.[279] Subtle seizures include activities such as abnormal oral–buccal–lingual movements; ocular movements; swimming, pedaling, or stepping movements; and occasionally apnea.[275] In addition, autonomic nervous system signs such as changes in HR, BP, respirations, skin color, oxygenation, salivation, or pupil size may occur.[280] Clinical neonatal seizures may or may not be associated with EEG changes.[280]

Neonatal seizure activity is a common manifestation of a life-threatening underlying neurologic process (Table 94-10); therefore, initial efforts may not include antiepileptic drug therapy. Definitive treatment is directed toward specific identified etiologies. The acute evaluation of neonatal seizures includes assessment of the infant's airway, breathing, and circulation and a review of the infant's history, physical examination, and laboratory studies. Every neonate with seizure activity should have a bedside determination of glucose; laboratory determinations of serum electrolytes, including sodium, BUN, glucose, calcium (Ca), and magnesium (Mg); blood gases; bilirubin; and an infectious disease workup, including CBC with platelets, blood culture, urine culture, lumbar puncture with CSF analysis (cell count, protein, glucose), and CSF culture.[275,279] Treatment with antiepileptic drugs is indicated after correction of known electrolyte abnormalities. Antiepileptic drug therapy can be initiated (after correction of hypoglycemia) while laboratory test results are pending.

If these tests do not reveal any abnormalities, an EEG, metabolic disease workup (e.g., serum ammonia, lactate, pyruvate; serum and urine amino and organic acids), and screening of blood and urine for drugs can be performed.[275,279,280]

Table 94-10 Causes of Neonatal Seizures

Metabolic

- Hypoxic—ischemia (i.e., asphyxia)
  - Hypoxia
  - Hypoglycemia
  - Hypocalcemia
- Hypoglycemia
  - Intrauterine growth retardation
  - Infant of a diabetic mother
  - Glycogen storage disease
  - Galactosemia
  - Idiopathic
- Hypocalcemia
  - Hypomagnesemia
  - Infant of a diabetic mother
  - Neonatal hypoparathyroidism
  - Maternal hyperparathyroidism
  - High phosphate load
- Other electrolyte imbalances
  - Hypernatremia
  - Hyponatremia

Cerebrovascular Lesions (other than trauma)

- Cerebral infarction (thrombotic versus embolic) ischemic versus hemorrhagic
- Cortical vein thrombosis

Trauma

- Subarachnoid hemorrhage
- Intracranial hemorrhage
- Subdural/epidural hematoma
- Intraventricular hemorrhage

Infections

- Bacterial meningitis
- Viral-induced encephalitis
- Congenital infections
  - Herpes
  - Cytomegalovirus
  - Toxoplasmosis
  - Syphilis
  - Coxsackie meningoencephalitis
  - AIDS
- Brain abscess

Brain Anomalies (cerebral dysgenesis from either congenital or acquired courses)

Drug Withdrawal or Toxins

- Prenatal substance: methadone, heroin, barbiturate, cocaine, etc.
- Prescribed medications: propoxyphene, isoniazid
- Local anesthetics
- Bilirubin

Hypertensive Encephalopathy

Amino Acid Metabolism

- Branched-chain amino acidopathies
- Urea-cycle abnormalities
- Nonketotic hyperglycinemia
- Ketotic hyperglycinemia

Pyridoxine Dependency

Familial Seizures

- Neurocutaneous syndromes
- Tuberous sclerosis
- Incontinentia pigmenti
- Autosomal-dominant neonatal seizures

Selected Genetic Syndrome

- Zellweger syndrome
- Neonatal adrenal leukodystrophy
- Smith-Lemli-Opitz syndrome

Adapted with permission from reference 280.

Intrauterine infections associated with congenital neurologic abnormalities and seizures can be identified by obtainment of TORCH titers (see Question 37). Cranial ultrasounds, CT scans, and MRIs may be obtained to identify infarcts, hemorrhages, calcifications, or cerebral malformations that may cause seizure activity.[275,281]

47. The physician assesses F.H. as having adequate ventilation and circulation. She establishes an IV line and sends blood samples for electrolytes, Ca, and Mg. A Chemstrip reveals a blood glucose of 20 mg/dL. What is your assessment and recommendation at this time?

Hypoglycemia seems to be the cause of F.H.'s seizure activity. Hypoxic ischemic encephalopathy (secondary to asphyxia), however, is the most common cause of neonatal seizures. Hypoxic ischemic encephalopathy can be associated with metabolic abnormalities such as hypoglycemia, hypocalcemia, and hyponatremia (owing to inappropriate secretion of antidiuretic hormone). Hypocalcemia may also be accompanied by hypomagnesemia.[280] Hypoglycemia is defined as a whole blood glucose <20 mg/dL for premature infants and <30 mg/dL for term infants during the first 72 hours of life and <40 mg/dL for any neonate after 72 hours of age. In clinical practice, however, a glucose <40 mg/dL in a neonate of any age would be treated.[282]

F.H. should receive an IV bolus dose of 7 to 14 mL (2–4 mL/kg) of dextrose 10% (200–400 mg/kg) given over 2 to 3 minutes, followed by a continuous infusion of dextrose 10% at an initial dose of 12.6 to 16.8 mL/hour (6–8 mg/kg/minute or 3.6–4.8 mL/kg/hour).[281] Serum glucose levels should be monitored, and the dextrose infusion should be titrated as needed. If hypoglycemia persists, possible causes such as islet tumor of the pancreas, adrenal insufficiency, and inborn errors of metabolism should be investigated. Corticosteroids, glucagon, and diazoxide have been used to treat persistent hypoglycemia.[282]

Treatment of Hypocalcemia and Hypomagnesemia

48. The physician administers 10 mL (1 g) of 10% dextrose solution IV and starts an IV infusion of glucose at 8 mg/kg/min. A repeat Chemstrip reveals a blood glucose of 80 mg/dL, but F.H. continues to have seizure activity. F.H.'s laboratory results come back with the following results: Na, 137 mEq/L; K, 4.3 mEq/L; CO_2, 22 mEq/L; Cl, 104 mEq/L; BUN, 7 mg/dL; SrCr, 0.7 mg/dL; glucose, 25 mg/dL; Mg, 1.0 mEq/L; and Ca, 5 mg/dL. What should be done next to control F.H.'s seizures?

[SI units: Na, 137 mmol/L; K, 4.3 mmol/L; CO_2, 22 mmol/L; Cl, 104 mmol/L; BUN, 2.5 mmol/L of urea; SrCr, 61.9 μmol/L; glucose, 1.4 mmol/L; Mg, 0.5 mmol/L; Ca, 1.25 mmol/L]

F.H. also has hypocalcemia and hypomagnesemia, both of which may cause seizure activity. Neonatal hypocalcemia is defined as a serum calcium <7.5 mg/dL in preterm and <8 mg/dL in term infants[280] or an ionized serum calcium <3 mg/dL.[281] Hypomagnesemia (defined as a serum magnesium <1.5 mEq/L) is rare but may coexist with hypocalcemia. Hypomagnesemia should be suspected when hypocalcemia cannot be corrected despite large doses of calcium.[283]

F.H. should receive calcium gluconate 700 mg (200 mg/kg) given slowly intravenously as a 10% solution[280] and magnesium sulfate 25 to 50 mg/kg/dose (0.2–0.4 mEq/kg/dose) IM as a 50% solution or intravenously as a dilute solution (maximum concentration, 100 mg/mL) administered over 2 to 4 hours.[8] Doses of calcium gluconate and magnesium sulfate may be repeated based on serum determinations. If IV calcium is administered too quickly, vasodilation, hypotension, bradycardia, and cardiac arrhythmias may occur. Calcium gluconate may be administered intravenously at a maximum rate of 50 mg/min while monitoring HR, BP, and electrocardiogram (ECG).[8] To avoid IV extravasation with resultant severe dermal necrosis, calcium salts should be administered through a properly working IV line, and the IV site should be monitored for signs of infiltration.

Treatment With Antiepileptic Drugs

49. Despite normalization of her laboratory tests, F.H. continues to have seizure activity. Phenobarbital 35 mg IV push over 1 minute is administered. Ten minutes later, F.H. continues to have intermittent seizure activity. Describe a pharmacotherapeutic plan to control F.H.'s seizure activity.

Phenobarbital is the initial antiepileptic drug of choice for neonatal seizures; phenytoin and lorazepam usually are considered the second and third drugs of choice.[284] Because of the large Vd of phenobarbital in neonates (approximately 1 L/kg), large initial loading doses of 20 mg/kg are required to produce therapeutic serum concentrations (Table 94-11). Because F.H. received only a 10-mg/kg dose (35 mg) of phenobarbital, an additional 10 mg/kg should be given now. Phenobarbital should be administered IV at a rate of ≤1 mg/kg/minute,[8] so a 35-mg dose should be given over at least 10 minutes, not over 1 minute. Rapid administration of phenobarbital may cause respiratory depression, apnea, or hypotension. If F.H. continues to have seizure activity after a total phenobarbital loading dose of 20 mg/kg, additional 5- to 10-mg/kg loading doses may be given every 15 to 20 minutes as needed up to a total loading dose of 40 mg/kg. Ventilatory support may be required when using these higher doses, and serum phenobarbital concentrations should be monitored. Phenobarbital's therapeutic effect of controlling neonatal seizures plateaus at serum concentrations of 40 mcg/mL; adverse effects increase at higher serum concentrations.[285]

If seizure activity is not controlled in F.H. (despite optimal phenobarbital loading doses), a phenytoin loading dose of 70 mg (20 mg/kg) should be administered IV at a rate ≤0.5 mg/kg/minute.[8,279] Rapid IV administration of phenytoin may cause cardiac arrhythmias, bradycardia, or hypotension. Phenytoin also may cause severe damage to tissues if extravasation occurs. Therefore, BP, HR, ECG, and the IV site of infusion should be monitored. Recently, fosphenytoin, the diphosphate ester salt of phenytoin, became available in the United States for IV and IM use in adults.[8] Fosphenytoin is a water-soluble prodrug of phenytoin that undergoes conversion by plasma and tissue esterases to phenytoin, phosphate, and formaldehyde. Fosphenytoin has several advantages over phenytoin. Because of its greater water solubility, the IV preparation does not contain propylene glycol, and thus fosphenytoin may have fewer cardiovascular adverse effects associated

Table 94-11 Pharmacotherapy of Neonatal Seizures[a,8]

Drug	Loading Dose	Maintenance Dose	Therapeutic Concentration
Phenobarbital	*IV: Initial:* 20 mg/kg then 5–10 mg/kg Q 15–20 min if needed until total load of 40 mg/kg	*IV PO: Initial: Premature:* 3 mg/kg/day Term: 4 mg/kg/day May need to ↑ to 4–5 mg/kg/day by 2–4 weeks of therapy	20–40 mcg/mL
Phenytoin	*IV:* 15–20 mg/kg	*IV: Initial:* 5 mg/kg/day May need to ↑ to ≥10 mg/kg/day by 2–4 weeks of therapy	8–15 mcg/mL
Lorazepam	*IV:* 0.05–0.1 mg/kg	May repeat doses if needed Q 10–15 min	
Diazepam	*IV:* 0.1–0.3 mg/kg	May repeat doses if needed Q 10–15 min	
Midazolam	*IV:* Initial bolus dose of 0.15 mg/kg has been used in some studies; however, for safety reasons, this bolus dose should not be given if the neonate has received an IV dose of a benzodiazepine	*IV continuous infusion: Initial:* 0.05 mg/kg/hr; ↑ by 0.025 mg/kg/hr increments; usual maximum 0.4 mg/kg/hr; some studies reported neonates who required doses up to 1 mg/kg/hr	
Pyridoxine	*IV:* 50–100 mg	*IV* PO: 20–50 mg/day; ↑ dose PRN with age	
Valproic acid	*PO:* 20 mg/kg	*PO:* 10 mg/kg/dose Q 12 hr	40–50 mcg/mL

[a] See text for comments on appropriate IV administration and monitoring.
IV, intravenous; PO, oral.

with IV administration. Unlike phenytoin, fosphenytoin's more neutral pH also allows for IM administration. Unfortunately, appropriate clinical studies of fosphenytoin in neonates have not yet been conducted. Unanswered concerns about the neonatal handling of formaldehyde also exist. Currently, routine use of fosphenytoin in neonates cannot be recommended. Studies assessing the safety, efficacy, and optimal dosing are needed.

Lorazepam or diazepam may be used to treat F.H.'s seizures if they are unresponsive to phenobarbital and phenytoin.[286,287] Although lorazepam offers the advantage of a longer duration of effect than diazepam, the use of either agent (especially in combination with phenobarbital) may cause respiratory and CNS depression. RR, BP, and HR should be monitored. Both IV preparations contain propylene glycol and benzyl alcohol. Although these substances have been reported to cause toxicities in newborns, the actual amount administered when using appropriate benzodiazepine doses is minimal and should not pose a significant risk.[286] Doses of lorazepam should be diluted with an equal volume of D_5W, normal saline, or sterile water for injection before IV use and administered slowly over 2 to 5 minutes. The relatively high concentration of diazepam injection (which results in <0.1-mL doses) and its physical incompatibility with most diluents, make it impractical to use in small neonates. As a result, lorazepam has become the preferred benzodiazepine in many neonatal ICUs.

If seizure activity continues in F.H., continuous IV infusion of midazolam, or oral levetiracetam should be considered.[280,288–290] An IV formulation of levetiracetam is commercially available in the United States. Although not approved for use in neonates, some neonatal centers use the oral dosing recommendations for the IV formulation because the two forms are bioequivalent.[8] However, the optimal neonatal dose of levetiracetam has not been established. Neonatal case reports have used doses from studies in pediatric patients.[290] Given that levetiracetam is primarily excreted via the kidney (66% of a dose is excreted as unchanged drug in the urine) and that the renal function of neonates is decreased compared with older infants, prudence dictates using conservative dose titration and close monitoring of adverse effects. Oral carbamazepine, primidone, lamotrigine, or valproic acid (IV, oral) have also been used to treat neonatal seizures in limited numbers of patients.[279,291,292] Because the risk of valproic acid-associated hepatotoxicity is higher for patients <2 years of age, this drug is not a preferred agent for use in neonates.[8] IV pyridoxine should be considered when seizure activity persists. Pyridoxine is a cofactor required for the synthesis of the inhibitory neurotransmitter γ-aminobutyric acid (GABA). Patients with pyridoxine dependency require higher amounts of pyridoxine for proper GABA synthesis. Pyridoxine dependency is a rare disorder, but should be considered in neonates with seizure activity unresponsive to antiepileptic drug therapy. Lifelong supplementation of pyridoxine is required in these patients.[280]

Antiepileptic Drug Maintenance Doses

50. F.H.'s seizure activity stopped after receiving a total loading dose of 105 mg of phenobarbital and 70 mg of phenytoin. A serum phenobarbital concentration of 35 mcg/mL and a phenytoin concentration of 17 mcg/mL were measured 1 hour after the phenytoin loading dose (2 hours after the last phenobarbital loading dose). How should maintenance doses of antiepileptic drugs be instituted in F.H.?

It is not surprising that F.H. required both phenobarbital and phenytoin to control her seizures. Although phenobarbital and phenytoin are equally effective, neonatal seizures are controlled in fewer than 50% of neonates with either agent alone. When both agents are used together, neonatal seizures are controlled in approximately 60% of neonates.[293]

F.H. should be placed on maintenance doses of both phenobarbital and phenytoin because both drugs were needed to control her seizure activity. Because the half-life of phenobarbital is prolonged in neonates (about 100–150 hours), maintenance doses can be instituted 24 hours after the loading dose at 3 to 4 mg/kg/day[280,294] as a single daily dose (Table 94-11). Although this newborn is term, she should receive a lower dose of phenobarbital (2.5–3 mg/kg/day) because of her history of asphyxia. Asphyxiated neonates have impaired phenobarbital clearance and therefore require lower maintenance doses than nonasphyxiated neonates to achieve similar phenobarbital serum concentrations.[43] Maintenance doses of phenytoin (3–4 mg/kg/day given in divided doses Q 12 hours) may be initiated 12 to 24 hours after the loading dose. Serum concentrations of these agents should be monitored periodically because maintenance dose requirements increase over time (usually by week 2–4 of therapy).[294] This may be due to a normal maturation of hepatic enzyme systems with age or induction of P450 enzymes. In neonates, oral phenytoin is poorly absorbed and should be avoided in the acute setting. A routine 25% increase in the dose is needed when converting IV phenytoin to oral to attain similar serum concentrations. In addition, after 2 to 4 weeks of age, dosing intervals of every 8 hours may be needed.

The optimal duration of anticonvulsant treatment of neonatal seizures has not been clearly established. Typically, anticonvulsants are continued for approximately 6 months in neonates with persistently abnormal neurologic examinations. Because of the potential long-term toxicities of these medications and the low risk of seizure recurrence, anticonvulsants are generally discontinued before discharge if the neonate's neurologic examination and EEG are normal.[295] However, the duration of anticonvulsant medications should be individualized.

NEONATAL ABSTINENCE SYNDROME

A disturbing incidence of maternal substance abuse and associated obstetric and neonatal complications exists.[296,297] Drugs such as alcohol, opiates, barbiturates, and benzodiazepines readily cross the placenta and may induce fetal dependency. In addition to the neonatal abstinence syndrome (NAS), other problems seen in infants of addicted mothers must be recognized to optimize patient care. In utero exposure to drugs of abuse may have serious short- and long-term consequences on fetal growth, physiological functions, and neurologic development. The use of cocaine during pregnancy may cause complications such as fetal distress, preterm labor, spontaneous abortion, abruptio placentae, stillbirths, or congenital malformations and may place the infant at a higher risk for IVH and NEC.[296,298] Intrauterine growth retardation and sudden infant death syndrome have been associated with heroin, methadone, and cocaine abuse during pregnancy.[296,297] Neonatal systolic hypertension, abnormal thyroid function, hyperbilirubinemia, thrombocytosis, and increased platelet aggregation have been reported with maternal methadone use.[296] The increase of polydrug abuse during pregnancy also may complicate treatment.

Although environmental, familial, and neonatal coexisting factors (such as prematurity and low birth-weight) need to be considered, investigations assessing neurobehavioral development suggest that drug-exposed infants may be at a greater risk for certain learning, developmental, and behavioral problems.[296] For example, infants born to narcotic-dependent mothers may have later difficulties with short-term memory, attention, concentration, and general processing of perception. Delayed language development has been noted for methadone- and cocaine-exposed infants. Hyperactivity, aggressiveness, impulsiveness, uncontrollable temper, and other behavioral problems have been reported in follow-up studies of infants of drug-dependent mothers.[296] Investigations that control for confounding factors are needed to fully assess the long-term neurobehavioral outcomes of drug-exposed infants and the long-term effects of currently recommended therapies.[299]

Adverse neonatal effects from the maternal use of selective serotonin reuptake inhibitors (SSRIs) during pregnancy have been reported. First trimester exposure to SSRIs may increase the risk of congenital cardiovascular malformations; antenatal exposure to paroxetine has been associated with an increased risk of cardiac defects (e.g., ventricular or atrial septal defects).[300,301] Late pregnancy SSRI exposure is associated with an increased risk for persistent pulmonary hypertension of the newborn and the neonatal behavioral syndrome.[302,303] This syndrome includes respiratory distress, tremors, jitteriness, increased muscle tone, feeding difficulties, seizures, and temperature instability. However, it is unknown whether these symptoms are due to toxic effects of SSRIs or drug withdrawal.[302] To help reduce the incidence of neonatal behavioral syndrome, physicians should try to taper maternal SSRIs in late pregnancy. Unfortunately, it is unknown whether tapering of SSRIs in high-risk patients could complicate labor and delivery. Therefore, it is important to assess the risks and benefits and use SSRIs with caution during pregnancy.

Clinical Presentation

51. A.K., a 38-week gestation, 2,000-g, small-for-gestational-age female, was born to a gravida 3 para 2 mother with a history of frequent heroin use during pregnancy. A.K.'s mother was enrolled in a methadone maintenance program 1 month ago, and her last dose of methadone was 12 hours before delivery. On further questioning, A.K.'s mother admits to the continued use of heroin and occasional use of crack cocaine. Her last "fix" was 3 hours before delivery. On the first day of life, A.K. became restless, irritable, and tachypneic, and displayed spontaneous tremors and a high-pitched cry. A.K. developed vomiting and diarrhea on day 2 of life after starting feedings with a standard formula. Although A.K. frequently suckled on her fist, she was not able to suckle properly while feeding. A.K.'s drug screen was positive for cocaine, opiates, and methadone. What clinical symptoms of NAS does A.K. demonstrate? How do the onset, severity, and duration of NAS vary with various commonly abused substances?

Symptoms of drug withdrawal occur in 30% of infants exposed to SSRIs in utero and 50% to 90% of infants born to narcotic-dependent mothers, with a higher incidence for methadone (70%–90%) compared with heroin (50%–75%).[296,304] NAS is a generalized disorder characterized by CNS hyperirritability (e.g., hyperactivity, irritability, high-pitched or prolonged cry, hyperreflexia, fist sucking, abnormal sleep pattern, tremor, myoclonic jerks, and rarely, seizures), respiratory difficulties (e.g., stuffy nose, rhinorrhea, respiratory distress, tachypnea, respiratory alkalosis, and apnea), GI dysfunction (e.g., regurgitation, drooling, vomiting, diarrhea, hyperphagia, uncoordinated suck and swallow reflex, and poor feeding), and vague autonomic symptoms (e.g., sneezing, yawning, hiccups, sweating, lacrimation, hyperthermia or hypothermia, and skin mottling).[296,297,299]

The onset, severity, and duration of NAS may be influenced by many factors, including the specific drug(s) abused, duration of drug exposure, timing and amount of the mother's last dose before delivery, elimination of the drug by the infant, and the gestational age of the infant at birth.[297–299,305] Preterm infants display a less severe abstinence syndrome compared with term infants, possibly because of their CNS immaturity or a decreased total in utero drug exposure.[306] Neonatal methadone withdrawal may be more severe than heroin withdrawal and is associated with a higher incidence of seizures (10%–20%).[296] Withdrawal from non-narcotic drugs usually is less severe, but can also be associated with seizures.[307] Typically, the cocaine-exposed newborn is hypertonic when alert, irritable, and tremulous. Infants may display decreased interactive behavior, disorganized sleeping and feeding patterns, abnormal cry patterns, seizures, and may be intermittently lethargic. These symptoms are considered to be signs of cocaine toxicity rather than withdrawal.[297,307]

The onset of narcotic drug withdrawal ranges from minutes after delivery to 2 weeks of age, with most symptoms appearing within 72 hours.[297–299] Withdrawal from methadone, however, may be delayed in some infants, with symptoms presenting as late as 2 to 4 weeks of age.[296,298] Similarly, symptoms of barbiturate withdrawal can appear as late as 10 to 14 days.[298,299,305] The long elimination half-life of these abused substances contributes to the delayed onset of drug withdrawal (and possibly a greater duration of symptoms). Major symptoms of opiate withdrawal usually continue for 2 to 3 weeks, but subacute signs may persist for 2 to 6 months.[297–299,307] In mild cases, significant symptoms may subside within a week. The onset of SSRI withdrawal ranges from birth to 3 weeks of life with duration ranging from 2 days to 2 weeks.[302] Maternal polydrug abuse, as seen in A.K., may result in biphasic patterns or recurrence of abstinence syndrome.[299]

A.K.'s presentation is consistent with neonatal narcotic abstinence syndrome. However, clinical manifestations of NAS are similar to other serious neonatal diseases. Disorders such as infection (sepsis, meningitis), metabolic abnormalities (hypoglycemia, hypocalcemia, hypomagnesemia, hypothermia), endocrine dysfunction (adrenal insufficiency, hyperthyroidism), and CNS abnormalities (hemorrhage and anoxia) must be ruled out before specific neonatal abstinence therapy is begun.[297,307] Failure to recognize and treat these diseases would have dire consequences for A.K. A.K. also may be at risk for hepatitis and sexually transmitted diseases, including the HIV. Therefore, an accurate maternal history or testing also should be performed.

Treatment

52. What initial therapy is recommended for A.K.'s narcotic withdrawal symptoms?

Supportive Care

Because pharmacologic therapy may prolong A.K.'s hospital stay or expose her to unnecessary adverse effects, initial treatment should include nonpharmacologic measures directed at decreasing sensory stimulation. Provision of a quiet, dark, warm environment, gentle handling, and swaddling can be beneficial. Use of a pacifier for non-nutritive, excessive sucking also may help. Hypercaloric formulas (24 cal/oz) should be given as frequent small feedings to supply the additional calories that these infants require (150–250 cal/kg/day).[307] Changes in severity of symptoms, vital signs, sleeping and feeding patterns, and weight loss or gain should be monitored.

Successful management of 40% to 50% of symptomatic infants can be accomplished with supportive care alone.[297] In addition, most infants who are exposed to cocaine as the primary drug of abuse can be managed successfully without pharmacologic intervention.[297] Although most infants exposed to SSRIs require no pharmacologic treatment, some infants may benefit from supportive care measures that are commonly used to treat infants with neonatal opioid withdrawal. However, this intervention has not been evaluated in a controlled trials. Infants who have severe signs of SSRI-related withdrawal/toxicity may require pharmacologic therapy including anticonvulsants, fluid replacement, and respiratory support.[306]

Monitoring and Indications for Pharmacologic Treatment

An abstinence scoring system (e.g., Finnegan) should be used to more objectively assess symptoms of withdrawal and the need for pharmacologic treatment or dosage adjustment. The abstinence scoring sheet lists common signs and symptoms of neonatal opiate withdrawal. The infant is monitored and a number score that indicates severity is assigned to each observed symptom. A "total score" is calculated for each 2- or 4-hour observation period and is used to initiate, increase, decrease, or discontinue pharmacologic therapy.[297] Standardized scoring systems currently are used for all neonates regardless of gestational age; however, studies suggest the need for development of specific scoring systems for preterm newborns.[306] In addition, the scoring systems have not been validated for nonopioid drug exposure. Also, a potential for bias and subjectivity may affect the scores and thresholds for treatment. In general, indications for pharmacologic treatment include seizures; excessive weight loss or dehydration owing to diarrhea, vomiting, or poor feeding; severe hyperactivity, irritability, tremors, or tachypnea that interferes with feeding; inability to sleep; and significant hypothermia or hyperthermia.[296,307] If the Finnegan scoring system is used, pharmacologic treatment is generally initiated when the average of three scores is higher than 7.[298]

A.K. should be monitored closely and, if her symptoms are not controlled with supportive care, pharmacologic therapy is indicated. Pharmacologic therapy is needed in approximately 30% to 91% of infants with NAS.[306] The most common agents used to treat neonatal narcotic or CNS depressant withdrawal are phenobarbital, paregoric (camphorated tincture of opium), diluted tincture of opium, and diazepam. The choice of agent depends on the specific nursery, the predominant symptoms displayed, and the substance of abuse. For example, diazepam is the preferred agent in neonatal withdrawal from maternal benzodiazepine abuse. Doses of these agents should be initiated at lower amounts and titrated upward to a dose that controls withdrawal symptoms but does not produce toxicity. Once A.K. is symptom free for 3 to 5 days, the dose should be decreased gradually by 10% to 20% of the dose every 2 to 3 days with close patient monitoring.[298] The goals of pharmacologic therapy are to control the symptoms of withdrawal and wean the patient completely off therapy.

53. A.K.'s laboratory tests were within normal limits and other diseases have been ruled out. Her symptoms have worsened despite supportive care and pharmacologic therapy for NAS is initiated. Phenobarbital was started on day 3 of life with an IV dose of 10 mg Q 12 hours for four doses, followed by 3 mg Q 8 hours. This morning's phenobarbital serum concentration was 27 mcg/mL.

A.K. is less irritable today (day 6 of life) and no longer tachypneic. Her tremors have decreased significantly and she no longer has a high-pitched cry. She continues to have significant diarrhea and is feeding poorly. A.K. has not gained weight in the past 4 days. Evaluate A.K.'s therapy. What are your recommendations?

Phenobarbital

Phenobarbital is the drug of choice for NAS due to non-narcotic (e.g., barbiturate, alcohol) and polydrug abuse[297,298,305] and because it is a second-line agent for treatment of seizures due to withdrawal. Phenobarbital is effective in approximately 50% of neonates exposed to methadone in utero, but it is effective in approximately 90% of infants exposed to multiple drugs in utero.[307] Phenobarbital is especially useful (as demonstrated in A.K.) for controlling symptoms of CNS hyperirritability.[297] GI symptoms of withdrawal, however, do not respond well to phenobarbital. A.K. received the proper phenobarbital total loading dose (20 mg/kg) and maintenance therapy (4.5 mg/kg/day). Although generally reserved for more symptomatic patients, a loading dose of phenobarbital may decrease the duration of treatment when phenobarbital is used as a single agent.[298] The recommended loading dose is 15 to 20 mg/kg and can be given as a single dose or in divided doses.[305] A single IV, IM, or oral loading dose may be given when rapid control of symptoms is desired. However, single loading doses may be associated with CNS and respiratory depression (e.g., sedation, apnea, or an increase in periodic breathing). Maintenance doses range from 2 to 6 mg/kg/day.[297] Doses should be adjusted according to symptoms, and serum concentrations should be monitored to avoid toxicity. High dosages of phenobarbital may result in oversedation and impairment of the suck reflex. Other disadvantages of phenobarbital include development of tolerance to the sedative effects, induction of drug metabolism, and oral availability as an elixir containing 14% to 25% alcohol.[305,307] The therapeutic serum concentration for control of withdrawal symptoms has not been clearly identified; however, 20 to 30 mcg/mL has been suggested.[299,305] Although A.K.'s serum phenobarbital concentration is within the normal range, she continues to have diarrhea and has not gained weight. Because GI symptoms do not respond well to phenobarbital, an alternative agent (preferably a narcotic) should be selected.

Narcotic Agents

Because paregoric (0.4 mg/mL anhydrous morphine), tincture of opium (10 mg/mL morphine), morphine, and methadone are narcotics, they may have a physiological advantage over non-narcotics in the treatment of neonatal opiate withdrawal syndrome.[298,299,306] In addition, the constipating side effects of narcotics may be advantageous when diarrhea is part of the withdrawal symptoms. Although any narcotic theoretically could be used, most studies assessing opioid treatment have used paregoric. Paregoric is easy to administer and controls withdrawal symptoms in 90% of infants. In comparative studies, paregoric improved sucking coordination, nutrient ingestion, and weight gain better than diazepam or phenobarbital. Infants treated with paregoric also may have a lower incidence of seizure episodes than those treated with phenobarbital or diazepam. Unfortunately, large doses of paregoric often are needed and the duration of treatment usually is longer than with other agents.[297,307] In addition to opium alkaloids, paregoric contains unwarranted compounds such as antispasmodics (noscapine, papaverine), camphor (a CNS stimulant that is eliminated slowly), high concentrations of alcohol (44%–46%), anise oil, benzoic acid, and glycerine. Because some of these substances may have adverse effects on the newborn, a 25-fold dilution of tincture of opium with water (final concentration 0.4 mg/mL morphine) now is preferred.[307] The dilution of tincture of opium is free of unnecessary ingredients and has a lower alcohol concentration. It is stable for 2 weeks after dilution.[305] For term infants, the dose of paregoric (or a 25-fold dilution of tincture of opium) is 0.1 mL/kg or 2 drops/kg (0.04 mg/kg morphine)[307] given orally with feedings every 3 to 4 hours until control of withdrawal symptoms. A.K.'s dose may be initiated at 0.2 mL/dose (or 4 drops/dose) and titrated upward as needed by 0.1 mL/kg/dose every 3 to 4 hours until withdrawal symptoms are controlled. Once symptoms are controlled for 3 to 5 days, the dosage can be tapered gradually (keeping the same dosing interval).[307] A.K. also should be monitored for signs of overtreatment such as hypotonia, lethargy, irregular respirations, and bradycardia.[297]

Oral morphine (in concentrations of 2 and 4 mg/mL) may be a preferred agent when treating NAS due to opioid withdrawal. Oral morphine preparations contain less alcohol than paregoric and do not contain unwanted additives. In addition, medication errors may occur during the dilution and dosing of tincture of opium. Parenteral morphine has been used in infants to treat narcotic withdrawal seizures[298] and vasomotor collapse secondary to heroin withdrawal.[307] Parenteral morphine, however, may contain sodium bisulfite and phenol, substances that have been associated with adverse effects in newborns when given at higher doses.[307] Parenteral morphine may be used if A.K. is unable to take oral medications and a narcotic agent is desired. Methadone also may be used, but the prolonged elimination half-life (26 hours) makes tapering the dosage difficult. Initial methadone doses of 0.05 to 0.1 mg/kg given every 6 hours are recommended. Doses may be increased by 0.05 mg/kg/dose until control of withdrawal symptoms. Methadone can be administered every 12 to 24 hours once signs of withdrawal are controlled and can be discontinued once doses are weaned down to 0.05 mg/kg/day.[307]

Diazepam, Chlorpromazine, and Clonidine

Diazepam (0.3–0.5 mg/kg Q 8 hours) has been used to control the CNS hyperactivity associated with neonatal narcotic withdrawal symptoms.[296] However, diazepam may be less effective than paregoric or phenobarbital in treating symptoms of NAS. Adverse effects, which may be related to prolonged elimination and accumulation of diazepam and metabolites, can limit the drug's usefulness (e.g., depression of the suck reflex, sedation, late-onset seizures, and bradycardia).[298,299] In addition, the parenteral formulation contains substances (benzyl alcohol, sodium benzoate, ethanol, propylene glycol) known to cause problems in the newborn (see Question 49).[307]

Chlorpromazine (0.5–0.7 mg/kg Q 6 hours) controls the CNS and GI symptoms of neonatal withdrawal.[299] Disadvantages of chlorpromazine include a wide spectrum of pharmacologic effects such as cerebellar dysfunction, decreased seizure threshold, prolonged elimination in the neonate (half-life, 3 days), hypothermia, hematologic problems such as eosinophilia, and lack of long-term studies on behavioral outcomes.[299,307] As a result, chlorpromazine rarely is used to treat NAS.

Clonidine is commonly used in adults to treat narcotic withdrawal symptoms. One pilot study in neonates ($n = 7$) used oral clonidine at an initial single dose of 0.5 to 1 mcg/kg. Doses were then increased slowly over 1 to 2 days to 3 to 5 mcg/kg/day divided every 4 to 6 hours.[308] Clonidine controlled most neonatal methadone withdrawal symptoms except for poor sleeping. Hypotension and other cardiac adverse effects did not occur. Transient mild metabolic acidosis, however, was reported in two patients. Mean duration of clonidine treatment (13 days) was shorter than phenobarbital treatment (27 days) in a retrospective comparative group. Further clinical trials are needed before clonidine can be routinely recommended for treatment of NAS.

A.K. should receive long-term follow-up to monitor for potential developmental problems. Because A.K. is at risk for recurrence of drug withdrawal, her parents should receive information on recognition of symptoms. Her parents need instructions on how to care for this drug-exposed infant as well as counseling for drug addiction.

SEDATION AND PARALYSIS DURING VENTILATION

Pharmacology and Monitoring Parameters

54. M.M., a 42-week-gestation (post-term), 3,500-g male, is born with a history of meconium-stained amniotic fluid. At birth, meconium was removed by suction from M.M.'s nose and mouth. M.M. was tachypneic (RR, 80 breaths/minute) and cyanotic and had decreased peripheral perfusion. His Apgar score at 1 minute was 5. M.M. was intubated shortly after delivery and his trachea was suctioned to remove meconium. Immediate ABGs, obtained while M.M. was intubated and ventilated with an Ambu bag at 60 breaths/minute and 100% oxygen, revealed the following: pH, 7.18; P_{CO_2}, 55 mmHg; and PO_2, 50 mmHg. M.M.'s clinical condition and ABG results (acidosis, increased P_{CO_2}, and hypoxia) were consistent with persistent pulmonary hypertension of the newborn and appropriate tests confirmed the diagnosis. He currently is receiving mechanical ventilation using hyperoxia and hyperventilation to achieve a target P_{CO_2} of 30 mmHg and pH of 7.5. M.M. had been "fighting the ventilator" and pancuronium bromide 0.35 mg IV every 30 to 60 minutes as needed for spontaneous movement was initiated. M.M.'s other medications are ampicillin and gentamicin to rule out sepsis, and dopamine, dobutamine, and sodium bicarbonate for his persistent pulmonary hypertension of the newborn. After evaluating M.M.'s paralysis therapy, what medications should be started immediately for him?

[SI units: P_{CO_2}, 7.33 kPa, 4.0 kPa, respectively; P_{O_2}, 6.7 kPa]

Neonates with severe lung disease (e.g., RDS, persistent pulmonary hypertension of the newborn, pneumonia) may require mechanical ventilation with high ventilatory settings (high rates or pressures). Ineffective mechanical ventilation results when neonates fight the ventilator (i.e., spontaneously breathe asynchronously or out of phase with mechanical ventilation). Advancements in ventilator technology (e.g., synchronized ventilation or patient-triggered ventilation) may help to decrease asynchronized breathing. However, sedation generally is indicated when high ventilator settings are used or when patients fight the ventilator after ventilator adjustments. Paralysis usually is reserved for cases when sedation alone does not improve the effectiveness of mechanical ventilation. Typically, paralysis is required in severely ill, hypoxic neonates such as M.M. Paralysis increases chest wall compliance and allows for adequate oxygenation and ventilation.[309,310] It also decreases oxygen consumption, improves blood gases, and may decrease the risk for pneumothorax.[309,311] In addition, paralysis of neonates with persistent pulmonary hypertension of the newborn (like M.M.) indirectly decreases right-to-left shunting through the ductus arteriosus and foramen ovale and results in increased oxygenation.[312]

Pancuronium bromide causes skeletal muscle paralysis by competitively blocking acetylcholine at postsynaptic nicotinic cholinergic receptors located on the muscle fiber (motor endplate) of the neuromuscular junction.[311,313] At normal clinical doses, pancuronium has minimal ganglionic blocking effects and possesses little histamine-releasing activity.[311,313] Onset of effect occurs within minutes and duration, which typically lasts 30 to 60 minutes after a single dose, increases with incremental dosing. Like pancuronium, vecuronium is also a nondepolarizing neuromuscular blocking agent commonly used in neonates.[8] Each agent may offer certain advantages in specific neonatal patients. Pancuronium is primarily eliminated via the kidneys (60%). Thus, without a dosage adjustment, patients with decreased renal function have a prolongation of pancuronium's neuromuscular blocking effect. Vecuronium, however, is excreted primarily via biliary elimination (50%) and, therefore, dosage reduction in hepatic (but not renal) dysfunction is required. Many neonatal centers prefer vecuronium because a dosage adjustment is not needed in patients with renal dysfunction. M.M.'s dose of pancuronium is appropriate. Pancuronium and vecuronium can be dosed at 0.05 to 0.1 mg/kg every 30 to 60 minutes IV as needed for spontaneous movement. Some neonates require a continuous infusion, using doses of either agent of 0.02 to 0.05 mg/kg/hour. Many factors (e.g., serum electrolytes, acid–base balance, concomitant medications) can affect the duration of action of neuromuscular blocking agents and dosage needs to be individualized.[8]

The greatest danger of using any neuromuscular blocking agent is inadvertent disconnection from the ventilator with resultant apnea. When paralytic agents are initiated, adjustments in ventilator settings usually are required to avoid hypoventilation. Clinically important adverse effects include tachycardia and fluid retention with significant edema.[311,314] Although pancuronium usually does not have a significant effect on BP,[314] hypertension[315] and occasional reports of hypotension[316] (usually in marginally hypovolemic neonates) have been reported. Ventilatory settings, blood gases, spontaneous movements, daily weights, fluid intake and output, HR, and BP should be monitored. If tachycardia becomes serious, another nondepolarizing neuromuscular blocking agent with fewer cardiovascular effects, such as vecuronium, can be used.

Paralysis, as well as intubation and mechanical ventilation, may be extremely stressful to the neonate. Neuromuscular blocking agents do not possess any analgesic, sedative, or amnestic effects.[311,313] Therefore, sedation therapy should be instituted as soon as possible in M.M. Neonates and even premature newborns have the anatomical structures and physiological capacity to sense pain.[317,318] Because clinical symptoms of pain may go undetected in paralyzed neonates, a sedative/analgesic such as morphine may be preferred for sedation. In fact, preliminary data suggest that poor neurologic outcomes may occur less frequently in mechanically ventilated neonates who receive continuous low-dose morphine infusions compared with those who receive infusions of midazolam or placebo.[319] In addition, administration of analgesics for painful procedures may be easily forgotten when neonates are sedated with nonanalgesics such as phenobarbital, benzodiazepines, or chloral hydrate. Because paralysis masks the clinical symptoms of seizures,[311] M.M. should be monitored carefully for rhythmic fluctuations in HR, BP, ECG, and oxygenation. These rhythmic changes may indicate seizure activity in a paralyzed neonate and, if observed, EEG testing is indicated.[320] The EEG also may be monitored in paralyzed newborns who are at high risk for seizure activity (e.g., asphyxiated neonates). Alternatively, some clinicians advocate routine sedation with phenobarbital (rather than morphine), which also would treat any clinically inapparent seizure activity.

Morphine usually is administered by slow IV push over 1 to 2 minutes at initial doses of 0.05 to 0.1 mg/kg every 2 to 4 hours.[321] The dose is then titrated according to clinical symptoms. A continuous morphine infusion may be preferred for patients with persistent pulmonary hypertension or in infants requiring intermittent morphine doses every 2 hours or less. Clinically, a bolus infusion of 0.05 mg/kg can be given, followed by a continuous infusion at an initial dose of 0.02 mg/kg/hour (20 mcg/kg/hour). The infusion should be carefully titrated. Morphine clearance in neonates, especially premature neonates, is greatly reduced but increases with PCA.[322] Adverse effects of morphine include hypotension, decreased GI motility, respiratory depression, tolerance, and physiological dependence with prolonged use. The use of morphine in neonates may be limited by histamine release and the development of hypotension.

Fentanyl, a synthetic opiate with less histamine-releasing activity and fewer cardiovascular effects, may be used as an alternative agent. Fentanyl is 50 to 100 times more potent than morphine, but has a shorter duration of action and therefore usually is administered by continuous IV infusion (0.5–2 mcg/kg/hour).[8,323] Continuous infusion of fentanyl, however, may be associated with a greater development of tolerance and physical dependence compared with intermittent morphine administration.[324,325] Continuous fentanyl infusions of 5 and 9 or more days have been associated with a >50% and a 100% chance, respectively, of developing withdrawal symptoms,[326] and withdrawal has been reported after as few as 3 days.[327]

At this time, recommendations for M.M. should include the addition of morphine as a sedative agent (initial bolus infusion of 0.18 mg, followed by a continuous infusion starting at 0.07 mg/hr [70 mcg/hour]) and an ocular lubricant to prevent corneal abrasions. Neuromuscular blocking agents prevent blinking, and corneal abrasions may occur. Because tolerance to opiates develops, the morphine dose needs to be increased with continued use. Determination of adequate sedation is difficult in paralyzed infants, but increases in HR and BP or decreases in oxygenation may indicate inadequate sedation. M.M. may also require additional sedation/anxiolytic therapy with benzodiazepines such as lorazepam or midazolam. Diazepam is not a preferred agent for sedation in neonates owing to its long half-life and accumulation of its active metabolite (*N*-desmethyldiazepam).

Drug/Disease Interactions

55. Morphine and an ocular lubricant (as an ophthalmic ointment applied to both eyes Q 6 hours PRN) were added to M.M.'s therapy. On day 2 of life, M.M. continues on mechanical ventilation with hyperoxia and hyperventilation. His ABG is pH, 7.5; P_{CO_2}, 30 mmHg; and P_{O_2}, 55 mmHg. M.M. continues to receive IV ampicillin, gentamicin, dopamine, dobutamine, sodium bicarbonate, and pancuronium. What factors may influence the neuromuscular blocking effect of pancuronium in M.M.? What adjustments to his dosing schedule should be made?

[SI units: P_{CO_2}, 4.0 kPa; P_{O_2}, 7.33 kPa]

Both alkalosis and gentamicin may potentiate the neuromuscular blocking effects of pancuronium in M.M.[311] Although alkalosis may potentiate and acidosis may antagonize the effects of pancuronium, the opposite effects have been reported with vecuronium.[311] Pancuronium already is being dosed in M.M. on an "as-needed" basis. Monitoring for spontaneous movement should continue, and a longer required dosing interval may be noted. If gentamicin then is discontinued or pH is normalized, the duration of effect may shorten. Other factors such as electrolyte status, disease states, and other medications may influence the pharmacodynamics of neuromuscular blocking agents.[311] For instance, renal or hepatic impairment (such as cholestasis) may result in accumulation of drug or active metabolite (3-hydroxypancuronium) and a prolonged effect.

Toxicity

56. Sodium bicarbonate, dobutamine, and dopamine were discontinued on day 3 of life. On day 4 of life, M.M.'s antibiotics were discontinued after culture results ruled out infection. On Friday (day 5 of life), pancuronium was discontinued and M.M. remained intubated. Concerns about morphine "addiction" resulted in the discontinuation of morphine and the initiation of chloral hydrate 250 mg NG Q 4 hours for sedation. On Monday morning, M.M. was noted to have severe lethargy, decreased deep tendon reflexes, and respiratory depression requiring an increase in ventilator settings. Bowel sounds were absent and M.M. had marked abdominal distention. Is M.M. experiencing prolonged paralysis from pancuronium? What is your assessment of this situation?

Administration of opiates for sedation or analgesia does not cause addiction.[328] The term "addiction" should be used only to describe complex behavioral patterns characterized by a preoccupation with obtainment of a drug (drug-seeking behavior) and compulsive drug use. Prolonged administration of opiates may cause tolerance (i.e., a decreased effect after repeated administration of the original dosage or an increasing dosage requirement to attain the original effect) or physical dependence. Physical dependence requires the continued administration of a medication to prevent symptoms of withdrawal. Although symptoms of withdrawal may occur when opiates are discontinued, careful weaning of the opiate and appropriate monitoring of symptoms using an abstinence scoring method lessen withdrawal severity. Opioids may be weaned in <72 hours when low to moderate doses have been used for <1 week. Typically, the dose is decreased by 25% to 50% initially (and by 20% subsequently) every 6 to 8 hours. If opioids are used for >1 week, smaller decreases in doses, a longer total weaning time, and conversion to an oral agent usually are required.[328] In M.M.'s case, IV morphine could have been continued for sedation or an appropriate oral agent could have been used if normal bowel function was apparent.

Disuse atrophy, muscle weakness, joint contractures, and prolonged paralysis have been reported after discontinuing neuromuscular blocking agents.[311] Prolonged neuromuscular blockade may be more common in patients with renal or hepatic dysfunction or with the use of continuous infusion, prolonged therapy, or certain concomitant medications. In particular, prolonged paralysis may be seen after discontinuation of steroidally based neuromuscular blocking agents (e.g., pancuronium, vecuronium) when these agents have been administered with corticosteroids.[329] In this case, M.M. did not have any apparent renal or hepatic disease, was treated with intermittent "as-needed" doses, received short-term paralysis, and did not receive corticosteroids. Therefore, M.M. would be at a low risk for developing prolonged paralysis after discontinuation of pancuronium.

The most likely cause of M.M.'s current symptoms is chloral hydrate intoxication. The recommended initial dose of chloral hydrate for prolonged sedation in neonates is 10 to 30 mg/kg/dose given every 6 to 8 hours on an as-needed basis.[330] Although some clinicians recommend 20 to 40 mg/kg/dose every 4 to 6 hours as needed (80–240 mg/kg/day),[321] toxicity has been reported in a term infant with persistent pulmonary hypertension of the newborn receiving doses of 44 to 50 mg/kg every 6 hours (176–200 mg/kg/day).[330] M.M. received approximately 70 mg/kg/dose every 4 hours around the clock for 3 days.

Chloral hydrate is metabolized quickly in erythrocytes and the liver by alcohol dehydrogenase to trichloroethanol, an active metabolite. Trichloroethanol is metabolized to trichloroacetate and to trichloroethanol glucuronide in the liver and renally eliminated. The conversion of chloral hydrate to trichloroethanol may not be as rapid in neonates,[331] and both chloral hydrate and trichloroethanol may be responsible for the sedative effects seen in neonates.[332] The parent drug (chloral hydrate) may be responsible for the immediate short-term sedative effects, whereas trichloroethanol may be responsible for long-term effects. The short duration of sedation (2 hours) necessitates frequent repeated dosing that unfortunately results in accumulation of the active metabolite, trichloroethanol, and toxic effects. The half-life of trichloroethanol is prolonged in preterm (40 hours) and term neonates (28 hours).[331] Because trichloroethanol may accumulate, chloral hydrate should be used only on an as-needed basis for long-term sedation in neonates. The lower end of the recommended dosage range should be used for preterm newborns, and all neonates, especially those who require frequent repeated doses, should be monitored for toxic effects.

Toxicities of chloral hydrate include CNS, respiratory, and myocardial depression; gastric irritation; adynamic ileus; cardiac arrhythmias; hypotension; renal impairment; bladder atony; and direct hyperbilirubinemia.[330] Although M.M. is showing signs of CNS depression (lethargy, decreased deep tendon reflexes), respiratory depression (increased ventilator settings), and GI effects (absent bowel sounds, abdominal distention), a physical examination and appropriate laboratory tests should be performed to identify other known toxicities (e.g., serum BUN and SrCr to detect renal impairment). In addition, other causes of M.M.'s current condition also should be ruled out (e.g., sepsis, meningitis, intracranial hemorrhage, metabolic disorder). Chloral hydrate should be discontinued and trichloroethanol serum concentrations determined, if available. Supportive care should be given and severe toxicities may require exchange transfusions.[330]

USE AND ADMINISTRATION OF MEDICATIONS

Drug Formulation Problems

57. What problems are encountered with the use of commercially available medications in the neonate?

The lack of appropriate enteral and parenteral formulations results in many unique problems of drug use and administration in the neonatal population.

Lack of Nonsolid Enteral Dosage Formulations

Many drugs used in neonates and infants are not commercially available in an enteral liquid dosage form, including acetazolamide, captopril, enalapril, rifampin, spironolactone/hydrochlorothiazide, and ursodiol. For some medications, such as sodium chloride, the liquid injectable form can be given enterally. Otherwise, extemporaneous powder formulations or liquid preparations must be made from the solid dosage forms.[8,333]

Little information exists regarding the preparation and stability of extemporaneous formulations.[334] Formulations intended for neonates should limit the use of pharmaceutical adjuvants, unnecessary ingredients (e.g., flavoring agents for drugs administered via nasogastric tubes), and other substances that would increase osmolality.

Inappropriate Concentrations

Most drugs are formulated for use in the adult population. As a result, the available concentrations of liquid formulations result in appropriate volumes for adult doses, but extremely small volumes for the doses required by neonates. Frequently, these volumes are too small to accurately measure (i.e., <0.1 mL). Therefore, dilutions of commercially available injections (e.g., aminophylline, digoxin, morphine, phenobarbital) are necessary to accurately measure the small doses required by neonates. Proper diluents and dilutional techniques must be ensured because inappropriate dilutions are a common source of potentially fatal medication errors (Table 94-12).[321,335] In addition, the sterility and stability of these diluted injections need to be documented before being used in neonates.[334]

Hypertonicity

In the neonate, parenteral and enteral administration of hypertonic medications may result in severe adverse effects.[336,337] NEC and IVH have been associated with IV administration of hyperosmolar drugs, such as radiographic contrast media or sodium bicarbonate. Infusions of hypertonic medications directly into the umbilical or portal vein have resulted in severe hepatic injury. In addition, enteral administration of hyperosmolar medications and feedings have been associated with NEC.[336,337] Therefore, appropriate dilutions of hypertonic medications should be made before administration to neonates.

Pharmaceutical Adjuvants

Ingredients used for the enhancement of bioavailability, stability, taste, or appearance of medications can cause adverse

Table 94-12 Potential Errors in Drug Administration Techniques

Factors Involving Drug (Dose) Preparation
Inappropriate dilutions
Similarity in appearance of dose units
Loss of potentially large amounts of drug dose in the dead space of a syringe or infusion Y site
Unsuitable drug formulations for administration
Unlabeled or undesirable ingredients in dosage forms
Undesirable drug concentrations and/or osmolalities
Errors in interpreting drug orders and/or dose calculations
Factors Involving IV Drug Administration
Loss of drug consequent to routine changing of IV sets
Reduction in serum concentrations for drugs with rapid plasma clearance that are infused slowly
Extreme ↑in plasma concentrations consequent to rapid infusion of drugs with small central compartment Vd
Delayed infusion of total dose when IV line is not flushed
Inadvertent admixture of drugs by the manual IV retrograde method
Large distance between the site of drug infusion into an IV line and the insertion of the line into the patient
Potential loss of large-volume doses in the overflow syringe with the IV retrograde technique
Possible loss of drug because of binding to IV tubing
Use of large intraluminal diameter tubing for small patients
Infiltrations not detected by pump alarms
Infusion of multiple medications/fluids at different rates by means of a common "hub"
Oscillations in fluid/dose rate of potent medications infused with piston-type pumps
Factors Involving Other Routes of Drug Administration
Loss of delivery (NG tube dead space) or from oral cavity
Leakage of drug from IM or SC injection site
Expulsion of drug from the rectum
Misapplication to external sites (i.e., ophthalmic ointment in young infants)

IM, intramuscular; IV, intravenous; NG, nasogastric; SC, subcutaneous; Vd, volume of distribution.

Reproduced with permission from Blumer JL, Reed MD. Principles of neonatal pharmacology. In: Yaffe SJ, Aranda JV, eds. Neonatal and Pediatric Pharmacology: Therapeutic Principles in Practice, 3rd ed. Philadelphia: Lippincott Williams & Wilkins; 2005:152. 1992;168.

effects in neonates.[338] Preservatives such as benzyl alcohol or methylparaben may displace bilirubin from albumin-binding sites.[23] Benzyl alcohol also may cause the potentially fatal "gasping syndrome" (see the Neonatal Pharmacokinetics, Metabolism section). Propylene glycol, a solubilizing agent, may cause several toxicities in neonates, including hyperosmolality, lactic acidosis, seizures, CNS and respiratory depression, hypotension, and arrhythmias.[338] Emulsifiers, such as Polysorbate 20 and Polysorbate 80, have been associated with hypotension, renal dysfunction, hepatotoxicity, and death in low-birth-weight infants.[339] Sorbitol, a poorly absorbed sweetener, may cause osmotic diarrhea, intestinal gas, bloating, and abdominal pain when administered enterally in large doses. A report of sorbitol-induced pneumatosis intestinalis in a child underscores the serious consequence of receiving multiple liquid medications containing sorbitol.[340] Unfortunately, these undesired substances are currently not required by law to be listed in the package insert of oral medications.[338] The safety of pharmaceutical adjuvants should be examined thoroughly before these substances are used in the neonatal population. In addition, further studies are required to identify other pharmaceutical ingredients that may be potentially toxic to the neonate.

Drug Administration

58. D.S., a 4-day-old female neonate born at 30 weeks' gestational age with a current weight of 1,200 g, has a birth history of prolonged rupture of membranes and a difficult delivery. Her current problems include rule out sepsis and apnea of prematurity. D.S. receives the following: ampicillin, 60 mg IV Buretrol Q 12 hours at 2 am and 2 pm (100 mg/kg/day); gentamicin, 3.6 mg IV Buretrol Q 24 hours at 7 am (3 mg/kg/day); aminophylline, 1.2 mg IV Buretrol Q 12 hours at 10 am and 10 pm (2 mg/kg/day); and dextrose, 5% NaCl 0.2% with KCl 1.8 mEq/day and calcium gluconate 250 mg/day at 6 mL/hr. Gentamicin serum concentrations were obtained today (day 4 of antibiotic therapy) and reported as a trough of 1.2 mcg/mL at 6:50 am and a peak of 2.8 mcg/mL at 8 am. Using standard pharmacokinetic equations you calculate a Kd of 0.037 hr^{-1}, half-life of 18.7 hours, and Vd of 1.8 L/kg. What should be done next for D.S.?

Serum concentrations of aminoglycosides and other drugs can be affected significantly by the IV drug delivery system.[341,342] The low IV infusion rates required by neonates significantly delay drug delivery, especially if medications are administered via volumetric chamber devices (e.g., Buretrol or Metriset) or via the Y-site injection port distal to the patient. Even when factors such as injection site, infusion rate, drug volume, and tubing diameter are considered, actual drug delivery may be delayed up to 2 hours using volumetric chamber devices.[341] If aminoglycosides are administered by Y-site injection, peak concentrations can be decreased by a mean of 2.5 mcg/mL and delayed by 1.5 hours compared with IV syringe pump administration.[343] Trough concentrations, however, are not significantly affected. As a result of inappropriate administration methods, a larger Vd and prolonged half-life would be calculated, as demonstrated in D.S.

D.S.'s unbelievably large Vd should lead to suspicion of the method of drug administration. At this time, no dosage change can be recommended for D.S. Serum aminoglycoside concentrations should be repeated after an appropriate IV administration method is instituted. This method should include the use of a neonatal syringe pump, low-volume IV tubing, and drug injection into the port most proximal to the neonate.[341,342]

Other potential neonatal IV drug administration errors are listed in Table 94-12. Additional problems include significant overdoses resulting from the unintended delivery of residual drug from the hub or needle of syringes (i.e., dead spaces), and underdosages due to trapping of medications in IV filters.[321,335] In addition, the neonate's limited ability to tolerate excess fluid prohibits drug delivery via IV riders or "piggybacks," which significantly increase fluid administration. Neonates also require special IV rates of drug infusion (i.e., mg/kg/minute) to avoid significant adverse effects. Appropriate references should be consulted for drug-specific methods and rates of infusion, appropriate final concentrations, and other special neonatal considerations.[8]

REFERENCES

1. Shirkey H. Editorial comment: therapeutic orphans. *Pediatrics* 1999;104:583.
2. Gilman JT, Gal P. Pharmacokinetic and pharmacodynamic data collection in children and neonates: a quiet frontier. *Clin Pharmacokinet* 1992; 23:1.
3. Wilson JT. An update on the therapeutic orphan. *Pediatrics* 1999;104:585.
4. Pediatric studies of drugs, Section 111, FDA Modernization Act of 1997, Public Law 105–115, 105th Congress of the United States.
5. Best Pharmaceuticals for Children Act, Public Law, 107–109, 107th Congress of the United States.
6. Fletcher MA. Physical assessment and classification. In: Avery GB et al., eds. *Neonatology: Pathophysiology and Management of the Newborn,* 5th ed. Philadelphia: Lippincott Williams & Wilkins; 1999:301.
7. MacDonald MG et al. *Avery's Neonatology: Pathophysiology and Management of the Newborn,* 6th ed. Philadelphia: Lippincott Williams & Wilkins; 2005:1501.
8. Taketomo CK et al. *Pediatric Dosage Handbook,* 14th ed. Hudson, OH: Lexi-Comp; 2007.
9. Yahav J. Development of parietal cells, acid secretion, and response to secretagogues. In: Lebenthal E, ed. *Human Gastrointestinal Development.* New York: Raven Press; 1989:341.
10. Hyman PE et al. Gastric acid secretory function in preterm infants. *J Pediatr* 1985;106:467.
11. Morselli PL. Clinical pharmacology of the perinatal period and early infancy. *Clin Pharmacokinet* 1989;17(Suppl 1):13.
12. Besunder JB et al. Principles of drug disposition in the neonate. A critical evaluation of the pharmacokinetic-pharmacodynamic interface. Part I. *Clin Pharmacokinet* 1988;14:189.
13. Radde IC. Mechanisms of drug absorption and their development. In: Radde IC, MacLeod SM, eds. *Pediatric Pharmacology and Therapeutics.* St. Louis: Mosby-Year Book; 1993:16.
14. Heimann G. Enteral absorption and bioavailability in children in relation to age. *Eur J Clin Pharmacol* 1980;18:43.
15. Stewart CF, Hampton EW. Effect of maturation on drug disposition in pediatric patients. *Clin Pharm* 1987;6:548.
16. Seigler RS. The administration of rectal diazepam for acute management of seizures. *J Emerg Med* 1990;8:155.
17. Wu PYK et al. Peripheral blood flow in the neonate. 1. Changes in total, skin, and muscle blood flow with gestational and postnatal age. *Pediatr Res* 1980;14:1374.
18. Barrett DA, Rutter N. Transdermal delivery and the premature neonate. *Crit Rev Ther Drug Carrier Syst* 1994;11:1.
19. Radde IC. Growth and drug distribution. In: Radde IC, Macleod SM, eds. *Pediatric Pharmacology and Therapeutics.* St. Louis: Mosby-Year Book; 1993:43.
20. Friis-Hansen B. Water distribution in the foetus and newborn infant. *Acta Paediatr Scand* 1983; 305(Suppl):7.
21. Morselli PL et al. Clinical pharmacokinetics in newborns and infants. *Clin Pharmacokinet* 1980;5: 485.
22. Besunder JB et al. Principles of drug disposition in the neonate. A critical evaluation of the pharmacokinetic-pharmacodynamic interface. Part II. *Clin Pharmacokinet* 1988;14:261.
23. Radde IC. Drugs and protein binding. In: Radde IC, Macleod SM, eds. *Pediatric Pharmacology and Therapeutics.* St. Louis: Mosby-Year Book; 1993:31.
24. Aranda JV et al. Pharmacokinetic aspects of theophylline in premature newborns. *N Engl J Med* 1976;295:413.
25. Rane A et al. Plasma protein binding of diphenylhydantoin in normal and hyperbilirubinemic infants. *J Pediatr* 1971;78:877.
26. Cashore WJ. Hyperbilirubinemia. In: Pomerance JJ, Richardson CJ, eds. *Neonatology for the Clinician.* Norwalk, CT: Appleton & Lange; 1993:231.
27. Robertson A, Brodersen R. Effect of drug combinations on bilirubin-albumin binding. *Dev Pharmacol Ther* 1991;17:95.
28. Martin E et al. Ceftriaxone-bilirubin-albumin interactions in the neonate: an in vivo study. *Eur J Pediatr* 1993;152:530.
29. Stutman HR et al. Potential of moxalactam and other new antimicrobial agents for bilirubin-albumin displacement in neonates. *Pediatrics* 1985; 75:294.
30. Springer C, Eyal F. Pharmacology of trimethoprim-sulfamethoxazole in newborn infants. *J Pediatr* 1982;100:647.
31. Kearns GL. Pharmacogenetics and development: are infants and children at increased risk for adverse outcomes? *Curr Opin Pediatr* 1995;7:220.
32. Radde IC, Kalow W. Drug biotransformation and its development. In: Radde IC, Macleod SM, eds. *Pediatric Pharmacology and Therapeutics.* St. Louis: Mosby-Year Book; 1993:57.
33. Leeder JS, Kearns GL. Pharmacogenetics in pediatrics: implications for practice. *Pediatr Clin North Am* 1997;44:55.
34. de Wildt SN et al. Cytochrome P450 3A: ontogeny and drug disposition. *Clin Pharmacokinet* 1999;37:485.
35. Aranda JV et al. Hepatic microsomal drug oxidation and electron transport in newborn infants. *J Pediatr* 1974;85:534.
36. Kraus DK et al. Alterations in theophylline metabolism during the first year of life. *Clin Pharmacol Ther* 1993;54:351.
37. de Wildt SN et al. Glucuronidation in humans: pharmacogenetic and developmental aspects. *Clin Pharmacokinet* 1999;36:439.
38. LeBel M. Benzyl alcohol metabolism and elimination in neonates. *Dev Pharmacol Ther* 1988;11:347.
39. Gershanik J et al. The gasping syndrome and benzyl alcohol poisoning. *N Engl J Med* 1982;307:1384.
40. Food and Drug Administration. Benzyl alcohol may be toxic to newborns. *FDA Drug Bull* 1982;12:10.
41. Morselli PL et al. Diazepam elimination in premature and term infants and children. *J Perinat Med* 1973;1:133.
42. Sereni F et al. Induction of drug metabolizing enzyme activities in the human fetus and in the newborn infant. *Enzyme* 1973;15:318.
43. Gal P et al. The influence of asphyxia on phenobarbital dosing requirements in neonates. *Dev Pharmacol Ther* 1984;7:145.
44. Radde IC. Renal function and elimination of drugs during development. In: Radde IC, Macleod SM, eds. *Pediatric Pharmacology and Therapeutics.* St. Louis: Mosby-Year Book; 1993:87.
45. Vanpee M et al. Renal function in very low birthweight infants: normal maturity reached during early childhood. *J Pediatr* 1992;121:784.
46. Rodvold KA et al. Bayesian forecasting of serum vancomycin concentrations in neonates and infants. *Ther Drug Monit* 1995;17:239.
47. Rodvold KA et al. Pharmacokinetics and administration regimens of vancomycin in neonates, infant and children. *Clin Pharmacokinet* 1997;33:32.
48. Rodvold et al. Prediction of gentamicin concentrations in neonates and infants using a Bayesian pharmacokinetic model. *Dev Pharmacol Ther* 1993;20:211.
49. Kildoo C et al. Developmental pattern of gentamicin kinetics in very low birthweight (VLBW) sick infants. *Dev Pharmacol Ther* 1984;7:345.
50. Kasik JW et al. Postconceptional age and gentamicin elimination half-life. *J Pediatr* 1985;106:502.
51. Phelps SJ. Pediatric Injectable Drugs, 6th ed. Bethesda: *American Society of Health-System Pharmacists*: 2002:180.
52. Prober CG et al. The use of antibiotics in neonates weighing less than 1200 grams. *Pediatr Infect Dis J* 1990;9:111.
53. Friedman CA et al. Gentamicin disposition in asphyxiated newborns: relationship to mean arterial pressure and urine output. *Pediatr Pharmacol* 1982;2:189.
54. Zarfin Y et al. Possible indomethacin-aminoglycoside interaction in preterm infants. *J Pediatr* 1985;106:511.
55. Koren G et al. Effects of indomethacin on digoxin pharmacokinetics in preterm infants. *Pediatr Pharmacol* 1984;4:25.
56. Hook JB, Hewitt WR. Development of mechanisms for drug excretion. *Am J Med* 1977;62:497.
57. Notter RH. Lung surfactants. In: Lenfant C, ed. *Lung Biology in Health and Disease.* New York: Marcel Dekker; 2000:233.
58. Whitsett JA et al. Acute respiratory disorders. In: Avery GB et al., eds. *Neonatology: Pathophysiology and Management of the Newborn,* 5th ed. Philadelphia: Lippincott Williams & Wilkins; 1999: 485.
59. Hagedorn MI et al. Respiratory diseases. In: Merenstein GB, Gardner SL, eds. *Handbook of Neonatal Intensive Care,* 4th ed. St. Louis: Mosby-Year Book; 1999:437.
60. Stark AR, Frank ID. Respiratory distress syndrome. *Pediatr Clin North Am* 1986;33:533.
61. Jobe AH. Lung development and maturation. In: Martin RJ et al., eds. *Neonatal-Perinatal Medicine: Diseases of the Fetus and Infant,* 8th ed. Philadelphia: Mosby-Elsevier; 2006:1069.
62. Rodriguez RJ et al. The respiratory distress syndrome and its management. In: Martin RJ, Fanaroff AA, Walsh MC, eds. *Neonatal-Perinatal Medicine: Diseases of the Fetus and Infant,* 8th ed. Philadelphia: Mosby Elsevier; 2006:1097.
63. Goldenberg RL, Rouse DJ. Medical progress: prevention of premature birth. *N Engl J Med* 1998;339: 313.
64. National Institutes of Health (NIH) Consensus Development Panel. Effect of corticosteroids for fetal maturation on perinatal outcomes. *JAMA* 1995;273: 413.
65. Crowley PA. Antenatal corticosteroid therapy: a meta-analysis of the randomized trials, 1992–1994. *Am J Obstet Gynecol* 1995;173:322.
66. Aghajafari F et al. Multiple courses of antenatal corticosteroids: a systematic review and meta-analysis. *Am J Obstet Gynecol* 2001;185:1073.
67. French H et al. Repeated antenatal corticosteroids: size at birth and subsequent development. *Am J Obstet Gynecol* 1999;180:114.
68. Vermillion ST et al. Neonatal sepsis and death after multiple courses of antenatal betamethasone therapy. *Am J Obstet Gynecol* 2000;183:810.
69. National Institutes of Health Consensus Development Panel. Antenatal corticosteroids revisited: repeat courses. *Obstet Gynecol* 2000;98:144.
70. Guinn DA et al. Single vs weekly courses of antenatal corticosteroids for women at risk of preterm delivery. *JAMA* 2001;286:1581.
71. Crowther CA et al. Neonatal respiratory distress syndrome after repeat exposure to antenatal corticosteroids: a randomised controlled trial. *Lancet* 2006;367:1913.
72. Wapner RJ et al. Single versus weekly courses of antenatal corticosteroids: evaluation of safety and efficacy. *Am J Obstet Gynecol* 2006;195:633.
73. Baud O et al. Antenatal glucocorticoid treatment and cystic periventricular leukomalacia in very premature infants. *N Engl J Med* 1999;341:1190.
74. Lee BH et al. Adverse neonatal outcomes associated with antenatal dexamethasone versus antenatal betamethasone. *Pediatrics* 2006;117:1503.
75. Spinillo A et al. Two-year infant neurodevelopmental outcome after single or multiple antenatal courses of corticosteroids to prevent complications of prematurity. *Am J Obstet Gynecol* 2004; 191:271.
76. Hallman M et al. The fate of exogenous surfactant in neonates with respiratory distress syndrome. *Clin Pharmacokinet* 1994;26:215.

77. Crowther CA et al. Prenatal thyrotropin-releasing hormone for preterm birth. *Cochrane Database Syst Rev, The Cochrane Library* 2003;1:CD000019.
78. Walti H, Monset-Couchard M. A risk-benefit assessment of natural and synthetic exogenous surfactants in the management of neonatal respiratory distress syndrome. *Drug Saf* 1998;18:321.
79. Stevens TP, Sinkin RA. Surfactant replacement therapy. *Chest* 2007;131:1577.
80. Curley AE, Halliday HL. The present status of exogenous surfactant for the newborn. *Early Hum Dev* 2001;61:67.
81. Survanta intratracheal suspension package insert. Columbus, OH: Ross Products Division, Abbott Laboratories Inc.; 2004 May.
82. Infasurf intratracheal suspension package insert. St. Louis, MO: Forest Pharmaceuticals, Inc.; 2003 June.
83. Curosurf intratracheal suspension package insert. Napa, CA: Dey; 2002 February.
84. Bloom BT et al. Comparison on Infasurf (calf lung surfactant extract) to Survanta (beractant) in the treatment and prevention of respiratory distress syndrome. *Pediatrics* 1997;100:31.
85. Kattwinkel J. Surfactant: evolving issues. *Clin Perinatol* 1998;25:17.
86. Speer CP et al. Randomised clinical trial of two treatment regimens of natural surfactant preparations in neonatal respiratory distress syndrome. *Arch Dis Child* 1995;72:F8.
87. Soll RF. Surfactant therapy in the USA: trials and current routines. *Biol Neonate* 1997;71(Suppl 1):1.
88. Kattwinkel J et al. High-versus low-threshold surfactant retreatment for neonatal respiratory distress syndrome. *Pediatr* 2000;106:282.
89. Soll RF, Morley CJ. Prophylactic versus selective use of surfactant in preventing morbidity and mortality in preterm infants. *Cochrane Database Syst Rev* 2001:2:CD000510.
90. Yost CC, Soll RF. Early versus delayed selective surfactant treatment for neonatal respiratory distress syndrome. *Cochrane Database Syst Rev* 2000:2: CD001456.
91. Sitler CG et al. Pump administration of exogenous surfactant: effects on oxygenation, heart rate, and chest wall movement of premature infants. *J Perinatol* 1993;13:197.
92. Attar MA. Immediate changes in lung compliance following natural surfactant administration in premature infants with respiratory distress syndrome: a controlled trial. *J Perinatol* 2004;24:626.
93. Sinha SK et al. A multicenter, randomized, controlled trial of lucinactant versus poractant alfa among very premature infants at high risk for respiratory distress syndrome. *Pediatrics* 2005;115: 1030.
94. American Academy of Pediatrics. Committee on Fetus and Newborn. Surfactant replacement therapy for respiratory distress syndrome. *Pediatrics* 1999; 103:684.
95. Zola EM et al. Comparison of three dosing procedures for administration of bovine surfactant to neonates with respiratory distress syndrome. *J Pediatr* 1993;122:453.
96. Tran JH, Raju TNK. Cost-analyses from repackaging of expensive drugs: An example using an exogenous surfactant preparation [Abstract]. *Pediatr Res* 1999;40:220A.
97. Green TP et al. Furosemide promotes patent ductus arteriosus in premature infants with the respiratory distress syndrome. *N Engl J Med* 1983;308: 743.
98. Jobe AH, Bancalari E. NICHD/NHLBI/ORD workshop summary: bronchopulmonary dysplasia. *Am J Respir Crit Care Med.* 2001;163:1723.
99. Davis JM, Rosenfeld WN. Chronic lung disease. In: Avery GB et al., eds. *Neonatology: Pathophysiology and Management of the Newborn,* 5th ed. Philadelphia: Lippincott Williams & Wilkins; 1999:509.
100. Ehrenkranz RA et al. Validation of the National Institutes of Health consensus definition of bronchopulmonary dysplasia. *Pediatrics* 2005;116: 1353.
101. Oh W et al. Association between fluid intake and weight loss during the first ten days of life and risk of bronchopulmonary dysplasia in extremely low birth weight infants. *J Pediatr* 2005;147:786.
102. Banks-Randall BA, Ballard RA. Bronchopulmonary dysplasia. In: Taeusch HW et al., eds. *Avery's Diseases of the Newborns,* 8th ed. Philadelphia: Elsevier Saunders; 2005:723.
103. Bhandari A, Bhandari V. Bronchopulmonary dysplasia: an update. *Indian J Pediatr* 2007;74:73.
104. Farrell PA, Fiascone JM. Bronchopulmonary dysplasia in the 1990s: a review for the pediatrician. *Curr Probl Pediatr* 1997;27:133.
105. Cafcit injection and oral Solution package insert. Bedford, OH: Mead Johnson & Company; 2003, May.
106. Barrington KJ, Finer NN. Treatment of bronchopulmonary dysplasia: a review. *Clin Perinatol* 1998;25:177.
107. Brion LP, Primhak RA. Intravenous or enteral loop diuretics for preterm infants with (or developing) chronic lung disease. *Cochrane Database Syst Rev* 2002:1:CD001453.
108. Brion LP et al. Aerosolized diuretics for preterm infants with (or developing) chronic lung disease. *Cochrane Database Syst Rev* 2006:3:CD001694.
109. Schmidt B et al. Caffeine therapy for apnea of prematurity. *N Engl J Med* 2006;354:2112.
110. Pantalitschka T, Poets CF. Inhaled drugs for the prevention and treatment of bronchopulmonary dysplasia. *Pediatr Pulmonol* 2006;41:703.
111. De Boeck K et al. Response to bronchodilators in clinically stable 1-year-old patients with bronchopulmonary dysplasia. *Eur J Pediatr* 1998;157: 75.
112. Brundage KL et al. Bronchodilator response to ipratropium bromide in infants with bronchopulmonary dysplasia. *Am Rev Respir Dis* 1990;142:1137.
113. Ng GY, Ohlsson A. Cromolyn sodium for the prevention of chronic lung disease in preterm infants. *Cochrane Database Syst Rev* 2001:1:CD003059.
114. Ward RM, Lugo RA. Drug therapy in the newborn. In: Avery GB et al., eds. *Neonatology: Pathophysiology and Management of the Newborn,* 5th ed. Philadelphia: Lippincott Williams & Wilkins; 1999:1363.
115. Khalaf MN et al. A prospective controlled trial of albuterol aerosol delivered via metered dose inhaler-spacer device (MDI) versus jet nebulizer in ventilated preterm neonates. *Am J Perinatol* 2001;18:169.
116. Bancalari E. Corticosteroids and neonatal chronic lung disease. *Eur J Pediatr* 1998;157(Suppl 1):S31.
117. Halliday H et al. Moderately early (7–14 days) postnatal corticosteroids for preventing chronic lung disease in preterm infants. *Cochrane Database Syst Rev, The Cochrane Library* 2003;1:CD001144.
118. Halliday HL et al. Delayed (>3 weeks) postnatal corticosteroids for chronic lung disease in preterm infants. *Cochrane Database Syst Rev, The Cochrane Library* 2003;1:CD001145.
119. Halliday HL et al. Early postnatal (<96 hours) corticosteroids for preventing chronic lung disease in preterm infants. *Cochrane Database Syst Rev, The Cochrane Library* 2003;1:CD001146.
120. Barrington KJ. The adverse neuro-developmental effects of postnatal steroids in the preterm infant: a systematic review of RCTs. *BioMed Central Pediatr* 2001;1:1.
121. Doyle LW, Davis PG. Postnatal corticosteroids in preterm infants: systematic review of effects on mortality and motor function. *J Paediatr Child Health* 2000;36:101.
122. American Academy of Pediatrics. Committee on Fetus and Newborn. Canadian Paediatric Society. Fetus and Newborn Committee. Postnatal corticosteroids to treat or prevent chronic lung disease in preterm infants. *Pediatrics* 2002;109:330.
123. Doyle LW et al. Low-dose dexamethasone facilitates extubation among chronically ventilator-dependent infants: A multicenter, international, randomized, controlled trial. *Pediatrics* 2006;117: 75.
124. Doyle LW et al. Outcome at 2 years of age of infants from the DART study: a multicenter, international, randomized, controlled trial of low-dose dexamethasone. *Pediatrics* 2007;119:716.
125. van der Heide-Jalving M et al. Short-and long-term effects of neonatal glucocorticoid therapy: is hydrocortisone an alternative to dexamethasone? *Acta Paediatr* 2003;92:827.
126. Watterberg KL et al. Prophylaxis of early adrenal insufficiency to prevent bronchopulmonary dysplasia: a multicenter trial. *Pediatrics* 2004;114:1649.
127. Watterberg KL et al. Growth and neurodevelopmental outcomes after early low-dose hydrocortisone treatment in extremely low birth weight infants. *Pediatrics* 2007;120:40.
128. Rademaker KJ et al. Neonatal hydrocortisone treatment: neurodevelopmental outcome and MRI at school age in preterm-born children. *J Pediatr* 2007;150:351.
129. Grier DG, Halliday HL. Management of bronchopulmonary dysplasia in infants: guidelines for corticosteroid use. *Drugs* 2005;65:15.
130. Shah V et al. Early administration of inhaled corticosteroids for preventing chronic lung disease in ventilated very low birth weight preterm neonates. *Cochrane Database Syst Rev* 2003:1:CD001969.
131. Shah SS et al. Inhaled versus systemic corticosteroids for preventing chronic lung disease in ventilated very low birth weight preterm neonates. *Cochrane Database Syst Rev* 2003:1:CD002058.
132. Shah SS et al. Inhaled versus systemic corticosteroids for the treatment of chronic lung disease in ventilated very low birth weight preterm infants. *Cochrane Database Syst Rev* 2003:1:CD002057.
133. Cole CH et al. Early inhaled corticosteroid therapy to prevent bronchopulmonary dysplasia. *N Engl J Med* 1999;340:1005.
134. Ng PC et al. Pituitary-adrenal suppression in preterm, very low birthweight infants after inhaled fluticasone propionate treatment. *J Clin Endocrinol Metab* 1998;83:2390.
135. Yeh TF et al. Outcomes at school age after postnatal dexamethasone therapy for lung disease of prematurity. *N Engl J Med* 2004;350:1304.
136. Biniwale MA, Ehrenkranz RA. The role of nutrition in the prevention and management of bronchopulmonary dysplasia. *Semin Perinatol* 2006;30:200.
137. Darlow B, Graham P. Vitamin A supplementation to prevent mortality and short and long-term morbidity in very low birthweight infants. *Cochrane Database Syst Rev* 2007:4:CD000501.
138. Wardle SP et al. Randomised controlled trial of oral vitamin A supplement in preterm infants to prevent chronic lung disease. *Arch Dis Child Fetal Neonatal Ed* 2001;84:F9.
139. Berstein D. The fetal to neonatal circulatory transition. In: Behrman RE et al., eds. *Nelson Textbook of Pediatrics,* 16th ed. Philadelphia: WB Saunders; 2000:1341.
140. Hammerman C. Patent ductus arteriosus: clinical relevance of prostaglandins and prostaglandin inhibitors in PDA pathophysiology and treatment. *Clin Perinatol* 1995;22:457.
141. Brook MM, Heymann MA. Patent ductus arteriosus. In: Emmanouilides G et al., eds. *Moss and Adam's Heart Disease in Infants, Children, and Adolescents: Including the Fetus and Young Adults,* 5th ed. Baltimore: Williams & Wilkins; 1995:746.
142. Bell SG. Neonatal cardiovascular pharmacology. *Neonatal Network* 1998;17:7.
143. Clyman RI. Patent ductus arteriosus in the premature infant. In: Taeusch HW et al., eds. *Avery's Diseases of the Newborn,* 8th ed. Philadelphia: Elsevier Saunders; 2005:816.
144. Clyman RI. Recommendations for the postnatal use of indomethacin: an analysis of four separate treatment strategies. *J Pediatr* 1996;128:601.
145. Gersony WM et al. Effects of indomethacin in premature infants with patent ductus arteriosus: results of a national collaborative study. *J Pediatr* 1983;102:895.
146. Clyman RI. Medical treatment of patent ductus arteriosus in premature infants. In: Long WA, ed. *Fetal*

and Neonatal Cardiology. Philadelphia: WB Saunders; 1990:682.
147. Shaffer CL et al. Effect of age and birth weight on indomethacin pharmacodynamics in neonates treated for patent ductus arteriosus. *Crit Care Med* 2002;30:343.
148. Brion LP, Campbell DE. Furosemide in indomethacin-treated infants–systematic review and meta-analysis. *Pediatr Nephrol* 1999;133:212.
149. Gal P, Gillman JT. Drug disposition in neonates with patent ductus arteriosus. *Ann Pharmacother* 1993;27:1383.
150. Pham JT, Carlos MA. Current treatment strategies of symptomatic patent ductus arteriosus. *J Pediatr Health Care* 2002;16:306.
151. Van Overmeire B et al. A comparison of ibuprofen and indomethacin for closure of patent ductus arteriosus. *N Engl J Med,* 2000;343:674.
152. Aranda JV, Thomas R. Systematic review: intravenous ibuprofen in preterm newborns. *Semin Perinatol* 2006;30:114.
153. Ohlsson A et al. Ibuprofen for the treatment of patent ductus arteriosus in preterm and/or low birth weight infants. *Cochrane Database of Syst Rev* 2005;4:CD003481.
154. Van Overmeire B al. Early versus late indomethacin treatment for patent ductus arteriosus in premature infants with respiratory distress syndrome. *J Pediatr* 2001;138:205.
155. Hammerman C, Aramburo MJ. Prolonged indomethacin therapy for the prevention of recurrences of patent ductus arteriosus. *J Pediatr* 1990; 117:771.
156. Weiss H et al. Factors determining reopening of the ductus arteriosus after successful clinical closure with indomethacin. *J Pediatr* 1995;127:466.
157. Tammela O et al. Short versus prolonged indomethacin therapy for patent ductus arteriosus in preterm infants. *J Pediatr* 1999;134:552.
158. Fowlie PW. Prophylactic indomethacin: systematic review and meta-analysis. *Arch Dis Child* 1996; 74:F81.
159. Gournay V et al. Pulmonary hypertension after ibuprofen prophylaxis in very preterm infants. *Lancet* 2002;359:1486.
160. De Carolis MP et al. Prophylactic ibuprofen therapy of patent ductus arteriosus in preterm infants. *Eur J Pediatr* 2000;159:364.
161. Van Overmeire B et al. Prophylactic ibuprofen in premature infants: a multicentre, randomized, double-blind, placebo-controlled trial. *Lancet* 2004;364:1945.
162. Bellini C et al. Pulmonary hypertension following L-lysine ibuprofen therapy in a preterm infant with patent ductus arteriosus. *CMAJ* 2006;174:1843.
163. Stoll BJ. Epidemiology of necrotizing enterocolitis. *Clin Perinatol* 1994;21:205.
164. Holman RC et al. Necrotising enterocolitis hospitalisations among neonates in the United States. *Paediatr Perinat Epidemiol* 2006;20:498.
165. Crouse DT. Necrotizing enterocolitis. In: Pomerance JJ, Richardson CJ, eds. *Neonatology for the Clinician*. Norwalk, CT: Appleton & Lange; 1993:363.
166. Berseth CL, Poenaru D. Necrotizing enterocolitis and short bowel syndrome. In: Taeusch HW et al., eds. *Avery's Diseases of the Newborn,* 8th ed. Philadelphia: Elsevier Saunders; 2005:1123.
167. Pierro A. Necrotizing enterocolitis: pathogenesis and treatment. *Br J Hosp Med* 1997;58:126.
168. Walsh MC, Kliegan RM. Necrotizing enterocolitis: treatment based on staging criteria. *Pediatr Clin North Am* 1986;33:179.
169. Edelson MB et al. Circulating pro-and counterinflammatory cytokine levels and severity in necrotizing enterocolitis. *Pediatrics* 1999;103:766.
170. Boccia D et al. Nosocomial necrotising enterocolitis outbreaks: epidemiology and control measures. *Eur J Pediatr* 2001;160:385.
171. Guillet R et al. Association of H2-blocker therapy and higher incidence of necrotizing enterocolitis in very low birth weight infants. *Pediatrics* 2006; 117:e137.
172. Pietz J et al. Prevention of necrotizing enterocolitis in preterm infants: a 20-year experience. *Pediatrics* 2007;119:e164.
173. McKeown RE et al. Role of delayed feeding and of feeding increments in necrotizing enterocolitis. *J Pediatr* 1992;121:764.
174. Caple J et al. Randomized controlled trial of slow versus rapid feeding volume advancement in preterm infants. *Pediatrics* 2004;114:1597.
175. Salhotra A, Ramji S. Slow versus fast enteral feed advancements in very low birth weight infants: a randomized controlled trial. *Ind Pediatr* 2004;41: 435.
176. Kennedy KA et al. Early versus delayed initiation o progressive enteral feeding for parenterally fed low birth weight or preterm infants. *Cochrane Database Syst Rev* 2000:2:CD001970.
177. Moss RL et al. Laparotomy versus peritoneal drainage for necrotizing enterocolitis and perforation. *N Engl J Med* 2006;354:2225.
178. Scheifele DW et al. Comparison of two antibiotic regimens for neonatal necrotizing enterocolitis. *J Antimicrob Chemother* 1987;20:421.
179. Bury RG, Tudehope D. Enteral antibiotics for preventing necrotizing enterocolitis in low birthweight or preterm infants. *Cochrane Database Syst Rev, The Cochrane Library* 2003;1:CD000405.
180. Faix RG et al. A randomized trial of parenteral clindamycin in neonatal necrotizing enterocolitis. *J Pediatr* 1988;112:271.
181. Horwitz JR et al. Complications after surgical intervention for necrotizing enterocolitis: A multicenter review. *J Pediatr Surg* 1995;30:994.
182. Vanderhoof JA. Short bowel syndrome in children and small intestinal transplantation. *Pediatr Clin North Am* 1996;43:533.
183. Synder CL et al. Survival after necrotizing enterocolitis in infants weighing less than 1,000 gm: 25 years' experience at a single institution. *J Pediatr Surg* 1997;32:434.
184. Schulzke SM et al. Neurodevelopmental outcomes of very low-birth-weight infants with necrotizing enterocolitis. *Arch Pediatr Adolesc Med* 2007;161: 583.
185. Thureen PJ, Hay WW. Early aggressive nutrition in preterm infants. *Semin Neonatol* 2001;6:403.
186. Tyson JE, Kennedy KA. Trophic feedings for parenterally fed infants. *Cochrane Database Syst Rev* 2005:3:CD000504.
187. Lucas A, Cole TJ. Breast milk and neonatal necrotizing enterocolitis. *Lancet* 1990;336:1519.
188. Agostoni C et al. Probiotic bacteria in dietetic products for infants: a commentary by the ESPGHAN Committee on Nutrition. *J Pediatr Gastroenterol Nutr* 2004;38:365.
189. Deshpande G et al. Probiotics for prevention of necrotising enterocolitis in preterm neonates with very low birthweight: a systematic review of randomised controlled trials. *Lancet* 2007;369:1614.
190. Perez EM, Weisman LE. Novel approaches to the prevention and therapy of neonatal bacterial sepsis. *Clin Perinatol* 1997;24:213.
191. Vergano S et al. Neonatal sepsis: an international perspective. *Arch Dis Child Fetal Neonatal Ed* 2005;90:F220.
192. Stoll BJ et al. Late-onset sepsis in very low birth weight neonates: the experience of the NICHD Neonatal Research Network. *Pediatrics* 2002;110: 285
193. Polin RA et al. Bacterial sepsis and meningitis. In: Taeusch HW et al., eds. *Avery's Diseases of the Newborn,* 8th ed. Philadelphia: Elsevier Saunders; 2005:551.
194. Gerdes JS. Diagnosis and management of bacterial infections in the neonate. *Pediatr Clin North Am* 2004;51:939.
195. Philip AGS. The changing face of neonatal infection: experience at a regional medical center. *Pediatr Infect Dis J* 1994;13:1098.
196. Freij BJ, McCracken GH. Acute infections. In: Avery GB et al., eds. *Neonatology Pathophysiology and Management of the Newborn,* 5th ed. Philadelphia: WB Saunders; 1999:1189.
197. McManus MC. Prudent selection of antimicrobials for neonatal sepsis. *Am J Health-Syst Pharm* 1996;53:1956.
198. Gaynes RP et al. Nosocomial infections among neonates in high-risk nurseries in the United States. *Pediatrics* 1996;98:357.
199. Krediet TG et al. Clinical outcome of cephalothin versus vancomycin therapy in the treatment of coagulase-negative Staphylococcal septicemia in neonates: relation to methicillin resistance and mec A gene carriage of blood isolates. *Pediatrics* 1999; 103:E29.
200. Patrick CC et al. Persistent bacteremia due to coagulase-negative staphylococci in low birthweight neonates. *Pediatrics* 1989;84:977.
201. Harvey D et al. Bacterial meningitis in the newborn: a prospective study of mortality and morbidity. *Semin Perinatol* 1999;23:218.
202. Norris CMR et al. Aseptic meningitis in the newborn and young infant. *Am Fam Physician* 1999; 59:2761.
203. Payne NR et al. Selecting antibiotics for nosocomial bacterial infections in patients requiring neonatal intensive care. *Neonatal Network* 1994;13:41.
204. Matrai-Kovalskis Y et al. Positive blood cultures for coagulase-negative Staphylococci in neonates: does highly-selective vancomycin usage affect outcome? *Infection* 1998;26:85
205. Deville JG et al. Linezolid versus vancomycin in the treatment of known or suspected resistant gram-positive infections in neonates. *Pediatr Infect Dis J* 2003;22:S158.
206. Manzoni P et al. A multicenter, randomized trial of prophylactic fluconazole in preterm neonates. *N Engl J Med* 2007;356:2483.
207. Bradley JS, Nelson JD. *Nelson's Pocket Book of Pediatric Antimicrobial Therapy,* 16th ed. Buenos Aires, Argentina: Alliance for World Wide Editing; 2006:23.
208. Fanos V, Dall'Agnola A. Antibiotics in neonatal infections: a review. *Drugs* 1999;58:405.
209. Kraus DM et al. Efficacy and tolerability of extended-interval aminoglycoside administration in pediatric patients. *Pediatr Drugs* 2002;4: 469.
210. Rodvold KA et al. Single daily doses of aminoglycosides. *Lancet* 1997;350:1412.
211. Parker SE, Davey PG. Once-daily aminoglycoside administration in gram-negative sepsis. *PharmacoEconomics* 1995;7:393.
212. Rao SC et al. One dose per day compared to multiple doses per day of gentamicin for treatment of suspected or proven sepsis in neonates. *Cochrane Database Syst Rev* 2006:1:CD005091.
213. Rastogi A et al. Comparison of two gentamicin dosing schedules in very low birth weight infants. *Pediatr Infect Dis J* 2002;21:234.
214. Hansen A et al. Once-daily gentamicin dosing for the preterm and term newborn: proposal for a simple regimen that achieves target levels. *J Perinatol* 2003;23:635.
215. Garcia B et al. Population pharmacokinetics of gentamicin in premature newborns. *J Antimicrob Chemo* 2006;58:372.
216. Heath PT et al. Neonatal meningitis. *Arch Dis Child Fetal Neonatal Ed* 2003;88:173.
217. Shah S et al. Intraventricular antibiotics for bacterial meningitis in neonates. *Cochrane Database Syst Rev* 2004:4:CD004496.
218. Schelonka RL, Infante AJ. Neonatal immunology. *Semin Perinatol* 1998;22:2.
219. Jenson HB, Pollock BH. Meta-analyses of the effectiveness of intravenous immune globulin for prevention and treatment of neonatal sepsis. *Pediatrics* 1997;99:E2.
220. Ohlsson A, Lacy JB. Intravenous immunoglobulin for preventing infection in preterm and/or low-birth-weight infants. *Cochrane Database Syst Rev, The Cochrane Library* 2004:1:CD000361.
221. Ohlsson A, Lacy LB. Intravenous immunoglobulin for suspected or subsequently proven infection in neonates. *Cochrane Database Syst Rev, The Cochrane Library* 2004:1:CD001239.

222. Faranoff AA et al. A controlled trial of intravenous immune globulin to reduce nosocomial infections in very-low-birth-weight infants. *N Engl J Med* 1994;330:1107.
223. Weismann LE, Lorenzetti PM. High intravenous doses of human immune globulin suppress neonatal group B streptococcal immunity in rats. *J Pediatrics* 1989;115:445.
224. Gotoff SP. Pathogenesis and epidemiology. In: Behrman RE et al., eds. *Nelson Textbook of Pediatrics,* 16th ed. Philadelphia: WB Saunders; 2000:538.
225. Burchett SK. Infections: viral infections. In: Cloherty JP, Stark AR, eds. *Manual of Neonatal Care,* 4th ed. Philadelphia: Lippincott-Raven, 1998:239.
226. Hollier LM, Cox SM. Syphilis. *Semin Perinatol* 1998;22:323.
227. Yudin MH, Gonik B. Perinatal infections. In: Martin MJ et al., eds. *Neonatal-Perinatal Medicine: Diseases of the Fetus and Infant,* 8th ed. Philadelphia: Mosby Elsevier; 2006:429.
228. American Academy of Pediatrics; Pickering LK, ed. *2006 Red Book: Report of the Committee on Infectious Diseases,* 27th ed. Elk Grove Village, IL: American Academy of Pediatrics; 2006.
229. Brown ZA et al. Effects of serologic status and cesarean delivery on transmission rates on herpes simplex virus from mother to infant. *JAMA* 2003; 289:203.
230. Kimberlin DW. Herpes simplex virus infections of the newborn. *Semin Perinatol* 2007;31:19.
231. Brown Z. Preventing herpes simplex virus transmission to the neonate. *Herpes* 2004;11:175A.
232. Kimberlin DW et al. Safety and efficacy of high-dose intravenous acyclovir in the management of neonatal herpes simplex virus infections. *Pediatrics* 2001;108:230.
233. Kimberlin D et al. Administration of oral acyclovir suppressive therapy after neonatal herpes simplex virus disease limited to the skin, eyes, and mouth: results of a Phase I/II trial. *Pediatr Infect Dis J* 1996;15:247.
234. Fonseca-Aten M et al. Herpes simplex virus encephalitis during suppressive therapy in a premature infant. *Pediatrics* 2005;115:804.
235. Montoya JG, Rosso F. Diagnosis and management of toxoplasmosis. *Clin Perinatol* 2005;32:705.
236. Centers for Disease Control and Prevention. Congenital syphilis—United States, 2002. *MMWR* 2004;53:716.
237. Chang M. Hepatitis B virus infection. *Semin Fetal Neonatal Med* 2007;12:160.
238. Brown HL, Abernathy MP. Cytomegalovirus infection. *Semin Perinatol* 1998;22:260.
239. Adler SP, Marshall B. Cytomegalovirus infections. *Pediatr Rev* 2007;28:92.
240. Galli L et al. Valganciclovir for congenital CMV infection: a pilot study on plasma concentration in newborns and infants. *Pediatr Infect Dis J* 2007;26: 451.
241. Poets CF et al. Epidemiology and pathophysiology of apnoea of prematurity. *Biol Neonate* 1994;65: 211.
242. Barrington K, Finer N. The natural history of the appearance of apnea of prematurity. *Pediatr Res* 1991;29:372.
243. Consensus Statement. National Institutes of Health Consensus Development Conference on Infantile Apnea and Home Monitoring, Sept. 29 to Oct. 1, 1986. *Pediatrics* 1987;79:292.
244. Martin GI. Infant apnea. In: Pomerance JJ, Richardson CJ, eds. *Neonatology for the Clinician.* Norwalk, CT: Appleton & Lange; 1993:267.
245. Miller MJ, Martin RJ. Apnea of prematurity. *Clin Perinatol* 1992;19:789.
246. Martin RJ et al. Pathogenesis of apnea in preterm infants. *J Pediatr* 1986;109:733.
247. Finer NN et al. Obstructive, mixed, and central apnea in the neonate: physiologic correlates. *J Pediatr* 1992;121:943.
248. Darnall RA. Aminophylline reduces hypoxic ventilatory depression: possible role of adenosine. *Pediatr Res* 1985;19:706.
249. Myers TF et al. Low-dose theophylline therapy in idiopathic apnea of prematurity. *J Pediatr* 1980; 96:99.
250. Kritter KE, Blanchard J. Management of apnea in infants. *Clin Pharm* 1989;8:577.
251. Lopes JM et al. The effects of theophylline on diaphragmatic fatigue in the newborn. *Pediatr Res* 1982;16:355A.
252. Tang-Lui DDS et al. Nonlinear theophylline elimination. *Clin Pharmacol Ther* 1982;31:358.
253. Tang-Lui DD, Reigelman S. Metabolism of theophylline to caffeine in adults. *Res Commun Chem Pathol Pharmacol* 1981;34:371.
254. Muttitt SC et al. The dose response of theophylline in the treatment of apnea of prematurity. *J Pediatr* 1988;112:115.
255. Hendeles L et al. Revised FDA labeling guideline for theophylline oral dosage forms. *Pharmacotherapy* 1995;15:409.
256. Kraus DM et al. Pharmacokinetic evaluation of two theophylline dosing methods for infants. *Ther Drug Monit* 1994;16:270.
257. Eichenwald EC et al. Apnea frequently persists beyond term gestation in infants delivered at 24 to 28 weeks. *Pediatrics* 1997;100:354.
258. Aldridge A et al. Caffeine metabolism in the newborn. *Clin Pharmacol Ther* 1979;25:447.
259. LeGuennec JC et al. Maturational changes of caffeine concentration and disposition in infancy during maintenance therapy for apnea of prematurity: influence of gestational age, hepatic disease, and breast-feeding. *Pediatrics* 1985;76:834.
260. Aranda JV et al. Maturation of caffeine elimination in infancy. *Arch Dis Child* 1979;54:946.
261. Larsen PB et al. Aminophylline versus caffeine citrate for apnea and bradycardia prophylaxis in premature neonates. *Acta Paediatr* 1995;84: 360.
262. Davis JM et al. Use of caffeine in infants unresponsive to theophylline in apnea of prematurity. *Pediatr Pulmonol* 1987;3:90.
263. Schmidt B et al. Long-term effects of caffeine therapy for apnea of prematurity. *N Engl J Med* 2007;357:1893.
264. Eyal F et al. Aminophylline versus doxapram in idiopathic apnea of prematurity: a double-blind controlled study. *Pediatrics* 1985;75:709.
265. Peliowski A, Finer NN. A blinded, randomized, placebo-controlled trial to compare theophylline and doxapram for the treatment of apnea of prematurity. *J Pediatr* 1990;116:648.
266. Barrington KJ et al. Dose-response relationship of doxapram in the therapy for refractory idiopathic apnea of prematurity. *Pediatrics* 1987;80:22.
267. Tay-Uyboco J et al. Clinical and physiological responses to prolonged nasogastric administration of doxapram for apnea of prematurity. *Biol Neonate* 1991;59:190.
268. Papageorgiou A, Bardin CL. The extremely-low-birth-weight infant. In Avery GB et al., eds. *Neonatology: Pathophysiology & Management of the Newborn,* 5th ed. Philadelphia: Lippincott Williams & Wilkins; 1999:445.
269. De Villiers GS et al. Second-degree atrioventricular heart block after doxapram administration. *J Pediatr* 1998;133:149.
270. de Vries L. The central nervous system, part three: intracranial hemorrhage and vascular lesions. In: Martin RJ et al., eds. *Neonatal-Perinatal Medicine: Diseases of the Fetus and Infant,* 8th ed. Philadelphia: Mosby Elsevier; 2006:924.
271. Hill A. Intraventricular hemorrhage: emphasis on prevention. *Semin Pediatr Neurol* 1998;5:152.
272. Wells JT, Ment LR. Prevention of intraventricular hemorrhage in preterm infants. *Early Hum Dev* 1995;42:209.
273. Roland EH, Hill A. Intraventricular hemorrhage and posthemorrhagic hydrocephalus: current and potential future interventions. *Clin Perinatol* 1997;24:589.
274. Chang GY et al. Heparin and the risk of intraventricular hemorrhage in premature infants. *J Pediatr* 1997;131:361.
275. Moe P, Paige PL. Neurologic disorders. In: Merenstein GB, Gardner SL, eds. *Handbook of Neonatal Intensive Care,* 4th ed. St. Louis: Mosby-Year Book; 1998:571.
276. Ment LR et al. Low-dose indomethacin and prevention of intraventricular hemorrhage: a multicenter randomized trial. *Pediatrics* 1994;93:543.
277. Ment LR et al. Neurodevelopmental outcome at 36 months' corrected age of preterm infants in the multicenter indomethacin intraventricular hemorrhage prevention trial. *Pediatrics* 1996;98: 714.
278. Dani C et al. Prophylactic ibuprofen for the prevention of intraventricular hemorrhage among preterm infants: a multicenter, randomized study. *Pediatrics* 2005;115:1529.
279. Hill A, Volpe JJ. Neurological and neuromuscular disorders. In: Avery GB et al., eds. *Neonatology: Pathophysiology & Management of the Newborn,* 5th ed. Philadelphia: Lippincott Williams & Wilkins; 1999:1231.
280. Scher MS. Seizures in the newborn infant: diagnosis, treatment, and outcome. *Clin Perinatol* 1997; 24:735.
281. Morrison A. Neonatal seizures. In: Pomerance JJ, Richardson CJ, eds. *Neonatology for the Clinician.* Norwalk, CT: Appleton & Lange; 1993:411.
282. Haymond MW. Hypoglycemia in infants and children. *Endocrinol Metab Clin North Am* 1989;18:221.
283. Stafstrom CE. Neonatal seizures. *Pediatr Rev* 1995; 16:248.
284. Massingale TW, Buttross S. Survey of treatment practices for neonatal seizures. *J Perinatol* 1993; 13:107.
285. Gilman JT et al. Rapid sequential phenobarbital treatment of neonatal seizures. *Pediatrics* 1989;83: 674.
286. Deshmukh A et al. Lorazepam in the treatment of refractory neonatal seizures: a pilot study. *Am J Dis Child* 1986;140:1042.
287. McDermott CA et al. Pharmacokinetics of lorazepam in critically ill neonates with seizures. *J Pediatr* 1992;120:479.
288. Conde JRC et al. Midazolam in neonatal seizures with no response to phenobarbital. *Neurology* 2005;64:876.
289. Shany E et al. Comparison of continuous drip of midazolam or lidocaine in the treatment of intractable neonatal seizures. *J Child Neurol* 2007;22: 255.
290. Shoemaker MT, Rotenberg JS. Levetiracetam for the treatment of neonatal seizures. *J Child Neurol* 2007;22:95.
291. Gal P et al. Valproic acid efficacy, toxicity, and pharmacokinetics in neonates with intractable seizures. *Neurology* 1988;38:467.
292. Singh B et al. Treatment of neonatal seizures with carbamazepine. *J Child Neurol* 1996;11:378.
293. Painter MJ et al. Phenobarbital compared with phenytoin for the treatment of neonatal seizures. *N Engl J Med* 1999;341:485.
294. Painter MJ et al. Phenobarbital and phenytoin in neonatal seizures: metabolism and tissue distribution. *Neurology* 1981;31:1107
295. Levene M. The clinical conundrum of neonatal seizures. *Arch Dis Child Fetal Neonatal Ed* 2002; 86:F75.
296. Bandstra ES, Accorneo VH. Infants of substance-abusing mothers. In: Martin RJ et al., eds. *Neonatal-Perinatal Medicine: Diseases of the Fetus and Infant,* 8th ed. Philadelphia: Mosby Elsevier; 2006:733.
297. Weiner SM, Finnegan LP. Drug withdrawal in the neonate. In: Merenstein GB, Gardner SL, eds. *Handbook of Neonatal Intensive Care,* 4th ed. St. Louis: Mosby-Year Book; 1998:129.
298. Oei J, Lui K. Management of the newborn infant affected by maternal opiates and other drugs of dependency. *J Pediatr Child Health* 2007;43:9.
299. Levy M, Spino M. Neonatal withdrawal syndrome: associated drugs and pharmacological management. *Pharmacotherapy* 1993;13:202.

300. Kallen B, Otterblad Olausoon P. Antidepressant drugs during pregnancy and infant congenital heart defect. *Reprod Toxicol* 2006;21:221
301. Wogelius P et al. Maternal use of selective serotonin reuptake inhibitors and risk of congenital malformations. *Epidemiology* 2006;17:701.
302. Moses-Kolko et al. Neonatal signs after late in utero exposure to serotonin reuptake inhibitors: literature review and implications for clinical applications. *JAMA* 2005;293:237.
303. Chambers CD et al. Selective serotonin-reuptake inhibitors and risk of persistent pulmonary hypertension of the newborn. *N Engl J Med* 2006;354:579.
304. Levinson-Castiel et al. Neonatal abstinence syndrome after in utero exposure to selective serotonin reuptake inhibitors in term infants. *Arch Pediatr Adolesc Med* 2006;160:173.
305. Tran JH. Treatment of neonatal abstinence syndrome. *J Pediatr Health Care* 1999;13:295.
306. Kuschel C. Managing drug withdrawal in the newborn infant. *Semin Fetal Neonat Med* 2007;12:127.
307. American Academy of Pediatrics, Committee on Drugs. Neonatal drug withdrawal. *Pediatrics* 1998; 101:1079.
308. Hoder EL et al. Clonidine treatment of neonatal narcotic abstinence syndrome. *Psychiatry Res* 1984;13:243.
309. Stark AR et al. Muscle relaxation in mechanically ventilated infants. *J Pediatr* 1979;94:439.
310. Crone RK, Favorito J. The effects of pancuronium bromide on infants with hyaline membrane disease. *J Pediatr* 1980;97:991.
311. Buck ML, Reed MD. Use of nondepolarizing neuromuscular blocking agents in mechanically ventilated patients. *Clin Pharm* 1991;10:32.
312. Carlo WA et al. Assisted ventilation and complications of respiratory distress. In: Martin RJ et al., eds. *Neonatal-Perinatal Medicine: Diseases of the Fetus and Infant,* 8th ed. Philadelphia: Mosby Elsevier; 2006:1108.
313. Taylor P. Agents acting at the neuromuscular junction and autonomic ganglia. In: Hardman JG et al., eds. *Goodman and Gilman's The Pharmacological Basis of Therapeutics,* 9th ed. New York: McGraw-Hill, 1996:177.
314. Greenough A et al. Investigation of the effects of paralysis by pancuronium on heart rate variability, blood pressure and fluid balance. *Acta Paediatr Scand* 1989;78:829.
315. Cabal LA et al. Cardiovascular and catecholamine changes after administration of pancuronium in distressed neonates. *Pediatrics* 1985;75:284.
316. Piotrowski A. Comparison of atracurium and pancuronium in mechanically ventilated neonates. *Intensive Care Med* 1993;19:401.
317. Menon G et al. Practical approach to analgesia and sedation in the neonatal intensive care unit. *Semin Perinatol* 1998;22:417.
318. Abu-Saad HH et al. Assessment of pain in the neonate. *Semin Perinatol* 1998;22:402.
319. Anand KJS et al. Analgesia and sedation in preterm neonates who require ventilatory support: results from the NOPAIN trial. *Arch Pediatr Adolesc Med* 1999;153:331.
320. Goldberg RN et al. Detection of seizure activity in the paralyzed neonate using continuous monitoring. *Pediatrics* 1982;69:583.
321. Zenk KE. Practical pharmacology for the clinician caring for the newborn. In: Pomerance JJ, Richardson CJ, eds. *Neonatology for the Clinician.* Norwalk, CT: Appleton & Lange; 1993:59.
322. Scott CS et al. Morphine pharmacokinetics and pain assessment in premature newborns. *J Pediatr* 1999;135:423.
323. Roth B et al. Analgesia and sedation in neonatal intensive care using fentanyl by continuous infusion. *Dev Pharmacol Ther* 1991;17:121.
324. Norton SJ. After effects of morphine and fentanyl analgesia: a retrospective study. *Neonatal Network* 1988;7:25.
325. Arnold JH et al. Changes in the pharmacodynamic response to fentanyl in neonates during continuous infusion. *J Pediatr* 1991;119:639.
326. Katz R et al. Prospective study on the occurrence of withdrawal in critically ill children who receive fentanyl by continuous infusion. *Crit Care Med* 1994;22:763.
327. Lane JC et al. Movement disorder after withdrawal of fentanyl infusion. *J Pediatr* 1991;119:649.
328. Anand KJS, Arnold JH. Opioid tolerance and dependence in infants and children. *Crit Care Med* 1994;22:334.
329. Watling SM, Dasta JF. Prolonged paralysis in intensive care unit patients after the use of neuromuscular blocking agents: a review of the literature. *Crit Care Med* 1994;22:884.
330. Anyebuno MA, Rosenfeld CR. Chloral hydrate toxicity in a term infant. *Dev Pharmacol Ther* 1991;17: 116.
331. Mayers DJ et al. Chloral hydrate disposition following single-dose administration to critically ill neonates and children. *Dev Pharmacol Ther* 1991; 16:71.
332. Mayers DJ et al. Sedative/hypnotic effects of chloral hydrate in the neonate: trichloroethanol or parent drug? *Dev Pharmacol Ther* 1992;19:141.
333. Nahata MC et al. *Pediatric Drug Formulations,* 5th ed. Cincinnati, OH: Harvey Whitney Books Company; 2003.
334. Nahata MC. Lack of pediatric drug formulations. *Pediatrics* 1999;104:607.
335. Blumer JL, Reed MD. Principles of neonatal pharmacology. In: Yaffe SV, Aranda JV, eds. *Neonatal and Pediatric Pharmacology: Therapeutic Principles in Practice,* 3rd ed. Philadelphia: Lippincott Williams & Wilkins; 2005:146. 1992: 164.
336. Ernst JA et al. Osmolality of substances used in the intensive care nursery. *Pediatrics* 1983;72:347.
337. White KC, Harkavy KL. Hypertonic formula resulting from added oral medications. *Am J Dis Child* 1982;136:931.
338. American Academy of Pediatrics, Committee on Drugs. "Inactive" ingredients in pharmaceutical products: update (subject review). *Pediatrics* 1997; 99:268.
339. Balistreri WF et al. Lessons from the E-Ferol tragedy. *Pediatrics* 1986;78:503.
340. Duncan B et al. Medication-induced pneumatosis intestinalis. *Pediatrics* 1997;99:633.
341. Nahata MC. Intravenous infusion conditions: implications for pharmacokinetic monitoring. *Clin Pharmacokinet* 1993;24:221.
342. Roberts RJ. Issues and problems associated with drug delivery in pediatric patients. *J Clin Pharmacol* 1994;34:723.
343. Nahata MC et al. Effect of infusion methods on tobramycin serum concentrations in newborn infants. *J Pediatr* 1984;104:136.
344. Halliday H. Synthetic or natural surfactants. *Acta Pediatr* 1997;86:233.

CHAPTER 95

Pediatric Immunizations

Sherry Luedtke, Michelle Condren, and Mark Haase

The use of immunizations to control common childhood infectious diseases has been one of the most important medical developments to date. Children are now routinely immunized against 13 infectious diseases.[1] Immunization rates are at an all-time high in the United States with >80% of children 3 years of age receiving all the recommended vaccines. As a result, cases of diphtheria, tetanus, mumps, measles, rubella, polio, and *Haemophilus influenzae type b* are at record-low levels. Despite the overall high rates of immunization coverage, however, only 9% of infants 24 months of age have received all the vaccines at the recommended ages,[2] thus putting infants at risk for disease. The need for timely immunization administration is key to preventing disease resurgences.[2] As the incidence of vaccine-preventable disease continues to decrease, however, parents are becoming less aware of the significance and severity of the diseases that could be prevented. This, along with the parental concerns regarding vaccine safety, may jeopardize the vaccination coverage achievements. Health care providers play a vital role in clarifying misconceptions and educating parents and health care practitioners about the importance of proper and complete immunizations. Any contact with a pediatric patient represents an opportunity to promote immunization. Every medication history should include a complete immunization history, and the child's vaccination card should be used to detect any deficiency in immunization status.[3,4–6]

GUIDELINES

Schedule for Immunizations

1. K.C., a 2-month-old baby girl, is brought to the clinic for a scheduled well-baby visit. K.C.'s mother inquires about immunizations for her daughter. What are the current recommendations for immunizing pediatric patients? When should these immunizations be given to K.C.?

The goal of pediatric immunization is to prevent specific infectious diseases and their sequelae. For maximal effectiveness, a vaccine must be administered to the susceptible population before anyone has been exposed to the pathogen. The age at which immunizations are administered to specific individuals depends, however, on several factors (e.g., age-specific risks of the disease, risks of complications, presence of maternal antibodies transferred through the placenta, maturity of the immune system). Usually, immunizations are administered at the youngest age that the child is able to develop an adequate antibody response.

The recommended childhood and adolescent immunization schedules (Fig. 95-1)[7] are reviewed annually in *Morbidity and Mortality Weekly Reports* by the Centers for Disease Control and Prevention (CDC) and are available on-line through their website. The minimal immunization requirements for entry into public schools and daycare centers, however, vary with each state and the departments of health of individual states need to be consulted for these guidelines.

Immunization schedules can be adjusted to meet individual needs and may begin at any time of the year. Vaccines should not be administered at time intervals shorter than those recommended to allow for maximal immune responses before the administration of subsequent doses.[3] A CDC administration schedule for immunizations of children and adolescents who begin their immunizations late or who are >1 month behind schedule in their immunizations, and recommendations for minimal intervals between doses for the administration of various vaccines are depicted in Figure 95-2.[7] An interruption or delay in the recommended schedule does not interfere with the final immunity gained.

Contraindications

2. K.C. was exposed to a viral upper respiratory tract infection a few days before her scheduled well-baby visit. What immunizations should K.C. receive at this visit, or should her immunizations be delayed?

DEPARTMENT OF HEALTH AND HUMAN SERVICES • CENTERS FOR DISEASE CONTROL AND PREVENTION

Recommended Immunization Schedule for Persons Aged 0–6 Years—UNITED STATES • 2007

Vaccine ▼ Age ▶	Birth	1 month	2 months	4 months	6 months	12 months	15 months	18 months	19–23 months	2–3 years	4–6 years
Hepatitis B[1]	HepB	HepB		*see footnote 1*	HepB				HepB Series		
Rotavirus[2]			Rota	Rota	Rota						
Diphtheria, Tetanus, Pertussis[3]			DTaP	DTaP	DTaP		DTaP				DTaP
Haemophilus influenzae type b[4]			Hib	Hib	*Hib*[4]	Hib		Hib			
Pneumococcal[5]			PCV	PCV	PCV	PCV				PCV PPV	
Inactivated Poliovirus			IPV	IPV	IPV						IPV
Influenza[6]					Influenza (Yearly)						
Measles, Mumps, Rubella[7]						MMR					MMR
Varicella[8]						Varicella					Varicella
Hepatitis A[9]						HepA (2 doses)				HepA Series	
Meningococcal[10]										MPSV4	

Legend: Range of recommended ages; Catch-up immunization; Certain high-risk groups

This schedule indicates the recommended ages for routine administration of currently licensed childhood vaccines, as of December 1, 2006, for children aged 0–6 years. Additional information is available at http://www.cdc.gov/nip/recs/child-schedule.htm. Any dose not administered at the recommended age should be administered at any subsequent visit, when indicated and feasible. Additional vaccines may be licensed and recommended during the year. Licensed combination vaccines may be used whenever any components of the combination are indicated and other components of the vaccine are not contraindicated and if approved by the Food and Drug Administration for that dose of the series. Providers should consult the respective Advisory Committee on Immunization Practices statement for detailed recommendations. Clinically significant adverse events that follow immunization should be reported to the Vaccine Adverse Event Reporting System (VAERS). Guidance about how to obtain and complete a VAERS form is available at http://www.vaers.hhs.gov or by telephone, 800-822-7967.

A

DEPARTMENT OF HEALTH AND HUMAN SERVICES • CENTERS FOR DISEASE CONTROL AND PREVENTION

Recommended Immunization Schedule for Persons Aged 7–18 Years—UNITED STATES • 2007

Vaccine ▼ Age ▶	7–10 years	11–12 YEARS	13–14 years	15 years	16–18 years
Tetanus, Diphtheria, Pertussis[1]	*see footnote 1*	Tdap	Tdap		
Human Papillomavirus[2]	*see footnote 2*	HPV (3 doses)	HPV Series		
Meningococcal[3]	MPSV4	MCV4	MCV4[3] MCV4		
Pneumococcal[4]	PPV				
Influenza[5]	Influenza (Yearly)				
Hepatitis A[6]	HepA Series				
Hepatitis B[7]	HepB Series				
Inactivated Poliovirus[8]	IPV Series				
Measles, Mumps, Rubella[9]	MMR Series				
Varicella[10]	Varicella Series				

Legend: Range of recommended ages; Catch-up immunization; Certain high-risk groups

This schedule indicates the recommended ages for routine administration of currently licensed childhood vaccines, as of December 1, 2006, for children aged 7–18 years. Additional information is available at http://www.cdc.gov/nip/recs/child-schedule.htm. Any dose not administered at the recommended age should be administered at any subsequent visit, when indicated and feasible. Additional vaccines may be licensed and recommended during the year. Licensed combination vaccines may be used whenever any components of the combination are indicated and other components of the vaccine are not contraindicated and if approved by the Food and Drug Administration for that dose of the series. Providers should consult the respective Advisory Committee on Immunization Practices statement for detailed recommendations. Clinically significant adverse events that follow immunization should be reported to the Vaccine Adverse Event Reporting System (VAERS). Guidance about how to obtain and complete a VAERS form is available at http://www.vaers.hhs.gov or by telephone, 800-822-7967.

B

FIGURE 95-1 **2007 Recommended Immunization Schedules (A) 0–6 years of age (B) 7–18 years of age.** The reader should refer to the links above or go to www.cdc.gov/mmwr and follow the appropriate links to obtain further information on immunization guidelines which are updated annually and to view the detailed footnotes indicated in these tables.

Catch-up Immunization Schedule

UNITED STATES • 2007

for Persons Aged 4 Months–18 Years Who Start Late or Who Are More Than 1 Month Behind

The table below provides catch-up schedules and minimum intervals between doses for children whose vaccinations have been delayed. A vaccine series does not need to be restarted, regardless of the time that has elapsed between doses. Use the section appropriate for the child's age.

Vaccine	Minimum Age for Dose 1	Minimum Interval Between Doses: Dose 1 to Dose 2	Dose 2 to Dose 3	Dose 3 to Dose 4	Dose 4 to Dose 5
CATCH-UP SCHEDULE FOR PERSONS AGED 4 MONTHS–6 YEARS					
Hepatitis B[1]	Birth	4 weeks	8 weeks (and 16 weeks after first dose)		
Rotavirus[2]	6 wks	4 weeks	4 weeks		
Diphtheria, Tetanus, Pertussis[3]	6 wks	4 weeks	4 weeks	6 months	6 months[3]
Haemophilus influenzae type b[4]	6 wks	4 weeks if first dose administered at age <12 months 8 weeks (as final dose) if first dose administered at age 12-14 months No further doses needed if first dose administered at age ≥15 months	4 weeks[4] if current age <12 months 8 weeks (as final dose)[4] if current age ≥12 months and second dose administered at age <15 months No further doses needed if previous dose administered at age ≥15 months	8 weeks (as final dose) This dose only necessary for children aged 12 months–5 years who received 3 doses before age 12 months	
Pneumococcal[5]	6 wks	4 weeks if first dose administered at age <12 months and current age <24 months 8 weeks (as final dose) if first dose administered at age ≥12 months or current age 24–59 months No further doses needed for healthy children if first dose administered at age ≥24 months	4 weeks if current age <12 months 8 weeks (as final dose) if current age ≥12 months No further doses needed for healthy children if previous dose administered at age ≥24 months	8 weeks (as final dose) This dose only necessary for children aged 12 months–5 years who received 3 doses before age 12 months	
Inactivated Poliovirus[6]	6 wks	4 weeks	4 weeks	4 weeks[6]	
Measles, Mumps, Rubella[7]	12 mos	4 weeks			
Varicella[8]	12 mos	3 months			
Hepatitis A[9]	12 mos	6 months			
CATCH-UP SCHEDULE FOR PERSONS AGED 7–18 YEARS					
Tetanus, Diphtheria/ Tetanus, Diphtheria, Pertussis[10]	7 yrs[10]	4 weeks	8 weeks if first dose administered at age <12 months 6 months if first dose administered at age ≥12 months	6 months if first dose administered at age <12 months	
Human Papillomavirus[11]	9 yrs	4 weeks	12 weeks		
Hepatitis A[9]	12 mos	6 months			
Hepatitis B[1]	Birth	4 weeks	8 weeks (and 16 weeks after first dose)		
Inactivated Poliovirus[6]	6 wks	4 weeks	4 weeks	4 weeks[6]	
Measles, Mumps, Rubella[7]	12 mos	4 weeks			
Varicella[8]	12 mos	4 weeks if first dose administered at age ≥13 years 3 months if first dose administered at age <13 years			

FIGURE 95-2 Catch-Up Immunization Schedule. The reader should refer to the links above or go to www.cdc.gov/mmwr and follow the appropriate links to obtain further information on immunization guidelines which are updated annually and to view the detailed footnotes indicated in these tables.

Misconceptions about contraindications and precautions for immunization often result in missed opportunities to provide needed immunizations. Acute, severe febrile illness; history of anaphylaxis to the vaccine or vaccine components; and history of a severe reaction to an immunization are clear contraindications to immunizations. Immunizations, however, should not be delayed in a child who has a minor illness (e.g., upper respiratory tract infection, otitis media, diarrhea) even in the presence of a low-grade fever. A family history of seizures, allergies, and sudden infant death syndrome are not contraindications for immunizations. Immunization of a child with a history of anaphylaxis to a vaccine or vaccine component should be withheld until the child has undergone desensitization.[3] Preterm infants should begin to receive routine immunizations based on their chronological age for all vaccines, although initiation of the hepatitis B series should begin at 1 month of age.[8]

Allergic reaction to previous exposure to vaccine components, immunosuppression (e.g., immunosuppressive therapy, immunodeficiencies), encephalopathy, recent administration of blood products, and pregnancy (although the risk in pregnancy is largely theoretic) are contraindications to live-attenuated virus or live-bacterial vaccines. Pooled blood products (e.g., immunoglobulins, packed red blood cells, platelet transfusions) can impair the immune response to a live vaccine because these products contain antibodies, which can prevent an infant's immune system from mounting an adequate response. The impairment of an immune response to an immunization varies, depending on the type and amount of blood product administered and immunizations may need to be delayed for up to 12 months if pooled blood products have been administered recently.[3] With any question about immune response, antibody titers can be obtained to determine if a patient needs to be reimmunized.[3]

Because K.C. does not have any contraindications, she can continue her active immunization series at this visit. She should receive her first doses of diphtheria, tetanus, acellular pertussis (DTaP), *H. influenzae type b* (Hib), inactived polio (IPV), hepatitis B, conjugated pneumococcal, and rotavirus vaccines.

Adverse Effects

3. K.C.'s mother is very concerned about the potential adverse effects of vaccines. How should parents evaluate the balance between the benefits and the risks of immunizations?

Immunizations have had a dramatic impact on several once common childhood infections. For example, smallpox has been eradicated from the world, polio is moving toward global eradication, and invasive *H. influenzae type b* disease among children has declined 95%.[9] Vaccines, however, have potential side effects that often cause concern for parents.

Adverse reactions to inactivated vaccines include pain at the injection site (also see Question 4) and fever within 48 to 72 hours of administration. In contrast, adverse effects from live-attenuated vaccines occur 7 to 10 days after immunization, after the virus has replicated and the immune system has responded. Adverse reactions to live-attenuated vaccines mimic the symptoms of disease. Transient rash occurs in 5% of patients receiving measles, mumps, rubella (MMR) immunizations, and a mild varicella-like rash (median of five lesions) occurs in fewer than 5% of patients receiving the varicella vaccine. Syncope, usually occurring within 30 minutes of immunization, has been reported.[10] Although anaphylactic reactions to vaccines are rare, an allergic reaction may occur as a result of specific allergy to the vaccine itself or to trace components in the vaccine (e.g., preservatives, antibiotics). Children with egg allergy can receive vaccines produced in chick-embryo-fibroblast tissue culture (e.g., MMR) because the risk for serious reaction to these vaccines in egg-allergic children is very low.[11–13] MMR should be used cautiously in individuals with a history of a severe reaction to gelatin, which is a stabilizer in the MMR vaccine. Trace amounts of streptomycin, bacitracin, and neomycin are present in oral polio virus vaccine (OPV), IPV, and MMR; therefore, these vaccines should not be administered to individuals with a history of an anaphylactic reaction to these antibiotics.[14]

Overall, vaccinations are safe, especially when compared with the risks of the diseases that these vaccines prevent, and the safety of immunizations are scrutinized continually. In response to concerns about vaccine safety, the National Vaccine Injury Compensation Act mandated an ongoing review of evidence regarding the possible adverse effects of vaccines and established a no-fault injury compensation program for selected vaccines.[9,14,15]

COMMON PARENT CONCERNS

4. K.C.'s mother is very concerned about the pain associated with immunization and the number of injections K.C. is to receive at each office visit. How can the pain associated with immunization injections be minimized? Can immunizations be given together in the same syringe to lessen the number of injections?

The pain associated with injection of immunizations is typically brief and often more upsetting for the parent than the child. The need for multiple injections can result, however, in an unhappy baby, especially by the third or fourth injection. Administration of an oral sucrose solution during the injection may help alleviate pain.[16,17] Topical anesthetics containing prilocaine and lidocaine can reduce pain and crying associated with immunization; however, high cost and the time required between application and injection have limited the use of these agents. More importantly, the use of topical anesthetics does not seem to modify the fear of injection or post-immunization discomfort.[18]

Ideally, pediatricians and parents would like to be able to deliver all needed vaccines with the fewest number of injections; however, admixing various vaccines in the same syringe is strongly discouraged. Commercially prepared combinations of immunizations (e.g., DTaP with Hib; DTaP with hepatitis B [HepB] and IPV; HepB with Hib) are available to reduce the number of injections and can be used after 6 weeks of age.[19] It is preferred that the same manufacturer of acellular pertussis vaccines be used for the first three doses to ensure adequate immune responses. The recommended number of injections of a specific antigen is acceptable if a commercially available combination vaccine will reduce the number of injections.[19] If combination products are not used, the vaccines should be administered at different sites. If more than one injection must be administered in the same limb, the thigh is the preferred location because of the greater muscle mass.[3]

5. Some opponents to immunizations have raised the questions of whether immunizations can cause autism or weaken a child's immune system. What is the basis for these concerns?

Some parents are concerned that the MMR vaccine, in particular, might cause autism. Because of a rise in the prevalence of autism and the development of autistic symptoms around the time of vaccination, some suggested that MMR vaccination might cause autism.[20,21] Multiple epidemiologic studies, however, have shown no correlation between vaccination and the development of autism.[22–25]

In a National Network for Immunization Information Steering Committee survey, 25% of parents believe that administering "too many" immunizations at one time can weaken a child's immune system.[24] While children now receive at least 20 immunizations by 2 years of age, the number of antigens to which they are exposed is far less than children received in the 1980s. Only an estimated 0.1% of the immune system would be affected if 11 immunizations are given simultaneously.[24] Current studies do not support the hypothesis that multiple immunizations weaken the immune system.[25]

HEPATITIS B

6. K.C.'s mother was hepatitis B-surface antigen (HBsAg) negative before delivery, and her baby received Engerix-B shortly after birth. When should K.C. receive her next immunization for hepatitis B?

Hepatitis B virus (HBV) can be transmitted via exposure to contaminated blood (e.g., blood products, on medical instruments, on nonsterilized needles used in intravenous drug abuse or tattooing), exposure to body fluids (e.g., sexual intercourse), and transplacentally from an HBsAg-positive mother. The prevention of HBV maternal transmission to an infant is essential because acute disease can progress to a chronic carrier state, which can lead to chronic liver disease and primary hepatocellular carcinoma. Children acquiring HBV infection before 5 years of age are at an especially high risk of developing chronic infection.[26] All pregnant women should be tested for

HBsAg and infants born to HBsAg-positive mothers should receive their first vaccine dose within 12 hours of birth.[27] The vaccination of infants born to HBsAG-negative mothers may be delayed only in rare circumstances and in accordance with appropriate documentation. Subsequent vaccine doses should be administered at age 1 to 2 months if the mother is HBsAg negative and again at age 6 months. Hepatitis B immunoglobulin (HBIG) should be administered as soon as possible for infants born to HBsAg-positive mothers. If the mother's HBsAg status is unknown, the infant should be also immunized within 12 hours of birth. Infants born to HBsAg-negative mothers should begin their immunization series before hospital discharge. All unimmunized children should receive HBV vaccine as soon as they are identified.[27]

Two hepatitis B (HepB) vaccines are currently available for use in the United States. Recombivax-HB™ and Engerix-B™ are yeast-derived recombinant vaccines administered as a three-dose series. Adolescents and adults also should follow a three-dose schedule at 0, 1, and 6 months apart. As an option, adolescents may receive a two-dose schedule of the adult formulation of Recombivax-HB.[7] Patients on dialysis and other immunocompromised patients may require a fourth dose if the anti-HBs level is <10 mIU/mL 2 months after the third dose.[28] Antibody screening following immunization is only recommended in high-risk groups. HBV vaccine is combined with *Haemophilus influenzae* type b vaccine in Comvax. PEDIARIX is a combination of DTaP, hepatitis B, and IPV. Monovalent vaccines are preferred for the initial vaccination; however, combination vaccines can be used to complete the series after 6 weeks of age.[7,19]

K.C.'s immunization against hepatitis B at birth was appropriate based on current national guidelines, and HBIG was not needed because her mother is HBsAg negative. K.C. can receive her subsequent doses of HBV vaccine according to the schedule in Table 95-1. Either formulation can be used because the immune response from an immunization series using different vaccines is comparable to that of a full series using a single vaccine.[3,19]

ROTAVIRUS

7. J.M., a 24-year-old mother, presents her 2-month-old infant to receive immunizations. She is concerned about the administration of the RotaTeq vaccine because the infant's grandmother is undergoing chemotherapy for breast cancer and she is concerned that the vaccine may put her mother at risk for infection as well as "bowel problems" for her baby.

Rotavirus is a major cause of gastroenteritis and subsequent dehydration in the United States. Almost all children in the United States will develop rotavirus gastroenteritis within the first 5 years of their lives and up to 50% of hospitalizations secondary to gastroenteritis in children are caused by rotavirus infection.[29,30] The American Academy of Pediatrics and CDC currently recommend the routine immunization of infants with RotaTeq, a live-attenuated, pentavalent oral vaccine against rotavirus.[7] This immunization regimen calls for a three-dose series at 2, 4, and 6 months, with the initial vaccination at 6 to 12 weeks of age and repeat doses at 4- to 10-week intervals. Rotavirus immunization should not be initiated for infants >12 weeks of age and should not be administered after age 32 weeks. Although immunization against rotavirus does not prevent all future episodes of rotavirus infection, it can reduce significantly the severity of infections and reduce hospitalization rates.

Because the rotavirus vaccine is a live-attenuated vaccine and infants can shed the virus for up to 1 week after administration, the immunocompromised person (the grandmother) should avoid contact with the infant's feces and adhere to good handwashing procedures, particularly during the first week after vaccine administration.[29] Although an immunized infant can spread the rotavirus to an immunocompromised person, the risk is believed to be small relative to the benefits and risks to the immunocompromised individual. Rotavirus immunization of infants under this circumstance still is strongly encouraged.[29] The immunization of infants, who themselves are immunocompromised, is more controversial: rotavirus immunization in this circumstance remains with the medical practitioner to discuss risks and benefits with the infant's parents.

The routine implementation of a rotavirus immunization policy was halted a few months after implementation because of an increased rate of intussusception. Intussusception, a form of bowel obstruction, can occur either spontaneously or after natural rotavirus infections in an infant. In postmarketing studies, an increased incidence of intussusception was noted with the RotaShield vaccine, which was subsequently withdrawn from the market. Studies with the new RotaTeq vaccine did not find an increased risk of intussusception; however, reports of intussusception around the time of immunization have been documented.[29,30] At present, the number of cases of intussusception in rotavirus-immunized children is not more than is expected to occur naturally; therefore, the CDC continues to support routine immunizaiton.[31] After rotavirus immunization, infants should be observed for signs and symptoms of intussusception (constipation, diarrhea, bloody stools, abdominal pain).

PERTUSSIS

Pertussis ("whooping cough"), an infectious disease caused by *Bordetella pertussis,* is characterized by a paroxysmal cough with a whooplike, high-pitched inspiratory noise, vomiting, and lymphocytosis. It is a highly communicable infection, which can affect 90% of infants and young children in nonimmunized households, and it can be associated with serious sequelae, particularly in young infants. An estimated 0.3% to 14% of patients with pertussis experience encephalopathy, 0.6% to 2% have permanent neurologic damage, and about 0.1 to 4% die.[32] This serious childhood infection has been mitigated with the availability of a pertussis vaccine, which commonly is administered in combination with diphtheria and tetanus vaccines (i.e., DTP). The efficacy of the DTP vaccines against pertussis after primary immunization (three doses) is greater than 80%.[33] Protection increases to 90% after the last booster (age 4–6 years) and then decreases over the next 12 years, after which protection is minimal.[34]

Despite the availability of an effective vaccine and a high rate of vaccine coverage, reports of pertussis continue to rise.[35] Decreased immunity in adolescents and adults is believed to contribute to this problem. About 12% of adult patients with a cough lasting >2 weeks have pertussis.[36] Although the illness is typically mild in adults and adolescents, they serve as a source of transmission to unprotected infants. This has led to the development and recommendation of pertussis booster vaccines for adolescents and adults.[37]

The association of serious adverse events with whole-cell pertussis vaccine generated considerable controversy on whether the risk-to-benefit ratio was sufficient to warrant routine immunization. As a result, vaccines containing whole-cell pertussis have been withdrawn and replaced with acellular pertussis. Despite a much more favorable adverse effect profile, the DTaP vaccine is contraindicated in any child experiencing an anaphylactic reaction or encephalopathy within 7 days of immunization with DTaP when these symptoms cannot be attributed to another cause.[33] In addition, careful consideration of subsequent doses should be given to infants experiencing a temperature of 105°F (not resulting from another cause) or persistent, inconsolable crying lasting >3 hours within 48 hours after the administration of a pertussis-containing vaccine.[33] The pertussis component of the DTaP vaccine should be eliminated (i.e., continue vaccination with DT) in any child experiencing collapse or a hypotonic-hyporesponsive episode. If an evolving neurologic disorder is present, pertussis immunization should be deferred until the neurologic problem has been fully evaluated. Pre-existing, stable neurologic conditions (e.g., well-controlled seizures) are not contraindications because the benefits of pertussis immunization outweigh the risks. A family history of seizures or other central nervous system (CNS) disorder is not a contraindication.

The recommended schedule for DTaP immunization is shown in Figure 95-1. Acetaminophen or ibuprofen should be administered at regular intervals for 24 hours after immunization to minimize the possibility of postvaccination fever and pain associated with the local reaction.

Three DTaP vaccines (Infanrix, Tripedia, and Daptacel) are approved for the primary vaccination series. The combination product of DTaP-HepB-IPV (PEDIARIX) is also approved for the primary vaccination series, whereas the combination vaccine DTaP-HIB (TriHIBit) is approved for the 15- to 18-month vaccination. If possible, the same DTaP product should be used for all five doses because the immunity, safety, and efficacy associated with the interchanging of different DTaP vaccines are unknown.[3,19] If the product information is unknown or unavailable from prior vaccinations, however, any licensed DTaP vaccine can be used to complete the vaccination series.[3,10,19] Two pertussis vaccine (Tdap) formulations (BOOSTRIX and ADACEL) have been U.S. Food and Drug Administration (FDA) approved for use as a booster dose for children 11 to 18 years of age. This dose should be given at least 5 years from a previous DTaP or Td dose.[37]

POLIO

Polio, an infectious disease caused by a highly contagious enterovirus, can strike at any age, but primarily affects children younger than 3 years of age (>50% of cases). The three identified serotypes of poliovirus are transmitted person to person by direct fecal–oral contact or indirect exposure to infectious saliva, feces, or contaminated water. After household exposure, 90% of susceptible contacts become infected. The poliovirus enters through the mouth and then multiplies in the throat and intestines. Once established in the intestines, poliovirus can enter the bloodstream and invade the CNS. As it multiplies, the virus destroys nerve cells, which cannot be regenerated. As a result, muscles no longer function because of the lack of electrical stimuli from affected nerve cells and paralysis is permanent. The muscles of the legs are affected more often than arm muscles; however, when trunk muscles and muscles of the thorax and abdomen are affected, quadriplegia can be the result. The polio virus also can attack the motor neurons of the brainstem and, thereby, cause difficulty in speaking, swallowing, and breathing.

Immunity to polio can be achieved following natural infection with poliovirus; however, infection by one serotype of the poliovirus does not protect an individual against infection from the other two serotypes. Immunity also can be achieved through immunization, and the development of effective vaccines to prevent paralytic polio was one of the major medical breakthroughs of the 20th century. Since the advent of the trivalent OPV and IPV, the incidence of paralytic poliomyelitis has been reduced dramatically. Inspired by the success of the smallpox initiative, a global poliomyelitis eradication initiative has been inaugurated by the World Health Assembly. As a result of exclusive use of OPV, the Americas, Europe, and the western Pacific regions have been certified free of indigenous wild poliomyelitis. The resurgence of polio, however, can be affected by religious, economic, or political factors (e.g., Africa, Middle East), and the possibility for importation of wild virus still exists unless worldwide eradication is achieved. To prevent a polio epidemic in the United States, high levels of immunization for children during the first year of life are essential.

8. K.C.'s mother is surprised when the nurse brings in a polio injection because her son received an oral form of the vaccine when he was a baby. Why is KC receiving a different form of polio vaccine than her older brother received?

Until recently, the OPV or Sabin vaccine has been the vaccine of choice in the United States. Its advantages include low cost and ease of administration. OPV induces lifelong immunity similar to that observed after natural infection. In addition, OPV provides a high level of gut immunity, thus preventing the carrier state. Finally, the fecal shedding of vaccine virus after Sabin vaccine administration is an effective way to immunize or boost the pre-existing immunity in close contacts.[38] Despite these benefits, OPV carries the risk of vaccine-associated paralytic polio (VAPP), especially after the first dose. In the United States, 8 to 10 cases of VAPP occur each year. The current overall rate of paralytic disease is approximately 1 case per 2.4 million doses distributed, or 1 case per 1.4 million doses for immunologically normal children receiving OPV for the first dose.[39] The risk of VAPP is greater for immunocompromised patients, especially those with B-lymphocyte disorders (e.g., agammaglobulinemia, hypogammaglobulinemia).[40]

In contrast to OPV, the Salk vaccine (IPV) has not been associated with VAPP or other reactions. Enhanced-potency IPV (IPOL, POLIOVAX), with an improved immunogenic response, has been available in the United States since 1987.[41] IPV provides the same systemic immunity as OPV. IPV also induces some immunity of the gastrointestinal tract mucosa, however, less than OPV.[42] Intestinal immunity improves when two doses of OPV follow the first two doses of IPV.[43] IPV is administered only by injection, however.

Considerable debate has raged over which immunization, OPV or IVP, should be used in the United States. OPV is necessary for global eradication and should be used in countries endemic for poliovirus. Because of the reduced threat of wild poliovirus, however, the risks associated with OPV have become less acceptable. In 1997, the Advisory Committee on Immunization Practices (ACIP) provided three options for poliovirus vaccination: sequential use of IPV and OPV, OPV alone, and IPV alone.[44] In 1999, as the global polio initiative progressed and the likelihood of importing wild polio into the United States greatly decreased, the ACIP modified the polio vaccination recommendations to include only an all-IPV schedule. Based on these revised recommendations, all children will receive four doses of IPV (ages 2 months, 4 months, 6 to 18 months, and 4 to 6 years).[45] Currently, OPV may be used only in special circumstances, such as vaccination to control outbreaks of paralytic polio, unvaccinated children traveling in <4 weeks to areas endemic for polio, and children of parents who reject the number of vaccine injections (these children should receive IPV for the first two doses followed by OPV for doses three and four).[45] This revised strategy provides protection against poliomyelitis while minimizing the possibility of VAPP among OPV recipients as well as household and community contacts. IPV is the only poliovirus vaccine that should be used in patients with an immunodeficiency disorder, those receiving immunosuppressive chemotherapy, or children living with a person who is known or suspected to have these conditions.

9. A 28-year-old patient is planning extensive travels through the African continent and is concerned about polio because she had not been immunized as a child. What would be a prudent immunization schedule for her if her trip includes travel to a polio-endemic area?

Routine poliovirus vaccination of persons older than 18 years of age is not necessary in the United States because U.S. residents are at minimal risk of exposure. Vaccination, however, should be considered for adults at high risk of polio exposure (e.g., travel to an area endemic for polio, close contact with children who will be receiving OPV, close contact with patients who may be excreting wild polioviruses, work that requires handling poliovirus specimens). IPV is the vaccine of choice because it has not been associated with VAPP and adults have a higher incidence of VAPP than do children. Ideally, nonimmunized persons anticipating exposure should receive two doses of IPV, administered 4 to 8 weeks apart followed by a third dose 6 to 12 months later. If exposure is likely in <8 weeks, two doses of IPV should be administered at least 4 weeks apart.[45] If this patient's travel must be undertaken on short notice, the patient and physician must weigh the risk of OPV use against the risk of infection abroad. Adults who have completed a primary series of OPV or IPV can receive another dose of OPV or IPV before travel.[39,45] In domestic outbreaks of polio, OPV is routinely given to adult contacts because the risk of natural disease is much greater than the risk of paralysis from OPV. Pregnancy is not a contraindication to OPV immunization when protection is needed (i.e., during an epidemic).

HAEMOPHILUS INFLUENZAE TYPE b

Haemophilus influenzae type b (Hib) was the most common cause of bacterial meningitis and a leading cause of serious, systemic bacterial diseases in children <5 years of age until an effective vaccine was added to the routine immunization schedule.[46–48] The mortality rate associated with Hib meningitis was approximately 5%, with neurologic sequelae observed in 25% to 35% of survivors.[49,50] Epiglottitis, cellulitis, septic arthritis, osteomyelitis, pericarditis, and pneumonia also were commonly caused by *H. influenzae.* Although *H. influenzae* is commonly associated with otitis media and respiratory tract infections, type b strains account for only 5% to 10%.[51]

10. K.C. will be attending day care. Which of the available Hib immunizations should be administered to K.C.?

The first Hib polysaccharide vaccine could elicit an adequate immune response in children >2 years of age; however, in children 18 to 23 months of age, the immune response was only partial and a booster dose was required at 24 months of age.[52,53] The polysaccharide vaccine was replaced by conjugate Hib vaccines to improve the immune response in younger children. It has led to a 95% reduction in the incidence of Hib disease in children <5 years of age.[9] The four currently available Hib polysaccharide conjugate vaccines (HbCV) are as follows: Hib diphtheria toxoid conjugate vaccine or PRP-D (ProHIBiT), Hib meningococcal protein conjugate vaccine or PRP-OMP (PedvaxHIB), Hib tetanus toxoid conjugate vaccine or PRP-T (ActHIB, OmniHIB), and Hib diphtheria CRM197 protein conjugate vaccine or HbOC (HibTITER).[9] As with the original polysaccharide vaccine, immunogenicity of the conjugate vaccines are age dependent (i.e., older children have an improved immune response).[49,54] These four conjugated vaccines have been approved for use in infants, the group at greatest risk for *H. influenzae* infection.[55,56] The HbCV immunization series requires a priming series followed by a booster dose at 12 to 18 months. PRP-OMP (PedvaxHIB) follows a slightly different priming series schedule compared with the other HbCV; the primary series is administered at 2 and 4 months of age in contrast to the schedule of 2, 4, and 6 months' primary series for the other vaccines. Ideally, the primary series should be completed with the same HbCV; however, data support the interchangeability of the products for the priming and booster doses.[57] If PRP-OMP (PedVaxHIB) is used in a priming series with another HbCV, the number of doses necessary to complete the series for the other product should be administered.[57] K.C. could be immunized with any of these four Hib immunizations.

The number of doses of HbCV vaccine needed in older infants and children depends on their age at presentation. Children who begin HbCV at 7 to 11 months of age should receive a primary series of two doses of an HbOC-, PRP-T-, or PRP-OMP-containing vaccine followed by a booster dose at 12 to 18 months of age administered at least 2 months after the previous dose. Children ages 12 to 15 months should receive a primary series of one dose followed by a booster dose 2 months later. If a child reaches 15 months of age without receiving HbCV, only one dose is necessary. HbCV is not indicated in children >5 years of age unless special circumstances place a child at an increased risk of infection.[55,58] The ACIP suggests considering immunization of children >5 years of age who have functional asplenia, sickle cell anemia, or human immunodeficiency virus (HIV) infection. Although the combination vaccine TETRAMUNE (DTwP-Hib) is available to reduce the number of injections, it is preferred to utilize an accellular from of pertussis for childhood immunization.

Availability of HbCV for infants and children has dramatically reduced the incidence of invasive Hib infections. K.C. should start her primary series with an HbCV approved for young infants.

VARICELLA VACCINE

11. A working mother of two children has learned of a case of chickenpox at their elementary school. Her children are 7 and 10 years of age, respectively, and have both been previously immunized with the varicella vaccine. Will her children be protected from a breakthrough infection or would additional immunization be indicated?

Varivax, a live attenuated vaccine against varicella-zoster (chickenpox), is the first herpesvirus vaccine to be widely tested in healthy and high-risk children and adults.[59–61] Chickenpox is a highly contagious, mild childhood disease in healthy children, but it can be severe and even fatal, especially in the immunocompromised patient. Unusual complications (e.g., severe bacterial superinfections, Reye's syndrome, encephalopathies) are worth preventing with an immunization program. Before the vaccine was available, approximately 4 million cases of chickenpox were reported annually, with 4,000 to 9,000 hospitalizations and 100 deaths. Historically, 55% of varicella-related deaths occur in adults, many of whom are infected by exposure to unvaccinated preschool-aged children with typical cases of varicella.[62] Although most children with chickenpox have a self-limited disease lasting 4 to 5 days, many direct and indirect costs are involved. Direct costs include nonprescription and prescription (e.g., acyclovir) medications used to treat the illness, whereas indirect costs are those associated with missed work to be home to care for an ill child.[63]

Previously, a single dose of the vaccine was recommended for children 12 months to 12 years of age who lacked a reliable history of varicella infection: two injections 4 to 8 weeks apart were recommended for children > 13 years of age.[64] Although the vaccine was effective in preventing severe cases of chickenpox, the single-dose immunization of children resulted in only 85% efficacy in preventing disease overall.[65] Despite high vaccine coverage rates, outbreaks of breakthrough varicella continued to occur. As a result, current guidelines recommend a two-dose series for all children.[7,65] The current immunization schedule recommends administration of the first varicella vaccine dose at 12 to 15 months of age, followed by the second dose at 4 to 6 years of age. For persons 7 to 13 years of age who have not received varicella vaccine, two doses of varicella vaccine should be administered at least 3 months apart. For persons > 13 years of age, administer two doses of varicella vaccine at least 4 weeks apart. The varicella vaccine may be given to healthy varicella-susceptible children, such as those described in this case who already have been exposed. Chickenpox can be prevented if varicella vaccine is administered within 3 days of exposure, and might be prevented if administered within 5 days.[66] If the exposure does not cause infection, the vaccination will provide protection for future exposures. In this case, this parent's 7- and 10-year-old children should receive a second dose of varicella vaccine, and if administered within 5 days of exposure, it can prevent a break-through infection. If her children also are in need of their second dose of MMR vaccine, the quadrivalent combination vaccine ProQuad (MMRV) containing measles, mumps, rubella, and varicella antigens, can be used because it can be interchanged with the single entity vaccines.[65]

The most common adverse effect associated with varicella vaccine administration is rash. Transmission of the virus from the vaccine has been documented in only 3 of 15 million doses administered, all of which occurred in the presence of a vesicular rash after vaccination.[64] Salicylates should not be used for 6 weeks after administration of the varicella vaccine because of its association with Reye's syndrome: nonsalicylate analgesics can be used.

Although varicella vaccine might not entirely prevent the occurrence of chickenpox in the immunocompromised patient, it can modify the disease. In the National Institutes of Health's Collaborative Varicella Vaccine Study, a seroconversion rate of only 85% was observed after a single dose in adults, compared with 95% in healthy children and 90% in children with leukemia.[67] Varicella vaccine is generally not recommended in children who have cellular immunodeficiencies, but it can be used in those with impaired humoral immunity.[64] The vaccine should be avoided in children with symptomatic HIV, but may be considered in asymptomatic or mildly symptomatic patients.[64] Although the vaccine is not licensed for routine use in children with acute lymphocytic leukemia, immunization is available for patients enrolled in specific research protocols.

12. What is the recommended dosage and role of varicella zoster immune globulin (VZIG) in children who have been exposed to chickenpox?

Prepared from plasma of healthy volunteer donors with high varicella-zoster virus (VZV) titers, VZIG can decrease the incidence of varicella in selected individuals. It is not useful for treatment of varicella or herpes zoster. VZIG, distributed by the American Red Cross, can prevent clinical varicella if administered within 72 to 96 hours of exposure. Direct contact with an infected person or continuous household exposure carries the greatest risk of infection.

Varicella zoster immune globulin is recommended for individuals at high risk for serious complications following exposure to varicella. Those at risk include immunocompromised children or adults (e.g., acquired or congenital immunodeficiency, immunosuppressive therapy, cancer) and premature infants <28 weeks' gestation or <1,000 g at birth. Pregnant women, who have not had chickenpox, are at high risk of severe varicella complications (e.g., disseminated infection, pneumonia, death) and should receive VZIG within 72 hours of exposure of varicella. Neonates born to women with symptoms of varicella within 5 days before, or 2 days after, delivery should receive VZIG regardless of whether the mother received VZIG.

Varicella zoster immune globulin is administered intramuscularly at a dose of 125 U/10 kg of body weight up to a maximum of 625 U. The minimal dose is 125 U, and fractional doses are not recommended. Protection is thought to last approximately 3 weeks. To limit the need for VZIG in the hospital setting, all susceptible personnel (including health profession students) should be immunized with varicella virus vaccine.[68]

MEASLES/MUMPS/RUBELLA

13. At 15 months, K.C. (Question 1) is scheduled to receive her MMR (a combination vaccine containing live attenuated measles, mumps, and rubella viruses). K.C.'s mother, who has never received MMR, is pregnant with her third child. Should K.C.'s immunization be delayed because of her mother's pregnancy? Should K.C.'s mother be immunized?

Measles, a highly contagious and common disease of childhood historically, often is associated with symptoms, such as high fever, rash, cough, rhinitis, and conjunctivitis. Complications, although uncommon, can include pneumonia and encephalitis. Live-attenuated measles virus vaccine produces a benign infection that is thought to produce lifelong immunity. Despite the availability of the vaccine, measles is responsible for approximately 10% of deaths among children <5 years of age in developing countries. The United States is currently in its third attempt to eliminate measles infection. The most significant decrease in the incidence of measles occurred when U.S. children were required to receive the vaccine before entering school.[69] During the 1985–1988 epidemic, most measles transmission occurred in areas with 95% immunization rates, thereby, indicating that some children fail to respond adequately to the initial vaccine dose.[70] In addition, up to 47% of reported cases of measles in the United States result from international importation; the remaining cases result from outbreaks in school-age children who did not receive a second dose of the vaccine.[71]

The first dose of the MMR vaccine should be administered in children 12 to 15 months of age, and followed by a second dose of MMR at entrance to grade school (age 4 to 6 years).[7,72] The combination vaccine MMRV (ProQuad) should be administered when both MMR and varicella vaccinations are required.[7,72] During an epidemic outbreak, infants can be immunized at 6 to 9 months of age with single-antigen measles, followed by a dose of MMR at 12 months of age, and a dose of MMR at 4 to 6 years of age; older children should receive an additional vaccine dose.[69,73] Adults should receive a second dose of MMR if they were born between 1963 and 1967, previously vaccinated with killed measles vaccine, are students in postsecondary institutions, work in health care facilities, travel internationally, or were recently exposed to a measles outbreak.[74] Persons born after 1968 should receive one dose of a measles-containing vaccine.[75,76]

Mumps immunization remains controversial in childhood because mumps illness in children rarely produces complications. Meningoencephalitis generally is a benign meningitis, and postinfectious encephalitis, a serious complication, is extremely rare (1 of 6,000). Deafness, commonly considered a risk of mumps, occurs rarely (1 of 15,000) and usually is unilateral. Orchitis, another complication, affects adult men. Mumps vaccination at 12 to 15 months of age may not protect male children into their adult years. Although administration of a second dose of MMR at age 4 to 6 years may provide longer protection, current immunization practices are aimed at eliminating the mumps virus from the pool of young children, thereby, minimizing the exposure of nonimmunized adults.[72,76]

Tuberculin-skin testing, when necessary, should be performed before, simultaneously with, or 6 weeks after administration of mumps vaccine because the vaccine can temporarily suppress the skin reaction to the tuberculin.

Rubella, another historically common childhood infection, often is misdiagnosed because its signs and symptoms (e.g., postauricular and suboccipital lymphadenopathy, arthralgia, transient erythematous rash, low-grade fever) vary widely. The most significant consequences of rubella occur in pregnant women (e.g., abortions, miscarriages, still births, fetal anomalies), especially when rubella infection occurs during the first trimester. Preventing congenital rubella through elimination of the viral pool is the primary objective of rubella immunization programs because about 10% to 20% of women of child-bearing age have not acquired natural immunity.

Live-rubella virus vaccination is recommended for all children at 12 to 15 months of age.[72] Immunization or rubella antibody titer screening of women at premarital examinations and postpartum also is recommended. Women of childbearing age receiving the rubella vaccine should use contraception for at least 28 days after immunization.[77] Antibody titers should be measured 3 months after immunization to evaluate antibody response in individuals who have received blood products or immunoglobulin within 8 weeks of immunization because the latter may inhibit antibody stimulation.[78,79]

Before reformulation of the rubella vaccine in 1979, rubella immunization in women who were unknowingly pregnant, resulted in congenital rubella infection in about 10% of fetuses. The current RA27/3 vaccine has reduced dramatically the risk of fetal infection.[73,80] Data from the U.S. Rubella Vaccine in Pregnancy Registry and the UK National Congenital Rubella Surveillance Programme found no evidence of congenital rubella syndrome in 680 women who were inadvertently administered rubella vaccine 3 months before or during pregnancy.[77] Current recommendations are to avoid pregnancy for 28 days following vaccination with a rubella-containing vaccine because of the theoretic risk of contracting disease from the vaccine.[77]

K.C.'s mother should have rubella antibody titers measured. If she does not have natural immunity to rubella, she should receive MMR postpartum. Because the vaccine presents no risk to nonimmunized close contacts, K.C. should receive MMR vaccination at this visit.

TETANUS TOXOID AND RABIES VACCINE

14. A.R., a 9-year-old boy, presents to the emergency department 3 hours after being bitten by a neighbor's dog. He has two deep lacerations and one puncture wound on his right hand. The wounds are cleaned and he is given amoxicillin-clavulanic acid. The neighbor claims that the dog has been vaccinated against rabies but has no proof. The county health department is notified, and the dog is placed in quarantine. A.R.'s immunizations are up to date (verified by card) and his last tetanus shot (DTP) was 4 years ago. Should A.R. receive tetanus immunoglobulin (TIG) or tetanus toxoid (Td)? What is the role of rabies immunoglobulin (RIG) and rabies vaccine in animal bites?

Tetanus (lockjaw) is a highly fatal, noncommunicable disease that is most notably manifested by generalized, board-like muscular rigidity. It results from wounds (including animal bites) infected by *Clostridium tetani,* an anaerobic, gram-positive rod that exists in nature as an extremely resistant spore. Prophylaxis can be achieved by actively stimulating antibody formation against the toxin by immunization with Td. Passive immunity can be achieved by administrating TIG. Because A.R.'s immunizations are up to date and <5 years have elapsed since his last dose of Td, he does not need to receive Td or TIG.[81,82]

Rabies is an important concern in any patient presenting with an animal bite. Wild animals serve as reservoirs for rabies and may infect domestic animals. All wild animals should be considered rabid until such is proved otherwise. In the United States, domestic dogs and cats have a low incidence of rabies, but must be quarantined for 7 to 10 days and monitored for signs and symptoms of rabies unless proof of vaccination is available.

Infection with rabies virus produces an acute illness with rapid, progressive encephalitis. Once the onset of symptoms occurs, the prognosis is extremely poor; therefore, emphasis is placed on prevention. Following exposure, rabies prophylaxis includes passive immunization with RIG (20 U/kg) as soon as possible and active immunization with rabies vaccine on days 0, 3, 7, 14, and 28.[83,84] Because the dog that attacked A.R. was a family pet and in good health, A.R. does not need to receive rabies prophylaxis at this time. Postexposure prophylaxis will need to be initiated immediately if the dog develops any sign of rabies.[82–87]

PNEUMOCOCCUS

15. The pneumococcal, influenza, and hepatitis A vaccines have been added to the pediatric immunization schedule. What is the role of the pneumococcal and influenza vaccines in children? Should all children receive these vaccines?

Streptococcus pneumoniae (pneumococcus) is responsible for meningitis, pneumonia, and otitis media.[88] Children <2 years of age and adults >65 years are at highest risk for developing pneumococcal infections. The risk for disseminated pneumococcal infections is increased by some underlying medical conditions (heart failure, chronic obstructive pulmonary diseases), chronic liver disease (e.g., cirrhosis), functional or anatomic asplenia (e.g., sickle cell disease, splenectomy), and acquired or inherited immunosuppressive conditions (e.g., HIV, cancer, immunosuppressive therapy). *S. pneumoniae* is a common pathogen in children with HIV, often presenting as one of the first manifestations of HIV infection.

Two pneumococcal vaccines are available: the original polysaccharide vaccine (Pneumovax) and the conjugate-pneumococcal vaccine (Prevnar). Pneumovax contains 23 purified capsular-polysaccharide antigens of *S. pneumoniae.* Antibody response to the Pneumovax is inconsistent in children <2 years of age, and the antigens included in Pneumovax protect against strains that typically cause adult disease. The conjugate pneumococcal vaccine (Prevnar) improves immunogenicity and efficacy in infants and toddlers. This vaccine protects against the seven strains of pneumococcus that cause 80% of all pneumococcal invasive disease in children <6 years of age. The ACIP recommends giving the conjugate vaccine to all children <24 months of age to prevent invasive pneumococcal disease (e.g., meningitis, pneumonia); and to any child <5 years of age who is at high risk of pneumococcal disease.[88] The polysaccharide vaccine is recommended as a supplement to the conjugate vaccine for some high-risk children (e.g., sickle cell anemia).[88]

Immunocompromised patients typically have an unreliable response to vaccines, but because of the potential benefits, the pneumococcal vaccines should be administered. Some studies have found transient elevation of plasma HIV levels after pneumococcal vaccination, although this has not been associated with decreased patient survival.[89,90] To maintain immunity, revaccination with the 23-valent polysaccharide vaccine is recommended after 3 years in high-risk children <10 years of age and after 5 years in older patients.

HEPATITIS A

Viral hepatitis can be caused by at least six hepatotrophic viruses (identified by letters A through G) and can present as either an acute or chronic illness (see Chapter 73, Viral Hepatitis). Typically, the course of hepatitis A includes an incubation phase, an acute hepatitis phase, and a convalescent phase. Symptoms often include fever, malaise, anorexia, nausea, abdominal discomfort, and jaundice. Clinical illness typically lasts 1 to 2 months. More than 70% of older children and adults have symptomatic infection, but just as many children <6 years of age are asymptomatic. Asymptomatic children serve as a source of infection, especially for household or other close contacts.

About one-third of hepatitis A cases occur in children <5 years of age.[91] Among all reported cases, the most common source of infection is household or sexual contact, followed by day care attendance or employment, international travel, and food or waterborne outbreak.

The ACIP had previously (1987–1997) recommended routine vaccination of children 2 years of age and older in communities with an average incidence of >20 cases per 100,000 population.[92] Rates of disease in these areas has dramatically decreased to at or below rates in areas where vaccination was not recommended; therefore, the ACIP now recommends routine vaccination for all persons >1 year of age.[93] Vaccination programs targeting toddlers and young children are important because children are often asymptomatic and unwittingly transmit the virus to adolescents and adults. In addition, data suggest a "herd effect" when vaccination of children is widespread.[94] A program aimed exclusively at toddlers in an endemic area reduced the prevalence of hepatitis A by >90%, not only in the 2- to 4-year-old vaccine recipients, but in all age groups.

Havrix and Vaqta, two hepatitis A vaccines with adult and pediatric formulations, are indicated for adults and children 1 year of age or older. Two doses are recommended, the second dose should be administered 6 to 18 months after the initial dose, depending on the formulation (see Chapter 73: Viral Hepatitis). The pediatric formulations of each product are indicated for those 1 to 18 years of age and contain half the antigen of adult formulations. Twinrix, a combination hepatitis A and B vaccine, is indicated in individuals >18 years of age on a three-dose schedule.

INFLUENZA

The influenza vaccine is currently recommended for anyone older than 6 months of age who is at increased risk for complications secondary to influenza. The American Academy of Pediatrics and the CDC also recommend that healthy children 6 to 59 months of age receive the influenza vaccine. This age recommendation was recently expanded from children 6 to 23 months of age because although children <24 months of age have increased hospitalization rates, healthy children from 24 to 59 months of age also experience significant morbidity resulting in increased use of health care resources.[95] Additional target groups for the influenza vaccine include the following[96]:

- Any household contact or caregiver of high-risk individuals or children <5 year of age
- People 50 or more years of age
- Residents of chronic care facilities
- Adults and children with chronic pulmonary or cardiovascular disorders, diabetes mellitus, renal dysfunction, hemoglobinopathies, or immunosuppression
- Children <18 years of age receiving aspirin therapy (because of an increased risk of Reye's syndrome after influenza)
- Adults and children who have any condition predisposing to respiratory complications, such as aspiration
- Women who will be pregnant during the influenza season
- Household members and care providers in close contact with high-risk patients

Each year, the influenza vaccine includes three inactivated influenza-18 virus strains (usually, two type A and one type B) thought to be circulating in the United States during the upcoming winter. The vaccine is available as both a split- and whole-virus preparation. The split-virus vaccine is used in children <12 years of age to decrease the likelihood of a febrile reaction. Immunocompetent children and young adults typically develop high postvaccination antibody titers. Elderly patients and some people with chronic disorders have lower antibody titers and may remain susceptible to influenza despite vaccination.[96]

Influenza vaccine should be administered annually for adequate protection. Children <9 years of age require two doses of the vaccine administered 1 month apart to achieve adequate antibody response. If these children received influenza vaccination in a previous season, however, only one dose is required. One dose of the vaccine is indicated for individuals >9 years of age. Influenza vaccine contains a small amount of egg protein and historically has been contraindicated in patients with a severe egg allergy. Evidence indicates, however, that even patients with severe egg allergies can safely receive the influenza vaccine.[97,98]

A live, attenuated trivalent intranasal influenza vaccine (FluMist) is available for use in healthy, nonpregnant patients 5 to 49 years of age. After administration, recipients become infected with attenuated virus strains, which stimulate both local IgA and circulating IgG antibodies.[99–102] Live vaccine may be especially useful for healthy individuals, including health care workers, during periods when supply of inactivated vaccine may be low, potentially increasing availability of the inactivated product for those unable to receive the live vaccine. Individuals should not receive the live vaccine if any of the following apply[95]:

- Age <5 years
- Moderate to severe illness
- Received another live vaccine within 4 weeks
- Severe allergy to eggs
- Currently taking salicylates
- Known or suspected immunodeficiency
- History of Guillain-Barré syndrome
- Asthma or reactive airway disease or other condition conferring high risk of severe influenza

Although the health and economic benefits of protecting targeted groups of adults from influenza are well documented, the cost-effectiveness of routine immunization for children is not known at this time.

ADOLESCENT IMMUNIZATIONS

Meningococcus

16. J.C. is a 12-year-old girl who presents for a check-up with her pediatrician. In discussion, it is found that her cousin attends a university where an outbreak of meningococcal disease recently occurred. What are current recommendations for children and adolescents regarding administration of meningococcal vaccine?

Until recently, the ACIP has recommended meningococcal vaccination for special populations, such as travelers to endemic areas, those with certain immunodeficiencies (i.e., terminal complement deficiency), those with functional or anatomic asplenia, and laboratory personnel who may come in contact with aerosolized meningococus.[103] With the use of the *H. influenzae type b* and pneumococcal conjugate vaccines, however, *Neisseria meningitidis* has become a more prominent cause of bacterial meningitis.

The two available meningococcal vaccines, a polysaccharide preparation and a conjugated vaccine, cover the serotypes A, C, Y, and W-135 of *N. meningitidis*. The polysaccharide preparation (Menomune), or MPS4, is indicated for persons 2 to 10 years of age with the risk factors mentioned above. It is important to note that polysaccharide vaccines such as this only stimulate B-lymphocytes, not T-lymphocytes, and thus do not produce a memory response. As a result, the effectiveness wanes over time. In addition, nasopharyngeal colonization of meningococcus is not reduced, so person-to-person transmission continues, blocking the development of herd immunity.[103]

The conjugate vaccine (Menactra), or MCV4, is indicated for individuals 11 to 55 years of age. ACIP recommends administration of this vaccine to all persons at 11 to 12 years of age (or at high school entry if there is no history of vaccination) and to unvaccinated college freshmen residing in dormitories.[103]

Adverse effects (e.g., fever, headache, chills, malaise, and arthralgias) from both vaccines are similar and relatively rare; however, in October 2006, the CDC and FDA issued a warning regarding the potential for increased risk of Guillain Barré syndrome in patients receiving the conjugate vaccine. Over a 16-month period beginning in June of 2005, 15 cases were reported in the 11- to 19-year age group, and 2 cases in those >20 years of age. All patients recovered. Despite this apparent small increased risk of Guillain Barré syndrome, current recommendations remain the same, but monitoring of this development will continue.[104] At this time, J.C. should receive the MCV4 vaccine.

Human papilloma Virus (HPV)

17. What is the role of the HPV vaccine and who should be targeted for immunization?

The human papilloma virus (HPV), a virus that commonly infects the genital tract, is primarily transmitted by sexual contact. Infection with HPV has been associated with cervical cancer as well as other anogenital cancers, anogenital warts, and recurrent respiratory papillomatosis.[105,106] Acute infections with HPV typically resolve without clinical complications within 1 year; however, 10% to 15% of infections remain persistent and pose a risk of invasive cervical carcinoma and other anogential carcinomas.[106] Although not all HPV infections cause cervical cancer, almost all (99%) of cervical cancer in women is associated with a previous HPV infection.[105,106] Two strains of HPV, HPV 16 and 18, have been associated with 70% to 80% of what are referred to as "high grade" or precancerous cervical lesions[105,106] and are the targets of the currently marketed HPV vaccine (Gardisil). The vaccine also protects against HPV strains 6 and 11, which have been associated with >90% of all genital warts and 10% of "low grade" or low risk cervical lesions. Infection with one strain of HPV does not prevent infection from other strains; thus, repeated infections can occur through one's lifetime[106] and those with prior HPV infections benefit from immunization as well.

Routine vaccination with the HPV vaccine is recommended for female patients at 11 to 12 years of age.[105] Vaccination at this age attempts to achieve an immune response before the sexual debut[105] and involves a three-dose series administered at intervals of 0, 2, and 6 months.[105,107] The vaccine can also be administered from 9 to 26 years of age.[105] Immunization against HPV is 90% effective in reducing persistent HPV infections and 100% effective in preventing HPV-related diseases, such as genital warts or lesions.[105–107]

The mandatory requirement for immunization against HPV is controversial and debated in many state legislatures because of ethical and social concerns. The CDC and AAP recommend immunization for adolescent females, regardless of current sexual activity, to decrease the lifetime risk of cervical cancer and to protect against infection when the time comes that an individual chooses to become sexual active.

PEDIATRIC IMMUNIZATIONS FOR IMMUNOCOMPROMISED PATIENTS

18. B.R., a 15-month-old boy who is HIV positive, lives with foster parents taking care of two other immunocompromised children. He is taking zidovudine 180 mg/m² PO QID, didanosine 120 mg/m² PO BID, trimethoprim-sulfamethoxazole (TMP-SMX) 75 mg/m² PO BID three times weekly, and intravenous immunoglobulin (IVIG) 400 mg/kg once monthly. His recent CD4 T-lymphocyte counts were 976 g/L (23%). Currently, he is asymptomatic and has not received any immunizations. What immunizations are recommended for immunocompromised children and their close contacts?

Immunocompromised children (e.g., those with acquired or congenital immunodeficiencies, leukemia, lymphoma, generalized malignancies, and those receiving cancer chemotherapy or other immunosuppressive agents) should be immunized with all of the regularly scheduled inactivated vaccines, although an adequate immune response cannot be guaranteed. Previously, vaccination of these children with live-attenuated virus vaccines was deemed to be contraindicated because of possible infection from uncontrolled viral replication; however, the risk of disease often outweighs the risk of vaccination. Patients receiving high-dose corticosteroids (>2 mg/kg/day of prednisone or its equivalent) for >2 weeks; however, should not receive live-attenuated vaccines for at least 3 months after the discontinuation of the corticosteroid.[3] In patients infected with HIV, transient increased viremia from immune activation is of concern and has been reported in adults so infected after a booster dose of Td, although the clinical significance is unclear.[3,108]

The MMR vaccine, a live-virus vaccine, should not be administered to severely immunocompromised patients.[3,109] Because the risk of developing illness from the vaccine is low, MMR can be administered to patients with HIV who are not severely immunocompromised (as determined by age-appropriate CD4 lymphocyte counts and percentage).[3,75,110] Response to the vaccine declines as HIV progresses; therefore, susceptible individuals should be vaccinated as soon after diagnosis as possible.[75] Infants infected with HIV should be vaccinated at 12 months of age with a second dose administered 1 month later rather than waiting to give the booster dose at 5 years of age. Immunization of children who are asymptomatic and mildly symptomatic HIV infected against varicella should be considered[64]; however, varicella vaccine continues to be contraindicated in patients with cellular immunodeficiencies.[3]

Although B.R.'s ability to mount an antibody response cannot be determined, he should receive all inactivated vaccines as scheduled, including pneumococcal and influenza vaccinations. Because he is asymptomatic and has an adequate CD4 lymphocyte count for his age, varicella and MMR vaccines also should be considered. His monthly administration of IVIG, however, may compromise his ability to respond to the MMR and varicella vaccines.[75,111] If B.R. is exposed to chickenpox or measles, passive prophylaxis with VZIG and IG, respectively, should be instituted if it has been >3 weeks since his last dose of IVIG. Specific recommendations for immunization of children with varying degrees of immunodeficiency are available from the CDC.[3,111]

REFERENCES

1. Centers for Disease Control and Prevention. National, state, and urban area vaccination coverage levels among children aged 19–35 months—United States, 2005. *MMWR* 2006;55:988.
2. Luman ET et al. Timeliness of childhood immunizations. *Pediatrics* 2002;110:935.
3. Centers for Disease Control and Prevention. General recommendations on immunizations. *MMWR* 2006;55(RR-15).
4. Watson MA et al. Inadequate history as barrier to immunization. *Arch Pediatr Adolesc Med* 1996;150:135
5. Moneymaker CS et al. Missed opportunities to immunize in public, private and military primary care settings in Norfolk, VA [Abstract]. *Pediatr Res* 1996;39:96A.
6. Zell E et al. Reliability of vaccination cards and parent-derived information for determining immunization status: lessons from the 1994 National Health Interview Survey (NHIS) provider record check (PRC) study. *Pediatr Res* 1997;41:101A.
7. Committee on Infectious Diseases Recommended Childhood and Adolescent Immunization Schedule-United States, 2007. *Pediatrics* 2007;119:207.
8. American Academy of Pediatrics Committee on In-

fectious Disease. Immunization of preterm and low birth weight infants. *Pediatrics* 2003;112:193.
9. Centers for Disease Control and Prevention. Progress toward elimination of Haemophilus influenzae type b disease among infants and children—United States, 1987–1995. *JAMA* 1996;276:1542.
10. Braun MM et al. Syncope after immunization. *Arch Pediatr Adolesc Med* 1997;151:255.
11. Kemp A et al. Measles immunization in children with clinical reactions to egg protein. *Am J Dis Child* 1990;144:33.
12. Fasano MB et al. Egg hypersensitivity and adverse reactions to measles, mumps, rubella vaccine. *J Pediatr* 1992;120:878.
13. James JM et al. Safe administration of the measles vaccine to children allergic to eggs. *N Engl J Med* 1995;332:1262.
14. Centers for Disease Control and Prevention. Update: vaccine side effects, adverse reactions, contraindications and precautions. Recommendations of the Advisory Committee on Immunization Practices (ACIP). *MMWR* 1996;45:RR–12.
15. Smith M. National childhood vaccine injury compensation act. *Pediatrics* 1988;82:264.
16. Allen KD et al. Sucrose as an analgesic agent for infants during immunization injections. *Arch Pediatr Adolesc Med* 1996;150:270.
17. Lewindon PJ et al. Randomised controlled trial of sucrose by mouth for the relief of infant crying after immunization. *Arch Dis Child* 1998;78:453.
18. Uhari M et al. A eutectic mixture of lidocaine and prilocaine for alleviating vaccination pain in infants. *Pediatrics* 1993;92:719.
19. American Academy of Pediatrics. Combination vaccines for childhood immunization: recommendations of the Advisory Committee on Immunization Practices (ACIP), the American Academy of Pediatrics (AAP), and the American Academy of Family Practice (AAFP). *Pediatrics* 1999;103:1064.
20. Wakefield AJ et al. Ileal-lymphoid-nodular hyperplasia, non-specific colitis, and pervasive developmental disorder in children. *Lancet* 1998;351:637.
21. Madsen KM et al. A population-based study of measles, mumps, and rubella vaccination and autism. *N Engl J Med* 2002;347:1477.
22. Taylor B et al. Autism and measles, mumps, and rubella vaccine: no epidemiological evidence for a causal association. *Lancet* 1999;353:2026.
23. Taylor B et al. Measles, mumps, and rubella vaccination and bowel problems or developmental regression in children with autism: population study. *BMJ* 2002;324:393.
24. Offit PA et al. Addressing parents' concerns: do multiple vaccines overwhelm or weaken the infant's immune system? *Pediatrics* 2002;109:124.
25. Francois G et al. Vaccine safety controversies and the future of vaccination programs. *Pediatr Infect Dis J* 2005;24:953.
26. Margolis HS et al. Hepatitis B: evolving epidemiology and implications for control. *Semin Liver Dis* 1992;11:84.
27. Advisory Committee on Immunization Practices (ACIP). Hepatitis B virus: a comprehensive strategy for eliminating transmission in the United States through universal childhood vaccination; Part I: Immunization of infants, children, and adolescents. *MMWR* 2005;54(No RR-16):1.
28. Hollinger FB. Factors influencing the immune response to hepatitis B vaccine, booster guidelines and vaccine protocol recommendations. *Am J Med* 1989;87(S-3A):36S.
29. American Academy of Pediatrics Committee on Infectious Diseases. Prevention of rotavirus disease: guidelines for the use of rotavirus vaccine. *Pediatrics* 2007;119:171.
30. Centers for Disease Control and Prevention Advisory Committee on Immunization Practices. Prevention of rotavirus gastroenteritis among infants and children: recommendations of the Advisory Committee on Immunization Practices. *MMWR* 2006;55(RR-12):1.
31. A public health notification: information on RotaTeq and intussusception. Accessed May 23, 2007 at: http://www.fda.gov/cber/safety/phnrota021307.htm.
32. Katz SL. Controversies in immunization. *Pediatr Infect Dis J* 1987;6:607.
33. Centers for Disease Control and Prevention. Pertussis vaccination: use of acellular pertussis vaccines among infants and young children. Recommendations of the Advisory Committee on Immunizations Practices (ACIP). *MMWR* 1997; 46:RR-7.
34. Bass JW et al. Return of epidemic pertussis in the United States. *Pediatr Infect Dis J* 1994;13:343.
35. Centers for Disease Control and Prevention. Pertussis vaccination: acellular pertussis vaccine for reinforcing and booster use. Supplementary ACIP statement. *MMWR* 1992;41:1.
36. Nenning ME et al. Prevalence and incidence of adult pertussis in an urban population. *JAMA* 1996;275:1772.
37. Centers for Disease Control and Prevention. Preventing tetanus, diphtheria, and pertussis among adolescents: use of tetanus toxoid, reduced diphtheria toxoid, and acellular pertussis vaccines: Recommendations of the Advisory Committee on Immunization Practices. *MMWR* 2006;55(RR-3)1.
38. Ogra PL et al. Poliovirus vaccine: live or dead. *J Pediatr* 1986;108:1031.
39. National Immunization Program, Department of Health and Human Services. Epidemiology and Prevention of Vaccine-Preventable Diseases, Poliomyelitis. Atlanta, GA: Centers for Disease Control and Prevention; 2001.
40. Sutter RW et al. Vaccine associated paralytic poliomyelitis among immunodeficient persons. *Infect Med* 1994;190:41.
41. Faden H et al. Comparative evaluation of immunization with live attenuated and enhanced-potency inactivated trivalent poliovirus vaccines in childhood: systemic and local immune responses. *J Infect Dis* 1990;162:1291.
42. Onorato IM et al. Mucosal immunity induced by enhanced-potency inactivated and oral polio vaccines. *J Infect Dis* 1991;163:1.
43. Modlin JF et al. Humoral and mucosal immunity in infants induced by three sequential inactivated poliovirus vaccine-live attenuated poliovirus vaccine immunization schedules. *J Infect Dis* 1997; 175(Suppl 1):S228.
44. Centers for Disease Control and Prevention. Poliomyelitis prevention in the United States: introduction of a sequential vaccination schedule of inactivated poliovirus vaccine followed by oral poliovirus vaccine. Recommendations of the Advisory Committee on Immunizations Practices (ACIP). *MMWR* 1997;46:RR-3.
45. Centers for Disease Control and Prevention. Poliomyelitis prevention in the United States: updated recommendations of the Advisory Committee on Immunization Practices (ACIP). *MMWR* 2000;49(RR-5)1.
46. Fraser DW. Haemophilus influenza in the community and the home. In: Sell SH et al., eds. *Haemophilus Influenzae: Epidemiology, Immunology, and Prevention of Disease.* New York: Elsevier Science 1982:11.
47. Schlech W et al. Bacterial meningitis in the United States, 1978 through 1981. *JAMA* 1985;253:1749.
48. Dajani AS et al. Systemic Haemophilus influenzae disease: an overview. *J Pediatr* 1979;98:355.
49. Taylor HG et al. Intellectual, neuropsychological, and achievement outcomes in children six to eight years after recovery from *Haemophilus influenzae* meningitis. *Pediatrics* 1984;74:198.
50. Peltoa H et al. Prevention of Haemophilus influenzae type b bacteremic infections with the capsular polysaccharide vaccine. *N Engl J Med* 1984;310:1566.
51. Anonymous. Polysaccharide vaccine for prevention of *Haemophilus influenzae* type b disease. *JAMA* 1985;253:2630.
52. Black SB et al. Efficacy of *Haemophilus influenzae* type b capsular polysaccharide vaccine. *Pediatr Infect Dis* 1988;7:149.
53. Harrison LH et al. *Haemophilus influenzae* type b polysaccharide vaccine: an efficacy study. *Pediatrics* 1989;84:255.
54. Lepow ML et al. Safety and immunogenicity of *Haemophilus influenzae* type b diphtheria toxoid conjugate vaccine (PRP-D) in infants. *J Infect Dis* 1987;156:591.
55. American Academy of Pediatrics Committee on Infectious Diseases. *Haemophilus influenzae* type b conjugate vaccines: update. *Pediatrics* 1989;84:386.
56. U.S. Food and Drug Administration approval of use of Haemophilus b conjugate vaccine for infants. *MMWR* 1990;39:698.
57. Centers for Disease Control and Prevention. Notice to readers: recommended childhood immunization schedule-United States, 1998. *MMWR* 1998;47:8.
58. Schaffer SJ et al. Immunization status and birth order. *Arch Pediatr Adolesc Med* 1995;149:792.
59. Centers for Disease Control and Prevention. Prevention of varicella. Recommendations of the Advisory Committee on Immunization Practices. *MMWR* 1996;45:RR-11.
60. Gershon AA. Live attenuated varicella vaccine. *Pediatr Ann* 1984;13:653.
61. Arbeter AM et al. Immunization of children with acute lymphoblastic leukemia with live attenuate varicella vaccine without complete suspension of chemotherapy. *Pediatrics* 1990;85:338.
62. Centers for Disease Control and Prevention. Varicella-related deaths among adults-United States 1997. *MMWR* 1997:46:409.
63. Lieu AT et al. The cost of childhood chickenpox: parents' perspective. *Pediatr Infect Dis J* 1994; 13:173.
64. Centers for Disease Control and Prevention. Prevention of varicella: updated recommendations of the Advisory Committee on Immunization Practices (ACIP) *MMWR* 1999;48(RR-06):1.
65. American Academy of Pediatric Committee on Infectious Diseases. Policy Statement. Prevention of varicella: recommendations for use of varicella vaccines in children, including a recommendation for a routine two-dose varicella vaccine immunization schedule. Accessed at http://www.cispimmunize.org/pro/pdf/Varicella-040907.pdf May 14, 2007.
66. Arbeter AM et al. Varicella vaccine studies in healthy children and adults. *Pediatrics* 1986;78:748.
67. Gershon A et al. NIAID Varicella Vaccine Collaborative Study Group: live attenuated varicella vaccine in immunocompromised children and healthy adults. *Pediatrics* 1986;78:757.
68. Centers for Disease Control and Prevention. Varicella zoster immune globulin for the prevention of chickenpox. *MMWR* 1984;33:84.
69. Robbins KB et al. Low measles incidence: association with enforcement of school immunization laws. *Am J Public Health* 1981;71:270.
70. Gustafson TL et al. Measles outbreak in a fully immunized secondary-school population. *N Engl J Med* 1987;316:771.
71. Centers for Disease Control and Prevention. Measles outbreak among internationally adopted children arriving in the United States, February–March 2001. *MMWR* 2002;51:1115.
72. Centers for Disease Control and Prevention. Measles, Mumps, and Rubella-Vaccine Use and Strategies for Elimination of Measles, Rubella, and Congenital Rubella Syndrome and Control of Mumps: Recommendations of the Advisory Committee on Immunization Practices (ACIP). *MMWR* 1998;47(RR-8);1.
73. Bernstein DI et al. Fetomaternal aspects of immunization with RA 27/3 live attenuated rubella virus vaccine during pregnancy. *J Pediatr* 1980;97:467.
74. Centers for Disease Control. Clarification: Vol 51, No. 40 Recommended Adult Immunization Schedule-United States, 2002–2003. *MMWR* 2003; 52:345.

75. Centers for Disease Control and Prevention. Measles, mumps, and rubella-vaccine use and strategies for elimination of measles, rubella, and congenital rubella syndrome and control of mumps: recommendations of the Advisory Committee on Immunization Practices (ACIP). *MMWR* 1998;47(RR-8):1.
76. American Academy of Pediatrics Committee on Infectious Disease. Measles: reassessment of the current immunization policy. *Pediatrics* 1989;84:1110.
77. Centers for Disease Control and Prevention. Notice to Readers: Revised ACIP Recommendation for avoiding pregnancy after receiving a rubella-containing vaccine. *MMWR* 2001;50:1117.
78. Landes RD et al. Neonatal rubella following postpartum maternal immunization. *J Pediatr* 1980;97:465.
79. Centers for Disease Control and Prevention. Rubella prevention recommendation of the immunization practices advisory committee. *MMWR* 1990;39:RR-15.
80. Balfour HH et al. RA 27/3 rubella vaccine: a four-year follow up. *Am J Dis Child* 1980;134:350.
81. American Academy of Pediatrics. Tetanus. In: Pickering LK, ed. *2000 RedBook: Report of the Committee on Infectious Disease.* 25th ed. Elk Grove Village, IL: American Academy of Pediatrics; 2000:563.
82. Centers for Disease Control and Prevention (CDC). Tetanus: United States 1987 and 1988. *MMWR* 1990;39:37.
83. American Academy of Pediatrics. Rabies. In: Pickering LK, ed. *2000 Red Book: Report of the Committee on Infectious Diseases.* 25th ed. Elk Grove Village, IL: American Academy of Pediatrics; 2000:475.
84. Centers for Disease Control and Prevention. Human rabies prevention-United States, 1999 recommendations of the Advisory Committee on Immunization Practices (ACIP). *MMWR* 1999;48(RR-1):1.
85. Griego RD et al. Dog, cat and human bites: a review. *J Am Acad Dermatol* 1995:1019.
86. Centers for Disease Control and Prevention (CDC). Rabies postexposure prophylaxis—Connecticut 1990–1994. *MMWR* 1996;45:232.
87. Centers for Disease Control and Prevention. Human rabies prevention-United States, 1999 recommendations of the Advisory Committee on Immunization Practices (ACIP). *MMWR* 1999; 48(RR-1):1.
88. Centers for Disease Control and Prevention. Preventing pneumococcal disease among infants and children: recommendations of the Advisory Committee on Immunization Practices (ACIP). *MMWR* 2000;49:RR-9.
89. Brichacek B et al. Increased plasma HIV-1 burden following antigenic challenge with pneumococcal vaccine. *J Infect Dis* 1996;174:1191.
90. Katzenstein TL et al. Assessment of plasma HIV RNA and CD4 counts after combined Pneumovax and tetanus toxoid vaccination: no detectable increase in HIV replication 6 weeks after immunization. *Scand J Infect Dis* 1996;28:239.
91. National Immunization Program, Department of Health and Human Services. Epidemiology and prevention of vaccine preventable diseases. Hepatitis A. Atlanta, GA: Centers for Disease Control and Prevention; 2001.
92. Centers for Disease Control and Prevention. Prevention of hepatitis A through active or passive immunization: recommendations of the Advisory Committee on Immunization Practices (ACIP). *MMWR* 1999;48(RR-12):1.
93. Centers for Disease Control and Prevention. Prevention of hepatitis A through active or passive immunization: recommendations of the Advisory Committee on Immunization Practices (ACIP). *MMWR* 2006;55(RR07):1.
94. Dagan R et al. National hepatitis A (HAV) immunization program aimed exclusively at toddlers in an endemic country resulting in >90% reduction in morbidity rate in all ages. (Abstract) Infectious Disease Society Association 40th Annual Meeting, Chicago, IL; October 27, 2002.
95. Committee on Infectious Disease. Prevention of influenza: recommendations for influenza immunization of children, 2006–2007. *Pediatrics* 2007;119:846.
96. Centers for Disease Control and Prevention. Prevention and control of influenza. Recommendations of the Advisory Committee on Immunization Practices (ACIP). *MMWR* 2006;55(RR-10):1.
97. Murphy KR et al. Safe administration of influenzae vaccine in asthmatic children hypersensitive to egg proteins. *J Pediatr* 1985;106:931.
98. James JM et al. Safe administration of influenza vaccine to patients with severe allergy. *J Pediatr* 1998;133:624.
99. Belshe RB et al. The efficacy of live attenuated, cold-adapted, trivalent, intranasal influenza virus vaccine in children. *N Engl J Med* 1998;338:1405.
100. Edwards KM et al. A randomized controlled trial of cold-adapted and inactivated vaccines for the prevention of influenza A disease. *J Infect Dis* 1994;169:68.
101. Nichol KL et al. Effectiveness of live, attenuated intranasal influenza virus vaccine in healthy, working adults. *JAMA* 1999;282:137.
102. Belshe RB et al. Efficacy of vaccination with live attenuated, cold-adapted, trivalent, intranasal influenza virus vaccine against a variant (A/Sydney) not contained in the vaccine. *J Pediatr* 2000;136:168.
103. Centers for Disease Control and Prevention. Prevention and control of meningococcal disease: recommendations of the Advisory Committee on Immunization Practices (ACIP). *MMWR* 2005;55(RR-07):1.
104. Centers for Disease Control and Prevention. Update: Guillain-Barre syndrome among recipients of Menactra Meningococcal Conjugate Vaccine—United States, June 2005–September 2006. *MMWR* 2006;55:1120.
105. Centers for Disease Control and Prevention. Quadravalent human papillomavirus vaccine. Recommendations of the Advisory Committee on Immunization Practices. *MMWR* 2007; 56(RR02).
106. Saslow D et al. American Cancer Society guideline for human papillomavirus (HPV) vaccine use to prevent cervical cancer and its precursors. *CA Cancer J Clin* 2007;57:7.
107. Siddiqui MAA et al. Human papillomavirus quadrivalent (types 6, 11, 16, & 18) recombinant vaccine (Gardisil). *Drugs* 2006;66:1263.
108. Recommendations of the Advisory Committee on Immunization Practices (ACIP). Use of vaccines and immune globulins for persons with altered immunocompetence. *MMWR* 1993; 42(RR-4):1.
109. Committee on Pediatric AIDS. Evaluation and medical treatment of the HIV-exposed infant. *Pediatrics* 1997;99:909.
110. Stanley SK et al. Effect of immunization with a common recall antigen on viral expression in patients infected with human immunodeficiency virus type 1. *N Engl J Med* 1996;334:1222.
111. American Academy of Pediatrics Committee on Infectious Diseases. Recommended timing of routine measles immunizations for children who have recently received immune globulin preparations. *Pediatrics* 1994;93:682.

CHAPTER 96

Pediatric Infectious Diseases

Irving Steinberg

OVERVIEW

Infectious diseases account for the vast majority of annual visits to the pediatrician. Acute febrile illnesses, either viral or bacterial, occur in children on average six to eight times a year. For this reason, the management of pediatric infectious diseases remains a significant component of care.

Several host and microbial factors contribute to the relatively high incidence of infectious diseases in pediatric patients. Deficiencies in both cellular and humoral immunity have been described in the immediate newborn period as well as in the first several years of life. Concentrations of all the immunoglobulins (IgG, IgM, IgD, IgE, and IgA) are diminished at birth, particularly in the premature neonate. Although some IgG is transferred to the newborn from the mother via the placenta, this is generally a short-lived effect that dissipates during the first year of life. Deficits in complement and C-reactive protein (CRP) decrease opsonization, and the phagocytic and intracellular killing functions of neutrophils and macrophages are depressed. The microbial naivety of children also has a significant impact on their ability to fight infection. Potential pathogens are able to colonize and cause clinical infection more readily in newborns and infants because the full complement of normal flora bacteria has not been fully developed. Children begin acquiring their own immunity to organisms by becoming exposed to antigens, developing an immune response, and generating lasting memory immunity cells.

Children are increasingly exposed to potential pathogens at an earlier age, placing them at greater risk of infection. Societal and family reliance upon formal or informal child care arrangements is more prevalent often exceeding 20 to 30 hours per week of outside care in groupings of children larger than six.[4] As a result, more children are attending day care and school environments, where they are more likely to come in contact with an infected child or caregiver.[1]

The age of the child and the site of infection, implicate different potential pathogens; however, there is significant overlap. *Streptococcus pneumoniae, Moraxella catarrhalis,* and *Hemophilus influenzae* are the most common pathogens. Antimicrobial therapy in pediatric patients almost always includes an agent that is active against these organisms, especially when the organism is unknown. Many different viruses cause respiratory infections in children, but these are not cultured clinically because treatments are not readily available.

OTITIS MEDIA

Otitis media, an inflammation of the middle ear, is one of the most common childhood illnesses. Acute otitis often has been treated with an antibiotic, despite controversial evidence in support of the routine use of antibiotics for this condition.[2] About a decade ago, about half of all prescriptions written for children in the United States were for the treatment of otitis media; however, more recent data from the Centers for the Disease Control and Prevention note a 42% reduction in the number of ambulatory visits and antibiotic prescriptions for acute otitis media (AOM) in children younger than 2 years over a 7-year period.[3] These decreases probably can be attributed to increased immunizations with the seven-valent pneumocococcal conjugate vaccine and more appropriate use of antibiotics.

The middle ear is the anatomical location of the hearing apparatus. It is separated from the outer ear canal by the tympanic membrane (eardrum) and drains into the nasopharynx via the Eustachian tubes. The presence of a dull, red, bulging, tympanic membrane that shows no movement during insufflation (application of slight changes in air pressure in the ear canal) on otoscopic examination is diagnostic of AOM. Otitis media peaks between 6 months and 3 years of age and is thought to be most likely due to Eustachian tube obstruction and secondarily to the decreased immunocompetence present in young children. Eustachian tube dysfunction has been associated with upper respiratory tract infections (URIs) and allergies.[4–6] Some children may have three or four infections per year, whereas others suffer from continuous chronic otitis media for prolonged periods (>3 months). Viruses cause many otitis media infections alone or together with bacteria[7]; however, it is difficult to distinguish viral from bacterial etiology based solely on clinical presentation and otoscopic examination.

Clinical Presentation

1. T.T., a 20-month-old male, is seen in the urgent care clinic with a fever that began about a day and a half ago. He is pulling on his right earlobe, has purulent nasal drainage, and a moderately wet cough. His temperature currently is 101.2°F. He has had a runny nose and cough for 4 days and the daycare center director called to bring this to the attention of T.T.'s mother. He has had several episodes of wheezing over the last 5 months, which now is considered to be asthma by his pediatrician. He now uses a nebulizer (PulmoAide) at home when needed. As a result of this diagnosis, T.T.'s father has discontinued his smoking of cigars in the house. T.T.'s immunizations are up to date. According to his mother, T.T. had experienced one case of otitis media when he was 8 months old, which responded to amoxicillin; another one at 15 months of age after a bout of the flu; and has had two URIs. What is the relationship between T.T.s URI and a potential bacterial infection? Why should (or should not) he be treated with medications?

The need for restraint in managing URIs with medications in pediatric patients is increasingly advocated, especially because of recent scientific panel evaluations. Although cold symptom control medications (e.g., decongestants, antihistamines) have been widely used, the U.S. Food and Drug Administration (FDA) recommends avoidance of their usage in children younger than 6 years of age because of the potential for significant adverse effects (see Chapter 93). In addition, the treatment of URIs with antimicrobials should be individualized for specific situations and should be prescribed judiciously.

Avoidance of antibiotic management of viral URIs is critical in efforts to limit the clonal expansion and spread of antibacterial-resistant organisms. Parents (or guardians) often have expectations of antibiotic treatments when their child is brought to a clinician for evaluation, and clinicians often presume such expectations.[8] In videotaped encounters with 38 pediatricians, 64% of parents of children who were experiencing cold symptoms expected an antibiotic to be prescribed. In addition, 22% of the physicians perceived that the child's parents wanted antibiotics, resulting in more than a 32% increase in the likelihood of inappropriate prescribing. When information about bacterial resistance, antibiotic use, and nonantibiotic alternatives to treatment were offered by the physician, parental demands for antibiotic treatment from the physician were decreased. In contrast, perceived school or daycare pressures for antibiotic therapy increased parental demands for antimicrobial treatment from the physician. Low socioeconomic status of the parents also contributed to a greater likelihood of inappropriate prescribing.[9]

The relationship between antibiotic utilization and subsequent development of microbial resistance is complex; however, this relationship has been supported by large multinational data as well as by data from individual patient cohorts.[10] The temporal onset, and offset, of antibiotic-resistance selection pressure for *S. pneumoniae* and *H. influenzae* have been noted in cohorts of children exposed to β-lactam antibiotics.[11] Increases in the mean inhibitory concentrations (MICs) associated with enhancement of resistance mechanisms that are chromosomally mediated, or mediated via mobile-exchange elements (and temporally correlated to antibacterial usage) have been demonstrated for both of these pathogens. Clonal dissemination of resistant organisms is more likely in close contact or overcrowded environments (e.g., daycare centers, homes with multiple siblings). Although the diagnostic distinction between viral and bacterial URI can be difficult, clinicians, nevertheless, need to utilize appropriate diagnostic criteria to minimize the indiscriminant use of antibiotics.

Some success already has been achieved in reducing the burden of antibiotic use in pediatric patients in outpatient and emergency room settings.[12] More specifically, the use of antibiotics for URIs in emergency rooms decreased from 55% in 1993 to 35% in 2004,[13] and a greater percentage of decrease in antibiotic use was noted in patients who are white, from the southern states in the United States, or who were dwelling in nonurban areas.[14] Ongoing applied vigilance has been advocated and standards have been developed to minimize the misuse of antibiotics for viral URIs. In 2004, the National Committee for Quality Assurance initiated Health Plan Employer Data and Information Set (HEDIS) measures to be used as benchmarks for a variety of chronic and acute disease states, including appropriate testing and treatment of pharyngitis and URIs in children and adolescents. These newly instituted benchmarks are significant because individual states and large health plans use HEDIS measures to optimize diagnosis, treatment, and resource utilization, and as a component of pay-for-performance incentives. The need for HEDIS measures was supported by data that antibiotics were prescribed for 51.2% of office visits for URIs out of 69,936 Pennsylvania Medicaid recipients, and for 44.9% of the 20,213 children younger than 5 years.[13] Moreover, 77.3% of these patients received the antibiotic on the same day as the index URI. The URI diagnosis of acute bronchitis drove prescribing of antibiotics about threefold more than that for the common cold. Amoxicillin and advanced-generation macrolides were most often prescribed.

The concern for inappropriate use of antibiotics for viral URIs, however, is juxtaposed with the well-recognized relationship between viral infections, either concurrent with, or as a prelude to, bacterial infection. In an evaluation of 709 URI episodes over a 1-year period in 198 children 6 to 35 months of age, 35% of episodes were complicated by AOM. The adjusted odds ratio of AOM was 1.8, 2.2, and 1.9 for *S. pneumoniae*, *H. influenza*, and *M. catarrhalis* isolates, respectively, compared with no bacteria isolated at the time of the URI (after controlling for breast-feeding, daycare center attendance, and cigarette smoke exposure).[15] The odds ratio was 2.6 if two or more of these pathogens were found. Similarly, an AOM complication rate of 33% was noted in a longitudinal study that followed a cohort of families through a winter season using weekly pneumatic otoscopy.[7] In this latter study, intrafamilial transmission of coldlike illnesses was an associated risk factor.[9]

T.T. has had an URI for several days and has a clinical indication of an AOM with new onset of fever and ear pulling. This child's physical examination should be directed toward the proper middle ear examination, and possible initiation of antimicrobial therapy that depends on the nature of the otitis media.

Diagnostic Findings

2. Further examination, including pneumatic otoscopy, reveals bulging and red tympanic membranes in both ears (right greater than left). Upon injecting air, the child cries more intensely; the left tympanic membrane is somewhat mobile, but the right is not. T.T. is sent home with a provisional diagnosis of AOM. Antibiotics were not prescribed, and the patient's parent was instructed to observe the patient for the next 48-hours. What diagnostic findings of otitis media are evident in T.T.?

The diagnostic distinction between AOM and otitis media with effusion (OME) is one of the first steps in the determination of whether antibiotic use is appropriate. The judicious use of antibiotics in children initially was recommended by the American Academy of Pediatrics (AAP) in 1996, with an emphasis on reducing antibiotic use both for the treatment of OME and for the prophylaxis of recurrent otitis. AOM features rapid onset of acute illness (i.e., fever, irritability, otalgia) along with signs of middle ear inflammation and effusion. In contrast, OME features signs of middle ear inflammation and effusion in the absence of acute illness. T.T.'s fever, irritability, otalgia, and red, bulging tympanic membranes (Table 96-1) are consistent with a diagnosis of AOM.

Otoscopic findings of middle ear disease use the color, anatomical position and mobility of the tympanic membrane to establish the presence of AOM. Meta-analysis suggests that tympanic membrane findings of distinct redness (likelihood ratio [LR] = 8.4), bulging (LR = 51), and distinctly impaired mobility (LR = 31) are the most important diagnostic indicators of AOM.[8] In addition, criteria for the otologic diagnosis of AOM utilizing pneumatic otoscopy have been established (Table 96-1). Yet, despite these clinical and otoscopic hallmarks (similar to those reemphasized by the AAP and American Academy of Family Practitioners (AAFP) in their joint 2004 guidelines), the application of these diagnostic criteria in clinical trials has been inconsistent. Only 17 and 20 of 88 studies from 1994 through 2005 utilized all three AAP and Hoberman criteria (i.e., rapid onset, middle ear effusion, erythema, otalgia), respectively.[16] The prime concern is that lack of diagnostic stringency, in combination with a high spontaneous resolution rate, can contribute to the conclusion of a good cure rate, even though a relatively microbiologically ineffective antibiotic was used.[17] These factors create difficulty in evaluating and comparing antibiotics within and between therapeutic trials. Despite apparently large numbers of patients, the clinical trials using endpoints without culture evidence often lack sufficient statistical discriminating power. Studies in which tympanocentesis is used to screen patients with bacterial AOM, and trials where tympanocentesis is done on entry and at 3 to 5 days of antibiotic therapy (i.e., double tympanocentesis), require fewer patients to statistically discriminate between superior and inferior antibiotics.

Table 96-1 Diagnostic Criteria for Acute Otitis Media[16]

American Academy of Pediatrics and the American Academy of Family Practitioners (AP/AAFP) Subcommittee on Management of Acute Otitis Media
A diagnosis of AOM requires a history of recent, usually acute, onset of signs and symptoms of middle ear inflammation and effusion in the presence of either distinct erythema of the tympanic membrane or distinct otalgia (discomfort clearly referable to the ear that results in interference with, or precludes, normal activity or sleep). The presence of middle ear effusion can be present as bulging of the tympanic membrane, limited or absent mobility of the tympanic membrane, air–fluid level behind the tympanic membrane, or otorrhea.
Consensus Recommendations
A diagnosis of otitis media can be established if purulent otorrhea of <24 hours (not otitis externa), or if two of four tympanic membrane abnormalities (i.e., middle ear effusion) are present as: (a) Marked decrease or absent mobility; (b) Yellow/white discoloration; (c) Opacification (other than from scarring); (d) Air–fluid interfaces
WITH
One indicator of inflammation as: (a) New ear pain (± unaccustomed ear pulling); (b) Marked tympanic membrane redness; or (c) bulging tympanic membrane

Viral infection of the middle ear can occur in 30% to 40% of cases in the absence of bacteria, and cannot easily be discriminated from bacterial disease. Moreover, the spontaneous resolution rate for AOM is suggested to be high (somewhat organism dependent; lower with pneumococcus). Therefore, a concern for indiscriminant antibiotic prescribing is logical, as the number needed to treat to cure one case of AOM or to prevent complications is high.

Immediate versus Delayed Treatment

3. Why is the recommendation of a short period of observation for T.T. more appropriate (or less appropriate) than the initiation of antibiotics when the diagnosis already has been established?

The wait-and-see or safety-net prescription approach to treatment has been utilized in several respiratory tract infections. The underlying assumption of this strategy is based on the expectation that the likelihood of a spontaneous resolution of an infection is deemed to be highly likely. In these situations, an antibiotic prescription is issued, but the parent is instructed not to fill the prescription unless the respiratory infection persists or worsens over the ensuing 2 to 3 days. This practice has been applied to AOM with favorable acceptance by parents and clinicians, and about two-thirds of the time the prescription has not been filled.[18] This strategy, however, may not be applicable

Table 96-2 Nonqualifiers for Delayed Prescription for Acute Otitis Media

- Symptoms suggestive of AOM for >48 hours.
- Antibiotic therapy within past 7 days for any reason.
- Infant ≤6 months of age.
- Toxic-appearing child.
- Tympanic membrane perforation or impending perforation.
- Tympanostomy tubes.
- Hearing impairment.
- Chronic condition that may impede the child's immunity or ability to clear the infection.
- Another episode of AOM within the past 3 months.
- Coexisting bacterial infection.
- Family unable to access prompt medical follow-up if child deteriorates.
- The child's parent/guardian cannot gain an acceptable understanding of the protocol (according to the parent/guardian or the clinician).

to the majority of patients with otitis media. In a randomized study of 776 children who presented to an emergency room with AOM, 64% of the children were excluded from participating because of clinical or other discretionary reasons. The remaining children included for randomization were older (i.e., 3.2 vs. 2.3 years of age for the exclusions) and predominantly (84%) had unilateral disease, thereby, suggesting milder infection in a less vulnerable age group. The 38% of the wait-and-see group who eventually filled the antibiotic prescription at the parents' discretion had statistically longer periods of pain and fever, requiring more symptom-relieving medications, and experienced more episodes of vomiting.[18a] Therefore, although the delayed treatment strategy, with caregiver acceptance, can successfully reduce antibiotic use in children with AOM, care must be taken in appropriate patient selection, diagnosis, and follow-up. Criteria for the exclusion of children who could participate in a delayed treatment plan are listed in Table 96-2.

More precision in defining demographic and clinical predictors of patients with AOM who would most benefit from antibiotic therapy is a continuing focus of clinical studies. In recent studies, children younger than 2 years or those with bilateral disease generally experience longer periods of fever and pain, and generally do not experience spontaneous resolution of AOM if antibiotic therapy is delayed or not given. In one study of 824 untreated children with AOM, approximately 70% of children younger than 2 years with bilateral disease, and 60% of those with unilateral disease, would continue to experience ear pain and/or fever for 2 days after diagnosis. In comparison, only 40% of those older than 2 years with unilateral or bilateral disease, in this same study, would have these symptoms still present at 2 days.[18a] Given that children over than 2 years of age with AOM account for 60% of all visits to an emergency department, and because more than 50% of these patients are prescribed antibiotics,[19] these age-specific criteria and clinical findings help to identify patients who would benefit from prompt antibiotic treatment and those who would benefit from a strategy involving delayed treatment. The successful application of these criteria (i.e., age specificity, clinical findings) can help to reduce inappropriate antibiotic use and decrease the development of microbial resistance to antibiotics.

Laterality (i.e., unilateral or bilateral ear involvement) is an additional variable in the selection of patients to receive prompt treatment, rather than delayed treatment, because patients with bilateral ear involvement experience more severe disease.[20,21] Bilateral disease also correlates with younger age[21] and the presence of *H. influenzae* as the primary pathogen[20,21]; therefore, the selection of an antibiotic that is effective against this organism would be an important consideration for treating children younger than 2 years, and those with bilateral disease. In addition, otitis-prone children, children enrolled in a daycare facility, and children with more severe signs and symptoms are candidates for early antimicrobial therapy. In T.T.'s case, age, recurrent fever, bilateral middle ear inflammation, and 4 days of URI symptoms preclude watchful waiting, and prompt antibiotic therapy would have been more appropriate.

Risk Factors

4. What are risk factors for the development of AOM in T.T.?

T.T.'s gender puts him at greater risk for the development of otitis because infections of the middle ear occur with greater prevalence in boys.[22] His attendance in a daycare facility also is a risk factor because it subjects him to greater risk of viral and bacterial-communicable infections (e.g., AOM), and especially to the acquisition and dissemination of antibiotic-resistant organisms. T.T.'s atopy (asthma), can contribute to altered local immunity, especially in the handling of nontypeable *H. influenzae*. Another risk factor is that T.T., at 15 months of age, experienced a previous episode of AOM after a bout of influenza. The association of the flu with AOM does decrease subsequent to influenza vaccination in infants.[23] T.T.'s father has discontinued his cigar smoking in the house. Nevertheless, passive exposure to cigarettes has been related to increases in URIs, AOM, and OME in children. The use of a pacifier, being fed in a horizontal position or by bottle propping, or being breast-fed for fewer than 6 months are other risk factors for otitis; however, information about these details were not solicited during the taking of the medical history. Anatomical factors such as craniofacial malformation, adenoids, and horizontal Eustachian tube–middle ear disposition (infants and American Indian and Eskimo ethnicities) can increase risk. Winter or early spring season, siblings with URIs, household overcrowding, and exposure to pollutants are additional risk factors for AOM.[9] Recurrence has also been associated with recent antibiotic use (≤3 months), and this temporal relationship convenes added risk of reinfection or relapse with resistant pathogens. Lack of influenza and conjugate pneumococcal vaccine inoculations can be considered risk factors in light of the reductions of AOM incidence when the vaccinations are provided. In addition to clinical and demographic risk factors, genetic susceptibility via overrepresentation of polymorphisms in genes coding for proinflammatory cytokines (e.g., interleukin [IL]-6, IL-10, and tumor necrosis factor-α)[24,25] have been associated with an otitis-prone state, and may contribute to lower capsular-antibody response after antipneumococcal vaccination. In summary, T.T. has a number of risk factors for AOM (gender, age, attendance at daycare, asthma, history of AOM).

Pathogens

The majority of cases of AOM are caused by *S. pneumoniae*, *H. influenza*, and *M. catarrhalis*. Regional, seasonal, and clinical variances of the pathogen and its resistance pattern are recognized, but a priori determination of the organism without benefit of a tympanocentesis and culture is difficult. A proposed clinical scoring system based on severity of symptoms (temperature, irritability, ear tugging) and otoscopic signs (redness, bulging) can statistically differentiate tympanocentesis-proven bacterial AOM from culture-negative disease.[26] This clinical scoring system can associate the benefits of antibiotics in reducing severity scores, but it cannot identify the responsible bacterial pathogen. In a study of 929 tympanocentesis-proven cases of AOM caused by the three major pathogens, a higher percentage of children with high fever correlated with infection by *S. pneumoniae*; however, more than half of the patients did not experience any fever. There was no difference in other signs and symptoms within the three groups, except for the known relationship of the conjunctivitis–otitis syndrome and *H. influenzae*.[27]

5. T.T. returns to the pediatrician's office with a temperature of 103°F and severe conjunctival injection. He has continued to pull on his right ear and cries when trying to be put to sleep. What is the likely organism in addressing the empiric treatment T.T. should receive?

The likely organism for T.T. is *H. influenzae* for several reasons. As mentioned, bilateral disease has been associated with *H. influenzae* more than with the other pathogens,[20,21] and the conjunctivitis is indicative of AOM with *H. influenzae*. Additionally, because T.T. most likely already would have been immunized with all four doses of conjugate pneumococcal vaccine (Prevnar), infection with *H. influenzae* is more likely than with pneumococcus. Since the addition of the conjugate pneumococcal vaccine to the childhood immunization schedule, *H. influenzae* has been more commonly associated with AOM, with 57% of these middle ear isolates expressing β-lactamase.[28] Finally, the presence of asthma could loosely reflect the relationship of atopy and OME,[29] and that could, in turn, influence the development of persistent and recurrent bacterial AOM. *H. influenzae* was the most isolated pathogen in a large study of patients who underwent tympanostomy tube placement.[30] In other patients, recent treatment with amoxicillin could select for early relapse or reinfection with *H. influenzae*.[31]

Although *H. influenzae* is the most likely causative organism, the pathogen could still be pneumococcus, which likely would be amoxicillin resistant. Although the pneumococcal vaccine has reduced the prevalence of *S. pneumoniae*–associated AOM by a third, non–vaccine-susceptible serotypes of pneumococci have been observed to be increased in AOM. Serotype 19A in particular, which is not handled well by the conjugate pneumococcal vaccine, might become more prevalent in AOM, and the inherent penicillin resistance of this serotype can be troubling.[32] *M. catarrhalis*, which accounts for 5% to 20% of AOM episodes, is another pathogen that may not have been eradicated by prior treatment with amoxicillin because 90% to 100% of these isolates are β-lactamase producers. Fortunately, high spontaneous resolution rates are associated with *M. catarrhalis* AOM. Group A streptococci are less of a concern in T.T. because of the absence of concomitant sore throat symptoms. Nevertheless, group A streptococci are implicated in 3% to 5% of all AOM cases, and are associated with older age and a higher risk of mastoiditis.[33] Staphylococci can be the pathogenic organism in recurrent infections, and methicillin-resistant strains have been identified in recurrent and chronic infection, as well as in patients with otorrhea from tympanostomy tubes.[34] Additionally, trends toward greater isolation of staphylococcus in the postpneumococcal vaccine era have been associated with the development of mastoiditis and sinusitis.[35,36]

6. When would tympanocentesis have a role in establishing the microbiologic etiology of T.T.'s AOM?

Tympanocentesis can be useful, but seldom is indicated for first-time or infrequent middle ear infections. In the absence of an organism to be obtained in another way, direct access to the infected body fluid is important, particularly in the face of repeated or relapsing infection. Results from culture and sensitivity testing could be especially useful, for example, when a clinician is faced with the consideration of using an antibiotic such as clindamycin for highly penicillin-resistant pneumococcus (given its absence of coverage for *H. influenzae* and *M. catarrhalis*), or whether a macrolide might be more acceptable. Tympanocentesis would be more urgent in a young infant with otitis, particularly in the presence of concurrent signs of sepsis; other organisms (including enteric gram-negative rods) could be the otitis-producing pathogens. Tympanocentesis can be of benefit not only for diagnostic purposes, but also for the benefits associated with drainage of infected middle-ear fluid.

Treatment

Empiric Antibiotic Selection

7. What empiric antibiotic therapy should be initiated for T.T.? What are some of the selection/dosing issues involved in treatment selection?

As with other infectious diseases, therapy without the benefit of culture and sensitivity tests must be based on clinical and demographic variables that point the clinician toward the most likely pathogen(s). If *H. influenzae* is the organism in T.T.'s case for the reasons enumerated previously, then the choice of a β-lactamase–stable cephalosporin (e.g., cefpodoxime, cefdinir, cefuroxime) or a β-lactam/β-lactamase inhibitor combination (e.g., amoxicillin-clavulanate) are effective choices. In contrast, the AAP/AAFP empirically recommends high-dose amoxicillin if the patient has no fever and mild pain, and high-dose amoxicillin-clavulanate if high temperature ($\geq$39°C) or severe pain is present. Cephalosporins or macrolides are recommended by AAP/AAFP if penicillin hypersensitivity is present (non–type 1 and type 1, respectively). As discussed, fever and pain may not reliably indicate the pathogen, and high fever might be more reflective either of infection with *S. pneumoniae*[27] or from a coexisting viral infection. Therefore, more information on the patient's history of recent antibiotic usage and vaccination, additional clinical/demographic variables, as well as regional and patient-specific expectations for bacterial resistance must be assessed. Although regular or high-dose amoxicillin should be among the first choices for a first-time infection, modifying factors might encourage a broader range of choices if organisms other than *S. pneumoniae* are potentially involved because amoxicillin probably would

Table 96-3 Modifying Factors for Consideration of Alternatives to Amoxicillin in Treating Acute Otitis Media

	First Infection, No Modifying Factors	Modifying Factors Present (See Table 96-4)
First-line therapy	Amoxicillin (40–45 mg/kg/day) or high-dose amoxicillin (80–90 mg/kg/day) (**dose selection depends on patient experience and regional resistance prevalence)	High-dose amoxicillin (80–90 mg/kg/day); high-dose amoxicillin/clavulanate (80–90/6.4 mg/kg/day), cefuroxime, cefpodoxime, cefdinir
Treatment failure at day 3	High-dose amoxicillin-clavulanate, cefuroxime, cefpodoxime, cefdinir; ceftriaxone IM (if compliance problems or seriously ill)	Ceftriaxone IM, levofloxacin, clindamycin; (tympanocentesis for culture)
Treatment failure at day 10–28	High-dose amoxicillin/clavulanate, cefuroxime, cefpodoxime, cefdinir IM ceftriaxone, levofloxacin	High-dose amoxicillin/clavulanate, cefuroxime, cefpodoxime, cefdinir, IM ceftriaxone, levofloxacin; tympanocentesis for culture

not be effective against β-lactamase–producing pathogens.[37] The recommendations for alternatives to amoxicillin (Tables 96-3, 96-4, and 96-5) are consistent with the modified Centers for the Disease Control and Prevention guidelines for AOM treatment in 1999.[38] Ten days of antibiotic treatment is recommended for patients who are younger than 2, otitis prone, or in a daycare facility.

The specific antibiotic choice is affected by multiple variables (e.g., past history of antibiotic use by the patient; past patient history of success with antibiotics and consideration of microbial resistance; previous history of adherence to therapy; interactions of patient with multiple siblings or in a daycare facility). T.T. has previously been treated with antibiotics for two previous episodes of otitis, has been on prophylaxis, and has been successfully treated instead of selection of resistant strains. Although T.T. also had two more recent cases of URI (presuming that they were viral), they are spaced apart sufficiently in time for the label of recurrent or otitis prone not to apply. However, other factors (e.g., bilateral disease, conjunctivitis, conjugate pneumococcal vaccination) in the case suggest that T.T. may have β-lactamase producing pathogens or penicillin-nonsusceptible *S. pneumoniae* for which alternatives to amoxicillin should be sought.

The dosing regimens for the antibiotic treatment of AOM are based on the doses that have been associated with the most positive outcomes in clinical studies. For example, ceftriaxone has been evaluated in single-dose regimens; however, the three-dose regimen showed greater efficacy in young children with recurrent disease.[39] High-dose regimens of amoxicillin and amoxicillin-clavulanate are recommended to enhance efficacy against nonsusceptible strains of *S. pneumoniae.* In another example, once-daily dosing of cefdinir 14 mg/kg/day was associated with 80% middle-ear fluid eradication of pneumococcus and statistically better clinical resolution in children younger than 2 years versus 55% for the twice-daily dosing regimen.[40] Similarly, twice daily dosing of cefdinir was less effective in a comparison with high-dose amoxicillin-clavulanate in a subgroup of patients younger than 2 years, but equivalent in older patients.[41] A non–FDA-approved dose of cefdinir 25 mg/kg once daily in patients with recurrent AOM eradicated less susceptible middle ear pathogens in North and Central American children. The magnitude of the dose in the presence of bacterial infection might have assisted the penetration of the

Table 96-4 Modifying Factors and Useful Antibiotics

Modifying Factors	Useful Antibiotics When Modifying Factors Present
• Daycare center attendance • Recent antibiotic use (within 30–60 days) • Resistance suspected/documented • Bilateral disease • Conjunctivitis-otitis syndrome • Recurrent AOM/otitis prone • Past/current amoxicillin failure • AOM in patient with chronic OME • TM perforation/tympanostomy tubes • Immunosuppression • Infant <6 months old	Cefpodoxime 10 mg/kg/day PO BID Cefdinir 14 mg/kg/day QD Cefuroxime 30 mg/kg/day PO BID Amoxicillin/clavulanate 90/6.4 mg/kg/day PO BID Ceftriaxone 50 mg/kg/dose IM ×3 days Levofloxacin 10 mg/kg/day PO BID (not FDA-approved for AOM)[180] Clindamycin 30 mg/kg/day PO TID (lacks activity against *H. influenzae* and *M. catarrhalis*)

AOM, acute otitis media; BID, twice a day; IM, intramuscularly; OME, otitis media with effusion; PO, orally; QD, daily; TID, three times a day; TM, tympanic membrane. Adapted from reference 180.

Table 96-5 Drugs With Less Reliability in the Management of Acute Otitis Media

- Cefixime and Ceftibuten: Good for once daily dosing against β-lactamase–producing *H. influenzae* and *M. catarrhalis*, but low activity against nonsusceptible *S. pneumoniae*
- Loracarbef and Cefaclor: Achieves high concentrations in the middle ear, but MICs prohibitively high; substantial failure data, serum sickness-like syndrome.
- Cefprozil: High *H. influenzae* MICs compared to other second- and third-generation cephalosporins.[176]
- Trimethoprim-Sulfamethoxazole: BID dosing and inexpensive, but high resistance rates for susceptibility *S. pneumoniae*, *H. influenzae*, GABHS; lacks clinical success in culture-positive AOM.[177]
- Azithromycin: Intracellular drug disposition for mostly extracellular bugs, failures in younger children; unacceptably poor eradication of *H. influenzae* and nonsusceptible *S. pneumoniae*[178]; may be useful when coexistent atypical pneumonia (clarithromycin likely better for AOM). However, good activity on biofilm-producing organisms in chronic/recurrent otitis.[179]

AOM, acute otitis media; BID, twice a day; GABHS, group A β-hemolytic streptococcus; MIC, minimum inhibitory concentration.

β-lactams,[42] and could have disproportionately increased middle ear fluid levels than lower doses.[43] Additionally, middle ear fluid half-lives for β-lactams are more prolonged than serum half-life in pharmacokinetic studies using the of chinchilla model of otitis.[44]

The adverse effect profiles of antibiotics also must be considered in the choice of an antibiotic for treatment of AOM. High-dose amoxicillin-clavulanate has not caused more diarrhea than a more modest dose, but it is associated with more diarrhea than with most cephalosporins.[41] Products containing probiotics (e.g., lactobacillus, saccharomyces) can lessen antibiotic-associated diarrhea.[45] The pain from ceftriaxone intramuscular injections can be lessened with lidocaine, but large doses might need to be divided and injected into more than one anatomical site in older or larger-sized patients. Clindamycin has not been formally evaluated in the management of AOM, is poor tasting, and has a greater potential for inducing antibiotic-associated diarrhea than other antibiotics. Poor taste also reduces the ease of use of cefuroxime and cefpodoxime in comparison with cefdinir.

Failed Treatment Sequelae

Failed or inadequately treated otitis can result in hearing impairment and subsequent learning difficulties,[22] or possibly more serious sequelae (e.g., mastoiditis, labyrinthitis, ossicle sclerosis, sinus thrombosis, meningitis, brain abscess). Mastoiditis can present with postauricular swelling and protrusion of the pinna with redness over the mastoid prominence. Extension of disease results in opacification and coalescence of the mastoid air cells and subperiosteal abscess. *S. pneumoniae*, *S. aureus,* and *P. aeruginosa* are the common pathogens in cases of acute mastoiditis, whereas *P. aeruginosa* is the primary pathogen in cases of chronic mastoiditis (≥3 weeks of symptoms).[35] Pediatric mastoiditis in the pneumococcal conjugate vaccine era has not changed from the prevaccination period, but ceftriaxone nonsusceptibility significantly increased from 7% to 30% (all but one isolate being highly resistant).[35] Although methicillin-resistant *Staphylococcus aureus* (MRSA) was not frequently isolated, vancomycin, clindamycin, or linezolid might be needed to treat some cases of acute mastoiditis. Intravenous antibiotics should be sufficient for treatment of milder cases of acute mastoiditis; however, they might need to be supplemented with tympanostomy tube insertions, abscess drainage, and mastoidectomy for progressively severe mastoiditis.[46]

OME can develop in 40% of the cases of AOM at 1 month after appropriate treatment, 20% by 2 months, and 10% by 3 months. Patients with continued otitis for longer than 3 months are deemed to have chronic OME. A 10-day trial of a β-lactamase–resistant antibiotic and prednisone 1 mg/kg/day can be helpful in the treatment of chronic OME, and might be sufficient to delay or avoid the need for tympanostomy tube insertion.

Preventive Treatment

When three distinct AOM episodes occur within 6 months (or four within 1 year), prophylactic treatment with sulfisoxazole (50 mg/kg/day) might be effective. Influenza vaccine can prevent the development of AOM cases subsequent to an episode of influenza, and oseltamivir treatment of influenza also can reduce secondary AOM.[47] Adherence to pediatric immunization schedules (see Chapter 95) is essential in minimizing the potential of chronic OME and minimizing other risk factors (see Question 4) also can be useful. Oral xylitol solution has had some benefit in trials. If the patient has tympanostomy tubes already inserted and if these tubes appear to have increased purulent drainage, antibiotic eardrops (e.g., ciprofloxacin/hydrocortisone 3 drops BID or ofloxacin 5 drops BID) can be initiated.

PHARYNGITIS AND GROUP A β-HEMOLYTIC STREPTOCOCCAL IN FECTION

Standard of Practice

In an effort to limit the overuse of antibiotics within health care organizations, HEDIS measures were developed to assess children 2 to 18 years of age who received an antibiotic prescription for the management of pharyngitis and who also were tested for group A β-hemolytic streptococcus (GABHS). Although the probability of bacterial infection only is about 15% to 36% in children seen as outpatients for a sore throat, the antibacterial prescription rates in the United States varied from 47% to 54% from 1998 to 2003.[48] Testing to identify a bacterial cause for pharyngitis was performed in 57%, with a higher percentage of testing in private plans as compared to Medicaid plans. These numbers are similar to the 43% antibiotic prescription rate among more than 125,000 pharyngitis visits from five health plans, where 75% of children underwent testing.[49] The national HEDIS data for 2006 was 70.7% appropriate diagnostic testing and antibiotic prescribing for pharyngitis.

Practice perspective contributes to the misuse of antibiotics for pharyngitis. Of 948 family medicine and pediatric practitioners responding to a survey, 401 (42%) would initiate antibiotics before knowing the results of diagnostic tests and continue them despite negative results. About 27% of practitioners prescribed antibiotics in this manner often or almost always. Family practice physicians were significantly more likely than pediatricians to initiate antibiotics before learning the test results (76% vs. 57%; $p < .01$), less likely than pediatricians to perform in-office throat cultures (13% vs. 32%; $p < .01$), and more likely than pediatricians to admit that parent expectations might have an effect on their decision to provide antimicrobial treatment (90% vs. 58%; $p < .01$). Overall, the stated reasons for prescribing antibiotics were to prevent acute rheumatic fever (95%), prevent local suppurative complications (71%), shorten clinical course (70%), decrease contagiousness (70%), and prevent acute glomerulonephritis (57%).[50] The incidence of acute rheumatic fever, poststreptococcal glomerulonephritis and other nonsuppurative complications actually have been decreasing in children in the United States, whereas suppurative complications (e.g., retropharyngeal abscess) have increased.[51,52]

Throat culture is the standard for determining the presence of GABHS pharyngitis, as many other viral and bacterial etiologies exist for pharyngitis. Nevertheless, the rapid-antigen-determination test (RADT) is commonly used within office, urgent care, and emergency room practice in determining the need for antibiotics. These RADT have acceptable although not high sensitivity (70%–90%).[53,54] However, 6.8% (range, 3.5%–9.8%) of patients with negative RADT have a positive throat culture for GABHS; therefore, culture confirmation has been advocated.[54]

Testing and Initial Treatment

8. M.G., a 14-year-old female, comes to the urgent care center complaining of fatigue, a sore throat, and tender cervical adenopathy for the past 2 days. She reports that she had been studying with two classmates who had complained of similar symptoms. On physical examination, her temperature is 101°F and her other vital signs are normal. Her pharynx is beefy red, with petechiae on the palate and pus on the tonsils. She denies sexual activity or tampon use. She has been self-administering ibuprofen every 6 hours for pain relief for the past 2 days. What testing should be undertaken for this patient?

This sore throat case scenario describing M.G. is often met with an unnecessary antibiotic prescription. She could be treated with antibiotics justifiably in the following four situations: (a) Initiate an antibiotic if the RADT is positive. If the RADT is negative, obtain a throat culture and start antibiotics, but discontinue the antibiotic if the culture is negative. (b) As in the first situation, initiate an antibiotic if the RADT is positive. If the RADT is negative, obtain a throat culture and, unlike the first situation, start antibiotics only if culture is positive. (c) Initiate an antibiotic without undertaking a RADT, but obtain a throat culture and discontinue the antibiotic if the culture result is negative. (d) Initiate an antibiotic only if a throat culture is positive. Although these guidelines are well-supported in the literature, only two-thirds of physician respondents agreed with these management options; 36% of family practitioners would start and continue antibiotics either without testing or regardless of the test results.[50] Appropriate clinical and diagnostic assessment is crucial to appropriate antibiotic use in pharyngitis.

Adolescents, who had recent close physical contact with individuals with pharyngitis, also should be tested with a monospot for infectious mononucleosis (an Epstein-Barr virus infection) because the latter can present with similar symptoms (fever, exudative pharyngitis, lymphadenopathy). A culture for *N. gonorrhoeae* also might be considered for M.G.; however, it would be unnecessary because other hallmarks of gonococcal disease (e.g., tenosynovitis, vulvovaginitis, sexual history) are absent.

9. On the assumption that M.G. had been tested appropriately and an antibiotic should be initiated, what would be a reasonable treatment initiative?

Because GABHS resistance to penicillin is minimal, a 10-day course of penicillin or ampicillin is the option of choice. A 5-day course of therapy with a β-lactamase stable cephalosporin is equally effective, possibly superior, and supported by studies and meta-analyses.[55] M.G. does not have a history of a penicillin allergy; however, patients with a non–type 1 penicillin allergy can be treated with a cephalosporin (e.g., cephalexin). A macrolide should be prescribed if a type 1 allergy exists. The dosing regimen for azithromycin in children with streptococcal pharyngitis is different than for other indications. The azithromycin should be dosed at 12 mg/kg PO once daily for 5 days for a total course of 60 mg/kg, based on a meta-analysis that supports the superiority of this regimen over a 3-day course of 10 mg/kg/day.[56]

Recurrent and Systemic Group A β-Hemolytic Streptococcus Infection

10. M.G. completes a 10-day course of ampicillin after testing positive for GABHS, and returns to her usual state of good health for several weeks. About 4 days ago, she again developed a sore throat, fever, nonproductive cough, and rhinorrhea. Two days ago, she felt dizzy when she walked, and her symptoms worsened the next day. She developed left upper quadrant, sharp abdominal and epigastric pain, especially prominent at the lower left costal margin, which she rated as an 8 (on a 10-point scale) and worse with inspiration and movement. Her temperature is 103.8°F, and she is unable to swallow liquids. She has no neck stiffness, headache, or dysuria, but feels dizzy. On presentation to the pediatric ED, she had a heart rate of 124 beats/minute; blood pressure of 90/50 mm Hg, and respiratory rate of 38 breaths/minute. Her O_2 saturation was 93%. Her breath excursions are asymmetric and she splints her inspirations on the left. On auscultation, she has egophony at the left lower base, and occasional crackles on the right. She has a sandpaperlike rash on her anterior neck, chest, and arms, but no areas of cellulitis or abscess. Her white blood cell (WBC) count is 4,700/mm^3 with, 88% polymorphonuclear neutrophilic leukocytes, and >50% band forms. Her CRP is 32.5 mg/dL, blood urea nitrogen is 14 mg/dL, creatinine 0.8 mg/dL. Her antistreptolysin-O titer is mildly elevated. Coagulation parameters were within normal limits, except for a slightly elevated fibrinogen level. Her weight is 49.5 kg. She had a lactate level of 4.5 mmol/L. She received normal saline boluses of 20 mL/kg × 3, and her blood pressure increased to 110/66 mm Hg, and her heart rate decreased to 96 beats/minute. Treatment with pressor drugs were not begun. Her urine is nitrite and leukocyte negative, blood culture is pending. Her chest x-ray (anteroposterior and lateral view) shows a left lower lobe consolidation and a large pleural effusion. Her brother had strep throat after M.G. finished her initial treatment. The throat culture is positive for a pathogen. Why could this be a recurrence of GABHS infection?

M.G. presents now with a clinical picture consistent with toxic shock syndrome. Although many organisms can cause systemic inflammatory response syndrome, which then can progress to septic shock, the slow onset of M.G.'s symptoms is more suggestive of infection with a gram-positive organism. The nonpetechial rash and presence of a pleural effusion make meningococcus less likely. The elevated antistreptolysin O titer is suggestive of recent infection and will peak in another 2 to 3 weeks.[51] The high CRP level supports the presence of an encapsulated organism and potential for producing a superantigen response. The superantigens activate large populations of T cells without the typical antigen presentation through histocompatibility complex molecules. This leads to a massive overproduction of proinflammatory cytokines (e.g., tumor necrosis factor, IL-6) producing the systemic inflammatory response syndrome (vasodilatation, capillary leak, and hypoperfusion).[57] The hemodynamic abnormalities and lactate level in M.G. also is compatible with systemic inflammatory response syndrome. Although no history is provided regarding a recent varicella infection in M.G., varicella is a recognized risk for invasive GABHS infection. A relationship between nonsteroidal anti-inflammatory use and invasive GABHS infection has some weak epidemiologic support[57]; however, support is somewhat stronger for non-necrotizing invasive disease in patients taking ibuprofen combined with acetaminophen.[57–59]

Pneumococcus is certainly a consideration for M.G., particularly given the greater number of cases of empyema in children despite the routine use of 7-valent conjugate-pneumococcal vaccine, which does not protect against serotypes 1, 3, and 19A. The likelihood of bacteremia and dissemination with this organism shortly after a full course of ampicillin is unlikely, but infection with a penicillin-resistant strain of *S. pneumoniae* is a possibility.[60] Staphylococcal toxic shock is possible, but absence of tampon use, influenza, recent surgery, and premorbid cutaneous lesions or burns reduce the likelihood of infection with this pathogen. More common in children is streptococcal toxic shock syndrome (STSS) and invasive GABHS infection, which can be associated with necrotizing fasciitis, myositis, and septic arthritis, but mostly with infections of sterile sites, including the lung and pleural space. The described rash is very consistent with STSS and production of pyrogenic exotoxins from M1 and M3 strains of GABHS,[61] as is the presence of a large pleural effusion. These strains are also common in asymptomatic carriers of *Streptococcus pyogenes*. Genetically low levels of protective antibodies to the M proteins and family of superantigens places the patient at risk for STSS, and a variety of other invasive disease manifestation (including the more benign scarlet fever).[61] M.G.'s low WBC and profound left shift indicate peripheral consumption of neutrophils, most likely from chemotaxis, sequestration, and destruction within the pleural empyema.

11. What additional empiric treatment should be initiated in M.G.?

Ampicillin can eradicate *S. pyogenes* pharyngitis, but failures do occur on a number of pharmacologic grounds. The carrier state and spread from close contacts may cause for repeated cases. Importantly, other pathogens and commensals in the nasopharynx have a protective/enhancing effect on local GABHS, and ampicillin/penicillin may select for these. Among 548 cases of GABHS tonsillophayngitis, β-lactamase producing organisms (e.g., *H. influenzae*, *M. catarrhalis*, *S. aureus)* were cocultured in 39%, 22%, and 17% cases, respectively. These pathogens, therefore, can inactivate the penicillins in situ and cause clinical failures. This is reflected in the widening efficacy differences observed between cephalosporins and penicillin over a 30-year period,[62] and in the greater number of symptomatic relapses seen in patients treated for GABHS pharyngitis with penicillin and amoxicillin compared with treatment with β-lactamase stable cephalosporins and amoxicillin-clavulanate.[63] Additionally, under the concept of bacterial interference, penicillins eradicate commensal α-hemolytic streptococci, which are natural competitors of GABHS occupancy in the mucosa; cephalosporins spare this organism. This contributes to increased GABHS carriage in patients treated with penicillin. Differences in cultures of protective α-hemolytic streptococcus, β-lactamase producing penicillin-inactivating copathogens and GABHS from tissue obtained at the time of tonsillectomy in patients pretreated with cefdinir or penicillin have been demonstrated.[64] Cephalosporins have also been more effective in prophylaxis of intrafamilial transmission of GABHS.[65] Therefore, oral cefuroxime or cefdinir should be considered if relapse or past failure to eradicate occurs (particularly if copathogens are isolated), or if a higher rate of microbiologic failures and clinical relapses are recognized within a family or local community.[66]

Beside the fluid boluses for hemodynamic support for M.G., with the necessary monitoring for response for further intervention, antibiotic management must be promptly begun. With concerns for pneumococcus, staphylococcus, and GABHS infection, cell wall active agents and protein synthesis agents are needed. Although penicillins, cephalosporins, and vancomycin can be used depending on the risk assessed for penicillin-resistant *S. pneumoniae* and MRSA, use of protein-synthesis inhibitors is critical for the treatment of invasive GABHS infection. Clindamycin, a ribosome-bound agent, can decrease exotoxin, superantigen, and cytokine production, and, thereby, the clinical effects of toxic shock syndrome, while eliminating this pathogen. Clindamycin added to a β-lactam enhances the clinical outcome of invasive *S. pyogenes*.[67] Therefore, IV clindamycin (40 mg/kg/day divided into three to four doses) should be added to empiric coverage with a cephalosporin effective against GABHS, nonsusceptible *S. pneumoniae*, and β-lactamase–producing pathogens (e.g., cefotaxime at 200 mg/kg/day divided into four doses). Clindamycin will additionally cover community-acquired MRSA if this pathogen is considered as an etiology for the pleural effusion, and cover cephalosporin-resistant *S. pneumoniae*. Vancomycin (40–60 mg/kg/day divided into three to four doses) alternatively can be used to cover MRSA, resistant pneumococcus, and GABHS. Vancomycin, however, is a cell wall active agent and will not confer protection against GABHS toxin production, and may act like a β-lactam in disseminating preformed toxin. Intravenous immunoglobulin is often added to bind circulating exotoxin and superantigens, and has improved clinical outcomes,[57] although different brands have varying efficacy in these neutralizing properties.[68]

Pleural Empyema

12. Three days after admission to the pediatric intensive care unit, M.G.s throat culture grew *S. pyogenes*. Vancomycin, clindamycin, and cefotaxime were started upon her admission to the pediatric intensive care unit. The rash is fading, but pleuritic chest pain remains, and the patient is placed on patient-controlled analgesia with morphine. The lactate level is now normal, but the CRP is still 30.5 mg/dL. Thoracentesis of the pleural effusion yields 300 mL of exudate, which shows gram-positive cocci, but the culture is negative. The fluid reaccumulated after 24 hours, but the patient is breathing more comfortably, and she is weaned to room air with O_2 saturation remaining above 95%. Her CRP is still 27 the next day, and her temperature remains at 101.8°F. What further interventions in M.G.'s care should be implemented?

The throat culture, the pleural fluid Gram stain, and clinical course denote the most likely pathologic entity is STSS, with recurrence of GABHS from an earlier pharyngitis or familial reacquisition. The vancomycin can be discontinued, but treatment should continue with both the clindamycin and the cefotaxime. The sustained CRP elevation is concerning, and the reaccumulated pleural fluid remains a pyrogenic source, although the pleural fluid culture being negative in the face of a positive Gram's stain may represent dead organisms. Pleural fluid often reaccumulates after thoracentesis.[69] Ultrasound or computed tomography can help to determine whether the loculated areas of pus exist that must be drained. Thick pleural fluid and loculation in the presence of unremitting fever, pain, and respiratory difficulty may require surgical decortication of the pleura.[69] More conservative management can be attempted with placement of a chest tube, with injection into the pleural space of tissue plasminogen activator (2 mg in 20 mL normal saline) if drainage is inadequate. Antibacterials should be continued for 2 to 4 weeks depending on M.G.s clinical progress and whether surgical intervention is employed. Management with early decortication for pediatric empyema has been advocated for more rapid and definitive resolution, and shortening of length of stay (LOS) and overall cost of care.[70] Monitoring lung function recovery for M.G. to rule out restrictive disease should be long-term.

CROUP

Clinical Presentation

13. Y.M., a 3-year-old male who attends daycare, developed a cold at the end of the school week. According to his mother, his cold was accompanied by coughing and post-tussive emesis of whitish, thick phlegm. Overnight on Saturday, his cough, which had become harsher through the day, now sounded like a seal, and he continued to have emesis in an attempt to clear his airway. He did not turn blue, but his mother became concerned when he became inconsolable and seemed not to be able to catch his breath. When brought to the emergency department at his local hospital, he was not toxic appearing, but had audible inspiratory stridor and a barking cough. His temperature was 104°F, his respiratory rate was 38 breaths/minute and shallow, his heart rate was 142 beats/minute. He exhibited perioral cyanosis, retractions, and seemed tired and somewhat listless. His oxygen saturation was 97%. He was placed on 30% oxygen by mask with nebulized medication, and was able to take sips of fluid after his respirations became deeper and slower, although he still had stridor and harsh coughing. Direct fluorescence antibody test for influenza was negative. Why is this clinical picture consistent with croup?

Croup, or acute laryngotracheitis, is a viral upper airway infection that can affect the structures that the anatomical name suggests. It has an annual prevalence of about 3% and occurs predominantly between 6 months and 3 years of age, primarily during the cold weather months.[71] Males have 1.5 times the prevalence over females. Symptoms include hoarseness, barking cough and a high-pitched audible inspiratory stridor, that are caused by subglottic inflammation, edema, and narrowing. In-drawing of the chest wall and respiratory muscle retractions can be seen. Greater work of breathing from increased inspiratory airway resistance coupled with lower lung volumes generated for the effort made creates perceived air hunger.[72] The rapid respiratory rate and increased intrathoracic pressure attempt to maintain the necessary minute inspiratory volume, but with steadily increasing fatigue of the child and potentially altered sensorium. Parainfluenza virus and respiratory syncytial virus (RSV) are the usual viral etiologic agents, but rhinovirus, adenovirus, and mycoplasma can also cause croup; influenza can cause the most severity.[71] High fever, toxic appearance, and concurrent bronchitis are more indicative of secondary bacterial tracheitis (e.g., *S. aureus*, streptococci), and often requires intensive care admission.[73] Spasmodic croup is distinguished from acute laryngotracheitis by the suddenness of onset, but with noninflammatory subglottic edema and the lack of fever and coryza; this can occur more in atopic children. Recurrent croup also can have some of the components of allergy or gastroesophageal reflux.[74]

About 85% of croup cases in the emergency department are mild.[75] A validated croup scoring system based on the degree of stridor, intercostal respiratory muscle retractions, air entry, level of consciousness, and cyanosis in room air, has been used in clinical studies of severity and response to therapy, but seldom is utilized in routine clinical practice.[71] Anteroposterior view on x-ray of the neck shows a steeple sign with the column of air narrowing proximally.

Initial Treatment

Bronchodilators

The great majority of cases of croup are managed at home (<5% need hospitalization). Caregivers generally are instructed to provide warm ambient humidification, despite the absence of sound evidence as to its efficacy, with the hope of a possible marginal benefit from a rather risk-free intervention.[76] Enhanced humidification might serve to relax the child and, thereby, lessen the risk of respiratory muscle fatigue. Mucolytics have essentially no role and the ability to administer aerosolized bronchodilators in a home situation to a child with upper airway inflammation and stridor is difficult and might delay more beneficial therapy. In moderate to severe disease, the patient should be administered nebulized racemic epinephrine 2.25% (0.25–0.5 mL diluted with normal saline to a 3 mL volume), which decreases capillary hydrostatic pressure via precapillary arteriolar vasoconstriction leading to diminished laryngeal edema.[71,75] The β-agonist effect can relax bronchial smooth muscle, but this is secondary to the larger airway effects. Doses of racemic epinephrine can be repeated every 2 to 3 hours if needed. L-Epinephrine (1:1,000 diluted in 5 mL of saline) can alternatively be used, and repeated doses can diminish the potential need for intubation.[77]

Corticosteroids

Because edema and inflammation are the main pathophysiological factors in the development of symptoms of croup, corticosteroids have long been utilized in the management of moderate-to-severe disease. In addition, meta-analysis of clinical trials has supported the benefit of steroids in croup.[78] Corticosteroids also have been used increasingly for the treatment of mild croup. Even a single oral dose of dexamethasone 0.6 mg/kg can significantly hasten symptom resolution, and reduce sleep disturbance, parental stress, and revisits for medical care.[79] Smaller oral doses have also been very successful, and intramuscular administration has been especially useful for use in children with emesis.[80,81] Prednisone 1 mg/kg can be used with similar effect,[82] but the longer half-life and greater potency of dexamethasone may be advantageous. Although budesonide in 2 to 4 mg doses can be administered via nebulizer, it is doubtful whether it provides additive effects to the systemic dexamethasone.[83] Budesonide also can be nebulized together with epinephrine for severe cases. Repeated doses of steroids are not advocated because of the risk of bacterial and fungal complications.[71] Influenza vaccination should help to prevent the most severe cases of croup. If testing for influenza is positive in the presence of severe croup, neuraminidase inhibitors should be considered along with the above specified treatments. The patient should be observed and monitored for 2 to 4 hours, and hospitalization should be considered if the steroids and repeated epinephrine doses are not resolving stridor at rest or chest wall in-drawing. Secondary bacterial infection and empiric antibiotic therapy with vancomycin and cefotaxime should be considered at that point.

14. What pharmacologic treatment should be initiated for Y.M.?

This child should be treated with a single oral dose of dexamethasone of 0.6 mg/kg (presuming oral tolerance continues after being able to take small volumes of liquid), and supported with oxygen by mask. The treating clinician can administer an additional dose of racemic epinephrine for the continued stridor, but consideration should be given to not administering additional doses if the normal oxygen saturation is maintained because the already rapid heart rate is likely to increase more with continued catecholamine use. The dose of racemic epinephrine should be repeated if the stridor or oxygen saturation worsens (or cannot be maintained once off oxygen), or if the response to the dose of dexamethasone is lacking after four hours of monitoring. Acetaminophen (15 mg/kg) should be given for fever and any intercostal or upper airway pain due to the vigorous cough.

BRONCHIOLITIS

Etiology

Bronchiolitis is a common illness of the small airways (bronchioles) caused by an infection, usually from a virus, resulting in inflammation of the bronchioles and subsequent mucus production. It is the most common lower respiratory tract infection in infants, and is the top primary diagnosis among hospitalized infants younger than 1 year.[84] It most commonly occurs in the winter months and usually is caused by RSV, which can be isolated in 75% of children younger than 2 years who are hospitalized with this airway disease.[85] Rhinoviruses have also been implicated.[86] It is estimated that 22.8 per 1,000 emergency department visits by children during RSV season can be attributable to bronchiolitis. Reinfections within or during subsequent seasons are not unusual given the lack of lasting immunity and the high communicability of this infection. As with other respiratory viruses, dissemination of this infection is through aerosolization and touch. Hand washing is mandatory for caregivers to minimize the spread of this disease. Specific genetic susceptibility may also play because four single-nucleotide polymorphisms in innate immune genes are strongly associated with RSV bronchiolitis susceptibility.[87]

The infection causes edema, inflammation, mucus production, necrosis, and cell sloughing within small airway epithelium, resulting in bronchospasm. Infants younger than 6 months are at highest risk of hospitalization, which occurs in 0.5% to 2.0% of all RSV infections. Premature neonates, infants with chronic lung disease, and children with congenital heart disease and heart failure are at added risk for morbidity and mortality from bronchiolitis.[88] Hypoxia can develop from ventilation/perfusion mismatching. Gas exchange is further compromised by the mucus plugging, airway obstruction, and subsequent air trapping distal to the narrow airways.

Clinical Presentation

15. M.V., a 3-month-old male born at 31 weeks of gestation, is admitted for poor feeding and respiratory distress. M.V.'s mother relates that the infant had been fussy for the past 2 days, had a runny nose, and was stopping feeds prematurely and tiring. His respirations had gone from panting to grunting over the last 12 hours, and he was turning blue around the mouth. His temperature was 101°F, with a respiratory rate of 82 breaths/minute and a heart rate of 180 beats/minute. On physical examination, nasal congestion was seen in one nare and he had crackles and occasional wheezing bilaterally on chest auscultation. His tympanic membranes are clear. His oxygen saturation was 88% on the pulse oximeter and his venous blood gas showed a pH of 7.35, P_{CO_2} of 56 mm Hg, and a P_{O_2} of 50 mm Hg. He received a dose of nebulized albuterol and more wheezing was heard bilaterally. Continuous albuterol was applied, but the oxygen saturation went only to 90%. M.V. has a WBC of 8,700/mm^3, with 42% neutrophils (<10% band forms), 50% lymphocytes, 6% monocytes, and 2% eosinophils; few atypical lymphocytes were seen on the smear. His CRP was 1.3 mg/dL. A chest x-ray was obtained and a diagnosis of bronchiolitis was made. The patient was transferred to the pediatric intensive care unit for close monitoring.

M.V.'s coryza and rhinorrhea are common clinical findings, and can occur with or without fever. Normal respiratory rates are age dependent; M.V.'s high respiratory rate is within the expected range for young infants with bronchiolitis (can exceed 70–90 breaths/minute), and his respirations that sound like panting is common with this illness. His difficulties with feeding and sleeping result from the rapid respiratory rate that is required for adequate minute ventilation. At this point, sedating medications must be avoided because these can slow the respiratory rate and potentially compromise his minute ventilation. As his condition worsens, his respirations progressed from panting to grunting because he closes his glottis against exhaling pressure as a means of keeping his alveoli open for gas exchange, a process known as "auto–peak end-expiratory pressure." Nasal congestion is important to identify and treat because young infants tend to be obligate nose breathers, and nasal obstruction can cause respiratory impairment. Wheezing, nasal flaring, increased intercostal muscle retractions, and cyanosis can result if treatment is not promptly instituted or if treatment fails. When apnea is present, immediate attention is paramount, and increases the need for mechanical ventilation, especially in infants younger than 8 weeks old and in premature infants. Pulse oximetry should be used to assess the degree of oxygen saturation. Blood gases also should be obtained to monitor oxygen content for deteriorating or mechanically ventilated patients. Both the low oxygen saturation and elevated P_{CO_2} reflect M.V.'s significant respiratory distress. Peribronchiolar infiltration of lymphocytes can be appreciated on the chest x-ray as peribronchial cuffing. Lobar atelectasis can occur due to the cell sloughing, and hyperinflation on the chest x-ray results from air trapping. WBC count and CRP are most often normal,[89] as they are in M.V., and bacterial cultures generally can be avoided because the development of concurrent bacterial infection is very low in bronchiolitis.[90] Nevertheless, bacterial colonization of endotracheal tube aspirates is common in ventilated patients.[91]

Laboratory Testing

16. What testing should be done on M.V. to identify the causative agent?

Rapid RSV-antigen testing using direct immunofluorescent antibody staining or enzyme-linked immunosorbent assay of a nasal aspirate or wash, or a deep nasopharyngeal swab sample, reliably detect active viral shedding with sensitivity and specificity of nearly 90%. A simple nasal mucus swab does not obtain sufficient epithelial cells, and leads to increased false-negative results. During the season when influenza is endemic, the obtained specimen should be tested for both viruses. The availability of effective testing for RSV and influenza with rapid turnaround times has enhanced the ability to distinguish serious bacterial infections from viral infections in young infants; thereby, decreasing extensive laboratory testing, time in the emergency department, and needless antibiotic exposure.[92]

Treatment

17. What available treatments should be used to M.V.?

As with croup, the treatment of bronchiolitis is controversial when evidence-based benefit is balanced against risk, and recommendations for treatment often fly against practice traditions. More than 50% of bronchiolitis episodes are treated with bronchodilators, corticosteroids, or antivirals despite only limited supportive evidence for such treatments.[93]

Bronchodilators

The use of bronchodilators has been declining because the literature does not support their routine use, and they do not seem to decrease LOS in hospitals or prevent the need for hospitalization. Some individual infants, however, seem to experience early benefit based on scores of clinical improvement.[94] Aerosolized administration of bronchodilators by mask or hood to infants with bronchiolitis also results in similar outcomes. The hood generally is the preferred aerosolized method of administration because the mask or nasal prongs often become displaced with the head movements of young infants.[95] Additionally, nebulized epinephrine, in contrast with placebo or albuterol, has been beneficial in some outpatients; however, epinephrine can promote adverse increases in heart rate.[96] Several international studies have demonstrated decreased hospital LOS for infants with moderate viral bronchiolitis when treated with nebulized 3% saline. Nevertheless, formal recommendations for the use of nebulized saline are lacking.[97] Therefore, an aerosolized bronchodilator should not be used in treating M.V. because he already has an increased heart rate and it would unnecessarily expose him to potential adverse effects from a treatment with unproven efficacy.

Corticosteroids

A variety of corticosteroid have been studied in the treatment of RSV bronchiolitis; however, the routine use of these drugs has not been endorsed by the AAP.[85] Corticosteroids might prove to have a role in early or later disease course. In a randomized, placebo-controlled trial of 174 children (<2 years old), a single dexamethasone 0.6 mg/kg dose decreased duration of symptoms, decreased the need for oxygen, and decreased hospital LOS.[98] In a larger, multicenter trial, 600 infants (2–12 months old) randomly received 1 mg/kg of oral dexamethasone or placebo in the emergency department to treat moderate to severe bronchiolitis; outcome measures of hospitalization and clinical score were evaluated over a 4-hour observation period. The mean improvement of symptom scores and in the LOS for those hospitalized were not different, and the hospital admission rates also did not differ for the steroid (39.7%) and placebo (41%) groups.[99] These results do not exclude the possibility that corticosteroids, used later in the course of the disease, might decrease residual inflammation, wheezing, and bronchial remodeling. The prevention of the development of pulmonary dysfunction with corticosteroids has been studied with mixed results.[100] Therefore, unlike for croup where the benefit of corticosteroids is seen within 4 hours, the use of a corticosteroid in M.V. must be predicated on his clinical course. M.V.'s worsening wheezing provides justification for early use of methylprednisolone (2 mg/kg loading dose, and 0.5 mg/kg Q 6 hr for maintenance).

Supportive Care

The mucolytic recombinant human deoxyribonuclease (e.g., Dornase) had no effect on LOS, supplemental oxygen needs, or symptom scores.[101] Intravenous fluids should be given as needed because infants may not be feeding adequately and insensible losses may be increased with the higher respiratory rates. Nasal suctioning and 0.0625% to 0.125% phenylephrine every 4 to 6 hours should be applied to keep M.V.'s nasal passage patent. Higher concentrations or more frequent administration of phenylephrine should be avoided because catecholamine-induced hypertension has been observed owing to the nasal vascular (mainly arterial) uptake. Supplemental oxygen should be continued for M.V. if an oxygen saturation of <90% is sustained.

Antivirals

The antiviral, ribavirin, generally is delivered by mist tent as 6 g over 12 hours for 3 consecutive days when used for treatment of bronchiolitis. The airborne spread of ribavirin is of concern during administration of ribavirin, and safety policies need to be established to minimize healthcare worker exposure because of potential adverse effects. Although initial studies of ribavirin efficacy were positive, other larger cooperative clinical trial results have been mixed and its use has decreased, even among patients at significant clinical risk.[102] Out of 11 heterogeneously designed trials, 7 were associated with patient benefits, and 4 noted no benefit. Ribavirin might be of value in immunocompromised or cardiovascular-impaired patients with severe disease,[85] but should be deferred in M.V.

Antibacterials

The empiric use of antibacterials is not at all common because concurrent bacterial pneumonia is not an expectation, despite the occasional appearance of pulmonary infiltrates and atelectasis on chest x-ray. Acute otitis media can certainly be caused by RSV, but it can difficult to differentiate viral from bacterial etiologies. Although some evidence suggest that more than 50% of hospitalized children with bronchiolitis develop AOM, antibacterials should not be administered to M.V. empirically in the absence of a specific diagnosis.[85] Macrolide antibiotics might have benefit in RSV-associated bronchiolitis that some speculate might be attributable to their immunomodulatory effects; however, the needed 3-week course of therapy cannot be supported based on present data.[103]

18. Is M.V. a candidate to receive RSV prophylaxis?

Palivizumab

A polyclonal RSV immunoglobulin was utilized for the prevention of RSV infection, but interest waned because increased mortality was noted in patients with congenital heart disease. A humanized monoclonal anti-RSV antibody, palivizumab (Synagis) is available for clinical use. When monthly palivizumab intramuscular injections of 15 mg/kg were administered during the RSV seasonal months to high-risk infants and children with hemodynamically significant congenital heart disease, RSV hospitalizations were decreased.[104] Table 96-6 identifies patients who could benefit from palivizumab administration. M.V. is eligible for palivizumab, despite his current infection, because there is a lack of durable immunity against RSV. M.V. should have received his first dose of palivizumab before discharge from the hospital after birth. This medication is costly and cost-effectiveness strategies should be considered. Opportunities for greater use of palivizumab are notable; only half of the children presenting to an ED with bronchiolitis who met AAP criteria for palivizumab prophylaxis received it.[105] In 2-year follow-up studies, the incidence of recurrent wheezing decreased in infants who received this drug compared to those who did not.[106] A more potent second-generation monoclonal antibody, motavizumab, is currently undergoing phase III clinical trials.[107] Although palivizumab is FDA approved for prophylaxis against RSV, it also has been used intravenously for the treatment of severe upper and lower respiratory RSV infection in high-risk patients, including those with malignancy.[108,109] Efforts to develop an appropriately attenuated and immunogenic live RSV vaccine are ongoing.[110]

Table 96-6 Indications for Palivizumab

- Infants and children <24 months old with chronic lung disease of prematurity who have required medical therapy within 6 months of RSV season (including diuretics or corticosteroids or supplemental oxygen)
- Infants born at ≤32 weeks gestation, with or without chronic lung disease:
  - ≤28 weeks gestation during the first 12 months of life
  - 29–32 weeks gestation during the first 6 months of life (if overlapping with the start of RSV season
- Infants 32–35 weeks of gestation with ≥2 of the following risk factors:
  - child care attendance, school-aged siblings
  - exposure to environmental air pollutants
  - congenital abnormalities of the airways
  - severe neuromuscular disease
- Children ≤24 months old with hemodynamically significant cyanotic and acyanotic congenital heart disease
  - Infants who are receiving medication to control congestive heart failure
  - Infants with moderate to severe pulmonary hypertension
  - Infants with cyanotic heart disease

RSV, respiratory syncytial virus.

KAWASAKI DISEASE

Kawasaki disease (KD), also known as mucocutaneous lymph node syndrome, is an inflammatory vasculitis with multiple clinical features. Although it is one cause of fever of unknown origin in children, Kawasaki syndrome or KD is unique. It occurs in children younger than 5 years, has a slight male predominance, and occurs more frequently in children of Asian descent.[111]

Diagnosis

The diagnosis of KD is based on a constellation of symptoms, including a fever of at least 5 days' duration in the absence of an alternative diagnosis and with at least four of the following five features:[111]

a. bilateral bulbar conjunctival injection;
b. oral mucous membrane changes (e.g., injected or fissured lips, injected pharynx, strawberry tongue, periungual desquamation during the subacute and convalescent phases);
c. peripheral extremity changes (e.g., painful erythema of palms or soles, edema of hands or feet) especially during the acute phase;
d. polymorphous rash; and
e. cervical lymphadenopathy (at least one lymph node >1.5 cm in diameter).

Atypical or incomplete KD refers to cases in which fever is accompanied by three or fewer of these features. These cases occur more in infants and in chemically induced KD (e.g., carbamazepine, griseofulvin, mesalamine, carpet shampoo exposure). Additional clinical findings of KD may include hepatic dysfunction, gallbladder hydrops, pseudo-obstruction, urethritis, aseptic meningitis, arthralgia, and arthritis.

Etiology

The etiology of KD is not well defined, but it has been linked to viral (coronavirus), bacterial, and rickettsial exposures. KD mimics a number of infectious diseases, including toxic shock syndrome, Rocky Mountain spotted fever, scarlet fever, bacterial cervical adenitis, and staphylococcal scalded skin syndrome. It also has been linked to a superantigen hypothesis, in which proinflammatory cytokines advance vascular inflammation in the acute phase (first 10 days). In this hypothesis, vascular endothelial factors are released and stimulate myointimal proliferation and medial thinning, leading to local dilatation, ectasia, and aneurysm formation. This occurrence in the coronary arteries of the affected child represents the most concerning, and potentially life-threatening, complication of this disease. Myocarditis and pericarditis can also present during this period as early complications.

19. J.H., a 4-year-old Korean male, is in a kindergarten class where several children have come down with the flu. J.H. has been febrile with respiratory symptoms, but his fever has lasted for 9 days and had been as high as 104.6°F. On physical examination, J.H.'s hands and feet are swollen and red, his tongue is red and pimply, and his lips show small fissures. His conjunctiva are red bilaterally without discharge, and there is a maculopapular rash with irregular borders on the chest. He has a 2-cm mobile cervical node on the left side of his neck and a few shoddy inguinal nodes. He has an I/VI systolic ejection murmur, and the point of maximal impulse is normally located. His abdominal examination is benign. He complains of burning on urination. He has quadriceps muscle and knee pain, and his parents suspected that this was the influenza that had spread among his classmates. His parents have not given him antibiotics and deny any other drug use except for ibuprofen for the fever. The laboratory results show a WBC count of 27,500 cell/mm^3 with 12% band forms, and 50% lymphocytes with atypical lymphocytes and toxic granulation seen on smear. His platelet count is 325,000 cells/mm^3, and his hemoglobin is 10.7 gm/dL, with a mean corpuscular volume of 89 μm^3. He has a CRP of 12.7 mg/dL, an erythrocyte sedimentation rate (ESR) of 88 mm/hr, an albumin of 2.9 g/dL, and an alanine aminotransferase of 102 IU/mL with normal ammonia. Urinalysis shows 5 to 10 WBC per high-power field (hpf), but nitrite negative. Blood and urine cultures are negative. Antibiotics are not started. What diagnostic findings and considerations in J.H. are consistent with KD?

J.H. has a fever of unknown origin for more than a week, and his age (<5 years) and nationality (Korean) fit the typical profile of a patient with KD. More important, J.H. has some signs and symptoms referable to influenza, but the presence of the prominent swelling of the hands and feet (criterion C); a maculopapular versus an urticarial rash (criterion D); and the unilateral cervical adenopathy (criterion E) and the high fever for 9 days differentiates this illness from the usual flu symptom pattern. In addition, J.H.'s conjunctiva are red bilaterally (criterion A); his tongue is red and pimply in appearance (criterion B).

The laboratory test results of J.H. also are consistent with those commonly noted in patients with KD. Leukocytosis (J.H.'s is 27,500 cells/mm^3), anemia (J.H.'s hemoglobin is 10.7 and normocytic), elevations in CRP (J.H.'s CRP is 12.7 mg/dL) and ESR (88 mm/hour in J.H.), transaminasesemia (alanine aminotransferase in J.H. is 102 IU/mL), and sterile pyuria (5–10 WBC/hpf in J.H.) are present. J.H.'s platelet count is normal, but the platelet count can rise to more than 1 million/mm^3 during the subacute phase (days 11–21) of KD, when fever often dissipates and toes and fingers desquamate. During the convalescent phase (days 21–60), the development and presence of coronary artery aneurysms are prominent concerns. J.H.'s ESR and CRP are increased and in the ranges (>50 and 10, respectively) where coronary aneurysms are observed more frequently.[112]

Treatment

20. What treatment should be offered to J.H. during the acute phase?

Medications to provide a measure of comfort for the patient (e.g., analgesics and antipyretics) are essential, but the need for treatment to minimize the potential for coronary aneurysms, as detected by echocardiography, is paramount. The risk of coronary artery ectasia and aneurysm is higher if treatment is delayed beyond 10 days from initial symptoms. In one study, 7% of patients with complete KD had an aneurysm on the initial echocardiogram versus 30% of those with incomplete KD.[113] KD patients treated by day 7 of illness had 6% occurrence of aneurysm versus 27% among those treated at days 8 to 10. A delay in diagnosis of KD, whether due to the lack of access to health care or to the lack of health insurance, or more than one visit to a health care provider before establishment of the diagnosis, increases the risk of the development of coronary aneurysms. Patients younger than 6 months, and those with atypical KD, who have diagnosis and treatment delay of 10 days or more after fever onset, also are at higher risk of developing aneurysms.[114,115]

Intravenous immunoglobulin has become the mainstay of treatment to minimize the risk of aneurysm in patients with KD. The recommended doses of IV immunoglobulin has been modified over time from 400 mg/kg/day for 5 days to 1 g/kg for 2 days to the current regimen of a single dose of 2 g/kg, delivered as a 12-hour infusion.[111] An additional dose of IV immunoglobulin at the same dose is warranted if defervescence of fever and clinical indications of improvement have not occurred by 36 to 48 hours after the first dose of IV immunoglobulin. A third dose can be given if necessary with the addition of 1 to 3 days of pulse methylprednisolone at 30 mg/kg/dose.[116]

Corticosteroids are appropriate if refractory fever continues after two doses of IV immunoglobulin, but the effect on coronary artery dilatation and aneurysm is uncertain.[117] The use of methylprednisolone combined with first-dose IV immunoglobulin does not add to the cardiac efficacy of prompt IV immunoglobulin treatment given alone, although greater reductions were observed with ESR, CRP, and febrile days with the combination.[118] In contrast, a meta-analysis of eight KD studies showed improved coronary protective efficacy in regimens that included corticosteroids, which were the mainstays of therapy with aspirin before the emergence of IV immunoglobulin.

An antiplatelet drug such as aspirin is still used during the febrile phase at doses of 80 to 100 mg/kg/day divided every 4 or 6 hours. Once the patient's fever diminishes, the dose of aspirin is reduced to 3 to 5 mg/kg/day (especially important if the platelet count is very high in the subacute phase) and continued for 6 to 8 weeks until evidence of no development of coronary aneurysms; treatment length is indefinite if coronary aneurysms form, because these can rupture during adulthood. J.H., still with the potential for influenza to have been a trigger for KD, should have an enzyme immunoassay for influenza to assess the risk of Reye syndrome because of the intent to prescribe aspirin. Clopidogrel can be used as an alternative to aspirin, or for persistent platelet counts higher than 1 million/mm^3, with doses of 0.2 mg/kg/day for children younger than 2 years and 1 mg/kg/day for older children being well-tolerated and effective.[119] The rare occurrence of coronary thrombosis in patients with KD could be treated with medications (e.g., thrombolytics, heparin, warfarin), similar to treatment algorithms in adults. Revascularization and coronary bypass surgery have been performed in severe cases.

PEDIATRIC URINARY TRACT INFECTION

Urinary tract infections (UTIs) in children are common causes of febrile illness in infants, children and adolescents.[120] Up to 7% of girls and 2% of boys will have a symptomatic, culture-confirmed UTI by 6 years of age; and more so with younger age (7% of febrile newborns). The yearly prevalence of UTIs in children is estimated to be 2.4% to 2.8%. In a large cohort of febrile children younger than 2 years, 2.1% were diagnosed with UTI; and in 13% of Caucasian girls younger than 6 months of age.[121] The prevalence in that age group presenting to the pediatric emergency room was 3.3%.[122] Among 1,025 febrile infants evaluated during seasons where bronchiolitis is prevalent, 9% were diagnosed with a UTI.[123]

The importance of UTIs in children is not limited to the need for prompt diagnosis and treatment, but also concern for the potential ramifications of prolonged untreated, poorly treated, and repeated infection. The relationship of UTI to loss of nephron mass with consequent decrease in glomerular function, childhood hypertension, reflux nephropathy, and renal scarring is well-established; the needs for treatment and prophylaxis are important pediatric issues.

Clinical Features and Risk Factors

21. K.P., a 2-month-old male, presents to the emergency department with fever and a small amount of blood in his diaper. The mother claims to be changing the infant's diaper with the usual frequency, but noticed over the last 2 days the urine was malodorous. Although somewhat irritable, the infant has been behaving otherwise normally. Birth history was unremarkable, although the mother had a case of acute pyelonephritis during the second trimester, and had two more such cases in the past. On examination, the child is flushed in appearance, but otherwise normal appearing and responsive. His temperature is 103.8°F and his heart rate is 180 beats/minute; other vital signs are normal for age. He is uncircumcised, but no outward anomalies (e.g., abnormal urethral opening, spina bifida) are noted. Crying is elicited on abdominal palpation, but no organomegaly is appreciated, nor is pain elicited on palpation of the flank area. A urinalysis and urine culture was obtained via a collection bag (the infant is noted to cry while urinating). A blood culture is obtained, but a lumbar puncture is deferred due to the lack of significant mental status change. Stool was also obtained for microscopy and culture. What demographic and clinical features of childhood UTI are relevant to this patient's UTI?

This patient demonstrates some salient demographic and clinical features of pediatric UTIs, which differ from the UTIs experienced by adolescents and adults. Serious bacterial infection can be identified in 7% to 12% of febrile infants younger than 3 months old, and 67% to 85% of these can be attributed to UTIs.[121,124,125] The incidence of UTIs in males is much higher during early infancy than in later childhood and adolescence. The incidence of UTI during the first year of life is 2.7% in males versus 0.7% in females. This gender difference for UTI reverses to 0.1 to 0.2% in males and 0.9 to 1.4% in females 1 to 5 years old, and 0.04 to 0.2% in males and 0.7 to 2.3% in females 6 to 16 years old.[120] UTIs in adults most commonly result from ascending infection from the lower urinary tract, whereas in young infants the UTI often results from a hematogenous spread to the urinary tract. As a result, concern for the possibility of sepsis in young infants is important, and a blood culture is essential in the face of K.P.'s clinical findings.

Family history also might be of relevance because the children of mother's with a history of pyelonephritis have a higher incidence of acute pyelonephritis, although pyelonephritis during pregnancy has no inheritability impact. Of interest, K.P.'s mother had experienced a bout of pyelonephritis during her second trimester. Lower human IL-8 CXCR1 receptor expression has been noted in both of these family patient groups compared with children without UTIs.[126] Adolescents who self-catheterize because of spina bifida or severe bladder dysfunction are at higher risk for recurrent UTIs, particularly if poor catheterization routines are employed.[127]

An anatomical urologic anomaly, or the presence of renal stones, is commonly associated with UTIs in male infants; therefore, a thorough clinical and radiologic search for these etiologies is prudent. The gross hematuria in the case of K.P. more predominantly occurs in males with UTI, and is often observed in concert with vesicoureteral reflux (VUR), or with other urinary tract anomalies found more often in boys (e.g., posterior urethral valves, ureteropelvic junction obstruction, hypospadias, ureterocele).[128] The hematuria in K.P. also can be indicative of hypercalciuria, which can increase the potential for nephrocalcinosis and urolithiasis (seen more typically in low-birth-weight premature infants). Medical trauma, particularly if this patient had multiple prior urethral catheterization attempts, could also cause hematuria, and heighten the risk of subsequent UTI. The lack of organomegaly in K.P. tends to exclude polycystic kidney disease as causative or associated with UTI.

The clinical risk factors associated with UTIs in young children are summarized in Table 96-7. Uncircumcised boys harbor significantly higher concentration of uropathogens that may ascend into the urinary tract than in circumcised infants; bacteriuria is 10- to 12-fold more common during the first 6 months of life among uncircumcised males than in those circumcised. Lack of circumcision was the highest multivariate predictor of UTI in 1,025 febrile infants who were more than 60 days old.[123] In this same study, a temperature exceeding 39°C (102.2°F) also provides high predictive value. K.P.'s heart rate is appropriately elevated in the presence of a high fever and potential serious bacterial infection. His crying on abdominal palpation is common but nonspecific, and eliciting true flank pain in infants with pyelonephritis is more elusive than in adults. K.P.'s dysuria needs to be observed at the time of his urination because discomfort in the infant during

Table 96-7 Urinary Tract Infection Risk Factors for Young Children

- Known urinary tract abnormalities
- Uncircumcised boys
- History of urinary tract infection
- Temperature >39°C
- Fever >24 hr
- No apparent source for fever
- Ill appearance
- Suprapubic tenderness
- Nonblack race

urination might be attributable to other causes. K.P.'s decreased feeding, along his vomiting, diarrhea, and signs of dehydration often are noted in infants with pyelonephritis. Systemic signs and symptoms of hesitancy, dysuria, frequency, anorexia, and abdominal or flank pain are most easily noted in older verbal children. Because K.P. is uncircumcised, a baseline probability of UTI would about 6%, but the addition of one or more of the factors in Table 96-7 increases the probability to 10 to 25% before any urine testing.[129]

Urinalysis

22. The dipstick of K.P.'s urine is positive for nitrites and leukocyte esterases. Microscopy of his urine shows 10 WBCs/hpf, and the initial urine culture has grown 10^4 gram-negative rods/mL. The patients CRP is 5.5 mg/dL, and the WBC count is 15,500/mm^3 with a differential showing 82% neutrophils (20% band forms). What is the diagnostic value of these tests for UTI? Can cystitis and pyelonephritis be clinically discriminated in a similar fashion as in adults?

Individually, these urine tests contribute varying amounts of information to the diagnosis of UTI in children. Overall for children, a positive urinalysis for leukocyte esterases, nitrites, or pyuria has a sensitivity of 82%, and a specificity of 92%.[130] The positive LR of a nitrites and leukocyte esterases present on urinalysis in a young child suspected of a UTI is 28, and the probability of UTI in K.P. with his test results is about 75 to 90%.[129]

K.P. does have pyuria (i.e., ≥5 WBCs/hpf). In one study, infants 3 months old or younger seen in the emergency room with fever and pyuria had a positive yield on urine culture of 81%.[131] The combination of pyuria and bacteriuria has a positive predictive value as high as 85%,[132] yet 10% of infants can have a negative urinalysis in presence of a culture- and nuclear scan-proven UTI.

As with adults, the validity of any of these tests depends on the method of urine collection. Urine can be collected for study in infants or children by clean-void catch, suprapubic aspiration, bag specimen, and urethral catheterization. Suprapubic aspiration is utilized more commonly in septic neonates and occasionally in infants when contamination using other collection methods is suspect; however, suprapubic aspiration is invasive and is more painful than catheterization.[133] The threshold of organisms needed for a positive urine culture (≥100 CFU/mL) is much lower when urine is obtained by suprapubic aspiration than other methods of urine collection because sterility of the bladder urine is assumed. The more common methods of bag collection, catheterization, and clean-void catch have been compared. In over 1,500 young infants (0–3 months old), leukocyte esterases tested from bag specimens showed somewhat lower sensitivity (76% vs. 86%) and statistically lower specificity (higher false-positive rate) than urine from catheterization (84% vs. 94%), although these were not from matched specimens.[134] Specificity using nitrites testing was nearly 100% by either collection method, but the sensitivity was unacceptably low for both collection methods (25% and 43%, respectively). Diagnostic yield was also lower for bag specimens at various cutoff points for white cell counts in urine microscopy relative to the presence of infection. No statistical differences were detected in infection rates by urine culture (8.5% vs. 10.8%, respectively),[134] although it is usually accepted that bag specimens will have a higher false-positive rate and more multiorganism and contaminated urine cultures than catheterization specimens.

These differences in technique probably are smaller in males than females. In a study using matched specimens in 303 children at risk for UTI, dipstick testing from bag specimens had higher sensitivity in girls but lower specificity than catheter-obtained specimens.[135] Only in the subset of boys 90 days old or younger were both sensitivity and specificity statistically similar between urine sampling methods. Therefore, bag urine testing for leukocyte esterases and white cells can be used a screening method toward more selective catheterization strategy in young infant boys, but this would not be applicable for girls or older children, in whom urinary catheterization is the preferred collection method for urine testing. Urine for urinalysis and culture of a catheterized urine specimen should generally be collected from non–toilet trained children with symptoms of UTI.[129] In toilet-trained children, the collection of a midstream urine sample after thorough cleaning of the perineum with soap reduces the culture contamination rate by two-thirds.[136]

As with other serious bacterial infections, K.P. demonstrates an elevated peripheral WBC count, with a left shift; the CRP is also elevated. Although these tests have significantly higher values in infants with pyelonephritis than cystitis, their diagnostic accuracy (around 50%) in localizing the infection suffers from poor specificity.[137] Procalcitonin, although not routinely measured, has been shown to have the highest accuracy among blood measurements in differentiating upper from lower UTI. The most accurate method in children to distinguish pyelonephritis from cystitis is using technetium-labeled dimercaptosuccinic acid renal scan, which shows irregularly patterned and incomplete uptake into the kidney cortex in the presence of pyelonephritis, and detects pyelonephritis in 60% to 70% of infants with UTI.[138,139]

Urinary Pathogens and Susceptibility

23. What could be anticipated from K.P.'s urine culture and sensitivity tests? Are there pathogen susceptibility differences between children and adults?

As always, the urine collection technique is important in the proper interpretation of the urine cultures. The magnitude of bacteriuria in K.P.'s case is significant, particularly in boys, if the urine was obtained via a clean catch method or obtained from a urine bag or pad; however, a urine collection bag that has been attached for a prolonged period can cause false-positive results from colonizing skin organisms in the introitus. A single organism, excluding typical skin commensals, can be noted to be potentially pathogenic. *Escherichia coli* is the expected pathogen in 60% to 90% of cases of childhood UTI, although strain differences exist in toxins, uroepithelial receptor binding and adhesions, fimbriation, and antibiotic resistance.[120] Specific urovirulence gene expression in *E. coli* is associated with lobar nephronia (focal abscess) in children.[140]

Antimicrobial susceptibility data for urinary isolates from children differ somewhat from adults, and can be age, acuity, and gender dependent. When compared to adults, tested outpatient isolates were overall less susceptible to ampicillin, trimethoprim-sulfamethoxazole, and nitrofurantoin in children younger than 14 with UTI; antimicrobial resistance increased through the years of study.[141,142] Comparative data specific for *E. coli* showed similar child–adult differences.[143] Susceptibility was comparatively higher for ciprofloxacin and levofloxacin in children.[141] Regional differences in gram-negative rod susceptibility among children are also observed.[141]

The susceptibility of *E. coli* to ampicillin and amoxicillin continues to decrease throughout the world, and the resistance of this organism to these aminopenicillins is estimated to be about 50% to 70%. These penicillins should not be selected for the initial management of pediatric UTI.[141,143,144] In one study, the susceptibility of 11,341 urinary *E. coli* isolates collected in children with UTI demonstrated pansusceptibility to tested antibiotics in only 41.8% to 59.4% within four different age groupings, with the lowest susceptibility noted in children 1 to 24 months of age.[145] Similar data on resistance to at least one tested antibiotic (48%) have been observed by others.[144] Resistance to two or more antibiotics ranged from 15.9% to 27.3% among the groups, with the most common co-resistance being observed with ampicillin and trimethoprim-sulfamethoxazole (10.5%–18.3%).[145] Resistance to three or more antibiotics was low in all age groups (3.1%–5.2%). The range of intermediate and full resistance combined for cefazolin and amoxicillin-clavulanate was 5.7% to 11.8% and 13.3% to 22.5%, respectively. Although improved activity over ampicillin is observed with the inclusion of a β-lactamase inhibitor (e.g., clavulanate), the inhibitor does not fully prevent resistance. In a study of 77 gram-negative rods from children with UTI (72 of which were *E. coli*), resistance to ampicillin was 46% and to ampicillin-sulbactam was 28%.[144] The first-generation cephalosporin, cephalexin, was associated with more bacterial resistance than second or third-generation oral cephalosporins.[142]

Non–*E. coli* gram-negative rods (e.g., *Klebsiella pneumoniae*, *Pseudomonas aeruginosa*, *Enterobacter* spp., and enterococci), are encountered more often in males, neonates, children with reflux and underlying renal or urinary abnormalities, and children who have received antibiotics in the month before the UTI.[146–148] Additionally, a greater proportion of these organisms are found in UTIs with lower colony counts ($\leq$50,000 CFU/mL).[149] These gram-negative organisms also tend to be more resistant to the antibiotics typically recommended for initial treatment (e.g., aminoglycosides, cephalosporins). This led to inappropriate initial therapy for these non–*E. coli* infections (19% vs. 2% for *E. coli*; $p = .0001$), resulting in longer hospitalizations.[146,150] Higher rates of resistance to multiple antibiotics have been noted by other investigators, with children younger than 4 years having a greater incidence of antibiotic resistance. *P. aeruginosa* often is the pathogenic organism in children with chronic pyelonephritis.

Among 361 pediatric patients hospitalized for UTI over a 5-year period, statistically lower susceptibility was observed for parenteral penicillins, cephalosporins, and trimethoprim-sulfamethoxazole in patients with a history of UTIs, and lower still in patients receiving antibiotic prophylaxis.[150] This pattern was consistent with the finding of more non–*E. coli* UTI in these patients, and the greater likelihood of those organisms being more resistant. The sensitivity to the aminoglycosides and aztreonam, however, did not vary among these groups and was at least 95% (carbapenems were not tested). Pseudomonas resistance patterns resemble those of adults, except that less resistance is seen for the fluoroquinolones.[143,151] This is understood as being a function of much lower volume of usage of this class of antibiotics in children, and therefore, less selective pressure toward enzyme target and efflux expression of resistance. Pediatric urinary bacterial isolates have lower susceptibility to trimethoprim-sulfamethoxazole, with *E. coli* susceptibility of 70% to 75%.[152,153] High susceptibility is still maintained for *E. coli* for nitrofurantoin (<3% resistance), but its use is limited in infants to prophylaxis, given the high percentage of cases of pyelonephritis among UTIs in infants, the lack of localizing signs and symptoms distinguishing upper tract infection in this age group, and the absence of effective serum and tissue concentrations of this drug.

Treatment Selection

24. K.P. has been febrile for 48 hours and the culture and sensitivity are pending. What should be the therapeutic approach, anticipated response and follow-up monitoring?

K.P.'s treatment should begin promptly because delays in initiation of the antibiotic management enhance the risk of renal scarring or abscess formation. The use of a cephalosporin as initial therapy in an outpatient setting is reasonable, provided follow-up of the culture and sensitivity report is ensured. Ampicillin/amoxicillin or trimethoprim-sulfamethoxazole cannot be relied upon empirically, given the baseline resistance rates that now exist. A variety of treatment regimens and approaches have been evaluated in managing pediatric UTIs. A 10-day course of an appropriate oral antibiotic can be as effective as parenteral antibiotics, even in the management of pyelonephritis.[154] However, use of parenteral antibiotics is recommended if patients are toxic in appearance, dehydrated, or have decreased oral intake. Cefixime, cefpodoxime, and cefdinir are potent single daily-dose oral agents for *E. coli* and non–*E. coli* UTIs, although cefdinir does not have an FDA indication for UTI.[155] Multiple daily doses of amoxicillin-clavulanate, cephalexin, cefprozil, and cefuroxime are alternative choices pending culture and sensitivity reporting. Experience with fluoroquinolones has been limited; however, these can be used to treat complicated UTIs in children with multi-resistant urinary isolates, despite the relative contraindications to the use of fluoroquinolones in children (see Question 21).[156]

K.P. would likely require hospitalization and therapy should be initiated with either a parenteral cephalosporin (e.g., cefotaxime 100–200 mg/kg/day or ceftriaxone 50–100 mg/kg/day) or an aminoglycoside, with dosage adjustments to achieve targeted serum levels, depending on severity of infection and/or simultaneous infection at other sites. Alternatively, the less ill infant could be treated in an outpatient health care facility with daily intravenous injections of an aminoglycoside.[157] Intravenous therapy should be continued for at least 3 to 7 days, and should be followed by a course of therapy with an appropriate oral antibiotic (assuming an uncomplicated clinical course). The AAP has recommended a 7- to 14-day course of antibiotic therapy for all children 2 months to 2 years of age with UTI based on comparative data, which showed better efficacy with this 1- to 2-week course of treatment than with shorter treatment courses. This treatment regimen can utilize a combination of parenteral and oral therapy. Meta-analysis supports this recommendation for longer treatment lengths for pediatric UTIs, with lower failure rates observed even in the absence of evidence of pyelonephritis.[158] A good treatment response for K.P. would be anticipated with the correct antibiotic selection. Generally, fever resolves within 48 hours in approximately 90% of infants. Few failures are reported, and the need for follow-up cultures for proof of effect may be dubious.[159] For lobar nephronia, 3 weeks of therapy (IV and oral) has proven better than shorter courses.[160]

Recommended follow-up testing and treatment traditionally includes a renal ultrasound or renal scan of the UTI diagnosis to detect anomalies, structural lesions, calculi or obstruction, and a voiding cystourethrogram or renal scan within 3 months to evaluate for VUR, with antibiotic prophylaxis until the voiding cystourethrogram is performed.[161]

Complications of Urinary Tract Infections in Children and Prophylaxis

25. K.P. is discharged from the hospital after responding well to 6 days of intravenous cefotaxime for *K. pneumoniae* (10^5 CFU/mL). He also has completed 14 days of therapy with oral cefixime (8 mg/kg once daily), which was continued until the voiding cystourethrogram performed a month later revealed grade III reflux of the left collecting system. What therapeutic initiatives should be considered?

VUR is the most common urologic abnormality in children, with a 1% to 2% incidence, and is discovered in 30% to 50% of children with one or more episodes of UTI.[139,162] Higher prevalence exists in offspring of those previously affected (via autosomal-dominant inheritance). VUR occurs when the high pressure in the bladder produces a breakdown of normal ureterovesicular junction barriers to retrograde urinary flow. This creates an increased risk of ascending travel of contaminated urine and repeated upper tract infections, delaying resolution of VUR and furthering the risk of renal scarring and damage.

VUR (grades I–V) is classified by the extent of dilatation and tortuosity of the ureters, ascending toward deformity of the kidney calyces and papillary structures.[162] VUR should be treated either medically or surgically to prevent further damage to the kidney parenchyma (primarily scarring) and avoid progression to hypertension and renal insufficiency. Spontaneous resolution of VUR is affected by age, severity grade, and whether it is unilateral or bilateral. Children receiving long-term antimicrobial prophylaxis who are younger than 2 years, who have a lower severity grade, and who have only unilateral reflux have higher rates of spontaneous resolution.[162,163]

Although some investigations suggest that antibiotic prophylaxis may not be necessary for the prevention of reinfection and scarring when managing patients with lower grades of reflux,[164] long-term antimicrobial prophylaxis has been the standard approach endorsed by several medical societies.[165] Longitudinal studies with 10-year follow-up suggest that antimicrobial prophylaxis is as effective as surgical approaches in patients with grades III and IV VUR in preventing new scarring, although more febrile UTIs can occur in the prophylaxis group.[163,164] Boys with grade III VUR given prophylaxis with trimethoprim-sulfamethoxazole showed reduction in further UTIs.[166]

Antibiotic doses for prophylaxis usually are to the usual daily treatment doses. Nitrofurantoin, trimethoprim, trimethoprim-sulfamethoxazole, cephalexin, cefixime, and amoxicillin are the most commonly utilized antibiotics for this indication. Although prophylaxis with antibiotics is considered to be safer in children than in adults, long-term prophylaxis can result in adverse effects. Even with these lower doses, antibiotic use was modified in nearly 10% of children. Severe or life-threatening complications from low-dose antibiotic prophylaxis have been rare.[167,168] When antibiotics for prophylaxis in children were compared, fewer adverse reactions were associated with nitrofurantoin than for cefixime. Although nitrofurantoin was associated with more adverse effects than trimethoprim, it was more effective than trimethoprim.[169]

All of these antibiotics can facilitate the growth of resistant bacteria over time, especially for non–*E. coli* isolates, which pose a greater risk for children with urologic abnormalities.[165,170] In K.P., reinfection with *Klebsiella* may occur with the development of an expressed extended-spectrum β-lactamase if a low-dose cephalosporin is utilized chronically. An organized strategy for continuing with the same antibiotic, changing to a different one, or otherwise modifying prophylactic regimens based on other parameters, requires study.

Table 96-8 Selected Uses of Fluoroquinolones in Children

- Urinary tract infections caused by *P. aeruginosa* or other multidrug-resistant, gram-negative bacteria (FDA licensed for complicated *E. coli* urinary tract infections and pyelonephritis attributable to *E. coli* in patients 1–17 years of age)
- Complicated acute otitis media failing to respond to initial antibiotic treatment[180]
- Chronic suppurative otitis media or malignant otitis externa caused by *P. aeruginosa*
- Exacerbation of pulmonary disease in patients with cystic fibrosis who have colonization with *P. aeruginosa* and can be treated in an ambulatory setting
- Gastrointestinal tract infection caused by multidrug resistant *Shigella* species, *Salmonella* species, *Vibrio cholerae*, or *Campylobacter jejuni*
- Gram-negative bacterial infections in immunocompromised hosts in whom oral therapy is desired or resistance to alternative agents is present
- Serious infections attributable to fluoroquinolone-susceptible pathogen(s) in children with life-threatening allergy to alternative agents
- Documented bacterial septicemia or meningitis attributable to organisms with in vitro resistance to approved agents or in immunocompromised infants and children in whom parenteral therapy with other appropriate antimicrobial agents has failed
- Chronic or acute osteomyelitis or osteochondritis caused by *P. aeruginosa* (not for prophylaxis of nail puncture wounds to the foot)
- Mycobacterial infections caused by isolates known to be susceptible to fluoroquinolones
- Treatment exposure to aerosolized *Bacillus anthracis* to decrease the incidence or progression of disease (FDA licensed)

Adapted from reference 156.

Fluoroquinolone Usage in Pediatrics

26. **K.P., now 14 months old, is continued on prophylactic doses of nitrofurantoin, but has his third infection over the past 6 months. The last urine culture showed 10^5 CFU/mL *P. aeruginosa*, which is resistant to cephalosporins and penicillins. K.P. has had a number of courses of aminoglycosides to treat acute infection, and the MICs of the organism have risen. Because there is concern for aminoglycoside-induced nephrotoxicity, ciprofloxacin 15 mg/kg/day divided into two doses a day is prescribed because the organism on sensitivity testing is sensitive to the fluoroquinolones. Why do the benefits of fluoroquinolone therapy to K.P. outweigh the well-publicized contraindication to use this class of agents in children?**

The contraindications for the use of fluoroquinolones in pediatric patients have been based largely on juvenile animal cartilage toxicity studies (species- and dose-dependent toxicity). When benefits of therapy outweigh concerns for the musculoskeletal adverse effect of fluoroquinolones, these drugs should be prescribed. In one study, myalgias and arthralgias of large joints occurred in 3.8% of patients treated with a fluoroquinolone versus 0.4% of controls who received other antibiotics (odds ratio = 3.7). The musculoskeletal adverse effect was evident during the first week of therapy, but was transient. The risk of this adverse effect was greatest with pefloxacin, a quinolone not available in the United States.[171] In a review of database-assessed claims, <1% of 6,000 fluoroquinolone-treated children experienced tendon or joint disorders.[172] The fluoroquinolone-induced arthropathy was judged not a permanent adverse effect based on the absence of MRI changes in children who received fluoroquinolones for a prolonged period for the treatment of cystic fibrosis.[173,174] K.P. has a complicated UTI with a multiresistant organism. The use of ciprofloxacin for K.P. in this situation is reasonable, despite the potential for toxicity to cartilage. Table 96-8 lists clinical situations when fluoroquinolones can be considered on the basis of clinical and literature support. Nevertheless, the use of fluoroquinolones in children should not be encouraged for common childhood infections because of this adverse effect and because of the need to discourage the development of bacterial resistance to these drugs, particularly when first- and second-line alternatives are available. Although nalidixic acid was not associated with arthropathy in one study when used for the treatment of recurrent UTIs, this drug has not been as effective as others for the treatment of UTIs (Chapter 64: Urinary Tract Infections).[175]

REFERENCES

1. Bradley RH, Vandell DL. Child care and the well-being of children. *Arch Pediatr Adolesc Med* 2007;161:669.
2. Hedley JO. Otitis Media. *N Engl J Med* 2002;347:1169
3. Zhou F et al. Trends in acute otitis media-related health care utilization by privately insured young children in the United States, 1997–2004. *Pediatrics* 2008;121:253.
4. Winther B et al. Temporal relationships between colds, upper respiratory viruses detected by polymerase chain reaction, and otitis media in young children followed through a typical cold season? *Pediatrics* 2007;119:1069.
5. Singh A, Bond BL. Evidence-based emergency medicine/rational clinical examination abstract. Does this child have acute otitis media? *Ann Emerg Med* 2006;47113.
6. Alper CM et al. Temporal relationships for cold-like illnesses and otitis media in sibling pairs. *Pediatr Infect Dis J* 2007;26:778.
7. Chonmaitree T et al. Viral upper respiratory tract infection and otitis media complication in young children. *Clin Infect Dis* 2008;46:815.
8. Mangione-Smith R et al. Ruling out the need for antibiotics: are we sending the right message? *Arch Pediatr Adolesc Med* 2006;160:945.
9. Kuzujanakis M et al. Correlates of parental antibiotic knowledge, demand, and reported use. *Ambul Pediatr* 2003;3:203.
10. Goossens H et al. Outpatient antibiotic use in Europe and association with resistance: a cross-national database study. *Lancet* 2005;365:579.
11. Chung A et al. Effect of antibiotic prescribing on antibiotic resistance in individual children in primary care: prospective cohort study *BMJ* 2007;335:429.
12. McCaig LF et al. Antimicrobial drug prescription in ambulatory care settings, United States, 1992–2000. *Emerg Infect Dis* 2003;9:432.
13. Vanderweil SG et al. Declining antibiotic prescriptions for upper respiratory infections, 1993–2004. *Acad Emerg Med* 2007;14:366.
14. Zuckerman IH et al. Concurrent acute illness and comorbid conditions poorly predict antibiotic use in upper respiratory tract infections: a cross-sectional analysis. *BMC Infect Dis* 2007;30:47.
15. Revai K et al. Association of nasopharyngeal bacterial colonization during upper respiratory tract infection and the development of acute otitis media. *Clin Infect Dis* 2008;46:e34.
16. Chandler SM et al. Consistency of diagnostic criteria for acute otitis media: a review of the recent literature. *Clin Pediatr (Phila)* 2007;46:99.
17. Marchant CD et al. Measuring the comparative efficacy of antibacterial agents for acute otitis media: the "Pollyanna phenomenon." *J Pediatr* 1992;120:72.
18. Spiro DM, Arnold DH. The concept and practice of a wait-and-see approach to acute otitis media. *Curr Opin Pediatr* 2008;20:72.

18a. Rovers MM et al. Predictors of pain and/or fever at 3 to 7 days for children with acute otitis media not treated initially with antibiotics. A meta-analysis of individual patient data. *Pediatrics* 2007;119:579.

19. Fischer T et al. National trends in emergency department antibiotic prescribing for children with acute otitis media, 1996–2005. *Acad Emerg Med* 2007;14:1172.
20. Leibovitz E et al. Is bilateral acute otitis media clinically different than unilateral acute otitis media? *Pediatr Infect Dis J* 2007;26:589.
21. McCormick DP et al. Laterality of acute otitis media: different clinical and microbiologic characteristics. *Pediatr Infect Dis J* 2007;26:583.
22. Powers JH. Diagnosis and Treatment of Acute Otitis Media: Evaluating the Evidence. *Infect Dis Clin North Am* 2007;21:409.
23. Hambidge SJ et al. Safety of trivalent inactivated influenza vaccine in children 6 to 23 months old. *JAMA* 2006;296:1990.
24. Emonts M et al. Genetic polymorphisms in immunoresponse genes TNFA, IL6, IL10, and TLR4 are associated with recurrent acute otitis media. *Pediatrics* 2007;120:814.
25. Patel JA et al. Association of proinflammatory cytokine gene polymorphisms with susceptibility to otitis media. *Pediatrics* 2006;118:2273. Erratum in: Pediatrics 2007;119:1270.
26. Satran R et al. Clinical/otologic score before and during treatment of acute otitis media. *Acta Paediatr* 2007;96:1814.
27. Palmu AA et al. Association of clinical signs and symptoms with bacterial findings in acute otitis media. *Clin Infect Dis* 2004;38:234.
28. Pichichero ME. Evolving shifts in otitis media pathogens: relevance to a managed care organization. *Am J Manag Care* 2005;11:S192.
29. Umapathy D et al. A community based questionnaire study on the association between symptoms suggestive of otitis media with effusion, rhinitis and asthma in primary school children. *Int J Pediatr Otorhinolaryngol* 2007;71:705.
30. Ford-Jones EL et al. Microbiologic findings and risk factors for antimicrobial resistance at myringotomy for tympanostomy tube placement—a prospective study of 601 children in Toronto. *Int J Pediatr Otorhinolaryngol* 2002;66:227.
31. Leibovitz E et al. Recurrent acute otitis media occurring within one month from completion of antibiotic therapy: relationship to the original pathogen. *Pediatr Infect Dis J* 2003;22:209.
32. Pichichero ME, Casey JR. Emergence of a multiresistant serotype 19A pneumococcal strain not included in the 7-valent conjugate vaccine as an otopathogen in children. *JAMA* 2007;298:1772.
33. Segal N et al. Acute otitis media caused by Streptococcus pyogenes in children. *Clin Infect Dis* 2005;41:35.
34. Coticchia JM, Dohar JE. Methicillin-resistant *Staphylococcus aureus* otorrhea after tympanostomy tube placement. *Arch Otolaryngol Head Neck Surg* 2005;131:868.
35. Roddy MG et al. Pediatric mastoiditis in the pneumococcal conjugate vaccine era: symptom duration guides empiric antimicrobial therapy. *Pediatr Emerg Care* 2007;23:779.
36. Brook I, Gober AE. Frequency of recovery of pathogens from the nasopharynx of children with acute maxillary sinusitis before and after the introduction of vaccination with the 7-valent pneumococcal vaccine. *Int J Pediatr Otorhinolaryngol* 2007;71:575.

37. Piglansky L et al. Bacteriologic and clinical efficacy of high dose amoxicillin for therapy of acute otitis media in children. *Pediatr Infect Dis J* 2003;22:405.
38. Bauchner H et al. Effectiveness of Centers for Disease Control and Prevention recommendations for outcomes of acute otitis media. *Pediatrics* 2006;117:1009.
39. Leibovitz E et al. Bacteriologic and clinical efficacy of one day vs. three day intramuscular ceftriaxone for treatment of nonresponsive acute otitis media in children. *Pediatr Infect Dis J* 2000;19:1040.
40. Block SL et al. Comparative safety and efficacy of cefdinir vs. amoxicillin/clavulanate for treatment of suppurative acute otitis media in children. *Pediatr Infect Dis J* 2000;19:S159.
41. Block SL et al. Efficacy, tolerability, and parent reported outcomes for cefdinir vs. high-dose amoxicillin/clavulanate oral suspension for acute otitis media in young children. *Curr Med Res Opin* 2006;22:1839.
42. Canafax DM et al. Amoxicillin middle ear fluid penetration and pharmacokinetics in children with acute otitis media. *Pediatr Infect Dis J* 1998;17:149.
43. Harrison CJ, Welch DF. Middle ear effusion amoxicillin concentrations in acute otitis media. *Pediatr Infect Dis J* 1998;17:657.
44. Cheung BW et al. The chinchilla microdialysis model for the study of antibiotic distribution to middle ear fluid. *AAPS J* 2006;8:E41.
45. Johnston BC et al. Probiotics for the prevention of pediatric antibiotic-associated diarrhea. *Cochrane Database Syst Rev* 2007;18:CD004827.
46. Ho D et al. The relationship between acute mastoiditis and antibiotic use for acute otitis media in children. *Arch Otolaryngol Head Neck Surg* 2008;134:45.
47. Gums JG et al. Oseltamivir and influenza-related complications, hospitalization and healthcare expenditure in healthy adults and children. *Expert Opin Pharmacother* 2008;9:151.
48. Linder JA et al. Antibiotic treatment of children with sore throat. *JAMA* 2005;294:2315.
49. Mangione-Smith R et al. Measuring the quality of care for group A streptococcal pharyngitis in 5 U.S. health plans. *Arch Pediatr Adolesc Med* 2005;159:491.
50. Park SY et al. Clinicians management of children and adolescents with acute pharyngitis. *Pediatrics* 2006;117;1871.
51. Hahn RG et al. Evaluation of poststreptococcal illness. *Am Fam Physician* 2005;71:1949.
52. Abdel-Haq NM et al. Retropharyngeal abscess in children: the emerging role of group A beta hemolytic streptococcus. *South Med J* 2006;99:927.
53. Alcaide ML, Bisno AL. Pharyngitis and epiglottitis. *Infect Dis Clin North Am* 2007;21:449.
54. Mirza A et al. Throat culture is necessary after negative rapid antigen detection tests. *Clin Pediatr* 2007;46:241.
55. Casey JR, Pichichero ME. The evidence base for cephalosporin superiority over penicillin in streptococcal pharyngitis. *Diagn Microbiol Infect Dis* 2007;57(3 Suppl):39S.
56. Casey JR, Pichichero ME. Higher dosages of azithromycin are more effective in treatment of group A streptococcal tonsillopharyngitis. *Clin Infect Dis* 2005;40:1748.
57. Burnett AM, Domachowske JB. Therapeutic considerations for children with invasive group a streptococcal infections: a case series report and review of the literature. *Clin Pediatr (Phila)* 2007;46:550.
58. Wright AD, Liebelt EL. Alternating antipyretics for fever reduction in children: an unfounded practice passed down to parents from pediatricians. *Clin Pediatr (Phila)* 2007;46:146.
59. Lesko SM et al. Invasive group A streptococcal infection and nonsteroidal antiinflammatory drug use among children with primary varicella. *Pediatrics* 2001;107:1108.
60. Byington CL et al. Impact of the pneumococcal conjugate vaccine on pneumococcal parapneumonic empyema. *Pediatr Infect Dis J* 2006;25:250.
61. Chuang YY et al. Toxic shock syndrome in children: epidemiology, pathogenesis, and management. *Pediatr Drugs* 2005;7:11.
62. Casey JR, Pichichero ME. Meta-analysis of cephalosporin versus penicillin treatment of group A streptococcal tonsillopharyngitis in children. *Pediatrics* 2004;113:866.
63. Casey JR, Pichichero ME. Symptomatic relapse of group A beta-hemolytic streptococcal tonsillopharyngitis in children. *Clin Pediatr (Phila)* 2007;46:307.
64. Brook I. Overcoming penicillin failures in the treatment of Group A streptococcal pharyngotonsillitis. *Int J Pediatr Otorhinolaryngol* 2007;71:1501.
65. Kikuta H et al. Efficacy of antibiotic prophylaxis for intrafamilial transmission of group A beta-hemolytic streptococci. *Pediatr Infect Dis J* 2007;26:139.
66. Brook I. Cephalosporins in overcoming beta-lactamase-producing bacteria and preservation of the interfering bacteria in the treatment of otitis, sinusitis and tonsillitis. *Expert Rev Anti Infect Ther* 2007;5:939.
67. Zimbelman J et al. Improved outcome of clindamycin compared with beta-lactam antibiotic treatment for invasive Streptococcus pyogenes infection. *Pediatr Infect Dis J* 1999;18:1096.
68. Schrage B et al. Different preparations of intravenous immunoglobulin vary in their efficacy to neutralize streptococcal superantigens: implications for treatment of streptococcal toxic shock syndrome. *Clin Infect Dis* 2006;43:743.
69. Sonnappa S, Jaffe A. Treatment approaches for empyema in children. *Paediatr Respir Rev* 2007;8:164.
70. Li ST, Gates RL. Primary operative management for pediatric empyema: decreases in hospital length of stay and charges in a national sample. *Arch Pediatr Adolesc Med* 2008;162:44.
71. Cherry JD. Croup. *N Engl J Med* 2008;358:384.
72. Argent AC et al. The mechanics of breathing in children with acute severe croup. *Intensive Care Med* 2008;34:324.
73. Hopkins A et al. Changing epidemiology of life-threatening upper airway infections: the reemergence of bacterial tracheitis. *Pediatrics* 2006;118:1418.
74. Kwong K et al. Recurrent croup presentation, diagnosis, and management. *Am J Otolaryngol* 2007;28:401.
75. Bjornson CL, Johnson DW. Croup-treatment update. *Pediatr Emerg Care* 2005;21:863.
76. Moore M, Little P. Humidified air inhalation for treating croup: a systematic review and meta-analysis. *Fam Pract* 2007;24:295.
77. Argent AC et al. The effect of epinephrine by nebulization on measures of airway obstruction in patients with acute severe croup. *Intensive Care Med* 2008;34:138.
78. Russell K et al. Glucocorticoids for croup. The Cochrane Database of Systematic Reviews 2004. Issue 1. Art No.: CD001955.pub2. DOI: 10.1002/14651858.CD001955.pub2.
79. Bjornson CL et al. A randomized trial of a single dose of oral dexamethasone for mild croup. *N Engl J Med* 2004;351:1306.
80. Chub-Uppakarn S, Sangsupawanich P. A randomized comparison of dexamethasone 0.15 mg/kg versus 0.6 mg/kg for the treatment of moderate to severe croup. *Int J Pediatr Otorhinolaryngol* 2007;71:473.
81. Donaldson D et al. Intramuscular versus oral dexamethasone for the treatment of moderate-to-severe croup: a randomized, double-blind trial. *Acad Emerg Med* 2003;10:16.
82. Fifoot AA, Ting JY. Comparison between single-dose oral prednisolone and oral dexamethasone in the treatment of croup: a randomized, double-blinded clinical trial. *Emerg Med Australas* 2007;19:51.
83. Geelhoed GC. Budesonide offers no advantage when added to oral dexamethasone in the treatment of croup. *Pediatr Emerg* Care2005;21:359.
84. Sangare et al. Hospitalization For respiratory syncytial virus among California infants: disparities related to race, insurance, and geography. *J Pediatr* 2006;149:373.
85. American Academy of Pediatrics Subcommittee on Diagnosis and Management of Bronchiolitis. Diagnosis and management of bronchiolitis. *Pediatrics* 2006;118:1774.
86. Brownlee JW, Turner RB. New developments in the epidemiology and clinical spectrum of rhinovirus infections. *Curr Opin Pediatr* 2008;20:67.
87. Janssen R et al. Genetic susceptibility to respiratory syncytial virus bronchiolitis is predominantly associated with innate immune genes. *J Infect Dis* 2007;196:826.
88. Leader S, Kohlhase K. Recent trends in severe respiratory syncytial virus (RSV) among U.S. infants, 1997–2000. *J Pediatr* 2003;143:S127.
89. Purcell K, Fergie J. Lack of usefulness of an abnormal white blood cell count for predicting a concurrent serious bacterial infection in infants and young children hospitalized with respiratory syncytial virus lower respiratory tract infection. *Pediatr Infect Dis J* 2007;26:311.
90. Levine DA et al. Risk of serious bacterial infection in young febrile infants with respiratory syncytial virus infections. *Pediatrics* 2004;113:1728.
91. Thorburn K et al. High incidence of pulmonary bacterial co-infection in children with severe respiratory syncytial virus (RSV) bronchiolitis. *Thorax* 2006;61:611.
92. Antonyrajah B, Mukundan D. Fever without apparent source on clinical examination. *Curr Opin Pediatr* 2008;20:96.
93. Christakis DA et al. Variation in inpatient diagnostic testing and management of bronchiolitis. *Pediatrics* 2005;115:878.
94. Gadomski AM, Bhasale AL. Bronchodilators for bronchiolitis. *Cochrane Database Syst Rev* 2006;3:CD001266.
95. Amirav I et al. Aerosol delivery in respiratory syncytial virus bronchiolitis: hood or face mask? *J Pediatr* 2005;147:627.
96. Wainwright C et al. A multicenter, randomized, double-blind, controlled trial of nebulized epinephrine in infants with acute bronchiolitis. *N Engl J Med* 2003;349:27.
97. Tal G. Hypertonic saline/epinephrine treatment in hospitalized infants with viral bronchiolitis reduces hospitalization stay: 2 years experience. *Isr Med Assoc J* 2006;8:169.
98. Teeratakulpisarn J et al. Efficacy of dexamethasone injection for acute bronchiolitis in hospitalized children: a randomized, double-blind, placebo-controlled trial. *Pediatr Pulmonol* 2007;42:433.
99. Corneli HM et al. A multicenter, randomized, controlled trial of dexamethasone for bronchiolitis. *N Engl J Med* 2007;357:331.
100. Hall CB. Therapy for bronchiolitis: when some become none. *N Engl J Med* 2007;357:402.
101. Boogaard R et al. Recombinant human deoxyribonuclease in infants with respiratory syncytial virus bronchiolitis. *Chest* 2007;131:788.
102. Purcell K, Fergie J. Driscoll Children's Hospital respiratory syncytial virus database: risk factors, treatment and hospital course in 3308 infants and young children, 1991 to 2002. *Pediatr Infect Dis J* 2004;23:418.
103. Tahan F et al. Clarithromycin in the treatment of RSV bronchiolitis: a double-blind, randomized, placebo-controlled trial. *Eur Respir J* 2007;29:91.
104. Parnes C et al. Palivizumab prophylaxis of respiratory syncytial virus disease in 2000–2001: results from The Palivizumab Outcomes Registry. *Pediatr Pulmonol* 2003;35:484.

105. Mansbach J et al. Evaluation of compliance with palivizumab recommendations in a multicenter study of young children presenting to the emergency department with bronchiolitis. *Pediatr Emerg Care* 2007;23:362.
106. Simoes EA et al. Palivizumab prophylaxis, respiratory syncytial virus, and subsequent recurrent wheezing. *J Pediatr* 2007;151:34.
107. Wu H. Immunoprophylaxis of RSV infection: advancing from RSV-IGIV to palivizumab and motavizumab. *Curr Top Microbiol Immunol* 2008; 317:103.
108. Chvez-Bueno S et al. Intravenous palivizumab and ribavirin combination for respiratory syncytial virus disease in high-risk pediatric patients. *Pediatr Infect Dis J* 2007;26:1089.
109. Khanna N et al. Respiratory syncytial virus infection in patients with hematological diseases: single-center study and review of the literature. *Clin Infect Dis* 2008;46:402.
110. Wright PF et al. The absence of enhanced disease with wild type respiratory syncytial virus infection occurring after receipt of live, attenuated, respiratory syncytial virus vaccines. *Vaccine* 2007;25:7372.
111. Satou GM et al. Kawasaki disease: diagnosis, management, and long-term implications. *Cardiol Rev* 2007;15:163.
112. Anderson MS et al. Erythrocyte sedimentation rate and C-reactive protein discrepancy and high prevalence of coronary artery abnormalities in Kawasaki disease. *Pediatr Infect Dis* J2001; 20:698.
113. Baer AZ et al. Prevalence of coronary artery lesions on the initial echocardiogram in Kawasaki syndrome. *Arch Pediatr Adolesc Med* 2006; 160:686.
114. Wilder MS et al. Delayed diagnosis by physicians contributes to the development of coronary artery aneurysms in children with Kawasaki syndrome. *Pediatr Infect Dis J* 2007;26:256.
115. Minich LL et al. Delayed diagnosis of Kawasaki disease: what are the risk factors? *Pediatrics* 2007;120:e1434.
116. Newburger JW et al. Diagnosis, treatment, and long-term management of Kawasaki disease. *Circulation* 2004;110:2747.
117. Lang BA et al. Corticosteroid treatment of refractory Kawasaki disease. *J Rheumatol* 2006;33:803.
118. Newburger JW et al. Randomized trial of pulsed corticosteroid therapy for primary treatment of Kawasaki disease. *N Engl J Med* 2007;356:663.
119. Li JS et al. Dosing of clopidogrel for platelet inhibition in infants and young children: Primary Results of the Platelet Inhibition in Children On cLOpidogrel (PICOLO) Trial. *Circulation* 2008;117:553.
120. Chang SL, Shortliffe LD. Pediatric urinary tract infections. *Pediatr Clin North Am* 2006;53:379.
121. Bachur RG, Harper MB. Predictive model for serious bacterial infections among infants younger than 3 months of age. *Pediatrics*. 2001;108:311.
122. Shaw KN et al. Prevalence of urinary tract infection in febrile young children in the emergency department. *Pediatrics* 1998;102:e16.
123. Zorc JJ et al. Clinical and demographic factors associated with urinary tract infection in young febrile infants. *Pediatrics* 2005;116:644.
124. Levine DA et al. Risk of serious bacterial infection in young febrile infants with respiratory syncytial virus infections. *Pediatrics* 2004;113:1728.
125. Byington CL et al. Serious bacterial infections in febrile infants younger than 90 days of age: The importance of ampicillin-resistant pathogens. *Pediatrics* 2003;111:964.
126. Lundstedt AC et al. Inherited susceptibility to acute pyelonephritis: a family study of urinary tract infection. *J Infect Dis* 2007;195:1227.
127. Holmdahl G et al. Self-catheterization during adolescence. *Scand J Urol Nephrol* 2007;41:214.
128. Greenfield SP, Williot P, Kaplan D. Gross hematuria in children: a ten-year review. *Urology* 2007;69:166.
129. Shaikh N et al. Does this child have a urinary tract infection? *JAMA* 2007;298:2895.
130. Bachur RG, Harper MB. Reliability of the urinalysis for predicting urinary tract infections in young febrile children. *Arch Pediatr Adolescent Med* 2001;155:60.
131. Goldman RD et al. What is the risk of bacterial meningitis in infants who present to the emergency department with fever and pyuria? *CJEM* 2003;5:394.
132. Hoberman A et al. Is urine culture necessary to rule out urinary tract infection in young febrile children? *Pediatr Infect Dis J* 1996;15: 304.
133. Kozer E et al. Pain in infants who are younger than 2 months during suprapubic aspiration and transurethral bladder catheterization: a randomized, controlled study. *Pediatrics* 2006;118:e51.
134. Schroeder AR et al. Choice of urine collection methods for the diagnosis of urinary tract infection in young, febrile infants. *Arch Pediatr Adolesc Med* 2005;159:915.
135. McGillivray D et al. A head-to-head comparison: "clean-void" bag versus catheter urinalysis in the diagnosis of urinary tract infection in young children. *J Pediatr* 2005;147:451.
136. Vaillancourt S et al. To clean or not to clean: effect on contamination rates in midstream urine collections in toilet-trained children. *Pediatrics* 2007;119:e1288.
137. Garin EH et al. Diagnostic significance of clinical and laboratory findings to localize site of urinary infection. *Pediatr Nephrol* 2007;22:1002.
138. Tseng MH et al. Does a normal DMSA obviate the performance of voiding cystourethrography in evaluation of young children after their first urinary tract infection? *J Pediatr* 2007;150: 96.
139. Hoberman A et al. Imaging studies after a first febrile urinary tract infection in young children. *N Engl J Med* 2003;348:195.
140. Cheng CH et al. Comparison of urovirulence factors and genotypes for bacteria causing acute lobar nephronia and acute pyelonephritis. *Pediatr Infect Dis J* 2007;26:228.
141. Zhanel GG et al. Antibiotic resistance in outpatient urinary isolates: final results from the North American Urinary Tract Infection Collaborative Alliance (NAUTICA). *Int J Antimicrob Agents* 2005;26:380.
142. Prais D et al. Bacterial susceptibility to oral antibiotics in community acquired urinary tract infection. *Arch Dis Child* 2003;88:215.
143. Abelson Storby K et al. Antimicrobial resistance in *Escherichia coli* in urine samples from children and adults: a 12 year analysis. *Acta Paediatr* 2004;93:487.
144. McLoughlin TG Jr, Joseph MM. Antibiotic resistance patterns of uropathogens in pediatric emergency department patients. *Acad Emerg Med* 2003;10:347.
145. Gaspari RJ et al. Multidrug resistance in pediatric urinary tract infections. *Microb Drug Resist* 2006;12:126.
146. Marcus N et al. Non-*Escherichia coli* versus *Escherichia coli* community-acquired urinary tract infections in children hospitalized in a tertiary center: relative frequency, risk factors, antimicrobial resistance and outcome. *Pediatr Infect Dis J* 2005;24:581.
147. Kanellopoulos TA et al. First urinary tract infection in neonates, infants and young children: a comparative study. *Pediatr Nephrol* 2006;21:1131.
148. Friedman S et al. Clinical and laboratory characteristics of non-*E. coli* urinary tract infections. *Arch Dis Child* 2006;91:845.
149. Kanellopoulos TA, Vassilakos et al. Low bacterial count urinary tract infections in infants and young children. *Eur J Pediatr* 2005164:355.
150. Lutter SA et al. Antibiotic resistance patterns in children hospitalized for urinary tract infections. *Arch Pediatr Adolesc Med* 2005;159:924.
151. Karlowsky JA et al. Fluoroquinolone-resistant urinary isolates of *Escherichia coli* from outpatients are frequently multidrug resistant: results from the North American Urinary Tract Infection Collaborative Alliance-Quinolone Resistance study. *Antimicrob Agents Chemother* 2006;50: 2251.
152. Noel G et al. Fluoroquinolone susceptibility profiles of recent urinary tract isolates obtained from pediatric patients [abstract #282]. 44th Annual Meeting Infectious Disease Society of America, October 2006, Toronto, Canada.
153. Jones ME et al. Rates of antimicrobial resistance among common bacterial pathogens causing respiratory, blood, urine, and skin and soft tissue infections in pediatric patients. *Eur J Clin Microbiol Infect Dis* 2004;23:445.
154. Baumer JH, Jones RW. Urinary tract infection in children, National Institute for Health and Clinical Excellence. *Arch Dis Child Educ Pract Ed* 2007;92:189.
155. Bonsu BK et al. Susceptibility of recent bacterial isolates to cefdinir and selected antibiotics among children with urinary tract infections. *Acad Emerg Med* 2006;13:76.
156. Committee on Infectious Diseases, American Academy of Pediatrics. The use of systemic fluoroquinolones. *Pediatrics* 2006;118:1287.
157. Gauthier M et al. Treatment of urinary tract infections among febrile young children with daily intravenous antibiotic therapy at a day treatment center. *Pediatrics* 2004;114:e469.
158. Keren R, Chan E. A meta-analysis of randomized, controlled trials comparing short- and long-course antibiotic therapy for urinary tract infections in children. *Pediatrics* 2002;109:E70.
159. Oreskovic NM, Sembrano EU. Repeat urine cultures in children who are admitted with urinary tract infections. *Pediatrics* 2007;119:e325.
160. Cheng CH et al. Effective duration of antimicrobial therapy for the treatment of acute lobar nephronia. *Pediatrics* 2006;117:e84.
161. Cohen AL et al. Compliance with guidelines for the medical care of first urinary tract infections in infants: a population-based study. *Pediatrics* 2005;115:1474.
162. Bundy DG. Vesicoureteral reflux. *Pediatr Rev* 2007;28:e6.
163. Jodal U et al. Ten-year results of randomized treatment of children with severe vesicoureteral reflux. Final report of the International Reflux Study in Children. *Pediatr Nephrol* 2006;21:785.
164. Garin EH et al. Clinical significance of primary vesicoureteral reflux and urinary antibiotic prophylaxis after acute pyelonephritis: a multicenter, randomized, controlled study. *Pediatrics* 2006; 117:626.
165. Mattoo TK. Medical management of vesicoureteral reflux. *Pediatr Nephrol* 2007;22:1113.
166. Roussey-Kesler G et al. Antibiotic prophylaxis for the prevention of recurrent urinary tract infection in children with low grade vesicoureteral reflux: results from a prospective randomized study. *J Urol* 2008;179:674.
167. Karpman E, Kurzrock EA. Adverse reactions of nitrofurantoin, trimethoprim and sulfamethoxazole in children. *J Urol* 2004;172:448.
168. Uhari M et al. Adverse reactions in children during long-term antimicrobial therapy. *Pediatr Infect Dis J* 1996;15:404.
169. Williams GJ et al. Long-term antibiotics for preventing recurrent urinary tract infection in children. *Cochrane Database Syst Rev* 2006;3: CD001534.
170. Conway PH et al. Recurrent urinary tract infections in children: risk factors and association with prophylactic antimicrobials. *JAMA* 2007;298: 179.
171. Chalumeau M et al. Pediatric Fluoroquinolone Safety Study Investigators. Fluoroquinolone safety in pediatric patients: a prospective, multicenter, comparative cohort study in France. *Pediatrics* 2003;111:e714.

172. Yee CL et al. Tendon or joint disorders in children after treatment with fluoroquinolones or azithromycin. *Pediatr Infect Dis J* 2002;21:525.
173. Redmond A et al. Oral ciprofloxacin in the treatment of pseudomonas exacerbations of paediatric cystic fibrosis: clinical efficacy and safety evaluation using magnetic resonance image scanning. *J Int Med Res* 1998;26:304.
174. Richard DA et al. Oral ciprofloxacin vs. intravenous ceftazidime plus tobramycin in pediatric cystic fibrosis patients: comparison of antipseudomonas efficacy and assessment of safety with ultrasonography and magnetic resonance imaging. Cystic Fibrosis Study Group. *Pediatr Infect Dis J* 1997;16:572.
175. Schaad UB. Fluoroquinolone antibiotics in infants and children. *Infect Dis Clin North Am* 2005;19:617.
176. Pottumarthy S et al. Susceptibility patterns for amoxicillin/clavulanate tests mimicking the licensed formulations and pharmacokinetic relationships: do the MIC obtained with 2:1 ratio testing accurately reflect activity against beta-lactamase-producing strains of *Haemophilus influenzae* and *Moraxella catarrhalis*? *Diagn Microbiol Infect Dis* 2005;53:225.
177. Soley C et al. An open-label, double tympanocentesis, single-center study of trimethoprim sulfamethoxazole in children with acute otitis media. *Pediatr Infect Dis J* 2007;26:273.
178. Hoberman A et al. Large dosage amoxicillin/clavulanate, compared with azithromycin, for the treatment of bacterial acute otitis media in children. *Pediatr Infect Dis J* 2005;24:525.
179. Starner TD et al. Subinhibitory concentrations of azithromycin decrease nontypeable Haemophilus influenzae biofilm formation and diminish established biofilms. *Antimicrob Agents Chemother* 2008;52:137.
180. Noel GJ et al. A randomized comparative study of levofloxacin versus amoxicillin/clavulanate for treatment of infants and young children with recurrent or persistent acute otitis media. *Pediatr Infect Dis J* 2008;27:483.

CHAPTER 97

Pediatric Nutrition

Michael F. Chicella and Jennifer W. Chow

Adequate nutrition is an essential component of the health maintenance of children, and, in part, has been responsible for the dramatic reduction of infant mortality seen in the United States during the 20th century. Clinical experience has confirmed the value of optimal nutrition in resisting the effects of disease and trauma and in improving the response to medical and surgical therapy. The metabolic demands of rapid growth and maturation, in addition to the low nutritional reserves present during infancy, make the potential benefit of good nutrition to critically ill pediatric patients even greater.

Breast-feeding is the ideal method of feeding an infant up to 1 year of age. When this is not feasible, a wide variety of infant formulas are available that provide appropriate nutrients for infants using the oral route. A pediatric patient who has a functioning intestinal tract, but is unable to achieve adequate oral intake, can be fed enterally using a tube inserted into the stomach or small intestine. Indications for providing specialized enteral nutrition include malnutrition, malabsorption, hypermetabolism, failure to thrive, prematurity, and disorders of absorption, digestion, excretion, or utilization of nutrients.

Despite the many formulas and feeding techniques available, several medical and gastrointestinal (GI) dilemmas arise in infants and children that limit the use of the GI tract for nutritional support. Premature infants with severe respiratory disease, congenital abnormalities of the GI tract, or necrotizing enterocolitis are typical candidates for support with parenteral nutrition (PN). Older children with short bowel syndrome, severe malnutrition, intractable diarrhea, or inflammatory bowel disease have been treated successfully with PN therapy. Pediatric patients receiving chemotherapy for the treatment of malignancies or bone marrow transplant, and children with severe cardiac failure, also have been successfully rehabilitated with PN.

Many disorders that adversely affect nutrient intake or absorption also have an adverse impact on fluid and electrolyte status. Consequently, fluid, electrolyte, and nutrient management should be approached in an integrated manner. This chapter reviews selected aspects of fluid and electrolyte management and nutrition therapy for the pediatric population.

FLUID AND ELECTROLYTE MAINTENANCE

Management of fluid and electrolyte disturbances involves providing normal daily maintenance requirements, and replacing deficits and ongoing losses. To design rational fluid therapy, it is necessary to know the normal composition of body water, and to understand the routes through which water and solutes are lost from the body and the effects of disease and medications on water and electrolytes. Sodium-containing fluids are often referred to as fractions of normal saline (NS) (0.9% NaCl). Normal saline contains 154 mEq/L of sodium chloride.

Requirements

The general recommendations for calculating maintenance fluid, electrolyte, and nutrient requirements on the basis of weight are provided in Table 97-1. These requirements can be altered when fluid and electrolyte losses are increased or when excretion is impaired.

When abnormal fluid losses are present from any of the sources listed in Table 97-2, they must be added to the patient's daily fluid and electrolyte formula. Replacement fluid is generally 1 mL for every 1 mL lost, but can be replaced as 0.5 mL for every 1 mL lost. In general, a solution of one-half NS with 20 mEq of KCl/L is used to replace upper GI tract losses; however, the electrolyte content of GI secretions varies widely. The composition of a replacement fluid can be estimated based on knowledge of the usual electrolyte distribution of the fluid type being lost. Estimates are listed in Table 97-3. If serum electrolyte concentrations are abnormal, indicating that the replacement fluid is not appropriate, a sample of the fluid lost from the patient can be analyzed for electrolyte content, and electrolyte replacement fluid can be individualized.

The requirements for fluid and calories normalized to body weight are much greater in very small children than in older children and adults as can be seen in Table 97-1. This is because infants have a much larger body surface area relative to weight, lose more fluid through evaporation, and dissipate more heat per kilogram than their older counterparts. Furthermore, very low-birth-weight (VLBW) infants cannot concentrate urine and are at increased risk for dehydration if inadequate fluids are provided.

Calculation of Maintenance Fluid and Electrolyte Requirements

1. P.J., a 2-day-old, 3.5-kg term female infant has developed abdominal distention, and her oral feedings have been stopped. Calculate a maintenance fluid and electrolyte prescription for her. Her admission serum electrolytes include the following: sodium (Na), 137 mEq/L (normal, 135–145 mEq/L); potassium (K), 4.2 mEq/L (normal, 3.5–5 mEq/L); chloride (Cl), 105 mEq/L (normal, 102–109 mEq/L); and bicarbonate (HCO_3^-), 23 mEq/L (normal, 22–29 mEq/L). While P.J. receives nothing by mouth (NPO), her fluid and electrolyte needs must be met intravenously. Estimate her requirements.

[SI units: Na, 137 mmol/L (normal, 135–145); K, 4.2 mmol/L (normal, 3.5–5.0); Cl, 105 mmol/L (normal, 102–109); HCO_3^-, 23 mmol/L (normal, 22–29)]

Although a commercially available intravenous (IV) solution will be used, each component of the solution can be calculated separately. Using the guidelines in Table 97-1, P.J.'s maintenance requirements can be estimated as follows:

Fluid	100 mL/kg × 3.5 kg = 350 mL/day or 15 mL/hour	
Sodium	2–4 mEq/kg/day × 3.5 kg = 7–14 mEq/day	(97-A)
Potassium	2–3 mEq/kg/day × 3.5 kg = 7–10.5 mEq/day	

Fluid and electrolyte requirements can be met by infusing a solution of 5% dextrose with one-quarter NS (38 mEq/L) and 20 mEq/L of KCl at 15 mL/hour. This provides 12 mEq (3.4 mEq/kg/day) of NaCl and 7 mEq (2 mEq/kg/day) of KCl in 360 mL (103 mL/kg/day) of fluid per day.

Adjustment for Ultraviolet Light Therapy

2. On the third day of life, P.J.'s indirect bilirubin is 15.2 mg/dL (normal, 0.6–1.05 mg/dL). It is decided to use phototherapy lights to treat her hyperbilirubinemia. How will this modify her maintenance fluid needs?

[SI unit: bilirubin, 259.92 μmol/L (normal, 10.3–179.5)]

Table 97-2 details situations that alter maintenance fluid needs. Phototherapy lights will increase P.J.'s insensible losses and will increase her maintenance fluid needs by 10% to 20%. This can be met by increasing her IV fluid rate to 17 mL/hour (116 mL/kg/day). Although her increased fluid loss will be free from solutes and the solution she is receiving contains sodium and potassium, the electrolytes she receives still will be within the range of normal, and her kidneys should be able to compensate for the small increase.

Dehydration

Clinical Presentation: Vomiting

ACUTE MANAGEMENT

3. H.S., a 2-year-old lethargic girl, is seen in her pediatrician's office with a 2-day history of vomiting and minimal oral intake. Yesterday, she required only three diaper changes instead of her usual eight and has needed only one change today. Her vital signs are as follows: temperature, 39°C; pulse, 140 beats/minute (normal, 80–130 beats/minute); respiratory rate, 30 breaths/minute (normal, 30–35 breaths/minute); and blood pressure (BP), 80/45 mmHg (normal, 80–115 mmHg systolic and 50–80 mmHg diastolic). On physical examination, her eyes appear sunken, her mucous membranes are dry, and her skin is dry and cool to touch. Although she is crying, there are no tears and the skin over her sternum tents when pinched. Her weight today is 11.4 kg; 3 weeks ago, it was 12.9 kg. What do these findings represent? What immediate treatment should be provided?

H.S.'s lethargy, decreased urine output, tearless crying, dry mucous membranes, dry skin with fever, sunken eyes, mild tachycardia with low normal blood pressure, and poor skin turgor are all signs of dehydration. This is consistent with her 2-day history of vomiting and poor intake. Her weight loss of 1.5 kg gives a further clue to the extent of dehydration. Dehydration or fluid loss is determined most accurately by weight loss. Because 1 g of body weight is approximately equal to 1 mL, her fluid deficit is estimated to be 1,500 mL. The percentage dehydration is estimated using the following formula:

$$\%\ \text{Dehydration} = \frac{\text{Normal body weight} - \text{Actual body weight}}{\text{Normal body weight}} \times 100 \qquad (97\text{-}1)$$

If recent weights are unavailable, the extent of dehydration can be approximated from physical findings as described in Table 97-4. Tachycardia and marginal blood pressure dictate

Table 97-1 Daily Parenteral Nutrient Requirements in Children

Nutrient	Weight/Age	Requirement
Macronutrients		
Fluid	<1.5 kg	150 mL/kg
	1.5–2.5 kg	120 mL/kg
	2.5–10 kg	100 mL/kg
	10–20 kg	1,000 mL + 50 mL/kg for each kg >10 kg
	>20 kg	1,500 mL + 20 mL/kg for each kg >20 kg
Calories	Up to 10 kg	100 kcal/kg
	20 kg	1,000 kcal + 50 kcal/kg for each kg >10 kg
	>20 kg	1,500 kcal + 20 kcal/kg for each kg >20 kg
Protein[a]	Infants	2–3 g/kg
	Older children	1.5–2.0 g/kg
	Adolescents and older	1.0–1.5 g/kg
Fat[b]	Infants and children	Initially: 0.5–1 g/kg then increase by 0.5–1 g/kg (maximum of 3 g/kg in preterm neonates, 4 g/kg older infants and children) (≥4% of calories as linoleic acid)
	>50 kg	One 500 mL bottle (100 g fat)
Electrolytes and Minerals[c]		
Sodium	Infants and children	2–4 mEq/kg
Potassium	Infants and children	2–3 mEq/kg
Chloride	Infants and children	2–4 mEq/kg
Magnesium	Preterm and term infants	0.25–0.5 mEq/kg
	Children >1 yr (or >12 kg)	4–12 mEq
Calcium	Preterm and term infants	2–3 mEq/kg
	Children >1 yr (or >12 kg)	10–20 mEq
Phosphorus	Preterm and term infants	1.0–1.5 mmol/kg
	Children >1 yr (or >12 kg)	10–20 mmol
Trace Elements		
Zinc	Preterm Infants	400 mcg/kg
	Term Infants	
	<3 mos	250 mcg/kg
	>3 mos	100 mcg/kg
	Children	50 mcg/kg (up to 5 mg)
Copper	Infants and children	20 mcg/kg (up to 300 mcg)
Manganese	Infants and children	1 mcg/kg (up to 50 mcg)
Chromium	Infants and children	0.2 mcg/kg (up to 5 mcg)
Selenium	Infants and children	2 mcg/kg (up to 80 mcg)

Vitamins	Preterm Infants <2.5 kg (2 mL/kg MVI[e] Pediatric)	Term Infants/Children <11 yrs (5 mL MVI Pediatric)	Children >11 yrs (10 mL MVI-12)
Vitamin A	280 mcg/kg	700 mcg	1 mg
Vitamin D	160 IU/kg	400 IU	200 IU
Vitamin E	2.8 mg/kg	7 mg	10 mg
Vitamin K[d]	80 mcg/kg	200 mcg	None
Thiamine	0.48 mg/kg	1.2 mg	3 mg
Niacin	6.8 mg/kg	17 mg	40 mg
Riboflavin	0.56 mg/kg	1.4 mg	3.6 mg
Pyridoxine	0.4 mg/kg	1 mg	4 mg
Vitamin B_{12}	0.4 mcg/kg	1 mcg	5 mcg
Biotin	8 mcg/kg	20 mcg	60 mcg
Vitamin C	32 mg/kg	80 mg	100 mg
Folic acid	56 mcg/kg	140 mcg	400 mcg

[a] "Infant" amino acids contain histidine, taurine, tyrosine, and cysteine, which are essential in infants but not older patients.

[b] Because linoleic acid represents 54% of the fatty acid in soy bean oil and 77% in safflower oil, 7% to 10% of calories must be provided as fat emulsion. This can be given daily over 24 hours (preferred in patients predisposed to sepsis and preterm infants) or two to three times weekly.

[c] These doses are guidelines and all patients should be evaluated individually for appropriateness of dosing. For example, patients with short bowel syndrome may require large doses of magnesium and patients with renal insufficiency may require none to low amounts of potassium, calcium, phosphorous, and magnesium.

[d] For patients receiving MVI-12, it may be desirable to add vitamin K.

[e] MVI, multivitamin.

Adapted from references 1, 41, 87.

Table 97-2 Situations That Alter Maintenance Fluid Requirements

Situation	Mechanism	Extent of Change (%)
Extreme prematurity	↑Skin losses	Varies
Radiant warmer use	↑Insensible water loss	20–40
Croup tent	↓Evaporative water loss	20–50
Diarrhea or vomiting	↑GI loss	Varies
Fever	↑Insensible water loss	10–15/°C
Renal dysfunction	↑Or ↓renal loss	Varies
Hyperventilation	↑Pulmonary evaporative loss	Varies
Phototherapy for hyperbilirubinemia	↑Insensible water loss	10–20
GI tract suction or ostomy	↑GI loss	Varies
Mechanical ventilation	↓Insensible water loss	20–30

GI, gastrointestinal.

the need for immediate IV rehydration. Normal serum sodium concentration ranges from 135 to 145 mEq/L of sodium; thus, normal saline approximates the sodium concentration of plasma and is often used as a volume expander. In this patient, 10–20 mL/kg of normal saline (12.9 kg × 10–20 mL/kg = 129–258 mL) should be infused as rapidly as possible to establish normal blood pressure. For symptomatic patients, including those with seizures, the serum sodium concentration should be increased acutely only to the degree necessary to abate symptoms.

CALCULATION OF REQUIREMENTS

4. Calculate H.S.'s fluid and electrolyte needs. Her serum electrolyte results were as follows: Na, 128 mEq/L (normal, 135–145 mEq/L); K, 3.1 mEq/L (normal, 3.5–5 mEq/L); Cl, 88 mEq/L (normal, 102–109 mEq/L); and HCO_3^-, 30 mEq/L (normal, 22–29 mEq/L).

[SI units: Na, 128 mmol/L (normal, 135–145); K, 3.1 mmol/L (normal, 3.5–5); Cl, 88 mmol/L (normal, 102–109); HCO_3^-, 30 mmol/L (normal, 22–29)]

In addition to normal maintenance fluids, H.S. must be provided with fluids and electrolytes to replace her deficit secondary to dehydration and compensate for increased insensible water loss because of fever. Each component of the fluid can be calculated separately, using Equations 97-2 to 97-4.

$$\text{Fluid deficit} = \text{Weight loss (kg)} \times 1{,}000\ \text{mL/kg} \quad \textbf{(97-2)}$$

$$\text{Fever adjustment} = 10\% \times \text{Maintenance for each } ^\circ\text{C} > 30^\circ\text{C} \quad \textbf{(97-3)}$$

$$(CD - CO) \times F_d \times \text{Weight} = \text{mEq required} \quad \textbf{(97-4)}$$

where *CD* is the concentration of sodium desired (mEq/L), *CO* is the concentration observed (mEq/L), F_d is the apparent distribution factor as a fraction of body weight (Table 97-5), and weight is the baseline weight before illness (kg). In consideration of both maintenance needs and current deficits, fluid and electrolyte requirements for H.S. would be estimated as follows.

Fluid

Maintenance	1,000 mL + (50 × 2.9) = 1,145 mL	
Fever	2°C × 0.1 (1,145) = 229 mL	**(97-B)**
Deficit	1.5 kg × 1,000 mL/kg = 1,500 mL	
	Total fluid = 2,874 mL	

Sodium

Maintenance	3 mEq/kg × 12.9 kg = 38.7	
Deficit	(135 − 128 mEq/L) × 0.6 L/kg × 12.9 kg = 54.2	**(97-C)**
	Total sodium ~ 93 mEq	

Chloride

H.S. has a mild metabolic alkalosis as evidenced by her serum chloride of 88 mEq/L and her serum bicarbonate of 30 mEq/L. This is most likely because of the loss of hydrogen and chloride in her vomitus. Thus, both the sodium and potassium replacements should be administered as chloride salts.

Potassium

Potassium is primarily an intracellular ion. It moves in and out of cells in exchange for hydrogen ions to maintain a normal blood pH. Therefore, in metabolic alkalosis, the intracellular shift of potassium will decrease the serum potassium concentration. When the pH normalizes, as will occur with rehydration, the hydrogen ions will move intracellularly and the potassium will move extracellularly, thus causing the serum potassium concentration to increase. Additionally, potassium is also excreted by the kidney in exchange for hydrogen ion conservation. These factors make the serum potassium concentration difficult to interpret. Intravascular volume depletion causes hypoperfusion of the kidney and can result in acute renal failure; therefore, the prudent approach is to give no potassium until urine output is clearly established. Then, only maintenance doses of potassium should be administered until a normal acid

Table 97-3 Body Fluid Volumes and Electrolyte Content

Source	Volume (L/day)	Na^+ (mEq/L)	K^+ (mEq/L)	Cl^- (mEq/L)	HCO_3^- (mEq/L)
Salivary glands	1.5 (0.5–2)	10 (2–10)	26 (20–30)	10 (8–18)	30
Stomach	1.5 (0.1–4)	60 (9–116)	10 (0–32)	130 (8–154)	—
Duodenum	(0.1–2)	140	5	80	—
Ileum	3 (0.1–9)	140 (80–150)	5 (2–8)	104 (43–137)	30
Colon	—	60	30	40	—
Pancreas	(0.1–0.8)	140 (113–185)	5 (3–7)	75 (54–95)	115
Bile	(0.05–0.8)	145 (131–164)	5 (3–12)	100 (89–180)	35

Table 97-4 Clinical Signs of Dehydration

Severity	Dehydration (%)	Psyche	Thirst	Mucous Membranes	Tears	Anterior Fontanel	Skin	Urine-Specific Gravity
Mild	<5	Normal	Slight	Normal to dry	Present	Flat	Normal	Slight change
Moderate	6–10	Irritable	Moderate	Dry	±	±	±	Increased
Severe	10–15	Hyperirritable to lethargic	Intense	Parched	Absent	Sunken	Tenting	Greatly increased

base and fluid status are established and the serum potassium can be assessed more accurately. Hence, H.S. should receive approximately 26 to 39 mEq of potassium (2–3 mEq/kg 12.9 kg) once urine flow is established.

ADMINISTRATION OF FLUID REQUIREMENTS

5. How should these calculated needs be given?

Requirements for the first 24 hours of parenteral fluid therapy should provide approximately 2,875 mL of fluid (maintenance fluid, fever replacement, and deficit replacement). In addition to fluid, at least 93 mEq of sodium (maintenance needs and deficit replacement) should be provided in the first 24 hours. It is important to provide sufficient amounts of sodium and water.

Rehydration fluids are usually dispensed in volumes less than the 24-hour requirement. This is to prevent wasting IV fluids caused by changes in electrolyte needs during replacement therapy. Because this patient requires approximately 3 L of fluid, only 1 L would be prepared initially, and this would likely consist of dextrose 5% and 0.2% NS (or greater). Approximately 15 mEq/L of potassium would be added to the next liter of IV solution if the patient had a reasonable urine output.

The infusion rate should be calculated to provide one-third of the daily maintenance fluid plus one-half of the deficit replacement during the first 8 hours. The remainder of the maintenance fluid (adjusted for fever) and deficit replacement should be administered over the next 16 hours. Usually, serum electrolytes are monitored every 6 to 8 hours during rehydration therapy to ensure that appropriate electrolytes are being provided. Usually, the concentration of serum electrolytes is monitored frequently during fluid replacement therapy of deficits. In general, the serum sodium concentration should not be increased >10 to 12 mEq/L/day. After the initial fluid deficits are replaced, the infusion rate of the IV fluid would be decreased to 48 mL/hour (1,152 mL or approximately maintenance fluid rate).

Clinical Presentation: Diarrhea

6. S.B., a 4-month-old, 5.9-kg boy, is seen in his pediatrician's office because of a 4-day history of diarrhea (five to eight large, liquid stools each day). On a well-child visit 4 weeks ago, his weight was 6 kg. Since the onset of diarrhea, he has only been receiving oral rehydration fluids. Physical examination reveals the following: temperature, 39.8°C; pulse, 110 beats/minute (normal, 80–160 beats/minute); respirations, 45 breaths/minute (normal, 20–40 breaths/minute); and BP, 100/58 mmHg (normal, 75–105 mmHg systolic and 40–65 mmHg diastolic). His skin is pale, warm, and dry. He is very irritable, and his mucous membranes are dry. S.B.'s serum electrolytes are as follows: Na, 159 mEq/L (normal, 135 to 145 mEq/L); K, 3.3 mEq/L (normal, 3.5–5.0 mEq/L); Cl, 114 mEq/L (normal, 102–109 mEq/L); and HCO_3^-, 12 mEq/L (normal, 22–29 mEq/L). Correlate S.B.'s history and physical findings with the reported laboratory values.

[SI units: Na, 159 mmol/L (normal, 135–145); K, 3.3 mmol/L (normal, 3.5–5.0); Cl, 114 mmol/L (normal, 102–109); HCO_3^-, 12 mmol/L (normal, 22–29)]

Table 97-5 Electrolytes and Apparent Distribution

Electrolyte	F_d (L/kg)
Sodium	0.6–0.7
Bicarbonate	0.4–0.5
Chloride	0.2–0.3

F_d, apparent distribution factor as a fraction of body weight.

Diarrheal fluid losses commonly contain high concentrations of bicarbonate, accounting for S.B.'s metabolic acidosis. This, in turn, has resulted in a rapid respiratory rate as the body attempts to compensate for the acidosis by eliminating carbon dioxide. The increased insensible water losses of fever and tachypnea have resulted in the loss of water in excess of sodium, producing hypernatremia.

ACUTE MANAGEMENT

7. How will S.B.'s management differ from that of H.S. (see Questions 3–5)?

Unlike H.S., S.B. has relatively normal vital signs and will not require rapid fluid replacement to correct hypotension. Hypernatremia in S.B. indicates fluid losses in excess of sodium and this should be corrected. With hypernatremia, the central nervous system (CNS) increases intracellular osmolarity load to prevent intracellular dehydration of cells in the CNS. Rapid correction of hypernatremia can cause excessive movement of water into the cells of the CNS and has been associated with seizures. Therefore, S.B.'s fluid and electrolyte deficits should be corrected over 2 to 3 days at a consistent rate, rather than rapidly. In general, serum sodium should not be decreased >2 mEq/hour (maximum, 15 mEq/L/day).

CALCULATION OF REQUIREMENTS

8. Estimate S.B.'s fluid and electrolyte requirements to correct his deficits.

S.B.'s requirements are estimated using the same methods described in Question 4. First, the approximate extent of dehydration must be estimated. S.B.'s weight of 6 kg at the time of his well-child visit at 3 months of age was at the 50th percentile. If his growth has continued at this rate, his current pre-illness weight should be approximately 6.5 kg. This weight should be used to calculate his maintenance requirements. Thus, his water deficit is approximately 0.6 L, or 9%. Using this approximation, his fluid and electrolyte requirements can be estimated as follows.

Fluid

Maintenance	6.5×100 mL/kg = 650 mL/24 hour	
Fever	2.8°C × 0.1 (650 mL) = 182 mL/24 hour	(97-D)
Deficit	600 mL/3 days = 200 mL/24 hour	
	Total daily needs = 1,032 mL or 43 mL/hour	

Sodium

Maintenance	3 mEq/kg × 6.5 kg = 19.5 mEq/24 hr	
Deficit	This is calculated at total body deficit (normal – actual)	
Normal	145 mEq/L × 0.6 L/kg × 6.5 kg = 566 mEq	(97-E)
Actual	159 mEq/L × 0.6 L/kg × 5.9 = 563 mEq	
Deficit	= 3 mEq	
	or 1 mEq/day	

Potassium

As noted in Question 4, the serum potassium value of 3.3 mEq/L may not be indicative of S.B.'s total body potassium status. A metabolic acidosis in S.B. should have facilitated the movement of hydrogen ions into the cells and the movement of potassium from the intracellular to the extracellular space. Thus, the serum potassium of 3.3 mEq/L probably indicates a total body deficit. Therefore, a maintenance potassium dosage of 13 to 20 mEq/day (~2 to 3 mEq/kg) of potassium should be given. Serum electrolytes should be measured every 8 to 12 hours and the intake of all electrolytes should be readjusted based on the results.

Bicarbonate

With metabolic acidosis, bicarbonate should be administered as well. No maintenance amount is customarily given, but deficit replacement is calculated in a manner similar to that used for sodium (Table 97-5). The volume of distribution of bicarbonate is 0.5 L/kg. For S.B. the bicarbonate deficit is as follows:

$$\begin{aligned}\text{Calculated Deficit Requirment} &= (\text{Normal} - \text{Actual}) \times \text{Vd} \times \text{Wt}\\ &= (23 - 12)\ \text{mEq/L} \times 0.5\ \text{L/kg} \times 65\ \text{kg}\\ &= 36\ \text{mEq}\end{aligned} \qquad \text{(97-F)}$$

Initially, about half this amount should be replaced over the first 8 to 12 hours. His serum electrolytes then should be reassessed, and the dosages adjusted accordingly. The entire bicarbonate deficit need not be replaced at once because other compensatory mechanisms will contribute to endogenous bicarbonate sparing.

REPLACEMENT FLUID COMPOSITION

9. Recommend an appropriate replacement fluid for S.B.'s therapy.

S.B.'s fluid and electrolyte maintenance requirements and deficits should be corrected with dextrose 5% and approximately 0.2% NS with half as the chloride salt and half as $NaHCO_3$. An infusion of this solution at 43 mL/hour should correct approximately half the calculated fluid and bicarbonate deficits within 24 hours in addition to his normal daily doses. After he urinates, 15 mEq/L KCl can be added to the next liter of solution to provide approximately 2.6 mEq/kg/day to this patient. The concentration of serum electrolytes should be measured often and the concentration of electrolytes in the replacement fluid should be adjusted every 8 to 12 hours based on laboratory results. The amount of fluid replacement should be modified based on whether this patient's diarrhea has resolved and fever has subsided.

ADMINISTRATION OF REQUIREMENTS

10. By what route should the fluid calculated above be administered?

Rehydration of the dehydrated patient may be achieved by either the oral or intravenous route. In some patients, vomiting may preclude effective oral rehydration. If the losses are diarrheal and no problem with vomiting exists, the oral route may be a cost-effective alternative to the parenteral route. Various solutions have been used to rehydrate children orally. In an asymptomatic dehydrated child, the sodium concentration of an oral rehydration fluid should contain at least 70 mEq/L of sodium.[2–4]

The composition of several products is shown in Table 97-6. A glucose concentration of 2% optimizes water and electrolyte absorption from the GI tract[5]; more concentrated glucose solutions can worsen rather than ameliorate diarrhea. Use of the oral route and the more concentrated sodium solutions may allow safe rehydration of hypernatremic dehydration in a shorter time frame than the 2 to 3 days previously noted.[5,6]

S.B.'s output must be measured to account for ongoing fluid loss. This often is accomplished by weighing the baby's diapers when they are dry and again when they are full. Composition of additional replacement fluids can be determined by using the average composition of the patient's losses (Table 97-3). As an alternative, the composition of the losses can be determined by actual laboratory measurement. If prolonged therapy is necessary, specific analyses are recommended because of the wide range of normal values for diarrheal stool and other GI tract fluids. Because frequent adjustments may be necessary, replacement fluid should be administered separately if PN is being used as a maintenance solution.

INFANT NUTRITION

Growth assessment is an important focus of pediatric health care during the first year of life. With the exception of the intrauterine period, the most rapid growth occurs during the

Table 97-6 Composition of Oral Rehydration Products

Product	Na^+ (mEq/L)	K^+ (mEq/L)	Cl (mEq/L)	Bicarbonate Source (mEq/L)	Carbohydrate (%)
Gastrolyte	90	20	80	30 citrate	2
Rehydrate	75	20	65	30 citrate	2.5
Lytren	50	25	45	30 citrate	2
Pedialyte	45	20	35	30 citrate	2.5
WHO salts	90	20	80	30 bicarbonate	2

WHO, World Health Organization.

first year. On average, a normally growing infant gains approximately 30 g/day. Typically, healthy infants weigh approximately three times their birth weight by their first birthday. Caloric requirements can be estimated using the formula provided in Table 97-1.

The American Academy of Pediatrics (AAP) has suggested that infant feeding be divided into three stages.[7] In the nursing period, only liquids are provided. During the transitional period, solid foods are introduced, but human milk, or commercially prepared infant formula, still provides the major source of the infant's caloric and nutrient supply. In the modified adult period, most nutrition is derived from the solid foods consumed by other household members.

At birth, the human GI tract is adapted for the consumption of a human milk-based diet. Intestinal lactase is present from 36 weeks' gestation and exhibits its maximal activity during infancy. Pancreatic amylase secretion is low, and the bile salt pool is decreased relative to older persons, resulting in decreased fat absorption.[8] Human milk provides nutrients in their most usable form for the developing GI tract.

Human Milk Feeding

11. M.E.'s mother will breast-feed her infant. What are the nutritional implications of this decision for M.E.?

Human milk is the ideal food for a human infant. There are three phases to human milk production. During the first 5 days of lactation, a viscous, yellow liquid known as *colostrum* is produced. Colostrum is rich in protein, minerals, and other substances (e.g., immunoglobulins). During the next 5 days, transitional milk is produced; in the last phase, mature human milk is produced. The exact nutritional content of human milk varies from mother to mother; however, mature human milk provides sufficient protein, minerals, and calories regardless of the mother's nutritional status.[9] Mature human milk generally provides 70 kcal/100 mL and fat accounts for >50% of the caloric content.[10] The fat in human milk is highly digestible and absorbable.[11] An additional 40% of calories is provided as carbohydrates, primarily in the form of lactose, and the remaining 10% is provided as protein. Whey and casein are the two primary proteins in mature human milk, with whey being the major protein component (whey-to-casein ratio of 55:45).[8] Human milk is of such biologic quality and bioavailability that adequate growth can be attained with a lower overall intake of protein than is provided by commercially prepared infant formulas, which contain lower whey-to-casein ratios.[9,11]

The iron content of human milk is inadequate for term infants; however, supplementation generally is unnecessary in the breast-fed infant.[12] Regardless of maternal status, the vitamin D and fluoride contents of human milk are inadequate. Thus, M.E. will require 400 IU of vitamin D and 0.25 mg/day of fluoride while she is exclusively breast-fed.[9,13]

12. Aside from nutrients, what other benefits are associated with human milk and breast-feeding?

Human milk provides the infant with protection against a wide variety of infectious diseases, including otitis media, diarrhea, pneumonia, and bronchiolitis. Evidence further suggests that human milk provides protection against noninfectious disorders, such as allergies, inflammatory bowel disease, insulin-dependent diabetes mellitus, and sudden infant death syndrome.[14] Human milk contains immunologically active cellular components and antibodies. These include secretory IgA, both T- and B-lymphocytes, macrophages, and neutrophils.[9,11] The lipases and amylase present in human milk may facilitate digestion of fat and carbohydrates in the still developing GI tract. Proteins present in human milk serve as carriers for trace minerals and facilitate their absorption.[9] Oligosaccharides and glycopeptides may promote the colonization of the GI tract by *Lactobacilli* and decrease colonization by *Bacteroides, Clostridia,* enterococci, and gram-negative rods, all of which may be pathogenic.[11]

13. What potential complications are associated with breast-feeding? What instructions should be given to M.E.'s mother?

Complications associated with breast-feeding are few; however, there are some potential problems. "Breast milk jaundice" associated with an indirect (unconjugated) hyperbilirubinemia can occur in the breast-fed infant during the first week of life, and generally resolves by the fourth week of life. Although the infant's skin, sclera, and palate become yellow, this is generally not a dangerous condition. Nevertheless, if the bilirubin level becomes too high, the infant could develop an encephalopathy known as kernicterus. Therefore, the mother should temporarily stop breast-feeding and feed the infant formula until the jaundice starts to resolve.

Some maternal infections have the potential to be transmitted to the infant during breast-feeding. Human immunodeficiency virus (HIV) and human T-lymphotropic virus 1 (HTLV-1) can be transmitted via breast milk and, therefore, maternal infections with these viruses are contraindications to breast-feeding.[15] Other viruses, such as herpes simplex virus, can be transmitted if contact with active lesions occurs during breast-feeding. Similarly, some medications taken by the mother are detectable in her breast milk. Only a few agents (e.g., antineoplastics, radiopharmaceuticals, ergot alkaloids, iodides, atropine, lithium, cyclosporine, chloramphenicol, bromocriptine), however, are absolute contraindications to breast-feeding.[15] (See Chapter 46, Obstetric Drug Therapy for additional information concerning the transfer of medications and chemicals into breast milk.)

14. E.R.'s mother decides not to breast-feed her infant. She received a sample package of infant formula at the time of her discharge from the hospital. How are these products prepared and how do they differ from human milk?

Examples of infant formulas and their individual components are provided in Table 97-7. According to AAP guidelines for commercially prepared infant formula composition, formula should provide 20 kcal/oz; osmolality should be between 300 and 400 mOsm/L; protein quantity should be a minimum of 1.8 g/100 kcal and should not exceed 4.5 g/100 kcal; and fat quantity should be between 3.3 and 6 g/100 kcal, supplying between 30% and 54% of calories. Infant formulas generally begin with a cow's milk base; however, intolerance to pure cow's milk has resulted in several modifications. The predominant protein in cow's milk is casein, which is more difficult for infants to digest than the human milk protein, whey. Consequently, infant formulas generally have less casein than cow's

Table 97-7 Infant Formulas and Their Individual Components

Product	Calories per 100 mL	Carbohydrate (g/100 mL)	Carbohydrate Source	Protein (g/100 mL)	Protein Source	Fat (g/100 mL)	Fat Source
Human milk	70	7.2	Lactose	1	Whey 55%, casein 45%	4	Human milk fat
Cow's Milk-Based Formulas							
Enfamil with iron[a]	67	7.5	Lactose	1.4	Whey 50%, casein 50%	3.6	Palm, soy, coconut, safflower oil
Similac with iron[a,b]	68	7.2	Lactose	1.5	Nonfat milk, whey	3.6	Soy, coconut oil
Carnation Good Start	67	7.5	Lactose	1.5	Whey 100%	3.4	Palm, soy, safflower
Soy-Based, Lactose-free Formulas							
Isomil	67	6.8	Corn syrup, sucrose	1.7	Soy, L-methionine	3.7	Soy, coconut, safflower oil
Nursoy	68	6.9	Sucrose	2.1	Soy, L-methionine	3.6	Soy, coconut, safflower oil
ProSoBee	67	7.2	Corn syrup	1.8	Soy, L-methionine	3.7	Palm, soy, coconut, safflower oil
Alsoy	67	7.5	Maltodextrin, sucrose	1.9	Soy, L-methionine	3.3	Palm, soy, coconut, safflower oil
Carnation Follow Up	67	8.8	Corn syrup	1.7	Nonfat milk	2.8	Palm, soy, coconut, safflower oil
Similac Lactose Free	68	7.2	Maltodextrin, sucrose	1.5	Milk protein isolates	3.6	Soy, coconut oil
Enfamil LactoFree	67	7.3	Corn syrup	1.4	Milk protein isolates	3.5	Palm, soy, coconut, safflower oil
Elemental, Premature Infant Formulas							
Alimentum	68	6.7	Sucrose, modified tapioca starch	1.9	Hydrolyzed casein	3.7	MCT, safflower, soy oil
Nutramigen	67	9.1	Corn syrup, modified corn starch	1.9	Hydrolyzed casein	2.6	Corn oil
Pregestimil[b]	67	9.1	Corn syrup, modified corn starch	2.4	Hydrolyzed casein	2.7	MCT, corn, soy oil
NeoCate	67	7.1	Corn syrup	1.9	Free amino acids	2.8	Soy, safflower, coconut oil
Neosure Advance	75	7.7	Maltodextrin, lactose	1.9	Nonfat milk, whey	4.1	MCT, soy, coconut oil
Enfamil Premature with Lipil[b]	67	7.3	Corn syrup, lactose	2	Nonfat milk, whey	3.4	MCT, soy, sunflower, safflower, crypthecodinium, mortierella alpina oil
Similac Special Care[a,b]	68	7.2	Corn syrup, lactose	1.8	Nonfat milk, whey	3.7	MCT, soy, crypthecodinium, mortierella alpina oil

Product	Osmolality (mOsm/L)	Sodium (mEq/100 mL)	Potassium (mEq/100 mL)	Chlorid (mEq/100 mL)	Calcium (mg/100 mL)	Phosphorus (mg/100 mL)	Iron (mg/100 mL)
Human milk	300	0.7	1.3	1.2	32	14	0.03
Cow's Milk-Based Formulas							
Enfamil with iron[a]	300	0.8	1.9	1.2	53	36	1.3
Similac with iron[a,b]	290	1	2.1	1.5	57	37	1.2
Carnation Good Start	265	0.3	0.9	1.1	43	24	1
Soy-Based, Lactose-free Formulas							
Isomil	180	1.3	1.9	1.1	71	51	1.2
Nursoy	296	0.9	1.8	1.1	60	42	1.2
ProSoBee	200	1	2.1	1.5	71	56	1.2
Alsoy 2	200	0.9	2	1.3	71	41	1.2

Continued

Table 97-7 Infant Formulas and Their Individual Components *(Continued)*

Product	Osmolality (mOsm/L)	Sodium (mEq/100 mL)	Potassium (mEq/100 mL)	Chlorid (mEq/100 mL)	Calcium (mg/100 mL)	Phosphorus (mg/100 mL)	Iron (mg/100 mL)
Carnation Follow Up	326	0.4	1.2	1.6	80	54	1.2
Similac Lactose Free	180	0.9	1.8	1.2	57	38	1.2
Enfamil LactoFree	200	0.3	1	1.9	54	37	1.2
Elemental, Premature Infant Formulas							
Alimentum	333	1.3	2	1.6	71	50	1.2
Nutramigen	320	1.4	1.9	1.6	62	42	1.2
Pregestimil[b]	350	1.4	1.9	1.6	62	50	1.2
NeoCate	342	0.9	2.4	1.4	83	62	1.2
Neosure Advance	250	1	2.7	1.6	78	46	1.2
Enfamil Premature with Lipil[b]	260	0.6	0.9	1.7	110	55	1.8
Similac Special Care[a,b]	211	1.3	2.2	1.6	122	68	1.8

[a] Also available as a low iron formula.
[b] Also available as a 24 kcal/oz formula.
MCT, medium-chain triglyceride.

milk, although not to the level of human milk. Casein-to-whey ratios of infant formulas and human milk are compared in Table 97-7. The casein present in cow's milk formulas also may be heat denatured to improve its digestibility. In addition, the fat source in cow's milk is replaced by one of several vegetable oils allowing for easier digestion. Last, the carbohydrate source in cow's milk-based formula is supplemented with lactose or sucrose because the lactose content of cow's milk is only 50% to 70% of that in human milk. Soy-based and protein hydrolysate formulas are available for infants who are intolerant of cow's milk-based formulas.

Soy-based formulas use soybean as the protein source. The soy is heat treated to enhance protein digestibility and improve the bioavailability of some nutrients. Although nutrients, such as methionine, zinc, and carnitine, are still present, their concentrations are relatively low. Therefore, methionine is routinely added to all soy-based formulas by the manufacturer. Zinc and carnitine may not be added and exogenous supplementation may be necessary. Soy-based formulas substitute sucrose, corn syrup, or a combination of the two for lactose as the carbohydrate source. Additionally, soy protein formulas are more expensive than cow's milk-based formulas. The AAP recommends that the use of soy-based formula be limited to patients with primary lactase deficiency (galactosemia); patients with secondary lactose intolerance from enteric infections or other causes; vegetarian families in which animal protein formulas are not desired; and infants who are potentially cow milk protein allergic, but who have not demonstrated clinical manifestations of allergy. Long-term use of soy-based formulas in premature and low birth weight infants should not be recommended. Soy-based formulas have aluminum contamination, and have been associated with the development of rickets. Soy-based formulas are also not recommended for infants with documented allergic reactions to cow's milk protein because of the potential for cross-antigenicity between the two proteins. Soy protein formulas are not recommended for the routine management of colic.[16]

Elemental formulas, made with hydrolysate formulas, are another option for infants who are intolerant of cow's milk-based formulas. The milk proteins (i.e., casein and whey) are heat treated and enzymatically hydrolyzed to enhance digestibility of protein hydrolysate formulas, which are fortified with additional amino acids that are lost during processing. As with soy protein formulas, protein hydrolysates substitute sucrose, tapioca, or corn syrup for lactose as the carbohydrate source. Protein hydrolysate formulas often include significant amounts of medium-chain triglycerides (MCT) because they are easily absorbed. Because the proteins are extensively hydrolyzed, these formulas probably are the least allergenic of the infant formulas and, therefore, may be appropriate for infants with true allergy to cow's milk protein. Nevertheless, prospective studies on the safety of such a substitution in human infants have not been undertaken because it would be unethical to intentionally expose infants with documented allergies to a potential allergen. Protein hydrolysate formulas are the least palatable of the available pediatric formulas, and are more costly than other formulas.[17]

Infant formula is available from the manufacturer in three forms: ready-to-feed form, reconstitutable powder, and concentrated liquid. The ready-to-feed form is the most convenient but also the most expensive. The powder and the concentrated liquid are less expensive; however, both require that predetermined amounts of boiled water be added before use. To save money, some parents will dilute infant formula to a greater extent than is recommended to make the formula last longer. This practice should be discouraged because excessive free water intake by infants <1 year of age may result in hyponatremia and, ultimately, seizures. Similarly, supplementing an infant's diet with free water, for whatever reason, may also result in hyponatremia and seizures and should be discouraged. Recently, use of dry powder formula in the neonatal intensive care unit has been associated with severe bacterial infection. Because of this, dry powder formula in neonatal intensive care patients should be used cautiously.[18]

Introduction of Pure Cow's Milk

15. At her 2-month-old, well-child checkup, E.R. is found to have a hematocrit (Hct) of 33% (normal, 35%–45%). After questioning her mother, the pediatrician learns that E.R. was taken off infant formula 1 month ago and changed to whole cow's milk to decrease food costs. How are these two findings related? What should be added to E.R.'s diet?

[SI unit: hematocrit, 0.35 (normal, 0.35–0.45)]

Pure cow's milk, straight from the dairy counter in the grocery store, is not recommended for infants <1 year of age. Unlike human milk, the iron in cow's milk is present in inadequate concentrations and absorbed poorly from the human GI tract. For this reason, most infant formulas are fortified with iron. Cow's milk has been associated with GI blood loss in infants <140 days of age.[19] When the milk is heated to a higher temperature than the usual pasteurization temperature, as it is in formula preparation, the association of cow's milk with GI bleeding is no longer present; therefore, the component responsible for the blood loss appears to be a heat-labile protein. Furthermore, cow's milk contains excessive amounts of solute that cannot be eliminated by the immature kidney. Also, cow's milk does not contain taurine, an amino acid that is important in retinal development.

To treat E.R.'s anemia, iron should be added to her diet. This can be done by changing back to an iron-fortified infant formula, feeding her an iron-fortified cereal, or giving a therapeutic ferrous sulfate liquid medication. The appropriate iron replacement dose for severe anemia is 4–6 mg/kg/day of elemental iron in divided doses with follow-up of the infant's hemoglobin and hematocrit.

Introduction of Solid Foods

16. At her 4-month-old, well-child checkup, M.E.'s mother asks her pediatrician about the introduction of "baby foods" into M.E.'s diet. When and how should solids be introduced?

Human milk or commercially prepared infant formula provides adequate nutrition for an infant for the first 12 months of life. Introduction of solid foods before the age of 4 months, although common in the past, is discouraged because the younger infant is unprepared to swallow foods other than liquids. Solids (first cereals, then fruits and vegetables) should be introduced when the child has good control of the head and neck movements (i.e., usually at the age of 4–6 months).[7] Preferably, one new food should be introduced at a time, at 1-week intervals, to allow assessment of food allergy.

Therapeutic Formulas

Phenylketonuria

17. L.B. is a 2-week-old infant whose newborn screen is positive for phenylketonuria (PKU). Discuss the concepts behind the production of therapeutic formulas and the dietary management of patients with inborn errors of metabolism. How must L.B.'s diet be modified?

Inborn errors of metabolism are disorders in which an enzyme or its cofactor is absent or insufficient to meet metabolic demands. As a result, one or more precursor compounds in a metabolic pathway can accumulate before the defective step. Correspondingly, one or more metabolic products that normally would have been generated after the defective step in the metabolic pathway are not sufficiently available.

The dietary management of metabolic errors is based on the following strategies:

- Reduce the intake of a precursor compound that cannot be metabolized.
- Supplement the deficient compounds that would have been produced if the normal metabolic pathway had not been blocked.
- Add a substrate that provides an alternative pathway for elimination of an accumulated toxin.

Therapeutic formulas are designed to reduce the intake of precursor compounds or to provide the deficient metabolic end product.

When hydroxylation of phenylalanine to tyrosine does not take place, phenylalanine accumulates in the blood and results in mental retardation. Because PKU has been diagnosed in L.B., his diet should be modified using a formula containing little or no phenylalanine (e.g., Lofenalac, Phenex-1, Phenyl-Free). The tyrosine deficiency of PKU also can be managed by the addition of tyrosine to the phenylalanine-free therapeutic formulas that are available for patients with PKU. When L.B. progresses to solid foods, protein must be provided from predominately phenylalanine-free sources; therefore, patients with PKU should take in only minimal protein from table foods.[20]

Other Metabolic Errors

18. What other metabolic errors present in infancy require a specialized diet?

Other metabolic errors present in infancy include galactosemia (galactose cannot be metabolized to glucose), homocystinuria (methionine is not converted to cysteine), urea cycle disorders (ammonia detoxification is impaired), and maple syrup urine disease (metabolism of the branched chain amino acids, leucine, isoleucine, and valine is blocked).

These metabolic errors are managed by manipulating the diet.[21] In galactosemia, the carbohydrate source should not contain galactose or lactose. In homocystinuria, methionine should be present only in quantities sufficient to meet basic requirements, and cysteine should be supplemented. In the urea cycle disorders, protein often is provided only as essential amino acids, and a high-energy diet is provided to maximize the formation of nonessential amino acids from nitrogen and to minimize ammonia production. In maple syrup urine disease, natural protein is fed in small quantities to provide the minimal requirement of branched chain amino acids, and a branched chain-free supplement is added to provide adequate protein intake.

Route of Administration

Nutritional support using the GI tract is the preferred approach when possible. Enteral nutrition provides several advantages. First, interposition of the GI mucosa between the nutrient supply and the circulation allows absorptive function to provide a homeostatic control. Second, the flow of nutrients from the GI tract to the liver via the portal circulation before reaching the systemic circulation also assists homeostatic control. Third, the lack of enteral nutrition allows normal GI tract flora to overgrow and translocate into the blood, ultimately resulting in bacteremia. Finally, the intestinal mucosa depends on intraluminal absorption for much of its energy supply. Hence, provision of at least a small amount of enteral feeding, referred to as trophic feeds, helps to ensure a healthy GI tract and may facilitate advancement to full enteral feedings at the appropriate time.[22,23]

Normal oral feeding is the most basic method for patients who are willing and able to eat or drink. Patients whose GI motility, structure, and function are normal but whose oral feeding is prevented by an altered state of consciousness, incoordination of sucking and swallowing, or other conditions that prevent adequate oral ingestion can be fed by a GI tube in intermittent boluses or by continuous infusion.

Bolus tube feedings more closely mimic the normal state. They periodically distend the stomach, which aids in gastric secretion and emptying. When bolus tube feeding is undertaken, the volume of formula required to provide sufficient calories for a 24-hour period is administered through the tube in equal aliquots every 2, 3, 4, or 6 hours. The frequency of administration depends on the patient's age, gastric capacity, and the infant's ability to maintain a normal serum glucose concentration between feedings. In general, younger and more premature infants require more frequent feedings. Intolerance to bolus tube feedings can be manifested as diarrhea, gastroesophageal reflux with emesis, or poor motility. Poor motility usually is apparent when large volumes of feeding, referred to as residuals, remain in the stomach when the next feeding is due.

Continuous tube feedings can be given at a constant rate of infusion by pump into the stomach or duodenum when bolus feedings have failed. This approach may be better tolerated by premature infants and children with diarrhea.[24]

Patients with intrinsic GI disease (Table 97-8) or malabsorption may require total or supplemental PN. Concurrent administration of low-volume, trophic enteral feedings may provide important nutrients to the gut mucosa even when the parenteral route supplies all of the necessary systemic nutrients.[22,23] Administration of PN into a peripheral vein is limited to those patients expected to require parenteral feeding only for a short time (i.e., 2 weeks) because the amount of nutrients that can be safely infused peripherally is limited. In patients who require long-term PN, the IV solution is more concentrated and must be administered into a central vein.

Nutritional Assessment

The patient's nutritional status should be assessed before beginning a nutritional support regimen and reassessed at regular intervals during the course of treatment. If the patient previously was well nourished, the goal is to maintain that status until a normal diet can be resumed. In a child who was previously malnourished, an effort should be made to promote "catch-up" growth and to normalize the biochemical nutritional measures. About one-third of children admitted to the hospital are malnourished at the time of their admission.[25] Malnutrition in children is a risk factor for decreased social skills and impaired intellectual development.[26–28]

Table 97-8 Indications for Parenteral Nutrition Support

- Extreme prematurity
- Respiratory distress
- Congenital GI anomalies
  - Duodenal atresia
  - Jejunal atresia
  - Esophageal atresia
  - Tracheoesophageal fistula
  - Pyloric stenosis
  - Congenital webs
  - Hirschsprung's disease
  - Malrotation
  - Volvulus
- Abdominal wall defects
  - Omphalocele (herniation of viscera into the umbilical cord base)
  - Gastroschisis (defect of abdominal wall, any location except umbilical cord)
  - Congenital diaphragmatic hernia
- Necrotizing enterocolitis
- Chronic diarrhea
- Inflammatory bowel disease
- Chylothorax
- Pseudoobstruction
- Megacystic microcolon
- Abdominal trauma involving viscera
- Adverse effects of treating neoplastic disease
  - Radiation enteritis
  - Nausea and vomiting
  - Stomatitis, glossitis, and esophagitis
- Anorexia nervosa
- Cystic fibrosis
- Chronic renal failure
- Hepatic failure
- Metabolic errors

GI, gastrointestinal.

Factors used to determine nutritional status in children include dietary history, weight, height, and visceral protein measurements (e.g., albumin, prealbumin, retinol binding protein, transferrin). Other measurements used in adults, such as 24-hour creatinine excretion, 24-hour nitrogen excretion, and nitrogen balance, are reserved for older children because complete collections of urine are difficult to obtain and because the percentage of nonurea nitrogen present in urine is variable in infants.

Anthropometric Measurements

Height, weight, and head circumference are used to determine nutritional status in infants and children. Standards for these measurements have been derived from pediatric patients in the United States and compiled into graphs referred to as growth curves (http://www.cdc.gov/growthcharts).[29] An individual patient's measurements are compared with the graph of normal values for that specific age group. As prematurely born infants age, a standard growth curve adjusted for prematurity can be used. Using these measurements, comparisons with standards are possible: weight for age, height for age, and weight for height.[29] A weight that is below the fifth percentile for the patient's height is considered an indication of acute malnutrition. Similarly, a height and weight that are below the fifth percentile for the patient's age indicates chronic malnutrition. It is important to consider the height and weight of the child's parents because genetics are important determinants of the height and weight that a child may ultimately achieve. Additionally, the revised growth charts include the body mass index (BMI) for age for children >2 years. The BMI helps identify children at risk for obesity and type 2 diabetes, two problems that have recently become a concern in children.[29]

Biochemical Measurements

Numerous biochemical indices are used in the assessment of nutritional status. Several, such as the quantitative excretion of compounds such as 3-methyl-histidine and creatinine, are difficult to use in children because they require cumbersome 24-hour urine collections. Also, reliable standards for very young children are unavailable.

Of the biochemical markers of nutritional status, the most readily available and widely used is the serum albumin concentration. Although a low serum albumin can be a specific indicator of protein-calorie malnutrition, albumin's long half-life (20 days)[30] makes it an insensitive indicator for developing and resolving malnutrition.

Prealbumin, fibronectin, transferrin, and retinol-binding protein are plasma transport proteins that also can function as biochemical markers of nutritional status.[30–33] They have the advantage of being more sensitive than albumin to acute nutritional changes because their half-lives are shorter, and they are useful when exogenous albumin infusions are given.[34] Nevertheless, transferrin, fibronectin, and retinol-binding protein are influenced by factors other than nutrition (e.g., stress), and are less specific indicators of nutritional status.[35,36]

Laboratory and Clinical Assessments

The nutritional status of a patient receiving PN should be evaluated at regular intervals (e.g., weekly). The adverse effects of enteral and PN should include evaluations of the patient for signs and symptoms of fluid overload, GI losses (e.g., stool, emesis, ostomy output), and metabolic imbalances. The patient should be weighed and the fluid intake, urine output, and GI losses assessed daily.

Blood and urine glucose concentrations initially should be monitored daily until the patient is stable on a formulation; subsequently, the frequency of monitoring can be reduced. Several laboratory tests also should be monitored routinely in those receiving PN (Table 97-9). The frequency of monitoring the subjective and objective data of a patient should be modified based on the clinical condition of the patient.

Table 97-9 Routine Laboratory Monitoring of Pediatric and Neonatal Parenteral Nutrition[a]

Test	*Frequency*
Electrolytes, glucose, BUN, SrCr	Daily until stable, then 2–3 times/wk
Calcium	1–2 times/wk
Phosphorus	1–2 times/wk
Magnesium	1–2 times/wk
Triglycerides	QOD until stable on maximal fat dose, then weekly
PA or RBP	Weekly
Total protein, albumin	Weekly if PA, RBP not available
Alkaline phosphatase	Weekly
Bilirubin (total, direct)[a]	Weekly
Hgb, WBC count	Weekly
AST, ALT, GGT	Monthly

[a] Bilirubin (indirect) daily in the newborn, until normal.

ALT, alanine aminotransferase; AST, aspartate aminotransferase; BUN, blood urea nitrogen; GGT, γ-glutamyl transpeptidase; Hgb, hemoglobin; PA, prealbumin; RBP, retinol binding protein; SrCr, serum creatinine; WBC, white blood cell.

Clinical Presentation: Nutritional Assessment

19. T.C., a 4-month-old, lethargic boy, is seen in his pediatrician's office for routine well-baby care. At examination, he has a moderately distended abdomen and dry mucous membranes. No other remarkable abnormalities are noted. His weight is 6.5 kg (50th–75th percentile for age). At a previous well-baby visit when he was 2 months old, T.C. weighed 5.6 kg (75th percentile for age), and his length was 57 cm (50th percentile for age). His mother reports that for the past 5 to 7 days, he has had five to eight large, liquid stools per day. His diet has not been changed and consists of 5 to 6 oz of a commercial, infant formula every 4 hours around the clock. He is to be hospitalized for evaluation of his diarrhea and weight loss and for fluid and nutritional management.

After correction of his initial fluid and electrolyte deficits, an assessment of his nutritional status shows the following: weight, 6.5 kg (50th–75th percentile); length, 62 cm (50th percentile); albumin, 3.8 g/dL (normal, 4–5.3 g/dL); and prealbumin, 7 mg/dL (normal, 20–50 mg/dL). What do these data suggest about the nature of T.C.'s malnutrition?

[SI units: albumin, 38 g/L (normal, 40–53); prealbumin, 70 mg/L (normal, 200–500 mg/L)]

If T.C. had continued to gain weight at his previous rate, his weight, extrapolated from the appropriate growth chart, should be approximately 7.2 kg. His growth in length has continued to progress at the same rate. Thus, the decrease in weight for age with a normal progression in length for age indicates malnutrition of a relatively short duration. This is further validated by a near-normal serum concentration of albumin with a decrease in prealbumin.

Role of Enteral Nutrition in Chronic Diarrhea

20. After initial IV rehydration and receiving nothing by mouth (NPO) for 48 hours, T.C.'s stool output has decreased dramatically. Is this characteristic of infants with chronic diarrhea? Should enteral intake be initiated?

A prompt decrease in stool output when enteral intake is stopped is typical of infants with chronic diarrhea. Nonetheless, evaluation of bowel function and adaptation has shown that enteral nutrition is superior to PN with regard to histologic recovery, improvement of D-xylose absorption,[37] protein absorption, and disaccharidase activity.[38–40] In fact, improvement in histology or absorptive function might not occur until enteral nutrients are given.[38,39] Thus, for T.C., every effort should be made to provide some nutrition enterally, whether this route is used exclusively[38] or in combination with supplemental PN.[40]

Choice of Formula

21. What type of enteral formula should be chosen for T.C.?

The enteral regimen should be initiated with a lactose-free formula, such as an elemental formula or a soy-based formula. Although any soy-based formula would be appropriate, Isomil DF is a soy-based formula with added fiber that is indicated for infants with diarrhea. Infants with chronic diarrhea can have small bowel mucosal damage and decreased disaccharidase activity.[39,40] Carbohydrate absorption depends on digestion of disaccharides and polysaccharides to monosaccharides through disaccharidase activity in the intestinal lumen. Substitution of free glucose orally may overcome the problem of carbohydrate digestion and absorption. Administration of large amounts of oral glucose should be limited, however, because of its osmotic effect and potential to worsen diarrhea. Furthermore, incompletely absorbed carbohydrate is available to colonic bacteria for fermentation, the end products of which can produce diarrhea through colonic irritation.

Unlike carbohydrate, protein rarely causes diarrhea, but the mucosal damage present in patients with chronic diarrhea, such as T.C., can reduce the absorptive surface area so that protein malabsorption may occur. This can be minimized through the administration of a formula containing protein in the form of dipeptides and tripeptides, which are absorbed more efficiently than free amino acids.[41]

Dilution of hypertonic formulas to half strength may improve formula tolerance.[38] The concentration is increased in a step-wise fashion to full strength if there is no carbohydrate malabsorption and if stool output is not excessive (defined by Orenstein as $\geq$40% of enteral intake).[38] Tolerance may be improved by continuous infusion of the enteral product.[24] If enteral refeeding results in the return of diarrhea, fluid and electrolytes must be replaced with an equal volume of an IV solution of similar electrolyte composition to the stool loss.[38]

Monitoring

22. How can T.C.'s tolerance to the formula and his recovery of intestinal function be assessed?

Malabsorption or formula intolerance can be assessed by stool studies, which would include assessing for the presence of reducing substances and stool pH. Lactose is a reducing sugar and its presence in stool is an assessment of carbohydrate absorption. The bacterial fermentation products of malabsorbed carbohydrates can result in a decreased stool pH, which suggests malabsorption. To further evaluate carbohydrate absorption D-xylose may be given orally; a blood sample is drawn 4 to 5 hours later to determine the amount absorbed. This test may be of initial prognostic value in predicting which patients will require prolonged courses of treatment.[37] More than 5% of ingested fat in a stool collection (usually 3 days) is indicative of fat malabsorption. All these tests can be followed serially during treatment to help guide the refeeding process.

Reinstitution of Standard Formula

23. Once the diarrhea has resolved and the enteral diet is well tolerated, how should standard infant formula be reinstituted for T.C.?

Standard formula feedings are restarted somewhat arbitrarily in patients such as T.C., although the D-xylose absorption test may be a useful guide.[37,38] The diarrhea should have resolved completely, and full maintenance fluid and caloric intake should be established using an enteral elemental or soy-based formula. Regardless of the time chosen, a gradual step-wise conversion is suggested. A small volume of standard formula is substituted for an equal volume of elemental or soy-based formula and the substitution volume is increased daily until the elemental or soy-based formula is eliminated completely from the regimen.

If a specific nutrient intolerance has been identified, a standard formula that does not contain that nutrient must be selected. For example, a patient with cow's milk protein intolerance may require a soy protein formula or an elemental formula.

Pediatric Parenteral Nutrition

Nutrient Requirements

The basic requirements for a parenteral nutrient regimen are listed in Table 97-1. These guidelines for the initiation of a nutrient regimen should be individualized to specific patient needs because requirements can vary from patient to patient. The correct regimen for any specific patient is that which supplies sufficient nutrients to promote a normal rate of growth without toxicity. In particular, patients with ongoing, abnormal nutrient losses may require much larger doses of certain nutrients. Individualization of the nutrient prescription cannot be overemphasized.

Many of the requirements listed in Table 97-1 apply to nutrients administered by the enteral route as well. In some instances, the absorption of a particular nutrient from the GI mucosa is incomplete and enteral requirements are substantially higher. This is particularly true of the major minerals (calcium, magnesium, and iron) and trace elements.[42] In some cases, parenteral doses may be greater than enteral doses to achieve the same blood concentration.[41]

Indications

Parenteral nutrition is indicated for any patient unable to take in sufficient nourishment to maintain normal growth. Some specific indications are listed in Table 97-8.

Very Low-Birth-Weight Infants

Extremely premature infants require specialized nutritional support for two distinct reasons. First, the third trimester in utero is a time of rapid growth and accumulation of protein, glycogen, fat, and minerals.[43] The infant born in the very early stages of the third trimester does not accumulate these stores and, therefore, must receive nutrients earlier than a more mature infant. Second, extreme prematurity is associated with poor coordination of the suck and swallow reflex, poor GI motility, and incomplete absorption.[44] Therefore, enteral nutrients may need to be administered via an orogastric or nasogastric tube, and PN supplementation probably will be needed. PN, especially amino acids, should be initiated soon after birth to duplicate intrauterine growth and prevent a catabolic state in the first few days of life. The fetus in utero has a continuous supply of amino acids that is immediately stopped after preterm birth.[45,46] On the first day of life, a type of PN called "vanilla" PN may be started. "Vanilla" PN does not actually contain vanilla, but the name relates to the colorless solution. Most PN formulations have multivitamins added that give the solution a yellow coloring, whereas "vanilla" PN does not contain multivitamins. It is prepared as a standardized solution containing amino acids and dextrose and is used for infants weighing <1 kg in the first 24 hours of life. There has been some reluctance to administer amino acids this soon after birth because of increased risk of hyperammonemia, uremia, and metabolic acidosis. Several studies, however, have shown early introduction of amino acids is safe, provides a positive nitrogen balance, and promotes better health outcomes.[47,48]

Respiratory Distress

Respiratory distress may preclude the ability to consume sufficient nutrients enterally because high respiratory rates prevent coordinated breathing and swallowing. In infants who are hypoxic, or at high risk for hypoxia, aggressive enteral feedings during the acute phase of their illness can increase the likelihood of bowel ischemia. Often, these situations are resolved in 3 to 5 days, but this can rarely be predicted at the outset. Trophic feedings (1–5 mL/hour) are often implemented to maintain GI tract integrity. Nutritional support in such cases is initiated by giving parenteral fluids, which provide dextrose as a caloric source. This allows the infant to conserve endogenous energy substrates, an important consideration for the VLBW infant whose entire body composition may contain a 3- to 4-day energy supply.[43] PN should be initiated as soon as it becomes clear the enteral feeding will be impossible for 3 to 5 days or when several days have elapsed and no clear time frame can be determined for the establishment of enteral feeding. Although a short course (5 days) of PN may be used, the quantity of nutrients supplied during the process of initiation and gradual increase to full requirements is so low that extremely short courses may be difficult to justify. Peripheral PN using fat emulsion as a significant source of calories, however, can provide up to 70 kcal/kg and, with appropriate types and amounts of protein, can result in modest weight gain and nitrogen equilibrium.

Gastrointestinal Anomalies

Infants with GI anomalies often require PN because the implementation of enteral feedings may be delayed. For example, GI tract atresias or stenosis can obstruct, or partially obstruct, the lumen of the GI tract. This prevents or slows the passage of fluids and nutrients and can result in vomiting, depending on the location of the obstruction. Similarly, infants with necrotizing enterocolitis have zones of ischemic bowel and are at risk for bowel perforation if fed enterally.[49] Infants with these disorders need PN until the viability of the entire GI tract can be assured.

Chronic Renal Failure and Hepatic Disease

Chronic renal or hepatic disease requires modification of a normal diet to account for the impaired elimination of nitrogenous waste or impaired protein metabolism. Careful caloric supplementation with a reduced amount of protein may permit normal growth while minimizing excess urea production in an infant with renal failure.

24. Approximately 48 hours after discharge from the hospital, T.C. returns to the emergency department (ED) with abdominal distention and bloody diarrhea. He is diagnosed with postgastroenteritis syndrome. T.C. cannot receive nutrients enterally, and PN is to be initiated because he is nutritionally depleted. Describe how a regimen of PN should be instituted in T.C. What aspects of his disease may alter specific nutrient needs?

When initiating PN, the protein (amino acids), glucose (dextrose), fat (lipids or fat emulsion), fluid and electrolyte, mineral, and vitamin components of the regimen are managed as separate entities. In addition, the route of PN delivery is important to consider because the amount of glucose, potassium, and calcium must be limited if the infusion is given peripherally. In general, 12.5% dextrose, 40 mEq/L potassium, and 10 mEq/L calcium are the maximal amounts that should be provided by infusion into a peripheral vein. These nutrients can be increased if a central venous line is placed. The fluids, electrolytes, minerals, and vitamins are initiated at full daily maintenance doses after correction of any pre-existing abnormalities. Protein should be initiated at full daily doses in term infants and children with normal renal and hepatic function. Glucose and fat are started at lower doses and increased daily until requirements are reached. Forgetting to increase doses in T.C. will lead to underfeeding.

Protein should be started in T.C. at full daily requirements of 2 to 3 g/kg/day. Azotemia and acidosis have occurred in infants receiving >4 g/kg/day of protein; however, these complications are rare at the recommended dosage.

Parenteral glucose administration is initiated at 5 to 8 mg/kg/minute (7.2–11.5 g/kg/day). This closely approximates normal endogenous glucose production[50] and should be tolerated. At normal maintenance fluid rates, 10% glucose represents a generally well-tolerated starting solution for patients of virtually any age or size, except the VLBW infant. In T.C.'s case, the glucose concentration will begin and continue at 10% because of the peripheral line limitations. This concentration of glucose will provide 7.3 mg/kg/minute. If a central line later becomes necessary, the concentration of glucose can be increased by 5% each day until the caloric requirement is met. This glucose increment should be accompanied by blood and urine glucose monitoring. If the blood glucose is ≥150 mg/dL or if the urine glucose exceeds "trace" amounts, the PN infusion rate should be decreased by at least 25% and a second IV solution should be added to provide needed fluids and electrolytes. Alternatively, the dextrose concentration can be decreased or insulin can be infused concomitantly and titrated to a desired serum glucose concentration of 120 to 140 mg/dL.

Fat should be initiated at 1 g/kg/day and increased daily by 0.5 to 1 g/kg/day until the maximal dosage of 3 g/kg/day is reached. The daily fat dose should be infused at a constant rate because fats are better tolerated when infused over 24 hours.[51] Serum triglycerides should be monitored every other day while the dose of fat is being increased. Patients with a fasting triglyceride concentration of 150 mg/dL or less may have their fat dose increased. In patients who are receiving inadequate calories, triglycerides may be elevated because endogenous fats are being mobilized. If the triglyceride concentration is >150 mg/dL, the serum sample must be examined visually. A clear sample with a mildly elevated triglyceride concentration probably indicates the use of endogenous fat stores for energy. Conversely, a turbid or lipemic sample indicates the patient's inability to use the amount of intravenous fat administered. In this case, further increases in the fat dose should be delayed until triglyceride concentrations decrease.[52]

25. **T.C. has a single peripheral IV line. Can the glucose–amino acid solution and the IV fat emulsion be infused through the same IV line?**

Not only can they be infused through the same peripheral IV line, but doing so may prolong the patency of the IV site and reduce the likelihood of local complications, such as phlebitis.[53,54] Lipids dilute the hypertonic glucose–amino acid solution. The fat, however, has two more important effects. It acts as a mechanical barrier to the vascular endothelium and has a local modulating effect on prostaglandin and leukotriene mediators of inflammation.[54]

Special Considerations and Complications

26. **J.H., a 4-day-old boy, was born at 31 weeks' gestation. His birth weight was 1,950 g, and he now weighs 2,000 g. On the first day of life, he was given a commercial preterm infant formula by orogastric tube in gradually increasing quantity with supplemental IV fluids. Now, on the fourth day of life, he has developed a distended abdomen and his stools contain bright red blood. An abdominal radiograph shows pneumatosis intestinalis (gas within the intestinal wall). All enteral feedings are stopped (NPO). What do these findings represent? What are the implications for J.H.'s nutritional management?**

Abdominal distention, bloody stools, and pneumatosis intestinalis are characteristic of necrotizing enterocolitis.[49] The causes of this disorder are unclear, but it occurs more often in premature than in term infants; it can occur in clusters of cases, rarely is seen before enteral feeding is instituted, and can be associated with rapid increases in enteral intake.[55] Because J.H. will receive antibiotics for 10 to 14 days and remain NPO, he requires PN. The planned duration of the regimen makes central venous access a necessity.

Parenteral Nutrition

Goals of Long-Term Support

27. **The following day, intestinal perforation requires the resection of two-thirds of J.H.'s distal jejunum and one-third of his ileum, with creation of a jejunostomy. The ileocecal valve and the entire colon are left intact. During the operation, a central venous catheter is placed. What is the goal of PN for J.H.?**

J.H. will be NPO for a prolonged time. Therefore, the goals of his PN must be to promote normal growth as well as healing of his diseased gut and surgical wounds.

Because J.H. is a premature infant, it will be difficult to predict how well he will tolerate PN. VLBW infants tolerate normal doses of pediatric amino acids without difficulty; however, some clinicians initiate protein at a lower daily dose (e.g., 1.0 g/kg/day) and advance by 0.5 g/kg/day each day until a goal of 2 to 3 g/kg/day is achieved. The problem with this approach is that it is easy to forget to advance the protein, which leads to underfeeding. Fat should be started at 0.5 to 1 g/kg/day and increased by 0.5 g/kg/day up to 3 g/kg/day. Glucose should be initiated at 5 to 10 g/kg/day and increased by 2 to 3 g/kg until the desired caloric intake is achieved. Appropriate doses of electrolytes and minerals may be started immediately using the guidelines listed in Table 97-1.

Fat Emulsions: Complications

28. **What must be considered in making decisions regarding fat administration in J.H.?**

Although J.H. can receive adequate calories using only glucose and crystalline amino acids, he will require fat to provide a more physiologic diet and to prevent essential fatty acid deficiency (EFAD), which develops quickly in low birth weight infants who have little fat reserve.[56] J.H. should receive a minimum of 5% of his total caloric requirement as fat emulsion to minimize the risk of EFAD.[52] Ideally, his nutrition regimen will provide approximately 40% of calories from fat, which is similar to what is provided by human milk.

Infusions of fat emulsions have been associated with impaired oxygen transport and pulmonary ventilation-perfusion mismatch. This adverse effect generally occurred when the dose of fat was $\geq$4 g/kg and infused over a relatively short (4 hours) period. Current practice is to increase gradually the doses of fat from 0.5 to 1 g/kg/day up to a maximum of 4 g/kg/day and to infuse the fat emulsion over 24 hours to minimize the likelihood of pulmonary problems and to promote clearance.

It is unclear if IV fat administration is detrimental to patients with sepsis. Rapid IV infusion of fat and in vitro incubation of leukocytes with fat emulsion has resulted in impaired leukocyte chemotaxis and phagocytosis.[57] On the other hand, the linoleic acid in IV fat is the precursor to arachidonic acid, prostaglandins, thromboxane, interleukins, and immune-mediating cells. Theoretically, this may minimize bacteremia. Necrotizing enterocolitis, intestinal perforation, and surgery predispose J.H. to sepsis. Therefore, he should have his IV fat infused at an appropriate dose over 24 hours. Because fat clearance can be impaired during infection, it is also prudent to monitor his triglyceride concentrations.

Free fatty acids can displace bilirubin from its albumin binding sites, thereby placing the infant at risk for kernicterus.[58] Therefore, before advancing the fat dose, the total bilirubin and direct bilirubin should be measured. Patients with an indirect bilirubin (total bilirubin–direct bilirubin) $\leq$10 mg/dL whose albumin levels are normal are at low risk for kernicterus. Indirect bilirubin usually peaks before 1 week of age. After the risk for indirect hyperbilirubinemia has passed, the fat dose can be increased as recommended in Table 97-1. The infusion of 1 g/kg over 24 hours is associated with minimal risk for decreased bilirubin binding;[58] however, rapid infusion of this same dose can displace bilirubin from albumin binding sites. Given the low level of indirect bilirubin found on routine monitoring (see Question 36) and the planned fat infusion rate, J.H. should not be at risk for kernicterus.

Egg phospholipids are used to emulsify fats; therefore, patients with a known allergy to eggs (e.g., fever, chills, urticaria, dyspnea, bronchospasm, chest pain) should not receive fat emulsion.[52]

Glucose Intolerance

29. **Because J.H is a premature infant, PN should be initiated using 5% glucose, 2.5 g/kg/day of amino acids, and 0.5 g/kg/day of fat emulsion. The volume of PN should be 240 mL based on a maintenance fluid requirement of 120 mL/kg (Table 97-1). On the second day, he receives 10% glucose and 2.5 g/kg/day of amino acids and 1 g/kg/day of fat. On the third day, glucose is increased**

to 15%, amino acids remain at 2.5 g/kg, and fat emulsion is increased to 1.5 g/kg/day. On the fourth day, glucose is increased to 20%, amino acids remain at 2.5 g/kg, and fats are increased to 2 g/kg/day. After this solution has infused for 8 hours, his urine tests 1% for glucose (normal, no glucose) and his blood glucose level is 210 mg/dL (normal, 120 mg/dL). Explain this new finding and the problems it may cause. How should hyperglycemia be managed?

[SI unit: blood glucose, 11.7 mmol/L (normal, 6.66)]

Maximal glucose oxidation rates in milligrams per kilograms per minute are inversely related to age, and decrease from 15 to 18 mg/kg/minute in neonates and young infants to 4 to 5 mg/kg/minute in adults. In full-term neonates and infants receiving maintenance fluids (100 mL/kg), glucose concentrations can be started at 10 g/kg/day (equivalent to dextrose 10%) and advanced by 5 g/kg (equivalent to dextrose 5%) every 24 hours up to approximately 25 g/kg/day (equivalent to dextrose 25%).

In preterm neonates, such as J.H., dextrose is started at a lower dose and advanced at smaller increments, usually 2 to 3 g/kg/day. Glucose tolerance varies significantly, so each patient should be considered individually.

At J.H.'s prescribed fluid rate of 10 mL/hour, 20% glucose represents 16.7 mg/kg/minute of glucose. The hyperglycemia and glycosuria probably have occurred because the increases in the infusion rate have exceeded J.H.'s ability to adapt to the glucose dose. Patients who have been euglycemic on their glucose dose and then become glucose intolerant should be evaluated, however, for other causes, such as infection.[59]

Hyperglycemia and glycosuria can result in serum hyperosmolarity, osmotic diuresis, and dehydration. Regardless of the cause, the hyperglycemia should be treated by reducing the glucose administration rate. The rate of the PN infusion can be decreased further if hyperglycemia continues or increased if the hyperglycemia resolves.

When the PN order is written for the subsequent days, the glucose increases should be made in smaller amounts up to the maintenance calorie requirements per day. Frequent blood and urine glucose monitoring must be continued. Severe glucose intolerance in patients who require PN can be managed with insulin to normalize serum glucose. Although insulin is compatible with PN solutions, it does adsorb to glass, polyvinyl chloride, and filters, resulting in decreased delivery of insulin.[60] The addition of albumin can decrease the binding of insulin to solution containers.[61] Frequently, pediatric patients have changing insulin requirements that prevent the addition of insulin to PN solutions. A separate continuous infusion of regular insulin (initial dose: 0.05 to 0.1 units/kg/hour) titrated to control serum glucose concentrations offers a practical solution to minimize waste of the PN solution.[62] It is essential to discontinue the insulin infusion if the PN solution is discontinued to avoid hypoglycemia.

Effects of Bronchopulmonary Dysplasia and Mechanical Ventilation

30. J.H. remains dependent on a ventilator because of his immature lungs. How could J.H.'s respiratory disease influence his nutritional regimen?

At older than 28 days of age, J.H.'s ventilator dependence defines him as having bronchopulmonary dysplasia (BPD), a chronic lung disease of infancy. BPD is characterized by an increase in resting energy expenditure, increased work of breathing, and growth failure.[63,64] Therefore, J.H.'s caloric requirement may be higher than expected. Additionally, J.H.'s ventilator may also alter the approach to his caloric supply. Very high carbohydrate loads have been associated with an increase in carbon dioxide production.[65] This, in turn, may make it difficult to wean J.H. from the mechanical ventilator. As discussed, rapid infusions of fat emulsion can also have a detrimental effect on pulmonary function. Fat emulsion should not be omitted from J.H.'s PN regimen; rather, a slower infusion rate, with gradual dose increases, while monitoring pulmonary function is appropriate.

Pediatric Amino Acid Formulations

31. Why would a specialized pediatric amino acid solution be preferable to a standard adult formulation for J.H.?

Patients 1 year of age or older tolerate standard adult amino acid preparations (e.g., Aminosyn [Abbott Laboratories] and Travasol [Baxter Healthcare]) well. For infants <1 year of age, two specifically designed pediatric amino acid formulations (PAAF)–TrophAmine (B. Braun) and Aminosyn PF (Abbott Laboratories)–are available. PAAF were developed in response to the abnormal plasma amino acid patterns noted in infants receiving adult amino acid formulations. The products were designed with the goal of producing plasma amino acid patterns closely matching those of 2-hour postprandial, human-milk–fed infants. Theoretically, normal plasma amino acid patterns will promote normal protein synthesis in growing infants.

Pediatric amino acid formulation differ from conventional amino acid formulations in several ways. First, they contain a higher content of branch chain amino acids (leucine, isoleucine, and valine), and a lower content of glycine, methionine, and phenylalanine (Table 97-10). In addition, PAAF have a higher percentage of essential amino acids with a wider distribution of the nonessential amino acids. Finally, PAAF are unique in that they contain three essential amino acids for neonates: taurine, tyrosine (as *N*-acetyl-L-tyrosine), and cysteine (added as L-cysteine HCl). Adult solutions contain little if any of these amino acids. Neonates have immature liver functions. This results in decreased levels of both hepatic cystathionase and phenylalanine hydroxylase enzymes. Without these enzymes, neonates cannot adequately convert methionine to cysteine or phenylalanine to tyrosine or synthesize taurine from cysteine. Deficiencies in these amino acids can have a significant impact on the health of the neonate. For example, taurine has a role in retinal development, protection and stabilization of cell membranes, neurotransmission, regulation of cell volume, and bile acid conjugation. Taurine also may be important in decreasing or preventing cholestasis associated with long-term PN.

Several investigators have studied the clinical, nutritional, and biochemical effects of TrophAmine in term and preterm infants.[66,67] The use of TrophAmine was found to result in nearly normal amino acid patterns. In addition, patients receiving TrophAmine had greater weight gain and significantly better nitrogen utilization than similar groups using the adult formulations. TrophAmine and Aminosyn-PF, given over a 7-day period, produced comparable weight gain and nitrogen retention.[68] In one study, some of the VLBW infants

Table 97-10 Pediatric Amino Acid Solutions

	TrophAmine 6%	Aminosyn-PF 7%
Essential Amino Acids (EEA) (mg/1 g Total Amino Acids)		
Isoleucine	81.7	76.3
Leucine	140.0	118.7
Lysine	81.7	67.9
Methionine	33.3	17.9
Phenylalanine	48.3	42.9
Threonine	41.7	51.4
Tryptophan	20.0	17.9
Valine	78.3	64.6
Cysteine HCl[a]	3.3	0
Histidine	48.3	31.4
Tyrosine	23.3	6.3
Taurine	2.5	7.1
Nonessential Amino Acids (mg/1 g Total Amino Acids)		
Alanine	53.3	70.0
Arginine	121.7	123.0
Proline	68.3	81.4
Serine	38.3	49.6
Glycine	36.7	38.6
L-aspartic acid	31.7	52.9
L-glutamic acid	50.0	82.3
Sodium (mEq/L)	5.0	0
Acetate (mEq/L)	56.0	32.5
Chloride (mEq/L)	<3	0
% essential amino acid	60.1	50.2
% branched chain amino acid (g amino acid/1 g nitrogen)	30.0	26.0

[a] 40 g of cysteine syringe available.

experienced metabolic acidosis.[66] L-cysteine, an HCl salt, provides an additional 5.7 mEq Cl/100 mg and may have contributed to the acidosis. Whereas the manufacturer's recommended dose of 40 mg L-cysteine per gram of amino acid may be too much for the VLBW infant; the most appropriate dose of L-cysteine for the VLBW infant has not been determined.

To date, PAAF have been effective in producing a positive weight gain, positive nitrogen balance, and normalizing amino acid patterns in preterm neonates. They also allow for the provision of larger doses of calcium and phosphorus because PAAF lower the pH of the final PN solution. Providing greater amounts of calcium and phosphorus, in appropriate ratios, should minimize metabolic bone disease. Further evaluation of these products is needed to determine the magnitude of the proposed benefits (i.e., improved nitrogen retention, better weight gain, enhanced bone growth, and decreased cholestasis) and the most appropriate L-cysteine dose to use in VLBW infants. In any event, these potential benefits, and clinical experience with these products, have resulted in the use of PAAF as the standard of care in infants requiring PN.

Carnitine

32. Why would carnitine supplementation be warranted in J.H.?

Carnitine has many functions within the body, but it primarily serves to transport long-chain fatty acids (LCFA) across the mitochondrial membrane where they undergo β-oxidation to produce energy. Deficiency in carnitine lessens LCFA availability for oxidation, resulting in the accumulation of LCFA and a decrease in ketone and adenosine triphosphate (ATP) production. This can adversely affect the CNS and skeletal and cardiac muscles. Carnitine deficiency in premature infants also has been linked to disorders such as GI reflux, apnea, and bradycardia.[69]

Whereas carnitine is a nonessential nutrient in adults and is readily available from a diet that includes meat and dairy products, it appears to be an essential nutrient in neonates and infants. This population has low body stores of carnitine and a decreased ability to synthesize it on their own. The premature infant has even lower stores of carnitine because carnitine accumulation occurs during the third trimester. Human milk and most cow's milk-based infant formulas contain carnitine. Some soy-based formulas have additional carnitine added during manufacturing. PN, however, is not routinely supplemented with carnitine. Therefore, infants who are exclusively fed by PN are at risk for developing complications associated with carnitine deficiency.[69]

Because J.H. has two risk factors for the development of carnitine deficiency (prematurity and exclusive use of PN), and because carnitine has little or no adverse effects associated with its use, it is appropriate to provide J.H. with a carnitine supplement. Carnitine is available as both an oral and IV formulation. The recommended dose in J.H. is 10 to 20 mg/kg/day. The addition of carnitine directly to PN improves carnitine plasma concentrations and nutritional status.

Septicemia

33. J.H. was diagnosed with necrotizing enterocolitis and received 14 days of antibiotics. On his sixth day off antibiotics, he begins having 15 to 20 episodes of bradycardia per day. His physical examination is remarkable for cold extremities and slow capillary refill, but his chest radiographs show no acute change. Laboratory evaluation at this time includes electrolytes, blood glucose, complete blood count, and blood cultures, which are reported as follows: Na, 139 mEq/L (normal, 135–145 mEq/L); K, 4.7 mEq/L (normal, 3.5–5.0 mEq/L); Cl, 112 mEq/L (normal, 102–109 mEq/L); HCO_3^-, 17 mEq/L (normal, 22–29 mEq/L); glucose, 164 mg/dL (normal, 70–105 mg/dL); platelet count, 36,000/mm^3 (normal, 150,000–450,000/mm^3); and white blood cell (WBC) count, 24,300/mm^3 (normal, 5,500–18,000/mm^3). WBC differential includes 52% segmented neutrophils (normal, 20%–50%) and 27% immature neutrophils (normal, 3%–5%). Blood cultures are drawn; results will be unavailable for at least 24 hours. What is the likely cause of these findings? How might J.H.'s nutrition regimen affect the diagnostic evaluation and treatment selected?

[SI units: Na, 139 mmol/L (normal, 135–145); K, 4.7 mmol/L (normal, 3.5–5.0); Cl, 112 mmol/L (normal, 102–109); HCO_3^-, 17 mmol/L (normal, 22–29); glucose, 9.1 mmol/L (normal, 3.9–5.8); platelet count, 36 × 10^5/L (normal, 150–450); WBC count, 24.3 × 10^2 cells/L (normal, 5.5–18.0)]

This constellation of findings (metabolic acidosis, hyperglycemia, thrombocytopenia, leukocytosis, bradycardia, and poor perfusion) is nonspecific but could represent septicemia.

The presence of a central venous catheter predisposes J.H. to infection with gram-negative bacteria and bacteria normally found on the skin (e.g., coagulase-negative staphylococci).[70]

Cultures growing coagulase-negative staphylococci must not be presumed to be the result of contamination in symptomatic patients. The typical antimicrobial sensitivities of this organism dictate that vancomycin be among the empiric antibiotics. A third-generation cephalosporin to cover gram-negative organisms should be added empirically as well.

The central venous catheter and the use of broad-spectrum antibiotics also predisposes J.H. to fungal infection.[71] Candidal infection can occur and, when fat emulsions are used, as in J.H., systemic infection with *Malassezia furfur* must be considered. *M. furfur* is a normal skin fungus that requires an exogenous source of fatty acids. The empiric use of antifungal drugs is not indicated in patients with *M. furfur*; however, the clinician should screen specifically for this fungus by culture.

Metabolic Bone Disease (Rickets)

34. On the chest radiograph taken to evaluate the septic episode just described, the radiologist notes that J.H. has two rib fractures and that the bones appear undermineralized. The most recent laboratory values show a serum calcium (Ca) of 9.3 mg/dL (normal, 8.5–10.5 mg/dL), a serum phosphorus of 3.6 mg/dL (normal, 4.0–8.5 mg/dL), and an alkaline phosphatase of 674 U/L (normal, 350 U/L). What diagnosis is suggested by these findings? How and why has J.H.'s nutrition regimen placed him at risk for this disease?

[SI units: Ca, 2.3 mmol/L (normal, 2.1–2.6); phosphorus, 1.16 mmol/L (normal, 1.3–2.7); phosphatase, 674 U/L (normal, 350)]

During the last trimester of pregnancy, bone accretion is accelerated reaching its peak at about 36 weeks. Premature infants, therefore, require larger calcium and phosphorous doses. Limitations to venous access, however, may preclude the infusion of concentrated calcium solutions peripherally, and the patient's end-organs may be resistant to vitamin D. Thus, metabolic bone disease is not unexpected in a premature infant such as J.H.

Aluminum, a contaminant in some parenteral salt products (particularly calcium), also may play a role in impaired bone mineralization.[72] Low serum phosphorus with high alkaline phosphatase, undermineralized bones, and fractures resulting from routine handling are consistent with a diagnosis of rickets.

Parenteral nutrition solutions provide calcium and phosphorus in much smaller amounts than the infant would accumulate in utero.[73] Solution pH, temperature, calcium salt, and final calcium and phosphorus concentrations influence their solubility in PN solutions. An acidic PN solution favors the solubility of these salts. The pH of commercially available amino acid preparations ranges from 5.4 (in the PAAF) to 7 (in adult amino acid formulations). The addition of L-cysteine, with a pH of 1.5, also makes the solution more acidic. Because dextrose also is acidic, solutions with higher dextrose concentrations are more acidic. Of note, colder storage temperatures promote calcium and phosphorus solubility. Therefore, refrigerated PN solutions may appear to be free of precipitate on visual inspection. Calcium and phosphate can precipitate, however, when warmed to room temperature, or when infused into patients with fever or in incubators. Calcium salt selection is another important consideration because the chloride salt dissociates rapidly and favors precipitation, whereas the gluconate and gluceptate salts dissociate less quickly.

Serum phosphorus concentrations should be monitored several times per week and phosphorus intake adjusted to prevent symptomatic hypophosphatemia. Serum calcium is not useful as an indicator of disease activity because it will remain normal at the expense of bone mineralization. This is demonstrated by J.H.'s serum calcium at the time of diagnosis (see Question 33).

Liver Disease Associated With Parenteral Nutrition

35. On the 56th day of life, J.H. is noted to be mildly jaundiced. A review of his laboratory tests reveals the following:

	Age (days)				
Test	22	29	36	43	50
Aspartate aminotransferse (AST) (U/L) (normal, <40)	14	17	15	20	25
Alanine aminotransferse (ALT) (U/L) (normal, <28)	6	7	10	10	11
Alkaline phosphatase (IU/L) (normal, <350)	103	158	345	506	695
Bilirubin	—	—	—	—	—
Indirect (normal, <1 mg/dL)	0.9	0.9	0.8	0.8	0.9
Direct (normal, <0.2)	0.1	0.1	0.8	1.6	3

Could this be related to his PN?

In past decades, hepatic damage has been reported in up to one-third of infants receiving PN,[74] with a higher prevalence (up to 50%) in VLBW infants such as J.H.[75] Although it is still a concern today, hepatic damage is less prevalent because of current better understanding of how to treat infants requiring long-term PN. The laboratory abnormalities reported in J.H. are typical of this complication. The first change observed is usually an elevated direct (conjugated) bilirubin, which can occur as early as 2 weeks after beginning PN.[76] Increases in the serum concentrations of the hepatic enzymes, AST and ALT, lag 2 weeks or more behind the rise in direct bilirubin.[76] Alkaline phosphatase also can rise, but it is a nonspecific indicator of liver disease. Alkaline phosphatase is produced by the liver, GI tract, and bones.[76] Although the laboratory results observed in J.H. are consistent with the pattern associated with liver disease induced by PN, PN-associated cholestasis is a diagnosis of exclusion; therefore, other causes, such as viral hepatitis, must be ruled out.

RISK FACTORS

36. What clinical factors placed J.H. at high risk for developing cholestatic liver disease secondary to PN?

Although components of PN solutions are commonly blamed for the development of cholestasis, many potential causes exist.[77] J.H. has several other risk factors for developing cholestasis, and prolonged enteral fasting may be the most significant.[78] Stimulation of bile flow and gallbladder contraction depend on GI hormones, which depend on enteral feeding for their release.[79] Absence of these secretogogues, therefore, can promote cholestasis.[80–82] Immature hepatic function secondary to prematurity also places J.H. at risk, as does the duration of PN therapy. As the duration of PN use increases, so does the prevalence of hepatic disease in premature infants;

25% of infants nourished in this manner for ≥30 days show evidence of cholestasis.[75] Surgical patients have a greater likelihood of developing hyperbilirubinemia than medical patients, especially those requiring GI surgery.[83,84] Many surgical procedures are associated with a higher risk of jaundice.[78] Finally, J.H.'s infection increases his risk for cholestasis.[85]

The use of adult amino acid preparations in infants increases the risk of cholestasis. In one study, the incidence of cholestasis in VLBW infants receiving TrophAmine was reduced to 23% relative to historical controls of 30% to 50%.[86] In another study comparing the two PAAF mentioned above, no difference in the incidence of cholestasis was found in infants 1 year of age, and the overall incidence of cholestasis was 27%.[87] These investigators did not assess whether or not the patients were provided with L-cysteine, which may be important because L-cysteine is a precursor for taurine and taurine forms the water-soluble nontoxic bile acid, taurocholate.

An additional risk factor for cholestasis not present in J.H. is the administration of large amounts of protein or dextrose. Because amino acids are actively transported in hepatocytes, it is important to provide appropriate types and amounts of amino acids to minimize the development of cholestasis. In one study, a high-protein regimen (3.6 g/kg/day) was associated with an earlier onset and greater degree of cholestasis than a low-protein regimen (2.3 g/kg/day).[88] Similarly, dextrose overload is a known cause of hepatic steatosis and has been shown to decrease bile flow.[89] Therefore, overly aggressive feeding of J.H. with PN should be avoided.

In addition to the hepatic damage, gallstones have been reported in infants and children receiving PN.[90,91] The ileal resection performed during the acute phase of his necrotizing enterocolitis may put J.H. at increased risk for this hepatobiliary complication as well.[90]

37. What modifications can be made in J.H.'s regimen in the presence of cholestasis?

First, the institution of enteral feeding must be considered. Even low-volume trophic feeding may help alleviate the condition and should be attempted in cholestatic patients. Next, the protein and glucose dose provided by the PN should be evaluated. During cholestasis, calories should be provided using an appropriate mix of protein, carbohydrate, and fat.

Although the effect of cycling a patient off PN has not been evaluated in clinical trials, this should be considered. Cycling PN, when the infusion rate is gradually decreased to off for a period and then restarted and gradually increased to the desired rate, will decrease the length of time the liver is exposed to PN. VLBW infants, however, may become hypoglycemic even with very gradual decreases in infusion rate, so this option should be used with care. In any event, a short time off PN (e.g., 2 hours) should be attempted.

The trace elements provided by the formulation should be examined. Both copper and manganese are enterohepatically recycled and may accumulate in liver disease. Manganese can also contribute to hepatotoxicity and should be removed from J.H.'s PN solutions. Studies have not established when removal of copper and manganese is warranted. The inappropriate removal of copper could lead to anemia, osteopenia, and neutropenia.[92] Therefore, decreasing the copper dose and monitoring serum concentrations of both copper and manganese should guide therapy.

Pharmacologic interventions have had limited success in the management of PN-associated cholestasis. Neither phenobarbital nor bile acid binding agents, such as cholestyramine, are effective in reducing or reversing PN-associated cholestasis.[93,94] Ursodiol 10 to 20 mg/kg/day has been used successfully in the treatment of other cholestatic liver diseases, and preliminary reports indicate that it may also improve PN-associated cholestasis in children.[95] Ursodiol, a naturally occurring nontoxic bile acid, presumably works by displacing and replacing the endogenously produced, potentially toxic bile salts that accumulate with cholestasis.

Sincalide, is part of the endogenous hormone cholecystokinin (CCK), and may improve signs of PN-associated cholestasis. CCK is secreted in the small intestine in response to meals and stimulates gallbladder contraction and increases intestinal motility. In PN-dependent patients, such J.H., endogenous CCK secretion is diminished. For J.H., the dose of sincalide would be 0.12 mcg/kg/day.[96]

The antibiotic, metronidazole, also appears promising in the prevention of PN-associated cholestasis in adults. Metronidazole inhibits the bacterial overgrowth in the GI tract that occurs with intestinal stasis. The bacteria are responsible for increased formation of hepatotoxic bile acids such as lithocholate; 15 mg/kg/day of metronidazole has been shown to prevent lithocholate accumulation.[97]

PROGNOSIS

38. Project the course of J.H.'s liver disease if PN is discontinued and enteral feedings are instituted within 2 weeks. What may occur if enteral feedings cannot be instituted?

If PN can be discontinued soon after the onset of cholestasis, the prospects for J.H. to recover normal hepatic function are good. Jaundice usually resolves within 2 weeks after PN is discontinued, and the biochemical abnormalities normalize soon thereafter.[98] The pathologic changes observed on biopsy resolve even more slowly. Biopsy evidence of cholestasis has been observed for up to 40 weeks after resolution of clinical and serologic evidence of hepatic disease.[98,99]

If enteral feedings cannot be instituted successfully, the prognosis for J.H.'s liver function is not as good. Studies have demonstrated that infants receiving PN for ≥90 days had biopsy evidence of irreversible liver damage.[81] Thus, it clearly is advantageous to convert J.H.'s nutrition to the enteral route as soon as he tolerates such a change.

REFERENCES

1. Holliday MA et al. The maintenance need for water in parenteral fluid therapy. *Pediatrics* 1957;19:823.
2. Santoshm M et al. Oral rehydration therapy of infantile diarrhea: a controlled study of well-nourished children hospitalized in the United States and Panama. *N Engl J Med* 1983;306:1070.
3. Santosham M et al. Oral rehydration therapy for acute diarrhea in ambulatory children in the United States: a double-blind comparison of four different solutions. *Pediatrics* 1985;76:159.
4. Pizzaro D et al. Oral rehydration in hypernatremic and hyponatremic diarrheal dehydration. *Am J Dis Child* 1983;137:730.

5. Meeuwisse GW. High sugar worse than high sodium in oral rehydration solutions. *Acta Paediatr Scand* 1983;72:161.
6. Guzman C et al. Hypernatremic diarrheal dehydration treated with oral glucose-electrolyte solution containing 90 or 75 mEq/L of sodium. *J Pediatr Gastroenterol Nutr* 1988;7:694.
7. American Academy of Pediatrics, Committee on Nutrition. On the feeding of supplemental foods to infants. *Pediatrics* 1980;65:1178.
8. Bucuvalas JC et al. The neonatal gastrointestinal tract. In: Fanaroff AA, et al., eds. *Neonatal-Perinatal Medicine: Disease of the Fetus and Infant.* St. Louis: Mosby; 1987:894.
9. Anderson GH. Human milk feeding. *Pediatr Clin North Am* 1985;32:335.
10. Yom HC et al. Genetic engineering of milk composition: modification of milk components in lactating transgenic animals. *Am J Clin Nutr* 1993;58(Suppl):299.
11. Garza C et al. Special properties of human milk. *Clin Perinatol* 1987;14:11.
12. Oski FA. Iron deficiency—facts and fallacies. *Pediatr Clin North Am* 1985;32:493.
13. American Academy of Pediatrics, Committee on Nutrition. Fluoride supplementation. *Pediatrics* 1986;77:758.
14. Dewey KG et al. Differences in morbidity between breast-fed and formula-fed infants. *J Pediatr* 1995;126.
15. Churchill RB et al. The pros (many) and cons (a few) of breastfeeding. *Contemp Pediatr* 1998;15:18.
16. Committee on Nutrition. Soy-protein formulas: recommendations for use in infant feeding. *Pediatrics* 1983;72:359.
17. Committee on Nutrition. Hypoallergenic infant formulas. *Pediatrics* 1989;83:1068.
18. Anonymous. Enterobacter sakazakii infections associated with the use of powdered infant formula—Tennessee 2001. *MMWR* 2002;51:298.
19. Fomon SJ et al. Cow milk feeding in infancy: gastrointestinal blood loss and iron nutritional status. *J Pediatr* 1981;98:540.
20. Crump IM. Selected inborn errors of metabolism. In: Kelts DG, Jones EG, eds. *Manual of Pediatric Nutrition.* Boston: Little, Brown; 1984:211.
21. Collins JE et al. The dietary management of inborn errors of metabolism. *Human Nutrition Applied Nutrition* 1985;39:255.
22. Dunn L et al. Beneficial effects of early hypocaloric enteral feeding on neonatal gastrointestinal function: preliminary report of a randomized trial. *J Pediatr* 1988;112:622.
23. Slagle TA et al. Effect of early low-volume enteral substrate on subsequent feeding tolerance in very low-birth-weight infants. *J Pediatr* 1988;113:526.
24. Parker P et al. A controlled comparison of continuous versus intermittent feeding in the treatment of infants with intestinal disease. *J Pediatr* 1981;99:360.
25. Leleiko NS et al. Nutritional assessment of pediatric patients admitted to an acute-care pediatric service utilizing anthropometric measurements. *JPEN* 1986;10:166.
26. Georgieff MK et al. Effect of neonatal caloric deprivation on head growth and 1-year developmental status in preterm infants. *J Pediatr* 1985;107:581.
27. Galler JR et al. Long-term effects of early kwashiorkor compared with marasmus. II. Intellectual performance. *J Pediatr Gastroenterol Nutr* 1987;6:847.
28. Galler JR et al. Long-term effects of early kwashiorkor compared with marasmus. III. Fine motor skills. *J Pediatr Gastroenterol Nutr* 1987:6:855.
29. 2000 CDC growth charts: United States. Retrieved April 1, 2003 from the World Wide Web: http://www.cdc.gov/growthcharts.
30. Thomas MR et al. Evaluation of transthyretin as a monitor of protein-energy intake in preterm and sick neonatal infants. *JPEN* 1988;12:162.
31. Yoder MC et al. Comparison of serum fibronectin, prealbumin and albumin concentrations during nutritional repletion in protein calorie malnourished infants. *J Pediatr Gastroenterol Nutr* 1987;6:84.
32. Georgieff MK et al. Serum transthyretin levels and protein intake as predictors of weight gain velocity in premature infants. *J Pediatr Gastroenterol Nutr* 1987;6:775.
33. Moskowitz SR et al. Prealbumin as a biochemical marker of nutritional adequacy in premature infants. *J Pediatr* 1983;102:749.
34. Vanlandingham S et al. Prealbumin: a parameter of visceral protein levels during albumin infusion. *JPEN* 1982;6:230.
35. Ramsden DB et al. The interrelationship of thyroid hormones, vitamin A and the binding proteins following acute stress. *Clin Endocrinol* 1978;8:109.
36. Sandstedt S et al. Influence of total parenteral nutrition on plasma fibronectin in malnourished subjects with or without inflammatory response. *JPEN* 1984;8:493.
37. Hill R et al. An evaluation of D-xylose absorption measurements in children suspected of having small intestinal disease. *J Pediatr* 1981;99:245.
38. Orenstein SR. Enteral versus parenteral therapy for intractable diarrhea of infancy: a prospective, randomized trial. *J Pediatr* 1986;109:277.
39. Rossi TM et al. Extent and duration of small intestinal mucosal injury in tractable diarrhea of infancy. *Pediatrics* 1980;66:730.
40. Green HL et al. Protracted diarrhea and malnutrition in infancy: changes in intestinal morphology and disaccharidase activities during treatment with total intravenous nutrition or oral elemental diets. *J Pediatr* 1975;87:695.
41. Greene HL et al. Guidelines for the use of vitamins, trace elements, calcium, magnesium, and phosphorus in infants and children receiving total parenteral nutrition: report of the subcommittee on pediatric parenteral nutrient requirements from the committee on clinical practice issues of the American Society for Clinical Nutrition. *Am J Clin Nutr* 1988;48:1324.
42. Hambridge M. Trace element deficiencies in childhood. In: Suskind RM, ed. *Textbook of Pediatric Nutrition.* New York: Raven; 1981:163.
43. Heird WC et al. Intravenous alimentation in pediatric patients. *J Pediatr* 1972;80:351.
44. Topper WH. Enteral feeding methods for compromised neonates and infants. In: Lebenthal E, ed. *Textbook of Gastroenterology and Nutrition in Infancy.* New York: Raven, 1981:645.
45. American Academy of Pediatrics-Committee on Nutrition. Nutritional needs of low-birth-weight infants. *Pediatrics* 1985;75:976.
46. Thureen PJ et al. Protein balance in the first week of life in ventilated neonates receiving parenteral nutrition. *Am J Clin Nutr* 1998;68:1128.
47. Hay WW et al. Workshop summary: Nutrition of the extremely low birth weight infant. *Pediatrics* 1999;104:1360.
48. Te Braake FWJ et al. Amino acid administration to premature infants directly after birth. *J Pediatr* 2005;147:457.
49. Kleigman RJ et al. Necrotizing enterocolitis. *N Engl J Med* 1984;310:1093.
50. Pildres RS et al. Carbohydrate metabolism in the fetus and neonate. In: Fanaroff AA et al., eds. *Behrman's Neonatal-Perinatal Medicine.* St. Louis: Mosby; 1983;845.
51. Kao LC et al. Triglycerides, free fatty acids, free fatty acids/albumin molar ratio and cholesterol levels in serum of neonates receiving long-term lipid infusions: controlled trial of continuous and intermittent regimens. *J Pediatr* 1984;104:429.
52. Cochran EB et al. Parenteral nutrition in pediatric patients. *Clin Pharm* 1988;7:351.
53. Phelps SJ et al. Effect of the continuous administration of fat emulsion on the infiltration of intravenous lines in infants receiving peripheral nutrition solutions. *JPEN* 1989;13:628.
54. Pineault M et al. Beneficial effect of coinfusing a lipid emulsion on venous patency. *JPEN* 1989;13:637.
55. Zabielski PB et al. Necrotizing enterocolitis: feeding in endemic and epidemic periods. *JPEN* 1989;13:520.
56. Friedman Z et al. Rapid onset of essential fatty acid deficiency in the newborn. *Pediatrics* 1976;58:640.
57. Herson VC et al. Effect of intravenous fat infusion on neonatal neutrophil and platelet function. *JPEN* 1989;13:620.
58. Andrew G et al. Lipid metabolism in the neonate: II. The effect of Intralipid in bilirubin binding in vitro and in vivo. *J Pediatr* 1976;88:279.
59. Beisel WR. Metabolic response of the host to infections. In: Feigin RD et al., eds. *Textbook of Pediatric Infectious Disease.* Philadelphia: WB Saunders; 1981:1.
60. Weber SS et al. Availability of insulin from parenteral nutrient solutions. *Am J Hosp Pharm* 1977;34:353.
61. Niemiec PW et al. Compatibility considerations in parenteral nutrient solutions. *Am J Hosp Pharm* 1984;41:893.
62. Sajbel TA et al. Use of separate insulin infusions with total parenteral nutrition. *JPEN* 1987;11:97.
63. Yeh TF et al. Metabolic rate and energy balance in infants with bronchopulmonary dysplasia. *J Pediatr* 1989;114:448.
64. Kurzner SI et al. Growth failure in infants with bronchopulmonary dysplasia: nutrition and elevated resting metabolic expenditure. *Pediatrics* 1988;81:379.
65. Covelli HD et al. Respiratory failure precipitated by high carbohydrate loads. *Ann Intern Med* 1981;95:579.
66. Heird WC et al. Pediatric parenteral amino acid mixture in low birth weight infants. *Pediatrics* 1988;81:41.
67. Helms RA et al. Comparison of a pediatric versus standard amino acid formulation in preterm neonates requiring parenteral nutrition. *J Pediatr* 1987;110:466.
68. Adamkin D et al. Comparison of two neonatal intravenous amino acid formulations in preterm infants: a multicenter study. *J Perinatol* 1991;11:375.
69. Crill CM et al. Carnitine: a conditionally essential nutrient in the neonatal population? *Journal of Pediatric Pharmacy Practice* 1999;4:127.
70. Baumgart S et al. Sepsis with coagulase-negative staphylococci in critically-ill newborns. *Am J Dis Child* 1983;137:461.
71. Johnson DE. Systemic candidiasis in very low-birth-weight infants (1500 grams). *Pediatrics* 1984;73:138.
72. Koo WWK et al. Response of preterm infants to aluminum in parenteral nutrition. *JPEN* 1989;13:516.
73. Ziegler EE et al. Body composition of the reference fetus. *Growth* 1976;40:329.
74. Postuma R et al. Liver disease in infants receiving total parenteral nutrition. *Pediatrics* 1979;63:110.
75. Pereira GR et al. Hyperalimentation-induced cholestasis: increased incidence and severity in premature infants. *Am J Dis Child* 1981;135:842.
76. Vileisis RA et al. Laboratory monitoring of parenteral nutrition-associated hepatic dysfunction in infants. *JPEN* 1981;5:67.
77. Merritt RJ. Cholestasis associated with total parenteral nutrition. *J Pediatr Gastroenterol Nutr* 1986;5:22.
78. Drongowski RA et al. An analysis of factors contributing to the development of total parenteral nutrition-induced cholestasis. *JPEN* 1989;13:586.
79. Lucas A et al. Metabolic and endocrine consequences of depriving preterm infants of enteral nutrition. *Acta Paediatr Scand* 1983;72:245.
80. Enzenauer RW et al. Total parenteral nutrition cholestasis: a cause of mechanical biliary obstruction. *Pediatrics* 1985;76:905.
81. Cohen C et al. Pediatric total parenteral nutrition: liver histopathology. *Arch Pathol Lab Med* 1981;105:152.
82. Benjamin DR. Hepatobiliary dysfunction in infants and children associated with long-term total

parenteral nutrition: a clinicopathologic study. *Am J Clin Pathol* 1981;76:276.
83. Kattwinkel J et al. The effects of age on alkaline phosphatase and other serologic liver function tests in normal subjects and patients with cystic fibrosis. *J Pediatr* 1973;82:234.
84. Bell RL et al. Total parenteral nutrition-related cholestasis in infants. *JPEN* 1986;10:356.
85. Kubota A et al. Hyperbilirubinemia in neonates associated with total parenteral nutrition. *JPEN* 1988;12:602.
86. Mauer E. Incidence of cholestasis in low birth weight neonates on TrophAmine. *JPEN* 1991; 15(Suppl):25S.
87. Gura K et al. Incidence of cholestasis in infants receiving parenteral nutrition: comparison of Aminosyn-PF and TrophAmine. *JPEN* 1992; 16(Suppl):28S.
88. Vileisis RA et al. Prospective controlled study of parenteral nutrition-associated cholestatic jaundice: effects of protein intake. *J Pediatr* 1980; 96:893.
89. Hira Y et al. High caloric infusion induced hepatic impairment in infants. *JPEN* 1979;3:146.
90. Roslyn JJ et al. Increased risk of gallstones in children receiving total parenteral nutrition. *Pediatrics* 1983;71:784.
91. Suita S et al. Cholelithiasis in infants: association with parenteral nutrition. *JPEN* 1984;8:568.
92. Knight P et al. Calcium and phosphate requirements of preterm infants who require prolonged hyperalimentation. *JAMA* 1980;2432:1244.
93. Gleghorn EE et al. Phenobarbital does not prevent total parenteral nutrition-associated cholestasis in non-infected neonates. *JPEN* 1986;10:282.
94. Levy JS et al. Prolonged neonatal cholestasis: bile acid patterns and response to cholestyramine [Abstract]. *Mount Sinai J Med* 1979;46:169.
95. Sandler RH et al. Use of ursodeoxycholic acid (UDCA) for children with severe liver disease from total parenteral nutrition (TPN): report of three cases [Abstract]. *Pediatr Res* 1989;25:124.
96. Prescott WA et al. Sincalide in patients with parenteral nutrition-associated gallbladder disease. *Ann Pharmacother* 2004;38:1942.
97. Lambert JR et al. Metronidazole prevention of serum liver enzyme abnormalities during total parenteral nutrition. *JPEN* 1985;9:501.
98. Dahms BB et al. Serial liver biopsies in parenteral nutrition-associated cholestasis of early infancy. *Gastroenterology* 1981;81:136.
99. Suita S et al. Follow-up studies of children treated with long-term intravenous nutrition (IVN) during the neonatal period. *J Pediatr Surg* 1982;17:37.

CHAPTER 98

Cystic Fibrosis

Sandra B. Earle

Cystic fibrosis (CF) is a severe, complex, hereditary disease that affects 1 of every 3,200 live births, or approximately 30,000 children and adults in the United States. One in 31 Americans carry the autosomal recessive gene for CF, which arises from a mutation in coding for the cystic fibrosis transmembrane regulator protein (CFTR). This genetic mutational error results in the complex, multisystem disease of CF, which is characterized by malabsorption and a state of chronic lung inflammation and infection.

The course and severity of cystic fibrosis are variable and unpredictable. The median life expectancy (i.e., about 40 years) for a child born with CF in 1990 was about double what would have been expected for a child diagnosed with CF 20 years earlier because of advances in the management of this disorder.[1] Although therapy continues to rely on treatment of symptoms rather than the underlying pathologic causes, continuing improved understanding of CF is likely to result in better control and perhaps a cure. CF is still a lethal disease, but aggressive therapy can decrease the morbidity of this disease and increase the life expectancy of the patient.[2]

HISTORY

In early history (~3,000 BC), the forehead of a newborn was licked crosswise for cleaning, and if a salty taste was perceived, the baby was considered "bewitched" and expected to soon die.[3] This early observation is consistent with the later discovery that patients with CF lose excess chloride "salt" in their sweat and with the subsequent establishment of the "sweat chloride test" for the diagnosis of CF.[4] The term "cystic fibrosis" was first used in 1938 to describe "cystic fibrosis of the pancreas" from postmortem pancreatic lesions.[5] Cystic fibrosis, therefore, is a relatively newly described disease. As a result, most patients cannot relate a long family history of this disease.[6]

GENETIC BASIS

Cystic fibrosis is caused by mutations in the CFTR, which is a member of the ATP binding cassette (ABC) family. CFTR is dependent on cyclic adenosine monophosphate (cAMP) for chloride transport: defective coding for CFTR inhibits the normal regulation of ion transport in and out of the cell on the apical surface of secretory epithelial cells.[7] CFTR also regulates the transport of bicarbonate and sodium ions, mucous rheology, pulmonary inflammation, and bacterial adherence.[8–12]

Approximately 5% of Caucasians are asymptomatic carriers of the CF mutation. The high frequency of this mutation has been attributed to a heterozygote-selective advantage that presumably protected the carrier against dehydration from cholera, cancer, and other disease.[13–21]

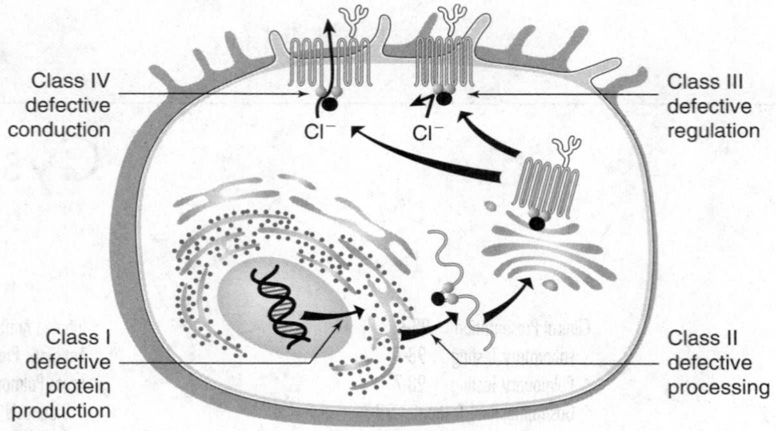

FIGURE 98-1 Classification of mutations: Class I mutations include those in which the production of the cystic fibrosis transmembrane regulator (CFTR) protein is blocked. These are called *stop mutations*. Defective protein processing is responsible for the class II mutations. In this class, the protein is made, but it is unable to make its way from the point of origin on the endoplasmic reticulum to the apical membrane, where it is needed for proper operation. This includes the most common, ΔF508, mutation, which is caused by improper folding of the protein. Class III mutations cause the disruption of the channel to open properly. Class IV mutations are unable to achieve proper ion conduction. Class V is a milder form of class I mutations and includes mutations that cause reduced production of functional CFTR. (From ref. 25, with permission.)

Almost two decades have passed since the identification and cloning of the gene responsible for CF, and >1,000 new CFTR mutations have been discovered.[22–24] These mutations have been grouped into five major classes according to the functional consequence of the defect (Fig. 98-1).[25,26] The most common variant is ΔF508, representing 66% of all mutations. Approximately 90% of all patients with CF have at least one copy of this mutation.[27] Interestingly, even among individuals with identical genotypes, a broad spectrum of disease severity is seen.[28,29] The contribution of genetic factors other than the misfunctioning CFTR can have a great influence on disease severity.[30–37] For example, an increased expression of transforming growth factor $\beta 1$ is associated with a poorer clinical outcome.[38] Another potentially important modifier may be an anti-inflammatory mediator, macrophage inhibitory factor.[39] As genetic modifiers are better understood, more effective therapies can be developed.[40,41]

CLINICAL MANIFESTATIONS

Genotype, environmental factors, and modifier gene status all contribute to the highly variable clinical course of CF. The linking of the loss of CFTR function to clinical manifestations of the disease, however, has been central to gaining an understanding of the disease and in the discovery of new therapies. Normally, CFTR is highly expressed on the membranes of epithelial cells of the lungs, sweat glands, salivary glands, and male genital ducts as well as the pancreas, kidney tubules, and digestive tract. The CFTR performs different functions in specific tissues; therefore, a dysfunctional or absent CFTR has different effects on different organs resulting in the multiorgan clinical manifestations of CF (Table 98-1).

Sweat Glands

Fluid secreted by the sweat glands in patients with CF is normal, but a defect in the reabsorption of electrolytes leads to sweat with a high salt content. CFTR, in the apical membrane of the resorptive area of the sweat gland, functions as an ion channel for chloride transport and also activates an associated epithelial sodium channel (ENaC).[42] Normally, these channels efficiently reabsorb sodium chloride from sweat. In patients with CF, loss of these functioning channels blocks the ability of the sweat ducts to reabsorb salt, leading to sweat sodium chloride (NaCl) concentrations of >100 mM (Fig. 98-2). The loss of these sodium and chloride ion channels serves as the basis for the diagnostic sweat chloride test and as the scientific basis for the "infant who tastes of salt" in folklore.

Sinus Involvement

Nasal polyps, which are outgrowths of normal sinus epidermis, can be found in up to 20% of older patients with CF and may become sufficiently large to block nasal passages. The pathogenesis of these polyps is unknown, but the obstruction of nasal passages can lead to infection. The faulty ionic transport of chloride across the apical membrane of epithelial cells lining exocrine glands leads to dehydration of extracellular fluids and the development of thickened inspissated mucus in nasal and sinus passages. Most patients with CF develop sinus disease with pan-opacification of the sinuses in 90% to 100% of patients >8 months of age. On radiographic examination, >90% of adult-age patients have pansinusitis, which can contribute to pulmonary exacerbations.[43,44] The impact of sinusitis on the CF population is significant.

Pancreatic Involvement

The exocrine and ultimately the endocrine function of the pancreas are affected in CF. Pancreatic enzymes normally are secreted into bicarbonate-rich fluid from the pancreatic duct, and CFTR is needed to secrete the bicarbonate into the lumen. The loss of CFTR function inhibits secretion of digestive enzymes and bicarbonate into the duodenum, and the enzymes are

Table 98-1 Clinical Manifestations of Cystic Fibrosis[234]

	Approximate Incidence (%)		
Manifestation	*Infants*	*Children*	*Adults*
Pancreatic			
Insufficiency	80–85	85	90
Pancreatitis		1–2	2–4
Abnormal glucose tolerance		5/yr[a]	30
Diabetes mellitus		2–4	8–15
Hepatobiliary			
Biliary cirrhosis		10–20	>20
Cholelithiasis		5	5–10
Biliary obstruction		1–2	5
Intestinal			
Meconium ileus	10–15		
Meconium ileus equivalent		1–5	10–20
Rectal prolapse		10–15	1–2
Intussusception		1–5	1–2
Gastroesophageal reflux		1–5	>10
Appendiceal abscess		0–1	1–2
Respiratory			
Upper			
Nasal polyps	<1	4–10	15–20
Pansinusitis			90–100
Lower			
Bronchiectasis		30–50	>90
Pneumothorax		1–2	10–15
Hemoptysis[b]		5–15	50–60
Genitourinary			
Delayed puberty			85
Infertility			
Males			98
Females			70–80

[a] ↑ in glucose intolerance of approximately 5% per year.
[b] Percentage includes both major and minor hemoptysis.

trapped in the pancreas by ductal obstruction. Over time, these enzymes (lipase, protease, amylase) accumulate and eventually begin to digest the pancreatic tissue.[12,45] The term *cystic fibrosis* arises from the fibrotic scar tissue that replaces the destroyed pancreas. Without these enzymes, there is poor digestion of fats and, to a lesser extent, proteins and carbohydrates are absorbed poorly. As a result, 90% of patients with CF experience pancreatic insufficiency characterized by steatorrhea (fatty stools), decreased absorption of the fat-soluble vitamins (A, D, E, and K), malnutrition, and failure to thrive. Early in life, serum concentrations of amylase and lipase are increased secondary to pancreatic autodigestion. This destructive process can result in either painful or asymptomatic chronic pancreatitis.

Eventually, the progressive destruction of the pancreas affects its endocrine function, leading to glucose intolerance in about 17% of children and 75% of adults.[46,47] Diabetes mellitus occurs in approximately 40% of adult patients with CF.[48] The additional diagnosis of diabetes in CF is associated with significantly increased morbidity and mortality,[49,50] and

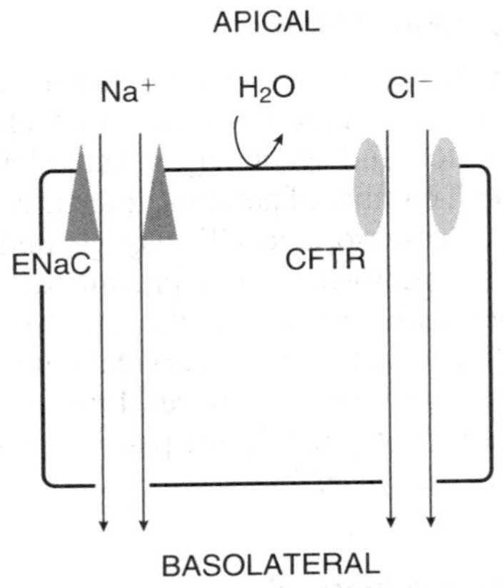

FIGURE 98-2 Normal salt (NaCl) absorption in the sweat duct with working epithelial sodium channel (ENaC) and cystic fibrosis transmembrane regulator (CFTR).

a decrease in insulin sensitivity is associated with pulmonary exacerbations.[51] Early aggressive insulin therapy can result in improved clinical outcomes.[52]

Intestinal Involvement

Meconium ileus, an intestinal obstruction at birth, occurring in 20% of newborns with CF, is an inheritable trait of this disease.[53] Outside the neonatal period, distal intestinal obstruction syndrome (DIOS, also called *meconium ileus equivalent*) can occur at any age and results from the complete or partial obstruction of the intestine. Intestinal obstruction occurs in 10% to 20% of patients and results from the inspissation of intestinal secretions and incompletely digested intestinal contents. A right lower quadrant mass, abdominal distention, failure to pass stools, and vomiting can accompany DIOS.

Gastrointestinal reflux disease (GERD) is common in both children and adults with CF.[54–56] Children with CF should be screened for GERD and treated, if diagnosed. Other intestinal complications include rectal prolapse, intussusception, and appendiceal abscesses.

Hepatic Involvement

Located on the apical surfaces of the cells lining the intrahepatic and extrahepatic bile ducts and the gallbladder, CFTR functions to facilitate ion transport.[57] In patients with CF, the abnormal chloride efflux across the cells results in the reduction in water and sodium movement into the bile. The resulting decrease in the volume and flow of bile leads to stasis and obstruction of the biliary tree. With chronic obstruction, there is inflammation, giving rise to the characteristic lesion of focal biliary cirrhosis.[58]

Liver disease develops in the first decade of life. Significant liver disease is seen in 13% to 25% of children with CF.[59–61] Prevalence rates may be underestimated. Progressive cirrhosis is associated with portal hypertension, hypersplenism, esophageal varices, ascites, and, in a small number of patients, complete hepatic failure requiring transplantation. Approximately 30% of adult patients with CF have abnormal gallbladder function and size (absent or small gallbladder) with 5% to 10% of patients developing gallstones.[62]

Genitourinary Involvement

Approximately 98% of males with CF are infertile secondary to *in utero* obstruction of the vas deferens or related structures. Hormonal secretion and secondary sexual characteristics are normal. In a small number of patients, infertility can be the only manifestation of disease, and CF may go undiagnosed until fertility testing is performed. The prevalence of infertility is higher in women with CF and hypothesized to be related to the production of thick and tenacious cervical mucus. Hundreds of pregnancies have been carried successfully to term, but these are not without risk, especially for patients with moderate to severe pulmonary disease.[63]

Bone and Joint Involvement

Patients with CF have low bone mineral density, slower rate of bone formation, high rate of bone loss, accelerated rate of bone loss, and arthritis.[64,65] Osteoclastic precursors are elevated during acute pulmonary exacerbation.[66] Although early, aggressive treatment of pulmonary exacerbations can improve bone health, sufficient intake and absorption of the fat-soluble vitamins, D and K, are important, and oral bisphosphonates may also be indicated.[65,67–73]

Patients with CF often suffer from intermittent arthritis symptoms, but only about 2% of patients have persistent symptoms. The three types of intermittent CF arthritis are (a) hypertrophic osteoarthropathy, (b) immunoreactive, and (c) CF arthropathy. The first two types are associated with pulmonary disease flare-up. The third type, CF arthropathy, affects large joints and may be accompanied by fever and erythema nodosum.[74–78]

Pulmonary Involvement

The relationship of ion-channel disruption (resulting from CFTR dysfunction) to lung tissue destruction has yet to be firmly established. Presently, the CF gene mutation is believed to cause CFTR dysfunction, which in turn causes ion transporter defects, and subsequent changes in the airway secretions. The changes in airway secretions promote the infection-inflammation-tissue damage cycle (Fig. 98-3). Chronic infection combined with inflammation has been the hallmark of lung disease in CF. The cycle of unchecked inflammation and infection has been the focus of much investigation and ongoing debate to "Which came first—infection or inflammation."[79] Although the inflammatory response appears to set up bacterial colonization in the airways, infection also can stimulate an inflammatory response. In either case, the cycle of inflammation and infection eventually leads to lung tissue damage and bronchiectasis.[80]

This pattern of inflammation and infection has not been observed in any other tissue where CFTR is expressed. Differences in the airway surface liquid, mucus, and other protective mechanisms in the lung of the patient with CF are being studied, and some of these differences may help explain the inflammation–infection cycle (Table 98-2).

Infection

Despite repeated courses of aggressive antibiotic therapy, patients with CF eventually develop endobronchial bacterial colonization and infection. Understanding why bacteria seldom are eradicated is important to treating this disease.

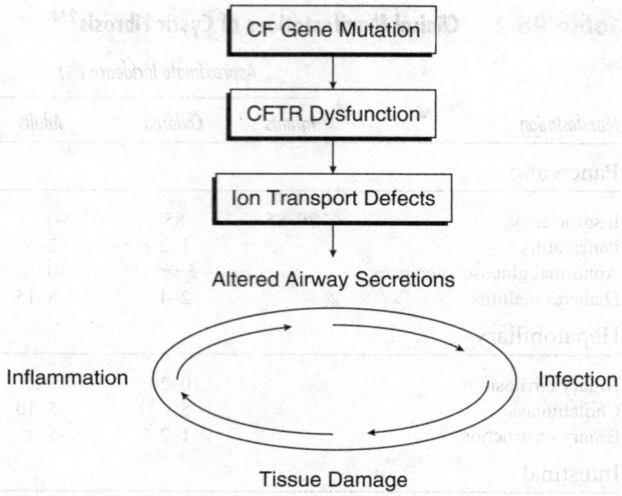

FIGURE 98-3 Pathologic cycle in lung disease. CFTR, cystic fibrosis transmembrane regulator. (From ref. 235, with permission.)

The lower airways of a normal lung are always maintained free of pathogens through various lung defense mechanisms. For example, a thin film of liquid on the airway surfaces called the *airway surface layer* (ASL) contains antimicrobials, antioxidants, proteases, and other substances that work to eliminate pathogens. The ASL also signals molecules to turn on the cellular immune system by recruiting neutrophils and macrophages to the site of microbe invasion. In addition, the ASL can remove invading microbes from the lung by moving a mucous gel toward the mouth through ciliary motion. Mucociliary clearance of microbes and debris is aided by the cough reflex to keep the airways clean. Because coughing is an important defense mechanism necessary for patients with CF, cough suppressants should not be prescribed or taken by them.

Local antibacterial peptides in the ASL are inactivated by high concentrations of salt similar to the concentrations found in CF ASL.[81,82] The ion channel dysfunction associated with CF can dehydrate and thicken mucus as well as deplete periciliary fluid and collapse cilia.[83,84] Thick mucus, which is not easily cleared, serves as a nidus for bacterial growth and, when combined with impaired mucociliary clearance, promotes chronic bacterial infection.[85]

Cystic fibrosis epithelial tracheal cells express high numbers of surface receptors for *Pseudomonas aeruginosa* and *Staphylococcus aureus*.[86] *S. aureus* is frequently responsible for the initial bacterial colonization, whereas *P. aeruginosa* is the most common pathogen isolated in chronically colonized patients.

The oxygen radicals produced by the inflammatory response in infected CF airways induce bacterial mutations of *P. aeruginosa* that lead to production of alginate, a biofilm that allows the organism to become more resistant to antibiotics. Mucoid *P. aeruginosa* bacteria also produce exotoxin A, protease, and elastase, which damage lung tissue and decrease the effectiveness of the neutrophils (polymorphonuclear leukocytes [PMN]) and macrophages.[87,88] *Burkholderia cepacia,* another

Table 98-2 Host Abnormalities That Predispose to Chronic Lung Infection

Abnormality	Proposed Impact	Proposed Intervention(s)
Abnormal cystic fibrosis transmembrane regulator (CFTR)	Altered secretions (low volume of airway surface fluid and hypertonicity) lead to thick dehydrated mucus, impairment of mucociliary escalator, and impaired defensin-mediated antimicrobial activity	• Chest physiotherapy • Inhaled deoxyribonuclease (DNase) • Gene therapy[a] • Alter electrolyte and water balance by aerosolized hypertonic saline, amiloride (block Na^+ uptake)[a] uridine triphosphate (UTP) (increase Cl efflux),[a] or provide novel peptides[b]
Increased expression of asialoganglioside (aGMI)	Increased *P. aeruginosa* and *St. aureus* binding to respiratory epithelial cells	• Anti-aGMI blocking antibody[b]
Defective CFTR-mediated uptake of *P. aeruginosa* by respiratory epithelial cells	Decreased clearance of internalized *P. aeruginosa* with sloughed epithelial cells	• Gene therapy[a]
Abnormal regulation of proinflammatory cytokines	• Hyperexuberant neutrophil recruitment and release of neutrophil oxidants	• Anti-inflammatory therapy (e.g., steroids or ibuprofen) beneficial, but associated with side effects such as cataracts, poor growth, or gastrointestinal bleeding
Increased IL-8 expression and tumor necorosis factor (TNF)-α	• Upregulation of human mucin genes	• More selective anti-inflammatory agents[b]
Variant mannose-binding lectin (MBL)	Polymorphisms may differentially bind bacterial surface carbohydrates	• MBL replacement[b]

[a]Investigational intervention.
[b]Theoretic intervention.
Adapted from Saiman L, Siegel J. Infection control recommendations for patients with cystic fibrosis: microbiology, important pathogens and infection control practices to prevent patient-to-patient transmission. *Am J Infect Control* 2003;31(3 Suppl):S1, with permission.

opportunistic pathogen found in patients with CF, is highly resistant to virtually all antibiotics. Patients may be asymptomatic or may have a fulminant infection leading to death. Such patients infected with mucoid strains of *P. aeruginosa* and *B. cepacia* experience increased morbidity and mortality.[89–91]

Viruses, fungi, and mycobacteria are also potential pathogens. Viruses can predispose patients to subsequent bacterial infection and may be responsible for activating the inflammation cycle. *Aspergillus fumigatus,* a fungus, has been associated with allergic bronchopulmonary aspergillosis (ABPA) in 5% to 25% of patients with CF. ABPA is an immunologic reaction to *Aspergillus,* which can lead to progressive pulmonary fibrosis if left undiagnosed and untreated. Nontuberculous mycobacteria have emerged as pathogens in the CF population.[92,93] The clinical course associated with nontuberculous mycobacteria infection is variable and it complicates the diagnosis and treatment of the patient with CF.

Inflammation

Inflammation is the lung's response to chronic infection.[86,94] Neutrophils (PMN) are "called" to the site of an infection by interleukin-1 (IL-1), interleukin-8 (IL-8), leukotriene (LTB_4), endotoxin, and tumor necrosis factor (TNF-α).[95] IL-8 is a major chemoattractant, and when bound to heparan sulfate-containing proteoglycans, its activity is prolonged.[95] When neutrophils arrive at the site, they release proteases, oxidants, elastases, and cytokines. Antiproteases and interleukin-10 (IL-10), an anti-inflammatory cytokine, subsequently are released in an effort to counterbalance the inflammatory system. Platelets also are dysfunctional and can contribute to inflammation through nitric oxide pathway.[96] Anti-inflammatory compounds are relatively low in patients with CF, and levels of neutrophils, proteases, elastases, oxidants, and cytokines all are increased.[97–99] These abnormalities lead to a sustained and destructive cycle of unchecked inflammation that begins at a very early age.[94]

Arachidonic acid (AA), an agonist in the inflammation pathway, is increased, and docosahexaenoic acid (DHA), a down-regulator of AA, is decreased in the bronchial lavage fluid in patients with CF. This imbalance of fatty acids favors the inflammatory and mucus-producing AA, and, therefore, provides an explanation for the role of CFTR in causing inflammation and increased mucus production in the airways.[100]

DIAGNOSIS

Diagnostic Criteria

Most children with CF are diagnosed in the first year of life (median age at diagnosis, 6 months), but 8% are not diagnosed until later (>18 years of age).[101] A positive diagnosis of CF is contingent on having one or more of the characteristics listed in Table 98-3, a history of CF in a sibling, or a positive newborn screening test result. These must then be accompanied by two positive sweat chloride tests, two positive nasal potential differences (NPD) tests, or identification of two CF mutations.[102,103] The classic triad of clinical signs and symptoms for the diagnosis of CF are a positive sweat chloride test, gastrointestinal (GI) malabsorption, and chronic pulmonary disease. With the discovery of the *CF* gene, DNA typing is now available for 95% of the CF mutations.

When the pilocarpine iontophoresis test (i.e., sweat chloride test) is conducted at a certified CF center and is positive (>60 mEq/L) on two different days, the diagnosis of CF can be applied.[104] Sweat collection amounts may be inadequate in a preterm or neonate <1 week of age. Currently, a sweat chloride

Table 98-3 Phenotypic Features Consistent With Diagnosis of Cystic Fibrosis (CF)

1. Chronic sinopulmonary disease manifested by:
   - Persistent colonization or infection with typical CF pathogens (e.g., *St. aureus*, nontypeable *H. influenzae,* mucoid and nonmucoid *P. aeruginosa,* and *B. cepacia*
   - Chronic cough and sputum production
   - Persistent chest radiograph abnormalities (e.g., bronchiectasis, atelectasis, infiltrates, hyperinflation)
   - Airway obstruction manifested by wheezing and air trapping
   - Nasal polyps; radiographic or computed tomographic abnormalities of paranasal sinuses
   - Digital clubbing
2. Gastrointestinal and nutritional abnormalities including:
   - *Intestinal:* meconium ileus, distal intestinal obstruction syndrome, rectal prolapse
   - *Pancreatic:* pancreatic insufficiency, recurrent pancreatitis
   - *Hepatic:* chronic hepatic disease manifested by clinical or histologic evidence of focal biliary cirrhosis or multilobular cirrhosis
   - *Nutritional:* failure to thrive (protein–calorie malnutrition), hypoproteinemia and edema, complications secondary to fat-soluble vitamin deficiency
3. Salt loss syndromes: acute salt depletion, chronic metabolic alkalosis
4. Male urogenital abnormalities resulting in obstructive azoospermia (CBAVD)

CBAVD, congenital bilateral absence of the vas deferens.
From ref. 103, with permission.

value of >40 mmol/L is required for the diagnosis of CF in the newborn period; infants with values >30 mmol/L, require follow-up. In programs that perform mutation analysis, confirmatory sweat testing should be obtained even in infants who test positive for two mutations. A false–positive sweat chloride test finding for CF can result from glucose-6-phosphate dehydrogenase deficiency, hypothyroidism, glycogen storage disease, untreated adrenal insufficiency, and malnutrition.[105]

A second diagnostic test for CF evaluates the pattern of increased NPD. Abnormalities of ion transport in respiratory epithelia results in patients with CF having a higher basal NPD, which reflects enhanced Na^+ transport across a relatively Cl^- impermeable barrier. This test can be effective in diagnosing CF in infants in the first few hours of life. Older children may need mild sedation before initiating the test for NPD. Inflamed mucosa or nasal polyps can generate a false–negative NPD finding. The NPD test should be repeated on a separate day at a reputable CF center if the first test is positive for CF.[106]

Genetic Testing

Prenatal Screening

If both parents are known to be carriers of CF, the American College of Medical Genetics (ACMG) and the American College of Obstetrics and Gynecology (ACOG) recommend prenatal screening.[107] Amniocentesis, chorionic villus sampling (CVS) and pancreatitis-associated protein (PAP) all have been used to diagnose CF *in utero*. Genetic testing for CF should be conducted at a center that has knowledgeable genetic counselors who understand the validity and reliability of the tests as well as the sociomedical implications for a child diagnosed with CF.

Neonatal Screening

Growing consensus is that early aggressive therapy improves the quality of life and extends the life-span of patients with CF.[108,109] CF is included on the 2006 newborn screening list released by the American Academy of Pediatrics and is advocated by many clinicians.[105,110–115] Early diagnosis is associated with improved height and weight, likely owing to early introduction of nutritional interventions, and improved survival.[116,117] Immunoreactive trypsinogen (IRT) concentration is high in the blood of infants with CF. If elevated in a blood-spot screen, the IRT may be repeated or a mutation analysis for genotype can be performed. Newborns who present with meconium ileus are always suspected of having CF; however, in this subset of patients, for reasons not understood, IRT has a high prevalence of false–negative results.[118] If neonatal screening is to be effective, an infrastructure must be in place to provide education and counseling for families.[119,120]

Clinical Presentation

1. L.T., a 9-month-old male, is brought to the pediatric primary care clinic. His mother states, "He can't seem to eat enough food and cries constantly." She says that he has 8 to 10 stools per day, but she thought this was because he ate so much. On further questioning, she says that the stools are large, greasy, and foul smelling. He has never been hospitalized, but has had three ear infections and three chest colds, which were treated with antibiotics. When plotted on a standard growth curve, L.T. is found to be in the fifth percentile for both weight and height (7.5 kg and 68 cm). The pregnancy and delivery were uncomplicated, and L.T.'s medical history is otherwise unremarkable. Physical examination shows a poorly nourished, small-for-age infant in no apparent distress. Family history is unremarkable. Review of systems reveals diffuse crackles in the lower lung fields; all other systems are within normal limits. A sweat chloride test is ordered and the results are a chloride concentration of 110 mEq/L (normal, <60 mEq/L). L.T.'s chest x-ray study shows mild peribronchial thickening of both upper lobes. What subjective and objective data for L.T. are suggestive of the diagnosis of CF?

L.T. fulfills the classic triad for the diagnosis of CF: elevated sweat chloride, chronic recurrent pulmonary infections, and apparent pancreatic insufficiency. Although not showing symptoms of pulmonary infection at present, the baby has had several chest colds, and chest x-ray study indicates chronic inflammation. As illustrated by L.T., the earliest chest x-ray study shows peribronchial thickening in the upper lung fields. As the lung disease progresses, hyperinflation, as evidenced by increased anteroposterior diameter of the chest (barrel chest) and flattening of the diaphragm, is evident. Eventually, areas of collapse, consolidation, and abscess formation and bronchiectasis develop, indicating severe pulmonary tissue destruction. L.T.'s pancreatic insufficiency is suggested by his multiple daily fatty stools and failure to thrive despite a voracious appetite. In summary, a positive sweat test, evidence of GI malabsorption, and pulmonary involvement support the probable diagnosis of CF in L.T.

Laboratory Testing

2. What further testing can be done to confirm the diagnosis of CF in L.T.?

The sweat chloride test should be repeated on another day to affirm laboratory testing reliability and to rule out other conditions that can cause an elevated sweat chloride level (see Diagnostic Criteria above). Genetic testing can be done to identify CFTR mutations. Because genetic testing cannot identify all the possible mutations that can cause CF, it is not the diagnostic test of choice. A diagnosis of CF is likely if the second sweat chloride test is positive, especially in light of L.T.'s clinical presentation.

Pulmonary Testing

3. What testing and follow-up should be completed to define L.T.'s pulmonary involvement?

Baseline pulmonary function tests, chest x-ray studies, oxygen saturation, and sputum cultures are a part of the normal workup. Spirometry should be performed at least every 6 months, and complete pulmonary function tests should be performed once a year. The percent of the predicted forced expiratory volume in 1 second (FEV_1) stratifies the level of lung disease. Greater than 90% is considered normal; between 70% and 89% is mildly impaired, 40% to 69% is moderate impairment and <40% is severely impaired. Arterial blood gases or pulse oximetry need to be completed on patients with severe disease. Children such as L.T., who are younger than 5 years of age, are unable to perform the tasks associated with pulmonary function testing adequately. Chest x-ray studies should be obtained annually, whenever the patient has a pulmonary-related hospital admission, and before any surgery. Respiratory tract cultures and sensitivities should be completed annually and before initiation of antibiotic therapy. Because obtaining a voluntary sputum sample from an infant is difficult, an oropharyngeal swab can be used to initiate a gag reflex and cough, and then a sputum sample is collected. The sputum sample obtained actually may contain only normal upper airway flora rather than bacteria colonizing the lower airway; therefore, it is important to interpret persistently normal flora from a sputum culture of an infant with caution.[108] The need for a smoke-free environment for L.T. should be emphasized to the family.[121]

Gastrointestinal Testing

4. What testing and follow-up should be completed in L.T. to define GI and nutritional involvement?

L.T.'s head circumference, height, and weight should be plotted on standard growth charts every 3 months for the first year. An experienced, knowledgeable registered dietician should meet with the family to help them understand the importance of appropriate nutrition and help develop a plan for L.T. Nutritional assessments should be completed annually, or more often if L.T. shows evidence of weight loss or poor weight gain. Serum lipase and amylase, fasting blood glucose, liver function tests, albumin, prealbumin, serum electrolytes, iron, and vitamins A, D, and E levels should be determined at least annually. An abdominal examination should be done to determine liver and spleen size and consistency at each office visit. Although quantification of fecal fat content may assist in the titration of pancreatic enzyme doses, an accurate dietary fat intake history is needed for accurate quantification. Many CF centers undertake this assessment only in patients who have demonstrated excessive pancreatic enzyme dose requirements.

THERAPY

The management of a case of CF is costly and complex. In addition, the emotional, physical, and social effects of caring for a chronically ill child can be overwhelming. Family socioeconomic status also seems to be a predictor of the health of a child with CF. The risk of death in the lowest income group (<$20,000/year) increased by 44%, and patients in this group had consistently lower pulmonary functions and body weights than those with higher income.[122,123]

In a review of more than 18,000 patients with CF, those who were monitored frequently and treated aggressively had better lung health as measured by FEV_1.[124] Aggressive preventive therapies, therefore, apparently result in better outcomes than treating problems as they arise.[108,125–127] Although a cure for CF is still the ultimate goal, new therapies to target malabsorption and the infection–inflammation cycle are being vigorously studied.

Control of Malabsorption

Patients with untreated CF have pancreatic insufficiency and are malnourished. Early diagnosis and treatment of malabsorption (i.e., meeting caloric needs, providing vitamin, mineral, and digestive enzymes) are beneficial to the patient.

Caloric Needs

Poor nutrition correlates with negative prognosis; therefore, maximizing the nutritional status of the patient with CF is important. CF patients are hypermetabolic and do not absorb fats and proteins normally. Therefore, the CF diet must be high in calories, fat, and protein. An infant at diagnosis may need a total daily caloric goal of 120 to 150 kcal/kg to make up for lost time. Weight gain, fat stores, and growth then drive the daily caloric goal. When a patient has a significant weight loss or falls below the tenth percentile for weight or height for age, it is indicative of nutritional failure, which requires therapeutic intervention.[128] Supplementation does not seem to be of benefit.[129] Some patients at nutritional risk benefit from night-time enteral feedings.[130,131]

Vitamin and Mineral Supplementation

The malabsorption of fats in patients with CF with pancreatic insufficiency also results in decreased GI absorption of the fat-soluble vitamins (A, D, E, and K). Approximately 45% of the CF population is deficient in one of these vitamins, even when pancreatic enzymes are being used appropriately.[132] The current recommendations for replacement therapy are listed in Table 98-4.[128] Concerns about inadequate supplementation of vitamins D and K resulting in poor bone health have arisen.[67,68,133–135] Calcium, sodium, and iron supplements might also be needed. A new vitamin supplement AquADEK has been formulated for patients with CF as a soft gel, rather than a chewtab, with added antioxidants, selenium, and more

Table 98-4 Daily Recommended Doses of Fat-Soluble Vitamins for Patients with Cystic Fibrosis (CF) and Vitamin Content in ADEK and AquADEK Formulations

Age	Vitamin A (IU)	Vitamin E (IU)	Vitamin D (IU)	Vitamin K (mg)
0–12 mon	1,500	40–50	400	0.3–0.5
1–3 yr	5,000	80–150	400–800	0.3–0.5
4–8 yr	5,000–10,000	100–200	400–800	0.3–0.5
>8 yr	10,000	200–400	400–800	0.3–0.5
Vitamin Content				
ADEK Chew Tab	9,000 (60% as β carotene)	150	400	0.15
ADEK drops	3,170	40	400	0.1
AquADEK liquid 1 mL	5751 (87% as β carotene)	50	400	0.4
AquADEK softgels	18,167 (92% as β carotene)	150	800	0.7

Adapted from ref. 128, with permission.

zinc, vitamin D and K.[128,136,137] Some patients purportedly have experienced a "niacin flush"-like reaction to AquADEK.

Enzyme Supplementation

The mainstay of treatment for pancreatic insufficiency is exogenous replacement of pancreatic digestive enzymes. The goals of pancreatic enzyme supplementation are to (a) improve weight gain, (b) minimize steatorrhea, and (c) eliminate abdominal cramping and bloating. Supplementation with currently available therapies does not fully restore fat absorption and the absorption of sufficient fat-soluble vitamins continues to be problematic.[138] The digestive enzymes (lipase, protease, amylase) are available in a mixture of approximately one part amylase to three parts protease and three parts amylase in capsules that contain enteric-coated microspheres of these enzymes (Table 98-5). The enteric coating protects these enzymes from gastric acid. Because the breakdown of fat is the most important function of these enzymes, dosing is based on the lipase content, and the dose varies according to weight, age, dietary fat intake, and symptom severity. The initial dose for

Table 98-5 Selected Pancreatic Enzymes

	Microencapsulated Enzymes		
Product[a]	Lipase	Protease	Amylase
Creon 5	5,000	18,750	16,600
Creon 10	10,000	37,500	33,200
Creon 20	20,000	75,000	66,400
Pancrease	4,500	25,000	20,000
Pancrease MT 4	4,000	12,000	12,000
Pancrease MT 10	10,000	30,000	30,000
Pancrease MT 16	16,000	48,000	48,000
Pancrease MT 20	20,000	44,000	56,000
Ultrase	4,500	25,000	20,000
Ultrase MT 12	12,000	39,000	39,000
Ultrase MT 18	18,000	58,500	58,500
Ultrase MT 20	20,000	65,000	65,000

[a]Dosing and comparison of products based on lipase content.
Adapted from Drug Facts and Comparisons, Inc., 2007, with permission.

infants is 2,000 to 2,500 units of lipase/kg per breast-feeding or per 120 mL of bottle-feeding: the dose is decreased to 1,000 units/kg/meal when infants begin to eat solid food. For children >4 years of age, 500 units of lipase/kg/meal is the empiric dose for enzyme supplementation.[139] A full dose is taken with meals, and half the prescribed dose is taken with snacks. Subsequent dosing adjustments are titrated to response.

Although enzyme dose is not correlated with growth or GI symptoms, lack of weight gain; smelly, greasy stools; and abdominal pain or bloating might be indicative of insufficient enzyme supplementation.[140,141] Generic substitutions of pancreatic enzymes have resulted in therapeutic failure and are not recommended.[142]

High-strength pancreatic enzymes have been associated with colonic strictures, which are accompanied by symptoms similar to that of DIOS and which must be differentiated from DIOS by ultrasound or x-ray study.[143] Although cause and effect have not been firmly established, doses >6,500 units lipase/kg/meal have been associated with stricture formation. As a result, most recommend that the daily dose of lipase not exceed 10,000 units of lipase/kg.[144]

When patients require unusually high doses of enzyme supplements, it sometimes can be attributable to high gastric acidity. The enteric coating on the pancreatic enzyme microspheres dissolves at a pH of 5.8, and the enzymes are destroyed at a pH of 4.0. Patients with CF have longer postprandial periods of time when the pH is <4.0 in the bowel and also have significantly less time when the pH is >5.8. Because enzymes may be less effective when the bowel pH is very low,[145,146] adding an H_2-antagonist or a proton-pump inhibitor to increase gastric pH might help lower the enzyme dosing requirement.[147–149]

5. Significant laboratory findings for L.T. include the following: serum vitamin E, 2.5 mg/L (normal, 3–15.8 mg/L); vitamin A, 26 mcg/dL (normal, 30–90 mcg/dL); lipase, 47 U/L (normal, 0.1–208 U/L); amylase, <30 U/L (normal, 0–110); albumin, 2.7 g/dL (normal, 3.4–5.1 g/dL); all other laboratory values are within normal limits. Pancreatic enzymes are to be started in L.T. What would be a reasonable dosing and monitoring plan for his pancreatic enzyme therapy?

The dosing of pancreatic enzymes is empirically started at 1,000 U/kg based on the lipase component. The initial dose for

L.T., who weighs 7.5 kg, would be 7,500 U, with a full dose for meals and a half-dose for snacks. To simplify drug therapy, it is best to select a single capsule strength that can be used for both meals and snacks. Therefore, a product with close to the desired amount (e.g., Creon 10) should be selected and dosed as one capsule with meals, and half a capsule with light meals or snacks. For the best result, the supplements should be given at the beginning of the meal or snack.[150] This is challenging, especially for an infant. Capsules can be opened and the microspheres put on the nipple of a mother nursing her infant or on the nipple of a bottle. Alternatively, the capsules can be opened and added to a spoonful of cereal or applesauce and given just before nursing or giving a bottle. The microspheres should not be chewed or put on hot food or liquid because the coating can be destroyed. The dose of the pancreatic enzymes should be adjusted to minimize steatorrhea, and the dose increased as needed. L.T.'s family should also be taught the signs of constipation or stomach pain in an infant.

L.T.'s weight gain and growth should be assessed every 3 months for the first year. As L.T. grows, his enzyme requirements will change and eventually he will need to become responsible for taking them on his own before eating. Neighbors, friends, and teachers should store a few supplements for L.T. to accommodate spontaneous eating of snacks.

6. In addition to enzyme replacement, what fat-soluble vitamin supplementation is appropriate for L.T.?

L.T.'s laboratory evaluation reveals vitamin A and E deficiencies, which are relatively common in patients with malabsorption. The long-term effects of inadequate fat-soluble vitamin intake are unclear. Vitamins A, D, E, and K, however, should be prescribed for L.T. because of the theoretic benefits, low cost, and low risk. L.T. should be started on 1 mL of AquADEK or ADEK drops daily (Table 98-4). Vitamins A, D, and E should be monitored yearly: his vitamin K need not be monitored unless risk factors are present or clotting difficulties are suspected.[128]

Control of Infection

Mucocilliary Clearance

Sputum in patients with CF is difficult to mobilize because pulmonary secretions are thick as a result of both the CFTR defect and the large amounts of viscous DNA from the breakdown of white blood cells and the bacterial debris left over from chronic infections. Mechanical clearance methods and inhaled mucolytics can be helpful in mobilizing pulmonary secretions.

MECHANICAL METHODS

Methods used to mechanically break up and mobilize mucus in the pulmonary tree include traditional hand percussion and postural drainage (P&PD); oscillating positive-end pressure (OPEP) with the flutter valve; high-frequency chest-wall oscillation (HFCWO) with the ThAIRapy vest; intrapulmonary percussive ventilation (IPV); and autogenic drainage (a technique of deep breathing exercises). These mechanical approaches for mobilizing mucus are about equal in efficacy, and the selection of the most appropriate one for a patient depends on the ability, motivation, preference, and resources of the patient.[151] When the traditional P&PD was compared with HFCWO and OPEP, clinical efficacy and safety were comparable, but 50% of patients preferred the HFCWO, 37% preferred OPEP, and 13% preferred P&PD.[152]

DORNASE ALFA

Dornase alfa (Pulmozyme) is an inhaled recombinant form of human deoxyribonuclease I, which breaks up the DNA formed by the PMN that block airways in the patient with CF. It has a beneficial effect on neutrophilic airway inflammation when compared with controls and reduces exacerbation frequency in patients.[153–157] It is safe for use in infants, but does not seem to be of benefit in an acute exacerbation.[158] Dornase alfa is very expensive, with costs averaging about $1,200/month; and the cost:benefit ratio for its use continues to be debated.[159,160] Nevertheless, this medication improves lung function, reduces exacerbations of patients >6 years of age, and is recommended.[161] More than 50% of patients with CF use dornase alfa.[101]

HYPERTONIC SALINE

Inhalation of hypertonic saline (IHS) also improves mucocilliary clearance. When twice-daily inhaled normal saline was compared with 7% (hypertonic) sodium chloride, the IHS-treated patients experienced better overall lung function and fewer exacerbations.[162,163] In another study, IHS also improved lung function and mucociliary clearance.[164] Although not compared in a head-to-head trial with IHS, dornase alpha seems to increase lung function more, but at a much higher financial cost than IHS. A short-acting β_2-agonist should be given before IHS treatment because IHS has been associated with bronchospasm.[165] IHS is available commercially and is recommended to improve lung function and reduce exacerbations in all patients >6 year of age.[161]

BRONCHODILATION

The chronic use of inhaled β_2-agonists improves lung function in patients with bronchial hyperresponsiveness or a positive bronchodilator response, and is recommended for use.[161] No clear consensus exists for the use of other bronchodilators. Although leukotriene modifiers have improved lung function in small studies, the overall data are insufficient to support a recommendation.[166] Studies in support of inhaled anticholinergic medications for the treatment of CF also are limited, and the results have been mixed.[167] Cromolyn use also is not routinely recommended because of limited evidence of positive outcomes with this drug.[161]

7. What mucus clearance methods would be appropriate for L.T.'s therapy?

Methods of mechanical assistance to remove pulmonary secretions are all equally effective, but hand P&PD would be the method of choice for L.T. because he is only 9 months of age. His parents should be taught the method of using a cupped hand or a vibrator device to shake loose the secretions that have accumulated in L.T.'s lungs. The other methods of chest physiotherapy can be used when L.T. is older and better able to participate.

Dornase alfa improves sputum viscosity in patients with CF and they are able to benefit from this drug early in the course of their lung disease.[153] In the Pulmozyme Early Intervention Trial (PEIT), the risk of pulmonary exacerbations was reduced by 34% in young patients with mild lung function abnormalities, and pulmonary function tests also were improved in patients with close to normal pulmonary function. The addition of dornase alfa is a viable consideration if the cost and scheduling of regular treatments are not issues for L.T.

Patient counseling is important if dornase alfa is prescribed for L.T. Dornase alfa should not be mixed with other drugs because it is an enzyme that can be denatured. Only approved nebulizers can be used because of the variability of delivery of aerosolized medications from different nebulizers. Baseline pulmonary function tests should be obtained, and L.T. should be re-evaluated in 6 weeks. Evidence of improvement should include the following: diminished dyspnea and cough, increase in sputum production, increased appetite, improved subjective measures (e.g., perception of energy, ability to sleep), and improvement in pulmonary function tests. Dornase alfa should be discontinued if the patient does not appear to be benefiting from therapy.[160]

Immunizations

8. A Gram's stain of L.T.'s sputum reveals normal respiratory flora, and the throat culture is pending. What immunizations should be considered for L.T. at this time?

L.T. has no evidence of a pulmonary infection at this time. He should receive all childhood immunizations at the usual recommended times (see Chapter 95: Pediatric Immunizations) and an annual flu vaccine as well. Prevention of influenza may help avoid the onset of a bacterial infection. When an immunization for *P. aeruginosa* is available, it will be essential for patients with CF.[168]

Antibiotic Therapy

Antibiotics are commonly used for the patient with CF to improve or delay the decline of pulmonary function. The indications for antimicrobial use include (a) treatment for an exacerbation, (b) prevention of colonization with *P. aeruginosa,* and (c) maintenance therapy for chronic *P. aeruginosa.* Bacterial resistance to antibiotics commonly develops in the patient with CF because pathogens often are not eradicated from the patient's airway. As a result, such patients probably need to receive broad-spectrum antibiotics more often than might be indicated in other populations.[169–172]

DIFFERENCES IN KINETICS

The physiologic changes in the patient with CF affects how the body absorbs, distributes, and clears drugs. Lack of bicarbonate secretion in the GI tract and prolonged GI transit times can affect the rate and extent of absorption of some drugs (e.g., oral ciprofloxacin). In addition, the apparent volume of distribution of drugs that are distributed in total body water can be increased because patients with CF have alterations in their body water:mass ratio.[173,174] For example, the volume of distribution is typically increased for aminoglycosides and β-lactams.

Both hepatic and renal clearances are increased for many drugs in patients with CF. *N*-acetyltransferase activity is increased,[173] but the P450 system does not seem to be greatly affected and remains isoenzyme dependent (i.e., CYP1A2, CYP2A6, CYP2C9, and CYP3A4 enzyme activity is not changed in these patients).[174–176] CYP2C8 activity and biliary secretion, however, may be enhanced.[177] The malfunctioning CFTR is hypothesized to increase the renal tubular clearance of organic anion drugs in these patients (e.g., penicillins and trimethoprim).[173,178–180]

These increases in clearance and volume of distributions make it necessary to adjust doses of some antibiotics for patients with CF. Increased clearance requires larger daily doses and possibly shorter dosing intervals. Table 98-6 contains an abbreviated list of suggested dosage regimens.

MONITORING AND ADVERSE EFFECTS

The prolonged, repeated use of aminoglycosides in patients with CF increases the risk for drug-related toxicity; however, the nephrotoxicity, ototoxicity, and vestibular damage associated with aminoglycosides seem to be less common in these patients than in the rest of the population.[181] Nevertheless, diligence in monitoring for these adverse effects are essential. The Cystic Fibrosis Center recommends urinalysis and assessment of the blood urea nitrogen (BUN) and creatinine serum concentrations after each course of aminoglycosides. Some clinicians suggest audiometric assessments for patients who have had 10 or more courses of intravenous (IV) aminoglycosides.[181] The adverse effects most often encountered with β-lactams are elevated liver enzymes, diarrhea, hypersensitivity reactions, and fungal overgrowth.

Broad-spectrum antibiotics can cause overgrowth of *Clostridium difficile* in the gut lumen or fungus in the oropharyngeal cavity. Patients should be instructed to report any episodes of diarrhea, difficulty in swallowing, or white plaques in their mouth.

INHALED ANTIBIOTICS

Patients with CF frequently receive large doses of systemic antibiotics to treat lung infections. The site of infection in CF is the airway lumen, not the lung parenchyma, however. Aerosolized administration of an antibiotic delivers the drug directly to the site of infection and, theoretically, should improve drug concentrations in the airway lumen and decrease the risk of systemic toxicity. Aerosolized tobramycin and colistin have been the most studied antibiotics for inhalation in patients with CF, but other antibiotics are also administered via this route.[182,183] Chronic inhalation of tobramycin reduces exacerbations, improves lung function, and is recommended for use in patients with persistently positive *P. aeruginosa* cultures and mild or moderate-to-severe lung disease.[162] Other inhaled antibiotics (e.g., colistin, gentamicin) do not have sufficient evidence to support a recommendation for use in patients with CF with positive cultures for pseudomonas.[161,184] More than 40% of all such patients in the United States are prescribed inhaled tobramycin.[101]

ANTIBIOTIC PROPHYLAXIS

9. When is it appropriate to give L.T. antibiotics to prevent lung infection and colonization?

Some clinicians prescribe prophylactic antibiotics in an effort to prevent *S. aureus* infections in young children and subsequent pseudomonas infections. In one randomized study, cephalexin significantly decreased colonization with *S. aureus,* but it also increased *P. aeruginosa* infections.[186] Thus, routine

Table 98-6 Antibiotic Doses For Cystic Fibrosis

Systemic Antibiotics

Drug	Daily Dosage (mg/kg)	Frequency	Maximal Individual Dose (mg)
Amikacin	30	Divided Q 8, 12, 24 hr	TDM
Ceftazidime	150–225	Divided Q 8 hr	2,000
Cefuroxime	150–225	Divided Q 8 hr	1,500
Ciprofloxacin IV	30	Divided Q 8 hr	400
Ciprofloxacin PO	40	Divided Q 12 hr	1,000
Gentamicin	10–15	Divided Q 8, 12, 24 hr	TDM
Imipenem	40–80	Divided Q 6 hr	1,000
Oxacillin	200	Divided Q 6 hr	2,000
Piperacillin	200–400	Divided Q 6 hr	4,000
Ticarcillin/clavulanate	200–400	Divided Q 6 hr	3,100
Tobramycin	10–15	Divided Q 8, 12, 24 hr	TDM

Inhaled Antibiotics

Drug	Dosage	Interval	
Amikacin	7.5 mg/kg/dose	BID–TID	
Gentamicin	2.5 mg/kg/dose	BID–TID	
TOBI	300 mg	BID	30 days on, 30 days off
Colistin	37.5–75 mg	BID–QID	

BID, twice daily; Q, every; TID, three times daily; TDM, therapeutic drug monitoring (gentamicin/tobramycin desired C_{max} 12–15 mg/L multiple daily dosing, C_{max} >20 mg/L once daily dosing); TOBI, tobramycin for inhalation.
Adapted from ref. 210, with permission.

antistaphylococcal prophylaxis is not recommended for young children with CF and would not be recommended for L.T.[161]

ACUTE PULMONARY EXACERBATION

Diagnosis

10. B.W., a 19-year-old woman, was diagnosed with CF at 3 years of age after a history of chronic pneumonias. She presents to the pulmonary clinic with increasing cough and sputum production over the past 2 weeks, with a change in sputum color from white to green. She currently weighs 45.2 kg and states she has lost 4 pounds. B.W. is a slightly thin adult woman whose breathing is labored. Pulmonary function tests reveal an FEV_1 of 65% of predicted normal and a forced vital capacity (FVC) of 60% (her usual baselines are FEV_1, 85%, and FVC, 80%). *P. aeruginosa* grew out of her sputum sample taken at the clinic 4 weeks ago for the first time. Other pertinent laboratory findings: white blood cell (WBC) count, 17,000/mm^3 (normal, 4,500–11,000/mm^3) with 4% bands (normal, 0%–11%), 35% segmented neutrophils (normal, 36%–66%), 50% lymphocytes (normal, 24%–44%), 11% eosinophils (normal, 1%–4%); BUN, 7 mg/dL (normal, 5–18 mg/dL); and creatinine, 0.5 mg/dL (normal, 0.6–1.3 mg/dL). All other blood work, liver function tests, and electrolytes are within normal limits. Heart rate and blood pressure are normal. Temperature is 99.2°F, respiratory rate is 25 breaths/minute (normal, 12–16) with an oxygen saturation of 95% (normal, 97%–100%). A number of new pulmonary infiltrates are seen on chest radiograph. Her current medications include the following: one multiple vitamin every day (QD), two microencapsulated pancreatic enzyme capsules (16,000 U lipase/capsule) with meals, and one or two capsules with snacks as needed.

What subjective and objective findings does B.W. exhibit that would lead to the diagnosis of a pulmonary exacerbation?

The onset of a pulmonary exacerbation of CF usually is marked by an increase in symptoms, such as an increase in sputum production (usually purulent), increased cough, dyspnea, weight loss, and a 15% to 20% decline in pulmonary function tests over baseline. All these findings are present in B.W. An increase in WBC count, fever, or appearance of a new infiltrate on chest radiograph may or may not be present. Traditional management for an acute CF exacerbation includes nutritional repletion, antibiotics, and chest physiotherapy.[171]

Early Treatment of *Pseudomonas aeruginosa*

11. B.W. is admitted to the hospital for a "cleanout," consisting of aggressive chest physiotherapy, aggressive nutritional repletion, and antipseudomonal antibiotics. Because *P. aeruginosa* was found in her sputum 4 weeks ago, the following sensitivities to antibiotics were tested and noted: *P. aeruginosa* strain resistant to all antibiotics except tobramycin and ceftazidime. What is the value in giving antibiotics at this time?

If given in the early phase of colonization, antibiotics can prevent the switch to a chronic mucoid infection. A combination of inhaled tobramycin with oral ciprofloxacin (see Question 14 on restricted use of quinolones), or inhaled antibiotics alone, are used to treat early pseudomonas infection.[186,187] In 14 of 15 patients treated with inhaled tobramycin for 1 year, colonization was not only prevented, but pseudomonas was eradicated.[188] Because pulmonary tissue damage probably is related to bacterial load because of the infection–inflammation cycle, decreasing bacterial burden might slow the progression of lung disease. Therefore, it would be beneficial to treat B.W. aggressively with antipseudomonal therapy.

Aminoglycoside Dosing

12. B.W. is admitted to the hospital for a course of antibiotic treated because of her clinical presentation. What would be a good antimicrobial treatment plan for B.W. based on her current laboratory data? Why might an extended-interval dosing regimen for aminoglycoside therapy be of potential advantage for B.W.?

In patients with CF, *P. aeruginosa* infection should be treated with a combination of two antibiotics (e.g., an aminoglycoside with a β-lactam) to lessen the risk of bacterial resistance to antimicrobials. Given the aforementioned sensitivities for B.W., ceftazidime plus tobramycin would be a good initial choice of antibiotics for this exacerbation. B.W.'s renal and liver functions are normal, therefore, standard CF dosing can be prescribed.

Ceftazidime 2 g IV every 8 hours could be administered to B.W. by continuous infusion because the β-lactams are time-dependent bactericidal antibiotics and the administration of ceftazidime, as a constant infusion, in a patient with CF is likely to be safe and effective.[189]

Extended-interval dosing of aminoglycosides (i.e., Q 12 hr or Q 24 hr compared with Q 8 hr) is easier and less costly to administer, and potentially it limits toxicity. The efficacy of extended-interval dosing of aminoglycosides, however, needs to be studied further in the CF population because of the altered pharmacokinetics in patients with CF. Nevertheless, several studies with small sample sizes suggest that the use of extended-interval dosing of aminoglycosides is safe and effective for both children and adults with CF.[190–196] A large, multicenter trial investigating this issue more fully is currently underway.

In B.W., the initial dosing regimen of IV tobramycin would be 225 mg (5 mg/kg) every 12 hours. Target peak concentrations of 12 to 15 mg/L should be verified on the third dose. Target trough concentrations should be <2 mg/L. A serum trough tobramycin level should be measured at least every 7 days while B.W. is on therapy, along with serum concentrations of BUN and creatinine.

The antibiotics should be administered for 2 weeks, and extended for an additional 7 days if B.W. fails to reach specified endpoints at day 14. After the initiation of antibiotics in this hospitalization, IV home-antibiotic therapy should be a consideration for B.W.[197] The duration of B.W.'s antibiotic therapy should be based on her clinical response. Ideally, her pulmonary function (e.g., FEV_1) should improve by 10% to 20% and should be evaluated weekly. The purulent nature and volume of the sputum should decrease and a gradual overall improvement in subjective feeling should be noted. Improved appetite and increased weight gain should be assessed daily with the goal of reaching baseline weight.

Inhaled Tobramycin

13. Why should (or should not) inhaled aminoglycosides be added to the parenteral regimen of B.W.?

Tobramycin for inhalation (TOBI) is a special formulation of tobramycin for inhalation. Aerosolized antibiotics have been used in combination with IV antibiotics for treatment of acute exacerbations. Although eradication of *P. aeruginosa* from the sputum might be enhanced with these combined routes of therapy, the response could be only temporary.[198] The evidence for the addition of inhaled antibiotics to parenteral therapy is not strong, but the evidence for using inhaled tobramycin prophylactically to reduce bacterial load and avoid future exacerbations is getting stronger. Improved pulmonary function, along with a decrease in exacerbations or hospitalizations, has been demonstrated with TOBI prophylactic regimens.[170,198–201] TOBI can be prescribed as twice-daily inhalations (300 mg) administered as a 30-day on and 30-day off schedule. Although this is a time-consuming and expensive therapy, it has been deemed cost-effective.[202,203] B.W. should be discharged on TOBI 300 mg twice daily (BID) prophylactic cycle schedule.

ORAL ANTIBIOTICS

14. B.W. reaches her clinical endpoints and is sent home on TOBI therapy. Six months later, she calls the clinic from her college dorm. She has signs of an exacerbation, but refuses IV antibiotics or hospitalization, because she is in the middle of final exams. What alternative to IV therapy is available to treat B.W.? She now weighs 53 kg.

The quinolone family of antibiotics is currently the only option for oral coverage of *P. aeruginosa*. Emergence of resistant strains of staphylococcal and pseudomonas species have led the CF medical community to restrict the use of quinolones to the treatment of acute CF exacerbations.[204,205] Oral fluoroquinolones (e.g., ciprofloxacin) have become widely used in patients with CF, because they are less expensive, easy to administer, and as effective as IV therapy in an acute exacerbation.[206,207]

Quinolones are not approved for use in patients <18 years of age because of the risk of arthropathy. One study of 634 children failed, however, to demonstrate any arthropathy in the patients, although reversible arthralgias were noted.[208] This risk is further complicated by the underlying problems with bone metabolism seen in CF. Although this issue has not been fully resolved, quinolones are used with caution in certain pediatric populations. In addition, B.W. is of childbearing age and quinolones are relatively contraindicated because of possible effects on cartilage development in the fetus. If a quinolone is used, B.W. should be counseled to use appropriate birth-control techniques.

Because of the past sensitivities of B.W.'s organisms and her refusal to be admitted to the hospital, ciprofloxacin 1,000 mg orally twice daily for 1 week can be initiated in addition to the aerosolized tobramycin.[209] After 1 week of the combined aerosol and oral therapies, B.W. should be re-evaluated for hospital admission if her condition worsens, or her therapy can be continued if her condition improves.

Control of Inflammation

The inflammatory response in CF airways can be treated with drugs that block PMN chemotaxis, proinflammatory cytokines, or any other step in the inflammatory cascade. Corticosteroids, nonsteroidal anti-inflammatory agents (NSAID), and macrolides all have been used to control the inflammation seen in CF lung disease.

Corticosteroids

15. J.J., an 18-year-old young man with CF, returns to the clinic for a routine 6-month visit. He now has severe pulmonary disease as reflected by his pulmonary function tests (FEV_1 is 39% of

predicted normal and FVC is 37%) and marked chest radiographic changes that include areas of bronchiectasis and hyperinflation. He is chronically colonized with a resistant strain of *P. aeruginosa* and has a chronic productive cough, which currently is at baseline. Because the lung damage in CF is from inflammation secondary to the bacterial infection, what anti-inflammatory therapies might be considered for use in J.J.?

Oral corticosteroids are not recommended in the treatment of CF. Although prednisone 1 to 2 mg/kg every other day can reduce the decline of lung function and decrease pulmonary exacerbations in patients with pseudomonas infections, it also can result in cataracts, glucose intolerance, and persistent growth retardation.[210–212] Inhaled steroids do not show an improvement in pulmonary function in patients with CF when used alone.[213] Many such patients with concurrent reactive airway disease, asthma, or ABPA in addition to CF respond to corticosteroids.

Nonsteroidal Anti-Inflammatory Agents

Nonsteroidal anti-inflammatory drugs have been used to slow lung function decline. High-dose ibuprofen (20–30 mg/kg BID with doses titrated to a therapeutic range of 50–100 mg/L) can significantly slow the annual rate of FEV_1 decline in children between 6 and 13 years of age.[214] Ibuprofen serum concentrations must be measured and monitored closely to stay in the therapeutic window because lower concentrations can increase PMN infiltration. Because these doses are much higher than the recommended doses to treat pain or fever, concerns about long-term side effects, including GI bleeding and renal toxicity, together with the need for frequent blood draws have not made this method of treatment common. For patients $\geq$6 years of age with an FEV_1 >60% of predicted, chronic oral ibuprofen is recommended to reduce the loss of lung function.[161] Less than 5% of the CF population is using ibuprofen.[101,215]

16. Is J.J. a candidate for high-dose ibuprofen? He has refused routine blood draws in the past and worries about the side effects of medication.

For maximal benefit, ibuprofen therapy must be started early, before the disease is as advanced as J.J.'s. Because J.J. does not like having to come in for blood draws or the having possible side effects of GI distress or renal impairment, and his lung disease is too advanced, high-dose ibuprofen should not be recommended.

Macrolide Antibiotics

17. When and why would azithromycin be indicated for J.J.?

Macrolide antibiotics, which have both immunomodulatory properties and antimicrobial activity, have been shown to improve pulmonary function tests, reduce exacerbations, and improve quality of life in children and adults with end-stage disease.[216,217–220] In a 3-month prospective, randomized, double-blind, placebo-controlled study of azithromycin (250 mg/day) in 60 adults with CF, FEV_1 improved, C-reactive protein decreased, and fewer IV antibiotics were needed in the azithromycin group.[219] In a 15-month, randomized, double-blind, placebo-controlled, crossover trial, 41 children with CF received azithromycin. FEV_1 improved by 5.4% in the treatment group, and most patients required fewer courses of antibiotics while on azithromycin. No changes in sputum bacterial density, inflammation markers, exercise tolerance, or quality of life were detected.[218] Patients improve on long-term azithromycin therapy regardless of whether they had a positive pseudomonas culture.[221] The development of bacterial resistance with long-term use of azithromycin is of genuine concern, and patients should be followed up closely if azithromycin is initiated on this basis.[223,224] Recommendation is that patients with persistent *P. aeruginosa* sputum cultures receive chronic azithromycin to improve lung function and reduce exacerbations.[161]

In recent long-term studies, azithromycin had a definite role for use in a patient with *P. aeruginosa* and possibly also a role in patients before pseudomonas is cultured. J.J. should be started on 500 mg azithromycin thrice weekly and monitored for improvement of his lung function and a decrease in exacerbations.

Other Strategies

18. What other approaches may be tried to modify the course of CF in B.W. and J.J.?

J.J. and B.W. are both colonized with pseudomonas in their lungs. J.J. should be started on a trial of azithromycin, TOBI, and both patients may be candidates for hypertonic saline and dornase alfa inhalation therapy. Re-evaluation of the type of mechanical clearance method, nutritional status, exercise regimen, and enzyme dose should be considered. J.J. and B.W. should also be tested for liver disease, bone disease, and insulin resistance. J.J. and B.W.'s disease course and weight history should be carefully evaluated along with a fasting blood glucose, HbA_{1c}, and oral glucose tolerance test.

FUTURE THERAPIES

19. What kind of treatments might be available to help patients with CF in the future?

Many drugs are being evaluated to intercede at various levels of the pathologic cascade (Fig. 98-3) seen in CF. Fixing the inactive or malfunctioning CFTR by repairing the mutant gene would be a cure for CF. Much research is focused on developing new therapies for CF, as can be seen in Figure 98-4.

Correcting the Gene

Gene therapy to correct the CFTR in the lungs is being actively pursued. CFTR is expressed in low levels in the lungs so that only 6% to 10% of the cells need active CFTR to correct the chloride channel deficiency. Several vectors are being developed to deliver the good gene and allow it to be incorporated into these cells, including several viruses, a new compacted DNA and lipid DNA complex.[222–225] Viral vectors in general are problematic because they do not allow for repeated administration. Two nonviral vectors that have found some success are DNA nanoparticles and lipid DNA complexes. Nanotechnology has been used to "compact" or tightly bind strands of DNA, making it sufficiently tiny to pass through a cell membrane and into the nucleus. Four of the 12 patients receiving the nanoparticles via the nose exhibited some normal chloride response during the 2-week period studied.[226] Although each of these vectors needs work, real hope exists for a gene transfer to the lung in the not too distant future.

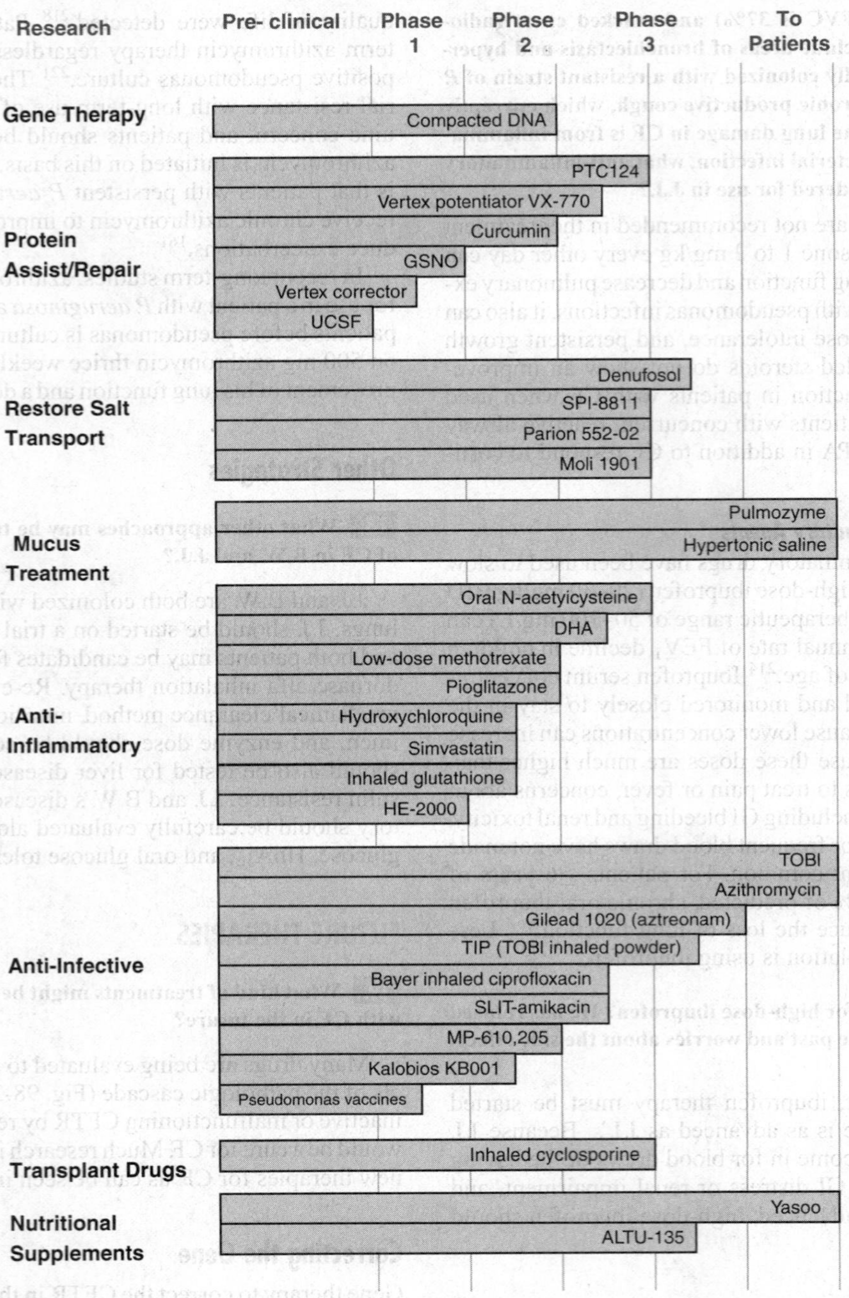

FIGURE 98-4 Drug pipeline for cystic fibrosis. (Reprinted with permission from the Cystic Fibrosis Foundation.)

Restoring Salt Transport

Several therapies are directed at restoring CFTR function from a mutation-specific standpoint. The most common mutation, ΔF508, is caused by a misfolding of the responsible protein. Several "chemical chaperones," such as cellular osmolytes and low-molecular-weight compounds, when added to cells, rescue the folding of mutated proteins such as ΔF508 CFTR.[227,228] Gentamicin has been shown to restore a class I mutation in vitro, and genistein has been shown to correct the G551D mutation.[229] Restoring normal ion transport (Na channel blockers, Cl channel activators) would also be an effective cure for CF. At this point, short-acting sodium channel blockers are of no benefit.[228,230–232] Alternative molecules are in phase II clinical trials and research stages.

Other

Drugs to combat the inflammation–infection cycle of CF, drugs to improve the outcome from lung transplants, new therapies, and rapidly improving scientific understandings of CF provide much hope for more effective treatment of this disease, and even perhaps a cure.

REFERENCES

1. Yankaskas JR et al. Cystic fibrosis adult care: consensus conference report. *Chest* 2004;125:1S.
2. Davis B. Cystic fibrosis since 1938. *Am J Respir Crit Care Med* 2005;173:475.
3. Busch R. On the history of cystic fibrosis. *Acta Univ Carol [Med] (Praha)* 1990;36:13.
4. di Sant'Agnese PA et al. Abnormal electrolyte composition of sweat in cystic fibrosis of the pancreas. *Pediatrics* 1953;12:549.
5. Andersen DH. Cystic fibrosis of the pancreas and its relation to celiac disease, a clinical and pathological study. *Am J Dis Child* 1938;56:344.
6. Kubba AK, Young M. The long suffering of Frederic Chopin. *Chest* 1998;113:210.
7. Welsh MJ. Abnormal regulation of ion channels in cystic fibrosis epithelia. *FASEB J* 1990;4:2718.
8. Boucher RC et al. Na+ transport in cystic fibrosis respiratory epithelia. Abnormal basal rate and response to adenylate cyclase activation. *J Clin Invest* 1986;78:1245.
9. Smith JJ et al. cAMP stimulates bicarbonate secretion across normal, but not cystic fibrosis airway epithelia. *J Clin Invest* 1992;89:1148.
10. Ballard ST et al. CFTR involvement in chloride, bicarbonate, and liquid secretion by airway submucosal glands. *Am J Physiol* 1999;277(Pt 1):L694.
11. Schwiebert EM et al. CFTR is a conductance regulator as well as a chloride channel. *Physiol Rev* 1999;79(Suppl):S145.
12. Lee MG et al. Cystic fibrosis transmembrane conductance regulator regulates luminal Cl-/HCO3-exchange in mouse submandibular and pancreatic ducts. *J Biol Chem* 1999;274:14670.
13. Rodman DM et al. The cystic fibrosis heterozygote–advantage in surviving cholera? *Med Hypotheses* 1991;36:253.
14. Romeo G et al. Why is the cystic fibrosis gene so frequent? *Hum Genet* 1989;84:1.
15. Gabriel SE et al. Cystic fibrosis heterozygote resistance to cholera toxin in the cystic fibrosis mouse model. *Science* 1994;266:107.
16. Padua RA et al. The cystic fibrosis delta F508 gene mutation and cancer. *Hum Mutat* 1997;10:45.
17. Warren N et al. Frequency of carriers of cystic fibrosis gene among patients with myeloid malignancy and melanoma. *BMJ* 1991;302:760.
18. Neglia JP et al. The risk of cancer among patients with cystic fibrosis. Cystic Fibrosis and Cancer Study Group. *N Engl J Med* 1995;332:494.
19. Abraham EH et al. Cystic fibrosis hetero- and homozygosity is associated with inhibition of breast cancer growth. *Nat Med* 1996;2:593.
20. Laniado ME et al. Expression and functional analysis of voltage-activated Na+ channels in human prostate cancer cell lines and their contribution to invasion in vitro. *Am J Pathol* 1997;150:1213.
21. Southey MC et al. CFTR delta F508 carrier status, risk of breast cancer before the age of 40 and histological grading in a population-based case-control study. *Int J Cancer* 1998;79:487.
22. Rommens JM et al. Identification of the cystic fibrosis gene: chromosome walking and jumping. *Science* 1989;245:1059.
23. Kerem B et al. Identification of the cystic fibrosis gene: genetic analysis. *Science* 1989;245:1073.
24. Riordan JR. Identification of the cystic fibrosis gene: cloning and characterization of complementary DNA. *Science* 1989;245:1066.
25. Welsh MJ et al. Research on cystic fibrosis: a journey from the Heart House. *Am J Respir Crit Care Med* 1998;157(Pt 2):S148.
26. Zielenski J et al. Cystic fibrosis: genotypic and phenotypic variations. *Annu Rev Genet* 1995;29:777.
27. Consortium TCFGA; Cystic Fibrosis Mutation Data Base, in http://www.genet.sickkids.on.ca/cftr. 1998, The Cystic Fibrosis Genetic Analysis Consortium.
28. Kerem E et al. The relation between genotype and phenotype in cystic fibrosis: analysis of the most common mutation (delta F508). *N Engl J Med* 1990;323:1517.
29. Zielenski J. Genotype and phenotype in cystic fibrosis. *Respiration* 2000;67:117.
30. Grasemann H et al. Endothelial nitric oxide synthase variants in cystic fibrosis lung disease. *Am J Respir Crit Care Med* 2003;167:390.
31. Merlo CA et al. Modifier genes in cystic fibrosis lung disease. *J Lab Clin Med* 2003;141:237.
32. Bronsveld I et al. Chloride conductance and genetic background modulate the cystic fibrosis phenotype of Delta F508 homozygous twins and siblings. *J Clin Invest* 2001;108:1705.
33. Hull J et al. Contribution of genetic factors other than CFTR to disease severity in cystic fibrosis. *Thorax* 1998;53:1018.
34. Drumm ML. Modifier genes and variation in cystic fibrosis. *Respir Res* 2001;2:125.
35. Arkwright PD et al. End-organ dysfunction in cystic fibrosis: association with angiotensin I converting enzyme and cytokine gene polymorphisms. *Am J Respir Crit Care Med* 2003;167:384.
36. Henrion-Caude A et al. Liver disease in pediatric patients with cystic fibrosis is associated with glutathione S-transferase P1 polymorphism. *Hepatology* 2002;36:913.
37. Garred P et al. Association of mannose-binding lectin gene heterogeneity with severity of lung disease and survival in cystic fibrosis. *J Clin Invest* 1999;104:431.
38. Drumm ML et al. Genetic modifiers of lung disease in cystic fibrosis. *N Engl J Med* 2005;353:1443.
39. Plant BJ et al. Cystic fibrosis, disease severity, and a macrophage migration inhibitory factor polymorphism. *Am J Repir Crit Care Med* 2005;172:1412.
40. Boyle MP. Strategies for identifying modifier genes in cystic fibrosis. *Proceeding of the American Thoracic Society* 2007;4:52.
41. Garred P et al. Mannose-binding lectin (MBL) therapy in an MBL-deficient patient with severe cystic fibrosis lung disease. *Pediatr Pulmonol* 2002; 33:201.
42. Reddy MM et al. Activation of the epithelial Na+ channel (ENaC) requires CFTR Cl–channel function. *Nature* 1999;402:301.
43. Ramsey B et al. Impact of sinusitis in cystic fibrosis. *J Allergy Clin Immunol* 1992;90(Pt 2):547.
44. Umetsu DT et al. Sinus disease in patients with severe cystic fibrosis: relation to pulmonary exacerbation. *Lancet* 1990;335:1077.
45. Sohma Y et al. HCO_3-transport in a mathematical model of the pancreatic ductal epithelium. *J Membr Biol* 2000;176:77.
46. Hardin DS et al. Diabetes mellitus in cystic fibrosis. *Endocrinol Metab Clin North Am* 1999;28:787, ix.
47. Solomon MP et al. Glucose intolerance in children with cystic fibrosis. *J Pediatr* 2003;142:128.
48. Moran A et al. Abnormal glucose metabolism in cystic fibrosis. *J Pediatr* 1998;133:10.
49. Finkelstein SM et al. Diabetes mellitus associated with cystic fibrosis. *J Pediatr* 1988;112:373.
50. Lanng S et al. Influence of the development of diabetes mellitus on clinical status in patients with cystic fibrosis. *Eur J Pediatr* 1992;151:684.
51. Hardin DS et al. Insulin resistance is associated with decreased clinical status in cystic fibrosis. *J Pediatr* 1997;130:948.
52. Dobson L et al. Clinical improvement in cystic fibrosis with early insulin treatment. *Arch Dis Child* 2002;87:430.
53. Blackman SM et al. Relative contribution of genetic and nongenetic modifiers to intestinal obstruction in cystic fibrosis. *Gastroenterology* 2006;131:1030.
54. Brodzicki J et al. Frequency, consequences and pharmacological treatment of gastroesophageal reflux in children with cystic fibrosis. *Med Sci Monit* 2002;8:CR529.
55. Ledson MJ et al. Prevalence and mechanisms of gastro-oesophageal reflux in adult cystic fibrosis patients. *J R Soc Med* 1998;91:7.
56. Heine RG et al. Gastro-oesophageal reflux in infants under 6 moths with cystic fibrosis. *Arch Dis Child* 1998;78:44.
57. Cohn JA et al. Localization of the cystic fibrosis transmembrane conductance regulator in human bile duct epithelial cells. *Gastroenterology* 1993;105:1857.
58. Kopelman H. Cystic fibrosis. Gastrointestinal and nutritional aspects. *Thorax* 1991;46:261.
59. Akata D et al. Liver manifestations of cystic fibrosis. *Eur J Radiol* 2006;61:11.
60. Gaskin KJ et al. Liver disease and common-bile-duct stenosis in cystic fibrosis. *N Engl J Med* 1988; 318:340.
61. Colombo C et al. Analysis of risk factors for the development of liver disease associated with cystic fibrosis. *J Pediatr* 1994;124:393.
62. Sokol RJ et al. Recommendations for management of liver and biliary tract disease in cystic fibrosis. Cystic Fibrosis Foundation Hepatobiliary Disease Consensus Group. *J Pediatr Gastroenterol Nutr* 1999;28:S1.
63. Geddes DM. Cystic fibrosis and pregnancy. *J R Soc Med* 1992;85:36.
64. Elkin SL et al. Histomorphometric analysis of bone biopsies from the iliac crest of adults with cystic fibrosis. *Am J Respir Crit Care Med* 2002;166:1470.
65. Haworth CS et al. A prospective study of change in bone mineral density over one year in adults with cystic fibrosis. *Thorax* 2002;57:719.
66. Shead EF et al. Osteoclastogenesis during infective exacerbations in patients with cystic fibrosis. *Am J Respir Crit Care Med* 2006;174:306.
67. Conway SP et al. Vitamin K status among children with cystic fibrosis and its relationship to bone mineral density and bone turnover. *Pediatrics* 2005;115:1325.
68. Boyle MP et al. Failure of high-dose ergocalciferol to correct vitamin deficiency in adults with cystic fibrosis. *Am J Respir Crit Care Med* 2005;172:212.
69. Boyle MP. Update on maintaining bone health in cystic fibrosis. *Curr Opin Pulm Med* 2006;12: 453.
70. Cawood TJ et al. Oral bisphosphonates improve bone mineral density in adults with cystic fibrosis. *Ir Med J* 2005;98:270.
71. Brenckmann C et al. Bisphosphonates for osteoporosis in people with cystic fibrosis. *Cochrane Database Syst Rev* 2001;4.
72. Haworth CS et al. Low bone mineral density in adults with cystic fibrosis. *Thorax* 1999;54:961.
73. Sood M et al. Bone status in cystic fibrosis. *Arch Dis Child* 2001;84:516.
74. Dixey J et al. The arthropathy of cystic fibrosis. *Ann Rheum Dis* 1988;47:218.
75. Rush PJ et al. The musculoskeletal manifestations of cystic fibrosis. *Semin Arthritis Rheum* 1986;15:213.
76. Newman AJ et al. Episodic arthritis in children with cystic fibrosis. *J Pediatr* 1979;94:594.
77. Phillips BM et al. Pathogenesis and management of arthropathy in cystic fibrosis. *J R Soc Med* 1986;79(Suppl 12):44.
78. Pertuiset E et al. Cystic fibrosis arthritis. A report of five cases. *Br J Rheumatol* 1992;31:535.
79. Hoiby N. Inflammation and infection in cystic fibrosis–hen or egg? *Eur Respir J* 2001;17:4.
80. Elborn JS et al. Host inflammatory responses to first isolation of *Pseudomonas aeruginosa* from sputum in cystic fibrosis. *Pediatr Pulmonol* 1993; 15:287.
81. Smith JJ et al. Cystic fibrosis airway epithelia fail to kill bacteria because of abnormal airway surface fluid. *Cell* 1996;85:229.
82. Travis SM et al. Activity of abundant antimicrobials of the human airway. *Am J Respir Cell Mol Biol* 1999;20:872.
83. Matsui H et al. Evidence for periciliary liquid layer depletion, not abnormal ion composition, in the pathogenesis of cystic fibrosis airways disease. *Cell* 1998;95:1005.
84. Trout L et al. Disruptive effects of anion secretion inhibitors on airway mucus morphology in isolated perfused pig lung. *J Physiol (Lond)* 2003;549:845.

85. Ballard ST et al. Liquid secretion inhibitors reduce mucociliary transport in glandular airways. *Am J Physiol Lung Cell Mol Physiol* 2002;283:L329.
86. Scheid P et al. Inflammation in cystic fibrosis airways: relationship to increased bacterial adherence. *Eur Respir J* 2001;17:27.
87. Mahadeva R et al. Anti-neutrophil cytoplasmic antibodies (ANCA) against bactericidal/permeability-increasing protein (BPI) and cystic fibrosis lung disease. *Clin Exp Immunol* 1999; 117:561.
88. Tager AM et al. The effect of chloride concentration on human neutrophil functions: potential relevance to cystic fibrosis. *Am J Respir Cell Mol Biol* 1998;19:643.
89. Henry RL et al. Mucoid *Pseudomonas aeruginosa* is a marker of poor survival in cystic fibrosis. *Pediatr Pulmonol* 1992;12:158.
90. Soni R et al. Effect of *Burkholderia cepacia* infection in the clinical course of patients with cystic fibrosis: a pilot study in a Sydney clinic. *Respirology* 2002;7:241.
91. Konstan MW et al. Current understanding of the inflammatory process in cystic fibrosis: onset and etiology. *Pediatr Pulmonol* 1997;24:137; discussion 159.
92. Olivier KN et al. Nontuberculous mycobacteria. II: nested-cohort study of impact on cystic fibrosis lung disease. *Am J Respir Crit Care Med* 2003;167:835.
93. Olivier KN et al. Nontuberculous mycobacteria. I: multicenter prevalence study in cystic fibrosis. *Am J Respir Crit Care Med* 2003;167:828.
94. Armstrong DS et al. Lower airway inflammation in infants and young children with cystic fibrosis. *Am J Respir Crit Care Med* 1997;156(Pt 1):1197.
95. Solic N et al. Endothelial activation and increased heparin sulfate expression in cystic fibrosis. *Am J Respir Crit Care Med* 2005;172:892.
96. O'Sullivan BP et al. The inflammatory role of platelets in cystic fibrosis. *Am J Respir Crit Care Med* 2006;173:483.
97. Bonfield TL et al. Inflammatory cytokines in cystic fibrosis lungs. *Am J Respir Crit Care Med* 1995; 152(Pt 1):2111.
98. Bonfield TL et al. Normal bronchial epithelial cells constitutively produce the anti-inflammatory cytokine interleukin-10, which is downregulated in cystic fibrosis. *Am J Respir Cell Mol Biol* 1995;13: 257.
99. Bonfield TL et al. Altered respiratory epithelial cell cytokine production in cystic fibrosis. *J Allergy Clin Immunol* 1999;104:72.
100. Freedman SD et al. A membrane lipid imbalance plays a role in the phenotypic expression of cystic fibrosis in cftr(−/−) mice. *Proc Natl Acad Sci USA* 1999;96:13995.
101. Foundation CF. Patient Registry 2001 Annual Data Report, in epidemiology. 2002: Bethesda, MD.
102. Parad RB. Buccal cell DNA mutation analysis for diagnosis of cystic fibrosis in newborns and infants inaccessible to sweat chloride measurement. *Pediatrics.* 1998;101:851.
103. Rosenstein BJ et al. The diagnosis of cystic fibrosis: a consensus statement. Cystic Fibrosis Foundation Consensus Panel. *J Pediatr* 1998;132: 589.
104. Gibson L et al. A test for concentration of electrolytes in sweat in cystic fibrosis of the pancreas utilizing pilocarpine iontophoresis. *Pediatrics* 1959;23:545.
105. Farrell PM et al. Sweat chloride concentrations in infants homozygous or heterozygous for F508 cystic fibrosis. *Pediatrics* 1996;97:524.
106. Knowles MR et al. In vivo nasal potential difference: techniques and protocols for assessing efficacy of gene transfer in cystic fibrosis. *Hum Gene Ther* 1995;6:445.
107. Farrell PM et al. Prenatal screening for cystic fibrosis: where are we now? *J Pediatr* 2002;141: 758.
108. Conway SP. Evidence-based medicine in cystic fibrosis: how should practice change? *Pediatr Pulmonol* 2002;34:242.
109. Grosse SD et al. Newborn screening for cystic fibrosis: evaluation of benefits and risks and recommendations for state newborn screening programs. *MMWR Recomm Rep* 2004;53:1.
110. Hammond KB et al. Efficacy of statewide neonatal screening for cystic fibrosis by assay of trypsinogen concentrations. *N Engl J Med* 1991;325:769.
111. Merelle ME et al. Newborn screening for cystic fibrosis. *Cochrane Database Syst Rev* 2000: CD001402.
112. Farrell PM et al. Nutritional benefits of neonatal screening for cystic fibrosis. Wisconsin Cystic Fibrosis Neonatal Screening Study Group. *N Engl J Med* 1997;337:963.
113. Wagener JS et al. A debate on why my state (province) should or should not conduct newborn screening for cystic fibrosis (14th Annual North American Cystic Fibrosis Conference). *Pediatr Pulmonol* 2001;32:385.
114. Farrell PM et al. Early diagnosis of cystic fibrosis through neonatal screening prevents severe malnutrition and improves long-term growth. Wisconsin Cystic Fibrosis Neonatal Screening Study Group. *Pediatrics* 2001;107:1.
115. Kaye CI et al. Introduction to the newborn screening fact sheets. *Pediatrics* 2006;118:1304.
116. Farrell PM et al. Early diagnosis of cystic fibrosis through neonatal screening prevents severe malnutrition and improves long-term growth. Wisconsin Cystic Fibrosis Neonatal Screening Study Group. *Pediatrics* 2001;107:1.
117. Grosse SD et al. Potential impact of newborn screening for cystic fibrosis on child survival: a systematic review and analysis. *J Pediatr* 2006;149:362.
118. Hammond KB et al. Efficacy of statewide neonatal screening for cystic fibrosis by assay of trypsinogen concentrations. *N Engl J Med* 1991;325:769.
119. Farrell M et al. Genetic counseling and risk communication services of newborn screening programs. *Arch Pediatr Adolesc Med* 2001;155:120.
120. Wheeler PG et al. Genetic counseling after implementation of statewide cystic fibrosis newborn screening: two years' experience in one medical center. *Genet Med* 2001;3:411.
121. Kovesi T et al. Passive smoking and lung function in cystic fibrosis. *Am Rev Respir Dis* 1993;148:1266.
122. Schechter MS et al. The association of socioeconomic status with outcomes in cystic fibrosis patients in the United States. *Am J Respir Crit Care Med* 2001;163:1331.
123. O'Connor GT et al. Median household income and mortality rate in cystic fibrosis. *Pediatrics* 2003;111(Pt 1):e333.
124. Johnson C et al. Factors influencing outcomes in cystic fibrosis: a center-based analysis. *Chest* 2003;123:20.
125. Corey M. Modelling survival in cystic fibrosis. *Thorax* 2001;56:743.
126. Fiel SB. Early aggressive intervention in cystic fibrosis: is it time to redefine our "best practice" strategies? *Chest* 2003;123:1.
127. Koch C. Early infection and progression of cystic fibrosis lung disease. *Pediatr Pulmonol* 2002;34: 232.
128. Borowitz D et al. Consensus report on nutrition for pediatric patients with cystic fibrosis. *J Pediatr Gastroenterol Nutr* 2002;35:246.
129. Kalnins D et al. Failure of conventional strategies to improve nutritional status in malnourished adolescents and adults with cystic fibrosis. *J Pediatr* 2005;147:399.
130. Rosenfeld M et al. Nutritional effects of long-term gastrostomy feedings in children with cystic fibrosis. *J Am Diet Assoc* 1999;99:191.
131. Steinkamp G et al. Improvement of nutritional status and lung function after long-term nocturnal gastrostomy feedings in cystic fibrosis. *J Pediatr* 1994;124:244.
132. Feranchak AP et al. Prospective, long-term study of fat-soluble vitamin status in children with cystic fibrosis identified by newborn screen. *J Pediatr* 1999;135:601.
133. Rashid M et al. Prevalence of vitamin K deficiency in cystic fibrosis. *Am J Clin Nutr* 1999;70:378.
134. Wilson DC et al. Treatment of vitamin K deficiency in cystic fibrosis: effectiveness of a daily fat-soluble vitamin combination. *J Pediatr* 2001;138:851.
135. Beker LT et al. Effect of vitamin K1 supplementation on vitamin K status in cystic fibrosis patients. *J Pediatr Gastroenterol Nutr* 1997;24:512.
136. Back EI et al. Antioxidant deficiency in cystic fibrosis: when is the right time to take action? *Am J Clin Nutr* 2004;80:374.
137. Conway SP et al. Vitamin K status among children with cystic fibrosis and its relationship to bone mineral density and bone turnover. *Pediatrics* 2005;115:1325.
138. Littlewood JM. Diagnosis and treatment of intestinal malabsorption in cystic fibrosis. *Pediatr Pulmonol* 2006;41:35.
139. Borowitz DS et al. Use of pancreatic enzyme supplements for patients with cystic fibrosis in the context of fibrosing colonopathy. Consensus Committee. *J Pediatr* 1995;127:681.
140. Borowitz D. Update on the evaluation of pancreatic exocrine status in cystic fibrosis. *Curr Opin Pulm Med* 2005;11:524.
141. Baker SS et al. Pancreatic enzyme therapy and clinical outcomes in patients with cystic fibrosis. *J Pediatr* 2005;146:189.
142. Hendeles L et al. Treatment failure after substitution of generic pancrelipase capsules. Correlation with in vitro lipase activity. *JAMA* 1990;263:2459.
143. Smyth RL et al. Strictures of ascending colon in cystic fibrosis and high-strength pancreatic enzymes. *Lancet* 1994;343:85.
144. FitzSimmons SC et al. High-dose pancreatic-enzyme supplements and fibrosing colonopathy in children with cystic fibrosis. *N Engl J Med* 1997;336:1283.
145. Guarner L et al. Fate of oral enzymes in pancreatic insufficiency. *Gut* 1993;34:708.
146. Robinson PJ et al. Duodenal pH in cystic fibrosis and its relationship to fat malabsorption. *Dig Dis Sci* 1990;35:1299.
147. Heijerman HG. Ranitidine compared with dimethylprostaglandin E2 analogue enprostil as adjunct to pancreatic enzyme replacement in adult cystic fibrosis. *Scand J Gastroenterol Suppl* 1990;178:26.
148. Heijerman HG et al. Omeprazole enhances the efficacy of pancreatin (Pancrease) in cystic fibrosis. *Ann Intern Med* 1991;114:200.
149. Hendriks JJE et al. Changes in pulmonary hyperinflation and bronchial hyperresponsiveness following treatment with lansoprazole in children with cystic fibrosis. *Pediatr Pulmonol* 2001;31:59.
150. Brady MS et al. Effectiveness of enteric coated pancreatic enzymes given before meals in reducing steatorrhea in children with cystic fibrosis. *J Am Diet Assoc* 1992;92:813.
151. Varekojis SM et al. A comparison of the therapeutic effectiveness of and preference for postural drainage and percussion, intrapulmonary percussive ventilation, and high-frequency chest wall compression in hospitalized cystic fibrosis patients. *Respir Care* 2003;48:24.
152. Oermann CM et al. Comparison of high-frequency chest wall oscillation and oscillating positive expiratory pressure in the home management of cystic fibrosis: a pilot study. *Pediatr Pulmonol* 2001;32:372.
153. Quan JM et al. A two-year randomized, placebo-controlled trial of dornase alfa in young patients with cystic fibrosis with mild lung function abnormalities. *J Pediatr* 2001;139:813.
154. Fuchs HJ et al. Effect of aerosolized recombinant human DNase on exacerbations of respiratory symptoms and on pulmonary function in patients with cystic fibrosis. The Pulmozyme Study Group. *N Engl J Med* 1994;331:637.
155. Harms HK et al. Multicenter, open-label study of recombinant human DNase in cystic fibrosis patients with moderate lung disease. DNase International Study Group. *Pediatr Pulmonol* 1998;26:155.

156. McCoy K et al. Effects of 12-week administration of dornase alfa in patients with advanced cystic fibrosis lung disease. Pulmozyme Study Group. *Chest* 1996;110:889.
157. Paul K et al. Effect of treatment with dornase alpha on airway inflammation in patients with cystic fibrosis. *Am J Respir Crit Care Med* 2004;169:719.
158. Wilmott RW et al. Aerosolized recombinant human DNase in hospitalized cystic fibrosis patients with acute pulmonary exacerbations. *Am J Respir Crit Care Med* 1996;153:1914.
159. Grieve R et al. A cost-effectiveness analysis of rhDNase in children with cystic fibrosis. *Int J Technol Assess Health Care* 2003;19:71.
160. Cramer GW et al. The role of dornase alfa in the treatment of cystic fibrosis. *Ann Pharmacother* 1996;30:656.
161. Flume PA et al. Cystic fibrosis pulmonary guidelines, chronic medications for maintenance of lung health. *Am J Respir Crit Care Med* 2007;176: 957.
162. Wark PA et al. Nebulised hypertonic saline for cystic fibrosis. *Cochrane Database Syst Rev* 2003:CD001506.
163. Elkins MR et al. A controlled trial of long-term inhaled hypertonic saline in patients with cystic fibrosis. *N Engl J Med* 2006;354:229.
164. Donaldson SH et al. Mucus clearance and lung function in cystic fibrosis with hypertonic saline. *N Engl J Med* 2006;354:241.
165. Taylor LM, et al. Hypertonic Saline treatment of cystic fibrosis. *Ann Pharmacother* 2007;41:481.
166. Conway SP et al. A pilot study of zafirlukast as an anti-inflammatory agent in the treatment of adults with cystic fibrosis. *Journal of Cystic Fibrosis* 2003;2:25.
167. Ziebach R et al. Bronchodilatory effects of salbutamol, ipratropium bromide and their combination: double-blind, placebo-controlled cross-over study in cystic fibrosis. *Pediatr Pulmonol* 2001;31: 431.
168. Zuercher AW. Antibody responses induced by long-term vaccination with an octovalent conjugate Pseudomonas aeruginosa vaccine in children with cystic fibrosis. *FEMS Immunol Med Microbiol* 2006;47:302.
169. Saiman L et al. Infection control recommendations for patients with cystic fibrosis: microbiology, important pathogens, and infection control practices to prevent patient-to-patient transmission. *Am J Infect Control* 2003:S1.
170. Ramsey BW et al. Intermittent administration of inhaled tobramycin in patients with cystic fibrosis. Cystic Fibrosis Inhaled Tobramycin Study Group. *N Engl J Med* 1999;340:23.
171. Ramsey BW. Management of pulmonary disease in patients with cystic fibrosis. *N Engl J Med* 1996; 335:179.
172. Frederiksen B et al. Changing epidemiology of *Pseudomonas aeruginosa* infection in Danish cystic fibrosis patients (1974–1995). *Pediatr Pulmonol* 1999;28:159.
173. Hutabarat RM et al. Disposition of drugs in cystic fibrosis. I. Sulfamethoxazole and trimethoprim. *Clin Pharmacol Ther* 1991;49:402.
174. Wang JP et al. Disposition of drugs in cystic fibrosis. VI. In vivo activity of cytochrome P450 isoforms involved in the metabolism of (R)-warfarin (including P450 3A4) is not enhanced in cystic fibrosis. *Clin Pharmacol Ther* 1994;55:528.
175. O'Sullivan TA et al. Disposition of drugs in cystic fibrosis. V. In vivo CYP2C9 activity as probed by (S)-warfarin is not enhanced in cystic fibrosis. *Clin Pharmacol Ther* 1993;54:323.
176. Hamelin BA et al. Caffeine metabolism in cystic fibrosis: enhanced xanthine oxidase activity. *Clin Pharmacol Ther* 1994;56:521.
177. Kearns GL et al. Hepatic drug clearance in patients with mild cystic fibrosis. *Clin Pharmacol Ther* 1996;59:529.
178. Woodland C et al. Hypothetical framework for enhanced renal tubular secretion of drugs in cystic fibrosis. *Med Hypotheses* 1998;51:489.
179. Wang JP et al. Disposition of drugs in cystic fibrosis. IV. Mechanisms for enhanced renal clearance of ticarcillin. *Clin Pharmacol Ther* 1993;54:293.
180. Weber A et al. Probenecid pharmacokinetics in cystic fibrosis. *Dev Pharmacol Ther* 1991;16:7.
181. Tan KH et al. Aminoglycoside prescribing and surveillance in cystic fibrosis. *Am J Respir Crit Care Med* 2003;167:819.
182. Kuhn RJ. Pharmaceutical considerations in aerosol drug delivery. *Pharmacotherapy* 2002;22:80S.
183. Kuhn RJ. Formulation of aerosolized therapeutics. *Chest* 2001;120:94S.
184. Hodson ME et al. A randomised clinical trial of nebulised tobramycin or colistin in cystic fibrosis. *Eur Respir J* 2002;20:658.
185. Stutman HR et al. Antibiotic prophylaxis in infants and young children with cystic fibrosis: a randomized controlled trial. *J Pediatr* 2002;140:299.
186. Nixon GM et al. Clinical outcome after early *Pseudomonas aeruginosa* infection in cystic fibrosis. *J Pediatr* 2001;138:699.
187. Wiesemann HG et al. Placebo-controlled, double-blind, randomized study of aerosolized tobramycin for early treatment of *Pseudomonas aeruginosa* colonization in cystic fibrosis. *Pediatr Pulmonol* 1998;25:88.
188. Ratjen F et al. Effect of inhaled tobramycin on early *Pseudomonas aeruginosa* colonisation in patients with cystic fibrosis. *Lancet* 2001;358:983.
189. Bosso JA et al. A pilot study of the efficacy of constant-infusion ceftazidime in the treatment of endobronchial infections in adults with cystic fibrosis. *Pharmacotherapy* 1999;19:620.
190. Contopoulos-Ioannidis DG et al. Extended-interval aminoglycoside administration for children: a meta-analysis. *Pediatrics* 2004;114:111.
191. Smyth AR et al. Once-daily versus multiple-daily dosing with intravenous aminoglycosides for cystic fibrosis. *Cochrane Database Syst Rev* 2006;3.
192. Aminimanizani A. Distribution and elimination of tobramycin administered in single or multiple daily doses in adult patients with cystic fibrosis. *J Antimicrob Chemother* 2002;50:553.
193. Master V et al. Efficacy of once-daily tobramycin monotherapy for acute pulmonary exacerbations of cystic fibrosis: a preliminary study. *Pediatr Pulmonol* 2001;31:367.
194. Vic P et al. Efficacy, tolerance, and pharmacokinetics of once daily tobramycin for pseudomonas exacerbations in cystic fibrosis. *Arch Dis Child* 1998;78:536.
195. Whitehead A et al. Once-daily tobramycin in the treatment of adult patients with cystic fibrosis. *Eur Respir J* 2002;19:303.
196. Bragonier R et al. The pharmacokinetics and toxicity of once-daily tobramycin therapy in children with cystic fibrosis. *J Antimicrob Chemother* 1998;42:103.
197. Marco T et al. Home intravenous antibiotics for cystic fibrosis. *Cochrane Database Of Syst Rev* 2000;4.
198. Ramsey BW et al. Efficacy of aerosolized tobramycin in patients with cystic fibrosis. *N Engl J Med* 1993;328:1740.
199. Gibson RL et al. Significant microbiological effect of inhaled tobramycin in young children with cystic fibrosis. *Am J Respir Crit Care Med* 2003;167:841.
200. Steinkamp G et al. Long-term tobramycin aerosol therapy in cystic fibrosis. *Pediatr Pulmonol* 1989;6: 91.
201. Moss RB. Long-term benefits of inhaled tobramycin in adolescent patients with cystic fibrosis. *Chest* 2002;121:55.
202. Hagerman JK. Tobramycin solution for inhalation in cystic fibrosis patients: a review of the literature. *Expert Opin Pharmacother* 2007;8:467.
203. Heinzl B et al. Effects of inhaled gentamicin prophylaxis on acquisition of *Pseudomonas aeruginosa* in children with cystic fibrosis: a pilot study. *Pediatr Pulmonol* 2002;33:32.
204. Blumberg HM et al. Rapid development of ciprofloxacin resistance in methicillin-susceptible and -resistant *Staphylococcus aureus*. *J Infect Dis* 1991;163:1279.
205. Radberg G et al. Development of quinolone-imipenem cross resistance in *Pseudomonas aeruginosa* during exposure to ciprofloxacin. *Antimicrob Agents Chemother* 1990;34:2142.
206. Bosso JA et al. Ciprofloxacin versus tobramycin plus azlocillin in pulmonary exacerbations in adult patients with cystic fibrosis. *Am J Med* 1987;82: 180.
207. Hodson ME et al. Oral ciprofloxacin compared with conventional intravenous treatment for *Pseudomonas aeruginosa* infection in adults with cystic fibrosis. *Lancet* 1987;1:235.
208. Chysky V et al. Safety of ciprofloxacin in children: worldwide clinical experience based on compassionate use. Emphasis on joint evaluation. *Infection* 1991;19:289.
209. Rubio TT et al. Pharmacokinetic disposition of sequential intravenous/oral ciprofloxacin in pediatric cystic fibrosis patients with acute pulmonary exacerbation. *Pediatr Infect Dis J* 1997;16:112; discussion 123.
210. Eigen H et al. A multicenter study of alternate-day prednisone therapy in patients with cystic fibrosis. Cystic Fibrosis Foundation Prednisone Trial Group. *J Pediatr* 1995;126:515.
211. Auerbach HS et al. Alternate-day prednisone reduces morbidity and improves pulmonary function in cystic fibrosis. *Lancet* 1985;2:686.
212. Lai, HC et al. Risk of persistent growth impairment after alternate-day prednisone treatment in children with cystic fibrosis. *N Engl J Med* 2000;342:851.
213. Dezateux C et al. Inhaled corticosteroids for cystic fibrosis. *Cochrane Database Syst Rev* 2000; CD001915.
214. Konstan MW et al. Effect of high-dose ibuprofen in patients with cystic fibrosis. *N Engl J Med* 1995;332:848.
215. Dezateux C et al. Oral non-steroidal anti-inflammatory drug therapy for cystic fibrosis. *Cochrane Database Syst Rev* 2000;55:CD001505.
216. Saiman L et al. Heterogeneity of treatment response to azithromycin in patients with cystic fibrosis. *Am J Respir Crit Care Med* 2005;172:1008.
217. Jaffe A et al. Long-term azithromycin may improve lung function in children with cystic fibrosis. *Lancet* 1998;351:420.
218. Equi A et al. Long term azithromycin in children with cystic fibrosis: a randomised, placebo-controlled crossover trial. *Lancet* 2002;360:978.
219. Wolter J et al. Effect of long term treatment with azithromycin on disease parameters in cystic fibrosis: a randomised trial. *Thorax* 2002;57:212.
220. Gaylor AS et al. Therapy with macrolides in patients with cystic fibrosis. *Pharmacotherapy* 2002; 22:227.
221. Clement A et al. Long term effects of azithromycin in patients with cystic fibrosis: a double blind, placebo controlled trial. *Thorax* 2006;61:895.
222. Alton EW et al. Cationic lipid-mediated CFTR gene transfer to the lungs and nose of patients with cystic fibrosis: a double-blind placebo-controlled trial. *Lancet* 1999;353:947.
223. Konstan MW. Gene transfer using novel compacted DNA. In 6th Annual American Society of Gene Therapy Meeting. 2003; Washington, DC.
224. Aitken ML et al. A phase I study of aerosolized administration of tgAAVCF to cystic fibrosis subjects with mild lung disease. *Hum Gene Ther* 2001;12:1907.
225. Moss R. Respiratory tract: planning and executing a gene therapy trial for the respiratory tract. In 6th Annual American Society of Gene Therapy Meeting. 2003; Washington, DC.
226. Konstan MW et al. Compacted DNA nanoparticles administered to the nasal mucosa of cystic fibrosis subjects are safe and demonstrate partial to complete cystic fibrosis transmembrane regulator reconstitution. *Hum Gene Ther* 2004;15:1255.
227. Zeitlin PL et al. Evidence of CFTR function in cystic fibrosis after systemic administration of 4-phenylbutyrate. *Mol Ther* 2002;6:119.
228. Jiang C et al. Partial restoration of cAMP-stimulated CFTR chloride channel activity in

DeltaF508 cells by deoxyspergualin. *Am J Physiol* 1998;275:C171.
229. Hamilton JW. Gentamicin in pharmacogenetic approach to treatment of cystic fibrosis. *Lancet* 2001;358:201.
230. Pons G et al. French multicenter randomized double-blind placebo-controlled trial on nebulized amiloride in cystic fibrosis patients. The Amiloride-AFLM Collaborative Study Group. *Pediatr Pulmonol* 2000;30:25.
231. Burrows E. Sodium channel blockers for cystic fibrosis. *Cochrane Database Syst Rev* 2006;3.
232. Zegarra-Moran O et al. Correction of G551D-CFTR transport defect in epithelial monolayers by genistein but not by CPX or MPB-07. *Br J Pharmacol* 2002;137:504.
233. MacLusky L. Spectrum of clinical manifestations of cystic fibrosis. *Pediatr Ann* 1993;22:544.
234. Gardiner-Caldwell. Cystic fibrosis: pathogenesis and therapies. In major pathogenic events in cystic fibrosis lung disease. Monterey Park, CA: Synermed Communications; 1994.
235. Ramsey BW et al. Predictive value of oropharyngeal cultures for identifying lower airway bacteria in cystic fibrosis patients. *Am Rev Respir Dis* 1991;144:331.
236. Wood DM et al. Antibiotic strategies for eradicating Pseudomonas aeruginosa in people with cystic fibrosis. *Cochrane Database Syst Rev* 2006;1.
237. Valerius NH et al. Prevention of chronic *Pseudomonas aeruginosa* colonisation in cystic fibrosis by early treatment. *Lancet* 1991;338: 725.
238. Prunier AL et al. Clinical isolates of *Staphylococcus aureus* with ribosomal mutations conferring resistance to macrolides. *Antimicrob Agents Chemother* 2002;46:3054.
239. Phaff SJ. Macrolide resistance of *Staphylococcus aureus* and *Haemophilus species* associated with long-term azithromycin use in cystic fibrosis. *J Antimicrob Chemother* 2006;57:741.
240. Scott CS et al. Cystic fibrosis. In: Carter BL et al., eds. *Pharmacotherapy Self-Assessment Module.* Kansas City, MO. ACCP 1999:109.

SECTION TWENTY ONE

GERIATRIC THERAPY

Bradley R. Williams
SECTION EDITOR

CHAPTER 99

Geriatric Drug Use

Jiwon Kim and May Mak

Demographic and Economic Considerations

Demographic changes and U.S. medical progress in the last half of the 20th century have created imperatives to improve our knowledge about the health care and drug therapy of older adults. The Federal Interagency Forum on Aging-Related Statistics recently published an updated chart book, which provides the most current information on the health and well-being of older Americans in the United States (Table 99-1).[1]

The oldest-old category (i.e., those older than 85 years of age) is going to have the greatest impact on the health care system because the number of people in this group has increased faster than any other age category, and many are physically and medically frail. This group will triple its size by 2040, which is more than double the growth rate of the next fastest-growing category.[2] By 2050, at least half of Americans will live to age 85; they will number almost 21 million and comprise 5% of the total U.S. population.[3] Because the frail elderly are often dependent and in ill health, they require the highest level of health services. They have the highest health care expenditures, hospitalization rates, and home health visits.[1]

Approximately 4% of the 35 million U.S. residents 65 years of age or older in 1999 resided in long-term care facilities (LTCFs).[4] Elderly LTCF residents are predominantly women, 75 years and older, white non-Hispanic, and widowed. Although the prevalence of functional disability in the elderly is expected to be reduced,[5] the national expenditure for long-term care services for the elderly is expected to grow through the year 2040.[4] Of older adults who live at home, about 10% in the 65- to 74-year-old age group and up to 50% in the over 85 age group require assistance with everyday activities.[2] Up to 64% of those who receive care rely on informal care from children and other relatives.[1] Thus, it is important to include the caregiver in the counseling and monitoring of activities when feasible.

Health care for the elderly is increasingly based on a prospective reimbursement system in institutional settings. Managed care practices aim to minimize high-cost hospitalizations by shifting care to lower-cost alternatives, such as home health care, assisted living, and hospice care. The escalating costs and affordability of medications is a national concern, especially in the Medicare population. As reforms are put in place to enhance access to drugs, it is especially important to keep in mind that this population is particularly vulnerable to drug-related morbidity and mortality, which costs the U.S. health care system at least $30.1 billion annually.[6]

Table 99-1 Profile of Older Americans

Current Status of the Older Population

- The older population, persons age 65 years and older, numbered 35 million in 2000, representing 13% of the U.S. population. This means that since 1900, the percentage of Americans age 65 years and older tripled (4.1% in 1900 to 13% in 2000), and their numbers have increased 10-fold (from 3.1 million to 35 million in 2000).
- There are more women than men in the older population. Among persons 65 years old in 2000, 58% were women. In the oldest old group, 70% of persons age 85 years and older were women.
- The older population is getting older. In 2000, the 85 and older age group (4 million) was 31 times larger than in 1900.
- The expected number of years of life increased by approximately 60% since 1900. In 2003, life expectancy was 79.8 years for women and 76.8 years for men.
- In 2003, the most common and costly health conditions among all persons age 65 and older were heart disease, diabetes, stroke, and cancer.
- Among all persons age 65 and older, the five leading causes of death are heart disease, cancer, stroke, chronic obstructive pulmonary diseases, and pneumonia and influenza.

Future Growth of the Older Population

- Although the rate of growth slowed during the 1990s because of the relatively small number of births during the Great Depression of the 1930s, the most rapid increase is expected between the years 2010 and 2030, when the baby boom generation reaches age 65.
- By 2030, there will be about 70 million older persons, 2.7 times their number in 1980. If current fertility and immigration levels remain stable, the only age groups to grow significantly will be those older than 55 years of age.
- By 2030, persons age 65 and older are expected to represent 20% of the population; the population age 85 years and older will more than double to approximately 9.6 million persons.

From reference 1.

Table 99-2 Factors That May Influence Functional Age

Poor vs. good or adequate nutrition
Smoking vs. quit smoking vs. never a smoker
Acute or chronic diseases vs. good health
Acute or chronic drug therapy vs. no drug use
"Couch potato" vs. lifelong habit of exercise
Institutionalized vs. living independently at home

Age-Related Physiological, Pharmacokinetic, and Pharmacodynamic Changes

An important determinant of drug-related problems in the elderly is an increased physiological vulnerability to medication adverse effects and an impaired ability to recover from drug-induced insults. The progressive decrease in the ability of each organ system to maintain homeostasis in the face of challenge is a definition of physiological aging.[7] Disruption of homeostatic "balance" predisposes an older adult to disease or medication side effects. Homeostatic mechanisms in the cardiovascular and nervous systems are less efficient, drug metabolism and excretion decrease, body tissue composition and drug volume of distribution change, and drug receptor sensitivity may be altered. Age-associated changes are progressive, occurring gradually over a lifetime, rather than abruptly at any given age (e.g., 65 years of age). The physiological processes of aging often result in an increased susceptibility to many diseases. However, older people remain a heterogeneous group, with chronologic age not always reflecting "functional age" (Table 99-2). Distinct separation of these interrelated factors is difficult because all may contribute to variability in drug response. In particular, pharmacodynamic changes in the aging population is a research topic fraught with many methodological and logistic constraints, as evidenced by the scarcity of information on aging and pharmacologic effects. Resnick and Marcantonio summarized six geriatric clinical care principles in Table 99-3.[7]

Absorption

Changes in the gastrointestinal (GI) tract with age may influence drug absorption. Gastric pH increases, intestinal blood flow diminishes, and some impairment of both active and passive transport mechanisms occurs.[8] However, the significance of these changes is not clear. One study found nearly 90% of healthy, independently living elders were able to acidify gastric contents (pH 3.5), even in the basal unstimulated state (ages, 65–96 years).[9] However, these volunteers were "functionally" young (Table 99-2), with an average of only 2.1 self-reported disease states and 1.6 over-the-counter (OTC) and prescription medications. Assessment of age-associated changes in absorption requires careful attention to methodology. For example, samples must be collected for four to six half-lives in older subjects to obtain a complete area under the time-concentration curve (AUC). Also, intravenous (IV) and oral (PO) data must be compared in the same subject to validate the assumption that clearance is constant:

$$AUC = \frac{(S)(F)(Dose)}{Cl} \qquad \textbf{(99-1)}$$

where *(S)(F)* is the fraction of dose administered that will reach systemic circulation and *Cl* is clearance.

Transdermal administration is becoming increasingly common and is used for several medications taken by older adults. Alterations in the stratum corneum, lipid composition of the skin, changes in sebaceous gland activity, and changes in the dermis and epidermis may affect drug absorption.[10] Lipophilic drugs (e.g., estradiol) appear to be less affected by aging than do hydrophilic compounds (e.g., acetylsalicylic acid).[11]

The following generalizations can be concluded: the extent of absorption via the oral route is similar in older patients and in young adults, the rate of absorption is reduced or unaltered in older patients, and drugs that undergo first-pass metabolism are absorbed more completely in the older patient. Changes in transdermal absorption of drugs have not been sufficiently studied; thus, close monitoring is warranted.

1. I.W., a 75-year-old woman, 5′4″, 120 lb, serum creatinine (SrCr) of 1.9 mg/dL, has an acute exacerbation of heart failure (HF). She is given furosemide 40 mg orally, but this produces little increase in urine output or resolution of her symptoms. What might be an explanation for I.W.'s lack of response to furosemide? How might the desired response to furosemide be achieved?

The extent of furosemide (Lasix) absorption is not changed in older patients, but the rate of absorption is slowed. This results in a diminished efficacy of the drug because active secretion into the urine (rate of entry) must reach the steep portion

Table 99-3 Geriatric Clinical Care Principles

Care Principle	Outcome/Example
Because of impaired physiological reserve in older patients, disease often presents at an earlier stage.	• Mild disease may tip the "balance." • Drug side effects may occur with agents and doses unlikely to be toxic in younger people. • Stoic elderly may be less likely to seek help for dysfunction until symptoms are advanced.
Presentation of a new disease depends on the organ system made most vulnerable by previous changes, and this "weak link" often differs from the organ newly diseased.	• Presentation is often atypical, with the "weakest link" being the brain (confusion), lower urinary tract (incontinence), musculoskeletal system (falling), or cardiovascular system (fainting).
Clinical findings abnormal in younger patients are common in older people and may not be responsible for a particular symptom.	• An elderly patient with syncope due to medications and dehydration, but with ventricular ectopy on a cardiac monitor, may be harmed by misdirected antiarrhythmic therapy.
Because comorbid disease and drug use are common, symptoms are often due to multiple causes.	• Incontinence may involve a combination of fecal impaction, drugs inducing confusion, and impaired mobility due to arthritis.
Because many homeostatic mechanisms may be compromised concurrently, multiple abnormalities can be amenable to treatment, and small improvements in several areas may yield dramatic benefits to overall function.	• Falls associated with diabetic polyneuropathy are exacerbated by concomitant drug use, arthritis, and orthostatic hypotension, which are more easily treated than the underlying disease.
Because older patients are more likely to suffer adverse consequences of disease, treatment and prevention may be equally or more effective.	• Thrombolytics for AMI. • β-Blockers after MI. • Hypertension treatment. • Immunization (influenza, pneumococcal pneumonia). • Fall prevention (modify drugs that induce orthostasis or confusion, remove environmental hazards, address balance, peripheral edema, nocturia).

AMI, acute myocardial infarction; MI, myocardial infarction.

of the sigmoid dose–response curve for maximal effect of the drug.[12] I.W. should be given a 40-mg dose of furosemide intravenously to bypass the problem of decreased rate of absorption. High sodium intake or concurrent use of nonsteroidal anti-inflammatory drugs (NSAIDs) can also decrease the effectiveness of furosemide. Further increases in the dose of furosemide may be necessary, with consideration of a continuous infusion in patients with severe chronic renal insufficiency (see Chapter 19).[12]

Distribution

A number of changes that can affect the distribution of drugs in the body may occur with aging. Cardiac output decreases about 1% per year from ages 19 to 86.[13] In many older patients, this decline in cardiac output is accompanied by an increase in peripheral vascular resistance and a proportional decrease in hepatic and renal blood flow. However, noninstitutionalized older adults who are free of coronary artery disease or other debilitating health problems exhibit little age-related declines in cardiac output (functionally young).[14] Body composition undergoes changes during normal aging. Total body water and lean body mass both decline with age, and total fat content increases between ages 18 and 85 years from 18% to 36% in men and from 33% to 48% in women.[15,16] Thus, the volume of distribution (Vd) of drugs that are distributed primarily in body water or lean body mass (e.g., lithium, digoxin) is decreased in older adults; unadjusted dosing can result in higher blood levels. Conversely, the Vd of highly lipid-soluble drugs, such as long-acting benzodiazepines (e.g., diazepam), may be increased, thereby delaying maximal effects or leading to accumulation with continued use.[17] Factors with special applicability in older patients that may affect binding include protein concentration, disease states, coadministration of other drugs, and nutritional status. Serum albumin concentrations fall progressively for each decade beyond 40 years of age, reaching a mean of 3.58 g/dL (normal, 4 g/dL) in those older than 80 years of age.[18] Decreased albumin concentrations are important because albumin is a major site of drug binding. Increases in α_1-acid glycoprotein in older patients[19] affect the binding of weak bases such as lidocaine and propranolol. Data are lacking concerning age-related changes in tissue protein binding of drugs. However, the Vd of digoxin decreases in subjects with impaired renal function, as does the myocardial-to-serum concentration ratio.[20] Finally, an important factor in determining the significance of changes in protein binding status is whether a drug is restrictively or nonrestrictively cleared.[21]

Altered Protein Binding

2. O.T., a 90-year-old woman, 5′8″, 132 lb, is brought to the emergency department (ED) for evaluation of a "shaking spell." In the ED, another "spell" is observed, starting with shaking of the left arm and progressing into a generalized tonic-clonic seizure. A loading dose of phenytoin (Dilantin) 1,000 mg is given IV over 30 minutes. O.T. is admitted to the neurology unit for further evaluation and given phenytoin 300 mg QHS. What is your assessment of O.T.'s phenytoin therapy given her age? What laboratory tests should be ordered, and how often should these be monitored?

O.T. received an average phenytoin loading dose of 17 mg/kg (normal, 15–20 mg/kg) and is receiving the average daily maintenance dose. A sodium serum concentration should be obtained to rule out a hyponatremia-induced seizure, and an albumin serum concentration should be obtained because of phenytoin's high (90%) protein binding. A phenytoin serum concentration should be measured before O.T. is discharged from the hospital to document that the desired therapeutic serum concentration has been achieved. The serum phenytoin concentration should be obtained whenever an adverse drug reaction or seizure occurs. A follow-up, steady-state phenytoin serum concentration should be obtained in 10 to 14 days to determine if the current dose is appropriate.

3. The serum albumin concentration is 2.2 g/dL (normal, 3.2–5.2 g/dL), Na is 140 mEq/L (normal, 138–145 mEq/L), and the phenytoin serum concentration is 15 mcg/mL (normal, 10–20 mcg/mL). O.T. complains of drowsiness and has a wide-based, unsteady gait. What is the likely cause of her symptoms?

[SI units: albumin, 22 g/L (normal, 32–52); phenytoin, 59.5 mmol/L (normal, 40–80)]

O.T. could have a phenytoin free-fraction percentage of up to 18%, compared with the normal value of 10%, because of her low albumin serum concentration.[21] This would produce a free phenytoin concentration of 27 mcg/mL (normal, 10–20 mcg/mL), explaining O.T.'s symptoms (assuming O.T.'s serum phenytoin concentration is at steady state). In O.T.'s case, free phenytoin concentration monitoring would be appropriate, if available, and her dosage should be adjusted accordingly. A dietary consultation to examine the reason for her low albumin may contribute to her overall health.

Metabolism

O.T.'s phenytoin metabolism may be affected due to factors shown to influence hepatic drug metabolism, which include disease states, concurrent drug use, nutritional status, environmental compounds, genetic differences, gender, liver mass, and blood flow. Hepatic microsomal enzyme activity is reduced with increasing age in animals, but the clinical significance of this is controversial in humans. Large interindividual variation in liver metabolism exists for any given drug and, in most cases, may be more important than the changes associated with aging.[8,22–25] Also, liver mass declines and hepatic blood flow decreases 45% between the ages of 25 and 65.[26] Unfortunately, clinical tools for the assessment of hepatic metabolism are not readily available. Age-related changes in the liver metabolism of warfarin and long-acting benzodiazepines have been reported in humans.[27–29] Compounds undergoing phase I metabolism (reduction, oxidation, hydroxylation, demethylation) have a decreased or unchanged clearance, whereas compounds metabolized by phase II processes (conjugation, acetylation, sulfonation, glucuronidation) have no change in clearance with age. Drugs with high hepatic-extraction ratios, such as the nitrates, barbiturates, lidocaine, and propranolol, may have reduced hepatic metabolism in older adults.[30]

Reduction in Hepatic Reserve

4. D.A., an independently living 65-year-old man, 5′10″ tall and weighing 260 lb, has a chief complaint of severe shortness of breath (SOB; respirations, 26 breaths/minute), palpitations (heart rate [HR], 120 beats/minute), and nausea. He has a history of chronic obstructive pulmonary disease (COPD) and HF. D.A.'s current medications are theophylline-SR (Theo-Dur) 450 mg Q 8 h, captopril (Capoten) 12.5 mg TID, and furosemide (Lasix) 20 mg QD. At his last visit to his physician 2 months ago, his theophylline serum concentration was 15 mcg/mL (therapeutic range, 8–12 mcg/mL). After a long history of heavy smoking, D.A. finally took his physician's advice and abruptly quit. The diagnosis of acute HF is made on the basis of the chest radiograph, 2% pitting edema, and "junky" sounding lungs. Based on the information given, what potential problems should be added to the list of differential diagnoses to be considered?

Theophylline toxicity should be suspected for two reasons: (a) lack of hepatic microsome/enzyme stimulation from his recent smoking cessation, and (b) the known reduction of theophylline hepatic metabolism secondary to acute HF.[21] The theophylline dose should be held until the serum theophylline concentration is within the desired therapeutic range. In patients who are at high risk of developing theophylline toxicity, other treatment options such as an inhaled anticholinergic agent (e.g., tiotropium) with or without an inhaled β_2-agonist should be considered in place of theophylline (see Chapter 24).

Although the potential for theophylline toxicity can be predicted reasonably in D.A., the sudden onset of clinical deterioration or an adverse effect often arises unexpectedly in many older patients. Patients often do well while medically stable only to abruptly experience a "cascade of disasters" when hospitalized or when they begin taking additional medications. As presented in the answer to question 3, the process of aging can be associated with declining liver mass, decreased hepatic blood flow, altered nutritional status, and a host of other physiological changes. These alterations result in a loss of "hepatic reserve," making the patient susceptible to adverse effects because new drugs compete for the same metabolic enzymes. The concept of a lost "reserve" in the elderly applies to other organ systems as well. Therefore, D.A.'s response to renally excreted drugs (e.g., captopril, furosemide) should also be considered during this episode of acute HF.

Excretion

Age-related changes in renal function result in more adverse drug events (ADEs) than any other age-related physiological alterations. Compounding these changes in the kidney are the arteriosclerotic changes and a declining cardiac output that decrease renal perfusion by 40% to 50% between the ages of 25 and 65. This is accompanied by a corresponding decrease in glomerular filtration and urea clearance.[31] Urine concentrating ability declines with age, as does renal sodium conservation.[32,33] Tubular secretory capacity and creatinine clearance (ClCr) may also be reduced.[34,35] The kidney loses functioning cells with age, and histologic studies reveal a decline in the absolute number of nephrons.[36] All these measures of kidney function decline uniformly, leading to the concept of the "intact nephron." Significant variability can occur in the rate of decline in renal function in a minority of elderly patients[37] (Table 99-2).

The plasma half-life is prolonged for a number of renally excreted drugs in "healthy" older adults. The highest-risk drugs are those that depend entirely on the kidney for elimination. Examples of these are listed in Table 99-4.

Age-related changes in renal function are evaluated using the ClCr, an estimate of glomerular filtration rate. The Cockcroft-Gault equation is used most commonly to estimate ClCr.[38] Many controversies exist with regard to the use of this equation. One relates to whether the actual or lean body weight (LBW) should be used.[39,40] The use of LBW may reflect SCr

Table 99-4 Drugs Highly Dependent on Renal Function for Elimination[a]

Acetazolamide	Diflunisal	Metoclopramide
Acyclovir	Digoxin	Nadolol
Allopurinol	Enalapril	Nitrosourea
Amantadine	Ethambutol	Penicillamine
Amiloride	Fluconazole	Pentamidine
Aminoglycosides	Flucytosine	Phenazopyridine
Amphotericin B	Fluoroquinolones (most)	Plicamycin
Atenolol		Probenecid
Aztreonam	Furosemide	Procainamide
Bleomycin	Gallamine	Pyridostigmine
Bretylium	Gold sodium thiomalate	Spironolactone
Captopril		Sulfamethoxazole
Cephalosporins (most)	H_2 blockers (most)	Sulfinpyrazone
	Imipenem	Thiazides
Chlorpropamide	Lisinopril	Ticarcillin
Cisplatin	Lithium	Trimethoprim
Clonidine	Methenamine	Vancomycin
Colistimethate	Methotrexate	

[a]This list is not comprehensive; see references 156 and 157 for additional details.

production more accurately because creatinine is produced in muscle mass, which is decreased in older patients. There is also a question of whether one should use the actual creatinine value when it is <1.0 mg/dL or whether it should be rounded to 1.0. Finally, for certain subpopulations of older patients (i.e., ambulatory and healthy vs. hospitalized, malnourished, and/or critically ill), other methods may produce more accurate estimates of renal function.

Table 99-5 provides a composite picture of the age-related physiological changes, disease states, and pharmacologic factors that affect pharmacokinetic processes in older adults.

Pharmacodynamic Changes

Homeostasis and Postural Hypotension

D.A. is susceptible not only to decreased clearance (i.e., hepatic metabolism, renal elimination), but also to pharmacodynamic changes. Pharmacodynamic changes are defined loosely in this chapter as alterations in concentration–response relationships or receptor sensitivity. Drug side effects that are mild or nonexistent in younger patients may be significant in older adults due to inefficient homeostatic adjustments. For example, the higher rate of orthostatic hypotension observed in older patients is often the result of impaired baroreceptor function and a failure of cerebral blood flow autoregulation. Orthostatic hypotension occurs in 20% of ambulatory patients older than 65 years of age and in 30% of those older than 75,[41] and it is often aggravated by drugs with sympatholytic activity (e.g., α-adrenergic blocking agents, phenothiazines, tricyclic antidepressants [TCAs]), volume-depleting drugs (e.g., diuretics), and vasodilating agents (e.g., nitrates, alcohol).[42] In one study of 100 geriatric psychiatric outpatients, almost 40% complained of dizziness and falling, which were attributed to psychiatric medications.[43] Patients with impaired cardiac output and patients taking concurrent diuretic therapy (e.g., patient D.A.) are especially vulnerable. Also, aging impairs balance and posture maintenance, and drug effects on posture control may contribute to drug-induced falls in older adults.[44] Table 99-6 reviews the therapeutic agents commonly associated with adverse drug reactions that may affect the mobility of older patients.

Receptor Sensitivity

An exaggerated response to some drugs (e.g., nitrazepam, heparin [in females], warfarin) may reflect an intrinsic, age-related change in receptor sensitivity.[45,46] The aging central nervous system (CNS) is particularly vulnerable to qualitative

Table 99-5 Changes Affecting Pharmacokinetic Parameters

Parameter	*Physiological Changes*	*Disease States*	*Pharmacologic Factors*
Absorption (bioavailability, first-pass metabolism)	Gastric pH Absorptive surface Splanchnic blood flow GI motility Gastric emptying rate	Achlorhydria, diarrhea, gastrectomy, malabsorptive syndromes, pancreatitis	Drug interactions, antacids, anticholinergics, cholestyramine, food
Distribution	Cardiac output TBW Lean body mass Serum albumin α_1-Acid glycoprotein Body fat Altered relative tissue perfusion	CHF; dehydration; edema, ascites; hepatic failure; malnutrition; renal failure	Drug interactions, protein binding displacement
Metabolism	Hepatic mass Enzyme activity Hepatic blood flow	CHF, fever, hepatic failure, malignancy, malnutrition, thyroid disease, viral infection or immunization	Dietary makeup, drug interactions, insecticides, alcohol, smoking, induction of metabolism, inhibition of metabolism
Excretion	Renal blood flow GFR Tubular secretion Renal mass	Hypovolemia, renal insufficiency	Drug interactions

GI, gastrointestinal; TBW, total body water; CHF, congestive heart failure; GFR, glomerular filtration rate.

Table 99-6 Adverse Drug Reactions That May Affect Mobility of the Older Patient

Medication Class	Adverse Drug Reaction
TCAs	Orthostatic hypotension, tremor, cardiac arrhythmias, sedation
Benzodiazepines and sedative hypnotics	Sedation, weakness, coordination, confusion
Narcotic analgesics	Sedation, coordination, confusion
Antipsychotics	Orthostatic hypotension, sedation, extrapyramidal effects
Antihypertensives	Orthostatic hypotension
β-Adrenergic blockers	Ability to respond to work load

TCAs, tricyclic antidepressants.

and quantitative alterations in drug response. The aging brain, like the aging kidney, loses a significant number of active cells during later life, and some brain atrophy is a common, although not necessarily pathological, finding in older adults. Normal aging also involves a reduction in cerebral blood flow and oxygen consumption, and increased cerebrovascular resistance.[47] Older adults often have cerebral blood flow rates that are as much as 20% lower than those of younger persons.[13] In addition, inhibitory and excitatory pathways in the CNS are delicately balanced to modulate cognitive functions and behavior. With aging, there is a selective decline in some pathways and the preservation of others. For example, cholinergic neurons in the neocortex and hippocampal areas of the brain normally decrease with age. Pathological cholinergic deficits are associated with memory loss, confusion, and other cognitive impairments.[48] Drugs with anticholinergic properties are particularly notorious for inducing mental fuzziness and confusion in older patients. Several examples of therapeutic classes with anticholinergic properties are listed in Table 99-7.

Table 99-7 Categories of Anticholinergic Drugs That Can Induce Confusion in Older Patients

Therapeutic Class	Examples (Brand Name)
Antispasmodic	Belladonna (Generic) Dicyclomine (Bentyl) Propantheline (Pro-Banthine)
Antiparkinson	Benztropine (Cogentin) Trihexyphenidyl (Artane)
Antihistamine	Diphenhydramine (Benadryl) Chlorpheniramine (Chlor-Trimeton)
Antidepressant	Amitriptyline (Elavil) Imipramine (Tofranil)
Antiarrhythmic	Quinidine Disopyramide (Norpace)
Neuroleptic	Thioridazine (Mellaril) Chlorpromazine (Thorazine)
Hypnotic	Hydroxyzine (Vistaril)
OTC agents	Antidiarrheals Doxylamine Cold remedies

OTC, over the counter.

Both central and peripheral responsiveness of adrenergic receptors decline with aging.[49] Monoamine-oxidase activity increases with normal aging, and this is reflected by a decline in norepinephrine and dopamine levels in aging brains.[50] The decline in CNS dopamine synthesis is associated with increased sensitivity to dopamine blocking agents (e.g., neuroleptics, metoclopramide). However, β-receptor sensitivity to both β-agonists and β-antagonists decreases, even if the number of β-receptors does not decrease in older patients.[51,52] Because these neurologic and biochemical reserves are reduced as a normal consequence of aging, iatrogenic behavioral disorders are relatively common in older adults, and drugs are one of the most common causes of sudden, unexplained mental impairment in the older adult. For example, in one study, 11% of 300 patients older than 65 years of age experienced cognitive impairment as a result of an adverse drug reaction, and the risk increased ninefold when patients were taking four or more prescription drugs.[53]

In conclusion, D.A. is susceptible to significant variations in response to his medications and needs to be monitored carefully because of both pharmacokinetic and pharmacodynamic alterations attributable to aging. His theophylline therapy, in particular, should be evaluated.

Problems Associated With Drug Use in Older Adults

Polymedicine

Multiple medication use is the primary cause of drug-related adverse events in the older population according to the Centers for Disease Control and Prevention.[54] Polydrug therapy thrives under conditions in which multiple chronic diseases exist in patients with communication problems, especially when the physician is under pressure to be time efficient. These factors can lead to misdiagnoses and unclear drug indications. For these reasons, monitoring drug therapy in these patients is not only challenging but imperative. Busy health care providers often assign a low priority to nursing home patients in terms of individual attention, and much of the prescribing of medications and follow-up is done by telephone. Duplicative prescribing within the same drug class often occurs, and unrecognized drug side effects are treated with more drugs. With minimal actual patient contact, prescribers may continue drugs in patients long after the original problem has resolved to avoid the inconvenience of meticulous dosage adjustments and follow-up monitoring. Careful drug regimen review is essential to identify potentially unnecessary or inappropriate medications and to systematically taper and discontinue these agents, with attentive monitoring of the older person.[55–57]

Adverse Drug Events

An ADE includes preventable and nonpreventable events and accounts for errors related to prescribing and administration. The combining of several medications can also increase the risk of clinically significant drug interactions and subsequent ADEs in the elderly. Age per se is not an independent risk factor for ADEs, but rather, increased risk is derived from age-related factors (e.g., physiological changes), chronic disease states, use of different health care providers, and inappropriate prescribing.[58]

Twenty-eight percent of hospitalizations of older persons are a result of ADEs and poor medication adherence.[59]

Table 99-8 Predictors of Adverse Drug Events

- More than four prescription medications
- Length of stay in hospital longer than 14 days
- More than four active medical problems
- Admission to a general medical unit vs. a specialized geriatric ward
- History of alcohol use
- Lower mean Mini-Mental Status Examination score (confusion, dementia)
- Twenty-four new medications added to medication regimen during hospitalization

Adapted from references 61 and 63.

Adverse drug reactions in older patients cared for in the community may be as high as 35%.[60] An estimated 32,000 hip fractures, 163,000 cases of drug-induced cognitive impairment, and 61,000 cases of neuroleptic-induced Parkinsonism occur annually.[59]

ADEs can be difficult to detect in older patients because they often present atypically and with nonspecific symptoms, such as lethargy, confusion, lightheadedness, or falls. Nevertheless, most adverse reactions represent extensions of a drug's pharmacologic effect, have identifiable predictors, and are preventable (Table 99-8).[61–63] Adverse drug reactions remain a significant problem, with some experts placing the direct health care costs for adverse drug reactions at $3.6 billion annually.[64]

ADVERSE DRUG REACTIONS IN OLDER PATIENTS

5. S.E., an 85-year-old woman, 5′2″ and 102 lb, with a SrCr of 1.6 mg/dL, is admitted for chest pain, SOB, and to rule out myocardial infarction (MI). Her physician is concerned about oversedation with narcotics and prescribes ketorolac (Toradol) 30 mg Q 6 h IV. She has a history of severe HF and angina for which she takes lisinopril 10 mg QD, furosemide 40 mg QD, aspirin 81 mg QD, and nitroglycerin SR 6 mg BID. The lisinopril dosage is increased to 20 mg QD, and the furosemide dosage is also increased to 40 mg BID. Her BP is 110/66 mm Hg, and her urine output has been 20 to 30 mL/hour for 4 hours since ketorolac was initiated. What risk factors are present in S.E. for drug-induced renal problems?

[SI unit: SrCr, 141.4 mol/L]

S.E. has a number of risk factors for the development of drug-induced acute renal failure (ARF). Angiotensin-converting enzyme (ACE) inhibitors are indicated for HF management and improve renal function by increasing cardiac output. However, they can diminish efferent arteriole glomerular capillary filtration pressure and precipitate ARF in predisposed patients. A 13% incidence of azotemia has been reported in LTCF residents started on a short course of NSAID treatment.[65] A low serum sodium concentration, high-dose diuretics, diabetes, severe HF (i.e., New York Heart Association [NYHA] class IV), use of a long-acting ACE inhibitor, and concurrent NSAID use are all risk factors for drug-induced ARF (see Chapter 31). Patients with these risk factors should be monitored closely when an ACE inhibitor is initiated and when the dosage of an ACE inhibitor is increased (see Chapter 19). Renal prostaglandins (PGE_2, PGI_2) increase or help maintain renal blood flow when renal function is compromised by intrinsic renal disease, HF, liver disease with ascites, or hypertension; therefore, the use of a prostaglandin inhibitor such as ketorolac places S.E. at an increased risk for ARF. Furthermore, the ketorolac dose is excessive for S.E. based on the recommended maximum dose of 15 mg every 6 hours for elderly patients.[66]

Disease-Specific Geriatric Drug Therapy

Cardiovascular Disease in the Ambulatory Older Patient

6. T.M. is a 78-year-old woman who presents to a "brown bag" session being sponsored by the local senior center and school of pharmacy. She reports that recently she has begun to feel "sluggish" and fainted a few times. She lives at home alone on a modest, fixed retirement income. She has a number of chronic medical problems, including coronary artery disease (CAD), congestive heart failure (CHF), hypertension, diabetes, and hyperlipidemia. She visits different specialists on a sporadic basis for management of her various disease states and takes "a lot of medications," the names of which she does not know. She admits to skipping her medications periodically. T.M. usually maintains a fairly active social life, hosting and visiting her elderly friends regularly and attending the local seniors' lunch social three times a week. She is highly interested in matters relating to her health, and she often self-medicates with nonprescription medications and herbal remedies she hears about through her peers. Because of the recent weakness, however, she is now afraid to attend social gatherings. Review of her "brown bag" reveals the following items: glyburide 2.5 mg BID, HCTZ 25 mg QD, propranolol 20 mg QID, niacin 500 mg TID, ASA 325 mg PRN, digoxin 0.25 mg QD, isosorbide dinitrate (ISDN) 20 mg QID, NTG 0.4 mg SL PRN, captopril 25 mg TID, furosemide 40 mg BID, acetaminophen 500 mg PRN, verapamil 60 mg QID, multivitamins with minerals, calcium carbonate 500 mg TID, hawthorn tincture 20 drops BID, ibuprofen 200 mg PRN, rosiglitazone 2 mg BID, and dandelion 10 mL BID. She also drinks a glass of red wine with dinner and several cups of licorice tea with breakfast and lunch. What initial steps are necessary for safe and effective management of T.M.'s drug therapy?

Like many ambulatory older patients who are being treated for multiple chronic medical conditions, T.M. is at high risk for drug-induced problems secondary to nonadherence, medication errors, inappropriate prescribing, self-medicating, and polymedicine. She is representative of more than 9 million older adults who live at home alone. The isolated community-dwelling older patient is typically female, 75 years of age or older, has multiple medical issues, and takes multiple medications.[67] Many of these individuals lack close support and a daily routine, and may not be fully aware of the time of day or the day of the week. Limited time awareness makes adherence to complex medication regimens more difficult in this population. In addition to older people like T.M., a second high-risk group of older persons consists of those individuals who were recently discharged from the hospital. The postdischarge period can be a time of confusion for these patients, who often must cope with new drugs or replacement drugs added to an already complex prehospitalization regimen. A summary of the various factors contributing to nonadherence in the older patient is presented in Table 99-9.[68]

T.M. needs a primary care provider to coordinate her medical care and to follow-up on her new-onset "sluggishness and fainting." She should also be advised to establish a relationship at one pharmacy that can monitor all her medications.

Table 99-9 Factors Influencing the Inability to Comply With a Medication Regimen

Three chronic conditions
More than five prescription medications
Twelve medication dosages per day
Medication regimen changed four times during the past 12 months
Three prescribers involved
Significant cognitive or physical impairments (e.g., memory, hearing, vision, color discrimination, child-resistant containers)
Living alone in the community
Recently discharged from the hospital
Reliance on a caregiver
Low literacy
Medication cost
Demonstrated poor compliance history

Adapted from references 68 and 68.

Furthermore, T.M. should be counseled to discontinue alcohol, which can interact with several of her current medications and worsen her conditions. Finally, assessment of the risk for medication-related problems (MRPs) is highly recommended by doing a drug regimen review such as with the brown bag event, medication therapy management,[69] and/or using validated tools such as a self-administered questionnaire to identify potential for MRPs.[70]

7. T.M. presents to the multidisciplinary geriatric care team on the advice of pharmacists and students at the "brown bag" session. During the pharmacy intake interview, she admits to selective adherence with many medications based on how they make her feel and their cost. Her "glass" of wine with dinner is 32 oz, four times a week. She also reveals that she has not been taking her furosemide and potassium supplement because she feels that they were contributing to her "sluggishness" and fainting. She is using hawthorne and dandelion instead. The geriatrician's summary of T.M.'s history and physical examination reads as follows: 78-year-old white female, 5′6″, 189 lb. Vital signs: BP, 168/82 mm Hg; HR, 54 beats/minute; temperature, 98.7°F; and respiratory rate, 18/minute. Pertinent laboratory values: SCr, 1.5 mg/dL (nl 0.6–1.2 mg/dL); BUN, 35 mg/dL (nl 8–18 mg/dL); Na, 153 mEq/L (nl 138–145 mEq/L); K, 3.1 mEq/L (nl 3.5–5 mEq/L); Mg, 1.5 mEq/L (nl 1.6–2.4 mEq/L); glucose, 250 mg/dL (nl 70–110 mg/dL); A1c, 9.5%, cholesterol, 259 mg/dL; low-density lipoprotein (LDL), 140 mg/dL; high-density lipoprotein (HDL), 40 mg/dL; triglycerides (TG), 200 mg/dL; proteinuria; and digoxin level, 1.5 ng/mL. Electrocardiogram showed sinus bradycardia with an old anterior MI. Echo: EF 25%. Problem list: new-onset sluggishness and fainting, chest pain/SOB on exertion, 3(+) pitting edema bilaterally, NYHA class II–III HF, hypertension, type 2 diabetes, obesity, excessive alcohol intake, CAD, and hyperlipidemia. What factors may be contributing to T.M.'s feeling of sluggishness and fainting?

T.M's sluggishness and fainting are most likely due to her low heart rate, somewhat dehydrated state, and multiple medications that have the potential for producing weakness. Specifically, digoxin 0.25 mg daily is considered a high dose for an elderly patient who has moderate kidney compromise. A level of 1.5 ng/mL is excessive for the CHF condition (therapeutic range 0.5–1.2 ng/mL for HF); therefore, one or two doses should be held, and then the dose should be lowered to 0.125 mg daily. Her condition on the new dose should be re-evaluated after about 2 weeks.[71] After stabilization of the current exacerbation, one can try discontinuing digoxin to evaluate whether T.M. is actually benefiting from this agent. Dizziness can result from T.M.'s use of supplements. Although hawthorn has been approved for use by the German Commission E in NYHA class II HF, it may increase digoxin's toxicity and should be discontinued.[72,73] Dandelion can also produce mild diuretic, hypokalemic, and hypoglycemic effects. Therefore, its use needs to be monitored closely.[74] In addition, the licorice tea T.M. drinks has mineral corticoid properties and may cause blood pressure elevation, salt and water retention, as well as low potassium levels, all of which are already present in T.M.[75] In general, elderly patients should be advised not to self-medicate with supplements without clear indication and cautioned against potential drug interactions with their prescription medications. Furthermore, T.M. is also taking propranolol and verapamil, which may lower the heart rate and contribute to the sluggishness. Switching propranolol to an extended-release β-blocker should help, and verapamil can be discontinued at this point because it may not have benefits toward T.M.'s other medical problems.

HEART FAILURE

8. What is appropriate management for T.M.'s stage of HF?

HF is a common cause of morbidity and mortality in older patients. The standard therapy for HF typically consists of three or more medications (diuretics, β-blockers, and ACE inhibitors, with or without digoxin and spironolactone). Standard use of multiple medications in the treatment of HF makes close monitoring of drug therapy essential. T.M. has stage II–III HF. Based on her history of an old MI and low EF, she is also in stage B of the American College of Cardiology/American Heart Association classification scheme. Although such a patient is symptomatically relieved with diuretics, the recommended therapy for stage B includes an ACE inhibitor or ARB, and a β-blocker. Concurrent behavioral modification with weight loss and salt restriction will also allow this medical therapy to be more effective.[76]

9. What factors should be considered for the selection of a diuretic in HF?

Two diuretics were prescribed for T.M., although she is taking only the HCTZ. Loop diuretics are generally more effective than thiazides; furosemide is also preferred in her case because HCTZ is generally ineffective in moderate to severe renal compromise (CrCl <30 mL/minute).[77] It should be explained to T.M. that the HCTZ is duplicative in its action and needs to be replaced with furosemide, which is the more effective diuretic in her case. It will help resolve her current HF exacerbation and bilateral edema. Potassium supplementation will depend on current potassium level and the potential of hyperkalemia with a concurrent ACE inhibitor, which T.M. will be maintained on. Regular monitoring of SCr and potassium is essential, and K+ supplementation should be given if necessary. Elderly patients often dislike taking diuretics due to the frequent need to urinate. In the case of T.M., she may be advised to take the furosemide later on during the day after her outings when she is home.

ACE INHIBITORS AND ANGIOTENSIN RECEPTOR BLOCKERS

10. T.M. has been taking captopril 25 mg TID. Why is this an inappropriate choice of ACE inhibitor for T.M.?

ACE inhibition is essential in the management of HF due to its benefits in ventricular remodeling.[78,79] The current ACE inhibitor in T.M.'s regimen is captopril 25 mg TID, which is inconvenient and may contribute to poor adherence. A more suitable ACE inhibitor may be ramipril, initiated at 1.25 to 2.5 mg daily. Alternatively, fosinopril 5–10 mg QD may also be desirable based on its 50% hepatic and 50% renal elimination profile.[80] So far, T.M. has not complained of any cough, so she may tolerate a long-acting ACE inhibitor such as ramipril or fosinopril. However, if an intolerable cough develops or if she does not respond to an ACE inhibitor, then an ARB such as candesartan can be substituted and initiated at 4 mg daily and titrated up as needed. Recent studies have also supported the addition of an ARB to ACE inhibitor therapy based on a lower mortality and hospitalization rate compared to an ACE inhibitor alone.[81]

β-BLOCKERS

11. T.M. is being treated with propranolol 20 mg QID. Why is this an inappropriate choice of β-blocker for T.M.?

The β-blockers carvedilol, metoprolol, and bisoprolol have been proven to reduce morbidity and mortality in patients with HF.[82–84] One of these agents should be considered in patients with HF, unless the patient is in stage IV CHF, where there is no evidence of benefits. In T.M.'s case, propranolol should be discontinued for several reasons. It is probably contributing to her feeling of sluggishness because it is a nonselective β-blocker; she may also be taking it inconsistently due to the four-times-daily regimen. Extended-release forms of metoprolol (Toprol XL 25 mg daily)[85] and carvedilol (Coreg CR 10 mg daily) that require only one daily dose are available.[86] An appropriate β-blocker should be substituted for propranolol and initiated when her current exacerbation of HF has resolved.

CORONARY HEART DISEASE/HYPERLIPIDEMIA

12. T.M. does not take her niacin because she experienced unbearable facial flushing. Despite her history of MI, she does not believe that cholesterol and "heart disease" are major health concerns for her because she is a woman. Is it important to manage cholesterol in an elderly woman with coronary heart disease (CHD)? Are women older than age 65 at greater, lower, or equal risk of death due to CHD compared with their male counterparts?

Elevated cholesterol levels have been shown to increase the risk for CHD in older adults.[87] This increased risk is statistically significant, even after adjusting for indicators of frailty and poor health.[80] Furthermore, CHD is the number one cause of death in women older than age 65.[88] Serum total cholesterol levels >240 mg/dL are present in 42% of women older than 65 years of age compared with just 25% of men older than 65 years of age.[89] After age 65, the mortality from CHD is equal in men and women.[90] T.M. has a history of MI with multiple CHD risks and risk equivalents; therefore, her LDL goal should be <100 mg/dL with a more aggressive option of <70 mg/dL. The American Diabetes Association (ADA) has also recommended that the TG goal for a patient with diabetes be <150 mg/dL.[91] Therefore, T.M. needs to be aggressively treated to lower her LDL and TG levels in light of her risk category, which confers a 10-year CHD risk of >20%.[87,91]

13. What is an optimal therapeutic plan for management of T.M.'s hyperlipidemia?

T.M.'s treatment plan should begin with lifestyle and dietary modifications. However, her history of MI places her at extremely high risk, so she should be started with aggressive lipid-lowering therapy. Statins are the drugs of choice for lowering LDL and should also be considered in the elderly population as they are effective and well tolerated. An adequate dose of a statin is able to lower the LDL up to 60% and the TG up to 35%.[89] Monotherapy with statins, therefore, should be adequate to bring her LDL and TG to target levels. Clinicians will need to titrate up to effective dosages with effective education and monitoring of liver function. Elderly patients are likely to be nonadherent due to the fear of myopathy and rhabdomyolysis, and counseling needs to be done to validate the fear, as well as the relatively low risk, of these adverse effects.[90] If combination therapy is indicated, then addition of niacin is reasonable because it may also raise the HDL level. The strategy of taking an aspirin (indicated for her CAD and diabetes mellitus [DM]) half an hour before taking the niacin may prevent the flushing syndrome. Fibrates or the cholesterol absorption inhibitor ezetimibe can also be combined with statins to further reduce the levels of LDL and TG, if necessary. Discontinuation of alcohol would be beneficial because it can increase triglycerides by as much as 50%.[92]

14. What other interventions should be implemented to optimize management of T.M.'s CAD?

Any strategy to optimize her CAD management should take into consideration her functional status, comorbidities, and risks versus benefits. T.M. is still experiencing anginal pain on her current regimen, possibly due to her inability to adhere to the four-times-daily regimen of ISDN. A once daily long-acting nitrate preparation (ISMN) may be better suited for her, with sublingual NTG available as needed. Calcium channel blockers such as verapamil, like nitrates, may relieve anginal symptoms but have not been shown to improve survival.[93] Therefore, verapamil may be discontinued. However, the other mainstays of angina therapy, aspirin and β-blockers, have proven to increase survival in patients with CHD and should be considered because aspirin is also indicated for MI prevention and β-blockers may be beneficial for CHF. To prevent further endothelial injury from the atherosclerosis that leads to plaque rupture, statins are indicated as described previously. Interestingly, ACE inhibitors (ramipril) have also been shown to reduce mortality and improve secondary prevention of CAD, particularly in the age group 65 years or older.[94]

HYPERTENSION

15. T.M. has uncontrolled hypertension. How should this be managed in light of her advanced age?

T.M.'s blood pressure is well above the goal of <130/80 mm Hg for diabetic patients as set forth by the ADA and the Seventh Report of the Joint National Committee on

Prevention, Detection, Evaluation, and Treatment of High Blood Pressure (JNC VII).[91,95] Hypertension is present in more than two-thirds of individuals older than 65 years of age. Despite having the highest prevalence of hypertension, this population is the least likely to have their blood pressures adequately treated and controlled.[96] Treatment of elderly patients, such as T.M., should be based on the same guidelines published for the general care of hypertension. Standard doses of antihypertensive drugs and multiple-drug therapy are needed in the majority of older patients. However, in many of these patients, lower initial doses are needed to minimize the risk of adverse effects such as postural hypotension. T.M. is taking furosemide, propranolol, isosorbide dinitrate, captopril, and verapamil, all of which have hypotensive effects. T.M. is also a patient with compelling indications as defined by JNC VII, such as DM, HF, and CAD. In such a patient, the use of a diuretic, ACE inhibitor or ARB, and/or β-blocker in appropriate combination may improve morbidity and mortality outcomes. Although adequate dosing and combination therapy are essential in achieving blood pressure control in the elderly population, close monitoring is also necessary. With moderate doses of diuretics, potential of hypokalemia and insulin resistance require frequent monitoring of potassium and glucose status. The use of ACE inhibitors or ARBs, however, raises the risk of hyperkalemia and renal failure. β-blockers, although indicated for earlier stages of CHF and high coronary risk associated with DM and HTN, are not generally desired due to multiple undesired effects, such as reduced insulin sensitivity, erectile dysfunction, depression, and lack of energy, all of which are more likely in an elderly patient. Therefore, it is recommended for T.M. that adequate doses of furosemide, benazepril, or candesartan with close monitoring be the main therapeutic approaches for her hypertension. Extended- or controlled-release formulations of metoprolol and carvedilol may be considered if deemed beneficial for CHF and if tolerated. Verapamil should be reserved as second-line treatment in this patient due to a lack of benefit in CHF.[95]

Diabetes in the Elderly

16. T.M. reports that she frequently feels light headed and shaky after she takes the glyburide. She admits to not taking glyburide regularly because it also causes fast heartbeats. What is an optimal therapeutic plan for the management of T.M.'s diabetes?

Comprehensive diabetes education needs to be initiated, stressing the importance of weight loss, self-monitoring of blood glucose, alcohol abstinence, and medication adherence. A 5% to 10% weight loss will improve her glucose control and cardiovascular status.[91] T.M.'s alcohol consumption and self-reported erratic meal schedule may be contributing to the hypoglycemia (in addition to the glyburide), as well as to the worsening of her HTN and CHF. The daily allowance of alcohol recommended is 1.5 oz of distilled alcohol for men and women, respectively. In T.M.'s case, this would be one small glass of wine (3–4 oz).[92] Glyburide is also a long-acting sulfonylurea and is associated with severe hypoglycemia more commonly than other sulfonylureas due to its active metabolites. In general, the elderly are more susceptible, even at low doses, to hypoglycemia. The incidence of hypoglycemia in the elderly population is high, and symptoms may be unrecognized.[97] Among the second-generation sulfonylureas, glipizide or glimepiride are better choices. Alternatively, T.M. could be treated with a meglitinide, such as repaglinide, which does not require dose adjustment in elderly patients. Use of a meglitinide also allows for a more flexible meal pattern because it is taken with each meal and can be skipped if a meal is skipped. Any new diabetes medication should be initiated in low doses and gradually titrated upward to avoid hypoglycemic episodes and to achieve glycemic goals in accordance with ADA guidelines.[91] Current treatment algorithm states that metformin with lifestyle modification is the initial management approach. However, metformin is contraindicated in T.M. due to SCr >1.4 mg/dL. When metformin is contraindicated, glitazones, sulfonylureas, and/or basal insulin can be used to achieve a hemoglobin A1c goal of <7%. Because the glitazones are also contraindicated in T.M. due to CHF, a combination of repaglinide plus basal insulin is reasonable to bring her diabetes under control. Recent new incretin mimetics may work to prevent progressive β-cell exhaustion and insulin deficiency, and should be considered early on during the disease state. Both exenatide (glucagon like peptide analog) and sitagliptin (dipeptidyl peptidase inhibitor) do not promote hypoglycemia: exenatide has the advantage of inducing weight loss, and the dosage of sitagliptin may have to be adjusted when CrCl <50 mL/minute.[98,99] In general, the priority of diabetes management in the elderly population should be on reduction of cardiovascular risks with strict control of blood pressure and lipids in addition to avoidance of hypoglycemia events. Therefore, an A1c goal of <8% may be acceptable in some elderly patients who are prone to have hypoglycemia.[100] Comprehensive screening of diabetic complications should be done routinely to decrease morbidity and mortablity.[91]

Depression and the Older Patient

Significant depression is the most common mental illness among older adults, occurring in about 15%; it is a source of significant morbidity and mortality in this population.[101] Unfortunately, depression remains underrecognized and undertreated, even though it is a major risk factor for suicide in the elderly, who have a suicide rate that is more than five times the national average.[102,103] Older patients may be at increased risk of depression due to the high prevalence of comorbid medical conditions (i.e., stroke, cancer, MI, rheumatoid arthritis, dementia, Parkinson disease, DM).[104] Refer to Chapter 79 for further discussion of risk factors for depression and potential drug-induced causes. Most patients are treated in the primary care setting.[103]

17. J.W. is a married, 5′8″, 110-lb, 79-year-old woman who presents for a psychiatric evaluation. Her husband says she just has not been herself lately. The changes in J.W. began on a family vacation 6 months earlier when she got lost on the cruise ship. Since that incident, she has become increasingly anxious and has developed insomnia. Although she does not feel sad or "depressed," she generally does not feel well. J.W.'s normally positive attitude toward life has become pessimistic. Her husband confirms that she has become more forgetful and no longer enjoys eating. In fact, she has lost 18 lb over the past 2 months. J.W. no longer does her volunteer work at the local children's center. She says she wants to die because she is no longer the person she used to be, but she denies having any specific suicidal thoughts. Her medical history is significant for diabetes and hypertension,

which are both well controlled on glipizide 5 mg QAM and HCTZ 25 mg QD. Her medical evaluation and physical examination are unremarkable. Laboratory results and head CT scan are within normal limits. J.W. is diagnosed as having a major depressive episode. What symptoms of depression are present in J.W.?

J.W.'s presenting symptoms are quite typical of major depression in an older patient, which is commonly quite different than that of younger depressed patients. Criteria set forth in the *Diagnostic and Statistical Manual of Mental Disorders, Fourth Edition*, for diagnosing depression were developed using younger subjects and may not be applicable to the older depressed patient.[105,106] Older patients are less likely to report suicidal thoughts, but are more likely to experience weight loss as a symptom of depression. Anxiety, irritability, somatic complains, or a change in functional ability may be more significant features in late-life depression than depressed mood. Memory problems, such as J.W.'s forgetfulness, may be due to a lack of concentration or effort stemming from her depression. This is distinct from dementia, which manifests itself prominently with impairment in short- and long-term memory (see Chapter 100). Therefore, depressed mood cannot be relied on for determining whether an older patient has a depressive disorder.[102] Table 99-10 lists atypical depressive symptoms that may be found in older adults. The presence of any one of these symptoms should be considered a red flag and should prompt further evaluation for major depression.

18. J.W.'s physician decides to prescribe antidepressive medication. Which antidepressants are preferred for use in older adults?

Selection of an antidepressant drug for elderly patients must take into consideration age-related changes in pharmacokinetic, pharmacodynamic, and physiological parameters that make this population more vulnerable to adverse effects. Although the available antidepressants are about equally effective, selective serotonin reuptake inhibitors (SSRIs) are better tolerated than older agents, such as the tricyclic antidepressants. Therefore, low-dose SSRIs should be considered first-line therapy for most older patients. Of course, this does not preclude the use of sound clinical judgment that incorporates the patient's history of response, comorbidities, and the drug's side effect profile. J.W. should start taking a low-dose SSRI with gradual dose titration to achieve control of her depressive symptoms. Table 99-11 lists recommended starting doses for antidepressants in older patients. Full antidepressant response may take twice as long in older patients compared with younger patients; it may take 8 to 12 weeks before assessment of J.W.'s full response can be made.[107]

Table 99-10 Atypical Depressive Symptoms in the Older Adult

Agitation/anxiety/worrying
Reduced initiative and problem-solving capacities
Alcohol or substance abuse
Paranoia
Obsessions and compulsions
Irritability
Somatic complaints
Excessive guilt
Marital discord
Social withdrawal
Cognitive impairment
Deterioration in self-care

Adapted from reference 102.

Table 99-11 Antidepressant Dosing in Older Adults

	Initial Dosage	*Maximum Dosage*
Citalopram HBr	10 mg QD	40 mg QD
Escitalopram Oxalate	5 mg QD	20 mg QD
Fluoxetine HCL	5 mg QD	40 mg QD
Fluvoxamine	25 mg QHS	200 mg QHS
Paroxetine HCL	10 mg QD	40 mg QD
Sertraline HCL	25 mg QD	150 mg QD
Mirtazapine	7.5 mg QD	45 mg QD
Bupropion	37.5 mg BID	75 mg BID
Duloxetine	20 mg QD	40 mg QD
Venlafaxine	25 mg BID	N/A

Asthma and Chronic Obstructive Pulmonary Disease in the Elderly

Epidemiologic studies estimate the prevalence of asthma in the elderly to be between 6.5% and 17% and even higher for COPD.[108,109] Although many patients have a history of childhood asthma that persists into adulthood, a significant proportion (up to 48%) are diagnosed with asthma after age 65.[110] Rates of hospitalization for asthma are highest in the older population, and asthma-related mortality for adults age 65 to 74 years is higher compared with younger adults, possibly due to underdiagnosis and undertreatment of the disease.[111] Symptoms of asthma, including wheezing, cough, chest tightness, and dyspnea are similar in both older and younger patients (see Chapter 23). However, because the elderly are more likely to have coexisting medical conditions (e.g., HF, angina, COPD, gastroesophageal reflux disease [GERD]) with symptoms that mimic asthma, accurate diagnosis and assessment of severity is often more difficult.[113]

COPD is a lung disease caused by chronic bronchitis and/or emphysema seen largely in those older than 65 years. This chronic condition is a major cause of morbidity and mortality in the older population,[112,113] but it is often undiagnosed because patients tend to accept worsening pulmonary function as part of the "normal" aging process or may be less aware of the symptoms of airflow obstruction.[114,115] Drug therapy for COPD in the elderly does not differ significantly from standard management regimens (see Chapter 24). However, older patients with pulmonary disease and coexisting medical problems may be more sensitive to the adverse effects of pharmacologic agents.

19. J.C., a 67-year-old woman, 5′6″, 145 lb, presents to the ED with complaints of SOB for the past 2 days. She was in her usual state of health until 4 days ago when she developed flulike symptoms consisting of fever, cough, and mild wheezing. J.C. has a history of asthma, diabetes, hypertension, headache, and GERD. Her current medications include glipizide 5 mg QD, lisinopril 10 mg QD, metoprolol 50 mg BID, lansoprazole 30 mg QD, ibuprofen 200 mg Q 6 h PRN for headache, albuterol metered-dose inhaler (MDI) 2 puffs QID PRN for SOB, and fluticasone (44 g) MDI 2 puffs BID. Her drug regimen has been unchanged for the past

2 years, and she reports taking all medications as prescribed. The only recent change has been the need for albuterol every 3 to 4 hours for coughing and wheezing over the past few days. What factors (including medications) may have contributed to her acute asthma exacerbation?

Management of acute asthma exacerbations in previously stable elderly asthmatics should begin with a review of the medication history for asthma-inducing agents. Aspirin and other NSAIDs are known to induce acute bronchoconstriction in approximately 3% to 5% of adult asthmatics.[116] J.C. should be queried about her previous (especially recent) use of ibuprofen in relation to her asthma symptoms. If she reports worsening of her asthma following ingestion of ibuprofen, further use of aspirin and NSAIDs should be avoided. Alternative agents for pain control include acetaminophen or selective cyclo-oxygenase (COX)-2 inhibitors (e.g., celecoxib). Nonselective β-blockers, including topical ophthalmic formulations, can precipitate acute bronchoconstriction and should be avoided in patients with reactive airway disease. Although cardioselective β-blockers are generally considered safe for use in patients with asthma, it is important to recognize that cardioselectivity may be lost with higher dosages. Because J.C. has been taking low-dose metoprolol (a cardioselective agent) for years without problem, this medication is unlikely to be contributing to her current asthma exacerbation. One of the most important triggers for asthma exacerbations is respiratory infection (particularly viral). J.C. reports the recent onset of symptoms consistent with influenza, and this is likely precipitating her current pulmonary symptoms. As a future prophylactic measure, J.C. should be counseled to receive the influenza vaccine annually. In addition, because she is older than 65 years, she should receive a one-time pneumococcal vaccine to reduce the risk of developing pneumococcal pneumonia.

20. Are the medication regimens used to treat asthma in elderly patients different from those used in children and younger adults? Should J.C.'s asthma regimen be changed?

Medications used in the management of persistent form of asthma in the elderly are similar to those used in younger patients and consist of bronchodilators in combination with anti-inflammatory agents (see Chapter 23). The primary difference relates to drug selection and monitoring, which may be more complicated in the elderly because of the greater likelihood of coexisting medical conditions and increased potential for drug–disease and drug–drug interactions.

Inhaled β_2-agonists are an important class of drugs used to treat asthma in all age groups. The low incidence of drug interactions and reduced side effect profile make inhaled β_2-agonists ideal for use in the older asthmatics. However, both inhaled and oral β_2-agonists can cause dose-dependent systemic side effects, such as tremor, tachycardia, hypokalemia, and arrhythmias, which are of particular concern in patients with cardiac conditions.[117] Inhaled corticosteroids are the preferred treatment for all forms of persistent asthma and, in general, are well tolerated by older patients. However, elderly patients receiving high dose therapy are at an increased risk for osteoporosis, cataracts, skin thinning, and bruising.[118] In addition to the well-known complications associated with systemic corticosteroid use (see Chapter 44), these agents can acutely cause confusion, agitation, and hyperglycemia. Theophylline should be used with caution in the elderly because of the potential for CNS stimulation, nausea, vomiting, and, in higher doses, arrhythmias and seizures.

J.C. is currently maintained on low doses of an inhaled corticosteroid (fluticasone) in combination with a short-acting β_2-agonist (albuterol), and this is an appropriate regimen for a patient with mild-persistent asthma. J.C.'s asthma control should be re-evaluated within the next 3 months. If her asthma symptoms are not well controlled, she may benefit from an increase in her fluticasone dose or the addition of a long-acting inhaled β_2-agonist (salmeterol or formoterol). Because J.C. is postmenopausal, she is at risk for osteoporosis; calcium and vitamin D supplementation should be initiated.

21. J.C. was admitted to the hospital and given intravenous methylprednisolone for 4 days. She is discharged home with glipizide 5 mg QD, lisinopril 20 mg QD, fluticasone HFA (44 g) 2 puffs BID, albuterol 2 to 4 puffs Q 4 hours PRN, and prednisone 40 mg QD 7 days. What are some of the important counseling points for J.C. regarding her discharge medications?

Appropriate use of MDIs is difficult for most patients, but may be particularly problematic in the elderly population because of decreased hand strength or arthritis, difficulty timing actuation to inhalation, or impaired mental function. The use of spacer/holding chamber devices can alleviate this problem by minimizing the coordination necessary for proper use of an MDI, resulting in improved pulmonary drug delivery. In addition, spacers may reduce the incidence of systemic and local (cough, hoarseness, thrush) side effects associated with inhaled corticosteroids. J.C. should be discharged with a spacer device to use with her albuterol and fluticasone MDIs. Even though J.C. previously used an MDI, she should be asked to demonstrate her MDI technique and reinstructed, if necessary, to ensure she is using the inhaler and spacer correctly. If J.C. is unable to correctly use her MDIs with a spacer, use of nebulized solutions, breath-activated inhalers, or dry-powdered delivery devices should be considered. Although J.C. is prescribed prednisone for a short course, counseling for J.C. should also include more frequent monitoring of blood glucose while she is taking systemic corticosteroid therapy because of her diabetes.

Infectious Diseases in the Elderly

Infections are among the most common problems in the elderly and are a significant cause of morbidity and mortality. Infections are also one of the most frequent reasons for hospitalization of older ambulatory persons.[119] Antibiotic therapy for an infection in the elderly is often delayed because they present with atypical signs and symptoms. The older population is also more likely to have polymicrobial infections than younger people, and treatment duration is usually longer because of other comorbidities present in this population.[120]

PNEUMONIA

22. Three days after J.C. is discharged from the hospital, she presents again to the ED. This time, she is accompanied by a neighbor who noted that J.C. suddenly became forgetful and confused and continued to have difficulty breathing. Her neighbor reports that J.C. has been staying in bed the past 2 days and has not eaten much. J.C. has a low-grade fever, and chest examination reveals faint breath sounds with light crackling rales over

her right lung base. A chest radiograph confirms the diagnosis of pneumonia. How is J.C.'s clinical presentation consistent with community-acquired pneumonia in the elderly? How should she be treated for her respiratory infection?

Pneumonia is the leading infectious cause of mortality in the elderly, who have a 5- to 10-fold increased risk of developing pneumonia compared with younger adults.[121] Most patients admitted to hospital for the treatment of community-acquired pneumonia (CAP) are elderly.[122] Risk factors for CAP in the elderly include alcoholism and asthma, but other medical conditions common in older population, such as dementia, CHF, cerebrovascular disease, and chronic obstructive lung disease, can also increase the risk of pneumonia in this population.[123] *Streptococcus pneumoniae,* the most common cause of CAP in the elderly, is responsible for up to 50% of cases.[124–126] Viral pneumonia is the second most common cause of lower respiratory infection in older ambulatory patients. Respiratory symptoms and fever are often subtle or absent in older patients with pneumonia; instead, like J.C. they may present only with altered mental status (delirium, acute confusion, memory problems) or a decline in functional status. Delirium or acute confusion is a common presentation in elderly patients who may have new-onset lower respiratory infection. In many cases, management of pneumonia in the elderly requires hospitalization because they are at greater risk for mortality and complications. Early empiric antibacterial therapy is particularly important for older patients with pneumonia (see Chapter 60). J.C. should be hospitalized again and treated aggressively for pneumonia with broad-spectrum IV antibiotics.

PREVENTION

23. After 7 days of hospitalization, J.C. is discharged home with an oral antibiotic to finish the 14-day course of therapy. What preventive measures are available to J.C. after she is discharged?

Both influenza and pneumococcal vaccinations are beneficial in the prevention of pneumonia in the older population.[127,128] Among the elderly residents of nursing homes, influenza vaccine was found to be up to 60% effective in preventing pneumonia and hospitalization, and it was up to 70% effective in preventing hospitalization of ambulatory older adults. Among the respiratory viruses, influenza virus causes the greatest morbidity and mortality.[129] Influenza virus damages respiratory epithelial cells, decreases cell-mediated immunity, and exacerbates or worsens many chronic underlying medical conditions common to the older population. A yearly influenza vaccine is therefore recommended for all persons age 65 years and older. Amantadine, rimantadine, or oseltamivir are effective for the early treatment of influenza and for prophylaxis against influenza. Unlike oseltamivir, which is active versus both influenza A and B, amantadine and rimantadine are only active versus influenza A. If amantadine or rimantadine are selected, they should be given at a reduced dose of 100 mg orally per day in older patients; the dose of amantadine should be further reduced in patients with renal impairment to avoid CNS adverse effects. Although the previous agents are effective in the prevention of influenza, vaccination should be the primary prophylactic intervention. The pneumococcal vaccine has been shown to be up to 80% effective in preventing pneumococcal bacteremia in those older than 65 years of age,[130] although the reduction in the risk of pneumonia with pneumococcal vaccine is questionable.[131] Pneumococcal vaccine is nonetheless recommended in all adults age 65 and older to prevent bacteremia. Pneumococcal vaccination is generally given one time; if the vaccination was administered before the age of 65, however, another pneumococcal vaccine should be given. J.C. should be offered both influenza and pneumococcal vaccines after she is discharged from the hospital.

URINARY TRACT INFECTION

24. A.H. is a 72-year-old Hispanic woman who is currently wheelchair-bound because of pain in her right hip. Her granddaughter brings A.H. to the geriatric clinic because she has recently developed urinary incontinence. Her granddaughter reports that A.H. has been feeling weak the past 2 days and fell while getting out of the wheelchair. A urinalysis indicates the presence of a urinary tract infection (UTI), and A.H. is prescribed a 7-day course of ciprofloxacin 500 mg PO BID. Is this therapy appropriate?

UTI is the most common bacterial infection in the elderly.[132] The frequency of bacteriuria in ambulatory older adults is 10% to 30% in women and 5% to 10% in men. These figures are even higher in elderly people residing in LTCFs. Impaired voiding with residual urine in older women and obstructive uropathy from prostatic disease in older men predispose them to bacteriuria. The severity of UTI in the older population ranges from mild cystitis to life-threatening urosepsis; both are more difficult to treat because of resistant organisms and age-related decreases in host defenses. The majority of UTIs in the older population do not present typically, but there are often nonspecific manifestations such as decline in functional status, cognitive impairment, weakness, falls, and urinary incontinence.[133] A.H.'s presentation (weakness, urinary incontinence, and a recent fall) is consistent with this pattern. As with most UTIs, those in the elderly are caused primarily by *Escherichia coli.* However, other species of bacteria such as *Klebsiella* sp., *Proteus* sp., and *Enterococcus* sp. are also frequently involved (see Chapter 64).[134]

Oral antibiotics are appropriate for most elderly patients with symptomatic UTI.[135] One study suggests that fluoroquinolones are significantly better tolerated than trimethoprim-sulfamethoxazole for the treatment of UTI in elderly women.[136] There was better clinical resolution at the end of the therapy, and the incidence of drug-related adverse events was significantly lower in women treated with a fluoroquinolone. This study suggests that a fluoroquinolone may be the preferred agent for a broad range of UTIs in the elderly and should be considered as initial therapy in the majority of the older population. Ciprofloxacin is a reasonable choice for A.H. because *E. coli* is the most likely causative agent and fluoroquinolones are well tolerated in the elderly.

The most important effect of age on antibiotic therapy for UTI is impaired renal function. Many older patients have limited renal function reserve due to prostatic disease or chronic UTIs.[137] Nitrofurantoin should not be used in those patients with significantly impaired renal function due to increased risk of peripheral neuropathy and acute pneumonitis, which may occur more frequently in geriatric patients. For those patients requiring IV therapy for UTI, aminoglycosides pose a distinct disadvantage in older patients due to their drug-related nephrotoxicity and the need for serum drug–level monitoring.[137]

Osteoarthritis Pain

Arthritis is the most common cause of disability in people older than 75 years of age, with prevalence rates up to 30%.[138] It is also the most common cause of immobility in the older population, resulting in confinement in bed or to the house. Osteoarthritis, also called degenerative joint disease, is the most common type of joint disease in the older population. Its prevalence increases with age. Nonpharmacologic management of osteoarthritis, such as physical therapy and occupational therapy, have been shown to decrease pain and improve function in patients with osteoarthritis, both alone or in combination with appropriate analgesics.[139]

25. C.W., a 71-year-old retired school teacher, has been suffering from osteoarthritis of his hands for 5 years. He is an active older adult who enjoys volunteer work at the local hospital. He presents to the geriatric clinic with increased arthritis pain, which is uncontrolled by his current pain medication. He also complains of increased heartburn and gastric reflux symptoms. He also takes several other medications for his diabetes, hypertension, hypercholesterolemia, and GERD. C.W.'s current medications include glipizide 10 mg QD, verapamil sustained-released 240 mg QD, atorvastatin 10 mg QD, famotidine 20 mg BID, docusate sodium 100 mg BID, and ibuprofen 200 mg QID PRN. What modifications can be made to his drug regimen to better control his arthritis pain and minimize side effects from his pain medication?

Acetaminophen is the drug of choice for mild to moderate arthritis pain (see Chapter 43). For elderly patients with reduced hepatic function or for those who drink more than two alcoholic beverages a day, the recommended maximum daily dose is 2.5 g/day.[139] Acetaminophen is preferred over NSAIDs in the elderly because of its low renal and GI toxicity. C.W.'s past medication history should be reviewed. If he has not tried acetaminophen in the past for his arthritis pain, acetaminophen 1 g TID should be initiated. Older patients suffering from osteoarthritis pain often find relief from NSAIDs, which should be used with caution because of their potential GI side effects and renal toxicity. In a group of UK population age 65 or older, for example, the risk of GI complications was found to be 4.03 per 1,000 patient-years, compared to 1.36 for all individuals 25 or older.[140] Up to 2% of older persons maintained on NSAID therapy are hospitalized due to serious GI complications, and up to 30% of all peptic ulcer–related hospital admissions and mortality in those older than 65 years are associated with chronic NSAID use. NSAID-associated renal toxicity is not as common as GI toxicity, but advanced age is one of the major risk factors.[140] Renal toxicities of NSAIDs in the elderly include sodium and water retention and increased risk for hypertension.[141] Thus, ibuprofen may be contributing to C.W.'s increased GERD symptoms and to his hypertension. Nonacetylated salicylates, such as salsalate, can be used if acetaminophen does not provide adequate pain relief. Compared to NSAIDs, nonacetylated salicylates have fewer renal and GI side effects. Currently available selective COX-2 inhibitor celecoxib is preferred in older patients because it is less likely to cause GI side effects than nonselective agents; however, the risk of adverse renal events is equivalent.[141] A COX-2 inhibitor or an addition of more potent gastroprotective agent such as a proton pump inhibitor to ibuprofen are options for C.W., who may experience reduced GI symptoms with equally effective pain relief.

26. C.W. reveals that he has tried acetaminophen without much relief of his pain. He is prescribed celecoxib and tries it for several months, but his pain continues and he is still experiencing GI distress. What other pain medication options does C.W. have?

For moderate to severe chronic pain due to osteoarthritis, the topical analgesic, capsaicin, has been shown to provide temporary pain relief. However, capsaicin requires multiple daily applications for effective management of pain, and optimal efficacy takes 4 to 6 weeks of continued use. Glucosamine and chondroitin have also been shown to decrease osteoarthritis pain and delay progression of the disease.[142] Glucosamine 1,500 mg combined with 1,200 mg chondroitin daily is recommended and is well tolerated by most elderly patients. However, glucosamine might increase the insulin resistance in diabetic patients, and C.W. should be counseled to monitor his blood glucose more closely when initiating this agent.

Another option for C.W. is a long-acting opioid medication combined with acetaminophen, which can provide relief from pain with minimal side effects (see Chapter 9). Codeine and tramadol are "weak" opioids that have ceiling effects and generally do not provide adequate analgesia. The use of propoxyphene should be avoided in the elderly because of its limited efficacy and the risk for neural and cardiac toxicity.[143] Meperidine should also be avoided in older adults because of its high potential for CNS side effects, especially in those with reduced renal function. C.W. is a candidate for opioid therapy. He should be started on the lowest dose of a short-acting formulation on a scheduled regimen and counseled on the side effects. Constipation may be a particular problem because he is also taking verapamil, which can also cause significant constipation. The elderly are also at increased risk for constipation due to age-related reduced bowel motility. To prevent opioid-associated constipation in C.W., prophylactic laxatives and stool softeners should be started at the initiation of opioid therapy. Bulk laxatives are ineffective and should be avoided. He should be counseled to drink adequate fluids as well.[143]

Rehabilitative Geriatric Medicine

The geriatric population forms a major part of rehabilitative medicine. Relative to persons younger than 65 years of age, people 65 and older have more than twice as much disability, four times the activity limitation, and about twice as many hospital stays lasting about 50% longer.[144] The goal of all rehabilitation programs is to develop a person to the fullest physical, psychological, social, vocational, avocational, and educational potential consistent with his or her physiological, anatomical, and environmental limitations. Realistic goals based on functional activities that are essential to the independence and well-being of the individual should be established. The patient, family, and interdisciplinary rehabilitation team should work together to establish these goals. In the older person, rehabilitation often means working to obtain optimal function, despite residual disability caused by an irreversible medical condition. Rehabilitation can take place in the home, hospital, or nursing home setting.

Functional Assessment

Meticulous clinical evaluation of the patient's medical and functional status is the first step in a rehabilitation program.[145] The functional status evaluation should include an assessment of age, gender, and environment-appropriate activities of daily living (ADLs). According to the National Center for Health Statistics, more than 25% of noninstitutionalized persons at least 65 years of age are unable to perform one or more ADLs due to chronic health condition.[146] ADLs include dressing, eating, bathing, grooming, using the toilet, and moving around within the home. Instrumental activities of daily living (IADLs) are other activities that determine an individual's functional independence. IADLs include food preparation, laundry, housekeeping, shopping, the ability to use the telephone, use of transportation, medication use, financial management, and child care, if appropriate. Leisure and recreational activities important to a person's physical and psychological well-being can also be considered IADLs. A disability or dysfunction is defined as any deviation from the normal or characteristic ability of a person to perform tasks of living. Impairments are defined as abnormalities in organs or body systems that can lead to dysfunction. When the inability to perform tasks results in social disadvantage, the condition is viewed as a handicap.[147]

Pharmacists' Role in Geriatric Rehabilitation

27. B.L., a 5′10″, 180-lb, 78 year-old man, experienced an embolic stroke 7 days before transfer to the rehabilitation unit. His medical history is significant for atrial fibrillation and GERD. Medications at the time of transfer are digoxin 0.25 mg QD, warfarin 5 mg QD except 2.5 mg on Monday/Thursday, ranitidine 150 mg BID, metoclopramide 10 mg QID, metoprolol 50 mg BID, and milk of magnesia PRN for constipation. His laboratory values are as follows: Na, 135 mEq/L; K, 4.2 mEq/L; SCr, 1.5 mg/dL; BUN, 23 mg/dL; and digoxin level, 1.2 ng/mL. His vital signs are BP, 110/70 mm Hg; HR, 60 beats/minute; and temperature, 98.4°F. What is the pharmacist's role in the initial evaluation of B.L.?

[SI units: Na 135 mmol/L; K 4.2 mmol/L; SrCr 132.6 mmol/L; BUN 8.2 mmol/L]

An interdisciplinary "geriatric assessment" team is essential to accomplishing a comprehensive functional evaluation of the rehabilitation patient. These teams, including a pharmacist member as the pharmacotherapy specialist, significantly reduce length of stay, readmissions, drug costs, and patient mortality.[148,149] A physician trained and certified in rehabilitation medicine (i.e., a physiatrist) usually leads the team. Other disciplines represented on the team are physical therapy, occupational therapy, speech therapy, recreational therapy, behavioral medicine (psychologist, social worker), and nursing. The pharmacist's role in the initial assessment is to obtain a complete medication history so that an accurate assessment of drug therapy can be made. Adverse reactions to medications can be detrimental to the functional capacity of the geriatric patient by worsening cognition, psychological state, vascular reflexes, balance, bowel and bladder control, muscle tone, and coordination, any of which may already be impaired by the present illness or injury. It is the responsibility of the team pharmacist to alert the rest of the team to drug-induced problems, facilitate medication adherence, provide medication education, advocate to discontinue unnecessary medications, screen for drug interactions, and recommend appropriate changes in therapy based on the physiological effects of aging. The team pharmacist should also make some assessment of the individual's ability to self-medicate. Table 99-12 lists conditions and skills that have been identified as possible indicators of an older person's ability to self-medicate.

Table 99-12 Indicators of the Inability to Self-Medicate

Cognitive impairments
More than five prescription medications
Inability to read prescription and auxiliary labels
Difficulty opening nonchildproof containers
Problems removing small tablets from containers
Inability to discriminate between medication colors and shapes

Adapted from references 158 and 159.

Drug Effects on Functional Ability

28. During the initial team meeting to discuss B.L., the physical therapist mentions that the patient walks with a stooped posture and has a shuffling gait and poor balance. The speech therapist reports that B.L. has difficulty in swallowing, noting that the problem is out of proportion for the location of his stroke. A flat affect, crying episodes, fatigue, and drowsiness are reported by the occupational therapist. The psychologist notes confusion and possible dementia on neuropsychological testing. Can any of B.L.'s problems be attributed to his current medication regimen?

Functional impairments in older adults can be medication induced.[150] Table 99-13 lists several examples of drugs that can interfere with the functional, physical, social, and psychological assessment of the older patient. Dopamine-depleting drugs may produce extrapyramidal side effects and interfere with physical and occupational therapy goals. Neuroleptics, tricyclic antidepressants, and excessive doses of antihypertensives can increase the risk of falls by causing orthostatic hypotension. Problems with balance and/or tinnitus may be precipitated by drugs that affect the vestibular system and cause damage to the eighth cranial nerve (e.g., aminoglycosides, loop diuretics, high serum concentrations of aspirin). Long-term corticosteroid use may lead to proximal muscle wasting and slow the recovery of strength, even when patients are undergoing aggressive rehabilitative therapy.

CNS medications may lead to oversedation and decrease the capability to learn, ambulate, eat, or use the toilet, as well as increase the risk of falls. Drugs such as benzodiazepines, antihypertensives, neuroleptics, H_2 blockers, and analgesics have been reported to cause reversible cognitive impairment. Digoxin toxicity in the elderly may initially manifest as confusion, delirium, nightmares, or hallucinations. Medications that cause a relative dominance of dopamine over acetylcholine in the brain may produce psychosis, hallucinations, or delirium.

Depression is an important adverse reaction to look for in patients undergoing rehabilitation because it may mimic dementia on neuropsychological testing. Depression may be worsened or induced by some antihypertensives (e.g., central agonists, highly lipophilic β-blockers). Metoclopramide is an important yet often overlooked potential contributor to depression.

Table 99-13 Drug Effects on Other Assessments

Assessments	*Drug Effects*	*Drug Examples*
Functional	Movement disorders (extrapyramidal, tardive dyskinesia)	Neuroleptics, metoclopramide, amoxapine, methyldopa
	Balance (neuritis, neuropathies, tinnitus, dizziness, hypotension)	Metronidazole, phenytoin, aspirin, aminoglycosides, furosemide, ethacrynic acid, β-blockers, calcium channel blockers, neuroleptics, antidepressants, diuretics, vasodilators, benzodiazepines, levodopa, metoclopramide
Physical	Supporting structures (arthralgias, myopathies, osteoporosis, osteomalacia)	Corticosteroids, lithium, phenytoin, heparin
	Incontinence (urinary retention, secondary oversedation)	Anticholinergic agents, TCAs, neuroleptics, antihistamines, smooth muscle relaxants, nifedipine, phenylpropanolamine, prazosin; benzodiazepines, sedatives, hypnotics
	Sexual dysfunction	Hypotensive agents, CNS depressants, SSRI antidepressants
Social	Malnutrition	Drugs affecting appetite
	Poor dental health	Anticholinergic agents, glucose-containing oral liquid/chewable dosage forms
Psychological	Cognitive impairment (metabolic alterations; memory loss, dementia)	β-Blockers, corticosteroids, diuretics, sulfonylureas, methyldopa, propranolol, hydrochlorothiazide, reserpine, neuroleptics, opiates, cimetidine, amantadine, benzodiazepines, anticonvulsants
	Behavioral toxicity (insomnia, nightmares, sedation, agitation, delirium, psychosis, hallucinations)	Anticholinergics, cimetidine, ranitidine, famotidine, digoxin, bromocriptine, amantadine, baclofen, levodopa, opiates, sympathomimetics, corticosteroids
	Depression	Reserpine, methyldopa, β-blockers, metoclopramide, corticosteroids, CNS depressants

TCA, tricyclic antidepressant; CNS, central nervous system; SSRI, selective serotonin reuptake inhibitors.
Adapted from reference 150.

B.L. is receiving several medications that may be contributing to the functional impairments found during the initial assessment. Metoclopramide has dopamine-blocking activity and can produce pseudo-Parkinson symptoms like those reported by the physical therapist. Dopamine blockers can cause swallowing difficulties. Metoclopramide has also been known to produce mental depression in some patients that may or may not recur when the drug is reinstituted at lower dosages. B.L. is at even greater risk for these adverse effects from metoclopramide because it is primarily renally excreted and B.L. has reduced renal function, with an estimated ClCr of 42 mL/minute. H_2 blockers, such as ranitidine, can cause confusion and agitation in older patients with decreased renal function. Metoclopramide and ranitidine should be discontinued at this time. B.L.'s GERD should be reassessed, and if chronic therapy is needed, a proton pump inhibitor (e.g., rabeprazole, others) is an appropriate choice because there is a low likelihood that it will cause functional impairment.

B.L.'s problem of depressive symptoms reported by the occupational therapist and potential dementia reported by his psychologist are compatible with CNS effects of metoprolol, a highly lipophilic β-blocker. Metoclopramide may also be a contributor to these findings. If B.L. must continue taking a β-blocker for additional rate control, he should be switched to an agent with low-lipid solubility, such as atenolol, which has a lower likelihood of producing CNS side effects. Otherwise, the dose of metoprolol should be reduced immediately and then tapered.

B.L.'s digoxin level is currently within normal limits, and he does not have any clinical signs of digoxin toxicity. However, the pharmacist team member should monitor B.L. for signs and symptoms of digoxin toxicity and make appropriate dose adjustments as necessary. Finally, B.L. should have an INR drawn to ensure that the dose of warfarin is correct.

The contribution of medication to functional deficits must not be overlooked when assessing patients undergoing rehabilitation. Defined criteria for determining medications that are potentially inappropriate in the elderly has been published by Beers and recently updated.[151] When using these criteria, it is important to keep in mind that these are "potentially" inappropriate medications. The pharmacotherapy specialist trained in geriatric care is responsible for applying patient-specific criteria, such as history of use and response, when evaluating the appropriateness of a drug in a particular patient.

Long-Term Care Facility

The LTCF environment is governed in part by the Omnibus Budget Reconciliation Act (OBRA), as well as by numerous other laws and regulations. Table 99-14 summarizes the mandated responsibilities of the "supervising pharmacist" in a LTCF. The completion of these responsibilities must include monthly review of each resident's medication profile to determine the following:

1. Is each drug clearly indicated?
2. If indicated, is it being dosed and administered appropriately?
3. Are the laboratory results and vital signs being done appropriately, and are they available for adequate evaluation of therapy?
4. Are any real or potential problems with drug side effects or interactions present?

Table 99-14 Basic Requirements of OBRA 1990 Legislation

Prospective DUR
Retrospective DUR
Education and intervention programs
Patient counseling and provision of information to patients/caregivers
Documentation of DUR and educational activities

OBRA, Omnibus Budget Reconciliation Act; DUR, drug utilization review.
From reference 160.

5. What specific recommendations can be made to optimize this resident's drug therapy?
6. If neuroleptic agents are being prescribed, has their use been justified and is the therapy being monitored?
7. Have therapeutic goals been established for chronic drug therapies?
8. Are any unnecessary drugs present?

OBRA regulations require inclusion of a pharmacist on the pharmaceutical and infection control committees. The pharmacist is also required to participate in drug use evaluations. All medication errors and adverse drug reactions must be reported to the patient's physician and documented by the pharmacist or the nurse. The American Society of Consultant Pharmacists publishes detailed information concerning standards of practice in the LTCF environment.[152]

29. As a new consulting pharmacist to a 60-bed, skilled nursing facility, several multiple drug use problems become apparent during initial chart reviews. A typical case is D.M., an 82-year-old man who has resided there for the past month. D.M.'s past medical history is significant for hypertension, depression, constipation, long-standing mild cognitive impairment that is now worsening, and dizziness. In the nurses' notes, it is documented that D.M. had a fall when getting out of bed last week.

At admission, D.M.'s weight was 165 lb; BP, 100/60 mm Hg; pulse, 85 beats/minute; and temperature, 98.6°F. Subsequent vital signs are not recorded systematically into his medical record. Sporadic documentation in the nurses' notes indicate little change from admission values. No laboratory information is available at this time. D.M. has no known allergies.

Current medications include felodipine 10 mg QD, diltiazem CD 240 mg QD, HCTZ 25 mg QD, nortriptyline 150 mg QHS, thioridazine 25 mg TID, haloperidol 0.5 mg BID, benztropine 1 mg BID, docusate sodium 100 mg BID, milk of magnesia 30 mL QD, flurazepam 15 mg QHS, and acetaminophen one to two 325-mg tablets Q 4 to 6 h PRN pain. D.M. follows a 2-g sodium diet.

D.M. is ambulatory and takes his meals in the facility's cafeteria. He is not in any acute distress, but the nurses' notes indicate that D.M. is often confused and complains of dizziness when ambulating. His weight has decreased 4 lb since being admitted. What should be expected of this LTCF with respect to medication monitoring, and what OBRA deficiencies can be found in the review of D.M.'s case?

Under OBRA, the establishment of goals of antihypertensive therapy and monitoring for these goals are required. D.M.'s blood pressure should be measured and documented in his medical record with a signature and date on a regular basis. D.M.'s dizziness, a symptom of orthostatic hypotension, may be due to overtreatment of his hypertension as evidenced by his low admission blood pressure. Orthostatic hypotension occurs in more than half of frail, elderly LTCF residents and is most common when patients first arise, indicating that this may have been the cause of D.M.'s recent fall. D.M. is currently being inappropriately treated with two calcium channel blockers. Discontinuation of one of them should reduce this patient's dizziness and help prevent future falls. Preferably, felodipine should be discontinued because dihydropyridine calcium channel blockers are known to cause orthostasis. The use of antipsychotic and anti-Parkinson agents have also been associated with orthostatic hypotension. Because D.M. is being treated with a diuretic, he should have a chemistry panel drawn to check for electrolyte abnormalities.

In the admission workup, D.M. was described as having a long-standing history of mild cognitive impairment, but subsequent nursing notes suggest that his symptoms of disorientation and confusion worsened quickly after admission. Chronic dementia is not normally characterized by rapid deterioration of mental acuity (see Chapter 100). This should raise the suspicion that a reversible factor could be responsible for D.M.'s mental decline. Overprescribing of psychotropic drugs in institutionalized elderly patients is well documented.[153,154] The cognitive impairment of chronic degenerative dementia can be greatly exaggerated by D.M.'s treatment with flurazepam, nortriptyline, thioridazine, haloperidol, and benztropine.

Neuroleptics are some of the most commonly prescribed drugs in nursing home residents. It is only appropriate to use these drugs in elderly patients with documented psychotic behavioral disturbances or in those with impulsivity and agitation associated with functional or organic disorders, such as degenerative dementia. Unfortunately, neuroleptics are often unnecessarily prescribed for anxiety, insomnia, confusion, "senility," and failure to conform to the institution's standards for behavior. OBRA regulations require that these drugs be used for a specified condition, at the lowest possible dosage, and for the shortest possible time. The regulations also mandate tapering of the dose and careful documentation of all clinical assessments that justify the ongoing need for neuroleptics. Even when a neuroleptic agent is indicated, the use of two or more, as in D.M., is irrational. Unless extrapyramidal symptoms have been clearly documented, D.M.'s treatment with benztropine is not indicated.

Antidepressant treatment may not be indicated for D.M., but if it is, nortriptyline is a poor choice because it has significant anticholinergic and sedating side effects (see prior discussion of depression in this chapter). D.M. is being treated with several sedating medications (flurazepam, haloperidol, and thioridazine). These agents may induce pseudodepression, which should resolve by reducing the number of sedating drugs. Flurazepam, a long-acting benzodiazepine, may increase the risk of falls and bone fractures in the geriatric population. Continuous nightly use of long-acting benzodiazepines increases the relative risk of hip fractures by 50% compared with shorter-acting benzodiazepines.[155] Elderly patients naturally sleep for shorter periods with a shallower sleep that is subject to frequent awakenings. Thus, the need for scheduled bedtime sleep agents must always be evaluated critically (see Chapter 77).

In light of the atypical deterioration of D.M.'s cognitive function, the doses of all psychotropic medications should be gradually tapered down and then discontinued. A baseline assessment of D.M.'s cognitive function and psychiatric status should be performed by a geriatrician, psychiatrist, or clinical psychologist to establish the presence or absence of psychotic behavioral disturbances or depression. If any of these disorders are present, then each should be managed with a single drug, titrated to the appropriate therapeutic dose. In accordance with established immunization practices, D.M., other LTCF residents, and staff members should receive an annual influenza vaccine. A pneumococcal vaccination should also be administered to D.M. if he has not previously received one.

REFERENCES

1. Federal Interagency Forum on Aging-Related Statistics. Older Americans update 2006: key indicators of well-being. *Federal Interagency Forum on Aging-Related Statistics.* Washington, DC: U.S. Government Printing Office; July 2006.
2. Congressional Budget Office. Financing Long-Term Care for the Elderly. 2004.
3. U.S. Bureau of the Census. Current population reports, special studies. P23-209. 65+ in the United States: 2005. Washington, DC: U.S. Government Printing Office; 2005.
4. Jones A. The National Nursing Home Survey: 1999 summary. National Center for Health Statistics. *Vital Health Stat* 2002;13.
5. Singer BH. Manton KG. The effects of health changes on projections of health service needs for the elderly population of the United States. *Proc Natl Acad Sci U S A* 1998;95:15618.
6. Johnson JA, Bootman JL. Drug-related morbidity and mortality; a cost of illness model. *Arch Intern Med* 1995;155:1949.
7. Resnick NM, Marcantonio DR. How should clinical care of the aged differ? *Lancet* 1997;350:1157.
8. Swift CG. Clinical pharmacology in the older patients. *Scott Med J* 1979;24:221.
9. Hurwitz A et al. Gastric acidity in older adults. *JAMA* 1997;278:659.
10. Cusack BJ. Pharmacokinetics in older persons. *Am J Geriatr Pharmacother* 2004;2:274
11. Roskos KV et al. The effect of aging on percutaneous absorption in man. *J Pharmacokin Biopharm* 1989;17:617.
12. Rudy DW et al. Loop diuretics for chronic renal insufficiency. *Ann Intern Med* 1991;115:360.
13. Bender AD. The effect of increasing age on the distribution of peripheral blood flow in man. *J Am Geriatr Soc* 1965;13:192.
14. Riesenberg DE. Studies reshape some views of the aging heart. *JAMA* 1986;255:871.
15. Shock NW et al. Age differences in the water content of the body as related to basal oxygen consumption in males. *J Gerontol* 1963;18:1.
16. Novak IP. Aging, total body potassium, fat-free mass, and cell mass in males and females between ages 18 and 85 years. *J Gerontol* 1972;27:438.
17. Greenblatt DJ et al. Toxicity of high-dose flurazepam in the elderly. *Clin Pharmacol Ther* 1977; 21:355.
18. Greenblatt DJ. Reduced serum albumin concentration in the older patients: a report from the Boston Collaborative Drug Surveillance Program. *J Am Geriatr Soc* 1979;27:20.
19. Israili ZH, Dayton PG. Human alpha-1 glycoprotein and its interactions with drugs. *Drug Metab Rev* 2001;33:161.
20. Jusko WJ, Weintraub M. Myocardial distribution of digoxin and renal function. *Clin Pharmacol Ther* 1974;16:449.
21. Mayersohn MB. Special pharmacokinetic considerations in the elderly. In: Evans WE, et al., eds. *Applied Pharmacokinetics: Principles of Therapeutic Drug Monitoring.* 3rd ed. Vancouver, WA: Applied Therapeutics; 1992.
22. Farah F et al. Hepatic drug acetylation and oxidation: effects of aging in man. *Br Med J* 1977;2: 255.
23. O'Malley K, et al. Effect of age and sex on human drug metabolism. *Br Med J* 1971;3:607.
24. Thompson EN et al. Effect of age on liver function with particular reference to bromsulphalein excretion. *Gut* 1965;6:266.
25. Triggs EJ et al. Pharmacokinetics in the older patients. *Eur J Clin Pharmacol* 1975;8:55.
26. Geokas MC et al. The aging gastrointestinal tract. *Am J Surg* 1969;117:881.
27. Hewick DS et al. The effect of age on sensitivity to warfarin sodium. *Br J Pharmacol* 1975;2:189P.
28. Shader RI et al. Absorption and disposition of chlordiazepoxide in young and older patients male volunteers. *J Clin Pharmacol* 1977;17:709.
29. Klotz U et al. Effects of age and liver disease on disposition and elimination of diazepam in adult man. *J Clin Invest* 1975;55:347.
30. Nies AS et al. Altered hepatic blood flow and drug disposition. *Clin Pharmacokinet* 1976;1:125.
31. Rowe JW et al. The effect of age on creatinine clearance in man: a cross sectional and longitudinal study. *J Gerontol* 1976;31:155.
32. Rowe JW et al. The influence of age on renal response to water deprivation in man. *Nephron* 1976;17:270.
33. Epstein M et al. Age as a determinant of renal sodium conservation. *J Lab Clin Med* 1976;87: 411.
34. Baylis EM et al. Effects of renal function on plasma digoxin levels in elder ambulant patients in domiciliary practice. *Br Med J* 1972;1:338.
35. Leikola E et al. On oral penicillin levels in young and geriatric patients. *J Gerontol* 1957;12:48.
36. Palmer BF, Moshe L. Effect of aging on renal function and disease. In: Brenner BM, Rector FC, eds. *Brenner and Rector's The Kidney.* 5th ed. Philadelphia: WB Saunders; 1996:2274.
37. Lindeman RD et al. Longitudinal studies on the rate of decline in renal function with age. *J Am Geriatr Soc* 1985;33:278.
38. Cockcroft DW, Gault MH. Prediction of creatinine clearance from serum creatinine. *Nephron* 1976;16:31.
39. O'Connell MB, et al. Predictive performance of equations to estimate creatinine clearance in hospitalized elderly patients. *Ann Pharmacother* 1992;26:627.
40. Smythe M et al. Estimating creatinine clearance in elderly patients with low serum creatinine concentrations. *Am J Hosp Pharm* 1994;51:198.
41. Lipsitz LA. Orthostatic hypotension in the older patients. *N Engl J Med* 1989;321:952.
42. Davis TA et al. Orthostatic hypotension: therapeutic alternatives for geriatric patients. *DICP Ann Pharmacother* 1989;23:750.
43. Blumenthal MD et al. Dizziness and falling in elderly outpatients. *Am J Psychiatry* 1980;137:203.
44. Overstall PW et al. Falls in the older patients related to postural imbalance. *Br Med J* 1977;1:261.
45. Anonymous. Drugs in the older patients. *Med Lett Drugs Ther* 1979;21:43.
46. Castleden CM et al. Increased sensitivity to nitrazepam in old age. *Br Med J* 1977;1:10.
47. Smith BH et al. Aging and the nervous system. *Geriatrics* 1975;30:109.
48. Roth M. Senile dementia and its borderlands. *Proc Annu Meet Am Psychopathol Assoc* 1980;69:205.
49. Heinsimer JA et al. The impact of aging on adrenergic receptor function: clinical and biochemical aspects. *J Am Geriatr Soc* 1985;33:184.
50. Samorajski T. Age-related changes in brain biogenic amines. In: Schneider EL, ed. *Aging: Clinical, Morphologic and Neurochemical Aspects in the Aging Central Nervous System.* New York: Raven Press; 1975;1:199.
51. Fleg JL et al. Age-related augmentation of plasma catecholamines during dynamic exercise in healthy males. *J Appl Physiol* 1985;59:1033.
52. Vestal RE et al. Reduced beta-adrenergic sensitivity in the elderly. *Clin Pharmacol Ther* 1979;26: 181.
53. Larson EB et al. Adverse drug reactions associated with global cognitive impairment in older patients persons. *Ann Intern Med* 1987;107:169.
54. Anonymous. Surgeon General's workshop on health promotion and aging: summary recommendations of the medication working group. *JAMA* 1989;262:1755.
55. Simon SR, Gurwitz JH. Drug therapy in the elderly: improving quality and access. *Clin Pharmacol Ther* 2003;73:387.
56. Zermansky AG et al. Randomized controlled trial of clinical medication review by a pharmacist of elderly patients receiving repeat prescriptions in general practice. *Br Med J* 2001;323:1.
57. Zhan C et al. Potentially inappropriate medication use in the community-dwelling elderly. *JAMA* 2001;286:2823.
58. Yoshikawa TT et al. *Practical Ambulatory Geriatrics.* St. Louis, MO: Mosby; 1998:23.
59. American Society of Consultant Pharmacists. Senior care pharmacy: the statistics. *Consult Pharm* 2000;15:310.
60. Hanlon JT et al. A randomized, controlled trial of a clinical pharmacist intervention to improve inappropriate prescribing in elderly outpatients with polypharmacy. *Am J Med* 1996;100:428.
61. Riedinger JL, Robbins LJ. Prevention of iatrogenic illness: adverse drug reactions and nosocomial infections in hospitalized older adults. *Clin Geriatr Med* 1998;14:681.
62. Gray SL et al. Adverse drug events in hospitalized elderly. *J Gerontol* 1998;53A:M59.
63. Gurwitz JH et al. Incidence and preventability of adverse drug events among older persons in the ambulatory setting. *JAMA* 2003;289:1107.
64. Bates DW et al. The costs of adverse drug events in hospitalized patients. *JAMA* 1997;277:307.
65. Beyth RJ, Shorr RI. Epidemiology of adverse drug reactions in the elderly by drug class. *Drugs Aging* 1999;14:231.
66. Roche Laboratories. *Toradol package insert.* Nutley, NJ: Roche Laboratories; September 2002.
67. Lamy PP. The elderly, communications, and compliance. *Pharm Times* 1992;58:33.
68. Bero LA et al. Characterization of geriatric drug-related hospital readmissions. *Med Care* 1991;29:989.
69. American Pharmacists Association. Medication Therapy Management in Community Pharmacy Practice, core elements of an MTM service. version 1.0. April 29, 2005.
70. Barenholtz Levy H. Self-administered medication-risk questionnaire in an elderly population. *Ann Pharmacother* 2003;37:982.
71. Terra SG et al. Therapeutic range of digoxin's efficacy in heart failure: what is the evidence? *Pharmacotherapy* 1999;19:1123.
72. Natural Medicines Comprehensive Database. Hawthorn monograph. Available at: http://www.naturaldatabase.com. Accessed February 9, 2007 (subscription required).
73. Valli G, Giardina EGV. Benefits, adverse effects, and drug interactions of herbal therapies with cardiovascular effects. *J Am Coll Cardiol* 2002;39:1083.
74. Dandelion, hawthorne, and herbal diuretics

monographs. *Review of Natural Products, Facts and Comparisons,* 1998.

75. National Center for Complementary and Alternative Medicine. Herbs at a Glance: Licorice Root. Available at: http://nccam.nih.gov/health/licoriceroot. Accessed January 9, 2008.
76. AHA/ACC Guideline Update for the Evaluation and Management of Chronic Heart Failure in the Adult. A report of the American College of Cardiology/American Heart Association Task Force on Practice Guidelines (Writing committee to update the 2001 guidelines for the evaluation and management of heart failure): Developed in collaboration with the American College of Chest Physicians and the International Society for Heart and Lung Transplantation: endorsed by the Heart Rhythm Society. *Circulation* 2005;112:e154.
77. Carter BL. Dosing of antihypertensive medications in patients with renal insufficiency. *J Clin Pharmacol* 1995;35:81.
78. Heart Outcomes Prevention Evaluation (HOPE) study investigators. Effects of ramipril on cardiovascular and microvascular outcomes in people with diabetes mellitus: results of the HOPE study and MICRO-HOPE sub-study. *Lancet* 2000;355;253.
79. The Studies of Left Ventricular Dysfunction (SOLVD) Investigators. Effect of enalapril on survival in patients with reduced ventricular ejection fraction and congestive heart failure. *N Engl J Med* 1991;325:293.
80. Williams BR, Kim J. Cardiovascular drug therapy in the elderly: theoretical and practical considerations. *Drugs Aging* 2003;20:445.
81. McMurray JJV et al. Effects of candesartan in patients with chronic heart failure and reduced left-ventricular systolic function taking angiotensin-converting-enzyme inhibitors: the CHARM-Added trail. *Lancet* 2003;362:761.
82. Funck-Bretano C, et al. Predictors of medical events in patients enrolled in the Cardiac Insufficiency Bisoprolol Study (CIBIS): a study of the interactions between beta blocker therapy and occurrence of critical events using analysis of competitive risks. *Am Heart J* 2000;139:262.
83. MERIT-HF Study Group. Effect of metoprolol CR/XL in chronic heart failure: metoprolol CR/XL randomized intervention trial in congestive heart failure (MERIT-HF). *Lancet* 1999;353:2001.
84. Krum H et al. Carvedilol Prospective Randomized Cumulative Survival (COPERNICUS) Study Group. Effects of initiating carvedilol in patients with severe chronic heart failure: results from the COPERNICUS Study. *JAMA* 2003;289:712.
85. AstraZeneca. *Toprol XL prescribing information.* Wilmington, DE: AstraZeneca; September 2006.
86. GlaxoSmithKline. *Coreg CR prescribing information.* Research Triangle Park, NC: GlaxoSmithKline; October 2006.
87. National Cholesterol Education Program (NCEP) Expert Panel on Detection, Evaluation, and Treatment of High Blood Cholesterol in Adults. Executive summary of the third report of the NCEP. *JAMA* 2001;285:2486.
88. Grundy SM et al. Cholesterol lowering in the elderly population. *Arch Intern Med* 1999;159:1670.
89. National Lipid Education Council. Treating dyslipidemia in the elderly: are we doing enough? *Lipid Manage Newslett* 1999;4:1.
90. Dalal D, Robbins JA. Management of hyperlipidemia in the elderly population: an evidence-based approach. *South Med J* 2002;95:1255.
91. American Diabetes Association. Clinical practice recommendations. *Diab Care* 2007;30:s15.
92. U.S. Department of Health and Human Services. Dietary Guidelines for Americans, 2005. Available at: http://www.health.gov/dietaryguidelines/dga2005/document/default.htm. Accessed January 9, 2008.
93. Grundy SM. The role of cholesterol management in coronary heart disease risk reduction in elderly patients. *Endocrinol Metab Clin North Am* 1998;27:655.
94. Talbert RL. Safety issues with statin therapy. *J Am Pharm Assoc* 2006;46:479.
95. Chobanian AV et al. The seventh report of the joint national committee on prevention, detection, evaluation, and treatment of high blood pressure: The JNC 7 Report. *JAMA* 2003;289:2560.
96. Hyman DJ, Pavlik VN. Characteristics of patients with uncontrolled hypertension in the United States. *N Eng J Med* 2001;345:479.
97. Shorr RI et al. Incidence and risk factors for serious hypoglycemia in older persons using insulin or sulfonylureas. *Arch Intern Med* 1997;157:1681.
98. Amylin Pharmaceuticals, Inc. Byetta package insert. San Diego, CA: Amylin Pharmaceuticals, Inc.; February 2007.
99. Merck & Co., Inc. Januvia package insert. Whitehouse Station, NJ: Merck & Co., Inc.; 2007.
100. California Healthcare Foundation/American Geriatric Society Panel on Improving Care for Elders with Diabetes. Guidelines for improving the care of the older person with diabetes mellitus. *J Am Geriatr Soc* 2003;51:s265.
101. Jeste DV et al. Consensus statement: the upcoming crisis in geriatric mental health: challenges and opportunities. *Arch Gen Psychiatry* 1999;56:848.
102. Sable JA et al. Late-life depression: how to identify its symptoms and provide effective treatment. *Geriatrics* 2002;57:18.
103. Centers for Disease Control and Prevention, Department of Health and Human Services. WISQARS (Web-based Injury Statistics Query and Reporting System). Available at: www.cdc.gov/NCIPC/wisqars/default.htm. Accessed January 9, 2008.
104. Reynolds CF, Kupfer DJ. Depression and aging: a look to the future. *Psychiatr Serv* 1999;50:1167.
105. American Psychiatric Association. *Diagnostic and Statistical Manual of Mental Disorders.* 4th ed. Washington, DC: American Psychiatric Association; 1994.
106. Blazer DG. Depression in the elderly: Myths and misconceptions. *Psychiatr Clin North Am* 1997;20:111.
107. Mulsant BH et al. Pharmacological treatment of depression in older primary care patients: the PROSPECT algorithm. *Int J Geriatr Psychiatry* 2001;16:585.
108. Renwick DS, Connolly MJ. Prevalence and treatment of chronic airflow obstruction in adults over the age of 45. *Thorax* 1996;51:164.
109. Parameswaran K et al. Asthma in the elderly: underperceived, underdiagnosed and undertreated: a community survey. *Respir Med* 1998;92:573.
110. Burr ML et al. Asthma in the elderly: an epidemiological survey. *Br Med J* 1979;1:1041.
111. Enright PL et al. Underdiagnosis and undertreatment of asthma in the elderly: Cardiovascular Health Study Research Group. *Chest* 1999;116:603.
112. Claessens MT et al. Dying with lung cancer or chronic obstructive pulmonary disease: insights from SUPPORT. *J Am Geriatr Soc* 2000;48:S146.
113. Renwick DS, Connolly MJ. Impact of obstructive airways disease on quality of life in older adults. *Thorax* 1996;51:520.
114. Petheram IS et al. Assessment and management of acute asthma in the elderly: a comparison with younger asthmatics. *Postgrad Med J* 1982;58:149.
115. Connolly MJ et al. reduced subjective awareness of bronchoconstriction provoked by methacholine in elderly asthmatic and normal subjects as measured on a simple awareness scale. *Thorax* 1992;47:410.
116. Szczeklik A, Stevenson DD. Aspirin-induced asthma: advances in pathogenesis and management. *J Allergy Clin Immunol* 2003;111:913.
117. National Asthma Education and Prevention Program. Considerations for Diagnosing and Managing Asthma in the Elderly, 1997. NIH Publication No. 97-4051.
118. National Institutes of Health. Expert Panel Report 2. Guidelines for the Diagnosis and Management of Asthma, 1997. NIH Publication No. 97-4051.
119. Ruben FL et al. Clinical infections in the noninstitutionalized geriatric age group: methods utilized and incidence of infections. The Pittsburgh Good Health Study. *Am J Epidemiol* 1995;141:145.
120. Miller RA. The aging immune system: primer and prospectus. *Science* 1996;273:70.
121. Jokinen C et al. Incidence of community-acquired pneumonia in the population of four municipalities in Eastern Finland. *Am J Epidemiol* 1993;137:977.
122. Marrie TJ. Community-acquired pneumonia in the elderly. *Clin Infect Dis* 2000;31:1066.
123. Lipsky BA et al. Risk factors for acquiring pneumococcal infections. *Arch Intern Med* 1986;146:2179.
124. Porth A et al. The epidemiology of community-acquired pneumonia among hospitalized patients. *J Infect* 1997;34:41.
125. Burman, et al. Diagnosis of pneumonia by cultures, bacterial and viral antigen detection tests, and serology with special references to antibodies against pneumococcal antigen. *J Infect Dis* 1991;163:1087.
126. Kauppienen MT et al. the etiology of community-acquired pneumonia among hospitalized patients during a *Chlamydia pneumoniae* epidemic in Finland. *J Infect Dis* 1995;172:1330.
127. Gross PA et al. The efficacy of influenza vaccine in elderly persons: a meta-analysis and review of the literature. *Ann Intern Med* 1995;123:518.
128. Ortqvist A et al. Swedish pneumococcal vaccination study group. Randomized trial of 23-valent pneumococcal capsular polysaccharide vaccine in prevention of pneumonia in middle-aged and elderly people. *Lancet* 1998;351:399.
129. Couch RB et al. Influenza: its control in persons and populations. *J Infect Dis* 1986;153:431.
130. Shapiro ED et al. The protective efficacy of polyvalent pneumococcal polysaccharide vaccine. *N Engl J Med* 1991;325:1453.
131. Jackson LA et al. Effectiveness of pneumococcal polysaccharide vaccine in older adults. *N Engl J Med* 2003;348:1747.
132. Nicolle LE. Urinary tract infections in the elderly. *J Antimicrob Chemother* 1994;33:99.
133. Raz P. Urinary tract infection in the elderly women. *Int J Antimicrob Agents* 1998;10:177.
134. Ackermann RJ, Monroe PW. Bacteremic urinary tract infection in older people. *J Am Geriatr Soc* 1996;44:927.
135. Eykyn SJ. Urinary tract infections in the elderly. *Br J Urol* 1998;82:79.
136. Gomolin IH et al. Efficacy and safety of ciprofloxacin oral suspension versus trimethoprim:sulfamethoxazole oral suspension for treatment of older women with acute urinary tract infection. *J Am Geriatr Soc* 2001;49:1606.
137. McEvoy GK et al., eds. *AHFS Drug Information.* Bethesda: American Society of Health-System Pharmacists, Inc.; 2002:838.
138. Felson DT. The course of osteoarthritis and factors that affect it. *Rheum Dis Clin North Am* 1993;19:607.
139. American Geriatrics Society Panel on Pain in Older Persons. The management of persistent pain in older persons. *J Am Geriatr Soc* 2002;50:S205.
140. Chou R et al. Comparative effectiveness and safety of analgesics for osteoarthritis. Comparative effectiveness review no. 4 (Prepared by the Oregon Evidence-based Practice Center under Contract No. 290-02-0024). Rockville, MD: Agency for Healthcare Research and Quality; September 2006.
141. Aw TJ et al. Meta-analysis of cyclooxygenase-2 inhibitors and their effects on blood pressure. *Arch Intern Med* 2005;165:490.
142. Richy F et al. Structural and symptomatic efficacy of glucosamine and chondroitin in knee osteoarthritis: a comprehensive meta-analysis. *Arch Intern Med* 2003;163:1514.
143. Davis MP, Srivastava M. Demographics, assessment and management of pain in the elderly. *Drugs Aging* 2003;20:23.

144. Brotman HB. Every ninth American: an analysis for the chairman of the Select Committee on Aging, House of Representatives. Comm publication no. 1-97-332. Washington, DC: U.S. Government Printing Office; 1982.
145. DeLisa JA et al. Rehabilitation medicine, past, present, and future. In: DeLisa JA, ed. *Rehabilitation Medicine: Principles and Practice.* Philadelphia: Lippincott; 1988:3.
146. U.S. Department of Health and Human Services, Centers for Disease Control and Prevention, National Center for Health Statistics. Health, United States, 2006, with Chartbook on Trends in the Health of Americans. Hyattsville, MD: Author; 2006.
147. World Health Organization. International Classification of impairments, Disabilities, and Handicaps: A Manual of Classification Relating to the Consequences of Disease. Geneva: WHO; 1980.
148. Thomas DR et al. Inpatient community-based geriatric assessment reduces subsequent mortality. *J Am Geriatr Soc* 1993;41:101.
149. Bjornson DC, Hiner WO Jr. Evaluation of the effects of clinical pharmacists on inpatient health-care outcomes. Presented at AJHP Midyear Clinical Meeting; Orlando, Florida; December 1992.
150. Owens NJ et al. The relationship between comprehensive functional assessment and optimal pharmacotherapy in the older patient. *DICP Ann Pharmacother* 1989;23:847.
151. Fick DM et al. Updating the Beers criteria for potentially inappropriate medication use in older adults. *Arch Intern Med* 2003;163:2716.
152. American Society of Consultant Pharmacists. ASCP Policies, Standards, and Guidelines 2002.
153. Aparasu RR, Mort JR. Inappropriate prescribing for the elderly: Beers criteria-based review. *Ann Pharmacother* 2000;34:338.
154. Liu GG, Christensen DB. The continuing challenge of inappropriate prescribing in the elderly: an update of the evidence. *J Am Pharm Assoc* 2002;42:847.
155. Ray WA et al. Benzodiazepines of long and short elimination half-life and the risk of hip fracture. *JAMA* 1989;262:3303.
156. Arnoff GR et al. *Drug Prescribing in Renal Failure: Dosing Guidelines for Adults.* 4th ed. Philadelphia: American College of Physicians; 1999:18.
157. Swan SK, Bennett WM. Drug dosing guidelines in patients with renal failure. *West J Med* 1992;156:633.
158. Murray MD et al. Factors contributing to medication noncompliance in older patients public housing tenants. *Drug Intell Clin Pharm* 1986;20:146.
159. Meyer ME et al. Assessment of geriatric patients' functional ability to take medication. *Drug Intell Clin Pharm* 1989;23:717.
160. Canaday BR. *OBRA '90: A Practical Guide to Effecting Pharmaceutical Care.* Washington, DC: American Pharmaceutical Association; 1994.

CHAPTER 100

Geriatric Dementias

Bradley R. Williams and Nicole J. Brandt

With the continuing growth in the elderly population, the incidence and prevalence of cognitive disorders continues to rise.[1,2] Alzheimer disease (AD) is the most common cause of dementia, accounting for approximately half of all diagnosed cases.[3] Vascular dementias (VaDs), dementia with Lewy bodies (DLB), and Parkinson disease with dementia (PDD) are the next most common dementias, with frontotemporal dementia, pseudodementia, and other forms occurring less often.[3,4] Dementia is currently the fifth leading cause of death in the United States.[5]

Incidence and Prevalence

The exact incidence and prevalence of dementia are difficult to determine for several reasons, including a lack of universally accepted diagnostic criteria, demographic variables, and well-designed epidemiologic studies.[6–9] Prevalence estimates have ranged from 2.5% in Great Britain to 24.6% in the former Soviet Union.[7] Studies in the United States have estimated the prevalence of dementias to be from 3.5% to 16.1% for the population age 65 years and older.[10,11] The worldwide prevalence of AD appears to be about 1% of the elderly population, with an exponential age-related increase.[9,12] AD currently affects approximately 2.3 million Americans.[2] The prevalence in the United States may be more than 10% of those age 65 and older, increasing sharply with age, from 3% among those 65 to 74 years of age to as much as 47.2% of those older than 85 years.[13,14] The incidence of dementia for people age 50 and older in the United States has been estimated at 527 new cases/100,000 population per year, with 437/100,000 diagnosed as AD.[15] The incidence increases with age, and women may be at a slightly higher risk than men.[1,16]

Life expectancy following a diagnosis of AD is reduced by as much as 69% for those diagnosed before age 70 years and by 39% for those diagnosed after age 90 years.[17]

The cost of dementia is staggering. The annual direct and total costs of treating a dementia patient are estimated to be almost $48,000 and $174,000, respectively.[18] Managed care organizations spend 1.5 times more on patients with dementia than on nondemented enrollees.[19] The cost to society in the United States of treating dementia is approximately $148 billion annually.[20]

Clinical Diagnosis

Dementia is a syndrome that exhibits impaired short- and long-term memory as its most prominent feature. Multiple cognitive deficits that compromise normal social or occupational function must be present before dementia can be diagnosed (Table 100-1).[21] Commonly, forgetfulness is the primary complaint of patients or the first symptom noted by the family.[21] Family members or others may note several symptoms that should prompt a medical evaluation (Table 100-2).[22] Memory loss often accompanies several diseases or disorders in elderly individuals. Therefore, a medical history, physical examination, and medication history are essential in excluding systemic illness or medication toxicity as causes of the dementia (Table 100-3).[23] Laboratory and other tests to assist in differentiating

Table 100-1 Diagnostic Criteria for Alzheimer-Type Dementia

1. The presence of multiple cognitive deficits manifested by both
   - Impaired memory (ability to learn new information or to retrieve information previously learned), and
   - At least one of the following:
     Aphasia (language difficulties)
     Apraxia (diminished ability to perform motor activities in the presence of intact motor function)
     Agnosia (inability to recognize or name objects despite intact sensory function)
     Disruption of executive function (diminished ability to plan, organize)
2. The previous deficits significantly interfere with normal work or social activities and represent a decline from previous ability to function
3. The previous deficits cannot be attributed to any of the following:
   - Central nervous system conditions that cause progressive cognitive or memory impairment (e.g., cerebrovascular disease)
   - Systemic conditions known to cause dementia (e.g., hypothyroidism, neurosyphilis, HIV infection)
   - Substance-induced conditions (e.g., drug toxicity)
4. The deficits do not occur exclusively during the course of a delirium
5. The disturbance is not better accounted for by another Axis I disorder (schizophrenia, major depressive disorder)

Adapted from reference 21, with permission.

dementia from other disorders are listed in Table 100-4. In patients with primary degenerative dementia, or AD, test results will generally be normal; evidence of cerebrovascular disease is present in patients with VaDs.

Brain imaging, such as a computed tomography (CT) scan or magnetic resonance imaging (MRI), can be useful in establishing the presence of a dementia, but neither is diagnostic. A CT scan is useful when a space-occupying lesion, such as a tumor, is suspected as a possible cause. An MRI scan is capable of identifying small infarcts, such as those found in some VaDs, and atrophy of subcortical structures such as the brainstem.[23]

The initial test in mental status screening is generally the Folstein Mini-Mental Status Exam (MMSE).[24] This test rapidly assesses orientation, registration, attention and calculation, recall, and language. Patients with dementia exhibit deficits in multiple areas. Those who score below the normal range on the MMSE or who exhibit symptoms characteristic of dementia receive further testing (Tables 100-1 and 100-2). The Blessed Dementia Scale evaluates daily functional capacity (e.g., shopping, performing household tasks), activities of daily living (e.g., eating, dressing, toileting), and personality. The Blessed Information-Memory-Concentration Test evaluates orientation, memory, and concentration.[25] All screening tests are subject to limitations. Therefore, additional psychometric testing is often ordered to further establish the presence and type of dementia.[22]

Dementias may be classified as cortical or subcortical, according to the areas of the brain preferentially affected by the

Table 100-2 Symptoms Suggesting Dementia

Symptom	Evidence
Difficulty learning or retaining new information	Repeats questions; difficulty remembering recent conversations, events, etc.; loses items
Unable to handle complex tasks	Cannot complete tasks that require multiple steps (e.g., difficulty following a shopping list)
Impaired reasoning	Difficulty solving everyday problems; inappropriate social behavior
Impaired spatial orientation and abilities	Gets lost in familiar places; difficulty with driving
Language deficits	Problems finding appropriate words (e.g., difficulty with naming common objects)
Behavior changes	Changes in personality; suspiciousness

Adapted from reference 22.

Table 100-3 Causes of Dementia Symptoms

Central Nervous System Disorders	*Systemic Illness*	*Medications*
Adjustment disorder (e.g., inability to adjust to retirement)	Cardiovascular disease	Anticholinergic agents
Amnestic syndrome (e.g., isolated memory impairment)	Arrhythmia	Anticonvulsants
Delirium	Heart failure	Antidepressants
Depression	Vascular occlusion	Antihistamines
Intracranial causes	Deficiency states	Anti-infectives
Brain abscess	Vitamin B12	Antineoplastic agents
Normal pressure	Folate	Antipsychotic agents
Hydrocephalus	Iron	Cardiovascular agents
Stroke	Infections	Antiarrhythmics
Subdural hematoma	Metabolic disorders	Antihypertensives
Tumor	Adrenal	Corticosteroids
	Glucose	H_2-receptor antagonists
	Renal failure	Immunosuppressants
	Thyroid	Narcotic analgesics
		Nonsteroidal anti-inflammatory agents
		Sedative hypnotics and Anxiolytics
		Skeletal muscle relaxants

Table 100-4 Dementia Screening Tests

Test	*Rationale for Testing*
Complete blood count with sedimentation rate	Anemic anoxia, infection, neoplasms
Metabolic screen	
Serum electrolytes	Hypernatremia, hyponatremia; renal function
Blood urea nitrogen, creatinine	Renal function
Bilirubin	Hepatic dysfunction (e.g., portal systemic encephalopathy, hepatocerebral degeneration)
Thyroid function	Hypothyroidism, hyperthyroidism
Iron, B12, folate	Deficiency states (B_{12}, folate neuropathies), anemias
Stool occult blood	Blood loss, anemia
Syphilis serology	Neurosyphilis
Urinalysis	Infection, proteinuria
Chest roentgenogram	Neoplasms, infection, airway disease (anoxia)
Electrocardiogram	Cardiac disease (stagnant anoxia)
Brain scan	Cerebral tumors, cerebrovascular disease
Mental status testing	General cognitive screen
Depression testing	Depression, pseudodementia

disorder. AD, a typical cortical dementia, disrupts the cerebral cortex. Patients with cortical dementias display impaired language rather than impaired speech, a learning deficit (amnesia), reduced higher cortical functions (e.g., inability to perform calculations, poor judgment), and an unconcerned or disinhibited affect. Subcortical dementias such as PDD primarily affect the basal ganglia, thalamus, and brainstem. Deficits include abnormal motor function, disrupted speech patterns rather than language difficulties, forgetfulness (impaired recall), slowed cognitive function, and an apathetic or depressed affect.[26]

ALZHEIMER DISEASE

Etiology

A definitive cause for AD has yet to be determined. Although elevated aluminum concentration has been noted in patients with Alzheimer-type dementia, this finding has not been consistent.[27–29] For example, patients with aluminum toxicity, as seen in dialysis dementia, do not exhibit AD-type lesions.[30] Increased concentrations of cerebral aluminum may be a secondary process resulting from an underlying pathological condition.[31] Other reported risk factors for AD include young (15–19 years) or old (older than 40 years) maternal age,[32–34] head trauma,[34,35] small head circumference and brain size,[36,37] and low intelligence.[38]

Genetics play a significant role in the development of Alzheimer-type dementia. The high familial occurrence of Alzheimer dementia has been linked to autosomal-dominant traits on chromosomes 21, 14, and 1.[39] The risk to first-degree relatives of patients with AD is 24% to 48% and may be as high as 64% for offspring.[40–43] Familial dementia of the Alzheimer type is associated with an early onset, faster progression, family history of psychiatric problems, and more prominent language difficulties.[40,44–46] However, there is some association between changes on chromosome 14 and late-onset AD.[47,48]

In families with a history of Down syndrome or other defects on chromosome 21, the prevalence of Alzheimer-type dementia is increased significantly. AD affects virtually all Down syndrome patients who survive into old age.[45,49,50] Mutations on chromosome 14 are responsible for most cases of familial early-onset AD, whereas chromosome 1–associated mutations account for cases in only a small cohort of families.[51,52] However, differences in risk based on age at onset and discordance for the disease among monozygotic twins indicate some heterogeneity in the genetic etiology.[43,45,53] Clinically, patients with familial dementia of the Alzheimer type are indistinguishable from those with nonfamilial, or sporadic, forms of the disease, suggesting a combination of genetic and environmental causes.[32,46] Despite the familial patterns, these mutations account for only approximately 5% of all cases of AD.[54]

Abnormalities in serum protein and alterations in immune function are often found among patients with AD. Amyloid precursor protein (APP), a normal protein found throughout the body (e.g., platelets and peripheral lymphocytes),[55] maps on chromosome 21 and is produced in excess in patients with Down syndrome.[49] Because of overproduction or transcription errors, an abnormal subunit (i.e., β-amyloid) is produced.[49,56] This finding is consistent in families with a high incidence of Alzheimer-type dementia, especially those with early-onset (before age 65) forms.[45,49,56]

Mutations on chromosome 14 occur in the presenilin-1 gene, and mutations on chromosome 1 occur in the presenilin-2 gene.[51,52,57] These mutations also code for alterations in the processing of APP. The abnormal cleavage of APP produces a 42–amino acid form of β-amyloid that demonstrates a higher toxicity than other amyloid forms.[39]

Apolipoprotein E (ApoE), a protein that is involved in cholesterol and phospholipid metabolism, plays a role in the development of sporadic, late-onset AD.[58] The ApoE gene resides on chromosome 19 and possesses three alleles: $\varepsilon 2$, $\varepsilon 3$, and $\varepsilon 4$. The $\varepsilon 3$ allele is most common, the $\varepsilon 2$ allele appears to be protective against AD, and the $\varepsilon 4$ allele increases the risk for AD.[59,60] The presence of ApoE-4, the protein coded for by the $\varepsilon 4$ allele, appears to increase the deposition of β-amyloid and promote its change to a more pathological configuration.[39] Measurable memory decline in people with either one or two copies of the $\varepsilon 4$ allele occurs much earlier than in those with no copies and well in advance of the first clinical symptoms of AD.[61,62] The risk for developing AD by age 80 years has been estimated at 47% for people with one copy of ApoE-$\varepsilon 4$ and at 91% for those who carry two copies. In contrast, the risk is approximately 20% for those with no ApoE-$\varepsilon 4$ copies.[59]

Amyloid protein can commonly be found in the neuritic plaques, which occur in Alzheimer-type dementia; and cerebral amyloid angiopathy occurs in 50% to 90% of patients with progressive dementia and neurofibrillary degeneration.[63,64] Amyloid protein is also noted in blood vessel walls of patients with AD.[55] β-Amyloid protein deposits occur early in the course of Alzheimer dementia and are distinct from the amyloid proteins found in other amyloid disorders, such as primary amyloidosis or multiple myeloma.[31,55]

Neuropathology

Although brain atrophy is the most obvious finding among patients with Alzheimer-type dementia, it is not diagnostic for AD or other dementias because some degree of atrophy accompanies normal aging.[65] Atrophic changes induced by AD are found primarily in the temporal, parietal, and frontal areas of the brain; the occipital region, primary motor cortex, and somatosensory areas are generally unaffected (Fig. 100-1).

Neuronal changes in the cerebral cortex associated with AD include neurofibrillary tangles, neuritic plaques, amyloid angiopathy, and granulovacuolar degeneration. These changes lead to loss of neurons and synapses (Fig. 100-2).[39] Neurofibrillary tangles (NFTs) are found primarily in the pyramidal regions of the neocortex, hippocampus, and amygdala, but they are also noted in areas of the brainstem and locus ceruleus.[39,66] Tangles are a prominent feature of Alzheimer-type dementia, but can be found in several other brain disorders (e.g., Down syndrome, postencephalitic Parkinson disease) and even in normally aging brains, although they are generally less numerous and histologically different.[39,67] Conversely, Alzheimer-type dementia may also occur in the absence of NFTs.[67]

NFTs are composed of paired helical filaments, combinations of fibrils with a characteristic width and contour, containing a tau protein with an abnormal pattern of phosphate deposition.[39,68,69] They are highly immunoreactive and are most likely to form in large pyramidal neurons. NFTs typically begin in the transentorhinal cortex and spread to the limbic cortex and the neocortex.[39] Although the nerve structures (axons,

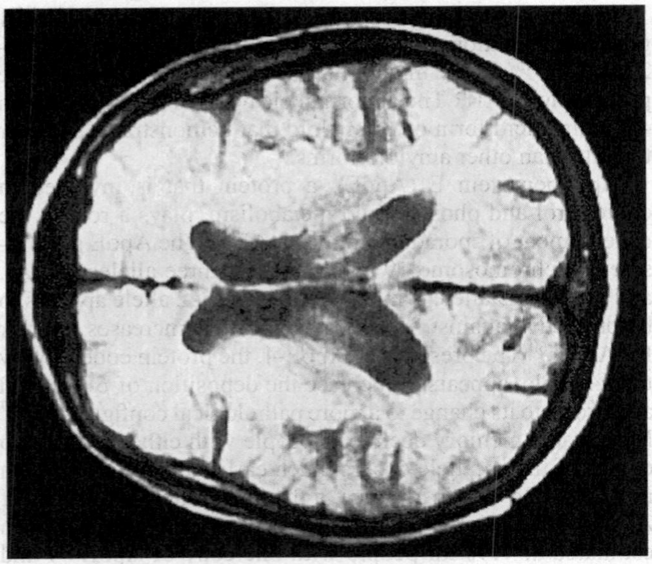

FIGURE 100-1 Alzheimer disease: MRI scan. Ventricles are enlarged, and there is generalized atrophy, with greater atrophy present near the temporal areas.

dendrites, and nerve terminals) found within NFTs contain amyloid deposits, abnormal axons may occur independently of amyloid deposition. Thus, the presence of amyloid protein is not required for the development of tangles.[70] The presence of NFTs in the neocortical areas is associated with the presence of Alzheimer-type dementia, and their number in the nucleus basalis is correlated with the severity and duration of the disease.[71,72]

Neuritic plaques are spherical bodies of tissue composed of granular deposits and remnants of neuronal processes.[3] Diffuse plaques, considered to represent the early stage of plaque formation, contain no amyloid core. They have been found in areas in the cerebellum and throughout cerebral hemispheres that are not related to AD symptoms.[39] The typical neuritic plaques of AD may develop from preamyloid deposits with subsequent deposition of amyloid protein and accumulation

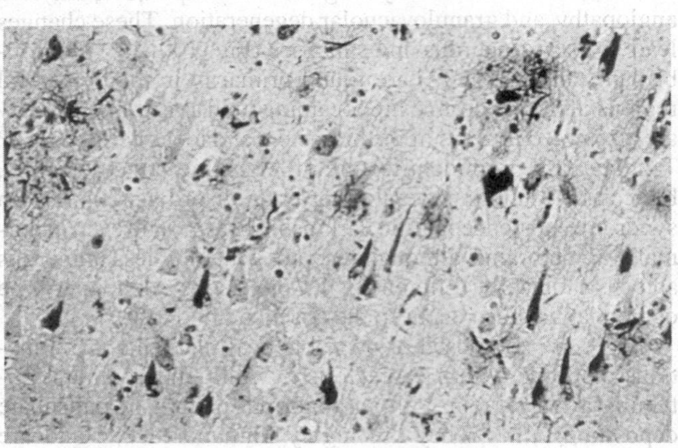

FIGURE 100-2 Numerous plaques (large, round bodies) and tangles (tear-shaped bodies) are found throughout the cortex in Alzheimer-type dementia.

of oligosaccharide, aggregation of amyloid subunits, and β-pleating of the protein.[73,74] They are spherical structures between 50 and 200 μm wide and exhibit a three-tiered structure: a central amyloid core, a middle region of swollen axons and dendrites, and an outer zone containing degenerating neuritic processes.[39] The plaques are concentrated in the cerebral cortex and hippocampus, but they are also found in the corpus striatum, amygdala, and hypothalamus.[75] Rare plaques have also been found in nondemented elderly patients.[71]

Plaques contain APP, which can be cleaved by a defective metabolic process to form β-amyloid.[76–78] In addition to β-amyloid, plaques also contain protein, apolipoprotein E, and acute phase inflammatory proteins such as α_1-chymotrypsin and α_2-macroglobulin.[39,79] Although β-amyloid is found in both normal and AD subjects, NFTs occurring in the plaques of nondemented subjects do not contain the abnormal protein seen in individuals with dementia.[71] The deposition of amyloid in neuritic plaques correlates with the severity of AD, and the density of cortical plaques is associated with decreased choline acetyltransferase and the severity of cognitive impairment.[76,80] β-Amyloid has been identified in plaques associated with Down syndrome and in both familial and sporadic forms of dementia of the Alzheimer type.[76,81] The process of development from the time of amyloid deposition to plaque formation may take as long as 30 years.[76,82]

In addition to neuritic plaques, APP and β-amyloid produce an amyloid angiopathy outside brain tissue. APP has been located in the adenohypophysis, adrenal gland, cardiac muscle, and peripheral nervous system.[77] Amyloid deposits, identical to those found in neuritic plaques, have been found in cerebral blood vessels as well as in the vasculature of skin, subcutaneous tissue, and intestine.[39,76,83]

Granulovacuolar degeneration is the other major histologic finding in AD. It consists of clusters of intracytoplasmic vacuoles that contain tiny granules. The vacuoles appear to be specifically located in the pyramidal neurons of the hippocampus. Granulovacuolar degeneration can also occur, albeit rarely, in individuals without dementia.[39]

The loss of cortical neurons that originate in the nucleus basalis and project into the cerebral cortex is the most significant histopathological consequence of AD.[39,80,84,85] Cell loss, granulovacuolar degeneration, and neurons with NFTs are concentrated in this area.[39]

Accompanying these changes are decreased concentrations of several neurotransmitters and enzymes. Choline acetyltransferase levels are reduced 60% to 90% in the cortical and hippocampal regions.[39,80] Acetylcholine and acetylcholinesterase (AChE) are also decreased, whereas muscarinic receptors in the cortex and hippocampus remain at normal levels or are moderately decreased.[80,86] Nicotinic receptor proteins are also reduced in patients with Alzheimer-type dementia when compared with age-matched controls.[87,88] Decreased choline acetyltransferase activity has been correlated with plaque density and disease severity.[80] Cortical synapse loss, especially in the midfrontal region, is associated with disease severity.[89]

Changes affecting AChE have significant implications for the management of AD symptoms. Many isoforms of AChE have been identified; they possess identical amino acid sequences, but display different posttranslational modifications, predominate at diverse anatomical and microanatomical locations, and function in different ways.[90] The predominant form of AChE in the cortical and hippocampal regions of humans is G4, a tetrameric form that is membrane bound. The monomeric form, G1, is found in a much lower concentration. There is a selective loss of the G4 form in patients with AD, allowing the G1 form to assume greater importance.

Although cholinergic activity is most significantly affected by Alzheimer-type dementia, other neurochemical systems are also altered. Norepinephrine, serotonin, and γ-aminobutyric acid levels may be normal or moderately decreased.[39] Somatostatin and corticotropin-releasing factor are also reduced in patients with Alzheimer-type dementia.[80,91]

Clinical Presentation and Diagnosis

1. C.L., a 63-year-old woman, complains of increasing memory problems over the past 2 years. She states that she began writing reminder notes to herself, but she often forgot to look at them. Eventually, she began to lose items around her house, forget appointments, and fail to pay some important bills. During the past 2 to 3 months, she has had difficulty following a shopping list and has become disoriented in the store. One week ago, she became agitated when she heard the low-battery alarm in her smoke detector. C.L. admits to becoming increasingly depressed over her memory problems but denies appetite or sleep changes or suicidal ideation. She also denies hallucinations, delusional thoughts, or symptoms of anxiety. C.L.'s medical history is significant for type 2 diabetes mellitus, which is diet controlled, and bilateral open-angle glaucoma, treated with dipivefrin 0.1%, one drop twice daily. Her family history is negative for stroke and positive for diabetes mellitus and hypertension. She reports that two or three of her maternal relatives had "memory problems" and that one aunt was diagnosed with AD 5 years ago.

Physical examination reveals a moderately obese woman who is well dressed and groomed. Her blood pressure (BP) is 140/86 mmHg supine and 132/82 mmHg standing, with pulse rates of 74 beats/minute and 78 beats/minute, respectively. She is awake and oriented to place and person. During the interview, she is reserved but becomes easily irritated with the physician.

The Folstein MMSE score was 23/30, with errors in orientation, attention, and calculation (inability to spell "world" backward), recall, and language (difficulty with word finding). Her score on the Blessed Dementia Scale was 25/33, with deficits in personality, memory, concentration, and habits. Neurologic examination revealed no deficits. The rest of the physical examination was within normal limits.

Laboratory tests performed include renal and liver chemistries, thyroid function tests, glycosylated hemoglobin, vitamin B12 and folate levels, syphilis and HIV tests, complete blood count (CBC) with sedimentation rate, and urinalysis. All results were normal with the exception of a fasting glucose level of 150 mg/dL (normal, <126 mg/dL) and a glycosylated hemoglobin of 8.4% (normal, 4%–6%). Chest radiograph and electrocardiogram (ECG) were normal. Depression testing revealed a sad, mildly anxious individual who was not depressed. What is the most probable diagnosis for C.L.?

[SI units: fasting glucose, 8.3 mmol/L; glycosylated hemoglobin, 0.084%]

C.L. is in the early stages of AD. She displays several trigger symptoms associated with dementia, including problems learning new information, difficulty with complex tasks (shopping), impaired reasoning (recognizing the smoke alarm battery warning), and increased irritability.[22] Her score of 23/30 on the Folstein MMSE indicates a mild stage of the dementia as evidenced by errors in orientation, calculation, recall, and language.[24] Personality and habit changes and deficits in memory and concentration are revealed in C.L.'s score on the Blessed Dementia Scale.[25] Secondary medical causes of cognitive impairment can be eliminated by C.L.'s generally normal physical examination and laboratory test results. C.L.'s fasting glucose and glycosylated hemoglobin levels are mildly elevated, but cannot account for her significant cognitive decline. MRI or CT scanning may be useful in many cases to help eliminate brain pathology, such as stroke, but the lack of any abnormal neurologic findings renders imaging in C.L. unnecessary.

Secondary psychiatric causes for C.L.'s decline can also be discounted. Although she is sad and anxious, the absence of alterations in appetite or sleep patterns, absence of suicidal thoughts, and the results of psychologic testing indicate C.L. is not depressed. She is fully conscious, alert, and oriented to place and person. She exhibits no psychotic behavior and no evidence of delirium.

C.L.'s slowly progressive decline, its impact on her social and occupational function (forgetting appointments, failing to pay bills), normal physical examination and laboratory findings, and family history meet the *Diagnostic and Statistical Manual of Mental Disorders,* Fourth Edition (DSM-IV) criteria for AD (Table 100-1). Because she is younger than 65 years, she also may be classified as early-onset type.[21] Her history and course to date satisfy the criteria for Alzheimer-type dementia and do not indicate a likely alternative explanation for her condition. Thus, C.L. can be classified as probable AD according to the criteria established by the National Institute of Neurological and Communicative Disorders-Alzheimer's Disease and Related Disorders Association Task Force (Table 100-5).[92]

2. C.L.'s children are very concerned about the family history for dementia. They ask if there are any tests they should receive at this time to determine their risk. What should they be told?

Although there is a strong genetic association with AD, such instances account for a small minority of cases.[54] There is no apparent family history of Down syndrome. Mutations in the presenilin-1 and presenilin-2 genes have been documented in only a few families worldwide.[93] The test that would most likely be performed is ApoE-4 genotyping, but this is not recommended because the sensitivity and specificity of the test is not yet known.[93,94]

Prognosis

3. What is the likely prognosis for C.L.?

AD follows a predictable course that may progress over 10 years or more.[17,95] Two common rating scales for dementia are the Global Deterioration Scale and the Clinical Dementia Rating Scale. According to the Global Deterioration Scale (Table 100-6), C.L.'s impaired social functioning, anxiety, and objective cognitive decline as well as her continued ability to concentrate and perform some complex skills, combined with her preserved affect and social interaction, are consistent with

Table 100-5 National Institute of Neurological and Communicative Disorders-Alzheimer's Disease and Related Disorders Association Criteria for Dementia of the Alzheimer Type (DAT)

Definite DAT
- Clinical criteria for probable DAT
- Histopathological evidence for DAT (autopsy or biopsy confirmed)

Probable DAT
- Dementia established by clinical examination and documented by mental status testing (e.g., history and physical examination, Folstein Mini-Mental Status Exam)
- Confirmation of dementia by neuropsychologic tests (e.g., Blessed Dementia Scale and other tests)
- Deficits in at least two areas of cognitive function (e.g., language, memory)
- Progressive deterioration of memory and other cognitive function
- Undisturbed consciousness
- Onset between the ages of 40 and 90 yrs
- Absence of systemic or other brain disease capable of producing dementia

Possible DAT
- Atypical onset, presentation, or progression of dementia with an unknown etiology
- Presence of a systemic or other brain disease capable of producing dementia, but not believed to be the cause of the dementia
- Gradually progressive decline in one intellectual function in the absence of another identifiable cause

Unlikely DAT
- Sudden onset
- Focal neurologic findings (e.g., deep tendon reflexes, hemiparesis)

Adapted from reference 92.

the features of stage three dementia of the Alzheimer type. This stage of AD is generally associated with a period of mild cognitive decline.[96] The more general Clinical Dementia Rating Scale also places C.L. in the category of mild dementia.[97] Clinical diagnoses of AD using clinical criteria for probable AD have a sensitivity of approximately 85% when compared with autopsy-confirmed cases.[93,98]

Table 100-6 Stages of Dementia of the Alzheimer Type

Stage of Cognitive Decline	*Features*
No cognitive decline	Normal cognitive state
Very mild cognitive decline	Forgetfulness, subjective complaints only; no objective decline
Mild cognitive decline	Objective decline through psychiatric testing; work and social impairment; mild anxiety and denial
Moderate cognitive decline	Concentration, complex skills decline; flat affect and withdrawal
Moderately severe cognitive decline	Early dementia; difficulty in interactions; unable to recall or recognize people or places
Severe cognitive decline	Requires assistance with bathing, toileting; behavioral symptoms present (agitation, delusions, aggressive behavior)
Very severe cognitive decline	Loss of psychomotor skills and verbal abilities; incontinence; total dependence

Adapted from reference 96.

Because of technologic advances, it is possible to diagnose dementia earlier and to keep patients alive into the final stages of the disease. The early diagnosis of AD in C.L. will allow her condition to be followed closely. Although it is less expensive to maintain a patient at home, caregiver burden can become a significant consideration.[99,100] Eventually, C.L. should be moved into a sheltered environment (e.g., a relative's home, residential care facility, or nursing home) before suffering an injury caused by her poor judgment (e.g., failing to dress properly for the weather, falling). In the later stages, interventions ranging from tube feedings to life support may prolong life, yet prove to be controversial.[101] Death in the late stage of AD is commonly associated with the development of infections such as pneumonia, urinary tract infections, or decubitus ulcers.

Treatment

4. What is an appropriate initial treatment strategy for C.L.?

Maintaining independence as long as possible is an important goal in treating a patient with dementia. Keeping patients in familiar surroundings allows them to function without the added burden of having to attempt to adapt to a strange environment. C.L. appears to be functioning reasonably well at home, although her forgetfulness is causing some problems for her. She is still eating well (her laboratory testing indicated no deficiencies in total protein or albumin, vitamin B12, or folic acid) and performing normal daily activities such as dressing, grooming, bathing, and toileting. Some regular supervision from family members, neighbors, or household help will ensure that C.L. remains safe in her own home.

C.L.'s diabetes mellitus and general medical condition should also be monitored closely. Because both hyperglycemia and hypoglycemia can impair cognitive processes, either complication can exacerbate her memory problems. Concurrent diseases and many medications can reduce function and increase cognitive impairment in demented patients, so any new findings in C.L. must be evaluated carefully to distinguish new problems from a worsening of her dementia.

C.L.'s family needs to be educated about what to expect as her dementia progresses. They should be referred to the Alzheimer's Association Website. Results of trials investigating precursor loading and agonists have been disappointing. Moderate success has been demonstrated with cholinesterase inhibitors[102] (Fig. 100-3). However, the long-term value of this strategy is limited by the fact that the disease process is unaltered and neuronal degeneration continues.[103]

TACRINE

Tacrine, the first agent approved for the symptomatic treatment of mild to moderate AD, is an aminoacridine derivative that reversibly inhibits both AChE and butyrylcholinesterase (BChE).[104] It has a relatively low bioavailability, which is further decreased when the drug is taken with meals. Multiple daily doses are required because tacrine's half-life is short (Table 100-7).[104] Significant cholinergic adverse effects, primarily nausea, vomiting, diarrhea, and abdominal pain, and a high risk of hepatotoxicity have rendered this agent obsolete.[105,106]

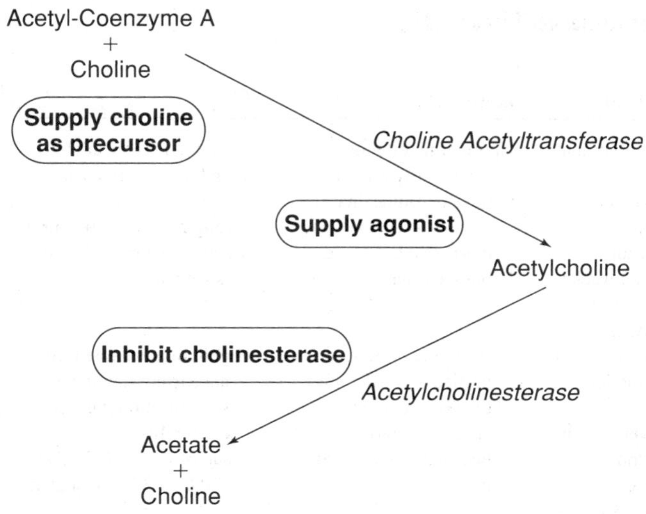

FIGURE 100-3 Potential strategies for cholinergic manipulation.

DONEPEZIL

Donepezil represents the first of what has been termed the "second-generation" cholinesterase inhibitors.[102] It is a piperidine derivative that is more selective for AChE than BChE and, like tacrine, it reversibly inhibits cholinesterase activity. Donepezil is completely bioavailable and exhibits a long half-life, allowing it to be given as a single daily dose.[107] It is highly protein bound, primarily to albumin (Table 100-7).[108]

Donepezil may improve cognition, global function, and behavioral symptoms across all stages (mild, moderate, and severe) of AD. In a multicenter, double-blind, placebo-controlled trial, subjects with mild to moderately severe AD improved over a 12-week treatment period.[109] Subjects taking 10 mg of donepezil at bedtime improved their cognitive function as measured by the Alzheimer's Disease Assessment Scale-Cognitive Subscale (ADAS-Cog), and their overall function as measured by the Clinician's Interview-Based Impression of Change with caregiver input (CIBIC-Plus).[110,111] A 24-week multicenter, placebo-controlled trial using dosages of 5 mg/day and 10 mg/day demonstrated similar results. Both 5 and 10 mg doses were superior to placebo; adverse effects were less common with the 5 mg dose.[112] A long-term, open-label follow-up study to these trials demonstrated that donepezil effects may persist for almost 3 years.[113] Interruption or discontinuation of donepezil treatment was followed by a return of cognition and function to baseline or below.

Donepezil is the only cholinesterase inhibitor currently indicated for the severe stage of AD. A 6-month, double-blind, parallel group, placebo-controlled study in patients with severe AD (MMSE 1–10) showed at 6 months an improvement in the severe impairment battery (SIB) and Modified Alzheimer's Disease Cooperative Study activities of daily living inventory for severe AD (ADCS-ADL-severe).[114] The domains that showed a significant improvement over placebo were language, praxis, visuospatial, bowel/bladder function, and ability to get dressed. There were no differences noted in the neuropsychiatric inventory for behavioral issues associated with dementia.

The most common adverse effects of donepezil are associated with cholinergic activity. They tend to be mild to moderate in nature and resolve with stabilization of the dose.[109,112] In a 144-week extension trial of donepezil, the most frequently encountered adverse effects were nausea, diarrhea, and headache.[113]

RIVASTIGMINE

Rivastigmine is a carbamate derivative that inhibits both AChE and BChE activity. BChE provides an alternate pathway for acetylcholine metabolism. Rivastigmine inhibits the activity of both cholinesterases, primarily in the central nervous system (CNS).[115] Its AChE inhibition is greater for the G1 as compared to the G4 form.[116] The drug binds to the esteratic site of the AChE and BChE molecule and slowly dissociates. Because of this, it is often referred to as a "pseudoirreversible" inhibitor.[117] Rivastigmine's biological half-life is approximately 1 hour, but because its slow dissociation extends its activity for at least 10 hours, it can be dosed twice daily. Rivastigmine is bound approximately 40% to serum proteins and is metabolized via hydrolysis to renally excreted inactive compounds.[116] Rivastigmine absorption is nearly complete, but because it undergoes a significant first-pass effect, the resultant bioavailability is approximately 36% (Table 100-7).

In two large clinical trials conducted in patients with mild to moderately severe AD, rivastigmine improved cognition, the ability to perform daily activities, and global function over 24 weeks.[118,119] In each multicenter, double-blind, placebo-controlled trial, subjects were randomized to receive placebo or low-dose (1–4 mg/day) or high-dose (6–12 mg/day) rivastigmine in two divided doses during a 26-week period. In one study, subjects in both dosage groups demonstrated statistically significant improvement after 26 weeks on the ADAS-Cog and CIBIC-Plus scales.[118] In the other trial, only those subjects taking 6 to 12 mg/day improved on the same scales.[119] An open-label extension study that included subjects from both previous studies found that subjects taking 6 to 12 mg/day of rivastigmine had significantly better cognitive function after 1 year than did subjects who had originally received placebo.[120]

Adverse effects typically included nausea, vomiting, diarrhea, and other cholinergically mediated gastrointestinal (GI) effects.[121] They are most common when rivastigmine is taken on an empty stomach or when the dose escalation is too rapid. Headache, dizziness, and fatigue are also common adverse effects. Increasing the dose by 1.5 mg twice daily at 4-week intervals increases drug tolerability and reduces the frequency and severity of GI side effects.

GALANTAMINE

Like other agents used to treat AD, galantamine enhances cholinergic activity by inhibiting AChE. However, it also stimulates nicotinic receptors at a site distinct from that stimulated by acetylcholine, an action that does not rely on the presence of acetylcholine.[122] This action is referred to as allosteric modulation. Galantamine is rapidly and completely absorbed, reaches peak serum levels in <2 hours, and has a half-life of approximately 5 hours. It exhibits low protein binding and has a large volume of distribution. Galantamine is metabolized primarily by CYP2D6 and CYP3A4, and is eliminated in the urine (Table 100-7).[123,124]

Clinical trials have shown galantamine to be effective for the symptomatic treatment of mild to moderate AD. Doses of 16 and 24 mg/day produced clinically meaningful improvement

Table 100-7 U.S. Food and Drug Administration–Approved Drugs for Alzheimer Disease (AD)

Generic Drug (Brand Name) and Mechanism	Dosage Form and Dosage	Indication and Effect	Adverse Effects	Other
Donepezil HCl (Aricept) Reversibly inhibits acetylcholinesterase (AChE), primarily in central nervous system (CNS)	5-, 10-mg tablets 5, 10 mg ODT 1 mg/mL oral solution 5 mg daily, usually at bedtime Dose may be increased to 10 mg after 4–6 weeks	Symptomatic treatment of mild to severe AD Small improvements in cognition and function occur within 12–24 weeks; benefits may last for at least 2 years	Cholinergic effects, particularly affecting the gastrointestinal (GI) tract (nausea, anorexia, diarrhea); headache; bradycardia may occur	Completely bioavailable and may be given as a single daily dose due to long half-life (70 hours) Metabolized by CYP3A4 isoenzymes
Galantamine HBr (Razadyne and Razadyne ER) Reversibly inhibits AChE, primarily in CNS; also stimulates nicotinic receptors at a site distinct from that of acetylcholine	4-, 8-, 12-mg tablets 4 mg/mL oral solution 8, 16, 24 mg extended release capsule 4 mg BID, with food Dose may be increased every 4–6 weeks in 4 mg BID increments, to a maximum dose of 12 mg BID Extended-release (ER) formulation can be given once daily starting at 8 mg daily and increasing as noted previously	Symptomatic treatment of mild to moderate AD Small improvements in cognition and function occur within 12–24 weeks. Benefits may last for more than 1 year	Cholinergic effects, particularly affecting the GI tract (nausea, anorexia, diarrhea); headache; bradycardia may occur	Highly bioavailable Initial dose is not therapeutic; slow titration increases tolerability Metabolized by CYP2D6 and CYP3A4 isoenzymes
Rivastigmine tartrate (Exelon) Reversibly inhibits AChE and butyrylcholinesterase (BChE), primarily in CNS	1.5-, 3-, 4.5-, 6-mg tablets 4.6, 9.5 mg/24 hr extended release patch 2 mg/mL solution 1.5 mg BID, with food Dose may be increased every 4–6 weeks in 1.5 mg BID increments, to a maximum dose of 6 mg BID	Symptomatic treatment of mild to moderate AD Small improvements in cognition and function occur within 12–24 weeks. Benefits may last for more than 1 year	Cholinergic effects, particularly affecting the GI tract (nausea, anorexia, vomiting, diarrhea); headache; bradycardia may occur	Highly bioavailable Therapeutic effect greatly exceeds biological half-life (1 hour), allowing for twice daily dosing Metabolized by hydrolysis Initial dose is not therapeutic; administration with food and slow titration are necessary to increase tolerability
Tacrine (Cognex) Reversibly inhibits AChE and BChE, in CNS and periphery	10-, 20-, 30-, 40-mg tablets Initially 10 mg QID, with increases of 10 mg QID every 4 weeks; maximum dose is 40 mg QID	Symptomatic treatment of mild to moderate AD Small improvements in cognition and function occur within 12–24 weeks	Cholinergic effects, particularly affecting the GI tract (nausea, anorexia, vomiting, diarrhea); abdominal pain; headache; bradycardia may occur. Increases in ALT levels require frequent monitoring	Poor bioavailability, further reduced by giving with food Adverse effects limit patient tolerability Multiple daily doses require frequent dosing Metabolized by CYP1A2, CYP2D6 Initial dose is not therapeutic
Memantine (Namenda) Uncompetitive antagonist of the N-methyl-D-aspartate type of glutamate receptors	5- and 10-mg tablets and solution, oral: 5 mg/day for 1 week; 5 mg BID for 1 week; 15 mg/day given in 5 mg and 10 mg separated doses for 1 week; then 10 mg BID Severe impairment: Creatinine clearance 5–29 mL/min): 5 mg BID	Symptomatic treatment of moderate to severe AD Small improvements in cognition and function as well as less burden on caregivers	Well tolerated, yet can cause headaches and dizziness	Can be used as monotherapy or in conjunction with cholinesterase inhibitors

Adapted from references 104, 105, 107, 109, 113, 115, 116, 120–123, 127, and 245–248.
BID, twice daily; QID, four times daily; ODT, orally disintegrating tablets.

in ADAS-Cog and CIBIC-Plus scores during a 5-month, randomized, placebo-controlled trial.[125] A similar trial conducted in Europe and Canada that evaluated patients over 6 months used doses of 24 and 32 mg/day. Both doses were more effective than placebo, but patients in the 32 mg/day group exhibited more adverse effects.[126] A 6-month, open-label extension trial showed that patients treated with galantamine 24 mg/day maintained ADAS-Cog scores throughout the entire 12 months of the study.[127]

As with the other cholinesterase inhibitors, cholinergic effects in the GI tract are the most commonly encountered adverse effects. Nausea, diarrhea, vomiting, and anorexia were the most frequent events encountered during clinical trials.[124] They were typically present during the dose escalation phases of the studies. A dose titration interval of 4 weeks reduces the severity of adverse effects and increases tolerability.

C.L. is in the mild stage of the disease, so a cholinesterase inhibitor would be the first choice. It is unlikely that a cholinesterase inhibitor will produce a dramatic or long-lasting improvement in C.L.'s cognitive abilities. Systematic reviews of cholinesterase inhibitor therapy have consistently concluded that these agents provide modest benefits, at best, in the majority of patients.[128,129] Treatment, however, may slow her cognitive decline, help maintain her ability to care for herself for 1 year or more, and reduce the risk for nursing facility placement for as much as 2 years.[130] The choice of drug is based on the agent most likely to produce a positive response with the fewest adverse effects. Ease of adherence must also be considered. All agents exhibit similar adverse effect profiles. Rivastigmine may be less prone to drug interactions because of its metabolic pathway. It is also available as a patch that is applied daily. Donepezil and galantamine can be given as a single daily dose. They can be given at bedtime, which may make cholinergic side effects less troublesome. We decide to start C.L. on donepezil.

6. How should treatment with donepezil be instituted in C.L., and how should therapy be monitored?

C.L. should receive donepezil 5 mg at bedtime. She should be monitored for cholinergic side effects (particularly nausea and diarrhea), insomnia, headache, and dizziness, the adverse effects most commonly reported in clinical trials.[109,112] Her family and physician should look for improvements in her memory, orientation, and ability to concentrate on complex tasks, such as shopping. She may also become less irritable. If she has not improved noticeably after 4 to 6 weeks, the dose of donepezil may be increased to 10 mg at bedtime.

If her condition does not respond to donepezil after a trial of 3 to 6 months or she is unable to tolerate the donepezil, it is reasonable to switch C.L. to another cholinesterase inhibitor. Both rivastigmine and galantamine have additional mechanisms of action that might prove beneficial. Rivastigmine is started at a dose of 1.5 mg twice daily with meals to slow absorption and improve tolerability. The dose may be increased at 4-week intervals by 1.5 mg twice daily, up to the maximum dose of 6 mg twice daily. Galantamine can be started at 4 mg twice daily or 8 mg daily and increased every 4 weeks by 8 mg, up to a maximum dose of 24 mg daily. Taking galantamine with meals may improve tolerability of GI effects. If a trial of a second agent does not improve or stabilize a patient's condition, there is no value in attempting a third agent.

MEMANTINE

7. C.L. tolerated donepezil well, with the exception of some mild nausea and occasional loose stools. She was once again able to engage in normal activities with the help of reminder notes and became much less irritable, according to her family.

One year later, C.L. is exhibiting some decline in her cognition and is becoming more disoriented, particularly in the afternoon and evening. Her physician considers her to now be in the moderate stage of AD. What other drug therapy strategies may be appropriate for C.L.'s worsening AD?

Evidence that release of glutamate in the CNS can lead to excitotoxic reactions and cell death has led to research into the use of N-methyl-D-aspartate (NMDA) antagonists to treat AD and other neurodegenerative disorders.[131] Memantine is an uncompetitive NMDA receptor antagonist with moderate affinity and voltage-dependent binding. It is completely absorbed after oral administration, reaches peak serum concentrations in 3 to 8 hours, and is moderately protein bound (Table 100-7).[130]

Two large clinical trials have evaluated memantine in subjects with moderate to severe AD. A dose of 10 mg/day for 12 weeks increased functional ability (e.g., dressing, toileting, participating in group activities) and reduced care dependence compared with placebo.[132] A 28-week trial using a dose of 20 mg/day improved CIBIC-Plus scores, activities of daily living, and global function compared with placebo.[133] Overall, the benefits of memantine are modest.[134] Common adverse effects include diarrhea, insomnia, dizziness, headache, and hallucinations.[131] The combined use of memantine and a cholinesterase inhibitor has been shown to be superior to a cholinesterase inhibitor alone in individuals with moderate to severe dementia.[135,136] C.L. should be started on memantine 5 mg daily, with the dosage increased in weekly intervals by 5 mg/day, up to a dose of 10 mg twice daily.[137]

Investigational Agents

Several medications are being studied for the management of dementia at various stages. Some are medications already approved for other uses, and others are new and investigational agents. The Alzheimer's Association and clinicaltrials.gov are great resources to find and gather additional information on investigational treatments.

ESTROGEN

Estrogen has several beneficial effects on the brain, including improved cerebral blood flow, increased glucose transport and metabolism, and facilitated repair of damaged neurons.[138] Retrospective studies have demonstrated a link between postmenopausal estrogen replacement and improved performance on memory testing in older women.[139] A reduced risk for dementia has been found among postmenopausal estrogen users in some studies but not in others.[140] The Women's Health Initiative Study found that women taking combined estrogen and progestin were more likely to develop dementia than those who had not taken these hormones. The hazard ratio for developing dementia was 2.05.[140] One recent study found no link between estrogen and AD among nonsmokers, but an elevated risk among smokers.[141]

NONSTEROIDAL ANTI-INFLAMMATORY DRUGS

The recognition that acute phase inflammatory proteins are present in neuritic plaques has led to the investigation of nonsteroidal anti-inflammatory drugs (NSAIDs) for the treatment or prevention of AD.[79] In retrospective studies, people who took NSAIDs had a lower prevalence of AD when compared with nonusers.[142–145] Acetaminophen did not appear to have any protective effects.[145] Prospective pilot studies using indomethacin and diclofenac/misoprostol in patients with mild to moderate AD produced promising but inconclusive results.[146,147] Although an epidemiologic study demonstrated reduced risk for AD with NSAID use,[148] clinical trials of naproxen, rofecoxib, and celecoxib showed no effect on cognition when compared with placebo.[149,150]

MONOAMINE OXIDASE INHIBITORS

Findings of decreased central norepinephrine and increased monoamine oxidase type B (MAO-B) among patients with Alzheimer-type dementia led to the investigation of the MAO-B inhibitor, selegiline (Eldepryl), as a potential treatment.[66,151] Improvement in memory, attention, and social interaction, as well as reductions in anxiety, depression, and tension, were demonstrated in some clinical trials, although others found no significant benefit.[151–154] An investigation that evaluated selegiline and vitamin E (2,000 IU/day), alone and in combination, found that each agent independently delayed the progression of AD longer than did the combination.[155] However, concerns with vitamin E in doses >400 IU/day in individuals with cardiovascular disease has been associated with increased mortality.[156]

ALTERNATIVE MEDICINES

Extract of ginkgo biloba has been used for many years in Europe to improve memory performance. Although its mechanism is not well understood, it may function as an antioxidant and may increase cholinergic activity.[157–159] Increasing interest in alternative medicines in the United States has led many people to use the crude extract. Three published trials have evaluated EGb 761, a specific combination of constituents, as a treatment for AD. Two trials found modest improvement in memory without significant adverse effects,[158,159] whereas the third found no benefit after 24 weeks of treatment (see Chapter 3).[160]

Two factors must be considered when referring C.L. for investigational treatments. The first is the appropriateness of individual therapies for her, and the second is the likelihood that she will be able to comply with a research protocol. The most recent evidence regarding hormone replacement therapy suggests that the benefits may not outweigh the potential risks. Likewise, NSAID therapy poses significant GI, renal, and cardiovascular risks; therefore, neither should be used solely for the treatment of AD (see Chapter 43). Any decision to pursue investigational therapy should be discussed fully by C.L., her family, and her physician.

LEWY BODY DEMENTIAS

Etiology

Lewy bodies are hyaline-containing inclusion bodies typically found in people with Parkinson disease. Recently, attention has been given to distinguish DLB and PDD to help further research.[161] It is known that up to 25% of patients with dementia have Lewy bodies in the brainstem and cortex.[162] Many of these patients display extrapyramidal signs without the classic presentation of Parkinson disease.[163] The role of α-synuclein is a common biological theme in both DLB and PDD, with α-synuclein aggregates found in Lewy bodies and neurites.

Clinical Presentation

8. J.F. is a 72-year-old woman who was diagnosed with mild cognitive impairment 6 months ago. She had been increasingly forgetful and confused for about 1 year before the diagnosis. Approximately 3 months ago, J.F. and her family decided that J.F. should move in with them so she would not be left alone. Since moving in with the family, her son has noted that she seems "spaced out" at times. Some days, she appears to be very clear and not confused; other days she is very forgetful and requires assistance with daily tasks. Her daughter-in-law reported that J.F. has been unsteady on her feet at times and has fallen twice. She notes at times she moves very slowly and has difficulty initiating movement. Recently, J.F. reported seeing people coming out of the painting on the wall (a European street scene), stating that "they were walking all through the house trying to steal anything that can be hidden in a coat pocket."

At the physician visit, J.F. was found to be medically stable. Vital signs, serum chemistries, and CBC were within normal limits. Her MMSE score was 21/30. During the review of systems, J.F.'s daughter-in-law had to answer some questions because J.F. appeared either not to not hear them or to ignore them. On physical examination, she demonstrated mild cog-wheeling rigidity bilaterally, bradykinesia, and masked facies; she did not display a resting tremor. What is the most likely explanation for J.F.'s presentation?

Given her physical health, inability to live by herself because of impaired cognition, and MMSE score, J.F. meets the criteria for dementia. Her rigidity, bradykinesia, and masked facies may be consistent with early Parkinson disease (see Chapter 53). There have been revised criteria for the clinical diagnosis of DLB[164] (Table 100-8). J.F. exhibits all the central features, two core features, and the supportive feature of repeated falls. Her presentation is consistent with probable DLB versus PDD due to her temporal sequence and lack of well-established diagnosis of Parkinson disease.

Treatment

9. What is an appropriate treatment for J.F.?

To date, cholinesterase inhibitors are the only treatment strategy for the cognitive symptoms of both PDD and DLB. The largest randomized, placebo-controlled trials have used rivastigmine (up to 12 mg/day) in subjects with mild to moderate disease, and this medication has received U.S. Food and Drug Administration indication for PDD. Rivastigmine was reported to worsen tremor in 10% of the patients with PDD, yet overall there was not a statistically significant difference between groups.[161]

Levodopa/carbidopa therapy should be started to help the symptoms of Parkinsonism, yet it is important to monitor for

Table 100-8 Revised Diagnostic Criteria for Dementia with Lewy Bodies (DLB)

1. *Central features (essential for a diagnosis of possible or probable DLB):* Dementia is defined as a progressive cognitive decline that interferes with normal social or occupational function. There is prominent or persistent memory impairment usually evident with progression but not necessarily present in the early stages. Deficits on tests of attention, executive function, and visuospatial ability may be especially prominent.
2. *Core features (two core features are sufficient for diagnosis of probable DLB, one for possible DLB):* (a) Fluctuating cognition with pronounced variations in attention and alertness, (b) recurrent visual hallucinations that are typically well formed and detailed, and (c) spontaneous features of parkinsonism.
3. *Suggestive features (if one or more is present in the presence of one or more core features, a diagnosis of probable DLB can be made. In the absence of core features, one or more suggestive features are sufficient for possible DLB. Probable DLB should NOT be diagnosed on the basis of suggestive features alone):* (a) Rapid eye movement sleep behavior disorder, (b) severe neuroleptic sensitivity, and (c) low dopamine transporter uptake in basal ganglia demonstrated by single-photon emission computed tomography (SPECT) or positron emission tomography imaging (PET).
4. *Supportive features (commonly present but not proven to have diagnostic specific):* (a) Repeated falls and syncope; (b) transient, unexplained loss of consciousness; (c) severe autonomic dysfunction; (d) hallucinations in other modalities; (e) systematized delusions; (f) depression; (g) relative preservation of medial temporal lobe structures with reduced occipital activity; (h) generalized low uptake on SPECT/PET perfusion scan with reduced occipital activity; and (i) abnormal (low uptake) MIBG myocardial scintigraphy.
5. A diagnosis of DLB is less likely in the presence of cerebrovascular disease, presence of any other physical illness or brain disorder, or if Parkinsonism only appears for the first time at stage of severe dementia.
6. Need to evaluate the temporal sequence of symptoms to differentiate between DLB and Parkinson disease dementia (PDD). DLB should be diagnosed when dementia occurs before or concurrently with Parkinsonism. PDD should be used to describe dementia that occurs in the context of well-established Parkinson disease (generally the 1 year rule between the onset of dementia and Parkinsonism should be followed in the diagnosis).

Adapted from reference 164.

adverse effects such as worsening psychosis and cognition. Typical antipsychotics, such as haloperidol, may worsen her extrapyramidal symptoms (EPS) and should be avoided. Novel atypicals, namely, quetiapine and clozapine, may be less likely to exacerbate the Parkinsonism but should be instituted after a trial of a cholinesterase inhibitor or if more acute symptom control of behaviors are required.[161,164]

VASCULAR DEMENTIAS

Etiology

VaD is a broad classification of cognitive disorders caused by vascular disease. The most common cause of VaD is occlusion of cerebral blood vessels by a thrombus or embolus, leading to ischemic brain injury.[165] The term multi-infarct dementia (MID) refers specifically to the cognitive decline that follows multiple small or large cerebrovascular occlusions.[166] A number of diseases, including atherosclerosis, arteriosclerosis, and vasculitis, lead to the production of emboli and thrombi that potentially occlude brain vessels. Hemorrhagic phenomena and disorders such as hypertension or cardiac disease can produce episodes of cerebral ischemia or hypoxia and are responsible for some cases of VaD.[23,165] Specific risk factors for VaDs include advancing age, diabetes mellitus, small vessel cerebrovascular disease, hypertension, heart disease, hyperlipidemia, cigarette smoking, and alcohol use.[167–170]

Neuropathology

VaDs are typically subcortical. Most patients with MID have blockage of multiple blood vessels and infarction of the cerebral tissue supplied by those vessels. When the distribution of a large artery or medium-size arteriole is blocked, focal neurologic deficits can result (see Chapter 55). Depending on the area affected, there may be significant cognitive impairment. More often, however, a patient may have suffered transient ischemic attacks (TIAs) or multiple microinfarcts that have remained unrecognized.[171,172] Patients with subcortical VaDs often exhibit small, deep ischemic infarcts in arterioles of the basal ganglia, thalamus, and internal capsule.[6,173] A history of atherosclerosis, diabetes mellitus, or hypertension is often present without a history of stroke.[171,174,175] MRI scans can be very useful in diagnosing VaDs because areas of cerebral infarction are easier to visualize than they are with CT scanning (Fig. 100-4). Lesions in white matter may occur in as many as 85% of patients with VaD.[176] Deep white matter lesions known as leukoaraiosis often include demyelination and may represent early changes in dementia.[175,177,178] Although patients with Alzheimer-type dementia may also exhibit leukoaraiosis, it is much more prevalent in those with MIDs.[6,179] Blood flow in patients with leukoaraiosis is reduced in all brain regions except parietal white matter, especially in the putamen and

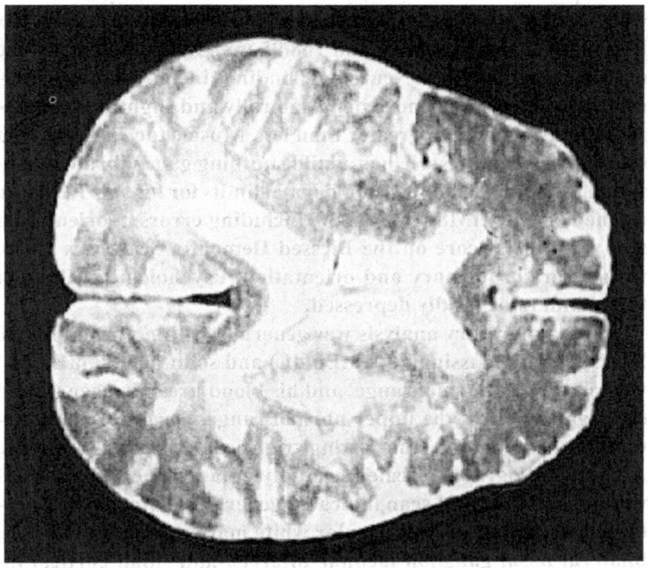

FIGURE 100-4 A large stroke is visible to the right of the ventricles. There is evidence of atrophy in the right temporal area.

thalamus.[180] Patients with long-standing uncontrolled hypertension often develop multiple leukoaraiosis lesions, leading to ischemic periventricular encephalopathy.[175] The lesions are too small to be visualized grossly but are evident on MRI scans.[165] Known as Binswanger disease, this disorder is characterized by focal neurologic deficits, emotional lability, gait disturbances, and urinary incontinence.[175,181] Patients with Binswanger disease exhibit activation of the coagulation-fibrinolysis pathway, which may lead to microthrombi and microcirculatory disturbances.[182]

VaDs typically have an earlier onset than dementia of the Alzheimer type.[95] Unlike AD, males are affected more often than females, and survival is shorter for VaD patients.[95,183]

Clinical Presentation

10. D.V., a 73-year-old man, is accompanied by his daughter for evaluation of "fuzzy thinking." Although his chief complaint is impaired memory, he denies significant impact on his daily routine. D.V. states his memory problem began 2 years ago after a dizzy spell and subsequent fall. However, his daughter states that the impairment began approximately 1 year before that episode. The memory loss has been slowly progressive. D.V. states that he feels useless because of his memory problems and his "boring" daily routine. Although D.V. is generally independent, he relies on his daughter for assistance with most financial matters. He has voluntarily quit driving because of a lack of confidence in his abilities. D.V.'s daughter reports that according to her mother, D.V. is sometimes disoriented at night when he awakens to urinate. He has no history of urinary incontinence. D.V. has a questionable history of TIAs, but no focal neurologic deficits. He has a long history of mild hypertension, which is treated with a diuretic. He drinks alcohol occasionally and smokes about half a pack of cigarettes per day. His medical history is unremarkable except for the possible TIAs, hypertension, and a mildly enlarged prostate. His family history is positive for diabetes and heart disease.

On physical examination, D.V. is found to be a mildly obese man who is well dressed and groomed, alert, and oriented to person. His BP is 160/92 mmHg sitting and 168/95 mmHg standing. Cardiac examination is normal. Neurologic findings include somewhat diminished extraocular movements laterally and slightly asymmetric reflexes, with right greater than left. Muscle tone is normal in the lower extremities. He has a mild shuffling gait. Vibratory sensation is diminished but within normal limits for his age. His score on the Folstein MMSE was 22/30, including errors in orientation and recall. His score on the Blessed Dementia Scale was 16/33, with errors in memory and orientation. Psychologic evaluation found him to be mildly depressed.

A full laboratory analysis was generally within normal limits. D.V.'s serum potassium (3.8 mEq/dL) and sodium (138 mEq/dL) were in the low normal range, and his blood urea nitrogen (BUN) (18 mg/dL) was in the upper normal range. Serum total cholesterol was 246 mg/dL, and fasting triglycerides were 230 mg/dL. A chest radiograph revealed a mildly enlarged heart; his ECG was normal. An MRI scan indicated generalized atrophy with enlarged ventricles, periventricular white matter ischemic changes, bilateral basal ganglion lacunar infarcts, and small cortical infarcts in the right parietal lobe. What subjective and objective evidence exists for a diagnosis of dementia in D.V.?

[SI units: BUN, 6.4 mmol/L of urea; total cholesterol, 6.36 mmol/L; triglycerides, 2.60 mmol/L]

D.V.'s major complaint is "fuzzy thinking" and impaired memory that he attributes to his dizzy spell and fall. However, his family began to note problems a full year before that episode, with progression over time. Although D.V. denies that his impairment significantly affects his daily routine, he has voluntarily stopped driving and relies on his daughter for assistance with financial matters. His memory difficulties appear to have affected his mood and made him feel useless. D.V. is disoriented at night when he awakens to urinate. These factors satisfy the DSM-IV criteria for interference with normal activities.[21]

Multiple deficits are present on both the Folstein MMSE[24] (orientation, recall) and on the Blessed Dementia Scale[25] (memory, orientation), indicating impaired short- and long-term memory. D.V.'s inability to drive reflects poor judgment behind the wheel of a car; a disturbance of higher cortical function is indicated by his need for assistance with financial matters. There is no evidence of a delirium being present. Evidence of an organic cause is provided by the MRI scan.

Diagnosis

11. What type of dementia does D.V. have?

There is sufficient evidence to indicate that D.V. suffers from a VaD. Although DSM-IV provides diagnostic criteria for VaD (Table 100-9), it is not clear that D.V. satisfies the requirements.[21] VaDs commonly present suddenly after a cerebrovascular insult. This is followed by a period of stability and further declines after additional episodes, in a stepwise pattern. Cognitive impairments are variable and depend on the area of the brain affected by the insult.[21]

With the exception of the dizzy spell and fall, D.V.'s deterioration has had a pattern that resembles a downhill slide rather than stepwise decline. Although his cognitive deficits

Table 100-9 *Diagnostic and Statistical Manual of Mental Disorders*, Fourth Edition, Criteria for Vascular Dementia

1. The presence of multiple cognitive deficits manifested by both
   - Impaired memory (ability to learn new information or to retrieve information previously learned)
   - At least one of the following:
     Aphasia (language difficulties)
     Apraxia (diminished ability to perform motor activities in the presence of intact motor function)
     Agnosia (inability to recognize or name objects despite intact sensory function)
     Disruption of executive function (diminished ability to plan, organize)
2. The previous deficits significantly interfere with normal work or social activities and represent a decline from previous ability to function
3. Focal neurologic deficits (e.g., hyperactive deep tendon reflexes, gait disturbances, weak extremities) or laboratory evidence indicating cerebrovascular disease (e.g., multiple infarctions of the cortex or white matter) judged to be etiologically linked to the disorder
4. The deficits do not occur exclusively during the course of a delirium

Adapted from reference 21.

are "patchy" (e.g., he appears to have no language difficulty), they are not particularly prominent. D.V. displays some neurologic signs and symptoms, including diminished extraocular movements, asymmetric reflexes, and a mild shuffling gait, but they are subtle and might be easily missed by an untrained observer as being related to a dementia. Reliance solely on the clear presence of diagnostic criteria may often lead to a missed diagnosis.[184] The Hachinski Ischemic Scale ranks signs and symptoms associated with cognitive impairment of cerebrovascular origin and is used to help differentiate between AD and MID.[185] According to this scale, D.V.'s nocturnal confusion, depression, hypertension history, and focal neurologic signs and symptoms are sufficient to indicate VaD.

D.V.'s history and clinical presentation do not suggest dementia caused by a single large stroke or several small strokes. Large strokes produce significant motor damage, typically on one side of the body (the side contralateral to the stroke). Multiple smaller strokes cause prominent motor deficits in discrete areas controlled by the affected areas. Neither of these patterns describes D.V.'s condition. However, he is clearly exhibiting signs of dementia and has significant cerebrovascular disease. He possesses several risk factors for a VaD, including hypertension, smoking, and hyperlipidemia. His MRI indicates a lacunar state, with multiple small infarcts in the deep penetrating arterioles at the base of the brain, particularly in the basal ganglia, internal capsule, thalamus, and pons (see Chapter 55). These MRI findings are consistent with D.V.'s long-standing hypertension and neurologic presentation. The absence of a significant gait disturbance and urinary incontinence argues against Binswanger disease.

Because diagnostic criteria for VaDs are vague, arriving at a specific diagnosis is difficult. Therefore, diagnostic criteria (Table 100-10) have been proposed for ischemic VaD, providing a structure for the most common type of these disorders.[165]

Table 100-10 Proposed Diagnostic Criteria for Ischemic Vascular Dementia (IVD)

Definite IVD (Requires Histopathological Examination of the Brain)

Clinical evidence of dementia

Pathological confirmation of multiple infarcts, some extracerebellar

Probable IVD

Dementia

Evidence of at least two ischemic strokes by history, neurologic signs, or neuroimaging, or a single stroke with clearly documented temporal relationship to the dementia onset

Supporting evidence of multiple infarcts in regions affecting cognition, history of transient ischemic attacks or vascular risk factors, elevated Hachinski score

Possible IVD

Dementia, plus one or more of the following:

- History or evidence of a single stroke (but not multiple strokes) without clearly documented temporal relationship to dementia onset
- Binswanger disease (without multiple strokes), including all of the following:
  - Early-onset urinary incontinence unexplained by urologic disease, or gait disturbance not explained by peripheral cause
  - Vascular risk factors
  - Extensive white matter change on neuroimaging

Adapted from reference 165.

According to this diagnostic scheme, D.V. suffers from probable ischemic VaD.

Treatment

12. How should D.V. be managed?

Several treatment options that modify risk factors for VaDs are available.

Smoking Cessation

D.V. should be counseled to stop smoking because cigarette smoking reduces cerebral blood flow and increases the risk for stroke.[186] Among smokers with MID, cessation of cigarette use improves cognitive performance.[187]

Antihypertensive Therapy

Hypertension and hyperlipidemia, both present in D.V., are additional risk factors for stroke and MID. Control of systolic hypertension reduces the risk of stroke by 36% in elderly patients,[188] and maintaining the systolic BP between 135 and 150 mmHg is associated with improved cognition among MID patients. A systolic BP that exceeds 150 mmHg indicates inadequate control, whereas a systolic BP below 135 mmHg may lead to inadequate cerebral perfusion.[187] As in nondemented individuals, nonpharmacologic treatment (e.g., diet, weight loss, exercise) is an essential component. The antihypertensive agent must be chosen carefully in this population to maximize compliance and minimize adverse reactions.[189] Both thiazide diuretics and β-adrenergic blockers may increase lipid levels, a potential complication in D.V. α-Adrenergic blockers and sympatholytic agents may cause depression or impair cognitive activity. Calcium channel blockers or angiotensin-converting enzyme (ACE) inhibitors are acceptable because they are well tolerated by elderly patients and may help preserve renal function in patients with diabetes mellitus (see Chapter 13). Dihydropyridine calcium channel blockers have been shown to improve cognition in patients with dementia[190] and reduce the risk of dementia in elderly patients with isolated systolic hypertension.[191] Because D.V. has benign prostatic hyperplasia, he may benefit from the use of an α-adrenergic blocking agent, such as doxazosin (Cardura) 1 mg at bedtime or terazosin (Hytrin) 1 mg at bedtime (see Chapter 101). Evidence indicating an increased risk for negative cardiac outcomes, however, makes the α-adrenergic blocking agents less attractive choices.[192] The use of a vasodilating calcium channel blocker, such as amlodipine 5 mg/day, is an appropriate first choice. An ACE inhibitor such as benazepril (Lotensin) 10 mg/day is an appropriate alternative. Both agents exhibit the advantage of once-daily dosing over some other agents within their respective classes. This feature is important for maximizing adherence in patients with declining memory.

Antiplatelet Therapy

Prophylaxis against future cerebrovascular events is indicated in MID, but few studies that have looked specifically at individuals with dementia are available. Cerebral perfusion and cognitive performance were improved in MID patients receiving aspirin 325 mg/day for 1 year when compared with a control population.[193] Aspirin dosages as low as 30 mg/day reduce the incidence of TIAs and are associated with fewer adverse effects than higher dosages.[194]

Other agents that affect the coagulation process include clopidogrel (Plavix), ticlopidine (Ticlid), aspirin/dipyridamole (Aggrenox), and warfarin (Coumadin). None of these agents has been evaluated specifically in people with VaDs. Guidelines from the American College of Chest Physicians recommend the use of antiplatelet therapy in patients with a history of TIA or atherothrombotic stroke that is not of cardiogenic origin. Warfarin is recommended after cardioembolic cerebral ischemic events. According to those guidelines, aspirin 25 mg/dipyridamole extended-release 200 mg twice daily is recommended as the first-line agent.[195]

Cholinesterase Inhibitors

Deficits in cholinergic transmission and nicotinic receptor binding abnormalities have been noted in VaD.[196] Early clinical trials with donepezil,[197] galantamine,[198] and rivastigmine[199] have demonstrated improvement in cognition and daily function among patients with VaD. As of yet, however, the use of these agents remains investigational and controversial.

BEHAVIORAL DISTURBANCES IN DEMENTIA

Several types of behavioral disturbances may develop during the course of a dementia, particularly during the later stages (Table 100-11).[96] The disturbances can be classified into two broad categories: psychologic behavior and nonpsychologic behavior. Psychologic behavior includes agitation and anxiety, depression, withdrawal, psychotic behaviors, and aggression. Agitation and anxiety are often managed best with nonpharmacologic treatment. Pharmacologic interventions are appropriate when nondrug therapies are unsuccessful or the behavior is severe. Nonpsychologic behaviors such as wandering, inappropriate motor activity, shouting, and incontinence respond better to environmental modification than to drug therapy.[200,201] The first step in evaluating altered behavior in patients with dementia is to ensure that the problem is not the result of an unrecognized medical problem or to an adverse effect of a medication (see Chapter 99).

Agitation

13. T.G., a 62-year-old man, has recently been diagnosed with AD, for which he takes donepezil 10 mg at bedtime. He also has hypertension that is treated with hydrochlorothiazide 12.5 mg daily and amlodipine 5 mg daily. He no longer takes his daily walks around the neighborhood because he is afraid he will get lost; instead, he follows his wife around the house as she does her daily chores. Other times, he paces throughout the house. He also expresses worry about the burden he will place on his family as his condition worsens. Recently, he has had episodes of incontinence and awakens four to five times during the night to urinate. His concerns contribute to his nighttime awakenings, making him quite tired during the day. How should T.G.'s agitation and anxiety be managed?

Agitation and anxiety are common problems in the early stages of dementia. Patients are aware of their progressive cognitive decline and have sufficient insight to understand the consequences. T.G.'s shadowing of his wife and pacing through the house are examples of agitated behavior. T.G. is exhibiting anxiety, as evidenced by his worry about placing a burden on his family. His poor sleep is due both to nocturia and anxiety.

His behaviors should first be addressed with nonpharmacologic treatments. Although T.G. has been taking hydrochlorothiazide without difficulty, he may no longer be recognizing the cues to urinate. The drug should be discontinued; if his blood pressure rises, the amlodipine dose can be increased. Shadowing and pacing are demonstrations of unfocused energy. T.G.'s wife can give him simple tasks to perform, such as drying dishes, folding laundry, or simple gardening, to help channel his energy. She also could accompany him on walks to alleviate his fear of getting lost. Appropriate strategies to manage agitated behaviors without medication are listed in Table 100-12.

When nonpharmacologic interventions are not successful in reducing problem behaviors, medications can be considered. Benzodiazepines are the most commonly used anxiolytics and will address T.G.'s insomnia and anxiety. However, they are associated with several negative outcomes in the elderly, including confusion, amnestic syndromes, ataxia, and falls.[202] Long-acting benzodiazepines are generally considered

Table 100-11 Behavior Disturbances in Dementia

Behavior	Typical Presentation	Treatment
Anxiety	Excessive worrying, sleep disturbances, rumination	Trazodone Buspirone (if no insomnia) Short-acting benzodiazepine Selective serotonin reuptake inhibitor (SSRI) antidepressant
Depression	Withdrawal, loss of appetite, irritability, restlessness, sleep disturbances	Trazodone SSRI antidepressant
General agitation	Repeated questions, wandering, pacing	Often unresponsive to medications; redirecting activity may be effective; safety-proofing the residence reduces wandering
Psychotic behaviors	Delusions (often of theft), hallucinations, misperceptions	Atypical antipsychotic, if associated with paranoid features SSRI antidepressant, if associated with withdrawal, tearfulness, themes of loss
Aggressive behaviors	Physical or verbal aggressiveness toward others, excessive yelling and screaming, manic features	Anticonvulsant, such as divalproex or carbamazepine, possibly in combination with an atypical antipsychotic

Adapted from references 200, 201, 202, 249, and 212.

Table 100-12 Nonpharmacologic Behavior Management Strategies

General strategies	Safety-proof living areas.
	Issue one-step commands for directions.
	Maintain a daily routine of activities.
	Avoid arguing incorrect statements.
	Avoid startling the patient.
	Limit unusual or overly stimulating environments.
Anxiety	Listen to and acknowledge frustrations.
	Provide reassurance.
	Engage the patient in enjoyable activities.
	Limit noise and distractions.
Aggression	Identify the precipitating cause or situation.
	Focus on the patient's feelings and concerns.
	Avoid getting angry or upset.
	Maintain a simple, pleasant, and familiar environment.
	Employ music, exercise, etc., as a calming activity.
	Shift the focus to another activity.

Adapted from references 200, 201, and 250–252.

inappropriate for geriatric patients because age-associated accumulation increases the risk of acute toxicity.[203] Benzodiazepines with short half-lives, such as lorazepam (Ativan) or oxazepam (Serax), may be used, if necessary, but only for a short term and with caution.

Trazodone is a sedative antidepressant that is effective for insomnia and agitated behaviors in patients with AD.[202,204] Treatment is started at 25 mg at bedtime (HS) and may be increased to a dose of 250 mg/day in divided doses. Another alternative treatment is buspirone, which does not cause the cognitive impairments associated with the benzodiazepines. Dosage begins at 5 mg three times daily and may be increased up to 15 mg three times daily. However, buspirone requires 3 to 4 weeks to become fully effective and will not concurrently manage T.G.'s insomnia because it has no sedative effect.[205] Citalopram has been shown to reduce agitated behaviors in people with dementia and could be used.[205]

If the nondrug strategies are ineffective in reducing T.G.'s insomnia and agitation, trazodone should be initiated at a dose of 25 mg HS. It may be increased by 25 mg/day at 5- to 7-day intervals, up to 100 mg. Doses above 100 mg/day should be split into two daily doses.

Psychosis

14. T.G.'s mental status continues to decline to the point that he requires help with bathing and dressing. During a physician visit, he accuses his wife and children of stealing from him. He also cannot locate his coin collection, which he placed in a "safe" location when his memory began to decline; during the night, he rummages through the house looking for it. He believes his family has been plotting to steal his assets and then turn him out onto the street. T.G.'s son reports that T.G. has been verbally abusive and has threatened several members of the family recently. How should T.G.'s psychotic behavior be managed?

Delusions and hallucinations are common among demented individuals. Paranoid ideation or delusions have been reported in up to half of dementia patients.[206–208] Delusions typically involve suspicion of theft by family members, which may be secondary to the patient's inability to remember where valuable items were placed and incorrectly concluding that they were stolen.[207] Another common delusion is the misidentification of people or objects. Capgras syndrome, the belief that a person has been "replaced" by an identical-looking impostor or the belief that photographs or television pictures are real individuals, may occur in almost half of demented individuals.[207,209,210]

Psychotic symptoms respond best to antipsychotic agents, although these are not highly effective, and no single antipsychotic is more effective than any other. Delusions, hallucinations, aggression, and uncooperativeness symptoms respond best, but overall improvement occurs in only about 18% of patients.[210,211]

The choice of an antipsychotic agent is determined by the symptoms displayed by the patient as well as the potential for adverse effects. First, it is important to evaluate the target symptoms to determine whether they will respond to pharmacotherapy. Then, an appropriate agent that has a relatively low risk for adverse effects can be chosen.[212] The atypical antipsychotic agents are better tolerated by older adults than are the conventional neuroleptics (see Chapter 78).[202,212,213]

T.G. is experiencing a delusion of theft, suspiciousness, and aggressive behavior. It is possible that the verbal abuse and threats are consequences of fear brought on by the false belief that his family is stealing from him and plans to abandon him. The delusions and suspiciousness may respond to the use of an antipsychotic agent, which may then diminish his aggression as well.

T.G. has no major contraindications to the use of any antipsychotic agent, and his target symptoms will probably respond to any of the available agents. Therefore, the choice can be made according to which antipsychotic agent is least likely to cause intolerable adverse effects. Risperidone has been evaluated in a case series and in a large double-blind, placebo-controlled trial.[214,215] In the case study series, symptoms improved in half of the patients taking dosages ranging from 0.5 mg every other day to 3 mg twice daily. However, 50% also experienced EPS, even at the lowest dosage used.[214] Subjects in the double-blind trial received either placebo or risperidone at dosages of 0.5 mg/day, 1 mg/day, or 2 mg/day for 12 weeks. Daily doses of 1 or 2 mg reduced psychosis and improved behavior, but extrapyramidal symptoms (EPS) and somnolence were common adverse effects.[215] Low doses of olanzapine, 5 to 15 mg/day, were superior to placebo for reducing agitation, aggression, and psychosis during a 6-week study among nursing facility residents.[216] Somnolence and gait disturbances were the most common adverse effects. Quetiapine has been shown to reduce agitated and psychotic behaviors at doses of 100 to 200 mg/day.[217] Clozapine poses significant toxicity risks and requires careful monitoring.[212] Significant concerns exist regarding marginal benefit with an increased risk for serious adverse effects, including stroke and mortality among patients with dementia who take either conventional or atypical antipsychotics.[218–220] Because T.G. does not have cardiovascular or cerebrovascular risk factors and does not have gait or balance problems, either risperidone 0.25 mg HS or quetiapine 25 mg HS can be initiated. Doses of risperidone may be increased by 0.25 mg/day in weekly intervals, up to 2 mg/day; quetiapine doses can be increased by 25 mg/day, up to 200 mg/day in divided doses. Once his behavior has stabilized, the medication should be continued for about 3 months. At that time, the dose should be decreased in weekly intervals to determine whether the medication is still required. T.G. should be monitored closely for adverse effects, including EPS, which can occur with the atypical antipsychotics.[212,221]

Aggressive Behaviors

15. After 3 months, T.G.'s delusions have subsided, but he continues to be verbally abusive and often displays angry, emotional outbursts, especially when he requires help with bathing or toileting. At other times, he is withdrawn and apathetic. He has also been found wandering in the neighborhood on three occasions. These behaviors persist despite treatment with quetiapine 100 mg twice daily. What alternative treatments can be attempted?

Although psychotic symptoms respond to antipsychotic agents, many other behaviors do not. More than 80% of patients with dementia exhibit at least one disruptive behavior such as angry outbursts, screaming, and abusive language, and more than 50% display multiple aggressive behaviors.[206,222,223] About 21% display assaultive or violent behavior.[206] Such behaviors are typically directed at caregivers, precipitated by receipt of assistance with activities of daily living such as bathing and toileting, and increase in frequency with dementia severity.[206,222,224] Several of these behaviors may be merely defensive responses to perceived threats in cognitively impaired individuals.[224] Behavioral disturbances must be addressed because they can have a negative effect on the patient's ability to perform activities of daily living.[225]

Some behaviors exhibited by T.G. are not likely to respond to medications. Wandering is typically unaltered by the use of medications unless the patient is oversedated. Nonpharmacologic treatments, such as periods of physical exercise and rest, or environmental modification are much more effective.[201,226] T.G.'s reactions to assistance with bathing and toileting may be caused by confusion and fear. Breaking the tasks down to step-by-step procedures, accomplished individually, often helps modify aggressive behaviors.[226]

Verbal abuse and aggressiveness place both the patient and the caregiver at risk for injury. Anticonvulsant agents have been shown to reduce rage and aggressive behaviors in patients resistant to treatment with antipsychotics.[227] Carbamazepine and valproic acid (including divalproex) are the most well-studied agents.[228,229] Carbamazepine (Tegretol) 200 to 1,000 mg/day, titrated to a serum level of 5 to 8 mcg/mL, reduces severe agitation in dementia patients.[228–230] Significant adverse effects include dizziness, drowsiness, ataxia, and agranulocytosis. Patients should be monitored for CNS effects (e.g., increased confusion, daytime drowsiness) and require baseline and periodic CBCs with differentials. Carbamazepine also induces hepatic microsomal enzymes, causing more rapid metabolism of several drugs.

Valproic acid and divalproex, alone and in combination with an antipsychotic, are also effective in managing acute aggressive behaviors.[231–233] Common adverse effects are nausea, vomiting, and dizziness. They do not produce blood dyscrasias and are subject to fewer drug interactions than carbamazepine.[201] This makes these agents a better choice for the treatment of T.G.'s symptoms, and they may be added to his quetiapine treatment unless his symptoms are determined to be caused by depression (see the following). The initial dosage of divalproex should be 125 mg/day; it may be increased by 125 mg/day every 3 to 6 days until the behavior improves or until a maximum therapeutic serum level is reached.[227] When his behavior has stabilized, the quetiapine dose should be reduced, and if T.G.'s psychotic symptoms do not recur, the drug may be discontinued. Likewise, divalproex treatment should be re-evaluated after 2 to 3 months.

Depression

16. How should T.G.'s social withdrawal and apathy be treated?

Depression often accompanies dementia and may significantly impair a patient's functional capacity, cognitive abilities, and communication.[234,235] T.G. is withdrawn and apathetic, symptoms suggestive of depression. Screaming and irritability are also believed to be a symptom of depression in individuals with dementia, perhaps reflecting feelings of loneliness, boredom, or the need for attention.[222,236] Because a definite diagnosis of depression relies heavily on a patient interview and response to questions, a formal diagnosis in patients with dementia is difficult, if not impossible. Therefore, one must rely on patient observation to make a clinical evaluation.

The selective serotonin reuptake inhibitors have not been well studied in patients with dementia, but are effective antidepressants with adverse effects that are better tolerated than those of the tricyclic antidepressants. Sertraline, in doses of 50 to 150 mg/day, was superior to placebo in reducing depression in AD patients during a 12-week trial.[237] Citalopram has also demonstrated effectiveness in small trials; in contrast, fluoxetine and fluvoxamine have not demonstrated benefit.[202]

Trazodone (Desyrel) reduces disruptive and aggressive behaviors in cognitively impaired patients and thus is a reasonable choice for treatment of depression in T.G.[201,238,239] This drug is sedating, may help with sleep disorders, and is free of anticholinergic effects. It does, however, possess α-adrenergic blocking activity, which may cause orthostasis. If it is determined that T.G. is depressed, trazodone may be initiated at 50 mg HS and increased to 100 mg HS after several days. If necessary, dosages for T.G. can be increased by 50 mg/day every 5 to 7 days. If further dosage increases are needed, the total daily dose should be divided into two or three doses up to a maximum daily dose of 300 mg.[201] The trazodone should induce a restful sleep at night, increase T.G.'s sociability, and decrease his abusive behaviors. If he does not respond to trazodone, either sertraline 50 mg/day or citalopram 10 mg/day may be tried. Dosages may be increased weekly up to a maximum of 150 mg/day or 40 mg/day, respectively.

Social Support

17. T.G.'s family indicates that caring for him at home has become so burdensome that they are considering placing him in an institution. What social support services are available to families facing this decision?

Institutionalization is a typical outcome for patients in the late stages of dementia. The total care required to manage a dementia patient usually becomes unmanageable for most families as the disease progresses. Caregiver stress is often exacerbated by the patient's declining memory, inability to communicate, physical decline, and incontinence, as well as the caregiver's loss of freedom and depression.[240] Caregivers commonly experience anger, helplessness, guilt, and worry, and suffer from physical stressors such as fatigue and illness.[226]

Outside assistance is essential to families caring for a patient with dementia. Families should be referred to the Alzheimer's Association as soon as a diagnosis of dementia is received. The association has local affiliates in most major cities. The book *The 36-Hour Day* is a valuable resource for families as well.[226] It describes the symptoms, behaviors, and problems that can be encountered when caring for a patient with dementia.

Support groups, individual and family counseling, and other sources of support are useful and may help families cope for a longer period.[241] However, the key intervention to reduce caregiver stress is respite care, which allows a family time away from the responsibilities of taking care of a frail individual.[242] Respite care brings a person into the home or allows the patient to go to a day care center or similar environment on a regular schedule. Such programs may delay the need to institutionalize a patient.

PSEUDODEMENTIA

Clinical Presentation and Diagnosis

18. G.Y., an 86-year-old woman, lives alone in a low-income housing unit. Over the past 6 weeks, she has become disoriented and confused. A neighbor brought her to the hospital after finding her wandering through the neighborhood in her nightclothes. She eats only one meal a day—a frozen pot pie—because she generally forgets to eat her other meals. Several bills remain unpaid. She has difficulty sleeping and expresses little desire to live because "all my friends are gone." Her score on the Folstein MMSE is 18/30 with multiple deficits. Most errors are attributable to answers of "I don't know" or "I can't." She currently takes propranolol 40 mg three times daily for high BP, cimetidine 400 mg twice daily for gastroesophageal reflux disease, and temazepam 15 mg HS PRN for insomnia. What subjective and objective data support a diagnosis of pseudodementia in G.Y.?

Depression

G.Y. clearly exhibits cognitive impairment as evidenced by her symptoms of confusion and disorientation, forgetting to eat, wandering, and a low score on the Folstein MMSE.[24] However, the rapid course of her decline, her lack of effort on mental status testing, and the medications she is taking suggest that her impairment might be secondary to causes other than true dementia.[243]

Depression is the most common cause of pseudodementia, accounting for at least 50% of cases. Depressive symptoms in G.Y. include self-neglect, insomnia, loss of desire to live, and lack of effort on mental status testing. When given a mental status screening test, depressed patients tend to give "I don't know" answers, which reflect dysphoria or an inability to cooperate, whereas demented patients typically provide incorrect answers.[243]

Medications

Medications are often responsible for cognitive impairment in older adults, accounting for dementia symptoms in approximately 12% of patients with cognitive impairment. Psychotropic medications, analgesics, antihypertensives, corticosteroids, and cimetidine are often implicated (see Chapter 79).[23,203,244]

Treatment

19. What is the proper treatment for G.Y.'s pseudodementia?

Initial therapy should consist of the discontinuation of her medications, all of which may be contributing to her cognitive decline. Because the medications are relatively short acting, her mental status should improve significantly within 48 hours. At that time, her hypertension and gastroesophageal reflux disease can be re-evaluated and more appropriate therapy instituted, if warranted.

G.Y. should be evaluated for depression, and psychotherapy should be initiated if she is in fact depressed. She should also be referred to a social services agency or senior center to provide her with assistance and to offer her opportunities for social interaction.

REFERENCES

1. Jorm AF, Jolley D. The incidence of dementia: a meta-analysis. *Neurology* 1998;51:728.
2. Brookmeyer R et al. Projections of Alzheimer's disease in the United States and the public health impact of delaying onset. *Am J Public Health* 1998;88:1337.
3. Dickson DW. Neuropathology of Alzheimer's disease and other dementias. *Clin Geriatr Med* 2001;17:209.
4. Knopman DS. An overview of common non-Alzheimer dementias. *Clin Geriatr Med* 2001;17:281.
5. Minino A et al. Deaths: Preliminary Data for 2004. *National Vital Statistics Reports*. Hyattsville, MD: National Center for Health Statistics; 2006.
6. Cummings J et al. Reversible dementia: illustrative cases, definition, and review. *JAMA* 1980;243:2434.
7. Ineichen B. Measuring the rising tide: how many dementia cases will there be by 2001? *Br J Psychiatry* 1987;150:193.
8. Larson EB. Alzheimer's disease in the community [editorial]. *JAMA* 1989;262:2591.
9. Henderson AS. The epidemiology of Alzheimer's disease. *Br Med Bull* 1986;42:3.
10. Kokmen E et al. Prevalence of medically diagnosed dementia in a defined United States population: Rochester, Minnesota, January 1, 1975. *Neurology* 1989;39:773.
11. Weissman MM et al. Psychiatric disorders (DSM-III) and cognitive impairment among the elderly in a U.S. urban community. *Acta Psychiatr Scand* 1985;77:366.
12. Rocca WA et al. Frequency and distribution of Alzheimer's disease in Europe: a collaborative study of 1980–1990 prevalence findings. *Ann Neurol* 1991;30:381.
13. Evans DA et al. Prevalence of Alzheimer's disease in a community of older persons: higher than previously reported. *JAMA* 1989;262:2551.
14. Wernicke TF, Reischies FM. Prevalence of dementia in old age: clinical diagnoses in subjects aged 95 years and older. *Neurology* 1994;44:250.
15. Rocca WA et al. Incidence of dementia and Alzheimer's disease. *Am J Epidemiol* 1998;148:51.
16. Gao S et al. The relationship between age, sex and the incidence of dementia and Alzheimer's disease. *Arch Gen Psychiatry* 1998;55:809.
17. Brookmeyer R et al. Survival following a diagnosis of Alzheimer disease. *Arch Neurol* 2002;59:1764.
18. Ernst RL, Hay JW. The U.S. economic and social costs of Alzheimer's disease revisited. *Am J Public Health* 1994;84:1261.
19. Gutterman EM et al. Cost of Alzheimer's disease and related dementia in managed-Medicare. *J Am Geriatr Soc* 1999;47:1065.
20. Anonymous. Alzheimer's Disease Facts and Figures 2007. Chicago: Alzheimer's Association; 2007.
21. American Psychiatric Association (APA). *Diagnostic and Statistical Manual of Mental Disorders*. 4th ed. Washington, DC: APA; 1994.
22. Costa PT Jr et al. Recognition and Initial Assessment of Alzheimer's Disease and Related Dementias. Clinical Practice Guideline No. 19. AHCPR Publication No. 97-0702. Rockville, MD: US DHHS, PHS, AHCPR; November 1996.
23. Small GW et al. Diagnosis and treatment of

Alzheimer disease and related disorders. *JAMA* 1997;278:1363.
24. Folstein MF et al. "Mini-mental state": a practical method for grading the mental state of patients for the clinician. *J Psychiatr Res* 1975;12:189.
25. Blessed G et al. The association between quantitative measures of dementia and of senile change in the cerebral grey matter of elderly subjects. *Br J Psychiatry* 1968;114:797.
26. Geldmacher DS. Differential diagnosis of dementia syndromes. *Clin Geriatr Med* 2004;20:27.
27. Shore D et al. Serum aluminum in primary degenerative dementia. *Biol Psychiatry* 1980;15:971.
28. Markesbery WR et al. Instrumental neutron activation analysis of brain aluminum in Alzheimer disease and aging. *Ann Neurol* 1981;10:511.
29. Good PF et al. Selective accumulation of aluminum and iron in the neurofibrillary tangles of Alzheimer's disease: a laser microprobe (LAMMA) study. *Ann Neurol* 1992;31:286.
30. Glenner GG. The pathobiology of Alzheimer's disease. *Ann Rev Med* 1989;40:45.
31. Selkoe DJ. Alzheimer's disease: insights into an emerging epidemic. *J Geriatr Psychiatry* 1992;25:211.
32. Edwards JK et al. Are there clinical and epidemiological differences between familial and nonfamilial Alzheimer's disease? *J Am Geriatr Soc* 1991;39:477.
33. Rocca WA et al. Maternal age and Alzheimer's disease: a collaborative re-analysis of case-control studies. *Int J Epidemiol* 1991;20:S21.
34. Chandra V et al. Head trauma with loss of consciousness as a risk factor for Alzheimer's disease. *Neurology* 1989;39:1576.
35. Mortimer JA et al. Head trauma as a risk factor for Alzheimer's disease: a collaborative re-analysis of case-control studies. *Int J Epidemiol* 1991;20:S28.
36. Graves AB et al. Head circumference as a measure of cognitive reserve: association with severity of impairment in Alzheimer's disease. *Br J Psychiatry* 1996;169:86.
37. Mori E et al. Premorbid brain size as a determinant of reserve capacity against intellectual decline in Alzheimer's disease. *Am J Psychiatry* 1997;154:18.
38. Snowden DA et al. Linguistic ability in early life and cognitive function and Alzheimer's disease in late life. *JAMA* 1996;275:528.
39. Cummings JL et al. Alzheimer's disease: etiologies, pathophysiology, cognitive reserve, and treatment opportunities. *Neurology* 1998;51(Suppl 1):S2.
40. Huff FJ et al. Risk of dementia in relatives of patients with Alzheimer's disease. *Neurology* 1988;38:786.
41. Farrer LA et al. Assessment of genetic risk for Alzheimer's disease among first-degree relatives. *Ann Neurol* 1989;25:485.
42. Hoffman A et al. History of dementia and Parkinson's disease in 1st-degree relatives of patients with Alzheimer's disease. *Neurology* 1989;39:1589.
43. Farrer LA et al. Transmission and age-at-onset patterns in familial Alzheimer's disease: evidence for heterogeneity. *Neurology* 1990;40:395.
44. Chui HC et al. Clinical subtypes of dementia of the Alzheimer type. *Neurology* 1985;35:1544.
45. Van Duijn CM et al. Familial aggregation of Alzheimer's disease and related disorders: a collaborative re-analysis of case-control studies. *Int J Epidemiol* 1991;20:S13.
46. Luchins DJ et al. Are there clinical differences between familial and nonfamilial Alzheimer's disease? *Am J Psychiatry* 1992;149:1023.
47. Devi G et al. Validity of family history for the diagnosis of dementia among siblings of patients with late-onset Alzheimer's disease. *Gen Epidemiol* 1998;15:215.
48. Hayashi Y et al. Evidence for presenilin-1 involvement in amyloid angiopathy in the Alzheimer's disease-affected brain. *Brain Res* 1998;789:307.
49. St. George-Hyslop PH et al. The genetic defect causing familial Alzheimer's disease maps on chromosome 21. *Science* 1987;235:885.
50. Lai F, Williams RS. A prospective study of Alzheimer disease in Down syndrome. *Arch Neurol* 1989;46:849.
51. Mann DMA et al. Amyloid β protein (Aβ) deposition in chromosome 14-linked Alzheimer's disease: predominance of A–42(43). *Ann Neurol* 1996;40:149.
52. Levy-Lahad E et al. Candidate gene for the chromosome 1 familial Alzheimer's disease locus. *Science* 1995;269:973.
53. Creasey H et al. Monozygotic twins discordant for Alzheimer's disease. *Neurology* 1989;39:1474.
54. Whitehouse PJ. Genesis of Alzheimer's disease. *Neurology* 1997;48(Suppl 7):S2.
55. Joachim CL, Selkoe DJ. The seminal role of β-amyloid in the pathogenesis of Alzheimer's disease. *Alzheimer Dis Assoc Disord* 1992;6:7.
56. Murrell J et al. A mutation in the amyloid precursor protein associated with hereditary Alzheimer's disease. *Science* 1991;254:97.
57. Gustafson L et al. A 50-year perspective of a family with chromosome-14–linked Alzheimer's disease. *Hum Genet* 1998;102:253.
58. Poirier J et al. Apolipoprotein E4 allele as a predictor of cholinergic deficits and treatment outcome in Alzheimer disease. *Proc Natl Acad Sci USA* 1995;92:12260.
59. Corder EH et al. Gene dose of apolipoprotein E type 4 allele and the risk of Alzheimer's disease in late onset families. *Science* 1993;261:921.
60. Farrer LA et al. Effects of age, sex, and ethnicity on the association between apolipoprotein E genotype and Alzheimer's disease. *JAMA* 1997;278:1349.
61. O'Hara R et al. The ApoE e4 allele is associated with decline on delayed recall performance in community-dwelling older adults. *J Am Geriatr Soc* 1998;46:1493.
62. Caselli RJ et al. Preclinical memory decline in cognitively normal apolipoprotein E-e4 homozygotes. *Neurology* 1999;53:201.
63. Glenner GG. Current knowledge of amyloid deposits as applied to senile plaques and congophilic angiopathy. In: Katzman R et al, eds. *Alzheimer's Disease, Senile Dementia and Related Disorders*. New York: Raven Press; 1978:493.
64. Chui HC. The significance of clinically defined subgroups of Alzheimer's disease. *J Neural Transm* 1987;24(Suppl):57.
65. Poirier J, Finch CE. Neurochemistry of the aging human brain. In: Hazzard WR et al., eds. *Principles of Geriatric Medicine and Gerontology*. New York: McGraw-Hill; 1990:905.
66. Bondareff W et al. Loss of neurons of origin of the adrenergic projection to cerebral cortex (nucleus locus ceruleus) in senile dementia. *Neurology* 1982;32:164.
67. Khachaturian ZS. Diagnosis of Alzheimer's disease. *Arch Neurol* 1985;42:1097.
68. Grundke-Iqbal I et al. Abnormal phosphorylation of the microtubule-associated protein tau in Alzheimer cytoskeletal pathology. *Proc Natl Acad Sci USA* 1986;83:4913.
69. Lee VMY et al. A68: a major subunit of paired helical filaments and derivatized forms of normal tau. *Nature* 1991;251:675.
70. Tabaton M et al. The widespread alteration of neurites in Alzheimer's disease may be unrelated to amyloid deposition. *Ann Neurol* 1989;26:771.
71. McKee AC et al. Neuritic pathology and dementia in Alzheimer's disease. *Ann Neurol* 1991;30:156.
72. Samuel WA et al. Severity of dementia in Alzheimer disease and neurofibrillary tangles in multiple brain regions. *Alzheimer Dis Assoc Disord* 1991;5:1.
73. Bugiani O et al. Preamyloid deposits, amyloid deposits, and senile plaques in Alzheimer's disease, Down syndrome, and aging. *Ann NY Acad Sci* 1991;640:122.
74. Mann DM. Neuropathology of Alzheimer's disease: towards an understanding of the pathogenesis. *Biochem Soc Trans* 1989;17:73.
75. Lassman H et al. Synaptic pathology of Alzheimer's disease. *Ann NY Acad Sci* 1993;695:59.
76. Beyreuther K et al. Mechanisms of amyloid deposition in Alzheimer's disease. *Ann NY Acad Sci* 1991;640:129.
77. Arai H et al. Expression patterns of β-amyloid precursor protein (β-APP) in neural and nonneural human tissues from Alzheimer's disease and control subjects. *Ann Neurol* 1991;30:686.
78. Haass C et al. Normal cellular processing of the β-amyloid precursor protein results in the secretion of the amyloid β peptide and related molecules. *Ann NY Acad Sci* 1993;695:109.
79. Aisen PS. Inflammation and Alzheimer's disease: mechanisms and therapeutic strategies. *Gerontology* 1997;43:143.
80. Coyle JT et al. Alzheimer's disease: a disorder of cortical cholinergic innervation. *Science* 1983;219:1184.
81. Rumble BR et al. Amyloid A4 protein and its precursor in Down's syndrome and Alzheimer's disease. *N Engl J Med* 1989;320:1446.
82. Davies LB et al. A4 amyloid protein deposition and the diagnosis of Alzheimer's disease: prevalence in aged brains determined by immunocytochemistry compared with conventional neuropathologic techniques. *Neurology* 1988;38:1688.
83. Joachim CL et al. Amyloid β-protein deposition in tissues other than brain in Alzheimer's disease. *Nature* 1989;341:226.
84. Whitehouse PJ et al. Alzheimer's disease and senile dementia: loss of neurons in the basal forebrain. *Science* 1982;215:1237.
85. Whitehouse PJ et al. Alzheimer disease: evidence for selective loss of cholinergic neurons in the nucleus basalis. *Ann Neurol* 1981;10:122.
86. Weinberger DR et al. The distribution of cerebral muscarinic acetylcholine receptors in vivo in patients with dementia. *Arch Neurol* 1991;48:169.
87. Schroder H et al. Cellular distribution and expression of cortical acetylcholine receptors in aging and Alzheimer's disease. *Ann NY Acad Sci* 1991;640:189.
88. Ladner CJ, Lee JM. Pharmacological drug treatment of Alzheimer disease: the cholinergic hypothesis revisited. *J Neuropathol Exp Neurol* 1998;57:719.
89. Terry RD et al. Physical basis of cognitive alterations in Alzheimer's disease: synapse loss is the major correlate of cognitive impairment. *Ann Neurol* 1991;30:572.
90. Krall WJ et al. Cholinesterase inhibitors: a therapeutic strategy for Alzheimer's disease. *Ann Pharmacother* 1999;33:441.
91. Nemeroff CB et al. Recent advances in the neurochemical pathology of Alzheimer's disease. *Ann NY Acad Sci* 1991;640:193.
92. McKhann G et al. Clinical diagnosis of Alzheimer's disease: report of the NINCDS-ADRDA Work Group, Department of Health and Human Services Task Force on Alzheimer's Disease. *Neurology* 1984;34:939.
93. The Ronald and Nancy Reagan Research Institute of the Alzheimer's Association and the National Institute on Aging Working Group. Consensus report of the Working Group on: Molecular and biochemical markers of Alzheimer's disease. *Neurobiol Aging* 1998;19:109.
94. Farlow MR. Alzheimer's disease: clinical implications of the apolipoprotein E genotype. *Neurology* 1997;48(Suppl 6):S30.
95. Barclay LL et al. Survival in Alzheimer's disease and vascular dementias. *Neurology* 1985;35:834.
96. Riesberg B et al. The global deterioration scale for assessment of primary degenerative dementia. *Am J Psychiatry* 1982;139:1136.
97. Hughes CP et al. A new clinical scale for the staging of dementia. *Br J Psychiatry* 1982;140:566.
98. Morris JC. Clinical and neuropathological findings from CERAD. In: Becker R, Giacobini E, eds. *Alzheimer Disease: From Molecular Biology to Therapy*. Boston: Birkhauser; 1996:7.
99. Ernst RL et al. Cognitive function and the cost of Alzheimer's disease. *Arch Neurol* 1997;54:687.
100. Gwyther LP. Social issues of the Alzheimer's

disease patient and family. *Am J Med* 1998; 104:17S.
101. Finucane TE et al. Tube feeding in patients with advanced dementia: a review of the evidence. *JAMA* 1999;282:1365.
102. Schneider LS. Treatment of Alzheimer's disease with cholinesterase inhibitors. *Clin Geriatr Med* 2001;17:337.
103. Brinton RD, Yamazaki RS. Advances and challenges in the prevention and treatment of Alzheimer's disease. *Pharmaceut Res* 1998;15:386.
104. Crismon ML. Pharmacokinetics and drug interactions of cholinesterase inhibitors administered in Alzheimer's disease. *Pharmacotherapy* 1998;18:47S.
105. Farlow M et al. A controlled trial of tacrine in Alzheimer's disease. *JAMA* 1992;268:2523.
106. Watkins PB et al. Hepatotoxic effects of tacrine administration in patients with Alzheimer's disease. *JAMA* 1994;271:992.
107. Mihara M et al. Pharmacokinetics of E2020, a new compound for Alzheimer's disease, in healthy male volunteers. *Int J Clin Pharmacol Ther Toxicol* 1993;31:223.
108. Rho JP, Lipson LG. Focus on donepezil. *Formulary* 1997;32:677.
109. Rogers SL et al. Donepezil improves cognition and global function in Alzheimer's disease. *Arch Intern Med* 1998;158:1021.
110. Rosen WG et al. A new rating scale for Alzheimer's disease. *Am J Psychiatry* 1984;141:1356.
111. Knopman DS et al. The clinician interview-based impression (CIBI): a clinician's global change rating scale in Alzheimer's disease. *Neurology* 1994;44:2315.
112. Rogers SL et al. A 24-week, double-blind, placebo-controlled trial of donepezil in patients with Alzheimer's disease. *Neurology* 1998;50:136.
113. Doody RS et al. Open-label, multicenter, phase 3 extension study of the safety and efficacy of donepezil in patients with Alzheimer disease. *Arch Neurol* 2001;58:427.
114. Winblad B et al. Donepezil in patients with severe Alzheimer's disease: double-blind, parallel-group, placebo-controlled study. *Lancet* 2006;367:1057.
115. Cutler NR et al. Dose-dependent CSF acetylcholinesterase inhibition by SDZ ENA 713 in Alzheimer's disease. *Acta Neurol Scand* 1998;97:244.
116. Polinsky RJ. Clinical pharmacology of rivastigmine: a new-generation acetylcholinesterase inhibitor for the treatment of Alzheimer's disease. *Clin Ther* 1998;20:634.
117. Anand R et al. Clinical development of Exelon (ENA-713): the ADENA programme. *J Drug Dev Clin Pract* 1996;8:117.
118. Corey-Bloom J et al. A randomized trial evaluating the efficacy and safety of ENA 713 (rivastigmine tartrate), a new acetylcholinesterase inhibitor, in patients with mild to moderately severe Alzheimer's disease. *Int J Geriatr Psychopharmacol* 1998;1:55.
119. Rösler M et al. Efficacy and safety of rivastigmine in patients with Alzheimer's disease: international randomized controlled trial. *BMJ* 1999;318:633.
120. Farlow M et al. A 52-week study of the efficacy of rivastigmine in patients with mild to moderately severe Alzheimer's disease. *Eur Neurol* 2000;44:236.
121. Williams BR et al. A review of rivastigmine. *Clin Ther* 2003;25:1634.
122. Maelicke A et al. Allosteric sensitization of nicotinic receptors by galantamine, a new treatment strategy for Alzheimer's disease. *Biol Psychiatry* 2001;49:279.
123. Mihailova D et al. Pharmacokinetics of galanthamine hydrobromide after single subcutaneous and oral dosage in humans. *Pharmacology* 1989;39:50.
124. Scott LJ, Goa KL. Galantamine: a review of its use in Alzheimer's disease. *Drugs* 2000;60:1095.
125. Tariot PN et al. A 5-month, randomized, placebo-controlled trial of galantamine in AD. *Neurology* 2000;54:2269.
126. Wilcock GK et al. Efficacy and safety of galantamine in patients with mild to moderate Alzheimer's disease: multicentre randomized controlled trial. *BMJ* 2000;321:1.
127. Raskind MA et al. Galantamine in AD: a 6-month randomized, placebo-controlled trial with a 6-month extension. *Neurology* 2000;54:2261.
128. Birks J. Cholinesterase inhibitors for Alzheimer's disease. *Cochrane Database Syst Rev* 2006:1.
129. Kaduszkiewicz H. Cholinesterase inhibitors for patients with Alzheimer's disease: systematic review of the literature. *BMJ* 2005;331:321.
130. Becker M et al. The effect of cholinesterase inhibitors on risk of nursing home placement among Medicaid beneficiaries with dementia. *Alzheimer Dis Assoc Disord* 2006;20:147.
131. Cacabelos R et al. The glutamatergic system and neurodegeneration in dementia: preventive strategies in Alzheimer's disease. *Int J Geriatr Psychiatry* 1999;14:3.
132. Jarvis B, Figgitt DP. Memantine. *Drugs Aging* 2003;20:406.
133. Winblad B et al. Memantine in severe dementia: results of the M-BEST study (benefit and efficacy in severely demented patients during treatment with memantine). *Int J Geriatr Psychiatry* 1999;14:135.
134. McShane R et al. Memantine for dementia. *Cochrane Database Syst Rev* 2006;2.
135. Reisberg B et al. Memantine in moderate-to-severe Alzheimer's disease. *N Engl J Med* 2003;348:1333.
136. Farlow MR et al. Memantine/donepezil dual therapy is superior to placebo/donepezil for treatment of moderate to severe Alzheimer's disease [abstract]. *Neurology* 2003;60(Suppl 1):A412.
137. Namenda package insert. St. Louis, MO: Forest Labs, Inc.; 2005.
138. Birge SJ. The role of estrogen in the treatment of Alzheimer's disease. *Neurology* 1997;48(Suppl 7):S36.
139. Robinson D et al. Estrogen replacement therapy and memory in older women. *J Am Geriatr Soc* 1994;42:919.
140. Yaffe K et al. Estrogen therapy in postmenopausal women: effects on cognitive function and dementia. *JAMA* 1998;279:688.
141. Roberts RO et al. Postmenopausal estrogen therapy and Alzheimer's disease: overall negative findings. *Alzheimer Dis Assoc Disord* 2006;20:141.
142. Breitner JCS et al. Inverse association of anti-inflammatory treatments and Alzheimer's disease: initial results of a co-twin control study. *Neurology* 1994;44:227.
143. Anderson K et al. Do nonsteroidal anti-inflammatory drugs decrease the risk for Alzheimer's disease? *Neurology* 1995;45:1441.
144. Rich JB et al. Nonsteroidal anti-inflammatory drugs in Alzheimer's disease. *Neurology* 1995; 45:51.
145. Stewart WF et al. Risk of Alzheimer's disease and duration of NSAID use. *Neurology* 1997;48:626.
146. Rogers J et al. Clinical trial of indomethacin in Alzheimer's disease. *Neurology* 1993;43:1609.
147. Scharf S et al. A double-blind, placebo-controlled trial of diclofenac/misoprostol in Alzheimer's disease. *Neurology* 1999;53:197.
148. in t'Veld BA et al. Nonsteroidal antiinflammatory drugs and the risk of Alzheimer's disease. *N Engl J Med* 2001;345:1515.
149. Aisen PS et al. Effects of rofecoxib or naproxen vs. placebo in Alzheimer disease progression. *JAMA* 2003;289:2819.
150. Soininen H et al. Long-term safety and efficacy of celecoxib in Alzheimer's disease. *Dement Geriatr Cogn Disord* 2007;23:8.
151. Tariot PN et al. L-deprenyl in Alzheimer's disease. *Arch Gen Psychiatry* 1987;44:427.
152. Piccinin GL et al. Neuropsychological effects of L-deprenyl in Alzheimer's type dementia. *Clin Neuropharmacol* 1990;13:147.
153. Burke WJ et al. L-deprenyl in the treatment of mild dementia of the Alzheimer type: results of a 15-month trial. *J Am Geriatr Soc* 1993;41:1219.
154. Freedman M et al. L-deprenyl in Alzheimer's disease. *Neurology* 1998;50:660.
155. Schneider LS et al. A double-blind crossover pilot study of L-deprenyl (selegiline) combined with cholinesterase inhibitor in Alzheimer's disease. *Am J Psychiatry* 1993;150:321.
156. Miller ER et al. Meta-analysis: high-dosage vitamin E supplementation may increase all-cause mortality. *Ann Intern Med* 2005;142:1.
157. Tyler V. Herbs of Choice: The Therapeutic Use of Phytomedicinals. New York: Pharmaceutical Products Press; 1994.
158. Le Bars PL et al. A placebo-controlled, double-blind, randomized trial of an extract of *Ginkgo biloba* for dementia. *JAMA* 1997;278:1327.
159. Maurer K et al. Clinical efficacy of *Ginkgo biloba* special extract EGb 761 in dementia of the Alzheimer type. *J Psychiatric Res* 1997;31:645.
160. van Dongen MCJM et al. The efficacy of *Ginkgo* for elderly people with dementia and age-associated memory impairment: new results of a randomized clinical trial. *J Am Geriatric Soc* 2000;48:1183.
161. Lippa CF et al. DLB and PDD boundary issues. Diagnosis, treatment, molecular pathology and biomarkers. *Neurology* 2007;68:812.
162. McKeith IG et al. Consensus guidelines for the clinical and pathological diagnosis of dementia with Lewy bodies (DLB): report of the consortium on DLB international workshop. *Neurology* 1996;47:1113.
163. Knopman DS. An overview of common non-Alzheimer dementias. *Clin Geriatr Med* 2001;17: 281.
164. McKeith IG et al. Diagnosis and management of dementia with Lewy Bodies: third report of the DLB consortium. *Neurology* 2005;65:1863.
165. Chui HC et al. Criteria for the diagnosis of ischemic vascular dementia proposed by the State of California Alzheimer's Disease Diagnostic and Treatment Centers. *Neurology* 1992;42:473.
166. Hachinski VC et al. Multi-infarct dementia: a cause of mental deterioration in the elderly. *Lancet* 1974;2:207.
167. Tresch DD et al. Prevalence and significance of cardiovascular disease and hypertension in elderly patients with dementia. *J Am Geriatr Soc* 1985;33:530.
168. Meyer JS et al. Aetiological considerations and risk factors for multi-infarct dementia. *J Neurol Neurosurg Psychiatry* 1988;51:1489.
169. Zimetbaum P et al. Lipids, vascular disease, and dementia with advancing age. *Arch Intern Med* 1991;151:240.
170. Ross GW et al. Characterization of risk factors for vascular dementia. *Neurology* 1999;53:337.
171. Pullicino P et al. Small deep infarcts diagnosed on computed tomography. *Neurology* 1980;30:1090.
172. Goto K et al. Diffuse white-matter disease in the geriatric population. *Radiology* 1981;141:687.
173. Ishii N et al. Why do frontal lobe symptoms predominate in vascular dementia with lacunes? *Neurology* 1986;36:340.
174. Donnan GA et al. A prospective study of lacunar infarction using computerized tomography. *Neurology* 1982;32:49.
175. Roman GC. Senile dementia of the Binswanger type: a form of vascular dementia in the elderly. *JAMA* 1987;258:1782.
176. Wallin A, Blennow K. Pathogenetic basis of vascular dementia. *Alzheimer Dis Assoc Disord* 1991;5:91.
177. Hachinski VC et al. Leuko-araiosis. *Arch Neurol* 1987;44:21.
178. Munoz DG. The pathological basis of multi-infarct dementia. *Alzheimer Dis Assoc Disord* 1991;5:77.
179. Inzitari D et al. Vascular risk factors and leuko-araiosis. *Arch Neurol* 1987;44:42.
180. Kawamura J et al. Leukoaraiosis correlates with cerebral hypoperfusion in vascular dementia. *Stroke* 1991;22:609.
181. Babikian V, Ropper AH. Binswanger's disease: a review. *Stroke* 1987;18:2.
182. Tomimoto H et al. Coagulation activation in patients with Binswanger disease. *Arch Neurol* 1999;56:1104.

183. Rocca WA et al. Prevalence of clinically diagnosed Alzheimer's disease and other dementing disorders: a door-to-door survey in Appignano, Macerata Province, Italy. *Neurology* 1990;40:626.
184. Nussbaum M et al. DSM-III criteria for primary degenerative dementia and multi-infarct dementia. *Alzheimer Dis Assoc Disord* 1992;6:111.
185. Hachinski VC et al. Cerebral blood flow in dementia. *Arch Neurol* 1975;32:632.
186. Rogers RL et al. Cigarette smoking decreases cerebral blood flow suggesting increased risk for stroke. *JAMA* 1983;250:2796.
187. Meyer JS et al. Improved cognition after control of risk factors for multi-infarct dementia. *JAMA* 1986;256:2203.
188. SHEP Cooperative Research Group. Prevention of stroke by antihypertensive drug treatment in older persons with isolated systolic hypertension. *JAMA* 1991;265:3255.
189. Williams BR, Kim J. Cardiovascular drug therapy in the elderly: theoretical and practical considerations. *Drugs Aging* 2003;20:445.
190. Tollefson GD. Short-term effects of the calcium channel blocker nimodipine in the management of primary degenerative dementia. *Biol Psychiatry* 1990;27:1133.
191. Forette F et al. The prevention of dementia with antihypertensive treatment: new evidence from the Systolic Hypertension in Europe (Sys-Eur) study. *Arch Intern Med* 2002;162:2046.
192. The ALLHAT Officers and Coordinators for the ALLHAT Collaborative Research Group. Major cardiovascular events in hypertensive patients randomized to doxazosin vs. chlorthalidone: the Antihypertensive and Lipid-Lowering Treatment to Prevent Heart Attack Trial (ALLHAT). *JAMA* 2000;283:1967.
193. Meyer JS et al. Randomized clinical trial of daily aspirin therapy in multi-infarct dementia: a pilot study. *J Am Geriatr Soc* 1989;37:549.
194. Dutch TIA Trial Study Group. A comparison of two doses of aspirin (30 mg vs. 283 mg a day) in patients after a transient ischemic attack or minor ischemic stroke. *N Engl J Med* 1991;325:1261.
195. Albers GW et al. Antithrombotic and thrombolytic therapy for ischemic stroke. *Chest* 2001;119:300S.
196. Erkinjunti T. Cognitive decline and treatment options for patients with vascular dementia. *Acta Neurol Scand* 2002;106(Suppl 178):15.
197. Meyer JS et al. Donepezil treatment of vascular dementia. *Ann NY Acad Sci* 2002;977:482.
198. Erkinjuntti T et al. Efficacy of galantamine in probable vascular dementia and Alzheimer's disease combined with cerebrovascular disease: a randomized trial. *Lancet* 2002;359:1283.
199. Moretti R et al. Rivastigmine in subcortical vascular dementia: an open 22-month study. *J Neurol Sci* 2002;141:203.
200. Maletta GJ. Management of behavior in elderly patients with dementias. *Clin Geriatr Med* 1988;4:719.
201. Tariot PN. Treatment of agitation in dementia. *J Clin Psychiatry* 1999;60(Suppl 8):11.
202. Tariot PN et al. Pharmacologic therapy for behavioral symptoms of Alzheimer's disease. *Clin Geriatr Med* 2001;17:359.
203. Beers MH et al. Explicit criteria for determining potentially inappropriate medication use by the elderly. *Arch Intern Med* 1997;157:1531.
204. Aultzer DL et al. A double-blind comparison of trazodone and haloperidol for treatment of agitation in patients with dementia. *Am J Geriatr Psychiatry* 1997;5:60.
205. Pollock BG et al. Comparison of citalopram, perphenazine and placebo for the acute treatment of psychosis and behavioral disturbances in hospitalized, demented patients. *Am J Psychiatry* 2002;159:460.
206. Swearer JM et al. Troublesome and disruptive behaviors in dementia. *J Am Geriatr Soc* 1988;36:784.
207. Binetti G et al. Delusions in Alzheimer's disease and multi-infarct dementia. *Acta Neurol Scand* 1993;88:5.
208. Hirono N et al. Factors associated with psychotic symptoms in Alzheimer's disease. *J Neurol Neurosurg Psychiatry* 1998;64:648.
209. Neitch SM, Zarraga A. A misidentification delusion in two Alzheimer's patients. *J Am Geriatr Soc* 1991;39:513.
210. Rapp MS et al. Behavioural disturbances in the demented elderly: phenomenology, pharmacotherapy and behaviour management. *Can J Psychiatry* 1992;37:651.
211. Schneider LS et al. A meta-analysis of controlled trials of neuroleptic treatment in dementia. *J Am Geriatr Soc* 1990;38:553.
212. Schneider LS. Pharmacologic management of psychosis in dementia. *J Clin Psychiatry* 1999; 60(Suppl 8):54.
213. Kumar V et al. Pharmacologic management of Alzheimer's disease. *Clin Geriatr Med* 1998;14:129.
214. Herrmann N et al. Risperidone for the treatment of behavioral disturbances in dementia: a case series. *J Neuropsychiatry Clin Neurosci* 1998;10:220.
215. Katz I et al. Comparison of risperidone and placebo for psychosis and behavioral disturbances in dementia: a randomized, double-blind trial. *J Clin Psychiatry* 1999;60:107.
216. Street JS et al. Olanzapine treatment of psychotic and behavioral symptoms in patients with Alzheimer disease in nursing care facilities. *Arch Gen Psychiatry* 2000;57:968.
217. Zhong KX et al. Quetiapine to treat agitation in dementia: a randomized, double-blind, placebo-controlled study. *Curr Alzheimer Res* 2007;4:81.
218. Wooltorton E. Risperidone (Risperdal): increased rate of cerebrovascular events in dementia trials. *Can Med Assoc J* 2002;167:1269.
219. Schneider LS et al. Effectiveness of antipsychotic drugs in patients with Alzheimer's disease. *N Engl J Med* 2006;355:1525.
220. Gill SS et al. Antipsychotic drug use and death in older adults with dementia. *Ann Intern Med* 2007;146:775.
221. Maixner SM et al. The efficacy, safety, and tolerability of antipsychotics in the elderly. *J Clin Psychiatry* 1999;60(Suppl 8):29.
222. Cohen-Mansfield J et al. Screaming in nursing home residents. *J Am Geriatr Soc* 1990;38:785.
223. Cariaga J et al. A controlled study of disruptive vocalizations among geriatric residents in nursing homes. *J Am Geriatr Soc* 1991;39:501.
224. Bridges-Parlet S et al. A descriptive study of physically aggressive behavior in dementia by direct observation. *J Am Geriatr Soc* 1994;42:192.
225. Freels S et al. Functional status and clinical findings with Alzheimer's disease. *J Gerontol* 1992;47:M177.
226. Mace NL, Rabins PV. The 36-Hour Day. Baltimore: The Johns Hopkins University Press; 1981:64.
227. Grossman F. A review of anticonvulsants in treating agitated demented elderly patients. *Pharmacotherapy* 1998;18:600.
228. Gleason RP, Schneider LS. Carbamazepine treatment of agitation in Alzheimer's outpatients refractory to neuroleptics. *J Clin Psychiatry* 1990;51:115.
229. Tariot PN et al. Efficacy and tolerability of carbamazepine for agitation and aggression in dementia. *J Clin Psychiatry* 1998;155:54.
230. Essa M. Carbamazepine in dementia. *J Clin Psychopharmacol* 1986;6:234.
231. Hass S et al. Divalproex: a possible treatment alternative for demented, elderly aggressive patients. *Ann Clin Psychiatry* 1997;9:145.
232. Porsteinsson AP et al. Placebo-controlled study of divalproex sodium for agitation in dementia. *Am J Geriatr Psychiatry* 2001;9:1.
233. Narayan M, Nelson JC. Treatment of dementia with behavioral disturbance using divalproex or a combination of divalproex and a neuroleptic. *J Clin Psychiatry* 1997;58:351.
234. Salzman C. Treatment of agitation, anxiety, and depression in dementia. *Psychopharmacol Bull* 1988;24:39.
235. Fitz AG, Teri L. Depression, cognition, and functional ability in patients with Alzheimer's disease. *J Am Geriatr Soc* 1994;42:186.
236. Carlyle W et al. ECT: an effective treatment in the screaming demented patient [letter]. *J Am Geriatr Soc* 1991;39:637.
237. Lyketsos CG et al. Randomized, placebo-controlled, double-blind clinical trial of sertraline in the treatment of depression complicating Alzheimer's disease: initial results from the Depression in Alzheimer's Disease Study. *Am J Psychiatry* 2000;157:1686.
238. Simpson DM, Foster D. Improvement in organically disturbed behavior with trazodone treatment. *J Clin Psychiatry* 1986;47:191.
239. Pinner E, Rich C. Effects of trazodone on aggressive behavior in seven patients with organic mental disorders. *Am J Psychiatry* 1988;145:1295.
240. Williamson GM, Schulz R. Coping with specific stressors in Alzheimer's disease caregiving. *Gerontologist* 1993;33:747.
241. Mittelman MS et al. An intervention that delays institutionalization of Alzheimer's disease patients: treatment of spouse-caregivers. *Gerontologist* 1993;33:730.
242. Knight BG et al. A meta-analytic review of interventions for caregiver distress: recommendations for future research. *Gerontologist* 1993;33:240.
243. Cole JO et al. Tricyclic use in the cognitively impaired elderly. *J Clin Psychiatry* 1983;44:14.
244. Larson EB et al. Adverse drug reactions associated with cognitive impairment in elderly persons. *Ann Intern Med* 1987;107:169.
245. Parke-Davis. Cognex package insert. Morris Plains, NJ: Parke-Davis; November 1993.
246. Reisberg B et al. Memantine in moderate-to-severe Alzheimer's disease. *N Engl J Med* 2003;348:1333.
247. Tariot PN et al. Memantine treatment in patients with moderate to severe Alzheimer disease already receiving donepezil: a randomized controlled trial. *JAMA* 2004;291:317.
248. Dantoine T et al. Rivastigmine monotherapy and combination therapy with memantine in patients with moderately severe Alzheimer's disease who failed to benefit from previous cholinesterase inhibitor treatment. *Int J Clin Pract* 2006;60:110.
249. Burke WJ et al. Effective use of anxiolytics in older adults. *Clin Geriatr Med* 1998;14:47.
250. Gray KF. Managing agitation and difficult behavior in dementia. *Clin Geriatr Med* 2004;20:69.
251. Logsdon RG et al. Evidence-based psychological treatments for disruptive behaviors for individuals with dementia. *Psychol Aging* 2007;22:28.
252. Lyketsos CG et al. Position statement of the American Society for Geriatric Psychiatry regarding principles of care for patients with dementia resulting from Alzheimer disease. *Am J Geriatr Psychiatry* 2006;14:561.

CHAPTER 101

Geriatric Urologic Disorders

Michael R. Brodeur and John F. Thompson

SEXUAL DYSFUNCTION

Sexual dysfunction has been described as a public health concern by a National Institutes of Health Consensus Panel.[1,2] Sexual dysfunctions are highly prevalent in both sexes, ranging from 10% to 52% in men and from 25% to 63% in women.[3,4] In addition, advancing age is accompanied by a decrease in sexual function. Intercourse decreases from an average of once a week at the age of 65 to once every 10 weeks at the age of 80.[5] The frequency of sexual intercourse among the elderly actually has increased over the past 40 years, but still is substantially less than in younger individuals.[5–8] Although individual variations in frequency are large, most studies show that sexual activity among the elderly depends on the life pattern and past experiences of good or poor sexual function in each patient. Elderly patients may experience physiologic changes and encounter additional interference with sexual activity because of disability, disease, and medications. Furthermore, interest in sexual activity declines with aging.[9]

Poor health often is cited by elderly women as a reason for not participating in sexual activity, and among men, erectile dysfunction is the leading cause of decline in activity.[5,10] The major factors that correlate with reduced sexual activity include an older spouse, poor mental or physical health, marital difficulties, previous negative sexual experiences, and negative attitudes toward sexuality in the aged.[11] During the postmenopausal years, women undergo substantial physiologic change. The major physiologic event of natural menopause is a decrease in estrogen production. Little doubt exists that a decline in estrogen production is associated with many of the physiologic changes causing elderly women to report a low interest in sexual activity. The medical literature is replete with research and data on elderly male sexual dysfunction, but little, if any, data exist on female sexual dysfunction.

Male Sexual Dysfunction

Aging men may experience andropause, a syndrome consisting of weakness, fatigue, reduced muscle and bone mass, impaired hematopoiesis, oligospermia, sexual dysfunction, and psychiatric symptoms.[12] The relationship between declining testosterone and andropause is not firmly established. Free testosterone levels begin to decline at the rate of 1% per year after age 40 years. By the age of 60 years, 20% of men have levels below the lower limit of normal.[13] The physiologic and psychological effects of declining hormone levels in men are less dramatic than those experienced by women.

Sexual function is considered an interaction among motivation, drive, desires, thoughts, fantasies, pleasures, experiences (referred to as the *libido*), penile vasocongestion, erection, orgasmic contractions, and ejaculations (referred to as *potency*).[14,15] Testosterone plays an important role in male libido and sexual behavior, and may play some role in penile erection. Elderly men show a strong correlation between advancing age and diminishing bioavailable serum testosterone levels.[16,17] Testosterone progressively declines after the seventh decade, partly because of testicular and hypothalamic-pituitary dysfunction.[18]

Male sexual dysfunction, denoting the inability to achieve a satisfactory sexual relationship, may involve inadequacy of erection or problems with emission, ejaculation, or orgasm. *Erectile dysfunction* is the inability to achieve and maintain a firm erection sufficient for satisfactory sexual performance.[19] *Premature ejaculation* refers to uncontrolled ejaculation before or shortly after entering the vagina. *Retarded ejaculation* usually is synonymous with delayed ejaculation. *Retrograde ejaculation* denotes backflow of semen into the bladder during ejaculation caused by an incompetent bladder neck mechanism.

The neurologic structures in the brain most closely associated with sexual function and arousal are the limbic system and the hypothalamus. The psychogenic sexual arousal mechanism involving sensory organs (e.g., vision, auditory, olfactory, tactile) and imaginative stimuli participate in sexual function through the hypothalamus and limbic systems. Subsequent nerve transmission down the spinal cord to the autonomic nervous system and sacral and thoracolumbar centers mediates the penile erection. Furthermore, the reflexogenic mechanism of penile erection (stimulation of the genital area) also involves nerve transmission by the pudendal nerve to the sacral erection center. Neurotransmission in the peripheral nervous system is mediated by adrenergic and cholinergic stimulation and may be diminished in advanced age.[20] Neurochemical mediators also are involved with sexual function. For example, dopamine is associated with sexual arousal (stimulation), whereas serotonin has an inhibitory effect.[21,22] In the elderly, reduced onset of sexual arousal may be attributed to global cerebrovascular disease and diminished sensory input to the central nervous system (CNS). Peripheral mechanisms of sexual arousal also may be affected by aging.

Erectile dysfunction (ED), once regarded as a psychosocial disorder, today is regarded as caused by a variety of medical, psychological, and lifestyle factors. According to data from the Massachusetts Male Aging Study (MMAS), the combined prevalence of minimal, moderate, and complete erectile dysfunction among all elderly men is 52%.[23,24] According to the Baltimore Longitudinal Study of Aging, ED was a problem in 8% of all healthy men by age 55, and its prevalence increased to 25%, 55%, and 75% for men 65, 75, and 80 years of age, respectively.[25] Erectile dysfunction is estimated to affect as many as 30 million men in the United States. Of males aged 45 years or older in the United States, 5% seek prescription drug therapy for ED, on an annual basis.[26]

Approximately 80% of all cases of ED now are thought to be related to organic disease and subject to numerous influences.[14,27–29] In one study,[17] neurologic and vascular disorders were the primary causes of ED among elderly men, and psychogenic factors were the cause in <10%. The single most common etiology for erectile failure in the elderly is severe atherosclerosis (e.g., vascular disease and diabetes mellitus).[17] Cardiovascular disease, hypertension, diabetes mellitus, elevated low-density lipoprotein cholesterol, and cigarette smoking are associated with a greater probability of complete erectile dysfunction in men.[23] Therefore, prevention of cardiovascular disorders by interventions such as low-fat and low-cholesterol diets and abstinence from tobacco should minimize the development of geriatric sexual erectile dysfunction.

Different physiologic mechanisms are involved in erection, emission, ejaculation, and orgasm. Except for nocturnal emissions, ejaculation requires stimulation of the external genitalia. Ejaculation occurs in three phases. The first phase is termed *emission*. Efferent signals traveling in the hypogastric nerve activate secretions and transport sperm from the distal epididymis, vas deferens, seminal vesicles, and prostate to the prostatic urethra (Fig. 101-1). The second phase is the coordinated closing of the internal urethral sphincter and the relaxation of the external sphincter to direct the semen into the bulbous urethra. The coordinated closing of the internal sphincter and relaxation of the external sphincter is mediated by α- and β-adrenergic stimulation. The third phase, *external ejaculation*,

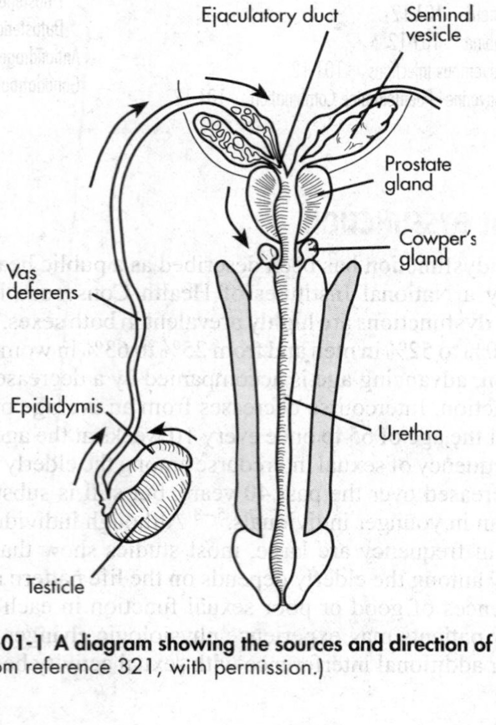

FIGURE 101-1 A diagram showing the sources and direction of seminal flow. (From reference 321, with permission.)

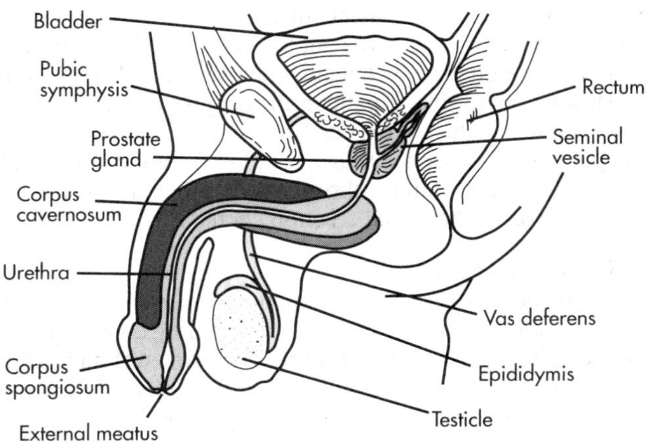

FIGURE 101-2 A diagram showing the relations of the bladder, prostate, seminal vesicles, penis, urethra, and scrotal contents. (From reference 321, with permission.)

involves the somatomotor efferent segment of the pudendal nerve to contract the bulbocavernosus muscle, which forces the semen through a pressurized conduit, the much-narrowed urethral lumen compressed by the engorged corpora cavernosa and corpus spongiosum (Fig. 101-2), to produce 2 to 5 mL of ejaculate.[28] In the elderly male, ejaculation is less vigorous and the total ejaculate is likely to be reduced.[30]

The hemodynamics of penile erection involve the pudendal artery (the major blood supply to the penis), of which the terminal portion divides into three branches: (a) the bulbourethral artery, (b) the dorsal artery, and (c) the cavernous artery. The cavernous artery supplies the corpora cavernosa; the dorsal artery, the glans penis; and the bulbourethral artery, the corpus spongiosum. The corpora cavernosa and the corpus spongiosum (also referred to as *corporal smooth muscle*) are the erectile muscle tissues, which appear to be under β-adrenergic control.[14,28] Thoracolumbar or sacral erection-center stimulation shunts the blood to these structures and an erection ensues. The sympathetic nervous system also is involved in the constriction of veins in the erectile tissue that diminishes venous outflow. The resultant high intracavernous (IC) pressure converts a soft, flaccid organ to a blood-distended erect penis. Distention of the erectile tissue further results in compression of the venules, reducing the venous capacity to minimum, which allows full erection of the penis. These actions maintain erection in the corpora cavernosa without diverting too much cardiac output for penile erection.[31]

The biochemical basis of erection is simply an extension of the neuronal physiologic mechanisms. The erectile system involves neural initiation, cellular translation, and vascular transduction. Central initiation of an erection involves erectogenic stimuli (tactile), erotic imagery at the cerebral cortex, or both. The nuclei that integrate erectile signaling are highly specific.[32] The medial preoptic area (MPOA) of the hypothalamus may be the integration for the central control of erection. It receives sensory impulses from the amygdala that have inputs from cortical association areas.[33] The signals generated follow the spinal pathways and create an erection through receptor interaction and cellular mechanisms in the vasculature in the periphery. As a result of erectogenic or erotic activity, dopamine, acting via the D_2-receptor, is the initiating neurotransmitter. Inhibitory stimuli such as anxiety can dampen the response of the dopaminergic system.

The cellular mechanisms that control the vascular response necessary for penile erection are similar to equivalent mechanisms elsewhere in the vasculature. Cellular mechanisms are designed to induce vascular relaxation and thus cause an erection. Essentially, two cellular factors are believed to induce vascular relaxation. The first factor, prostaglandin E_1, is released at the local level as a result of the spinal pathway message; it causes adenyl cyclase to accelerate the production of cyclic adenosine monophosphate (cAMP) and results in intracellular release of potassium, a known vasodilator. A second factor involves the release of nitric oxide from local neuronal tissue. Nitric oxide is the main neurotransmitter mediating erection. Once called endothelium-derived relaxing factor, nitric oxide has been shown to induce relaxation of vascular smooth muscle.[6] Nitric oxide induces the formation of cyclic guanosine monophosphate (cGMP) in the vascular system; cGMP is postulated to activate protein G, leading to the phosphorylation of proteins regulating corporal smooth muscle through ion channel changes.[34] This results in the opening of potassium channels and hyperpolarization of the muscle cell membrane, sequestration of intracellular calcium by the endoplasmic reticulum, and blocking of calcium influx by calcium channel inhibition.[35] Nitric oxide is released by endothelial cells and efferent neuronal cells in response to erectogenic stimuli.

The major arteries needed for an erection are the feeder pelvic vessels and the penile vessels themselves. In all of these components, multiple competing systems exist in a state of balance. The final vascular consequence of these actions depends on the intracellular response and the interaction of the vascular wall complex (smooth muscle, endothelium, nerves plus the effects of stromal and luminal blood pressure). The vascular wall complex is the interplay of vasodilators (prostaglandin E_1, nitric oxide, potassium), the inhibition of the vasoconstrictor mechanisms, and the resultant relaxation of the vascular wall.[36]

The process of orgasm is the least understood sexual process. Simultaneous with emission and ejaculation are involuntary rhythmic contractions of the anal sphincter, hyperventilation, tachycardia, and blood pressure elevation. Because erectile dysfunction is more likely in male patients with coronary artery disease, the understanding of the cardiovascular stresses involved with sexual intercourse can aid in patient management. Cardiac and metabolic expenditures during sexual intercourse vary depending on the type of sexual activity. Healthy males with their usual female partners generally achieve a peak heart rate of 110 beats/minute with woman-on-top coitus and an average peak heart rate of 127 beats/minute with man-on-top coitus.[37] There is significant individual variation in cardiovascular response, when measured as oxygen uptake and metabolic expenditures, for male-on-top coitus.

In a study of medication-free patients with coronary artery disease who were in the New York Heart Association functional class I or II, sexual activity was compared with near-maximal exercise treadmill test.[38] Electrocardiographic changes representing ischemia during intercourse were found in one-third of the patients; however, two-thirds of these patients remained asymptomatic. All patients with ischemia during coitus also demonstrated ischemia during exercise treadmill testing. The average heart rate during coitus was 118 beats/minute, with some patients attaining a heart rate of 185 beats/minute at orgasm. Intercourse in patients with coronary artery disease may provoke increased ventricular ectopic activity that is not necessarily elicited by other stimuli.[39] These electrocardiographic changes and associated symptoms can be abolished with the use of β-blockers.[40] Sexual activity is a likely contributor to the onset of myocardial infarction only 0.9% of the time.[41] Coital death is rare, accounting for 0.6% of sudden death cases.[42] The hemodynamic changes associated with sexual activity may be far greater with an unfamiliar partner, in unfamiliar settings, and after excessive eating and alcohol consumption.

Erectile Dysfunction

Pathogenesis

Erection involves the neurologic, psychological, hormonal, arterial, and venous systems. In a study of 1,500 elderly men over a period of 10 years, organic erectile dysfunction was diagnosed in >1,050 subjects.[43] As a result of research in vascular physiology, neurophysiology, and neuropharmacology of the penis, most urologists today believe that up to 80% of elderly erectile dysfunction cases are organic in origin and that the remainder are owing to psychological factors[44] (Table 101-1). In most elderly male sexual dysfunction studies, 50% involve vascular problems, and 30% relate to diabetes mellitus.[45]

NEUROGENIC DISORDERS

Erectile dysfunction can be caused by damage to the brain, spinal cord, cavernous or pudendal nerves, terminal nerve endings, and the receptors. Neurogenic erectile dysfunction can be caused by diabetes, spinal cord injury, cauda equina lesions, polyneuropathy, myelopathy, multiple sclerosis, dorsal nerve dysfunction from alcohol abuse or parkinsonism, and radical pelvic surgery.[44] Erectile dysfunction was the presenting symptom in 12% of males with unrecognized diabetes mellitus.[46] Similarly, erectile dysfunction can be the presenting symptom of temporal lobe epilepsy.[47]

Approximately 95% of patients with upper motor neuron lesions resulting from spinal injury are capable of erection through the reflexogenic mechanism,[48] whereas only 25% of patients with complete lower motor neuron lesions can have erections through the psychogenic mechanism.[48] With incomplete lesions, up to 90% of patients in both groups retain erectile ability. Patients who have a cerebrovascular accident, dementia, epilepsy, Parkinson disease, or a brain tumor most likely experience erectile failure through loss of sexual interest or overinhibition of the spinal erection centers.[44]

Table 101-1 Causes of Erectile Disfunction

Vascular	Iatrogenic
Atherosclerosis	Pelvic radiation
Penile Raynaud's phenomenon	Lumbar sympathectomy
Neurologic	Prostatectomy
	Renal transplantation
Cerebrovascular accident	Spinal cord resection
Spinal cord damage	**Psychogenic**
Autonomic neuropathy	
Peripheral neuropathy	Performance anxiety
Endocrine	Depression
	Widower's syndrome
Diabetes mellitus	
Hypogonadism	
Prolactinomas	
Hyperthyroidism	
Hypothyroidism	

Adapted from reference 79, with permission.

HORMONAL DISORDERS

The incidence of erectile dysfunction with a hormonal cause has been estimated to be 5% to 35%, depending on which medical specialty is reporting the finding.[49] The most common hormonal disorder associated with ED in the elderly is diabetes mellitus. Approximately 75% of elderly male diabetics experience ED owing to a combination of vascular, neurologic, and psychological factors.[50] Insulin dosage, duration, and glycemic control are unrelated to sexual dysfunction.

Other hormonal disorders, such as hypothyroidism, hyperthyroidism, Addison's disease, and Cushing's syndrome, are associated with erectile dysfunction. Patients with hypogonadism due to pituitary or hypothalamic tumors, antiandrogen therapy, or orchiectomy experience ED. These patients can have a normal erection from visual stimulation, however, indicating that the erectile mechanism is intact.[51]

VASCULAR DISORDERS

Atherosclerosis is the leading vascular disease associated with male erectile dysfunction. The age of onset of coronary artery disease parallels the onset of ED, indicating a generalized atherosclerotic etiology for the erectile dysfunction.[52] The degree of arteriolar narrowing and clinical presentation, however differ from patient to patient. Some patients can have severe coronary artery disease but retain the capability of a full erection. As long as the arterial flow into the penis exceeds the venous outflow, the patient can be potent. Narrowing of the arterial lumen lowers pressure in the cavernous arteries, and poor arterial flow can only partially fill the sinusoidal system. Overall, the partial filling of the sinusoidal system causes inadequate expansion of the sinusoidal wall, resulting in partial compression of the venules. The net effect is a partial erection, difficulty in maintaining an erection, or the most common complaint, early detumescence. Intrapenile arterial disease resulting from diabetes mellitus, atherosclerosis, or aging does not respond to present surgical techniques.

Signs and Symptoms

1. F.M., a 66-year-old man, was referred to a urologist because he was experiencing a loss of interest in sexual activity. He describes the inability to maintain a firm erection for the past 6 months in >75% of sexual attempts with his sexual partner. Physical examination was unremarkable except for an enlarged prostate gland and evidence of pubic and axillary hair loss. Vital signs were as follows: blood pressure (BP), 160/95 mmHg; pulse, 88 beats/minute; respirations, 14 breaths/minute; and temperature, 98.7°F. Current medications include ramipril 5 mg/day and glyburide 5 mg/day. F.M.'s medical history is positive for cigarette smoking, hypertension, and diabetes mellitus. Significant laboratory results include the following: random blood sugar, 200 mg/dL (normal, 70–110); serum creatinine (SrCr), 1.5 mg/dL (normal, 0.6–1.2); blood urea nitrogen (BUN), 22 mg/dL (normal, 8–18);

free testosterone level, 30 pg/mL (normal, 52–280); luteinizing hormone (LH), 4 mU/mL (normal, 1–8); follicle-stimulating hormone (FSH) level, 40 mIU/mL (normal, 4–25); and serum prolactin level, 28 ng/mL (normal, <20). What signs and symptoms does F.M. have that would suggest the need for a complete medical workup for erectile dysfunction?

[SI units: glucose, 11.1 mmol/L (normal, 3.9–6.1); SrCr, 132.6 μmol/L (normal, 50–110); BUN, 7.9 mmol/L urea (normal, 3.0–6.5); LH, 4 IU/L (normal, 1–8); FSH, 40 IU/L (normal, 4–25); serum prolactin, 28 mg/L (normal, <20)]

F.M. presents with the complaint of loss of interest in sexual activity and the inability to maintain a full erection during >75% of sexual encounters with his partner. On physical examination, F.M. is found to have a noticeable loss of pubic and axillary body hair. With longstanding androgen deficiency, there may be loss of hair in the androgen-dependent areas of the body, fine wrinkling of the skin around the mouth and eyes, noticeable loss of muscle mass and strength, altered body-fat distribution, and osteoporosis. In contrast, overt hypogonadism results in a change in the pattern of pubic hair from the male diamond shape to the female inverted triangle appearance. At this point, it appears that F.M.'s loss of pubic and axillary hair is the result of androgen deficiency, with the cause yet to be determined. The laboratory results for gonadal function coincide with what is expected in an elderly male with erectile dysfunction (see Question 4).

Urologic Workup

2. What clinical evaluations and laboratory tests should be included in the medical workup of F.M. to determine the cause of his erectile dysfunction?

A detailed medical and sexual history and thorough physical examination are essential in the evaluation of sexual dysfunction. General medical history and physical examination should consider drug-induced erectile dysfunction (Table 101-2); cigarette smoking (cigar and pipe tobacco have not been associated with sexual dysfunction); prior surgery (e.g., transurethral resection of prostate [TURP], aortoiliac bypass, prostatectomy); prior physical trauma (e.g., herniated disc, testicular trauma); voiding dysfunction; visual field defects (visual field changes may be one of the first presenting symptoms of diabetes mellitus, the most common endocrine abnormality associated with male sexual dysfunction and may be associated with pituitary tumor pressure on the optic nerve); femoral artery bruits; testicular atrophy; Peyronie's plaques (a fibrous palpable plaque along the shaft of the penis, causing penile curvature and poor erection distal to the plaque, thought to be caused by atherosclerosis or severe vasculitis); pedal pulses; and neurologic examination. Hormonal and metabolic screening should be included with the history and physical examination.

Although laboratory-based diagnostic procedures are available, it is proposed that sexual function is best assessed in a naturalistic setting with patient self-report techniques. One such self-reporting tool, the International Index of Erectile Function (IIEF), has been demonstrated to address the relevant domains of male sexual function (erectile function, orgasmic function, sexual desire, intercourse satisfaction, and overall satisfaction), is psychometrically sound, and has been linguistically validated in 10 languages.[53]

F.M.'s endocrine status should include assessment of his diabetes, thyroid function tests, and a serum lipid profile. Neuropathy and atherosclerosis are common findings among male patients with diabetes mellitus, and both are potential causes of ED. Patients experiencing hypothyroidism may have decreased libido, and hypothyroidism is associated with hyperprolactinemia, which can result in an inhibition in the release of testosterone. Elevated serum lipids (e.g., total cholesterol, triglycerides) may be associated with significant vascular damage that could contribute to erectile dysfunction. Diabetes mellitus is best evaluated with a hemoglobin-A1_c and a fasting blood glucose tests.[54]

The serum concentrations of free testosterone, prolactin, and LH should be evaluated. Testosterone, as with all other hormones secreted into the plasma, is available to tissues only in the free form (i.e., unbound to serum proteins, particularly the sex hormone-binding globulin). Only 1% to 2% of testosterone is free and physiologically active; therefore, measurement of the unbound serum testosterone provides the best estimate of biologically available testosterone. Low testosterone serum concentrations are associated with primary and secondary hypogonadism. Primary hypogonadism is associated with testicular disease (e.g., Leydig cell tumors), whereas secondary hypogonadism is the result of pituitary or hypothalamic disease.

The serum prolactin concentration should be determined, because a high serum concentration of prolactin inhibits release of testosterone from the testes. Therefore, a low serum testosterone concentration may be caused by hyperprolactinemia. Hyperprolactinemia may be caused by prolactin adenomas, diabetes mellitus, or drug therapy (e.g., neuroleptics, metoclopramide).

LH stimulates testicular steroidogenesis and secretion of testosterone. LH increases the conversion of cholesterol to pregnenolone, a precursor of testosterone. FSH is required for spermatogenesis in early puberty, but is not a required gonadotropin for the maintenance of spermatogenesis in adult men. Normal testicular function depends on stimulation by the gonadotropin LH, which is secreted by the anterior pituitary gland. Consequently, a low normal serum concentration of LH is associated with secondary hypogonadism.

In patients with symptoms of prostatic disease, expressed prostatic secretions (EPS) should be examined because prostate inflammation has been associated with ejaculatory dysfunction. During prostatic inflammation, the EPS contains leukocytes and macrophages, and microscopic examination of the EPS can determine the degree of prostate inflammation. The presence of >20 white blood cells (WBC) per high-powered field (HPF) in the EPS is abnormal, and indicative of prostatitis. Only about 5% of prostatitis can be attributed to a bacterial infection; the remaining 95% is owing to unknown etiologies.

Ideally, assessment of erectile dysfunction should include urologic, endocrinologic, psychiatric, and neurologic evaluations as close together as possible. The chief complaint of ED must be identified carefully and described, because medical intervention is indicated if it occurs over a 6-month period and in >50% of attempts.[28] A detailed history should determine whether ED varies with partners, sexual settings, position, and

Table 101-2 Common Drug-Induced Alterations in Sexual Response

Drug Categories	*Clinical Considerations*
Antihypertensives	
Diuretic	
Thiazides	Temporal association with sexual dysfunction. Reported incidence varies between 0 and 32%[307–311]; however, impotence generally is not considered common. Mechanism believed to be a "steal syndrome" whereby blood is routed from erectile tissues to skeletal muscle.[89]
Spironolactone	Associated with ↓ libido, impotence, and gynecomastia. Mechanism may be hormone related. Incidence is dose related and reported to be 5%–67%[89,312,313] and much more commonly encountered than with the thiazides. May be owing to antiandrogen effects of drug.
Sympatholytics	
Methyldopa	Central action mediated causing vasodilation resulting in erectile dysfunction. Reported incidence: 10%.[89,92] Also ↓ libido.
Clonidine	Induces erectile dysfunction. Mechanism similar to methyldopa and other central α_2-agonists. Incidence reported to be 4%–70% and dose related.[314–316] Also ↓ libido.
Guanabenz, guanfacine	Incidence and mechanism believed to be similar to other central α_2-agonists.
Nonselective β-Blockers	
Propranolol	Associated with erectile dysfunction and ↓ libido. Mechanism believed to be caused by ↓ vascular resistance and central effects. Erectile dysfunction reported to begin at doses of 120 mg/day. Incidence may be as high as 100% at higher dosages.[86,92,317]
Selective β-Blockers	
Atenolol, metoprolol, pindolol, timolol (drops)	Incidence of erectile dysfunction is significantly less than nonselective β-blockers.[318]
α-Blockers	
Doxazosin, prazosin, terazosin	Associated with erectile dysfunction and priapism.[92,315] Reported incidence: 0.6%–4%.[320] Mechanism is local α_1-blockade resulting in vasodilation. Erectile dysfunction and priapism appears to be unique to the nonspecific α_1-antagonists.
Phenoxybenzamine	Associated with priapism, retrograde ejaculation, and inhibited emissions during erection. Effects are dose related.[321,322]
Direct Vasodilators	
Hydralazine	Associated with erectile dysfunction. Mechanism is vascular smooth muscle relaxation. Incidence not reported.[321]
Calcium Channel Blockers	
Nifedipine	Associated with erectile dysfunction. Mechanism believed to be vasodilation and possibly muscle relaxation. Reported incidence: <2%.[79]
Diltiazem, verapamil	Similar to nifedipine. Reported incidence: <1%.
Antiarrhythmics	
Class 1A	
Disopyramide	Associated with erectile dysfunction in patients treated for ventricular arrhythmias. Incidence not reported. Mechanism believed to be caused by strong anticholinergic effect.[89,321]
Anticonvulsants	
Carbamazepine, phenytoin	May be associated with sexual dysfunction through decreasing DHEA, which is a precursor to testosterone, estrogen, and pheromones.[267]
Antidepressants	
Selective serotonin reuptake inhibitors	Drugs with prominent serotonin agonist effects commonly cause delayed ejaculation and anorgasmia. The reported incidence for delayed ejaculation among men is 2% to 12%; for anorgasmia among women users, the incidence appears to be <3%. This adverse effect is directly dose related.[267]
Tricyclic antidepressants (TCA), monoamine oxidase inhibitors	Associated with impairment of sexual performance in both male and female: ↓ libido, anorgasmia, retrograde ejaculation, erectile dysfunction. Mechanism believed to be caused by anticholinergic and serotonergic effects. Incidence not reported; several case studies in the literature.[20]
Trazodone	Associated with priapism in men and ↑ libido in women. Mechanism similar to TCA. Incidence not reported but believed to be dose related.[20] (Note: The literature reports that overall there is less sexual dysfunction with desipramine than with other antidepressants.)
Antipsychotics	
Phenothiazines	Frequently associated with sexual dysfunction. Commonly, ↓ libido is reported. Mechanism is due to hyperprolactinemia secondary to central dopamine antagonism. Thioridazine is the most often reported offender. Erectile and ejaculatory pain are very common with this drug class; the α-antagonism and anticholinergic effects are responsible. Priapism is common with this drug group, owing to the peripheral α-blockade property. Incidence for all sexual dysfunction with this drug class: approximately 50% of users.[20]

Table 101-2 Common Drug-Induced Alterations in Sexual Response (*Continued*)

Drug Categories	*Clinical Considerations*
Anxiolytics	
Short-acting barbiturates	Biphasic effect. At low doses, libido ↑, similar to ethanol, and at higher doses, CNS depression causes ↓ libido and performance.[20]
Benzodiazepines	Biphasic effect. At low doses, ↑ libido, whereas at higher dosages, CNS depression causes performance failure. Some reports of anorgasmia (men and women) and ejaculatory failure.[20]
Substances of Abuse	
Alcohol	Alcohol is thought to impair sexual function through its chronic effects on the nervous system. Short-term use of alcohol can induce erectile dysfunction through its sedative effects. More than 600 mL/wk of alcohol increases the probability of erectile dysfunction.[222]
Cocaine	Biphasic effect. At low doses, there is enhanced sexual desire (similar to amphetamines) and possibly performance. At higher dosages, there may be arousal dysfunction, ejaculatory dysfunction, anorgasmia. Freebasing has been associated with spontaneous orgasm. Continued use ("on a run") causes significant loss of sexual interest and performance ability. Chronic use associated with hyperprolactinemia resulting in ↓ libido.[20]
Ethanol	At low doses actually may enhance libido. Sexual dysfunction is dose related and caused by CNS depressant effects.[89,92,319]
Hallucinogens	Biphasic effect for most drugs in this category. At low doses, libido is enhanced; at higher doses, libido is severely ↓. No reports on chronic use.[20]
Marijuana	Biphasic effect similar to ethanol. With chronic use there is a ↓ in libido. Mechanism may be due to ↓ testosterone. Incidence not reported. [20]
Opioids	Associated with sexual dysfunction: erection lubrication, orgasm, and ejaculation. Chronic use associated with ↓ libido. Mechanism may be owing to α-antagonism, alterations in testosterone, and the intoxicating effects. Incidence not reported.[88,92,319,323]
Miscellaneous	
Amyl nitrate	Associated with intense and prolonged orgasms in both male and female. Impotence has been reported in some cases owing to vasodilation.[20]
Cimetidine, ranitidine	Associated with ↓ libido and erectile dysfunction. Mechanism due to antiandrogen qualities and drug-induced elevation of prolactin. May be dose related.[92,324]
Metoclopramide	Associated with ↓ libido and erectile dysfunction. Mechanism is through CNS dopamine antagonism, resulting in hyperprolactinemia. Incidence not reported.[92]

CNS, central nervous system; DHEA, dehydroepiandrosterone; SSRI, selective serotonin reuptake inhibitors; TCA, tricyclic antidepressants.

masturbation, and if morning and nocturnal erections are impaired.

Clinicians should ask the patient to estimate the degree of penile rigidity, especially with regard to the ability for vaginal penetration, and ask about nocturnal penile tumescence to differentiate psychogenic from organic causes of ED. The examiner should ascertain the presence of associated problems (e.g., atherosclerosis, diabetes mellitus) and attempt to correlate these problems to identified concerns with libido, orgasm, and ejaculation. Ideally, the sexual partner should be present during history taking. A pattern of progressive erectile dysfunction often indicates organic cause, whereas a pattern of intermittent episodes of ED with an abrupt onset suggests a psychogenic cause.

Relationship of Medical History and Erectile Dysfunction

3. What is the relationship among hypertension, cigarette smoking, diabetes mellitus, and F.M.'s erectile dysfunction?

HYPERTENSION

Among elderly men, erectile dysfunction most often is caused by neurovascular diseases.[17] The high degree of arteriosclerosis among elderly American men is the leading cause of ED.[17,55,56] In the MMAS, heart disease with hypertension and low serum high-density lipoprotein correlated with erectile dysfunction.[14] The hemodynamics of erection can be impaired in patients with myocardial infarction, coronary bypass surgery, cerebrovascular accidents, and peripheral vascular disease.[57–60] In several studies of impotent men, the number of abnormal penile vascular findings significantly increased when the history included hypertension and cigarette smoking.[61–63] In one report, 8% to 10% of all untreated hypertensive elderly males were impotent at the time of diagnosis of hypertension.[64] Control of blood pressure among hypertensive male patients does not necessarily improve erectile function, and antihypertensive medications can have a significant effect on erectile dysfunction and sexual performances (Table 101-2).[65–67]

CIGARETTE SMOKING

The prevalence of cigarette smoking among men with erectile dysfunction is higher than in the general population.[62,68,69] When the relation between cigarette smoking and erectile physiology was studied in 314 men with ED,[70] smoking was noted to further compromise penile physiology in men experiencing difficulty maintaining erections long enough for satisfactory intercourse. Several investigators report lower penile blood pressure indices, penile arterial insufficiency, and abnormal blood perfusion associated with cigarette smoking.[62,71] Clearly, cigarette smoking is counterproductive in men with existing ED.

DIABETES MELLITUS

Diabetes mellitus has been associated with erectile dysfunction. In the MMAS, male patients with diabetes mellitus were three times more likely to have ED than patients without diabetes.[14] Other investigators using exclusively diabetic populations have found a prevalence of ED as high as 75% among subjects.[72,73] The onset of ED in the diabetic patient occurs at an earlier age when compared with the general population. In a few cases, it may be the presenting symptom of diabetes mellitus and, in most cases, ED follows within 10 years of the diagnosis, regardless of insulin-dependence status.[74,75] Researchers disagree as to the exact contribution of diabetes mellitus to erectile dysfunction, but most of the literature supports an atherosclerotic etiology.[76,77] Other possible causes also include autonomic neuropathy and gonadal dysfunction.[74]

Gonadal Function in Erectile Dysfunction

4. What is the significance of the gonadal function results for F.M.?

GONADOTROPINS

Abnormalities of primary or secondary hypogonadism must be ruled out, particularly in patients with a decreased libido with or without erectile dysfunction. The results of F.M.'s gonadal function tests are relatively normal for an aged male. Testosterone serum levels decline with aging as a result of hypothalamic-pituitary changes or Leydig cell dysfunction. The understanding of changes that take place in the hypothalamic-pituitary level with advancing age is in a state of flux. For some time, most investigators focused on the increased serum concentration of male gonadotropins (LH, FSH), believing that all elderly males had some degree of primary hypogonadism.[78] Other studies have shown, however, that LH levels in elderly males are lower than the median of that in younger patients.[79] These findings show that LH levels do not increase in response to the decrease in testosterone serum concentrations in the aged male, indicating a defect in the hypothalamic-pituitary axis, leading to secondary hypogonadism.[80] Secondary hypogonadism results when there is a dysregulation of pituitary LH release, resulting in low serum testosterone levels.[44]

TESTICULAR SIZE AND AGING

Testicular size decreases with age; however, the testicular degeneration is sporadic, thereby allowing most elderly men to maintain a normal or slightly decreased sperm output.[78] Overall, spermatogenesis decreases and is accompanied by an increase in serum concentration of FSH. FSH elevation correlates well with a decline in the number of Sertoli cells that secrete inhibin. Inhibin normally decreases FSH.[81]

TESTOSTERONE

As a result of primary or secondary hypogonadism in the elderly male, available testosterone declines. Approximately 60% to 75% of circulating serum testosterone is bound to a β-globulin known as sex hormone-binding globulin or testosterone-binding globulin. Approximately 20% to 40% of testosterone is bound to serum albumin, and 1% to 2% is unbound, or free. The unbound portion of testosterone is the only active portion of the total serum testosterone concentration. Testosterone serum concentrations are 20% higher in the morning than in the evening, and this should be taken into consideration when evaluating laboratory results. In virtually all cases of male erectile dysfunction, the serum concentration of testosterone should be measured in the morning.

Testosterone production is regulated by feedback with the hypothalamus and pituitary. The hypothalamus produces gonadotropin-releasing hormone (Gn-RH) in response to low testosterone levels. Gn-RH induces the pituitary to secrete LH and FSH, which in turn stimulate the Leydig cells of the testes to secrete testosterone. Less than 10% of cases of erectile dysfunction studied are caused strictly by hypogonadism.[17,82] The role of testosterone in ED is complex. After testosterone production decreases, libido eventually declines and precedes the decrease in frequency of erections.[83] Men given antiandrogens maintain their erectile capacity but have a decreased libido.[84] On the other hand, high dosages of androgens given to hypogonadal men increase both the frequency of erections and libido.[85] It would seem reasonable to postulate that at physiologic levels, testosterone modulates the cognitive processes associated with sexual arousal more than it contributes to erectile capability.

ENDOCRINE DISORDERS

Many endocrine disorders can result in erectile dysfunction. Patients with prolactinomas commonly have ED, but prolactinomas account for <1% of erectile dysfunction cases.[86] Prolactin inhibits the release of testosterone, resulting in secondary hypogonadism. Hyperprolactinemia may be more prevalent in diabetic patients.[87] In the elderly, however, hyperprolactinemia often is secondary to the use of medications. F.M.'s serum prolactin level is elevated, most likely because of his diabetes mellitus.

In summary, aged males have a decrease in testosterone because of defects in testicular and hypothalamic-pituitary function. Secondary hypogonadism in elderly males is common, and the point at which this becomes pathologic has not yet been established. Correspondingly, the use of hormonal therapy to treat physiologic secondary hypogonadism is extremely controversial. Therefore, the gonadal function tests for F.M. are normal for his age and do not provide an explanation for his ED.

Medications That Cause Erectile Dysfunction

5. What medications are known to contribute to male erectile dysfunction? Is it likely that a medication is causing F.M.'s erectile dysfunction?

Several general statements can be made regarding sexual function and medications. Drugs that affect libido generally have a central mode of action. For example, medications that block central dopamine transmission can decrease libido, and opiates have an antiandrogen effect.[88] Drugs that alter hemodynamics may interfere with erection. Excessive sympathetic tone is thought to cause the "steal syndrome," which increases blood flow to muscles, drawing blood away from the erectile tissue.[89] Drugs that block the peripheral sympathetic system can cause retrograde ejaculation, or no ejaculation at all.

Numerous drugs have been associated with altered sexual function[90] (Table 101-2).

Few studies exist in the literature solely devoted to drug-induced erectile dysfunction or sexual dysfunction.[66,67] A few studies and review articles, however, list medications as one of many potential causes for ED.[14,21,25,44,91]

Most studies documenting drug-induced erectile dysfunction have been subjective and based on case reports, uncontrolled studies, and clinical impressions. In a study (MMAS) from the New England Research Institute at Boston University Medical Center, complete erectile dysfunction was most significant for smokers being treated with cardiac drugs.[14] In this study, erectile dysfunction was statistically correlated with antihypertensive, vasodilator, cardiac, and hypoglycemic drugs. The probability of moderate as well as complete ED was particularly high for vasodilator drugs.[14] Although the MMAS is one of the most well-designed studies to date, the medications reported are not considered to be the universe of all medications associated with ED. Diagnosis of drug-induced sexual dysfunction should be restricted to a reproducible dose-related effect that disappears on discontinuation of the drug.[92] A much larger survey of a controlled study in a clinical population would be required to establish any suspect medication as causative, rather than temporal.

F.M.'s sexual dysfunction (e.g., loss of interest in sexual activity and erectile dysfunction) is not caused by his current drug regimen, ramipril and glyburide. Although the MMAS[14] reported a correlation between the use of antihypertensives and hypoglycemic drugs with erectile dysfunction, clinicians must look at the individual drugs themselves and the conditions for which they are prescribed. Sexual dysfunction has not been reported for ramipril, or any of the other angiotensin-converting enzyme (ACE) inhibitors, or for the hypoglycemic agent, glyburide. Although ramipril is an antihypertensive, its pharmacologic effects do not contribute to a decline in libido or cause ED (an advantage that ACE inhibitors have over other antihypertensive medications). Similarly, the pharmacologic action of glyburide does not contribute to F.M.'s decreased libido or ED. In most sexual dysfunction cases, it is less likely that the medication is the direct cause of the problem; rather, it is the medical condition for which the drugs were prescribed. The ability of a drug to induce sexual dysfunction simply is an extension of its pharmacologic actions. As a general rule, drugs that manipulate the sympathetic or the parasympathetic system, both centrally and peripherally, are associated with sexual dysfunction.

F.M. is a patient with hypertension and diabetes who smokes cigarettes. Those three factors are more likely to be the cause of F.M.'s sexual dysfunction than are his medications. Again, in the MMAS[14] study, cigarette smoking combined with hypertension was determined to be the most significant cause of ED. Diabetes mellitus is the most common hormonal disorder associated with ED in the elderly population.[50] The continued loss of interest in sexual activity experienced by F.M. most likely is the result of having experienced ED during past and present sexual events.

F.M.'s subjective and objective findings are common among elderly men. His sexual dysfunction is caused by atherosclerosis and possible neuropathy secondary to diabetes mellitus. Because cigarette smoking is no doubt contributing to F.M.'s ED, cessation should be encouraged; some improvement can be expected.[20] There is no need to alter F.M.'s drug regimen.

Management

Essentially, there are three levels to the management of erectile dysfunction. Level I mandates lifestyle and drug therapy modifications. Specifically, the patient should be instructed to modify smoking and alcohol use. The patient's drug regimen should be checked periodically to ensure that drugs associated with ED are not being prescribed. If necessary, psychosocial counseling should be provided. After careful consideration, oral medications for management of ED should be instituted. If level I therapies have failed or are not acceptable to the patient, then level II therapy is instituted. These interventions include a vacuum construction device to elicit an erection, intracavernosal injections, or transurethral inserts. Level III management involves placement of a penile prosthesis.

Pharmacotherapy

Any therapy directed at male sexual dysfunction must include the elimination of drugs causing adverse sexual effects. Drug therapy is directed primarily toward treatment of erectile dysfunction and includes hormonal therapy, bromocriptine, yohimbine, prostaglandin E_1, sildenafil, tadalafil, vardenafil, and apomorphine.

TESTOSTERONE

6. Should F.M. be treated with testosterone?

Primary hypogonadism with severely deficient serum levels of bioavailable testosterone is the only appropriate indication for the use of androgen hormone therapy.[93] The goal of androgen replacement therapy is to restore potency and libido by maintaining normal serum levels of testosterone.[94] Testosterone has no benefit in the treatment of eugonadal or mildly hypogonadal elderly men and actually may enhance the growth of undiagnosed adenocarcinoma of the prostate or cause further erectile dysfunction.[27] In eugonadal men, testosterone enhances the rigidity of the erection, but does not change the penile circumference.[95] F.M. would not be a candidate for testosterone therapy.

7. Which type of patient would benefit from testosterone therapy?

Unless testosterone deficiency is severe, for example, if free testosterone serum levels are <7 to 8 pg/mL, testosterone replacement therapy will not improve the success rate of intercourse.[96] Testosterone replacement in patients with primary hypogonadism generally restores libido and potency. In some patients with secondary hypogonadism caused by disorders of the hypothalamus or pituitary, Gn-RH analogs can be administered to differentiate between hypothalamic and pituitary abnormalities and to correct testosterone deficiency.[94] Libido and potency then are restored.

8. How should testosterone be used as a treatment for erectile dysfunction?

Testosterone replacement therapy is available in several formulations, including gels, topical body or scrotal patches, and intramuscular injection. In a study by Monga et al.,[97] transdermal testosterone system (Testoderm-TTS) nonscrotal application was determined to provide improved erections and intercourse when compared with Testoderm scrotal patches. In this study, intramuscular testosterone or transdermal testosterone was favorably accepted by the study patients.

Because of poor drug bioavailability, oral testosterone replacement therapy is less effective than parenteral testosterone in achieving normal serum testosterone levels. Oral administration also is associated with a higher incidence of hepatotoxicity and adverse serum lipid effects.[27,98] A long-acting testosterone intramuscular formulation, such as the enanthate or the cypionate ester, is still considered the regimen of choice for the treatment of primary hypogonadism. A dose of 50 to 400 mg should be administered intramuscularly every 2 to 4 weeks. Side effects of testosterone therapy include early gynecomastia, increases in hematocrit (sometimes to the point of polycythemia), and fluid retention that may worsen hypertension or congestive heart failure (CHF).

Results of several studies have demonstrated that serum testosterone levels are normalized while using transdermal testosterone applications.[99–102] The system normalizes dihydrotestosterone:testosterone ratios and reduces LH levels toward the normal range. The testosterone transdermal system (TTS) is well tolerated, with application site reactions such as pruritus, burnlike blisters, and erythema being the most commonly reported events. Nightly applications of the TTS patch in men with hypogonadism results in a 24-hour serum testosterone concentration profile that mimics the circadian pattern observed in healthy young men.[83] The adhesive side of the TTS patch should be applied to a clean, dry area of the skin on the back, abdomen, upper arms, or thighs. The patient should be instructed to avoid application over bony prominences or on a part of the body that may be subject to prolonged pressure during sleep or sitting (e.g., the deltoid region of the upper arm, the greater trochanter of the femur, and the ischial tuberosity); do not apply to the scrotum. The sites of application should be rotated, with an interval of 7 days between applications to the same site. The area selected should not be oily, damaged, or irritated.

Topical testosterone gel should be applied once daily in the morning to clean, dry skin on the upper arms, shoulders, or abdomen. Topical testosterone gel is available as a 1% gel in unit-dose packets containing a 25- or 50-mg dose. The dose can be as high as 100 mg/24 hours. After the gel has dried on the site of application, it should be protected with clothing to prevent transfer to a nonuser. The patient's hands should be washed.

Commonly reported adverse effects in chronic users include acne, edema, gynecomastia, and dermatologic reactions to injections or transdermal applications of testosterone. The most serious risk of prolonged testosterone use is prostate carcinoma, although the association between high concentrations of testosterone and the risk of prostate carcinoma is controversial.[103,104] Three studies suggest that testosterone replacement therapy is relatively safe in hypogonadism.[105–107] Baseline assessment of the prostate should be done before starting testosterone replacement therapy. This should consist of a transrectal ultrasound, digital palpation of the prostate gland, and analysis of the total and free prostate-specific antigen (PSA) levels. Fine-needle biopsy of the prostate gland may be necessary in some hypogonadal men, because the PSA analysis may not be completely reliable.[108]

BROMOCRIPTINE

9. Because F.M.'s prolactin serum concentration is 28 ng/mL, should bromocriptine (Parlodel) be prescribed to decrease his hyperprolactinemia and treat his erectile dysfunction?
[SI unit: prolactin, 28 mcg/L]

Hyperprolactinemia may be treated with the ergot alkaloid, bromocriptine. Normalization of the serum prolactin level is mandatory if potency is to be restored. Even with normalization of prolactin levels, approximately 50% of elderly male patients are unable to achieve erectile function and desire.[94,98] Bromocriptine therapy may be initiated with twice-daily 1.25-mg doses taken with meals to minimize gastrointestinal upset. Thereafter, doses may be increased weekly, at a rate of no more than 2.5 mg/day. Because bromocriptine is associated with dizziness, drowsiness, hypotension, and cerebrovascular accidents, the patient should be forewarned.[27,94]

F.M. is not a candidate for treatment with bromocriptine because he does not have secondary hypogonadism, and his ED probably is secondary to atherosclerosis associated with his hypertension, diabetes, and cigarette smoking. Normalizing the prolactin serum level in F.M. would not correct his problem. Furthermore, the elevation of F.M.'s serum prolactin concentration is not significant to warrant drug therapy. With only a 50% (or less) response rate to bromocriptine in elderly men, the risk of adverse reactions (e.g., dyskinesia, dizziness, hallucinations, dystonia, confusion, cerebrovascular accidents) outweighs the benefit of this drug therapy.

SILDENAFIL

10. Would sildenafil citrate (Viagra) be appropriate for F.M.? What are its side effects and contraindications? Does it interact with other drugs?

F.M. has diabetes mellitus and atherosclerosis and therefore is a candidate for sildenafil. In a multicenter, randomized, double-blind, placebo-controlled, flexible dose-escalation study, sildenafil was shown to be effective and well tolerated for erectile dysfunction in men with diabetes.[109] Sildenafil citrate is an orally active and selective inhibitor of cGMP-specific phosphodiesterase type 5, the predominant phosphodiesterase isoenzyme metabolizing cGMP in the corpus cavernosum. Sildenafil facilitates an erection in response to sexual stimulation by enhancing the nitric oxide-induced relaxation of corpus cavernosal smooth muscle. The results of double-blind, placebo-controlled clinical trials in men with ED of various causes have demonstrated that sildenafil significantly improves erectile function and the rate of successful sexual intercourse, with therapeutic outcomes approaching those of normal men of the same age.[110]

The typical dose of sildenafil is 50 mg orally, taken 1 hour before sexual activity. Sildenafil citrate may be taken anywhere from 4 hours to 0.5 hour before sexual activity, however. The maximal recommended dosing frequency is once per day. The following factors are associated with increased plasma levels of sildenafil: age >65 years (40% increase in area under the curve [AUC]), hepatic impairment (e.g., cirrhosis, 80% increase), severe renal impairment (creatinine clearance <30 mL/minute,

100% increase), and concomitant use of potent cytochrome P450 (CYP) 3A4 inhibitors (erythromycin, ketoconazole, itraconazole, 200% increase). Because higher plasma levels may increase both the efficacy and the incidence of adverse events, a starting dose of 25 mg should be considered in these patients. The dose may be increased to 100 mg or reduced to 25 mg. Because F.M. is >65 years of age, he should be started on 25-mg tablets of sildenafil. The dose may be increased under strict supervision.

F.M. should be counseled on the adverse effects of sildenafil. The vasodilating action of sildenafil affects both the arteries and the veins, so the most common side effects are headache and facial flushing.[111] Sildenafil causes small decreases in both systolic and diastolic blood pressures, but clinically significant hypotension is rare. Studies of sildenafil and nitrates taken together show much greater drops in blood pressure. For that reason, sildenafil is contraindicated in patients taking long-acting nitrates or short-acting, nitrate-containing medications.[27] In phase II/III studies before U.S. Food and Drug Administration (FDA) approval, >3,700 patients received sildenafil and almost 2,000 received placebo in double-blind and open-label studies. Approximately 25% of patients had hypertension and were taking antihypertensive medications, and 17% were diabetic. In these studies, the incidence of serious cardiovascular adverse effects was similar to the double-blind sildenafil group, the double-blind placebo group, and the open-label group. Twenty-eight patients had experienced a myocardial infarction. When adjusted for patient-years of exposure, no significant differences were seen in the myocardial infarction rates between the sildenafil and the placebo group, and no deaths were attributed to sildenafil.[112,113] Nevertheless, several deaths caused by myocardial infarction or arrhythmia have been associated with the use of sildenafil.[114] Deaths associated with sildenafil (and presumably other PDE5 inhibitors) are most likely caused by increased cardiac workload in patients with unstable angina.[115]

Transient visual anomalies (mostly blue-green color-tinged objects, increased perception of light, and blurred vision) have been reported in patients taking sildenafil, especially at higher dosages (>100 mg). These visual effects appear to be related to the weaker inhibiting action of sildenafil on the enzyme, phosphodiesterase-6 (PDE-6), which regulates signal transduction pathways in the retinal photoreceptors. Sildenafil is 10-fold selective for PDE-5 over PDE-6. In patients with inherited disorders of retinal PDE-6, such as retinitis pigmentosa, sildenafil should be administered with extreme caution.

The vasodilator actions of nitrates are profoundly amplified with concomitant use of sildenafil. This interaction likely applies to all nitrates and nitric oxide donors, regardless of their predominant hemodynamic site of action. Sildenafil also may potentiate the inhaled form of nitrate, such as amyl nitrite, and therefore is contraindicated in patients using this product. Dietary sources of nitrates, nitrites, and L-arginine (the substrate from which nitric oxide is synthesized) do not contribute to the circulating levels of nitric oxide in humans and therefore are unlikely to interact with sildenafil. The anesthetic agent, nitrous oxide, is eliminated unchanged from the body, mostly via the lungs, within minutes of inhalation. It does not form nitric oxide in the human body and does not itself activate guanylate cyclase. As such, no contraindication exists to its use after administration of sildenafil.

It is unknown how much time must elapse from the time a patient takes sildenafil before a nitrate-containing medication might be given without the marked hypotensive effect being produced. On the basis of the pharmacokinetic profile of sildenafil, it can be assumed that the coadministration of a nitrate within 24 hours is likely to produce an exaggerated hypotensive response and therefore is contraindicated. After 24 hours, the administration of nitrates can once again be considered. In patients in whom sildenafil may have a prolonged half-life, the nitrate-free period must be extended. All patients taking nitrates must be warned of the contraindications and the potential consequences of taking sildenafil in the 24-hour interval after taking a nitrate preparation, including sublingual nitroglycerin. Although sublingual nitroglycerin is short-acting, its use within a 24-hour time period before sexual relations does suggest that it may be needed again after sildenafil-enhanced sexual activity.

Sildenafil is metabolized by both the CYP 2C9 pathway and the CYP 3A4 pathway. Thus, inhibitors of the CYP 3A4 isoenzyme, such as erythromycin or cimetidine, may lead to competitive inhibition of its metabolism; however, CYP 3A4 is a high-capacity pathway. The effects of erythromycin or cimetidine on the half-life and physiologic effects of sildenafil are not known, but clinicians should be warned about the potential interaction.

Inadequate physical sexual stimulation while using any of the PDE-5 inhibitors can lead to treatment failure. Adequate sexual stimulation is needed to trigger the events leading to erection.[116] PDE-5-inhibitors cannot initiate an erection, they can only assist in the process. Some patients may need several attempts at sexual stimulation before they are successful with intercourse.

11. Is F.M. a candidate for tadalafil or vardenafil?

TADALAFIL

Similar to sildenafil, tadalafil (Cialis) is a selective inhibitor of phosphodiesterase-5 (PDE-5). Tadalafil has several times more affinity for PDE-5 than sildenafil.[117] The clinical significance of this increased affinity for PDE-5 is unknown because comparative clinical trials between the PDE-5-inhibitors (sildenafil, tadalafil, and vardenafil) have not been conducted. Tadalafil and vardenafil, however, have minimal or no effect on visual disturbance (impairment of blue-green color discrimination), which is a well recognized side effect of sildenafil.[118] Tadalafil's extended half-life of 17.5 hours relative to sildenafil most likely precludes its use in patients with angina or hypertension. Tadalafil is metabolized by the hepatic CYP 3A4 isozyme. Food has no effect on the oral absorption of tadalafil in contrast to sildenafil (bioavailability decreased by 29%). Tadalafil may be advantageous in a subset of patients, based on its shorter onset of action (16 minutes) and 24-hour duration of action.[119] Specifically, patients with psychogenic or neurogenic ED and those with stable cardiovascular systems may prefer tadalafil because it offers the potential for multiple sessions of intercourse encounters with a single daily dose. F.M. has hypertension that most likely would be affected by tadalafil; therefore, extreme caution is advised. Perhaps the shorter-acting sildenafil would be the PDE-5-inhibitor drug of choice for F.M. The warnings regarding the use of nitrates while taking tadalafil are similar to the warnings for sildenafil.

VARDENAFIL

Vardenafil (Levitra) is the third FDA-approved oral PDE-5 inhibitor for treatment of erectile dysfunction. Vardenafil, as with the other PDE-5-inhibitors, has an affinity for PDE-6 and will therefore cause ocular adverse effects. The warnings regarding the use of nitrates while taking vardenafil are similar to the warnings for sildenafil. Patients using vardenafil may experience headache, flushing, or rhinitis; the incidence of these side effects are dose related.[120] Vardenafil is metabolized by the hepatic CYP 3A4 isozyme and has a reported half-life of 5 hours.[121] Thus, drugs known to inhibit the CYP 3A4 isozyme have the potential to prolong its half-life. Vardenafil 10 mg does not impair the ability of patients with stable coronary artery disease to exercise at levels equivalent to or greater than that attained during sexual intercourse.[122]

12. What other drug therapy is available for F.M.?

YOHIMBINE

Yohimbine, an indole alkaloid derived from the bark of the West African yohimbine tree, has been classified as an aphrodisiac in many pharmacopoeias. Yohimbine hydrochloride is an α_2-adrenergic antagonist that decreases the outward blood flow from the penile corporal tissue. The effectiveness of yohimbine relies on an adequate penile blood supply. It has been used in treating ED among diabetics with some degree of success.[123] In a trial of men with psychogenic ED, yohimbine produced a 47% response rate versus 28% among placebo users.[124] This finding was affirmed in a subsequent study.[125] Men with psychogenic or neurogenic ED have some response.[123–125] Despite its modest efficacy, yohimbine is used in patients who do not accept more invasive methods because it is safe, available, and easy to use. Because F.M. is experiencing vasculogenic, neurogenic, and psychogenic ED, his response to yohimbine may be none to slight, at best, owing to his atherosclerosis and resultant low penile blood supply. Again, the risk of side effects compared with the slight benefit that F.M. may experience suggests that other therapies be considered.

In some patients, yohimbine has been associated with nausea, tachycardia, a slight elevation in blood pressure, anxiety, and panic attacks.[98] The drug regimen used in clinical trials is 6 mg orally three times a day, and beneficial effects usually become apparent within 2 to 3 weeks.[21,123,124] In some of the trials, the point was made that the dose of 18 mg/day may be too low; however, dose-response trials would be necessary before higher doses could be recommended.

INTRACAVERNOUS INJECTIONS

In 1982, inadvertent injection of papaverine into the penis was found to produce an erection.[126] This landmark observation ushered in a new methodology for the diagnosis and therapy of erectile dysfunction. By 1986, papaverine injection into the penis had gained worldwide popularity for the treatment of ED.[127] In 1983, the α-blocker, phenoxybenzamine, also was noted to be effective.[128] Shortly thereafter, the combination of papaverine with another vasodilator, phentolamine, reportedly enhanced and prolonged erection duration.[129] These vasoactive drugs, when injected into the cavernosa, cause prolonged penile arterial vasodilation and venous compression, thus allowing the patient to achieve and maintain an erection. Erectile dysfunction responds favorably to the self-injection of vasoactive drugs into the penis.[127,130,131] Originally, the IC regimen of papaverine with phentolamine was prescribed as a short-term measure taken while patients were awaiting the results of counseling or a penile implant. Currently, self-injection of vasoactive drugs has become accepted as a nonsurgical method of treating ED (Table 101-3).

Table 101-3 Agents Used to Treat Vasculogenic Erectile Dysfunction

Drugs	Route	Mechanism
Papaverine	ICI	Phosphodiesterase inhibitor; penile arteriolar vasodilator
Phentolamine	ICI	α-Adrenergic blockade; direct vasodilator
Prostaglandin E_1	ICI	α-Blockade; vasodilator
Atropine	ICI	Antimuscarinic; smooth muscle relaxant

ICI, intracavernous injection.

Papaverine–Phentolamine Combination

Papaverine, a nonspecific phosphodiesterase inhibitor, increases the serum concentration of cAMP, resulting in penile arteriolar and corporal sinusoidal smooth muscle relaxation. In laboratory studies, papaverine blocks voltage-operated calcium channels, inhibits the release and storage of intracellular calcium, increases calcium efflux, and inhibits calcium-activated chloride and potassium currents in vascular smooth muscle.[132–134] Papaverine also may relax an elastic venous valve mechanism that is kept open by an α-adrenergically mediated smooth muscle contraction.[135–137]

Phentolamine exerts its relaxant effects by α-adrenergic receptor blockade of both α_1- and α_2-adrenoceptors. In addition, phentolamine also may have a direct, nonspecific relaxant effect on vessels.[138] The combined use of papaverine with phentolamine exerts a greater effect than would be experienced with either drug alone.[139] The use of alprostadil (prostaglandin E_1) by IC injection is addressed in Question 19.

Candidates for Intracavernous Injection Therapy

13. What objective data must be obtained to ensure that F.M. can receive IC injections safely?

Patients who have failed to obtain a satisfactory erection while on oral drug therapy, such as sildenafil, tadalafil, yohimbine, or sublingual apomorphine (available in Europe), are candidates for the IC injections of vasoactive drugs. The patient must have a complete medical workup to include assessment of the penile arterial system. Doppler sonography of the penis identifies penile architecture, defines the thickness of any plaques, measures the diameter of cavernous arteries (before and after vasodilation), and allows visualization of the penile arteries. This noninvasive assessment of the individual penile arteries is much more accurate than the penile brachial pressure index (PBI). The PBI is the ratio of the penile systolic blood pressure (measured by continuous-wave Doppler analysis) to the brachial artery systolic pressure. This method of assessment measures all the penile arteries rather than signals from a single penile artery. PBI ratios that are normal (i.e., >0.6) do not always indicate normal penile blood flow, because the PBI is obtained while the penis is flaccid. F.M. should have sonography combined with Doppler analysis to assess the adequacy of his penile arterial blood flow.

In some urologic practices, the functional evaluation of penile arteries is obtained by IC injection of vasoactive drugs at the office. If the patient develops a fully rigid erection within 12 minutes of injection of papaverine hydrochloride 30 to 60 mg or prostaglandin E_1 10 to 20 mg and maintains a rigid erection for 30 minutes, adequate arterial flow and an intact venous mechanism can be assumed.[28] The patient then is a candidate for at-home IC injection of vasoactive drugs.

14. The Doppler sonography analysis of F.M.'s penile arteries showed severe atherosclerosis, indicating a vasculogenic etiology for his erectile dysfunction. Is F.M. still a candidate for IC injection therapy?

Patients with psychogenic or neurogenic erectile dysfunction who respond to test doses of IC injections of a vasoactive drug are optimal candidates for IC injection therapy.[140] Patients with vasculogenic ED are less responsive to the IC injections of vasoactive drugs, and corporeal veno-occlusive dysfunction is the primary potential obstacle to this treatment.[141,142]

An abnormal veno-occlusive mechanism can result in penile venous incompetence, causing rapid detumescence or partial erection (referred to as venogenic erectile dysfunction). The veno-occlusive mechanism of the corpora cavernosa can be assessed through an elaborate and quite painful invasive process, using angiocatheters and iodinated contrast media. In a study to determine the effectiveness and safety of IC therapy in vasculogenic impotent men, 40% of the participants had arteriovenogenic ED, and 32% had venogenic ED (i.e., they had a dysfunctional veno-occlusive mechanism), with only 28% of participants having pure arteriogenic ED.[143] Only 4% of the participants failed to achieve a sustained rigid erection, however; massive veno-occlusive mechanism dysfunction was cited as the reason. At a mean follow-up of 20 months, the remaining 96% of patients (including those with some degree of veno-occlusive mechanism dysfunction) still were using the IC injection therapy. Given these findings, F.M. has a good chance of responding to IC injection therapy, even if it is determined that he has some veno-occlusive disease. Absolute contraindications to IC injection therapy are anticoagulant therapy, Peyronie's disease, and idiopathic priapism.

Dosing

15. What is the protocol for starting a patient on an IC injection therapy program for home use?

The initial dose of the papaverine–phentolamine combination should take into consideration the underlying etiology for the erectile dysfunction, the findings of the Doppler sonography, and the patient's response to a test dose of the IC injection. Generally, patients with neurogenic ED are started on the lowest doses (usually 0.5 mL), whereas patients with severely compromised penile arterial blood flow would receive larger doses (e.g., 1.0 mL). It should be kept in mind that there may be excessive sympathetic stimulation in an anxious patient while at the physician's office, and more drug may be required to overcome the vasoconstriction.[144] This implies that at-home use may require a lower dose. The standard mixture for the most common vasoactive IC injection solution is 30 mg/mL of papaverine and 1 mg/mL of phentolamine, for a total volume of 10 mL. The initial test dose administered in the physician's office generally is 0.5 mL (but may be as low as 0.25 mL) of the 30:1 mixture, using a tuberculin syringe with a 26-gauge needle. The patient is observed for both therapeutic and adverse effects, such as bradycardia, hypertension, dizziness, or flushing. If any of these adverse effects are observed, atropine should be injected IC.[145] In the event that the patient's erection becomes prolonged beyond 30 to 60 minutes, the subsequent dose of papaverine–phentolamine should be reduced. Prolonged erection, which may progress to a pulsatile priapism, is the most significant complication of IC injections of vasoactive drugs. Treatment should be instituted immediately with epinephrine 1 mg/mL, 10 to 20 mL injected IC as an irrigant, and then aspirated.[140] Prolonged erections can lead to intracorporeal hypoxia, resulting in corporeal fibrosis.[145] In some cases, the physician may choose single-drug IC injection with papaverine 25 to 60 mg, or prostaglandin E_1 10 or 20 mg/dose.

Extemporaneous Compounding

16. What procedures should be taken when extemporaneously compounding a papaverine–phentolamine injectable solution, and what expiration date is acceptable?

The method used to extemporaneously compound the papaverine–phentolamine mixture was developed in the early 1980s without consideration of pharmaceutical product stability. Nevertheless, the compounding of the papaverine–phentolamine solution has not changed much from those early days. The final product usually consists of a 10-mL vial of papaverine and phentolamine in a ratio of 30:1 mg/mL. Papaverine hydrochloride is available in a 30-mg/mL, 10-mL multidose vial that also contains 0.5% chlorbutanol as a preservative. Phentolamine mesylate (Regitine) is available in vials containing 5 mg of active drug and 25 mg of mannitol, in a sterile lyophilized form. Extemporaneous compounding of this product requires sterile technique. One vial of papaverine and two vials of phentolamine are needed to make the final product. Using a small-gauge needle and 3-mL syringe, remove 2 mL (i.e., 60 mg) from the papaverine vial and use 1 mL to reconstitute the first vial of phentolamine. With the remaining 1 mL of papaverine solution in the syringe, reconstitute the second vial of phentolamine. Using the empty syringe, remove the solution from both phentolamine vials and instill this volume into the 10-mL papaverine multidose vial. Each milliliter of the final concentration in the papaverine vial should contain 30 mg of papaverine hydrochloride with 1 mg of phentolamine mesylate (plus 0.5% chlorbutanol and 5 mg of mannitol).

Currently, the FDA has not approved either papaverine or phentolamine alone or in combination as a treatment modality for erectile dysfunction. The addition of phentolamine mesylate to a multidose vial of papaverine hydrochloride for at-home patient use is not mentioned in the respective manufacturers' package inserts.[146,147] In a product-stability study, the combination of papaverine and phentolamine was stable for at least 40 days when stored at room temperature.[148] In this study, the concentration of papaverine hydrochloride was 25 mg/mL and phentolamine mesylate was 0.83 mg/mL. Thus, the common practice of using a 30-day expiration date on extemporaneously prepared papaverine–phentolamine multidose preparations is justified.

Patient Instructions

17. What instructions should be provided to the patient for IC injection therapy?

Once the dose of IC injection vasoactive drug is determined for the patient at the physician's office, the patient then is taught self-injection using a 26-gauge needle, 1-mL syringe.

Patients should be instructed to inject into the right side of the penis (lateral aspect), approximately 4 cm from the glans after the area has been cleaned with an alcohol swab. The tip of the needle should be placed into the center of the right corpus cavernosum with a quick jab. The injection is administered within a 1- to 2-minute period. If pain is felt in the glans penis, the rate of injection should be slowed (next time) to perhaps 3 or 4 minutes. On withdrawal of the needle, the puncture site is compressed and the penis should be massaged gently by squeezing intermittently for approximately 3 minutes to distribute the drug throughout the shaft. A tourniquet at the base of the penis is not necessary. Sterile technique should be stressed when discussing this procedure with patients.

The number of injections per month is limited by a 10-mL supply to prevent long-term complications. The 10-mL volume allows patients to have intercourse 10 to 20 times per month if doses of 0.5 to 1 mL are used.

Adverse Effects

18. F.M. has been using papaverine–phentolamine 30:1 mixture at a dose of 1.0 mL per sexual episode over the past 6 months. He has injected himself 32 times. For the past month, he has noticed a lateral deviation of his penis when rigid, and now he feels a "hard spot" (induration) below the surface of the skin on the shaft. What are the adverse effects associated with repeated use of papaverine–phentolamine IC injections?

Penile induration and corporeal fibrosis are complications of IC injections, particularly when papaverine hydrochloride is used. The appearance of induration or fibrosis significantly correlates to the number of injections administered.[149] Men with penile induration or fibrosis injected the papaverine–phentolamine mixture two and one-half times more often than those who did not experience this side effect. Similarly, men who administered higher doses also were more likely to develop penile induration or fibrosis ($p < 0.01$). Hence, a 10-mL solution of the papaverine–phentolamine combination should be dispensed on a monthly basis to manage both the frequency of use and the total dose. The patient should be educated about the complications and side effects of penile injection with vasoactive drugs (Table 101-4).

Corporeal fibrosis, which can result in Peyronie disease, is the limiting factor with any combination of papaverine, because the relative acidity of the drug (pH, 3–4) is associated with sclerosis.[150–153] The frequency of IC papaverine injections should be limited. At least 94% of patients using IC self-injection experience at least one complication, with 70% of users reporting at least two to three complications.[154] Injection site pain is related more to the injection of the drugs than to the insertion of the needle.[155] The pain is described as a burning sensation in the glans penis occurring 30 seconds after the injection begins and lasting for 1 to 2 minutes after the injection is stopped. The most devastating complication, priapism, is experienced by approximately 4% of patients and requires treatment. Of interest, none of the patients who experienced priapism had vasculogenic impotence. Self-administration side effects, such as pain, bruising, and swelling, usually do not occur when physicians inject the vasoactive drugs into the penis.[149]

Systemic effects of papaverine–phentolamine initially were believed to be insignificant. The use of this mixture has been associated, however, with abnormal liver function tests (LFT) in 40% of recipients, mostly involving mild to moderate elevations of serum alkaline phosphatase and serum lactic dehydrogenase.[149] Hepatotoxicity, which may have an immune mechanism, has been associated with papaverine injection infrequently. A patient may be advised to discontinue the use of this medication if the LFT are indicative of hepatocellular injury.

The adverse effects from the use of papaverine–phentolamine generally do not prevent continued use of this therapy. After an episode of priapism, patients are instructed not to use the injection for at least 1 month.[154] Most patients who have experienced one or more adverse effects (e.g., bruising, pain, fibrosis, priapism) from the papaverine–phentolamine injections generally still resist penile implantation for as long as possible and continue the injection therapy.[154]

Several studies have reported various degrees of satisfaction among users of IC self-injection.[130,131,154] Eventually, most users discontinue the use of IC injection and consider a penile implant. Complications resulting from IC injection of vasoactive drugs do not prevent successful prosthetic implantation.[154]

Table 101-4 Side Effects of Papaverine-Phentolamine ICI for Vasculogenic Impotence

Prolonged erection	Penile induration
Priapism	Pain at injection site
Painless penile nodules	Bruising or bleeding at injection site
Peyronie's disease	Abnormal LFT

ICI, intracavernous injection; LFT, liver function tests.

Alprostadil

19. What other drugs can be used by IC injection in patients who are unresponsive to the papaverine–phentolamine mixture? How is alprostadil used to treat erectile dysfunction?

Patients with vasculogenic erectile dysfunction are less likely to respond to papaverine–phentolamine by IC injection. These patients generally require larger doses of papaverine–phentolamine and thus are more likely to develop penile induration. However, 96% of patients with vasculogenic ED responded to a four-drug vasoactive mixture of papaverine hydrochloride 12.1 mg/mL, prostaglandin E_1 10.1 mg/mL, phentolamine mesylate 1.01 mg/mL, and atropine sulfate 0.15 mg/mL. The solution was obtained by mixing 250 mg papaverine hydrochloride (14.4 mL), 200 mg of prostaglandin E_1 (0.4 mL), 20 mg of phentolamine mesylate (2 mL), and 3 mg of atropine sulfate (3 mL), for a total of 19.8 mL.[143] Doses administered were from 0.1 to 1.0 mL via a 27-gauge self-injection device.

Prostaglandin E_1 (alprostadil) is available for IC injection, as a urethral insert (referred to as *medicated urethral system for erection* [MUSE]) and as a topical cream. All of these pharmaceutical preparations have been shown to be efficacious for men with ED,[19,156,157] with users reporting successful intercourse 65% of the time. The efficacy of alprostadil was similar, regardless of the patient's age or the cause of ED, which included vascular disease, diabetes, surgery, and trauma. Prostaglandin E_1 has α-blocking properties mediated through a membrane receptor. It relaxes the cavernous and arteriolar smooth muscle while restricting venous outflow.[140] The addition of an oral α-blocker may have a beneficial effect in patients with ED for whom IC injection therapy alone fails. The synergistic effects of vascular dilation and blockade of sympathetic inhibition may explain this response.[158] Prostaglandin E_1 is an acceptable alternative to papaverine and patients experience few side effects.[159,160] The use of IC papaverine with prostaglandin E_1 has proved, however, to be superior to prostaglandin E_1 alone.[161] Prostaglandin is metabolized in the local tissue and is unlikely to cause any systemic effects.[162] The most common side effects of urethral alprostadil inserts are penile pain, which occurs in 29% to 49%[163] of users, and hypotension within 1 hour of use, which occurs in 3.3% of users. Urethral bleeding has been reported in 5% of users. Patients should be advised about hypotension, particularly if they also are using nitrates or antihypertensive medications. Less than 2% of users have reported swelling of leg veins, leg pain, perineal pain, and rapid pulse. Penile induration has not yet been reported with use of prostaglandin E_1.

BENIGN PROSTATIC HYPERPLASIA

Benign prostatic hyperplasia (BPH), a common cause of urinary dysfunction symptoms in elderly men, results from proliferation of the stromal and epithelial cells of the prostate gland.[164,165] There is both a static and a dynamic component to prostate enlargement. The static component increases the prostate size by smooth muscle cell proliferation in the prostate stroma, whereas the dynamic component contributes to an enlarged prostate through an increase in smooth muscle tone in the prostate and bladder neck. The term *benign prostatic hypertrophy* often is used inappropriately because the prostate gland pathology results from hyperplasia rather than hypertrophy. BPH rarely is detected in men <40 years of age. After age 40, the prevalence of BPH is age dependent.[166] Approximately 75% of men who live to the age of 70 develop clinical symptoms of BPH that are sufficiently severe to necessitate medical attention, and approximately 90% of octogenarians have evidence of BPH. Essentially, all men will develop BPH if they live long enough. The microscopic incidence of BPH is fairly constant among several Western and developing countries,[167] suggesting that the initiation of BPH may not be environmentally or genetically influenced. Although BPH and prostatic cancer often coexist, no compelling evidence indicates that BPH predisposes patients to the development of prostate cancer.[168] The appearance of atypical prostatic hyperplasia correlates, however, with the presence of latent prostatic carcinoma.[169]

The cause of BPH is unclear; however, most hypotheses are based on hormonal and aging processes. This is because intact, normally functioning testes are essential for BPH to develop,[170] and castration before puberty prevents the development of BPH. The prostate is dependent on androgens both for embryologic development and maintenance of size and function in the mature male.[171] Testosterone, the major circulating androgen, is metabolized to dihydrotestosterone (DHT) by 5 α-reductase. The two isoenzymes of 5 α-reductase are designated type I and type II. Type II is found predominantly in the prostate and other genital tissues, whereas type I is found throughout the body, as well as in the prostate.[172] For testosterone to be active in the prostate, it must be converted to DHT; therefore, DHT is the obligate androgen responsible for normal and hyperplastic prostate growth. Within the prostate, DHT initiates RNA synthesis, protein synthesis, and cell replication. The exact role of testosterone may be only to initiate fibroadenomatous hyperplasia, eventually resulting in glandular enlargement.

Stromal hyperplasia in the prostate periurethral glands is one of the earliest microscopic findings in men with BPH.[167] As men increase in age, testosterone serum concentrations decrease and the peripheral conversion of testosterone to estrogen increases. At one time, estrogens were thought to initiate stromal hyperplasia, which in turn induces epithelial hyperplasia. It is now known, however, that estrogens do not have a direct effect on the development of BPH and prostatic carcinoma, but progesterone does play a role in their pathogenesis. Progesterone receptors have been shown to exist in prostate stromal cells, whereas estrogen receptors were essentially nonexistent.[173]

Pathophysiology and Clinical Presentation

20. G.M., a 72-year-old man, presents to the emergency department with severe lower abdominal discomfort of 4 days' duration. His history consists of having increasing difficulty initiating urination, a significant decrease in the force of his urinary stream, occasional midstream stoppage, and postvoid dribbling. Physical examination is unremarkable except for the abdominal and rectal examination. Abdominal examination reveals distention, tenderness, and increased dullness in the hypogastrium with a large mass, believed to be the bladder. On rectal examination, the prostate is found to be severely enlarged, firm, and rubbery without nodules or undue hardness. G.M. gives a history of nocturia (approximately four to five times a night) and daytime urinary frequency (eight to ten times a day). G.M. indicates that when he is able to urinate he does not feel relieved. Laboratory findings are as follows: BUN, 45 mg/dL (normal, 8–18); SrCr, 3.2 mg/dL (normal, 0.6–1.2); serum prostatic acid phosphatase, 3 U/L; and serum PSA, 7.1 ng/mL (normal, 0.1–4.0). A urethral catheter was inserted, and 900 mL of urine was obtained. G.M. subsequently was scheduled for a urologic workup. What is the pathophysiologic basis for G.M.'s symptoms?

[SI units: BUN, 16.1 mmol/L urea; SrCr, 282.9 μmol/L; serum prostatic acid phosphatase, 3 U/L (normal, 2.5–11)]

Symptoms of BPH can be both obstructive and irritative, and descriptions of the symptoms need a frame of reference for standardization. The Boyarsky index, a questionnaire consisting of nine questions to quantify the severity of BPH,[174] has been developed. Five questions are designed to assess obstructive symptoms and four to assess irritative symptoms. Although some limitations to the use of this questionnaire (Table 101-5) may exist, it is one of the most common measures used to quantify symptoms in BPH studies[167] and it correlates well with the pathophysiology of BPH. The format of the Boyarsky

Table 101-5 BPH Symptom Scoring System (Boyarsky Index)[a]

Nocturia	
0	Absence of symptoms
1	Urinates 1 time/night
2	Urinates 2–3 times/night
3	Urinates ≥4 times/night
Daytime Frequency	
0	Urinates 1–4 times/day
1	Urinates 5–7 times/day
2	Urinates 8–12 times/day
3	Urinates ≥13 times/day
Hesitance (lasts ≥1 min)	
0	Occasional (≤20% of the time)
1	Moderate (20%–50% of the time)
2	Frequent (≥50% of the time)
3	Always present
Intermittency (lasts ≥min)	
0	Occasional (≤20% of the time)
1	Moderate (20%–50% of the time)
2	Frequent (≥50% of the time)
3	Always present
Terminal Dribbling (at end of voiding)	
0	Occasional (≤20% of the time)
1	Moderate (20%–50% of the time)
2	Frequent (≥50% of the time)
3	Always present (may wet clothes)
Urgency	
0	Absence
1	Occasionally difficult to postpone urination
2	Frequently difficult to postpone urination
3	Always difficult to postpone urination
Impairment of Size and Force of Urinary Stream	
0	Absence
1	Impaired trajectory
2	Most of the time size and force are restricted
3	Urinates with great effort and stream is interrupted
Dysuria	
0	Absence
1	Occasional burning sensation during urination
2	Frequent (>50% of the time) burning sensation
3	Frequent and painful burning sensation during urination
Sensation of Incomplete Voiding	
0	Absence
1	Occasional sensation
2	Frequent (>50% of the time) sensation
3	Constant and urgent sensation, no relief on voiding

[a]Symptom scoring provides the clinician with a tool to measure the relative need for, and efficacy of, different interventions. No specific score is associated with the need for a specific intervention. A low symptom score in the absence of significant urine retention generally indicates that medical management can be attempted before considering surgical intervention.[174] BPH, benign prostatic hyperplasia.

index is designed to help the clinician educate the patient about the obstructive and irritative symptoms of BPH. The Boyarsky index was the first of three patient questionnaires developed to quantitatively assess BPH and the effectiveness of individual treatment.[171] As such, this questionnaire has been used in numerous clinical trials to measure the outcome of interventions. The Boyarsky index is not useful in comparing different treatment therapies among BPH patients, because it has not been sufficiently validated for this purpose; rather, it is useful in evaluating an individual's response to therapy.

The Multidisciplinary Measurements Committee of the American Urologic Association (AUA) also has published a Urinary Symptom Index for Prostatism[175] (Table 101-6). The AUA recognized the importance of a validated symptom index for assessing the baseline severity of prostatism, disease progression, and the effectiveness of different therapies. The AUA symptom index allows comparison between therapies and is the preferred questionnaire for BPH research. It has been validated through internal consistency reliability, constructive reliability, test-retest reliability, and criterion reliability.[171] The AUA index, however, may not be BPH specific.[176] When 101 men and 96 women between the ages of 55 and 79 used the AUA index, urinary symptoms and severity of urinary symptoms were similar in both groups. Therefore, symptoms associated with prostatism can be associated with aging as well as BPH. The National Institutes of Health (NIH) convened a chronic prostatitis workshop to come to consensus on a new classification system for the diagnosis and management of prostatitis.[177] This group developed a symptom index that provides a valid outcome measure for men with prostatitis. This index attempts to quantify the pain and discomfort associated with prostatism, and should help differentiate prostatism from prostatic hyperplasia. The symptom index is self-administered.

G.M. presents with obstructive symptoms consistent with BPH as follows: (a) a history of difficulty in initiating urination (hesitancy), (b) a decrease in urinary force, (c) occasional midstream stoppage, (d) postvoiding dribbling, and (e) a feeling of incomplete bladder emptying. The common obstructive symptom of decreased force and size of urine stream is caused by urethral compression from prostate gland hyperplasia. Hesitancy, another obstructive symptom, is the result of the bladder detrusor muscle taking a longer time to generate the initial increased pressure to overcome urethral resistance. Urinary stream intermittency is caused by the inability of the bladder detrusor muscle to sustain the increased pressure until the end of voiding. Terminal dribbling and incomplete emptying occur for the same reason, but also may be caused by obstructive prostatic tissue at the bladder neck, causing a "ball valve" effect.

G.M. also has a history of classic irritative symptoms that are consistent with BPH as follows: (a) nocturia approximately four to five times a night and (b) daytime urinary frequency of 8 to 10 times a day. Incomplete emptying of the bladder results in shorter intervals between voiding, explaining the complaint of frequency. Also, a large prostate gland provokes the bladder to trigger a voiding response more frequently. This response is more pronounced if the prostate is growing intravesically and compromising the bladder volume. Bladder detrusor muscle becomes hypertrophied as a result of the greater bladder residual urine volume, which can result in increased detrusor muscle excitability. Clinically, this excitability may result in bladder instability. The symptoms of urinary frequency are

Table 101-6 American Urological Association (AUA) Urinary Symptom Index for Prostatism

Symptom	Score: Not at All	<1 in 5 Times	<1/2 the Time	=1/2 Time	>1/2 the Time	Almost Always
1. Over the past month or so, how often have you had a sensation of not emptying your bladder completely after you finished urinating?	0	1	2	3	4	5
2. Over the past month or so, how often have you had to urinate again <2 hr after you finished urinating?	0	1	2	3	4	5
3. Over the past month or so, how often have you found you stopped and started several times when you urinated?	0	1	2	3	4	5
4. Over the past month or so, how often have you found it difficult to postpone urination?	0	1	2	3	4	5
5. Over the past month or so, how often have you had a weak urinary stream?	0	1	2	3	4	5
6. Over the past month or so, how often have you had to push or strain to begin urination?	0	1	2	3	4	5
7. Over the past month or so, how many times did you most times typically get up to urinate from the time you went to bed at night until the time you got up in the morning?	0 times	1 time	2 times	3 times	4 times	5 times

Interpretation of AUA Symptom Index

AUA Symptom Score = Sum of questions 1–7 = ____________

Mild prostatism ≤7
Moderate prostatism 8–18
Severe prostatism >18
Highest possible score 35

Reprinted from reference 325, with permission.

more pronounced at night because cortical inhibitions are lessened and bladder sphincter tone is more relaxed during sleep. Obstructive symptoms are associated more with an enlarged prostate, and the predominance of irritative symptoms could suggest voiding dysfunctions in addition to those of BPH.

Urinary incontinence is not a common symptom of BPH. With advanced BPH, a large residual volume of urine in the bladder weakens the bladder sphincter and allows the escape of small amounts of urine when the bladder is full. As the residual bladder volume increases, the ureters will dilate, resulting in stasis of urine in the ureters. The end result may be ascending hydronephrosis caused by the transmission of high pressure to nephrons, which produces renal damage (Fig. 101-3). This can account for abdominal discomfort and flank pain during voiding and ascending urinary tract infections.

Acute urinary retention in BPH can occur as a result of increasing size of the prostate gland. Independent of gland size, drugs may precipitate acute urinary retention. Drugs, such as alcohol, anticholinergic agents, α-adrenergic agents, and neuroleptics, all have been associated with acute urinary retention in men with BPH. Commonly, when advanced BPH is present, acute urinary retention is exacerbated if the patient does not void at the first sign of urgency. G.M. is not taking any drugs commonly associated with urinary retention.

Clinical Findings

21. What objective findings in G.M. are associated with BPH?

G.M. presents with classic symptoms of BPH. The increasingly severe symptoms culminated in an episode of acute urinary retention as evidenced by inability to void and lower abdominal discomfort. Objective symptoms associated with G.M.'s BPH include: (a) abdominal tenderness with increased dullness in the hypogastrium; (b) the finding of an enlarged bladder; (c) an enlarged, firm, and rubbery prostate gland; and (d) a return of 900 mL of urine via urinary catheter. The normal serum acid phosphatase, slightly elevated PSA, and digital rectal examination of the prostate suggest that G.M. does not have prostatic carcinoma at this time (see following section). The elevated BUN and serum creatinine may suggest hydronephrosis as a result of his BPH.

Urinalysis

Because patients with BPH also may have a urinary tract infection, a urinalysis with microscopic examination is essential. It is mandatory that G.M. give a urine specimen for urinalysis before the digital rectal examination of the prostate gland, because examination of the prostate causes prostatic secretions to be expelled into the urethra, which may contaminate the urine specimen and make it difficult to determine the source of an infection. The presence of WBC and bacteria in the urine necessitates a workup for infection. Similarly, hematuria requires a workup for urinary tract pathology other than BPH. Because BPH also can cause hydronephrosis, renal function and serum electrolytes should be evaluated.

Digital Rectal Examination

A serum PSA followed by a digital rectal examination of the prostate remains a fundamental part of evaluating a man with prostatism. The prostate examination should determine the size, shape, consistency, and nodularity of this gland. Prostatic

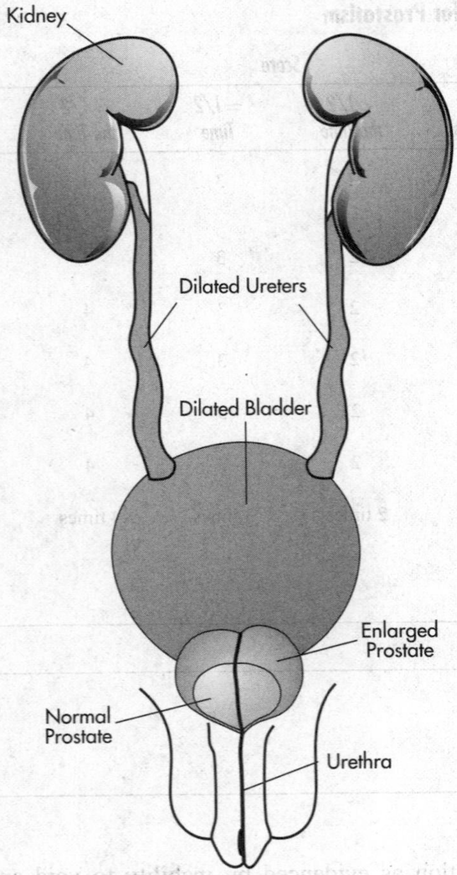

FIGURE 101-3 Flow of urine is interrupted by compression from a prostate that has enlarged from normal size. In this diagram, the ureters and bladder are dilated by backed-up urine.

hyperplasia results in a large, palpable prostate with a smooth mucosal surface rectally. The discernment of the right and left prostate lobes is lost in BPH. The digital rectal examination of a patient with BPH commonly finds asymmetry of the prostate, with one side being larger than the other. Prostatic enlargement can be in both an anteroposterior and a superoinferior direction. As a result, on digital rectal examination, the upper extent of prostate hyperplasia is not palpable. Occasionally, the degree of enlargement felt by digital rectal examination may be misleading, because a substantial portion of enlargement may be intravesical. The consistency of the gland may be soft or firm, depending on the predominance of glandular or fibromuscular elements.[178] The presence of firm-to-hard nodules; irregularities; induration; or a stony, hard prostate suggests possible prostate cancer. In those cases in which the prostate gland size or shape may be questioned, the patient should have a transrectal ultrasound (TRUS) to determine the gland volume.

Prostate-Specific Antigen

Prostate-specific antigen is a glycoprotein enzyme (molecular weight, 33,000) that is secreted in the cytoplasm of the prostatic cells; it aids in the liquefaction of semen. Some claim that this enzyme is specific for prostate origin, although a few isolated instances of elevation in nonprostate tumors have been reported. PSA correlates reasonably well, on average, with prostate weight owing to benign prostate glandular

Table 101-7 Age-Adjusted PSA Values

Age Range (yr)	PSA Upper Limit (ng/mL)	PSA Density
40–49	2.5	0.08
50–59	3.5	0.10
60–69	4.5	0.11
70–79	6.5	0.13

PSA, prostate-specific antigen.

hyperplasia.[179] Prostate cancer, however, produces approximately 10 times the amount of PSA on a tissue volume basis than does BPH.[180] For the past decade, men 50 years of age or older have been encouraged to have an annual measurement of serum PSA and a digital rectal examination, as a basic screen for prostate cancer and to monitor the growth of the prostate gland. Several investigators have proposed age-adjusted PSA reference ranges, which reflect the size of the prostate gland[181–183] (Table 101-7). Studies have resulted in several formulas that try to adjust the PSA for the effect of BPH. The best-known formula for predicting the PSA level (PSA serum density) is as follows[184]:

$$\text{PSA (in ng/mL or mcg/mL)} = 0.12 \times \text{gland volume (in cubic centimeters [cc] by transrectal ultrasound [TRUS])}$$

$$\text{TRUS gland volume} = \text{prostate height} \times \text{width} \times \text{length} \times 0.523$$

The PSA result for G.M. is slightly above the upper limit for his age. As such, he should have a TRUS to determine the prostate gland volume and hence, the PSA density. Once the prostate gland volume is determined, the significance of his PSA level of 7.1 can be determined.

Radiologic and Imaging Studies

22. Why should G.M. have his urinary tract evaluated with radiologic and imaging studies?

Visualization of the kidneys, ureters, and bladder (KUB) with intravenous pyelography (IVP) is commonly used to evaluate BPH in some institutions. The routine use of IVP is being questioned, however, because this procedure does not visualize the bladder outlet during voiding and therefore cannot be used to detect obstruction directly. As noted, G.M. is suspected of having hydronephrosis because his BUN and serum creatinine are elevated. Thus, the nephrotoxic risk of IVP may outweigh its potential benefit.[185–187] Furthermore, when hydronephrosis is a concern, ultrasound is the preferred diagnostic maneuver, because it spares the patient exposure to radiation and possible adverse reactions to the contrast agent.[188] Presently, the consensus is that IVP is warranted only if hematuria is present.[178] Computed tomographic (CT) scanning and magnetic resonance imaging (MRI) have little value in BPH assessment.

Urodynamic Evaluation and Cystoscopy

23. Why should G.M. have urodynamic evaluation and cystoscopy for his BPH?

Because G.M. may be scheduled for a surgical procedure, it is important to determine the extent of urinary flow obstruction and the urinary flow rate. An accurate determination of the urinary peak flow rate and the voided volume correlated with G.M.'s history will be useful in determining the degree of his urinary obstruction. Urodynamic evaluation involves assessing the urinary flow rate, bladder volume, detrusor pressure, and visualization of voiding. Peak *urinary flow rate* to assess prostatism is a useful method because it is noninvasive and requires only simple and inexpensive equipment.

The urinary flow rate depends on bladder volume,[189] and a nomogram that corrects for age has been developed.[190,191] Flow rate represents the contributions of bladder contraction and outlet opening during voiding. A low flow rate may reflect diminished bladder contractility (e.g., owing to aging, disease, medications) or outlet obstruction. Thus, a low flow rate is not specific and cannot differentiate bladder outlet obstruction from an underactive detrusor muscle, nor does it discriminate well between those who will and those who will not benefit from surgery.[190–192] The use of urinary flow rates as predictors of surgery outcomes is controversial. Kadow et al.[193] found no significant difference in symptomatic outcomes from surgery when comparing pre-surgery urinary flow rates. In addition, although flow rates tend to improve after surgery, wide individual variation is seen, and an increased postoperative peak flow does not always correlate with symptom relief.[194]

Voiding cystourethrography involves retrograde filling of the bladder with a contrast agent, followed by visualization of the bladder and urethra during the resting, voiding, and postvoiding phases. Although this procedure has the same problems as the IVP, it does have the advantage of providing a dynamic evaluation of the urethral outlet during micturition.[178] Voiding cystourethrography often is performed by technicians and read by radiologists who might not be well trained in lower urinary tract physiology and who therefore do not provide sensitive analyses.

Despite its utility, pressure–flow analysis is not widely used in the evaluation of prostatism because the patient must be able to forestall voiding during bladder filling, and then void on command. As a result, interpretable data are obtained in only 60% to 86% of cases analyzed in optimal laboratory settings.[195]

Cystoscopy is used in prostatism to rule out intravesical pathology such as tumors or stones that also cause voiding symptoms and to evaluate bladder trabeculation, prostatic length and size, the presence of an enlarged median lobe, and the degree of obstruction. As with an IVP, cystoscopy is required if hematuria is present and also should be considered whenever there is pelvic pain with voiding.

In making treatment decisions, the roles of intravenous urography, the visual appearance of the prostate via cystoscopy, urodynamic studies, urine flow measurements, and the degree of obstructive and irritative voiding symptoms, collectively, remain controversial and do not provide data sufficient to dictate the best treatment for the patient.[196,197] Therefore, these tests are not necessary for G.M.

Nonpharmacologic Treatment

Transurethral Resection of the Prostate

24. What nonpharmacologic treatment is best for G.M.? When should prostate surgery be undertaken in general?

G.M.'s subjective and objective findings, particularly the acute urinary retention and hydronephrosis, collectively indicate the need for a transurethral resection of the prostate gland. G.M. has been advised by his urologist that a TURP is the treatment of choice given the severity of his presentation (e.g., large prostate gland with acute urinary retention) and that the procedure will relieve his symptoms, allow him to lead a relatively normal life, and avoid sequelae of prolonged obstruction.

Transurethral resection of prostate provides significant relief of BPH symptoms in 86%, 83%, 75%, and 75% of patients at 3 months, 1 year, 3 years, and 7 years, respectively.[197] Of patients with severe BPH, 93% report reduced symptoms 1 year after a TURP.[196] The TURP is considered the "gold standard" for the treatment of BPH and is used in 90% of patients with symptoms of residual urine or acute urinary retention.[167] As a result, surgical alternatives are always compared with the outcome studies of TURP.

The need for a TURP in G.M.'s situation is fairly clear. In most cases, however, the need for a TURP is less clear because the symptoms do not inevitably worsen and men often are willing to live with their symptoms. Therefore, clinicians need to be able to talk with patients and help them answer the question of whether the discomfort, risk, and problems during the postsurgical recovery period are outweighed by the high probability that surgery will relieve symptoms. After conditions that clearly require surgery have been ruled out, the severity of a patient's symptoms and the degree to which they interfere with living a normal life are the dominant factors in any decision to proceed with prostate surgery. Because surgery for prostate enlargement most often is performed to improve the patient's quality of life, clinicians must counsel patients and help them make the decision. For a comparison of common surgical treatments please refer to Table 101-8.

Drug Therapy

α_1-Adrenergic Receptor Antagonists

25. What drug therapy should be prescribed to treat G.M.'s prostatic hyperplasia?

G.M. most likely will be scheduled for a TURP, because he presents with acute urinary retention and hydronephrosis owing to a moderately enlarged prostate gland (i.e., >40 g and <80 g). He should be started and maintained on an α_1-adrenergic receptor antagonist to reduce the tension of the bladder neck, the prostate adenoma, and the prostatic capsule. Similarly, he should receive finasteride to induce atrophy of the prostate gland and halt progression of the disease.

The prostatic capsule and BPH adenoma have plentiful α_{1A}-adrenergic receptors. The three known subtypes of the α_1-adrenergic receptor are α_{1A}, α_{1B}, and α_{1D}. Inhibiting the α_{1A}-adrenergic receptors can reduce the smooth muscle tone of the prostatic urethra, thereby reducing the functional component of urethral constriction and obstruction.

Phenoxybenzamine (Dibenzyline), a nonselective α-antagonist, has been 80% effective in increasing urinary flow rates, but its use is hampered by a 30% incidence of side effects (fatigue, dizziness, hypotension), which are exacerbated by its long half-life.[198,199] The dose of phenoxybenzamine is 5 to 20 mg/day orally. Prazosin (Minipress) 2 to 4 mg/day is more α_{1A}-selective and is less likely to cause side effects compared

Table 101-8 Common Procedures

Therapy	Brief Description	Comments
Transurethral resection of the prostate (TURP)	A resectoscope is inserted into the urethra and obstructing tissue is removed a piece at a time.	Post-TURP syndrome: potentially life threatening, caused by the absorption of irrigating fluid. Cerebral edema and seizures may result from hypervolemia and hyponatremia. Late complications: erectile dysfunction (up to 30%), urinary incontinence, and bladder neck contractures, retrograde ejaculation.
Transurethral incision of the prostate (TUIP)	Shallow incisions in the prostatic urethra area relieve bladder outflow obstruction.	Advantageous in high-risk patients such as the elderly because it can be performed under local anesthesia.
Transurethral dilation of the prostate (TUDP)	Balloon catheter is positioned in the prostatic urethra and inflated.	Appropriate for men with smaller prostates who wish to avoid potential side effects of other procedures.
Visual laser ablation of the prostate gland (VLAP)	Laser is used to partially remove obstructing prostate.	Used in men with smaller prostates.
Transurethral microwave hyperthermia	Local microwave hyperthermia, delivered transurethrally or transrectally.	Not as effective as surgical therapy but can be completed as an outpatient in 1 hour.

with phenoxybenzamine. The clinical efficacy of prazosin in improving urinary flow rates is somewhat less impressive.[199] Prazosin should be avoided in elderly patients because of its side effect profile, including high risk for first-dose syncope, and need for multiple daily doses.

TERAZOSIN

Terazosin (Hytrin), a long-acting α_{1A}-adrenergic receptor antagonist, has significantly reduced obstructive symptoms and improved urinary flow rates at doses of 1 to 5 mg/day (Table 101-9).[171,200] The α_{1A}-blockade alone does not account for the long-term clinical responses exerted by this drug in the treatment of benign prostatic hyperplasia. Terazosin has been shown to induce prostate smooth muscle cell apoptosis resulting in reducing urinary symptoms. Terazosin (and doxazosin) has a quinazoline nucleus, which may account for this effect. Tamsulosin, which is not a quinazoline, does not induce prostate smooth muscle cell apoptosis.[203]

In most patients, the dose of terazosin will need to be increased to 5 to 10 mg/day to obtain desired results. Orthostatic hypotension, however, may occur in the beginning days of therapy or during dosage adjustment periods. In patients who, for whatever reason, stop their terazosin therapy for 2 or more days, therapy should be reinstituted cautiously to avoid the "first-dose" adverse effect of syncope.

Terazosin maintained the level of improvement in BPH symptom scores over a 30-month period. Only 10% of the patients experienced treatment failure.[171] In this long-term study, the systolic blood pressure in normotensive and hypertensive patients was decreased by 4 and 18 mmHg, respectively. Apparently, terazosin typically only lowered the blood pressure significantly in the hypertensive patients.

Terazosin commonly is prescribed with finasteride to control the progression and symptoms of BPH despite the lack of adequate clinical studies.[204] The mechanisms of action for both of these drugs are different, and the combined use of both produces a synergistic effect. When combined with finasteride, a smaller terazosin maintenance dose (1–5 mg/day) can be used, resulting in fewer dose-related side effects (e.g., orthostatic hypotension and dizziness).

Table 101-9 Drug Therapy of Persistent Urinary Incontinence

Type	Treatment With Initial Doses
Urge	Oxybutynin 2.5 mg QD–TID; 5–30 mg XL Tolterodine 1–2 mg QD; 2–4 LA QD Trospium 20 mg BID Darifenacin 7.5 mg QD Solifenacin 5 mg QD
Stress	Pseudoephedrine 15–30 mg BID–TID Imipramine 25 mg QD Vaginal estrogen cream 0.5–1.0 g two times/wk
Overflow	Terazosin 1–5 mg QD (usually at HS) Doxazosin 1–8 mg QD Tamsulosin 0.4–0.8 mg QD Alfuzosin 10 mg QD Bethanechol 10 mg TID
Functional	None

BID, twice daily; HS, at bedtime; LA, long acting; QD, every day; TID, three times daily; XL, extended release.

DOXAZOSIN

Doxazosin (Cardura), another quinazoline derivative, is a long-acting selective α_{1a}-adrenergic receptor antagonist structurally related to prazosin and terazosin (Table 101-9). Doxazosin originally was prescribed primarily for hypertension and currently is not considered a first-line antihypertensive agent. (For a discussion of the current use of α-blocker in hypertension, see Chapter 13 Essential Hypertension.) Hypertension and BPH are linked by the sympathetic nervous system. As with terazosin, doxazosin improves urinary flow rates and symptoms in patients with BPH. These effects have been demonstrated in controlled clinical studies, within weeks, and over the long term. Doxazosin should be started at 1 mg/day. After 1 to 2 weeks, the dose can be increased over several weeks to 8 mg/day. As with other long-acting α_1-adrenergic receptor antagonists, the first dose should be taken at bedtime to minimize lightheadedness and syncope (the first-dose effect), and the blood pressure of the patient should be monitored periodically during therapy. Most patients require between 4 and 8 mg/day for effective control of the urinary symptoms of BPH. Dosages >4 mg/day are associated with a greater frequency of dizziness, orthostatic hypotension, and syncope.[200,201]

TAMSULOSIN

Tamsulosin, a nonquinazoline, is a long-acting α_{1A}-adrenergic receptor antagonist similar to doxazosin, terazosin, and prazosin. Tamsulosin and its metabolites are more specific for the prostatic α_{1A}-adrenergic receptors than any of the other α_{1A}-adrenergic receptor antagonists.[205] Apparently, tamsulosin and its metabolites are less specific for the vascular α_{1A}-adrenergic receptors, and therefore cause less orthostatic hypotension than the other agents in the class. Consequently, no need exists to titrate tamsulosin to the recommended daily dose range of 0.4 to 0.8 mg. Coadministration of tamsulosin with antihypertensives does not require dosage adjustment of the antihypertensives. Tamsulosin is very effective in treating bladder outlet obstruction associated with BPH.[206,207]

More than 90% of tamsulosin is absorbed following oral administration of a 0.4-mg dose under fasting conditions. Administration with food decreases the bioavailability by 30% and increases time to peak plasma concentration. Tamsulosin is hepatically metabolized by CYP isozymes, CYP 3A4 and CYP 2D6.[208] Impaired renal function increases total tamsulosin plasma concentration by approximately 100% during steady-state administration. Because active, unbound drug levels are not affected, no dose modification is required in renally impaired patients with symptomatic BPH.[209] As with all α_{1A}-adrenergic receptor antagonists, tamsulosin does not affect the PSA and must be taken indefinitely to maintain its therapeutic effect.[210]

ALFUZOSIN

Alfuzosin is a quinazoline α_1-adrenergeric receptor antagonist that is selective the for the α_{1A} receptor in the lower urinary tract. Because of alfuzosin's uroselectivity, it has a lower rate of hypotensive effects than doxazosin and terazosin. A lack of penetration of alfuzosin into the brain has been hypothesized to contribute to the decreased CNS effects such as somnolence. Unlike tamsulosin, alfuzosin will not cause ejaculatory dysfunction; the incidence is comparable to placebo.[210]

Androgen Suppression

Considerable information has accrued concerning the endocrine basis for control of BPH (Fig. 101-4), the effect of age on hormone dynamics in men, and the hormonal changes in the hyperplastic human prostate. Maintenance of morphology and functional activity of the adult human prostate is controlled by, and dependent on, androgens. Prostatic regression after androgen deprivation is an active process that requires the synthesis of macromolecules.[211] As a result of androgen deprivation,[212] the loss of stromal and epithelial prostate cells is disproportionate, with four times greater loss of epithelial cells. Testosterone serves as the pro-hormone for the two active metabolites, DHT and 17-β-estradiol. Testosterone is metabolized to DHT by the enzyme 5α-reductase (type I and type II). Thus, conversion of testosterone to DHT precludes its conversion to estrogen by the enzyme, aromatase, and the relative activity of these two enzymes is of paramount importance in prostate homeostasis.[213]

Although the mean plasma testosterone level in men falls after the age of 60, the level of testosterone in subjects with BPH and age-matched controls is not different.[214] Moreover, the onset of BPH starts some 10 to 20 years before the plasma testosterone levels decrease. The serum concentration of DHT is increased, however, in men with BPH.[211,215,216] The mechanism responsible for accumulation of DHT has not been established, but a significant increase in 5α-reductase activity occurs, which is known to produce DHT.[217,218]

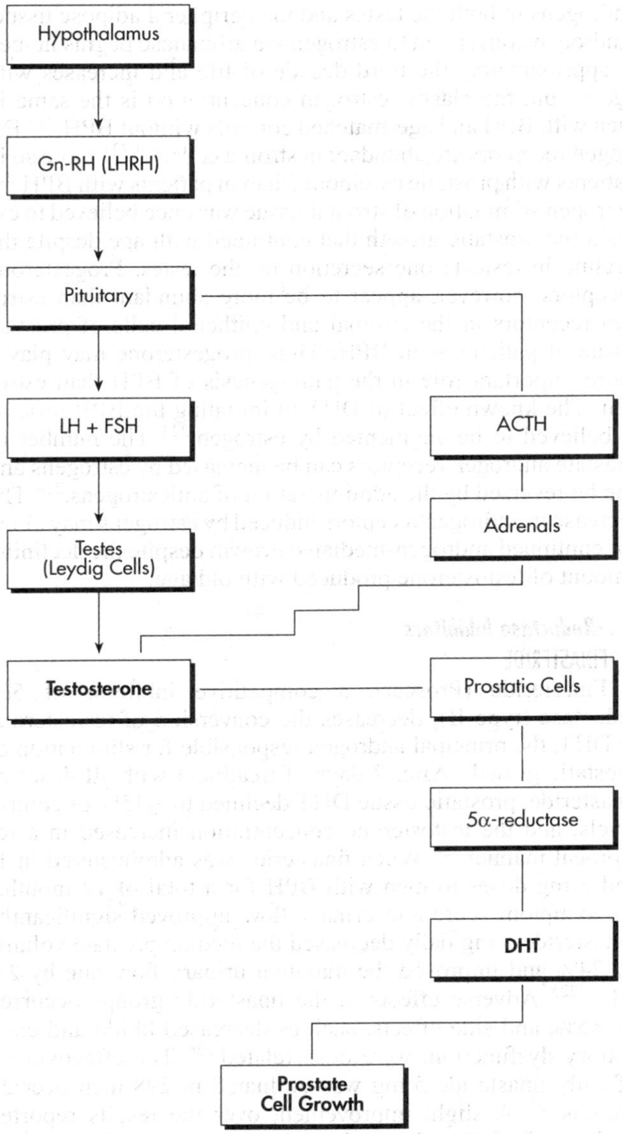

FIGURE 101-4 Pituitary-gonadal axis: endocrine basis for control of benign prostatic hyperplasia (BPH). The pituitary-gonadal axis plays an important role in prostatic growth. Neurons in the preoptic area of the hypothalamus secrete gonadotropin-releasing hormone (Gn-RH), also known as luteinizing hormone-releasing hormone (LHRH). LHRH is a small peptide that interacts with surface receptor sites on the plasma membrane of the pituitary cells. LHRH stimulates the pituitary to release both luteinizing hormone (LH) and follicle-stimulating hormone (FSH). LH secretion causes the Leydig cells of the testicle to produce testosterone. Testosterone appears to inhibit LHRH at the hypothalamic level and LH at the pituitary level. The adrenals only contribute approximately 1% of circulating testosterone. Testosterone diffuses into the prostatic cells, where it is converted to dihydrotestosterone (DHT) by 5—reductase. DHT binds to steroid receptor complexes in the nucleus of the prostate, which causes cell growth. ACTH, corticotropin; DHT, dihydrotestosterone; FSH, follicle-stimulating hormone; Gn-RH, gonadotropin-releasing hormone; LH, luteinizing hormone. (From reference 166, with permission.)

One other major hormonal change associated with aging is the increased formation of estrogen from circulating androgens in both the testes and the peripheral adipose tissue. Androgen conversion to estrogen via aromatase begins in men at approximately the third decade of life and increases with age,[219] but the plasma estrogen concentration is the same in men with BPH and age-matched controls without BPH.[215] Estrogen receptors are abundant in stroma cells,[220,221] more so in patients with prostatic carcinoma than in patients with BPH.[222] Estrogen stimulation of stromal tissue was once believed to explain the prostatic growth that continued with age despite the decline in testosterone secretion by the testes. Progesterone receptors, however, appear to be more abundant than estrogen receptors in the stromal and epithelial cells of prostate tissue of patients with BPH. Thus, progesterone may play a more important role in the pathogenesis of BPH than estrogen. The known effect of DHT in initiating the BPH process is believed to be augmented by estrogen.[223] The number of prostate androgen receptors can be increased by estrogens and can be reversed by the administration of antiestrogens.[214] The increase in androgen receptors induced by estrogens may allow for continued androgen-mediated growth despite the declining amount of testosterone produced with old age.

5α-Reductase Inhibitors

FINASTERIDE

Finasteride (Proscar), a competitive inhibitor of 5α-reductase (type II), decreases the conversion of testosterone to DHT, the principal androgen responsible for stimulation of prostatic growth. After 7 days of treatment with all doses of finasteride, prostatic tissue DHT declined to $\leq$15% of control levels, and the testosterone concentration increased in a reciprocal manner.[224] When finasteride was administered in 1- and 5-mg doses to men with BPH for a total of 12 months, the symptom score and urinary flow improved significantly. Finasteride 5 mg daily decreased the median prostate volume by 24% and improved the maximal urinary flow rate by 2.9 mL/s.[225] Adverse effects in the finasteride groups occurred in <5%, and side effects, such as decreased libido and ejaculatory dysfunction, were dose related.[226] The effectiveness of daily finasteride 5 mg was evaluated in 298 men over 24 months.[227] A slight improvement over the results reported at the end of the 12-month period was noted. The median DHT levels had declined by 74.5% compared with 69.3% at 12 months, and prostate volume declined by 25.2% compared with 21.2% at 12 months. Patient symptom scores indicated slightly more improvement at 24 months, compared with 12 months. Obstructive symptom scores were responsible for most of the improved symptoms reported. The prevalence of sexual adverse experiences at 24 months was similar to that at 12 months. In those men who experienced finasteride-induced sexual dysfunction, 50% will experience resolution after discontinuing the medication.[228] Inhibition of DHT by 5α-reductase inhibitors does not affect testosterone-mediated functions on muscle mass, libido, or spermatogenesis. Thus, finasteride has an acceptable safety profile, halts disease progression, and improves the quality of life in patients with moderate BPH disease (i.e., enlarged prostate with symptoms of urinary obstruction, but not acute urinary retention). Finasteride improves objective pressure flow parameters after 1 year of therapy, and efficacy appears to be greatest in patients with large prostates (>40 g).[229] For those who do respond, the drug must be continued indefinitely because DHT serum concentrations return to pretreatment levels within 14 days of discontinuing finasteride, and prostate size returns to pretreatment levels within 4 months.[230,231]

Unlike leuprolide, finasteride does not affect the histologic features of BPH and prostate cancer.[232] Morphologic evaluation of patients treated with finasteride with symptomatic BPH having adenectomy showed a reduction in the size of the prostate and an increase in the stroma:epithilial and stroma:lumen ratios.[233]

DUTASTERIDE

Dutasteride (Avodart) is a competitive and specific inhibitor of both type I and type II 5α-reductase isoenzymes. An advantage of dutasteride over finasteride is the additional inhibition of 5α-reductase (type I) in the peripheral tissues, which produces a further decline in serum DHT. In a prospective study of 2,951 men with moderate to severe BPH, dutasteride 0.5 mg/day decreased DHT serum levels by 90% at 1 month in 58% of patients. At 24 months, 85% of those treated with dutasteride were noted to have a 90% reduction of serum DHT.[234] Correspondingly, the patients noted reduction in urinary symptoms as early as 3 months after treatment and a significant (p <0.001) reduction in symptoms by the sixth month when compared with those treated with placebo. Common side effects of dutasteride are similar to those of finasteride: impotence (4.7%), decreased libido (3.0%), ejaculation disorder (1.4%) and gynecomastia (1.0%).

Antiandrogens: Flutamide

Flutamide (Eulexin) is an orally administered nonsteroidal antiandrogen that inhibits the binding of androgen to its receptor. The safety and efficacy of flutamide were evaluated in a double-blind, placebo-controlled study of 31 male patients with symptomatic BPH.[235] Patients received a daily dose of 375 mg of flutamide for 12 weeks. No significant differences were noted in the treatment and placebo groups with regard to any symptoms of prostatism (force of stream, frequency, nocturia). Based on the digital rectal examination, patients receiving flutamide had a significant reduction of prostate size. Of 15 patients treated with flutamide, 7 developed nipple tenderness and decreased libido. In another study, no significant difference was seen between flutamide and placebo.[236] In this same study, which used flutamide 250 mg three times daily, 53% of the patients experienced breast tenderness and 11% experienced diarrhea. Because flutamide is a potent hepatotoxin in certain patients, serial blood aminotransferase levels should be monitored during the first few months of therapy.[237] Flutamide also is associated with a 50% reduction in the serum concentration of PSA.[204,236] In summary, flutamide results in toxicity with limited effectiveness; however, its use may be justified in patients who are unable to tolerate a 5α-reductase inhibitor with or without an α_1-adrenergic blocker.

Gonadotropin-Releasing Hormone: Leuprolide

Analogs of Gn-RH can cause regression of BPH. Leuprolide acetate (Lupron) is a synthetic nonpeptide analog of natural-occurring Gn-RH. It desensitizes LH-releasing hormone receptors (when given continuously and in therapeutic doses), thereby preventing the release of gonadotropin. Chronic leuprolide acetate therapy will suppress testicular testosterone production, causing a "chemical-like" castration. Because it reversibly binds to Gn-RH receptors, testosterone production resumes when it is discontinued. In a double-blind, placebo-controlled study, patients with BPH received leuprolide 3.75 mg intramuscularly monthly for 24 weeks.[238] No statistically or clinically significant differences were noted in the percentage change in total, obstructive, or irritative symptoms at 24 weeks between the placebo and leuprolide groups. Detrusor muscle pressure at maximal urine flow was improved at 24 weeks, and prostate volume was reduced. Of those patients receiving leuprolide acetate, 92% developed hot flashes, and of the sexually active patients, 95% experienced a loss of potency.

Leuprolide should be reserved for patients with prostate cancer. Its high cost, questionable effectiveness, and castrationlike adverse effects make it an undesirable choice for treatment of BPH.

Effect of Androgen Suppression on Prostate-Specific Antigen

26. What effect does androgen suppression have on PSA?

The possibility that antiandrogen treatment of BPH could adversely affect the interpretation of the PSA screening test for prostate cancer is of concern. For example, androgen suppression with leuprolide acetate reduces prostate volume primarily by inducing involution of the epithelial elements of the prostate.[239] Because PSA primarily is produced by the epithelial cells of the prostate, these drugs can alter serum and prostate concentrations of PSA.[240] Finasteride 5 mg/day also can reduce the serum PSA level by 50%.[241] Dutasteride reduces total serum PSA by ~40% after 3 months of treatment and by ~50% after 24 months.[234] The serum PSA level reduction is predictable, however, and serum PSA levels can be recalculated during hormonal treatment for BPH. Nevertheless, patients receiving a 5α-reductase inhibitor should have (a) a digital rectal examination of their prostate periodically, (b) a PSA level measured, and (c) any suspicious findings investigated immediately.[227] Androgen suppression therapy is not contraindicated in BPH solely on the basis of its effect on serum PSA levels.[242]

27. What over-the-counter medications are available for prostate disorders?

Two agents, saw palmetto and pygeum, have been promoted for the treatment of BPH. Saw palmetto is an herbal product obtained from the fruit of the *Serenoa repens* tree. The active ingredients are phytosterols; β-sitosterol and β-sitosterol-3-O-glucosides are the most abundant. Saw palmetto has antiandrogen activity. Several trials have shown that it significantly improves benign prostatic hyperplasia symptoms,[243–246] to a degree similar to finasteride.[247] Pygeum (*P. africanum* bark extract) has been observed to moderately reduce urinary symptoms associated with enlargement of the prostate gland.[248] Pygeum has been well tolerated in most studies; however, the safety has not been extensively or systematically studied.

URINARY INCONTINENCE

Urinary incontinence, both acute and chronic, is a common disorder among elderly individuals, affecting ~50% of the institutionalized elderly and 20% of the community-dwelling elderly.[249,250] Neurologic impairment, immobility, female gender, and history of hysterectomy are independent risk factors for incontinence, but neither advanced age nor chronic bacteriuria seem to be. Incontinence has economic costs, and medical (e.g., cystitis, urosepsis, pressure sores, perineal rashes, falls) and psychosocial (e.g., embarrassment, isolation, depression, predisposition to institutionalization) consequences. Nevertheless, incontinence often is a neglected condition. Only a few patients whose lives are seriously disrupted seek medical attention; when they do, their incontinence often is attributed to aging and not evaluated further.[249,251] Incontinence is not an inevitable consequence of aging. It is a pathologic condition that, when rationally approached, usually can be ameliorated or cured, often without invasive tests or surgery and almost invariably without an indwelling catheter (Table 101-10).[252,253]

Table 101-10 Causes of Incontinence

	Resnick's Mnemonic: DIAPPERS
D	Delirium and dementia
I	Infections
A	Atrophic vaginitis, atrophic urethritis, atonic bladder
P	Psychological causes, depression
P	Pharmacologic agents
E	Endocrine (diabetes, hypercalcemia, hypothyroidism)
R	Restricted mobility
S	Stool impaction

Adapted from reference 262, with permission.

Neurophysiologic Considerations

The bladder can be thought of as a "balloon" with a narrow outlet, wrapped with a muscular layer, the detrusor muscle. The detrusor and the bladder outlet functions are coordinated neurologically to allow for storage and expulsion of urine.[254] The detrusor muscle is innervated by the parasympathetic nervous system, and the bladder neck is innervated by the sympathetic nervous system (α-adrenergic) (Fig. 101-5). The proximal smooth muscle (internal) sphincter in the bladder neck also is innervated through the sympathetic nervous system (α-adrenergic). The distal striated muscle (external) sphincter of the urethra is supplied by the somatic nervous system.

Urine storage is the result of detrusor muscle relaxation and closure of both the internal and external sphincters. Detrusor relaxation is accomplished by CNS inhibition of the parasympathetic tone; sphincter closure is mediated by a reflex increase in α-adrenergic and somatic activity. Voiding occurs when detrusor contraction is coordinated with sphincter relaxation. Detrusor contraction is mediated by the parasympathetic nervous system, and relaxation requires inhibition of somatic and sympathetic nerve impulses to the outlet. The bladder capacity is ~300 mL in the elderly and ~400 mL in young adults. The relationship between the detrusor and the outlet is coordinated by a micturition center located in the CNS, perhaps the pons.[255] The cortex and diencephalon also permit inhibition of what would otherwise be a reflex contraction of the detrusor muscle in response to bladder distention.

Age-Related Changes

Aging affects the lower urinary tract in several ways (Table 101-11). Structural and functional changes have been observed. Bladder capacity, the ability to postpone voiding, urethral and

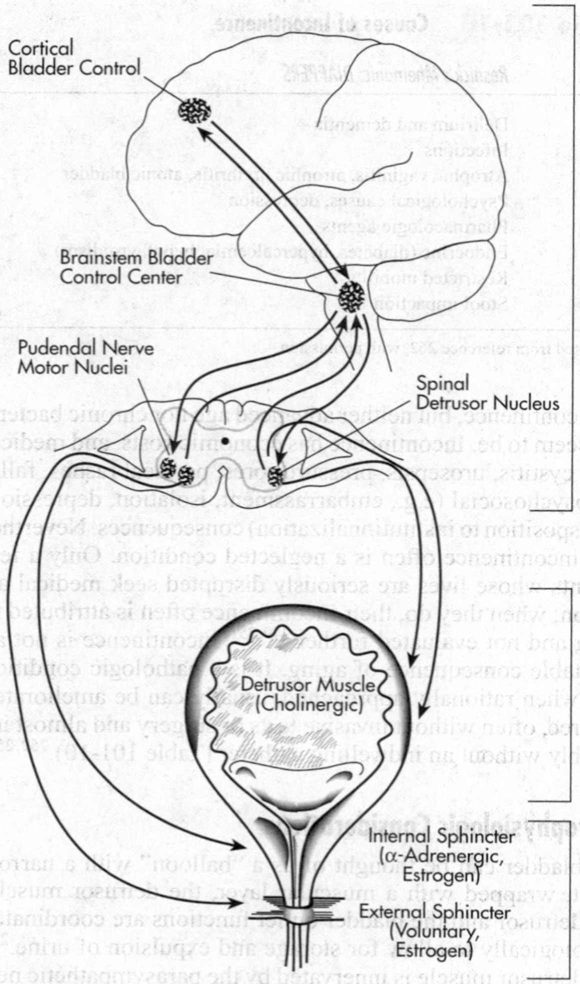

FIGURE 101-5 Neurologic bladder control. Three major components are involved in urine storage and release. (1) Central nervous system: Inhibition from the frontal lobe (cortical) micturition center permits bladder relaxation and filling, and sphincter closure to prevent leakage of urine. When cortical inhibition ceases (i.e., the patient wants to urinate), the brainstem (pontine) micturition center sends impulses down the spinal cord to the detrusor muscle, resulting in muscle contraction. (2) Bladder: Increase in bladder volume stimulates proprioception receptors in the bladder wall and sensory impulses are transmitted through the sacral nerves (S_2–S_4 roots) to trigger bladder contraction. This stimulus for bladder contraction is under inhibitory control by the central nervous system frontal lobe as described previously. Cholinergic stimulation results in bladder contraction. (3) Bladder outlet: The two major factors in maintaining urethral pressure are the internal and external sphincters. Internal sphincter: α-Adrenergic stimulation causes muscle contraction, preventing flow of urine. External sphincter: It consists of striated muscle under voluntary control. Contraction prevents flow of urine. Estrogen deficiency in women can result in decreased competence of the internal and external sphincters. (From reference 326, with permission.)

bladder compliance, maximal urethral closure pressure, and urinary flow rate all are reduced with normal aging.[255,256] For women, these changes are correlated with the postmenopausal decline of estrogen production. Estrogen has trophic effects on the epithelium and on tissues lining and surrounding the urethra, bladder outlet, and vagina. Atrophy of these tissues can result in friability, inflammation, susceptibility to infection, diminished periurethral blood flow, and prolapse of pelvic structures. All of these effects can precipitate symptoms of urinary incontinence. For men, the age-related changes in the prostate gland are responsible for many of the changes in urination. The most common age-related change, in both women and men, is involuntary bladder contractions (detrusor motor instability). These involuntary bladder contractions occur in up to 20% of asymptomatic, neurologically normal, continent elderly patients.[257–260]

Table 101-11 Age-Related Changes in Urologic Function

↓ Bladder capacity
↑ Residual urine
↑ Uninhibited bladder contractions
↑ Nocturnal sodium and fluid excretion
↓ Urethral resistance in women
↑ Urethral resistance in men
Weakness of pelvic floor muscles in women

In many elderly persons, nocturia is a common complaint and may stem from age-related increases in nocturnal urine production.[261] Each of these changes predisposes people to incontinence, but none alone precipitates it. This predisposition to incontinence, together with the increased likelihood that an older person will be subjected to additional pathologic, physiologic, or pharmacologic insults, underlies the higher incidence of incontinence in the elderly. The onset or exacerbation of incontinence in an older person is likely to be caused by a precipitating factor outside the lower urinary tract.[262] Correspondingly, reversal of the precipitating factor may be sufficient to restore continence without correction of the underlying urologic abnormality.

Drug-Induced Urinary Incontinence

Occasionally, reports of female stress incontinence from α_1-adrenergic receptor antagonists, which have a relaxant effect on urethral smooth muscle, have appeared in the medical literature.[263–265] In one study, the incidence of genuine stress incontinence was significantly higher in women taking prazosin (86.2%) than in the nonprazosin group (65.7%) ($p < 0.01$). In 55% of the women contacted in the prazosin group, urinary incontinence was reduced or cured by prazosin withdrawal.[266] There was a significant increase in functional urethral length, maximal urethral closure pressure, and abdominal pressure transmission to the urethra after prazosin withdrawal. In one case report, switching from doxazosin to enalapril briefly reduced the female patient's stress incontinence; however, she developed a persistent dry cough (from the enalapril) that continued to cause episodic stress incontinence. Her cough and stress incontinence resolved when she was switched to amlodipine.[267]

Classification

Urinary incontinence can be classified several different ways. The two most basic types of urinary incontinence are *acute (or transient) and reversible* or *chronic and persistent*. Persistent urinary incontinence (PUI), which refers to incontinence that is not acute and occurs over a long period of time, can be classified further into four subgroups: (a) urge, (b) stress, (c) overflow, and (d) functional.

Acute Incontinence

Urinary incontinence that is of relatively recent onset or associated with an acute medical problem should prompt a review for reversible factors. These include the following: (a) cystitis, atrophic vaginitis, and urethritis; (b) CHF; (c) polyuria from diabetes; (d) delirium and acute confusional states; (e) immobility; and (f) medication side effects. The following medications are associated with acute onset urinary incontinence: diuretics; α-adrenergic agonists (e.g., pseudoephedrine); α-adrenergic antagonists (e.g., terazosin); anticholinergics; and neuroleptics. The management of acute forms of urinary incontinence depends on the identification and elimination of the reversible factor.

For women with urethritis and atrophic vaginitis with irritative voiding symptoms, estrogen replacement can be very helpful. An intravaginal estrogen cream is administered nightly for 7 days, followed by at least once-a-week application.[268] For women with an intact uterus, the conjugated estrogen should be given in a cyclic manner with a progestational agent. In keeping with the Women's Health Initiative Trial, serious risks, including breast cancer and cardiovascular disease, appear, however, to outweigh long-term benefits of this combination of hormone therapy.[269]

Persistent Urinary Incontinence

URGE INCONTINENCE

Urge incontinence, the most common form of incontinence affecting the elderly, occurs when involuntary voiding is preceded by a warning of a few seconds to a few minutes. Urge PUI is characterized by precipitous urine leakage, most often after the urge to void is perceived. Urge PUI can be caused by a variety of genitourinary and neurologic disorders. It most often, but not always, is associated with detrusor motor instability (involuntary contraction of the bladder) or detrusor hyperreflexia (detrusor motor instability caused by a neurologic disorder). The most common causes are local genitourinary conditions, such as cystitis, urethritis, tumors, stones, bladder diverticula, and outflow obstruction. Neurologic disorders, such as stroke, dementia, parkinsonism, and spinal cord injury, can be associated with urge PUI.[270]

STRESS INCONTINENCE

Stress incontinence, the involuntary leakage that occurs only during stress, is common in elderly women but uncommon in men (unless the sphincter has been damaged during a TURP or prostatectomy). Stress incontinence occurs when an abrupt increase in intra-abdominal pressure (e.g., coughing, sneezing, laughing, lifting) overcomes urethral resistance. Typical stress PUI is characterized by daytime loss of small to moderate amounts of urine, infrequent nocturnal incontinence, and a low postvoiding residual volume in the absence of a large cystocele. The usual cause of stress PUI is urethral hypermobility owing to weakness and laxity of pelvic floor musculature, but other conditions, such as sphincter incompetence, urethral instability, or stress-induced detrusor instability, occasionally are responsible.[255] Obesity or TURP in men also can predispose individuals to stress incontinence. Many factors have been suggested to contribute to the development of urinary stress incontinence in women, including estrogen deficiency and a genetic defect in the connective tissue in such patients. The prevalence of urinary stress incontinence among first-degree relatives of patients with urinary incontinence is three times ($p < 0.005$) that of matched control groups of women without micturition disorders.[271]

OVERFLOW INCONTINENCE

Overflow incontinence occurs when the weight of urine in a distended bladder overcomes outlet resistance. Leakage of small amounts of urine is common throughout the day and night. The patient may complain of hesitancy, diminished and interrupted flow, a need to strain to void, and a sense of incomplete emptying. The bladder usually is palpable, and the residual urine volume is large. If the cause is neurologically mediated, control of the perianal sphincter may be impaired.[272]

Overflow incontinence results from an anatomic outlet obstruction or an acontractile bladder.[270] Common causes are BPH, urethral stricture, bladder-sphincter dyssynergia, diabetic neuropathy, fecal impaction, and anticholinergic medication use.

FUNCTIONAL INCONTINENCE

Functional incontinence occurs when a continent individual is unable or unwilling to reach the toilet to urinate. Common causes are musculoskeletal disorders, muscle weakness, impaired mental status, use of physical restraints, psychological impairment, environmental barriers, and medications (e.g., sedatives, neuroleptics).

Clinical Presentation and Evaluation

28. H.K., an 83-year-old female resident of a nursing facility, developed urinary incontinence 3 years before admission. She has been managed with adult diapers and bladder training. What objective and subjective data are needed to determine the pathophysiology (and hence the classification) of H.K.'s urinary incontinence?

The rationale for the clinical evaluation of H.K. is to classify the imbalance between bladder pressure and bladder sphincter resistance and, as a result, institute appropriate medical or surgical management of her urinary incontinence.

Documentation of H.K.'s urinary incontinence is accomplished most easily by having her or one of her nurses keep an incontinence record. Observations should be recorded every 2 hours regarding whether the patient is wet or dry, as well as associated symptoms or circumstances. A record maintained over 3 to 4 days will facilitate assessment of the voiding pattern. Knowledge of the voiding pattern can be used to design bladder training programs and to detect iatrogenic causes (e.g., diuretic ingestion, use of restraints). Successful bladder training relies on estimating when the bladder is full.

Physical examination of H.K. is paramount in determining the cause and classification of her urinary incontinence. A complete neurologic examination is mandatory. Clinical findings may identify specific pathophysiologic abnormalities. H.K. should have a thorough pelvic examination to determine the contribution of atrophic vaginitis, uterine prolapse, and bladder anatomy. Funneling of the bladder neck suggests stress incontinence, and palpation of the bladder suggests overflow incontinence. The presence of physical restraints or musculoskeletal disability would suggest functional incontinence.

H.K.'s bladder should be catheterized immediately after urination to determine residual urine volume. Volumes >50 mL are abnormal and may indicate obstruction or an adynamic detrusor muscle. Although urodynamic studies are widely recommended and used, little evidence suggests that these produce clinically useful data for institutionalized geriatric patients. A urinalysis, blood chemistries, renal function, and glucose tolerance test should be performed. An abnormal urinalysis may suggest pathology (e.g., infection) that can be managed medically. Urinary tract infection is common in the incontinent patient.

Treatment options exist for each type of urinary incontinence (Table 101-9). Proper evaluation should guide the clinician in choosing the optimal course of drug therapy. Drug therapy should be based on sound principles of neurophysiology, urology, and pharmacology. Basically, drug therapy is directed at decreasing bladder contractility (detrusor instability) and increasing outlet obstruction (bladder neck and proximal urethra).

29. The incontinence record maintained by the nursing staff indicates that H.K. has urinary urges quite frequently, resulting in urine leakage. Throughout the day and night, H.K. urinates four to five times. Physical examination reveals atrophic vaginitis, no funneling of the bladder neck, and no bladder distention. H.K. does have a history of stroke. The urinalysis is normal, as are the blood chemistries. Postvoiding bladder catheterization produced a residual urine volume of 30 mL. What is the pathophysiology and classification of H.K.'s incontinence?

Most neuropathic disease processes can change bladder function. As illustrated by H.K., a cerebrovascular accident is commonly associated with bladder dysfunction and incontinence in the elderly. Neurologic injury above the level of the micturition center in the spinal cord, in most cases, results in bladder spasticity. Sacral reflexes are intact, but loss of inhibition from higher CNS centers results in spastic bladder and inappropriate sphincter behavior. The degree of spasticity varies between the bladder and sphincter, as well as from patient to patient with the same CNS lesions. H.K. has a spastic detrusor muscle resulting from an unchecked sacral reflex. H.K.'s bladder dysfunction is classified as urge urinary incontinence of the persistent type.

Drug Therapy

Anticholinergic Agents

30. What drug therapy should be prescribed for H.K.?

H.K. has detrusor instability and requires anticholinergic drug therapy. Detrusor muscle stabilization through pharmacologic intervention and behavioral modification is the treatment of choice for urge PUI. The major neurohormonal stimulus for physiologic bladder muscle contraction is acetylcholine-induced stimulation of postganglionic parasympathetic cholinergic receptor sites on bladder smooth muscle.[273] Atropine and atropinelike substances depress true involuntary bladder contractions of any etiology.[274] Other drugs with anticholinergic properties also have local anesthetic and smooth muscle relaxant effects. These include tolterodine, flavoxate, oxybutynin, and dicyclomine. These drugs act directly on smooth muscle at a site that is metabolically distal to the cholinergic receptor. Because their effectiveness in treating urge incontinence is owing to their muscle relaxant property, rather than their anticholinergic effects, they are classified as antispasmodics.[274] All agents in this group should be prescribed for a 2-week trial period. If no improvement has been observed with one drug, trial with another may be appropriate.

OXYBUTYNIN CHLORIDE

Oxybutynin (Ditropan, Generic) is available as an oral immediate-release tablet, an extended-release tablet, or a transdermal system. Oxybutynin is commonly used to produce an anticholinergic effect in the lower urinary tract. The transdermal system contains 36 mg of active drug and delivers 3.9 mg of oxybutynin per day when dosed twice a week.[275] The transdermal system should be protected from moisture and humidity. Common side effects from the transdermal system at the application site are pruritus (14%) and site redness (8.3%). A comparison study of immediate-release oxybutynin and the transdermal system indicated that patients using the transdermal system experienced fewer side effects. Dry mouth was reported in 38% of the oxybutynin transdermal system users in contrast to 94% of those who used immediate-release tablets.[276]

Oxybutynin has been described as a strong independent smooth muscle relaxant with local anesthetic activity that has minor anticholinergic effects.[274,277] This agent has been used successfully to depress uninhibited detrusor contractions in patients with and without neurogenic bladder dysfunction. Oxybutynin improves total bladder capacity, neuropathic voiding dysfunction, and bladder filling pressure.[278,279] The dosage of oxybutynin chloride suggested for the elderly is 2.5 mg up to three times a day; in some cases, the dosage may need to be increased to 5 mg three times a day. Because oxybutynin is a tertiary-amine anticholinergic compound, the potential for CNS toxicity increases as the dose is increased. Compared with oral propantheline bromide 15 mg three times a day, a full dose of oral oxybutynin (5 mg three times a day) in one study produced a good response more frequently.[280] Once-daily, controlled-release oxybutynin at doses of 5 to 30 mg reduced the number of incontinence episodes.[16,281] Maximal benefit was demonstrated by maintenance week 4 and was sustained as long as the patient continued therapy.[282]

TOLTERODINE TARTRATE

Tolterodine (Detrol, generic Detrol LA) is a competitive muscarinic receptor antagonist (anticholinergic) indicated for the treatment of overactive bladder symptoms of urinary frequency or urge incontinence. At doses of 1 to 2 mg twice a day, compared with a placebo, the number of urinary voids per 24 hours decreased ($p = 0.0045$), the volume of urine per void increased ($p < 0.001$), and the mean number of incontinence episodes decreased by 50% ($p < 0.19$).[283] No clinical or electrocardiographic evidence was seen of significant cardiac adverse events in the group studied. Tolterodine has greater selectivity for the bladder than the salivary glands in vivo, which is not attributable to muscarinic receptor subtype selectivity.[284]

Thus, tolterodine is much less potent in inhibiting salivation, suggesting that it may have less propensity to cause dry mouth in clinical use. The onset of pharmacologic action of tolterodine is <1 hour, and therapeutic efficacy is maintained during long-term treatment. In comparative trials, tolterodine and oxybutynin are equivalent in terms of efficacy, but tolterodine is better tolerated.

Despite short terminal half-lives of 2 to 3 and 3 to 4 hours for tolterodine and its active 5-hydroxy metabolite, respectively, twice-daily dosing is effective because of the drug's long pharmacodynamic effects.[285] Dosage adjustment is recommended in the presence of hepatic impairment and during concurrent therapy with drugs that inhibit CYP 2D6 and CYP 3A4 isozymes.

TROSPIUM CHLORIDE

Trospium (Sanctura) is a quaternary ammonium antimuscarinic agent used for the management of overactive bladder and urge incontinence. The hydrophilic properties of trospium minimize the passage of the drug through the blood–brain barrier, thereby causing fewer CNS and cognitive adverse events.[286] The long-term efficacy of trospium has been compared with oxybutynin in a 52-week study.[287] No significant differences were found in urodynamic outcomes. In addition, the reduction in 24-hour micturition frequency and urgency episodes at 26 and 52 weeks of treatment was not significant. The incidence of dry mouth and gastrointestinal adverse events was significantly lower in the trospium group. The medication should be administered at a dose of 20 mg twice daily and for those patients with severe renal insufficiency (creatinine clearance <30 mL/minute), the dose should be reduced to 20 mg daily.

DARIFENACIN

Darifenacin (Enablex) is a selective M_3 muscarinic receptor antagonist indicated for the treatment of overactive bladder with symptoms of urinary incontinence, urgency, and frequency. A pooled analysis of three 12-week, double-blind, placebo-controlled trials ($N = 1{,}059$) demonstrated that darifenacin reduced the median number of incontinence episodes per week ($p < 0.01$) versus placebo.[289] Dry mouth and constipation were the most common reasons for discontinuation. The recommended starting dose is 7.5 mg once daily. Based on the individual response, the dose may be increased to 15 mg daily after 2 weeks.

SOLIFENACIN

Solifenacin (Vesicare) is a competitive muscarinic receptor antagonist used for the treatment of overactive bladder with symptoms of urinary incontinence. In clinical trials solifenacin showed significant reduction in the symptoms of urinary frequency, urgency, and urge incontinence compared with placebo.[290,291] Safety concerns with solifenacin include an increased risk of QT interval prolongation in patients with a known history of QT interval prolongation or patients who are taking medications known to prolong the QT interval. The recommended dose of solifenacin is 5 mg once daily. If the 5-mg dose is well tolerated, it may be increased to 10 mg once daily.

PROPANTHELINE BROMIDE

Propantheline bromide (Pro-Banthine, generics) is an oral agent prescribed to produce an anticholinergic effect in the lower urinary tract. The adult dose is 15 to 30 mg every 4 to 6 hours. Higher doses sometimes are necessary and are well tolerated. Propantheline bromide is a quaternary ammonium anticholinergic compound that does not cross the blood–brain barrier.[274] As such, CNS side effects are insignificant. Oral administration of propantheline in the fasting state is preferred to improve bioavailability. The anticholinergic effects of propantheline on the detrusor muscle when compared with other anticholinergic agents are similar.[277] These anticholinergic agents differ primarily in their frequency of dosing and their side effect profiles. No other oral drug, however, is available whose direct anticholinergic binding potential approximates that of atropine.[292]

DICYCLOMINE HYDROCHLORIDE

Dicyclomine hydrochloride (Bentyl) is a tertiary-amine and has dose-related CNS effects.[274] An oral dose of 20 mg three times a day will increase bladder capacity in patients with detrusor hyperreflexia. The dose for elderly patients is listed as 10 to 20 mg three times a day, but it may need to be increased to 30 mg three times a day.[277,288] As the dose is increased, anticholinergic side effects become prominent.

FLAVOXATE HYDROCHLORIDE

Evidence for the efficacy of flavoxate hydrochloride (Urispas) is weak. The recommended adult dose is 100 to 200 mg three to four times a day.

β-Adrenergic Agents: Terbutaline

Terbutaline (Brethine) 5 mg orally three times a day reportedly benefits select patients with urge PUI and does not have significant effects on the bladders of healthy persons.[293] The human bladder muscle has β-adrenergic receptors that, when stimulated, will increase the capacity of the bladder. The effect of β-adrenergic stimulation in patients with detrusor hyperactivity is inadequately studied, however.

Although any of the aforementioned drugs would be useful for H.K., oxybutynin is considered the drug of choice for the elderly. Oxybutynin has fewer anticholinergic effects and a more prominent detrusor relaxation effect than any of the other drugs except tolterodine. Tolterodine is a much more expensive agent when compared with oxybutynin and is best reserved for patients who are intolerant of, or fail, oxybutynin. Oxybutynin can be dosed once a day in some cases and, in most cases, twice a day. Flavoxate, dicyclomine, and propantheline require at least three doses a day. The systemic anticholinergic side effects from oxybutynin, tolterodine, flavoxate, and dicyclomine are relatively mild compared with propantheline. A beginning dose of oxybutynin for H.K. would be 2.5 mg/day; the dose can be increased by increments of 2.5 mg/day, not to exceed 5 mg three times a day.

Monitoring H.K. necessitates evaluating her urinary frequency through patient (and where possible, nurse or caregiver) interviews. Specifically, a reduction in the urinary urgency sensation is the desired outcome. Too much anticholinergic therapy can result in urinary hesitancy and possibly urinary retention. If the patient has to concentrate on the act of micturition, the anticholinergic drug dose should be reduced. CNS and systemic side effects should be assessed as often as possible. As with all patients with urge incontinent, urinary tract infection is common. If symptoms of dysuria appear, or if urinary urgency reappears, a urinalysis should be obtained.

Increasing Bladder Outlet Resistance

31. M.K., a 68-year-old woman, has been diagnosed with urinary stress incontinence. What drug therapy would be appropriate for this classification of PUI?

IMIPRAMINE HYDROCHLORIDE

Imipramine hydrochloride (Tofranil, generics) is useful for increasing bladder capacity and increasing bladder outlet resistance.[294] The pharmacologic mechanism of tricyclic antidepressants (TCA) in treating PUI has been studied extensively.[295] The results and conclusions of the data reported demonstrate that, at best, the mechanism of action on the lower urinary tract is speculative. All the TCA have some degree of anticholinergic effect, both centrally and peripherally, but not at all sites. These drugs block the active transport system in the presynaptic nerve ending and prevent the uptake of norepinephrine and serotonin; they produce varying degrees of CNS sedation. All the TCA antagonize histamine receptors, both H_1 and H_2, to some degree, and they desensitize some α_2-adrenergic receptors.[295,296] Imipramine has significant systemic anticholinergic effects, but it has weak anticholinergic effects at the detrusor muscle.[297] Imipramine has a significant inhibitory effect on the detrusor muscle, however, which is neither anticholinergically nor adrenergically mediated. Its detrusor inhibitory effect may be the result of peripheral blockade of norepinephrine reuptake. The ability of imipramine to increase bladder outlet resistance is believed to be owing to enhanced α-adrenergic effects in the smooth muscle of the bladder base and proximal urethra, where α-receptors outnumber β-receptors. Imipramine 75 mg/day produced continence in 68% of women with stress PUI within 4 weeks.[298]

The initial dose for imipramine is 25 mg orally at bedtime. The dose can be increased every third day by 25 mg until the patient is continent, side effects occur, or a dose of 150 mg/day is reached.[294] Most patients become continent within 7 to 10 days, and some patients may become continent in as few as 3 to 5 days. The usual adult dose for voiding dysfunction is 25 mg four times a day, and for geriatric patients the dose is 25 mg twice a day, because the serum half-life is prolonged in the elderly.[299] Weakness, fatigue, and postural hypotension are significant problems associated with imipramine. A threefold increase in hip fractures was reported among elderly patients taking imipramine.[300]

α-Adrenergic receptor stimulation at the detrusor muscle and proximal urethra will increase the maximal urethral pressure (MUP) and the maximal urethral closure pressure (MUCP).[301] Oral α-adrenergic agonist agents should be used cautiously in the elderly because of side effects, which include anxiety, insomnia, blood pressure elevation, headache, tremor, weakness, palpitations, cardiac arrhythmias, and respiratory difficulties.[302]

ESTROGENS

Estrogens affect many aspects of uterine smooth muscle, including excitability, receptor density, and transmitter metabolism, especially adrenergic nerves.[303] The detrusor and urethra are embryologically related to the uterus, and significant work has been done on estrogenic hormone effects on the lower urinary tract. α-Adrenergic stimulation of the urethra is estrogen dependent,[304] and several studies have demonstrated the relationship of estrogen to α-adrenergic receptor density in the lower urinary tract.[305] Estrogen therapy, in the form of vaginal suppositories (1 mg/day), facilitates urinary storage in some postmenopausal patients by increasing urethral outlet resistance and it has an additive effect with α-adrenergic therapy (pseudoephedrine 20 mg three times daily).[263] The use of estrogen in the treatment of stress PUI requires further study. The use of long-term estrogen treatment must be considered carefully in light of the controversy over whether estrogen therapy predisposes to the development of endometrial carcinoma. If estrogen is combined with α-adrenergic agonist therapy, the lowest effective maintenance dose should be prescribed.

Decreasing Bladder Outlet Resistance

Overflow incontinence in female patients resulting from outlet obstruction or weak detrusor muscle is now being treated with α_{1A}-blockers by many urologists. Traditional treatments include cholinergic agents (e.g., bethanechol), Foley catheter, surgical procedures, or urethral caps. α_{1A}–Blockers, such as prazosin, terazosin, or doxazosin, are certainly not the drugs of choice, but they can decrease outflow resistance by decreasing sphincter tone.[305] Most α_{1A}-receptors are found in prostate tissue; however, these same receptors are also located in the spinal cord, bladder neck, urethra, and periurethral tissue in women.[306] The urinary symptoms suggestive of prostatism are not gender specific. Well-controlled, randomized, cross-over studies are needed to determine the efficacy of α_{1A}-blockers in overflow incontinence.

REFERENCES

1. Lauman EO et al. Sexual dysfunction in the United States. *JAMA* 1999;281:537.
2. NIH Consensus Conference. Impotence. National Institutes of Health Consensus Development Panel on Impotence. *JAMA* 1993;270:83.
3. Rosen RC et al. Prevalence of sexual dysfunction in women: results of a survey study of 329 women in an outpatient gynecological clinic. *J Sex Marital Ther* 1993;19:171.
4. Spector IP. Incidence and prevalence of the sexual dysfunctions: a critical review of the empirical literature. *Arch Sex Behav* 1990;19:389.
5. Kinsey A et al., eds. *Sexual Behavior in the Human Male*. Philadelphia: WB Saunders; 1984.
6. Pfieffer E et al. Sexual behavior in aged men and women. *Arch Gen Psychiatry* 1986;19:735.
7. Bretschneider JG et al. Sexual interest and behavior in healthy 80 to 102 year olds. *Arch Sex Behav* 1988;17:109.
8. Diokno AC et al. Correlates of sexual dysfunction in the elderly. *J Urol* 1988;139:496A.
9. Tordarello O et al. Sexuality in aging: a study of a group of 300 elderly men and women. *J Endocrinol Invest* 1985;8(Suppl 2):123.
10. Starr BD et al. *The Starr-Weiner Report on Sex and Sexuality in the Mature Years*. New York: Stein and Day; 1981.
11. Persson G. Sexuality in a 70-year-old urban population. *J Psychosom Res* 1980;24:137.
12. Sternbach H. Age-associated testosterone decline in men: clinical issues for psychiatry. *Am J Psychiatry* 1998;155:1310.
13. Vermeulen A et al. Ageing of the hypothalamopituitary-testicular axis in men. *Horm Res* 1995;43:25.
14. Feldman HA et al. Impotence and its medical

and psychosocial correlates: results of the Massachusetts Male Aging Study. *J Urol* 1994;151:54.
15. Melman A. Evaluation of the first 70 patients in the center for male sexual dysfunction of Beth Israel Medical Center. *J Urol* 1984;131:53.
16. Shrom SH et al. Clinical profile of experience with 130 consecutive cases of impotent men. *Urology* 1980;13:511.
17. Mulligan T et al. Why aged men become impotent. *Arch Intern Med* 1989;149:1365.
18. Hsueh WA. Sexual dysfunction with aging and systemic hypertension. *Am J Cardiol* 1988;61(Suppl):18H.
19. Padam-Nathan H et al. Treatment of men with erectile dysfunction with transurethral alprostadil. *N Engl J Med* 1997;336:1.
20. McWaine DE et al. Drug-induced sexual dysfunction. *Medical Toxicology* 1988;3:289.
21. Deamer RL et al. The role of medications in geriatric sexual function. *Clin Geriatr Med* 1991;7:95.
22. Mooradian AD et al. Endocrinology in aging. *Dis Mon* 1988;34:398.
23. Wein AJ et al. Drug-induced male sexual dysfunction. *Urol Clin North Am* 1988;15:23.
24. Johannes CB et al. Incidence of erectile dysfunction in men 40 to 69 years old: longitudinal results from the Massachusetts Male Aging Study. *J Urol* 2000;163:460.
25. Morley JE. Impotence. *Am J Med* 1986;80:897.
26. Hatzichristou DG. Sildenafil citrate: lessons learned from 3 years of clinical experience. *Int J Impot Res* 2002;14(Suppl 1);43.
27. Krane RJ et al. Impotence. *N Engl J Med* 1989;321:1648.
28. Lue TF. Male sexual dysfunction. In: Tanagho EA et al., eds. *Smith's General Urology*. Norwalk: Appleton & Lange; 1992:696.
29. Deslypere JP et al. Leydig cell function in normal men: effect of age, life-style, residence, diet, and activity. *J Clin Endocrinol Metab* 1984;59:955.
30. Tesitouras PD. Effects of age on testicular function. *Endocrinol Metab Clin North Am* 1987;16:1045.
31. Lue TF et al. Physiology of erection and pharmacological management of impotence. *J Urol* 1987;137:829.
32. Heaton JPW et al. Recovery of erectile function by the oral administration of apomorphine. *Urology* 1995;45:200.
33. Shabsigh R et al. Erectile dysfunction. *Annu Rev Med* 2003;54:153.
34. Lincoln TM et al. Towards an understanding of the mechanism of action of cyclic AMP and cyclic GMP in smooth muscle relaxation. *Blood Vessels* 28;128:1991.
35. Lue TF. Erectile dysfunction. *N Engl J Med* 2000;342:1802.
36. Burnett AL. Nitric oxide in the penis: physiology and pathology. *J Urol* 1997;157:320.
37. Bohlen JG et al. Heart rate, rate-pressure product, and oxygen uptake during four sexual activities. *Arch Intern Med* 1984;144:1745.
38. Drory Y et al. Myocardial ischemia during sexual activity in patients with coronary artery disease. *Am J Cardiol* 1995;75:835.
39. Johnson BL et al. Dynamic electrocardiographic recording during sexual activity in recent post-myocardial infarction and revascularization patients. *Am Heart J* 1979;98:736.
40. Jackson G. Sexual intercourse and angina pectoris. *International Rehabilitation Medicine Association* 1981;3:35.
41. Muller JE et al. Triggering myocardial infarction by sexual activity: low absolute risk and prevention by regular physical exertion. Determinants of Myocardial Infarction Onset Study. *JAMA* 1996;275:1405.
42. Ueno M. The so-called coital death. *Japanese Journal of Legal Medicine* 1963;17:330.
43. Padam-Nathan H et al. Evaluation of the impotent patient. *Semin Urol* 1986;4:225.
44. Whitehead ED et al. Diagnostic evaluation of impotence. *Postgrad Med* 1990;88:123.
45. Goldstein I and The Working Group for the Study of Central Mechanisms in ED. Male sexual circuitry. *Sci Am* 2000;283:70.
46. Deutsch S et al. Previously unrecognized diabetes mellitus in sexually impotent men. *JAMA* 1980;244:2430.
47. Spark RF et al. Hypogonadism, hyperprolactinaemia, and temporal lobe epilepsy in hyposexual men. *Lancet* 1984;1:413.
48. Gerstenberg TC et al. Nerve conduction velocity measurement of dorsal nerve of the penis in normal and impotent men. *J Urol* 1985;21:90.
49. Spark RF et al. Impotence is not always psychogenic: newer insights into hypothalamic-pituitary-gonadal dysfunction. *JAMA* 1980;243:750.
50. Rubin A et al. Impotence and diabetes mellitus. *JAMA* 1958;168:498.
51. Bancroft J et al. Changes in erectile responsiveness during androgen therapy. *Arch Sex Behav* 1983;12:59.
52. Michal V et al. Arterial lesions in impotence: phalloarteriography. *Int Angiol* 1984;3:247.
53. Rosen RC et al. The international index of erectile function (IIEF): a multidimensional scale for assessment of erectile dysfunction. *Urology* 1997;49:822.
54. Jardin A et al. Recommendations of the First International Consultation on Erectile Dysfunction. In: Jardin A et al., eds. *Erectile Dysfunction*. Plymouth: Plymbridge Distributors; 2000:711.
55. Spina M et al. Age-related changes in the composition of and mechanical properties of the tunica media of the upper thoracic human aorta. *Arteriosclerosis* 1983;3:64.
56. Smulyan H et al. Effect of age on arterial distensibility in asymptomatic humans. *Arteriosclerosis* 1983;3:199.
57. Wabrek AJ et al. Male sexual dysfunction associated with coronary heart disease. *Arch Sex Behav* 1980;9:69.
58. Gundle MJ et al. Psychological outcome after aorto-coronary artery surgery. *Am J Psychiatry* 1980;137:1591.
59. Agarwal A et al. Male sexual dysfunction after stroke. *J Assoc Physicians India* 1989;37:505.
60. Ruzbarsky V et al. Morphologic changes in the arterial bed of the penis with aging. Relationship to the pathogenesis of impotence. *Invest Urol* 1977;15:194.
61. Morley JE et al. Relationship of penile brachial pressure index to myocardial infarction and cerebrovascular accidents in older men. *Am J Med* 1988;84:445.
62. Virag R et al. Is impotence an arterial disorder? *Lancet* 1985;1:181.
63. Shabsigh R et al. Cigarette smoking and other vascular risk factors in vasculogenic impotence. *Urology* 1991;38:227.
64. Oaks WW et al. Sex and hypertension. *Medical Aspects of Human Sexuality* 1972;6:128.
65. Bulpitt CJ et al. Changes in symptoms of hypertensive patients after referral to hospital clinic. *Br Heart J* 1976;38:121.
66. Report of Medical Research Council Working Party on Mild to Moderate Hypertension. Adverse reaction to bendroflumethiazide and propranolol for the treatment of mild hypertension. *Lancet* 1981;2:539.
67. Veterans Administrative Cooperative Study Group on antihypertensive agents. Comparison of prazosin with hydralazine in patients receiving hydrochlorothiazide: a randomized double blind clinical trial. *Circulation* 1981;64:722.
68. Wabrek AJ et al. Noninvasive penile arterial evaluation in 120 males with erectile dysfunction. *Urology* 1983;22:230.
69. Condra M et al. Prevalence and significance of tobacco smoking in impotence. *Urology* 1986;27:495.
70. Hirshkowitz M et al. Nocturnal penile tumescence in cigarette smokers with erectile dysfunction. *Urology* 1992;34:101.
71. DePalma RG et al. A screening sequence for vasculogenic impotence. *J Vasc Surg* 1987;5:228.
72. Zemel P. Sexual dysfunction in the diabetic patient with hypertension. *Am J Cardiol* 1988;61:27H.
73. Rubin A et al. Impotence and diabetes mellitus. *JAMA* 1958;168:498.
74. Whitehead ED et al. Diabetes-related impotence in the elderly. *Clin Geriatr Med* 1990;6:771.
75. McCulloch DK et al. The prevalence of diabetic impotence. *Diabetologia* 1980;18:279.
76. Kannel W et al. The role of diabetes in congestive heart failure: the Framingham study. *Am J Cardiol* 1974;34:29.
77. Lehman TP et al. Etiology of diabetic impotence. *Urology* 1983;129:291.
78. Morley JE et al. Testicular function in the aging male. In: Armbrecht HJ, ed. *Endocrine Function and Aging*. New York: Springer-Verlag; 1989:456.
79. Morely JE et al. Sexual function with advancing age. *Med Clin North Am* 1989;73:1483.
80. Snyder PJ et al. Serum LH and FSH response to synthetic gonadotropins in normal men. *J Clin Endocrinol Metab* 1975;41:938.
81. Tenover JS et al. Decreased serum inhibin levels in normal elderly men: evidence for a decline in Sertoli cell function with aging. *J Clin Endocrinol Metab* 1988;67:455.
82. Kaiser FE et al. Impotence and aging: clinical and hormonal factors. *J Am Geriatr Soc* 1988;36:511.
83. Skakkeback N et al. Androgen replacement with oral testosterone in hypogonadal men: a double-blind controlled study. *Clin Endocrinol (Oxf)* 1981;14:49.
84. Bancroft J. Endocrinology of sexual function. *Clin Endocrinol Metab* 1980;4:253.
85. Davidson JM et al. Hormonal changes and sexual function in aging men. *J Clin Endocrinol Metab* 1983;57:71.
86. Morley JE. Impotence. *Am J Med* 1986;80:897.
87. Mooradian AD et al. Hyperprolactinemia in male diabetics. *Postgrad Med J* 1985;61:11.
88. Mirin SM et al. Opiate use and sexual function. *Am J Psychiatry* 1980;137:909.
89. McWaine DE et al. Drug-induced sexual dysfunction. *Med Toxicol* 1988;3:289.
90. Bissada NK et al. Urologic manifestations of drug therapy. *Urol Clin North Am* 1988;15:725.
91. Crenshaw TL et al. *Sexual Pharmacology: Drugs That Affect Sexual Function*. New York: WW Norton; 1996.
92. Wein AJ et al. Drug-induced male dysfunction. *Urol Clin North Am* 1988;15:23.
93. Morley JE. Impotence. *Am J Med* 1986;80:897.
94. Whitehead ED et al. Treatment alternatives for impotence. *Postgrad Med* 1990;88:139.
95. Scruti A et al. The effects of testosterone administration and visual erotic stimuli on nocturnal penile tumescence in normal men. *Horm Behav* 1990;24:435.
96. Guay AT et al. Efficacy and safety of sildenafil for treatment of erectile dysfunction in a population with associated organic risk factors. *J Androl* 2001;22:793.
97. Monga M et al. Patient satisfaction with testosterone supplementation for the treatment of erectile dysfunction. *Arch Androl* 2002;48:433.
98. Morley JE et al. Sexual function with advancing age. *Med Clin North Am* 1989;73:1483.
99. Yu Z et al. Transdermal testosterone administration in hypogonadal men: comparison of pharmacokinetics at different sites of application and at the first and fifth days of application. *J Clin Pharmacol* 1997;37:1129.
100. McCellan KJ et al. Transdermal testosterone. *Drugs* 1998;55:253.
101. Winters SJ. Current status of testosterone replacement therapy in men. *Arch Fam Med* 1999;8:257.
102. Parker S et al. Experience with transdermal testosterone replacement therapy for hypogonadal men. *Clin Endocrinol (Oxf)* 1999;50:57.
103. Gann PH et al. Prospective study of sex hormone levels and risk of prostate cancer. *J Natl Cancer Inst* 1996;88:1118.
104. Nomura A et al. Serum androgens and prostate

cancer. *Cancer Epidemiol Biomarkers Prev* 1996;5: 621.

105. Sih R et al. Testosterone replacement in older hypogonadal men: a 12 month randomized controlled trial. *J Clin Endocrinol Metab* 1997;82: 1661.
106. Hajjar R et al. Outcomes of long-term testosterone analysis. *J Clin Endocrinol Metab* 1997;82:3793.
107. Zgliczynski S et al. Effect of testosterone replacement therapy on lipids and lipoproteins in hypogonadal and elderly men. *Atherosclerosis* 1996;121: 35.
108. Morgentaler A et al. Occult prostate cancer in men with low serum testosterone levels. *JAMA* 1996;276:1904.
109. Rendell MS et al. Sildenafil for treatment of erectile dysfunction in men with diabetes: a randomized controlled trial. *JAMA* 1999;281:421.
110. Cheitlin MD et al. ACC/AHA Expert Consensus Document: use of sildenafil in patients with cardiovascular disease. *J Am Cardiol* 1999;33:273.
111. Goldstein I et al. Oral sildenafil in the treatment of erectile dysfunction. *N Engl J Med* 1998;538: 1397.
112. Morales A et al. Clinical safety of oral sildenafil citrate (Viagra) in the treatment of erectile dysfunction. *Int J Impot Res* 1998;10:69.
113. Mitka M. Viagra leads as rivals are moving up. *JAMA* 1998;280:119.
114. Cohen JS. Comparison of FDA reports of patient deaths associated with sildenafil and with injectable alprostadil. *Ann Pharmacother* 2001;35:285.
115. Arruda-Olson AM et al. Cardiovascular effects of sildenafil during exercise in men with known or probable coronary artery disease. A randomized crossover trial. *JAMA* 2002;287:719.
116. Sadovsky R et al. Three-year update of sildenafil citrate efficacy and safety. *Int J Clin Pract* 2001;3:196.
117. Angulo J et al. Tadalafil enhances NO-mediated relaxation of human arterial and trabecular penile smooth muscle. *Annual Meeting of the European Association for the Study of Diabetes;* 2001; Glascow, Scotland [Abstract].
118. Vickers MA et al. Phosphodiesterase type 5 inhibitors for the treatment of erectile dysfunction in patients with diabetes mellitus. *In J Impot Res* 2002;14:466.
119. Padma-Nathan H. Cialis–(tadalafil) provides prompt response and extended period of responsiveness for the treatment of men with erectile dysfunction (ED). *J Urol* 2001;(Suppl):165:224.
120. Porst H et al. The efficacy and tolerability of vardenafil, a new, oral, selective phosphodiesterase type 5 inhibitor, in patients with erectile dysfunction: the first at home clinical trial. *Int J Impot Res* 2001;13:192.
121. Steidle CP et al. Pharmacokientics of vardenafil in the elderly and subgroup data on efficacy and safety in elderly patients with erectile dysfunction [Abstract]. *J Am Geriatr Soc* 2001;49:S103.
122. Thandani U et al. The effect of vardenafil, a potent and highly selective phosphodiesterase-5 inhibitor for the treatment or erectile dysfunction, on the cardiovascular response to exercise in patients with coronary disease. *J Am Coll Cardiol* 2002;40:2006.
123. Morales A et al. Is yohimbine effective in the treatment of organic impotence? Results of a controlled trial. *J Urol* 1987;137:1168.
124. Morales A et al. Oral and transcutaneous pharmacological agents in the treatment of impotence. *Urol Clin North Am* 1988;15:87.
125. Reid K et al. Double blind trial of yohimbine in treatment of psychogenic impotence. *Lancet* 1987;2:421.
126. Virag R. Intracavernous injection of papaverine for erectile failure. *Lancet* 1982;2:328.
127. Sidi AA et al. Intracavernous drug-induced erections in the management of male erectile dysfunction: experience with 100 patients. *J Urol* 1986;135: 704.
128. Brindley GS. Cavernosal alpha-blockade: a new technique for investigating and treating erectile impotence. *Br J Psychiatry* 1983;143:332.
129. Zorgniotti AW et al. Auto-injection of the corpus cavernosum with a vasoactive drug combination for vasculogenic impotence. *J Urol* 1985;133:39.
130. Nelson RP. Injections of papaverine and Regitine into the corpora cavernosa for erectile dysfunction: clinical results in 60 patients. *South Med J* 1989;82:26.
131. Watters GR et al. Experience in the management of erectile dysfunction using the intracavernosal self-injection of vasoactive drugs. *J Urol* 1988;140:1417.
132. Brading AF et al. The effects of papaverine on the electrical and mechanical activity of the guinea pig ureter. *J Physiol* 1983;334:79.
133. Huddart H et al. Inhibition by papaverine of calcium movements and tension in the smooth muscle of rats vas deferens and urinary bladder. *J Physiol* 1984;349:183.
134. Wang Q et al. Modulation of noradrenaline-induced membrane currents by papaverine in rabbit vascular smooth muscle cells. *J Physiol* 1991;439:501.
135. Brindley GS. Neurophysiology of erection. In: *Proceedings of the First World Meeting on Impotence*. Paris, France; 1984:39.
136. Brindley GS. New treatment for priapism. *Lancet* 1984;2:220.
137. Juenemann KP et al. Hemodynamics of papaverine and phentolamine induced penile erection. *J Urol* 1986;136:158.
138. Juenemann KP et al. Further evidence of venous outflow restriction during erection. *Br J Urol* 1986;58:320.
139. Keogh E et al. Treatment of impotence by intrapenile injections: a comparison of papaverine versus papaverine and phentolamine: a double-blind crossover study. *J Urol* 1989;142:726.
140. Lue T et al. Physiology of erection and pharmacological management of impotence. *J Urol* 1987;137:829.
141. Lue T et al. Functional evaluation of penile veins by cavernosography in papaverine induced erections. *J Urol* 1986;135:479.
142. Wespes E et al. Systemic complications of intracavernous papaverine injections in patients with venous leakage. *Urology* 1988;31:114.
143. Montorsi F et al. Effectiveness and safety of multidrug intra-cavernous therapy for vasculogenic impotence. *Urology* 1993;42:554.
144. Katlowitz N et al. Effect of multidose intracorporeal injection and audiovisual sexual stimulation in vasculogenic impotence. *Urology* 1993;42:695.
145. Nelson RP. Injections of papaverine and Regitine into the corpora cavernosa for erectile dysfunction: clinical results in 60 patients. *South Med J* 1989;82:26.
146. Papaverine Hydrochloride USP Injection, package insert. Indianapolis, IN: Eli Lilly and Company; April 1994.
147. Phentolamine Mesylate USP package insert. Woodbridge, NJ: Ciba Pharmaceuticals; April 1994.
148. Benson G, Seifert W. Is phentolamine stable in solution with papaverine? *J Urol* 1988;140:970.
149. Levine SB et al. Side-effects of self-administration of intracavernous papaverine and phentolamine for the treatment of impotence. *J Urol* 1989;141:54.
150. Larsen EH et al. Fibrosis of corpus cavernosum after intra-cavernous injection of phentolamine/papaverine. *J Urol* 1987;137:292.
151. Malloy TR et al. Pharmacologic treatment of impotence. *Urol Clin North Am* 1987;14:297.
152. Abozeid M et al. Chronic papaverine treatment: the effect of repeated injections on the simian erectile and penile tissue. *J Urol* 1987;138:1263.
153. Fuchs M et al. Papaverine-induced fibrosis of the corpus cavernosum. *J Urol* 1989;141:125.
154. Girdley FM et al. Intracavernous self-injection for impotence: a long-term therapeutic option? *Experience in 78 patients. J Urol* 1988;140:972.
155. Keogh EJ et al. Treatment of impotence by intrapenile injections. A comparison of papaverine versus papaverine and phentolamine: a double-blind, crossover trial. *J Urol* 1989;142:726.
156. Kunelius P et al. Intracavernous self-injection of prostaglandin E_1 in the treatment of erectile dysfunction. *Int J Impot Res* 1999;11:21.
157. Steidle C et al. Topical alprostadil cream for the treatment of erectile dysfunction: a combined analysis of the phase II program. *Urology* 2002; 60:1077.
158. Kaplan SA et al. Combination therapy using oral alpha-blockers and intracavernosal injection in men with erectile dysfunction. *Urology* 1998;52:739.
159. Ishii N et al. *Therapeutic trial with prostaglandin E_1 for organic impotence. Abstract presented at Second World Meeting on Impotence*. Prague, Czechoslovakia; 1986.
160. Sarsody M et al. A prospective double-blind trial of intra-corporeal papaverine versus prostaglandin E_1 in the treatment of impotence. *J Urol* 1989;141:551.
161. Zaher TF. Papaverine plus prostaglandin E_1 versus prostaglandin alone for intracorporeal injection therapy. *Int Urol Nephrol* 1998;30:193.
162. Hedlund H et al. Contraction and relaxation induced by some prostanoids in isolated human penile erectile tissue and cavernous artery. *J Urol* 1985;134:1245.
163. Hellstrom WJ et al. A double-blind placebo controlled evaluation of the erectile response to transurethral alprostadil. *Urology* 1996;48:851.
164. Walsh PC. Benign prostatic hyperplasia. In: Walsch PC et al., eds. *Campbell's Urology*. 5th ed. Philadelphia: WB Saunders; 1986:1248.
165. Standberg JD. Comparative pathology of benign prostatic hypertrophy. In: Lepor H et al., eds. *Prostatic Diseases*. Philadelphia: WB Saunders; 1993:212.
166. Berry SJ et al. The development of human benign prostatic hyperplasia with age. *J Urol* 1984; 132:474.
167. Narayan P. Neoplasms of the prostate. In: Tanago EA et al., eds. *Smith's General Urology*. Norwalk: Appleton & Lange; 1992:378.
168. Greenwald P et al. Cancer of the prostate among men with benign prostatic hyperplasia. *J Natl Cancer Inst* 1970;53:335.
169. Takahashi S et al. Latent prostatic carcinomas found at autopsy in men over 90 years old. *Jap J Clin Oncol* 1992;22:117.
170. Issacs JT et al. Etiology and disease process of benign prostatic hyperplasia. *Prostate Suppl* 1989;2:34.
171. Lepor H. Medical therapy for benign prostatic hyperplasia. *Urology* 1993;42:483.
172. Bartsch G et al. Dihydrotestosterone and the concept of 5-alpha reductase inhibition in human benign hyperplasia. *Eur Urol* 2000;37:367.
173. Hiramatsu M et al. Immunolocalization of oestrogen and progesterone receptors in prostatic hyperplasia and carcinoma. *Histopathology* 1996;28: 163.
174. Boyarsky S et al. A new look at bladder neck obstruction by the U.S. Food and Drug Administration regulators: guidelines for the investigation of benign prostatic hypertrophy. *Transactions of the American Association of Genito-Urinary Surgeons*. 1977;68:29.
175. Barry MJ et al. The American Urological Association symptom index for benign prostatic hyperplasia. *J Urol* 1992;148:1549.
176. Lepro H et al. Comparison of AUA Symptom Index in unselected males and females between fifty-five and seventy nine years of age. *Urology* 1993;42:36.
177. Litwin M et al. The National Institutes of Health chronic prostatitis symptom index: development and validation of a new outcome measure. *J Urol* 1999;162:369.
178. DuBeau CE et al. Controversies in the diagnosis and management of benign prostatic hypertrophy. *Adv Intern Med* 1991;37:55.
179. Dalkin BL et al. Prostate specific antigen levels in men older than 50 years without clinical evidence of prostatic carcinoma. *J Urol* 1993;150:1837.
180. Reissigl A et al. Comparison of different prostate-specific antigen cutpoints for early detection of prostate cancer: results of a large screening study. *Urology* 1995;46:662.

181. Borer JG et al. Age specific prostate-specific antigen reference ranges: population specific. *J Urol* 1998;159:444.
182. Slovacek KJ et al. Use of age-specific normal ranges for serum prostate-specific antigen. *Arch Pathol Lab Med* 1998;122:330.
183. Richardson TD et al. Age-specific reference ranges for serum prostate-specific antigen. *Urol Clin North Am* 1997;24:339.
184. Ravel R. Laboratory aspects of cancer. In Ravel R, ed. *Clinical Laboratory of Medicine*. 6th ed. St Louis: CV Mosby; 1995:566.
185. Talner LB. Specific causes of obstruction. In: Pollack HM, ed. *Clinical Urology*. 2nd ed. Philadelphia: WB Saunders; 1990:1629.
186. Mushlin AI et al. Intravenous pyelography. The case against its routine. *Ann Intern Med* 1989;111:58.
187. Wasserman NF et al. Assessment of prostatism: role of intravenous urography. *Radiology* 1987;165:831.
188. Webb JAW. Ultrasonography in the diagnosis of renal obstruction. Sensitive but not very specific. *BMJ* 1990;301:944.
189. Siroky MB et al. The flow rate nomogram: I. Development. *J Urol* 1979;122:665.
190. Haylen BT et al. Maximum and average urine flow rates in normal male and female populations. *Br J Urol* 1989;64:30.
191. Marshall VR et al. The use of urinary flow rates obtained from voided volumes less than 150 mL in the assessment of voiding ability. *Br J Urol* 1983;55:28.
192. Lepor H et al. The efficacy of transurethral resection of the prostate in men with moderate symptoms of prostatism. *J Urol* 1990;143:533.
193. Kadow C et al. Prostatectomy or conservative management in the treatment of benign prostatic hypertrophy. *Br J Urol* 1988;61:432.
194. Bruskewitz RC et al. 3 year follow-up of urinary symptoms after transurethral resection of the prostate. *J Urol* 1989;142:1251.
195. Chancellor MB et al. Bladder outlet obstruction and impaired detrusor contractility: a blinded comparison of the video-urodynamic diagnosis versus the diagnosis based on a detrusor contractility parameter, a urethral resistant parameter, and a sustained/fade index. *Neurourol Urodyn* 1990;9:209.
196. Fowler FJ et al. Symptom status and quality of life following prostatectomy. *JAMA* 1988;259:3018.
197. Bruskewitz RC et al. Critical evaluation of transurethral resection and incision of the prostate. *Prostate* 1990;3:27.
198. Lepor H. The role of alpha-adrenergic blockers in the treatment of benign prostatic hypertrophy. *Prostate Suppl* 1990;3:75.
199. Caine M. The present role of alpha-adrenergic blockers in the treatment of benign prostatic hypertrophy. *J Urol* 1986;136:1.
200. Fulton B et al. Doxazosin: an update of its clinical pharmacology and therapeutic applications in hypertension and benign hyperplasia. *Drugs* 1995;49:295.
201. Pool JL. Doxazosin: a new approach to hypertension and benign prostatic hyperplasia. *Br J Clin Pract* 1996;50:154.
202. Dunzendorfer U. Clinical experience: symptomatic management of BPH with terazosin. *Urology* 1988;32(Suppl):27.
203. Kyprianou N. Doxazosin and terazosin suppress prostate growth by inducing apoptosis: clinical significance. *J Urol* 2003;169:1520.
204. Lepor H et al. The relative efficacy of terazosin versus terazosin and flutamide for the treatment of symptomatic BPH. *Prostate* 1992;20:89.
205. Taguchi K et al. Effects of tamsulosin metabolites at alpha-1 adrenoceptor subtypes. *J Pharmacol Exp Ther* 1997;280:1.
206. Chapple CR et al. Tamsulosin, the first prostate selective alpha-1a-adenoceptor antagonist–a meta analysis of two randomized, placebo controlled, multicenter studies in patients with benign prostatic obstruction. *Eur Urol* 1996;29:145.
207. Murayama K et al. Clinical evaluation of tamsulosin hydrochloride on bladder outlet obstruction associated with benign prostatic hyperplasia; effect on urethral pressure profile and cystometrogram. *Hinyokika Kiyo* 1997;43:799.
208. Kamimura H et al. Identification of cytochrome P450 involved in metabolism of the alpha-1 adrenoceptor blocker tamsulosin in human liver microsomes. *Xenobiotica* 1998;28:909.
209. Wolzt M et al. Pharmacokinetics of tamsulosin in subjects with normal and varying degrees of impaired renal function: an open-label single-dose and multiple-dose study. *Eur J Clin Pharmacol* 1998;54:367.
210. Narayan P. Tamsulosin: the United States trials. *Geriatrics* 1998;53:S29.
211. Isaacs JT et al. Changes in the metabolism of dihydrotestosterone in the hyperplastic human prostate. *J Clin Endocrinol* 1983;56:139.
212. DeKlerk DP et al. Quantitative determination of prostatic epithelial and stromal hyperplasia by a new technique: biomorphometrics. *Invest Urol* 1978;16:240.
213. Matzkin H et al. Endocrine treatment of benign prostatic hypertrophy: current concepts. *Urology* 1991;37:1.
214. Wilson JP. The pathogenesis of benign prostatic hyperplasia. *Am J Med* 1980;68:745.
215. Bartsh W et al. Hormone blood levels and their interrelationships in normal men and men with benign prostatic hypertrophy. *Acta Endocrinol* 1979;90:727.
216. Ghanadian et al. Serum dihydrotestosterone in patients with benign prostatic hypertrophy. *Br J Urol* 1977;49:541.
217. Siiteri PK et al. Dihydrotestosterone in prostatic hypertrophy, the formation and content of DHT in the hypertrophic prostate of man. *J Clin Invest* 1970;49:1737.
218. Bruchovsky N et al. Increased ration of 5-alpha reductase: 3-alpha (Beta)-hydroxysteroid dehydrogenase activities in the hyperplastic human prostate. *J Endocrinol* 1979;80:289.
219. Habenicht UF et al. Development of a model for the induction of estrogen-related prostatic hyperplasia. *Prostate* 1986;6:181.
220. Geller J et al. BPH and prostate cancer: results of hormonal manipulation. In: Bruchovsky N et al., eds. *Regulation of Androgen Action*. Berlin: Congessdruck R. Bruckner; 1985:51.
221. Charisiri N et al. Examination of the distribution of estrogen receptor between the stromal and epithelial compartments of the prostate. *Prostate* 1980;1:357.
222. Feldman HA et al. Impotence and its psychological correlates: results of the Massachusetts male aging study. *J Urol* 1994;151:54.
223. DeKlerk DP et al. Comparison of spontaneous and experimentally induced canine prostatic hypertrophy. *J Clin Endocrinol Metab* 1979;64:842.
224. McConnell JD et al. Finasteride, an inhibitor of 5 alpha-reductase, suppresses prostatic dihydrotestosterone in men with benign prostatic hyperplasia. *J Clin Endocrinol Metab* 1992;74:504.
225. Lowe FC et al. Long-term 6-year experience with finasteride in patients with benign prostatic hyperplasia. *Urology* 2003;61:791.
226. Gormley GJ et al. The effect of finasteride in men with benign prostatic hyperplasia. The finasteride study group. *N Engl J Med* 1992;327:1185.
227. Stoner E et al. Maintenance of clinical efficacy with finasteride therapy for 24 months in patients with benign prostatic hyperplasia. *Arch Intern Med* 1994;83:154.
228. Weeslls H, et al. Incidence and severity of sexual adverse prostatic hyperplasia. *Urol* 2003;61:579.
229. Abrams P et al. Improvement of pressure flow parameters with finasteride is greater in men with large prostates. *Urology* 1999;161:1513.
230. Anonymous. Finasteride for benign prostatic hypertrophy. *Med Lett Drugs Ther* 1992;34:83.
231. MK-906C Finasteride Study Group. One year experience in the treatment of benign prostatic hyperplasia with finasteride. *J Androl* 1991;12:372.
232. Yang XJ et al. Does long-term finasteride therapy affect the histological features of benign prostatic tissue and prostate cancer on needle biopsy? *PLESS Study Group (Proscar Long-Term Efficacy and Safety Study). Urology* 1999;53:696.
233. Montironi R et al. Treatment of benign prostatic hyperplasia with 5-alpha-reductase inhibitor: morphological changes in patients who fail to respond. *J Clin Pathol* 1996;49:324.
234. Roehrborn C et al. Efficacy and safety of a dual inhibitor of 5-alpha-reductase types 1 and 2 (dutasteride) in men with benign prostatic hyperplasia. *Urology* 2002;60:434.
235. Caine M et al. The treatment of benign prostatic hypertrophy with flutamide (SCH 13521): a placebo-controlled study. *J Urol* 1975;114:564.
236. Stone NN. Flutamide in treatment of benign prostatic hypertrophy. *Urology* 1989;34(Suppl):64.
237. Wysowski DK et al. Flutamide hepatotoxicity. *J Urol* 1996;155:209.
238. Eri LM et al. A prospective placebo controlled study of the luteinizing hormone releasing hormone agonist leuprolide as a treatment for patients with benign prostatic hyperplasia. *J Urol* 1993;150:359.
239. Keane PF et al. Response of the benign hypertrophied prostate to treatment with an LHRH analogue. *Br J Urol* 1988;62:163.
240. Oesterling JE. Prostate specific antigen: a critical assessment of the most useful tumor marker for adenocarcinoma of the prostate. *J Urol* 1991;145:907.
241. Guess HA et al. The effect of finasteride on prostate specific antigen in men with benign prostatic hyperplasia. *Prostate* 1993;22:31.
242. Lepor H. Medical therapy for benign prostatic hyperplasia. *Urology* 1993;42:483.
243. Wilt TJ et al. Saw palmetto extracts for treatment of benign prostatic hyperplasia: a systematic review. *JAMA* 1998;280:1604.
244. Bent S et al. Saw palmetto for benign prostatic hyperplasia. *N Eng J Med* 2006;354:557.
245. Bayne CW et al. Serenoa repens: a 5 alpha-reductase type I and II inhibitor–new evidence in a coculture model of BPH. *Prostate* 1999;40:232.
246. Gordon AE et al. Saw palmetto for prostate disorders. *Am Fam Physician* 2003;67:1281.
247. Carraro JC et al. Comparison of phytotherapy (Permixon) with finasteride in the treatment of benign prostate hyperplasia: a randomized international study of 1,098 patients. *Prostate* 1996;29:231.
248. Wilt T. Pygeum africanum for benign prostatic hyperplasia. Cochrane Database. *Syst Rev* 2002;(1):CD001044.
249. Ouslander JG et al. Urinary incontinence in elderly nursing home patients. *JAMA* 1982;248:1194.
250. Mohide EA. The prevalence and scope of urinary incontinence. *Clin Geriatr Med* 1986;2:639.
251. Thomas TM et al. Prevalence of urinary incontinence. *BMJ* 1980;281:1243.
252. Marron et al. The nonuse of urethral catheterization in the management of urinary incontinence in the teaching nursing home. *J Am Geriatr Soc* 1983;31:278.
253. Colling J et al. The effects of patterned urge-response toileting (PURT) on urinary incontinence among nursing home residents. *J Am Geriatr Soc* 1992;40:135.
254. Gosling JA et al. The anatomy of the bladder, urethra, and pelvic floor. In: Mundy AR et al., eds. *Urodynamics: Principles, Practice, and Application*. New York: Churchill Livingstone; 1984:3.
255. Resnick NM et al. Management of urinary incontinence in the elderly. *N Engl J Med* 1985;313:800.
256. Rud T. Urethral pressure profile in continent women from childhood to old age. *Acta Obstet Gynecol Scand* 1980;59:331.
257. Jones KW et al. Comparison of the incidence of bladder hyperreflexia in patients with benign prostatic hypertrophy and age-matched female controls. *J Urol* 1985;133:425.
258. Ouslander JG et al. Genitourinary dysfunction in a geriatric outpatient population. *J Am Geriatr Soc* 1986;34:507.

259. Castleden CM et al. Clinical and urodynamic studies in 100 elderly incontinent patients. *BMJ* 1981;282:1103.
260. Overstall PW et al. Experience with an incontinence clinic. *J Am Geriatr Soc* 1980;28:535.
261. Ouslander JG et al. Disorders of micturition in the aging patient. *Adv Intern Med* 1989;34:165.
262. Resnick NM. Voiding dysfunction in the elderly. In: Yalla SV et al., eds. *Principles and Practice of Urodynamics and Neuro-Urology*. New York: Macmillan; 1986:180.
263. Marshall HJ et al. Alpha-adrenoceptor blocking drugs and female urinary incontinence: prevalence and reversibility. *Br J Clin Pharmacol* 1996;42:507.
264. Menefee SA et al. Stress urinary incontinence due to prescription medications: alpha-blockers and angiotensin converting enzyme inhibitors. *Obstet Gynecol* 1998;91:853.
265. Dwyer PL et al. Prazosin: a neglected cause of genuine stress incontinence. *Obstet Gynecol* 1992;79:117.
266. Montejo-Gonzales AL et al. SSRI-induced sexual dysfunction: fluoxetine, paroxetine, sertraline and fluvoxamine in a prospective, multicenter, and descriptive clinical study of 344 patients. *J Sex Marital Ther* 1997;23:176.
267. Crenshaw TL et al. *Sexual Pharmacology: Drugs That Affect Sexual Function*. New York: WW Norton; 1996.
268. Mandel FP et al. Biological effects of various doses of vaginally administered conjugated equine estrogens in postmenopausal women. *J Clin Endocrinol Metab* 1983;57:133.
269. Writing Group for The Women's Health Initiative Investigators. Risks and benefits of estrogen plus progestin in healthy postmenopausal women: principal results from the Women's Health Initiative randomized controlled trial. *JAMA* 2002;288:321.
270. Ouslander JG. Causes, assessment, and treatment of incontinence in the elderly. *Urology* 1990; 36(Suppl):25.
271. Mushkat Y et al. Female urinary stress incontinence—does it have familial prevalence? *Am J Obstet Gynecol* 1996;174:617.
272. Blaivas JG et al. The bulbocavernous reflex in urology: a prospective study of 299 patients. *J Urol* 1981;126:197.
273. Jensen D Jr. Pharmacological studies of the uninhibited neurogenic bladder. *Acta Neurol Scand* 1981;64:175.
274. Brown JH et al. Muscarinic receptor agonists and antagonists. In: Brunton LL et al., eds. *Goodman and Gilman's The Pharmacological Basis of Therapeutics*. New York: McGraw-Hill; 2006:183.
275. Product Information for Oxytrol. Corona, CA 92880: Watson Pharmaceuticals; February 14, 2003.
276. Davila GW et al. A short-term, multicenter, randomized double-blind dose titration study of the efficacy and anticholinergic side effects of transdermal compared to immediate release oral oxybutynin treatment of patients with urge urinary incontinence. *J Urol* 2001;166:140.
277. Wein AJ. Pharmacological treatment of incontinence. *J Am Geriatr Soc* 1990;38:317.
278. Moisey CU et al. The urodynamic and subjective results of the treatment of detrusor instability with oxybutynin chloride. *Br J Urol* 1980;52:472.
279. Hehir M et al. Oxybutynin and the prevention of urinary incontinence in spina bifida. *Eur Urol* 1985;11:254.
280. Gajewski JB et al. Oxybutynin versus propantheline in patients with multiple sclerosis and detrusor hyperreflexia. *Urology* 1986;135:966.
281. Goldenberg MM. An extended-release formulation of oxybutynin chloride for the treatment of overactive urinary bladder. *Clin Ther* 1999;21:634.
282. Gleason DM et al. Evaluation of a new once-daily formulation of oxybutynin for the treatment of urinary urge incontinence. Ditropan XL Study Group. *Urology* 1999;54:420.
283. Millard R et al. Clinical efficacy and safety of tolterodine compared to placebo in detrusor overactivity. *J Urol* 1999;161:1551.
284. Hills JC et al. Tolterodine. *Drugs* 1998;55:813.
285. Guay DR. Tolterodine, a new antimuscarinic drug for treatment of bladder overactivity. *Pharmacotherapy* 1999;19:267.
286. Zinner N et al. for the Trospium Study Group. Trospium chloride improves overactive bladder symptoms: a multicenter phase II trial. *J Urol* 2004;171:2311.
287. Halaska M, et al. Controlled, double-blind, multicentre clincial trial to investigate long-tern tolerability and efficacy of trospium chloride in patients with detrusor instability. *World J. Urol* 2003;20:392.
288. Bentyl package insert. Kansas City, MO: Marion Merrel Dow; April 1994.
289. Chapple CR et al. A polled analysis of three phase III studies to investigate the efficacy, tolerability and safety of darifenacin, a muscarinic M3 selective receptor antagonist, in the treatment of overactive bladder. *BJU Int* 2005;95:993.
290. Cardozo L et al. Randomized, double-blind placebo controlled trial of once daily antimuscarinic agent solifenacin succinate in patients with overactive bladder. *J Urol* 2004;172:1919.
291. Chapple C et al. Randomized, double-blind placebo and tolterodine controlled trial of once daily antimuscarinic agent solifenacin in patients with symptomatic overactive bladder. *BJU Int* 2004;93:303.
292. Levin RM et al. The muscarinic cholinergic binding kinetics of the human urinary bladder. *Neurourol Urodyn* 1982;1:122.
293. Norlen L et al. Beta-adrenoceptor stimulation of the human urinary bladder in vivo. *Acta Pharmacol Toxicol* 1981;43:5.
294. Castleden CM et al. Imipramine—a possible alternative to current therapy for urinary incontinence in the elderly. *J Urol* 1981;125:218.
295. Hollister LE. Current antidepressants. *Ann Rev Pharmacol Toxicol* 1986;26:23.
296. Baldessarini RJ. Drugs and the treatment of psychiatric disorders. In: Gilman AG et al., eds. *Goodman and Gilman's The Pharmacological Basis of Therapeutics*. New York: Pergamon Press; 1990:383.
297. Levin RM et al. Analysis of the anticholinergic and musculotropic effects of desmethylimipramine on the rabbit urinary bladder. *Urol Res* 1983;11:259.
298. Gilja I et al. Conservative treatment of female stress incontinence with imipramine. *J Urol* 1984;132:909.
299. Abernethy DR et al. Imipramine and desipramine disposition in the elderly. *J Pharmacol Exp Ther* 1985;232:183.
300. Ray WA et al. Psychotropic drug use and the risk of hip fracture. *N Engl J Med* 1987;316:363.
301. Wein AJ et al. *Voiding function and dysfunction: a logical and practical approach*. Chicago: Year Book Medical Publishers; 1988:195.
302. Hoffman BB et al. Catecholamines and sympathomimetic drugs. In: Gilman AG et al. eds. *Goodman and Gilman's The Pharmacological Basis of Therapeutics*. New York: Pergamon Press; 1990:187.
303. Gibson A. The influence of endocrine hormones on the autonomic nervous system. *J Auton Pharmacol* 1981;1:331.
304. Batra SC et al. Female urethra: a target for estrogen action. *J Urol* 1983;129:418.
305. Lepor H et al. Randomized double-blind study comparing the efficacy of terazosin versus placebo in women with prostatism-like symptoms. *J Urol* 1995;154:116.
306. Sivkov AV et al. Use of alpha 1-adrenergic blockers in voiding disorders in women [Abstract]. *Urologica* 2002;5(Suppl):52.
307. MRC Working Party on Mild to Moderate Hypertension. Adverse reactions to bendroflumethiazide and propranolol for the treatment of hypertension. *Lancet* 1981;2:539.
308. Bulbitt DJ et al. Drug treatment and quality of life in the elderly. *Clin Geriatr Med* 1990;6:309.
309. Bauer GE et al. Side-effects of antihypertensive treatment: a placebo-controlled study. *Clin Sci Mol Med* 1978;55:341s.
310. Bulpitt CJ et al. Side-effects of hypotensive agents evaluated by self-administered questionnaire. *Am J Cardiol* 1973;3:485.
311. Hogan MJ et al. Antihypertensive therapy and male sexual dysfunction. *Psychosomatics* 1981;21:234.
312. Mallett EC et al. Sexuality in the elderly. *Semin Urol* 1987;5:141.
313. Zarren HS et al. Unilateral gynecomastia and impotence during low dose spironolactone administration in men. *Mil Med* 1975;140:417.
314. Ebringer A et al. The use of clonidine in the treatment of hypertension. *Lancet* 1970;1:524.
315. Laver MC. Sexual behavior patterns in male hypertensives. *Aust NZ J Med* 1974;4:29.
316. Onesti G et al. Clonidine: a new antihypertensive agent. *Am J Cardiol* 1971;28:74.
317. Burnett WG et al. Sexual dysfunction as a complication of propranolol therapy in men. *Cardiovasc Med* 1979;4:811.
318. Buffum J. Pharmacosexology: the effects of drugs on sexual function: a review. *J Psychoactive Drugs* 1982;14:5.
319. Troutman WG. Drug-induced sexual dysfunction. In: Knoben JE, Anderson PO, eds. *Handbook of Clinical Drug Data*. 6th ed. Hamilton, IL: Drug Intelligence Publications; 1988:112.
320. Amery A et al. Double-blind crossover study with a new vasodilator–prazosin—in the treatment of mild hypertension. *Excerpta Medica International Congress Series* 1974;331:100.
321. Van Arsdalen KN et al. Drug induced sexual dysfunction in older men. *Geriatrics* 1984;39:63.
322. Caine M et al. Phenoxybenzamine for benign prostatic obstruction. *Urology* 1981;17:542.
323. Buffum JC. Pharmacosexology update: heroin and sexual function. *J Psychoactive Drugs* 1983;15:317.
324. Beeley L. Drug-induced sexual dysfunction and infertility. *Adverse Drug React Acute Poisoning Rev* 1984;3:23.
325. Longe RL et al. *Physical Assessment: A Guide for Evaluating Drug Therapy*. Vancouver, WA: Applied Therapeutics; 1994.
326. Ferri FF et al. Practical Guide to the Care of the Geriatric Patient. St. Louis: CV Mosby; 1992.

CHAPTER 102

Osteoporosis

Rebecca A. Rottman

OSTEOPOROSIS

The term osteoporosis is derived from the Greek words osteon (bone) and poros (pore).[1] Although osteoporosis has many definitions, the World Health Organization (WHO) defines it as a disease "characterized by low bone mass and microarchitectural deterioration of bone tissue, leading to enhanced bone fragility and a consequent increase in fracture risk."[2] Other definitions have been developed to help clinicians diagnose osteoporosis. For example, a WHO working group defined osteoporosis as "the presence of bone mineral density (BMD) or a T score that is 2.5 standard deviations (SD) or more below the mean peak value in young, healthy adults."[3,4] Osteopenia, a lesser degree of bone loss, is defined as a T score that is between 1 and 2.5 SD below the mean peak value in young, healthy adults. A *Z* score (mean value for BMD in normal subjects of the same age and sex) can aid in the diagnosis of osteoporosis. For example, a *Z* score <−1 at the lumbar spine or proximal femur indicates "a value in the lowest 25% of the reference range, a value at which the risk of fracture is approximately double. A *Z* score <−2 indicates a value in the lowest 2.5% of the reference range, a level associated with a considerably greater increase in the risk of fracture."[4]

Incidence and Fracture Sites

Osteoporosis is a major health problem that affects approximately 10 million people in the United States, with 80% of the affected population being women 50 years of age and older. Another estimated 34 million Americans, 50 years and older, are at increased risk for osteoporosis, according to the National Osteoporosis Foundation.[5] Estimates suggest that by 2010, 52 million Americans will have low bone mass and by 2020 the number may exceed 60 million.[6] The incidence for osteoporosis increases with age; 30% of women 80 years of age or older develop osteoporosis without medical intervention.[7]

Annually, more than 1.5 million osteoporosis-related fractures occur in elderly Americans.[5,8] Osteoporosis-related fracture sites predominantly include the vertebrae, distal radius (Colles' fracture), and hips. Approximately 50% of women age 50 years and older will sustain an osteoporosis-related fracture (i.e., fractures of spine, distal forearm, or hip) in their lifetime.[5] Worldwide disability from hip fracture is projected to exceed 2.5 million people by the year 2025, with a projected 700,000 deaths. Patients who suffer hip fractures have a 12% to 20% higher mortality rate relative to persons of the same sex and similar age without fractures.[9] In addition, hip fractures result in a multitude of complications for the elderly, including prolonged hospitalization, decreased independent living, depression, fear of future falls, and lifelong disability. Vertebral fractures may be painless or result in pain that usually lasts <3 months. The initiating injury may be as minor as a cough or turning over in bed. Vertebral collapse or deformity can result in loss of height, kyphosis (dowager's hump), abdominal protuberance, decreased pulmonary function, and chronic back pain.

The annual direct cost for treating osteoporosis and osteoporosis-related fractures in the United States is estimated at $14 billion per year, compared with $7.5 billion for heart failure and $6.2 billion for asthma. This figure will continue to rise in the next 20 years if prevention and early intervention measures do not reduce the incidence of osteoporosis.[6,10,11] Thus, the impact of osteoporosis on the health care system as the baby-boom generation ages and lifespan increases is potentially staggering.

Physiology

Structurally, bone is either cortical or cancellous (trabecular), with the adult skeleton containing 80% cortical and 20% cancellous bone. Dense cortical bone forms the outer shell of the skeleton, whereas porous cancellous bone forms the interior structures in a honeycombed fashion. The proportions of cortical and cancellous bone vary at different sites in the skeleton, with cortical bone predominating in long bones (~90%) except at their ends, which are predominantly cancellous. This type of bone is also found in the vertebrae and distal forearms. A balance between osteoblast and osteoclast activity results in a continuous remodeling process; osteoclasts resorb bone, whereas osteoblasts help reform bony surfaces and fill bony cavities.

Bone remodeling normally is a continuous process that occurs in discrete skeletal foci called *bone-remodeling units.* This process begins with bone resorption that is initiated by osteoclasts excavating lacuna found on the surface of cancellous bone, or it occurs when cavities are formed in cortical bone (Fig. 102-1). Enzymes produced in this process dissolve bone mineral and proteins. Thereafter, bone formation occurs as osteoblasts gradually refill spaces created during the resorption process. This occurs as collagen fills in bone cavities, which then are calcified.

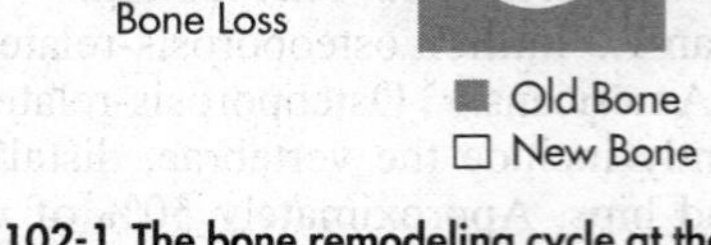

FIGURE 102-1 The bone remodeling cycle at the cellular level. In normal young adults *(top panels)*, the bone removed by the osteoclasts *(left)* is replaced completely by the osteoblasts *(right)*. In high-turnover bone loss *(middle panels)*, such as that which occurs in women soon after menopause, the osteoclasts create a deeper resorption cavity that is not refilled completely. In low-turnover bone loss *(bottom panels)*, such as that which occurs with aging, the osteoclasts create a resorption cavity of normal or decreased depth, but the osteoblasts fail to refill it. (From the *New England Journal of Medicine* 1992;372:621, with permission.)

Calcium and vitamin D are important nutrients required for bone growth. Parathyroid hormone, glucocorticoid hormones, calcitonin, estrogen, and testosterone are all factors involved in bone remodeling.[12] Parathyroid hormone (PTH) and glucocorticoid hormones have been associated with bone resorption, whereas calcitonin, estrogen, and testosterone have been associated with bone formation.[13] The small intestine is the site for the absorption of dietary calcium; the kidneys reabsorb calcium in the tubular system; and the skeletal system serves as a reservoir for calcium. Calcium is primarily regulated by the actions of PTH, vitamin D, and calcitonin. The parathyroid gland releases PTH in response to low serum calcium levels, which in turn facilitates the mobilization of calcium and phosphate from bone and stimulates reabsorption of calcium through the tubular system in the kidneys.[14] Vitamin D aids in intestinal absorption of calcium as well as phosphorous and magnesium. Increases in vitamin D levels decreases PTH levels. Vitamin D also increases bone resorption to prevent symptomatic hypocalcemia.[15] Calcitonin is released in response to high serum calcium levels. Calcitonin decreases intestinal absorption of calcium and phosphorous, inhibits calcium excretion in the kidneys, and prevents bone resorption (Fig. 102-2).[16]

Changes in Bone Mass

Bone mass peaks during the third decade of life. At about 35 years of age, cortical bone gradually begins to decrease 0.3% to 0.5% yearly in both women and men.[17] With menopause, the decline in 17β-estradiol concentrations further accelerates cortical bone loss by 2% to 3% per year that is superimposed on age-related bone loss. This loss gradually decreases over the next 8 to 10 years.[17] This hormone-related, accelerated bone loss can also occur after surgical oophorectomy. Longitudinal data suggest that estrogen may play an important role in the development of osteoporosis in men as well.[18] Serum testosterone concentration has been evaluated in many studies that have failed to connect a strong association between testosterone levels and bone density.[19,20]

Cancellous bone loss begins between the ages of 30 and 35 with yearly decreases in women of 0.6% to 0.8% (linear decrease) or 2.4% (curvilinear decrease).[17,21] Age-related cancellous losses in women appear to begin up to a decade earlier than cortical bone loss. The effect of menopause on cancellous bone loss is controversial; some studies indicate an increased rate of loss, whereas others do not.[21] Thus, early cancellous bone loss in conjunction with postmenopausal decreases in cortical and possibly cancellous bone may lead to increased vertebral and distal forearm fractures, which predominate early after menopause.[17] Men begin to lose bone mass after 30 years of age. Cortical bone in the proximal radius, as well as cortical and trabecular bone in the distal radius, lose content at a rate of approximately 1% annually.[22] Spine and hip density also decline with increasing age.[23,24] Women may lose as much as 50% of cancellous and 30% of cortical bone over their lifetimes, whereas men may lose only 30% and 20%, respectively.[8,25] In addition, women may have an increased risk for osteoporosis because throughout life they have 30% less bone mass than men of a similar age.[26]

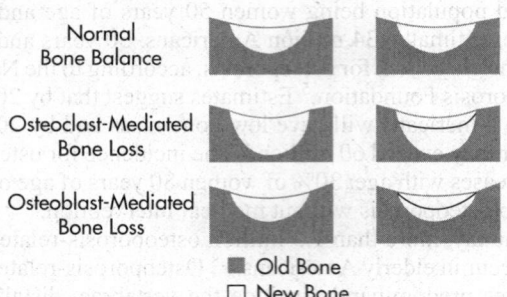

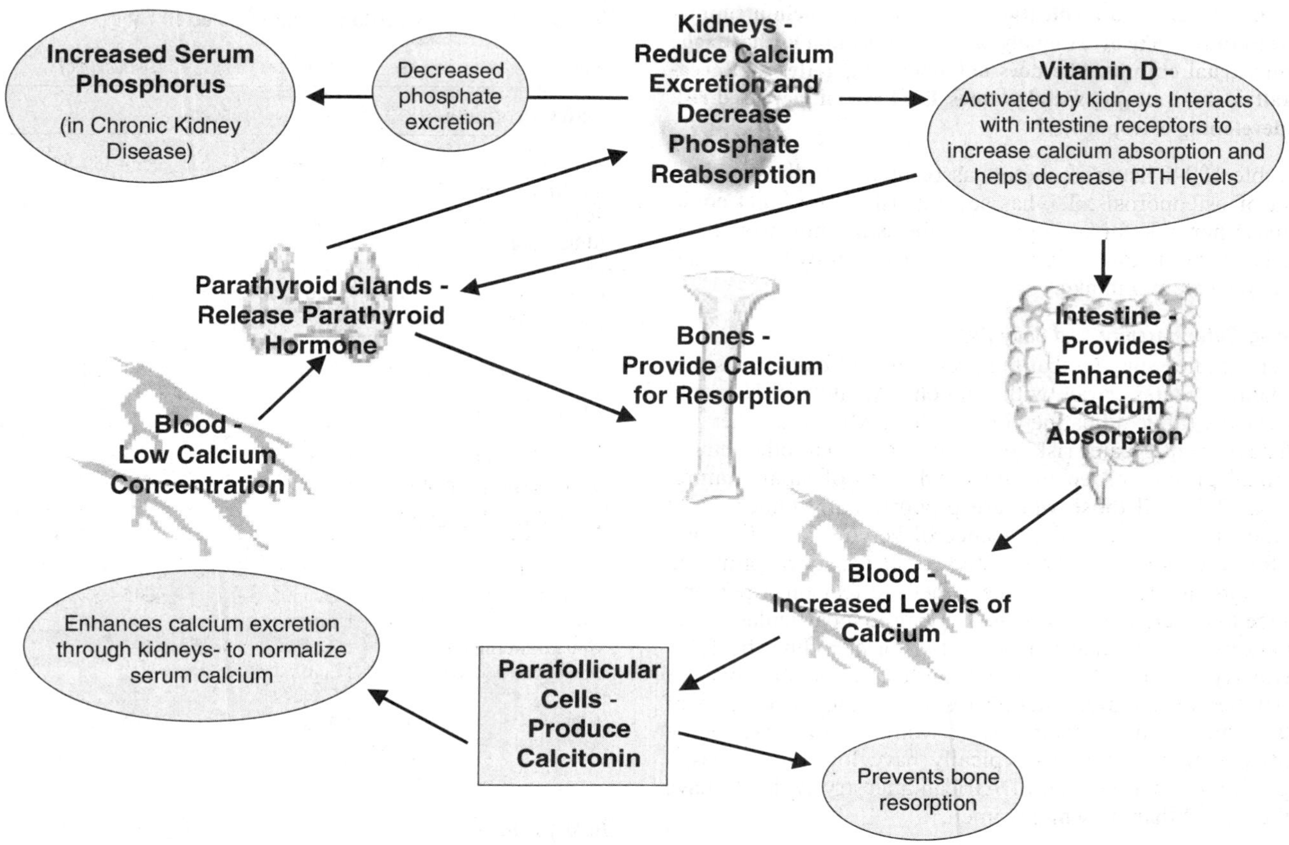

FIGURE 102-2 Pathway for calcium homeostasis with involvement from parathyroid hormone, vitamin D, and calcitonin.

Classification

Osteoporosis can be defined as primary or secondary. Sometimes primary osteoporosis is further classified as type I or II. Type I, *postmenopausal osteoporosis*, is associated with increased cortical and cancellous bone loss resulting from increased bone resorption. It typically occurs in women during the first 3 to 6 years after menopause. Postmenopausal osteoporosis is manifested by vertebral fractures, distal radius fractures, hip fractures, and even an increased tooth loss secondary to osteoporosis of the mandible. Postmenopausal osteoporosis can occur earlier in women who have had an oophorectomy. Type II, *senile osteoporosis*, occurs in both women and men 75 years of age and older with a female:male ratio of 2:1.[21] Cortical and cancellous bone losses are proportional. These persons are at greatest risk for hip, pelvic, and vertebral fractures.

Secondary osteoporosis results from the use of various medications or the presence of particular disease states (Table 102-1). This type of osteoporosis can occur at any age and is equally common in men and women.

Risk Factors

1. T.J., a 28-year-old, thin white woman, is worried about developing osteoporosis. Her 75-year-old maternal grandmother has osteoporosis and recently her postmenopausal mother (age 53) was told that she was at increased risk for osteoporosis. T.J. is 5 ft 2 in, weighs 108 lbs, and is in good health. She jogs and occasionally does aerobic exercise. Her diet typically consists of cereal for breakfast, a sandwich for lunch, and meat with vegetables for dinner. Her only milk consumption consists of 1 cup of skim milk on her cereal. She occasionally has a dairy product for lunch or

Table 102-1 Risk Factors Associated with the Development of Osteoporosis

↑Age Female gender Caucasian or Asian Family history Small stature Low weight	Predisposing medical problems (e.g., chronic liver disease, chronic renal failure, hyperthyroidism, primary hyperparathyroidism, Cushing's syndrome, insulin dependent diabetes, gastrointestinal resection, malabsorption, irritable bowel disease, chronic obstructive pulmonary disease, and acquired immune deficiency syndrome or human immunodeficiency virus)
Early menopause or oophorectomy Sedentary lifestyle ↓Mobility Low calcium intake Excessive alcohol problems Cigarette smoking	Drugs (e.g., corticosteroids, long-term anticonvulsant therapy [e.g., phenytoin or phenobarbital], excessive use of aluminum-containing antacids, long-term high-dose heparin, furosemide, excessive levothyroxine therapy)

dinner. T.J. takes no medications, vitamins, or calcium supplement routinely. She occasionally takes a medication for headache or menstrual cramps. She does not smoke cigarettes and occasionally drinks alcohol socially. Does T.J. have an increased risk for developing osteoporosis?

Table 102-1 lists risk factors associated with the development of osteoporosis. T.J. has several risk factors that could increase her risk for osteoporosis. She is a white woman of small stature and low weight, has a positive family history, and has a low calcium intake.

Gender, Race, Heredity, and Body Build

Recent studies suggest that the prevalence of osteoporosis in the United States varies with ethnicity. White and Hispanic Americans (after adjusting for weight, BMD, and other covariates) are at greater risk for osteoporosis than other ethnic or racial groups, especially those who are of small stature, such as T.J., and those who are proportionally underweight for their height.[27] The significance of heredity as a risk factor for osteoporosis is being studied. It has been proposed that approximately 75% of the genetic effect on a person's chance to develop osteoporosis is owing to a particular allelic variant in the gene that is responsible for encoding the 1,25-dihydroxyvitamin D receptor.[26] Data from a meta-analysis of 16 studies revealed conflicting results on the association of polymorphisms and fracture risk.[28] Women with a first-degree relative with osteoporosis typically have low bone mass.[29] In addition, black women of African ancestry typically have higher BMD than do white women.[27]

Mobility and Physical Activity

Immobility owing to prolonged bedrest (especially in the elderly) has been associated with decreased bone mass. Conversely, weight-bearing exercise (e.g., walking, running, step aerobics, lifting weights) helps prevent bone loss. Exercise throughout life helps maintain skeletal mass and may help reduce bone loss in postmenopausal women. Exercise appears to stimulate osteoblastic activity to help maintain bone mass.[30] Thirty minutes of weight-bearing exercise three times weekly has been associated with improvements in bone density and a reduced hip fracture risk in older women.[31]

Cigarette Smoking and Alcohol Ingestion

Although T.J. does not smoke and only occasionally ingests alcohol, it is important to include questions concerning cigarette and alcohol use when obtaining a medication history from a person at risk for osteoporosis. Women who smoke, especially those who are thin, have an increased risk for fractures compared with nonsmokers.[32] Cigarette smokers may have impaired calcium absorption and lower 17β-estradiol levels, however, the mechanisms are unknown for affects on bone mass.[27]

Excessive alcohol use by both women and men may predispose them to low BMD, but it is unclear whether moderate alcohol consumption has an effect on bone mass. Consuming as few as two alcoholic drinks daily significantly increases the fracture risk.[33] The proposed mechanism may be a direct effect of alcohol on osteoblasts, or it may be secondary to nutritional compromise that could result in impaired calcium and vitamin D intakes with subsequent decreased in bone formation.[34] Alcoholics also may be at risk for increased falls.

Table 102-2 Calcium Content of Selected Foods

Food	Serving Size	Calcium (mg)
Dairy Products		
Milk, dry nonfat	1 cup	350–450
Yogurt, low fat	1 cup	345
Milk, skim	1 cup	300
Milk, whole	1 cup	250–350
Cheese, cheddar	1 oz	211
Cheese, cottage	1 cup	211
Cheese, American	1 oz	195
Cheese, Swiss	1 oz	270
Ice cream or ice milk	1/2 cup	50–150
Fish		
Sardines, in oil	8 med	354
Salmon, canned (pink)	3 oz	167
Fruits and Vegetables		
Calcium fortified juices	1 cup	100–350
Spinach, fresh cooked	1/2 cup	245
Broccoli, cooked	1 cup	100
Collards, turnip greens	1/2 cup	175
Soy beans, cooked	1 cup	131
Tofu	1 oz	75
Kale	1/2 cup	50–150

Dietary Intake

Calcium, in conjunction with vitamin D, is needed to strengthen bones, increase bone mass, and decrease fracture rates. Girls and women such as T.J. need an adequate calcium intake to achieve and help maintain optimal bone mass, but the typical American diet is low in calcium. The National Academy of Sciences published recommendations for calcium intakes based on age. For example, they recommended 1,000 mg/day of elemental calcium for women <51 years of age.[35] The National Institutes of Health (NIH) recommend the same amount of calcium for women in this age group.[36] Calcium is best ingested from the diet (Table 102-2 lists the calcium content of various foods), but if the diet is low in calcium, supplements can be used (Table 102-3; see Questions 2 and 3). A diet high in caffeine, protein, phosphorous and sodium has been associated with an increased risk of fractures by adversely effecting calcium balance.[37] Many studies have, however, found conflicting results. Patients with adequate calcium intake may negate the effects of these dietary risks.[37–42]

Table 102-3 Percentage of Calcium in Various Salts

Salt	% Calcium
Calcium carbonate	40
Tricalcium phosphate (calcium phosphate, tribasic)	39
Calcium chloride	27
Dibasic calcium phosphate dihydrate	23
Calcium citrate	21
Calcium lactate	13
Calcium gluconate	9

Other Potential Risks

DRUGS

Various medications that may be associated with the development of secondary osteoporosis are listed in Table 102-1.

DISEASES

Patients with various diseases may be at higher risk than the general population for secondary osteoporosis (see Table 102-1 for specific diseases). In addition, women who have undergone oophorectomy before menopause have a high risk for developing osteoporosis at a younger age.

Prevention

Premenopausal Women

2. Although T.J. is premenopausal, what recommendations could be made to decrease her future risk of developing osteoporosis?

T.J.'s course of action should be to maximize her peak bone mass and prevent or decrease bone loss. This may be accomplished by ingesting a nutritious diet with adequate calcium and vitamin D intake and developing a lifelong exercise program.

EXERCISE

T.J. should be encouraged to participate regularly in weight-bearing exercises such as jogging, walking, running, biking, tennis, or weight lifting and to continue exercise appropriate for her age throughout life. Weight-bearing exercise is important for the maximization and maintenance of bone. Aerobic training is important in controlling weight, increasing cardiorespiratory endurance, and decreasing the risk for cardiovascular disease (CVD).

Young women such as T.J. should be informed that excessive exercise can cause amenorrhea. Women with exercise-induced amenorrhea have been reported to have decreased bone mineralization and an increased risk for fractures.[43]

VITAMIN D INTAKE

Vitamin D helps regulate calcium by a complex interaction that involves PTH (also see Chapter 32 Chronic Kidney Disease) and by having a direct effect on bone. Studies have shown noted improvement in muscle strength and balance as well as reduced risk of falls with vitamin D supplementation.[27] Adult requirements for vitamin D range from 200 to 600 IU daily (200 IU daily for nonpregnant women ages 19–50 years). The North American Menopause Society (NAMS) recommends vitamin D doses of 700 to 800 IU daily in women at high risk of deficiency.[27] T.J should be able to obtain adequate vitamin D intake from her diet and exposure to sunlight. Other sources of vitamin D include liver and fatty fish. She could also take a multivitamin daily that contains at least vitamin D 200 IU. Studies have found that when vitamin D is used in conjunction with calcium supplementation, bone loss can be reduced; however, the effectiveness of vitamin D alone for fracture prevention is unclear.[27,44] Higher-than-recommended doses could lead to increased risks, including hypercalciuria and hypercalcemia.[27]

CALCIUM INTAKE

T.J.'s diet should be calcium-enriched to ensure that she receives 1,000 mg/day of elemental calcium. Optimally, calcium should be from dietary sources. Because dairy products are the major source of dietary calcium in the United States, T.J. should select low- or non-fat dairy products to decrease her caloric intake and minimize her fat intake when possible. If T.J. were lactose intolerant, she could select dairy products containing lactase. Although nondairy sources may contain lower amounts of calcium, they may be included in a diet plan to increase calcium content, especially when a woman cannot or will not use dairy products (see Table 102-2 for the calcium content of selected foods). The ingestion of foods rich in phytates (i.e., cereal grains, legumes, and nuts) may decrease calcium absorption.

If T.J. cannot meet her daily calcium requirement from dietary sources, she can use a calcium supplement. Table 102-3 lists the percentage of elemental calcium available from selected calcium salts. (See Question 50 for further information on calcium supplements.)

MAGNESIUM

Currently, no evidence exists that magnesium supplementation is needed to prevent osteoporosis. People who might need extra magnesium beyond that found in their diets most likely are elderly women or individuals with gastrointestinal (GI) disease.[27]

ISOFLAVONES

Isoflavones are a class of phytoestrogens found in soybeans, soy products, and red clover. Although some promote their use for the prevention or treatment of osteoporosis, the current data, mostly from small studies of short duration, are insufficient to support the use of isoflavones for this purpose.[27]

SMOKING CESSATION

A woman who smokes should be encouraged to stop because cigarette smoking is associated with lowered BMD and increased fracture risk as well as other health problems.[27]

3. If T.J. needs a calcium supplement, which calcium salt should be recommended?

Calcium carbonate is usually the calcium salt recommended for women such as T.J. because it is reasonably priced and contains the highest percentage of elemental calcium (40%); this allows fewer tablets per day to meet daily calcium requirements. If T.J. needs a calcium supplement, she should be advised to take it in divided doses (e.g., 500–600 mg/dose) to maximize absorption. In addition, calcium should be taken with fluids during or after meals that are low in fiber to increase absorption. Because their absorption may be decreased, medications such as tetracyclines, iron, quinolones, and atenolol should not be taken concomitantly with calcium. T.J. should be informed that the most common adverse effects associated with calcium are constipation, GI irritation, and flatulence. Doses exceeding 2,500 mg/day of elemental calcium can result in hypercalcemia, hypercalciuria, and, possibly, urinary stones. If T.J. or any family member has a history of urinary stones, she should be under medical supervision while taking calcium.

Table 102-4 Techniques for Measuring Bone Mineral Density

Technique	Abbreviation	Measurement Sites
Dual-energy x-ray absorptiometry	DXA	Hip, spine, total body bone mineral density
Peripheral dual-energy x-ray absorptiometry	PDXA	Forearm, fingers, heel
Peripheral quantitative computed tomography	PQTC	Forearm
Quantitative ultrasound	QUS	Heel, shin
Quantitative computed tomography	QCT	Spine
Single-energy x-ray absorptiometry	SXA	Heel

Postmenopausal Women

4. T.J.'s mother, M.J., age 53, also is a woman of small stature and low weight. She occasionally walks in the evenings, but otherwise exercises little. She currently is taking a calcium supplement to maintain her total calcium intake (dietary plus supplementation) of about 1 g/day. She takes no medications except omeprazole (OTC) for her gastroesophageal reflux disease (GERD) and occasional acetaminophen for headaches. M.J. was a cigarette smoker but stopped in her late twenties; she rarely drinks alcohol. She is in good health and has had no gynecologic surgery or major diseases. M.J. does admit to having a strong family history of breast cancer. Her last menstrual period was approximately 6 months ago, but she began experiencing menstrual irregularity 2 years ago. M.J. has been experiencing some menopausal symptoms, such as hot flushes, but states that these are mild and occur only at night. M.J., worried about developing osteoporosis, decided to make an appointment with her gynecologist to discuss preventive measures. A dual-energy x-ray absorptiometry (DXA), formerly DEXA, measurement of her spine was administered, which noted her T score to be a –2 and a Z score of –1. In addition to the DXA, what other information should be obtained to determine whether she is at risk for developing osteoporosis or already has osteoporosis?

A medical history (including a medication history) and physical examination are needed in addition to a risk factor analysis. Other diagnostic tests should be obtained if needed.

From her history and risk factor analysis, it is determined that M.J. shares similar risk factors for osteoporosis with her daughter. In addition, she is early in the postmenopausal phase, has GERD and was a previous smoker. M.J. has no loss of height, does not complain of back pain, and does not have signs of kyphosis (abnormal curvature of the spine in the thoracic region), all of which may be signs of osteoporosis. (Women can lose 1 to 1.5 inches in height as part of the normal aging process, secondary to shrinking of intervertebral disks.[27]) Biochemical markers of bone turnover are not needed for M.J. at this time (i.e., alkaline phosphatase, calcium and phosphorous levels).

The NAMS recommends a BMD measurement in women such as M.J., who are <65 years of age if risk factors for osteoporosis are present (e.g., body weight <127 lbs, fracture [other than skull, facial bone, ankle, finger or toe] after menopause, first-degree relative with a history of a vertebral or hip fracture), and smoking.[27] The National Osteoporosis Foundation (NOF) recommends BMD testing for women <65 years of age when risk factors for osteoporosis are present and for women >65 years of age, in the absence of risk factors for osteoporosis, and postmenopausal women who present with fractures to confirm diagnosis and severity of disease.[5] Medicare has specific guidelines for covering BMD testing and physicians should refer to the most recent guidelines.

Differential absorption of x-rays from two different energies determines the amount of mineral in a given region with a DXA. One x-ray energy source is blocked by the patient with the other x-ray energy source passing completely through the patient, with higher density bone blocking both x-rays. Lower density bone or soft tissue allows x-rays to be transmitted. X-ray energies completely transmitted are sent to a computer which then translates compiled data into an image with density measurements in grams per centimeter squared (g/cm^2), with pencil beam and fan beam DXA machines being the most commonly used.[45] Central DXA of hip or spine remain the preferred measurement for definitive diagnosis.[5]

Although DXA is the gold standard for determining BMD, other methods can be used for screening but should not be used for diagnosis or to follow a patient's response to therapy[27] (Table 102-4). For postmenopausal women who are not receiving medications for osteoporosis prevention, a DXA may be useful no more frequently than every 3 years because it takes approximately 3 to 5 years for a 0.5 change in SD from the mean in either T or *Z* scores to occur.[27] T-score values are supported by both the NOF and NAMS for diagnosis. The Z score can be useful when looking for secondary causes of osteoporosis, with a Z score of <-1.5 suggesting secondary causes for osteoporosis.[5,27,45] In addition, it has been estimated that for every one point decrease in SD from the mean T score, a 10% to 12% change can occur in BMD. The magnitude of this change can be translated into a 1.5-fold change in risk for fractures.[27] As a result, a BMD determination should be obtained no more frequently than every 2 years to assess the effectiveness of pharmacologic interventions for the prevention or treatment of osteoporosis in a postmenopausal woman.[27]

5. What preventive measures would help decrease M.J.'s likelihood of developing osteoporosis?

EXERCISE

Although M.J. goes for walks occasionally, she should begin an aerobic and weight-bearing exercise program appropriate for her age and physical condition because exercise (particularly weight-bearing exercise) in conjunction with appropriate calcium and vitamin D intake is important for maintaining healthy bones. Weight-bearing exercise improves muscular function and agility, whereas aerobic exercise helps improve cardiovascular health (also see Question 2).

VITAMIN D INTAKE

As with T.J., it is important for M.J. to have an adequate vitamin D intake for her diet and from exposure to sunlight.

The recommended daily allowance (RDA) for vitamin D for women between 51 and 70 years of age is 400 IU/day, and those >70 years of age an intake of 700 to 800 IU/day may be needed.[27] This may be achieved from ingesting foods that contain vitamin D (e.g., vitamin D fortified milk, fatty fish) or from ingesting a daily multiple vitamin containing vitamin D. For elderly persons who have limited exposure to sunlight because of minimal outdoor activities or because they live in areas where winters are long, vitamin D supplementation may be needed. Patients with renal or hepatic disease may need supplementation with active vitamin D metabolites, which are available by prescription only. (For further information about vitamin D, see Question 2.)

CALCIUM INTAKE

Because of her postmenopausal status and other risk factors, M.J. should increase her current intake of elemental calcium to at least 1,200 mg/day to prevent bone loss.[35] The NIH Consensus Development Panel on Optimal Calcium Intake recommended that postmenopausal women who do not receive EPT (estrogen-progestin therapy–formerly called hormone replacement therapy or HRT) or ET (estrogen therapy) should have a daily elemental calcium intake of 1,500 mg. Although calcium has antiresorptive activity, its use alone by postmenopausal women is not an alternative to ET, EPT, bisphosphonates, or a selective estrogen receptor modulator (SERM) for osteoporosis prevention. Calcium supplementation, however, helps delay BMD loss in postmenopausal women, and its use reduces the risk of hip fractures by 25% to 70%.[46] (Also see Questions 2 and 3.)

Estrogen-Progestin Therapy

Previously, EPT would have been considered first-line prevention for osteoporosis in a postmenopausal woman such as M.J., who has an intact uterus and is at risk for osteoporosis (Table 102-1) based on her risk factors and T score. Approved indications for use of these products include prevention of postmenopausal osteoporosis; however, not for the treatment of postmenopausal osteoporosis, with the recommendation that the agents are used for the shortest possible time (i.e., duration of menopausal symptoms).[47] Studies have not been conducted to evaluate fracture rate reduction in lower than standard doses of ET or EPT[27] (also see Chapter 48 Gynecologic and Other Disorders of Women). Since the publication of the Heart and Estrogen/Progestin Replacement Study (HERS) I[48] and HERS II[49] and the NIH Women's Health Initiative (WHI),[50] health care providers are less likely to prescribe ET or EPT for the sole purpose of osteoporosis prevention or to continue its use after a woman no longer needs ET or EPT for postmenopausal symptoms such as hot flushes. Table 102-5 lists oral and transdermal estrogens approved for the prevention of osteoporosis.

ESTROGEN EFFECTS ON BMD AND FRACTURE RATE

6. M.J. is considering hormone therapy. What effect does estrogen have on BMD in a postmenopausal woman such as M.J.? Can EPT or ET decrease fracture rates?

The primary effect of estrogen on BMD is related to its antiresorptive activity, which decreases bone loss and lowers fracture rates. Estrogen receptors (ER) are proteins that bind estrogens with high affinity and specificity.[51] Researchers have identified different ER, including α, β, and γ.[52] ER act on the reproductive organs, however, α and β also have a role on cardiovascular organs and bone.[53] Although not fully understood, the interplay between estrogens and their receptors may stimulate osteoblast activity and the secretion of insulinlike growth factor 1 and transforming growth factor-β. In addition, estrogens possibly inhibit interleukin-1 (IL-1), IL-6, and the release of tumor necrosis factor. Both ER-α and ER-β have been isolated from primary osteoblastic cells of neonatal rats, which if it can be translated to humans, shows that both ER may have beneficial effects on BMD.[54] Estrogen may also affect calcium absorption and vitamin D receptors in osteoblasts.

An estimated 10% to 15% of a woman's bone mass is estrogen dependent[55]; therefore, estrogen (oral or transdermal) appears to effectively delay or prevent osteoporosis in postmenopausal women.[27] The addition of a progestin to ET for women with a uterus does not appear to decrease estrogen efficacy as an osteoporosis preventative. More than 50 randomized, placebo-controlled clinical trials have shown that ET or EPT can increase BMD by 4% to 6% in the spine and 2% to 3% in hips.[27] These levels of BMD also have been noted to be maintained after 3 years of therapy.[27]

In the Postmenopausal Estrogen/Progestin Interventions (PEPI) trial, a randomized, placebo-controlled, multicenter 3-year study of 875 postmenopausal women averaging 56 years of age, BMD increased in the spine 3.5% to 5% and in the hips at an average of 1.7% in all groups who received oral conjugated equine estrogens (CEE) 0.625 mg with or without a progestin (MPA or micronized progesterone [MP]).[56]

In observational studies, ET or EPT appears to reduce fracture rates in postmenopausal women. In one meta-analysis, hip fracture risk was reduced by 25% for postmenopausal women who had used ET or EPT.[57] A second meta-analysis found that the use of ET or EPT for at least 1 year significantly reduced nonvertebral fracture risk (relative risk [RR] 0.73, 95%; confidence interval [CI] 0.56 to 0.94). This effect on fracture rate was somewhat reduced in women who began ET or EPT after age 60 years.[58]

The Study of Osteoporotic Fractures, a large prospective cohort study, showed decreased risks for wrist and nonspinal fractures in estrogen users who were >65 years of age and decreased risks in the incidence of hip fractures in those >75.[59] The relative risk for nonspinal fractures in postmenopausal women who were current estrogen users versus those not receiving ET or EPT was 0.66 and 95% CI was 0.24 to 0.64. Vertebral bone mass increases in women with known osteoporosis who receive ET or EPT, which can then decrease fracture rates.[60]

In a randomized, placebo-controlled trial that enrolled 2,763 postmenopausal women (HERS), a different outcome was noted. No reduction in fracture risk was observed, even after 4 years of EPT (CEE 0.625 mg/day and MPA 2.5 mg/day). Women enrolled in HERS had histories of cardiac disease, but many were at low risk for fractures because they did not have osteoporosis. Women were enrolled in HERS to determine whether EPT use would decrease the incidence of CVD whereas fracture risk was a secondary observation.[48]

The National Osteoporosis Risk Assessment Study and the Million Women Study, both large observational studies by design, found that ET or EPT provided significant relative risk reductions in fracture.[61,62] These results were confirmed by the

WHI with both the ET and EPT arms, showing significant risk reductions in hip, vertebral, and total fractures compared with placebo.[50,63]

CONTRAINDICATIONS TO ESTROGEN USE

7. What are contraindications to the use of ET or EPT in a postmenopausal woman?

Contraindications to ET or EPT include pregnancy; active deep vein thrombosis, pulmonary embolism, or a history thereof; active or recent (e.g., within the past year) arterial thromboembolic disease (e.g., stroke, myocardial infarction); undiagnosed abnormal genital bleeding; known, suspected, or a history of breast cancer; known or suspected estrogen-dependent neoplasia; liver dysfunction or disease; or known hypersensitivity to the product or any of its ingredients.[64] In addition, women with a history of asthma, diabetes mellitus, migraine, epilepsy, systemic lupus erythematous, porphyria, and hepatic hemangiomas may have their disease exacerbated by the use of ET or EPT. Thus, women with any of the previously mentioned diseases who receive ET or EPT should be monitored closely by their physicians for potential problems.[64] ET or EPT therapy is associated with risks. Patients on ET or EPT are at increased risk for cancer, including endometrial (if not on EPT), breast (for EPT), and ovarian cancer as well as increased cardiovascular events, thromboembolic disease, stroke, gallbladder disease, and dementia (also see Chapter 48 Gynecologic and Other Disorders of Women). M.J. has a strong family history of breast cancer and starting her on EPT therapy may not be the treatment of choice for her to prevent osteoporosis.

ADVERSE EFFECTS

8. What are the potential adverse effects of estrogens and progestins administered to a postmenopausal woman such as M.J.?

Such a postmenopausal woman should be made aware of estrogen-related adverse effects, such as nausea, vomiting, dizziness, weight gain, breast tenderness, and breast enlargement. She must also be educated about the possible return of uterine bleeding if she begins using ET or EPT. Used alone, estrogens produce dose-dependent uterine bleeding; women who received 0.625 mg/day of CEE had a 1% to 4% incidence.[64] The addition of a progestin cyclically increases the incidence of uterine bleeding, normalizes the bleeding pattern, and reduces breakthrough bleeding. The continuous administration of both hormones decreases the incidence of bleeding, but breakthrough bleeding may continue for 6 months to 1 year until the endometrium becomes atrophic.

Adverse effects associated with progestin use may depend on the type of progestin prescribed, but typically these effects include edema, increased breast size, mastalgia, rash, acne, hirsutism, alopecia, headaches, and psychological effects (e.g., irritability, fatigue, mood swings, depression).[64] Edema and mastalgia may be more commonly noted with MPA or gestodene use. Alopecia, acne, and hirsutism may be more commonly noted with the use of the more androgenic agents, norethindrone and levonorgestrel.

Other Prevention Modalities

Selective Estrogen Receptor Modulators

9. Should a selective estrogen receptor modulator (SERM), such as raloxifene, be considered for the prevention of osteoporosis in M.J.?

RALOXIFENE

Raloxifene (Evista), a SERM, may be an alternate therapeutic choice for M.J. SERM are pharmaceutical agents that are "hormone-related" or "designer estrogens" that have estrogen agonist, antagonist, or both activity in various tissues where estrogen receptors are present. These compounds are also structurally diverse. For example, benzothiophene analogs, such as raloxifene, have agonistic (estrogenic) effects on bone and serum lipid profiles and antagonistic (antiestrogenic) effects on endometrial and breast tissues. Triphenylethylene analogs, such as tamoxifen (Nolvadex), have agonistic effects on bone, serum lipid profiles, and endometrial tissue, and antagonistic effects on breast tissue.

Raloxifene at a dose of 60 mg/day is the only SERM currently approved by the U.S. Food and Drug Administration (FDA) for the prevention and treatment of postmenopausal osteoporosis.[65] SERM are used for various health problems and disease states. For example, tamoxifen is used as an adjuvant for axillary node-negative or node-positive breast cancer in women, for metastatic breast cancer in women and men, and for the prevention of breast cancer in high-risk women. Clomiphene (Clomid) is used for ovulatory dysfunction and toremifene (Fareston) is used to treat metastatic breast cancer in postmenopausal women.

Raloxifene's agonist activity on bone tissue is believed to occur through a reduction in bone resorption and a decreased rate of bone turnover, which then results in increased BMD. The effects appear to be mediated through action as an estrogen agonist at ER in bone. Raloxifene activity may be mediated through transforming growth factor-β3 (TGF-β3) and suppression of cytokinase IL-6.[66]

Data supporting raloxifene's effect on BMD were collected in three clinical osteoporosis prevention trials that were conducted in North America (544 women), Europe (601 women), and internationally (619 women, all of whom had undergone hysterectomy).[65,66] The trials were all randomized, double-blind, placebo-controlled studies that lasted 2 years. Participants were postmenopausal women 45 to 60 years of age. All received calcium supplementation, and women in the treatment groups received raloxifene 60 mg/day; in the international study also had a CEE arm (0.625 mg/daily). The results of these studies showed loss of approximately 1% BMD in the women in the placebo groups. In contrast, those in the raloxifene groups had an increase in BMD of 1.3% to 2.4% in the hips, 1.6% to 2.5% in femoral neck, 1.3% to 2.7% in the trochanter, 1.3% to 2.4% in the intertrochanter, and 1.8% to 2.4% in the lumbar spine. The increase in BMD in the hips of women in the CEE arm of the international study was two times that noted for raloxifene.

The Multiple Outcomes of Raloxifene Evaluation (MORE) trial enrolled 7,705 postmenopausal women 31 to 80 years of age. Of these women, 5,129 were randomized to either a

60 mg/day or 120 mg/day raloxifene group and the remainder were in the placebo group.[67] MORE trial outcomes after 3 years were as follows for BMD: increases in femoral neck BMD were 2.1% (60 mg/day group) and 2.4% (120 mg/day group) compared with placebo, with spinal BMD increases of 2.6% and 2.7% in the raloxifene groups, respectively, compared with placebo. The RR for vertebral fractures was 0.7, 95% CI 0.5 to 0.8 for those in the 60 mg/day group, whereas those in the 120 mg/day group had an RR of 0.5, 95% CI 0.4 to 0.7. This translates into a 38% and 41% reduction in vertebral fracture rate for the 60 mg/day and 120 mg/day groups, respectively.[68] No significant difference in nonvertebral fractures was noted among groups.

Differences in BMD, bone architecture, and bone turnover were determined in a 6-month study in which raloxifene 60 mg/day was compared with CEE 0.625 mg/day in 51 white women ages 55 to 85 years.[69] During this short, randomized, double-blind study, most of the markers of bone resorption or formation were decreased in both groups, but to a greater extent in those receiving CEE. Total body and lumbar spine BMD increased in both groups with a greater increase in women receiving CEE. Hip BMD was similar for both groups. Overall, CEE had a greater effect on BMD, but effects were positive for raloxifene users. It should be remembered that study results were determined after only 6 months and that the number of women enrolled was small.

Sambrook, et al.[70] conducted the EFFECT (EFficacy of FOSAMAX versus EVITSA Comparison Trial), a randomized, double-blind, double dummy multicenter international study including 487 postmenopausal women with low bone density of the spine or hip (T score ≤2) to determine efficacy and tolerability of alendronate and raloxifene. Patients were randomized to either alendronate or raloxifene. After 1 year, BMD increased in both the alendronate and raloxifene groups in the lumbar spine (4.8% vs. 2.2%, respectively) and total hip (2.3% vs. 0.8%, respectively). Tolerability and GI effects were similar in both groups; however, significantly higher reports of vasomotor symptoms came from the raloxifene group.[70]

The CORE Study assessed the effects of raloxifene on breast cancer for an additional 4 years beyond the 4-year MORE trial. A substudy assessed lumbar spine and femoral neck BMD at 7 years, including 386 women (127 placebo, 259 raloxifene) who did not take other bone-active agents from the fourth year of MORE and who were ≥80% compliant with the study medication in CORE. When comparing MORE baseline BMD, after 7 years, raloxifene significantly increased lumbar spine (4.3% from baseline, >2.2% than placebo) and femoral neck (1.9% from baseline, >3% than placebo) BMD, with BMD significantly above MORE baseline at all time-frames observed at both sites with raloxifene.[71]

A paradox exists about how raloxifene can decrease vertebral fractures by up to 41% while increasing BMD by only 2% to 3%, rates that are lower than those noted for ET, EPT, or alendronate. In addition, raloxifene has not been observed to have a positive effect on hip fractures. It has been postulated that the antifracture effect of raloxifene on vertebral fractures occurs secondary to its normalization of the high turnover rate of cancellous bone, which then prevents further disruption of bone microarchitecture.[72,73] This probably occurs through raloxifene binding at estrogen β-receptor sites that are predominant in cancellous bone.[72,73] In addition, a less potent antiresorptive agent, such as raloxifene, may help prevent vertebral fractures but not hip fractures because the threshold for preventing osteoclastic activity in cancellous bone, which is predominant in vertebrae, may be lower than in cortical bone, which predominates in hips. It should also be noted that ER in cortical bone are predominantly α, whereas those in cancellous bone are typically β. Thus, bone type and estrogen receptors are different in the hips compared with vertebrae. For these reasons, it may require a more potent antiresorptive agent to increase BMD in the hips.

Raloxifene might be considered for osteoporosis prevention in a woman such as M.J., even with her strong family history of breast cancer. This latter recommendation is based on results from the MORE trial. A 76% decrease was noted in risk for invasive breast cancer in postmenopausal women with osteoporosis (mean age, 66.5 years) who received raloxifene for 3 years.[74] A total of 7,705 women were assigned to raloxifene groups (60 mg twice daily or 60 mg daily) or a placebo group. Of those enrolled in either raloxifene group (n = 5,129), only 13 cases of breast cancer were reported versus 27 that occurred in the 2,576 women in the placebo group.

M.J would be a candidate for raloxifene for prevention of osteoporosis, because her T score of <2 indicates that she is currently osteopenic.[5,22] M.J. should speak with her physician before stopping raloxifene if her vasomotor symptoms worsen. Studies have shown that discontinuing raloxifene therapy resumes bone loss.[71,75]

Dosing and Pharmacokinetics

If M.J. is to use raloxifene, she should take 60 mg once daily without regard for food.[65] Raloxifene is approximately 60% absorbed after oral ingestion and then undergoes extensive glucuronide conjugation, resulting in a 2% absolute bioavailability. Some circulating raloxifene glucuronide conjugates are converted back to the parent compound.[65] Raloxifene and its monoglucuronide conjugates are highly protein bound. Raloxifene is primarily excreted in feces, with <0.2% excreted unchanged and <6% eliminated in urine as glucuronide conjugates.[65] There appear to be no differences in pharmacokinetics based on age or gender. Raloxifene has a mean half-life of 27.7 hours after a single dose and 32.5 hours after multiple doses.[65]

Contraindications and Potential Drug Interactions

Raloxifene is contraindicated for administration to women who are pregnant or who may become pregnant. It is also contraindicated for women with an active or previous history of venous thromboembolic events.[65] Hypersensitivity to raloxifene or any constituent in Evista tablets is also a contraindication to its use. Patients with hepatic dysfunction may need dosage adjustments, although more information is needed to clarify doses needed.[65] Cholestyramine, when coadministered with raloxifene, may decrease raloxifene absorption by 60% because of its effects on enterohepatic cycling.[65] Women who may be receiving warfarin as well as raloxifene should be monitored closely.[65] This may also be true for some other highly protein-bound medications. It does not appear that M.J. has any contraindication to the use of raloxifene.

Adverse Effects

M.J. should be counseled about adverse effects of raloxifene that might pertain to her if she begins the medication. Adverse effects include an increased risk for venous thromboembolic disease and an increase in hot flushes (25% in postmenopausal raloxifene users versus 18% in those receiving placebo).[65] The greatest risk for thromboembolic events is during the first 4 months of therapy.[65] To decrease the risk of thrombosis associated with immobilization, raloxifene should be discontinued for at least 72 hours before immobilization such as that associated with surgery. M.J. is still experiencing hot flushes which could be exacerbated by raloxifene, so she should be counseled extensively on this potential side effect.

Other Potential Effects of Raloxifene

10. What are other effects of raloxifene?

In addition to antagonist effects on breast tissue, raloxifene is an antagonist in the uterus. Therefore, vaginal bleeding is not likely to occur nor is endometrial hyperplasia and the risk for endometrial cancer.[65,66] A decreased incidence of breast pain, flatulence, and abdominal pain have also been reported in women with an intact uterus who were administered raloxifene versus those receiving continuous EPT.[65]

Raloxifene was thought to have benefits in the prevention of CVD. Most studies that have evaluated the effects of raloxifene on CVD have reported surrogate markers such as lipid serum concentrations rather than cardiovascular outcomes. For example, in the MORE study, postmenopausal women who received raloxifene had significantly fewer reports of hypercholesterolemia.[74] Total cholesterol and low-density lipoprotein cholesterol (LDL-C) concentrations in women who were using raloxifene were reduced significantly compared with those receiving placebo.[74] When compared with EPT, raloxifene showed similar reductions in LDL-C. Only EPT significantly increased high-density lipoprotein cholesterol (HDL-C), but it also elevated triglyceride concentrations.[76] It is currently unknown whether or not these effects translate into a reduction in mortality from CVD.

The RUTH trial was conducted to determine the effects of raloxifene on coronary heart disease (CHD) and breast cancer. The study included 10,101 postmenopausal women with CHD or multiple risk factors for CHD and had a mean follow up of 5.6 years. Raloxifene was found to have no significant effect on the risk of primary coronary events when compared with placebo. Invasive breast cancer risk was reduced with raloxifene versus placebo (absolute risk reduction of 1.2 cases per 1,000 women treated for 1 year). No significant death from any cause or total stroke was found; however, raloxifene was associated with an increased risk of fatal stroke (HR 1.49) and thromboembolism (HR 1.44).[77]

Vogel, et al.[78] conducted the STAR trial to evaluate the relative effects and safety of raloxifene and tamoxifen on the risk of developing invasive breast cancer and other disease outcomes. They conducted a prospective, double-blind, randomized trial in 19,747 postmenopausal women of mean age 58.5 years with an increased 5-year breast cancer risk. No statistically significant difference was noted between tamoxifen and raloxifene (163 vs. 168 cases respectively, RR 1.02) and fewer cases of noninvasive breast cancer in the tamoxifen group (57) versus the raloxifene group (80) with a RR of 1.4. No differences were found in other cancer sites, with the exception of uterine cancer, which was found to be more prevalent in the tamoxifen group (36 cases) versus the raloxifene group (23 cases) with a RR 0.62. No differences were found for ischemic heart disease, stroke, or death, with fewer cases of thromboembolic events and cataracts occurring in the raloxifene group.[78]

Bisphosphonates

ALENDRONATE, RISEDRONATE, AND IBANDRONATE

11. Why should bisphosphonates be considered for the prevention of osteoporosis in a woman such as M.J.?

Another alternative treatment option for M.J. would be a bisphosphonate, such as alendronate sodium (Fosamax), risedronate sodium (Actonel), or the newest agent on the market, ibandronate (Boniva). Alendronate, risedronate, and ibandronate are approved for both the prevention and treatment of osteoporosis in postmenopausal women. Alendronate and risedronate are also approved for osteoporosis in men, glucocorticoid-induced osteoporosis prevention and treatment, and in Paget's disease.[79–81] Alendronate, an aminobisphosphonate, decreases bone resorption, resulting in decreased fracture rates in postmenopausal women who are at risk for osteoporosis. The amino group on alendronate appears to increase selectivity for the antiresorptive surfaces of bone. Alendronate and risedronate have high affinities for bone hydroxyapatite and can be incorporated into bone; in doing this, they can then interfere with osteoclast-mediated bone resorption. Because of their incorporation into bone, bisphosphonates have long half-lives, estimated to be 1 to 10 years. Unlike etidronate (another bisphosphonate), alendronate, risedronate, and ibandronate do not inhibit bone mineralization, which could lead to osteomalacia.[79–81]

Effects on Bone Mineral Density

A study of the efficacy and safety of oral alendronate (5 mg/day) for osteoporosis prevention in early postmenopausal women[82] showed BMD increases in the spine of 2.9% (range 2.3%–3.5%) at 5 years for women receiving alendronate, whereas total body density was increased only 0.3%. In a 2-year prevention study in postmenopausal women <60 years,[83] placebo, 2.5 mg/day alendronate, 5 mg/day alendronate, and EPT were compared. An increased BMD in the spine, total hip, and total body were observed in the alendronate groups versus the placebo group. Results from the 5-mg group were as follows: lumbar spine, 3.5% (range 3.3%–3.7%); hip, 1.9% (range 1.8%–2.0%); and total body, 0.7% (range 0.6%–0.8%). These results were better than for those in the 2.5-mg group but lower than those who received estrogen; BMD for the HRT group was 1% to 2% greater than for the alendronate 5-mg group.

Another study found that women (ages 55–81 years) diagnosed with postmenopausal osteoporosis who were in an alendronate study group (alendronate 5 mg/day for 2 years followed by 10 mg/day for 1 year) had reduced risk for fractures at various anatomic sites compared with those in the placebo group.[84] For new vertebral fractures, the RR was 0.53 (95% CI 0.41–0.68); hip, 0.49 (95% CI 0.23–0.99); and wrist, 0.52 (95% CI 0.31–0.87). The Fracture Intervention Trial (FIT) was a multicenter, placebo-controlled trial that enrolled 2,027 women between the ages of 55 and 81 years who had vertebral fractures and reduced BMD.[85] These women received placebo or alendronate 5 mg/day for 2 years and 10 mg/day during the third year. Relative to the placebo group, BMD increased by 6.2% in the spine and 4.7% in the total hip region after 3 years. Over 3 years, 18.2% of the placebo group and 13.6% of the alendronate group had fractures.

In 2000, Black, et al.[86] combined the data from the previous two studies to give overall information from the FIT. These investigators believed this was appropriate because fracture reduction rates in both studies with the use of alendronate were similar. The pooled information from 3 to 4 years of alendronate versus placebo use resulted in the following fracture risk data: hip RR 0.47 (95% CI 0.26–0.79); radiographic vertebral RR 0.52 (95% CI 0.42–0.66); clinical vertebral RR 0.55 (95% CI 0.36–0.82); and all clinical fractures RR 0.70 (95% CI 0.59–0.82). The investigators concluded from these data that women with osteoporosis (T score <–2.5), with or without previous vertebral fractures who took alendronate, had reduced risk for fractures.

A meta-analysis was used to determine the nonvertebral fracture rate in postmenopausal women with osteoporosis who had been treated for at least 3 years with placebo or alendronate (doses used in the five trials ranged from 1–20 mg/day).[87] The overall results showed a 12.6% incidence of nonvertebral fracture in the placebo groups and a 9.0% incidence in the alendronate groups. This resulted in a RR of 0.71 (95% CI 0.502–0.997) for those receiving alendronate.

Several studies have addressed the effects of risedronate on BMD. In a study of women 40 to 60 years of age (early postmenopausal) who had normal BMD for age, those receiving risedronate 5 mg/day for 2 years had BMD increases of 5.7% in lumbar spine and 5.4% in the hip compared with women taking placebo.[88] In another study, postmenopausal women (mean age 69 years) who were older than those mentioned in the previous study had increases in BMD of 4.3% in the spine and 2.8% in the femoral neck when risedronate use was compared with placebo over 3 years.[89]

Ibandronate has been shown to have beneficial effects on BMD. McClung, et al.[90] evaluated the effects of ibandronate in early postmenopausal women resulting in a significantly increased BMD in the lumbar spine (1.9%) versus placebo (–1.9%) and total hip (1.2%) versus placebo (–0.6%) after 2 years. Follow-up from the Mobile Study revealed that the monthly ibandronate dose of 150 mg significantly improved BMD over the 2.5-mg daily dose in the lumbar spine (6.6% vs. 5%) after 2 years of treatment.[91] Ibandronate is also available as an IV formulation of 3 mg administered every 3 months. One-year results from the Dosing Intravenous Administration (DIVA) study improved BMD in the lumbar spine (4.5% vs. 3.5%) and the total hip (2.1% vs. 1.5%) to a similar if not greater degree than daily oral tablets.[92]

Many studies show the benefits of bisphosphonates in not only the prevention of osteoporosis-related fractures by increasing BMD, but also for the treatment of osteoporosis. Many of these studies have been conducted for 3 years with at least one of 7 years,[93] with a 3-year extension.[94] This latter study extension noted that during years 8 through 10, a total of 247 women receiving either alendronate 5 mg/day or 10 mg/day had similar safety and tolerance profiles as women in placebo groups. They noted that spinal BMD increased by 2.3% for those in the 10 mg/day group and 1.20% for the 5 mg/day group; hip and total body BMD was maintained, if not slightly improved, at levels that were noted at 7 years; and forearm BMD was maintained in the 10 mg/day group but decreased slightly in the 5 mg/day group. Women who took alendronate for 5 years, but thereafter were in a placebo group, maintained their spinal and total body BMD over 5 years. Ten-year cumulative spinal BMD was 13.7% for the 10 mg/day group and 9.8% for the 5 mg/day group. Rates for nonvertebral fractures between years 8 and 10 were 8.1% for the 10 mg/day group, 11.5% for the 5 mg/day group, and 12.0% for the group who had been on alendronate for 5 years and off alendronate for 5 years. In addition, most bisphosphonate studies have been randomized, double-blind, and placebo-controlled with large sample sizes.

No consensus is currently available on how long to continue with bisphosphonate therapy. In the Fracture Intervention Trial Long-term Extension (FLEX) trial, 1,099 of the original FIT trial participants, did not have extremely low T scores (<–3.5) or BMD lower than their FIT baseline levels. Statistically significant bone loss occurred (2%–3% more than those who took alendronate for 10 years) when women were switched to placebo after 5 years of alendronate therapy; however, BMD remained well above FIT baseline. A gradual rise was seen in biochemical markers of bone turnover as well as a slightly higher risk of clinically detected vertebral fractures, suggesting that women at high risk for vertebral fracture or have T scores <–3.5 may benefit from continued bisphosphonate therapy. The FLEX study results suggest that women with good response to bisphosphonate therapy who are not at high risk for fracture may be able to take a "drug holiday" after 5 years of treatment.[95,96]

Contraindications and Precautions

Although no dosage change is recommended for a patient with mild to moderate renal failure, alendronate, risedronate, and ibandronate use are not recommended for patients with significant renal insufficiency (e.g., creatinine clearance <35 mL/minute for alendronate and <30 mL/minute for risedronate and ibandronate). Hypocalcemia, if it exists, should be corrected before beginning therapy. Caution is warranted in patients who have any upper GI problem, such as esophageal disease, dysphasia, duodenitis, or ulcers. Sitting upright after ingesting alendronate is necessary to decrease the possibility of reflux into the esophagus and to decrease esophageal irritation as well as to ensure the absorption of oral bisphosphonates, which have low bioavailability. A patient who cannot sit upright for at least 30 minutes (60 minutes for ibandronate) after ingesting the drug should not use oral bisphosphonates.[79–81] M.J.'s diagnosis of GERD (on omeprazole) may preclude her use of bisphosphonate therapy for prevention of osteoporosis.

Adverse Effects

Common adverse effects associated with the use of bisphosphonates include GI symptoms, such as acid regurgitation, dysphagia, abdominal distention, gastritis, nausea, dyspepsia, flatulence, diarrhea, and constipation. Although rare, esophageal adverse effects, such as esophagitis, esophageal ulcers, and erosions, have occurred and have been followed by esophageal stricture.[79–81] The latter adverse effect is one of the reasons a patient should sit upright for 30 to 60 minutes after ingestion. In addition, musculoskeletal pain, headaches, and rash have been noted. Increasing concern over osteonecrosis of the jaw (ONJ) or "death of tissue" or "dead jaw" can occur if blood loss in bone tissue is temporarily or permanently impaired, resulting the eventual collapse of the bone. Patients taking oral bisphosphonates are at risk for the development of ONJ; however, most patients with ONJ are cancer patients receiving chemotherapy and concurrent IV bisphosphonate therapy. A fewer number of cases have been reported in patients on oral bisphosphonate therapy with active dental disease and recent dental procedures.

Dosing

For prevention of osteoporosis, alendronate and risedronate can be prescribed 5 mg daily or 35 mg once weekly or ibandronate 2.5 mg daily or 150 mg once monthly. It might be more convenient to take the medication once weekly or once monthly, and this might also increase adherence to therapy. Patients should be instructed to take their medication with 6 to 8 ounces of water early in the morning on arising and at least 30 minutes (60 minutes for ibandronate) before ingesting food, beverage, or other medications. Patients should not lie down, but should stay fully upright for at least 30 minutes (60 minutes for ibandronate) after ingesting an oral bisphosphonate to prevent esophageal irritation or ulceration and to ensure appropriate bioavailability. Patients should ingest adequate calcium and vitamin D, but should not take the calcium or vitamin D at the same time as the alendronate. Alendronate is available in a formulation with vitamin D (Fosamax Plus D) and risedronate is available in a formulation with calcium (Actonel with Calcium).[79–81]

Treatment

12. T.J.'s 75-year-old grandmother, M.B., was diagnosed with osteoporosis 5 years ago when she broke her distal forearm. In addition, she has lost 2 inches in height (current height 5 ft and weight 100 lb) and has mild kyphosis. M.B. denies severe back pain but occasionally uses acetaminophen or ibuprofen for mild back pain. A recent bone scan revealed significantly decreased vertebral and forearm bone mass. M.B. had her last menstrual period before her hysterectomy approximately 25 years ago. Her only major medical problem is mild congestive heart failure (CHF) for which she receives hydrochlorothiazide 25 mg daily and enalapril 10 mg daily. In addition, M.B. takes CEE 0.625 mg daily and calcium carbonate 1,200 mg/day in divided doses with meals. Does M.B. have any clinical signs of osteoporosis? What changes, if any, should be made in her treatment plan? What other medications might be considered for the treatment of osteoporosis?

Clinical signs of osteoporosis exhibited by M.B. include a loss of 2 inches in height and the presence of mild kyphosis. She also has mild back pain that may be associated with osteoporosis. (See Question 4 for further information about osteoporosis clinical signs and symptoms.)

A treatment plan for M.B. should be aimed at preventing further bone loss and minimizing falls, which could lead to fractures.

Calcium and Vitamin D Intake

Calcium supplementation can slow or prevent further bone loss. M.B.'s calcium intake, which should be at least 1,200 mg/day of elemental calcium, is adequate according to National Academy of Sciences,[35] but information from the NIH recommends 1,500 mg/day of elemental calcium for women such as M.B. who are age 65 and older.[36] Calcium absorption may be decreased in older people because of lower gastric acid secretion, decreased 1,25-dihydroxyvitamin D_3 serum concentration, and decreased endogenous estrogen serum concentration. To overcome this problem, M.B. should continue taking her calcium in divided doses with meals or use a more soluble calcium product such as calcium citrate. (Questions 2, 3, and 5 further discuss calcium requirements, supplementation, and product selection and the use of vitamin D for postmenopausal women.)

Estrogens

In light of the results from the WHI for both the ET and EPT arms and the previously published HERS, estrogen use is in question, especially if used long term.[48,50] As discussed in Question 6, ET or EPT has positive effects on BMD and fracture rates but does not appear to prevent CHD[50] nor prevent further cardiovascular events in individuals with a history of heart disease.[48] Thus, M.B. and her physician should discuss whether she should continue ET or be switched to another drug for treatment of her osteoporosis.

Exercise and Prevention of Falls

M.B. should continue an exercise routine (particularly a weight-bearing exercise) that is appropriate for her age and physical condition. Exercise helps maintain bone mass, function, and agility. The prevention of falls, which often result in fractures, also should be considered part of M.B.'s therapy.

Fall prevention measures should be adopted in the elderly because nearly 90% of fractures are precipitated by falling.[97] These measures should include intrinsic (e.g., balance and gait problems, visual impairments, impaired cognition), extrinsic (inappropriate footwear, polypharmacy, sedatives, and so forth), and environmental factors (e.g., bad lighting in home, loose rugs, uneven pavement, lack of safety equipment). Fall risks should be evaluated at least annually and should be conducted to determine if underlying factors or medical conditions are associated with the falls.[98] Removal of contributing factors and treating underlying medical conditions with the fewest medications possible can reduce the risk of falling. The Assessing Care of Vulnerable Elders (ACOVE) project to improve patient outcomes suggests documentation and evaluation for falls and osteoporosis and the need for proper workup to improve quality of life and survival.[99]

Thiazides

M.B. currently is receiving hydrochlorothiazide for mild heart failure, but thiazides may also increase calcium retention. Whether this effect has a long-term benefit on calcium balance is debatable. Data from a meta-analysis of 11 studies (none were prospective) established an RR of 0.82 (95% CI 0.73–0.91) for hip fractures and 0.88 (0.77–1.02) for all fractures related to osteoporosis in people taking thiazides.[100] In most of these studies, patients were age 65 years or older. It also appears that longer use of thiazides had a greater effect on the prevention of fractures. Thus, M.B.'s thiazide therapy may have a positive effect on her BMD; however, no randomized clinical trials are available that have evaluated thiazides' effects on BMD. NAMS does not believe that thiazides prevent bone loss or fracture risk, although in the elderly there may be some benefit.[27]

Because M.B. has a history of fractures, she should continue calcium supplementation (possibly increasing it to 1,500 mg/day), hydrochlorothiazide (as long as it is needed for another health problem), and an adequate vitamin D intake. A decision needs to be made about her ET. If it is decided that she should not continue ET, then a decision should be made whether a bisphosphonate or raloxifene might be an alternative. If ET is discontinued, it would most likely be best to taper her off estrogen and not stop it abruptly. No guidelines show to how to taper estrogen, but NAMS recommends one of the following two ways: either skip progressively more days between doses or lower the dose of estrogen every 4 to 6 weeks until the hormone has been successfully tapered.[101]

Selective Estrogen Receptor Modulators

Raloxifene might be considered for M.B. because of her need for osteoporosis treatment and her history of CVD (see Question 10). Raloxifene is FDA approved for the prevention and treatment of postmenopausal osteoporosis. Ettinger, et al.[67] noted that at 3 years, women (ages 31–80) with postmenopausal osteoporosis who received raloxifene (60 mg or 120 mg daily) had increased BMD in the femoral neck (2.1% and 2.4%, respectively) compared with placebo. Subjects also had increased BMD in their spines of 2.6% and 2.7%, respectively, compared with placebo, but they also had an RR of 3.1 (95% CI 1.5–6.2) for venous thromboembolism versus those in the placebo group. In another study that compared raloxifene 60 and 120 mg/day with placebo,[102] increases in BMD were noted in the total hip and ultradistal radius in the 60 mg/day group. Nonsignificant trends over placebo were noted for the lumbar spine, total body, and total hip in the 120 mg/day group. In addition, results showed a lower increase in BMD when compared with estrogen studies. (See Questions 9 and 10 for additional information about raloxifene.)

Another study was undertaken to ascertain whether raloxifene prescribed with alendronate would have an additive effect on biochemical markers for bone remodeling and BMD in postmenopausal women with osteoporosis.[103] Postmenopausal women (N = 331) who were 75 years of age or younger were divided into four groups: placebo; raloxifene 60 mg/day only; alendronate 10 mg/day only; or raloxifene plus alendronate (combination group) at 30 study sites worldwide. Markers of bone turnover (serum osteocalcin, bone-specific alkaline phosphatase, and urinary N- and C-telopeptide) were measured, as was BMD at baseline, at 6 months, and then 12 months later. In the final time period, markers of bone turnover were decreased in all groups except the placebo group. These markers were reduced 1.6-fold in the alendronate-only group compared with the raloxifene-only group. No differences were noted in marker reduction at 12 months between the alendronate-only and the combination groups, but lumbar spine BMD increased by 2.1%, 4.3%, and 5.3% from baseline for raloxifene-only, alendronate-only, and combination therapy, respectively. The increase in femoral neck BMD in the combination group was 3.7% above baseline compared with the alendronate-only (2.7%) and raloxifene-only (1.7%) groups. Total hip BMD and total body BMD were not determined. Overall, combination therapy was better at increasing BMD at some sites than either raloxifene or alendronate alone. Thus, combination therapy could be considered for individuals who do not respond to either therapy alone. In addition, markers of bone turnover and BMD appear to respond better to alendronate alone than to raloxifene alone. The study did not address fracture rates.

Bisphosphonates

ALENDRONATE, RISEDRONATE, AND IBANDRONATE

A bisphosphonate, such as alendronate, risedronate, or ibandronate, can be an alternative to ET if another benefit of HRT (e.g., genitourinary) is not needed or can be provided by another medication.

In addition to the alendronate, risedronate, and ibandronate clinical studies described in Question 11, the following studies address the use of alendronate, risedronate, and ibandronate in the treatment of postmenopausal osteoporosis. In 1995, Liberman, et al.[104] performed a multicenter, double-blind, placebo-controlled study in which 994 postmenopausal women, ages 45 to 80 years with osteoporosis were enrolled. Alendronate 5 or 10 mg or placebo was administered daily for 3 years followed by 20 mg daily for 2 years, and then 5 mg/day for 1 year. All study participants received calcium 500 mg/day. Increases in BMD of 8.8 ± 0.4% were noted in lumbar spine, 5.9 ± 0.5% in the femoral neck, and 7.8 ± 0.6% at the trochanter in the alendronate 10 mg daily group. Vertebral fractures occurred in 6.2% of those receiving placebo and in 3.2% of those receiving alendronate (48% reduction in fracture rate). In another study, increases in lumbar spine BMD of 0.65%, 3.5%, and 5.7% were noted in elderly women who received 1, 2.5, or 5 mg of alendronate daily over 2 years with calcium supplements versus those receiving placebo.[105] A meta-analysis that compared the results of five studies performed in postmenopausal women between the ages of 42 and 85 years documented that alendronate, when given in doses of 10 mg/day for 3 years, increased BMD over placebo administration as follows: spine 8.8%, femoral neck 5.9%, and trochanter 7.8%.[79]

In two clinical trials,[89,106] the use of risedronate 5 mg daily for 3 years reduced vertebral fractures in postmenopausal women with osteoporosis by 41% and 49%, respectively. The incidence of nonvertebral fractures was reduced by 39% over the same time period.[89] McClung, et al.[107] studied two groups of women (5,445 women ages 70–79 with confirmed osteoporosis and 3,886 women age 80 years or older who had risk factors for osteoporosis or low BMD at the femoral neck) to determine whether risedronate could decrease the risk for hip fractures. All women were randomly assigned to receive risedronate 2.5 mg/day, 5 mg/day, or placebo for 3 years. In the osteoporosis group (i.e., women 70–79 years of age), the overall incidence of hip fracture in the risedronate groups was 1.9% with a rate of 3.2% among those in the placebo group (RR 0.6, 9% CI 0.4–0.9). Among the women age 80 years and older, the incidence of hip fractures was 4.2% among risedronate users and 5.1% in those in the placebo group. Thus, risedronate significantly reduced the risk of hip fracture in women diagnosed with osteoporosis but not in the women over age 80 who had risk factors for osteoporosis and low BMD but not osteoporosis.

A study to investigate the use of alendronate 70 mg once weekly for the treatment of osteoporosis showed that its effects on BMD in the lumbar spine and total hip were similar to that produced by alendronate 10 mg daily after 1 year.[108] The study addressed convenience of therapy while making sure that efficacy was not diminished. Alendronate is approved for the treatment of postmenopausal osteoporosis in doses of 10 mg daily or 70 mg once weekly. Risedronate is approved for the treatment of osteoporosis in doses of 5 mg daily or 35 mg once weekly. Alendronate and risedronate are discussed in detail in Question 11. Risedronate has been shown to be effective and well tolerated in postmenopausal women with osteoporosis after 7 years of treatment.[109]

In a study looking at older women, mean age 69 years, oral ibandronate significantly increased BMD in the spine and femoral neck when compared with placebo after 3 years of treatment.[110] Daily oral ibandronate therapy has been associated with a decrease in morphometric vertebral fracture by over 52% over 3 years; however, no significant effect on decreasing nonvertebral fractures has been shown.[110] Current studies do not show that ibandronate decreases nonvertebral fractures and, with significant data supporting use of alendronate and risedronate, careful consideration should be taken for ibandronate use in patients at high risk.

Combination therapy of ET and bisphonates has not been evaluated specifically for the treatment of osteoporosis. M.B. has been diagnosed with osteoporosis despite receiving ET. Further disease progression in M.B. may be prevented by switching to a bisphosphonate, because bisphosphonates have shown to have a greater effect on BMD then does raloxifene.

ZOLEDRONIC ACID

Zoledronic acid (Reclast) is the first IV bisphosphonate FDA approved for the treatment of postmenopausal osteoporosis. Zoledronic acid is approved as a single 5-mg infusion given once yearly over no <15 minutes through a separate vented infusion line.[111]

In a randomized, double-blind, placebo-controlled trial, zoledronic acid was administered for 1 year to 351 postmenopausal women who had low BMD.[112] The study population was divided into five treatment groups and a placebo group. Doses of zoledronic acid 0.25 mg, 0.5 mg, 1 mg, or placebo were administered at 3-month intervals, whereas 4 mg of the drug was administered as a single dose or as two doses of 2 mg at 6-month intervals. Increases in BMD were as follows: spine BMD for treatment patients ranged from 4.3% to 5.1% above placebo; femoral neck BMD was 3.1% to 3.5% greater than placebo. When looking at nonvertebral BMD, results were not as good as those noted for vertebral BMD. In the distal radius, BMD was only slightly greater for the treatment groups than for the placebo group at 1 year (range 0.8%–1.6% compared with placebo, which decreased about 0.8%). Differences between treatment groups and the placebo group in terms of total body BMD were 0.9% to 1.3% higher for the treatment groups (significant for all except the 0.5 mg every-3-month group). No vertebral fractures were noted during the study period. Two nonvertebral fractures were noted in the group receiving four doses of 1 mg and one fracture was noted in each of the other groups, except the group receiving four doses of 0.25 mg of zoledronic acid. Dropout rates were similar for treatment and placebo groups. Because the duration of the study did not extend beyond 1 year, data from longer term studies are needed.

Black, et al.,[113] in their report on the Health Outcomes and Reduced Incidence with Zoledronic Acid Once Yearly (HORIZON) Pivotal Fracture Trial, conducted as double-blind, placebo-controlled trial including 7,765 women, of which 3,889 patients were randomized to receive a single 15-minute infusion of 5 mg zoledronic acid and 3,876 patients were randomized to placebo. Patients received doses at baseline, and at 12 and 24 months and were followed until 36 months. Zoledronic acid decreased the risk of vertebral fractures by 70% (RR 0.3; 95% CI 0.24–0.38). Hip fractures were reduced by 41% (RR 0.59; 95% CI 0.42–0.83). BMD significantly increased in the lumbar spine by 6.71% (95% CI 5.69–7.74), total hip 6.02% (95% CI 5.77–6.28) and femoral neck 5.06% (95% CI 4.76–5.36).[113]

Adverse event reported have been similar to that of oral bisphosphonates, with decreased incidence of GI adverse events. Acute phase reactions including fevers, flulike symptoms, headache, and arthralgias primarily occur within the first 3 days following the infusion and the incidence decreases with subsequent doses. Increased incidence of atrial fibrillation was noted to be greater than placebo in clinical trials. ONJ has been reported once during clinical trials. Patients with creatinine clearance <30 mL/minute should not receive zoledronic acid.[111]

ETIDRONATE

Etidronate (Didronel), another bisphosphonate available in the United States, inhibits bone resorption mediated by osteoclasts. It is not FDA approved for the treatment (nor for the prevention) of postmenopausal osteoporosis, but it is approved for the treatment of Paget's disease in the United States and for the treatment of osteoporosis in Canada. Studies have shown that, although etidronate has positive effects on fracture prevention, concern exists about the development of osteomalacia. To overcome this potential problem, alternating regimens of etidronate 400 mg/day for 2 weeks followed by a 13-week (3 months) course of calcium and vitamin D have been used.[114] The cyclical regimen was chosen owing to daily high dose use possibly interacting with bone mineralization.[115]

A meta-analysis was used to evaluate 13 clinical trials of etidronate administration in an intermittent, cyclical fashion as therapy for postmenopausal osteoporosis (administered daily for 2 weeks, every 3 months).[116] Results showed that, relative to controls, with 1 to 2 years of etidronate therapy at 400 mg/day, BMD was increased by 4.1% in the lumbar spine and 2.3% in the femoral neck. It was suggested that use of etidronate could reduce vertebral fractures by 37%, but not the risk for nonvertebral fractures.

Calcitonin

Calcitonin acts directly on osteoclasts to inhibit bone resorption primarily from vertebral and femoral sites. Both the injection and the intranasal spray are approved for the treatment, but not the prevention, of postmenopausal osteoporosis for those who have been diagnosed for at least 5 years.[117] It also is effective in reducing corticosteroid-induced osteoporosis.

Calcitonin may increase BMD in the lumbar spine (cancellous bone) by 1% to 3%, but its use has little effect on cortical bone. In one study, new fractures were reduced. This resulted in an RR of 0.23 (CI 0.7–0.77).[118] Various intermittent regimens of calcitonin are being used investigationally to see whether they can help prevent a decrease in effectiveness that occurs after 1 to 2 years. Calcitonin is used in some patients because of its analgesic effects on bone pain, especially for those who suffer from vertebral compression fractures.[27] Although the mechanism of pain relief is unclear, a small study of 56 osteoporotic women who sustained atraumatic vertebral fractures reported decreased pain scores and analgesic use in the calcitonin group versus placebo.[119]

A large, randomized, double-blind, placebo-controlled study (Prevent Recurrence of Osteoporotic Fracture [PROOF]) explored the effectiveness of intranasal calcitonin at a dose of 200 IU/day for 5 years versus other doses.[120] Calcitonin decreased the risk of developing new vertebral fractures in women with osteoporosis by 33%. Doses of 100 and 400 IU/day administrated in this same trial did not result in positive results. No significant effect on hip BMD occurred at any dose.[101] When compared with alendronate therapy, intranasal calcitonin 200 IU daily was inferior to alendronate 10 mg daily, only increasing BMD in the lumbar spine (1.18% vs. 5.16%), trochanter (0.47% vs. 4.73%), and the femoral neck (0.58% vs. 2.78%) after 12 months of therapy. Fracture data were not evaluated in this study.[121]

When used intranasally, calcitonin (Miacalcin) is dosed at 200 IU daily in alternating nares; given subcutaneously or intramuscularly (Calcimar) the dose is 100 IU/day.[117] A patient using calcitonin should have adequate intake of calcium and vitamin D.

Adverse effects associated with intranasal calcitonin include nasal symptoms, such as rhinitis and epistaxis. Other adverse effects include arthralgia, headache, and back pain. When calcitonin therapy is administered by injection, adverse effects, such as flushing, nausea, and vomiting, as well as local irritation at the injection site (10%) can occur.[117,122] Flushing typically occurs on the hands and face and is noted in approximately 2% to 5% of patients. Nausea and vomiting occur in about 10%. These latter reactions most commonly occur when therapy is initiated and usually subside with time. Injectable calcitonin should be refrigerated when not in use. The intranasal preparation should be refrigerated until it is opened for use; thereafter, it is stable for 30 days at room temperature.[122]

Other Therapies

13. What other agents (both FDA approved and investigational) are possible alternative or additive therapies for the treatment of postmenopausal osteoporosis?

PARATHYROID HORMONE

Parathyroid hormone works differently from other medications discussed thus far because it stimulates new bone formation and activates remodeling, which then results in increased BMD and connectivity in trabecular bone more than cortical bone. This can be accomplished by administration of recombinant human PTH in women with postmenopausal osteoporosis.[27,123,124] Despite an incomplete understanding of the mechanisms for PTH, it is known that PTH stimulates the interaction of preosteoblasts to osteoblasts within the first month of treatment, peaking 6 to 9 months after daily administration.[125] For example, in one study of 1,637 postmenopausal women who had previously sustained vertebral fractures, therapy (19 months of PTH 20 or 40 mcg daily subcutaneously) resulted in a reduction of new vertebral fractures by 65% and 69%, respectively, and a reduction of new nonvertebral fractures by 53% and 54%, respectively.[126]

The FDA has approved the PTH derivative teriparatide (Forteo) for use by women and men with osteoporosis who do not adequately respond to other therapies. In addition, those diagnosed as having severe osteoporosis and who are at an increased risk for fracture may be considered for therapy. Teriparatide 20 mcg should be given once daily subcutaneously in the thigh or abdomen. Initial administration should be given when the patient can sit or lie down. Teriparatide pens are stable for up to 28 days, including the first injection from the pen. The remaining medication after 28 days should be discarded and teriparatide should never be shared. Teriparatide should be stored under refrigeration 2°C to 8°C (36°F–46°F) and injected immediately on removal from refrigeration. After use, the pen should be recapped and protected from light. Safety and efficacy with teriparatide have not been studied beyond 2 years and therapy is not recommended after 2 years.[127]

Because osteosarcomas were noted in study animals that received teriparatide, the FDA has required a black box warning for this medication even though no osteosarcomas have been observed in patients.[127] This information may also be found in a medication guide that should be given to all patients receiving teriparatide. Children, adolescents, and individuals with Paget's disease are not candidates for teriparatide because those with growing bones are at increased risk for developing osteosarcomas. Studies have confirmed that BMD gains noted in the hip and spine decline after discontinuation with an approximate 2% loss in spinal BMD and 17% loss in trabecular BMD.[125,128] Women who were randomized to the alendronate group of the Black, et al. study,[128] had a further increase of approximately 6% during the first year of therapy with alendronate. Similar effects were noted when estrogen therapy was started after discontinuing PTH,[129] suggesting that antiresorptive therapy should be started after discontinuation of PTH to preserve BMD.

Adverse effects that have been noted to be associated with teriparatide use include hypercalcemia, leg cramps, nausea, and dizziness. Orthostatic hypotension may occur within 4 hours of administration and spontaneously resolves after a few minutes to hours for the first several doses. Patients should immediately sit or lie down if symptoms occur.[127]

Glucocorticoid-Induced Osteoporosis

14. T.J.'s father, D.J, age 56, was diagnosed with rheumatoid arthritis (RA) 10 years ago. The RA has progressed over the past 2 years, with increased swelling and tenderness in his hands and feet. D.J. made an appointment with his physician who noted that D.J.'s laboratory finding and imaging were suggestive of further progression of his RA. D.J. has been maintained on methotrexate, sulfasalazine, and hydroxychloroquine for the past 5 years. D.J. is not interested in starting injectable therapy at this time and would like to try an alternative treatment that will help alleviate his pain quickly. D.J.'s physician would like to have BMD testing performed on D.J. before initiating prednisone 10 mg daily. D.J. is curious about why he will need a DXA test. What should D.J.'s physician tell him?

Prednisone is classified as a glucocorticoid steroid. Glucocorticoids have several possible mechanisms that contribute to bone loss resulting in osteoporosis. Glucocorticoids have been linked to decreases in serum estrogen and testosterone and increases in bone urine calcium excretion and decreased calcium absorption, which are proposed to increase bone resorption. Glucocorticoids have direct action on bone cells, decrease serum testosterone, and decrease muscle, which results in decreased bone formation. Both the increase in bone resorption and decrease in bone formation lead to decreased bone volume, resulting in a more rapid bone loss than other medications that have been associated with bone loss.[130,131] Glucocorticoids are not thought to affect bone-resorbing activity of mature osteoclasts, because they do not have functioning glucocorticoid receptors.[132] Decreases in BMD can be seen as soon as 3 to 6 months after glucocorticoid initiation; however, fracture risk appears to be contributed to by glucocorticoid duration and dose, but is independent of BMD.[133,134] After discontinuation of glucocorticoid therapy, BMD begins to increase.[135]

15. Are any medications available to prevent osteoporosis in D.J.?

Bisphosphonates

Alendronate and risedronate are FDA approved for the prevention and treatment of glucocorticoid-induced osteoporosis. They are thought to prevent glucocorticoid-induced osteoclast apoptosis, however, this theory has been challenged suggesting that glucocorticoids may overcome the proapoptotic effects of bisphosphonates. Another thought is that bisphosphonates may prolong the life of osteoblasts.[136,137]

Saag, et al.[138] looked at alendronate 5- and 10-mg doses versus placebo and found that BMD in the lumbar spine increased in both alendronate groups and BMD declined in the placebo group 2.1%, 2.9% and −0.4%, respectively, over 48 weeks. Total body, trochanter, and femoral neck bone mass also increased in the alendronate groups. Vertebral fractures were lower in the alendronate groups versus placebo (2.3 vs. 3.7%),[138] with benefits of alendronate seen after 2 years.[139] Risedronate is also effective in the prevention and treatment of glucocorticoid-induced osteoporosis. Reid, et al.[140] conducted a 1-year study with risedronate versus placebo in patients taking >7.5 mg of prednisone daily for 6 or more months. They found increases in both lumbar spine and femoral neck (2.7% and 1.8%, respectively), with no change in BMD in patients taking placebo.[140] A study with IV pamidronate 30 mg every 3 months with oral calcium versus calcium alone also had promising results in patients taking glucocorticoids long-term. Spine and hip BMD increased in the pamidronate–calcium group (2.3% and 2.6%, respectively) and decreased in the calcium alone group (−4.6% and −2.2%, respectively).[141]

Calcitonin

Calcitonin has been studied for the prevention of glucocorticoid-induced osteoporosis as well. Luengo, et al.[142] conducted a 2-year study in patients with asthma who had become glucocorticoid dependent. Patients were randomized to calcitonin nasal spray plus calcium or calcium alone. BMD increase was seen in the calcitonin–calcium group (2.7%) in year 1 versus a decrease in BMD seen in the calcium alone group (−2.8%). BMD preservation was also noted after the second year of the study.[142]

Other Therapies

Researchers have conducted small studies to evaluate the prevention of glucocorticoid-induced osteoporosis. Thiazide diuretics with salt restrictions, estrogen and testosterone replacement, as well as PTH are agents undergoing investigation.

16. What recommendations should D.J.'s physician inform him of to prevent osteoporosis?

The American College of Rheumatology (ACR) recommends preventative therapy in patients taking prednisone 5 mg daily or higher (including therapeutic equivalents) for more than 3 months. The ACR recommends the following:

- Calcium 1,500 mg daily
- Vitamin D 800 IU daily
- Bisphosphonate therapy
- Replacement of gonadal steroids in men (if deficient)
- Exercise program (appropriate for individual patient)
- BMD screen if >3 months of glucocorticoid therapy will be needed
- Smoking cessation

Calcitonin can be considered for patients who have contraindications to bisphosphonates. ACR recommends 24-hour urine collections for all patients because glucocorticoids can cause hypercalciuria. The recommendation of a thiazide diuretic plus salt restriction may be implemented if significant hypercalciuria is present.[143]

D.J. does not currently have any contraindications to bisphosphonate therapy. Alendronate 70 mg weekly or risedronate 35 mg weekly plus adequate calcium (1,500 mg daily) and vitamin D (800 IU daily) in divided doses could be used to prevent glucocorticoid-induced osteoporosis if he is to take prednisone 10 mg daily for an extended period. D.J should be counseled on the proper administration and adverse effects of bisphosphonates (see Questions 11 and 12). D.J. should be encouraged to incorporate 30 minutes of weight-bearing exercise into his daily routine.

Osteoporosis in Men

17. D.J presents to his physician 1 year later and finds himself in good health. D.J. is concerned about the development of osteoporosis in his wife's father. J.B., age 77, has become more frail and is falling occasionally. His wife, M.J., is osteopenic and his wife's mother, M.B., has osteoporosis. D.J. knows that osteoporosis occurs often in women, but was not aware that osteoporosis (excluding drug-induced) can occur in men. Should D.J. be concerned about osteoporosis in J.B.?

Osteoporosis is less common in men than in women; however, about 1.5 million men in the United States have osteoporosis with another 3.5 million at risk.[144] Projections suggest that 17% of men who reach 90 years of age will develop osteoporosis.[145] Although reasons are still unknown, mortality rates after hip fracture are higher in men than in women, with patient having a previous distal radius fracture correlating with a high absolute risk for hip fractures in men.[146]

18. D.J. knows that BMD loss in both his wife and her mother has been attributed to a decrease in hormones. Is hormone loss the same cause of osteoporosis in men?

Bone loss for men may begin in their 30s with an estimated 1% loss of BMD occurring at the distal radius, with spinal content decreasing more quickly.[22,23] Many risk factors contribute to osteoporosis in men (Table 102-1), however, androgen and estrogen production are the primary hormonal contributors to the development of osteoporosis in this population.

Androgens and Estrogens

Androgen production, more specifically serum testosterone concentrations, is known to decrease with age. These decreased concentrations are thought to decrease bone formation and increase resorption. Testosterone has been linked to decreases in BMD versus dihydrotestosterone.[147] Despite testosterone's importance for skeletal health in men, research is now suggesting that estrogen may play a more important role in skeletal biology.[148] Khosla, et al.[149] found two genes required for estrogen effects; estrogen receptor α and aromatase. ER-α are found on osteoblasts, osteoclasts, and stem cells in bone. Aromatase is present in osteoblasts and stem cells in bone.[150] The absence of these genes results in an inability to convert androgen into estrogen.[151,152] Replacement of estrogen in aromatase deficiency showed significant increases in bone mass and markers of bone turnover normalized.[152] Further research is still needed to delineate the role of estrogen in hypogonadal osteoporosis.

19. Should J.B. be given supplementation for hypogonadism if his testosterone levels are low?

Hypogonadism may be a major contributor of bone loss in men with low serum estradiol being the main contributor.[18] It would be appropriate for J.B.'s physician to order serum testosterone levels. Snyder et al.[153] found that replacing testosterone (then converted to estrogen), increased bone density by 5.9% when pretreatment serum testosterone levels were below 200 ng/dL (normal 300–1,000 ng/dL).

20. How is osteoporosis diagnosed in men?

The WHO criteria were established for diagnosing postmenopausal women with osteoporosis.[2] To date, no specific diagnostic criteria have been established for men. Currently, diagnosis of osteoporosis in men can be made when a T score is <-2.5 until further definitions of osteoporosis are established by the National Osteoporosis Foundation and the International Osteoporosis Foundation.

Investigational Agents

In the next few years, new agents should be approved for the prevention and treatment of diseases such as osteoporosis that affect postmenopausal women; an example of these new agents is the SERM bazedoxifene (Viviant).

In a randomized, double-blind, placebo-controlled trial, zoledronic acid was administered for 1 year to 351 postmenopausal women who had low BMD.[112] The study population was divided into five treatment groups and a placebo group. Doses of zoledronic acid 0.25 mg, 0.5 mg, 1 mg, or placebo were administered at 3-month intervals, whereas 4 mg of the drug was administered as a single dose or as two doses of 2 mg at 6-month intervals. Increases in BMD were as follows: spine BMD for treatment patients ranged from 4.3% to 5.1% above placebo; femoral neck BMD was 3.1% to 3.5% greater than placebo. When looking at nonvertebral BMD, results were not as good as those noted for vertebral BMD. In the distal radius, BMD was only slightly greater for the treatment groups than for the placebo group at 1 year (range 0.8%–1.6% compared with placebo, which decreased about 0.8%). Differences between treatment groups and the placebo group in terms of total body BMD were 0.9% to 1.3% higher for the treatment groups (significant for all except the 0.5 mg every-3-month group). No vertebral fractures were noted during the study period. Two nonvertebral fractures were noted in the group who received four doses of 1 mg and one fracture was noted in each of the other groups except the group who received four doses of 0.25 mg of zoledronic acid. Dropout rates were similar for treatment and placebo groups. Because the duration of the study did not extend beyond 1 year, data from longer term studies are needed.

STRONTIUM RANELATE

Strontium ranelate has antiresorptive and mild anabolic effects. The exact mechanism of action remains unknown. Strontium has been shown to decrease the risk of spine and nonspine fractures (35%–49%), as well as increase BMD in the spine and femoral neck (14% and 8%, respectively). Studies have been conducted for up to 3 years. Nausea and vomiting have been associated with oral dissolved strontium, which abated after 3 months of therapy.[154,155]

DENOSUMAB

Denosumab is a human monoclonal antibody that targets the receptor activator of nuclear factor κB ligand (RANKL), which has been shown to be a necessary part of bone-resorbing osteoclasts. Initial studies show statistically significant increases in BMD when compared with both placebo and alendronate. Denosumab, being a monoclonal antibody, does function with the immune system, increasing the potential infectious complication.[156]

STATINS

When it was discovered that bisphosphonates might suppress osteoclastic activity by inhibiting a step in the cholesterol synthesis pathway, speculation followed to whether agents, such as hydroxymethylglutaryl-coenzyme A (HMG CoA)-reductase inhibitors (i.e., statins) might display similar effects. In laboratory studies, statins inhibit osteoclastic-related bone resorption. It is unknown whether lipid-reducing doses of statins, which are used clinically, can have an effect on bone. Study results thus far have not presented consistent results and prospective clinical trials are needed.[157,158]

REFERENCES

1. Health Evidence Network (HEN). What evidence is there for prevention and screening of osteoporosis. 2006; http://www.euro.who.int/HEN/Synthesis/osteoporosis/20060504_1.
2. World Health Organization. Assessment of Fracture Risk and Its Application to Screening for Postmenopausal Osteoporosis: report of a WHO Study Group. Geneva, Switzerland: World Health Organization; 1994:2. Technical Report Series 843.
3. Kanis JA et al. The diagnosis of osteoporosis. *J Bone Miner Res* 1994;9:1137.
4. Eastell R. Treatment of postmenopausal osteoporosis. *N Engl J Med* 1998:338;736.
5. National Osteoporosis Foundation 2007. www.nof.org/osteoporosis/diseasefacts.htm.
6. National Osteoporosis Foundation. 8 Common Myths About Osteoporosis. 2002. www.nof.org.

7. Prestwood KM et al. Osteoporosis: up-to-date strategies for prevention and treatment. *Geriatrics* 1997;52:92.
8. Riggs BL et al. The prevention and treatment of osteoporosis. *N Engl J Med* 1992;327:620.
9. Cummings SR et al. Epidemiology of osteoporosis and osteoporotic fractures. *Epidemiol Rev* 1985;7:178.
10. Gold DT et al., eds. *Working with Patients to Prevent, Treat and Manage Osteoporosis: A Current Guide for the Health Professions.* 3rd ed. Durham, NC: Center for the Study of Aging and Human Development, Duke University Medical Center; 2001.
11. Majumdar SR et al. Persistence, reproducibility and cost effectiveness of an intervention to improve the quality of osteoporosis care after a fracture of the wrist: results of a controlled trial. *Osteoporosis Int* 2007;18:261.
12. The North American Menopause Society (NAMS). The role of calcium in peri- and postmenopausal women. 2006 position statement. *Menopause* 2006; 13:862.
13. Seeman E et al. Differential effects of endocrine dysfunction on the axial and the appendicular skeleton. *J Clin Invest* 1982;69:1302.
14. Brown EM. PTH secretion in vivo and in vitro. Regulation by calcium and other secretagogues. *Miner Electrolyte Metab* 1982;8:130.
15. Reichel H et al. The role of vitamin D endocrine system in health and disease. *N Engl J Med* 1989;320:980.
16. Austin LA et al. Calcitonin: physiology and pathophysiology. *N Engl J Med* 1981;304:269.
17. Riggs BL et al. Involutional osteoporosis. *N Engl J Med* 1986;314:1676.
18. Khosla S et al. Relationship of serum sex steroid levels to longitudinal changes in bone density in young versus elderly men. *J Clin Endocrinol Metab* 2001;86:3555.
19. Center JR et al. Hormonal and biochemical parameters on the determination of osteoporosis in elderly men. *J Clin Endocrinol Metab* 1999;84:3626.
20. Amin S et al. Association of hypogonadism and estradiol level with bone mineral density in elderly men from the Framingham Study. *Ann Intern Med* 2000;133:951.
21. Willhite L. Osteoporosis in women: prevention and treatment. *JAPhA* 1998;38:614.
22. Orwoll ES et al. The rate of bone mineral loss in normal men and the effects of calcium and cholecalciferol supplementation. *Ann Intern Med* 1990;112:29.
23. Meier DE et al. Marked disparity between trabecular and cortical bone loss with age in healthy men. Measurement by vertebral computed tomography and radial photon absorptiometry. *Ann Intern Med* 1984;101:605.
24. Jones G et al. Progressive loss of bone in the femoral neck in elderly people: longitudinal findings from the Dubbo Osteoporosis Epidemiology Study. *BMJ* 1994;309:691.
25. Gallagher JC. Pathophysiology of osteoporosis. *Semin Nephrol* 1992;12:109.
26. Morrison NA et al. Prediction of bone density from vitamin D receptor alleles. *Nature* 1994;367:284.
27. The North American Menopause Society (NAMS). Management of Postmenopausal Osteoporosis: 2006 position statement of the North American Menopause Society. *Menopause,* 2006;13:340.
28. Cooper GS et al. Are vitamin D receptor polymorphisms associated with bone mineral density? A meta-analysis. *J Bone Miner Res* 1996;11:1841.
29. Kanis JA et al. A meta-analysis of previous fracture and fracture risk. *Bone* 2004;35:375.
30. Gutin B et al. Can vigorous exercise play a role in osteoporosis prevention? A review. *Osteoporos Int* 1992;2:55.
31. Feskanick D et al. Walking and leisure-time activity and risk of hip fracture in postmenopausal women. *JAMA* 2002;288:2300.
32. Baron JA et al. Cigarette smoking, alcohol consumption, and risk for hip fracture in women. *Arch Intern Med* 2001;161:983.
33. Kanis JA et al. Alcohol intake as a risk factor for fracture. *Osteoporos Int* 2005;16:737.
34. Moniz C. Alcohol and bone. *Br Med Bull* 1994; 50:67.
35. Institute of Medicine, National Research Council. Summary statement on calcium and related nutrients. 1997:S1. Available from http://www.nas.edu/new.
36. NIH Consensus Development Panel on Optimal Calcium Intake. Optimal calcium intake. *JAMA* 1994;272:1942.
37. NIH Consensus Development Panel on Osteoporosis Prevention, Diagnosis and Therapy. Osteoporosis prevention, diagnosis and therapy. *JAMA* 2001;285:785.
38. Cummings SR et al. Risk Factors for hip fracture in white women. *N Engl J Med* 1995;332:767.
39. Barrett-Conner E et al. Coffee-associated osteoporosis offset by daily milk consumption. The Rancho Bernardo Study. *JAMA* 1994;271:280.
40. Tucker KL et al. Colas, but not other carbonated beverages, are associated with low bone mineral density in older women: The Framingham Osteoporosis Study. *Am J Clin Nutr* 2006;84:936.
41. Wengreen HJ et al. Dietary protein intake and risk of osteoporotic hip fracture in elderly residents of Utah. *J Bone Miner Res* 2004;19:537.
42. Kerstetter JE et al. Changes in bone turnover in young women consuming different levels of dietary protein. *J Clin Endocrinol Metab* 1999;84:1052.
43. Cummings DC. Exercise induced amenorrhea, low bone density and estrogen replacement therapy. *Arch Intern Med* 1996;156:2193.
44. The Cochrane Collaborative Group in Vitamin D and Vitamin D analogues for preventing fractures associated with involutional and post-menopausal osteoporosis. 2007(2), www.thecochranelibrary.com.
45. Trent J et al. Bone mineral density testing: an update. *Federal Practitioner* 2006;23:42.
46. Cummings RG et al. Calcium for prevention of osteoporotic fractures in postmenopausal women. *J Bone Miner Res* 1997;12:1321.
47. Kusiak V. FDA approves prescribing information for postmenopausal hormone therapies. Wyeth Pharmaceuticals: Philadelphia; January 6, 2003 (letter to health care professionals).
48. Grady D et al. Heart and estrogen/progestin replacement study (HERS): design, methods and baseline characteristics. *Control Clin Trials* 1998; 19:314.
49. Grady D et al. Cardiovascular disease outcomes during 6.8 years of hormone therapy: heart and estrogen/progestin replacement study follow-up (HERS II). *JAMA* 2002;288:49.
50. Cauley JA et al. For the Women's Health Initiative Investigators. Effects of estrogen plus progestin on risk of fracture and bone mineral density: The Women's Health Initiative Randomized Trial. *JAMA* 2003;290L1729.
51. McEwan IJ. Sex, drugs, and gene expression: signaling by members of the nuclear receptor superfamily. *Essays Biochem* 2004;40:1.
52. Gao M et al. Expression of estrogen receptor-related receptor isoforms and clinical significance in endometrial adenocarcinoma. *Int J Gynecol Cancer* 2006;16:827.
53. Deroo BJ et al. Estrogen receptors and human disease. *J Clin Invest* 2006;111:561.
54. Kuiper GGJM et al. The estrogen receptor beta subtype: a novel mediator of estrogen action in neuroendocrine systems. *Front Neuroendocrinol* 1998;19:253.
55. Ettinger B et al. The waning effect of postmenopausal estrogen therapy on osteoporosis. *N Engl J Med* 1993;329:1192.
56. The Writing Group for the PEPI. Effects of hormone therapy on bone mineral density: results from the Postmenopausal Estrogen/Progestin Interventions (PEPI) Trial. *JAMA* 1996;276:1389.
57. Grady D et al. Hormone therapy to prevent disease and prolong life in postmenopausal women. *Ann Intern Med* 1992;117:1016.
58. Torgerson DJ et al. Hormone replacement therapy and prevention of nonvertebral fractures: a meta-analysis of randomized trials. *JAMA* 2001; 285:2891.
59. Cauley JA et al. Estrogen replacement therapy and fractures in older women: Study of Osteoporotic Fracture Research Group. *Ann Intern Med* 1995;122:9.
60. Lufkin EG et al. Treatment of postmenopausal osteoporosis with transdermal estrogen. *Ann Intern Med* 1992;117:1.
61. Sirus ES et al. Identification and fracture outcomes of undiagnosed low bone mineral density in postmenopausal women: results from the National Osteoporosis Risk Assessment. *JAMA* 2001;286:2815.
62. Banks E, et al. For the Million Women Study Collaborators. Fracture incidence in relation to the pattern of use of hormone therapy in postmenopausal women. *JAMA* 2004;291:2212.
63. Anderson GL et al. For the Women's Health Initiative Steering Committee. Effects of conjugated equine estrogen in postmenopausal women with hysterectomy: the Women's Health Initiative randomized controlled trial. *JAMA* 2004;291:1701.
64. PremproTM and Premphase-package insert. Wyeth Pharmaceuticals: Philadelphia; May 23, 2003.
65. Evista package insert. Eli Lilly and Company. Indianapolis; 1997 (revised 2007).
66. Delmas PD et al. Effects of raloxifene on bone mineral density, serum cholesterol concentrations, and uterine endometrium in postmenopausal women. *N Engl J Med* 1997;337:1641.
67. Ettinger B et al. Reduction of vertebral fracture risk in postmenopausal women with osteoporosis treated with raloxifene: results from a 3-year randomized clinical trial. *JAMA* 1999;282:637.
68. Sarkar S et al. Relationships between bone mineral density and incident of vertebral fracture risk with raloxifene therapy. *J Bone Miner Res* 2002;17:1.
69. Prestwood KM et al. A comparison of the effects of raloxifene and estrogen on bone in postmenopausal women. *J Clin Endocrinol Metab.* 2000;85:2197.
70. Sambrook PN et al. Alendronate produces greater effects than raloxifene on bone density and bone turnover in postmenopausal women with low bone density: results of the EFFECT (EFficacy of FOSAMAX vs. EVITSA Comparison Trial) International. *J Intern Med* 2004:255:503.
71. Siris ES et al. Skeletal effects of Raloxifene after 8 years: results from the Continuing Outcomes Relevant to Evista (CORE) study. *J Bone Miner Res* 2005;20:1514.
72. Riggs L et al. Selective estrogen-receptor modulators-mechanisms of action and application to clinical practice. *N Engl J Med* 2003;348:618.
73. Riggs BL et al. Bone turnover matters: the raloxifene treatment paradox of dramatic decreases in vertebral fractures without commensurate increases in bone density. *J Bone Miner Res.* 2002;17:11.
74. Cummings SR et al. The effect of raloxifene on risk of breast cancer in postmenopausal women: results from the MORE Randomized Trial. *JAMA* 1999;281:2189.
75. Nale SJ et al. Effect of 1 year discontinuation of raloxifene or estrogen therapy on bone mineral density after 5 years of treatment in healthy postmenopausal women. *Bone* 2003;30:599.
76. Walsh BW et al. Effects of raloxifene on serum lipids and coagulation factors in healthy postmenopausal women. *JAMA* 1998;279:1445.
77. Barnett-Conner E et al. Effects of raloxifene on cardiovascular events and breast cancer in postmenopausal women. *N Engl J Med* 2006;355:125.
78. Vogel VG et al. Effects of tamoxifen versus raloxifene on the risk of developing invasive breast cancer and other disease outcomes: the NSABP Study of Tamoxifen and Raloxifene (STAR) P-2 trial. *JAMA* 2006;295:2727.
79. Fosamax Package Insert. Merck and Co. Inc. Whitehouse Station, NJ; 2006 (revised).
80. Actonel Package Insert. Proctor and Gamble Pharmaceuticals, Inc. Cincinnati, OH; 2007 (revised).

81. Ibandronate Package Insert. Roche Pharmaceuticals. Nutley, NJ; 2006.
82. Weiss et al. Five-year efficacy and safety of oral alendronate for prevention of osteoporosis in early postmenopausal women [Abstract]. *J Bone Min Res* 1997;12 (Suppl 1):165.
83. Hosking MD et al. Prevention of bone loss with alendronate in postmenopausal women under 60 years of age. *N Engl J Med* 1998;338:485.
84. Black DM et al. Randomised trial of effect of alendronate on risk of fracture in women with existing vertebral fractures. *Lancet* 1996;348:1535.
85. Cummings S et al. Effect of alendronate on risk of fracture in women with low bone density but without vertebral fractures: results from the Fracture Intervention Trial. *JAMA* 1998;280:2077.
86. Black DM et al. Fracture risk reduction with alendronate in women with osteoporosis: the fracture intervention trial. *J Clin Endocrinol Metab* 2000;85:4118.
87. Karpf DB et al. Prevention of nonvertebral fractures by alendronate: a meta-analysis. *JAMA* 1997;277:1159.
88. Mortensen L et al. Risedronate increases bone mass in an early postmenopausal population: two years of treatment plus one year of follow-up. *J Clin Endocrinol Metab* 1998;83:396.
89. Harris ST et al. Effects of risedronate treatment on vertebral and nonvertebral fractures in women with postmenopausal osteoporosis: a randomized controlled trial. *JAMA* 1999;282:1344.
90. McClung MR et al. For the Oral Ibandronate Study Group. Oral daily ibandronate prevents bone loss in early postmenopausal women without osteoporosis. *J Bone Miner Res* 2004;19:120.
91. Reginster JY et al. Efficacy and tolerability of once-monthly oral ibandronate in postmenopausal osteoporosis: 2 year results from the MOBILE study. *Ann Rheum Dis* 2006;65:654.
92. Delmas PD et al. Intravenous ibandronate injection in postmenopausal women with osteoporosis: one-year results from the dosing intravenous administration (DIVA) study. *Arthritis Rheum* 2006;54:1838.
93. Tonino RP et al. Skeletal benefits of alendronate: 7-year treatment of postmenopausal osteoporotic women. *J Clin Endocrinol Metab* 2000;85:3109.
94. Bone HG et al. Ten year's experience with alendronate for osteoporosis in postmenopausal women. *N Engl J Med* 2004;350:1189.
95. Black DM et al. Effects of continuing or stopping alendronate after 5 years of treatment: the Fracture Intervention Trial Long-Term Extension (FLEX): a randomized trial. *JAMA* 2006;296:2927.
96. Colon-Eneric CS. Ten vs. five years of bisphosphonate treatment for postmenopausal osteoporosis: enough of a good thing. *JAMA* 2006;296(24):2968.
97. Cummings SR et al. Epidemiology and outcomes of osteoporotic fractures. *Lancet* 2002;359:1761.
98. Woolf AD et al. Preventing fractures in elderly people. *BMJ* 2003;327:89.
99. Higashi T et al. Quality of care is associated with survival in vulnerable older patients. *Ann Intern Med* 2005;143:274.
100. Jones G et al. Thiazide diuretics and fractures: can meta-analysis help? *J Bone Miner Res* 1995;10:106.
101. The North American Menopause Society. Amended report from the NAMS Advisory Panel on Postmenopausal Hormone Therapy. *Menopause* 2003;12:10.
102. Lufkin EG et al. Treatment of established postmenopausal osteoporosis with raloxifene: a randomized trial. *J Bone Miner Res* 1998;13:1747.
103. Johnell O et al. Additive effects of raloxifene and alendronate on bone density and biochemical markers of bone remodeling in postmenopausal women with osteoporosis. *J Clin Endocrinol Metab* 2002;87:985.
104. Liberman UA et al. Effect of oral alendronate on bone mineral density and the incidence of fractures in postmenopausal osteoporosis. *N Engl J Med* 1995;333:1437.
105. Bone HG et al. Dose-response relationships for alendronate in osteoporotic elderly women. *J Clin Endocrinol Metab* 1997;82:265.
106. Reginster J et al. Randomized trial of the effects of risedronate on vertebral fractures in women with established postmenopausal osteoporosis. Vertebral Efficacy with Risedronate Therapy (VERT) Study Group. *Osteoporos Int* 2000;11:83.
107. McClung MR et al. Effect of risedronate on the risk of hip fracture in elderly women. *N Engl J Med* 2001;344:333.
108. Schnitzer T et al. Therapeutic equivalence of alendronate 70 mg once weekly and alendronate 10 mg daily in the treatment of osteoporosis. *Aging Clin Exp Res* 2000;12:1.
109. Mellstrom DD et al. Seven years of treatment with risedronate in women with postmenopausal osteoporosis. *Calcif Tissue Int* 2004;75:462.
110. Chestnut CH III et al. Effects of oral ibandronate administered daily or intermittently on fracture risk in postmenopausal osteoporosis. *J Bone Miner Res* 2004;19:1241.
111. Reclast package insert. Novartis Pharmaceuticals Corporation. East Hanover, NJ; 2007.
112. Reid IR et al. Intravenous zoledronic acid in postmenopausal women with low bone mineral density. *N Engl J Med* 2002;346:653.
113. Black DM et al. Once-yearly zoledronic acid for the treatment of postmenopausal osteoporosis. *N Engl J Med* 2007;356:1809.
114. Storm T et al. Five years of clinical experience with intermittent cyclical etidronate for postmenopausal osteoporosis. *J Rheumatol* 1996;23:1560.
115. Hodsman A et al. Use of bisphosphonates in the treatment of osteoporosis: prevention and management of osteoporosis: consensus statements from the scientific advisory board of the Osteoporosis Society of Canada. *Can Med Assoc J* 1996;155(Suppl):S945.
116. Cranney A et al. A meta-analysis of etidronate for the treatment of postmenopausal osteoporosis. Osteoporosis Research Advisory Group. *Osteoporos Int* 2001;12:140.
117. Miacalcin Package Insert. Novartis Pharmaceuticals Corp., East Hanover, NJ; 2006 (revised).
118. Silverman SL. Calcitonin. *Am J Med Sci* 1997;313:13.
119. Lyritis GP et al. Analgesic effect of salmon calcitonin in osteoporotic vertebral fractures: a double blind, placebo-controlled clinical study. *Calcif Tissue Int* 1991;49:369.
120. Chesnut CH III et al. A randomized trial of nasal spray salmon calcitonin in postmenopausal women with established osteoporosis: the Prevent Recurrence of Osteoporotic Fractures Study. PROOF study group. *Am J Med* 2000;109:267.
121. Downs RW et al. Comparison of alendronate and intranasal calcitonin for treatment of osteoporosis in postmenopausal women. *J Clin Endocrinol Metab* 2000;85:1783.
122. Miacalcin Injection Package Insert. Novartis Pharmaceuticals. East Hanover, NJ; 2000 (revised).
123. Jerome CP et al. Treatment with human parathyroid hormone (1–34) for 18 months increases cancellous bone volume and improves trabecular architecture in ovariectomized cynomolgus monkeys (Macaca faseicandaris). *Bone* 2001;28:150.
124. Rosen CJ. The cellular and clinical parameters of anabolic therapy for osteoporosis. *Crit Rev Eukeryot Gene Expr* 2003;13:25.
125. Black DM et al. The effects of parathyroid hormone and alendronate alone or in combination in postmenopausal osteoporosis. *N Engl J Med* 2003;349:1207.
126. Neer RM et al. Effect of parathyroid hormone (1–34) on fractures and bone mineral density in postmenopausal women with osteoporosis. *N Engl J Med* 2001;344:1434.
127. Forteo Package Insert. Eli Lilly Company. Indianapolis, IN; 2004 (revised).
128. Black DM, et al. One year of alendronate after one year of parathyroid hormone (1–84) for osteoporosis. *N Engl J Med* 2005;353:555.
129. Lane NE et al. Bone mass continues to increase at the hip after parathyroid hormone treatment is discontinued in glucocorticoid-induced osteoporosis: results of a randomized controlled clinical trial. *J Bone Min Res* 2000;15:944.
130. Libanati CR et al. Prevention and treatment of glucocorticoid-induced osteoporosis. A pathogenic perspective. *Chest* 1992;102:1426.
131. Reid IR et al. Determinants of vertebral mineral density in patients receiving long-term glucocorticoid therapy. *Ann Intern Med* 1990;150:2545.
132. Zelissen PM et al. Effect of glucocorticoid replacement therapy on bone mineral density in patients with Addison's disease. *Ann Int Med* 1994;120:207.
133. Kanis JA et al. A meta-analysis of prior corticosteroids and risk of fracture risk. *J Bone Miner Res* 2004;19:893.
134. Van Staa TP et al. The epidemiology of corticosteroid-induced osteoporosis: a meta-analysis. *Osteoporosis Int* 2002;13:777.
135. Pocock NA et al. Recovery from steroid-induced osteoporosis. *Ann Intern Med* 1987;107:319.
136. Plotkin LI et al. Prevention of osteocyte and osteoblast apoptosis by bisphosphonate and calcitonin. *J Clin Invest* 1999;104:1363.
137. Weinstein RS et al. Promotion of osteoclast survival and antagonism of bisphosphonate-induced osteoclast apoptosis by glucocorticoids. *J Clin Invest* 2002;109:1041.
138. Saag KG et al. Alendronate for the prevention and treatment of glucocorticoid-induced osteoporosis. *N Engl J Med* 1998;339:292.
139. Adachi JD et al. Two-year effects of alendronate on bone mineral density and vertebral fracture in patients receiving glucocorticoids: a randomized, double-blind, placebo-controlled extension trial. *Arthritis Rheum* 2001;44:202.
140. Reid DM et al. Efficacy and safety of daily risedronate in the treatment of corticosteroid-induced osteoporosis in men and women: a randomized trial. European Corticosteroid-Induced Osteoporosis Treatment Study. *J Bone Miner Res* 2000;15:1006.
141. Bousten Y et al. Primary prevention of glucocorticoid-induced osteoporosis with intravenous pamidronate and calcium: a prospective controlled 1-year study comparing a single infusion, an infusion given every 3 months, and calcium. *J Bone Miner Res* 2001;16:104.
142. Luengo M et al. Prevention of further bone mass loss by nasal calcitonin in patients on long term glucocorticoid therapy for asthma: a two year follow-up study. *Thorax* 1994;49:1099.
143. Recommendations for the prevention and treatment of glucocorticoid-induced osteoporosis: 2001 update. American College of Rheumatology Ad Hoc Committee on Glucocorticoid-Induced Osteoporosis. *Arthritis* 2001;44:1496.
144. Sidoligui NA et al. Osteoporosis in older men: discovering when and how to treat it. *Geriatrics* 1999;54:20.
145. Melton LJ III et al. How many women have osteoporosis. *J Bone Miner Res* 1992;7:1005.
146. Haentjens P et al. Evidence from data searches and lifetable analyses for gender-related differences in absolute risk of hip fracture after Colles' or spine fracture: Colles' fracture as an early and sensitive marker of skeletal fragility in white men. *J Bone Miner Res* 2004;19:1993.
147. Matzkin H et al. Prolonged treatment with finasteride (a 5 alpha-reductase inhibitor) does not affect bone density and metabolism. *Clin Endocrin (Oxf)* 1992;37:432.
148. Orwoll ES. Men, bone and estrogen: unresolved issues. *Osteoporosis Int* 2003;14:93.
149. Khosla S et al. Estrogen and the male skeleton. *J Clin Endocrinol Metab* 2002;87:1443.
150. Marcus R et al. *Osteoporosis.* 2nd ed. San Diego: Academic Press; 2001.
151. Smith EP et al. Estrogen resistance caused by a

mutation in the estrogen receptor in a man. *N Engl J Med* 1994;331:1056.
152. Bilezikian JP et al. Increased bone mass as a result of estrogen therapy in a man with aromatase deficiency. *N Engl J Med* 1998;339:599.
153. Snyder PJ. Effect of testosterone treatment on bone mineral density in men over 65 years of age. *J Clin Endocrinol Metab* 1999;84:1966.
154. Meunier PJ et al. The effects of strontium ranelate on the risk of vertebral fracture in women with postmenopausal osteoporosis. *N Engl J Med* 2004;350:459.
155. Reginster JY et al. Strontium ranelate reduces the risk of nonvertebral fractures in postmenopausal women with osteoporosis: treatment of peripheral osteoporosis (TROPOS) study. *J Clin Endocrinol Metab* 2005;90:2816.
156. McClung MR et al. Denosumab in postmenopausal women with low bone mineral density. *N Engl J Med* 2006;354:821.
157. LaCroix AZ et al. Statin use, clinical fracture and bone density in postmenopausal women: results from the Women's Health Initiative Observational Study. *Ann Intern Med* 2003;139:97.
158. Rejnmark L et al. Effects on simvastatin on bone turnover and bone mineral density: a 1-year randomized controlled trial in postmenopausal osteopenic women. *J Bone Miner Res* 2004;19:737.

DRUG INDEX

Page numbers followed by *f* denotes figure and page numbers followed by *t* denotes table.

INDEX

Page numbers followed by *f* denotes figure and page numbers followed by *t* denotes table.